MASSRY & GLASSOCK'S TEXTBOOK OF NEPHROLOGY

FOURTH EDITION

MASSRY & GLASSOCK'S TEXTBOOK OF NEPHROLOGY

FOURTH EDITION

EDITORS

SHAUL G. MASSRY, MD

Professor Emeritus
Keck School of Medicine
University of Southern California School of Medicine
Los Angeles, California

RICHARD J. GLASSOCK, MD

Professor Emeritus
Department of Internal Medicine
UCLA School of Medicine
Los Angeles, California

LIPPINCOTT WILLIAMS & WILKINS
A Wolters Kluwer Company
Philadelphia • Baltimore • New York • London
Buenos Aires • Hong Kong • Sydney • Tokyo

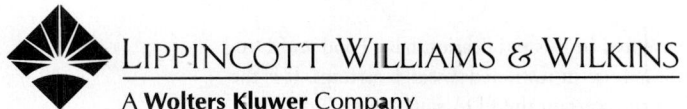

Acquisitions Editor: Timothy Y. Hiscock
Developmental Editor: Glenda Insua/Delois Patterson
Production Editor: Tony DeGeorge
Manufacturing Manager: Colin Warnock
Cover Designer: Christine Jenny
Compositor: Graphic World
Printer: Courier Westford

530 Walnut Street
Philadelphia, PA 19106 USA
LWW.com

Printed in the USA

Library of Congress Cataloging-in-Publication Data
Massry & Glassock's textbook of nephrology / [edited by] Shaul G. Massry, Richard J. Glassock.—4th ed.
p. ; c.m.
Includes bibliographical references and index.
ISBN 0-683-30488-7 (alk. paper)
1. Kidneys—Diseases. 2. Nephrology. I. Title: Textbook of nephrology. II. Title: Massry & Glassock's textbook of nephrology. III. Massry, Shaul G. IV. Glassock, Richard J.
[DNLM: 1. Kidney Diseases. 2. Kidney—anatomy & histology. 3. Kidney—physiology. WJ 300 M421 2000]
RC902.T48 2000
616.6'1—dc21 00-040541

---

10 9 8 7 6 5 4 3 2 1

TO OUR PATIENTS
Whose experiences have allowed us to enrich our knowledge of Nephrology

TO OUR TEACHERS
Who introduced us to Nephrology and nurtured our abilities in the practice of Nephrology

TO OUR WIVES
Meira Massry and Jo-Anne Glassock for their unflagging support

TO OUR CHILDREN
Guy, Lisa, Alexis, Yael, and Dina Massry, and Efrat, Ram, Raef, and Emma Cogan
Ellen, Ric, Max, and Naomi Reiner, and Sharon, Colin, Sarah, Kirsten and Blake
Anderson, and Scott, Aurora, Brian, Erin Glassock, and Mark Glassock
For their patience and understanding

CONTENTS

SECTION VIII: UREMIA AND THE EFFECTS OF DIALYSIS 1201

FOREWORD TO THE FOURTH EDITION

World War II began on September 1, 1939. A librarian at the National Library of Medicine could find in its computerized card catalog only three medical books on the kidney in 1939 and none for 1938. One of these was by my mentor, Homer W. Smith (*Physiology of the Renal Circulation*). Perhaps the most widely used text on medical physiology was *MacLeod's Physiology and Biochemistry in Modern Medicine*, whose first edition was in 1918. Its popularity prompted new editions in 1919, 1920, 1922, 1926, 1930, and 1935, when Biochemistry was removed from the title. Macleod died. Philip Bard brought out the eighth and ninth editions and changed the title for the tenth edition to Medical Physiology. In a 1421-page text, kidney physiology was allotted thirty pages (pp. 780–810). This is 2.11% of the text for a vital organ, the kidney, which gets a major share of the cardiac output and is the master chemist of the body. Of course J.P. Peters published his notable book *Body Water—The Exchange of Fluids in Man* in 1935. He trained and stimulated some Nephrology pioneers such as the late Lou Welt and Donald Seldin, who wrote the foreword to the first Edition of this great Textbook of Nephrology. Their careers facilitated the integration of related metabolism into the mainstream of Nephrology.

Nephrology was a useless key word prior to WWII. Very few academic departments of medicine in the United States had such a division. If so, they were generally called Renal Medicine, Renal & Electrolyte, Medical Kidney, and so on. The late Jean Hamburger started a Nephrology service at the Necker Hospital in Paris and with colleagues founded a French Society of Nephrology in 1959. As a true classicist, he preferred the Greek root *nephros* to the Latin *renalis* or the French alternative, *renes* or *reins*. The counterpart in the United Kingdom was the British Renal Society. An International Society of Nephrology (ISN) was formed and its First Congress held at Evian, France, September 1–4, 1960. About a hundred participants attended the opening session and there were 217 names in the author index of the printed transactions. The Second Congress in Prague had limited attendance behind the "iron curtain." Preparations for the Third Congress in Washington were grounded in anxiety. How many "nephrologists" were there? Who were they? How would we reach them? Based on "expert guesses," we reserved 1000 rooms at the Washington Hilton, at that time only an excavation on Connecticut Avenue. I researched all appropriate journals at the Georgetown and National Medical Library for the current three years and recorded all authors on every paper in my eclectic horizon. When selected members were added from related societies such as clinical investigation, physiology, pharmacology, and biochemistry, we had a mailing list of over 10,000! It was unprecedented to have over half responding to the first announcement. Paid attendance for the full week of the Third ISN Congress was 2134 scientists, and some sessions had over 3500!

The growth of Nephrology after WWII has been described with adjectives like "explosive" and "meteoric." It is now not unusual for the American Society of Nephrology (ASN) to register over 10,000 at its Congress. The National Kidney Foundation (NKF) Clinical meetings are huge as are related meetings in transplantation, hemodialysis, peritoneal dialysis, pediatric nephrology, and sub-sub specialties like vascular-access, hemoperfusion, polycystic and genetic diseases, and even nephro-psychiatry and nephro-ethics.

Some of the growth hormones for the clinical explosion in Nephrology came out of Washington, D.C. Leaders of the NKF held a prolonged strategic planning session culminating in a five-year plan to 1) amend the Vocational Rehabilitation Act to include kidney patients, 2) add kidney to the regional medical program, 3) increase pediatric funds through the Crippled Children's Act, 4) expand authority of the Chronic Disease Control Program, 5) triple NIH research funds in Nephrology 6) have representation as an Institute [now NIDDK], 7) open VA Hospitals to nonveterans for dialysis when needs are unmet, especially in remote communities. The culmination of their plan was enactment of Public Law 92-603, the ESRD legislation establishing a national program which has kept nearly a million Americans alive on renal replacement and renal therapies. NKF leaders at that session included Welt, Seldin, Bricker, Scribner, Teschan, and myself with perhaps some others and congressional input from Charles Plante, Dr. James Mongan, and Senator Russell Long.

This very fast growth of Nephrology was perhaps greater than any other new medical specialty. Some pundits speculate that textbooks are facing a sunset in their traditional role of basic education and as a ready reference for clinicians. It is true that Internet E-mail programs such as "NEPHROL" are wonderful for reaching remote places, sharing anecdotes, collecting experience on rare diseases, adverse reactions to therapies, and so on. Some even share experimental data. My own views are 180 degrees opposite such pundits, although their enthusiasm for learning is most welcome.

Clinical anecdotes are experiences but not necessarily science or truth. Experiments properly done are facts but not truth. That requires systematization and the crucible of organized trials in which extraneous elements can be reduced systematically or excluded. I like *scientia* in the classic Latin sense. And I like

Sir W. Hamilton's definition "science is a complement of cognition, having, in point of form, the character of logical perfection, and in point of matter, the character of real truth." It logically follows that more and better rather than less or no textbooks are needed in the face of expanding anecdotes and experimental data. No one person can authoritatively write a textbook on what Nephrology has become today. The strategic planning is enormous to define such a book and to organize and systematize its sections, chapters, and interrelations. The *sine qua non* of execution by chapter authors is to be very knowledgeable about the particular subject chosen or assigned **and they must be good teachers and good writers.** Shaul Massry and Richard Glassock have clearly excelled at such strategy. You can see the organization simply by scanning the table of contents and noting the clarity of interrelations between topics. They have labored at both ends of this fine textbook. Dr. Massry has written sixteen chapters, Dr. Glassock has written seventeen, and the two have formally collaborated on three.

If you are a student seeking to scope a specialty or decide on elective clerkships, student fellowships, or the site of postgraduate training, this great Fourth Edition of *Massry and Glassock's Textbook of Nephrology* will be here for you. If you are a new Nephrology fellow searching for questions to answer and subfields on which to focus your research questions, such as salt, water and potassium or calcium, phosphorus, and bone metabolism, or infection or immunology or genetics or transplantation or dialysis, this textbook is here for you. If you are a general practitioner or general internist, you will want to know how other diagnoses and treatments are affected by kidney failure, acid-base disturbances, or the loss of circulating albumin function by nephrotic range proteinuria. This book will be here for you. If you are treating a wide variety of disease entities, you must be aware that almost every potent medicine can be a nephrotoxin under certain conditions, this book will tell you what, when, and why. When the kidney, as our master chemist, is deranged, it can affect the selection, dosage, efficacy, mode of administration, or side effects of many medicines used for almost any disease from acne to Alzheimer's. Toxic nephropathy, defined as any functional or morphologic change in the kidney produced by a drug, chemical, or biologic agent that is ingested, injected, inhaled, or absorbed can damage or destroy kidney function. The concept is also valid for normal ions or molecules circulating in abnormal concentrations such as hypokalemic, hypomagnesemic, or hyperuricemic nephropathy. To understand the mechanisms and the management, this book is here for you. And it works when the hard drive has crashed, the surge protector has failed or the virus has landed!

Shaul Massry and Richard Glassock have both had excellent training coupled with experience both broad and long at both the bench and the bedside. They are esteemed by their peers as teachers and lecturers. They are good writers and editors and have had time to hone their skills on three previous successful editions. They have done a fine job editing this excellent Fourth Edition of a great textbook of Nephrology simply because they "have been there and done that"!

George E. Schreiner, A.B., M.D., M.A.C.P., F.R.C.P.S.
Distinguished Professor of Medicine,
Georgetown University School of Medicine,
Washington, D.C.

FOREWORD TO THE FIRST EDITION

Nephrology is a young discipline. It had its origins before World War II in the studies of renal function and renal disease undertaken by a relatively small number of physiologists and clinicians scattered in basic science and clinical departments.

At the time, the principal concern of the renal physiologist was a static portrayal of the chemical composition of the body fluids and urine. The analytical methods were painfully cumbersome and time-consuming and usually required substantial amounts of material; moreover, many critical constituents of blood and urine could not be measured at all. Conceptual formulations, such as those emerging from the analysis of renal hemodynamics, were largely at a stage of description. In a real sense, the normal function of the kidney as a regulatory organ responsible for the maintenance of the volume and composition of the body fluids was only dimly perceived; therefore, the description of renal function under the impact of physiological derangements or renal disease was almost wholly unknown. Consequently, the therapeutic armamentarium, given this primitive theoretic base, was pitifully inadequate. The administration of water or isotonic or hypertonic saline constituted the principal therapeutic modality at the disposal of the renal physician.

The study of renal disease was also in its infancy. Light microscopy, simple roentgenographic examinations, and the life history of a disease constituted virtually the only investigative tools. Almost nothing could be said about the pathogenesis of the major renal diseases because the disciplines underpinning the exploration of tissue injury were themselves weak and had hardly been applied to the kidney.

The physician interested in renal medicine was thus functioning without any significant framework for the understanding of either normal or deranged renal function or the pathogenesis or treatment of the significant renal diseases, and therefore was reduced to the role of a sympathetic and concerned but virtually powerless spectator.

After World War II, the application of the methods and principles of the generalizing sciences, physics, and chemistry to medicine transmuted the study of renal function and renal disease into a discipline of formidable explanatory power and technical sophistication. The development of powerful analytic tools—typified early by the flame photometer and later by exquisitely sensitive micromethods involving microchemistry, enzymatic assay, immunoassay, microelectrodes, and nuclear magnetic resonance—furnished the methodology for the explosive advance of renal physiology. At first, the newer analytical tools were used in balance and clearance studies to examine changes in organ function under the impact of physiological and pathological disturbances. Then, the reintroduction of micropuncture and the development of microperfusion of isolated tubules permitted an assessment of the function of nephron segments. Still later, the availability of isolated membrane vesicles coupled with micromethods of greater sensitivity facilitated the analysis of cellular and epithelial function. As a result, a broad, although admittedly incomplete, progression of the investigation of organ function to that of the nephron and finally to epithelial and cellular levels began to be elaborated. The functions of the kidney could now be embraced in dynamic theories of regulation.

The study of renal disease was similarly transformed. The electron microscope and immunofluorescent techniques resulted in burgeoning advances in immunological theory fostering the evolution of the new domain of immunonephrology. Theories of the pathogenesis of the major renal diseases began to emerge. Rational therapy, aimed at suppressing injurious processes originating in disturbances of immunological mechanisms, coagulation, and inflammation, was now designed.

The appreciation of the role of the kidney as an endocrine organ served to expand the study of the kidney outside its traditional domain of renal physiology and renal disease. The kidney was initially recognized to be the target of circulating hormones, such as antidiuretic hormone, aldosterone, and parathyroid hormone; in addition, it was shown to secrete hormones that acted at such distant sites as bone, blood vessels, and bone marrow; and it produced hormones acting at intrarenal loci.

It was the integration of the rapidly advancing conceptual systems of renal physiology, immunonephrology, and renal endocrinology that transformed the study of renal function from tentative beginnings into the new discipline of nephrology.

The *Textbook of Nephrology*, edited by Drs. Shaul G. Massry and Richard J. Glassock, fully embraces the broad domain of the new specialty. The first two sections are devoted to an analysis of the normal anatomy and function of the kidney and urinary tract. Integrated organ function is explored in the chapters on renal hemodynamics and urinary concentration and dilution. Nephron function is examined by a consideration of the transport of a variety of solutes. The endocrine function of the kidney, as both the target as well as the source of hormones, is treated in detail. In Sections 3, 4, and 5, a thorough examination of the deranged physiology of water and electrolytes, immunological renal injury, and impaired renal hemodynamics is undertaken. It is particularly noteworthy that in these sections extensive treatment is given to physiological derangements rather than specific diseases. As a consequence, a broad background is furnished for the subsequent analysis of disease states. The following Section 6 treats the various forms of glomerular and tubular syndromes and diseases. The failure of renal function, its manifestations and treatment by dietary management, dialysis, and transplantation, are meticulously explored in Chapters 7, 8, and 9. Finally, the book concludes with an unusually thorough description of the clinical and laboratory procedures available for the diagnosis and follow-up of patients with renal disease.

Drs. Massry and Glassock are distinguished investigators who have made extensive contributions to the study of normal and deranged electrolyte metabolism, the elucidation of the clinical features of uremia, and the relatively new fields of renal endocrinology and immunonephrology. Their interests are as deep as they are broad. Their editing of the textbook as well as their own chapters reflect this by providing an elaborate conceptual framework of basic nephrology which then functions as a foundation for the detailed consideration of the pathogenesis and treatment of both discrete forms of renal disease and overall failure of renal function. They have been able to accomplish this while discharging extensive teaching, clinical, and investigative responsibilities. This impressive achievement is a tribute to their high competence in nephrology, their energy, and their dedication to academic medicine.

Donald W. Seldin, M.D.
Dallas, Texas

PREFACE TO THE FOURTH EDITION

After devoting a major portion of our professional careers to the preparation and publication of the *Textbook of Nephrology*, we have both gained an immense respect for the diversity and vitality of the discipline of Nephrology. Starting from an already enormous base of knowledge, remarkable changes have occurred in the field even over the short period of time that has elapsed since the Third Edition was published.

As with prior editions, we have endeavored to provide in the Fourth Edition a volume that matches the extraordinary breadth, depth, and intellectual richness of the field of Nephrology, while retaining the virtues of practicality, readability, and usefulness as distinguishing characteristics.

The reader will recognize that the Fourth Edition adds many new authors and introduces many novel topic areas, which we hope will add to the value of the textbook for practitioners, scientists, and students.

The distinguished authors who have contributed to the Fourth Edition continue a tradition of outstanding scientific and medical writing. We are greatly indebted to them for their efforts, without which this edition could not have been produced according to our high standards of excellence.

We sincerely hope that this edition will be received by readers with the same or greater enthusiasm with which it was conceived and developed.

We are deeply grateful to Rhonda Wood, Mary Benson, Nancy Stinnett, and Charlotte Hatton for their invaluable assistance. We are also very appreciative of the strong and continued support of the publishers.

Shaul G. Massry, M.D.
Richard J. Glassock, M.D.

PREFACE TO THE FIRST EDITION

The publication of the *Textbook of Nephrology* represents the culmination of a labor of love. Both of us have been nurtured, professionally and personally, by the field of nephrology since we began to work in this new specialty over 20 years ago.

The changes which have occurred over this period of time have been dramatic, exciting, and far reaching. Nephrology has emerged as one of the few disciplines which encompasses the vast and broad array of medicine in all of its vagaries and complexities. Indeed, a nephrologist is a consummate internist.

Many excellent volumes dealing with the kidney and its diseases have appeared in recent years. These treatises have represented either single-authored personalized monographs or detailed multi-authored reference books. In our view, a gap exists and remains unfilled for those who wish to have a systematic, comprehensive, and concise presentation of the current knowledge to enable them to learn the art and the practice of nephrology. The *Textbook of Nephrology* has been specifically designed to meet these objectives.

A large number of clinician-scientists in various fields of nephrology contributed succinct essays in specific areas of their expertise. Their contributions provide the state of the art and their personal experience in the physiology of the kidney and in the pathophysiology, pathology, clinical features, diagnosis, prognosis, and management of a wide array of disorders related to the general scope of nephrology.

The *Textbook of Nephrology* is a "horn of plenty" which will appeal to all audiences of nephrology and medicine irrespective of the level of their training or experience. We hope it will be received with the same excitement and enthusiasm with which it was conceived and developed.

We wish to give special thanks and appreciation to Ms. Jamie Jimenez for her valuable assistance which she performed with patience, dedication, and devotion during the preparation of this book.

Shaul G. Massry, M.D.
Richard J. Glassock, M.D.

CONTRIBUTING AUTHORS

Mauro Abbate, M.D., Head, Unit of Pathology and Immunopathology, Negri Bergamo Laboratories, "Mario Negri" Institute for Pharmacological Research, Bergamo, Italy

Christine K. Abrass, M.D, Professor, Department of Medicine, University of Washington, Seattle, Washington

Stefan Aczel, M.D., Research Assistant, Department of Medicine, Academic Teaching Hospital, Feldkirch, Austria

John W. Adamson, M.D., Professor, Department of Medicine (Hematology/Oncology), Medical College of Wisconsin, Milwaukee, Wisconsin

Sharon G. Adler, M.D., Professor, Department of Medicine, University of California, Los Angeles, School of Medicine, Los Angeles, California

Horacio J. Adrogue, M.D., F.A.C.P., Professor, Department of Medicine, Baylor College of Medicine, Houston, Texas

Tejinder S. Ahuja, M.B.B.S., Assistant Professor, Department of Medicine, University of Texas Medical Branch, Galveston, Texas

Mohammad Akmal, M.D., Professor, Department of Medicine, Division of Nephrology, Keck School of Medicine, University of Southern California, Los Angeles, California

Qais Al-Awqati, M.D., Robert F. Loeb Professor of Medicine, Division of Nephrology, Columbia University, College of Physicians and Surgeons, New York, New York

Robert J. Alpern, M.D., Professor, Dean, Southwestern Medical School, University of Texas, Southwestern Medical Center, Dallas, Texas

Fred K. Alavi, Ph.D., Research Assistant Professor, Department of Internal Medicine, University of South Dakota School of Medicine, Sioux Falls, South Dakota

William J.C. Amend, Jr., M.D., Professor of Clinical Medicine, Department of Medicine, University of California, San Francisco, San Francisco, California

Richard Amerling, M.D., Assistant Professor, Department of Medicine, Albert Einstein College of Medicine, Bronx, New York

A.R. Amir, M.D., Staff Nephrologist, ARAMCO, Dhahran Health Clinic, Dhahran, Saudi Arabia

Sharon Anderson, M.D., Professor of Medicine, Interim Chief, Division of Nephrology, Oregon Health Sciences University, Portland, Oregon

Thomas E. Andreoli, M.D., Professor and The Nolan Chair, Department of Internal Medicine, University of Arkansas College of Medicine, Little Rock, Arkansas

Michael S. Anger, M.D., Clinical Professor of Medicine, Department of Medicine, Division of Nephrology, University of Colorado Health Sciences Center, Denver, Colorado

Gerald B. Appel, M.D., Professor of Clinical Medicine, Department of Medicine, Columbia University, College of Physicians and Surgeons, New York, New York

Alexandr Arakelov, M.D., Research Fellow, Department of Medicine, Emory University School of Medicine, Decatur, Georgia

Allen I. Arieff, M.D., Professor of Medicine, University of California, San Francisco, San Francisco, California

George R. Aronoff, M.D., F.A.C.P., Professor, Department of Medicine and Pharmacology, Chief, Division of Nephrology, University of Louisville, Louisville, Kentucky

Robert C. Atkins, M.D., Professor of Medicine, Director, Nephrology, Monash Medical Center, Clayton, Australia

Steven A. Atlas, M.D., Associate Professor, Department of Medicine, Mount Sinai School of Medicine, New York, New York

Morell M. Avram, M.D., F.A.C.P., Professor, Department of Medicine, Chief, Division of Nephrology, Long Island College Hospital, Brooklyn, New York

G. Reza Babapour, M.D., Dermatologist, Beverly Hills; Clinical Faculty, University of California, Los Angeles, Los Angeles, California

Kamal F. Badr, M.D., Professor, Chair, Department of Internal Medicine, American University of Beruit, Beruit, Lebanon

George L. Bakris, M.D., Professor, Vice Chairman, Department of Preventive Medicine, Director, Hypertension Clinical Research Center, Rush University, Chicago, Illinois

Lise Bankir, Ph.D., Director of Research, INSERM, Unit 367, Paris, France

Rashad S. Barsoum, M.D., Professor and Chair, Department of Internal Medicine, Cairo University School of Medicine, Cairo, Egypt

Bryan N. Becker, M.D., Assistant Professor, Department of Medicine, University of Wisconsin, Madison, Wisconsin

Gavin J. Becker, M.D., F.R.A.C.P., Professor and Director, Department of Nephrology, The Royal Melbourne Hospital, Victoria, Australia

Guido Bellinghieri, M.D., Professor and Chief of Nephrology, Poli Clinico Universitario Gazzi, Messina, Sicily

Julio E. Benabe, M.D., Professor, Department of Medicine, Director, University of Puerto Rico Medical Science Campus, San Juan, Puerto Rico

William M. Bennett, M.D., Professor of Medicine, Nephrology, Department of Medicine, Oregon Health Sciences University, Portland, Oregon

Carl J. Bentzel, M.D., Department of Medicine, East Carolina University School of Medicine, Greenville, North Carolina

Jonas Bergström, M.D., Ph.D., Professor Emeritus and Baxter Novum, Karolinska Institute, Stockholm, Huddinge, Sweden

Tomas Berl, M.D., Professor, Department of Medicine, University of Colorado, Denver, Colorado

Gordon R. Bernard, M.D., Professor, Department of Medicine, Vanderbilt University School of Medicine, Nashville, Tennessee

Paul Bernstein, M.D., Section of Nephrology, Rochester General Hospital, Rochester, New York

Giuseppe Bianchi, M.D., Professor of Nephrology, Universitá Vita E Salute, Milan, Italy

Jürg J. Biber, M.D., Titular Professor, Institute of Physiology, University of Zürich, Zürich, Switzerland

Daniel J. Birmingham, Ph.D., Associate Professor, Department of Internal Medicine, The Ohio State University Medical Center, Columbus, Ohio

Roland C. Blantz, M.D., Professor, Department of Medicine, University of California, San Diego, La Jolla, California

Paola Boccardo, Biol. Sci.D., Clinical Research Center for Rare Diseases, Aldo e Cele Dacco "Mario Negri" Institute for Pharmacological Research, Bergamo, Italy

Bernard H. Bochner, M.D., Assistant Professor, Department of Urology, University of California, Los Angeles, School of Medicine, Los Angeles, California

Mirian Aparecida Boim, Ph.D., Associate Researcher, Department of Medicine, Escola Paulista de Medicina, Sao Paulo, Brazil

W. Kline Bolton, M.D., Professor, Department of Medicine, University of Virginia, Charlottesville, Virginia

Dorin-Bogdan Borza, Ph.D., Department of Biochemistry, University of Kansas Medical Center, Kansas City, Kansas

William D. Boswell, Jr., M.D., F.A.C.R., Associate Professor, Department of Radiology, University of California, Los Angeles, California

Nadine Bouby, Ph.D., Chargé de Racherche, INSERM, Unit 367, Paris, France

D. Craig Brater, M.D., Chairman and Professor, Department of Medicine, Indiana University School of Medicine, Indianapolis, Indiana

William E. Braun, M.D., Clinical Professor of Medicine, University of Pennsylvania, Hershey, Pennsylvania

Michael E. Brier, Ph.D., Associate Professor, Department of Medicine, University of Louisville School of Medicine, Louisville, Kentucky

Kenneth L. Brigham, M.D., Professor, Department of Medicine, Vanderbilt University School of Medicine, Nashville, Tennessee

Alex J. Brown, Ph.D., Research Assistant Professor of Medicine, Department of Internal Medicine, Renal Division, Washington University School of Medicine, St. Louis, Missouri

David W. Butterly, M.D., Assistant Professor, Department of Medicine, Duke University Medical Center, Durham, North Carolina

Vito M. Campese, M.D., Professor of Medicine, Chief, Division of Nephrology, Keck School of Medicine, University of Southern California, Los Angeles, California

Giovanni C. Cancarini, M.D., Associate Professor, Chair of Nephrology, University of Brescia, Brescia, Italy

Thomas G. Cangiano, Attending Urologist, Florida Hospital Orlando, Orlando, Florida

J. Michael Cecka, Ph.D., Clinical Research Director, Immunogenetics Laboratory, University of California, Los Angeles, School of Medicine, Los Angeles, California

Laurence Chan, M.D., Ph.D., F.R.C.P., F.A.C.P., Professor, Department of Medicine, Director, Transplant Nephrology, University of Colorado Health Sciences Center, Denver, Colorado

Lucienne Chatenoud, M.D., D.Sc., Professor, Department of Immunology, Hospital Necker, Paris, France

Russell W. Chesney, M.D., Le Bonheur Chair and Professor, Department of Pediatrics, University of Tennessee, Memphis, Memphis, Tennessee

Karpal S. Chugh, M.D., National Kidney Clinic and Research Center, Chandigarh, India

Carol Clayberger, Ph.D., Associate Professor, Departments of Cardiothoracic Surgery and Pediatrics, Stanford University School of Medicine, Stanford, California

Jack W. Coburn, M.D., Professor, Department of Medicine, University of California, Los Angeles, School of Medicine, Los Angeles, California

Fredric L. Coe, M.D., Professor, Department of Medicine and Physiology, University of Chicago, Chicago, Illinois

Arthur H. Cohen, M.D., Professor, Departments of Pathology and Medicine, University of California, Los Angeles, School of Medicine, Los Angeles, California

Lewis M. Cohen, M.D., Associate Professor, Department of Psychiatry, Tufts University School of Medicine, Boston, Massachusetts

Patrick M. Colletti, M.D., Professor, Department of Radiology, University of Southern California, Los Angeles, California

Fernando G. Cosio, M.D., Professor, Department of Medicine, Division of Nephrology, The Ohio State University Medical Center, Columbus, Ohio

John J. Curtis, M.D., Professor, Department of Medicine, Division of Nephrology, University of Alabama at Birmingham, Birmingham, Alabama

William C. Cushman, M.D., Professor, Departments of Preventive Medicine and Medicine, University of Tennessee Health Science Center, Memphis, Tennessee

Daniele Cusi, Associate Professor of Nephrology, Department of Sciences and Medical Technologies, University of Milano, Segrate—Milano, Italy

Ralph E. Cutler, M.D., Professor, Department of Medicine, Pharmacology, Loma Linda University, Loma Linda, California

Vivette D. D'Agati, M.D., Professor, Department of Pathology, Columbia University College of Physicians and Surgeons, New York, New York

Giuseppe D'Amico, M.D., F.R.C.P., Professor of Medicine, Postgraduate School of Medicine, University of Milan, Milan, Italy

Eugene Dafnis, M.D., Assistant Professor, Department of Nephrology, University of Crete Medical School, Heraklion, Crete, Greece

Prasun K. Datta, Ph.D., Department of Medicine, Division Nephrology, Robert Wood Johnson Medical School, University of Medicine and Dentistry New Jersey, New Brunswick, New Jersey

Jean B. deKernion, M.D., The Fran and Ray Stark Professor of Urology, University of California, Los Angeles, School of Medicine, Los Angeles, California

Frederick C. De Beer, M.D., Department of Internal Medicine, University of Kentucky, Lexington, Kentucky

Peter Deetjen, M.D., Professor, Chairman, Department of Physiology, University of Innsbruck, Innsbruck, Austria

Thomas A. Depner, M.D., Professor of Medicine, Department of Internal Medicine, University of California, Davis, Sacramento, California

Béatrice Descamps-Latscha, M.D., Ph.D., Director of Research, Hospital Necker, Paris, France

José A. Diaz-Buxo, M.D., F.A.C.P., Clinical Professor of Medicine, University of North Carolina at Chapel Hill, Chapel Hill, North Carolina

Susan A. Dilly, M.B., B.S., F.R.C.Path., Dean of Health, Faculty of Health, Keele University, Staffordshire, United Kingdom

Leslie P. Dornfeld, M.D., Clinical Professor of Medicine and Nephrology, University of California, Los Angeles, School of Medicine, Los Angeles, California

James F. Douglas, M.D., Senior Nephrologist, Department of Nephrology and Transplantation, Belfast City Hospital, Belfast, Northern Ireland, United Kingdom

Heinz Drexel, M.D., Head, Department of Medicine, Academic Teaching Hospital, Feldkirch, Austria

Tilman B. Drüeke, M.D., Director of Research, INSERM, Unit 507, Necker Hospital, Paris, France

Thomas D. DuBose, Jr., M.D., Peter T. Bohan Professor, Chair, Department of Internal Medicine, University of Kansas Medical School, Kansas City, Kansas

Matthew D. Dunn, M.D., Assistant Professor, Department of Urology, Keck School of Medicine, University of Southern California, Los Angeles, California

Adriana S. Dusso, Ph.D., Research Assistant Professor of Medicine, Department of Internal Medicine, Renal Division, Washington University School of Medicine, St. Louis, Missouri

John B. Eastwood, M.D., F.R.C.P., Reader in Medicine, Department of Renal Medicine, St. George's Hospital and Medical School, London, United Kingdom

Glenn R. Ehresmann, M.D., Associate Professor of Rheumatology, Department of Medicine, Hoffman Research Center, Los Angeles, California

Somchai Eiam-Ong, M.D., Professor, Division of Nephrology, Department of Medicine, Coordinating Kidney Center, Chulalongkorn University Hospital, Bangkok, Thailand

Garabed Eknoyan, M.D., Professor, Department of Medicine, Baylor College of Medicine, Houston, Texas

Marlies Elger, Ph.D., Department of Internal Medicine, Division of Nephrology, Medizinische Hochschule Hanover, Hanover, Germany

Bryan T. Emmerson, M.D., Ph.D., Professor Emeritus, Honorary Research Consultant, Department of Medicine, University of Queensland, Brisbane, Queensland, Australia

Lea Emmett, R.N., M.S., Research Administrator, Department of Pediatrics, New York Medical College, North American Pediatric Renal Transplant Cooperative Study, Hawthorne, New York

Hitoshi Endou, M.D., Ph.D., Professor, Department of Pharmacology and Toxicology, Kyorin University School of Medicine, Tokyo, Japan

Murray Epstein, M.D., F.A.C.P., Professor, Department of Medicine, University of Miami School of Medicine, Miami, Florida

Kenneth F. Fairley, M.D., Epworth Hospital, Richmond, Victoria, Australia

Ronald J. Falk, M.D., Professor, Department of Medicine, Chief, Division of Nephrology and Hypertension, University of North Carolina at Chapel Hill, Chapel Hill, North Carolina

Nicolette E. Farman, M.D., Ph.D., Director, INSERM, Unit 478, Bichat Medical School, Paris, France

Robert G. Fassett, M.B., B.S., Associate Professor and Director of Medicine, University of Tasmania, Launceston General Hospital, Launceston, Tasmania, Australia

Hervé Favre, M.D., (deceased) Fondation pour Rechercle Médicale, University of Geneva, Geneva, Switzerland

Eric Féraille, M.D., Ph.D., Laboratory of Nephrology, Fondation pour Rechercle Médicale, University of Geneva, Geneva, Switzerland

Richard N. Fine, M.D., Professor and Chairman, Department of Pediatrics, University Medical Center at Stony Brook, Stony Brook, New York

M. Roy First, M.D., Professor, Department of Internal Medicine, University of Cincinnati Medical Center, Cincinnati, Ohio

Robert C. Flanigan, M.D., Chairman and Albert J. Sr. and Claire R. Spech Professor, Department of Urology, Loyola University Medical Center, Maywood, Illinois

Agnes B. Fogo, M.D., Professor of Pathology and Medicine, Associate Professor of Pediatrics, Vanderbilt University Medical Center, Nashville, Tennessee

Robert N. Foley, M.B., M.Sc, Consultant Renal Physician, Department of Renal Medicine, Hope Hospital, Salford, United Kingdom

Steven C. Forland, Pharm D, Department of Pharmacy and Clinical Pharmacology, Loma Linda University, Loma Linda, California

Alessandro Fornasieri, M.D., Division of Nephrology, San Carlo Hospital, Milan, Italy

Harris E. Foster, Jr., M.D., Associate Professor, Section of Urology, Yale University School of Medicine, New Haven, Connecticut

Chris N. Fotiadis, M.D., Department of Nephrology, Carolina Medical Center, Charlotte, North Carolina

Harold A. Franch, M.D., Assistant Professor, Renal Division, Emory University School of Medicine, Atlanta, Georgia

Martina Franz, M.D., Division of Nephrology, Department of Medicine III, University Hospital, Vienna, Austria

Cosmo L. Fraser, M.D., Associate Professor of Medicine, University of California, San Francisco, San Francisco, California

João M. Frazão, M.D., Ph.D., Assistant Professor, Department of Medicine, Medical School of Porto, University of Porto, Porto, Portugal

Gerard Friedlander, M.D., Ph.D., Professor INSERM, Unit 426, Department of Physiologie, Faculté de Médecine Xavier Bichat, Paris, France

Michael M. Friedlaender, F.R.C.P. (UK), Associate Professor of Medicine, Department of Nephrology and Hypertension, Hadassah University Hospital, Jerusalem, Israel

Aaron L. Friedman, M.D., Professor and Chairman, Department of Pediatrics, University of Wisconsin—Madison, Madison, Wisconsin

Francis B. Gabbai, M.D., Associate Professor, Department of Medicine, University of California, San Diego, La Jolla, California

John H. Galla, M.D., Professor, Department of Medicine, University of Cincinnati Medical Center, Cincinnati, Ohio

Gill Gaskin, Ph.D., F.R.C.P., Senior Lecturer, Department of Medicine, Imperial College School of Medicine, London, United Kingdom

Robert S. Gaston, M.D., Professor, Department of Medicine, University of Alabama at Birmingham, Birmingham, Alabama

Joel Gelman, M.D., Assistant Professor, Department of Surgery, Division of Urology, University of California, Irvine, Orange, California

F. John Gennari, M.D., Professor, Department of Medicine, Division of Nephrology, University of Vermont College of Medicine, Burlington, Vermont

Gerhard Giebisch, M.D., Sterling Professor, Department of Cellular and Molecular Physiology, Yale University School of Medicine, New Haven, Connecticut

Richard J. Glassock, M.D., M.A.C.P., Professor Emeritus, Department of Internal Medicine, University of California, Los Angeles, School of Medicine, Los Angeles, California

Ram Gokal, M.D., Honorary Reader, Department of Medicine, Manchester University, Manchester, United Kingdom

Harvey C. Gonick, M.D., Adjunct Professor, Department of Medicine, University of California, Los Angeles, Los Angeles, California

Mahendra V. Govani, M.D., M.R.C.P. (UK), Clinical Assistant Professor, Department of Medicine, Division of Nephrology, Indiana University School of Medicine, Indianapolis, Indiana

John M. Grange, M.Sc., M.D., Reader in Clinical Microbiology, National Heart and Lung Institute, Imperial College School of Medicine, London, United Kingdom

Jared J. Grantham, M.D., Distinguished Professor, Department of Medicine, Kansas University of Kansas, Kansas City, Kansas

Arthur Greenberg, M.D., Professor of Medicine, Division of Nephrology, Duke University Medical Center, Durham, North Carolina

Suzanne Greenberg, M.D., Assistant Professor, Department of Obstetrics and Gynecology, University of Cincinnati, College of Medicine, Cincinnati, Ohio

Antonio Guasch, M.D., Associate Professor, Department of Medicine, Emory University, Atlanta, Georgia

Arnold W. Gurevitch, M.D., Professor, Department of Medicine, Keck School of Medicine, University of Southern California, Los Angeles, California

Raymond M. Hakim, M.D., Ph.D., Adjunct Professor of Medicine, Department of Nephrology, Vanderbilt University, Nashville, Tennessee

Phillip M. Hall, M.D., Department of Nephrology and Hypertension, Cleveland Clinic foundation, Cleveland, Ohio

Leah A. Haseley, M.D., Division of Nephrology, University of Washington School of Medicine, Seattle, Washington

Michael J. Hausmann, M.D., M.Sc., Lecturer, Faculty of Health Sciences, Ben-Gurion University, Beer-Sheva, Israel

George B. Haycock, M.B., F.R.C.P., Professor, Department of Pediatrics, University of London, London, United Kingdom

Lee A. Hebert, M.D., Professor of Medicine, Director, Division of Nephrology, Department of Internal Medicine, The Ohio State University, Columbus, Ohio

August Heidland, M.D., Professor, Department of Internal Medicine, University of Würzburg, Würzburg, Germany

J. Harold Helderman, M.D., Professor of Medicine, Microbiology and Immunology, Department of Medicine, Vanderbilt University Medical School, Nashville, Tennessee

William L. Henrich, M.D., Professor and Chairman, Department of Medicine, University of Maryland School of Medicine, Baltimore, Maryland

Raimund Hirschberg, M.D., Division of Nephrology and Hypertension, Harbor-University of California, Los Angeles Medical Center, Torrance, California

Robert W. Hoffman, D.O., Professor and Director, Department of Medicine, Division of Immunology and Rheumatology, University of Missouri, Columbia, Missouri

Walter H. Hörl, M.D., Ph.D., Professor, Department of Medicine, Chief, Division of Nephrology, University Hospital, Vienna, Austria

Robert G. Horn, M.D., Pathologist and Owner, Laboratory for Renal Biopsy Pathology, Nashville, Tennessee

Keith A. Hruska, M.D., Ira M. Lang Professor, Department of Medicine and Cell Biology, Washington University, St. Louis, Missouri

Billy G. Hudson, Ph.D., Professor and Chair, Department of Biochemistry and Molecular Biology, University of Kansas Medical Center, Kansas City, Kansas

Jeffry L. Huffman, M.D., Professor, Department of Urology, University of Southern California School of Medicine, Los Angeles, California

H. David Humes, M.D., John G. Searle Professor, Department of Internal Medicine, University of Michigan Medical School, Ann Arbor, Michigan

Michael H. Humphreys, M.D., Professor, Department of Medicine, University of California, San Francisco, San Francisco, California

Tracy E. Hunley, M.D., Assistant Professor, Department of Pediatrics, Division of Pediatric Nephrology, Vanderbilt University Medical Center, Nashville, Tennessee

Niilo-Pekka Huttunen, M.D., Ph.D., Senior Lecturer, Department of Pediatrics, University of Oulu, Oulu, Finland

Edwin K. Jackson, M.D., Ph.D., Professor of Pharmacology and Medicine, Department of Pharmacology, University of Pittsburgh School of Medicine, Pittsburgh, Pennsylvania

Claude Jacobs, M.D., Professor of Nephrology, UFR Pitie-Salpetriere, Paris, France

Michel Jadoul, M.D., Assistant Clinical Professor, Department of Internal Medicine, Universite Catholique de, Louvain, Brussels, Belgium

J. Ashley Jefferson, M.D., M.R.C.P., Chief Fellow, Department of Medicine, Division of Nephrology, University of Washington Medical Center, Seattle, Washington

J. Charles Jennette, M.D., Brinkhous Distinguished Professor and Chair, Department of Pathology and Laboratory Medicine, University of North Carolina School of Medicine, Chapel Hill, North Carolina

Vivekanand Jha, M.D., D.M., Associate Professor, Department of Nephrology, Postgraduate Institute of Medical Education and Research, Chandigard, India

Richard J. Johnson, M.D., Professor, Division of Nephrology, Baylor College of Medicine, Houston, Texas

Valerie L. Johnson, M.D., Ph.D., Associate Professor of Clinical Pediatrics, Department of Pediatrics, Weill Medical College of Cornell University, New York, New York

Jaap A. Joles, D.V.M., Ph.D., Associate Professor, Department of Nephrology and Hypertension, University Medical Center, Utrecht, The Netherlands

Andre A. Kaplan, M.D., F.A.C.P., Professor, Department of Medicine, University of Connecticut Health Center, Farmington, Connecticut

Bernard S. Kaplan, M.D., Professor, Department of Pediatrics, University of Pennsylvania, Philadelphia, Pennsylvania

Neil Kaplowitz, M.D., Professor and Chief, Department of Medicine, GI/Liver Division, University of Southern California, Los Angeles, California

Clifford E. Kashtan, M.D., Associate Professor, Department of Pediatrics, University of Minnesota, Minneapolis, Minnesota

Charles J. Kaupke, M.D., Associate Adjunct Professor of Medicine, Department of Nephrology, University of California, Los Angeles, Los Angeles, California

Laurie H. Kayne, Ph.D., C.N.S., Research Consultant, Department of Medicine, Division of Nephrology, University of California, Los Angeles, Los Angeles, California

George A. Kaysen, M.D., Ph.D., Professor of Medicine, Department of Internal Medicine, Chief, Division of Nephrology, University of California, Davis, Davis, California

William F. Keane, M.D., Professor, Department of Medicine, University of Minnesota Medical School, Minneapolis, Minnesota

Francis J. Kelly, M.B, M.R.C.P.I., Assistant Professor of Medicine, Division of Nephrology, Oregon Health Sciences University, Portland, Oregon

David B. Kershaw, M.D., Pediatric Nephrology, University of Michigan Medical Center, Ann Arbor, Michigan

Naseeruddin Khan, M.D., Fellow of Nephrology, Renal Division, Washington University School of Medicine, St. Louis, Missouri

Rizwan Z. Khan, M.D., Attending Nephrologist, Department of Nephrology and Hypertension, Baylor University Medical Center, Dallas, Texas

Ramesh Khanna, M.D., F.A.C.P., Professor of Medicine, Department of Internal Medicine, Director, Division of Nephrology, University of Missouri School of Medicine, Columbia, Missouri

Fernando J. Kim, M.D., Chief Resident, Department of Urology, Loyola University Medical Center, Maywood, Illinois

Paul L. Kimmel, M.D., Professor, Department of Medicine, George Washington University Medical Center, Washington, DC; and Director, Diabetic Nephropathy and HIV Programs, Division of Kidney Urology and Hematologic Diseases, National Institute of Diabetes and Digestive and Kidney Diseases, Bethesda, Maryland

Mark S. Kindy, M.D., Associate Professor, Department of Biochemistry, University of Kentucky, Lexington, Kentucky

Saulo Klahr, M.D., John E. and Adaline Simon Professor of Medicine, Department of Medicine, Washington University School of Medicine, St. Louis, Missouri

Charles R. Kleeman, M.D., Factor Family Foundation Emeritus Professor of Medicine and Nephrology, Department of Medicine, University of California, Los Angeles, School of Medicine, Los Angeles, California

David C. Kluth, B.Sc., M.B., B.S., M.R.C.P., Clinical Lecturer, Department of Medicine and Therapeutics, University of Aberdeen, Aberdeen, Scotland

Valentina Kon, M.D., Associate Professor, Division of Pediatric Nephrology, Vanderbilt University Medical Center, Nashville, Tennessee

Hein A. Koomans, D.V.M., Ph.D., Professor of Nephrology, Department of Nephrology and Hypertension, University Medical Center, Utrecht, The Netherlands

Joel D. Kopple, M.D., Professor, Medicine and Public Health, Chief, Division of Nephrology, Harbor-University of California, Los Angeles Medical Center, Torrance, California

Stephen M. Korbet, M.D., F.A.C.P., Professor of Medicine, Department of Internal Medicine, Rush Medical College, Chicago, Illinois

Jeffrey A. Kraut, M.D., Professor, Department of Medicine, University of California, Los Angeles, School of Medicine, Los Angeles, California

Alan M. Krensky, M.D., Shelagh Galligan Professor, Department of Pediatrics, Stanford University Medical Center, Stanford, California

Wilhelm Kriz, M.D., Professor and Chairman, Departments of Anatomy and Cell Biology, University of Heidelberg, Heidelberg, Germany

Kiyoshi Kurokawa, M.D., M.A.C.P., Professor, Department of Internal Medicine, Tokai University School of Medicine, Kanagawa, Japan

Ira Kurtz, M.D., Professor, Department of Medicine, Chief, Division of Nephrology, University of California, Los Angeles, School of Medicine, Los Angeles, California

Neil A. Kurtzman, M.D., F.A.C.P., University Distinguished Professor, Arnett Professor of Medicine, Professor of Physiology, Department of Internal Medicine, Texas Tech University Health Sciences Center, Lubbock, Texas

Eduardo K. Lacson, Jr., M.D., M.P.H., Medical Director for Research, Home Dialysis Therapies, Fresenius Medical Care North America, Lexington, Massachusetts

Bernard Lacour, Ph.D., Professor, Laboratory of Physiology, Faculté de Pharmacie, Malabry, France

Fadi G. Lakkis, M.D., Associate Professor, Department of Medicine, Emory University, Atlanta, Georgia

Florian Lang, M.D., Chair, Department of Physiology, University of Tübingen, Tübingen, Germany

M. Chris Langub, Ph.D., Research Assistant Professor, Department of Internal Medicine, Division of Nephrology, Bone and Mineral Metabolism, University of Kentucky Medical Center, Lexington, Kentucky

Sandra M. Rodrigues Laranja, M.D., Associate Researcher, Department of Medicine, Escola Paulista de Medicina, Sao Paulo, Brazil

Marc A. Lavine, M.D., Chief Resident in Urology, Department of Urology, Brown University, Rhode Island Hospital, Providence, Rhode Island

David B. N. Lee, M.B., B.S., Professor of Medicine, University of California, Los Angeles, School of Medicine, Los Angeles, California

Jacob Lemann, Jr., M.D., (retired) Professor of Medicine, Nephrology Division, Medical College of Wisconsin, Milwaukee, Wisconsin

Andrew S. Levey, M.D., Dr. Gerald J. and Dorothy R. Friedman Professor of Medicine, Tufts University School of Medicine, Boston, Massachusetts

Barton S. Levine, M.D., Professor, Department of Medicine, University of California, Los Angeles, School of Medicine, Los Angeles, California

Nathan W. Levin, M.D., F.A.C.P., Professor, Department of Clinical Medicine, Albert Einstein College of Medicine, Bronx, New York

Norman B. Levy, M.D., Adjunct Professor of Medicine and Clinical Professor of Psychiatry, State University of New York Health Science Center at Brooklyn, Brooklyn, New York

Elias A. Lianos, M.D., Professor of Medicine, Robert Wood Johnson Medical School, New Brunswick, New Jersey

Ellin Lieberman, M.D., Professor, Department of Pediatrics, Division of Nephrology and Transplantation, University of Southern California, Los Angeles, California

Gary Lieskovsky, M.D., Professor, Department of Urology, University of Southern California School of Medicine, Los Angeles, California

Victoria S. Lim, M.D., Professor, Department of Medicine, University of Iowa College of Medicine, Iowa City, Iowa

Robert G. Luke, M.D., Chairman, Department of Internal Medicine, University of Cincinnati Medical Center, Cincinnati, Ohio

A. Peter Lundin, M.D., Professor of Clinical Medicine, State University of New York Health Science Center at Brooklyn, Brooklyn, New York

Thomas Maack, M.D., Ph.D., Professor of Physiology, Department of Physiology, Weill Cornell Medical College, New York, New York

Robert Mactier, M.D., F.C.R.P., Honorary Senior Lecturer, University of Glasgow, Glasgow, Scotland, United Kingdom

David A. Maddox, Ph.D., Professor, Department of Internal Medicine, University of South Dakota School of Medicine, Sioux Falls, South Dakota

Nicolaos E. Madias, M.D., Executive Academic Dean, Professor of Medicine, Tufts University School of Medicine, Boston, Massachusetts

Rosario Maiorca, M.D., Chairman, Chair of Nephrology, University of Brescia, Brescia, Italy

Deepak K. Malhotra, M.D., Ph.D., Associate Professor, Chief, Department of Medicine, Division of Nephrology, Medical College of Ohio, Toledo, Ohio

Hartmut H. Malluche, M.D., F.A.C.P., Professor of Medicine, Chief, Division of Nephrology, Bone and Mineral Metabolism, University of Kentucky Medical Center, Lexington, Kentucky

Harry S. Margolius, M.D., Ph.D., Professor of Pharmacology and Medicine, Medical University of South Carolina, Charleston, South Carolina

Pierre-Yves Martin, M.D., Medecin Adjoint, Privat Docent, Department of Medicine, Geneva University, Geneva, Switzerland

Arturo Martinez, M.D., F.A.C.S., Sharp Memorial Medical Center, San Diego, California

Manuel Martínez-Maldonado, M.D., President and Dean, Ponce School of Medicine, Ponce, Puerto Rico

Shaul G. Massry, M.D., Professor Emeritus, Keck School of Medicine, University of Southern California School of Medicine, Los Angeles, California

Ziad Massy, M.D., Research Associate, INSERM, Unit 507, Necker Hospital, Paris, France

Philip R. Mayeux, Ph.D., Associate Professor, Department of Pharmacology and Toxicology, University of Arkansas, Little Rock, Arkansas

Mary G. McGeown, M.D., Ph.D., Professional Fellow, Faculty of Medicine, Queen's University, Belfast, Northern Ireland, United Kingdom

Robert Mendez, M.D., Professor of Urology and Surgery, University of Southern California, Los Angeles, California

Catherine M. Meyers, Department of Medicine, Renal-Electrolyte and Hypertension Division, University of Pennsylvania School of Medicine, Philadelphia, Pennsylvania

Jeffrey H. Miner, M.D., Department of Medicine, Renal Division, Washington University School of Medicine, St. Louis, Missouri

William E. Mitch, M.D., Garland Herndon Professor of Medicine, Director, Renal Division, Emory University School of Medicine, Atlanta, Georgia

Toshio Miyata, M.D., Ph.D., Associate Professor, Department of Internal Medicine, Tokai University School of Medicine, Kanagawa, Japan

Stephen K.L. Mo, M.B., M.R.C.P., Specialist in Medicine/ Senior Medical Doctor, Department of Medicine, Pamela Youde Nethersole Eastern Hospital, Hong Kong, China

Kulwant Singh Modi, M.D., F.R.C.P., F.A.C.P., Associate Professor, Department of Medicine, Division of Nephrology, Medical College of Ohio, Toledo, Ohio

András Mogyorósi, M.D., Assistant Professor, Department of Medicine, Virginia Commonwealth University, Medical College of Virginia, Richmond, Virginia

Bruce A. Molitoris, M.D., Professor of Medicine, Director, Division of Nephrology, Indiana University Medical Center, Indianapolis, Indiana

Marie-Claude Monier-Faugere, M.D., Research Professor of Medicine, Department of Internal Medicine, Division of Nephrology, Bone and Mineral Metabolism, University of Kentucky, Lexington, Kentucky

John Moran, M.D., VASCA Inc., Tewksbury, Maine

R. Scott Morehead, M.D., Associate Professor, Department of Internal Medicine, Division of Pulmonary and Critical Care Medicine, University of Kentucky School of Medicine, Lexington, Kentucky

Peter E. Morris, M.D., Department of Medicine, Pulmonary and Critical Care Medicine, University of Kentucky, Lexington, Kentucky

Heini Murer, M.D., Professor and Chief, Department of Physiology, University of Zürich, Zürich, Switzerland

Shigeaki Muto, M.D., Assistant Professor, Department of Nephrology, Jichi Medical School, Minamikawachi, Tochigi, Japan

Bryan D. Myers, M.D., Professor, Department of Medicine, Stanford University Medical Center, Stanford, California

Catherine M. Myers, M.D., Department of Medicine, Renal-Electrolyte and Hypertension Division, Penn Center for Molecular Studies of Kidney Diseases, University of Pennsylvania School of Medicine, Philadelphia, Pennsylvania

Joseph V. Nally, Jr., M.D., Director of Fellowship Training, Department of Nephrology and Hypertension, The Cleveland Clinic Foundation, Cleveland, Ohio

Robert G. Narins, M.D., Director of Postgraduate Education, American Society of Nephrology, Washington, D.C.

Cynthia C. Nast, M.D., Professor of Pathology, University of California, Los Angeles, School of Medicine, Los Angeles, California

Karl A. Nath, M.B., Ch.B., Professor, Department of Medicine, Mayo Clinic, Rochester, Minnesota

Nicholas J. Nickl, M.D., Associate Professor of Internal Medicine, Director of Endoscopy, University of Kentucky School of Medicine, Lexington, Kentucky

David J. Nikolic-Paterson, D.Phil., Honorary Lecturer, Department of Medicine, Monash University, Clayton, Victoria, Australia

Toshimitsu Niwa, M.D., Ph.D., Associate Professor and Deputy Director, Department of Preventive Medicine, Nagoya University Daiko Medical Center, Nagoya, Japan

Karl D. Nolph, M.D., Professor Emeritus, Department of Medicine, Nephrology, University of Missouri Health Science Center, Columbia, Missouri

Irene Noronha, Department of Nephrology, University of Sao Paulo School of Medicine, Sao Paulo, Brazil

Antonia C. Novello, M.D., M.P.H., Commissioner of Health, New York, New York, 14th Surgeon General of the United States, Visiting Professor of Health Policy and Management, Johns Hopkins School of Hygiene and Public Health, Baltimore, Maryland

Hiroaki Oda, M.D., Ph.D., Lecturer, Second Department of Medicine, Hiroshima University School of Medicine, Hiroshima, Japan

Unini Odama, M.D., Fellow, Department of Preventive Medicine, Rush Presbyterian-St. Luke's Medical Center, Chicago, Illinois

Michael O'Donnell, Ph.D., Nephrology Research Laboratory, Minneapolis Medical Research Foundation, Minneapolis, Minnesota

Jeffrey L. Osborn, M.D., Professor, Department of Biology and Neuroscience Program, Trinity College, Hartford, Connecticut

William F. Owen, Jr., M.D., Associate Professor, Department of Medicine, Duke University School of Medicine, Durham, North Carolina

Paul M. Palevsky, M.D., Renal Section, Veterans Affairs Pittsburgh Healthcare System, Pittsburgh, Pennsylvania

Mark S. Paller, M.D., Professor, Department of Medicine, University of Minnesota, Minneapolis, Minnesota

Biff F. Palmer, M.D., Professor of Internal Medicine, Director of Clinical Nephrology, University of Texas Southwestern Medical School, Dallas, Texas

Patrick S. Parfrey, M.D., F.R.C.P.C., Research Professor, Department of Medicine, Memorial University of Newfoundland, St. John's, Newfoundland, Canada

Yuri R. Parisky, M.D., Associate Professor, Department of Radiology, University of Southern California, Norris Cancer Center, Los Angeles, California

Gustavo Parra, M.D., Professor and Nephrologist, Department of Medicine, La Universitario de Zulia Hospital Universitario de Marcaibo, Zulia, Venezuela

Patrizia Passerini, M.D., Assistant in Nephrology, Division of Nephrology and Dialysis, Ospedale Maggiore Policlinico IRCCS, Milan, Italy

Richard V. Paul, M.D., Associate Professor, Department of Medicine, Medical University of South Carolina, Charleston, South Carolina

Oscar Fernando Pavão dos Santos, M.D., Associate Professor, Department of Medicine, Escola Paulista de Medicina, Sao Paulo, Brazil

V. Ram Peddi, M.D., Associate Professor, Department of Medicine, University of Cincinnati College of Medicine, Cincinnati, Ohio

Israel Penn, M.D., (deceased) Professor, Department of Surgery, Transplantation Division, University of Cincinnati College of Medicine, Cincinnati, Ohio

Guido O. Perez, M.D., Professor, Department of Medicine, University of Miami School of Medicine, Miami, Florida

Alessandra F. Perna, M.D., Ph.D., Assistant Professor, Department of Pediatrics, Division of Nephrology, Second University of Naples, School of Medicine, Naples, Italy

Phuong-Chi T. Pham, M.D., Assistant Clinical Professor of Medicine, Department of Medicine, Division of Nephrology, Olive View—University of California, Los Angeles Medical Center, Sylmar, California

Phuong-Thu T. Pham, M.D., Clinical Instructor, Department of Medicine, Division of Nephrology, Kidney and Pancreas Transplantation, University of California, Los Angeles Medical Center, Los Angeles, California

Jeffrey L. Platt, M.D., Professor of Surgery, Immunology and Pediatrics, Department of Transplant Biology, Mayo Clinic Rochester, Rochester, Minnesota

Craig F. Plato, M.D., Hypertension Research Division, Henry Ford Hospital, Detroit, Michigan

David W. Ploth, M.D., Arthur V. Williams Professor of Medicine, Director, Division of Nephrology, Medical University of South Carolina, Charleston, South Carolina

Marc A. Pohl, M.D., Ray W. Gifford Endowed Chair, Section Head in Clinical Hypertension, Department of Nephrology and Hypertension, The Cleveland Clinic Foundation, Cleveland, Ohio

Claudio Ponticelli, M.D., Chief, Division of Nephrology and Dialysis, Ospedale Maggiore, Milan, Italy

Mordecai M. Popovtzer, M.D., F.A.C.P., Professor of Medicine, Chief, Department of Nephrology and Hypertension, Hebrew University-Hadassah Medical Organization, Jerusalem, Israel

Jerome G. Porush, M.D., Professor, Department of Medicine, State University of New York Health Science Center at Brooklyn, Brooklyn, New York

John B. Pritchard, Ph.D., Chief, Laboratory of Pharmacology and Chemistry, National Institute of Environmental Health Sciences, Research Triangle Park, North Carolina

Jules B. Puschett, M.D., Professor, Chief, and The Harry B. Greenberg Chair in Internal Medicine, Department of Medicine, Tulane University School of Medicine, New Orleans, Louisiana

Charles D. Pusey, F.R.C.P., F.R.C.Path., Professor of Renal Medicine, Department of Medicine, Imperial College School of Medicine, London, United Kingdom

Gary A. Quamme, D.V.M., Ph.D., Professor, Department of Medicine, Vancouver Hospital and Health Sciences Center, University of British Columbia, Vancouver, British Columbia, Canada

Hamid Rabb, M.D., Associate Professor, Division of Nephrology, Hennepin County Medical Center, Minneapolis, Minnesota

Ralph Rabkin, M.D., Professor, Department of Medicine, Stanford University, Stanford, California

Jacob Rajfer, M.D., Professor, Department of Urology, University of California, Los Angeles, School of Medicine, Los Angeles, California

Juhani Rapola, M.D., Ph.D., Chief Emeritus, Pathology Unit, Hospital for Children and Adolescents, University of Helsinki, Oulu, Finland

Andrew J. Rees, M.D., Regius Professor of Medicine, Department of Medicine and Therapeutics, University of Aberdeen, Aberdeen, Scotland

W. Brian Reeves, M.D., Associate Professor, Department of Medicine, University of Arkansas for Medical Sciences, Little Rock, Arkansas

Max C. Reif , M.D., Professor, Department of Medicine, University of Cincinnati, Cincinnati, Ohio

Ira W. Reiser, M.D., Assistant Professor, Department of Medicine, State University of New York Health Science Center at Brooklyn, Brooklyn, New York

Giuseppe Remuzzi, M.D., Director, Negri Bergamo Laboratories, "Mario Negri" Institute for Pharmacological Research, Bergamo, Italy

Jeffrey M. Rimmer, M.D., Professor, Department of Medicine, University of Vermont, Burlington, Vermont

Eberhard Ritz, M.D., Head, Division of Nephrology, Department of Internal Medicine, Ruperto Carola University, Heidelberg, Germany

Bernardo Rodríguez-Iturbe, M.D., Professor, Department of Medicine, La Universidad del Zulia, Maracaibo, Venezuela

Diane Rouse, Ph.D., Assistant Professor, Department of Medicine, Baylor College of Medicine, Houston, Texas

Robert H. Rubin, M.D., F.A.C.P., Gordon and Marjorie Osborne Professor of Health Sciences and Technology, Professor of Medicine, Harvard—MIT Division of Health Sciences and Technology, Harvard Medical School, Boston, Massachusetts

Robert K. Rude, M.D., Professor, Department of Medicine, Division of Endocrinology, Keck School of Medicine, University of Southern California, Los Angeles, California

Piero Ruggenenti, M.D., Head, Department of Renal Medicine, Mario Negri Institute for Pharmacological Research, Assistant Professor of Nephrology, Department of Nephrology and Dialysis/Ospedali Riuniti di Bergamo Istituto Di Ricerche Farmacologiche "Mario Negri" Institute for Pharmacological Research, Bergamo, Italy

Sandra Sabatini, M.D., Ph.D., F.A.C.P., Professor, Departments of Internal Medicine and Physiology, Texas Tech University Health Sciences Center, Lubbock, Texas

Robert L. Safirstein, M.D., Professor, Vice-Chair, Department of Medicine, University of Arkansas for Medical Sciences, Little Rock, Arkansas

Yahya Sagliker, M.D., Professor, Department of Medicine, Cukurova University School of Medicine, Adana, Turkey

Jeff M. Sands, M.D., Professor, Department of Medicine, Renal Division, Emory University, Atlanta, Georgia

Dianne Sandy, M.D., Lecturer in Adult Medicine, Department of Clinical Medical Sciences, Faculty of Medical Sciences, University of The West Indies, St. Augustine, Trinidad, West Indies

Steven C. Sansom, Ph.D., Associate Professor, Department of Physiology and Biophysics, University of Nebraska Medical Center, Omaha, Nebraska

Mark J. Sarnak, M.D., Assistant Professor, Department of Medicine, Division of Nephrology, Tufts University School of Medicine, Boston, Massachusetts

Vincenzo Savica, M.D., Associate Professor of Nephrology, Poli Clinico Universitario Gazzi, Messina, Sicily

Sabine Schmaldienst, M.D., Division of Nephrology, Department of Medicine III, University Hospital, Vienna, Austria

Eva Schnabel, M.D., Department of Radiology, Staedtisches Krankenhaus Bietigheim, Bietigheim, Gemany

Michael Schoemig, M.D., Department of Internal Medicine, Division of Nephrology, Ruperto Carolina University, Heidelberg, Germany

Nestor Schor, M.D., Professor, Department of Medicine, Escola Paulista de Medicina, Sao Paulo, Brazil

Robert W. Schrier, M.D., Professor and Chair, Department of Medicine, University of Colorado Health Sciences Center, Denver, Colorado

Gerald Schulman, M.D., Associate Professor and Director, End Stage Renal Diseases, Department of Medicine, Vanderbilt University Medical Center, Nashville, Tennessee

Steve J. Schwab, M.D., Professor and Vice Chair, Department of Medicine, Duke University Medical Center, Durham, North Carolina

Khaled Selim, M.D., Assistant Professor of Medicine, Division of Gastroenterology, Hepatology, and Nutrition, The University of Texas Houston Medical Center, Houston, Texas

Stuart I. Senkfor, M.D., Chief, Section of Nephrology, St. Joseph Hospital, Denver, Colorado

Sudhir V. Shah, M.D., Professor and Director, Division of Nephrology, University of Arkansas for Medical Sciences, Little Rock, Arkansas

Kumar Sharma, M.D., Associate Professor of Medicine, Director of Center for Diabetic Kidney Disease, Department of Medicine, Thomas Jefferson University, Philadelphia, Pennsylvania

Hamid Shidban, M.D., Assistant Professor, Department of Medicine and Urology, University of Southern California, Los Angeles, California

Cathryn L. Shuler, M.D., Assistant Professor, Division of Nephrology, Oregon Health Sciences University, Portland, Oregon

Miles H. Sigler, M.D., F.A.C.P., Clinical Professor, Department of Medicine, Thomas Jefferson University Medical College, Philadelphia, Pennsylvania

Eric E. Simon, M.D., Associate Professor, Department of Medicine, Section of Nephrology, Tulane University School of Medicine, New Orleans, Louisiana

Raja Sinniah, M.D., Professor, Department of Pathology, National University Hospital, Singapore

Visith Sitprija, M.D., Ph.D., Emeritus Professor, Department of Medicine, Chulalongkorn University Hospital and Director, Queen Saovabha Memorial Institute, Bangkok, Thailand

Eduardo Slatopolsky, M.D., Joseph Friedman Professor of Renal Diseases in Medicine, Department of Internal Medicine, Renal Division, Washington University School of Medicine, St. Louis, Missouri

Caroline Slive, M.D., INSERM, Unit 426, Faculté de Medicine Xavier Bichat, Paris, France

Miroslaw J. Smogorzewski, M.D., Ph.D., Associate Professor, Department of Medicine, Division of Nephrology, University of Southern California, Los Angeles, California

Hans W. Sollinger, M.D., Folkert O. Belzer Professor of Surgery, Department of Surgery, University of Wisconsin, Madison, Wisconsin

Rajanna Sreedhara, M.D., Associate Professor of Clinical Medicine, Department of Internal Medicine, State University of New York Health Science Center at Brooklyn, Brooklyn, New York

Barry S. Stein, M.D., Professor and Chief, Division of Urology, Brown University School of Medicine, Providence, Rhode Island

Peter Stenvinkel, M.D., Ph.D., Associate Professor, Department of Renal Medicine, Karolinska Institute, Huddinge, Sweden

Richard H. Sterns, M.D., Professor of Medicine, University of Rochester, Rochester, New York

C. Frederic Strife, M.D., Professor, Department of Pediatrics, University of Cincinnati College of Medicine, Cincinnati, Ohio

Wadi N. Suki, M.D., Professor of Medicine and Physiology and Molecular Biophysics, Department of Medicine, Baylor College of Medicine, Houston, Texas

Victoria L. Szatalowicz, M.D., Clinical Instructor, Department of Family Medicine, University of Southern California School of Medicine, Los Angeles, California

Michio Takeda, M.D., Department of Pharmacology and Toxicology, Kyorin University School of Medicine, Tokyo, Japan

Adina Tanasescu, M.D., Division of Nephrology, Keck School of Medicine, University of Southern California, Los Angeles, California

Richard L. Tannen, M.D., Professor, Department of Medicine, University of Pennsylvania School of Medicine, Philadelphia, Pennsylvania

Nauman Tarif, M.D., Instructor, Department of Preventive Medicine, Rush Presbyterian-St. Luke's Medical Center, Chicago, Illinois

Brendan P. Teehan, M.D., F.R.C.P., Clinical Professor, Department of Medicine, Jefferson Medical College, Philadelphia, Pennsylvania

Amir Tejani, M.D., Professor, Department of Pediatrics and Surgery, New York Medical College, North American Pediatric Renal Transplant Cooperative Study, Hawthorne, New York

Scott C. Thomson, M.D., Associate Professor, Department of Medicine, University of California, San Diego, San Diego, California

Nina E. Tolkoff-Rubin, M.D., Associate Professor of Medicine, Harvard Medical School, Boston, Massachusetts

Vicente E. Torres, M.D., Ph.D., Professor of Medicine, Department of Internal Medicine, Chair, Division of Nephrology, Mayo Clinic/Mayo Foundation, Rochester, Minnesota

Norishi Ueda, M.D., Assistant Professor, Department of Medicine, Division of Nephrology, University of Arkansas for Medical Sciences, Little Rock, Arkansas

Jean-Pierre Valentin, Ph.D., Principal Safety Pharmacologist, Department of Safety Pharmacology, Astrazeneca Research and Development Charnwood, Loughborough, Leics, United Kingdom

Spiros Vamvakas, M.D., Institute for Pharmacology and Toxicology, University of Würzburg, Würzburg, Germany

L. A. van Es, M.D., Professor of Medicine, Department of Nephrology, Leiden University Medical Center, Leiden, The Netherlands

Charles van Ypersele de Strihou, M.D., Professor of Medicine, Department of Internal Medicine, University of Louvain Medical School, Brussels, Belgium

David B. Van Wyck, M.D., Professor of Medicine and Surgery, Department of Medicine, University of Arizona College of Medicine, Tucson, Arizona

Nosratola D. Vaziri, M.D., Professor, Department of Internal Medicine, University of California, Irvine, Irvine, California

Edward F. Vonesh, Ph.D., Professor, Department of Clinical Preventive Medicine, Northwestern University Medical School, Chicago, Illinois

Thomas Waid, M.D., M.S., Associate Professor of Medicine, Department of Internal Medicine, Division of Nephrology, Bone and Mineral Metabolism, University of Kentucky College of Medicine, Lexington, Kentucky

Wei Wang, M.D., Instructor, Department of Medicine, Division of Renal Diseases and Hypertension, University of Colorado Health Sciences Center, Denver, Colorado

Florence L. Watts, M.D., Staff Physician, Department of Anesthesiology, Kennestone Hospital, Marietta, Georgia

Robert M. Weiss, M.D., Professor and Chief, Section of Urology, Department of Surgery, Yale University School of Medicine, New Haven, Connecticut

Donald E. Wesson, M.D., Professor of Medicine and Physiology, Chief of Nephrology and Renal Physiology Chairman, Department of Internal Medicine, Texas Tech University Health Sciences Center, Lubbock, Texas

Clark D. West, M.D., Professor Emeritus, Division of Pediatrics, University of Cincinnati College of Medicine, Cincinnati, Ohio

Roger C. Wiggins, M.B., B.Chir., Professor, Department of Internal Medicine, University of Michigan Medical School, Ann Arbor, Michigan

Christopher S. Wilcox, M.D., Ph.D., George E. Schreiner Professor of Nephrology, Division of Nephrology and Hypertension, Department of Medicine, Georgetown University, Washington, D.C.

James F. Winchester, M.D., Professor, Department of Medicine, Division of Nephrology and Hypertension, Georgetown University Medical Center, Washington, D.C.

Robert L. Winer, M.D., Adjunct Professor, Department of Medicine, University of California, Irvine, Irvine, California

Franz T. Winklhofer, M.D., Assistant Professor, Department of Medicine, University of Kansas, Kansas City, Kansas

Elaine M. Worcester, M.D., Assistant Professor, Department of Medicine, Medical College of Wisconsin, Milwaukee, Wisconsin

Robert L. Wortmann, M.D., Professor and Chair, Department of Internal Medicine, University of Oklahoma College of Medicine, Tulsa, Tulsa, Oklahoma

Nabil A. Yassa, M.D., Radiologist, Good Samaritan Hospital, Los Angeles, California

Jerry Yee, M.D., Division of Nephrology and Hypertension, Henry Ford Hospital, Detroit, Michigan

Luciano Zamboni, M.D., Emeritus Professor, Pathology and Laboratory Medicine, University of California, Los Angeles, School of Medicine, Los Angeles, California

Edward T. Zawada, Jr., M.D., Freeman Professor and Chairman, Department of Internal Medicine, University of South Dakota School of Medicine, Sioux Falls, South Dakota

Fuad N. Ziyadeh, M.D., Professor of Medicine, Division of Renal Electrolyte and Hypertension, University of Pennsylvania, Philadelphia, Pennsylvania

Carla Zoja, Biol.Sci.D., Head, Laboratory of Experimental Models of Kidney Diseases, Department of Molecular Medicine, "Mario Negri" Institute for Pharmacological Research, Bergamo, Italy

Fabio Zorzi, M.D., Assistant, Institute of Dermatological Science, IRCCS Ospedale Maggiore di Milan, Milan, Italy

SECTION I

Normal Anatomy, Physiology, and Metabolism of the Kidney

CHAPTER 1

Embryology and Structure of the Kidney

PART 1
Embryology of the Urinary System

Luciano Zamboni

The development of the organs of the definitive urinary system is the final stage of a long and continuous process that begins in the third week of fetal life (VIII to IX somite embryos) and results in the development of (a) the pronephros, (b) the mesonephros, and then (c) the metanephros. A detailed analysis of the first two stages (pronephric and mesonephric) of this continuous morphogenetic process is beyond the scope of this chapter; thus the following description will be concerned exclusively with the complex events that accompany the development of the definitive urinary organs, from the fifth to the thirty-fourth or thirty-sixth week of fetal life.

At the end of the fourth week of fetal life, the nephrogenic ridge (where most of the changes associated with urinary tract development are to occur) appears as a voluminous elongated body consisting of two main regions: a posterior region predominantly made up of undifferentiated mesenchymal cells in a primitive stroma and an anterior region occupied by the highly organized structures of the mesonephros. These highly organized structures are the mesonephric nephrons (glomeruli and excretory tubules) disposed in craniocaudal array and the collecting tubules draining into the wolffian duct; the wolffian duct runs in a craniocaudal direction along the entire length of the ridge and empties into the allantois, the embryonal transitory bladder, which in humans is rudimentary. The allantois voids in the cloaca, which the mesonephros shares with the primitive gut.

The development of the urinary bladder and urethra initiates with the formation of a membrane, the *urorectal septum*, which divides the cloaca into two distinct compartments: a dorsal or rectal compartment into which the primitive intestine empties and a ventral or urogenital compartment in communication with the allantois. The most caudal portion of the mesonephros, now separated from the terminal segment of the primitive intestine, soon assumes the configuration of an elongated tubular cavity, the *urogenital sinus*, opening to the exterior in a caudal and ventral direction and continuing with the allantois in a cranial and dorsal direction. In subsequent stages, the most caudal and ventral portions of the urogenital sinus differentiate into the urethra, whereas the cranial and dorsal segments give rise to the pavement of the bladder (i.e., the portion situated beneath and ventral to the orifices of the ureters). The trigonal region of the bladder derives from the transformation of the most caudal segment of the wolffian duct, whereas the upper portion of the bladder originates from the lower segment of the allantois.[1]

Considerably more complex are the morphogenetic events associated with the development of the ureter and kidney. These events begin with the formation of a diverticulum of the wolffian duct, the *ureteric bud*, which is first seen at the beginning of the fifth week of fetal life as a small evagination of the duct, close to its opening into the allantois. The diverticulum soon develops into a prominent tubular structure, which for the first week after it appears continues to elongate into the mesenchyme of the nephrogenic cord along a dorsocranial direction forming the rudiment of the ureter. From the sixth week on, the elongation of the diverticulum is accompanied by repeated branching; this process of elongation and division is responsible for the development of the kidney and its components, from the pelvis to the nephrons. The complex patterns of ureteric bud elongation and division were clarified by microdissection procedures. These studies demonstrated that the ureteric bud consistently divides dichotomously, either symmetrically or asymmetrically. In the first case, the branches arising from a division are of the same caliber and elongate at the same rate and for the same distance before the next division. In the second case, the branches are of different caliber and display different rates of growth and/or different attitudes toward division. Each branch consists of a main tubular segment and an advancing extremity, referred to as an *ampulla* because of its bulbous shape.

The first division of the ureteric bud is symmetrically dichotomous; it produces two branches (the rudiment of the pelvis) that elongate in a craniocaudal direction, determining the future shape and orientation of the kidney. These branches soon divide asymmetrically, each producing one long and one short branch. The long branches are directed toward the poles

[1] The upper segment of the allantois obliterates and is transformed into a fibrous, cordlike structure, the urachus, reaching to the umbilicus.

of the kidney, and the short branches are directed toward the interpolar region at right angles to the others. The next divisions are usually asymmetrical, with branching at the poles of the developing kidney occurring more rapidly than in the interpolar regions, where, because of the slower divisional rate, the tubules generally elongate more than the polar ones. The branches from these successive generations of divisions are those from which calyces, papillary ducts, and collecting tubules originate. The major calyces develop from the second to the third generation of branches, and the minor calyces develop from a single division that can occur at any time between the third and the sixth generation. These branches soon attain their definitive configuration as they become rapidly distended by the urine produced in the developing nephrons and prevented from easily flowing out of the calyces by the restricted lumen of the ureter. The papillary ducts develop from subsequent generations of branches (up to the ninth or the tenth), and the collecting tubules develop from still later generations.

Beginning with the tenth and eleventh generations, any further branching of the ureteric bud results in the development of nephrons, which become organized from the mesenchymal elements of the nephrogenic ridge under the inductive influence of the ampullar extremities of the advancing collecting tubules (Fig. 1.1).

The complex events that accompany the development of each nephron and its various components initiate with the condensation of the undifferentiated mesenchymal cells of the nephrogenic ridge around the ampullar extremity of each collecting tubule; thus crescentic bodies (called *metanephric caps*) made up of several concentric cellular layers form (Fig. 1.2). Owing to the direction of growth of the ureteric bud branches, the metanephric caps are found at any given time just beneath the capsule of the developing kidney (Figs. 1.1 and 1.3). Each time an ampulla expands and begins to flatten in preparation for another division and formation of another generation of collecting tubules, an ovoidal nest of cells, representing the precursor of

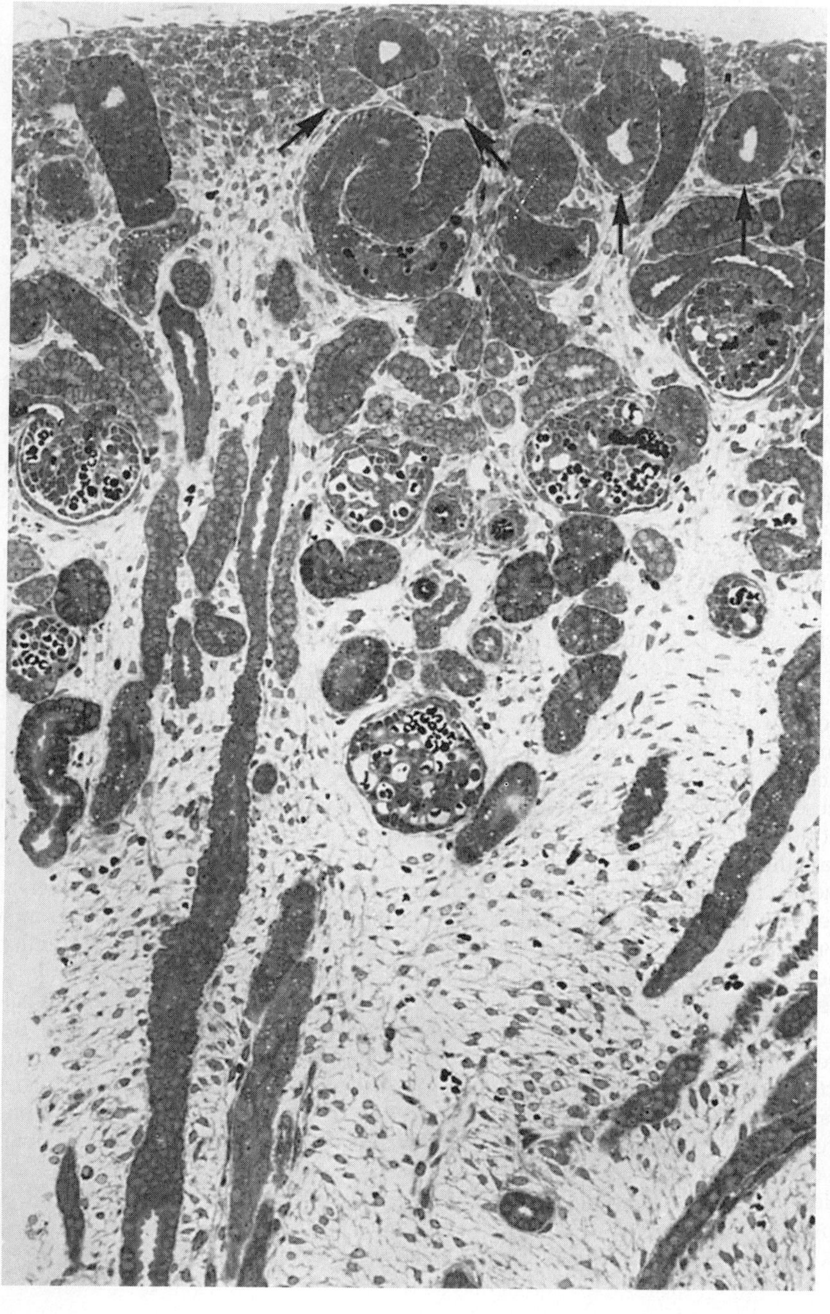

Figure 1.1. Nephron formation in the developing kidney of a 12-week-old human fetus. Notice the condensation of the mesenchyme around the most superficial extremities of the branches of the ureteric bud just below the surface of the organ; metanephric vesicle formation *(arrows)* is also shown. A 1-μm thick plastic section stained with toluidine blue. ×220.

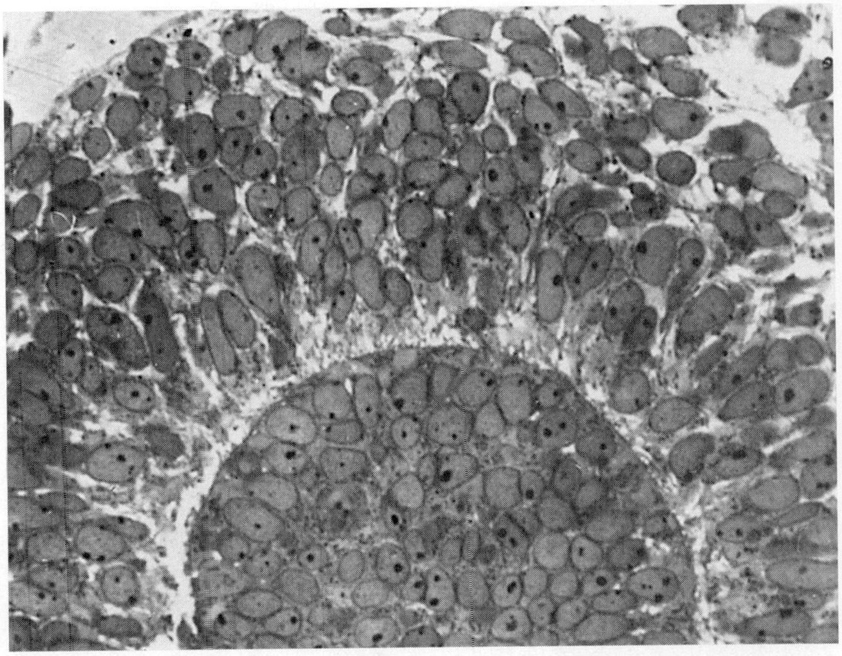

Figure 1.2. Metanephric cap forming around the ampullar extremity of a ureteric bud branch (collecting tubule). A 1-μm thick plastic section stained with toluidine blue. ×900.

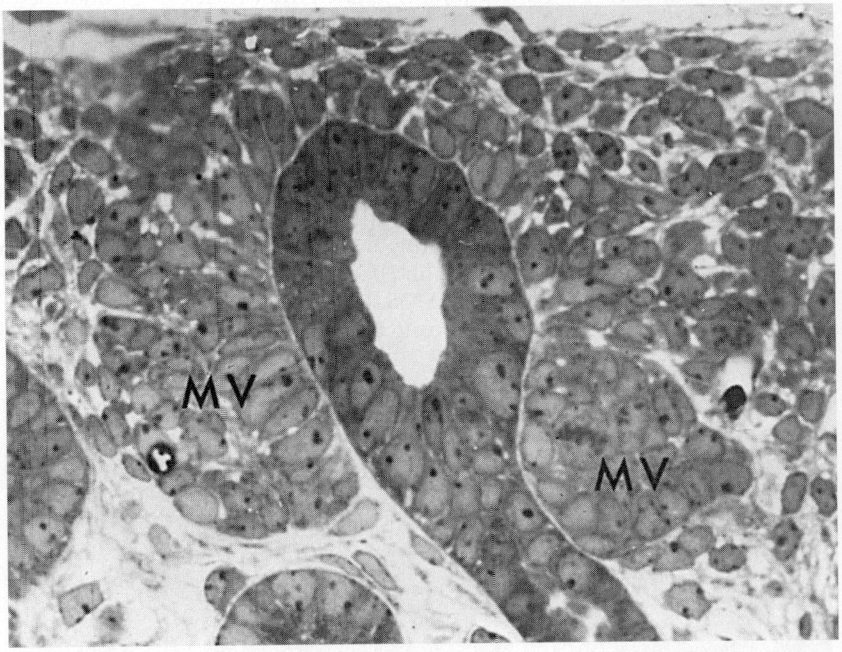

Figure 1.3. Early stage of metanephric vesicle *(MV)* formation from a metanephric cap around the ampullar extremity of a collecting tubule just below the surface of the developing kidney. A 1-μm thick plastic section stained with toluidine blue. ×750.

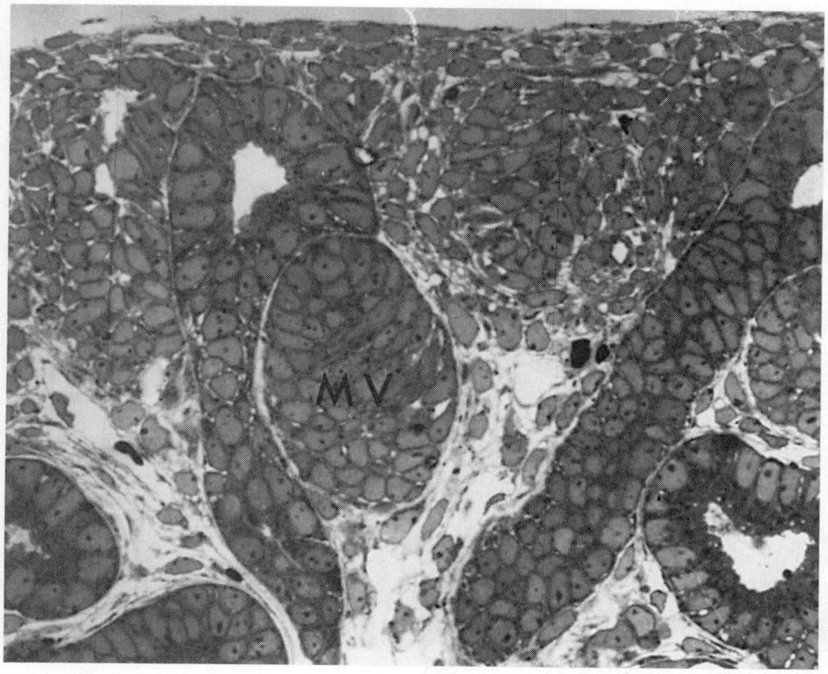

Figure 1.4. A later stage of metanephric vesicle *(MV)* formation than that shown in Fig. 1.3. The vesicle, the lumen of which is not visible in this plane of section, has become separated from the metanephric cap and appears already to be demarcated by a basal lamina. A 1-μm thick plastic section stained with toluidine blue. ×600.

the various segments of the nephron, separates from each extremity of the metanephric cap and remains localized in the angle between the ampulla and the collecting tubule (Figs. 1.3 and 1.4). Almost immediately, this cellular mass becomes surrounded by a basal lamina (Fig. 1.4) and is provided with a central cavity (Fig. 1.1), the presence of which justifies the term *metanephric vesicle* used to designate this hollow nest of cells. The cavity of the vesicle soon establishes communication with the lumen of the collecting tubule. Through intense cell multiplication, the metanephric vesicle elongates rapidly, and as a consequence of differential growth, its original outline becomes modified by two indentations or clefts (Fig. 1.5): one on the lower third of the outer surface of the vesicle (i.e., opposite the collecting tubule) and the other on the inner surface just below the upper third. The vesicle thus assumes the shape of a letter "S" consisting of three limbs: an upper limb situated above the upper cleft and communicating with the collecting tubule, a middle limb between upper and lower clefts, and a lower limb below the lower cleft on the outer surface of the vesicle. Each of these limbs differentiates into one or more segments of the nephron. The upper and middle limbs, which remain tubular, produce distal and proximal tubules and the thin limb of Henle's loop. The lower limb expands, assuming a cuplike shape (see Fig. 1.5). Its cells become organized into two layers: an upper layer of cuboidal cells and a lower layer of flattened cells (Figs. 1.6 and 1.7), which soon become separated by a slitlike space, part of the original

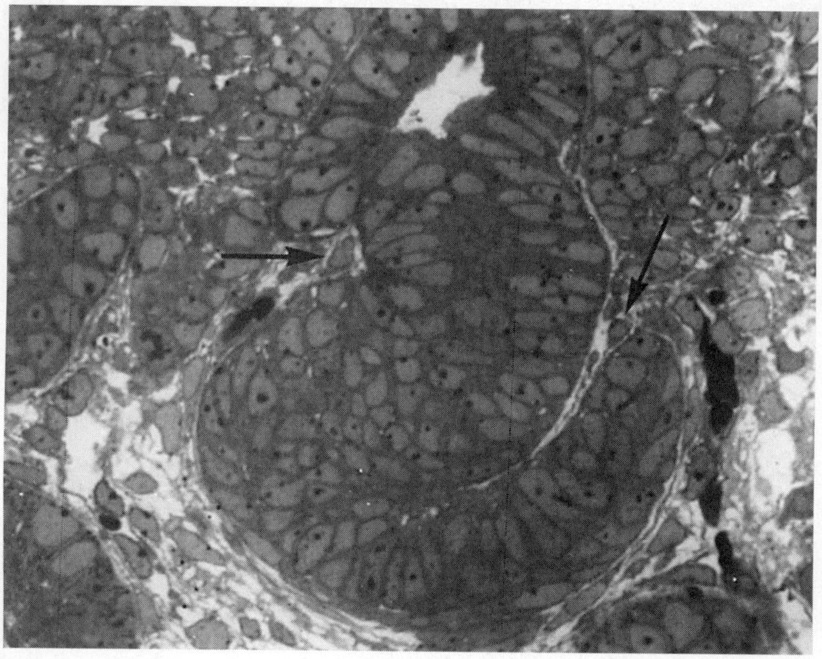

Figure 1.5. The "S" stage of metanephric vesicle development. Owing to formation of two clefts *(arrows)* as a result of differential growth, the vesicle now consists of three limbs. The blood capillary at the mouth of the lower cleft *(center right)* will later develop into glomerular vessels. A 1-μm thick plastic section stained with toluidine blue. ×750.

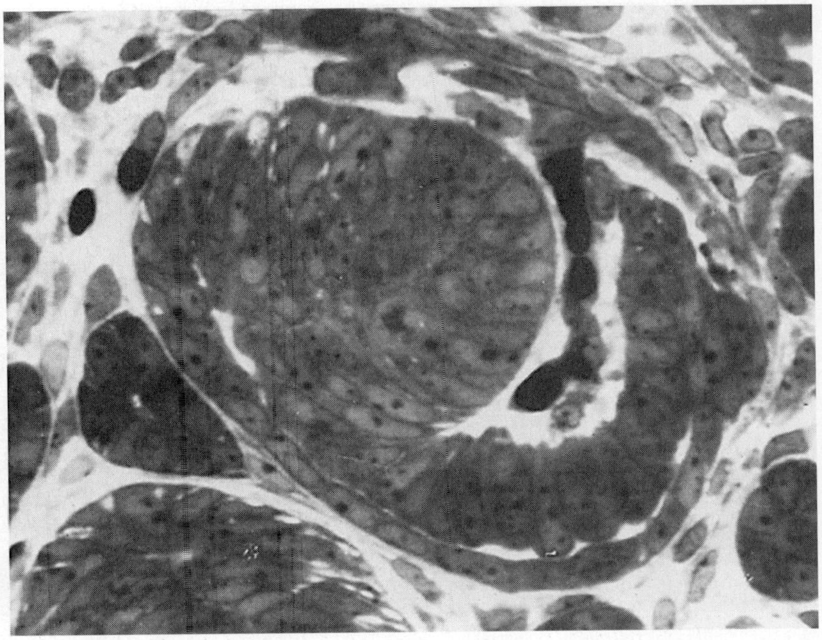

Figure 1.6. Sequential stages in the development of the lower limb of the S-shaped metanephric vesicle; the upper layer of cuboidal cells (the future visceral epithelial cells of the glomerulus) and the lower layer of flattened cells (the future parietal epithelium) are separated by a narrow space that will become the glomerular space. Notice the deepening into the cleft between the vesicle's lower and middle limbs of the blood capillary from which glomerular vessels will later develop. ×900.

vesicle lumen. The cells of the upper layer differentiate into the visceral epithelium, and those of the lower layer differentiate into the parietal epithelium; the narrow space between the two layers represents the future glomerular space.

The vascular elements of the glomerulus derive from a blood capillary that is first seen at the mouth of the lower cleft at the time the metanephric vesicle begins to elongate (Fig. 1.5); subsequently, the vessel deepens into the cleft (Figs. 1.6 and 1.7), increases in extension, and splits repeatedly within the confined cleftal space, gradually differentiating into glomerular arterioles and capillaries (Fig. 1.8). The myoepithelial cells of the arteriolar tunica media and the mesangial cells of the capillaries originate from a few primitive mesenchymal cells accompanying the capillary during its penetration into, and development within, the lower cleft of the S-shaped vesicle (Figs. 1.7 and 1.8). The changes responsible for the development of the epithelial and vascular elements of the glomerulus occur simultaneously with continuous elongations of the upper and middle limbs of the original S-shaped vesicle and their differentiation into the various tubular segments of the nephron (Fig. 1.9).

The pattern by which different nephrons attach to their collecting tubules varies considerably. It has been shown that these anatomic variations are the expression of the different activities of the ampullar portions of the collecting tubules in subsequent stages of nephron development. In an early stage, from the fifth to the fifteenth week, communication between the developing

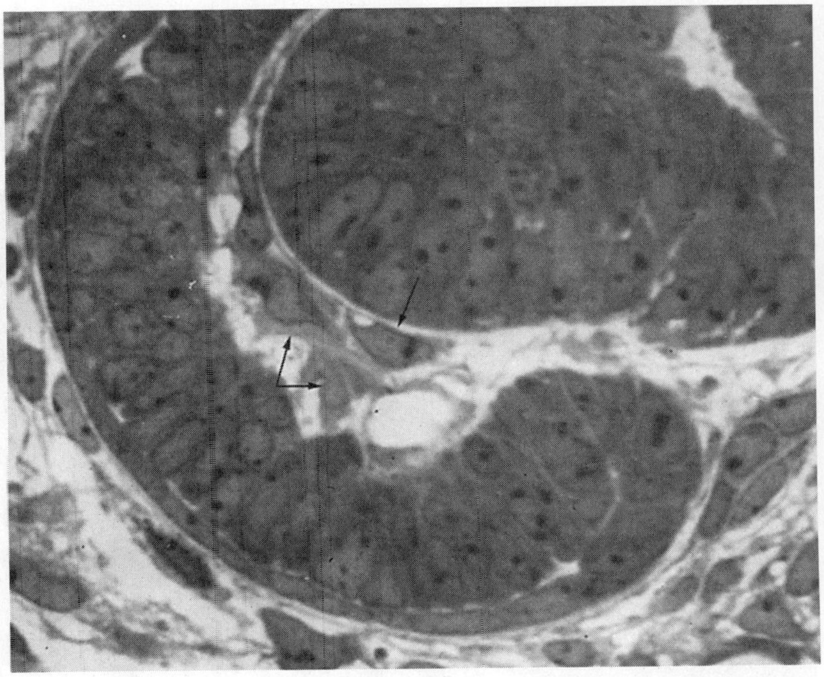

Figure 1.7. The intracleftal portion of the capillary is associated with a few mesenchymal cells *(arrows),* which will later differentiate into mesangial cells. A 1-μm thick plastic section stained with toluidine blue. ×900.

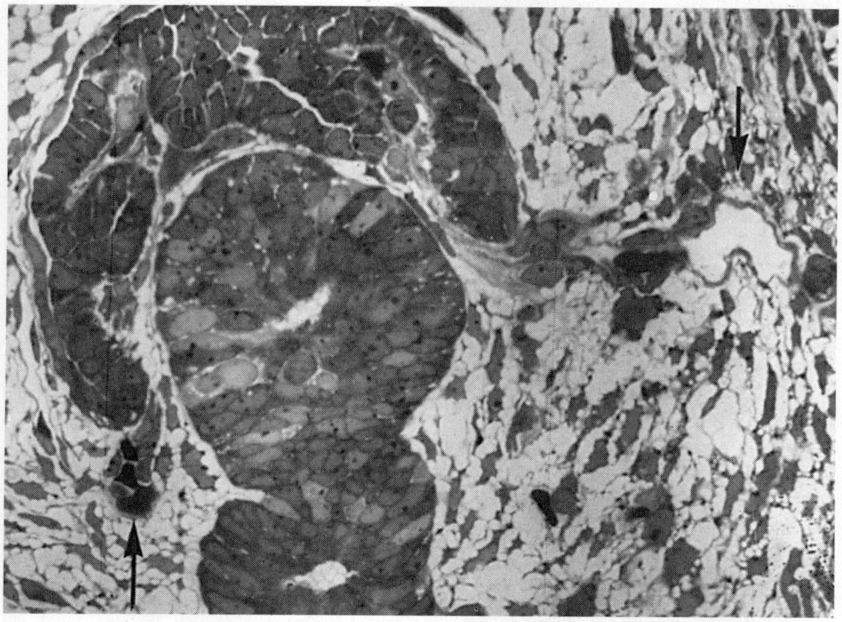

Figure 1.8. A later stage of glomerulus formation from the lower limb of the metanephric vesicle. Afferent and efferent vessels can be seen on each side of the limb *(arrows)* while capillaries are developing in a tortuous pattern within the narrow cleftal space. The separation between the lower limb of the vesicle and the tubular middle and upper limbs is only apparent and is caused by the plane of the section. A 1-μm thick plastic section stained with toluidine blue. ×750.

nephron and the ampulla is within the zone of ampullar growth. At this stage, ampullae can induce new nephron formation only when they are not already carrying a nephron. Consequently, as newer generations of collecting tubules are formed, the nephrons remain attached to the ampullae of origin and are transferred from one generation of collecting tubules to the next; thus irrespective of the generation of collecting tubules to which they belong, all nephrons induced during this stage come to be permanently attached to the last collecting tubule formed in this period. From the fifteenth to the twenty-second week, the communication between a nephron and its inducing ampulla continues to be within the area of growth; to compensate for the decreased branching activity of this period, however, the ampullae acquire the capability of inducing new nephron formation even when they are already carrying nephrons. Nephrons of successive generations formed during this period do not attach individually to their collecting tubules but become attached to one another via a connecting tubule, with only the nephron of the last generation attaching directly to the ampulla of the collecting tubule from which it was induced. Such a succession of nephrons draining into a single collecting tubule via a common connecting tubule is know as an *arcade.* From the twenty-second to the thirty-sixth week, ampullae no longer branch but are still able to grow and induce new nephron formation. Each nephron induced during this period attaches to the ampulla behind the zone of growth (i.e., at the junction of the ampulla with the main segment of the collecting tubule). As the ampullae advance, these nephrons are left behind, resulting in an orderly succession of nephrons of different generations attached to the terminal unbranched segments of the collecting tubules. From the thirty-

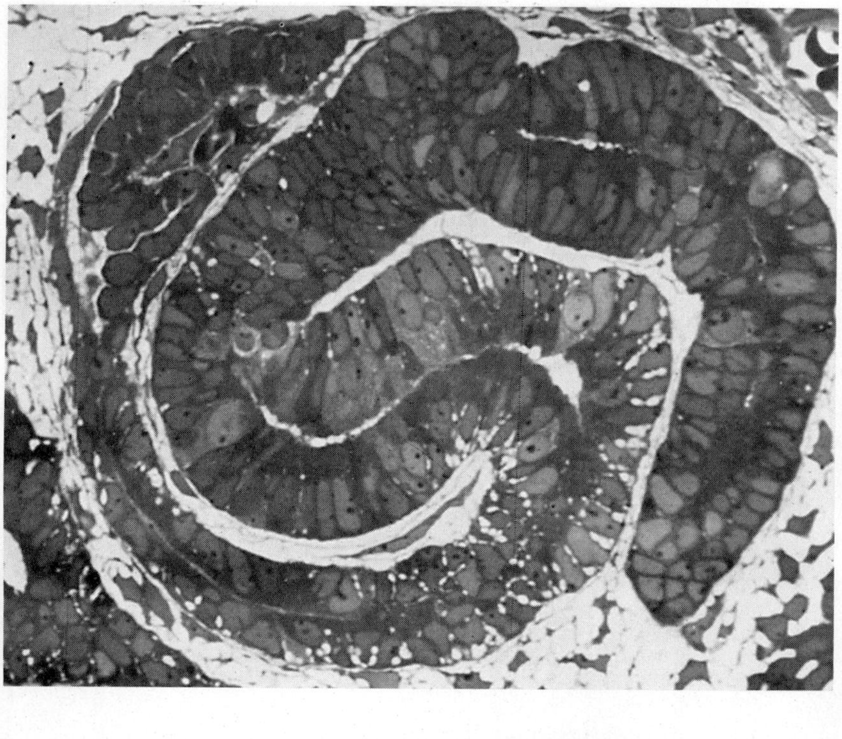

Figure 1.9. Progressive elongation of the upper and middle limbs of the metanephric vesicle to form the various tubular segments of the nephron. The developing glomerulus is toward the *upper-left corner* of the micrograph. A 1-μm thick plastic section stained with toluidine blue. ×850.

sixth week on, ampullar activity ceases and there is no further production of collecting tubules and nephrons. The last nephron induced by each collecting tubule represents the termination of that tubule, which now has 10 to 15 nephrons attached to it according to different patterns.

Selected Readings

Osathanondh V, Potter EL. Development of human kidney as shown by microdissection. III. Formation and interrelationship of collecting tubules and nephrons. *Arch Pathol* 1965;76:290–302.

The first study to clarify the structural (embryologic) bases for the variable patterns by which different nephrons become connected to their collecting tubules and for the different lengths of the Henle's loops in cortical and juxtamedullary nephrons.

Saxen L. *Organogenesis of the kidney.* Cambridge: Cambridge University Press, 1987:1–173.

This is a classic monograph on the ontogenesis of vertebrae excretory system. It discusses in detail the experimental methods used for the study of kidney development, interaction between epithelial and mesenchymal components of the kidney, and inductive signals for the establishment of the structure of the nephron.

PART 2

Molecular and Cellular Events During Kidney Development

Qais Al-Awqati

The mature mammalian kidney develops when an outgrowth of the wolffian duct, the ureteric bud, induces the metanephric mesenchyme to differentiate into the nephron. The ureteric bud in turn is induced to branch by the mesenchyme to form the collecting system. As contact is established between these two cell types, a complex transformation occurs whereby the mesenchymal cells convert to an epithelial type and form the renal vesicle. The renal vesicle then undergoes a morphologic transformation into a comma-shaped body. It develops a slit, the glomerular crevice, and undergoes asymmetric elongation to form a structure termed the *S-shaped body,* which upon being connected to the ureteric bud branch forms the primitive nephron. Endothelial cells invade the glomerular crevice located at the pole farthest away from the ureteric bud branch and form the glomerular capillaries. Epithelial cells of the glomerulus, proximal and distal tubules, and loop of Henle are derived from the mesenchyme; the papillary, medullary, and cortical collecting tubules are derived from the ureteric bud.

The early critical events in nephrogenesis involve a number of rate-limiting steps. Some of these steps may require diffusible factors such as growth factors. Others may involve the expression of surface proteins, which in the right three-dimensional context will act as the agent for cell-to-cell contact, leading to the conversion of mesenchymal cells to epithelial cells and the further development of epithelial cells to segmented nephrons.

STEM CELLS IN THE KIDNEY

The mature nephron of mammals is composed of at least 13 epithelial cell types derived from the mesenchyme and several others derived from the ureteric bud. In addition, the kidney contains endothelial cells (probably of different types), interstitial cells, and vascular smooth muscle cells, including mesangial cells. A metanephric mesenchymal cell must undergo a phenotype conversion to these different cell types, a process that is then followed by further differentiation into one or another of the terminally differentiated renal cells. To study the path that the mesenchymal cell takes toward becoming a differentiated tubule cell, the "fate map" of these cells must be known. Two potential schemes can be postulated. Figure 1.10, which for simplicity, shows only that of the epithelial cell lineage. A similar one could be constructed for the stromal lineage, which produces endothelia, smooth muscle, and interstitial cell types.

In one scheme, the mesenchyme is made up of multipotent stem cells, each of which can generate all of the cell types (Fig. 1.10, *right*). Alternatively, the cells of the mesenchyme have already been committed to a developmental pathway and induction allows association of the requisite types of cells into the renal vesicle (Fig. 1.10, *left*). To distinguish between these two models, it was necessary to develop a system that will allow the explicit determination of the progeny of a single cell. We used a method that introduced a reporter gene (β-galactosidase) by means of a replication defective retrovirus. Clonal dilution is eventually reached by reducing the titer of the infecting virus. Poisson statistics showed that only a single cell must have been infected. When rat mesenchymal cells were infected at clonal dilution before induction by ureteric bud, tagged cells appeared in all identifiable segments of one individual nephron. These results demonstrate the presence of stem cells in the metanephric mesenchyme similar to the predictions of the right panel in Fig. 1.10. Interestingly, labeled cells derived from a single progenitor cell were found in two adjacent nephrons. The most likely interpretation of the latter studies is that the daughters of a stem cell were mobile and able to insert themselves into adjacent renal vesicles. This demonstrates that a nephron is not clonally derived. Only about 5% to 10% of the cells of the nephron were derived from a single progenitor implying that it takes several (10 to 100) stem cells to form a single nephron. Half of the studies generated stromal cells and not epithelial cells.

When the mesenchyme was first induced and then labeled at clonal dilution, the results were dramatically different. The progeny of a single cell populated only one segment of a single nephron. Hence, the developmental potential of a metanephric cell is restricted after it has been induced. Individual blue cells are seen in single nephron segments but are not present in the adjacent segment of the same nephron. The most likely reason is that the location of a cell in a renal vesicle or S-shaped body exposes it to the effect of neighboring cells, which guide or force it into a specified developmental pathway.

Conversion of induced mesenchyme into the different segments can follow two potential pathways. In one pathway, induction allows all segment progenitors to be "born" at the same

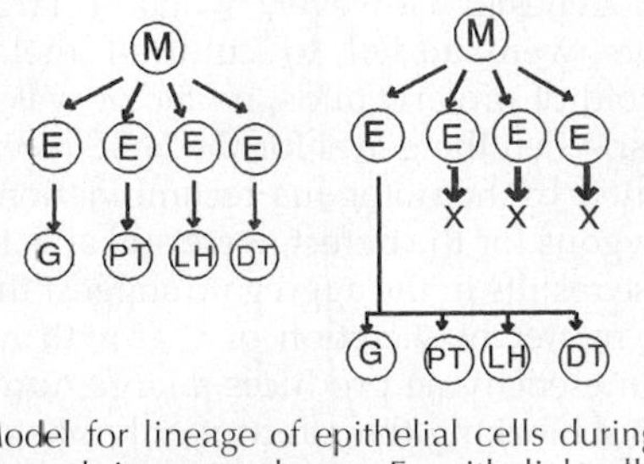

Figure 1.10. Model for lineage of epithelial cells during kidney development. *M,* metanephric mesenchyme; *E,* epithelial cell; *G,* glomerular epithelium; *PT,* proximal tubule; *LH,* loop of Henle; *DT,* distal tubule.

time. Here the segment progenitors will proceed to produce all the nephron segments simultaneously. In another model, after induction, a cascade of development is initiated in which one segment of the nephron develops first and perhaps influences the adjacent segment to develop. When nephron progenitors were infected 24 hours after induction, it was found that most positive colonies were in proximal tubules and distal tubules with very few glomerular colonies. These studies suggest that the proximal and distal progenitor cells are undergoing a burst of proliferation. The low number of glomerular colonies suggests either the glomerular progenitors have already completed their proliferation or they are yet to start it. This demonstrates that proliferation of induced progenitors does not occur at the same time, implying that segmentation of the nephron occurs in some kind of ordered cascade. The conclusion is that the segmental progenitors are not all "born" at the same time.

Other studies have highlighted the role of stromal cells in kidney development. Deletion of the gene BF2 resulted in gross defects in kidney development, with a drastic reduction in the number of nephrons formed. BF2 is a transcription factor that is expressed only in stromal cells. Furthermore, others have shown that deletion of retinoic acid receptor (RARβ2) also resulted in gross malformation of the epithelial lineage. Remarkably, they showed that this transcription factor was also expressed in stromal cells, but its pattern of expression did not overlap with that of BF2, implying that at least two lineages of stromal cells exist, each of which expresses a different activity that controls epithelial development.

APOPTOSIS IN RENAL DEVELOPMENT

When metanephric mesenchyme was cultured *in vitro* without an inducer, the cells fragmented, with the condensed nuclear appearance characteristic of apoptosis. DNA was rapidly degraded in these rudiments such that by 24 hours, very little high-molecular-weight DNA remained. Incubation with an inducer such as embryonic spinal cord prevented the DNA degradation. These results suggest that induction of metanephric mesenchyme involves at least two stages: Rescue of the cells from programmed cell death must precede the other steps of proliferation and mesenchymal to epithelial conversion. It has been demonstrated that the ureteric bud secretes into the medium a large number of activities that rescue the metanephric mesenchyme from apoptosis. One of these factors, when purified and sequenced, was found to be basic fibroblast growth factor (bFGF); another was tissue inhibitor of metalloproteinase 2 (TIMP2). These activities were able to prevent apoptosis but did not result in conversion of the mesenchyme to epithelia.

To examine the roles of growth factors in kidney development, investigators have inactivated these factors by adding either antibodies or antisense DNA for their receptors in *in vitro* organ culture. Inhibition of the effect of insulinlike growth factors (IGFI or II), nerve growth factor (NGF), hepatocyte growth factor (HGF), and transforming growth factor α (TGFα) prevented tubulogenesis. However, when a large number of growth factors were added to cultured metanephric mesenchyme devoid of ureteric buds, no factor was able to induce tubulogenesis. When the genes for the NGF receptor and IGFII were inactivated by homologous recombination, the progeny, when homozygous for the defect, were still able to form normal kidneys. These results in the aggregate suggest that induction is not simply a matter of secretion of a growth factor. That the metanephric mesenchyme produces a large number of growth factors and that blocking the effect of only one of these factors can stop development implies that there must be a number of rate-limiting steps in nephrogenesis, each requiring at least one growth factor. The role of these factors will have to be examined using assays that identify these steps.

RECIPROCAL INTERACTIONS BETWEEN MESENCHYME AND URETERIC BUD

Conversion of mesenchyme to epithelial cells is the most dramatic effect of induction. During this process, epithelial proteins such as collagen IV and uvomorulin appear and mesenchymal proteins such as vimentin and N-CAM are no longer expressed by these cells. The induction of several genes and the repression of others implies that a critical transcription factor is being activated. Identification of this transcription factor is one of the most important aims of developmental nephrology. Once the metanephric mesenchyme has been induced, it induces the ureteric bud to divide, making each tip of the branch capable of inducing another cluster of mesenchymal cells. Several transcription factors have been genetically deleted, leading to a variety of renal developmental anomalies. Deletion of Pax2 and Lim-1, which are expressed in mesenchyme, led to widespread abnormalities in development, suggesting that these factors are critical for specification of the epithelial progenitors of the kidney. Deletion of WT1 (the Wilms' tumor gene) prevented the ureteric bud from its initial branching. Deletion of the homeobox gene Emx-2 allowed the ureteric bud to invade the mesenchyme, but then no epithelia developed even though the mesenchyme continued to express WT1. Although the latter finding suggests that Emx-2 is downstream from WT1, at present, it is not clear whether these transcription factors form a cascade of events in a single pathway.

Classic experiments have demonstrated that when the metanephric mesenchyme was cocultured with the ureteric bud, it underwent all the developmental changes seen *in vivo*, including the formation of primitive nephrons. This *in vitro* system has allowed the study of the initial events in morphogenesis. Some heterologous tissues, such as the embryonic spinal cord, can also induce the mesenchyme *in vitro*. That induction occurred when the target and the inducer were separated by a filter paper suggested initially that a diffusible substance is secreted by the inducer. However, morphologic analysis using the spinal cord as an inducer showed that this tissue sent out processes that contacted the mesenchyme through the pores of the filter. When the contact was prevented by using filters with small pore sizes, the induction was prevented. Although these results were widely interpreted as showing that cell-to-cell contact was necessary, they are not by themselves decisive. Barasch recently showed that factors secreted by a ureteric bud cell can convert metanephric mesenchyme to epithelia, provided the medium contained basic FGF (FGF2). These important results demonstrate that conversion of mesenchyme to epithelia requires a combinatorial system of two proteins: bFGF and leukemia inhibitory factor.

The dramatic discovery by Herzlinger that fibroblasts expressing WNT1 genes induced tubulogenesis in metanephric mesenchyme focused attention on WNT genes whose prototype encodes a secreted protein that specifies the fate of cells in Drosophila. Mammalian embryos contain at least 13 WNT genes, and two of them, WNT4 and WNT11, are expressed in embryonic kidneys. McMahon et al found that the knockout of WNT4 results in a massive abnormality in kidney development, whereas deletion of WNT11 has more subtle effects. WNT4 is expressed in early metanephric mesenchyme and may specify the cells that will respond to the inductive ureteric signals. Kidneys from mice lacking WNT4 form a ureteric bud that invades the metanephric mesenchyme, but no tubules are formed. However, a few nephrons are formed; hence, at present, it is unclear at what step this important gene is working.

One of the most satisfying discoveries in renal development has been the identification of an important pathway that mediates reciprocal interaction between the ureteric bud and the metanephric mesenchyme. Metanephric mesenchyme express glial-derived neurotrophic factor (GDNF), whereas the tips of the ureteric bud express its receptor RET, which is a tyrosine kinase. Deletion of either of these genes (or the coreceptor, GDNFRα) results in the same phenotype, no branching of the ureteric bud, and therefore no induction and no kidneys develop. Hence, this ligand receptor pathway represents the first authentic pathway of reciprocal induction in kidney development.

Other proteins have been identified as being involved in kidney development, but their exact role or the stage at which they work is less clear. The integrin α8β1 is expressed by the metanephric mesenchyme and presumably binds to a ureteric bud extracellular matrix protein. Deletion of this integrin disrupts ureteric bud branching and development. In embryonic kidneys taken from mice lacking BMP-7, a TGF-β family member the ureteric bud can invade and induce the mesenchyme and several tubules form before nephrogenesis ceases. These results suggest that this ureteric bud protein is required somewhat later than the initial inductive events. Many of the studies described earlier have assumed that the reciprocal interaction of the mesenchyme and ureteric bud occurs without the involvement of the stromal cell lineages. However, newer experiments have demonstrated that factors produced by two types of stromal cells are absolutely critical for nephrogenesis. Deletion of either BF2 or the retinoic acid receptors RARα and RARβ2 results in severe abnormalities in nephrogenesis. Because these two are transcription factors expressed solely in different populations of stromal cells but not in epithelial cells, it follows that they control the synthesis or function of secreted factors that affect epithelial mesenchymal interaction. Hence, a complete picture of a pathway will require inclusion of products of these nonepithelial cells.

The preceding summary of the genetic information available demonstrates that the state of this field is exciting specifically because there is no single overarching hypothesis or pathway that can explain reciprocal interaction between the ureteric bud and metanephric mesenchyme. Hence, the field is ripe for a major discovery. The renal results have been accumulated in an "opportunistic" manner; largely as a byproduct of gene deletion (for other reasons) and because the kidney is a large organ whose absence from the abdominal cavity is not easy to miss. Hence, the field will benefit from these accidental discoveries of critical genes for kidney development. One hopes that we will soon reach the stage at which informed and targeted (in more than one sense of the word) mutations will be performed to examine the many interacting steps that force the ureteric bud and metanephric mesenchyme into their exquisitely choreographed dance.

BRANCHING OF THE URETERIC BUD

Most organs are composed of units, be they nephrons in the kidney or lobules in exocrine glands. The arborization is stereotyped in each organ, resulting in a set number of divisions and a defined number of units. However, the branching patterns are specific to the organ. The development of the renal pattern was analyzed by Jean Oliver using dissections of the branching tree in human kidneys of different embryonic ages in a classic monograph, *Nephrons and Kidneys*.

All branching patterns consist of only two structural elements: branch points and stems. Two types of branches can be differentiated. *Lateral* branches (also termed *monopodial*) originate from a main stem at equally spaced or random intervals. Lateral branches often determine a lobule of an organ, for instance, in the breast, salivary glands and pancreas. This kind of pattern is also commonly found during the development of the blood vessels, including capillary networks. In *bifid* (or *dipoidal*) branches, the main stem divides into two daughter branches similar in size to each other. Each daughter branch can divide in a bifid manner until a terminal set of branches is reached. The angle of bifurcation is variable, in the first bifurcation of the ureteric bud, it is as large as 180 degrees. The analysis of these two types of branches is often difficult and is ideally performed in a time-lapse study of an individual branch. This problem was solved when a mouse that expresses green fluorescent protein in the ureteric bud was generated. Isolation of the kidney and its growth in culture allowed frequent analysis of the branching pattern in the same kidney. A time-lapse analysis is posted on the Internet by F. Costantini's laboratory (http://cpmcnet.columbia.edu/dept/genetics/kidney and click on movie).

Formation of the characteristic system of the kidney requires both lateral and bifid branches to form three different patterns of branching that unfold one after the other. Each pattern bears a specific quantitative relation to the others. The number of branches in a tree made up of a simple repeating unit of bifid branches, where the tip of each bifid branch divides into another bifid branch is equal to 2^n, where *n* is the number of bifid divisions; we term this an *iterative bifid branching system* (Fig. 1.11). However, microdissection of human embryonic kidneys have shown that this simple pattern does *not* occur in the kidney. This follows from the fact that each tip of the branch induces and becomes connected to a nephron; this connection removes the tip from the possibility of further branching. The growth and division of the ureteric bud proceeds in two steps that occur in rapid succession; first a lateral branch, which then divides into two terminal branches (Fig. 1.11). We refer to this as a *terminal bifid branching system*. It is referred to as *terminal* because each tip does not generate a further bifid branch. This type of branching process is unique to the kidney and is repeated 15 times during human nephrogenesis. The same pattern is seen from

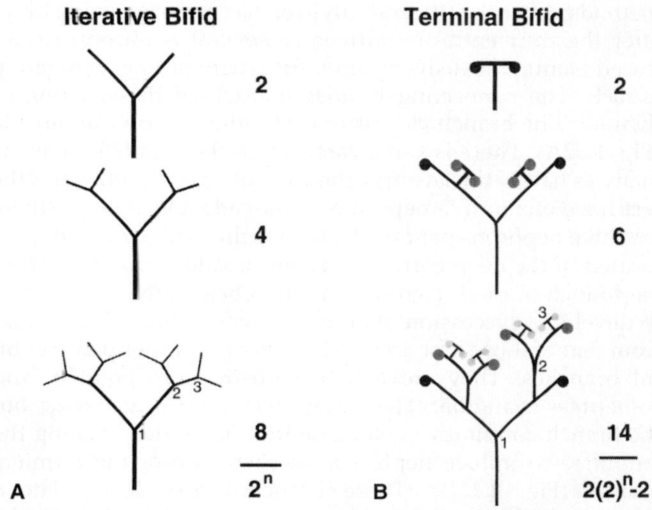

Figure 1.11. Types of branching iterative bifid branching. Terminal bifid system, a unique renal type of branching; a lateral branch followed by a terminal bifid branch. *n*, number of bifid branches. (Reproduced with permission from Al-Awqati Q, Goldberg MR. Architectural patterns in branching morphogenesis in the kidney. *Kidney Int* 1998;54:1832–1842.)

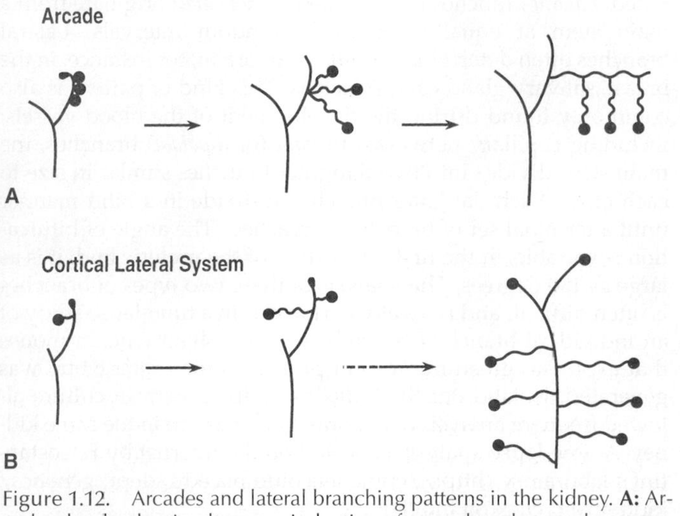

Figure 1.12. Arcades and lateral branching patterns in the kidney. **A:** Arcades develop by simultaneous induction of several nephrons whose connecting tubules fuse and then elongate to form the arcade. **B:** The final branch continues to induce as it elongates toward the cortex, generating laterally situated nephrons. (Reproduced with permission from Al-Awqati Q, Goldberg MR. Architectural patterns in branching morphogenesis in the kidney. *Kidney Int* 1998;54:1832–1842.)

the beginning; the budding of the ureteric bud from the wolffian duct is the first lateral branch that then divides into two, producing the first bifid branch point.

The stem carrying each tip elongates, transporting it and its induced nephron toward the developing cortex. From the shaft of the elongated branch, a new ampulla appears, which first grows to form a lateral branch that then eventually is transformed into the yoke of a new bifid division capable of inducing two new nephrons (Fig. 1.11B). As can be shown in Fig. 1.11B, the number of branches (nephrons) that results from this pattern would be equal to $2(2^n)$-2, where n is again the number of bifid branches. This pattern has been called the *closed divided system of branching* by Oliver. For 15 of these terminal bifid divisions, the number of resulting branches is only 65,534 nephrons, clearly much lower than the number of nephrons in one human kidney.

The remainder of the nephrons develop by two additional methods. After the fifteenth division has occurred (sometimes after the thirteenth or fourteenth) several nephrons are induced simultaneously around the stem of the elongating branch. The connecting tubules of each of these nephrons then join the branch closest to each other to form an arcade (Fig. 1.12A). There is some variation in the arcade system; as many as half of the late branches do not have arcades, and the rest have one to five nephrons per arcade. On average, there are three nephrons per arcade. In the adult kidney, arcades are located in the deep cortex. After the arcades form, the terminal branch of the fifteenth generation begins to elongate and to develop a succession of ampullae whose shape is different from that of those that occurred during the earlier phase of bifid branches: They are less ballooned, more pointed, and sometimes triangular. These ampullae occur near the tip, but the branch continues to elongate into the cortex, leaving the ampullae to induce nephrons on each side of the terminal branch (Fig. 1.12B). These branches are clearly lateral (monopodial) branches and have been termed the *open divided system* by Oliver. By the time this branch terminates in two final branches, an average of 10 nephrons have been induced per cortical system. When these numerical averages are used, 1 million nephrons per kidney are generated, which is the expected number (see the following section for a further discussion of the number of nephrons).

The molecular and cellular basis of the three mechanisms of branching in the kidney require elucidation. Whether the differences among them represent minor variations on one general theme or are the consequences of three fundamentally different mechanisms remains to be determined.

DEVELOPMENT OF THE BLOOD VESSELS

Development of an organ requires that morphogenesis of its parenchymal cells be synchronized with proliferation, migration, and morphogenesis of the endothelial cells of its vasculature. Anatomic examination of mature organs illustrates the complexity of this process. For example, the kidney has three morphologically and functionally distinct capillary beds (glomerular, peritubular, and vasa recta), each in close contact with, and functionally linked to, a different nephron segment. An additional level of complexity arises from the fact that each nephron possesses its own vascular supply, requiring that morphogenesis of its parenchymal and vascular components occur simultaneously. Endothelial cells of the kidney develop *in situ* from progenitor cells termed *angioblasts* (as shown by Abrahamon); and they invade the kidney from the outside. It was found that as the ureteric bud generates new branches, each of these ampullae becomes tightly surrounded by endothelial cells, thereby providing a potential targeting mechanism for the vascularization of individual nephrons. This suggests that cells of the renal anlage might synthesize molecules regulating endothelial cell migration and location. Indeed, with monoclonal antibodies, we found an antigen synthesized by embryonic kidney parenchymal cells that colocalizes with migrating endothelial cells. This antigen likely provides embryonic renal endothelial cells with directional cues because addition of the antibody to developing kidney rudiments *in vitro* inhibited localization of these cells around ureteric bud ampulla. Although endothelial cells synthesize their own basement membrane, others found in chimeric embryonic kidneys that endothelial cells arriving to the glomerulus are surrounded by a basement membrane whose collagen IV is of endothelial and epithelial origins. Similarly, fusion of endothelial and epithelial basement membranes during the early phase of glomerular capillary basement membrane development further suggests that epithelial cells play a role in the morphogenesis of the mature renal capillary bed.

Renal embryonic parenchymal cells also synthesize endothelial growth and chemotactic factors as well as molecules capable of regulating their phenotype. Some epithelial cells of the renal anlage synthesize vascular endothelial growth factor/vascular permeability factor (VEGF), a restrictive endothelial mitogen. Furthermore, although synthesis of VEGF greatly decreases as the kidney matures, synthesis continues in the glomerular epithelial cells of the adult kidney, likely contributing to the high permeability of the glomerular capillary. Similarly, a new endothelial growth factor, HDGF (hepatoma-derived growth factor) was found to be synthesized by ureteric bud and mesenchymal cells during embryonic growth, but its expression was also turned off during maturation. The intricate arrangement between endothelial and epithelial cells in the adult kidney makes it likely that during its development, a complex reciprocal interaction exists between these parenchymal cells and endothelial cells that guarantees the correct association of the two cell types.

HOW MANY NEPHRONS ARE THERE?

The number of generations and divisions is the ultimate determinant of the number of nephrons. Two issues are critical here: How stereotyped is this, and what possible mechanism could account for a constant or near constant number of generations? As discussed, the ureteric bud undergoes 15 bifid divisions, followed by the formation of arcades and lateral branching. Quantitative analyses have confirmed much older studies that the number of nephrons in the human kidney is more variable than the "1 million per kidney." Using different methods of quantitative morphology, the same investigator found a variety of nephron numbers with a spread of values probably greater than can be accounted for by methodologic error. Numbers as low as 300,000 and as high as 1,780,000 have been found, with averages of about 600,000. Different animals vary in their nephron numbers, from 30,000 in the rat to almost 200,000,000 in the whale. Unfortunately, little is known about the quantitative architecture of these animals. At least in the 50,000 nephrons of the rabbit kidney, the nephrons are generated by all three mechanisms of branching: terminal bifid, arcades, and cortical lateral. What is unclear is whether the number of the initial wave of terminal bifid branches, the average number of nephrons on an arcade, or the number of lateral cortical nephrons are lower in rabbits compared with humans.

An important hypothesis proposed by Brenner suggested that the number of nephrons in humans is associated with or may even be an important cause of many diseases of the kidney. These include hypertension and the genetic propensity to develop glomerulosclerosis in response to renal injury. The kidneys of individuals with reduced glomeruli are normal by the usual criteria of histopathology. Because the ultimate determinant of nephron number is the number of branches, it is likely that the cause of fewer nephrons in some individuals is premature cessation of branching and induction. Alternatively, its tempo may have been slower, and then the program of branching was turned off (perhaps in response to birth) before a large number of nephrons was made. Because branching occurs in bursts, drugs and other intrauterine events might interfere with the ultimate number of nephrons. Some literature suggests that premature birth is associated with a decreased number of nephrons. Nephrogenesis in humans continues until the eighth month of embryonic life; hence, it may not be surprising that birth, with its attendant changes in circulation, oxygenation, and a variety of humoral factors, interrupts this late phase of nephrogenesis. These considerations add an urgency to examination of the molecular basis of determination of the control of branching during kidney development.

Selected Readings

Al-Awqati Q, Goldberg MR. Architectural patterns in branching morphogenesis in the kidney. *Kidney Int* 1998;54:1832–1842.
An excellent review on the molecular control of renal morphogenesis.

Davie J. *The Kidney Development Database*, http://www.ana.ed.ac.uk/anatomy/database/kidbase/kidhome.html
This important resource contains a catalog of all genes expressed in the kidney during kidney development. It also includes a superb reference list and updated tables regarding the expression of genes, knockout with their kidney phenotypes (if any), and the ability to submit new data and publications. Most of the publications referred to in this chapter can be found in this database.

Oliver J. *Nephrons and kidneys: a quantitative study of developmental and evolutionary mammalian renal architectonics.* New York: Harper and Row, 1968.
A classic description of renal development that is invaluable.

Saxen L. *Organogenesis of the kidney*. Cambridge: Cambridge University Press, 1987.
An important and critical summary of the field until 1987. Comprehensive analysis of the "older" literature that is still valuable despite the passage of a decade.

PART 3
Structure of the Kidney

Marlies Elger, Eva Schnabel, and Wilhelm Kriz

The basic architecture of a mammalian kidney is best understood by examining the unipapillary kidney of the rat or rabbit. This type of kidney corresponds to a renculus of the human kidney, which is a compound multilobar kidney (Figs. 1.13 and 1.14). From a longitudinal section, one can discern two major areas: the cortex and the medulla. The cortex, which surrounds the medulla like a cup with inverted margins, is divided into the cortical labyrinth and the medullary rays. The medulla, with its tip, the papilla, projecting into the renal pelvis, can be described as roughly pyramid shaped. It is divided into an outer medulla and an inner medulla with the papilla. The renal papilla is surrounded by the pelvic cavity. The renal pelvis may be regarded as a dilation of the ureter. It is located within the renal sinus, which opens through the renal hilum to the medial surface of the kidney.

THE NEPHRON: AN OVERVIEW

The nephron is the specific structural unit of the kidney. A human kidney has about 1 million nephrons, but there are wide

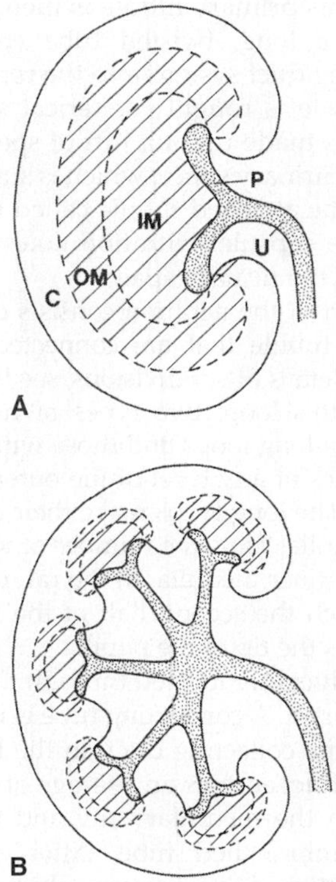

Figure 1.13. Different types of mammalian kidneys. **A:** Unipapillary rat kidney showing three major zones: cortex *(C)*, outer medulla *(OM)*, inner medulla *(IM)*, pelvis *(P)*, and ureter *(U)*. **B:** A compound multilobar human kidney. Individual medullary pyramids are shaded; calyces, pelvis, and ureter are stippled. In contrast to what is shown, the human kidney generally exhibits fusion of individual medullary pyramids terminating in a compound papilla.

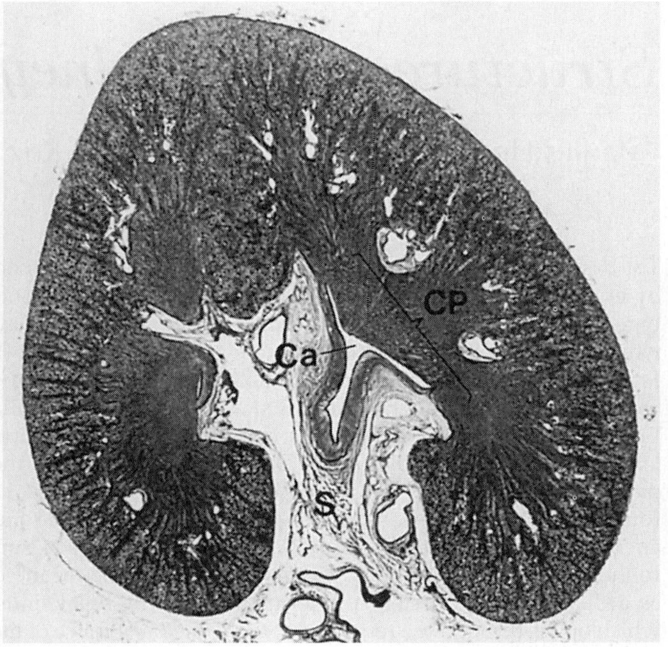

Figure 1.14. Cross section through a human kidney showing the continuous cortex covering three medullary pyramids; at least one of them is a compound papilla *(CP)*. *Ca,* calyx; *S,* renal sinus. The stripes within the cortex correspond to the medullary rays of the cortex; in between is the cortical labyrinth.

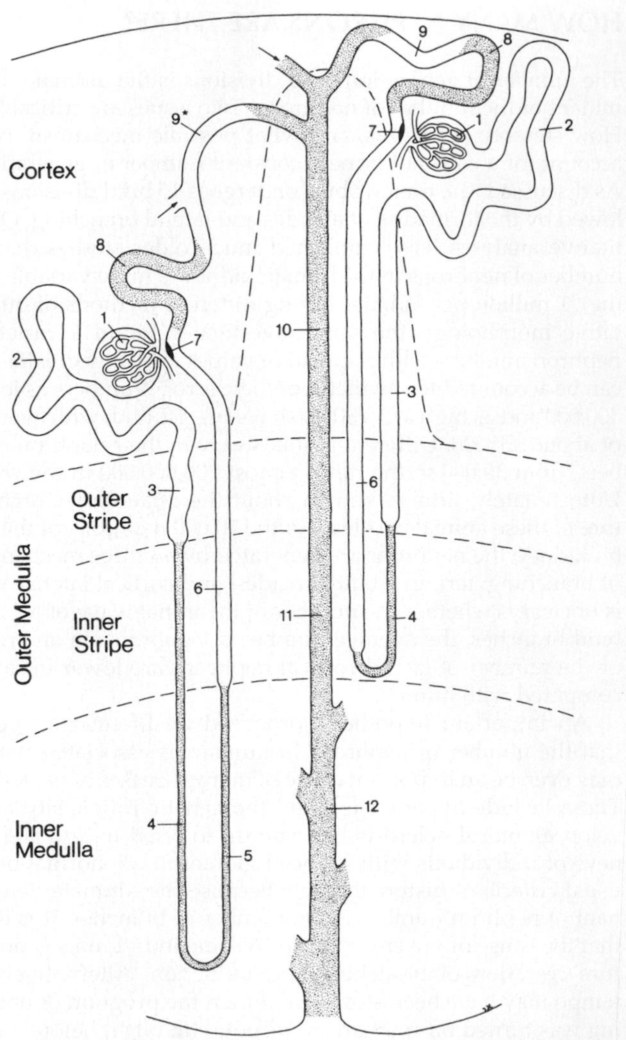

Figure 1.15. Schematic of nephrons and collecting duct. This scheme depicts a short-looped and a long-looped nephron together with the collecting system. It is not drawn to scale. Within the cortex, a medullary ray is delineated by a dashed line. *1:* Renal corpuscle including Bowman's capsule and the glomerulus (glomerular tuft); *2:* proximal convoluted tubule; *3:* proximal straight tubule; *4:* descending thin limb; *5:* ascending thin limb; *6:* distal straight tubule (thick ascending limb); *7:* macula densa located within the final portion of the thick ascending limb; *8:* distal convoluted tubule; *9:* connecting tubule; *9*:* connecting tubule of the juxtamedullary nephron that forms an arcade; *10:* cortical collecting duct; *11:* outer medullary collecting duct; *12:* inner medullary collecting duct. [Reprinted with permission from Kriz W, Bankir L. A standard nomenclature of the kidney. The renal commission of the International Union of Physiological Sciences (IUPS). *Pfluegers Arch* 1988;411:113–120.]

variations in the number of nephrons per kidney. Each nephron starts with a renal corpuscle, where the primary urine is filtered from the blood. This primary filtrate is then modified and concentrated within a long, twisted tube and finally drained through a collecting duct system into the renal pelvis.

A renal corpuscle is roughly spherical with a diameter of about 200 μm. It is made up of a tuft of specialized capillaries projecting into the urinary space, which is surrounded by a cup-like extension of the attached tubule called the parietal epithelium of Bowman's capsule. Filtration takes place through the capillary wall into the urinary space.

The tubular part of the nephron consists of a proximal and a distal convoluted tubule that are connected by a loop called Henle's loop. For details of subdivisions, see Fig. 1.15. Depending on the length of this loop, two types of nephrons are distinguished: those with long loops and those with short loops. Short loops may turn back at any level of the outer medulla and even within the cortex. The long loops make their bend at various levels within the medulla. Thus the number of loops is successively reduced along the inner medulla. In the rat, roughly one-sixth of the long loops reach the second half of the inner medulla, and only 1 of 40 reaches the tip of the papilla.

The collecting ducts are formed through the joining of several nephrons in the cortex. A connecting tube is interposed between the nephron and the collecting duct. In the human kidney, one cortical collecting duct accepts an average of 11 nephrons before it descends within the medullary ray and traverses the outer medulla as an unbranched tube. After entering the inner medulla, the collecting ducts successively fuse with each other. On average, eight fusions take place. Thus in humans one papillary duct drains a total of 2,500 to 3,000 nephrons.

The medullary rays of the cortex are given their characteristically striped appearance by the straight parts of proximal and distal tubules and by the cortical collecting ducts. Within a medullary ray, the straight tubules of superficial nephrons generally occupy a central position, and those of deeper (midcortical) nephrons occupy a peripheral position. The collecting ducts are situated between the superficial and midcortical nephrons. The straight tubular parts of juxtamedullary nephrons do not enter the medullary rays at all, but rather descend directly into the outer medulla.

The four major zones of the kidney—cortex, outer medulla with outer and inner stripes, and inner medulla—correlate to the presence or absence of certain parts of the nephron. The renal corpuscles are characteristic for the cortex; they are exclusively found in the cortical labyrinth together with the convoluted parts of proximal and distal tubules (Fig. 1.16).

In contrast to the cortex, the medulla does not contain any renal corpuscles or convoluted tubules. Three regions of the medulla are distinguished according to their different populations of nephron segments (Fig. 1.17). The outer stripe contains straight parts of the proximal tubule (S3 segments) and of the

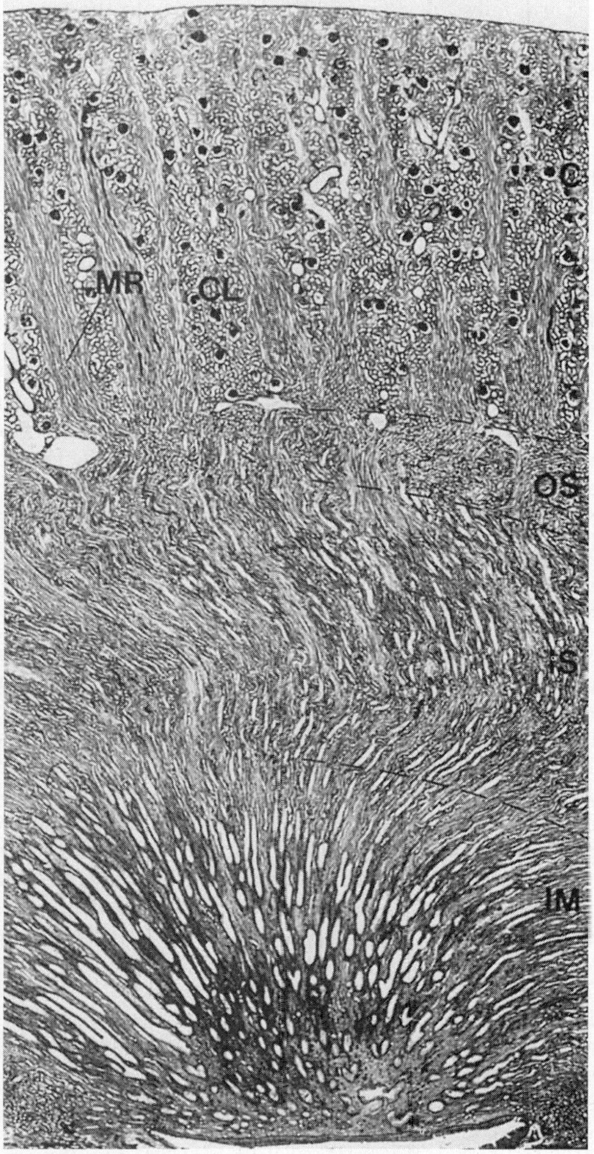

Figure 1.16. Longitudinal section through a human kidney showing the cortex *(C)* composed of cortical labyrinth *(CL)* and the medullary rays *(MR)*, the outer stripe *(OS)*, the inner stripe *(IS)*, and the inner medulla *(IM)* terminating in a papilla. Note the large vessels at the cortical medullary border. *Ca,* calyx. LM ×~16.

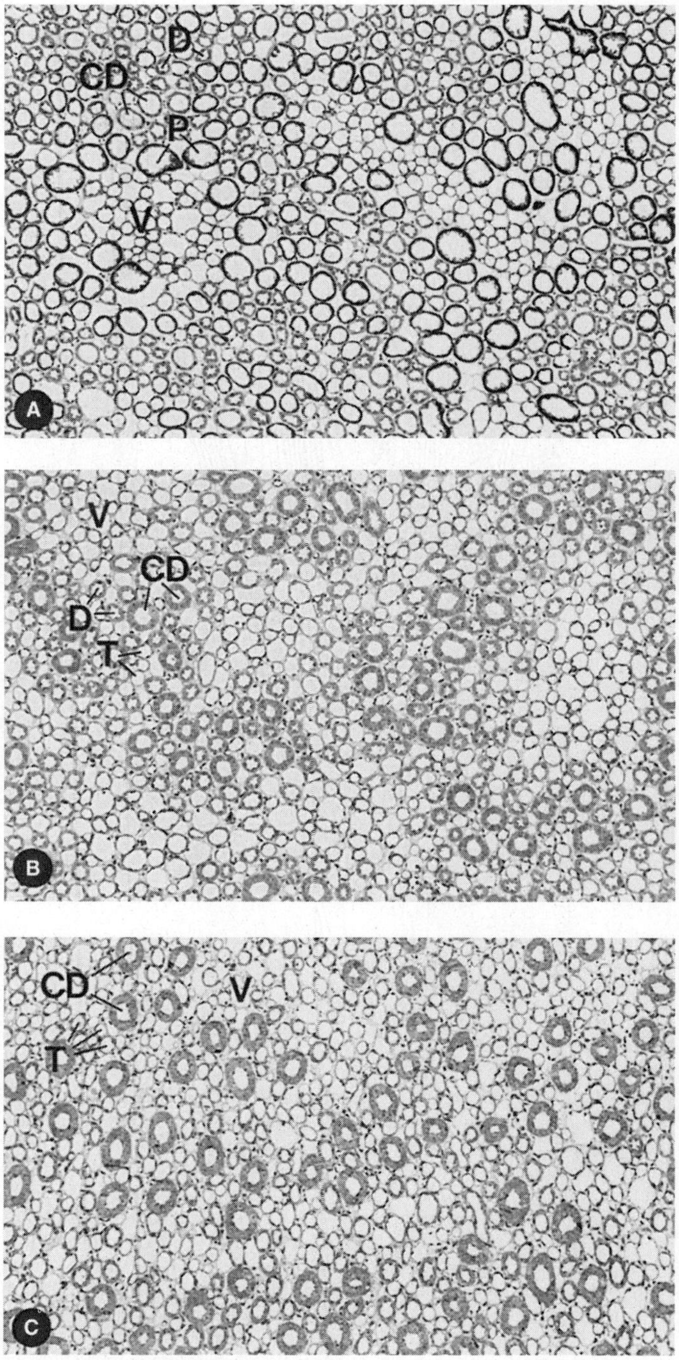

Figure 1.17. Cross sections through three medullary zones. **A:** Outer stripe. The proximal tubules *(P)*, the distal tubules *(D)*, and the collecting ducts *(CD)* are arranged around the vascular bundles *(V)*. **B:** Inner stripe. Vascular bundles are most prominent with descending and ascending vasa recta. Thin descending limbs *(T)*, distal tubules *(D*; thick ascending limbs), and collecting ducts *(CD)* are seen around them. **C:** Inner medulla. The organization of the inner medulla is dominated by collecting ducts *(CD)*, which are arranged in groups. Small vascular bundles *(V)* and thin limbs of Henle's loop *(T)* are seen between them. Human kidney, LM ×~90.

distal tubule (thick ascending limbs). The border between the outer and inner stripe is marked by the abrupt ending of the proximal straight tubules and the beginning of the thin descending limbs. In the inner stripe, only the thick ascending limbs and thin descending limbs remain. In the inner medulla, only the thin descending and ascending limbs of Henle's loop remain. Because the collecting ducts start within the medullary rays of the cortex and run to the tip of the papilla, they are present in all four zones of the kidney.

RENAL VASCULATURE AND ARCHITECTURAL ORGANIZATION

Vasculature of the Cortex

Close to the renal hilus, the renal artery divides into several branches from which the interlobar arteries branch off to enter the actual renal parenchyma at the border between the cortex and medulla (Fig. 1.18). From there they continue in an arch-like fashion, hence the name *arcuate arteries.* From these arteries, the cortical radial arteries, formerly called interlobular arteries, ascend radially within the cortical labyrinth. The renal corpuscles, which are supplied from the cortical radial artery by the *afferent arterioles,* and the corresponding convoluted

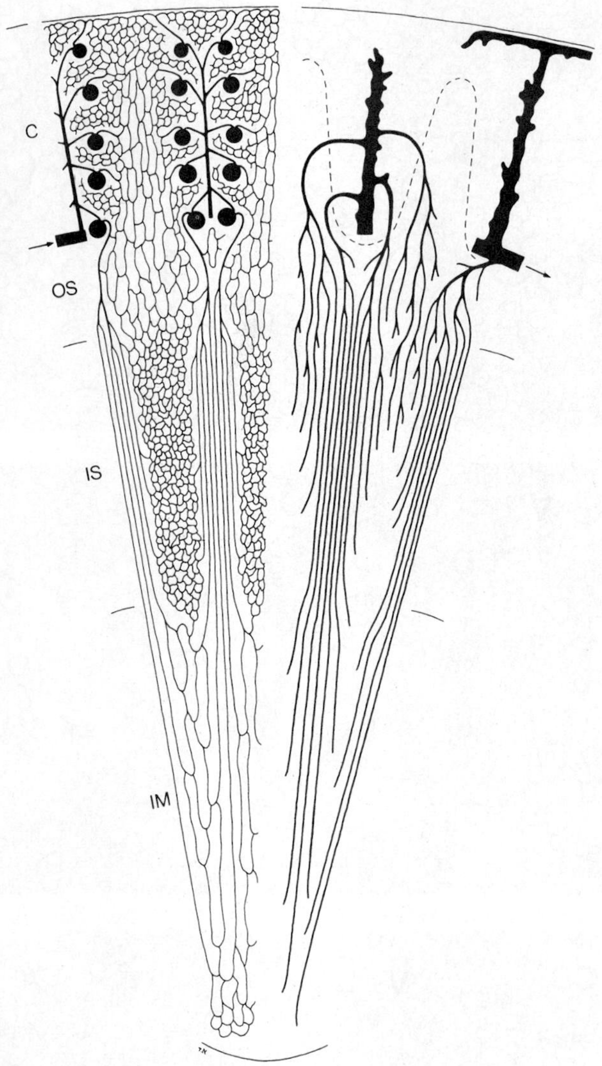

Figure 1.18. Organization of the intrarenal vasculature (basic pattern). The left half of the drawing shows the arterial vessels and the capillaries, the right half shows the venous vessels. The dashed line within the cortex **(right)** indicates the medullary rays. *C,* cortex; *OS,* outer stripe; *IS,* inner stripe; *IM,* inner medulla. At the corticomedullary border, a short segment of an arcuate artery is shown giving rise to a cortical radial artery. This, in turn, gives off afferent arterioles to superficial, midcortical, and juxtamedullary glomeruli. The efferent arterioles of superficial and midcortical glomeruli supply the dense capillary plexus of the cortical labyrinth and the looser, long-meshed plexus of the medullary rays. The efferent arterioles of juxtamedullary glomeruli descend into the outer stripe and divide into descending vasa recta. At intervals, descending vasa recta leave the vascular bundles to supply the adjacent capillary plexus. Note the different appearance of the capillary plexus in the outer stripe, inner stripe, and inner medulla. The cortex is drained by interlobular veins, some of which begin as stellate veins at the renal surface. The medulla is drained by ascending vasa recta. (From Rollhäuser H, Kriz W, Heinke W. Das Gefässsystem der Rattenniere. *Z Zellforsch* 1964;64:381–403.)

tubules are arranged around these vascular axes. The efferent arterioles leave the renal corpuscles to supply the peritubular capillaries.

Depending on the location of the glomeruli within the cortex, three different types of efferent arterioles can be distinguished: juxtamedullary, superficial, and midcortical. The efferent arterioles of juxtamedullary renal corpuscles turn toward the medulla and are the supplying vessels of the medulla. The superficial efferent arterioles extend to the kidney surface before they divide into peritubular capillaries. The midcortical efferent arterioles are defined by exclusion. Both the superficial and midcortical efferent arterioles supply the cortical peritubular capillaries. These capillaries form two plexuses: one dense network within the cortical labyrinth and a second, less dense network within the medullary rays. Efferent arterioles do not enter the medullary rays but often break off into capillaries just at the border to the medullary rays.

The renal veins, cortical radial veins and arcuate veins, accompany the corresponding arteries. In humans, like in cats and dogs, the venous blood from the outer cortex is drained in veins called stellate veins on the renal surface. These veins are connected to the arcuate veins by additional cortical radial veins called interlobular veins. The interlobular veins, which extend through the entire cortex, are not accompanied by arteries. The venous drainage of the two cortical capillary plexuses is different. The plexus of the cortical labyrinth drains directly into the cortical radial veins that run through the labyrinth. The blood from the medullary ray capillary plexus must first pass the plexus of the cortical labyrinth to gain access to the cortical radial veins.

Vasculature of the Medulla

In contrast to the dense arterial supply of the cortex, no arteries enter the medulla, nor does any vein originate in the medulla. The medulla is supplied exclusively by the efferent arterioles of juxtamedullary glomeruli (Figs. 1.18 and 1.19). These vessels descend into the outer stripe and divide into the descending vasa recta, which then penetrate the inner stripe of the outer medulla in cone-shaped vascular bundles. Descending vasa recta leave the bundles to join the capillary plexus of the adjacent medullary parenchyma at intervals. Most leave the bundle within the inner stripe. Only a small proportion of the descending vasa recta enters the inner medulla, and even fewer reach the tip of the papilla.

The capillary plexuses of the renal medulla differ in the three regions. The plexus of the outer stripe, which is supplied by few direct branches of efferent arterioles, is sparse. In contrast, the capillary plexus of the inner stripe is very dense and round meshed. The plexus of the inner medulla is even less dense and long meshed.

The drainage of the renal medulla is affected by the ascending vasa recta. In the inner medulla, the vasa recta are present at every level and ascend as unbranched vessels to the border between inner and outer medullary zones. Here they join the vascular bundles to traverse the inner stripe inside the bundles. Apart from those draining the lower-most part of the inner stripe, the ascending vasa recta draining the inner stripe do not join the bundles but ascend directly within the interbundle regions to the outer stripe. Within the outer stripe, the vasa recta ascending within the bundles spread out and, together with those directly ascending from the inner stripe, traverse the outer stripe as individual tortuous channels with wide lumina.

All descending vasa recta servicing the inner medulla already exist as individual vessels in the outer stripe and traverse the inner stripe within the bundles. All ascending vasa recta from the inner medulla traverse the inner stripe within the bundles without joining ascending vasa recta from the inner stripe. The blood flow of the inner stripe and of the inner medulla are separate from each other.

Architecture of the Medulla

Outer Stripe

The architectural organization of the medulla is best described by considering the vascular bundles as central axes around

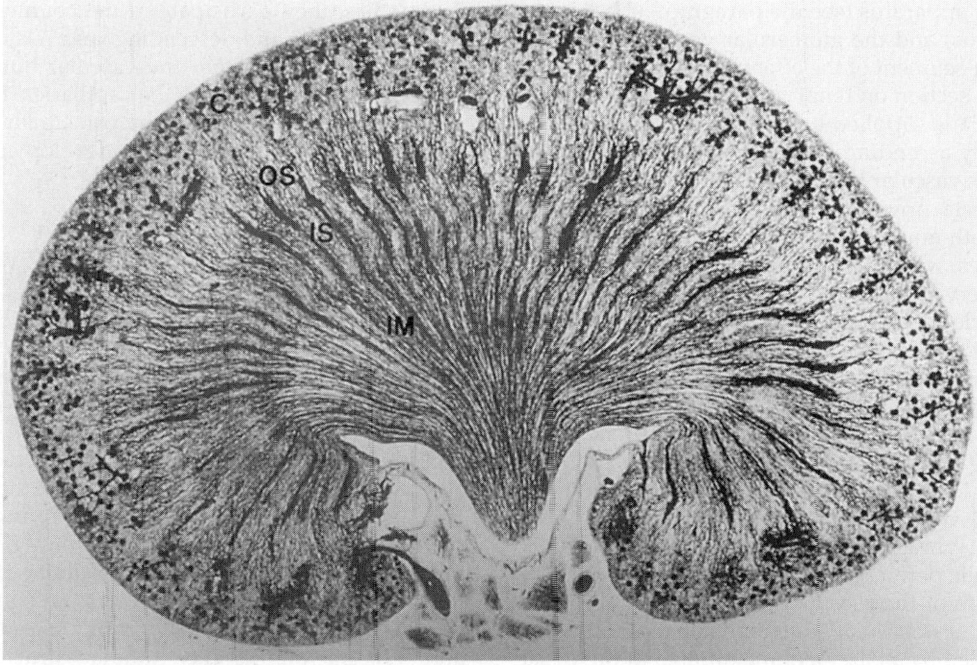

Figure 1.19. Microvasculature of the rat kidney. Filling of the arterial vessels with indian ink. Cortex *(C)*, outer stripe *(OS)*, inner stripe *(IS)*, and inner medulla *(IM)* are clearly distinguishable by their vessel patterns. The vascular bundles take shape along the OS and are best developed within the IS. Only a minor part of the descending vasa recta of each bundle enter the IM, where they gradually decrease in number toward the papilla. Note the lack of true capillaries in the OS. ×~8.

which the tubules are arranged. In a cross section of the outer stripe (Fig. 1.17A), the vascular bundles are small. They are surrounded by prominent proximal tubule profiles, the straight parts (pars recta) of the juxtamedullary nephrons, with the distal straight parts between. The tubules of superficial and midcortical nephrons, together with the collecting ducts, are grouped around the medullary rays.

A very specific capillary plexus supplies the tubules of the outer stripe. True capillaries, derived from direct branches of the efferent arterioles, are few. The dominating vessels are the ascending vasa recta, which traverse the outer stripe as wide, tortuous channels, meeting the tubules in a manner similar to that of capillaries. Because these vessels carry the entire venous blood from the medulla, the outer stripe tubules are supplied with venous blood mainly from deeper parts of the medulla. In the proximal tubules, tubular fluid descends into the medulla, whereas in the adjacent vasa recta, blood ascends out of the medulla. This countercurrent system makes possible the exchange between the urine in the proximal tubules and the venous blood from the medulla. This tubular-vascular relationship may be interpreted as a trap that prevents the renal medulla from losing solutes via the venous outflow.

Inner Stripe

The inner stripe of the outer medulla is the most constant part of the renal medulla. Similar to the pattern found in the outer stripe, the tubules are arranged around vascular bundles (Fig. 1.17B). Henle's loops, which originate from juxtamedullary nephrons, lie nearest the bundles, whereas those loops from superficial and midcortical nephrons lie most distant from the bundles. The collecting ducts generally are arranged in distant rings around the bundles and are intermingled with loops derived from superficial and midcortical nephrons. Together they are perfused by the dense capillary plexus of the inner stripe. In several rodent species with a high urine-concentrating ability, such as rats and mice, the architectural organization of the inner stripe is more complex. In these species, the descending limbs of short loops exclusively are incorporated into the vascular bundles. Consequently, the bundles within the inner stripe change from the classic countercurrent arrangement, consisting of descending and ascending vessels, to a system in which one ascending tube, the ascending vasa recta, is arranged together with two descending tubes: the descending vasa recta and the short descending thin loop limbs.

Inner Medulla

An architectural pattern is less apparent in the inner medulla than in the outer medulla (Fig. 1.17C). The vascular bundles have significantly fewer vasa recta when entering the inner medulla. Toward the papilla, they are further diminished until finally they are totally absent. Descending vasa recta continue as individual vessels to the tip of the papilla. In most cases, ascending vasa recta ascend independently of the bundles, which they finally join at the border of the inner stripe. At the beginning of the inner medulla, the collecting ducts and the ascending and descending limbs of the loops are still arranged in groups around the vascular bundles that reflect their grouping within the medullary rays of the cortex. Toward the tip of the papilla, cross sections appear homogenous because the spaces between the regularly distributed collecting ducts are filled evenly with descending and ascending loop limbs as well as individually running vasa recta. All of this is embedded into wide, interstitial spaces that increase toward the papillary tip.

Wall Structure of Intrarenal Vessels

Compared with arterial vessels of the same size in other organs, the intrarenal arteries and arterioles do not show any peculiarities in their wall structure. The exceptions are the terminal portion of the afferent arteriole (granular cells) as part of the juxtaglomerular apparatus (see the paragraph about juxtaglomerular apparatus) and the glomerular vessels (capillaries and intraglomerular segment of the efferent arteriole) as part of the glomerulus (see section on renal corpuscle).

The renal medulla is supplied by descending (arterial) vasa recta and drained by ascending (venous) vasa recta. The vasa recta are arranged as vascular bundles (Figs. 1.19 and 1.20). The descending vasa recta originate from the efferent arterioles. Gradually, the smooth muscle cells of the efferent arterioles are replaced by pericytes, which form an incomplete layer around the vessels. The innervation of the vasa recta ends with the loss of the smooth muscle cell layer because in contrast to smooth muscle cells, pericytes are not innervated by nerve endings. Arterial vasa recta are a specialized form of precapillary arterioles.

The ultrastructure of the peritubular capillaries is similar in both the cortex and medulla. The capillaries are the fenestrated type, surrounded by a thin basement membrane. Except for the perinuclear region, the endothelium is extremely flat. It contains regularly and densely arranged fenestrations that are bridged by a thin diaphragm. The diaphragm is considered an area of high hydraulic permeability.

The wall structure of the ascending vasa recta is similar to that of capillaries. The walls show the same flat, fenestrated endothelium surrounded by a basement membrane. In the vascular bundles, they participate in the countercurrent system between ascending and descending vasa recta. In the outer stripe, they run separately from the vascular bundles to supply the tubules in a way similar to the capillaries. Even the cortical radial veins show a wall structure principally the same as that of renal capillaries. The renal veins develop an adventitia only as arcuate veins.

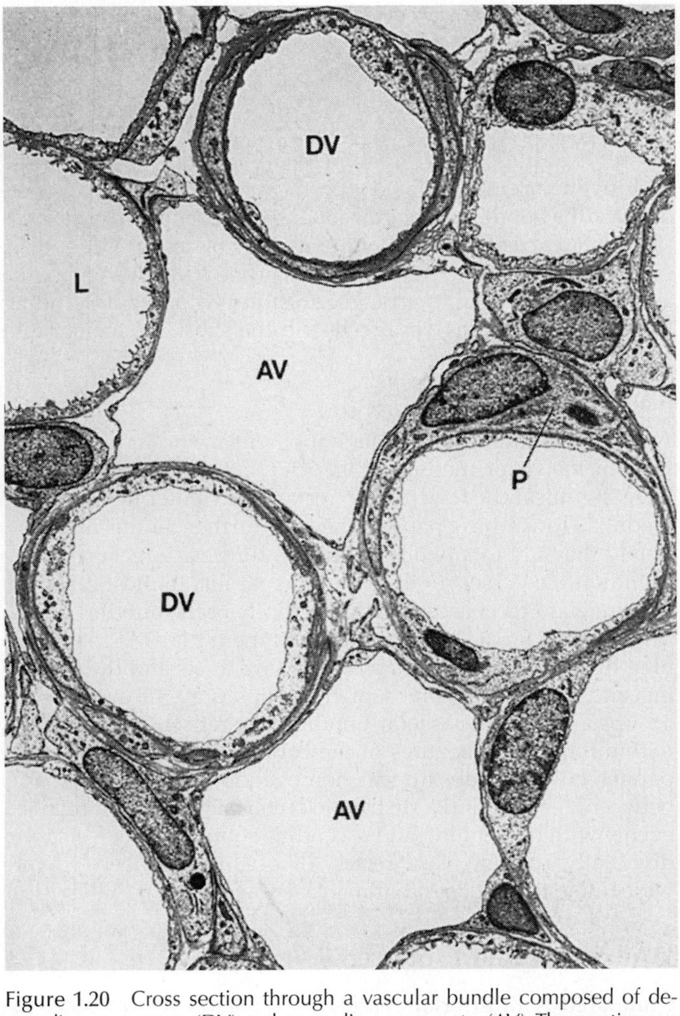

Figure 1.20 Cross section through a vascular bundle composed of descending vasa recta *(DV)* and ascending vasa recta *(AV)*. The continuous endothelium of the DV is surrounded by pericytes *(P)*. The endothelium of the AV is highly fenestrated *(arrows)*. *L*, thin descending limb of Henle's loop. Rabbit; TEM, ×~2,500.

INTERSTITIUM AND LYMPHATIC VESSELS

The interstitium of the kidney may be divided into a cortical and a medullary part. Within the cortex a peritubular interstitium must be distinguished from the periarterial interstitium; only the latter contains lymphatic vessels. In all renal zones, the cellular constituents of the interstitium are (a) resident fibroblasts, which establish the scaffolding frame for tubules, renal corpuscles, and blood vessels and maintain the three-dimensional architecture of the tissue, and (b) varying amounts of bone marrow–derived migrating cells (Fig. 1.21). The spaces between the cells are filled with an extracellular matrix consisting of ground substance (i.e., proteoglycans and glycoproteins, such as fibronectin and laminin), collagenous fibers (collagen types I, III, and VI), microfibrils (i.e., tubular structures approximately 15 nm in diameter), and interstitial fluid.

Fibroblasts

Fibroblasts are connected by attachment plaques to the basement membranes of epithelia and vessels and are interconnected by intermediatelike junctions. They are in close contact with nerve terminals and with all types of migrating interstitial cells. The ultrastructure of renal fibroblasts is similar to that of fibroblasts elsewhere in the body. They possess a well-developed apparatus for protein synthesis (rough endoplasmic reticulum, ri-

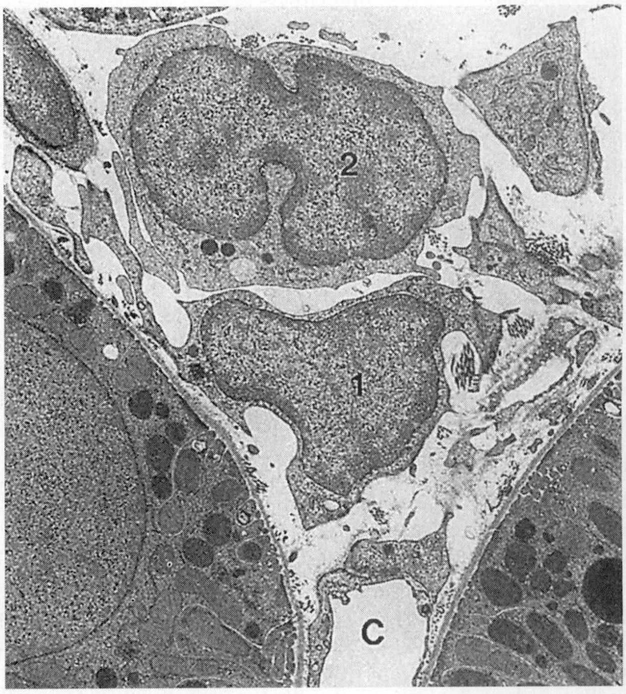

Figure 1.21. Peritubular interstitium of the cortex. Interstitial cells are of two types: *(1)* fibroblasts and *(2)* a second type of branched cells, which are lighter in appearance and probably represent dendritic cells. *C*, capillary. Rat; TEM, ×~7,100.

bosomes, and Golgi apparatus) and extensive formation of cell processes with prominent bundles of microfilaments. The long lamellar processes extend along the tubules even into the narrow peritubular spaces, where they may be interposed between the capillary endothelium and the tubular basement membrane.

Extensive phenotypical modulations of fibroblasts *in vivo* occur under the influence of environmental factors such as extracellular matrix composition, cytokines, and growth. Under pathologic conditions, such as interstitial inflammation and fibrosis, the fibroblasts can transform into myofibroblasts with upregulated cytoskeletal elements (α-smooth muscle actin, vimentin, and desmin), formation of gap junctions, and altered extracellular matrix production.

Bone Marrow–Derived Cells

In healthy kidneys, most of the bone marrow–derived interstitial cells are major histocompatibility complex (MHC) class II positive and have been identified as dendritic cells. These cells regularly are found close to the fibroblasts. Under inflammatory conditions, monocytes/macrophages and lymphocytes may invade the interstitial spaces and spotlike contacts between fibroblasts and bone marrow–derived cells, lymphocytes and dendritic cells in particular, are frequent.

Interstitium of the Cortex

Peritubular Interstitium

The peritubular interstitium (Fig. 1.21) of healthy rats makes up only 7% to 9% of the cortical volume. In humans, the cortical interstitial volume ranges from 5% to 37%, with a tendency to increase with age.

Immunocytochemistry facilitates the distinction between fibroblasts and dendritic cells. Among all interstitial cells, only fibroblasts exhibit the enzyme ecto-5′-nucleotidase (5′NT), whereas dendritic cells express MHC class II. The enzyme 5′NT is a source of extracellular adenosine. The cortical radial vessels, the glomerular arterioles, the renin-containing granular cells, and the nerve endings along the arteries and adjacent tubules are known targets for extracellular adenosine.

Normally, the activity of 5′NT is highest in fibroblasts in the deep cortex. However, under anemic conditions, the activity of the enzyme is strongly upregulated in fibroblasts in the superficial cortex and to a lesser extent in the medullary rays. Similar distribution patterns displaying mRNA for erythropoietin (EPO) under anemic and hypoxic conditions were observed for cells, suggesting a link between the expression of 5′NT and the synthesis of EPO. Colocalization of 5′NT and EPO mRNA demonstrated that 5′NT-positive fibroblasts synthesize renal EPO. Transformation of cortical fibroblasts into myofibroblasts is associated with an increased potential for matrix production but a reduced potential for EPO gene expression and a progressive loss of 5′NT activity.

Periarterial Interstitium

The periarterial interstitium is a layer of loose connective tissue that surrounds the arcuate arteries and cortical radial arteries and diminishes along the afferent arterioles (Fig. 1.22). It is continuous with the peritubular interstitium and with the connective tissue underlying the epithelium of the renal pelvis and ureter. The renal veins are apposed to this sheath. The lymphatic vessels originate in the vicinity of the afferent arterioles and leave the kidney through the periarterial sheaths toward the renal hilum.

The scaffold of the periarterial sheath is constituted by 5′NT-negative, but weakly α-smooth, muscle-positive fibroblasts with thin lamellar processes that form a three-dimensional net. The extracellular spaces are filled with thick bundles of collagenous fibers, interstitial fluid, dendritic cells, and monocytes/macrophages. During inflammation, lymphocytes accumulate in the periarterial sheath.

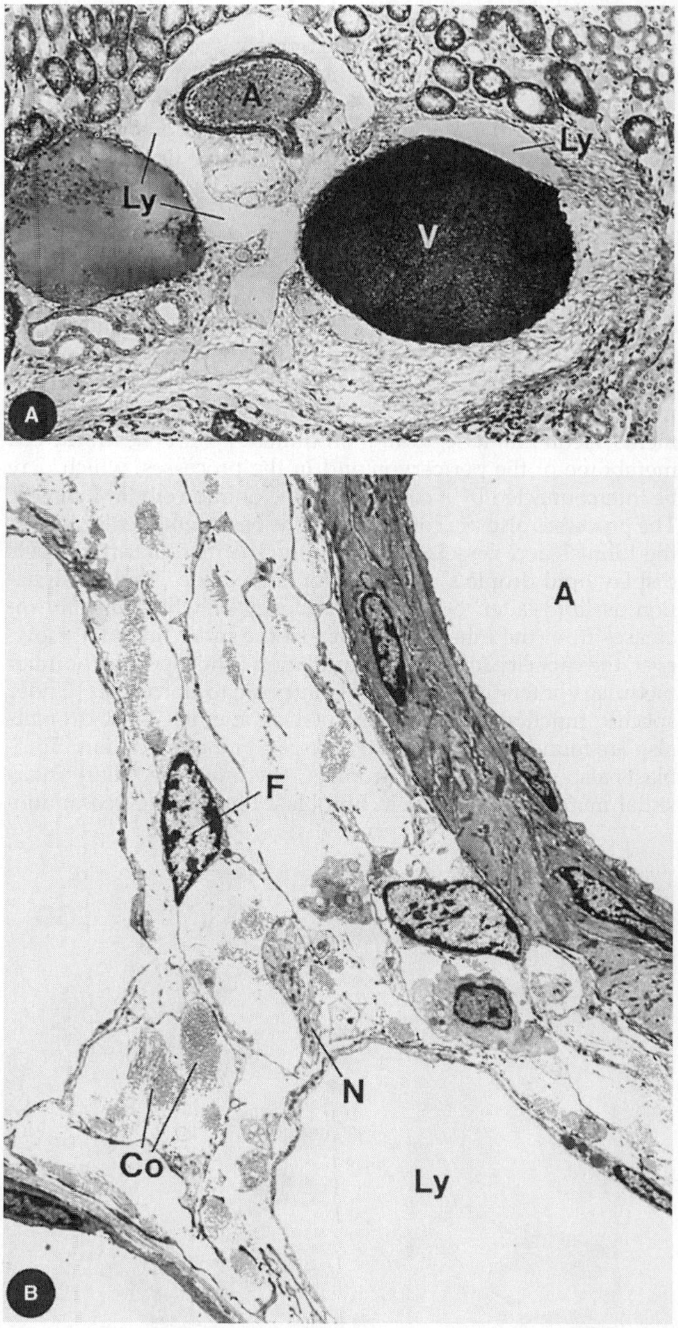

Figure 1.22. Periarterial interstitium with lymphatic vessels of the kidney. **A:** Several lymphatics *(Ly)* are seen with the periarterial loose connective tissue sheath alongside an arcuate artery *(A)* and vein *(V)*. Feline kidney; paraffin section, Azan stain; ×~120. **B:** Electron micrograph of the periarterial loose connective tissue sheath of an interlobular artery. Note the fibroblasts *(F)*, collagenous fiber bundles *(Co)*, and a nerve *(N)* passing through this tissue. Rat. ×~4,000.

Interstitium of the Medulla

The medullary interstitial volume is developed differently in the three medullary zones. In the outer stripe of the outer medulla and in the vascular bundle compartment of the inner stripe, the interstitial tissue is extremely sparse, with a fractional volume of 3% to 5%. In the interbundle compartment of the inner stripe, the fractional volume is up to 10% in rats. In the inner medulla, the fractional volume continuously increases from the base of the papilla (10% to 25%) to the tip of the papilla (30% to 40%). The medullary interstitium has no drainage by lymphatics.

The medullary fibroblasts do not display 5′NT nor mRNA for EPO. The inner medullary fibroblasts are oriented perpendicularly, like rungs of a ladder, to the longitudinally running tubules and vessels (Fig. 1.23). The phenotype of the medullary fibroblasts shows progressive transformation from the cortical phenotype into the so-called lipid-laden cell located in the inner medulla. One striking change is the increase in cytoskeletal elements. Actin filaments form a prominent layer beneath the cell membrane of the pericaryon and in the processes, which may be interconnected by a composite type of intercellular junction. The processes also are connected to the basement membranes of the tubules and vessels. Furthermore, the medullar fibroblasts display lipid droplets in their cytoplasm (hence, their designation as lipid-laden cells), the frequency of which usually increases from the inner stripe toward the inner medulla. However, the capacity for lipid accumulation is not specific for inner medullary interstitial cells but is intrinsic to fibroblasts. Under specific functional conditions such as anemia, lipid droplets also are found in cortical fibroblasts, and inner medullary fibroblasts also may lack lipid droplets. The inner medullary interstitial matrix is abundant in fibroblast-produced glycosaminoglycans. Furthermore, the cells secrete vasoactive substances, particularly prostaglandin E_2.

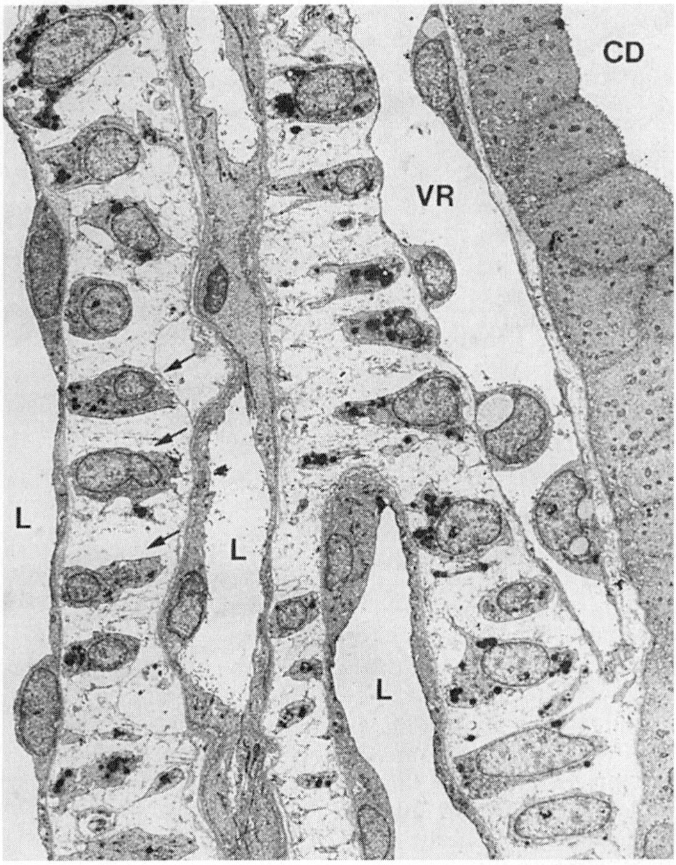

Figure 1.23. Lipid-laden fibroblasts in the interstitium of the inner medulla, demonstrated in a longitudinal section. The interstitial cells *(arrows)* are arranged like the rungs of a ladder between parallel running tubules or vessels. The fibroblasts contain numerous lipid granules *(black)*. *L*, loop limb; *VR*, vas rectum; *CD*, collecting duct. Rat; TEM, ×~1,250.

Bone marrow–derived cells with a high expression of MHC II are numerous in the inner stripe of the outer medulla and, like in the cortex, are narrowly associated with fibroblasts. In the inner medulla, they progressively disappear in the healthy kidney.

INNERVATION OF THE KIDNEY

The kidney is innervated by the autonomous nervous system. Most of the efferent nerves are postganglionic sympathetic nerves. They accompany the intrarenal arteries and the afferent and efferent arterioles. Afferent nerve fibers are found, but little is known about their origin or function. They might originate from mechanoreceptors of the arterial walls.

The distribution of the sympathetic nerves has been studied intensively. The nerve fibers run in the loose connective tissue around the arteries and arterioles. The descending vasa recta within the medulla are innervated by adrenergic nerve terminals as far as they are enveloped by smooth muscle cells. A dense assembly of nerves and terminal axons is found around the juxtaglomerular apparatus (JGA), especially around granular, renin-producing cells. Renin secretion can be stimulated by nerve excitation.

Many tubules do not have any direct contact with nerve terminals. Only those located around arteries or arterioles or adjacent to the JGA are touched by terminal axons. Tubular portions located within the medullary rays of the cortex, as well as most of the tubules in the medulla, are not reached by nerve terminals. Additional discussion of renal nerves and their effect on renal function is found in Chapter 5.

THE RENAL CORPUSCLE (GLOMERULUS)

The renal corpuscle (Figs. 1.24 and 1.25) is made of a tuft of specialized capillaries, the glomerulus, surrounded by a cup-shaped extension of the proximal tubulus, called Bowman's capsule. The term *glomerulus* also is widely used for the entire corpuscle.

The afferent and efferent arterioles, which supply and drain the capillary tuft, enter and leave the glomerulus at the vascular pole. The entire tuft is covered by epithelial cells called podocytes, which represent the visceral layer of Bowman's capsule. At the vascular pole, the visceral layer of Bowman's capsule turns into the parietal layer, a simple squamous epithelium. At the urinary pole opposite the vascular pole, where the urinary space (i.e., the space between both Bowman's layers) continues into the lumen of the proximal tubule, the parietal epithelium of Bowman's capsule abruptly transforms into the high epithelium of the proximal tubule.

The glomerular basement membrane (GBM) lies between the glomerular capillaries and the epithelial (i.e., visceral) layer of Bowman's capsule and continues into the basement membrane of the parietal layer at the vascular pole.

The Glomerular Tuft

At the entrance to Bowman's capsule, the afferent arteriole divides into several primary capillary branches. Each of these branches forms an anastomosing capillary network that runs toward the urinary pole and turns back toward the vascular pole. As a result, the glomerular tuft is subdivided into two to five lobules, each containing both an afferent and an efferent capillary portion. This separation into lobules is not strict. Anasto-

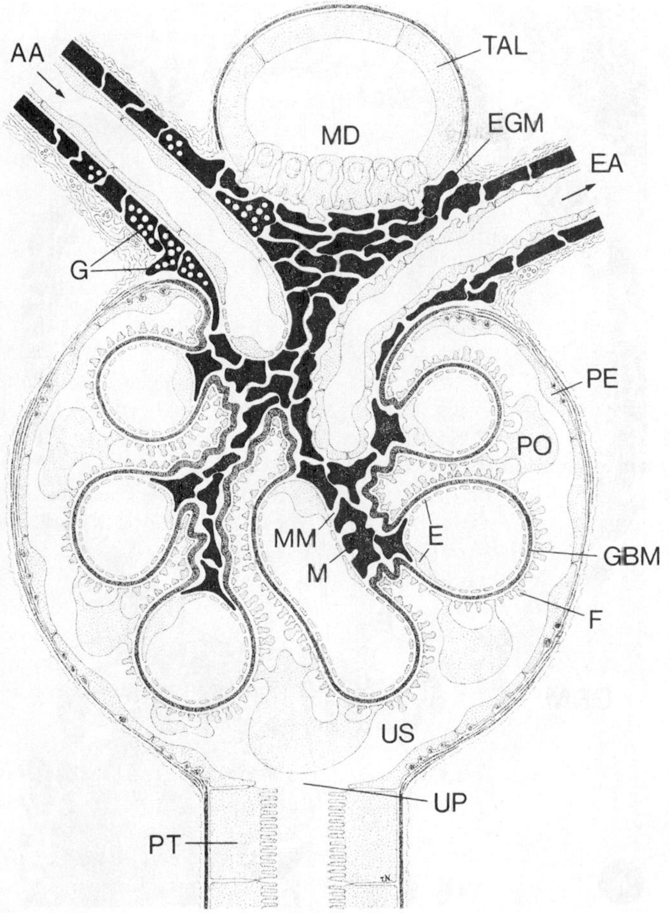

Figure 1.24. Diagram of a longitudinal section through a glomerulus and its juxtaglomerular apparatus (JGA). The capillary tuft consists of a network of specialized capillaries, which are outlined by a fenestrated endothelium (*E*). At the vascular pole, the afferent arteriole (*AA*) enters, branching into capillaries immediately after its entrance; the efferent arteriole (*EA*) is established inside the tuft and passes through the glomerular stalk before leaving at the vascular pole. The capillary network and the mesangium (cells, *M;* matrix, *mm*) are enclosed in a common compartment bound by the glomerular basement membrane (*GBM*). Note that there is no basement membrane at the interface between the capillary endothelium and the mesangium. The glomerular visceral epithelium consists of highly branched podocytes (*PO*), which, in a typical interdigitating pattern, cover the outer aspect of the GBM. At the vascular pole, the visceral epithelium and the GBM are reflected into the parietal epithelium (*PE*) of Bowman's capsule, which passes over into the epithelium of the proximal tubule (*PT*) at the urinary pole (*UP*).
At the vascular pole, the glomerular mesangium is continuous with the extraglomerular mesangium (*EGM*) consisting of extraglomerular mesangial cells and an extraglomerular mesangial matrix. The EGM together with the granular cells (*G*) of the AA and the macula densa (*MD*) establish the JGA. All cells that are suggested to be of smooth muscle origin are shown in black. *F,* podocyte foot processes; *TAL,* thick ascending limb; *US,* urinary space. (Adapted with permission from Kriz W, Sakai T, Hosser H. Morphological aspects of glomerular function. In: Davison AM, ed. *Nephrology,* Vol 1. London: Bailliere Tindàl, 1988:3–23.)

moses between lobules may be found, especially in regions near the vascular pole.

The efferent arteriole develops deep within the glomerular tuft (Figs. 1.24 and 1.25) by the confluence of tributaries from all lobules. This intraglomerular segment of the efferent arteriole continues into a segment that is closely associated with the extraglomerular mesangium (EGM). Both parts are also called the outflow segment of the efferent arteriole. The intraglomerular segment of the efferent arteriole is made up of a continuous endothelium that is strictly separated from the GBM by mesangial cell processes and matrix. These mesangial cells become extraglomerular mesangial cells on their course through the EGM.

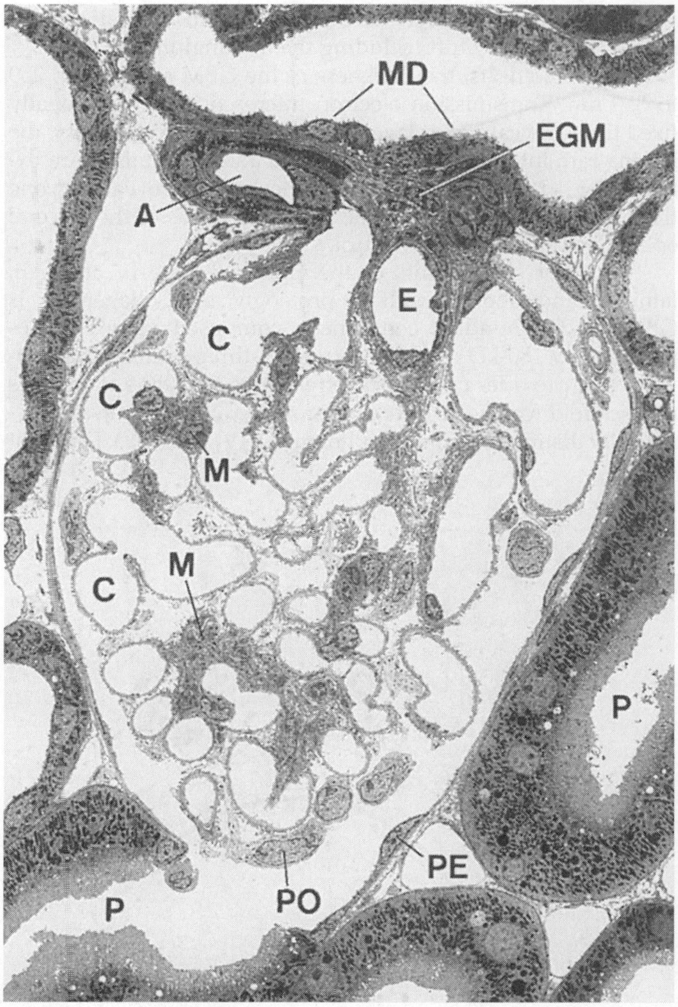

Figure 1.25. Longitudinal section through a glomerulus. The afferent arteriole (*A*), the intraglomerular segment of the efferent arteriole (*E*), the extraglomerular mesangium (*EGM*), and the macula densa (*MD*) are seen at the vascular pole. The tuft consists of capillaries (*C*), the mesangium (*M*), and podocytes (*PO*). The beginning of the proximal tubule is seen (*P*) at the urinary pole. *PE,* Parietal epithelium of Bowman's capsule. Rat; TEM, ×~750.

Smooth muscle cells then gradually replace mesangial and extraglomerular mesangial cells. When leaving the EGM, the efferent arteriole is established as a proper arteriole with a continuous layer of smooth muscle cells.

The glomerular capillaries are made up of only an endothelial tube (Figs. 1.26 and 1.27). A small portion of this tube is in direct contact with the mesangium, the axis of each glomerular lobulus. This small juxtamesangial portion attaches the capillaries to the glomerular lobule. Here they are not underlaid by a basement membrane. The major part of the endothelial tube is surrounded by the GBM (pericapillary) and the layer of interdigitating podocyte foot processes (visceral epithelium of Bowman's capsule). This part of the capillary wall represents the actual filtering area.

The pericapillary GBM continues into the GBM overlying the mesangium, where it is not in contact with capillaries. Like the paracapillary GBM, the paramesangial GBM is covered on its outer surface by a layer of interdigitating podocyte foot processes.

Glomerular Basement Membrane

The GBM serves as the skeleton of the glomerular tuft. In the mature glomerulus, the GBM is produced mainly by the visceral epithelium. Together with the podocytes, it encompasses the capillary tuft including the mesangium.

In human adults, the thickness of the GBM amounts to 250 to 350 nm. Transmission electron microscopy of traditionally fixed tissue reveals three layers of different electron density: the lamina rara interna, the lamina densa, and the lamina rara externa (Fig. 1.28). Studies using freeze techniques reveal only one thick, dense layer directly attached to the bases of the visceral epithelium and the endothelium.

The major components of the GBM are type IV collagen, laminin, and heparan sulfate proteoglycan. Collagen IV is GBM's most abundant component, composed mainly of approximately 180-kD α chains forming a three-dimensional network that provides mechanical strength to the GBM and serves as a scaffold for alignment of other matrix components. Six genetically distinct α chains are known, α1(IV) to α6(IV). Different

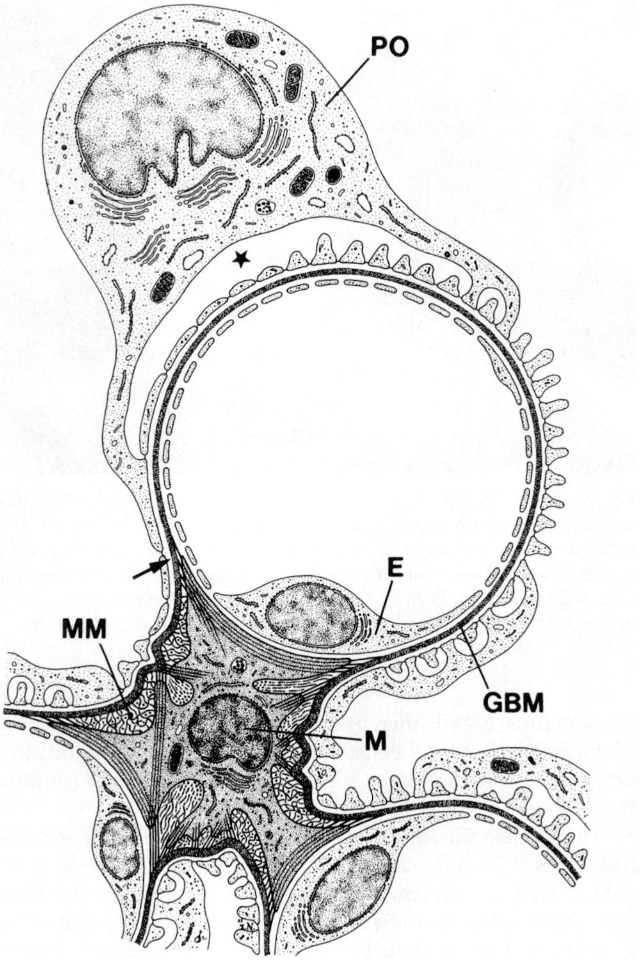

Figure 1.26. Schematic to show the arrangement of the structures in the glomerular tuft. Part of a glomerular lobule is shown with three glomerular capillaries (two are only partly shown) attached to a mesangial center. The glomerular capillary is made up of a fenestrated endothelium *(E)*. The peripheral part of the endothelial tube is surrounded by the glomerular basement membrane *(GBM)* which, at the mesangial angles *(arrow)*, deviates from a pericapillary course and covers with the mesangium. The interdigitated pattern of the podocyte *(PO)* foot processes form the external layer of the filtration barrier. Note the subcell-body space *(star)*. PO are also found covering the paramesangial GBM. In the center, a mesangial cell *(M)* is shown. Its many processes contain microfilament bundles and run toward the GBM to which they are connected. The mesangial matrix *(MM)* contains an interwoven network of microfilaments. (Reprinted with permission from Kriz W, Kaissling B. Structural organization of the mammalian kidney. In: Seldin DW, Giebisch G, eds. *The Kidney: Physiology and Pathophysiology,* 2nd ed. New York: Raven Press, 1992:707–777.)

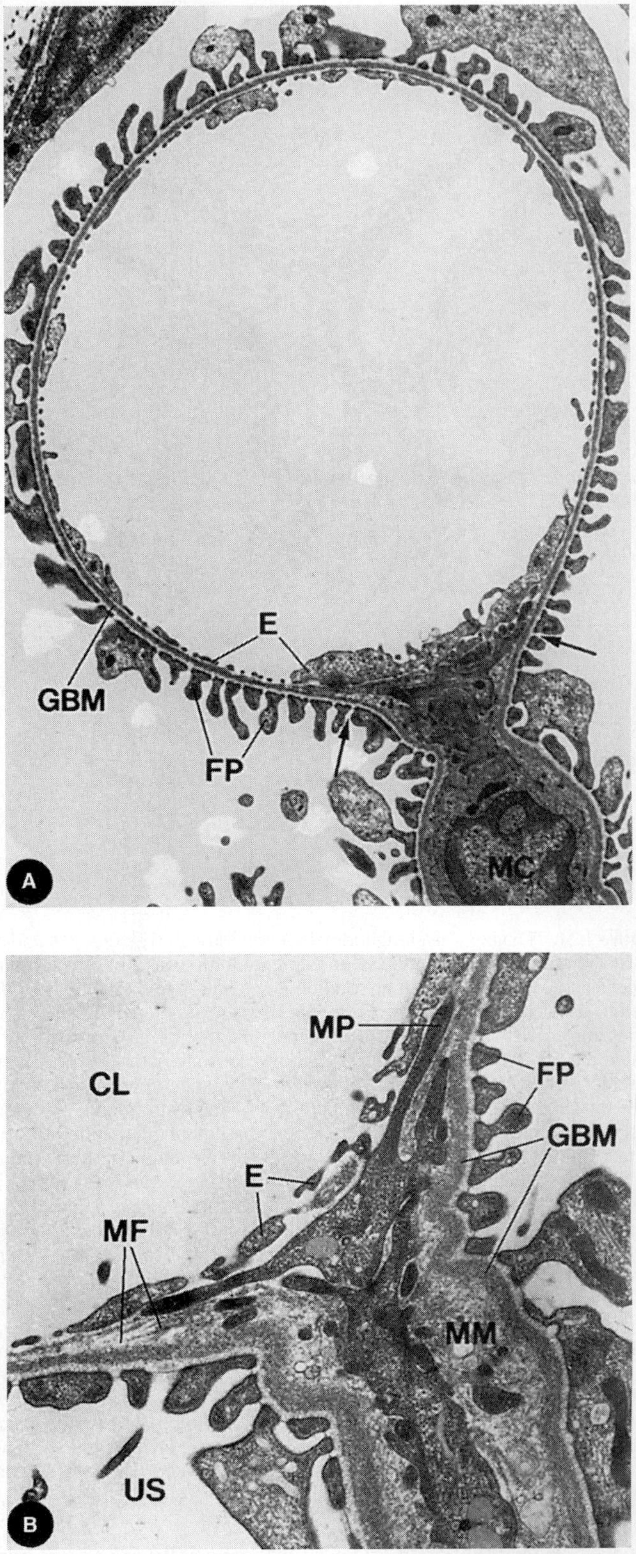

Figure 1.27. Overview of glomerular capillary. **A:** The peripheral wall of the glomerular capillary is made up of the fenestrated endothelium *(E)*, the glomerular basement membrane *(GBM)*, and the layer of interdigitating foot processes *(FP)* of podocytes. This wall constitutes the filtration barrier. At the mesangial angles *(arrows)*, the GBM deviates from a pericapillary course and covers the mesangium, where a mesangial cell *(MC)* is seen. **B:** The juxtamesangial part of the endothelium shown from another capillary profile is underlaid by mesangial cell processes *(MP)* that contain microfilament bundles and interconnect the GBM from the two opposing mesangial angles. The mesangial matrix *(MM)* contains microfibrills *(MF)*, which frequently interconnect mesangial cell processes and the GBM. *CL*, capillary lumen; *US*, urinary space. Rat; TEM, **(A)** ×~7,500, **(B)** ×~21,000.

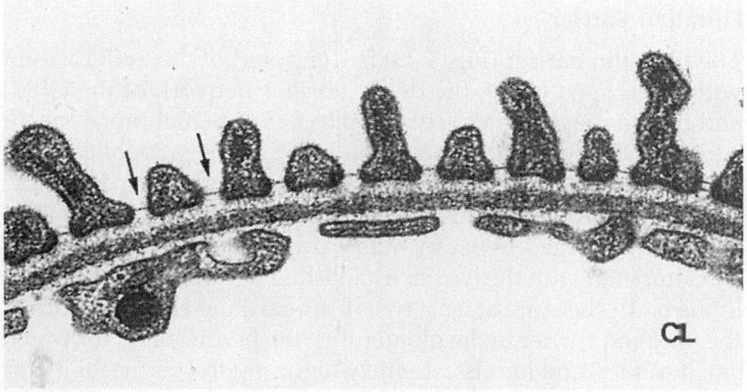

Figure 1.28. Filtration barrier. The peripheral part of the glomerular capillary wall comprises three layers: the endothelium with large open pores, the glomerular basement membrane *(GBM)*, and the layer of interdigitating podocyte foot processes. The GBM consists of a lamina densa, a lamina rara interna toward the endothelium, and a lamina rara externa toward the epithelium. Note the slit diaphragms bridging the filtrations slits *(arrows)*. *CL*, capillary lumen. Rat; TEM, ×~33,400.

from most other basement membranes, the adult GBM contains very little α1 and α2(IV) but many α3-α5(IV) chains. Mutations in any of the collagen α3-α5(IV) genes are responsible for Alport syndrome. In this disease, the mature GBM lacks the collagen α3-α5(IV) chains, and the α1 and α2(IV) chains are retained. See Chapter 43.2 for further discussion on Alport syndrome.

The major glycoproteins of the GBM are laminin and nidogen (entactin). Laminin consists of three polypeptide chains (α, β, and γ) and is thought to bind directly or via nidogen to type IV collagen as well as to integrin and nonintegrin cell surface receptors of endothelial and epithelial cells (podocytes). Currently, several forms of the α, β, and γ chains can assemble into at least 11 laminin trimers called laminin 1 to 11. Laminin 11 (α5β2γ1) is the major laminin of the adult GBM. Expression of laminin chains changes during embryogenesis. Laminin α1 and β1 chains are expressed transiently in early GBM development, and β2 chains and the newly described α5 chain appear later. Nidogen/entactin is a 150-kD polypeptide that serves as a link between the laminin network (specifically the γ1 chain) and the collagen IV network.

The ubiquitous heparan sulfate proteoglycans contribute by their polyanionic glycosaminoglycan side chains to the net negative charge of the GBM, and, therefore, are partly responsible for its impermeability to anionic plasma proteins. Agrin binds to several different laminin trimers and is the major heparan sulfate proteoglycan in the human GBM. Perlecan, containing a 400- to 500-kD core protein, is expressed only weakly in the adult GBM.

Glomerular Endothelium

The endothelial cells are large, flat cells. Together they form the endothelial tube of the capillaries (Fig. 1.27). Their cell bodies are located near the mesangial axes. The flat peripheral parts contain large fenestrations of 50 to 100 nm in diameter (Figs. 1.27 and 1.28). Unlike peritubular capillaries, most of these fenestrations lack a diaphragm; they are true pores. Furthermore, the endothelium is different than other capillaries because micropinocytosic vesicles are rare in glomerular endothelial cells. The endothelial cell bodies contain all the usual cell organelles. A well-developed cytoskeleton consists of intermediate filaments and microtubuli. The luminal cell surface of endothelial cells is highly negatively charged because its cell coat contains several polyanionic glycoproteins, including the sialoglycoprotein, podocalyxin.

The Podocytes

The visceral epithelial cells of Bowman's capsule, the podocytes, are highly differentiated cells. They have a very low potential for cell multiplication. Consequently, only cell hypertrophy can compensate for cell loss. Under stimulation, podocytes may undergo nuclear division (mitosis) but are unable to perform cell division (cytokinesis). The result is maladapted binucleated cells.

Podocytes have a large cell body with long cytoplasmic processes that connect them to the GBM (Figs. 1.26, 1.27, and 1.29). The cell bodies are not in direct contact with the basement membrane but rather float freely within the urinary space. The large nucleus sits peripherally within the cell body, close to the cell membrane facing the urinary space. The cytoplasm contains a well-developed Golgi apparatus, abundant cisternae of smooth and rough endoplasmic reticulum, and many lysosomes. In contrast to the cell bodies, the cell processes contain only a few organelles.

Long primary processes emerge from the cell bodies and extend toward the capillaries to which they are affixed by numerous secondary processes in a specific interdigitating pattern. The foot processes of neighboring cells interdigitate with one another, sparing between them meandering slits (Fig. 1.28). These filtration slits have a depth of 300 to 500 nm and a width of 20 to 30 nm.

Near the GBM, the slits are spanned by a 4-nm thick extracellular structure, called slit membrane or slit diaphragm, that has a regular substructure. The slit membrane consists of small rodlike subunits that extend alternately from both sides of the foot processes to the center of the slit, where the subunits are linked by a central bar. This arrangement forms a zipperlike structure. The rectangular spaces between the subunits and the central bar have dimensions of about 4 × 40 nm, approximately the size of an albumin molecule.

The composition of the slit membrane is not completely understood. Certain data suggest that it represents a modified adherens junction. P-cadherin may represent the essential membrane-spanning protein making up the subunits and being anchored in the adjacent cytoplasm to ZO-1 and thus to the cytoskeleton. In addition, a 51-kD protein is found specifically at the slit membrane, but the character of this protein is not yet known.

The luminal cell membrane of podocytes (i.e., the membrane above the slit diaphragm, facing the urinary space) is covered by a thick surface coat rich in sialoglycoproteins, which are responsible for the high negative surface charge of podocytes. This cell coat also bridges the slits and covers the urinary side of the slit diaphragm. Podocalyxin was identified as the major sialoglycoprotein of this glycocalyx. This surface charge contributes decisively to the maintenance of the interdigitating pattern of the foot processes and the width of the filtration slits. The abluminal membrane contains a podocyte-specific 120-kD protein called A13, and nephrin, probably a specific cell-adhesion protein of the immunoglobulin family. The major podocyte antigen of rat Heymann nephritis, gp330/megalin, is present on the entire surface of podocytes.

Cytoskeleton of Podocytes

Within the cell body and the primary cell processes, microtubules and intermediate filaments dominate, whereas within the foot processes, longitudinally running bundles of microfilaments are encountered. The prominent bundles of microtubules in the large cell process are accompanied by microtubule associated proteins (MAPs), especially MAP 3 and MAP 4. In addition, these large processes contain an abundance of the intermediate filament protein vimentin. In the foot processes, there is a complete, microfilament-based contractile apparatus. This system is composed of actin, myosin II, α-actinin, talin, and vinculin. The microfilaments form loop-shaped bundles, with their limbs running in the longitudinal axis of the foot processes. The bends of these loops are located centrally at the transition to the large processes and appear to be connected to the microtubules by the microtubule-associated protein τ, which is also known from other sites as a mediator connecting microtubules and microfilaments. The role of synaptopodin, a podocyte-specific actin-associated protein, in the cytoskeletal organization and function of podocytes is still unknown. Peripherally, the actin bundles appear to anchor in the dense cytoplasm that is associated with the basal cell membrane of podocytes (i.e., the sole plates of the foot processes). The anchoring of the sole plates to the GBM is achieved by a specific $\alpha3\beta1$-integrin. Within the dense cytoplasm of the sole plates, integrins interact with the actin cytoskeleton via talin and vinculin. It has been proposed that the cytoskeleton of the foot processes is responsible not only for mediating the fixation of these cells to the basement membrane but also for contributing to the tone of the capillary wall. Based on the finding that the GBM is an elastic expandable structure, it is suggested that the contractile apparatus of podocyte foot processes counteracts the actual expansion of the pericapillary wall brought about by the hydrostatic pressure difference across this wall.

Podocytes respond to many vasoactive substances, and several receptors have been localized by immunocytochemistry to these cells. At present, the growing list includes angiotensin II, atrial natriuretic peptide, bradykinin, nitric oxide, parathyroid hormone and parathyroid hormone–related peptide, and acetylcholine.

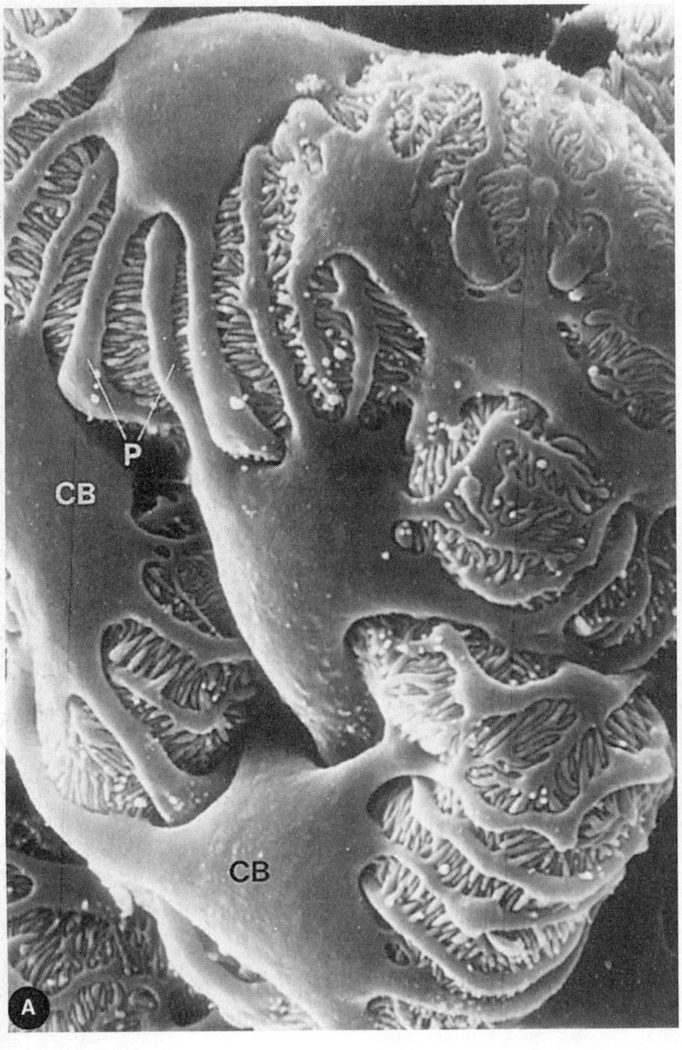

Filtration Barrier

The filtration barrier (Fig. 1.28) is composed of the endothelium with large open pores, the dense fibrillar network of the GBM, and the slit diaphragms between the podocyte foot processes. In addition, the whole filtration area is highly negatively charged because of the negatively charged glycocalyx of both the podocytes and the endothelial cells as well as the high content of negatively charged heparan sulfate proteoglycans of the GBM.

Compared with the barrier established in capillaries elsewhere in the body, there are at least two distinguishing characteristics of the filtration barrier in the glomerulus: the permeability for water, small solutes, and ions is extremely high, and the permeability for plasma proteins and other macromolecules is low. No cell membrane or lipid layer is part of the barrier, which explains the high permeability for water and ions. The major hydraulic barrier is thought to be established by the slit membranes, which cover only about 2% to 3% of the wall surface of the capillaries.

The barrier function for macromolecules is selective for size and charge. The charge selectivity is based on the dense accumulation of negatively charged molecules throughout the entire depth of the filtration barrier, including the surface coats of endothelial and epithelial cells and all three layers of the GBM. These assemblies of negative charges appear to establish an electronegative shield, repelling polyanionic macromolecules in the plasma, such as plasma proteins. This mechanism obviously is important to minimizing the clogging of the filter.

A debate as to the morphologic correlation for the size selectivity of the barrier is ongoing; both the GBM and the slit membrane appear to be relevant, with the slit membrane establishing the main barrier for molecules larger than albumin. Uncharged macromolecules with an effective radius of 1.8 nm or less pass freely through the filter. Larger compounds are increasingly more restricted until an absolute barrier is reached by a radius of about 4 nm. The term *effective radius* is an empirical value (measured in artificial membranes) that takes into account the shape of macromolecules and attributes a radius to nonspherical molecules. Plasma albumin has an effective radius of 3.6 nm. Without the repulsion caused by the negative charge, plasma albumin would pass through the filter in considerable amounts. The fate of macromolecules that enter the filter is unknown. They probably pass through the filter slowly and are then phagocytized by podocytes. Mesangial cells may also contribute to the phagocytosis of those molecules to keep the filter clean.

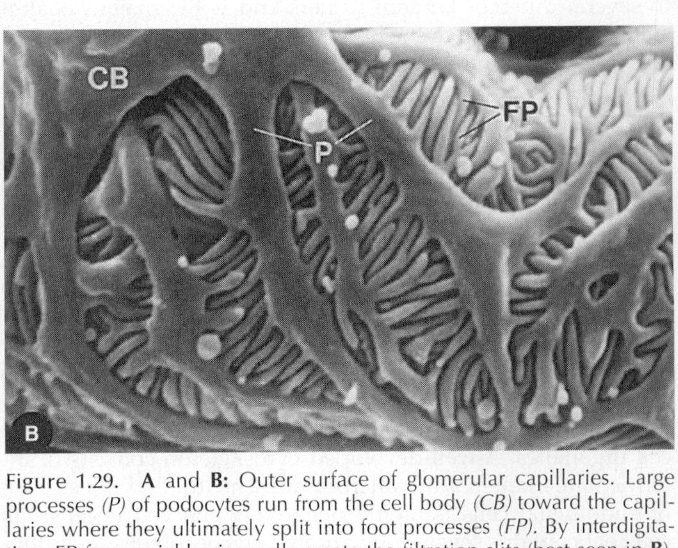

Figure 1.29. **A** and **B:** Outer surface of glomerular capillaries. Large processes *(P)* of podocytes run from the cell body *(CB)* toward the capillaries where they ultimately split into foot processes *(FP)*. By interdigitation, FP from neighboring cells create the filtration slits (best seen in **B**). Rat; SEM, **(A)** ×~2,200, **(B)** ×~4,300.

The Mesangium

The mesangium consists of mesangial cells and mesangial matrix (Figs. 1.26 and 1.27). The mesangium generally is believed to form a supporting framework that maintains the structural integrity of the glomerular tuft. It occupies the axial region of a glomerular lobule and continues into the glomerular stalk, where it is connected to the EGM, which fills the conical space between afferent and efferent arterioles. Together with the glomerular capillaries, the mesangium fills the space inside the GBM.

Mesangial cells are considered contractile cells, representing modified smooth muscle cells. They are irregular in shape, with numerous cytoplasmic processes extending from the cell body toward the GBM. Mesangial cells contain bundles of contractile microfilaments, particularly within their processes. These microfilament bundles contain actin, myosin, and α-actinin, thus creating a complete actin-based contractile apparatus. A small population (3% to 7%) of cells is bone marrow derived; they are macrophages that have invaded the mesangium.

In the mesangial matrix, collagen types IV [α1 and α2(IV) chains], V, and VI have been demonstrated. As opposed to the GBM, the mesangial matrix is abundant in the glycoprotein fibronectin.

Stability of the Glomerular Tuft

Glomerular capillaries are constantly exposed to high transmural pressure gradients of up to 40 mm Hg, which is considerably higher than pressure gradients in capillaries elsewhere in the body. The major structure providing stability to glomerular capillaries is the GBM. In cooperation with two contractile systems—that of mesangial cells and that of podocytes—the GBM appears to be capable of developing the necessary wall tension to counteract the distending forces, thus preventing capillary dilation.

The first stabilizing system consists of the GBM and the mesangium. Mesangial cells are connected with the GBM either by direct apposition of mesangial cell processes or by the interposition of the matrix elements. The mesangial matrix consists of densely interwoven microfibrils that connect the entire paramesangial part of the GBM to mesangial cells. Distinct bundles of microfibrils often are found in the juxtacapillary region and are regarded as microtendons, which allow the transmission of the contractile force of mesangial cells to specific sites of the GBM. Microfibrils are noncollagenous, nonbranching tubes that are approximately 15 nm thick. They contain the protein fibrillin and are associated with the 31-kD glycoprotein MAGP.

The actin filament bundles are particularly well developed in the processes surrounding the attachment site of the glomerular capillaries to the mesangium, that is, the underlying juxtamesangial part of the endothelium. Mesangial cell–GBM connections are especially prominent in the juxtacapillary region. At this site, tonguelike mesangial cell processes densely filled with microfilament bundles run underneath the capillary endothelium toward the mesangial angles of the GBM where they are anchored. The contractile forces of these mesangial processes appear to stabilize the folding pattern of the GBM and thus the shape of the capillaries.

There is no hydraulic barrier between capillary lumen and mesangium, and therefore no pressure barrier exists. As a result, hydrostatic pressure gradients similar to those existing across the capillary wall also may exist across the paramesangial wall. These differences are balanced by contractile forces of mesangial cells pulling the paramesangial walls centripetally to the mesangial axis.

The second structure-stabilizing system superimposed on the mesangial cell–GBM system is the podocytes. Two mechanisms appear to be involved. First, podocytes stabilize the folding pattern of glomerular capillaries by fixing the points of inflection of the GBM between neighboring capillaries. The narrow angles between neighboring capillaries generally are filled by conspicuous terminal portions of podocyte processes attaching to the GBM. These terminal-process portions contain dense accumulations of microfilaments and the specific podocyte protein synaptopodin. The relevance in maintaining such angles is seen clearly in experiments in which the mesangium is totally dissolved after being treated with antibodies against Thy-1. Even after total mesangiolysis, those angles are maintained, stabilizing the folding pattern of the GBM. Second, podocytes are attached to the GBM by foot processes over almost its entire external surface. It is suggested that foot-process attachments act on the GBM as a large number of small stabilizing patches by locally counteracting the elastic distension of the GBM.

The Parietal Epithelium

The parietal layer of Bowman's capsule consists of squamous epithelial cells resting on a basement membrane (Figs. 1.24 and 1.25). The flat cells are polygonal with a central cilium and few microvilli. They contain bundles of actin filaments that are particularly prominent at the vascular pole, where they run in a circular direction around the glomerular entrance. At the urinary pole, the flat, parietal epithelial cells transform into the typical proximal tubule cells.

The parietal epithelium basement membrane (PBM) has a specific structure. At the transition from the GBM, it splits into several dense layers separated by translucent layers. The transitional region between the GBM and the PBM is mechanically connected to extraglomerular mesangial cells and to smooth muscle cells of both glomerular arterioles. In the PBM, collagen IV is characterized by the α6(IV) chain.

THE RENAL TUBULES

The glomerular filtration is selective for size and charge of macromolecules but does not show any specificity for other plasma compounds. The final composition of the urine is a result of reabsorption and secretion processes along the uriniferous tubule.

The tubule is established by a single-layered epithelium anchored to a basement membrane. The epithelium is of the transporting type, consisting of flat or cuboidal epithelial cells connected apically by a junctional complex. As a result of this organization, two different pathways through the epithelium exist: a transcellular pathway, including the transport across the luminal and basolateral cell membranes and through the cytoplasm, and a paracellular pathway through the junctional complex and the lateral intercellular spaces.

The tight junction determines the paracellular permeability of an epithelium, whereas the other parts of the junctional complex (i.e., zonula adherens and desmosomes) serve as mechanical connections of the cells. The tight junctions are not impenetrable seals but rather gates that selectively regulate the passage of ions between the cells; that is, they regulate the amount of paracellular transport. Depending on the type of epithelium, a zonula occludens may be too narrow for ions to pass, as is the case in the collecting duct, where it consists of multiple anastomosing junctional strands. By contrast, the proximal tubule has a leaky epithelium; its cells are connected by shallow occluding junctions with only one interrupted junctional strand. Tight junctions also serve as a fence to limit the diffusion of membrane constituents between the apical and lateral membranes. This is essential for the maintenance of cell-surface polarity.

The transcellular transports are defined by the composition of the luminal and basolateral cell membranes (i.e., by the specific channels, carriers, and transporters in these membranes). In general, a membrane's surface area determines the quantity of transport through a membrane; the receptor and transport proteins can be incorporated only to a certain density in the membrane. Microvilli and brush border formations enhance the membrane surface on the luminal side of an epithelial cell. Brush borders are characteristic of reabsorbing epithelia. They are highly specific formations rather than dense arrays of microvilli.

On the basolateral cell surface, two forms of cell-surface amplification are found: (a) infolding of the basal cell membrane and (b) interdigitations of cells by lateral cell processes. Cellular interdigitations are developed in salt-transporting epithelia. The amount of mitochondria found in the interdigitating cell processes correlates with the enhancement of the membrane surface. The close association between transporting membranes and mitochondria is found only in interdigitating epithelia; it is lacking in epithelia with mere basal infoldings. Basal infoldings create narrow extracellular spaces deep within the cell, but these spaces do not communicate with the lateral intercellular spaces. In contrast, the extracellular spaces created by interdigitations communicate with each other and can be considered lateral interstitial spaces that participate in paracellular transport.

Proximal Tubule

Histologically, the proximal tubule is divided into a straight part and a convoluted part. Ultrastructurally, three segments—S1, S2, and S3—generally are distinguished. Within the second half of the convoluted part, S1 cells are gradually replaced by S2 cells. Thus S2 begins within the cortical labyrinth. The transition from S2 to S3 occurs along the straight part within the medullary ray. The S3 segments continue into the lower portions of the medullary ray and into the outer stripe. In humans, only two segments corresponding to S1 and S3 have been ultrastructurally characterized.

The proximal tubule epithelium is characterized by a prominent brush border at its luminal side and, basolaterally, by extensive interdigitation of lateral cell processes that are filled with large mitochondria (Figs. 1.30, 1.31, and 1.32). This organization considerably increases both the luminal and basolateral membrane areas of the epithelium. The lateral cell interdigitation extends up to the tight junction, thus increasing the tight junctional belt in length and providing increased passage for passive transports.

As in every other tubular segment, the transcellular transports are governed by the Na^+-K^+-ATPase, which is located within the basolateral cell membranes and associated with large mitochondria. Most other transport systems are coupled in secondary transport fashion to the work of Na^+-K^+-ATPase. The luminal transporter for Na^+ entry specific for the proximal tubule is the Na^+-H^+ exchanger. Other secondary transport systems of the luminal membrane are the Na^+-glucose symport and several Na^+–amino acid symport systems, which are responsible for the reabsorption of glucose and amino acids from the tubular urine. The apical and the basolateral cell membrane contain the constitutive water channel aquaporin 1 (AQP 1), which is present in both membranes in high amounts, accounting for the high water permeability of the proximal tubule. The leaky tight junctions are responsible for a low-resistance shunt pathway parallel with the high-resistance pathway across the membranes of the tubule. The proximal tubule cells are the only ones among the renal epithelial cells that are electrically coupled by gap junctions.

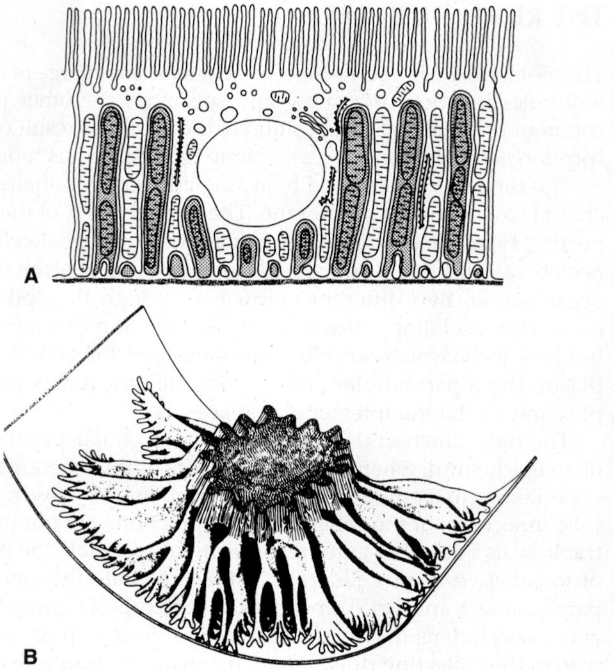

Figure 1.30. Schematics of proximal tubule epithelium. **A:** Apicobasal section showing the apical brush border and the interdigitation of the cell bodies by large lateral processes. To demonstrate the cellular interdigitation, neighboring cells and their processes are stippled. The interdigitating processes are filled with mitochondria. **B:** Three-dimensional model of a proximal tubule cell showing the large lateral processes. (Reprinted with permission from Welling LW, Welling DJ. Shape of epithelial cells and intercellular channels in the rabbit proximal tubule. *Kidney Int* 1976;9:385–394.)

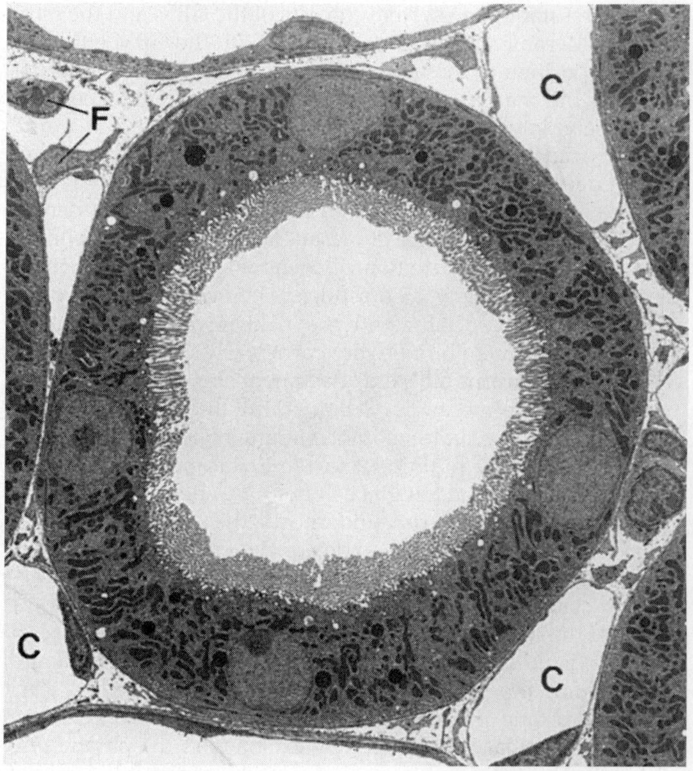

Figure 1.31. Cross section of a proximal tubule (S1 segment). Note the apical brush border, the vesicular zone beneath the brush border, and the zone of interdigitating cell processes filled with mitochondria. Note the sparse peritubular interstitium and narrow relationships of proximal tubule epithelium to peritubular capillaries *(C)*. *F*, fibroblasts. Rat; TEM, ×~1,800.

A prominent lysosomal system is the apical vacuolar endocytotic apparatus, which is responsible for the reabsorption of macromolecules (polypeptides and proteins up to the size of albumin) that have passed through the glomerular filter along with filtration. The trafficking of internalized material from the vacuolar apparatus to degrading lysosomes, which are generally situated in deeper regions of the cells, critically depends on the microtubular system. Recent data suggest that in addition to processing proteins endocytosed from the tubular fluid, the vacuolar apparatus may serve as a transient store for intrinsing membrane proteins (e.g., Na^+-phosphate transporter) recycled from the apical cell membrane. The extent of the endocytotic apparatus and its capacity for protein degradation diminishes from S1 to S3. In S3 cells, it is only slightly apparent, corresponding to the lack of proteins within the tubular fluid under healthy conditions at this site.

The previously mentioned characteristics of the proximal tubule epithelium are best developed in S1 segments. The brush border in S2 segments is not as high as that in S1 segments. Furthermore, the complexity of the lateral cell processes decreases. Thus the surface area of both apical and basolateral cell membranes is smaller than the surface area in S1 segments and decreases further along S3 segments. This is associated with a decrease in mitochondrial density and in the elaboration of vacuolar apparatus. In contrast, smooth endoplasmic reticulum and peroxisomes are more abundant in S3 than in the preceding segments. Chapter 6 discusses the principles of renal tubular transport, Chapter 15.1 details water transport, and Chapter 15.2 discusses sodium transport.

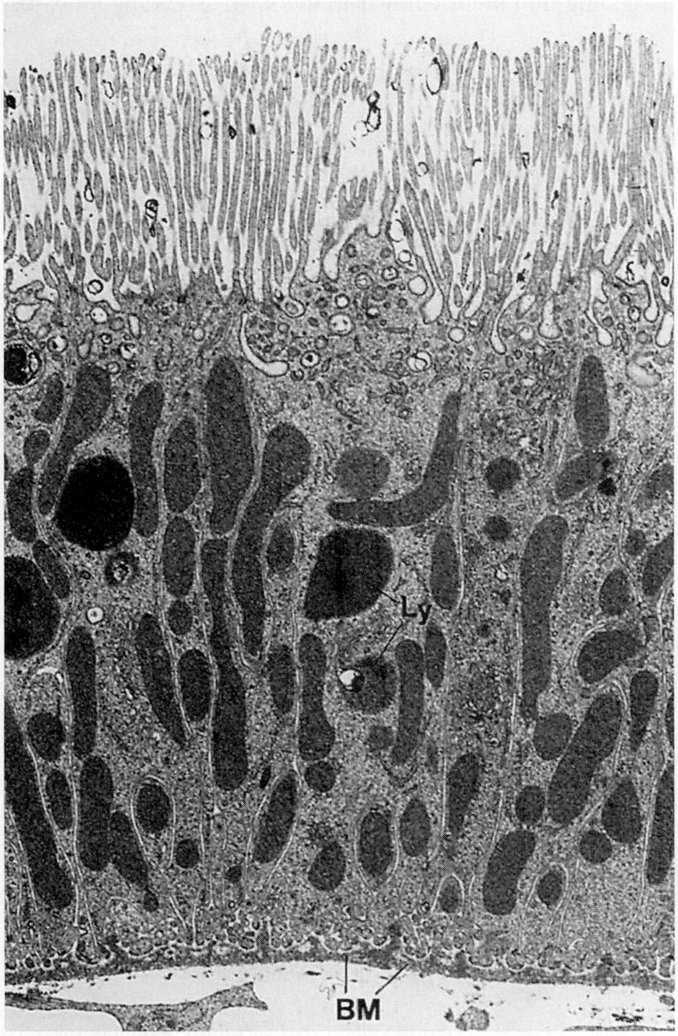

Figure 1.32. Proximal tubule epithelium, S1 segment. Beneath the brush border (made up of densely arranged long microvilli) in the apical cytoplasm, a well-developed vacuolar apparatus is seen. The mitochondria are aligned along the lateral cell membranes of interdigitating cell processes. *BM,* basement membrane; *Ly,* lysosomes. Rat; TEM, × ~20,000.

Thin Limb of Henle's Loop (Intermediate Tubule)

The transition from the proximal tubule to the intermediate tubule (thin descending limb of Henle's loop) is abrupt. Ultrastructurally, the thin limbs of Henle's loop are made up of four segments (Fig. 1.33): the descending thin limbs of short loops

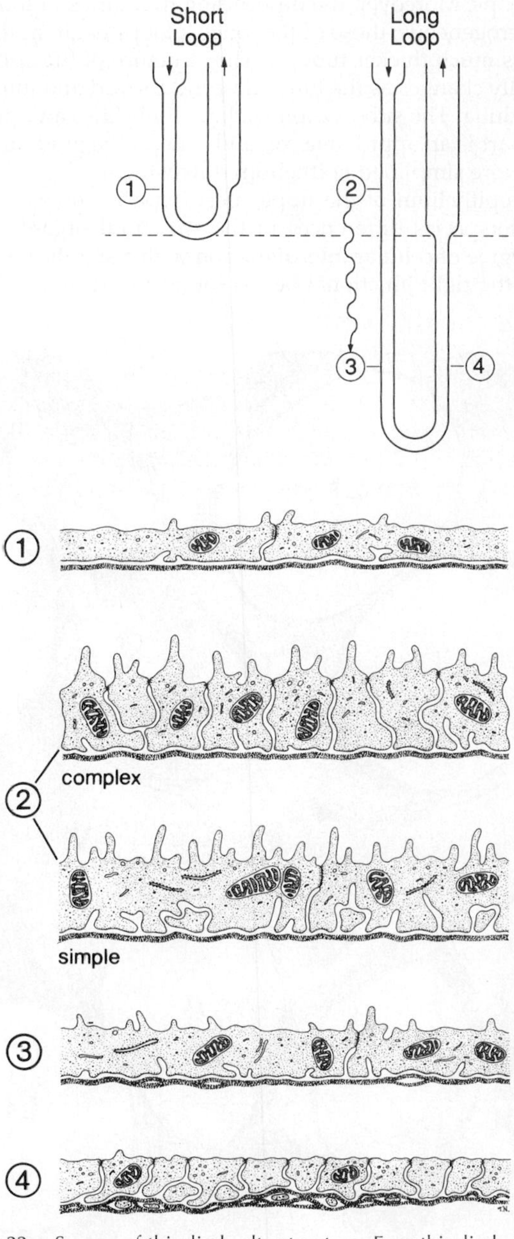

Figure 1.33. Survey of thin limb ultrastructure. Four thin limb segments are discernible: *1:* Thin descending limb of short loops. *2* and *3:* Thin descending limbs of long loops, subdivided into an upper part and a lower part. The upper part is developed differently among species: A complex type **(upper panel)** found for example in rats, mice, and probably humans, is distinguished from a simple type **(lower panel)** found for example in rabbits and guinea pigs. The transition between upper and lower parts is gradual. *4:* Thin ascending limb. (Reprinted with permission from Welling LW, Welling DJ. Shape of epithelial cells and intercellular channels in the rabbit proximal nephron. *Kidney Int* 1976;9:385–394.)

(type 1 epithelium); the descending thin limbs of long loops, which are subdivided into an upper (type 2) and a lower part (type 3); and the ascending thin limbs (type 4). The long loops generally belong to the juxtamedullary renal corpuscles, whereas the short loops are part of the more superficially situated corpuscles.

The descending thin limbs of short loops show a simple and uniform epithelial organization. The epithelium (type 1) is made up of flat, noninterdigitating cells. The luminal cell membrane bears only a few short microvilli. The tight junction consists of several anastomosing junctional strands, and desmosomes are common.

The descending limbs of long loops generally are much larger in diameter and have a thicker epithelium than those of short loops. Moreover, the descending thin limbs of long loops are heterogeneous; those of the longest loops begin in the inner stripe as much thicker tubules. The structure of the epithelium gradually changes as the limbs descend toward and into the inner medulla. The subdivision of these limbs into an upper and lower part is an approximation and reflects the gradual change into a more simplified epithelium downstream.

The epithelium of the upper part (type 2) shows considerable interspecies differences in the structural organization. A high degree of cellular interdigitation with a significant elongation of the tight junctional belt is found in rats and mice. The tight junctions are shallow, consisting usually of one strand. In other species (e.g., rabbit, minipig), the cells do not interdigitate and the tight junctions are deeper. As a consistent feature, apical and basolateral membranes of type 2 epithelial cells are densely studded with integral proteins, including basolateral Na^+-K^+-ATPase.

The epithelium of the lower part (type 3) of long descending thin limbs is comparatively simple (Fig. 1.34). It consists of flat, noninterdigitating cells bearing some sparse microvilli. The tight junctions are of an intermediate apicobasal depth consisting of several junctional strands.

The epithelium of the ascending thin limbs (type 4) is different from that of the descending thin limb in the inner medulla. The transition from the descending type of epithelium to the ascending type occurs a short distance before the bend. The ascending type of epithelium is characterized by flat but heavily interdigitating cells. The tight junctions are elongated and shallow, consisting of only one uninterrupted strand. This organization of the paracellular pathway corresponds to the high permeability of the ascending limb for ions. The epithelia types 1, 2, and 3—all descending limb segments—are highly water permeable because of the abundance of AQP 1 in their membranes. The epithelia 1 and 3 display the urea transporter UT-A2 and have high urea permeability. In contrast, the epithelium 4 of the ascending thin limbs (similar to the thick ascending limb; dis-

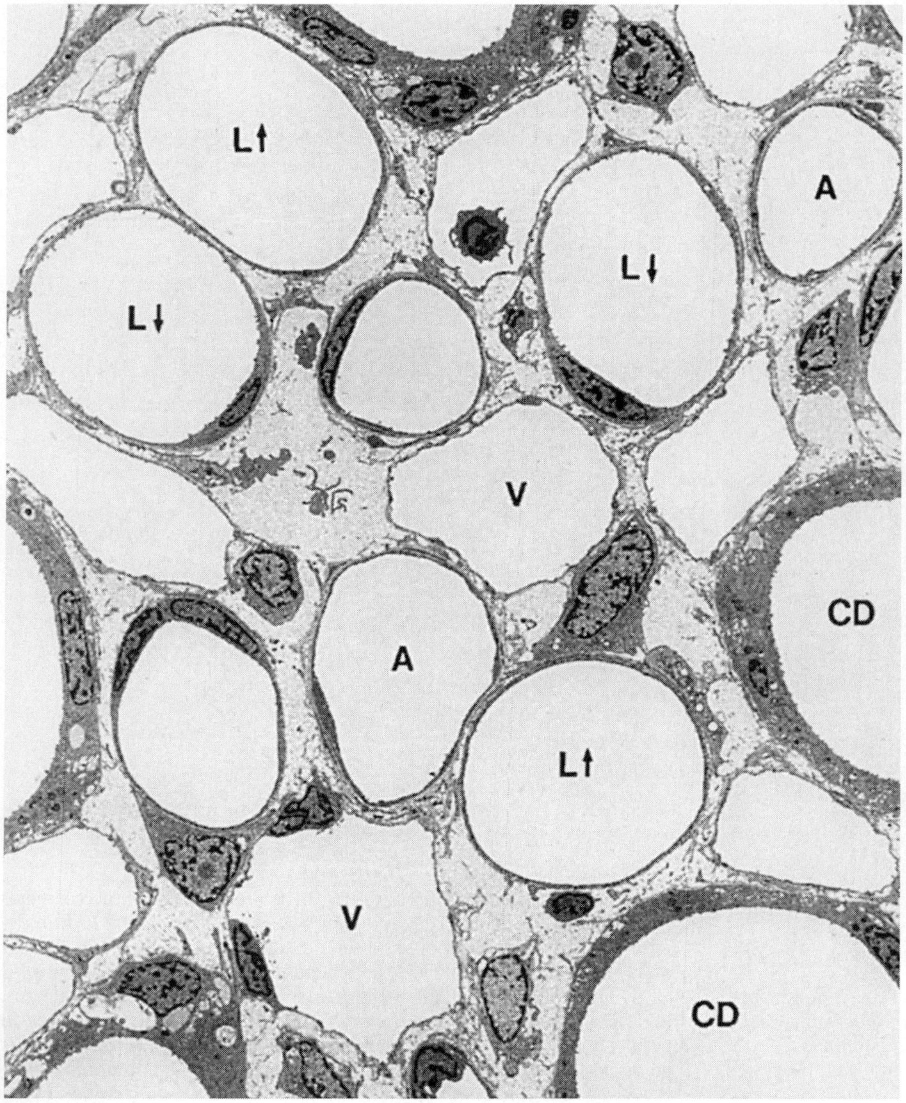

Figure 1.34. Cross section of the inner medulla. Collecting ducts *(CD)*, thin descending limbs *(L↓)*, thin ascending limbs *(L↑)*, and venous *(V)* and arterial *(A)* vasa recta are seen. Note the wide interstitium with many interstitial cells. Rat; TEM, ×~1,750.

cussed later in this chapter) lack any water channels or urea transport proteins and are impermeable for transepithelial water flow.

Distal Straight Tubule (Thick Ascending Limb of Henle's Loop)

The transition from the thin ascending limb to the thick ascending limb is abrupt. The level of this transition defines the border between the inner medulla and the inner stripe of the outer medulla. The medullary part of the thick ascending limb begins here. The cortical part ends shortly beyond the macula densa in the cortex.

The length of the thick ascending limb depends on the location of the respective renal corpuscle from which the tubule originates. The superficial renal corpuscles are associated with the longest cortical part and therefore have the longest thick ascending limbs. In contrast, juxtamedullary nephrons have the shortest distal straight tubule.

The medullary thick ascending limb is composed of tall cells (Figs. 1.35 and 1.36). In the basal three quarters, the cells are ramified into lamellalike lateral cell processes. The large lateral cell processes completely interdigitate with those of neighboring cells and are filled with large mitochondria. In contrast, the apical portions of the cells exhibit a simple, polygonal outline. The tight junctional belt that seals the intercellular spaces from the luminal space consists of several tightly arranged parallel strands. The apical cytoplasm is abundant in smooth vesicles and profiles of smooth endoplasmic reticulum. Immunocytochemical studies show that the Tamm-Horsfall protein is associated with these vesicles and with the apical and lateral cell membrane.

The structural differences between the medullary part and the cortical part of the thick ascending limb are considerable, but the differences develop gradually. The most obvious change

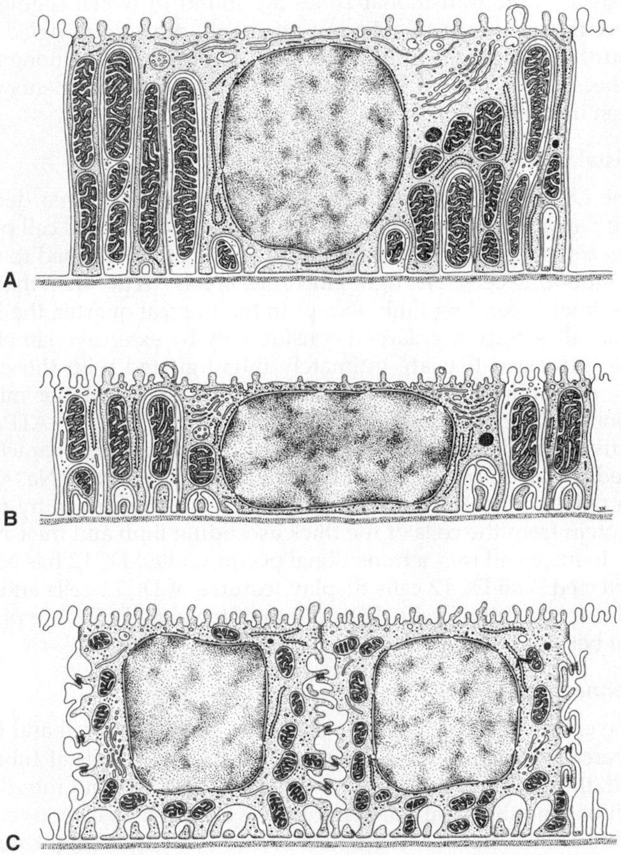

Figure 1.35. Survey of ultrastructure of distal straight tubule cells (thick ascending limb) and macula densa. The homogeneous epithelium of the medullary **(A)** and the cortical part **(B)** is heavily interdigitated by large lateral cell processes. Neighboring cells and their cell processes are unstippled. The cells of the macula densa **(C)** do not interdigitate with each other but are separated by conspicuous intercellular spaces. (Reprinted with permission from Kaissling B, Kriz W. Morphology of the loop of Henle, distal tubule and collecting duct. In: Windhager EE, ed. *Handbook of Physiology,* 2nd ed. New York: Oxford Press, 1992:41–108.)

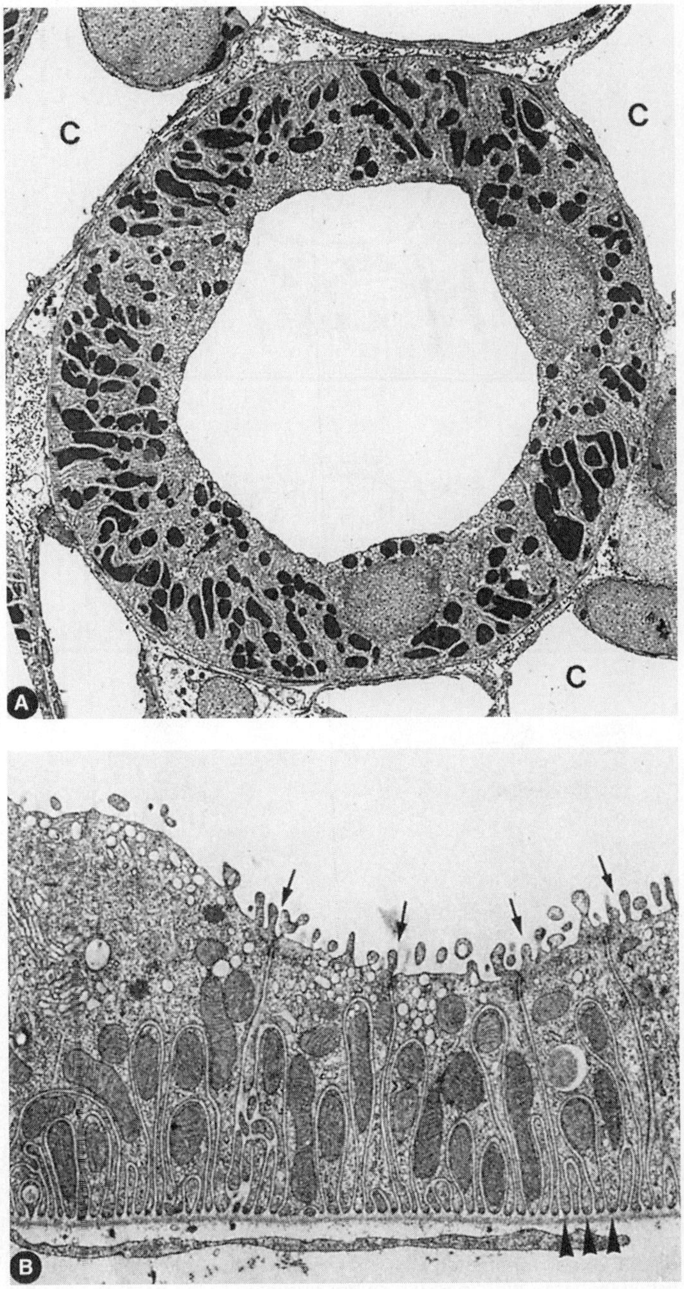

Figure 1.36. Distal straight tubule (thick ascending limb), medullary part. **A:** Entire tubule profile, showing the dense mitochondrial content of this epithelium. Note the narrow relationships to peritubular capillaries *(C).* **B:** The cellular interdigitation in the outer medullary part comprises the apical cell portions; therefore numerous tight junction profiles are seen *(arrows).* The mitochondria are closely associated with lateral interdigitated cell membranes. Note the thin basal ridges *(arrowheads)* resting on the basement membrane. In the apical cytoplasm, many vesicles are seen. Rat, TEMs, **(A)** ×~2,500, **(B)** ×~12,000.

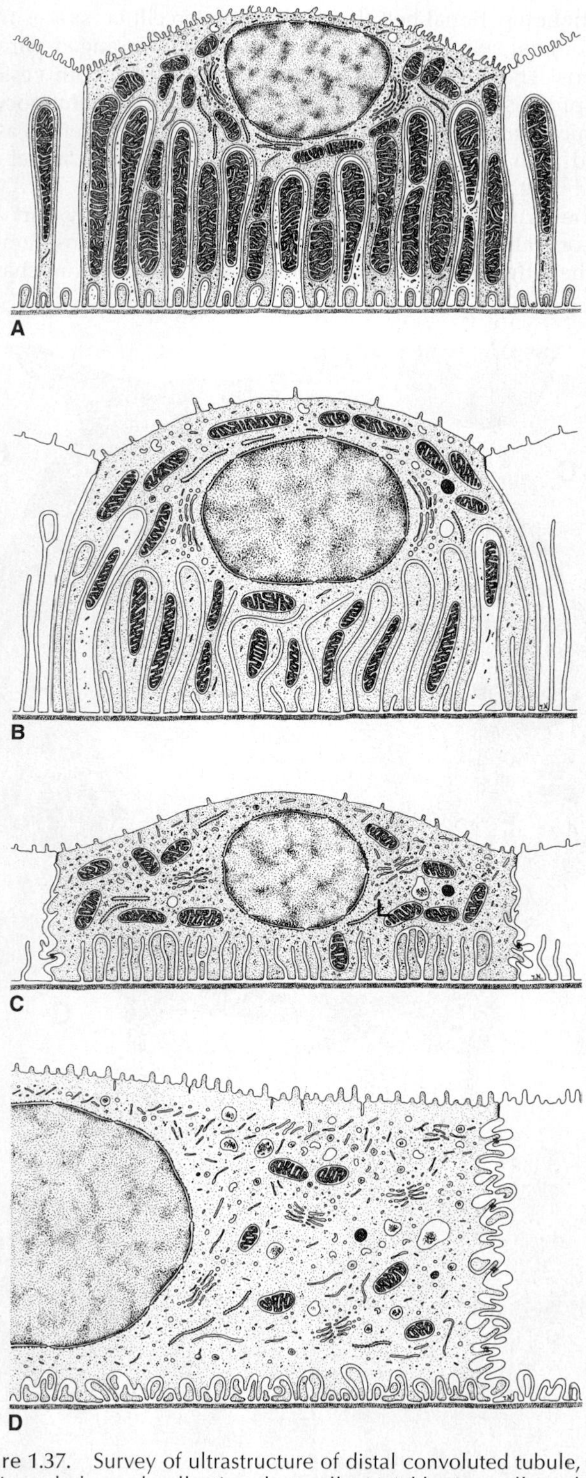

Figure 1.37. Survey of ultrastructure of distal convoluted tubule, connecting tubule, and collecting duct cells. Neighboring cells and their processes are unstippled. **A:** Distal convoluted tubule (DCT) cell. The membranous labyrinth is established by cellular interdigitation. **B:** Connecting tubule (CNT) cell. The membranous labyrinth is established predominantly by infoldings of the basal cell membrane. **C:** Collecting duct (CD) cell (principal cell). The basal labyrinth is exclusively established by basal infoldings, which are restricted to the basal third of the cell. **D:** Inner medullary collecting duct (IMCD) cell; the basal infoldings occupy a narrow rim. Note the many lateral microplicae. (Reprinted with permission from Kriz W, Kaissling B. Structural organization of the mammalian kidney. In: Seldin DW, Giebisch G, eds. *The Kidney: Physiology and Pathophysiology,* 2nd ed. New York: Raven Press, 1992:707–777.)

is the decrease in cell height toward the cortex (Fig. 1.35). The apical cell pole increasingly becomes as foliated as the basal cell portion so that eventually the lateral interdigitations extend from the base up to the lumen. This is associated with a considerable elongation of the tight junctional belt. The basolateral cell membrane area, the high Na^+-K^+-ATPase activity, and the mitochondrial number all decrease toward and within the cortex. In contrast, apical microvilli become more numerous.

The epithelium is characterized by a low permeability for water but a high reabsorptive capacity for salt. The apical Na^+-K^+-$2Cl^-$ symport system is most important for salt transport in the distal straight tubule. The respective transport protein (NKCC2), called bumetanide-sensitive cotransporter 1 (BSC-1), has been localized in the kidney to this segment exclusively. Na^+-H^+ exchangers such as the NHE3 protein and epidermal growth factor, also are located in the apical cell membrane. The role of this segment in the concentration of urine is discussed in detail in Chapter 8.

Distal Convoluted Tubule and Collecting Duct System

Downstream from the thick ascending limb of Henle's loop are three more segments: (a) the distal convoluted tubule (DCT), (b) the connecting tubule (CNT), and (c) the collecting duct (CD) (Fig. 1.37). In most species, including humans, the different segments are not clearly marked by abrupt changes in cell type. Instead, large transitional zones are found in which segment-specific cell types of adjacent segments are intermingled. A fourth cell type, the intercalated cell, is interspersed among the other cells. Clear-cut borders between the three segments are seen in rabbits.

Distal Convoluted Tubule

The DCT (Fig. 1.38) begins shortly beyond the macula densa with an abrupt increase in epithelial height. The apical cell pole has a simple polygonal outline and is smoothly apposed to the neighboring cells. The tight junctional belt is deeper than that in the thick ascending limb. Except in their apical quarter, the lateral cell surface is enlarged considerably by extensive lamella-like processes that are intimately interdigitated with those of the neighboring cells. This and the considerably higher mitochondrial density coincides with the highest Na^+-K^+-ATPase activity of all other tubule segments. DCT cells were characterized by the apical localization of the thiazide-sensitive Na^+-Cl^- cotransporter (NCC or TSC) and may be distinguished by this protein from the cells of the thick ascending limb and the CNT.

In mice and rats, a transitional portion called DCT2 has been detected. The DCT2 cells display features of DCT1 cells and of connecting tubule cells. In addition, intercalated cells are present between the DCT2 cells.

Connecting Tubule

The epithelium consists of two cell types, the CNT cell and the intercalated cell (Figs. 1.37 and 1.39). Unlike the distal tubule cell, the CNT cell has a smooth lateral border without interdigitation, and the basal cell membrane is enlarged by elaborate infoldings associated with mitochondria. The apical tight junctions are composed of several anastomosing strands. CNT cells have been the only cell type within the kidney that shows immunoreactivity for kallikrein. It is assumed that the cells synthesize and secrete this proteolytic enzyme. Kallikrein is found in apical vesicles, in the Golgi apparatus, and also in small endocytotic vesicles along the basal infoldings.

The amiloride-sensitive Na^+ channel ENaC and the secretory ATP-sensitive K^+ channel ROMK in the apical membrane

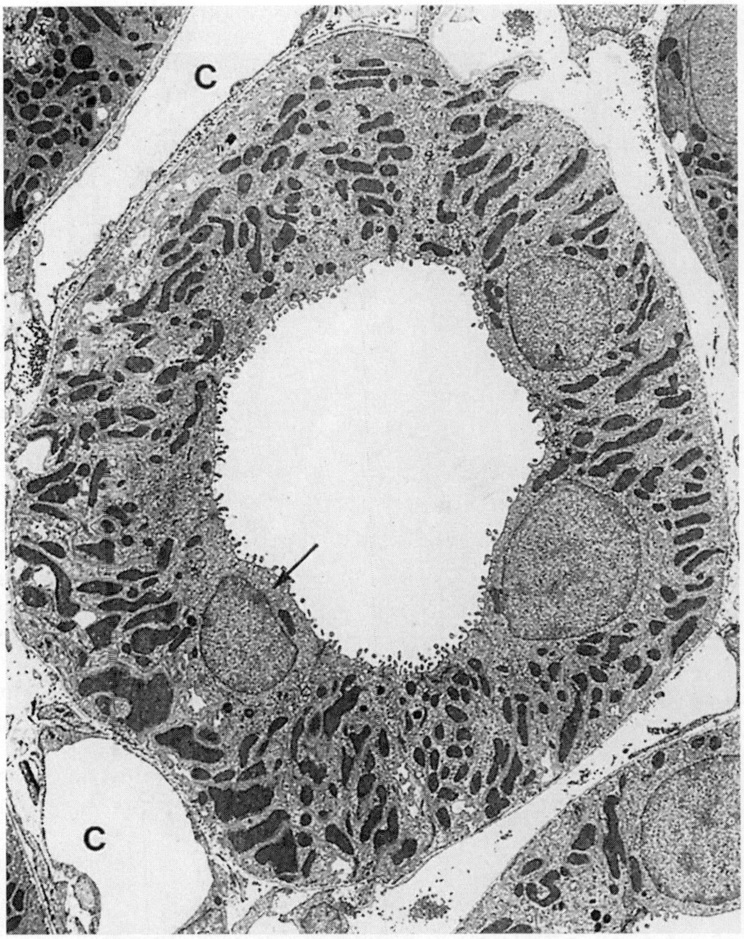

Figure 1.38. Distal convoluted tubule, cross section. The homogeneous epithelium is densely stuffed with mitochondria associated with interdigitated lateral cell membranes. The cell nuclei lie in the apical cell portion. Note the many vesicles in the apical cytoplasm *(arrow)*. *C,* peritubular capillaries. Rat; TEM, ×~3,000.

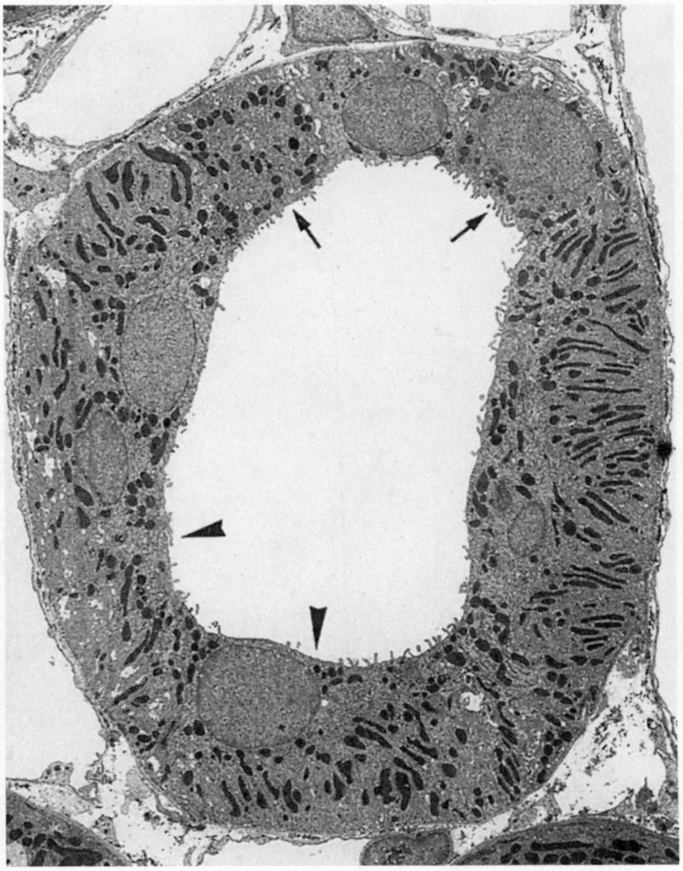

Figure 1.39. Connecting tubule, cross section. The epithelium is made up of connecting tubule cells *(arrowheads)* and of intercalated cells *(arrows)*. Rat; TEM, ×~2,300.

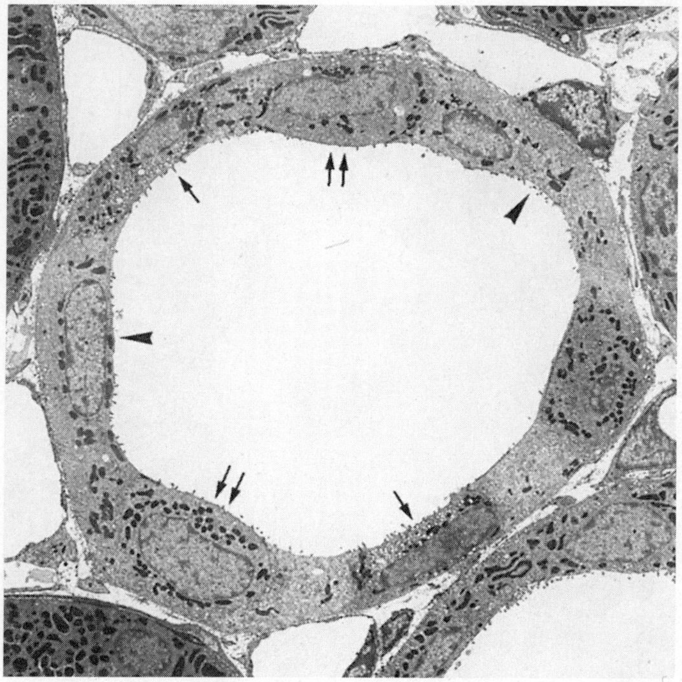

Figure 1.40. Cortical collecting duct, cross section. The epithelium is made up of collecting duct (CD) cells *(arrowheads)* and intercalated cells, type A *(single arrows)* and type B *(double arrows)*. Rat; TEM, ×~2,100.

appear to be involved in sodium reabsorption and potassium secretion in CNT cells. This function is apparently regulated by mineralocorticoids. The CNT cells further express an apical H^+-ATPase, a basolateral Ca^{2+}-Mg^{2+}-ATPase, a Na^+-Ca^{2+} exchanger, and an extracellular Ca^{2+}-sensing receptor, which suggests a prominent role in calcium reabsorption of this segment.

Collecting Duct

Depending on its location, the CD is divided into a cortical, outer medullary portion and an inner medullary collecting duct (IMCD) portion. Intercalated (IC) cells are interposed between the segment-specific cells (the CD cells) from the cortex to the first portion of the inner medullary duct (Fig. 1.40).

Collecting Duct Cells. The basic organization of the CD cells is similar to that of CNT cells (Figs. 1.37 and 1.41). The lateral cell surface is rather smooth without interdigitation with the neighboring cells. Instead, numerous microvilli and microfolds are formed and are connected to microvilli of adjacent cells by abundant desmosomes. The width of the intercellular spaces vary in relation to vasopressin-dependent transepithelial water flow. The basal cell membrane forms lamellar infoldings into the cell. The infoldings are densely arranged without mitochondria and are restricted to the basal third of the cell.

Similar to CNT cells, CD cells express the apical amiloride-sensitive Na^+ channel ENaC for sodium reabsorption. Beneath the apical cell membrane of CD cells, microtubules and micro-

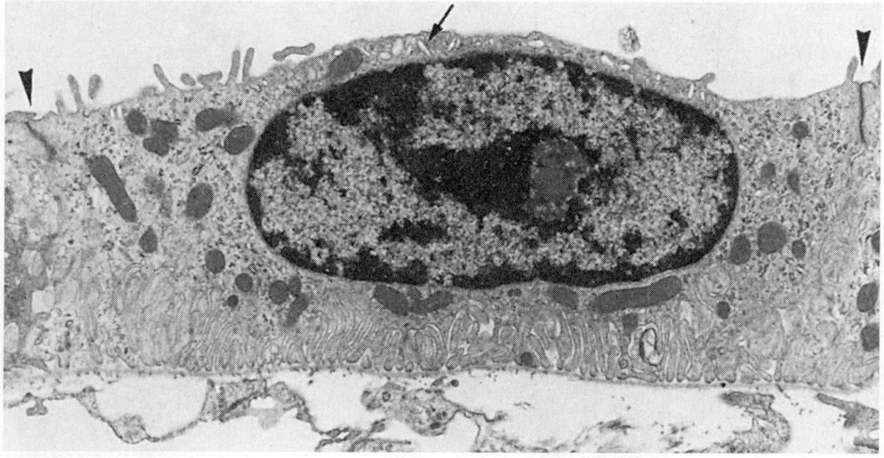

Figure 1.41. Collecting duct (CD) cell (principal cell) of a cortical collecting duct. Note the basal rim of infoldings of the basal cell membrane. Note also the elongated vesicles (aggrephores) in the apical cytoplasm *(arrows)*. The tight junctions are deep *(arrowheads)*. Rabbit; TEM, ×~4,900.

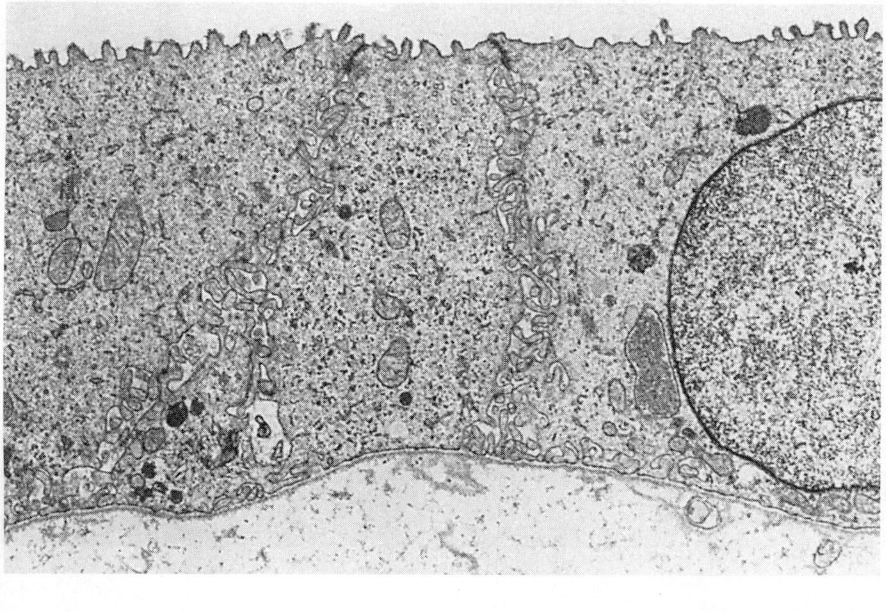

Figure 1.42. Inner medullary collecting duct; epithelium of the middle portion. The epithelium is homogeneously composed by one cell type. Note the conspicuous intercellular spaces and the deep tight junctions. Rat; TEM, ×~11,000.

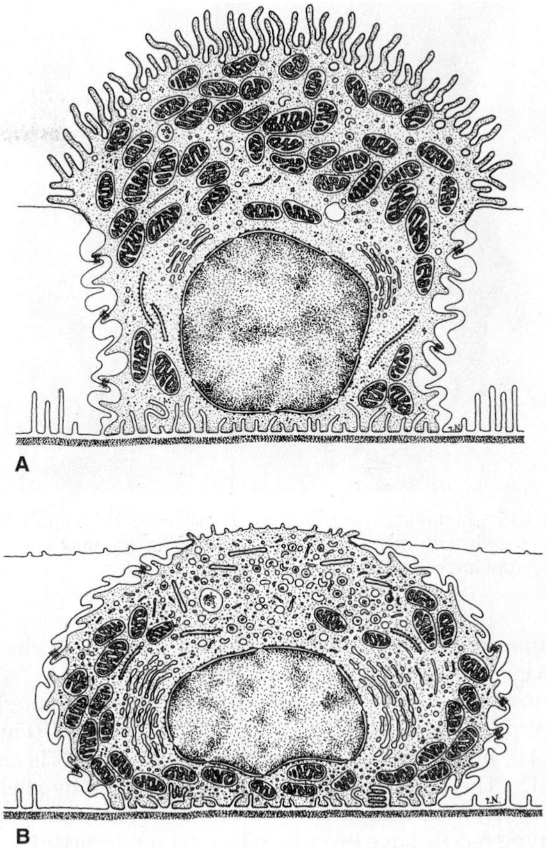

Figure 1.43. Survey of ultrastructure of intercalated cells. **A:** Type A. **B:** Type B. (Adapted with permission from Kriz W, Kaissling B. Structural organization of the mammalian kidney. In: Seldin DW, Giebisch G, eds. *The Kidney: Physiology and Pathophysiology,* 2nd ed. New York: Raven Press, 1992:707–777.)

filaments form a dense network. Among them, small, elongated vesicular profiles are common. These profiles are oriented either perpendicular to or in an oblique angle to the luminal membrane (Fig. 1.31). These so-called aggrephores contain water-permeable channels, namely aquaporin 2, which are activated for water reabsorption by the antidiuretic hormone (ADH). ADH is linked to specific receptors (V2) at the basolateral cell membrane, using cyclic adenosine monophosphate (cAMP) as a second messenger. This triggers a number of intracellular actions that finally lead to the fusion of the apical vesicles with the cell membrane and thus to the insertion of the water channels into the luminal membrane. In the basolateral membrane of CD cells from the cortex to the papillary tip, aquaporin 3 was found, whereas the basolateral aquaporin 4 (which is also permeable for urea) appears to be limited to the inner stripe and the first portion of IMCD. The IMCD further expresses the apical ADH-regulated urea transporter UT-A1. A well-developed cytoskeleton serves to counteract and limit cytoplasmic swelling during water reabsorption.

Differences in the relative amount of cell organelles and cell membrane specializations were found along the CD in most species, namely a gradual decrease in mitochondria, an increase in lateral microvilli and lysosomes, and a more elaborate subapical network of microtubules and microfilaments. The tight junctional belt consists of several anastomosing strands, corroborating with the high electrical resistance of the CD. In several species, including humans, a drastic alteration in cell size (up to a 20-fold increase in height) is observed along the IMCD (Figs. 1.37 and 1.42).

Intercalated Cells. IC cells (Figs. 1.43, 1.44, and 1.45) are interspersed as single cells among the segment-specific cells of DCTs, CNTs, and CDs. The luminal cell surface carries microvilli or microfolds, and it lacks the central cilium. In contrast to the more polygonal shape of the surrounding cells, the luminal outline is rounded. The lateral cell faces usually are covered by numerous small microprojections that are connected to those of the CD cells by desmosomes.

A striking feature of IC cells are membrane domains (apical or basolateral cell membranes and apical vesicles) that, on their cytoplasmic side, carry a specific coat of densely arranged particles, so-called studs, of 10 nm. The electrogenic V-type H^+-ATPase, the proton pump, is associated with the studs. This H^+-ATPase, as well as the carbonic anhydrase II, are present in IC cells in higher abundance than in other tubular cells. In many cases, the H^+-ATPase colocalizes with the phosphatidyl-inositol–anchored ectoenzyme 5′ectonucleotidase. In addition, IC cells express a gastric-type K^+-H^+-ATPase for

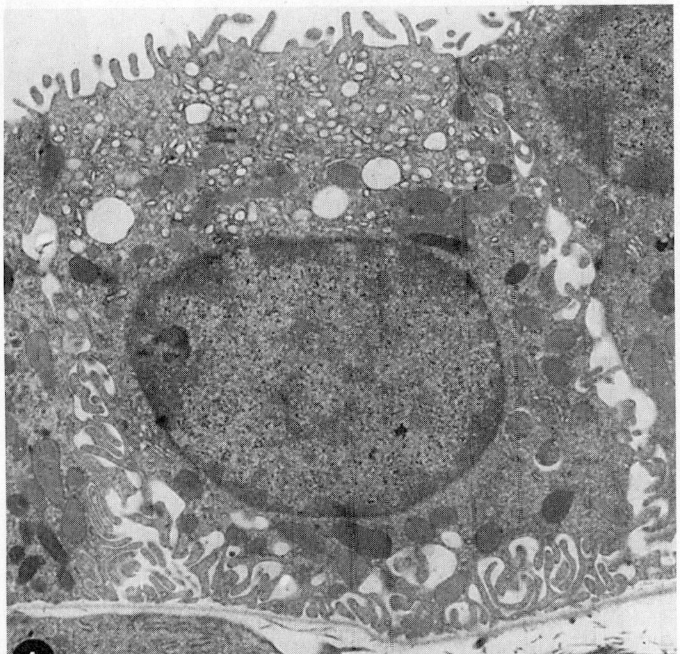

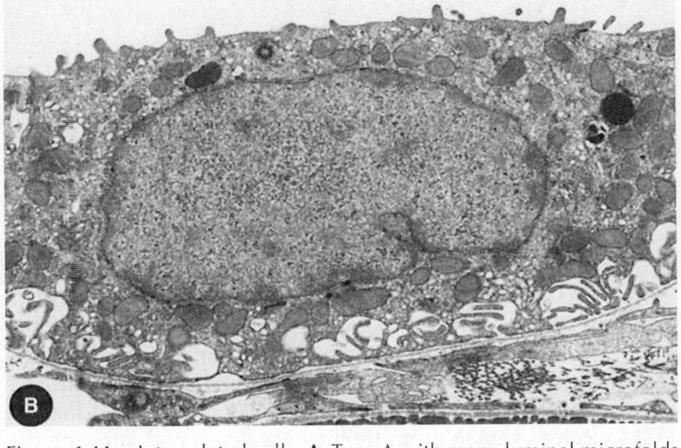

Figure 1.44. Intercalated cells. **A:** Type A with many luminal microfolds and numerous apical vesicles. **B:** Type B with lack of apical vesicles. Instead, vesicles are seen in the basal cell parts. Rat; TEM **(A)** ×~9,100, **(B)** ×~8,100.

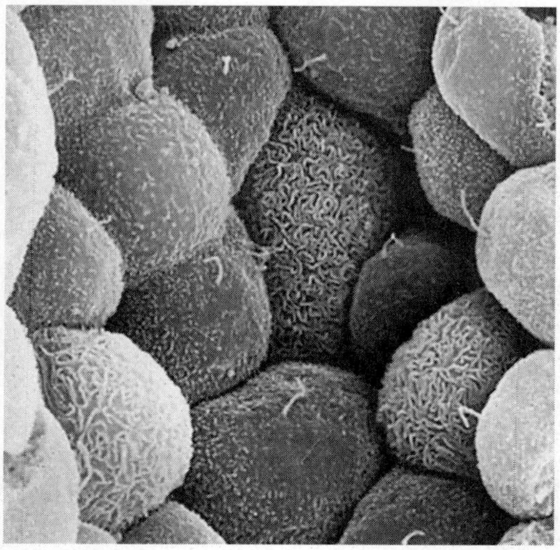

Figure 1.45. Luminal aspect of cortical collecting duct epithelium. Intercalated cells with many apical folds and collecting duct cells with an apical cilium are seen. Rat; SEM, ×~4,000.

potassium reabsorption, apparently associated with clusters of rod-shaped particles in the cell membrane.

Two subtypes of IC cells can be distinguished, although transitional phenotypes between both may be revealed (Figs. 1.43 and 1.44). Both type A and type B are present in CNTs and cortical CDs. Their number appears to be influenced by alterations in the acid–base status and also varies between animal species. Only type A cells have been found in the outer medulla.

Type A IC cells show a broad apical cell pole with elaborate microfolds. Mitochondria and vesicles usually abound in the apical cell pole. The H^+-ATPase (associated with the studs) is located in the apical cell membrane and apical vesicles. In the basolateral cell membrane, the anion (Cl^--HCO_3^-) exchanger AE1 is present and considered a decisive criterium for identifying type A cells. In addition, type A cells display the chloride channel CIC 5 in the apical membrane. Type B IC cells have a rather narrow apical pole with only a few short microvilli. The mitochondria and the H^+-ATPase accumulate along the basolateral cell membrane. An anion exchanger has not been found in these cells. Functionally, type A cells have been associated with proton secretion and bicarbonate reabsorption, whereas type B cells may be involved in the opposite processes, namely proton reabsorption and bicarbonate secretion.

THE JUXTAGLOMERULAR APPARATUS

The juxtaglomerular apparatus is made up of the macula densa, the terminal portion of the afferent arteriole with its renin-producing granular cells, the initial portion of the efferent arteriole, and the extraglomerular mesangium (EGM) (Figs. 1.24 and 1.25).

The structural organization of the juxtaglomerular apparatus strongly suggests a regulatory function. It is widely agreed that some component of the distal urine is sensed by the macula densa and that this information is used to adjust the tonus of the glomerular arterioles, resulting in a change in glomerular blood flow and filtration rate. This mechanism is known as the tubuloglomerular feedback. The juxtaglomerular apparatus is also the main site for the regulation of renin secretion. Little is known about the relevance of the EGM. It is suggested that the EGM receives signals from the macula densa and, after modulation and integration with other signals, transfers them to the granular cells and the ordinary smooth muscle cells for the glomerular arterioles.

The Macula Densa

At the point where the thick ascending limb returns to its parent renal corpuscle, the limb firmly attaches to the EGM between afferent and efferent arterioles (Fig. 1.46). At this point of attachment, the epithelium of the thick ascending limb changes its character and forms a plaque of specialized cells, the macula densa. The most obvious structural features of the cell plaque are the large, narrowly packed cell nuclei, which account of the term *macula densa*.

In contrast to the surrounding cells of the thick ascending limb, the macula densa cells (Fig. 1.47) do not interdigitate with each other but display a fairly polygonal outline. The luminal surface is studded with stubby microvilli and lacks the Tamm-Horsfall protein characteristic of thick ascending limb epithelium. Macula densa cells are joined by tight junctions consisting of several junctional strands similar to those of the thick ascending limb. The lateral membranes bear folds and fingerlike villi that often are connected to those of neighboring cells by desmosomes. The lateral intercellular spaces are a prominent

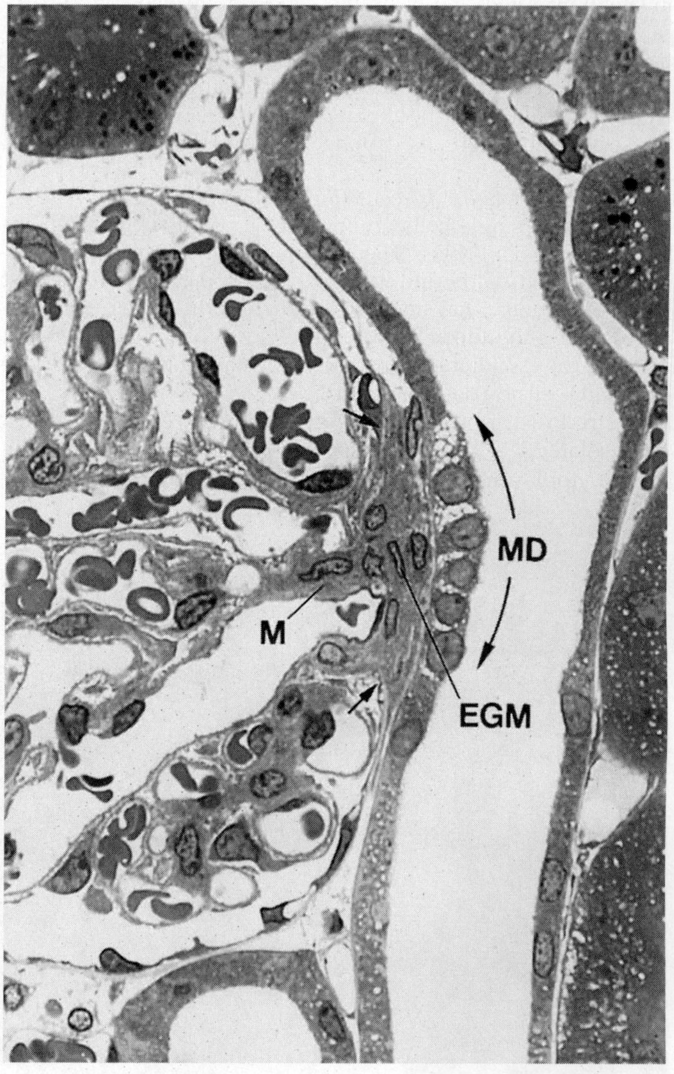

Figure 1.46. Meridional section through a glomerulus running in between both arterioles. The macula densa *(MD)* is a prominent cell plaque within the thick ascending limb. It covers the extraglomerular mesangium *(EGM)*. Within the glomerular stalk the EGM continues into the mesangium *(M)*. The EGM interconnects opposing parts of the reflection of the GBM to the basement membrane of Bowman's capsule (BCBM) *(arrows)*. Note the dilated intercellular spaces between MD cells. TEM, ×~8,100.

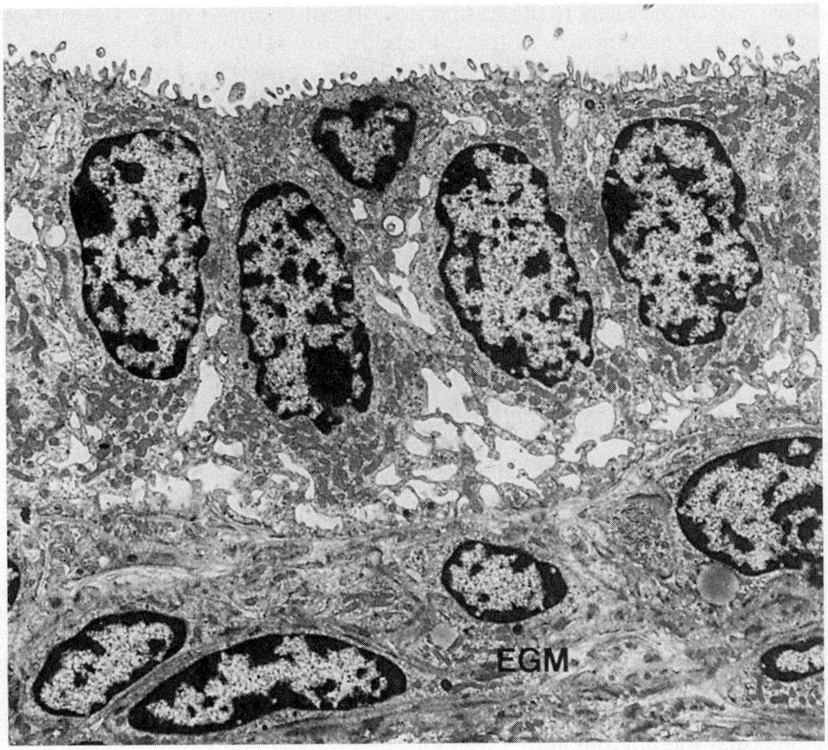

Figure 1.47. The macula densa is conspicuous because of its densely arranged and large cell nuclei and its prominent intercellular spaces. Macula densa cells are closely apposed to the extraglomerular mesangium *(EGM)*. Rabbit; TEM, ×~15,000.

feature of the macula densa. They resemble those between CD cells. The width varies under different functional conditions. The spaces are dilated under most physiologic conditions. Compounds such as furosemide, which block sodium transport, are associated with the narrowing of the intercellular spaces. Water flow through the macula densa is secondary to active sodium reabsorption. At the very base, the cells ramify into slender processes. The basal surface of the macula densa attaches to the EGM. The attachment of the macula densa cells to the underlying basement membrane and to the matrix of the EGM is mediated by αvβ6 integrin, a fibronectin-binding heterodimer that, in kidney tissue, is found in the macula densa exclusively. In addition, the macula densa touches various portions of the afferent and efferent arterioles. However, the only consistent histotopographic relationships of the macula densa are established with the EGM.

Granular Cells

The granular cells are assembled in clusters with up to 15 cells within the terminal portion of the afferent arteriole, replacing ordinary smooth muscle cells in the vessel wall (Fig. 1.48). The

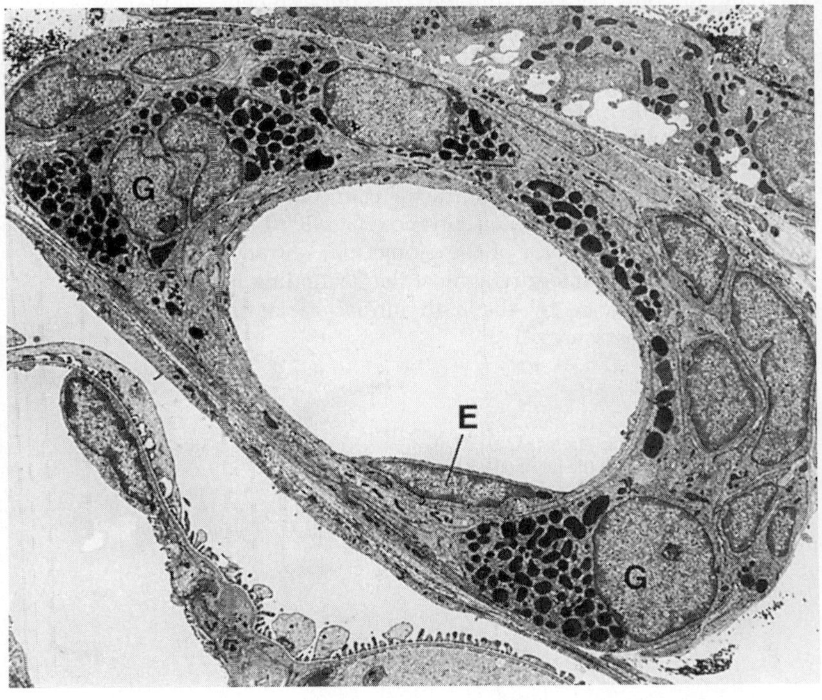

Figure 1.48 Juxtaglomerular portion of an afferent arteriole. Smooth muscle cells are replaced by granular cells *(G)*. Note the dense accumulation of granules within the cytoplasm. *E*, endothelial cell. Rat; TEM, ×~2,700.

term *granular cell* refers to the specific cytoplasmic granules that may densely accumulate in the cytoplasm. The granules are dark, membrane-bound, and irregular in shape and size. Renin, the major secretion product, is stored in these granules. Small granules with crystalline substructures represent protogranules containing both renin prosegment and mature renin. The amorphous, mature granules contain only mature renin. Renin is released by exocytosis into the surrounding interstitium and may then be distributed within the periarterial connective tissue sheaths retrogradely along the intrarenal arterioles and arteries.

Granular cells are modified smooth muscle cells. Under conditions requiring enhanced renin synthesis (e.g., volume depletion or stenosis of the renal artery), additional smooth muscle cells located upstream in the wall of the afferent arteriole (and in the wall of the cortical radial artery) transform into granular cells. Like the smooth muscle cells, granular cells are extensively coupled by gap junctions to adjacent granular cells, smooth muscle cells, extraglomerular mesangial cells, and endothelial cells. Granular cells are densely innervated by sympathetic nerve terminals.

The Extraglomerular Mesangium

The EGM is a dense cell cluster filling the cone-shaped space between the two glomerular arterioles and the macula densa (Figs. 1.24, 1.46, and 1.47). It is in continuation with the intraglomerular mesangium and is well attached to Bowman's capsule. EGM cells form a solid cell complex that is not penetrated by blood or lymphatic vessels.

EGM cells are flat, elongated cells arranged in several layers parallel to the base of the macula densa. The cells nearest the glomerular stalk continue into the intraglomerular mesangium. The cells are embedded in a matrix that differs in its composition from the intraglomerular matrix; microfibrils, in particular, are rarely found in the EGM matrix.

EGM cells are characterized by their sparse cytoplasm and their extensive ramification at both cell poles. These cell processes contain a considerable amount of microfilaments. Strong structural similarities are found among arteriolar smooth muscle cells, granular cells, intraglomerular mesangial cells, and EGM cells, suggesting that they are all of the same origin. EGM cells are strongly interconnected by gap junctions that are found not only between different cells but also between individual cell processes of the same cell. Gap junctional contact exists between all other cells of the juxtaglomerular apparatus except for the macula densa.

The contractile processes of EGM cells are connected to the basement membrane of Bowman's capsule and to the walls of both glomerular arterioles. From a structural viewpoint, the EGM represents a spiderlike contractile clamp interconnecting all structures of the glomerular entrance. The EGM may be regarded as a closure device of the glomerular entrance, maintaining its structural integrity against the distending forces exerted on the entrance by the high intraarteriolar and high intraglomerular pressures.

Selected Readings

Barajas L, Powers K, Carretero OA, et al. Immunocytochemical localization of renin and kallikrein in the rat renal cortex. *Kidney Int* 1986;29:965–970.

This original paper emphasizes the narrow spatial relationships between the connecting tubule and the afferent arteriole and the possibility of interactions of kallikrein, which is synthesized in the connecting tubule, with the renin-angiotensin system.

Elger M, Sakai T, Kriz W. The vascular pole of the renal glomerulus of rat. *Adv Anat Embryol Cell Biol* 1998;139:1–98.

This monograph investigates the topography of the vascular pole, focusing on biochemical and geometrical aspects. In addition, the study provides new data on the structure of the efferent arteriole and the assemblage between afferent and efferent arterioles.

Fourman J, Moffat DB. *The blood vessels of the kidney.* Oxford: Blackwell Scientific, 1971.

This basic monography presents a detailed description of the renal vasculature, the arrangement within the renal tissue, the relationship to the nephron and collecting duct system, and the cellular organization of the vessels.

Kaissling B, Hegyi I, Loffing J, et al. Morphology of interstitial cells in the healthy kidney. *Anat Embryol* 1996;193:303–318.

This review provides a detailed description of the morphologic characteristics of the various cell types of the interstitium in the healthy kidney. The data are a guideline for identifying the cell types representing resident fibroblasts or members of the immune system by electron microscopy and by immunocytochemistry and for the understanding of the distribution of the cells within the renal zones under different experimental or pathologic conditions.

Kaissling B, Stanton BA. Structure-function correlation in electrolyte transporting epithelia. In: Seldin DW, Giebisch G, eds. *The kidney: physiology and pathophysiology, 2nd ed.* New York: Raven Press, 1992:779–802.

This review on transporting epithelia correlates the elaboration of specific structural components, such as the zonula occludens, the structure and mode of amplification of plasma membrane domains with specific cellular mechanisms involved in transepithelial transport processes.

Kriz W, Elger M, Lemley KV, et al. Structure of the glomerular mesangium: a biomechanical interpretation. *Kidney Int* 1990;38(Suppl 30):S2–S9.

This paper summarizes the current knowledge of the structural details and functional significance of the system of contractile filaments in the glomerular mesangium. In conjunction with the glomerular basement membrane, the mesangial contractile apparatus seems capable of supporting sufficient wall tension to counteract the distending forces acting across glomerular capillary walls.

Kriz W, Elger M, Mundel P, et al. Structure-stabilizing forces in the glomerular tuft. *J Am Soc Nephrol* 1995;5:1731–1739.

The glomerular tuft is constantly exposed to considerable expansile forces, resulting from high capillary pressures. This review addresses the general problem of which components in the glomerulus contribute to the structural stability of the tuft and how they may contribute to acute or chronic regulation of glomerular function. Two systems are described: a basic system consisting of the glomerular basement membrane and the mesangium, and a superimposed contractile system in the foot processes of the podocytes.

Kriz W, Kaissling B. Structural organization of the mammalian kidney. In: Seldin DW, Giebisch G, eds. *The kidney: physiology and pathophysiology, 3rd ed.* New York: Raven Press, 2000.

This is a comprehensive and updated review on the cellular organization of the nephrons and collecting duct system, the glomerulus, the renal vasculature, the renal interstitium, and the topographic arrangement of these systems within the kidney.

Lemley KV, Kriz W. Cycles and separations: the histotopography of the urinary concentrating process. *Kidney Int* 1987;31:538–548.

This article presents a number of features of the histotopography of the renal medulla, that is, the relative spatial configurations of vessels, interstitium, and tubular segments, which may be important in the process of urinary concentration. Possible recycling routes for solutes and urea and functionally separated domains (compartmentalization) within the medulla, based on spatial incontiguity and on special characteristics of the interstitium and the blood supply, are suggested, paying attention to local membrane characteristics.

Madsen KM, Verlander JW, Tisher CC. Relationship between structure and function in distal tubule and collecting duct. *J Electr Microsc Tech* 1988;9:187–208.

Morphometric analysis combined with micropuncture and microperfusion studies has provided evidence that the CNT and CCD cells are responsible for potassium secretion. This review emphasizes the role of morphometric analysis in establishing the relationship between structure and function in the distal tubule and collecting duct.

Mundel P, Kriz W. Structure and function of podocytes: an update. *Anat Embryol* 1995;192:385–397.

The general structure of the highly specialized epithelial cell of the glomerular filtration membrane, the methods used to investigate podocytes (especially recent approaches in podocyte culture), and a survey of podocyte functions are presented. Aspects of podocyte development, inclusive of the capacity for cell replication, are discussed.

Taugner R, Hackenthal E. *The juxtaglomerular apparatus.* Berlin, Heidelberg: Springer-Verlag, 1989.

This monograph is a comprehensive overview of the research of the juxtaglomerular apparatus (JGA) and accommodates most of the essential original information. In addition to the description of the components of the JGA (glomerular arterioles, extraglomerular mesangium, and macula densa), this volume provides a flood of information on the renin-angiotensin system, carrying with it several aspects of broader interest, such as general questions of cell differentiation and adaptation, structural and biochemical mechanisms of the secretory processes, and integrated control mechanisms of secretion. A chapter on the pathology of the human JGA is included.

PART 4
Basement Membrane and Cellular Components of the Nephron

Dorin-Bogdan Borza, Jeffrey H. Miner, and Billy G. Hudson

COMPOSITION OF RENAL BASEMENT MEMBRANES

The basement membrane, also known as basal lamina, is a specialized form of extracellular matrix that underlies epithelial and endothelial cells and surrounds muscle, peripheral nerve, and adipose cells. It has the appearance of an amorphous, porous, sheetlike structure. Basement membranes fulfill several important functions: (a) they play a structural role by providing mechanical support for cells and compartmentalizing tissues, (b) they act as selective permeability barriers by restricting the free diffusion of macromolecules and the passage of cells, and (c) they actively interact with neighboring cells to regulate growth, differentiation, and cell migration.

Reflecting particular adaptations to specific functions, the morphology, structure, and composition of basement membranes may differ between different tissues, during development, and under particular physiologic circumstances. In kidneys, the nephrons and collecting ducts are enveloped in basement membranes whose molecular heterogeneity corresponds to the segmental nature of the nephron and may reflect specific functions of different segments (Fig 1.49, *right*). For instance, the glomerular basement membrane (GBM), a relatively thick (250 to 300 nm) structure formed by fusion of epithelial and endothelial basement membranes during kidney development (Fig. 1.49, *top left*), has a distinct molecular composition (Table 1.1) closely related to its specialized plasma ultrafiltration function. Alteration of GBM components in humans or in experimental animals can compromise the structural or functional integrity of the GBM.

Despite their diversity, all basement membranes contain four major components: type IV collagen, laminin, entactin/nidogen, and heparan sulfate proteoglycans (Fig. 1.49, *bottom left*). The heterogeneity of basement membranes arises from the presence of multiple molecular isoforms of the components and from variations in the stoichiometric relationships among these components. This chapter describes the major basement membrane components, their structure, their function, and the way they interact to form a supramolecular structure, with a particular focus on renal basement membranes.

Type IV Collagen

Genetic Isoform and Tissue-Specific Distribution

Type IV collagen is the most abundant component of basement membranes. It forms a meshlike network whose building block is the trimeric collagen protomer containing three chains of approximately 180 kD each. Each α chain has a short (approximately 15 residues), noncollagenous amino terminus, a long (approximately 1,400 residues), triple-helical collagenous domain consisting of Gly-X-Y triplet repeats interrupted at multiple sites by short noncollagenous sequences, and a globular noncollagenous (NC1) carboxy terminal domain of approximately 230 residues. There are six genetically distinct but highly homologous chains of type IV collagen, designated α1(IV)-α6(IV). The α1(IV) and α2(IV) chains are ubiquitous, but α3(IV)-α6(IV) chains have a tissue-restricted distribution. In the human kidney, the mesangial matrix and proximal tubule basement membrane contain primarily α1/α2(IV), whereas Bowman's capsule contains α5/α6(IV) and the GBM is rich in the α3/α4/α5(IV) chains. Distal tubule collecting duct basement membranes contain all six α(IV) collagen chains.

The genes for α1(IV) and α2(IV), COL4A1 and COL4A2, are located head-to-head on chromosome 13 and share a common promoter. This arrangement is thought to ensure the coordinated expression of the two chains, and, indeed, the ratio of α1(IV):α2(IV) is close to 2:1 in most tissues. The COL4A3/COL4A4 pair of genes is similarly positioned on chromosome 2, and the COL4A5/COL4A6 pair is likewise on the X chromosome. This suggests that the family of α(IV) collagen genes came from an initial duplication and inversion of an ancestral gene, followed by two more duplication events.

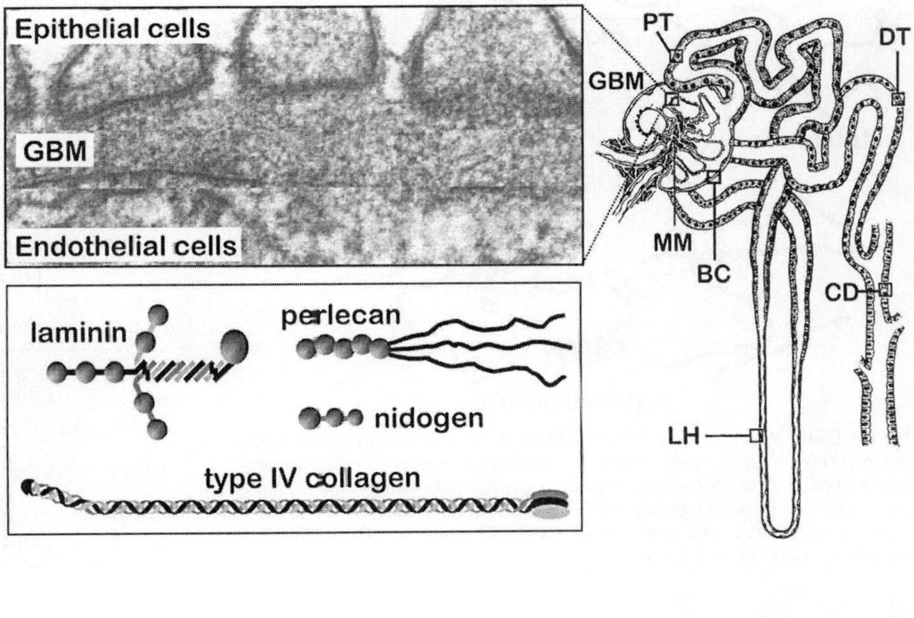

Figure 1.49. **Right:** Localization of basement membranes in the nephron. GBM, glomerular basement membrane; MM, mesangial matrix; BC, Bowman's capsule; PT, proximal tubule; LH, Henle's loop; DT, distal tubule; CD, collecting duct. **Left, top:** The GBM as seen by electron microscopy. **Left, bottom:** The major molecular components of basement membranes.

TABLE 1.1. Distribution of Basement Membrane Components in Human Kidneys

	Type IV Collagen						Laminin				E/N	PG		
	α1	α2	α3	α4	α5	α6	−1	−2	−10	−11		P	A	B
Glomerular basement membrane	+	+	+	+	+					+	+	±	+	
Bowman's capsule	+	+			+	+	+		+		+	+	±	+
Mesangial matrix	+	+					+	+	+		+	+		+
Proximal tubule	+	+					+	±	+		+	+	±	+
Henle's loop	+	+					+	±	+		+	+	±	+
Distal tubule	+	+	±	±	±	±		±	+		+	+	±	+
Collecting duct	+	+	±	±	±	±		±	+		+	+		+

A, agrin; B, bamecan; P, perlecan; PG, proteoglycans.

Molecular Structure

The type IV collagen protomer appears in electron microscopy as a flexible, threadlike structure 400 nm long with a 15-nm globular (NC1) domain. It is formed by intertwining three α chains in a process that starts at the C-terminus and proceeds in a zipperlike fashion toward the N-terminus (Fig. 1.50, *top*). The NC1 domain appears to be important for the proper alignment of the collagenous region. Isolated cysteine residues are widespread throughout the collagenous domain, and they form interchain disulfide bonds to prevent melting of the triple helix. The flexibility of the collagenous domain, resulting from numerous noncollagenous interruptions, is an important structural feature of type IV collagen that distinguishes it from other types of collagen. The repertoire of six α chains allows for 56 protomer isoforms that differ in the type and stoichiometry of chains. However, only a few isoforms, such as [$\alpha1(IV)_2\ \alpha2(IV)$], have been demonstrated to date. There is evidence that chain selection (i.e., the specificity for assembly of triple helical protomers) is a nonrandom process driven by the NC1 domains.

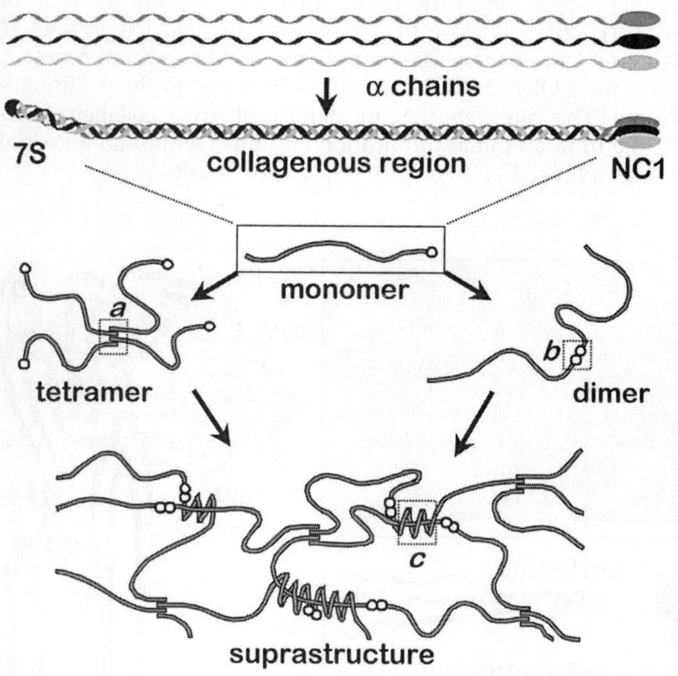

Figure 1.50. Structure of type IV collagen. Three α chains make up a collagen protomer *(top)*. From amino to carboxyl terminus, a collagen protomer consists of a 7S domain, a long, triple helical collagenous domain, and a globular noncollagenous NC1 domain *(middle)*. The protomers associate head-to-head **(A)**, end-to-end **(B)**, and laterally **(C)** to form a supramolecular network *(bottom)*.

The type IV collagen protomers self-associate to form an irregular polygonal network that is the structural backbone of basement membranes. Three different types of supramolecular interactions can be distinguished (Fig 1.50, *bottom*): tetramerization at the amino terminus, dimerization at the carboxyl terminus (through the NC1 domains), and lateral associations between the triple helical and NC1 domains. The interactions at the amino termini are stabilized by intramolecular and intermolecular disulfide bonds to form a collagenase resistant 7S region. Dimerization at the carboxyl terminus produces a hexamer of NC1 domains (three from each protomer) that may be further stabilized by disulfide exchange between subunits. The extent of disulfide cross-linking of the NC1 domains varies with the tissue, being low (less than 10%) in the lens capsule but relatively high (approximately 75%) in the GBM.

Like chain selection, the specificity of end-to-end associations also appears to reside in the NC1 domains. Because of these discriminatory molecular interactions, type IV collagen can form networks with distinct chain composition and properties. At least two different networks have been demonstrated in the GBM: one formed by α1/2(IV) chains and another containing predominantly by α3-5(IV) chains. The latter network is missing in Alport syndrome. Unlike the α1/2(IV) network, the α3-5(IV) network features interprotomer disulfide crosslinks that produce loops and supercoiling of the triple helices and is more resistant to digestion with proteases.

Function and Disease

Self-association of the flexible type IV collagen protomers at both ends of the molecule followed by covalent cross-linking produces a strong but resilient chicken wire–like network. This network forms the scaffolding of the basement membrane, conferring it mechanical strength, supporting its other component molecules, and providing a substrate for cell attachment. The importance of type IV collagen for proper kidney structure and function is well illustrated in several kidney diseases, including Alport syndrome, Goodpasture syndrome, and diabetic nephropathy (Table 1.2).

TABLE 1.2. Type IV Collagen Genes, Their Chromosomal Location, and Associated Diseases

α Chain	Gene	Location	Disease
α1(IV)	COL4A1	13q34	None (probably lethal)
α2(IV)	COL4A2	13q34	None (probably lethal)
α3(IV)	COL4A3	2q35-37	Autosomal-recessive Alport Goodpasture autoantigen
α4(IV)	COL4A4	2q35-37	Autosomal-recessive Alport Benign familial hematuria
α5(IV)	COL4A5	Xq22	X-linked Alport syndrome
α6(IV)	COL4A6	Xq22	Diffuse leiomyomatosis

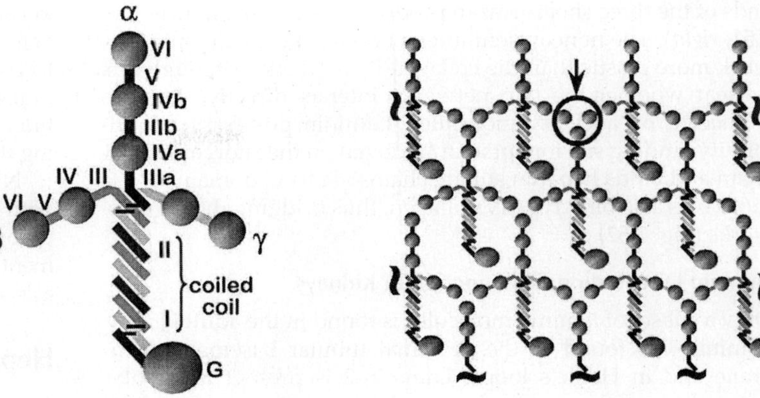

Figure 1.51. Structure of laminin. Laminin is an αβγ heterotrimer consisting of three globular short arms and a long arm **(left).** The domain structure of α and β chains is shown; γ chain is similar to β chain. In the presence of calcium, laminin polymerizes to form a network in which all three short arms interact with one another **(right).**

Alport syndrome is a hereditary progressive form of glomerulonephritis characterized by hematuria, hearing loss, and ocular lesions. Ultrastructurally, the GBM is thickened and split irregularly. The autosomal form of the disease is caused by mutations in COL4A3 and COL4A4 genes. The more common X-linked form affects primarily males and is caused by mutations in the COL4A5 gene. More than 200 different mutations in COL4A5 genes have been identified to date, including point mutations, deletions, insertions, duplications, and transpositions. Although the severity of disease and the pattern of organ involvement vary among patients, no correlation has been found so far between the Alport phenotype and the type of mutation, and "hot spots" have not been identified in the COL4A5 gene. Interestingly, a defect in *any* of the α3, α4, or α5(IV) collagen chains prevents the accumulation of *all* three chains in the GBM. This indicates that the synthesis, secretion, and/or assembly of these chains are coordinated, which is consistent with the existence of a separate α3-5(IV) collagen network. Despite containing only the α1/2(IV) collagen chains, the GBM from Alport patients is structurally and functionally normal for a while but then becomes gradually damaged, presumably because of its higher sensitivity to proteases. Detailed discussion of Alport syndrome is found in Chapter 43.2.

Goodpasture syndrome (also known as anti–basement membrane disease or pulmonary-renal syndrome) is an autoimmune disorder characterized by circulating anti–basement membrane autoantibodies, pulmonary hemorrhage, and rapidly progressive glomerulonephritis leading to renal failure and end-stage renal disease. Although relatively rare, the disease is important because it takes a fatal course unless diagnosed early and treated promptly. The primary autoantigen, shared by all patients, has been identified as the NC1 domain of the α3(IV) chain. The epitopes for Goodpasture autoantibodies are predominantly conformational and have been mapped to two short amino acid sequences within the α3(IV) NC1 domain. The Goodpasture epitope is sequestered within the NC1 hexamer, being reversibly exposed upon dissociation of subunits under denaturing conditions. Unmasking of the auto-epitope *in vivo* from its immunologically privileged site is believed to precede the onset of the disease. Detailed discussion of Goodpasture syndrome is found in Chapter 42.6.

A related condition afflicts 5% to 10% of Alport patients after kidney transplantation because of the production of antibasement membrane alloantibodies to the NC1 domain of the α3(IV) and α5(IV) collagen chains. Goodpasture disease has been experimentally induced in animals (rats, mice, rabbits, and sheep) by passive transfer of autoantibodies or by immunization with purified Goodpasture antigen.

Laminin

Molecular Structure

Laminin is the major noncollagenous component of basement membranes. Each molecule is a 600- to 800-kD heterotrimer consisting of α, β, and γ chains (formerly known as A, B1, and B2 chains, respectively). In electron microscopy laminin looks like a cross-shaped molecule with three short (35 to 50 nm) arms and a long (75 nm) arm. The short arms represent the N-termini of the α, β, and γ chains and consist of two (β and α chains) or three (α chain) globular domains connected by flexible rodlike segments. The long arm is a coiled-coil structure formed by the three chains and stabilized at its ends by disulfide bonds. The longer α chain also has a globular G domain at the C-terminus (Fig. 1.51, *left*).

There are five genetically distinct isoforms of α chains (α1-α5), three isoforms of β-chains (β1-β3), and two isoforms of γ chains (γ1,γ2). Thus, 30 different types of laminin are theoretically possible. However, only 11 have been identified to date. Under a new nomenclature system, laminin trimers are numbered sequentially in the order they were discovered (Table 1.3). Notably, β3 and γ2 chains are found (along with α3 chain) only in one trimer, laminin-5. Mutations in any of the chains comprising laminin-5 lead to Herlitz's junctional epidermolysis bullosa, a skin blistering disease.

In the presence of calcium ions and above 30°C, laminin polymerizes reversibly in a concentration-dependent manner. Laminin is probably secreted as trimers that self-associate in the extracellular space, which contains much higher concentrations of calcium. The current three-arms model for laminin self-assembly, consistent with electron microscopy and biochemical data, involves interactions between the globular domains at the

TABLE 1.3. Nomenclature of Laminin Trimers

Chains		α1	α2	α3	α4	α5
γ1	β1	Laminin-1	Laminin-2	Laminin-6	Laminin-8	Laminin-10
	β2	(Laminin-3)	Laminin-4	Laminin-7	Laminin-9	Laminin-11
γ2	β3	—	—	Laminin-5	—	—

Note: Laminin-3 has not been formally identified.

ends of the three short arms to produce a hexagonal lattice (Fig. 1.51, *right*). The noncovalent interactions make the laminin network more plastic than the collagen IV network. Although it is unclear whether the two networks interact directly, they are connected by ancillary molecules. Laminin possesses a high-affinity binding site for entactin/nidogen on the short arm of γ1 chain and binds heparan sulfate chains via its G domain. These molecules also bind type IV collagen, thus bridging the two networks (Fig. 1.52).

Laminin Distribution and Function in Kidneys

Only a subset of laminin molecules is found in the adult kidney. Laminin-1 is found in the proximal tubular basement membrane and in Henle's loops. Laminin-2 is present in tubular basement membranes and mesangial matrix. Laminin-5 is found in the epithelial basement membrane of the papilla. Laminin-10 is abundant in tubular and collecting duct basement membranes. Laminin-11, the only β2-containing laminin in the kidney, is restricted to the GBM.

Most knowledge about the specific function of laminins in the kidney comes from animal models. Only laminin-11 has been demonstrated to be important for renal function. Mice lacking β2 exhibit massive proteinuria at one week after birth and die at around 4 weeks of age, despite substitution of β2 chain by β1. Laminin-1 plays a role in kidney development since antibodies to laminin α1 chain inhibit the mesenchyme to epithelium transition. The role laminin-10 plays in the kidneys is more difficult to assess since mice with a defective α5 gene (thus lacking both laminin-10 and laminin-11) die *in utero* with multiple defects. Last, laminin-2 does not appear to be important for normal kidney development and function since patients with merosin-deficient congenital muscular dystrophy, a disease caused by mutations in the laminin α2 gene, have normal kidneys.

Entactin/Nidogen

Nidogen, also known as entactin, is a ubiquitous component of basement membranes. It is a dumbbell-shaped molecule approximately 30 nm long. It is a sulfated glycoprotein of about 150 kD, composed of three globular domains (G1 to G3) connected by linker segments (Fig. 1.49). Nidogen forms a tight complex with laminin. The interaction involves the G3 domain of nidogen and the short arm of the laminin γ1 chain, and consequently, all known laminins except laminin-5 should bind to nidogen. Nidogen also binds to type IV collagen and the core protein of perlecan via its G2 domain, as well as to cellular receptors. Thus, nidogen plays a central role in the architecture of basement membranes by interacting with all its components and interconnecting the type IV collagen and laminin networks (Fig. 1.52).

Nidogen-2/entactin-2 has been identified as a 200-kD protein with 46% homology to nidogen-1. It was found to colocalize with nidogen-1 in most basement membranes, including renal basement membranes. Nidogen-2 binds type IV collagen and perlecan as strongly as nidogen-1 but has lower affinity for laminin-1.

Heparan Sulfate Proteoglycans

Proteoglycans consist of a protein core to which one or more glycosaminoglycan chains are covalently attached. In basement membranes, heparan sulfate proteoglycans (HSPGs) are predominant. The overall properties of HSPGs are conferred by the heparan sulfate chains, which are long, linear sulfated copolymers of glucosamine and glucuronic or iduronic acid. The negatively charged heparan sulfate brings a major contribution to the charge selective permeability of basement membranes by repelling anionic proteins because the removal of the glycosaminoglycan chains increases the permeability of the GBM. The heparan sulfate chains bind numerous ligands, largely by electrostatic interactions that are sensitive to the local charge density but less influenced by the primary sequence. Interaction of proteoglycans with other basement membrane components may contribute to the stabilization of the supramolecular network, whereas their binding to cellular receptors further anchors the cells to the matrix. Heparan sulfate chains also bind tightly various soluble proteins, including growth factors and cytokines (acidic and basic fibroblast growth factors, interleukin-3, and interferon-γ), serum proteins (fibronectin), and enzymes. Basement membrane proteoglycans may act as a reservoir of growth factors, which are trapped, protected from degradation, and slowly released to cells in a controlled fashion.

The best-characterized basement membrane proteoglycan is perlecan. Its core protein (molecular weight approximately 400 to 470 kD) consists of five domains, which resemble a string of beads approximately 80 nm long (Fig 1.49). Up to three heparan sulfate chains may be attached to the N-terminal domain, and in some tissues, these may be substituted by chondroitin sulfate chains. The core protein binds entactin/nidogen and is in-

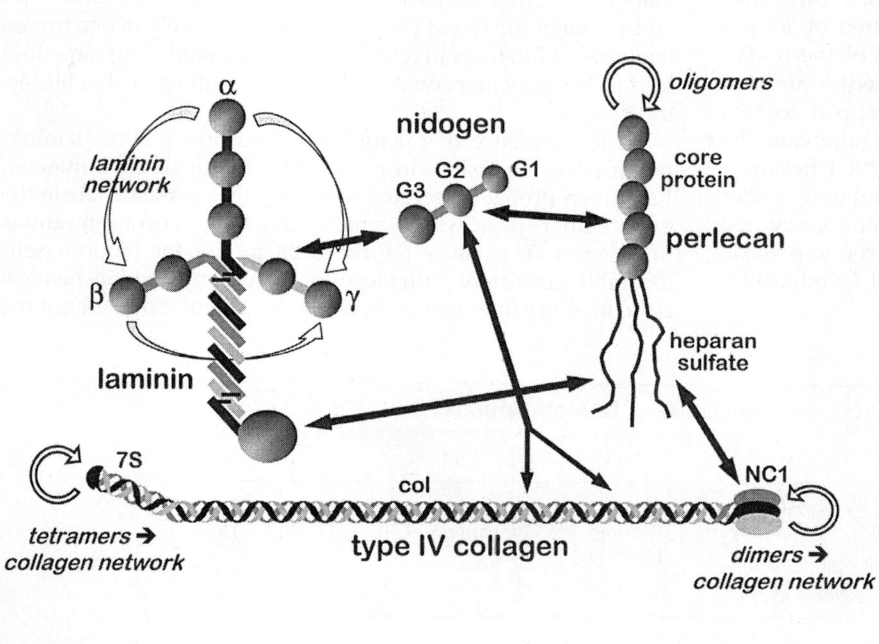

Figure 1.52. Interactions between basement membrane components. The white arrows indicate self-association. The solid arrows point to the domains involved in heterologous interactions.

volved in the formation of oligomers (dimers, trimers, and tetramers). The heparan sulfate chains bind laminin, type IV collagen, and cell surface receptors. Perlecan is found throughout the nephron basement membranes except the GBM, where it is restricted to the subendothelial aspect.

Agrin is a 220-kD heparan sulfate proteoglycan with a tissue-restricted distribution. Its distribution in the nephron is complementary to that of perlecan, being abundant in the GBM. In the tubular basement membranes, it exists mostly in a truncated form lacking the C-terminus. Agrin binds both laminin and α-dystroglycan and thus may function as a cell-matrix linker. The only agrin function demonstrated to date is clustering the acetylcholine receptors in the neuromuscular junction. Mice with a mutation in agrin gene die at birth because of lack of neuromuscular transmission. As the major heparan sulfate proteoglycan in the GBM, agrin may play a role in ultrafiltration due to its negative charge.

Type XVIII collagen is the first type of collagen found to harbor heparan sulfate proteoglycan side chains. It is widespread in basement membranes, including those in the kidney. Its NC1 domain is identical to endostatin, an angiogenesis inhibitor.

Bamacan is a basement membrane–associated chondroitin sulfate proteoglycan. In kidneys, its distribution pattern is similar to that of perlecan, being found in all basement membranes except the GBM.

INTERACTION WITH CELLS

All basement membrane components are produced by the neighboring cells and secreted into the extracellular space as protomers, which self-assemble into supramolecular structures in a process driven by the law of mass action. The basic information needed to assemble a basement membrane is encoded in the structure of its building blocks, which produce a basement membrane–like gel *in vitro* under certain experimental conditions. The interactions between the various components described above are summarized in Fig. 1.52. The structural complexity of native basement membranes is increased by spatial and temporal variations in the type and amount of the isoforms produced and by cell receptors, which provide nucleation centers for matrix assembly.

Integrins occupy a prominent place among cellular receptors for basement membrane components. They consist of two transmembrane chains associated noncovalently. Integrins α1β1, α2β1, and α3βv bind type IV collagen. Integrin α6β1 is the high-affinity laminin receptor, binding to the G domain of laminin trimers. Other integrins, such as α1β1 and α2β1, are specific for certain laminin isoforms. Additional cell–matrix interactions include those between laminin and sulfated glycolipids, agrin and α-dystroglycan, and perlecan and selectins.

Besides providing mechanical support, basement membranes can modulate the phenotype of neighboring cells. These effects are generally mediated by integrins, whose cytoplasmic tail connects to intracellular signaling pathways. Basement membranes influence cell polarity, shape, differentiation, migration, and so on. The activity of extracellular signaling molecules is also modulated by basement membrane components; for instance, heparan sulfate chains act as a reservoir of basic FGF.

BASEMENT MEMBRANE DYNAMICS

Although basement membrane components have a low turnover rate and are relatively long lived, there is a dynamic equilibrium between degradation of old chains and synthesis of new chains. Degradation is performed by specialized matrix metalloproteinases (MMPs), whose activity is kept in check by tissue inhibitors of metalloproteinases (TIMPs). Other proteases such as plasmin, cathepsins, and neutrophil elastase may also play a role in basement membrane degradation under certain circumstances. For instance, in inflammation and metastasis, activated immune cells or tumor cells secrete matrix-degrading proteases to bore their way through the basement membrane, which otherwise prevents the passage of cells. After passage of these cells, the basement membrane seals itself.

Basement membrane dynamics are an important part of kidney development. Kidney development involves mesenchyme to epithelium transformations and complex morphologic changes. Coincident with these morphologic changes are molecular transitions in the basement membrane components that are found in various parts of the developing nephron. Changes in the developing GBM's composition, in terms of laminin and type IV collagen isoforms that are deposited there, demonstrate these morphologic changes best. At the S-shaped stage of nephrogenesis, the future GBM contains the α1 and α2 chains of collagen IV and laminins 1, 8, and 10. At the capillary loop stage, the laminin β2 chain appears, probably as part of laminin-11. As the glomerular capillaries are maturing, the collagen α3-5(IV) chains begin to be deposited into the GBM and form a network separate from that composed of α1/α2(IV) chains. The α1/2(IV) network becomes confined to the subendothelial aspect of the GBM. Laminin-11 continues to be deposited into the GBM, and the other laminins are gradually eliminated by an unknown mechanism.

In Alport syndrome, mutations in any of the COL4A3, COL4A4, or COL4A5 genes prevent the developmental switch from the fetal α1/2(IV) chains to the mature α3-5(IV) collagen network. The following two animal models of Alport syndrome have been instrumental in learning the molecular basis of Alport syndrome: a COL4A3 gene knockout mouse and a dog strain harboring a nonsense COL4A5 mutation. The affected GBMs retain the α1 and α2(IV) chains throughout the width of the GBM. However, although these chains function properly initially, they eventually fail to maintain proper structure and function of the GBM, leading to a delayed onset of glomerulonephritis. This indicates that the α1/2(IV) network is important during the development of the glomerulus, whereas the α3-5(IV) network is important long term.

Likewise, laminin transitions that occur in the developing GBM have been experimentally prevented by mutating the laminin β2 chain gene in mice. These mice retain β1-containing laminins in their GBMs. Although these GBMs appear ultrastructurally normal, they do not function properly; these mice exhibit severe proteinuria by 1 week of age and die by 4 weeks of age. These results show that laminin β2 has an important role for which the β1 chain cannot compensate.

Selected Readings

Groffen AJ, Ruegg MA, Dijkman H, et al. Agrin is a major heparan sulfate proteoglycan in the human glomerular basement membrane. *J Histochem Cytochem* 1998;46:19–27.

A remarkable finding that agrin, not perlecan, is the most abundant HSPG in GBM.

Gunwar S, Ballester F, Noelken ME, et al. Glomerular basement membrane: identification of a novel disulfide-cross-linked network of α3, α4, and α5 chains of type IV collagen and its implications for the pathogenesis of Alport syndrome. *J Biol Chem* 1998;273:8767–8775.

The discovery and characterization of distinct networks of type IV collagen in the GBM.

Harvey SJ, Zheng K, Sado Y, et al. Role of distinct type IV collagen networks in glomerular development and function. *Kidney Int* 1998;54:1857–1866.

Recent work illustrating the role of α3-5(IV) collagen network for glomerular structure and function in an experimental model of Alport syndrome.

Hudson BG, Reeders ST, Tryggvason K. Type IV collagen: structure, gene organization, and role in human diseases. *J Biol Chem* 1993;268:26033–26036.

A review of type IV collagen with focus on the newly discovered α3(IV)-α6(IV) collagen chains and their role in kidney pathology.

Kalluri R, Shield CF, Todd P, et al. Isoform switching of type IV collagen is developmentally arrested in X-linked Alport syndrome leading to increased susceptibility of renal basement membranes to endoproteolysis. *J Clin Invest* 1997;99:2470–2478.

The identification of the developmental switch from α1/2(IV) to α3-5(IV) collagen in humans and its implications for the pathogenesis of Alport syndrome.

Miner JH. Developmental biology of glomerular basement membrane components. *Curr Opin Nephrol Hypertens* 1998;7:13–19.

A review highlighting the distinct compositions of the glomerular basement membrane and its developmental transitions.

Miner JH. Renal basement membrane components. *Kidney Int* 1999; S6: 2016–2024.

A review of the principal basement membrane components and their localization in kidneys.

Miner JH, Patton BL, Lentz SI, et al. The laminin alpha chains: expression, developmental transitions, and chromosomal locations of alpha1-5, identification of heterotrimeric laminins 8-11, and cloning of a novel alpha3 isoform. *J Cell Biol* 1997;137:685–701.

A study of the distribution of laminin α chains in the developing and adult kidney and identification of novel laminin heterotrimers.

Timpl R, Brown JC. Supramolecular assembly of basement membranes. *Bio Essays* 1996;18:123–132.

A good introduction to basement membrane components and their interactions.

Tryggvason K. Mutations in type IV collagen genes and Alport phenotypes. *Contrib Nephrol* 1996;117:154–171.

An overview of mutations linked to Alport syndrome.

Yurchenco PD, O'Rear JJ. Basal lamina assembly. *Curr Opin Cell Biol* 1994;6:674–681.

A review of the basement membrane structure and assembly.

CHAPTER 2

The Renal Circulation

Richard V. Paul and David W. Ploth

The renal circulation is anatomically and functionally unique. Its organization and regulation are highly specialized to meet the organism's need to eliminate large quantities of metabolic wastes while conserving vital constituents of the body fluids. Although much has been learned after several decades of research, the renal circulation remains an active focus of investigation in nephrology. Interest has been sustained by the unusually direct connection between bench research and clinical medicine in this field.

Many techniques have been used in the investigation of renal hemodynamics. Classical whole-organ clearance techniques, the isolated perfused kidney, and renal micropuncture have been available for decades and are still being successfully applied to study the effects of newly discovered vasoactive mediators and pharmacologic compounds. Newer techniques that permit direct observation of functioning renal microvasculature (Figs. 2.1 and 2.2), along with studies of cultured smooth muscle and endothelial cells, have been responsible for most of the more recent advances in the normal physiology of the renal circulation. The ongoing revolution in molecular biology also has contributed heavily to current knowledge in the area. The accelerating pace of cloning of ion channels, receptors, and other regulatory molecules continues to produce unprecedented insights into their functions.

One defining characteristic of kidney circulation is the low resistance and high flow relative to other major organs. Renal structures contain less than 0.5% of the adult body weight yet normally receive approximately 20% of the cardiac output. Because disturbances in renal hemodynamics invariably manifest as disturbances in renal function, the maintenance of normal body fluid homeostasis requires flexible, capable mechanisms to direct and regulate the torrent of renal circulation. After covering the important anatomic relationships, this chapter reviews the current knowledge of these normal mechanisms. This chapter also addresses the influences of the major known local and systemic humoral mediators on renal vascular function. In addition, this chapter highlights those aspects of renal circulatory regulation that remain incompletely understood or controversial. Last, the renal hemodynamic effects, desirable and undesirable, of some therapeutic agents are considered.

VASCULAR ANATOMY OF THE KIDNEY

Major Renal Arteries

Functional renal tissue is supplied by main renal arteries, most commonly one to each kidney, which branch from the abdominal aorta. In most cases, the renal arteries divide into posterior and anterior main branches just before entering the renal hilus. Classically, the anterior branch immediately subdivides into segmental branches. Although many normal variants of this structure exist, the main and segmental renal arteries are always functional end arteries, therefore having no anastomotic connections between them. As a result, sudden occlusion of a main or segmental artery invariably leads to infarction of tissue. In occasional cases of gradually progressive arterial obstruction, collateral circulation can develop, for example from an adrenal vessel to maintain viability, if not function, of some of the downstream renal mass. The anteroposterior division of the renal circulation was considered to give rise to Brödel's line, a relatively bloodless sagittal plane along the posterolateral margin of the kidney. In fact, individual anatomic variability may obviate any consistent advantage to the urologic surgeon in using this approach to remove tumors or staghorn calculi.

Interlobar arteries arise from the segmental branches and course along the columns of Bertin between the renal pyramids. Branches of the interlobar arteries that curve to follow the corticomedullary junction are known as arcuate arteries. The location of the arcuate arteries dictates the preference of the nephrologist to avoid crossing the corticomedullary junction with a biopsy needle. Interlobular arteries branch from the arcuate arteries and through the cortex toward the renal capsule, creating afferent arterioles and their glomeruli at all levels of the cortex. Occasional interlobular branches have been observed to empty directly into medullary vessels, but most medullary blood flow comes from the cortical (postglomerular) circulation.

Glomerular Circulation

Glomerular capillaries are unique among the capillaries of the body because they have variable resistance elements (i.e., the afferent and efferent arterioles) at both ends. The long, narrow,

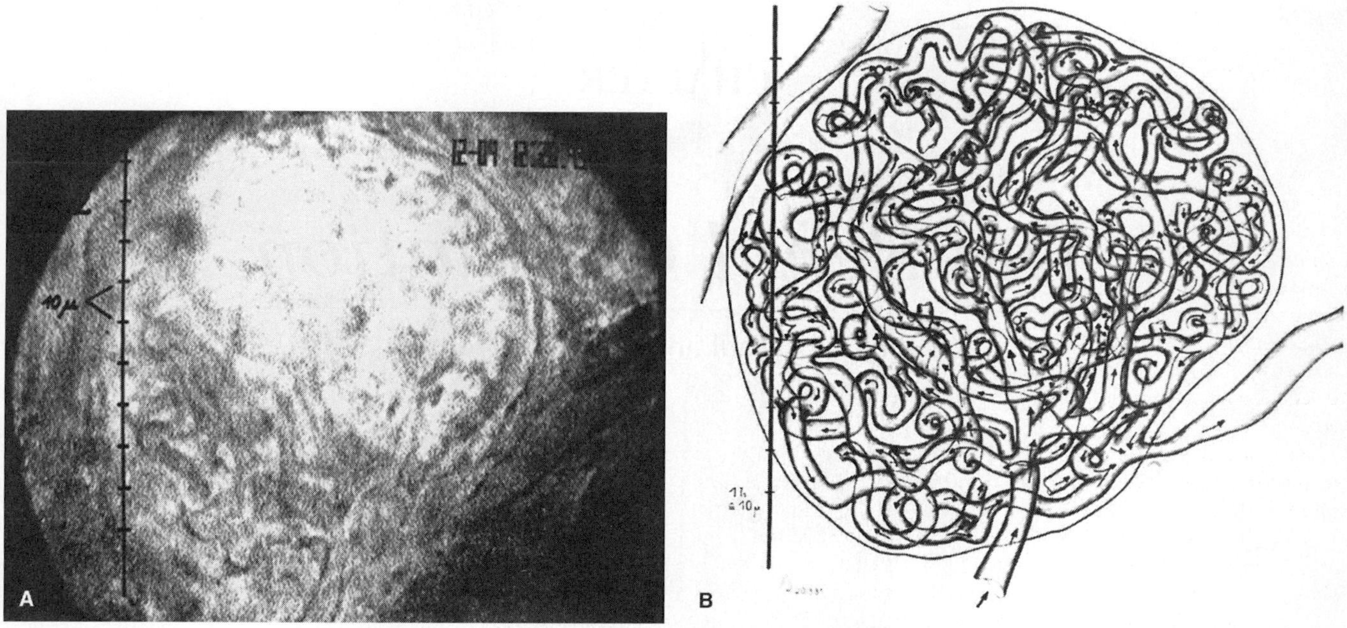

Figure 2.1. **A:** Video image of functioning glomerulus *in vivo* revealed by the split hydronephrotic kidney preparation described by Steinhausen et al. (*Kidney Int* 1983;23:794–806.) **B:** Analysis of video information obtained by following the paths of red blood cells as the plane of focus is moved up and down through the glomerulus reveals the complexity of the flow. This painstaking analysis demonstrates the degree of oversimplification that may be involved in the currently available mathematic models of glomerular ultrafiltration, which consider flow to occur along a single dimension.

afferent arteriole provides the primary regulatory site of the composite preglomerular resistance. Upon entering Bowman's capsule, the arteriole abruptly divides into numerous capillaries, whose much larger total luminal diameter provides minimal impediment to flow.

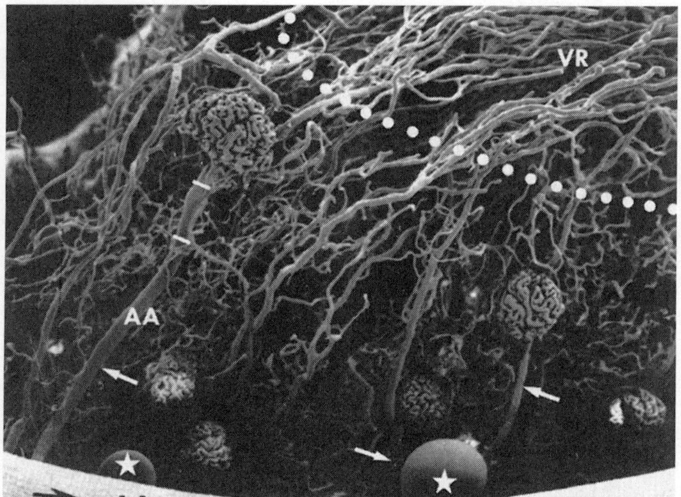

Figure 2.2. Investigator's view of the isolated perfused juxtaglomerular nephron preparation described by Casellas and Navar (*Am J Physiol* 1984;246:F349.) Vascular structures have been filled with resin for this photograph; the *stars* label resin droplets that have escaped the vascular compartment. The *large, dark arrow* indicates the direction of flow in the arcuate artery *(ArA)*. The *dotted line* represents the corticomedullary junction, where postglomerular vessels form the bundles of vasa recta *(VR)*. Several afferent arterioles *(AA)* are seen perfusing their respective glomeruli; the light arrows indicate afferent arterioles that branch directly from the arcuate artery at the bottom of the picture. This anatomic relationship is unusual in other regions of the renal cortex. The arteriolar segment between the dashes is the terminal segment of the afferent arteriole, the primary site of autoregulatory-resistance adjustments.

As the afferent arteriole enters the glomerulus, surrounded by the extraglomerular mesangial cells of the juxtaglomerular apparatus, it uniformly passes in close apposition to the thick ascending limb of the Henle's loop of the same nephron. At this point and immediately upstream, many of the smooth muscle cells have lost their contractile apparatus and have acquired secretory granules, which contain renin. The site of contact between the thick ascending limb and the juxtaglomerular apparatus is characterized by a morphologically distinctive patch of tubular epithelium known as the macula densa. This site is the anatomic substrate for the functional connection between distal tubular fluid composition, afferent arteriolar tone, and renin release.

The treelike structure of the mesangium provides structural support for the glomerulus. In addition to anchoring glomerular capillary loops, the contractile cells of the mesangium may also provide some of the functional postglomerular resistance. Blood proceeds through the glomerulus from the vascular pole toward Bowman's capsule, then back toward the vascular pole through the mesangium to coalesce abruptly into an efferent arteriole.

Efferent arterioles generally are much shorter than afferent arterioles. However, they also provide a significant resistance element because they narrow to a smaller diameter than corresponding afferent arterioles after leaving the immediate vicinity of the glomerulus. The outlet of efferent arterioles varies, depending on their location within the cortex. Outer cortical efferent arterioles branch quickly into myriad peritubular capillaries, which often rise to supply the proximal convoluted tubules of the same or neighboring nephrons. Midcortical efferent arterioles either descend or ascend before dividing into anastomotic peritubular capillary networks that supply the tubules of many nephrons, particularly in the medullary rays. Inner cortical efferent arterioles may descend to the corticomedullary junction to form the vascular bundles and capillary networks of the outer medulla and, ultimately, the descending vasa recta.

Medullary Circulation

The organization of the medullary circulation differs greatly from that of the cortex, reflecting divergent functional requirements. Blood flow to the cortex must be exuberant to provide a high rate of glomerular filtration, whereas blood flow to the inner medulla must be restricted to avoid dissipation of the solute gradients that enable urinary concentration. However, the descending proximal straight tubules and thick ascending limbs of Henle's loop in the outer medulla have considerable requirements for metabolic substrates to fuel active transport functions. Therefore capillary networks arise from the outer medullary vascular bundles to supply these structures. Their blood supply is collected into venous channels that rise toward the corticomedullary junction without entering the inner medulla.

The specific measurement of medullary blood flow is fraught with technical difficulties, but estimates converge on a total medullary flow that is approximately 10% to 15% of cortical blood flow. Most of this is restricted to the outer medulla. Outer medullary blood flow, expressed as mL/min/g tissue weight, is still higher than blood flow of most extrarenal organs.

The vascular bundles of the outer medulla separately give rise to the vasa recta, unbranched capillarylike vessels that course toward the papillary tip, only to make hairpin turns and rise back toward the outer medulla. The side-by-side arrangement of the blood supply and drainage of the inner medulla enables countercurrent exchange, an adaptation that permits the maintenance of an osmotic gradient across the medulla for urinary concentration. Nevertheless, vasodilator administration, which results in diversion of a higher-than-usual blood supply to the inner medulla, can dissipate the gradient and result in diuresis.

Renal Veins

Unlike their arterial counterparts, frequent anastomosis occurs between renal veins at various levels. In small animals such as rodents, the renal venous drainage from the cortex and medulla tends to congregate in arcuate-level vessels at the corticomedullary junction. Larger animals such as humans possess subcapsular venous networks that ultimately drain the cortex through the medullary rays toward the hilus. In most people, a single renal vein returns blood from each kidney into the inferior vena cava; however, renal vein obstruction, unless it occurs very abruptly, seldom causes infarction because of potential alternative drainage through other routes.

INTRINSIC CONTROL MECHANISMS OF THE RENAL VASCULATURE

Signal Transduction of Smooth Muscle Cell Contraction

The slow, long-lived contraction of circumferentially oriented smooth muscle in the vascular wall controls segmental vascular resistance. This is the final effector pathway for the myriad influences that regulate glomerular filtration and the distribution of blood flow to the kidney versus other organs. Glomerular mesangial cells possess contractile filaments and other phenotypic similarities to vascular smooth muscle cells, and their contraction is thought to be regulated in a similar manner.

In keeping with the need for rapid contraction and relaxation, skeletal and cardiac muscles are activated by direct interaction of intracellular calcium with the contractile apparatus. Smooth muscle contraction also responds to intracellular calcium flux, but in contrast to striated muscle, the use of intermediary signaling molecules ensures slower activation and deactivation of contraction (Fig. 2.3). In smooth muscle cells, free intracellular calcium exerts its downstream signaling effects through a specific binding protein, calmodulin. The calcium–calmodulin complex activates myosin light-chain kinase, and it is the phosphorylation of myosin light chain that initiates movement of actin filaments relative to myosin. Free intracellular calcium is the limiting reagent in this process; therefore its availability is the major determinant of smooth muscle cell contractile tone. The resting concentration of free calcium in smooth muscle cell cytoplasm is maintained lower than that of the extracellular fluid by four orders of magnitude through active transport of calcium into both extracellular and intracellular compartments.

Depolarization of the plasma membrane occurs by gating of ions (Na^+, Ca^{2+}, Cl^-) through channels responsive to hormones, second messengers, or mechanical forces. Depolarization causes the opening of voltage-activated calcium channels in the plasma membrane, which leads to calcium influx and cell contraction. Calcium also is released into the cytoplasm from the sarcoplasmic reticulum through the action of second messengers such as inositol trisphosphate or calcium itself. Different vascular segments may have different mechanisms controlling these processes. For example, experiments with calcium channel blockers indicate that vascular tone in afferent arterioles depends largely on calcium entry from the extracellular

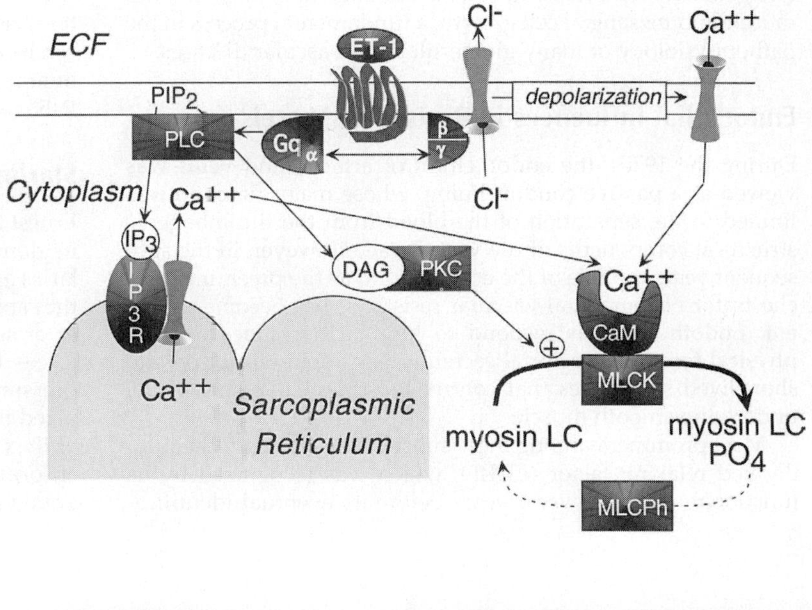

Figure 2.3. Model of some of the signaling cascade leading to smooth muscle contraction in response to endothelin-1. The activated α subunit of the receptor-coupled GTP-binding protein G_q is thought to activate phospholipase C, which hydrolyzes membrane phospholipids to release intermediate signaling molecules as shown. Free β/γ subunits may activate plasma membrane chloride channels to depolarize the membrane. Concerted liberation of Ca^{2+} ions into the cytoplasm from intracellular and extracellular sources activates calmodulin, favoring myosin light-chain phosphorylation. *ET-1,* endothelin-1; *ECF,* extracellular fluid; *GC,* guanylate cyclase; *GTP,* guanosine triphosphate; *CaM,* calmodulin; *IP_3,* inositol 1,4,5-trisphosphate; *PIP_2,* phosphatidylinositol 4,5-biphosphate; *DAG,* diacylglycerol; *PKC,* protein kinase C; *IP_3R,* inositol 1,4,5-trisphosphate receptor; *LC,* light chain; *MLCK,* myosin light-chain kinase; *MLCPh,* myosin light-chain phosphatase.

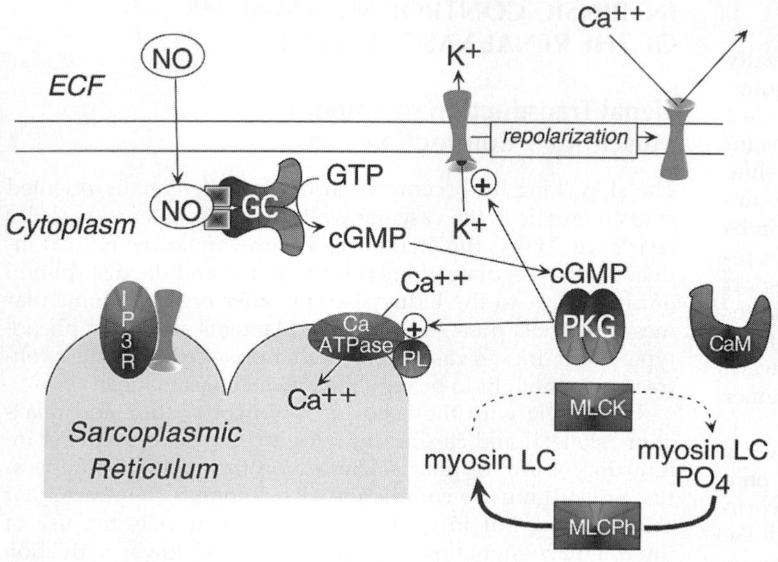

Figure 2.4. Model of the signaling events leading to smooth muscle relaxation after exposure to nitric oxide *(NO)*. Interaction of NO with the soluble guanylate cyclase leads to generation of cGMP. Two intracellular targets of cGMP are shown: the calcium-activated large conductance potassium channel and the cGMP-dependent protein kinase *(PKG)*. One known target of PKG is phospholamban *(PL)*, which, when activated by phosphorylation, promotes active calcium uptake from the cytoplasm into the sarcoplasmic reticulum. Low cytoplasmic calcium leads to low calmodulin activity, which favors myosin light chain dephosphorylation. *NO*, nitric oxide; *ECF*, extracellular fluid; *GC*, guanylate cyclase; *GTP*, guanosine triphosphate; *cGMP*, 3′,5′-guanosine cyclic monophosphate; *PKG*, cGMP-dependent protein kinase; *CaM*, calmodulin; *IP_3R*, inositol 1,4,5-trisphosphate receptor; *LC*, light chain; *MLCK*, myosin light-chain kinase; *MLCPh*, myosin light-chain phosphatase.

fluid, whereas efferent arteriolar tone is controlled mainly by calcium release from intracellular stores.

Contraction is terminated by dissipation of membrane depolarization through the eventual opening of potassium channels. One major class of potassium channels that participates in repolarization is directly responsive to intracellular calcium release. With restoration of resting membrane potential, voltage-gated calcium channels close, calcium is again transported out of the cytoplasm, myosin light chain is dephosphorylated, and relaxation occurs (Fig. 2.4). Opposition between vasoconstrictor and vasodilator influences may be exerted at the level of receptors, ion channels, second messengers, protein phosphorylation, or virtually anywhere else along the signal transduction pathway just outlined.

The major endogenous humoral influences on renal vascular tone are discussed individually, later in this chapter, in terms of their mechanisms of interaction with the signaling of smooth muscle cell contraction. Although this discussion must be confined to the renal vasculature, nearly all of these substances have important interactions with extravascular elements of the kidney as well, often through distinct signaling pathways. In addition, the signals that cause smooth muscle or mesangial cell contraction strongly overlap with those that produce cell growth, either hypertrophy or hyperplasia. Thus vasoconstrictors generally tend to favor, and vasodilators to oppose, smooth muscle and mesangial cell growth, a fundamental process in the pathophysiology of many glomerular and vascular diseases.

Endothelial Influences in Resistance Vessels

During the 1970s, the endothelium of arteries and veins was viewed as a passive conduit lining, whose major function was limited to the separation of the blood from the thrombogenic structural components of the vessel wall. However, in the subsequent years the role of the endothelium as the preeminent orchestrator of segmental vascular resistance has become apparent. Endothelial cells respond to luminal hormones or local physical forces by vectorial secretion of a repertoire of potent, short-lived substances that control the contractile state of the underlying smooth muscle.

Most prominent among these substances is the endothelium-derived relaxing factor (EDRF), which was recognized by its functional activity several years before its eventual identification as nitric oxide (NO). The importance of the discovery and identification of NO as the EDRF was recognized with the 1998 Nobel Prize in Physiology or Medicine. This small, freely diffusible molecular species is synthesized from L-arginine and released immediately as needed. There appears to be a tonic or baseline level of secretion at all times, as indicated by the appearance of increased renal vascular resistance and accelerated hypertension in animal models in which NO synthesis is blocked. NO has an affinity for heme prosthetic groups and a half-life in aqueous solution of approximately 6 seconds. During this brief existence, NO affects vascular tone by diffusing from the endothelium into nearby smooth muscle cells. Hemoglobin immediately captures any NO that escapes into the circulation, thereby limiting its action to paracrine or autocrine modes.

Conversely, endothelium is also the major source of the most potent known vasoconstrictor, the peptide hormone endothelin-1 (ET-1). Because of preferential secretion in the abluminal direction, the actions of ET-1 are thought to be exerted mostly at a paracrine level. The mechanisms of the opposing and interacting vascular effects of NO and ET-1 are discussed in more detail later in this chapter.

In many experimental circumstances, the effects of endothelium-derived vasoactive factors that are neither NO nor endothelins can be observed. Although the nature of these factors has not been completely explained, some of their activities can be abolished by pharmacologic blockade of the metabolism of arachidonic acid through the cyclooxygenase or cytochrome P450 monooxygenase pathways.

Starling Forces in Capillaries

Ernest Starling first articulated the factors controlling filtration in glomerular capillaries and reabsorption in peritubular capillaries approximately 100 years ago. Hydrostatic pressure within the capillary and the oncotic pressure generated by the presence of proteins outside the capillary favor filtration. The opposing forces favoring reabsorption include plasma colloid osmotic pressure and interstitial hydrostatic pressure. Starling recognized that these forces do not remain constant along the length of the capillary and that therefore the rate of net filtration or reabsorption along a given capillary bed depends on the integrated algebraic sum of forces along its length.

Although the principles elucidated by Starling apply to all capillaries, several characteristics quantitatively distinguish the Starling forces acting on renal capillaries from those in all other vascular beds. First, in glomerular capillaries, there is no need to consider interstitial colloid osmotic pressure because of the absence of proteins in Bowman's space under normal conditions. Second, the presence of a downstream resistance element ensures a high capillary hydrostatic pressure. Third, large volume filtration from glomerular capillaries results in a significant increase in plasma colloid osmotic pressure along the length of the capillaries. This increase is aided by the nonlinear relationship between plasma protein concentration and colloid osmotic pressure.

Because the peritubular capillaries are downstream from glomeruli, the initial plasma colloid osmotic pressure in these capillaries is higher than that of any other capillaries in the body. This anatomic arrangement results in a reabsorptive capability of the peritubular capillaries that matches the magnitude of the upstream glomerular filtration.

Autoregulation in the Renal Circulation

Nearly all regions of circulation are characterized by some degree of autoregulation, that is, the capability to maintain constant flow in the face of changes in perfusion pressure. With the possible exception of the brain, the autoregulatory capability of the kidney is superior to that of all other major vascular beds. Because most of the renal blood flow passes through the glomeruli, the exquisite autoregulation of renal blood flow may be conceptualized as a byproduct of the need to maintain the glomerular filtration rate. Without autoregulation, fluctuations in renal perfusion pressure might expose the organism to inadequate clearance function or to failure of sodium and water conservation. Because autoregulatory adjustments in renal blood flow and glomerular filtration rate (GFR) are always exerted in the same direction, the primary autoregulatory-responsive elements must occur at preglomerular sites. Indeed, direct observation of autoregulation in the renal microvasculature *in situ* indicates that the distal afferent arteriole is the primary site of the autoregulatory mechanisms. Efficient autoregulation occurs in the isolated perfused kidney and isolated perfused juxtamedullary nephron preparations, which indicates that all necessary components of autoregulatory mechanisms are intrinsic to the kidney and not dependent on external neurohormonal influences.

The enhanced autoregulatory capability of the kidney likely results from two mutually reinforcing mechanisms of autoregulation: tubuloglomerular feedback, which is unique to the kidney, and the myogenic response, which is present in other tissues.

The tubuloglomerular feedback (TGF) response originates at the macula densa. The phenomenon is activated by an increase in the osmolality and/or chloride concentration of the tubular fluid at the macula densa, which under physiologic conditions is a consequence of a flow increase through Henle's loop. A vasoconstricting mediator, whose nature is still uncertain, is generated in response to the macula densa signal and transmitted to the afferent arteriole, resulting in a lower GFR and diminished flow through the tubule. Ideally, the result is restoration of the fluid at the macula densa to its original composition. It is unclear whether an opposing vasodilatory mediator is released in response to a decrease in distal tubular fluid chloride or osmolality or whether the resulting afferent arteriolar dilation is the consequence of a decrease in vasoconstrictor tone.

The myogenic response refers to an intrinsic capability of the vascular smooth muscle of resistance vessels to contract when stretching forces are increased. The proximate cause of this phenomenon appears to be stretch-induced depolarization of smooth muscle cells through the opening of nonselective cation channels. The depolarization results in calcium entry through voltage-dependent calcium channels and consequent contraction. Although the endothelium may modulate myogenic response, this response is intrinsic to the vascular smooth muscle because it can be demonstrated in deendothelialized vessels. Myogenic responses can propagate for long distances along arterial resistance vessels, partly because arteriolar smooth muscle cells can be linked by gap junctions that presumably allow for the cell-to-cell transmission of electrical and/or calcium signaling.

These two component mechanisms of renal autoregulation can be separated to some extent by their time course. The myogenic response is complete within seconds, whereas the response time of TGF is limited by the transit time of fluid through Henle's loop. Frequency-domain analysis of renal autoregulatory responses has demonstrated both fast and slow components that presumably correspond to these two mechanisms. Mathematic modeling also indicates that the fine accuracy of autoregulation results from synergy between TGF and the myogenic response. For example, TGF-mediated constriction of terminal afferent arteriolar segments can lead to elevated transmural pressure of upstream segments, thereby eliciting a myogenic response. Although autoregulatory capability is a property of each individual nephron, some cooperation between adjacent nephrons also may contribute to whole-kidney autoregulatory efficiency. Coupling between autoregulatory responses of nephrons perfused by a common interlobular artery can be demonstrated experimentally. Arterial branch points appear to have a high density of calcium channels and may be initiating points for the myogenic response to propagate down both branches. It is also possible that soluble mediators or modulators of TGF responses not only can affect the nephron of origin but also can diffuse far enough to affect the function of neighboring nephrons.

Research into the mechanisms by which the macula densa transmits the signal that elicits TGF has been hampered by difficulty in distinguishing mediators of the response from substances that merely affect its sensitivity. The initial step in TGF, detection of the tubular fluid composition, depends largely on the Na-K-2 Cl cotransporter because loop diuretics, such as furosemide, that inhibit this transporter also inhibit TGF. Chloride concentration in the distal tubular fluid appears to be the rate-limiting component for the activity of this transporter. Distal tubular fluid osmolality also may be an important signal to elicit the TGF response. The macula densa is the only part of the thick ascending limb of Henle's loop, which is permeable to water.

Angiotensin II might be considered a logical candidate for the vasoconstrictor mediator of TGF. However, when pharmacologic tools to manipulate the renin-angiotensin system became available, it quickly became clear that TGF still occurs in the presence of angiotensin II–receptor blockers or converting enzyme inhibitors, albeit at reduced sensitivity and intensity. Vasoconstrictor arachidonate metabolites such as thromboxane A_2 appear to exert similar effects as those of angiotensin II. In fact, the release of thromboxane A_2 may contribute to the effects of angiotensin II on TGF. Adenosine also has been proposed as a possible TGF mediator, partly because increased metabolic work of active transport by macula densa cells would result in increased adenosine release as a byproduct of adenosine triphosphate (ATP) consumption. The renal hemodynamic effects of adenosine and related purinergic compounds are complex; vasodilation and vasoconstriction can both be observed, depending on receptor subtype, distribution, and the presence or absence of endothelium. Specific pharmacologic desensitization of P_2 purinergic receptors, which respond to ATP much better than to adenosine itself, completely abolishes autoregulatory responses in directly visualized afferent arterioles. However, appropriate physiologic modulation of local nucleotide release, which would be a necessary attribute of any putative mediator of TGF, has yet to be demonstrated at the time of this writing.

Another observation of potential interest is the macula densa's dense immunostaining for a nitric oxide synthase (NOS) isoform. This gene is expressed at much lower levels in the other cells of the thick ascending limb and medullary collecting duct and is not significantly expressed in other renal cells. This NOS isoform is known as the neuronal NOS because it is also highly expressed in the cerebellum. The role of NO in TGF is unclear. Initial studies suggest that NOS inhibitors increase the sensitivity of TGF responses, whereas NO donors mitigate but do not abolish TGF-mediated vasoconstriction. Autoregulation persists in the presence of either NO donors or NOS inhibitors. However, NO may play a much larger role in the macula densa regulation of renin release because the effect of a low-salt diet to stimulate renin can be nearly abolished by chronic NOS inhibition.

Medullary Circulation and Pressure Natriuresis

The tendency of the kidney to increase sodium excretion when perfusion pressure is increased is known as pressure natriuresis. This phenomenon is seen in the isolated perfused kidney, indicating that its mechanism is intrinsic to the kidney. Numerous experimental animal and computer-modeling studies have shown pressure natriuresis as a mechanism of primary importance for controlling blood pressure and extracellular volume. Despite its critical physiologic role, much remains to be learned about the mechanism of pressure natriuresis.

Others have emphasized the role of the medullary circulation in pressure natriuresis. Their studies on rats have used acutely or chronically implanted miniature devices to demonstrate increased blood flow and interstitial hydrostatic pressure in the inner medulla when renal perfusion pressure is increased. This mechanism requires the autoregulation of inner medullary blood flow to be less efficient than the autoregulation of cortical blood flow. Because most medullary blood flow is postglomerular and glomerular blood flow to both superficial and deep nephrons is efficiently autoregulated, it has been difficult to envision how changes in renal perfusion pressure are transmitted to the medulla. Indeed, studies of dogs indicate that medullary blood flow is autoregulated as efficiently as in that of the cortex. These results have been confirmed at the microvascular level in the isolated perfused rat juxtaglomerular nephron preparation.

As noted previously, careful anatomic studies demonstrate occasional direct shunts between the interlobular arteries and the medullary circulation. It is possible that these bypass pathways transmit some portion of a change in systemic arterial pressure to the medullary circulation. Exactly how these relatively small increases in medullary blood flow and interstitial hydrostatic pressure could influence tubular sodium reabsorption has yet to be determined. Another possibility is that blood is diverted from outer medullary capillary networks to the inner medulla during periods of increased perfusion pressure, although no mechanism for sensing and initiating this diversion has been identified. Alternatively, some investigators have hypothesized that a soluble mediator, such as NO, could inhibit medullary tubular sodium transport in response to increased perfusion pressure.

HUMORAL REGULATION OF RENAL BLOOD FLOW

Maintenance of a steady state often is required of the renal circulation; however, various endogenous and exogenous vasoactive mediators can affect kidney function in appropriate or inappropriate directions by perturbing segmental or global vascular tone. In this section, we briefly review the mechanisms of action of the major hormones and autocoids that affect the renal vasculature.

Nitric Oxide

NO is short lived but freely diffusible. Within the smooth muscle cells, NO binds to the heme-containing enzyme soluble guanylate cyclase, leading to generation of the vasodilating second messenger guanosine 3′, 5′-cyclic monophosphate (cGMP). cGMP relaxes smooth muscle by increasing plasma membrane–potassium conductance and stimulating calcium uptake or extrusion from the cytoplasm. These effects are produced through concerted interactions of cGMP with several different smooth muscle and mesangial cell proteins, including ion channels, phosphodiesterases, and the type I cGMP-dependent protein kinase (Fig. 2.4).

Other potential molecular targets of NO include heme-containing enzymes of the cytochrome P450 system, which may lead to inhibition of the synthesis of vasoconstrictor arachidonic acid metabolites in either endothelial or smooth muscle cells. In addition, NO can combine with the superoxide anion, a short-lived product of some cellular oxidases, to form a highly reactive molecular species, peroxynitrite ($ONOO^-$). This species can affect protein function via nitrosylation of tyrosine residues.

NOS, the enzyme that generates NO from L-arginine, exists in several isoforms in various tissues. The endothelial isoform is activated by the release of calcium and its interaction with calmodulin in endothelial cell cytoplasm. Under pathologic circumstances such as the presence of endotoxin or certain cytokines, another isoform of NOS (known as inducible NOS, or iNOS) is highly expressed in the smooth muscle cells themselves. The consequent release of large quantities of NO may produce refractory vasodilation and the clinical syndrome of septic shock.

Nitric Oxide–Dependent Vasodilators

Certain vasodilators such as the peptide hormone bradykinin, exert their effects only in the presence of an intact endothelium. Bradykinin's seven-transmembrane-domain B_2-receptor couples with guanosine triphosphate (GTP)-binding proteins of the G_q family in both endothelial and smooth muscle cells, leading to the release of calcium into the cytoplasm from extracellular and/or intracellular sources. This stimulus in the endothelium leads to the elaboration and release of NO. Through this indirect mechanism, bradykinin is a potent vasodilator in the intact vessel. However, in the absence of endothelium, bradykinin receptors on vascular smooth muscle promote cytoplasmic calcium release and vasoconstriction when exposed to their ligand. Acetylcholine, serotonin, and histamine are also examples of substances that exert their vasodilatory effects by stimulating endothelial NO release.

Renin-Angiotensin System

Tigerstedt and Bergmann first reported in 1898 that an extract of kidney cortex could raise blood pressure in experimental animals and named the active principle of this response renin.

Renin, a proteolytic enzyme with highly defined substrate specificity, is not a hormone itself. It specifically cleaves angiotensinogen to produce angiotensin I. Angiotensin I, an inactive compound, is then further processed by angiotensin-converting enzyme (ACE), which is highly expressed on endothelial cells and in the renal intersititium. The product is angiotensin II, a potent vasoconstrictor. Angiotensin II promotes calcium entry into and vasoconstriction of smooth muscle cells through its G_q-coupled AT_1-receptor subtype, which is highly expressed in these cells. Under most physiologic circumstances, the cleavage of angiotensinogen is the rate-limiting processing step; ACE becomes rate limiting only if its action is pharmacologically inhibited. In the absence of ACE inhibitors, the rate of renin release is considered the proximate regulator of angiotensin II activity.

The renin-angiotensin system is a major mediator of sodium conservation in land animals through its multifarious actions in the kidney. Angiotensin II is generated locally within the renal interstitium and as a result is present in the kidney in much higher concentrations than it is in systemic circulation. Both tubular and vascular actions contribute to its sodium- and water-retaining effects. It has been widely disseminated that angiotensin II exerts preferential vasoconstrictor effects on efferent, as opposed to afferent, arterioles, but this is an oversimplification. Both preglomerular and postglomerular arterioles are visibly responsive, to an approximately equal degree, to application of angiotensin II in the isolated perfused juxtamedullary nephron preparation. However, during exogenous angiotensin II administration *in vivo*, GFR can be relatively protected from preglomerular vasoconstriction by compensatory mechanisms involving prostaglandins and NO, as well as by postglomerular vasoconstriction. Therefore, at the cost of an increase in filtration fraction, GFR tends to be preserved during angiotensin II infusion at low to moderate dosages, even with increased renal vascular resistance and decreased renal blood flow. Similar mechanisms presumably act to preserve GFR during activation of endogenous angiotensin II generation.

During the administration of high dosages of exogenous angiotensin II, its preglomerular vasoconstrictor effect may overwhelm these compensatory mechanisms, causing GFR to fall. Under conditions in which the endogenous renin-angiotensin system is activated, a similar filtration failure can be produced by inhibiting the vasodilatory compensatory mechanisms within the afferent arteriole, for example, by inhibiting the synthesis of prostaglandins with nonsteroidal antiinflammatory drugs. In experimental animals, acute administration of NOS inhibitors during angiotensin II administration produces a similar effect.

Other Peptide Hormones

Bradykinin

As noted previously, bradykinin is a classic example of an NO-dependent vasodilator. Its mechanism of activation is similar to that of angiotensin II in that bradykinin and related peptides are cleaved from much larger protein substrates by local release of the relevant protease within the kidney. In the case of bradykinin, the activating protease is tissue kallikrein, large amounts of which are synthesized in certain nephron segments, particularly in the connecting segment between the distal convoluted tubule and the collecting duct, for release into the renal interstitium and the tubular lumen. Low urinary kallikrein excretion appears to be a marker for salt-sensitive hypertension in humans and certain animal models. Kininogens, the precursors of kinins, may originate in the liver and travel to the kidney through the circulation, or they may be synthesized locally within the vascular and/or extravascular compartments of the kidney.

Once released from kininogen, the half-life of bradykinin is limited in either the circulation or the interstitium. It is subjected to further proteolysis to yield metabolites, some of which may contain biologic activity. One of the primary proteases that inactivates bradykinin within the kidney is ACE. Therefore some renal functional consequences of ACE inhibitors may be ascribed to prolonging bradykinin's effects, instead of, or in addition to, diminishing activation of angiotensin II. For example, an efferent arteriolar vasodilating effect, which might produce acute loss of filtration function after ACE inhibition in states of diminished renal perfusion, has recently been ascribed to bradykinin. The role of bradykinin in the effects of ACE inhibitors is expected to be clarified in future studies by comparing the effects of ACE inhibitors, angiotensin II receptor blockers, and the recently available, more specific kinin-receptor blockers.

Endothelins

Endothelins are tremendously potent vasoconstrictor peptides that are secreted in a regulated manner from endothelial cells in response to hypoxia, growth factors, or other humoral or mechanical stimuli. Of the three known endothelins, ET-1 has the most potent vasoconstrictor activity and constitutes the major isoform secreted by endothelial cells in culture. Endothelins may be released in excessive quantities in diseases causing endothelial cell injury, thereby decreasing GFR and renal blood flow. On the other hand, ET-1 secretion is inhibited by NO in an autocrine fashion and (at least *in vitro*) by atrial natriuretic peptide. Exposure to ET-1 increases NOS activity in endothelial cells, presumably generating a negative-feedback response that may limit its vasoconstrictor effects *in vivo*.

Like other peptide hormones, ET-1 is generated from a larger precursor. This precursor, known as "big" ET-1, is cleaved by a specific endothelial cell protease called endothelin-converting enzyme (ECE), which has become a target for experimental pharmacologic manipulation. Endothelin secretion is vectorially directed toward nearby vascular smooth muscle. If ET-1 escapes into the circulation, its half-life is brief. Therefore it is uncertain whether increased circulating endothelin concentration in certain disease states has pathophysiologic significance. In contrast, once ET-1 binds to vascular smooth muscle cells and vascular rings *in vitro*, its action is uniquely prolonged, compared with that of other vasoconstrictors such as angiotensin II, which are terminated rapidly by desensitization mechanisms.

The known endothelin receptors fall into two pharmacologically and molecularly distinct isoforms: ET_A and ET_B. ET_A receptors predominate on vascular smooth muscle cells and are coupled to calcium entry and subsequent vasoconstriction through G-proteins of the G_q/G_{11} family. The ET_B receptor predominates on endothelial cells and appears to be the receptor that stimulates NO release. Specific pharmacologic blockers of these receptors are available. The effects of global blockade of endothelin receptors or ECE on the hemodynamic status of normal experimental animals generally are minimal, although some human studies suggest that endothelin contributes to the normal maintenance of vascular tone in forearm and dermal resistance vessels. Studies of endothelins' role in normal renal blood flow regulation in animals have produced variable results. This variability may be related to species differences, differential subtype-specific activities of the antagonists, prolonged residual action of ET-1 after initiation of receptor blockade, or balance of the vasoconstrictor effects of ET-1 by NO release. Nevertheless, the use of selective ET_A antagonists has suggested that ET-1 participates in the abnormal regulation of the renal circulation in various pathophysiologic states, including contrast nephrotoxicity, cyclosporine nephrotoxicity, congestive heart failure, and transplant rejection.

Adrenomedullin

Adrenomedullin, a 52–amino acid peptide, was identified originally in extracts from a human pheochromocytoma through its adenylate cyclase-stimulating activity. It is now known to be synthesized locally within several organs, including the kidney. When administered to conscious rats, an increase in renal blood flow was observed, despite a decrease in systemic blood pressure, indicating a pronounced renal vasodilatory effect. Adrenomedullin is also a potent natriuretic and diuretic agent. Despite producing substantial increases in renal blood flow in rats and dogs, its effects on GFR generally are minimal or variable. Some of the vasodilator effect of adrenomedullin on the systemic and renal vasculature may be endothelium dependent because it can be partially blocked by NOS inhibition. There also appears to be some pharmacologic overlap with the calcitonin gene-related peptide (CGRP). CGRP administration can block some adrenomedullin effects, although it does not block its renal vasodilator effect.

An orphan receptor with the typical seven-transmembrane-domain topology of the G-protein–coupled receptor family has been identified as an adrenomedullin receptor. It stimulates cyclic adenosine monophosphate (cAMP) production, presumably through interaction with the adenylate cyclase-activating, GTP-binding protein G_s. CGRP is a weak antagonist of the receptor when the receptor is expressed in COS cells. In view of the sensitivity of some adrenomedullin effects to NO inhibition, it is also of interest that adrenomedullin has been reported to stimulate NO production through intracellular calcium release and calcium entry pathways in cultured endothelial cells.

Natriuretic Peptides

The existence of apparent secretory granules in cardiac atrial myocytes was recognized some 40 years ago; however, the natriuretic and diuretic activity of atrial, as compared with ventricular, extracts was first reported by deBold in 1981. This activity eventually was determined to be caused by atrial natriuretic peptide (ANP), a 28–amino acid peptide cleaved from a larger precursor and released into the circulation in response to atrial stretch. Subsequent investigation has revealed that ANP and two related peptides, brain natriuretic peptide (BNP) and C-type natriuretic peptide (CNP), are expressed in multiple tissues besides the heart. Three natriuretic peptide receptors (NPRs) also have been identified, with differential but overlapping specificities for the various peptides: They are NPR-A, NPR-B, and NPR-C. The genes for ANP, CNP, and all three receptors are expressed in various locations within the kidney.

The vasodilator actions of natriuretic peptides are due to the distinctive signal transduction mechanism of NPR-A and NPR-B, which are membrane-bound guanylate cyclases, entirely unrelated to the NO-dependent cytoplasmic guanylate cyclase. NPR-A, which is activated by both ANP and BNP, is expressed in glomeruli and vascular smooth muscle, as well as in vascular endothelium and various epithelial cells within the nephron. Infusion of moderate dosages of ANP or BNP in whole animals results in hypotension but, nevertheless, produces renal vasodilation and natriuresis. The increase in renal blood flow tends to be transient because ANP does not affect renal autoregulation and GFR is unaffected by concentrations of ANP within the physiologic range. During administration of pharmacologic doses of ANP, a sustained increase in GFR can be seen, which is due to a combination of afferent arteriolar vasodilation and efferent vasoconstriction. The cellular signaling mechanism that produces efferent vasoconstriction is unknown. The natriuretic response to very large doses of ANP is abrogated by the decrease in systemic blood pressure.

NPR-B appears to be a specific receptor for CNP. Immunostaining in the vascular structures of the kidney can detect the expression of this receptor. It also is present in cultured human glomerular mesangial cells and rat vascular smooth muscle cells, although in the latter cell type it is induced by passage in culture and expressed only at low levels in quiescent cells *in vivo*. Exogenously infused CNP is not natriuretic, but it is a potent renal and systemic vasodilator. Secretion of CNP by cultured endothelial cells has been described; therefore CNP may be a component of a NO-independent, endothelium-dependent, guanylate cyclase–coupled vasodilator system.

NPR-C is highly expressed on endothelial cells and may be expressed on vascular smooth muscle as well, although its expression becomes more prominent in the latter cell type as the cells are cultured. NPR-C binds and internalizes all of the natriuretic peptides and many synthetic peptides, with little or no affinity for NPR-A or NPR-B. NPR-C is not coupled to guanylate cyclase, and its role, if any, in regulating vascular tone, other than participating in the prompt clearance of circulating natriuretic peptides, is not clear.

Arachidonic Acid Metabolites

Arachidonate is released from membrane lipids by hormone-responsive phospholipases, the most prominent of which is cytoplasmic phospholipase A_2. An enormous variety of signaling lipids from arachidonate are produced through one of three metabolic pathways: cyclooxygenase, lipoxygenase, or cytochrome P450 monooxygenase. Many of the resulting signaling molecules have prominent vasoconstrictor or vasodilator effects, most of which are thought to be mediated by various G-protein–coupled receptors in the membrane of vascular smooth muscle and/or endothelial cells. Receptors for direct vasodilator arachidonate metabolites are coupled to G_s (the activator of adenylate cyclase) in smooth muscle cells, whereas receptors for vasoconstrictor metabolites couple to activation of various isoforms of phospholipase C, through G_i or G_q/G_{11} family proteins, with subsequent intracellular calcium liberation. Progress in understanding the role of arachidonate metabolites in the renal vasculature and elsewhere has been impeded by the simultaneous production of a multitude of chemically similar molecules, their sometimes conflicting properties, and their frequently short half-lives. Stable synthetic analogs of many natural arachidonate metabolites, as well as more or less selective inhibitors of arachidonate metabolism, have been useful tools in physiologic studies. Further progress can be expected as compounds of increased potency and specificity are discovered.

Cyclooxygenase Metabolites

The most prominent cyclooxygenase metabolites that normally participate in renal vascular regulation are the prostaglandins, notably PGE_2 and PGI_2. Vasoconstrictor mediators such as angiotensin II normally induce secondary prostaglandin release in vascular smooth muscle cells and glomeruli, which appear to exert important protective effects on GFR by limiting constriction of preglomerular vascular-resistance elements. In rat glomeruli, PGE_2 synthesis predominates, whereas in human glomeruli and microdissected rabbit cortical microvasculature, PGI_2 is the major prostaglandin synthesized.

Four pharmacologically distinct PGE_2 receptors are produced from different genes and differ in their spectrum of G-protein coupling. The EP_2 subtype of PGE_2 receptor is most prominent in the glomerular circulation. This receptor couples preferentially with G_s and adenylate cyclase and is the presumed mediator of PGE_2 vasodilation. EP_1- and EP_3-receptor subtypes can couple with G_i and G_q/G_{11}, respectively, but these receptors are expressed mainly in tubular segments rather than in the vasculature. Nevertheless, exogenous PGE_2, when administered experimentally, has not been a universal vasodilator. Vasoconstrictor responses under certain experimental circumstances may reflect the activation of receptor subtypes other than EP_2 or the secondary release of vasoconstrictor mediators. PGE_2 is a notably potent and physiologically relevant agonist of renin release. The effect of PGE_2 may also depend on the underlying vasoconstrictor tone. In contrast, PGI_2 (i.e., prostacyclin) seems to exert straightforward actions as a cAMP-coupled vasodilator in the renal and systemic circulation.

Another cyclooxygenase metabolite of pathophysiologic importance is the evanescent but extremely potent vasoconstrictor and platelet-aggregating agent thromboxane A_2 (TXA_2). Produced by a specific synthase from PGH_2, this enzyme is normally highly expressed in platelets and activated macrophages but not in the renal vasculature. Unfortunately, blocking this synthase generally is ineffective in abrogating the effects of TXA_2 because its precursor PGH_2 is an agonist of the same receptors. Receptors for PGH_2/TXA_2 are expressed in vascular smooth muscle and mesangial cells and appear to be coupled mainly to G_q in vascular smooth muscle. Although production of TXA_2 in the kidney appears to be minimal under normal circumstances, there is experimental evidence for the involvement of increased TXA_2 synthesis and/or action in the abnormal hemodynamic states produced by ureteral obstruction, cyclosporine nephrotoxicity, and renovascular hypertension. Like the prostaglandins, TXA_2 production can be stimulated by angiotensin II, an effect that can be shown under certain conditions to constitute a significant contribution to the effects of angiotensin II on renal vascular resistance and tubuloglomerular feedback.

Various other prostaglandins, such as $PGF_{2\alpha}$, 8-epi-$PGF_{2\alpha}$, PGD_2, and PGJ_2, can be produced in the kidney *in vivo* or by renal cells in culture; their physiologic role in the renal circulation remains unknown.

Lipoxygenase and Monooxygenase Pathways

Arachidonate is metabolized by lipoxygenase to the precursor of leukotrienes C_4, D_4, and E_4, and the hydroxyeicosatetraenoic acids (HETEs). Other HETEs, epoxyeicosatetraenoic acids (EETs), and dihydroxyeicosatetraenoic acids (DIHETES) are produced by the epoxygenase and hydroxylase components of the cytochrome P450–monooxygenenase pathway. Various compounds in these groups induce vasoconstriction, endothelium-dependent vasodilation, or both. Some also inhibit renin release.

A series of studies has implicated monooxygenase metabolites, in particular 20-HETE, in renal autoregulation. Although considerable controversy exists in this technically complex area, there is evidence for involvement of the cytochrome P450 system in modulating both myogenic- and tubuloglomerular-feedback responses. In a patch clamp study of rat preglomerular vascular smooth muscle cells, 20-HETE decreased and cytochrome P450 inhibition increased the opening of large conductance Ca-activated K channels (which hyperpolarize the cell and inhibit contraction). The signaling mechanism by which this change occurred has yet to be determined.

Adenosine and Adenosine Nucleotides

The ubiquitous purine adenosine is generated in both the renal cortical and the medullary interstitium, albeit at a higher concentration in the medulla under basal conditions. During ischemia or hypoxia, the release of adenosine by renal tissue increases greatly, presumably reflecting the dephosphorylation of cellular ATP stores. Adenosine also can be generated from cAMP by the sequential action of phosphodiesterase and 5′-nucleotidase.

P_1 purinergic receptors for adenosine on vascular smooth muscle can be pharmacologically resolved into A_1 and A_2 receptors, which are seven-transmembrane-domain receptors that preferentially couple to G_i and G_s, respectively. Thus adenosine has the capability to mediate either vasoconstriction or vasodilation. During renal arterial adenosine infusion in dogs, both responses are observed. There is an initial decrease, then increase past the baseline, in renal blood flow. There appears to be some selectivity within the various regions of the kidney to the vasodilatory response because blood flow through deep cortical nephrons and the renal medulla preferentially increases during the vasodilatory phase. The propensity of A_1 receptors to inhibit and A_2 receptors to stimulate renin release further complicates the interpretation of whole-organ studies.

In previous years, several investigators hypothesized that adenosine might mediate tubuloglomerular feedback, based on the idea that adenosine release from the macula densa would depend on the metabolic work of transport in the thick ascending limb of Henle's loop. Thus high-salt delivery to this segment would result in increased consumption of ATP, release of adenosine, and preglomerular vasoconstriction. Unfortunately for this hypothesis, the effects of various adenosine agonists and antagonists on tubuloglomerular feedback and renal autoregulation have been inconsistent. Consequently, the role of adenosine in these responses is still controversial.

Intact ATP also can be released into the renal interstitium from intrinsic cells or possibly from nerve terminals. P_2 purinergic receptors share the pharmacologic characteristic of high selectivity for ATP or adenosine diphosphate (ADP) over adenosine. The P_2 receptor family has multiple members, some of which are G-protein–coupled receptors and some of which are putative calcium channels. When infused into renal arteries of dogs, ATP produces an endothelium-dependent vasodilation that can be reversed or converted to vasoconstriction by NOS inhibitors. Directly applying ATP to mesangial cells results in contraction. Direct superfusion of ATP analog in the isolated perfused juxtamedullary nephron preparation has consistently demonstrated prompt, profound, and reversible vasoconstriction of directly visualized preglomerular segments. Interestingly, desensitization of P_2 receptors in this preparation abolished autoregulator afferent arteriolar vasoconstriction in response to increased perfusion pressure, raising the possibility that a P_2-receptor ligand, presumably ATP rather than adenosine itself, could be a long-sought mediator of tubuloglomerular feedback and renal autoregulation.

Renal Nerves and Catecholamines

Renal sympathetic nerve activity affects the renal circulation, either directly through α-adrenergic terminals on the vasculature or indirectly through stimulation of renin release. Under basal conditions in conscious animals, efferent renal sympathetic activity generally appears to be too low to exert significant direct vasoconstrictor effects. When nerve stimulation is artificially applied, there is a frequency-dependent increase in renal vascular resistance. Micropuncture data indicate that this vasoconstrictor response is exerted on both preglomerular and postglomerular resistance elements. Single-nephron GFR is well preserved with moderate frequency stimulation but falls significantly when high-intensity stimulation is applied. Anesthesia and other physiologic stress cause overt effects of endogenous renal nerve activity on renovascular tone. In anesthetized, hypovolemic rats, micropuncture experiments have shown that angiotensin II receptor blockade increases single-nephron GFR and plasma flow and that renal denervation increases it further, indicating a direct effect of the renal nerves on renal microvascular resistance, at least in preglomerular segments in these circumstances.

Nevertheless, some vascular resistance changes after renal nerve stimulation appear to reflect intrarenal angiotensin II activation. GFR, which is ordinarily maintained under mild to moderate renal nerve stimulation, can be decreased by simultaneously administering ACE inhibitors, which suggests that at least some of the increase in postglomerular resistance seen after renal nerve stimulation is mediated by angiotensin II. Conversely, angiotensin II is thought to facilitate norepinephrine release from adrenergic nerve terminals in the kidney, possibly through prejunctional receptors. Thus the renal vasoconstrictor response to angiotensin II infusion in the rabbit is significantly blunted by renal denervation.

Circulating epinephrine secreted from the adrenal gland also can facilitate norepinephrine release from adrenergic terminals, probably through presynaptic β_2-receptors. On the other hand, evidence for presynaptic inhibition of norepinephrine release exists for several other vasoactive compounds, including prostaglandins, adenosine, dopamine, neuropeptide Y, NO, ANP, and norepinephrine itself, the latter through α_2-receptors.

Dietary Protein

In experimental animals and humans, ingestion of a protein meal is followed within a few minutes by the onset of a renal vasodilatory response, which results in increases in renal blood flow and GFR, which are sustained for several hours (Fig. 2.5). In healthy humans, the GFR can rise 20% or more after a protein load; this response has been referred to as the renal reserve. Vegetarians with no clinical renal disease characteristically have a lower 24-hour creatinine clearance than meat eaters, which is at least partly caused by decreased activation of the renal reserve over the course of the day. Renal reserve is diminished or lost early in the course of renal disease; therefore, its absence has been suggested as a potential marker for subclinical renal insufficiency. In animal models, the involvement of hormones derived from the portal circulation, such as glucagon or secretin, is suggested by the ability of somatostatin or hepatectomy to blunt the renal vasodilatory response to a protein load. Nevertheless, a qualitatively similar response is noted after intravenous amino acid infusion. Although the response may be attenuated by inhibitors of NOS, it is not necessary that the infused amino acids contain L-arginine, the precursor of NO, to produce renal vasodilation. The detailed mechanism of renal reserve is still unknown.

Micropuncture studies in rats have demonstrated that the rise in GFR after protein loading is associated with preglomerular vasodilation and a rise in glomerular capillary pressure, factors that have been correlated in various rodent models of renal disease with more rapid progression of glomerulosclerosis and uremia. Consequently, protein restriction has attracted considerable investigative interest as a potential method of delaying renal failure. The mixed results of clinical trials in this area are covered in more detail in Chapter 67.1 and Chapter 83.2.

PHARMACOLOGY OF RENAL BLOOD FLOW

Numerous drugs in clinical use can modify renal function, either as a desired therapeutic outcome or an unwanted side effect. In view of the complex network of endogenous agents that participate in renal hemodynamic regulation, it is not surprising that some of the most clinically important effects of numerous pharmacologic agents are exerted through the renal vasculature. A brief review of the renal hemodynamic effects of some widely used therapeutic agents is presented next.

ACE Inhibitors and Angiotensin II Receptor Blockers

The identification of an important role for glomerular capillary hydrostatic pressure in the progression of experimental renal failure led to an explosion of investigative and clinical interest in agents that are capable of decreasing this pressure. The most intensively investigated of these agents are the ACE inhibitors. Although most renal vasoconstrictors decrease glomerular capillary hydrostatic pressure, the balanced preglomerular and postglomerular constrictor effects of angiotensin II can lead to stable or even increased glomerular capillary pressure when the renin-angiotensin system is stimulated. Conversely, blockade of the renin-angiotensin system in the remnant kidney rat model

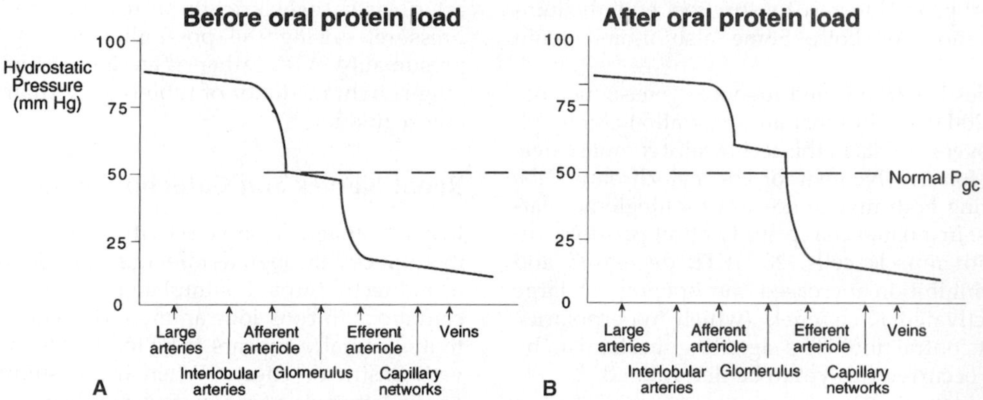

Figure 2.5. Profiling of hydrostatic pressure changes across the renal circulation. **A:** Preprandial renal hemodynamics. A glomerular capillary hydrostatic pressure (P_{gc}) of 50 mm Hg is depicted in this and subsequent figures. The exact value of this parameter in humans has not been determined. **B:** Activation of renal reserve after a protein meal. The increase in renal blood flow and GFR results from decreased preglomerular resistance.

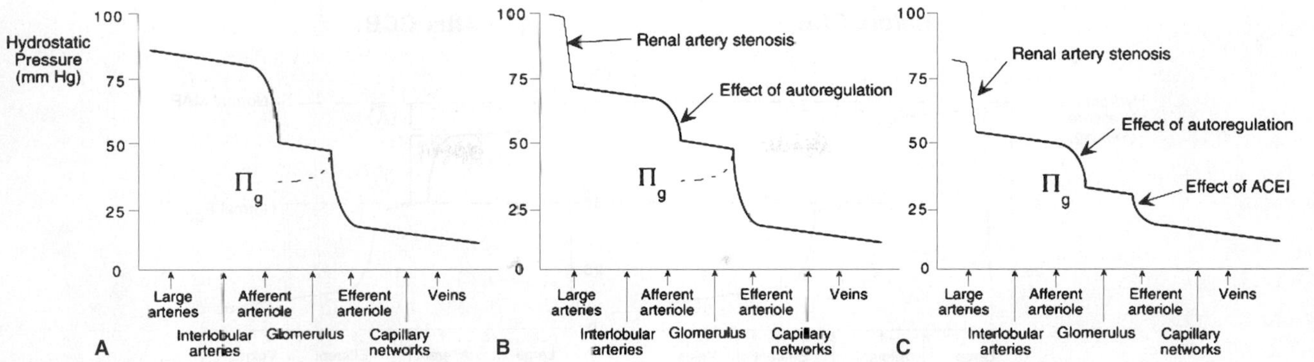

Figure 2.6. Profiling of hydrostatic pressure changes across the renal circulation. The dotted line labeled Πg represents the colloid osmotic pressure in glomerular capillaries, which opposes filtration and rises as ultrafiltrate along the length of the capillaries. **A:** Normal renal hemodynamics. **B:** Subcritical renal artery stenosis. The drop in renal perfusion pressure across the stenosis has been offset by an autoregulatory vasodilation in the afferent arteriole, resulting in preservation of glomerular capillary hydrostatic pressure. **C:** After institution of converting enzyme inhibitor treatment, loss of postglomerular vasomotor tone results in a glomerular capillary hydrostatic pressure that drops below Πg, resulting in filtration failure. It is assumed that preglomerular autoregulatory capability has been exceeded at this point.

decreases glomerular capillary pressure more than the administration of less specific antihypertensive agents; this property was found to be associated with protection from glomerular injury in the renal ablation model in rats. Numerous subsequent investigations generally have confirmed these findings in other disease models and, to the extent possible, in clinical disease states. Other studies have revealed qualitatively similar cortical hemodynamic effects of angiotensin II AT_1-receptor blockade. Medullary blood flow appears to be influenced by endogenously generated bradykinin to a greater extent than cortical blood flow. Because ACE inhibitors potentiate the action of kinins and receptor blockers do not, the hemodynamic effects of these agents may be less equivalent in the medulla.

Shortly after captopril (the first clinically available ACE inhibitor) was released in the United States, a high incidence of acute filtration failure with this agent, in the setting of renal artery stenosis, was recognized. When a high-grade, fixed structural obstruction of a renal artery exists, the autoregulatory response produces afferent vasodilation to maintain glomerular capillary pressure, and renin release is stimulated by the decreased renal perfusion pressure. At this point, administration of diuretics in an attempt to control volume retention and blood pressure further stimulates the renin-angiotensin system. Angiotensin II can actually be critical to the maintenance of GFR under these circumstances through at least two mechanisms. First, angiotensin II released into the circulation raises the systemic blood pressure, thereby tending to normalize the perfusion pressure distal to the renal artery stenosis. Second, intrarenal angiotensin II will increase the glomerular capillary pressure by continuing to constrict the efferent arteriole, while afferent vasoconstriction is offset by autoregulatory vasodilation. If ACE inhibitors are administered in this situation, the combination of decreased renal perfusion pressure and release of efferent vasoconstriction may lead to cessation of GFR (Fig. 2.6). This may occur even though renal blood flow is maintained or even increased by the decrease in total renal vascular resistance.

Calcium Channel Blockers

Patch-clamp studies have characterized voltage-sensitive calcium channels in vascular smooth muscle as T-type or L-type. T-type channels are short-acting channels that are highly sensitive to depolarization; L-type channels have longer opening times and, although less sensitive overall to depolarization, are thought to account for the major component of calcium flux across the plasma membrane. The calcium channel blockers, which are currently available in the United States for clinical use, decrease the conductance of L-type calcium channels. Because the constriction of afferent arterioles strongly depends on extracellular calcium, administering drugs such as nitrendipine or verapamil produces preglomerular vasodilation and inhibition of autoregulatory responses. Efferent arteriolar vasoconstriction is much less affected by L-type calcium channel blockade than is vasoconstriction in preglomerular segments. The effects of more recently developed T-type calcium channel blockers, such as mibefradil, on renal segmental microvascular resistance is unknown.

Whether glomerular capillary hydrostatic pressure rises or falls after administration of calcium channel blockers depends on the balance between the drug effects on renal perfusion pressure and preglomerular vasodilation; the latter effect depends on baseline preglomerular vascular tone. Selective infusion of verapamil into the renal artery of an anesthetized dog, with appropriate dosage adjustment to preclude any large change in blood pressure, significantly increases GFR and decreases renal vascular resistance, an effect consistent with the elevation of glomerular capillary hydrostatic pressure through afferent vasodilation. Systemic administration of calcium channel blockers generally results in a lesser increase or no change in GFR and renal blood flow because renal perfusion pressure also diminishes significantly in this setting (Fig. 2.7). Nevertheless, stable renal blood flow in the setting of a lower blood pressure indicates a significant decrease of renal vascular resistance with calcium channel blockers.

Nonsteroidal Antiinflammatory Drugs

There are several mechanisms by which nonsteroidal antiinflammatory drugs (NSAIDs) can produce a decrease in renal function, but the most common is functional interference with the normal regulatory mechanisms of the renal circulation. In the presence of stimulation of the renin-angiotensin systems by actual or functional blood volume depletion, the patency of the afferent arteriole can be protected by endogenous vasodilating mechanisms. Among these mechanisms is the generation of the

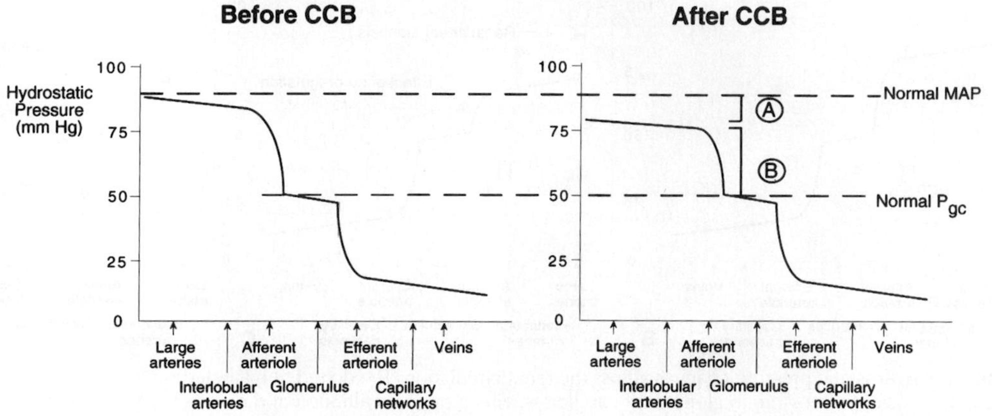

Figure 2.7. Profiling of hydrostatic pressure changes across the renal circulation. **Left panel:** Normal renal hemodynamics. **Right panel:** Hypothetical changes after administration of a calcium channel blocker. The drop in systemic arterial pressure *(A)* has been offset by a drop in preglomerular resistance *(B)*, resulting in no change in glomerular capillary hydrostatic pressure. The glomerular capillary hydrostatic pressure in a given individual after treatment with calcium channel blockers could rise, fall, or remain unchanged, depending on the relative magnitudes of *(A)* and *(B)*. MAP, mean arterial blood pressure; P_{gc}, glomerular capillary hydrostatic pressure.

vasodilatory prostaglandins PGE_2 and PGI_2, which are blocked by NSAIDs. Therefore, in circumstances in which there is activation of angiotensin II generation, renal function is uniquely vulnerable to the induction of unopposed preglomerular vasoconstriction by NSAIDs. For this reason, doses of NSAIDs that produce no detectable alterations in renal function in some patients may produce oliguric acute renal failure in others. Examples of patients who may manifest this pathophysiology include diuretic-treated or otherwise volume-depleted patients and those with congestive heart failure or hepatic cirrhosis.

The rate-determining step in prostaglandin synthesis is the step catalyzed by cyclooxygenase, which is inhibited by NSAIDs. Molecular cloning studies reveal the existence of two isoforms of cyclooxygenase. The isoform constitutively expressed in renal tissue and other organs under basal conditions is known as COX1, whereas COX2 was believed to be a more inducible isoform that is preferentially expressed at sites of inflammation and cell activation. More recently, COX2 is now recognized to be constitutionally expressed in the macula densa and medulla. Several pharmacologic agents that selectively inhibit COX2 are under active clinical investigation in the hope that they will exhibit improved specificity at sites of inflammation without affecting the normal renal homeostatic mechanisms presumably mediated by COX1. However, at the time of this writing, preliminary clinical data indicate that administration of COX2-selective inhibitors also can be associated with acutely decreased renal function.

Catecholamines

α-Adrenergic receptors on vascular smooth muscle, which primarily consist of the α_1 subtype, are coupled to calcium entry and intracellular calcium release. Norepinephrine is a powerful α-adrenoreceptor agonist that increases blood pressure by increasing peripheral vascular resistance during systemic administration. Renal vascular smooth muscle is also highly sensitive to norepinephrine. In fact, administering norepinephrine to experimental animals is a reliable method of producing ischemic acute renal failure. Therefore norepinephrine is considered a therapy of last resort. In the desperate clinical circumstances in which norepinephrine administration is necessary, acute renal failure is a serious hazard.

Epinephrine is released into the systemic circulation from the adrenal medulla and is used clinically as an inotropic and pressor agent. Its major effect on the renal circulation appears to be indirect. Epinephrine potentiates norepinephrine release from sympathetic nerve terminals through stimulation of presynaptic β_2-receptors. These receptors couple preferentially with G_s and cAMP generation and therefore are vasodilating when expressed on vascular smooth muscle. However, in the renal vascular smooth muscle, α-adrenergic receptors far outnumber β-receptors, as assessed by autoradiography. In most circumstances, the net effect of epinephrine in the renal circulation during systemic administration is vasoconstriction.

Dopamine is the metabolic precursor of norepinephrine, as well as a neurotransmitter, with its own set of specific receptors. Therapeutic dopamine in small doses exerts a potent vasodilator effect in the normal kidney, accompanied by diuresis and natriuresis. Although a D_1-receptor subtype can be pharmacologically demonstrated in the preglomerular vasculature, the vasodilation may be predominantly caused by a presynaptic inhibitory effect on α-adrenergic nerve terminals. When dopamine is clinically used in small doses to support the systemic circulation, renal function generally is not adversely affected. A selective D_1 agonist, fenoldopam, is capable of exerting potent systemic and renal vasodilatory effects (as well as a natriuretic effect mediated by proximal tubule receptors) and therefore has been approved for the treatment of hypertensive emergencies.

Despite its effects in the normal kidney, dopamine is generally not an effective vasodilator in the postischemic acute renal failure kidney. Furthermore, increasing the rate of dopamine infusion beyond a low level can result in α-adrenergic stimulation and renal vasoconstriction, through either a direct α-agonist effect of dopamine or uptake by nerve terminals and conversion to norepinephrine.

Cyclosporine and Tacrolimus

Cyclosporine and tacrolimus are potent, immunosuppressive agents whose major adverse effect is nephrotoxicity, which is mediated primarily in the short term through the promotion of vasoconstriction by these drugs in the renal circulation. Long-term administration results in structural changes in the walls of the preglomerular vessels, with downstream glomerulosclerosis and tubular atrophy. Despite intensive study, the mechanisms by which either vasoconstriction or structural lesions in renal vessels are induced by cyclosporine are not entirely understood.

The mechanism of action of both cyclosporine and tacrolimus in immunosuppression is signal transduction interference through the calcium-dependent phosphatase calcineurin in T lymphocytes. The contribution of this mechanism in vascular cells to subsequent nephrotoxicity is controversial; however, some contribution seems likely because cyclosporine and tacrolimus are structurally distinct and use different intracellular proteins as receptors, yet they exert similar degrees of nephrotoxicity at therapeutically equivalent dosages. There appear to be some significant differences between the high-dose, acute preparations often studied in animal models and the clinical manifestations of nephrotoxicity, which may be manifested either acutely or in the long term. For example, there is no evidence that the renin-angiotensin system plays a significant role in the short-term changes in renal blood flow and GFR seen in cyclosporine-treated patients, but acute activation of the renin-angiotensin system has been observed in some animal models.

One common thread in certain animal models and clinical nephrotoxicity with these agents is endothelial cell dysfunction. There is evidence for both enhanced release of endothelin and inhibition of NO production in cyclosporine-exposed endothelium. Increased sensitivity to endothelin and other vasoconstrictors in vascular smooth muscle cells also may be present. Alterations in arachidonate-metabolite production also appear to play a role because pharmacologic antagonists of the TXA_2/PGH_2 receptor can ameliorate cyclosporine-induced renal vasoconstriction in experimental animals. The vasoconstrictor effect of cyclosporine appears to be exerted preferentially in the preglomerular circulation, an effect that has been observed by scanning electron micrography in the rat. Acute and chronic decreases in GFR and renal blood flow in animal models can also be ameliorated by antagonists of endothelin receptors, and to some extent by calcium channel blockers.

Selected Readings

Carmines PK, Ohishi K, Ikenaga H. Functional impairment of renal afferent arteriolar voltage-gated calcium channels in rats with diabetes mellitus. *J Clin Invest* 1996;98:2564–2571.
An example of bench research with straightforward clinical implications that illustrate the power of the isolated juxtaglomerular nephron technique.

Casellas D, Carmines PK. Control of the renal microcirculation: cellular and integrative perspectives. *Curr Opin Nephrol Hyperten* 1996;5:57–63.
Brief review article that centers on the role of ion channels in regulating arteriolar tone.

Cowley AW. Role of the renal medulla in volume and arterial pressure regulation. *Am J Physiol* 1997;273:R1–R15.
Review that advocates the position that incomplete autoregulation of the medullary circulation is primarily responsible for pressure natriuresis.

DiBona GF, Kopp UC. Neural control of renal function. *Physiol Rev* 1997;77:75–197.
Exhaustively detailed review of the actions of renal nerves, including details of recently recognized neurotransmitters, such as neuropeptide Y, not covered in this chapter.

Inscho EW. Purinoreceptor-mediated regulation of the renal vasculature. *J Autonomic Pharmacol* 1996;16:385–388.
Review that summarizes the role of purinergic receptors in the renal circulation, including evidence from the author's laboratory for P_2-receptor mediation of tubuloglomerular feedback.

Ito S, Abe K. Contractile properties of afferent and efferent arterioles. *Clin Exp Pharmacol Physiol* 1997;24:532–535.
Brief review that emphasizes the different contractile mechanisms and mediators that control the preglomerular and postglomerular resistance segments.

Iversen BM, Arendshorst WJ. ANG II and vasopressin stimulate calcium entry in dispersed smooth muscle cells of preglomerular arterioles. *Am J Physiol* 1998;274(3 Pt 2):F498–F508.
The most direct evidence available for a major role of calcium entry, rather than release from intracellular stores, in contractile function of afferent arteriolar smooth muscle.

Katz AM. Protein families that mediate Ca^{2+} signaling in the cardiovascular system. *Am J Cardiol* 1996;78:2–6.
Brief review of the structure and function of calcium channels and binding proteins in contractile cells, including some projected therapeutic implications.

Kone BG. Nitric oxide in renal health and disease. *Am J Kidney Diseases* 1997;30:311–333.
Detailed review of the vascular and extravascular actions of NO in the kidney that pays particular attention to signaling pathways and the control of expression of the various isoforms of NOS.

Navar LG, Inscho EW, Majid DSA, et al. Paracrine regulation of the renal microcirculation. *Physiol Rev* 1996;76:425–536.
Scholarly monograph that summarizes and reconciles the results of more than 1,200 primary studies in this field.

Navar LG, Majid DS. Interactions between arterial pressure and sodium excretion. *Curr Opin Nephrol Hypertens* 1996;5:64–71.
Balanced summary of current knowledge and lack of knowledge about the mechanism of pressure natriuresis.

O'Bryan GT, Hostetter TH. The renal hemodynamic basis of diabetic nephropathy. *Semin Nephrol* 1997;17:93–100.
Illustration of important clinical implications of some of the concepts covered in this chapter.

Owens GK, Vernon SM, Madsen CS. Molecular regulation of smooth muscle cell differentiation. *J Hypertens Suppl* 1996;14:S55–S64.
Review of pathophysiologic changes in smooth muscle phenotype and their relationship to disease.

Savineau JP, Marthan R. Modulation of the calcium sensitivity of the smooth muscle contractile apparatus: molecular mechanisms, pharmacological and pathophysiological implications. *Fund Clin Pharmacol* 1997;11:289–299.
Integrative review of current understanding of the mechanisms of intracellular interaction between vasodilator and vasoconstrictor signal transduction.

Schnackenberg CG, Granger JP. Verapamil abolishes the preglomerular response to ANG II during intrarenal nitric oxide synthesis inhibition. *Am J Physiol* 1997;272:R1670–R1676.
Example of the continuing contributions of whole-animal studies. Pharmacologic tools are used to explore interactions between NO and angiotensin II signaling upstream and downstream of the glomerulus.

Singh I, Grams M, Wang WH, et al. Coordinate regulation of renal expression of nitric oxide synthase, renin, and angiotensinogen mRNA by dietary salt. *Am J Physiol* 1996;F1027–F1037.
An example of the ongoing trend toward integration of molecular biology techniques into whole-animal physiology. The study supports an important role for NO in macula densa function by demonstrating that the expression of neuronal NOS from renal cortex (presumably mostly from macula densa) is specifically regulated by dietary salt in conjunction with renin-angiotensin system components.

Vaandrager AB, de Jonge HR. Signalling by cGMP-dependent protein kinases. *Mol Cell Biochem* 1996;157:23–30.
Review that explores the incompletely understood but increasingly important signaling mechanisms downstream of cGMP in response to nitrovasodilators in the cardiovascular system.

CHAPTER 3

Glomerular Filtration

Francis B. Gabbai and Roland C. Blantz

The kidneys constitute 0.5% of total body mass and receive 20% of the cardiac output, approximately 1 L of blood per minute. This large perfusion volume leads to blood flows per gram of tissue which are 40-fold higher than the average tissue in the body. Such a high perfusion rate per gram of kidney in the presence of normal systemic blood pressure can be achieved only with low vascular resistances, which result from the large number of vascular units packed into the kidney. There are approximately 0.8 to 1.2 million glomeruli, or capillary units, per kidney. This number of glomeruli, or nephron units, is established by about 36 weeks' gestation, cannot increase but only decrease throughout the life time of an individual.

High renal blood flow and plasma flow rates are critical to maintain the glomerular filtration rate (GFR) necessary to allow adequate clearance of nitrogen waste products and other toxic substances. Of plasma flow, 20% to 30% normally passes across the glomerular capillary membrane barrier as plasma or glomerular ultrafiltrate, generating approximately 150 to 200 L of glomerular ultrafiltrate in 24 hours. Taking into consideration that a normal individual weighing 70 kg has a total water weight of 42 L, a normal GFR of 140 L constitutes more than three times the entire total body water. Production of such large volumes of glomerular filtrate has important implications for the overall body homeostasis. Although it provides ample opportunity to eliminate nitrogen waste products and toxic substances, it also constitutes a major threat to volume and pressure homeostasis if not tightly regulated. Production of glomerular ultrafiltrate is tightly coupled to the process of tubular reabsorption to allow excretion of maximum amounts of waste products in the minimum required volume. Uncoupling of these two processes with an error in either one, be it excess filtration and reduced reabsorption or vice versa, could lead to disastrous consequences for the individuals. Therefore it is critical for both processes to be highly regulated to avoid significant problems.

DETERMINANTS OF THE GLOMERULAR ULTRAFILTRATION PROCESS

Production of plasma ultrafiltrate at the levels of the glomerulus follows the same general principle as any other capillary system in the body with some unique characteristics which are specific to the glomerular capillary bed. Fluid movement across the glomerular capillary membrane is governed by the Starling's forces (i.e., glomerular hydrostatic pressure and glomerular oncotic pressure) and the permeability of the membrane.

$$\mathrm{GFR} = \mathrm{LpA}\,(\Delta \mathrm{P} - \Delta\pi)$$

where ΔP corresponds to the transcapillary hydrostatic pressure gradient, $\Delta\pi$ corresponds to the transcapillary oncotic pressure gradient, and *LpA* corresponds to the ultrafiltration coefficient. The transcapillary hydrostatic pressure gradient (ΔP) is equal to the glomerular capillary hydrostatic pressure (P_{GC}) minus the hydrostatic pressure in Bowman's space (P_{BS}), and $\Delta\pi$ is equal to glomerular capillary oncotic pressure (π_{GC}) minus the oncotic pressure in Bowman's space (π_{BS}). Because π_{BS} is negligible, $\Delta\pi$ is equal to π_{GC}. The ultrafiltration coefficient is equal to the product of the permeability constant of the glomerular capillary multiplied by the filtering surface area. One of the important characteristics of the glomerular capillary bed is that the ultrafiltration coefficient is 50 to 100 times greater than that of a muscle capillary.

Another characteristic that makes the glomerular capillary bed unique is its location between two arterioles. The glomerular capillary network is located between the afferent and efferent arteriole and is constituted by 20 or more parallel capillary units that freely communicate with one another. Glomerular capillary hydrostatic pressure is determined by the transmission of the systemic blood pressure to the glomerular capillary and the tone of the afferent and efferent arterioles. The combination of vasoconstriction or vasodilation in both arterioles allows for increases and reductions in the glomerular capillary pressure, which becomes, to a certain extent, independent of the systemic blood pressure. This unique capacity of the glomerular capillary network to regulate glomerular capillary pressure independent of systemic blood pressure is known as autoregulation. The autoregulatory capacity of the glomerulus is critical to maintain high GFR levels around the clock independent (within physiologic limits) of the individual's condition.

Glomerular capillary hydrostatic pressure has been measured in individual glomeruli of rodents by direct puncture of glomerular capillaries with micropipettes in the range of 45 to 50 mm Hg for P_{GC}. The urinary's space pressure has been measured at 10 to 15 mm Hg such that ΔP values range between 34 to 40 mm Hg. Multiple punctures of the same glomerulus

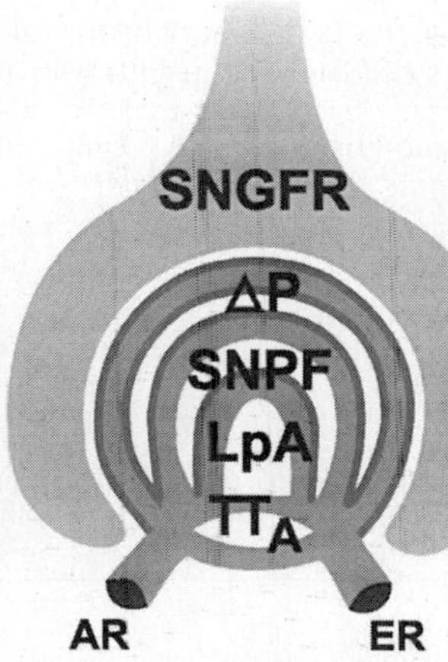

Figure 3.1. Schematic representation of a glomerulus depicting the major determinants of the glomerular ultrafiltration process which include the transcapillary hydrostatic pressure gradient *(ΔP)*, single nephron plasma flow *(SNPF)*, the glomerular ultrafiltration coefficient *(LpA)*, and the plasma oncotic pressure *(πA)*. SNGFR single nephron glomerular filtration rate; AR, afferent arteriolar resistance; ER, efferent arteriolar resistance.

have shown similar values for P_{GC}, demonstrating that P_{GC} is constant throughout the glomerulus. Oncotic pressure is derived from the proteins in plasma, estimated values at the afferent site are approximately 20 to 25 mm Hg. The gradient of hydrostatic and oncotic pressure at the afferent site favors filtration by a value of approximately 13 to 15 mm Hg. As protein-free ultrafiltrate enters the urinary space, protein concentration in the glomerular capillary progressively increases up to the point at which filtration stops when oncotic pressure is equal to ΔP. Depending on the plasma flow rate, the filtration pressure equilibrium ($\Delta P = \pi$) can be reached early after the afferent arteriole (low plasma flow rate) or at the level of the efferent arteriole (high plasma flow rate). Under the conditions of filtration pressure equilibrium, increases in plasma flow lead to increases in GFR and maintenance of the filtration fraction (GFR/RPF). In certain experimental conditions (high plasma flow rate in rodents) and in some species (like the dog), π is not equal to ΔP at the efferent site leading to what is known as filtration pressure disequilibrium. Under filtration pressure disequilibrium, changes in ΔP and LpA constitute the major factors influencing GFR with changes in plasma flow being less important in this condition. In summary, there are four major determinants of the glomerular ultrafiltration process, which include nephron plasma flow, ΔP, the ultrafiltration coefficient (LpA), and the afferent oncotic pressure (π_A) (Fig. 3.1).

REGULATION OF GLOMERULAR FILTRATION RATE

We have previously mentioned that maintenance of GFR is critical to maintain water, electrolyte, acid–base homeostasis, and elimination of waste products. Experimental studies demonstrate that GFR remains within normal ranges despite changes in sodium and water intake and physiologic changes in systemic blood pressure. Maintenance of GFR under these variety of conditions requires the interaction of several systems and mechanisms, including the autoregulation process, tubuloglomerular feedback system, and the intervention of neurohumoral factors. The multiplicity and variety of systems that affect the glomerulus demonstrate that the glomerulus is an active organ as opposed to a passive system submitted to filtration forces.

Autoregulation

Studies performed in dogs 30 to 40 years ago demonstrate that renal blood flow is maintained within normal limits despite changes in mean systemic blood pressure in the range of 70 to 140 mm Hg. Similar studies performed in rats confirmed not only the presence of renal blood flow autoregulation but also the presence of GFR autoregulation. Careful examination of critical glomerular capillary pressures in the latter experiments also revealed the presence of autoregulation of glomerular capillary hydrostatic pressure. Autoregulation of blood flow and glomerular hydrostatic pressure requires changes in afferent and efferent arteriolar resistances during variations in systemic blood pressure. Increases in systemic blood pressure produce afferent arteriolar constriction, which limits the transmission of the systemic blood pressure to the glomerular capillary. In contrast, reductions in systemic blood pressure dilate the afferent arteriole and constrict the efferent arteriole to maintain glomerular capillary hydrostatic pressure. Systemic blood pressure values above or below the autoregulatory range lead to directly proportional changes in glomerular capillary hydrostatic pressure and significant changes in GFR.

The mechanism by which autoregulation is mediated remains incompletely understood. Two different components seem to participate in renal autoregulation. A rapid component at the afferent arteriole appears to be dominantly myogenic in character while a slower component, which is unique to the kidney, involves the participation of the tubuloglomerular feedback system as described in detail later in this chapter. The myogenic component is similar to the response that is observed in other vascular beds in which changes in blood flow produce arteriolar changes capable of restoring blood flow to baseline conditions. Several mechanisms have been proposed to explain the myogenic response, they include the presence of a stretch receptor in the arteriolar wall as well as increased or reduced delivery of oxygen or nutrients to the tissue. In the specific situation of the kidney, there is no evidence that changes in oxygen delivery or nutrients play a major role in autoregulation, implying that stretch receptors are responsible for changes in afferent arteriolar tone. Changes in afferent tone involve changes in intracellular calcium concentration. Interestingly, efferent arterioles do not seem to respond to changes in stretch and therefore do not participate in the myogenic response. The tone of the efferent arteriole is in large part dictated by neurohumoral factors and possibly P_{GC} in a counterautoregulatory manner, for example, increased P_{GC} causes reduction in tone.

Tubuloglomerular Feedback System

The large volume of glomerular filtrate produced in 24 hours needs to be tightly coupled to the tubular reabsorptive process to avoid catastrophic change in extracellular volume. A normal individual produces approximately 140 L/day of glomerular filtrate and eliminates between 1 and 1.5 L of urine per day in physiologic conditions, reabsorbing 99% of the filtered load. Such tight coupling between filtration and reabsorption depends upon two mechanisms, glomerulotubular balance and tubuloglomerular feedback system. The interaction of these two mechanisms explains how increases in GFR do not produce significant extracellular fluid losses, whereas reductions in GFR are not associated with significant fluid retention. Glomerulotubular balance adapts tubular reabsorption to filtered load. As the filtered load increases, tubular reabsorption increases while reductions in the filtered load is associated with reduction in tubular reabsorption. Multiple factors are involved in the glomerulotubular balance process, including intraluminal factors (e.g., glucose, amino acids, sodium chloride) and extraluminal factors (e.g., peritubular physical factors, neurohumoral factors). Although glomerulotubular balance is critical to prevent large changes in extracellular fluid content, this process is inflexible if the filtered load is the only element that dictates tubular reabsorption. The flexibility in the tight coupling of the filtration-reabsorption process is provided by the tubuloglomerular feedback system.

The tubuloglomerular feedback system is constituted by an afferent or sensing mechanism (macula densa cells in the cortical thick ascending limb of Henle's loop are located near the vascular pole, i.e., afferent and efferent arterioles of the same nephron) and an effector system that is responsible to change the GFR. In this system, increases in Henle's loop delivery of sodium chloride to the macula densa lead to reduction in nephron filtration rate, whereas decreases in delivery to the macula densa increase the nephron filtration rate. The effector mechanism includes the afferent arteriole, and some experimental evidence indicates that changes in the ultrafiltration coefficient may also participate as secondary efferent arteriolar participation. Increased distal delivery activates tubuloglomerular feedback, which leads to afferent arteriolar constriction and reductions in nephron plasma flow, glomerular capillary hydrostatic pressure, and nephron filtration rate. In contrast, decreased delivery to the macula densa leads to afferent arteriolar dilation and increases in plasma flow, glomerular capillary hydrostatic pressure, and nephron filtration rate.

The mediator(s) of the tubuloglomerular feedback system still remain(s) undefined. Although the proximity of the tubuloglomerular feedback system (TGF) to the juxtaglomerular apparatus makes renin and angiotensin II likely candidates, studies demonstrate that angiotensin II is a modulator of the TGF and not the mediator. The most compelling argument against angiotensin II as mediator comes from the fact that increases in distal delivery of sodium chloride suppress renin secretion while activating TGF. There is recent evidence to suggest a role for adenosine as a mediator of TGF because adenosine increases afferent arteriolar tone and adenosine-receptor blocker largely inhibits TGF responses in some, but not all, experimental conditions. Other proposed mediators include thromboxane and alternatively changes in chloride concentration in the interstitial region bordered by the macula densa and the glomerular arterioles.

TGF is important because it brings important flexibility to the glomerulotubular balance process, and it acts as a potential safety device in certain pathophysiologic conditions. TGF activity provides important flexibility to glomerulotubular balance because it can modulate and adapt to various stimuli including volume expansion, volume contraction, and reduction in renal mass. Under these various stimuli, increased or reduced TGF activity allows small adjustments in the coupling of filtration-reabsorption, leading to increased or reduced water and sodium excretion. In pathophysiologic states such as acute tubular necrosis, in which the reabsorptive process is greatly reduced, increased TGF activity reduces GFR, thereby preventing catastrophic losses in water and electrolytes.

Neurohumoral Control of Glomerular Filtration Rate

Several neurohumoral factors, including angiotensin II, renal nerves, prostaglandins, endothelin, and atrial natriuretic peptide, modulate GFR. Their effect on the determinants of the glomerular ultrafiltration process are summarized in Tables 3.1 and 3.2.

TABLE 3.1. Effects of Neurohumoral Factors on Determinants of Glomerular Ultrafiltration Process

	Angiotensin II	RNS	Endothelin	ANP	PG
ΔP	↑	↑	↓	↑	=
Single-nephron plasma flow	↓	↓	↓↓	↑	↑
LpA	↓	↓	↓	±	↓
SNGFR	=↓	=↓	↓	↑	↓=↑

ANP, atrial natriuretic peptide; PG, prostaglandin (in this case vasodilatory prostaglandin PGE_2 or PGI_2); RNS, renal nerve stimulation; SNGFR, single nephron glomerular filtration rate.

Angiotensin II

Initial studies based on exogenous administration of angiotensin II (AII) demonstrated that AII exerts rather complex effects on the glomerular ultrafiltration process. AII increases both afferent and efferent resistances and decreases plasma flow. A somewhat larger effect on the efferent arteriole explains the increases in glomerular capillary hydrostatic pressure and the transcapillary hydrostatic gradient during AII infusion. AII also decreases the ultrafiltration coefficient. The interaction of positive (increases ΔP) and negative (decreased plasma flow and ultrafiltration coefficient) influences explains why GFR is relatively well maintained during AII infusion, although at the expense of a higher filtration fraction. Endogenous generation of AII in models of chronic salt depletion and congestive heart failure results in almost identical changes in glomerular hemodynamics as during exogenous administration.

The decrease in the ultrafiltration coefficient during endogenous or exogenous elevations in AII suggests the presence of target cells other than vascular smooth muscle cells, which respond to AII. These cells include the glomerular mesangial cell, which exhibits modest contractile properties, and probably the visceral epithelial cell acting in concert to mediate the decrease in the ultrafiltration coefficient. Recent studies demonstrate a large capacity for the kidney to generate high levels of AII because measurements of AII in the early proximal tubule and efferent arteriole reveal values up to 1,000 times higher than plasma.

Renal Adrenergic Activity

Renal nerve stimulation or increases in circulating norepinephrine result in renal vasoconstriction. The presence of multiple adrenergic receptor subtypes (α_1, α_2, and β with their respective subtypes) complicates the analysis of the norepinephrine effects on the renal vasculature. Moreover, the interaction of the renal adrenergic system with other vasoconstrictor system makes this analysis even more complex. In general, α-adrenergic activity

TABLE 3.2. Effects of Neurohumoral Factors on Afferent and Efferent Glomerular Resistances

	Angiotensin II	RNS	Endothelin	ANP	PG
Afferent	↑	↑	↑↑	↓	↓
Efferent	↑↑	↑↑	↑↑	↑	=

ANP, atrial natriuretic peptide; PG, prostaglandin (PGE_2 or PGI_2); RNS, renal nerve stimulation.

produces renal vasoconstriction, whereas β-adrenergic activity stimulates renin and AII generation. Low-frequency renal nerve stimulation (3 Hz) produces renal vasoconstriction, largely mediated by AII because AII suppression under these conditions removes approximately 75% of the vasoconstrictive effect. Alternatively, acute renal denervation does not produce a major increase in renal plasma flow unless AII is inhibited. Subacute renal denervation results in modest nephron plasma flow increases that most likely are caused by an increase in AII receptor number and heightened AII sensitivity.

The application of specific receptor agonists to investigate the role of the various receptor subtypes is also complex. Administration of α_2-agonists in innervated kidney results in vasodilation, whereas similar experiments in a denervated kidney reduces the nephron filtration rate primarily by producing a reduction in the ultrafiltration coefficient. AII and α_2-adrenoreceptors are synergistic in that the effects of α_2-adrenergic agonists are enhanced by increased AII activity and are blocked by AII-receptor blockers. Levels of α_2-adrenergic agonists, which do not affect glomerular hemodynamics, amplify the effects of AII on the ultrafiltration coefficient.

Endothelin

Endothelin 1 (ET-1) is produced by endothelial cells, mesangial cells, and epithelial cells in the glomerulus. ET-1 infusion reduces renal plasma flow and GFR. At the single nephron level, ET-1 increases afferent and efferent resistance and decreases nephron plasma and the ultrafiltration coefficient, leading to a reduction in nephron GFR. ET-1–induced vasoconstriction is mediated by increases in intracellular calcium concentration secondary to release from intracellular stores by the inositol triphosphate pathway and by receptor-operated and voltage-gated channels in the plasma membranes.

Three major categories of stimuli lead to increased renal ET-1 production, including vasoconstrictors/thrombogenic agents (AII, vasopressin, 8-epi-prostaglandin $F_{2\alpha}$, and thrombin), physical factors (mechanical strain), and inflammatory cytokines (tumor necrosis factor-α and interleukin-1). Nitric oxide (NO), prostacyclin, atrial natriuretic peptide (ANP), prostaglandin E_2, bradykinin, and heparin inhibit ET-1 production. Additional details on endothelin and its interaction with the kidney are found in Chapter 13.5.

Prostaglandins

Prostacyclin (PGI_2) is the most abundant prostaglandin in the renal cortex and is synthesized by glomeruli and arterioles, whereas PGE_2 is the most abundant prostaglandin produced by the tubules, although it is also produced in the glomerulus. Systemic and intrarenal administration of prostaglandins reduces afferent and efferent resistance and increases plasma flow. The increase in plasma flow is associated with variable changes in GFR, probably a reflection of the hypotension associated with these agents and the activation of other neurohumoral systems. Micropuncture studies have demonstrated that prostaglandin administration is associated with decreases in the ultrafiltration coefficient secondary to increased AII activity.

Prostaglandins are not major regulators of GFR or renal plasma flow in normal conditions because acute or chronic prostaglandin blockade with nonsteroidal antiinflammatory drugs (NSAIDs) does not modify GFR or renal plasma flow in euvolemic animals or normal volunteers. In contrast, conditions associated with increased neurohumoral activity in the kidney such as congestive heart failure, cirrhosis with ascites, nephrotic syndrome, and acute volume depletion demonstrate significant reductions in GFR and renal plasma flow after NSAID administration. Such conditions clearly stress the importance of renal prostaglandin generation as antagonists or modulators of the intrarenal vasopressor hormones. Additional information on prostaglandins and their interaction with the kidney are found in Chapter 13.1 and Chapter 47.3.

Atrial Natriuretic Peptide

ANP is released by the left atrium in the presence of volume expansion. In contrast to the previous neurohumoral factors, ANP raises GFR through the unusual combination of decreased afferent resistance with increased efferent constriction leading to increased P_{GC} and ΔP. ANP also affects tubular reabsorption such that increased ANP levels, either through endogenous or exogenous mechanisms, raise GFR and increase sodium excretion. For further details, see Chapter 13.8.

Nitric Oxide

The kidney contains the three different isoforms of nitric oxide synthase (eNOS, bNOS, and iNOS), the enzyme required to generate NO from the amino acid L-arginine. eNOS is found in glomeruli and renal vessels, whereas bNOS is localized at the level of the macula densa and efferent arteriole. Both isoforms are considered constitutive and require intracellular calcium mobilization for activation. Localization of eNOS and bNOS suggests that both enzymes play an important role in the regulation of renal blood flow and GFR. In contrast, iNOS is inducible and has been detected in almost all the structures, both vascular and tubular, within the kidney.

Using various inhibitors of NOS, a large number of studies demonstrate that NOS blockade is associated with increased systemic blood pressure, and at the kidney level, it increases afferent and efferent resistance and decreases the ultrafiltration coefficient, leading to reductions in renal plasma flow and variable effects on GFR. AII suppression negates most of the effects of NOS blockade on glomerular hemodynamics (the exception being the increase in afferent resistance, which most likely reflects the myogenic response of this vessel to the increase in systemic blood pressure), suggesting that NO functions primarily in the kidney as a tonic antagonist of AII. This functional antagonism between NO and AII appears to occur not only at the level of the vasculature and glomerulus but also at the proximal tubular level where AII blockade can reverse the reduction of proximal tubular reabsorption induced by NOS blockade.

Renal adrenergic innervation modifies the effects of acute NOS blockade in that subacute renal denervation eliminates the effects of NOS blockade on glomerular hemodynamics. The effects of denervation can be reversed by the concurrent administration of α_2-adrenergic agonists, which restore the reduction in plasma flow and ultrafiltration coefficient observed during NOS blockade. In innervated kidneys, administration of an α_2-adrenergic antagonist, yohimbine, prevents the glomerular and tubular effects of NOS blockade. Therefore these studies suggest a complex three-way interaction between NO, AII, and α_2-adrenergic activity in the control of renal plasma flow and GFR.

Interactions Between the Various Neurohumoral Factors

As mentioned, there are significant interactions between the various neurohumoral factors which regulate GFR (Fig. 3.2). AII and renal nerves have synergistic effects in which adrenergic activity increases renin and AII generation, whereas increased AII activity heightens the response to renal nerve stimulation. AII and prostaglandins are also closely linked. AII stimulates the generation of prostaglandins, which limit the vasoconstrictive effects of AII, whereas some of these prostaglandins (PGI_2) are directly involved in the secretion of renin. AII and NO share similarities with the AII-prostaglandin interaction in which NO

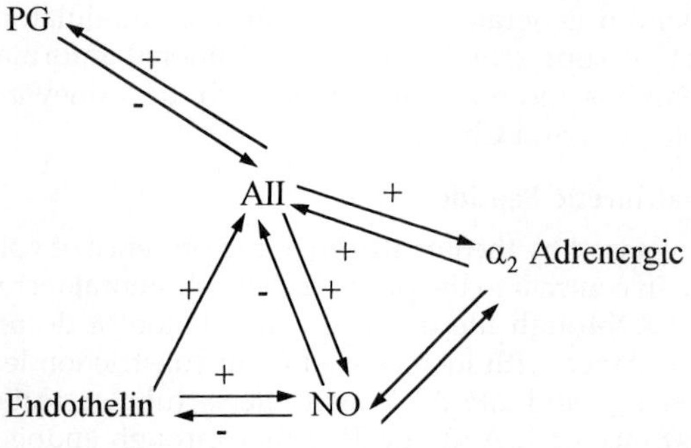

Figure 3.2. Interaction between renal neurohumoral mediators, which include prostaglandins *(PG)*, angiotensin II *(AII)*, α_2-adrenergic activity, nitric oxide *(NO)*, and endothelin. The plus (+) and minus (−) refer to stimulatory and inhibitory effects, respectively.

is a tonic antagonist of AII and NO is involved in renin secretion. Another example of this bidirectional effect is the interaction between endothelin and NO in which increased endothelin levels stimulate generation of NO through the endothelin type B receptor, which limits the vasoconstrictive effects of endothelin. The multiplicity of these interactions clearly demonstrate the complexity of factors capable of modifying renal plasma flow and GFR under normal conditions but more importantly in pathophysiologic conditions. The interactions between NO and the kidney are further discussed in Chapter 13.6.

CHANGES IN THE DETERMINANTS OF THE GLOMERULAR ULTRAFILTRATION PROCESS IN VARIOUS PATHOPHYSIOLOGIC CONDITIONS

It is not within the scope of this chapter to extensively review the effects of renal disease processes on glomerular hemodynamics. However, we would like to review some examples to demonstrate how various physiologic and disease conditions affect the determinants of the glomerular ultrafiltration process. As shown in Table 3.3, we have included chronic salt depletion, hypertension (contralateral or exposed kidney in a model of two one-clip Goldblatt hypertension), acute glomerulonephritis (intravenous administration of antiglomerular basement membrane antibody), and reduction in renal mass (5/6 nephrectomy). Chronic salt depletion is characterized by increased afferent and efferent resistance, decreased nephron plasma flow, and the ultrafiltration coefficient. Despite the increase in P_{GC} and ΔP, nephron filtration rate is low normal because of the opposing action of the reduction in nephron plasma flow and ultrafiltration coefficient. In contrast, glomerular hemodynamics in the contralateral kidney of two kidney one-clip hypertension are characterized by increased nephron filtration rate. The increase in SNGFR is secondary to increases in nephron plasma flow, P_{GC}, and ΔP, despite the reduction in the ultrafiltration coefficient. Afferent and efferent resistances are also mildly increased in this model.

Administration of antiglomerular basement membrane antibody leads to severe reductions in nephron filtration rate secondary to severe reductions in nephron plasma flow and the ultrafiltration coefficient. Increases in P_{GC} and ΔP partially counteract the severe effects of reductions in plasma flow and the ultrafiltration coefficient in this experimental model.

Renal ablation is associated with afferent and efferent vasodilation leading to large increases in nephron plasma flow. Predominance of afferent over efferent dilation increases P_{GC} and ΔP. Increased SNGFR values in this model result from the combination of high nephron plasma flow and high $P_{GC}/\Delta P$ in spite of mild reductions in the ultrafiltration coefficient.

The examples described demonstrate how changes in one or more of the major determinants of the glomerular ultrafiltration process (nephron plasma flow, ΔP, and the ultrafiltration coefficient) can produce a major impact on the rate at which glomerular ultrafiltrate is produced. The success of any therapeutic intervention will depend on its capacity to restore one or more of these parameters back to normal.

TABLE 3.3. Determinants of Glomerular Ultrafiltration Process in Various Pathophysiologic Conditions

	Chronic Salt Depletion	Two Kidney Goldblatt Hypertension	AntiGBM-Ab GN	Renal Ablation
ΔP	↑	↑↑	↑	↑
Single-nephron plasma flow	↓	↑	↓↓	↑↑
LpA	↓	↓	↓↓	=↓
SNGFR	↓=	↑↑	↓↓	↑↑

AntiGBM Ab Gn, antiglomerular basement membrane antibody glomerulonephritis; SNGFR, single nephron glomerular filtration rate.

Selected Readings

Baylis C. Glomerular filtration dynamics. In: Lote CJ, ed. *Advances in renal physiology.* London: Grune & Stratton, 1986:33–83.

A comprehensive review of the glomerular ultrafiltration process with emphasis on the changes in GFR during experimental manipulations of the various determinants. Examines the effects of AII and other hormones on GFR.

Blantz RC, Thomson SC, Peterson OW, Gabbai FB. Physiologic adaptations of tubuloglomerular feedback system. *Kidney Int* 1990;38:577–583.

A review of the role of tubuloglomerular feedback system in the control of the GFR. Various physiologic and pathophysiologic conditions lead to adaptations of the tubuloglomerular feedback system.

De Nicola L, Blantz RC, Gabbai FB. Nitric oxide and angiotensin II. Glomerular and tubular interaction in the rat. *J Clin Invest* 1992;89:1248–1256.

A study demonstrating the interaction between NO and AII in the control of both glomerular and tubular function. The changes in glomerular and tubular function induced by NOS blockade can be prevented by AII-receptor blockers.

Dunn BR, Ichikawa I, Pfeffer JM, et al. Renal and systemic hemodynamic effects of synthetic atrial natriuretic peptide in the anesthetized rat. *Circ Res* 1986;59:237–253.

A study to examine the effects of atrial natriuretic peptide on glomerular hemodynamics. Atrial natriuretic peptide has the unique property of producing afferent arteriolar vasodilation and efferent arteriolar vasoconstriction, leading to increased glomerular filtration rate.

Kon V, Yoshioka T, Fogo A, et al. Glomerular actions of endothelin in vivo. *J Clin Invest* 1989;83:1763–1770.

An experimental study to investigate the effects of endothelin on glomerular hemodynamics. Endothelin produces severe reduction in nephron filtration as a result of glomerular arteriolar vasoconstriction and decrease in the ultrafiltration coefficient. Administration of endothelin antibody reverses renal vasoconstriction in an ischemia model.

Kone BC, Baylis C. Biosynthesis and homeostatic roles of nitric oxide in the normal kidney. *Am J Physiol* 1997;272:F561–F578.

A comprehensive review of the different isoforms of NOS in the kidney and their potential regulation. Extensive analysis of the role of NO in the regulation of the GFR and renal plasma flow.

Navar LG, Inscho EW, Majid SA, et al. Paracrine regulation of the renal microcirculation. *Physiol Rev* 1996;76:425–536.

A comprehensive review of the role of AII and other paracrine systems in the control of renal plasma flow and the GFR. Concentrations of AII up to 1,000 times higher than plasma are found in proximal tubules and peritubular capillaries.

Schnermann J, Weihprecht H, Briggs J. Inhibition of tubuloglomerular feedback during adenosine$_1$ receptor blockade. *Am J Physiol* 1990;258:F553–F561.

An experimental study to determine the role of adenosine in tubuloglomerular feedback activity. Specific blockade of the adenosine$_1$ receptor inhibit the normal tubuloglomerular feedback response.

CHAPTER 4

Determinants of the Glomerular Filtration of Macromolecules

Bryan D. Myers

FUNCTIONAL PROPERTIES OF GLOMERULAR CAPILLARY WALLS

The walls of glomerular capillaries behave as high-capacity, ultrafiltration membranes. In humans, for example, a very rapid rate of ultrafiltration (approximately 150 L/day) is achieved, despite a pressure for ultrafiltration that is estimated to be below 20 mm Hg. Despite its remarkably low resistance to water flow, the glomerular capillary wall imposes an extremely efficient barrier to the passage of proteins the size of albumin and larger. Fluid sampled by micropuncture techniques from the first part of the proximal tubule conforms closely to that of an ideal ultrafiltrate of plasma. The concentration of inulin (molecular radius of 1.6 nm, or 16Å) and substances smaller than inulin in Bowman's space fluid are essentially identical to that in plasma. In contrast, the corresponding Bowman's space concentration of albumin (molecular radius of 36Å) is below 1 mg/dl, a value 3 to 4 orders of magnitude lower than plasma albumin concentration (typically 4 g/dl). The Bowman's space-to-plasma concentration ratio of a given macromolecule is known as a sieving coefficient and provides a precise measure of the permeability of the glomerular filtration barrier to the macromolecule.

The mechanisms whereby the normal glomerular capillary wall restricts the transmural passage of large plasma proteins, while offering little resistance to the filtration of water and small solutes, have been extensively explored. The relation between the molecular properties of several proteins and glomerular barrier selectivity is illustrated in Fig. 4.1. In these examples, either direct sampling of the first part of the proximal tubule by the micropuncture technique or the urinary clearance corrected for tubular protein reabsorption has been used to determine the glomerular sieving coefficients of various proteins in the rat. Each sieving coefficient is plotted as a function of the effective molecular radius of the protein. Transmural transport of the largest proteins (albumin and IgG) is considerably more restricted than that of the smallest proteins (monomeric immunoglobulin light chains). However, a trend toward progressive restriction of transmural transport with increasing size of the test protein becomes obvious only when the molecular charge of each protein is taken into account. Thus the inverse relation between the sieving coefficient and molecular radius of either anionic or cationic proteins indicates that the glomerular capillary wall has the properties of a size-selective filter (Fig 4.1). On the other hand, the greater restriction of anionic than cationic proteins of equivalent or similar radius points to the existence within the glomerular capillary wall of an electrostatic barrier that also functions as a charge-selective filter.

Because of the inaccessibility of Bowman's space and the technical limitations to accurate measurement of protein concentration of nanoliter samples of Bowman's space fluid, the number of observations of the type shown in Fig. 4.1 is limited. However, glomerular permeability to macromolecules has been extensively studied with the use of the fractional clearance technique. The fractional clearance of a test macromolecule (M) is defined as the clearance of M divided by the glomerular filtration rate of water. With the clearance of inulin used to measure the latter, fractional clearance is calculated from the urine (U) and plasma (P) concentration of M and inulin (in) as follows:

$$\text{Fractional clearance of M} = (U/P)_m/(U/P)_{in}$$

If, like inulin, the test macromolecule is neither reabsorbed nor secreted by the tubule, the fractional clearance of M will be exactly equal to the Bowman's space-to-plasma concentration ratio of M, or the sieving coefficient (θ). Thus, for a test macromolecule with these special properties $(\theta) = (U/P)_m/(U/P)_{in}$, and only urine and plasma samples are required to calculate the sieving coefficient.

BARRIER SELECTIVITY BASED ON SIZE, SHAPE, AND CHARGE

Because endogenous proteins undergo extensive proximal tubular reabsorption, they are unsuitable as test macromolecules when fractional clearances are used to probe the glomerular filtration barrier. Instead, three nonprotein polymers, namely polyvinylpyrrolidone, dextran (a polymer of glucopyranose), and Ficoll (a polymer of sucrose), all of which are neither reabsorbed nor secreted by the tubule, have been used for this

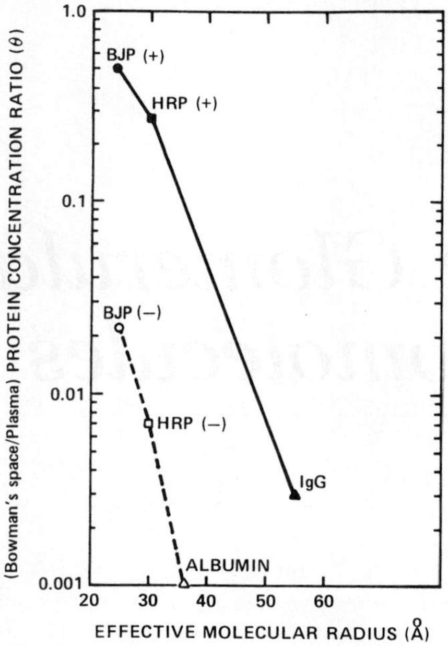

Figure 4.1. Sieving coefficients for several proteins plotted as a function of effective molecular radius. Closed symbols, cationic proteins; open symbols, anionic proteins; *BJP,* Bence Jones protein (IgG light chains); *HRP,* horseradish peroxidase; *IgG,* immunoglobulin G.

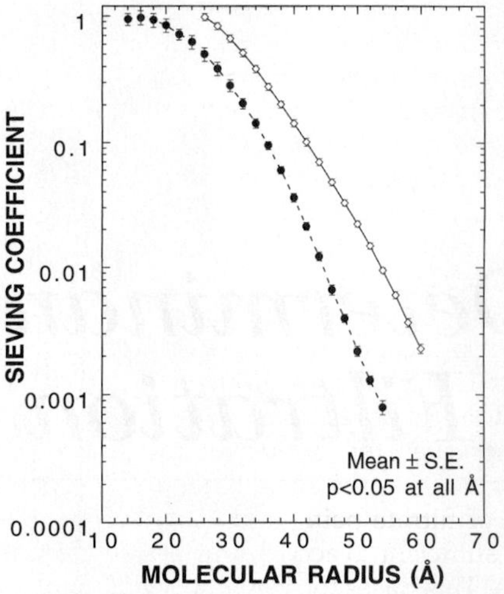

Figure 4.2. Glomerular sieving by the healthy human kidney. Sieving coefficients for dextran *(open symbols)* and ficoll *(closed symbols)* are plotted as a function of molecular radius.

purpose. The size-selective properties of the glomerular capillary wall have been elucidated by using uncharged, polydisperse preparations of these polymers. The absence of charge eliminates the consequences of electrical interaction between the permeating macromolecule and charged sites within the glomerular capillary wall; the use of preparations of broad size distribution permits sieving coefficients to be determined over a wide range of molecular radii.

Whereas dextran behaves as a random coil in solution, it becomes uncoiled under shear during transglomerular permeation. The conformational alteration results in facilitated transport of dextran across the glomerular barrier and leads to an overestimation of the effective radii presented by glomerular "pores" to permeating proteins. In contrast, Ficoll behaves as a rigid sphere during permeation across synthetic membranes. Its transport during transglomerular permeation is also consistent with that of a spherical molecule, as envisioned in the theory of hindered transport through pores. The effect of these differences in shape on transglomerular sieving has been demonstrated by the simultaneous infusion of dextran and Ficoll. In an experiment on healthy human volunteers, the sieving coefficients of each macromolecular species have been plotted as a function of molecular radius, with the latter determined by elution from calibrated gel chromatographic columns (Fig. 4.2). Discrimination based on size is evident from the finding that sieving coefficients of each macromolecule species decline in monotonic fashion with increasing radii. The fact that the transport of Ficoll is restricted (as judged by a lower sieving coefficient) compared with that of dextran of an equivalent gel chromatographic radius demonstrates the effect of molecular shape on glomerular sieving.

An abnormality of glomerular size selectivity has been demonstrated consistently in nephrotic subjects with heavy proteinuria. The abnormality is qualitatively similar for dextran and Ficoll, which is illustrated for the latter barrier probe in a group of nephrotic subjects with membranous nephropathy in Fig. 4.3. Whereas sieving coefficients at the low-radius end of the nephrotic sieving curve tend to be depressed, those at the high-radius end are significantly elevated. Furthermore, whereas Ficoll of radius greater than 56Å was undetectable in the urine of the healthy volunteer control group, larger Ficoll molecules of up to 68Å were easily measurable in the urine of the nephrotic group (Fig. 4.3); the progressive elevation of the sieving coefficients for large, nearly impermeant Ficoll molecules of above 50Å radius, indicates a glomerular membrane with a less sharp cut-off than normal.

The most widely used descriptions of macromolecule transport across the glomerular capillary wall are based on a hydrodynamic theory of hindered solute transport through water-filled pores. A variety of distributions that are commonly used in probability analysis has been examined by a curve-fitting technique so as to select the pore-size distributions that best replicate the observed sieving coefficients. Although several heteroporous membrane models can satisfactorily represent the glomerular capillary wall, the best fit has been a model with a bimodal pore-size distribution. The lower mode is composed of restrictive pores with a continuous lognormal distribution of radii. The upper mode is composed of very large and nondiscriminatory pores, which serve as a shunt pathway (Fig. 4.4).

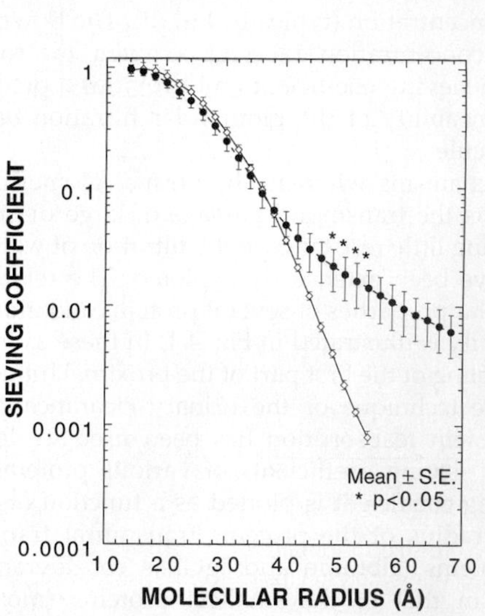

Figure 4.3. Ficoll sieving profile in a group of nephrotic subjects with membranous nephropathy *(closed symbols)* is compared with that in a group of healthy control subjects *(open symbols).*

According to this model, the peak radius of the restrictive pores in the lower distribution is paradoxically lower in nephrotic subjects that in nonproteinuric controls, 36Å versus 44Å, respectively. However, the distribution of restrictive pores is broader in nephrotics than in control subjects, such that a higher fraction of the largest, restrictive pores (60 to 70Å) is found in nephrotic rather than control subjects. The model reveals there is also a large excess of the shuntlike pores of the upper mode in nephrotic subjects. Thus, whereas the fraction of filtrate permeating shunt-like pores in control subjects is only 0.1×10^{-3} on average, it is increased by more than three orders of magnitude to 2.8×10^{-3} on average in the nephrotic subjects (Fig. 4.4, *right panel*). Using mass balances, we calculate that the shuntlike pores can serve as the exclusive portal through which IgG reaches Bowman's space in our nephrotic subjects. However, the fraction of filtrate being shunted through these very large pores is not sufficient to account for the magnitude of observed albuminuria. This raises the possibility that depletion of anionic glomerular sites with a loss of electrostatic barrier function could permit albumin (radius of approximately 36Å) to also be lost in large quantities via the largest pores of the lower distribution of restrictive pores (Fig. 4.4, *left panel*).

We have proven this by infusing a narrowly dispersed preparation of anionic dextran sulfate into nephrotic patients with either membranous or minimal change nephropathies and into healthy nonproteinuric control subjects. The sieving coefficient for dextran sulfate of radius 16Å was determined by separating this fraction of the preparation by size exclusion chromatography of urine and an ultrafiltrate of plasma. In healthy control subjects it was 0.63 ± 0.03 (Fig. 4.5). In comparison, uncharged dextran molecules of similar radii were unrestricted; that is, the sieving coefficient was 1.0 ± 0.04. Thus we demonstrated for the first time that the glomerular capillary wall in humans normally exhibits charge-selectivity similar to that reported for experimental animals. In our nephrotic subjects, the charge discrimination was lost. The sieving coefficient for the 16Å radius dextran sulfate fraction was 0.91 ± 0.05 (p less than .001 vs. controls). The latter value was not significantly different from unity, or from the corresponding sieving coefficient for uncharged dextran molecules of similar radii (Fig. 4.5). From these findings, we infer that the albuminuria observed in membranous and minimal change nephropathies reflects a combination of size- and charge-selective defects. Because dextran overestimates the effective pore size of the glomerular capillary wall, it is not yet possible to calculate the relative importance of the two types of defects. We must wait for similar studies with charged species of a more ideal macromolecular probe, one such as Ficoll, that behaves as a sphere during transglomerular permeation to make this determination.

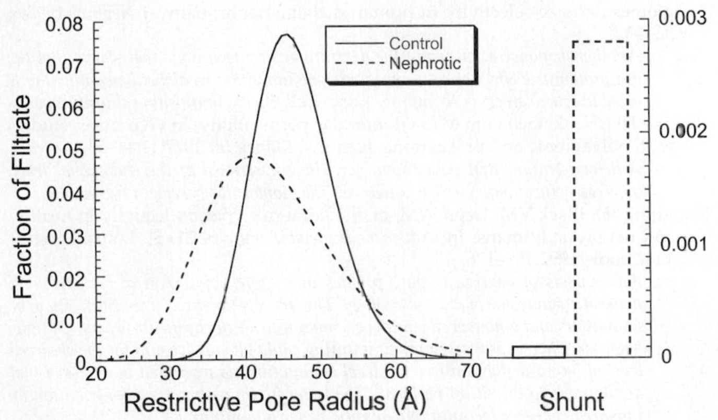

Figure 4.4. Pore-size distribution in glomerular capillary walls of subjects with nephrotic syndrome *(dashed)* versus control subject *(solid)*. Distributions have been computed from ficoll sieving profiles in Fig. 4.3. Fraction of filtrate permeating pores of each interval is plotted as a function of pore radius in the restrictive **(left)** and shunt-like portions **(right)** of the filtration barrier (see text).

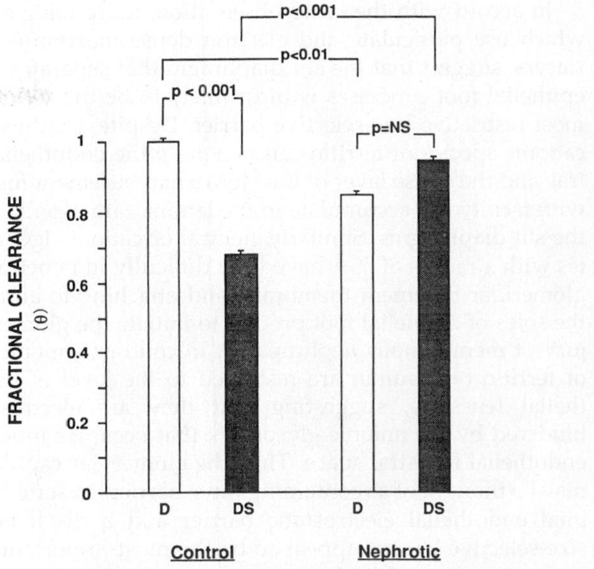

Figure 4.5. The sieving coefficient for anionic dextran sulfate *(DS, solid bars)* and neutral dextran of similar radius *(D, open bars)* in healthy controls **(left)** and nephrotic subjects **(right)**.

STRUCTURAL-FUNCTIONAL RELATIONSHIPS

The computation of effective pore radii from the sieving coefficients of probe macromolecules is mainly useful for making comparisons within the context of a particular model. The definition of structural counterparts to these "functional" pores has proven elusive. A large body of literature has long implied that the extracellular matrix of the glomerular basement membrane provides the barrier to the passage of proteins. However, most available evidence points away from a prominent role for the glomerular basement membrane in filtration barrier function. It has been shown that glomerular sieving coefficients for albumin and large dextran molecules are orders of magnitude lower *in vivo* in the rat with an intact glomerular capillary wall than are corresponding values *in vitro* for an isolated preparation of rat glomerular basement membrane (Fig. 4.6).

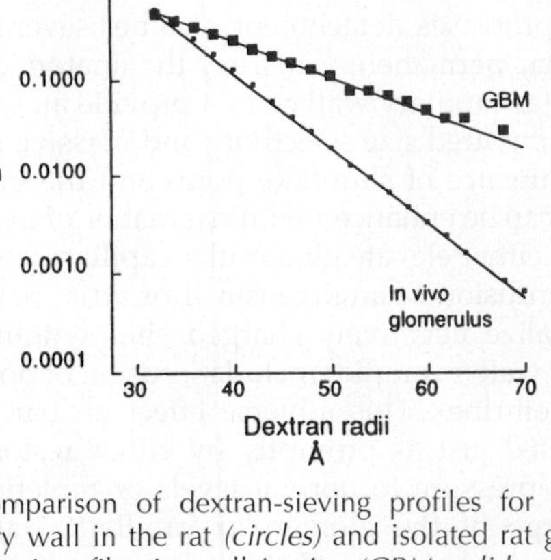

Figure 4.6. A comparison of dextran-sieving profiles for the intact glomerular capillary wall in the rat *(circles)* and isolated rat glomerular basement membrane in a filtration cell *in vitro (GBM, solid squares)*.

In accord with the latter observation, morphologic studies, which use particulate and electron dense macromolecules as tracers, suggest that the slit diaphragm that separates adjacent epithelial foot processes is most likely to be the ultimate and most restrictive size-selective barrier. Despite a radius of 61Å, cationic species of ferritin can penetrate the endothelial fenestrae and the dense layer of the glomerular basement membrane with facility but accumulate in the lamina rara externa beneath the slit diaphragms. Similarly, neutral or cationic IgG antibodies with a radius of 55Å have little difficulty in penetrating the glomerular basement membrane and attaching to antigens on the soles of epithelial foot process to initiate the glomerular injury of membranous nephropathy. In contrast, anionic species of ferritin or albumin are restricted to the level of the endothelial fenestrae, suggesting that they are electrostatically hindered by the anionic glycocalyx that occupies much of the endothelial fenestral space. Thus the glomerular capillary wall may be thought of as containing three barriers in series. A proximal endothelial electrostatic barrier and a distal epithelial size-selective barrier appear to be the most important. An intermediate barrier of less quantitative importance but with both size- and charge-selective properties is provided by the glomerular basement membrane.

The slit diaphragms that separate adjacent epithelial foot processes are, in fact, modified tight junctions. Evidence of a role for these structures as tight junctions is provided by the finding that they are richly endowed with proteins of the zona occludens complex. The slit diaphragms constitute a distal size-selective barrier, which is also consistent with the ultrastructural finding of rectangular apertures, the dimensions of which would prevent the passage of proteins the size of albumin are larger into Bowman's space. The ubiquitous deformation (or so-called effacement) of adjacent foot processes that accompanies all nephrotic disorders could alter the shape and size of the apertures, causing a few to become enlarged and permeable to proteins. Another potential size defect is the complete detachment of some foot processes and their slit diaphragms from the lamina rara externa of the basement membrane. It is precisely at such sites of basement membrane denudation that ferritin particles have been demonstrated to penetrate into Bowman's space in various rat models of proteinuric glomerular injury. However, the latter usually are associated with focal and segmental glomerulosclerosis, and comparable defects are rarely apparent in nephrotic humans with nonsclerosing glomerular injuries such as membranous or minimal change nephropathies. Because our ability to detect an alteration in the dimensions of slit diaphragmatic apertures is beyond the resolution of conventional electron microscopy, the precise structural basis of impaired barrier size-selectivity in membranous and minimal change nephropathy and other nephrotic disorders of humans remains unknown.

Foot processes detachment or other severe structural alterations that permanently disrupt the anatomic integrity of the glomerular capillary wall cannot provide an exclusive explanation for impaired size selectivity and massive proteinuria. Both the prominence of shuntlike pores and the magnitude of proteinuria can be enhanced within a matter of minutes by maneuvers that either elevate glomerular capillary pressure (examples include infusion of angiotensin II or atrial natriuretic peptide) or neutralize negatively charged sites within the glomerular capillary wall (examples include infusion of polycations such as hexadimethrine). This adverse effect on barrier function can be reversed just as promptly by either restoring glomerular-capillary pressure to normal levels or repleting the net negative charge of the glomerular capillary wall. Similarly, the administration of drugs that block the intrarenal production of prostaglandins or angiotensin II can reduce the size of the shunt pathway and the level of proteinuria within a matter of days in nephrotic patients. Withdrawal of these agents promptly restores barrier size-selectivity and proteinuria to pretreatment levels. Morphologic studies suggest that the aforementioned perturbations of barrier function and the filtered protein load are accompanied by alterations in the conformation of epithelial foot processes. Thus at least some of the changes in glomerular capillary wall structure that attend the phenomenon of massive proteinuria are temporary in nature. They likely represent a reversible and nonspecific response by glomerular epithelial cells to a variety of glomerular injuries.

Selected Readings

Blouch K, Deen WM, Fauvel J-P, et al. Molecular configuration and glomerular size selectivity in healthy and nephrotic humans. *Am J Physiol (Renal Physiol)* 1997;42:F430–F437.

An analysis of ficoll sieving in humans with the nephrotic syndrome. It suggests that about 0.3% of plasma filtered into Bowman's space passes unrestricted through large, nondiscriminatory pores. Shunting through such size defects accounts for part but not all of the observed proteinuria.

Bridges CR, Rennke HG, Deen WM, et al. Reversible hexadimethrine-induced alterations in glomerular structure and permeability. *J Am Soc Nephrol* 1991;1: 1095–1108.

Infusion of the polycation hexadimethrine caused immediate proteinuria, effacement of epithelial foot processes, and a dextran-sieving defect indicative of impaired barrier size-selectivity. The entire barrier injury was reversed during infusion of polyanionic heparin sulfate.

Daniels BS, Deen WM, Mayer G, et al. Glomerular permeability barrier in the rat. Functional Assessment by in vitro methods. *J Clin Invest* 1993;92:929–936.

Glomerular basement membrane was isolated and its permeability studied in an ultrafiltration cell in vitro. It was found to be much more permeable to dextrans and albumin than the intact glomerular capillary wall.

Deen WM, Bridges CR, Brenner BM, et al. A heteroporous model of size-selectivity: application to normal and nephrotic humans. *Am J Physiol* 1985;249:F347–F389.

A theoretical analysis of hindered solute transport through a porous membrane applied to dextran filtration data.

Guasch A, Deen WM, Myers BD. Charge-selectivity of the glomerular filtration barrier in healthy and nephrotic humans. *J Clin Invest* 1993;92:2274–2282.

A study showing that the normal glomerular capillary wall of humans functions as a negatively charged electrostatic barrier and that this property is lost in disorders causing the nephrotic syndrome.

Morelli E, Loon N, Meyer T, et al. Effects of converting-enzyme inhibition on barrier function in diabetic glomerulopathy. *Diabetes* 1990;39:76–82.

The use of the dextran-sieving technique demonstrates that therapy with a converting-enzyme inhibitor in diabetic nephropathy causes a parallel decline in the level of proteinuria and the magnitude of the shunt pathway.

Oliver JD, Anderson S, Troy JL, et al. Determination of glomerular size-selectivity in the normal rat with ficoll. *J Am Soc Nephrol* 1992;3:214–228.

Ficoll, an uncharged polymer of sucrose, was shown to behave like a spherical molecule during transglomerular permeation. It exhibited a substantially lower sieving coefficient than uncharged dextran of an equivalent radius. It should prove to be a better probe of the filtration barrier than dextran in studies designed to elucidate the mechanisms of proteinuria.

Remuzzi A, Ruggenenti P, Mosconi L, et al. Effect of low-dose enalapril on glomerular size-selectivity in human diabetic nephropathy. *J Nephrol* 1993;6: 36–43.

Another demonstration using the dextran-sieving technique that shows that the antiproteinuric effect of converting-enzyme inhibition in diabetic nephropathy is attributable to an effect to improve size-selectivity by diminishing shuntlike pores.

Rennke HG, Venkatachalam MA. Glomerular permeability: in vivo tracer studies with polyanionic and polycationic ferritins. *Kidney Int* 1977;11:44–53.

A demonstration that polyanionic ferritin is restricted at the endothelial level, whereas polycationic ferritin penetrates the glomerular basement membrane.

Scandling JD, Black VM, Deen WM, et al. Glomerular permselectivity in healthy and nephrotic humans. In: *Advances in nephrology*, vol 21, St. Louis: Mosby–Year Book, 1992:159–176.

An analysis of dextran-sieving profiles in a large population of patients with nephrotic syndrome of diverse etiology. This reveals impaired size-selectivity to be ubiquitous and a nonspecific finding common to all nephrotic disorders. Of note, however, whereas transmembrane shunting could always account for the observed level of immunoglobulinuria, the level of albuminuria was often in excess of that attributable to the shunt pathway. The latter finding supports a contribution by impaired charge-selectivity to nephrotic-range albuminuria.

Schneeberger EE, Level RH, McCluskey RT, et al. The isoporous substructure of the human glomerular slit diaphragm. *Kidney Int* 1975;8:48–52.

A morphometric examination of 'porelike' apertures in the slit diaphragm.

Tojo A, Endou H. Intrarenal handling of proteins in rats using fractional micropuncture technique. *Am J Physiol 263 (Renal Fluid Electrolyte Physiol 32)* 1992; F601–F606.

A micropuncture study quantifying the filtered protein load and proximal tubule protein handling in the rat.

CHAPTER 5

The Neural Control of Renal Function and Extracellular Fluid Volume

Jeffrey L. Osborn, Suzanne Greenberg, and Craig F. Plato

The regulation of extracellular fluid volume encompasses an ongoing relationship between sodium and water intake and excretion. As humans, we exist as intermittent sodium and water consumers, leaving the bulk of the task of regulating our constant expansion and contraction of extracellular fluid volume to renal excretory mechanisms. Over the past decade, numerous discoveries have been made regarding the influence of afferent extracellular fluid volume sensors and efferent renal nerve activity on renal function. The control of adrenergic receptor expression in the kidneys, as a mediator of renal functional responses, has made recognition of the neural control of renal function a key factor in the overall control of extracellular fluid volume. In this chapter, we describe the basic mechanisms by which the renal nerves participate in the regulation of extracellular fluid volume.

RENAL EFFERENT SYMPATHETIC NERVE ACTIVITY AND RENAL FUNCTION

The nerve traffic emanating from the central nervous system (CNS) to the kidneys is sympathetic in nature and terminates in catecholaminergic nerve terminals. Other neurotransmitters that colocalize with intrarenal norepinephrine now have been identified. These include substance P, neuropeptide Y, serotonin, and adenosine triphosphate (ATP).

Renal Hemodynamics

Renal vasoconstriction during intense stimulation of the renal nerves either experimentally or via reflex activation of endogenous sympathetic outflow is well documented, and this vascular response is mediated by α_1-adrenoceptors. Experiments have provided the basis for examining the influence of low frequencies (i.e., less than 2.0 Hz) of renal nerve activity on renal function and renal hemodynamics. The early neurogenic studies almost exclusively used high frequencies of nerve stimulation or large baroreflex stimuli, which elicited renal vasoconstriction. Important influences of low frequencies of renal nerve activity that do not alter total renal blood flow (RBF) selectively affect other parameters of renal function, including intrarenal hemodynamics. Although changes in extracellular fluid volume will increase or decrease basal renal nerve traffic, in normal hydration states, basal renal nerve activity is approximately 1.5 to 2.0 Hz.

Numerous attempts have been made to determine the intrarenal distribution of blood flow and the influence of many perturbations on intrarenal blood flow distribution. Initial studies of intrarenal hemodynamic responses to adrenergic stimulation were conducted using radioactive microspheres. However, a subsequent elegant series of studies by Aukland and coworkers showed that axial streaming within the architecture of the renal vasculature make interpretation of these data impossible.

Laser Doppler flowmetry has provided the technology necessary to evaluate the neurogenic control of intrarenal blood flow distribution. Early studies with ^{86}Rb uptake identified intrarenal redistribution of blood flow away from the renal medulla over a wide range of renal nerve stimulation frequencies (0 to 10 Hz). Using laser Doppler flowmetry, renal nerve stimulation of less than 2.0 Hz has been shown to shift blood flow from the medulla to the cortex. This new technology allows chronic, repetitive determinations of intrarenal hemodynamics. During ultralow frequencies of renal nerve stimulation in rats (less than 0.5 Hz), the renal medullary circulation is preferentially constricted compared with the cortical circulation. In both dogs and rats, endogenous renal sympathetic nerve activity exists in the range of 1 to 2 Hz at rest. Therefore intrarenal regional hemodynamics are likely modulated by physiologic levels of renal sympathetic nerve activity. Thus increases in renal sympathetic nerve activity beyond 0.5 Hz may significantly alter intrarenal medullary blood flow. Higher frequencies of electrical renal nerve stimulation (greater than 2.0 Hz) abolish deep medullary blood flow and begin to decrease significantly measurable whole kidney blood flow via vasoconstriction in the renal cortex. Because medullary blood flow represents only a fraction (approximately 5%) of the total renal circulation, selective medullary vasoconstriction is not manifested in measurable changes in whole kidney flow at the renal artery. However, this medullary vasoconstriction may be critical to numerous aspects of renal function, including urinary concentration and dilution and control of blood pressure.

Tubular Transport

Histochemical and autoradiographic methods have demonstrated renal sympathetic nerve fibers located in direct apposition to basement membranes of proximal tubules, Henle's loops and distal and cortical collecting tubules. Direct electrical stimulation of the renal nerves at low frequencies decreases urinary sodium excretion without changing renal perfusion pressure, RBF, or glomerular filtration rate (GFR). The advent of tubular micropuncture techniques allowed for more direct assessment of the renal nerves on tubular sodium reabsorption. Proximal tubular sodium and water transport decreased following acute renal nerve stimulation without changing single nephron GFR. Thus low-frequency renal nerve stimulation causes antinatriuresis and antidiuresis without changing whole kidney hemodynamics or filtration rate via direct activation of tubular sodium and water transport.

The mechanism of renal neurogenic tubular sodium reabsorption has been identified as a direct adrenergic response to activating tubular transport by Na^+-H^+ exchange and Na^+-K^+-ATPase mediated 2Cl-Na^+ cotransport. The antinatriuretic response to renal nerve stimulation is blocked by intrarenal arterial infusion of α-adrenergic antagonists phentolamine (α_1/α_2) and prazosin (α_1). However, this does not occur with yohimbine (α_2), rauwolscine (α_2), or β-adrenergic antagonists d,l-propranolol (β_1/β_2) or atenolol (β_1). Thus antinatriuresis during 1.0-Hz renal nerve stimulation is mediated predominantly by renal, α_1-adrenoceptors and not by α_2- or β-adrenoceptors. Newer studies have shown α_2-adrenoceptor–mediated activation of tubular sodium transport in suspensions and primary cultures of distal tubular cells. These findings have led to a renewed interest in identifying the physiologic role for α_2-adrenoceptors in the control of Na^+ balance.

Renin Release

Autoradiographic localization of innervation at juxtaglomerular granular cells implies a direct physiologic role for renal sympathetic nerves in the regulation of renin release. Electrical stimulation of renal nerves increases renin secretion even at frequencies as low as 0.5 Hz. These very low levels of nerve stimulation do not change either whole kidney blood flow or tubular sodium reabsorption, suggesting that this low stimulus is a direct effect of adrenergic neurotransmitter on the juxtaglomerular granular cells. Other indirect neurogenic methods of activating renin release include decreased perfusion pressure at the aortic or carotid baroreceptors, head-up tilt, and nonhypotensive blood volume depletion. Under each of these conditions, renal sympathetic nerve activity is increased leading to renin release that can be abolished by renal denervation. Therefore the renal nerves appear to be a physiologic controller of renin release by reflex response to stimuli such as posture and decrements in blood volume. The adrenergic mechanism(s) underlying neurally stimulated renin release have been determined as β. The nonselective β-adrenergic receptor antagonist d,l propranolol blunts the renin release response to intrarenal NE infusion. The selective β_1-receptor antagonists atenolol and metroprolol abolish the renin release response to low-level (0.5 to 1.0 Hz) renal nerve stimulation. Furthermore, the effects of renal nerve stimulation on renin release can occur at β_1 receptors located on juxtaglomerular granular cells but not indirectly via changes in macula densa sodium chloride delivery. At higher frequencies of nerve stimulation, which invoke proximal tubular sodium reabsorption by α_1-adrenoceptor stimulation, renin release is increased further as a result of decreased sodium chloride delivery to the macula densa. Thus activation of renal sympathetic nerves may directly stimulate juxtaglomerular cell renin release via β_1-adrenoceptor mechanisms. As renal nerve activity summarily increases, other nonneural mechanisms are activated at tubular (macula densa) and vascular (afferent arteriole) sensors, which serve to stimulate further the release of renin from juxtaglomerular granula cell stores.

INTRARENAL ADRENERGIC RECEPTOR MODULATION OF RENAL NEUROGENIC CONTROL OF RENAL FUNCTION

Adrenergic receptors have been identified classically as α_1-, α_2-, β_1-, and β_2-adrenoceptors. However, newer work has allowed further subclassification of α-adrenergic receptors to α_{1A}, α_{1B}, α_{1C}, and α_{1D}, as well as α_{2A}, α_{2B}, α_{2C}, and α_{2D}. Although subclassification of β-adrenoceptors have also been identified, the subclassified α-adrenergic receptors have been the primary adrenergic receptors located to date within the kidney. Classical homogenate ligand-binding techniques have been used to identify some of the subtypes of adrenoceptors in the kidney. The recent advent of microdissection of intrarenal structures and molecular techniques has provided new and useful information regarding the specific localization of the adrenoceptor subtypes in nephron segments.

By combining immunohistochemical autoradiographic techniques with ligand binding, a high density of β-adrenoceptors were identified within renal arteries and arterioles, juxtaglomerular granular cells, and proximal and distal convoluted tubules in frozen kidney sections. The renal veins contain fewer β-adrenoceptors, whereas no fluorescence was found in the glomerulus, Henle's loop, or collecting tubules. Radioligand binding has localized renal tubular β-adrenoceptors more concentrated within distal rather than proximal tubular segments. Newer autoradiographic studies with ^{125}I cyanopindolol confirm this pattern of distribution for β-adrenoceptors. The highest receptor density is located within the juxtamedullary region and in distal tubular cells of the renal cortex.

Similar radioligand-binding techniques have been used for intrarenal localization and characterization of α-adrenoceptor subtypes. Original kidney homogenate studies showed the presence of both α_1- and α_2-adrenoceptors in rat renal cortex, and α_2-adrenoceptor binding sites have been found in the glomeruli, proximal tubules, and collecting ducts. However, α_1-adrenoceptors seem to be present predominantly in the arteries and arterioles, proximal tubules, and medullary thick ascending limbs but not in the glomeruli.

The discovery of adrenergic receptor subtype-selective ligands and availability of rat adrenoceptor cDNAs has provided preliminary identification of α_1-receptor subtypes in different regions of the kidney, along with different nephron segments. Approximately 50% of the rat cortical α_1-adrenergic receptors are composed of a mixture of α_{1B} and/or α_{1D} subtypes. Using quantitative RT-PCR to evaluate different tubular α_1-receptor subtypes, approximately 66% of the α_{1A}-receptors are localized in proximal tubules and medullary thick ascending limb segments. The remaining 33% are composed of α_{1B} and α_{1D} receptors throughout the various tubular structures. Therefore the kidney exhibits a wide diversity of α_1-receptor subtypes whose expression is heterogeneous throughout nephron segments. The specific functional correlates of these subtypes remain to be conclusively identified.

AFFERENT NEUROGENIC MECHANISMS MODULATING NEURAL CONTROL OF EXTRACELLULAR FLUID VOLUME

Low-Pressure Baroreflex Regulation of Efferent Renal Sympathetic Nerve Activity

Mechanoreceptors in the cardiopulmonary region have been linked to changes in efferent renal sympathetic outflow for more than 35 years. Activation of left atrial receptors at the pulmonary vein–atrial junction via balloon distention decreases efferent renal sympathetic nerve activity via vagally mediated projections to the CNS. These receptors, located in the left atria, are capable of responding to changes in pressure and/or vascular volume via medullated and nonmedullated afferent nerve fibers such that changes in circulating blood volume modulate extracellular fluid volume via appropriate reflex increases and decreases in renal sympathetic nerve activity. Stimulation or unloading of low-pressure baroreflexes mediate modest but significant changes in renal efferent sympathetic nerve activity. As described, increased right atrial pressure will increase afferent impulses from atrial receptors and decrease renal efferent sympathetic outflow. Conversely, decreased right atrial pressure will decrease afferent nerve activity from the atrial regions and increase renal sympathetic nerve activity. Although these changes in efferent renal nerve traffic are of modest magnitude, they do provide sufficient renal neurogenic responses to change directly renin secretion via β_1 adrenoceptor stimulation and/or tubular sodium reabsorption via α_1-adrenoceptor stimulation. Thus extracellular fluid volumes may be altered directly by changing sympathetic outflow to the kidneys mediated by sensory mechanisms of vascular volume in the atria and vena cava sinus in juxtaposition with the right atrium.

High-Pressure Baroreflex Regulation of Efferent Renal Sympathetic Nerve Activity

The relationship between carotid sinus pressure and renal sympathetic nerve activity is the other major pathway by which blood volume is sensed and the neural output to the kidney can importantly alter renal function. Bursting of renal sympathetic nerve activity is synchronous with the rise and fall of arterial pressure. Thus the basal level of tonic renal nerve activity is maximal at the nadir of each arterial wave and minimal at the peak of each arterial wave. In conscious animals ingesting a normal or high-salt diet, renal nerve activity is inhibited completely during peak systole by carotid sinus and aortic arch baroreflex mechanisms. As carotid sinus pressure varies, renal nerve activity appropriately increases and decreases.

High-pressure baroreceptor modulation of renal function is mediated by reduction of carotid sinus pressure, eliciting reflex activation of efferent renal sympathetic nerve activity coupled with concomitant decreases in the renal excretion of sodium. The antinatriuretic response occurs in the absence of measurable changes in renal perfusion pressure, RBF, or GFR. Renal excretion of sodium also decreases after 60-degree head-up tilt. This antinatriuresis was not mediated by low-pressure baroreflexes traversing vagal afferents, as is evidenced by the failure of bilateral vagotomy to attenuate or prevent the response. In both cases, bilateral renal denervation did abolish the antinatriuresis, verifying the neurogenic nature of the reflex. Thus the neural control of renal function is under the constant influence of high-pressure baroreflex modulation of renal sympathetic outflow. High-pressure baroreflexes not only maintain basal renal nerve traffic but also are critical to the upregulation and downregulation of overall renal neurogenic tone.

RENORENAL REFLEXES AND RENAL AFFERENT NERVES

The renorenal reflexes represent a large class of neurogenic functions of the kidney where responses occurring in one kidney result from direct neural actions mediated by mechanisms derived from the same (ipsilateral) or opposite (contralateral) kidney. The kidneys contain both mechanoreceptors, which respond to changes in intrarenal pressure, and chemoreceptors, which sense renal ischemia and/or changes in the chemical environment of the renal interstitium. Stimulation of both mechanoreceptors and chemoreceptors may mediate reflex neurogenic changes in renal function of either the ipsilateral and/or the contralateral kidney. These changes directly influence the control of extracellular fluid volume. Functional existence of the renorenal reflexes was first demonstrated by unilateral renal denervation eliciting an ipsilateral diuresis and natriuresis, and a simultaneous contralateral antidiuresis and natriuresis associated with an increase in contralateral efferent renal nerve activity. The sodium and water conserving effects of the contralateral kidney were abolished by subsequent contralateral renal denervation. This indicated that the response elicited by unilateral renal denervation caused neurogenic contralateral sodium and water retention.

Many of the renorenal reflex responses to unilateral renal denervation have been corroborated by direct electrical stimulation of afferent nerve fibers from one kidney. The sum of evidence to date documents that afferent renal nerves exert a tonic inhibition of contralateral renal nerve activity promoting sodium and water retention from the opposite kidney.

SODIUM INTAKE AND NEUROGENIC REGULATION OF EXTRACELLULAR FLUID VOLUME

The physiologic consequences of maintaining normal extracellular fluid balance contain a significant and critical neurogenic component. Renal efferent nerve activity responses to increased or decreased sodium intake are associated with inverse changes in urinary sodium excretion. Following a step-decrease in sodium intake in conscious dogs, renal efferent nerve activity increases within 8 hours. This neurogenic activation is associated with a simultaneous and inverse decrease in urinary sodium excretion (Fig. 5.1). The renal neurogenic response to a step-decrease in sodium intake becomes maximal within 10 hours. This is approximately the same time period in which the antinatriuretic response is also maximal. The rapid changes in urinary sodium excretion are abolished by bilateral renal denervation. In the absence of renal nerve traffic, regulation of urinary sodium excretion is mediated solely by long-term controllers of extracellular fluid volume, including humoral factors, RBF, GFR, and physical forces (i.e., oncotic pressure).

In similar studies using step increases in sodium intake, the neural and nonneural factors mediating the rate of achieving sodium balance and regulation of extracellular fluid volume have been semiquantitated. These quantitative effects are calcu-

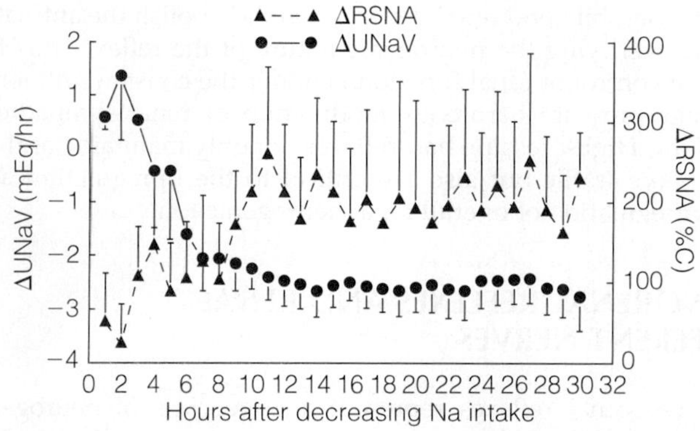

Figure 5.1. Hourly changes in urinary sodium excretion *(UNaV)* and renal sympathetic nerve activity *(RSNA)* during the first 30 hours after a step decrease in Na intake. Changes in RSNA are depicted by triangles and changes in UNaV by circles.

lated by comparing the rate of achieving sodium balance of conscious animals with innervated and denervated kidneys in the first 72 hours after a step increase in sodium intake. In the absence of renal neurogenic controllers of urinary sodium excretion, the rate of achieving sodium balance is significantly delayed (Fig. 5.2). The neural component of the summed controllers of sodium balance (and consequently extracellular fluid volume) has been estimated at approximately 35% of the total sodium intake. Thus the central-neural regulation of extracellular fluid volume is critical to the overall rate of achieving sodium balance. Because the regulation of extracellular fluid volume is vital to the functioning of the organism, in particular the cardiovascular system, numerous other intrinsic and extrinsic renal factors mediate changes in urinary sodium excretion and contribute substantially to the overall sodium balance. The sum total of these controllers thereby provides important redundancy to this regulatory system (Fig. 5.3). Thus renal efferent nerve traffic is primarily critical to the control of the rate at which sodium balance is achieved during increases and decreases in sodium intake, whereas other long-term controllers of sodium excretion maintain the appropriate level of sodium excretion.

The multiple effects of dietary sodium intake on the controllers of arterial blood pressure have been the subject of myriad investigations. In addition to the assorted individual

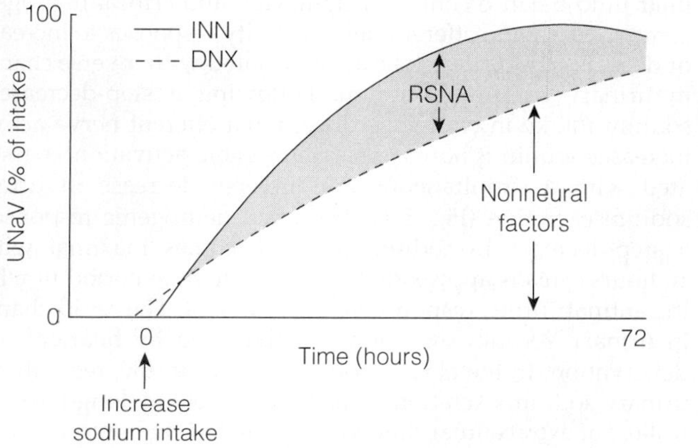

Figure 5.2. Hourly changes in urinary sodium excretion *(UNaV)* in rats with innervated *(INN)* and denervated *(DNX)* kidneys for 72 consecutive hours after a step increase in sodium intake. Stippled area represents sodium excretion response that can be attributed to inhibition of renal

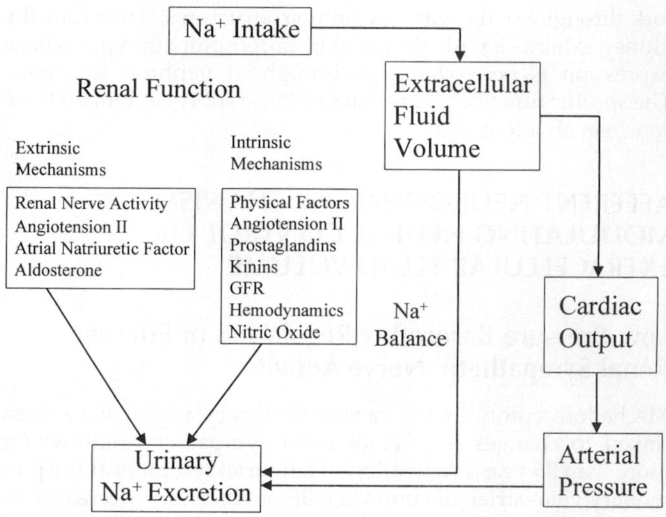

Figure 5.3. Major factors modulating urinary sodium excretion as a function of the regulation of extracellular fluid volume. *GFR,* glomerular filtration rate.

effects of sodium intake on arterial pressure controllers, complex interactions exist between sodium intake, angiotensin II, and renal sympathetic nerve activity in the control of extracellular fluid volume and, consequently, arterial blood pressure (Fig. 5.3). In view of this complexity, many studies have restricted their focus to a particular organ system (e.g., CNS, kidney, baroreceptors) in sodium deplete or replete animal models. Excess sodium intake impairs reflex chronotropic responses to intravenous phenylephrine infusions and diminishes low-pressure cardiopulmonary receptor gain during volume expansion. Thus renal sympathetic nerve activity is already elevated in animals with low dietary sodium intake to such an extent that the overall baroreflex control of renal sympathetic nerve activity is critically altered. In this regard, renal nerve stimulation at 0.5, 1.0, and 2.0 Hz elicits an exaggerated renin release response in sodium restriction and an attenuated renin release response in sodium excess. Thus, under conditions in which humoral factors are maximized for sodium retention (i.e., low sodium), renal nerve stimulation enhances renin release. Conversely, under conditions that lead to sodium loss (i.e., high sodium intake), the renin release during renal nerve stimulation is suppressed.

There are several pathophysiologic conditions in which altered control of renal efferent sympathetic nerve activity contributes significantly to an imbalance in the regulation of sodium excretion. This consequently leads to excess fluid and water retention. These diseases that represent major edema-forming states include congestive heart failure, cardiac tamponade, nephrotic syndrome, and cirrhosis of the liver. In each of these pathophysiologic conditions, one or a combination of the controllers of urinary sodium excretion identified in Fig. 5.3 may contribute to the overall extracellular fluid volume status. Activation of renal sympathetic outflow has been identified as a significant factor in promoting sodium and water retention, edema formation, and further pathogenesis of all of these conditions. The activation of renal sympathetic outflow functions as a consequence of afferent sensory signals, which are responding to overall cardiovascular dysfunction. In this regard, the rate of preventing complete cardiovascular collapse may be increased significantly under conditions in which renal sympathetic outflow is substantially elevated. Thus, even in conditions in which overall cardiovascular function is declining, activation of renal sympathetic nerve activity may importantly circumvent more rapid dysfunction and loss of blood pressure and/or cardiac output.

Selected Readings

DiBona GF. Role of renal nerves in edema formation. *News Physiol Sci* 1994; 9:183–188.

This basic review provides primary documentation that several pathophysiologic states resulting in extracellular fluid volume expansion and edema formation contain significant aberrations in the control of renal sympathetic outflow. Furthermore, studies describe how altered reflex regulation of renal nerve traffic may contribute to the retention of salt and water and ultimately influence overall cardiovascular function.

DiBona GF, Kopp UC. Neural control of renal function. *Physiol Rev* 1997;77:75–197.

This comprehensive review of the neural control of renal function provides up-to-date information on the critical nature of renal sympathetic nerve activity and its effects on the overall regulation of tubular and vascular function. The review not only provides an exhaustive description of the early work of neurogenic factors mediating kidney function but also presents up-to-date examples of current research areas. The review presents the most comprehensive synopsis of the control of afferent and efferent renal neurogenic mechanisms.

Osborn JL. Relation between sodium intake, renal function and the regulation of arterial pressure. *Hypertension* 1991;17(Suppl I):I91–I96.

The hypothesis that important interactions exist between renal nerve traffic, sodium and water balance, and the pathology of hypertension is presented in this review. Sodium intake is described as a critical controller of renal sympathetic nerve traffic and as a potential mediator of renal neurogenic hypertension. The review also surveys the importance of renal sympathetic outflow as an influence on the development of chronically elevated blood pressure.

Osborn JL, Plato CF, Gordin E, et al. Long-term increases in renal sympathetic nerve activity and hypertension. *Clin Exp Pharmacol Physiol* 1997;24:72–76.

This original manuscript provides the evidence that chronic and selective elevation of renal neurotransmitters will increase arterial pressure. The hypertension is sustained and does not result in expansion of extracellular fluid volume. The study presents primary evidence for the development of renal neuroadrenergic hypertension.

CHAPTER 6

General Principles of Renal Tubular Transport

W. Brian Reeves and Thomas E. Andreoli

The homeostatic role of the kidney in regulating the volume and composition of body fluids is the net result of discrete transport processes that occur in series along the length of individual nephrons. Thus, despite large temporal variations in the intake and generation of solutes and water, the kidney is able to regulate the osmotic and solute concentrations of body fluids within the narrow range compatible with life. This regulatory capacity proceeds from the ability of the mammalian kidney to elaborate a final urine that is either dilute or concentrated relative to plasma and that contains regulated quantities of solutes and buffers.

Three basic processes are involved in the formation of urine: glomerular filtration, tubular reabsorption, and tubular secretion. Glomerular filtration has been dealt with in Chapter 3. As a result of glomerular filtration, the fluid that enters the initial portions of the nephron represents an ultrafiltrate of plasma. The composition of the final urine results from serial absorptive and secretory processes across the tubular epithelium. We shall direct our attention to a necessarily brief overview of the cellular components of, and the mechanisms involved in, these tubular transport processes, and to the driving forces responsible for transepithelial transport of electrolytes and nonelectrolytes. The general principles of transport discussed in the following paragraphs apply equally well to a variety of transporting epithelia in addition to the renal tubular epithelium. The interested reader is invited to consult the selected references cited at the end of this chapter for a more complete discussion.

BIOMEMBRANES

Transepithelial tubular transport involves the movement of substrates either through the paracellular pathway or transcellularly. Transcellular transport processes necessitate the movement of these substrates across the plasma membrane barriers that function to bound, and maintain constant, the internal composition of the cell. Transcellular movement of substrates also provides the driving force for transepithelial transport that occurs via paracellular pathways. The capabilities of biologic membranes to participate in transport functions derive from specialized permeability characteristics of membranes and from specialized membrane transport proteins. A logical starting point for the description of the principles involved in the translocation of substrate across membranes is a brief exposition of the anatomy of biologic membranes and the central role played by water in the formation and function of biomembranes.

Characteristics of Water

Two particular features of liquid water contribute to its unique suitability as a biologic solvent. As shown in Fig. 6.1, the water molecule assumes isosceles triangular rather than planar geometry. The hydrogen–oxygen bond angle of 104.5 degrees is the consequence of asymmetric charge distribution. Specifically, the distribution of electrons results in a positive charge near each hydrogen atom, and the oxygen atom contains a lone pair of unshared electrons. Thus the electrically neutral water molecule is endowed with a relatively high dipole moment, which reflects this highly polarized configuration.

In an applied electric field, water molecules orient themselves, thereby dissipating in part the external field. The large dipole moment for water also gives rise to a high dielectric constant for liquid water. The dielectric constant is a measure of the forces between charged particles of a particular medium. As the dielectric constant increases, there is a reduction in the force between charged particles.

Liquid water is an effective solvent for electrolytes partly because it damps, because of its high dielectric constant, and because of electrostatic interactions between oppositely charged groups. Sodium and chloride, for example, are strongly ionized in water, which forms hydration shells around individual ions and acts as an insulator separating Na^+ and Cl^-. Thus water is eminently suitable as a biologic solvent. In contrast, charged species will be virtually insoluble in liquids with very small dielectric constants (e.g., the interior of a pure lipid bilayer) because of the lack of similar offsetting effects on their electrostatic interactions.

A second property of liquid water relevant to a consideration of membrane transport processes is the so-called hydrophobic effect. The hydrophobic effect refers to the tendency for nonpolar hydrocarbon tail groups of phospholipids, which lack significant hydrogen binding capability, to be expelled from liquid water, that is, to be squeezed out of solution. Biomembranes are composed primarily of lipids and proteins. Lipids such as phos-

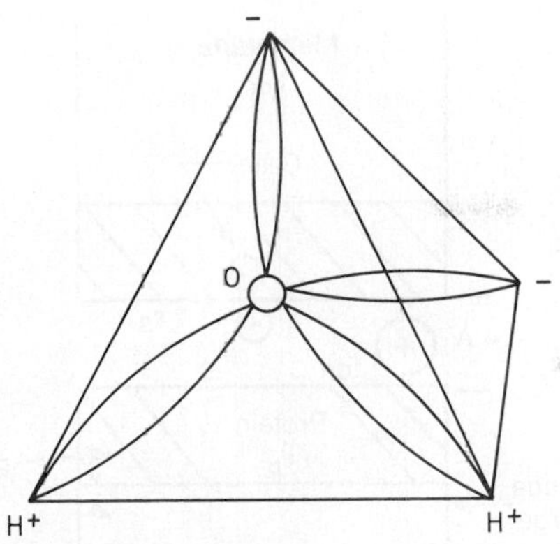

Figure 6.1. Schematic representation of the tetrahedral structure of water and consequent charge polarization. Two sets of electron orbitals are involved in the covalent O-H bond. The remaining two orbitals each contain a pair of unshared oxygen electrons.

phoglycerides and sphingolipids are amphipathic because they contain a polar head group, which is soluble in water, and a hydrophobic tail, which is not water soluble. As a consequence of this polarity, amphipathic substances tend to orient themselves so as to form hydrogen bonds with water. One orientation that phospholipids adopt is that of a bilayer in which the hydrophobic polar tails form the core of a lamella; the hydrophilic head groups, situated at the lipid–water interface, form hydrogen bonds with water. This lipid bilayer configuration serves as the fundamental structural unit for biological membranes.

Organization of Biomembranes

A theoretical scheme that can account for many of the physical, chemical, and physiologic properties of biomembranes is the fluid mosaic model of membrane structures. The essential features of the fluid mosaic model are that the lipid components of the membranes are structured as a bilayer; that the protein constituents are largely amphipathic; and that the membrane constituents are arranged in a fluid array and, hence, may be subject to structural changes.

The first requirement is fulfilled as a direct physical consequence of phospholipid dispersion in aqueous media. The requirement that membrane proteins be amphipathic suggests that the hydrophobic portion of membrane proteins will be anchored partially within the membrane within the domain of the hydrophobic lipid tail. It also suggests that the hydrophilic portions of the protein molecule will project into the aqueous medium surrounding the membrane. Certain proteins are sufficiently large to span the membrane, and thus contain hydrophilic portions within both the cytoplasm and the extracellular aqueous environments, and a hydrophobic portion spanning the membrane.

A lipid bilayer constitutes a huge energy barrier to the transmembrane flow of hydrophilic species. The magnitude of this barrier is greater than the energy required for the free diffusion of a solute in an aqueous environment. It therefore follows that transport across biomembranes occurs principally via specialized aqueous pathways. The proteins contained within the lipid bilayer are important mediators of transmembrane transport and provide an ideal locus for the regulation of transport.

Transport can occur also via bulk movement of quanta of aqueous solutions through the processes of exocytosis and endocytosis. The former can accomplish the expulsion into the extracellular fluid of substances stored within cytoplasmic organelles; the latter might trap a quanta of extracellular fluid or an extracellular ligand and transport it into the cell. These processes, which involve primarily rearrangements of portions of the lipid bilayer, appear to be dependent on the segregation of lipids within the membrane, which are initiated by specialized membrane proteins (e.g., clathrin) and directed by the intracellular cytoskeleton. Of the three principal mediators of transport, proteins, lipids, and cytoskeleton, we discuss in detail only the proteins.

Membrane Proteins

Membrane proteins can be categorized as peripheral or integral according to the ease with which they dissociate from membrane lipid constituents. This biochemical differentiation of membrane protein subtypes is physiologically relevant. Peripheral and integral proteins appear to perform different functions as determined by their association with different domains within the lipid bilayer. Proteins can associate with the lipid bilayer in a number of ways. Transmembrane proteins extend through the lipid membrane as one or more α helices. Other proteins may attach to the lipid bilayer via covalent linkage to fatty acid chains or phosphatidylinositol, and some are associated indirectly via noncovalent interactions with other membrane proteins.

Peripheral proteins may be found on either the cytoplasmic or noncytoplasmic surfaces of plasma and mitochondrial membranes, are easily dissociated from the lipid constituents of membranes, and are associated preferentially with the hydrophilic domains (polar head groups) of lipid bilayers or with other integral membrane proteins. Only certain peripheral proteins on the cytoplasmic surfaces of membranes have been well characterized to date. The latter most notably include the proteins of the cytoplasmic surface of the red blood cell plasma membrane and the clathrin proteins associated with coated pits.

The cytoplasmic peripheral membrane proteins of the red blood cell function either as sites of attachment for certain cytoplasmic structures, such as the cytoskeleton, or as enzymes involved exclusively in intracellular processes. Spectrin, for example, forms the infrastructure of the red blood cell cytoskeleton. Spectrin is bound via attachment proteins, such as ankyrin and actin, to the integral red blood cell membrane proteins band 3 and band 4.1.

Similar cytoskeleton-associated proteins have been identified in other cell types, including epithelial cells. None of these proteins seems to operate directly as a transporter. However, the interaction of cytoskeleton-associated proteins with certain integral membrane transport proteins, such as Na^+-K^+-ATPase, may have important effects on the function of the transport protein. In addition, cytoskeleton-associated proteins are important participants in endocytotic and exocytotic processes that involve organellar and tubular structures. Similarly, the peripheral protein clathrin appears to participate in receptor-mediated endocytosis and has been identified in more than 25 such systems in many cell types.

In contrast to peripheral proteins, integral proteins either span the membrane and therefore contain a hydrophobic portion that is tightly associated with the hydrophobic domain (nonpolar tail groups) of the lipid bilayer or they are covalently attached to moieties within the lipid bilayer (e.g., fatty acids or phosphatidylinositol). Isolation of these proteins requires detergents that disrupt the integrity of the lipid bilayer. Integral, or intrinsic, proteins may represent receptors for hormone recognition or pathways for transmembrane transport of hydrophilic solutes that would otherwise be excluded from the membrane. According to this view, water and electrolytes move through the α-helical structures and interspaces within proteins traversing the hydrophobic lipid domain.

Included among integral membrane proteins are most proteins known to subserve major transport functions, such as

Na^+-K^+-ATPase, Ca^{2+}-ATPase, band 3 of the erythrocyte membrane (an anion exchange protein), and channels for both water and electrolytes.

Transport of substrates by integral membrane proteins may proceed via discrete conformational alterations in the protein (carrier mode) or via potential-driven diffusion through large aqueous pores, or channels, established by the protein (pore mode). A channel may be thought of as an intrinsic membrane protein that creates a transmembrane hydrophilic pathway distinguished by its high dielectric constant, thereby permitting energy-efficient transfer of substrate between two extramembranous aqueous phases. A carrier protein may be defined similarly. Channels are operationally distinguished from carriers by their higher maximal transport rates (10^6 ions/sec versus 10^3 to 10^5 ions/sec).

The Na^+-K^+-ATPase is an imperfect paradigm for the carrier mode of operation. Occupancy by the substrate ions Na^+ and K^+ and the phosphorylation-dephosphorylation of the Na^+-K^+-ATPase protein complex produces a series of conformational alterations in the complex, which results in net transmembrane flux of Na^+ and K^+. The cations move in the aqueous environment created by the complex, and these ions are accumulated against their respective electrochemical gradients.

Diptheria toxin is a paradigm for the pore mode of transport. The pore created by diptheria toxin is sufficiently large to allow nonselective transmembrane flux of water and electrolytes. An idealized model of a membrane channel is shown in Fig. 6.2. Most channels are sufficiently narrow that free diffusion of substrate is partially limited by ion–ion interactions within the aqueous channels. The distribution of charge at the channel openings or along the length of the channel, as well as the actual physical size of the channel, will selectively favor the passage of certain ions. These features will confer on the channel the property of selectivity, that is, the tendency to allow only certain ionic species to pass through the channel. Furthermore, changes in the transmembrane potential, or changes in the nature of the charged species binding to or in the vicinity of the pore, will influence the charge distribution of the channel protein. The resultant conformational shifts and hence changes in pore configuration, may influence closing or opening of the channel to the transported substrate. This property of channels is known as gating. Gating may be determined by transmembrane potential, the presence of competing ions, or the binding of certain ions to sites on the channel, such as calcium gating of the potassium channel.

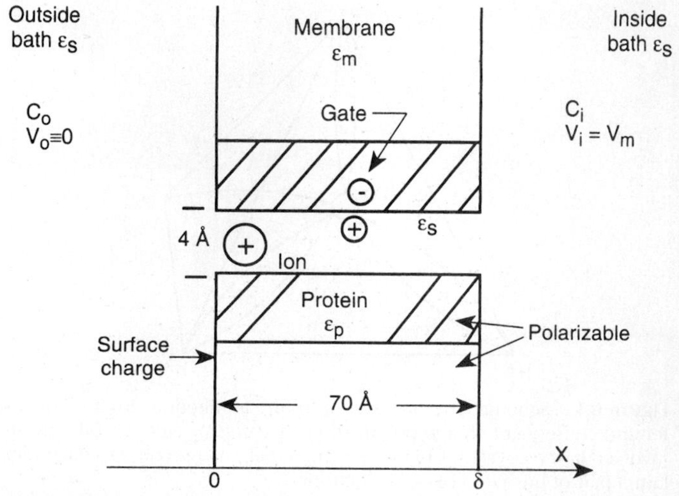

Figure 6.2. Idealized representation of a membrane channel. Permeation of the ion will be determined by (a) pore size relative to ion size and charge density, (b) surface charge and polarity of the channels, and (c) the gating characteristics of the channel. (From Cooper K, Jakobsson E, Wolynes P. *Prog Biophys Molec Biol* 1985;46:51–96.)

In conclusion, the bilayer configuration of lipid membranes follows as a direct consequence of the molecular properties of water on amphipathic molecules. Specific transport functions are imparted to the lipid bilayer as a result of the insertion of proteins with unique and specialized characteristics. The function of the protein can be modulated under the influence of lipid–lipid, lipid–protein, and protein–protein interactions.

Finally, it should be mentioned that the synthesis of membrane proteins is under genetic control. Thus alterations in an amino acid sequence, for instance, may have clinically important consequences if the protein containing the altered or deleted amino acid sequence is involved in the recognition of a hormone or the transport of ions or metabolic substrates. A growing number of disorders are now known to be caused by mutations in hormone receptors or transport proteins within the kidney (Table 6.1).

TABLE 6.1. Genetic Diseases of Renal Epithelial Transport

Disease	Affected Gene Product(s)	Primary Transport Defect	Clinical Features
Bartter syndrome	ROMK potassium channel Na-K-Cl cotransporter ClC-K2 Cl^- channel	Decreased TAL NaCl absorption	Hyperreninemia, hypotension, hypokalemia, metabolic alkalosis
Gittleman syndrome	NaCl cotransporter	Decreased DCT NaCl absorption	Hypotension, hypokalemia, hypocalciuria
Liddle syndrome	ENaC sodium channel	Increased CCT sodium reabsorption	Hypertension, hypokalemia, metabolic alkalosis
Pseudohypoaldosteronism, type I	ENaC sodium channels Mineralocorticoid receptor	Decreased CCT sodium reabsorption	Hypotension, hyperkalemia, metabolic acidosis
Distal renal tubular acidosis	AE1 Cl^--HCO_3 exchanger	Decreased H^+ secretion in collecting duct	Metabolic acidosis, hypokalemia
Nephrogenic diabetes insipidus	V_2 vasopressin receptor Aquaporin 2 water channel	Decreased CCT water permeability	Polyuria, hypernatremia
Cystinuria	D2H dibasic amino acid transporter	Decreased proximal reabsorption of cystine	Urinary tract calculi
Dent's disease	ClC-5 Cl^- channel	Unclear	Hypercalciuria, renal stones, low molecular weight, proteinuria

CCT, cortical collecting tubule; DCT, distal convoluted tubule; TAL, thick ascending limb.

EPITHELIAL CELL STRUCTURE AND TRANSPORT

The operation of the mechanisms responsible for fluid and solute transport by the kidney depends on the nature of the cells that comprise the nephron. Each nephron segment is composed of a single layer of lining epithelial cells. The differences in the cells lining the various nephron segments impart each segment with distinct transport capabilities. Renal epithelial cells, like other epithelia, are inherently polarized. The properties of the membranes that face the urinary space (apical) differ from the membranes that face the interstitium (basolateral). It is precisely this asymmetry in the transport properties of the two sides of the cell that enables the renal epithelium to perform vectorial transport of solutes, that is, the net transport of a solute either from the urinary space to the blood or vice versa. By contrast, nonpolarized cells, such as nerve, muscle, or red blood cells, are capable of cellular accumulation and extrusion only. The fundamental anatomic features of a prototypical epithelial cell are shown in Fig. 6.3. They include a luminal (apical or mucosal) membrane facing the urinary surface and a basolateral (serosal, peritubular, or contraluminal) membrane facing the interstitium. Tight junctions connect adjacent cells near their apical poles and prevent the movement of lipids and proteins between the apical and basolateral membrane domains.

Although luminal and basolateral cell membranes are similar in overall lipid and protein composition, they differ strikingly in the array of transport proteins they contain. The sodium–potassium exchange pump Na^+-K^+-ATPase, for instance, is located exclusively along basolateral cell membranes. This asymmetric distribution of Na^+-K^+-ATPase plays a critical role in energizing transcellular transport.

Transport may proceed either through cells or between adjoining cells. Transcellular transport is conservative. Substrates are transported by either primary active or secondary active transport pathways. The second major transport pathway is paracellular. When tight junctions are permeable to a given solute, that solute may gain direct access to the lateral intercellular space without traversing the luminal cell membrane. The paracellular pathway is the major route for passive ion transport. The electrical resistance offered by tight junctions is generally much less than that of the individual cell membranes. By providing this low-resistance or shunt pathway, high electrical voltages against which sodium, for instance, must be transported do not develop. That is, the electrogenic effect of rheogenic transport may be dissipated through a shunt pathway. Similarly, in hydraulically leaky epithelia, such as the proximal renal tubule, the gallbladder and the ileum, water flow proceeds primarily via a paracellular route.

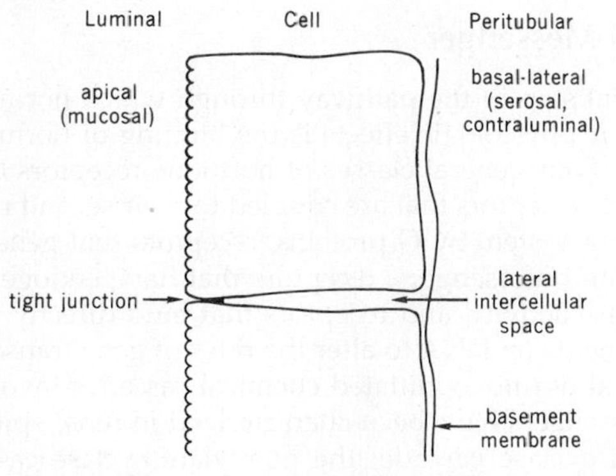

Figure 6.3. Diagrammatic representation of an epithelial cell with salient topographic features.

Net transport also can be regulated by adjusting the rate of solute backleak across the tight junction into the tubular lumen. Furthermore, as a consequence of the differential permeability for anions and cations across the tight junction, an electrical diffusion potential will develop what, depending on its magnitude and orientation, may either accelerate or retard the movement of other ions. Finally, different reflection coefficients among solute components on either side of the membrane (tight junction) may lead to osmotic water flow across the junctional complex. Conversely, the hydraulic permeability of the tight junction may influence solute flow by solvent drag, that is, the net transport of solutes coupled to the bulk movement of solution.

Although the same general principles govern solute movement in the nephron as in other transporting epithelia, the particular geometry of the renal tubule imposes important constraints on these processes. As a consequence of its cylindrical geometry, the luminal volume is small relative to the apical membrane surface area containing it. In the proximal tubule, this surface area-to-volume ratio is further amplified by the presence of a prominent microvillar brush border. Consequently, the axial luminal fluid composition can be modified dramatically as a result of radial transepithelial transport events occurring over a short length of renal tubule. Bicarbonate, glucose, and amino acids, for instance, are normally absorbed from the proximal tubular fluid within a short distance of the glomerulus. However, because the rate of absorptive transport is limited, the axial flow rate can alter the rate of radial solute transport significantly. Thus, as glomerular filtration rate and hence axial flow increase, a greater portion of the nephron is exposed to a luminal concentration of solute above the maximal absorptive capacity of that segment. Therefore the absolute quantity of substrate that can be absorbed by the proximal convoluted tubule is increased.

HORMONAL REGULATION AND TRANSPORT

The net transport of water and solutes across renal epithelia depends on two features of cell function that can be exploited precisely because of the arrangement of these specialized cells into ordered epithelial structures. These two features, the polarity of the cells and the activity (or number) of transport proteins (transport units), are to a large degree under hormonal control. Transport of a particular substrate may be increased or decreased by two general processes. These are either insertion of additional, fully functional, substrate-specific transport units into membranes, or modification of preexisting transport units that increase the functional activity of each unit.

These two processes may be initiated by hormones or other biochemical signals either directly as a consequence of hormone binding to, activation of, or induction of the mRNA for the proteins responsible for the physiologic effect; or via a second messenger released as a consequence of hormone binding to its receptor. The messenger subsequently promotes a physiologic response at a site physically distinct from the hormone–receptor complex.

The wide spectrum of hormone-mediated physiologic responses characteristic of epithelia are mediated through a limited number of signal transduction pathways. The major signal transduction pathways that have been studied in renal epithelial cells include (a) the adenyl cyclase–cyclic adenosine monophosphate (cAMP) pathway; (b) the guanylate cyclase–cyclic guanosine monophosphate (cGMP) pathway; (c) the phosphoinositide pathway; (d) the receptor tyrosine kinase pathway; (e) the direct regulation of gene expression produced by hormone–receptor binding to regulatory elements on DNA; and (f) receptor–ligand

TABLE 6.2. Hormone-Receptor–Mediated Processes in Renal Epithelia

Class	Second Primary Effect	Primary Effect of Messenger	Second Messenger	Example	Physiologic Effect
Membrane receptor–adenyl cyclase	Stimulates or inhibits production of cAMP via G_s and G_i proteins	cAMP	Promotes cAMP-dependent phosphorylation of effector proteins	ADH (V_2 receptor)	Increases water permeability of CCT
Membrane receptor–guanylate cyclase	Stimulates production of cGMP	cGMP	Promotes cGMP-dependent phosphorylation of effector proteins; direct effects on effector proteins	ANP	Inhibits sodium absorption in the medullary collecting duct
Membrane receptor–phophoinositide cascade	Activates PLC to release DAG and IP_3	DAG IP_3	Activates protein kinase C; phosphorylation of effector proteins; stimulates release of intracellular calcium	PGE_2	Inhibits sodium transport in CCT
Membrane receptor–tyrosine kinase	Activates kinase activity of receptor	?	Cascade of phosphorylation—eventually phosphorylation of effector proteins (e.g., transcription factors)	Insulin	Stimulates Na^+-K^+-ATPase activity
Cytosolic or nuclear receptors	Activated receptors bind to DNA, alter gene transcription	None	None	Aldosterone	Increases synthesis of Na^+-K^+-ATPase

ADH, antidiuretic hormone; ANP, atrial natriuretic peptide; cAMP, cyclic adenosine monophosphate; CCT, cortical collecting duct; cGMP, cyclic guanosine monophosphate; DAG, diacylglycerol; IP3, inositol 1,4,5-triphosphate; PLC, phospholipase C.

mediated endocytosis. Some of the features of these pathways are listed in Table 6.2.

Several of these pathways involve the activation of specific protein kinases, such as cAMP-dependent protein kinase, and result in the phosphorylation of specific proteins. The resultant physiologic response is not specific to the second messenger, but rather is specified by the cell in which the response occurs. That is, in a given cell, a second messenger will produce a given response. For example, the antidiuretic hormone–induced production of the second messenger cAMP in the medullary thick ascending limb cell stimulates net transepithelial sodium chloride transport, whereas in the cortical collecting tubule, cAMP permits increased osmotic water flux.

These six signal transduction pathways, and the manner in which they influence renal epithelial transport, are discussed in the following paragraphs. We begin our discussion with an examination of endocytosis and exocytosis, because these processes may alter directly the surface area available for transport, as well as the basic lipid and protein composition of the membrane upon which all other types of regulation ultimately depend.

Endocytosis and Exocytosis

Membrane transport may be regulated by altering the number of transport proteins present in the cell membrane via vesicular trafficking. Such a mechanism, in which cytoplasmic tubulovesicular structures laden with membrane transport proteins fuse with the plasma membrane, plays a key role in the short-term regulation of collecting duct water permeability by vasopressin. Studies have demonstrated that in the hydrated state, aquaporin 2, the water channel of the collecting duct apical membrane, resides in vesicular structures located beneath the apical plasma membrane. Upon stimulation with vasopressin, these vesicles fuse with the apical membrane such that the aquaporin 2 molecules become integrated into the plasma membrane, thereby increasing its water permeability. At the end of the vasopressin stimulation, the process is reversed and the aquaporin 2 molecules are retrieved from the plasma membrane and recycled into the vesicular structures. A similar process serves to regulate proton transport in the distal nephron. In the mammalian collecting tubule and in the turtle bladder, for example, physiologic perturbations that increase the rate of acidification (i.e., hydrogen ion transport) also stimulate the insertion of tubulovesicular structures into the apical membrane by the process of exocytosis. The tubulovesicular structures contain hydrogen ion transporters (the H^+-ATPase) that may mediate the increased rate of hydrogen ion secretion. In response to an alkaline shift in pH, the reverse process is initiated in the turtle bladder and mammalian collecting tubule. That is, endocytotic removal of H^+-ATPase transporters from the apical membrane. The targeting and fusion of vesicles with the plasma membrane appears to be mediated through specific proteins known as SNAREs on both the target membrane and the vesicle membrane. The interactions between the target membrane SNAREs (t-SNARE) and the vesicular SNAREs (v-SNARE) are believed to ensure that vesicles dock and fuse at the appropriate sites.

Second Messenger

The initial step in the pathway through which hormones produce their physiologic effects is the binding of hormone to its receptor. Four general classes of hormone receptors have been described: receptors that are coupled to their second messenger generating system by G proteins, receptors that generate their own second messengers, receptors that have endogenous protein kinase activity, and receptors that bind directly to regulatory elements on DNA to alter the rates of gene transcription.

Several hormone-initiated chemical cascades involving second messengers have been characterized in renal epithelia: the adenylyl cyclase cascade; the guanylate cyclase cascade; the phosphoinositide cascade; and the protein tyrosine–kinase cascade (Fig. 6.4). Some examples of the various pathways in renal

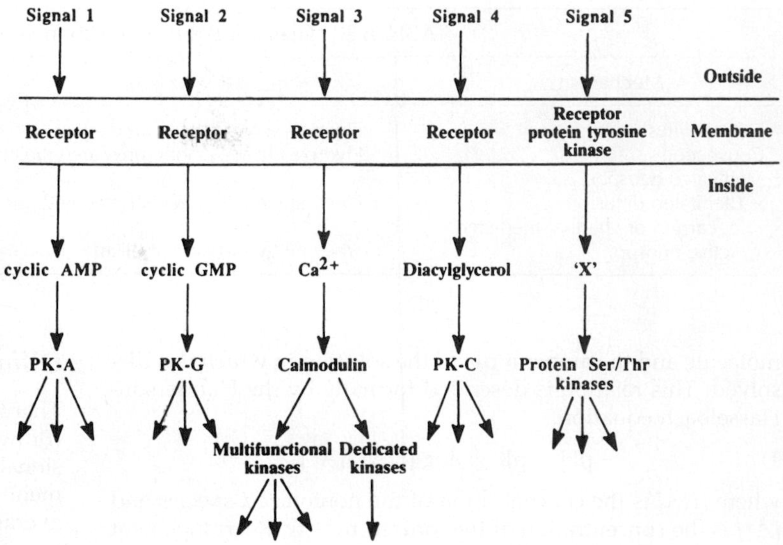

Figure 6.4. Five of the signal-transduction pathways that operate in renal epithelial cells. *PK-A,* cAMP-dependent protein kinase; *PK-G,* cGMP-dependent protein kinase; *PK-C,* protein kinase C; *"X,"* phosphorylated intermediates that vary depending on the particular receptor. (From Cohen P. *Trends Biochem Sci* 1992;17:408–414, with permission.)

epithelia include the stimulation of cAMP production in proximal tubule cells by parathyroid hormone, the stimulation of cGMP production by atrial natriuretic peptide in inner medullary-collecting duct cells, and the activation of phosphoinositide hydrolysis by vasopressin in medullary-collecting duct cells.

A number of important features are common to these hormone-induced second messenger cascades. First, these cascades have stimulatory and inhibitory elements that may be induced separately by different hormones or that may act directly as negative effectors on the opposite limb. Second, the second messengers function in part through activation of specific protein kinases that catalyze the phosphorylation of specific protein substrates. In addition, some receptors, such as the insulin receptor and the epidermal growth factor receptor, are themselves protein kinases that become activated upon binding to hormone. As a consequence of phosphorylation, a protein substrate will undergo a conformational change in structure and a shift in functional activity. The protein substrates may be the actual transport proteins or may be associated effector proteins that, once activated, secondarily alter the related transport protein. Third, the second messenger may cause either an increase or a decrease in the activity of a particular transporter. The effect of the second messenger is cell type specific. Fourth, activation by phosphorylation consumes energy as adenosine triphosphate (ATP). Fifth, the net activity of the phosphorylated proteins will be related directly to the degree of phosphorylation, which is a function of the relative rates of phosphorylation and dephosphorylation. The rate of phosphorylation is under hormonal control; the rate of dephosphorylation may also be under hormonal control. Sixth, hormones that regulate function by way of a second messenger cascade will effect a physiologic response relatively rapidly because activation and deactivation involve preformed constituents. In other words, activation does not require the production of new protein.

In contrast to the extracellular location of receptors for hormones that operate via second messengers, steroid hormones, either glucocorticoid or mineralocorticoid, and thyroid hormone bind to intracellular receptors. As a consequence of receptor binding, these hormones directly induce a change in gene expression as reflected in the increased production of specific messenger RNA. Therefore drugs that interfere with gene translation or protein production will inhibit the physiologic effects of these hormones. Furthermore, as protein production continues even in the relative absence of these hormones, the latter can often function as potentiators of other hormone responses.

Therefore a single transport process in a given cell might be regulated by multiple hormones. In the proximal convoluted tubule, for example, glucocorticoids increase the observed V_{max} for the Na^+-H^+ antiporter indicating a probable increase in the density of this transporter per unit area of apical plasma membrane. Conversely, parathyroid hormone, which modulates proximal convoluted tubule Na^+-H^+ antiporter activity via the second messenger cAMP, a cAMP-dependent protein kinase, and a Na^+-H^+ regulatory protein, inhibits the apparent transport rate per apical membrane antiporter. Thus two hormones regulate the same transport protein at two distinct loci. Such multitiered regulation is characteristic of virtually all major renal epithelial transport processes.

FACTORS AFFECTING TRANSPORT

Four characteristics of a molecule affect its ability to penetrate a membrane: (a) lipid solubility, as reflected in its partition coefficient; (b) molecular size; (c) size of the hydration shell; and (d) degree of ionization. Thus the rate of entry of nonelectrolytes into a pure lipid membrane is correlated directly with the lipid solubility of the dissolved species. This is referred to as Overton's rule. Nonpolar (hydrophobic) compounds that have a high lipid solubility penetrate faster than polar (hydrophilic) compounds. Accordingly, hydrophobic solutes traverse the lipid phase of the membrane, whereas small charged ions, such as sodium and potassium, pass through aqueous pores within the lipid matrix.

Second, the larger the molecular radius of a solute, the more restricted its penetration will be. In the case of univalent ions, the smaller the unhydrated ionic radius, the greater the associated charge density. Thus more water molecules will be held in hydration shells. Consequently, the smaller the unhydrated ionic radius, the larger the hydrated radius; therefore the more restricted its penetration.

Finally, if an electrolyte is in a nonionized form, permeation through the hydrophobic core of the membrane will be enhanced. This consideration is of particular importance for the transport by nonionic diffusion of weak organic electrolytes, such as ammonia, and for many endogenous metabolites and drugs. The degree of ionization depends on the pK_a of the

TABLE 6.3. Classification of Mechanisms of Membrane Transport

Mechanism	Driving Force	Kinetics
Simple diffusion	Electrochemical potential gradient	Proportional to concentration difference, nonsaturable
Convection	Hydrostatic or osmotic pressure gradient	Proportional to pressure difference, nonsaturable
Medicated transport		
Facilitated diffusion (carrier- or channel-mediated)	Electrochemical potential gradient	Saturable, independent of intensity of metabolism
Active transport	Free energy from metabolism	Saturable, dependent on intensity of metabolism

molecule and the ambient pH of the solution in which it is dissolved. This relation is described formally by the Henderson-Hasselbach equation.

1) $$pH = pK_a + \log [HA]/[A^-]$$

where *[HA]* is the concentration of the nonionized species and *[A⁻]* is the concentration of the ionized moiety. Rearrangement of this equation yields the following:

2) $$[A^-]/[HA] = 10^{(pH - pKa)}$$

from which it is apparent that small differences in the pH near the pK_a will effect an appreciable change in the extent to which a substance is ionized. The pK_a values for many substances of biologic importance are close to the pH encountered within the cell. Under conditions in which a pH gradient exists across a cell membrane, weak organic anions tend to accumulate in the relatively alkaline compartment whereas cations are accumulated in the relatively acidic compartment.

BASIC TRANSPORT PROCESSES

In general, basic transport mechanisms in biologic membranes can be divided into those that are primarily dissipative and those that are conservative. Diffusion, convection, and facilitative diffusion are essentially dissipative. Endocytosis/exocytosis and active transport are conservative. Table 6.3 illustrates this classification of transport mechanisms, their respective driving forces, and kinetic manifestations. A sample of the most commonly encountered terms in membrane transport, their abbreviations and dimensional units, is given in Table 6.4.

TABLE 6.4. Common Symbols Used in Transport Physiology

Symbol	Definition	Unit
J_v	Net volume flux	$cm^3\ sec^{-1}\ cm^{-2}$
J_i	Net solute flux	$mole\ sec^{-1}\ cm^{-2}$
R	Gas constant	8.314 joules $mole^{-1}$ deg K^{-1}
T	Absolute temperature	deg K (=273+degC)
ΔP	Hydrostatic pressure difference	atm
$\Delta\pi_s$	Osmotic pressure difference	atm
L_p	Hydraulic membrane permeability	cm sec^{-1} atm^{-1}
σ_s	Reflection coefficient	
P_i	Permeability coefficient	Eq sec^{-1} cm^{-1}
Ψ	Electrical potential	volt
V_e	Transepithelial electrical potential difference ($\Delta\Psi$)	volt
g	Electrical conductance	S cm^{-2}
Z	Valence	
F	Faraday constant	96,500 coulomb $mole^{-1}$

Diffusion

Thermal kinetic energy exhibited by molecules in solution (Brownian movement) provides the required energy for diffusional motion. In the absence of a vectorial driving force, movement from one side of the membrane to the other will, on the average, equal movement in the opposite direction. Thus no net transfer will occur. The driving force for net diffusional transport of nonelectrolytes is provided by the concentration gradient of the solute across the membrane. Therefore diffusion can be regarded as an equilibration process in which thermal kinetic energy dissipates a concentration gradient. Simple diffusion involves no specific interaction of the solute with the membrane.

Movement of small electrolytes via membrane channels may be thought of as primarily diffusive and can be described, in the aggregate, by the general formulations that describe simple diffusion across an epithelium. The character of ion movement through a channel will deviate from this model to the degree that movement through the channel is constrained, as might occur if ions were forced by the narrowness of the channel to move through the channel in single file. The major characteristics of selected channels that are important in renal epithelial transport are shown in Table 6.5.

For a molecule bearing a charge, the driving force for transport will be the combined chemical and electrical potential gradients. The rate of diffusional flux ($J^d{}_i$) at a given point is a product of the solute mobility (u_i), the area available for diffusion (A), the concentration (C_i), and the electrochemical potential (μ_i). Thus the generalized diffusion flux equation is as follows:

3) $$J_i{}^d = -u_i\, A\, C_i\, d(\mu_i)/dx$$

The electrochemical potential is given by the following formula:

4) $$\mu_i = RT\ln C_i + Z\, F\, \Psi$$

where *R* is the gas constant, *T* the absolute temperature, *Z* the valence of the ion, Ψ the voltage, and *F* the Faraday constant. The first term on the right side of the equation describes the chemical potential, and the second term, the electrical potential. Substituting equation 4 into equation 3 and rearranging with consideration of the Einstein relationship, $D_i = RTu_i$ (where D_i is the diffusion coefficient within the membrane), yields the following:

5) $$J^d{}_i = -D_iAC_i\,[(d\ln C_i/dx) + (Z_iF/RT)\, d\Psi/dx]$$

which is the differential form of the Nernst-Planck equation. According to this relation, diffusion is directly proportional to the coefficient of diffusion within the membrane, the concentration gradient of the solute within the membrane, and the electrical potential gradient if the solute is an electrolyte or if its transport is coupled to that of an electrolyte. The expression in brackets in equation 5 is regarded, in the terminology of irreversible thermodynamics, as the conjugate force responsible for

TABLE 6.5. Selected Characteristics of Several Renal Epithelial Ion Channels

Channel	Example	Conductance	Gating/Regulation	Selectivity	Inhibitors
Sodium	Apical membrane CCT	5–10 pS	pH, voltage, sodium, PKA	$H^+ > Na^+ >> K^+$	Amiloride
CFTR-like	Apical membrane IMCD	10 pS	ATP, PKA	$Cl^- > I^- > F^-$	Glibenclamide
Chloride	Basolateral membrane TAL	40–80 pS	ATP, PKA, Cl^-	$NO_3^- > Cl^- > I^-$	DPC, SITS
Potassium	Apical membrane TAL, CCT	20–30 pS	ATP, PKA, pH	$K^+ = Rb^+ > Na^+$	Barium, glibenclamide

CFTR, cystic fibrosis transmembrane conductance regulator; DPC, diphenylamine carboxylate; IMCD, inner medullary collecting duct; PKA, protein kinase A; pS, picosiemens; SITS, 4-acetamide-4′-isothiocyanato stilbene-2,2′disulfonic acid; TAL, thick ascending limb.

producing the flux $J^d{}_I$. Simple diffusional transport follows first-order reaction kinetics. That is, it does not exhibit saturation.

Solution of equation 5 requires explicit values for either the intramembrane chemical or electrical potential gradients. By assuming that the electrical gradient ($d\Psi/dx$) is linear, Goldman was able to integrate the Nernst-Planck flux equation to give the following:

6) $$J_i = -P_i(Z_iF/RT)V_e\,[(C^o - C^i\exp(-Z_iFV_e/RT))/ 1 - \exp(-Z_iFV_e/RT)]$$

where V_e is the transmembrane potential, $\Delta\Psi$ (where $\Delta\Psi = \Psi^i - \Psi^o$), and C^o, C^i are the solute concentrations in the two bulk phase solutions. In the absence of external current sources and where sodium, potassium, and chloride carry the bulk of the electrical current, the transmembrane electrical potential is given by the following relationship, known as the Goldman-Hodgkin-Katz (GHK) equation.

7) $$V_e = RT/F\ \ln[(P_{Na}C^o{}_{Na} + P_KC^o{}_K + P_{Cl}C^i{}_{Cl})/ (P_{Na}C^i{}_{Na} + P_KC^i{}_K + P_{Cl}C^o{}_{Cl})]$$

where the P terms are the passive permeability coefficient for the respective ions and the C terms are the ion concentrations on the two sides of the membrane.

At equilibrium, that is, in the absence of a net flux, the contribution to transepithelial electrical potential for a single electrolyte is given by the Nernst equation.

8) $$V_e = -RT/ZF\ \ln(C^o/C^i)$$

Conversely, if the transepithelial voltage is known, the equilibrium solute concentration may be calculated. This relationship defines the mutual dependence of the concentration difference and the electrical potential difference for an ion at electrochemical equilibrium. If an ion is distributed at equilibrium across a membrane, it will not participate in the generation of a voltage. Clearly, a nonelectrolyte will be at equilibrium when there is no concentration difference across the membrane.

A third approach may be applied to describe diffusive electrolyte flux. A useful equation derives directly from Ohm's Law, where the current flux (i) will be equal to the electrical driving force divided by the resistance. For an electrolyte, therefore:

9) $$i_i = g_i\,(V_m - E_i)$$

where g_i, the conductance of the membrane to the ith ion, is the inverse of the membrane resistance and where ($V_m - E_i$), the driving force, represents the displacement of the actual transmembrane voltage (V_m) from E_i, the equilibrium voltage for that ion.

This formulation of the flux equation is useful when studying ion channels because current and conductance can be measured explicitly. In that regard, Table 6.5 lists electrical parameters for selected channels. The patch clamp technique has proven to be a valuable tool to study membrane ion channels. In this technique, a small patch of plasma membrane is sealed onto the tip of a polished glass electrode. The high electrical and physical resistance of the seal between the membrane and the glass permits the detection of the very low amounts of current that pass through individual ion channels. The physical stability of the membrane–electrode seal also permits access to the cytoplasmic surface of the membrane.

By clamping the voltage across the membrane and measuring the corresponding single channel current amplitude, the conductance of the channel can be calculated using equation 9. Likewise, by determining the zero current potential in the presence of asymmetric salt solutions, the ion selectivity of the channel is given by equation 7. Ion channels also exhibit the tendency to alternate between open, or conducting, states and closed states, a process referred to as gating. Analysis of the lifetimes of the open and closed states can provide information about the mechanisms underlying channel gating. Channels may exhibit complex patterns of gating with multiple open and closed states.

In addition, the gating kinetics for a channel may be affected by the membrane voltage, permeant ion concentration, calcium ion concentration, the state of phosphorylation of the channel, the presence of regulatory substances, such as ATP, or the presence of channel inhibitors. The overall current flowing across a cell membrane through a given class of ion channels is a function of the number of active channels present (N), the open probability of each channel (P_o), the conductance of the channel (g), and the driving force for that ion:

$$I_i = N \cdot P_o \cdot g\,(V_m - E_i)$$

Accordingly, the ion current across a particular cell membrane is subject to multiple levels of regulation, such as by changes in channel density, changes in individual channel activity (e.g., produced by changes in voltage, pH, Ca^{++}, or phosphorylation), and changes in membrane voltage or in permeant ion concentration.

Convection

In contrast to simple diffusion, convective transport describes the bulk flow of solvent and solute in a given direction as a consequence of an imposed driving force, such as hydrostatic pressure. Thus convection can be regarded as an equilibration process in which hydrodynamic flow dissipates a pressure gradient; consequently, a hydrostatic or osmotic pressure gradient will drive net water movement. When the same principles described for the general case in equation 3 are applied, hydrodynamic flow may be expressed quantitatively as follows:

10) $$J_v = -L_pA\,(\Delta P + \Delta\pi)$$

where J_v is the volume flow, L_p is the hydraulic permeability of the membrane, ΔP is the hydrostatic gradient, $\Delta\pi$ is the osmotic pressure gradient, and A the effective membrane area available for volume flow. Equation 10 is the Starling equation. According to equation 10, an osmotic pressure difference is formally identical to a hydrostatic pressure difference. This equivalence is indicated in the van't Hoff relation:

11) $$\Delta\pi = -\Delta P = RT(C^{\circ} - C^{i})$$

when the solute in question is absolutely impermeant. However, solutes will exert varying degrees of osmotic pressure depending on the degree to which they penetrate membranes. The ratio of the observed osmotic pressure to that predicted from equation 11 is given by the reflection coefficient, σ, introduced by Staverman:

12) $$\sigma = \Delta\pi_{observed}/\Delta\pi_{theoretical}$$

For an absolutely impermeant solute, $\sigma = 1$, the solute is completely reflected by the membrane. By contrast, for a solute whose permeability approaches that of water, $\sigma = 0$.

Clearly, for solutes with a reflection coefficient less than unity, solute flow through an aqueous channel will be accelerated in the direction of water flow. Conversely, solute flow through a membrane will be retarded by water flow in the opposite direction. This modulation of solute flow has been termed solvent drag. The quantity of solute displaced by solvent drag (J_{SD}) may be estimated in terms of the sieving coefficient ($1 - \sigma$, the reflection coefficient) and the mean pore concentration, c, for that solute:

13) $$J_{SD} = J_v (1 - \sigma) c$$

Finally, a serious factor that may complicate the determination of permeability coefficients arises from the fact that areas immediately adjacent to a membrane are not, in general, well stirred. In the absence of complete convective mixing, the solute concentration in the unstirred region next to the membrane will be different than that in bulk solutions. Consequently, solute movement toward a membrane or away from a membrane will depend, at least in part, on diffusion within unstirred layers. Therefore the effect of an unstirred layer is to alter the actual concentration gradient across the membrane with respect to that in bulk solutions; consequently, unstirred layers may lead to inaccurate estimates of permeability coefficients.

Mediated Transport

Facilitated Diffusion

For solutes traversing large aqueous membrane pores or channels by simple diffusion, the ease of movement is regulated by the relation between molecular size and pore diameter. However, there are biologically important solutes for which transport is much faster than would be predicted on the basis of their molecular size or lipid solubility. For this reason, it has been proposed that some of these substances are transported by facilitated diffusion. This mechanism differs from simple diffusion in both its kinetics and its molecular mechanism. However, like simple diffusion, facilitated diffusion is an equilibrating process driven by an electrochemical potential gradient and is unable to effect transport against this gradient. Thus facilitated diffusion can be classified as a dissipative transport process. The membrane permeation mechanisms of facilitative diffusion involve specific interactions between the solute and the permeation site, rather than exclusively steric interactions.

Facilitated diffusion is thought to be mediated by membrane components endowed with a high degree of specificity for the transported substrate. As a consequence, facilitated transport mechanisms exhibit competitive inhibition by structurally related compounds. Furthermore, the rate of transport will not increase linearly as the solution concentration of transported solute increases; rather, transport will manifest saturation.

Finally, under conditions approaching saturation, part of the movement of the transported species will involve exchange for molecules in the opposite direction. The free energy accumulated by the movement of a molecule in one direction is dissipated by movement in the opposite direction. This phenomenon has been termed exchange diffusion. Thus, with increasing solute concentrations on both sides of the membrane, the carrier or channel will saturate at both boundaries and net transport will cease. However, even in the absence of net movement, exchange diffusion will continue. Finally, as a consequence of the interaction of the transported solute with discrete membrane components, these mediated transport processes will exhibit the potential to be subject to genetic and hormonal feedback regulation as noted.

Active Transport

Active transport effects movement against an electrochemical gradient. By this definition, endocytosis and exocytosis may be considered as active transport processes. In the following discussion, however, we restrict our remarks to those active transport processes mediated by the intrinsic plasma membrane proteins. The energy required to achieve net transport against an electrochemical gradient may derive directly from cellular metabolism, in which case the process is known as primary active transport (e.g., movement of sodium and potassium by the Na^+-K^+-ATPase pump). Alternatively, movement may be energized by coupling the flux of one solute with that of another species whose transport, in turn, depends on cellular metabolism. In this case, the process is called secondary active transport, a mechanism by which cellular metabolic energy, accumulated by the active transport of one solute, is stored in a concentration gradient that is dissipated in driving the transport of a second solute in the same or opposite direction. These latter two processes are called symport and antiport, respectively.

Active transport processes share some of the same kinetic characteristics as facilitated diffusion: stereochemical specificity, saturation, competitive inhibition by other transported species, and noncompetitive inhibition by carrier poisons. Moreover, as a reflection of its energy dependence, an active transport process is substrate and oxygen dependent, inhibited by metabolic poisons such as cyanide and dinitrophenol, and profoundly inhibited by lowering the ambient temperature.

In classic studies on the origin of the electrical potential difference across frog skin, Ussing and his co-workers demonstrated that sodium was transported actively while chloride movement was passive and followed the positive potential generated by active transport of sodium. This conclusion was reached by placing the isolated skin between identical bathing solutions and abolishing the spontaneous electrical potential difference across the membrane. This short-circuiting was accomplished by applying an external voltage of equal magnitude but opposite polarity to that of the spontaneous membrane potential. Under these conditions, any current passing through the tissue (short-circuit current) was caused by active ion transport.

As noted earlier, to effect net transport across a cell, the two membranes must be functionally polarized. Based on this premise and on the observation that sodium transport was active while chloride transport was passive, as well as on the cellular ion distribution of sodium (low intracellular and high extracellular) and potassium (high intracellular and low extracellular), Koefoed-Johnsen and Ussing proposed a fundamental cell model for the transport of sodium across epithelial cells.

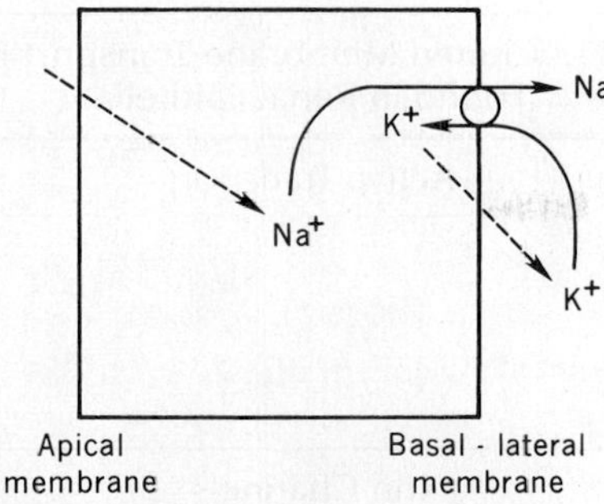

Figure 6.5. Cellular model of epithelial sodium transport proposed by Koefoed-Johnsen and Ussing. *Dotted lines* denote passive ion movements, and *solid lines* indicate energy-dependent active transport. The apical cell membrane is selectively permeable to sodium and the basolateral membrane is selectively permeable to potassium. (From Koefoed-Johnsen V, Ussing HH. *Acta Physiol Scand* 1958;42:298–308.)

This scheme is illustrated in Fig. 6.5. This model predicts that the apical membrane is selectively permeable to sodium and impermeable to potassium, whereas the basolateral cell membrane is selectively permeable to potassium but virtually impermeable to sodium.

The observed properties of the basolateral membrane are common not only to epithelial cells but also to electrically excitable cells and, in fact, to nearly all somatic cells. They are relatively high potassium and chloride permeabilities, low sodium permeability, and the presence of a Na^+-K^+-ATPase. The unique permselective properties of apical cell membranes characterize epithelial cells with respect to other cell types and determine their polarity.

Linked transport of sodium and potassium can be attributed to the Na^+-K^+-ATPase located in the basolateral cell membrane. In this system, ATP hydrolysis is the source of energy, and sodium efflux is linked to potassium influx, generally with a coupling ratio that is $3Na^+$:$2K^+$. If the coupling ratio of sodium to potassium were equal, no net movement of charge would occur, and the pump would be electroneutral. However, when more than one sodium is extruded for each potassium ion taken up by the cell, there is a net transfer of positive charge out of the cell, leaving the cell interior electrically negative. Such transport is said to be rheogenic.

The rheogenic nature of the sodium–potassium pump results in a sodium distribution between cells and extracellular fluid that is remote from electrochemical equilibrium. Both the cellular electronegativity and the low cytosolic sodium concentration, resulting from the active extrusion of sodium across the basolateral cell membrane, contribute to the generation of an appreciable gradient favoring the passive influx of sodium across the apical cell membrane. This sodium gradient from extacellular to intracellular fluids provides an energy source for the movement of sugars, amino acids, chloride, lactate, and many other organic and inorganic solutes across the apical membrane against an electrochemical gradient into the cell. The selected cotransporters and countertransporters shown in Table 6.6 all include sodium as one of the transported species. They are all driven by dissipation of the sodium gradient established by the Na^+-K^+-ATPase pump.

A composite cell model illustrating several sodium-dependent cotransport and countertransport processes is shown in Fig. 6.6. The cotransport of hexose sugars and sodium across the apical cell membrane, for example, demonstrates considerable specificity not only for sodium but also with respect to the steric requirements for individual sugars. Transcellular transport results from the passive movement of these sugars across the basolateral cell membrane. In the initial portions of the proximal convoluted tubule, lumen-negative electrical potentials are observed only when D-glucose and amino acids are available for cotransport with sodium across the luminal membrane, suggesting that sodium-dependent cotransport is a dominant mechanism for organic solute reabsorption in this nephron segment. By contrast, in the proximal straight tubule, a lumen-negative potential persists even in the absence of these organic solutes. Similarly, the electrochemical gradient for sodium entry into the cell is responsible for coupled chloride and potassium entry into cells of the thick ascending limb of Henle via the tritransporter. The energy required to transport chloride into the cell against its electrochemical gradient is derived from the movement of sodium down its electrochemical gradient and thus ultimately on the continued active extrusion of sodium from the cell by the sodium pump.

TABLE 6.6. Selected Renal Epithelial Cotransporters and Antiporters

	Transport Substrates	Location	Stoichiometry	Charge Carried
Cotransporters				
	Na^+-glucose	BBM-PCT	1:1	Electrogenic: positive
		BBM-PST	1:2	
	Na^+-phosphate	BBM-PCT	2:1	Electroneutral
	Na^+-Cl^-	apical membrane DCT	1:1	Electroneutral
	Na^+-K^+-Cl^+	apical membrane TAL	1:1:2	Electroneutral
	Na^+-HCO_3^-	BLM-PCT	1:3	Electrogenic: negative
Antiporters				
	Na^+-H^+	BBM-PCT	1:1	Electroneutral
		apical membrane TAL		
	Na^+-Ca^{2+}	BLM-PCT	3:2	Electrogenic: positive

BBM, brush border (apical) membrane; BLM, basolateral membrane; DCT, distal convoluted tubule; PCT, proximal convoluted tubule; PST, proximal straight tubule; TAL, thick ascending limb.

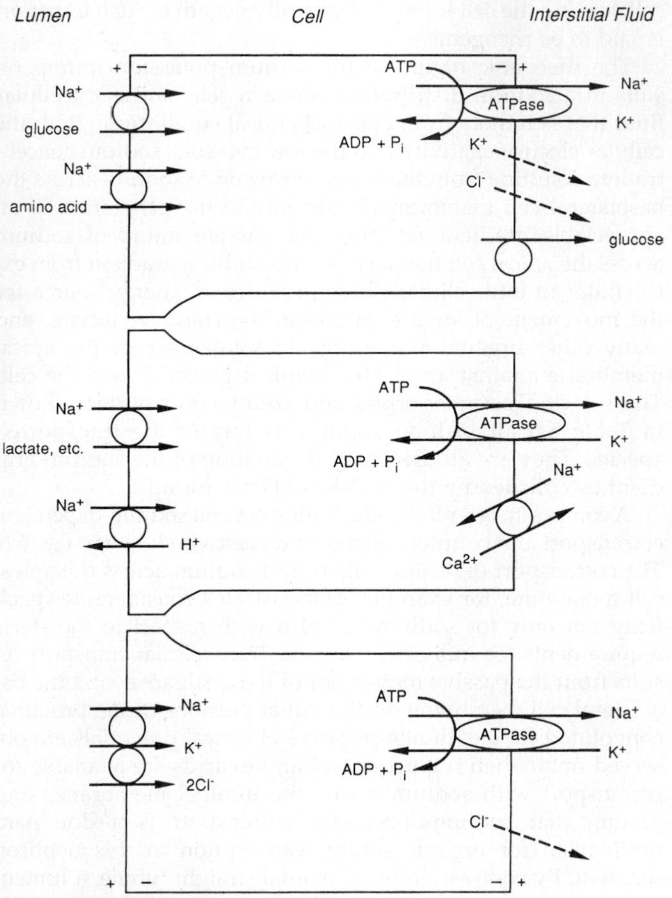

Figure 6.6. Composite cell depicting a variety of coupled cotransport and countertransport schemes. Sodium entry across the luminal cell membrane is enhanced by cotransport with many organic solutes and possibly by countertransport with protons. Sodium–calcium countertransport across the basolateral cell membrane is also indicated. The Na^+-K^+-ATPase located in the basolateral cell membrane facilitates Na-K exchange and is responsible for maintaining the intracellular sodium activity at low levels remote from equilibrium. This extracellular to intracellular sodium gradient supplies the energy for the sodium-coupled transport events.

Secondary active transport may also occur as a result of countertransport. In this situation, the downhill movement of one species along its electrochemical gradient provides the driving force for the uphill movement of a second solute against its electrochemical gradient. Acidification of the proximal tubular fluid may arise, at least in part, from sodium for hydrogen countertransport. In isolate brush border membrane vesicles, for example, the imposition of an outwardly directed sodium gradient leads to acidification of the intravesicular space. Sodium–calcium countertransport across the basolateral cell membrane of the proximal tubule and the collecting tubule may represent an important mechanism for the regulation of intracellular calcium concentration. According to this model, a small but finite entry of sodium into the cell across the basolateral cell membrane provides the energy to drive, in part, the extrusion of calcium from the cell against its electrochemical gradient.

With the explosion in the application of molecular biologic techniques to the study of membrane transport processes, a number of important transport proteins have been cloned (Table 6.7). Already, the information and tools provided by such molecular approaches have led to important advances in our understanding of the function and regulation of membrane transport in health and disease. In this regard, the genetic bases for a number of fluid and electrolyte transport disorders have now been determined (Table 6.1). For example, disorders characterized by excessive sodium reabsorption as well as sodium wasting have been found to be due to activating and inactivating mutations in some of the major sodium-transport proteins.

TABLE 6.7. Cloned Membrane Transport Proteins Found in Renal Epithelia

Active Transport
Na^+-K^+-ATPase
H^+-ATPase
Ca^{2+}-ATPase
P-glycoprotein
H^+-K^+-ATPase
Ion Channels
Inward rectifying K^+ channels (e.g., ROMK)
CFTR/CFTR-like channels
Aquaporin family of water channels
Amiloride sensitive Na^+ channel (ENAC)
ClC Cl^- channel family (CLC-2, CLC-K1, CLC-K2, CLC-5)
P64 Cl^- channel
cGMP-gated cation channel
Voltage-dependent calcium channels
Other Transport Proteins
Na^+-K^+-$2Cl^-$ cotransporter
NaCl cotransporter
Sodium-proton antiporter
Dibasic amino acid transporter
Sodium-glucose cotransporter
Sodium-phosphate cotransporter
Sodium bicarbonate cotransporter
Urea transporter
Sodium-dicarboxylate cotransporter

Selected Readings

Benga G, Holmes RP. Interactions between components in biological membranes and their implications for membrane function. *Prog Biophys Molec Biol* 1984;43: 195–257.

An extensive review of the lipid composition of submembrane domains, the effects of the relative lipid composition on membrane behavior, membrane fluidity, and the differential characteristics of the inner and outer leaflets of the lipid bilayer.

Cooper K, Jakobsson E, Wolynes P. The theory of ion transport through membrane channels. *Prog Biophys Molec Biol* 1985;46:51–96.

A review of the mathematical models that describe the transport of ions through membrane channels. The authors discuss and critique three distinct approaches to a description of ion transport. They review existing membrane transport theory, notably the Nernst-Planck theory and the Eyring-Rate theory. Furthermore, they develop an alternate approach that uses a computer simulation of Brownian dynamics to describe membrane ion transport.

deRouffinac C, Elalouf JM. Hormonal regulation of chloride transport in the proximal and distal nephron. *Ann Rev Physiol* 1988;50:123–140.

This text offers a thorough discussion of the known effects of hormones in the regulation of salt transport throughout the nephron.

Hille B. *Ionic channels of excitable membranes.* Sunderland, MA: Sinauer Associates, 1992.

A clearly written text covering the basic principles of ion channel function and structure. Although slanted toward voltage-gated ion channels, the discussions of ion permeation, selectivity, channel blockade, and structure–function relations will appeal to those studying epithelial ion transport.

Giebisch G, Boulpaep E. Symposium on contrasport mechanisms in renal tubules. *Kidney Int* 1989;36(3):333–496.

This symposium issue contains short research and review articles that deal with various cotransport systems in renal epithelia. A discussion of the general aspects of cotransport processes is followed by sections on sodium symporters, Na-K-2Cl cotransport, and cotransporters involved in volume regulation.

Hebert SC, Reeves WB. Symposium on ion channels. *Kidney Int* 1995;48(4). 917–1346.

This symposium issue contains excellent reviews of the physiology and molecular biology of renal water and ion channels.

Knepper MA. Molecular physiology of urinary concentrating mechanism: regulation of aquaporin water channels by vasopressin. *Am J Physiol: Renal Physiol* 1997;272:F3–F12.

This review discusses recent advances in our understanding of the regulation of water permeability by vasopressin, including its effects on membrane trafficking and gene transcription.

Schultz SG. *Basic principles of membrane transport.* New York: Cambridge University Press, 1980.

A now classic monograph, this text sets forth the principal mathematic and theoretic formulations upon which membrane transport theory is based. The principles governing both passive and active transport processes are discussed. This monograph would be particularly helpful to readers as an adjunct to understanding the most current research on the biophysical and electrical properties of membranes.

Trends Biochem Sci 1992;17(10).

This issue contains several excellent reviews that cover different aspects of signal transduction pathways.

CHAPTER 7

Renal Handling of Organic Compounds

PART 1
Renal Excretion of Urea

Lise Bankir and Nadine Bouby

Urea, a small molecule (MW = 60) with two nitrogen atoms, is the main end product of protein catabolism in mammals and is the most abundant solute in urine in omnivores and carnivores but usually not in herbivores. Because of its high solubility in water, urea can be highly concentrated in urine without risk of precipitation (and stone formation), and this property enables the excretion of relatively large amounts of nitrogen wastes in modest amounts of water. This is especially important in terrestrial and marine mammals in which water conservation is a crucial necessity. However, excreting nitrogenous wastes in the form of urea is costly since the synthesis of each urea molecule consumes three adenosine triphosphate (ATP), and its concentration in urine imposes an additional cost to the kidney. The complete synthesis of urea from ammonia occurs only in the liver and involves five successive enzymatic reactions, using ornithine as a nitrogen carrier in a cycle called the ornithine cycle. The last enzymatic step, hydrolysis of arginine (containing four nitrogen atoms) into urea and ornithine (two nitrogen atoms each) catalyzed by arginase, is also found in other organs (kidney, brain, white blood cells, and testis), but the amount of urea formed in these organs is very small compared with that released by the liver.

Urea diffuses freely through biologic membranes, and in a steady state, its concentration in all extracellular and intracellular fluids is equal to that in plasma. However, this equilibration is slow (in the order of minutes through a simple epithelium) because urea permeability through biologic membranes is quite low as a result of its poor solubility in lipids. In some cells, such as erythrocytes, hepatocytes, and some renal vascular and tubular structures, this equilibration is much more rapid (in the order of seconds) because of the presence of facilitated urea transporters in the plasma membrane of the cells.

Urea was the first organic molecule that was isolated, characterized, and quantitated in blood and urine at the end of the 18th century. Only several decades later was the kidney's involvement in urea excretion and the significance of uremia understood. During the first half of the 20th century, the evaluation of renal function was mainly based on blood urea concentration and on urea clearance from blood until better endogenous and exogenous markers were discovered. Although urea clearance and excretion were no longer of much interest for nephrologists, renal physiologists turned their attention to the movements of urea along the nephron, trying to understand the role of this solute in the urine concentrating mechanism. The recent cloning of several urea transporters has brought a new insight into this complex function of the mammalian kidney.

EXCRETION OF UREA AND ITS CONCENTRATION IN URINE

Urinary excretion of urea in humans varies from 300 to 600 mmol/day according to protein intake. Fecal excretion of urea is negligible, except during administration of some antibiotics because urea is hydrolyzed in the gut by bacteria possessing intense urease activity. Even though urea represents only 2% of plasma solutes, it represents 40% to 50% of urinary solutes in humans and laboratory rats. In humans, urea is concentrated in urine 20 to 100 times more than in the plasma (and even more in rodents and carnivores). Because of this low plasma concentration and the large amount of urea excreted (Table 7.1), urea is by far the solute that imposes the largest effort for water conservation on the body. Other solutes, like ammonia, or protons may reach much higher urea-to-plasma ratios than urine, but they represent a much smaller fraction of the total excreted osmoles.

Influence of Urine Flow Rate on Fractional Excretion of Urea

Urea excretion depends on filtration of plasma through glomeruli and reabsorption by diffusion along the nephrons and collecting ducts (CDs). Reabsorption of urea along the proximal convoluted tubule amounts to about 50% of the filtered load and apparently is not influenced by any regulatory factor or by urinary flow rate. In contrast, urea reabsorption in the distal nephron is greatly influenced by urinary flow rate. This explains the significant decline in urea clearance and its fractional excretion when urinary flow rates fall below 2 ml/min (Fig. 7.1). This large fall has been described for more than fifty years and was mentioned in every book of nephrology until the 70s. Thereafter, the notion seems to have been neglected. However, in normal life, spontaneous urinary flow rate usually varies between 0.5 and 2 ml/min, which is exactly the range in which fractional excretion of urea (FE_{urea}) is greatly influenced by urinary flow rate.

TABLE 7.1. Concentration of Total Osmoles and of the Three Main Solutes in Plasma and Urine, Their Daily Excretion, and Their Urine-to-Plasma Concentration Ratio in Healthy Humans

	Concentration in Plasma	Concentration in Urine	Daily Excretion	Urine/ Plasma
	mOsm/kg H_2O	*mOsm/kg H_2O*	*mOsm/day*	
Total osmoles	289 ± 3	660 ± 49	890 ± 51	2.29 ± 0.18
	mmol/L	*mmol/L*	*mmol/day*	
Sodium	141 ± 1	144 ± 9	195 ± 14	1.02 ± 0.07
Potassium	4.2 ± 0.2	54 ± 7	72 ± 7	12.4 ± 1.2
Urea	5.7 ± 0.5	275 ± 26	368 ± 21	51.3 ± 5.7

Means ± SEM of 8 male healthy subjects (22–35 years of age, mean body weight of 68 ± 2 kg) on a normal Western-type diet.
Water excretion (or urine flow rate) was 1420 ± 130 ml/day.
Adapted from Choukroun et al. *Am J Physiol,* 1977;273:R1726–R1733.

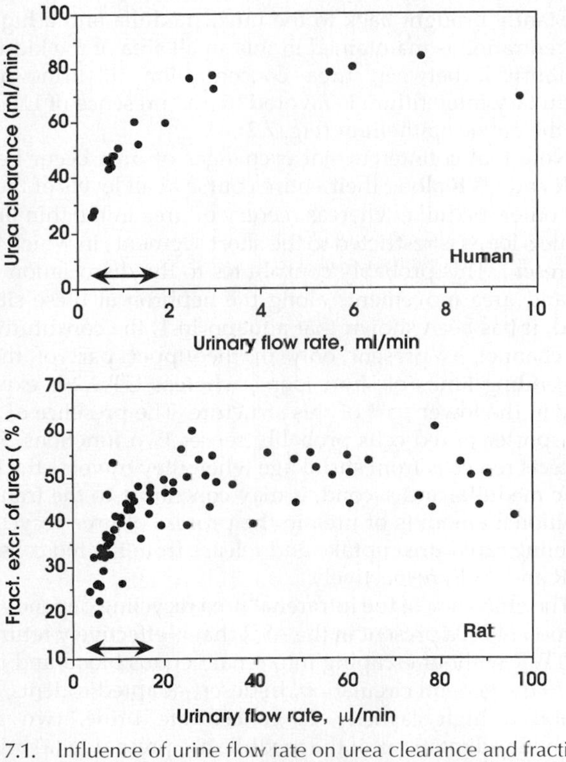

Figure 7.1. Influence of urine flow rate on urea clearance and fractional excretion in humans **(top)** and rats **(bottom).** Note that for low urine flows, the efficiency of urea excretion decreases dramatically. The *double arrow* shows the range of urinary flow rates observed during normal life in each species. (From Bankir. In: Brenner BM, Rector FC, eds. *The Kidney.* Philadelphia: WB Saunders, 1996:571–606, with permission.)

The decline in the fractional excretion during a low urine flow is the result of two additive reabsorptive processes, both influenced (indirectly or directly) by vasopressin. First, a passive diffusion of urea occurs along the entire distal nephron (including the distal tubular and collecting system). Although the permeability of these nephron segments to urea is relatively low, the long length of these structures, traversing the entire cortex and medulla, enables significant amounts of urea to be reabsorbed when vasopressin is present. Vasopressin promotes water removal from these segments, resulting in slowing urine flow, increasing contact time, and enhancing the transepithelial urea concentration difference. All of these events favor passive urea diffusion. Second, in the terminal part of the CD in the inner medulla, vasopressin is known to selectively increase the permeability of the epithelium to urea. A vasopressin-dependent facilitated urea transporter, UT-A1, is expressed in the luminal membrane of these cells. As a result, urea, which was concentrated upstream by water reabsorption, diffuses out of the CD in the interstitium of the deep medulla. Afterward, its excretion in the urine falls.

Intrarenal Urea Recycling and Urea Transporters

Vasopressin-dependent urea diffusion in the terminal inner medullary collecting duct (IMCD) represents an essential element in the process of water conservation by the kidney. Bringing a concentrated urea solution to the interstitium of the deep inner medulla enhances the local osmotic pressure (which is ensured by sodium chloride*) and enables more intense, osmotically-driven water reabsorption and better concentration of all urinary solutes, including urea itself. However, urea brought this way into the inner medulla is constantly taken up by the ascending venous vasa rectae (AVR) and could be rapidly removed from the medulla. However, urea ascending in AVR returns, at least in part, to the inner medulla by countercurrent exchange with the surrounding descending structures. The descending vasa recta in the inner and outer medulla are equipped along their whole length with the facilitated urea transporter UT-B1, and the thin descending limbs of Henle's loops are equipped along some of their length with the facilitated urea transporter UT-A2.

Figure 7.2 displays both the sites along the nephron and renal vessels where urea transporters have been located and also the pathways of intrarenal urea recycling. All urea transporters cloned so far are transmembrane proteins which increase approximately 50- to 1,000-fold the passive permeability of cell membranes to urea, thus enabling a much faster equilibration of urea concentration in different compartments. UT-A1 is present in the luminal membrane of the terminal inner medullary CD, and it is the limiting factor for urea permeability in the CD. The function of this transporter is vasopressin dependent. The mechanism by which vasopressin influences UT-A1 permeability remains unclear. It does not follow the same pattern as that of aquaporin 2, the vasopressin-dependent water channel,

*This accumulation of sodium results from countercurrent multiplication in the outer medulla involving active sodium reabsorption in the thick ascending limbs of Henle's loops, coupled with sodium secretion in and/or water removal from the surrounding thin descending limbs. For further details, see Chapter 8.

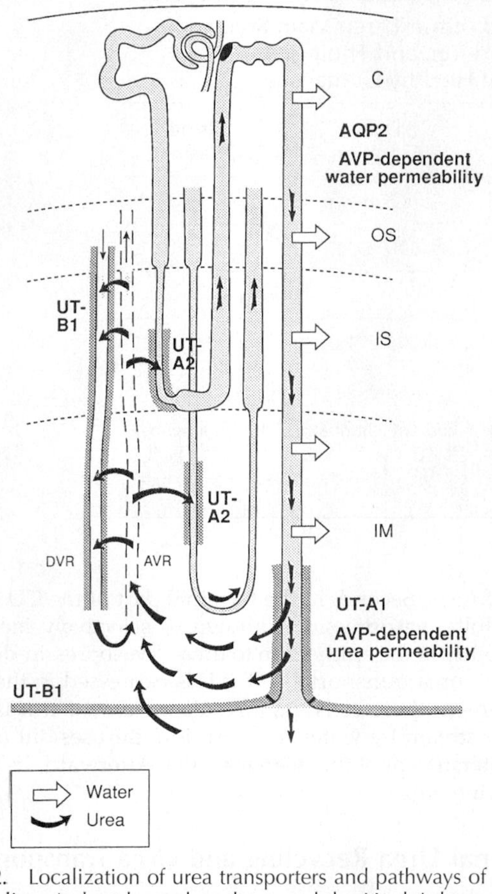

Figure 7.2. Localization of urea transporters and pathways of intrarenal urea recycling. A short-looped nephron and the Henle's loop of a long-looped nephron are shown, together with a collecting duct (CD) (not drawn to scale). Under the influence of vasopressin, urea is concentrated in the CD lumen by water reabsorption *(white arrows)* and can diffuse into the insterstitium of the deep inner medulla because of the presence of UT-A1. Urea *(black arrows)* is taken up by ascending vasa recta, and some of it does not return to the general circulation but is recycled by countercurrent exchange in descending structures in which urea permeability is high because of UT-A2 (in thin limbs) and UT-B1 (in vasa recta). Some urea exchanges are also possible between urine and medullary interstitium because of UT-B1 lining the pelvic epithelium (see text).

which is included in subapical vesicles and is shuttled to the cell surface under the influence of vasopressin or its second messenger cyclic adenosine monophosphate (cAMP).

Another urea transporter UT-A2 is derived from the same gene as UT-A1 through alternative splicing and has been found only in the thin descending limbs of Henle's loops on both sides of the cell. It is more abundant in the short loops of Henle than in long loops, where its expression seems to vary with the intensity of the urinary concentrating activity.

UT-B1 is a more ubiquitous UT, expressed in a number of organs and tissues (such as bone marrow, kidney, brain, thymus, testis, and spleen). This transporter is abundant in red cells and is responsible for their long-known high permeability to urea. In the kidney, UT-B1 is localized exclusively in the endothelium of descending vasa recta and in the pelvic epithelium. No urea transporters or aquaporin are present in the AVR. However, the endothelium of these vessels is highly fenestrated and this, together with the slow transit time because of the large total cross-sectional area of these vessels, probably ensures a high permeability to water and small solutes such as urea and electrolyte.

Functional studies performed with micropuncture or microperfusion techniques showed physiologists that urea undergoes a complex intrarenal recycling, which contributes to its accumulation in the inner medulla and to the more efficient water reabsorption in the CD. In particular, the reentry of urea into Henle's loops of superficial nephrons was deduced from the observation of a much higher delivery of urea in the early distal tubule than in the late proximal tubule with the difference increasing with increasing urinary osmolality. Molecular biology has enabled the identification of the precise location of the urea transporters and thus a more precise characterization of these intrarenal movements. The first and limiting step in this urea recycling is the vasopressin-dependent increase in urea permeability of the terminal CD. This enables urea, concentrated upstream by water abstraction, to diffuse in the inner medulla interstitium. Though urea is taken up by the AVR and flows toward the cortex, a variable fraction of it will diffuse, along a favorable concentration gradient, into the descending vasa rectae (DVR) and thin segments of Henle's loops. Thereafter, urea will mostly remain in the lumen of the nephron, traversing segments with a low urea permeability until it reaches again the terminal inner medulla CD and can be recycled again. In the same way, urea recycled through the DVR will return to the inner medulla, where it can be recycled again. In this way, urea is constantly brought back to the inner medulla and a high urea concentration is maintained in this small area of the kidney. An equilibrium between urea concentration in urine and in medullary interstitium is favored by the presence of UT-B1 lining the pelvic epithelium (Fig. 7.2).

Note that countercurrent exchanges of urea occur between AVR and DVR along their entire course at all levels of the inner and outer medulla, whereas reentry of urea in the thin limbs of Henle's loops is restricted to the short segments in which UT-A2 is present. This probably contributes to the dissociation of water and urea movements along the nephron at these sites. Indeed, it has been shown that aquaporin 1, the constitutive water channel, is present only in the upper part of the thin descending limbs of short loops, whereas UT-A2 is expressed only in the lower part of this structure. The presence of a urea transporter in red cells probably serves two functions. First, it protects red cells from shrinkage when they traverse the hypertonic medulla, and second, it may contribute to the transfer of additional amounts of urea in the process of urea recycling by enabling rapid urea uptake and release from the red cells in the DVR and AVR, respectively.

The efficiency of the intrarenal urea recycling depends on the fraction of urea present in the AVR that is effectively returned to the DVR without escaping into renal venous blood and returning to the general circulation. In desert-adapted rodents, which exhibit a high capacity to concentrate urine, two special anatomic adaptations of the medulla are present to (a) bring the descending and ascending medullary structures involved in countercurrent exchanges in closer contact by increasing the number of vessels in vascular bundles in the inner stripe and incorporating the thin, descending limbs of short Henle's loops in these bundles, and (b) lengthen the distance over which these exchanges take place by lengthening the renal papilla.

MAIN FACTORS INFLUENCING UREA EXCRETION AND UREA HANDLING BY THE KIDNEY

Influence of Diet on Urea Excretory Needs

The rate of urea synthesis, urea turnover, and urea handling by the kidney differ widely among mammals according to the dietary regimen and its influence on the amount of urea they need to excrete (Fig. 7.3). In carnivores, most of the energy supply

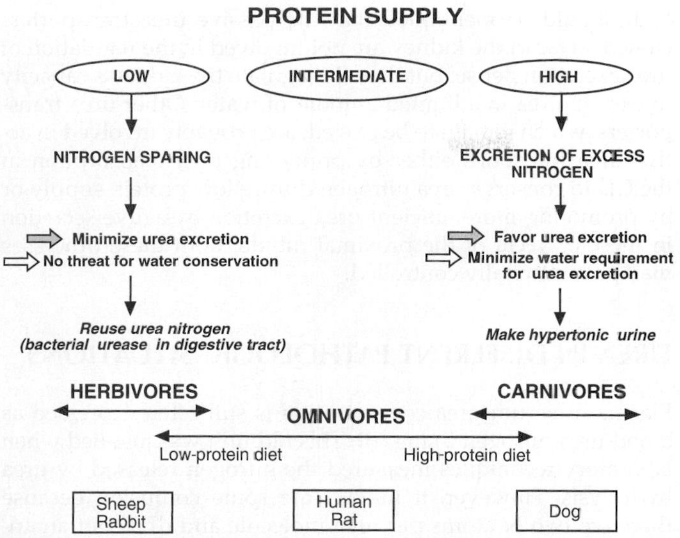

Figure 7.3. Protein supply and corresponding needs with regard to urea and water excretion according to diet in different mammalian groups. (From Bankir L, Bouby N, Trinh-Trang-Tan MM, et al. Direct and indirect cost of urea excretion. *Kidney Int* 1996;49:1598–1607, with permission.)

comes from protein-rich food, and accordingly, the need to excrete urea is high. In these animals, urea accounts for about 70% to 80% of all urinary solutes. The kidney of the dog, and probably that of other carnivores, seems to be specially adapted to an efficient urea excretion because urea clearance per unit kidney weight is about twice that of rats, rabbits, or humans. This may be because of active urea secretion that occurs in a special subsegment of the pars rectae described in the dog kidney.

In herbivores, protein intake is relatively low and nitrogen supply is only close to the minimal needs. Urea excretion is minimized by a special interorgan cycle that enables reuse of urea nitrogen. Filtered urea is largely reabsorbed along the nephron and the inner medullary CD, which is assumed to possess an active urea transport process. This explains the very low urea concentration in urine and urea excretion. Blood urea diffuses passively into the gut (or rumen in ruminants), whereas a urease-rich microflora can break down urea into ammonia and carbon dioxide. Ammonia can then be reused for nitrogen metabolism in the intestinal epithelium and/or liver. This allows the substitution of urea to more expensive nutrients in cattle feeds. In this context UT-A1, the urea transporter present in the inner medulla CD, has also been identified in the colon of the rabbit (herbivore) but not in that of the rat (omnivore).

In omnivores, like humans and rats, urea excretory needs vary widely according to the proportion of proteins in the total energy supply (Fig. 7.3). With high protein intake, some urea secretion may take place along the nephron and improve the efficiency of urea excretion. However, this possibility is not yet firmly established. With low protein intake, sustained for several weeks, urea excretion becomes extremely low in rats because of an active Na-coupled urea reabsorption that has been shown to appear in the inner medullary CD. In this situation, rats may develop the same adaptation that normally is present in herbivores, interorgan nitrogen recycling. If this is the case, they should also exhibit a facilitated urea permeability in some segment of the lower digestive tract to enable the diffusion of urea and the action of intestinal bacteria. However, this has not yet been demonstrated. Whether humans can develop such adaptations to reduce urea excretion and favor the reuse of urea nitrogen through intestinal bacteria is not well established. Some studies of normal individuals suggest that, on a low-protein diet sustained for several weeks (or during lactation in women), as much as 30% of urea synthesized in the liver may be reused in this way. In contrast, studies of renal patients conclude that the possibility to reuse urea nitrogen is very small. However, these studies may have been too short to reveal full adaptation.

Active Secretion of Urea

Urea excretion is controlled by filtration at the glomerulus and by reabsorption along the nephron. Other nitrogenous wastes like creatinine and uric acid are secreted in the pars recta, and several findings suggest that this may also be the case for urea. Twenty years ago, when rabbit tubules were studied *in vitro* because nephron segments were easier to dissect in this species, a modest but significant active urea secretion was demonstrated in the pars recta, but other studies did not confirm this finding. Unfortunately, no other species was investigated. Yet, even if mammals do secrete urea, this process must be negligible in herbivores and more significant in omnivores or carnivores. Several findings in whole animals and humans suggest that urea secretion probably takes place in some segment of the nephron, most likely in the pars rectae. The existence of a special subsegment of the proximal tubule in dogs, a species with highly efficient urea excretion, favors this hypothesis, as does the occurrence of a rare disease, familial azotemia, which could be explained by the inability to secrete urea. If urea secretion did take place in the pars recta, hormonal regulation of this secretion could influence the kidney's capacity to improve urea excretion to compensate for some of the urea reabsorption linked to the process of water conservation.

Regulation of Urea Excretion at the Tubular Level

It is generally accepted that urea excretion is not regulated and that its excretion depends on the difference between the amount filtered and the amount that is passively reabsorbed along the nephron. Accordingly, the glomerular filtration rate (GFR) represents a main determinant of urea excretion, and in the absence of changes in tubular reabsorption, urea excretion will vary in proportion to the GFR. However, as already pointed out in 1958 by Bodil Schmidt-Nielsen, this currently accepted concept does not explain a number of observations. It is possible that urea excretion is controlled by some regulation taking place at the tubular level.

Apart from vasopressin, which influences renal handling of urea through its action on water conservation, several hormones have actually been shown to affect urea excretion by a tubular action, thus modifying the fraction of filtered urea excreted by the kidney. The most important are glucocorticoids and glucagon. In a relatively old study, glucocorticoids were shown to increase FE_{urea}. The decrease in plasma corticosterone concentration, which occurs in rats when their protein supply is reduced, was thought to contribute to the reduction in FE_{urea} observed in this situation. In adrenalectomized rats, as well as in rats fed a protein-poor diet, chronic glucocorticoid administration significantly increased FE_{urea}. These effects took several days to reach their full intensity. The influence of glucocorticoids on FE_{urea} was thought to result from a decrease in urea permeability of the CD. Because a Na-dependent active reabsorption of urea has now been found in rats fed a low-protein diet, it may be assumed that this transport, if present constitutively in the CD, is inhibited by glucocorticoids and that its full expression appears in situations in which cortisol secretion is reduced.

Like glucocorticoids, glucagon has also been shown to increase FE_{urea} but more rapidly. Besides its well-known role in the maintenance of plasma glucose concentration, glucagon also plays a major role in controlling protein catabolism and urea excretion, although this role often is not clearly appreciated or recognized. Glucagon is secreted either after the ingestion of proteins (or an experimental infusion of amino acids) or during a fast. At first glance, these two situations appear to be opposite. However, in both cases, glucagon similarly stimulates gluconeogenesis and ureagenesis. In the first case (protein meal), the amino acids of exogenous origin need to be deaminated so as to excrete the nitrogen they contain independent of the body's glucose needs. In the other case (fast), glucagon stimulates the break down of endogenous amino acids to maintain normoglycemia during shortage of substrates resulting from fasting, but the nitrogen atoms of these amino acids also need to be excreted in the form of urea. Glucagon has been shown to stimulate the first, rate-limiting step of the ornithine–urea cycle, thus stimulating ureagenesis in the liver. Therefore, whether amino acids originate from an exogenous or an endogenous source, glucagon is an essential hormone regulating the body's nitrogen metabolism (Fig. 7.4).

Parallel to its effects on hepatic urea synthesis, glucagon also increases the renal excretion of urea through two additive mechanisms. First, it increases glomerular filtration, and second, it induces an increase in FE_{urea} by decreasing its tubular reabsorption (and/or possibly by increasing its secretion). This tubular effect of glucagon probably results from an indirect action on the pars recta of the proximal tubule of extracellular (hepatically-derived) cAMP, and from a direct effect of glucagon on the CD. Insulin, which counteracts the effects of glucagon on the liver by reducing glucagon-dependent cAMP production, also most likely counteracts the indirect effects of glucagon on the kidney. Thus glucagon is responsible for a coordinated action on the liver and kidney, regulating in parallel the synthesis and excretion of urea. These effects limit the rise in plasma urea concentration that follows protein ingestion (Fig. 7.4).

In summary, two hormonal systems seem to regulate urea excretion by modulating its tubular reabsorption (or secretion): glucocorticoids and glucagon. The time scales of these two systems are quite different. Glucagon plays a role in the rapid adaptation to changes in urea excretion linked to feeding and fasting, whereas glucocorticoids play a role in the chronic adaptation that occurs after prolonged changes in the level of protein intake.

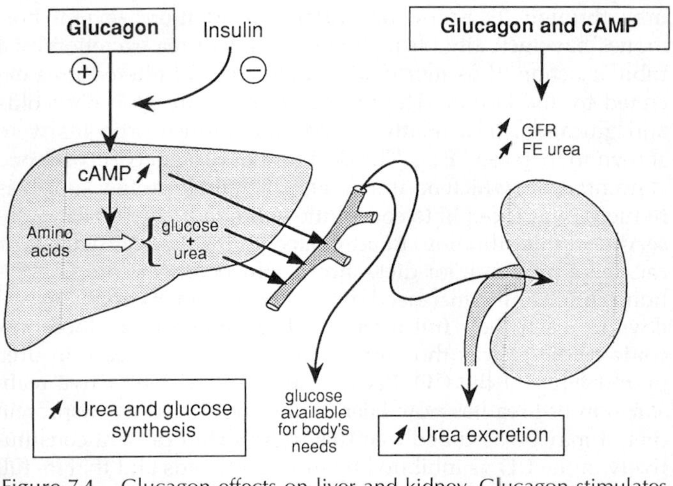

Figure 7.4. Glucagon effects on liver and kidney. Glucagon stimulates, by a cyclic adenosine monophosphate *(cAMP)*-dependent pathway, gluconeogenesis and ureagenesis in the liver. The combined effects of glucagon and hepatically-derived cAMP on the kidney contribute to increase the glomerular filtration rate and urea excretion (see text).

It should be mentioned that the passive urea transporters cloned so far in the kidney are not involved in the regulation of urea excretion per se, but they do regulate the kidney's capacity to excrete urea in a limited amount of water. Other urea transporters, which remain to be cloned, are probably involved in active urea transport, either by promoting urea reabsorption in the CD to conserve urea nitrogen during low protein supply or by promoting more efficient urea excretion by active secretion in the pars recta of the proximal tubule. Both these processes may be hormonally controlled.

UREA IN DIFFERENT PATHOLOGIC SITUATIONS

Plasma or serum urea concentration is still often expressed as blood urea nitrogen in mg/dl. This old unit was justified when laboratory techniques measured the nitrogen released by urea hydrolysis. However, it may create some confusion because there are two N atoms per urea molecule and dL is not an appropriate unit in the International Unit system. Moles of urea per liter should now be preferred (1 mg/dl BUN = 0.35 mmol/L urea). Normal urea plasma (or blood) concentration ranges from 4 to 8 mmol/L (corresponding to 11.5 to 23 mg/dl urea nitrogen or 24 to 48 mg urea/dl). Values in females are usually about 10% to 20% lower than in males.

In chronic renal failure (CRF), plasma urea increases gradually with the progressive deterioration of renal function, thus maintaining urea excretion to an appropriate level despite the reduction of GFR. Because the urea-to-creatinine ratio (10 : 1) remains fairly constant during the course of CRF and because secretion of creatinine increases in this condition, it can be assumed that urea secretion also takes place and is increased in parallel, although urea secretion has not been demonstrated yet. Apart from acute or chronic renal failure, plasma urea and urea excretion are also elevated in subjects with unusually high protein intake, in severe catabolic states and in uncontrolled diabetes mellitus.

Azotemia may occur in some instances in the absence of any sign of renal dysfunction. This is the case in subjects with bleeding of the upper but not lower gastrointestinal tract because upper bleeding results in an increased hepatic urea synthesis from the nitrogen load absorbed downstream in the gut. In contrast, an hemorrhage arising distal to the absorptive surface does not increase plasma urea concentration. A marked and selective increase in plasma urea, called diuretic-induced azotemia, is often observed during administration of loop diuretics. Plasma urea can be elevated about three-fold above normal in familial azotemia, a rare genetic anomaly leading to a selective marked reduction in urea clearance and urea fractional excretion with unaltered GFR and creatinine clearance. Several studies have shown that the defect originates at the level of the proximal tubule. The most likely explanation is a dysfunction or absence of a urea transporter involved in urea secretion in the proximal tubule pars recta. In all these conditions, the urea to creatinine ratio in plasma is higher than 10.

In a few physiologic and pathologic conditions, plasma urea concentration is below normal, in relation to an increase in fractional urea clearance. This is the case in pregnancy, in sickle cell anemia, and in the syndrome of inappropriate secretion of antidiuretic hormone.

Acknowledgments

The authors thank Marie-Marcelle Trinh-Trang-Tan, and Mina Ahloulay for their collaboration in several of the studies mentioned in this chapter.

Original diagrams (Figs. 7.2 and 7.4) were drawn by Martine Netter, INSERM, Hôpital Necker, Paris.

Selected Readings

Ahloulay M, Déchaux M, Laborde K, et al. Influence of glucagon on GFR and on urea and electrolyte excretion: direct and indirect effects. *Am J Physiol (Renal Fluid and Electrolyte Physiol 38)* 1995;269:225–235.

An original paper describing how glucagon stimulates urea synthesis in the liver and urea excretion by the kidney by an indirect effect involving cAMP release by the liver.

Bankir L. Urea and the kidney. In: Brenner BM, Rector FC, eds. *The kidney*, 6th Ed. Philadelphia: WB Saunders, 2000:637–679.

Probably the first extensive chapter about urea handling by the kidney in a nephrology book in several decades. It covers hepatic urea synthesis, urea formation, and compartmentation in the kidney; and the influence of protein intake, of glucagon, and of vasopressin on urea excretion. In addition, it includes a comparative section explaining differences between dogs, rats, and humans in renal handling of urea and also some information about urea in diverse pathologic situations.

Bankir L, Bouby N, Trinh-Trang-Tan MM, et al. Direct and indirect cost of urea excretion. *Kidney Int* 1996:49:1598–1607.

A short review focusing on the links between urea concentration in urine and GFR. It explains why urea excretion can be more costly for the kidney than usually assumed.

Bouby N, Ahloulay M, Nsegbe E, et al. Vasopressin increases GFR in conscious rats through its antidiuretic action. *J Am Soc Nephrol* 1996;7:842–851.

An original paper describing the influence of urinary concentration (and vasopressin) on GFR and explaining how the concentration of urea in urine is probably responsible for this not yet well recognized influence.

Marsh DJ, Knepper MA. Renal handling of urea. In: Windhager EE, ed. *Handbook of physiology. Section 8: renal physiology.* New York, Oxford: Oxford University Press, 1992:1317–1348.

A good survey of the renal handling of urea, focusing mainly on the role of urea in the urinary concentrating mechanism, with a physiologist's view but also including information about regulation of urea synthesis and excretion and theoretical aspects of urea transport.

Sands JM, Timmer RT, Gunn RB. Urea transporters in kidney and erythrocytes (editorial review). *Am J Physiol* 1997 *(Renal Physiol 42)*;273:F321–F339.

An extensive review of our present knowledge of urea transport in red cells and renal epithelia and of the facilitated urea transporters that had been cloned until 1997, including their molecular structure and their contribution to the urinary concentrating process.

Schmidt-Nielsen B. Urea excretion in mammals. *Physiol Rev* 1958;38:139–164.

An extensive review presenting the current knowledge about renal handling of urea on a comparative physiologic basis, based on 20 years of intense physiologic research, at a time when mostly whole animal studies were performed. The author suggested the existence of a specific regulation of tubular handling of urea, which unfortunately received little attention thereafter.

Schmidt-Nielsen B, Kerr DWS, eds. *Urea and the kidney.* Amsterdam: Excerpta Medica Foundation, 1970.

This book contains a number of contributions describing urea synthesis, urea transport through membranes, and renal urea handling in vertebrates from fish to humans. Other sections deal with the influence of protein intake and the urinary concentrating mechanism. Although about 30 years old, most of the information included in this book is still of interest because little new information has been obtained in these fields since then.

PART 2
Renal Handling of D-Glucose and Other Sugars

Peter Deetjen, Heinz Drexel, and Stefan Aczel

Among the functions of the kidney, reabsorption of D-glucose from the glomerular filtrate has attracted the interest of nephrologists ever since Cushny introduced the conceptual framework of the filtration-reabsorption theory of urine formation. The hallmarks of our present understanding of the renal handling of D-glucose are the definition of a tubular transport maximum (T_mG), identification of the proximal tubule as the major site of D-glucose transport, and description of the sodium-D-glucose cotransport system across the epithelial cell layer.

GLUCOSE TRANSPORT ACROSS MEMBRANES

Diffusion of the polar molecule glucose through lipid layers such as cell membranes is negligible. Therefore transmembrane glucose flux must be facilitated to meet cellular glucose demands.

D-glucose transport is accomplished by membrane-bound proteins. Functionally, two families of such D-glucose carriers can be distinguished: proteins that bind both D-glucose and sodium (termed sodium-D-glucose transporter, or SGLT), which take part in an energy-dependent, active transport system; and proteins that bind solely D-glucose (termed glucose transporters, or GLUT), which mediate facilitated diffusion driven by a transmembrane concentration difference for D-glucose.

SGLT is abundant at the apical membrane of enteric cells and the brush border membrane of proximal tubular epithelia (i.e., at the site of Na^+ entrance into the cell). SGLT also is found in other tissues capable of transepithelial Na^+ transport, such as salivary and mammary glands. Consistent with the direction of the Na^+ flux across parotid acinar cells and milk-producing mammary cells, SGLT is located in these organs on the basolateral membrane, which is, again, the site of Na^+ entrance into the cell.

Five isoforms of SGLT (SGLT1 to SGLT5) have been described. In the proximal tubule, two isoforms are present: SGLT1 operates with high affinity, whereas SGLT2 has lower affinity (by one order of magnitude). SGLT1 couples Na^+ and D-glucose at a molar ratio of 2:1, whereas SGLT2 couples Na^+ and D-glucose at a ratio of 1:1.

All isoforms of SGLT are folded across the membrane and possess a core of 13 membrane-spanning helices with 1 additional span at the C-terminus in the case of SGLT1. A monomer with about 84 kD is able to carry only D-glucose but not Na^+, whereas sodium–D-glucose cotransport activity is mediated by a tetramer with about 294 kD.

SGLT molecules are structurally unrelated to GLUT molecules. GLUT molecules are located at the membranes of almost all eukaryotic cells. They are also folded across the membrane bilayer and possess 12 membrane-spanning helices. Their N- and C-termini are located on the cytoplasmic side of the plasma membrane. A loop of 33 amino acids located between the first and second membrane-spanning segment is the site for D-glucose addition. Five structurally related subtypes (GLUT1 through GLUT5) with a tissue-specific pattern of distribution have been described. In addition to the two types of SGLT (SGLT1 and SGLT2, *vide supra*), the kidney contains at least four types of GLUT (GLUT1, GLUT2, GLUT3, and GLUT5). Phlorizin specifically blocks SGLT1, whereas phloretin inhibits D-glucose transport by GLUT. Besides phlorizin, atrial natriuretic peptides also have been found to block SGLT1 activity and thus to decrease sodium absorption in the intestine and kidney. Recently, the pharmaceutical industry has gained interest in SGLT1 because inhibition of the system by specific blockers is promising as an antidiabetic strategy both by lowering blood D-glucose levels as well as by promoting D-glucose (i.e., energy) loss via the urine.

Renal proximal tubule cells contain the SGLT1 protein at the apical membrane and the GLUT1 and GLUT2 molecules at the basolateral membrane; the convoluted part of the proximal tubule contains GLUT2, whereas the straight part expresses GLUT1. The glucose affinity is 10-fold higher for GLUT1 than for GLUT2. Anatomic distribution of GLUT molecules thus predicts some biochemical properties of the different nephron segments: The convoluted part of the proximal tubule with high intracellular glucose levels because of high capacities for glucose reabsorption and gluconeogenesis expresses GLUT2 and therefore offers relatively low glucose affinity. In contrast, nephron segments that are active in glycolysis but less active in glucose transport or in glyconeogenesis (e.g., the straight part of the proximal tubule or the collecting duct) have low intracellular glucose levels and thus express the GLUT1 type that offers high glucose affinity. The convoluted part with its high rate of glucose transport and gluconeogenesis and the preferential expression of GLUT2 therefore is remarkably similar to the liver, whereas the straight part behaves similarly to erythrocytes and brain tissue with a high rate of glycolysis and preferential expression of GLUT1.

GLUCOSE TRANSPORT ACROSS CELLS

The sequence of events in transcellular transport of glucose involves three steps (Fig. 7.5): creation of an inward-oriented Na^+ gradient; binding of Na^+ and glucose to SGLT1 and transport across the brush border membrane; and glucose transport across the basolateral membrane by GLUT.

Hydrolysis of adenosine 5′-triphosphate (ATP) supplies the energy required to drive the electrogenic sodium pump located at the basolateral membrane (Na^+-K^+-ATPase). By pumping sodium out of the cell into the interstitium, the pump decreases the intracellular sodium concentration and thus establishes an inward-oriented sodium gradient across the brush border membrane. This gradient is the direct driving force for the sodium-D-glucose cotransport.

The D-glucose molecule can cross the brush border membrane only in a transporter complex together with sodium. SGLT1 forms a pore that allows the transmembrane passage of Na^+ and D- glucose. Water accompanies the solutes in the same pore via osmotic force.

At the inner side of the brush border membrane, in the cytosolic compartment, the SGLT–sodium–D-glucose complex dissociates into its reactants, and the SGLT cycles back to the luminal side to close the circle.

The sodium–D-glucose cotransport system increases the cytosolic D-glucose concentration to a level that activates the GLUT system at the basolateral membrane. With the extrusion of D-glucose into the interstitium, the transcellular movement of D-glucose and Na^+ is completed. Thus D-glucose reabsorption requires the coordinated activity of three membrane proteins: basolateral Na^+-K^+-ATPase, apical SGLT1, and basolateral GLUT2; SGLT-mediated D-glucose flux is a secondary active transport, whereas GLUT-mediated flux represents facilitated diffusion.

Final uptake of D-glucose from the peritubular fluid into blood capillaries accompanies fluid uptake mediated by Starling forces of peritubular capillary pressure and plasma proteins (see Chapter 14.2). The entire process of D-glucose absorption requires about 9 seconds, which seems to be a long time when one considers that the anatomic distance is only about 20 μm.

Because the transport process is accompanied by generation of a transmembrane electrical current (resulting from the positive charge of Na^+), absorption of D-glucose is electrogenic ("rheogenic").

The chair configuration of the sugar molecule and a free hydroxyl group in the C_2 position are prerequisites for proximal tubular D-glucose transport via SGLT (Fig. 7.6, Table 7.2). Thus, in addition to D-glucose, three other structurally related monosaccharides can use the sodium cotransport system: D-galactose, α-methyl-D-glucoside, and 6-deoxy-D-glucose.

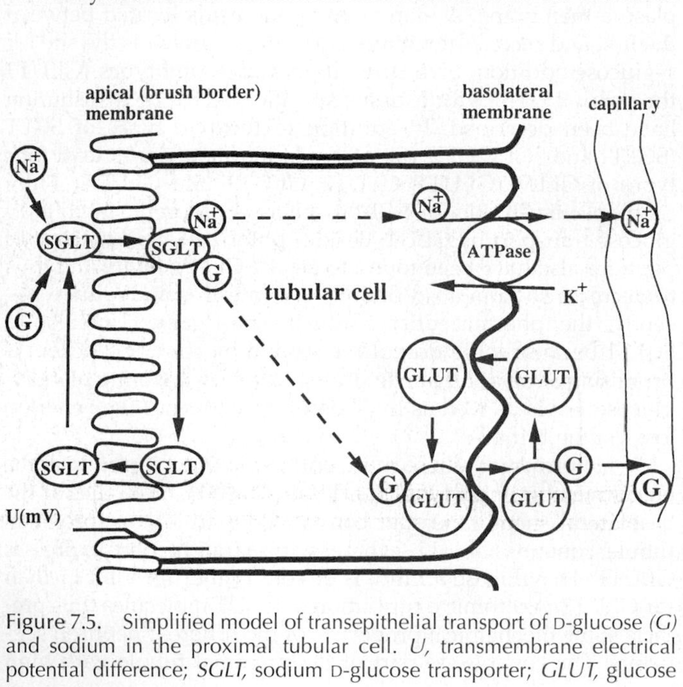

Figure 7.5. Simplified model of transepithelial transport of D-glucose *(G)* and sodium in the proximal tubular cell. *U,* transmembrane electrical potential difference; *SGLT,* sodium D-glucose transporter; *GLUT,* glucose transporter.

NEPHRON SITES OF D-GLUCOSE REABSORPTION

Walker introduced micropuncture techniques in renal physiology and paved the way for extensive investigation of the function of nephron segments. His data, later confirmed by many others, established that D-glucose is almost completely reabsorbed in the first 30% of the proximal tubule of a mammalian kidney. Under normal conditions, the proximal convoluted segment lowers the D-glucose concentration far below the plasma level. In the distal segments of the nephron, D-glucose has no specific transport system, and only a small amount of passive diffusion occurs. Consequently, the concentration increases again in a manner similar to that of inulin. Consequently, there is some physiologic glucose excretion. In the healthy human, this normal baseline glucosuria amounts to approximately 75 mg/day (0.4 mmol per 24 hours). Rats have greater baseline glucosuria than humans.

CONCEPT OF T_mG

Shannon has outlined the still valid concept of saturable reabsorption of D-glucose in the kidney, which works below capacity at physiologic blood sugar levels (Fig. 7.7). As outlined previously, baseline glucosuria of approximately 75 mg/day

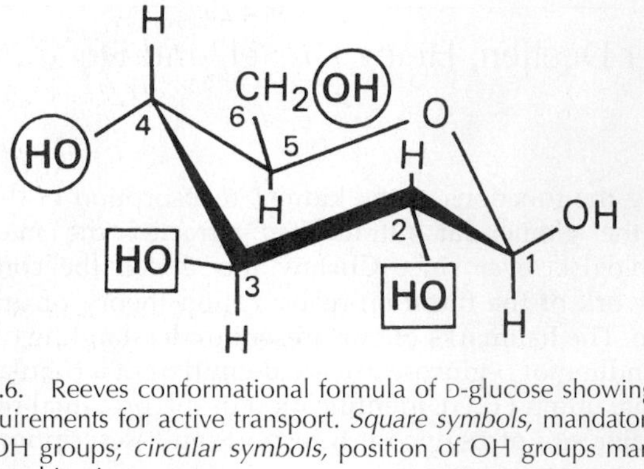

Figure 7.6. Reeves conformational formula of D-glucose showing structural requirements for active transport. *Square symbols,* mandatory position of OH groups; *circular symbols,* position of OH groups mandatory only in combination.

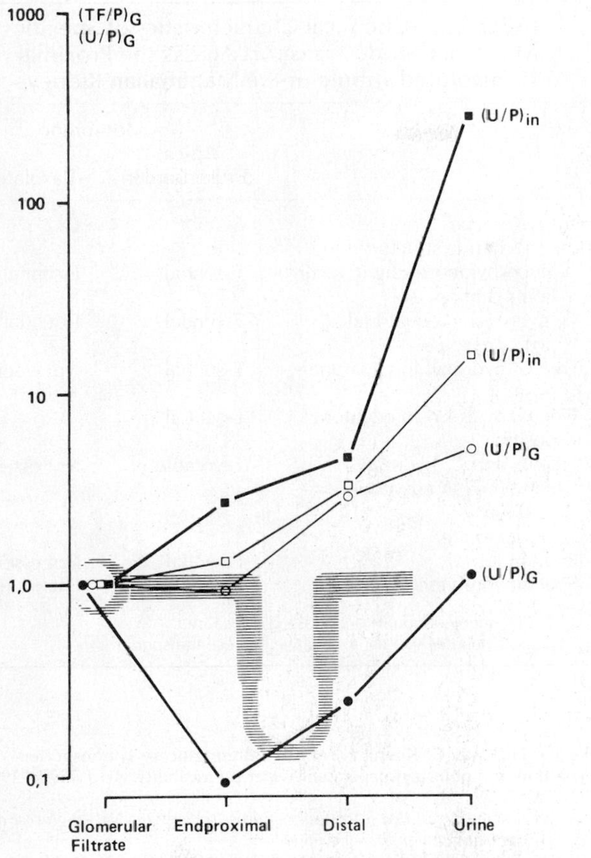

Figure 7.7. Experimental data for D-glucose reabsorption along the nephron in the mammalian kidney (rat model). **Ordinate:** Concentration quotient: tubular fluid/plasma *(TF/P)* and urine/plasma *(U/P)* for glucose *(G)* and inulin *(in)*, an indicator of fluid reabsorption. **Abscissa:** anatomic site of determination. *Solid symbols*, normoglycemia; *open symbols*, hyperglycemia, D-glucose infusion.

occurs at normal blood glucose levels. If the blood sugar level rises above 140 mg/dl, this excretion value increases (minimal threshold). Above a blood sugar concentration of 260 mg/dl, excretion becomes a linear function of the amount filtered (or the plasma level of D-glucose). Consequently, a plot of urinary D-glucose excretion rate against plasma D-glucose concentration yields maximal renal D-glucose transport. T_mG is found by extrapolation of the linear part of the urinary D-glucose excretion curve to its intercepts with the negative ordinate. The curvilinear segment between the minimal threshold and the linear part of the D-glucose excretion curve is termed *splay.* The determination of such a curve is called *D-glucose titration of the kidney.* This relationship is expressed by the following equation:

$$T_mG = GFR \times P_G - U_G \times V$$

where U_G is D-glucose concentration in urine, V is urine flow rate, P_G is D-glucose concentration in plasma, and *GFR* is glomerular filtration rate. It is evident that both P_G and GFR are determinants of renal D-glucose handling. The application of microperfusion techniques has clarified some characteristics of D-glucose handling in the proximal nephron. These techniques make it clear that transport is flow dependent, which is similar to "glomerulotubular balance," and that the transport obeys Michaelis Menten kinetics. This interrelation between GFR and T_mG is in humans described by the following ratio:

$$T_mG/GFR = 2.56 \text{ mg/ml}$$

This ratio transforms the tubular transport rate to a concentration and implies the maximal concentration difference that can be achieved between glomerular filtrate and tubular fluid after D-glucose reabsorption (when concomitant volume reabsorption is corrected for mathematically). This dependence of T_mG from GFR is evident in renal insufficiency, in which the GFR is permanently reduced. Concomitantly, the kidney's capacity to reabsorb D-glucose is reduced. The baseline D-glucose excretion is about sevenfold larger in this condition because the curvilinear segment of the titration curve (the so-called splay) is enlarged. Although in modern clinical nephrology the determination of a D-glucose titration curve for demonstration of a dysfunction of tubular reabsorption is no longer used, the described relationship helps illustrate how tubular transport mechanisms work.

Under normal conditions, D-glucose reabsorption represents a very potent transport mechanism in the kidney. The urinary content of D-glucose is negligible in comparison with the amount filtered. Approximately 99.7% of the filtered amount (130 g/day = 0.72 mol/24 hr) is reabsorbed. In extreme hyperglycemia, transport capacity in humans can be increased by a factor of 3.5.

HYPERGLYCEMIC GLUCOSURIA

In clinical practice, the most common cause for hyperglycemia is intravenous glucose administration. The only other cause is diabetes mellitus. In the nephron, hyperglycemia induces a cascade of three events.

First, the filtered glucose load increases above the capacity of the proximal tubule to reabsorb glucose (T_mG). It should be noted that the concept of glomerulotubular balance implies that increasing the filtered glucose load by a rise in GFR will not result in glucosuria. However, if the glucose load is increased by raising the plasma glucose concentration, glucosuria eventually will occur. In diabetic patients, glucose loss by excretion is beneficial because more severe hyperglycemia is prevented and glucose-related hyperosmolality with osmotic dehydration of cells is limited. Thus glucosuria can be considered as a protective overflow valve in hyperglycemia.

Second, once the absorptive capacity of the proximal convoluted tubule is exceeded, glucose gains access to more distal parts of the nephron. The latter is still able to concentrate the urinary solutes. Therefore D-glucose concentration in the final urine exceeds the plasma concentration in a manner similar to inulin (Fig. 7.7); however, the increase in inulin concentration is far less than that during normoglycemia. This indicates an increase in free water clearance and therefore net suppression of fluid reabsorption. In clinical practice, this condition is termed "osmotic diuresis" of uncontrolled severe diabetes mellitus.

Third, if osmotic diuresis is sustained, chronic sodium loss occurs. If fluid and sodium loss are not counterbalanced by fluid intake, GFR eventually decreases. This leads to a parallel reduction of T_mG due to glomerulotubular balance. Because of the reduced glomerular filtration of glucose, more severe hyperglycemia develops, leading to glucose-related hyperosmolality; cells dehydrate and hyperosmolar coma develops.

NORMOGLYCEMIC GLUCOSURIA

Abnormalities in renal glucose transport, which may be either congenital or acquired, also may lead to glucosuria. This type of glucosuria is of renal origin and is called *renal glucosuria.* It is defined as glucosuria that occurs independent of food intake and in the absence of hyperglycemia. Patients with renal glucosuria have normal blood glucose levels, have normal glucose tolerance tests, can store and use carbohydrates normally, and do not display other derangements in tubular function.

Two major forms of hereditary glucosuria exist: the A and the B types. The model of inheritance is autosomal dominant in both. Patients with type A renal glucosuria excrete glucose at low plasma glucose concentration and have a low T_mG with little splay in the titration curve. The term *type O glucosuria* refers to a state of virtual absence of proximal tubular D-glucose reabsorption. The defect is an extreme of type A glucosuria, with a T_mG of practically O. However, it is extremely rare. Individuals with type B renal glucosuria also excrete glucose at low plasma glucose levels but have normal T_mG with exaggerated splay. These two conditions are not of great clinical importance except that patients with renal glucosuria may be misdiagnosed as having diabetes mellitus if blood sugar levels are not measured. Occasionally, these patients develop mild symptoms of osmotic diuresis. Further discussion of renal glucosuria is provided in Chapter 26.

Fanconi syndrome is a generic term used to describe a clinical disorder with defects in the proximal tubular transport mechanisms for various substances, including phosphate, uric acid, bicarbonate, and amino acids, in addition to glucose. Fanconi syndrome may be observed in certain hereditary diseases such as tyrosinuria, cystinosis, Wilson's disease, fructose intolerance, galactosemia, Lowe's syndrome, and at times, glycogen storage disease. There are also acquired forms of Fanconi syndrome that could be secondary to the toxic effects of abnormal proteins in multiple myeloma, heavy metals such as lead and cadmium, or other chemical toxins such as outdated tetracycline, streptozotocin, and Lysol A. Discussion of glucosuria in pregnancy is found in Chapter 58.

RENAL EXCRETION OF SUGARS OTHER THAN D-GLUCOSE

Our knowledge of renal handling of other monosaccharides is far less complete and consists of little more than renal excretion data. Galactose is absorbed by the same system as D-glucose; however, because plasma levels are very low, galactosuria is uncommon.

With the exception of D-glucose and D-galactose, the origin of sugars found in urine remains unclear; however, comparison between excretion and filtration data reveals that a renal transport system must be operative in the case of D-fructose and D-mannose because the amount excreted is only a small percent of the amount filtered. Maximum fructose reabsorption rate is about 10% of the maximum capacity to reabsorb glucose. The reabsorptive mechanism of fructose appears to be independent of that for glucose. Because plasma levels like D-xylose, D-fucose, D-arabinose, or D-ribose of fructose are very low, fructosuria is uncommon. For other sugars, especially those with undetectable plasma levels, one may speculate that these substances do not have a specific transport system and that the concentration change along the nephron attributable to volume reabsorption may raise the extremely small amount presented to the tubular system to a concentration that can be detected with sensitive tools such as high-pressure liquid chromatography. The same considerations seem to apply to disaccharides like lactose, saccharose, or maltose.

TABLE 7.2. Chemical Characteristics of Specific Monosaccharide Transport Across the Proximal Convoluted Tubule of the Mammalian Kidney

	Membrane	
	Apical (Brush Border)	Basolateral
Transporter type	SGLT[a]	GLUT[b]
Monosaccharide structure		
D-glucospyranose ring in chair configuration	Essential	Essential
C_1 hydroxyl in equatorial position	Essential	Essential
Free C_2 hydroxyl in equatorial position	Essential	Not essential
Free C_3 hydroxyl in equatorial position	Essential	
Free C_4 and C_6 hydroxyls combined in equatorial position	Favorable	Not essential
Ionic requirement		
Sodium ions	Essential	Not essential
Specific inhibitors	Phlorizin	Phloretin

[a]SGLT denotes sodium D-glucose cotransporter.
[b]GLUT denotes specific facilitative glucose transporter.

Selected Readings

Gould GW, Bell GI. Facilitative glucose transporters: an expanding family. *TIBS* 1990;18–23.
A review of the molecular biology of glucose transporters.

Jette M, Vachon V, Potier M, Beliveau R. Radiation-inactivation analysis of the oligomeric structure of the renal sodium/D-glucose symporter. *Biochim Biophys Acta* 1997;1327:242–248.
Studies about the functional size of the Na⁺–D-glucose cotransporter SGLT1.

Loike JD, Hickman S, Kuang K, et al. Sodium-glucose cotransporters display sodium- and phlorizin-dependent water permeability. *Am J Physiol* 1996;271: C1774–C1779.
Studies to suggest that water and D-glucose traverse the Na^+–D-glucose cotransport protein through the same pore.

Mackenzie B, Loo DDF, Panayotova-Heiermann M, Wright EM. Biophysical characteristics of the pig kidney Na^+/glucose cotransporter SGLT2 reveal a common mechanism for SGLT1 and SGLT2. *J Biol Chem* 1996;271:32678–32683.
Biophysical properties of SGLT2 compared with SGLT1.

Oulianova N, Berteloot A. Sugar transport heterogeneity in the kidney: two independent transporters or different transport modes through an oligomeric Protein? 1. Glucose transport studies. *J Membr Biol* 1996;153:181–194.
Studies about kinetics and heterogeneity of sodium-D-glucose cotransporters.

Shannon JA, Farber S, Troast L. The measurement of glucose T_m in the normal dog. *Am J Physiol* 1941;133:752–761.
The first report to demonstrate a tubular transport maximum for D-glucose.

Thorens B, Lodish HF, Brown D. Differential localization of two glucose transporter isoforms in rat kidney. *Am J Physiol* 1990;259:C286–C294.
Detailed studies of glucose metabolism and glucose transporter types in different nephron segments.

Walker AM, Bott PA, Oliver J, MacDowell MC. The collection and analysis of fluid from single nephrons of the mammalian kidney. *Am J Physiol* 1941;134:580–595.
Studies demonstrating that the proximal tubule is the major site for D-glucose transport.

PART 3
Renal Handling of Uric Acid

Robert L. Wortmann and Carl J. Bentzel

The purine base, uric acid, is the final product of all purine nucleotide, nucleoside, and base degradation in humans (Fig. 7.8). Uric acid is a weak organic acid with a pKa of 5.75. It exists in the nonionized form in the urine, where the pH is generally less than 5.0. In the serum and extracellular fluids at a pH of 7.4, more than 98% of uric acid exists in the more soluble salt form, monosodium urate. In human disease, uric acid, which normally is supersaturated in urine, is a component of some renal

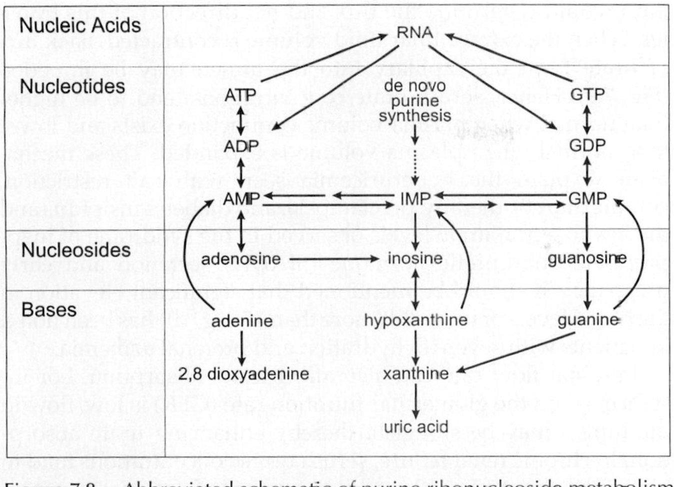

Figure 7.8. Abbreviated schematic of purine ribonucleoside metabolism in humans. Purine nucleosides are composed of a purine base joined to a sugar component. If the sugar is ribose, the nucleoside is a ribonucleoside (adenosine, inosine, and guanosine); if the sugar is deoxyribose, deoxynucleosides (deoxyadenosine, deoxyinosine, and deoxyguanosine) are formed. The addition of phosphorus moiety to a nucleoside results in nucleotide formation. These can be either ribonucleotides (ATP and GTP), the building blocks for ribonucleic acids *(RNA)*, or deoxynucleotides (deoxy ATP and deoxy GTP), the purine constituents of DNA. Uric acid is the final degradation product of purine metabolism in humans. *ADP,* adenosine dephosphate; *AMP,* adenosine monophosphate; *ATP,* adenosine triphosphate; *GDP,* guanosine diphosphate; *GMP,* guanosine monophosphate; *GTP,* guanosine triphosphate; *IMP,* inosine monophosphate.

calculi (see Chapter 53) and is the pathologic agent in acute uric acid nephropathy (tumor lysis syndrome). In this syndrome, uric acid precipitates in collecting ducts, where the pH is lowest and the solute concentration is highest. Monosodium urate is elevated in the serum of individuals with gout, is present in crystalline form in synovial fluid during acute gouty attacks, and is the major constituent of gouty tophi. The renal syndromes associated with gout and hyperuricemia are discussed in Chapter 44.

Uric acid may derive from the breakdown of exogenous, dietary purines or from purines produced endogenously by either *de novo* purine synthesis or nucleic acid turnover. The exogenous contribution to the total body urate pool and urinary uric acid excretion is often significant and varies with the amount and type of purine in the diet. The endogenous component is determined by measuring urinary uric acid excretion on a diet free of purines. After 1 week of dietary purine elimination, a 24-hour urine collection contains between 300 and 500 mg of uric acid in normal individuals.

Most uric acid is eliminated through the kidney. Tissue uricolysis is minimal. Some extrarenal elimination occurs through the alimentary tract with up to one-third of the daily uric acid excreted in saliva, gastric fluids, bile, pancreatic fluids, and intestinal juices. In renal failure, elimination of uric acid through the intestines greatly increases. The combination of renal and intestinal excretion of uric acid is quite effective. In fact, serum urate levels above 14.0 mg/dl are rarely encountered except when these routes are overwhelmed such as in cases of acute renal failure with uric acid nephropathy (tumor lysis syndrome), rhabdomyolysis, or severe acute pancreatitis.

Renal Handling of Uric Acid

The renal handling of uric acid includes glomerular filtration, early proximal tubular reabsorption, secretion into the proximal tubule, and postsecretory proximal tubular reabsorption (Fig. 7.9). A small percentage of filtered uric acid is also transported out of the distal nephron passively. The amount of uric acid that appears in the urine is the net result of reabsorptive and secretory processes and generally equals 8% to 12% of the filtered urate load.

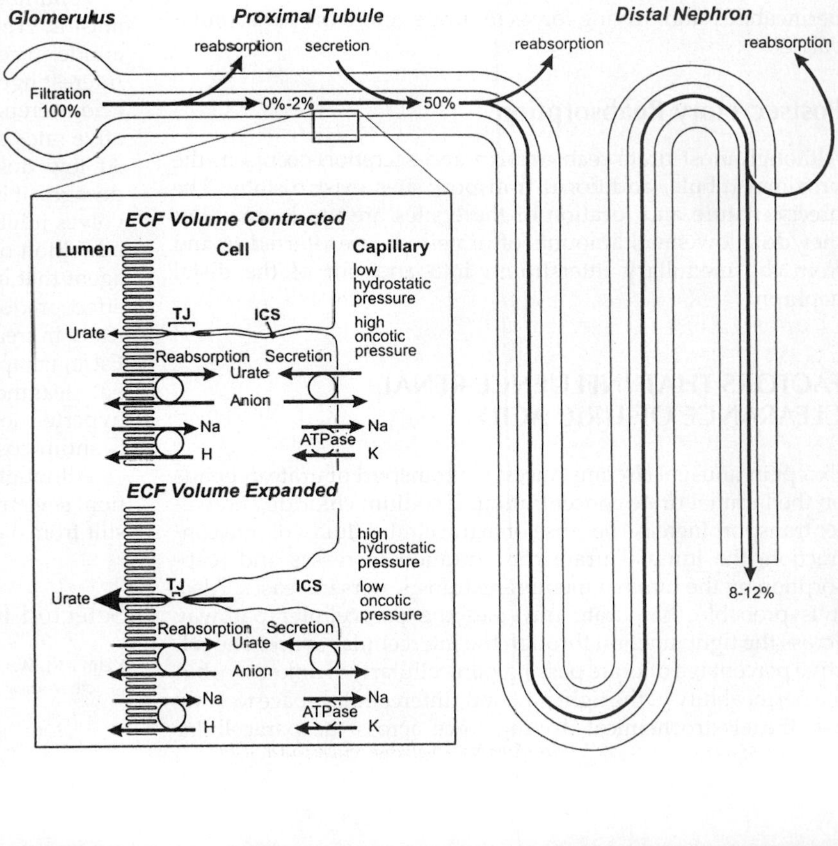

Figure 7.9. Schematic representing the renal handling of uric acid. The *arrows* represent the net direction of flux with the percentage of filtered urate. Insert represents activities at the proximal tubule cell level relative to extracellular fluid volumes.

Urate is both reabsorbed and secreted across the proximal tubule cell. A urate transporter is located in the luminal membrane, where urate is exchanged for another anion such as OH^- generated by the Na^+-H^+ exchanger. The initial step in secretion is via an anion exchanger located within the basolateral cell membrane domain. Transporters and exchangers are represented by *circles* and *arrows*.

When extracellular fluid volume is contracted (salt depletion), shown at the upper section, intercellular spaces *(ICS)* are collapsed due to low hydrostatic and high oncotic pressures in the peritubular capillary. Under these conditions more tight junctional elements are inserted into the membrane, thereby decreasing permeability to small molecules such as urate *(thin arrow)*. Thus net urate (and NaCL) absorption into the capillary is favored, which leads to a relative hyperuricemia.

In the volume expanded state (NaCL excess), shown in the lower section, peritubular factors restrict net NaCl and urate movement out of the more fluid-filled ICS. Because of the larger backflux across a more permeable tight junction *(heavy arrow)*, net urate absorption decreases, which leads to a relative hypouricemia. This is a hypothesis, and several alternative mechanisms can be invoked to explain the inverse relationship between extracellular fluid volume and serum uric acid concentration.

Glomerular Filtration

In the bloodstream, less than 5% of urate is bound to plasma proteins. This degree of binding is offset by the Donnan-Gibbs potential generated across the glomerular membrane such that urate is freely filtered at the glomerulus.

Proximal Tubular Reabsorption

Entering the proximal tubule, urate is reabsorbed across the luminal membrane into the cell by an active transport process in exchange for other anions. This is a saturable process, but it usually operates below its maximum capacity. The major driving force for urate reabsorption comes from Na^+-K^+-ATPase activities located in the basolateral membrane domain. Studies using isolated luminal membrane vesicles from dogs, rats, and humans indicate that the proximal tubular cells contain a specific urate transporter that is located in the luminal membrane. The urate transporter moves urate into the cell in exchange for hydroxyl, chloride, and bicarbonate ions generated by a hydrogen-sodium exchanger (Fig. 7.9). Organic anions such as pyruvate, lactate, b-hydroxybutyrate, pyrazinoate, and *p*-aminohippurate can also substitute for the anion in the exchanger, thereby increasing urate absorption. The luminal anion exchanger is inhibited by probenecid, furosemide, and stilbene derivatives. Once inside the cell, urate probably moves across the basolateral membrane in response to its electrochemical gradient.

Tubular Secretion of Urate

Studies of isolated basolateral membranes indicate that urate can move intracellularly through an anion exchange mechanism with affinities similar to the luminal exchanger except that lactate and *p*-aminohippurate have no effect. Probenecid and stilbene derivatives also inhibit the secretory basolateral exchanger. Although there is a complex bidirectional movement across both the cellular and paracellular pathways, the net direction for urate transport in humans, rats, and dogs is reabsorption. This is determined by the relative affinities of the luminal and basolateral transporters, as well as the passive permeability and driving forces for urate across the paracellular barrier.

Postsecretory Reabsorption

Although most urate reabsorption and secretion occurs in the proximal tubule, additional transport sites exist distally. The precise nature and location of these sites are not known, but they do allow small amounts of urate to be transferred to and from the medullary interstitium into and out of the distal nephron.

FACTORS THAT INFLUENCE RENAL CLEARANCE OF URIC ACID

Except in unusual circumstances, the transport of urate depends on the luminal urate concentration. If sodium chloride and water transport increase because of extracellular fluid volume contraction, the luminal urate concentration increases and reabsorption by the luminal membrane transporters increases. Also, it is probable that urate traverses the paracellular pathway across the tight junction through the intercellular space. The relative percentage of urate passing paracellularly is unknown, but the permeability of the tight junction/intercellular space to urate and the electrochemical driving force across the paracellular path would determine the flux and net direction of this transfer. When the extracellular fluid volume is contracted, back flux of urate from the capillary into the lumen may be impeded (Fig. 7.9). Hence, serum urate concentrations tend to be higher than normal when plasma volume contraction exists and lower than normal when plasma volume is expanded. These mechanisms explain the hyperuricemia seen with salt restriction, chronic diuretic therapy, preclampsia, and diabetes insipidus and the lower serum urate levels observed in the syndrome of inappropriate antidiuretic hormone (SIADH) secretion and early pregnancy. It should be mentioned that significant elevation in the blood levels of uric acid (more than 15 mg/dl) has been noted in patients with severe dehydration and prerenal azotemia.

Luminal flow rate can also affect urate absorption. For instance, when the glomerular filtration rate (GFR) is low, flow in the lumen may be sluggish, thereby enhancing urate absorption. In chronic renal failure, serum urate concentrations tend to plateau at about 12 to 13 mg/dl because the fractional excretion of urate increases with decreasing GFR and intestinal excretion increases. In contrast, hypouricemia may develop in diabetic patients with poor glycemic control because the fractional excretion of urate increases secondary to the osmotic diuresis caused by hyperglycemia.

Gout is the most common clinical condition associated with hyperuricemia. More than 95% of gouty patients are hyperuricemic as a result of altered renal handling of urate. A comparison of uric acid clearances and excretion rates over a wide range of filtered urate loads between gouty and healthy subjects showed a lower $C_{urate}/C_{insulin}$ in gouty subjects. This ratio increases in each group when the serum urate increases, but higher serum urate values are required in those with gout to reach the uric acid excretion rates observed in healthy subjects. This abnormality is attributed to diminished renal urate secretion per nephron, but the precise nature of the defect(s) is unknown.

Any accumulation of organic acids can be associated with hyperuricemia. This may result from a competitive inhibition of urate secretion. This is the case with starvation or alcoholic ketosis, diabetic ketoacidosis, maple syrup urine disease, and lactic acidosis of any cause.

A number of drugs can cause hyperuricemia by renal mechanisms. These drugs include low-dose salicylates, pyrazinamide, nicotinic acid, ethambutol, ethanol, and cyclosporine. Interestingly, salicylates produce a biphasic response in uric acid excretion, undoubtedly because of the drug's effect on relative rates of reabsorption and secretion in the proximal tubule. At low dosages, urate excretion is decreased, and at higher dosages, it is increased. An explanation for this phenomenon involves inhibition of secretion by low dosages of salicylate and inhibition of reabsorption by higher dosages. Probenecid is an agent that inhibits both secretion and absorption, but the latter effect predominates. Accordingly, this medication is useful clinically in treating hyperuricemia by promoting hyperuricosuria. Estrogen appears to lower serum urate levels by increasing renal clearance. In diabetic patients with insulin resistance and hypertension, serum urate levels may be elevated. Insulin itself is antiuricosuric.

Although little is known about distal sites of urate reabsorption, several cases of familial hypouricemia are believed to result from a defect in these mechanisms.

Selected Readings

Kahn AM, Weinman EJ. Urate transport in the proximal tubule: in-vivo and vesicle studies. *Am J Physiol* 1985;249:F789–F798.

Review of techniques use to study uric acid handling by the kidney with correlations and interpretations.

Kelley WN, Wortmann RL. Gout and hyperuricemia. In: Kelley WN, Harris ED Jr, Ruddy S, et al. eds. *Textbook of Rheumatology*, 5th ed. Philadelphia: WB Saunders, 1997:1313–1351.

Detailed review of purine metabolism, hyperuricemia, and diseases related to uric acid.

Quinones-Galvan A, Ferrannini E. Renal effects of insulin in man. *J Nephrol* 1997;10:188–191.

Review of the effects of insulin on glomerular and tubular functions, including the antinatruretic and antiuricosuric response. State of insulin resistance with hypertension and hyperuricemia is discussed.

Roch-Ramel F, Guisan B, Diezi J. Effects of uricosuric and antiuricosuric agents on urate transport in human brush border membrane vesicles. *J Pharm Exp Ther* 1997;280:839–845.

Because there is so much species variation even among mammals with respect to urate handling by the kidney, studies in human kidney are most sought. Brush border vesicles from the human kidney were used to study anion exchange mechanisms and the affinities of various organic anions on urate transport.

Simkin PA. Gout and hyperuricemia. *Curr Opin Rheumatol* 1997;9:268–273.

Review with 64 references on metabolism, transport, and clinical aspects of gout and management of hyperuricemia.

Ter Maaten JC, Voorburg A, Heine RJ, et al. Renal handling of urate and sodium during acute physiologic hyperinsulinemia in healthy subjects. *Clin Sci* 1997; 92:51–58.

Thirteen healthy subjects were studied with clearance techniques during exogenous insulin infusions. Insulin caused a decline in both fractional sodium and urate excretion.

PART 4
Renal Handling of Organic Acids and Bases

John B. Pritchard

Organic acids and bases are ingested with our food, consumed as drugs, and absorbed from our environment. In addition, many foreign chemicals are metabolized to charged products, and many endogenous compounds are converted to anionic or cationic metabolites. These compounds are eliminated from the body by the liver and kidney, with the kidney serving as the major route for the smaller (500 D or smaller), more water-soluble molecules. Examples are shown in Table 7.3. A number of factors, including plasma protein binding, changes in glomerular filtration rate (GFR) or in peritubular blood flow, and active or passive tubular reabsorption, have an impact on the kidney's ability to excrete charged organic compounds. However, for most organic ions, the primary determinant of excretion rate is secretion via the renal organic anion and organic cation transport systems. Both systems are strikingly effective, capable of clearing the renal plasma of a good substrate such as the anion *p*-aminohippurate (PAH) or the cation, tetraethylammonium (TEA) in a single pass through the kidney. This ability underlies the use of PAH clearance to estimate the effective renal plasma flow. Equally important for their excretory role, unlike many transport systems, which are highly specific, both systems are capable of transporting a remarkably diverse group of substrates, requiring only the presence of an appropriate charge and a hydrophobic region. Together, their capacity for effective transport and ability to handle structurally diverse compounds make the organic anion and organic cation secretory systems extremely effective in their primary role—protection of the body from the toxic effects of both endogenous and foreign chemicals.

TABLE 7.3. Classes of Organic Anions and Cations Secreted by the Proximal Tubule

Organic Anion System		
Antibiotics	Analgesics	Benzoates
Bile acids	Cyclic nucleotides	Corticosteroids
Decarboxylates	Glucuronides	Heterocyclic acids
Hippurates	Monocarboxylates	Oligopeptides
Penicillins	Phenols	Phenoxyacetates
Phenylpropionates	Prostaglandins	Sulfate esters
Sulfonamides	Sulfonic acids	
Organic Cation System		
Acridines	Aliphatic amines	Aminoindoles
Anilines	Benzodiazepines	Benzylamines
Catecholamines	Cephalosporins	Corticosteroids
Cyanine dyes	Ephedrines	Guanidines
Imidazoles	Morphines	Piperidines
Pyridines	Quaternary bases	Quinolines
Tetraacylammoniums	Thiazoles	

GENERAL FEATURES

History

Study of the organic anion system played a major role in the early development of renal physiology and medicine, thanks to the efficacy of transport and the ease of measuring urinary and plasma concentrations of colored organic anions. Thus secretion of an organic anion was first reported by Heidenhain more than a century ago. The importance of renal tubular secretion was hotly debated for 50 years until secretion of phenol red by *Lophius,* an aglomerular teleost incapable of glomerular filtration, provided definitive proof that tubular secretion was of fundamental importance in determining urinary solute composition. Soon thereafter, it was shown that the renal clearance of PAH could be used as a quantitative estimate of renal plasma flow and that secretion was a saturable process, with a definite transport maximum (T_m) *in vivo*. In contrast, the organic cation system was first observed in 1947 by Rennick in dog and Sperber in chicken. Organic cation secretion was also shown to be a saturable process *in vivo*, with T_m that often approached that of PAH.

Sites

Studies using stop flow and micropuncture *in vivo* and isolated tubular segments perfused *in vitro* demonstrated that transport of both organic anions and cations takes place in the proximal tubule. In most species, organic anions are transported by the entire proximal segment, but transport is most effective in the early portion of the pars recta (S_2 region). In contrast, organic cation secretion is most effective in the S_1 region of the tubule (pars convoluta). Nevertheless, both early and late portions (S_2 and S_3) of the pars recta are also capable of organic cation secretion. For both systems, greater carrier density, rather than differences in carrier affinity or function, appears to underlie regional differences in transport activity.

Specificity

The capillary microperfusion studies of Ullrich have greatly refined our understanding of the structural characteristics preferred by these systems. Optimal organic anion substrates have two negative (or partial negative) charges located 6 to 7 Å from each other and an 8- to 10-Å hydrophobic region (often aromatic). Singly charged anions are also transported by this carrier, provided they have the required hydrophobic region. Within a series of related molecules, their effectiveness as inhibitors of organic anion uptake increases as their pK_a falls and the degree of ionization increases. In general, the same principles hold for organic cations (i.e., the greater the lipid solubility and the higher the pK_a, thus the greater the ionization of the base at physiologic pH, the stronger the interaction with the organic cation carrier).

Binding

Protein binding of organic anions and organic cations reduces their free concentration in plasma, thus decreasing their availability for filtration or secretion. However, if the carrier proteins have a high affinity for the substrate, transport may compete effectively and the agent may still be secreted at rates approaching the renal plasma flow. Conversely, for a lower-affinity substrate (e.g., phenol red on the organic anion system), transport cannot proceed rapidly enough to deplete the plasma and changes in binding may greatly alter the efficacy of transport.

Reabsorption

Reabsorption may also impact the efficiency of excretion. For some compounds, such as urate, ascorbate, and choline, carrier-mediated pathways may return luminal organic ions to the blood. For most organic anions and organic cations, reabsorption is passive, driven by the lumen-to-blood concentration gradient produced by secretion and the concurrent reabsorption of tubular fluid. The primary determinant of passive reabsorption is lipid solubility, which permits diffusion through the plasma membrane of the tubular cells. Thus PAH is negligibly reabsorbed; whereas salicylate, which is nearly 300 times more lipid soluble, is reabsorbed extensively. Characteristic of passive reabsorption is a strong dependence of clearance on urine flow rate (i.e., the longer the contact time with the tubule, the greater the reabsorption and the lower the clearance). Furthermore, because the free acids and bases are the primary lipid-soluble forms, changes in luminal pH greatly alter their clearance. For example, reducing luminal pH will increase the concentration of the uncharged free acid, increasing lumen-to-cell flux. Once the acid reaches the higher pH of the cell interior, it is converted to the anion, effectively preventing diffusion back into the tubular lumen. This phenomenon, termed *pH trapping,* may greatly facilitate passive reabsorption. Clinically, urinary pH can be an important factor when excretion of anionic or cationic drugs must be accelerated after an overdose. If the urine is alkalinized, excretion of lipid-soluble weak acids will be favored (by reducing passive reabsorption). Conversely, an acid urine will favor elimination of basic drugs.

ORGANIC ANION TRANSPORT

Secretion of organic anions is a multistep process (Fig. 7.10). Basolateral entry takes place against a steep electrochemical gradient because the anion must move against a concentration gradient into the electrically negative interior of the cell. Thus uptake must be coupled to metabolic energy (i.e., active transport). As such, it must be carrier mediated, saturable, and inhibited competitively by other substrates. In contrast, luminal exit is energetically downhill, although it is also carrier mediated.

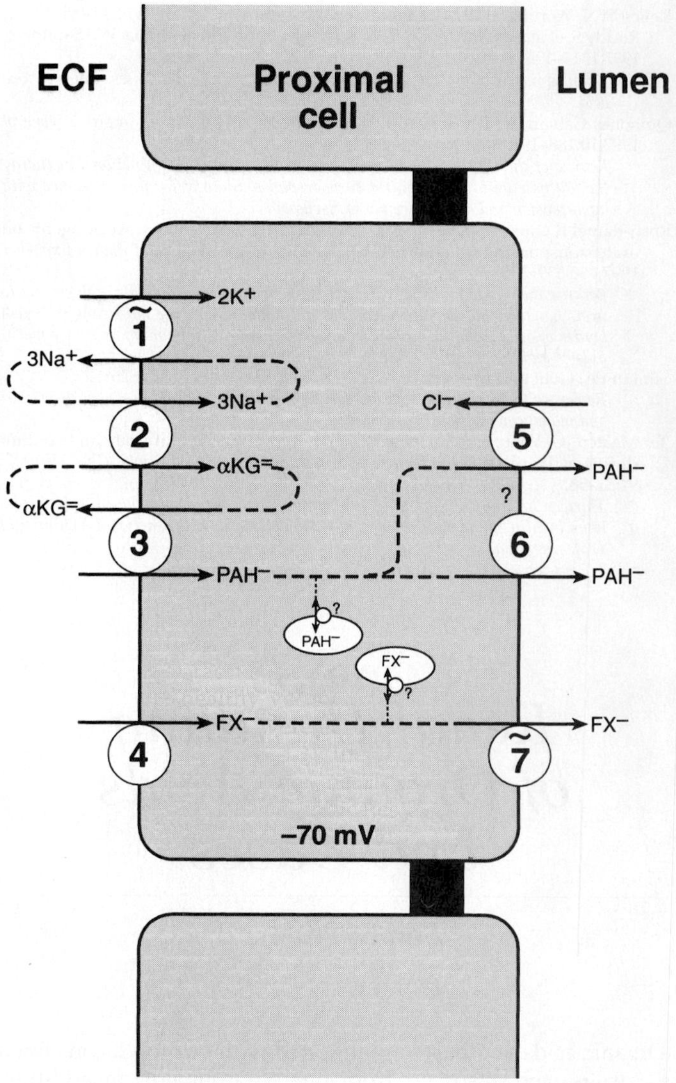

Figure 7.10. Schematic diagram showing the major components of renal organic anion transport. *Open circles* denote carrier proteins, the symbol ~ within a circle indicates an ATPase, and *arrows* indicate the preferred direction of transport. Individual transport components are numbered. At the basolateral membrane, uptake is uphill. Coupling of secretion of small organic anions (e.g., PAH) to ATP is tertiary, via Na^+-K^+-ATPase (#1), Na-αKG cotransport (#2), and αKG–organic anion exchange (#3). Metabolism supplies both the counterion (αKG) and the ultimate energy source, ATP. Large, lipophilic weak acids (e.g., FX) may enter via a Na-independent path (#4) or by simple diffusion. Intracellular organic anion may diffuse to the luminal membrane, bind to macromolecules, or be transported into vesicular structures. Uptake into vesicles is carrier mediated, but the mechanisms are unknown. Upon reaching the luminal membrane, organic anion efflux into the lumen is mediated by facilitated diffusion (#6) down its electrochemical gradient. The luminal anion exchanger (#5) may also play a role in secretion but is more likely responsible for mediated reabsorption of urate. Finally, larger lipophilic anions (e.g., FX) are actively transported to the lumen by the drug transporting ATPase, MPR2 (#7). *ECF,* extracellular fluid; *PAH, p*-aminohippurate; *FX,* fluorescein-methotrexate; *αKG,* α-ketoglutarate. (See text for a more complete discussion.)

Basolateral Mechanism

Basolateral organic anion uptake is inhibited by any maneuver that disrupts cellular energy production, including anoxia, cold, and metabolic inhibitors. As depicted in Fig. 7.10, coupling of basolateral organic anion uptake to Na is indirect—a tertiary active process in which coupling to metabolic energy is achieved through two intervening steps. Adenosine triphosphate (ATP) is hydrolyzed to drive the Na pump, creating the out > in Na gradient; Na entry down this gradient drives the uptake of α-ketoglutarate (αKG), creating an in > out αKG gradient; and the organic anion is taken up in exchange for αKG. Thus the αKG is recycled, and the overall process yields net uptake of Na and organic anion. Inhibitors of either organic anion-αKG exchange (e.g., probenecid) or Na-αKG cotransport (e.g., lithium or fumarate) inhibit the coupled system. Its abundance *in vivo* and the impact of changes in αKG concentration and gradient on organic anion transport in the intact tissue indicate that αKG is the physiologic counterion for organic anion secretion. Metabolic changes that alter αKG production also have an impact on organic anion secretion. Unlike the organic anion site on the exchanger, which accepts a broad range of substrates, the dicarboxylate site is very specific. Only glutarate, suberate, or adipate can substitute for αKG.

Imaging studies indicate that, at least for larger (500 to 1000 D) anions, additional basolateral pathways participate in secretion. For example, basolateral fluorescein-methotrexate (923 D; FX) uptake is independent of the Na gradient and is not be inhibited by the Na^+-K^+-ATPase inhibitor ouabain. Both treatments abolish uptake of substrates secreted via the tertiary active classical system (e.g., PAH). The quantitative importance of this alternative system is as yet unknown.

Intracellular Events

Secreted anions are not uniformly distributed within the tubular cells. They are subject to extensive intracellular binding. Moreover, imaging studies using fluorescein (332 D), a fluorescent organic anion, have shown that a portion of the intracellular organic anion is sequestered within vesicular structures via a specific uptake process that is inhibited by microinjection of PAH or probenecid into the cells. The physiologic roles of binding and sequestration, if any, remain to be established. However, two possibilities are likely. First, both processes decrease the free concentration of intracellular organic anions during secretion, perhaps reducing the likelihood of toxicity. Second, intracellular trafficking of vesicular structures, known to occur in many cell types, including kidney cells, could play a role in transcellular organic anion movement.

Luminal Mechanism

As shown in Fig. 7.10, two potential pathways for exit of secreted organic anions have been observed in luminal, or brush border, membrane (BBM) vesicles. The first is an organic anion exchanger, which is shared by PAH, lactate, and urate, as well as several inorganic anions (Cl^-, HCO_3^-, OH^-). However, this transporter has been described only in urate reabsorbers (dogs, rats) and is absent in urate secretors (rabbits, pigs). Because both groups secrete organic anions, this exchanger does not appear to be an obligatory component in secretion. Furthermore, the presence of luminal Na-H antiport, which will make the cell interior more alkaline than tubular fluid, favors reabsorptive (lumen-to-cell) flux. Thus it appears that the BBM exchanger may be more important in urate reabsorption than in organic anion secretion. Both urate secretors (pigs) and reabsorbers (rats) also have a probenecid-sensitive, potential-driven carrier in the luminal membrane. Given the steep electrochemical gradient favoring cell-to-lumen flux of anions across the BBM, such an electrogenic carrier would be sufficient to account for luminal efflux of secreted organic anions. Other data indicate the presence of a third luminal transporter, the drug transporting ATPase, MRP2 (*m*ultidrug *r*esistance–associated *p*rotein). The leukotrienes anionic prostaglandin metabolites are particularly well transported by the MRP system at extrarenal sites. They also block luminal transport of the larger organic anions (e.g., FX) in the proximal tubule. Once again, the quantitative significance of this newly discovered mechanism has not been established.

Bidirectional Transport (Urate)

Renal transport of urate also takes place in the proximal tubule. However, its handling is complex. Some species (humans, chimpanzees, rats, and mongrel dogs) show net reabsorption; whereas others (rabbits, Dalmatian dogs, and pigs) show net secretion. The simplest case is for urate secretors such as the pig. In these species, PAH and urate are handled similarly at both basolateral membrane (BLM) and BBM. BLM urate uptake is indirectly coupled to Na via αKG-urate exchange and Na-αKG cotransport. However, transport is poorly inhibited by PAH and, unlike PAH, has little Cl^- dependence. Thus the two mechanisms seem parallel but are apparently mediated by separate carriers. Luminal exit of secreted urate is mediated by the potential driven carrier discussed previously. Urate reabsorbers, like the dog, use the luminal anion exchanger to take up urate in exchange for various internal inorganic and organic anions. The required in > out gradients for counterions are maintained through the Na gradient (e.g., the Na-H antiporter or Na-lactate cotransporter). Basolateral efflux of reabsorbed urate is potential driven and probenecid inhibited, but this pathway is not shared by PAH. A number of uncertainties remain, for example, the extent to which reabsorption occurs in secreting species and vice versa, but overall a clearer picture of urate handling is now emerging. The renal handling of urate is discussed in detail in Part 3 of this chapter.

ORGANIC CATION TRANSPORT

Many commonly used drugs, including local anesthetics, antihistamines, anticholinergics, and neuromuscular blockers, are substrates for the organic cation system (Table 7.3). Thus competition for excretion via the organic cation system may be very important in drug interactions, decreasing excretory efficiency and elevating plasma and tissue levels. Nicotine and certain abused drugs (e.g., cocaine, morphine) are also organic cation system substrates, further complicating this issue. In mammals, most of these organic cations are handled by similar transport mechanisms. However, it appears that organic cation transport is not a single monolithic system. Several renal organic cation transporters have now been cloned. The precise role of each is unknown, but by analogy with the drug metabolizing enzymes (e.g., cytochrome P450), each may handle a subset of the cationic agents reaching the kidney. The major features of organic cation transport are depicted in Fig. 7.11. Secretion is a multistep process. Peritubular (BLM) uptake of the positively charged organic cations is energetically downhill, apparently driven by the potential difference across the membrane. Luminal exit is uphill, opposed by the membrane potential and must be coupled to metabolic energy.

Basolateral Mechanism

BLM uptake of the model substrates TEA and N^1-methylnicotinamide (NMN) is inhibited by other organic cations. Thus uptake is carrier mediated. In both membrane vesicles and intact tissue, basolateral organic cation transport is driven by membrane potential. Because the basolateral potential difference is

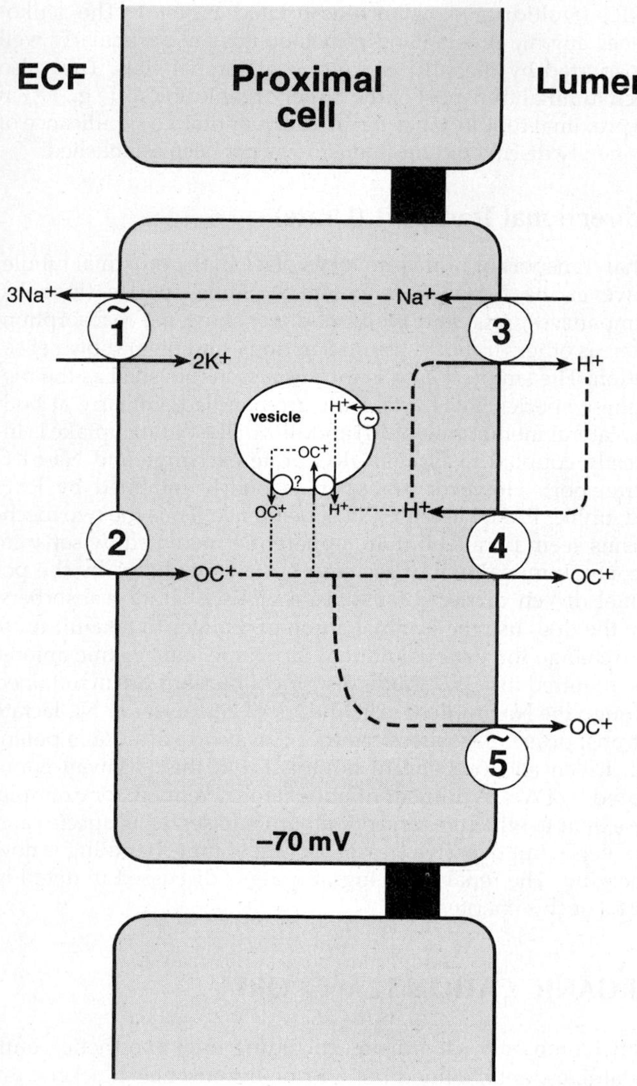

Figure 7.11. Schematic diagram of the major components of renal organic cation transport. Symbols have the same meaning as in Fig. 7.10. At the basolateral membrane, organic cations enter the cell by facilitated diffusion (#2) down the electrochemical gradient supplied by the inside negative membrane potential. Larger, more lipid-soluble weak bases may also enter by diffusion. Some of the internal organic cation is bound, and some is taken up into vesicular organelles via proton–organic cation exchange driven by the proton gradient created by the vacuolar H^+-ATPase. The functional role of sequestration, if any, has not yet been established. At the luminal membrane, exit may occur by two paths. The major pathway transports small organic cations (e.g., TEA, NMN) and is mediated by proton–organic cation exchange (#4). Exchange is driven by the pH gradient (lumen acidic) maintained by luminal Na-proton exchange (#3). Thus this pathway is indirectly coupled to the out > in Na gradient, maintained by the Na pump (#1). The second possible route for larger, lipophilic cations is mediated by the multidrug transport ATPase (MDR) (#5). *ECF,* extracellular fluid; *TEA,* tetraethylammonium; *NMN,* N^1-methylnicotinamide. (See text for details.)

about −70 mV, facilitated diffusion alone could account for the 10- to 12-fold (cells > medium) gradients seen in most species without additional energy input. TEA and NMN appear to share the same basolateral mechanism in most species, as judged by their mutual inhibition *in vivo* and *in vitro.* Their affinities vary from species to species, but TEA is the better substrate with a K_m of approximately 100 μM, as compared with NMN, which has one-fifth to one-tenth the affinity.

Intracellular Events

Some species (e.g., rabbits, snakes) show intracellular TEA concentrations as great as 100 times the peritubular bathing medium. If this TEA were free in the cytoplasm, its accumulation could not be accounted for by potential-driven transport alone. However, no additional active mechanisms have been detected in these species, suggesting that free intracellular TEA must be much lower than its total concentration, that is, that a substantial fraction must be bound to macromolecules or sequestered within intracellular compartments. Indeed, as for organic anions, both processes may contribute. Uptake into acidic subcellular organelles (e.g., endosomes, lysosomes, Golgi vesicles) may be particularly important. Proton-cation exchange and/or pH trapping lead to extensive accumulation of organic cations within these organelles. The precise roles of organic cation sequestration and binding are yet to be resolved. However, it is clear that these processes are found in all species, not just the rabbit and snake. Thus sequestration may be important in protecting the tubule from organic cation toxicity and/or in transit of organic cations across the tubular cells.

Luminal Mechanism

Luminal exit of organic cations is opposed by the same potential gradient that drives BLM entry. Thus additional energy input is required. As demonstrated in isolated BBM vesicles from several species, luminal membranes have a proton–organic cation antiporter. In concert with the Na-proton antiporter, this antiporter is poised to couple luminal organic cation efflux to the Na gradient (Fig. 7.11). Na-proton exchange keeps the luminal proton concentration higher than the tubular cells, enabling proton–organic cation exchange to mediate luminal efflux of intracellular organic cations. In addition, the multidrug-resistance transport ATPase (called *MDR, p-glycoprotein,* or *gp-170*) is able to transport many drugs (mostly larger organic cations) across the luminal membrane. This system is distinct from the organic cation–proton exchanger, and its physiologic role has yet to be determined, but it has the potential to transport organic cations in the secretory direction. Thus, like MRP2, which transports larger organic anions, MDR may be an important alternative pathway for the luminal step in organic cation secretion.

Bidirectional Transport (Choline)

Carrier-mediated reabsorption of choline was described many years ago, but its mechanism was unknown. Wright showed that luminal membranes transport choline via two paths. One is a low-affinity system, shared with TEA and NMN, and appears to be the proton–organic cation antiporter discussed previously. The second has a high affinity for choline, is driven by membrane potential, and is not shared by TEA or NMN. Thus, at low choline concentrations, reabsorption from the lumen is driven by the high-affinity carrier. Basolateral exit of reabsorbed choline apparently is mediated by the organic cation carrier mentioned earlier. At higher concentrations, secretion is mediated by the BBM proton-choline antiporter.

MOLECULAR BIOLOGY

Several of the transport proteins that contribute to renal organic anion and cations secretion have now been cloned, including the basolateral αKG–organic anion exchanger (Fig. 7.10) and several potential-driven facilitated diffusion carriers for organic cations (Fig. 7.11). The luminal ATP-driven transporters (MRP2 and MDR) have also been cloned. Attempts are currently under way to clone the luminal transporters for both classical systems. Further progress in this area should yield much information about the biochemical determinants of transport and regulatory mechanisms controlling secretory activity. However, at present, there are many questions and few answers. Already, it is clear that there are more transport proteins than were previously anticipated and that organic anion and cation carriers share substantial sequence homology, but the functional significance of these observations is uncertain.

PERSPECTIVES

Together, the organic anion and organic cation transport systems mediate the excretion of myriad foreign and endogenous anions and cations, particularly drugs and their metabolites. This constitutes a primary line of defense against their systemic toxicity. However, it also means that competition for excretory transport is an important site of drug interactions. Likewise, the extensive intracellular accumulation of organic anions and organic cations, which occurs during secretion, makes the kidney an important target for expression of the toxicity of both foreign and endogenous chemicals. Finally, new insights from cellular and molecular biology indicate the participation of multiple systems of differing specificity. It will be a major challenge to assess the partitioning of drugs between these systems and predict its consequences in terms of drug interactions and toxicity.

Selected Readings

Burckhardt G, Pritchard JB. Organic anion and cation antiporters. In: Seldin DW, Giebisch G, eds. *The kidney: physiology and pathophysiology*, 3rd ed. New York: Raven Press, 2000 (in press).

A comprehensive review of the mechanisms, specificity and molecular biology of the organic anion and cation secretory systems.

Miller DS, Pritchard JB. Dual pathways for organic anion secretion in renal proximal tubule. *J Exptl Zool* 1997;279:462–470.

Reviews evidence for transport pathways in addition to the classical sodium-dependent, αKG-coupled renal organic anion secretory system.

Pritchard JB, Miller DS. Intracellular compartmentation of organic anions and cations during renal secretion. *Cell Physiol Biochem* 1996;6:50–59.

Reviews mechanisms and potential roles of vesicular accumulation and intracellular compartmentation in renal organic anion and cation secretion.

Ullrich KJ. Renal transporters for organic anions and cations. Structural requirements for substrates. *J Membrane Biol* 1997;158:95–107.

Summarizes extensive studies combining molecular modeling and transport measurement to define the structural requirements for organic ion transport.

PART 5
Renal Tubular Handling of Proteins and Peptides

Valerie L. Johnson and Thomas Maack

The kidney plays an important role in the stabilization of the concentration and turnover of oligopeptides and proteins in the extracellular fluid (ECF). For intermediate and large proteins, the kidney acts essentially as a passive barrier against their loss to the external environment. Nevertheless, even under normal circumstances, a small proportion of these proteins are filtered by the kidney and absorbed by the renal tubular cells. For these proteins, the kidney's conservative role becomes apparent only when the glomerular barrier loses its effectiveness. When this occurs, plasma levels decrease and turnover in plasma proteins, particularly albumin, increases, leading to a major imbalance of the internal environment.

On the other hand, under normal conditions, the kidney plays an essential role in the regulation of the concentration and turnover rates of low-molecular-weight proteins (LMWPs). LMWPs are a heterogeneous group of proteins and polypeptides of various molecular structure, physiochemical properties, and biologic functions. They constitute a small but biologically important fraction of the total plasma protein mass. Whereas the plasma half-life of albumin and globulins is days or weeks, the plasma half-life for LMWPs is measured in terms of hours or, in many instances, minutes. One of the main reasons for the short plasma half-life of LMWPs is that they are extensively filtered, absorbed by the tubular epithelium, and eventually hydrolyzed within the renal tubular cells to their constituent amino acids. As a consequence, when glomerular filtration is impaired, the plasma half-life and plasma levels of LMWPs increase. This chapter reviews the pathways and mechanisms of the renal handling of LMWPs and peptides.

RENAL ACCUMULATION OF PROTEINS

Administration of LMWPs to intact animals leads to preferential accumulation of these proteins in the kidneys. For several LMWPs, up to 30% to 60% of the administered dose is accumulated by the kidney. On a weight basis, the kidney accumulates LMWPs to a much larger degree than any other organ in the body. This process is due to filtration of the administered protein with subsequent tubular absorption. Indeed, when filtration is experimentally abolished or tubular absorption is inhibited by metabolic inhibitors, renal accumulation of administered LMWPs is greatly impaired.

For a number of administered LMWPs, a linear relationship exists between the administered dose and the renal tissue content of the protein over a wide range of doses, indicating that the accumulation process is not readily saturable. Nevertheless, saturation has been shown to occur with lysozyme and cytochrome-c. Interestingly, much higher dosages of lysozyme than of cytochrome-c are necessary to saturate the accumulation process. This particular characteristic of high and differential capacity of accumulation of administered LMWPs is due to the particular kinetics of tubular absorption of proteins.

RENAL EXTRACTION OF PROTEINS

The kidney's role in the turnover of circulating LMWPs was initially inferred from results of experiments in which the plasma half-lives of these proteins were compared in the presence and absence of kidneys. More reliable determinations of the renal extraction rates for proteins are obtained by measuring the organ clearance of these substances either in intact animals or in an isolated kidney preparation. For example, the determination of the renal extraction rate for rat growth hormone (rGH) in the isolated perfused rat kidney shows that the perfusate disappearance rate for ^{125}I-rGH is less than that of a glomerular filtration marker, indicating that renal extraction of rGH can be accounted for by its filtration. This conclusion is further strengthened by the finding that the renal extraction of rGH in the nonfiltering isolated perfused kidney is negligible. From the data on the renal extraction of rGH in the isolated rat kidney and the total plasma disappearance rate for rGH in the rat, it can be calculated that renal extraction accounts for approximately 70% of the total metabolic clearance rate (MCR) for this protein in the intact rat. As with rGH, renal extraction accounts for the major proportion of the metabolic clearance for many LMWPs examined thus far. Of note is the finding that the renal extraction rates are not related to the biologic activity of the protein in the kidney itself. Moreover, the process of renal extraction does not necessarily depend on the presence of specific renal receptors for LMWPs or polypeptide hormones. A notable exception in this regard occurs with atrial natriuretic peptide (ANP), whose extraction by the kidney is determined by its binding to a specific class of receptors, named clearance (C) receptors of ANP. However, these receptors are mostly distributed in glomerular and vascular structures of the kidney rather than in tubular cells. Other work has identified megalin, belonging to the low-density lipoprotein (LDL) receptor family, as a putative receptor in the proximal tubule mediating endocytosis of a large variety of macromolecules. In addition, Pept-1 and Pept-2 have been identified as transporters of oligopeptides (dipeptides and tripeptides).

FILTRATION OF PROTEINS

Filtration is the initial and rate-limiting step in the renal turnover of many circulating proteins. Figure 7.12 represents schematically the major factors that determine the degree of filterability of circulating proteins and polypeptide hormones.

The glomerular sieving coefficient (GSC; concentration of protein in glomerular filtrate/concentration of protein in plasma water) for albumin has been the subject of numerous investigations. Initial micropuncture studies in the rat would have albumin concentrations in the glomerular filtrate of 10 to 20 mg/dl with a GSC of 0.001 to 0.005. As methodology improved, values for albumin concentration in glomerular filtrate became smaller (less than 1 mg/dl to 3 mg/dl). Because of the very low degree of albumin filterability under normal conditions, the kidney does not play an important role in the turnover of this protein or of proteins with larger molecular size. With renal disease, however, filtration of albumin and larger proteins becomes considerable, and tubular absorption, renal catabolism, and urinary excretion become significant.

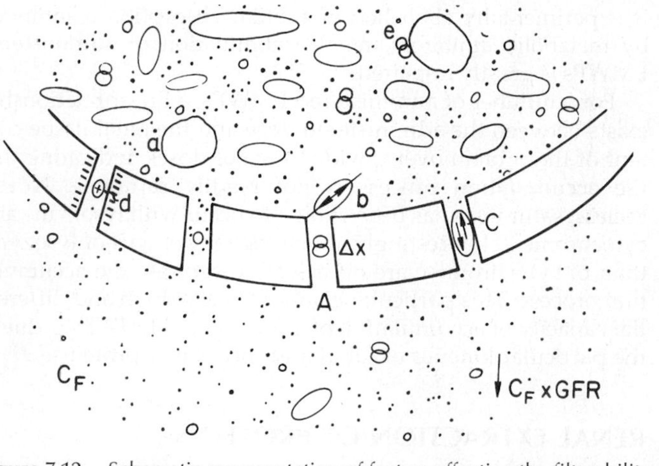

Figure 7.12. Schematic representation of factors affecting the filterability of proteins. Glomerular barrier is represented with hypothetic pores communicating between the lumen of capillaries and Bowman's space. C_P, protein concentration in plasma water; C_F, protein concentration in filtrate; *GFR,* glomerular filtration rate; *a,* molecular dimension hindrance; *b,* steric hindrance; *c,* viscous drag; *d,* electrical hindrance; *e,* protein–protein interaction. Proteins with dimensions larger than the size of "pores" or bound to larger proteins are not filtered *(a, e)*. Proteins in which at least one of the diameters is smaller than the diameter of the "pores" are restricted by steric hindrance, viscous drag, and electrical hindrance *(b, c, d)*. Electrical hindrance retards the passage of negatively charged proteins and favors passage of positively charged proteins. Steric hindrance, viscous drag, and electrical hindrance affect mainly intermediate proteins (e.g., albumin) and have little influence on filtration of low-molecular-weight proteins. (Reprinted from Heinemann HO, Maack T, Sherman RI. Proteinuria. *Am J Med* 56: 71–81. Copyright 1974 with permission from Excerpta Medica Inc.)

Proteins smaller than albumin appear in significant quantity in the glomerular filtrate relative to their plasma concentration. Table 7.4 shows GSC values for several LMWPs together with their respective molecular weights and Stokes-Einstein radii. As can be seen from this table, the degree of sieving is inversely related to the molecular size of the protein. Furthermore, renal filtration of intermediate proteins such as horseradish peroxidase (Table 7.4) and albumin are greatly influenced by the net charge of the protein.

This is because negative charges in the glomerular basement membrane hinder the filtration of anionic and enhance the filtration of cationic macromolecules. However, the influence of charge becomes significant only as the Stokes-Einstein radii of the protein approaches the radius of the "filtration pores."

TUBULAR ABSORPTION OF PROTEINS

Reabsorption of macromolecules by the renal proximal tubule is mediated by an extensive apical endocytic apparatus consisting of an elaborate network of coated pits and small coated and noncoated endosomes. The renal tubular cells also contain a large number of late endosomes/prelysosomes, lysosomes, and so-called dense apical tubules involved in recycling membrane from the endosomes to the apical plasma membrane. As a result of this uptake process, normally, urinary excretion of proteins is negligible compared with their total filtered load. Taking β_2-microglobulin (β_2M) as an example, it can be seen in Fig. 7.13 that the fractional clearance ($C_{\beta 2M}$/GFR) of this protein is quite small. Because the GSC for β_2M is close to 1 (Table 7.4), the low

TABLE 7.4. Glomerular Sieving Coefficients (GSC) for Some Low-Molecular-Weight Proteins

Protein	Molecular Weight	Molecular Radius (Å)	GSC
Cytochrome-c	12,400	15	0.93
Insulin	6,000	15	0.89
β_2-Microglobulin	11,600	16	0.94
Myoglobulin	16,900	19	0.75
Lysozyme	14,600	19	0.75
Rat GH	20,000	20	0.60
Bovine PTH	9,000	21	0.65
Horseradish peroxidase	40,000		
Anionic		32	0.007
Neutral		30	0.06
Cationic		30	0.34
Bence Jones			
(λ light chain)	44,000	28	0.09
Albumin	66,000	36	<0.0005

GH, growth hormone; PTH, parathyroid hormone.

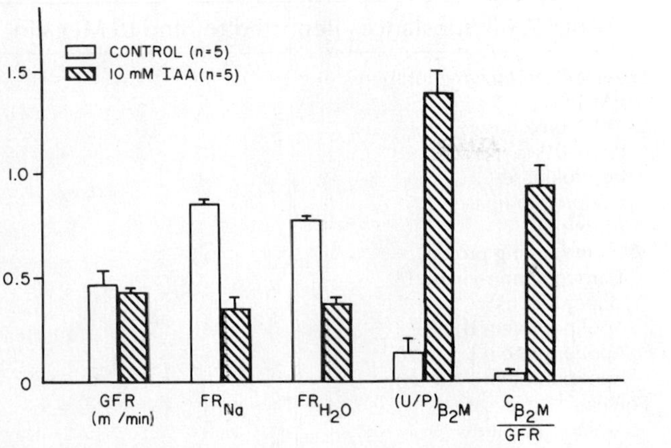

Figure 7.13. Renal handling of β_2-microglobulin (β_2M) in isolated perfused rat kidney showing the influence of the metabolic inhibitor iodoacetate *(IAA)*. *GFR*, glomerular filtration rate; *FR_{Na}*, fractional reabsorption of sodium; *FR_{H_2O}*, fractional reabsorption of water; *$(U/P)_{\beta_2M}$*, urine-to-perfusate concentration ratio of β_2M; *C_{β_2M}/GFR*, fractional clearance of β_2M. (Based on data from Sumpio BE, Maack T. Kinetics, competition and selectivity of tubular absorption of proteins. *Am J Physiol* 1982;243:F379–F392.)

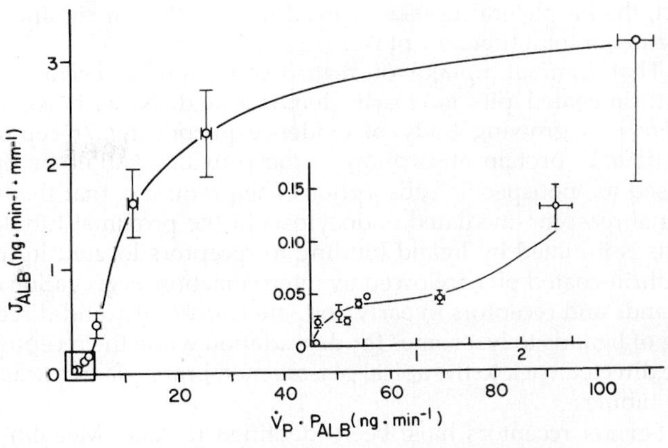

Figure 7.14. Kinetics of albumin *(ALB)* absorption in isolated perfused proximal convoluted tubules of the rabbit kidney. **Abscissa:** Perfused loads of albumin, where V_p is tubular flow rate and P_{ALB} is albumin in tubular fluid. **Ordinate:** Albumin absorption rates *(J)*. The absorption curve has two components: a high-capacity, low-affinity component (J max ALB = 3.7 ng/min/mm tubule length; K_m 1.2 mg/ml); and a low-capacity, higher-affinity component (inset, J max ALB = 0.0064 ng/min/mm tubule length; K_m = 0.031 mg/ml). (Reprinted from Park CH, Maack T. *J Clin Invest* 1984;73:767–777. Copyright by permission of the American Society for Clinical Investigation.)

fractional clearance indicates that the bulk of the filtered load of this protein has been absorbed by the renal tubular cells. Results similar to these have been found for a number of other LMWPs and polypeptides/peptides.

Renal uptake of proteins occurs predominantly in the pars convoluta or S_1 and S_2 segments of the proximal tubules and, to a lesser extent, in the pars recta or late S_2 and S_3 segments. Up to the present, it has been held that proteins are largely absorbed by nonspecific adsorptive endocytosis. Tubular absorption is thought to be initiated by an electrostatic interaction between positively charged groups on the protein and anionic sites on the luminal membrane or membrane coat. The results of a number of studies indicate that the net charge of a protein is a main determinant of its uptake kinetics. However, there is not a simple relationship between the number and density of the net positive charges of a macromolecule and the selectivity, capacity, and efficiency of its absorption. For example, highly cationic DEAE-dextran is not absorbed to any appreciable degree by the tubular cells.

The protein adsorbed at the luminal membrane is endocytosed and concentrated within vesicles at the apical border of tubular cells (endocytic vesicles). These endocytic vesicles fuse with acidic organelles that belong to the endosomal compartment. The endosomes (also called *phagosomes*), containing the segregated protein, then migrate to the cell interior, where they fuse with lysosomes, cell organelles that contain acid hydrolases. As is discussed in the following sections, absorbed proteins are eventually hydrolyzed to completion within lysosomes and the resulting amino acids cross the contraluminal membrane to return to the circulation.

The abundance of available morphologic and qualitative data prompted further studies defining the quantitative aspects of this process. The evidence demonstrates that tubular uptake of proteins is a high-capacity, low-affinity transport system localized mostly in proximal tubular cells. Figure 7.14, which shows the titration curve of albumin absorption by isolated perfused proximal tubules of the rabbit, provides an example of the quantitative aspects of the tubular absorption of proteins. The kinetics of albumin absorption by proximal tubules are characterized by an overall high capacity and relatively low affinity compared with the normal filtered loads of this protein. This kinetic characteristic is universal among all proteins tested to date. In addition to the high-capacity transport, the albumin titration curve also reveals a low-capacity system, with a maximal capacity that is approximately two orders of magnitude lower than that of the high-capacity system. This low-capacity system is therefore operational in the lower ranges of tubular fluid albumin concentration (0.1 to 0.2 mg/dl), which includes near physiologic tubular fluid concentrations of this protein and those observed in mild albuminuria. One possible explanation for the dual kinetics of albumin uptake is that it is caused by a combination of adsorptive endocytosis (low-capacity system) and bulk incorporation of albumin aggregates by fluid endocytosis. The low overall affinity rather than low capacity of albumin uptake explains why small increases in albumin filtered loads lead to significant increases in albuminuria.

Although the uptake process has been interpreted to be a nonspecific adsorptive endocytic mechanism, the kinetic parameters of tubular absorption differ significantly even for proteins of similar size and net charge, as is the case for lysozyme and cytochrome-c, two cationic proteins of similar pI and molecular radius. Therefore there is some selectivity for tubular absorption, whose mechanism is not well understood. Selectivity for tubular absorption, however, does not mean that proteins do not compete for tubular absorption. Thus cytochrome-c has been shown to competitively inhibit the tubular absorption of lysozyme and vice versa. Similarly, tubular absorption of the anionic protein cadmium metallithione has been shown to be inhibited by a large excess of myoglobin, a slightly anionic protein. On the other hand, proteins of net opposite charge (e.g., lysozyme, myoglobin) do not readily compete for the tubular absorption process. Under pathologic conditions, in view of the high capacity of absorption, it is unlikely that proteins compete for tubular absorption, even when filtered loads are significantly elevated. This explains why elevations of plasma levels or filtered loads of a particular protein do not necessarily lead to increased urinary excretion of other proteins.

Basolateral endocytic uptake in the proximal tubule is insignificant for most proteins. However, for certain hormones and growth factors for which receptors may be localized to the basolateral membranes, it can be of quantitative importance. In fact, the basolateral uptake of insulin constitutes a significant portion of total tubular uptake.

That luminal uptake of reabsorbed proteins occurs via clathrin-coated pits is clearly demonstrated. Now, however, there is a growing body of evidence purporting "receptor-mediated" protein absorption in the proximal tubule as opposed to "nonspecific" absorption. The premise is that the luminal receptor–mediated endocytosis in the proximal tubular cells is initiated by ligand binding to receptors located in the clathrin-coated pits, followed by internalization, segregation of ligands and receptors in early and late endosomes, and directing of ligands to lysosomes for degradation while the receptors are directed back to the apical plasma membrane via dense apical tubules.

Several receptors have been identified to date. Megalin is probably the most important receptor in the proximal tubule. In addition, there are more specific receptors such as the folate receptor, the insulinlike growth factor II/Man-6-P, and the intrinsic factor receptor.

Megalin, previously called gp330 or the Heymann nephritis antigen, is a large-molecular-weight membrane protein first localized to glomerular epithelial cells and proximal tubule cells. The receptor constitutes a significant portion of the total membrane protein in the proximal tubule. However, the kidney is not the only membrane site (i.e., it is also found in the parathyroids, epididymis, type II pneumocytes, ependyma and ciliary epithelium of the eye, and inner ear epithelium). Megalin is a 600-kD protein, and the largest known single-chain membrane receptor. The protein belongs to the low-density lipoprotein receptor family. In the renal proximal tubule cells, megalin has been shown to be present in the clathrin-coated pits at the base of the microvilli, as well as apical endocytic vacuoles, and dense apical tubules. Variable degrees of brush border labeling are seen in the late S_1, S_2, and S_3 segments of the proximal tubule.

The early studies showing its location in coated pits first suggested that megalin might function as an endocytic receptor. Several functional studies have supported its ability to bind a wide variety of macromolecules, including albumin in the proximal tubule. The one common feature of a ligand's ability to bind to megalin is the presence of basic patches on the surface of the macromolecule. The distribution of the surface charges rather than the isoelectric point seems to determine the efficiency of binding. Although a putative receptor, megalin does not appear to be very selective. The list of substances that have been demonstrated to bind to megalin are shown in Table 7.5. As a result of the fact that so many ligands bind to megalin, it has been called a scavenger receptor. In view of megalin's lack of selectivity, it would be more appropriate to characterize it as a "binding protein" rather than as a "receptor." In this sense, megalin-mediated endocytosis in proximal tubular cells does not differ substantially from the concept of nonselective absorptive endocytosis described previously. Of note, the binding capacity and thus role of megalin under pathophysiologic conditions have not been evaluated.

TABLE 7.5. Substances Reported to Bind to Megalin

Enzymes and enzyme inhibitors
PAI-1
PAI-1-urokinase
PAI-1-tPA
Prourokinase
Lipoprotein lipase
Aprotinin
Vitamin-binding protein
Transcobalmin-vitamin B_{12}
Apolipoproteins
Apolipoprotein B
Apolipoprotein E
Apolipoprotein J/clusterin
Polybasic drugs
Aminoglycosides
Polymyxin B
Aprotinin
Low-molecular-weight proteins
Insulin
Prolactin
EGF
Cytochrome-c
Lysozyme
Other
Plasminogen
Albumin
Lactoferrin
RAP

PAI, plasminogen activator-inhibitor; EGF, epidermal growth factor; RAP, receptor-associated protein.

TUBULAR ABSORPTION OF PEPTIDES

Recent advances have been made in our understanding of the renal reabsorption of oligopeptides (dipeptides and tripeptides) as well. This transport process is distinct from those available for free amino acids. Until now, it was believed that oligopeptides were poorly utilized if they are infused intravenously. However, it has become increasingly clear that they rapidly disappear from plasma with only trace amounts being lost in the urine. As in the case of LMWPs, the kidney is also the tissue with the greatest cytoplasmic dipeptidase activity. Two transporters have been identified and cloned (Pept-1 and Pept-2). These transporters are responsible for the intracellular accumulation followed by hydrolysis and again release of constituent amino acids to the circulation. Pept-1 is a low-affinity, high-capacity transporter, and Pept-2 is a high-affinity, low-capacity transporter. Pept-1 is expressed in the intestine and kidney, whereas Pept-2 is expressed only in the kidney. These receptors rely on protons and membrane potential for their driving force. This transport system also accepts as substrates several pharmacologically active compounds such as β-lactam antibiotics, which possess peptidelike chemical structures.

METABOLISM OF ABSORBED PROTEINS

As indicated, absorbed proteins are hydrolyzed to completion within lysosomes. The characteristics of the renal disposal of proteins are qualitatively and quantitatively similar for all the proteins tested to date. Figure 7.15 illustrates the results of studies in which metabolism of administered ^{125}I-rGH by the rat kidney was examined. Within 10 minutes after the intravenous administration of ^{125}I-rGH, the rat kidney accumulated approximately 30% of the administered dose (Fig. 7.15, *A*). The radioactivity accumulated by the kidney eluted from Sephadex as intact ^{125}I-rGH (Fig. 7.15, *B*). Upon isolation of the kidney and closed-circuit perfusion, the radioactivity was released from the kidney with a half-life of approximately 20 minutes (Fig. 7.15, *C*). The radioactivity released to the perfusate eluted in Sephadex as ^{125}I-monoiodotyrosine (Fig. 7.15, *D*), demonstrating that the hormone absorbed by the kidney cells was hydrolyzed to amino acids, which were then returned to the circulation. The amino acids resulting from lysosomal hydrolysis are not reused by the renal cells and do not accumulate within these

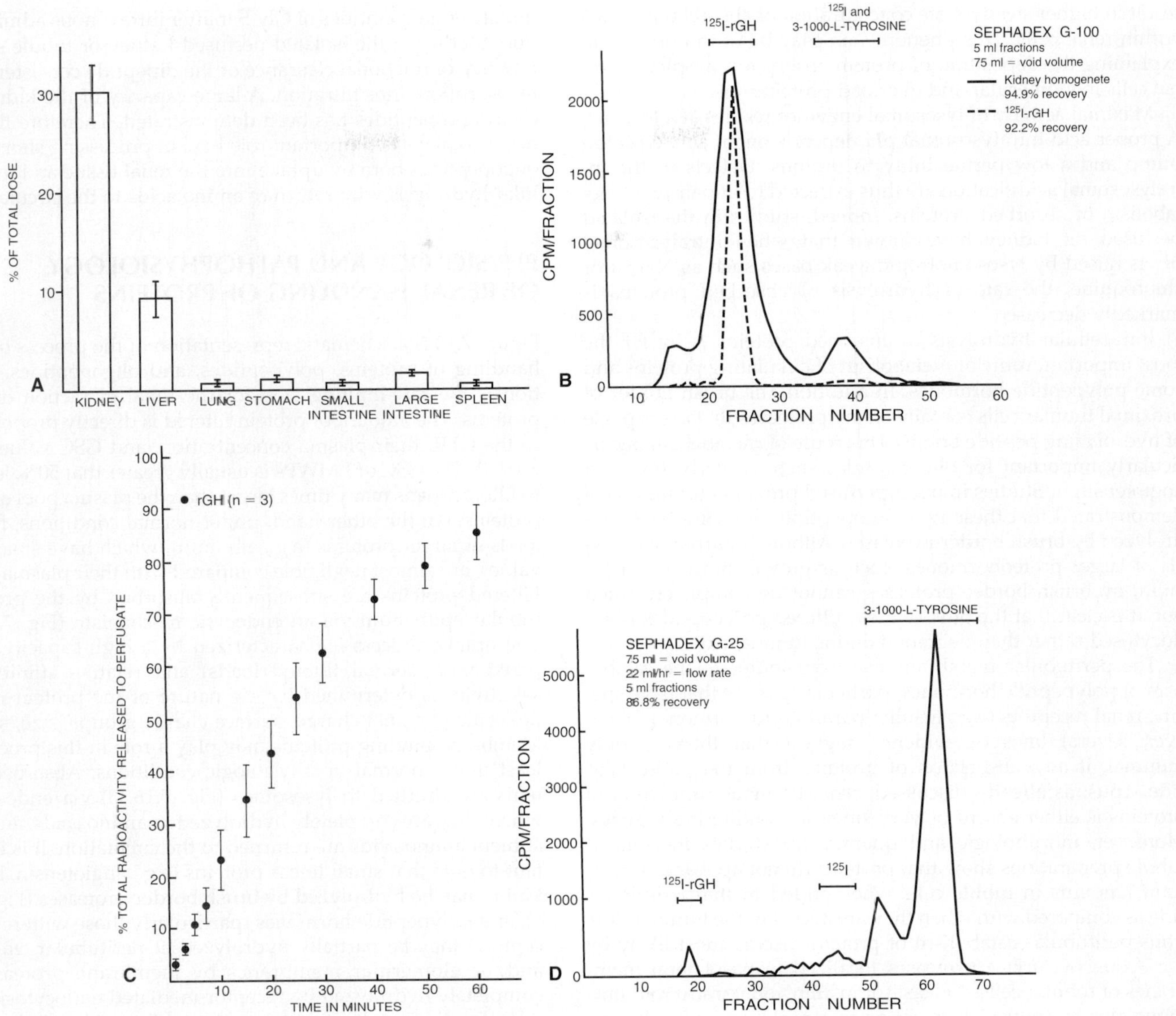

Figure 7.15. Accumulation and disposal of rat growth hormone *(rGH)* by the isolated perfused rat kidney. **A:** Relative distribution of administered ^{125}I-rGH in several organs in rat. **B:** Chromatogram of radioactivity in rat kidney tissue after administration of ^{125}I-rGH. **C:** Efflux of radioactivity from isolated rat kidney preloaded with ^{125}I-rGH label to the perfusate. **D:** Chromatogram of radioactivity released to the perfusate. These experiments demonstrate that the kidney is the major organ to accumulate administered rGH and that the accumulated hormone is hydrolyzed to amino acids, which are then returned to the circulation. (Reprinted with permission from Johnson V, Maack T. Renal extraction, filtration, absorption, and catabolism of growth hormone. *Am J Physiol* 1977;233:F185–F196.)

cells. Consequently, the rate of efflux of radioactivity to the perfusate (Fig. 7.15, C) essentially measures the rate of hydrolysis of the absorbed protein within lysosomes.

The rate of hydrolysis for different absorbed proteins varies greatly, being faster for polypeptide hormones and slower for other circulating LMWPs. This selectivity in renal disposal of proteins is probably based on the degree of resistance of the absorbed protein to the hydrolytic action of lysosomal enzymes. In most studies to date, lysosomal hydrolysis of absorbed proteins has been shown to proceed to completion. One exception is that of the renal handling of very high dosages of lysozyme. Experiments in flounder renal tubules and in the isolated perfused rat kidney suggested that at high dosages, part of the absorbed lysozyme was released intact to the medium. The pathways for the transport of intact lysozyme are unknown but may occur by disruption of lysosomes overloaded with a poorly hydrolyzable protein with subsequent spillage of lysozyme from the cytosol into the peritubular circulation. Alternatively, overloaded lysosomes may fuse with basolateral membranes, releasing lysozyme directly into the peritubular spaces. This phenomenon may be of importance in explaining tubular lesions in overload proteinurias.

Particularly for polypeptide hormones, the rate of intracellular catabolism increases in proportion to the absorption rate over a wide range of protein filtered loads. In the case of lysozyme, as the concentration of absorbed protein in lysosomes increases, there is a concomitant increase in the activity of cathepsin D, a powerful protease, which leads to a compensatory increase in the rate of lysozyme hydrolysis within these cell organelles. In the case of cytochrome-c, the catabolic process tends to saturate at rates near the transport maximum (T_m) of the absorption for this protein. Saturation of the catabolic process will result in higher steady-state concentration of absorbed proteins within renal cells. This phenomenon may be of importance in explaining the deposition of protein absorption droplets in renal cells in glomerular and overload proteinurias.

Maximal activity of lysosomal enzymes resides at a low pH. A proper acid intralysosomal pH depends on an active proton pump and a low permeability to protons. Defects in the intralysosomal acidification are thus expected to impair renal metabolism of absorbed proteins. Indeed, studies in the isolated perfused rat kidney have shown that when intralysosomal pH is raised by lysosomotropic weak bases such as NH_4Cl or chloroquine, the rate of hydrolysis of absorbed proteins is markedly decreased.

Intracellular hydrolysis of absorbed proteins is by far the most important route of metabolism of circulating proteins and some polypeptide hormones. In addition, the brush border of proximal tubular cells contains many proteases that are capable of hydrolyzing peptide bonds. This route of metabolism is particularly important for oligopeptides such as bradykinin and angiotensin II. Studies in microperfused proximal tubules have demonstrated that these two oligopeptides are completely hydrolyzed by brush border proteases. Although partial hydrolysis of larger proteohormones, such as growth hormone or insulin, by brush border proteases cannot be completely ruled out, it is clear that the bulk of these filtered polypeptides is endocytosed rather than degraded on the luminal side.

The peritubular membrane also contributes to the catabolism of polypeptide hormones, particularly those that have specific renal receptors (e.g., insulin, parathyroid hormone). However, several lines of evidence suggest that there is only minimal, if any, absorption of proteins from the peritubular side. Thus, as already discussed, renal tissue accumulation of proteins is either absent or very small in nonfiltering kidneys. Moreover, morphologic and quantitative studies in isolated tubule preparations show that proteins do not appear in significant amounts in tubule cells when added to the peritubular side as compared with when they are added to the luminal side. Thus peritubular catabolism of proteins occurs most likely by the action of surface proteases localized in basolateral membranes of tubular cells. At least for insulin and parathyroid hormone, this hydrolysis does not go to completion and rather results in large polypeptide fragments. Some of these fragments are biologically inactive, but it cannot be completely ruled out that biologically active fragments may result from the peritubular metabolism of these hormones.

Finally, the process of receptor-mediated internalization and lysosomal hydrolysis may be of significance for termination of hormonal responses and plasma homeostasis of some polypeptide hormones. Thus it is likely that the termination of parathyroid and insulin actions on the kidney is the result of endocytosis of receptor-ligand complexes. In the case of atrial natriuretic factor, there is even a specific class of receptors (C-ANP receptors) whose major function is not to mediate the main effects of this hormone on the kidney but to clear the hormone from the circulation by receptor-mediated internalization and lysosomal hydrolysis of the ligand.

The kidney also plays an important role in the removal of oligopeptides. In addition to short-chain peptides in the tubular system because of the action of brush border proteases, considerable quantities of dipeptides and tripeptides for reabsorption enter by glomerular filtration. Evidence for the importance of the kidney in removing these oligopeptides from circulation comes from studies on the clearance of hydrolysis-resistant dipeptides such as glycyl-L-sarcosine (Gly-Sar). Following nephrectomy, the elimination of Gly-Sar is reduced compared with that of controls. The kidney tissue has also been shown to accumulate large quantities of Gly-Sar after intravenous administration. Studies in the isolated perfused kidney or tubule show a low rate of fractional clearance of the dipeptide consistent with reabsorption after filtration. A large capacity of the kidney for clearing dipeptides has been demonstrated. Therefore the kidney also plays an important role here in processing short-chain oligopeptides both by uptake into the renal tissue and intracellular hydrolysis with return of amino acids to the circulation.

PHYSIOLOGY AND PATHOPHYSIOLOGY OF RENAL HANDLING OF PROTEINS

Figure 7.16 is a schematic representation of the process of renal handling of proteins, polypeptides, and oligopeptides. Filtration is the rate-limiting step for the renal extraction of most proteins. The amount of protein filtered is directly proportional to the GFR, their plasma concentration, and GSC values (Fig. 7.16, *1*). The GSC of LMWPs is usually greater that 50%, leading to filtered loads many times larger than the plasma pool of these proteins. On the other hand, under normal conditions, filtered loads of larger proteins (e.g., albumin), which have small GSC values, are almost negligible compared with their plasma pools. Filtered proteins are subsequently absorbed by the proximal tubular epithelium via an endocytic mechanism (Fig. 7.16, *2*). The uptake process is characterized by a high capacity (compared with normal filtered loads) and relative affinity. The selectivity is determined by the nature of the protein macromolecule (e.g., net charge, surface charge groups, size, shape). Membrane-binding proteins may play a role in this process, at least under normal or physiologic conditions. Absorbed proteins are shuttled to lysosomes (Fig. 7.16, *3*) via endosomes, where they are completely hydrolyzed to amino acids, and constituent amino acids are returned to the circulation. It is important to note that small linear proteins (e.g., angiotensin, bradykinin) may be hydrolyzed by brush border proteases (Fig. 7.16, *5*), and polypeptide hormones (particularly those with renal receptors) may be partially hydrolyzed at peritubular, vascular, and/or glomerular membranes by membrane proteases or completely hydrolyzed by receptor-mediated endocytosis (Fig. 7.16, *6*). The resultant oligopeptides (dipeptides and tripep-

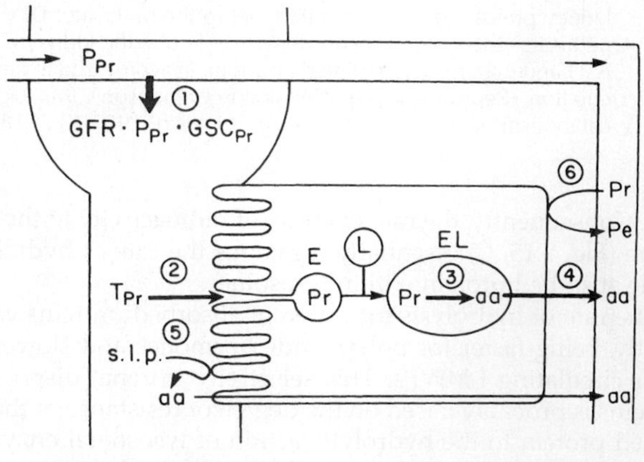

Figure 7.16. Schematic representation of renal handling of proteins and peptides. See text for discussion of steps 1 to 6. *GFR*, glomerular filtration rate; P_{Pr}, plasma protein concentration; GSC_{Pr}, glomerular sieving coefficient of protein; T_{Pr}, tubular protein; *s.l.p.*, small linear polypeptide; *aa*, amino acids; *Pr*, protein; *E*, endosome; *L*, lysosome; *EL*, endolysosome; *Pe*, peptide fragment. (Reprinted with permission from Maack T, Park CH, Camargo MJF. Renal filtration, transport, and metabolism of proteins. In: Seldin DW, Giebisch G, eds. *The kidney: physiology and pathophysiology.* New York: Raven Press, 1992.)

tides) are then reabsorbed by the peptide transport system, and amino acids are reabsorbed by the amino acid transport system.

Therefore increases in the urinary excretion of proteins result from increases in their filtered loads or from defects in their tubular uptake. An increase in the permselectivity of the glomerular barrier leads to proportionately greater increases in the filtered loads of albumin and larger anionic proteins than of LMWPs. This is because GSC values for LMWPs are already very high and cannot increase further, whereas even a small increase in glomerular permeability to macromolecules leads to very significant increases in the filtered loads of larger proteins, leading to albuminuria and proteinuria. On the other hand, increases in urinary excretion of LMWPs occurs when their plasma concentration increases, such as is the case for lysozyme in myelocytic leukemias and Bence Jones proteinuria in multiple myeloma.

Tubular proteinurias result from renal tubular lesions, which lead to impaired tubular uptake of proteins (e.g., heavy metal poisoning, Fanconi syndrome, Wilson's disease). Tubular proteinurias are associated with a proportionately greater urinary excretion of LMWPs because of the larger GSC for these proteins compared with that of albumin or larger proteins. However, in view of the greater plasma concentration of albumin compared with that of LMWPs, the filtered load of the former may actually exceed that of the latter. Consequently, even in the tubular proteinurias, the absolute amount of albumin excreted in urine may be greater than that of LMWPs.

In almost every case of proteinuria, protein absorption droplets (hyaline droplets) can be detected in proximal tubular cells. However, there is no clear correlation between proteinuria and the presence of hyaline droplets within tubular cells. The deposition of filtered protein in tubular cells depends on the balance between absorption and catabolic rates. In turn, the latter depends on the integrity of intralysosomal pH, which may be impaired when tubular lesions are present, resulting in a greater probability of intracellular accumulation of absorbed protein even at relatively low rates of proteinuria. On the other hand, high absorption rates of proteins may lead to striking changes in tubular morphology, including dramatic enlargement of protein absorption droplets and loss of brush border structure, suggesting pathologic injury. Tubular damage with impairment of lysosomal function occurs as part of this process. Consequently, the degree of deposition of absorption droplets within tubular cells results from a complex process that is not simply related to the rate of proteinuria.

One of the major consequences of a decrease in renal function, particularly a decrease in GFR such as occurs in renal failure, is the increased plasma levels of LMWPs that result from this process. In the absence of filtration, a major pathway for the metabolic clearance of LMWPs and polypeptide hormones is lost, resulting in an increase in their plasma concentration. Moreover, for some polypeptide hormones (e.g., parathyroid hormone) the decrease in renal function will indirectly contribute to an increase in its synthesis, further compounding the decrease in metabolic clearance. The increase in plasma concentration of LMWPs, particularly polypeptide hormones, contributes to the kaleidoscopic nature of symptoms in uremic syndrome. On the other hand, the capacity of the kidney to actively transport oligopeptides and peptidomimetic drugs enables the kidney to play major roles in pharmacologic and nutritional therapies such as the addition of dipeptides to amino acid solutions used for parenteral nutrition or design of drugs with less nephrotoxicity.

Selected Readings

Camargo MJF, Sumpio BE, Maack T. Kinetics of renal catabolism of absorbed proteins: influence of load and lysosomal pH. *Am J Physiol* 1984;247:F656–F664.

Studies demonstrating the importance of the acid environment of lysosomes for the renal catabolism of absorbed proteins. This study indicates that increases in the filtered loads of proteins and alkalinization of intralysosomal pH may lead to the deposition of protein absorption droplets in tubular cells.

Christensen EI, Birn H, Verroust P, Moestrup SK. Membrane receptors for endocytosis in the renal proximal tubule. *Int Rev Cytol* 1998;180:237–284.

A recent extensive review of the membrane receptors for endocytosis in the proximal tubule, including megalin.

Daniel H, Herget M. Cellular and molecular mechanisms of renal peptide transport. *Am J Physiol* 1997;273:F1–F8.

An in-depth review of the renal peptide transporters bringing out their importance from a nutritional as well as pharmacological standpoint.

Johnson V, Maack T. Renal extraction, filtration, absorption and catabolism of growth hormone. *Am J Physiol* 1977;233:F185–F196.

Studies examining the renal handling of rat growth hormone in the intact rat and in filtering and nonfiltering isolated perfused kidneys. It was found that the kidney accounts for a major fraction of the total plasma turnover of growth hormone. Similar findings were subsequently found for other polypeptide hormones and circulating low-molecular-weight proteins.

Maack T. Renal handling of proteins and polypeptides. In: Windhager EE, ed. *Handbook of physiology.* New York: Oxford University Press, 1992:2039–2118.

An inclusive review on the renal transport and metabolism of proteins and polypeptides with 281 references. It includes a review of studies showing the various biologic processes of protein uptake and metabolism in epithelial cells and of receptor-mediated endocytosis and metabolism of atrial natriuretic factor.

Maack T, Park CH, Camargo MJF. Renal filtration, transport, and metabolism of proteins. In: Seldin D, Giebisch G, eds. *The kidney: physiology and pathophysiology,* vol 3, ed 2. New York: Raven Press, 1992:3005–3038.

An extensive review on the renal handling of proteins.

Park CH, Maack T. Albumin absorption and catabolism by isolated perfused proximal convoluted tubules of the rabbit. *J Clin Invest* 1984;73:767–777.

In vitro *studies describing the kinetics of albumin absorption by proximal tubular cells and factors that influence this process. The study demonstrates the existence of a dual system for albumin absorption by the proximal tubule.*

CHAPTER 8

Urinary Concentration and Dilution

Jeff M. Sands

Terrestrial mammals do not have continuous access to water. As a result, their kidneys have developed mechanisms that allow them to regulate water excretion in response to intermittent water consumption. These regulatory mechanisms must be able to respond rapidly to acute water boluses followed by longer periods without water intake. They also must be able to regulate water excretion independently of sodium excretion. Otherwise, it would be impossible to excrete urine, which is either concentrated or diluted relative to plasma osmolality. These mechanisms are located in the renal medulla. The mechanisms responsible for concentrating and diluting the urine in the outer medulla are well defined. However, controversy remains regarding the concentrating mechanisms in the inner medulla, even though many of the transport proteins involved in concentration and dilution of urine have been cloned in recent years.

ANATOMIC CONSIDERATIONS

The mammalian kidney generally consists of two populations of nephrons: short-loop nephrons and long-loop nephrons. Both types of loops are arranged in a hairpin or U-shape configuration. Short-loop nephrons originate from superficial glomeruli, whereas long-loop nephrons originate from juxtamedullary glomeruli. Short-loop nephrons have Henle's loop, which turn at the inner-outer medullary border and consist of a proximal straight tubule, a thin descending limb, and a thick ascending limb. Long-loop nephrons extend into the inner medulla and contain a thin ascending limb in addition to segments found in short-loop nephrons. Thin ascending limbs are located exclusively in the inner medulla and become thick ascending limbs at the inner-outer medullary border. Thus, regardless of the type of loop, only thick ascending limbs are found in the outer medulla.

The vasa recta form the blood supply to the medulla. Like Henle's loops, vasa rectae are arranged in a hairpin configuration. Blood enters the medulla through a descending vasa recta, passes through a capillary plexus located at various depths within the medulla, then joins to form an ascending vasa recta.

The collecting duct (CD) is the final structure in the medulla. In the cortex, distal convoluted tubules merge to form cortical CDs that descend through the cortex and the outer medulla. In the inner medulla, these collecting ducts continually merge, ultimately forming the ducts of Bellini, which open into the renal pelvis at the papillary tip. The renal pelvis is continuous with the ureter.

COUNTERCURRENT MULTIPLICATION

Countercurrent multiplication by Henle's loops is the critical mechanism for generating a concentrated urine. Isosmotic fluid enters the thin descending limbs and is concentrated as it flows down to the bend of Henle's loop. As it flows up the ascending limbs of Henle's loops, it is diluted so that the fluid that emerges is hypotonic to plasma.

This U-shaped counterflow arrangement allows relatively small osmolality gradients generated near the top of the U to be multiplied down the length of the U, resulting in an enormous increase in osmolality at the bend of the U. Countercurrent multiplication depends on the U-tube having the following transport properties in the outer medulla: (a) the descending limb is permeable to water but impermeable to sodium, (b) the ascending limb is permeable to sodium but impermeable to water, and (c) the ascending limb contains an active (energy-dependent) transport mechanism that allows the ascending limb to pump NaCl out of the lumen. Active NaCl reabsorption from the ascending limb will draw water out of the sodium-impermeable descending limb by osmosis.

Figure 8.1 illustrates how countercurrent multiplication allows the outer medulla to generate an axial osmotic gradient that exceeds the osmotic gradient at any level in the medulla. Figure 8.1, *A* shows a U-tube with isosmolar fluid throughout. Next, the active transport mechanism pumps enough NaCl to establish a gradient of 20 mOsm/kg H_2O between the lumens of the ascending and descending limbs at any level of the U-tube (Fig. 8.1, *B*). Third, the fluid flows half-way down the descending limb and up the ascending limb (Fig. 8.1, *C*). Now, when the active transport mechanism reestablishes the gradient of 20 mOsm/kg H_2O, as shown in Fig. 8.1, *D*, the luminal fluid near the bend of the U achieves a higher final osmolality. As this iterative process is repeated, the bend of the U achieves a progressively higher osmolality (Fig. 8.1, *E*). The final axial osmotic gradient far exceeds the original gradient of 20 mOsm/kg H_2O generated at any level in the U-tube. Thus the 'single-effect' of establishing a gradient of 20 mOsm/kg H_2O by active NaCl reabsorption has been multiplied axially down the length of the U-tube by countercurrent multiplication.

Outer Medulla

The U-tube is a good model for the actual physiology in Henle's loops within the outer medulla. The nephron segments

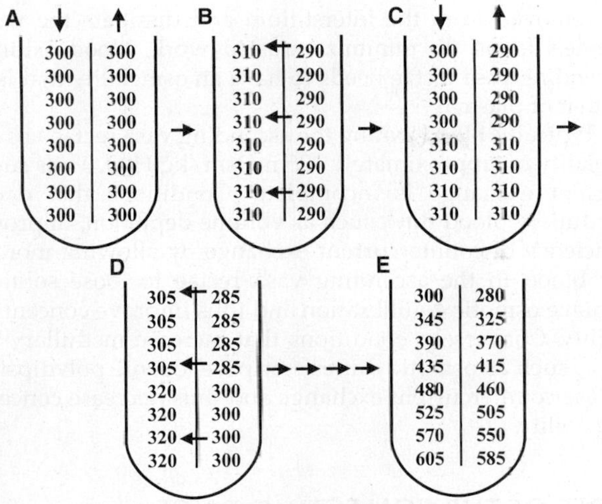

Figure 8.1. Countercurrent multiplication. **A:** U-tube begins with isosmolar fluid throughout. **B:** Active NaCl transport establishes a 20 mOsm/kg H_2O gradient between the lumens of the ascending and descending limbs at each level of the U-tube. **C:** Fluid flows half-way down the descending limb and up the ascending limb. **D:** Active transport reestablishes a 20 mOsm/kg H_2O gradient between the lumens of the ascending and descending limbs at each level of the U-tube. Note that the luminal fluid near the bend of the loop achieves a higher final osmolality than in B. **E:** As the processes in **C** and **D** are repeated, the bend of the loop achieves a progressively higher osmolality so that the final axial osmotic gradient far exceeds the original 20 mOsm/kg H_2O gradient generated at any level in the U-tube.

in the outer medulla have the necessary transport properties described in the U-tube. Both the proximal straight tubule, located in the outer stripe of the outer medulla, and the thin descending limb, located in the inner stripe of the outer medulla, are highly permeable to water because of the presence of aquaporin-1 (AQP1) water channels in both the apical and basolateral membranes.

The thick ascending limb cell generates the single-effect by active NaCl reabsorption using the mechanism illustrated in Fig. 8.2. The thick ascending limb cell contains a furosemide-inhibitable Na^+-K^+-$2Cl^-$ cotransporter (called NKCC2 or BSC1) in its apical membrane and Na^+-K^+-ATPase in its basolateral membrane. The Na^+-K^+-ATPase expends energy (ATP) to lower intracellular Na^+, thus generating a favorable electrochemical gradient for the luminal uptake of NaCl via the Na^+-K^+-$2Cl^-$ cotransporter. The K^+ that enters the cell on the Na^+-K^+-$2Cl^-$ cotransporter is recycled into the luman via a K^+ secretory channel (ROMK1), generating a lumen-positive voltage that drives paracellular Na^+ reabsorption. The net result is reabsorption of 2 Na^+ and 2 Cl^- rather than 1 Na^+, 1 K^+, and 2 Cl^-.

Because the thick ascending limb is water impermeable, NaCl reabsorption results in a hypertonic medullary interstitium and dilutes the luminal fluid. Both of these results are physiologically important because they establish conditions necessary for excreting concentrated or diluted urine. During antidiuresis, the hypertonic medullary interstitium will draw water out of the sodium-impermeable thin descending limb, thus concentrating the fluid in its lumen. During diuresis, NaCl removal from the lumen of the thick ascending limb generates a tubular fluid, which is dilute relative to plasma. In the absence of vasopressin (AVP, also called *antidiuretic hormone*, ADH), this dilute fluid can be excreted as dilute urine. Furosemide inhibits both the generation of a hypertonic medulla and the generation of a dilute tubular fluid by inhibiting the Na^+-K^+-$2Cl^-$ cotransporter. Thus patients treated with furosemide will be unable to

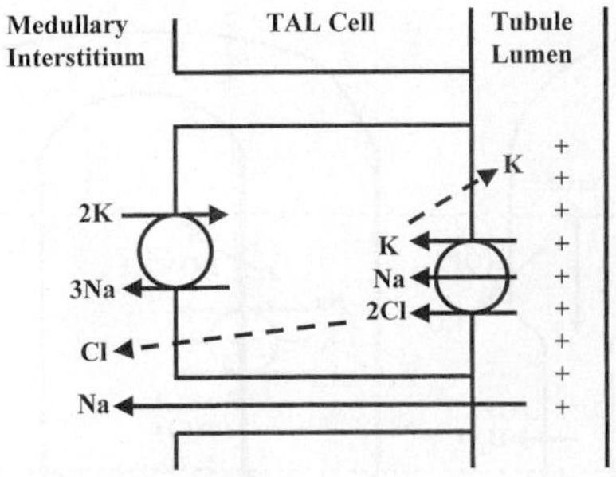

Figure 8.2. NaCl reabsorption by thick ascending limb *(TAL)* cells. The apical membrane contains the furosemide-inhibitable Na^+-K^+-$2Cl^-$ cotransporter (NKCC2, BSC1). The basolateral membrane contains Na^+-K^+-ATPase, which expends energy (ATP) to lower intracellular Na^+, thus generating a favorable electrochemical gradient for the luminal uptake of NaCl via the Na^+-K^+-$2Cl^-$ cotransporter. The K^+, which enters the cell on the Na^+-K^+-$2Cl^-$ cotransporter, is secreted into the lumen via the ROMK1 K^+ channel, generating a lumen-positive voltage that drives paracellular Na^+ reabsorption.

either concentrate or dilute their urine and will produce urine with an osmolality of approximately 300 mOsm/kg H_2O.

Inner Medulla

As described, Henle's loop segments in the inner medulla are different from those in the outer medulla. The inner medullary thin descending limb has similar properties to the outer medullary thin descending limb: it is highly water permeable because of the presence of AQP1 water channels but is sodium impermeable. However, the thick ascending limbs are replaced by thin ascending limbs. Like the thick ascending limb, the thin ascending limb is water impermeable and sodium permeable. Unlike the thick ascending limb, the thin ascending limb cannot actively reabsorb NaCl. It also has a moderate permeability to urea.

The single-effect in the inner medulla is different from the single-effect in the outer medulla because the thin ascending limb cannot actively reabsorb NaCl. Instead, the thin ascending limb passively reabsorbs NaCl by taking advantage of the chemical disequilibriums for NaCl and urea that exist between the lumen of the thin ascending limb and the inner medullary interstitium.

Animal cells cannot maintain an osmotic gradient across their cell membrane, requiring that intraluminal, intracellular, and interstitial osmolality be equal at any given level in the inner medulla. However, the composition of the osmotically active particles does not have to be equal. Comparing the fluid within the lumen of the thin ascending limb with the inner medullary interstitial fluid, the thin ascending limb fluid has a higher concentration of NaCl and a lower concentration of urea. Thus chemical gradients favor passive NaCl reabsorption and urea secretion. Because the thin ascending limb has a higher permeability to NaCl than to urea, NaCl reabsorption exceeds urea secretion, resulting in dilution of the luminal fluid as it ascends toward the outer medulla.

This passive-equilibration mechanism for concentrating urine in the inner medulla (Fig. 8.3) was proposed in 1972 by Kokko and Rector and by Stephenson. It is currently considered the best model for explaining urine concentration within the inner medulla. However, computer simulations of medullary function using the passive mechanism are unable to reproduce the degree of hyperosmolality found *in vivo*, causing some investigators to question whether the passive mechanism is sufficient to explain urine concentrating ability in the inner medulla. This

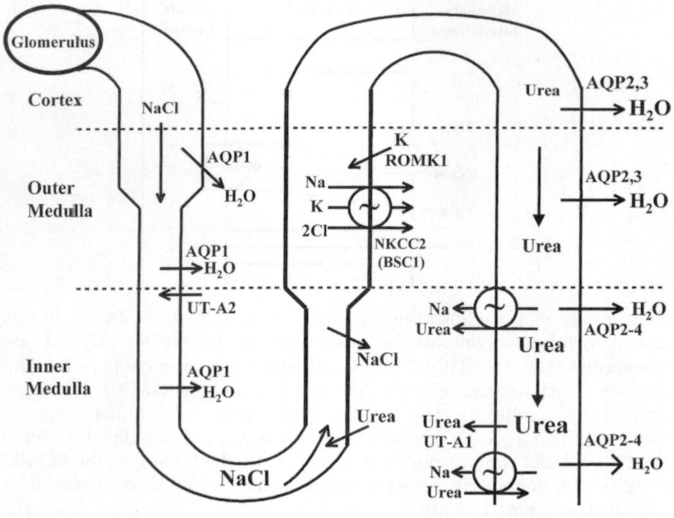

Figure 8.3. Passive equilibration model of countercurrent multiplication system. Active NaCl reabsorption from the thick ascending limb generates a hypertonic medullary interstitium, which concentrates NaCl in the thin descending limb fluid by the osmotic removal of water. In the inner medulla, the NaCl concentration in the thin ascending limb fluid exceeds the interstitial NaCl concentration, while the urea concentration gradient is oriented in the opposite direction. Because the thin ascending limb NaCl permeability exceeds its urea permeability, these opposite gradients result in greater amounts of passive NaCl reabsorption than urea secretion and dilution of the fluid within the thin ascending limb. In the presence of vasopressin, water is reabsorbed from the collecting duct by AQP2 water channels in the apical membrane and AQP3 and AQP4 water channels in the basolateral membrane and returned to the systemic circulation. Water reabsorption also concentrates urea in the collecting duct lumen until the fluid reaches the urea-permeable terminal inner medullary collecting duct where urea is recycled into the inner medullary interstitium by the vasopressin-regulated urea transporter UT-A1. Also shown are two sodium-coupled active urea transport pathways in the inner medullary collecting duct, AQP1 water channels in the proximal straight tubule and thin descending limb, and UT-A2 urea transporter in the thin descending limb.

discrepancy may result from simplifications inherent in the computer simulations, or it may indicate that additional concentrating mechanisms are present in the inner medulla. Thus additional studies are needed to understand completely this interesting question in renal physiology.

COUNTERCURRENT EXCHANGE

The vasa rectae, which supply blood to the medulla, are arranged in a hairpin configuration, similar to Henle's loops. As the arterial blood in the descending vasa rectae descends into the hypertonic medulla, it must come into osmotic equilibrium with the medullary interstitium. Because the vasa rectae are freely permeable to water, sodium, and urea, osmotic equilibration is achieved by a combination of water reabsorption and solute secretion. This process is reversed in the venous or ascending vasa rectae. The ascending blood must loose solute and gain water as it ascends through progressively lower osmolalities. This overall process is called *countercurrent exchange,* in other words, the exchange of water and solute between the descending and ascending vasa rectae.

Countercurrent exchange is essential for producing concentrated urine. Concentrating ability depends on the generation of a hypertonic medulla by countercurrent multiplication. The descending vasa rectae take up solute as they come into osmotic equilibrium with the medullary interstitium. If this solute were carried out of the medulla by the vasa rectae, this solute would be removed from the interstitium and dissipate the work of Henle's loops. To minimize wasted work, blood exiting the ascending vasa rectae needs to have an osmolality that is close to that of plasma.

Typically, blood exiting the ascending vasa rectae has an osmolality of approximately 325 mOsm/kg H_2O. Thus countercurrent exchange is incomplete. Conditions that decrease medullary blood flow, such as volume depletion, improve the efficiency of countercurrent exchange by allowing more time for blood in the ascending vasa rectae to loose solute and achieve osmotic equilibration and thus improve concentrating ability. Conversely, conditions that increase medullary blood flow, such as osmotic diuresis or psychogenic polydipsia, decrease countercurrent exchange and thus decrease concentrating ability.

ROLE OF THE COLLECTING DUCT

Countercurrent multiplication in Henle's loops generates a hypertonic medulla. Countercurrent exchange in the vasa rectae minimizes the dissipation of this gradient. However, neither of these processes results in water excretion. This function, as well as the regulation of water excretion, is performed by the CDs. The CDs form from the merger of several distal convoluted tubules in the cortex and extend distally to the papillary tip. The fluid that enters the CDs is dilute relative to plasma. The entire CD is very water impermeable in the absence of vasopressin. However, the CD becomes highly water permeable when stimulated by vasopressin.

During conditions of water depletion, plasma osmolality increases. An increase of 2 mOsm/kg H_2O is sensed by the hypothalamic osmoreceptors and results in vasopressin secretion by the posterior pituitary. Vasopressin binds to V_2-receptors in the basolateral membrane of principal cells in the CDs, stimulates adenylyl cyclase to produce cyclic adenosine monophosphate (cAMP), activates protein kinase A, and ultimately inserts aquaporin-2 (AQP2) water channels into the apical membrane (Fig. 8.4). The result is a significant increase in CD water permeability.

AQP2 is the vasopressin-regulated water channel (Table 8.1). In the absence of vasopressin, AQP2 resides in vesicles below the apical membrane (subapical vesicles). When vasopressin

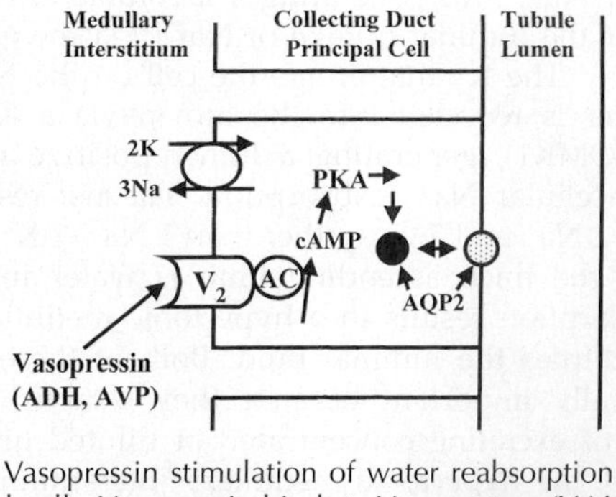

Figure 8.4. Vasopressin stimulation of water reabsorption in collecting duct principal cells. Vasopressin binds to V_2-receptors *(V_2)* in the basolateral membrane, stimulates adenylyl cyclase *(AC)* to produce cyclic adenosine monophosphate *(cAMP)*, activates protein kinase A *(PKA)*, and ultimately inserts AQP2 water channels *(closed circle)* into the apical membrane *(open circle with dots)*. The result is a significant increase in collecting duct water permeability. When vasopressin is removed, AQP2 water channels are removed from the apical membrane and remain in the cytoplasm until the cell is stimulated again by vasopressin. Thus AQP2 recycles between the cytoplasm and apical membrane in response to vasopressin stimulation and withdrawal *ADH,* antidiuretic hormone; AQP, aquaporin; *AVP,* vasopressin.

TABLE 8.1. Comparison of Renal Aquaporins

Aquaporin	Renal Localization
AQP1	Proximal tubule, thin descending limb
AQP2	Collecting duct apical membrane and subapical vesicles, regulated by vasopressin
AQP3	Collecting duct basolateral membrane
AQP4	Inner medullary collecting duct basolateral membrane

AQP, aquaporin.

stimulates a principal cell, the AQP2-containing vesicles fuse with the apical membrane. Transepithelial water reabsorption is accomplished by the combination of AQP2 water channels in the apical membrane and AQP3 and AQP4 water channels in the basolateral membrane; AQP3 is found along the entire CD, whereas AQP4 is present only in the inner medullary CD. When vasopressin stimulation ends, AQP2 is reendocytosed and remains in the subapical vesicles until the cell is stimulated again by vasopressin.

In addition to this acute regulatory role, vasopressin regulates the amount of AQP2 long term. Treating rats with central diabetes insipidus (Brattleboro rats) with vasopressin increases the amount of AQP2 protein in the kidney and restores the ability to concentrate urine. Conversely, AQP2 protein is reduced in several experimental models of acquired nephrogenic diabetes insipidus, including hypokalemia, hypercalcemia, treatment with lithium, treatment with a V_2-receptor antagonist, and feeding a low-protein diet.

The vasopressin-stimulated increase in water permeability allows water to be reabsorbed from the collecting duct lumen until the luminal fluid achieves osmotic equilibration with the hypertonic medullary interstitium (Fig. 8.3). The reabsorbed water is returned to the systemic circulation by the ascending vasa recta. Most water reabsorption occurs in the cortex and outer medulla. The inner medulla has the highest osmolality and is important for reabsorbing the remaining water when maximal water conservation is required. Further discussion on the role of vasopressin in the renal handling of water is found in Chapter 15, Part 1.

ROLE OF UREA

Urea plays a special role in the urinary concentrating mechanism. The passive mechanism requires that the inner medullary interstitial urea concentration exceed the urea concentration in the lumen of the thin ascending limb. If inadequate quantities of urea are delivered to the deep inner medulla, the chemical gradients necessary for passive NaCl reabsorption are not established and the concentrating ability is reduced. Studies show that patients fed a low-protein diet or showing signs of protein or protein-calorie malnutrition are unable to concentrate their urine maximally; urea replacement improves their ability to concentrate their urine.

The kidney has several urea-recycling pathways that serve to maintain high urea concentrations within the inner medullary interstitium. The major urea-recycling pathway involves the thin ascending limb and the terminal inner medullary CD. The urea that is secreted into the thin ascending limb is carried distally as the luminal fluid moves along the nephron. The nephron segments distal to the thin ascending limb are all impermeable to urea except for the last nephron segment, the terminal inner medullary CD. When the urea reaches the terminal inner medullary CD, it is reabsorbed by a specialized, vasopressin-regulated, urea transport protein (UT-A1, Table 8.2). Thus the urea secreted from the interstitium into the thin ascending limb is recycled back to the interstitium by reabsorption from the terminal inner medullary CD.

The only portion of the CD that is permeable to urea in animals fed a normal-protein diet is the terminal inner medullary CD, even though the entire CD is permeable to water when vasopressin is present. As water is reabsorbed from the cortical outer medullary and initial inner medullary CDs, urea is trapped within the CD lumen. When the luminal fluid finally reaches the urea-permeable terminal inner medullary CD, the intraluminal urea concentration is very high and urea can be rapidly reabsorbed into the interstitium by the vasopressin-regulated urea transporter UT-A1.

This schema separates the primary sites of urea and water reabsorption. Water is primarily reabsorbed in the cortex and outer medulla where the blood supply is greatest. The reabsorbed water can be returned to the circulation without diluting the deep inner medulla. Urea is primarily reabsorbed in the deep inner medulla, where it is needed to generate the chemical gradients necessary for passive NaCl reabsorption from the thin, ascending limb. Little water remains to be reabsorbed from the terminal inner medullary collecting duct, thus, the inner medullary interstitium is not diluted significantly. Moreover, the blood supply to this region of the kidney is quite poor, making it difficult to return the reabsorbed water to the circulation.

Two families of urea transporters have been reported (Table 8.2): the UT-A and UT-B families. The UT-A family was originally cloned from rabbit inner medulla. The UT-A1 urea transporter is present in the apical membrane of principal and inner medullary CD cells in the inner medullary CD. UT-A1 is regulated acutely by vasopressin; the mechanism by which this

TABLE 8.2. Comparison of Cloned Urea Transporters

UT Name*	Original name	Tissue†	Molecular Weight‡	Renal Localization
UT-A1	UT1	Kidney	95.9	Inner medullary CD
UT-A2	UT2	Kidney	43.1–43.4	Thin descending limb
UT-A3	UT-A3, UT4	Kidney	44.5	Outer and inner medulla
UT-A4	UT-A4	Kidney	43.3	Outer and inner medulla
UT-B1	HUT11, UT3, Rach1	Bone marrow, kidney	42.1–42.7	Vasa recta
UT-B2	UT11	Brain	45.2	Vasa recta

*The urea transporter names used in this chapter are based on the systematic nomenclature proposed in Sands JM, Timmer RT, Gunn RB. Am J Physiol 1997.
†Indicates the tissue used for the original cDNA cloning of this isoform.
‡Predicted molecular weight (in kD) based on the deduced amino acid sequence.
CD, collecting duct; UT, urea transporter.

occurs is not presently known. Thus, both AQP2 and UT-A1 are regulated acutely by vasopressin.

Three other isoforms of the UT-A family have been identified to date. The UT-A2 urea transporter is present in the thin descending limb and is not stimulated by vasopressin. Both UT-A3 and UT-A4 only recently have been cloned and are present in the outer and inner medulla. Immunohistochemical studies using the UT-A1 antibody show staining of the inner medullary CD apical membrane but no staining of the basolateral membrane. Because functional studies show that there are urea transporters in both the apical and basolateral membranes, the molecular identity of the basolateral membrane urea transporter is presently unknown. However, the UT-A3 protein has a carboxy-terminal sequence which is unique from UT-A1, UT-A2, and UT-A4, making it the only currently identified isoform that would not be detected by the available antibodies to UT-A1 and thus a potential candidate for the basolateral membrane urea transporter.

The inner medullary CD also expresses two sodium-coupled active urea-transport mechanisms. A sodium-urea countertransporter is present in the terminal inner medullary CD of normal rats (Fig. 8.3). This sodium–urea antiporter is upregulated fivefold by water diuresis. A second active urea transport mechanism, a sodium–urea cotransporter, is present in the initial inner medullary CD in rats fed a low-protein diet but not in rats fed a normal-protein diet. The precise role of these active urea transporters in the urinary concentrating mechanism remains to be determined.

The UT-B family of urea transporters (Table 8.2) was originally cloned from an erythrocytelike cell line. UT-B1 and UT-B2 differ by only a few amino acids and have been found in red blood cells and the vasa rectae. The critical importance of urea transport for producing maximally concentrated urine in humans was shown in a study of people whose erythrocytes lacked a urea transporter. People who lack the Kidd antigen (Jka-b-), a minor blood group antigen, also lack the UT-B urea transporter in their red blood cells. Unlike normal individuals who are able to concentrate their urine to approximately 1,200 mOsm/kg H_2O, these Jka-b- individuals are only able to concentrate their urine to approximately 800 mOsm/kg H_2O, even following overnight water deprivation and exogenous vasopressin administration.

Urea also serves another function in the medulla. Because urea is the major source for waste nitrogen excretion, large quantities of urea need to be excreted daily. If urea could not be concentrated in the CD lumen, far more water would need to be excreted. Also, the high interstitial urea concentration is able to osmotically balance the urea within the CD lumen. If interstitial urea were unavailable to offset the osmotic effect of the luminal urea destined for excretion, the interstitial NaCl concentration would have to be much higher. This would require an increase in NaCl reabsorption from the thick ascending limb with an accompanying increase in work (ATP consumption). Thus, as Gamble reported in 1934, there is an "economy of water referable to urea." Additional information on the renal handling of urea is found in Chapter 7, Part 1.

URINARY DILUTION

The portions of the kidney that are responsible for urinary concentration are also responsible for urinary dilution. During conditions of water excess, the osmoreceptors sense a reduction in plasma osmolality and signal the posterior pituitary to decrease or stop vasopressin secretion. In the absence of vasopressin, the entire CD becomes highly impermeable to water due to the absence of AQP2 water channels from the apical membrane.

The thick ascending limb reabsorbs enough NaCl to dilute the luminal fluid even in the absence of vasopressin. Thus the thick ascending limb is often called the *diluting segment.* The fluid delivered to the distal convoluted tubule typically has an osmolality of approximately 50 mOsm/kg H_2O. In the absence of vasopressin, this dilute fluid passes through the CD and is excreted. Humans are able to lower urine osmolality to approximately 50 mOsm/kg H_2O.

Another mechanism that promotes urinary dilution is the moderate water permeability of the terminal inner medullary CD in the absence of vasopressin. This moderate permeability allows some water reabsorption into the deep inner medulla, thereby diluting the inner medulla and promoting excretion of dilute urine. Interestingly, urea permeability increases in the inner medullary collecting duct during long-term water or furosemide diuresis. The increase in urea permeability is accompanied by an increase in UT-A1 urea transporter protein abundance. The physiologic importance of this finding is unclear.

OSMOPROTECTIVE OSMOLYTES

Urine and inner medullary osmolality vary widely in response to changes in water intake. Following a prolonged period without water intake, such as when an individual sleeps, inner medullary osmolality rises to produce a concentrated urine of approximately 1,200 mOsm/kg H_2O. Urine and inner medullary osmolality may decrease quite rapidly to approximately 50 mOsm/kg H_2O if the water deprivation is followed by a large ingestion of water, which commonly occurs at breakfast. These large and rapid changes in osmolality require that the inner medullary cells are able to withstand such changes without undergoing osmotic damage.

One possible mechanism for achieving osmotic balance is for the inner medullary cells to accumulate the same osmotically active compounds (osmolytes) as are found in the urine and interstitium (i.e., NaCl and urea). However, these compounds perturb protein function. If inner medullary cells accumulated such perturbing osmolytes, these cells would need special mechanisms to allow their proteins to function over a wide range of intracellular composition.

Another possible mechanism is for inner medullary cells to accumulate nonperturbing osmolytes—substances that are osmotically active but do not alter protein function. This second approach is used in the inner medulla. Inner medullary cells accumulate nonperturbing or organic osmolytes such as sorbitol, glycerylphosphorylcholine, betaine, taurine, and inositol.

These organic osmolytes are divided into two classes: compatible osmolytes and counteracting osmolytes. The compatible osmolytes (sorbitol and inositol) have no effect on protein function and are accumulated intracellularly to osmotically balance extracellular NaCl. The role of the counteracting osmolytes (glycerylphosphorylcholine, betaine, and taurine) is more complex. In addition to being osmotically active, these compounds have stabilizing effects on protein function. They counteract the destabilizing effects of urea on protein function when they are accumulated intracellularly at a ratio of 1 mole of counteracting osmolyte to 2 moles of urea.

Organic osmolytes are regulated to respond to acute intermittent water ingestion between more prolonged periods without water ingestion. During periods between water ingestions, inner medullary cells maintain high concentrations of organic osmolytes to match extracellular osmolality. When water is ingested, these cells rapidly transport the organic osmolytes into the urine by increasing their cell membranes' permeabilities to these osmolytes, thus decreasing intracellular osmolality. However, they continue to produce the osmolytes while they are being secreted. Although continued osmolyte production may appear to be inefficient, it enables the cell to respond rapidly to the cessation of water ingestion. When the water bolus ceases, cell membrane permeability decreases, and because the osmolytes are still being produced, intracellular osmolyte concentration is rapidly restored. If the water infusion is prolonged for days, inner medullary cells downregulate osmolyte production and increase cell permeability. In this case, osmolyte concentrations cannot be rapidly restored because upregulating osmolyte production requires new protein synthesis. This mechanism may contribute to the inability of patients with psychogenic polydipsia to concentrate their urine normally for several days after ceasing their excessive water intake. Further details on cell volume regulation during osmotic stresses are found in Chapter 14, Part 3.

PATHOPHYSIOLOGIC CONDITIONS

In recent years, the mechanism(s) underlying several pathophysiologic conditions associated with reductions in urine concentrating ability have been studied. Interestingly, certain patterns of changes in water and urea permeabilities are common to multiple pathophysiologic states. Rats made hypercalcemic by vitamin D treatment and rats fed a low-protein diet have a reduction in urine concentrating ability. In both conditions, water permeability and the amount of AQP2 protein are reduced in the inner medulla, and urea permeability and UT-A1 protein are increased. Thus, the concentrating defect in these conditions is related to changes in both water and urea transport.

Adrenalectomized rats also have less ability to concentrate urine, which can be corrected by glucocorticoid replacement. Adrenalectomy increases urea permeability and UT-A1 protein in the inner medulla, whereas dexamethasone replacement decreases them. Further evidence for the role of glucocorticoids in regulating UT-A1 urea transporter protein abundance in the inner medulla was obtained by studying rats with uncontrolled diabetes mellitus caused by streptozotocin. Uncontrolled diabetes mellitus is associated with elevated levels of glucocorticoids in both rats and humans. Rats with diabetes mellitus have reduced expression of UT-A1 protein in their inner medulla, consistent with their elevated levels of glucocorticoids. Control studies showed that the reduction in UT-A1 protein was independent of insulin.

Acknowledgments

The author's research is supported by National Institutes of Health grants R01-DK41707 and P01-DK50268, and the American Heart Association Grant-in-Aid 96006090.

Selected Readings

Garcia-Perez A, Burg MB. Renal medullary organic osmolytes. *Physiol Rev* 1991; 71:1081–1115.

A thorough and well-written review of the role of organic osmolytes in the kidney. This review covers in vivo *studies and studies of cultured cells exposed to hypertonicity.*

Kato A, Sands JM. Evidence for sodium-dependent active urea secretion in the deepest subsegment of the rat inner medullary collecting duct. *J Clin Invest* 1998;101:423–428.

This paper contains the original experiments describing an active sodium-urea countertransporter in the terminal inner medullary collecting duct and reviews other active urea transport mechanisms in mammals.

Knepper MA. Molecular physiology of urinary concentrating mechanism: regulation of aquaporin water channels by vasopressin. *Am J Physiol* 1997;272: F3–F12.

A recent review of water channels in the kidney emphasizing their acute and long-term regulation by vasopressin and their role in producing concentrated urine.

Sands JM, Gargus JJ, Fröhlich O, et al. Urinary concentrating ability in patients with Jk(a-b-) blood type who lack carrier-mediated urea transport. *J Am Soc Nephrol* 1992;2:1689–1696.

This clinical study demonstrates that humans who do not have a UT-B urea transporter in their erythrocytes are unable to concentrate their urine maximally.

Sands JM, Kokko JP. Current concepts of the countercurrent system. *Kidney Int* 1996;50:S93–S99.

This review contains a more detailed description of the transport properties of Henle's loop and collecting duct segments involved in the concentrating and diluting processes.

Sands JM, Timmer RT, Gunn RB. Urea transporters in kidney and erythrocytes. *Am J Physiol* 1997;273:F321–F339.

A recent review of urea transporters in the kidney and erythrocytes with an emphasis on the molecular structure of urea transporters and their role in producing concentrated urine.

CHAPTER 9

Renal Cell Metabolism

Michio Takeda and Hitoshi Endou

Because the kidney is a heterologous organ, each nephron segment has its own distinct morphologic and functional characteristics. Table 9.1 shows the anatomic, physiologic, and biochemical heterogeneity along the nephron segments. Among the renal biochemical characteristics, we focus in particular on adenosine triphosphate (ATP) turnover, glucose metabolism, and ammoniagenesis. ATP synthesized in individual nephron segments provides energy for various transport processes in the kidney. Renal gluconeogenesis had been thought to contribute significantly to the maintenance of glucose homeostasis only under specific conditions, such as metabolic acidosis and starvation. However, studies in humans and dogs using a combination of net balance and isotopic techniques have revealed that renal gluconeogenesis plays an important role in the maintenance of glucose homeostasis, even under physiologic conditions. Renal ammonia production and excretion are closely associated with the maintenance of acid–base balance. Thus renal metabolism plays an important role in the maintenance of physiologic conditions not only within the kidney but also in the body at large. Production of erythropoietin, prostaglandin, renin, and vitamin D metabolites as listed in Table 9.1; their regulation is described in other chapters in this book.

ATP TURNOVER IN THE KIDNEY

Energy-Consuming Processes in the Kidney

Although the kidney mass occupies only about 0.5% of the total body weight, the renal blood flow rate is about 20% of the cardiac output. Of renal blood flow, 20% is filtered through the glomerulus, and more than 99% of the filtrate is reabsorbed in the tubule. In general, active ionic transport is mediated by specific plasma membrane–bound enzymes known as *ion-transporting ATPases,* including Na^+-K^+-ATPase, Ca^{2+}-ATPase, H^+-ATPase, H^+-K^+-ATPase, and HCO_3^--ATPase. These ATPases are coupled to an energy-yielding reaction, namely, the hydrolysis of ATP: ATP $\rightarrow$ ADP + P_i (inorganic phosphate). Among these ATPases, Na^+-K^+-ATPase consumes the largest amount of ATP (60% to 80% of the total). Na^+-K^+-ATPase activities in the rabbit, rat, and mouse kidneys are the highest in the medullary and cortical thick ascending limb of the loop of Henle (MTAL and CTAL) and the distal convoluted tubule (DCT). In contrast, the thin descending and ascending limbs of Henle's loop exhibit a very low activity. Ca^{2+}-ATPase is detected in all rabbit nephron segments, with the highest activity in the DCT and cortical collecting tubule (CCT). H^+-ATPase was also recognized in all rabbit nephron segments, with the highest activity in the DCT and connecting tubule (CNT). HCO_3^--ATPase activity is the highest in the pars recta, DCT, CCT, and outer medullary collecting tubule (OMCT), whereas the lowest activities are found in the MTAL and CTAL in rabbit. H^+-K^+-ATPase is mainly localized in the distal nephron segments, with the highest activity in the CNT in rabbit. In addition, organic anion uptake in the basolateral membrane and organic cation uptake in the apical membrane of the proximal tubule (PT) are also ATP-dependent processes.

Thus ATP is a major source of fuel for cellular functions. Lack of intracellular ATP causing disturbances in intracellular homeostasis and derangement of phospholipid metabolism is a critical factor in numerous pathogenic events. To maintain a continuous supply of ATP and meet the energy demands of transport processes as described, the renal cells metabolize substrates and generate ATP. The generation of cellular ATP in renal cells depends on the metabolic processes such as oxygen delivery, transport of substrates, distribution of various enzymes to be related to use of endogenous and/or exogenous substrates, and the concentrations of endogenous substrates. As shown in Table 9.2, net ATP production or consumption depends on the metabolic pathways and substrate use.

ATP Synthesis in the Kidney

In the kidney, ATP is produced not only by mitochondrial oxidative phosphorylation but also by aerobic and anaerobic glycolysis, as described next.

Mitochondrial Oxidative Phosphorylation

The kidney cell generates about 95% of its intracellular ATP content by mitochondrial oxidative phosphorylation. Metabolic substrates, including pyruvate, and fatty acids enter the mitochondria, where they are oxidized to form acetyl-CoA. Acetyl-CoA is further oxidized in the tricarboxylic acid (TCA) cycle to yield two CO_2, one $FADH_2$, one GTP, and three NADH molecules. NADH generated by cytosolic enzyme reactions can also be used for mitochondrial oxidative phosphorylation. Because the mitochondrial membrane is impermeable to NADH, several electron shuttle systems, including the glycerol–phosphate and malate–asparate shuttle systems exist to facilitate the transfer of NADH into the mitochondria. The metabolic processes involved in mitochondrial oxidative phosphorylation are illustrated in Fig. 9.1. The oxidation of NADH by O_2 is coupled to electron transfer along the

TABLE 9.1. Heterogeneity along Nephron Segments

Anatomic	Physiologic	Biochemical
Glomerulus		
Epithelium	Constant filtration rate	Renin production
Endothelium	Ultrafiltration	PGE_2 synthesis
Mesangium	Mesangial contraction	
Proximal tubule		
S_1	Constant reabsorption	Ammoniagenesis
S_2	Isotonic reabsorption	Gluconeogenesis
S_3	Organic substance reabsorption	Erythropoietin synthesis
	Organic ion secretion	1α25-$(OH)_2$ D_3 production
		Cytochrome P450
Henle's loop		
Thin segment	Water permeable (thin)	Tamm-Horsfall glycoprotein production
Thick segment	Water-impermeable (thick)	
	Na-K-2Cl transport	
Distal tubule		
Distal convoluted tubule (single cell type)	K secretion	Kallikrein production
	Na-K cotransport	
Connecting tubule (multiple cell type)	Aldosterone action	
Collecting tubule		
Cortical collecting duct	Vasopressin action	PGE_2 synthesis
Outer medullary collecting duct	Aldosterone action	
	ANP action	
Inner medullary collecting duct		

mitochondrial respiratory chain. The respiratory chain is located in the inner mitochondrial membrane and consists of three large membrane-spanning multimeric protein complexes and two smaller mobile protein complexes. The transfer of electrons from NADH to O_2 results in loss of energy. This energy is used by the transmembrane protein complexes of the respiratory chain to release H^+ across the inner mitochondrial membrane, which leads to the generation of a H^+ electrochemical gradient across the inner mitochondrial membrane. The transmembrane mitochondrial F_0-F_1 type of H^+-ATPase (ATP synthase) uses the H^+ electrochemical gradient to catalyze the formation of ATP from adenosine diphosphate (ADP) and P_i. In summary, oxidation of one molecule of NADH with the consumption of one atom of oxygen generates three molecules of ATP.

Glycolysis

Glucose is metabolized under either aerobic or anaerobic conditions to produce ATP. Glucose is converted to pyruvate under aerobic conditions and converted to lactate under anaerobic conditions. During both processes, two molecules of ATP and two molecules of NADH are produced. NADH synthesized during aerobic metabolism provides energy for the production of ATP, whereas that produced under anaerobic conditions does not.

TABLE 9.2. ATP Synthesis (+) or Use (−) by Major Pathways of Renal Metabolism

Reaction	Net ATP
1 palmitate → 16 CO_2	+129
1 glucose → 6 CO_2	+36
1 glutamine → 5 CO_2	+27
1 lactate → 3 CO_2	+18
2 glutamine → glucose + 4 CO_2	+14
2 lactate → 1 glucose	−6

Reprinted with permission from Simpson DP. Renal metabolism. In: Schrier, Gottschalk, eds. *Diseases of the kidney.* Boston: Little, Brown, 1988:241.

Characteristics of ATP Synthesis in Individual Nephron Segments

There is considerable heterogeneity in the pathways and rates of ATP metabolism along the various nephron segments. The cortex has a high rate of aerobic metabolism. TCA cycle enzymes, including citrate synthase, isocitrate dehydrogenase, and α-ketoglutarate dehydrogenase (α-KGDH), are present in all nephron segments, with the highest activities noted in the thick ascending limb of the loop of Henle (TAL), DCT, and CCT. In contrast, the medulla is characterized by a high rate of glycolysis. The activities of enzymes involved in glycolysis—namely hexokinase, phosphofructokinase, and pyruvate

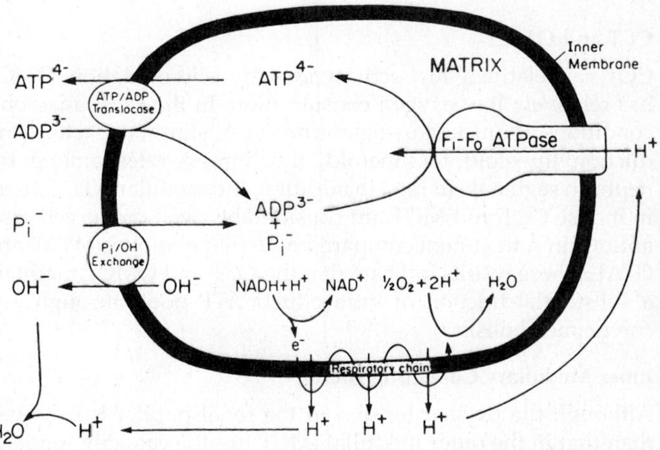

Figure 9.1. Mitochondrion showing the basic elements that participate in oxidative phosphorylation. ADP and P_i enter in exchange for ATP and OH^-, respectively. Electrons (e^-) are transferred by the respiratory chain from NADH to O_2. The extrusion of H^+ by the respiratory chain generates a transmembrane H^+ gradient that drives H^+ entry through the F_1-F_0 ATPase to generate ATP. The newly synthesized ATP exits to the cytosol in exchange for ADP. (Reprinted with permission from Gullans SR, Hebert SC. Metabolic basis of ion transport. In Brenner BM, Rector FC Jr, eds. *The kidney.* Philadelphia: WB Saunders, 1991, p. 76.)

kinase—are abundant in the distal nephron segments, whereas PT shows the lowest activities. In the distal nephron segments, glycolysis could be dramatically stimulated by inhibition of oxidative metabolism, which may be important for the maintenance of cell viability in this region of the kidney where oxygen tension is low. However, when oxidative metabolism is abolished, glycolysis alone cannot sustain normal functions in any of the renal segments. The characteristics of ATP production processes in individual nephron segments are described later.

PT

ATP production in the PT is mediated predominantly by mitochondrial oxidative phosphorylation, whereas glycolytic activity is low in this nephron segment. Consistent with this, the PT is generally more susceptible to ATP depletion or ischemic renal injury than other nephron segments. There is also intersegmental heterogeneity among PT. As shown in Fig. 9.2, ATP production from glucose is minimal in the first portion of PT (S_1), but it is substantial in the third portion of PT (S_3) in mice. This is consistent with the results of studies on the enzyme distribution, which revealed that hexokinase activity was low in S_1, whereas it was slightly higher in S_3. This may also be related to the finding that S_1 is much more susceptible to anoxic injury than S_3.

MTAL and CTAL

Na^+ is actively transported in TAL at a rate exceeding that in the PT. To meet the energy demand, TAL has a high density of mitochondria and the highest level of oxygen consumption among the nephron segments. Lactate production in the rat CTAL increases about 2-fold when mitochondrial ATP production is inhibited, whereas that in the rat MTAL increases 15-fold. However, antimycin A treatment significantly depleted intracellular ATP both in the mouse MTAL and CTAL. Thus, ATP production in these nephron segments appears to be mainly the result of mitochondrial oxidative phosphorylation.

DCT

DCT is relatively rich in mitochondria and Na^+-K^+-ATPase activity, and it largely depends on oxidative metabolism for its ATP production, whereas anaerobic metabolism appears to make little contribution to the maintenance of ATP content in the DCT.

CCT and OMCT

CCT has relatively low activity for fatty acid oxidation. OMCT has relatively low oxygen consumption. In the CCT, anaerobic conditions, mimicked using antimycin A, stimulate lactate production threefold to ninefold, the highest rates among the nephron segments in rats. In addition, intracellular ATP content in mouse CCT and MCT are considerably well conserved after antimycin A treatment compared with that in mouse MTAL and CTAL. These results indicate that the CCT and OMCT maintain a substantial fraction of intracellular ATP pools through glycolytic metabolism.

Inner Medullary Collecting Tubule

Although the oxygen tension in the renal papilla is even less than that in the outer medulla, IMCT has the capacity for aerobic mitochondrial metabolism as well as aerobic glycolytic metabolism. The inner medullary collecting tubule (IMCT) is the only segment of the nephron where the rate of anaerobic glycolysis is comparable with that of aerobic glycolysis. Although IMCT cells have such a large capacity to metabolize glucose under anaerobic conditions, anaerobic glycolysis could support most, if not all, of the ATP demand.

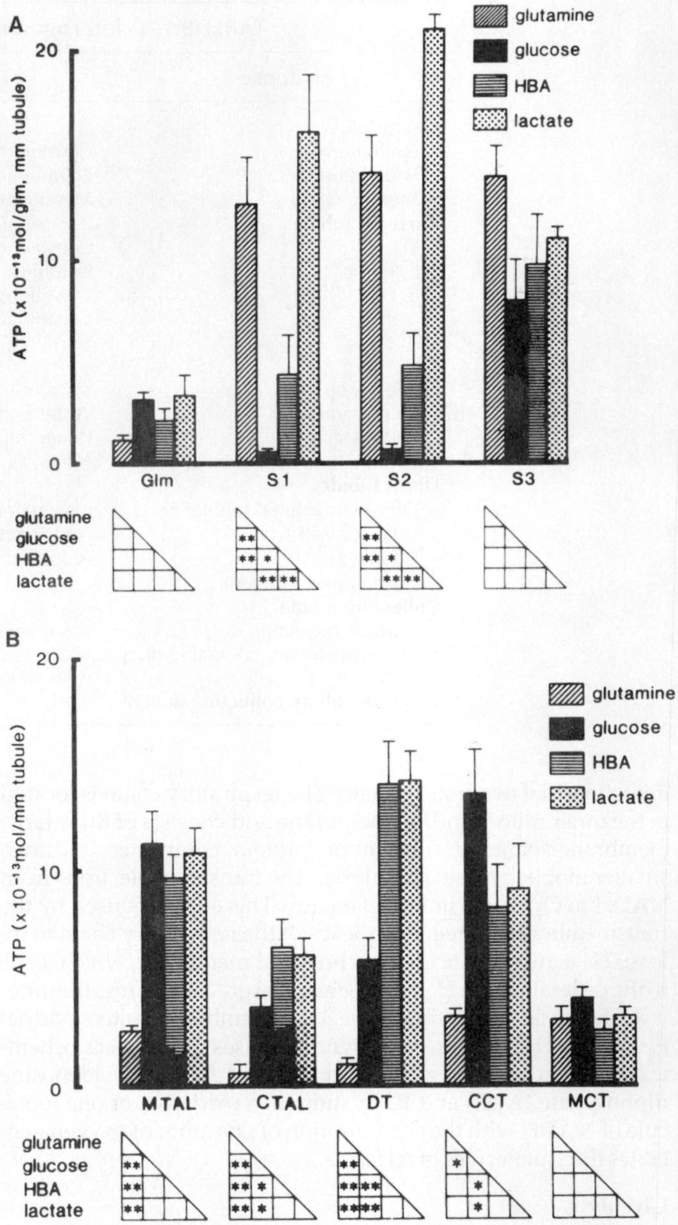

Figure 9.2. ATP production in glomeruli and proximal tubule segments (**A**) and distal tubule segments (**B**) as a function of substrates. **A:** Values are difference in ATP content between samples incubated with and without each substrate for 30 minutes. **B:** Values are difference in ATP content between samples incubated with and without each substrate for 15 minutes in the presence of monensin (10 μg/mL). Values are means ±SE of at least five experiments. Statistical significance was evaluated by analysis of variance (ANOVA). *$P < .05$. **$P < .01$. (Reprinted with permission from Uchida S, Endou H. Substrate specificity to maintain cellular ATP along the mouse nephron. *Am J Physiol* 1988;255:F981.)

Transport of Substrates across Cytoplasmic and Mitochondrial Membranes

Because substrate uptakes generally are not saturated at physiologic concentrations, renal metabolism is modulated by substrate availability. A relatively low concentration of substrates (10^{-4} M) is sufficient to maintain the cellular ATP pool in almost all segments of the nephron. Considering the physiologic concentrations of these substrates, glomerulus and tubules normally should be continuously surrounded by sufficient concentrations of metabolic substrates *in vivo*. Most substrates are thought to cross the luminal membrane into the cells via a Na-coupled mechanism, using the Na electrochemical gradient set up by Na^+-K^+-ATPase. Subsequently, these metabolic substrates enter the mitochondria via at least 12 specific transporters in the inner mitochondrial membrane and are oxidized by intramitochondrial enzymes. However, it is unclear whether all these transporters exist in renal mitochondria. On the basolateral membrane, the same substrates are transported by different, generally Na^+-independent mechanisms. It is generally considered that the substrate specificity of each nephron segment largely depends on the presence or absence of specific organic substrate transport in the plasma and/or mitochondrial membranes. It remains unknown whether they are rate-determining for the metabolism.

Substrate Specificity for ATP Production in Individual Nephron Segments

The preferred substrates used to supply energy needs vary from organ to organ. The brain uses glucose almost exclusively, whereas the heart and kidney use a mixture of substrates, including glucose, fatty acids, lactate, amino acids (glutamate, glutamine, and proline), citrate, and ketone bodies. The substrates used preferentially by the kidney may vary with the metabolic state. For example, during metabolic acidosis, the preferred substrate in the kidney changes from lactate to glutamine. In rats with diabetic ketoacidosis, ketone bodies and glutamine substitute for lactate. The substrate specificities for ATP production in the mouse nephron segments are demonstrated in Fig. 9.2. Glutamine and lactate are the preferred substrate in the PT. In contrast, ATP production from glutamine is less than that from the other substrates in distal nephron segments. Lactate and β-hydroxybutyrate (β-HBA) are preferred substrates for maintenance of the ATP pool in the CTAL, MTAL, and DCT. Glucose is the preferred substrate in the CCT. The substrate specificity in the short- and long-loop nephron segments (SDL and LDL, respectively) was determined in rats. Glucose and pyruvate were the preferred substrates in both SDL and LDL. ATP production from glutamine, β-HBA, and lactate is substantial in LDL. In SDL, glutamine is the preferred substrate, whereas β-HBA and lactate are minimally used. These results indicate that each nephron segment has its own distinct ability to use specific substrates for ATP production.

When the substrate specificities for ATP production were compared among rabbits, rats, and mice, different PT substrate specificities were noted. In contrast, in distally located nephron segments, similar substrate specificities among mice, rats, and rabbits were observed, and glucose was a useful substrate for cellular ATP production in these species.

Fatty Acids and Ketone Bodies as the Metabolic Substrates for ATP Production

Fatty Acids

As shown in Table 9.2, fatty acids, including oleate, palmitate, and linoleate, are considered the major substrates for ATP production in the kidney. Fatty acids enter the basolateral side of the PT in a linear correlation with their arterial concentrations. However, only a small proportion of the fatty acids taken up are oxidized, whereas most are incorporated into triacylglycerol. β-oxidation of fatty acids is important for ATP production in the cortex and outer medulla, whereas in the inner medulla, carbohydrates play a major role in this process. β-oxidation of fatty acids appears to be saturated at physiologic concentrations of fatty acids. β-oxidation of fatty acids to acetyl-CoA occurs in both the mitochondria and peroxisomes. In the cytosol, fatty acids are converted to fatty acyl-CoA. Because the mitochondrial membrane is impermeable to fatty acyl-CoA, fatty acyl-CoA has to be transesterified to the carnitine derivative to be transported through the mitochondrial membrane. Fatty acyl-CoA is metabolized to acetyl-CoA by hydroxyacyl-CoA dehydrogenase, and acetyl-CoA is then introduced into the TCA cycle. On the other hand, in the peroxisomes of the cytosol, fatty acids are converted to acetyl-CoA by fatty acyl-CoA oxidase, whereas this pathway may be of only minor importance in the kidney. β-oxidation of fatty acids occurs in all nephron segments. The distribution of hydroxyacyl-CoA dehydrogenase activities also parallels the known distribution of these enzymes in the mitochondria, with the highest activity in the DCT, relatively high activity in both the PCT and TAL, and relatively low activity in the glomerulus and CCT. On the other hand, the distribution of fatty acyl-CoA oxidase activity parallels that in the peroxisomes and is highest in the proximal straight tubule (PST).

Ketone Bodies

During ketoacidosis resulting from starvation or uncontrolled diabetes, basolateral uptake as well as apical reabsorption of 3-hydroxybutyrate (3-HBA) and acetoacetate are increased. In this regard, the kidney plays a significant role in ketone body turnover. 3-HBA is catalyzed to acetoacetate by 3-HBA dehydrogenase. Acetoacetate is further converted to acetoacetyl-CoA by 3-oxoacid-CoA transferase. Acetoacetyl-CoA is split into acetyl-CoA by a specific thiolase, and acetyl-CoA enters the citric acid cycle to be oxidized to CO_2. All these reactions occur in the mitochondrial matrix. 3-hydroxybutyrate dehydrogenase is abundant in both proximal and distal nephrons. 3-oxoacid-CoA transferase activity is highest in the TAL and DCT, significant in the PT, and lowest in the glomerulus, CCT, and thin limbs of Henle's loop.

Endogenous Substrates for Renal ATP Production

In addition to the substrates transported via luminal membrane transporters, endogenous substrates also play a role in energy metabolism. The amount of glycogen stored in the kidney is small, but it has been shown that the TAL and papilla have a 10-fold larger glycogen content than the PT. When isolated nephron segments from rabbits, rats, and mice were incubated at 37°C in the absence of exogenous substrates for 30 minutes, the cellular ATP decreased drastically in the PT. However, it did not decrease so conspicuously in the lower nephron segments, indicating that the distal nephron segments may contain higher concentrations of endogenous substrates than the PT. In addition, cellular ATP content in rat and mouse PT was in the order S_3 > the second portion of PT (S_2) > S_1. This may be related to the finding that S_3 is the most vulnerable to ischemia.

Creatine-Phosphate as a High-Energy Phosphate Donor for ATP Production in the Kidney

The energy demand within cells is sustained in part through the availability of alternative storage forms of energy, such as creatine phosphate. The use of this stored energy for the replenishment of ATP occurs by transphosphorylation of ADP through the action of creatine kinase as follows.

$$\text{Creatine phosphase} + \text{ADP} \rightleftarrows \text{Creatine} + \text{ATP}$$

Although this reaction occurs mainly in the skeletal muscle, various observations suggest that the creatine phosphate and kinase system also play a role in the kidney. The process of creatine biosynthesis is as follows. Guanidinoacetic acid (GAA) is synthesized from arginine by glycine-amidinotransferase, which is localized exclusively in the S_1 and S_2 segments of PTs. GAA is transported to the liver, where it is methylated to creatine by GAA-methyltransferase. Although no creatine synthetic activity was recognized in rat nephron segments, all nephron segments contained a significant amount of creatine, and the glomerulus, MTAL, CTAL, and DCT showed the highest creatine content. In addition, the levels of creatine kinase were highest in the TAL and DCT. These results suggest that the creatine phosphate and kinase system is involved in ion transport and oxidative phosphorylation in the distal nephron segments of the kidney, as it is in the skeletal muscle. Creatine is nonenzymatically converted to creatinine. Creatinine is further catalyzed to methylguanidine, a uremic toxin, by methylguanidine synthetase, the cDNA of which was cloned and shown to be identical to long-chain L-2 hydroxy acid oxidase.

Effects of Nephrotoxins on the ATP Content in the Individual Nephron Segments

The measurement of intracellular ATP content in individual nephron segments is an efficient method for evaluating the intrarenal toxic site and potency of various nephrotoxins. Ochratoxin A (OTCA) is a mycotoxin, produced by several species of *Aspergillus* and *Penicillium*, and it has been assumed to be the causative agent of Balkan endemic nephropathy. OCTA has been shown to affect liver mitochondrial respiration and oxidative phosphorylation, and it also act as a competitive inhibitor of mitochondrial transport carrier proteins. Among the various nephron segments tested, OCTA at 5×10^{-5} M significantly decreased the cellular ATP content only in S_2 and S_3 segments of the PT, suggesting that these segments are the specific target sites for OCTA-induced nephrotoxicity. On the other hand, mercuric chloride ($HgCl_2$) at concentrations higher than 10^{-6} M caused an abrupt and significant decrease in ATP content in the S_2 segment of the PCT, whereas 10^{-4} M $HgCl_2$ was required to significantly reduce the ATP content in the MCT, suggesting that S_2 is the segment most sensitive to $HgCl_2$ within the nephron.

Role of Extracellular ATP in the Kidney

The concentration of ATP within the cells is in the millimolar range, and a significant amount of cytoplasmic ATP could be released from renal cells during activation of cells by physiologic and pathophysiologic stimuli. Since P2 purinoceptor subtypes have been successively cloned, much attention has been focused on the role of ATP as a ligand for the P2 purinoceptor family, which is subdivided into $P2X_{1\text{-}7}$ and $P2Y_{1\text{-}8}$ purinoceptors. Among these, $P2Y_1$, $P2Y_2$, $P2Y_3$, and $P2X_4$ purinoceptor mRNA have been shown to be expressed in the kidney. The roles of ATP actions in the kidney clarified so far are limited and include gluconeogenesis in S_1 segments via the P2Y purinoceptor, mitogenesis in mesangial cells and tubular cells via the $P2Y_2$ purinoceptor, and inhibition of the increase in vasopressin-induced hydrostatic pressure in the collecting duct via the $P2Y_2$ purinoceptor. The development of an efficient P2 purinoceptor antagonist would lead us to a better understanding of the actions of extracellular ATP in the kidney.

Intracellular and Extracellular ATP Degradation in the Kidney

Intracellular ATP Degradation

Oxygen deprivation resulting from ischemia, hypoperfusion, or hypoxia in the kidney results in a rapid decrease in the intracellular ATP content and an increase in the concentration of ATP degradation products such as ADP, adenosine monophosphate (AMP), adenosine, inosine, and hypoxanthine, which can serve as a substrate for xanthine oxidase. The xanthine–xanthine oxidase system has been postulated as being one of the potential sources of reactive oxygen species (ROS). ROS have been shown to cause tissue injury in the kidney. Most mammalian cells contain enzymes capable of degrading AMP to nucleoside and purine bases. The breakdown of adenine nucleotides (ATP, ADP, and AMP) may result in the formation of adenosine by 5′-nucleotidase. Adenosine is deaminated to inosine by adenosine deaminase, and inosine is cleaved by purine nucleoside phosphorylase to hypoxanthine and ribose-1-phosphate. This process may operate either to transfer purines among cells or to prevent intracellular accumulation of AMP during a fall of ATP. Microdissection studies have demonstrated that the specific activity of 5′-nucleotidase is highest in the PT and CCT but low in the glomerulus. In contrast, the highest activity of adenosine deaminase is found in the glomerulus. The distribution pattern of purine nucleoside phosphorylase was similar to that of adenosine deaminase. These results suggest that adenosine can be synthesized in various nephron segments and that the glomerulus possesses the highest capacity to metabolize this nucleotide. Others postulated that the glomerular injury associated with puromycin aminonucleoside (PAN) may be mediated by the generation of ROS because hypoxanthine, an intermediate metabolite of PAN, can be used as a substrate for xanthine oxidase in this model. Thus, the high purine-catabolizing activity in the glomerulus, as described, may be related to the finding that renal injury from PAN is predominant in the glomerulus, both morphologically and functionally.

Extracellular ATP Degradation

Degradation of extracellular ATP is also mediated by extracellular ATPases and nucleotidases. For instance, an ecto-5′-nucleotidase, ectophosphodiesterase, ectoadenosinetriphosphatase (ecto-ATPase), and ectonucleotide pyrophosphatase have been found in the brush border of cells of PT. The concentrations of these enzymes are sufficient for the degradation of all adenine nucleotides to adenosine. These extracellular ATPases and nucleotidases presumably serve at least two important functions: (a) to terminate the ATP-induced signal transduction through P2-purinoceptors and (b) to catalyze the generation of adenosine that then acts on P1-purinoceptors.

GLUCOSE METABOLISM

To meet the energy requirements of tissues such as brain and erythrocytes, which use only glucose as fuel, glucose has to be continuously released into the circulation in the postabsorptive state. Release of glucose into the circulation occurs via two processes: (a) gluconeogenesis, which is defined as the *de novo* synthesis of glucose from noncarbohydrate precursors, and (b) glycolysis, characterized by the formation of lactate from glucose or glycogen. Only the liver and kidney are capable of both producing glucose (gluconeogenesis) and consuming glucose (glycolysis). Although parallels exist in the regulation of gluconeogenesis between the kidney and liver, several important differences are recognized. In the liver, the coexistence of glucose-consuming and glucose-producing pathways in the same cells suggests the presence of so-called futile cycles. In contrast, in the kidney, glucose use occurs predominantly in the medulla, whereas glucose production is confined to the cortex. In addition, differences between the kidney and liver also exist with respect to substrate use, pathway stimulation, and hormonal regulation of glucose production.

Metabolic Pathways of Gluconeogenesis and Glycolysis

As shown in Fig. 9.3, the pathways of gluconeogenesis and glycolysis share many enzymatic steps, but key regulatory steps are distinct between the two processes. Glucose-6-phosphatase, fructose bisphosphatase, and phosphoenolpyruvate carboxykinase (PEPCK) are specific for gluconeogenesis, whereas hexokinase, phosphofructokinase, and pyruvate kinase are specific for glycolysis. Gluconeogenesis within the mammalian liver or renal proximal tubular cells is highly compartmentalized. The coordinated synthesis of glucose from noncarbohydrate precursors requires the participation of enzymes localized in the mitochondria, cytoplasm, and endoplasmic reticulum. The primary substrates for renal gluconeogenesis are lactate, pyruvate, glutamine, and α-ketoglutarate. Glucose production from these substrates requires the formation of oxaloacetate as an intermediate. For example, pyruvate is converted to oxaloacetate by pyruvate carboxylase, an intramitochondrial enzyme. Oxaloacetate cannot cross the mitochondrial membrane. To cross the mitochondrial membrane, oxaloacetate is converted to malate by malate dehydrogenase, and it is then transported out of the mitochondrion via the malate–aspartate shuttle. Oxaloacetate is then converted into phosphoenolpyruvate by PEPCK. A series of enzymes that subsequently convert phosphoenolpyruvate to glucose-6-phosphate are localized in the cytosol, whereas the final step in the pathway, catalyzed by glucose-6-phosphatase, occurs in the endoplasmic reticulum.

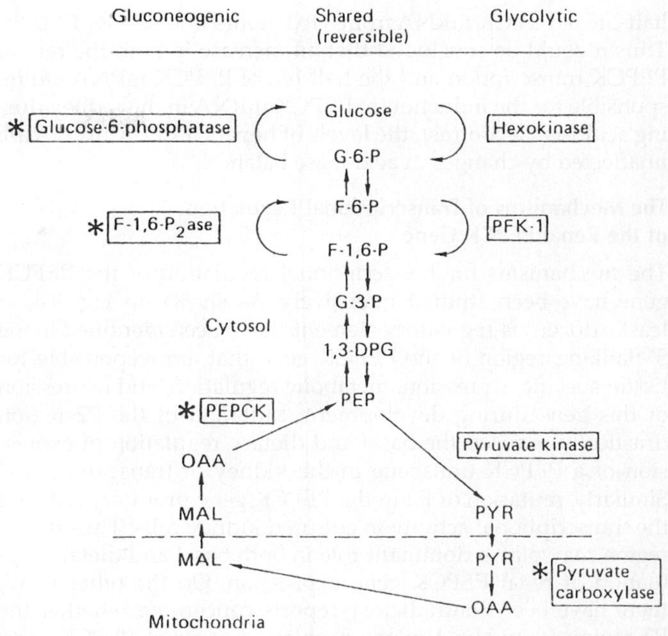

Figure 9.3. Metabolic pathways of gluconeogenesis and glycolysis in the kidney. G-6-P, glucose-6-phosphate; F-6-P, fructose-6-phosphate; F-1, 6-Pase, fructose-1,6-bisphosphatase; F-1,6-P, fructose-1,6-bisphosphate; G-3-P, glycerol-3-phosphate; 1,3-DPG, 1,3-diphosphoglycerate; PEPCK, phosphoenolpyruvate carboxykinase; PEP, phosphoenolpyruvate OAA, oxaloacetate; MAL, malate; PYR, pyruvate. *Enzymes unique to gluconeogenesis. (Reprinted with permission from Schoolwerth AC, Smith BC, Culpepper RM. Renal gluconeogenesis. *Miner Electrolyte Metab* 1988; 14:347.)

Intranephron and Internephron Heterogeneity of Gluconeogenesis

Among the individual nephron segments, only the PT possesses three gluconeogenic enzymes both in rabbits and in rats. The order of these enzyme activities in the rat was $S_1 > S_2 > S_3$. Consistent with the intranephron distribution of gluconeogenic enzymes, the site of gluconeogenic activity from pyruvate and glutamine in control rats was limited to the PT. The gluconeogenic activity from pyruvate and glutamine in the rat was in the order $S_1 > S_2 >> S_3$. This extremely low level of gluconeogenic activity in S_3 suggests the existence of glycolytic activity in this portion of the nephron segment, as described. Gluconeogenic activity from glutamine in superficial (SF) nephrons was significantly higher than that in juxtamedullary (JM) nephrons; no differences were seen in the activity from pyruvate. In acidotic and K^+-depleted rats, a significant increase in gluconeogenic activity could be seen in both S_1 and S_2, but not in S_3, segments of the PCT. In acidosis, glucose production from pyruvate and glutamine in SF nephrons and that from glutamine in JM nephrons was elevated significantly compared with control, but that from pyruvate in JM nephrons did not change. Thus S_1 of the SF nephrons may play the most important role in gluconeogenesis under control conditions, whereas the S_1 segment of the JM nephrons as well as the S_2 segments may contribute to gluconeogenesis in acidotic and/or possibly K^+-depleted rats.

Regulation of Renal PEPCK Activity and Gene Expression

Because the step catalyzed by PEPCK is generally accepted to be the rate-limiting step, the regulation of PEPCK activity and gene expression have been studied intensively. PEPCK exists in two forms: the cytosolic and mitochondrial forms. This localization is species specific. PEPCK is almost exclusively cytosolic in the rat, but it is present in both cytosol and mitochondria in most other mammalian species. The mitochondrial PEPCK is constitutive, whereas the gene for cytosolic PEPCK is stimulated by glucocorticoid and metabolic acidosis but inhibited by metabolic alkalosis, insulin, and a high-carbohydrate diet. Moreover, the intracellular location of PEPCK has important metabolic consequences. Mitochondrial PEPCK is involved in gluconeogenesis from lactate, whereas the cytosolic form may operate gluconeogenesis from lactate, pyruvate, and amino acids.

Regulation of Expression of the PEPCK Gene in Acidosis

A number of studies have demonstrated that metabolic as well as respiratory acidosis stimulate renal gluconeogenesis. In the rat kidney, PEPCK activity associated with PEPCK mRNA expression is stimulated during acidosis. In contrast, neither glucose-6-phosphatase nor pyruvate carboxylase shows any significant change in activity. Reverse transcription and polymerase chain reaction studies have demonstrated that PEPCK mRNA is localized in the PT and the amount in the order $S_3 > S_2 > S_1$ in control rats. Ten hours after NH_4Cl feeding in rats, an increase in PEPCK mRNA expression, limited to S_1 and S_2, was recognized. This was consistent with the change in the enzyme activity. *In situ* hybridization and immunohistochemical studies confirmed that PEPCK mRNA and protein expressions were confined to medullary rays under normal conditions, whereas enhanced expression was noted throughout the cortex after the induction of NH_4Cl acidosis in rats. Nuclear run-on experiments showed that stimulation of renal PEPCK mRNA expression during acute and chronic metabolic acidosis is primarily caused by an increased rate of transcription. In addition, acidosis also exerts its effect by stabilizing PEPCK mRNA against degradation. It has been demonstrated that a change in pH of the culture medium from 7.4 to 6.9 alters the half-life of PEPCK mRNA from 3 to 9 hours in LLC-PK_1-F^+ cells. Thus it could be concluded that an increase in both the rate of PEPCK transcription and the half-life of PEPCK mRNA are responsible for the induction of PEPCK mRNA in the kidney during acidosis. In contrast, the levels of hepatic PEPCK mRNA are unaffected by changes in acid–base balance.

The Mechanisms of Transcriptional Regulation of the Renal PEPCK Gene

The mechanisms for transcriptional regulation of the PEPCK gene have been studied intensively. As shown in Fig. 9.4, at least a dozen *cis*-regulatory elements have been identified in the 5′-flanking region of the PEPCK gene that are responsible for tissue-specific expression, metabolic regulation, and expression of this gene during development. Mutation of the P2 region drastically reduced the basal and dietary regulation of expression of a PEPCK transgene in the kidney of transgenic mice. Similarly, mutation of P2 in the PEPCK gene promoter reduced the transcriptional activity in cultured kidney cells. Thus the P2 region may play a dominant role in both basal and dietary regulation of renal PEPCK gene expression. On the other hand, there have been contradictory reports concerning whether the P2 region is involved in the regulation of renal PEPCK gene during acidosis. In contrast, the P3 region was required for basal expression of the PEPCK gene in the liver but not in the kidney. In LLC-PK_1-F^+ cells, mutation of the P3 or CRE-1 region (cAMP-responsive element), had little effect on basal PEPCK transcriptional activity but caused a 50% decrease of the activity during acidosis. The P3 and CRE-1 regions were shown to be involved in cAMP activation of the PEPCK gene in LLC-PK_1-F^+ cells.

Hormonal Regulation of Renal Gluconeogenesis

As shown in Table 9.3, many factors, including hormones, have been shown to regulate renal glucose production. In normal dogs, physiologic hyperinsulinemia suppressed renal glucose production by 75% and stimulated renal glucose uptake by 75%, resulting in a net change in the renal glucose balance from zero to net uptake. This insulin-mediated increase in renal glucose uptake may occur in the distal nephron segments and may reflect an increase in both glycogen synthesis and glucose oxidation. Infusion of epinephrine, which results in circulating insulin concentrations similar to those observed in hypoglycemia, increased renal glucose production by 100% in healthy humans.

Physiologic Significance of Renal Gluconeogenesis

Renal gluconeogenesis has a physiologic significance in the maintenance of glucose homeostasis and the regulation of intracellular ATP content.

Glucose Homeostasis

In *in vitro* experiments, the gluconeogenic capacity of the kidney exceeds that of the liver on a gram-for-gram tissue basis. However, until recently, the human kidney generally has been regarded as contributing insignificantly to postabsorptive glucose production. This contention is based on the observation that the difference in renal arterial and venous glucose concentrations was not significant except in patients with respiratory acidosis and in obese individuals after prolonged fasting. By merely representing the differences between uptake and release of a substrate, net balance measurements could not evaluate the contribution of a particular organ to the entry and removal of a substrate from the systemic circulation. In this context, a combination of net balance measurements and isotopic techniques, with measurements of substrate as well as tracer concentrations, has been recently introduced and has made it possible to assess individually the uptake and release of glucose in the kidney. The studies using this technique have revealed that in humans, renal glucose production contributes to approximately 25% of the systemic glucose production and renal glucose uptake accounts for 20% of systemic glucose removal. These results indicate an important role for the human kidney in the maintenance of glucose homeostasis. Because the normal human kidney does not contain appreciable glycogen stores, it is likely that release of glucose by the kidney is mainly, if not exclusively, the result of gluconeogenesis. Consistent with this notion, the net renal uptake of key gluconeogenic precursors such as lactate, glycerol, glutamine, and other amino acids was sufficient to account for the entire observed release of glucose by the kidney.

Regulation of Intracellular ATP Content

Apart from glomerular filtration rate and tubular transport of sodium, there is the factor of oxygen consumption by the kidney. Of the energy-requiring processes, gluconeogenesis is

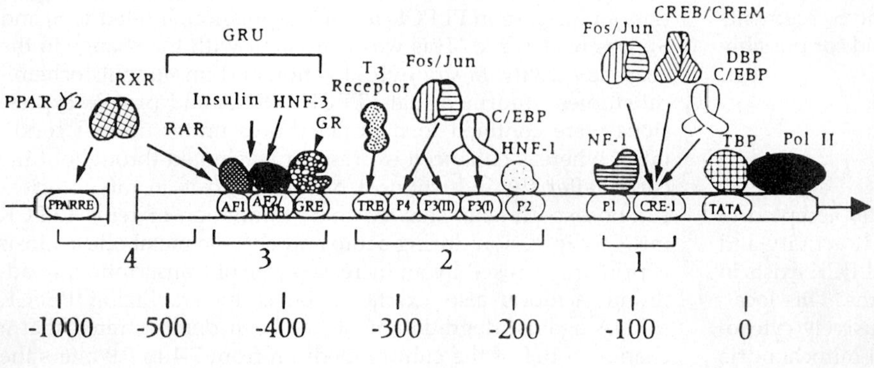

Figure 9.4. Transcriptional regulatory elements of the PEPCK-C gene promoter. The positions of the regulatory elements in the PEPCK-C gene promoter are represented by ovals, and the various proteins that regulate transcription of the PEPCK gene are shown relative to their binding sites on the promoter. CRE, cAMP regulatory element; TRE, thyroid hormone regulatory element; GRE, glucocorticoid regulatory element; TBP, TATA-binding protein; IRE, insulin regulatory element; PPARRE, peroxisome proliferator-activated receptor regulatory element; AF-1, accessory factor-1; C/EBP, CAAT/enhancer binding protein; CREB, cAMP regulatory element binding protein; DBP, D-binding protein; NF-1, nuclear factor-1; HNF-1, hepatic nuclear factor-1; HNF-3, hepatic nuclear factor-3; GRU, glucocorticoid regulatory unit; GR, glucocorticoid receptor; RAR, retinoic acid receptor; RXR, retinoic X receptor; PPARγ2, peroxisome proliferator-activated receptor γ2. (Reprinted with permission from Nizielski SE, Lechner PS, Croniger CM, et al. Transcriptional regulatory elements the P-enolpyruvate carboxykinase promoter. *J Nutr* 1996;126:2699.)

TABLE 9.3. Factors Affecting Renal Gluconeogenesis

	Stimulation	Inhibition
Hormones	Catecholamines	Adrenalectomy
	Glucocorticoids	
	Aldosterone	
	Insulin deficiency (diabetes mellitus)	Insulin
	Parathyroid hormone	Calcitonin
	Vitamin D	
	Thyroxine	
	Growth hormone	
	Angiotensin	
Acid–base balance	Acidosis	Alkalosis
Others	Prolonged fasting	
	Exercise	
	High protein diet	Branched-chain amino acids
	Liver failure	
	Nonesterified fatty acids	

Reprinted with permission from Stumvoll M, Meyer C, Mitrakou A, et al. Renal glucose production and utilization: new aspects in humans. *Diabetologia* 1997;40:752.

clearly the most important. When gluconeogenesis is stimulated, it can account for as much as 25% of the oxygen consumed by the kidney, whereas triglyceride synthesis does not account for more than 1% of the oxygen consumption. In addition, there are many indications that gluconeogenesis and the reabsorption of sodium are reciprocally related as they compete for a limited pool of cellular ATP, although this is not always the case. In contrast, no consistent correlation is recognized between gluconeogenesis and phosphate or glucose transport. Thus gluconeogenesis may be involved in the regulation of ATP content in proximal tubules.

AMMONIAGENESIS

The urinary excretion of ammonia (free-base ammonia, NH_3; and ammonium ion, NH_4^+) plays a central role in the maintenance of acid–base balance because the bicarbonate necessary to neutralize the daily hydrogen ion load is derived from the production of ammonia in the PT and excretion into the urine.

Glutamine Metabolism

Glutamine

Plasma glutamine plays an important role as a carrier of amino nitrogen, carbon, and energy between organs; in addition, it is used for hepatic urea synthesis and renal ammoniagenesis and is a major respiratory fuel in many cells. Glutamine is synthesized primarily in skeletal muscle, lung, and adipose tissue. Glutamine is released during stress and hypercatabolic states, including metabolic acidosis, cancer, trauma, and injection of endotoxin. Glutamine is the most abundant single amino acid in the plasma (0.5 mM) in dogs and the third highest in abundance (0.29 mM) in rats. Glutamine is taken up from the basolateral side of the PT or reabsorbed from the first third of the PT. As shown in Fig. 9.5, glutamine is taken up into the cytosol and transported to the intramitochondrial space for ammoniagenesis. Glutamine is the most important substrate for ammoniagenesis in the kidney. Glutamine metabolism is tightly coupled to the regulatory function of the organ in acid–base homeostasis. In normal acid–base balance, the kidney extracts and metabolizes very little glutamine. However, metabolic acidosis is associated

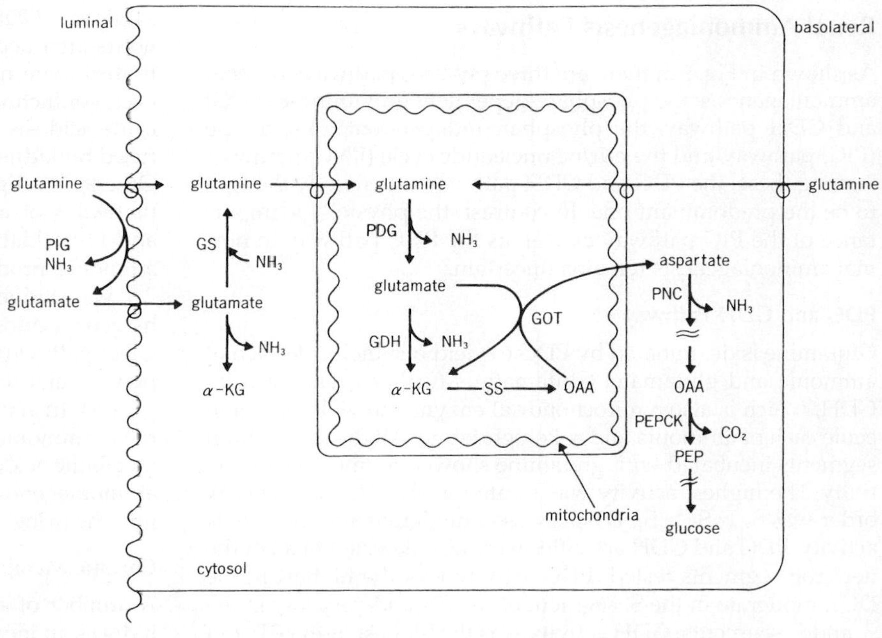

PDG : phosphate dependent glutaminase
GS : glutamine synthetase
GOT : glutamate oxaloacetate transaminase
PNC : purine nucleotide cycle
OAA : oxaloacetate
PIG : phosphate independent glutaminase
GDH : glutamate dehydrogenase
PEPCK : phosphoenolpyruvate carboxykinase
α-KG : α-ketoglutarate
PEP : phosphoenolpyruvate

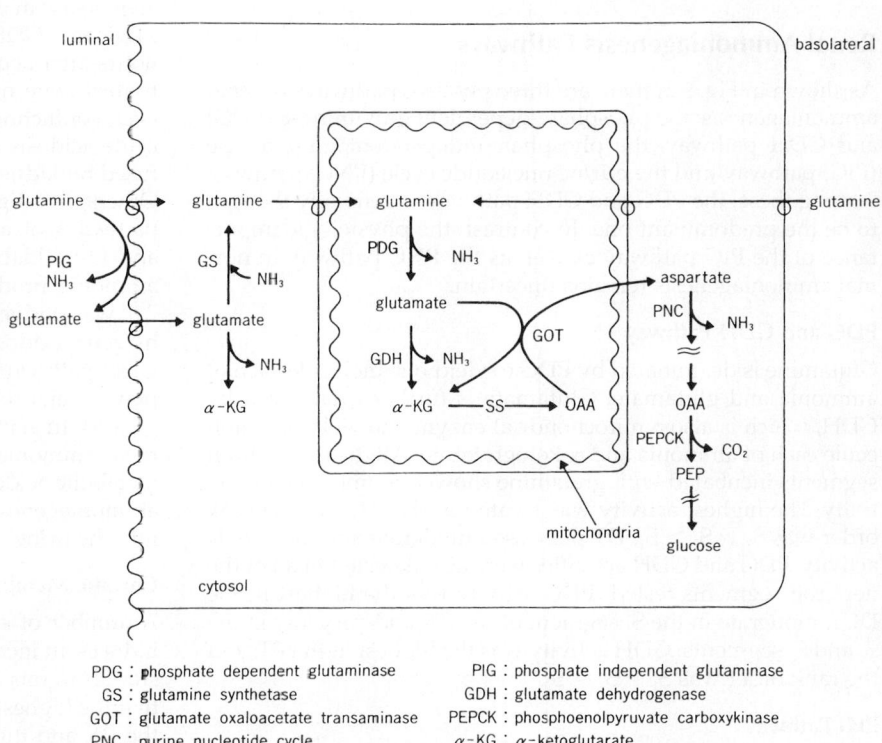

Figure 9.5. Metabolic pathways of ammoniagenesis.

with increased renal excretion of plasma glutamine in humans, dogs, and rats.

Glutaminase

Glutaminase exists in two isoforms: the kidney-type and the liver-type. Kidney-type glutaminase is abundant in kidney, brain, intestine, fetal liver, lymphocytes, and transformed cells, whereas liver-type glutaminase is expressed only in the periportal hepatocytes of the postnatal liver. Kidney-type glutaminase is localized within the mitochondrial matrix. It requires a polyvalent anion for activity. The most common activator is phosphate. Kidney-type glutaminase activity increases only in response to metabolic acidosis, whereas hepatic glutaminase increases under conditions of starvation, diabetes, and intake of a high-protein diet. Kidney-type glutaminase activity is regulated at the posttranscriptional level, whereas hepatic glutaminase activity is mediated by changes in the rate of transcription.

Glutamine and Glutamate Transport across the Mitochondrial Membrane

The transport of glutamine and glutamate across the inner mitochondrial membrane is closely related to flux through enzymes located within the mitochondrial matrix space. Several transporters regulate glutamate movement across the inner mitochondrial membrane in the kidney. These transporters, which are also found in the mitochondria in other tissues, include the glutamate hydroxyl transporter and the glutamate–asparate antiporter. The glutamate hydroxyl transporter is functionally linked to the metabolism of glutamate dehydrogenase (GDH); although an insignificant amount of glutamate enters the renal mitochondria via this transporter, a decrease in glutamate flux from the matrix space via this transporter during metabolic acidosis could contribute to an accelerated GDH flux. On the other hand, glutamine is also transported into mitochondria via a specific transporter. The transport of glutamine across the inner mitochondrial membrane has been proposed to be the rate-limiting step in glutamine metabolism during acidosis.

Renal Ammoniagenesis Pathways

As shown in Fig. 9.5, there are three possible pathways of renal ammoniagenesis: the phosphate-dependent glutaminase (PDG) and GDH pathway, the phosphate-independent glutaminase (PIG) pathway, and the purine nucleotide cycle (PNC) pathway. Among these, the PDG and GDH pathway is generally thought to be the predominant one. In contrast, the physiologic importance of the PIG pathway as well as the PNC pathway in normal ammoniagenesis remains uncertain.

PDG and GDH Pathway

Glutamine is deaminated by PDG to yield one molecule each of ammonia and glutamate. Glutamate is further catabolized by GDH, which is also a mitochondrial enzyme, to yield one molecule each of ammonia and α-ketoglutarate. All the rat nephron segments incubated with glutamine showed ammoniagenic activity. The highest activity was located in the PT, and the rank order was $S_2 > S_3 > S_1$. DT possessed moderate ammoniagenic activity. PDG and GDH activities were also detected in all of the nephron segments tested. PDG activity was the highest in the DCT, moderate in the S_1 segment of the PT, and very low in the S_2 and S_3 segments. GDH activity was the highest in the PT, and the rank order was $S_1 > S_2 > S_3$.

PIG Pathway

PIG has been shown to be identical to γ-GT (γ-glutamyl-transpeptidase) and is localized in the brush border membrane of the S_3 segment of the PT in rats. Glutamine is hydroxylated extracellularly by γ-GT, resulting in the generation of one molecule each of ammonium and glutamate. Ammonia production from glutamate was recognized in a rat cortical tubular suspension, whereas the ammonia production from glutamate was about 10% of that from glutamine. However, because glutamine is removed almost completely from the glomerular filtrate in the S_1 and S_2 segments of the PT, no substrate is available for ammonia formation in the brush border of the S_3 segment of the PT, where PIG activity is localized.

PNC Pathway

In the PNC pathway, aspartate is metabolized to one molecule each of ammonia and fumarate. This reaction is catalyzed by adenylic acid deaminase, adenylosuccinate synthetase, and adenylosuccinase. Microdissection studies have revealed ammoniagenesis from aspartate in all of the nephron segments tested, with the highest activity in the S_1 segment and intermediate activity in the S_2 segment and CCT. However, the kidney has not been found to extract aspartate from the blood in either control and chronically acidotic rats.

Regulation of Renal Ammoniagenesis

Metabolic acidosis and K^+ depletion are two major stimuli for renal ammoniagenesis. Although the adaptive changes in renal ammoniagenic pathways under these two conditions were not identical, as described next, the PCT is the primary site of the regulation under both conditions.

Acute Metabolic Acidosis

Acute acid load results in a large increase in ammonia excretion in rats. The increased concentrations of hydrogen ions activates renal cortical α-KDGH. The activation of α-KGDH results in a decrease in mitochondrial matrix α-ketoglutarate content, which leads to glutamate deamination and ammonia production by flux through GDH. Glutamate deamination by GDH precedes an increase in glutamine deamination by PDG in rats. Although PDG and GDH mRNA expressions were induced within 24 hours after acute acid load in rats, PDG and GDH enzyme activities were not significantly increased until 48 hours. However, conflicting results were reported. One study showed that acute acidosis stimulated ammoniagenesis in the isolated perfused rat kidney entirely as a result of enhanced flux from PDG. Others investigated the effect of intensity of the acidosis on the pathways of ammoniagenesis in LLC-PK_1 cells using [5-^{15}N] and [2-^{15}N]-labeled glutamine. They found that the increased ammonia production under conditions of acute acidosis (pH 7.0) was derived entirely from GDH flux, whereas that induced by acute acidosis (pH 6.8) was derived from both the PDG and GDH pathways. Thus the severity of acute acidosis appears to play a major role in the regulation of the pathways of ammoniagenesis. In acute metabolic acidosis in humans, the response of renal ammonia production was slow and renal adaptation to metabolic acidosis was characterized by not only an increase in ammoniagenesis but also a preferential excretion of ammonia into the urine.

Chronic Metabolic Acidosis

A number of studies have demonstrated that chronic acidosis induces an increase in ammoniagenesis in rats. Microdissection studies in rats during chronic metabolic acidosis demonstrated that the highest level of ammoniagenic activity was localized in the PT, and the rank order was $S_1 > S_2 > S_3$. Although no difference in ammonia production was noted between SF-S_1 and JM-S_1 in control rats, ammonia production in SF-S_1 was significantly higher than that in JM-S_1 during chronic metabolic acidosis. Thus the SF-S_1 nephron segment but not JM-S_1 is reactive to acidosis. Consistent with the pattern of ammoniagenic activities, an increase in PDG and GDH activities limited to S_1 and S_2 was recognized in the rat kidney during chronic metabolic acidosis. In contrast to rats, the long-term ammoniagenic response in dogs is not associated with an increase in either PDG or GDH activity. This is thought to be due to an increase in glutamine uptake by mitochondria or increased PDG flux. *In situ* hybridization and immunohistochemical studies demonstrated that NH_4Cl acidosis induced the increased mRNA and protein expressions of both PDG and GDH in rats, and the increases in expression were confined to the PT. During chronic metabolic acidosis, under which condition the decrease in plasma pH is largely compensated, sustained induction of PDG and GDH mRNA may be mediated primarily by the decreased bicarbonate concentration. Nuclear run-on assays have indicated that the rate of transcription of PDG is unaffected by alterations in the acid–base balance. The 3′-nontranslated region of rat PDG mRNA, which contains the sequence AUUUA, was related to the stability of this mRNA. The studies with transfection of a chimeric gene construct containing nearly 1 kb of the 3′-nontranslated region of the rat PDG mRNA revealed that this region of PDG mRNA contains a pH-responsive stability element that mediates its cell-specific induction during acidosis. Thus the increase in PDG mRNA expression is now thought to result from the increase in stability of its mRNA. Similarly, the increase in GDH mRNA expression also may be caused by an increase in the stability of its mRNA. Because no significant increase in PIG activity was recognized during chronic metabolic acidosis, PIG activity is generally considered insignificant in ammoniagenesis in acidotic states.

Other Acid–Base Disturbances

Other types of acid–base disorders have also been shown to be associated with the alterations in ammonia metabolism. In acute respiratory acidosis in dogs, renal glutamine extraction and ammoniagenesis increased and the latter reached levels comparable with those seen in chronic metabolic acidosis. In a rat chronic chrolide depletion alkalosis model, ammonium excretion decreased, largely because of a decrease in net ammonium secretion by the PCT. In addition, there was no detectable change in renal ammonia production, presumably because the inhibitory influence of alkalemia on ammoniagenesis was offset by the stimulatory influence of hypokalemia. There was a species difference with respect to the adaptive responses in chronic respiratory acidosis. Ammonia excretion increased in dogs, but no response was observed in rats.

Changes in Extracellular K^+ Concentration

It is well known that K^+ is an important regulator of ammonia production. In dogs and rats, an acute increase in ambient K^+ concentration suppresses ammonia production, whereas it remains unknown whether an acute decrease in ambient K^+ concentration would stimulate ammonia production. In patients with chronic potassium depletion caused by primary aldosteronism, renal ammonia production was significantly increased. In rats fed with a diet low in K^+ for 2 weeks, a K^+-depleted model, extracellular pH increased (alkalosis) and the intracellular pH decreased (acidosis). The ammoniagenic activity in microdissected nephron segments from K^+-depleted rats showed a similar pattern to that in acidotic rats (i.e., the rank order was $S_1 > S_2 > S_3 >$ DT). Similar to changes observed during chronic metabolic acidosis, the SF-S_1 segment was reactive to K^+ depletion, but JM-S_1 did not respond to K^+-depletion. In K^+-depleted rats, a significant increase in PDG activity was recognized in the PT, CCT, and MCT. Because CCT and MCT were hypertrophied under K^+-depleted conditions, the increase in PDG activity in these two nephron segments was not significant when the enzyme activity was represented as activity per tissue protein. K^+-depleted rats also showed a significant increase in GDH flux without any change in GDH activity or mRNA level. Thus increased PDG activity and GDH flux may be responsible for the increased ammonia production in K^+-depleted rats. In addition, taking together the results of mechanisms of ammoniagenesis in acidotic and K^+-depleted rats, it could be concluded that the ammoniagenic activity from glutamine depends on a decrease in intracellular pH but not extracellular pH.

Other Factors Influencing Renal Ammoniagenesis

Ammoniagenesis is regulated by several endogenous peptide hormones. Angiotensin II, α-adrenergic agonists, parathyroid hormone (PTH), insulin, dopamine, and glucocorticoids stimulate ammoniagenesis. The overall effect of angiotensin II on PT function may result from a combination of luminal and basolateral angiotensin II effects on the PT. It has been demonstrated that luminal angiotensin II stimulates ammonia production as well as luminal ammonia secretion in the mouse PT, whereas basolateral angiotensin II stimulates ammonia production but inhibits luminal ammonia secretion.

It has also been shown that acute metabolic acidosis results in a significant increase in prostaglandin (PG) synthesis, which inhibits an increase in ammonia production in response to acidosis. The mechanisms whereby $PGF_{2\alpha}$ inhibits the renal ammoniagenic response to acute metabolic acidosis appear to inhibit flux through PDG and GDH, which is the result of an increase in intracellular pH secondary to the activation of the Na^+-H^+ antiporter. In contrast, PGE_2 showed no significant effect on ammoniagenesis under either basal or acidotic conditions in the isolated perfused rat kidney and rat cortical tubules. However, we have reported that the PG synthetase inhibitors meclofenamate and indomethacin increased ammoniagenesis mainly in the S_3 segment of rats and mice, whereas PGE_2 inhibited ammoniagenesis in all of the nephron segments except the glomerulus. Thus the effect of PGE_2 on ammonia production remains undetermined.

Ammoniagenesis and Diseases

Polycystic Kidney Disease

The metabolic processes linked to renal ammoniagenesis are now thought to play a role in the pathogenesis of polycystic kidney disease (PKD) in animals and humans. In Han: SRPD rats (a PKD model), administration of sodium bicarbonate decreased the urinary excretion of ammonia and inhibited tubular dilatation, enlargement of cysts, and progression of renal dysfunction. In patients with autosomal-dominant who had a normal glomerular filtration rate, the urinary excretion of ammonia was reduced. This reduction could not be explained either by a lower production of ammonia in the renal cortex or by a defect of proton secretion in the collecting ducts. It is likely to result from impaired urinary concentration mechanisms and reduced trapping of ammonia in the renal medulla.

Progression of Renal Disease

With the progressive reduction in the number of nephrons, during progressive renal insufficiency, metabolic acidosis ensues. The burden of net acid excretion evokes an increase in ammonia production and excretion per nephron in humans, dogs, and rats. This adaptive response may prevent severe

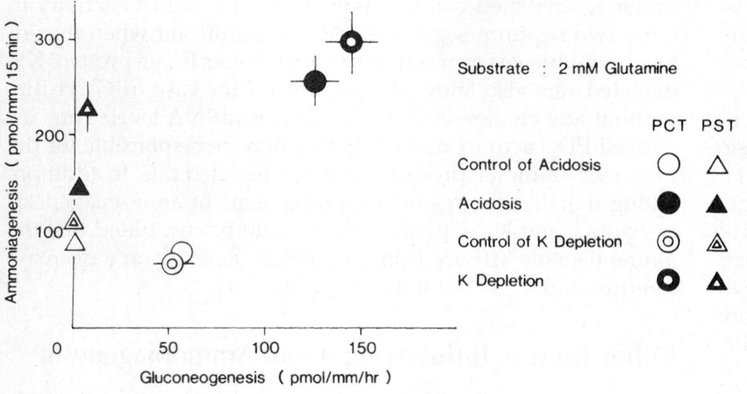

Figure 9.6. Relationship between gluconeogenesis and ammoniagenesis in the PCT and PST of rats under various conditions. (Reprinted with permission from Endou H, Nonoguchi H, Takehara Y, et al. Intranephron heterogeneity of ammoniagenesis and gluconeogenesis in rats. Ammonia production and transport. In: Berlyne GM and Giovannetti S, eds: Karger: Basel, 1985:103.)

metabolic acidosis from occurring early in the course of progressive renal disease, whereas progressive reduction in renal mass ultimately limits ammonia production and results in well-recognized metabolic acidosis of chronic renal failure. Ammonia can activate the alternative complement pathway by amidation, and this activation could lead to tissue injury in the form of tubulointerstitial disease. Chronic bicarbonate supplementation reduces renal ammonia production, renal growth, and tubulointerstitial injury in hypokalemic nephropathy in rats. In addition, increased renal ammoniagenesis contributes to the enhanced renal growth of remnant kidney tissue and hypokalemic nephropathy models. Accelerated renal growth is thought to be a prerequisite for the development of progressive renal injury. Thus the sustained increase in ammoniagenesis may be involved in the progression of various chronic renal diseases.

Relationship between Ammoniagenesis and Gluconeogenesis in the Kidney

As shown in Fig. 9.6, ammoniagenesis from glutamine increases in parallel with gluconeogenesis from glutamine in the PCT of acidotic and K^+-depleted rats, suggesting that the two reactions may be serial, whereas no such relationship was observed in the PST and the other nephron segments. Therefore ammoniagenesis and gluconeogenesis from glutamine may be interrelated only in the PCT of rats. This has been confirmed by the result that 3-mercaptopicolinate (3-MP), a specific inhibitor of PEPCK, inhibited ammoniagenesis from glutamine in S_1. However, contradictory results of the effect of 3-MP on ammoniagenesis in a rat kidney tubular suspension were also presented.

Cysteine S-Conjugate β-Lyase

Nephrotoxic haloalkenes, including volatile halogenated anesthetics, are metabolized via two pathways: (a) oxidation, catalyzed by cytochrome P450, and (b) conjugation with glutathione (GSH), catalyzed by GSH S-transferase. GSH conjugation is an important step for both detoxication and bioactivation of a variety of xenobiotics and occurs predominantly in the liver. The resultant GSH S-conjugates are subsequently metabolized to the corresponding cysteine S-conjugates, mainly in the kidney and, to a lesser extent, in the small intestine, by the brush border membrane enzymes, γ-glutamyltransferase, aminopeptidase M, and cysteinylglycine dipeptidase. The GSH S-conjugates filtered through the glomeruli may be metabolized to the corresponding cysteine S-conjugates by γ-glutamyltransferase, aminopeptidase M, and cysteinylglycine dipeptidase in the renal brush border membrane. The resultant cysteine S-conjugates may be transported into the renal epithelial cells via sodium-dependent or sodium-independent transport systems. On the other hand, the GSH S-conjugates in the peritubular capillaries may be metabolized to cysteine S-conjugates by γ-glutamyltransferase present in the renal vasculature or basolateral membrane. A probenecid-sensitive organic anion transporter present on the basolateral side of the proximal tubular cells has been shown to play a primary role in the accumulation of cysteine S-conjugates. The cytotoxicity of cysteine S-conjugates depends on the efficiency of their transport. Recently, a rat organic anion transporter 1 (OAT1), which is localized in the S_2 segment of the proximal tubule, has been cloned. This transporter has been shown to be at least partly responsible for the uptake of cysteine S-conjugates. Within the proximal tubular cells, the nephrotoxic cysteine S-conjugates formed as metabolic products of halogenated xenobiotics are metabolized by cysteine S-conjugate β-lyase to pyruvate, ammonia, and thiols. Cysteine S-conjugate β-lyase is a pyridoxal phosphate-dependent enzyme found in the cytosolic and mitochondrial fractions of the renal cortex. Microdissection studies have demonstrated that cysteine S-conjugate β-lyase activity is localized in the proximal tubule in order of $S_1 \doteqdot S_2 > S_3$. The thiols formed by the enzymatic cleavage of cysteine S-conjugates and their interaction with cellular macromolecules are associated with mitochondrial dysfunction and ATP depletion.

Acknowledgments

This study was supported in part by grants from the Ministry of Education, Science, Sports and Culture of Japan (11671048, 11694310); the Ministry of Health and Welfare of Japan; the Suzuken Memorial Foundation; Research on Health Sciences Focusing on Drug Innovation from the Japan Health Sciences Foundation; and the Science Research Promotion Fund of the Japan Private School Promotion Foundation.

Selected Readings

Curthys NP, Watford M. Regulation of glutaminase activity and glutamine metabolism. *Ann Rev Nutr* 1995;15:133–159.

Review describing biochemical and molecular biologic aspects of regulation of glutaminase activity and glutamine metabolism.

Hansen WR, Barsic-Tress N, Taylor L, et al. The 3′-nontranslated region of rat renal glutaminase mRNA contains a pH-responsive stability element. *Am J Physiol* 1996;271:F126–F131.

Studies revealing that the 3′-nontranslated region of rat renal glutaminase mRNA contains a pH-responsive stability element, using LLC-PK$_1$ cells.

Hanson RW, Reshef L. Regulation of phosphoenolpyruvate carboxykinase gene expression. *Ann Rev Biochem* 1997;66:581–611.

Review article describing the mechanisms of regulation of phosphoenolpyruvate carboxykinase gene expression.

Kim HS, Cha SH, Abraham DG, et al. Intranephron distribution of cysteine S-conjugate β-lyase activity and its implication for hexachloro-1,3-butadiene-induced nephrotoxicity in rats. *Arch Toxicol* 1997;71:131–141.

The first report demonstrating the intranephron distribution of cysteine S-conjugate β-lyase activity.

Nonoguchi H, Takehara Y, Endou H. Intra- and internephron heterogeneity of ammoniagenesis in rats: effects of chronic metabolic acidosis and potassium depletion. *Pfluegers Arch* 1986;407:245–251.

The first report concerning the effects of chronic acidosis and potassium depletion on ammoniagenic activity using microdissected nephron segments.

Sekine T, Watanabe N, Hosoyamada M, et al. Expression cloning and characterization of a novel multispecific organic anion transporter. J Biol Chem 1997;272: 18526–18529.

The first report of isolating organic anion transporter cDNA.

Scoolwerth AC, DeBoer PA, Moorman AFM, et al. Changes in mRNAs for enzymes of glutamine metabolism in kidney and liver during ammonium chloride acidosis. *Am J Physiol* 1994;267:F400–F406.

The first report describing changes in the distribution pattern of mRNAs and proteins involved in the enzymes of glutamine metabolism (phosphoenolpyruvate carboxykinase, glutaminase and glutamate dehydrogenase) in the rat kidney.

Stumvoll M, Meyer C, Mitrakou A, et al. Renal glucose production and utilization: new aspects in humans. *Diabetologia* 1997;40:749–757.

Review article describing the current progress in renal production and use in humans.

Uchida S, Endou H. Substrate specificity to maintain cellular ATP along the mouse nephron. *Am J Physiol* 1988;255:F977–F983.

The first description of heterogeneity of substrate specificity in ATP production along the microdissected nephron segments.

Yamada H, Nakada J, Aizawa C, et al. Intra- and internephron heterogeneity of gluconeogenesis in the rat: effects of chronic metabolic acidosis and potassium depletion. *Pfluegers Arch* 1986;407:1–7.

The first report demonstrating the effects of chronic metabolic acidosis and potassium depletion on gluconeogenic activity using microdissected nephron segments.

CHAPTER 10

Physiology of Ureter, Bladder, and Urethra

Robert M. Weiss and Harris E. Foster, Jr.

Urine transport from the kidneys begins with the origin of electrical activity at pacemaker sites located in the proximal portion of the upper urinary tract. Electrical activity is propagated distally and gives rise to the mechanical contractile events of peristalsis that propel the urine distally from the kidney to the bladder. Urine passes into the bladder via the ureterovesical junction, which, under normal conditions, acts as a one-way valve, permitting urine passage in an antegrade but not in a retrograde direction. Efficient transport of urine into the bladder depends on the maintenance of relatively low intravesical pressures. During the storage phase, the bladder adapts to increasing volumes of urine with the maintenance of low intravesical pressures, while the urethra provides continence by maintaining a higher pressure than the bladder. Voiding is heralded by a drop in intraurethral pressure, which precedes the rise in intravesical pressure and urine flows until the bladder is emptied. An appropriate interaction between ureteral, bladder, and urethral function is required for adequate urine transport, preservation of renal function, and the maintenance of continence.

UPPER URINARY TRACT

Functional Anatomy

The ureteral smooth muscle cell, which is the primary functional anatomical unit of the ureter, is extremely small, approximately 250 to 400 μm long and 5 to 7 μm wide. The cell consists of a nucleus surrounded by cytoplasm or sarcoplasm, which contains the structures involved in cell function. The nucleus contains a darkly staining body, the nucleolus, and the genetic material of the cell. Dispersed within the sarcoplasm are the contractile proteins actin and myosin, which interact in the presence of calcium to result in contraction. Increases in calcium concentration in the region of the contractile proteins result in contraction; conversely, decreases in calcium concentration, in the region of the contractile proteins, result in relaxation. The small size of the ureteral muscle cell permits a significant proportion of the calcium involved in contraction to enter the cell from the extracellular fluid at the time of excitation. Intracellular calcium storage sites, namely the endoplasmic or sarcoplasmic reticulum, and certain sites on the internal surface of the cell membrane also provide a source of calcium for the contractile process.

The ureter lacks discrete neuromuscular junctions. Propagation of peristaltic activity appears to depend on the direct spread of excitation from one muscle cell to another. The ureteral cell is surrounded by a double-layered cell membrane. The inner plasma membrane surrounds the entire cell, whereas the outer basement membrane surrounds the periphery of the cell except at areas of close cell-to-cell contact, referred to as *intermediate junctions*. These areas of close cellular apposition may provide low-resistance pathways for the conduction of excitation from one muscle cell to another.

Pacemaker Activity

In species with a multicalyceal system, such as the pig and the human, there is morphologic and physiologic evidence to suggest that the origin of peristaltic activity begins in the region of the calyces. It has been postulated that ureteral peristalsis could be accounted for either by activity from a single pacemaker site or more probably by the discharge of electrical activity from multiple pacemaker sites, the summation of whose effect is sufficient to induce a peristaltic contraction wave.

At low levels of urine output, propagation of electrical activity arising from pacemaker sites in the region of the calyces is often blocked in the renal pelvis or at the ureteropelvic junction. With increasing urine flow, there is a cessation of this block and a 1:1 relationship is observed between pacemaker and ureteral contractions. Thus, at low flows, the frequency of calyceal contractions is greater than that of the ureter, whereas at high flows, ureteral and calyceal contractions occur at the same frequency.

Although the "primary" pacemaker, which accounts for the antegrade propagation of peristalsis under normal conditions, is located in the proximal portion of the collecting system, other areas in the ureter possess potential or "latent" pacemaker properties. Under normal conditions, these latent pacemaker areas are dominated by activity arising at the primary pacemaker site; however, if these latent pacemaker sites are freed of their domination by the primary pacemaker, they may in turn act as the pacemaker. This may account for the retrograde propagation of peristalsis observed in certain pathologic conditions.

Excitation, Contraction, and Excitation–Contraction Coupling

As with all other excitable tissues, the electrical activity of the ureter depends on the distribution of ions across the cell membrane and the relative permeability of the cell membrane to these ions. In the nonexcited or resting state, the electrical potential across the cell membrane is primarily determined by the distribution of potassium ions across the cell membrane and the permeability of the cell membrane to potassium. The transmembrane potential of the resting ureteral cell ranges between −40 and −70 mV, with the inside of the cell membrane being negative with respect to its outer surface.

With excitation by an external stimulus, whether it be electrical, mechanical (stretch), or chemical or by conduction of electrical activity from an already excited adjacent cell, depolarization occurs, with the inside of the cell membrane becoming less negative than it was before excitation. If a sufficient area of the cell membrane is depolarized rapidly enough to reach a critical level of transmembrane potential (referred to as the threshold potential), a regenerative depolarization is initiated. The excited cell loses its preferential permeability to potassium and becomes more permeable to sodium (Na^+) and calcium (Ca^{2+}) ions, which move inward across the cell membrane and give rise to the upstroke of the action potential; this, in turn, is the primary event in conduction of electrical activity in the ureter and gives rise to the contractile event of peristalsis. The rate of rise of the upstroke of the ureteral action potential is relatively slow (1.2 ± 0.6 V/sec in the cat), and this is an important determinant of the slow rate of conduction of peristalsis (2 to 6 cm/sec in the ureter). After reaching the peak of its action potential, the ureteral cell membrane maintains its potential for a period of time (plateau of the action potential) before the transmembrane potential returns to its resting level (repolarization). The plateau of the action potential appears to result from the persistence of inward Ca^{2+} and Na^+ currents, and the repolarization phase is at least in part caused by an outward Ca^{2+}-dependent K^+ current.

Every contractile event of peristalsis is preceded by an electrical event, an action potential. The exact mechanism for this excitation–contraction coupling in the ureter is unknown; however, it is apparent that the electrical event leads to an increase in the sarcoplasmic calcium concentration in the region of the contractile proteins. The most widely accepted theory suggests that phosphorylation of myosin is involved in the contractile process. It is suggested that with excitation, there is a transient increase in the sarcoplasmic calcium concentration from its steady-state concentration of 10^{-8} to 10^{-7} M to a concentration of 10^{-6} M or higher and that at this higher concentration, calcium forms an active complex with the calcium-binding protein calmodulin. Calmodulin without calcium ions is inactive. The calcium–calmodulin complex activates a calmodulin-dependent enzyme, myosin light-chain kinase, which in turn catalyzes the phosphorylation of the 20,000-D light chain of myosin. Phosphorylation of the myosin light chain allows activation by actin of myosin Mg^{2+}-ATPase activity, leading to hydrolysis of adenosine triphosphate (ATP) and the development of smooth muscle tension or shortening. Actin cannot activate ATPase activity of the dephosphorylated myosin light chain.

Propulsion of Urinary Bolus

As the renal pelvis fills with urine, renal pelvic pressure rises and urine extrudes from the renal pelvis into the ureter. Because the ureter, before being filled with urine from the renal pelvis, is in a collapsed state, a bolus of urine forms in the proximal ureter. Contraction waves originating in the most proximal portion of the ureter move the bolus of urine, which lies in front of it within a passive, noncontracting part of the ureter, in a distal direction toward the bladder. For efficient propulsion of the urinary bolus, the peristaltic contraction wave must completely coapt the ureteral wall. Baseline (resting) ureteral pressure is approximately 0 to 5 cm H_2O, and peristaltic contraction waves of 20 to 60 cm H_2O are superimposed on this baseline pressure at 10- to 30-second intervals.

To enter the bladder, the urine traverses the ureterovesical junction (UVJ), which when functioning properly permits only one-way urine transport. The bolus of urine is forced into the bladder by the advancing contraction wave that dissipates at the UVJ. For efficient transport of urine across the UVJ into the bladder, the magnitude of the ureteral contractile pressure wave must exceed the magnitude of the intravesical pressure. The UVJ does not act as a typical valve in that it does not relax, although telescoping and shortening of the distal ureteral segment aids in the transport of urine across the UVJ.

Peristaltic contraction waves pushing a urinary bolus in front of it provide the usual means of urine transport. When transport becomes inadequate, urinary stasis results, with resultant ureteral dilation. Finally, peristaltic activity becomes overwhelmed and ceases. Under such conditions, urine flows from the kidney to the bladder in a continuous column rather than as a series of boluses. As with any tubular structure, the ureter can efficiently transport a set maximum amount of fluid per unit of time. Inadequate transport can result from either too much fluid entering the ureter per unit of time or from too little fluid exiting the ureter per unit of time. Thus ureteral dilation, impairment of peristaltic activity, and stasis may result either from excessive diuresis or from obstruction to outflow (Table 10.1). When predicting whether ureteral dilation and impairment of peristaltic activity will occur, one must consider both the input and the output. For instance, a minor degree of obstruction to outflow will cause more dilation at high flow rates than at low flow rates. Even a normal nonobstructed ureter will impede urine transport if the rate of flow is great enough.

The functional response of the ureter to obstruction, bladder filling, or diuresis are similar. With increasing degrees of diuresis, peristaltic frequency increases until a maximum frequency is achieved and further increases in urine transport are achieved by increases in bolus volume. With further increases in urine flow, several boluses coalesce, and finally the ureter becomes filled with a column of urine and dilates. At high flow rates, urine transport is through an open tube.

Because the UVJ does not relax, the relationship between ureteral pressure and intravesical pressure is important in determining the efficacy of urine passage across the UVJ into the

TABLE 10.1. Upper Urinary Tract Dilatation

Excessive Input
Diuresis: excess fluid input from above
Vesicoureteral reflux: excess fluid input from below
Decreased Output
Anatomic or functional obstruction (e.g., UPJ obstruction, UVJ obstruction, ureteral calculi, retrocaval ureter, ureteroceles, retroperitoneal fibrosis, pregnancy)
Elevated intravesical pressures
Functional Dilation
Congenital Megaureter
Infection
Pregnancy

UPJ, ureteropelvic junction; UVJ, ureterovesical junction.

bladder. Urine passes from the ureter into the bladder because intraureteral pressure is higher than intravesical pressure. Under normal circumstances, intraureteral contractile pressures exceed intravesical pressures and this accounts for the transport of urine into the bladder. In the dilated, poorly contracting ureter or in the normal ureter at extreme flow rates, the ureter does not coapt its walls to form boluses and the baseline pressure in the column of urine within the ureter must exceed the intravesical pressure for urine to pass into the bladder.

As the relationship between ureteral intraluminal pressure and intravesical pressure determines the efficacy of urine passage across the UVJ, increases in intravesical pressure with bladder filling may act as an obstructive factor. The pressure within the bladder during the storage phase is most important in determining the efficacy of urine transport into the bladder because this is the pressure that the ureter needs to work against for the longest period of time. During filling of the normal bladder, sympathetic impulses, which excite β-adrenergic receptors in the bladder dome, and the viscoelastic properties of the bladder wall inhibit the magnitude of the intravesical pressure rise with the maintenance of a relatively low intravesical pressure during the storage phase. The low intravesical pressure facilitates urine transport across the UVJ and prevents ureteral dilation. In the noncompliant fibrotic bladder and in some forms of neurogenic vesical dysfunction, the bladder is autonomous, and relatively small increases in bladder volume result in large increases in intravesical pressure, with resultant impairment of ureteral emptying. Under these circumstances, as with diuresis, the ureter initially responds to bladder filling and its decreased ability to empty, with an increase in peristaltic frequency. Ultimately, stasis occurs and ureteral dilation results. The ureter has been shown to decompensate when intravesical pressure approaches 40 cm H_2O.

In addition to diuresis and obstructive factors, several other conditions may result in impairment of peristaltic activity and ureteral dilatation. Nonobstructed dilated ureters are seen in certain disease states such as vesicoureteral reflux and the syndrome of absence of abdominal musculature (prune belly syndrome), and with nonobstructive congenital megaureters. Infection also may inhibit ureteral activity and result in ureteral dilation. Finally, although the major factor in hydroureteronephrosis of pregnancy appears to be obstruction, hormonally induced changes in ureteral function may be contributory.

Neurophysiology

Multiunit smooth muscles have a specific innervation for each smooth muscle fiber, whereas syncytial-type smooth muscles, such as those of the ureter, lack discrete neuromuscular junctions and depend on the diffuse release of transmitter from nerve bundles with subsequent spread of excitation from one muscle cell to another. Because ureteral peristalsis may persist after transplantation and antegrade propagation of peristaltic waves persist after *in situ* reversal of a ureteral segment, it is evident that innervation is not an absolute requirement for peristalsis. However, available data suggest that although the antonomic nervous system is not required for peristalsis, it can affect ureteral function.

Both α- and β-adrenergic receptor mechanisms are present in the ureter. α-Adrenergic receptors appear to be predominant and are excitatory. Although both α_1- and α_2-adrenergic receptors are present in the ureter, α_1-adrenergic agonists are more potent than α_2-adrenergic agonists in increasing the force and frequency of ureteral contractions. Some of the actions of α_1-adrenergic agonists are related to changes in inositol lipid metabolism. The interaction of the α_1-agonist with a receptor located on the outside of the cell membrane activates the enzyme phospholipase C, which hydrolyzes polyphosphatidylinositol 4,5-biphosphate (PIP_2) with the formation of two second messengers—1,4,5-inositol trisphosphate (IP_3) and diacylglycerol (DG). IP_3 is involved in calcium mobilization from intracellular stores, such as the endoplasmic reticulum, and DG increases calcium influx across the cell membrane via a process that involves the activation of protein kinase C and a cascade of protein phosphorylations.

β-Adrenergic agonists, on the other hand, are inhibitory, causing a decrease in contractile force and relaxation. β-Adrenergic agonist–induced relaxation in the ureter is mediated by cyclic adenosine 3′,5′-monophosphate (cAMP). In this signal transduction pathway, the β-adrenergic agonist combines with a receptor on the outer surface of the cell membrane and the agonist–receptor complex activates the enzyme adenylyl cyclase, located on the inner surface of the cell membrane. A guanine nucleotide regulatory protein (G protein) acts as a functional communicator between the agonist–receptor complex and the catalytic or active component of the adenylyl cyclase enzyme. Both adenylyl cyclase and phosphodiesterase, the enzymes involved in the synthesis and degradation of cAMP, respectively, have been demonstrated in the ureter. Adenylyl cyclase activity can be stimulated by isoproterenol, and phosphodiesterase activity can be inhibited by theophylline. These two agents, which relax ureteral smooth muscle, could at least in part exert their effect by increasing cAMP levels within the ureteral muscle, isoproterenol by increasing synthesis and theophylline by decreasing degradation.

The role of the parasympathetic nervous system in the control of ureteral function is less well understood. Available data suggest that cholinergic agonists can increase the amplitude of ureteral contractions either by directly stimulating cholinergic receptors or by indirectly causing the release of catecholamines. Some of the actions of muscarinic cholinergic agonists are related to the activation of phospholipase C and an increase in inositol lipid metabolism. Other actions of muscarinic cholinergic agonists appear to be related to inhibition of adenylyl cyclase activity. Some of the actions of α_2-adrenergic agonists also involve inhibition of adenylyl cyclase activity.

The demonstration of adrenergic and cholinergic receptor mechanisms in the ureter by classic pharmacologic and receptor-binding methodologies does not in itself prove that the ureter is innervated. However, electrical field stimulation has been demonstrated to release a neurotransmitter, presumably from intrinsic neural tissue within the wall of the ureter and renal calyx, that can stimulate α-adrenergic receptors. Furthermore, acetylcholine release from the ureter has been demonstrated during electrical field stimulation. Thus, although innervation is not necessary for ureteral peristalsis, the autonomic nervous system would appear to have at least a modulating function.

Other studies have demonstrated the presence of nitric oxide synthase activity in the ureter. Nitric oxide synthase converts L-arginine to L-citrulline and nitric oxide in a reaction that requires nicotinamide-adenine-dinucleotide phosphate (NADPH). Nitric oxide can activate the enzyme guanylyl cyclase with the resultant production of cyclic guanosine 3′,5′-monophosphate (cGMP), which is a potent ureteral relaxant. Thus nitric oxide may be involved in ureteral relaxation.

Capsicin-sensitive sensory nerves are located in the ureter. Release of the tachykinins, substance P, neurokinin A, and neuropeptide K from these capsaicin-sensitive sensory nerves has an excitatory effect on ureteral peristalsis, whereas release of calcitonin gene-related peptide (CGRP) from these nerves has an inhibitory effect on ureteral peristalsis. Peptidergic neurons containing neurtopeptide Y (NPY) and vasoactive intestinal polypeptide (VIP) also have been demonstrated in the ureter, with VIP inhibiting ureteral activity.

LOWER URINARY TRACT

Urinary storage and micturition are basic functions of the lower urinary tract. The ability to provide an adequate low-pressure reservoir for urine storage and, when socially appropriate, the ability to empty the reservoir completely requires a complex interaction of anatomic, physiologic, and biochemical events. A detailed discussion of this topic is beyond the scope of this chapter, but the following discussion should provide a sufficient overview for the reader to begin to understand the rationale behind the pharmacologic and surgical management of neurourologic dysfunctions of the lower urinary tract.

Anatomy

The anatomy of the lower urinary tract provides a useful framework on which one can build an understanding of lower urinary tract function. The lower urinary tract consists of a reservoir, the bladder, and a complex sphincteric mechanism that is made up of (a) the bladder neck, (b) the smooth and specialized striated muscles intrinsic to the urethra, and (c) the striated skeletal muscle of the pelvic floor extrinsic to the urethra (extrinsic rhabdomyosphincter) (Table 10.2 and Fig. 10.1). During the storage phase, approximately 350 to 400 ml of urine is stored at pressures under 10 cm H_2O by passive and active relaxation of the bladder and by contraction of the various components of the urinary sphincter. During the voiding phase, there is active and passive relaxation of the bladder neck and urethra, which is coordinated with an effective sustained contraction of the bladder. Effective coordination of these processes results in complete emptying of the bladder.

The Bladder

The bladder is an extraperitoneal pelvic organ that consists primarily of smooth muscle, the detrusor, which histologically consists of randomly intertwined muscle fibers. The outer surface of the detrusor is covered by an adventia of loose connective tissue, except on its dome and upper posterior surface, where it is densely adherent to the peritoneum. Transitional cell epithelium lines the inner surface of the bladder. This specialized epithelium is capable of stretching as the bladder distends, prevents the passive transfer of electrolytes and water between the urine and the blood, and secretes a layer of glycosaminoglycans that reduces bacterial adherence.

The trigone represents an embryologically and anatomically distinct area of the bladder. The trigone begins cranially at the level of the ureteral orifices and tapers as it extends caudally to the junction of the bladder and urethra, the bladder neck. The superficial smooth muscle layer of the trigone extends distally,

TABLE 10.2. Components of the Urinary Sphincter
Internal Sphincter
Bladder neck
External Sphincter (Distal Sphincter Mechanism)
Intrinsic to the urethra
Longitudinal smooth muscle
Circular slow-twitch striated muscle (intrinsic rhabdomyosphincter)
Extrinsic to the urethra
Levator ani (extrinsic rhabdomyosphincter)

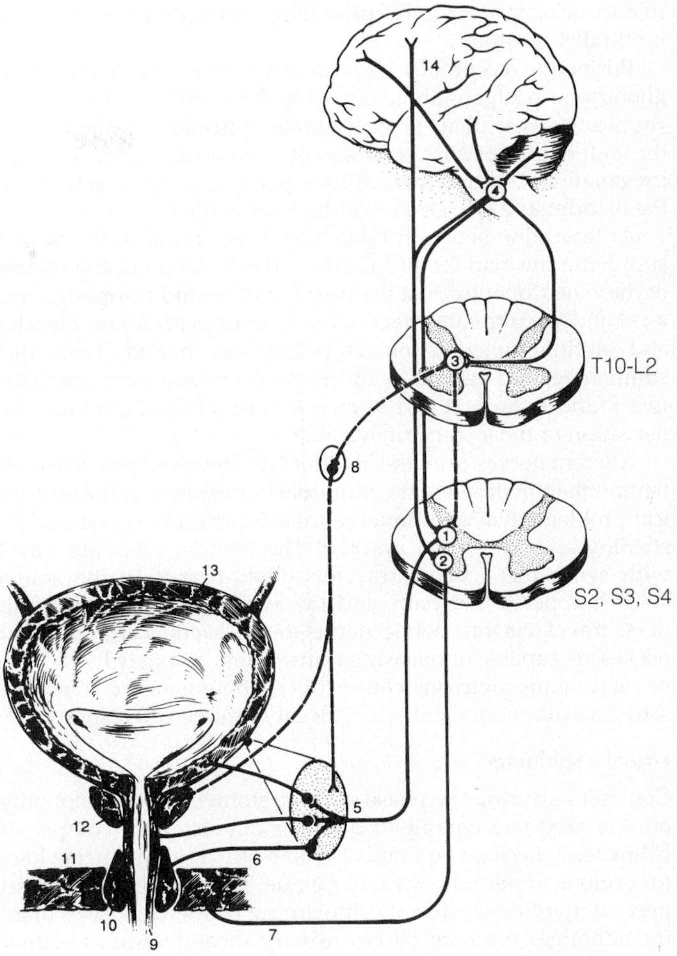

Figure 10.1. Schematic diagram of the neurologic control of the lower urinary tract. *1,* Detrusor motor nucleus; *2,* pudendal motor nucleus; *3,* thoracolumbar sympathetic nucleus; *4,* pontine micturition center (locus ceruleus); *5,* expanded representation of a pelvic nerve parasympathetic ganglion; *6,* postganglionic parasympathetic fibers; *7,* pudendal nerve; *8,* inferior mesenteric sympathetic ganglion and postganglionic hypogastric nerve; *9,* longitudinal smooth muscle intrinsic to the urethra; *10,* circular striated muscle intrinsic to the urethra; *11,* extrinsic rhabdomyosphincter; *12,* circular smooth muscle of the bladder neck; *13,* detrusor muscle; *14,* supraportine centers.

forming the inner longitudinal smooth muscle of the urethra. Deeper layers of the trigone appear to be a continuation of the detrusor muscle and do not extend into the urethra.

Parasympathetic nerves arising from the sacral spinal cord provide the predominate innervation to the detrusor (Fig. 10.1). Stimulation of postganglionic parasympathetic nerves causes the release of the neurotransmitter acetylcholine, which results in a detrusor contraction. Although the predominant muscarinic cholinergic receptor is of the M2 subtype, cholinergic-induced contractions result from activation of the M3 subtype. Parasympathetic stimulation plays an important role in micturition. Sympathetic nerves also innervate the lower urinary tract. β_2-Adrenergic receptors are found throughout the detrusor and, when stimulated, result in detrusor relaxation. α_1-Adrenergic receptors are concentrated predominantly in the bladder base, bladder neck, and urethra, although they also sparsely exist in the detrusor of the bladder body. Activation of α_1-adrenergic receptors results in smooth muscle contraction and thus facilitates sphincter closure. α_2-Adrenergic receptors also are present in the urethra, especially in females. In summary, stimulation of the sympathetic system plays an important role in urinary storage by promoting detrusor relaxation and urethral closure.

Purinergic receptors are found at the termination of preganglionic and postganglionic nerves to the bladder. Experimental studies suggest that postganglionic purinergic stimulation, through release of ATP, enhances bladder contractility, whereas preganglionic stimulation inhibits parasympathetic activity to the bladder and decreases bladder contractility.

At least nine neuropeptides have been found in the nerves supplying the bladder and urethra. The inducers of the release of these neuropeptides at the preganglionic and postganglionic level and the ultimate effect of these neuropeptides on bladder and urethral function remain poorly understood. Table 10.3 summarizes the various neurotransmitters and neuromodulators found in animal and human studies of the peripheral innervation of the lower urinary tract.

Afferent nerves from the bladder have received much less attention than their efferent counterparts, despite significant clinical problems that may involve their function (i.e., sensory instability and interstitial cystitis). The bladder afferents travel with sympathetic and parasympathetic nerves to the spinal cord. It appears that pain, and the awareness of bladder fullness, travel via the pelvic nerve to the sacral cord. Afferent nerves are capable of releasing transmitters and may be capable of modulating detrusor contractility, efferent nerve transmission, vascular permeability, and local immune cell responses.

Urinary Sphincter

Continence during the phase of urine storage depends not only on a relaxed and compliant detrusor but also on a competent sphincteric mechanism that is capable of preventing urine loss, for prolonged periods, without fatigue. The sphincter also must prevent involuntary loss of urine during sudden increases in intraabdominal pressure (stress urinary incontinence). Urethral pressure recordings localize the zone of maximal urethral closure pressure to the midportion of the urethra in women and to a site distal to the apex of the prostate in men. Normal maximal urethral closure pressures range from 35 to 120 cm H_2O. The zone of maximal urethral closure pressure is confined to a relatively short, approximately 1.5-cm, segment of urethra.

In the zone of maximal urethral closure pressure, there is an inner longitudinal layer of smooth muscle originating from the trigone and an outer circular layer of specialized striated muscle. Both layers are "intrinsic" to the urethra (Table 10.2 and Fig. 10.1). External to these "intrinsic" layers and "extrinsic" to the urethra is the striated skeletal muscle of the pelvis, known as the extrinsic rhabdomyosphincter. Collectively, these intrinsic and extrinsic muscular sphincters are referred to as the distal sphincter mechanism or external sphincter. The precise neural control of the distal sphincter mechanism remains controversial.

The muscles of the pelvic floor (i.e., extrinsic rhabdomyosphincter) are innervated by somatic efferent fibers that arise from α-motor neuron cells in the anterior horn of S2, S3, and S4 and that coalesce into the pudendal nerve. Bilateral ablation of the pudendal nerves does not impair continence, suggesting that the rhabdomyosphincter is not a critical component of the distal sphincter mechanism. However, the extrinsic rhabdomyosphincter does help maintain adequate urethral closure during rapid increases in the intravesical pressure, such as may accompany coughing or straining. The extrinsic rhabdomyosphincter is under volitional control and, when contracted, produces reflex inhibition of detrusor activity at the level of the sacral spinal cord. This mechanism enables one to stop micturition on demand. Therapeutically, this inhibitory reflex occasionally has been exploited by electrically stimulating the pelvic floor, pudendal nerve, and sacral nerves as they exit their respective sacral foramina to control refractory detrusor instability.

TABLE 10.3. Transmitters and Neuromodulators Found in the Peripheral Innervation of the Lower Urinary Tract of Humans and Animals

Acetylcholine
Amines and aminoacids (serotonin, dopamine, histamine, GABA)
Norepinephrine
Peptides (enkephalins, neuropeptide Y, substance P, VIP)
Prostaglandins ($PGF_{2\alpha}$, PGE_1, PGE_2)
Purines (ATP)
Nitric oxide

ATP, adenosine triphosphate; GABA, γ-aminobutyric acid.

The remaining components of the distal sphincter mechanism, the inner longitudinal smooth muscle and the outer specialized circular striated muscle, are intrinsic to the wall of the urethra. It appears that the outer circular layer, consisting of slow-twitch striated muscle fibers, is most responsible for the zone of maximal urethral closure pressure and corresponds to it anatomically. This striated circular muscle, intrinsic to the urethra (intrinsic rhabdomyosphincter), is distinct from the striated skeletal muscle that makes up the pelvic floor (extrinsic rhabdomyosphincter). The intrinsic rhabdomyosphincter has a predominance of small diameter (15 to 20 μm) slow-twitch muscle fibers, whereas the extrinsic rhabdomyosphincter has a predominance of fast-twitch, easily fatigued fibers. In contrast to the extrinsic rhabdomyosphincter, the intrinsic rhabdomyosphincter has an abundance of sympathetic nerve endings, receives its innervation via the pelvic nerve rather than the pudendal nerve, and is controlled by sacral motor neurons distinct from the α-motor neurons of the anterior horn that control the extrinsic rhabdomyosphincter.

The inner longitudinal smooth muscle of the urethra is believed to be an extension of the trigone. It does not play a major role in the maintenance of continence but may provide an active mechanism to facilitate opening of the bladder neck and proximal urethra during voiding. Lack of correlation between anatomic and physiologic studies, differences between species, and the inability to isolate the various components of the distal sphincter mechanism in human studies makes the neurologic control of the human continence mechanism difficult to understand. Preservation of continence in acquired motor neuron disease of the sacral anterior horn cells and after bilateral ablation of the pudendal nerves support the hypothesis that continence is a visceral efferent function. Histologically, postganglionic cholinergic and adrenergic nerve endings are found in the anatomic region of the intrinsic rhabdomyosphincter. The neuropeptides VIP, NPY, and serotonin are found in association with these nerves. The role of each in controlling the tone of the intrinsic rhabdomyosphincter is not known.

In addition to the external sphincter, or distal sphincter mechanism, there exists yet another sphincter at the junction of the bladder and urethra, the bladder neck (Table 10.2 and Fig. 10.1). This area is referred to as the internal or proximal urinary sphincter, and in men is referred to as the preprostatic sphincter. Anatomically, in men, the bladder neck consists of a prominent bundle of circularly oriented smooth muscle with rich α-adrenergic innervation. In women, the bladder neck is much less prominent and histologically is noted to have a relatively scant supply of adrenergic nerves. These differences suggest that the primary role of the bladder neck may be a sexual one, the prevention of retrograde ejaculation. Indeed, after retroperitoneal lymph node dissection for testicular cancer, retrograde ejaculation may occur as a result of resection of the sympathetic ganglia around the aorta. Men have no problems with urinary control after retroperitoneal lymph node dissection or prostate surgery, indicating that the bladder neck, or internal sphincter, is not critical for continence. However, the bladder neck may be sufficient to provide continence for men with acquired defects of the distal sphincter mechanism, such as may occur after traumatic disruption of the membranous urethra. Conversely, dysfunction of the bladder neck and proximal urethra in females, termed intrinsic sphincter deficiency (ISD), results in stress urinary incontinence. Generally, ISD is caused by fibrosis around the bladder neck secondary to prior surgery and/or radiation therapy, and the incontinence that results can be severe.

Central Nervous System Control of the Lower Urinary Tract

Urine storage and voiding are neurologically complex events that involve virtually all levels of the nervous system. The peripheral innervation of the lower urinary tract has been discussed, and the focus now turns toward the central nervous system (CNS) control of the lower urinary tract. It is useful to consider CNS control of the lower urinary tract in three separate but intimately related parts: the spinal cord, the pons, and the supraponline/cortical centers (Fig. 10.1). CNS control of micturition is discussed primarily from an anatomic perspective because the neurotransmitters involved in the central regulation of the micturition reflex are largely unknown. Enkephalinergic mechanisms have received the most attention. In the future, selective opioid drugs may provide a practical means of modulating CNS control of the sacral micturition reflex.

The Spinal Cord

The spinal cord supplies parasympathetic, sympathetic, and general somatic efferent nerves to the bladder, bladder neck, and distal sphincter mechanism and receives afferent fibers from these structures via the pelvic, hypogastric, and pudendal nerves, respectively. With the exception of the hypogastric nerve and its sympathetic fibers, most of the control of the lower urinary tract is located in the sacral spinal cord (S2, S3, S4). Anatomically, this portion of the spinal cord is located at the level of the twelfth thoracic and first lumbar vertebrae.

The sacral detrusor nucleus is a cluster of preganglionic parasympathetic neurons located in the intermediolateral gray matter of S2, S3, and S4 (Fig. 10.1). The primary function of the sacral detrusor nucleus is to excite the smooth muscle fibers of the detrusor to contract during voiding. Axons from these preganglionic neurons leave the cord ventrally and exit the spinal canal via the sacral foramina. Lateral to the rectum, they coalesce to form the pelvic nerve, which also picks up adrenergic fibers from the hypogastric nerve. The parasympathetic fibers terminate on ganglia near the bladder or in the wall of the bladder and urethra. Sympathetic and peptidergic fibers influence parasympathetic transmission at the level of the parasympathetic ganglia and possibly at the neuromuscular junction.

The sacral pudendal nucleus is a collection of neurons found in the ventrolateral gray matter of S2 and, to a lesser extent, at S3 and S4. As previously noted, these neurons are α-motor neurons that, via the pudendal nerve, excite the striated skeletal muscle of the extrinsic rhabdomyosphincter (Fig. 10.1).

The sacral detrusor nucleus, the sacral pudendal nucleus, and their afferent and efferent connections to the lower urinary tract make up the micturition reflex. Thus, if the sacral cord is isolated from the brain, as may occur with a complete suprasacral spinal cord injury, stimulation of the sacral micturition reflex by progressive accumulation of urine in the bladder will eventually trigger a reflex detrusor contraction. However, in the absence of pontine influences, there is loss of coordination between the detrusor motor nucleus and the pudendal motor nucleus, leading to a loss of coordination of detrusor and extrinsic rhabdomyosphincter activity (detrusor-sphincter dyssynergia). Thus the sacral micturition reflex is inadequate by itself to provide for physiologically normal voiding.

The thoracolumbar sympathetics (T10-L2) influence the micturition reflex via two mechanisms. The first mechanism has been described earlier and consists of adrenergic modulation of parasympathetic ganglia in the pelvic nerve as well as postganglionic parasympathetic fibers. The second mechanism appears to be exerted through intraspinal pathways between the sympathetic neurons in the intermediolateral gray matter of the thoracolumbar cord and the sacral micturition reflex. These intraspinal pathways appear to inhibit the micturition reflex within the cord, complementing the effects of peripheral pelvic sympathetic activity.

The Pontine Micturition Center

The pontine micturition center (PMC) is the second level of the CNS to exert significant influence on lower urinary tract function (Fig. 10.1). Anatomically, it corresponds to the locus ceruleus of the rostral pons. Functionally, it is the center of CNS control over the lower urinary tract. The PMC receives input from the cortex, cerebellum, and other suprapontine centers. Through the reticulospinal tracts of the spinal cord, the PMC exerts control over the thoracolumbar sympathetics and sacral micturition reflex. Coordinated activity of the sacral detrusor nucleus, the pudendal motor nucleus, and the sympathetic nucleus depends on an intact PMC. A lesion involving the PMC, or suprasacral cord, may cause profound physiologic changes in lower urinary tract function. Such lesions will lead to a limited storage phase, an incomplete voiding phase, and a lack of coordinated relaxation of the distal sphincter mechanism. It is this detrusor-sphincter dyssynergia that produces the serious urologic/renal complications associated with suprasacral spinal cord injuries and other types of neurovesical dysfunction. The pontine micturition center coordinates voiding events, ensuring coordinated activity of detrusor and sphincter functions.

Suprapontine Control of the Lower Urinary Tract

The third level of CNS control over the lower urinary tract is the suprapontine and cortical areas. Although an intact PMC is essential for coordinated, physiologically normal voiding, intact suprapontine centers are required to facilitate urine storage and ensure complete emptying of the bladder. At the cortical level, studies support the existence of a detrusor motor area in the medial frontal lobe and genu of the corpus callosum. Neurons in the medial central sulcus are believed to exert control over the striated muscle of the urinary sphincter. In general, the cerebrum is believed to exert primarily an inhibitory influence on the sacral micturition reflex. The theory of cerebral inhibition assumes a constant inhibition of the sacral micturition reflex. Thus uninhibited detrusor activity, which may result in incontinence, might be expected after a cerebrovascular accident or traumatic brain injury, and indeed, this is commonly observed clinically.

The basal ganglia also appear to exert a predominantly inhibitory influence on the micturition reflex. Stimulation of the basal ganglia appears to facilitate the storage phase. Clinically, dysfunction of the basal ganglia, such as seen in Parkinson's disease, often leads to uninhibited detrusor activity and subsequent incontinence. The thalamus may function to relay autonomic and somatic afferent input from the bladder and urethra, but its precise effect on lower urinary tract function is unclear. The limbic system provides an anatomic link for emotion and lower urinary function. The influence of the limbic system is generally believed to be primarily excitatory, but the neural mechanisms are largely unknown.

In summary, cortical and suprapontine centers, with the exception of the limbic system, appear to provide an inhibitory function on the micturition reflex. Through the PMC, detrusor and sphincteric function is coordinated, urine is stored at low pressure and adequate volume, and complete bladder emptying during the voiding phase is facilitated.

URINE STORAGE AND MICTURITION

Urine filling the bladder during the storage phase leads to increased awareness of bladder distension and is probably the key factor leading to the voiding phase in the neurologically intact mature human. Learned behavioral control of the sacral micturition reflex prevents initiation of voiding until socially appropriate. During the storage phase, visceral afferent stimulation from detrusor stretch receptors travels via the pelvic nerve to the sacral cord, as well as to the thoracolumbar, pontine, and suprapontine centers. As the bladder reaches maximal filling, an awareness of abdominal distension develops through increased activity of afferent fibers that travel to the thoracolumbar spinal cord via the hypogastric nerve. Despite a progressive increase in afferent nerve activity, the bladder maintains a low intravesical pressure. This is accomplished through inhibition of sacral parasympathetic activity by inhibitory interneurons in the sacral cord and by inhibition of parasympathetic ganglionic activity via peripheral sympathetic, purinergic, and peptidergic pathways. Urine storage also may be facilitated by reflex inhibition of bladder activity resulting from volitional contraction of the extrinsic rhabdomyosphincter.

The voiding phase is heralded by the combination of a voluntary relaxation of the extrinsic rhabdomyosphincter and a fall in the maximal urethral closure pressure generated by the intrinsic rhabdomyosphincter. Relaxation of the internal sphincter (bladder neck) follows. Whether the bladder neck opens actively or by passive responsive to other anatomic events during voiding is debated. Afferents arising from the proximal urethra sense the presence of urine, and via the pelvic nerve and lateral columns of the spinal cord give rise to cortical awareness of imminent voiding. A detrusor contraction occurs with the release of the central (pontine and suprapontine) inhibition of the sacral detrusor nucleus and with the release of peripheral parasympathetic nerve transmission.

Clinically, the events occurring during the storage and voiding phases of lower urinary tract function can be evaluated by urodynamic testing. Techniques used in the urodynamic assessment of neurologic dysfunction are listed in Table 10.4. The International Continence Society has standardized these techniques and the terminology used to report urodynamic findings. Accurate interpretation of urodynamic results depends on a thorough understanding of the normal events of bladder storage and micturition, as described previously, and an appreciation of how a patient's underlying disease may alter these events. Such evaluation permits classification of voiding/storage dysfunction as outlined in Table 10.5 and provides a rational basis for the pharmacologic electrophysiologic behavioral and surgical treatment of voiding dysfunction. Some of the drugs commonly used to treat disorders of lower urinary tract function and their indications are listed in Table 10.6.

TABLE 10.4. Components of the Urodynamic Examination of Lower Urinary Tract Function

Determination of residual urine
Quantification of urine loss (pad test)
Cystometry (filling, voiding, and ambulatory)
Urethral pressure profilometry
Measurement of leak point pressure (Valsalva and detrusor)
Noninvasive urinary flow rate
Pressure/flow studies
Electromyography
Nerve conduction studies
Reflex latencies
Sensory testing
Provocative pharmacologic testing
Videofluoroscopic monitoring

TABLE 10.5. Urodynamic Classification of Voiding Dysfunction

Detrusor motor instability: spontaneous involuntary detrusor contractions during the storage phase
Idiopathic
Neurogenic (e.g., postcerebrovascular accident, SCI)
Detrusor sensory instability: urinary frequency and urgency associated with involuntary detrusor activity or inflammatory conditions
Detrusor-sphincter dyssynergia: inappropriate contraction of sphincter mechanism during voiding phase
Volitional (e.g., the "nonneurogenic" neurogenic bladder of childhood)
Reflex (e.g., multiple sclerosis, suprasacral spinal cord injury)
Detrusor areflexia
Normal compliance (e.g., sacral spinal injury, diabetes)
Decreased compliance (hypertonic) (e.g., myelodysplasia)
Motor paralytic bladder: sensation intact, bladder paralyzed (e.g., posthemorrhoidectomy retention)
Sensory paralytic bladder: sensation absent, motor nerves intact (e.g. diabetes mellitus, tabes dorsalis)
Urethral incompetence (ISD) (e.g., nerve injury during abdominal-perineal resection, inadequate urethral closure)
Stress urinary incontinence (e.g., postpartum female)

SCI, spinal cord injury.

TABLE 10.6. Pharmacologic Treatment of Lower Urinary Tract Dysfunction

Drugs That Improve Urine Storage
Inhibition of detrusor contractility
Anticholinergic drugs
Propantheline HCl
Smooth muscle depressants
Oxybutynin chloride
Flavoxate HCl
Dicyclomine HCl
Imipramine HCl
Tolterodine HCl
Enhancement of urethral tone
α-Adrenergic agonists
Phenylpropanolamine HCl
Imipramine HCl
β-Adrenergic antagonists
Propranolol HCl
Drugs That Facilitate the Voiding Phase
Enhancement of detrusor contractility
Cholinergic drugs
Bethanechol chloride
Inhibition of sphincter tone
α-Adrenergic antagonists
Prazosin HCl
Phenoxybenzamine HCl
Terazosin
Tamsulosin
Skeletal muscle relaxants
Diazepam
Dantrolene sodium
Baclofen

Selected Readings

Abrams P, Blaivas JG, Stanton SL, Anderson JT. Standardisation of lower urinary tract function. *Neurourol Urodynam* 1988;7:403–427.

Outlines standards approved by the International Continence Society for the performance and reporting of urodynamic tests of the bladder and urinary sphincter. Provides the definition of terms commonly used to describe lower urinary tract functions in clinical and experimental studies.

Biancani P, Hausman M, Weiss RM. Effect of obstruction on ureteral circumferential force-length relations. *Am J Physiol* 1982;243:F204–F210.

The obstructed ureter develops an increase in dimensions, muscle hypertrophy, and an increase in developed force. As there is an increase in force per unit area of muscle, the obstructed ureter actually develops an increase in contractility. From the force-length data obtained on circumferential ureteral rings, calculations of pressure–diameter relationships show that despite the muscle hypertrophy and increased contractility, the obstructed ureter is unable to generate intraluminal pressures required for coaptation of the ureteral walls and efficient transport of urine.

Elbadawi A. Neuromorphologic basis of veiscourethral function: I. Histochemistry, ultrastructure and function of the intrinsic nerves of the bladder and urethra. *Neurourol Urodynam* 1982;1:3–50.

A detailed presentation of histochemical data that support the current concepts of the innervation of the lower urinary tract; includes data to support the innervation of the urinary sphincter and a detailed review of afferent and efferent detrusor innervation.

Wein AJ, Van Arsdalen KN. Nonsurgical management of neuropathic voiding dysfunction. *Semin Urol* 1985;3:216–237.

An article focusing on the pharmacologic manipulation of disorders of bladder and urethral function. It is primarily clinical in orientation, emphasizing a functional approach to the treatment of voiding disorders, and contains an excellent discussion of the drugs commonly used to treat voiding disorders.

Weiss RM. Physiology of the upper urinary tract. *Semin Urol* 1987;5:148–154.

Weiss RM. Effect of pathologic processes and pharmacologic interventions on ureteral function. *Semin Urol* 1987;5:167–175.

Basic physiology of the ureter is reviewed and correlated with clinical states and the effects of diuresis, bladder filling, neurogenic vesical dysfunction, vesicoureteral reflux, infection, and obstruction on ureteral function. Includes a discussion of the diagnostic modalities used for differentiating obstructive from nonobstructive etiologies of hydroureteronephrosis. Includes review of pharmacologic modalities used in the treatment of pathologic states affecting the upper urinary tract.

CHAPTER 11

Renal Growth and Hypertrophy

Agnes B. Fogo

Renal growth occurs normally during development and maturation, and pathologically either as an initial response to injury or loss of nephrons from various insults. This chapter reviews the various mechanisms and stimuli for normal and abnormal renal growth, and their consequences for renal function and structure.

RENAL GROWTH IN DEVELOPMENT AND MATURATION

The embryology of the kidney is discussed in Chapter 1, Part 1. Complex interactions of undifferentiated cells allow development of the highly specialized subunits of the nephron. After term birth, no new nephrons are formed in humans. However, maturational growth continues until adulthood, with increases in total renal mass resulting largely from tubular growth. Glomerular size and glomerular basement membrane (GBM) thickness increase with maturation. Glomeruli also undergo qualitative changes. The immature glomerulus is a simply branched capillary structure with cuboidal glomerular visceral epithelial cells, evolved from the S-shaped body. During maturation, complex capillary branching occurs, and the glomerular visceral epithelial cells become flattened and restricted in their ability to proliferate. This limitation may have profound consequences for responses to some glomerular injuries. Maturation proceeds in a centripetal pattern, with juxtamedullary glomeruli maturing first, and maintaining a larger size than the more superficial glomeruli until adulthood.

Analysis of genetically engineered mice has begun to shed light on the role of specific factors in various stages of renal development. For instance, platelet-derived growth factor (PDGF) B is necessary for vascularization of glomeruli, and the renin-angiotensin system (RAS) appears necessary for normal glomerular as well as for papillary growth. However, findings from genetically engineered mice must be analyzed with caution. The absence of a gene from the earliest point in development may lead to adaptations or structural or even lethal phenotypes that obscure or make difficult interpretation of a specific gene's role during development or disease processes in humans. Complex interactions and feedbacks can result in surprising phenotypes in gene-manipulated animals. For instance, both the total lack of angiotensin, induced in the angiotensinogen knockout mouse ($Atg^{-/-}$), and its overabundance, either by infusion or genetic manipulation, result in vascular sclerosis and mesangial increase, with hypotension in the former setting and hypertension in the latter.

RENAL GROWTH

Adaptations to increase renal mass and function presumably occur in attempts to restore renal function toward normal after injury. Renal growth occurs by both hyperplasia (increase in cell number) and hypertrophy (increase in cell size). Increases in renal mass primarily reflect tubular growth. However, glomerular growth also occurs in response to some injuries or reduced nephron mass. The glomerular growth occurred primarily by lengthening of the capillaries without significant increase in diameter after loss of renal parenchyma or in children with reflux nephropathy. In contrast, growth was accomplished by new capillary branching in experimental diabetes and in toxic nephropathy as a result of lithium (Fig. 11.1). With more extreme hemodynamic abnormalities, dilation of capillaries may occur and contribute to increased glomerular size.

Size

Hyperplasia is the response to a mitogenic signal that results in cell division. The initial stimulus is followed by a complex cascade, each of which is regulated by specific proteins, and governs the progression through the cell cycle from resting G0 to G1, S, G2, and M phases. The cell cycle is regulated by interactions of cyclins with their catalytic cdk (cyclin dependent kinases) subunits, and cyclin inhibitors. Cyclin D and E govern the rate of progression through G1 into S phase. Different family members of each of these cyclins modulate cell proliferation in differing cell types. The p21/Kip family inhibits both cyclin D and E, whereas the INK4 family affects only cyclin D. Hyperplasia is associated with activation of both cyclin D and E and inactivation of retinoblastoma protein (pRB), a key inhibitor of cell proliferation. Numerous growth factors promote proliferation either by directly inducing these events or by playing a permissive role in responsiveness to mitogenic stimuli. Hypertrophy occurs when cells grow without division, with resulting increased cellular protein-to-DNA ratio. In cell cycle–dependent hypertrophy, cells enter the cell cycle but arrest at G1. In tubular cells undergoing hypertrophy, pRB protein remains active. Cyclin D is activated, but there appears to be insufficient activation of cyclin E. The result is arrest at G1/S and hypertrophy. Transforming growth factor-β (TGF-β) is one key mediator of this hypertrophic response. Tubular cells may also undergo hypertrophy independent of the cell cycle via inhibition of pH-sensitive lysosomal enzymes, which lead to decreased intracellular protein degradation. This results in in-

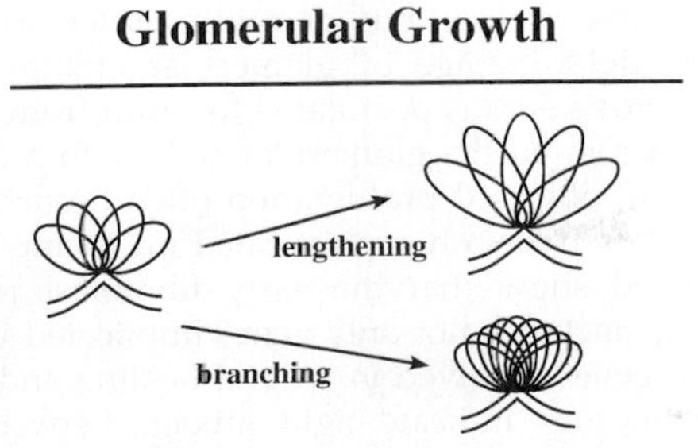

Figure 11.1. Schema illustrating documented mechanisms of glomerular hypertrophy due to capillary growth by either branching or lengthening of capillaries.

creased cell protein content without changes in DNA (i.e., hypertrophy).

Ammonia and acidification are strong stimuli for tubular cell hypertrophy. Ammonia generation varies both with pH and single-nephron glomerular filtration rate (SNGFR), and therefore may be the mediator of hypertrophy in many conditions. For instance, ammoniagenesis appears to be the underlying mechanism for hypertrophy induced by potassium depletion because bicarbonate administration concurrently decreases ammoniagenesis and ablates the effect of potassium depletion on renal growth. In diabetes, polyamines are implicated in tubular hypertrophy. The intracellular mechanisms of tubular cell hypertrophy vary in different settings. In the metabolically induced conditions of diabetes and acidosis, there is attenuated proteolysis and accelerated protein synthesis. High-protein dietary intake, angiotensin, and TGF-β induce cellular hypertrophy by reducing proteolysis both *in vitro* and *in vivo.* In contrast, in compensatory growth following nephrectomy, the increase in cell protein content results entirely from increased protein synthesis. These differences could have pathogenic implications for subsequent cell adaptations and fibrosis. Hypertrophy after unilateral nephrectomy also appears to be a malleable event, with reversal occurring readily upon restoration of renal mass.

Whole kidney weight increases shortly after ablation as a result of adaptive growth of tubules and glomeruli via hyperplasia and hypertrophy. Tubular hypertrophy and hyperplasia are demonstrable at 2 days after 5/6 nephrectomy before increases in α1(IV) collagen mRNA. Of note, later increases in this collagen mRNA occurred predominantly in proximal tubules in the deep cortex and outer medullary stripe but was dissociated from tubular enlargement. So-called glomerular hypertrophy, that is, an increase in glomerular size, represents both cellular hypertrophy and hyperplasia (Fig. 11.2). Glomerular hypertrophy can be detected biochemically and morphologically by electron microscopy as early as 2 days after 5/6 nephrectomy. Increased glomerular volume at 2 days was attributable to increased glomerular visceral epithelial cell expansion, likely hypertrophy in view of this cell's limited mitogenic capacity. Later increases in glomerular volume were contributed to by mesangial cell increase, likely both hypertrophy and hyperplasia. The relative contributions of cellular hyperplasia and hypertrophy to the increase in glomerular size depend on both the amount of renal mass lost and age. Hyperplasia occurred to greater extent after subtotal (5/6) nephrectomy, whereas hypertrophy was the predominant form of growth after uninephrectomy. Glomerular hypertrophy was much greater after 5/6 nephrectomy and was associated with later sclerosis. Glomerular and tubular proteinase and cathepsin activities, possible modulators of matrix accumulation, were lower after 5/6 nephrectomy than after uninephrectomy.

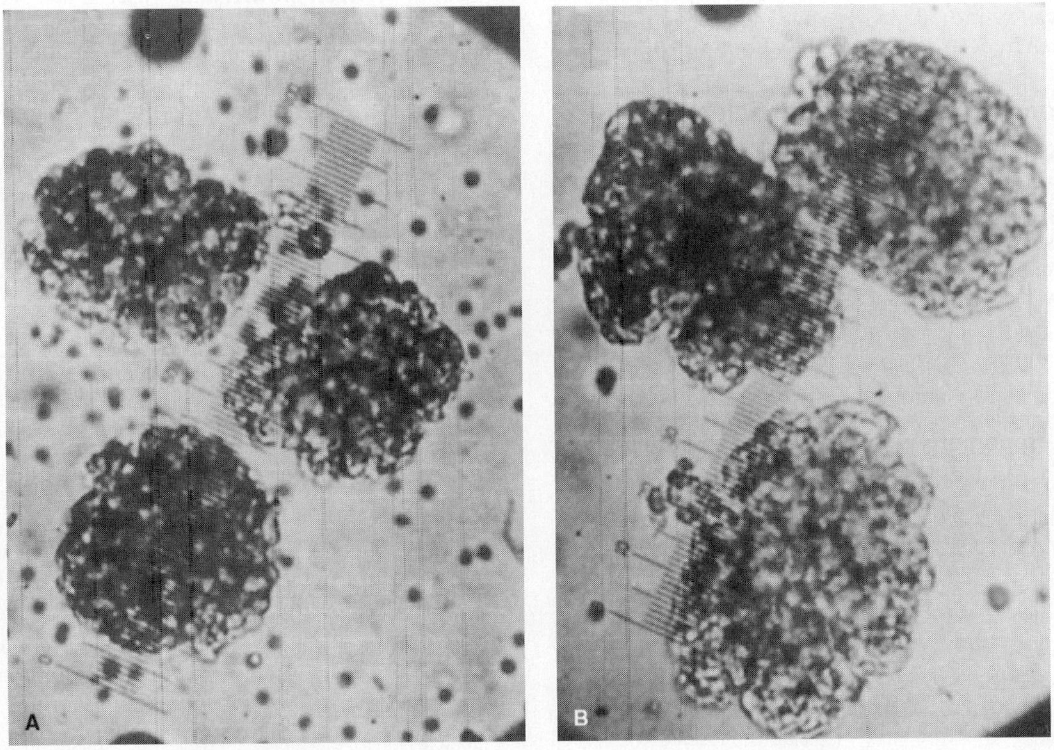

Figure 11.2. Normal glomeruli from the rabbit kidney **(A)** versus hypertrophied glomeruli from the remnant kidney **(B)** photographed at the same magnification. Glomeruli are isolated from their vascular supply, and the enlargement thus cannot reflect vascular engorgement, but rather increase in cell mass and/or number.

Interestingly, although angiotensin is strongly implicated with normal maturational growth and abnormal growth linked to sclerosis, it does not appear to be necessary for compensatory growth after unilateral nephrectomy. Thus no changes in the RAS were detected after unilateral nephrectomy in adult rats, and compensatory growth occurred even in the presence of angiotensin I–converting enzyme (ACE) inhibitor. In young rats, ACE inhibitors inhibited maturational growth of glomeruli, although catch-up growth normalized glomerular size after discontinuation of ACE inhibitors.

The precise trigger(s) for initiation of growth response remain undetermined. Early work proposed that renal growth after uninephrectomy was merely in response to increased workload. In the early 1970s, the concept of "renotropic" factor(s) was formulated as the alternative explanation based on observations of renal growth in normal animals connected by parabiosis with an anephric partner. Extracts from tubules from a model of tubular cell regeneration, gentamicin toxicity, readily induced tubular cell growth, attributable to IGF-1 activity. A possible quantitative trait locus (QTL) linked to genetic modulation of the compensatory growth response has been identified in the mouse on chromosome 11. This marker maps near the genes for ACE, growth hormone and neural growth factor receptor (NGFR), all of which have known influences on growth responses in the kidney.

Hypertrophy of remnant glomeruli was previously thought to be the consequence of the abnormal hemodynamics developing within these glomeruli or merely to represent engorgement. However, the increased growth in the remnant kidney model in the rat where $1^2/_3$ kidney are removed (total 5/6 nephrectomy) occurred before increases in SNGFR and are present even when glomeruli are isolated (Fig. 11.2). The patterns of gene expression were also significantly different in hypertrophy versus hyperplasia, with a rapidly, transiently increased expression of the protooncogenes c-fos, c-myc, and c-Ha-ras in hyperplasia, with c-fos and c-jun also elevated at day 14 after 5/6 nephrectomy. In contrast, there was a gradual, progressive increase in these protooncogenes when hypertrophy occurred after uninephrectomy.

Abnormal Glomerular Growth and Sclerosis

Glomerular hypertrophy and sclerosis are linked in numerous diseases in humans and in experimental animal models (Table 11.1). The association of abnormal glomerular growth and sclerosis is also seen in human diseases. *In vivo* and *in vitro* experimental evidence point to the capability of many cytokines to promote growth of glomerular cells and also to enhance extracellular matrix release, thus promoting sclerosis as well as growth. The tight linkage of glomerular enlargement with glomerulosclerosis is thus postulated to result from the actions of multiple factors on the glomerular cells with a response of matrix, hypertrophy, and proliferation often occurring in concert. *In vitro* data based on sophisticated microchip gene array analysis indeed show that the early fibroblast response to growth factors includes not only genes implicated in cell division but also genes involved in wound healing and angiogenesis. These findings indicate tight linkage between growth, differentiation, and wound healing/remodeling responses. Stimuli to abnormal growth noted in humans include hypoxia, as seen in cyanotic heart disease, sickle cell disease, and obesity-associated sleep apnea, and limited renal mass, as in transplantation, nephrectomy of more than one kidney, and unilateral renal agenesis. All of these conditions have also been associated with focal segmental glomerular sclerosis (FSGS). Other stimuli that have been shown in experimental conditions to promote growth and glomerulosclerosis include high-protein or high-salt diet, various hormones (e.g., growth hormone, insulinlike growth factor, androgens, glucocorticoids), and vasoactive molecules such as angiotensin or endothelin (Table 11.2). In diabetic nephropathy and idiopathic FSGS, the glomerular enlargement appears to result from primary pathogenic mechanisms; it is not secondary to nephron loss or hypoxia. Although hypertrophic stimuli accelerate the glomerulosclerosis, the converse is also true; decreasing the hypertrophic response is associated with decreased glomerulosclerosis. Interventions that ameliorate glomerulosclerosis and dampen glomerular hypertrophy include low-protein, low-salt, or low-phosphate diet; ablation of androgen effects by castration; antagonism of growth hormone with octreotide, a somatostatin analog; or inhibition of angiotensin or endothelin.

Glomerular Hypertrophy in Experimental Models

This link between growth and sclerosis has been demonstrated at the single-nephron level as well. In the subtotally nephrectomized rat, a strong correlation was found between the degree of total glomerular sclerosis and the maximum glomerular planar area, determined by serial section analysis (Fig. 11.3). Furthermore, a biphasic population of glomeruli was observed. For the severely sclerotic glomeruli, a negative correlation with glomerular area was seen, in keeping with the well-known clinical observation of small, shrunken hyalinized glomeruli in the end-stage human kidney. Development of mild to moderate

TABLE 11.1. Conditions with Glomerular Hypertrophy and Sclerosis

Animal Models	Human Diseases
Remnant kidney	Focal segmental glomerular sclerosis
Puromycin nephropathy	Unilateral renal agenesis
$Bc12^{-/-}$ mice	Extensive loss of renal mass
$Os^{+/+}$ mice	Oligomeganephronia
Diabetic models*	Diabetic nephropathy
High-protein diet	Reflux nephropathy
Angiotensin infusion	Sickle cell disease
Growth hormone or insulinlike growth factor-1 administration	Cyanotic heart disease
	Obesity/sleep apnea

*Associated with mesangial expansion only in rodent models.
Os, oligosyndactyly mouse.

TABLE 11.2. Modulators of Renal Growth *In Vivo*

Stimulators*	Inhibitors
TGF-β†	TGF-β
VEGF	Angiostatin
Angiotensin II	Angiotensin-converting enzyme inhibitor
Growth hormone or insulinlike growth factor = I	Octreotide (somatostatin analog)
K^+ depletion	Concurrent bicarbonate and K^+ depletion
High-protein diet	Low-protein diet
High-salt diet	Low-salt diet
Androgens	Castration
Diabetes	Insulin treatment or pancreas transplant

*Stimulators of growth and inhibitors of their actions are listed pairwise.
†TGF-β stimulates or inhibits growth depending on cell cycle.
TGF, transforming growth factor.

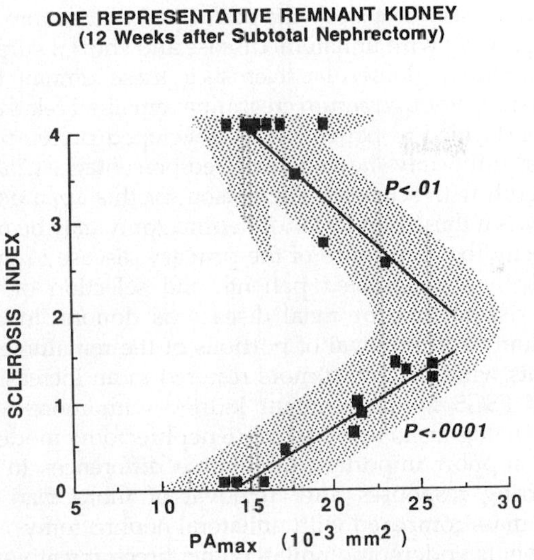

Figure 11.3. Relationship of glomerular hypertrophy and sclerosis in individual glomeruli within one kidney at 12 weeks after 5/6 nephrectomy. When sclerosis index (0 to 4 scale by serial section) and maximum planar area (PA_{max}) were evaluated for each of 22 glomeruli in a single remnant rat kidney 12 weeks after subtotal nephrectomy, a significant correlation with a biphasic pattern was found between these parameters. Thus there was a negative correlation for the glomeruli with advanced sclerosis and a positive correlation for the glomeruli with early-stage sclerosis, pointing to a potential linkage between the pathogenesis of glomerular hypertrophy and sclerosis. (Reprinted with permission from Fogo A, Ichikawa I. Evidence for the central role of glomerular growth promoters in the development of sclerosis. *Semin Nephrol* 1989;9:329–342.)

sclerosis was seen in close association with enlargement of the glomerular size. The sclerosis and hypertrophy were decreased in parallel by ACE inhibitors, further pointing to a link between the two processes. In the ureter diversion model in the rat, the ureter of one kidney is diverted into the peritoneum with 2/3 ligation of the contralateral kidney. Renal or glomerular hypertrophy are not induced, despite equally severe hemodynamic perturbation as in the 5/6 nephrectomy model. The lack of significant glomerular hypertrophy was associated with absence of sclerosis, further pointing to a link between these two processes. These experiments also indicate that hyperfiltration alone is insufficient to induce pathogenic glomerular hypertrophy and subsequent sclerosis.

Of note, ACE inhibitors were not equally effective at all stages of glomerular growth and sclerosis: glomeruli with more advanced sclerosis showed continuous progression, whereas progression of early-stage sclerosis was inhibited. These findings indicate that different mechanisms of cell growth and matrix accumulation are predominant among the heterogeneously affected glomeruli, with differing potential for response to treatment and remodeling.

Significant glomerular hypertrophy and accelerated glomerulosclerosis also occur in response to excess growth hormone, whether endogenously produced (i.e., transgenic mice) or exogenously administered (i.e., growth hormone administration). Growth hormone accelerated growth and sclerosis in uremic young rats. Even in normal young rats with intact kidneys, treatment with recombinant human growth hormone resulted in glomerular hypertrophy and sclerosis. In contrast, dwarf rats with a defect in growth hormone or with a specific growth hormone receptor deletion are resistant to the development of glomerulosclerosis after renal ablation. A rat strain characterized by a larger number of small glomeruli and a minimal hypertrophic response to loss of nephrons, the PVGc strain, has proved resistant to the development of glomerulosclerosis after the removal of one kidney. Other studies in mice have indicated that the hypertrophic response and subsequent development of sclerosis depend on the genetic background, suggesting that complex genetic traits modulate the response of glomerular cells to pathogenic stimuli. Mice with reduced nephron number as a result of a radiation-induced mutation, which results in about a 50% nephron reduction in association with oligosyndactyly ($Os^{+/+}$), developed severe glomerular enlargement and sclerosis when this abnormality occurred on the sclerosis-prone ROP genetic background but not in C57 mice. The interplay of genetic background and response to injury is also well recognized in humans, in whom only about 40% of patients with type 1 diabetes mellitus develop diabetic nephropathy.

The age of the injury also modifies the growth response to renal ablation. In young animals in which maturational growth is occurring, injury after renal ablation was more severe than in adults. Detailed analysis of the distribution of this glomerular injury revealed more focal and severe glomerulosclerosis in the deep versus superficial glomeruli in the young rats. Hemodynamic factors were not different among the two age groups. Although glomerular enlargement occurred to a greater degree in the young compared with the adult rat after renal ablation, glomerular enlargement occurred proportionally in both superficial and deep nephron populations. The more severe injury of the deep glomeruli in the young immature rat was therefore postulated to be related to factors unique in the young growing kidney, which is characterized by centripetal growth and differentiation. The mechanisms that promote hyperplasia rather than hypertrophy in the accentuated growth and wound healing in response to nephron loss may also promote scarring.

Glomerular Hypertrophy and Human Disease

Some human conditions associated with enlarged glomeruli include solitary kidney (renal agenesis or postnephrectomy), congenital cyanotic heart disease, sickle cell disease, diabetes, oligomeganephronia, and significant obesity (all of which may be associated with FSGS). In human FSGS, increased glomerular size precedes development of the sclerotic lesions. Pediatric patients who have nephrotic syndrome and apparent minimal change disease on initial biopsies and who display subsequent progression to overt FSGS had significantly enlarged glomerular areas in those first biopsies (Fig. 11.4). These findings have been confirmed in adult patients and in different ethnic groups in Sweden, Korea, and the United States. Similarly, adult patients with existing FSGS had significantly larger glomerular size than adult patients with minimal change disease. Thus, in cases of nephrotic syndrome without evident segmental glomerular sclerosis, patients with normal glomerular size appear to have a good prognosis. In contrast, patients with significantly enlarged glomerular size have a high risk of subsequent progression to overt FSGS.

A genetic analysis of children with nephrotic syndrome found FSGS patients to have a higher prevalence of the ACE deletion (D) polymorphism compared with the insertion (I) polymorphism than patients with minimal change disease. This D allele has been associated with higher activity of the RAS, which may influence both renal growth and scarring responses. These findings also support that MCD and FSGS are different diseases from the earliest stage.

Conversely, glomerular hypertrophy was not found in patients with glomerular tip lesions (i.e., segmental sclerosis only at the tubular pole of the glomerulus). In this entity, prognosis is thought to be similar to that of minimal change disease. Of interest, the association of increased glomerular size and subsequent evolution of glomerular sclerosis was also seen in the setting of recurrent FSGS in the transplant. Children who received an adult kidney transplant who did not develop FSGS in their

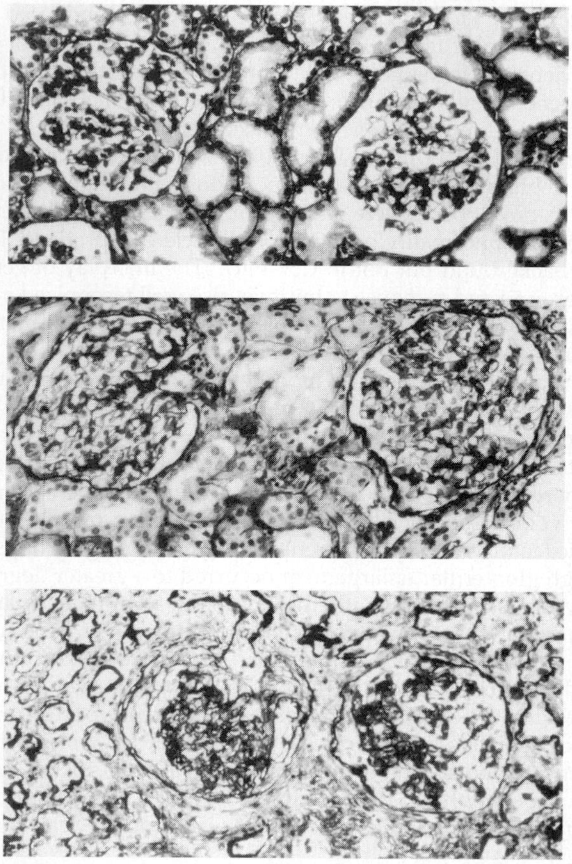

Figure 11.4. Glomerular size in FSGS versus MCD. The two *top panels* show initial biopsies from patients with apparent MCD. The 5-year-old girl's initial biopsy in the *middle panel* was indistinguishable from age-matched typical MCD *(top panel),* except for marked glomerular enlargement. Her subsequent biopsy *(bottom panel),* 50 months later, showed FSGS. (Jones' silver stain, ×160.) (Reprinted with permission from Fogo A, Hawkins ETP, Berry PL, et al. Glomerular hypertrophy in minimal change disease predicts subsequent progression to focal glomerular sclerosis. *Kidney Int* 1990;38:115–123.)

transplants did not show increased glomerular size over the initial months after transplantation. In contrast, those who developed recurrent FSGS had significant, abnormal glomerular growth in their transplant, preceding overt structural manifestation of FSGS.

Loss of Renal Mass in Humans

Response to decreased renal mass in humans varies according to age at loss, underlying condition, and extent of tissue loss. Several follow-up studies conducted on renal transplant donors and nephrectomized individuals secondary to trauma and unilateral diseases suggest a relatively benign course after unilateral nephrectomy. Although none of the patients in these studies reached a stage of chronic renal failure as a result of nephrectomy, an increased incidence, by some twofold, of hypertension has been reported in some of the groups. The majority of more than 2,000 U.S. Armed Forces personnel who were nephrectomized as a result of trauma during World War II, the Korean war, and Vietnam war have not been evaluated and are presumed to not have overt manifestations of renal damage up to 55 years after nephrectomy. In a series of 78 follow-up cases of transplant donors, two patients with FSGS were found on renal biopsy of the remnant kidney. These relatively benign trends are in contrast to series of patients with nephrectomy for unilateral disease. Biopsies were performed much more liberally in these patients with unilateral disease and show a surprisingly high incidence of glomerular sclerosis in these remnant kidneys. In one series, although serum creatinine remained relatively low, biopsy performed in patients who developed proteinuria (3 to 4 g/24 hr) uniformly showed increased percentages (2% to 20%) of glomeruli with sclerosis. The reason for this apparent difference between these two forms of nephrectomy may be multifactorial, including recurrence of the primary disease in the therapeutically nephrectomized patients and selection of patients without risk factors for renal disease as donors. In contrast, nephrectomy and removal of portions of the remaining kidney in patients with bilateral tumors resulted in an increasing incidence of FSGS in the remnant kidney with more extensive surgery, analogous to the rodent 5/6 nephrectomy model. These findings support important qualitative differences in growth and scarring responses after removal of more than 50% of nephron mass compared with unilateral nephrectomy.

In patients undergoing unilateral nephrectomy at young age for Wilms' tumor, kidney size by ultrasound increased most in those who had surgery at a younger age. Microalbuminuria developed in 11 of 34 patients and was associated with increased kidney growth. In another series of 29 patients with a single kidney (5 of them as a result of agenesis), only 1 patient with renal agenesis had elevated albuminuria. The remaining 4 patients with renal agenesis (ages 22 to 58 years at follow-up) and the patients with surgical removal of the kidney had no evidence of decreased renal function. Blood pressure was slightly elevated in only 3 patients. A review of 9,200 autopsy cases from a tertiary hospital documented 7 cases of solitary kidney as a result of unilateral renal agenesis. Of those, 2 (29%) died of chronic renal failure with FSGS lesions. In this series, 10 patients were autopsied 8 to 46 years after surgical unilateral neprhectomy, none of whom had clinical sign of renal disease or FSGS histologic pattern in the remnant kidneys. This retrospective study from the tertiary-care hospital may still overestimate the true incidence of FSGS in solitary kidney as a result of renal agenesis as indicated by a Swedish report. In this latter report, 15 patients with a solitary kidney were followed from their early childhood for up to 47 years. The mode of initial detection of the patients was not documented (i.e., whether the solitary kidney was discovered incidentally or because of renal-related symptoms). These patients showed a gradual but significant decline in inulin and PAH clearance rates compared with age-matched controls. Forty-seven percent of them had microalbuminuria, but no patients had renal insufficiency or hypertension.

Oligomeganephronia is another congenital condition of reduced nephron population in humans characterized by, as expected from its name, few but significantly enlarged nephrons. The histologic pattern of the glomerulus includes not only an impressive hypertrophy but also severe FSGS. This condition presents clinically with proteinuria and progressive renal failure, although again, the true incidence of this disease and the probability of developing renal failure remain undetermined.

The nephron number has not been established in various human populations, but interestingly, glomerular size in normal African Americans is larger than in Caucasians. These differences in glomerular size may reflect factors that have an impact on glomerular/renal development. Decreased nephron number has been postulated to occur secondary to low birth weight. The latter is associated with increased risk for progressive renal disease in adulthood. Other possible mechanisms that could underlie these differences in normal glomerular growth and also relate to the well-documented increased incidence of end-stage renal disease in the African-American population include polymorphisms of genes involved both in renal/glomerular development and in scarring mechanisms, such as the RAS.

These reports support the overall trend found in the literature that congenital unilateral absence of a kidney has poorer prognosis than acquired loss and that loss of a kidney at younger age has worse long-term prognosis than when it occurs in adults. Animal and human studies indicate that in response to unilateral nephrectomy, greater compensatory hypertrophy and hyperfunction are achieved in immature than in adult remnant kidneys, suggesting that immature remnant kidneys are more predisposed to glomerular damage. It is also conceivable that the number of remnant nephrons in the congenital solitary kidney may, in fact, be decreased (i.e., hypogenesis), thereby representing a more severe form of reduction in nephron population than surgical unilateral nephrectomy. The possibility that the remnant glomeruli of congenital solitary kidney are under greater hypertrophic stress is indeed supported by quantitative morphometric studies. The volume of each glomerulus in solitary kidneys was found to be five to six times normal, a value closer to that found in oligomeganephronia than that seen in postnephrectomized adults. Thus abnormal glomerular growth may be taken as an indicator of abnormal growth stimuli, which ultimately result in the maladaptive responses of augmented cell growth, matrix accumulation, and then sclerosis.

Factors Mediating Growth

In vivo and *in vitro* evidence point to the capability of many cytokines to promote growth of glomerular cells and also to enhance extracellular matrix release, thus promoting sclerosis and growth in tandem. Several growth factors appear to play key roles in progression of glomerular and tubulointerstitial scarring. The specific factor(s) and the roles they play may differ at the various stages of injury. The mechanisms that underlie the differential effect of growth factors on cell cycling may relate to altered cell–cell or cell–matrix interaction, which profoundly modulate growth responses. Multiplication of cells *in vitro* in response to any stimuli is avid until the cells reach confluency. In quiescent cells, stimuli generally augment extracellular matrix accumulation over cell growth. For example, TGF-β is growth stimulatory or inhibitory *in vitro,* largely depending on the degree of confluency of cells and cell origin. The local matrix environment also modifies the response to growth factors. Mesangial cells in routine culture readily proliferate in response to PDGF-B and express PDGF-B receptors, whereas culture under three-dimensional conditions within a matrix network renders mesangial cells of a distinctly different phenotype: The PDGF-B receptor is downregulated, and the cells do not proliferate in response to PDGF. Enhanced matrix accumulation in even a segment of the glomerulus *in vivo* similarly could lead to downregulation of PDGF expression in later stages of sclerosis, when other growth factors are activated. This may result in a loss of response to maneuvers that target PDGF. The possibility exists that the state of differentiation and receptor modulation may be greatly altered locally at a site of injury, with resultant augmented local response to specific growth factors.

Specific Growth Factors

Altered gene expressions in pathophysiologic settings implicate many factors, including the following: PDGF, TGF-β, TGF-α, insulinlike growth factor-1 (IGF-1), growth hormone, epidermal growth factor (EGF), interleukins 1 and 6, tumor necrosis factor-α (TNF-α), angiotensin II, hepatocyte growth factor (HGF) and its receptor c-myc, and endothelin (Table 11.2). Several growth factors, including angiotensin II, PDGF, and TGF-β, are now considered to play key causal roles in glomerulosclerosis, based on results of infusion, transfection, and inhibition of these factors. Other data implicate vasopressin in renal and glomerular growth, although its effects on sclerosis have not been documented. Manipulations of the RAS, whether direct or indirect via furosemide-induced volume depletion, implicate the RAS in renal hypertrophy. Of interest, HGF treatment significantly augmented tubular hyperplasia in a mouse model of chronic renal disease and suppressed TGF-β and PDGF expression. This augmented tubular growth was associated with inhibition of renal scarring both in the tubulointerstitial compartment and in the glomeruli. These findings indicate that augmented growth of tubules, in contrast to the accelerated growth of glomeruli, may have a salutary effect on end organ damage, perhaps by minimizing activation of other profibrotic mechanisms. To date, the relative importance of these specific growth factors in development of FSGS or in remodeling and restoration of function and structure in humans is not defined.

In vitro studies have demonstrated that angiotensin II, a potent vasoconstrictor, also induces the smooth muscle cell c-fos oncogene. Infusion of angiotensin II *in vivo* also activates the early growth response genes c-fos and Egr-1. Although implications for long-term structural effects of these early protooncogene changes have not yet been delineated, the induction of protooncogenes may be a common pathway for hypertrophic agents, allowing transition from a quiescent to an active state. The activity of the transcription factor NF-kappaB is also induced by angiotensin, thus possibly directing coordinated expression of a number of genes that together promote growth and sclerosis. Some of the lipid-lowering drugs, the HMG coA reductase inhibitors (so-called statins), also may affect cell proliferation by their effects on farnesylation and activity of transcription factors, thereby possibly decreasing cell proliferation and matrix production.

Angiotensin II actions in addition to vasoconstriction include effects on mesangial muscle, vascular smooth muscle, and tubular cell growth and matrix production, implicating it as a key factor promoting sclerosis. Therefore therapies that inhibit its actions are of particular interest. Animal models have shown efficacy of antihypertensive drugs that inhibit angiotensin II, either ACE inhibitors, or a newly developed angiotensin II–type 1 receptor antagonist. These agents not only are effective systemic antihypertensives but also appear to be more efficacious than other, nonspecific antihypertensives in protecting against progressive renal injury. Therefore inhibition of angiotensin II actions on cell growth and matrix accumulation is postulated to be involved in the effect of these drugs on sclerosis. Angiotensin induces tubular gluconeogenesis and ammoniagenesis, products of which also affect cell growth. Angiotensin also influences transport and acidification in proximal and distal tubules.

Proximal tubular cells exposed to angitensin II progress from G0 to G1, where they remain, thus undergoing hypertrophy, whereas distal tubules can proliferate in response to angiotensin II. The hypertrophic angiotensin II effect is transduced by the AT1 receptor and appears to be mediated by oxygen radical induction of the cyclin-dependent kinase inhibitor p27Kip1. Whereas this may be an initial beneficial response to injury, ongoing hypertrophy likely promotes fibrotic mechanisms. Transformation of injured tubular cells to myofibroblast-like interstitial cells which can avidly contribute to interstitial fibrosis, has been proposed. Whether hypertrophic/hyperplastic stimuli also are involved in transformation has not been proven.

In vitro studies suggest that TGF-β effects may depend on the cell cycle and that TGF-β acts synergistically with some growth factors. For example, epidermal growth factor alone had no effect on mesangial cell matrix production, whereas the combination of TGF-β and epidermal growth factor doubled matrix production versus TGF-β alone. TGF-β is also a potent inducer of PDGF-β receptor and thus could enhance responsiveness to PDGF. Elevated expression of TGF-β has been found in numerous animal models associated with renal scarring. Conversely, pretreatment of rats with antibody to TGF-β in the anti-Thy1 model, characterized by mesangial proliferation and increased production and activity of TGF-β, dramatically attenuated injury, and antibody to TGF-β also inhibited growth in the streptozotocin diabetic mouse model. Studies in human renal diseases have begun to map some of these key growth factors, showing upregulation in some settings. Direct extrapolation from expression studies to functional significance cannot be made. The complex interactions of growth factors make it difficult to predict cell responses. Moreover, even a given growth promoter may affect different cells differently, inducing proliferation or hypertrophy or even inhibiting growth, depending on the host cells' milieu and phenotype status.

Metabolic Factors Promoting Renal Growth

Only 40% of all patients with diabetes develop diabetic nephropathy. The primary morphologic abnormality in diabetic nephropathy is marked mesangial expansion with increased cellularity and matrix. However, predictors of development of diabetic nephropathy have not been identified. As in FSGS, abnormal renal growth precedes development of sclerosis in diabetic nephropathy. Patients with diabetic nephropathy showed significantly larger mean glomerular size and mesangial volume compared with both normal controls and diabetic patients without nephropathy. In addition, a strong correlation existed between the severity of glomerular sclerosis and glomerular hypertrophy. However, biopsies performed during the early stages of microalbuminuria showed variable lesions. The potential importance of the diabetic milieu in promoting the glomerular hypertrophy and mesangial matrix expansion of diabetic nephropathy was evident in a study of diabetic patients with renal and pancreas transplants. Patients with the combined transplants who achieved a metabolic cure of their diabetes had only minimal mesangial expansion in their transplant kidneys. Long-term follow-up showed reversal of sclerosis in some of these patients. The pancreas transplant patients also had smaller mean glomerular volume and mesangial volumes than control patients. In contrast, diabetic patients receiving only a kidney transplant and who therefore remained diabetic, showed more severe diabetic renal lesions. Although the lesions in type I and type II diabetes may be caused by a similar pathogenetic mechanism, the glomerular volume remains normal in type II diabetic patients, contrasting enlarged glomeruli in type I diabetic patients. There are currently no long-term studies establishing whether the degree and/or presence of glomerular hypertrophy or mesangial expansion are reliable markers of long-term progression.

Control of glucose has always been advocated to minimize complications of diabetes, and certain data have indicated that tight control of glucose decreases the rate of glomerular filtration rate loss. Reversal of mesangial matrix expansion was even achieved with pancreas transplantation in patients with diabetic nephropathy. Hyperglycemia results in accumulation of other metabolic products that can also modulate glomerular cell growth and glomerulosclerosis. Thus both polyamines and glucose levels affect mesangial cell growth and matrix accumulation. Increased polyamines are implicated in the tubular hypertrophy of diabetes. Increased ornithine decarboxylase appears crucial in this step because its inhibitors prevent this hypertrophic response. Advanced glycosylation end products (AGEs) are formed by effects of increased glucose on proteins. The glycosylated products can form stable adducts (AGEs) via protein cross-linking and polymerization. AGEs are increased in diabetes and also in aging. AGEs have direct effects to upregulate multiple cytokines, which in turn augment matrix production. Furthermore, AGEs may prevent normal protease digestion of collagens to which they bind. Infusion of AGEs into normal mice lead to glomerular hypertrophy and increased expression of matrix genes. Conversely, inhibition of AGE cross-linking with aminoguanidine significantly blunted these effects. Longer courses of administration of AGEs resulted in significant glomerulosclerosis and proteinuria, ameliorated by cotreatment with aminoguanidine. Aminoguanidine had a similar beneficial effect on mesangial expansion in diabetic animal models without altering glucose levels.

IGF-1 is one key growth factor altered in progressive renal diseases, including diabetes. The circulating level is under the control of growth hormone, although many factors may affect its biologic actions. IGF-1 induces renal and glomerular hypertrophy *in vivo* as demonstrated in transgenic mice and causes mesangial cell hyperplasia *in vitro;* however, it may require synergistic actions of other cytokines to result in a sclerotic lesion. Specific receptors for IGF show increased expression in diabetic rat mesangial cells. Puberty influences the growth response of the kidney in adolescents with diabetes. With the onset of puberty, kidney volume increased significantly, apparently preceding the development of microalbuminuria. Increases in urinary IGF-1 correlated with increased kidney volume, and both urinary IGF-1 and growth hormone correlated with microalbuminuria.

Several other growth factors, including basic fibroblast growth factor, PDGF, and EGF, may be altered in diabetes and affect glomerular growth and sclerosis. Treatment in experimental models with ocetreotide, a somatostatin analog, inhibited early diabetic renal hypertrophy but was ineffective in reversing existing abnormal growth. In contrast, insulin treatment, which normalized glucose levels, was effective in reversing existing renal hypertrophy.

Cell-Specific Growth Responses

Growth may occur in any of the cellular components of the kidney, including glomerular resident and/or infiltrating cells, tubules, and interstitial cells. Differences in the renal cell populations affected by different primary injuries may dictate the subsequent response. The glomerular resident cells are highly specialized and include the endothelial, epithelial, and mesangial cells, each with unique adaptations and growth responses after injury. These alterations in response to either the initial injury or to a decrease in remaining renal mass after initial injury, contribute to maintaining renal function in the short term. However, in the long term, these adaptive changes promote matrix accumulation and thereby renal malfunction.

Endothelial Cell

The glomerular endothelial cell has a long half-life, approximately 100 days. Endothelial cell apoptosis as well as proliferation and migration also occur in several animal models of glomerular injury. The balance between endothelial cell growth and death appear to be crucial for determining whether healing or scarring will result after injury. Specific angiostatins that inhibit angiogenesis thus retarded healing in the anti-Thy1 mesangial proliferation model of glomerular injury.

Normally, endothelial cells inhibit smooth muscle cell migration and proliferation. Endothelial cells produce numerous factors that modulate mesangial or vascular smooth muscle cell growth (e.g., vascular endothelial growth factor, VEGF; nitric oxide; endothelin, PDGF). Some endothelial-derived factors act in synergy with heparinlike substances. VEGF is an endothelial cell–specific mitogen that, within the kidney, originates largely from epithelial cells and may mediate physiologic and pathologic angiogenesis. VEGF gene expression is induced by hypoxia and has been implicated in the pathogenesis of diabetic retinopathy. Of note, new capillary growth also occurs in the glomerulus in diabetes, for example, suggesting an analogous role for VEGF in glomerular, as well as ocular, lesions with abnormal growth of vessels. Nitric oxide results in significant inhibition of mitogen-induced mesangial cell proliferation. Endothelin, a powerful vasoconstrictor, is released from endothelial cells in response to various stimuli and also after injury. Endothelin results in the adaptive responses of hyperplasia, hypertrophy, and increased matrix in mesangial cells in culture. Endothelin also enhances PDGF release, another key factor augmenting these processes. Thus endothelial cell damage potentially may have profound consequences on collagen production, both directly via elaboration of the aforementioned substances and by loss of synergistic inhibition of mesangial cell production of collagen. Subtle differences in baseline expression of basement membrane collagen in different portions of the kidney and even within a glomerulus may then result in differential growth and matrix responses at these sites to injury. Normal glomerular endothelial cells show heterogeneous expression of mRNAs for GBM components. For example, $\alpha 1$(IV) and $\alpha 2$(IV) collagen mRNAs are localized to endothelial cells in small-diameter capillary loops. During development, a shift occurs from a GBM network of $\alpha 1$(IV) and $\alpha 2$(IV) collagen and to the mature GBM with prominence of $\alpha 3,4,5$(IV) collagen.

Several anticoagulant agents and platelet inhibitors have been shown to regulate glomerular cell proliferation and also ameliorate glomerular sclerosis. Inhibition of platelet aggregation prevents release of PDGF and other active substances. Heparin, which is released locally within the glomerulus, suppresses the growth of, as well as extracellular matrix accumulation from, mesangial cells in a dose-dependent manner. Of note, a nonanticoagulant heparin fraction is equally potent in this regard. Heparin also modulates other growth factor activities. Endothelial cell growth factor (ECGF) and heparin together, but not ECGF alone, significantly inhibit vascular smooth muscle cell collagen I and IV gene expression. Conversely, the plasminogen activator-inhibitor-1, PAI-1, has been linked to not only thrombosis but also fibrosis through its effects to inhibit matrix degradation. PAI-1 induction occurs in response to several growth factors and cytokines, which play key roles in renal growth and fibrotic responses, including TGF-β and angiotensin. Thus PAI-1 may be an additional target for antifibrotic therapies.

Glomerular Visceral Epithelial Cell

The glomerular visceral epithelial cell is highly specialized. It not only serves as part of the capillary wall barrier but also contributes extracellular matrix to the normal GBM and is a source of increased matrix in pathologic settings. Glomerular visceral epithelial cells have limited capacity for hyperplasia. Mesangial and endothelial cells do not show similar limitations and can rapidly increase turnover in response to injury. Glomerular growth and sclerosis are accelerated when renal ablation is superimposed on adriamycin injury. The increased glomerular size occurs in this model without proportional increase in number of glomerular visceral epithelial cells. Consequentially, epithelial cells often are detached from the underlying basement membrane, especially in areas of hyalinosis. These epithelial cell defects are postulated to play an important role in progressive scarring due to injury from exudation of plasma proteins. Because increased glomerular growth occurs after many injuries, leading to glomerulosclerosis, this mechanism may be important for initiating glomerular injury. The exciting discoveries of specific cyclin-dependent kinase inhibitors expressed in mature (but not in immature) glomerular visceral epithelial cells suggest a possible mechanism for this limitation of this highly specialized cell. Manipulations of one of these inhibitors, p27Kip-1, in experimental mice models illustrated that abnormal glomerular visceral epithelial cell proliferation, whether too little or too much, resulted in augmented glomerular injury. These results indicate the normally tightly controlled fine balance of cell turnover necessary for normal glomerular function and structure.

Glomerular visceral epithelial cell injuries also result in dedifferentiation and altered expressions of integrins, which affect cell–matrix interactions and potentially growth and sclerosis responses. The Wilms' tumor gene WT1, is expressed in mature, differentiated visceral epithelial cells, but is decreased in injured glomerular visceral epithelial cells in collapsing or HIV-associated forms of FSGS. The function of WT1 in normal kidneys is unknown, but these recent genetic findings implicate it in a wide spectrum of functions, including renal development, glomerular permselectivity, and sclerosis.

Glomerular visceral epithelial cells interact with other glomerular cells and modulate cell growth and matrix synthesis/degradation by elaboration of growth factors and cytokines, such as heparin (inhibits mesangial cell growth) and VEGF (stimulates endothelial cell growth and increases permeability). Nephrin, expressed in glomerular visceral epithelial cell, has recently been identified as the gene that is mutated in congenital nephrotic syndrome, and localizes it to the slit diaphragm, implicating it in both proteinuria and sclerosis. The structure of nephrin suggests that it may affect permselectivity and matrix accumulation by modulating epi-thelial cell–matrix interactions.

Mesangial Cell

Many growth factors initially may be released from infiltrating macrophages, platelets, or resident glomerular cells (i.e., endothelial and epithelial cells, see previous discussion), which affect the mesangial cells. The RAS has been studied extensively, not only because of its influences on other key factors but also because of the readily available clinically used inhibitors of its activity. Angiotensin II induces mesangial cell hypertrophy and increases matrix production from mesangial cells *in vitro* and induces the smooth muscle cell c-fos oncogene. TGF-β increases both collagen and proteoglycan production by mesangial cells and, depending on the cell cycle stage, acts synergistically with other growth factors. Mesangial cells in culture release both interleukin-1 and a PDGF-like factor, and proliferate in response to these substances, suggesting both autocrine and paracrine regulation of mesangial cell proliferation. PDGF-B is increased in several models of glomerulosclerosis, especially at early points after injury. PDGF increases both matrix and proliferation of mesangial cells in culture and *in vivo* and has been implicated in several settings of renal injury (see previous discussion).

The mesangial cells share many characteristics with vascular smooth muscle cells. After initial injury, the activated mesangial cell changes phenotype, expressing fibroblastlike myosin. This wound healing phenotype is associated with increased matrix generation. α-Actin expression is also increased after injury, along with increased PDGF-B, recapitulating their developmental patterns of expressions in mesangial cells.

Tubular Epithelial Cell

Tubular hyperplasia and hypertrophy are the major contributors to increased renal mass in response to removal of nephron mass or injury. Numerous factors, including EGF, HGF, IGF-1, endothelin-1, acidic fibroblast growth factor (FGF), and TGF-β, have been implicated in tubular hyperplasia after injury. In the normal kidney, there is low level turnover of tubular cells. Various segments of the tubule show heterogeneity both in structural and in biochemical responses to stimuli and injuries. Cell turnover is prominent after tubulointerstitial injury. In a study of acute tubular necrosis (ATN) in native kidneys due to various causes, either ischemic or toxic, most tubules with regenerating morphologic features showed distal tubule phenotype marking. In the ischemia-reperfusion injury model of ATN, egr-1 protein, an early response gene, increased significantly in the thick ascending limb and principal cells of the collecting ducts, whereas proximal tubular cells showed no egr-1. In kidney transplants with ATN, particularly after cyclosporine treatment, there was an equal distribution of distal and proximal tubules with apparent regenerating change. These findings suggest that different mechanisms operate in ATN due to various injuries and that cell-specific expression of genes after injury may have an impact on this response.

Tubular responses to injury, whether regeneration or transformation, may directly contribute to chronic renal injury. Evidence suggests that transformation of injured tubular cells to a fibroblastlike phenotype may occur, with migration of these fibrogenic cells into the interstitial compartment. A fibroblast-specific protein, FSP1, related structurally to the S100 protein family, has been described. Although its function is not yet elucidated, its expression was highly restricted to fibroblasts, and its *de novo* expression localized to atrophic injured tubular segments. This molecule may therefore serve as a marker or even target for fibrogenic processes in the tubulointerstitium. *In vitro* results suggest that altered surrounding matrix may allow this process to reverse, possibly leading to therapies directly aimed at healing interstitial injuries. Interactions of cells with matrix and altered adhesion molecules, such as β1 integrins, are possible modulators of these processes of growth and differentiation.

After injury, tubules undergo adaptations of metabolism and structural changes. For example, oxygen consumption is increased, antioxidant enzymes are induced in some segments, cell hyperplasia and hypertrophy occur in some segments, whereas other segments respond to injury, particularly ischemia, by undergoing atrophy.

Cell Proliferation Versus Apoptosis

Cell turnover is an ongoing event affected by different mediators over the course of the disease. Markers for cell proliferation, such as Ki-67, PCNA, and bromodeoxyuridine incorporation, are increased in tissue repair and remodeling. This increased turnover and increased extracellular matrix mRNA persists at the same high levels even in late-stage glomerulosclerosis, indicating that ongoing remodeling can occur. Growth factors affect cell cycle events other than those related to hypertrophy or proliferation. TGF-β may directly cause apoptosis, an active form of cell death that does not elicit an inflammatory response. Angiotensin mediates apoptosis via the AT2 receptor. Withdrawal of some growth factors, including PDGF or IGF-1, may activate apoptosis. Apoptosis and necrosis occur with acute tubular injury, and growth factor therapies may diminish this injury. Increased cell growth was accompanied by increased apoptosis both in proliferative and in sclerotic human glomerular diseases. In experimental mesangial proliferative glomerulonephritis, apoptosis of the mesangial cells was associated with healing and return of structure to normal. Studies of polycystic kidney disease have shown increased apoptosis in this setting of renal injury as well. Apoptosis may serve as a healing mechanism, eliminating injured cells with minimal stimulation of immune/inflammatory mechanisms and cytokines. However, apoptosis in disproportionate amounts of cells that cannot regenerate may have deleterious consequences. Thus far, the ultimate effect on organ function of apoptosis of a cardiac myocyte versus a renal tubular epithelial cell, for example, has not been established.

Selected Readings

Fine LG. Biology of renal hypertrophy. *Kidney Int* 1986;29:619–634.

An excellent overview of the history, pathophysiology, and cell biology of renal hypertrophy.

Fogo A, Hawkins EP, Berry PL, et al. Glomerular hypertrophy in minimal change disease predicts subsequent progression to focal glomerular sclerosis. *Kidney Int* 1990;38:115–123.

This study shows that glomerular hypertrophy precedes development of FSGS in children with nephrotic syndrome.

Gassler N, Elger M, Inoue D, et al. Oligonephronia, not exuberant apoptosis, accounts for the development of glomerulosclerosis in the bcl-2 knockout mouse. *Nephrol Dial Transplant* 1998;13:2509–2518.

This study demonstrates a link between decreased nephron number and sclerosis in the genetically manipulated mouse devoid of bcl-2.

Ichikawa I, Ikoma M, Fogo A. Glomerular growth promoters, the common key mediator for progressive glomerular sclerosis in chronic renal diseases. *Adv Nephrol Necker Hosp* 1991;20:127–148.

This review article details mechanisms implicated in the linkage of glomerular growth and sclerosis.

Iyer VR, Eisen MB, Ross DT, et al. The transcriptional program in the response of human fibroblasts to serum. *Science* 1999;283:83–87.

These in vitro studies using microchip gene array analysis of fibroblasts exposed to growth factors in vitro demonstrate early responses of groups of genes temporally linked to growth, as well as those linked to wound healing and angiogenesis. These studies provide important molecular evidence that processes of growth and repair are interconnected.

Kujubu DA, Norman JT, Herschman HR, Fine LG. Primary response gene expression in renal hypertrophy and hyperplasia: evidence for different growth initiation processes. *Am J Physiol* 1991;260:F823–F827.

These interesting studies show differences in the expression of several primary-response genes in various mitogenic and differentiation cell models in vivo.

Lee GS, Nast CC, Peng SC, et al. Differential response of glomerular epithelial and mesangial cells after subtotal nephrectomy. *Kidney Int* 1998;53:1389–1398.

This paper illustrates the differential cellular growth response after subtotal nephrectomy, showing early expansion of glomerular visceral epithelial cells and later expansion of mesangial cells.

Safirstein R, DiMari J, Megyesi J, Price P. Mechanisms of renal repair and survival following acute injury. *Semin Nephrol* 1998;18:519–522.

An excellent review of the heterogenous reaction of the renal epithelium to injury and the role of kinases, their molecular targets, as well as cell cycle–specific factors that determine whether a cell survives the injury.

Wolf G, Neilson EG. Cellular biology of tubulointerstitial growth. *Curr Top Pathol* 1995;88:69–97.

The cell biology of tubular hypertrophy and hyperplasia is reviewed, including growth factors and various second messengers.

Wolf G, Ziyadeh FN. Renal tubular hypertrophy induced by angiotensin II. *Semin Nephrol* 1997;17:448–454.

This review details the role of angiotensin in renal tubular growth, including the response in differing nephron segments, the receptor and signal transduction mechanisms, and implications for matrix production and renal disease.

SECTION II

The Kidney and Endocrine System

CHAPTER 12

Role of the Kidney in Hormone Metabolism

Michael J. Hausmann and Ralph Rabkin

The endocrine and metabolic aspects of renal function have received increasing attention in recent years. This is in part because of the progress achieved in the management of patients with advanced renal failure. Patients whose lives have been prolonged by means of conservative treatment, dialysis, and transplantation have developed several disturbances that indicate the kidney has certain metabolic and endocrine functions not previously apparent. It is now well established that the kidney is an important site of hormone metabolism. A further stimulus to the study of renal hormone metabolism has been the development of sensitive, reliable, and specific tests for measuring trace amounts of hormone in plasma and urine and advances in molecular and cellular biology. Our subsequent increase in understanding of hormone metabolism has lead to novel strategies that by prolonging the action of short-lived peptide hormones improve their therapeutic efficacy. These strategies include the development of potent long-acting analogs of naturally occurring hormones and inhibitors of peptide hormone degradation.

The kidney may interact with hormones in several ways (Table 12.1). Perhaps the best studied of these are the many diverse actions that hormones have on the kidneys (see Chapter 1). Also of major importance is the role of the kidney in producing hormones such as erythropoietin (see Chapter 13, Part 2), 1,25-dihydroxyvitamin D_3 (see Chapter 13, Part 11), growth factors such as epidermal growth factor (EGF) and insulinlike growth factor-1 (IGF-1), and autocoids such as the prostaglandins, kinins, and adenosine (see Chapters 1, 4, 12, and 13). Finally, the kidney is the site of inactivation and elimination of many circulating hormones, especially polypeptide hormones. This chapter is concerned with this latter aspect of renal function. The disturbances of polypeptide hormone metabolism occurring in renal failure is also briefly reviewed.

Research into the renal metabolism of hormones has involved the use of radiolabeled hormones, unlabeled exogenous and endogenous hormones, and more recently, molecular biologic approaches. Many animal species have been studied both *in vivo* and *in vitro;* when possible, the data reviewed in this section are derived from studies in humans. The use of iodine-labeled hormones and sensitive assay techniques has simplified the study of polypeptide hormone metabolism. However, iodohormones, especially the heavily iodinated species, may suffer radiation damage and may lose biologic activity, factors that can alter their metabolism. Thus studies with recombinant, unlabeled hormones or analogs thereof are generally preferable. Nevertheless, even the study of endogenous polypeptide hormones is not without potential error because the presence of immunoreactivity or the lack thereof does not always correlate with biologic activity. Thus the measurement of endogenous hormones by radioimmunoassay may not distinguish between circulating heterogeneous forms of the hormones (e.g., precursor molecules, active hormone, protein-bound hormone, immunoreactive degradation products). This is a particular problem when evaluating hormone metabolism during renal failure, when there is often differential accumulation of various immunoreactive forms. Despite these potential pitfalls, much is now known about the renal metabolism of several important hormones.

The most informative studies have involved the direct measurement of arterial and renal venous hormone concentrations with simultaneously measured renal blood flow. This allows quantitation of the amount of hormone removed by the kidney and estimation of the renal contribution to peripheral metabolism of the hormone. The role of glomerular filtration in the renal removal of non–protein-bound hormones may be determined from the measured glomerular filtration rate (GFR) and the sieving coefficient of the hormone. If the total amount of a hormone removed by the kidney is greater than can be accounted for by glomerular filtration alone, this indicates that filtration-independent removal is occurring. In general, this represents removal from the postglomerular peritubular circulation. The presence of tubular absorption or secretion of a hormone may be determined from the rate of filtration and urinary excretion of the hormone.

METABOLISM OF POLYPEPTIDE HORMONES

The kidney is a major site of polypeptide hormone metabolism, and together with the liver, the kidney is responsible for most of the metabolism of these hormones. Some hormones and hormone fragments, such as growth hormone (GH), calcitonin,

TABLE 12.1. Relation Between the Kidney and Various Hormones

Hormones with Major Renal Action	Hormones Produced by the Kidney	Hormones Metabolized by the Kidney
Parathyroid hormone	1,25-Dihydroxyvitamin D_3	Polypeptide hormones
Vasopressin	Prostaglandins	Parathyroid hormone
Angiotensin	Erythropoietin	Insulin
Atrial natriuretic peptide	Renin	Glucagon
Calcitonin	Kinins	Growth hormone
Insulin	Angiotensin	Prolactin
Insulinlike growth factor-1	Insulinlike growth factor-1	Gastrointestinal hormones
1,25-Dihydroxyvitamin D_3	Epidermal growth factor	Calcitonin
Prostaglandins		Vasopressin
Aldosterone		Angiotensin
Thyroid hormones		Atrial natriuretic peptide
Catecholamines		Kinins
		Glycoprotein hormones
		Steroid hormones
		Adrenocortical hormones
		Sex hormones
		Thyroid hormones
		Catecholamines

C-peptide, and the COOH-terminal fragment of parathyroid hormone (PTH), are metabolized predominantly or exclusively by the kidney. Measured extraction ratios across the kidney indicate that the kidney removes between 16% and 45% of polypeptide hormone present in the renal circulation and contributes up to 80% of the total metabolic clearance rate, depending on the particular hormone. The metabolic clearance rate represents the volume of plasma from which the circulating hormone is irreversibly removed per unit time. The renal removal system is a high-capacity system, and unlike the liver, it is difficult to saturate. This largely reflects the predominance of glomerular filtration as a means of hormone removal. Consequently, the kidney clears the hormone from a constant volume of plasma per minute over a wide range of plasma hormone concentration. This in effect helps regulate plasma hormone levels because when the hormone concentration rises, a greater quantity is removed. This does not, however, constitute a true feedback system.

Removal of polypeptides from the glomerular circulation is determined by factors such as the size, shape, and charge of the molecule; the permeability properties of the glomerular filtration barrier; and glomerular plasma flow. Obviously, binding to a larger protein further restricts passage of the molecule—this occurs, for example, with IGFs. The sieving coefficient of most polypeptide hormones has not been directly measured; however, indirect measurements indicate that the glomerular sieving coefficient of free GH, with a molecular weight (MW) of 22,000 kDa, is approximately 0.7. The estimated sieving coefficient of insulin (MW = 6,000) is 0.9. Smaller peptide hormones such as angiotensin, vasopressin, and oxytocin are probably filtered without restriction. Once filtered, polypeptides are efficiently absorbed in the proximal tubule and relatively little intact hormone is excreted in the urine, usually less than 1% to 2% of the filtered load. Tubular absorption is by endocytosis. This process is largely initiated by binding to the endocytic membrane receptor megalin, originally named *gp330.* Megalin has been identified as a Heymann nephritis antigen present in the proximal tubular brush border and coated pits. It mediates endocytosis of several ligands including insulin and prolactin as well as albumin, EGF, and aminoglycosides. To a much lesser extent, endocytosis may be initiated by charge-related brush border membrane binding. The internalized hormone is transported within endocytotic vesicles (endosomes) until fusion with lysosomes occurs. Enzymatic degradation then follows, and the liberated amino acids diffuse across the basolateral cell membrane, eventually entering the peritubular circulation (Fig. 12.1). In some cases, degradation begins in endosomes, before fusion with lysosomes takes place. Trace amounts of hormone also may be transported in endosomes in intact and partially cleaved form to the opposite or same side of the cell where it is released extracellularly. The fate of filtered, small simple peptides such as the atrial natriuretic peptide (ANP), angiotensin, and bradykinin differs somewhat from that of larger complex polypeptides. These simple peptides are degraded at the enzyme-rich luminal surface of the brush border membrane by a process of membrane or contact degradation with near-complete absorption of the breakdown products. This process is similar to that of ingested peptides that come into contact with the intestinal brush border membrane. However, although it is useful conceptually to think of simple peptides as being degraded at the proximal tubule brush border and larger, more complex polypeptides as being catabolized within the proximal tubule cell after endocytosis, in fact, for many hormones, there is likely a good deal of overlap between these two pathways. A major benefit to the body attributable to this system of proximal tubular uptake and metabolism of polypeptide hormones is the deactivation of bioactive material that might exert unwanted effects on the more distal nephron segments. Understanding this process has led to the development of selective enzyme inhibitors that, by blocking proximal hydrolysis, enhance the distal action of a specific peptide. This novel strategy is discussed later in the context of ANP.

In addition to their removal from the glomerular circulation by means of filtration, it is evident that the kidney also removes polypeptide hormones from the peritubular circulation. The peritubular process in humans is most clearly demonstrated by the handling of insulin because glomerular filtration can account for only 60% of the insulin the kidneys remove. The bulk of insulin removed from the peritubular circulation is probably taken up by the contraluminal aspect of the tubules; lymphatic flow can account for only a small amount removed. In the best-studied cases, contraluminal uptake is initiated by hormone binding to specific receptors. This is followed by endocytosis of the hormone–receptor complex and subsequent degradation of hormone in endosomes and lysosomes. The major importance of this peritubular removal process appears to be the delivery of

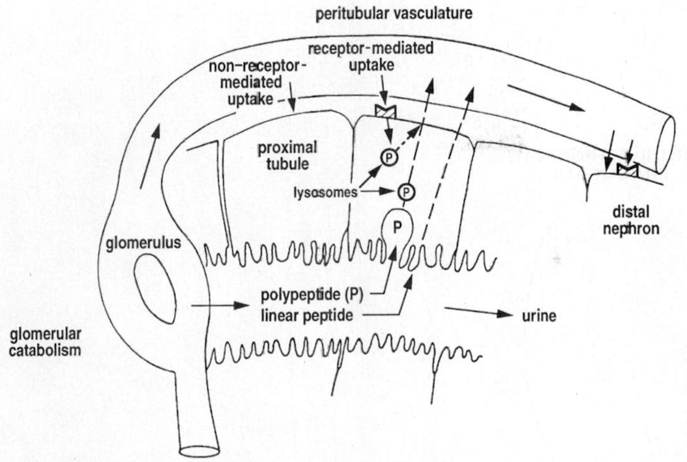

Figure 12.1. Diagrammatic representation of the renal handling of polypeptide and peptide hormones. Glomerular filtration, the major pathway of removal, is followed by avid absorption of polypeptides; this occurs by endocytosis. Internalized polypeptide is largely degraded in lysosomes, with return of end products to the circulation. By contrast, small, simple peptides undergo surface hydrolysis after contact with the brush border membrane, and the liberated amino acids are transported across the cell. Peritubular extraction of polypeptide and peptide hormones, which may involve specific receptor binding, is followed by degradation. Glomeruli have the potential to locally degrade certain simple peptide hormones.

renotropic hormones to their site of action. It is by this process that hormones such as PTH, calcitonin, and vasopressin are delivered to their receptor sites. Some polypeptide hormones, including PTH, ANP, angiotensin, vasopressin, and insulin, are also removed from the glomerular circulation by binding to hormone-specific receptors in the glomerulus. Although glomerular receptors are important in mediating hormone-induced alterations in glomerular contractility, permeability, and metabolism, they appear to have little quantitative importance in the overall removal of most hormones.

Effect of Renal Failure on Polypeptide Hormone Metabolism (Table 12.2)

In advanced renal failure, the plasma levels of most polypeptide hormones are elevated. This may be a consequence of several factors, including impaired renal and extrarenal degradation and abnormal patterns of hormone secretion. In early kidney failure, the rate of hormone removal falls secondary to the reduction of renal blood flow. As renal failure advances, this is compounded by a decrease in the capacity of the residual tissue to extract the hormone. Tubular absorption of filtered hormone usually is impaired, and fractional clearance of the hormone rises. Indeed, fractional clearance of filtered polypeptides may be used as a sensitive indicator of proximal tubular function. In addition to the loss of the kidney as a site of polypeptide hormone degradation, the accompanying uremia may depress extrarenal sites of hormone degradation, further elevating the plasma hormone level. As hormone levels are determined by both the rate of secretion and the rate of removal, it is obvious that if excessive secretion of hormone is present, this will by itself elevate the plasma concentration. Indeed, excessive secretion of PTH, prolactin, GH, and perhaps luteinizing hormone (LH) is seen in uremia. On the other hand, if hormone secretion is depressed in the presence of impaired degradation, plasma levels may be normal.

The nature of the hormones accumulating in uremia is of particular interest because they may be in heterogeneous forms. Usually, these heterogeneous forms consist of low-molecular-weight structures, presumably hormonal fragments; high-molecular-weight structures, either polymers or prohormones; and normal-molecular-weight structures, presumably the active specific hormones. Although they may cross-react with the hormone-specific antibody that is used to measure the plasma hormone concentration, not all these forms are biologically active. The heterogeneity in large part results from the accumulation of forms largely dependent on renal metabolism (e.g., proinsulin, C-terminal fragment of PTH).

A common and important consequence of uremia is an altered response to hormone action, usually in the form of resistance (e.g., GH, insulin, PTH). However, increased sensitivity occasionally may occur, as is the case with glucagon. The abnormal response may result from a reduction in receptor protein, a change in hormone–receptor interaction, altered postreceptor events, the presence or absence of counterregulatory hormones, or reduced hormone bioavailability resulting from increased association with circulating binding proteins as occurs with IGF-1. This increase in protein-bound hormone is largely the result of an increase in the level of circulating binding proteins, in part a consequence of impaired renal clearance.

TABLE 12.2. Effect of Renal Failure on Kidney-Polypeptide Hormone Interrelationships

Impaired hormone metabolism with consequent plasma hormone accumulation, often in heterogenous form
Renal mechanism: decreased delivery, impaired filtration, impaired cellular uptake, impaired degradation
Extrarenal mechanisms: impaired degradation by peripheral tissues (e.g., insulin by muscle, parathyroid hormone by liver)
Increased secretion
Abnormal feedback and control (e.g., prolactin, growth hormone)
Adaptive response to renal failure (e.g., parathyroid hormone, atrial natriuretic peptide)
Abnormal action
Reduced bioavailability (e.g., insulinlike growth factor-1)
Diminished tissue response (e.g., insulin, parathyroid hormone)
Increased tissue response (e.g., glucagon)

Metabolism of Individual Polypeptide Hormones in Health and in Renal Failure

Parathyroid Hormone (MW = 9,500)

PTH contains 84 amino acids and is normally found in the circulation (Fig. 12.2) both in the intact form and C-terminal metabolite. In renal failure, the N-terminal fragment may also be detected. These metabolic fragments are derived from enzymatic cleavage of the intact molecule in the liver and, to a lesser extent, the kidney and the parathyroid glands. The liver and the kidneys are the principal sites of intact PTH metabolism, accounting for 61% and 31%, respectively, of intact hormone removal. Although Kupffer cells in the liver remove the intact hormone and cleave it, hepatic removal of circulating C-terminal fragments occurs more slowly, if at all. In contrast, bone, which does not remove the intact hormone, avidly removes the N-terminal fragment that mediates PTH action in this tissue. Intact hormone, and N- and C-terminal fragments are removed by the kidney by glomerular filtration and tubular absorption. In addition, the biologically active intact hormone and the N-terminal fragment, but not the C-terminal fragment, are removed from the peritubular circulation by means of contraluminal uptake. This process involves receptor binding, activation of the

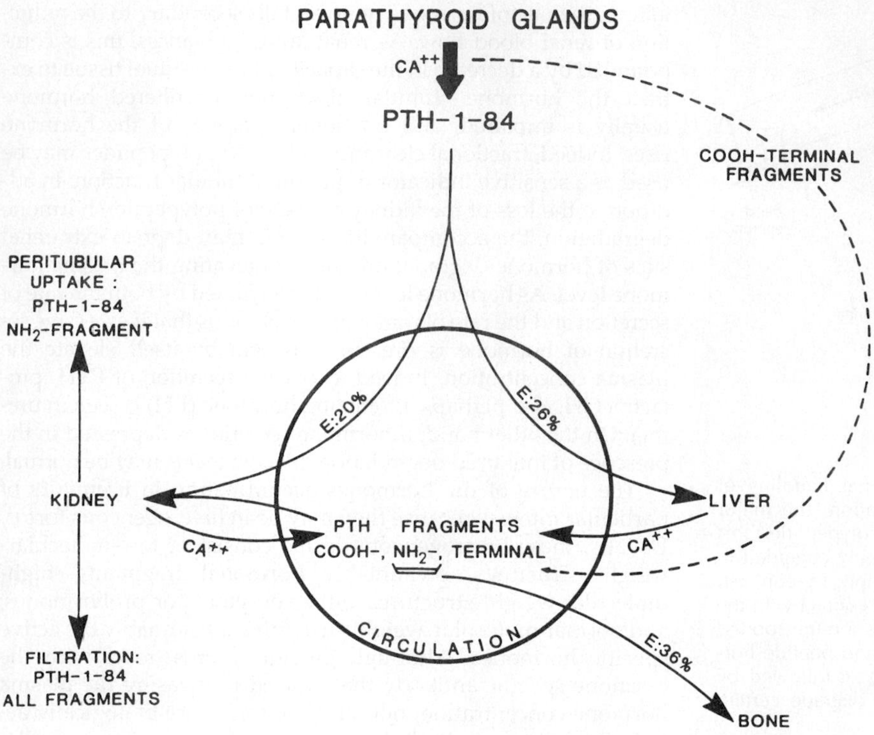

Figure 12.2. Metabolism of parathyroid hormone. E, arteriovenous extraction; PTH-1-84, the intact hormone.

signal transduction pathway, and degradation. The C- and N-terminal fragments are released into the renal circulation, probably as products of the peritubular processing of intact hormone. PTH-specific receptors are also present in glomeruli and may play a role in modulating the GFR. Despite the presence of these receptors, glomerular degradation is negligible. Interestingly evidence is accumulating that in addition to PTH, other humoral factors (phosphatonin) may regulate proximal tubular phosphate transport. This is highlighted by patients with X-linked hypophosphatemic rickets who have been found to carry a mutated gene (PEX gene) with endopeptidase homology. The renal phosphate wasting characteristic of these patients is possibly the result of impaired degradation of phosphatonin.

Advancing renal failure is accompanied by a rise in circulating PTH levels, which is a consequence of a varying combination of impaired degradation and increased secretion. In addition to impaired renal degradation of intact PTH and its major fragments, depression of extrarenal degradation of the intact hormone and N-terminal fragment occurs. In particular, the hepatic removal of the intact hormone is depressed. As the kidney is the major site of C-terminal fragment removal, the elevated plasma PTH levels, as measured by C-terminal immunoreactivity, are largely attributable to the impaired removal of this moiety. This is not the same for N-terminal immunoreactivity because of extrarenal sites of degradation. Accordingly, N-terminal immunoreactivity, which reflects both the N-terminal fragment and intact hormone, is not as dramatically elevated and is more reflective of increases in secretion. As outlined in Chapter 77, the secretion of PTH is increased in renal failure as a consequence of altered calcium, phosphorus, and vitamin D metabolism. Despite the consequences of increased PTH activity, which contribute to the uremic syndrome (see Chapter 68, Part 1), there is a degree of resistance to hormone action, especially action on bone. This may be attributed largely to altered vitamin D metabolism and perhaps also in part to a numerical downregulation of PTH receptors in response to high circulating hormone levels.

Calcitonin (MW = 3,500)

The kidney is the major site of calcitonin metabolism, accounting for approximately 65% of the total metabolic clearance rate of the hormone. In humans, the renal extraction of calcitonin is 17%, which is similar to that of insulin, suggesting that removal is largely via the glomerular filtration pathway. However, a significant peritubular process for the removal of calcitonin has been observed in the isolated perfused rat kidney. In addition to degrading the hormone, the kidney is a calcitonin target organ and possesses peritubular hormone-specific receptors; hormone binding to these receptors activates adenylate cyclase. In humans, the excretion of solute, especially calcium and phosphorous, is increased by large doses of calcitonin. However, smaller doses in some experimental animals decrease renal calcium excretion, and the true physiologic role of calcitonin remains unsettled. Calcitonin-binding sites are also found in tubular brush border membranes. These binding sites do not appear to mediate hormonal action and presumably participate in the internalization of filtered hormone; less than 2% of filtered calcitonin is excreted intact in the urine. *In vitro,* major subcellular sites of calcitonin degradation in the proximal tubule include the brush border membrane, lysosomes, and cytosol, although all of these sites may not be important *in vivo.* Proximal tubule basolateral membranes do not possess significant calcitonin degrading activity; presumably filtration-independent calcitonin degradation takes place after internalization by endocytosis, or at other nephron segments. Glomeruli contain the necessary enzymes to degrade calcitonin, but the role of glomerular calcitonin degradation *in vivo* has not been established. In renal failure, the metabolic clearance rate of calcitonin is decreased and the plasma level of the immunoreactive hormone rises; this is due predominantly to a high-molecular-weight species with unknown biologic activity. The metabolic consequences of the elevated hormone levels, if any, are unknown.

Insulin (MW = 6,000)

After being released from the pancreas into the portal circulation, approximately 40% of the insulin is extracted by the liver during fasting and less than half that amount during feeding (Fig. 12.3). Of the insulin reaching the systemic circulation, at least a third is removed by the kidney; other important peripheral sites of insulin metabolism include muscle and liver. Small amounts of the insulin precursor proinsulin also reach the systemic circulation, and the kidney accounts for the destruction of approximately 55% thereof. C-peptide, the peptide cleaved from proinsulin during insulin formation in the pancreas, is not removed by the liver; the kidney accounts for approximately 70% of its metabolism. In diabetic patients receiving insulin by injection, the importance of the kidney in insulin metabolism is enhanced because the hormone enters the systemic circulation directly without first passing through the liver. Insulin, proinsulin, and C-peptide are removed from the renal circulation by glomerular filtration and by extraction from the peritubular vessels; the latter accounts for 40% of the total renal insulin removal. A portion of the insulin removed by this pathway undergoes partial degradation and is released back into the circulation. Some intact insulin is transported to the lumen while the remainder is completely hydrolyzed. Whether the partially degraded insulin still retains bioactivity is unknown. Insulin-specific receptors are present on the contraluminal plasma membranes, and binding is followed by receptor phosphorylation and initiation of action. Filtered insulin is avidly absorbed by endocytosis in the proximal renal tubule and degraded in the endolysosomal compartment. Fractional urinary clearance of filtered insulin is less than 1%. Degrading activity is present along the length of the nephron but predominates in the proximal tubule, where filtered insulin is absorbed. The subcellular sites that possess insulin-degrading activity have been identified in the proximal tubules and include cytosol, endosomes, and lysosomes. The respective contributions of these various subcellular sites to *in vivo* insulin metabolism has not been completely established. However, it appears likely that most degradation occurs within lysosomes, with initial cleavage beginning in the endosomes involving the insulin degrading enzyme. Although this enzyme has also been located in cytosol it is still unknown how endocytosed insulin would come into contact with it. Trace amounts of insulin may escape intracellular degradation to be released from the endosomes to the cell exterior.

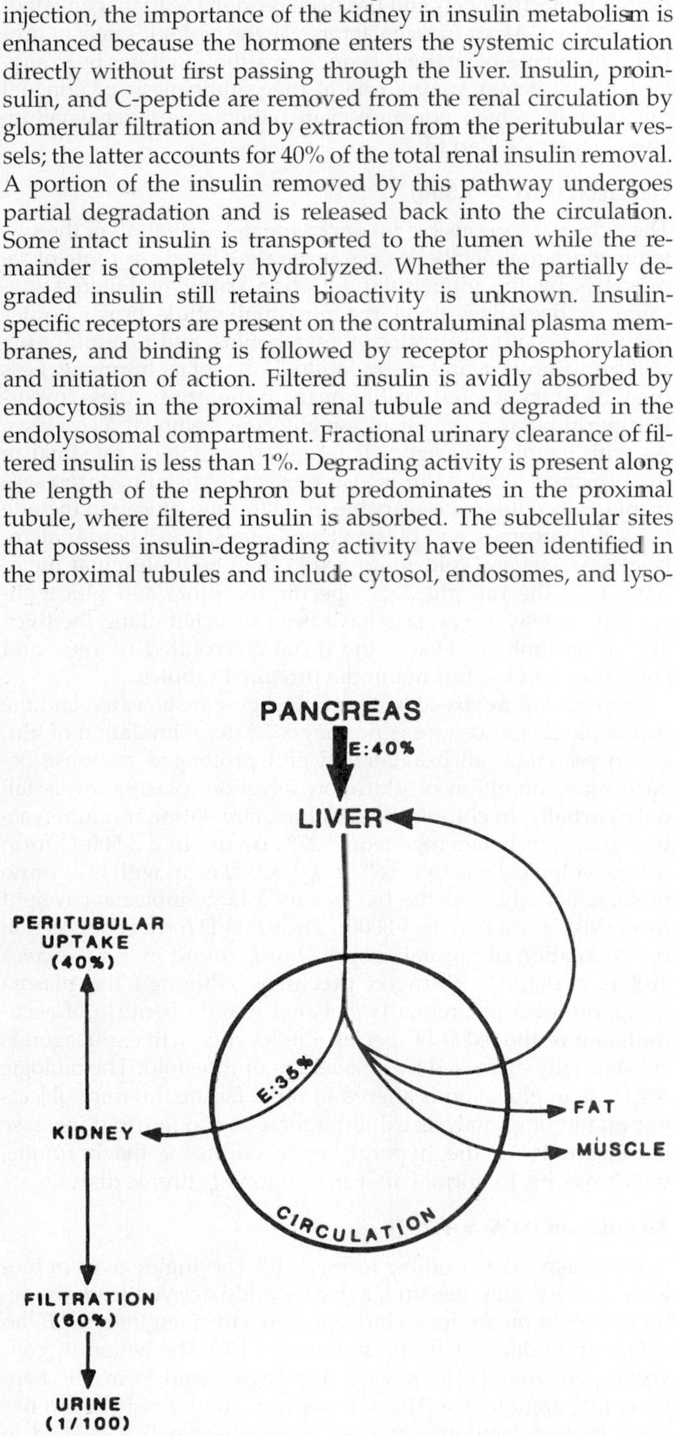

Figure 12.3. Metabolism of insulin. E, arteriovenous extraction.

In renal failure, basal insulin, proinsulin, and C-peptide levels are all elevated. However, the normal relationship between insulin and C-peptide levels whereby C-peptide may be used as a measure of insulin release is lost. This is consequent to the larger role the kidney plays in C-peptide metabolism and hence greater alteration in its metabolism in uremia. In renal failure, the total metabolic clearance rate of insulin is prolonged, mainly because of the loss of kidney as a site of degradation but also because of the inhibitory effect of uremia on degradation by muscle. Prolongation of insulin half-life in uremic diabetic patients often necessitates the reduction or discontinuation of administered insulin. Paradoxically, with the advent of renal failure, resistance to insulin develops, manifesting as carbohydrate intolerance in previously tolerant patients.

Insulinlike Growth Factor-1 (MW = 7,500)

IGF-1 mediates most of the growth-promoting actions of GH and causes an increase in renal blood flow, GFR, and tubular reabsorption of phosphate. This peptide growth factor is produced locally by most tissues, including the kidneys, but the liver is the main source of the circulating hormone. In the circulation, most IGF-1 is complexed with several high-affinity IGF-binding proteins (IGFBPs), especially IGFBP-3, which together with an acid–labile subunit forms a 150-kD complex. Altogether, six different IGFBPs have been identified. Less than 1% of the IGF-I is present as free hormone. Because of the large size of the IGF-1–IGFBP complexes (32 to 150 kD), glomerular filtration of IGF-1 is severely restricted and the kidney's role in its disposal is limited. This has been confirmed in human studies that found the serum clearance of IGF-1 to be similar in patients with advanced chronic renal failure and normal controls. Tissue IGFBPs also limit the uptake of IGF-1 at a cellular level. The free circulating IGF-1 that is filtered is absorbed in the proximal tubule by endocytosis, followed by intracellular degradation, which proceeds at a much slower rate than occurs with insulin. IGF-1–specific receptors are present throughout the kidney. In the proximal tubules, they are far more abundant in the contraluminal plasma membranes than in the brush border membranes.

Urinary excretion of IGF-1 tends to be higher in the young, reflecting the higher serum levels, and declines with age. It is increased threefold in acromegalics. In nephrotic syndrome, with lessening of the restrictive glomerular filtration barrier, the filtration of the smaller IGF-1–IGFBP complexes increases and urinary IGF-1 excretion increases fivefold. This may contribute to the slightly decreased serum IGF-1 levels seen in nephrotic children, although serum IGF-1 levels do not correlate with urinary excretion rate. It has also been suggested that the subsequent increase in tubular cell exposure to the bioactive growth factor may play a role in mediating the progression of renal disease. In subjects with normal renal function, IGFBP-2 and IGFBP-3 are the major urinary IGFBPs. In patients with acute or chronic renal failure, urinary IGFBP-3 protease activity is increased and IGFBP-3 almost disappears from urine while urinary IGFBP-1 levels increase, presumably resulting from increased tubular secretion. In nephrotic children, urinary IGFBP-1 excretion increases 12-fold, whereas IGFBP-2 and IGFBP-3 excretion increase twofold. Urinary IGFBP-3 excretion correlates with the degree of proteinuria, but no correlation exists between serum levels of IGFBPs and their urinary excretion, serum levels being well above normal. In renal failure, the serum IGF-1–binding capacity increases by an order of magnitude and is likely caused by the increased levels of IGFBP-1 and IGFBP-2 and partially degraded IGFBP-3. Reduced renal clearance accounts for the increase in IGFBP-3 fragments and in part for the increase in intact IGFBPs. The overall effect of the increase in serum-binding capacity is to maintain the circulating IGF-1 concentration at a relatively normal level despite reduced hepatic IGF-1 production. However, because the complexed IGF-1 is not readily bioavailable, this contributes to the growth retardation seen in uremia.

Growth Hormone (MW = 22,000)

The clearance of GH from the circulation is complicated by the presence of heterogeneous circulating forms and the presence of serum GH–binding proteins (GHBPs). Whereas most (approximately 85%) of circulating GH consists of a 22-kD form, the rest consists of a 20-kD form, dimers, aggregates, and large fragments. One GHBP (61 kD) corresponds to the extracellular domain of the GH receptor and binds with high affinity as a dimer to GH. The other, non–receptor-related GHBP forms a monomeric low-affinity complex with GH. Approximately 50% of the 22-kD form of GH circulates bound to GHBPs, mostly the high-affinity form. Protein binding reduces the volume of distribution and the metabolic clearance rate of GH. In humans, the kidney is the major site of GH clearance, accounting for half of the total serum GH metabolic clearance rate. The renal handling of free GH resembles that of other polypeptides with the glomerular filtration–tubular reabsorption pathway predominant; a minor peritubular removal process does exist. Animal studies have indicated that the hormone is avidly reabsorbed by endocytosis from the proximal tubular lumen with subsequent lysosomal degradation, and only 1% of the filtered hormone appears in the urine. Although urinary GH excretion rates have been used to assess GH secretion, even minimal tubular dysfunction can reduce GH absorption and thus alter urinary excretion.

In advanced renal failure, the metabolic clearance rate of GH falls significantly and is often associated with elevated plasma GH levels. Abnormal secretion of GH occurs, and this may also contribute to the elevated plasma hormone concentration. Indeed, after the administration of thyroid-stimulating hormone or glucose, a paradoxical rise in GH levels occurs and an exaggerated rise is seen after the administration of L-Dopa. In humans, renal GHBP excretion is not affected by renal failure because their size precludes filtration even by the healthy kidney. However, GHBP levels fall, and this likely reflects reduced production because of a fall in the number of tissue GH receptors from which the GHBP is derived. It is thought that this reduction in GH receptors is a cause of GH resistance in uremia.

Prolactin (MW = approximately 23,000)

Similar in structure to GH, prolactin circulates predominantly in a monomeric free form of 23 kD and is largely removed from the circulation by glomerular filtration. In normal subjects, the renal extraction is approximately 16%. This is less than the filtration fraction indicating that filtration of the molecule is restricted. After glomerular filtration, the hormone is absorbed by the proximal tubular cells with less than 1% of the filtered load being excreted in the urine. The exact contribution of the kidney to prolactin metabolism in humans is unknown but is presumably considerable. Animal studies indicate the presence of hormone-specific receptors in the kidneys and in lower species prolactin plays an important role in sodium and water metabolism. However, in humans, a prolactin effect on renal electrolyte and water excretion has not been established.

In many patients with chronic renal failure, basal plasma prolactin levels rise and are elevated in approximately 80% of females and more than 30% of males. The hyperprolactinemia is not acutely suppressed by the administration of dopamine or bromocriptine, and after administration of thyroid-releasing hormone, a suboptimal and prolonged rise in prolactin levels occurs. These findings suggest both a disorder at the level of the pituitary and a defect in the peripheral metabolism of the hormone. Indeed, the measured total metabolic clearance rate of prolactin is reduced by a third in renal failure. On the other hand, long-term administration of bromocriptine suppresses elevated prolactin levels and has been used in the management of galactorrhea. Apart from galactorrhea, the biologic effect of prolactin in the uremic patient is unclear, although it has been suggested that it may play a role in the pathogenesis of gonadal dysfunction, which is common in patients with renal failure (see Chapter 74, Part 6).

Glucagon (MW = 3,500)

The kidney is responsible for approximately one third of the systemic glucagon metabolic clearance rate. The major route of removal is by the glomerular filtration pathway. Filtered glucagon is degraded along the proximal tubule brush border membrane, with absorption of metabolites, and to a minor extent by absorption and degradation of the intact hormone. Less than 2% of the filtered load appears in the urine. A less important peritubular mechanism for glucagon removal also exists. As with insulin, glucagon degradation activity is maximal in the proximal tubules but is also present in distal nephron segments. Subcellular sites capable of degrading glucagon include cytosol, lysosomes, and plasma membranes. Brush border membranes are several-fold more active than contraluminal membranes. In the rat, glucagon-specific receptors and glucagon-sensitive adenylate cyclase have been detected along the thick ascending limbs of Henle, the distal convoluted tubules, and collecting tubules, but not in the proximal tubules.

In renal failure, basal levels of glucagon are elevated and the metabolic clearance rate is prolonged. After stimulation of glucagon secretion, an exaggerated and prolonged response occurs; after inhibition of glucagon secretion, plasma levels fall only partially. In chronic renal failure, circulating immunoreactive glucagon is heterogeneous: 27% occurs in a 3,500-D form that is biologically active, 56% in a 9,000-D form with little or no biologic activity, and the balance as a large-molecular-weight form (MW = more than 40,000). The 9,000-D form is not seen in the circulation of normal subjects but is found in the pancreas and is perhaps a glucagon precursor. Although the plasma glucagon level in uremia is elevated mainly because of accumulation of the 9,000-D species, the level of active glucagon is substantially increased by an average of threefold. The biologic response to glucagon is altered in renal failure: uremic subjects not undergoing dialysis exhibit a threefold to fourfold increase in sensitivity to the hyperglycemic effects of the hormone, which returns to normal after institution of chronic dialysis.

Angiotensin (MW = 1,297)

Angiotensin exists in three forms, with varying degrees of biologic activity: angiotensin I, a decapeptide derived from the action of renin on angiotensinogen, is inactive; angiotensin II, an octapeptide derived from angiotensin I by the action of converting enzyme, is the most active angiotensin form; the heptapeptide angiotensin III is formed from angiotensin II and has some biologic activity. Circulating angiotensin II is formed in the pulmonary vascular bed. Many tissues, however, including the kidney (especially in proximal tubules and to a lesser extent arterioles and glomeruli), possess the necessary enzymes for the local generation of angiotensin II and local renin-angiotensin systems are likely as important as the circulating system. The half-life of circulating angiotensin II is very short (less than 1 minute). Several organs extract the hormone, including the kidney, liver, and muscle. This is followed by rapid destruction by peptidases present in their vascular beds and tissues. In the kidney, angiotensin enters the proximal tubule by glomerular filtration and by secretion of locally generated hormone or its precursor, which is converted to angiotensin in the tubule lumen. In the proximal tubule, angiotensin is handled as are other simple linear peptides; it is degraded at the brush border, and the constituent amino acids are then reabsorbed. Angiotensin-converting enzyme (ACE) is present in abundance in the brush border membrane. In addition to activating angiotensin I at this location, it may participate in the degradation of other filtered peptides such as the kinins. Moreover, ACE is secreted by tubular cells in the collecting duct, where it presumably inactivates kinins generated in the distal nephron.

The kidney degrades about 70% of angiotensin II circulating through it. Because this is more than can be accounted for by glomerular filtration, filtration-independent pathways for catabolism of angiotensin must exist. Within the kidney, angiotensin II binds to specific receptors in the glomerular mesangium, where it stimulates contraction of the mesangial cells. In glomerular diseases with mesangial proliferation, angiotensin II acts as a growth factor, contributing to the mitogenic response of the mesangial cell. AT1 receptors for angiotensin II have been identified on both the afferent and the efferent arteriole mediating local vasoconstriction. The effect of angiotensin II on glomerular microcirculation is further compounded by the presence of vasodilatory AT2 receptors on the afferent and efferent arterioles. Receptors are also present in cortical brush border and contraluminal tubular membranes. Contraluminal receptors are present along the length of the nephron, especially the proximal tubule. Receptor binding initiates the tubular action of the hormone, namely enhanced NaCl and $NaHCO_3$ transport at physiologic dosages; higher dosages inhibit transport. Apical binding is followed by endocytosis; however, non–receptor-mediated degradation by brush border membrane peptidases (aminopeptidase A and meprin A) probably accounts for most of the luminal degradation. There is growing evidence that angiotensin II is accumulated intracellularly in tissues, including kidney tissues, with a much longer half-life of 15 minutes as compared with less than 1 minute for circulating angiotensin. Accumulated angiotensin may be of significance for its growth-promoting effect. Angiotensin II–induced proliferative response of mesangial cells is abolished by transfection with aminopeptidase.

Atrial Natriuretic Peptide (MW = 3,080)

ANP is a potent hormone with natriuretic, diuretic, and vasodilator properties. Although ANP is found in many tissues, its predominant site of synthesis and storage is the cardiac atria. ANP is the best studied member of a larger family of peptides. Brain natriuretic peptide (BNP) was first described in the central nervous system, but it is now known that the heart is an important source of circulating BNP. C-type natriuretic peptide (CNP) is the most recently discovered of the three natriuretic peptides. Originally isolated from porcine brain tissue, it is widely distributed within the vascular endothelium. Furthermore, a specific CNP receptor has been identified on vascular smooth muscle cells, and CNP immunoreactivity has been found in plasma from dogs and humans. Finally, urodilatin, or renal natriuretic peptide (RNP), is found in the urine, presumably a result of renal synthesis, and it is not found in the plasma. Thus far, three receptors that bind natriuretic peptides have been identified. Two of these receptors are guanylate cyclase linked and mediate the natriuretic and vascular actions of the natriuretic hormones. There are two subtypes of these guanylate cyclase (GC) receptors: GC-A receptors and GC-B receptors, which differ in their ligand specificity and tissue distribution. The third receptor is termed the clearance or C-receptor. It does not mediate any hemodynamic or natriuretic actions and is not linked to guanylate cyclase. However, there is recent evidence that the C-receptor may inhibit adenyl cyclase and may also mediate other ANP actions such as inhibition of cell proliferation or antagonism of other hormone effects.

The plasma half-life of ANP is very short (2.5 to 4 minutes), and in end-stage renal failure, the half-life is prolonged by a third. Plasma ANP levels are increased in patients receiving hemodialysis, possibly because of increased secretion secondary to volume overload. However, increased ANP levels are found in patients with chronic renal failure even when cardiac filling pressures and intravascular volume are reduced. In humans, the renal extraction ratio for ANP is 35%, and the renal extraction is 78 ml/min per kidney in patients with creatinine clearance rates of 69 ml/min per kidney. Because vasculature at many sites can clear ANP from plasma, glomerular filtration accounts for only 30% of the total renal clearance of ANP and the kidney accounts for only 14% of the total metabolic clearance of the hormone in dogs. Filtered ANP is degraded by renal tubular cells, most likely predominantly by proximal tubular brush border peptidases, although all portions of the nephron possess ANP-degrading activity. In the kidney, endopeptidase 24.11 is located most significantly in the proximal tubule brush border. This enzyme hydrolyzes specific bonds within the ring portion of ANP, and the hormone thus loses biologic activity. Orally active specific inhibitors of endopeptidase 24.11 have been developed and are being evaluated in humans. When given to human volunteers, these inhibitors can increase plasma ANP levels and urinary excretion of intact ANP. Under some circumstances, endopeptidase 24.11 inhibitors can produce a natriuresis and reduce elevated blood pressure. The natriuretic effect of endopeptidase inhibitors is significant even in patients with chronic renal failure and may also benefit patients with congestive heart failure or cirrhotic ascites. Endopeptidase inhibitors may produce their natriuretic effect by preventing the degradation of filtered ANP at the proximal tubule, thus allowing ANP to act more distally within the lumen of the nephron. However, because endopeptidase 24.11 is found at many sites in the body and is not specific for ANP but also degrades BNP, bradykinin, angiotensin, and other small peptides, the precise mechanism by which inhibition of this enzyme leads to physiologic alterations is unknown.

The kidney also possesses non–filtration-dependent pathways for ANP metabolism. Because only insignificant ANP-degrading activity exists in basolateral membrane fractions of homogenized kidney cortex, ANP is unlikely to be degraded at the contraluminal surface of the proximal tubule cell. Of great interest, however, is the observation that more than 95% of renal cortical ANP receptors are C-receptors. On binding to C-receptors, ANP is internalized by receptor-mediated endocytosis and delivered to lysosomes, where it is degraded to amino acids. C-receptors have been hypothesized to regulate plasma ANP concentration by binding ANP without producing a physiologic effect. ANP analogs that bind to clearance receptors but not to GC-receptors have been developed. When these ligands have been administered to laboratory animals, ANP is displaced from clearance receptors, plasma ANP levels increase, and the actions of ANP are enhanced.

Vasopressin (MW = 1,084)

The metabolism of vasopressin occurs mainly in the kidney, liver, and prehepatic tissues (intestines). The kidney is responsible for about two thirds of the total metabolic clearance rate of the hormone. Vasopressin is removed from the renal circulation mainly by glomerular filtration but also by extraction from the peritubular circulation. The kidney has a large capacity for removing the hormone, and removal by the whole organ is not saturated over a wide range of vasopressin concentrations. Most filtered vasopressin is hydrolyzed at the proximal tubule brush border with absorption of the degradation products. However, this cyclic peptide can also be absorbed by the proximal tubule after filtration and subsequently degraded in lysosomes. Although whole organ clearance is not saturable, tubular uptake of vasopressin is, and the percentage of filtered vasopressin excreted in the urine varies from 6% at basal plasma levels to 60% at supraphysiologic levels. Hormone-specific receptors (V2 receptors) are present on basolateral plasma membranes of the renal tubular epithelium, and receptor binding is followed by activation of adenylate cyclase with measurable formation of cyclic adenosine monophosphate (cAMP) in the collecting tubules. Binding of vasopressin to its renal V2 receptor induces proteolytic cleavage of the receptor by a coexpressed plasma membrane metalloendoproteinase. V1 receptors are present in glomerular mesangial cells, and binding to these receptors stimulates mesangial contraction and may thereby modulate GFR.

Renal failure is associated with reduced renal removal of the hormone, and whereas tubular uptake of filtered hormone is unaltered in chronic renal failure, it is impaired in acute renal failure. In patients receiving regular hemodialysis treatment, plasma vasopressin levels are usually elevated. Although this correlates well with plasma osmolality in the patient not receiving dialysis, vasopressin levels do not fall during dialysis despite a fall in osmolality. This may be related in part to impaired hormone metabolism, but other factors operative during dialysis therapy, including volume removal, which acts as a stimulus to vasopressin release, and changes in hemodynamics and solute content, make interpretation difficult.

METABOLISM OF GLYCOPROTEIN HORMONES

The renal metabolism of glycoprotein hormones is less well understood than that of peptide hormones. However, it is recognized that the kidney is a major site of clearance of several glycoprotein hormones and their metabolites, including LH, follicle-stimulating hormone (FSH), human gonadotropin, and thyroid-stimulating hormone (TSH). The role the kidney plays differs with each hormone, in part resulting from differences in the structure, conformation, and charge of the molecule. Indirect estimates in animals indicate that the kidney accounts for 95% and 78% of the total metabolic clearance of LH and FSH, respectively. Renal failure is associated with a decrease in the total metabolic clearance of most glycoprotein hormones. Clearance of TSH is reduced by 43% in patients with renal failure. In part, this may be accounted for by altered TSH glycosylation. Depending on the balance between hormone secretion and metabolism, the plasma levels may not be elevated. Erythropoietin (EPO, 34 kD) is produced by the kidney but is largely cleared through extrarenal pathways. Elimination of EPO in the sheep is unchanged by nephrectomy, although in healthy humans, an estimated 3% to 10% of EPO is cleared by the kidneys. In general, the renal clearance of glycoprotein hormones is relatively slow compared with that of nonglycosylated polypeptide hormones. This may be attributed to restricted glomerular filtration due to the large size (MW = more than 25,000 kDa) and the structure of the glycoprotein hormone. Also, the lack of peritubular hormone-specific receptors excludes a receptor-mediated pathway of removal from the postglomerular circulation. It is noteworthy that the urinary excretion of EPO is increased in nephrotic syndrome, whereas less than 10% of endogenous erythropoietin is excreted unchanged in the urine of healthy individuals. Tubular absorption of filtered glycoprotein hormones is generally less efficient than that of the nonglycosylated polypeptide hormones, hence the finding that the urinary clearance of most glycoproteins is high. For example, the urinary clearance of FSH is 43% of the total FSH cleared by the kidney, whereas for peptide hormones the fractional urinary excretion is usually less than 1%.

METABOLISM OF STEROID HORMONES

Whereas the liver is the major site of steroid hormone inactivation, the kidney is the major site of steroid metabolite excretion. With a few important exceptions, metabolism of intact steroid hormone by the kidney is minimal. This is because steroid hormones circulate bound to plasma proteins, namely albumin and certain globulins, with high affinity for specific steroid hormones. A relatively small quantity of intact hormone, that which is not bound to plasma protein, is freely filtered or removed from the postglomerular peritubular circulation. Steroid hormones are lipid soluble, so they enter the tubular epithelial cells where they bind to receptors and undergo metabolic transformation. In contrast to the bound, intact hormone, circulating metabolites, largely derived from hepatic metabolism, are freely filtered and readily eliminated by the kidney.

Glucocorticoids

The liver is the major site of glucocorticoid inactivation, being responsible for 90% of the metabolism. The kidney also inactivates glucocorticoids but serves mainly as a site of elimination of hepatic metabolites, excreting approximately 90% of these products in the urine in the form of sulfate and glucuronic acid conjugates; conjugation of metabolites does not occur in the kidney. Less than 1% of the glucocorticoids excreted in urine is intact hormone. In humans, cortisol is the most prevalent corticosteroid synthesized by the adrenal gland. Ninety percent of the serum cortisol is bound with high affinity to the steroid-binding globulin transcortin or, to a lesser extent, albumin. Free cortisol is readily filtered and between 60% and 90% is absorbed, especially in the distal tubule. The kidney is the major site where the active hormone cortisol is transformed into the inactive metabolite cortisone and as discussed next, abnormalities in this process may lead to pronounced clinical manifestations. This conversion is accomplished by 11β-hydroxysteroid dehydrogenase (11β-OHSD) expressed in two forms: 11β-OHSD1 and 11β-OHSD2. In the proximal tubule, 11β-OHSD1 regulates the glucocorticoid level to control exposure of tubular epithelial cells to glucocorticoids. This conversion appears to be important for the kidney, given that glucocorticoids are known to induce experimental polycystic kidney disease in rodent neonates and low enzymatic activity of 11β-OHSD1 has been implicated in the development of renal cysts in cpk mice with hereditary polycystic renal disease.

In the distal nephron, the isoenzyme 11β-OHSD2, localized in aldosterone-sensitive cells of the collecting duct, is important because mineralocorticoid receptors do not distinguish between cortisol and aldosterone. Because plasma cortisol concentrations are several orders of magnitude greater than those of aldosterone, renal inactivation of cortisol by metabolism to cortisone allows aldosterone to act independently of glucocorticoids in the kidney. When the kidney does not convert cortisol to cortisone, either because of congenital absence of 11β-OHSD2 (syndrome of apparent mineralocorticoid excess) or because of inactivation of this enzyme (as with glycyrrhetinic acid, a component of licorice), cortisol can then act on renal mineralocorticoid receptors and hypertension, hypokalemia, and sodium retention ensue. Similarly, kaliuresis consequent to furosemide therapy may in part be due to inactivation of 11β-OHSD2. Also, the synergistic action of vasopressin and aldosterone on sodium reabsorption in the collecting duct has been explained by the stimulation of 11β-OHSD2 by vasopressin. Endogenous inhibitors of 11β-OHSD have been extracted from urine but not yet identified; they have been termed *glycyrrhetinic acidlike factors,* or GALF. The kidney (collecting duct) also possesses 6β-hydroxylase and is an important source of urinary 6β-hydroxycortisol and 6β-hydroxycortisone. Although this enzyme is mainly active during fetal life and infancy, renal 6β-hydroxycortisol may be important in certain hypertensive states by resulting in an increase in tubular sodium reabsorption.

In advanced renal failure, urinary excretion of conjugated 17-hydroxcorticosteriods decreases and plasma levels rise. Accumulation of cortisol metabolites in renal failure may interfere with radioimmunoassays of plasma cortisol concentration. Total and free cortisol levels are elevated, and the mean 24-hour plasma total cortisol level is double that seen in normal subjects. However, this is not associated with clinical features of hyperadrenocorticism. In patients with end-stage renal failure who are receiving hemodialysis therapy, the cortisol half-life averages 115 minutes, being prolonged from the normal value of 55 minutes. This prolongation is presumably in part caused by the loss of functioning renal tissue and in part secondary to the effect of uremia on hepatic cortisol metabolism. The normal diurnal rhythm of cortisol secretion is not disturbed in these patients, although during dialysis treatments, secretory activity does occur. Because cortisol is largely protein bound, little (less than 3%) of the total daily production of the hormone is removed during dialysis. Resistance to dexamethasone suppression is common, suggesting some hypothalamic-pituitary-adrenal dysfunction. However, it has been reported that the metabolism of dexamethasone is significantly increased in renal failure, particularly in patients receiving hemodialysis therapy. Therefore, resistance to dexamethasone suppression may in part result from rapid inactivation of the administered dexamethasone.

Aldosterone

The plasma half-life of aldosterone is approximately 30 minutes. As with other steroid hormones, the kidney is of secondary importance to the liver in removing and inactivating aldosterone. This is well illustrated by studies in animals: 30 minutes after the intravenous injection of radiolabeled aldosterone, 40% localizes in the liver and 2.5% in the kidneys. Aldosterone circulates less tightly bound to plasma proteins than are glucocorticoids, hence it is more rapidly cleared from plasma than glucocorticoids and renal extraction is more prominent. Ten percent of the aldosterone passing through the kidney is extracted, compared with 92% passing through the liver. The kidney's major role is to eliminate hepatic metabolites of aldosterone in the urine, which it achieves by glomerular filtration and tubular secretion. Unbound aldosterone is freely filtered at the glomerulus, and although some is excreted in the urine, 80% to 95% of the filtered hormone is absorbed by the tubular cells, both proximal and distal. Absorption appears to be a passive process influenced by sodium and water transport. Aldosterone is also removed from the peritubular circulation. Metabolic transformation of aldosterone in the kidney is rapid; accordingly, metabolites present in this organ are derived from both local and hepatic metabolism. Aldosterone metabolism in both the liver and the kidney is sex dependent and influenced by sodium intake; both the amount and nature of renal metabolites differ according to sex and dietary salt intake. In general, the bulk of the aldosterone metabolites in the kidney consist of polar-neutral hydroxylated compounds (nonconjugated) and nonpolar reduced compounds. Sulfates and carboxylic acid products are also found. Animal studies suggest that the nonpolar ring-A–reduced metabolites may be important in the regulation or mediation of aldosterone action. Indeed, several of the reduced metabolites have demonstrable bioactivity, albeit less than that of the parent hormone.

In advanced renal failure, aldosterone metabolites accumulate and the plasma aldosterone concentration, largely determined by its rate of secretion, is often elevated. Under these circumstances, aldosterone secretion is mainly influenced by the renin-angiotensin system and is modulated by the plasma potassium concentration. In anephric humans, plasma aldosterone levels tend to be low, perhaps in part because of an increase in the hepatic metabolic clearance rate. In these subjects, the various stimuli known to increase plasma aldosterone are effective, although the response is qualitatively different from the normal, being largely modified by the basal aldosterone level and sodium balance. In particular, potassium is an important determinant of aldosterone secretion in anephric humans. In some patients with renal failure, aldosterone levels may be low, but these patients have an isolated deficiency in aldosterone production, usually secondary to hyporeninemia.

Estrogens

Although quantitatively of minor importance, the kidney does inactivate and conjugate estrogens. Circulating non–protein-bound estrogens undergo glomerular filtration, followed by tubular absorption of approximately 90% of the filtered hormone; only small amounts of unaltered hormone appear in the urine. Thus, after the intravenous administration of radiolabeled estrone or estradiol, less than 4% appears in the urine in the unconjugated form. However, urinary excretion of estrogen metabolites is of major importance. Conjugated estrogen metabolites undergo glomerular filtration, and there is tubular secretion of estradiol-16-glucuronide, estradiol-17-glucuronide, and estradiol-3-glucuronide.

In preeclamptic toxemia, the urinary clearance of several of the estrogen conjugates is depressed, the decrease in estradiol-16-glucuronide correlating with the decrease in creatinine clearance. In renal failure, the kidney's ability to conjugate estrogens is impaired. Nevertheless, estrogen levels in premenopausal females with chronic renal failure are similar to those found in normal women during the follicular phase of the ovarian cycle. In most females receiving dialysis treatment, menstrual disturbances are present and are associated with an anovulatory hormonal pattern with estrogen, progesterone, and FSH levels at low-normal concentrations. LH levels may be elevated, however. The abnormal hormone pattern seen in chronic renal failure probably results from a defect at the hypothalamic-pituitary level because primary ovarian failure is uncommon; altered metabolism does not appear to be a factor. In advanced renal failure, fecal elimination of estrogen metabolites increases considerably and accounts for 60% to 80% of the metabolites. These products are effectively removed by hemodialysis.

Testosterone

Testosterone is metabolized in several tissues. Two metabolic pathways exist. The first involves the enzyme 17β-hydroxysteroid dehydrogenase; oxidation occurs at the 17-position, and the hormone is inactivated. This process produces 17-ketosteroids and occurs in several tissues, including, to a minor extent, the kidney. The second metabolic pathway occurs primarily in target tissues; it requires the enzyme 5α-reductase and results in the formation of active products, including dihydrotestosterone. The importance of the kidney in testosterone metabolism is in the elimination of metabolites, especially androsterone and etiocholanolone, the major urinary 17-ketosteroid. Although fecal elimination is usually small, in patients with end-stage renal failure who are receiving hemodialysis, the gastrointestinal route becomes preeminent and accounts for excretion of 60% to 80% of the metabolites; in addition, there is considerable removal by hemodialysis. In chronic renal failure, plasma testosterone levels fall, apparently secondary to the effects of uremia on the testes and perhaps in some instances because of impaired hypothalamic-pituitary function and increased testosterone metabolism. Oligospermia or azoospermia is common.

METABOLISM OF THYROID HORMONES

Thyroid hormones, iodinated amino acids, may undergo several metabolic transformations in the body, including conjugation, oxidative deamination, decarboxylation, and deiodination. The latter is the major pathway for thyroid hormone metabolism and accounts for approximately 75% of hormone disposal. Iodothyronines can be deiodinated at either the phenolic (outer) ring or the tyrosyl (inner) ring, and these reactions are catalyzed by 5′-deiodinases and 5-deiodinases, respectively. The 5′-deiodination of thyroxine (T_4) yields triiodothyronine (T_3), the metabolically most active thyroid hormone. Kidney and liver are important sites for this conversion, with the greatest 5′-deiodinase activity per tissue weight found in the kidney. Renal 5′-deiodinase has been localized to the basolateral membrane of the proximal convoluted tubule. About half of the daily thyroid gland iodothyronine production is excreted in the urine as the completely deioninated derivative thyronine or its acetic acid analog. Thyroid hormones are bound to cytosolic proteins and nuclear receptors in renal cells, accounting for their effect on renal growth and function. Both unbound T_4 and T_3 are filtered, and although approximately 65% of the T_4 is subsequently reabsorbed by the tubules, secretion of T_3 occurs. This T_3 may be in part derived from the renal conversion of T_4. However, because thyroid hormones are largely protein bound, the extent of removal of T_4 and T_3 by the kidney is small, and an arteriovenous concentration difference cannot be measured. Thus only small amounts of thyroid hormones are excreted unaltered in the urine. Renal excretion of thyroid hormones is increased in nephrotic urine, however. The kidneys also provide the major pathway for iodide elimination from the body: iodide is filtered at the glomerulus, then a portion is passively reabsorbed by the tubules, so the renal iodide clearance is about 30 to 40 ml/min. Thyroid hormone metabolism in chronic renal failure is discussed in detail in Chapter 74, part 4.

Selected Readings

Christensen EI, Birn H. Hormone, growth factor, and vitamin handling by proximal tubule cells. *Curr Opin Nephrol Hypertens* 1997;6:20–27.
Reviews the metabolism of protein hormones by proximal tubule.

Egfjord M. Corticosteroid metabolism in isolated perfused rat liver and kidney. *Acta Physiol Scand* 1995;155(S627):7–42.
A detailed review of steroid metabolism with emphasis on aldosterone metabolism.

Kaptein EM. Thyroid hormone metabolism and thyroid diseases in chronic renal failure. *Endocr Rev* 1996;17:45–63.
Reviews the impact of renal failure on thyroid hormone metabolism.

Markham A, Bryson HM. Epoetin alfa. *Drugs* 1995;49(2): 232–254.
A review of its pharmacodynamic and pharmacokinetic properties and therapeutic use in nonrenal applications.

Mellor JD, Hobkirk R. In vitro synthesis of estrogen glucuronides and sulfates by human renal tissue. *Can J Biochem* 1975;53(7):779–783.

Morris DJ, Brem AS. Metabolic derivatives of aldosterone. *Am J Physiol* 1987; 252:F365–F373.
An overview of aldosterone metabolism in the kidney.

Rabkin R, Dahl DC. Renal uptake and disposal of proteins and peptides. In: Audus KL, Raub TJ, eds. *Biologic Barriers to Protein Delivery.* New York: Plenum Publishing Company, 1993.
A comprehensive review of the renal handling of low-molecular-weight proteins and peptides, particularly hormones.

Rabkin R, Fervenza FC, Maidment H, et al. Pharmacokinetics of insulin-like growth factor-1 in advanced chronic renal failure. *Kidney Int* 1996;49: 1134–1140.
A description of the impact of renal failure on the insulinlike growth factor–binding proteins and the disposal of IGF-1.

Reams G, Villarreal D, Bauer JH. Intrarenal metabolism of angiotensin II. *Am J Physiol* 1990;258:F1510–F1515.
An in vivo study of the renal metabolism of angiotensin II in dogs. Provides evidence for the intrarenal production of angiotensin II.

Ruskoaho H. Atrial natriuretic peptide: synthesis, release, and metabolism. *Pharmacol Rev* 1992;44(4):479–602.
An extensive review of ANP metabolism.

White PC, Mune T, Agarwal AK. 11β-hydroxysteroid dehydrogenase and the syndrome of apparent mineralocorticoid excess. *Endocr Rev* 1997;18:135–156.
Excellent review of abnormalities of mineralocorticoid metabolism.

Wolf G, Mentzel S, Assmann KJM. Aminopeptidase A: a key enzyme in the intrarenal degradation of angiotensin II. *Exp Nephrol* 1997;5:364–369.
Reviews biochemistry, renal distribution, and pathophysiologic significance of aminopeptidase in the kidney.

CHAPTER 13

Kidney and Endocrine System

PART 1
Eicosanoids

Rizwan Z. Khan and Kamal F. Badr

Eicosanoids are oxygenated derivatives of arachidonic acid (AA), a polyunsaturated essential fatty acid with 20 carbon atoms and 4 double bonds (C20:4).It is formed in the liver by elongation and desaturation of its precursor, linoleic acid (C18:2). There are three different enzymatic pathways through which oxidation of AA can occur. Oxidation of AA by the cyclooxygenase (COX) enzyme system results in the formation of prostaglandins (PGs) and thromboxanes. These eicosanoids are involved in the regulation of renal vascular tone and tubule function under normal conditions and in mediating alterations in glomerular function during injury. The second pathway involves the lipoxygenase (LO) group of enzymes, products of which participate in the mediation of renal inflammatory injury. Products of the third pathway of oxidation of AA, the cytochrome P450 enzyme system, are synthesized in the normal kidney and appear to regulate renal vascular tone and salt and water transport. AA is also subjected to free radical attack, with subsequent nonenzymatic oxidation and generation of isomeric eicosanoid species, the isoprostanes. Some of these compounds express significant biologic activities *in vitro* and *in vivo*.

We review advances in understanding the biology and roles of these enzymatic and nonenzymatic derived lipid mediators in the regulation of renal function under normal and pathologic conditions.

CYCLOOXYGENASE PATHWAY

PGs and thromboxanes, collectively called *prostanoids*, are a unique group of cyclic fatty acids with diverse biologic effects. They are produced throughout the body; the kidney is a major site of PG production, metabolism, and action. PGs are important modulators of renal function in both physiologic and pathophysiologic settings. The spectrum of their effects in the kidney encompasses modulation of renal blood flow (RBF), glomerular filtration rate (GFR), salt and water transport, and the release of renal hormones. It is within the setting of compromised renal status that maintenance of renal function is most dependent on PGs. Under these circumstances, inhibition of PG synthesis with nonsteroidal antiinflammatory drugs (NSAIDs) is likely to impair renal function.

Cyclooxygenase 1 and 2 (Prostaglandin Endoperoxide H Synthases)

The COX enzyme system is the major pathway for AA metabolism in the kidneys. It was assumed that only one COX gene and protein exists, an enzyme that is now called *cyclooxygenase-1* (COX-1). In 1991, however, by virtue of its molecular cloning, the existence of a second isoform, called *cyclooxygenase-2* (COX-2), was confirmed. COX-1 and COX-2 proteins have roughly a 60% homology in amino acid sequence and appear to have similar affinity and capacity to convert AA to PG and thromboxanes. Despite this, the two isoforms exhibit notable differences in several respects. COX-1 is present in most tissues, performing a "housekeeping" function by synthesizing PGs that regulate normal cell activity and maintain cellular homeostasis. COX-2, on the other hand, is almost undetectable in most tissues, but its expression can be induced rapidly in response to inflammation and several cytokines, mitogenic stimuli, hormones, and other factors.

In the kidney, COX-1 is constitutively present in arterial and arteriolar endothelial cells, mesangial cells, glomerular epithelial cells, renal interstitial cells, and in most segments of the tubule, although in markedly varying concentrations. By contrast, the expression of COX-2 under basal conditions in rats has been demonstrated in medullary interstitial cells, macula densa cells, and in adjacent epithelial cells of the nearby cortical thick ascending limb. In human kidneys, expression of COX-2 was localized to endothelial cells and smooth muscle cells of renal arteries and veins and intraglomerularly to podocytes, whereas no COX-2 expression was found in the macula densa.

In addition to these roles for COX-1 and COX-2, there is evidence for a role of COX-2 in the postnatal development of the kidneys. Postnatally and increasing with age of the animals, COX-2-deficient mice developed severe renal abnormalities. Only few functioning nephrons with immature, small glomeruli and dysplastic tubules grew in underdeveloped mesenchymal tissue.

In view of all these features, significant interest has been shown in the differential pharmacologic properties of COX-1 and COX-2 enzymes and their inhibitors. Most NSAIDs are better inhibitors of murine COX-1 than COX-2. However, it is clear that COX-2 as well as COX-1 can be inhibited by NSAIDs. Similar results have been obtained with human COX isozymes. Because COX-2 plays a major role in inflammation, selective inhibitors of this isozyme will probably be more potent antiinflammatory agents and lack the undesirable effects of NSAIDs by virtue of not inhibiting COX-1 and hence not inhibiting its important physiologic functions.

Biosynthesis and Metabolism

Prostanoid synthesis is initiated by the interaction of a stimulus with the cell surface. This stimulus typically takes the form of hormones such as angiotensin, bradykinin, or thrombin, or even nonspecific stimuli such as cell ischemia, free radical injury, or calcium ionophore. This stimulus leads to the activation of one or more lipase systems, which in turn cause the hydrolysis of the AA moiety from the sn2 position of phospholipids. This stimulus-lipase activation process is called the *arachidonate release step.* At least acutely, this is the major site of regulation of prostaglandin formation as the rate of prostanoid production is dependent on the release of free AA from tissue stores by phospholipases. In principle, there are a variety of phospholipases, though predominantly one or more phospholipase A_2 (PLA_2) and in certain conditions phospholipase C, which participate in mobilizing arachidonate from cellular lipids. Current evidence suggest that Ca^{2+}-dependent cytosolic PLA_2 and secretory PLA_2 are more widely involved with cardiac PLA_2 being involved under special Ca^{2+}-independent conditions. PLA_2 activity is influenced by a large number of agents, such as hormones and growth factors (Table 13.1). Arachidonate tissue stores vary with dietary intake of essential fatty acids and can be depleted when intake is deficient. Fish-oil diets (rich in omega-3 polyunsaturated fatty acids will compete for the arachidonate oxidation process and inhibit formation of active products).

Once arachidonate is released in its free form, it can be acted upon by one of the COX isozymes. Each of these isozymes, as an initial step, catalyzes the insertion of molecular oxygen into the carbon backbone structure of AA, with the concomitant cyclization of carbons 8 to 12 to form a cyclic endoperoxide PGG_2 (15-hydroperoxide). In the presence of reduced glutathione-dependent peroxidase, PGG_2 is converted to the 15-hydroxy derivative PGH_2. These unstable endoperoxide intermediates (PGG_2 and PGH_2) have a half-life of about 5 minutes. PGH2 is further transformed to yield the biologically active PGs and thromboxane (Fig. 13.1). In the presence of isomerase and reductase enzymes, PGH_2 is converted to PGE_2 and PGF_2, respectively. Thromboxane synthase converts PGH_2 into thromboxane A_2 (TXA_2). Prostacyclin synthase, abundant in vascular endo-

TABLE 13.1. Modulators of Prostaglandin Synthesis*

Modulator	Site of Action
Promoters	
Angiotensin II	PLA_2
AVP	PLA_2
Bradykinin	PLA_2
Norepinephrine	PLA_2
PAF	PLA_2
Interleukin-1	PLA_2 and COX
TNF-α	PLA_2
PDGF	COX
EGF	COX
Calcium	PLA_2
Diabetes	PLA_2
Ischemia	PLA_2
Chronic AVP therapy	COX
Ureteral obstruction	COX and TX synthase
Venous obstruction	COX
Glomerulonephritis	COX
Nephrotic syndrome	TX synthase
Inhibitors	
Glucocorticoids	PLA_2 and COX
Potassium	PLA_2
Urea	PLA_2
Mepacrine	PLA_2
NSAID	COX

*Note that hormones are important physiologic modulators of prostaglandin production.

EGF, epidermal growth factor; NSAIDS, nonsteroidal antiinflammatory drugs; PAF, platelet-activating factor; PDGF, platelet-derived growth factor; TNF-α, tumor necrosis factor α.

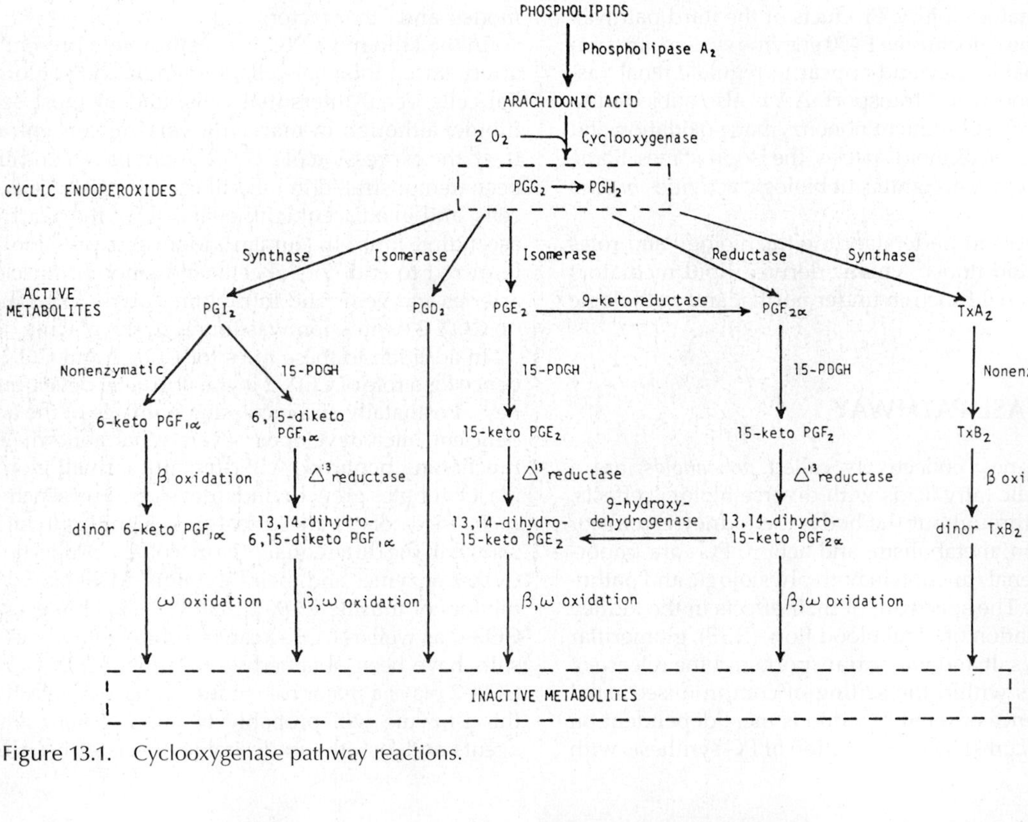

Figure 13.1. Cyclooxygenase pathway reactions.

thelial cells, catalyzes the biosynthesis of PGI_2 (prostacyclin). PGD_2 formation in the kidney is uncertain.

COX gene expression and biologic activity are up-regulated by cytokines and growth factors such as interleukin-1 and platelet-derived growth factor. On the other hand, corticosteroids inhibit PLA_2 and COX gene expression. Several renal pathophysiologic states, such as glomerulonephritis and ureteral obstruction, are associated with increased prostanoid production. Table 13.1 lists several modulators of the key steps involved in PG synthesis.

Prostaglandin endoperoxide (PGH_2) can be converted to one of many different biologically active prostanoid derivatives, including PGE_2, $PGF_{2\alpha}$, TXA_2, or PGI_2, although in general a given cell type forms only one of these prostanoids as its major product. PGI_2 is the major bioactive product released by renal arterial and arteriolar endothelial cells. Whole glomeruli generate several prostanoids; the predominant product varies among species, but in humans it appears to be PGI_2, rather that PGE_2, as seen in rats and rabbits. Cultured human mesangial cells are capable of generating PGE_2 as well as $PGF_{2\alpha}$ and PGI_2 ($PGE_2 > PGF_{2\alpha} > PGI_2 = TXA_2$). Glomerular epithelial and endothelial cells generate PGs, but the pattern of the products remains controversial. Intraglomerular macrophages, localized in the mesangium, are a potential source of prostanoids and other eicosanoids, particularly after glomerular injury. In the rest of the nephron, the collecting tubule, particularly its medullary portion, is a predominant site of PG synthesis, where PGE_2 is the major prostanoid synthesized. Table 13.2 lists the different cyclooxygenase products generated in response to various stimuli at different sites of the nephron.

The PGs and TXA_2 undergo rapid destruction and inactivation within the kidney by cytosolic degradative enzymes. Elimination of PGE_2, $PGF_{2\alpha}$, and PGI_2 proceeds through enzymatic oxidation and nonenzymatic hydrolysis, whereas that of TXA_2 is exclusively nonenzymatic. The initial degradative step is catalyzed by 15-hydroxyprostaglandin dehydrogenase (15-PGDH), with formation of biologically inactive 15-keto-PGs. These metabolites are further degraded by a PG reductase. PGI_2 and TXA_2 undergo rapid nonenzymatic degradation to 6-keto-PGF_1 (and TXB_2, respectively). Because the kidney metabolizes and also excretes circulating PGs, it is difficult to evaluate the net rate of renal production of a particular PG. Intact PGs and stable hydrolysis products are excreted in the urine and largely reflect the rate of renal PG production. Excretion of PGE_2 in the urine probably reflects renal production, although a number of variables can cause measurement errors, including contamination with seminal fluid. Urinary excretion of 6-keto-$PGF_{1\alpha}$, the hydrolytic product of PGI_2, may reflect both augmented systemic and local PGI_2 synthesis. Active PGs are also detected in the renal venous effluent, but apart from PGI_2, they are destroyed in the lungs and do not enter the systemic circulation.

Biologic Actions of COX Products in the Kidney

PGs have diverse actions, in part related to their site of synthesis and the cells on which they act. Their principal physiologic role is mediation and modulation of hormone action. Thus cortical production by arterioles and glomeruli is related to regulation of RBF, GFR, and renin release. Medullary PG production is

TABLE 13.2. AA-CO Products Generated by Various Hormones and Other Stimuli at Different Sites of the Nephron

Hormone/Stimulus	Site/Species	Product
Angiotensin II	Glomerulus/human	$PGI_2 > PGE_2$
	Mesangial cell/human	PGI_2
	Glomerulus/rat	$PGE_2 > PGF_{2\alpha}$
	Mesangial cell/rat	$PGE_2 > PGF_{2\alpha}$
	Glomerular epithelial cell/rat	$PGE_2 > PGF_{2\alpha}$
	Proximal tubule/rabbit	$PGE_2 > PGF_{2\alpha}$, PGI_2
Arginine vasopressin	Mesangial cell/rat	PGE_2
	CCT/rabbit	PGE_2
Bradykinin	Proximal tubule/rabbit	$PGF_{2\alpha}$
	Perfused kidney/rat	PGE_2
Norepinephrine	Mesangial cell/rat	PGE_2
	Glomer/rat	PGE_2, $PGF_{2\alpha}$
	MDCK cells	PGE_2
Serotonin	Mesangial cell/rat	PGE_2/PGI_2
Interleukin-1	Mesangial cell/rat	$PGF_{2\alpha}$
Epidermal growth factor	Glomerulus/rat	$PGF_{2\alpha}$
	Mesangial cell/rat	PGE_2
PAF-acether	Glomerulus/rat	TXA_2
	Mesangial cell/rat	TXA_2/PGE_2
U-44069	Mesangial cell/rat	PGE_2
Estradiol	Papilla/rat	PGE_2
A23187	Glomerulus/rat	$PGE_2 > PGF_{2\alpha} > PGI_2 > TXA_2$
	Mesangial cell/rat	$PGE_2 > PGF_{2\alpha} > PGI_2 > TXA_2$
	CCT/rat	PGE_2
Endotoxin	Cortical slices/rat	$PGE_2 > PGI_2 > TXA_2$
Reactive oxygen species	Glomerulus/rat	PGE_2
	Mesangial cells/rat	PGE_2/TXA_2
	Interstitial cells/rat	PGE_2
Ischemia/hypoxia	Glomerulus/rat	$PGE_2/PGF_{2\alpha}/PGI_2$
	Mesangial cell/rat	PGE_2
Membrane fluidity	MDCK cells	PGE_2
PKC activation	MDCK cells	PGE_2
Endocytosis	Mesangial cells/rat	PGE_2

CCT, cortical collecting tubules; MDCK, Madin-Darby canine kidney; PAF, platelet activating factor; PKC, protein kinase C.

directed to regulating vasa recta blood flow, tubular sodium (Na), chloride transport, and the response of the collecting duct to AVP. Inhibition of COX activity in the absence of exogenous administration or endogenous release of hormones such as angiotensin II or AVP has little effect on renal functional parameters. Once their local release is enhanced, COX products may themselves stimulate the local generation of other hormones. PG-stimulated renin release is an example of this mode of action. Under pathophysiologic conditions such as inflammatory injury, local release of prostanoids may mediate some of the functional derangement that characterizes these conditions.

Prostanoids act through specific and distinct receptors. The cDNAs for numerous prostanoid receptors, including receptors for TXA_2, $PGF_{2\alpha}$, and PGE_2, have now been cloned and sequenced. All these receptors are members of the G-protein–coupled family of receptors. Multiple subtypes of each of these prostanoid receptors may exist, as in the case with the PGE_2 receptor (EP receptor), thus explaining the apparently contrasting effects mediated by PGE_2 on smooth muscle and collecting duct permeability to water. All the four proposed PGE_2 receptor subtypes (EP-1, EP-2, EP-3, and EP-4) have been cloned, sequenced, and expressed. The EP-1 and EP-3 receptors mediate smooth muscle constriction, whereas the EP-2 and EP-4 receptors mediate smooth muscle relaxation. Activation of the EP-1 receptor causes an increase in intracellular Ca2+ (accounting for smooth muscle constriction), presumably phosphatidylinositol-mediated. The EP-3 receptor predominantly signals through the inhibitory G-protein (Gi), diminishing hormone-stimulated cyclic adenosine monophosphate (cAMP) generation. In contrast, EP-2 receptors display dose-dependent stimulation of cAMP generation with PGE_2 concentrations above 10^{-8} M. In mesangial cells the $PGF_{2\alpha}$ receptor (FP receptor) seems to be coupled to increased intracellular Ca^{2+} At higher concentrations $PGF_{2\alpha}$ also stimulates EP receptors. The TXA_2 receptor (TP receptor) appears to signal via phosphatidylinositol hydrolysis, leading to increased intracellular Ca^{2+}. The PGI_2 receptor (IP receptor) signals via stipulations of cAMP generation. PGI_2 has been shown to play an important vasodilator role in the glomerular microvasculature, where the effects of PGI_2 and PGE_2 to stimulate cAMP generation were distinct and additive.

Renal Hemodynamics

There are some species differences in the renal actions of PGs, and this must be taken into account when extrapolating data from animals to humans. In general, PGE_2 and PGI_2 are vasodilators in most species, whereas TXA_2, $PGF_{2\alpha}$, and PGE_2 (in certain circumstances) are vasoconstrictors. PGE_2 relaxes rat and rabbit afferent arterioles. PGI_2 is a potent vasodilator in both humans and dogs. It is also a highly potent relaxant of rabbit afferent, efferent and interlobular arteriolar smooth muscle, but has little intrinsic vasoactive properties in rat kidney. $PGF_{2\alpha}$ is without effect on any arterial segment in rabbit kidney but is a mild vasoconstrictor in dogs. TXA_2 analogs exert constrictor effects on rat arteriolar smooth muscle and cause renal vasoconstriction accompanied by a severe reduction in filtration fraction, suggesting a predominant preglomerular action. The contribution of these vasoactive properties of COX products to the regulation of renal vascular tone under normal physiologic conditions is probably minimal. This is best exemplified by the minimal change or absence of change in RBF and GFR in euvolemic rats or humans following COX inhibition or selective antagonism of TXA_2 synthesis or actions.

By contrast, the local release of vasodilator PGs (PGE_2 and PGI_2) in response to renal vasoconstrictors plays an important role in maintaining RBF and GFR. There is compelling evidence indicating that mesangial cell synthesis and release of PGE_2 and PGI_2 modulate the constrictor actions of angiotensin II, norepinephrine, and AVP. Activation of the renin-angiotensin and sympathetic nervous systems leading to enhanced release of angiotensin, catecholamines, and AVP occurs in conditions such as hemorrhage, volume depletion, general anesthesia and cardiac failure. While serving to maintain the systemic blood pressure, these hormones constrict mesangial cells and glomerular arterioles. Fortunately, their enhancement of renal PG release locally opposes their constrictor effects. The vasodilatory action of PGs on the afferent arteriole serves to maintain renal perfusion, whereas their relaxant effects on mesangial cells maintains the effective surface area for filtration. Inhibition of PG generation in these circumstances is associated with a dramatic fall in RBF and GFR. Vasodilator PGs, in particular PGI_2, may also counteract the vasoconstrictor responses to calcium in humans.

In addition to modulating the effects of vasoconstrictors, endogenous PGs mediate the actions of some vasodilator agents. These include a role for PGI_2 in mediating the vasorelaxant actions of dopamine and magnesium in humans, and of hydralazine and epidermal growth factor in dogs. PGs may also mediate the renal vasodilatory response to a protein meal in humans. Conversely, TXA_2, whose synthesis is increased in experimental glomerular immune injury and ureteral obstruction, may cause glomerular contraction.

Effects on Salt and Water Transport

It is now well established that arachidonate metabolites of the COX pathway have important effects on salt and water transport in the kidney through direct actions on the epithelial cells that line the nephron independently of any hemodynamic changes produced by these compounds. It is important to reiterate that these arachidonic acid metabolites are predominantly autocoids and therefore their locus of action will be close to their point of generation. Thus direct epithelial effects of these compounds will result when they are produced by the tubule cells themselves or the neighboring interstitial cells.

Salt Excretion

Neither the proximal convoluted tubule nor the proximal straight tubule are significant sources for biologically active COX metabolites of arachidonic acid. PGE_2 may block the activation of adenyl cyclase by parathyroid hormone (PTH) through interaction at the inhibitory guanine nucleotide regulatory protein Gi. This effect of PGE_2 is also observed in other renal epithelial cells and is discussed later. There is very little data on the actions of other COX metabolites in proximal tubules. *In vitro* microperfusion studies with $PGF_{2\alpha}$ failed to show an effect on sodium chloride or phosphate transport.

The nephron segments making up Henle's loop also displayed limited metabolism of AA through the COX pathway. However, in many mammalian species, the collecting ducts and the medullary thick ascending limb express the majority of receptors for PGE_2 in the kidney. This is consistent with prior studies that suggest that PGE_2 inhibits salt reabsorption in this nephron segment. However, under normal circumstances, inhibition of COX does not result in alteration of Na delivery out of Henle's loop to the early distal tubule. There is evidence that inhibition of COX either augments sodium chloride reabsorption in Henle's loop or blocks inhibition of sodium chloride reabsorption in Henle's loop by other agents, such as furosemide. The inhibitory effect of PGE_2 on sodium chloride transport in the thick ascending limb probably involves inhibition of adenyl cyclase activation.

In almost all mammalian species studied to date, the collecting ducts are the major nephron segments responsible for PG synthesis. Medullary collecting ducts produce greater amounts of COX products than do cortical collecting ducts. The predominant COX metabolite produced by collecting ducts is PGE_2. Infusion of AA or the COX product PGE_2 directly into the renal artery results in natriuresis. Although hemodynamic changes probably contribute, as mentioned, earlier studies ruled out the contribution of the proximal tubule and Henle's loop to this increased natriuresis. Various studies have confirmed the role of PGE_2 on this natriuresis by virtue of its action on the collecting ducts—medullary more than cortical. There is evidence that PGE_2 exerts its inhibitory effect on rabbit cortical collecting duct Na transport by two mechanisms. The first involves inhibiting principal cell basolateral Na^+-K^+-ATPase activity, the second by directly decreasing the open probability of the apical amiloride-sensitive Na channel. PGE_2 uses multiple signal transduction pathways in the cortical collecting duct. These include increase of intracellular Ca^{2+}, activation of protein kinase C, and modulation of cAMP levels. Inhibition of COX with ibuprofen produces antinatriuresis and increased accumulation of sodium in the renal papillae.

Water Excretion

PGs, especially PGE_2, affect water transport in the collecting duct in many ways. Although the direct effect of either PGE_1 or PGE_2 is to stimulate basal hydraulic conductivity of isolated perfused collecting tubules, PGs of the E series blunt the hydraulic conductivity response of the collecting duct to AVP. In fact, *in vivo* infusions of arachidonic acid or PGE_2 induce a water diuresis, while inhibition of PG synthesis potentiates the urinary hyperosmolality caused by AVP. These effects on water conductivity in the collecting ducts have been explained by changes in cAMP accumulation. AVP mediates the increase in water conductivity in the collecting duct through increased cAMP accumulation.

Studies on the effect of PGE_2 on cAMP metabolism in this nephron segment demonstrated that PGE_2 can both stimulate basal cAMP generation and suppress AVP-stimulated cAMP generation. The inhibitory effects of PGE_2 on AVP-stimulated cAMP generation and water conductivity in the collecting duct are probably mediated through the EP-3 receptor via the pertussis toxin-sensitive inhibitory guanine nucleotide–binding protein Gi. In addition to affecting water flow via modulation of cAMP levels, PGE_2 has been shown to inhibit AVP-induced water conductivity by activation of protein kinase C and elevation of intracellular calcium.

Another facet of PGE_2–AVP interactions is that AVP acutely stimulates endogenous PGE_2 production by the collecting duct. This effect suggests that PGE_2 participates in a negative feedback loop, whereby endogenous PGE_2 production dampens the action of AVP. However, there is still controversy about the physiologic relevance of AVP-induced PGE_2 production, especially the finding that the concentration of AVP necessary to stimulate PGE_2 synthesis in the collecting duct *in vitro* is at least 1 or 2 log orders of magnitude higher than the AVP concentration that allows maximal water conductivity in the isolated collecting tubule.

Other Effects on Renal Function

Extensive evidence supports the capacity of PGs, particularly PGE_2 and PGI_2, to release renin. By contrast, TXA_2 exerts a negative effect on renin release. Inhibition of COX activity reduces plasma renin activity, suggesting that the predominant influence of prostanoids is stimulatory. PG-mediated renin release is independent of α-adrenergic mechanisms. Conflicting evidence exists regarding the involvement of prostanoids, particularly TXA_2, in the mediation of tubuloglomerular feedback responses.

Role of COX Metabolites in Renal Pathophysiology

Acute Renal Failure

The pathophysiologic significance of COX metabolites has been investigated in various models of prerenal, intrinsic and postrenal (obstructive) acute renal failure (ARF). Of the major causes of ARF, an important homeostatic and pathophysiologic role of PGs and TXA_2 has been established during hemodynamic prerenal failure, endotoxin-induced ARF, and obstructive injury.

When cardiac output is compromised, as in extracellular fluid volume depletion or congestive heart failure, and systemic blood pressure is preserved by the action of high circulating levels of systemic vasoconstrictors (norepinephrine, angiotensin II, AVP), amelioration of the effects of these vasoconstrictors on the renal vasculature by PGs serves to blunt the development of otherwise concomitant marked depression of RBF. As noted earlier, the intrarenal generation of vasodilator products of AA, including PGE_2 and PGI_2 is a central part of this protective adaptation. The increase in renal vascular resistance (RVR) induced by exogenously administered angiotensin II or renal nerve stimulation (increased α-adrenergic tone) is exaggerated during concomitant inhibition of prostaglandin synthesis. Studies in patients with congestive heart failure have confirmed that enhanced PG synthesis is crucial in protecting kidneys from various vasoconstrictor influences in this condition. Fig. 13.2 schematizes the role of vasoconstrictor–PG interactions in the preservation of renal perfusion when systemic hemodynamics are compromised. Should renal hypoperfusion be sufficiently severe, intrinsic (structural) ischemic acute renal failure will develop. Evidence from animal studies suggests that augmented synthesis of TXA_2 may exacerbate postischemic renal failure, and elevated levels of PGI_2 may exert a cytoprotective effect, limiting renal structural and functional deterioration. The clinical relevance of these findings remains uncertain.

Endotoxin-induced ARF is characterized by progressive reduction in RBF and GFR before the onset of hypotension. A number of reports have provided evidence for a role for TXA_2-induced renal vasoconstriction in this model of renal dysfunction. In addition the literature abounds with isolated reports regarding the roles of PGs and TXA_2 in modulating or modifying renal injury in a number of models of toxin-mediated acute tubular injury, including those induced by uranyl nitrate, aminoglycosides, glycerol, oxygen radicals and analgesics.

After induction of chronic (more than 24 hours) ureteral obstruction in animals or humans, renal PG and TXA_2 synthesis is markedly enhanced. Enhanced prostanoid synthesis likely arises from infiltrating mononuclear cells, proliferating fibroblastlike cells, interstitial macrophages, and interstitial medullary cells.

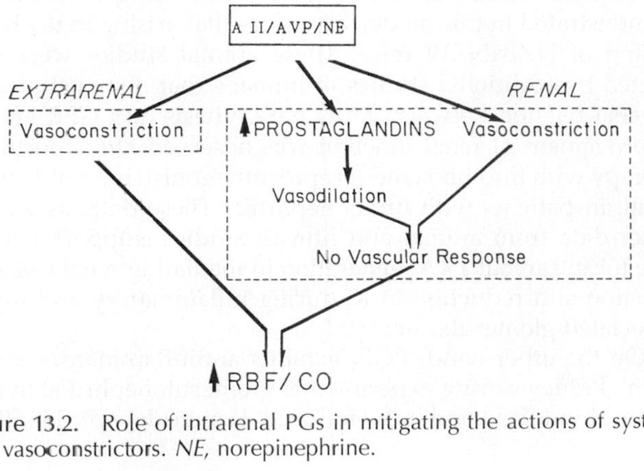

Figure 13.2. Role of intrarenal PGs in mitigating the actions of systematic vasoconstrictors. *NE*, norepinephrine.

Considerable evidence, derived form studies using specific enzyme inhibitors, suggest a casual relationship between increased renal generation of this eicosanoid (TXA_2) and the intense vasoconstriction that characterizes a kidney after removal of an obstruction or a hydronephrotic kidney.

Experimental and Human Glomerular Injury

Because of their synthesis by glomerular mesangial and epithelial cells, possible local generation and release by infiltrating leukocytes and platelets, and potent effects of renal vascular tone and mesangial cell function, the involvement of COX products in the mediation of glomerular injury has been the subject of vigorous research.

In examining the role of COX products in the mediation of inflammatory glomerular injury, investigators have focused their attention on two models: experimentally induced antiglomerular basement membrane antibody (anti-GBM Ab)–induced glomerulonephritis [often referred to as *nephrotoxic serum* (NTS) *nephritis*] and the naturally occurring model of lupuslike disease in the F_1 hybrid of NZBxNZW mice.

NTS-induced glomerulonephritis, produced in the rat by administration of antibody directed against glomerular basement membrane antigens has proven to be a useful tool for evaluating the pathogenesis of glomerulonephritic injury. The principal factor accounting for the falls in filtration rates in this model of injury is a marked reduction in the glomerular capillary ultrafiltration coefficient (K_f or Lp). Although K_f is low throughout both phases of the disease process, the acute (heterologous) and the delayed (homologous) phases, RVR is initially elevated during the heterologous phase but eventually falls as the lesion transforms into the autologous phase at 10 to 14 days after the initial injury. RVR may be equal or even less than that observed in control animals. Studies have established an important role for TXA_2 release in mediating the increase RVR observed during the early phase of this disease. These studies also suggest an increasing role for PGE_2 generation, by day 1, accounting for the progressive dilation of renal arterioles leading to progressive increase in RBF at this stage and during later stages. In these studies, TXA_2 antagonism appeared to ameliorate the falls in RBF and GFR 2 hours after NTS, but not at day 1. During the heterologous phase, the weight of current evidence favors a predominant role of COX products in mediating both the renal vasodilation and the reduction in K_f that characterizes this phase. The net functional result of COX inhibition during this phase of experimental glomerulonephritis, therefore would depend on the relative importance of renal perfusion versus the preservation of K_f for the maintenance of GFR.

Studies have also reported a beneficial effect for fish oil diets on the course of genetic murine lupus (MRL-lpr mice) and an accompanying reduction in the generation of COX products. In subsequent studies, enhanced TXA_2 and PGE_2 generation was demonstrated in this model, as well as that arising in the F_1 offspring of NZBxNZW mice. These animal studies were supported by additional studies in humans that demonstrated an inverse relation between TXA_2 biosynthesis and GFR and an improvement of renal function was observed after short-term therapy with thromboxane-receptor antagonist, but not with aspirin, in patients with lupus nephritis. These data, as well as other data from animal and human studies, support a major role for intrarenal TXA_2 generation in mediating renal vasoconstriction and reduction in K_f during inflammatory and lupus-associated glomerular injury.

On the other hand, PGE_1 exhibits antiinflammatory effects in the kidney during experimental glomerulonephritis. In rats, in antithymocyte antibody–induced glomerulonephritis, PGE_1 has been demonstrated to inhibit the expression of monocyte-chemoattractant protein-1 (MCP-1) and ameliorate the glomerular infiltration of monocytes at 24 hours and at day 5. In other studies, PGE_1 administration has attenuated the increase in mRNA levels of type III and type IV collagens and deposition of extracellular matrix in rat glomeruli with antithymocyte antibody–induced glomerulonephritis. The aforementioned evidence and data from numerous other studies assign a role for COX products in modifying the nature of the pathologic lesion and the extent of accompanying proteinuria.

Finally, it should be emphasized, that the model studied, the potency and dose of the antibody, the time at which measurements are performed, and the nature of the histopathologic lesion present, are all determinants of the prevailing functional parameters and, presumably, of their modification by COX inhibitors.

Diabetes Mellitus

Numerous studies in patients with insulin-dependent diabetes have demonstrated elevated urinary excretion rates of vasodilatory PGs and TXA_2 and reductions in the abnormally high values of GFR and RBF in patients receiving treatment with COX inhibitors. In patients with hyporeninemic hypoaldosteronism, deficient basal, as well as stimulated, PGI_2 production has been proposed as an underlying mechanism for the low active renin concentration and the altered vasomotor tone. The roles played by COX products in mediating diabetic nephropathy, however, remain controversial. Beneficial clinical responses to platelet inhibitory therapy (aspirin/dipyridamole) raise the possibility that the effect of COX inhibition may well relate to inhibition of platelet, rather than renal, thromboxane generation.

Hypertension

Several lines of evidence suggest the involvement of COX products in accentuating the salt-retaining stimuli that characterize patients with some forms of essential hypertension. This derives mainly from studies of salt balance and blood pressure measurements in hypertensive individuals receiving NSAIDs. These agents lead to increase salt retention in hypertensive patients, but not in normal individuals. In particular, COX inhibition is associated with resistance to the diuretic actions of thiazides and furosemide, and responsiveness to the blood pressure-lowering effects of beta-blockers. For this reason, the hypertensive patient tolerates better NSAIDs associated with lesser inhibition of renal COX, such as sulindac. The extent to which sulindac spares renal COX, however, is probably dose dependent.

In patients with renal artery stenosis, increased renal venous PG secretion is observed from the stenotic side, probably reflecting renin-stimulated synthesis. This local release of PGs in such patients maintains a relatively low RVR, thereby mitigating against the effects of decreased perfusion pressure on ipsilateral renal perfusion.

Attempts at treating hypertension with PG analogs have generally been disappointing, and those involving dietary manipulations have achieved only modest results.

Hepatorenal Syndrome

A number of clinical studies have documented diminished renal synthesis of vasodilator PGs, in particular PGI_2, in patients with liver cirrhosis complicated by functional (vasoconstrictive) renal failure. Diminished renal PG synthesis has also been implicated in the pathogenesis of the severe sodium retention in these patients, as well as their resistance to diuretic therapy. The sodium-retaining properties of NSAIDs are particularly exaggerated in patients with cirrhosis of the liver, attesting to the dependence of renal salt excretion on vasodilatory PGs. These drugs may also cause an acute rise in serum creatinine and potassium when given to patients with cirrhosis of the liver. It is unlikely that the severe degree of renal vasoconstriction seen in these patients is due solely to absence of renal synthesis of a vasodilator in the absence of an active vasoconstrictor stimulus. The overall mechanisms of the hepatorenal syndrome are discussed in chapter.

Allograft Rejection and Cyclosporine Nephrotoxicity

Acute administration of a TXA_2 synthesis inhibitor is associated with significant improvement in rat renal allograft function, leading some to suggest that increased urinary TXA_2 excretion may be an early indicator in renal and cardiac allograft rejection. Repeated observations in clinical and experimental models of cyclosporine nephrotoxicity have established the presence of a significant component of intrarenal vasoconstriction in its pathogenesis. In a number of cell systems, addition of cyclosporine has been shown to increase intracellular calcium concentrations and to augment receptor-mediated cellular calcium fluxes, a condition that may lead to stimulation of COX activity. Addition of cyclosporine to human peripheral blood monocytes increases PGE_2 synthesis. Furthermore, cyclosporine administration has been associated with activation of the renin-angiotensin system, a signal for intrarenal PG production. Numerous investigators have demonstrated effects of cyclosporine on renal PG/TXA_2 synthesis and provided evidence for a major role for renal and leukocyte TXA_2 synthesis in mediating acute and chronic cyclosporine nephrotoxicity in rats. Diets rich in fish oil and TXA_2 antagonists have been shown to reduce renal TXA_2 synthesis and afford protection against nephrotoxicity. The clinical applicability of these observations has, however, not yet been tested.

Pregnancy

Studies in pregnant rats and humans have documented increased glomerular synthesis and urinary excretion of PGE_2, PGF_2, and PGI_2 without significant changes in TXA_2 generation. The increased renal levels of these COX products may well relate to the documented decrease in the activity of 15-PGDH, the principal enzyme involved in the metabolism of PGs, likely resulting from the elevated levels of estrogen, which selectively decreases the V_{max} for this enzyme in the kidney (but not the lung). Augmented PG synthesis in gravid animals and humans has therefore been postulated as the basis for the increased levels of GFR and RBF normally seen during pregnancy. PG inhibition, however, is without effect on these parameters in anesthetized or conscious rats. Stimulated vasodilator PG synthesis does not appear to contribute to the regulation of GFR and RBF in normal pregnancy; however, diminished synthesis of PGI_2 has been demonstrated in human and animal models of pregnancy-induced hypertension. A beneficial effect of reducing TXA_2 generation, while preserving PGI_2 synthesis, by low-dose (60 to 100 mg/day) aspirin therapy, has been demonstrated in recent studies in patients at risk for pregnancy-induced hypertension.

Chronic Renal Insufficiency

Following experimental reduction in renal mass, glomerular and urinary excretion of PGs and TXA2 increases several fold, particularly when factored for the number of remaining nephrons. Inhibition of COX activity leads to reductions in perfusion rate and the K_f in remnant kidneys, but not in intact controls. Selective inhibition of TXA_2 synthesis is associated with an increase in GFR and, in chronic studies, with improvement in GFR, lessening of proteinuria, and preservation of renal histology.

LIPOXYGENASE (LO) PATHWAY

Biosynthesis

Enzymatic lipoxygenation of arachidonic acid leads to the generation of leukotrienes (LTs), lipoxins (LXs), and hydroxyeicosatetraenoic acids (HETEs). Formation of these compounds is initiated by 5-, 12-, or 15-lipoxygenase, whereby a hydroperoxyl group is introduced onto arachidonic acid at carbon 5, carbon 12, or carbon 15, respectively, to yield the corresponding 5-, 12-, or 15-hydroperoxytetraenoic acid (HPETE). HPETEs are unstable compounds that are transformed into the corresponding 5-, 12-, and 15-HETE, which undergo enzymatic modification, leading to the generation of these various LTs and LXs (Fig. 13.3). The 5-lipoxygenase pathway is a major route of arachidonic acid metabolism in the polymorphonuclear cells and macrophages leading to the formation of 5-HETE and LTs; 5-lipoxygenase requires activation by a cell-membrane-bound protein called the 5-lipoxygenase–activating protein (FLAP). Leukotriene A4 is an early pivotal intermediate in the 5-lipoxygenase pathway whose metabolism leads to the production of the LT series of metabolites. Formation of LTB4 requires LTA4 hydrolase activity, whereas generation of the cysteinyl-leukotrienes (LTC4, LTD4, and LTE3) requires the enzymatic action of glutathione-S-transferase. Unlike 5-lipoxygenase, which is largely restricted to cells of myeloid lineage, these enzymes are widely distributed among different cell types. The 15-lipoxygenase enzyme catalyzes the production of 15-HETE and initiates another major pathway of arachidonic acid metabolism in leukocytes. In activated neutrophils and macrophages, sequential lipoxygenation of arachidonic acid at carbons 15 and 5 yields trihydroxy derivatives, the LXs. LX synthesis can also occur in other cells, such as mesangial cells and platelets, by uptake of leukocyte-generated LTA4 and its transformation to LXs by either 15- or 12-lipoxygenase. The main LXs derived from 15-HETE are designated LXA4, LXB4, and 7-cis-11-trans-LXA4. In the kidney, lipoxygenase products are largely generated by infiltrating leukocytes or resident cells of macrophage–monocyte origin, but there is increasing evidence that intrinsic renal cells are capable of generating LTs and LXs either directly or through transcellular metabolism of intermediates.

Renal Metabolism of Leukotrienes

LTC4 is converted rapidly to LTD4 and LTE4 in rat glomeruli and papilla by sequential peptide cleavage. *N*-acetylation of LTE4 leads to loss of biologic activity. The renal metabolism of LTB4 proceeds via conversion to the 6-transisomer (biologically inactive), as detected in rat kidney homogenates, or by primary reduction of double bonds leading to the formation of 5,12-diHETE in mesangial cells, the biologic activity of which is undefined. The renal metabolism of LXs is unexplored.

Renal Receptors and Intracellular Signals for LO Products

Specific high-affinity LTD4 receptors have been identified on rat and human glomerular mesangial cells. The dissociation constants in both species are remarkably close (10 and 12 nM, respectively), as is the rank order of potency for binding competition by other LTs (LTD4 > LTE4 = LTC4 > LTB4). Of interest, a crucial stereochemistry requirement for LTD4 binding appears to be the S, R orientation of the polar substituents at C5 and C6, such that the 5R, 6S-LTD4 competes for binding with very low potency (=LTB4). LXA4, which posses similar

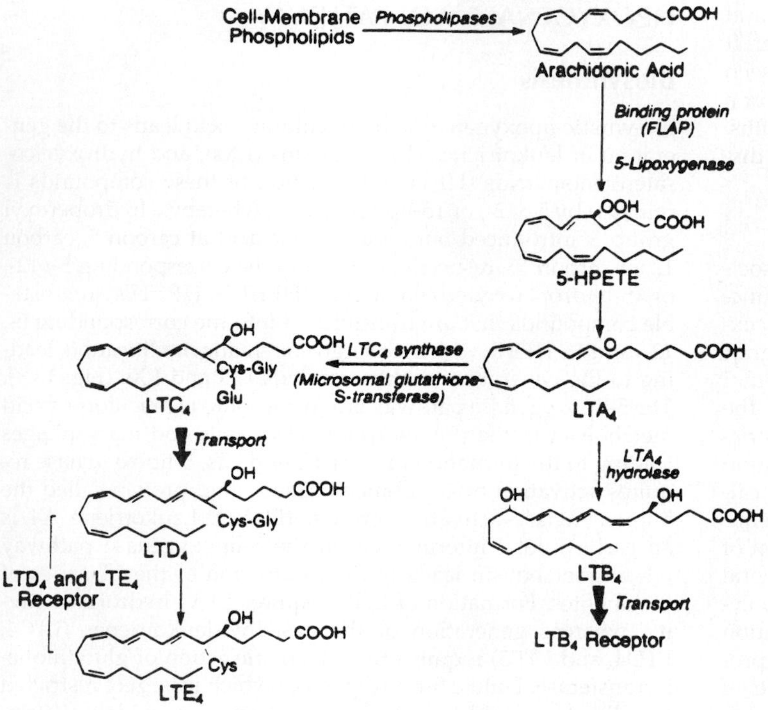

Figure 13.3. 5-LO pathway reactions leading to the formation of LTs.

stereochemistry at these carbons competes well for 3H-LTD4 binding to rat mesangial cells and elicits weak agonist activity. Intracellular signaling for LTD4 in human and rat mesangial cells involves receptor-activated phosphatidylinositol 4,5-biphosphate (PIP2) hydrolysis, release of inositol phosphates and increased intracellular calcium concentrations. Recently, the complementary DNAs for LTB4 and LXA4 receptors have been cloned and sequenced. The receptors for cysteinyl-leukotrienes are yet to be cloned.

Biologic Effects of Lipoxygenase Products

The LTs are potent proinflammatory molecules. LTB4 has minimal spasmogenic properties but is the most potent chemotactic substance yet described for polymorphonuclear cells, and it promotes their activation and adhesion to the endothelium. It has no significant effects on renal hemodynamics in normal animals, but it amplifies glomerular inflammation and proteinuria in animals with glomerulonephritic injury. The cysteinyl LTs contract vascular, pulmonary, and gastrointestinal smooth muscle and increase vascular permeability to macromolecules. LTC4 and LTD4 exert potent effects on glomerular hemodynamics. In rats, systemic administration of LTC4 leads to reduction in RBF and GFR. Similarly, infusion of either LTC4 or LTD4 in the isolated perfused kidney results in dramatic increase in RVR and reduction in GFR. LTD4 mediates these effects by causing a significant increase in efferent arteriolar resistance, leading to a fall in glomerular plasma flow rate (Qa), and a rise in glomerular capillary hydraulic pressure (PGC). In addition, it significantly reduces the glomerular capillary ultrafiltration coefficient (K_f); therefore its overall effect is to decrease single-nephron GFR. LTC4 and LTD4 contract mesangial cells, and LTD4 stimulates neutrophil adhesion to these cells. In both rats and humans, specific mesangial cell LTD4 receptors have been identified. Intracellular signaling for LTD4 in these cells involves receptor-activated phosphatidyl inositol diphosphate (PIP2) hydrolysis, release of inositol phosphates, and increased intracellular calcium concentrations.

15-S-HETE and LXA4 antagonize some of the actions of LTs. 15-S-HETE decreases LTB4 generation by leukocytes, antagonizes neutrophil chemotaxis to LTB4, and suppresses leukocyte activation in response to ionophore or other activators. These effects probably result from the incorporation and storage of 15-S-HETE in the phosphatidylinositol fraction of membrane lipids, with subsequent release and generation of structurally altered second messenger diacylglycerol. LXA4 attenuates LTB4-induced neutrophil chemotaxis and inhibits natural killer cell cytotoxicity. The effects of LXA4 are mediated primarily by functional high-affinity LXA4 receptors. In rat glomerular mesangial cells, LXA4 competes with LTD4 at a common receptor whereby LXA4 mediates partial agonist-antagonist effects. Different lipoxins display distinct effects on renal hemodynamics. In rats, LXA4 causes a selective decrease in afferent arteriolar resistance, thereby increasing RBF, PGC, and GFR. The LXA4-induced increase in GFR, however, is partially offset by its mild effect in decreasing K_f. The vasodilator actions of LXA4 are mediated by prostaglandins. LXB4 and 7-cis-11-trans-LXA4 display vasoconstrictive effects on renal hemodynamics in rats that are independent of COX activity. Recently, a new series of bioactive eicosanoids, 15-epi-lipoxins formed during aspirin triggered interactions between COX-2 and 5-LO, in leukocytes, have been shown to be potent inhibitors of neutrophil adhesion and inhibit cell proliferation.

Aspirin-Triggered 15-Epi-lipoxins

The interest in the role of 15-LO products during inflammation has been heightened by the discovery of the effect of aspirin on the catalytic activity of cyclooxygenase-2 (COX-2), also called *PGH synthase II (PGHS-II).* This enzyme, when induced by proinflammatory cytokines such as IL-1b, LPS, or TNF and, in presence of aspirin, switches its activity, generating 15-R HETE. Given this scenario, aspirin inhibits prostaglandin synthesis by PGH-I and PGH-II and acetylates PGH-II, which converts endogenous arachidonic acid into 15-R-HETE, which is then released and transformed via transcellular routes, to form

15-epi-LXs by adherent leukocytes. This pathway represents the third biochemical route for the synthesis of LXs. These compounds have biologic activities similar to those of lipoxins. 15-epi-LXA4 is more potent than LXA4 in inhibiting neutrophil adhesion, and 15-epi-LXB4 acts as an inhibitor of cell proliferation. The interest of this pathway is that COX-2 (or PGHS-II) is present in abundance in inflammatory reactions and in disease states. In fact, we have described an increased expression of RNA encoding for COX-2 in glomeruli isolated from rats with experimental glomerulonephritis, these levels being unaffected by pretreatment with aspirin. Glomeruli from nephritic rats also presented higher levels of LXs, and aspirin pretreatment further increased glomerular LXs synthesis by NTS treated rats. These findings suggest an endogenous antiinflammatory pathway triggered by aspirin treatment and revealed a new role for aspirin therapy in glomerular injury.

Role of Lipoxygenase Products in Kidney Disease

LTs are increasingly recognized as major mediators of glomerular hemodynamic and structural deterioration during the early phases of experimentally induced glomerulonephritis. Increased glomerular generation of LTB4 probably worsens glomerular injury by augmenting leukocyte recruitment and activation, and the cysteinyl LTs, by depressing K_f and GFR. In certain studies, there has been evidence supporting the involvement of 5-LO products in the mesangioproliferative phase of injury in both antiglomerular basement (NTS) model and anti-Thy1 model of renal glomerular injury. Selective blockade of the 5-lipoxygenase pathway in the course of glomerular injury is associated with significant amelioration of the deterioration of renal hemodynamic and structural parameters. In addition, dietary deprivation of essential fatty acids, which results in arachidonic acid and eicosanoid deficiency, confers protection against the histopathologic and the functional consequences of immune-initiated injury in the glomerulus. LTs are probably involved in the pathophysiology of human glomerulonephritis. In this regard, 5-lipoxygenase and FLAP mRNA expression have been detected in kidney biopsy specimens from patients with IgA nephropathy and mesangial proliferative glomerulonephritis, and were associated with clinically worse renal status. Also, urinary LTE4 levels have been found to be elevated in patients with active systemic lupus erythematosus. A pathophysiologic role for LTs has also been described in experimental acute allograft rejection, cyclosporine toxicity, and acute ureteral obstruction. Evidence suggests a potential role of 15-LO and its products as endogenous LT antagonists, exerting anti-inflammatory actions (Fig. 13.4).

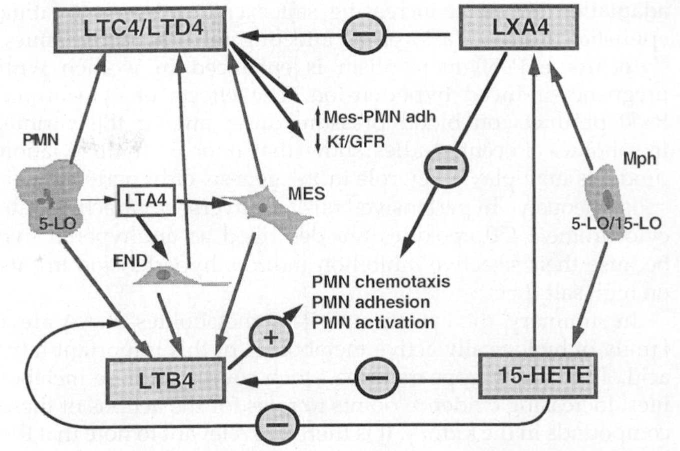

Figure 13.4. Proinflammatory and antiinflammatory actions of lipoxygenase-derived products.

CYTOCHROME P450 PRODUCTS

The microsomal NADPH-dependent cytochrome P450 enzyme system metabolizes arachidonic acid to a wide variety of oxygenated products. Three types of reaction can take place: (a) allylic oxidation leading to the formation of HETEs; (b) epoxidation resulting in the formation of epoxyeicosatrienoic acids (EETs) or epoxides, which can be hydrolyzed to their respective dihydroxyeicosatrienoic acids or vicinal diols; and (c) monooxygenation yielding α and α_1 hydroxylated acids. The kidney is a rich source of cytochrome P450 metabolites; cytochrome P450 activity resides mostly in the proximal tubule, thick ascending limb, and cortical collecting tubule. Cytochrome P450 enzymes constitute a multigene superfamily. Recent evidence suggest that the major arachidonate epoxygenase in the kidney is a member of the cytochrome P450 2C family, whereas α or α_1 hydroxylation appears to be mediated primarily by members of the cytochrome P450 4A gene family. Hormones such as epidermal growth factor, AVP, angiotensin II, calcitonin, and corticosteroids modulate activity of the cytochrome P450.

In the kidney, arachidonate cytochrome P450 metabolites have been assigned several biologic properties, including vasoactivity, effects on tubular water and ion transport, and local modulation or mediation of the activity of the renin-angiotensin system and other peptide hormones. The vasoactivity of the various metabolites varies among different species. Both vasoconstrictor and vasodilator effects have been described. For example, 5,6-EET and 20-HETE are vasodilatory in rabbit kidney but constrict rat blood vessels. The effects of the most potent vasoactive cytochrome P450 metabolites-5,6-EET and 20-HETE are COX dependent. In fact, the cytochrome P450 and the COX enzyme systems appear to interact transcellularly. In this manner, the COX pathway may modify the products of cytochrome P450 and vice versa. Such transcellular metabolism of 5,6-EET and 20-HETE by the COX pathway appears to be essential for expression of their vasoactive effects. With regard to their effects on salt and water balance, the cytochrome P450 metabolites are capable of inhibiting both ion transport in the medullary thick ascending limb and the hydraulic conductivity of AVP in the cortical collecting tubules. Intrarenal administration of 20-HETE, one of the major cytochrome P450 metabolites formed in cells of the medullary thick ascending limb, resulted in natriuretic and diuretic responses in rats. In addition all EETs and their corresponding dihydrotestosterone metabolites acted as inhibitors of the hydroosmotic effect of AVP in rabbit cortical collecting tubules. With regard to their interaction with the renin-angiotensin system, the cytochrome P450 metabolites 12(R)HETE and 14,15-EET inhibit renin release by rat kidney. On the other hand, angiotensin II stimulates the release of 5,6-EET from isolated rat proximal tubules, which mediates angiotensin II–induced increases in cytosolic calcium and Na absorption.

Overall, it appears that the cytochrome P450 pathway may have a role in modulating renal function both in health and disease. In this regard, dietary sodium loading has been demonstrated to selectively induce the renal excretion of cytochrome P450 metabolites. Induction of the cytochrome P450 enzyme system has also been observed after unilateral nephrectomy and experimental diabetes mellitus. The induction of cytochrome P450 in all these conditions may serve as a physiologic adaptation aimed at increasing salt excretion by modulating epithelial transport as well as affecting renal hemodynamics. Cytochrome P450 metabolism is enhanced in women with pregnancy-induced hypertension. The effects of cytochrome P450 products on blood pressure differ among the various metabolites. Recent studies show that α or α_1 hydroxylation products may play a key role in the genesis of hypertension in spontaneously hypertensive rats. Conversely, arachidonate cytochrome P450 epoxides are described as antihypertensive because their selective inhibition induces hypertension in rats on high salt diets.

In summary, the cytochrome P450 metabolites of AA are a family of biologically active metabolites of this important fatty acid. The kidney appears to be a rich source of these metabolites. Increasing evidence points to roles for the actions of these compounds in the kidney. It is therefore relevant to note that the levels of these compounds identified in normal human urine (using gas chromatographic–mass spectrometric techniques) are equivalent to those of COX metabolites.

THE ISOPROSTANES

Isoprostanes are prostaglandinlike compounds formed by free radical-catalyzed peroxidation of AA, independent of the cyclooxygenase enzyme. These compounds are easily detected in normal human plasma and urine and their production is enhanced markedly in animal models of free radical-induced injury. One of these, an F_2-isoprostane, 8-epi-prostaglandin $F_{2\alpha}$ (8-epi-$PGF_{2\alpha}$), is a potent renal vasoconstrictor and has been shown to have significant other biologic activities *in vivo* and *in vitro*.

Existing evidence, related to the formation of isoprostanes, suggests that these compounds are initially formed in situ esterified to phospholipids *in vivo*. Many different normal animal tissues, including the kidneys, have been shown to have detectable levels of these esterified isoprostanes.

Levels of isoprostanes in normal human plasma and urine exceed levels of cyclooxygenase derived PGs and thromboxanes by more than an order of magnitude, suggesting that the formation of isoprostanes is a major pathway of AA disposition. Also, given the fact, that the levels of unmetabolized isoprostanes in urine are very high, we initially examined whether 8-epi-$PGF_{2\alpha}$ exerted any biologic effects on renal function. Intrarenal arterial infusion of 8-epi-$PGF_{2\alpha}$-induced dose-dependent reductions in GFR and renal plasma flow, with renal function ceasing at the highest dose. Micropuncture measurements revealed a predominant increase in afferent compared with efferent arteriolar resistance, resulting in a significant fall in transcapillary hydraulic pressure difference and leading to reductions in single-nephron GFR and plasma flow. The 8-epi-$PGF_{2\alpha}$-induced changes in renal hemodynamics were completely abolished in the presence of the TXA_2 receptor antagonist SQ 29548. In addition, SQ 29548 completely reversed acute reductions in RBF induced by 8-epi-$PGF_{2\alpha}$, even during the continued administration of 8-epi-$PGF_{2\alpha}$. Using cultured rat aortic smooth muscle cells, we found specific binding sites for [≥H]SQ 29548 and for iodine 125 (^{125}I)– labeled BOP, a TXA_2 agonist. Both ligands were displaced from these binding sites by 8-epi-$PGF_{2\alpha}$, although with significantly less potency than nonlabeled SQ 29548, ^{125}I-labeled BOP, or U-46619, a TXA_2 agonist. In contrast, 8-epi-$PGF_{2\alpha}$ stimulated inositol 1,4,5-trisphosphate production and DNA synthesis in these cells with significantly greater potency than any TXA_2 agonist, effects only partially inhibited by SQ 29548. Thus 8-epi-$PGF_{2\alpha}$ probably exerts its biologic actions in vascular smooth muscle through activation of receptor sites related to, but distinct from TXA_2 receptors; 8-iso-$PGE_{2\alpha}$, an E_2-isoprostane, also showed similar renal hemodynamic effects with its renal vasoconstriction action completely abolished by SQ 29548. However, binding studies, as in the case of 8-epi-$PGF_{2\alpha}$, show that these effects were mediated by receptors related to, but distinct from, TXA_2 receptors.

A pathophysiologic role for isoprostanes has been suggested in quite a few conditions affecting the kidney. In a rat model of renal ischemia-reperfusion urinary excretion of these compounds was markedly enhanced. In a different study, circulating plasma concentrations of F_2-isoprostanes were selectively increased a mean of 7.8-fold in patients with hepatorenal syndrome, compared with those of the control group. Enhanced production of isoprostane has also been reported to occur in other disorders, like scleroderma and diabetes mellitus, in which free radicals have been thought to play a role.

In summary, isoprostanes are a recently described family of potentially important biologically active metabolites of AA which not only serve as a marker of oxidant stress, but by virtue of its significant biologic activities *in vivo* and *in vitro,* may play an important role in the pathophysiology of a spectrum of disorders affecting the kidney.

Selected Readings

Badr K, Breyer MD. Arachidonic acid metabolites and the kidney. In: Brenner BM. *The Kidney*, ed 5, WB Saunders, Philadelphia, 1997.

A comprehensive review of the chemistry, cellular signaling, and integrated function of eicosanoids in the kidney, including basic experimental and clinical information.

Badr KF, Ichikawa I. Prerenal failure: a deleterious shift from renal compensation to decompensation. *N Engl J Med* 1988;319:623.

An analysis of the role of PGs in the regulation of renal vascular tone and GFR during reductions in renal perfusion pressure in experimental and human situations.

Badr KF, Schreiner GF, Wasserman MA, Ichikawa I. Preservation of the glomerular capillary ultrafiltration coefficient during rat nephrotoxic serum nephritis by a specific leukotriene D4 receptor antagonist. *J Clin Invest* 1988; 81:1702.

The first description, using micropuncture techniques, of the functional significance of LTD_4 in reducing the glomerular capillary ultrafiltration coefficient, and hence GFR, in acute experimental glomerulonephritis.

Benigni A, Gregorini G, Frusca T, et al. Effect of low-dose aspirin on fetal and maternal generation of thromboxane by platelets in women at risk for pregnancy-induced hypertension. *N Engl J Med* 1989;321:357.

Further evidence in humans for the importance of TXA_2 generation in the pathophysiology of pregnancy-induced hypertension. Use of low-dose aspirin therapy extends the already established power of this treatment modality in cardiovascular thrombosis to pregnancy-associated disorders of vascular function.

Bonvalet JP, Pradelles P, Farman N. Segmental synthesis and actions of prostaglandins (PGs) along the nephron. *Am J Physiol* 1987;253:F377.

An excellent study on the qualitative and quantitative distribution of CO derivatives along the mammalian nephron.

Kelley, V E, Sneve S, Musinski S. Increased renal thromboxane production in murine lupus nephritis. *J Clin Invest* 1986;77:252.

Extension of the observations regarding the role of TXA_2 in glomerular immune injury to a clinically common disorder, lupus nephritis, by demonstrating increased production and functional significance for TXA in a murine model of this disorder.

Pierucci A, Simonetti BM, Pecci G, et al. Improvement of renal function with selective thromboxane antagonism in lupus nephritis. *N Engl J Med* 320:421.

A description of studies in humans that provide the first demonstration that rat and mouse studies can serve as excellent models for human disease. The studies reveal significant improvement in renal function on administration of TXA_2 receptor antagonists to patients with active lupus nephritis.

Samuelsson B. An elucidation of the arachidonic acid cascade: discovery of prostaglandins, thromboxane and leukotrienes. *Drugs* 1987;33(Suppl 1):2.

A comprehensive and authoritative account of the discovery of PGs and LTs, detailing their chemical properties.

Yared A, Albrightson-Winslow C, Griswold D, et al. Functional significance of leukotriene B4 in normal and glomerulonephritic kidneys. *J Am Soc Nephrol* 1991;2:45-56.

Evidence is presented in an experimental model of glomerulonephritis for increased production and functional relevance of LTB4. In addition, presence of infiltrating neutrophils as a source and target for LTB4 is established.

PART 2
Erythropoietin

John W. Adamson

The concept of a humoral regulator of red blood cell production has existed for more than a century. In the late 1800s, Paul Bert noted increased red cell numbers in individuals who lived at high altitude. Early in the twentieth century, Carnot and Deflandre provided physiologic observations in both humans and experimental animals that supported the concept that in response to hypoxemia or anemia, a factor circulated in the plasma to effectively increase red blood cell production. In 1906, Carnot and Deflandre published the results of their experiments, in which plasma from anemic rabbits stimulated new red cell formation (reticulocytosis) in recipient rabbits. These investigators postulated that a humoral factor was responsible; they named the factor *hemopoietin.* Although the timing of the increase in red cell production in these experiments defies understanding according to our current knowledge, these investigators nevertheless established a principle against which the results of subsequent experiments could be judged. Remarkably, nearly 50 years passed before other investigators took up the issue of the regulation of red cell production. In a classic series of experiments using parabiotic rats, Reissmann demonstrated that exposing one of two animals to hypoxia resulted in increased red cell production in both. Shortly after that, Erslev repeated the experimental strategy of Carnot and Deflandre and showed that the infusion of plasma from severely anemic rabbits resulted in an increase in reticulocytes in recipient animals; this was followed by an increase in hematocrit levels. The infusion of normal rabbit plasma had no such effect. Soon after, a group at the University of Chicago, headed by Leon Jacobson, confirmed not only that such a humoral factor existed but that its production likely resided in the normal kidney, a critical association. The early activity was called *erythropoietic stimulating factor;* only later was it known as *erythropoietin* (Epo).

These early physiologic studies, which seem crude in light of modern technologies, nevertheless provided the foundation for the work that followed. Ultimately, Goldwasser was able to purify trace amounts of human Epo from the urine of patients with aplastic anemia. The primary amino acid sequence information led to the design of degenerate primers that were then used to screen a cDNA library made from anemic rat kidneys. Identified sequences that hybridized to the probes were then used to design more specific primers, which led to the final isolation of Epo-specific mRNA and ultimately the cloning of the human Epo gene—a feat reported in 1983.

MOLECULAR BIOLOGY OF EPO

Human Epo is the product of a single gene that maps to the long arm of chromosome 7. The gene is made up of 4 introns and 5 exons. In addition to the structural gene, a number of regulatory elements are found in both the 3′ and 5′ untranslated regions. It has been reported that there are both enhancers and suppressors of transcription in the 5′ untranslated region of the Epo gene. Others have reported a steroid response element and a hypoxia inducible factor-1 (HIF-1) binding site in the 3′ flanking sequence.

The coding region of the gene predicts that the gene product would be a polypeptide of 193 amino acids, which includes a 27-member secretory leader sequence. The leader sequence is responsible for transporting the polypeptide to the endoplasmic reticulum.

Before the secretion of the molecule from the cell, further processing takes place and the carboxy-terminal arginine is cleaved off, leaving the mature polypeptide of 165 amino acids, as shown in Fig. 13.5.

The Epo molecule has four conserved cysteine residues at positions 7, 29, 33, and 161. Disulfide bridges are formed between 7 and 161, and between 29 and 33. These bridges are important for Epo's biologic activity and are found in many mammalian forms of Epo.

Human hepatoma cell lines (HepG2 and Hep3B), which produce Epo in response to induced hypoxia, have contributed substantially to our understanding of Epo gene regulation. These cell lines produce little Epo under normoxic conditions but increase Epo production significantly with hypoxic (Po_2 values less than 15 mm Hg) stimulus. This system has been exploited to demonstrate that the oxygen sensing mechanism involves a heme protein and that displacement of oxygen from the protein results in upregulation of Epo gene expression. Binding to a number of compounds, including cobalt, resulted in increased Epo production. Not only has this cellular system been useful for studying the molecular and chemical signals involved in Epo gene regulation, but also the observations have formally demonstrated that, at least for liver cells, the same cell that can sense a hypoxic stimulus can produce Epo.

Human Epo is a glycoprotein with a molecular weight of about 30.4 kD. The molecule is heavily glycosylated; there are 3 N-linked and 1 O-linked glycosylation sites on the molecule. Thus about 40% of the molecular size of Epo results from the addition of carbohydrates at these specific sites. The carbohydrate structures described for human urinary Epo are shown in Fig. 13.6. Approximately 65% of the oligosaccharides found on either purified human urinary Epo or Chinese hamster ovary (CHO) cell–derived recombinant human (rh) Epo are tetraantennary, with a small proportion containing one or two additional lactosamine repeats. The remaining carbohydrate (or sugar) additions are triantennary or biantennary structures. Both the terminal sialic acids and the degree of branching of the oligosaccharides have an important role in determining the level of *in vivo* bioactivity. RhEpo, enriched in tetraantennary oligosaccharides, has greater *in vivo* bioactivity and lower *in vitro* bioactivity than rhEpo enriched in biantennary structures. Polylactosamine repeats may decrease the *in vivo* activity of Epo because of more rapid clearance of the molecule from the circulation.

Although the carbohydrate additions to the molecule are not required for its bioactivity *in vitro,* or binding of the molecule to its receptor, the presence of the carbohydrates is critical to its biosynthesis, secretion, and bioactivity *in vivo.* The presence of the carbohydrates is also critical for the *in vivo* circulating half-life of the molecule. If the sialic acid residues are removed from the carbohydrates on Epo and desialated Epo is injected intravenously, Epo rapidly disappears from the circulation—probably as the result of uptake by galactose receptors in the liver. The requirement for the carbohydrates for *in vivo* bioactivity dictates the necessity for the production of rhEpo by mammalian cell expression systems.

The glycosylation of Epo—both native and recombinant—results in a number of isoforms of the molecule having different amounts of carbohydrate. When the different isoforms were isolated and studied for their bioactivity, it was found

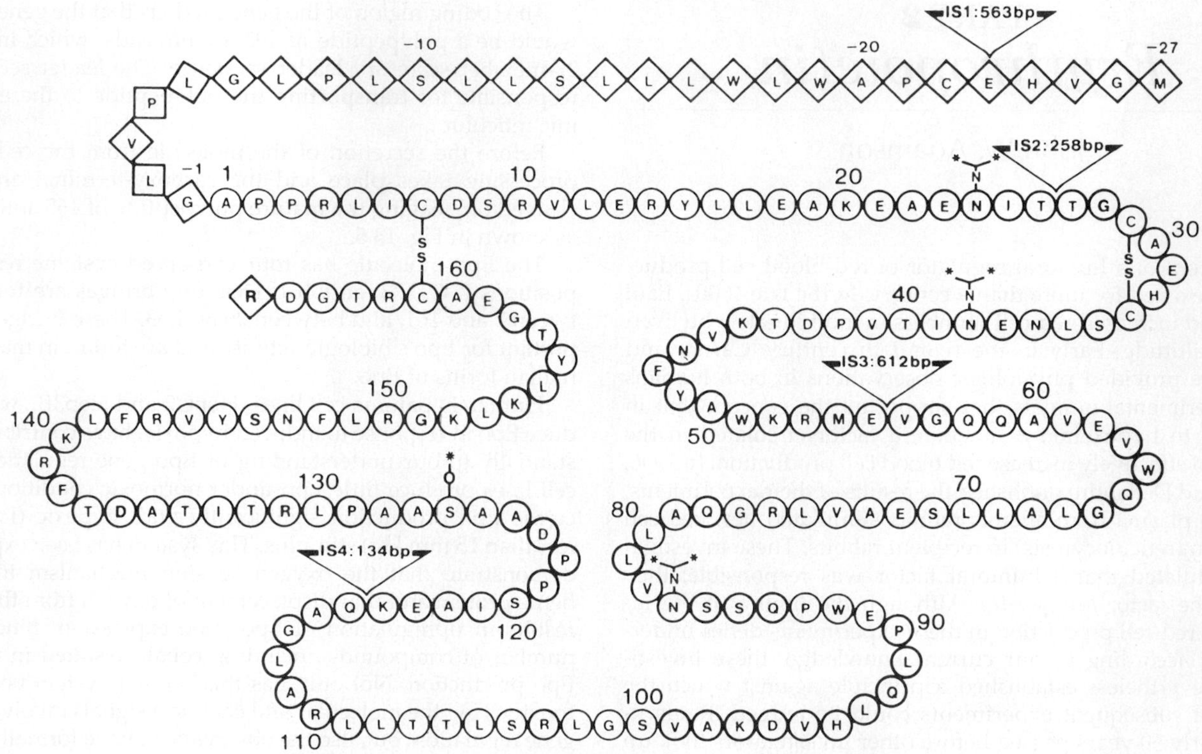

Figure 13.5. The amino acid sequence of the translation product of the human erythropoietin gene presented in one-letter code. The 27 amino-terminal amino acids of the putative signal peptide are boxed, and the residues in the 165–amino acid mature polypeptide are circled. Also boxed is the terminal arginine at position 166 that is removed posttranslationally. Positions of the two disulfide bonds (S-S), the three N-linked (Y), and the one O-linked (at position 126) glycosylation sites are shown. Positions at which the four intervening sequences (IS) interrupt the coding sequences of the gene are given, along with the length of each IS sequence. (Reproduced with permission from Egrie JC, Browne JK. The molecular biology of erythropoietin. In: Erslev AJ, Adamson AJ, Eschbach JW, et al, eds. *Erythropoietin. Molecular, cellular and clinical biology.* Baltimore: The Johns Hopkins Press, 1991:21–40.)

that those having the greatest number of sialic acids had a longer circulating half-life *in vivo* and greater biologic activity. This led to the development of a new therapeutic molecule that, by site-directed mutagenesis, contained additional N-linked glycosylation sites, increasing the number of sialic acid residues from the usual 9 to14 to as many as 20. The effect of these additional structures was to increase the circulating half-life 3-fold and the biologic activity 20-fold compared with rhEpo when dosing on a once-weekly basis was studied. This novel form of rhEpo is now in early clinical trials.

EPO PHYSIOLOGY

Epo is made largely by the kidney in adult mammals. There is no prohormone form of Epo, nor does a storage form exist. Consequently, in times of physiologic stimulus, new protein synthesis is required for increased Epo production and the resulting elevated levels of Epo in the circulation. A small amount (perhaps 5% to10%) of residual Epo production may come from the liver. In humans and several other species, including the sheep and rat, the liver is the major organ of Epo production in embryonic life. Sometime around birth, through mechanisms that are not well understood, the primary site of Epo production shifts to the kidney.

The site of Epo production within the kidney has been studied by a number of groups, sometimes with conflicting results. Thus renal glomeruli, mesangial cells, and tubular cells have all been proposed as the source of Epo production. While some controversy continues, the preponderance of evidence favors the conclusion that Epo production originates not in tubular or glomerular cells but in highly specialized epithelioid cells lining the capillaries surrounding proximal tubular cells. This has been shown by several groups using *in situ* hybridization techniques to localize Epo mRNA. It has been demonstrated that it is not an increased amount of Epo produced per cell that results in increased Epo production, but rather the number of Epo-producing cells recruited by the stimulus. In these studies, the kidneys from normal and anemic mice were harvested, fixed, and the number of cells positive for Epo mRNA determined. As shown in Fig. 13.7, there was an increase in cells containing Epo mRNA as a result of increasing anemic stimulus while the amount of Epo produced per cell, as judged by the density on autoradiograms, remained unchanged. Thus, at least in this species, cells appear to be "triggered" into Epo production.

These studies also provided information about the distribution of Epo-producing cells within the kidney. In response to moderate anemia, Epo-producing cells appeared in small clusters, and the clusters were largely found in the inner aspect of the cortex near the corticomedullary junction and were adjacent to proximal convoluted tubules rather than to other segments of the nephron. Under conditions of severe anemia, Epo-producing cells were more uniformly distributed throughout the inner cortex and outer medulla. These observations are consistent with other studies that have shown that Epo production is directly related to proximal tubular function. The studies also led to the conclusion that only a fraction of the total interstitial cell population participated in Epo production, suggesting that the Epo-

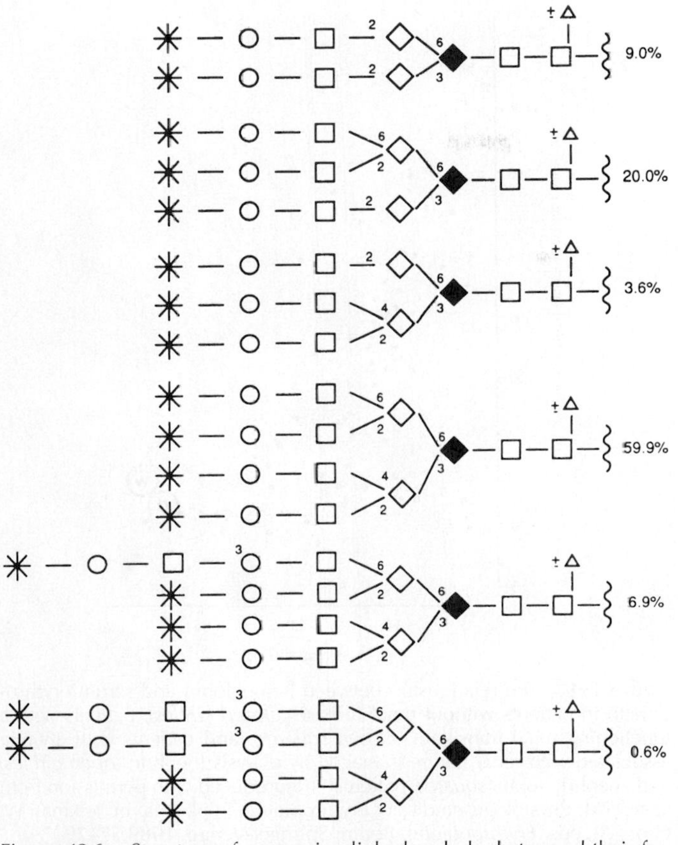

Figure 13.6. Structure of asparagine-linked carbohydrates and their frequency in human urinary erythropoietin. (Reproduced with permission from Egrie JC, Browne JK. The molecular biology of erythropoietin. In: Erslev AJ, Adamson AJ, Eschbach JW, et al, eds. *Erythropoietin. Molecular, cellular and clinical biology.* Baltimore: The Johns Hopkins Press, 1991; 21–40, with original data from Takeuchi M, Takasaki S, Miyazaki H, et al. Comparative study of the asparagine-linked sugar chains of human erythropoietins purified from urine and the culture medium of recombinant Chinese hamster ovary cells. *J Biol Chem* 1988;263:3657–3663.)

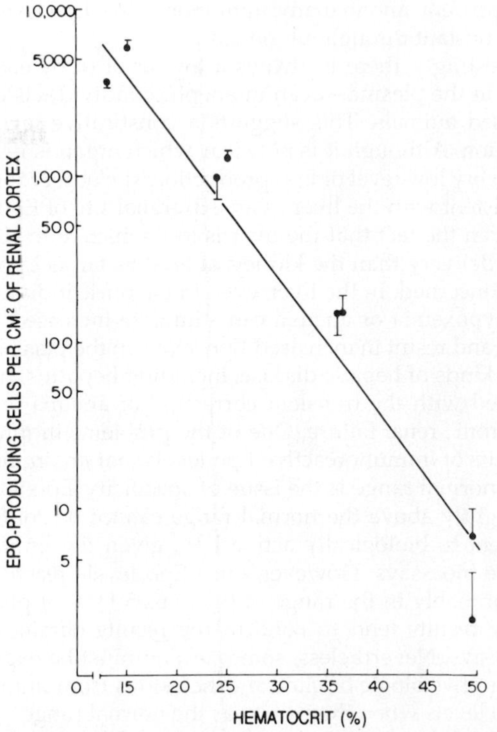

Figure 13.7. The exponential increase in the number of erythropoietin-producing cells with decreasing hematocrit. Erythropoietin-producing cells were identified as those positive for erythropoietin-specific mRNA. The data represent the mean ±SEM of quadruplicate experiments per mouse. (Reproduced with permission from Koury ST, Koury JM, Bondurant MC, et al. Quantitation of erythropoietin-producing cells in the kidney of mice by in situ hybridization: correlation with hematocrit, renal erythropoietin messenger RNA, and serum erythropoietin concentration. *Blood* 1989; 74:645–651.)

producing cells were a specialized cell type within the cortical interstitium. The fact that not only individual cells, but also regions of the interstitium, are recruited for Epo production suggested differences in vascular supply to these areas. However, whether Epo-producing cells are also those which "sense" the anemic stimulus is not known, but it is likely that they are.

In the liver, both hepatocytes and nonepithelial cells have been proposed as Epo-producing cells, with the bulk of Epo coming from hepatocytes. When hepatic Epo production was analyzed in a series of transgenic mice expressing the human Epo gene, hepatocytes carrying the Epo signal were found primarily around the central vein; Epo-producing cells were generally absent from the portal areas. This pattern of Epo production follows the known oxygen gradients within the liver, with the portal areas having the highest oxygen concentrations and the central veins the lowest. In contrast to the kidney, hepatocytes apparently increase Epo production on a per-cell basis rather than by the recruitment of additional Epo-producing cells.

It has been estimated that the liver normally contributes some 10% to 15% of Epo production in the basal state and that with renal failure, the liver is responsible for the majority of Epo production. Why the liver does not produce sufficient Epo to maintain a normal hematocrit level in patients with renal failure probably lies in the fact that the Epo-producing cells in the liver are far less sensitive to mild or moderate hypoxic stress than cells in the kidney.

Finally, although Epo mRNA has been found in the brain, testis, spleen, and lung—and the Epo-specific mRNA signals in these organs increase with hypoxia, the contribution to the overall production of Epo is negligible. What role locally expressed Epo might have in these tissues is entirely unknown.

The availability of rhEpo has led to the development of a number of sensitive immunoassays for the hormone. The data obtained from such measurements of plasma Epo levels have provided a number of insights into the relationship of circulating Epo levels in various experimental manipulations and clinical conditions.

The range of normal values for immunoreactive Epo in human plasma is 4 to 25 U/L. However, there is wide individual-to-individual variation within the normal range and neither sex nor age differences explain the variability. That there is no obvious difference in basal Epo levels between men and women is somewhat at variance with results obtained with older bioassays for Epo which suggested Epo levels were lower in women than in men. The difference was explained by the effects of estrogens and androgens on Epo production and was thought to account for the slight differences in mean hemoglobin levels between men and women in the childbearing age. With loss of estrogen production in the postmenopausal period, it was believed that the suppressive effect of estrogen on Epo production and erythropoiesis was lifted, allowing the hemoglobin concentrations of postmenopausal women to approach those of men.

There is also a diurnal variation in circulating Epo levels that is most apparent in anemic or hypoxic individuals whose baseline Epo levels are already above normal. Peak values are found in the evening hours. In normal individuals, the diurnal variation is less apparent, and in many, immunoreactive Epo levels are relatively constant throughout the day.

Interestingly, there is always a low level of detectable Epo present in the plasma—even in anephric individuals or hypertransfused animals. This suggests a constitutive level of Epo production. Although it is not clear which organ is responsible for this very low level of Epo production, the observation might be consistent with the liver as an extrarenal site of Epo production, given the fact that the liver is less sensitive to changes in oxygen delivery than the kidney, at least as far as Epo production is concerned. In the liver, even in anephric individuals, extreme hypoxemia or anemia can stimulate increased Epo production and result in increased Epo levels in the plasma. In fact, various kinds of hepatic disease, including hepatitis, have been associated with the transient correction of anemia in patients with chronic renal failure. One of the problems in interpreting the results of immunoreactive Epo levels that are in the normal or near-normal range is the issue of specificity. Epo levels in or even slightly above the normal range cannot be confirmed as equivalent to biologically active Epo, given the limitations of available bioassays. However, once Epo levels reach a certain value, probably in the range of 0.1 to 0.25 U/L of plasma, the bioassay results tend to confirm the results obtained by immunoassays. Nevertheless, some caution must be expressed in drawing physiologic or clinical conclusions from immunoreactive Epo levels when they are near the normal range.

In the circulation, the clearance (half-life) of Epo follows a monoexponential curve. The half-life is variable, ranging in some studies from a low of 3 hours to a high of 11 hours. The average is about 6 hours. Limited studies indicate that the half-life is the same for native Epo as it is for rhEpo. The half-life appears to be the same in individuals with active erythropoiesis as it is in individuals with suppressed red cell production, including those with renal failure who are undergoing dialysis. These and other experiments have led to the conclusion that very little of the clearance of Epo from the circulation is associated with the degree of erythroid marrow function. The reasons for the differences in Epo clearance times remain unexplained, and it is not clear how, or if, these differences are related to red cell production.

In studies of Epo metabolism, few clear answers emerge. Based on calculations of Epo turnover in the circulation and the amount that can be accounted for that appears in the urine over a 24-hour period, only 5% to 10% of the Epo produced is excreted. There is little evidence that the kidney actively metabolizes Epo. A small fraction of the Epo produced may be taken up by the liver or bone marrow, but the amount cannot be readily calculated as a percentage of overall Epo production. Although Epo, bound to its receptor, is known to be internalized in erythroid cells in the marrow, the amount that can be accounted for is extremely small, probably less than 1%. If rhEpo is radioactively labeled and the tracer followed to different tissues, no single obvious site of catabolism can be found. Thus the ultimate metabolic fate of most of the Epo produced remains unknown.

Circulating levels of Epo in normal individuals are related to the degree of anemic or hypoxic stress. Thus, in individuals with intact renal function, a decrease in hemoglobin or hematocrit is associated with a logarithmic increase in measurable Epo levels in the circulation, as shown in Fig. 13.8. This relationship is strikingly similar to the proposed model of cellular recruitment for the production of Epo shown in Fig. 13.7.

However, relatively modest changes in hemoglobin and hematocrit around the normal range do not result in substantial increases in Epo levels. This was demonstrated by measuring plasma Epo levels in normal individuals who were phlebotomized. While 1- or 2-unit blood donations led to a change in Epo levels, the changes were small, and the values remained

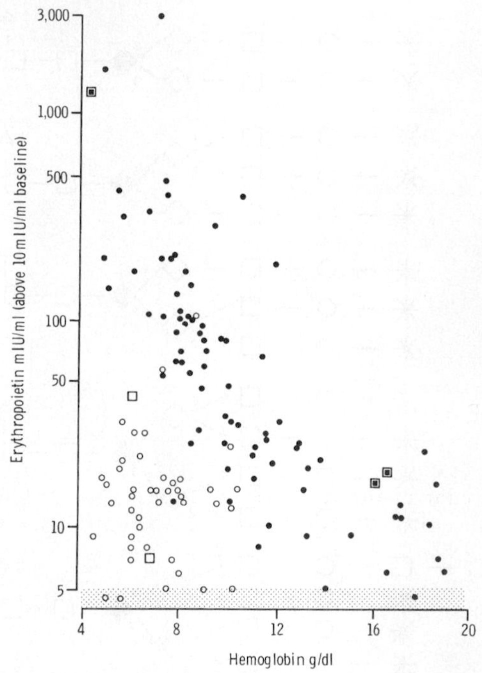

Figure 13.8. The relationship between hemoglobin and serum erythropoietin in patients without renal disease *(closed circles),* patients with a functioning renal transplant *(closed squares),* and patients with anemia associated with renal failure managed by dialysis [nephric *(open circles)* and anephric *(open squares)* patients]. (Reproduced with permission from Cotes PM. Physiologic studies of erythropoietin in plasma. In: Jelkman W, Gross AJ, eds. *Erythropoietin.* Berlin: Springer-Verlag, 1989:57–79.)

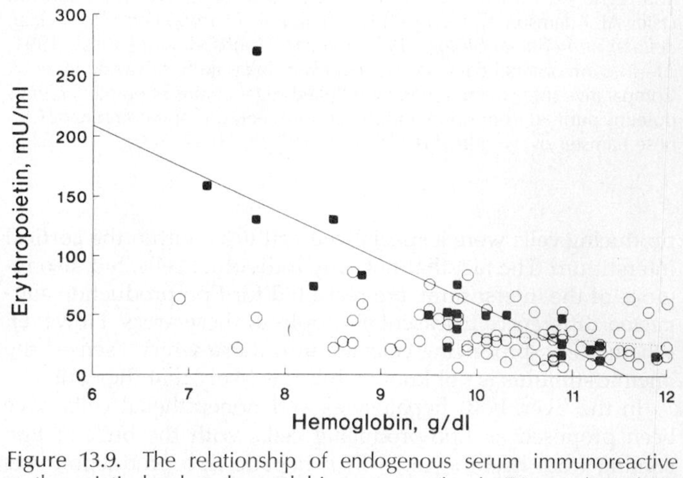

Figure 13.9. The relationship of endogenous serum immunoreactive erythropoietin levels to hemoglobin concentration in 74 anemic patients with cancer *(open circles)* and 24 patients with uncomplicated iron deficiency anemia *(closed squares).* There was no significant correlation between serum erythropoietin levels and hemoglobin concentration in the patients with cancer ($P = .48$) while a highly significant correlation was found for patients with iron deficiency ($P = .001$). (Reproduced with permission from Miller CB, Jones RJ, Piantadosi S, et al. Decreased erythropoietin response in patients with anemia of malignancy. *N Engl J Med* 1990;322:1689–1692.)

within the normal range. Thus the concept was advanced that there was a threshold effect for increasing Epo production and that major increases in Epo levels were associated with hemoglobin concentrations of 10 g/dl or less.

The relationship between stimulus and Epo production is lost in several disease states associated with chronic anemia, including renal failure (Fig. 13.9) and malignancy. In renal failure, the impaired renal function underlies the impaired production of Epo, resulting in what many believe to be a classic hormone deficiency state.

THE CELLULAR ANATOMY OF ERYTHROPOIESIS

All hematopoiesis begins at the level of the pluripotent stem cell. This cell is capable of undergoing lineage commitment to erythroid, myeloid, or lymphoid development through a series of steps that are poorly understood. The process of commitment or lineage restriction is not dictated by any of the known growth factors or hormones, such as Epo.

Epo stimulates erythropoiesis through its effects on Epo-responsive cells. The response is mediate by Epo-specific receptors (Epo-R) on the surface of the cells, and the appearance of Epo-R is part of the expression of the already committed or predetermined program of erythroid development.

The cellular anatomy of erythropoiesis has been defined using tissue culture techniques that permit different classes of erythroid progenitor cells to proliferate and form colonies of hemoglobinized red cells in semisolid medium. The growth factors required for colony formation, the size of the colonies, and the time of their appearance in culture have been used to distinguish the various classes of progenitors.

In the hierarchy of committed erythroid progenitor cells, as shown schematically in Fig.13.10, the earliest recognizable class is made up of erythroid burst-forming cells (BFU-E). This cell has the greatest proliferative capacity, often forming large colonies with 5,000 to 10,000 cells. When grown in semisolid medium in the presence of appropriate growth factors, the BFU-E initially gives rise to daughter cells that outmigrate from the parent cell and then undergo terminal differentiation and maturation to form clusters of well-hemoglobinized red cells. The appearance of this complex, multicentered colony is one of a "burst," hence the name *burst-forming cell.*

The BFU-E has very few Epo-R on its surface, but more Epo-R appear as the BFU-E undergoes several cell divisions to give rise to the erythroid colony-forming cell (CFU-E). The CFU-E is a cell with more restricted proliferative capacity, able to undergo no more than four or five cell divisions. Thus the erythroid colonies that arise from the CFU-E contain only 100 to 150 cells, at most. The CFU-E has up to 1,000 Epo-R per cell, and the numbers decline rapidly as CFU-E give rise to pronormoblasts and more mature erythroblasts.

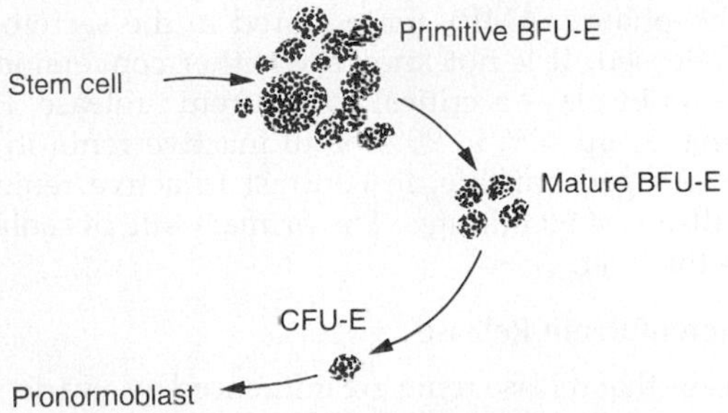

Figure 13.10. The cellular anatomy of erythropoiesis. Beginning with the pluripotent stem cell, erythropoiesis can be characterized by a series of cellular compartments that have different proliferative potentials and different growth factor requirements. The primitive BFU-E is the earliest recognizable progenitor cell committed to the erythroid lineage. Its numbers are unaffected by changes in ambient levels of erythropoietin. The CFU-E is further along the erythroid lineage pathway and its numbers are highly sensitive to changes in circulating levels of erythropoietin. (Reproduced with permission from Adamson JW. The relationship of erythropoietin and iron metabolism to red cell production in humans. *Semin Oncol* 1994;21:9–15.)

The differences in the erythroid cellular compartments are also brought out by studies of the numbers of the various progenitors under conditions of suppression or stimulation. Experimental hypertransfusion results in a 70% to 80% reduction in the number of CFU-E in the marrow, while an anemic or hypoxic stimulus (or administration of rhEpo) results in a threefold to fivefold increase in the number of CFU-E. Such manipulations have no effect on the absolute numbers of marrow BFU-E. Thus the numbers of CFU-E—but not BFU-E—in the animal are highly sensitive to changes in endogenous Epo levels.

In addition to erythroid progenitor cells, Epo-R are found on megakaryocytes, endothelial cells, and trophoblastic cells of the placenta. For some of these cell types, Epo has been shown to have a biologic effect—at least *in vitro.* Several investigators have demonstrated that endothelial cells will undergo a proliferative response in the presence of Epo under highly defined culture conditions. However, a physiologic role for Epo-endothelial cell interactions is unknown. Similarly, Epo-R have been well described on megakaryocytes, and several investigators have shown that Epo can act as a proliferative or maturation-inducing agent—again, under highly controlled culture conditions. Despite this latter observation, in numerous clinical studies with rhEpo, no consistent effect on platelet production has been found. The possible physiologic roles for Epo-R on the other cell types remain unexplained.

THE ERYTHROPOIETIN RECEPTOR

The human Epo-R is a polypeptide of 508 amino acids. It has a 22–amino acid transmembrane spanning region and almost equally sized cytoplasmic and extracellular domains. The Epo-R is a member of the hematopoietic growth factor receptor superfamily. Other members of the family include the receptors for interleukin (IL)-2 β and γchains, IL-3, IL-4, IL-7, IL-9, growth hormone, and prolactin, among others. Characteristic of this family is the presence of four conserved cysteine residues in the extracellular domain and a WSxWS motif.

Epo-R lack an intrinsic tyrosine kinase domain. For signal transduction, ligand (Epo)-receptor binding induces dimerization of the receptor. This in turn activates the JAK-STAT pathway, with phosphorylation of STAT-5 and JAK-3 being part of the signal transduction mechanism. How these signals are ultimately related to the induction of gene expression in the nucleus remains to be elucidated.

On ligand binding, Epo and the EpoR complex are internalized by the cell and the Epo degraded. Despite this fairly classic pathway of ligand-receptor metabolism, the actual amount of Epo consumed in the process is minute when compared with the overall amount of Epo produced per day.

Selected Readings

Erslev AJ, Adamson JW, Eschbach JW, et al, eds. *Erythropoietin. Molecular, cellular and clinical biology.* Baltimore: The Johns Hopkins University Press, 1991.

This book provides a full range of topics related to erythropoietin, including a historical perspective of the evolution of the study of the regulation of red blood cell production.

Fukuda MN, Sasaki H, Lopez L, et al. Survival of recombinant erythropoietin in the circulation: the role of carbohydrates. *Blood* 1989;73:84–89.

A study of the carbohydrate additions to the erythropoietin molecule and the importance of the glycosylation to the in vivo bioactivity of the hormone.

Jones SS, D'Andrea AD, Haines L, et al. Human erythropoietin receptor: cloning, expression and biological characterization. *Blood* 1990;76:31–35.

This article follows the first report by this group on the cloning of the mouse erythropoietin receptor. The findings permit the initial studies of the functional regions of the receptor and place the receptor in the growing family of hematopoietic growth factor receptors.

Kickler TS, Spivak JL. Effect of repeated whole blood donations on serum immunoreactive erythropoietin levels in autologous donors. *JAMA* 1988;260: 65–67.

In this study, serum erythropoietin levels were shown to change only slightly in normal subjects despite multiple whole-blood donations over a relatively short period. In fact, serum erythropoietin levels, while increasing, stayed within the normal range until the hemoglobin level fell to about 10 g/dl. This led the authors to conclude that there was a threshold effect for more marked erythropoietin production, and that the logarithmic increase in circulating erythropoietin levels related to anemia did not apply to hemoglobin values within or near the normal range.

Koury ST, Koury MJ, Bondurant MC, et al. Quantitation of erythropoietin-producing cells in the kidneys of mice by in situ hybridization: correlation with hematocrit, renal erythropoietin messenger RNA and serum erythropoietin concentration. *Blood* 1989;74:645–651.

An interesting study in which erythropoietin-producing cells were "quantitated" in histologic sections of the kidneys of mice which had been made anemic to different degrees. In situ hybridization studies were performed to identify those cells having detectable erythropoietin mRNA. There were several important findings. First, the amount (strength of signal) of mRNA did not change on a per cell basis. Rather, the number of cells that were positive increased in a logarithmic manner as related to the degree of anemia. Second, the increase in the number of erythropoietin-producing cells mirrored the circulating levels of erythropoietin as measured by a sensitive immunoassay.

Lin F-K, Suggs S, Lin C-H, et al. Cloning and expression of the human erythropoietin gene. *Proc Nat Acad Sci USA* 1985;82:7580–7585.

One of the first two reports of the successful cloning and expression of the human erythropoietin gene. The cloning of this gene was a landmark event in terms of providing an important therapeutic agent for the treatment of many anemia conditions in humans.

Miller CB, Jones RJ, Piantadosi S, et al. Decreased erythropoietin response in patients with anemia of malignancy. *N Engl J Med* 1990;322:1689–1692.

This study joined previous studies that had linked inadequate endogenous erythropoietin production to anemia. Like patients with renal insufficiency, patients with malignancy—whether solid tumors or hematologic malignancies—had a blunted erythropoietin response to anemia. However, the mechanisms underlying the anemia are different than those thought to be most important in the anemia associated with renal failure.

PART 3
Renin-Angiotensin System

Julio E. Benabe and
Manuel Martinez-Maldonado

The renin-angiotensin system (RAS) has emerged as one of the most critical endocrine, paracrine, juxtacrine, and possibly, autocrine systems in the regulation of normal physiology and the mediation of pathologic states. The RAS is involved in the control of blood pressure, the regulation of body water and sodium, and thus intravascular volume, and it is a major determinant of growth and remodeling of cardiovascular and renal tissues. All but perhaps a minute fraction of circulating renin is synthesized and released by the kidney. The renin activity ultimately determines the level of plasma angiotensin II. Angiotensin II, acting through specific receptors, is the active component of the system and mediates most of the physiologic and pathophysiologic effects of the RAS. Although genes encoding for components of the RAS are expressed to variable extents outside the kidney and all the proteins encoded by these genes can be locally synthesized, they are powerfully expressed and produced within the kidney itself. The presence of a complete RAS in the kidney that can generate angiotensin II locally has great implications in the regulation of renal function in that it suggests a dual regulatory system: one systemic and one local, both under the influence of angiotensin II. Moreover, the capacity to synthesize all the components of the RAS in other tissues suggests that angiotensin II may mediate functional aspects of other organs and organ systems as well. The following discussion will focus on chemistry and molecular biology of the RAS, physiologic functions of angiotensin II in the kidney, and the role of the renal RAS in hypertension and renal disease.

COMPONENTS OF THE RAS

Renin

Renin is an aspartyl protease that specifically cleaves a decapeptide, angiotensin I, from angiotensinogen. It exists in two major forms in the kidney and plasma: the active enzyme, which has a molecular weight of 40,000, and the inactive biosynthetic precursor of the enzyme, *prorenin,* which has a molecular weight of 47,000. In normal subjects, 30% or less of the circulating renin is in the active form; a greater percentage of active renin relative to prorenin is found within the kidney itself.

The primary source of renin in the kidney is the juxtaglomerular (JG) cells that express the renin gene most intensely under normal and pathologic conditions. Renin gene expression and production also occurs in smooth muscle cells in the afferent arteriole up to the interlobular arteries in the fetal kidney or in the adult kidney when the animal is subjected to stimuli that enhance renin production, such as administration of angiotensin-converting enzyme (ACE) inhibitors. In addition, renin messenger ribonucleic acid (mRNA) has also been identified in proximal and distal tubule cells and in mesangial cells. The human renin gene is located on chromosome 1; a single gene codes for the enzyme. Preprorenin is the primary translation product of renin mRNA. A signal peptide of 20 amino acids is cleaved from it to form prorenin, as the protein enters the endoplasmic reticulum, where the prorenin is glycosylated at Asp 5 and 75 (numbered with respect to Leu 1 of renin). After traversing the Golgi apparatus, prorenin can be sorted to three sites:

1. To lysosomal granules, where it is metabolized (less than 5% of the prorenin is sorted to lysosomes)
2. To secretory granules, where prorenin is processed to renin by the enzyme cathepsin B (which cleaves the 46–amino acid prosegment)
3. To membrane-bound vesicles, where prorenin does not undergo processing and is constitutively secreted

Both of the secretory pathways are enhanced when there is an increase in transcriptional activity. When there is an acute stimulation, such as occurs with cyclic adenosine 3′,5′-monophosphate (cAMP), renin stored in the secretory granules is released. It is not known whether conversion of prorenin to renin plays a critical role in renin release. Prorenin, which makes up 50% to 90% of all inactive renin in plasma, has a prolonged half-life, in contrast to active renin, which has a half-life of 90 minutes. The primary site of renin metabolism is the liver.

Regulation of Renin Release

The JG cells that release renin are influenced by a variety of both stimulatory and inhibitory signals. Renin secretion is influenced by the following: (a) an intrarenal vascular receptor or baroreceptor, (b) the concentration of sodium (or possibly chloride) ion sensed by the macula densa segment of the distal tubule, (c) the sympathetic nervous system and humorally released catecholamines, (d) other hormonal factors [e.g., angiotensin II, prostaglandins, atrial natriuretic peptide (ANP)], and (e) ions. Paracrine growth factors have also been shown to play an important role in the regulation of the RAS. The final control mechanism that governs renin release processes these signals to produce an integrated response.

Intrarenal Vascular Receptor or Baroreceptor. Renal vasodilation or an increase in perfusion pressure stretches the wall of the afferent arteriole (and JG cells) and decreases renin secretion. A reduction in renal perfusion pressure increases renin secretion. The mechanism, location, and nature of the sensing activity of renal baroreceptors are still unknown. It is thought that the renin-secreting epithelioid cell itself is the sensor for changes in transmural pressure gradient or circumferential stretch, although polarization of the afferent arteriolar cells has also been proposed. *Renal prostaglandins* appear to be mediators of the baroreceptor response. Prostaglandins (e.g., PGE_2, PGI_2) are potent stimulators of renin secretion and are released from preglomerular vessels on reduction of renal perfusion pressure. Although in some studies with anesthetized animals, inhibitors of PG synthesis prevented or attenuated the baroreceptor response of renin secretion, no effect of PG inhibition on the pressure-renin release curves was seen in conscious dogs. Thus, although PGs may have a significant modulation function on the baroreceptor response of renin release (especially under conditions of an increased rate of synthesis such as seen during renal nerve stimulation or during anesthesia), they are apparently not essential for the expression of the baroreceptor response. Other studies have described stretch activation of calcium channels in vascular endothelial cells. *Endothelin* is a potent renal vasoconstrictor and an inhibitor of renin release in the isolated perfused rat kidney. It acts as a calcium channel-gating agent in vascular smooth muscle cells. Therefore the endothelium may also be a possible signal-transmitting system, both in the autoregulation of renal blood flow (RBF) and baroreceptor-mediated renin secretion.

Sodium Signal. In all species examined, an inverse relationship between dietary salt intake and plasma renin activity (PRA) has been documented. There is a close anatomic association of the distal tubule at the site of the macula densa with JG renin–producing cells of the afferent arteriole. A tubular control mechanism senses changes in the sodium chloride concentration in the tubular fluid and stimulates renin release when this concentration is decreased and inhibits renin secretion when this concentration is increased. The extent of tubular segments that participate in the control of renin secretion is unclear because morphologic studies demonstrate that not only the macula densa but up to 90% of all distal connecting tubules come into close contact with the afferent arteriole. Therefore the control of renin may not only depend on the various local or systemic mechanisms but also on the state of activity of the RAS that determines the localization, how the renin-producing cells are spread, and the degree of transformation from smooth muscle to epithelioid cells. It is still debated whether sodium or chloride or both are primarily sensed by macula densa. A number of studies indicate that the rate of delivery of chloride into the early distal tubule determines the magnitude of both tubular feedback and renin secretion. In rats, infusion of sodium salts other than sodium chloride failed to decrease renin release, whereas infusion of varying concentrations of chloride produced inverse changes in renin release.

Adenosine Signal. Adenosine has also been proposed as an additional tubular signal for the activation of the macula densa–mediated renin release. *In vitro* studies using kidney slices, isolated glomeruli, isolated JG cells, and afferent arterioles demonstrated that adenosine inhibits renin release. *In vivo,* exogenous adenosine leads to transient renal vasoconstriction, a sustained reduction in glomerular filtration rate (GFR) and inhibition of renin release. Thus adenosine has profound effects on both renal hemodynamics and renin secretion. However, whether adenosine plays an essential mediator role in macula densa–dependent renin release remains to be established.

Adrenergic Signal. Electrical stimulation of renal nerves or infusions of pharmacologic concentrations of epinephrine and norepinephrine stimulate renin secretion. JG cells are innervated by sympathetic fibers, and β-adrenoreceptors are present in the juxtaglomerular apparatus (JGA) and glomerulus. Earlier approaches to show a direct effect of renal nerve stimulation were complicated by the fact that renal nerves may also affect the baroreceptor and macula densa pathway. Using graded electrical stimulation of renal nerves in anesthetized dogs, it has been demonstrated that at very low stimulation frequency, renin release is increased without any changes in RBF, GFR, and sodium reabsorption. In addition to epinephrine and norepinephrine, specific dopaminergic innervation of the JGA has been identified. Intrarenal infusion of dopamine (DA) or its direct addition to renal cortical slices produces a dose-related increase in renin secretion that is blocked by dopaminergic blocking agents, suggesting that DA stimulates renin by specific DA_1 receptor activation.

Local Hormonal Factors. Locally produced and circulating substances critically influence renin secretion. They include angiotensin II, PGs, and other eicosanoids, antidiuretic hormone (ADH), ANP, NO, and ions.

- *Angiotensin II:* Circulating or locally produced angiotensin II directly inhibits renin release in different experimental models such as the nonfiltering dog kidney, the denervated dog kidney, the perfused rat kidney, kidney cortex slices, isolated cortical cells, and isolated glomeruli. Inhibition of the production of angiotensin II or blockade of its action leads to potent stimulation of renin release.
- *PGs and other eicosanoids:* PGE_2, prostacyclin (PGI_2) and their inactive precursors stimulate renin secretion *in vivo* and when directly added to renal cortical slices or to isolated JG cells. PG synthesis inhibition blocks renin release. PGI_2 and PGE_2 are equipotent in stimulating renin release, but PGI_2 has a more important physiologic role. Biochemical analysis and immunohistochemical studies have shown that cyclooxygenase, the major enzyme leading to prostaglandins synthesis, is present in endothelial cells of renal arteries and arterioles, in the glomerulus, interstitial cells, and in cells along the tubules. PGI_2 and PGE_2 are produced by isolated glomeruli in equal amounts. PGI_2 is the major cyclooxygenase product of the renal vasculature, whereas PGE_2 is synthesized predominantly along the tubules. Some studies suggest that other cyclooxygenase products, such as thromboxane A_2 (TXA_2), may inhibit renin release especially in abnormal conditions such as in local inflammation, renal ischemia, or ureteral obstruction. Other arachidonic acid (AA) metabolites of the lipoxygenase and epoxygenase pathways, may also play a role in renin secretion. In kidney and vessels, AA is also a substrate for lipoxygenase (LO), an enzyme that converts AA into 12- and 15-hydroperoxyeicosatetraenoic acids (HPETEs), and their respective 12- and 15-hydroxyeicosatetraenoic acids (HETEs). 12-HETE is the most abundant arachidonate product in rat glomeruli, whereas human glomeruli synthesize 12- and 15-HETEs in equivalent amounts. HETEs can be incorporated into membrane phospholipids, can alter calcium flux, and can activate the protein kinase C system. HETEs are potent inhibitors of renin release, both in renal cortical slices

and in isolated perfused rat kidneys. Picomolar concentrations of 12-HETE block the PGI_2 stimulatory effects on renin, suggesting that HETEs are not only potent inhibitors of renin secretion but also modulators of PGI_2 actions on renin. In isolated JG cells and in renal cortical slices, angiotensin II stimulates 12-HETE levels. Inhibitors of the LO pathway, such as BW755c and baicalein, block angiotensin II–induced renin inhibition as well as 12-HETE levels. Furthermore, 12-HETE reproduces angiotensin II action during LO blockade. HETEs have also been shown to play an important role in angiotensin II–induced aldosterone secretion and in angiotensin II–induced vascular effects.

AA can also be metabolized via the cytochrome P450 epoxygenase pathway in the kidney that leads to formation of epoxyeicosatrienoic acids (EETs) such as 5,6-, 8,9-, 11,12-, and 14,15-EET. The EETs can be further metabolized by cytosolic epoxide hydrolases to vic-diols (DHETs). EETs cause vasodilation, influence calcium release from aortic microsomes, reversibly inhibit vasopressin-stimulated osmotic water flow across the toad bladder, and have also been shown to suppress isoproterenol-stimulated renin release from rat renal cortical slices.

- *ADH:* ADH inhibits stimulated renin release. It is unclear whether this inhibition of renin release results from a direct action of the hormone on JG cells or from expansion of the plasma volume. Concentrations of ADH in the pathologic range, but possibly in the physiologic range as well, are involved in the control of renin secretion.
- *ANP:* High-affinity binding sites for ANP in the kidney have been localized to the glomerulus and the distal collecting tubules. The action of ANP, which could be mediated by stimulation of guanylate cyclase and intracellular cyclic guanosine 3′,5′-monophosphate (cGMP) formation, on renin secretion is controversial. In most *in vivo* studies, ANP decreases PRA; this action of ANP is mediated by multiple mechanisms including an increase in GFR, a direct inhibition of tubule sodium reabsorption, and a direct effect on JG cells. *In vitro* studies have not clarified the issue: both inhibition and stimulation of renin secretion have been reported. ANP stimulates renin secretion and cGMP formation in cortical kidney slices; however, 8-bromo-cGMP does not alter renin secretion, suggesting that ANP may stimulate renin release but not through cGMP. Other investigators using both cortical kidney slices and isolated JG cells in tissue culture have shown a direct inhibitory effect of ANP on renin secretion that could be reproduced with cGMP. Moreover, both sodium nitroprusside and ANP increased cGMP and decreased renin release. The inhibitory action over renin release was reproduced with 8-bromo-cGMP and abolished with a guanylate cyclase inhibitor. In summary, there are data to support an inhibitory action of ANP on renin secretion through a direct action on the JG cells or by activation of the macula densa inhibitory pathway. The former seems to predominate and is mediated by the formation of cGMP. Under certain physiologic conditions the activation of the baroreceptor stimulatory pathway by the vasodilator effects of ANP may stimulate renin release by antagonizing its direct inhibitory actions.
- *Nitric oxide (NO):* NO is a nitrogenous metabolite formed constitutively through two alternative enzymatic pathways: the endothelial and the neuronal isoform of the nitric oxide synthase (NOS). The endothelial isoform is primarily responsible for the production of NO in response to shear stress in a calcium-calmodulin–dependent process. In the renal cortex, it is found primarily in the endothelial lining of the blood vessels and glomeruli, from where it regulates renal hemodynamics. NO lowers renal vascular resistance, counteracts local endogenous vasoconstrictors, such as angiotensin II and endothelin, and can directly inhibit sodium reabsorption. *In vitro,* NO, like ANP, inhibits renin release through the formation of the inhibitory second messenger cGMP. *In vivo,* however, there is controversy over the ultimate role of NO on renin release. Some investigators have reported that when the influence of the renal baroreceptor or the renal nerves are eliminated, endothelial NO appears to inhibit renin release. On the other hand, other investigators have demonstrated that renin stimulation through the renal baroreceptor triggered by reducing renal perfusion pressure below the range of autoregulation, is blunted by the inhibition of NOS, suggesting that with decreased renal perfusion, NO may contribute to stimulation of renin secretion. These reports have led to the proposal that NO derived from endothelial NOS inhibits renin release while that derived from neuronal NOS stimulates renin secretion. In support for the latter is a study where 7-nitro indazole, a specific neuronal NOS inhibitor, blocked furosemide-induced increase in renin secretion. Thus, in contrast to the renin inhibitory role of endothelium derived NO, neuronal NOS may be an integral part of the macula densa pathway, and its NO production leads to stimulation of renin secretion.
- *Ions:* It is now clear that, in addition to Na^+ and Cl^-, changes in the extracellular concentrations of Ca^{2+}, Mg^{2+}, K^+, and H^+ alter renin release. Calcium plays a central role in controlling renin secretion, as it does in smooth muscle contraction and relaxation. Factors that physiologically stimulate renin secretion appear to do so by lowering cytosolic calcium ($Ca^{2+}i$), those that inhibit secretion do so by raising $Ca^{2+}i$. Renin secretion is increased when extracellular Ca^{2+} is reduced in renal cortical slice incubations, in cortical cell suspensions, in isolated perfused kidney, and in isolated glomeruli. Chelation of Ca^{2+} with ethylenediaminetetraacetic acid (EDTA) and/or ethyleneglycol-*bis*-(β-amino-ethyl ether)-N,N′-tetraacetic acid (EGTA) also stimulates renin release in *in vitro* preparations. Ca^{2+} channel blockers such as verapamil, diltiazem, or nifedipine, similarly stimulate renin secretion both *in vivo* and *in vitro.* The inhibition of renin by angiotensin II is also a Ca^{2+}-dependent process because EDTA can block the effects of angiotensin II in isolated perfused rat kidneys and the angiotensin II effect can be blocked with Ca^{2+} channel blockers.

Although raising extracellular Ca^{2+} inhibits renin, raising extracellular *magnesium* concentration stimulates renin secretion. High concentrations of Mg^{2+} hyperpolarize the cell membrane and inhibit net Ca^{2+} influx. Whether the hyperpolarization is the result of decreased Ca^{2+} influx or some other mechanism has not been established. However, increased Ca^{2+} and depolarization inhibit the stimulatory effect of high Mg^{2+} on renin.

A reciprocal relationship between *potassium* and renin release has been shown. Raising the K^+ depolarizes the cell membrane, increases the Ca^{2+} permeability of the cell and therefore allows a net influx of Ca^{2+}. This is based on the observations that removing extracellular Ca^{2+} makes high K^+ ineffective in inhibiting renin release. Also the Ca^{2+} channel blocker verapamil prevents the inhibitory effects of K^+ on renin. Lowering the K^+ concentration below physiologic levels also inhibits renin release, possibly by inhibiting the Na^+-K^+-ATPase and by increasing Ca^{2+}.

Growth Factors. Tumor necrosis factor (TNF) and interleukin-1 (IL-1) are potent secretogogues for renin but inhibit aldosterone secretion. These cytokines have been implicated in the genesis of the syndrome of hyperreninemic hypoaldosteronism seen in critically ill patients. In contrast, epidermal growth factor (EGF), which is a potent vasoconstrictor and shares many properties in common with angiotensin II, is a more potent inhibitor of renin than angiotensin II in rat renal cortical slices. Transforming growth factor-α (TGF-α), which binds to the EGF receptor, similarly inhibits renin secretion. Although the exact mechanism or mechanisms by which EGF affects renin secretion is not clear, indirect evidence suggests that tyrosine kinase activation participates in EGF-mediated renin release. EGF also stimulates basal and angiotensin II–induced aldosterone synthesis in the normal adrenal. Physiologic concentrations of insulin and insulinlike growth factor-1 (IGF-1) have also been shown to stimulate renin in normal rat renal cortical tissue.

TGF-β is colocalized with renin in JG cells. Both TGF-β1 and TGF-β2 (10^{-12} M) stimulate renin in rat renal cortical slice preparations, and their effects at low concentrations are mediated via PG synthesis. However higher concentrations (10^{-10} M) of both peptides are less stimulatory or do not alter renin release. Water deprivation in mice results in a selective increase in expression of TGF-β2 accumulation in JG cells and an increase in PRA. NOS mRNA is also expressed in the macula densa and JG cells suggesting that there may be a physiologic interrelationship among NO, TGF-β and renin release control, the nature of which remains to be elucidated.

A number of growth factors act through cAMP. In addition to Ca^{2+}, cAMP is an important second messenger in renin secretion. cAMP also appears to be the mediator of the β-adrenergic stimulation of renin release. In several *in vitro* and *in vivo* models, addition of cAMP or dibutyryl cAMP stimulates renin secretion. Forskolin, which is a stimulator of adenylate cyclase, potently induces renin release.

ANGIOTENSINOGEN

Human angiotensinogen, the specific substrate of renin, is a heterogeneous glycoprotein constitutively secreted by the liver. This organ is the primary source of angiotensinogen in the body although extrahepatic tissues such as the brain, kidneys, adrenal glands, lungs, heart, vascular tissues, testes, and gastrointestinal tract produce angiotensinogen. In the kidney, angiotensinogen mRNA has been identified in the proximal tubule, and other renal structures; renal angiotensinogen mRNA levels have been reported to increase in congestive heart failure. In the vasculature, angiotensinogen mRNA has been identified at low levels in smooth muscle and in relatively larger quantities in perivascular fat. Whether local production contributes to vascular angiotensin II formation is under investigation. Relatively abundant levels of angiotensinogen mRNA have also been identified in human and rat heart. The latter appears to be regulated by dietary sodium and other perturbations. In the perfused rat heart, angiotensinogen release has been identified in the perfusate, suggesting that tissue sources may also contribute to circulating angiotensinogen levels.

A single gene for angiotensinogen exists in man. Analysis of the 5′-flanking region of the angiotensinogen gene suggests that there are consensus sequences for three glucocorticoid response elements (GRE), a thyroid hormone response element (TRE), and an estrogen response element (ERE). These sequences are likely to be functional because glucocorticoid, thyroid hormone, and estrogen increase angiotensinogen mRNA in rat hepatocytes. There is also an acute-phase response element (APRE), which is consistent with the observation that plasma angiotensinogen levels rise during inflammation. The angiotensinogen gene has two different polyadenylation signals that result in two mRNA species of different lengths. The heterogeneity of angiotensinogen has been attributed to different glycosylation levels at four putative asparagine-linked glycosylation sites, which may regulate its kinetics in relation to renin.

Levels of angiotensinogen in the circulation are at the Michaelis-Menten constant (K_m), so that the changes in substrate concentration will influence the kinetics of the renin-angiotensinogen reaction. Angiotensin I is formed when renin cleaves a Leu-Val bond in the N-terminal region of human angiotensinogen or a Leu-Leu bond in other animal angiotensinogen species. In general, when angiotensinogen levels increase as occurs in pregnancy, estrogen administration, and Cushing's syndrome, plasma renin concentration decreases. After bilateral nephrectomy, liver angiotensinogen mRNA levels and circulating angiotensinogen levels increase. There are several different molecular weight forms of angiotensinogen, ranging from 50,000 to 100,000. The larger forms appear during pregnancy or oral contraceptive use.

Angiotensinogen-deficient mice (knockouts) have no detectable plasma angiotensinogen or angiotensin peptides and exhibit chronic hypotension. Although the brain and heart of these animals are essentially normal, the kidneys exhibit significant vascular hypertrophy, interstitial inflammation, atrophic changes in the tubules and papilla, and increased expression of growth factors and neuronal NOS genes. They also have increased urine output and decreased urine osmolality compared to normal mice. It is of interest that, despite the absence of circulating detectable angiotensin peptides, salt loading increased blood pressure in the angiotensinogen knockouts.

Angiotensin-Converting Enzyme

ACE is a dipeptidyl carboxypeptidase that converts angiotensin I to the potent vasoconstrictor angiotensin II and inactivates the vasodilator bradykinin. It is a member of the family of zinc metallopeptidases and contains a molar equivalent of zinc that is essential for the catalytic reaction. The enzyme consists of a single chain that is moderately hydrophobic and is predominantly membrane bound, anchored at the C-terminus. It is present in the circulation and in a variety of tissues including the endothelium of vascular beds, kidney, lung, brain, testis, and ciliated gut epithelium. The available evidence suggests that ACE is responsible for the conversion of both systemically delivered and intrarenally formed angiotensin I to angiotensin II. Because the kidney degrades more than 90% of the systemically delivered angiotensin II, most of the angiotensin II generated must exert an intrarenal paracrine or juxtacrine effect. A single gene encodes for ACE; however, two distinct mRNAs are transcribed from this gene from two distinct but overlapping transcription units by alternative initiation and splicing. The pulmonary ACE mRNA contains between 4.5 and 5.0 kb of sequence, while the testicular ACE mRNA is 2.6 kb long. Moreover, the gene has two polyadenylation signals; the proximal one encodes the termination signal for the testicular form while the distal adenylation site terminates the pulmonary sequence.

ACE knockout mice have 50% lower blood pressure readings than control animals and zero plasma enzyme activity. However, these mice exhibit abnormal kidneys with stunted renal papilla, renal vascular lesions, and tubulointerstitial infiltrates. ACE gene expression and ACE activity are critical for blood pressure regulation since, when only one functional ACE allele was left in these knockout mice, and despite a four-fold increase in renal renin mRNA and a 50% increase in ACE activity, blood pressure was normal.

AII Receptors

Two main classes of angiotensin II receptors (AT_1 and AT_2) have been identified by binding studies, principally defined by antagonist binding. Losartan is the prototype AT_1-receptor antagonist and PD-123177 is the prototype AT_2-receptor antagonist.

The AT_1-receptor mediates nearly all of the known physiologic functions of angiotensin II, including vasoconstriction, aldosterone secretion, thirst and drinking, growth, and proximal tubular sodium reabsorption. The precise function of the AT_2 receptor, however, is unknown. AT_1 receptors are widely distributed, but AT_2 receptors are widely distributed only in the fetus and localize to discrete brain nuclei, heart, uterus, adrenal, and renal locations in the adult. Although the abundance of this receptor in fetal tissue suggests it may play a role in growth and development, mice with targeted disruption of the AT_2 receptor gene demonstrate apparently normal embryogenesis, failing to support their essential nature in fetal development. Studies suggest that angiotensin II–mediated catecholamine secretion from the adrenal medulla are mediated through the AT_2 receptor. Retention of the AT_2 receptor in the heart of adults may contribute its antimitogenic effects on coronary arteries endothelium in opposition to AT_1-receptor–mediated mitogenesis. AT_2 receptors also appear to counteract classical pressor responses to angiotensin II because the pressor response to the peptide is significantly enhanced in AT_2-deficient transgenic mice. Other studies have suggested a cGMP-mediated pathway for the actions of angiotensin II through AT_2 receptors in the kidney. By contrast, AT_1-receptor–mediated actions lead to increments in PGE_2, an effect that is magnified by AT_2-receptor blockade. The full significance of these findings remains to be established, but we can begin to complete a picture in which the function of the AT_2 receptors is found to modulate the actions of angiotensin II mediated by the AT_1 receptor.

A unique angiotensin-binding site, specific for the hexapeptide angiotensin IV, has been identified in cultured vascular endothelial and smooth muscle cells. This AT_4 site has also been found in the cortex and inner medulla but not the outer medulla of rat kidney. The site does not bind either AT_1- or AT_2-specific antagonists. Angiotensin IV increases renal cortical blood flow, an action that was obliterated by NOS inhibitor, suggesting that the effects of angiotensin IV on renal cortical blood flow are mediated by NO. Stimulation of AT_4 subtypes by angiotensin IV also increases cerebral blood flow and opposes the actions of angiotensin II to cause cerebral vasoconstriction. Whether this action of angiotensin IV is also dependent on NO is unknown.

The AT_1 and AT_2 receptor genes have been cloned and sequenced (there is approximately 30% homology). The AT_1 receptor is a member of the seven-transmembrane G-protein–coupled receptor family. The receptor has a molecular weight of 41,000 and three potential glycosylation sites. In the rat, two AT_1 receptor subtypes have been identified, AT_{1A} and AT_{1B}, which have 94% sequence identity. These receptor subtypes appear to be encoded by two separate genes, which are similar in the coding sequences but are quite different in the 3′- and 5′-flanking regions. Studies of knockout mice have shown that complete absence of AT_{1A} receptors is associated with a mild survival disadvantage. Mice, however, grew normally, and as evaluated by light microscopy and immunohistochemistry, kidneys from these mice were essentially normal. Two major findings were observed: there was significant hypertrophy of the JGA and proximal expansion of renin-producing cells along the afferent arterioles, and some glomeruli showed evidence of mesangial expansion. The severe renal vascular lesions or papillary atrophy that have been observed in angiotensinogen-deficient or ACE-deficient animals are not seen in AT_{1A} receptor–deficient animals. Thus it appears that the AT_{1A} receptor is not essential for normal kidney organogenesis; however, its absence is associated with mild mesangial expansion and JGA hypertrophy.

AT_1-receptor mRNA has been identified in all tissues that respond to angiotensin II, including liver, kidney, uterus, adrenals, ovary, spleen, lung, brain, heart, and blood vessels. Angiotensin II acutely downregulates its receptor mRNA within hours of administration in cultured vascular smooth muscle cells, mesangial cells, and cardiac fibroblasts, but levels increase to basal by 24 hours. Growth factors such as EGF and cAMP acutely down regulate the AT_1-receptor mRNA. Whether these changes in message level contribute to regulation of angiotensin II action remains to be determined.

Renal Action of Angiotensin II

Receptor mapping by autoradiography has demonstrated an abundant and widespread distribution of angiotensin II receptors in the kidney. High concentrations are found in the glomerulus, the mesangial cells, the arterioles, the proximal tubule, and more recently, the interstitial medullary cells. Most of these angiotensin II receptors are of the AT_1 subtype.

Glomerular Basement Membrane

Angiotensin II affects pore size of the glomerular basement membrane and, therefore, has an impact on protein sieving. Increased pore size induced by high local levels of angiotensin II results in proteinuria. ACE inhibitors have been shown to decrease nephrotic range proteinuria associated with various renal diseases.

Mesangium

Angiotensin II promotes contraction, growth, and extracellular matrix production in cultured mesangial cells. The contraction response is accompanied by an increase in eicosanoids. Angiotensin II elicits a hypertrophic response in normal, adult rodent mesangial cells in culture and may induce a proliferative response in cultured fetal mesangial cells or in SV-40 transformed mesangial cells. Angiotensin II also stimulates endogenous growth factor production in mesangial cells, which includes TGF-β and platelet-derived growth factor (PDGF). The former may promote collagen production in mesangial cells, whereas the latter promotes growth. Extracellular matrix proteins produced by the mesangial cell include collagen I and IV, fibronectin and laminin. Mesangial expansion caused by cellular hypertrophy and increased extracellular matrix production is an important pathologic alteration in diabetic nephropathy. Angiotensin II is implicated directly and indirectly (through hemodynamic changes) to contribute to mesangial expansion in diabetes. The inhibition of angiotensin II in animal models of diabetic mesangial hypertrophy prevents or retards the progression of these morphologic lesions.

Proximal Tubule

Angiotensin II is an important regulator of both proximal tubular sodium chloride and bicarbonate absorption. Angiotensin II directly enhances sodium reabsorption throughout the proximal convoluted tubule, and increases bicarbonate absorption in the early proximal tubule, probably via a peritubular signal. These effects occur with subpressor doses of angiotensin II. The hormone also enhances the mitogenic effect of other growth factors in cultured proximal tubule cells and stimulates collagen production. Effects of angiotensin II on the proximal tubule epithelium are mediated by angiotensin II receptors on both the apical and basolateral membranes.

A complete RAS may exist within the proximal tubule. Both angiotensinogen protein and mRNA have been localized in the proximal tubule. An abundance of ACE activity is found in the apical brush border. Although renin has been localized by immunohistochemistry in subapical vesicles of proximal tubule cells, these observations could not distinguish synthesized renin from renin trapped after glomerular filtration. *In situ* hybridization studies were unable to demonstrate renin transcripts in these cells except after ACE inhibitor administration when it was easily detected in the S2 segment of the proximal tubule. Micropuncture studies have revealed high levels of angiotensin II (10^{-8}) in proximal tubular fluid that is higher than the filtered concentration.

Renal Vasculature

Studies in anesthetized dogs have demonstrated that intraarterial infusions of angiotensin can elicit decreases in both RBF and GFR. A number of studies have shown that infusion of angiotensin II or inhibition of its action in the kidney results in increased or decreased filtration fraction, respectively. Both efferent and afferent arterioles constrict following angiotensin II action. However, studies using isolated microvessels have demonstrated higher sensitivity of the efferent arteriole, but the mechanisms responsible for these differences in sensitivity are not well understood. NO may modulate the vasoconstrictor action of angiotensin II in afferent arterioles but not in efferent arterioles, contributing to differential sensitivity to angiotensin II.

THE RAS IN HYPERTENSION

Acute infusions of angiotensin II consistently increase blood pressure by vasoconstriction of vascular beds. Angiotensin II increases intravascular volume directly by enhancing proximal tubular sodium reabsorption and indirectly by stimulating adrenal aldosterone production, which enhances distal tubular sodium reabsorption and potassium secretion. Renin-dependent forms of hypertension primarily include renal artery stenosis and renin-secreting tumors. The former can involve constriction of a major renal artery or a segmental intrarenal artery (e.g., Ask-Upmark kidney). Renin-secreting tumors commonly arise from the kidney; the most common extrarenal site is the ovary. Malignant hypertension is associated with hyperactivity of the RAS. Excess renin is secreted from the kidney because of severe vasoconstriction of the intrarenal vasculature, leading to a significant decrease in RBF.

The RAS probably contributes to the development and maintenance of normal and high renin essential forms of hypertension. Approximately 60% and 15% of patients with essential hypertension fall into these categories, respectively. Collectively, these patients have relatively high PRA for their level of sodium excretion and blood pressure. In general, these patients manifest a decrease in blood pressure in response to inhibitors of the RAS, although patients with low renin essential hypertension have also been reported to respond to the blood pressure lowering effects of RAS inhibitors. The importance of high renin levels in determining the level of blood pressure can be adduced from the fact that normal rats made transgenic (by microinjection of the mouse renin-2 gene) have fulminant hypertension. On the other hand, although four restriction fragment length polymorphisms (RFLPs) have been identified in the human renin gene, none of these has been linked to hypertension. However, RFLPs of the rat renin gene have been linked to hypertension in the Dahl salt-sensitive model and in the spontaneously hypertensive rat (SHR). Renin locus analysis in humans has not revealed differences between hypertensive and normotensive subjects. The available data are not sufficient to exclude the renin locus, yet they are strongly against its involvement in human essential hypertension.

Polymorphisms of other RAS genes, however, have been linked to human and animal forms of hypertension. In one study, variants of the angiotensinogen gene were linked to hypertension in more than 400 families with essential hypertension. Families with these variants had higher circulating levels of angiotensinogen than those families without them. Linkage analysis has also demonstrated that polymorphisms in the ACE gene can be linked to blood pressure in the stroke-prone SHR, but no link has been found in human hypertension. The M235T polymorphism affects plasma angiotensinogen levels that are lowest in hypertensive individuals homozygous for the M235 variant, intermediate in heterozygotes and highest in homozygotes for the 235T variant. An association between 235T and hypertension has been confirmed in several populations.

Mice carrying excess functional copies of the murine wild-type angiotensinogen gene have increases in blood pressure and increases in plasma level of angiotensinogen that relate linearly to the number of copies. Mice carrying both the human renin and angiotensinogen genes have severe hypertension.

The AT_1 receptor gene has been studied as candidate locus for hypertension in humans with one negative and one positive case-control study and one negative linkage analysis. Interactions with angiotensinogen gene variants have not been detected so far.

INHIBITION OF THE RAS

ACE inhibitors prevent the generation of angiotensin II, thereby inhibiting some of the actions of the peptide. These compounds are useful as first-line therapy for hypertension and congestive heart failure; captopril, one of the first ACE inhibitors, has been demonstrated to be useful for slowing the progression of diabetic nephropathy in type I diabetes and for preventing ventricular dilation, which develops into a chronic condition following myocardial infarction. ACE inhibitors also enhance prostaglandin production and prolong the metabolism of kinins; these actions may also contribute to their therapeutic effects. Kinins, however, contribute to the cough associated with ACE inhibition. The various ACE inhibitors so far tested lead to lowering of blood pressure in hypertensive animals and humans.

Inhibition of the RAS by the administration of the nonpeptidic inhibitors of the AT_1 receptor lower blood pressure and inhibit angiotensin II–mediated aldosterone and vasopressin release, thus reducing extracellular fluid volume. Although the long-term effects of AT_1-receptor inhibitors on renal function in patients with renal disease are still not known, in animal models they exert renoprotective actions indistinguishable from those on ACE inhibitors. Even though human studies are few so far, those carried out have consistently reported antiproteinuric effects with AT_1-receptor inhibitors.

RAS IN RENAL DISEASE

Chronic Renal Disease

The RAS may play an important role in the pathogenesis and progression of chronic renal disease. The RAS is activated in cyclosporine nephropathy, polycystic kidney disease, and malignant hypertension. Studies in animals demonstrate that angiotensin II–mediated changes in intraglomerular capillary pressure are also accompanied by changes in excretion of protein in urine. In an animal model of renal vein constriction, the increase in endogenous angiotensin II was shown to be associated with a rise in intraglomerular capillary pressure and in proteinuria, which disappeared after infusion of the peptidic, competitive analog saralasin. In a renal ablation model both the increase in intraglomerular capillary pressure and the proteinuria is corrected after inhibition of angiotensin II generation.

Patients with renal artery stenosis and activated RAS exhibit increased urinary protein loss, but this disappears after either renal angioplasty or after pharmacologic blockade of the RAS. In addition, angiotensin II may also contribute to intraglomerular hypertension, a condition that participates in the progression of renal disease to its end stage.

ACE inhibitors have been shown to lower urinary protein excretion both in nondiabetic and diabetic renal disease. The antiproteinuric effects of ACE inhibitors is optimal if dietary sodium intake is restricted. ACE inhibitors appear to be more effective than other antihypertensive therapy in lowering proteinuria in normotensive or hypertensive patients with renal function loss. Several studies suggest that the antiproteinuric effects of ACE inhibition are the result of reduced systemic and intraglomerular blood pressure, and the reduction of glomerular basement membrane pore size, that is under the regulation of angiotensin II. Thus ACE inhibitors have been useful to improve or correct nephrotic syndrome secondary to multiple causes.

The ACE gene contains a polymorphism based on the presence (insertion [I]) or absence (deletion [D]) within an intron of a 287–base-pair nonsense DNA domain, resulting in three genotypes (DD and II homozygotes, and DI heterozygotes). A codominance association has been observed between the D and I polymorphism and plasma ACE activity. The values of ACE activity in people with DD genotype are approximately double the values of those with II; intermediate values are found in those with DI. However, the association between ACE polymorphism and increased risks for coronary artery disease, left ventricular hypertrophy, hypertension or progression of renal disease seems fairly well established and has been linked with declining renal function in patients with IgA nephropathy and diabetes mellitus. Large-scale prospective studies to further address this possible role of the ACE would be welcome.

The number of studies using AT_1-receptor inhibitors in renal disease patients or in those suffering from nephrotic syndrome is very small, but the results are similar to those of ACE inhibitors. The possibility that the AT_1 receptor gene locus may be linked to renal disease is being explored. In one study, AT_1 receptor gene polymorphism was not associated with progression of renal disease in focal segmental glomerulonephritis in children.

DIABETIC NEPHROPATHY

In diabetic patients, the PRA is generally low compared with matched nondiabetic controls. This occurs in hypertensive as well as nonhypertensive subjects. The cause of the low circulating renin has been postulated to result from volume expansion, abnormal autonomic nervous system function, the defect in renal processing of prorenin (the biosynthetic precursor of renin) to renin, and low renal prostacyclin and high lipoxygenase production. In 10% of diabetic patients, the low renin leads to the syndrome of hyporeninemic hypoaldosteronism. Low aldosterone production results in hyperkalemia and type IV tubular acidosis. Fludrocortisone of furosemide administration usually correct the acidosis and normalize serum potassium.

Although PRA is low in diabetes, angiotensin II appears to mediate some of the pathophysiologic changes associated with diabetic nephropathy. The potential role of the RAS in diabetic nephropathy is underscored by the observation that ACE inhibitors and AT_1-receptor antagonists decrease proteinuria associated with this disease as well as the progression of the disease in both human and animal models. Potential effects of angiotensin II on the kidney of patients with diabetes mellitus include increased intraglomerular pressure caused by relatively more efferent arteriolar vasoconstriction compared with the afferent arteriolar constriction, direct effect to stimulate mesangial cell hypertrophy and increased extracellular matrix production, and increased glomerular basement membrane pore size. The first two effects contribute to morphologic changes of diabetic nephropathy (i.e., glomerulosclerosis). Moreover, mesangial volume enlargement contributes to progressive decrease in GFR in diabetic nephropathy. Extracellular matrix expansion contributes to the proteinuria associated with diabetic nephropathy. Whether increased renal sensitivity to angiotensin II contributes to these changes in diabetic nephropathy remains to be determined. ACE inhibitors slow the progression of renal disease in the insulin-dependent diabetes mellitus patient.

Selected Readings

Antonipillai I, Horton R. Paracrine regulation of the renin-aldosterone system. *J Steroid Biochem Mol Biol* 1993;45:27–31.

Studies describing the potential effects of some cytokines and growth factors on renin-aldosterone systems.

Chung O, Kuhl H, Stoll M, et al. Physiological and pharmacological implications of AT_1 vs AT_2 receptors. *Kidney Int* 1998;67(Suppl):S95–S99.

Short review of angiotensin II receptors and their differences.

Churchill PC. Second messengers in renin secretion. *Am J Physiol* 1985;249: F175–F184.

Concise review of the role of important messengers in renin secretion.

Cusi D, Bianchi G. A primer on the genetics of hypertension. *Kidney Int* 1998; 54:328–342.

Excellent review on the role of the renin gene and other genetic loci in hypertension.

Griendling KK, Murphy TJ, Alexander RW. Molecular biology of the renin-angiotensin system. *Circ Res* 1993;87:1816–1828.

Review summarizing advances in molecular biology of renin, angiotensinogen, ACE, and angiotensin II receptors.

Hackenthal E, Paul M, Ganten D, et al. Morphology, physiology and molecular biology of renin secretion. *Physiol Rev* 1990;70:1067–1116.

Molecular biology, physiology, pharmacology and biochemistry of renin synthesis and secretion.

Hsueh WA. Role of the extrarenal renin-angiotensin system. *Curr Sci* 1992;7: 745–751.

Describes effects of angiotensin II, other vasoactive agents, and growth factors on the heart, kidney, and vasculature.

Hsueh WA, Anderson PW. Systemic hypertension and the renin-angiotensin system in diabetic vascular complications. *Am J Cardiol* 1993;72:14H–21H.

Brief review on the role of the RAS in the physiologic and pathologic conditions of the diabetic subject.

Keeton TK, Campbell WB. The pharmacologic alteration of renin release. *Pharmacol Rev* 1981;31:81–226.

Detailed overview of the factors that regulate renin secretion.

Lee MA, Bohm M, Paul M, et al. Tissue renin-angiotensin systems: their role in cardiovascular disease. *Circulation* 1993;87(Suppl): IV:7–13.

Discusses the tissue RAS system and the effect its inhibition on long-term cardiovascular and renal protection.

Perico N, Remuzzi G. Angiotensin II receptor antagonists and treatment of hypertension and renal disease. *Curr Opin Nephrol Hypertens* 1998;7:571–578.

Review of the effect of ACE inhibitors and AT_1-receptor blockers in the progression of renal disease and on proteinuria.

PART 4
Kallikrein-Kinin System

Harry S. Margolius

The roles of tissue kallikreins and kinins in renal function and as participants in the actions of drugs affecting the kidney are becoming clear. It is likely that this phylogenetically ancient system has significant responsibilities for the regulation of renal hemodynamics and for handling electrolyte and water movements across renal and other epithelial cells. These conclusions are the result of important discoveries concerning localization of system components in the kidney; regulation of their gene expression; the molecular characterization of system components, including the substrate kininogens, the formative and destructive proteases and peptidases, and the receptors; interrelations among these components and other renal regulatory hormones and mechanisms; and finally, new findings demonstrating system aberrancies during or before the appearance of systemic diseases or renal manifestations of diseases, including hypertension and diabetes mellitus. This chapter summarizes these findings.

COMPONENT CHARACTERIZATION, LOCALIZATION, AND REGULATION

The human kininogen (K) gene is localized to chromosome 3q 26-> qter close to two other related genes, the α-2-HS-glycoprotein and the histidine-rich glycoprotein. It codes for the production of both high-molecular-weight (HMW, 626 aa, 88 to 120 kD) and low-molecular-weight (LMW, 409 aa, 50 to 68 kD) kininogens through alternative splicing from 11 exons (the first 9 of which are common to both forms, as well as the part of exon 10 that codes for the kinins and the 12 subsequent amino acids after their carboxy terminus), spread over a 27-kb pair span. There is an interesting gene duplication in the rat that results in the K gene coding for HMW and LMW kininogens and a so-called T gene coding for T-kininogens. Although these rat genes are highly homologous (more than 90%), the production of T-kininogens and K-kininogens, and hence T-kinin (Ile-Ser-bradykinin) and K-kinins (Lys-bradykinin and bradykinin), are regulated differently in the rat by hormones or stress.

All kininogens are single-chain glycoproteins with constant amino-terminal heavy chains and smaller, variable carboxy-terminal light chains after the intervening kinin moiety. Separate functions are resident in each section of the molecules, including cysteine protease inhibition (heavy chains), binding regions for endothelial surfaces, and for plasma prekallikrein and factor XI, which promote contact activation (light chain of HMW), and of course, the binding to kinin receptors by kinins released by the proteolytic kallikreins.

The kidney is presented with kininogens that are synthesized elsewhere, primarily in the liver, then are secreted and transported in plasma as well as on platelet and neutrophil membranes. Human vascular endothelial cells contain mRNA for HMW kininogen, and kininogen is found in rat vascular smooth muscle cells grown in defined media containing no serum. In addition, mRNA for LMW kininogen, the preferred substrate for tissue (renal) kallikrein, is detectable in human kidney cortex and medulla. Studies using antibodies specific for human LMW kininogen and tissue kallikrein precisely described by immunohistochemistry the spatial relationships of kininogen and kallikrein in the human kidney (Fig. 13.11). This work demonstrates kallikrein in connecting tubule cells and kininogen in principal cells of the same transitional tubule just preceding the collecting duct. The site is juxtaposed to the afferent arteriole, where synthesized kallikrein, already known to traffic to basolateral membranes of these epithelial cells, might affect interstitial cell or vascular wall function through local kinin formation. Alternatively, known kallikrein trafficking to the apical membranes of these epithelial cells and subsequent tubular secretion might generate kininogen in the adjacent principal cells to locally generate kinin to affect tubular ion and water transport.

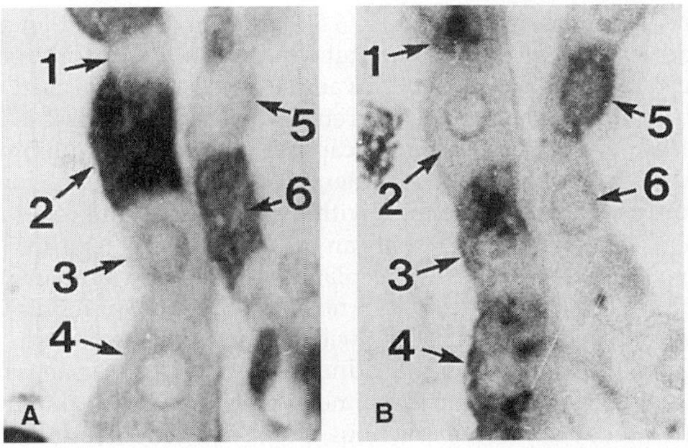

Figure 13.11. Serial sections of human renal connecting tubule immunostained for kininogen **(A)** and kallikrein **(B)**. Cells 2 and 6 show immunoreactive kininogen but not kallikrein. Cells 1, 3, 4, and 5 contain immunoreactive kallikrein but not kininogen. (× 3,000.) (Reprinted with permission from Figueroa CD, MacIver AG, Mackenzie JE, et al. Localisation of immunoreactive kininogen and tissue kallikrein in the human nephron. *Histochemistry* 1988;89:437–442.)

Renal kallikrein is a so-called true tissue kallikrein, a serine proteinase product of a gene in a small gene family of three in the human, but much larger families of up to 20 in the rat, of which 13 are characterized to date, and 24 in the mouse. The human genes are clustered on chromosome 19 at q13.2-13.4. The analogous locus in the mouse is on chromosome 7, but the locus is still not determined in the rat. The human gene is called *hKLK1* and is expressed in pancreatic and salivary duct cells as well as kidney and intestinal epithelial cells. The human neutrophil also contains tissue kallikrein mRNA showing that expression also occurs here. The closely related hKLK3 gene is of interest because it is expressed only in prostate and codes for the prostate-specific antigen (PSA). PSA has high sequence homology to tissue kallikrein, is also a serine proteinase, and is, of course, important to the detection of prostate carcinoma. The hKLK2 gene is also expressed in the prostate, but the product has as yet no defined function.

In the rat kidney, six kallikrein genes are expressed in addition to rKLK1, the "true" tissue kallikrein gene. All of these genes, regardless of species, consist of five exons and four introns; rKLK4, 7, and 9 are actually expressed at up to 10-fold higher levels in the rat kidney than rKLK1, but their functional importance, cellular localizations, and endogenous substrates are still unknown. The true tissue kallikreins of man and rodent are acidic glycoproteins of 24 to 45 kD. Most of the molecular weight variation results from variable glycosylation; for example, human urinary kallikrein is about 20% carbohydrate. The purified renal enzyme is synthesized as a zymogen called *prokallikrein* with an attached 17–amino acid signal peptide preceding a 7–amino acid activation sequence that must be cleaved to activate the enzyme. Several proteinases are capable of activating prokallikrein, including a human renal thiol proteinase, but the regulation of kallikrein activation and the identity of the specific activating enzyme *in situ* is still unclear.

Once activated, renal kallikrein cleaves LMW kininogen at a Met-Lys N-terminal bond and an Arg-Ser C-terminal bond to release Lys-bradykinin (kallidin). In most mammals, including humans, tissue kallikrein cleaves Lys-bradykinin from kininogens, whereas plasma kallikrein releases bradykinin. Conversion of Lys-bradykinin to bradykinin can occur through the action of aminopeptidases; however, the peptides are generally equipotent, and such conversion is considered important at present. Several inhibitors of the enzymatic activity of tissue kallikreins are known, including aprotinin, the bovine basic pancreatic trypsin inhibitor, a 6.5-kD, 58-aa polypeptide; and another serine proteinase inhibitor (a serpin) called *kallistatin.* The former is commercially available and is widely used experimentally as a tissue kallikrein inhibitor, although it is not specific in this regard and is capable of efficiently inhibiting other serine proteinases. The latter, a 58-kD acidic protein, slowly forms heat-stable complexes with active tissue kallikrein (and other serine proteinases) that can be blocked with heparin. The protein is measurable in the plasma of rats and humans. Its precise *in vivo* target is still unknown, and its role in regulating kallikrein activity locally is now beginning to be explored.

Kinin formed within the kidney is detectable in urine, renal interstitial fluid, and under some circumstances (i.e., kininase inhibition), even in renal venous blood. However, both the local and systemic half-life of kinins is widely considered to be very short, on the order of 10 to 30 seconds. Concentrations of kinins in biologic fluids are low (e.g., a few picograms per milliliter in human plasma), but for years kinin concentrations were overestimated by assays using inadequate inhibition of kinin-generating enzymes and by the use of nonspecific antisera that falsely elevated the estimates. On the other hand, the potency with which kinins exert a broad spectrum of effects on biologic targets has been underestimated, if anything, because an understanding of the contributors to kinin catabolism, particularly in the kidney, is still incomplete. Clear evidence for powerful effects of kinins on renal vascular resistance, electrolyte and water excretion, and interactions with other renal functional modulators such as renin and angiotensin, eicosanoids, catecholamines, nitric oxide (NO), atrial natriuretic peptide (ANP), vasopressin, and endothelin suggest strongly that the renal kallikrein-kinin system has important regulatory roles in renal function. Further support for this probability, in addition to the aforementioned localization information include the remarkably high daily turnover rate of mammalian renal kallikrein (estimated to be 3 hours in the rat), the high concentrations of renal kininases in discrete locales (e.g., proximal tubular brush borders), and the identification of kinin receptors on cortical and medullary collecting tubule cells, interstitial cells, cultured mesangial cells, and glomerular membranes. The effects of exogenous kinins to decrease afferent arteriolar resistance (and efferent resistance to a lesser degree) also affirms the existence of kinin receptors in renal vasculature.

These receptors are presently characterized as BK_1, BK_2, and perhaps, BK_3. BK_1 receptors are less prominent than BK_2 but are notably present in rabbit vasculature, especially after insult with, for example, *Escherichia coli* endotoxin or lipopolysaccharide. Then, the principal ligand for such entities, Des-Arg^9-bradykinin will produce significant vasodilation and hypotension, an effect not noted in normal tissue, although the peptide can also produce contraction of some vascular smooth muscle. These receptors have been described in several species and cell lines and have been cloned and characterized. There are now as many ligand-binding and second-messenger studies of these entities as of the previously more commonly studied BK_2 receptors. Of particular interest is work that has detected their coexistence with BK_2 receptors on rat mesangial cells.

The BK_2 receptors mediate most of the actions of kinins. The rat, mouse, and human BK_2 receptor genes have been cloned and expressed. The rat BK_2 receptor cDNA was obtained from a uterus library using Xenopus oocytes to assay for expression based on bradykinin-induced ion currents. Six rounds of clonal selection were required to obtain the single cDNA encoding this BK_2 receptor. The predicted protein sequence is 366 aa with a MW of 41,696 D and seven putative transmembrane domains. Strong homology is present to the histamine H_2 receptor, as well as to neurotensin and tachykinin receptors. As expected, the potency of bradykinin and Lys-bradykinin were equal (EC_{50} approximately equal to 1.9 to 2.9 nM) insofar as oocyte-induced currents and the BK_1-receptor agonist des-Arg^9-bradykinin had no effect on oocytes expressing the BK_2 receptor. Although the rat uterus has several times as much receptor message as any other tissue, the amounts in kidney are at least equivalent to that in heart, lung, testis, and brain.

cDNA or DNA encoding the human BK_2 receptor has been isolated. The predicted amino acid sequence from each is 81%, identical to the rat smooth muscle BK_2 receptor. Each could be transfected into CHO or COS cells, with resultant stable expression of high levels of kinin binding, high sensitivity to specific receptor blockade, and even coupling to the Ca^{2+}-phosphatidylinositol cascade. Interestingly, the level of human BK_2 receptor mRNA density was fivefold higher in kidney than in any other screened tissues, including uterus, lung, brain, heart, and testis. The isolation of these receptors from human and rodent are becoming very important to discerning kinin roles and to therapeutic advances based on receptor antagonism or stimulation.

The existence of additional BK receptors are being explored at various possible sites of expression, including bovine aortic endothelial cells, microvasculature of the hindbrain, and pulmonary smooth muscle of the guinea pig, and the smooth muscle of the opossum esophagus. At these and other sites, variant responses to BK_1 or BK_2 agonists and antagonists continue to suggest possible interaction with non-BK_1 or non-BK_2 receptors, now beginning to be called BK_3, BK_4, or BK_5 receptors. Full characterization of these binding sites remains to be accomplished.

The half-life of kinins is a function of both formation and destruction. Peptidases that hydrolyze kinins are known as *kininases,* although none is known to be specific for these peptides. Both aminopeptidases and carboxypeptidases can terminate kinin bioactivity, but the latter predominate; in rats, kininase II [angiotensin-converting enzyme (ACE)] and neutral endopeptidase 24.11 (enkephalinase) each removes COOH-terminal Phe^8-Arg^9, thus inactivating kinins. Both are present in high concentrations in proximal tubular brush borders and in urine, with the latter being the major kinin-destroying enzyme of rat urine. However, since the 1970s, ACE has been known to be bifunctional, either forming angiotensin II or hydrolyzing and destroying kinins. Although occurring as a soluble plasma enzyme, this kininase is highly concentrated on the luminal surface of the vascular endothelial cells as well as on the aforementioned renal proximal tubular cell apical membranes. The human lung vasculature is rich in this enzyme, but interestingly, levels the in kidney are about sixfold higher. For a considerable time, all therapeutic actions of converting enzyme inhibitors were considered to result from inhibition of angiotensin II formation. It is now clear that retardation of kinin destruction is likely to play a significant part in their efficacy, especially insofar as beneficial cardiac effects are concerned. For example, the ability of these inhibitors to reduce infarct size, left ventricular hypertrophy, or postischemic reperfusion injury is either attenuated or abolished by concomitant administration of the kinin BK_2-receptor antagonist, HOE 140 (icatibant) (Fig. 13.12). Such data, along with the corroborating kinin plasma level changes, suggest that locally produced kinins, at least in cardiac tissue, contribute to the beneficial effects of ACE inhibition. The data also continue to raise several questions about local kinin contributions to the function or dysfunction of other organs, including the kidney.

Any questions concerning local or systemic roles for kallikrein-kininogen-kinin systems ultimately reach the issue of system regulation *in situ.* The fact is that there is still little available information concerning the coordinate regulation of system com-

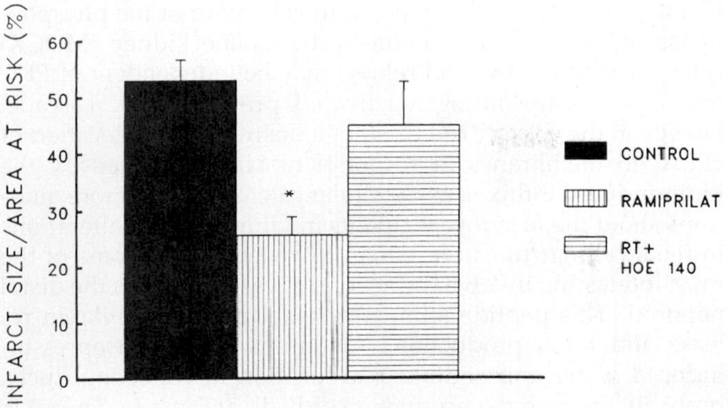

Figure 13.12. Reduction in infarct size, as a percentage of the area at risk, in control dogs ($n = 14$) and dogs treated with ramiprilat (40 ng/kg/min i.c.; $n = 8$) and ramiprilat plus HOE 140 (0.5 ng/kg/min i.c.; $n = 13$). Mean ±SEM. *$P < .05$ versus control dogs. (Reprinted with permission from Linz W, Schölkens BA. Role of bradykinin in the cardiac effects of angiotensin-converting enzyme inhibitors. *J Cardiovasc Pharmacol* 1992;20(Suppl 9): 583–590.)

ponents in response to various biochemical, physiologic, or pathologic stimuli. However, some information is beginning to appear at an increasing rate. For example, T-kininogen and HMW kininogen synthesis in cultured hepatocytes can be augmented by glucocorticoid, and maternal estrogen appears to be responsible for high circulating T-kininogen in neonatal rats or at puberty. Female rat liver kininogen mRNA levels are about fourfold higher than in male rats. Interestingly, estradiol and progesterone both increase renal kallikrein mRNA in the same animals. Whether these findings have relevance to cardiovascular or renal function still remains to be studied, and conspicuously unavailable are evaluations of the levels of gene expression and protein of multiple system components in relation to renal function and disease.

A great deal of data now describe the possible regulatory influences on tissue kallikrein. Both urinary and renal tissue kallikrein levels and synthesis rate can be increased by low-sodium, high-potassium diets, the first stimuli shown to change such levels in animals and humans. Chronic high levels of mineralocorticoids can increase renal kallikrein levels, and adrenalectomy reduces them. Female rat renal kallikrein mRNA is twice as high as in males. Various hormones affect these renal mRNA and protein levels, including testosterone, thyroxine, and insulin. Each significantly increases kallikrein synthesis and the level of enzyme activity. Vasopressin can also increase (but norepinephrine decreases) kallikrein release from rat renal cortical slices. This latter effect is accompanied by a reduction in *de novo* kallikrein synthesis and can be prevented by β_1-adrenergic blockade. These and other studies now provide ample opportunity to examine coordinate alterations in substrate and formative enzyme levels or gene expression in relation to pharmacologically induced or pathologic changes in renal function.

This conclusion has been reinforced dramatically by many studies of renal kinin receptors. These receptors were well characterized in earlier binding studies using ^{125}I-Tyr^8-BK, a partial BK agonist, and mesangial cell or glomerular membranes. In addition to describing both BK1 and BK_2 receptors in rat kidney and evaluating them in Goldblatt experiments, these studies showed that after 28 days of low sodium intake, there was a marked reduction in BK_2-binding site density, concomitant with increased renal and urinary kallikrein. Conversely, water deprivation resulted in a reduction in renal kallikrein level and an increase in BK_2 receptor density. This work suggests there is an inverse relation between presumptive renal kinin levels (inferred from augmented kallikrein activity) and BK-receptor density. These clues have been augmented by a series of studies using new technology that allows the direct measurement of renal interstitial kinin levels, which change markedly in response to various stimuli.

The contributions of kinin receptor–mediated events to early renal development and many aspects of renal function are being studied. Work in the developing rat kidney both postnatally and at early gestational ages have shown that renal kininogen and kallikrein are expressed early in development. There is a subsequent increased expression of kininase II in the postnatal preweaning period, and the striking finding that B_2 receptor gene expression is 10-fold higher during early renal development than in mature rat kidney. This latter receptor expression is preferential to immature glomeruli, distal tubules, and collecting ducts. The data gathered thus far support the notion that the renal kallikrein-kinin system plays a role in both renal development and homeostatic adaptation to postnatal life, and further work in this area is likely to reveal the extent to which components of this system participate in normal maturation of not only the kidney, but other organ systems, as well.

INTERRELATIONS OF KALLIKREIN AND KININS TO RENAL REGULATORY HORMONES

Renin-Angiotensin-Aldosterone

The only certain *in situ* biochemical connection is that ACE also efficiently catabolizes kinins. A great deal of data now document that converting enzyme inhibition by various drugs leads to changes in circulating or local kinin levels, which have significant functional consequences. It has established that these inhibitors also potentiate various effects of kinins (e.g., positive inotropy) by actions that are independent of converting enzyme inhibition, including an interesting blockade of kinin B_2 receptor desensitization. The widespread availability of an increasing spectrum of specific and potent antagonists of kinin receptors, most notably of the B_2 class, is allowing collection of data showing the specific biochemical or functional consequences that are due to the actions of either administered or accumulated kinins. Another connection previously suggested as a result of some *in vitro* work was that kallikreins might serve as prorenin activating enzymes. This possibility has not been reaffirmed by any *in vivo* studies, although extensive work has shown that some murine kallikrein gene family products, namely the enzymes called mK9 and mK13, but not mK1, the true tissue kallikrein, were reasonably efficient processing enzymes for prorenin *in vitro*. Similarly, because a tissue kallikrein was capable of generating angiotensin II from a plasma protein fraction *in vitro*, suggestions of alternative pathways for formation of the pressor peptide were made. Again, no convincing evidence for such a role *in vivo* has been generated in recent years.

Thus the two systems appear to function in concert but independently to maintain renal blood flow (RBF) and excretory capability. That is, although diets low in sodium (or high in potassium) or other systemic challenges (e.g., volume depletion) stimulate renin gene expression, renin synthesis, and increased systemic levels of angiotensin and aldosterone in defense of circulatory homeostasis, many of the same stimuli augment renal kallikrein and kinin production in what now appears to be a local defense of RBF and glomerular filtration rate (GFR) by vasodilator actions on renal cortical blood vessels, most particularly afferent arterioles. The explanations for changes in the two systems in opposite directions, such as occurs in the "two-kidney, one-clip" rat (with high renin and angiotensin levels but lowered renal kallikrein levels), are still not convincingly explained. The notion that such changes in kallikrein (among the earliest observed in the kidney enzyme) may only be a secondary response to a more important interstitial kinin level or kinin-receptor change (especially in the nonclipped kidney), which collectively promotes a compensatory excretory response to the contralateral insult, is now being explored given the availability of specific receptor blockers and other resources (e.g., Brown-Norway rats of the Katholiek strain), which produce no levels of functional LMW or HMW kininogen, the B_2 receptor knockout mice. These and other chemical and biologic resources are being more widely used to help unravel the related roles of these intertwined vasoactive peptide systems.

Atrial Natriuretic Peptide

Relations to other renal regulatory hormones continue to be sought. Tissue kallikrein is capable of forming ANP from its precursors as well as catabolizing the active peptide *in vitro*. Administration of this powerful natriuretic and diuretic agent affects urinary kallikrein excretion and conversely, cardiac tissue expresses and contains kallikreinlike enzyme that colocalizes in ANP-containing granules. Other work has localized the synthesis and secretion of an ANP from distal cortical connecting tubule cells of the mouse and rat, which also contain tissue kallikrein. Because ANP receptors—activation of which may modulate renal sodium reabsorption—exist downstream in the inner medullary collecting ducts, the hormone synthesized locally in the kidney may affect both tubular function and perhaps renin secretion through interstitial release from the same synthetic site. The role of renal tissue kallikrein produced in the same or adjacent cells in this local ANP production still requires further study, especially because certain work indicates that the proform of rat natriuretic peptide–mimicking peptides are good *in vitro* substrates for two members of the kallikrein family, rK2 (tonin) and rK9, but not for the kinin-releasing rK1 tissue kallikrein. It is also clear that additional members of the tissue kallikrein gene family are expressed in renal tissue, at least in rodents, but the actual roles of these proteases in processing other peptide hormone precursors are still undefined.

Eicosanoids

The renal kallikrein-kinin system activates eicosanoid synthesis in various renal cellular sites. Many studies show that kinins stimulate arachidonic acid release and subsequent eicosanoid synthesis in renal vasculature and interstitial and epithelial cells. Thus far, these all seem to occur through activation of BK_2 receptors and phospholipase A_2–mediated arachidonic acid release. Stimulation of PGE_2 production is known to occur in response to kinins added to the luminal surface of collecting duct cells (which conceivably enhances a kinin-induced natriuresis at this site) as well as in glomerular arterioles, mesangial and renomedullary interstitial cells. Vascular PGI_2 synthesis is powerfully stimulated by kinins, as is vascular or platelet synthesis of the vasoconstrictor thromboxane. Most studies attempting to interrupt these linkages with, for example, cyclooxygenase inhibitors or kinin-receptor blockers, or to modify putative relationships with converting enzyme inhibition or lipopolysaccharide-induced endotoxic shock, disclose a significant connection between kinins and prostaglandins, and especially their vasodilator and natriuretic properties.

The renal cellular biochemical participants in these relationships have been explored more extensively. For example, in rabbit cortical collecting duct cells, it has been shown that cytoplasmic phospholipase A_2 ($cPLA_2$) is the enzyme responsible for kinin-mediated arachidonic acid release and protein kinase C (PKC) is importantly involved in activation of the phospholipase, whereas in the Madin-Darby canine kidney (MDCK) cells, the arachidonic acid release may be independent of PKC and involves the mitogen-activated protein kinase cascade. However, these latter cells also demonstrate a translocation of $cPLA_2$ to membranes in response to kinin, initiated by the kinin-induced influx of extracellular calcium. Many more questions about the *in situ* participants in kinin-induced alterations in renal cellular function remain to be answered. Some of the most interesting involve the actions of vasopressin in the distal nephron. This peptide stimulates renal cellular kallikrein release and kinin production, but kinins inhibit vasopressin-induced water and sodium reabsorption in collecting ducts, probably through the production of PGE_2 at this site. Thus it is reasonable to consider that there is a local, negative feedback loop between kinins, eicosanoids, and vasopressin in the distal nephron.

Nitric Oxide

NO is another mediator now considered to be integral to kinin-induced vasodilation and hypotension. In the rat and dog renal vasculature, vasodilation produced by administered bradykinin is significantly but not totally dependent on NO synthesis and as such is markedly attenuated by either N^G-monomethyl-L-arginine or N^w-nitro-L-arginine, inhibitors of NO synthase. These studies brought consideration of endothelium-derived relaxing factor (EDRF, NO) known from the earliest studies of Furchgott to be a responsible mediator for kinin-induced vasodilation, to the renal circulation. Questions concerning this relation are still of great interest because there is a renal vascular hyperresponsiveness to bradykinin, particularly in the spontaneously hypertensive rat, insofar as both NO-dependent and NO-independent actions (Fig. 13.13). In addition, other work has begun to explain the long-observed but cryptic vasodilation produced by parenteral furosemide, as secondary to an enhanced endothelial synthesis of kinin with subsequent formation of NO and prostacyclin. Not only did furosemide enhance release of kinins from bovine aortic endothelial cells in culture, but the kinin antagonist icatibant (HOE 140) prevented the furosemide-induced release of NO and the eicosanoid. Studies such as these reinforce the likelihood that endogenous renal

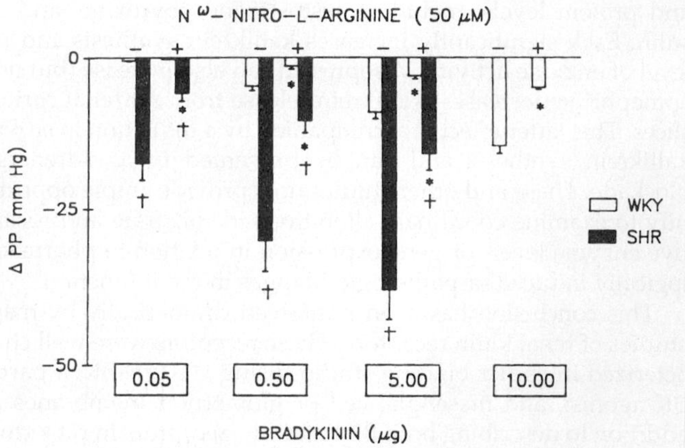

Figure 13.13. The effect on perfusion pressure (*PP*) of bolus injections of bradykinin in isolated kidneys of Wistar-Kyoto (W/Ky) rats and spontaneously hypertensive rats (SHR) perfused with (+) and without (−) N^w-nitro-L-arginine–containing media. Results are mean ±SEM of eight to nine experiments. *Significant difference ($P < .05$) relative to data in kidneys perfused without N^w-nitro-L-arginine. †Significant difference ($P < .01$) relative to data in W/KY rats. (Reprinted with permission from Cachofeiro V, Nasjletti A. Increased vascular responsiveness to bradykinin in kidneys of spontaneously hypertensive rats. *Hypertension* 1991;18(5):683–688.)

kallikrein or kinin production is reasonably likely to be involved in the mechanism of action of a spectrum of drugs or hormones which affect multiple aspects of renal vascular or epithelial cell function.

KALLIKREINS, KININS, AND RENAL FUNCTION

Speculations about the roles of the tissue kallikrein-kinin system in renal function, salt and water homeostasis, and blood pressure regulation began in 1909, when the hypotensive property of human urine, now known to represent excreted renal kallikrein, was discovered. The earliest definitive studies of the effects of kinins on renal function were carried out by Webster and Gilmore (1964) and Gill and associates (1965). They established the natriuretic/diuretic capabilities of a kinin in dog and humans and were soon followed by work showing that stimulation of water and electrolyte excretion was a function of increased RBF. Indeed, the most consistently observed renal effects of kinins is to reduce renal vascular resistance. Unlike other vasodilators, bradykinin can increase blood flow without significant change in GFR, but with a significant increase in fluid delivery to the distal nephron. This latter effect may contribute to the always observed increased urine volume and sodium excretion seen with exogenously administered kinin into kidneys. It appears that the natriuresis and diuresis results from an effect of kinins on renal papillary blood flow that inhibits sodium reabsorption distally secondary to a washout of the medullary solute gradient, rather than on cortical blood flow or, as mentioned earlier, GFR. Support for this contention is derived from several studies in which investigators used either inhibitors of renal kininases such as captopril and phosphoramidon (the latter, an inhibitor of neutral endopeptidase 24.11) or chronic treatment with desoxycorticosterone (DOC), also known to raise endogenous kinin levels, followed by various specific antagonists of renal kinin BK_2 receptors. The available data generally indicates that increases in papillary blood flow, urine volume, and sodium excretion induced by kininase inhibition or DOC can be either attenuated or abolished by kinin BK_2-receptor blockade. Thus it is now clear that *endogenously* produced kinin significantly affects renal hemodynamics and excretory function. What is still uncertain despite much additional work is whether the observed natriuretic/diuretic responses are all a result of effects on renal hemodynamics in the papilla or might include a component of distal tubular inhibition of electrolyte reabsorption. Although some studies showed clearly that kinin BK_2-receptor blockade greatly increased chloride and water absorption in the medullary collecting duct of the rat, the weight of present opinion suggests that intrarenal kinins modulate renal excretory function predominantly by effects on renal vasculature.

Among the most interesting possible assignments of a role in renal function for tissue kallikrein and kinins is that in tubuloglomerular feedback. Studies have established in either normal or hydronephrotic kidneys that bradykinin can differently reset tubuloglomerular feedback. The turning point is increased by kinin in control rats but is decreased in the hydronephrotic animals. Although concentrations of kinin used in the perfusates was rather high, no kininase inhibitors were used concomitantly. It was suggested that endogenously produced kinin might, through effects on prostaglandin production in the normal rats, lower tubuloglomerular feedback sensitivity or, through the effects on thromboxane synthesis in hydronephrotic rats, increase tubuloglomerular feedback sensitivity. In the hydronephrotic kidney, bradykinin is known to stimulate thromboxane synthesis. The work complements a previous study that showed the serine proteinase inhibitor aprotinin was able to diminish or prevent the attenuation of tubuloglomerular feedback induced by the converting enzyme/kininase II inhibitor captopril. This work suggested that endogenous renal kinin production might be reducing tubuloglomerular feedback (i.e., lowering sensitivity and increasing turning point). Another study characterized the effects of tubuloglomerular feedback inhibition by salt loading on the salt sensitivity of blood pressure in the spontaneously hypertensive rat (SHR). The results, including crossover studies that perfused tubules of the various groups of SHR and Wistar-Kyoto (W/Ky) control animals with previously collected tubular fluids from salt-loaded or control rats, showed that tubuloglomerular feedback was augmented in SHR and not affected by salt loading. It appeared that this resetting in SHR might be related to defective activation of a humoral feedback inhibitory substance in response to chronic salt load, resulting in a greater blood pressure increase in SHR versus control animals. Several working hypotheses can be formulated based on these findings and the renal kallikrein-kinin system abnormalities known to exist in SHR. Collectively, these studies still compel further evaluation of endogenous renal kallikrein-kinin system behavior in relation to this important connection between tubular and glomerular function, using newer models (e.g., kinin-receptor knockout or Brown-Norway kininogen-deficient animals) and the various kinin-receptor antagonists.

As stated earlier, the specific local roles of kinin generated from renal distal tubular kininogen by adjacent kallikrein in ion and water transport is still not fully defined. However, it is clear that kinin BK_2 receptors are coupled to cellular systems in polarized epithelia that lead to marked changes in vectorial ion and water transport. Many epithelia (e.g., rat colonic, porcine, or rat medullary or papillary collecting duct, guinea pig gallbladder) have been shown to secrete anions, predominantly chloride but also bicarbonate, in voltage clamp experiments in response to kinins; these effects are partially eicosanoid dependent and can be blocked by inhibitors of Na^+-K^+-Cl^--contransport such as furosemide or bumetanide. However, the actions of locally generated kinins on ion and water transport are less well defined. Some studies of isolated perfused rat medullary collecting ducts, mentioned above, have shown clearly that kinin BK_2-receptor blockade clearly enhances Cl^- and water absorption (Fig. 13.14), and along with previous work which suggested that kinin in-

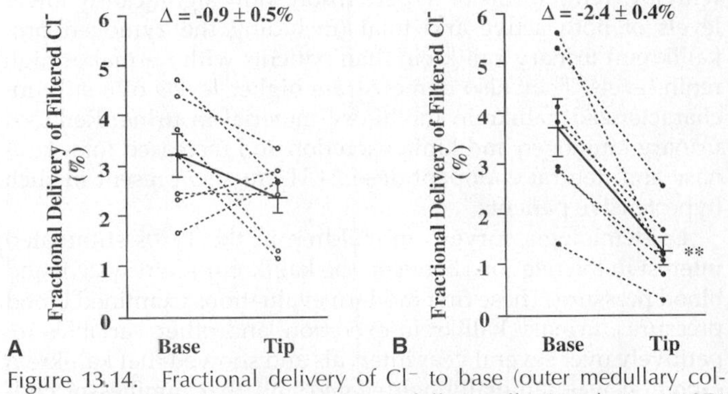

Figure 13.14. Fractional delivery of Cl^- to base (outer medullary collecting duct, OMCD) and tip (inner medullary collecting duct, t-IMCD) collection sites for individual rats treated with HOE 140. Individual and mean data for paired collections of tubular fluid from t-IMCD and OMCD taken during baseline **(A)** and HOE –140 treatment periods **(B)** are shown. Δ, Change. During baseline period, there is no significant change in fractional delivery of Cl^- between the two collection sites. By contrast, HOE 140 treatment resulted in significantly reduced fractional delivery of Cl^- to t-IMCD compared with that at OMCD (**$P < .01$). HOE 140 increased absorption of Cl^- along the medullary collecting duct. (Reprinted with permission from Mukai H, Fitzgibbon WR, Bozeman G, et al. Bradykinin β_2 receptor antagonist increases chloride and water reabsorption in rat medullary collecting duct. *Am J Physiol* 1996;271(2 Pt 2):R352–R360.)

hibited either electroneutral NaCl absorption or stimulated NaCl secretion, now challenge other earlier work that found no effects whatsoever of kinin on any electrophysiologic properties of this portion of the nephron. The continued study of this portion of the mammalian nephron, the site of expression of all tissue kallikrein-kinin system components, with more specific modulators, or kinin-receptor knockout animals will continue to shed light on system roles in the nephron.

KALLIKREIN-KININ SYSTEM IN RENAL AND SYSTEMIC DISEASES

Hypertension

The earliest evaluations of renal kallikrein in humans with arterial hypertension were carried out in the 1930s. Elliot and Nuzum found that urinary kallikrein excretion was significantly less than in comparable normotensive subjects. Even then, the notion that this finding might represent a deficiency in an endogenous renal vasodilator system that was contributory to the hypertensive state was prominently considered. Progress in addressing this possibility has been rather slow, unlike the enormous, sustained interest provoked on behalf of the renin-angiotensin system by the Goldblatt experiment. Today, interest in possible renal kallikrein-kinin contributions to the cause and pathogenesis of human hypertensive diseases is growing more rapidly because of a series of provocative findings reaching from epidemiologic surveys to gene knockout experiments. However, the case for involvement is still somewhat weak when compared with the easily demonstrable importance of vasoconstrictor influences in human hypertension.

Although it is clear that patients with essential hypertension excrete less urinary kallikrein than do normotensive subjects in general, there is much overlap in any of the population studies carried out over the past 30 years; that is, many hypertensive subjects show normal urinary kallikrein excretion. African-American adults and children excrete significantly less kallikrein than do whites, regardless of blood pressure. Hypertensive African-Americans generally show the lowest measured levels in many different surveys. Additional studies of kallikrein and other system components in more homogeneous human populations have now appeared. For example, Japanese patients with low-renin forms of hypertension show significantly lower levels of both active and total (including the zymogen prokallikrein) urinary kallikrein than patients with normal or high renin levels. They also demonstrate higher levels of a still uncharacterized kallikrein inhibitory material in urine. Reduced urinary kininogen and kinin excretion and increased total kininase and neutral endopeptidase 24.11 are also present in such hypertensive patients.

Epidemiologic surveys in children in the 1970s stimulated interest in the relations between the kallikrein-kinin system and blood pressure. These first modern evaluations examined blood pressures, urinary kallikrein excretion, and other variables repetitively over several year intervals and showed that kallikrein excretion was familially aggregated and that families of children with the lowest mean kallikrein excretions showed significantly higher blood pressures than did families of children with the highest kallikrein excretions. Additional surveys showed that urinary kallikrein and diastolic blood pressure are negatively correlated in newborn infants 2 to 4 days old, and such correlations are persistent in the same populations up to 18 months of age. In another important epidemiologic approach, examination of family history of hypertension in a large population (57 Utah pedigrees containing 391 youths and 405 adults) showed that youngsters with a higher urinary kallikrein excretion genotype were significantly less likely to have one or two hypertensive parents than those with a low kallikrein genotype, suggesting the higher excretion rate represents a genotype associated with a reduced risk of essential hypertension. Such studies, although serving as provocative landmarks, still require extension in various ways (including assessments of a spectrum of other components and markers of kallikrein-kinin system activity) before the case can be definitively established for a contributory role of renal kallikrein and kinins in the origins of some human forms of hypertension.

Work in rodent forms of hypertension has proceeded more rapidly. Goldblatt hypertensive rats were the first animal model shown to have reduced urinary kallikrein excretion and renal levels of the enzyme. This occurs principally in the compromised kidney, and levels in the contralateral kidney are either normal or reduced to a lesser extent. These changes have been studied in relation to the different salt-handling properties of the two kidneys. In addition, and as noted above, these differences are now being elaborated upon by examination of BK_2-receptor density, which is increased to a greater extent in the contralateral kidney that in the clipped one. These increases appear to signify an augmented kinin-induced PGE_2 release in compensatory response to the higher perfusion pressure this kidney faces. This contralateral kidney is already known to show higher RBF, GFR, and sodium excretion; characteristics that now deserve to be evaluated insofar as their continued existence or attenuation in kinin-receptor knockout rodents or after kinin-receptor blockade.

All genetic models of rat hypertension, including the SHR, Dahl, Milan, New Zealand, Fawn-hooded, and Sabra strains, have been evaluated for rate of urinary kallikrein excretion, and it is reduced in each. It is important to note that relatively few of these studies have been carried out longitudinally with respect to age, and it is still uncertain in many of the strains whether the urinary kallikrein abnormalities preceded or followed the appearance of hypertension. However, one of the earliest studies in Milan rats showed significantly lower levels in newborn animals of the hypertensive versus the control strain. Another study showed renal tissue active kallikrein in SHR was only 53% of values in W/Ky rats within 12 hours of birth, whereas total enzyme level (including the prokallikrein zymogen) was not different between strains. The difference was found to persist between SHR and W/Ky at 4, 8, and 12 weeks of age. This work suggested a possible defect in renal prokallikrein activation but not synthesis rate in the SHR.

Studies in Dahl salt-sensitive (SS/Jr) versus salt-resistant (SR/Jr) rats have provided some of the most interesting new information concerning renal kallikrein-kinin system and function in these highly inbred strains; renal kallikrein levels, renal kallikrein synthesis rate, and ureteral kinin excretion are increased and kininases reduced in young SR/Jr compared with SS/Jr. Some of these differences are detectable in 1-day-old newborn pups, and the rate of renal kallikrein synthesis in the SR/Jr is the highest ever observed in a rat population. Furthermore, BK_2-receptor blockade with icatibant (HOE 140) greatly reduces RBF and the GFR in SR/Jr, but not SS/Jr. In addition, chronic kinin B_2-receptor blockade produced the largest increase in blood pressure of young SR/Jr subjected to a high salt intake yet observed. This work supports the hypothesis that the high levels of renal kallikrein and renal kallikrein synthesis (and presumptively high endogenous kinin levels) contribute at least in part to the salt resistance of this strain. Finally, icatibant has also been used to show that chronic systemic BK_2-receptor blockade in rats treated long term with DOC results in an earlier and greater rise in blood pressure than is seen in rats treated with DOC alone. This and several other recent studies are providing additional evidence to support the hypothesis that endogenously produced kinins are indeed participating in arterial blood pressure regulation. However, and despite the strengthening data in this regard, the actual contributory sites of action of endogenously produced kinin are still quite uncertain.

Diabetes Mellitus

Rats with streptozotocin-induced diabetes mellitus have significantly altered renal kallikrein-kinin system function. Early in the course of the diabetic state, these animals treated with some insulin also show glomerular hyperfiltration along with increased renal kallikrein synthesis, levels, and urinary excretion. Treatment of such animals with aprotinin or a BK_2-receptor antagonist reduces GFR and renal plasma flow and increases renal vascular resistance to levels equal to those in normal rats. These earlier studies were confirmed in patients with type I (insulin-dependent) diabetes mellitus in whom filtration rate, blood flow, and renal tubular sodium reabsorption were measured. Patients with glomerular hyperfiltration showed greater urinary active kallikrein and PGE_2 excretion than patients with normal GFR or otherwise normal subjects. Both kallikrein and PGE_2 levels correlated directly with GFR, and the former also correlated directly with distal tubular sodium reabsorption as evidenced from lithium clearance. The possible contributions of renal kinins to the glomerular hemodynamic abnormalities associated with diabetes have been under intense investigation, and it has been shown that renal kinin production contributes to glomerulosclerosis characterized by mesangial cell proliferation and matrix expansion, possibly by tyrosine phosphorylation of tubulin and mitogen-activated protein kinase, as well as translocation of the latter to the nucleus, presumably leading to altered mesangial cell function. Such findings suggest that renal kallikrein and kinins may be significant contributors to the glomerular hyperfiltration of human diabetes.

Other Nephropathies

The ability of converting enzyme/kininase II inhibition to reduce proteinuria in nephrotic rats depends on the renal kallikrein-kinin system. Studies have shown that urinary kallikrein excretion as well as renal levels of kallikrein mRNA are reduced in passive Heymann nephritis. However, converting enzyme inhibition restores kallikrein mRNA levels to normal, increases urinary kallikrein excretion to some extent, and reduces urinary albumin excretion. The data suggest reversal of a transcriptional suppression of a renal kallikrein gene(s) without a concomitant effect on renin mRNA. Although the studies continue to implicate renal kallikreins and kinins in response to the insult, they are not yet coupled to the functional abnormalities of the disorder.

Over the past 30 years, hundreds of studies have disclosed abnormalities in components of this system in renal diseases or systemic diseases with renal features, including Bartter's syndrome, primary aldosteronism, pheochromocytoma, hepatic cirrhosis, hepatorenal syndrome, heavy metal poisoning, polycystic renal disease, end-stage renal disease, endotoxin shock, and others (Table 13.3). Many drugs or hormones affecting renal

TABLE 13.3. Human Kallikrein-Kinin System Abnormalities

	Urine			Plasma	
Disease	Kallikrein	Kininases	Kinin	Kininogen	Kinin
Disease					
Hypertension					
Essential	↓ or →	↑ Total and I	↓		
Primary aldosteronism	↑ or →	↑ Total, NEP	Normal		
Cushing's syndrome	↑	↑ I, II and ↑ NEP	—		
Pheochromocytoma	↑	—	—		
Preeclampsia	↓	—	—		
Renovascular	↓	↑ Total	—		
Bartter's syndrome	↑	—	↑		
Cirrhosis					
No renal failure	↑ or ↓	—	↓	↓	
Renal failure	↓	—	—		
Cadmium toxicity	↓	—	—		
Diabetes mellitus					
Type I—poor control	↑	—	—		
—good control	→	—	—		
with hyperfiltration	↑	—	—		
Diabetes insipidus	↓	—	↓		
Glomerulonephritis, chronic	↓	↑	↓		
Shock after trauma					↑
Drugs					
Diuretics					
Thiazides	↑ or →	—	—		
Spironolactone	↓	—	—		
Amiloride	↓	—	—		
Furosemide	↑	—	—		
ACE inhibitors	→	—	↑		↑
Insulin	↑	—	—		
Vasopressin	↑	—	↑		
β-Adrenergic blockers	↓	—	—		
Calcium channel blockers	→	—	↑		

PLASMA ↑, increased plasma level; Total, total kininase activity; I, kininase I; II, kininase II (angiotensin I converting enzyme); NEP, neutral endopeptidase 24.11.
URINE ↑, increased excretion rate; ↓, decreased excretion rate; →, no abnormality, —, not measured.

function also affect levels of the kallikrein-kinin system components, including the antihypertensive agents, diuretics, and cyclooxygenase inhibitors. With the significant advances of the last two decades in the understanding of renal kallikrein-kinin system gene families, sites of gene expression, component structural features, cellular localization, regulation, and the ability to manipulate the levels and activity of these components with various stimuli or inhibitors, it is now reasonable to conclude that the appreciated contributions of the system to either normal renal function or renal pathologic conditions will lead to new therapeutic strategies based on stimulation or interdiction of kinin actions.

Selected Readings

Bhoola KD, Figueroa CD, Worthy K. Bioregulation of kinins: kallikreins, kininogens, and kininases. *Pharmacol Rev* 1992;44:1–80.

A comprehensive review of the components of kallikrein-kinins systems; their structure, formation, regulation and roles in cellular processes and pathologic events. Coverage of renal kallikrein, kininases and kinin formation is still very adequate, but more recent information on kinin-receptor behavior and regulation is missing.

Jaffa AA, Miller BS, Rosenzweig SA, et al. Bradykinin induces tubulin phosphorylation and nuclear translocation of MAP kinase in mesangial cells. *Am J Physiol* 1997;273(Renal Physiol):F916–F824.

This group, among others, is characterizing second messenger and signal transduction events induced by kinin-receptor occupancy. They use immunofluorescence, immunoprecipitation, and immunoblotting techniques to identify tyrosine phosphorylation substrates in response to bradykinin in mesangial cells and have shown that bradykinin causes the phosphorylation of specific cellular proteins in these cells and suggest a role for both tubulin and mitogen-activated protein kinase in the signaling cascades by which bradykinin alters renal mesangial cell function.

Katori M, Majima M. Preventative role of renal kallikrein-kinin system in the early phase of hypertension and development of new antihypertensive drugs. *Adv Pharmacol* 1998;44:147–224.

This recent review summarizes the case for the renal kallikrein-kinin system having a role in attenuating the development and pathophysiologic consequences of hypertension and as a target for the development of new therapy.

Linz W, Weimer G, Gohlke P, et al. Contribution of kinins to the cardiovascular actions of angiotensin-converting enzyme inhibitors. *Pharmacol Rev* 1995;47:25–49.

This is a comprehensive review of the contributions of the kallikrein-kinin system and kinin peptides to the actions of converting enzyme inhibitors on the cardiovascular system. It includes summaries of data concerning the contributions of kinins to the antihypertensive actions of these compounds, as well as their more chronic effects on myocardial ischemia, myocardial hypertrophy, and experimental atherosclerosis.

Margolius HS. The Theodore Cooper Memorial Lecture. Kallikreins and kinins. Some unanswered questions about system characteristics and roles in human disease. *Hypertension* 1995;26:221–229.

This relatively short review focuses attention on areas of endeavor that are still relatively unexplored and important questions concerning kallikrein-kinin system characteristics, behavior, and roles in pathophysiologic circumstances.

Minshall RD, Erdös EG, Vogel SM. Angiotensin I-converting enzyme inhibitors potentiate bradykinin's inotropic effects independently of blocking its inactivation. *Am J Cardiol* 1997;80(3A):132–136.

The results of this surprising study in isolated guinea pig atrial preparations indicate that converting enzyme inhibitors, by both potentiating bradykinin effects and blocking bradykinin β_2 receptor desensitization, contribute to the beneficial cardiac effects of bradykinin, independently of blockade of its inactivation.

Mukai H, Fitzgibbon WR, Bozeman G, et al. Bradykinin B_2 receptor antagonist increases chloride and water reabsorption in rat medullary collecting duct. *Am J Physiol* 1996;271 (2 Pt 2):R352–R360.

This groups' study evaluated the role of intrarenal kinins in collecting duct chloride absorption and found that kinin β_2-receptor blockade markedly enhanced chloride and water absorption in the medullary collecting duct of Dahl/Rapp salt-resistant rats. Findings clearly supported a role for renal kinins in the regulation of renal sodium chloride and water excretion.

Mukai H, Fitzgibbon WR, Ploth DW, et al. Effect of chronic bradykinin β_2 receptor blockade on blood pressure of conscious Dahl salt-sensitive rats. *Br J Pharmacol* 1998;124:197–205.

In this chronic study, three separate protocols were used to determine the role of endogenous kinins in the striking resistance of the inbred Dahl/Rapp salt-resistant rats to high dietary salt intake. The studies showed that kinin activation of bradykinin β_2 receptors significantly contributes to early regulatory mechanisms that resist an increase in blood pressure, following exposure of these animals to a high-salt diet. The study serves to establish the potential preventative role of the kallikrein-kinin system in hypertension associated with excessive salt intake.

Yosipiv IV, Dipp S, El-Dahr SS. Role of bradykinin β_2 receptors in neonatal kidney growth. *J Am Soc Nephrol* 1997;8:920–928.

This study examined the role of bradykinin and kinin β_2 receptors in neonatal kidney growth. Treatment of newborn rats with the bradykinin β_2-receptor antagonist HOE 140 (icatibant) significantly reduced body weight, kidney to body weight ratios, and kidney DNA content. The growth retardation induced by bradykinin β_2-receptor blockade was observed only in the kidney, and to some extent in the heart. The results suggests that activation of bradykinin β_2 receptor expression in the neonatal kidney plays an important role in the regulation of renal DNA synthesis during nephrogenesis.

PART 5
Endothelins

Valentina Kon and Tracy E. Hunley

Endothelin (ET) was first recognized in culture media of porcine aortic endothelial cells. A description of its isolation, characterization, cloning, localization, and a putative biosynthetic pathway was all set forth in Yanagisawa's initial report in 1988. The paper went on to describe the physiologic effects of infusion of ET, showing it to be on an order of magnitude more potent than the most potent vasoconstrictors. In addition to its unparalleled vasoconstrictive potency, ET's effects were found to be exceptionally long-lasting, such that a single bolus produced a pressor response that lasted hours. ET was soon found to be one of a family of structurally and functionally related peptides. Within a year of its initial description, investigators had defined much of the structure of the isopeptides in various mammalian species, including humans, their genes, regulation of gene expression, and signal transduction. Cloning of ET's receptors, ETA and ETB, was achieved by 1990, and within the next 2 years there was extensive characterization of ET's synthetic pathway as well as the development of peptide and nonpeptide receptor antagonists. These discoveries permitted substantiation and characterization of the biologic importance of ETs in disease models of hypertension, ischemic heart disease, acute renal failure, cerebral vasospasm, and vascular remodeling. Indeed, within the decade of ET's discovery, pharmacologic antagonism of ET effects was shown to be beneficial in patients with cardiovascular disease and also with hypertension. The speed with which insights into ET have been made and brought to the bedside has been as unprecedented as the nature of its extraordinarily potent biologic effects.

BIOSYNTHESIS

The original ET, a 21–amino acid peptide, was soon recognized to be one of at least three isoforms, named endothelin-1 (ET-1), endothelin-2 (ET-2), and endothelin-3 (ET-3). ET-2 differs from ET-1 by two amino acids, and ET-3 differs from ET-1 in 6 of the 21 amino acid residues. All three members possess two intrachain disulfide bridges and a hydrophobic C-terminal tail. The structure of ET can be regarded in terms of two distinct subdomains: the N-terminal disulfide loop, which differs among the ET-isoforms, and the conserved C-terminal linear region. Removal of the Trp^{21} residue or cleavage of the disulfide bridges markedly reduces ET-1's vasoconstrictive potency. Modification of the N-terminus of ET-1 also lessens its vasoconstriction. These structural domains also dictate, at least in part, interactions of the ET peptide with the ET receptors. The C-terminal portion, particularly Glu^{10}- Trp^{21}, interacts with the relatively nonselective ETB receptor. On the other hand, the Cys^{1} residue and the N-terminal tertiary structure (including the disulfide bridges) are required for binding to the highly selective ETA receptor.

Not only are there specific domains within the ligands, but certain elements within the individual receptors also affect the ligand–receptor interactions. The isoforms of ET are widely distributed among various cells and tissues. Of the three isoforms, the most widely distributed, best studied, and most powerful is ET-1. In the kidney, besides endothelial cells, mesangial, glomerular, and tubule epithelial cells all produce ET-1. Circulating cells also secrete ET-1: macrophages are an important source for ET-1; neutrophils can convert ET's precursor, exogenous big ET-1, into the mature form and may, through this mechanism, contribute to pathophysiologic processes. The ET-2 isoform has been detected primarily in renal tissue and appears particularly abundant in renal adenocarcinoma. Finally, while ET-3 predominates in the brain, it is also found in various parts of the kidney. Its exact function is yet to be delineated.

Each of the mature ET peptides is sequentially processed from precursor peptides. The processing of proendothelin to big ET begins in a constitutive pathway. Both big ET and the mature ET are detected within endothelial cells. However, there is little intracellular storage of any of the isoforms, and while some ET is released into the circulation (plasma concentration of approximately 1 fmol/ml), more than 80% of synthesized ET is directed to the basolateral compartment. However, even in the interstitial space there is no accumulation of ET and its concentration approximates that of plasma. In tissues ET is some 100 times more concentrated than in plasma, probably reflecting the tight binding of the ligand to its receptors with only small amounts of free ligand. Another reason for the low levels of ET in plasma and interstitium is that enzymes such as neutral endopeptidase, enkephalinase-related proteases, and metalloproteases and nonmetalloproteases act as ET-degrading enzymes and contribute to the rapid clearance of the ligand. Because ET is not stored, its synthesis is regulated at the level of gene transcription with *de novo* synthesis of the precursor, cleavage, and release. There are numerous factors that stimulate ET production and may be classified into broad categories of vasoconstrictor/thrombogenics such as angiotensin II, vasopressin, adrenalin, thrombin, and prostaglandin F2α, as well as ET itself; inflammatory cytokines such as interleukin (IL)-1, transforming growth factor-β (TGF-β), and tumor necrosis factor; and physical factors such as mechanical strain, pressure, and low shear stress. ET synthesis is downregulated by vasodilators and anticoagulants [e.g., prostacyclin, nitric oxide (NO), atrial natriuretic peptide, and heparin], as well as physical factors such as high shear stress. Indeed, an important physiologic factor that regulates production and release of ET is blood flow. Increased blood flow is the result of shear stress–mediated decrease in production and release of the vasoconstrictor ET, while increasing production of the vasodilator NO.

The precursor of each isoform is encoded by a distinct gene: preproendothelin-1 (preproET-1) is on human chromosome 6p23-24, preproET-2 on human chromosome 1p34, and preproET-3 on human chromosome 20q13.2-13.3. The human ET-1 contains 5 exons and spans 6.8 kb of DNA. Several regulatory elements have been identified: the 5′-flanking region contains consensus binding sequence motifs for activation of protein-1 and nuclear factor-1, through which angiotensin II and TGF-β activate ET-1 expression, respectively. There are four copies of the hexanucleotide CTGGGA, the acute-phase reaction regulatory element that induces mRNA under stress conditions and has been postulated to be the mechanism for increased preproET-1 mRNA in disease states such as acute myocardial infarction. As described in more detail below, a potentially crucial component in fueling ET's effects in pathophysiologic settings is also under transcriptional regulation: thus, the ET peptide itself is a powerful stimulus for augmenting its own gene expression. Whether this autoinduction of ET synthesis is under the control of unique regulatory sites that are distinct from those regulating synthesis following non-ET stimuli (e.g., ischemia, thrombin) remains to be answered. In the 3′ region there are two AUUUA sequences, a feature that is conserved among different species. These sequences are known to mediate selective mRNA degradation and likely account for the short half-life of the ET mRNA and the ability of cycloheximide to cause superinduction.

Fig. 13.15 shows the three-step process by which the mature ET peptide is generated. Human preproET-1 gene encodes a 212–amino acid prepro peptide that undergoes proteolytic cleavage by an endopeptidase specific for a pair of dibasic amino acids to release a 38–amino acid intermediary structure, big ET-1. Subsequently, the intermediary big ET is cleaved into the mature ET-1 peptide by freeing the COOH terminus of the 21–amino acid residue. This step requires cleavage between Trp^{21}-Val^{22} of big ET-1 by endothelin-converting enzyme (ECE). It is noteworthy that the initial correct processing of preproET is just as essential as subsequent proteolysis by ECE. Thus the *lethal spotting mouse* has a point mutation in the ET-3 gene that

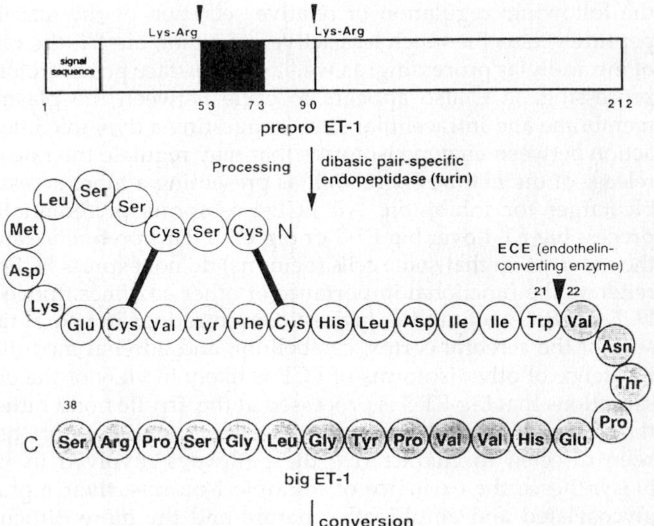

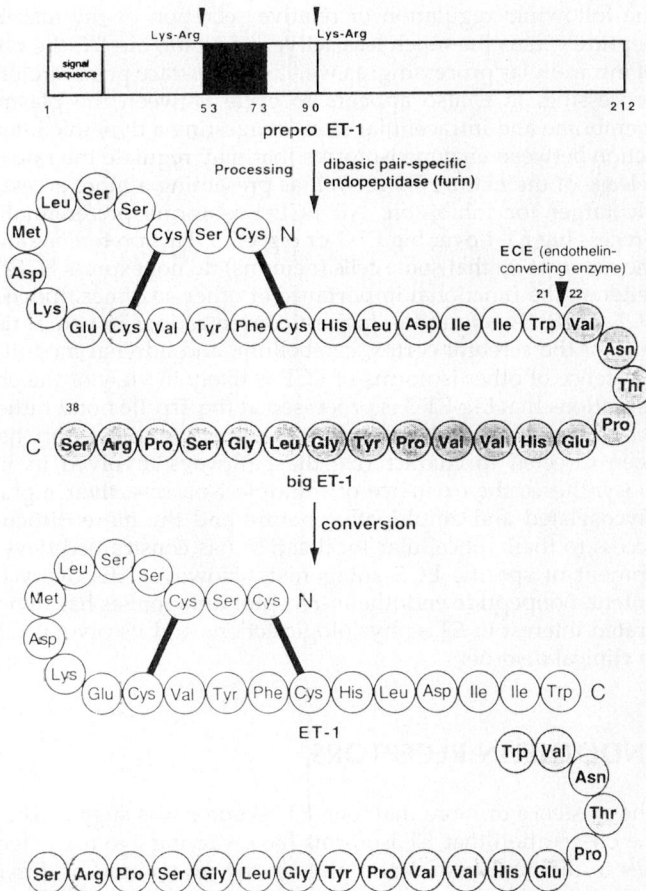

Figure 13.15. Biosynthesis of endothelin-1 (ET-1). The precursor prepro-ET is proteolytically cleaved by a dibasic pair-specific endopeptidase, probably furin, to form the intermediary form big ET-1. Big ET-1 is then specifically cleaved by endothelin-converting enzyme (ECE) to form the mature ET-1 peptide. (Reproduced with permission from Goto K, Hama H, Kasuya Y. Molecular pharmacological and pathophysiological significance of endothelin. *J Pharmacol* 1996; 72:261–290.)

disrupts the initial endopeptidase recognition site, thereby preventing production of big ET-3 and therefore, the mature peptide. As expected, the phenotype of this mouse recapitulates the appearance of the genetically engineered ET-3-knockout mouse that by design is devoid of ET-3, including aganglionic magacolon and pigmentary disorders.

ENDOTHELIN-CONVERTING ENZYME

In vivo, big ET has only 1% of the contractile activity of the mature peptide stressing ECE as an important activating protease in the biosynthetic pathway of ET and its expression of its full activity. Big ET-1 is cleaved both intracellularly and extracellularly by at least two ECE's (ECE1 and ECE2) which belong to a family of metalloprotease enzymes related to neutral endopeptidaes-24.11 (NEP) but not angiotensin converting enzyme. ECE-1 encoded on chromosome 1p36 appears to have three isoforms, ECE-1a, ECE-1b, and ECE-1c, which are derived from the same gene by alternative promoters and complex splicing. These isoforms have distinct cell and tissue distributions. ECE-1c mRNA appears the most predominant and together with ECE-1a localizes to the cell surface, while ECE-1b is found intracellularly colocalizing with markers for the Golgi apparatus. Although there is currently no evidence that ECE is a rate-limiting step in production of ET, it is possible that modulation of local ET levels depends on one or more of the following: regulation of relative secretion of the mature peptide versus the much less active precursor, big ET; the rate of intracellular processing; as well as cell surface postsecretory processing. ECE also appears to cycle between the plasma membrane and intracellular sites, suggesting a dynamic interaction between enzyme isoforms that may regulate the rate of release of the mature ET as well as presenting a more accessible target for inhibition. All ECE-1 isoforms preferentially process big ET-1 over big ET-2 or big ET-3. This preference and the observation that some cells (neurons) do not express ECE-1, reiterate the functional importance of other enzymes. Indeed, ECE-2 mRNA is found in highest concentrations in neural tissues of the cerebral cortex, cerebellum, and adrenal medulla. Existence of other isoforms of ECE is likely in view of the observations that big ET-3 is processed at the Trp-Ile bond rather than a Trp-Val bond. Overall, while considerable effort has been directed to characterize the pathways involved in ET biosynthesis, the existence of multiple isoforms, their highly glycosylated and amphipathic nature and the more difficult access to their subcellular localization has constrained development of specific ECE antagonists. However, discovery of potent, nonpeptide endothelin-receptor antagonists has invigorated interest in ET's physiologic actions and its pivotal role in clinical disorders.

ENDOTHELIN RECEPTORS

The existence of more than one ET receptor was suggested by the observation that ET isoforms have varying agonist potencies in different tissues and also by the recognition of differences in binding characteristics for the individual peptides. There are two receptors, ETA and ETB, and while several alternative human ETA- and ETB-receptor mRNA transcripts have been observed, their function remains uncertain. However, functional data indicate that the ETB receptor exists as ETB1 that is linked to NO release and ETB2 receptor responsible for smooth muscle contraction. In addition, pharmacologic studies imply other receptor subtypes, such as a putative ETC receptor cloned from *Xenopus laevis*, although mammalian counterparts to this isoform have not been found. Indeed, it is the consensus that another ET receptor gene would have little similarity to the two cloned receptors. The known receptors have homology with other heptahelical receptors of the rhodopsin superfamily, with seven transmembrane loops and intracellular actions mediated via G-proteins. ETA was originally cloned from bovine lung and subsequently from human tissue and contains 427 amino acids and binds with the rank order of affinities of ET-1 = ET-2 >> ET-3. The human gene for ETA is located on chromosome 4. The ETB receptor was originally cloned in the rat and later in humans, has 442 amino acids, and binds with the order of affinities of ET-1 = ET-2 = ET-3. There are distinct subdomains of the ET receptors that determine their relative selectivity for ETA antagonists and ETB agonists. For example, transmembrane domains (TMD) I, II, III, and VII, together with the intervening loops of the ETA receptor are selective for the ETA antagonist (BQ123), whereas TMD IV, V, and VI, with the adjacent loops of the ETB receptor, are selective for the ETB agonist (ET-3). These observations suggest that the ligand–receptor interaction of the ET system depends on both the ET peptide and receptor, so the N-terminal loop of the peptide and TMD IV through VI with adjacent loops determine isopeptide/subtype selectivity, while the C-terminal linear portion of the peptide and TMD I through III and VII, plus the adjacent loops, determine the binding.

Endothelins bind very tightly to their receptors and are slow to dissociate. Following binding, the ligand–receptor complex is internalized and sequestered into lysosomal compartments where an acidic environment leads to ligand dissociation. Notably, ET-1 can remain associated with ETA for up to 2 hours after endocytosis potentially continuing second messenger activation long after internalization. The biologic effects of endothelins are directed by the relative population of each receptor, which vary among tissues and cells types. The receptor number can be modulated and this is specific for the receptor and the modulator. For example, cyclosporine does not affect the ETA population in glomerular mesangial cells or whole kidney homogenates but increases ETB receptors. This may be functionally relevant because ETB receptor has been linked to autoinduction of ET-1 synthesis as well as to mitogenesis of renal tubular cells, and it has been postulated that it directs an autoregenerative system for restoring tubule integrity following injury. In this connection, the state of cellular differentiation also specifically and divergently affects each of the receptors, which in turn, can affect the magnitude of ET actions. Thus increasing passage of aortic vascular smooth muscle cells decreases ETA receptors while the ETB receptors are upregulated. This may facilitate the ETB receptor induced ET peptide production and mitogenesis.

Receptor Signaling

Both ETA and ETB are G-protein–coupled receptors that may lead to specific downstream signal transduction depending on the type of guanosine triphosphate (GTP)-binding protein coupled (Gq, Gs, Gi). There is little consensus regarding specific differences in signal transduction pathways between ETA and ETB. Both ETA and ETB receptors have potential SP-1 binding sites, four GATA motifs, an acute-phase reactant response element, and Ebox. The most generalized path following ET exposure is to activate phospholipase C, which hydrolyses phosphatidyl inositol into two products, inositol trisphosphate (IP3) and diacylglycerol (DAG). The exact G-protein coupling the receptor to phospholipase C differs among cells. There is an initial increase in intracellular calcium, which is caused by the rapid mobilization of calcium from the endoplasmic reticulum by IP3. This phase is not dependent on extracellular calcium. By contrast, the later, more sustained increase in calcium is linked to opening of membrane calcium channels and influx of extracellular calcium. This influx is mediated through pertussis toxin-sensitive GTP-binding protein. While it was originally proposed that ET-1 activates voltage-dependent L-type calcium channels, it is now appreciated that there are significant differences among cells and tissues in the ion channels through which ET promotes extracellular calcium entry, including dihydrosensitive and dihydroinsensitive ion channels as well as nonselective cation channels. Not only does ET activate several different channels, but ET-1 prolongs the mean duration of open time of ion channels that may further sustain its effects. As noted, phospholipase C activation causes a biphasic accumulation of DAG that in turn activates the key regulatory enzyme, protein kinase C (PKC), which phosphorylates specific proteins that regulate a array of different biologic effects, including potentiation of calcium mediated contraction and stimulation of the Na^+-H^+ exchange pump to alkalinize the intracellular pH.

Although ET-mediated increase in cyclic adenosine monophosphate (cAMP) appears limited to specific cell types, it is important as an unusual dual signaling mechanism by which ET induces mitogenesis as well as melanogenesis in human melanocytes. This dual action of ET is clearly different from other growth factors, such as basic fibroblast growth factor and hepatocyte growth factor, that mediate their proliferative effects through tyrosine kinase but that do not effect melanogenesis. On the other hand, melanocyte-stimulating hormone, which activates cAMP, induces melanization but does not have a significant effect on cell growth. ET signaling through cross-talk between protein kinases and tyrosine pathways induces dual cellular events. ET-1's activation of phospholipase D contributes to sustaining DAG accumulation, which leads to prolonged activation of PKC. ET-1 activates phospholipase A_2 and thus increases arachidonic acid metabolites, including leukotrienes, prostacyclin and thromboxane A_2, which occurs either through direct receptor–G-protein coupling or indirectly through intracellular calcium. An important signal transduction pathway that modulates the net ET effect relates to ET's stimulation of guanylate cyclase. This stimulation occurs through the ETB receptor (possibly an ETB_1 isoform) which potentiates NO-stimulated cGMP in vascular smooth muscle cells, including glomeruli. In some cells, such as neuroblastoma/glioma cells, this appears to be an NO-independent effect linked directly to the intracellular calcium surge. These effects of ET on NO/cGMP are pivotal in modulating ET effects on contraction, mitogenesis and aggregation. In addition, NO facilitates dissociation of ET and its ligand–receptor complex thereby directly terminating ET's effects. The long term control of ET effects of cell growth and differentiation is well recognized and has been confirmed in a variety of different cell lines. The mechanism for this effect includes induction of several protooncogenes, including *c-fos, c-myc,* and *c-jun;* VL-30; protooncogene–activator protein I complex; as well as stimulation of other growth factors, including platelet-derived growth factor (PDGF), epidermal growth factor (EGF), TGF-β, basic fibroblast growth factor (bFGF), insulin, insulinlike growth factor-I (IGF-I). Both ETA and ETB also increase collagen synthesis and attenuate collagenase activity, as well as inducing adhesion molecules (ICAM-1, VCAM-1, E-selectin) and chemotactic factors [tumor necrosis factor-α (TNF-α), MCP-1, IL-1b, IL-6, and IL-8]. It has been postulated that the intracellular pathways include sequential activation of *raf*-1, mitogen-activated protein kinase (MAPK), and in particular, extracellular signal-regulated kinase (ERK) subfamily, which is activated through both receptors. The ultimate phosphorylation of MAPK activates diverse intracellular protein targets involved in transcriptional activation, protein translation, and structural rearrangement of myelin and microtubule-associated protein, which leads to cell growth, proliferation and differentiation.

Receptor Distribution and Function

The distribution of the ET receptors is extensive and is paralleled by the multiple sources for ET production. This colocalization of peptide and receptors emphasizes the importance of paracrine/autocrine mechanisms for ET actions. As noted earlier, most of the endothelium-derived ET-1 peptide is directed to the basolateral side, providing an effective mechanism to localize ET's actions to discrete areas, regardless of the circulating levels of ET. Compartmentalization also suggests that susceptibility to ET-1 may vary among tissues and organs, depending on the ability of that tissue to increase or lessen ET production, as well as the distribution and the type of ET receptors possessed by the tissue. While some interspecies variability exists, ETA predominates in most vascular smooth muscle cells in most species, including humans. It is not detected in endothelial cells. The ETB receptor is found in endothelial cells and also in vascular smooth muscle cells and is prominent in aorta, brain, and lung. The ETB receptor is the major receptor subtype in the kidney tubule cells, while in many regions of the kidney, such as arterioles, glomerular capillaries, and inner medullary collecting ducts, the ETA and ETB receptors coexist. In general, the ETA receptor modulates vasoconstriction, cellular proliferation, and matrix deposition. Based on its prominent expression in the arterioles and glomerulus, the ETA receptor may modulate these processes at those sites. Our understanding of the function of the ETB receptor is evolving. Clearly, in some tissues of some species ETB has vasoconstrictive and proliferative actions. However, in endothelial cells, this receptor mediates the release of prostaglandins (PGI_2) and NO, which offset the vasoconstrictive and mitogenic effects of ET-1 through the ETA receptor. Finally, ETB appears to affect the synthesis of ET-1 itself, which is then available to interact with ETA or ETB, whereby the net effect is determined by the tissue-specific appearance of the receptor subtype (see the following).

Genetic engineering of ET receptor mutant mice has provided additional insights into receptor function. Targeted deletion of the ETB receptor causes aganglionic megacolon and white spotted coat pigmentation. The same phenotype was observed in mice whose ET-3 gene was disrupted and reiterates the close relationship of ET-3 and ETB. Interestingly, abnormalities in ET-3 or ETB receptor mutants have also been shown in patients with a hereditary form of Hirschsprung's disease that was mapped to human chromosome 13, which is the site of the human ETB receptor. These observations indicate that ET, in particular ET-3–ETB interaction, is an important regulator of mammalian neural crest development, specifically, the vagal neural crest enteric ganglion neurons and the trunk neural crest–derived epidermal melanocytes. These observations underscore the proliferative/differentiation and melanocytogenic functions of ET in these developing cells. ET-1 and ETA also play a major part in normal development of cells originating from the cephalic neural crest. Teratogenicity studies during the preclinical phase of ETA-receptor antagonists revealed developmental abnormalities that overlapped with the phenotype in mice with gene knockout for preproendothelin-1, namely, disturbed craniofacial, cardiovascular, and pharyngeal structures. Notably, defects in the ETA and ETB receptors have been linked to human Pierre-Robin and Treacher-Collins syndromes, which are characterized by craniofacial abnormalities. And although the exact disturbance in development has not been defined, a frameshift mutation of ET-3 has been reported in congenital central hypoventilation syndrome in humans. The mutation consisted of an insertion of a single nucleotide that caused a premature stop codon and the truncation of the last 41 amino acids of the protein. These studies therefore clearly implicate ET's importance in normal development.

EFFECTS ON RENAL PHYSIOLOGY

Various renal functions are affected by ET-1, including regulation of vasomotor tone of vessels and glomeruli, tubule reabsorption and secretion, as well as cellular proliferation and matrix deposition. Most conspicuously, endothelins constrict all segments of the renal microcirculation, and while ET is a powerful vasoconstrictor in all vascular beds, the renal circulation appears particularly susceptible to its effects. In early studies, measurement of blood flow in renal, bronchial, femoral, and coronary vessels revealed that the renal vasculature was some 10-fold more sensitive to ET than other vascular beds. The reasons for this sensitivity remain to be clarified but are not related to an overabundance of receptors and may instead relate to differences in the binding capacity or differences in ET production capabilities. The ETA receptor subtype mediates the vasoconstrictive actions in all species, including humans. The ETB receptor can also mediate constriction of vessels in some species, such as the rat. Infusing ET-1 into one of the branches of the main renal artery in a dose that has no effect on the systemic blood pressure or other circulatory parameters causes profound vasoconstriction. ET-mediated vasoconstriction is particularly long-lasting whereas afferent arteriole constricts more in response to ET than the efferent arteriole; both contribute to reducing the glomerular plasma flow rate and filtration. The glomerular capillary ultrafiltration coefficient also decreases in response to ET at a higher concentration of the peptide. While many studies described response to various doses and variously administered ET, data in humans clearly establish that endogenous ET-1 contributes to the maintenance of normal baseline vasomotor tone in humans.

Endothelin production and actions are not confined to the renal vascular tree. Tubules are both the source and an important target for ET's actions. While many tubular segments can produce endothelins, the inner medullary collecting duct is the predominant site of synthesis of both ET-1 and, to a lesser extent, ET-3, where they can regulate tubule function in an autocrine manner; that is, hemodynamically independent. The receptors parallel the sites of ET synthesis. Thus receptors are most prominent in the inner medullary collecting duct; somewhat less prominent in the outer medullary collecting duct and cortical collecting duct; and are even less abundant in the proximal tubule and thick ascending limb. Contrasting the vasculature and glomeruli where the ETA receptor predominates, it is the ETB receptor that predominates in the rest of the nephron. ET-1 has a biphasic effect of the proximal tubule. At low concentrations (0.1 pmol/L), ET-1 stimulates fluid reabsorption through PKC-mediated events. Conversely, higher dosages of ET-1 (1 nmol/L) decrease fluid reabsorption though PKC-, cyclooxygenase-, and lipoxygenase-mediated events. These concentration-dependent events may be relevant in that under normal conditions when ET-1 levels are low, there is enhanced tubule reabsorption of fluids. By contrast, under pathophysiologic settings, elevated local levels of intrarenal ET-1 promote natriuretic and diuretic effects in this segment. Distal nephron segments also show a biphasic but opposite response to ET-1, so that high levels enhance reabsorption in the collecting tubule, while low levels are inhibitory to sodium and water reabsorption. The inhibitory effects occur by dose-dependent reduction in arginine vasopressin (AVP)–stimulated cAMP accumulation and water flux by activation of PKC and is independent of dihydropyridine-type calcium channels and cyclooxygenase metabolites. Similar to the cortical collecting duct in the inner medullary collecting duct, ET-1 and ET-3 decrease water permeability by reducing AVP-stimulated cAMP accumulation, which is independent of dihydropyridine-type calcium channels and cyclooxygenase metabolites. These apparently opposing effects between the proximal tubule and the more distal nephron segments may be counterregulatory or may act in synchrony because of the difference in availability of the ligand along the nephron; that is, normal levels along the distal nephron are actually a "high dose" in the proximal tubule. In this regard, water loading in humans is associated with increased urinary concentration of ET (which is not linked to circulating ET and thus believed to represent *de novo* synthesis by renal tubular cells) and may well reflect the aforementioned ET-mediated decrease in reabsorption along the nephron. In addition, while some investigators have observed otherwise, hypotonicity per se appears to potentiate ET production by cells of renal origin while hypertonicity decreases it. Taken together, these data point to the idea that volume expanded, hypotonic conditions increase tubule ET-1 production, which promotes diuresis while volume-contracted, hypertonic settings rather lessen ET production by tubule cells and conserve salt and water. It is worth reiterating that the local concentration of ET appears pivotal in effecting the net physiologic response. ET interaction with primarily ETB receptors along the nephron complement the ETB effects in the vasculature toward vasodilation, whereas activation of ET around the vessels and glomeruli causes vasoconstriction and secondary increase in tubule reabsorption.

PATHOPHYSIOLOGIC IMPLICATIONS

The pathophysiologic implications of endothelins were apparent even from the first report: its powerful and long-lasting vasoconstrictive effects have provided the underpinnings for this idea. Indeed, the initial effects observed in rats have been reproduced in humans. Infusion of ET-1 into the brachial artery of normal men causes a slowly developing dose-dependent vasoconstriction and reduction in forearm flow that is sustained for more than 2 hours after the infusion is stopped. As previously noted, the potential importance of ET does not require demonstration of elevated circulating levels of ET, as it is primarily a paracrine system. However, many disease states are characterized by increased circulating levels of ET-1, including hypertension, ischemic cardiac dysfunction, primary pulmonary hypertension, acute and chronic renal failure, and preeclampsia. This elevation in circulating ET-1 reflects spillover of the activated synthesis in the affected organ system or damage to the clearance organs (lung or kidney). Indeed, in certain settings, the degree of elevation in plasma ET-1 is proportional to the extent of end-organ damage, such that the plasma ET-1 level has been shown to be good a predictor of outcome in patients with heart failure. It is therefore possible that ET levels in plasma or tissue may antedate detection of end-organ damage. Endothelins may contribute to the more severe organ damage even at similar levels of blood pressure in African-Americans compared with whites. In support of such an idea are the observations that young, healthy African-American men have almost twice as high plasma ET-1 concentrations as white Americans. Such an increase is sufficient to significantly increase systemic vascular resistance and decrease both heart rate and cardiac output and has been postulated to contribute to the racial differences in the prevalence and severity of hypertension and end-organ damage.

In addition to ET-1's direct effects, there is ample support that even subthreshold concentrations of ET-1 will augment vasoconstriction and mitogenic functions of other agents such as angiotensin II, norepinephrine, and serotonin, among others. Such cross-talk probably extends beyond vasoconstriction to other potentially important pathophysiologic processes such as enhancement of cellular proliferation and hypertrophy. Clearly, ET-1 and ET-3 each cause proliferation or hypertrophy in vascular smooth cells, cardiac myocytes, mesangial and tubulointerstitial cells, bronchial smooth muscle cells and fibroblasts. Notably, ET-1 also plays an important role in cellular transformation. Chicken embryonic ventricular myocytes, cultured in the presence of ET-1, converted into cells bearing Purkinje fiber–specific markers; that is, lost markers for contractile myocytes. This conversion from a contractile to a conductile phenotype was determined by tissue maturity and was specific to the ETA receptor.

ET-1 appears to be an important intermediary in the mitogenic effects of angiotensin II. For example, angiotensin II–induced hypertrophy of cultured myocytes was abolished by treatment with an ETA antagonist or exposure of the cells to antisense mRNA for endothelin. These hypertrophic effects of angiotensin II are now appreciated to be, at least in part, mediated through an AT_1-mediated stimulation of ET-1, which has a profound trophic effect on the nonmyocytes, that is, mainly cardiac fibroblasts. *In vivo* studies extend these observations by demonstrating that continuous exposure to angiotensin II not only increases plasma levels of ET-1 but significantly upregulates both the mRNA expression and tissue levels of ET-1. Notably, the vascular hypertrophy that characterizes this high angiotensin II state is lessened by antagonizing ETA receptors, indicating that ET is a pivotal mechanism in the hypertrophic vascular changes. In this connection, transgenic mice carrying the human renin and angiotensinogen genes reveal increased cardiac ET-1 mRNA and peptide levels and suggest that angiotensin II stimulation of ET-1 promotes cardiac hypertrophy in renin-angiotensin II–activated states. It is interesting that decreasing angiotensin II activity, such as by inhibiting angiotensin-converting enzyme (ACE), also lessens ET-1 production, an effect that may be channeled through ACE inhibitor's potentiation of bradykinin activity. From these findings it might be expected that therapy that inhibits ACE may, in addition to decreasing AII levels, have the additional potentially beneficial effect of reducing ET, thereby possibly having a synergistic effect on abnormalities of structure and function.

An important mechanism in ET's role in pathophysiologic settings may relate to autoinduction of ET-1 synthesis. The addition of ET-1 peptide caused a dramatic increase in preproET-1 gene expression in mesangial cells (Fig. 13.16). The increase was prompt, occurring within 30 minutes and became maximal at 60 minutes, at which time it was some 450% above baseline levels. This elevation was also persistent in that 24 hours later, the signal had not yet returned to prestimulated levels. The increase in gene expression was paralleled by a more than 600% increase in production of the mature peptide. It is noteworthy that autoinduction of ET synthesis also occurs in other cell types. Exogenous ET had previously been observed to increase preproET-1 mRNA in neonatal cardiac myocytes and umbilical endothelial cells. Taken together, these findings underscore the possibility that this contributes to the potent and long-lasting effects of ET wherever ET-1 is produced. Nuclear transcription run-off analyses revealed that ET-1 significantly increased transcription of the preproET-1 gene. Endothelin-1 stimulation also increased the stability of ET-1 transcripts. Normally, the half-life of preproET-1 mRNA is short, ~20 min, and has been attributed to the presence of two AUUUA sequences in the 3'-untranslated region thought to mediate selective mRNA degradation. Exposure of mesangial cells to ET-1 significantly increased stability of preproET-1 mRNA to a half-life of approximately 60 minutes. Although ET gene expression is primarily transcriptionally regulated, stabilization of preproET-1 mRNA in response to other cytokines also has been noted previously. Thus TGF-β has been noted to increase the half-life of preproET-1 mRNA in Madin-Darby canine kidney cells from 15 to 30 or 45 minutes. In bovine aortic endothelial cells, atrial natriuretic peptide increased the half-life of preproET-1 mRNA from 25 min to ≈ 70 min. It is possible then that increased transcription rate is a primary mechanism responsible for the early surge in the preproET-1 mRNA expression, while increased mRNA stability contributes more to the sustained elevation in ET gene expression observed in some pathophysiologic settings.

It is noteworthy that selective ETB-receptor antagonist abrogated the increase in preproET-1 mRNA expression occurring in mesangial cells exposed to ET-1. The ETB-receptor antagonist also squelched mature peptide production, completely abolishing the increased ET stimulation. Exposure to an ETB agonist, sarafotoxin S6c, increased preproET-1 mRNA expression. This potentiation in gene expression and peptide production were lessened by the ETB-receptor antagonist. Contrasting the results with the ETB-receptor antagonist, the selective ETA antagonist BQ123 did not affect preproET-1 mRNA expression. These findings have additional implications that, once stimulated to produce ET-1, those cells that have the ETB receptor could amplify and propagate ET-1 actions. Furthermore, the continued increase in ET-1 may contribute to the chronicity of functional and structural consequences of ET-1 activation. Indeed, persistent increases of ET gene expression and peptide synthesis have been documented in a variety of pathophysiologic settings. In addition, this autoinduction of ET-1 by ET-1 appears to play an important role in human renal tubular regeneration and restoration of

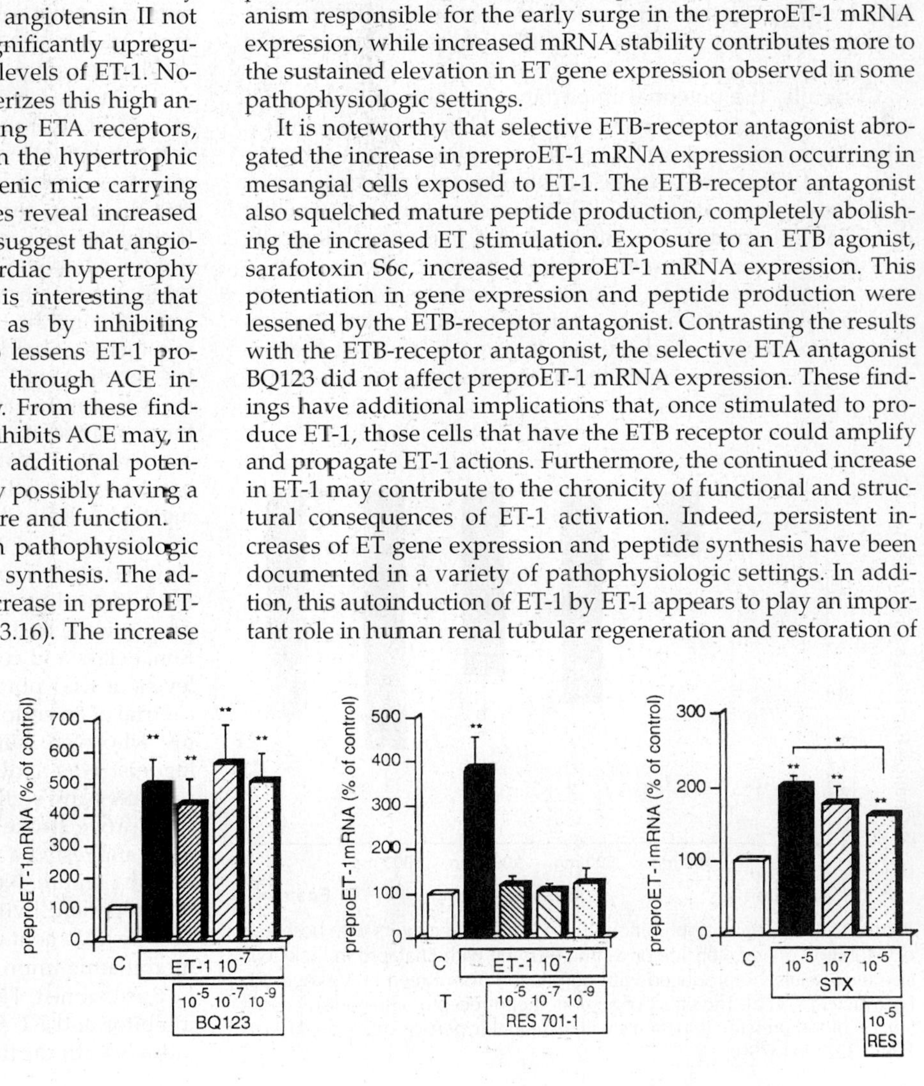

Figure 13.16. Stimulation of preproET-1 mRNA expression by ET-1 peptide and effects of antagonizing the ETA or ETB receptors. Vehicle *C* or ET-1 was added to mesangial cells with or without either the ETA-receptor antagonist (BQ123)(A) or ETB-receptor antagonist (RES701) (B). Cells were also exposed to the vehicle sarafotoxin S6c (STX) or STX-RES701-1. (Reproduced with permission from Kiowski W, Suetsch G, Hunziker P, et al. Evidence for endothelin-1 mediated vasoconstriction in severe chronic heart failure. *Lancet* 1995;346: 732–736.)

normal tubule integrity following injury. Moreover, similar to mesangial and endothelial cells, inhibition of the ETB, not the ETA receptor, markedly suppresses endogenous ET-1 synthesis and cellular proliferation by the human proximal tubule cells. By contrast, ET-1 synthesis is augmented by an agonist of the ETB receptor. These observations reiterate that autoinduction is a generalized function of the ETB receptor, which may be particularly important in the tubule cells because this is the primary receptor subtype along the postglomerular nephron segments.

Systemic Hypertension

Although there are inconsistent reports regarding circulating ET-1 levels in patients with hypertension, the vascular ET-1 concentration does associate with hypertension in animal models and also in humans. Antagonism of ET by ETA antagonists BQ123 and FR139317 lessens hypertension in deoxycorticosterone acetate (DOCA)–salt-induced hypertension and in hyperinsulinemic hypertensive rats. Moreover, enterally administered nonpeptide antagonists were effective in several different animal models, including sodium-depletion induced hypertension in squirrel monkeys, Goldblatt hypertension in dogs, and mouse (mRen-2)-transgenic rats. In the latter model, which is characterized by increase in angiotensin II, the hypertension was lessened by either AT_1-receptor antagonist, losartan, or the ETA/ETB antagonist, SB2099670, and these effects were additive. This reiterates the interconnection between ET and other cytokines in this setting, indicating that angiotensin II may potentiate endothelin production as noted previously.

Clinically, the potential importance of interrupting the ET system was recently shown in a group of hypertensive patients, whereby the orally active ETA-/ETB-receptor antagonist bosentan caused a sustained decrease in blood pressure over a 4-week period of observation (Fig. 13.17). It is unclear, however, whether the ETA/ETB antagonism interrupted a pathophysiologically specific mechanism or removed ET-1 ambient effects on vascular tone prevailing in humans. Nevertheless, these agents may provide an efficacious addition to our armamentarium of antihypertensive medications. In view of the fact that increasing doses of the combined antagonist was not associated

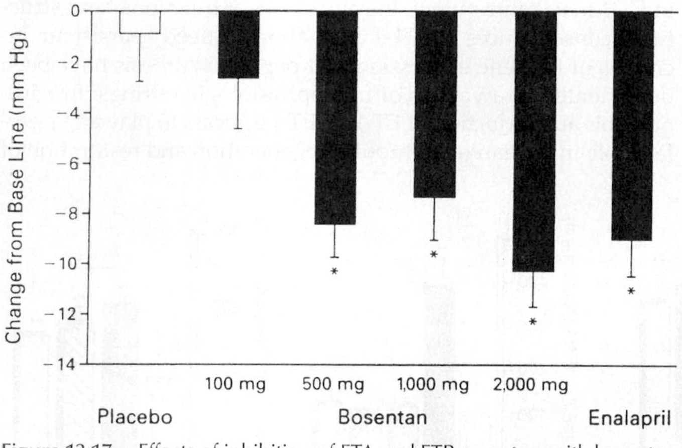

Figure 13.17. Effects of inhibition of ETA and ETB receptors with bosentan or inhibition of angiotensin-converting enzyme with Enalapril in hypertensive individuals. (Reproduced with permission from Kreen H, Viskoper RJ, Lacrouciere Y, et al. The effect of an endothelin-receptor antagonist, bosentan, on blood pressure in patients with essential hypertension. *N Engl J Med* 1998; 338:784–790.)

with additional antihypertensive effect, it is possible that the loss of the ETB function actually blunted the direct or indirect (NO, PGI_2-mediated) vasodilatory effects transduced by this receptor. In this connection, mice deficient in the ETB receptor have increased blood pressure at baseline and demonstrate salt-sensitive hypertension. These observations raise the possibility that while antagonism of the ETA receptor appears beneficial in cases of hypertension, antagonizing the ETB receptor might run counter to the goals of antihypertensive therapy.

Cardiac Dysfunction

Vasoconstriction, myocardial and vascular remodeling, and renal sodium retention characterize various forms of cardiac dysfunction. Each of these processes is regulated by ET and has thus provided the basis for the idea that ET in important in this setting. In addition, ET's potentiation of angiotensin II, aldosterone, adrenergic tone synergistically augments these processes. Animal data indicate that both circulating and tissue levels of ET-1 are increased in heart failure and that the magnitude of the increase parallels the degree of cardiac dysfunction. Levels of ET-1 in the tissue are increased, representing an increase in production by myocytes but not endothelial cells. This increase results from increased synthesis of ET-1, and solid data indicate that preproET-1 is elevated and this elevation persists. Interestingly, intrarenal ET-1 concentration increases in heart failure and thus may contribute to the renal constriction and sodium retention that typifies the kidney's response to heart failure and that has previously been ascribed to activation of the renin angiotensin system.

Pharmacologic inhibition of ET-1 actions ameliorates adverse cardiac events and improves survival in various settings of cardiac dysfunction. In coronary artery–ligated rats, there was a dramatic increase in the amount of cardiac ET-1 and of ET receptors. Continuous infusion of an ETA-receptor antagonist into these rats for 10 days produced improvement in left ventricular function and lessened ventricular dilation and hypertrophy. Moreover, there was substantial improvement in 12-week survival, from 43% to 85%. Evidence is accumulating that antagonizing the ETA receptor or ETA together with ETB receptors increases cardiac contractility, cardiac output, left ventricular function and reduces myocyte hypertrophy, ventricular mass expansion, and fibrous tissue formation. Notably, some of these changes occurred even with inhibition of angiotensin-converting enzyme; thus ET antagonism offers an additional benefit in this setting. Data from clinical studies are accumulating that solidify the importance of these observations in humans. Patients with ischemic or dilated cardiomyopathy have elevated levels of circulating and intracardiac endothelin, twofold to threefold higher than normal. The ET levels were proportional to the New York Heart Association (NYHA) functional class and correlated with mortality such that the highest levels of ET-1 portended the worst prognosis. In the first clinical trial of an endothelin antagonist in humans with cardiac failure who were withdrawn from ACE inhibitor, ETA/ETB antagonist was shown to reduce mean arterial and pulmonary pressures and right atrial and pulmonary wedge pressures and to improve stroke volume and cardiac output. These observations suggested a potentially additive effect of ET antagonism in heart failure. Notably, a 14-day trial of an ETA/ETB antagonist in patients with NYHA class III heart failure with dyspnea, despite treatment with ACEI, digoxin, and diuretics showed hemodynamic improvement following the addition of an ETA/ETB antagonist. These observations predict that benefits of ACE inhibitor and ET antagonism are indeed additive in such individuals with cardiac failure.

Acute Renal Failure

Ample evidence now points to an important role for ET in acute renal failure (ARF). Increased ET-1 gene expression and peptide production occur in response to a variety of injurious stimuli, including ischemia, radiocontrast, myoglobinuria, cyclosporine, and a number of toxins. Importantly, this activation persists for hours, days, and even weeks after resolution of the initial injury. Because the half-life for preproET-1 mRNA is very short (on the order of minutes), this long-term increase is clearly related to continuous production of new transcripts. In support of ET's importance in ARF are the numerous studies that show that antagonism of ET's actions lessens duration and severity of ARF. ECE inhibition by phosphoramidon improved ischemia-induced hypofiltration. Phosphoramidon reduced sodium wasting and proteinuria, even at doses that did not improve glomerular filtration rate (GFR) or renal plasma flow, implying direct protection of the tubule epithelium. An early study evaluated the role of endogenous ET in glomerular dysfunction following ischemic renal damage. ET antibody was able to increase the single nephron GFR by 40% and doubled the glomerular plasma flow above the ischemic level. This occurred primarily because of a decrease in both afferent and efferent arteriolar resistance. These observations make a strong point. A number of maneuvers can ameliorate ARF if initiated before or at the time of injury. However, these experiments reveal the unusual circumstance that even established renal failure can be lessened by antagonizing ET. Thus these studies indicate that ET has a role in maintaining postischemic glomerular dysfunction. However, ET is important not only in the initiation and maintenance of vasoconstriction but also in the tubule regeneration that follows ARF. Proximal tubule mitogenesis has been shown to be mediated by ET, and this effect occurs through the ETB receptor. The implication of these observations is that while early antagonism of ET action is desirable, ET inhibition after ARF is well established may confound tubule regeneration from surviving cells to reepithelialize the damaged nephron.

In addition to elevating the ET-1 peptide, ARF injuries also affect the ET receptors. Early studies showed increased the ligand-binding affinity of both the ETA and ETB receptors in the renal cortex following ischemia. Further, glycerol-induced ischemic renal failure has also been shown to significantly upregulate both ETA and ETB receptors in the cortex and the medulla, measured by ligand binding and RT-PCR assay for mRNA levels of the receptors. This effect was more pronounced in the medulla than in the cortex and affected ETB receptors more than ETA receptors. ETB, but not ETA mRNA, was also elevated in a postischemic model and again was particularly apparent in the renal medulla, although this is not a uniform finding. Nephrotoxicity from cyclosporine also appears to preferentially increase the ETB receptor in the renal medulla. Cultured mesangial cells exposed to cyclosporine also increased ETB but not the ETA mRNA. Taken together, it appears that injury particularly affects the ETB receptor and particularly the renal medulla. However, this does not mean that the ETA receptor is not functionally important. On the contrary, treatment with an ETA antagonist before or at the time of ischemia has been shown to lessen the glomerular dysfunction. In addition, ETA antagonism has been shown to lessen structural damage accompanying ARF and dramatically improve outcome of postischemic ARF. Forty-five minutes of ischemia caused uniform mortality in uninephrectomized, chronically instrumented rats. Treatment with an ETA-receptor antagonist 24 hours after the injury improved survival to 75% which the authors attribute to preservation of tubule function. Gradual recovery of the GFR was observed in the survivors. Overall, these observations have the implications that while early antagonism of ET actions is desirable, ET inhibition after ARF is well established may rather confound tubule regeneration from surviving cells to reepithelialize the damaged nephron. Thus, early inhibition of both ETA and ETB receptors may lessen vasoconstriction and autoinductive perpetuation of ET signal, while established renal failure may benefit from selective ETA inhibition allowing ETB to mediate tubule cell regrowth.

Chronic Renal Failure

Endothelin participates in all the processes known to be involved in renal parenchymal destruction of chronic renal failure, including cellular hypertrophy, proliferation, and collagen deposition. Findings in transgenic mice reiterate this point. It is notable that while exogenous ET-1 and also ET-2 are powerful *in vivo* vasoconstrictors, transgenic rat models overexpressing either the human ET-1 or the ET-2 gene were not found to be hypertensive. Thus, despite marked overexpression of the human ET genes and significant increase in the circulating precursors as well as the mature peptide in the blood, pressure of the transgenic animals was comparable with that of their nontransgenic littermates. Because no change in gene expression of the receptors for ET was detected, the surprising normotension is believed to result from counterregulation of other vasoactive substances, such as NO. Nevertheless, even with normal blood pressure, there was significant interstitial fibrosis and proteinuria, pointing to important direct and indirect effects of ET's that are independent of systemic blood pressure effects. In addition to its own direct effects of these processes, ET-1 also interacts synergistically with other growth factors, including EGF, TGF-α and TGF-β, and PDGF to potentiate cellular proliferation and matrix gene expression, thereby promoting the scarring process. ET-1 also increases expression or mRNA for collagen type I, II, IV, and laminin, and through the ETA receptor, ET-1 induces expression of c-*fos* and c-*myc* and *fra-1* immediate early genes. ET-1 stimulates MAP-kinases that have been proposed to mediate nuclear signaling and mesangial growth, as well as tyrosine kinases, which are believed to be important regulators of cellular growth and differentiation. Circulating and renal tissue levels of ET increase in chronic renal failure, and renal preproET-1 mRNA increases parallel the degree of progressive damage. Overexpression of ET-1 per se causes glomerular and interstitial scarring in animals that are not hypertensive. Similarly, ET-2 transgenic mice develop glomerulosclerosis and interstitial fibrosis without systemic hypertension. These observations reiterate the blood pressure–independent effects of ET in promoting scarring. These findings complement earlier data in nonhypertensive models, such as chronic cyclosporine nephrotoxicity, or Heymann nephritis, indicating that glomerular dysfunction is lessened by chronic antagonism of ET, specifically with the ETA receptor. This finding suggests that functional (reversible) ETA-mediated vasoconstriction is an important determinant of renal dysfunction with chronic renal failure. Studies in chronic cyclosporine nephrotoxicity—together with our previous observations that glomerular dysfunction following acute cyclosporine administration is lessened by acute antagonism of ETA receptor—imply that ET, through the ETA receptor, mediates glomerular dysfunction throughout the spectrum of cyclosporine toxicity. However, ETA antagonism did not normalize the GFR in these animals who underwent long-term treatment. ETA antagonism did not alleviate structural damage associated with chronic cyclosporine nephrotoxicity. Thus other factors affecting vasoconstriction and structural injury also contributed to glomerular dysfunction in this setting.

The beneficial effects of concurrent ETA/ETB antagonism offered remarkable benefit in protecting the GFR during chronic cyclosporine treatment evaluated over a 5-week treatment period. Notably, antagonizing both the ETA and ETB receptors in chronically NO-inhibited hypertensive mice resulted in marked diminution of collagen expression, glomerular sclerosis, and vascular injury. Hypertension is well recognized to be a cause and result of chronic renal failure and is associated with progression of renal failure. In this context inhibition of ET appears efficacious. Thus chronic ET antagonism lessens renal hypoperfusion and hypofiltration and spares the kidneys from structural damage in the renal ablation model in rats.

Importantly, even in the face of angiotensin II inhibition, ET antagonism offers additional benefit. Indeed, combination of angiotensin and ET antagonism effected less proteinuria and lower creatinine than either treatment alone. In this connection proteinuria per se is now believed to promote tubulointerstitial fibrosis. This may at least in part reflect the direct effect of proteinuria in stimulating ET synthesis by tubule cells.

Selected Readings

Bruzzi I, Corna D, Zoja C, et al. Time course and localization of endothelin-1 gene expression in a model of renal disease progression. *Am J Pathol* 1997;151:1241–1247.

Important observations focusing on the complicated role of endothelins in progressive renal destruction.

Goto K, Hama H, Kasuya Y. Molecular pharmacology and pathophysiological significance of endothelin. *Jpn J Pharmacol* 1996;72:261–290.

Thorough summary with poignant commentary of the evolution of endothelin research.

Hosoda K, Hammer RE, Richardson JA, et al. Targeted and natural (Piebald-lethal) mutations of endothelin-B receptor gene produce megacolon associated with spotted coat color in mice. *Cell* 1994;79:1267–1276.

Genetic engineering was used to persuasively demonstrate that the endothelin receptor (in this case the ETB) has important function particularly in normal development.

Iwasaki S, Homma T, Matsuda Y, et al. Endothelin receptor subtype B mediates autoinduction of endothelin-1 in rat mesangial cell. *J Biol Chem* 1995;270:6997–7003.

Observations which addressed the mechanisms for the much hailed long-term effects of endothelin actions.

Kiowski W, Suetsch G, Hunziker P, et al. Evidence for endothelin-1 mediated vasoconstriction in severe chronic heart failure. *Lancet* 1995;346:732–736.

The initial demonstration of benefit in antagonizing endothelin actions in human disease.

Kon V, Yoshioka T, Fogo A, Ichikawa I. Glomerular actions of endothelin in vivo. *J Clin Invest* 1989;. 83:1762–1767.

The first documentation of endothelin's importance in a pathophysiologic setting.

Krum H, Viskoper RJ, Lacrourciere Y, et al. The effect of an endothelin-receptor antagonist, bosentan, on blood pressure in patients with essential hypertension. *N Engl J Med* 1998;338:784–790.

The first demonstration that long-term endothelin receptor angatonism benefits patients with mild-to-moderate hypertension.

Yanagisawa M, Kurihara H, Kimura S, et al. A novel potent vasoconstrictor peptide produced by vascular endothelial cells. *Nature* 1988;332:411–415.

The landmark paper, not only in terms of originality but its completeness. A real treat!

PART 6
Nitric Oxide

Scott C. Thomson and Roland C. Blantz

In 1987, nitric oxide (NO) was identified as the elusive endothelium-derived relaxing factor (EDRF). Since then, NO has been confirmed to perform numerous signaling functions in cells throughout the body. Interest in the role of NO in the kidney led to the publication of more than 1,000 reports in the biomedical literature between January 1990 and March 1998.

NITRIC OXIDE BASICS

NO is synthesized from the terminal guanidino nitrogen of arginine, oxygen, and NADPH in the presence of tetrahydrobiopterin (BH_4). This reaction is catalyzed by nitric oxide synthases (NOSs). There are three principle classes of NOS, each composed of one or more isoforms. Several investigators have employed reverse-transcriptase polymerase chain reaction or *in situ* hybridization to localize NOS mRNA, or immunohistochemistry to localize NOS proteins in the kidney. Data suggest that each class, NOS I, II, and III, is differentially expressed in different parts of the kidney under different circumstances. NOS I, also known as *neuronal NOS* (nNOS or bNOS), is primarily expressed in the macula densa, where its content varies inversely with dietary salt levels. NOS II, initially known as *inducible* or *calmodulin-independent NOS* (iNOS), appears to be constitutively expressed in thick ascending limb cells of the outer medulla under the positive influence of dietary salt and may be induced in the glomerulus and other nephron segments by exposure to cytokines or lipopolysaccharide. NOS III, also known as *endothelial NOS* (eNOS), is constitutively expressed in endothelial cells to varying degrees throughout the renal vasculature. All NOSs are activated by binding to calcium-calmodulin. The binding affinity of calcium-calmodulin for NOS I and NOS III is within the range in which changes in intracellular free calcium constitute a main control point for NO production by NOS I and NOS III. The affinity for NOS II is much higher, to the extent that intracellular calcium is not rate limiting for NOS II activity. NOS is autoinhibited by NO and also inhibited by asymmetric dimethyl-arginine, which is generated endogenously. NO is a highly diffusible gas that moves freely through tissues. When NO is removed from tissue solely by autooxidation to biologically inert nitrite/nitrate, the diffusion distance of NO is calculated to be on the order of 100 to 200 μm. However, NO is also removed by rapid binding to scavengers, such as hemoglobin and superoxide anion. Thus its half-life is short, and the distance from its site of synthesis to its site of action may not exceed a few microns.

To date, most of the cellular functions attributed to NO have been ascribed to the direct activation of the soluble heme-containing enzyme, guanylyl cyclase, and the formation of cyclic-GMP. However, NO may also affect kidney function through binding to transition metal centers in other heme-containing enzymes, where the net effect of NO binding is to inhibit these enzymes. Examples include inhibition of cytochrome P450 oxidases, which convert arachidonic acid to HETEs and EETs in the renal tubule and microcirculation and autoinhibition of NOS itself. NO may also subserve cellular functions that do not directly involve heme proteins. For instance, one-electron oxidation of NO by molecular oxygen yields the nitrosating species NO^+, which readily reacts with thiolates (RS^-) to form nitrosothiols (RS-NO). RS-NOs are predisposed to heterolytic transfer of NO^+ to other sulfhydrils, leading to regulation of many membrane and cytosolic proteins by S-nitrosylation. One example of this that is potentially important to renal vascular tone is the hyperpolarization of arteriolar smooth muscle from enhanced activity of calcium-dependent membrane K-channels. Nitrosation reactions may also be sustained by non–thiol nucleophilic centers. For instance, NO generated in the macula densa can combine with superoxide anion to form peroxynitrite, leading ultimately to tyrosine nitr(os)ation of proteins around the glomerulus.

Electrodes are available that are capable of measuring the NO content of tissues, but these have not been employed widely to study the kidney. Most studies of NO in the kidney or in cells derived from the kidney have measured physiologic responses to NOS antagonists or NO donors or have measured the appearance of nitrite/nitrate or cyclic guanosine monophosphate (cGMP). Most NOS antagonists in common use are methylated arginine or citrulline compounds, which compete with arginine for binding to NOS. Most studies have used antagonists that inhibit all three NOS isoforms (L-NAME, L-NMMA), although agents are now available that are relatively specific for NOS I (s-methyl thiocitrulline and 7-nitroindazole) or NOS II (-N6-(1-iminoethyl)lysine). No compound that specifically inhibits endothelial NOS III is currently available. Examples of NO agonists in common usage include *S*-nitroso-*N*-acetyl-penicillamine (SNAP) and nonoate, which donate NO; 3-morpholinosydnonimine (SIN-1), which simultaneously donates NO and superoxide anion; and sodium nitroprusside, which directly activates soluble guanylyl cyclase. Putative roles for NOS have also been ascribed to the effects of exogenous L-arginine. However, most L-arginine metabolized in the kidney is converted to urea by arginase or to biologically active agmatine by arginine decarboxylase. Furthermore, L-arginine has profound effects on the release of several hormones, including glucagon, growth hormone, insulin, somatostatin, and catecholamines, which are not necessarily mediated through NO. This should be taken into account when assigning effects of exogenous L-arginine to NO.

NITRIC OXIDE AND HEMODYNAMICS IN THE RENAL CORTEX

The single-nephron glomerular filtration rate (SNGFR) is determined by glomerular capillary hydrostatic pressure, nephron plasma flow, glomerular capillary ultrafiltration coefficient, and plasma oncotic pressure. Among these determinants, there is the potential for endothelial NOS III to exert a direct tonic influence over nephron plasma flow and glomerular capillary pressure through effects on vascular smooth muscle and to alter the glomerular ultrafiltration coefficient through effects on mesangial cells. There is also the potential for macula densa NOS I to influence glomerular hemodynamics through tubuloglomerular feedback. Because NOS I is also an important downmodulator of sympathetic nerve traffic, there is the additional potential for systemically administered NOS blockers to influence renal hemodynamics through increased efferent sympathetic renal nerve activity.

The importance of NO as an endogenous renal vasodilator has been examined by measuring the acute effects of nonspecific NOS blockers on glomerular filtration rate (GFR) and renal blood flow (RBF) in conscious animals and in humans. The role of endogenous NO in the glomerular microvasculature has been studied by micropuncture in anesthetized rats. The effect of NOS inhibition on vascular function has been examined by changes in diameter of intrarenal arteries and glomerular arterioles in the split hydronephrotic rat kidney and glomerular arterioles of *in vitro* blood perfused juxtamedullary glomeruli. In addition, the renovascular effects of chronic NOS blockade have been investigated.

When infused in conscious humans, a subpressor dose of L-NMMA reduces RBF by 20% without affecting GFR, thus implying that basal RBF in humans is maintained by endogenous NO and that flow to the kidney might be more susceptible to NO inhibition than flow to other organs. While it is not possible to know how the individual determinants of SNGFR are affected by L-NMMA in humans, the fact that L-NMMA causes the filtration fraction to increase suggests that renal vasoconstriction induced by L-NMMA in humans is not limited to the preglomerular vasculature.

Several laboratory groups have performed micropuncture in rats to determine the effects of systemic NOS inhibition on the determinants of SNGFR. The earliest such experiments were reported in 1991 and showed that a pressor dose of L-NMMA increased preglomerular and postglomerular vascular resistances, reduced nephron plasma flow,and reduced the glomerular ultrafiltration coefficient. The efferent arteriole was primarily affected, such that the decrements in nephron plasma flow and ultrafiltration coefficient were fully offset by a substantial increase in glomerular capillar pressure, leaving SNGFR unaffected. In a nearly identical rat model, reductions in ultrafiltration coefficient and nephron plasma flow were described during L-NMMA, which, in the absence of a major increase in glomerular capillary pressure, caused SNGFR to decrease. Subsequently micropuncture results provided similar data with respect to the effect of L-NMMA on glomerular capillary pressure, as well as with respect to the effect on SNGFR. The data from these three studies are less discrepant than suggested by the differences in glomerular capillary pressures and SNGFR because each study demonstrated a tonic influence of endogenous NO over the preglomerular and postglomerular vasculature and over the glomerular ultrafiltration coefficient. The different pressure and SNGFR responses result from differences in the relative influence of endogenous NO over the various vascular elements rather from a qualitative disagreement as to which elements are under the influence of NO. When nonspecific NOS inhibitors are administered systemically, the acute renal hemodynamic effects are confounded by a simultaneous increase in systemic arterial blood pressure and by a disinhibition of sympathetic outflow from the central nervous system. The increase in renal vascular resistance that ensues results from a combination of autoregulation, increased renal nerve activity, and direct inhibition of NOS III in the kidney. Only one micropuncture study has been published in which a NOS inhibitor was infused directly into the renal artery. In this study, local endogenous NO seemed to exert no significant effect on the efferent arteriole, although neither was there a decline in glomerular capillar pressure as NOS blockade increased preglomerular resistance. Furthermore, the lack of a role for NO in the efferent arteriole is difficult to reconcile with other data from the split hydronephrotic kidney or blood perfused juxtamedullary nephron.

The split hydronephrotic rat kidney is an experimental preparation in which the renal tubules are chronically ablated rendering the cortical vessels amenable to study by transillumination *in vivo*. Intravenous infusion of L-NAME in this model was reported to constrict the arcuate artery and efferent arteriole. The juxtamedullary blood perfused nephron is an experimental preparation in which the glomerular microvasculature of a rat juxtamedullary glomerulus is exposed by dissection and subjected to videometric analysis while the kidney is mechanically perfused. Perfusion with L-NMMA in this model has revealed a vasodilatory influence of endogenous NO on the afferent and efferent arterioles.

NITRIC OXIDE AND HEMODYNAMICS IN THE RENAL MEDULLA

Vasa recta bundles contain minor amounts of NOS II mRNA and thick ascending limb cells contain greater amounts of NOS II mRNA and NOS II protein, which could influence the function of adjacent vasa recta. In dissected descending vasa recta preconstricted with norepinephrine and examined *in vitro*, L-NMMA prevents acetylcholine-induced vasodilation and abluminal L-arginine causes vasodilation. Examined in the rat *in vivo*, renal vasoconstriction by systemic L-NMMA may be more pronounced in the medulla than in the cortex and papillary blood flow may be reduced by infusion of L-NAME directly into the medullary interstitium. These limited data suggest that the medullary circulation is subject to the influence of NO.

NITRIC OXIDE AND TUBULAR FUNCTION

NOS can be expressed in several tubular segments. In particular, NOS II has been identified by immunohistochemistry in tubular epithelium of the proximal tubules, thick ascending limb of Henle's loop, distal convoluted tubule and intercalated cells of the collecting duct. Also, nephron segments containing guanylyl cyclase might be subject to influence from NO generated by NOS III in peritubular capillaries.

There is some confusion as to whether NO in the kidney acts to increase or to decrease epithelial transport. For example, it has been argued that NO-mediated increases in vasa recta blood flow are required for the increase in interstitial pressure that underlies the pressure-natriuresis phenomenon. According to this theory, NO acting on the vasa recta would create physical forces that oppose reabsorption in the proximal tubule and descending limb. However, several investigators have reported major natriureses/diureses along with reduced proximal reabsorption in response to hypertensive doses of intravenous L-NMMA. Furthermore, several lines of evidence suggest that NO generated within the peritubular capillary can lead to increased proximal reabsorption through cGMP-mediated activation of sodium-proton exchange in the proximal tubule brush border.

NITRIC OXIDE AND TUBULOGLOMERULAR FEEDBACK

Tubuloglomerular feedback is the term applied to a chain of physiologic processes that take place in the juxtaglomerular apparatus and that confer an inverse dependence of SNGFR on the salt content of fluid at the luminal macula densa. Tubuloglomerular feedback participates in autoregulation of RBF and stabilizes the amount of salt and water delivered to the distal nephron. Tubuloglomerular feedback is commonly studied by measuring changes in SNGFR or an index of glomerular capillary pressure during microperfusion of the loop of Henle. Tubuloglomerular feedback data are then depicted by an inverted hyperbolic tangent drawn in a plane in which the abscissa represents late proximal flow and the ordinate represents SNGFR or glomerular capillary pressure. NOS I is highly concentrated in the macula densa where it is strategically positioned to influence tubuloglomerular feedback. The tubuloglomerular feedback signal must transit the macula densa and extraglomerular mesangium to reach the vascular pole of the glomerulus and a variety of theories have been advanced as to the form assumed by this signal en route. Each of these theories is easily modified to accommodate a role for NO. In terms of actual data, several investigators have examined the effects on tubuloglomerular feedback when NOS inhibitors are delivered into the tubular lumen by microperfusion. The most consistent picture to be drawn from these data is one in which NO generated in the macula densa exerts a tonic upward pressure on SNGFR while causing the tubuloglomerular feedback curve to shift rightward relative to ambient late proximal flow and to become less steep. In other words, macula densa NO is a potent modulator of tubuloglomerular feedback, which may be responsible for maintaining coordination between the tubuloglomerular feedback curve and ambient tubular flow or for setting the gain of the tubuloglomerular feedback response. However, NO does not directly mediate the tubuloglomerular feedback GF response to minute-to-minute changes in tubular flow.

INTERACTION WITH OTHER SYSTEMS

In the kidney, NO functions as a counterregulatory influence to the vasoconstrictor effects of endothelin, angiotensin II, and renal adrenergic nerves. In the case of endothelin, endogenous NO not only mitigates the vasoconstrictor actions of endothelin but also suppresses its synthesis and release.

Depending on the experimental model, NO in the juxtaglomerular apparatus is reported to stimulate or to suppress renin synthesis and secretion. Several studies in the isolated perfused kidney have found NO donors to function as renin secretagogues, and NO blockers to suppress renin secretion. This role of NO appears to involve cGMP-mediated inhibition of phosphodiesterase III leading to accumulation of cyclic adenosine monophosphate (cAMP), a known stimulant to renin release. In contrast, several studies in cortical kidney slices have suggested that NO is a potent inhibitor of renin secretion. A tenable hypothesis to account for these latter observations is that NO, generated by Ca^{2+}-calmodulin binding to NOS, is an intermediary in the suppression of renin release by agents, such as angiotensin II, which increase cytosolic calcium. It is difficult to reconcile all the experimental results, but it is conceivable that NO will have opposing effects on renin secretion, depending on the prevailing balance between other systems that affect cAMP and cytosolic calcium. When renin is manipulated either by changes in dietary salt or by clipping the renal artery, NOS I and renin immunoreactivities tend to cosegregate. However, in these same models, NOS immunoreactivity is inversely related to the hemodynamic effects of NOS blockade. Therefore linkage between NOS I and renin by immunocytochemistry in the JGA should not be construed as evidence that increased NO causes increased renin.

Interactions between NOS and angiotensin II occur within both the glomerular microvasculature and proximal tubule. In a study in which acute NOS blockade in normal rats increased systemic blood pressure, constricted the afferent and efferent glomerular arterioles, reduced glomerular ultrafiltration coefficient, reduced nephron plasma flow, and reduced SNGFR, the effects of NOS blockade in animals pretreated with the angiotensin II–receptor antagonist losartan were limited to an increase in systemic arterial pressure and an autoregulatory increase in afferent resistance. Neither SNGFR nor any of its other determinants were affected by NOS blockade in losartan-treated rats. Angiotensin II exerts both stimulatory and inhibitory effects on proximal tubular reabsorption. Under normal circumstances, the stimulatory mechanism responds to subnanomolar angiotensin II, whereas the inhibitory mechanism responds to suprananomolar angiotensin II. Acute NO blockade sensitizes the inhibitory response rendering proximal reabsorption vulnerable to inhibition by ambient amounts of angiotensin II.

NO modulates the effects of renal sympathetic nerve activity on the glomerulus and proximal tubule, particularly under conditions of heightened sympathetic activity. In fact, all of the previously listed glomerular hemodynamic effects of acute NOS blockade are prevented by prior renal denervation. This link between the sympathetic-adrenergic and NO systems appears to be mediated by adrenoceptors of the α_2 subtype because studies using α_2-agonists and antagonists have demonstrated that the effects of acute NOS inhibition on SNGFR, nephron plasma flow, afferent and efferent arteriolar resistances, ultrafiltration coefficient, and proximal reabsorption all correlate with the amount of underlying α_2-adrenergic activity.

ROLE OF RENAL NITRIC OXIDE IN DISEASE STATES

Sepsis

Early in the sepsis syndrome, renal function deteriorates rapidly despite normal or increased cardiac output. Arterial hypotension may develop during this hyperdynamic stage of sepsis as the result of a generalized increase in NO production by cytokine-dependent NOS II. Despite the overall reduction in systemic vascular resistance during this stage of sepsis, there is severe renal vasoconstriction in which the local production of endothelin, angiotensin II, and various vasoconstrictor eicosanoids have been implicated. Nonselective NOS inhibitors administered to animals under these conditions can prevent hypotension, but exacerbate renal vasoconstriction leading to worsening renal failure or glomerular thrombosis. In contrast, specific inhibitors of NOS II prevent renal vasoconstriction from occurring in rats treated with bacterial lipopolysaccharide (LPS). Furthermore, in glomeruli from LPS-treated animals, the ability to stimulate cGMP formation via NOS III is suppressed and restored by NOS II blockade. It appears as though NO generated by NOS II during sepsis inhibits NOS III, thereby interfering with a normal cycling of NO production by NOS III, which is required to mitigate the effects of locally derived vasoconstrictors in the glomerular microvasculature. The manipulation of this pathway as a means for preventing renal failure has not yet been tested in patients with sepsis.

Ischemic Acute Renal Failure

Ischemic renal injury desensitizes the kidney to endothelium-dependent vasodilators and increases its vulnerability to subsequent ischemic insults. This condition was once suspected of arising from endothelial injury, leading to suppressed endothelial NOS activity. However, it has since been confirmed that endothelial NOS III is fully present and active in postischemic acute renal failure and cannot be further stimulated because of saturation. *In vitro* studies also suggest that NO generated in the proximal tubule may contribute to hypoxia/reoxygenation injury because of reactivity with the superoxide radical to yield peroxynitrite. Also, antisense oligonucleotides targeted to prevent induction of NOS II prevented lethal injury to the proximal tubule in rats subjected to renal ischemia and reperfusion. However, not all the effects of NOS II in acute renal failure are deleterious because NOS II activity may be required for normal cell migration to the basement membrane during the healing phase of epithelial injury.

Immune Renal Disease

In nephrotoxic serum, antimesangial cell antibody, and antimyeloperoxidase models of acute glomerulonephritis, NOS II is expressed in mesangial cells, intraglomerular mononuclear cells, or cells infiltrating into the urinary space. Elevated NO production in each of these models has been linked to both the exacerbation and mitigation of immune injury. Increased NOS II activity is reported to contribute to injury and cell death in these models by suppression of normal NOS III activity, leading to glomerular thrombosis through formation of peroxynitrite, which participates in mesangiolysis, or by activating p53-mediated apoptosis in native or infiltrating cells. Cytokine induction of NOS II may be less facile in the mesangium of humans than rats, and there may be interspecies differences in the role of NOS II in glomerulonephritis. Nonetheless, NOS II is expressed in the glomeruli and tubulointerstitium of patients with class IV lupus nephritis, where it correlates with apoptosis. However, in humans with IgA nephropathy and MPGN, NOS II immunoreactivity is elevated only in stimulated monocyte/macrophages.

T lymphocytes are sensitive to antiproliferative effects of NO, and in the Brown Norway rat model of autoimmune tubulointerstitial nephritis, a T cell–mediated disease, NOS II is expressed in tubular epithelial cells where its effects are host protective.

Hypertension

Inhibition or deficiency of NO is a potent stimulus to hypertension. Nonselective NOS inhibitors cause hypertension by a variety of mechanisms, depending on the dose and time course over which they are administered. For instance, acute inhibition will cause hypertension by direct inhibition of endothelial NO production and by disinhibition of sympathetic outflow from the central nervous system. Chronic NOS blockade has the additional effect on blood pressure of interfering with the normal relationship between dietary salt intake and NOS I activity in the macula densa and brain, which may be important for sodium homeostasis. In particular, increased NO generation by macula densa NOS I may mediate the resetting of tubuloglomerular feedback, which is required for SNGFR and late proximal flow to increase in animals fed a high-salt diet. In fact, an attenuated increase in renal NOS I activity during increased dietary salt is reported to account for salt-sensitive hypertension in the Dahl salt-sensitive rat.

In patients with essential hypertension, basal and stimulated endothelial-dependent relaxation are both impaired while the hypotensive response to exogenous nitro donors is enhanced. Among normotensive offspring with a hypertensive family history these traits are bimodally distributed, suggesting that some abnormality of endothelial function constitutes an intermediate phenotype for human essential hypertension. However, the inheritance of this phenotype is not linked to the NOS III gene. It has been suggested that endothelium-dependent vasodilation is impaired in high-renin hypertension, not from impaired NO production, but from increased decomposition of NO by superoxide resulting from angiotensin II induction of the NADPH oxidase system. Furthermore, a family history of hypertension is a strong predictor of hydrogen peroxide accumulation in the plasma of patients after blockade of endogenous catalase.

Diabetes Mellitus

Early diabetes is associated with glomerular hyperperfusion and hyperfiltration, raising the obvious suspicion that diabetes might be a state of renal NO excess. Most data addressing the role of NO in diabetic hyperfiltration have been obtained from studies in rats with streptozotocin diabetes. In fact, diabetic rats do excrete more NO oxidation products (NOx) in their urine, but in some studies this may be the consequence of hyperphagia and in other studies excess NOx excretion was not reversed with NOS blockers. Several groups have tested diabetic rats for an enhanced renal vasoconstrictor response to nonselective NO inhibition. The results reported are mixed. Others have employed isolated glomeruli or renal resistance vessels to study the effects of diabetes or ambient glucose concentrations on endothelial dependent relaxation. Based on the responsiveness to NOS blockers, NO activity in afferent arterioles appears to be suppressed in diabetes and restored by addition of exogenous superoxide dismutase. Analogous findings are reported for isolated glomeruli from diabetic rats, in which the capacity to increase cGMP through agonist stimulation of NOS III or with NO donors is impaired despite intact guanylyl cyclase. These findings point to increased quenching of NO in the diabetic glomerulus.

Feeding L-arginine to diabetic rats with low plasma L-arginine concentrations, paradoxically reverses hyperfiltration by reducing filtration fraction without restoring plasma L-arginine, altering hypertrophy, or affecting overall renal vascular resistance. Based on current understanding of L-arginine and NO in renal physiology, there is no easy way to account for this effect of L-arginine on the diabetic kidney. One possibility is that, lacking in the ability to normally modulate macula densa NO, the diabetic kidney, to coordinate ambient tubular flow to the tubuloglomerular feedback response, relies on other internal control mechanisms that are not sensitive to dietary salt. Providing the macula densa with L-arginine reduces the reliance on these other systems, enabling the diabetic kidney to modulate NO and effect tubuloglomerular feedback resetting. In other words, NO must be produced in the first place in order for the kidney to cause tubuloglomerular feedback resetting by reducing NO. This hypothesis is supported by immunohistochemical and histochemical findings that maculae densa of rats with established diabetes contain less NOS enzyme and manifest less NADPH diaphorase activity than normal subjects, whereas NADPH diaphorase activity in juxtaglomerular arterioles (which depends on NO generated in the upstream vasculature) is preserved.

Uremia

Deficient or excessive NO activity may contribute to various aspects of uremia. There are several potential pathways whereby NO activity might be altered in uremia or in patients receiving dialysis. Examples include defective endothelial NO production resulting from accelerated atherosclerosis; decreased L-arginine production resulting from loss of functioning renal mass; increased cytokine-mediated NOS II activity related to dialysis; increased generation or retention of the endogenous NOS inhibitor, asymmetric dimethyl arginine (ADMA); changes in the physical form of NO resulting from redox alterations. Overall, NO activity is difficult to quantify in patients or experimental animals and may not be relevant to the activity of NOSs in specific organs. Also, it is possible for changes in NO activity to exacerbate or to mitigate aspects of uremia.

Healthy blood exposed to a cellulosic hemodialysis membrane is rendered capable of inducing NOS II in transformed murine endothelial cells, which normally express NOS II and NOS III. However, predialysis plasma from most uremic patients or patients with moderate renal failure will inhibit NOS II expression in these cells, whereas plasma from a minority of uremic patients and from patients after dialysis will enhance NOS II expression. Therefore it appears that different constituents of uremic blood can induce or suppress NOS II activity, and that induction predominates after dialysis either because of lymphocyte activation during dialysis or because an endogenous NOS inhibitor is removed by dialysis. Indeed, ADMA accumulates in the plasma of uremic patients and is removed during dialysis. However, the concentration of ADMA in uremic patients (0.5 to 0.9 μm) is below the IC50 for NOSs. In addition, uremic plasma also contains elevated amounts of L-arginine and either stimulates or has no effect on NOS III activity in cultured endothelial cells. Furthermore, increased NO-mediated cGMP production by uremic platelets may contribute to uremic platelet dysfunction and several authors have argued that increased production of NO and its release into the circulation can mediate hypotension during hemodialysis.

In addition to the hemodynamic and hemostatic implications of NO in uremia, NO may alter the net effect of intradialytic oxidative stress. NO may suppress NADPH-oxidase and xanthine oxidase activities, thereby diminishing formation of superoxide anion. On the other hand, NO may combine with superoxide to form the potent oxidant, peroxynitrite with potentially nefarious long-term consequences for dialysis patients.

Selected Readings

DeNicola L, Blantz RC, Gabbai FB. Nitric oxide and angiotensin II: glomerular and tubular interactions in the rat. *J Clin Invest* 1992;89:1248–1256.

This paper describes the effects of NOS inhibition on glomerular hemodynamics and was the first to illustrate that the balance between NO and angiotensin II activities in the kidney has an impact on the normal modulation of glomerular hemodynamics.

Kone BC, Baylis C. Biosynthesis and homeostatic roles of nitric oxide in the normal kidney. *Am J Physiol* 1997;272:F561–F578.

This review summarizes the current state of knowledge regarding the regulation of NOSs and their role in kidney physiology.

Palmer RM, Ferrige AG, Moncada S. Nitric oxide release accounts for the biological activity of endothelium-derived relaxing factor. *Nature* 1987;327:524–526.

This landmark paper identifies nitric oxide as the endothelium-derived relaxing factor.

Reyes AA, Karl I, Klahr S. Role of arginine in health and in renal disease. *Am J Physiol* 1994;267:F331–F346.

L-arginine is also the substrate for synthesis of compounds other than NO that are important for vascular regulation, immune function, growth, and interorgan communication. This paper reviews L-arginine metabolism from a wider perspective.

Wilcox CS, Welch WJ, Murad F, et al. Nitric oxide synthase in macula densa regulates glomerular capillary pressure. *Proc Natl Acad Sci USA* 1992;89:11993–11997.

This group made the original observation that NOS I is present in high concentration in the macula densa, where it influences glomerular function. Since this paper was published, its message has been refined or embellished by several other groups of investigators. NOS I in the macula densa is unique outside of the nervous system and the role of NOS I in the juxtaglomerular apparatus is unique in physiology.

PART 7
Catecholamines

Alexandr Arakelov and Fadi G. Lakkis

The principal catecholamines that act on the kidney are epinephrine, norepinephrine, and dopamine. Their biosynthesis occurs in catecholamine-secreting adrenergic neurons (norepinephrine and to a lesser extent, dopamine), adrenal medullary cells (epinephrine and norepinephrine), and in renal proximal tubule cells (dopamine). Catecholamines therefore reach the kidney through the circulation, urine, or adrenergic nerve endings found in the afferent and efferent glomerular arterioles, proximal and distal tubules, thick ascending limb of the loop of Henle, and the juxtaglomerular apparatus.

Catecholamines affect renal blood flow, glomerular filtration rate, tubular function, and renin secretion by binding to high-affinity receptors. Norepinephrine and epinephrine actions are mediated by α- and β-adrenoreceptors. Norepinephrine binds preferentially to α-receptors, while epinephrine has the highest affinity to β-receptors. Dopamine actions are mediated by specific dopamine receptors (DA). At high concentrations, dopamine also activates α- and β-adrenoreceptors. Biochemical and molecular studies have identified several subclasses of catecholamine receptors with different pharmacologic actions. These subclasses include α_1, α_2, β_1, β_2, DA_1, and DA_2; α_1-receptors are present on postsynaptic sites such as smooth muscle cells, where they mediate vasoconstriction. Although α_2-receptors are predominantly presynaptic and are involved in feedback inhibition of norepinephrine release from nerve endings, postsynaptic expression also exists, and it mediates catecholamine-induced vasoconstriction. The site of β_1-receptors is cardiac tissue, whereas β_2-receptors are generally extracardiac. Stimulation of β_2-receptors causes relaxation of bronchial and vascular smooth muscle cells. Stimulation of either DA_1- or DA_2-receptors also leads to smooth muscle relaxation in vascular beds.

Catecholamine receptors are distributed throughout the renal vasculature, renal epithelial cells, and juxtaglomerular cells. The actions of catecholamines on the kidney are summarized in Table 13.4 and are described in further detail in the following section.

TABLE 13.4. Renal Actions of Catecholamines

	Renal Effects
Norepinephrine and epinephrine	Decrease renal blood flow Decrease glomerular filtration rate Antinatriuretic
Dopamine	Increase renal blood flow Increase glomerular filtration rate Natriuretic

EFFECTS OF CATECHOLAMINES ON THE KIDNEY

Effects of Renal Circulation

Knowledge of how adrenergic stimulation regulates renal perfusion is derived primarily from animal studies. Modest activation of sympathetic nerves has a minimal effect on renal blood flow, suggesting that renal sympathetic nerve activity does not play a significant autoregulatory role under normal physiologic conditions. However, more intense stimulation increases renal vascular resistance and decreases renal blood flow. Under these conditions, adrenergic stimulation induces vasoconstriction of the renal, arcuate, and interlobular arteries. It also constricts the afferent and efferent arterioles, leading to decreased glomerular capillary pressure and glomerular capillary ultrafiltration coefficient. The end result is reduction of the single-nephron glomerular filtration rate. The renal vasoconstrictive effect of catecholamines is mediated almost exclusively by α_1-adrenoreceptors. In fact, α_1-receptors are the predominant adrenergic receptors expressed on the renal vasculature; β-receptor expression on renal vessels is scarce.

Although dopamine-containing nerve endings are present in the kidney, their physiologic significance is unknown. Exogenous dopamine and dopamine produced by proximal tubule cells, on the other hand, increase renal blood flow and GFR. These effects result from DA_1-receptor–mediated vasodilation of the renal vasculature, including afferent arterioles. DA_2 receptors are present in glomeruli and may directly modulate the glomerular filtration rate. Supraphysiologic levels of dopamine lead to renal vasoconstriction, decreased renal blood flow, and a drop in GFR by stimulating α_1-adrenoreceptors.

Effects on Solute and Water Transport

High-density expression of α_1- and α_2-adrenoreceptors occurs on the basolateral membranes of proximal tubule cells. Activation of these receptors by norepinephrine leads to increased sodium and water reabsorption. Stimulations of α-receptors also increases sodium reabsorption in the thick ascending limb of Henle's loop and in the distal tubule. Conversely, administering α-receptor blockers to volume-overloaded experimental animals or humans induces natriuresis and diuresis. It is suggested that α-receptor–mediated renal vasoconstriction and sodium reabsorption occur under conditions of high frequency renal adrenergic nerve stimulation. In humans, these conditions include surgical stress, trauma, congestive heart failure, liver cirrhosis, and severe nephrotic syndrome. It is also postulated that an increase in renal α-adrenoreceptor number may play a role in genetic forms of hypertension. Studies in the spontaneously hypertensive rat (SHR) strain demonstrated increased density of renal α_1- and α_2-adrenoreceptors when compared with nonhypertensive rat strains. Upregulation of these receptors preceded elevation of blood pressure in SHR. On the other hand, renal α_1- and α_2-receptor expression is normal or decreased in animal models of acquired hypertension. Studies addressing the role of renal α-adrenoreceptors in the pathogenesis of human hypertension have yielded conflicting results.

Low-frequency stimulation of renal adrenergic nerve stimulates sodium and water reabsorption but does not cause renal vasoconstriction. The antinatriuretic effect is mediated mainly by β-receptor–induced renin release from the juxtaglomerular cells of afferent arterioles. β-receptor stimulation also increases sodium and water reabsorption in the proximal tubule and the thick ascending limb of Henle's loop independent of enhanced renin secretion. Although β-receptor agonists increase K^+ reabsorption by type A intercalated cells in the collecting duct, the effect of β-receptor stimulation on net potassium secretion in the nephron is unclear. There is evidence that β-receptor agonists increase calcium and magnesium reabsorption in the cortical segment of the thick ascending limb of the loop of Henle.

The main source of dopamine in the kidney is the proximal tubular epithelium. Renal nerve stimulation does not significantly alter urinary or interstitial fluid dopamine concentrations. Proximal tubule cells take up circulating and/or filtered L-dopa for dopamine biosynthesis. High salt intake increases dopamine synthesis possibly by enhancing sodium-coupled uptake of L-Dopa by proximal tubule cells. Dopamine synthesized by proximal tubule cells acts in an autocrine and paracrine fashion to induce natriuresis. It does so by inhibiting Na^+-K^+-ATPase activity, an effect mediated by dopamine binding to DA_1 and DA_2 receptors on the basolateral membranes of tubule cells in all segments of the nephron. However, the highest density of DA receptors is present in the proximal tubule. Dopamine binding to DA_1 receptors on the apical membrane further enhances natriuresis by inhibiting Na^+-H^+ exchange. Disturbances in the renal dopamine system may play an important role in the pathophysiology of hypertension. Studies in humans with essential hypertension have demonstrated decreased renal production of dopamine or impaired natriuretic response to endogenous dopamine. Abnormalities in the renal dopamine system have also been found in patients with diabetic nephropathy, a condition associated with sodium retention. The natriuretic and vasodilatory actions of dopamine have earned it a therapeutic role in patients with extracellular fluid volume expansion, particularly when administered at low dosages, which do not activate α-adrenoreceptors. Exogenous dopamine does not induce natriuresis in sodium-depleted subjects.

Selected Readings

Aperia A. Dopamine action and metabolism in the kidney. *Curr Opin Nephrol Hypertens* 1994;3:39–45.

Review focusing on the renal dopamine system. The renal actions of dopamine, particularly those leading to natriuresis, are discussed. Data linking abnormalities of the renal dopamine system to salt-sensitive hypertension are also summarized.

Aperia A, Fryckstedt J, Holtback U, et al. Cellular mechanisms for bi-directional regulation of tubular sodium reabsorption. *Kidney Int* 1996;49:1743–1747.
Review of the cellular and molecular mechanisms underlying the regulation of sodium excretion by dopamine and norepinephrine. It emphasizes how these two catecholamines exert opposite actions on Na⁺-K⁺-ATPase activity.

DiBona GF, Kopp UC. Neural control of renal function. *Physiol Rev* 1997;77:75–197.
Comprehensive review of renal sympathetic innervation. The role of sympathetic nerve activity in regulating renal blood flow, glomerular filtration rate, renal tubular solute and water transport, and hormonal release is summarized. The significance of renal innervation in physiologic and pathophysiologic conditions is discussed.

Goldstein DS. Catecholamine receptors and signal transduction. Overview. *Adv Pharmacol* 1998; 42:379–390.
This report provides an overview of catecholamine receptors and summarizes their structures, classification, tissue localization, signal transduction pathways, and pharmacologic functions.

Jeffries WB, Pettinger WA. Adrenergic signal transduction in the kidney. *Miner Electrolyte Metab* 1989;15:5–15.
This paper reviews the renal actions of catecholamines that are mediated via α- and β-adrenoreceptors. The renal distribution of these receptors and their intracellular signal transduction pathways are summarized.

PART 8
Natriuretic Peptides

Michael H. Humphreys

It is generally accepted that constancy of extracellular fluid and blood volumes is maintained by a close coupling of renal sodium excretion to dietary sodium intake. To do this, mammals have developed a number of complex and sometimes redundant systems that interact to regulate the rate of sodium excretion. When there is a sodium deficit, the renin-angiotensin, aldosterone, and sympathetic nervous systems are activated to promote renal sodium conservation. In circumstances of sodium surfeit, the activity of these antinatriuretic pathways is suppressed, and systems are activated that lead to natriuresis. Chief among these is the family of natriuretic peptides.

This section summarizes currently available information on the role of these peptides in the physiologic and pathophysiologic regulation of sodium excretion. and will also discuss the more controversial field of an endogenous digitalislike inhibitor of Na^+-K^+-ATPase. Sections on the renin-angiotensin system, aldosterone, the renal nerves, and the overall control of sodium excretion are found elsewhere in this textbook.

NATRIURETIC PEPTIDES

The Natriuretic Peptide Family

The observation that crude extracts of cardiac atria led to a massive natriuresis initiated a period of intense research that resulted in the identification of the active principle in the extracts as atrial natriuretic peptide (ANP). ANP is a 28–amino acid peptide; its gene is found on the short arm of chromosome 1. The gene contains three exons and two introns, and the mature RNA encodes a prohormone of 126 amino acids. At the time of secretion, this prohormone is cleaved into the C-terminal 28 amino acids constituting the active peptide, the structure of which is depicted in Fig. 13.18. A large N-terminal fragment is also cosecreted and found in the circulation. As will be discussed later, this fragment undergoes further processing into smaller peptides, three of which have been shown to possess actions on the vasculature and on electrolyte excretion. ANP is expressed in the cardiac ventricles, the brain, and a few other organs, but its major site of expression is in the atria, where its mRNA composes up to 5% of all mRNA. Circulating ANP derives, probably exclusively, from atrial secretion. The major stimulus for secretion is an increase in atrial pressure, which increases secretion through distension of the atrial myocytes. However, other factors have also been shown to influence ANP gene expression and peptide release. These include glucocorticoids, endothelin, vitamin D, prostaglandins, and, possibly, oxytocin. The physiologic significance of these other regulators is not yet clear but is probably minor in relationship to the role of atrial stretch.

Understanding the physiologic functions of ANP became complicated with the rapid discovery of B-type natriuretic peptide (BNP), C-type natriuretic peptide (CNP), and urodilatin or renal natriuretic peptide (RNP) (Fig. 13.18). Also called *brain natriuretic peptide* (BNP) because of its discovery from a porcine brain cDNA library, BNP is most prominently expressed in cardiac ventricles and, to a lesser extent, in cardiac atria. CNP was also isolated from brain, where it is the most abundant of the three natriuretic peptide gene products; it is also synthesized in endothelial cells. All three peptides share structural homology, chiefly in the form of a 17-member ring structure created by

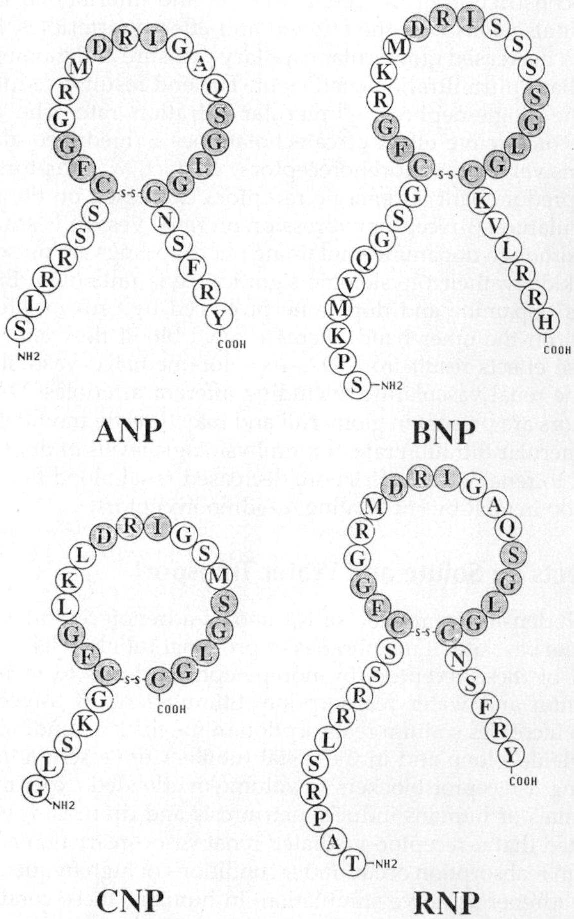

Figure 13.18. Amino acid structures of human atrial natriuretic peptide (ANP), B-type natriuretic peptide (BNP), C-type natriuretic peptide (CNP), and renal natriuretic peptide (RNP), showing the common 17-member ring structure formed by disulfide bonding of two cysteines. Shaded amino acids are universally shared among the four peptides.

sulfhydryl bonding of two cysteine residues. ANP and BNP have both N- and C-terminal extensions from this ring structure, whereas CNP has no C-terminal extension. RNP is identical to ANP, but with a four–amino acid N-terminal extension, identical to that found in the ANP prohormone. This has led to the belief that it represents a differently processed product of the ANP gene, expressed only in the kidneys and not found in the circulation.

Homologic correspondence is demonstrated not only among these members of the natriuretic peptide family but also among species. The one exception to this is BNP, which shows marked variability among mammalian species, not only with regard to amino acid sequence, but also in the length of the circulating peptide. The significance of this variability is not currently known. Interspecies homology is quite strong for ANP and CNP. Structure–function relationships have demonstrated that the ring structure is an absolute requirement for natriuretic peptide signaling. In the case of ANP and BNP, the C-terminal extension is also necessary for receptor activation. The absence of a C-terminal extension for CNP was an early hint that it might serve as a ligand for a receptor (or receptors) different from those activated by ANP and BNP.

Natriuretic Peptide Receptors

The alphabetized naming of the natriuretic peptides is matched by the confusing nomenclature used to describe the receptors so far identified, with which the peptides interact. Three such receptors are recognized to date (Fig. 13.19). Two of them, the natriuretic peptide A and B receptors (NPR-A, NPR-B) contain slightly more than 1,000 amino acids and consist of an extracellular ligand-binding domain, a short transmembrane sequence, and an intracellular portion characterized by a region of protein kinase homology adjacent to a region of guanylate cyclase activity. On occupancy of the binding site on the extracellular domain by the appropriate ligand, a conformational change is thought to occur that activates the intracellular guanylate cyclase region to produce cyclic guanosine-3′,5′-monophosphate (cGMP) from guanosine triphosphate (GTP). At present, cGMP is regarded as the exclusive intracellular second messenger for natriuretic peptide signaling via NPR-A and NPR-B.

The third member of the NPR family is NPR-C, also called the *clearance receptor.* It is a smaller molecule, possessing the external binding domain and transmembrane sequence, but containing only a short cytoplasmic "tail" lacking the protein kinase homology region or guanylate cyclase. It was originally thought that this receptor was silent with respect to intracellular signaling and served only to bind and internalize circulating natriuretic peptides, thereby acting as a buffer in situations where large concentrations of the peptides are released into the circulation. Subsequent studies have shown, however, that NPR-C may mediate a variety of effects in numerous tissues, including renal glomeruli, heart, brain, aorta, adrenal cortex, pheochromocytoma cells, and platelets. Activation of NPR-C inhibits neurotransmission in autonomic nerve terminals and proliferation of cultured smooth muscle cells. In general, these effects come about through inhibition of cellular cyclic adenosine-3′,5′-monophosphate (cAMP) accumulation. It thus appears that NPR-C may have many effects in addition to the proposed clearance of excess natriuretic peptide levels. By extension, it suggests that natriuretic peptides may have functions quite different from, and in addition to, their primary actions in cardiovascular homeostasis.

Homology among the NPRs is extensive, with the extracellular region exhibiting the most variability (Fig. 13.19). This presumably is related to the ligand specificities for the NPRs. NPR-A has highest affinity for ANP, with BNP showing slightly lower affinity; activation by CNP occurs only at pharmacologic concentrations of this peptide. NPR-B, on the other hand, interacts exclusively with CNP. NPR-C exhibits an affinity for each of the family members. Thus actions of the various natriuretic peptides are determined by a number of factors: the location of the receptor(s), the concentration of peptide(s), and the presence or absence of NPR-C. NPR-A is expressed in the kidney, in vascular smooth muscle, and in other organs, such as the adrenal glands, brain, and lungs. In the kidneys, the receptors are located in glomeruli, in vascular bundles, and on inner medullary collecting duct (IMCD) cells. NPR-C is also prominently expressed in glomeruli and constitute roughly two-thirds of renal cortical NPRs. However, IMCD cells express only NPR-A. Outside the kidney, NPR-C mRNA and protein are found in the heart, brain, adrenal cortex, platelets, aorta, and other tissues. NPR-B mRNA has been detected in the renal cortex, but only in such low abundance that its physiologic significance is probably minor, although CNP binds to cultured glomerular mesangial cells and stimulates the formation of cGMP. On the other hand, NPR-B is strongly expressed in vascular smooth muscle; because CNP is the natural ligand for NPR-B and is synthesized in endothelium, the concept has arisen that the peptide's interaction with its receptor permits local regulation of vascular tone in a paracrine manner. NPR-B has also been identified in the lungs, adrenal medulla, cerebellum, and pituitary; its function in these tissues is not known.

Several biochemical events have been identified that accompany the synthesis of cGMP by NPR-A. Mutant receptors lacking the protein kinase homology domain are constitutively activated and not influenced by ligand binding, indicating that this region is important in tonically suppressing guanylate cyclase activity. Adenosine triphosphate (ATP) binding and phosphorylation of serine and threonine are also important for maximum activity. The current model therefore suggests that ANP binding to the phosphorylated receptor in the presence of ATP

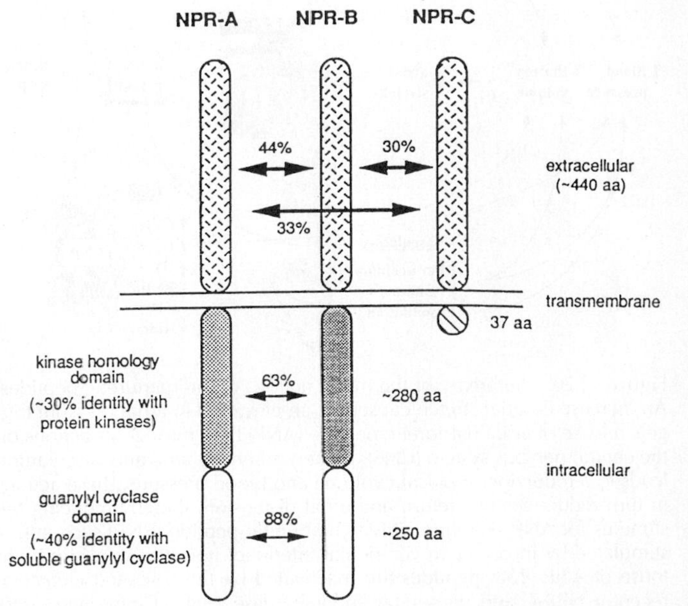

Figure 13.19. Diagrammatic structure of the three natriuretic peptide receptors. Numbers adjacent to arrows indicate the degree *(%)* of homology among the receptors for the extracellular domain, the protein kinase region, and the guanylate cyclase portion. Note that NPR-C has only a truncated intracellular domain of 37 amino acids. (From Koller KJ, Goeddel DV. Molecular biology of the natriuretic peptides and their receptors. *Circulation* 1992;86:1081–1086; reprinted with permission of the authors and the American Heart Association.)

induces a conformational change that removes inhibition of guanylate cyclase by the protein kinase–like domain. cGMP is then formed and produces the cellular actions associated with ANP signaling. Dephosphorylation of the receptor reduces its activity and renders it less sensitive to further stimulation by ANP. Although not yet studied in detail, it is presumed that NRP-B functions in a similar manner. Some evidence suggests that high levels of circulating ANP may downregulate NPR-A expression and activity in some tissues, although it is not yet possible to develop a detailed account of the mechanism or mechanisms by which this occurs.

Actions of Atrial Natriuretic Peptide

The synthesis and secretion of ANP by the heart and the predominant location of NPR-A in the kidneys, adrenal cortex, and vasculature provide a compelling rationale for the argument that the major functions of this hormonal system relate to cardiovascular homeostasis and volume regulation. As already mentioned, the primary stimulus for ANP release into the circulation is an increase in atrial stretch or distension, as would occur with an expanded blood or plasma volume. The actions of the peptide are shown in Fig. 13.20; in aggregate, they serve to reduce plasma volume, thereby operating as a closed feedback loop regulating plasma volume. Because expanded plasma volume can be accompanied by an elevation in blood pressure, the hormone's actions also are important in the regulation of circulatory hemodynamics (i.e., cardiac output, heart rate, and blood pressure). The peptide reduces plasma volume through its vascular and renal actions. Vascular actions include effects on capillary permeability and vascular smooth muscle.

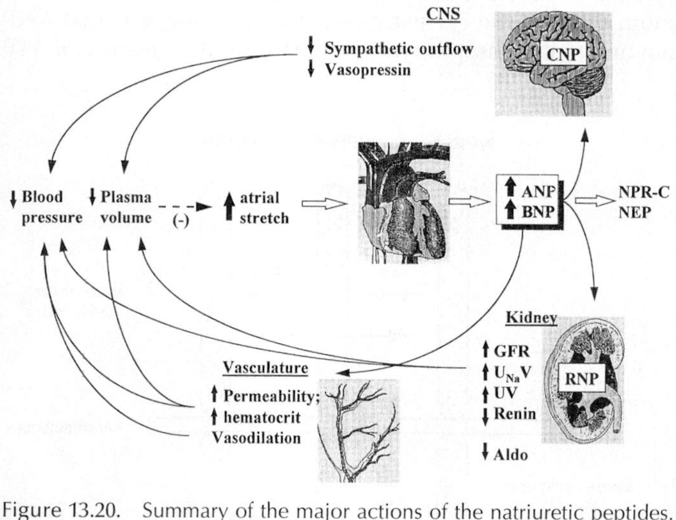

Figure 13.20. Summary of the major actions of the natriuretic peptides. An increase in atrial stretch caused by an elevation in atrial pressure triggers release of atrial natriuretic peptide (ANP) that, through its actions on the central nervous system (CNS), kidney, adrenal gland, and vasculature, leads to a reduction in plasma volume and blood pressure. These actions in turn reduce venous return and atrial distension, thereby reducing the stimulus for ANP secretion. B-type natriuretic peptide (BNP) secretion is stimulated by increases in ventricular afterload; its actions are similar to those of ANP. Both peptides are inactivated by the so-called clearance receptor NPR-C and by neutral endopeptidase (NEP). C-type natriuretic peptide (CNP) is found in high concentration in the CNS, where it may participate in the central control of the circulation, while renal natriuretic peptide (RNP) is localized to the kidney and functions as an intrarenal regulator of sodium excretion (*GFR,* glomerular filtration rate; *UV,* urine flow rate; *aldo,* aldosterone.) (From Humphreys MH, Valentin J-P. Natriuretic humoral agents. In: Seldin DW, Giebisch G, eds. *The kidney: physiology and pathophysiology,* 3rd ed, Philadelphia: Lippincott Williams & Wilkins, 2000:1375.)

Early studies using infusion of atrial extracts observed that the hematocrit level increased, and it has since been shown that this results from a specific effect of ANP to increase capillary permeability and promote the transfer of plasma water and proteins to the interstitial space in organs such as liver, intestine, and skeletal muscle, but not in lung or brain. This effect on vascular permeability is generally thought to be mediated by cGMP, although data on this point are equivocal. The result is a reduction in plasma volume, producing hemoconcentration and, to a lesser extent, an increase in plasma protein concentration because smaller plasma proteins such as albumin also escape into the interstitium. The mechanism of this selective increase in vascular permeability likely involves an interaction with angiotensin II because angiotensin-converting enzyme inhibitors or receptor antagonists prevent these ANP-mediated effects on hematocrit and plasma protein extravasation.

NPR-A is also expressed on vascular smooth muscle cells and mediate vasorelaxation and a reduction in peripheral vascular resistance through an increase in cGMP in these cells. Although this action by itself would lead to a direct reduction in blood pressure, data suggest that ANP's hypotensive action occurs indirectly through inhibition of autonomic reflexes. The decrease in blood pressure resulting from the ANP-induced increase in vascular permeability and decrease in plasma volume would normally elicit a reflex tachycardia and an increase in cardiac output, changes that should buffer the effects of the reduced plasma volume on blood pressure. However, reflex cardioacceleration does not occur because of central inhibition of these pathways by ANP, allowing the reduction in blood pressure to be more pronounced.

Studies in transgenic mice have emphasized the importance of the ANP system in blood pressure regulation: mice lacking ANP develop salt-sensitive hypertension, whereas mice overexpressing the ANP gene are hypotensive. Similarly, mice with the NPR-A gene knocked out are hypertensive, whereas transgenic mice expressing from one to four copies of the NPR-A gene have graded reductions in blood pressure. These observations indicate the dominance of this system because offsetting changes in vasodilatory pathways, such as nitric oxide or bradykinin, or in vasoconstrictor pathways, such as the renin-angiotensin system or endothelin, are unable to compensate fully for these ANP-related increases or decreases in blood pressure, respectively.

The hypotensive actions of ANP through increased vascular permeability and reduction in peripheral resistance are buttressed by its concurrent inhibition of renin secretion and increase in sodium excretion. These effects are part of the complex renal actions of the peptide, which include hemodynamic changes and inhibition of tubular transport of sodium and water as well as direct inhibition of renin secretion by the juxtaglomerular apparatus. Pharmacologic doses of ANP constrict the efferent arteriole and dilate the afferent arteriole to produce an increase in glomerular filtration rate (GFR) without overall change in renal plasma flow. These changes may not be as important at more physiologic levels of the peptide. Along the tubule, NPR-A is strongly expressed in IMCD cells, and there is now general agreement that ANP-stimulated natriuresis results from inhibition of sodium transport in this segment. This occurs through cGMP-mediated inhibition of the amiloride-sensitive sodium channel and is accompanied by a parallel reduction in oxygen consumption, as would be expected from inhibition of active sodium transport. Whether ANP has actions in other nephron segments has remained controversial. Functional data indicate that the peptide antagonizes angiotensin II–mediated sodium reabsorption in the proximal tubule, and interacts with dopaminergic inhibition of Na^{+}-K^{+}-ATPase to decrease reabsorption in this segment. However, to date, no evidence of proximal tubular NPR-A has been presented. ANP has also been shown to increase intracellular calcium concentration in cultured cortical thick ascending limb cells, and NPR-A have been demonstrated in cultured human cortical collecting duct cells. Thus multiple sites of action and effects on tubular transport may exist. ANP has been shown to inhibit vasopressin-stimulated water transport in cortical and medullary collecting ducts, contributing to the diuresis as well as the natriuresis caused by the peptide.

ANP inhibits renin secretion by a direct effect on renin-secreting juxtaglomerular cells through a mechanism involving increased cGMP. This reduction in renin secretion reduces circulating levels of angiotensin II, amplifying the vasodilator effect of ANP. Angiotensin II is also a potent secretagogue of aldosterone, and reduced levels would be expected to lead to reduced secretion of aldosterone. However, ANP inhibits aldosterone release more potently through a direct effect on zona glomerulosa cells. In these cells both NPR-A and NPR-C are expressed, and exposure to ANP increases cGMP accumulation, although the exact relationship of this increase in cellular cGMP to ANP's inhibition of aldosterone secretion is not fully understood. Some data suggest that signaling through NPR-C, with inhibition of adenylate cyclase and reduction of cellular cAMP, may be involved. The role of ANP-mediated reduction in aldosterone secretion on sodium and water balance is not completely clear, but it is to be expected that the reduced aldosterone would contribute to the decrease in distal nephron sodium reabsorption occurring in volume-expanded states with high levels of circulating ANP.

These multiple cardiovascular and renal actions all indicate an important role for ANP in the maintenance of sodium balance and regulation of body fluid volume. Plasma ANP concentration generally rises with consumption of a high-sodium diet, and interruption of the ANP system with monoclonal or polyclonal antibodies to ANP, atrial appendectomy to remove the source of circulating ANP, or antagonists of NPR-A in general produces an increase in blood pressure and a decrease in sodium excretion as well as blunted volume-expansion natriuresis. Consistent with these findings, evidence has pointed to the important role of ANP in maintaining sodium balance in such volume-expanded states as mineralocorticoid escape, the seven-eighths nephrectomized rat, and experimental diabetes mellitus. Despite this, however, the role of ANP as a natriuretic peptide has been questioned in view of the results of some studies, which failed to demonstrate activation of the ANP system in volume-expanded states. Such studies emphasize the role of ANP as a cardiovascular regulator, with renal actions attributed to its closely related family member RNP (urodilatin). This issue will be discussed in more detail later in this section.

The Role of ANP in Congestive Heart Failure

Much attention has been focused on the role of ANP in states of disturbed volume or cardiovascular regulation, such as congestive heart failure, cirrhosis of the liver, nephrotic syndrome, and hypertension. In heart failure, impaired left ventricular function leads to reflex activation of sympathetic nervous outflow, the renin-angiotensin system, and aldosterone secretion. Atrial pressures are high, and—as would be expected given the importance of atrial distension in triggering ANP release—plasma ANP concentrations are elevated in direct proportion to the severity of the heart failure. Similarly, therapies effective in ameliorating the heart failure reduce plasma ANP levels. Although the elevated plasma ANP in heart failure clearly is not able to fully correct the deleterious neurohumoral and renal functional patterns in this condition, it is evident that the peptide does attenuate some of the consequences of activation of these systems. Blockade of ANP in models of heart failure reduces sodium excretion and leads to further increases in plasma renin activity and aldosterone levels. Thus the peptide is important in a counterregulatory manner to oppose the vasoconstrictor/sodium-retaining stimuli so prominent in severe heart failure. Despite relative resistance to the effects of ANP, some studies indicate that further increases in plasma ANP concentration may lead to decreases in preload and afterload, enhancing myocardial performance.

As will be discussed shortly, such benefits are more pronounced with BNP. Resistance to the renal actions of ANP has been attributed to the predominance of opposing systems such as the renin-angiotensin pathway, endothelin, and sympathetic nervous system, to reduced binding of the peptide to its biologically active receptors (NPR-A), and to increased activity of phosphodiesterases, which inactivate cGMP formed on the interaction of ANP with NPR-A.

The Role of ANP in Hepatic Cirrhosis

Cirrhosis of the liver is another condition of pathophysiologic sodium retention characterized by renal resistance to ANP, although in contrast to heart failure, plasma ANP concentration is normal or only mildly elevated. The basis for this renal resistance is not fully understood, but it has been linked to heightened activity of a phosphodiesterase in renal target tissues, such as IMCD cells, in which cGMP produced as a consequence of normal ANP binding to NPR-A is rapidly catabolized. Increased enzyme activity occurs in IMCD cells, and blunted ANP responsiveness is corrected both *in vitro* and *in vivo* by selective inhibitors of this enzyme. Multiple pathways have been invoked to account for cirrhotic ascites and hemodynamic abnormalities, including the sympathetic nervous system, bradykinin, and the nitric oxide system. A completely integrated description of the interaction of these systems with the ANP pathway is not yet possible. Increasing plasma ANP concentration in cirrhosis is not a successful therapeutic intervention because hypotension develops, usually before any benefit on sodium excretion can be demonstrated.

The Role of ANP in Nephrotic Syndrome

Edema formation in the nephrotic syndrome has also been linked to renal resistance to ANP. Although debate continues over the importance of underfill versus overflow mechanisms in nephrotic edema, compelling evidence demonstrates the presence of a defect in tubular sodium handling that is intrinsic to nephrotic kidneys and is not related to abnormalities in the systemic circulation, such as hypoalbuminemia or reduced plasma volume. Micropuncture studies in experimental animals localize this defect to the collecting duct, the major tubular site of ANP action. As with experimental liver disease, plasma ANP concentration is usually normal, and ANP binding is normal. The transport defect can be corrected by selective inhibitors of the cGMP-specific phosphodiesterase; activity of this enzyme has been found to be elevated in IMCD cells in one model of experimental nephrosis in the rat. These findings argue that in nephrotic syndrome, heightened cGMP-phosphodiesterase activity accounts for ANP resistance and, by extension, participates in and possibly is entirely responsible for the sodium retention and edema associated with this condition. On the other hand, sodium metabolism in diabetes mellitus, another condition characterized by proteinuria, may become altered by another mechanism. In rats with diabetes induced by injection of streptozotocin, renal ANP resistance occurs, but this is related to diminished binding of ANP to renal NPR-A. This resistance is not affected by an inhibitor of cGMP-phosphodiesterase but is corrected by insulin administered to normalize blood glucose concentration. The mechanism by which insulin deficiency and hyperglycemia lead to this decrease in renal ANP binding is unknown. However, the hyperfiltration in experimental diabetes is blocked by a nonpeptide NPR-A/NPR-B–receptor antagonist, suggesting that the receptors mediating ANP hemodynamic actions may be affected in a different manner from those involved in inhibition of tubular sodium reabsorption.

The Role of ANP in Hypertension

The role of ANP in hypertensive states has also been evaluated. In volume-expanded hypertension, such as that resulting from DOCA-salt administration or subtotal nephrectomy, plasma ANP concentration is elevated, and antagonism of NPR-A exacerbates the hypertension. In humans with hypertension, plasma ANP and right atrial pressure correlate with arterial pressure, and some studies indicate that infusion of ANP lowers blood pressure. This cannot be taken to indicate that the hypertension results from deficiency of ANP, but merely that the vasculature is able to respond to the peptide infusion. In general, the ANP system appears to operate normally in hypertensive states; high plasma levels reflect a normal atrial secretory response to increased afterload on the one hand, and may help modulate or buffer the hypertension on the other.

ANP and Acute Renal Failure

Experimental studies of acute renal failure have indicated that ANP administration can improve the outcome. This has led to three randomized, prospective trials of the effect of ANP infusion in patients with acute renal failure. One trial suggested, by subgroup analysis, that there is a benefit in survival in patients with oliguric acute renal failure, but a prospective trial to address this question specifically was terminated for lack of efficacy. Similarly, a trial of ANP in contrast-induced acute renal failure also failed to find a beneficial effect.

B-Type Natriuretic Peptide

A second member of the natriuretic peptide is B-type natriuretic peptide (BNP). As noted, BNP originally stood for "brain natriuretic peptide," but the expression of this gene product, like ANP, is predominantly in the heart, and the awareness, again like ANP, that circulating BNP derives from cardiac secretion has given rise to the alternate name *B-type natriuretic peptide*. The structure of the BNP gene is similar to the ANP gene, with three exons and two introns. Within the heart, the distribution of BNP differs markedly from ANP. Whereas 95% of cardiac ANP is located in the atria, more than half of cardiac BNP is formed in the ventricles, and the bulk of circulating BNP is secreted from the ventricles. Levels in the circulation are lower than for ANP but are increased in conditions of ventricular abnormalities such as myocardial infarction, hypertension, and heart failure. Levels are also elevated in renal failure and cirrhosis with ascites, perhaps because of decreased metabolic clearance, as will be discussed later. Although the two peptides are cosecreted in many physiologic and pathophysiologic circumstances, evidence indicates that BNP can be secreted independently of ANP. Like ANP, active BNP is cleaved from proBNP at the time of secretion; unlike ANP, no biologic function of the cosecreted prohormone fragment has yet been identified. The structure of human BNP is illustrated in Fig. 13.18.

Actions of BNP in large measure resemble those of ANP (Fig. 13.20), and no receptor with unique affinity for BNP has been identified. On the other hand, human BNP binds with high affinity to human NPR-A and stimulates the production of cGMP. BNP infusions increase urinary cGMP excretion and plasma cGMP concentration, lower blood pressure, cause natriuresis, suppress renin and aldosterone secretion, and result in hemoconcentration, all actions duplicated by ANP. Consequently, prevailing thought is that BNP is acting through NPR-A. However, infusions of BNP result in increases in plasma ANP concentration, presumably due to displacement of ANP by BNP from sites of ANP catabolism. Thus, some actions attributed to BNP may actually reflect ANP acting through NPR-A. Moreover, the variability of BNP across species raises the possibility of an as yet undiscovered receptor that could mediate its actions. Compared with ANP, the half-life of BNP in the circulation is much longer, which is also likely to contribute to its actions.

Plasma BNP concentration is elevated in congestive heart failure, although the magnitude of this elevation relative to ANP is in dispute. It is also increased in cor pulmonale, suggesting that the right ventricle may contribute appreciably to circulating levels of BNP. As would also be expected, plasma BNP changes only sluggishly, if at all, in response to acute changes in blood volume, in contrast with the much more rapid change in plasma ANP concentration brought about by increases or decreases in blood volume. These characteristics have led to the hypothesis that the plasma BNP level may be a more sensitive and specific marker for disturbed left ventricular function in heart failure and myocardial infarction than plasma ANP is. Despite the already elevated plasma BNP concentration in patients with heart failure, infusion studies have demonstrated additional benefit in cardiac output, renal function, and sodium excretion, and at the time of this writing, application is before the Food and Drug Administration for approval to use the peptide in the treatment of congestive heart failure.

Plasma BNP concentration is also increased in patients with hypertension and left ventricular hypertrophy, and the magnitude of the increase correlates with left ventricular mass as assessed by echocardiography. This observation has led to the idea that plasma BNP reflects left ventricular mass in hypertensive patients. Infusion of a low dosage of BNP sufficient to achieve a plasma concentration in the pathophysiologic range in hypertensive subjects leads to natriuresis and an increase in plasma cGMP and reduction in plasma aldosterone without marked change in blood pressure. These results are similar to those observed with infusion of ANP at a comparable rate and raise the issue again of whether such infusion studies reflect the action of BNP itself, that of ANP as a result of prolongation of ANP's half-life, or a mixture of the two.

C-Type Natriuretic Peptide

CNP is a third member of the natriuretic peptide family. It is encoded by a separate gene, the structure of which bears some resemblance to the ANP and BNP genes. The initial gene product is a 103–amino acid prohormone whose sequence is highly conserved among mammalian species. The active peptide is the 22–amino acid C-terminal portion of the prohormone, probably cleaved from proCNP at the time of secretion (Fig. 13.18). CNP is widely expressed in the nervous system, leading to speculation that it may have an important role as a neurotransmitter involved in body fluid and blood pressure regulation (Fig. 13.20). Other sites of expression include the kidney, vascular endothelial cells, pituitary, and organs of the immune system. Lacking a C-terminal amino acid extension from the natriuretic peptide ring structure, CNP has a poor affinity for NPR-A but is a selective ligand for NPR-B. Binding to NPR-B stimulates the production of cGMP in all preparations yet studied, and cGMP is thought to be the major and perhaps exclusive intracellular second messenger of the peptide's actions, although one study showed that CNP suppressed peripheral sympathetic nerve transmission without activation of guanylate cyclase. This observation opens the possibility that some actions of CNP may occur through an as yet undiscovered receptor or receptors not linked to guanylate cyclase/cGMP. With this caveat, the bulk of CNP's actions are thus dictated by the location of NPR-B, chiefly in vascular smooth muscle and, to a small extent, within the kidney. The evidence for CNP gene expression in kidney tubular segments, along with NPR-B, has led to the idea that this peptide and receptor may function as a renal autocrine-paracrine system.

CNP is found in the circulation in low picomolar concentrations and could have endocrine functions as well. The source of circulating CNP is not established, but it could be secreted by endothelial cells, a major site of synthesis. The presence of endothelial CNP, with NPR-B on underlying vascular smooth muscle cells, suggests that this system may be an important local regulator of vascular tone and function. CNP shares routes of degradation with ANP and BNP, namely the neutral endopeptidase E.C. 24.11 and NPR-C. Thus, as we have seen with BNP, studies of CNP's actions from infusion studies may be confounded by competition for sites of ANP catabolism, with effects ascribed to CNP actually caused by higher concentrations of ANP (and/or BNP). Such considerations may account for the large variability in the actions of CNP, depending on species and experimental conditions. CNP infusion stimulates natriuresis in rats and sheep, but not in dogs or humans. The bases for these species differences in response are not yet understood but could relate to the issues just raised, and several studies have demonstrated that CNP infusion increases the concentration of ANP in the circulation. In any case, it may emerge that CNP is erroneously named as a natriuretic peptide. This possibility is supported by an observation that NPR mRNA expression in sheep kidneys was not affected by a high-sodium diet, but a selective increase in NPR-B mRNA levels occurred when a low-sodium diet was given.

Another caution in interpreting data from CNP infusion studies is that it has not been established that the peptide functions in a circulating, endocrine manner. CNP is a potent inhibitor of aldosterone by adrenal glomerulosa cells *in vitro*, although results of *in vivo* studies measuring plasma renin activity and aldosterone concentration have yielded equivocal results. As mentioned, NPR-B is expressed on vascular smooth muscle cells, and CNP is a potent vasodilator, signaling through cGMP. In contrast to ANP and BNP, CNP is also a strong venodilator, an action that contributes to its hypotensive action. Centrally administered CNP differs from ANP in that it stimulates rather than inhibits thirst. Like ANP and BNP, CNP exhibits antiproliferative actions in a variety of experimental circumstances.

Data on the CNP system in physiologic and pathophysiologic regulation are not yet available. Plasma concentration is elevated in patients with renal failure and in those with septic shock. The mechanism or mechanisms leading to these increases and their pathophysiologic significance are not known. Plasma levels are normal in patients with heart failure and hypertension.

It should be clear from this brief overview that it is not yet possible to develop an even rudimentary understanding of the role of CNP in body fluid homeostasis and cardiovascular regulation. An educated guess would be that its major function is as a local regulator of a vasomotor tone; however, it seems likely that other important functions will emerge after further study.

Renal Natriuretic Peptide

The biology of the natriuretic peptide family became even more complicated with the isolation in 1988 of an ANP-like peptide from human urine. Purification and sequencing disclosed that this peptide was identical to amino acids 95–126 of the ANP prohormone (i.e., ANP_{95-126}), rather than ANP itself (ANP_{99-126}) (Fig. 13.18). Earlier studies had shown the presence in kidney tissue of ANP-like immunoreactivity, but the techniques employed were not sensitive enough to distinguish *de novo* renal synthesis of the peptide from uptake of cardiac ANP from the circulation or tubular fluid by renal cells. Subsequently, renal transcription of the ANP gene was demonstrated by means of reverse transcription polymerase chain amplification, although the mRNA abundance observed was very low. Immunocytochemical staining indicated that the bulk of proANP was localized to the distal tubule and collecting duct. Although ANP_{99-126} is also found in urine, presumably as a result of filtration and tubular secretion, renal natriuretic peptide (RNP) must represent a separate product of processing of the prohormone because the addition of four N-terminal amino acids to circulating ANP would be a previously undescribed method of peptide metabolism. The current viewpoint holds that RNP represents a processing product of the ANP gene. Because it is not found in the circulation and has not been identified in any other tissue, it is thought to be expressed uniquely in the kidney.

Interest in RNP as a physiologic regulator of sodium excretion came from studies in humans and dogs that demonstrated a close correlation between urinary sodium excretion and excretion of RNP under diverse conditions, including diurnal variations, acute saline volume expansion, head-out water immersion, weightlessness in space flight, stepwise increases in daily sodium chloride intake in humans, and left atrial distension or intracarotid hypertonic saline infusion in dogs. These studies indicated that other mediators of natriuresis, including plasma ANP, plasma vasopressin, plasma renin activity, plasma aldosterone, and catecholamine concentration, correlated poorly or not at all with sodium excretion, leading to the hypothesis that RNP was responsible for the natriuresis in these various conditions rather than ANP. In this view, functions of ANP are largely confined to the cardiovascular system through its effects on blood pressure, vascular permeability, plasma renin activity, and plasma aldosterone. At present, data on the physiologic importance of RNP rest with the correlative observations mentioned previously, and it has not yet been possible to carry out specific interventions that could provide a more convincing picture of RNP's role. There is little information on the regulation of renal RNP production and its release into tubular fluid; this information is key to establishing the true place of RNP in sodium balance.

Infusion studies have been used to evaluate the actions of RNP, although the results must be viewed cautiously from the outset because the peptide is not found in the circulation and does not function as a circulating hormone. Be that as it may, the actions of RNP resemble with minor differences those of equimolar doses of ANP, including dose-dependent decreases in blood pressure and cardiac output and increases in GFR, urine flow rate, and sodium excretion. Plasma cGMP concentration and urinary cGMP excretion increase, as occurs with ANP infusion. *In vitro* studies have shown that RNP binds with high affinity to NPR-A and is as potent as ANP in generating cGMP in glomeruli and IMCD cells. These observations in aggregate suggest that infused RNP acts through NPR-A to produce actions by and large duplicating those of ANP, a conclusion not surprising in view of the identity of the two peptides in ring structure and C-terminal tail, two critical determinants for binding to and activation of NPR-A (Fig. 13.18).

As mentioned, within the kidney RNP is localized primarily to distal tubule and cortical collecting duct. In order to act in IMCD it must be secreted into the tubular lumen because abluminally secreted peptide in the cortex would be transported into renal venous blood and escape a medullary site of action. As also pointed out earlier, no circulating RNP has been detected. In the initial portion of the IMCD, NPR-A is located on the basolateral membrane of principal cells, but in deeper portions it appears on both luminal and basolateral surfaces, so luminal peptide could interact with luminally oriented NPR-A on these cells and increase sodium excretion. The factors regulating RNP synthesis and secretion remain to be elucidated.

As with the other natriuretic peptides, efforts have been made to determine whether RNP plays a role in various pathophysiologic conditions, or offers a therapeutic benefit. Nephrotic rat kidneys contain increased amounts of ANP prohormone as well as a smaller peptide (possibly RNP) compared to normal kidneys, observations suggesting that the RNP system could be activated in nephrotic syndrome and perhaps offer some defense against the sodium avidity of this condition. Prolonged infusion of RNP into patients with congestive heart failure improves both cardiac and renal function, paralleling the responses described earlier with infusion of BNP. Finally, several studies have demonstrated a favorable effect of RNP infusion in patients with various forms of acute renal failure. The success of RNP in this setting when ANP was not is perhaps noteworthy, although conditions studied and therapeutic protocols differed. RNP is resistant relative to ANP to degradation by neutral endopeptidase, and its longer half-life could contribute to greater efficacy when infused intravenously in these conditions. As is the case with CNP, extensive research is required in order to understand the role of RNP in the regulation of sodium excretion, and the mechanisms by which it is secreted and by which it inhibits sodium reabsorption in the inner medulla.

Other Peptides Derived from the ANP Prohormone

Circulating ANP is composed of the 28 C-terminal amino acids of proANP (i.e., ANP_{99-126}) cleaved at the time of secretion. The N-terminal fragment of proANP, ANP_{1-98}, is also found in the circulation, and early studies indicated that it too possessed natriuretic activity. It was subsequently shown to be further processed into three smaller peptides: ANP_{1-30}, ANP_{31-67}, and ANP_{79-98}. Each of these smaller peptides possesses natriuretic and/or kaliuretic activity and lowers blood pressure when infused intravenously. Their concentrations in plasma increase after maneuvers such as left atrial distension, or in conditions such as congestive heart failure in which ANP concentration is also elevated. Consequently, it has been argued that they may act in concert with ANP_{99-126} and even mediate some of the actions attributed to it.

It is clear, however, that these peptides act through a different cellular mechanism than ANP_{99-126} does. Their infusions do not increase plasma cGMP concentration, as is observed with infusion of ANP itself, and ANP_{31-67} fails to stimulate cGMP production by isolated IMCD cells. Rather, they appear to alter tubular function by inhibiting the basolateral Na^+-K^+-ATPase by a prostaglandin-dependent mechanism. The peptides stimulate prostaglandin E_2 production by kidney homogenates or isolated IMCD cells in parallel with their inhibition of Na^+-K^+-ATPase activity, and inhibition of this enzyme does not occur in the presence of prostaglandin synthesis inhibitors such as ibuprofen or naproxen. Because prostaglandin E_2 is a known inhibitor of the enzyme, the possibility has emerged whereby these N-terminal peptides may act in parallel with ANP_{99-126}, with the latter inhibiting apical sodium entry and the N-terminal peptides inhibiting basolateral sodium exit from the cell through prostaglandin-mediated Na^+-K^+-ATPase inhibition. The half-life of these smaller peptides in plasma is longer than that of ANP_{99-126}, and natriuresis lasts longer. Consequently, they may be acting in concert with ANP to achieve more sustained natriuresis than possible with ANP alone.

It is difficult at present to determine the role of these peptides in sodium homeostasis and cardiovascular regulation. The receptor(s) with which they interact have not been identified, and no inhibitors of their action are available, so it has not been possible to examine the effects of interruption of their action. This information should facilitate an awareness of their importance in the body fluid economy.

Other Natriuretic Peptides

A number of other peptide hormones have been shown to increase sodium excretion and could potentially play roles in the regulation of sodium balance. However, evidence to this effect is lacking, by and large, and the hormones will be mentioned only briefly. The pituitary hormones vasopressin and oxytocin are each natriuretic, and their cognate receptors are expressed in the kidney tubule. In addition, oxytocin has been suggested to be a stimulator of ANP release from the heart. Their roles in sodium balance are not known. Adrenomedullin is a 52–amino acid peptide originally isolated from human pheochromocytoma tissue. It is a potent vasodilator and is also natriuretic, although it is not yet clear if the natriuresis results from interaction with specific receptors or with receptors for the structurally related calcitonin gene–related peptide. Originally isolated from intestine, guanylin and uroguanylin are 15– and 16–amino acid peptides that are natriuretic, acting through a membrane guanylate cyclase, with some homology to the NPRs, to stimulate cGMP production. It has been argued that uroguanylin provides a link between intestinal sodium absorption and renal sodium excretion. Melanocyte-stimulating hormone (MSH) peptides are three structurally related sequences derived from the pituitary ACTH precursor proopiomelanocortin. All three peptides, α-, β-, and γ-MSH, are natriuretic, and both pituitary synthesis and plasma concentration of γ-MSH increase when a high-sodium diet is ingested. The natriuretic properties of these several other peptides suggest that there is still much to be learned regarding the maintenance of sodium balance through the regulation of sodium excretion.

ENDOGENOUS OUABAINLIKE FACTOR

The existence of an endogenous inhibitor of Na^+-K^+-ATPase has been suggested for several decades, but it was not until 1976 that the modern era of research in the field began. In that year, Haddy and Overbeck first developed the hypothesis that a circulating inhibitor of Na^+-K^+-ATPase could explain the pathogenesis of volume-dependent forms of hypertension. In the next year, Blaustein proposed a detailed cellular model that explained how inhibition of this enzyme in vascular smooth muscle cells could lead to contraction of these cells and result in the increased peripheral resistance of hypertension. There shortly followed reports of digitalislike material that could be extracted from guinea pig and bovine brain and of digitalislike activity in the plasma of volume-expanded dogs. However, despite these observations, the field has been beset by controversy, because precise characterization of the structure of ouabainlike factor (OLF) has proved elusive, and because it has not been possible to reproduce many of the experimental results designed to shed light on the physiology of OLF and its role in the pathogenesis of hypertension.

Evidence for Endogenous Ouabainlike Factor

Three experimental approaches have been employed to demonstrate OLF activity in plasma and tissue extracts. One is the inhibition of Na^+-K^+-ATPase activity of cell membrane preparations by the extracts. The second is inhibitory activity of the extract in one or more functional assays, such as inhibition of sodium transport by a transporting epithelium (e.g., toad bladder) or of ^{86}Rubidium uptake by intact cells, or stimulation of vascular smooth muscle contraction. The third approach measures immunoreactivity of the plasma or tissue extracts using (usually) polyclonal antisera raised against ouabain, digoxin, or another of the cardiac glycosides. Much of the conflicting data in the field emanates from the failure to apply these three measures of OLF uniformly to the extract being evaluated. It has become evident that multiple factors have inhibitory activity but are not ouabainlike. These include fatty acids, lysophospholipids, other steroids (including dehydroepiandrosterone, progesterone, and the amphibian steroids bufalin and 19-norbufalin), bile salts, and the vanadate ion. Thus a tissue extract containing vanadate will inhibit Na^+-K^+-ATPase activity in a biochemical assay and sodium transport in a functional assay; these observations could be interpreted to indicate "ouabainlike activity," even though an immunologic assay may not detect any such activity. Another confounding issue is the fact that Na^+-K^+-ATPase isoforms exhibit varying affinities for cardiac glycosides, so measures of enzyme activity or enzyme-linked cellular action can be influenced by the tissue, and Na^+-K^+-ATPase isoform, used in the assay. Also, few studies using an immunoassay of OLF have reported cross-reactivity of the antiserum with other structurally related compounds. Finally, some of the compounds reported to exhibit OLF do so only at concentrations far in excess of those likely to be achieved in plasma, making their role in physiologic regulation meaningless. These considerations make it obvious that research in this field requires multiple assays using standardized techniques and extraction procedures to clarify rather than confuse the role of OLF in fluid balance and hypertension.

These issues notwithstanding, considerable evidence documents the existence in plasma from humans and experimental animals of a compound closely related to, but probably not identical with, plant ouabain; rather, the current view is that it is an isomer of ouabain with identical molecular mass but with subtle intramolecular differences from ouabain. Tissue studies have indicated that the compound can be extracted from brain and adrenal gland, but it is not yet clear whether OLF from these two organs is identical, nor is the source of circulating OLF known. An adrenal source is suggested by observations indicating that adrenal OLF content is increased 500-fold over the plasma level, there is a step-up of OLF activity in adrenal venous plasma, and adrenalectomy reduces circulating activity. However, other studies cast doubt on an adrenal source of circulating OLF, because in at least one study, sodium loading led to increased plasma OLF in adrenalectomized rats, and in other studies adrenalectomy failed to reduce circulating OLF. As a result, it is not yet possible to assert the exact role of the adrenal in the synthesis and secretion of OLF. The hypothalamus is also regarded as a likely source of OLF, although evidence suggests that brain OLF may function in a local, paracrine manner to cause hypertension rather than do so after being secreted into the circulation. As with adrenal OLF, further research is required to characterize the role of brain OLF and its relationship to plasma ouabainlike activity.

Ouabainlike Factor in Normal Sodium Balance

Most studies examining tissue or circulating OLF have observed that plasma ouabainlike activity is increased in volume expanded states. Indeed, the first isolation of OLF was obtained from 85 L of plasma from volume expanded human subjects, and numerous other studies have shown increased activity in plasma or urine during ingestion of a high-sodium diet or in chronic renal failure, a condition usually accompanied by volume expansion. Such observations argue for a role in sodium homeostasis, but it has not been possible to establish this because the source of circulating or urinary OLF has not been determined, nor has it been possible to examine the consequences of sodium loading during blockade of OLF release or action. Rather, much more attention has focused on the relationship of OLF to the development of hypertension, particularly that which occurs with sodium loading, or salt-sensitive hypertension.

Ouabainlike Factor in the Pathogenesis of Hypertension

At least three lines of evidence argue for a role of circulating OLF in certain forms of hypertension. First, plasma ouabainlike activity, and in some cases tissue OLF levels, are increased in hypertensive animals or humans. Second, chronic infusion of ouabain leads to hypertension in experimental animals. Third, a digoxin antiserum, and active immunization against ouabain, mitigate volume expanded hypertension. These observations not only argue for a role of OLF in these forms of hypertension, but also implicate it as a circulating agent because at least exogenously administered antibodies would be unlikely to reach protected sites in the central nervous system. These data are buttressed by a cohesive model that integrates at the cellular level many of the observations that have been made in hypertension (Fig. 13.21). The model requires an intrinsic reduction of

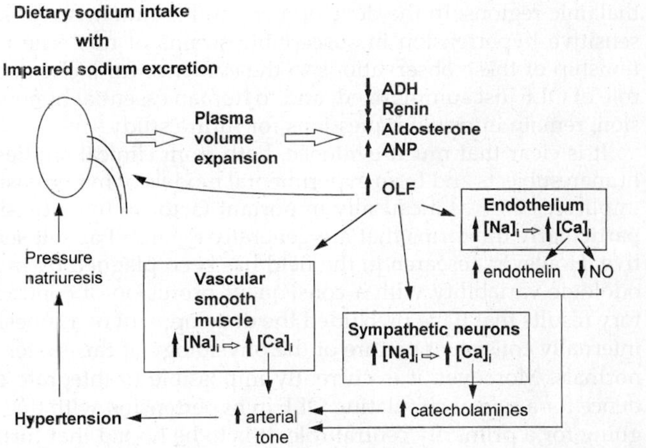

Figure 13.21. Proposed model to describe how an increase in circulating ouabainlike factor leads to sustained hypertension. A defect in renal sodium excretion results in plasma volume expansion. A variety of neurohumoral systems are then activated or suppressed to restore sodium balance; among them is elaboration of OLF. Through its inhibition of Na^+-K^+-ATPase, OLF increases intracellular calcium concentration in a variety of tissues. Chief among them is vascular smooth muscle, leading to sustained contraction and hypertension. Effects of OLF on nerve endings and the endothelium cause changes that contribute to elevation in blood pressure. Inhibition of renal tubular Na^+-K^+-ATPase, and pressure natriuresis, increase sodium excretion and help to restore sodium balance.

the ability of the kidneys to excrete sodium. In experimental animals, this results from maneuvers restricting sodium excretion, such as reduction in renal mass or DOCA-salt administration, although the nature of such an excretory defect in humans has not been characterized. In the face of a high dietary sodium intake, limited renal excretion leads to positive sodium balance and volume expansion. Through currently unidentified pathways, secretion of OLF increases and plasma OLF concentration rises. OLF then inhibits Na^+-K^+-ATPase in various tissues. This increases intracellular sodium and inhibits Na-Ca exchange, resulting in an increase in intracellular calcium. In arterial smooth muscle, the increase in calcium leads to contraction and an increase in arterial tone and blood pressure to produce hypertension. This action is complemented by effects of increased intracellular calcium in other tissues such as the endothelium, where an increase in the vasoconstrictor endothelin and decrease in the vasodilator nitric oxide occurs, and in sympathetic neurons, where increased catecholamine release takes place. These changes contribute to vascular smooth muscle contraction and hypertension. Inhibition of renal tubular Na^+-K^+-ATPase, and pressure natriuresis, lead to increased sodium excretion and restoration of sodium balance, but at the expense of an elevated OLF level. A variation on this model holds that plasma OLF is increased as a result of impaired renal OLF excretion. In either case, many features of the hypertensive state can be explained, and experimental data confirm many of the predictions of the model.

However, other compelling data argue for a central nervous system role of OLF in hypertension. Sodium-induced increases in brain OLF precede changes in plasma OLF activity, and intracerebroventricular injection of digoxin-specific antibody fragments corrects hypertension in Dahl salt-sensitive rats. Dietary sodium-induced increases in plasma and hypothalamic OLF activity occur in this strain, but not in the normotensive but genetically related Dahl salt-resistant strain. Microinjection of antibody fragments that bind ouabain with high affinity into the median preoptic nucleus reduces blood pressure in the spontaneously hypertensive rat. These and other observations support a central nervous system role of OLF, acting in specific hypothalamic regions, in the development and maintenance of salt-sensitive hypertension in susceptible strains of rats. The relationship of these observations to the evidence for a circulating role of OLF just summarized, and to human essential hypertension, remain intriguing questions for future study.

It is clear that much evidence, both from clinical studies in human subjects and from experimental models of hypertension, implicates OLF as a causally important factor in hypertension, particularly the forms that are generally regarded as salt sensitive. However, research in the field has been plagued by methodologic variability with a consequent profusion of contradictory results that have precluded the development of a cohesive, internally consistent picture of the physiology of this system in normals. Moreover, it is currently impossible to integrate evidence for a role of circulating OLF in hypertension with that arguing for a primarily central role. It is to be hoped that further research will resolve these ambiguities and permit a clear definition of the functions of OLF in normal homeostasis and in the pathophysiology of hypertension.

Selected Readings

Blaustein M. Endogenous ouabain: role in the pathogenesis of hypertension. *Kidney Int* 1996;49:1748–1753.
A concise summary of current information on OLF and its relationship to hypertension.

Drewett JG, Garbers DL. The family of guanylyl cyclase receptors and their ligands. *Endocrine Rev* 1994;15:135–162.
A comprehensive and scholarly review of guanylyl cyclase receptors, including the natriuretic peptide receptors.

Espiner EA, Richards AM, Yandle TG, et al. Natriuretic hormones. *Endocrinol Metab Clin North Am* 1995;24:481–509.
An excellent comprehensive review of natriuretic peptides and their receptors.

Ganguly A. Atrial natriuretic peptide-induced inhibition of aldosterone secretion: a quest for mediator(s). *Am J Physiol* 1992;263:E181–E194.
A detailed analysis of the cellular mechanisms likely to mediate inhibition of aldosterone release from the adrenal cortex by ANP.

Goetz KL. Renal natriuretic peptide (urodilatin?) and atriopeptin: evolving concepts. *Am J Physiol* 1991;261:F921–F932.
A review of similarities and differences in the actions of ANP and RNP, concluding that RNP is the mediator of natriuretic actions attributed to ANP and that ANP's role may be chiefly in the vasculature.

Hamlyn JM, Hamilton BP, Manunta P. Endogenous ouabain, sodium balance and blood pressure: a review and a hypothesis. *J Hypertens* 1996;14:151–167.
A comprehensive analysis of the controversies in this field, and the development of the hypothesis that elevated plasma ouabainlike activity may occur as a result of impaired renal excretion of such a compound.

Hollenberg NK, Graves SW. Endogenous sodium pump inhibition: current status and therapeutic opportunities. *Prog Drug Res* 1996;46:9–42.
A well-written review that seeks to make sense of the multiple conflicting observations regarding sodium transport inhibitors and hypertension.

Levin ER. Natriuretic peptide C-receptor: more than a clearance receptor. *Am J Physiol* 1993; 264:E483–E489.
A concise but complete summary of the evidence that intracellular signaling takes place through NPR-C.

Levin ER, Gardner DG, Samson WK. Natriuretic peptides. *N Engl J Med* 1998;339: 321–328.
A current brief overview of the family of natriuretic peptides and their receptors.

Marcus LS, Hart D, Packer M, et al. Hemodynamic and renal excretory effects of human brain natriuretic peptide infusion in patients with congestive heart failure. A double-blind, placebo-controlled, randomized crossover trial. *Circulation* 1996;94:3184–3189.
A well-designed trial demonstrating the efficacy of BNP infusion in patients with NYHA class III/IV congestive heart failure, even though preinfusion levels were already high.

Ruskoaho H. Atrial natriuretic peptide: synthesis, release, and metabolism. *Pharmacol Rev* 1992; 44:479–602.
An exhaustive review of the factors and mechanisms identified that regulate ANP synthesis and secretion from the cardiac atria.

Valentin J-P, Humphreys MH. Urodilatin: a paracrine renal natriuretic peptide. *Semin Nephrol* 1993;13:61–70.
A detailed review of the synthesis and actions of RNP.

PART 9
Glucocorticoids and Mineralocorticoids

Nicolette E. Farman

The corticosteroid hormones aldosterone and cortisol (or corticosterone in rodents) play a major role in the regulation of sodium excretion and blood pressure levels. Their mechanism of action is illustrated in Fig. 13.22. These steroid hormones enter the cell by diffusion and bind to intracellular receptors—the mineralocorticoid receptor (MR) or the glucocorticoid receptor (GR). The steroid–receptor complexes interact with the promoters of regulated genes, leading to changes in mRNA and protein expression. In the kidney, aldosterone action consists in an increase in transepithelial sodium reabsorption, through coordinate regulation of apical amiloride-sensitive sodium channels (ENaC) and basolateral Na^+-K^+-ATPase. The apical sodium channel represents the rate-limiting step for sodium reabsorption; its activity is tightly controlled by aldosterone and arginine-vasopressin. Stimulation of the Na^+-K^+-ATPase also

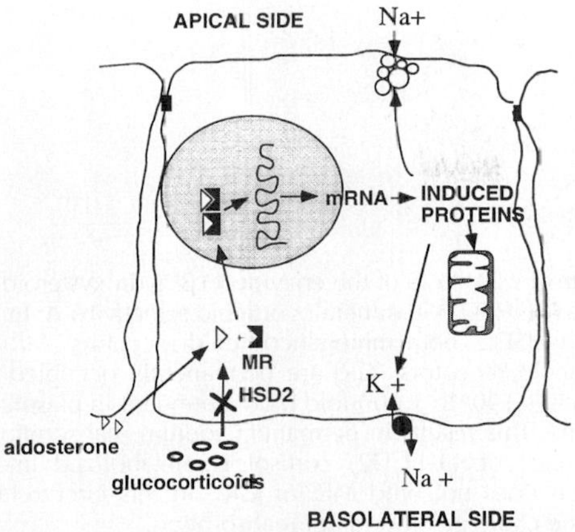

Figure 13.22. Corticosteroid regulation of sodium transport in the collecting duct principal cell. *MR,* mineralocorticoid receptor; *HSD2,* 11β hydroxysteroid dehydrogenase type 2.

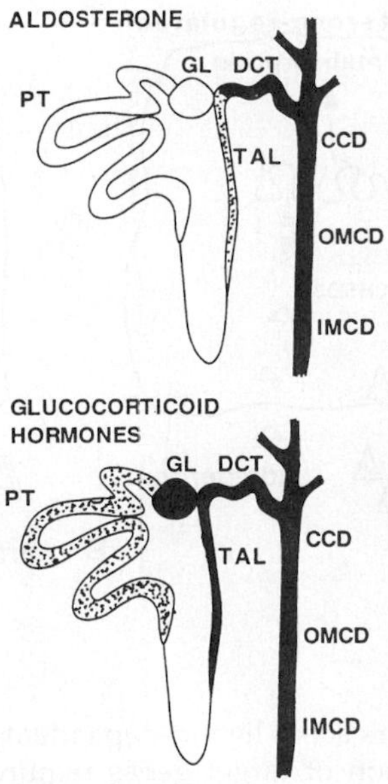

Figure 13.23. Sites of action of aldosterone and glucocorticoid hormones along the nephron. The nephron segments where corticosteroid hormone action has been clearly demonstrated by different approaches are shown in black; dotted areas represent tubular segments where this action is under discussion. *CCD,* cortical collecting duct; *DCT,* distal convoluted tubule; *Gl,* glomerulus; *IMCD,* inner medullary collecting duct; *OMCD,* outer medullary collecting duct; *PT,* proximal tubule; *TAL,* thick ascending limb of Henle's loop.

results in an increase in potassium entry from the interstitial space into the cell; as a result, potassium is secreted in the tubular lumen via K^+ channels, leading to the kaliuretic effect of aldosterone. Proton secretion is also stimulated by the hormone. Aldosterone acts (Fig. 13.23) in the terminal parts of the nephron, from the distal tubule to the papillary collecting duct; its effect on the loop of Henle is more controversial. These sites of action have been consistently documented by binding studies and evidence for expression of MR at the mRNA and at the protein level, by transport studies (micropuncture, isolated perfused tubules, rate of sodium fluxes), enzyme activity (upregulation of Na^+-K^+-ATPase) and regulation of some ion transporters, which will be detailed later. By contrast, much less is known about specific glucocorticoid effects in the kidney. Glucocorticoid hormones increase glomerular filtration rate; actions on tubular transport functions, such as proton and potassium movements, have been evoked, but may be secondary to the major effect on glomerular filtration rate and subsequent increase in fluid delivery to the various portions of the tubule. Glucocorticoid hormones increase ammoniogenesis and reduce phosphate reabsorption in the proximal tubule; this leads to an increase in urinary buffers and thus acid secretion is augmented. In addition, glucocorticoid hormones may also influence sodium reabsorption. Glucocorticoid receptors are present all along the nephron (Fig. 13.23), although the proximal tubule lacks nuclear binding and immunodetected GR.

Thus both MR and GR are coexpressed in the distal parts of the nephron and may function coordinately, as will be discussed later. In fact, it is often very difficult to discriminate between aldosterone and glucocorticoid hormone actions, because both hormones can bind both MR and GR and because of the lack of strictly specific ligands (agonists and antagonists).

MR and GR belong to the superfamily of nuclear steroid receptors, which share significant homologies in their DNA-binding domains and ligand-binding domains, explaining the cross-occupancy of each receptor by both ligands. However, *in vivo* effects of aldosterone and glucocorticoid hormones are at least partially distinct because molecular and cellular events confer mineralocorticoid selectivity to aldosterone target cells.

Plasma glucocorticoid concentrations are 100- to 1,000-fold higher than those of aldosterone; because the MR has the same affinity (10^{-9} M) for aldosterone and for glucocorticoid hormones, this should lead to permanent occupancy of MR by the latter hormones, leading to permanent maximal sodium retention, eliminating any regulatory role of aldosterone. Protection of the MR from illicit occupancy by glucocorticoid hormones is achieved by an enzyme, 11 β hydroxysteroid dehydrogenase (11-HSD). This enzyme metabolizes endogenous glucocorticoids (cortisol in humans, corticosterone in rodents) into 11-dehydro-derivatives (cortisone or 11-dehydro-corticosterone) with no affinity for MR (Fig. 13.24B). The MR-protecting form of the enzyme, 11-HSD2, is coexpressed with MR in aldosterone target cells, in particular in the collecting duct. The renal level of expression of MR, GR and 11-HSD2 is not (or very little) affected by the level of circulating corticosteroid hormones. The pivotal role of the 11-HSD2 in mineralocorticoid selectivity is illustrated by the consequences of inactivating mutations of 11-HSD2 identified in the syndrome of apparent mineralocorticoid excess (AME). AME is an inheritable form of severe hypertension with hypokalemia, suppressed renin and aldosterone levels, and reduced excretion of cortisone metabolites; in this syndrome, MR is permanently occupied by cortisol (Fig. 13.24A). Licorice intoxication leading to high blood pressure levels is also caused by dysfunction of 11-HSD2, which is inhibited by metabolites of licorice.

It is important to note that the 11-dehydro-derivatives of glucocorticoid hormones (cortisone) have no affinity for GR (in addition to MR). Thus this implies that 11-HSD2, when expressed in cells containing both MR and GR (as collecting duct cells), should impair binding of glucocorticoid hormones to GR (in addition to MR). This probably prevents most of specific glucocorticoid actions in the collecting duct and may explain why glucocorticoid effects have been difficult to demonstrate in this epithelium.

In addition to the major role of 11-HSD2, other factors probably contribute to the mineralocorticoid selectivity. The MR itself exhibits distinct properties (conformation, nuclear translocation, transactivation efficiency) that vary, depending on whether the ligand is aldosterone, antialdosterone molecules, or glucocorticoid hormones.

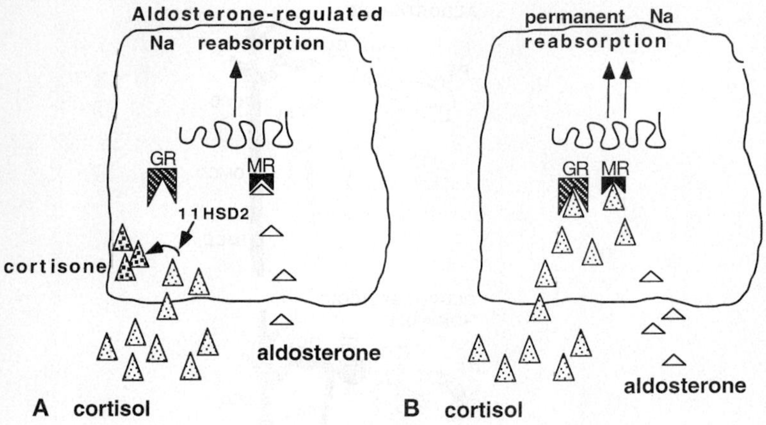

Figure 13.24: Role of the enzyme 11β hydroxysteroid dehydrogenase (11-HSD2) in mineralocorticoid selectivity. **A:** In the absence of 11-HSD2, both mineralocorticoid receptors *(MR)* and glucocorticoid receptors *(GR)* are permanently occupied by cortisol, which is 100- to 1,000-fold more abundant in plasma than aldosterone. This results in permanent sodium reabsorption. **B:** In the presence of 11-HSD2, cortisol is metabolized into cortisone, which does not bind MR (or GR). In this circumstance, aldosterone can regulate sodium reabsorption.

Steroid receptors act as ligand-dependent transcription factors. Transactivation of target genes requires the fixation of dimers on promoters of regulated genes. MR can form homodimers or heterodimers with GR; this results in different transactivation properties, depending on the relative proportion of each dimer and its ligands, leading to a great regulatory flexibility.

Interestingly aldosterone effects vary between tissues (e.g., in the collecting duct and in the colon), despite the presence of MR in each of these tissues. This points to the existence of tissue-specific transcription factors, not yet identified, that could interact with MR to yield different cellular responses.

Thus it is clear that aldosterone and glucocorticoid hormones have close interactions, leading the complementary effects through an overlapping network of gene expression. It is important to realize that all these events of mineralocorticoid selectivity form a series of successive selectivity filters (Table 13.5). An alteration in any of these steps will have important consequences on the events that follow in this cascade.

MR and GR are not redundant, as shown by the specificity of phenotypes yielded by gene-targeting experiments leading to their gene inactivation. Renal salt homeostasis is severely impaired in MR knockout mice (salt-wasting syndrome and death within 8 to 13 days after birth), despite the presence of GR. In humans, mutations of MR (resulting in loss of function) in some cases of autosomal dominant or sporadic pseudohypoaldosteronism type I also lead to neonatal renal salt-wasting syndrome, failure to thrive, and hypotension. The specific role of GR on kidney function cannot be elucidated at present from observation of GR knockout mice because of their early death (a few hours after birth) from severe lung atelectasis.

Several aldosterone-regulated genes have been identified and characterized at the molecular level. The upregulation of most of them is delayed for days beyond the observed physiologic response, such as the decrease in sodium excretion (1 to –2 hours). This suggests that they do not represent early induced proteins, but rather secondary effects of the hormone. Early effects may consist of the activation of preexisting channels or pumps (by unknown mechanisms) or the induction of factors (also unidentified as yet) that will then enhance the biosynthesis of the ion transporters.

In the collecting duct, aldosterone stimulates Na^+-K^+-ATPase activity (within hours) and the biosynthesis (within days) of its α subunit (α1 isoform). The amiloride-sensitive sodium channel ENaC is a major target of aldosterone. ENaC is located in the apical membrane of the distal tubule and the collecting duct principal cells (essentially in its cortical and outer medullary portions). Activation of ENaC occurs 1 to 2 hours after hormonal exposure, while induction of ENaC transcripts (α subunit) appears later. ENaC may be activated by an increase in channel density in the apical membrane (or decrease in its retrieval), or by a higher opening permeability of single channels. Phosphorylation state of the channels may also be important. These events may be caused by distinct effects of aldosterone or by coordinated effects with other factors. The aldosterone-mediated increase in K^+ secretion probably involves the apical ROMK potassium channels. Indeed, ROMK transcripts are upregulated in animals fed a low-salt diet, a condition that elevates plasma aldosterone levels without altering plasma glucocorticoid hormone concentration. In the distal tubule, besides ENaC, the thiazide-sensitive Na-Cl cotransporter controls sodium reabsorption, and evidence for its mineralocorticoid-dependent up regulation has been provided. Aldosterone and/or glucocorticoid hormones also control acid-base balance through direct or indirect effects on the Na^+/H^+ and the Cl^-/HCO_3^- exchangers. These rapid modulations may be indicative of nongenomic effects of aldosterone. Because sodium reabsorption requires energy, it has been proposed that aldosterone could stimulate the activity of mitochondrial enzymes, such as citrate synthase, which is enhanced in the collecting duct in the presence of aldosterone. Mineralocorticoid administration also results in cell swelling and multiplication of the infoldings of the basolateral membrane of the collecting duct principal cells.

Evidence is accumulating that aldosterone and arginine-vasopressin act in synergy to promote efficient sodium reabsorption. Such synergy may originate from rapid regulatory mechanisms; however cAMP-dependent transcription factors may also interact with the MR to regulate the expression of some transport proteins (e.g., the different subunits of ENaC or Na^+-K^+-ATPase). Arginine vasopressin also acts in synergy with glucocorticoid hormones to increase water permeability and urine concentration processes.

Altogether, it is clear that aldosterone regulates a number of determinants of sodium reabsorption, which will ultimately have important consequences on body sodium homeostasis and blood pressure levels. As an illustration of this concept, it is interesting to recall the pathologic situations that are linked to an abnormal functioning of this system.

Elevated plasma levels of aldosterone may result from inappropriate activation of the renin-angiotensin system or from aldosteronomas, both leading to hypertension. This is also the case when mineralocorticoid receptor selectivity is diminished (inhibition of 11-HSD2 after licorice ingestion or mutations in its gene in the syndrome of apparent mineralocorticoid excess) or

TABLE 13.5. Sequential Elements of Mineralocorticoid Selectivity

HSD2: Most of glucocorticoids entering the aldosterone target cell are metabolized into 11-dehydro-derivatives with no affinity for MR
MR properties differ in the presence of aldosterone, antialdosterone, or glucocorticoid hormones
MR can bind glucocorticoid-response elements (GRE) as homodimers (MR-MR) or heterodimers (MR-GR), resulting in distinct transactivation properties
MR can interact with other transcription factors: cAMP binding proteins; Tissue-specific factors; - Others; to modulate transcription in a tissue-specific manner, and to exert actions integrated in a multifactorial regulated environment

overwhelmed by excess glucocorticoid hormone secretion (as in Cushing's syndrome). Alternatively, mutations in MR leading to a truncated inactive receptor have been observed in some cases of autosomal dominant or sporadic forms of type I pseudohypoaldosteronism, characterized by salt-wasting syndrome. Genetic alterations of ENaC subunits may result in a loss of function as in autosomal recessive forms of type I pseudohypoaldosteronism, resulting in important sodium losses. Conversely, other mutations of ENaC, such as in Liddle's syndrome, lead to severe hypertension. In this case, hypertension results from an increased sodium reabsorption insensitive to MR antagonists. Mutations (loss of function) of the thiazide-sensitive Na-Cl cotransporter have been reported in Gitelman's disease, a variant of Bartter's syndrome in which inactive Na-Cl cotransport results in an hypokalemic metabolic alkalosis, accompanied by hypocalciuria and hypomagnesemia.

Drugs may alter the action of aldosterone. Some of them are used as diuretics, such as antagonists of the mineralocorticoid receptor (spironolactone) or blockers of aldosterone-regulated transporters (amiloride or triamterene, which inhibits ENaC, and thiazides as blockers of the Na-Cl transporter). Other drugs may also interfere with aldosterone action, leading to undesirable consequences (e.g., cyclosporine administration may lead to relative mineralocorticoid resistance of unknown pathogeny). Finally, it is important to note that aldosterone may participate in the development of cardiac fibrosis in cardiac failure. Whether the hormone is also involved in the development of renal fibrosis is not known at present.

Selected Readings

Bonvalet JP. Regulation of sodium transport by steroid hormones. *Kidney Int* 1998;53:S49–S56.

An integrated and comprehensive overview of aldosterone action in the kidney and other tissues.

Farman N. Molecular and cellular determinants of mineralocorticoid selectivity. *Curr Opin Nephrol Hypertens* 1999;8:45–51.

Summarizes the most recent knowledge of all steps involved in mineralocorticoid selectivity.

Garty H, Palmer L. Epithelium sodium channels: function, structure, and regulation. *Physiol Rev* 1997; 77:359–396.

A complete overview of the molecular and functional characteristics of the epithelial sodium channel ENaC. It integrates the molecular aspects of transepithelial sodium transport and its hormonal regulation.

Lifton R. Molecular genetics of human blood pressure variation. *Science* 1996;272: 676–680.

In this review the genetic disease of aldosterone biosynthesis and action are summarized, with special focus on their consequences on regulation of blood pressure.

Verrey F. Transcriptional control of sodium transport in tight epithelia by adrenal steroid. *J Membrane Biol* 1995;144:93–110.

A review of present knowledge of the mineralocorticoid receptor and aldosterone-regulated genes.

PART 10
Parathyroid Hormone and Calcitonin

Keith A. Hruska and Naseeruddin Khan

PARATHYROID HORMONE

Parathyroid hormone (PTH) is synthesized by the chief cells of the parathyroid glands as preProPTH and secreted as an 84–amino acid straight-chain polypeptide. The human PTH gene is located on the short arm of chromosome 11 at band 11p15. Its 5′ noncoding region contains a calcium response element, a vitamin D response element, and silencers that limit its transcription by the parathyroid gland chief cells.

In uremia, the double stimulus of hypocalcemia and low levels of $1,25(OH)_2D_3$ consistently lead to increased gene transcription and steady state levels of PTH mRNA. In chief cells, the "pre" or signal sequence directs the nascent peptide, preProPTH, into the endoplasmic reticulum where it is cleaved, leaving ProPTH to travel through the Golgi apparatus. Cleavage of the Pro sequence is accomplished before packaging the mature hormone in dense core secretory vesicles that fuse with the plasma membrane, releasing the hormone in response to a fall in blood calcium. PTH is also secreted through the constitutive pathway without packaging in the secretory granules. In mammalian circulation, PTH is the most important endocrine factor in the regulation of calcium and phosphorus metabolism. The key target organs of PTH are the kidneys and the skeleton. The intact biologically active hormone has a short half-life in the circulation of about 2 to 4 minutes, and its normal concentration range is approximately 10 to 55 ng/L (1 to 5 pmol/L). It is primarily cleared from the circulation by the kidneys and liver. In the serum, PTH exists as multiple fragments, including those of hepatic origin and parathyroid gland origin. The hepatic Kupffer cells and parathyroid cells cleave the hormone at amino acid 33–34, yielding an amino terminal biologically active fragment of the hormone that has a very short half-life and a carboxyl terminal fragment, 34–84, with a longer half-life because it is only cleared from the circulation by the renal proximal tubule. The amino terminal fragment is degraded within the parathyroid cells and by the Kupffer cells in the circulation and does not circulate in significant amounts. Secreted parathyroid hormone fragments arising from parathyroid chief cells are heterogeneous. Both classes of the PTH fragments are cleared by the kidneys, and in patients with renal insufficiency, PTH fragments accumulate in the blood.

The secretion of PTH is sensitive to serum calcium and phosphorus concentrations. There is a rapid rise in PTH secretion with hypocalcemia, and when the serum calcium is elevated, PTH secretion is suppressed. There is a sigmoidal relationship between calcium and parathyroid secretion, and the midpoint in the sigmoidal curve is often called the *setpoint* of PTH secretion. PTH secretion is pulsatile, and the pulses account for abrupt variations in PTH levels on a programmed basis. In addition, there is a circadian rhythm in PTH secretion.

Measurement Methods for PTH

There are different types of assays developed for PTH measurement, including traditional radioimmunoassays (RIAs) and two-site immunometric assays. RIAs are based on the development of antibodies against different segments of the PTH: namely, carboxyterminal middle region and amino terminal PTH epitopes. The most widely used two-site immunologic assays, IRMA (immunoradiometric assay) and ICMA (immunochemiluminometic assay), provide specific measurement of the intact PTH molecule. The modern two-site intact hormone assays have improved correlation with bone histology in renal failure and also aid in the detection of low values.

The carboxyl terminal and middle region PTH assays are always elevated in renal failure, because these assays measure not only the active hormone but also the inactive metabolites that are normally excreted by the kidneys. In case of renal failure, the PTH measured by these assays could be several times the upper limit of normal. Therefore, in cases of renal failure, measuring the intact PTH is a more accurate reflection of the parathyroid status of the patients. In cases of humoral hypercalcemia of malignancy (HHM) the intact hormone assay aids the differentiation between PTHrP-induced hypercalcemia versus ectopic PTH producing tumors. PTH levels are increased in cases of hyperparathyroid bone disease and renal osteodystrophy induced hypercalcemia, but they are suppressed in HHM. (For additional detailed discussion on HHM, see Chapter 17.)

Mechanism of PTH Action

PTH binds to the PTH1 receptor by the amino terminus of the molecule. Receptor binding activates heterotrimeric intracellular GTP-binding proteins; specifically Gs, which then stimulates membrane-bound adenylate cyclase, resulting in production of the second messenger cyclic adenosine monophosphate (cAMP). The cAMP thus produced binds to protein kinase A, which dissociates and phosphorylates proteins that carry out the actions of PTH. PTH binding to the PTH1 receptor also activates G-proteins of the Gq family in some circumstances, which activates phospholipase C or phospholipase D, causing increases in intracellular calcium and activation of protein kinases of the C family.

PTH regulates the level of calcium and phosphate in the blood and plays an important role in bone remodeling. The actions of PTH on the bone are complex but sustained elevations release calcium and phosphorus through stimulation of bone resorption. Its actions on the renal tubules are to cause an increase in tubular reabsorption of calcium and to inhibit the reabsorption of phosphate. In addition, it also causes renal hydroxylation of 25,OH vitamin D to its active form, 1,25 dihydroxyvitamin D, which in turn acts to increase the absorption of calcium and phosphate from the intestines and renal tubules (Fig. 13.25).

The net results of these actions are elevation of the blood levels of calcium and reduction in the levels of serum phosphate. Distal tubular calcium reabsorption and osteoclastic bone resorption are the major control points in minute-to-minute serum calcium homeostasis. The parathyroid gland chief cells are exquisitely sensitive to the ionized serum calcium concentrations and maintain a setpoint for the release or suppression of PTH. This setpoint is increased in response to renal disease, and it is decreased in treated postmenopausal women.

Also, with primary hyperparathyroidism the blood calcium level at which PTH secretion is one-half its maximum level is higher than in normal subjects, which is a setpoint error. The setpoint error for calcium regulated PTH secretion has long been demonstrated *in vitro*. The setpoint for ionized calcium in a normal parathyroid gland is approximately 1 mmol, whereas it is about 1.26 mmol in uremic patients with secondary hyperparathyroidism. The reports of this altered setpoint are variable

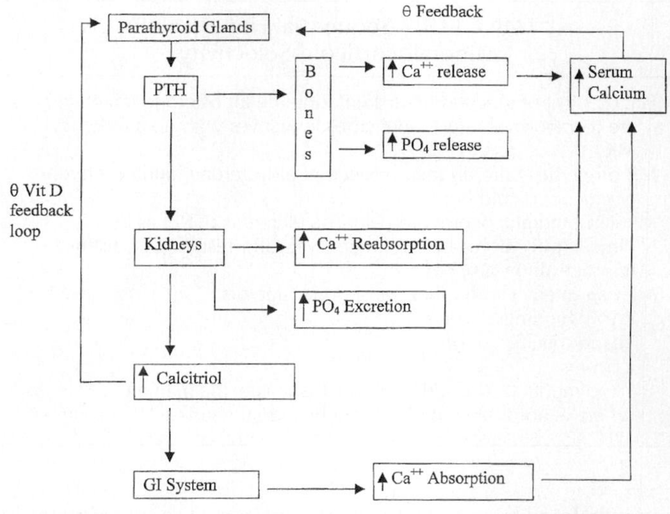

Figure 13.25. Renal, PTH, Ca^{++}, and [-] vitamin D feedback loop.

in different studies and it is reported that this alteration occurs only in a subgroup of uremic patients with severe refractory secondary hyperparathyroidism.

PTH regulates and acts through the calcium-phosphorus product, which is a biologic constant and a humoral factor that combats hyperphosphatemia. An acute rise in serum phosphorus produces a transient fall in the concentration of serum ionized calcium. The subsequent stimulation of PTH inhibits the transport of phosphorus and results in phosphaturia.

Aluminum and iron suppress PTH secretion, as does a high glucose concentration within parathyroid chief cells. The latter may relate to the functional hypoparathyroidism frequently observed in diabetic patients with end-stage renal disease (ESRD). Aluminum, iron, and hyperglycemia are all associated with low turnover osteodystrophy in patients with ESRD related in part to suppression of secondary hyperparathyroidism.

The histologic consequences of PTH action on the skeleton include an increase in osteoclast number and activity. PTH receptors are located in cells of the osteoblast lineage instead of osteoclasts (although this continues to be debated). When isolated osteoblasts are treated with PTH, they produce factors (especially osteoprotegrin ligand and IL-6) that stimulate osteoclastogenesis, activate existing osteoclasts and increase resorption of bone. The actions of PTH also increase osteoblast activity, which accompanies the increased osteoclast activity in hyperparathyroidism. In uremia the skeleton is resistant to the action of PTH and modest PTH elevations are required to maintain normal rates of bone remodeling. PTH directly stimulates osteoprogenitor cells in the bone and acts indirectly through substances such as 1,25-dihydroxyvitamin D and insulinlike growth factors. Osteoprogenitors differentiate to become osteoblasts capable of forming bone matrix. Sustained elevations of PTH interact with osteoblasts in such a way that production of type 1 collagen, osteocalcin, and osteopontin are inhibited. The latter two proteins have important roles in osteoid mineralization. PTH also stimulates cells of the bone remodeling microenvironment to secrete substances such as osteoprotegrin ligand, interleukin 6 and 11, and others, which in turn stimulate osteoclast precursor proliferation. Excess of secretion of PTH as in ESRD, results in osteitis fibrosa (renal osteodystrophy). The fibrosa component of the bone remodeling disorder is related to accumulation of a fibroblast phenotype of early osteoprogenitors with a fibroblast phenotype constrained from entering or blocked in their osteoblast differentiation.

Excess PTH and Nonclassic Target Organs

In 1977, Massry hypothesized that PTH may be a uremic toxin. Today we know that PTH in supraphysiologic concentrations affects target tissues other than kidney and bone through both the PTH1 and PTH2 receptors and that the PTH gene evolved from a primitive ancestor, which has led to the widespread expression of a sister gene, PTHrp, which shares the same PTH1 receptor for many of its functions. The function of the PTH1 receptor in nonclassic PTH target tissues is actually as the receptor for parathyroid hormone–related protein (PTHrp), but PTH binds to it in secondary hyperparathyroidism. The putative toxic triad is secondary hyperparathyroidism, chronic renal failure, and elevated cytosolic calcium levels. Several body systems may be affected, leading to a number of pathologic changes; of note are peripheral neuropathy, abnormal metabolism of phospholipids, changes in prolactin and aldosterone secretion, changes in insulin secretion, reduced serum testosterone levels, activation of proteolysis systems, induction of cytokine secretion, and inhibition of erythropoiesis. Moreover, the chronic uremic state, which is associated with an increased susceptibility to infection, may be contributed to by alterations in the immune system caused by elevated PTH levels. Animal studies demonstrate that verapamil treatment in animals with chronic renal failure and secondary hyperparathyroidism may improve the dysfunction of different systems as it blocks the PTH-induced elevations of cytosolic calcium. (Detailed discussion of the toxic effect of excess PTH in uremia is found in Chapter 68, Part 1.)

In 1987, PTHrp was discovered to be the factor responsible for humoral hypercalcemia of malignancy. Many tissues express PTHrp, especially breast, placenta, and smooth muscle. PTHrp is a key skeletal developmental morphogen involved in endochondral bone formation, and it is also involved physiologically with keratinocyte differentiation and smooth muscle relaxation. In addition to the widespread expression of the PTH1 receptor related to the physiologic role of PTHrp, the non–target organ actions of PTH are also accounted for, in part, by the concept that both PTH and PTHrp may be polyhormones. However, discovery of unique receptors for peptides derived from the PTH sequence will be required for physiologic demonstration of these concepts.

Primary Hyperparathyroidism

Primary hyperparathyroidism (PrHPT) is one of the two most common causes of hypercalcemia, the other being malignancy. Together they account for more than 90% of patients with hypercalcemia. The incidence of primary hyperparathyroidism varies between 1 in 500 and 1 in 1,000. It frequently presents in the sixth decade of life and has a female-to-male ratio of 3:1. Most cases involve postmenopausal women. PrHPT can also occur as a part of multiple endocrine neoplasia (MEN) syndrome, type I or type II. Most of the time, when it is not a part of MEN I or MEN II, it presents as a solitary adenoma in one of the four parathyroid glands; hyperplasia of all four glands is seen in about 15% to20% of patients with PrHPT. Rarely, PrHPT is seen with carcinoma of the parathyroid gland. In PrHPT, parathyroid hormone levels are very high despite elevations in the serum calcium. This is from an increase in number of the parathyroid gland cells with nonsuppressible PTH synthesis and secretion. The high levels of parathyroid hormone may be associated with skeletal and renal complications. In the skeleton the classic lesion is osteitis fibrosa cystica, with subperiosteal resorption of the distal phalanges, a salt and pepper type of appearance of the skull, a rugger jersey appearance of the spine, and brown tumors of the long bones.

There is an associated incidence of kidney stones with PrHPT reported to be about 24% in the late twentieth century. Nephrocalcinosis is also seen. Increased levels of blood calcium and PTH usually establish the diagnosis. The markers of bone resorption are also increased, while hypercalciuria resulting from increased filtered load of calcium is seen in about 30% of the patients. Other biochemical abnormalities include an increase in the circulating 1,25-dihydroxyvitamin D. Because PTH affects the cortical bone, reductions of bone mineral density in the cortical bone were observed with use of single-photon absorpiometry. More modern techniques demonstrate that bone mineral density of both trabecular and cortical bone may be reduced, although there is a relative preservation of the cancellous bone in the lumbar spine leading to the rugger jersey pattern of bone density in severe cases.

Treatment of Primary Hyperparathyroidism

The treatment of this condition depends on a number of factors and consists of observation, medical therapy and surgery. Indications for surgery may include serum calcium more than 12 mg/dl (greater than 3 mmol/L); patients with overt bone disease; nephrolithiasis; marked hypercalciuria (more than 400 mg/day); or bone mass more than 2 standard deviations below age- and sex-matched control subjects; age younger than 50 years (Table 13.6). In more than 90% of the cases, the parathyroid glands are located by surgeons accurately. Occasionally preoperative localization of parathyroid tissue is required. This is carried out by ultrasonography, CT scan, and MRI. There is an increasing emphasis on technetium-99m-sestamibi scans. Injected sestamibi persists in the parathyroid glands, which helps to localize the glands accurately. In difficult cases, arteriography and selective venous sampling for PTH may be required to locate the abnormal parathyroid tissue. The bone mass improves substantially in 2 to 3 years after surgery. Following surgery, there may be a transient period of hypocalcemia. This is especially the case in patients with overt skeletal disease resulting from a rapid deposition of calcium and phosphorus into the skeleton. During symptomatic hypocalcemia, or "hungry bone syndrome," patients frequently require parenteral calcium. If a patient is not a candidate for surgery, medical management is indicated; this would include adequate hydration and ambulation. A low-calcium diet should

TABLE 13.6. Potential Indications for Surgery in Primary Hyperparathyroidism

I. Overt manifestations of primary hyperparathyroidism
   a. Radiographic nephrolithiasis or otherwise documented kidney stone or stones
   b. Reduced creatinine clearance (not otherwise explained)
   c. Radiographically evident hyperparathyroid bone disease
   d. Classic hyperparathyroid neuromuscular disease
   e. Symptoms attributable to hypercalcemia per se
   f. Previous episode of life-threatening hypercalcemia
II. Serum calcium concentration greater than 3 mmol/L (12 mg/dl)
III. Urinary calcium excretion greater than 10 mmol/d (400 mg/d)
IV. Bone mineral density less than 2 SD below age-matched, sex-matched control
V. Age younger than 50
VI. Uncertain prospect for successful medical monitoring
   a. Patient requests surgery
   b. Consistent follow-up seems unlikely
   c. Coexistent illness that may contribute to, or confound detection of, disease progression

be avoided, because this could theoretically lead to augmentation of PTH secretion. In postmenopausal women, estrogen therapy has been considered useful. Bisphosphonates have also been considered for hypercalcemia. The role of a new class of drugs, which alter the function of the extracellular calcium sensing receptors of the parathyroid chief cells and renal tubular cells, is being investigated. Most patients who are not surgical candidates appear to do well with a twice a year follow-up. (For further discussion of primary hyperpathyroidism, see Chapter 17, Part 3.)

Familial Hyperparathyroid Syndromes

As many as 10% of cases of primary hyperparathyroidism are hereditary in origin. The most common type of familial hyperparathyroidism occurs in MEN type I syndrome along with pancreatic tumors, parathyroid glands, pituitary adenomas and sometimes adrenocortical hyperplasia. This syndrome is inherited in an autosomal-dominant pattern. PrHPT of MEN type I usually requires surgery, and it usually presents with hyperplasia of all four parathyroid glands. The current recommended therapy is dissection of three and a half glands, or autotransplantation of a glandular fragment into the forearm with removal of all four glands. First-degree relatives of individuals with MEN I syndrome should be screened for the disease.

MEN type II (aut-D) consists of hyperparathyroidism, medullary carcinoma of the thyroid, and up to 50% of cases also have pheochromocytoma or adrenal medullary hyperplasia. Most of the mortality associated with MEN type II results from unrecognized pheochromocytoma, which usually presents as bilateral adrenal hyperplasia. This is unlike the usual pheochromocytomas, which is usually unilateral. (The MEN I and MEN II syndromes are also discussed in Chapter 17, Part 3.)

Familial Hypocalciuric Hypercalcemia

Familial hypocalciuric hypercalcemia (FHH), also known as *familial benign hypercalcemia,* is transmitted as an autosomal-dominant inherited disease. It is caused by mutations of the calcium-sensor gene of the parathyroid glands and the kidney. In this disease, there is an alteration of renal tubular calcium reabsorption, and there is an increase in the parathyroid gland setpoint for calcium suppression of PTH secretion. As a result, higher than normal levels of serum calcium are needed to suppress PTH, and the tubular reabsorption of calcium is high, resulting in hypocalciuria. Serum calcium remains strikingly high, even after total parathyroidectomy. The net result is hypercalcemia and hypocalciuria and normal to slightly elevated PTH levels.

Patients should be advised that parathyroidectomy is not the appropriate treatment because the syndrome is asymptomatic, but it is often confused with PrHPT. Attempts to regulate serum calcium with medications such as diuretics, estrogen, and phosphates usually do not affect the serum calcium level. Pregnancy in individuals who are FHH carriers requires special consideration: affected offspring could show asymptomatic hypercalcemia associated with heterozygosity for FHH or severe neonatal hypercalcemia associated with homozygosity and intrauterine secondary hyperparathyroidism. In a patient with this diagnosis, the clinician must be alert for urinary calcium levels, and a parathyroidectomy would be inappropriate. (FHH is also discussed in Chapter 17, Part 3.) Other rare familial hyperparathyroidism syndromes include hyperparathyroidism–jaw tumor syndrome and familial isolated hyperparathyroidism.

Secondary Hyperparathyroidism

The term *secondary hyperparathyroidism* is used to describe a condition characterized by elevated levels of PTH hormone associated with reduced extracellular calcium levels, with hypertrophy of the parathyroid chief cells and hyperplasia. In some cases a single gland weighs 25 times the weight of a normal gland. These cells have a longer lifespan, with limited apoptosis resulting in persistently increased cell number. Hyperplastic glands sometimes have a nodular histologic pattern associated with clonality, and in those cases parathyroidectomy with autotransplantation may be associated with recurrent HPT. This type of disorder characteristically demonstrates nonsuppressible PTH secretion, even after treatment of the inciting metabolic abnormalities (e.g., hypocalcemia, hyperphosphatemia, and vitamin D deficiency). The levels of the vitamin D receptor and the calcium receptor are reduced in chief cells from nodular glands. The downregulation of vitamin D receptor number leads to impaired vitamin D receptor binding to the vitamin D response element. Abnormalities in the function of the vitamin D receptor and the calcium receptor are important factors in resistant hyperparathyroidism that may require parathyroidectomy. Uremia may also be associated with an impaired ability of calcitriol to induce the expression of vitamin D receptors.

End-stage Renal Disease

The incidence of HPT in ESRD, which is roughly 95%, is dependent on the duration of end-stage renal disease and on the duration of dialytic therapy. The uremic state presents multiple stimuli to the parathyroid glands that cause secondary HPT; these stimuli include hyperphosphatemia, 1,25-dihydroxyvitamin D deficiency, downregulation of vitamin D receptors, altered calcium-sensing, and hypocalcemia. In end-stage renal disease the target level of intact PTH is roughly three times higher than that of normal individuals (85 pg/ml), but PTH levels may not be suppressible; in such circumstances parathyroidectomy may be required.

PTH stimulates osteoblastic function in bone remodeling. Studies have shown that therapeutic suppression of PTH in the management of patients with chronic renal failure (CRF) results in deficiency in osteoblast precursor proliferation and conversion of high turnover renal osteodystrophy to an adynamic bone disorder. This indicates a deficiency in the osteoblast differentiation program inherent to chronic renal failure. One potential mechanism for such a constraint in osteoblast differentiation results from deficiency of bone morphogenetic proteins ([BMPs], especially BMP-7), a family of protein that regulates proliferation and differentiation of osteoblast precursors. Most of the BMP-7 made postnatally is synthesized in renal tubular cells. As renal failure progresses, BMP-7 production is reduced as well. To maintain rates of bone remodeling, PTH levels are elevated, resulting in secondary HPT. In the presence of high PTH and low BMP-7 uncommitted osteoprogenitors with a fibroblastic phenotype are overexpressed, resulting in osteitis fibrosa. PTH exerts its anabolic effect on bone formation through proliferation of progenitors, stimulation of insulinlike growth factor-I (IGF-I) production, and inhibition of osteoblast apoptosis. In CRF and ESRD, if PTH is suppressed, the resulting deficiency of osteoprogenitors, IGF-I, and osteoblast apoptosis contribute to the development of an adynamic bone remodeling disorder; hence levels of PTH above normal are needed to avoid adynamic bone disorder. In osteodystrophy associated with diabetic nephropathy, there are relatively low levels of PTH. Stimulation of osteoprogenitor differentiation toward adipocytes through the influence of PPARγ results in an adynamic bone disorder similar to other forms of ESRD, but with a slightly different pathogenesis.

The HPT of ESRD may be considered as responsive or refractory to suppression of PTH secretion. Refractory HPT is characterized by markedly elevated PTH levels and plasma phosphate levels and high-turnover metabolic bone disease. It also causes spontaneous hypercalcemia referred to by some as *tertiary hyperparathyroidism.* Responsive HPT is characterized by reduction of PTH levels with treatment to levels sufficient to maintain normal rates of bone remodeling associated with normal plasma Ca and P levels, usually requiring calcitriol therapy and careful management of phosphate binder therapy. After renal transplantation, 25% to33% of patients have transient hypercalcemia as a result of unresolved hyperparathyroidism. Patients with refractory HPT before transplant surgery are more likely to require parathyroidectomy.

Other Causes of Secondary Hyperparathyroidism

Disorders less common than ESRD are also associated with secondary hyperparathyroidism. Among these are X-linked hypophosphatemic (XLH) rickets. Patients with XLH are treated with large oral doses of phosphorus, which leads to chronic stimulation of PTH secretion. In chronic vitamin D deficiency states, especially in Asian individuals who are vegetarians, resistant HPT is observed. Another cause of PTH hypersecretion is observed in patients with primary biliary cirrhosis, which is characterized by low vitamin D levels secondary to the inability of the liver to convert vitamin D into 25-hydroxy vitamin D via 25-hydroxylase.

Treatment of Secondary HPT in CRF

PTH levels in secondary or tertiary hyperparathyroidism are treated by modulation of PTH levels through a step-wise approach.

1. Stage one: Prophylactic measures include phosphate control, calcium supplementation, calcitriol (oral or intravenous).
2. Stage two (with bone pain or fractures and renal osteodystrophy):
   - In hypocalcemic patients, institute prophylactic measures, as in stage one. Increase calcitriol doses to achieve normal calcium levels and monitor calcium levels weekly.
   - In normocalcemic patients, in addition to prophylactic measures, low calcium dialysate should be used and intravenous calcitriol therapy instituted. The target calcium should be less than 10.5 mg/dl and greater than 9 mg/dl.
   - In hypercalcemic patients, intravenous calcitriol and low calcium dialysate should be used as long as phosphorus levels are normal. Parathyroidectomy may be considered if phosphorus levels are elevated.
3. Stage three: Patients with hypercalcemia (without bone symptoms):
   - If calcium-phosphate product is greater than 65, consider parathyroidectomy.
   - If the calcium-phosphate product is less than 55, consider a trial of intravenous calcitriol and low calcium dialysate. If these two measures fail, consider parathyroidectomy.

(For a detailed discussion of secondary hyperparathyroidism of CRF and its treatment, see Chapter 77. Secondary hyperparathyroidism in renal transplant recipients is discussed in Chapter 89, Part 3.)

Hypoparathyroidism

Hypoparathyroidism is a clinical disorder manifested by either quantitative or functional deficiency of parathyroid hormone. It may result from a failure of the parathyroid glands to develop, destruction of the glands as a result of infiltrative processes, or resistance to PTH actions (Table 13.7). The common aspect of these conditions is decreased biologically active PTH. The clinical signs and symptoms of hypoparathyroidism result from hypocalcemia. The acute symptom is tetany, which may progress to seizures. Susceptibility to this symptom is increased during pregnancy, lactation, and in alkalotic states. Chronic hypocalcemia may be associated with muscle cramps, pseudopapilledema, extrapyramidal signs, mental retardation, and personality disorders. Other signs include abnormal dentition, alopecia, and cataracts. Because of abnormal calcium phosphate products, metastatic intracranial calcification may also be detected. The abnormalities found on laboratory evaluation include hypocalcemia and hyperphosphatemia in the presence of normal renal function. PTH levels are usually low, except in the PTH-resistant states, in which they are normal or elevated. 1,25-dihydroxyvitamin D levels are usually low, and alkaline phosphatase is normal. Nephrogenic cAMP excretion is low and the renal tubular reabsorption of phosphorus is increased. Urinary cAMP and phosphorus excretions are increased markedly after the administration of biologically active PTH except in the PTH resistant states.

The congenital causes of hypoparathyroidism are agenesis or hypoplasia of the parathyroid gland, which may be transmitted as an autosomal-dominant disorder, a recessive disorder, or as an X-linked recessive disorder. Embryologically, it may result from maldevelopment or underdevelopment of the third and fourth brachial pouches. The most common congenital abnormality is a group of diseases called the *DiGeorge syndrome*, related to the microdeletion of the long arm of chromosome 22. The conditions associated with the DiGeorge syndrome are chromosomal, monogenic, or teratogenic and result from diabetes, alcohol, or embryopathy. Other causes of hypoparathyroidism include destruction of the parathyroid gland as a result of hemorrhage, edema, or infiltrative diseases caused by iron intoxication, as in hematochromatosis and thalassemia, or destruction resulting from increased copper deposition, as in Wilson's disease.

There are other causes of hypoparathyroidism in which severe hypocalcemia is present following parathyroid surgery, hungry bone syndrome, and hypomagnesemia-associated

TABLE 13.7. Causes of Hypoparathyroidism

I. Congenital failure to develop parathyroid glands
   a. DiGeorge syndrome
II. Destruction of parathyroid glands
   a. Surgery
   b. Polyglandular autoimmune disease type I (PGA type I)
   c. Radiation
   d. Iron overload and infiltration (e.g., hemachromisis, thalassemia)
   e. Copper deposition (e.g., Wilson's disease)
   f. Neoplastic invasion
   g. Granulomatous infiltration (e.g., sarcoidosis)
   h. Amyloidosis
III. Impaired parathyroid hormone action/resistance in target organs
   a. Decreased Mg^{2+}, pseudohypoparathyroidism
IV. Altered parathyroid hormone secretion
   a. Altered Ca^{2+} sensor
      1. Mutation
      2. Acquired
   b. Decreased Mg^{2+}
   c. Maternal hyperparathyroidism

decreased secretion of PTH hormone. Still other causes of destruction of the glands include excessive neck radiation, the incidence of which has decreased. About 33% of these patients have idiopathic hypoparathyroidism, which could be related to polyglandular autoimmune deficiencies. Altered regulation of parathyroid gland function could be the result of maternal hyperparathyroidism. In addition, multiple rare genetic disorders of PTH gene-splicing and calcium-sensing receptor are also described that result in hypoparathyroidism. (For further discussion, see Chapter 17, Part 3.)

The primary goal of treatment is to keep calcium and phosphorus levels as close to normal as possible. The main agents available are supplemental calcium, vitamin D preparations, phosphate binders, and thiazide diuretics. The patient should be advised to avoid dairy products, which are high in phosphate.

Pseudohypoparathyroidism

The term pseudohypoparathyroidism (PHP) is applied to a group of disorders characterized by biochemical hypoparathyroidism, such as hypocalcemia and hyperphosphatemia, with an increased secretion of PTH and target tissue unresponsiveness. PHP consists of two types, type I (A and B) and type II. This syndrome was originally described by Fuller Albright. His observation was that these patients had resistance to the effects of PTH in the target organs, the skeleton, and the kidney.

Patients with PHP have neither a calcemic nor a phosphaturic response to exogenously administered PTH. This is the basis of the PTH infusion test to differentiate between the types.

Pseudohypoparathyroidism Type I

Patients with PHP type I do not show an appropriate increase in urinary excretion of cAMP and phosphate, whereas patients with type II show a normal increase in urinary cAMP but an impaired phosphaturic response. PHP type I is also called *Albright's hereditary osteodystrophy* (AHO). Phenotypically, it consists of short stature, round facies, obesity, brachydactyly, and subcutaneous ossifications.

There is a normocalcemic variant of PHP, which used to be called pseudohypoparathyroidism. These patients have the phenotype of PHP but have a normal urinary cAMP and phosphate response to PTH; this means that they do not have resistance to PTH and are able to maintain normal calcium levels without treatment. Patients with PHP type I have inactivating mutations in Gs, resulting in reduced hormone responsiveness to PTH, TSH, and gonadotropins. This form of PHP is called *type IA*. In *type IB* there is normal Gsα activity, but patients have PTH target organ resistance only. They have an abnormal cAMP response to a PTH infusion test and show skeletal lesions similar to those of patients with hyperparathyroidism. There are a few patients seen with PHP type I whose condition is labeled *type IC*. These patients are resistant to multiple hormones occurring in the absence of a demonstrable defect in Gs or Gi.

Pseudohypoparathyroidism Type II

In patients with PHP type II, there is a renal resistance to PTH manifested by reduced phosphaturic response to the administration of exogenous PTH despite a normal increase in urinary cAMP excretion. It results from an inability of intracellular cAMP to initiate the chain of metabolic events that results in the ultimate expression of PTH action.

Treatment

The basic principles of treatment of hypocalcemia and PHP are essentially those outlined in the section on hypoparathyroidism. The target is to maintain a low to mid-normal level of serum calcium. Patients with PHP type IA may have manifestations of other hormonal resistances, such as hypothyroidism or gonadal dysfunction. These patients should be treated as one would approach a patient with hypothyroidism or hypogonadism.

CALCITONIN

Calcitonin (CT) is a 32–amino acid peptide that is secreted primarily by the parafollicular or C cells of the thyroid gland in mammals. C cells are derived embryologically from neural crest cells. Calcitonin secretion is induced mainly by an acute increase in calcium concentration in the physiologic range. When blood calcium levels rise in an acute manner, there is a proportional increase in calcitonin secretion, leading to a decrease in blood calcium. Hypocalcemia produces a corresponding decrease in calcitonin secretion. A sigmoidal relationship between calcium concentration and calcitonin concentration just opposite in direction to the PTH-calcium curve has been described. The half-life of CT is small and is measured in minutes. CT is degraded in the liver, kidney, bone, and thyroid gland and is mainly excreted by the kidneys.

Biologic Effects

The calcitonin receptor belongs to the family of seven membrane-spanning domain receptors that include the PTH1 receptor and receptors for secretion of glucagon. They couple to heterotrimeric GTP-binding proteins—Gs and Gi in the case of calcitonin. The main biologiceffect of calcitonin is to inhibit osteoclastic bone resorption. CT acts by activating calcitonin receptors, producing an increase in cAMP and ultimately causing an increase in cytosolic calcium in the osteoclast cells. The osteoclasts respond by shrinkage in size and bone resorption activity. Newer data suggest that calcitonin may have an anabolic osteoblastic effect on the bone, which could improve bone quality and reduce the incidence of bone fracture. In normal physiologic conditions, however, the role of calcitonin on calcium homeostasis is still controversial.

Abnormalities of Calcitonin Secretion

Increased levels of calcitonin have been observed in medullary thyroid carcinoma and in acute and chronic renal failure. Increased levels could be caused by the immunologic heterogeneity of CT or measurement of inactive metabolites but also by its ineffective clearance. Studies have shown that in uremic patients with normal alkaline phosphatase, the PTH levels are relatively low, whereas CT levels are high. On the other hand, in uremic patients with high alkaline phosphatase and high PTH, the CT levels are low. From these studies it could be postulated that uremic patients with high CT levels have the ability to limit the bone resorptive capability of PTH, which is lacking in patients with high PTH and high bone turnover.

High calcitonin levels have been found in multiple neoplastic disorders. Of note is the medullary thyroid carcinoma, which although rare could present as part of the familial MEN type IIA and type IIB syndromes. Calcitonin is also increased in other neoplasms of neuroendocrine cell origin like small cell lung cancer, carcinoids and islet cell tumors of the pancreas.

Differentiation in ectopic CT production by tumors is by pentagastrin provocative test. In this test pentagastrin is injected intravenously and serum calcitonin is measured by a standard calcitonin RIA. In medullary thyroid carcinoma the calcitonin level secretion is usually very high when this stimulation technique is employed, while in other calcitonin-producing tumors, such as small cell carcinoma, the response is minimal with an elevated basal value.

Therapeutic Uses

Calcitonin has been available for clinical use since 1984, especially for the treatment of humoral hypercalcemia of malignancy and established osteoporosis. The skeletal effect of long-term calcitonin treatment is an increase in bone mineral density and a reduction in fracture risk; thus it is used to treat osteoporosis and Paget's disease. It has also been shown to relieve bone pain caused by tumor metastases, Paget's disease of bone, or osteoporosis, and nonbone pain caused by migraine or pancreatitis or following a thyroidectomy; the mechanism is possibly endorphins or inhibition of PGE_2. A nasal spray form of calcitonin has been approved for the treatment of established osteoporosis.

Selected Readings

Azria M, Avioli LV. Calcitonin. In: Bilezikian JP, Raisz LG, Rodan GA, eds. *Principles of bone biology.* San Diego: Academic Press, 1996:1083–1097.

Discusses the physiology of calcitonin in bone as well as its effects in other tissues.

Bilezikian JP, Marcus R, Levine MA, eds. *The parathyroids: basic and clinical concepts.* New York: Raven Press, 1994.

This textbook's chapters cover most, if not all, of the subject headings in this section. A few of them are specifically highlighted here.

Bro S, Olgaard K. Effects of excess PTH on nonclassic target organs. *Am J Kidney Dis* 1997;30:606–620.

Murray TM, Rao LG, Rizzoli RE. Interactions of parathyroid hormone, parathyroid hormone-related protein, and their fragments with conventional and nonconventional receptor sites. In: Bilezikian JP, Marcus R, Levine MA, eds. *The parathyroids: basic and clinical concepts.* New York: Raven Press, 1994: 185–211.

This review and chapter revisit the issue of PTH effects on multiple organs in uremia based on the discovery that PTHrp, which is widely expressed, uses the PTH1 receptor, which is therefore also widely expressed. In addition, there is accumulating evidence that PTH is a polyhormone and that 1–34, 28–48, and 53–84 are biologically active peptides.

Segre GV. Receptors for parathyroid hormone and parathyroid hormone-related protein. In: Bilezikian JP, Marcus R, Levine MA, eds. *The parathyroids: basic and clinical concepts.* New York: Raven Press, 1994:213–229.

This chapter examines the actions of PTH from the aspect of its PTH1 receptor, which it shares with PTHrp. Nontraditional PTH targets, the PTHrp knockout, and the actions of PTHrp and PTH are discussed.

PART 11
Vitamin D Metabolites

Alex J. Brown, Adriana S. Dusso, and Eduardo Slatopolsky

Vitamin D is essential for life in higher animals. It is one of the important regulators of calcium and phosphorus metabolism and is required for proper development and maintenance of bone. Vitamin D was first identified early in this century as the result of intensive research into the essential dietary components for growth and development. However, with adequate exposure to sunlight sufficient amount of vitamin D can be produced in the skin.

The structures of the two major forms of vitamin D, ergocalciferol (vitamin D_2) and cholecalciferol (vitamin D_3), are shown

This work was supported in part from a grant provided by the U.S.P.H.S. NIDDKD. Grants DK-07126, DK-09976 and DK-30178.

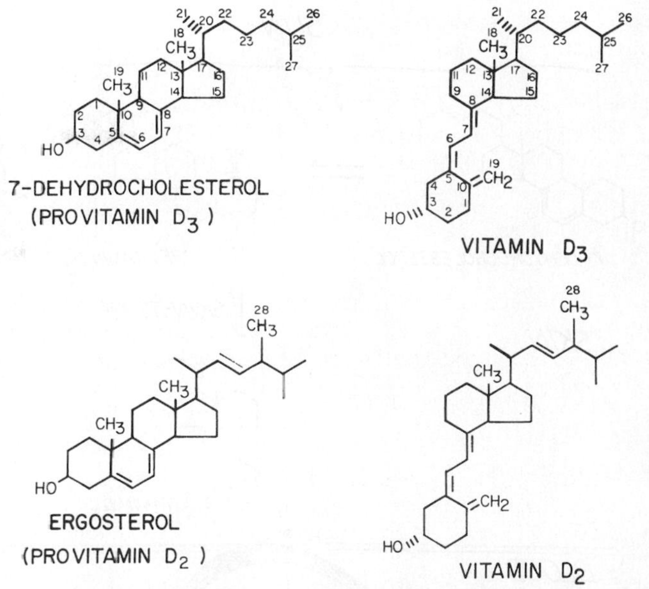

Figure 13.26. Structures of vitamins D_3 and D_2 and their respective precursors, 7-dehydrocholesterol and ergosterol. The only structural difference between vitamins D_2 and D_3 is in their side chains; vitamin D_2 has a double bond at carbon 22 and a methyl group on carbon 24. (Reproduced with permission from MacLaughlin JA, Holick MF. Photobiology of vitamin D_3 in the skin. In: Goldsmith LA, ed. *Biochemistry and physiology of the skin,* Vol. 2. New York: Oxford University Press, 1981:734–754.)

in Fig. 13.26. These compounds are steroids, or more precisely seco-sterols, derived from the photolytic cleavage of the B rings of ergosterol and 7-dehydrocholesterol respectively. They have little intrinsic antirachitic activity, they must be metabolized to the active form of vitamin D: 1,25-dihydroxyvitamin D_3 or calcitriol. It is now appreciated that 1,25-dihydroxyvitamin D_3 ($1,25\text{-}(OH)_2D_3$) is a hormone that acts via a specific cellular receptor to control not only mineral homeostasis but many other processes as well.

METABOLISM OF VITAMIN D

Photochemical Production of Vitamin D_3

Vitamin D_3 is produced in the skin from the provitamin D_3, 7-dehydrocholesterol. Exposure of skin to sunlight, specifically to the ultraviolet B portion of the spectrum (290 to 315 nm), causes photolytic conversion of the 7-dehydrocholesterol to previtamin D_3 (Fig. 13.27). Previtamin D_3 undergoes a thermally induced isomerization to vitamin D_3. Serum DBP, which preferentially binds vitamin D_3 over its precursor, may be responsible for the translocation of the vitamin from the epidermis into the circulation. The ability of the skin to produce vitamin D_3 is affected by a number of factors. There is a well-established inverse correlation between age and the provitamin D_3 levels in the epidermis. Sunscreens are also very effective in blocking the wavelengths of ultraviolet light necessary for previtamin D_3 formation. Similarly, melanin acts as a natural sunscreen and prevents photolysis of provitamin D_3, but other mechanisms may be more important in controlling the overproduction of vitamin D_3 in the skin. In addition to thermal isomerization to vitamin D_3, previtamin D_3 can absorb more ultraviolet light and be converted to the biologically inert products tachysterol and lumisterol as illustrated in Fig. 13.27. Thus, during prolonged exposure to sunlight, these reactions may limit the levels of previtamin D_3 and prevent overproduction of vitamin D_3.

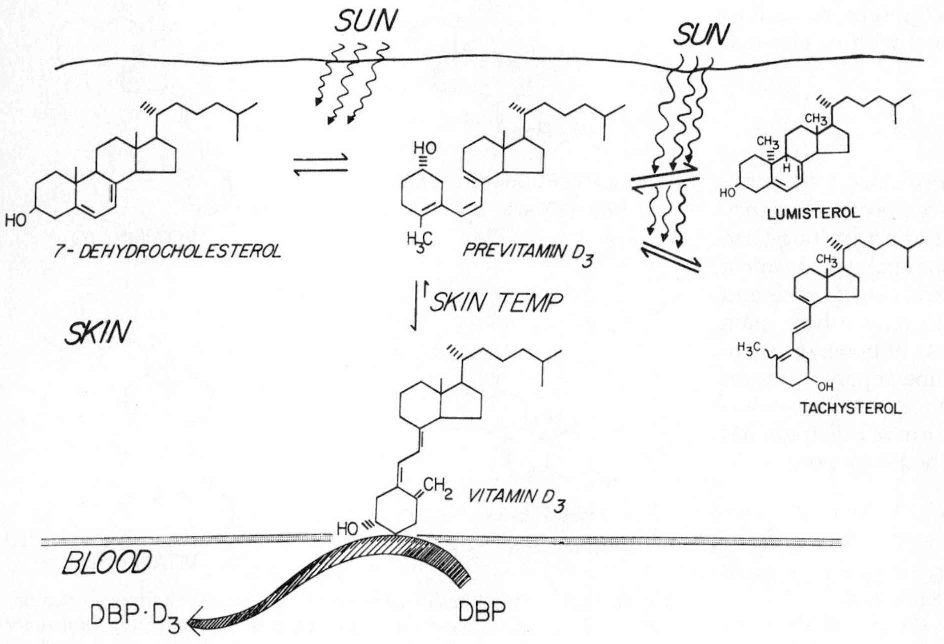

Figure 13.27. Schematic representation of the formation of previtamin D_3 in the skin during exposure to the sun and the thermal isomerization of pre–vitamin D_3 to vitamin D_3. (Reproduced with permission from Holick MF, MacLaughlin JA, Doppelt SH. Regulation of cutaneous previtamin D_3 photosynthesis in man: skin pigment is not an essential regulator. *Science* 1981;211: 590–593.)

Absorption of Vitamin D

In addition to its biosynthesis in the skin, vitamin D_3, along with vitamin D_2, can be obtained from the diet. Although only a few food sources such as fish oils, egg yolks, and liver contain significant amounts of vitamin D, many foods are now fortified with this vitamin. As with most fat-soluble compounds, vitamin D absorption takes place mainly in the upper part of the small intestine and requires bile salts, an intact absorptive surface, and an association with chylomicrons in lymph for its effective delivery into the blood. Patients with fat malabsorption syndromes, intestinal disease, or abnormalities in bile secretion may develop vitamin D deficiency as a result of malabsorption of this fat-soluble vitamin.

Metabolism of Vitamin D to 25-Hydroxyvitamin D

The first step in the metabolic activation of vitamin D, hydroxylation of carbon 25, occurs primarily in the liver, although other tissues may produce small amounts of 25-(OH)D_3. The 25-hydroxylase is a cytochrome P450 monooxygenase that requires molecular oxygen and a source of reducing equivalents that, in the mitochondria, are supplied by electron transfer from NADPH via ferredoxin reductase and ferredoxin as shown in Fig. 13.28.

The 25-hydroxylase has a relatively low affinity for vitamin D_3, and saturation is possible only at very high vitamin D concentrations. The activity of this enzyme is not tightly controlled, therefore the 25-(OH)D production would increase in proportion to vitamin D intake; plasma 25-(OH)D levels are often used as an indicator of vitamin D status.

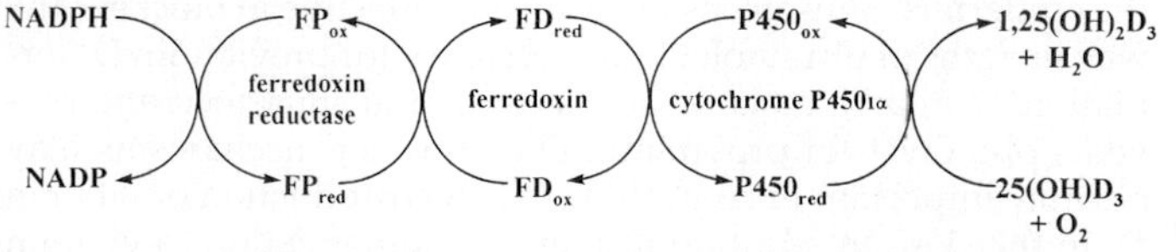

Figure 13.28. Mechanism of production of 1,25-$(OH)_2D_3$ by 25-hydroxyvitamin D_3 1α-hydroxylase. This enzyme is a mitochondrial cytochrome P450 that requires reducing equivalents supplied by NADPH via a flavoprotein (ferredoxin reductase) and an iron-sulfur protein (ferredoxin). This mechanism is used by the mitochondrial vitamin D 25-hydroxylase and 24-hydroxylase.

Formation of 1,25-Dihydroxyvitamin D from 25OHD$_3$ by the Kidney

It is generally accepted that 1,25-$(OH)_2D_3$ is the most active form of vitamin D. Early studies by Fraser and Kodicek indicated that the kidney is the major (if not exclusive) site of production of this metabolite. Therefore patients with severe renal failure often have a greatly reduced capacity for production of 1,25-$(OH)_2D_3$. However, a number of reports have demonstrated evidence for extrarenal synthesis of calcitriol. The contribution of these sources to 1,25-$(OH)_2D_3$ synthesis in healthy subjects is not known.

The renal enzyme responsible for producing 1,25-$(OH)_2D_3$ is the 25-(OH)D-1α-hydroxylase. Like 25-hydroxylase, this enzyme is located in the inner mitochondrial membrane, is a cytochrome P450 monooxygenase, and requires molecular oxygen, ferredoxin, and ferredoxin reductase. Other cytochrome P450s of the renal mitochondria are specific for other oxidations of vitamin D but use the same electron transport system.

The half-life of 1,25-$(OH)_2D_3$ in the circulation has been estimated to be approximately 6 to 8 hours. Because of the high potency of this hormone, its circulating levels are under very tight regulation, with normal values ranging from 25 to 50 pg/ml. It is transported primarily by the serum vitamin D–binding protein (DBP) with a smaller amount bound to albumin. Although more than 99% of the 1,25-$(OH)_2$D is bound *in vivo,* current evidence suggests that the unbound fraction of the hormone is biologically active. When DBP levels are altered, as in patients with liver disease (decreased DBP) or during estrogen therapy (increased DBP), there is a parallel change in total 1,25-$(OH)_2D_3$, but concentrations of the free hormone remain normal.

Extrarenal Production of 1,25-Dihydroxyvitamin D

The kidney is not unique in its ability to convert 25(OH)D to 1,25-$(OH)_2D_3$. Numerous cells and tissues express 1α-hydroxylase activity *in vitro.* Extrarenal synthesis of calcitriol in humans,

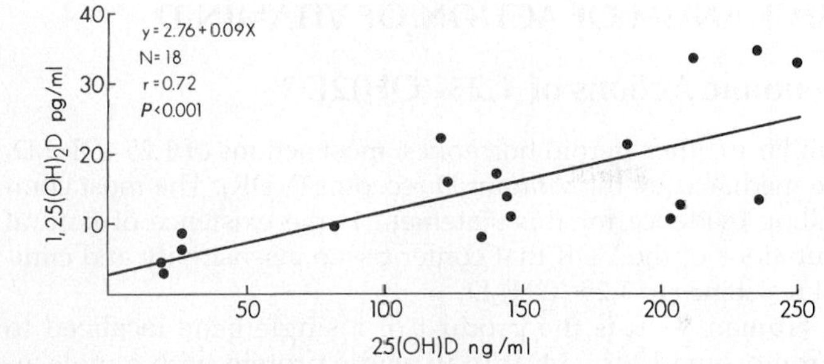

Figure 13.29. Correlation between serum levels of 25-(OH)D and 1,25-$(OH)_2D$ in anephric patients. (Reproduced with permission from Dusso A, Lopez-Hilker S, Rapp N, et al. Extra-renal production of calcitriol in chronic renal failure. *Kidney Int* 1988;34:368–375.)

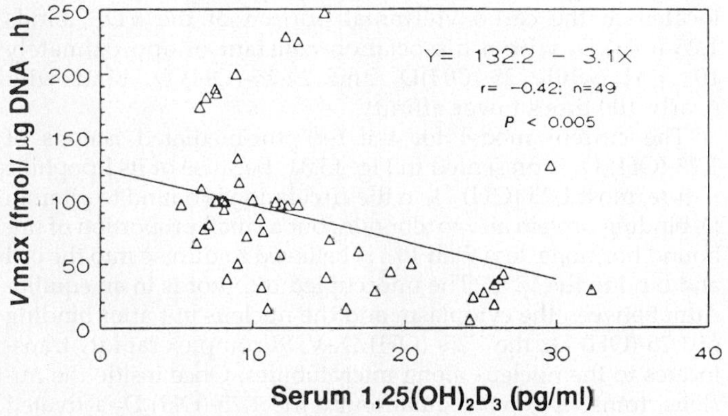

Figure 13.30. Correlation between 1α-hydroxylase activity (V_{max}) of peripheral blood monocytes and serum levels of 1,25-$(OH)_2D$ in hemodialysis patients. (Reproduced with permission from Gallieni M, Kaminmura S, Ahmed A, et al. Kinetics of monocytes 1-hydroxylase in renal failure. *Am J Physiol* 1995;268:F746–F753.)

however, only affects circulating calcitriol levels in pregnancy, sarcoidosis and other granulomatous diseases, and chronic renal failure.

In chronic renal failure, extrarenal 1,25-$(OH)_2D_3$ production can normalize the low serum 1,25-$(OH)_2D_3$ level only after 25(OH)D supplementation. Fig. 13.29 depicts a strong correlation between serum 25(OH)D and 1,25-$(OH)_2D_3$ levels in bilaterally nephrectomized patients undergoing hemodialysis. Peripheral blood monocytes were identified as a source of calcitriol. Monocyte 1,25-$(OH)_2D_3$ production in hemodialysis patients correlates inversely with serum 1,25-$(OH)_2D_3$ levels (Fig. 13.30), suggesting that extrarenal sources are induced to compensate for a defective renal 1α-hydroxylase. The need for supraphysiologic concentrations of 25(OH)D to normalize serum 1,25-$(OH)_2D_3$ levels in anephric patients demonstrates that substrate availability to extrarenal sources of calcitriol plays an important role in 1,25-$(OH)_2D_3$ production, thus providing an additional therapeutic tool to correct 1,25-$(OH)_2D_3$ deficiency in chronic renal failure.

Formation of 24,25-Dihyroxyvitamin D from 25-Hydroxyvitamin D

In normal subjects and experimental animals maintained on a diet containing adequate amounts of calcium and vitamin D, the major metabolite of 25-OH-D_3 is 24,25-$(OH)_2D_3$. The kidney is a major site of production of this metabolite, but its synthesis has been observed in nearly all target tissues for 1,25-$(OH)_2D_3$. The circulating levels of 24,25-$(OH)_2D_3$ are from 1 to 4 ng/ml. While it is controversial whether 24,25-$(OH)_2D_3$ is biologically active, 24-hydroxylation of vitamin D metabolites has been shown to be the first step in their degradation and excretion.

Metabolism of 1,25-Dihydroxyvitamin D

Metabolism of 1,25-$(OH)_2D_3$ is necessary to maintain steady-state levels of the hormone in the circulation and may play an important role in attenuating cellular responses, especially under conditions of excess 1,25-$(OH)_2D_3$. The side chain of 1,25-$(OH)_2D_3$ is the major site of metabolism with oxidation at carbons 23, 24, and 26. The two major end-products of side-chain metabolism of 1,25-$(OH)_2D_3$ are calcitroic acid (1-hydroxy-23-carboxy-24,25,26,27-tetranorvitamin D_3) and 1,25-$(OH)_2D_3$-23, 26-lactone. While calcitroic acid appears to be biologically inert, the lactone has been reported to antagonize the ability of 1,25-$(OH)_2D_3$ to promote the maturation of osteoclasts, the cells responsible for bone resorption. Most important is that this side chain metabolism is induced by 1,25-$(OH)_2D_3$, and may be a critical means of attenuating the actions of 1,25-$(OH)_2D_3$ in target cells, especially under conditions of vitamin D intoxication.

Regulation of Vitamin D Metabolism

The high potency of 1,25-$(OH)_2D_3$ in raising serum calcium and phosphate necessitates a stringent regulation of vitamin D metabolism. The most important regulators of calcitriol levels are parathyroid hormone (PTH), serum phosphorus, serum ionized calcium, and 1,25-$(OH)_2D_3$ itself. These factors have been demonstrated to affect both the synthesis and degradation of calcitriol. Many other regulators of calcitriol have been reported, but their contributions to 1,25-$(OH)_2D_3$ regulation are less well defined.

Hypocalcemia increases serum 1,25-$(OH)_2D_3$ levels by induction of renal 1-hydroxylase activity and decreasing 24-hydroxylase activity, but these effects are blunted by parathyroidectomy. Furthermore, patients with hypoparathyroidism have low 1,25$(OH)_2D_3$ levels despite low serum calcium. Cell culture experiments have implicated a direct action of PTH on vitamin D metabolism, presumably through cyclic AMP (cAMP) and other second messenger pathways, but the mechanism has not been fully elucidated.

Calcium may modulate 1,25-$(OH)_2D_3$ by PTH-independent mechanisms as well. When parathyroidectomized rats are repleted by PTH infusion, 1,25-$(OH)_2D_3$ levels decrease when serum calcium is raised by calcium chloride infusion and increase when serum calcium is lowered by infusion with EGTA, a calcium chelator. However, a direct effect of calcium on vitamin D metabolism on kidney proximal tubular cells *in vitro* has not been demonstrated.

Metabolic acidosis has also been shown to alter vitamin D metabolism. Acidosis blunts the action of PTH on the 1α-hydroxylase, and cAMP can restore this activity to normal in acidotic rats. Because loss of PTH responsiveness with acidosis is not due to a loss of renal PTH receptors, the blunted cAMP production is attributed to altered coupling of these receptors with adenylate cyclase. Acidosis also increases ionized calcium, which may be totally responsible for the altered vitamin D metabolism because EGTA can block the effect of acidosis on 1,25-$(OH)_2D_3$ levels without changing blood pH.

The importance of phosphorus as a regulator of renal vitamin D metabolism is well established. Dietary phosphate restriction increases serum 1,25-$(OH)_2D_3$ levels and renal 1α-hydroxylase activity. Small changes in dietary phosphorus within the normal range cause mild but significant alterations in serum calcitriol levels. The mechanism by which phosphorus controls the production of 1,25-$(OH)_2D_3$ is unclear, but it is independent of PTH and calcium. Direct effects of phosphate on 1α-hydroxylase activity on isolated kidney mitochondria, tubules, and cultured cells have not been demonstrated conclusively.

An interesting aspect of the regulation of 1,25-$(OH)_2D_3$ by hypophosphatemia is the role of somatomedins. The stimulatory action of dietary phosphate restriction on 1α-hydroxylase activity is prevented by hypophysectomy but can be restored by repletion with growth hormone or somatomedin C (IGF-I).

Perhaps the most important determinant of serum calcitriol is vitamin D status or, more specifically, the levels of 1,25-$(OH)_2D_3$. Calcitriol acts through a feedback mechanism to control its serum levels by inhibiting 1α-hydroxylase and stimulating enzymatic oxidation of its side chain. In vitamin D-deficient animals, 1α-hydroxylase activity is maximal and 24-hydroxylase is low or undetectable. Treatment with 1,25-$(OH)_2D_3$ reverses the expression of these two activities. These same effects are observed in kidney cell cultures, indicating that the effects of calcitriol are direct. The action of 1,25-$(OH)_2D_3$ on the vitamin D hydroxylases in cell culture is evident only after several hours, requires protein synthesis, and is reversed by removal of the hormone from the medium. It seems likely, then, that when the intake of calcium and phosphorus is adequate, regulation of vitamin D metabolism by 1,25-$(OH)_2D_3$ is the primary mechanism for maintaining proper circulating calcitriol levels. The extrarenal production of 1,25-$(OH)_2D_3$ could be attenuated by glucocorticoids; the effect of the latter explains the adequacy of small doses of glucocorticoids for the treatment of the hypercalcemia of sarcoidosis.

Transport of Vitamin D Metabolites

The hydrophobic nature of vitamin D metabolites requires carrier proteins for transport in the circulation. The most important of these carrier proteins is the serum vitamin D–binding protein (DBP), although albumin and lipoproteins are also important. All of the major vitamin D metabolites bind to DBP. The order of affinities are 25-$(OH)D_3$ = 24,25-$(OH)_2D_3$ > 1,25-$(OH)_2D_3$ > vitamin D_3. The dissociation constants for 25-$(OH)D_3$ and 1,25-$(OH)_2D_3$ differ by about tenfold. In mammals, vitamin D_2 compounds bind with the same relative affinities as the vitamin D_3 metabolites. DBP has a molecular weight smaller than albumin, and therefore it is lost in urine in proteinuric conditions, such as nephrotic syndrome.

DBP circulates in the plasma at a very high concentration, 400 mg/L or about 6 μm, 20 times higher than the total concentration of vitamin D metabolites. Because this protein has a single sterol-binding site, only about 5% of the total DBP in normal human plasma is occupied with vitamin D compounds. This differs from carrier proteins for other steroid hormones. The reason for this large excess of DBP is uncertain, although it probably functions to conserve vitamin D metabolites by increasing their half-lives in the circulation. DBP also buffers the free concentration of 1,25-$(OH)_2D_3$ to prevent vitamin D toxicity.

The plasma levels of DBP are not regulated by vitamin D. Pathologic conditions, such as liver disease, nephrotic syndrome, and malnutrition, can decrease DBP, while pregnancy and estrogen therapy increase DBP. In general, the concentration of the free, active form of 1,25-$(OH)_2D_3$ remains constant when DBP levels change, an example of the tight self-regulation of vitamin D metabolism. Numerous reports show that DBP retards the cellular uptake of vitamin D metabolites, including 1,25-$(OH)_2D_3$. Furthermore, the stimulation of 24- hydroxylase activity in keratinocytes and the inhibition of lymphocyte proliferation by calcitriol have been correlated with free, rather than total, concentration of the hormone.

MECHANISM OF ACTION OF VITAMIN D

Genomic Actions of 1,25-(OH)2D3

Similar to other steroid hormones, most actions of 1,25-$(OH)_2D_3$ are mediated by the vitamin D receptor (VDR). The most compelling evidence for this statement is the existence of natural mutations of the VDR that confer tissue insensitivity and clinical resistance to 1,25-$(OH)_2D_3$.

Human VDR is the product of a single gene localized to chromosome 12q13-14. It is an acidic protein with a molecular weight between 50 and 60 KD, with highly conserved DNA- and hormone-binding domains similar to all members of the steroid receptor superfamily. Two so-called zinc finger motifs in the DNA-binding domain mediate the high-affinity interactions of the VDR with specific DNA sequences in the promoter region of target genes. The ligand-binding domain, located in the carboxyterminal portion of the VDR, binds 1,25-$(OH)_2D_3$ with a dissociation constant of approximately 10^{-10} M, while 25-$(OH)D_3$ and 24,25-$(OH)_2D_3$ bind with nearly 100 times lower affinity.

The current model for the receptor-mediated actions of 1,25-$(OH)_2D_3$ is presented in Fig. 13.31. Because of its lipophilic nature, most 1,25-$(OH)_2D_3$ in the circulation is bound to vitamin D–binding protein and to albumin, but a small proportion of unbound hormone, less than 1%, is believed to diffuse into the cell and bind to the VDR. The unoccupied receptor is in an equilibrium between the cytoplasm and the nucleus but after binding of 1,25-$(OH)_2D_3$, the 1,25- $(OH)_2D_3$-VDR complex rapidly translocates to the nucleus along microtubules. Once inside the nucleus, transcriptional regulation by the 1,25-$(OH)_2D_3$-activated VDR involves multiple protein-protein and protein–DNA interactions. Heterodimerization of the VDR with the retinoid X receptor (RXR) is required to induce a VDR conformation that is competent to activate transcription. The VDR–RXR complex binds direct repeat vitamin D responsive elements (VDREs) upstream from vitamin D–controlled genes. Additional protein–protein interactions of the VDR with the transcription factor TFIIB and with coactivators facilitate the assembly of the transcription initiation complex and alter the rate of transcription of the target gene by RNA polymerase II. Interactions of the VDR partners RXR and SRC-1 with the CBP/p300 family of nuclear coactivators potentiate the transcriptional activity of various members of the steroid receptor superfamily and may certainly have synergistic effects on VDR-transactivating function.

Nongenomic Actions of 1,25-$(OH)_2D_3$

In addition to the genomic mechanism for vitamin D action, a number of nongenomic activities have been described. 1,25-$(OH)_2D_3$ rapidly increases calcium uptake, phosphoinositide metabolism, vesicular calcium transport, phosphate fluxes, alkaline phosphatase activity, and cyclic GMP in selected cells. These activities occur within seconds to minutes following the addition of 1,25-$(OH)_2D_3$ to the system, too rapid to involve changes in gene expression. A putative membrane receptor for 1,25-$(OH)_2D_3$ has been isolated from chicken intestine. It is structurally distinct from the VDR and displays a different ligand specificity. Of interest is the observation that the nongenomic pathway does not operate in states of vitamin D deficiency or when the VDR is absent or nonfunctional, suggesting that one or more components of the nongenomic pathway are induced by the genomic actions of 1,25-$(OH)_2D_3$.

The genomic and nongenomic actions of vitamin D combine to produce a multitude of responses in an ever-increasing list of target cells. In the following section, the actions of 1,25-$(OH)_2D_3$

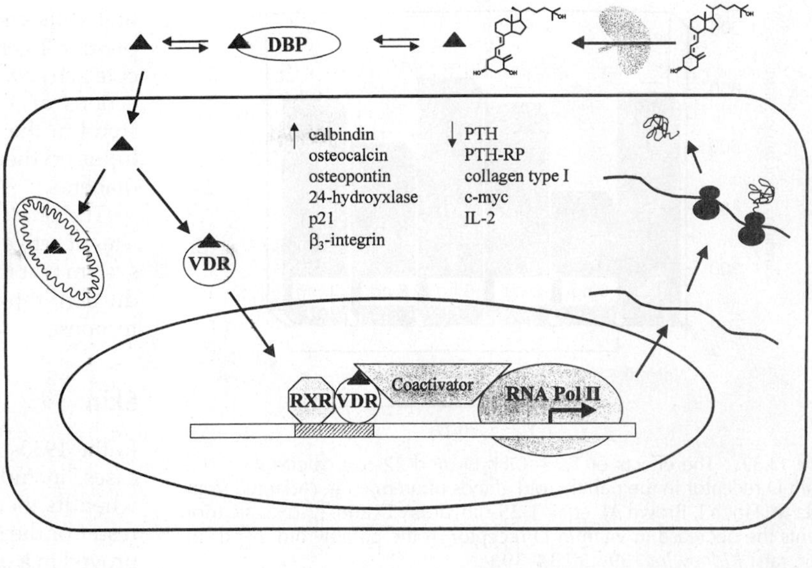

Figure 13.31. Model for the control of gene transcription by $1,25\text{-}(OH)_2D_3$. The activated vitamin D hormone is transported in the blood by serum DBP. $1,25(OH)_2D_3$ taken up by target cells is either degraded by the mitochondrial 24-hydroxylase or binds to the vitamin D receptor (VDR). The liganded VDR heterodimerizes with retinoid X receptor (RXR), enhancing the interaction with specific sequences in the promoter regions of target genes. The DNA-bound heterodimer attracts components of the RNA polymerase II (Pol II) preinitiation complex either by direct interactions or indirectly through coactivators, thereby altering the rate of gene transcription. The mRNA is processed and released to the cytoplasm, where it is translated into proteins. A list of gene products known to be upregulated or downregulated at the transcriptional level is shown.

on individual tissues and the physiologic consequences will be discussed in detail.

CLASSICAL ACTIONS OF VITAMIN D

Vitamin D is part of a stringent regulatory system that governs calcium and phosphorus homeostasis through specific actions in the classical mineral regulating organs: the intestine, bone, parathyroid glands and kidneys. This section summarizes our understanding of vitamin D actions in these tissues.

Intestine

The principal function of $1,25\text{-}(OH)_2D_3$ in mineral homeostasis is to enhance the efficiency of the small intestine in absorbing dietary calcium and phosphorus. $1,25\text{-}(OH)_2D_3$ increases the entry of calcium through the plasma membrane into the enterocyte, the movement of calcium through the cytoplasm, and the transfer of calcium across the basolateral membrane into the circulation. $1,25\text{-}(OH)_2D_3$ is the only hormone known to stimulate intestinal calcium transport directly. Other vitamin D metabolites can stimulate calcium transport, but only in supraphysiologic doses, consistent with their lower affinity for the VDR. Increasing evidence suggests that the VDR-mediated effects of $1,25\text{-}(OH)_2D_3$ may not be the only mode of action by which the hormone stimulates calcium absorption by the enterocyte. Rapid effects of calcitriol appear to mediate an increase in both the vesicular and paracellular pathways for intestinal calcium absorption. The actual contribution of these nongenomic pathways to intestinal calcium absorption *in vivo* is unclear.

In addition to its effects on calcium absorption, $1,25\text{-}(OH)_2D_3$ increases active phosphorus transport. The sterol directly stimulates the expression of the Na/Pi cotransporter and affects the composition of the enterocyte plasma membrane, increasing fluidity and phosphate uptake. Little is known, however, concerning the molecular mechanisms involved in the extrusion of phosphate across the basolateral membrane into the circulation. (For additional discussion on the effect of $1,25\text{-}(OH)_2D_3$ on the intestinal absorption of calcium and phosphorus, see Chapters 17 and 19, respectively.)

Skeleton

Vitamin D is essential for the development and maintenance of a mineralized skeleton. Vitamin D deficiency results in rickets in young growing animals and osteomalacia in adults. Several studies, however, have demonstrated that vitamin D is not absolutely essential for the ossification process. It is apparent, therefore, that vitamin D induces bone mineralization by increasing serum levels of calcium and phosphorus. The higher potency of $1,25\text{-}(OH)_2D_3$ in regulating mineral homeostasis makes calcitriol the most likely vitamin D metabolite involved in bone mineralization. Although controversial, $24,25\text{-}(OH)_2D_3$ appears to have synergistic effects with $1,25\text{-}(OH)_2D_3$ in bone formation.

In addition, to maintain calcium homeostasis, $1,25\text{-}(OH)_2D_3$ mobilizes calcium from bone by inducing the dissolution of bone and mineral matrix. $1,25\text{-}(OH)_2D_3$ induces bone resorption through enhancement of osteoclastogenesis and osteoclastic activity. Strong evidence suggests, however, that osteoblasts and osteoblast-derived substances are required for $1,25\text{-}(OH)_2D_3$ induction of osteoclastic bone resorption.

Parathyroid Glands

PTH is the principal hormone involved in the minute to minute regulation of ionized calcium levels in the extracellular fluid. Calcitriol plays a key role in the day to day maintenance of calcium balance. PTH stimulates the production of calcitriol by activating the renal 1α-hydroxylase enzyme and calcitriol suppresses the synthesis and secretion of PTH. Thus, both PTH and calcitriol directly affect calcium homeostasis, and each exerts important regulatory effects on the other. $1,25\text{-}(OH)_2D_3$ plays an important role in the regulation of PTH gene transcription *in vivo* in the rat. The $1,25\text{-}(OH)_2D_3$–vitamin D–receptor complex binds to its responsive element in the 5′-flanking region of the PTH gene decreasing the rate of transcription. Also, it has been shown that $1,25\text{-}(OH)_2D_3$ and its analog 22-oxacalcitriol upregulate the vitamin receptor in the parathyroid glands of uremic rats (Fig. 13.32).

Kidney

As described earlier, the most important effect of $1,25\text{-}(OH)_2D_3$ in the kidney is the suppression of 1α-hydroxylase activity and the stimulation of 24-hydroxylase activity. The role of vitamin D in the renal handling of calcium and phosphorus continues to be controversial. Even though the sterol increases calcium reabsorption, 99% of the calcium filtered by the kidney is reabsorbed, even in vitamin D deficiency. The effect of the sterol improving renal absorption of phosphate in the presence of PTH may not be a direct action on the kidney.

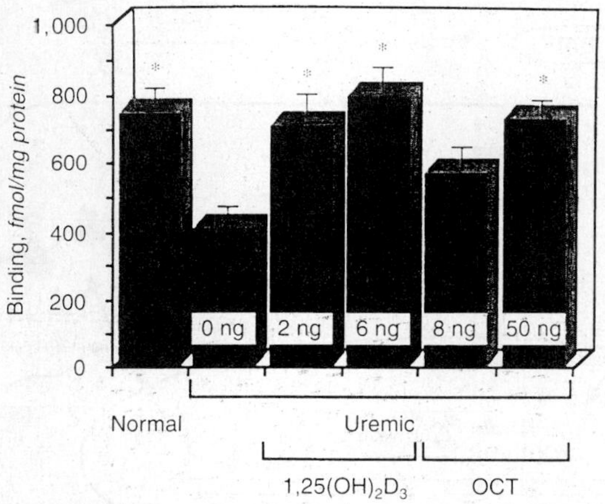

Figure 13.32. The effects of 1,25-$(OH)_2D_3$ and 22-oxa-calcitriol on the vitamin D receptor in the parathyroid glands of uremic rat. (Adapted from Denda M, Finch J, Brown AJ, et al. 1,25-dihydroxy D and 22-oxacalcitriol prevents the decrease in vitamin D receptor in the parathyroid glands in uremic rats. *Kidney Int* 1996;50:34–39.)

VITAMIN D ACTIONS ON NONCLASSICAL TARGET TISSUES

The VDR is expressed in tissues unrelated to mineral homeostasis, which respond to the sterol with a diverse range of biologic actions, including immunomodulation, the control of other hormonal systems, inhibition of cell growth, and induction of cell differentiation. The nonclassical actions summarized in this section have greatly expanded our understanding of the vitamin D endocrine system and have provided valuable clues for the therapeutic application of 1,25-$(OH)_2D_3$ in an increasing number of clinical disorders.

Hematopoietic Tissues

Anemia, decreased bone cellularity, extramedullary erythropoiesis, and a time-dependent reduction in spleen colony forming units have been reported in vitamin D deficiency and vitamin D–deficient rickets. Vitamin D administration rapidly improves the hematopoietic condition by unknown mechanisms.

1,25-$(OH)_2D_3$ inhibits clonal proliferation in a variety of human leukemia cell lines and promotes the differentiation of normal and leukemic myeloid precursors toward more mature, less aggressive phenotypes, thus rendering the sterol potentially useful in the treatment of leukemias and other myeloproliferative disorders.

Several clinical observations suggested a role for vitamin D in immunology before the discovery of the VDR in cells of the immune system. Recurrent infections are commonly associated with vitamin D–deficient rickets, and an impaired defense mechanism often accompanies chronic renal failure, a state of prolonged calcitriol deficiency. In both conditions, the impaired immunity can be improved with calcitriol therapy.

1,25-$(OH)_2D_3$ interacts with mature monocytes and macrophages enhancing their immune function, thus improving host defense against both bacterial infection and tumor cell growth. In addition, 1,25-$(OH)_2D_3$ promotes macrophage survival and function at the increased temperatures associated with tissue inflammation by inducing heat shock protein synthesis.

In contrast to the stimulatory effects of the hormone on monocytes and macrophages, the principal action of 1,25-$(OH)_2D_3$ in lymphocytes is to act as an immunosuppressive agent. It does so by decreasing both the rate of proliferation and the activity of T cells and B cells and by inducing the availability of suppressor T-cells, which further contributes to limiting lymphocyte activity. An important aspect of these immunosuppressive actions of 1,25-$(OH)_2D_3$ is the therapeutic application of the sterol in the control of autoimmune diseases such as systemic lupus erythematosus, rheumatoid arthritis, and juvenile (type I) diabetes.

The production of 1,25-$(OH)_2D_3$ by activated macrophages at sites of active inflammation may represent an autocrine-paracrine system that inhibits further T-cell activation and lymphokine production, thus preventing a potentially self-destructive immune response.

Skin

In the 1930s, vitamin D was used to treat a variety of skin diseases, including psoriasis. It was in the mid-1980s, however, when its therapeutic potential in skin diseases reemerged as a result of the observation that psoriatic lesions dramatically improved in a patient receiving oral 1α-hydroxyvitamin D_3 to treat severe osteoporosis. The antiproliferative and prodifferentiating effects of 1,25-$(OH)_2D_3$ in keratinocytes, melanocytes, and fibroblasts and its immunosuppressive properties on Langerhans cells, the antigen-presenting cells of the skin, have been exploited in the treatment of psoriasis, melanoma, and scleroderma. Alopecia in patients with hereditary vitamin D–resistant rickets and the high expression of VDR in the hair follicle suggest a potential use for vitamin D in the treatment of some forms of hair loss.

Muscle

Skeletal muscle weakness and atrophy, with electrophysiologic abnormalities in muscle contraction and relaxation, often occur in vitamin D deficiency, in calcitriol deficiency caused by chronic renal failure, and with the prolonged use of anticonvulsant agents, which decrease serum 25$(OH)D_3$. In the heart, vitamin D deficiency results in cardiomegaly. 1,25-$(OH)_2D_3$ and 25$(OH)D_3$ improve both the left ventricular function in patients with cardiomyopathies and the skeletal muscle weakness secondary to end-stage renal disease. The mechanisms involved are still unclear.

Pancreas

Vitamin D deficiency results in impaired glucose-mediated insulin secretion, which can be reversed by vitamin D repletion. In uremic patients, calcitriol therapy significantly increases serum insulin concentrations. It has been postulated that 1,25-$(OH)_2D_3$, through a VDR- mediated modulation of calbindin expression, controls intracellular calcium flux in the islet cells, which in turn affects insulin release. The immunomodulatory properties of the sterol have extended its therapeutic application to reducing the incidence of insulinitis and diabetes in animal models for type I diabetes and to preventing the recurrence of autoimmune diabetes after islet transplantation.

VITAMIN D ANALOGS WITH THERAPEUTIC POTENTIAL

The multitude of actions of 1,25-$(OH)_2D_3$ in both classical and nonclassical target cells has suggested potential therapeutic actions of this vitamin D hormone for the treatment of secondary hyperparathyroidism, for immunosuppression, and for hyperproliferative disorders, such as cancer and psoriasis. However,

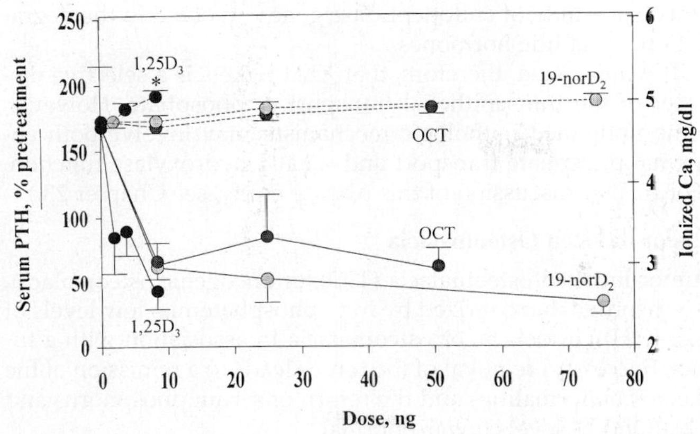

Figure 13.33. Effects of 1,25-$(OH)_2D_3$, OCT and 19-nor-1,25-$(OH)_2D_2$ on serum PTH *(solid lines)* and plasma ionized calcium *(dashed lines)* in uremic rats with secondary hyperparathyroidism. Both analogs effectively suppress PTH over a wide dose range without increasing serum calcium.

the potent calcemic activity of 1,25-$(OH)_2D_3$ has precluded its application in most instances. Advances in the development of vitamin D analogs have produced many compounds with enhanced or selective vitamin D activities, and many candidate analogs are in clinical trials, and one is already in use. Calcipotriol, developed by Leo Pharmaceuticals in Denmark, is now available, under the trade name Dovonex, for the treatment of psoriasis. Several analogs, 22-oxacalcitriol (OCT; Chugai Pharmaceuticals), 19-nor-1,25$(OH)_2D_2$ (Capthrol; Abbott Laboratories), and 1α$(OH)D_2$ (Bone Care International), have been approved for the treatment of secondary hyperparathyroidism. The selectivity of 22-oxacalcitriol and 19-nor-1,25$(OH)_2D_2$ for suppression of PTH in uremic rats with minimal calcemic activity is illustrated in Fig. 13.33. In addition, numerous analogs have shown promise in slowing the growth of tumors on their own, and may be especially useful in enhancing the actions of established anticancer drugs such as tamoxifen. Other analogs have shown impressive immunosuppressive activity in preclinical trials and may be useful, particularly in combination with other immunosuppressives such as cyclosporine, for treatment of autoimmune disorders and in transplantation. Table 13.8 lists analogs and their potential (or proven) application.

The mechanisms responsible for the selective actions of these "noncalcemic" analogs are being elucidated. Differences in pharmacokinetic properties, metabolism, VDR binding, and nongenomic activity have been demonstrated with various analogs. It is likely that one or more of these differences may be responsible for the unique biologic profiles of each analog observed *in vivo*.

CLINICAL DISORDERS OF VITAMIN D METABOLISM

Rickets and Osteomalacia

Osteomalacia and rickets are disorders of mineralization of bone and cartilage. Osteomalacia occurs in adults and is characterized by a defective mineralization of newly formed organic matrix (osteoid) in bones in which the epiphyseal plates have closed. In these patients, tetracycline labeling, an indicator of bone remodeling activity, usually shows a single band, no band, or an irregular and spotty uptake instead of the double bands seen in normal bone. (For further information on the use of bone biopsy for the diagnosis of osteomalacia, see Chapter 98.) In rickets, a disease of children, the growth plate at the epiphysis is also involved. This affects normal mineralization of cartilage, thus resulting in short stature and bone deformities.

A complete description of all causes of rickets and osteomalacia is beyond the scope of this chapter. In this section, the most important forms related to abnormalities in vitamin D metabolism will be described.

Nutritional Vitamin D Deficiency

After the discovery that rickets was caused by vitamin D deficiency, the addition of vitamin D to certain foods reduced the incidence of nutritional rickets in the United States to low levels. By the late 1940s, deficiency of vitamin D was no longer regarded as an important cause of osteomalacia and rickets.

The physiologic amount of vitamin D required in the diet is about 400 IU (10 μg) per day for children and pregnant women and 100 IU for adults. Nutritional deficiency of vitamin D results mainly from poverty, but ignorance and certain food habits (faddism) are also important factors to be considered. In addition, nutritional deficiency of vitamin D is frequently observed in alcoholics, institutionalized patients, and the elderly.

TABLE 13.8. Therapeutically Active Vitamin D Analogs

Application	Preclinical	Clinical	Approval	Source
Psoriasis				
Calcipotriol (Dovonex)	X	X	X	Leo Pharmaceuticals
22-oxacalcitriol (OCT)	X	X		Chugai Pharmaceuticals
Renal Osteodystrophy				
22-oxacalcitriol (OCT)	X	X	X	Chugai Pharmaceuticals
19-nor-1,25$(OH)_2D_2$	X	X	X	Abbott Laboratories
1α-$(OH)D_2$		X	X	Bone Care International
Cancer				
Calcipotriol		X		Leo Pharmaceuticals
EB1089	X			Leo Pharmaceuticals
22-oxacalcitriol (OCT)	X			Chugai Pharmaceuticals
1,25$(OH)_2$-16-ene-23-yne-F_6-D_3	X			Hoffmann-La Roche
1,25$(OH)_2$-16-ene-23-yne-D_3	X			Hoffmann-La Roche
1,22(S),25$(OH)_3$-24-homo-F_6-D_3	X			
Immunosuppression				
KH1060	X			Leo Pharmaceuticals
MC1288	X			Leo Pharmaceuticals
Osteoporosis				
ED-71	X			Chugai Pharmaceuticals

Vitamin D Malasorption

Intestinal malabsorption may result in a decreased absorption of vitamin D and calcium and depletion of endogenous 25-(OH)D stores. Ingested vitamin D is absorbed primarily in chylomicrons. Disorders that involve the biliary tract, the small intestine, and pancreas, resulting in an abnormal enterohepatic circulation, reduce the absorption of vitamin D. Clinical conditions, such as intestinal bypass surgery, adult celiac disease, regional enteritis, and cholestatic disease treated with cholestyramine, are frequently associated with vitamin D malabsorption. The majority of these patients, however, have asymptomatic bone disease. Characteristically, the levels of 25-(OH)D are very low in vitamin D malabsorption syndromes.

Liver Disease

The liver plays a key role in vitamin D metabolism. Because 25-(OH)D, the first metabolite in the activation of vitamin D, is synthesized in the liver, advanced liver disease may reduce the production of this metabolite. However, the low levels of 25-(OH)D found in patients with liver disease are usually attributed to reduced synthesis of DBP, poor nutrition, or malabsorption rather than to failure of the liver to metabolize vitamin D.

Nephrotic Syndrome

Abnormalities in vitamin D and calcium metabolism in patients with nephrotic syndrome are not uncommon. Patients with nephrotic syndrome and heavy proteinuria excrete a substantial amount of DBP in the urine. Consequently, they have a decrease in serum vitamin D metabolites. However, the concentration of the free, active form of 1,25-$(OH)_2D_3$ remains constant when DBP levels change, an indication of the tight self-regulation of vitamin D metabolism. Thus the measurement of the total concentration of calcitriol may be misleading in assessing the severity of vitamin D deficiency.

Occasionally, patients with nephrotic syndrome with very low levels of 25-(OH)D and evidence of secondary hyperparathyroidism or metabolic bone disease may require treatment with vitamin D metabolites. (For further discussion of vitamin D metabolism and calcium homeostasis, see Chapter 39.)

Anticonvulsant Osteomalacia

Anticonvulsant drugs (diphenylhydantoin and phenobarbital) are capable of inducing the activity of hepatic microsomal mixed function oxidases. Induction of this enzyme system leads to increased catabolism of vitamin D and 25-(OH)D to inactive metabolites. Thus long-term anticonvulsant drug therapy is associated with a marked decrease in the plasma half-life of vitamin D and an increased appearance of polar metabolites.

X-Linked Hypophosphatemic Rickets

Another form of osteomalacia, characterized by severe hypophosphatemia and alterations in vitamin D metabolism, is X-linked hypophosphatemic rickets. This is an X-linked dominant disorder of variable phenotypic expression (males are generally more severely affected than carrier females) that usually presents with bowed legs when ambulation begins. Hypophosphatemia is apparent in the first days of life.

Most patients with X-linked hypophosphatemic (XLH) rickets have normal serum values for 25-(OH)D and 1,25-$(OH)_2D_3$. However, in the presence of hypophosphatemia, an elevation in serum levels of 1,25- $(OH)_2D_3$ would be anticipated. Thus an abnormal response of the renal 1-hydroxylase to hypophosphatemia is seen in XLH rickets.

The gene responsible for this disorder (PEX) was isolated by positional cloning from Xp22.1 (the hyp locus). It is homologous to a family of endopeptidase genes involved in the degradation of peptide hormones.

It would seem, therefore, that XLH rickets is a selective disorder of the transepithelial transport of phosphate. However, some undefined pathologic mechanism may involve both abnormal phosphate transport and renal 1-hydroxylase function. (For further discussion of this disease entity, see Chapter 23.)

Tumor-Induced Osteomalacia

Tumor-induced osteomalacia (TIO), or oncogenic osteomalacia, is a disorder characterized by hypophosphatemia, low levels of 1,25-$(OH)_2D_3$, rickets, or osteomalacia in association with a tumor. Successful removal of the tumor leads to a remission of the skeletal abnormalities and the return of serum phosphorus and 1,25-$(OH)_2D_3$ levels toward normal.

Although the pathogenesis of TIO remains unknown, undoubtedly the tumor produces a factor that blocks the 25-(OH)D-1-hydroxylase enzyme, which explains the low levels of 1,25-$(OH)_2D_3$ in these patients. From the therapeutic point of view, complete resection of the tumor is generally accompanied by a correction of the biochemical and skeletal abnormalities.

Vitamin D–Dependent Rickets

Vitamin D–dependent rickets is a rare disorder characterized by symptoms and signs of rickets or osteomalacia. Currently, two main forms of vitamin D-dependent rickets have been characterized. The serum concentration of 1,25-$(OH)_2D_3$ serves to differentiate the two types of vitamin D-dependent rickets. Levels of 1,25-$(OH)_2D_3$ are low in type I and elevated in type II.

Vitamin D–dependent rickets type I (VDDR-type I) is a rare disease characterized by an autosomal recessive trait. At birth, affected children are healthy, but during the first years of life, they develop severe hypocalcemic episodes characterized by carpopedal spasm, laryngospastic crisis, and seizures. In addition to hypocalcemia, other biochemical abnormalities are hypophosphatemia and elevated plasma alkaline phosphatase. Secondary hyperparathyroidism resulting from hypocalcemia is present in the majority of these patients. There is now sufficient information to assign the cause of vitamin D dependency to an inborn error in conversion of 25-(OH)D to 1,25-$(OH)_2D_3$, resulting from deficiency of the renal 1-hydroxylase enzyme. The levels of 25-(OH)D are normal, whereas those of 1,25-$(OH)_2D_3$ are profoundly decreased. The 1α-hydroxylase gene has been cloned and shown to reside at the chromosomal locus to which this genetic disorder has been mapped. Furthermore, specific point mutations in the 1α-hydroxylase coding sequence have been identified in patients with VDDR- type I. Long-term administration of calcitriol (0.5 to 1.5 μg per day) is required to prevent the development of hypocalcemia and secondary hyperparathyroidism.

End-organ resistance to 1,25-$(OH)_2D_3$ caused by mutations in functional domains of the VDR has been proposed as the pathophysiologic mechanism involved in vitamin D–dependent rickets, type II (VDDR type II). The clinical features of VDDR type II appear early in life. Plasma levels of 1,25-$(OH)_2D_3$ are elevated. This finding, in association with radiographic and biochemical signs of rickets, implies resistance of the target tissue to calcitriol. This disease is more heterogenous than type I, but also appears to follow an autosomal recessive pattern of inheritance. Alopecia and abnormal teeth are frequently observed. Hypocalcemia, hypophosphatemia, and secondary hyperparathyroidism are commonly found. Plasma 25-(OH)D levels are normal. High levels of circulating 1,25-$(OH)_2D_3$ are critical in making the diagnosis.

Numerous mutations in the VDR gene have been identified. These mutations result in alterations in the functional domains of the VDR critical for 1,25-$(OH)_2D_3$ binding, cytoplasmic to nuclear translocation, heterodimerization with RXR, or interactions with vitamin D responsive elements in target genes. These defective VDRs result in various degrees of end-organ resistance to 1,25-$(OH)_2D_3$. The most severe clinical forms correspond to those mutations affecting the capability of the VDR to bind DNA.

The treatment of this condition requires large pharmacologic doses of vitamin D or calcitriol. The amount of 1,25-$(OH)_2D_3$ ranges between 5 to 30 μg per day. This disease entity is also discussed in Chapter 23.

Chronic Renal Failure

The kidney is the major site for conversion of 25-(OH)D to its active metabolite 1,25-$(OH)_2D_3$. Thus alterations in mineral homeostasis and skeletal disease can be expected in advanced renal failure. Because one of the main actions of vitamin D is to stimulate intestinal transport of calcium, it is easy to understand why the absorption of calcium from the intestine is decreased in patients with far-advanced renal insufficiency and low levels of 1,25-$(OH)_2D_3$. Increased levels of I-PTH have been found in patients with moderately abnormal renal function, as shown in Fig. 13.34.

Although the levels of 1,25-$(OH)_2D_3$ in most patients with advanced renal failure [glomerular filtration rate (GFR) less than 20 ml/min] are low, many patients lack histologic features of vitamin D deficiency. Thus reduced synthesis of 1,25-$(OH)_2D_3$ may not be the only factor responsible for the development of osteomalacia in this group of patients. Perhaps the normal to elevated serum phosphorus levels protect some uremic patients from osteomalacia. The role of decreased generation of other vitamin D metabolites, particularly 24,25-$(OH)_2D_3$, in the pathogenesis of osteomalacia remains uncertain. It should be emphasized, however, that the most common cause of osteomalacia in dialysis patients is aluminum accumulation and not lack of vitamin D. (For further discussion of the effect of aluminium on bone, see Chapter 68, Part 2.)

As described previously, 1,25-$(OH)_2D_3$ plays a key role in the regulation of the synthesis and secretion of PTH. An insensitivity to the suppressive effects of calcium on PTH secretion has been shown in glands obtained from patients with chronic renal failure. This observations suggests that one mechanism for increased PTH levels in chronic renal failure may be a decreased sensitivity for calcium-regulated PTH secretion in addition to an increase in the mass of parathyroid tissue. In part, this may result from decrease in the calcium receptor (CaR) that is localized in the membrane of the parathyroid cells and renal tubules.

It has been shown that uremic patients, dogs, and rats have low levels of vitamin D receptors in parathyroid glands. Because the VDR mediates the control of gene transcription by 1,25-$(OH)_2D_3$, the reduction in VDR levels in the parathyroid gland in CRF may determine the impaired response to calcitriol in these patients.

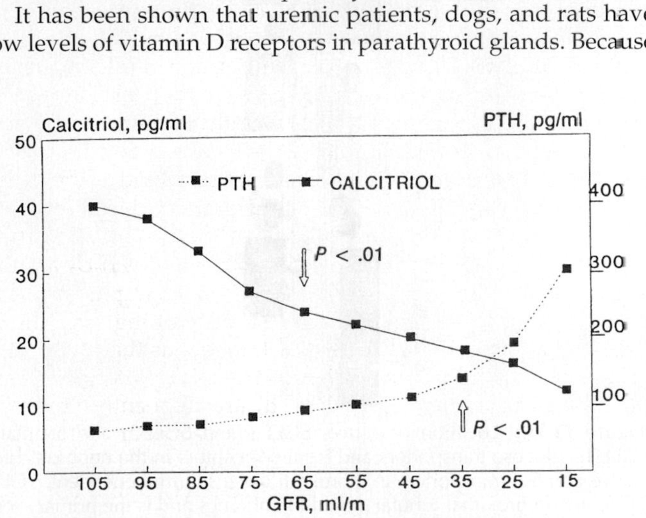

Figure 13.34. Calcitriol and PTH values in 150 patients with various levels of chronic renal failure. (Adapted from Martinez I, Saracho R, Montenegro J, et al. A deficit of calcitriol synthesis may not be the initial factor in the pathogenesis of secondary hyperparathyroidism. *Nephrol Dial Transplant* 1996; 53:22–28.)

Results of several clinical trials indicate the efficacy of 1,25-$(OH)_2D_3$ in treating patients with symptomatic renal osteodystrophy. These clinical evaluations have shown a decrease in bone pain, an improvement in muscle strength, and a decrease in plasma alkaline phosphatase. Studies of bone histology have revealed a prominent decrease in marrow fibrosis and other features of secondary hyperparathyroidism.

The intravenous administration of calcitriol markedly reduced the serum levels of PTH in hemodialysis patients. The suppression of PTH during intravenous administration of calcitriol was greater than that occurring after raising serum calcium levels with oral calcium carbonate. The possible greater suppressive effects of intravenous calcitriol versus oral calcitriol may relate to the high concentrations of calcitriol in serum following intravenous administration. Studies *in vitro* have clearly demonstrated that the suppression of PTH secretion by calcitriol is dose dependent. Studies on oral "pulse" calcitriol administration (2.0 to 3.0 μg twice per week) demonstrated significant suppression of PTH levels. (For further discussion on the abnormalities in phosphorus, calcium, vitamin D, PTH, bone and in the use of 1,25-$(OH)_2D_3$ in patients with chronic renal failure see Chapter 77.)

Sarcoidosis

Sarcoidosis, a granulomatous disease usually seen in young adults, is frequently associated with hypercalcemia and hypercalciuria caused by the endogenous overproduction of 1,25-$(OH)_2D_3$. In patients with sarcoidosis, mild elevations in serum 25-$(OH)D_3$ due to vitamin D administration or exposure to sunlight cause an increase in serum 1,25-$(OH)_2D_3$ to supraphysiologic levels. The extrarenal origin of the excessive calcitriol production was conclusively demonstrated by the finding of a high serum 1,25-$(OH)_2D_3$ level in an anephric patient with sarcoidosis. Disease-activated macrophages were identified as a source of the sterol in these patients.

Vitamin D–mediated hypercalcemia has also been documented in other granulomatous processes such as tuberculosis, disseminated candidiasis, ruptured silicone implants, and leprosy. The strong correlation between the concentrations of free 1,25-$(OH)_2D_3$ and γ-interferon in the pleural fluid of patients with tuberculosis suggests that γ-interferon stimulates the production of 1,25-$(OH)_2D_3$ by pleura-based macrophages.

Hypercalcemia of Malignancy

Primary hyperparathyroidism and malignancy are the two most important causes of hypercalcemia. The levels of 1,25-$(OH)_2D_3$ are usually elevated in hyperparathyroidism and low in humoral hypercalcemia of malignancy (HHM).

An elevation in the levels of serum 1,25-$(OH)_2D_3$ has been shown in some patients with HTLV-1–associated T-cell lymphoma or leukemia). PTH is normal or suppressed. In some patients, effective antitumor chemotherapy decreased the levels of 1,25-$(OH)_2D_3$ and calcium to normal. (For further discussion on hypercalcemia of malignancy, see Chapter 17, Part 3.)

Selected Readings

Brown AJ, Dusso A, Slatopolsky E. Selective vitamin D analogs and their therapeutic applications. *Semin Nephrol* 1994;14:156–174.

An overview of the development of selective vitamin D analogs, their biologic profiles in vivo, potential therapeutic applications, and possible mechanisms for their selectivity.

Denda M, Finch J, Brown AJ, et al. 1,25-dihydroxyvitamin D and 22-oxacalcitriol prevent the decrease in vitamin D receptor in the parathyroid glands of uremic rats. *Kidney Intern* 1996;50:34–39.

This article demonstrates that 1,25-$(OH)_2D_3$ and its analog, 22-oxcalcitriol, prevents decrease of the VDR in uremic rats.

Fraser DR, Kodicek E. Unique biosynthesis by kidney of a biologically active vitamin D metabolite. *Nature* 1970;228:764–766.

This paper was the first to demonstrate the production of the molecule later confirmed to be 1,25-$(OH)_2D_3$. Their data indicated that the kidney is the major site of 1,25-$(OH)_2D_3$ synthesis.

Lemire JM. Immunomodulatory role of 1,25-dihydroxyvitamin D_3. *J Cellular Biochem* 1992;49:26–31.

Review of the mechanisms involved in the modulation of the immune system by 1,25-dihydroxyvitamin D_3 and the potential of the sterol in immunosuppression and the control of autoimmune diseases.

Ozono K, Sone T, Pike JW. The genomic mechanism of action of 1,25-$(OH)_2D_3$. J Bone Mineral Res 1991;6:1021–1027.

This article reviews the vitamin D receptor–mediated actions of 1,25-$(OH)_2D_3$. The current mechanism for interactions of the receptor with 1,25-$(OH)_2D_3$, the newly described accessory factor and specific DNA sequences identified in several target genes is presented.

Silver J, Naveh-Many T, Mayer H, et al. Regulation by vitamin D metabolites of parathyroid gene transcription *in vivo* in the rat. *J Clin Invest* 1986;78:1296–1301.

This article describes the suppression of PTH gene transcription by calcitriol in vivo in rats.

Slatopolsky E, Weerts C, Thielan J, et al. Marked suppression of secondary hyperparathyroidism by intravenous administration of 1,25-dihydroxycholecalciferol in uremic patients. *J Clin Invest* 1984;74:2136–2143.

This article described for the first time the suppressive effects of intravenous calcitriol in dialyzed patients.

Suda T, Takahashi N, Abe E. Role of vitamin D in bone resorption. *J Cellular Biochem* 1992;49:53–58.

This article describes the direct role of 1,25-$(OH)_2D_3$ on osteoclast differentiation and its indirect action on osteoblastic activity modulating bone remodeling.

Walters M. Newly identified actions of the vitamin D endocrine system. *Endocrine Rev* 1992;13:719–764.

The various mechanisms, both genomic and nongenomic, for the actions of 1,25-$(OH)_2D_3$ are reviewed.

PART 12
Insulin, Insulin-like Growth Factor I, Somatostatin, and Glucagon

Raimund Hirschberg

Insulin, glucagon, insulinlike growth factor I (IGF-I), and somatostatin are peptide hormones with important metabolic activities that are relevant to renal physiology and pathophysiology. Moreover, in renal failure, there are alterations in the kinetics and/or activities of these hormones. This chapter reviews these issues as they relate specifically to the kidney and renal disease.

INSULIN

German pathologists first demonstrated the concept of an antidiabetic hormone of pancreatic origin more than a century ago. Several investigators contributed to the purification of pancreatic extracts until Banting, Best, and Collip filed a patent on insulin in 1923. J. Abel crystallized the hormone in 1926, and Sanger determined the primary structure in 1959. Proinsulin (86–amino acid residues) is synthesized in pancreatic islet β-cells and gives rise to insulin (molecular weight 5.8 kD) and C-peptide after proteolytic cleavage.

Insulin acts through specific, high-affinity tyrosine kinase receptors that are widely distributed in tissues. These receptors are heterodimers with two α- (extracellular binding domain) and two β-subunits (containing tyrosine kinase activity) of 135 and 95 kD, respectively. Binding of insulin causes autophosphorylation of the β-subunits, and activation of the receptor tyrosine kinase leads to activation of a series of tyrosine kinase signaling molecules in effector cells. Activation of transcription factors is associated with cell growth (insulin is a weak mitogen) and transcription of several other genes. Other signaling pathways regulate the activity of metabolic enzymes, resulting in glycogen synthesis, inhibition of lipolysis and β-oxidation of free fatty acids and ketogenesis, reduction in protein and amino acid catabolism, and an increase in protein synthesis and amino acid utilization.

One of the major functions of insulin is the regulation of glucose uptake into cells. Transmembranous glucose transport occurs through different isoforms of glucose transporters (GLUT-1 through GLUT-5). These facilitative transport proteins differ in their affinity for glucose, sensitivity to insulin (or lack thereof), and tissue distribution. In addition, two active, energy-dependent, insulin-independent sodium-glucose cotransporters, SGLT-1 and SGLT-2, are expressed in the gastrointestinal tract and in the kidney (Fig. 13.35).

GLUT-1 is found in brain, erythrocyte membranes, and fibroblasts and is weakly insulin sensitive. GLUT-3, which has similar tissue distribution GLUT-1, most likely facilitates basal glucose uptake. GLUT-2 (liver and islet β-cells) and GLUT-5 (kidney, small intestine, and brain) have low affinity for glucose. The Michaelis constant of GLUT-2 (Km = 7 to 17 mM) is higher than physiologic serum glucose levels and its transport capacity increases parallel to a rise in serum glucose. GLUT-2 in β-cells apparently serves as the glucose sensor important in the regulation

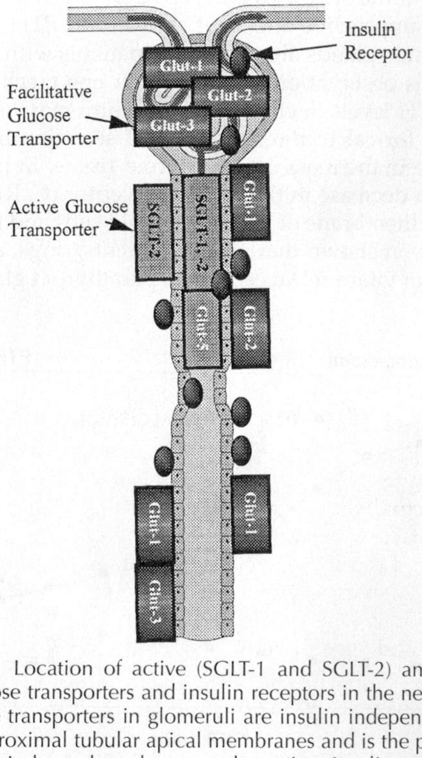

Figure 13.35. Location of active (SGLT-1 and SGLT-2) and facilitative (GLUTs) glucose transporters and insulin receptors in the nephron. Facilitative glucose transporters in glomeruli are insulin independent. SGLT-1 is located in proximal tubular apical membranes and is the primary regulator of insulin-independent glucose reabsorption. Insulin receptors in the apical and basolateral membranes in proximal tubules may primarily serve as scavenger receptors in the degradation of insulin.

of insulin release. GLUT-5 has a high affinity for fructose and probably functions in the facilitated uptake of this sugar. GLUT-4 is the high-affinity, highly insulin-sensitive glucose transporter in adipose tissue, skeletal muscle, and the heart. It is unclear how insulin regulates the activity of this transport protein. The Michaelis constant of high-affinity GLUTs is below normal serum glucose levels, resulting in near-maximal transport at euglycemia.

SGLT-1 and SGLT-2 are densely expressed in the intestine and proximal tubules in the kidney. SGLT-1, which has a high glucose affinity (Km = 0.12 mM) and a Na^+–D-glucose coupling ratio of 2:1, is located in the apical (brush border) membrane of proximal tubules in the kidney. There are also low-affinity transporters, SGLT-2, expressed in brush border membranes with a Km of 1.9 mM and a coupling ratio of 1:1. There is evidence for the expression of GLUT-5 in brush border membranes, but its role in glucose absorption is unclear. Because this protein has a high affinity for fructose, it may serve in the absorption of this latter hexose. Both SGLTs are not regulated by insulin and contribute to glucose homeostasis by gastrointestinal and renal tubular absorption from glomerular ultrafiltrate.

The basolateral expression of facilitative glucose transporters in renal tubules (Fig. 13.35) and their presence in glomerular tufts indicate their service in the provision of glucose as metabolic fuel. To satisfy the greater energy demand, the expression of GLUTs is greater in the medulla than in the cortex. However, the absorption of filtered glucose in proximal tubules follows active transport kinetics through apical SGLTs and is insulin independent. After uptake from tubular fluid, transport of glucose from tubular cells to peritubular capillary blood across the basolateral membrane occurs by concentration gradient-driven facilitated transport through high-affinity, low-capacity GLUT-1 and low-affinity, high-capacity GLUT-2. Hence, glucose absorption in proximal tubules is insulin independent.

GLUCAGON

Glucagon, a peptide hormone with 29 amino acid residues (molecular weight 3.5 kD), is secreted from α-cells in pancreatic islets but is also expressed in certain cells in the small intestine (enteroglucagon) and the hypothalamus. Pancreatic glucagon secretion is primarily glycemia regulated. Glucagon acts through G-protein–coupled glucagon receptors that are densely expressed in the liver but are also found in kidney. Glucagon generally opposes insulin actions.

IGF-I

IGF-I is a 7.5-kD peptide growth factor that is expressed in many tissues, circulates in serum, and acts in many target tissues by endocrine, paracrine, and/or autocrine modes. Growth hormone is the strongest secretagogue for IGF-I, and the peptide was actually discovered as a peripheral mediator of several biologic effects of growth hormone (somatomedin).

IGF-I acts through specific, high-affinity tyrosine kinase receptors that share functional and structural similarities with insulin receptors. IGF-I also binds with low affinity to insulin receptors, and insulin activates IGF-I receptors at high (pharmacologic) concentrations. IGF-I receptors are expressed in most segments of the nephron (Fig. 13.36). In several nephron segments, IGF-I and IGF-I receptors are coexpressed, giving rise to autocrine and paracrine modes of action (Fig. 13.36). However, in proximal tubules, IGF-I is not expressed, suggesting endocrine modes of actions in this part of the nephron.

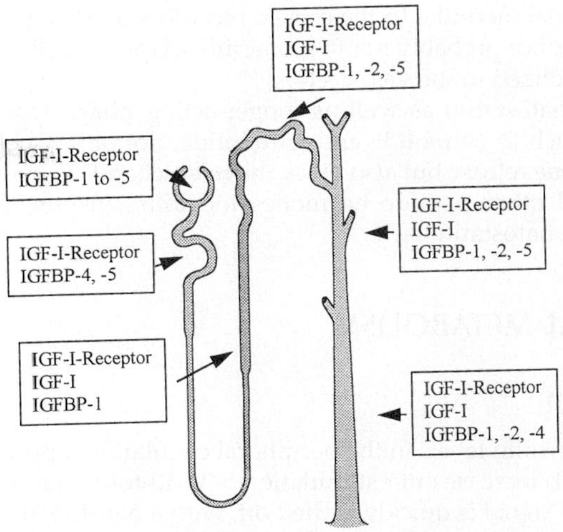

Figure 13.36. Expression of IGF-I receptors, IGF-I, and IGFBPs in the nephron. Note that proximal tubules express IGF-I receptors but lack the peptide. This suggests endocrine action of IGF-I in this part of the nephron. In most other nephron segments, IGF-I may act by paracrine/autocrine as well as by endocrine modes.

In serum, more than 99% of IGF-I is associated with IGF-binding proteins (IGFBPs) to form approximately 50- and 150-kD molecular forms of circulating IGF-I. Six different IGFBPs have been identified thus far. IGFBP-3 is the most abundant IGFBP in serum. This protein associates with another protein, the acid-labile subunit, to form a high-affinity complex with IGF-I of approximately 150 kD. As a rule, IGFBPs are coexpressed with IGF-I. Generally, IGFBPs compete locally with receptors for IGF-I binding and, hence, contribute to the regulation of IGF-I bioactivity. The kidney expresses at least IGFBP-1 through IGFBP-6, and IGFBP-5 is particularly abundant. This latter binding protein adheres to extracellular-matrix proteins and may provide a local reservoir for IGF-I. The regulation of IGF-I bioactivity is further complicated by the presence of specific (and possibly nonspecific) IGFBP-proteases that liberate IGF-I from binding protein complexes by proteolysis of IGFBPs.

IGF-I has many different biologic actions. As a (weak) mitogen, it accelerates the cell cycle at a G_1/S-transition point and promotes mitosis. IGF-I also induces cell and tissue growth by causing hypertrophy. The peptide raises protein synthesis and decreases protein degradation. It blocks apoptosis of injured cells. Moreover, in the kidney, IGF-I increases renal function and tubular transport of some solutes.

SOMATOSTATIN

Somatostatin was originally discovered in the hypothalamus as a 1.4-kD peptide that blocks pituitary growth hormone release. In addition to its synthesis in the hypothalamus and other parts of the brain (where the peptide may serve as a neurotransmitter), somatostatin is also expressed in the stomach, small intestine, and pancreas. The gastrointestinal tract is most likely the source for most of the circulating peptide. The kidney also may express somatostatin. Specific mRNA has been found in human renal cortex, and both somatostatin mRNA and secreted peptide are present in cultured mesangial cells.

Somatostatin acts through G-protein coupled receptors (SSTR). Five different receptors have been identified (SSTR-1 to SSTR-5) with broad distribution in peripheral tissues. High-affinity somatostatin receptors are expressed in renal cortex and renal medulla. In the cortex, receptors localize to proximal tubules but probably not to glomeruli. In the medulla, receptors are localized in the vasa recta.

Somatostatin, as well as longer-acting pharmacologic analogs such as octreotide and lantreotide, not only block growth hormone release but also block the release (and/or synthesis) of several other peptide hormones including insulin, glucagon, and somatostatin itself.

RENAL METABOLISM

Insulin

Basal insulin levels in the peripheral circulation (approximately 100 pM) increase after stimulation 5- to 10-fold. This stimulated insulin signal is quickly turned off, with a half-life of 5 minutes or less. The liver takes up about 50% of insulin from the portal circulation during the first pass, but the kidney accounts for as much as 40% of insulin degradation. Hence, the kidneys play a major role in regulating insulin bioactivity. In the kidney, insulin is eliminated from the circulation by glomerular ultrafiltration and subsequent uptake through proximal tubular apical membranes as well as by extraction from serum through basolateral uptake. Degradation occurs largely by internalization of occupied insulin receptors into endosomes and intracellular proteolysis by specific enzymes such as insulin-degrading enzyme (IDE, a metalloprotease) or glutathione-insulin-transhydrogenase (GIT).

About 30% of ultrafiltered insulin binds to low-affinity sites, probably megalin (gp500, formerly termed gp330), a scavenger receptor in coated pits of the brush border membrane. Megalin binds several ligands such as vitamins that are then recovered by transcytosis or undergo lysosomal degradation by fusion of the internalized receptor with lysosomes. Lysosomal degradation may account for one-third of insulin degradation in proximal tubules. In patients with chronic renal failure, the half-life of insulin is prolonged. This may account for the reduced dosage of exogenous insulin necessary to maintain euglycemia in diabetic patients with chronic renal failure.

Glucagon

The kidney's contribution to the degradation of glucagon appears less important. There is evidence for both luminal and basolateral uptake of glucagon in proximal tubules.

IGF-I

The serum half-life of free IGF-I is short, less than 5 minutes, but is prolonged by binding to IGFBPs. In normal subjects, IGF-I is excreted with urine. However, urinary IGF-I is most likely derived from collecting ducts, where the peptide is abundantly expressed, rather than from glomerular ultrafiltration. In contrast, in the nephrotic syndrome IGF-I/IGFBP complexes undergo glomerular ultrafiltration and the urinary excretion of IGF-I is increased.

IGF-I is taken up by proximal tubules through basolateral membranes. However, the contribution of the kidney to the degradation of this peptide is minimal. In patients with renal failure, the serum half-life of IGF-I is decreased rather than increased. Serum levels of IGF-I are also not different in renal failure patients compared with normal subjects. However, in a subgroup of malnourished, chronic maintenance dialysis patients, serum IGF-I levels are reduced, most likely a result rather than the cause of their catabolic and malnourished state.

In patients with chronic renal failure, there is increased activity of IGFBP-proteases, most notably for IGFBP-3, resulting in reduced serum levels of intact IGFBP-3 and increased levels of fragments with reduced IGF-I binding. Whether this results in increased or reduced IGF-I bioactivity is unknown.

In patients with nephrotic syndrome, there are complex abnormalities in the IGF/IGFBP system. Glomerular ultrafiltration of IGF-I–containing protein complexes results in approximately 30% reduced serum IGF-I levels. In nephrotic syndrome, IGFBP-3 undergoes proteolytic degradation and serum levels are reduced. High activities of the IGFBP-3 protease(s) are found in urine, suggesting renal origin of the enzyme(s). In contrast, liver synthesis and plasma levels of IGFBP-2 are increased more than twofold. Reduced serum IGFBP-3 and increased IGFBP-2 levels result in a shift of serum IGF-I from a high (approximately 150 kD) to lower (approximately 50 kD) molecular form, which may increase its availability to target tissues.

The ultrafiltration of IGF-I into tubular fluid in nephrotic syndrome exposes apical tubular membranes to abnormally great amounts of the peptide. Because specific IGF-I–signaling receptors are expressed in apical membranes in proximal and distal tubules, ultrafiltered IGF-I has pathophysiologic actions through this mode and may contribute to renal sodium retention, tubulointerstitial infiltration with monocytes/macrophages, and fibrosis.

Somatostatin

There is some evidence that somatostatin is, to a moderate extent, metabolized by the kidney. The kidney's overall contribution to somatostatin degradation is unclear.

RENAL ACTIONS

Effects on Renal and Nephron Growth

Nephron and kidney growth occur in many clinical and experimental settings. Kidneys undergo compensatory growth after unilateral or subtotal nephrectomy in humans or experimental animals as well as in individual surviving nephrons in chronic renal diseases. In patients with diabetes mellitus, kidney growth precedes the development of nephropathy and is associated with increased size and length of nephrons. Chronic potassium depletion also causes kidney hypertrophy. In all these conditions, increased renal expression of IGF-I has been associated with the initial, rapid phase of renal growth. Exogenous administration of rhIGF-I to rats causes (selective) renal growth.

Hyperinsulinemia has been implicated in the mechanisms that cause kidney growth in diabetes mellitus. Insulin is a weak mitogen and contributes to protein synthesis. Insulin has a low affinity to IGF-I receptors, and renal expression of IGF-I receptors is increased in diabetes. Hence, endogenous and/or exogenous insulin may contribute to renal hypertrophy in diabetes.

Longstanding renal/nephron hypertrophy may cause glomerular and tubulointerstitial fibrosis and chronic renal failure. *In vitro,* IGF-I increases the expression of extracellular-matrix proteins, which may contribute to the progression of chronic renal failure.

Several experimental studies have indicated that somatostatin or its analogs reduce the degree of renal growth after partial nephrectomy as well as in experimental diabetes in the rat. In rats, the analogs octreotide and lantreotide prevent or postpone the development of diabetic nephropathy. Somatostatin reduces renal (and systemic) IGF-I levels as well as growth hormone secretion, and the reduction in both hormones may be the major mechanisms through which somatostatin prevents renal growth in these disease settings. In cultured mesangial and proximal tubular cells, somatostatin is antiproliferative. Somatostatin may also reduce proliferation of monocytes/macrophages in glomeruli and interstitium.

Effects on Renal Hemodynamics and Glomerular Ultrafiltration

Administration of a protein-rich meal or intravenous infusions of amino acids cause a transient increase in glomerular filtration rate (GFR) of 15% to 20% in normal subjects. This rise is preceded by an amino acid–induced increase in serum insulin, glucagon (and growth hormone), and several other peptides mainly of gastrointestinal origin. Although insulin in very large doses was found to modestly increase GFR in rats, it is unlikely that this plays any regulatory role in humans. Insulin partially antagonizes the action of angiotensin II on smooth muscle cells or mesangial cell contraction *in vitro,* but this effect has no major significance *in vivo.*

Exogenous infusion of glucagon to mimic the postprandial rise in serum glucagon levels decreases renal vascular resistance and raises renal blood flow and GFR. In studies in dogs, infusion of glucagon into the portal circulation had a more dramatic effect on renal hemodynamics than direct intrarenal or systemic infusion. These findings suggest that glucagon induces a liver-borne substance that raises renal function. This mediator could be cyclic adenosine monophosphate (cAMP), which is induced by glucagon in the liver, circulates in serum, and raises renal hemodynamics.

Administration of somatostatin analogs increases renal vascular resistance and lowers GFR. Somatostatin analogs also reduce glomerular hyperfiltration in experimental diabetes in rats. Because somatostatin blocks the release of many peptide hormones, several of which have weak renal hemodynamic activity, the somatostatin-induced reduction in GFR may be a secondary effect. However, the peptide also has direct effects on the glomerulus, such as induction of prostaglandin E. It is unclear how this activity relates to the hemodynamic effects of somatostatin.

IGF-I reduces renal vascular resistance and raises GFR by reducing afferent and efferent arteriolar resistance and increasing the glomerular ultrafiltration coefficient. These actions are mediated through vasodilating prostaglandins and nitric oxide.

Exogenous rhIGF-I increases renal function in rats, in normal subjects, and in patients with chronic renal failure. This has led to open-label clinical studies of rhIGF-I in patients with advanced renal failure. Administration of rhIGF-I in patients with chronic renal failure raises GFR modestly, but the overall clinical benefit of such treatment is unclear.

In addition to its renal hemodynamic effects, rhIGF-I has further biologic activities that suggest its potential utility in the therapy of acute renal failure (ARF). IGF-I is mitogenic and reduces the incidence of apoptosis in injured cultured renal cells *in vitro* and in injured tubules *in vivo.* Moreover, the peptide increases protein synthesis and reduces protein degradation. In rats with experimental ARF, rhIGF-I accelerates the recovery of renal function and reduces mortality. However, in two clinical trials, its effects were far less impressive. In a single-center, blind, randomized clinical trial, rhIGF-I was given to patients shortly after abdominal aortic aneurysm surgery. The incidence of ARF was very low, and the study could not test the effects of rhIGF-I on the recovery from ARF. After 3 days of rhIGF-I therapy, subjects had a small increase in creatinine clearance, whereas patients treated with a placebo demonstrated a minor decline in creatinine clearance (Fig. 13.37). There was no difference in serum creatinine at hospital discharge, nor was there a difference in the length of hospital stay between the two groups. In another multicenter, blind, randomized clinical trial,

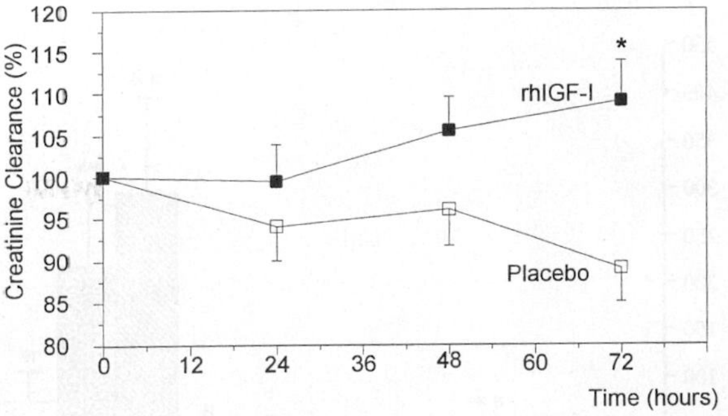

Figure 13.37. Change in creatinine clearance in patients who underwent abdominal aortic surgery and were treated with rhIGF-I or a placebo for the 3 days after the operation. *$p < .05$. However, there was no difference in serum creatinine at 3 days after surgery, and treatment with rhIGF-I did not affect mortality or length of hospital stay. (Reprinted with permission from Hammerman M, Miller S. Effects of growth hormone and insulin-like growth factor I on renal growth and function. J Pediatr 1997;131:S17–S19.)

patients with established ARF who were in the intensive care unit received rhIGF-I for up to 14 days. As compared with those patients treated with the placebo, subjects treated with rhIGF-I did not have accelerated recovery of renal function, improved urine excretion, or reduced mortality.

Effects on Renal Tubular Function

Sodium Absorption

Insulin, glucagon, and IGF-I affect renal sodium absorption. Administration of insulin decreases urinary sodium excretion and increases sodium absorption. In these studies, euglycemia was maintained by a glucose clamp. The effect of insulin on sodium absorption is not caused by increased proximal Na-linked glucose absorption, and insulin stimulated Na-Pi cotransport in proximal tubules is unlikely to account for the magnitude of the effect. There is evidence that insulin raises sodium absorption in the thick ascending limb of Henle's loop. Administration of IGF-I to (volume expanded) normal subjects very transiently and only to a minor extent decreases sodium excretion. Neither luminal perfusion nor basolateral perifusion of rabbit proximal tubules with rhIGF-I nor exposure of cultured proximal tubular cells to the peptide affects Na transport. However, there is experimental evidence suggesting IGF-I increases distal tubular sodium absorption. In some patients with type II diabetes and severe insulin resistance, administration of rhIGF-I is associated with severe sodium and fluid retention and edema formation.

Glucagon increases natriuresis, but this action of the peptide is indirect because infusion of glucagon directly into the renal artery does not affect urinary sodium excretion. Glucagon increases circulating cAMP, which may decrease tubular sodium absorption. Glucagon induces a rise in the release of cAMP in the liver. Perhaps, liver-derived, glucagon-induced cAMP reduces proximal tubular sodium absorption (Fig. 13.38). Although hypothetical, the insulin-induced reduction of glucagon release could reduce circulating cAMP, contributing to reduced natriuresis.

Phosphate Absorption

Both insulin and IGF-I increase proximal tubular phosphate absorption, and glucagon reduces phosphate absorption (Fig. 13.38). This apparently results from effects on the Na–P-1 cotransporter in proximal tubular cells. Insulin upregulates this transport protein, and both glucagon and cAMP downregulate it. However, another Na-P cotransporter isoform, Na–P-2, is not

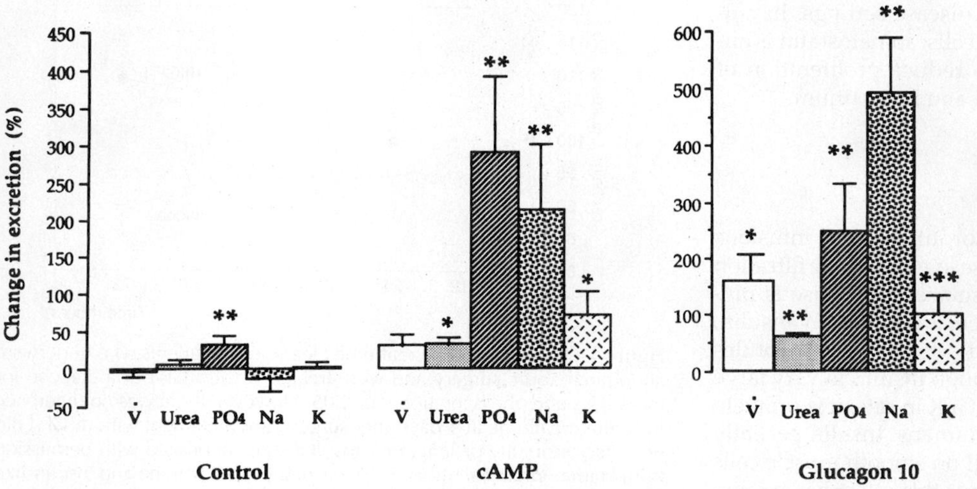

Figure 13.38. Effects of infusions of cAMP (5 nmol/min/100 gBW) or glucagon (120 ng/min/100 gBW) on urinary solute excretion in normal anesthetized rats. Cyclic adenosine monophosphate (cAMP), which is released from the liver upon stimulation with glucagon, as well as glucagon itself, reduce the tubular absorption of phosphate as well as sodium and may, in fact, mediate the effects of glucagon on Na and PO_4 absorption. *$p < .05$; **$p < .01$; ***$p < .001$. (Reprinted with permission from Ahlouly M, Dechauz M, Hassler C, et al. Cyclic AMP is a hepatorenal link influencing natriuresis and contributing to glucagon-induced hyperfiltration in rats. *J Clin Invest* 1996;98:2251–2258.)

affected by insulin. IGF-I is a strong upregulator of renal phosphate absorption. IGF-I acts on phosphate transport through IGF-I receptors in apical as well as basolateral membranes. Administration of rhIGF-I to normal subjects reduces urinary phosphate excretion by more than 50%, but the circadian rhythm of phosphaturia, which is possibly caused by parathyroid hormone (PTH), is maintained. Although IGF-I increases renal phosphate retention in normal subjects, serum levels of phosphate do not increase. This possibly results from an IGF-I–induced increased uptake of phosphate in bone.

Somatostatin and its analogs increase natriuresis in normal subjects and in patients with essential hypertension or type II diabetes (and hypertension) (Fig. 13.39). This effect may be direct, but it most likely results from the suppression of insulin secretion. Experimental data have suggested that somatostatin may increase calcium balance and may affect water permeability in the distal nephron. However, these findings are preliminary and require confirmation, especially in human studies.

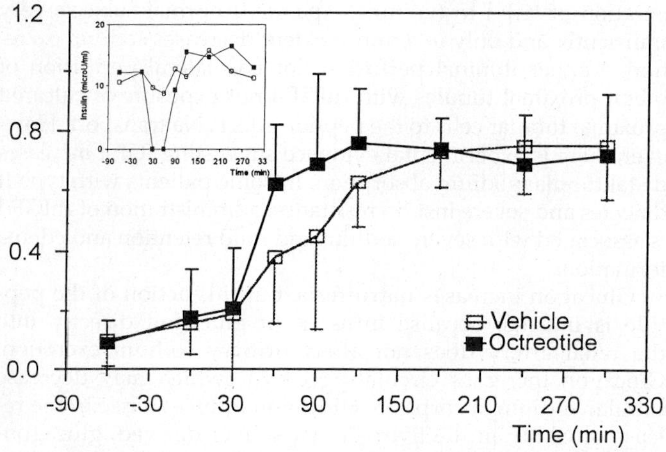

Figure 13.39. Acute effects of the somatostatin analog octreotide on urinary sodium excretion in lean patients with essential hypertension. At time 0, subjects received a single injection followed by a 30-minute infusion of octreotide or vehicle. Octreotide transiently blocked insulin release and reduced plasma insulin levels below detection limit *(insert)*. Octreotide (or somatostatin) acutely reduces renal sodium absorption either directly or secondary to reducing insulin activity. *$p < .05$ octreotide versus vehicle. (From Ferri C, De Mateia J, Bellini C, et al. Octreotide, a somatostatin analog, reduces insulin secretion and increases Na^+ excretion in lean essential hypertensive patients. *Am J Hypertens* 1993;6: 276–281.)

Insulin receptor–related receptors are orphan receptors with unknown ligands and functions that are structurally related to insulin receptors. These receptors are exclusively expressed in certain cells in cortical and medullary collecting ducts, suggesting a unique function in water or electrolyte transport. However, the physiologic function of these receptors or their ligand(s) are presently unknown.

RESISTANCE TO INSULIN AND IGF-I

Insulin resistance is an increased amount of insulin that is necessary to maintain euglycemia after a glucose load. By this somewhat stringent definition, insulin sensitivity has to be tested with gold standard methods, namely euglycemic insulin clamp studies. Hence, *insulin resistance* refers primarily to actions of insulin on glucose uptake and metabolism in tissues bearing insulin-sensitive, facilitative glucose transporters (skeletal muscle and adipose tissue) and not necessarily to other biologic actions of insulin. Severe insulin-resistant diabetes syndromes can be inherited due to mutations in the insulin receptor gene or signaling molecules or may be acquired as in the type B syndrome in which circulating antiinsulin-receptor antibodies neutralize receptor activation. Modest insulin resistance without diabetes mellitus can be acquired and occurs in chronic renal failure and in some patients with essential hypertension.

The high degree of correlation between non–insulin-dependent diabetes mellitus (NIDDM) and essential hypertension, which exceeds the expected probability based on the incidence of each disease, suggests a causal relationship. However, not all studies confirmed this hypothesis and a cause-and-effect relationship is still unproven. Insulin resistance in essential hypertension or in chronic renal failure appears to be associated with increased cytosolic Ca^{2+} levels in many cells such as adiposites. However, it is unclear whether increased cytosolic Ca^{2+} is a cause or a result of insulin resistance. Nevertheless, increased cell-free Ca^{2+} is also a common feature of essential hypertension.

There is also a close relationship between sodium intake and insulin resistance. High sodium intakes may reduce insulin receptor number under normal conditions but not in rat models

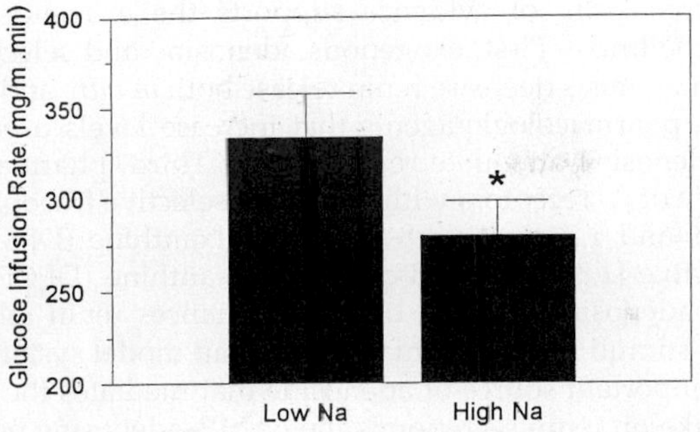

Figure 13.40. High-sodium, intake-induced insulin resistance in nondiabetic normal, white males. Subjects were maintained on low (10 mmol/day) or high (200 mmol/day) dietary sodium for the 5 days preceding the insulin clamp study. (Reprinted with permission from Donovan DS, Solomon CG, Seely EW, et al. Effect of sodium intake on insulin sensitivity. *Am J Physiol* 1993;264:E730–E734.)

of essential hypertension. Reduced receptor number may contribute to the renal excretion of sodium because it reduces the effect of insulin to increase renal sodium absorption. This would suggest that insulin resistance is not causally linked to sodium retention–induced hypertension. In dietary sodium-restricted subjects, a sodium load raises insulin resistance by as much as 20%, as measured by euglycemic insulin clamp (Fig. 13.40). In patients with essential hypertension, a similar Na challenge has virtually no effect on insulin sensitivity.

Insulin has also major effects on potassium homeostasis because it stimulates the Na^+-K^+-ATPase pump. By this means, insulin causes a shift of K from the extracellular to the intracellular compartment. This activity of insulin is independent of its activation of GLUT-4 and does not require enhanced cell uptake of glucose. The insulin-induced intracellular-K shift and resulting decline in serum K levels is associated with a significant increase in plasma renin activity and serum angiotensin II levels, but aldosterone levels fall in response to hypokalemia. Hypokalemia tends to worsen blood pressure control in hypertensive patients, and there is an inverse relationship between plasma K and systolic blood pressure control in patients with essential hypertension.

Clinical studies in patients with essential hypertension demonstrate that an octreotide-induced, short-term reduction in serum insulin levels has no effect on blood pressure. Similarly, a transient, acute rise in serum insulin (five times more than baseline) during euglycemic insulin clamp has no effect on blood pressure in these subjects. Although this data does not disprove a causative relationship between hyperinsulinemic insulin-resistant states and essential hypertension, it indicates that insulin does not regulate blood pressure acutely.

There is a relationship between glucagon and insulin and catecholamines. Activation of α-receptors by catecholamines reduces insulin release. At the same time, catecholamines cause increased glucagon secretion through β-receptors. These hyperglycemic effects of catecholamines explain why pheochromocytomas can cause diabetes. Thus patients with a pheochromocytoma may have hypertension and insulinopenic/hyperglucagonemic (not insulin-resistant) diabetes.

In nondiabetic chronic renal failure patients, there is moderately reduced insulin sensitivity. Experimental evidence suggests that chronic renal failure induces a postreceptor signaling defect, probably by a reduction in insulin-receptor kinase activity toward cellular substrates such as IRS-1. This may be caused by an unidentified uremic toxin. Elevations in counterregulatory hormones may also reduce glycemic response to insulin in chronic renal failure.

Selected Readings

Ahloulay M, Dechaux M, Hassler C, et al. Cyclic AMP is a hepatorenal link influencing natriuresis and contributing to glucagon-induced hyperfiltration in rats. *J Clin Invest* 1996;98:2251–2258.

An experimental study in rats giving support to the hypothesis that (glucagon-induced) hepatic cAMP release causes phosphaturia, natriuresis and contributes to a rise in GFR. Hepatic cAMP may mediate many of the renal effects of glucagon.

DeFronzo RA, Cooke CR, Andres R, et al. The effect of insulin on renal handling of sodium, potassium, calcium, and phosphate in man. *J Clin Invest* 1975;55: 845–855.

A "classic" clinical study of the effects of euglycemic insulin clamp on renal excretion of electrolytes. Insulin acutely caused an increase in renal sodium retention and an increase in free water clearance without a change in urine flow rate. Urinary potassium and phosphate excretion also decreased significantly.

Donovan DS, Solomon CG, Seely EW, et al. Effect of sodium intake on insulin sensitivity. *Am J Physiol* 1993;264:E730–E734.

An euglycemic insulin-clamp study in eight normal white males that high sodium intake reduces the sensitivity to insulin.

Fouque D, Peng SC, Kopple JD. Impaired metabolic response to recombinant insulin-like growth factor-1 in dialysis patients. *Kidney Int* 1995;47:876–883.

A short-term study on the metabolic effects of rhIGF-I in six normal subjects and twelve patients with end-stage renal disease (6 CAPD and 6 hemodialysis patients). The study demonstrates resistance to IGF-I in ESRD patients.

Hirschberg R, Brunori G, Kopple JD, et al. Effects of insulin-like growth factor I on renal function in normal men. *Kidney Int* 1993;43:387–397.

A study in 8 normal subjects of the effects of rhIGF-I on renal function. The study indicates the effects of the peptide to increase GFR and RBF, and renal retention of phosphate and, to a lesser extent, of sodium.

Ike JO, Fervenza FC, Hoffman AR, et al. Early experience with extended use of insulin-like growth factor-1 in advanced chronic renal failure. *Kidney Int* 1997; 51:840–849.

An open label clinical study of effects of treatment of eight patients with advanced CRF (GFR 17±3 ml/min/1.73 m²) with rhIGF-I for four weeks. This treatment resulted in a modest (14%) improvement in GFR, but BUN and serum creatinine levels did not change significantly.

Isaksson H, Nygren A, Ostergren J. Arterial pressure, plasma renin activity, atrial natriuretic factor, and sodium excretion during induced hyper- and hypoinsulinemia in therapy-resistant hypertensives. *Clin Exp Hypertens* 1993;15: 355–365.

A blinded, cross-over study of urinary Na excretion during euglycemic high- or low-serum insulin clamp in six patients with essential hypertension. Arterial pressure did not decrease during low insulin clamp. High insulin clamp induced natriuresis but did not affect blood pressure. These data suggest that hyperinsulinemia in insulin-resistance states does not cause hypertension.

PART 13
Adenosine

Edwin K. Jackson

Clinical and experimental investigations are revealing important roles for adenosine receptors in renal physiology and pathophysiology, and these new insights are leading to innovative drug development efforts. In this regard, adenomimetics and adenolytics (drugs that increase or decrease adenosine-receptor activation, respectively) may represent important new pharmacotherapeutic strategies for the treatment of renal disease. The purpose of this chapter is to summarize the state of knowledge regarding the role of adenosine in the kidneys and to indicate where new pharmacotherapeutic advances are imminent.

In mammals, four types of adenosine receptors exist: A_1, A_{2A}, A_{2B}, and A_3 adenosine receptors. Because so little is known about the function of A_3 receptors in the kidney, this receptor subtype is not discussed. Also, because it is difficult to distinguish A_{2A} and A_{2B} receptor subtypes using currently available adenosine-receptor agonists and antagonists, in this chapter, these receptor subtypes are consolidated under the rubric A_2 receptor and are discussed together.

RENAL A_1 RECEPTORS

A_1 Receptors in the Kidney

A_1 receptors are widely expressed in the kidney and exist in both vascular and tubular elements. Ligand-binding studies detect A_1 receptors in renal microvessels, glomeruli, collecting tubules, and cultured epithelial cell model systems with proximal or distal phenotype. *In situ* hybridization experiments demonstrate A_1-receptor mRNA expression in collecting tubules and in the juxtaglomerular apparatus, whereas reverse transcription polymerase chain reaction methods discern A_1-receptor mRNA expression in glomeruli, medullary collecting ducts, cortical and medullary thick ascending limbs, proximal convoluted and straight tubules, and the descending vasa recta of the outer medulla.

A_1 receptors modulate two important signal transduction systems. A_1 receptors inhibit adenylyl cyclase activity via coupling to the guanosine triphosphate (GTP)-binding protein G_i and stimulate phospholipase C activity via coupling to the GTP-binding protein $G_{q/11}$. The former pathway leads to a reduction in intracellular cyclic adenosine monophosphate (cAMP), and the latter pathway leads to increased intracellular levels of inositol trisphosphate and diacylglycerol.

Role of A_1 Receptors in Renal Physiology

Resistance of Preglomerular Microvessels

Administration of selective A_1 receptor agonists into the kidney interstitium reduces cortical and medullary blood flow, suggesting that A_1-receptor activation vasoconstricts the microcirculation supplying both superficial and deep nephrons. In this regard, an increase in the resistance of preglomerular microvessels mediates decreases in blood flow following A_1-receptor activation. However, increased resistance of the outer medullary descending vasa recta probably contributes to the decrease in blood flow to deeper nephrons.

The ability of A_1 receptors to constrict the preglomerular microcirculation is powerfully modulated by endogenous autocoids, most important of which are nitric oxide, prostaglandins, and angiotensin II. Nitric oxide and prostaglandins reduce A_1 receptor–induced preglomerular vasoconstriction, whereas angiotensin II enhances A_1 receptor–induced preglomerular vasoconstriction. However, not all studies report a positive synergy between angiotensin II and A_1 receptors, indicating that unknown factors that vary among model systems modulate this interaction. Such studies infer that the degree of renal vasoconstriction mediated by A_1-receptor activation may be importantly modulated by the disease state.

Renin Release

A_1 receptors are negatively coupled to adenylyl cyclase via G_i, and stimulation of renin release from juxtaglomerular cells generally entails activation of adenylyl cyclase. Therefore juxtaglomerular A_1 receptors function to restrain renin-release responses by limiting the cAMP production to any given stimulus. This mechanism is called the adenosine brake on renin release.

A large body of evidence supports the existence of the adenosine brake. First, exogenous adenosine and selective A_1-receptor agonists decrease renin release both *in vitro* and *in vivo*. Second, pharmacologic agents that increase levels of endogenous adenosine attenuate renin release. Third, pharmacologic blockade of A_1 receptors with either nonselective [theophylline, caffeine, and 1,3-dipropyl-8-sulfophenylxanthine (DPSPX)] or A_1-selective [1,3-dipropyl-8-cyclopentylxanthine (DPCPX) and FK453] adenosine-receptor blockers enhances renin release to various stimuli in both animal and human model systems.

An important source of adenosine that mediates the adenosine brake on renin secretion is the cAMP–adenosine pathway. Stimulation of adenylyl cyclase, for example by activation of prostaglandin receptors or β_1-adrenoceptors, causes transport of intracellular cAMP onto the cell surface. Extracellular cAMP is converted by ectophosphodiesterase to AMP, which in turn is converted to adenosine by ecto-5′-nucleotidase. Inasmuch as this sequence of enzymatic reactions occurs at the cell surface, activation of adenylyl cyclase causes adenosine biosynthesis in the biophase where the adenosine-binding domains of adenosine receptors reside. Consequently, the cAMP–adenosine pathway provides active concentrations of adenosine in an autocrine-paracrine fashion.

Tubuloglomerular Feedback

Tubuloglomerular feedback (TGF) is a process by which changes in flow rate to Henle's loop cause opposite changes in single-nephron glomerular filtration rate (SNGFR), thereby preventing the load of ultrafiltrate from exceeding the nephron's reabsorptive capacity. In this regard, when the SNGFR exceeds a critical threshold, the concentration of NaCl increases in the ultrafiltrate bathing the macula densa cells in the nephron. In response, the macula densa cells convey a signal to the afferent arteriole. This signal elicits constriction of the afferent arteriole and consequently reduces single nephron blood flow, glomerular capillary pressure, and SNGFR.

Adenosine may importantly participate in the mechanism of TGF. This hypothesis posits that increased NaCl presentation to Henle's loop enhances NaCl reabsorption by the macula densa, which augments adenosine triphosphate (ATP) breakdown and thereby increases adenosine biosynthesis from purine nucleotides. Adenosine diffuses from the macula densa cells to the nearby afferent arterioles, activates A_1 receptors, and induces afferent arteriolar vasoconstriction.

Several lines of evidence are consistent with this mechanism of TGF: (a) increases in renal energy demand decrease renal tissue ATP levels and augment adenosine levels in the kidney; (b) infusion of hypertonic saline into the renal artery increases adenosine release from thick ascending limbs; (c) a high-sodium diet significantly increases renal interstitial adenosine levels by as much as 18-fold and increases total tissue levels of adenosine in the renal cortex and medulla by approximately twofold; (d) nonselective and selective A_1 adenosine-receptor antagonists inhibit TGF; (e) blockade of A_1 receptors uncouples proximal reabsorption from SNGFR; (f) administration of exogenous adenosine deaminase, the enzyme that metabolizes adenosine to inosine, reduces TGF responses; (g) inhibition of adenosine transport or adenosine metabolism augments TGF; (h) intraluminal or peritubular infusions of selective A_1 receptor agonists decrease pressure in the glomerular capillaries; and (i) intrarenal infusion of hypertonic saline reduces renal blood flow (RBF) by activating TGF, and this response is inhibited by adenosine-receptor antagonists. However, the available evidence is also consistent with adenosine subserving a modulatory, rather than mediator, role in TGF.

Epithelial Transport

A_1 receptors regulate transport by renal proximal epithelial cells. Activation of A_1 receptors in cultured epithelial cells that express a proximal phenotype enhances Na^+-glucose and Na^+-phosphate symport, and stimulation of A_1 receptors increases basolateral Na^+-$3HCO_3^-$ symport in microperfused proximal convoluted tubules. The mechanism by which A_1 receptors stimulate transport in proximal epithelial cells probably involves the activation of G_i, which lowers cellular cAMP. Because cAMP inhibits luminal Na^+-H^+ antiport and basolateral Na^+-$3HCO_3^-$ symport, a reduction in cAMP would disinhibit Na^+-H^+ antiport and Na^+-$3HCO_3^-$ symport and thereby increase transepithelial ion transport.

Intravenous administration of nonselective and selective A_1 agonists decreases sodium excretion and urine volume. In humans, intravenous administration of adenosine reduces the urinary excretion of sodium, lithium, phosphate, uric acid, chloride, and urea. However, it is difficult to deduce from *in vivo* studies whether adenosine receptors have direct effects on tubular transport because changes in blood pressure, renal blood pressure (RBF), the intrarenal distribution of RBF, glomerular filtration rate (GFR), and renin release complicate interpretation of changes in urinary excretion of electrolytes induced by adenosine-receptor agonists. Moreover, renal levels of endogenous adenosine may saturate A_1 receptors on tubular epithelial cells, which also confounds the interpretation of the effects of exogenous adenosine-receptor agonists on renal excretory function. For these reasons, studies with adenosine-receptor antagonists provide more useful information regarding the role of A_1 receptors in renal physiology.

All *in vivo* studies with A_1 receptor antagonists support the conclusion that endogenous adenosine–A_1 receptor interactions enhance tubular reabsorption of sodium. In this regard, selective blockade of renal A_1 receptors induces diuresis and natriuresis with little effect on the potassium excretion rate. For example, intravenous infusions of equipotent doses of FK453 and DPCPX, two structurally dissimilar, highly potent and selective A_1 antagonists, cause similar increases in urine volume and sodium excretion, yet FR113452, the inactive enantiomer of FK453, does not alter renal excretory function, indicating that the effects of FK453 are mediated by blockade of A_1 receptors. The S-enantiomer of 1,3-dipropyl-8-[2-(5,6-epoxynorbornyl)] xanthine (CVT-124), an extremely potent and selective A_1 receptor antagonist, causes a maximum diuretic/natriuretic effect twice that of hydrochlorothiazide. Of potential clinical importance, CVT-124 potentiates the diuretic/natriuretic effect of furosemide without enhancing furosemide-induced potassium excretion. Direct intrarenal artery infusions of 8-(noradamantan-3-yl)-1,3-dipropylxanthine (KW-3902), another potent and selective A_1 receptor antagonist, greatly increase urine flow, sodium excretion, and osmolar clearance, indicating that the effects of A_1 receptor antagonists on renal excretory function are due to blockade of renal A_1 receptors. Because selective A_1 receptor antagonists have little effect on systemic or renal hemodynamics, the natriuretic and diuretic effects of these drugs most likely are the result of direct tubular actions.

The diuretic/natriuretic efficacy of selective A_1 receptor antagonists is due to actions of these drugs at three different intrarenal sites. Studies indicate that blockade of A_1 receptors in humans with FK453 causes diuresis/natriuresis mostly by interfering with proximal tubular transport but partly by reducing transport at more distal sites, probably the collecting tubules. A third important site of action of selective A_1-receptor antagonists is the renal microcirculation. By blocking A_1 receptors in the renal microcirculation, selective A_1-receptor antagonists inhibit TGF and thereby uncouple proximal reabsorption from SNGFR. Thus, unlike carbonic anhydrase inhibitors that diminish proximal transport and decrease SNGFR, selective A_1-receptor antagonists reduce proximal transport without decreasing SNGFR.

Role of A_1 Receptors in Renal Pathophysiology

Chronic Renal Failure

Nephron loss from any renal insult results in dilation of the afferent arterioles of the remaining nephrons. Although adaptive in the short term, in the long term, the increased glomerular pressure and hyperfiltration leads to glomerulosclerosis, further loss of nephron units, acceleration of chronic renal failure (CRF), and ultimately end-stage renal disease. Therefore pharmacotherapeutic agents that reduce glomerular pressure may cause an acute reduction in GFR and, more importantly, may delay or prevent the gradual progression to end-stage renal disease. On the other hand, drugs that increase glomerular pressure may increase GFR acutely but accelerate the rate of GFR decline.

It is possible that adenomimetics may find utility in the treatment of CRF. Activation of renal A_1-adenosine receptors on juxtaglomerular cells inhibits renin release and therefore angiotensin II formation. Because angiotensin II constricts postglomerular vessels, reducing the amount of angiotensin II decreases angiotensin II–mediated postglomerular vasoconstriction and thereby reduces glomerular hydrostatic pressure. Moreover, stimulation of renal A_1-adenosine receptors induces preglomerular microvascular vasoconstriction, a process that also decreases glomerular hydrostatic pressure. Thus activation of preglomerular microvascular and juxtaglomerular A_1 receptors with adenomimetics may reduce glomerular hydrostatic pressure and preserve renal function in CRF. In support of this concept, administration of selective A_1-receptor agonists to animals decreases stop-flow pressure (an index of glomerular pressure), and long-term administration of either an adenosine uptake or an adenosine deaminase inhibitor attenuates experimental CRF.

Conversely, adenolytics may be harmful in patients with CRF. Studies demonstrate that blockade of renal A_1 receptors increases glomerular capillary pressure, and long-term administration of caffeine accentuates angiotensin II–induced increases in filtration fraction. This indicates that blockade of renal adenosine receptors may augment angiotensin II–induced glomerular hypertension. Moreover, because angiotensin II constricts postglomerular microvessels and raises glomerular capillary pressure, activation of the renin-angiotensin system should be avoided in patients with CRF. This concept is underscored by several large clinical trails demonstrating that a blockade of the renin-angiotensin system with angiotensin-converting enzyme inhibitors decreases the rate of decline of renal function in patients with CRF. Because blockade of A_1 receptors enhances renin release, this is another reason to avoid adenolytic agents in patients with CRF. Indeed, newer studies demonstrate that blockade of A_1 receptors in humans augments renin release in patients with CRF. Animal experiments further support the negative impact of adenolytic drugs in patients with CRF. These experiments demonstrate that chronic caffeine (an adenosine-receptor blocker) administration worsens renal function in animals with renovascular hypertension or CRF. These considerations raise an important question. Does chronic caffeine ingestion exacerbate the rate of decline of renal function in patients with CRF? In modern societies plagued with obesity-induced, non–insulin-dependent diabetes mellitus in which CRF due to diabetic nephropathy increases at an alarming rate, it is conceivable that the prevalence of caffeine consumption is contributing to the increasing incidence of end-stage renal disease. Unfortunately, this hypothesis remains untested.

Radiocontrast-Induced Acute Renal Failure

Hypertonic radiocontrast media induces a decrease in GFR and RBF that is usually reversible but occasionally leads to acute renal failure (ARF) in some patients. The pathophysiologic mechanism of radiocontrast-induced nephropathy may involve A_1 receptors. The osmotic diuresis induced by hypertonic radiocontrast agents increases delivery of NaCl to the macula densa and triggers a TGF response. Because adenosine either mediates or modulates TGF responses, adenolytic drugs may be useful to prevent or treat radiocontrast-induced ARF.

Several experimental and clinical studies support the effectiveness of adenosine-receptor antagonists in radiocontrast-induced nephropathy. In both animals and humans, hypertonic radiocontrast media increases the urinary excretion of adenosine, and theophylline, an adenosine-receptor antagonist, reduces radiocontrast-induced decreases in RBF and GFR. However, the results with theophylline must be interpreted cautiously because theophylline is both a nonselective adenosine-receptor antagonist and a phosphodiesterase inhibitor. In animals, inhibition of adenosine uptake with dipyridamole augments the renal effects of hypertonic radiocontrast media, and selective blockade of A_1 receptors with either DPCPX or KW-3902 attenuates radiocontrast-induced reductions in RBF and GFR. Clinical trials are needed to ascertain whether adenolytic drugs besides theophylline, particular selective A_1-receptor antagonists, attenuate radiocontrast-induced nephropathy in humans.

Acute Tubular Necrosis

Theoretical considerations suggest that endogenous adenosine–A_1 receptor interactions may contribute functionally to acute tubular necrosis (ATN)-induced ARF. Inasmuch as injury to epithelial cells impairs energy production, depletion of ATP and accumulation of adenosine may occur in damaged epithelial cells. High levels of endogenous adenosine would stimulate A_1 receptors and thereby cause vasoconstriction of the preglomerular microcirculation, resulting in a functional reduction in GFR and RBF. Also, because cellular injury reduces the reabsorptive capacity of the proximal tubule epithelium, increased delivery of NaCl to the macula densa could reduce GFR and RBF by activating TGF, a mechanism mediated or modulated by endogenous adenosine–A_1 receptor interactions.

In support of the hypothesis that endogenous adenosine–A_1 receptor interactions play an important role in the mechanism of ATN-induced ARF, animal studies involving different adenosine-receptor antagonists and various nephrotoxins demonstrate that blockade of adenosine receptors does indeed attenuate ATN-induced reductions in GFR and RBF. For example, aminophylline, theophylline, 8-phenyl theophylline, DPCPX, 8-(dicyclopropylmethyl)-1,3-dipropylxanthine, FK453, and KW-3902 attenuate glycerol-induced ARF. Additional studies show that aminophylline, DPCPX, FK453, and KW-3902 reduce *cis*-platin–induced ARF, as do maneuvers that block TGF, such as a high-salt diet and furosemide. Also, FK453 and KW-3902 attenuate gentamicin-induced ARF, and KW-3902 attenuates cephaloridine-induced nephrotoxicity. Renal ischemia/hypoxia increases renal production of adenosine and can cause ARF, further suggesting a causal connection between adenosine and ARF. This inference is strengthened by the observations that theophylline and adenosine α,β-methylene diphosphate, an inhibitor of ecto-5′-nucleotidase, attenuate, and dipyridamole, an inhibitor of adenosine uptake, potentiates ischemia/hypoxia-induced ARF.

However, some studies challenge the view that adenosine–A_1 receptor interactions mediate functional changes in GFR and RBF in established ATN-induced ARF. For instance, in normal rats, intrarenal infusions of an A_1 agonist cannot mimic the magnitude of *cis*-platin–induced reductions in GFR and the increases in renal vascular resistance (RVR) that would be anticipated if endogenous adenosine played an important role in mediating the decreases in GFR and RBF in this form of ATN-induced ARF. Also, in rats with established *cis*-platin–induced ARF, the GFR and RVR responses to an A_1 agonist are not altered compared with control animals. This suggests that endogenous adenosine is not occupying A_1 receptors in established *cis*-platin–induced ARF. Moreover, renal cortical levels of adenosine, inosine, xanthine, and hypoxanthine are not elevated in established *cis*-platin–induced ARF, and selective blockade of A_1 receptors does not improve renal function in established *cis*-platin–induced ARF.

The observation that adenosine is not involved in established ATN-induced ARF necessitates a reevaluation of the hypothesis that adenosine participates in nephrotoxin-induced ARF by functionally constricting the preglomerular microcirculation. It is important to note that in all studies in which adenosine-receptor antagonists were shown to attenuate ATN-induced ARF, the antagonists were given before or very soon after the administration of the nephrotoxin. Because the diuretic site of action of A_1-receptor antagonists is predominantly the proximal tubule, A_1-receptor antagonists would decrease reabsorption of ultrafiltrate in the proximal tubule and thereby reduce the exposure of proximal tubular epithelial cells to high concentrations of nephrotoxins. This mechanism alone may be adequate to explain the renoprotection afforded by A_1-receptor antagonists in ATN-induced ARF. In support of this hypothesis, adenosine-receptor antagonists are much more effective against nephrotoxins that selectively injure the proximal nephron (e.g., glycerol, *cis*-platin, gentamicin, cephaloridine) compared with nephrotoxins that induce widespread tubular epithelial injury (e.g., amphotericin B, cyclosporine). Acetazolamide, a diuretic that inhibits transport in the proximal tubule, also attenuates *cis*-platin–induced ARF.

Further studies are required to elucidate the mechanism of renoprotection afforded by A_1-receptor antagonists. An increased understanding of the mechanism by which A_1-receptor antagonists attenuate ATN-induced ARF may determine how these drugs are applied clinically, for example, to prevent ARF as opposed to reversing it.

Fluid Retention

It is probable that adenolytics, particularly A_1-receptor antagonists, will be added to the pharmacotherapeutic armamentarium along side thiazide and loop diuretics in the management of edema. A_1-receptor antagonists have a unique triple effect on the nephron: (a) blockade of proximal tubular transport, (b) blockade of transport at more distal sites in the nephron, and (c) blockade of TGF responses that would normally be induced by increased delivery of NaCl to the macula densa. This unique combination of effects results in a brisk natriuresis/diuresis without triggering TGF and with little or no effect on potassium excretion. It is likely that adenolytic-based diuretic strategies will be useful in the treatment of edematous conditions such as heart failure, liver disease, and renal disease, particularly in patients with diuretic resistance or in patients that cannot tolerate other diuretics due to deteriorated renal function. It is hoped that ongoing clinical trials will soon establish the appropriate use of adenolytics in edematous states.

RENAL A_2 RECEPTORS

A_2 Receptors in the Kidney

Ligand-binding studies demonstrate A_2 receptors in kidney membranes, and *in situ* hybridization studies detect A_{2A}-receptor mRNA in the renal papilla and inner medulla outside the collecting duct. Reverse transcriptase polymerase chain reaction methods demonstrate A_{2A}- and A_{2B}-receptor mRNA in the outer medulla and outer medullary descending vasa recta. Activation of adenylyl cyclase via the stimulatory G protein G_s is the major signal transduction pathway used by renal A_2 receptors.

Role of A_2 Receptors in Renal Physiology

Evidence to date does not support an important role for A_2 receptors with regard to direct regulation of renal epithelial transport. For example, the diuretic efficacy of adenosine-receptor antagonists correlates with A_1-, but not with A_2-, receptor affinity. A_2 receptor–mediated renin secretion can be demonstrated, although this is of little physiologic significance. On the other hand, three renal systems may be importantly regulated by A_2 receptors: (a) postglomerular vascular tone, (b) neutrophil–endothelial cell interactions within the kidney, and (c) renal erythropoietin production.

Postglomerular Vascular Resistance

A_2-receptor activation in the renal microcirculation causes vasodilation of postglomerular vessels in the inner cortex and medulla but not in the outer cortex. This is in contrast to A_1-receptor activation, which leads to vasoconstriction of superficial and deep preglomerular microvessels. Intrarenal artery infusions of adenosine cause an immediate decrease in RBF that wanes in less than a minute, with RBF returning to or above baseline within a few minutes. This characteristic time course is due to the rapid onset of A_1 receptor–mediated preglomerular vasoconstriction followed by the slower onset of A_2 receptor–mediated postglomerular vasodilation. The rapid preglomerular vasoconstriction caused by adenosine-mediated A_1-receptor stimulation decreases RBF, and the delayed reduction in postglomerular resistance caused by A_2-receptor stimulation slowly restores RBF to or above the original baseline. Because vasoconstriction occurs in the outer renal cortex and vasodilation occurs in the inner cortex, adenosine redistributes RBF from the outer to the inner cortex. Selective A_2 agonists increase RBF without causing an initial reduction in RBF because the initial decline induced by adenosine is mediated by A_1 receptors.

The ability of A_2 receptors to vasodilate the renal medulla may participate importantly, albeit indirectly, in the regulation of sodium excretion. Chronic salt loading increases levels of adenosine in the renal medulla, and this may serve to dilate medullary vessels, an effect that would indirectly increase sodium excretion. Renal medullary interstitial infusions of adenosine increase medullary blood flow and sodium excretion, whereas renal medullary interstitial infusions of 3,7-dimethyl-1-propargylxanthine, a selective A_2-receptor antagonist, decrease medullary blood flow and sodium excretion.

Neutrophil–Endothelial Cell Interactions in the Kidney

Stimulation of A_2 receptors inhibits neutrophil–endothelial cell interactions *in vitro*, and A_2-receptor activation inhibits neutrophil–endothelial interactions following ischemic/reperfusion injury *in vivo*. Newer studies demonstrate that selective stimulation of A_{2A} receptors diminishes neutrophil infiltration into kidneys induced by ischemic/reperfusion injury of the kidneys.

Erythropoietin Synthesis

Adenosine receptors may regulate erythropoietin biosynthesis by peritubular fibroblasts. For example, in isolated, perfused kidneys, exogenous adenosine stimulates erythropoietin secretion. Inhibition of adenosine deaminase augments erythropoietin levels in hypoxic rats, whereas administration of adenosine deaminase has the opposite effect. In exhypoxic polycythemic mice, A_2-receptor stimulation increases erythropoietin levels. Moreover, anemia increases the expression of ecto-5′-nucleotidase on peritubular fibroblasts, and renal peritubular type I fibroblasts coexpress erythropoietin, 5′-nucleotidase, and an oxygen-sensing mechanism. However, not all studies support a role for adenosine in the regulation of erythropoietin production. For example, neither theophylline nor dipyridamole affect the increase in plasma erythropoietin levels caused by hemorrhage or hypobaric hypoxia in humans, and it appears that adenosine does not modulate carbon monoxide–induced erythropoietin production. Further investigations are required to resolve this controversy.

Role of A_2 Receptors in Renal Pathophysiology

Ischemia/Reperfusion Injury

In an animal model system of renal ischemia/reperfusion injury (45 minutes of ischemia followed by 48 hours of reperfusion), stimulation of A_{2A} receptors attenuates the increases in serum creatinine and blood urea nitrogen and reduces the extent of tubular epithelial necrosis, vascular congestion of the outer medulla, and neutrophil infiltration. It is possible that adenomimetics, particularly A_{2A}-receptor agonists, may have clinical usefulness in protecting the kidneys from ischemia/reperfusion injury.

Erythrocytosis

Approximately 15% of renal transplant recipients develop erythrocytosis. When administered for 8 weeks, theophylline, a nonselective adenosine-receptor antagonist, reduces erythropoietin levels, hematocrit, and red cell mass and eliminates the need for weekly phlebotomy in renal transplant patients that develop erythrocytosis. In this regard, more than 50% of patients appear to derive benefit from theophylline pharmacotherapy. Because A_2 receptors may regulate erythropoietin production, a strong rationale exists for clinical trials of selective A_2-receptor antagonists on red cell mass in renal transplant recipients with erythrocytosis.

Selected Readings

Gellai M, Schreiner GF, Ruffolo RR Jr, et al. CVT-124, a novel adenosine A_1 receptor antagonist with unique diuretic activity. *J Pharmacol Exp Ther* 1998;286:1191–1196.

This study demonstrates that A_1-receptor antagonists are efficacious diuretics that can be coadministered with loop diuretics to achieve sequential blockade of nephron segments without increasing potassium loss.

Jackson EK. Adenosine: a physiological brake on renin release. *Annu Rev Pharmacol Toxicol* 1991;31:1–35.

This review article summarizes data supporting the "adenosine-brake hypothesis" and the "cAMP–adenosine pathway."

Jackson EK, Mi Z, Herzer WA. Studies on the mechanism by which adenosine receptor antagonists attenuate acute renal failure. In: Belardinelli L, Pelleg A, eds. *Adenosine and Adenine Nucleotides: From Molecular Biology to Integrative Physiology.* Boston: Kluwer Academic Publishers, 1995:415–423.

This study challenges the received view regarding the mechanism by which A_1-receptor antagonists attenuate ARF induced by acute tubular necrosis.

Kuan CJ, Herzer WA, Jackson EK. Cardiovascular and renal effects of blocking A1 adenosine receptors. *J Cardiovasc Pharmacol* 1993;21:822–828.

This study firmly establishes that interactions of endogenous adenosine with A_1 receptors regulates sodium, but not potassium, excretion via a mechanism that does not involve changes in systemic or renal hemodynamics.

Osswald H, Muhlbauer B, Schenk F. Adenosine mediates tubuloglomerular feedback response: an element of metabolic control of kidney function. *Kidney Int* 1991;39:S128–S131.

This review article summarizes data supporting the hypothesis that adenosine mediates tubuloglomerular feedback.

Wilcox CS, Welch WJ, Schreiner GF, et al. Natriuretic and diuretic actions of a highly selective adenosine A_1 receptor antagonist. *J Am Soc Nephrol* 1999;10:714–720.

This study demonstrates that blockade of A_1 receptors uncouples proximal reabsorption of ultrafiltrate from SNGFR.

Zou AP, Nithipatikom K, Li PL, et al. Role of renal medullary adenosine in the control of blood flow and sodium excretion. *Am J Physiol* 1999;276:R790–R798.

This study demonstrates that interactions of endogenous adenosine with A_2 receptors in the outer and inner medulla dilate medullary vessels and consequently induce an indirect natriuretic response that overrides the direct tubular antinatriuretic effects of endogenous adenosine/A_1 receptor interactions.

SECTION III

Clinical Physiology of Fluid and Electrolyte Metabolism

CHAPTER 14

Body Fluid Compartments

PART 1
Volume Composition

Charles R. Kleeman

All vertebrates and invertebrates, with the exception of the most primitive unicellular organisms, have a distinct compartmentalization of their body water into intracellular and extracellular fluid (ICF and ECF, respectively). In those that have developed a recognized circulatory system (i.e., heart, arteries, capillaries, and veins), the ECF is further divided into intravascular and interstitial compartments. For absolute accuracy, in all complex organisms, we must further compartmentalize the fluid spaces as has been done in Table 14.1 for an idealized human subject. The fluid compartments are each in constant dynamic interchange and flux with each other, and the active and passive forces that regulate interchange between these various compartments, such as passive diffusion, osmotic equilibrium, active transport, and pressure gradients, are described elsewhere in this book. Despite the interchange and turnover, the homeostatic regulatory mechanisms of the body maintain the volume and composition of the various spaces at a remarkably constant level.

TOTAL BODY WATER

As the human embryo *in utero* develops into a fetus and then into the newborn child, it obviously passes through all phases of unicellular, multicellular, and then complex tissue, organ, and system development. With each of these changes, there is greater compartmentalization and greater development of the nonfluid or solid components of the organism. At birth, humans consist of at least 80% water, the percentage in males and females being approximately equal. The fat content is obviously extremely low, consisting almost entirely of essential cellular and extracellular lipids. By approximately age 15 years, both males and females have attained their adult proportions of total body water. Subsequently, as can be noted in Table 14.2, at each older age group, the percentage of body weight made up of total body water is significantly greater in the normal male than in the normal female. This difference is accounted for by the physiologic difference in fat content between males and females, which contributes significantly to the difference in body build and appearance of the sexes. Obviously, the fatter an individual, whether male or female, the smaller the percentage of total body water as a fraction of total body weight.

Today, total body water generally is measured by the technique of solute or isotope dilution:

where
C_1 = concentration of test substance administered
V_1 = volume of test substance administered
C_E = concentration of test substance lost in urine during equilibrium time
V_E = volume of urine excreted before equilibrium has been achieved
C_F = concentration of test substance after equilibrium has been achieved
V_F = amount of final volume of body water into which test substance has diffused or distributed at equilibrium

The labeled water, either tritium or deuterium, lost in urine is small, approximating 0.4% of the administered dose, and in practice, the term for urinary loss of labeled water is omitted, giving the following simplified equation:

TABLE 14.1. Body Water Distribution in a Healthy Young Adult Male, 70 kg of Body Weight[a]

Compartment	Percentage of Body Weight	Percentage of Total Body Water	Liters
Plasma	4.5	7.5	3
Interstitial fluid and lymph	12	20	8.5
Dense connective tissue and cartilage	4.5	7.5	3
Inaccessible bone water	4.5	7.5	3
Transcellular	1.5	2.5	1
Total extracellular	27	45	19
"Functional" extracellular[b]	21	35	14.5
Total body water	60	100	42
Total intracellular	33	55	23
Subcellular (mitochondrial, nuclear, other organelles)	?	?	?

Adapted from Edelman IS, Leibman J. Anatomy of body water and electrolytes. *Am J Med* 1959;27:256.
[a]All figures rounded to nearest 0.5.
[b]Minus bone water and transcellular water.

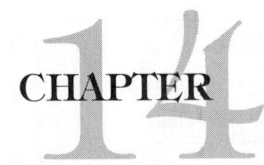

TABLE 14.2. Mean Values for Total Body Water in Normal Subjects

Age	Males	Females
yr	*% body weight*	
10-16	58.9	57.3
17-39	60.6	50.2
40-59	54.7	46.7
≥60	51.5	45.5

$$VF - \frac{C_1V_1 - C_EV_E}{C_F}$$

As shown in Table 14.2, total body water, as a percentage of body weight, falls with age after the adolescent period. This is a direct consequence of two factors: a progressive increase in fat mass and a reduction in muscle mass, the major contributor to the lean body mass and thus to total body water. The major fluid compartments of the total body water are ICF and ECF. As can be seen in Tables 14.2 and 14.3, water is the most abundant component of the human (and vertebrate) body.

EXTRACELLULAR FLUID VOLUME

By definition, ECF is body water that is external to the cells, thus including (1) plasma; (2) interstitial fluid and lymph; (3) the portion of the interstitial fluid in rapid exchange with plasma and that slowly exchanging with plasma, such as that in dense connective tissue and cartilage; (4) bone water; and (5) transcellular fluid. Any fluid under normal or abnormal conditions existing in the pleural, pericardial, peritoneal, and joint spaces should also be included in this definition.

Transcellular fluid, as defined by Edelman and Leibman, is "a variety of fluid collections which are not simple transudates and which have the common property of being formed by the transport activity of cells." These include the fluids of the salivary glands, pancreas, liver and biliary trees, gonads, skin, thyroid gland, kidneys, and mucous membranes of the respiratory and gastrointestinal tracts, in addition to the cavitary fluids of the eye, cerebrospinal fluid, and intraluminal fluid of the gastrointestinal tract.

The basic techniques and principles of measuring ECF again entail solute or isotope dilution as described previously. Many solutes, including inulin, mannitol, sucrose, thiosulfate, $^{35}SO_4$, bromide, ^{36}Cl, and ^{24}Na, have been used for this measurement. The "extracellular" space measured by these solutes varies from a low of 15% to 16% for inulin and mannitol to a high of 26% to 28% for sodium, chloride, and bromide. The large molecules such as inulin and sucrose seem most appropriate because they are completely, or almost completely, excluded from cells. However, they may also be excluded from a small portion of the total extracellular space within the reasonable time period of equilibrium. On the other hand, ions such as chloride or bromide may also penetrate the cell membrane of various tissues and thus give slightly higher values for ECF volume. It is probable that one of the best measures of ECF volume today is the distribution of inorganic radiosulfate. Studies carried out in humans with radiosulfate yield values of 17% to 19% of body weight. With all radioactive and nonradioactive substances used to measure a volume of distribution equivalent to that of the true extracellular compartment, varying degrees of error exist. It is probable that, in every case, it is far better to be able to compare a given human with himself or herself under certain

TABLE 14.3. Total and Exchangeable Sodium, Potassium, and Chloride in Healthy Subjects

Ion	Total Content	Exchangeable Men	Exchangeable Women
	mEq	*mEq*	
Sodium	3710 ± 7% SD	2835	2597
Potassium	3640 ± 8% SD	3367 (16–30 yr)	2681 (16–30 yr)
		2611 (61–90 yr)	2079 (61–90 yr)
Chloride	2147 ± 6%	2058	1869

From Hays RM. Dynamics of body water and electrolytes. In: Maxwell MH, Kleeman CR, eds. *Clinical Disorders of Fluid and Electrolyte Metabolism,* 3rd ed. New York: McGraw-Hill, 1979:1–36, with permission.

experimental or clinical conditions in which a change in the ECF volume is anticipated and being measured. In other words, intrapatient variability, in contrast to interpatient or interanimal variability, is most accurate. Changes in the volume of ECF have been measured with all these markers in states such as congestive heart failure, before and after therapy; chronic renal failure, before and after artificial dialysis; cirrhosis of the liver with ascites; and nephrotic syndrome—all in relatively large populations of both normal and sick individuals in every age group.

Plasma Volume

The plasma volume has generally been measured by determining the volume of distribution of labeled albumin. The label has been T-1824, a dye that combines with albumin, or the latter has been labeled with ^{131}I, ^{125}I, or ^{99m}Tc. Two techniques for plasma volume have been used: (a) the selection of a specific time after administration of a known amount of the labeled albumin (e.g., 10 to 15 minutes, at which time, under most circumstances, an insignificant quantity of albumin has left the vascular compartment but it has completely mixed with all the intravascular plasma volume). However, it is understood that albumin is not confined to the vascular compartment and has a certain finite escape or movement into the interstitial compartment and lymph. Therefore, for greatest accuracy in experimental and clinical situations, it is better to (b) take blood samples at 5-minute intervals for approximately 30 minutes and then extrapolate back to "zero time" or to the ordinate, rather than to pick a single specific time for a blood specimen after assumed equilibration. The second technique corrects for any loss of albumin from the vascular compartment during and subsequent to equilibration. It is of critical importance when there is any suspicion that conditions such as trauma, burns, profound hypoxemia, or vascular stasis have increased the permeability of the capillaries and allowed a greater than normal albumin leak from the vascular compartment.

Red Cell Mass and Whole Blood Volume

The red blood cell mass or whole blood volume has been measured for decades by labeling red blood cells with ^{51}Cr. Although other isotopes have been used, ^{51}Cr has been by far the most successful and practical. Plasma volume, total blood volume, or red blood cell mass can be estimated from the volume of distribution of either ^{51}Cr-red cells or labeled albumin and the simultaneous venous hematocrit. Obviously, the greatest degree of accuracy is attained when plasma volume and red blood cell mass are simultaneously measured by independent techniques. A slight error is introduced when the venous hematocrit is used because the "total body hematocrit" is not identical to the venous hematocrit. The whole body hematocrit is believed to be between 85% and approximately 90% of the peripheral large vein hematocrit.

INTRACELLULAR FLUID VOLUME

The volume of the intracellular space cannot be determined directly, but rather, it is determined by subtracting the measured ECF volume from that of total body water. This ICF volume may vary slightly depending on which measure is used for the ECF volume. As can be seen in Table 14.1, the total ICF volume in the adult male ordinarily represents 33% of the body weight or approximately 55% of the total body water. It is readily apparent that the single largest body fluid space is the ICF volume or intracellular component of the total body water.

TOTAL BODY SODIUM, POTASSIUM, AND CHLORIDE AND ELECTROLYTE COMPOSITION OF BODY FLUIDS

The techniques for isotope dilution are identical to those used in measuring the various body fluid spaces. Again, these electrolyte measurements may be of considerable value in intraanimal and intrapatient change brought about by some experimental or clinical intervention, or in the study of large groups of normal animals and humans, and to compare these values with those obtained in large groups of animals or humans with various abnormal states.

Table 14.4 lists the electrolyte composition of the ICF and ECF. Although the osmolalities of the ICF and ECF are identical, the striking differences in the composition of these two compartments are evident. These differences are maintained by both the active and passive transport processes responsible for solute and water movement (a) between the environment and the individual by way of the gastrointestinal tract, kidneys, skin, and liver and (b) across all body cells. The concentration gradients are completely dependent on hydrostatic, electrochemical, and energy-consuming forces. Various diseases can take a heavy toll on this ECF and ICF composition. These diseases and their consequences are discussed in detail in the other chapters dealing with abnormalities of water and electrolyte metabolism. Unfortunately, at present, we do not have a rapid, accurate, and practical methodology to measure simultaneously the major fluid compartment of the body. Such would greatly complement our clinical assessment of the patient.

Selected Readings

Barratt TM, Walser M. Extracellular fluid in individual tissues and in whole animals. The distribution of radiosulfate and radiobromide. *J Clin Invest* 1969;48:56–66.

A classic paper on the techniques for the practical measurements of a reliable extracellular volume in animals and humans.

Edelman IS, Leibman J. Anatomy of body water and electrolytes. *Am J Med* 1959;27:256–277.

The classic studies on the isotope dilution techniques and on the formulation of concepts of body fluid spaces.

Hays RM. Dynamics of body water and electrolytes. In: Maxwell MH, Kleeman CR. *Clinical Disorders of Fluid and Electrolyte Metabolism,* 3rd ed. New York: McGraw-Hill, 1979:1–36.

An in-depth review and discussion of body water, control of its transport, and analysis of techniques for its measurement in normal and disease states.

McCance RA, Widdowson EM. A method of breaking down the weight of living persons into terms of extracellular fluid, cell mass and fat and some applications to physiology and medicine. *Proc Soc Med (London)* 1951;138:115.

One of the classic in vivo studies of body fluid volumes and fat measurements.

PART 2
Transcapillary Fluid Exchange in Normal and Pathologic States

Jaap A. Joles and Hein A. Koomans

Fluid accumulates in the interstitial space when net capillary filtration (filtration − reabsorption) exceeds the volume of lymph

TABLE 14.4. Electrolyte Composition of the Body Fluids

Electrolytes	Serum	Serum Water	Interstitial Fluid	Intracellular Fluid (Muscle)
		mEq/liter		*mEq/kg H_2O*
Cations				
Sodium (Na^+)	142	152.7	145	10+
Potassium (K^+)	4	4.3	4	156
Calcium (Ca^{2+})	5	5.4		3.3
Magnesium (Mg^2)	2	2.2		26
Total cations	153	165	149	195
Anions				
Chloride (Cl^-)	102	109.7	114	2±
Bicarbonate (HCO_3^-)	26	28	31	8±
Phosphate (HPO_4^{2-})	2	2.2		95
Sulfate (SO_4^{2-})	1	1.1		20
Organic acids	6	6.5		
Protein	16	17.2		55
Total anions	153	165	145	180+

From Hays RM. Dynamics of body water and electrolytes, In: Maxwell MH, Kleeman CR, eds. *Clinical Disorders of Fluid and Electrolyte Metabolism,* 3rd ed. New York: McGraw-Hill, 1979:1–36, with permission.

exiting from the tissue and returning to the bloodstream. This is usually expressed as follows:

$$\Delta IFV = fL_pS[(P_c - P_i) - \sigma(\pi_p - \pi_i)] - fQ_L$$

where

ΔIFV = the change in interstitial fluid volume
L_p = the hydraulic conductivity of the capillary membrane
S = the surface area for exchange
L_pS = the filtration coefficient
P_c = capillary pressure
P_i = the interstitial fluid pressure (hydrostatic pressure gradient is determined by the difference between P_c and P_i)
σ = the capillary reflection coefficient for a certain protein
π = the colloid osmotic pressure
π_p = π in the capillary
π_i = π in the interstitium
fQ_L = the lymph flow out of the tissue into the bloodstream

Although this expression governs IFV in the whole body, the balance of forces in each tissue is determined by local parameters. Therefore some tissues are more susceptible to changes in IFV than others.

When excess IFV fluid becomes visually or manually detectable, it is termed *edema*. To understand how edema appears, is maintained, or disappears, we must therefore know which factors determine net capillary filtration, which factors determine lymphatic flow, and how both are related to local adaptations in the interstitial space. Subsequently, we will attempt to integrate what is known in nephrotic syndrome about changes of capillary filtration, lymphatic flow, and local interstitial adaptation.

CAPILLARY FILTRATION

A fall in arterial pressure will result in a fall in capillary pressure, which will decrease the filtration of fluid. Moreover, when blood pressure falls, baroperception immediately triggers precapillary arteriolar constriction, which facilitates hemodilution as a result of an increase in reabsorption of interstitial fluid. An increase in arterial pressure tends to have the reverse effect. Thus regulation of organ blood flow and IFV of that same organ are inextricably linked, although some sections of the vasculature are armored with autoregulatory capacity that dampens and delays this effect.

A much more serious threat to capillary pressure is an increase in venous pressure. Examples of conditions in which increases in venous pressure translate to increases in capillary pressure, and hence to edema, are backward failure (pulmonary edema), cirrhosis (hepatic edema and ultimately ascites) and standing (ankle edema). These examples also serve to illustrate that the interstitial space consists of separate compartments that communicate only via the circulating blood plasma. Decreases in venous pressure facilitate the rapid uptake of fluid from the interstitium. Of course, the most pertinent example in our field is ultrafiltration during hemodialysis.

Interstitial fluid pressure has a negative value in the skin and lung, is about 0 mm Hg in muscle, and is positive in tightly encapsulated organs such as the kidney. Interstitial fluid pressure is determined primarily by structural components, collagen and elastic fibres, as well as glycosaminoglycans. These are the structures that determine interstitial compliance, the relation between a change in interstitial fluid pressure and a change in IFV. This relation is steep during dehydration (i.e., when capillary pressure falls as in hemodialysis) but flat dur-

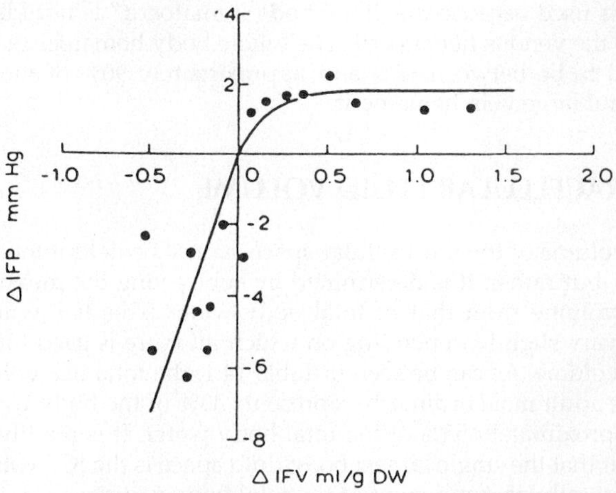

Figure 14.1. Changes in interstitial fluid volume (*ΔIFV*) and pressure (*ΔIFP*) in canine hind limb skin during overhydration and dehydration. The compliance curve is indicated as a solid line. (From Wiig H, Reed RK. Volume pressure relationship (compliance) of interstitium in dog skin and muscle. *Am J Physiol* 1987;253:H291–H298.)

ing overhydration (Fig. 14.1). Thus interstitial fluid pressure is not a powerful force in resisting an *increase* in IFV, and in that sense, edema is not self-limiting. However, absolute levels of interstitial fluid pressure can be very high, for instance, in the lower limbs of large ungulates.

Plasma π is about 25 mm Hg in humans, about half of which is accounted for by albumin. However, when albumin falls, increased levels of nonalbumin plasma proteins of hepatic origin rise, blunting the decrease in plasma π. A classic example of this is in analbuminemia. Even in the presence of proteinuria, if there are specific stimuli for increased globulin secretion (e.g., in HIV infection), plasma π can be close to normal, despite severe hypoalbuminemia.

The intravascular and extravascular albumin pools are in a dynamic equilibrium. Albumin continuously passes through the capillary wall from plasma to interstitium and returns via the lymph. In humans, the transcapillary albumin flux (TER_{alb}) is about 6% of the total pool, which implies that there is a complete exchange of intravascular and interstitial albumin every 24 hours. Interstitial π in healthy humans is about 15 mm Hg. Thus the transcapillary π gradient is about 10 mm Hg. Interstitial π is determined by protein molecules in solution in the free fluid surrounding the capillaries. Because the interstitial protein content is not regulated, a fall in plasma π inevitably results in an increase in net fluid filtration. However, two effects will limit such fluid filtration. Because the capillaries have a low permeability to macromolecules, the direct effect will be the dilution of interstitial proteins, so interstitial π falls and the gradient increases. A later effect is that increased IFV stimulates lymphatic flow, which results in a washout, or "wash-down," of interstitial protein and a decrease of interstitial π to a minimum of 2 to 3 mm Hg. This so-called osmotic buffering has a maximum capacity of about 10 mm Hg and will be exhausted when plasma π falls below about 12 mm Hg. However, it is a slow process, and rapid deceases in plasma π will result in transient decreases in transcapillary π. Such decreases can be expected to accompany sudden exacerbations of nephrotic syndrome in minimal change disease, specifically in children. In such patients, transient symptoms of hypovolemia and stimulated hormones are often observed, even though no differences in blood volume can actually be measured.

The filtration coefficient, L_pS, is the product of the hydraulic conductivity of the capillary membrane, L_p, and the surface area for exchange, S. Not much is known about active control of the hydraulic control of the capillary membrane, but clearly, precapillary vasoconstriction will reduce capillary filtration simply by reducing the surface area. Significant increases of L_pS have been found in frog mesentery when perfused in the practical absence of albumin (less than 1 g/L), but these observations have no relevance to hypoalbuminemia in the range seen in vertebrates.

The capillary reflection coefficient for (a certain) protein, σ, has often been measured for albumin during hypoalbuminemia. It is usually not reduced and hence the TER_{alb} is not or hardly elevated during hypoproteinemia *in vivo*. Thus, in most patients, this is not an important player at clinically relevant hypoalbuminemia, although we have observed an indication of increased TER_{alb} in a few children with severe hypoproteinemia. Moreover, it should be noted that under circumstances of significant hypoproteinemia, when the transcapillary colloid osmotic pressure gradient is slightly compromised, a 10% to 20% reduction in σ will at most reduce the gradient by 1 mm Hg.

LYMPHATIC FLOW

Hypoproteinemia (a reduction of plasma π) and venous stasis [an increase in capillary pressure (Pc)] increase both net fluid filtration and lymph flow. Hypoproteinemia has been studied with plasmapheresis in sheep. An acute reduction in plasma protein concentration resulted in an increase in lymph flow that was still elevated 24 hours after plasmapheresis, despite normalized transcapillary Starling forces. This increase was very pronounced in the lung, where a decrease in plasma π is twice as effective as a matched increase in hydrostatic pressure in increasing postnodal lymph flow. This may be the explanation for the characteristic absence of pulmonary edema in nephrotic subjects, in contrast to patients with renal failure. Long-standing hypoproteinemia induced by nephrotic syndrome also increases lymph flow. This has been measured indirectly in rats treated with puromycin aminonucleoside. The removal rate of radiolabeled albumin from the tail of a nephrotic rat was increased twice as much by a decrease in plasma π of 11 mm Hg than by an increase in tail venous pressure of 20 mm Hg. Recently, lymph flow, directly measured in the main intestinal lymph duct, was shown to be increased from 2.9 ml/hr in controls to 3.6 ml/hr in nephrotic rats (Fig. 14.2).

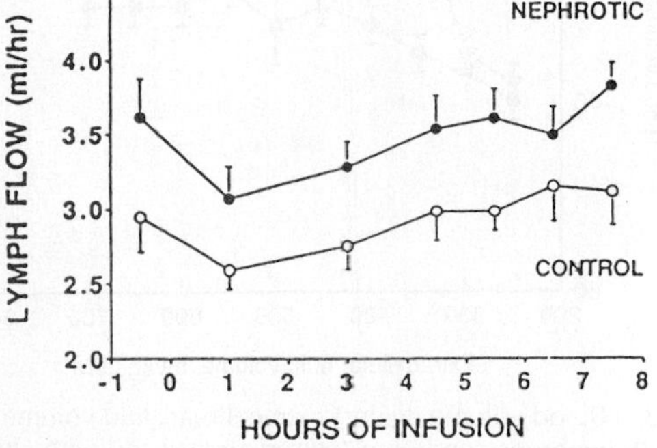

Figure 14.2. Intestinal lymph flow (mean ± SE) in nephrotic and control rats during 1-hour fasting and 8-hour intraduodenal lipid infusion. Lymph flow in the nephrotic group averaged 0.6 ml/hr higher than in the control group ($P = .015$). (From Paulson WD, Torres-Rivera CN, Gray L, Tso P. Intestinal lipid absorption in the nephrotic rat. *J Am Soc Nephrol* 1996; 7:431–436.)

LOCAL ADAPTATIONS IN THE INTERSTITIAL SPACE: SAFETY FACTORS

Tissue Compliance

As stated, the compliance of organs with a tight capsule is low. Such organs are relatively resistant against the formation of edema. On the other hand, when mild edema formation occurs in the kidney, this will raise interstitial hydrostatic pressure, thus decreasing reabsorption and facilitating natriuresis. However, severe intrarenal edema can increase tubular hydrostatic pressure to such an extent that glomerular filtration is impeded, thus eventually aggravate fluid retention.

Lymph Flow

Under steady-state conditions, net fluid flux out of the capillary is balanced by lymph flow back into the circulation. Consequently, lymph protein transport will also equal net transcapillary protein flux. The forces determining lymph transport to and in the initial lymphatics are elusive. Both intrinsic (constriction of the lymph vessel wall) and extrinsic (compression of tissues, muscle "pump") mechanisms play a role. It is plausible that in the presence of increased net filtration, extrinsic forces will be mobilized to enhance lymph flow and protein transport.

Transcapillary π

At the onset of low plasma π, when interstitial π has not yet adapted, the transcapillary π gradient will be reduced and signs of hypovolemia may occur. This phase can last 1 day or more. When lymphatic flow starts to increase, interstitial π will fall until the pool of interstitial protein is in equilibrium with the plasma pool. At this point, the transcapillary π gradient will be partially restored. However, restoration is rarely complete, and thus in this situation, some expansion of IFV is inescapable.

The combined effect of all the safety factors serve to buffer changes in intravascular volume, which is remarkably robust. This is presumably why despite signs of either hypovolemia or hypervolemia in patients with severe nephrotic syndrome, the measured blood volume as such is surprisingly constant.

CHANGES OF STARLING FORCES IN NEPHROTIC SYNDROME

A considerable effort has been invested over the last two or three decades in determining whether fluid retention in nephrotic syndrome is primarily caused by hypovolemia, and subsequent renal sodium retention ("underfill" hypothesis), or by a primary renal sodium retention ("overfill" hypothesis). Although we shall provide evidence in this chapter that both processes occur (albeit at different stages of the disease), it must be borne in mind that blood volume or renal sodium handling are not in themselves Starling forces. Thus changes in intravascular volume or renal sodium handling must translate to changes in Starling forces within a particular tissue to produce edema in this tissue. Moreover, in steady-state conditions, a certain constant amount of edema can be, and in fact often is, present without measurable changes in Starling forces, other than parallel decreases in plasma and interstitial π, being detectable at that time point.

Onset of Edema

Although the initial formation of edema usually escapes our attention in adults, we have recently had the opportunity to study a large cohort of children with minimal lesions nephrotic syndrome (MLNS). These patients often present with acute relapse of MLNS with abdominal pain, oliguria, cold extremities, and diarrhea—a constellation of symptoms suggestive of hypovolemia. Patients entered the study when their urinary dipsticks were positive for 3 consecutive days. Patients in stable remission served as controls. We identified a group of patients with moderate proteinuria and slight edema, but without hypovolemic symptoms. We called this *incipient proteinuria.* These patients had a normal plasma π and blood volume in the presence of a significant decrease of fractional sodium excretion, despite normal levels of renin, aldosterone, and noradrenaline. A second group of proteinuric patients presented with hypovolemic symptoms and edema, significantly reduced plasma π, normal blood pressure and volume, but decreases of glomerular filtration rate and sodium excretion, and stimulated renin, aldosterone, and adrenaline. This group was termed *nephrosis with hypovolemia.*

Our interpretation of these findings in terms of Starling forces is as follows:

- *Incipient proteinuria:* These patients clearly illustrate the "overflow" hypothesis, initial sodium and water retention without hypoproteinemia or hypovolemia. Presumably, these patients were in a phase of hypervolemia with increased capillary filtration, but these subtle changes could not be measured.
- *Nephrosis with hypovolemia:* These hypoproteinemic patients with sodium and water retention illustrate the "underfill" hypothesis. Presumably, these patients were in a phase of compensated hypovolemia with full mobilization of vasoconstrictors, causing peripheral and visceral hypoperfusion. The gradient between intracapillary and interstitial π was reduced to such an extent that capillary filtration is increased in many tissues, despite significant precapillary vasoconstriction. This is the category of patients who may benefit temporarily from infusion of hyperoncotic albumin. It is conceivable that this could help these otherwise hypotensive and frankly hypovolemic patients during the latent period needed to effectuate natriuresis by steroids or diuretics.

Once lymphatic flow is increased, both categories will progress toward a stable phase with a variable degree of edema, probably depending on the length of the period of onset. If the loss of plasma proteins is not very rapid, patients with incipient proteinuria can progress to the stable phase without experiencing any "underfill."

Maintenance of Edema

A third group of proteinuric patients with edema and equally significant reduction of plasma π, presented without hypovolemic symptoms with normal blood pressure and volume, and no change of glomerular filtration rate, renin, aldosterone, and adrenaline. Despite their edema, these patients were not actively retaining sodium. This group was termed *nephrosis without hypovolemia.* This situation was also observed in many adult nephrotic patients, in whom vasoconstrictor hormone levels are normal and a normal natriuretic response to atrial natriuretic peptide can be observed when baseline natriuresis is also normal. Moreover, in adult nephrotic patients, directly measured capillary pressure was found to be normal. Apparently, under these circumstances, a new homeostasis is achieved, which is characterised by decreased (but not decreasing) plasma and interstitial π and an expanded (but not expanding) interstitial fluid volume. The transcapillary pressure and π gradients are only mildly decreased, and homeostasis is not disturbed. If net capillary filtration is increased, it is apparently balanced by lymph flow. Nevertheless, although while in rest in this situation, homeostasis is preserved, it is more labile than in normoproteinemia, as can be ascertained by the exaggerated response to orthostasis, namely a much greater fall in plasma volume than in normals, and by the exaggerated increase in forearm volume during increases in venous pressure. Conversely, during hemorrhage in edematous dogs, we observed a more rapid shift of fluid into the circulation than in normoproteinemic dogs. Because the compliance curve is flat in edematous tissues, large changes in interstitial fluid volume can occur with little change in interstitial fluid pressure. Thus loss of edema-preventing (or "blood volume–maintaining") forces has as a direct consequence: the changes in capillary pressure result in enhanced transcapillary fluid flux, the direction depending on the direction of this change. In the light of this enhanced variability of the intravascular volume, it is clear that different interventions will have enhanced and variable effects on transcapillary fluid movements, and related vasoactive hormones in nephrotic subjects. This is the ideal setting for the generation of the conflicting results that can be found so abundantly in the literature. Moreover, under these conditions, hyperoncotic albumin infusion is contraindicated because it can cause congestive heart and respiratory failure. Sudden increases in plasma π will cause rapid mobilisation of large volumes of interstitial fluid, and nephrotic patients will shift from the "flat" compliance curve to the "steep" curve that is associated with the circulatory congestion common to patients with renal failure (Fig. 14.3).

Further abrupt increases in proteinuria will also destabilize the Starling equilibrium, and the patient can rapidly revert to

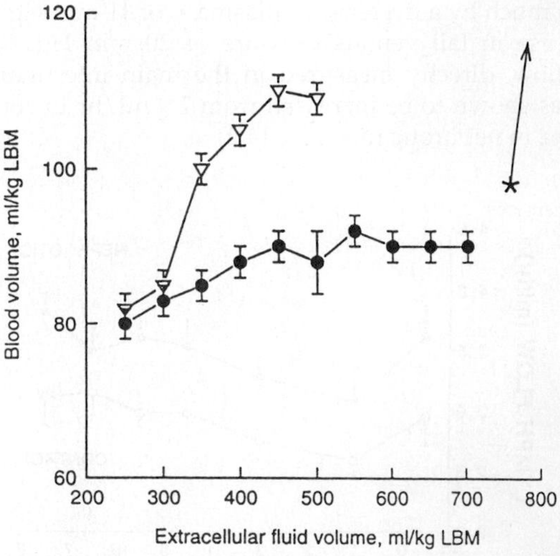

Figure 14.3. Blood volume against extracellular fluid volume *(ECFV)* for patients with nephrotic syndrome *(closed circles)* and with chronic renal failure *(open triangles)*. The data have been grouped in subsets of corresponding ECFV. The asterisk indicates a severely nephrotic subject who manifested frank pulmonary congestion after hyperoncotic albumin infusion *(arrow)*. (Modified from Koomans HA, Braam B, Geers AB, et al. The importance of plasma protein for blood volume and blood pressure homeostasis. *Kidney Int* 1986;30:730–735.)

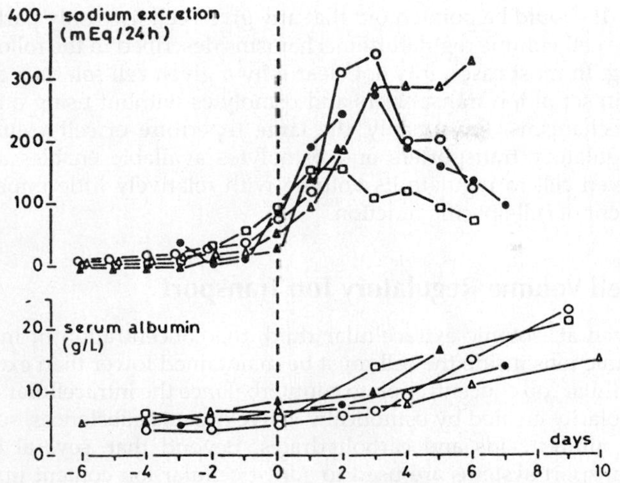

Figure 14.4. Sodium excretion and serum albumin in adults during steroid-induced recovery from nephrotic syndrome. Data from individual patients are represented with different symbols. (From Oliver WJ. Physiologic responses associated with steroid-induced diuresis in the nephrotic syndrome. *J Lab Clin Med* 1963;62:449–464.)

the situation described under Onset of Edema with hypovolemic symptoms. However, patients sometimes come into remission after a nephrotic episode, either spontaneously or after treatment, usually with glucocorticoids. This transition is discussed in the following section.

Disappearance of Edema

If an abrupt decrease in proteinuria occurs, one could expect plasma proteins to rise rapidly while interstitial protein concentrations lag behind. As a result, the transcapillary π gradient will increase, net filtration will become negative, hypervolemia will ensue, and natriuresis will be stimulated. However, the limited amount of information we have about this phase indicates that this is *not* the usual sequence of events. Proteinuria starts to fall within days after the first dose of prednisone, and within 1 to 3 days, a very abrupt increase in natriuresis occurs. However, at this stage, there was barely any increase in plasma protein and albumin concentrations, so this can hardly have been the driving force for the enhanced natriuresis (Fig. 14.4). Moreover, there were no consistent changes in PRA, aldosterone, or ANP before the onset of natriuresis. PRA decreases during peak natriuresis, but this relatively late event indicates an effect rather than a cause. A variable increase was noted in GFR, but this in itself cannot account for the very large increase in natriuresis. Clearly, there must be a natriuretic stimulus. However, its nature still remains unknown.

Thus nephrotic syndrome can be viewed as a contiguous spectrum of presentations. At one end, we can find patients, particularly children with MLNS during a precipitous severe exacerbation or infants with congenital "Finnish"-type nephrotic syndrome who lose huge amounts of albumin and are deeply hypoproteinemic. These patients can present with symptoms of hypovolemia and hypotension and may be temporarily supported by albumin infusion. At the other end, we can identify patients with a significant defect in sodium excretion in the presence of mild proteinuria and subnormal plasma π. Under these conditions, hypertension can be present and therapy should be directed toward suppression of sodium reabsorption. Albumin infusion is contraindicated because it can cause congestive heart and respiratory failure.

Selected Readings

Aukland K, Reed RK. Interstitial-lymphatic mechanisms in the control of extracellular fluid volume. *Physiol Rev* 1993;73:1–78.

In-depth review of all the factors affecting the Starling equilibrium in physiology and pathophysiology.

Brown EA, Markandu N, Sagnella GA, et al. Sodium retention in nephrotic syndrome is due to an intrarenal defect: evidence from steroid-induced remission. *Nephron* 1985;39:290–295.

To date, no consistent increase in any natriuretic (or decrease in any antinatriuretic) factor has been found that can explain why natriuresis occurs during early recovery from nephrotic syndrome.

Guardia JA, Ortiz-Butcher C, Bourgoignie JJ. Oncotic pressure and edema formation in hypoalbuminemic HIV-infected patients with proteinuria. *Am J Kidney Dis* 1997;30:822–828.

Novel observation on the effect of globulins on colloid osmotic pressure in a set of nephrotic subjects with chronic inflammation.

Joles JA, Koomans HA, Kortlandt W, et al. Hypoproteinemia and recovery from edema in dogs. *Am J Physiol* 1988;254:F887–F894.

Description of dynamics of changes in transcapillary colloid osmotic pressure and fluid volumes in dogs subjected to plasmapheresis and low-protein intake.

Joles JA, Rabelink AJ, Braam B, Koomans HA. Plasma volume regulation: defences against edema formation (with special emphasis on hypoproteinemia). *Am J Nephrol* 1993;13:399–412.

Comprehensive review of changes in the Starling equilibrium in hypoproteinemia.

Koomans HA, Braam B, Geers AB, et al. The importance of plasma protein for blood volume and blood pressure homeostasis. *Kidney Int* 1986;30: 730–735.

Analysis of the relation between blood volume and extracellular volume in hypoproteinemic and normoproteinemic patients with renal disease.

Koomans HA, Kortlandt W, Geers AB, Dorhout Mees EJ. Lowered protein content of tissue fluid in patients with the nephrotic syndrome: observations during disease and recovery. *Nephron* 1985;40:391–395.

Description of dynamics of changes in transcapillary colloid osmotic pressure in nephrotic subjects.

Lewis DM, Tooke JE, Beaman M, et al. Peripheral microvascular parameters in the nephrotic syndrome. *Kidney Int* 1998;54:1261–1266.

First report directly documenting normal capillary pressure in nephrotic syndrome.

Paulson WD, Torres-Rivera CN, Gray L, Tso P. Intestinal lipid absorption in the nephrotic rat. *J Am Soc Nephrol* 1996;7:431–436.

First report directly documenting increased lymph flow in the nephrotic syndrome.

Vande Walle JG, Donckerwolcke RAMG, Boer P, et al. Blood volume, colloid osmotic pressure and F-cell ratio in children with the nephrotic syndrome. *Kidney Int* 1996;49:1471–1477.

Separate measurement of red cell and plasma volumes; definition of normal ranges for children and comparison with blood volumes measured in children with minimal-change nephrosis.

Vande Walle JG, Donckerwolcke RAMG, van Isselt JW, et al. Volume regulation in children with early relapse of minimal-change nephrosis with or without hypovolaemic symptoms. *Lancet* 1995;346:148–152.

Description of dynamics of changes in plasma colloid osmotic pressure, fluid volumes, and hormones in children with minimal-change nephrosis.

Woolf AS, Lyson TL, Hoffbrand BI, et al. Effects of physiological infusion of atrial natriuretic factor on healthy subjects and patients with the nephrotic syndrome. *Nephron* 1989;52:244–250.

The renal and hormonal responses to infusion of ANF were normal in nephrotic subjects.

PART 3
Cell Volume Regulation

Florian Lang

One of the prerequisites for survival is the ability of cells to maintain their volume within certain limits. Obviously, gross alterations of cell volume will interfere with the integrity of cell membrane and cytoskeletal architecture. Moreover, cellular performance critically depends on the hydration of cytosolic proteins. Proteins and protein-bound water occupy a large portion of the cell interior (macromolecular crowding), leaving only a small fraction of cellular volume to free water. Abstraction or addition of cellular water to the extent of only a small percentage of cell volume thus has profound effects on protein function and cellular performance.

Water can freely enter or leave cells because the plasma membrane of most cells is highly permeable to water. In theory, driving forces for movement of water include hydrostatic and osmotic pressure gradients. However, the cell membrane is too fragile to withstand significant hydrostatic pressure gradients, and water movement across cell membranes usually is governed almost exclusively by osmotic gradients. Thus, to avoid swelling or shrinking, a cell has to achieve osmotic equilibrium across the cell membrane. If intracellular osmolarity exceeds extracellular osmolarity, water will enter following its osmotic gradient and the cell will swell. Conversely, when extracellular osmolarity exceeds intracellular osmolarity, water will leave and the cell will shrink. Myriad factors modify intracellular or extracellular osmolarity, and thus challenge the osmotic equilibrium across the cell membrane.

Cells use a multitude of mechanisms to maintain cell volume constancy, including altered transport across the cell membrane and altered metabolism. Hormones and mediators may influence these cell volume regulatory mechanisms, and thus cell volume participates in the regulation of cellular function. Beyond that, the interplay of cell volume regulatory mechanisms, cell hydration, and cell function participates in the pathophysiology of many diseases.

In the following, a description of cell volume regulatory mechanisms is followed by a synopsis of factors challenging cell volume constancy. Finally, examples are given illustrating the participation of cell volume regulatory mechanisms in disease.

CELL VOLUME REGULATORY MECHANISMS

Even in a perfectly isotonic environment, a number of cell volume regulatory mechanisms are operative to prevent osmotic disequilibrium across the cell membrane. Following cell swelling, these mechanisms concert to decrease intracellular osmolarity and cell volume, thus accomplishing regulatory cell volume decrease (RVD); upon cell shrinkage, the mechanisms achieve an increase of intracellular osmolarity and cell volume, thus accomplishing regulatory cell volume increase (RVI).

The most rapid and efficient mechanisms of cell volume regulation are ion transporters in the cell membrane. As outlined in the following, uneven ion composition of intracellular and extracellular fluid is one prerequisite for the establishment of osmotic equilibrium across the cell membrane. Furthermore, several ion transport systems in the cell membrane are modified upon alterations of cell volume. Following cell swelling, they mediate cellular ion release, and upon cell shrinkage, they allow cellular ion accumulation to reestablish osmotic equilibrium across the cell membrane. However, the use of ions in cellular osmoregulation is limited because high inorganic ion concentrations interfere with the proteins' stability. Beyond that, altered ion gradients across the cell membrane interfere with the function of gradient-driven transporters. For instance, an increase of intracellular Na^+ activity decreases the chemical gradient for Na^+ across the cell membrane, reduces the driving force for Ca^{2+} extrusion via the Na^+-Ca^{2+} exchanger, and thus increases intracellular Ca^{2+} activity.

To prevent excessive alterations of intracellular ion concentration, cells use organic osmolytes for osmoregulation. Moreover, cells adapt various metabolic functions and thus modify the cellular generation or disposal of osmotically active organic substances.

It should be pointed out that any given cell uses only part of the cell volume regulatory mechanisms described in the following. In most cases, it is not clear why a given cell selects a certain set of ion transporters and osmolytes without using other mechanisms. Presumably, the large repertoire of cell volume regulatory transporters and osmolytes available enables any given cell to regulate its volume with relatively little impairment of cell-specific function.

Cell Volume Regulatory Ion Transport

Even at isotonic extracellular fluid, the concentration of inorganic ions inside the cell must be maintained lower than extracellular ion concentration to counterbalance the intracellular osmolarity created by osmotically active organic substances, such as amino acids and carbohydrates. Beyond that, several ion transport systems are used to adjust cellular ion content upon alterations of cell volume.

Ions in the Maintenance of Cell Volume

To compensate for the cellular accumulation of substrates, cells maintain a low intracellular Cl^- concentration. Cl^- is not extruded directly but is driven out by the cell negative potential across the cell membrane, which is built up by asymmetric cation gradients: The cells extrude Na^+ in exchange for K^+ by the Na^+-K^+-ATPase. The cell membrane is less permeable to Na^+ than to K^+. K^+ tends to leave the cell through K^+ channels following its chemical gradient. The exit of K^+ creates a cell-negative potential difference across the cell membrane, which then drives anions such as Cl^- into the extracellular space. A cell membrane potential of only −18 mV allows a chloride gradient of 1:2 to be maintained, at an extracellular Cl^- concentration of 110 mmol/L intracellular Cl^- concentration is in electrochemical equilibrium at 55 mmol/L. In theory, such a Cl^- distribution would allow the excess accumulation of 55 mmol/L organic substances. In most cells, the potential difference across the cell membrane is more negative than −18 mV and intracellular Cl^- even lower than 55 mmol/L. As long as the cell membrane is not perfectly impermeable to Na^+, the maintenance of cell volume constancy requires expenditure of energy to fuel the operation of Na^+-K^+-ATPase (Fig. 14.5).

Ion Release Following Cell Swelling

Ion transport not only is crucial for the establishment of osmotic equilibrium across the cell membrane, but also is recruited for accomplishment of rapid cell volume regulation.

Following cell swelling, cells have to release ions to decrease their osmolarity. Most cells release ions by activation of K^+ channels and/or anion channels (Fig. 14.6). For cell volume regulation to occur, both ion channel types must be operative because neither K^+ nor anions can leave the cells without the respective counterion. Several cell volume regulatory ion channels have been identified at the molecular level: the K^+ channels Kv1.3, Kv1.5, and IsK, and the anion channels ClC-2 and ClC-3. The role of other ion channels [e.g., I_{Cln} and P-glycoprotein (MDR)] in cell volume regulation has been a matter of controversy. Clearly, many different ion channels are likely to contribute to cell volume regulation in different tissues, and the molecular identity of most of those channels is still elusive.

Swelling of some cells activates unspecific cation channels. Because the electrochemical gradient favours entry rather than exit of cations, these channels cannot directly serve cell volume regulation. Instead, the channels allow the entry of Ca^{2+}, which in turn activates Ca^{2+}-sensitive K^+ channels and/or Cl^- channels.

Besides ion channels, the most important mechanism contributing to regulatory cell volume decrease is KCl cotransport,

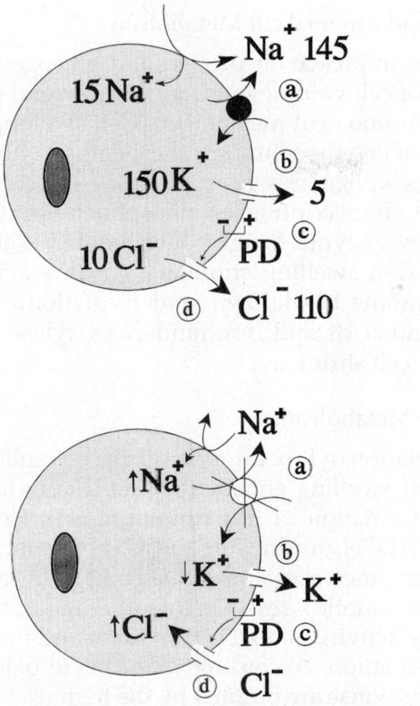

Figure 14.5. Maintenance of cell volume *(upper panel)* and the effects of energy depletion *(lower panel)*. *Upper panel:* The Na^+-K^+-ATPase extrudes Na^+ and accumulates K^+ *(a)*. The cellular accumulation establishes a chemical gradient for K^+, which tends to exit through K^+ channels *(b)*. The efflux of positively charged K^+ generates a cell-negative potential difference *(PD)* across the cell membrane *(c)*, which drives Cl^- out of the cells *(d)*. As a result, intracellular Cl^- activity is far lower than extracellular Cl^- activity. *Lower panel:* Energy depletion inhibits the Na^+-K^+-ATPase, and thus leads to dissipation of Na^+ and K^+ gradients; the decreased chemical driving force for K^+ efflux *(b)* depolarizes the cell membrane *(c)*, which in turn favors entry of Cl^- *(d)* and subsequent cell swelling *(b)*.

which allows coupled cellular release of both ions. Some cells release cellular KCl via parallel activation of K^+-H^+ exchange and Cl^--HCO_3^- exchange. The H^+ and HCO_3^- taken up in exchange for KCl react via H_2CO_3 to CO_2, which can easily leave the cell again.

Ion Uptake Upon Cell Shrinkage

Cell shrinkage activates the Na^+-K^+-$2Cl^-$ cotransport and/or Na^+-H^+ exchange in parallel to Cl^--HCO_3^- exchange. The latter tandem mediates the uptake of NaCl, because the H^+ and HCO_3^- lost in exchange for NaCl is replenished in the cell from CO_2 via H_2CO_3 (Fig. 14.7). The Na^+ accumulated by either Na^+-K^+-$2Cl^-$ cotransport or Na^+-H^+ exchange is extruded by the Na^+-K^+-ATPase in exchange for K^+. Accordingly, the transporters eventually lead to uptake of KCl. Several Na^+-K^+-$2Cl^-$ cotransporters and Na^+-H^+ exchangers have been cloned. Not all transporters need to serve cell volume regulation. Among the cloned Na^+-H^+ exchangers, NHE-1, NHE-2, and NHE-4 are activated following cell shrinkage, while the proximal tubular NHE-3 is inhibited.

A few cells activate Na^+ channels following cell shrinkage. The resulting depolarization drives Cl^- into the cell so that the net effect is cellular accumulation of NaCl. Other cells inhibit K^+ and/or Cl^- channels to prevent cellular ion loss.

Osmolytes

The most important osmolytes are polyols, such as sorbitol and myoinositol; methylamines, such as betaine and glycerophosphorylcholine (GPC); and amino acids and the amino acid derivative taurine. Unlike inorganic ions, organic osmolytes do not destabilize proteins. On the contrary, the organic osmolytes

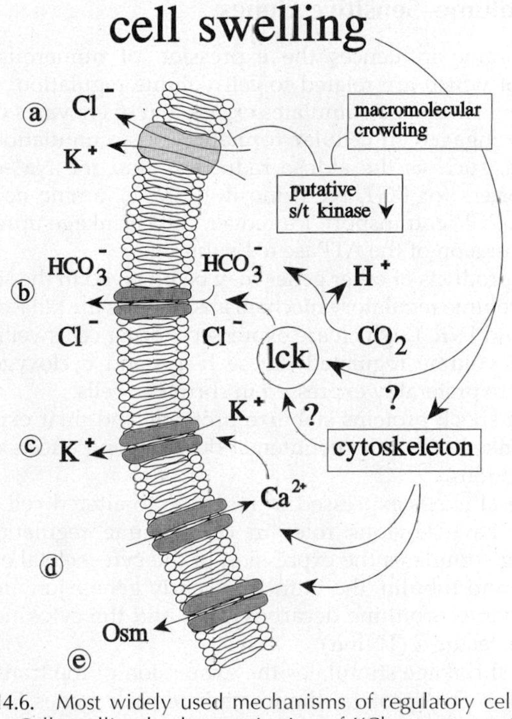

Figure 14.6. Most widely used mechanisms of regulatory cell volume decrease. Cell swelling leads to activation of KCl cotransport *(a)*, anion channels *(b)*, K^+ channels *(c)*, and channels releasing osmolytes such as sorbitol, inositol, taurine, and betaine *(e)*. The Ca^{2+}-permeable cation channels *(d)* do not directly serve cell volume regulation but mediate the stimulation of Ca^{2+}-sensitive K^+ channels. Among the many signaling mechanisms mediating activation of cell volume regulatory transport are Ca^{2+}, the tyrosine kinase lcK[56], and a putative serine/threonine kinase not yet identified at the molecular level.

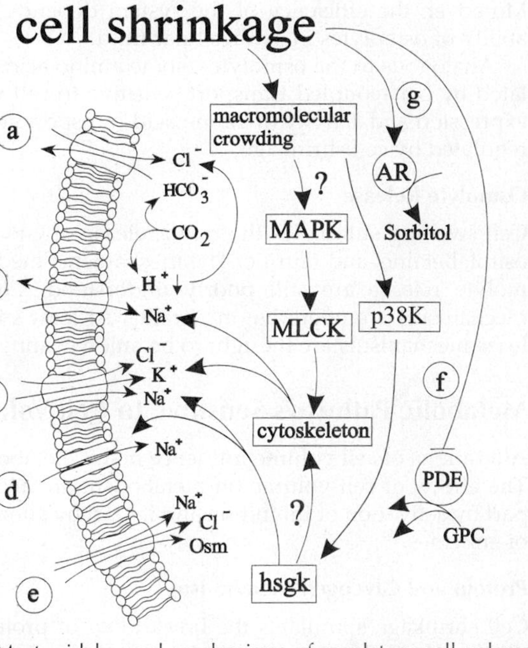

Figure 14.7. Most widely used mechanisms of regulatory cell volume decrease. Cell shrinkage leads to parallel activation of Na^+-H^+ exchange *(b)* and Cl^--HCO_3^- exchange *(a)*, of Na^+-K^+-$2Cl^-$ cotransport *(c)*; Na^+ channels *(d)*; and Na^+-coupled accumulation of inositol, taurine, and betaine *(e)*. Furthermore, cell shrinkage leads to cellular accumulation of glycerophosphorylcholine by inhibition of phosphodiesterase *(f)* and of sorbitol by activation of aldosereducase *(g)*. The carriers and enzymes are regulated by many signaling molecules, including the protein kinases p38K, MLCK, and hsgk.

serve to stabilize the proteins and in this respect to counteract the destabilizing effect of inorganic ions, some organic ions (spermidine), and urea. The stabilizing potency of the different organic osmolytes is not identical. For example, the effects of urea are best counteracted by betaine and GPC and to a lesser extent by myoinositol. The stabilizing effects of osmolytes not only are counteracting the destabilizing effects of ions but are further protecting against the destructive effects of heat shock, desiccation, and presumably radiation.

Osmolyte Accumulation by Metabolism

Sorbitol is generated from glucose under the catalytic action of aldose reductase. Stimulation of the transcription rate of the aldose reductase during osmotic cell shrinkage leads to cellular accumulation of sorbitol. The expression of the protein takes many hours, and the appropriate increase of sorbitol concentration requires hours to days.

GPC is produced from phosphatidylcholine under the catalytic action of a phospholipase A_2, which is distinct from the arachidonyl selective enzyme. GPC is degraded by a phosphodiesterase to glycerolphosphate and choline. Inhibition of the phosphodiesterase during cell shrinkage leads to cellular accumulation of GPC.

Osmolyte Accumulation by Transport

Myoinositol (inositol), betaine, and taurine are taken up by specific Na^+ coupled transporters. The transporters have been cloned (SMIT for myoinositol, BGT for betaine and NCT for taurine). In addition to Na^+ and organic osmolyte, BGT and NCT transport Cl^-. Moreover, the excess positive charge of the carriers depolarizes the cell membrane and thus favors entry of Cl^-. Those transporters mediate uptake of NaCl in parallel to organic osmolytes. The transcription rate of the transporters and the cellular accumulation of the respective osmolytes is stimulated by osmotic cell shrinkage. Because the expression of the transporters is slow, full adaptation requires hours to days. Moreover, the efficiency of the system depends on the availability of osmolytes in extracellular fluid.

Analogous to the osmolytes, some amino acids are accumulated by Na^+-coupled transport sensitive to cell volume. Thus expression and activity of amino acid transport system A is upregulated by cell shrinkage.

Osmolyte Release

Cell swelling stimulates the rapid release of GPC, sorbitol, inositol, betaine, and taurine. The mechanisms mediating the osmolyte release are still poorly understood. Clearly, several mechanisms are operative in parallel. At least some of the release mechanisms are thought to be anion channels.

Metabolic Pathways Sensitive to Cell Volume

Alterations of cell volume influence many metabolic pathways. The effects of cell volume on metabolism are accomplished in part by activation or inhibition and in part by altered expression of enzymes.

Protein and Glycogen Metabolism

Cell shrinkage stimulates the breakdown of proteins to amino acids and of glycogen to glucosephosphate. Furthermore, cell shrinkage inhibits protein and glycogen synthesis. Because the monomers are osmotically more active than the macromolecules, the net formation of macromolecules decreases cellular osmolarity. Cell swelling stimulates protein and glycogen synthesis and inhibits proteolysis and glycogenolysis, thus decreasing the intracellular concentration of amino acids and glucosephosphate.

Glucose and Amino Acid Metabolism

Besides its influence on protein and glycogen metabolism, alterations of cell volume interfere with several pathways of glucose and amino acid metabolism. Cell swelling inhibits glycolysis, stimulates flux through the pentose phosphate pathway, and favors lipogenesis from glucose—effects reversed by cell shrinkage. Transcription of phosphoenolpyruvate carboxykinase, a key enzyme for gluconeogenesis, is decreased by cell swelling. Cell swelling stimulates glycine and alanine oxidation, glutamine breakdown, and formation of NH_4^+ and urea from amino acids and ornithindecarboxylase, again effects reversed by cell shrinkage.

Oxidative Metabolism

The stimulation of flux through the pentose phosphate pathway during cell swelling enhances NADPH production, which favors the formation of glutathione (GSH). Cell shrinkage decreases NADPH production and GSH formation. Accordingly, cell swelling increases and cell shrinkage decreases cellular resistance to osmotic stress. On the other hand, cell shrinkage decreases the activity of NADPH-oxidase and thus impedes cellular O_2^- formation. Accordingly, leucocyte oxidative burst and immune response are blunted by the high osmolarity of the kidney medulla.

Other Metabolic Pathways

Cell swelling stimulates ketoisocaproate oxidation, acetyl-CoA carboxylase, and lipogenesis. In addition, it inhibits carnitine palmitoyltransferase I. It decreases cytosolic adenosine triphosphate (ATP) and phosphocreatine concentrations and increases respiration. Cell swelling stimulates RNA and DNA synthesis. All these effects are reversed by cell shrinkage.

Cell Volume–Sensitive Genes

Cell volume influences the expression of numerous genes, many of which are related to cell volume regulation. Accordingly, cell shrinkage stimulates expression of enzymes or transporters engaged in cellular formation or accumulation of osmolytes, such as the aldose reductase, and the Na^+-coupled transporters for BGT, NCT, inositol (SMIT), amino acids, and Na^+-K^+-$2Cl^-$ cotransport. Moreover, cell shrinkage upregulates the expression of the ATPase α 1 subunit.

The products of other genes may be involved in the signaling of cell volume regulatory mechanisms, such as the kinases ERK1, ERK2 and JNK-1, which are expressed during cell swelling, and the cell volume regulated kinase h-sgk and cycloxygenase-2, which are preferably expressed in shrunken cells.

Heat-shock proteins stabilize proteins, and their expression in shrunken cells may counteract destabilizing effects of accumulated ions.

Several genes expressed in response to altered cell volume do not have obvious roles in cell volume regulation. Cell swelling stimulates the expression of the cytoskeletal elements β-actin and tubulin, the immediate early gene c-jun and c-fos, the enzymes ornithine decarboxylase, and the cytokine tumor necrosis factor-α (TNF-α).

Cell shrinkage stimulates the expression of the transporters ClC-K1, P-glycoprotein, the immediate early genes Egr-1 and c-fos, the GTPase inhibitor α1-chimaerin, the CDβ antigen, the enzymes phosphoenolpyruvate carboxykinase (PEPCK), arginine succinate lyase, tyrosine aminotransferase, tyrosine hydroxylase, dopamin β-hydroxylase, matrix metalloproteinase-9, tissue plasminogen activator, and matrix proteins (including biglycan and laminin B_2).

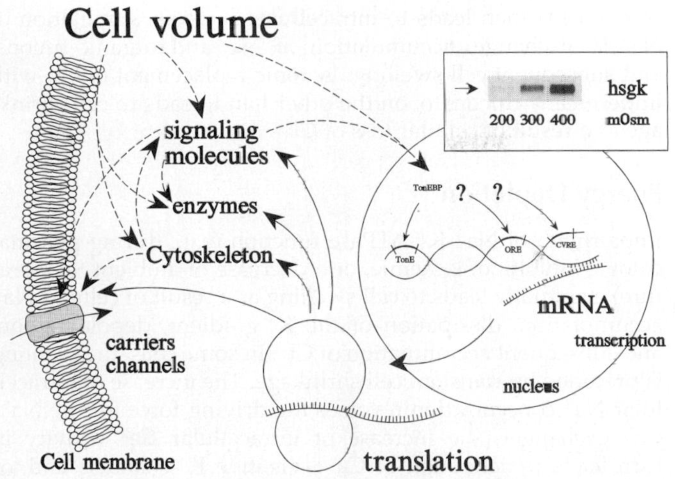

Figure 14.8. Regulation of gene expression by alterations of cell volume. Cell volume triggers the transcription of genes via tonicity-responsive elements *(TonE),* osmolarity-responsive elements *(ORE),* or cell volume–responsive elements *(CVRE).* In the case of TonE, a binding protein (TonEPB) that binds to TonE and thus stimulates transcription of the osmolyte transporter BGT has been identified. Other genes dependent on cell volume or ionic strength encode further transport proteins, cytoskeletal elements, enzymes, and signaling molecules. The insert illustrates the mRNA abundance of hsgk, a serine/threonine kinase at different ambient osmolarities.

Cell shrinkage stimulates both expression and release of antidiuretic hormone, which eliminates water and thus increases extracellular osmolarity.

The mechanisms mediating the altered gene expression are still poorly understood. The promoter region of the genes encoding aldose reductase and BGT have been described to contain osmolarity responsive (ORE), tonicity responsive (TonE), or cell volume–responsive (CVE) elements, which are required for osmolarity or cell volume–sensitive expression of the respective genes. As shown for the TonE governing BGT expression, the responsive element has been shown to bind a tonicity-responsive element binding protein TonEBP for stimulation of expression (Fig. 14.8). How this protein is regulated has remained elusive.

Signaling of Cell Volume Regulation

Alterations of cell volume or osmolarity must be perceived and stimulate a signaling cascade eventually leading to the triggering of cell volume regulatory mechanisms. Little is known about the mechanisms measuring alterations of cell size and hydration.

Circumstantial evidence points to the ability of cells to determine cellular protein content or macromolecular crowding. It has been speculated that a serine/threonine kinase sensitive to macromolecular crowding directly or indirectly regulates the activity of cell volume regulatory KCl- and Na^+-K^+-$2Cl^-$ cotransport.

Alterations of cell size are thought to impose stretch on the cytoskeleton and/or cell membrane, again leading directly or indirectly to activation of cell volume regulatory mechanisms.

Clearly, the mechanisms perceiving alterations of cell volume or cell hydration and the machineries transmitting the information to the cell volume regulatory mechanisms are far less defined than the cell volume regulatory mechanisms themselves. Nevertheless, a considerable body of information has been gathered about the effect of cell volume changes on certain elements of cellular signaling. As with the cell volume regulatory mechanisms, the effects of cell volume on signaling may vary considerably between different cells or a given cell in different functional states.

Intracellular Ca^{2+}

In many cells, swelling increases intracellular Ca^{2+} activity. Ca^{2+} may enter through Ca^{2+} channels in the plasma membrane or may be released from intracellular stores triggered by 1,4,5-inositol-trisphosphate. Ca^{2+} in turn activates some cell volume regulatory K^+ channels and Cl^- channels. However, in many cells, regulatory cell volume decrease is not paralleled by or does not require increase of intracellular Ca^{2+} activity.

Besides its involvement in regulatory cell volume decrease, intracellular Ca^{2+} may increase during and mediate some of the functional consequences of cell shrinkage.

Cytoskeleton

Alterations of cell volume modify the architecture of the cytoskeleton and the expression of cytoskeletal proteins. Both microtubules and actin filaments have been implicated in cell volume regulation. In several cells, disruption of actin filaments or microtubule network has been shown to interfere with cell volume regulation.

Protein Phosphorylation

Cell swelling and cell shrinkage have both been shown to modify the phosphorylation of many proteins. Kinases reported to be activated during cell swelling include tyrosine kinases, protein kinase C, adenylate cyclase, mitogen-activated protein (MAP) kinases, Jun-kinase, and focal adhesion kinase ($p121^{FAK}$). In Jurkat lymphocytes, for instance, cell swelling leads to activation of the src-like kinase lck^{56}, which activates the cell volume regulatory Cl^- channel ORCC. Genetic or pharmacologic knockout of the kinase abolishes the activation of ORCC and regulatory cell volume decrease of those cells.

Osmotic cell shrinkage has been shown to trigger several MAP kinase cascades, leading to activation of SAPK, p38 kinase, and myosin light-chain kinase (MLCK). The latter kinase may modulate the cytoskeleton and thus cell volume regulatory ion transport. Moreover, the kinase cascades lead to activation of transcription factors governing expression of cell volume–regulated genes. Among those is the serine/threonine kinase h-sgk (human serum and glucocorticoid-dependent kinase). Coexpression of h-sgk leads to activation of renal epithelial Na^+ channel ENaC and to thick ascending limb Na^+, K^+, $2Cl^-$-contransporter BSC-1. Both transport-proteins are expected to increase cell volume.

Eicosanoids

Cell swelling activates phospholipase A_2 and subsequently stimulates the formation of the 15-lipoxygenase product hepoxilin A_3 and the 5-lipoxygenase product leukotriene LTD_4. In some cells, these eicosanoids stimulate cell volume regulatory K^+ and/or Cl^- channels and/or taurine release. Enhanced formation of leukotrienes parallels decreased formation of PGE_2 and subsequent inhibition of PGE_2-sensitive Na^+ channels. In other cells, PGE_2 may activate volume regulatory K^+ channels.

pH of Acidic Cellular Compartments

In all cells studied thus far, swelling alkalinizes and cell shrinkage acidifies acidic cellular compartments, presumably including endosomes, lysosomes, and secretory granules. This effect is apparently mediated by the microtubules because it is abolished by disrupture of the microtubule network. The alkalinization of the acidic cellular compartments may contribute to the antiproteolytic action of cell swelling because the pH optimum of lysosomal proteases is in the acidic range and lysosomal alkalinization has indeed been shown to inhibit proteolysis.

CHALLENGES OF CELL VOLUME CONSTANCY

Many factors alter extracellular and/or intracellular osmolarity and thus cell volume. With cell function being highly sensitive to even minor alterations of cell volume, it is clear that alterations of cell volume participate in a wide variety of physiologic and pathophysiologic conditions.

Extracellular Osmolarity

In humans, most cells are normally bathed in well-controlled extracellular fluid. Gross alterations of extracellular osmolarity are encountered only in the kidney medulla, where extracellular osmolarity may approach 1,400 mOsm/L in humans. Renal medullary cells are exposed to this excessive extracellular osmolarity during antidiuresis and must cope with rapid changes of extracellular osmolarity during transition from antidiuresis to diuresis. Blood cells passing the kidney medulla experience high medullary osmolarity and a subsequent return to isoosmolarity within seconds.

During intestinal absorption, intestinal cells are exposed to anisosmotic luminal fluid and liver cells to minor alterations of portal blood osmolarity. Other tissues are exposed to moderately altered extracellular osmolarity during various disorders, as detailed next.

Extracellular Fluid Composition

Even at constant extracellular osmolarity, alterations of extracellular fluid composition may challenge cell volume control.

Extracellular K^+ Concentration

The potential difference across the cell membrane is maintained by K^+ flux through K^+ channels, which in turn depends on the electrochemical driving force for K^+. An increase of extracellular K^+ concentration decreases the chemical gradient for K^+ ions, impedes K^+ efflux, depolarizes the cell membrane, and thus favors Cl^- entry into the cell. The cellular accumulation of KCl eventually leads to cell swelling. Conversely, a decrease of extracellular K^+ may lead to cell shrinkage secondary to cellular loss of KCl.

H^+ and HCO_3^- Concentration

Upon increase of extracellular HCO_3^- concentration, cellular HCO_3^- release through anion channels and Na^+-HCO_3^- cotransport is blunted or even reversed, and the decreased efflux of negative charge hyperpolarizes the cell membrane and decreases the electrochemical gradient for K^+ efflux. As a result, the cell may swell by accumulation of K^+ and HCO_3^-.

An increasing extracellular pH favors the cellular H^+ elimination through the Na^+-H^+ exchanger and the resulting cellular Na^+ accumulation may lead to cell swelling.

During hypercapnea, cellular CO_2 dissociates to form H^+, which is subsequently extruded by the Na^+-H^+ exchanger. Again, cellular Na^+ accumulation is paralleled by cell swelling. Because of the sensitivity of the Na^+-H^+ exchanger to intracellular pH, cellular acidosis favors cell swelling, whereas cellular alkalosis has the opposite effect.

Organic Acids

Some organic anions, such as acetate, lactate, and proprionate, may enter the cell as un-ionized acids. Intracellular dissociation of the acids then leads to intracellular acidosis, stimulation of Na^+-H^+ exchange, accumulation of Na^+ and organic anions, and subsequent cell swelling. Isotonic replacement of Cl^- with impermeant gluconate, on the other hand, leads to cell shrinkage as a result of cellular loss of Cl^-.

Energy Depletion

Impairment of Na^+-K^+-ATPase function (e.g., during pharmacologic inhibition, ischemia, or a decrease of ambient temperature) eventually leads to cell swelling as a result of cellular Na^+ accumulation, dissipation of the K^+ gradient, depolarization, and subsequent accumulation of Cl^-. In some cells, the swelling is preceded by transient cell shrinkage. The increase of intracellular Na^+ concentration reverses the driving force for the Na^+-Ca^{2+} exchanger; the increase of intracellular Ca^{2+} activity in turn leads to activation of Ca^{2+}-sensitive K^+ channels and/or Cl^- channels as well as contraction of cytoskeletal elements.

Epithelial Transport

Most epithelial cells are faced with large transcellular fluxes of osmotically active substances. To cope with transcellular transport, the cells must coordinate the different transport systems at the apical and basolateral cell membranes. In both reabsorbing and secreting epithelia, cell volume participates in the coupling of these transport processes.

In proximal renal tubules and the intestine, for example, Na^+-coupled transport of substrates such as amino acids or glucose across the luminal cell membrane leads to cellular accumulation of Na^+ and substrate. Moreover, the entry of excess positive charge leads to depolarization, impeding the exit of Cl^- and HCO_3^- and thus favoring cell swelling. In Na^+-reabsorbing epithelia such as the renal collecting duct and colon, entry of Na^+ via Na^+ channels similarly challenges cell volume constancy. Limitation of cell swelling during stimulated Na^+ transport requires the operation of cell volume regulatory mechanisms, including activation of K^+ channels, which maintain the electrical driving force for Na^+ entry into the cell.

Activation of Cl^-- and/or K^+ channels in several Cl^--secreting epithelia is paralleled by decrease of intracellular Cl^- activity and cell shrinkage, which stimulate Na^+-K^+-$2Cl^-$ cotransport and/or Na^+-H^+ exchanger with the Cl^--HCO_3^- exchanger.

Substrate Transport

The influence of Na^+-coupled transport on cell volume is not limited to epithelial cells. In several epithelial and nonepithelial cells, concentrative uptake of substrates such as amino acids, glucose, taurine, and taurocholate increases cell volume.

Influence of Hormones and Transmitters on Cell Volume

Many hormones and other mediators have been shown to alter cell volume. Insulin swells liver cells by activating both Na^+-H^+ exchange and Na^+-K^+-$2Cl^-$ cotransport; glucagon shrinks hepatocytes, presumably by activation of ion channels (Fig. 14.9). The effect of these hormones on cell volume accounts for several of their metabolic effects. Notably, the swelling effect of insulin accounts for the antiproteolytic effect, and the shrinking effect of glucagon accounts for the proteolytic effect of the hormones.

Virtually all known growth factors increase cell volume by stimulation of Na^+-H^+ exchange and in some cases Na^+-K^+-$2Cl^-$ cotransport. As amplified in the following, an increase of cell volume appears to be required for cell proliferation.

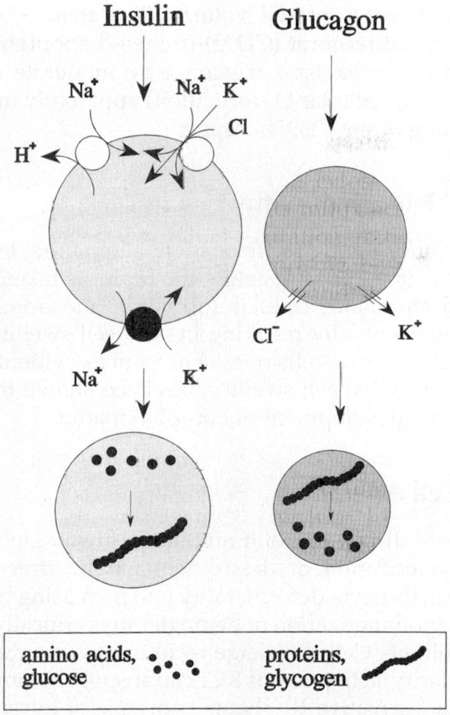

Figure 14.9. Cell volume in the regulation of metabolism by hormones. Insulin swells cells by KCl uptake via activation of Na^+-H^+ exchange, Na^+-K^+-$2Cl^-$ cotransport, and Na^+-K^+-ATPase. Glucagon shrinks cells by activation of K^+ and anion channels. The cell volume changes participate in the signaling of hormone action. Cell swelling stimulates protein and glycogen synthesis, and cell shrinkage stimulates proteolysis and glycogenolysis. The cell volume changes fully account for the effect of both hormones on proteolysis and contribute to the other effects on macromolecule metabolism.

Several excitatory neurotransmitters (e.g., glutamate) activate Na^+ channels or nonselective cation channels; the entry of Na^+ and the depolarization then favor cell swelling. Other neurotransmitters (e.g., GABA) activate K^+ channels and/or anion channels and thus induce cell shrinkage.

Mediators and hormones regulating epithelial transport, such as antidiuretic hormone, adrenaline, or acetylcholine, may either swell or shrink epithelial cells, depending on their effect on ion transport. Stimulation of Na^+-H^+ exchange, Na^+-K^+-$2Cl^-$ cotransport, or Na^+ channels tends to swell epithelial cells, whereas prevailing stimulation of Cl^- and/or K^+ channels shrinks epithelial cells.

Metabolism

Any reaction resulting in an increase of osmotically active substances, such as degradation of proteins to amino acids, glycogen to glucose phosphate, or triglycerides to glycerol and fatty acids, is expected to create intracellular osmolarity. The degradation of the substrates to CO_2 and H_2O then decreases intracellular osmolarity.

Enhanced glycolysis, as it occurs during forced exercise, for instance, leads to cellular accumulation of lactate and H^+, subsequent activation of Na^+-H^+ exchange, and cell swelling.

As explained in the following, diabetes mellitus may lead to either cell swelling or cell shrinkage.

Metabolic pathways may influence cell volume indirectly through alteration of transport across the cell membrane. A decrease of cellular ATP could activate ATP-sensitive K^+ channels, thus shrinking susceptible cells. Similarly, cellular formation of peroxides may shrink cells through activation of K^+ channels, as shown for hepatocytes, pancreatic β cells, and vascular smooth muscle cells. In endothelial cells, peroxides inhibit Na^+-K^+-$2Cl^-$ cotransport, an effect similarly expected to shrink the cells. On the other hand, oxidation leads to inhibition of n-type K^+ channels in lymphocytes and IsK K^+ channels in a variety of tissues, effects rather favoring cell swelling.

Others

Urea readily passes cell membranes and usually does not create osmotic gradients across the cell membrane. However, it has been shown that urea destabilizes proteins and thus shifts the cell volume regulatory set point toward smaller cell volume. Through activation of some cell volume regulatory mechanisms such as KCl cotransport, urea shrinks cells, as shown for erythrocytes, hepatocytes, renal cells, and vascular smooth muscle cells. Beyond that, cell volume is influenced by various drugs and toxins that interfere with cell volume regulatory mechanisms. For example, inhibition of K^+ channels leads to cell swelling, and inhibition of Na^+-K^+-$2Cl^-$ cotransport and/or Na^+-H^+ exchange leads to cell shrinkage.

PATHOPHYSIOLOGY OF CELL VOLUME REGULATION

Hyponatremia and Hypernatremia

A number of conditions alter extracellular Na^+ concentration. As Na^+ salts (mainly NaCl) normally contribute more than 90% to extracellular osmolarity, hypernatremia is necessarily paralleled by increase of extracellular osmolarity. However, because under pathophysiologic conditions osmotically active organic substances may accumulate in blood, hyponatremia may be associated with increased, normal, or even decreased extracellular osmolarity.

Hypernatremia

During hypernatremia, extracellular osmolarity is always enhanced and cells have to avoid cell shrinkage by triggering regulatory cell volume increase. Among those are accumulation of osmolytes. Owing to cell volume regulation, cell volume may become normal despite enhanced extracellular osmolarity. Rapid correction of chronically enhanced osmolarity may then lead to deleterious cell swelling, such as cerebral edema. Cerebral betaine, inositol, and glycerophosphorylcholine may remain enhanced for days following correction of extracellular hypertonicity.

Hyponatremia

As detailed in Chapter 15, hyponatremia may be caused by a surplus of water resulting from excessive oral load or impaired renal elimination of free water. Hyponatremia cannot be equated with hypoosmolarity but may occur in isoosmolar or even hyperosmolar states, as in hyperglycemia of uncontrolled diabetes mellitus and ethanol poisoning. When hyponatremia reflects a decreased extracellular osmolarity, it would be expected to induce cell swelling. However, hypoosmolar hyponatremia is observed following burns, pancreatitis, and crush syndrome, which are rather paralleled by cell shrinkage. It is tempting to speculate that in these conditions the primary event is cell shrinkage and the hyponatremia is the result of regulatory mechanisms to counteract cell shrinkage.

At decreased extracellular osmolarity, the cells must trigger regulatory cell volume decrease to prevent cell swelling. Among other mechanisms, the cells release organic osmolytes. Upon rapid correction of hyponatremia, the cells are unable to rapidly accumulate the osmolytes and the iatrogenic cell shrinkage may prove more harmful than the untreated hypoosmolarity.

Energy Depletion

As pointed out earlier, energy depletion impairs the function of the Na^+-K^+-ATPase, dissipates the Na^+ and K^+ gradients, depolarizes the cell membrane, and leads to cellular accumulation of Cl^- (Fig. 14.5). During ischemia, the cell membrane is further depolarized by increasing extracellular K^+ concentration. Cellular Na^+ and Cl^- accumulation eventually leads to cell swelling. Moreover, the excessive formation and reduced clearance of lactate during ischemia induces cellular acidosis and enhances Na^+-H^+ exchange activity, compounding cell swelling. In the brain, the depolarization triggers the release of glutamate, which activates unspecific cation channels and thus induces further cell swelling.

Cell Proliferation and Apoptotic Cell Death (Fig. 14.10)

Mitogenic factors are known to stimulate Na^+-H^+ exchange and in part Na^+-K^+-$2Cl^-$ cotransport. As shown in cell expressing ras oncogene, activation of those carriers leads to a shift of the set point for cell volume regulation toward greater volumes. In addition, activation of Na^+-H^+ exchange leads to cellular alkalinization. Apparently, the increase of cell volume is one of the prerequisites for cell proliferation, which is impeded by pharmacologic inhibition of Na^+-H^+ exchange and Na^+-K^+-$2Cl^-$ cotransport, as well as by osmotic cell shrinkage.

Cell shrinkage is one of the hallmarks of apoptotic cell death and marked osmotic cell shrinkage (more than 30%) has been shown to trigger apoptotic cell death. On the other hand, a

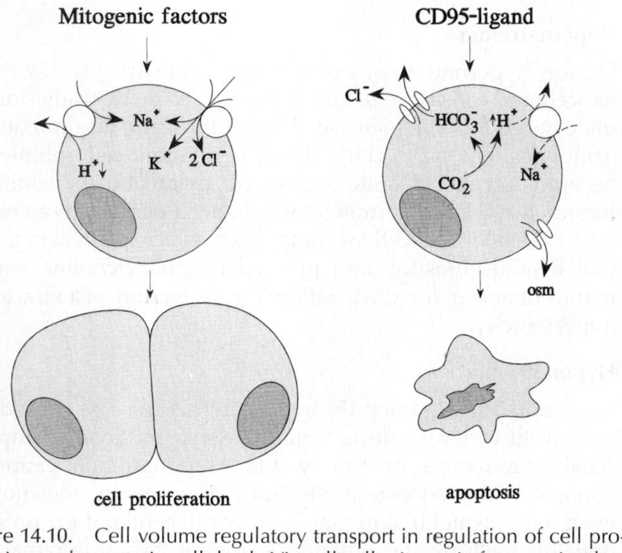

Figure 14.10. Cell volume regulatory transport in regulation of cell proliferation and apoptotic cell death. Virtually all mitogenic factors stimulate the Na^+-H^+ exchanger, and many activate the Na^+-K^+-$2Cl^-$ cotransporter. Among the consequences are cytosolic alkalosis and cell swelling, which are prerequisites for cell proliferation. CD95-induced apoptosis of Jurkat T lymphocytes is paralleled by inhibition of the Na^+-H^+ exchanger as well as activation of the anion channel ORCC and of an undefined osmolyte release mechanism. Cellular HCO_3^- lost is replenished from CO_2 under the generation of H^+. The altered transport eventually leads to cytosolic acidification and cell shrinkage. Again, these events are important for apoptotic cell death.

moderate decrease of cell volume (less than 30%) has been shown to blunt receptor (CD95)-triggered apoptotic cell death. The cellular mechanisms triggered by moderate osmotic cell shrinkage (e.g., cellular O_2-formation) apparently interfere with the signaling of the CD95-receptor.

Hepatic Encephalopathy

In liver insufficiency, urea formation is impaired, leading to accumulation of NH_3. NH_3 enters the brain, is taken up by glial cells, and stimulates cellular formation and accumulation of glutamine, eventually resulting in glial cell swelling. To counteract swelling, glial cells release inositol as evident from NMR spectroscopy. Glial cell swelling has been shown to be a major cause for the development of encephalopathy.

Sickle Cell Anemia

In sickle cell disease, a point mutation of hemoglobin (HbS) favors polymerization of desoxyhemoglobin, dramatically decreasing erythrocyte deformability and increasing blood viscosity. The depolymerization of hemoglobin is critically dependent on cell volume. Cell shrinkage resulting from enhanced ambient osmolarity, activation of KCl cotransport by urea, or activation of Ca^{2+}-sensitive K^+ channels by rise of intracellular Ca^{2+} activity potentiates polymerization of HbS. The high osmolarity and urea concentration in the kidney medulla thus contribute to the particular vulnerability of this tissue to ischemia in sickle cell anemia.

Diabetes Mellitus

Diabetic ketoacidosis is paralleled by cell swelling caused by cellular accumulation of organic acids and enhanced Na^+-H^+ exchange activity in response to cellular acidosis. Furthermore, the excessive glucose concentrations of hyperglycemia stimulate cellular formation and accumulation of sorbitol through aldose reductase. In an attempt to counteract swelling, cells decrease other osmolytes such as myoinositol, an effect that can be reversed by inhibition of aldose reductase with sorbinil. Moreover, hyperglycemia fosters the formation of advanced glycation end products, which have been shown to swell cells, thus leading to antiproteolysis.

On the other hand, hyperglycemia is paralleled by hyperosmolarity and intriguing evidence has been gathered pointing to cell shrinkage in hyperosmolar diabetes mellitus, which increases cellular Ca^{2+} concentration and thus induces cell injury.

Obviously, more experimental information is needed to clarify the role of cell volume changes in the pathophysiology of diabetic complications.

Chronic Renal Failure and Uremia

In uremia, extracellular osmolarity is usually enhanced because of accumulation of urea, which interferes with protein stability and cell volume regulation. The high urea concentrations in uremia stimulate the formation of methylamines, which counteract the perturbing effect of urea. Rapid alterations of urea concentration, as occurs during dialysis, presumably do not allow the osmolyte concentration to fully adjust and are thus expected to disturb the balance of stabilizing osmolytes and destabilizing urea.

Available evidence suggests that alterations of cell volume may participate in the progression of renal failure: Transforming growth factor-β1 (TGF-β1) has been postulated to accelerate renal fibrosis by inhibiting proteolysis and stimulating protein synthesis, leading to enhanced deposition of matrix proteins. Other evidence indicates that TGF-β1 stimulates Na^+-H^+ exchange and Na^+-K^+-$2Cl^-$ cotransport, thus leading to cell volume increase. Both inhibition of the carriers and osmotic cell shrinkage blunt the effects of TGF-β1 on proteolysis and protein synthesis.

Hypercatabolic States

In several hypercatabolic states (e.g., burns, acute pancreatitis, severe injury, liver carcinoma), a decrease of muscle cell volume is observed. This decrease correlates with urea excretion, an indicator of protein degradation. Because cell shrinkage is known to stimulate proteolysis, this correlation points to a causal role of altered cell volume in these hypercatabolic states. Conversely, hypercatabolism can be reversed by glutamine, which is known to swell cells by Na^+-coupled cellular accumulation.

Infection

Immune defense mechanisms are in many ways dependent on cell volume. Leucocyte proliferation, migration, O_2^- formation, phagocytosis, and matrix deposition are all mechanisms critically depending on cell volume regulatory mechanisms. Moreover, ample circumstantial evidence points to the involvement of cell volume regulatory mechanisms in host pathogen interaction. Thus deranged cell volume regulation is likely to affect the course of infectious diseases. For instance, the impaired immune defense in the hypertonic kidney medulla renders this tissue especially vulnerable for infections. Most recent observations indicate that the cell volume–regulated kinase hsgk is highly expressed in inflammatory tissues, such as enteritis, hepatitis, pancreatitis, and glomerulonephritis. Even though the precise functional role of the kinase in the inflammatory process is not yet known, this observation further underscores the role of cell volume regulatory mechanisms during inflammation.

Selected Readings

Burg MB, Kador PF. Sorbitol, osmoregulation, and the complications of diabetes. *J Clin Invest* 1988;81:635–640.

The case is made that high glucose concentrations lead to excessive cellular formation of sorbitol and subsequent detrimental cell swelling.

Burg MB, Kwon ED, Kultz D. Osmotic regulation of gene expression. *FASEB J* 1996;10:1598–1606.

A thorough discussion of the mechanisms involved in the regulation of gene expression during cell shrinkage.

Demerdash TM, Seyrek N, Smogorzewski M, et al. Pathways through which glucose induces a rise in $[Ca^{2+}]_i$ of polymorphonuclear leukocytes of rats. *Kidney Int* 1996;50:2032–2040.

Evidence is presented that high extracellular glucose concentrations impede leukocyte function by osmotic shrinkage and subsequent increase of intracellular Ca^{2+} activity.

Garcia-Perez A, Burg MB. Renal medullary organic osmolytes. *Physiol Rev* 1991; 71:1081–1115.

A most comprehensive review on osmolyte metabolism in renal medulla.

Häussinger D, Lang F. Cell volume: a "second messenger" in the regulation of metabolism by amino acids and hormones. *Cell Physiol Biochem* 1991;1:121–130.

Illustrates that hormones modify cell volume by regulating cell volume regulatory transport and that the respective alterations of cell volume mediate the hormonal actions.

Häussinger D, Roth E, Lang F, Gerok W. Cellular hydration state: an important determinant of protein catabolism in health and disease. *Lancet* 1993;341: 1330–1332.

It is shown that in several catabolic states, the excretion of urea as an indicator of protein degradation correlates with muscle cell volume. On the basis of experimental data, it is argued that hypercatabolism is caused by muscle cell shrinkage.

Hoffmann EK, Dunham PB. Membrane mechanisms and intracellular signalling in cell volume regulation. *Int Rev Cytol* 1995;161:173–262.

A careful review on cell volume regulatory mechanisms, with special emphasis on signaling of cell volume regulation.

Kinne RKH, Czekay R-P, Grunewald JM, et al. Hypotonicity-evoked release of organic osmolytes from distal renal cells: systems, signals, and sidedness. *Renal Physiol Biochem* 1993;16:66–78.

Describes mechanisms and regulation of osmolyte release.

Kwon HM, Handler JS. Cell volume regulated transporters of compatible osmolytes. *Curr Opin Cell Biol* 1995;7:465–471.

Discusses properties and regulation of Na^+-coupled osmolyte transporters.

Lang F, ed. Cell Volume Regulation. Contributions to Nephrology, Vol. 123. KARGER, 1998.

This collection of reviews outlines present knowledge on cell volume regulatory mechanisms, signaling, and the participation of cell volume in regulation of migration, cell proliferation, apoptosis, metabolism, urinary concentration, epithelial transport, metabolism, erythrocyte function, and glial cell function.

Lang F, Busch GL, Ritter M, et al. The functional significance of cell volume. *Physiol Rev* 1998;78:247–306.

This review describes mechanisms and signaling of cell volume regulation, challenges of cell volume maintenance, and the (putative) role of cell volume in erythrocyte function, epithelial transport, metabolism, receptor cycling, hormone and transmitter release, excitability and contraction, migration, pathogen–host interaction, cell proliferation, and cell death.

Lang F, Busch GL, Völkl H, Waldegger S. The diversity of cell volume regulatory mechanisms. *Cell Physiol Biochem* 1998;8:1–45.

A comprehensive list of cell volume regulatory mechanisms in different tissues.

Ling H, Vamvakas S, Busch GL, et al. Suppressing role of transforming growth factor-β1 on cathepsin activity in cultured tubule cells. *Am J Physiol* 1995; 269:F911–F917.

It is shown that TGF-β1 increases cell volume and that this effect correlates with the antiproteolytic effect of the hormone.

McManus ML, Churchwell KB, Strange K. Regulation of cell volume in health and disease. *N Engl J Med* 1995;333:1260–1266.

Reviews the role of deranged cell volume regulation in brain edema, complications of diabetes, and sickle cell anemia.

Ritter M, Woell E. Modification of cellular ion transport by the ha-ras oncogene: steps towards malignant transformation. *Cell Physiol Biochem* 1996;6:245–270.

A comprehensive list of mitogenic factors that influence individual cell volume regulatory mechanisms and a discussion of how mitogenic factors modify ion transport across the cell membrane.

Strange K, ed. *Cellular and Molecular Physiology of Cell Volume Regulation.* Boca Raton, FL: CRC Press, 1994.

A collection of reviews on cell volume regulatory mechanisms, organic osmolyte metabolism, sensing, and signaling of cell volume maintenance.

Waldegger S, Barth P, Raber G, Lang F. Cloning and characterization of a putative human serine/threonine protein kinase transcriptionally modified during anisotonic and isotonic alterations of cell volume. *Proc Nat Acad Sci USA* 1997; 94:4440–4445.

Describes the cloning, regulation, and tissue distribution of cell volume–dependent kinase hsg-k, which in later experiments turned out to play a striking role during inflammation.

CHAPTER 15

Water and Sodium Metabolism

PART 1
Control of Water Excretion

Michael S. Anger, Stuart I. Senkfor, and Tomas Berl

Water accounts for approximately 50% to 60% of an adult's body weight. Under normal physiologic conditions, the osmolality of body water is maintained within a remarkably narrow range, despite large variations of solute and water intake. This constancy is made possible by the active balance between intake and output, via enormous flexibility in the volume of water excreted daily. This range may be as low as 0.5 L to as high as 25 L in a normal adult. Renal water excretion is controlled by the interrelationship of thirst, the neurohypophysis, and the kidney. Central to the operation of this system is the appropriate release of vasopressin and its effect on its target organ, the kidney.

REGULATION OF THIRST

Under normal circumstances, the daily solute excretion in humans is approximately 600 mOsm per day. The volume that this is excreted in will depend on fluid intake. If the renal concentrating mechanism is fully activated and urine maximally concentrated (1,200 mOsm/kg water), there is an obligatory loss of about 500 ml per 24 hours. This volume represents the mandatory daily water intake to maintain water balance. Insensible losses are normally balanced by water produced in metabolic processes. Failure to ingest such a volume leads to progressive water depletion. Therefore it is not surprising that all terrestrial vertebrates possess a well-defined thirst mechanism. In fact, it is likely that the development of this mechanism along with the renal concentrating system were indispensable in the successful adaptation of living organisms in the transition from an aqueous to an arid environment. Water intake often exceeds the obligatory minimum because much drinking by humans is undertaken in response to habit rather than need. The water intake that follows the perception of thirst, however, is crucial in maintaining hydration in the face of threatened water deficit. Although thirst involves a decrease output of saliva and dryness of the mouth and throat, along with perception at the cortical level, its control appears to involve osmoreceptors located in the anterolateral hypothalamus, coincidentally near to those that regulate vasopressin release. This close proximity allows the integration of thirst and vasopressin secretion so that both are stimulated when water conservation is needed and both are suppressed in response to water excess. Despite their anatomic proximity, however, pathologic lesions to one nucleus tend to spare the other. Thus lesions that cause failure in vasopressin secretion often leave thirst regulation intact.

The major physiologic stimulus to thirst is a decrease in total body water and the increase in serum tonicity that accompanies it. Solutes to which these cell membranes are relatively *impermeable* (e.g., sodium chloride, mannitol, sucrose) result in dehydration of osmoreceptors, which in turn stimulate hypothalamic centers and thus thirst. Solutes to which these cell membranes are relatively *permeable* (e.g., glucose, urea) elevate extracellular fluid osmolality because they result in less osmoreceptor dehydration and do not stimulate thirst. The osmotic threshold for stimulation of thirst is reached at an osmolality at which vasopressin release is already maximal for antidiuretic effects at approximately 295 mOsm/kg water.

Nonosmolar pathways may stimulate water intake as well, the most potent of which is contraction of extracellular fluid volume. Any decrease in actual or effective blood volume may be accompanied by the sensation of thirst. The mechanism whereby nonosmolar-stimulated thirst is brought about is not well understood; the decrease in volume is detected by stretch receptors in the thoracic cavity, while baroreceptors in the arterial circulation may modulate thirst (by altering afferent parasympathetic tone). β-Adrenergic and cholinergic stimulation is associated with an increased water intake. The renin-angiotensin system is activated in all of the aforementioned settings in which nonosmolar thirst stimulation occurs, and there is compelling evidence for the dipsogenic properties of the octapeptide, angiotensin II. In addition, specific cerebral paraventricular structures, the subfornical organ, and the organum vasculosum laminae terminalis, in the walls of the third ventricle, have been found as sites involved in angiotensin II–induced drinking. These structures are vascular, and it is thought that the dipsogenic action of angiotensin II is related to its potent vasoconstrictor effect, producing mechanical deformation of the blood vessels in these structures. Reduced filling of the blood vessels in these regions stimulates drinking, whereas when the vasoconstrictive effects are blocked by vasodilators, thirst is also blocked. These observations may explain the intense thirst associated with disorders associated with high renin levels, such as chronic renal failure or malignant hypertension, and its abatement after bilateral nephrectomy.

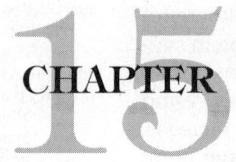

Other factors may also have a role in thirst (although less important than angiotensin II): low dosages of atrial natriuretic peptide appear to blunt thirst; vasopressin lowers the osmotic threshold for thirst in dogs. However, in Brattleboro rats with central diabetes insipidus, thirst remains intact, suggesting a limited role for vasopressin in the control of thirst. Dopamine exerts a permissive effect on the dipsogenic response to angiotensin, which is blocked by the dopamine antagonist haloperidol.

Clinical disturbances in thirst occasionally occur with no obvious underlying central nervous lesion, as in essential hypernatremia. However, most patients with hypodipsia or adipsia have either an organic hypothalamic lesion or even more often an alteration in the state of consciousness that impairs either their perception of thirst at a cortical level or their capacity to obtain water in response to it.

ANTIDIURETIC HORMONE (ARGININE VASOPRESSIN)

Arginine vasopressin (AVP), a cyclic octapeptide (molecular weight of 1,099) (Fig. 15.1) of 1,100 D, is the antidiuretic hormone (ADH) of humans and most mammals (except in pigs, which have lysine vasopressin). The vasopressin gene (Fig. 15.2) is located on chromosome 20, close to the oxytocin gene, and is about 2,000 base pairs long, including three exons and two introns. The promoter has *cis*-acting elements, including a glucocorticoid response element, a cyclic adenosine 3′,5′-monophosphate (cAMP) response element and 4 AP-2 binding sites.

Studies using histochemical techniques have conclusively demonstrated that all the cells of the supraoptic nucleus and most of the cells in the paraventricular nucleus are involved in the synthesis of ADH. Although oxytocin shows a similar anatomic localization, it is transcribed in a different subtype of magnocellular neurons in the SON and PVN. Experiments using a monoclonal antibody actually point to the paraventricular nucleus as the major site of AVP synthesis. With age, the weight of the neurohypophysis increases with an increase of connective tissue and a decrease of vasculature, yet there is no change in neurosecretory material.

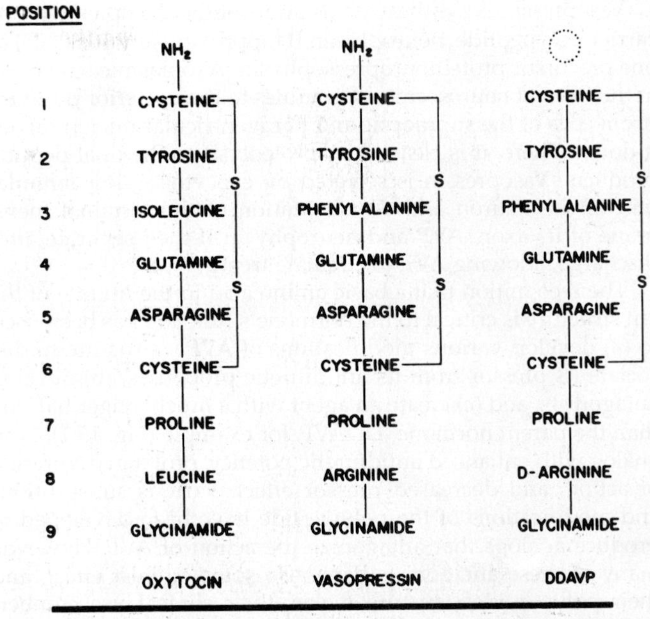

Figure 15.1. Primary structure of oxytocin, AVP, and DDAVP. (Reprinted with permission from Robertson GL, Berl T. Pathophysiology of water metabolism. In: Brenner BM, ed. *The Kidney,* Vol I, 5th ed. Philadelphia: WB Saunders, 1996.)

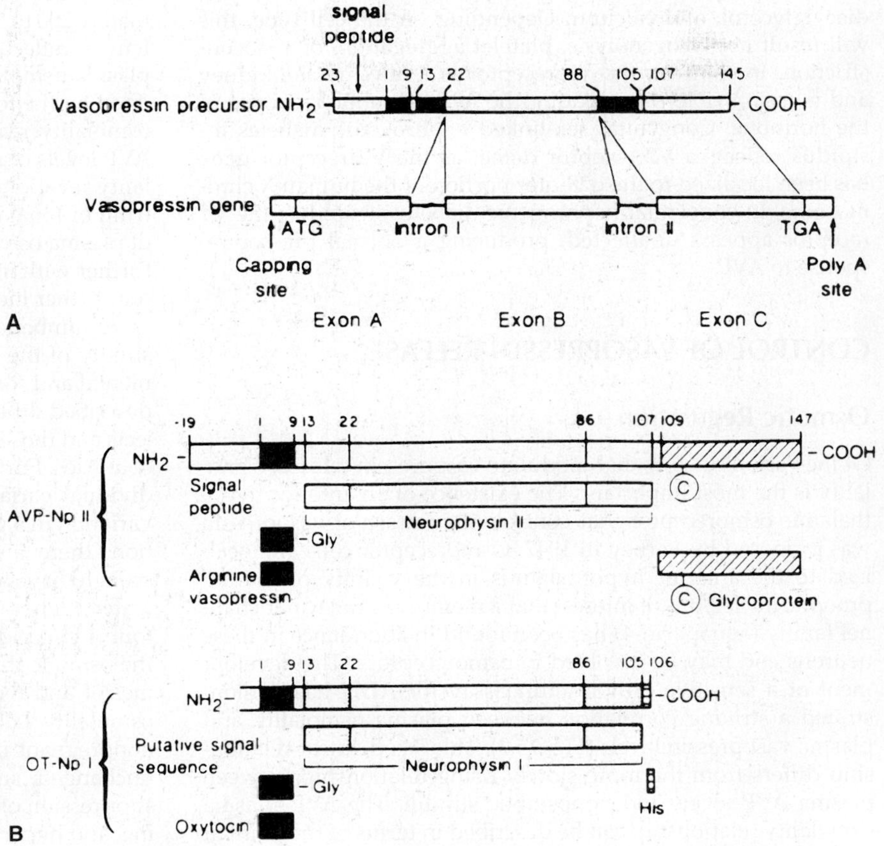

Figure 15.2. **A:** Structure of the gene that codes for the synthesis of propressophysin. **B:** The structure of the biosynthetic peptide precursors of arginine vasopressin (propressophysin) and oxytocin (pro-oxyphysin). (Reprinted with permission from Robertson G, Berl T. Pathophysiology of water metabolism. In: Brenner BM, Rector FC, eds. *The Kidney,* 4th ed. Philadelphia: WB Saunders, 1996:677–736.)

Vasopressin is synthesized as an insoluble complex with its carrier polypeptide, neurophysin II (approximately 10,000 D) as one precursor protein, propressophysin. Axoplasmic streaming in the form of neurosecretory granules to the posterior pituitary (from cells of the supraoptic and paraventricular nuclei) carries it down. There, it is cleaved by proteolysis to the final peptide products. Vasopressin is secreted by exocytosis after stimulation of the neuron and depolarization of the terminal membrane of its axon. AVP and neurophysin II then separate after discharge, allowing AVP to circulate freely.

The recognition that a basic amino acid in the middle of the tail structure is critical to the hormone's function has been used to (a) develop various modifications of AVP's structure to dissociate its pressor from its antidiuretic properties, (b) develop antagonists, and (c) create an agent with a much longer half-life than the parent hormone. DDAVP, for example (Fig. 15.1), is an analog with enhanced antidiuretic potency, prolonged duration of action, and decreased pressor effect. Various substitutions and modifications of the polypeptide have been developed to produce analogs that antagonize the action of AVP. However, many of these antagonists have also some agonist effect, and their polypeptide structure makes their clinical use cumbersome. More recently, orally active inhibitors of vasopressin receptors, such as the V1-receptor antagonist OPC-21268 and the V2-receptor antagonist OPC-31260, have been developed and are in clinical trials for human use.

VASOPRESSIN RECEPTORS

Three vasopressin receptors have been identified and cloned (V1a, V1b, and V2). They belong to the seven-membrane spanning receptor family. The V1a receptor is found in liver, platelets, and smooth muscle cells, and the V1b receptor is found in the pituitary. The V1 receptor transmits its extracellular signal via phospholipase C, resulting in release of phosphoinositide, diacylglycerol, and calcium. Depending on the cell type, this will result in glycogenolysis, platelet aggregation, or vasoconstriction. In contrast, the V2 receptor is limited to the kidney and is responsible for initiating the hydroosmotic response of the hormone. Congenital sex-linked nephrogenic diabetes insipidus reflects a V2 receptor defect as the V2 receptor gene has been localized to the q28-qter portion of the human X chromosome. In congenital nephrogenic diabetes insipidus, the V1 receptor appears unaffected, producing a normal pressor response to AVP.

CONTROL OF VASOPRESSIN RELEASE

Osmotic Regulation

Of the various factors that modulate vasopressin release, osmolality is the most important. The existence of an anterior hypothalamic osmoreceptor that controls the release of vasopressin was proposed by Verney in 1947. Osmoreceptor cells are localized to the anterior hypothalamus in the vicinity of the supraoptic nuclei. It is of interest that a member of the water channel family (aquaporin-4) has been found in abundance in these neurons and may be involved in osmoreceptors. The development of a sensitive radioimmunoassay for ADH has demonstrated a striking correlation between plasma osmolality and plasma vasopressin levels (Fig. 15.3). This steep, linear relationship differs from the more slowly rising relationship between plasma AVP levels and nonosmotic stimuli. The AVP–plasma osmolality relationship can be described in terms of the point at which detectable vasopressin levels appear in the circulation

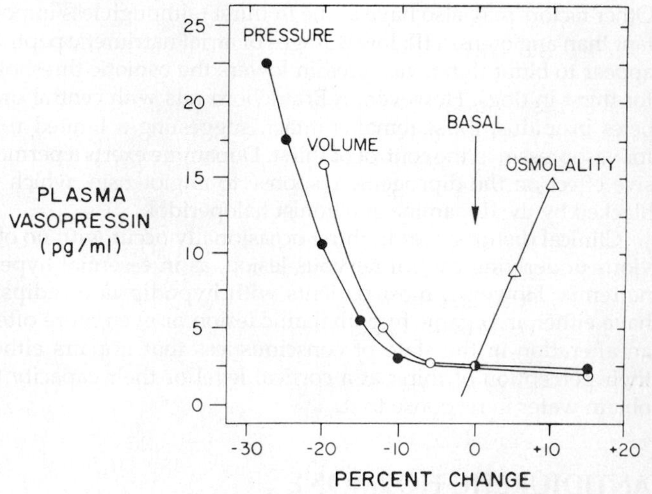

Figure 15.3. Relation of plasma vasopressin to the percent change in plasma osmolality *(triangles)*, volume *(open circles)*, and pressure *(solid circles)*. (Reprinted with permission from Robertson G, Berl T. Pathophysiology of water metabolism. In: Brenner BM, Rector FC, eds. *The Kidney,* 4th ed. Philadelphia: WB Saunders, 1996:677–736.)

(osmotic threshold) and the slope of the line (sensitivity) of the osmotic release of the hormone.

Although there are individual variations, at plasma osmolalities below 280 mOsm/kg, in humans, AVP is almost undetectable defining the osmotic threshold. At levels above this value, AVP concentrations are directly related to plasma osmolality. The relationship defining the osmotic sensitivity is such that changes of plasma osmolality of only 1% (approximately 3 mOsm/kg) are associated with changes of plasma AVP of approximately 1 pg/ml. There is also a close correlation between plasma AVP levels and urine osmolality. Thus, for each 1-pg/ml change in AVP levels, urinary osmolality increases by approximately 200 to 300 mOsm/kg. The high gain in this feedback system is reflected by the translation of very small changes in plasma osmolality into large changes in urinary osmolality defined by the following formula: Δ Uosm = 90 × Δ Posm. Urine osmolality reaches its maximum at about 1,200 mOsm/kg at AVP levels of about 5 pg/ml, corresponding to a plasma osmolality level of about 295 mOsm/kg. Therefore the entire spectrum of renal responsiveness to AVP occurs over a small range of plasma osmolality of 15 mOsm/kg. Plasma vasopressin rises further with increasing plasma tonicity beyond this point without further increment in urine osmolality.

A number of factors can alter the osmotic threshold and sensitivity of the osmoreceptor. There may be important environmental and/or genetic factors, for example, that account for the described difference between threshold values in Japanese subjects and those that have been reported in subjects from Western countries. Furthermore, it appears that there is considerable individual variation in osmotic threshold as well as significant variation in a given individual when repeatedly tested. In addition, there are species differences; most laboratory animals seem to have a threshold that is approximately 10 mOsm/kg of water higher than the mean value, 280 mOsm/kg of water, found in occidental humans. In addition, pregnancy decreases the osmotic threshold. Plasma volume increases in the first trimester and remains elevated until term. Concurrently, plasma osmolality falls to levels approximately 10 mOsm/kg below nonpregnant norms. Despite this, basal plasma AVP levels are unchanged, suggesting a change in the osmotic threshold for suppression of release. Following fluid deprivation, water loading, and hypertonic saline infusion, changes in plasma AVP parallel that seen postpartum. During the menstrual cycle, a small but significant fall in mean plasma osmolality occurs in the luteal phase. The mechanisms of this change in threshold remain unknown.

The sensitivity of the osmotic release of ADH can also be modified by a number of factors. The individual variations that occur in the threshold of vasopressin secretion are also found when the sensitivity of the osmoreceptor is assessed. However, in contrast to the threshold, the sensitivity of vasopressin release is fairly constant when a given individual is tested at various times. Age is another factor that alters osmoreceptor sensitivity; older subjects appear to have a steeper slope (i.e., more sensitive mechanism). The rate of increase in osmotic stimulus may also modify the relationship under discussion because AVP levels appear to be higher for any level of plasma tonicity if that level is arrived at in a shorter period. Whether the nature of the solute involved in the response is of importance has been a matter of controversy. Some investigators think that the concentration of sodium *per se* is critical. However, both Verney's original studies and later observations suggest that other solutes, such as mannitol, can produce a response of a magnitude indistinguishable from that of hypertonic saline. It appears that, although an increase in sodium concentration is not critical, the solute has to be one that does not readily cross cell membranes and thereby causes an alteration in the size of the osmoreceptor. The reflection coefficient for the cellular penetration of the solute will therefore determine its ability to release ADH. Although the role of angiotensin II in thirst control is incontrovertible, its role in modifying vasopressin release has been shrouded with some controversy. Although a physiologic role for this polypeptide in either directly stimulating vasopressin secretion or potentiating its osmotic release has not been convincingly demonstrated, *in vitro* studies suggest an important role for angiotensin II as a modifier of osmotic AVP release.

Whereas in pregnancy the osmotic threshold for AVP is changed, there is no alteration in the sensitivity for release. In contrast to this, during the luteal phase of the menstrual cycle, the sensitivity for AVP release appears to be reduced. The possibility that hypercalcemia and lithium increase the sensitivity of the osmoreceptor has also been suggested.

The effect of chronic hyponatremia on AVP synthesis has also been investigated. Following induction of hyponatremia in the rat by DDAVP, vasopressin synthesis is suppressed by the seventh day. In parallel, mRNA levels of the hormone decrease by 90%. Following correction of hyponatremia, mRNA levels return to normal in seven days. On the other hand, following chronic stimulation of AVP release, elevated mRNA levels decrease slowly over 2 to 4 weeks. Finally, nonosmotic factors not only alter the threshold for vasopressin release but also modify the sensitivity of the system. Thus volume contraction and hypotension increase while volume expansion presumably decreases the slope of the relation between plasma AVP levels and these nonosmotic stimuli.

TABLE 15.1. Nonosmotic Factors in the Control of Vasopressin Release

Blood volume
Left atrial pressure
Catecholamines
Angiotensin II
Atrial natriuretic factor
Nausea
Pain
Pharmacologic agents

Nonosmotic Regulation of Vasopressin Release

Some of the nonosmotic factors that alter vasopressin release are listed in Table 15.1. Of these, the most important is a change in blood volume. A decrease of approximately 7% to 10% in intravascular volume causes a prompt increase in AVP secretion. Once established, in contrast to osmolality, this relationship is not linear (Fig. 15.3). Osmotic control of AVP release and thirst may be overridden by nonosmotic stimuli in a number of pathologic and pharmacologic states. Thus, even if the tonicity of body fluids is decreased and would call for suppression of the hormone's release, alterations in systemic hemodynamics can maintain the secretion of the hormone to maximize water conservation. The homeostatic mechanism that maintains the integrity of circulatory volume takes precedence over mechanisms that maintain tonicity (law of circulating volume, Fig. 15.4).

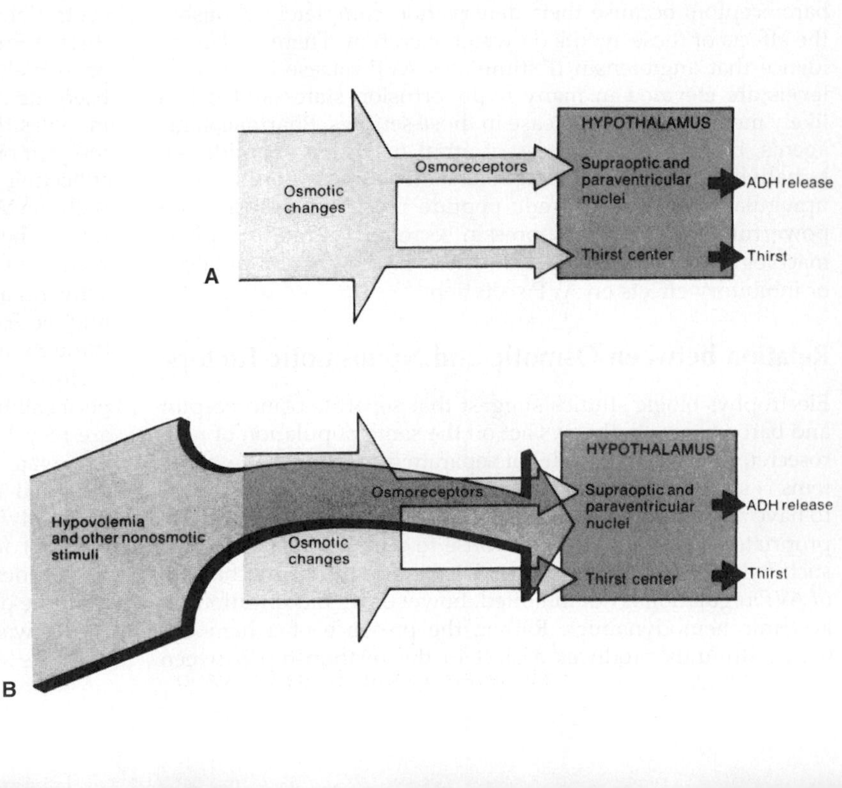

Figure 15.4. Graphic depiction of the law of circulating volume. Note that in the setting of volume deletion, this stimulus takes precedence over osmotic requirements. **A:** Osmotic changes in the extracellular fluid provide the normal stimulus for water control. **B:** Severe depletion of blood volume constitutes an overriding stimulus. Restoration of blood volume takes precedence over osmotic requirements. *ADH,* antidiuretic hormone. (Reprinted with permission from Goldberg M: Water control and the dysnatremias. In: Bricker NS, ed. *The Sea With Us.* New York: The Scientific Medical Publishing Co, 1975:14–25.)

Sensing receptors to volume changes that effect AVP release exist in the low-pressure areas of the circulation, likely the atria and intrathoracic veins. This is not surprising because the venous system contains approximately 85% of total blood volume at any given time. Maneuvers that decrease left atrial pressure, such as bleeding, acute pulmonary hypertension, and exposure of the lower body to negative pressure, result in AVP release. Conversely, maneuvers that increase left atrial pressure, such as volume expansion, atrial tachycardia, and water immersion, result in a fall in AVP levels. Because there is experimental evidence that atrial natriuretic peptide may inhibit dehydration and hemorrhage-induced AVP release, it is reasonable to postulate that a similar mechanism may be involved in the suppression of AVP release that accompanies atrial distension. Stretch receptors in the left atrium, aorta, and carotid sinuses respond to distension of the vessel by sending impulses through the vagus and glossopharyngeal nerves to the nucleus tractus solitarii of the medulla. From there, information is transmitted to the hypothalamus over postsympathetic pathways. Sensing receptors that can influence the secretion of AVP appear to be present in the high-pressure system of the circulation as well. Increased pressure in the arterial tree is associated with suppression of AVP release, whereas decreased pressure stimulates release of the hormone. In fact, denervation of the carotid sinus and the aortic arch baroreceptors is necessary to abolish the release of AVP in response to myriad nonosmotic stimuli, including thoracic caval constriction, nicotine use, anesthetic use, and hypoxia. It appears likely that both low- and high-pressure receptors act in concert and that afferent parasympathetic pathways that innervate them constitute the final common pathway for nonosmotic AVP secretion.

The sympathetic nervous system has a role in the regulation of water excretion. Supraoptic nuclei of the hypothalamus are heavily innervated by noradrenergic neurons. Stimulation of α-adrenergic receptors is associated with a diuresis, whereas β-adrenergic stimulation is antidiuretic; *in vitro* studies have demonstrated an effect of α_2-adrenergic agonists in inhibiting AVP action. It appears that the diuresis of α-adrenergic stimulation results from central suppression of AVP release and from a renal effect. In contrast, the antidiuretic effect of β-adrenergic stimulation is mediated via AVP release alone. Furthermore, these influences on AVP release also appear to be modulated by baroreceptors because their denervation completely abolishes the effects of these agents on water excretion. There is also evidence that angiotensin II stimulates AVP release because its levels are elevated in many hypoperfusion states and it is a likely mediator of AVP release in those settings. Pharmacologic agents, but not low dosages of atrial natriuretic peptide, alternatively inhibit AVP secretion. Water deprivation, in turn, upregulates atrial natriuretic peptide receptors. Nausea is a powerful stimulus to vasopressin secretion. Numerous pharmacologic agents have been shown to have either stimulatory or inhibitory effects on AVP secretion.

Relation between Osmotic and Nonosmotic Factors

Electrophysiologic studies suggest that separate osmoreceptor and baroreceptor pathways act on the same population of neurosecretory cells. The model of separate inputs for the two systems is supported by the observations in some humans shown to have absence of osmoreceptor-mediated AVP release, yet appropriate AVP secretion in response to a nonosmolar stimulus such as reduced blood volume. The osmoreceptor mechanism of AVP regulation is not inhibited, however, by modifications in systemic hemodynamics. Rather, the presence of a hemodynamic stimulus produces a shift in the relationship between plasma osmolality and AVP levels. In the presence of hypovolemia, AVP levels may be suppressed by a decrease in plasma osmolality, but this effect occurs at a lower plasma osmolality than in normal conditions. In most conditions, though, osmotic and nonosmotic stimuli act synergistically. As depicted in Fig. 15.3, the osmoreceptor is more sensitive, being activated by a 1% to 2% change in plasma osmolality, whereas a 5% to 10% change in blood volume is probably needed to activate the nonosmotic pathways. However, once these are activated, they are more potent than any conflicting input provided by the osmoreceptor pathway. Thus, in the face of significant volume depletion, both vasopressin secretion and thirst will be stimulated even in the hypoosmolar state. This phenomenon accounts for the abnormal excretion of water in a number of hyponatremic disorders.

Circulation and Metabolism of Vasopressin

Released AVP circulates essentially as a free peptide without significant protein binding and has a half-life of about 5 to 10 minutes in humans. The liver, kidney, and small intestine account for most of the degradation of the hormone. This appears to be linked to AVP's binding to its end-organ receptors. Diseases of the kidney, and especially the liver, increase the half-life in the blood. This impaired degradation likely plays little role in the abnormal water excretion seen in hepatic insufficiency, as AVP release is greatly increased. In pregnancy, the blood contains large quantities of a cystine aminopeptidase (of placental origin), which is capable of inactivating both AVP and oxytocin. Circulating levels of this vasopressinase are greatest in the second and third trimesters and can destroy AVP both *in vivo* and *in vitro.* It is important to recognize that despite the increased metabolic clearance rate found in pregnancy, the plasma levels of AVP are normal and not reduced, thus indicating the increased release of the hormone.

Mechanism of Action of Vasopressin

The aforementioned ability of normal humans to maintain water balance when imbibing as little as 0.5 L/day or as much as 20 to 25 L/day is critically dependent on the intact function of the renal concentrating and diluting mechanism. As mentioned earlier, vasopressin plays a critical role in the dilution and concentration of the urine by affecting water permeability in the distal tubule and collecting duct. The manner in which vasopressin alters the water permeability of the collecting duct has been the subject of considerable investigation. The initial step involves the binding of vasopressin to the aforementioned V2 receptor on the basolateral membrane of the principal cell of the collecting duct cell (Fig. 15.5). This interaction of vasopressin with the V2 receptor leads to increased adenylate cyclase activity via the stimulatory G-protein (Gs), which catalyzes the formation of cAMP from adenosine triphosphate. cAMP in turn activates a serine threonine kinase, protein kinase A. Cytoplasmic vesicles carrying the water channel proteins migrate through the cell and fuse with the apical membrane in response to increasing vasopressin binding, thereby increasing water permeability of the collecting duct cells. These water channels are recycled by endocytosis once the vasopressin is removed. The water channel that underlies water reabsorption in the proximal tubule and descending limb of Henle's loop is the originally described water channel [aquaporin-1 AQP-1)] (Table 15.2). Knockout mice lacking AQP-1 have a urinary concentrating defect reflecting the importance of water abstraction from the descending limb to the concentrating process.

The water channel responsible for the high water permeability of the luminal membrane in response to vasopressin has been

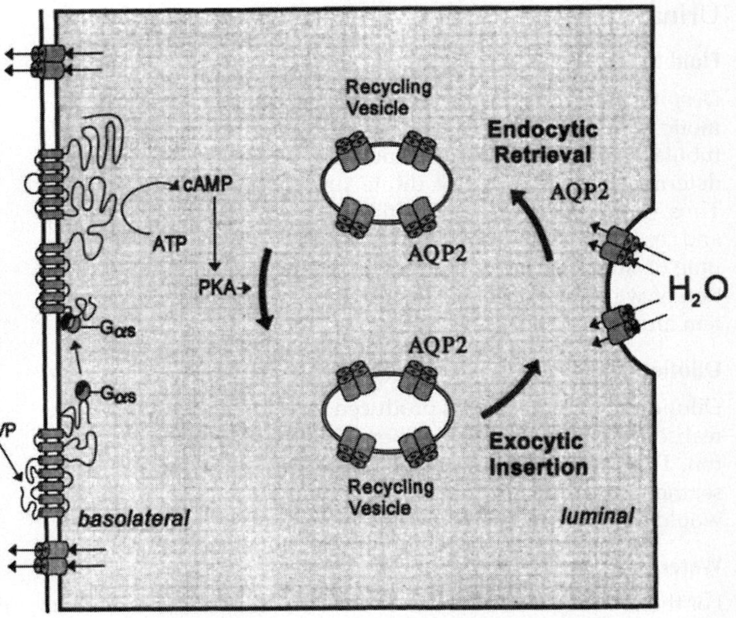

Figure 15.5. Schematic model of the cellular action of vasopressin in the principal cell of the collecting ducts. (Reprinted with permission from Bichet DG. Nephrogenic and central diabetes insipidus. In: Schrier RW, Gottschalk C, eds. *Diseases of the Kidney*, Vol III. Boston: Little Brown, 1997:2429.)

recently cloned and designated as aquaporin-2 (AQP-2). Immunolocalization place these channels solely to principal cells of the collecting duct. It is further localized to the apical plasma membrane and in intracellular vesicles of these cells. ADH appears to be involved in both the short- and long-term regulation of AQP-2. Short-term regulation, also described as the "shuttle hypothesis," includes a rapid increase (within minutes) in collecting duct water permeability. The process is mediated by the interaction of ADH with its receptor (V2), followed by a cAMP-generated cascade of cellular events, including fusing of AQP-2-containing intracellular vesicles with the apical plasma membrane, resulting in an increase in the number of water channels in the apical plasma membrane. This results in a rapid increase in apical membrane water permeability. The entire process is rapidly reversible. Long-term regulation of water permeability involves the conditioning effect seen in collecting ducts whereby elevated circulating ADH levels for 24 hours or more result in an increase in the maximal water permeability of the collecting duct epithelium, as a consequence of an increase in the total number of AQP-2 channels per cell. As opposed to the short-term regulation, the process is not readily reversible. Recessive forms of congenital nephrogenic diabetes insipidus are caused by mutation of the AQP-2 gene. Likewise, downregulation of AQP-2 has been described in various forms of acquired nephrogenic diabetes insipidus, including potassium depletion, lithium administration, ureteral obstruction, and protein deficient diets. A decrement in AQP-2 excreted has been shown to be a potential diagnostic tool in differentiating central and nephrogenic diabetes insipidus in humans. Conversely, increased AQP-2 expression has been described in some water-retaining states such as congestive heart failure, cirrhosis, and pregnancy.

The other members of the aquaporin family, AQP-3 and AQP-4, are located on the basolateral membranes (Table 15.2) and are probably involved in water exit from the cell. AQP-3 is also urea permeable and, under the stimulus of vasopressin, increases the permeability of the collecting duct to urea, resulting in its movement into the interstitium.

FACTORS INVOLVED IN NORMAL URINARY DILUTION AND CONCENTRATION

Although the process of urinary dilution and concentration is discussed in Chapter 8, a recapitulation of the factors involved will facilitate the understanding of disorders in the renal excretion of water.

TABLE 15.2. Aquaporins Expressed in the Kidney

	AQP-1	AQP-2	AQP-3	AQP-4
Size (amino acids)	269	271	285	301
Permeability to small solutes	No	No	Urea Glycerol	No
Regulation by ADH	No	Yes	No	No
Site	Proximal tubules Descending thin limb	Collecting duct—principal cells	Medullary collecting duct Colon	Hypothalamic—supraoptic, paraventricular nuclei Ependymal, granular and Purkinje cells
Cellular localization	Apical and basolateral membrane	Apical membrane and intracellular vesicles	Basolateral membrane	Basolateral membrane of the principal cells
Mutant phenotype	Normal (humans) Concentrating defect (mouse)	Nephrogenic diabetes insipidus	Unknown	Unknown

Urinary Dilution

Fluid Delivery from the Proximal Tubule

Despite the fact that reabsorption in the proximal tubule is isosmotic and therefore does not directly contribute to dilution of tubular fluid, the volume of fluid delivered to the distal tubule determines the volume of dilute urine that can be excreted. Thus, if the glomerular filtration rate is greatly diminished and/or proximal reabsorption is greatly enhanced, the low volume of fluid delivered to the distal nephron limits renal excretion of water even if the other components of the diluting system are normal.

Dilution of Tubular Fluid in the Ascending Limb of Henle's Loop

Dilution of tubular fluid is produced by active sodium chloride reabsorption in this water-impermeable segment of the nephron. Thus agents that impair sodium chloride transport in this segment, such as furosemide, ethacrynic acid, and thiazide, would interfere with diluting capacity.

Water Impermeability of the Collecting Duct

For the urine to be as dilute as or more dilute than the fluid that arrives at the early distal tubule, the reabsorption of water in the terminal segments of the nephron must be minimal. Therefore the collecting duct must remain water impermeable. The absence of vasopressin or of any other substance or drug that would render this epithelium permeable is therefore necessary for normal urinary dilution.

That the intact function of the diluting mechanism enables humans to ingest large amounts of water without adverse effects on body tonicity is perhaps best exemplified in patients who are compulsive water drinkers. However, continuous drinking from a shower hose or faucet, culminating in water intoxication, can occasionally exceed even this capacity. Much more commonly, however, the development of hyponatremia is a consequence of abnormal urinary dilution and can be ascribed to any one or a combination of the three factors just discussed.

Urinary Concentration

Generation of a Hypertonic Medullary Interstitium

As noted previously, this process primarily depends on the proper function of the ascending limb of Henle's loop. However, abnormalities in renal blood flow, glomerular filtration rate, and electrolytes (hypokalemia and hypercalcemia), as well as marked dietary aberrations (high water intake, low sodium and protein intake) can also interfere with the generation of interstitial tonicity.

Normal Secretion of Vasopressin

Abnormalities in the osmotic or nonosmotic release of the hormone will impair urinary concentration.

Normal Collecting Duct Responsiveness to Vasopressin

Urine cannot be maximally concentrated, even in the presence of vasopressin, if its target cells do not respond to it in a normal manner.

Abnormalities in the renal concentrating process obligate the excretion of a large volume of urine to maintain the daily solute balance. For example, if urine can be concentrated only to the level of plasma ((300 mOsm/kg of water), a urine flow of 2 L/day is needed to excrete the daily solute load of 600 mOsm/kg of water. If the concentrating defect is even more severe, to the level of 100 mOsm/kg of water for example, then 6 L need to be excreted. It should be noted, however, that as long as the thirst mechanism is intact and the renal losses are matched by appropriate intake, water homeostasis is maintained. However, if the concentrating defect also involves a state of hypodipsia or inability to replace obligatory renal losses, progressive water depletion and hypernatremia supervene.

Selected Readings

Berl T. Water channels in health and disease. *Kidney Int* 1998;53:1417–1418.

A review of the biology of water channels in water losing and retaining disorders.

Berl T, Robertson GL. Pathophysiology of water metabolism. In: Brenner BM, Rector FC, eds. *The Kidney*, 5th ed. Philadelphia: WB Saunders, 2000:866–924.

A thorough summary of vasopressin synthesis and action, water and thirst regulation, plus a detailed discussion of abnormalities in water metabolism.

Brown D. Structural-functional features of antidiuretic hormone-induced water transport in the collecting duct. *Semin Nephrol* 1991;11:478–501.

A detailed discussion of our current understanding of water transport, channel identification, insertion, and recirculation.

Gines P, Abraham WT, Schrier RW. Vasopressin in pathophysiological states. *Semin Nephrol* 1994;14:384–397.

A review of clinical conditions in which plasma AVP levels are abnormal, including current concepts on AVP secretion.

Knepper MA, et al. Mechanism of vasopressin action in the renal collecting duct. *Semin Nephrol* 1994;14:302–321.

A discussion on the regulation of water and urea transport in response to AVP, including signaling mechanisms and water channels.

Kovacs L, Robertson GL. Syndrome of inappropriate antidiuresis. *Endocrinol Metab Clin North Am* 1992;21:859–875.

The normal relationships between thirst and AVP in maintaining salt and water balance are reviewed, followed by a discussion of the syndrome of inappropriate secretion of ADH.

Lolait SJ, O'Carroll AM, McBride OW, et al. Cloning and characterization of a vasopressin V2 receptor and possible link to nephrogenic diabetes insipidus. *Nature* 1992;357:336–339.

The first successful identification, expression, gene localization, and sequencing of the V2 receptor along with mRNA distribution.

Poon WS, et al. Water and sodium disorders following surgical excision of pituitary region tumours. *Acta Neurochir (Wien)* 1996;138:921–927.

A prospective evaluation of the sodium and water disorders in patients with pituitary region tumors after surgical excision.

Schrier RW, Berl T, Anderson R. Osmotic and non-osmotic control of vasopressin release. *Am J Physiol* 1979;236:F321–F332.

A discussion of factors affecting the threshold and sensitivity of vasopressin release, as well as an electrophysiologic model of osmotic and non-osmotic interactions.

Zeidel ML, et al. Mechanisms and regulation of water transport in the kidney. *Semin Nephrol* 1993;13:155–167.

The examination of several aspects of the cellular and molecular biology of water reabsorption in the kidney, including structural features of apical membranes and water channels.

PART 2
Control of Sodium Excretion

Ira Kurtz

The excretion of sodium (Na^+) by the human kidney in relation to dietary Na^+ intake is a primary determinant of the circulating blood volume. Therefore disturbances in sodium balance are invariably associated with changes in the intravascular volume. Renal Na^+ excretion is determined by changes in the filtered load of Na^+ and by alterations in tubular reabsorption. The net effect of these two processes is to render the urine virtually Na^+ free (approximately 1 mEq/l) during volume depletion or a decrease in Na^+ intake. In contrast, during volume expansion or an increase in Na^+ intake, the urine Na^+ concentration can exceed 100 mEq/L.

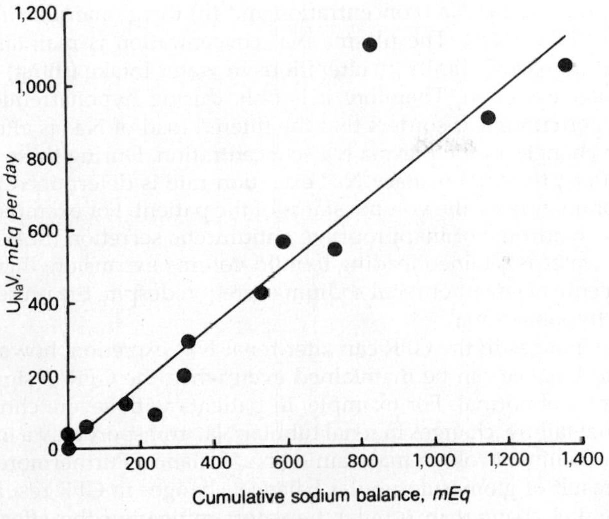

Figure 15.6. The effect of varying sodium intake on cumulative sodium balance. Increasing sodium intake (as reflected by sodium excretion) results in a progressive increase in sodium balance. (Adapted with permission from Walser M. Phenomenological analysis of renal regulation of sodium and potassium balance. *Kidney Int* 1985;27:837–841.)

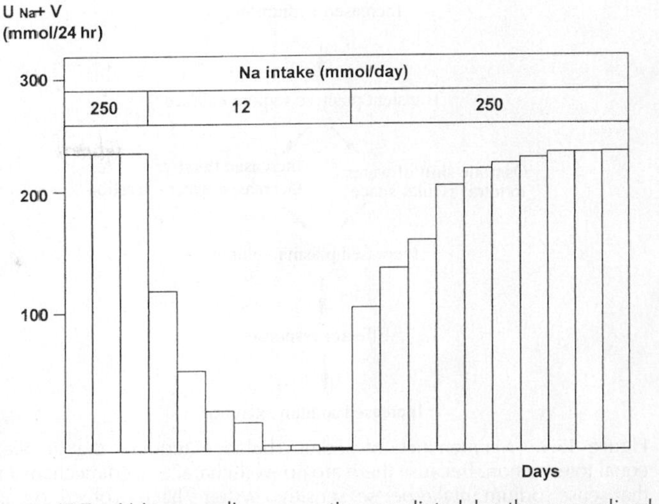

Figure 15.7. Urinary sodium excretion predicted by the generalized Strauss model following a step change in sodium intake from 250 mmol/day to 12 mmol/day and back to 250 mmol/day (it is assumed that 12 mmol/day is excreted by nonrenal routes. (Adapted with permission from Simpson FO. Sodium intake, body sodium, and sodium excretion. *Lancet* 1998;2:25–29.)

In general, we understand several of the individual factors controlling sodium excretion. How these factors are integrated to control the final output of sodium is not completely understood. The adaptation to different levels of sodium intake involves several neurohumoral mechanisms that minimize any alteration in extracellular fluid volume. In the steady state, a dynamic balance exists between sodium intake and excretion, and in normal individuals, on a constant intake, total body sodium and intravascular volume remain constant. When sodium intake is abruptly altered, however, a parallel change in intravascular volume/pressure occurs and it is this change which appears to be responsible for the subsequent change in urinary sodium excretion.

The evidence suggests that there is a minimum extracellular volume/pressure below which sodium excretion is extremely low and that the magnitude of sodium excretion normally is determined by the degree to which this minimum volume/pressure is exceeded. If sodium intake is changed suddenly, the rate of urinary sodium excretion changes gradually. The delay in achieving a new steady state (following an alteration in dietary intake) increases in proportion to the magnitude of the change in intake. This results in the relationship depicted in Fig. 15.6 between cumulative sodium balance and sodium excretion. After a sudden decrease in sodium intake, the excretion of sodium decreases with a half-life of about 24 hours. The half-life is shorter in the young, and increases in elderly people and in aldosterone-deficient states. Data calculated from a model of the temporal changes in sodium excretion in response to sudden changes in dietary intake is shown in Fig. 15.7. This model is based on the following equation: $Na_U(t) = Na_U(t_o) + (Na_{In}(1-e^{-kt})$, where $Na_U(t)$ is the urinary sodium excretion at time t, $Na_U(t_o)$ is the urinary sodium excretion at baseline (when $t = 0$), ΔNa_{In} is the step change in sodium intake, e is the base for the natural logarithms, and k is the rate constant. Half-life (h) is calculated as $0.693/k \times 24$. Integration of the exponential curve leads to the prediction that the cumulative change in sodium balance, after a new steady state has been achieved, is approximately 1.3 times the change in daily sodium intake. For example, a sustained increase in intake of 100 mmoles per day should result in a net positive sodium balance of about 130 mmoles, equivalent to a weight gain of about 1 kg. Actual balance studies are in agreement with this prediction (Fig. 15.8). Interestingly, a number of studies have shown that African-Americans have a delay in excreting a sodium load compared with whites. African-Americans had a longer half-life than whites at all levels of sodium intake. It has been suggested that this is in part due to the finding that African-Americans have fewer nephrons although other genetic factors affecting tubular transport processes may be involved.

Changes in sodium intake result in commensurate changes in sodium excretion. For the renal excretory mechanisms to "know" that a change in intake has occurred, a signal that alters efferent pathways that ultimately modify the rate of sodium excretion must have been sensed. It is currently thought that what is being sensed is a change in plasma volume/pressure. Therefore the regulation of sodium balance is coupled to changes in the intravascular volume/pressure status (Fig. 15.9).

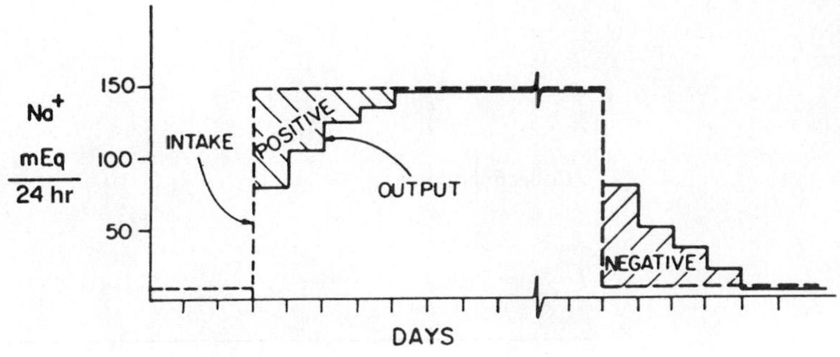

Figure 15.8. Effect of acute changes in sodium intake on body weight and sodium excretion. The delay in the excretory response results in a cumulative alteration in total body sodium content. (Adapted with permission from Reineck HJ, Stein JH. Regulation of sodium balance. In: Maxwell MH, Kleeman CR, eds. *Clinical Disorders of Fluid and Electrolyte Metabolism,* 3rd ed. New York: McGraw-Hill, 1980:89–112.)

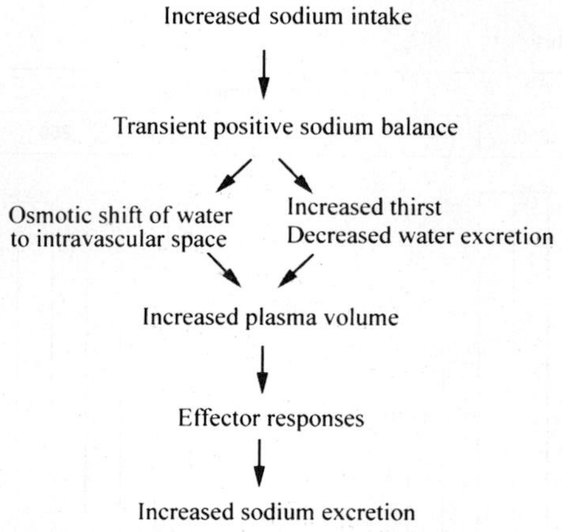

Figure 15.9. Maintenance of sodium balance requires that intake is equal to excretion. Because there are no well-characterized mechanism(s) that sense sodium intake *per se,* sensitive systems have evolved to transduce changes in sodium intake into changes in intravascular volume. Baroreceptors sense these changes in intravascular volume/pressure, which results in extrarenal and intrarenal neurohumoral responses that alter renal tubular sodium and water transport.

DETERMINANT OF RENAL SODIUM EXCRETION

Filtered Load of Sodium

The human kidneys filter approximately 150 to 180 L of fluid per day. Each liter of glomerular filtrate contains approximately 150 mEq of Na^+. Therefore approximately 24,750 mEq of Na^+ pass through all the glomeruli every 24 hours. Assuming an intake of 150 mEq of Na^+ per day, approximately 99.4% of this Na^+ load is absorbed. The filtered load of Na^+ is determined by (a) the plasma Na^+ concentration and (b) the glomerular filtration rate (GFR). The plasma Na^+ concentration is maintained within narrow limits by alterations in water intake (thirst) and water excretion. Therefore it is only during hyponatremic or hypernatremic disorders that the filtered load of Na^+ is altered by changes in the plasma Na^+ concentration. During these disorders, the final urinary Na^+ excretion rate is determined predominantly by the volume status of the patient. For example, in the syndrome of inappropriate antidiuretic secretion (SIADH), as water is retained leading to mild volume expansion, there is an enhancement of renal sodium excretion despite the presence of hyponatremia.

Changes in the GFR can alter renal Na^+ excretion; however, Na^+ balance can be maintained even when the GFR is significantly abnormal. For example, in patients with severe chronic renal failure, changes in renal tubular Na^+ transport play a more predominant role in maintaining Na^+ balance. Furthermore, as a result of glomerulotubular balance, changes in GFR result in parallel changes in tubular transport mitigating the effect of GFR on urinary Na^+ excretion.

Tubular Sodium Transport

In contrast to the filtered load, a change in the tubular transport of Na^+ is the primary adaptive mechanism that maintains sodium balance. In general, tubular Na^+ transport is modulated by hormonal, neurogenic, and physical factors. These determinants are nephron-segment specific, and it is the interplay of the changes in the transport of Na^+ in specific sites in the nephron that determines the final Na^+ excretion rate.

The contribution of individual nephron segments to tubular sodium transport is shown in Table 15.3. Variable sensitivity of each segment to various regulatory factors permits the kidney to modulate sodium excretion rapidly in response

TABLE 15.3. Mechanisms Responsible for Regulating Excretion of Sodium

Site	Percentage of Sodium Absorbed	Mechanism
Glomerulus	—	TG feedback Nitric oxide PGE_2, PGI_2 Angiotensin II Atrial natriuretic peptide Norepinephrine
Proximal tubule	60	Angiotensin II Atrial natriuretic peptide PGE_2 Parathyroid hormone Norepinephrine Dopamine Pressure natriuresis Peritubular oncotic pressure Luminal flow rate
Henle's loop	30	PGE_2 Antidiuretic hormone Pressure natriuresis β-agonists Peritubular tonicity Peritubular K^+ Peritubular Ca^{2+} Luminal delivery of NaCl
Collecting tubule	10	Atrial natriuretic peptide Aldosterone Dopamine PGE_2 Kinins Endothelin

to widely varying sodium intake. The neurohumoral regulation of Na^+ absorption occurs predominantly in the proximal tubule and collecting ducts. Proximal Na^+ absorption is stimulated by angiotensin II and norepinephrine. Collecting duct Na^+ transport is modulated by aldosterone and atrial natriuretic peptide (ANP). For example, mild volume depletion results in decreased Na^+ excretion that is predominantly caused by enhanced collecting duct transport as a result of increased circulating aldosterone and possibly caused by decreased ANP levels. More severe degrees of hypovolemia also enhance proximal tubule transport. Henle's loop transport may also be stimulated in part because of a decrease in medullary interstitial pressure. During volume expansion, these changes are reversed. Sodium absorption in the collecting duct is decreased and is possibly also decreased in the proximal tubule and Henle's loop. The factors reducing sodium absorption include decreased aldosterone and angiotensin II levels, increased ANP secretion, and possibly enhanced renal dopamine production.

SENSORS OF PLASMA VOLUME/PRESSURE

Baroreceptors

In general, changes in Na^+ balance (intake versus output) alter the intravascular volume because of secondary changes in water balance [thirst: water intake; antidiuretic hormone (ADH) secretion: water excretion]. Sensors, called baroreceptors, sense the change in intravascular volume and, via neurogenic mechanisms, alter renal tubular sodium transport. The information is processed by the hypothalamus and brainstem. Efferent responses adjust cardiac output, vascular resistances, and renal tubular Na^+ transport to maintain a constant intravascular volume.

An everyday example of this phenomenon is the increase in sodium excretion that occurs with recumbency. Moving from an erect to a recumbent position results in increased sodium excretion. A similar natriuresis occurs in individuals who are immersed in water or exposed to the weightlessness of outer space. Although the extracellular fluid volume is constant in these circumstances, the common feature is the increase in intravascular volume, which provides the signal(s) to increase sodium excretion.

Low-pressure venous baroreceptors are present in the atria. Upon stretching of the atria, afferent signals are sent via the vagus nerves to the brainstem. The brainstem then decreases sympathetic outflow, which (a) directly inhibits proximal tubular Na^+ transport, (b) causes arteriolar and venular dilation, and (c) inhibits renin secretion. Atrial stretch receptor stimulation also results in the inhibition of ADH release and the secretion of ANP.

High-pressure arterial baroreceptors are present in the aortic arch, the carotid sinus, and the afferent arteriole of the glomerulus. These baroreceptors sense the arterial pulse wave form. When the intravascular volume is increased, the wave form of the arterial pulse is altered. Altered baroreceptor activity changes sympathetic outflow as with the low-pressure baroreceptors. In addition to high- and low-pressure baroreceptors, other less well-characterized afferent pathways have been described. Afferent nerves have been described in the atria and ventricles. Renal afferent nerves that are regulated by the tonicity of the pelvic urine and by pelvic stretch stimulate the vasoregulatory areas of the brain. Furthermore, angiotensin II can stimulate the circumventricular organs in the brain, which lack a blood-brain barrier.

NEUROHUMORAL REGULATION OF TUBULAR TRANSPORT

Renin-Angiotensin-Aldosterone System

The renin-angiotensin system plays an important role in modulating renal tubular Na^+ transport. During renal hypoperfusion, renin is released from the juxtaglomerular apparatus. Renin cleaves angiotensinogen, which is produced in the liver into angiotensin I. Angiotensin I is converted into angiotensin II by a converting enzyme located in the endothelial cells of the lung and the glomerulus. Angiotensin II has multiple effects, including stimulating proximal tubule sodium transport, stimulating collecting duct water absorption, modulating glomerular and systemic hemodynamics, and stimulating adrenal aldosterone production.

Angiotensin II binds to apical and basolateral binding sites on the proximal tubule. At low concentrations, peritubular angiotensin II stimulates sodium transport, whereas at high concentrations, a decrease in sodium transport occurs. Angiotensin II stimulates sodium bicarbonate transport predominantly. This effect is mediated by a stimulation of apical Na^+-H^+ exchange and basolateral $Na(HCO_3)_n$ cotransport. The stimulation of bicarbonate transport is most pronounced in the earliest segment of the proximal tubule. In addition to stimulating proximal tubule transport, angiotensin II also alters the filtered load of sodium by modulating the GFR. During severe volume contraction and a concomitant decrease in systemic pressure, angiotensin II constricts the efferent arteriole of the glomerulus, resulting in an increase in glomerular hydrostatic pressure and a decrease in renal blood flow. An additional effect is the contraction of glomerular mesangial cells, resulting in a decrease in the surface area for filtration. The increase in filtration fraction raises the peritubular oncotic pressure, which favors enhanced tubular Na^+ absorption. In addition to these proximal tubular effects, angiotensin II, by decreasing inner medullary plasma flow, results in a decrease in the removal of osmoles from the inner medulla, thereby enhancing collecting duct water absorption.

There is increasing evidence that angiotensin-(1-7) has physiologic effects that are either identical or opposite to angiotensin II. Angiotensin-(1-7) is formed from the hydrolysis at Pro(7)-Phe(8) of angiotensin I by endopeptidases nephrolysin and prolyl endopeptidase. Angiotensin II may be converted to Angiotensin-(1-7) by carboxypeptidases and prolyl carboxypeptidase. Angiotensin-(1-7) is hydrolyzed to yield angiotensin-(1-5) by angiotensin-converting enzyme (ACE). Current evidence suggests that angiotensin-(1-7) modulates tubular sodium and bicarbonate absorption, diminishes Na^+-K^+-ATPase activity, induces a natriuresis, and is a vasodilator. In addition, angiotensin-(1-7) augments the actions of bradykinin and stimulates the synthesis and release of the vasodilatory prostaglandin PGI_2 and nitric oxide.

ACE inhibitors can lower systemic blood pressure in the presence of normal and decreased renin activity. It has been suggested that the effect of ACE inhibitors is in part mediated by an increase in tissue bradykinin levels. However, against this explanation is the finding that the specific β_2-receptor blocker HOE 140 does not reverse the antihypertensive effect of ACE inhibitors. Of interest is the finding that chronic ACE inhibition leads to an elevation of the plasma angiotensin-(1-7). Furthermore, the antihypertensive effect of ACE inhibitors is partially blocked by an angiotensin-(1-7) monoclonal antibody and an inhibitor of nephrolysin. These results suggest that the antihypertensive effect of ACE inhibitors is in part mediated by an increase in angiotensin-(1-7). Current data indicate that angiotensin-(1-7) acts via a novel non-AT_1/AT_2 receptor subtype and the signal transduction pathways remain unknown.

Aldosterone modulates Na^+ transport in the connecting tubule, cortical collecting ducts, and inner medullary collecting duct. The mechanism in the cortical collecting duct appears to be due to an increased number of active apical Na^+ channels and basolateral Na^+ pumps. An increase in intracellular calcium and methylation of channel proteins may be involved. Furthermore, an increase in apical Na^+ uptake is in part responsible for the increase in Na^+ pump activity.

Aldosterone acts on cells in the cortical collecting duct, where it binds to a specific basolateral receptor (the mineralocorticoid receptor), resulting in the enhanced absorption of Na^+ and increased secretion of K^+ and H^+. Following the binding to its receptor, the aldosterone–receptor complex is transported into the nucleus, where it stimulates specific genes that code for aldosterone-induced proteins (AIP). Examples of AIPs are subunits of the epithelial sodium channel (ENAC) and Na^+ pump. Two isoforms of the mineralocorticoid receptor (α and β) have been characterized in sweat glands, the colon, and the kidney. Regulation of β isoform expression may contribute to the regulation of mineralocorticoid activity in the kidney.

The most important factors modulating aldosterone secretion are angiotensin II and K^+. These factors enhance the conversion of cholesterol to pregnenolone and corticosterone to aldosterone. Other factors affecting aldosterone secretion are adrenocorticotropic hormone (ACTH), dopamine, ANP, and hyponatremia. Alterations in Na^+ balance induce a volume stimulus, which alters aldosterone levels via changes in renin-angiotensin II levels. Angiotensin II levels vary inversely with Na^+ balance. This feedback system permits angiotensin II to modulate Na^+ transport in the proximal tubule and aldosterone to alter Na^+ transport in the connecting tubule and collecting duct. Changes in volume status can also affect aldosterone secretion via a non–angiotensin II-mediated mechanisms by altering ANP and dopamine levels. Although aldosterone also plays an important role in K^+ balance, alterations in Na^+ balance do not appreciably alter K^+ balance. This results from the inverse relationship between volume-mediated aldosterone release and the luminal Na^+ concentration and flow rate in the cortical collecting duct. The latter factors are important mediators of cortical collecting duct K^+ secretion. Only in situations in which distal Na^+ delivery is maintained in the presence of high aldosterone levels (adrenal hyperplasia/adenoma) is renal K^+ secretion altered by changes in Na^+ balance.

Natriuretic Peptides

ANP is released from the atria in response to stretch and stimulation of baroreceptors in the afferent renal arteriole; however, the ventricles may also produce ANP following chronic congestive heart failure. ANP lowers the systemic vascular resistance and increases renal sodium and water excretion. Several actions of ANP contribute to the increase in renal sodium and water excretion: (a) an increase in GFR, (b) inhibition of sodium absorption in the inner medullary collecting duct, (c) decreased sodium absorption in the proximal tubule via a release of dopamine and inhibition of the stimulation of transport by angiotensin II, (d) inhibition of renin release, (e) inhibition of angiotensin II and potassium-induced aldosterone release, and (f) ADH-mediated water absorption. Most of the actions of ANP are mediated by the binding of ANP to the natriuretic peptide A receptor. An increase in cyclic guanosine monophosphate (cGMP) in the inner medullary collecting duct leads to the closure of apical Na^+ channels and inhibition of sodium absorption. The ANP C receptors mediate the clearance of ANP and limit the renal response.

ANP consists of amino acids 99-126 of pro-ANP. Other pro-ANP fragments are also natriuretic. When infused into normal subjects, peptide fragments 1-30 and 31-67 lower blood pressure by 5 to 10 mm Hg and cause a natriuresis. The 31-67 fragment inhibits inner medullary collecting duct sodium transport. This is mediated in part via prostaglandin-induced inhibition of the basolateral Na^+ pump. A separate pro-ANP C-terminal fragment, amino acids 95-126 called urodilantin, is produced in the kidney. Plasma urodilantin levels are negligible. Urodilantin excretion increases in response to volume expansion and binds to ANP receptors with the same activity as ANP itself. Urodilantin levels correlate with enhanced sodium excretion after a volume load more closely than ANP. Furthermore, urodilantin enhances renal sodium excretion at a concentration where ANP is without effect. This may be in part due to the fact that urodilantin is not catabolized by neutral endopeptidases. Brain natriuretic peptide (BNP) is moderately homologous to ANP. It is produced in the brain and ventricles. The level of BNP in blood is normally 20% of the ANP concentration; however, in congestive heart failure, it can exceed the ANP level. C-type natriuretic peptide (CNP) is produced by vascular endothelial cells in the kidney. CNP may have an autocrine or paracrine role in modulating sodium excretion.

The physiologic role of ANP in modifying renal sodium excretion is unclear. Some studies suggest that ANP accounts for about 40% of the increase in renal sodium excretion following a sodium load. Other studies suggest that the increment in ANP is insufficient to account for the rise in sodium excretion. The vasodilator effect of ANP may limit its natriuretic action. In particular, transgenic mice overexpressing ANP have a lower-than-normal blood pressure and are in sodium balance. When the blood pressure is normalized by volume expansion, an increase in sodium excretion ensues. Furthermore, in humans, in edematous disorders, ANP levels are increased, whereas sodium excretion is reduced. In patients with cirrhosis, mannitol restores the natriuretic response to ANP. In preliminary experiments, administration of anti-ANP antibodies have several interesting effects, including a decrease in steady-state urine Na^+ excretion, a decrease in the natriuretic response to volume expansion, and a further decrease in the rate of urine Na^+ excretion in heart failure. Similar results have been obtained in ANP-resistant animals using immunization. These results suggest that ANP contributes to the maintenance of sodium balance over a short time. More prolonged maintenance of sodium balance does not depend on ANP as in states of chronic volume expansion such as aldosterone administration and oral salt loading. In recent studies, knockout mice (homozygous or heterozygous) maintained on a low-salt diet had a greater natriuretic response to volume expansion than wild-type controls. However, animals maintained on a high-salt diet did not have a response that differed from controls. The results indicated that ANP lowers blood pressure in the absence of detectable changes in renal function and that ANP is required for the normal natriuretic response to acute volume expansion in mice maintained on a low-salt diet.

From experiments in animals and in preliminary results in humans, it appears that increasing the half-life of ANP (duration of action) may increase the natriuretic response with minimal hypotension. These studies have used an endopeptidase inhibitor or a cGMP phosphodiesterase inhibitor. The response to endopeptidase inhibition is enhanced by ACE inhibitors. Further information on ANP and its interaction with the kidney are found in Chapter 13, Part 8.

Digitalislike Hormones

Several circulating Na^+-K^+-ATPase inhibitors have been described. A ouabainlike compound is produced by the adrenal cortex and hypothalamus; however, its physiologic role in renal sodium handling has been questioned. It may contribute to the maintenance of vascular tone and systemic vascular resistance via its potential effect on intracellular calcium levels. Furthermore, it has been proposed that these compounds may play a role in the salt sensitivity seen in patients with essential hypertension. Possible mechanisms include the aforementioned effect on intracellular calcium and a stimulation by ouabainlike hormone in the brain of sympathetic outflow. In addition to ouabainlike compounds, nonesterified fatty acids and lysophospholipids can inhibit Na^+-K^+-ATPase activity. These compounds may be more involved with cell volume regulation than in the maintenance of sodium balance.

Sympathetic Nervous System

Tubule sodium reabsorption is increased during enhanced sympathetic outflow to the kidney. Several factors contribute to this response. First, there is a direct stimulation of proximal tubule transport mediated primarily by α_1-receptors. Second, peritubular hydrostatic pressure decreases as a result of vasoconstriction. Third, activation of β_1-adrenergic receptors stimulates renin production. Activation of α_2-receptors with clonidine or guanabenz increases sodium and water excretion. The increase in sodium excretion in part results from decreased proximal tubule transport, whereas the water diuresis results from the decreased ADH-mediated stimulation of collecting duct adenyl cyclase. The physiologic role of renal α_2-receptors remains unclear.

When systemic pressure is increased by enhanced sympathetic outflow, there are counteracting effects on renal Na^+ excretion. First, there is a direct stimulatory effect of norepinephrine on proximal tubule Na^+ transport. Second, an increase in systemic pressure favors a pressure natriuresis. These two effects counteract each other. With the administration of guanethidine, the interaction between these two opposing effects can be illustrated. When administered at dosages that do not decrease the systemic pressure, sodium excretion is increased. However, in hypertensive patients, guanethidine-induced Na^+ retention occurs because of the predominant effect of a reduction in renal capillary pressure to stimulate Na^+ transport. This is why diuretics should be used in combination with agents that block the sympathetic nervous system in the treatment of hypertension.

Sympathetic outflow to the kidney is modulated by pressure receptors in the left side of the heart. An increase in left-sided pressure decreases sympathetic outflow to the kidney despite the fact that total sympathetic outflow may be increased. For example, after an acute myocardial infarction, in the presence of an increased left-sided pressure, the decrease in systemic pressure reduces renal blood flow by a smaller extent than after an equivalent fall in blood pressure resulting from hemorrhage in which case left-sided cardiac pressures are also decreased. A cardiorenal reflex can explain the finding that ATN is uncommon after heart failure but is commonly observed after sepsis or hemorrhage.

Vasopressin (Antidiuretic Hormone)

Vasopressin is a peptide hormone that regulates intravascular volume by altering collecting duct water transport (V2 receptors) and systemic pressure by modulating the systemic vascular resistance (V1 receptors). As discussed previously, these changes in systemic hemodynamics affect baroreceptor function, which results in an alteration in renal Na^+ excretion. In addition, vasopressin directly modulates thick ascending limb Na^+ transport.

INTRARENAL FACTORS

Prostaglandins

Renal PGE_2 directly inhibits tubular Na^+ transport in the thick ascending limb of Henle's loop and the collecting duct. PGE_2 is also an important mediator of the natriuretic response to a pressure natriuresis. When administered to rats, PGE_2 enhances proximal tubular Na^+ transport. This effect is partially mediated by angiotensin II, demonstrating an interaction *in vivo* between the renin-angiotensin system and renal prostaglandin secretion. Furthermore, PGI_2 is thought to mediate baroreceptor-induced changes in renin secretion. In the steady state, prostaglandins have little effect; however, in hypovolemic states, prostaglandins modulate the hemodynamic and transport effects of endothelin, angiotensin II, and norepinephrine. The administration of nonsteroidal antiinflammatory drugs (NSAIDs) during volume depletion decreases sodium excretion by increasing tubular transport and decreasing the GFR.

In addition to directly affecting renal tubular sodium transport, prostaglandins indirectly alter Na^+ transport by altering renal hemodynamics, GFR, and intravascular volume. Specifically, PGE_2 and PGI_2 dilate the afferent renal arteriole during a decrease in systemic pressure, resulting in an increase in glomerular hydrostatic pressure and renal blood flow. Like angiotensin II, thromboxane constricts mesangial cells, whereas PGE_2 relaxes the mesangium. Finally, prostaglandins decrease the effect of ADH on collecting duct water permeability. The clinical importance of this effect is unclear.

Kallikrein-Kinin System and Endothelium-Derived Factors

Following the infusion of bradykinin into the renal artery, renin is released in addition to an increase in renal sodium excretion. Bradykinin is a potent vasodilator and possibly plays a role in modulating renal hemodynamics. Bradykinin binds to specific receptors on inner medullary collecting duct cells, where it inhibits sodium transport. The vasodilatory effect of bradykinin is mediated by nitric oxide (NO). Endothelium-derived NO modulates GFR, renal hemodynamics, and renal sodium excretion. Bradykinin and acetylcholine interact with receptors on endothelial cells to stimulate NO and prostaglandin production. These substances cause vasodilation and result in an inhibition of tubular sodium transport. When prostaglandin production is blocked, L-NMMA (N^{ω}-nitro-L-arginine methyl ester) prevents bradykinin from altering renal hemodynamics and tubular sodium transport. The NO precursor L-arginine restores the increase in renal sodium excretion and renal blood flow resulting from bradykinin administration. NO mediates an increase in renal sodium excretion in part via the pressure natriuretic response. In addition, NO is thought to play an important role in tubuloglomerular feedback. Endothelial cells also secrete endothelin, which is a potent vasoconstrictor. The role of endothelin in the maintenance of sodium balance is unclear; however, endothelin is known to inhibit sodium transport in the inner medullary collecting duct. Furthermore, endothelin stimulates cardiac ANP secretion.

There is increasing evidence that NO plays an important role in controlling renal function and blood pressure. NO buffers the influence of endogenous vasoconstrictor systems in the kidney. Renal vasoconstriction results in increased NO production, which diminishes the constrictor action of many control systems, such as the sympathetic nervous system. Despite the fact that most studies have reported that blockade of NO synthesis decreases renal sodium excretion and blunts pressure natriuresis, there are contradictory data suggesting that NO synthesis blockade may cause a natriuresis. It has been shown that inhibition of NO synthesis with low-dose NAME decreases renal sodium excretion and blunts pressure natriuresis only in rats with innervated kidneys, whereas it has no effect in denervated rats. High-dose NAME is effective in innervated and denervated rats. The results suggest that the natriuretic effect of NAME in innervated kidneys is in part attributed to inhibition of sympathetic outflow because of the rise in systemic pressure.

Dopamine

Dopamine is synthesized from circulating L-Dopa predominantly in the proximal tubule. In addition, dopaminergic nerves can be found in the kidney; however, their function is unclear. At low concentrations, dopamine increases renal blood flow by vasodilating both afferent and efferent arterioles. At higher concentrations, dopamine acts as a vasoconstrictor by activating α-adrenergic receptors. In addition to these hemodynamic effects, dopamine is a weak diuretic. It inhibits the apical Na^+-H^+ exchanger and the basolateral sodium pump in the proximal tubule and the cortical collecting duct. Furthermore, dopamine may decrease adrenal aldosterone. Administration of dopamine induces an increase in renal blood flow and sodium excretion. Modest volume expansion increases proximal tubule dopamine production. Dopamine receptor blockade impairs the natriuretic response to moderate volume expansion. A recent study of knockout mice lacking the dopamine D3 receptor, which is normally present in proximal tubule cells and juxtaglomerular cells, demonstrated failure to excrete a sodium load normally and elevated plasma renin levels.

Pressure Natriuresis

An important control mechanism for the regulation of systemic volume homeostasis and urinary sodium excretion is a phenomenon called pressure natriuresis (Fig. 15.10). Small changes in renal interstitial pressure results in the modulation of renal tubular Na^+ transport. An increase in blood pressure as a result of a disease process, aldosterone, or norepinephrine leads to an increase in renal capillary pressure and an ensuing increase in renal Na^+ excretion. The pressure natriuresis response is an important renal mechanism responsible for the long-term control of arterial pressure. The nephron sites and mechanisms involved are incompletely understood but appear to involve Henle's loop and the juxtamedullary proximal tubule. The mechanism of pressure-induced natriuresis may involve a direct effect of changes in systemic pressure on the hydrostatic pressure in the vasa recta capillaries of the medullary interstitium. Furthermore, prostaglandins and NO may, via renal vasodilation, increase intracapillary pressure. An elevation of intracapillary pressure would diminish the absorption of water via a hydrostatic effect. In addition, an increase in intracapillary pressure would be predicted to increase the flow of water into the thin descending limb, thereby diminishing the rise in intraluminal Na^+ concentration in the thin ascending limb required to drive passive Na^+ absorption.

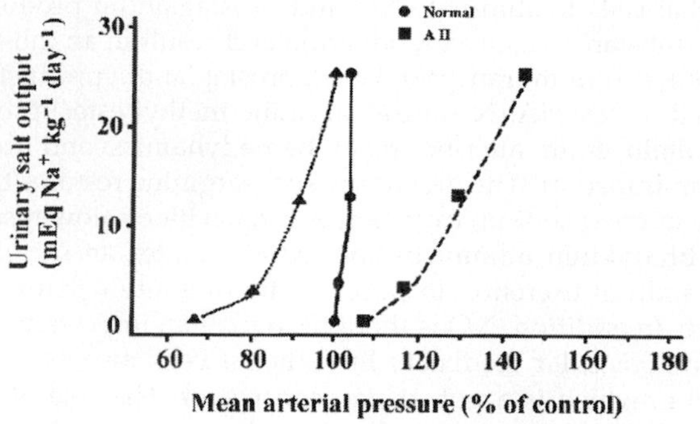

Figure 15.10. Pressure natriuresis. Sodium excretion as a function of mean blood pressure in normal dogs *(closed circles),* dogs treated with Captopril *(closed triangles),* and dogs infused with angiotensin II. (Adapted with permission from Guyton AC. Blood pressure control: Special role of the kidney and body fluids *Science* 1991;252:1813.)

In the presence of intact neurohumoral feedback mechanisms, pressure-induced changes in renal Na^+ excretion does not play a predominant role in acute sodium balance. However, when aldosterone and angiotensin II responses are impaired, Na^+ balance is maintained by the pressure natriuresis response. In the latter case, a new steady state is achieved following a greater-than-normal increase in systemic blood pressure.

MAINTENANCE OF SODIUM BALANCE—SUMMARY

To maintain Na^+ balance, minute changes in the fractional excretion of Na^+ are sufficient to handle the normal fluctuation of dietary Na^+ intake. The current data suggest that alterations in aldosterone release in response to small changes in Na^+ intake is responsible for the sensitivity of the excretory response. However, there is evidence that ANP levels increase in response to minor changes in Na^+ intake, although the significance of this finding is unclear. In ANP deficient animals, the natriuretic response to acute sodium loading is impaired. These findings suggest that the collecting duct may be the nephron segment that is primarily responsible for maintaining Na^+ balance on a day-to-day basis. In humans, there is also indirect evidence based on urate transport that the proximal tubule is involved in the acute regulation of sodium excretion. Urate is absorbed in the proximal tubule, and several studies have shown that proximal tubular urate transport appears to be modulated by volume status. For example, during volume depletion, urate excretion decreases, whereas enhanced urate excretion is associated with the syndrome of inappropriate ADH (SIADH).

Despite the importance of aldosterone to overall Na^+ balance, adrenalectomized patients on a fixed dose of mineralocorticoids are able to maintain Na^+ balance despite changes in dietary Na^+ intake. Furthermore, in patients with syndromes of mineralocorticoid excess, escape occurs because of decreased Na^+ transport in nephron segments outside the cortical collecting duct, in part mediated by ANP and by a pressure natriuresis. Interestingly, the cortical collecting duct still continues to respond to aldosterone. Similar to aldosterone, ANP does not appear to be essential for the maintenance of chronic Na^+ balance. In transgenic mice overexpressing ANP, plasma ANP levels are 10 times normal and yet sodium balance is maintained.

The pressure natriuretic response plays an important role in achieving a new steady state in the familiar aldosterone escape phenomenon. Following the administration of aldosterone, after an initial period of Na^+ retention wherein approximately 3 L of water is retained, Na^+ balance is achieved. The increase

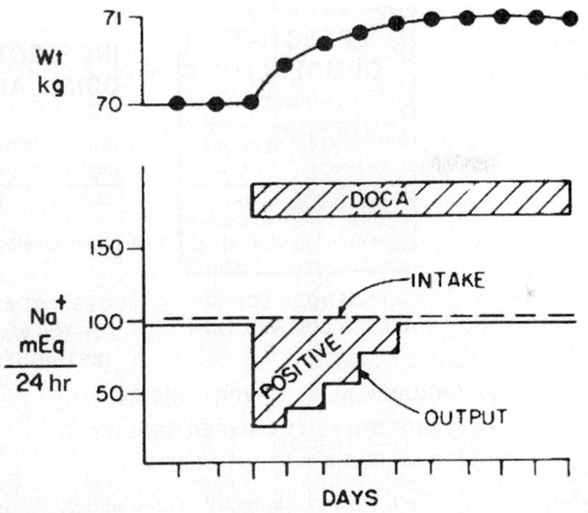

Figure 15.11. "Mineralocorticoid escape" phenomenon. During the administration of mineralocorticoid, positive sodium balance and weight gain occur. After a period of 3 to 5 days, a new steady state results, with sodium excretion again equal to intake. (From Reineck HJ, Stein JH. Sodium and water homeostasis. In: Brenner BM, Stein JH, eds. Renal regulation of extracellular fluid volume *Contemporary Issues in Nephrology.* Churchill Livingstone, 1978.)

in renal sodium excretion leading to a new steady state is called aldosterone or mineralocorticoid escape (Fig. 15.11). A rise in ANP levels precede the increase in renal sodium excretion by 1 to 2 days; however, the role of ANP in the mineralocorticoid escape phenomenon is unclear. ANP-deficient animals have a normal mineralocorticoid escape. Pressure natriuresis contributes to the escape phenomenon. A suprarenal aortic clamp prevents aldosterone escape by blocking the pressure natriuretic response, resulting in significant volume overload. Conversely, a decrease in renal interstitial pressure diminishes the pressure natriuretic response, resulting in a decrease in renal Na^+ excretion. A normal decrease in the pressure natriuretic response may mediate the increase in tubular Na^+ transport after diuretic therapy, the resistance to ANP in congestive heart failure, and the failure for Na^+ excretion to increase after neck immersion in cirrhotics.

Following a change in sodium intake, no one factor is responsible for the subsequent alteration in renal sodium excretion. Instead, these factors act in an integrated fashion to achieve the appropriate excretion rate of sodium. As is discussed in separate chapters, during certain pathologic states such as cirrhosis and congestive heart failure, the excretion rate of sodium is inappropriately decreased relative to the intake. In these diseases, the renal and extrarenal mechanisms responsible for increasing tubular sodium transport are stimulated, resulting in positive sodium balance and peripheral edema.

Acknowledgment

This work was supported by NIH grant DK46976, the Iris and B. Gerald Cantor Foundation, the Max Factor Family Foundation, the Verna Harrah Foundation, the Richard and Hinda Rosenthal Foundation, and the Fredericka Taubitz Foundation.

Selected Readings

Asico LD, Ladines C, Fuchs S, et al. Disruption of the dopamine D3 receptor gene produces renin-dependent hypertension. *J Clin Invest* 1998;102:493–498.
This study demonstrates the importance of dopamine D3 receptors in the maintenance of normal blood pressure and sodium balance.

Clavell AL, Burnett JC Jr. Physiologic and pathophysiologic roles of endothelin in the kidney. *Curr Opin Nephrol Hypertens* 1994;3:66–72.
Reviews the role of endothelin in modulating renal hemodynamics and sodium excretion.

Doris PA, Bargov AY. Endogenous sodium pump inhibitors and blood pressure regulation: an update on recent progress. *PNAS* 1998;218:156–167.
Reviews the evidence supporting endogenous ouabainlike compounds that control sodium pump activity and renal sodium excretion.

Ferraro CM, Chappell MC, Dean RH, Iyer SN. Novel angiotensin peptides regulate blood pressure, endothelial function, and natriuresis. *J Am Soc Nephrol* 1998; 9:1716–1722.
A comprehensive review of the physiologic actions of angiotensin-(1-7).

John SW, Veress AT, Honrath U, et al. Blood pressure and fluid-electrolyte balance in mice with reduced or absent ANP. *Am J Physiol* 1998;271:R109–R114.
This study examines the role of ANP in maintaining sodium balance in ANP knockout mice.

Madrid MI, Salom MG, Tornel J, et al. Interactions between nitric oxide and renal nerves on pressure-diuresis and natriuresis. *J Am Soc Nephrol* 1998;9:1588–1595.
The role of NO and the sympathetic nervous system in mediating the pressure natriuretic response is investigated.

Simpson FO. Sodium intake, body sodium, and sodium excretion. *Lancet* 1988;2:25–29.
An analysis of current views regarding the time dependence of renal sodium excretion after changes in intake.

PART 3
Dysnatremias

Jerry Yee, Richard H. Sterns, Paul Bernstein, and Robert G. Narins

Securely moored to the rigid confines of the cranial vault, the brain is vulnerable to forces that expand or contract its volume. Plasma hypotonicity from relative or absolute accumulation of water can passively inflate brain volume, causing fatal cerebral edema. By contrast, plasma hypertonicity from relative or absolute loss of water may shrink the brain, tearing it from its bony attachments and causing an equally tragic outcome. Thus survival is critically dependent on a regulatory system that prevents or minimizes osmotic stress on the brain. The remarkable stability of plasma tonicity, despite major challenges from the normal daily swings in water intake, and the durability of cerebral function seen in chronically hyponatremic or hypernatremic patients underscore the importance of the osmoregulatory system.

We first discuss the fundamental physiologic and pathophysiologic principles that underlie the cellular, hormonal, and renal aspects of the osmoregulatory system. Application of these principles toward establishing the diagnosis and therapy of the disorders of water balance follows.

BASIC PRINCIPLES

Water crosses cell membranes to equalize the opposing osmotic forces that impinge on cell membranes. Therefore the solute concentrations (osmolalities) of the extracellular fluid (ECF) and intracellular fluid (ICF) compartments are always equal. Transient inequalities are rapidly abolished by water movement. Although osmolalities are identical, the solute compositions of ECF and ICF are vastly different (Fig. 15.12).

Osmolality and Tonicity

Osmolality is defined by the number of solute particles (milliosmoles) dissolved in a kilogram of water (mOsm/kg). A colligative property of solutions, osmolality is linearly correlated with its freezing point; instruments that measure these properties (osmometers) are used to measure osmolality directly.

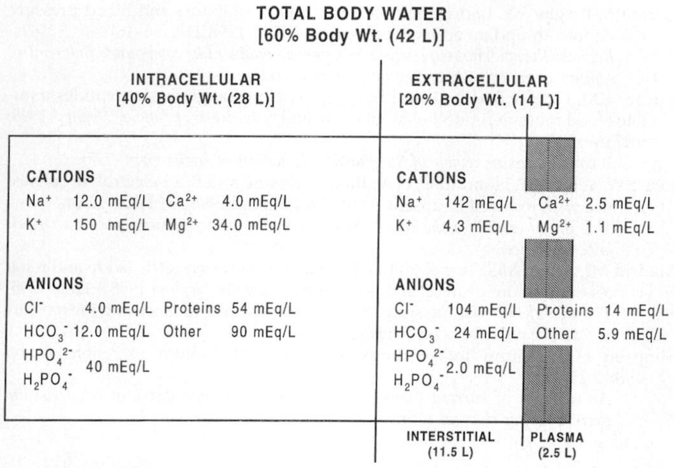

Figure 15.12. Distribution of body water and electrolytes. (Reproduced with permission from Narins RG, Krishna GC. Disorders of water balance. In: Stein JH, ed. *Internal medicine,* 2nd ed. Boston: Little Brown, 1987: 794–805.)

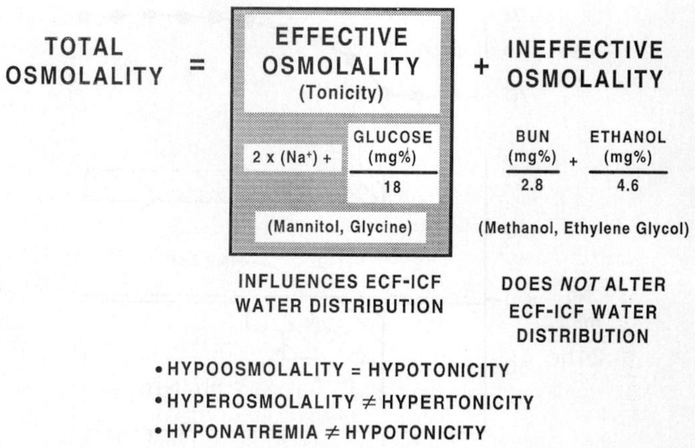

Figure 15.13. Total, effective, and ineffective osmolalities. (Reproduced with permission from Sterns RH, Ocdol H, Schrier RW, et al. Hyponatremia: pathophysiology, diagnosis and therapy. In: Narins RG, ed. *Clinical disorders of fluid and electrolyte metabolism,* 5th ed. New York: McGraw-Hill, 1984:583–615.)

Alternatively, osmolality can be estimated from the separately measured concentrations of the solutes making up the solution. The dissociability of each solute greatly influences its osmotic contribution. Thus a 150-mmol/L solution of NaCl, an admixture of the unionized molecule and its dissociated components (Na^+ and Cl^-), has an osmolality of approximately 275 mOsm/kg. A 150-mmol/L solution of glucose, a molecule that does not dissociate, has an osmolality of 150 mOsm/kg.

Normally, the major solutes present in the ECF are sodium salts, glucose, and urea. Therefore the plasma osmolality can be estimated by summing the osmotic contributions of these solutes.

$$\text{Calculated plasma osmolality} = 2 \times S_{Na} + \text{GLU (mg/dl)}/18 + \text{BUN (mg/dl)}/2.8$$

Because the concentrations of glucose (GLU) and urea nitrogen (BUN) are expressed in mg/100 ml, dividing the sugar concentration by one-tenth of its molecular weight (180) and dividing the concentration of the two nitrogens of urea by one-tenth of their summed atomic weights ($14 \times 2 = 28$), converts these solutes' concentrations to units of mmol/L, which is equivalent to mOsm/L. The equation overlooks the incomplete dissociation of sodium salts in solution, the fact that plasma is only 93% water, and the modest contribution of other cations (calcium, magnesium, and potassium) to plasma osmolality. Because these factors tend to offset each other, the calculated plasma osmolality normally varies by no more than 10 mOsm/L from the measured value. Calculated and measured values for plasma osmolality differ when exogenous low-molecular-weight solutes (mannitol, sorbitol, mannose, sucrose, glycine, glycerol, ethanol, methanol, ethylene glycol, or isopropyl alcohol) circulate in high concentrations, increasing the measured osmolality without altering the standard calculated value (Fig. 15.13). This difference between measured and calculated osmolalities is termed the *osmolal gap.*

Recognition of an osmolal gap is important in four situations: (a) the evaluation of suspected poisoning with substances such as ethanol, methanol, or ethylene glycol that raise the plasma osmolality without altering the serum sodium concentration; (b) the management of hyponatremia caused by systemic absorption of irrigants (e.g., glycine) during endoscopic prostate or uterine surgery; (c) the interpretation of the serum sodium concentration following therapeutic infusions containing impermeant sugars such as mannitol; and (d) the evaluation of possible pseudohyponatremia, associated with either severe hyperlipidemia or plasma cell disorders. These conditions are discussed later in the chapter.

Plasma osmolality is comprised of both "effective" and "ineffective" components (Fig. 15.13). Effective osmoles (e.g., Na^+, mannitol) are solutes that cannot freely permeate cell membranes and are therefore largely restricted to the ECF. Effective osmoles induce transcompartmental shifts in water. The effective osmolality of a solution is synonymous with its tonicity. Ineffective osmoles freely cross cell membranes and do not alter water distribution between fluid compartments. Such ineffective solutes (e.g., urea, ethanol) do not affect tonicity. Thus patients with renal failure whose blood urea concentrations are increased have hyperosmolality, but not hypertonicity.

When an effective solute such as sodium selectively accumulates at high concentrations in the ECF (hypertonicity), solute-free water will move down its concentration gradient from the ICF to the ECF, shrinking the ICF. Conversely, when the concentration of sodium and other extracellular solutes are reduced (hypotonicity), preservation of osmotic equilibrium requires that cells accumulate water and swell.

The cell membrane transporter Na^+-K^+-ATPase, which imports potassium and exports sodium from all body cells, ensures that potassium accounts for the vast bulk of cellular cations, whereas sodium serves as the dominant extracellular cation. Thus, by doubling the exchangeable sodium (Na^+_E) and potassium (K^+_E) content, and thereby accounting for the counterbalancing anions, one can approximate almost all total body solutes by estimating the extracellular and intracellular components. Division of this total body solute content by total body water (TBW) approximates the prevailing tonicity of all body fluids.

$$\text{Effective osmolality (ECF and ICF)} = 2 \times (Na^+_E + K^+_E)/\text{TBW}$$

Serum Sodium Concentration

In the absence of an osmolal gap, the serum sodium concentration is a more valid measure of body fluid tonicity than plasma osmolality, which includes the ineffective osmole urea. Because glucose contributes to tonicity, the serum sodium concentration can be interpreted only in the context of the prevailing blood glucose concentration. In diabetic hyperglycemia, glucose is an effective osmole that promotes electrolyte-free water movement from the ICF to the ECF, diluting the serum sodium concentration. With insulin therapy, glucose becomes an ineffective osmole as it enters cells and is metabolized. Thus the serum sodium concentration can be "corrected" for the effect of hyperglycemia by calculating what the serum sodium concentration would have been had the blood glucose been returned to normal and ECF water had returned to the ICF. The following equation is based on the observation that the serum sodium concentration is reduced by approximately 1.5 mEq/L for each 100-mg/dl increment above a baseline blood glucose value of 100 mg/dl.

$$\text{"Corrected" serum Na} = \text{Measured } S_{Na} + 1.5 \times [(\text{GLU} - 100)/100]$$

In this equation, blood glucose is expressed in milligrams per deciliter (mg/dl). For example, in a patient with a measured serum sodium concentration of 130 mEq/L and blood glucose of 900 mg/dl, the "corrected" serum sodium concentration equals 142 mEq/L [= 130 + 1.5 × (900 − 100)/100 = 130 + 12)].

Given that the corrected sodium concentration accounts for approximately half of the effective osmoles in the plasma, a relationship between Na^+_E , K^+_E, and TBW is apparent from the following equation:

$$S_{Na}\text{ (corrected)} = (Na^+_E + K^+_E)/\text{TBW}$$

This equation indicates that the serum sodium concentration changes when the ratio of total body cation content to body water content is altered.

Electrolyte-Free Water Balance and Tonicity

All of the fluids that we take in and excrete can conceptually be divided into two portions: isotonic fluid and electrolyte-free water. Isotonic fluid has a cation concentration equal to that of plasma; its gain or loss has no effect on body fluid tonicity. Electrolyte-free water contains no cations; the overall balance of electrolyte-free water determines what body tonicity will be. Accumulation (positive balance) of electrolyte-free water causes hyponatremia (hypotonicity), whereas negative-free water balance produces hypernatremia (hypertonicity).

Hypotonic fluid, which has a cation concentration lower than serum, can be thought of as an isotonic solution that has been diluted with electrolyte-free water. For example, 1 L of fluid with a total cation concentration ($Na^+ + K^+$) equaling 75 mEq/L (i.e., a 0.5 normal cation solution) can be conceptually partitioned into 500 ml of isotonic fluid and 500 ml of electrolyte-free water. Loss of 1 L of this 0.5 normal solution will alter body fluid as follows: the 500-ml isotonic component will shrink the ECF by 500 ml, without changing ICF volume and without altering the serum sodium concentration; the 500-ml electrolyte-free water component will shrink the ICF by 335 ml and the ECF by 165 ml. These volumes are derived from the normal partitioning of water between the ICF that comprises two-thirds of TBW and the ECF that comprises one-third of TBW.

Osmoregulation

The solute concentration of body fluids is held virtually constant by tightly regulating the ebb and flow of water. Water balance controls the concentration of solute in all body fluid compartments, whereas sodium balance with its link to water balance determines the volume of the ECF. The constancy of serum sodium concentration, despite minute-to-minute challenges from our capricious appetites for salt and water, underscores the vital importance of the osmoregulatory system (Fig. 15.14). Water retention, hypotonicity, and cellular swelling are averted by a prompt increase in the rate of renal water excretion. Water depletion, hypertonicity, and cell shrinkage are avoided by renal water conservation and thirst. Renal tubular water reabsorption and therefore water excretion are controlled by the antidiuretic hormone arginine vasopressin (AVP). Most cells, but especially those within the central nervous system (CNS), have the ability to discharge or accrue potassium and organic solutes (i.e., osmolytes), thereby controlling intracellular osmolality that, in turn, minimizes alterations of cellular volume. Thus the components of the osmoregulatory system are the thirst mechanism, vasopressin synthesis and release, the kidney, and the cellular balance of osmolytes (Fig. 15.14).

When plasma tonicity changes by as little as 1%, hypothalamic osmoreceptor cell volume is altered, triggering signals to neurons located in the supraoptic and paraventricular nuclei. These neurons then appropriately modify their secretion of vasopressin (see Chapter 15, Part 1). Under steady-state conditions of isotonicity (i.e., serum sodium concentration of 137 mEq/L osmolality of 285 mOsm/L), plasma vasopressin levels average 2.5 pg/ml. AVP levels are directly proportional to serum tonicity (Fig. 15.15). Normally, serum AVP levels are unmeasurable when serum osmolality falls below 280 mOsm/L (serum sodium 135 mEq/L). When serum osmolality rises to 295 mOsm/L (serum sodium 142 mEq/L), plasma vasopressin levels approximate 5.0 pg/ml.

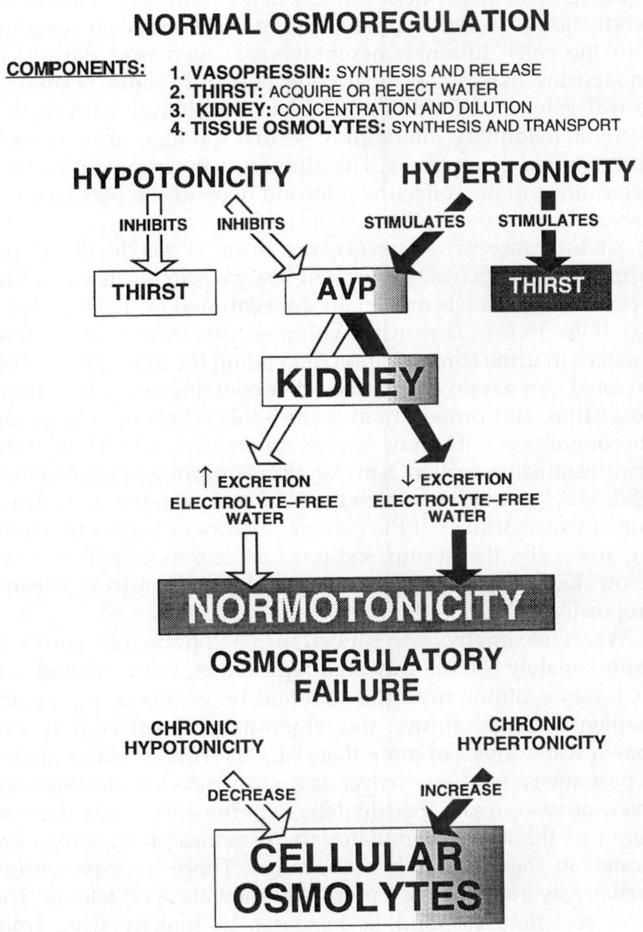

Figure 15.14. Osmoregulatory system. Interactions of the component parts of the system. *AVP*, arginine vasopressin.

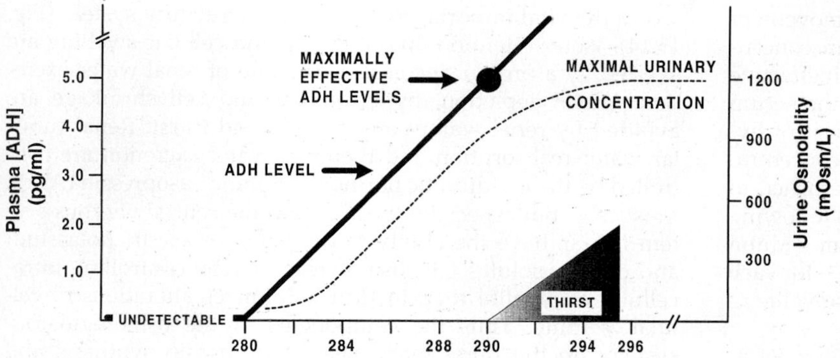

Figure 15.15. Antidiuretic hormone *(ADH)* levels, urinary osmolality, and thirst as functions of serum osmolality. Horizontal axis denotes plasma osmolality (mOsm/L). (Reproduced with permission from Narins RG, Krishna GC. Disorders of water balance. In: Stein JH, ed. *Internal medicine,* 2nd ed. Boston: Little Brown, 1987:794–805.)

Guided by the prevailing plasma vasopressin concentration, the kidney precisely excretes or retains the correct volume of water that prevents variation in serum sodium concentration by more than 1% or 2%. Glomerular filtrate that escapes isotonic reabsorption in the proximal tubule is delivered to diluting sites in the distal nephron (the ascending limb of Henle's loop and the distal convoluted tubule), where sodium chloride is selectively removed from the filtrate, leaving electrolyte-free water in the tubular lumen. Downstream from the diluting segments, the collecting duct is relatively "water proof." Here, when vasopressin is absent, electrolyte-poor fluid formed upstream may be excreted in the final urine. In the presence of vasopressin, V_2 receptors on the basolateral membrane of collecting duct cells are activated, initiating a cyclic adenosine monophosphate (cAMP)–dependent process that culminates in increased production of water channels (aquaporins) and their insertion into the cells' luminal membrane. An increased density of aquaporins makes the renal collecting duct more permeable to water; luminal fluid is then able to equilibrate with the hypertonic medullary interstitium so that the final urine is more concentrated than plasma. The ultimate urine osmolality is thus determined in the collecting duct and depends on plasma vasopressin levels.

At low vasopressin levels, the urine is maximally dilute (approximately 50 mOsm/kg). At vasopressin levels exceeding 5 pg/ml, the urine is maximally concentrated (= 1,200 mOsm/kg) (Fig. 15.15). The urine volumes that result from these changes in urine concentration depend on the amount of solute excreted. An average American diet contains enough sodium, potassium, and protein (that is metabolized to urea) to generate roughly 900 mOsm of urinary solute each day. Thus, if the urine osmolality is 50 mOsm/kg, urine output will be torrential (18 L/day), enough to match the intake of even the most determined water drinker. If the osmoregulatory system is functioning normally, the serum sodium concentration will not fall below 135 mEq/L, unless water intake reaches truly oceanic proportions.

When maximally concentrated, urine volume may shrink to approximately 500 ml/day on a typical diet, but unabated water losses continue from the skin and lungs. Fever, high environmental temperatures, and vigorous physical activity can spawn water losses of more than 1 L/hr. Without water intake, hypertonicity and hypernatremia rapidly develop, despite high levels of vasopressin. Fortunately, hypertonicity elicits the sensation of thirst and stimulates the osmoreceptors, which are located in the anterior hypothalamus. These tonicity sensors partially overlap with receptors that mediate AVP release. The thirst receptors respond to increases in tonicity (e.g., from sodium or mannitol), but not to increased concentrations of ineffective osmoles such as urea. Thirst is experienced at plasma osmolalities within the physiologic range. Regardless of the degree of water loss, an intact thirst response ensures that the serum sodium concentration will not exceed 142 mEq/L when water is sufficiently available. For example, patients with diabetes insipidus (DI), from either an inability to make vasopressin (central DI) or an insensitivity to the hormone (nephrogenic DI), maintain normonatremia, despite large urinary water losses. This remains true as long as the thirst center remains functional and the subject has access to water.

Hypotensive or volume-contracted subjects continue to retain proffered water, despite worsening hypotonicity. In teleologic terms, tonicity in this setting is sacrificed for maintenance of plasma volume, hemodynamic stability being the more vital function. Neural impulses from baroreceptors in the great vessels and atria, stimulated by an 8% to 10% reduction in ECF volume or by hypotension, are transmitted via afferent fibers of cranial nerves IX and X to the hypothalamus. A large hemodynamic stimulus elicits higher vasopressin levels than pathologically achievable osmotic stimuli. Thus, although vasopressin secretion is more sensitive to changes in tonicity, vasopressin release stimulated by volume contraction can greatly supersede the less potent inhibitory effect of hypotonicity on AVP secretion. Hypovolemia and hypotension also stimulate thirst, possibly through elevated plasma levels of angiotensin II. Various noxious stimuli, acting through higher centers, also stimulate AVP release. These secretagogues include pain, emotional stress, nausea, hypoxia, hypoglycemia, and various drugs. Excessive exposure to water when volume contraction or these other stimuli are present results in hypotonicity. The control of water excretion is discussed in detail in Chapter 15, Part 1.

Adaptations to Osmoregulatory Failure

When the interplay among thirst, vasopressin, and the kidney fails to maintain tonicity within the normal range, cells must adapt to the disturbance to preserve their volume (Fig. 15.16). Because intracellular osmolality must equal that of the ECF, extracellular hypotonicity causes cell swelling and hypertonicity causes cellular dehydration. Instead of maintaining osmotic equilibrium solely by gaining or losing water, many cells respond to osmotic disturbances by varying their solute content. Cells normally contain small, osmotically active organic molecules termed *osmolytes* (inositol, sorbitol, betaine, and glycerophosphocholine). Cells minimize volume loss in a hypertonic environment by accumulating more organic osmolytes. Cell swelling is limited in hypotonicity by extrusion of these same solutes. The flexible and protective balance of cellular osmolytes represents the final component of the osmoregulatory system.

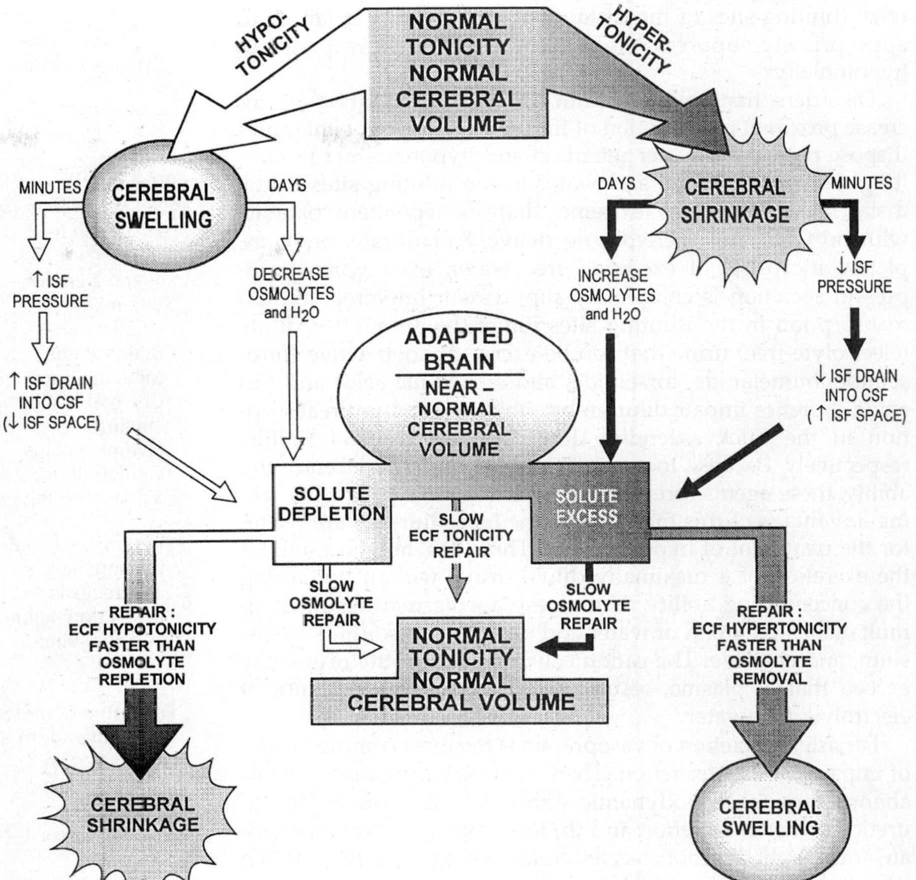

Figure 15.16. Abnormal extracellular fluid tonicity and cerebral adaptation. *ISF*, interstitial fluid.

The requirement for a volume regulatory adaptation to hyponatremia is most imperative in the brain. The rigid calvarium imposes sharp limits on the degree to which cerebral tissue may expand. Indeed, changes in brain water content of more than 10% are incompatible with life. Although the blood–brain barrier resists the permeation of most osmotically active solutes, it is water permeant. Thus, when the serum sodium concentration changes, a transient osmotic gradient forms between the systemic capillary blood and the brain, causing water to flow rapidly across the barrier with restoration of osmotic equilibrium. If the brain behaved in an osmotically perfect manner (i.e., swelling or shrinking in direct proportion to changes in tonicity), a reduction in sodium concentration from 140 to 127 mEq/L or an increase to 154 mEq/L (changes of 10%) would define the biologically tolerable range. The fact that humans may survive unharmed with serum sodium concentrations below 100 mEq/L (low enough to increase brain volume by 40%) and above 200 mEq/L (high enough to reduce brain volume by 50%) is living testimony to the resistance of the brain to osmotic stress.

Because adjustments in cell solute content require approximately 2 days to fully develop, the brain is imperiled by rapid osmotic changes. Thus acute hyponatremia and hypernatremia may be fatal, whereas similar changes in serum sodium concentration that develop chronically are usually well tolerated. Moreover, although the extrusion of organic osmolytes from brain cells ultimately protects against lethal cerebral edema, an accumulation of these compounds in the brain's interstitial space during the initial phase of cerebral osmotic adaptation may induce neurologic symptoms because many of these organic osmolytes are neurotransmitters. The adaptations that defend against cerebral edema in chronic hyponatremia and against brain shrinkage in chronic hypernatremia also predispose to brain injury when the electrolyte disturbance is corrected too rapidly (Fig. 15.16). In hyponatremia, solutes lost in the adaptive phase must be regained. Unless this process keeps pace with the rising serum sodium concentration, brain dehydration will result. Conversely, in hypernatremia, solutes gained during the adaptive phase must be extruded. It follows that inappropriately hasty correction of chronic hypernatremia causes cerebral edema.

HYPONATREMIA

Pathogenesis

Because the plasma sodium concentration is normally maintained within a narrow physiologic range by control systems that regulate water balance, hypotonic hyponatremia can occur only when water excretion is impaired or overwhelmed such that the intake of electrolyte-free water exceeds its losses. Thus it may be helpful to think of a low plasma sodium concentration as "hyperaquemia," rather than as a deficit of sodium, as the laboratory designation implies.

Occasionally, fluid intake can overwhelm normal mechanisms for water excretion (most often in patients with severe psychiatric disturbances). More often, hypotonic hyponatremia occurs in patients with impaired water excretion. Three basic mechanisms may limit electrolyte-free water excretion: (a) reduced glomerular filtration rate (GFR) and/or excessive proximal tubular reabsorption, (b) impaired NaCl reabsorption in the renal diluting sites of the distal nephron, and/or (c) failure to appropriately suppress vasopressin secretion in response to hypotonicity.

Disorders that severely limit glomerular filtration or increase proximal reabsorption of filtrate (e.g., hypovolemia) predispose patients to water retention and hyponatremia by limiting delivery of solute and water to the diluting sites of the distal nephron. At the extreme, dialysis-dependent patients with no GFR, and therefore no delivery of filtrate, are completely incapable of excreting free water, even when vasopressin secretion is completely suppressed. Impaired sodium reabsorption in the diluting sites limits the amount of dilute (electrolyte-free) urine that can be excreted. Loop-active (furosemide, bumetanide, torsemide, and ethacrynic acid) and thiazide diuretics impair dilution by inhibiting sodium reabsorption in the thick ascending limb and early distal tubule, respectively. Because loop diuretics also impair concentrating ability, these agents rarely cause hyponatremia. In fact, by taking advantage of this mechanism, the loop diuretics are useful for the treatment of hyponatremia. Thiazides, however, inhibit the excretion of a maximally dilute urine, without impairing the concentrating ability. Thus these agents may result in simultaneous retention of water and depletion of sodium, potassium, and chloride. The cation concentration of the urine may exceed that of plasma, resulting in a net positive balance of electrolyte-free water.

Persistent secretion of vasopressin is the most common cause of impaired water excretion. There are two basic causes for this abnormality: (a) hemodynamic stimuli for vasopressin (antidiuretic hormone) secretion and (b) the syndrome of inappropriate antidiuretic hormone secretion (SIADH) (Table 15.4). When a hemodynamic stimulus (hypovolemia, low cardiac output, or vasodilation) is responsible for nonosmotic release of vasopressin, urinary sodium excretion is generally reduced (except when urinary sodium wasting is the cause of hypovolemia). Sodium retention is a protective physiologic response to a perceived diminished effective circulating volume. In SIADH, water excretion is impaired but sodium excretion is normal, characteristically matching and sometimes exceeding sodium intake. Unimpaired sodium balance is underscored by normotension and lack of edema.

Although it is true that hyponatremia reflects disordered water balance, sodium and potassium losses often play an important role in the pathogenesis of the electrolyte disturbance. Recall that the serum sodium concentration is a ratio of solute to solvent. Therefore hyponatremia can result either from a decrease of sodium or potassium (numerator of the ratio) or from an increase in water (denominator of the ratio). Sodium depletion can be the primary disturbance, as in volume-depleted patients who secondarily retain water because of baroreceptor-mediated vasopressin secretion, or it may be a secondary physiologic response, as in patients who retain water in the ECF because of SIADH and secondarily lose sodium in their urine, which partially blunts the ECF volume expansion and further lowers the serum sodium concentration. Patients with severe chronic SIADH also lose potassium as an adaptive response to cell swelling. Thus the low serum sodium concentration in chronic SIADH stems from both water retention and cation depletion.

Primary potassium depletion from diuretics or gastrointestinal fluid losses may also contribute to a low serum sodium concentration. Because clinically significant potassium depletion generally entails loss of more than 100 mEq and because the entire ECF space contains only 55 to 65 mEq, it follows that the great bulk of shed cation must come from the ICF. Because potassium is the major intracellular osmole, its loss renders the ICF hypotonic, causing water to enter the normal, but now relatively more hypertonic, ECF space. Extracellular sodium enters cells in partial replacement of lost potassium. Furthermore, potassium depletion is dipsogenic. The additive effects of redistribution of water, entry of sodium into cells, and the increased acquisition of water should all favor the development of hyponatremia. The vasopressin-resistant polyuria that also characterizes potassium depletion tends to offset this predisposition to hyponatremia. However, potassium depletion is commonly associated with diuretic therapy and vomiting. The complicating hypovolemia may then minimize the polyuria and fully unmask the hyponatremic effects of hypokalemia. Just as potassium depletion can contribute to the pathogenesis of hyponatremia, replacement of potassium deficits contributes to the correction of hyponatremia.

TABLE 15.4. Common Causes of the Syndrome of Inappropriate Antidiuretic Hormone Secretion (SIADH)

Medical and Surgical Conditions	Pharmacologic Agents
Tumors	Direct Antidiuretic Action
Small cell lung cancer	Arginine vasopressin
Head and neck cancer	DDAVP
	Oxytocin
Central Nervous System Disorders	
Head trauma	Enhanced Vasopressin Action
Brain tumors	Chlorpropamide
Meningitis and encephalitis	Nonsteroidal antiinflammatory drugs
Cerebral hemorrhage and infarction	Carbamazepine (?)
Hydrocephalus	Oxcarbazepine (?)
Guillain-Barré syndrome	Cyclophosphamide (?)
Spinal cord injury	
	Enhanced Vasopressin Secretion
Pulmonary Disorders	Tricyclic antidepressants
Pneumonia	Selective serotonin reuptake inhibitors
Tuberculosis	Vincristine
Respiratory failure	Vinblastine
Severe asthma	Clofibrate
	Carbamazepine (?)
Endocrine Disorders	Oxcarbazepine (?)
Hypothyroidism	
Hypopituitarism	Vasopressin-Independent Action
Isolated adrenocorticotropic deficiency	Thiazide diuretics
Miscellaneous	
Nausea	
Surgery, pain, and stress	
Acquired immunodeficiency syndrome	
Alcohol withdrawal	

Etiology and Classification

The clinical approach to the hyponatremic disorders begins with their classification in terms of tonicity and then subclassification of the hypotonic forms of hyponatremia on the basis of clinically derived estimates of the volume of the ECF space (Fig. 15.17).

Isotonic and Hypertonic Hyponatremia

Patients with hypotonicity are always hyponatremic, but hyponatremia is not always synonymous with hypotonicity. Hypertonic hyponatremia caused by hyperglycemia was discussed earlier in this chapter.

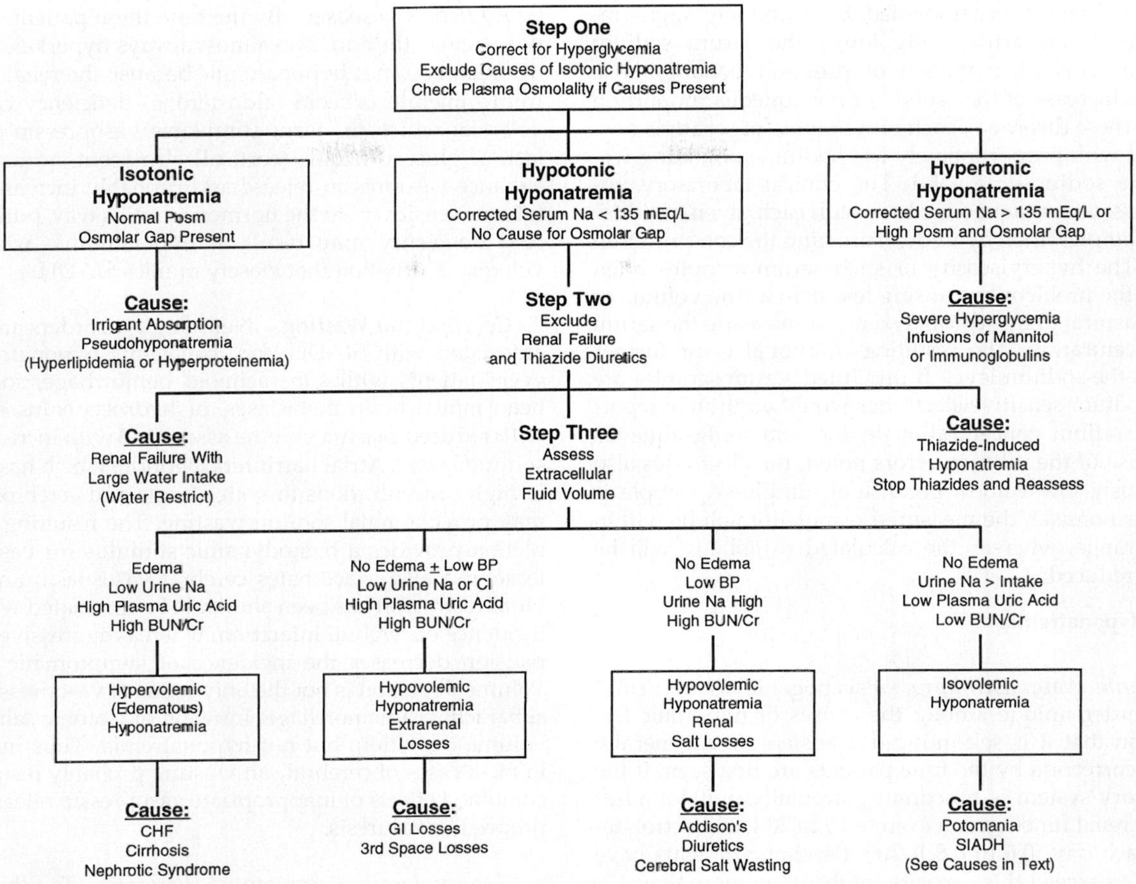

Figure 15.17. Approach to hyponatremic disorders.

Hypertonic Infusions. Infusion of hypertonic solutions of mannitol used to treat cerebral edema or to induce diuresis initially lowers the serum sodium concentration by osmotically attracting water from the ICF to the ECF. Thus the sodium concentration of the ECF is reduced while the osmolality of both the extracellular and intracellular compartments is increased. A similar phenomenon has been described after administration of immunoglobulin G solutions that contain high concentrations of the impermeant sugars, mannose, or sucrose. Retention of the infused sugars in patients with impaired renal function may create sustained hypertonic hyponatremia.

Irrigation Fluid Absorption Syndrome. Systemic absorption of isosmotic or moderately hypotonic solutions (glycine, sorbitol, or mannitol) that are used as nonelectrically conducting irrigants during endoscopic prostatic and gynecologic surgery is an important cause of isosmotic hyponatremia. The sodium-free solutions used in these procedures are initially confined to the ECF and, depending on the volume absorbed, may cause extraordinarily severe hyponatremia, with little or no change in plasma osmolality. Because of their restriction to the ECF, all of these irrigants reduce the serum sodium concentration to a much greater extent than a comparable volume of water (which distributes throughout body fluids). Mannitol, which is not metabolized, remains in the ECF until it is excreted in the urine. Sorbitol and glycine, which are metabolized, are only partially excreted. Sorbitol is rapidly converted to fructose and glucose and eventually to CO_2 and H_2O. Particularly when renal function is impaired, increasingly severe hypotonicity (comparable to that caused by an equal volume of water) and cerebral edema emerge as the absorbed sorbitol is metabolized, leaving solute-free water behind. Paradoxically, because of the intracellular migration of water, the serum sodium concentration increases as the plasma osmolality decreases, reflecting the migration of sorbitol into cells. Glycine is converted to serine and other amino acids that persist in the circulation. Because glycine does not readily cross the blood–brain barrier, early brain edema does not occur. However, glycine and its metabolites distribute in the cells of other tissues. The intracellular migration of the amino acids and the fluid associated with them increases the serum sodium concentration over the course of several hours. Glycine is eventually metabolized to urea and ammonia. The resulting hyperammonemia may equal or exceed that seen in advanced hepatic disease and may be associated with an equally severe encephalopathy. Glycine also inhibits neurotransmission in the retina, causing blurred vision, transient blindness, and dilated pupils. Fortunately, most patients recover, despite extraordinarily severe hyponatremia. Rational treatment requires frequent monitoring of plasma osmolality and serum sodium concentration. The osmolal gap is, of course, an indirect reflection of the concentration of the offending solute, and its change may be used to follow the redistribution, metabolism, or excretion of the agent. True symptomatic hypotonicity, which is particularly likely to emerge after absorption of sorbitol, should be treated like other causes of acute water intoxication. Severe symptoms in glycine-intoxicated patients may best be treated by dialysis, a procedure that will simultaneously remove the neurotoxic amino acid, prevent further ammonia production, and correct osmotic abnormalities and fluid overload.

Pseudohyponatremia. Hypertriglyceridemia, severe enough to produce plasma lactescence, and advanced multiple myeloma or macroglobulinemia accompanied by extremely high immunoglobulin levels artifactually lower the serum sodium concentration. This phenomenon of pseudohyponatremia is caused by an increase of the "solid" or nonaqueous proportion of serum. In these disorders, each unit volume of serum is now reconstituted with proportionately less sodium-containing water and more sodium-free solid. The clinical laboratory unknowingly assays less aqueous phase with each given milliliter of serum it samples, thereby underestimating the concentration of sodium. The hyperviscosity of such serum samples often compounds the problem by causing less than a true volume of serum to be aspirated by autoanalyzers that measure the serum sodium concentration. The resulting dilutional error further undervalues the sodium level. If undiluted serum samples are tested, the sodium-sensitive electrodes would accurately report the normal sodium concentration in the remaining aqueous phase. Because of the dilution errors noted, the electrodes also yield spuriously low values. Because an undiluted sample is used in an osmometer, the measured osmolality will be within the normal range, whereas the calculated osmolality will be erroneously reduced.

Hypotonic Hyponatremia

Psychogenic Water Drinking. Psychogenic water drinking is a disorder unique among the causes of hypotonic hyponatremia in that it is self-induced, transient, and generally undergoing correction by the time patients are first seen. If the osmoregulatory system is functioning normally, a 70-kg adult with normal renal function can excrete 15 to 20 L of electrolyte-free water each day (0.6 to 0.8 L/hr). Psychotic patients have been known to exceed this capacity by drinking more than 1 L of water per hour for several hours. The emotional trauma that drives such patients to drink may also prevent total suppression of vasopressin release, thereby reducing maximal urinary dilution and water excretion and reducing the amount of water that must be ingested to achieve serum sodium dilution. By the time they reach the hospital, most patients seem to have finally suppressed vasopressin secretion and are excreting very dilute urine. Whether transient abnormalities in the thirst mechanism underlie this syndrome in some patients is unknown. Several of these patients have an inability to inhibit vasopressin release at lower serum osmolality, thereby inhibiting appropriate urinary dilution. Other patients exhibit increased tubular sensitivity to low circulating levels of the hormone.

Hypovolemic Variants. The hypovolemic forms of hypotonic hyponatremia are characterized by baroreceptor-stimulated, or "appropriate," release of vasopressin. Hypovolemia can be secondary to the external loss of fluid and electrolytes or to the squandering of intravascular fluid to the interstitium, peritoneum, or other "third" spaces as with pancreatitis, burns, intestinal ileus, or rhabdomyolysis. These are isotonic "losses." Urinary salt wasting (e.g., diuretic-induced, *cis*-platinum nephrotoxicity, medullary cystic disease, and partial urinary tract obstruction) is another cause of hypovolemic hyponatremia. With rare exception, gastrointestinal, third space, and renal fluid losses are isotonic or hypotonic relative to the prevailing plasma tonicity. Such losses should cause isotonic contraction alone or hypernatremic hypovolemia. These patients become hyponatremic only if they replace their salt and water losses with electrolyte-free water. It follows that an individual almost never becomes hyponatremic unless that individual drinks or has water otherwise administered.

Addison's Disease. By the time these patients become hyponatremic, they are also almost always hyperkalemic. The addisonian becomes hyponatremic because the renal salt wasting from mineralocorticoid (aldosterone) deficiency causes hypovolemia, which, in turn, stimulates vasopressin release. The lack of glucocorticoids (cortisol) also seems to independently enhance vasopressin release and probably increases the distal tubular sensitivity to the hormone. In this way, pure glucocorticoid deficiency may result in hyponatremia without hypovolemia, a situation that closely mimics SIADH.

Cerebral Salt Wasting. Neurologic disorders are commonly associated with SIADH and isovolemic hyponatremia. However, patients with subarachnoid hemorrhage, some cases of head injury, brain metastases, or hydrocephalus may present with reduced plasma volume associated with increased urinary sodium losses. Atrial natriuretic peptide, which has been found in high concentrations in both plasma and cerebrospinal fluid, may provoke renal sodium wasting. The resulting volume depletion provides a hemodynamic stimulus for vasopressin release and also exacerbates cerebral vasospasm and ischemia. Fluid restriction has been shown to be associated with a greater incidence of cerebral infarction, whereas aggressive volume expansion decreases the incidence of symptomatic vasospasm. Volume depletion is not the only cause of vasopressin release in subarachnoid hemorrhage. Infusion of isotonic saline prevents volume depletion, but not hyponatremia. Thus hyponatremia in most cases of cerebral salt wasting probably results from the combined effects of inappropriate vasopressin release and inappropriate natriuresis.

Hypervolemic (Edematous) Variants. The hypervolemic forms of hypotonic hyponatremia are generally characterized by a reduction in the effective arterial blood volume (EABV), which triggers release of vasopressin. In congestive heart failure (CHF), large-vessel baroreceptors and those in the left ventricle stimulate vasopressin release. With right-sided heart failure and edema, EABV may be further compromised. Diminished renal perfusion, increased proximal tubular reabsorption, and limited delivery of filtrate to distal diluting sites further sensitize patients to developing hyponatremia. A low serum sodium concentration is generally taken as a poor prognostic sign in patients with chronic CHF. It apparently requires advanced degrees of myocardial compromise to elicit the pathophysiologic changes needed to render these edematous patients hyponatremic. As in CHF, when hyponatremia complicates hepatic cirrhosis, it usually reflects advanced disease and also signals a poor prognosis. Hyponatremia is also associated with increased levels of vasopressin, catecholamines, renin, angiotensin, and aldosterone. Advanced cirrhosis results in systemic vasodilation, most likely in response to increased production of nitric oxide by vascular endothelial cells. Systemic vasodilation causes relative underfilling of the arterial vascular compartment, triggering neurohumoral responses that promote salt and water retention. Nephrotic syndrome can cause hyponatremia, especially in children with minimal-change disease. Hypoalbuminemia and the displacement of plasma volume into the interstitial fluid (ISF) space causes the EABV to decline. The nonosmotic stimulation of vasopressin secretion is probably a root cause of water retention and hyponatremia. Because nephrotic adults tend to have ECF volume expansion and hypertension, hyponatremia appears to occur less often.

Isovolemic Variants. The isovolemic variants of hypotonic hyponatremia (Fig. 15.17) are usually associated with ECF spaces that are expanded or contracted but not altered enough to be clinically detected. At opposite ends of this spectrum are patients with SIADH and those with thiazide-induced hyponatremia. Patients with SIADH undergo secondary losses of both sodium and potassium, blunting ECF and ICF volume expansion. Many patients who become chronically hyponatremic while taking thiazide diuretics compensate for sodium and potassium depletion by retaining enough electrolyte-free water to sustain hemodynamic stability; therefore the fall in EABV is clinically undetectable. The syndromes accounting for isovolemic hypotonic hyponatremia are summarized in the following sections.

Beer Drinker's Potomania. Even if vasopressin secretion is totally suppressed and renal function is entirely normal, the urine cannot be diluted below 50 mOsm/L. Thus each liter of urine excreted by kidneys, under severe hypotonic challenge, must contain a minimum of 50 mOsm of solute. A normal diet that generates 900 mOsm of solute for excretion allows the kidney to excrete up to 18 L of 50 mOsm/L urine. Because beer does not contain much protein or salt, inveterate drinkers, who eat very little and imbibe very much, have reduced solute for excretion. Alcoholics who excrete only 200 mOsm of solute can excrete only 4 L of the most dilute urine (50 mOsm/L). They will become hyponatremic if they imbibe more than 6 L of beer each day. A similar dietary limitation of solute may contribute to the hyponatremia seen in other more common settings in which malnutrition and increased water ingestion coexist. An example of this is "the tea and toast syndrome" seen in nursing home residents.

Renal Failure. Residual nephrons in damaged kidneys retain their ability to reabsorb electrolytes without water and, in fact, excrete generous amounts of hypotonic urine until very late in the course of chronic renal failure. Patients in steady-state renal insufficiency continue to excrete approximately 900 mOsm/day of solute. The number of liters of glomerular filtrate formed each day at stable GFRs of 25 ml/min, 10 ml/min, and 5 ml/min are 36 L (25 ml/min × 1,440 min/day), 14 L, and 7.2 L, respectively. If one assumes that the total cation (sodium plus potassium) that is ingested and destined for excretion is 175 mEq/day, the isotonic component of the urine will be the 350 mOsm of electrolyte in 1.2 L (i.e., 292 mOsm/L). If we further assume that approximately 40% of the glomerular filtrate will be excreted, potential 24-hour urine volumes would be 14.4. L, 5.6 L, and 2.9 L, respectively. Subtracting the isotonic portion (1.2 L) of the urine from the total volume defines the maximal amount of electrolyte-free water that can be excreted, and these values for the aforementioned GFRs are 13.2 L/day, 4.4 L/day, and 1.7 L/day. Thus no serious threat of water retention and hyponatremia occurs until GFRs decline to values below 10 ml/min. Diabetic patients receiving dialysis may develop hyponatremia in association with marked hyperglycemia as a result of movements of water from the ICF to the ECF. The treatment of this hyponatremia is the control of blood glucose.

SIADH

SIADH is an isovolemic variant of hyponatremia. When vasopressin secretion persists despite normal intravascular volume, normal cardiac output, and the normally suppressive effects of hypotonicity, its continued release is considered inappropriate. This persistent abnormal secretion occurs in a reasonably well-defined group of clinical settings (Table 15.4). Four separate patterns of secretion have been described. In the type I pattern (37% of patients), vasopressin secretion is chaotic, oscillating independently of serum osmolality. This pattern is seen in active pulmonary tuberculosis and bronchogenic carcinoma. Individuals who manifest the type II pattern (33% of patients) secrete vasopressin in a manner that correlates with changes in serum osmolality, but the setpoint for tonicity-induced release is lower than normal. These patients mimic the *reset osmostat syndrome.* In this disorder, the osmoregulatory system behaves as if it were set to defend a lower serum sodium level than normal (e.g., 125 mEq/L instead of 140 mEq/L). Bronchogenic carcinoma and tuberculous meningitis are among the disorders causing these syndromes. Conceivably, these are one and the same disorder (i.e., type II SIADH and reset osmostat). In the past, the reset osmostat was known as *sick cell syndrome,* suggesting that it was caused by the accumulation of osmolytes (electrolyte and nonelectrolyte) in cells, especially those responsible for vasopressin release. Cell solute excess triggered those forces that provoked water acquisition and retention, thereby returning the misconceived "hypertonicity" to "normal." Type II SIADH may or may not be related to this speculative pathogenesis. In the type III pattern (16% of patients), vasopressin secretion correlates normally with serum osmolality but cannot be totally suppressed, despite even marked hypotonicity. A persistent "basal leak" occurs. In addition to the aforementioned etiologies, CNS disorders are also common in this group. The type IV pattern (14% of patients) is characterized by normal vasopressin secretion and plasma levels but inexplicably persistent renal water retention. Increased renal sensitivity to very low, unmeasurable vasopressin levels or to an undefined water-retaining material are two unproven postulates offered to explain the pathogenesis of this form of SIADH.

Clinical Conditions Associated with SIADH

Tumors

Small cell carcinoma of the lung is the tumor most commonly associated with SIADH. The syndrome also complicates a small percentage of head and neck tumors. Although many other malignancies have been linked to the disorder, such cases are extremely rare, appearing only in isolated case reports (Table 15.4). Immunoassayable vasopressin has been extracted from small cell tumors; secretory granules containing the hormone have been identified and cultured neoplastic cells have been shown to synthesize the hormone. However, because the hyponatremia of some patients with tumors occurs without demonstrable increases in circulating vasopressin, other antidiuretic substances are still being sought out. Malignancies have been identified wherein hyponatremia was the first clinical manifestation of the disorder. However, it is far more common for hyponatremia to appear well after the tumor has made its clinical appearance.

CNS Disorders

Virtually any disorder that can affect the CNS, except for those that also impair vasopressin synthesis, has been associated with SIADH (Table 15.4). These disorders range from head trauma (including "punch-drunk" boxers) to tumors to various infections. Increased vasopressin secretion, especially common in subarachnoid hemorrhage, may also be accompanied by the cerebral release of various natriuretic substances. In this setting, the ECF volume contraction from the natriuresis may cause or increase vasopressin release by triggering baroreceptor mechanisms.

Pulmonary Disorders

Pneumonia is arguably the most common cause of SIADH. Indeed some of the earliest cases that ultimately were defined as SIADH were encountered in patients with pneumococcal pneumonia. Hyponatremia, with increased circulating levels of vasopressin, is common during the first few days of most pneumonias. Increased insensible water loss and lack of access to water in the severely ill are obvious forces that limit the frequency of hyponatremia, despite increased vasopressin secretion. Fungi, viruses, and tuberculosis are other infective agents that have caused pulmonary disease and SIADH. In addition to tumors and infections of the lung, asthma and acute respiratory failure can also cause the nonosmotic release of vasopressin.

Endocrinopathies

Glucocorticoids and thyroid hormone exert effects on vasopressin secretion; SIADH is seen in states with deficiency of these hormones. Increased vasopressin levels have been identified in hyponatremic patients with hypothyroidism. Changes in cardiac output, cerebral perfusion, or systemic blood pressure may account for the increased neurohypophysial secretion. Because hypothyroidism also reduces renal blood flow and GFR, both central and peripheral forces may contribute to the hyponatremia. Anterior hypopituitarism or isolated deficiency of adrenocorticotropic hormone (ACTH) causes pure glucocorticoid deficiency, without the volume contraction that characterizes Addison's disease (combined glucocorticoid and mineralocorticoid deficiency). Inhibitory glucocorticoid receptors are present in the hypothalamic neurons that secrete vasopressin and cortisol deficiency provokes excess vasopressin release. Cortisol also directly enhances electrolyte-free water clearance by the kidney and the lack of hormone has the opposite effect. This phenomenon becomes evident when anterior pituitary deficiency develops in patients who had previously manifested pure central DI. Up to 28% of cortisol-deficient patients present with hyponatremia with features typical of SIADH. Administration of glucocorticoids promptly suppresses increased vasopressin levels, provoking a rapid diuresis.

Pharmacologic Causes

Direct stimulation of vasopressin release, hemodynamic changes (which, in turn, stimulate hormone secretion), or renal effects that enhance or directly mimic vasopressin action are the mechanisms by which various drugs cause water retention. The best-studied and more commonly encountered drugs associated with the syndrome are listed in Table 15.4.

Nausea

A very potent stimulus for vasopressin release, nausea is a symptom common to many diseases. Persistent nausea, with or without vomiting, can sustain high levels of vasopressin and promotes the appearance of hyponatremia. It should also be remembered that acutely hyponatremic patients become nauseated, which then closes the loop on a vicious circle that worsens retention of acquired water.

Surgical States

Anesthesia, nausea, vomiting, hypotension, pain, narcotics, hypoxia, are all-powerful nonosmotic stimuli to the release of vasopressin. It logically follows that increased circulating levels of vasopressin abound during the first postoperative week. Patients exposed to excessive amounts of dilute solutions, which they cannot excrete, routinely become hyponatremic. Although hypotonic fluid is the most common culprit in postoperative hyponatremia, excessive use of isotonic fluid can lower the sodium concentration as infused sodium is excreted in a hypertonic urine, essentially "desalinating" the infused saline solution.

Acquired Immunodeficiency Syndrome

Roughly a third to half of hospitalized patients with acquired immunodeficiency syndrome (AIDS) are hyponatremic. This population generally has all the possible infectious, hemodynamic, pulmonary, and CNS causes that sensitize them to hyponatremia. The "adrenalitis" complicating AIDS causes hyponatremia and hyperkalemia.

Diagnosis of Hyponatremia

The clinical and chemical steps needed to stratify the possible causes of hyponatremia are outlined in Fig. 15.17. A diagnosis of SIADH should be made only in nonhypovolemic patients who are free of edema (edema-forming states are associated with hemodynamic causes of vasopressin secretion). The major challenge comes in recognizing volume depletion. In addition to the history and physical examination, measurement of the urine sodium concentration and of blood urea nitrogen (BUN) and serum uric acid levels are helpful clues. A high BUN and elevated serum uric acid suggest a diagnosis of hypovolemia. Subtle, clinically apparent volume depletion may be identified by a low (less than 30 mEq/L) urinary sodium concentration (or chloride in alkalotic patients), provided that the patient's sodium intake is also not very low. The mild volume expansion in patients with SIADH is difficult to detect because two-thirds of retained water resides in the ICF and the initial water-induced volume expansion provokes a transient natriuresis, thereby minimizing ECF distension. This subclinical hypervolemia increases the renal clearance of urea and uric acid. When hyponatremia is associated with a BUN below 10 mg/dl and hypouricemia, SIADH is the likely cause.

In all patients with SIADH, a specific cause for excessive vasopressin secretion must be sought. Sometimes, particularly when hyponatremia develops in the hospital, the cause is obvious (e.g., pneumonia, subarachnoid hemorrhage, surgery), and further testing is unnecessary. In patients with no obvious cause, a search for an underlying malignancy, endocrine disorder, or neurologic condition is usually indicated. However, no study has satisfactorily defined the diagnostic yield of such workups. Idiopathic cases have been described, particularly in the elderly.

Clinical Consequences of Hyponatremia

When hyponatremia develops faster than the brain can adapt, cerebral edema and "water intoxication" results. The neurologic manifestations of this disorder include headache, nausea, vomiting, weakness, incoordination, tremors, delirium, and ultimately, seizures and coma. Fatalities have been reported, primarily in young women who become hyponatremic while receiving parenteral hypotonic fluids during and after surgical procedures. Deaths, caused by transtentorial herniation, and severe sequelae most commonly occur when the serum sodium concentration falls below 120 mmol/L at a rate that exceeds 1 mmol/L per hour.

When hyponatremia develops more gradually (over 2 days or more), the symptoms are more subtle, vague, and nonspecific than those of acute water intoxication and they tend to occur at lower serum sodium levels. Typically, symptoms include anorexia, nausea, emesis, muscular weakness, and cramps. The patient may also become irritable and may show striking personality changes, becoming depressed, uncooperative, confused, or hostile. With extremely low serum sodium concentrations, gait disturbances, stupor, and (more rarely) seizures may occur.

Patients with prolonged hyponatremia are susceptible to iatrogenic complications when their electrolyte disturbance is corrected too rapidly. The clinical manifestations of this injury are delayed, evolving one to several days after treatment in a characteristic fashion. The term *osmotic demyelination syndrome* has been coined to describe the disorder. Clinical and pathologic findings are attributable to disruption of myelin, with sparing of neurons and axons (myelinolysis). Classically, lesions are found in the center of the basal pons (central pontine myelinolysis, or CPM), but histologically similar lesions may also occur in a symmetric distribution in extrapontine areas of the brain, where there is a close admixture of gray and white matter. Affected patients have almost invariably undergone correction for hyponatremia at rates that exceed increments of 12 mEq/L or more in 24 hours and 18 mEq/L or more in 48 hours.

Treatment of Hyponatremia

Appropriate treatment should be crafted to the cause and to the demands of each clinical circumstance. The isotonic and hypertonic hyponatremias are special situations that have been discussed earlier. Also the approach to the management depends on the rapidity with which the hyponatremia has developed and on the state of ECF volume.

Acute Hyponatremia

Patients symptomatic from acute hyponatremia should be treated promptly to avoid injury from seizures or cerebral edema. Initial therapy should increase the serum sodium by 1 to 2 mEq/L per hour until symptoms begin to improve. Usually, an increase in sodium concentration of 6 to 8 mEq/L is sufficient. At this point, the rate of repair can be slowed.

Patients who are unable to excrete dilute urine should be treated promptly with intravenous hypertonic saline and furosemide. Diuretic-induced urinary sodium losses are replaced with intravenous hypertonic saline. Diuretic-induced urinary sodium losses are replaced with 3% saline (0.5 mmol/ml), returning the excreted salt milliequivalent for milliequivalent, in a smaller volume of water. Thus body sodium content is kept constant while electrolyte-free water is lost. Patients with acute hyponatremia who excrete maximally dilute urine (e.g., psychotic patients with self-induced water intoxication) need only be treated with water restriction because the water diuresis soon corrects the electrolyte disturbance.

Chronic Hyponatremia

Chronic hyponatremia should not be equated with *asymptomatic* hyponatremia. Very low sodium concentrations usually cause some neurologic symptoms even when the electrolyte disturbance has been present for several days. If there is an underlying neurologic problem or if there has been a recent abrupt decrease in sodium concentration, patients with longstanding hyponatremia may present with seizures and coma. If the electrolyte disturbance arose outside the hospital, it is best to assume that the disorder has been present long enough (more than 48 hours) to make excessively rapid correction potentially dangerous.

In severely symptomatic patients, treatment should be initiated in a similar fashion to that which is used for patients with known acute hyponatremia. However, because the risks of iatrogenic injury are much higher in chronic hyponatremia, extreme care is necessary to limit the rate of correction to less than 12 mEq/L on the first day and less than 6 mEq/L per day thereafter. Normonatremia should not be sought during the first week, and hypernatremia should be scrupulously avoided. In asymptomatic patients with longstanding hyponatremia, the dangers of the electrolyte disturbance are so minimal that the rate of correction can be maintained well below these limits.

Hypovolemic Hypotonic Hyponatremia

Hypovolemic patients should be treated with isotonic saline solutions along with potassium, bicarbonate, or steroids as indicated by the underlying condition. Improvement in hemodynamics, mentation, BUN, and serum creatinine serve as reasonable guideposts to judge the adequacy of therapy. Most of these patients will have been hyponatremic for at least 48 hours before hospitalization and therefore should be viewed as having an "adapted" brain tonicity (Fig. 15.16).

In each etiologic setting (Fig. 15.17), reexpansion of the ECF volume with 0.9% saline eliminates a hemodynamic stimulus to vasopressin and allows a water diuresis to occur. Thus the serum sodium concentration increases because of the combined effects of sodium repletion and elimination of electrolyte-free water. The contribution of potassium therapy to the reversal of hyponatremia must also be remembered as the physician attempts to govern the rate at which the serum sodium concentration is normalized. As volume contraction is corrected, retention of cations and excretion of water may normalize the serum sodium concentration much more rapidly than is desirable. The provision of glucocorticoids to patients with adrenal insufficiency can also lead to inappropriately rapid correction of the associated hyponatremia. Volume reexpansion and/or glucocorticoid replacement therapies have caused CPM when the serum sodium concentration was normalized too rapidly. Patients with thiazide-induced hyponatremia, usually present clinically as isovolemic hyponatremia and are similarly susceptible to complications from inadvertent rapid correction of hyponatremia when the diuretic is discontinued.

If a water diuresis emerges during therapy, it may become necessary to replace water losses to prevent iatrogenic complications. Alternatively, to gain control of water excretion, reexpansion of some volume-contracted patients may require use of aqueous pitressin, or DDAVP. If, during the repair of hypovolemic hyponatremia, the serum sodium concentration increases too quickly, continued reexpansion with 0.9% saline, combined with vasopressin administration, should allow for a more controlled titration. Frequent measurements of serum sodium concentration are mandatory. Some have found it easier to control the rate of rise of serum sodium concentration by using aqueous pitressin because of its much shorter duration of action.

Hypervolemic (Edematous) Hypotonic Hyponatremia

In addition to therapy directed at the underlying renal, hepatic, or cardiac disease, loop-active diuretics should be administered to promote excretion of hypotonic urine. As noted previously, loss of the two conceptual components of this urine (i.e., the isotonic portion and the remaining electrolyte-free water) will prove beneficial to these patients. Shedding of the isotonic portion facilitates the desired ECF volume contraction, and excretion of the water raises the serum sodium concentration. Saline infusion is obviously inappropriate in edematous patients, and oral fluids should be kept to a minimum (1 L/day).

Isovolemic Hypotonic Hyponatremia

Thiazide-induced hyponatremia can easily be treated by discontinuing the diuretic, restricting free water, and providing generous intake of salt and potassium. Isotonic saline infusions are usually unnecessary and may provoke excessively rapid correction of hyponatremia. In patients with SIADH, isotonic saline may actually worsen hyponatremia. The kidneys of patients with SIADH may excrete the infused sodium in hypertonic urine while retaining the infused water. However, the serum sodium concentration may increase extremely slowly when patients with SIADH are treated with water restriction alone.

For long-term therapy of SIADH, the combination of furosemide with high dietary salt intake or salt tablets can be effective. The increased salt intake replaces the diuretic-induced natriuresis while allowing the water to be lost. This treatment is especially useful for patients who cannot comply with water restriction. The patient's weight and serum sodium concentration must be followed carefully. Imbalances between diuretic action and sodium ingestion can lead to serious volume depletion or overload.

Demethylchlortetracycline, an antibiotic that blocks the effect of vasopressin on the collecting duct, may be useful in selected cases. It exerts its action by impairing cAMP production by antidiuretic hormone and its effect is achieved with a daily dose of 900 to 1,200 mg. However, the drug is expensive and has several other drawbacks: (a) its effects on water excretion do not begin for several days after the drug has been started, and the effect persists for several days after the drug has been withdrawn; (b) patients develop nephrogenic DI and must be healthy enough to seek water to avoid dehydration; and (c) it is nephrotoxic in patients with hepatic dysfunction. New agents have been developed that specifically block vasopressin's antidiuretic effect by antagonizing the hormone's action on collecting duct V2 receptors. Once these drugs, currently in clinical trials, become available, they are likely to supplant demethylchlortetracycline in the management of hyponatremia.

HYPERTONICITY

Etiology and Classification (Fig. 15.18)

Hypertonicity may arise separately from either one of two basic mechanisms or occasionally from a combination of the two: (a) water losses in excess of salt that are inadequately replaced or (b) salt accumulation in excess of water. Because thirst is such an important defense against hypertonicity, persistent hypernatremia cannot occur unless there is a defect in water intake. Most persistently hypertonic patients prove to be too ill, too young, or too old to obtain water by themselves or to ask for it. Less commonly, patients with hypertonicity are hypodipsic and do not become thirsty even when the serum tonicity increases above the normal range.

The state of ECF volume serves as a logical and clinically useful means of separating the causes of hypernatremia (Fig. 15.18). These disorders are briefly summarized in the following section.

Hypovolemic Hypernatremia

Because only one-twelfth of all electrolyte-free water that is lost derives from the intravascular space, it is most unusual for hemodynamically significant hypovolemia to complicate these losses. Thus the presence of hypovolemic hypernatremia almost always reflects the combined loss of sodium with disproportionately greater amounts of water. The underlying causes are essentially the same as those causing hypovolemic hyponatremia. In both settings, hypotonic fluid is lost. However, in one case, excessive electrolyte-free water is taken in replacement, whereas in the other setting, too little water is replaced. Patients with partial urinary tract obstruction, especially elderly men with prostatic enlargement, may excrete large volumes of hypotonic urine. Chronic back pressure in the distal nephron may also impair potassium secretion. Thus hyperkalemia, hypernatremia, and azotemia in an older man should suggest the need for renal ultrasonography. An osmotic urea diuresis can cause sustained hypernatremia when catabolic postoperative patients are fed excessive protein. Cathartic-induced gastrointestinal losses of hypotonic fluid causes hypernatremia in some patients being treated for hepatic encephalopathy.

Hypertonicity associated with diabetes mellitus is a complex disorder caused by excessive electrolyte-free water losses from glucose-induced osmotic diuresis and the accumulation of extracellular solute in the form of glucose. The osmotic diuresis causes negative sodium and water balance. Sodium losses nor-

CLINICALLY ASSESS EXTRACELLULAR FLUID VOLUME

DEPLETED → **HYPOVOLEMIC HYPERNATREMIA**

Loss of Water + Na; H_2O Loss > Na

CAUSES	BUN / Cr	U_{Na}	Uosm
Renal			
Diuretics	↑↑ / ↑	↑	↓
Glycosuria	↑ / N,↑	↑	↓
Urea Diuresis	↑↑ / N,↑	↑	↓
Acute, Chronic Renal Failure	↑↑ / ↑↑	↑	↓
Partial Obstruction	↑↑ / ↑↑	↑	↓
Adrenal			
Congenital, Acquired Deficiencies	↑↑ / ↑↑	↑	±↑
GI Losses	↑↑ / ↑	↓	↑
Respiratory Losses	↑↑ / ↑	↓	↑
Skin Losses	↑↑ / ↑	↓	↑

NORMAL → **ISOVOLEMIC HYPERNATREMIA**

Loss of Water

CAUSES	BUN / Cr	U_{Na}	Uosm
Diabetes Insipidus			
Central	↑ / N	N	↓
Nephrogenic	↑ / N	N	↓
Reset Osmostat	N / N	N	V
Skin Losses	↑ / N	↓	↑
Iatrogenic	N / N	V	↑

EXPANDED → **HYPERVOLEMIC HYPERNATREMIA**

Gain of Water + Na; Na Gain > H_2O

CAUSES	BUN / Cr	U_{Na}	Uosm
$NaHCO_3$ Therapy	N	↑	V
Salt Water Drowning	N	↑	V
Improperly Prepared Infant Formula	V	↑	V
Mineralocorticoid Excess			
Cushing's	N	N	V
Primary Aldosteronism	N	N	V
CAH	N	N	V
Exogenous	N	N	V

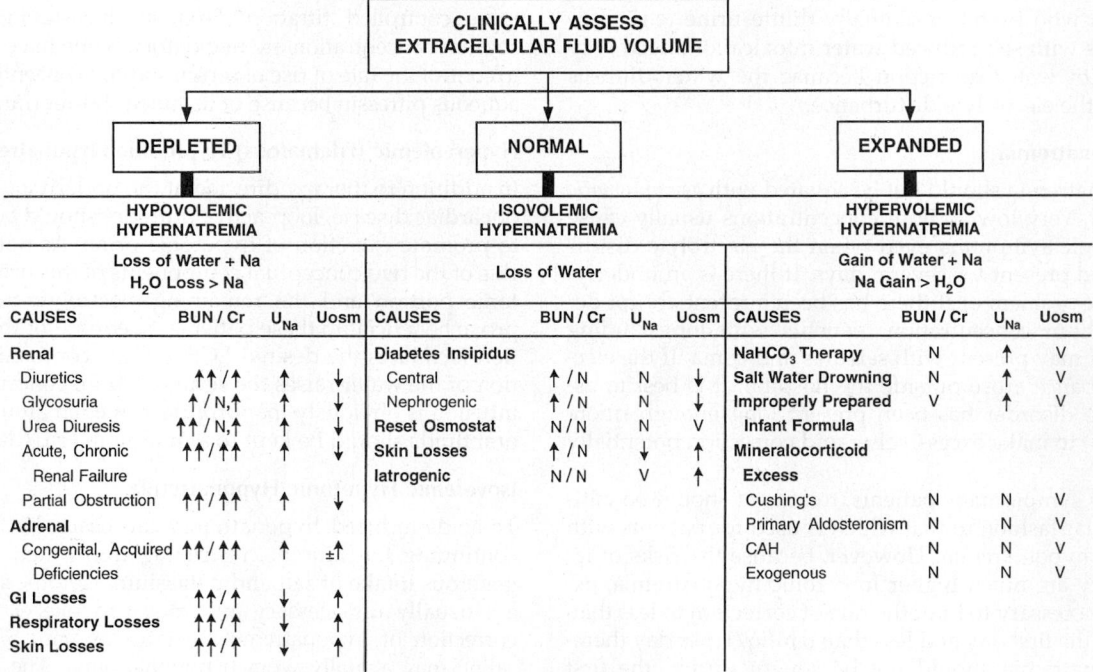

Figure 15.18. Approach to hypernatremic disorders. *N*, no change, *V*, variable.

mally cause extracellular volume depletion, but the hyperglycemia attracts and retains cellular water in the ECF. With correction of extremely severe hyperglycemia, marked hypovolemia may emerge as solute-free water reenters cells.

Hypervolemic Hypernatremia

Hypervolemic hypernatremic syndromes are conveniently subcategorized into acute and chronic forms.

Acute Hypervolemic Hypernatremia. Cellular dehydration and ECF volume expansion are the two immediate results of infusing hypertonic salt solutions. Brain volume may become so severely contracted that it disrupts the integrity of blood vessels coursing from the cerebrum to the surrounding cranial vault. Fatal intracerebral and pericerebral hemorrhage may occur.

Excessive salt ingestion is seen in the mentally disturbed, in those given table salt as an emetic, and when salt has been inadvertently substituted for sugar in infant formulas. A tablespoon of salt contains 15 g or 260 mEq of NaCl. Adults have died from rapid ingestion of 4 to 6 tablespoons of salt. The accidental ingestion of seawater may produce a similar picture.

Sodium excess from intravenous administration is commonly seen when hypertonic sodium bicarbonate solutions are used to treat metabolic acidosis. Each 50-ml ampule contains 50 mEq of sodium (1,000 mOsm/L). The severe acidemia from hypercapnia in patients with status asthmaticus, treated by controlled hypoventilation, is offset when pulmonologists administer hypertonic sodium bicarbonate. Abortions are induced by injection of 20% saline into the uterus. However, the inadvertent injection of the abortifacient directly into a uterine vein has caused sudden severe, and often fatal, hypernatremia.

Chronic Hypervolemic Hypernatremia. Edematous patients undergoing furosemide diuresis lose hypotonic fluid. If they are unable to gain access to water, hypernatremia will ensue. In normonatremic patients, approximately half of furosemide-induced urine losses should be replaced with water. The isotonic salt loss will therapeutically shrink the swollen ECF, but underreplaced free water losses will cause hypernatremia.

Comatose or severely ill patients who require intravenous fluids commonly receive fluids that are too hypertonic for their needs. Hypernatremia, mild ECF volume expansion, and hypertonicity occur when 0.9% saline is administered to patients who are losing hypotonic fluid (i.e., insensible loss and hypotonic urine). This is especially true of elderly persons whose renal concentrating and sodium excretory capabilities have declined with age.

Isovolemic Hypernatremia

Although ECF volume appears "clinically normal," patients with isovolemic hypernatremia have indeed lost several liters of electrolyte-free water. Evaporative losses of free water from the skin and lungs are increased by high environmental temperature, fever, and hypermetabolic states such as thyrotoxicosis. In susceptible individuals, several liters of water can be lost daily by the cutaneous route. Excessive unreplaced free water losses may also cause hypernatremia in patients with DI.

Diabetes Insipidus (Table 15.5)

Three types of DI have been identified. Central DI is brought on by partial or total failure of the hypothalamic synthesis of vasopressin in the first type, whereas nephrogenic DI, caused by renal tubular nonresponsiveness to normally secreted hormone, represents a second type. The third type, vasopressinase-induced DI, probably reflects a combination of partial central DI and increased catabolism of the hormone. Increased circulating vasopressinase destroys the circulating hormone and induces polyuria.

TABLE 15.5. Causes of Central Diabetes Insipidus (DI)

Central DI
Hereditary
Acquired
Posttrauma
Posthypophysectomy
Tumor
Pituitary adenoma
Craniopharyngioma
Pinealoma
Breast
Leukemia
Infections
Meningitis
Encephalitis
Guillain-Barré syndrome
Granulomata
Sarcoidosis
Tuberculosis
Eosinophilic granuloma
Histiocytosis X
Hand-Schüller-Christian disease
Vasculopathies
Nephrogenic DI
Intrinsic renal disease
Partial urinary tract obstruction
Electrolyte disorders
Hypokalemia
Hypercalcemia
Drug-induced DI
Lithium
Demeclocycline
Vasopressinase-induced DI
Pregnancy-related

Central Diabetes Insipidus

Central DI is caused by vasopressin deficiency; it may be transmitted as a heritable dominant trait or acquired as a result of head trauma or hypophysial surgery; much more rarely, it may result from a variety of pathologic conditions that affect the hypothalamus (Table 15.5). Patients complain of variable degrees of polyuria and polydipsia. In complete central DI, the onset is sharp and abrupt. The patient can precisely determine the time of onset of the polyuria. In severe cases, thirst is intense, and in this setting, a preference for ice-cold water is nearly pathognomonic for central DI. The only significant physical findings and routine laboratory abnormalities are those related to the underlying cause of DI and the hypertonicity. When deprived of water, patients with complete vasopressin deficiency continue to perniciously excrete large volumes of dilute urine, despite a rising serum osmolality and sodium concentration. Administration of exogenous hormone immediately reduces urine volume and increases urine osmolality to values exceeding plasma levels. Patients with partial vasopressin deficiency are unable to concentrate their urine maximally but have only mild polyuria. When urine osmolality has increased to its maximum after diagnostic water deprivation, administration of exogenous vasopressin evokes at least a 10% increase in urinary concentration in those with partial central DI.

Nephrogenic DI

Nephrogenic DI is a disorder of defective renal responsivity to vasopressin; it may be inherited as a rare X-linked trait (see Chapter 23) or acquired as a component feature of many diseases that cause structural renal damage. Because many patients with acquired nephrogenic DI can excrete isotonic urine, urine volumes tend to be in the range of 3 to 4 L/day. By contrast, the inherited defect is characteristically associated with severe polyuria. With prolonged water deprivation, plasma vasopressin levels increase appropriately for the level of serum sodium concentration, but the urine volume remains large. The urine osmolality increases by less than 10% in response to exogenous vasopressin. Patients who undergo surgical extirpation of craniopharyngiomas by the transfrontal route may develop an unusual form of nephrogenic DI. Apparently, after surgery, the plasma demonstrates immunoreactivity for an antidiuretic hormone–like precursor that does not activate V2 receptors. The exogenous administration of normal hormone results in submaximal antidiuresis, suggesting that the undefined precursor antagonizes the effect of the native hormone at the receptor level.

Vasopressinase-Induced DI

Vasopressinase-induced DI is a rare complication of pregnancy in which the usually modest increase in circulating vasopressinase is greatly exaggerated. Catabolism of circulating vasopressin, possibly combined with limited hypothalamic synthesis of the hormone, causes polyuria and polydipsia. The circulating vasopressinase is active enough to catabolize large amounts of administered hormone. Thus parenteral AVP does not alter urine volume. By contrast, the synthetic hormone DDAVP, which is unaffected by the enzyme, reduces urine volume and increases urine osmolality. This selective response to the vasopressin analog dually serves as a diagnostic test and a form of effective therapy.

Primary Polydipsia

It is possible to misdiagnose DI in patients who have a primary thirst disorder because both settings are associated with suppressed AVP secretion, polydipsia, and polyuria. Some well-defined conditions (most notably CNS sarcoid) can pathologically stimulate thirst. However, most patients with primary polydipsia are "driven to drink" by an underlying psychoneurotic need to cleanse and purge their bodies. Because patients with primary polydipsia secrete vasopressin normally, they do not become hypernatremic during diagnostic water deprivation (in fact, baseline serum osmolality and sodium concentrations are often mildly diminished). However, because chronic polyuria reduces the renal medullary concentration gradient, measured urine osmolality may not greatly exceed plasma levels, despite provocative water deprivation and exogenous vasopressin administration. Thus the results of these tests should be correlated with plasma vasopressin levels, particularly in borderline cases. The differential diagnosis of polyuric syndromes is discussed in detail in Chapter 26.

Clinical Consequences of Hypertonicity

Neurologic

Because sodium is confined to the ECF and because intracellular and extracellular osmolalities must be equal, a high serum sodium concentration causes water to leave cells. Clinical manifestations of cellular dehydration are most marked in the brain. The acute onset of hypernatremia (seen virtually exclusively with acute salt poisoning) causes the brain to shrink, leading to vascular injury (tears in veins) and intracranial bleeding (subdural hematoma). A characteristic neurologic syndrome results with seizures, coma, hyperventilation, hyperreflexia, hypertonia, and high fever. Fatalities are the rule in acutely hypernatremic patients with serum sodium concentrations exceeding 170 mEq/L.

When hypertonicity is sustained beyond 24 to 36 hours, brain cells accumulate organic osmolytes that minimize changes in cell volume, while facilitating osmotic equilibrium to occur between the ECF and ICF. Clinical manifestations that are less dramatic than those seen in acute salt poisoning range from lethargy to coma, depending on the severity of the hypernatremia. Brain hemorrhages generally do not occur when hypertonicity is slow to develop.

Hemodynamic

If pure water losses are responsible for hypertonicity, each body fluid compartment loses a volume of water correspondent to its proportion of the TBW. Plasma volume accounts for only about one-twelfth of total body water and is defended by oncotic pressure that increases with water loss, thereby minimizing circulating hypovolemia. Thus plasma volume contracts by less than 83 ml for each liter of water lost. Clinical signs of hypovolemia are unusual unless the water deficit is extremely large. It is instructive to note that if only pure water deficiency is responsible for serum sodium concentrations of 160 mEq/L, 170 mEq/L, and 180 mEq/L, the decrease in plasma volume would be 440 ml, 600 ml, and 755 ml, respectively. The amounts of intravascular volume lost are not dissimilar to those lost with blood donation.

Hypertonicity caused by hypotonic fluid losses (i.e., loss of sodium with proportionately more water) can be associated with substantial reductions in ECF volume. Complications attributable to hypotension and hemoconcentration (e.g., vascular occlusions, sagittal sinus thrombosis, renal vein thrombosis, and acute renal failure) contribute to the morbidity and mortality associated with hypertonic states.

Treatment of Hypernatremia

Once recognized, acute hypervolemic hypernatremia must be treated with the rapid administration of electrolyte-free water as 5% dextrose in water (D5W). Simultaneous induction of a hypotonic diuresis with furosemide should also be effected. Replacement of each milliliter of the approximately half-normal urine with 1 ml of water will lower serum concentration while ridding the cation from the body. Hemodialysis with a low sodium bath is, of course, indicated in those with renal failure.

In most cases, the onset of hypertonicity is slow enough to allow the brain to osmotically adapt itself, thereby minimizing cerebral dehydration. Organic osmolytes that accumulate during the adaptation to hypernatremia are slow to leave the cell during rehydration. If hypernatremia is corrected too rapidly, cerebral edema results as the relatively more hypertonic ICF accumulates water. To be safe, the rate of correction should not exceed 12 mEq/L per day.

Correction of hypertonicity should be postponed in patients with concurrent ECF volume depletion until reexpansion and hemodynamic stability are achieved. Hypotension and hypertonicity are particularly common in patients with hyperglycemic dehydration. Initial therapy for this condition should include an aggressive infusion of isotonic saline to achieve normotension and to replace the extracellular solute lost from preceding and ongoing glycosuria.

The pure water lost in patients such as those with DI should be replaced with pure water. In patients who are unable to drink, electrolyte-free water can be administered intravenously as D5W. Because D5W has the same osmolality as normal plasma, the infused solution does not induce hemolysis. Once the glucose has been metabolized, water remains in the ECF compartment. Dextrose solutions cannot be infused more rapidly than approximately 500 ml/hr. More rapid infusions supersede physiologic rates of glucose metabolism and therefore induce consequent hyperglycemia, glycosuria, and urinary water losses that are counterproductive to the correction of hypertonicity.

Hypernatremia and Water Deficit

The serum sodium concentration can be used to determine how much water is needed to restore isotonicity. The percentage increase in sodium concentration approximates the percentage decrease in TBW. More precisely, this estimate is expressed as follows:

$$\text{Water deficit} = \text{Normal TBW} \times [1 - (140\ \text{mEq/L}/\text{Current } S_{Na})]$$

TBW varies with body size and fat content (essentially nonaqueous). Thus, when considered in terms of body weight, body water content is influenced by age and gender. In young men, it approximates 60% of body weight, whereas in elderly men and young women, only 50% of body weight is water. In elderly women, body water content makes up just 40% of body weight. It is instructive to realize that an elderly 50-kg woman need lose only 2.85 L of water to raise her serum sodium level to 160 mEq/L. In patients with hyperglycemia, the magnitude of the water deficit is masked because glucose in the ECF osmotically attracts water from the ICF. The true water deficit can be estimated by using the corrected serum sodium concentration, as described previously. The calculated water deficit is the amount of water that will return the serum sodium concentration to normal. This deficit reveals nothing about the volume status of the ECF that must be estimated from the history and physical examination, never from the serum sodium concentration.

Selected Readings

Feig PU, McCurdy DK. The hypertonic state. *N Engl J Med* 1977;297:1444–1454.
Lucid review of hypertonic states with excellent diagrams.

Gullans SR, Verbalis JG. Control of brain volume during hyperosmolar and hypoosmolar conditions. *Annu Rev Med* 1993;44:289–301.
A good review of the forces governing the brain's responses to osmotic stress.

Laureno R, Karp BI. Myelinolysis after correction of hyponatremia. *Ann Intern Med* 1997;126:57–62.
A concise review of the neurologic complications that occur when chronic hyponatremia is corrected too rapidly.

Narins RG, Jones ER, Stom MC, et al. Diagnostic strategies in disorders of fluid, electrolyte and acid-base homeostasis. *Am J Med* 1982;72:496–520.
A good primer for the approach to fluid and electrolyte disorders.

Narins RG, Krishna GG. Disorders of water balance. In: Stein JH, ed. *Internal medicine.* St. Louis: Mosby, 1994:2655–2670.
A concise review of normal and disordered water balance.

Nielsen S, Marples D, Frokiaer J, et al. The aquaporin family of water channels in kidney: an update on the physiology and pathophysiology of aquaporin-2. *Kidney Int* 1996;49:1718–1723.
A review of the molecular mechanisms that underlie the kidney's regulation of electrolyte-free water excretion.

Palevsky PM, Bhagrath R, Greenberg A. Hypernatremia in hospitalized patients. *Ann Intern Med* 1996;124:197–203.
A fine insight into the demographics of inpatient hypernatremia.

Robertson GL. Differential diagnosis of polyuria. *Annu Rev Med* 1988;39:425–442.
A concise review outlining the diagnostic approach to patients with polyuria.

Schrier RW. Pathogenesis of sodium and water retention in high-output and low-output cardiac failure, nephrotic syndrome, cirrhosis, and pregnancy. *N Engl J Med 1988*;319:1127–1134.
A review article explaining the pathophysiology of the hypertonic state. Excellent diagrams provide a clear conceptual framework.

Seckl JR, Dunger DB, Bevan JS, et al. Vasopressin antagonist in early postoperative diabetes insipidus. *Lancet* 1990;335:1353–1356.
A good early study of the use of vasopressin antagonists.

Silver SM, Kozlowski SA, Baer JE, et al. Glycine-induced hyponatremia in the rat: a model of the post-prostatectomy syndrome. *Kidney Int* 1995;47:262–268.
A study of the pathogenesis of hyponatremia after irrigant absorption during endoscopic prostate and uterine surgery.

Sonnenblick M, Friedlander Y, Rosin AJ. Diuretic-induced severe hyponatremia. Review and analysis of 129 reported patients. *Chest* 1993;103:601–606.
A comprehensive review of thiazide-induced hyponatremia.

Sorensen JB, Andersen MK, Hansen HH. Syndrome of inappropriate secretion of antidiuretic hormone (SIADH) in malignant disease. *J Intern Med* 1995;238:97–110.
A comprehensive literature review of hyponatremia associated with malignancy. Cancers other than small cell carcinoma of the lung and head and neck tumors have been found to cause SIADH only in isolated case reports.

Steele A, Gowrishankar M, Abrahamson S, et al. Postoperative hyponatremia despite near-isotonic saline infusion: a phenomenon of desalination. *Ann Intern Med* 1997;126:20–25.
A prospective study of postoperative hyponatremia in young women emphasizing the important role of urinary cation losses in the pathogenesis of SIADH.

Sterns RH. Severe symptomatic hyponatremia: treatment and outcome. A study of 64 cases. *Ann Intern Med* 1987;107:656–664.
A retrospective study of 62 patients who collectively experienced 64 episodes of severe hyponatremia (serum sodium concentrations less than 110 mmol/L). Mortality was only 8%, and most deaths were caused by underlying disease. Adverse neurologic outcomes were limited to patients with chronic hyponatremia and were associated with more rapid rates of correction.

Sterns RH, Ocdol H, Schrier RW, et al. Hyponatremia: pathophysiology, diagnosis and therapy. In: Narins RG, ed. *Clinical disorders of fluid and electrolyte metabolism*, 5th ed. New York: McGraw-Hill, 1984:583–615.
A comprehensive review of the pathogenesis, diagnosis, and treatment of hyponatremia.

Sterns RH, Riggs JE, Schochet SS Jr. Osmotic demyelination syndrome following correction of hyponatremia. *N Engl J Med* 1986;314:1535–1542.
A report from two medical centers describing eight hyponatremic patients whose neurologic condition worsened a few days after their electrolyte disturbance was treated.

Verbalis JG. Pathogenesis of hyponatremia in an experimental model of the syndrome of inappropriate antidiuresis. *Am J Physiol* 1994;267:R1617–R1625.
A study of the pathogenesis of hyponatremia in the rat emphasizing the important role of cation depletion. Adaptive losses of extracellular sodium and intracellular potassium were found to markedly minimize the increase in body water in animals with severe, prolonged hyponatremia.

Vieweg WV, Karp BI. Severe hyponatremia in the polydipsia-hyponatremia syndrome. *J Clin Psych* 1994;55:355–361.
A review of self-induced water intoxication among institutionalized schizophrenic patients.

Zerbe RL, Robertson FL. Osmotic and nonosmotic regulation of thirst and vasopressin secretion. In: Narins RG, ed. *Clinical disorders of fluid and electrolyte balance*, 5th ed. New York: McGraw-Hill, 1984:81–100.
A review of the physiology and pathophysiology of thirst and vasopressin secretion.

CHAPTER 16

Potassium Homeostasis

PART 1
Control of Potassium Excretion

Steven C. Sansom, Shigeaki Muto, and Gerhard Giebisch

CONTROL OF INTERNAL AND EXTERNAL POTASSIUM BALANCE

Potassium is the most abundant cation in the intracellular fluid (ICF) and is required for many normal functions of the cell. Optimal potassium metabolism requires that both the intracellular and extracellular potassium concentrations be precisely regulated. This balance is delicate because 98% to 99% of total potassium is contained in cells. Accordingly, extracellular potassium concentration is highly sensitive to additions of potassium, either from localized tissue lesions or when intake is not matched by temporary uptake into cells and the appropriate excretory response.

Changes in total cell potassium not only control the volume and acid–base balance of cells but also affect protein synthesis, mitogenesis, growth, acid–base balance, and a host of other metabolic processes. Thus, for its survival, it is critical that each body cell autonomously regulate its internal potassium content and concentration. In addition, it is also critical for normal neuromuscular and cardiac activity that appropriate potassium concentration *gradients* be maintained across nerve and muscle cells so that electrical polarization of these cells is ensured. Thus it is vital that the extracellular potassium concentration, compared with that in the cytoplasm (120 to 140 mM), be stabilized at relatively low levels (3.5 to 5.0 mEq/L).

Two control mechanisms, extrarenal and renal, maintain potassium balance between the ICF and extracellular fluid (ECF) compartments, keeping plasma potassium levels within a narrow concentration range despite variations in potassium intake that may extend maximally over a 100-fold range. Figure 16.1 shows the interplay between extrarenal and renal regulation of potassium metabolism. Three aspects deserve mention: (a) most potassium resides within cells, (b) potassium uptake from the gastrointestinal tract is matched by renal and colonic excretion, and (c) uptake of potassium into body cells (e.g., muscle, liver, bone) is regulated by a pump-leak system in which active uptake of potassium by Na^+-K^+-ATPase is in balance with passive efflux through potassium channels. The interaction between controlled redistribution of potassium between cells and ECF on one hand, with renal (and colonic) excretion on the other safeguards potassium homeostasis.

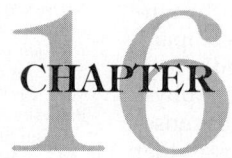

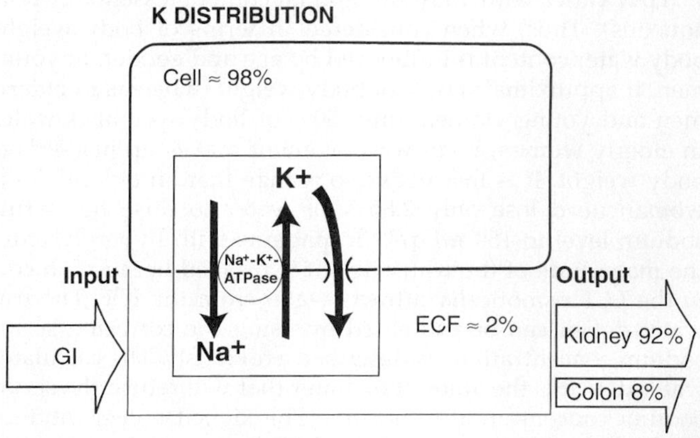

Figure 16.1. Elements of potassium balance. *External potassium balance* depends on potassium uptake by the gastrointestinal tract *(GI)* and the rate of renal and fecal (largely colonic) excretion. *Internal potassium balance* depends on the proper distribution of potassium between the extracellular fluid *(ECF)* and the multiorgan intracellular potassium pool. Internal distribution of potassium is regulated by the balance between the activities of Na^+-K^+-ATPase and potassium channels.

Extrarenal mechanisms include the effective although transitory movement of potassium into cell compartments when the extracellular potassium concentration rises. Factors involved in this type of potassium homeostasis ("internal potassium balance") are hormones such as insulin, epinephrine, and adrenal mineralocorticoids, all of which accelerate potassium uptake by cells. The extrarenal control of serum potassium is discussed in Chapter 16, Part 2.

The second mechanism responsible for controlling external potassium balance is the integrated regulation of the excretion of potassium by the kidney and, to a lesser extent, by the colon. So effective is the cooperative activity of extrarenal and renal mechanisms that even very large changes in potassium intake, over at least a 20-fold range, are tolerated with only small fluctuations of the plasma potassium level.

SINGLE-CELL POTASSIUM BALANCE

To understand how renal cells control body potassium content, it is first necessary to analyze how individual cells regulate their potassium content. Because blood cells are conveniently studied, much of our basic knowledge concerning single-cell potassium balance is based on research performed on these cells. They are also relatively unspecialized, but many regulatory processes in these cells are representative of general mechanisms for maintaining intracellular potassium.

In nonpolarized and polarized cells, potassium is kept high and sodium low by the membrane-bound Na^+-K^+-ATPase (sodium pump). The sodium pump is an enzyme that couples the energy from hydrolysis of adenosine 5′-triphosphate (ATP) to the transport of $3Na^+$ out of the cell in exchange for $2K^+$. It is the combination of the sodium pump carrying net positive charge out of the cell and potassium diffusing from the cell interior to the plasma through conductive pathways that imparts a negative electrical potential to the cell interior.

Although the Na^+-K^+-ATPase pump is responsible for the high potassium activity of cells, the leak pathway for potassium from cell to ECF is equally important for regulating cell potassium content. The leak pathway is a regulated ion channel with a high capacity for permitting the movement of potassium ions along a favorable concentration gradient. Normally, a steady state exists in cells, potassium being continually recycled across the membrane by pumps from outside into the cell and through channels in the opposite direction. Thus the resulting cell potassium depends on the combination of pump activity *and* leak conductance.

Two aspects of the potassium regulation of single cells are particularly relevant to renal tubule cells: (a) changes in potassium permeability that occur with changes in active Na^+-K^+ pumping and (b) changes in potassium transport associated with cell volume changes.

Several experimental situations reveal a tight relation between the rate of active Na^+-K^+ exchange and the passive leak permeability to potassium. In general, an increase in potassium permeability follows an increase in the activity of the pump. This important relationship is summarized in Fig. 16.2. The following points deserve mention. Many epithelial cells, including tubule cells, change their rate of net sodium transport by modulating sodium entry across the apical membrane followed by appropriate alterations in the rate of Na^+ pumping in the basolateral membrane. Such an increase of sodium pumping involves a simultaneous accelerated uptake of potassium that would increase cell potassium concentration and cell volume were it not for a rapid increase in the permeability of the membrane to potassium. Thus, adjusting the rate of potassium recycling allows cell potassium to remain constant despite alterations in active pump function and, in epithelial cells, despite changes in vectorial sodium transport. Figure 16.3 depicts a representative example, the mammalian proximal tubule. The mechanism of this type of coupling between *active* ATP-driven Na^+-K^+ transport and passive potassium leak may involve changes in cell calcium, pH, nitric oxide (NO), cell ATP, and/or other cellular messengers. An increase in cell volume and in basolateral membrane potential often accompanies stimulation of sodium reabsorption and has been implicated in the tight coupling between basolateral pump turnover and potassium "leak" conductance. It should be noted that coupling between Na^+-K^+-ATPase activity and potassium conductance is not confined to the basolateral membrane. Convincing evidence shows that activation of basolateral Na^+-K^+ transport also increases the apical potassium (and sodium) conductance. Such membrane "cross-talk" ensures that in potassium secreting cells the cell potassium concentration remains fairly constant with changes in basolateral Na^+-K^+ activity and alteration in potassium secretion.

Changes in potassium transport also occur when cells are exposed to either hypotonic or hypertonic media. Cells are normally bathed in plasma with relatively constant osmolalities. However, if challenged by exposure to either hypertonic or hypotonic solutions, cells initially shrink or swell. However, persistent changes in cell volume (i.e., in the total cell potassium and sodium content) are minimized by important modifications of both active and passive transport operations. Some of the potassium transport mechanisms that are normally dormant in *isotonic* media may be activated during cell volume regulation.

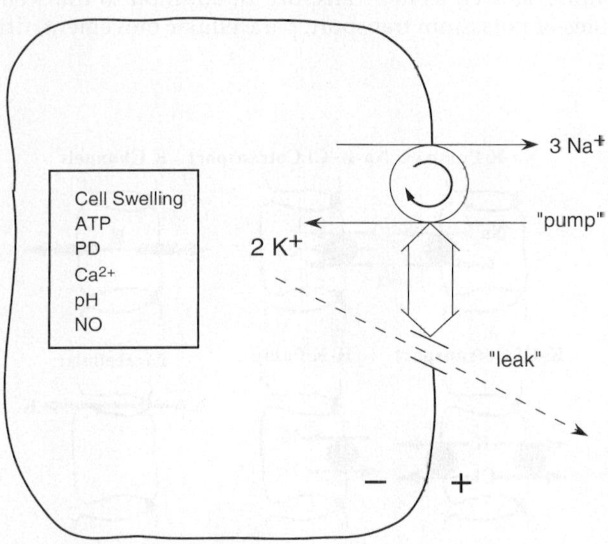

Figure 16.2. Relation of basolateral Na^+-K^+ pump to potassium conductance. Potassium uptake into the cell via the "pump" is exactly matched by a "leak" out of the cell through potassium channels. *PD*, potential difference; *NO*, nitric oxide. (Reprinted with permission from Giebisch G, Malnic G, Berliner RW. Renal transport and control of potassium excretion. In: Brenner BM, Rector FC Jr. *The kidney*, 3rd ed. Philadelphia: WB Saunders, 1999, in press.)

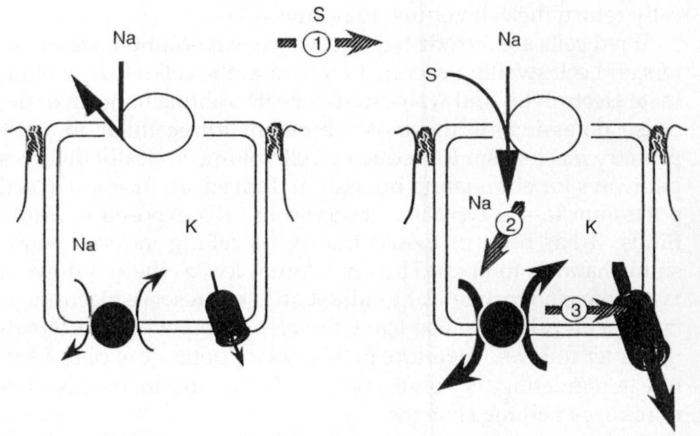

Figure 16.3. Coupling between Na^+-K^+-ATPase activity and K^+ recycling in the basolateral membrane of proximal tubule cells. Net rate of sodium transport was stimulated by addition of organic substrates (*S*, i.e., glucose or amino acid) to the lumen. Thus *(1)* apical Na entry via Na-dependent substrate cotransporters is stimulated in the presence of substrates (S). *(2)* The Na^+-K^+-ATPase subsequently increases so that active efflux of Na into the interstitium matches passive apical sodium entry. *(3)* K channel activity rises sharply and ensures that the increased active uptake of K^+ via the Na^+-K^+-ATPase will be efficiently recycled back across the basolateral membrane. (Reprinted with permission from Welling PA. Cross-talk and the role of K_{ATP} channels in the proximal tubule. *Kidney Int* 1995;48:1017–1023.)

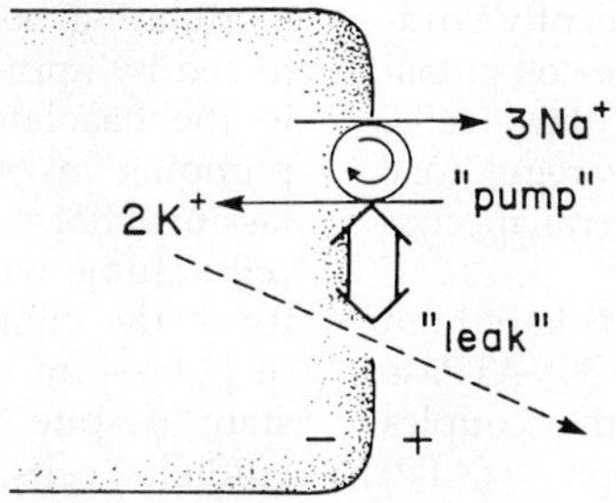

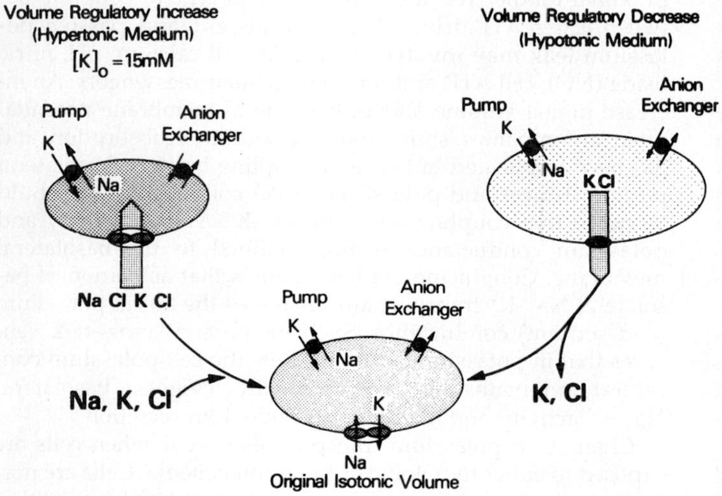

Figure 16.4. Illustration of the mechanism of volume regulation in the red blood cell. Cells initially swollen in hypotonic medium activate potassium and chloride conductive pathways. An outwardly directed gradient for potassium results in potassium, chloride, and water loss. Cells in a hypertonic medium initially shrink, whereupon a K^+-Na^+-$2Cl^-$ cotransporter is activated. A steep gradient for sodium allows these ions plus water to enter the cell and return volume toward normal. Sodium ions may also enter the cell by activation of sodium channels and by Na^+-H^+ exchanger. (Adapted with permission from Kregenow FM. Osmoregulatory salt transporting mechanisms: control of cell volume in anisotonic media. *Annu Rev Physiol* 1981;43:495. © 1980 by Annual Reviews Inc.)

Figure 16.4 is a general scheme of cell volume control. A red blood cell, introduced into a hypertonic solution, initially shrinks as cell water is lost. For cell volume to return to normal despite the hypertonicity of the surrounding medium, the cell must take up both electrolytes and water. One mechanism involved in this process is activation of a Na^+-K^+-$2Cl^-$ cotransporter. The large electrochemical gradient for sodium to enter cells provides the driving force for the simultaneous, carrier-mediated uptake of Na^+-K^+-$2Cl^-$ and water, which will typically return the cell volume to normal.

If red cells are introduced into a *hypotonic* solution, water enters and cell swelling occurs. In this case, the cell needs to eliminate electrolytes and water to reduce its volume to normal. Because potassium is the most abundant intracellular ion, the primary mechanism for reducing cell volume logically involves pathways for eliminating potassium. Indeed, an increase in cell potassium loss is typically observed in cells exposed to dilute fluids. It has been proposed that cell swelling induces potassium channels to open. Thus potassium leaves the cell down a favorable electrochemical gradient and, to preserve electroneutrality, chloride ions also leave the cell. To maintain isosmolality, water follows. Therefore pathways for potassium play a key role in regulating the solute content of cells, and their activation minimizes volume changes.

To transport ions unidirectionally (i.e., vectorially), renal epithelial cells are structurally and functionally polarized. The basolateral membrane, or the blood-facing membrane, is much like the membranes of nonpolarized cells such as red blood cells. It is the luminal membrane, which faces the tubular fluid, that confers directional transport characteristics on the epithelium. Furthermore, whereas neuromuscular and red cells are bathed in a medium of relatively constant osmolality, the apical membrane of tubule cells is faced with osmolar challenges. Many of the symmetric cell transport systems described previously, such as active Na^+-K^+ exchange, Na^+-K^+-$2Cl^-$ cotransport, and potassium channels, are the very same mechanisms used by kidney cells for regulating *unidirectional* transport of potassium. As shown in Figure 16.5, this is achieved by placing potassium channels and other potassium transporters selectively into the luminal or basolateral cell membranes. By this strategic placement of transport elements, kidney cells control their own potassium content and volume, as well as net transport. In addition to transcellular routes of potassium transport, paracellular movement, driven

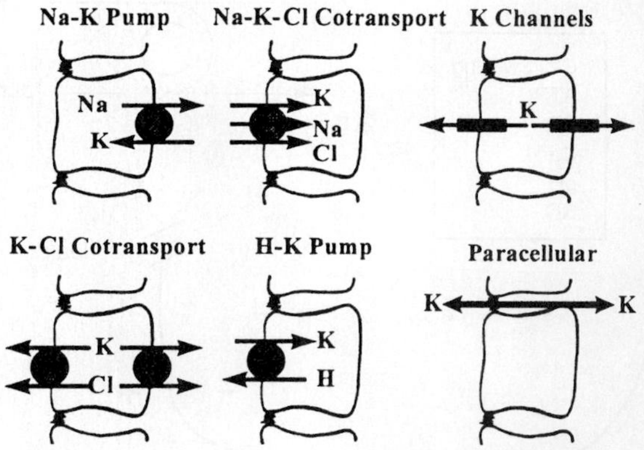

Figure 16.5. Potassium transporters in renal tubule cells. Direction and magnitude of potassium transport depends on the distribution of these transport proteins in apical and basolateral membranes. Na^+-K^+-ATPase is present in the basolateral membrane of all tubule cells. (Modified from Stanton BA, Giebisch GH. Renal potassium transport. In: Windhager E, ed. *Handbook of physiology,* Sect 8, Renal Physiology. New York: Oxford University Press, 1992:813.)

by transepithelial concentration and/or electrical gradients, also contributes to net potassium transport.

THE ROLE OF RENAL ION-SELECTIVE CHANNELS IN THE REGULATION OF POTASSIUM TRANSPORT

Potassium transport by renal cells involves ATPase-driven uptake of potassium, which must be balanced by passive pathways for cellular potassium exit. The passive pathways are potassium channels that are selectively conductive for potassium ions and play a major role in potassium homeostasis. Not only are they often regulated in tandem with the Na^+-K^+-ATPase, but as stated before, they participate in regulating renal cell volume. Importantly, they are also involved in potassium recycling in the thick ascending limb of Henle's loop; in the initial and cortical collecting duct, potassium channels play a major role in the regulated secretion of this ion.

The *patch clamp technique* has been instrumental in determining the single-channel properties of renal potassium-selective channels. By monitoring electrical events in a small membrane area, patch clamping has shown that the potassium conductive pathways are the result of rapidly gating channels that allow the selective permeation of potassium ions over Cl^-, Na^+, and other cations. Figure 16.6 shows the patch-clamp technique and a K^+-channel recording.

Potassium-selective channels in epithelial cells can either transport potassium unidirectionally or participate as "housekeeping" channels in a process of recycling that maintains constant cell volume or electrolyte content. For example, potassium channels that are contained in the same membrane as an H^+-K^+-ATPase, an Na^+-K^+-ATPase or an Na^+-2Cl-K^+ cotransporter, may function to recycle potassium to provide a continual supply of potassium to the respective pump or cotransport mechanism. In contrast, potassium channels in the apical membrane of principal tubule cells mediate unidirectional secretory transport of potassium.

The *proximal tubule* reabsorbs potassium both through paracellular and transcellular pathways and does not play a key role in regulation of potassium secretion. Fluid is driven by an osmotic gradient established by the basolateral Na^+-K^+-ATPase. It is therefore important that potassium recycle across the basolateral membrane in concert with the requirements of the Na^+-K^+ pump.

To achieve synchronous potassium recycling in the proximal tubule, the basolateral Na^+-K^+ pump and the potassium channels are directly coupled via ATP. When the Na^+ pump accelerates, the ratio of ATP to ADP (adenosine 5′-diphosphate) decreases as ATP supplies energy to the pump. Accordingly, the low ATP/ADP activates potassium channels, and potassium exits from the cell down an electrochemical gradient. In contrast, intracellular potassium is conserved with reduction of Na^+-K^+-ATPase turnover because the increase in ATP inhibits potassium channels and potassium leaking from the cell.

The *thick ascending limb* of Henle's loop, like the proximal tubule, contains a basolateral sodium pump and potassium channels that permit potassium to recycle across the apical membrane. Unlike other nephron segments, however, the thick ascending limb contains the luminal Na^+-K^+-$2Cl^-$ cotransporter, which together with apical potassium channels, allows this segment to mediate either potassium secretion or reabsorption. Because potassium is above electrochemical

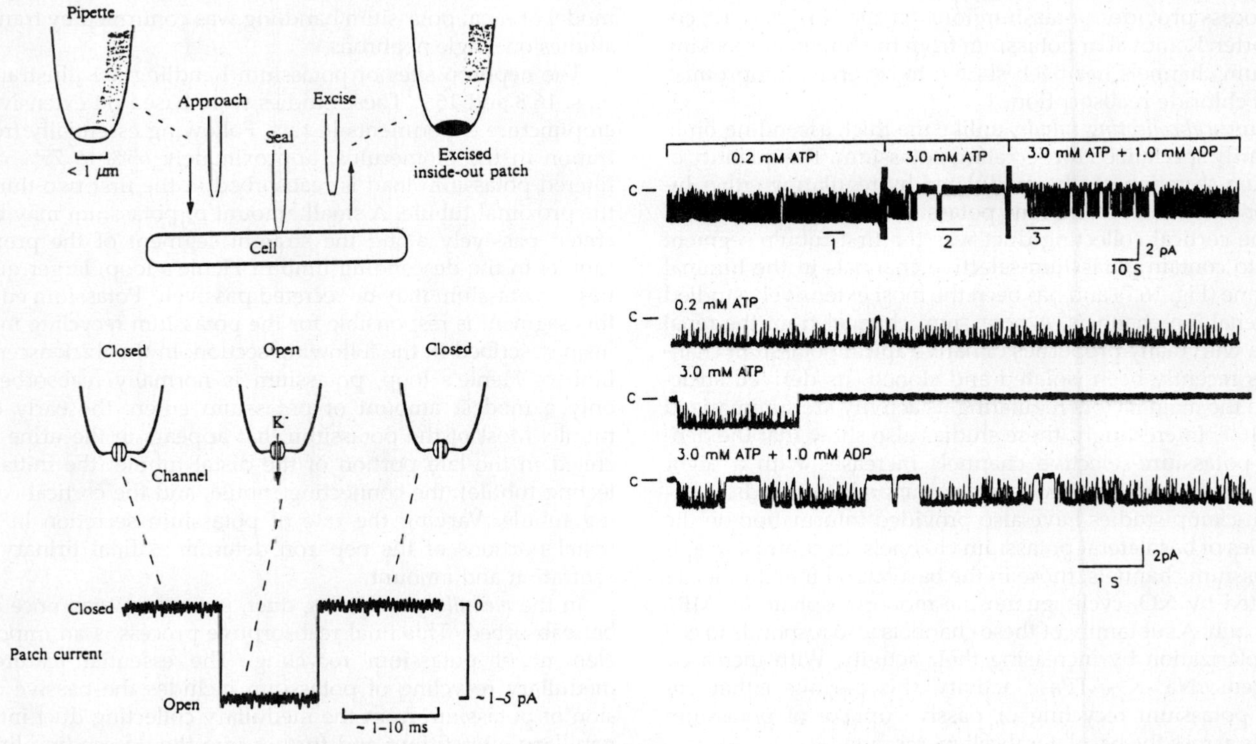

Figure 16.6. *Left*: Patch-clamp technique. Note formation of membrane patch in either cell-attached or excised mode. Single-channel currents are shown to coincide with channel openings. *Right:* Single-channel recording from an excised apical membrane patch of a principal tubule cell. Several channels are active initially, but channel activity ceases on elevation of adenosine triphosphate (ATP) on the cytosolic face of the membrane patch. Channel block is relieved by ADP. (Reprinted from Standen NB. Potassium channels, metabolism, and muscle *Exp Physiol* 1992;77:1–24; and Wang W, Giebisch G. Dual effect of adenosine triphosphate on the apical small conductance K+ channel of the rat cortical collecting duct. J *Gen Physiol* 1991;98:35–61.)

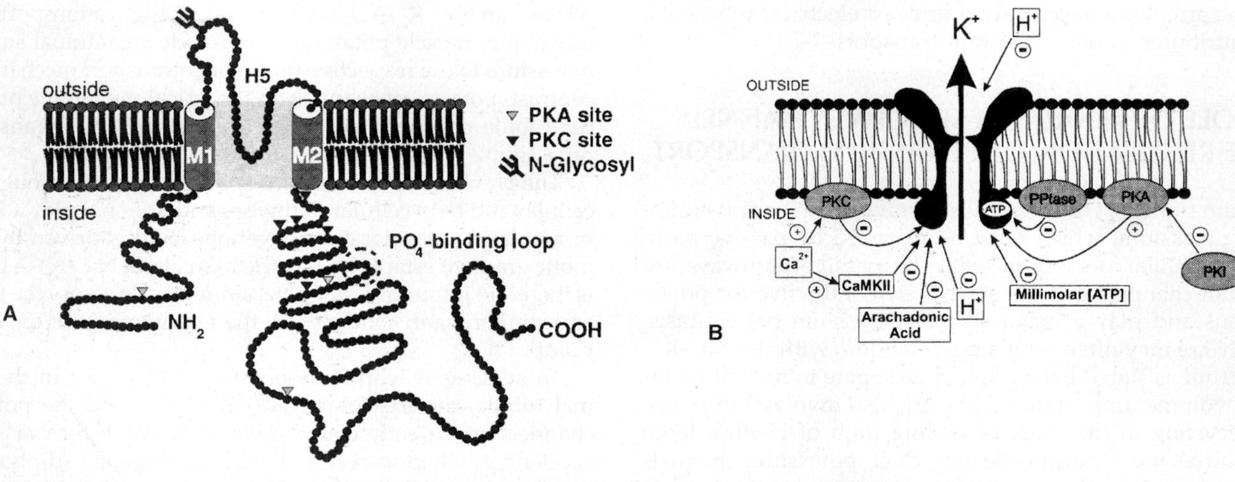

Figure 16.7. **A:** Topology of ROMK2. *Solid circles* represent individual amino acid residues, and the *cylinders* represent membrane-spanning helixes. Broken circumscription in the COOH terminus surrounds the location of the PO_4 binding loop or Walker A site proposed to be involved in Mg-ATP binding. Potential protein kinase A *(PKA)* and protein kinase C *(PKC)* phosphorylation sites, and the single *N*-glycosylation site (*N*-glycosyl) are indicated. **B:** Structural model of ROMK channel protein with factors modulating its activity. *CaMKII,* calcium-calmodulin activated kinase II; *PPT,* protein phosphatase; *PKI,* protein kinase inhibition.

equilibrium, potassium secretion will be enhanced by opening potassium channels in the luminal membrane and closing potassium channels in the basolateral membrane. Conversely, potassium reabsorption predominates when the potassium channels in the luminal membrane are closed and potassium channels in the basolateral membrane are open. It should be noted that potassium channels are also key elements of potassium recycling across the apical membrane. This process provides potassium ions for the Na^+-$2Cl^-$-K^+ cotransporter. Removal of potassium from the lumen or blocking potassium channels has been shown to severely compromise sodium chloride reabsorption.

The *cortical collecting tubule*, unlike the thick ascending limb, is primarily specialized for secreting potassium. The quantity of potassium secretion can be modulated by regulating either luminal or basolateral membrane potassium channels of *principal cells.* The cortical collecting duct was the first tubule segment shown to contain potassium-selective channels in the luminal membrane (Fig. 16.7) and has been the most extensively studied of the renal ion channels. A potassium channel from the renal medulla with many properties of native apical potassium channels has recently been isolated and cloned. Its derived structure and the main factors regulating its activity are summarized in Fig. 16.7. Interestingly, these studies also show that the density of potassium-selective channels increases with a high-potassium diet and elevated levels of mineralocorticoids.

Patch-clamp studies have also provided information on the properties of basolateral potassium channels. In contrast to apical potassium channels, those in the basolateral membrane are stimulated by NO, cyclic guanosine monophosphate (cGMP), and calcium. A subfamily of these channels also responds to cell hyperpolarization by increasing their activity. With increased electrogenic Na^+-K^+-ATPase activity, this permits either enhanced potassium recycling or passive uptake of potassium into cells across the basolateral cell membrane.

OVERVIEW OF RENAL POTASSIUM HANDLING

The pioneering clearance experiments of Berliner and Mudge and their associates provided important information on the mode and mechanisms of renal potassium excretion. These authors concluded that it was potassium secretion in distal nephron segment following extensive reabsorption in the proximal tubule and along Henle's loop that largely determined excretion of potassium into the urine. Moreover, they deduced that potassium secretion depended critically on the availability of sodium and that potassium secretion was strongly affected by acid–base changes, mineralocorticoids, and diuretics. This model of renal potassium handling was confirmed by transport studies on single nephrons.

The nephron sites of potassium handling are illustrated in Figs. 16.8 and 16.9. These studies were based on extensive micropuncture experiments in rats. Following essentially free filtration in the glomerulus, approximately 65% to 75% of the filtered potassium load is reabsorbed in the first two-thirds of the proximal tubule. A small amount of potassium may be secreted passively along the straight segment of the proximal tubule. In the descending limb of Henle's loop, larger quantities of potassium may be secreted passively. Potassium entry in this segment is responsible for the potassium recycling mechanism described in the following section. In the thick ascending limb of Henle's loop, potassium is normally reabsorbed, so only a modest amount of potassium enters the early distal tubule. Most of the potassium that appears in the urine is secreted in the late portion of the distal tubule (the initial collecting tubule), the connecting tubule, and the cortical collecting tubule. Varying the rate of potassium secretion in these distal portions of the nephron determines final urinary concentration and amount.

In the *medullary* collecting duct, potassium may once again be reabsorbed. This final reabsorptive process is an important element of potassium recycling. The essential features of medullary recycling of potassium includes the passive diffusion of potassium from the medullary collecting duct into the papillary interstitium and further into the descending limb of Henle's loop (Fig. 16. 8). An important consequence of this passive potassium movement and medullary potassium trapping is that the potassium concentration in the medullary interstitium will increase so that there would be only a small gradient for continued potassium reabsorption across the medullary collecting ducts. Thus the overall effect of recycling

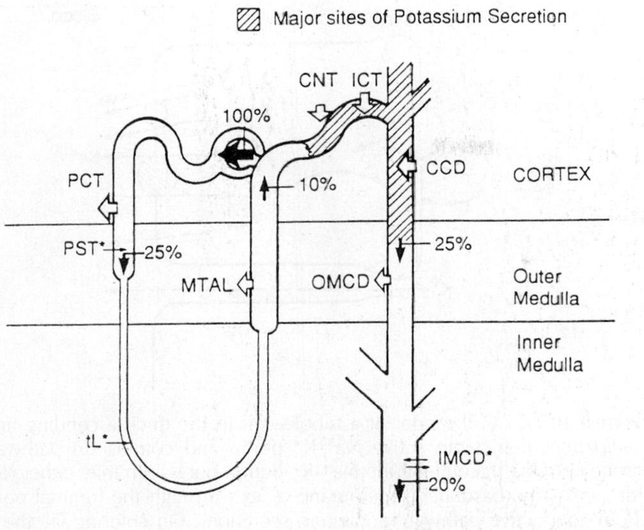

Figure 16.8. *Left:* Topography of potassium transport along the nephron in conditions of normal potassium intake. Indicated are changes in the amount of potassium remaining in the tubule. Numbers show percentage of filtered potassium. *Open arrows* show magnitude and direction of potassium flux. *CCD,* cortical collecting duct; *CNT,* connecting tubule; *ICT,* initial collecting tubule; *IMCD,* inner medullary collecting duct; *MTAL,* medullary thick ascending limb; *OMCD,* outer medullary collecting duct; *PCT,* proximal convoluted tubule; *PST,* proximal straight tubule; *tL,* thin descending limb of Henle's loop. *Right:* Medullary potassium recycling. (Modified from Peterson LN, Levi M. Disorders of potassium metabolism. In: *Renal and electrolyte disorders,* 1992.)

potassium is to increase the efficiency of potassium excretion. This is achieved by two processes: (a) preventing loss of potassium into the systemic circulation by trapping potassium lost from the collecting duct into Henle's loop and (b) increasing the papillary potassium concentration so that diffusional potassium loss from the medullary collecting duct is minimized.

Figure 16.9 depicts some additional features of potassium transport along the nephron. Inspection of distal nephron segments demonstrates that the initial and cortical collecting duct is the site of both potassium secretion and/or potassium reabsorption. Both processes are regulated by potassium and sodium uptake, acid–base status, tubule flow rate, and several hormones. Available evidence is consistent with the view that potassium secretion and sodium reabsorption take place in principal cells, whereas potassium reabsorption, in exchange for hydrogen ions, occurs in intercalated cells. Morphologic and functional heterogeneity of principal and intercalated cells is an important feature of the renal mechanism controlling potassium excretion.

CELL MECHANISMS OF POTASSIUM TRANSPORT

Proximal Tubule

The transport of potassium in the proximal tubules involves the reabsorption of a large fraction of the filtered potassium. Shown in Fig. 16.10 is a model of potassium transport pathways in the proximal tubule cell. As in all sodium-transporting epithelia, the basolateral membrane contains an Na^+-K^+-ATPase and a potassium conductive (channel) pathway. The apical membrane also contains a potassium-conductive pathway. Potassium concentration is kept above electrochemical equilibrium across both the basolateral and apical cell membranes by the basolateral Na^+-K^+ pumps. Because of the higher potassium permeability of the basolateral cell membrane, most intracellular potassium recycles across the *basolateral* membrane; only a small amount of potassium may leak from cell to lumen. Because net potassium secretion is not seen in the proximal tubule, the significance of the small apical membrane potassium conductance may be related to generating the electrical potential across this membrane. Apical potassium channels have also been shown to respond to cell volume increase with enhanced activity.

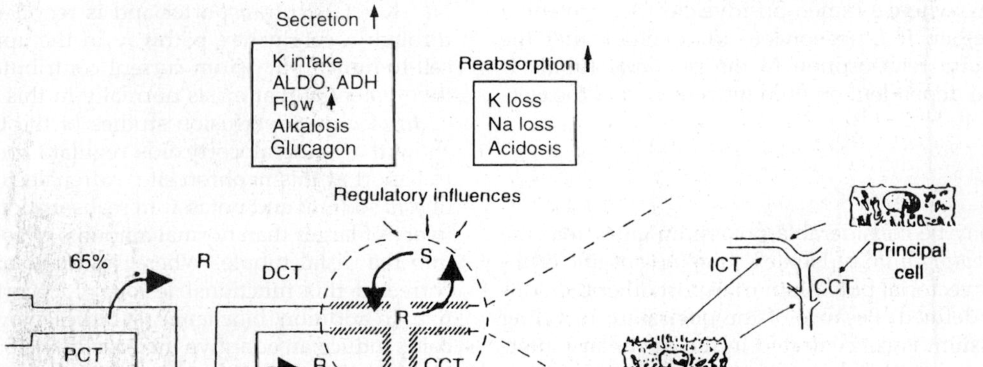

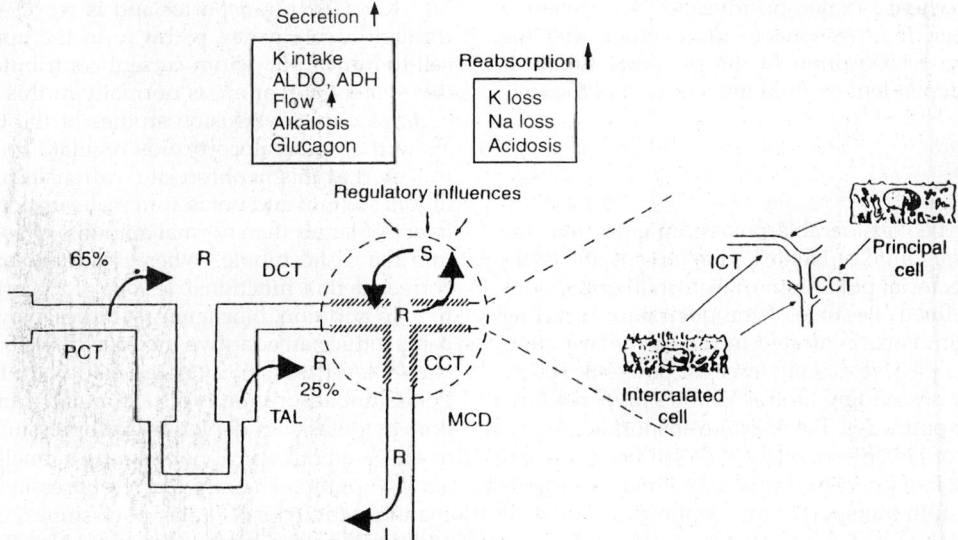

Figure 16.9. Potassium transport along the nephron. Note that secretion *(S)* in the distal nephron can be replaced by reabsorption *(R)* and that two cell types line the distal tubule and cortical collecting duct. The main factors regulating potassium secretion and potassium reabsorption are also shown. Following filtration, potassium is extensively reabsorbed along the proximal tubule and Henle's loop. Potassium is secreted along the initial and cortical collecting tubule. Net secretion can be replaced by net reabsorption in states of potassium depletion. Also shown are the two cell types lining the distal tubule and cortical collecting duct. Arrows show magnitude and direction of potassium flux. *ADH,* antidiuretic hormone; *ALDO,* aldosterone; *CCT,* cortical collecting tubule; *DCT,* distal convoluted tubule; *ICT,* initial connecting tubule; *MCD,* medullary collecting duct; *PCT,* proximal tubule; *TAL,* thick ascending limb. (Reprinted from Giebisch G. Renal potassium transport: mechanisms and regulation. *Am J Physiol* 1998;274:F817–F833.)

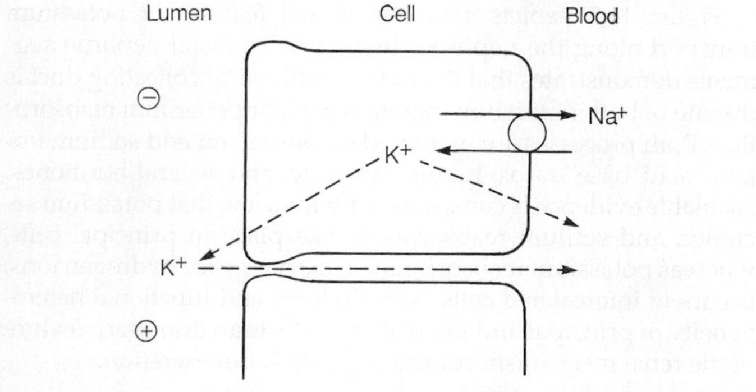

Figure 16.10. Cell model of the proximal tubule. *Solid arrows* depict the active Na^+-K^+-ATPase pump. *Broken arrows* depict conductive pathways for potassium. Because luminal potassium conductance is small, most intracellular potassium is recycled across basolateral membrane conductive pathways. Luminal potassium is reabsorbed largely through the paracellular pathway.

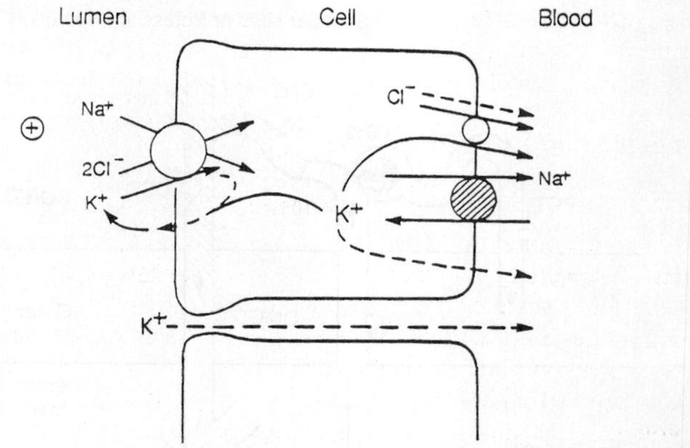

Figure 16.11. Cell model of a tubule cell in the thick ascending limb. *Solid lines* depict the active Na^+-K^+ pump and cotransport pathways. Once entering the cell via the Na^+-K^+ pump, potassium may either recycle across the basolateral membrane or exit through the luminal potassium conductive pathway (potassium secretion). On entering via the luminal Na^+-K^+-$2Cl^-$ cotransporter, potassium may recycle through the apical membrane conductive pathway or leave the cell across the basolateral membrane (potassium reabsorption). The lumen-positive potential normally constitutes a significant driving force for passive potassium reabsorption through the paracellular pathway. Breakdown of the potential difference after treatment with loop diuretics contributes to diminished potassium transport from lumen to peritubular fluid.

Many micropuncture studies indicate that the potassium concentration in the lumen of the first two-thirds of the proximal tubule is about equal to that of plasma. Because the proximal tubule is a relatively leaky epithelium, a large portion of fluid is reabsorbed isosmotically, through both transcellular and paracellular pathways. It is likely that potassium is entrained in the reabsorbate and transported passively across the tubule epithelium. Supporting this notion are microperfusion studies in which the net fluid transport was altered by applying different osmotic gradients across the proximal tubule. In such experiments, the luminal potassium concentration remains constant regardless of the direction of net water transport, and potassium movement is always in the same direction and proportional to transepithelial fluid transport. Also, proximal potassium is depressed when fluid reabsorption falls. In addition to such entrainment (solvent drag), potassium ions may also be reabsorbed by diffusion, particularly in those later segments of the proximal tubule where a lumen-positive electrical potential exists. Taken together, it is reasonable to conclude that the process of potassium reabsorption in the proximal tubule is largely passive and dependent on fluid movement and the electrical potential.

Henle's Loop

Although there may be considerable potassium entry into the lumen of the *descending* limb of Henle's loop, no specific cellular mechanisms of vectorial potassium transport other than diffusion have been defined. Because of the potassium recycling mechanism, potassium is concentrated in the medullary interstitium. This creates a passive driving force for potassium entry into the lumen of the descending limb of Henle's loop, possibly through paracellular pathways. Potassium transport across the thick *ascending* limb of Henle's loop has been studied more extensively with the isolated perfused tubule method; the essential features of potassium transport at this nephron site are well defined.

Shown in Fig. 16.11 is a model of potassium transport pathways in the thick ascending limb. Unlike the proximal tubule, the thick ascending limb is almost impermeable to water. Sodium is actively transported from cell to blood through the Na^+-K^+ pump in the basolateral membrane and cotransported as Na^+-K^+-$2Cl^-$ from lumen to cell across the apical membrane. The result is net transport of NaCl and K^+ while leaving water behind and diluting the fluid in the lumen. An additional driving force for potassium absorption through the paracellular pathway is the lumen-positive electrical potential.

Because multiple potassium transport pathways exist in both luminal and peritubular cell borders, these cells are able to adapt their rate and even direction of potassium transport. In the basolateral membrane, potassium is actively transported from the blood to the cell through the Na^+-K^+ pump. Because cell potassium is above electrochemical equilibrium, potassium can passively leak back from the cell to blood, either through a conductive pathway (potassium channels) or via electroneutral KCl or $KHCO_3$ cotransporter. In the luminal membrane, potassium is transported into the cell via an electrically neutral Na^+-K^+-$2Cl^-$ cotransporter and is recycled back to the lumen through a conductive pathway in the apical membrane. This cell-to-lumen potassium current contributes to the lumen positive potential that exists normally in this segment.

In vivo microperfusion studies of the thick ascending limb show that mineralocorticoids regulate sodium and potassium transport at this nephron site. Adrenalectomy reduces the rate of *both* sodium and potassium reabsorption and leads to the delivery of larger than normal amounts of sodium and potassium into the distal tubule. Whereas administration of aldosterone corrected this functional lesion, glucocorticoids were ineffective. In addition, biochemical studies show that mineralocorticoids induce an adaptive increase in the basolateral membrane Na^+-K^+-ATPase activity of the medullary thick ascending limb. Potassium absorption is also stimulated in the thick ascending limb by potassium depletion. Vasopressin has also been shown to activate both apical potassium channels and the basolateral Na^+-K^+ pump. The effect of vasopressin on apical potassium channel activity accelerates potassium recycling and provides additional potassium to the luminal Na^+-K^+-$2Cl^-$ cotransporter. Raising extracellular calcium has also been shown to decrease apical potassium channel activity and to reduce Na^+-$2Cl^-$-K^+ cotransport. This effect is the result of compromised potassium recycling and of physiologic significance because it provides a likely mechanism by which hypercalcemia lowers the urinary concentrating ability of the kidney.

It is also known that furosemide, bumetanide, and other loop diuretics act in the thick ascending limb to inhibit sodium, potassium, and chloride reabsorption. This results in an increase in the delivery of these ions into the distal nephron. By reducing potassium reabsorption, together with the large increase in sodium delivery and flow rate, large amounts of potassium may be excreted during diuretic therapy.[1]

Distal Nephron

Principal and Intercalated Cells of Cortical Collecting Ducts

Although both the "late" distal tubule (initial collecting duct) and the cortical collecting tubule are involved in regulation of potassium secretion, it is the potassium transport properties of the mammalian cortical collecting duct that have been most extensively studied. The cortical collecting tubule is composed of two distinctive cell types. The principal cells are primarily involved in sodium absorption and potassium secretion, whereas intercalated cells play a key role in hydrogen ion and bicarbonate transport. They also reabsorb potassium.

Models of principal and intercalated cells are shown in Fig. 16.12. In principal cells, sodium is actively transported from cell to blood via the Na^+-K^+ pump in the basolateral membrane. In the apical membrane, sodium is reabsorbed passively from lumen to cell along a favorable electrochemical gradient through a sodium channel. Potassium is transported actively from the blood into the cell, also via the Na^+-K^+ pump. Once in the cell, potassium can either recirculate through a conductive pathway in the basolateral membrane or be secreted through an apical membrane potassium-selective channel. Because the apical potassium-conductive pathway is much larger than that of the basolateral membrane, potassium transport, under almost all conditions, proceeds from cell to lumen. The principal cell is also ideally suited for potassium secretion because the apical sodium permeability and a lumen-to-cell–oriented sodium gradient depolarize the membrane and thereby generate a very favorable driving force for preferential potassium movement into the lumen.

Figure 16.13 shows a cell model of a principal cell, including two additional features. First, it includes an additional pathway for potassium secretion in the apical membrane. Perfusion studies with barium-containing solutions that block potassium channels have demonstrated continued potassium secretion, which was significantly enhanced when the concentration of chloride was lowered. These observations are best explained by an electroneutral K^+-Cl^- cotransporter in the apical membrane. The potential role of this pathway for potassium secretion, particularly during changes in net potassium transport, has yet to be explored. Second, as shown on the right of Fig. 16.13, electrical driving forces play an important role in regulating potassium movement. Because the magnitude of the electrical potential across the basolateral membrane is close to or slightly below the potassium equilibrium potential, loss of potassium into the peritubular blood is only modest under control conditions. The situation is quite different in the apical membrane. The much lower membrane potential, owing to the significant sodium permeability and sodium concentration gradient from lumen to cells, leads to a situation in which the potassium equilibrium potential greatly exceeds the membrane

[1] The delivery of increased amounts of fluid into the distal tubule after administration of loop diuretics is thought to result from reduced passive water reabsorption conditioned by a fall in NaCl transport in the thick ascending limb of Henle's loop. This leads to a decrease in renal papillary solute content and thus diminished passive fluid reabsorption across the thin descending limb of Henle's loop. Accordingly, more fluid enters the distal tubule, even though water movement per se is virtually uninfluenced by loop diuretics in the thick ascending limb of Henle's loop.

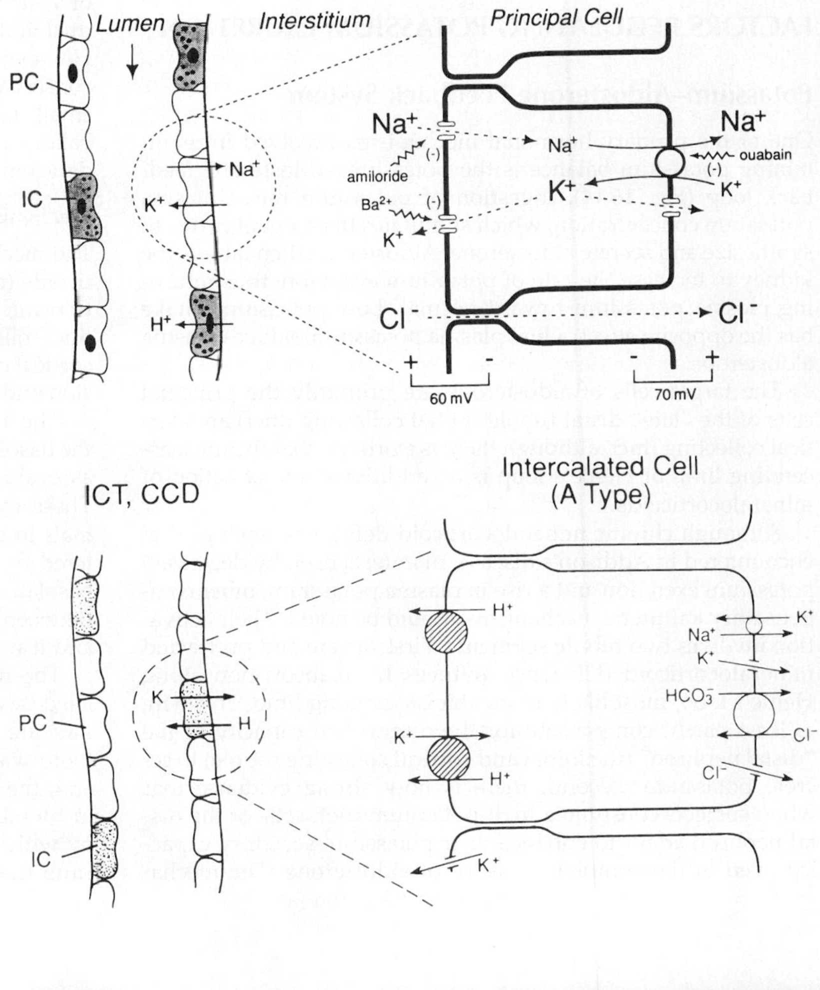

Figure 16.12. Models of principal and intercalated tubule cells. (From O'Neil RG. Adrenal steroid regulation of potassium transport. In: Giebisch G, ed. *Current topics in membranes and transport,* Vol 28, Orlando: Academic Press, 1987:185.)

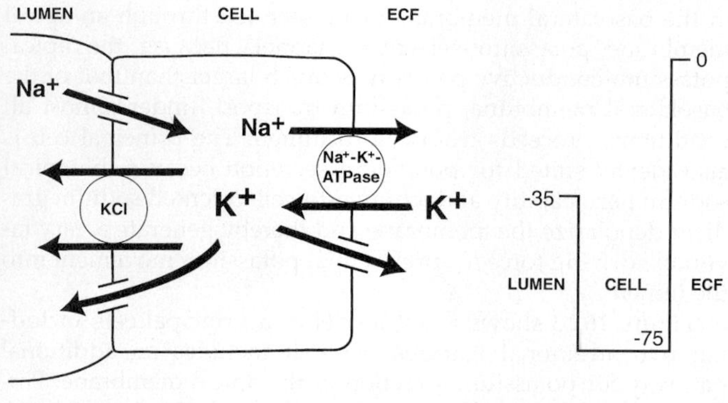

Figure 16.13. Model of principal tubule cell. *Left:* Apical and basolateral transporters. *Right:* Electrical profile showing marked asymmetry of cell polarization.

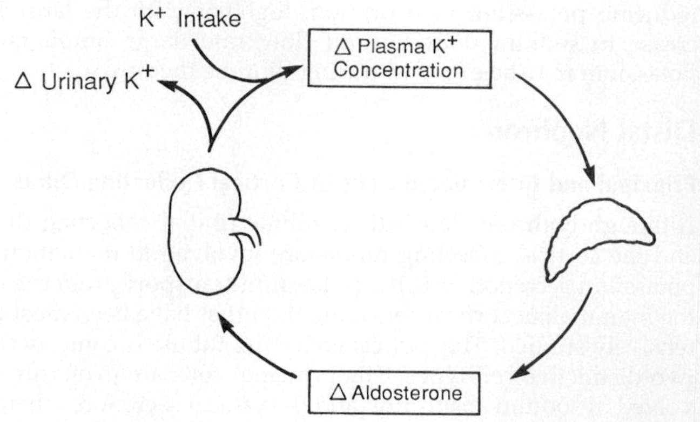

Figure 16.14. Feedback mechanism for control of urinary potassium excretion by aldosterone.

potential. As a consequence, potassium egress into the lumen greatly exceeds that across the basolateral membrane.

A model of an *intercalated* cell with K^+-H^+-ATPase in the apical membrane is also shown in Fig. 16.12. This transport mechanism resembles the ATP-dependent K^+-H^+ exchanger in the canalicular membrane of stomach parietal cells. Some of the renal isoforms of the enzyme are blocked by inhibitors of gastric acidification and have been shown to mediate during potassium depletion, both potassium and bicarbonate reabsorption in the initial and medullary collecting duct. Accordingly, potassium conservation is the result not only of depressed potassium secretion but also of activation of potassium reabsorption. Stimulation of this tubule K^+-H^+-ATPase explains both the observation of potassium conservation and the enhanced bicarbonate reabsorption during potassium depletion.

FACTORS REGULATING POTASSIUM EXCRETION

Potassium–Aldosterone Feedback System

One of the primary hormonal mechanisms involved in maintaining potassium balance is the potassium–aldosterone feedback loop (Fig. 16.14). Ingestion of potassium raises plasma potassium concentration, which stimulates the adrenal cortex to synthesize and secrete aldosterone. Aldosterone then targets the kidney to increase the rate of potassium excretion, thus returning plasma potassium toward normal. Low potassium intake has the opposite effect: a low plasma potassium reduces plasma aldosterone.

The target cells of aldosterone are primarily the principal cells of the "late" distal tubule (initial collecting duct) and cortical collecting duct, although there is evidence that the thick ascending limb of Henle's loop is an additional site of action of mineralocorticoids.

Although chronic mineralocorticoid deficiency, such as that encountered in Addison's disease, manifests itself by decreased potassium excretion and a rise in plasma potassium, other compensatory kaliuretic mechanisms should be noted. Their activation involves two tubule segments. First, severe and protracted mineralocorticoid deficiency reduces K^+ reabsorption along Henle's loop, most likely in the thick ascending limb. This will, at least partly, compensate for the diminished capacity of the "distal nephron" (the initial and cortical collecting tubule) to secrete potassium. Second, there is now strong evidence that when subjects consume a high-potassium diet, cells of the distal nephron adapt to enhance their potassium-secretory capacity, even in the complete absence of aldosterone. The mechanism of cellular adaptation to mineralocorticoids and to a high potassium intake alone is discussed later.

The renal response to a reduction of potassium intake is instructive, and several points deserve mention. Diminished distal potassium secretion, even activation of net potassium reabsorption along the distal tubule, is primarily responsible for the sustained fall in urinary potassium excretion. Two distinctive processes explain this response. First, an acute response, evolving within 24 hours of potassium restriction, is characterized by reduced mineralocorticoid levels. Second, if potassium deprivation continues, stimulation of potassium conservation follows with no further reduction in mineralocorticoids. There is convincing evidence that activation of a renal H^+-K^+-ATPase is responsible for potassium reabsorption in states of potassium depletion. According to this view, potassium ions are reabsorbed in exchange for hydrogen ions in the apical membrane of a subpopulation of intercalated cells of the cortical collecting duct and in the cells lining the outer medullary collecting duct. However, despite these efforts by the kidney, renal potassium conservation is insufficient to prevent the continued, albeit small, loss of potassium. Often, a state of negative potassium balance develops during prolonged consumption of a potassium-deficient diet.

Mechanism of Action of Mineralocorticoids

The mechanism by which principal cells adapt to mineralocorticoids (or to a high-potassium diet) has been studied by electron microscopy of morphologic changes in cortical collecting duct cells, by ultramicroassays of the Na^+-K^+-ATPase activity of cortical collecting tubules, and by a combination of microperfusion and microelectrode techniques.

The time course of mineralocorticoid-induced changes in the basolateral membrane area of the rat cortical collecting duct, as evaluated by electron microscopy, are shown in Fig. 16.15. These experiments were performed in adrenalectomized animals in which a physiologic dose of aldosterone was administered by osmotic minipumps for increasing time periods. The basolateral surface area increases with aldosterone treatment. Between 1 and 3 days, the surface area had sharply increased, and it was further amplified after 13 days.

The morphologic adaptation of the principal cell is paralleled by a similar time course of Na^+-K^+-ATPase activity. These data are summarized in Fig. 16.16. After a 1-day latent period, there was a large increase in Na^+-K^+-ATPase activity. In general, the magnitude of this increase was similar to the change in membrane area. These results show that one mechanism by which sustained aldosterone stimulates sodium and potassium transport is by increasing the number of Na^+-K^+ pumps

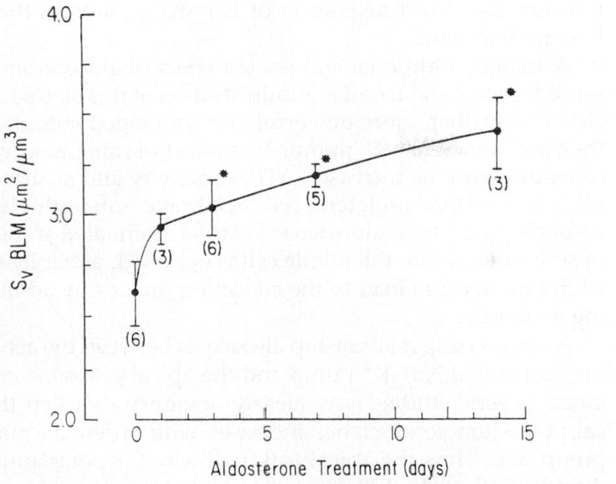

Figure 16.15 Time-dependent effects of aldosterone treatment on the ratio of basolateral membrane area to cell volume (*S_v BLM)* as measured by electron microscopy. Numbers in parentheses indicate the number of animals: asterisk indicates significant difference ($P < .05$) from the control group (0 day). (Reprinted with permission from Stanton B. Renal K adaptation: cellular mechanism and morphology. *Curr Top Membr Transport* 1987;28:185–206.)

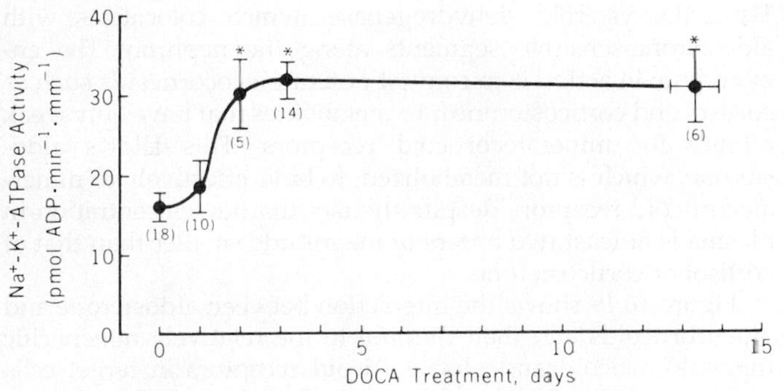

Figure 16.16. Time-dependent effects of deoxycorticosterone acetate *(DOCA)* on Na^+-K^+-ATPase activity. Similar to the increase in basolateral membrane area, full expression of increased pump activity is noted after a 1-day lag period. Numbers in parentheses indicate the number of animals; *asterisk* indicates significant difference ($P < .05$) from control (0 day). (Reprinted with permission from O'Neil RG, Hayhurst RA. Sodium dependent modulation of the renal Na^+-K^+-ATPase: influence of mineralocorticoids on the cortical collecting duct. *J Membr Biol* 1985;85:175.)

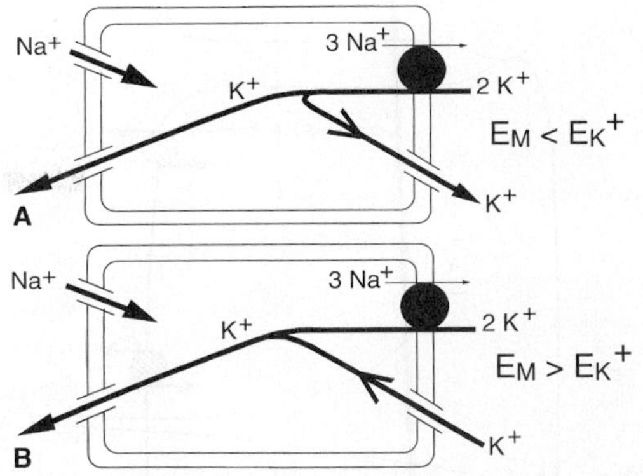

Figure 16.17. Schema of cortical collecting tubule cell with key sites of potassium transport. Depending on the magnitude of the electrical potential difference across the basolateral cell membrane, potassium ions may either leave the cell (recycle) *(top)* or be taken up into the cell in parallel with pump-mediated potassium transport *(bottom)*.

in the basolateral membrane. Because the basolateral membrane area of the principal cells, but not that of intercalated cells, was amplified by mineralocorticoid treatment, it is reasonable to conclude that mineralocorticoids induce an increase in Na^+-K^+-ATPase activity of principal cells only.

Because the basolateral membrane Na^+-K^+ pump transports $3Na^+$ from cell to blood and $2K^+$ from blood to cell, a net positive charge is carried from the cell to the blood across the basolateral membrane, a feature conferring "electrogenic" properties to this transport mechanism. This is partly responsible for a cell interior that is negative relative to the blood side and also for the observation that the magnitude of the cell-negative potential is set, at least partly, by the basolateral pump activity. Results from microelectrode studies, in which pump activity and cell potential were investigated, indicate that the potential across the basolateral membrane of adrenalectomized rats is less and that of mineralocorticoid-treated rabbits is more negative than normal. These results are consistent with a mineralocorticoid-induced increase of electrogenic sodium pump activity.

The sharp increase of the cell-negative transmembrane potential across the basolateral membrane has interesting consequences on potassium fluxes because they result in the reversal of the driving forces for passive potassium movement. As summarized in Fig. 16.17, potassium ions in chronically mineralocorticoid-treated animals move now from blood into the cell as the membrane potential exceeds the potassium equilibrium potential. Mineralocorticoids thus stimulate potassium uptake into principal cells across the basolateral membrane not only by upregulating Na^+-K^+-ATPase but also by accelerating passive potassium transport into the cell through conductive pathways.

An evaluation of the apical permeability properties in different states of mineralocorticoid activity has also been possible by the application of electrophysiologic techniques. Such experiments make use of electrical potential changes across the apical membrane of principal cells after substitution of luminal sodium and potassium by impermeant cations. In general, the magnitude of the potential change after an appropriate ion substitution is proportional to the relative sodium and potassium permeability. Another way to estimate specific ion permeabilities of renal cell membranes is to use substances that block ion channels. Such channel blockers will change the membrane potential in proportion to the contribution that diffusion potentials make to the transmembrane potential difference; they also prevent ion-induced voltage changes when luminal sodium and potassium concentrations are altered experimentally. Because apical membrane sodium channels are amiloride sensitive, addition of amiloride to the lumen can be used to quantify the specific sodium ion conductance. Similarly, barium is used to block potassium channels and to quantify the apical potassium ion conductance. Thus the partial conductances of the apical membrane for sodium and potassium can be monitored using microelectrodes and the blocking agents amiloride and barium.

Figure 16.18, depicts the model of mineralocorticoid (aldosterone) regulation of potassium transport in the principal cell of the rabbit cortical collecting duct. Two phases of mineralocorticoid action emerge. First, on entering the cell, aldosterone induces the synthesis of new proteins that stimulate both the basolateral Na^+-K^+ pump and the apical sodium permeability. This leads to enhanced early entry of sodium into the cell and to stimulation of the basolateral Na^+-K^+ pump. At the same time, another protein may be involved in the simul-

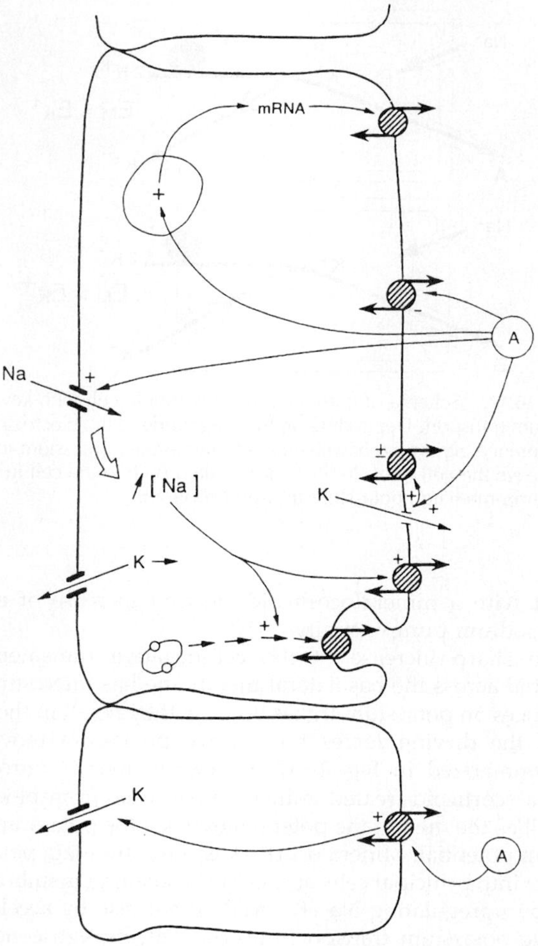

Figure 16.18. Summary of mechanisms involved in modulating basolateral Na^+-K^+-ATPase by aldosterone **(A)**. Changes in Na^+-K^+-ATPase activity in the basolateral membrane may be mediated by genomic factors leading to alteration in pump synthesis, effects on the pump turnover rate, substrate-related effects of cell Na concentration by primary effects of aldosterone on apical Na channels, or recruitment by cell Na concentration changes of latent pump units through exocytosis. Additional factors may involve changes in basolateral K conductance (recycling of K and effects of membrane voltage changes on electrogenic pump activity). Shown in **B** is the effect of changes in basolateral ATPase activity on apical K conductance. (Modified from Barlet-Bas C, Cheval L, Feraille E, et al. Regulation of tubular Na-K-ATPase. In: Hatano M, ed. *Nephrology, Proceedings of the XIth International Congress of Nephrology*. Berlin: Springer, 1991:419–434.)

taneous and direct activation of Na^+-K^+ pumps in the basolateral membrane.

A second, additional and *delayed* effect of aldosterone is observed some 24 hours after administration of this steroid. It consists of a further, more powerful and prolonged stimulation of the basolateral Na^+-K^+ pump. This effect of mineralocorticoids coincides with the increased ATPase activity and a surface amplification of the basolateral cell membrane. Interestingly, these secondary effects of aldosterone can be attenuated if the entry of sodium ions into the tubule cell is curtailed, either by diminishing the sodium load to the collecting duct or by administering amiloride.

An interesting relationship also exists between the activity of the basolateral Na^+-K^+ pump and the apical *potassium* conductance. Several studies have clearly demonstrated that the apical potassium conductance increases with an enhancement in pump rate. Thus the apical leak pathway for potassium is reduced in adrenalectomy or in states of low mineralocorticoid activity, whereas it is activated, in proportion to basolateral pump stimulation, in situations characterized by high aldosterone levels. An increase in basolateral Na^+-K^+-ATPase by increasing peritubular potassium concentrations, independent of mineralocorticoids, has also been shown to increase the apical potassium and sodium conductances.

Several studies have led to the recognition that target tissue specificity of mineralocorticoids depends, to a large extent, on 11β-hydroxysteroid dehydrogenase, which colocalizes with aldosterone-sensitive segments along the nephron. The enzyme's main action is to convert potent glucocorticoids such as cortisol and corticosterone into metabolites that have only weak affinity for mineralocorticoid receptors. This allows aldosterone, which is not metabolized, to bind effectively to mineralocorticoid receptors despite the fact that its concentration in plasma is at least two orders of magnitude smaller than that of cortisol or corticosterone.

Figure 16.19 shows the interaction between aldosterone and glucocorticoids and their binding to the relatively nonspecific mineralocorticoid and glucocorticoid receptors in target cells such as principal cells of the initial and cortical collecting tubule. The cell schema also highlight the important protective function of 11β-hydroxysteroid dehydrogenase. Inhibition of this regulatory enzyme leads to an apparent excess of mineralocorticoid effects such as sodium retention and potassium wasting because glucocorticoids are no longer prevented from effective binding to mineralocorticoid receptors.

Taken together, mineralocorticoids induce a series of integrated changes in the active and passive transport properties

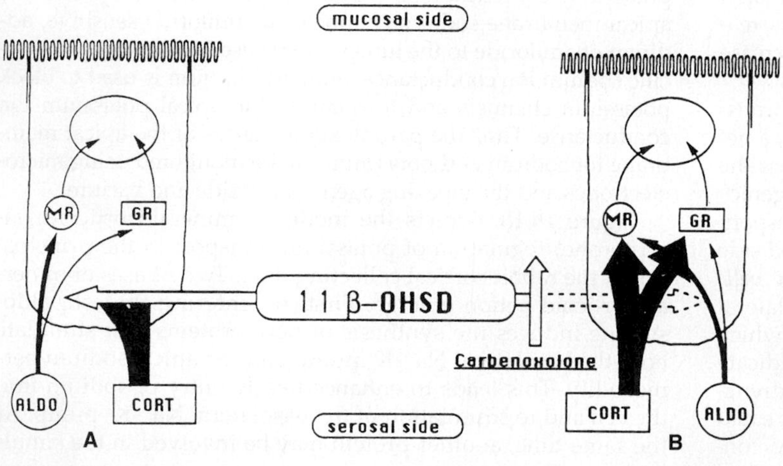

Figure 16.19. Cell models showing the effects of 11β-hydroxysteroid dehydrogenase on binding of aldosterone *(ALDO)* and cortisol or corticosterone *(CORT)* to mineralocorticoid and glucocorticoid receptors (*MR* and *GR*). The effects of carbenoxolone, an inhibitor of 11β-hydroxysteroid dehydrogenase, are also shown. Note that enzyme inhibition leads to mineralocorticoid receptor activation by glucocorticoids. (Reprinted from Rossier BC, Palmer LG. In: Seldin DW, Giebisch G, eds. *The kidney: physiology and pathophysiology*, 2nd ed. New York: Raven Press,

in principal cells of the cortical collecting tubule. These changes include (a) an increase in apical sodium permeability and depolarization of the apical electrical potential difference, (b) an increase in basolateral pump activity, and (c) an increase in the apical potassium leak that matches the rate at which potassium is actively pumped into the cell by the Na^+-K^+ exchanger. Provided the effect of mineralocorticoids is prolonged, additional pump recruitment is associated with a sharp rise in ATPase activity in basolateral membrane areas, as is increased sodium and potassium channel density in the apical membrane.

Finally, it is of interest that potassium secretion in the cortical collecting duct can also be stimulated by *mineralocorticoid-independent* factors. For instance, a high dietary potassium intake (about three times normal), even in the absence of steroids, leads to a significant rise in potassium excretion with only a modest rise in plasma potassium. Thus it has been demonstrated that the cortical collecting duct cells of adrenalectomized animals maintained on such a high-potassium diet underwent some of the very same changes seen in mineralocorticoid-treated animals, including increases in the Na^+-K^+-ATPase activity in the basolateral cell membrane area and in both sodium and potassium conductances of the apical cell membrane. It is likely that the high potassium intake induces these changes by stimulating basolateral Na^+-K^+-ATPase activity ("cross-talk" between basolateral and apical membranes).

It is worth noting that glucocorticoids also have a distinct stimulating effect on potassium secretion, particularly in the late distal tubule (initial collecting duct). However, this kaliuretic effect is not caused by a direct action of these steroids on tubular potassium transport but is related to the increased flow rate into the distal tubule that glucocorticoids induce by increasing glomerular filtration rate and water excretion. The full effect of steroid-induced stimulation of potassium excretion depends on the coordinated synergism of mineralocorticoids and glucocorticoids.

Plasma pH

Changes in acid–base balance have long been known to affect extrarenal and renal potassium balance. In general, metabolic or respiratory acidosis results in decreased potassium excretion and a high plasma potassium, whereas alkalotic conditions enhance potassium excretion and lower plasma potassium.

There are several possible explanations for the interaction between plasma pH and renal potassium excretion. First, lowering plasma pH reduces the ability of the distal tubule to secrete potassium as long as other factors, particularly distal flow rate, are unchanged. This fall in potassium excretion with acidosis is most likely related to the inhibitory effect of cell acidosis on basolateral active potassium uptake and to a reduction of the apical potassium permeability. The resulting fall of intracellular potassium in the distal tubule associated with a diminished apical potassium permeability would result in less favorable conditions for potassium secretion from the cell to the lumen. The opposite sequence of events would stimulate potassium secretion during alkalosis.

The complex interactions between H^+, NH_3, and K^+ are also of interest. As urine pH falls, NH_3 is trapped in the distal nephron and H^+ is eliminated in the urine as NH_4^+. This process is affected by potassium because hyperkalemia inhibits and hypokalemia stimulates renal NH_3 production. Accordingly, hyperkalemia tends to suppress NH_3 secretion and elimination of urinary H^+, a condition resulting in systemic acidosis. Potassium depletion, on the other hand, stimulates NH_3 production, promotes H^+ secretion, and raises blood pH. The changes in pH as a result of the effect on NH_3 secretion would then affect renal handling of potassium.

However, the development of hyperkalemia and acidosis also depends on the level of circulating mineralocorticoids. Their action is to increase H^+ secretion in the distal nephron. For instance, in severe dehydration, high plasma potassium induces acidosis because of its inhibition of NH_3 secretion. However, this tendency is opposed by the direct stimulating effect of mineralocorticoids on H^+ secretion. In the absence of appropriate adjustments in the aldosterone level (Addison's disease), high potassium levels (lack of distal K^+ secretion) and acidosis (suppression of NH_3 formation and of distal H^+ secretion) develop.

Volume Expansion–Increased Urinary Flow Rate

One of the most powerful stimuli of potassium secretion is the flow rate along the distal tubule and collecting tubule. Over a considerable flow range, potassium secretion is essentially flow-dependent, so the rate of potassium secretion increases as more fluid is delivered into the distal tubule. This feature of the potassium secretory mechanism is important because it accounts for the kaliuresis commonly observed after saline loading and for the increase in potassium excretion that follows all interventions that diminish fluid reabsorption upstream of the main site of potassium secretion. Several situations can affect potassium balance through changes in flow rate along the distal tubule and collecting tubule.

A relevant example is that of chronic mineralocorticoid administration. If mineralocorticoids such as aldosterone or deoxycorticosterone acetate are administered for prolonged periods, two responses can be distinguished. During the first day, sodium excretion is reduced and potassium excretion is enhanced. These are the typical effects to be expected of mineralocorticoid action on the distal nephron. However, after prolonged treatment with steroids, sodium retention stops, yet increased potassium excretion is maintained. This sodium "escape" phenomenon results from secondary volume expansion and the ensuing rise in glomerular filtration rate and inhibition of proximal sodium chloride and fluid reabsorption. As more sodium and fluid are delivered into the distal tubule, some sodium escapes reabsorption despite the high steroid levels. This tends to reestablish sodium balance, albeit at the expense of volume expansion. However, the high distal flow rate enhances the effect of mineralocorticoids on potassium excretion and results in sustained potassium loss. A gradual decline of potassium excretion may eventually occur and is initiated, no doubt, by activation of renal potassium reabsorption in response to hypokalemia.

For several years, it has been known that substances that increase urine flow, such as nonreabsorbable ions (high plasma levels of phosphate, sulfate, and bicarbonate, metabolic alkalosis and poorly reabsorbable sugars such as mannitol), have a strong kaliuretic effect. The kaliuresis that occurs from administration of many diuretics is also related to increased distal flow rate. Drugs such as furosemide, bumetanide, and thiazide enhance potassium excretion by stimulating potassium secretion as the flow rate along the distal tubule and the cortical collecting tubule increases.

Antidiuretic Hormone

The effects of antidiuretic hormone (ADH, vasopressin) include an increase in water permeability and a reduction in flow rate. Because ADH lowers volume delivery, decreased potassium secretion would be expected with high plasma ADH levels.

However, ADH administration actually increases fractional potassium excretion when care is taken to minimize the effects of ADH on distal flow rate.

Several mechanisms are responsible for the kaliuretic effect of ADH. First, as the flow rate in the distal tubule and cortical collecting tubule is reduced by ADH, sodium ions are concentrated in the tubular fluid. Hence, in the cortical collecting duct, where the sodium concentration is normally low and thus may limit potassium secretion, a rise in sodium concentration will facilitate potassium secretion. Second, there is evidence that ADH directly increases potassium secretion in the distal tubule and the cortical collecting ducts by activating apical potassium channels.

Interaction of Flow Rate with Other Regulatory Factors of Potassium Transport

Several examples of the complex interaction of factors that *directly* affect potassium transport at the site of potassium secretion and those factors that control potassium secretion *indirectly* are shown in Fig. 16.20. Extracellular volume expansion decreases proximal reabsorption of fluid and leads to increased distal flow rate. This would increase distal potassium secretion were it not for the simultaneous decrease in aldosterone, an effect tending to lower potassium secretion in the distal tubule. Under ideal conditions, these two opposing effects would cancel and dissociate potassium secretion from changes in ECF volume.

The situation during changes in water intake is also relevant. Water intake decreases ADH levels and, by diminishing distal water reabsorption, enhances distal flow rate and distal potassium secretion. However, as discussed, ADH directly increases potassium secretion in the distal nephron, and its decline would partly offset the increased potassium secretion that follows the increase in distal flow rate. What is common to the situations just described is the tendency to dissociate potassium balance from changes in sodium balance (volume of the ECF) and in water metabolism.

However, direct effects on potassium secretion and flow-related effects may not always be opposing each other. For instance, during high potassium intake, reduction in proximal fluid reabsorption and stimulation of potassium secretion in the distal tubule act to enhance potassium secretion. Similarly, during induction of metabolic alkalosis when large loads of bicarbonate reach the distal tubule, potassium secretion would be stimulated not only by the increase in distal flow rate but also by the direct effect of alkalosis to elevate potassium secretion along the distal tubule. Finally, the effects of diuretic treatment on potassium excretion can be best explained by the increase in distal flow rate and high aldosterone levels that follow contraction of the extracellular fluid volume.

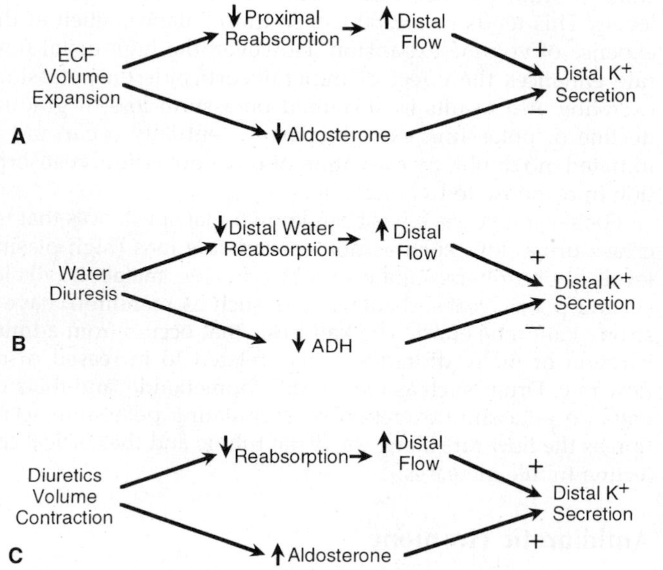

Figure 16.20. Proposed interactions between flow-related and hormonal effects on potassium excretion. (Modified from Giebisch G, Malnic G, Berliner RW. Renal transport and control of potassium excretion. In: Brenner BM, Rector FW Jr. *The kidney.* Philadelphia: WB Saunders, 1986:186.)

Selected Readings

Alpern RJ, Warnock DG, Rector FC Jr. Renal acidification mechanisms. In: Brenner BM, Rector FC Jr, eds. *The kidney.* Philadelphia: WB Saunders, 1986:206–249.

Description of the mechanism of the interaction between mineralocorticoids, acid, and potassium transport in the distal nephron. In hyperaldosteronism, potassium secretion is elevated, resulting in hypokalemia, which stimulates ammonia synthesis. High tubular fluid ammonia concentrations increase buffering capacity, thereby raising pH and stimulating acid secretion.

Field MJ, Giebisch G. Hormonal control of renal potassium excretion. *Kidney Int* 1985;27:379–387.

Review of the separate hormonal effects of ADH, aldosterone, and catecholamines. When the variable flow rate and distal sodium delivery are controlled, potassium secretion is increased by ADH and aldosterone but inhibited by catecholamines.

Giebisch G. Renal potassium transport: mechanisms and regulation. *Am J Physiol* 1998;274:F817.

Giebisch G, Wang W. Potassium transport: from clearance to channels and pumps. *Kidney Int* 1995;49:1624.

Both papers provide reviews of (a) the mechanisms by which potassium transport is mediated along the nephron and (b) the mechanisms by which regulation of potassium reabsorption and secretion occurs. Transport in analyzed in terms of net movement of potassium at specific tubule sites and in terms of specific transport properties of the cells lining the nephron. Analysis of the regulation of potassium transport includes such factors as potassium balance, control by hormones, by factors related to acid–base and distal fluid and sodium delivery.

Ho K, Nichols CG, Lederer WJ, et al. Cloning and expression of an inwardly rectifying ATP-regulated potassium channel. *Nature* 1993;362:31–37.

Describes the cloning, molecular structure, and the functional properties of a newly discovered renal potassium channel. It is expressed in several regions of the kidney, and many of its characteristics mimic the behavior of the potassium channel in the apical membrane of thick ascending limb cells and of the secretory potassium channel in the apical membrane of principal cells in the cortical collecting tubule.

Jamison RL. Potassium recycling. *Kidney Int* 1987;31:695–703.

A review of the evidence supporting the potassium recycling mechanism. The high potassium concentration can be accounted for by continued potassium reabsorption from the medullary collecting ducts after secretion in the cortical collecting tubule.

Morris DJ, Soundness GW. Protective and specificity-conferring mechanisms of mineralocorticoid action. *Am J Physiol* 1992;263:F759–F768.

Describes experiments that demonstrate the protective role of 11β-hydroxysteroid dehydrogenase in mineralocorticoid target tissues. This mechanism preserves distinct aldosterone effects in the presence of relatively high physiologic glucocorticoid concentrations. Additional mechanisms prevent extreme endogenous mineralocorticoid effects and appear to be mediated by additional steroid-metabolizing enzymes.

Muto S, Sansom SC, Giebisch G. Effects of high K^+ diet on the electrical properties of cortical collecting ducts from adrenalectomized rabbits. *J Clin Invest* 1988; 81:376.

Describes the electrophysiologic effects of an increase in potassium intake on apical sodium and potassium conductances. These observations indicate that a high-potassium diet induces in principal cells similar stimulation of apical cation permeabilities as those after administration of mineralocorticoids.

O'Neil RG. Aldosterone regulation of sodium and potassium transport in the cortical collecting duct. *Semin Nephrol* 1990;10:365–374.

A review of information on the cellular mechanism of action of mineralocorticoids. It summarizes the optical, electrical, and biochemical evidence for the role of the cortical collecting tubule principal cell in potassium secretion.

Rossier BC, Palmer LG. Mechanisms of aldosterone action on sodium and potassium transport. In: Seldin DW, Giebisch GH, eds. *The kidney: physiology and pathophysiology,* 2nd ed. New York: Raven Press, 1992:1373–1409.

An authoritative and up-to-date review on the role of aldosterone in regulation of sodium and potassium homeostasis.

Sansom SC, O'Neil RG. Mineralocorticoid regulation of apical cell membrane Na^+ and K^+ transport of the cortical collecting duct. *Am J Physiol* 1985;248: F858–F868.

Evidence that the early effects of mineralocorticoids on the cortical collecting tubule are an increase in apical membrane sodium conductance. Delayed or secondary effects include an increase of apical membrane potassium conductance and of basolateral membrane potential.

Stanton BA. Renal potassium transport: Morphological and functional adaptations. *Am J Physiol* 1989;257:R989.
Reviews the morphologic changes of specific renal cell types in potassium-adapted animals and correlating structure of cell types with potassium transport properties.
Tannen RL. Effect of potassium on renal acidification and acid-base homeostasis. *Semin Nephrol* 1987;7:263–272.
Description of the interaction between renal ammonia production and potassium secretion. Hyperkalemia suppresses renal ammonia production, resulting in depressed distal H⁺ secretion and systemic acidosis.
Wingo CS, Surolka AJ. Function and structure of H^+-K^+-ATPase in the kidney. *Am J Physiol* 1995;269:F1–F16.
Summarizes our present state of knowledge of the renal H^+-K^+-ATPase, its physiologic significance, and its role in potassium homeostasis. It emphasizes the importance of H^+-K^+-ATPase activity in states of potassium depletion and surveys the body of evidence that has recently emerged in support of the physiologic and pathophysiologic role of this transport protein.

PART 2

Extrarenal Control of Serum Potassium

Guido O. Perez

The maintenance of a normal serum potassium concentration depends on the kidney's ability to excrete potassium (external balance) and of extrarenal mechanisms (internal balance) to shift potassium in and out of cells. The latter constitutes the focus of this chapter; the excretion of potassium in sweat and feces is part of the external balance and is discussed separately. The importance of extrarenal mechanisms is illustrated by the events following ingestion of a potassium load (e.g., 60 mEq). After the load is absorbed, only half (30 mEq) of the ingested potassium is excreted in the urine during the subsequent 3 to 6 hours. Assuming that the volume of the extracellular fluid (ECF) compartment is 15 L, the retention of all 30 mEq in the extracellular compartment would result in an increase of 2 mEq/L in serum potassium concentration, an increment that might have pronounced effects on neuromuscular function. Fortunately, under normal conditions, approximately 80% of the retained potassium is shifted into cells and only 20% remains in the extracellular space. The retained potassium eventually is excreted in the urine over the next 24 hours.

POTASSIUM CONTENT OF THE INTRACELLULAR AND EXTRACELLULAR FLUID

Ninety-eight percent of the approximately 3,600 mEq of potassium in the body of a 70-kg person is located in the intracellular compartment (80% in muscle), and only 2% is found in the ECF (Fig. 16.21). The concentration of potassium in the former is 120 to 140 mEq/L, roughly 35-fold greater than that in the ECF (3.5 to 5.0 mEq/L). This asymmetric distribution of potassium in the different fluid compartments is maintained primarily by the Na^+-K^+-ATPase in the cell membrane, which pumps sodium out of and potassium into cells in a 3:2 ratio and offsets the diffusion of sodium into and potassium out of the intracellular compartment.

The ratio of potassium concentrations between the intracellular and the extracellular compartment is a major determinant of the resting membrane potential. This ratio is primarily influenced by the concentration of potassium in the ECF because

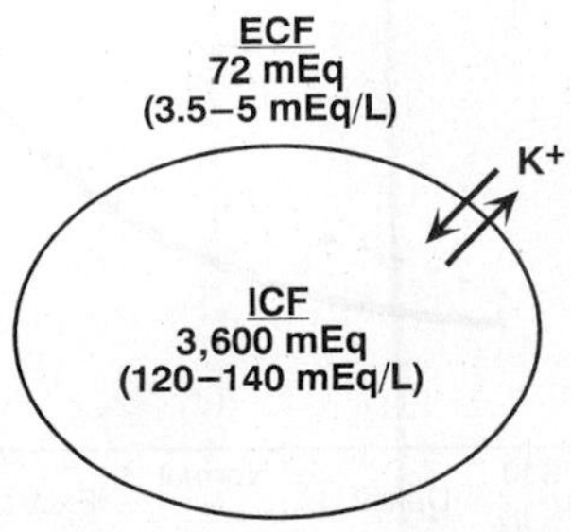

Figure 16.21. Distribution of potassium between the extracellular fluid *(ECF)* and intracellular fluid *(ICF)* in a typical 70-kg subject.

changes in total body potassium cause very little percentage change in the intracellular concentration. The resting membrane potential sets the stage for the generation of the action potential and is thus critically important for normal neural and muscular function.

PATHOPHYSIOLOGIC MECHANISMS THAT AFFECT POTASSIUM DISTRIBUTION

Several mechanisms affect the distribution of potassium between the intracellular and extracellular compartments. Most of these mechanisms influence either the electric gradient across cellular membranes or the permeability of membranes to potassium. For example, several hormones enhance cellular potassium uptake via stimulation of the Na^+-K^+-ATPase, whereas agents that block potassium channels may affect the permeability of cells to potassium. Changes in acid–base balance, anabolic or catabolic states, exercise, and cellular proliferation or necrosis may also result in transcellular potassium fluxes.

Potassium uptake and release varies considerably among different tissues and during the course of daily activities. A single class of hormones, such as catecholamines, may affect the activity of the sodium pump in opposite ways depending on the tissue involved. Furthermore, the same hormone may influence different types of potassium channels. Thus it is impossible to predict the magnitude of transcellular potassium shifts taking place continuously in the whole organism.

Effect of Changes in External Potassium Balance

Changes in external potassium balance may affect potassium distribution in the different body compartments and vice versa. The relationship between total body potassium and serum potassium concentration is almost linear during the initial phase of potassium depletion. In the face of more severe depletion of total body potassium, this relationship is lost because of the increasingly greater losses of potassium from the intracellular compartment (Fig. 16.22). The capacity for potassium reuptake by cells is impaired in potassium deficiency probably because of a reduction in the activity of the Na^+-K^+-ATPase. The latter effect may help prevent a fast decline in serum potassium levels. During the early phase of correction, serum levels usually increase slowly, reflecting the large volume of distribution of the administered potassium. Stimulation of the Na^+-K^+-ATPase during correction of the deficit may help prevent hyperkalemia by shifting potassium into cells. After potassium stores are replete, cellular uptake decreases and the serum potassium concentration may increase suddenly.

Adaptation to a high-potassium diet is mediated primarily by renal mechanisms, and it is associated with increased aldosterone production. Changes in the cells of the cortical collecting

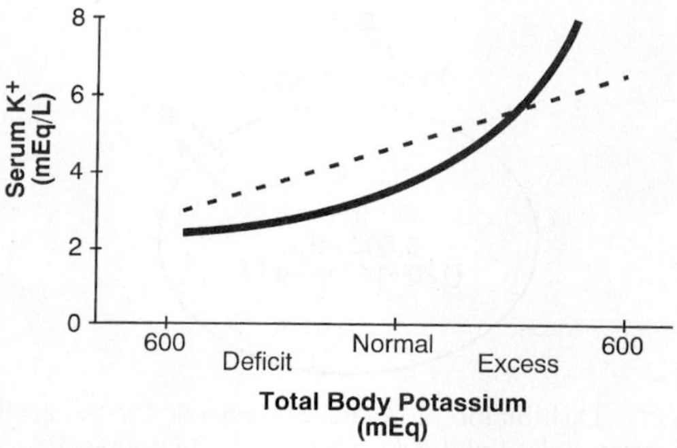

Figure 16.22. Relationship between serum potassium and total body potassium. Predicted *(dotted line)* and clinically observed *(solid line)* relationship between serum K^+ and total body K^+ content. In the early stage of potassium depletion, extracellular K^+ loss is proportionally greater than the loss of cellular K^+. Nevertheless, because the cells contain most of the total body K^+, almost all absolute losses originate from the intracellular fluid *(ICF)*. When K^+ loss is more severe, the curve becomes flatter, indicating a proportionally greater degree of K^+ loss from cells. This may help prevent a fast decline in serum K^+ levels. On the other hand, during early repletion, serum K^+ levels increase slowly, reflecting the large volume of distribution. During the late phase of correction, cellular uptake decreases and serum potassium increases. The stimulation of Na^+-K^+-ATPase induced by K^+ loading would be expected to facilitate K^+ uptake by cells and to prevent hyperkalemia.

duct include increased area of the basolateral membrane and increased content of Na^+-K^+-ATPase. Extrarenal mechanisms probably also contribute to such adaptation. As mentioned, shifts of potassium in and out of cells may influence external potassium balance. This is because of the resultant changes in potassium concentration in the cells of the cortical collecting duct, which is one of the factors that influence renal potassium secretion. In addition, changes in cellular potassium content may influence the secretion of aldosterone by the adrenal gland.

CAUSES OF INCREASED POTASSIUM SHIFT INTO CELLS (Table 16.1)

Hormones

Insulin

Insulin stimulates cellular potassium uptake, an effect that has been used therapeutically for many years for the treatment of hyperkalemia. It has been shown using the insulin-clamp technique that this effect is dose dependent, with a maximum effect (decrease in plasma potassium of approximately 1 mEq/L in 1 hour) approached at plasma insulin levels exceeding 20 to 40 times basal levels.

Under normal conditions, basal levels of insulin are needed to dispose of an acute potassium load. For example, studies in experimental animals have shown that pancreatectomy or inhibition of endogenous secretion with somatostatin impairs potassium tolerance. In healthy subjects, somatostatin infusion in the postabsorptive state results in a decline in plasma insulin levels and an increase of 0.5 to 0.7 mEq/L in potassium concentration. Insulinopenia may also contribute to the fasting hyperkalemia observed in patients receiving maintenance dialysis and to the normal or increased serum potassium levels observed in patients with diabetic ketoacidosis despite marked deficits in total body potassium.

The hypokalemic effect of insulin derives from its capacity to promote net potassium uptake by cells. Splanchnic uptake may be important during the first hour after insulin administration. Subsequently, there is a shift in potassium uptake to skeletal muscle, the main reservoir of potassium in the body. *In vitro* and *in vivo* studies have demonstrated that the effect of insulin on potassium uptake can be dissociated from its effect on glucose transport. This may explain the finding that uremic patients exhibit abnormalities in insulin-mediated glucose transport, whereas the hypokalemic effect of exogenous insulin is normal. An effect of hyperkalemia stimulating insulin secretion has been demonstrated consistently only after increases in serum potassium concentration greater than 1 mEq/L. Therefore it appears that a positive feedback loop does not exist at small, more physiologic, changes in serum potassium concentration.

There is strong evidence that insulin stimulates the activity of the Na^+-K^+-ATPase in skeletal as well as in other tissues. The hormonal stimulation of sodium and potassium transport develops within a few minutes and leads to a decrease in the ratio of intracellular sodium to potassium, as well as a decrease to hyperpolarization. This effect is blocked by ouabain. Studies in oxidative fiber-type skeletal muscle have shown that insulin induces a redistribution of the α_2 and β_1 isoforms of the Na^+-K^+-ATPase from an intracellular pool to the plasma membrane (Fig. 16.23). Increases in sodium uptake, increases in the affinity of the pump for sodium, and changes in phosphorylation of the pump may underlie the actions of insulin in other tissues.

β_2-Adrenergic Stimulation

Epinephrine induces hypokalemia in experimental animals after an initial (1 to 3 minutes) increase in serum potassium. Because epinephrine inhibits the renal excretion of potassium, the hypokalemic effect was attributed to net uptake by extrarenal tissues. The latter was confirmed during *in vivo* limb perfusion studies and *in vitro* studies in isolated skeletal muscle. It should be mentioned that β-adrenergic agents can raise plasma insulin secondary to either increases in plasma glucose or by directly stimulating pancreatic insulin release. However, the hypokalemic effects of epinephrine were also observed in pancreatectomized animals. This observation excludes an indirect effect resulting from insulin release.

Other studies have shown that stimulation of extrarenal disposal of potassium by epinephrine is mediated by β_2-adrenergic

TABLE 16.1. Factors that Influence Transcellular Distribution of Potassium

	Shifts into Cells	Shifts out of Cells
Hormones	Insulin, β_2-agonists	α-Agonists, parathyroid hormone
Acid–base status	Metabolic and respiratory alkalosis	Metabolic and respiratory acidosis
Anabolism/catabolism	Anabolism, cell proliferation	Catabolism, cell necrosis
Periodic paralysis	Hypokalemic form	Hyperkalemic form
Drugs/intoxications	Barium, chloroquine	Digitalis, fluoride

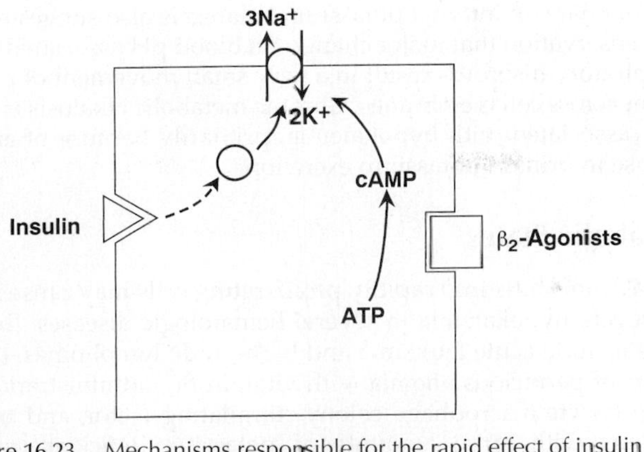

Figure 16.23. Mechanisms responsible for the rapid effect of insulin and β_2-agonists on serum potassium concentration. These agents induce rapid changes because they influence the phosphorylation state of the sodium pump (β_2-adrenergic agonists) or its cellular localization (insulin). More sustained changes in pump activity result from regulation of both transcriptional and posttranscriptional events, resulting in an increase in the number of pumps (e.g. aldosterone, thyroid hormone).

receptors. For example, the effects of epinephrine are prevented by nonselective β-blockers such as propanolol and the selective β_2-antagonist butoxamine. On the other hand, no effect on serum potassium concentration is produced by practalol, a specific β_1-antagonist. Furthermore, numerous studies have shown that several β_2-agonists (including albuterol, terbutaline, and ritodrine) lower potassium levels, whereas β_1-agonists have no effect.

The hypokalemic effect of β_2-agonists has been used for the treatment of hyperkalemia in patients with end-stage renal disease. Administration of albuterol intravenously (0.5 mg) or by inhalation of a nebulized solution (20 mg over 10 minutes) causes a reduction in potassium levels of approximately 1 mEq/L, with a peak effect at 30 minutes. Some albuterol-treated patients may experience modest tachycardia and increases in blood pressure. Thus these agents must be used with caution in patients with coronary artery disease. Of interest, the potassium-lowering effects of β_2-agonists are additive to those of insulin, suggesting different mechanisms of action. In patients receiving dialysis, concurrent administration of β_2-agonists may help prevent insulin-induced hypoglycemia.

The therapeutic use of β_2-adrenergic agonists for conditions other than hyperkalemia may cause profound decreases in serum potassium concentration. In patients with asthma or chronic obstructive lung disease, the effect of β_2-adrenergic agonists may be compounded by the administration of other potassium-lowering agents such as theophylline or diuretics. Ritodrine and terbutaline may induce hypokalemia in women treated with β_2-adrenergic agonists for preterm labor. Decreases in serum potassium concentration have been described in patients receiving adrenalin-containing local anesthetics.

It is unclear whether increases in serum potassium concentration within the physiologic range stimulate the endogenous secretion of catecholamines and thereby form a homeostatic feedback loop. A stimulatory effect of potassium on catecholamine release has been shown *in vitro* only when supraphysiologic levels of potassium are used. Nevertheless, it has been shown that infusion of epinephrine in amounts adequate to raise serum epinephrine concentrations to levels seen during stress results in a decrease of 0.4 to 0.6 mEq/L in serum potassium concentration. Indeed, hypokalemia may be associated with stressful conditions such as myocardial infarction (MI), surgery, head trauma, delirium tremens, and diabetic ketoacidosis. The combination of hypokalemia, with increased catecholamine levels, diuretic-induced hypomagnesemia, and the administration of drugs such as digitalis, may increase the susceptibility to arrhythmias in patients with acute MI. During insulin-induced hypoglycemia, increased catecholamine production potentiates the hypokalemic effect of insulin.

There are many common physiologic conditions in which catecholamines help defend against the development of hyperkalemia. Catecholamine release after meals may contribute, together with insulin, to the postprandial disposal of dietary potassium. During exercise, potassium is released by the contracting muscle. The resultant local increase in serum potassium concentration has been implicated in the pathogenesis of several related physiologic processes such as hyperemia and fatigue. The increased catecholamine levels during exercise and stimulation of the sodium pump help prevent hyperkalemia by shifting potassium intracellularly. Nevertheless, substantial elevations of serum potassium concentration occur during vigorous exercise, especially in untrained individuals, or after administration of β_2-adrenergic antagonists.

β_2-Adrenergic receptor stimulation initiates cyclic adenosine monophosophate (cAMP) formation, which leads to the activation of the sodium pump (Fig. 16.23). Theophylline, an inhibitor of phosphodiesterase, potentiates the effect of epinephrine on cation transport and membrane potential. The short-term regulation exerted by catecholamines is mediated by reversible phosphorylation of the pump catalytic subunit.

Other Hormones

The rapid changes in serum potassium concentration induced by insulin and β-adrenergic agonists depend on their ability to alter cellular localization or the phosphorylation state of the sodium pump. Hormones that cause sustained changes in pump activity usually act by increasing the number of pump units. This results from regulation of both transcriptional and posttranscriptional events. Thyroid hormone and aldosterone act on this posttranscriptional mechanism.

Aldosterone increases apical sodium conductance and stimulates Na^+-K^+-ATPase in the cortical collecting tubule, colon, and other epithelial cells. The resultant changes in urinary and fecal potassium excretion are very important in the regulation of external potassium balance. Several studies in humans and experimental animals have attempted to show an effect of aldosterone on the internal balance of potassium. Interpretation of these studies, however, is difficult because aldosterone also affects external potassium balance and acid–base metabolism. Of note, physiologic changes in serum potassium concentration influence the production of aldosterone by the adrenal glands.

Abnormal thyroid function may be associated with changes in muscle mass, and hence in total body potassium content. Serum potassium concentration is often lower than normal in patients with hyperthyroidism. Rarely, hypokalemic periodic paralysis occurs in thyrotoxic men, especially those of Asian or Latin-American origin.

Administration of growth hormone induces a positive nitrogen balance and could potentially affect extrarenal potassium uptake. It has not been determined whether this effect occurs with physiologic levels of the hormone. Serum and urinary potassium may increase if glucocorticoids are given rapidly as a bolus, suggesting a catabolic effect of steroids resulting in release of potassium from muscle. A specific effect of glucagon on extrarenal potassium metabolism has been difficult to demonstrate because the hormone also influences the secretion of insulin and catecholamines.

Increases in parathyroid hormone (PTH) worsen and calcium channel blockers improve tolerance to exogenous potassium loads in humans and in experimental animals. This effect of PTH is probably related to its ability to increase intracellular calcium, which is known to enhance potassium permeability *in vitro* in many cells, leading to potassium efflux. Indeed, excess PTH exaggerates hyperkalemia following a potassium load, and parathyroidectomy improves potassium tolerance in rats with chronic renal failure. Calcium channel blockers can reduce aldosterone production *in vitro,* but it has not been always possible to demonstrate an effect *in vivo.* Minor decreases in serum potassium levels have been observed in patients taking calcium channel blockers for hypertension. Of interest, magnesium deficiency is often associated with potassium deficiency, and the latter is not easily corrected until magnesium stores are replete. Although renal mechanisms are primarily involved in the generation of potassium deficits, magnesium deficiency reduces Na^+-K^+-ATPase activity and may inhibit the opening of ATP-sensitive potassium channels, thus affecting extrarenal potassium metabolism.

Metabolic and Respiratory Alkalosis

In metabolic disturbances of acid–base homeostasis, the concentration of potassium in plasma parallels the concentration of hydrogen ions, so acidosis is usually associated with increases and alkalosis with decreases in serum potassium levels. The explanation generally given for this observation is that during acidemia, intracellular buffering of hydrogen ions is accompanied by exit of potassium out of cells, whereas the reverse occurs during alkalemia. Nevertheless, a simple reciprocal exchange of hydrogen and potassium has not been described in muscle cells. Acidosis may directly or indirectly inhibit the activity of the Na^+-K^+-ATPase, reducing the uptake of potassium by cells. In addition to the effect of hydrogen ions, potassium fluxes are influenced by other numerous factors, including bicarbonate levels, the nature of the anion accompanying hydrogen ions, and the associated hormonal changes. Finally, acid–base disorders also influence external balance. Therefore it is difficult to design formulas that would accurately predict the associated changes in serum potassium concentration in the different acid–base disorders.

It is generally accepted that acute respiratory alkalosis results in minor changes in serum potassium concentration. Studies in humans during voluntary hyperventilation have shown both increases and decreases in serum potassium levels. For example, the plasma potassium response to hypocapnic hypocarbonatemic hyperventilation was compared with time control, isocapnic, and isobicarbonatemic hyperventilation; the former resulted in a signficant increase in plasma potassium and catecholamine concentrations. During recovery, a ventilation rate–dependent hypokalemic overshoot was observed. α-Adrenergic blockade obliterated the hyperkalemic response, whereas β-adrenergic blockade further increased the potassium levels. The hyperkalemia and catecholamine response did not occur during hypocapnic isocarbonatemic hyperventilation, suggesting that they were induced by the decrease in bicarbonate levels.

Production of metabolic alkalosis by infusion of sodium bicarbonate into nephrectomized animals results in modest decreases in serum potassium concentration, suggesting an effect on transcellular potassium distribution. In patients receiving dialysis who have modest acidemia, isotonic sodium bicarbonate infusion results in a decrease in serum potassium, but only 3 to 4 hours after the beginning of the infusion. These changes are not observed after infusions of isotonic saline or administration of a bolus of hypertonic sodium bicarbonate. As mentioned, several human and animal studies suggest that internal potassium balance is influenced by changes in serum bicarbonate even when ECF pH remains constant. An important effect of bicarbonate on internal potassium balance is also suggested by the observation that major changes in blood pH associated with respiratory disorders result in a very small movement of potassium across cell membranes. Chronic metabolic alkalosis is usually associated with hypokalemia, primarily because of an increase in urinary potassium excretion.

Anabolic States

Potassium shifts into rapidly proliferating cells may cause mild to severe hypokalemia in several hematologic diseases. Examples include acute leukemia and high-grade lymphomas, treatment of pernicious anemia with vitamin B_{12}, administration of granulocyte-macrophage colony-stimulating factor, and transfusions with large amounts of potassium-deficient frozen, washed, red blood cells.

By virtue of its anabolic effect, intravenous hyperalimentation could result in redistribution of potassium into cells. As mentioned, similar changes may take place during the administration of growth hormone. Recovery from hypothermia may be associated with increases in cellular potassium uptake and transient hypokalemia.

Periodic Paralysis

Hypokalemic periodic paralysis is an autosomal-dominant disorder characterized by episodic attacks of muscle weakness associated with hypokalemia. Symptoms begin during adolescence and are triggered by exercise, large carbohydrate meals, and medications such as insulin or epinephrine. Sporadic cases may occur, and they may be associated with thyrotoxicosis. Acute correction of the hypokalemia promptly improves the weakness and the frequency and severity of attacks are decreased by potassium, potassium-sparing diuretics, acetazolamide, and ammonium chloride. The only genetic abnormality described in these patients is in the gene encoding the α_1 subunit of the so-called L-type calcium channel, or voltage-gated dihydropyridine receptor.

Drugs/Intoxications

Poisoning with soluble barium salts may result in severe weakness and hypokalemia. Experimental studies have shown that infusions of barium chloride result in rapid decreases, followed by stabilization of serum potassium levels. Because renal potassium excretion does not increase, the effect must be caused by increased cellular uptake. In skeletal muscle, barium reduces potassium conductance because of competitive binding of barium to potassium channels. Blocking potassium efflux from cells leads to rapidly developing hypokalemia because of the unopposed ongoing activity of the sodium pump. The hypokalemia associated with chloroquine poisoning may also result from a block in potassium channels. Table 16.2 shows some of the drugs that may cause potassium shifts into cells.

CAUSES OF INCREASED POTASSIUM SHIFT OUT OF CELLS (Table 16.1)

Hormones

α-Adrenergic Stimulation

Pure α-adrenergic agonists such as phenylephrine impair potassium tolerance, an effect that is blocked by phentolamine. This effect is responsible for the *transient* increase in serum potassium after epinephrine administration and contributes to the impaired potassium tolerance in patients with chronic renal

TABLE 16.2. Drugs that Influence Extrarenal Potassium Homeostasis

K^+ Shifts into Cells	K^+ Shifts out of Cells
Albuterol, terbutaline, ritodrine	Propranolol (butoxamine)
Phentolamine	Phenylephrine
Theophylline*	Succinylcholine
Insulin	Digitalis*
Bicarbonate	Acidifying agents
Mineralocorticoids¶	Drugs that may cause: Malignant hyperthermia, muscle necrosis, hemolysis, and tumor lysis syndrome
Chloroquine*	Hypertonic, solutions
Calcium antagonists†	Glucocorticoids‡
Metroclopramide‡	Lithium,* Fluoride*
Dobutamine‡	
Hematinics	
Anabolic agents	

*Toxic doses.
†Slight effect.
‡Acute intravenous administration.
§Especially in patients with muscle disease.
¶Conflicting experimental results.

failure. In addition, increased α-adrenergic stimulation may help mitigate the expected fall in serum potassium concentration in potassium depletion and in clinical conditions associated with simultaneous α and β stimulation.

As mentioned, β-adrenergic blockade results in slight increases in serum potassium levels. The increases may be more marked in patients with impaired renal excretion of potassium caused by chronic renal failure or aldosterone deficiency. Strenuous exercise may cause release of potassium from muscle and hyperkalemia. During exercise, β-blockade induces greater increments in serum potassium levels than does exercise alone. Therefore cardioselective β_1-adrenergic blockers rather than nonselective β-antagonists should be used in patients with impaired renal excretion of potassium or those undergoing strenuous exercise.

Parathyroid Hormone

Several studies have shown that the increase in intracellular calcium induced by PTH enhances potassium efflux from cells. Hyperparathyroidism has been shown to impair potassium tolerance in patients with chronic renal failure, and the abnormality is improved by calcium channel blockers and by parathyroidectomy. Increased PTH levels also interfere with insulin release by the pancreas (see Chapter 74, Part 1), and this effect probably contributes to the impairment of potassium tolerance in patients with chronic renal failure. It may be prudent to take into consideration the severity of secondary hyperparathyroidism when prescribing potassium intake to patients with chronic renal failure.

Metabolic and Respiratory Acidosis

It must be emphasized that a fall in pH does not necessarily translate into a predictable rise in serum potassium. Acute respiratory acidosis is associated with very small incremental increases in serum potassium concentration, probably because carbon dioxide diffuses freely into cells. More severe respiratory acidosis, especially of more than 2 hours' duration, may result in more pronounced increases in potassium levels. Chronic respiratory acidosis in experimental animals is not associated with hyperkalemia.

The effects of metabolic acidosis on serum potassium concentration depend on the type of acidosis, its duration, the presence of prior total body potassium depletion, and associated complications such as renal failure and hypercatabolism. Acute "mineral acidosis" induced by infusing hydrochloric acid or ammonium chloride results in variable increases in potassium levels. Arginine or lysine hydrochloride in doses used for the treatment of metabolic alkalosis enhance potassium efflux from cells and may produce hyperkalemia, especially in patients with compromised renal function.

On the other hand, acute infusion of organic acids produces little or no increase in serum potassium. In organic acidoses, the anions of organic acids are transported into cells or are formed within cells, minimizing the need for potassium to leave the cells in exchange for hydrogen ions. In clinical states of organic acidosis, other factors may come into play. For example, ketonemia stimulates insulin release by the pancreas, and the sympathetic nervous system is activated in severe lactic or diabetic acidosis. The latter is often accompanied by potassium depletion, but serum potassium is usually normal or elevated at presentation because of the associated insulin deficiency, hypercatabolism, decreased glomerular filtration rate, and hyperosmolality.

Increases in plasma osmolality may cause modest increases in serum potassium levels. The release of potassium from cells has been attributed to the increased intracellular concentration of potassium due to cellular dehydration and to solvent drag. This phenomenon assumes clinical importance in insulin-deficient diabetic patients with hypoaldosteronism and/or renal failure. In this setting, administration of boluses of hypertonic glucose for the treatment of presumed hypoglycemia may result in severe hyperkalemia.

Cell Necrosis and Catabolism

Release of potassium from the intracellular compartment may occur in catabolic states and in conditions associated with cell necrosis. Clinically, significant hyperkalemia may occur when renal and/or extrarenal potassium homeostasis is also compromised. Catabolic states include sepsis, trauma, fractures, burns, and major surgery.

Tumor lysis syndrome usually occurs after chemotherapy for acute leukemia and high-grade lymphomas, especially Burkitt's lymphoma. It is often associated with hyperphosphatemia and hyperuricemia. Rhabdomyolysis can result in massive release of potassium from muscle. Life-threatening hyperkalemia may ensue rapidly when renal function is impaired. Intravascular hemolysis resulting from congenital or acquired hemolytic anemias and transfusion reactions may also cause transient elevations of serum potassium levels. Likewise, absorption of potassium from large hematomas or from blood in the gastrointestinal tract may cause hyperkalemia.

Periodic Paralysis

Hyperkalemic periodic paralysis is a rare autosomal-dominant disease characterized by sporadic attacks of weakness triggered by exercise, exposure to cold, or ingestion of large amounts of potassium. A defect in the skeletal muscle sodium channel α subunit has been demonstrated in patients with this disorder. The increase in the sodium content of cells would be expected to change the electric gradient across the membrane, thus favoring the efflux of potassium. Inhalation of albuterol has been introduced for the treatment and prevention of attacks.

Drugs/Intoxications

Hyperkalemia caused by inhibition of the Na^+-K^+-ATPase may occur in severe intoxications with substances such as digitalis or oleander tea. Impaired uptake of potassium by cells may be the cause of hyperkalemia in fluoride poisoning.

The syndrome of malignant hyperthermia after general anesthesia is postulated to result from increased levels of intracellular calcium, accelerated metabolism, and ATP depletion. The latter presumably impairs the sodium pump, resulting in an enhanced efflux of potassium from cells. In patients with an inherited predispostion for the development of this syndrome, the administration of dantrolene and the avoidance of triggering agents and stress is indicated. In large doses, depolarizing muscle relaxants such as succinylcholine may cause substantial increases in serum potassium concentration, especially in patients with renal failure. Massive release of potassium from muscle has been noted in patients with tetanus and other neuromuscular diseases. Other drugs that may cause a shift of potassium out of cells are listed in Table 16.2.

EXTRARENAL POTASSIUM HOMEOSTASIS IN CHRONIC RENAL FAILURE

In chronic renal failure, renal potassium homeostasis is maintained by an increase in potassium excretion per nephron. This adaptive mechanism is due in part to increased activity of Na^+-K^+-ATPase in the distal nephron. Enhanced colonic secretion of potassium mediated by aldosterone, and perhaps upregulation of angiotensin II receptors, also contributes to maintain external balance. Despite these adaptive mechanisms, the diseased kidney has little reserve with which to respond to an acute potassium load. The load could be disposed of initially by shifting potassium intracellularly. Nevertheless, available evidence suggests that a defect in internal potassium homeostasis is also present in these patients. Thus retention of potassium in the ECF is temporarily prolonged, which may increase the sensor-effector element of the control system until balance is restored, usually within 24 hours.

Extrarenal potassium homeostasis has been evaluated in humans and in experimental animals with chronic renal failure. In rats with chronic renal failure, several studies have shown impaired potassium tolerance, especially in animals consuming a high-potassium diet. On the other hand, a similar defect could not be demonstrated in uremic dogs receiving an acute potassium load. In patients with moderate renal insufficiency, potassium tolerance is normal. Internal potassium balance is abnormal, however, in patients who have end-stage renal disease and are receiving maintenance dialysis. Thus potassium supplements should be administered with extreme caution to these patients. The defect in these patients is not caused by increased intracellular potassium content because both total body potassium and intracellular potassium are decreased in uremia. Therefore it appears that impaired cellular potassium uptake is responsible for the aforementioned abnormality.

Several abnormalities in uremia might be responsible for the impaired extrarenal potassium homeostasis (Table 16.3). Resistance to insulin-mediated potassium uptake is not present in uremia. Nevertheless, insulinopenia induced by fasting may contribute to the fasting hyperkalemia observed in dialysis patients. This abnormality can be prevented by the administration of glucose/insulin in physiologic doses. On the other hand, uremic patients are resistant to the hypokalemic effect of epinephrine. Although a subset of dialysis patients are refractory to the hypokalemic effects of β_2-agonists, most patients respond to these agents and their effect is additive to that of insulin. Other studies indicate that the resistance to the potassium-lowering effect of epinephrine in dialysis patients is due primarily to an enhanced α-adrenergic response.

The role of mineralocorticoids in extrarenal potassium homeostasis has been investigated in humans and in experimental animals. In anephric patients treated with DOCA, spironolactone, or placebo, baseline serum potassium levels were similar. However, DOCA-treated patients exhibited an improved tolerance to potassium loads. Studies in experimental animals also suggest that administration of mineralocorticoids helps improve potassium tolerance. Secondary hyperparathyroidism has been shown to impair extrarenal potassium disposal as a result of an increase in intracellular calcium, leading to increased potassium efflux from cells and by inhibiting both glucose and potassium-stimulated insulin secretion, which leads to a decrease in calcium uptake by cells. Calcium channel blockers have been shown to ameliorate this abnormality. Other factors that may contribute to the potassium intolerance associated with uremia include metabolic acidosis and hyperosmolality. The latter may occur in decompensated diabetes, especially after administration of hypertonic glucose, and in patients receiving hypertonic saline or bicarbonate. Finally, the potassium intolerance in these patients can be attributed in part to the suppression of Na^+-K^+-ATPase activity associated with uremia.

TABLE 16.3. Factors that May Account for the Impaired Cellular K^+ Uptake in Chronic Renal Failure (CRF)

Factor	Defect in CRF	Clinical Relevance
Insulin	Increased levels, normal effect	Fasting may cause hyperkalemia in CRF; hypokalemic effect is additive to that of β_2-agonists
Catecholamines	Increased levels, decreased or increased effects	
β_2-Agonists	Decreased effect†	Cardioselective antagonists should be used in CRF; can be used to treat hyperkalemia
α-Agonists	Increased effect	May contribute to hyperkalemia especially after fasting or exercise
Aldosterone*	Variable levels	Contributes to renal and extrarenal balance; low levels or resistance may cause hyperkalemia
Parathyroid hormone	Increased levels	Calcium channel blockers have very little effect on serum K^+; parathyroidectomy may improve K^+ tolerance
Blood pH, HCO_3	Acidosis	Hypertonic HCO_3 does not correct hyperkalemia acutely
Osmolality	Increased (tonicity is normal)	Hyperglycemia may contribute to hyperkalemia in diabetes
Na^+-K^+-ATPase	Decreased activity	May contribute to decreased cellular uptake of K^+

*There is conflicting experimental evidence regarding the effect on extrarenal balance. Mineralocorticoid administration improves and spironolactone impairs potassium tolerance in dialysis patients.

†20%–40% of CRF patients receiving dialysis are resistant to the potassium-lowering effect of albuterol.

Selected Readings

Allon M. Hyperkalemia in end-stage renal disease: mechanisms and management. *J Am Soc Nephrol* 1995;6:1134–1142.

Review of the treatment of hyperkalemia in end-stage renal disease with emphasis on the effect of insulin and β_2-agonists and the lack of effectiveness of bicarbonate.

Antes LM, Kujubu DA, Fernandez PC. Hypokalemia and the pathology ion transport molecules. *Semin Nephrol* 1998;18:31–45.

A contemporary review of potassium channels and their abnormalities in cases of periodic paralysis and barium poisoning.

Bia MJ, DeFronzo RA. Extrarenal potassium homeostasis. *Am J Physiol* 1981;240: F257–F268.

A comprehensive review of extrarenal potassium homeostasis.

Brown RS. Extrarenal potassium homeostasis. *Kidney Int* 1986;30:116–127.

Presentation of a case and discussion of the determinants of extrarenal potassium metabolism.

Conte G, Canton AD, Imperatore P, et al. Acute increase in plasma osmolality as a cause of hyperkalemia in patients with renal failure. *Kidney Int* 1990; 38:301–307.

Shows that an increase in serum potassium correlates with elevation of plasma osmolality.

Epstein FH, Rosa RM. Adrenergic control of serum potassium. *N Engl J Med* 1983; 23:1450–1451.

Editorial review of clinical aspects of α- and β-adrenergic control of potassium balance.

Fernandez J, Oster JR, Perez GO. Impaired extrarenal disposal of an acute oral potassium load in patients with end stage renal disease on chronic hemodialysis. *Mineral Electrolyte Metab* 1986;12:125–129.

A study showing impaired extrarenal mechanisms of potassium disposal in patients receiving maintenance hemodialysis.

Perez GO, Oster JR, Vaamonde CA. Serum potassium concentration in acidemic states. *Nephron* 1981;27:233–243.

Detailed review of experimental and clinical studies on hyperkalemia and acidosis, emphasizing that hyperkalemia is not expected in organic acidosis and, if present, usually indicates complicating circumstances.

Spital A, Stern RH. Extrarenal potassium adaptation: review of a concept. *Am J Nephrol* 1995;15:367–373.

A reexamination of studies suggesting a nonrenal mechanism of potassium adaptation. The authors believe the prior potassium depletion is the cause of the enhanced potassium tolerance found in potassium-adapted animals.

Sterns RH, Cox M, Feig PU, Singer I. Internal potassium balance and the control of the plasma potassium concentration. *Medicine (Baltimore)* 1981;60:339–354.

Lengthy review of pathophysiologic processes affecting internal potassium homeostasis, emphasizing the relationship to external potassium balance.

PART 3
Dyskalemias

Richard L. Tannen

Potassium is located predominantly in the intracellular compartment, at a concentration of approximately 150 mEq/L under normal conditions. Total body potassium averages 58 mEq/kg in young adult males and 25% less in females. It decreases progressively with age because of a decrease in the ratio of muscle to fat and is approximately 20% lower in elderly individuals. *Potassium depletion* or *deficiency* refers to a loss of potassium that results in a decrease in intracellular potassium concentration. A decrease in total body potassium stores paralleled by a decrease in muscle mass (so that potassium concentration in the intracellular compartment is unaltered) does not represent potassium depletion.

Normal serum potassium concentration ranges from 3.5 to 5.0 mEq/L. *Hypokalemia* signifies a decrease below the normal range, whereas *hyperkalemia* refers to a serum potassium concentration above normal. In view of the trivial percentage of total body potassium located in the plasma compartment (approximately 0.4%), it is obvious that changes in serum (or plasma) potassium concentration need not reflect alterations in body potassium stores. Indeed, many factors can influence the distribution of potassium between the extracellular and intracellular compartments, thereby provoking hypokalemia or hyperkalemia without changes in body potassium stores (see Chapter 16, Part 2). On the other hand, pure potassium depletion in the absence of factors that alter transcellular potassium distribution is accompanied by hypokalemia. A close correlation exists between the magnitude of a potassium deficit and the fall in serum potassium concentration (Fig. 16.17, in Part 2 of this chapter). Over the range depicted, each 350-mEq deficit in potassium results in a decrement in serum potassium concentration of about 1 mEq/L. Precise data defining the relationship between potassium retention and hyperkalemia are unavailable. It appears that a 200 mEq or greater excess is required to raise serum potassium concentration by 1.0 mEq/L, but the slope is probably considerably steeper when potassium retention is of greater magnitude.

Daily potassium ingestion is 0.75 to 1.25 mEq/kg on a standard Western-civilization diet. Potassium balance is maintained by the kidney, which excretes approximately 90% of the ingested potassium and alters the excretory rate in response to the quantity of potassium ingested. Relatively normal potassium balance can be maintained with potassium intake varying from as low as 20 to 30 mEq/day to as high as 700 mEq/day. The normal kidney, aided by the endocrine system, can display multiple acute and very effective chronic adaptive mechanisms that permit these wide variations in excretory rates (see Chapter 16, Part 1).

HYPOKALEMIA

Clinical Sequelae

Hypokalemia results from an alteration in the transcellular distribution of potassium and/or from actual potassium depletion. Symptoms results from the increased ratio between intracellular and extracellular potassium concentration, which modifies membrane polarization and thereby alters the function of excitable tissues, including both nerve and muscle. A decrease in intracellular potassium concentration per se may also account for some of the manifestations of potassium depletion.

Mild hypokalemia (serum potassium between 3.0 and 3.5 mEq/L with a potassium deficit of 150 to 350 mEq) is often completely asymptomatic. Some patients may exhibit fatigue, weakness, muscle cramps, and rarely, myalgia. The most serious effects pertain to the heart. Digitalis toxicity can be provoked in patients treated with cardiac glycosides; there is an increased risk of ventricular arrhythmias, especially in patients with underlying heart disease, and the incidence of ventricular tachycardia or fibrillation is increased in patients who sustain an acute myocardial infarction. Mild glucose intolerance secondary to impaired pancreatic insulin release is commonly found with this degree of potassium depletion, and blood pressure is increased in both normotensive and hypertensive individuals.

Moderate depletion (serum potassium between 2.5 and 3.0 mEq/L with a deficit of 350 to 550 mEq) can result in rhabdomyolysis, in part because of the absence of exercise-induced vasodilation. Reduced gastrointestinal tract motility results in constipation; polyuria and polydipsia reflect a defect in renal concentrating ability. Encephalopathy can be provoked in patients with underlying hepatic disease as a result of a potassium-induced increase in renal ammonia production. Most patients with a serum potassium of less than 3.0 mEq/L will manifest electrocardiogram (ECG) changes typical of hypokalemia. These changes include a flattened T wave, a depressed ST segment, and the appearance of prominent U waves. Although these changes are indicative of potassium depletion, they do not signal a cardiac abnormality of clinical importance. Severe potassium depletion (serum potassium of less than 2.5 mEq/L and a potassium deficit of more than 550 mEq) can result in ileus. There is a risk of muscular paralysis with life-threatening respiratory insufficiency. Metabolic alkalosis and renal chloride wasting are also consequences of severe depletion. Longstanding severe potassium depletion can result in interstitial nephritis and rarely may lead to chronic renal failure. It also can impair growth.

Hypokalemic Nephropathy

Hypokalemic nephropathy is a term used to describe the abnormalities in renal structure and function associated with potassium depletion. The severity of the renal derangements depends on the duration and degree of the potassium depletion.

Structural Derangements

Potassium depletion is associated with structural changes in the kidneys of rats, mice, hamsters, gerbils, and humans, but not of dogs. The changes in animals appear to differ from those seen in humans.

In animals, potassium depletion is accompanied by striking renal hypertrophy. The histologic lesion, which is located primarily in the medulla, consists of two components: (a) With light microscopy, there are lesions that predominantly involve the medullary collecting duct and consist of a proliferative process with swelling, hyperplasia, and cytoplasmic granulation. Electron microscopic and morphometric analysis reveal hypertrophy and hyperplasia of both the principal and intercalated cells of the outer medullary collecting duct. However, the increase in apical and basolateral membrane area is much more striking in intercalated cells, which correlates with functional data suggesting that these cells exhibit increased potassium reabsorption and proton secretion via a luminal H^+-K^+-ATPase. (b) The second type of morphologic abnormality consists of distinctive periodic acid–Schiff positive droplets located in the medullary collecting duct epithelium and in medullary endothelial and interstitial cells. On electron microscopic examination, these droplets are multivesicular bodies surrounded by a single membrane and contain many membranous structures; they are cytoplasmic structures and not of mitochondrial origin.

These renal lesions are reversible with potassium repletion; however, when K^+ depletion is prolonged, permanent changes with interstitial scarring, glomerular sclerosis, and tubular dilation can result.

The renal lesions of potassium deficiency in humans differ from those in animals both in location and in appearance. The changes are seen primarily in the proximal tubule but may be noted in the distal convoluted tubule as well. There is intracellular vacuolization of the tubular epithelial cells, and the vacuoles may fill the cells, giving them a foamy appearance. The vacuoles may also be extracellular, located in between adjacent cells, but this cell separation stops at the tight junctions. The vacuolization may be severe, mild, or even absent in more than 50% of patients. In a few patients, droplet lesions of the medulla were noted; however, the amount of human material available for detailed medullary study is limited. The vacuolar changes of the tubular epithelium are reversible, as documented by repeat renal biopsies obtained from four patients during potassium depletion and several months after repletion. However, when potassium depletion is severe and prolonged, interstitial scarring, infiltration with lymphocytes, and tubular atrophy can occur. It has been suggested that this chronic interstitial nephritis might be secondary to either hypertensive disease or bacterial infection; however, the evidence points more strongly to a potassium-induced phenomenon. Chronic potassium depletion also predisposes patients to the development of renal cysts.

Functional Derangements

Potassium depletion can produce renal vasoconstriction with a reduction in renal blood flow in both animals and humans. Studies in the rat suggest that renal vasoconstriction is mediated both by vasoconstrictor prostaglandins and by increased levels of angiotensin II. Glomerular filtration rate (GFR) is also sometimes reduced. In humans, a fall in GFR appears to require severe and prolonged potassium depletion, and as in animals, GFR returns to normal with potassium repletion. However, severe, prolonged potassium depletion can produce chronic interstitial nephritis with permanent impairment of GFR, which occasionally is of sufficient degree to result in severe chronic renal failure.

A variety of alterations in renal tubular function accompany potassium depletion. There is an adaptation in the renal capacity to conserve potassium, which decreases urinary potassium excretion to less than 10 mEq/day. This adaptive phenomenon is reflected by a decrease in potassium secretion along with enhanced potassium reabsorption at distal nephron sites, which appears to be mediated by increased activity of H^+-K^+ -ATPase.

Sodium retention, of sufficient degree to expand the extracellular fluid space, accompanies even modest potassium depletion. The precise mechanism has not been elucidated. Renal chloride wasting occurs with severe potassium depletion. The defect in chloride reabsorption can involve the entire nephron but is most pronounced in the thick ascending limb and distal nephron, where it is accompanied by decreased expression of both Na-K-2Cl and NaCl cotransporters, respectively.

Potassium depletion can cause metabolic alkalosis in humans, as well as in rats. The propensity for humans to develop metabolic alkalosis is dramatically accentuated by a diet low in NaCl. By contrast, dogs develop metabolic acidosis mediated by the hypokalemia-induced decrease in plasma aldosterone. Factors that appear to account for the development and maintenance of metabolic alkalosis include a reduction in GFR, enhanced bicarbonate reabsorption by the proximal tubule, enhanced proton secretion by the collecting duct mediated by an increase in H^+-K^+-ATPase, and an increase in renal ammonia production. The defect in chloride reabsorption might also play a role.

The potassium depletion–induced increase in renal ammonia production exhibits a biochemical profile that is virtually identical to the changes seen with adaptation to chronic metabolic acidosis. Both phenomena may, in fact, be mediated by a persistent decrease in the intracellular pH of proximal tubular epithelium. However, there are some subtle differences in these two conditions, especially related to alterations in the activity of phosphate-dependent glutaminase, which raise the possibility that the potassium depletion–induced changes may involve more than the consequence of a decreased proximal tubular intracellular pH.

The increase in renal ammonia production accounts for the elevated urine pH observed with states of potassium depletion. Although it also has been suggested that the high urine pH under conditions of an acidifying stimulus might reflect a defect in proton transport, there is no convincing evidence to support this view.

Hypercalciuria, which is dependent on sodium retention, occurs with mild potassium depletion. The hypercalciuria is accompanied by hyperphosphaturia and increased 1-25-$(OH)_2$-D and parathyroid hormone (PTH) levels, presumably in response to a slight decrease in plasma calcium levels. These alterations in calcium homeostasis may predispose patients to renal nephrolithiasis and osteoporosis.

An impairment in urinary concentrating ability is perhaps the most consistent abnormality in renal function during potassium depletion. It is demonstrable in humans with potassium depletion of as little as approximately 250 mEq (i.e., a 6% to 7% deficit) and is completely reversible with K^+ repletion. Polyuria, which results from both the concentrating defect along with a potassium depletion–mediated stimulation of thirst, sometimes provides a clinical clue as to the presence of potassium deficiency. Although the renal concentrating defect has been appreciated for decades, the underlying mechanism has not been resolved definitively. Medullary tonicity is clearly decreased, which might result from a defect in chloride transport by the thick ascending limb, reduced delivery of filtrate to Henle's loop, impaired accumulation of medullary osmolytes secondary (in part because of a decrease in aldolase reductase), an increase in medullary blood flow, or some combination thereof. A defect in water transport by the collecting duct mediated by decreased expression of the aquaporin-2 water channel, also may contribute to the abnormality in urinary concentration. Abnormal vasopressin-mediated cyclic adenosine 3′,5′-monophosphate (cAMP) generation and also increased prostaglandins, which impair the hydrostatic effect of antidiuretic hormone (ADH), have been implicated as possible factors. In contrast to the defect in concentrating ability, urinary dilution is usually normal, except with very severe potassium depletion.

Hypokalemia without Potassium Depletion (Transcellular Redistribution)

Clinically significant hypokalemia without potassium depletion can be provoked by various factors that enhance net cellular potassium uptake. Although many of these phenomena are transient and do not require specific therapy, their recognition is important for diagnostic purposes, and in some circumstances (e.g., cardiac-related manifestations), therapeutic intervention may be appropriate. The identified causes of redistribution-mediated hypokalemia and the underlying mechanisms of the fall in serum potassium are listed in Table 16.4. This issue is discussed in detail in Part 2 of this chapter.

Hypokalemic periodic paralysis is a rare hereditary disorder with autosomal-dominant transmission. It is characterized by recurrent attacks of flaccid paralysis in association with a decline in serum potassium, usually to less than 3.0 mEq/L.

A mutation in the dihydropyridine (DHP) receptor gene, which functions as a voltage-gated calcium channel, accounts for the disorder, but the mechanism whereby it produces hypokalemia has not been elucidated. Acetazolamide is useful in eliminating attacks and in improving interattack weakness. Patients with thyrotoxicosis can develop episodes of periodic paralysis indistinguishable from the hereditary disease. Unlike the familial disease, the paralytic episodes in thyrotoxicosis are improved by therapy with β-blockers. The illness remits with adequate therapy of the thyrotoxicosis.

Hypokalemia with Potassium Depletion

It is useful to subdivide disorders resulting in hypokalemia and potassium depletion into those in which the deficit of potassium is based on extrarenal losses and those in which renal potassium losses are the primary cause. With potassium depletion of extrarenal cause, the kidney responds in an appropriate fashion to conserve potassium. Daily urinary potassium excretion is typically less than 20 mEq, while a spot urine potassium-to-creatinine ratio of less than 20 mEq/g and fractional excretion of less than 6% can be anticipated.

By contrast, when renal potassium loss accounts for the development of potassium depletion and the abnormality is still present at the time of evaluation, urinary values will exceed the guidelines that indicate appropriate renal potassium conservation.

TABLE 16.4. Hypokalemia Secondary to Transcellular Redistribution

Cause	Potential Mechanisms
Alkalemia	Stimulation of Na^+-K^+ pump
High plasma bicarbonate	Stimulation of Na^+-K^+ pump
Excess insulin (endogenous or exogenous)	Stimulation of Na^+-K^+ pump
β-Adrenergic agonists (e.g., salbutamol, terbutaline)	cAMP-dependent stimulation of Na^+-K^+ pump
Acute illiness (e.g., myocardial infarct, head injury, delirium tremens)	Catecholamine-mediated stimulation of Na^+-K^+ pump
Barium intoxication	Blockade of potassium channels
Acute chloroquine intoxication	Blockade of potassium channels
Toluene intoxication	?
Theophylline intoxication	Catecholamine, insulin, or direct cAMP stimulation of Na^+-K^+ pump
Hypokalemic periodic paralysis	?
hereditary	Mutated DHP receptor
thyrotoxicosis	Increased Na^+-K^+ ATPase
? Calcium channel blockade	Inhibition of calcium-activated potassium channel

cAMP, cyclic adenosine monophosphate.

Extrarenal Causes of Hypokalemia and Potassium Depletion (Table 16.5)

Severe dietary potassium restriction can result in potassium depletion, but the degree is mild as long as there are no accompanying abnormal losses of potassium. Thus the rare elderly patient consuming a "tea and toast" diet or the younger individual with anorexia nervosa can present with potassium depletion caused by dietary restriction, but abnormal losses of potassium should be sought, especially in the anorexic patient, who may simultaneously be vomiting or abusing laxatives and diuretics. Under circumstances of rapid cellular proliferation, potassium intake may be insufficient to meet the anabolic demand; this phenomenon has been described during the correction of severe megaloblastic and iron deficiency anemias, and supplemental potassium therapy may be required in these instances.

Intense physical conditioning in a hot climate can result in potassium depletion secondary to enormous losses of potassium

TABLE 16.5. Extrarenal Causes of Hypokalemia and Potassium Depletion

Inadequate potassium intake—absolute or relative
Copious sweat losses
Gastrointestinal tract losses
Geophagia
Laxative abuse
Villous adenoma of rectum
Diarrhea
Ureterosigmoidostomy

in sweat. Potassium depletion in this setting is unusual because serum potassium levels are normal and urinary excretion rates high, despite severe intracellular potassium deficits. Potassium depletion predisposes these individuals to the development of rhabdomyolysis and pathologic hyperthermia.

By far, the predominant cause of extrarenal potassium depletion is gastrointestinal tract losses, with diarrheal illnesses predominating. Most patients with diarrhea also have hyperchloremic metabolic acidosis concurrent with potassium depletion, although more rarely, the secretory diarrheas (e.g., gastrin and histamine-mediated hypersecretion), which cause massive chloride losses, can present with metabolic alkalosis. A rare cause of intestinal potassium loss is villous adenoma of the rectum, with a copious secretion high in potassium content. Individuals with ureterosigmoidostomies are subject to potassium depletion because of the potassium-secretory properties of the colon, and typically, they also develop metabolic acidosis. An uncommon, but important, cause of potassium depletion is chronic laxative abuse. These individuals typically deny laxative ingestion. They usually have a normal acid–base picture and potassium depletion associated with appropriate renal conservation, unless they are simultaneously abusing diuretics or surreptitiously vomiting. Identification of phenolphthalein in the stool or urine, by development of a pink color on alkalinization with sodium hydroxide, or the finding of melanosis coli on proctoscopy can help confirm the diagnosis.

Renal Causes of Hypokalemia and Potassium Depletion

Many disorders are associated with renal potassium losses and lead to hypokalemia and potassium depletion. These disorders may present with metabolic acidosis or with normal blood pH or metabolic alkalosis (Table 16.6). Hypokalemic patients with metabolic acidosis are usually normotensive; hypokalemic patients with normal pH or metabolic alkalosis either are normotensive or have high blood pressure.

Disorders Presenting with Metabolic Acidosis

Because potassium depletion tends to elevate plasma bicarbonate concentration, a presentation in combination with hyperchloremic metabolic acidosis is a helpful diagnostic clue. The renal potassium-wasting disorders that present with metabolic acidosis are distal renal tubular acidosis (RTA) (type I) and proximal renal tubular acidosis (type II). These disorders are discussed in Chapter 20, Part 5. Potassium depletion is a hallmark of distal RTA, but it can also accompany proximal RTA, especially when therapy with sodium bicarbonate is initiated. Potassium wasting in distal RTA may result from the combination of high aldosterone levels and increased distal sodium delivery secondary to the acidosis-mediated inhibition of proximal sodium reabsorption. Carbonic anhydrase inhibitors such as acetazolamide, which produce a drug-induced combination of proximal and distal RTA, also cause potassium depletion.

Patients with diabetic ketoacidosis always have potassium depletion, which results from the osmotic diuretic effect of glycosuria and the high rates of keto anion excretion. Serum potassium levels are often normal at the time of presentation, presumably because the combination of insulin deficiency, acidosis, and hyperosmolality results in a redistribution of potassium from the intracellular to extracellular fluid compartment. Initiation of insulin therapy promotes a dramatic fall in serum potassium levels, and adequate potassium replacement is an important component of therapy for diabetic ketoacidosis.

Disorders Presenting with a Normal pH or Metabolic Alkalosis

Most disorders that result in potassium depletion from renal losses are accompanied by metabolic alkalosis. One group of conditions causes hypokalemic metabolic alkalosis and typically is *associated with hypertension.* Patients with such conditions have an expanded extracellular volume and therefore do not exhibit renal chloride conservation; that is, urinary chloride excretion exceeds 10 mEq/day and is usually much higher. The hypertensive disorders associated with hypokalemia and potassium depletion encompass a variety of conditions characterized by increased levels of either mineralocorticoid or glucocorticoid hormones. The important points in differential diagnosis of these disorders are given in Table 16.7.

Primary hyperaldosteronism, secondary to an adenoma, hyperplasia, or rarely, carcinoma, is the most common entity with a primary excess of mineralocorticoid hormone. Renal potassium wasting results from increased delivery of sodium and fluid to a distal nephron that is primed by high levels of mineralocorticoid for potassium secretion. The mechanisms through which aldosterone augments potassium secretion in the distal nephron are discussed in Part 1 of this chapter.

Patients with primary aldosteronism have renal potassium wasting, hypokalemia, metabolic alkalosis, and hypertension. The plasma levels of aldosterone are elevated, whereas plasma renin activity is low, resulting in a high aldosterone-to-renin ratio. In patients with severe potassium depletion, plasma aldosterone may not be elevated because aldosterone production may be reduced in potassium depletion. Failure to suppress plasma levels of aldosterone by saline infusion (2 L in 4 hours)

TABLE 16.6. Hypokalemia and Potassium Depletion Secondary to Renal Losses

	Normal pH or Metabolic Alkalosis	
Metabolic Acidosis	Hypertensive	Normotensive

Renal tubular acidosis (RTA)
  Distal RTA (type I)
  Proximal RTA (type II)
  Carbonic anhydrase inhibitors
Diabetic ketoacidosis
	Mineralocorticoid-excess conditions
	  Primary hyperaldosteronism
	  Secondary hyperaldosteronism
	  Exogenous mineralocorticoid
	  Deoxycorticosterone acetate excess
	Cushing's syndrome
	Liddle's syndrome
	11β-hydroxysteroid dehydrogenase (11β-OHSD) deficiency
	  Congenital
	  Acquired (licorice, carbenoxolone, gossypol)
		Chloride-depletion syndrome
		  Vomiting/gastric drainage
		  Diuretic therapy
		Bartter's syndrome
		Gitelman's syndrome
		Magnesium depletion
		Antibiotics/chemotherapeutic drugs (penicillin, aminoglycosides, cisplatin)
		Leukemia

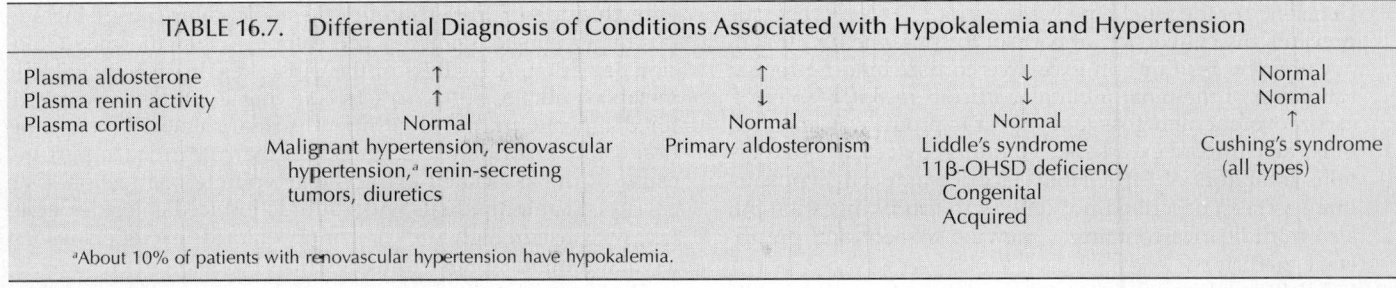

TABLE 16.7. Differential Diagnosis of Conditions Associated with Hypokalemia and Hypertension

Plasma aldosterone	↑	↑	↓	Normal
Plasma renin activity	↑	↓	↓	Normal
Plasma cortisol	Normal	Normal	Normal	↑
	Malignant hypertension, renovascular hypertension,[a] renin-secreting tumors, diuretics	Primary aldosteronism	Liddle's syndrome 11β-OHSD deficiency Congenital Acquired	Cushing's syndrome (all types)

[a]About 10% of patients with renovascular hypertension have hypokalemia.

or by administration of fludrocortisone (Florinef) at 0.2 mg twice a day for 3 days will establish the diagnosis. In normal subjects or patients with other causes of hypertension, the plasma levels of aldosterone will fall to less than 4 ng/dl after saline infusion or fludrocortisone administration. Patients with adrenal adenoma have more severe degrees of hypokalemia and significantly higher plasma levels of aldosterone. Computed tomography, radiolabeled scanning, and adrenal vein catheterization are used for the diagnosis of the tumor responsible for the disease. Magnetic resonance imaging is also very useful. The adenoma is best treated with surgery, whereas the treatment of choice for the hyperplasia is aldosterone antagonist (spironolactone); the latter is effective in reversing the electrolyte disturbances and in controlling the hypertension. Glucocorticoid remediable hyperaldosteronism, a rare autosomal-dominant inherited abnormality diagnosed by dexamethasone suppression or urinary excretion of excessive 18-hydroxy and 18-oxycortisol metabolites, results from a chimeric 11β-hydroxylase/aldosterone synthase gene, which renders aldosterone secretion adrenocorticotropic hormone (ACTH) responsive. These patients, who typically develop severe hypokalemia in response to thiazide diuretics, respond to treatment with low dosages of dexamethasone (0.75 mg/day).

Secondary hyperaldosteronism, commonly related to renal vascular disease that involves either the major renal arteries (renal artery stenosis) or small vessels (malignant hypertension or vasculitides) also results in hypokalemic alkalosis. It is important to appreciate that not all forms of secondary hyperaldosteronism cause potassium depletion. In secondary hyperaldosteronism associated with edematous states, reduced sodium and fluid delivery to the distal nephron counterbalances the stimulation of potassium secretion by the high aldosterone levels. The hypertensive forms of secondary hyperaldosteronism may be distinctive because salt and water delivery distally is sufficient to result in potassium depletion. Hemangiopericytoma (Robertson-Kihara syndrome) is a rare tumor of the juxtaglomerular apparatus. This benign tumor, as well as several nonrenal malignancies, can produce renin and cause secondary aldosteronism. Both plasma renin activity and plasma aldosterone are elevated, and hypokalemia and hypertension are present. Renal vein renin on the side of the tumor is elevated, and renal arteriogram reveals the tumor, whereas patients with extrarenal malignancies exhibit high plasma levels of inactive renin.

Primary and secondary forms of hyperaldosteronism are easily distinguished by measurements of plasma aldosterone and renin levels. Although aldosterone levels are elevated in both, primary aldosteronism is associated with suppressed and secondary aldosteronism with elevated levels of plasma renin activity.

Other mineralocorticoid excess states present with both suppressed renin and aldosterone levels. These include (a) excessive production of deoxycorticosterone (DOC), which occurs with the adrenogenital syndromes caused by 17α-hydroxylase or 11β-hydroxylase deficiencies (therapy with dexamethasone corrects the mineralocorticoid excess syndrome in these two hereditary disorders), and (b) ingestion of mineralocorticoid medication, such as Florinef, or of glucocorticoids, as well as use of topical or intranasal compounds containing 9α-fluoroprednisolone, which can produce a mineralocorticoid excess syndrome.

Two hereditary renal abnormalities that mimic the mineralocorticoid excess state have been defined (Table 16.8). They are as follows:

1. 11β-hydroxysteroid dehydrogenase-2 enzyme deficiency (11β-OHSD-2) accounts for the syndrome previously described as the *apparent mineralocorticoid excess syndrome.*

TABLE 16.8. Molecular Basis of Hereditary Renal Abnormalities of Potassium Handling

Disorder	Type Mutation	Target Gene
Hypokalemic Disorders		
Liddle's syndrome	Gain function	Epithelial Na^+ Channel
11β-OHSD deficiency	Loss function	11β-hydroxysteroid dehydrogenase-2
Bartter's syndrome	Loss function	Bumetanide sensitive Na-K-2Cl cotransporter
	Loss function	ROMK potassium channel
	Loss function	CLCNKB chloride channel
Gitelman's syndrome	Loss function	Thiazide-sensitive Na-Cl cotransporter
Hyperkalemic Disorders		
Pseudohypoaldosteronism		
Type I		
Autosomal-recessive	Loss function	Epithelial Na^+ Channel
Autosomal-dominant	Loss function	Mineralocorticoid receptor gene
Type II	?	Linkage to chromosome 1q31-42 and 17p11-q21 (specific gene still undefined)

Deficiency of the renal type 2 isoform of 11β-OHSD enzyme prevents the conversion of cortisol to cortisone by the kidney, thereby resulting in excessive cortisol binding to and activation of the renal mineralocorticoid receptor. Licorice, carbenoxolone, and gossypol appear to produce an acquired mineralocorticoid excess–like condition by acting as exogenous inhibitors of 11β-OHSD. Licorice-induced hypokalemia has been described not only with candy ingestion but also from licorice-containing chewing tobacco and proprietary medicines.

2. Liddle's syndrome, a rare cause of hypokalemia, results from mutations in the β or γ subunits of the renal epithelial sodium channel, producing constitutive overactivity of this sodium reabsorbing channel. Thus sodium reabsorption by the collecting duct is increased, leading to volume expansion and suppression of plasma renin activity and aldosterone along with hypertension. Increased renal potassium loss occurs in exchange for augmented distal sodium reabsorption and can lead to hypokalemic alkalosis; however, hypokalemia is not detected in all affected individuals. Administration of amiloride or triamterene, which inhibit the epithelial sodium channel, but not spironolactone, reverses the manifestations of this disorder.

Cushing's syndrome, which is characterized by high levels of glucocorticoids, also presents with hypertension, and about 30% of patients manifest hypokalemia. Patients with Cushing's syndrome secondary to ectopic ACTH production have a higher incidence of hypokalemia. Renal potassium wasting could result from glucocorticoid binding to the mineralocorticoid receptors, but the normal renin levels in most patients argue against this hypothesis. Animal studies suggest that high levels of glucocorticoids promote kaliuresis by increasing GFR and fluid delivery to the distal nephron.

Another group of disorders with renal potassium wasting and metabolic alkalosis is *not associated with hypertension.* However, it should be mentioned that hypokalemic alkalosis disorders may occur in patients with an underlying hypertension; under these circumstances, elevated blood pressure will be part of the clinical presentation. The important points for the differential diagnosis of normotensive hypokalemic patients with metabolic acidosis or alkalosis are given in Table 16.9.

The most important cause of hypokalemic alkalosis without hypertension is the *"syndrome of chloride depletion."* This pathophysiologic entity is most commonly induced by chloride losses from the upper gastrointestinal tract secondary to vomiting or gastric drainage or by renal losses secondary to diuretic therapy with thiazide or loop diuretics. Less common causes include posthypercapneic conditions and chloride-losing diarrhea. Chloride depletion, regardless of the cause, results in hypokalemic metabolic alkalosis. A characteristic that is particularly useful for diagnostic purposes is intense urinary chloride conservation. Daily chloride excretion is less than 10 mEq, in part because of the associated extracellular volume contraction. One caveat is that individuals with diuretic-induced chloride depletion will sustain high rates of urinary chloride excretion as long as they continue to take diuretics.

Potassium deficiency develops and is sustained during chloride depletion as a result of urinary potassium losses. Several mechanisms may account for the kaliuresis. Whereas high levels of aldosterone can play a role under some circumstances, as for example with continued diuretic ingestion, they are not required for the development of potassium depletion. Alkalosis promotes a kaliuresis, but its quantitative contribution is undefined. Finally, hypochloremia per se stimulates potassium secretion by the distal nephron, and this may be the predominant cause of inappropriate levels of renal potassium excretion. Another critical aspect of this syndrome is that significant potassium depletion can be corrected only by the provision of potassium in conjunction with chloride. Repair of the chloride deficit is an absolute requirement for correction of potassium depletion. Neither non–chloride-containing potassium salts such as citrate, gluconate, or phosphate nor high-potassium foods (which are also lacking in chloride) correct the potassium deficit. However, the potassium depletion can be corrected with administration potassium-sparing diuretics (spironolactone, triamterene, or amiloride) that directly inhibit potassium secretion by the distal nephron.

Diuretic-induced hypokalemia is probably the most common potassium abnormality encountered in clinical practice. When hypertensive patients are treated with standard doses of thiazides or chlorthalidone, serum potassium concentration decreases by an average of 0.6 mEq/L, whereas with furosemide, the decrement averages 0.3 mEq/L. Declines to levels below 3.0 mEq/L occur rarely (fewer than 5% of patients) and should trigger a concern about factors other than diuretics that might produce potassium depletion. The deficit of potassium with standard doses of diuretics averages 150 to 200 mEq. The degree of hypokalemia and potassium deficiency stabilizes in the first 1 to 2 weeks after initiating diuretic therapy, as long as the clinical situation is unaltered.

Considerable controversy exists regarding the appropriate management of diuretic-induced hypokalemia. Some argue that hypokalemia is usually mild and harmless, that its treat-

TABLE 16.9. Differential Diagnosis of Conditions Associated with Potassium Depletion and Normal Blood Pressure

Plasma bicarbonate	↓		Normal or ↑		↑	
Plasma chloride	↑		Normal or ↓		↓	
	Gastrointestinal Disorders	Renal Disorders	Gastrointestinal Disorders	Renal Disorders	Gastrointestinal Disorders	Renal Disorders
	Diarrhea Villous adenoma[a]	Renal tubular acidosis Acetazolamide Ketoacidosis Ureterosigmoidostomy	Laxative abuse	Magnesium depletion Penicillin Aminoglycosides	Vomiting Nasogastric suction Chloride-losing diarrhea	Bartter's syndrome Gitelman's syndrome Diuretics[b]
Urinary potassium	↓	↑	↓	↑	↑	↑
Urinary chloride	Variable	Variable	Variable	Variable	↓[c]	↑

[a] Villous adenoma sometimes presents with a normal pH or metabolic alkalosis.
[b] When diuretics have been discontinued before evaluation urine chloride will be low.
[c] Severe potassium depletion regardless of etiology can result in urinary chloride wasting and metabolic alkalosis.

ment is costly and has a risk of provoking hyperkalemia, and that routine therapy is therefore not warranted. Others are concerned about the propensity for ventricular arrhythmias both in stable ambulatory patients and after an acute myocardial infarction. In the absence of carefully controlled prospective trials, a definitive answer is unavailable. Most authorities recommend therapy of hypokalemia for all patients taking cardiac glycosides, for the rare patient whose serum potassium declines to less than 3.0 mEq/L, and for patients predisposed to hepatic coma. I also favor potassium maintenance therapy; that is, the maintenance of a normal serum potassium level (a) in patients with underlying cardiac disease, who it appears are at greater risk for potassium-induced ventricular arrhythmias; (b) in patients who develop diuretic-induced glucose intolerance; and (c) as trial therapy in patients who develop symptoms that may be ascribed to hypokalemia.

Adequate potassium maintenance therapy can be provided with KCl at dosages of at least 40 to 60 mEq/day or by the use of the potassium-sparing diuretics triamterene or amiloride. The potassium-sparing diuretics appear to be more effective than KCl in sustaining normal serum potassium levels. An alternative strategy in the therapy of hypertensive patients is to use lower dosages of diuretics, which are effective in lowering blood pressure and less likely to produce hypokalemia.

A rare but fascinating cause of renal potassium wasting and metabolic alkalosis is *Bartter's syndrome* (Table 16.8). These patients, described originally by Bartter in 1962, also manifest hyperreninemia, hyperaldosteronism, hyperplasia of the juxtaglomerular apparatus, and a normal blood pressure. Other characteristics include resistance to the pressor effects of angiotensin II and norepinephrine; increased urinary excretion of prostaglandins, kallikrein, and catecholamines; and a defect in platelet aggregation. These patients usually manifest the illness in childhood, exhibit stunted growth, and may develop interstitial nephritis, leading to progressive renal failure. In some patients, the illness may come to medical attention during adulthood. With the exception of hypokalemia, which is partially responsive, virtually all other manifestations of the syndrome can be corrected by using inhibitors of prostaglandin synthetase, suggesting that they are epiphenomena produced by excess prostaglandin production, which is probably secondary to potassium depletion.

Bartter's syndrome has been linked to three distinct genetic alterations, all of which result in impaired chloride reabsorption by the thick ascending limb: (a) a loss of function mutation of the bumetanide inhibitable Na^+-K^+-$2Cl^-$ cotransporter; (b) a loss of function mutation of the K^+ channel ROMK, which permits backleak of K^+ into the tubular fluid required for normal transport activity by the Na-K-2Cl cotransporter; and (c) a loss of function mutation of the renal chloride channel CLCNKB (Table 16.8). Potassium depletion in this syndrome results from the high rates of sodium and fluid delivery to the collecting duct in the presence of volume depletion–induced high levels of aldosterone.

Gitelman's syndrome has many features similar to Bartter's syndrome but differs by exhibiting hypocalciuria, whereas normocalciuria or hypercalciuria occurs with Bartter's syndrome. Hypomagnesemia can occur with both syndromes but is more common and typically more severe with Gitelman's syndrome, whereas the potassium wasting is generally less severe with Gitelman's syndrome. The genetic abnormality accounting for Gitelman's syndrome is a loss of function mutation of the thiazide-sensitive Na^+-Cl^- cotransporter. Thus NaCl reabsorption by the distal convoluted tubule is impaired, accounting for the features of this disorder.

Several other hereditary renal potassium-wasting syndromes have been described with many features similar to Bartter's syndrome but with subtle differences. They have not been characterized genetically to date.

The diagnosis of Bartter's and Gitelman's syndrome is straightforward. Both present with the combination of hypokalemic metabolic alkalosis, with a normal blood pressure, renal potassium wasting, and a high rate of urinary chloride excretion. The two are differentiated from each other by the presence or absence of hypocalciuria. It is apparent, however, that all these features are precisely those manifested by individuals taking either loop diuretics (Bartter's syndrome) or thiazide diuretics (Gitelman's syndrome). In fact, every patient who presents in adulthood with this diagnostic constellation should be considered a diuretic abuser until proven otherwise. Confirmation of this latter diagnosis requires screening the urine for diuretics and often, in my experience, careful observation of the patient in a metabolic ward. Other potential diagnoses that can be confused but readily delineated include laxative abuse, which should not exhibit renal potassium wasting, and surreptitious vomiting, which should exhibit intense urinary chloride conservation. Sometimes, several of these deviant behaviors are presented simultaneously, but careful dietary, stool, and urine electrolyte monitoring along with drug screening in a metabolic ward can sort them out.

Bartter's syndrome and other related primary potassium-wasting disorders, and to a lesser extent Gitelman's syndrome, present the most difficult management problems encountered in the treatment of hypokalemia. Potassium levels above 3.0 mEq/L represent a reasonable therapeutic objective. Oral KCl supplementation alone is usually inadequate to satisfy this goal, and the simultaneous use of a potassium-sparing diuretic is usually required. Amiloride appears to be the most useful agent. It is important to emphasize that the combination of potassium-sparing diuretics and KCl therapy is generally unwise because of the danger of hyperkalemia and should be reserved only for individuals with severe renal potassium-wasting abnormalities. If this therapeutic combination is inadequate, addition of a prostaglandin synthetase inhibitor can be efficacious, as long as the gastrointestinal side effects are tolerable.

Many other conditions that cause renal potassium wasting can present either with a normal pH or with metabolic alkalosis. Magnesium depletion secondary to acquired or hereditary disorders results in renal potassium wasting by mechanisms that have not been defined. Large doses of intravenous penicillins or penicillin derivatives promote potassium wasting because they are excreted in the urine as anions and thereby exhibit effects similar to those of a large sodium sulphate load. Aminoglycosides and the chemotherapeutic agent *cis*-platin can cause renal potassium and magnesium wasting by direct toxic effects on the renal tubule. Hypokalemia has been reported in 25% of cases of acute leukemia. Potential mechanisms include rapid cellular proliferation, therapy with antibiotics and tumoricidal drugs, and a direct effect of the leukemic process to promote renal potassium wasting, perhaps related in some fashion to lysozyme.

Drug-Induced Hypokalemia (Table 16.10)

It is apparent from the foregoing discussion that drugs can induce hypokalemia by every potential mechanism. Therefore, when a hypokalemic patient is seen, his or her medications should be reviewed. The medications that induce hypokalemia by redistribution, extrarenal potassium loss, and renal potassium wasting are categorized in Table 16.10.

TABLE 16.10. Drug-Induced Hypokalemia

Redistribution
$NaHCO_3$
Insulin
Glucose (normal pancreatic function)
β-Adrenergic agonists (epinephrine and selective β_2-agonists)
Theophylline intoxication
? Calcium channel blockers
Chloroquine intoxication
Extrarenal potassium losses
Laxatives
Renal potassium losses
Diuretics (thiazides, chlorthalidone, and loop diuretics)
Carbonic anhydrase inhibitors
Amphotericin B (produces distal renal tubular acidosis)
Florinef (other corticosteroids, including nasal sprays and topical)
Corticosteroids
Penicillins
Aminoglycosides (gentamicin)
Cis-platin

Therapy

Therapy for specific types of hypokalemia has been addressed in the preceding sections. However, there are some general principles applicable to the therapy of potassium depletion of most causes. As already noted, redistribution-induced hypokalemia is usually transient and does not require therapy, but when necessary, it can be treated with judicious administration of potassium. Potassium depletion of a significant degree, on the other hand, always requires potassium replacement. Decisions are required about the specific potassium salt, the route of administration, and the speed of administration. In addition, if oral therapy is used, the specific formulation of potassium must be chosen. Food stuffs can provide a good source of potassium to patients with clinical conditions predisposing them to potassium loss from the body. The potassium contents of various foods are listed in Table 16.11. KCl will correct potassium depletion regardless of the underlying cause, but it is an absolute requirement under conditions of chloride depletion. When metabolic acidosis and potassium depletion occur, potassium in combination with a bicarbonate precursor such as citrate, acetate, or gluconate is appropriate. If phosphate depletion accompanies a potassium deficit, as for example with diabetic ketoacidosis, potassium phosphate therapy is rational.

Oral replacement therapy is preferable when feasible, except in the setting of life-threatening abnormalities such as potassium depletion–induced malignant ventricular arrhythmias, digitalis intoxication, or paralysis. If rapid (more than 10 mEq/hr) potassium administration is given intravenously, cardiac monitoring in an intensive care unit is advisable. Under no circumstances should rates of administration exceed 40 mEq/hr. The quantity of potassium given is based on an estimate of the degree of depletion and on the symptoms of the patient. In general, it is wise to err on the side of slow replenishment and to monitor progress with repeated plasma potassium measurements. Oral therapy is usually given at dosages of 40 to 120 mEq/day. Oral potassium salts are available as a liquid (or as powders dissolved in liquid) or as wax matrix or microencapsulated slow-release forms of KCl. For short-term therapy, I generally recommend KCl solutions; however, for long-term treatment, slow-release forms are preferred by most patients. The risk posed by oral KCl is intestinal ulceration, which appears to occur rarely but is probably somewhat more common with slow-release than with liquid preparations.

The major risk of any potassium therapy is hyperkalemia, especially in patients with impaired renal function or those treated with intravenous potassium. Careful monitoring of serum potassium and an appreciation of those patients who are particularly at risk for this complication are essential.

TABLE 16.11. Potassium Content of Some Foods

	mEq
Orange juice	11–13/glass
Orange juice (crystals)	13–14/oz
Grapefruit juice	10–11/glass
Tomato juice	12–14/glass
Bananas	13–15 each
Avocados	25–30 each
Beans	12–14/cup
Cream of tartar (can be added to juice)	10–12/teaspoon
Bouillon cube (salt-free)	12–13 each
Milk	12–14/cup
Raisins	12–14½/cup
Salt substitute (KCl)	15–16½/teaspoon
Instant tea	9–11/teaspoon

HYPERKALEMIA

Clinical Sequelae

The manifestations of hyperkalemia result from the decrease in the ratio of intracellular to extracellular potassium. The alteration in membrane potential modifies cardiac conduction, which results in the ECG abnormalities depicted in Fig. 16.24. The earliest ECG abnormality is peaking of the T waves (serum potassium of 5.0 to 6.5 mEq/L). More severe hyperkalemia (serum potassium of 6.5 to 8.0 mEq/L) results in flattening of the P wave, prolongation of the PR interval, and widening of the QRS complex with development of a deep S wave. If hyperkalemia progresses further (more than 8 mEq/L), the widened QRS complex merges with the T wave into a biphasic sine wave pattern, and ventricular fibrillation or cardiac arrest is immi-

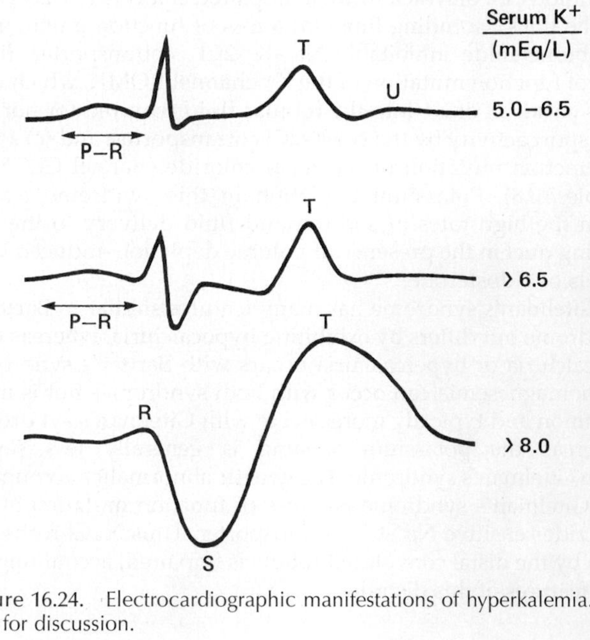

Figure 16.24. Electrocardiographic manifestations of hyperkalemia. See text for discussion.

nent. The cardiac effects of hyperkalemia are enhanced by hypocalcemia, hyponatremia, and acidosis.

Neurologic manifestations, including tingling, paresthesias, weakness, and even flaccid paralysis, can result from hyperkalemia, but severe cardiac toxicity typically precedes these symptoms. Involvement of respiratory muscles is very rare. Muscles innervated by cranial nerves are usually not affected, although impaired phonation and swallowing have been seen. In most patients, muscle weakness occurs with serum potassium levels of more than 8 mEq/L. However, patients with hyperkalemic periodic paralysis may develop muscle weakness with smaller elevations in serum potassium.

Spurious Hyperkalemia (Table 16.12)

Many factors can result in falsely elevated determinations of serum potassium. The most common culprit is a hemolyzed blood specimen, a problem that is readily appreciated because hemolysis of a sufficient degree to raise the serum potassium by 0.5 mEq/L is visible. More subtle leakage of potassium from erythrocytes with an abnormal membrane has been described in otherwise asymptomatic families (familial pseudohyperkalemia) and in acquired illness such as infectious mononucleosis. This problem can be obviated by prompt separation of serum from red blood cells. Similarly, high white blood cell counts (more than 200,000/mm^3) can elevate serum or plasma potassium levels because of leakage from the cells during storage in the cold. It is of interest that when cells are stored at room temperature, spurious hypokalemia can occur because the cells may take up potassium. Prompt separation of serum or plasma from the white blood cells solves the problem. Potassium release from platelets during clotting accounts for higher serum than plasma potassium concentration and can cause spurious hyperkalemia if platelet counts are elevated (greater than 1×10^6/mm^3). This problem can be circumvented by measuring plasma potassium concentration. If blood is drawn with excessively tight and prolonged tourniquet application, the potassium level can be increased by potassium release from the arm muscles and local hemoconcentration. One clue to spurious hyperkalemia is the presence of a completely normal ECG despite a high measured potassium level.

TABLE 16.12. Spurious Hyperkalemia

Hemolysis
Acquired
Familial pseudohyperkalemia
Leukocytosis (>2×10^5/mm^3)
Thrombocytosis (>1×10^6/mm^3)
Ischemic blood drawing

TABLE 16.13. Hyperkalemia Secondary to Redistribution

Cause	Potential Mechanisms
Acidosis	Inhibition of Na^+-K^+ pump and activation of K^+-ATP channels
Hyperosmolality (hyperglycemia)	Increase in intracellular potassium
β-Adrenergic blockade	Inhibition of Na^+-K^+ pump
Adrenergic agonists	?
Arginine HCl	?
Succinylcholine	Increase in potassium permeability
Digitalis intoxication	Inhibition of Na^+-K^+ pump
Periodic paralysis	Abnormal Na^+ channel with depolarization
Fluoride intoxication	Inhibition of glycolytic metabolism
Parathyroid hormone	Increased intracellular calcium with stimulation of calcium activated potassium channels
Intense exercise	Activation of K^+-ATP channels

Hyperkalemia Secondary to Redistribution from the Intracellular Compartment (Table 16.13)

Both acute respiratory acidosis and mineral acid–induced metabolic acidosis may result in hyperkalemia. The increment in plasma potassium is less with respiratory acidosis, and the magnitude of the change in serum potassium with changes in pH is variable and not predictable. Inhibition of the Na^+-K^+ pump and activation of muscle K^+-ATP channels by intracellular acidosis appear to account for the net efflux of potassium from cells. Acute acidosis secondary to organic acids does not appear to elevate serum potassium. It is possible that this divergent response might be explained by the insulin-stimulatory effect of ketoacids. Hyperosmolality provokes potassium exit from cells. It is estimated that each increase of 10 mOsm/kg in osmolality elevates serum potassium by 0.5 mEq/L. This phenomenon can result from the administration of hypertonic solutes, such as mannitol or glycerol, or from an increase in plasma glucose concentration in diabetic patients, who cannot increase insulin to counteract the cellular exit of potassium.

β-Adrenergic blockade elevates potassium by inhibiting the effects of the β_2-adrenergic system on potassium uptake. α-Adrenergic agonists promote potassium efflux from cells. An enhanced α-adrenergic response may explain why some patients with chronic renal failure do not lower serum potassium in response to epinephrine.

Administration of the cationic amino acid arginine hydrochloride elevates serum potassium by an unknown mechanism. Muscle-depolarizing relaxants, such as succinylcholine, elevate potassium by increasing the potassium permeability of the muscle. Severe digitalis intoxication poisons the Na^+-K^+ pump sufficiently to cause hyperkalemia; fluoride intoxication appears to cause hyperkalemia by inhibiting glycolytic metabolism. Hyperkalemic periodic paralysis is a rare autosomal-dominant disorder caused by mutation in the muscle sodium channel producing abnormal inactivation kinetics, which results in depolarization. It is characterized by intermittent paralytic attacks accompanied by hyperkalemia. Peaked T waves can be detected on the ECG, but other cardiac abnormalities do not occur. Therapy with β_2-agonists can abort paralytic attacks and is also useful as a preventive measure. A high concentration of PTH promotes cellular potassium efflux presumably by opening calcium-activated potassium channels secondary to an increase in intracellular calcium concentration. Exercise enhances potassium exit from skeletal muscle by opening potassium channels inhibited by adenosine 5′-triphosphate (ATP) and activated secondarily by intracellular acidosis. Both acute maximal physical performance and prolonged exhaustive exercise can increase plasma potassium above 7 mEq/L.

Hyperkalemia Secondary to Impaired Renal Excretion

Severe Compromise of Glomerular Filtration Rate

Potassium homeostasis is critically dependent on appropriate rates of renal elimination; therefore, as expected, a severe compromise in GFR predisposes patients to potassium retention and accompanying hyperkalemia. However, the kidneys possess a large capacity to excrete potassium. This adaptive increase in potassium-secretory capability, not only by the nephron but also by the colon, is similar to the adaptation observed when normal individuals are exposed to a high-potassium diet. Therefore, as long as potassium intake is normal, hyperkalemia is generally not a problem in patients with chronic renal insufficiency until the GFR declines to less than 5 ml/min. Nevertheless, a patient with a substantially compromised GFR is not able to eliminate a large potassium load effectively. Thus an increase in potassium ingestion or in endogenous release of potassium from tissue breakdown, such as rhabdomyolysis, tissue trauma, or red blood cell degradation in hematomas or following bleeding into the gastrointestinal tract, can provoke life-threatening hyperkalemia.

Surprisingly, patients with end-stage chronic renal failure generally manifest a decrease in total body potassium stores, which appears in part to reflect an actual decrease in intracellular potassium. Potential causes for this abnormality in cellular potassium accumulation include the effects of acidosis, of ouabainlike natriuretic factors that may be present in the blood, of uremia-induced defective transcription of the α_1 subunit of Na^+-K^+-ATPase, and of secondary hyperparathyroidism, which may activate calcium-dependent potassium channels by increasing intracellular calcium concentration. This defect in cellular potassium uptake might increase the susceptibility to hyperkalemia when these patients have an acute potassium load.

Acute oliguria, regardless of the cause, is likely to result in hyperkalemia. Even nonoliguric acute renal failure is accompanied by a high risk of potassium intoxication. The daily increase in plasma potassium in noncatabolic patients with acute renal failure averages 0.4 mEq/L, whereas it averages 0.7 mEq/L and can be substantially greater in patients with trauma or other catabolic conditions. An ECG to assess possible hyperkalemia should be obtained for any patient with acute renal failure.

Adequate Glomerular Filtration Rate (Table 16.14)

In patients with a GFR above 20 ml/min, the nephron mass is sufficient to deal with potassium loads and hyperkalemia is not expected. For example, if the normal kidney with a GFR of 100 ml/min can excrete 10 mEq/kg per day of potassium with a normal plasma potassium level, a kidney with one-fifth this level of function should be capable of excreting 2 mEq/kg per day of 140 mEq/day of potassium in a 70-kg individual. However, potassium excretion can be inadequate despite a sufficient number of functioning tubules in two general circumstances: (a) a deficiency in the kaliuretic hormone aldosterone and (b) a primary defect in the tubular potassium-secretory mechanisms, despite normal adrenal function.

Aldosterone deficiency (Table 16.14) can result from acquired adrenal abnormalities as in Addison's disease or from various hereditary enzymatic defects in aldosterone biosynthesis, including the adrenogenital syndrome (congenital adrenal hyperplasia) secondary to a C_{21}-hydroxylase or 3-β-hydroxysteroid dehydrogenase deficiency or to an isolated abnormality in aldosterone production caused by mutations in aldosterone synthetase, which can impair either corticosterone methyloxidase I or II activity. If salt intake is high, patients with hypoaldosteronism generally can maintain a normal serum potassium level. A low salt intake or hypovolemia precipitates hyperkalemia because decreased distal delivery of sodium and fluid in combination with low aldosterone levels compromises potassium excretion. Therapy of adrenal insufficiency requires sufficient replacement of mineralocorticoids (usually provided as Florinef) and glucocorticoids to maintain physiologic levels.

Aldosterone deficiency in association with chronic renal insufficiency has been recognized with increasing frequency. A small percentage of these patients with hyperkalemia have a *selective defect in aldosterone secretion* of unknown origin. Most of the patients (50% to 70%) who manifest hyperkalemia despite an adequate GFR have a *concurrent decrease in renin and aldosterone levels.* This syndrome of hyporeninemic hypoaldosteronism is found most often in patients with tubulointerstitial forms of renal disease and is especially prevalent in patients with diabetes mellitus. Hyporeninemic hypoaldosteronism has been reported in patients with acquired immunodeficiency syndrome (AIDS); however, hyperkalemia can also occur in these patients as a result of AIDS-related adrenal insufficiency or from the potential impairment of potassium excretion secondary to therapy with pentamidine or trimethoprim, which both inhibit the epithelial sodium channel in a fashion analogous to amiloride. There are also well-documented reports of hyporeninemic hypoaldosteronism in patients with primary glomerular disease. In addition to hyperkalemia, there is often a concurrent, mild hyperchloremic metabolic acidosis that results from the suppressive effects of hyperkalemia on renal ammonia production and the impairment of proton secretion secondary to aldosterone deficiency. In most of these patients, adequate prolonged mineralocorticoid replacement therapy normalizes both plasma potassium and bicarbonate levels.

Although it seems likely that the low aldosterone levels result from the defect in renal renin release, there may also be a primary abnormality in the adrenal gland because the aldosterone response to both exogenous adrenocorticotropic hormone and angiotensin II is often abnormal. The basis for the abnormality in renin secretion is also unclear. Hypotheses include damage to the juxtaglomerular apparatus; catecholamine, kallikrein, and prostaglandin deficiency; abnormal conversion of prorenin to renin, especially in diabetic patients; and renin suppression secondary to chronic volume expansion. High levels of atrial natriuretic peptide with suppression of both renin and aldosterone secretion have also been speculated but not proven. Possibly the syndrome is not a homogeneous entity but reflects a spectrum of several different pathophysiologic processes.

A practical approach to evaluate hyperkalemia in these patients includes measurement of potassium and creatinine in a 24-hour urine collection and in serum. The amount of potassium excreted reflects potassium ingestion and can uncover an unsuspected high potassium intake. An assessment of fractional potassium excretion [urine-to-plasma ratio (U/P) for potassium divided by U/P for creatinine] in relation to GFR de-

TABLE 16.14. Hyperkalemia with Adequate Glomerular Filtration Rate (>20 ml/min)

Aldosterone Deficiency	Normal Adrenal Function
Primary adrenal disease	Acquired disorders
Acquired	Renal transplants
Addison's disease	Lupus erythematosus
Isolated aldosterone deficiency	Amyloidosis
Hereditary enzymatic defects	Obstructive uropathy
Hyporeninemic hypoaldosteronism	Sickle cell nephropathy
Drug-induced	Hereditary
Prostaglandin synthetase inhibitors	Pseudohypoaldosteronism, types I and II
Angiotensin II–converting enzyme inhibitors	Potassium-sparing diuretics
Heparin	Epithelial Na^+ channel inhibitors
Cyclosporine, Tacrolemus	

termines whether renal tubular potassium secretion is impaired (Fig. 16.25). Alternatively, the distal transtubular K^+ concentration gradient (TTKG) can be assessed. This parameter, which is determined by dividing the U/P(K^+) concentration by the U/P osmolality, to correct for water abstraction by the medullary collecting duct, provides an indirect assessment of the K^+ concentration gradient and thereby K^+ transport by the cortical collecting duct. A low value reflects an impairment of K^+ secretion. The advantages of the TTKG are that it provides a more rational physiologic parameter than FEK and does not require comparison to a graphic display; however, there is no clear evidence that its diagnostic accuracy exceeds the assessment of FEK. These data combined with the measurement in an upright position of plasma renin and aldosterone will delineate whether hyporeninemic hypoaldosteronism accounts for the defect in potassium secretion or whether there is a primary defect in the tubular potassium-secretory mechanisms. If further confirmation of the diagnosis is required, a therapeutic trial of mineralocorticoid replacement (Florinef at 0.2 mg/day for 2 weeks) can be carried out to determine whether serum potassium levels return to normal.

Many therapeutic options exist for managing chronic hyperkalemia in these patients. If the elevation in serum potassium is mild (less than 5.8 mEq/L), no specific treatment may be required aside from dietary counseling against ingestion of a high-potassium diet and the avoidance of drugs that might further impair potassium homeostasis. Specific treatment to lower the serum potassium level can include mineralocorticoid replacement therapy, but this is usually ill advised because of the risk of salt retention with development of edema and the initiation or worsening of hypertension in individuals with underlying chronic renal disease. Therapy with furosemide or thiazide diuretics is often useful and well tolerated. Kayexalate provides an alternative mechanism for potassium elimination, but many patients dislike long-term use of this medication.

Many drugs used in therapeutic doses can induce hypoaldosteronism and associated hyperkalemia (Tables 16.14 and 16.15). Heparin directly impedes aldosterone biosynthesis by

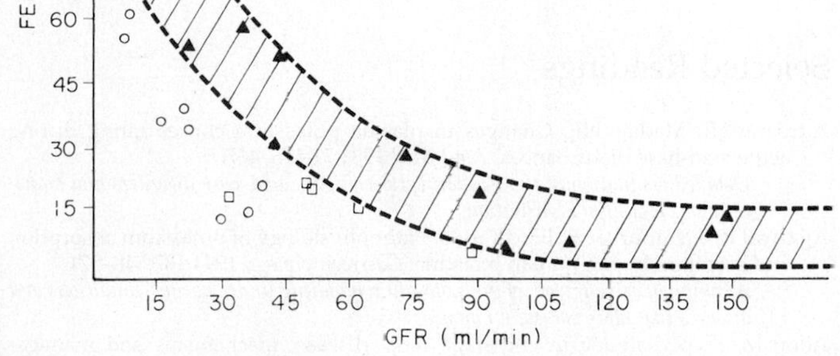

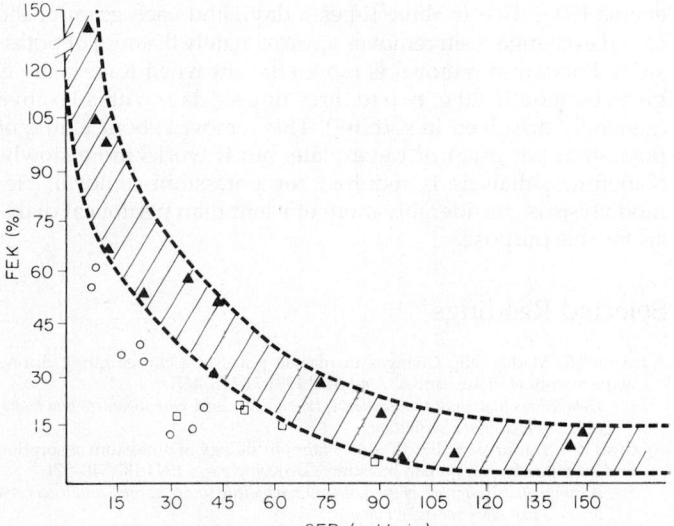

Figure 16.25. Relationships between fractional potassium excretion *(FEK)* and glomerular filtration rate *(GFR)*. Normal values fall within the *hatched area*, and the *open symbols* represent patients with abnormalities in potassium secretion. (Reprinted with permission from Batlle DC, Arruda JAL, Kurtzman NA. Hyperkalemic distal tubular acidosis associated with obstructive uropathy. *N Engl J Med* 1981;304:373–380.)

inhibition of the enzyme 18-hydroxylase. Indomethacin and other prostaglandin synthetase inhibitors, by diminishing prostaglandin production, reduce renin secretion and thereby induce the syndrome of hyporeninemic hypoaldosteronism. The angiotensin-converting enzyme inhibitors captopril and enalapril cause hypoaldosteronism by blocking angiotensin II–mediated aldosterone secretion. The immunosuppressive agents cyclosporine and tacrolimus (FK506) both produce hyperkalemia. Cyclosporine can reduce renin levels, but it also can interfere directly with tubular potassium secretion both by inhibiting Na^+-K^+-ATPase activity of the collecting duct and by inhibiting the apical K^+ channels of the principal cells. In general, drug-induced hyperkalemia is not a prominent clinical manifestation unless a defect in potassium excretion exists in addition to hypoaldosteronism. Thus it is usually unmasked in individuals with a concurrent reduction in GFR or some other abnormality that impairs potassium excretion.

Various acquired interstitial renal diseases, all of which can cause hyporeninemic hypoaldosteronism, can also induce hyperkalemia in the presence of *normal adrenal function* (Table 16.14). The clinical features of these patients are similar to those with hyporeninemic hypoaldosteronism, except that plasma renin and aldosterone levels are normal and the hyperkalemia is not corrected by mineralocorticoid replacement. In contrast to hypoaldosteronism, this entity commonly results in a concurrent defect in urinary acidification, manifested by an inability to lower urine pH below 5.5 in response to an acidifying stimulus such as acidosis. Clinically, the most important underlying cause is obstructive uropathy, which should be considered a potential problem in any patient with unexplained hyperkalemia. The potassium-secretory defect with obstruction results from a decrease in the activity of Na^+-K^+-ATPase coupled with decreased activity of both the apical sodium channel and potassium conductance. The precise mechanism whereby tubular potassium secretion is impaired by the other conditions is unclear. A similar clinical picture can be produced, however, by the potassium-sparing diuretic amiloride. This drug impairs both potassium secretion and urinary acidification by blocking the luminal epithelial sodium channel and thereby reducing sodium transport and transepithelial voltage. It has been hypothesized that the pathogenesis of the hyperkalemia in cases of normal adrenal function might be similar to the action of these

TABLE 16.15. Drug-Induced Hyperkalemia

Redistribution
Mannitol, glycerol
Glucose (diabetes mellitus)
β-Adrenergic blockage (e.g., propranolol)
Arginine HCl
Succinylcholine
Cardiac glycosides
α-Adrenergic agonists (?)
Excessive potassium intake
Potassium supplements
Salt substitutes
Potassium penicillin
Impaired renal excretion
Prostaglandin synthetase inhibitors (e.g., indomethacin)
Angiotensin converting enzyme inhibitors (captopril, enalapril)
Heparin
Cyclosporine
Spironolactone
Triamterene
Amiloride
Trimethoprim
Pentamidine
Nafamostat maleate

diuretics. The aldosterone antagonist spironolactone and the epithelial sodium channel inhibitor triamterene also can produce hyperkalemia with normal aldosterone levels.

In general, these potassium-sparing diuretics should not be given concurrently with potassium replacement because of the risk of serious hyperkalemia.

As noted previously, both trimethoprim and pentamidine, as well as nafamostat maleate, inhibit the epithelial sodium channel and can produce hyperkalemia. The hyperkalemic effects of trimethoprim can be minimized by urine alkalinization, which converts the drug to its inactive electroneutral form.

Two other abnormalities, called *pseudohypoaldosteronism,* cause hyperkalemia with normal renal function and normal aldosterone levels. *Type I pseudohypoaldosteronism* is evidenced in infants with classic signs of aldosterone deficiency, including salt wasting, acidosis, and hyperkalemia. The autosomal-recessive form of this disorder is produced by mutations of the α and β subunits of the epithelial sodium channel, resulting in loss of function. The autosomal-dominant form of this disorder results from loss of function mutations in the gene encoding the mineralocorticoid receptor. Salt supplementation is effective therapeutically, and these children usually manifest spontaneous recovery by the age of 2 years. *Type II pseudohypoaldosteronism,* which also has been called *Gordon's syndrome,* is evidenced in late childhood or adulthood with hyperkalemia, acidosis, and normal renal function, but in contrast to the infantile syndrome, these patients are not salt wasters and are usually hypertensive. The primary defect appears to be enhanced chloride reabsorption at a distal nephron site, which causes volume expansion, hypertension, often suppressed renin, and hyperkalemia, with aldosterone levels that are usually normal or slightly low. The genetic basis of this autosomal-dominant disorder has been localized to chromosomes 1 and 17 based on linkage analysis, but the precise molecular basis of the disorder has not been characterized. Thiazide diuretics are often effective in correcting the hyperkalemia, but the response to furosemide has been variable.

Drug-Induced Hyperkalemia (Table 16.15)

As with hypokalemia, any hyperkalemic patient should have a careful review of his or her medications to determine whether drugs can account for the development of hyperkalemia or be an exacerbating factor. This includes a consideration of the multiple agents that can interfere with potassium distribution between the intracellular and extracellular compartments, serve as hidden sources of potassium ingestion, and interfere with urinary potassium elimination.

Therapy (Table 16.16)

Acute hyperkalemia is a potentially life-threatening emergency because of the risk of cardiac arrest, and it requires prompt attention. The ECG abnormalities along with the level of serum potassium and the clinical situation guide the vigor of the therapeutic effort, but it is wise to err on the side of overtreatment in situations that are questionable. In general, when the ECG shows findings of hyperkalemia more serious than peaked T waves or when serum potassium exceeds 6.5 mEq/L, aggressive and prompt therapy should be instituted. The same holds true when the hyperkalemia is mild but the clinical situation suggests a potentially rapid increase in potassium, as for example in the patient with trauma and acute renal failure.

Therapy for hyperkalemia is twofold: (a) to actively mitigate the potential for cardiac toxicity, the effect of potassium is antagonized with calcium and potassium is driven into cells; and (b) simultaneously slower-acting measures are instituted to remove potassium from the body.

TABLE 16.16. Treatment of Acute Hyperkalemia

Rapid reversal of potassium toxicity	
Calcium gluconate	10–30 ml of 10% solution
Glucose and insulin	Glucose: 25–50 g/hr by continuous intravenous drip Regular insulin: 5 units intravenously every 15 min[a]
Albuterol	
Nebulized	20 mg in 4 ml normal saline over 10 minutes
Intravenous	0.5 mg in 100 ml 5% dextrose in water given over 10–15 minutes
Intravenous $NaHCO_3$	44–132 mEq
Potassium removal	
Kayexalate	Enema (50–150 g/day) Oral (40–60 g/day)
Hemodialysis	

[a]Usually 4–6 units of insulin with each 10 g of glucose.

As seen in Table 16.16, the acute measures include the use of intravenous calcium gluconate to counteract the effect of hyperkalemia on cardiac conduction; the effect of calcium lasts only a few minutes, and the calcium infusion may need to be repeated. Administration of insulin plus glucose is the most reliable treatment for driving potassium into cells. The effect on serum potassium is apparent within 20 to 30 minutes and lasts for up to 2 hours. β_2-Adrenergic agonists, such as albuterol, given either intravenously or by nebulizer, lower potassium in most patients. The time kinetics are similar to and the quantitative effects are additive to those of insulin. Although bicarbonate has been considered a mainstay of the treatment for hyperkalemia, other studies have not demonstrated significant efficacy of bicarbonate given alone; although it may enhance the potassium-lowering effect of insulin in hyperkalemic patients. When significant metabolic acidosis accompanies hyperkalemia, the use of bicarbonate seems reasonable.

Usually, Kayexalate is adequate therapy to remove excessive potassium from the body. It works most rapidly as a retention enema (50 g, two to three times a day), and each gram of the cation exchange resin removes approximately 0.5 mEq of potassium. Potassium removal is more efficient when Kayexalate is given by mouth (20 g, two to three times a day) with a laxative (generally dissolved in sorbitol). This removes about 1 mEq of potassium per gram of Kayexalate, but it works more slowly. Sometimes, dialysis is required for potassium removal. Hemodialysis is considerably more efficient than peritoneal dialysis for this purpose.

Selected Readings

Adrogue HJ, Madias NE. Changes in plasma potassium concentrating during acute acid-base disturbances. *Am J Med* 1981;71:456–467.

Detailed evaluation of the relation between acute acid–base disorders and transcellular potassium distribution.

Agarwal R, Afzalpurkar R, Fordtran JS. Pathophysiology of potassium absorption and secretion by the human intestine. *Gastroenterology* 1994;107:548–571.

A comprehensive review of gut potassium handling under normal conditions and diseases that alter potassium homeostasis.

Allon M. Hyperkalemia in end-stage renal disease: mechanisms and management. *J Am Soc Nephrol* 1995;6:1134–1142.

A review of the mechanisms of hyperkalemia in end-stage renal disease and of current views on therapy.

Battle DC, Arruda JAL, Kurtzman NA. Hyperkalemic distal renal tubular acidosis associated with obstructive uropathy. *N Engl J Med* 1981;304:373–380.

Clear proof for acquired primary disorders of tubular potassium secretion.

DeFronzo R. Hyperkalemia and hyporeninemic hypoaldosteronism. *Kidney Int* 1980;17:118–134.

An excellent review of hyporeninemic hypoaldosteronism.

DuBose TD Jr. Hyperkalemic hyperchloremic metabolic acidosis: pathophysiologic insights. *Kidney Int* 1997;51:591–602.

A review of the pathophysiology of hyperkalemic disorders.

Gennari FJ, Cohen JJ. Role of the kidney in potassium homeostasis: lessons from acid-base disturbances. *Kidney Int* 1975;8:1–5.

An analysis of the relation between potassium and chronic acid–base disorders.

Lifton RP. Molecular genetics of human blood pressure variation. *Science* 1996; 272:676–680.

A review of the molecular basis of several disorders associated with hereditary hypokalemia and hyperkalemia.

Salem MM, Rosa RM, Batlle DC. Extrarenal potassium tolerance in chronic renal failure: implications for the treatment of acute hyperkalemia. *Am J Kidney Dis* 1991;18:421–440.

A review of potassium metabolism in chronic renal failure with a discussion of therapy.

Schambelan M, Sebastian A, Biglieri EG. Prevalence, pathogenesis, and functional significance of aldosterone deficiency in hyperkalemic patients with chronic renal insufficiency. *Kidney Int* 1980;17:89–101.

An extensive analysis of hyperkalemia in patients with chronic renal failure and adequate levels of GFR.

Schwartz WB, Van Ypersele de Strihou C, Kassirer JP. Role of anions in metabolic alkalosis and potassium deficiency. *N Engl J Med* 1968;279:630–639.

The best description of the syndrome of chloride depletion.

Simon DB, Lifton RP. The molecular basis of inherited hypokalemic alkalosis: Bartter's and Gitelman's syndromes. *Am J Physiol* 1996;271:F961–F966.

A review of the clinical manifestations and molecular mechanisms in these two renal hereditary potassium-wasting disorders.

Tannen RL. Diuretic-induced hypokalemia. *Kidney Int* 1985;28:988–1000.

A detailed discussion of the risks and management of diuretic-induced hypokalemia.

Tannen RL, ed. Potassium metabolism. *Semin Nephrol* 1987;7:171–273.

Topics reviewed in this symposium include renal potassium handling, adaptation to potassium deprivation, disorders of internal potassium balance, renal hyperkalemia, hemodynamic effects of potassium, relationship between potassium and magnesium disorders, and potassium's effect on acid–base homeostasis.

Tannen RL. Potassium disorders. In: Kokko JP, Tannen RL, eds. *Fluids and electrolytes*, 2nd ed. Philadelphia: WB Saunders, 1990:195–300.

A detailed review of all aspects of clinical disorders.

Vallotton MB. Primary aldosteronism. Part I. Diagnosis of primary hyperaldosteronism. *Clin Endocrinol* 1996;45:47–52.

Valotton MB. Primary aldosteronism. Part II. Differential of primary hyperaldosteronism and pseudoaldosteronism. *Clin Endocrinol* 1996;45:53–60.

These two reviews address the diagnosis of primary aldosteronism and the pathophysiology and diagnosis of other hypokalemic hypertensive disorders.

17 CHAPTER

Calcium Metabolism

PART 1
Intestinal Absorption of Calcium

Phuong-Chi T. Pham, Phuong-Thu T. Pham, Laurie H. Kayne, and David B.N. Lee

Although calcium balance and homeostasis are intricately maintained by multiple mechanisms, intestinal calcium absorption is the only physiologic means through which *new* calcium can be translocated from the environment into the body to meet increases in calcium demand (e.g., for growth, during pregnancy and lactation, and to replenish calcium loss). We begin the discussion on the mechanism of calcium absorption at the level of intestinal epithelium.

TRANSEPITHELIAL CALCIUM TRANSPORT

Transepithelial calcium fluxes occur through two parallel processes: paracellular and transcellular. The three basic mechanisms involved are solvent drag, passive diffusion, and carrier-mediated active transport. The first two modes of transport occur almost entirely through a nonsaturable paracellular pathway, whereas the active transport is mediated via a saturable transcellular pathway.

Calcium Transport Through the Paracellular Pathway

The flow of water across the paracellular pathway can carry with it calcium in solution, a process termed *solvent drag* or *convection.* Under physiologic conditions, net water flow across the intestinal epithelium is in the absorptive (mucosal-to-serosal) direction. This sets up the condition for net calcium absorption by solvent drag.

A second mechanism that moves calcium across the shunt pathway is passive diffusion. The energy for this mode of transport is provided by the transepithelial electrochemical gradient, which can drive ions across the epithelium independent of water flow (Fig. 17.1). Assuming a transepithelial potential difference (PD) of 5 mV (serosal positive) and an ionized calcium concentration ([Ca^{2+}]) of 1.25 mM on the serosal or the extracellular fluid (ECF), it can be predicted (using the Ussing equation) that net diffusion in the absorptive (mucosal-to-serosal or lumen-to-ECF) direction will occur whenever luminal [Ca^{2+}] exceeds 2.0 mM. The [Ca^{2+}] in human digesta ranges from 0.5 to 10 mM, with the lower value being raised to 3.0 mM when 250 ml of milk is ingested. Thus, in adults who are in calcium balance and who consume a calcium-rich diet, calcium absorption across the intercellular conduit should be adequate to satisfy most physiologic needs.

Accumulating evidence suggests the flow of water and solutes across the paracellular pathway may be subjected to other forms of regulation. The tight junction at the apical end of this paracellular conduit may be populated by macromolecules that function like "channels" and "pores." Flux of solutes, including calcium, can therefore be regulated by variation in the insertion or removal of such units from the junction complex and also by altering the ratio of "open" versus "close" states of these units. Further modulation can be accomplished through changes in the internal characteristics of such molecules (e.g., changes in steric topography, charges, or degree of hydration).

Calcium Absorption Through the Transcellular Pathway

Active calcium absorption is most commonly studied and documented in the duodenum. However, in conditions of increased demand for calcium, such as those associated with growth and pregnancy or during periods of extremely low dietary calcium intake, active calcium absorption can occur in other segments of the intestine. The transcellular route of calcium absorption is a multistep process that involves the transport of luminal calcium

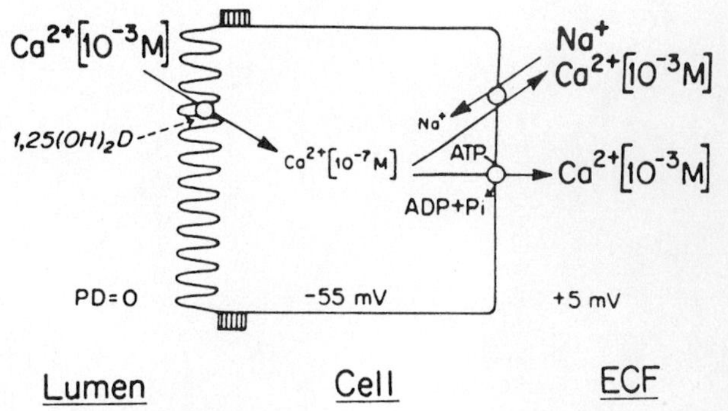

Figure 17.1. Thermodynamic considerations of transepithelial calcium absorption across intestinal epithelium.

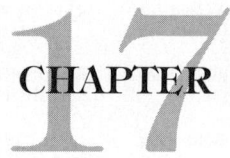

across the apical membrane into the enterocytes, the translocation of calcium across the cytoplasm, and the active extrusion of calcium from the basolateral membrane into the circulatory system.

Although the entry of cationic calcium into the enterocyte is favored by both electrical (cell interior is −55 mV) and chemical (luminal [Ca^{2+}] in the 10^{-3} range versus cytosolic [Ca^{2+}] in the 10^{-7} M range) gradients (Fig. 17.1), its influx across the apical brush border membrane exhibits saturation, rather than simple diffusional kinetics. This is not surprising because the lipid membrane is impermeable to calcium and its influx is most likely mediated by transporters or channels inserted in the lipid bilayers. Indeed, a dihydropyridine-sensitive cyclic adenosine monophosphate (cAMP)–dependent pathway for calcium influx in rat duodenal cells has been reported. Within 1 to 5 minutes, 1,25(OH)$_2$D stimulates calcium influx through this pathway in a dose-dependent manner.

After entry at the apical pole, calcium needs to be buffered so that the intracellular low [Ca^{2+}] environment is protected. It then has to traverse the cytoplasm to the basolateral pole of the cell for extrusion. Much interest has been focused on the vitamin D–dependent Ca^{2+}-binding proteins, the calbindin-Ds, as an intracellular system both for buffering and for ferrying calcium. Two types of calbindin-D have been described. The first one, with a molecular weight of 28,000 (calbindin-D_{28}) and four Ca^{2+}-binding sites, was originally found in avian intestine but was subsequently also found in a variety of mammalian tissue, including the kidney, brain, and placenta. The other calbindin-D, with a molecular weight of 9,000 (calbindin-D_9) and two Ca^{2+}-binding sites, was found in mammalian intestine. The dissociation constant (K_D) for calbindin-D_{28} found in rat kidney is estimated at 2.1×10^{-6} M and that for calbindin-D_9 found in rat intestine at 0.3 to 0.8×10^{-6} M, values within or close to the range of normal cytosolic [Ca^{2+}]. Current opinion suggests that the intestinal calbindin-D facilitates the diffusion of calcium within the enterocytes. A direct correlation between the amount of intestinal calbindin-D and the rate of transcellular intestinal calcium absorption has been documented in many physiologic conditions.

Calbindin-D can also influence apical calcium influx. Several studies suggest the calcium influxed across the apical microvillar membrane is bound to calmodulin, another calcium-binding protein, in the submembranous actin cytoskeleton. This accumulation of calcium leads to cytoskeletal remodelling and the closure of integral membrane channels. In the presence of 1,25(OH)$_2$D-induced calbindin-D, calcium is released from the cytoskeletal calmodulin and binds preferentially to the calbindin-D. The release of calcium from the calmodulin in turn leads to a sequence of events culminated in the reopening of the transmembrane calcium channels. In experimental studies, influxed calcium is localized and accumulated in the microvillar region in vitamin D–deficient enterocytes. With vitamin D repletion, the influxed calcium is diffused throughout the intestinal cells, instead of localizing in the microvillar region.

Thermodynamic considerations at the basolateral membrane are opposite to those at the apical membrane (Fig. 17.1). Exit of calcium requires movement of the cation against a potential difference of 60 mV (from −55 mV inside the cell to +5 mV in the ECF compartment) and a chemical concentration gradient of 10,000-fold (from 10^{-7} M inside the cell to 10^{-3} M in the ECF compartment). Two mechanisms may participate in this cellular expulsion of calcium: a Na^+-independent, calcium-sensitive, Mg^{2+}-dependent ATPase (Ca^{2+}-ATPase), and a Ca^{2+}-Na^+ exchange system. The calcium transporting Ca^{2+}-ATPase is a cAMP-dependent E_1E_2-type enzyme. In the presence of calmodulin, its K_m is about 0.5 μM, that is, the level of intracellular [Ca^{2+}]. 1,25(OH)$_2$D has been shown to stimulate the transcription and synthesis of this calcium pump in the enterocytes. However, even in the complete absence of vitamin D, calcium extrusion at the basolateral membrane is not a rate-limiting step in transepithelial calcium absorption. Calcium extrusion by the Na^+-Ca^{2+} exchanger depends on a favorable, inwardly directed Na^+ gradient. This transmembrane Na^+ gradient is maintained by the Na^+-K^+ pump. The physiologic role of this exchanger in normal calcium absorption is not well studied. The calcium-binding affinity of this exchanger in different systems has been reported to range between 0.1 and 8 μM. It has been predicted that calcium extrusion through this exchanger can be activated when intracellular [Ca^{2+}] is elevated to three times its normal level. The activity of this exchanger does not appear to be vitamin D dependent and has been estimated to account for 20% and 50% of the cellular calcium expelled in rat duodenum and ileum, respectively.

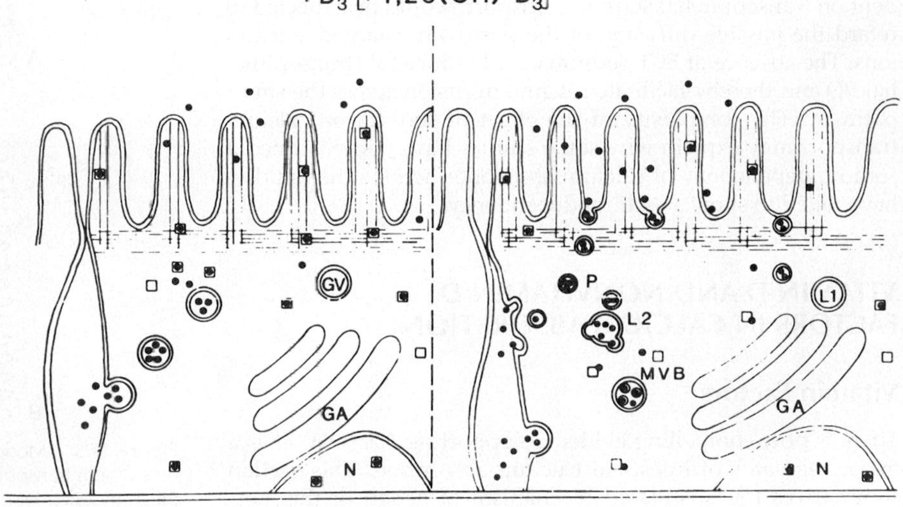

Figure 17.2. Calcium absorption through a postulated endocytic, vesicular pathway. •, Ca^{2+}; □▣, CaBP + Ca^{2+}; G, Golgi vesicle; GA, Golgi apparatus; L1, primary lysosome; L2, secondary lysosome; MVB, multivesicular body; N, nucleus; P, pinocytic vesicle. (Reproduced with permission from Nemere I, Norman AW. Vitamin D and intestinal cell membranes. *Biochem Biophys Acta* 1982;694:307–327.)

ENDOCYTOTIC, VESICULAR CALCIUM ABSORPTION (TRANSCALTACHIA)

Vesicular calcium transport in the intestine is schematized in Fig. 17.2. In the left panel, luminal Ca^{2+} enters the cell through the brush border Ca^{2+} channels. The internalized Ca^{2+} is first complexed to Ca-binding protein (CaBP), which then translocates the Ca^{2+} to the Golgi vesicles. Subsequent fusion of these vesicles with the basolateral membrane leads to the exocytosis of Ca^{2+} into the antiluminal side of the enterocyte. In the right panel, Ca^{2+} entry across the brush border membrane is postulated to occur through pinocytic vesicles. Transport is then completed through direct fusion of these vesicles with the basolateral membrane and exocytosis of Ca^{2+}. An alternative pathway requires the fusion of the pinocytic vesicles with primary lysosomes, packaged by the Golgi apparatus, to form secondary lysosomes, including multivesicular bodies. The fusion of these Ca^{2+}-bearing lysosomes with the basolateral membrane completes the transport process. Vesicular calcium transport has the virtue of moving significant quantities of calcium through the cell while imposing no threat to the fine-tuned homeostasis of the cellular calcium environment. Most studies in this area have been conducted in the bird, and the role of this process, particularly in mammalian intestinal calcium absorption remains to be established.

Sodium Dependence of Calcium Transport

Calcium entry across the brush border membrane does not depend on the presence of luminal sodium. In fact, calcium influx may even increase with replacement of luminal sodium by choline or mannitol. This is because the lowering of luminal sodium concentration reduces, or even reverses, the cell-ward directed sodium gradient, thus allowing maximal pumping of sodium out of the enterocytes. This causes greater intracellular negativity (hyperpolarization) and accelerates the cationic calcium across the apical membrane, down its electrochemical gradients. At the basolateral membrane, exit of calcium through the Ca^{2+}-Na^{+} exchange mechanism would be expected to depend on the presence of ECF sodium. In addition to its possible influence on transcellular calcium transport, sodium may also affect calcium transport across the paracellular pathway. The dependence of water absorption on sodium transport would predict that the portion of calcium absorbed through the solvent-drag effect would be indirectly dependent on net flux of sodium across the intestinal epithelium. Finally, the steady-state transepithelial PD (serosal-positive), which is critically dependent on transepithelial sodium transport, would be expected to retard the passive diffusion of the positively charged calcium ions. The absence of ECF sodium could reduce this transepithelial PD and thereby facilitate calcium diffusion across the shunt pathway. The complexity of the effect of sodium on calcium transport may explain why some studies have demonstrated a sodium dependency of calcium absorption while other studies have failed to show a sodium dependency.

VITAMIN D AND NONVITAMIN D FACTORS IN CALCIUM ABSORPTION

Vitamin Factors

There is now compelling evidence supporting $1{,}25(OH)_2D$ as a major regulator of intestinal calcium absorption. This section summarizes the postulated mechanism of action of this hormone on paracellular and transcellular transport of calcium. The possible influence of vitamin D–receptor polymorphism on intestinal calcium absorption is briefly mentioned.

$1{,}25(OH)_2D$ and Paracellular Calcium Absorption

Indirect evidence from studies three to four decades ago suggest that vitamin D, in addition to its better-known action on cellular calcium transport, also stimulates diffusional absorption of calcium. Since then, more direct evidence for a vitamin D–stimulated paracellular calcium flux has been reported. In rats treated with $1{,}25(OH)_2D$, calcium flux across the paracellular conduit was increased in all segments of the small intestine. $1{,}25(OH)_2D$ and its synthetic analogs also increased tight-junction conductance and paracellular calcium transport in Caco-2 cell cultures. The mechanism by which $1{,}25\text{-}(OH)_2D$ increases paracellular permeability and calcium flux is not known but may be mediated through its action on cytoskeletal remodeling, which is well known to modulate tight-junction structure and function. The traditional emphasis on the effect of vitamin D on active transcellular calcium transport has left the potentially more important calcium transport through the paracellular conduit relatively unexplored.

$1{,}25(OH)_2D$ and Transcellular Calcium Absorption: Nongenomic Pathway

$1{,}25(OH)_2D$ appears to have a direct, nongenomic, membrane effect (Fig. 17.3A), in addition to its classical steroid–hormone action that induces new protein synthesis (Fig. 17.3B), on transcellular calcium absorption. Studies have shown that the stimulation of calcium transport can occur under conditions in which new protein synthesis is completely inhibited. In addition, the stimulatory effect of $1{,}25(OH)_2D$ on apical calcium entry and transepithelial calcium absorption precedes the increment in synthesis of calbindin-D, a key marker of $1{,}25(OH)_2D$-induced gene expression in the intestine. A number of studies have demonstrated rapid $1{,}25(OH)_2D$-induced increases in calcium uptake in animals that are vitamin D replete. This rapid effect of $1{,}25(OH)_2D$ (within minutes of treatment) on intestinal calcium transport has been attributed to a direct effect of $1{,}25(OH)_2D$

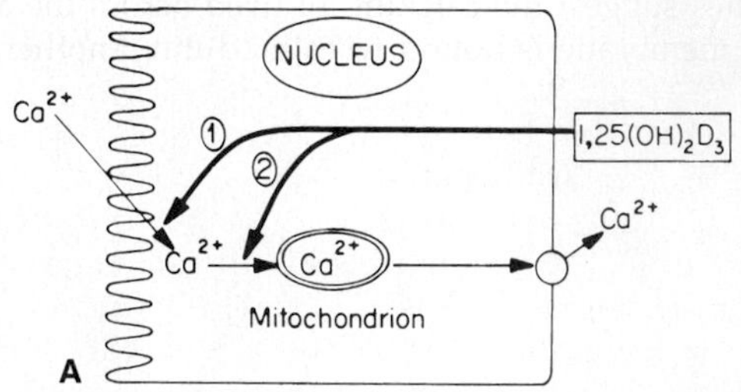

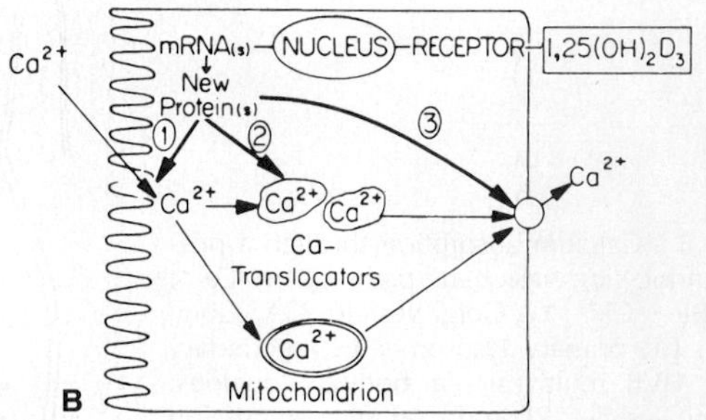

Figure 17.3. Model for short-term and long-term action of $1{,}25(OH)_2D$ on calcium transport across the intestinal cells. **A:** Short term, protein synthesis independent. **B:** Long term, protein synthesis dependent.

at the apical membrane domains (Fig 17.3A, *1*). One example is the stimulation of transcaltachia whereby calcium absorption is increased through increasing transcellular vesicular transport of this mineral. Another possible example is the effect of $1,25(OH)_2D$ on apical calcium influx not related to transcaltachia. As mentioned earlier, apical calcium influx responds rapidly (within minutes) to $1, 25(OH)_2D$ treatment. This has been attributed to a calcium channel–like pathway that is dihydropyridine sensitive and mediated through a cAMP-dependent pathway.

It needs to be pointed out that rapid induction of an hormonal action does not necessarily exclude possible dependence on new protein synthesis. Thus it is possible $1,25(OH)_2D$ may cause rapid shuttling of preformed "protein transporters" from an intracellular pool into the membrane. In addition, it has been proposed that $1,25(OH)_2D$ may induce changes in membrane lipid structure, leading to secondary changes in the functional activity of *in situ* membrane proteins, the so-called liponomic regulation of protein function. It is postulated that changing the lipid environment may render the protein functionally more efficient or activate previously hidden or nonfunctional proteins. Hard evidence for this theory remains to be demonstrated. Other proposed nongenomic, extranuclear pathways for $1,25(OH)_2D$ effect on calcium absorption include its action on cyclic nucleotides, protein kinase C, and cAMP-dependent protein kinase; phosphorylation of brush border membrane protein; and binding of calmodulin to brush border membrane proteins.

$1,25(OH)_2D$ also appears to have a stimulatory effect on mitochondrial calcium uptake, which is not dependent on new protein synthesis (Fig 17.3A, *2*). The mitochondrial uptake would prevent unchecked escalation in intracellular $[Ca^{2+}]$ during calcium transport across the enterocytes. This process ferries the influxed calcium across the cytosol and unloads it for efflux at the basolateral membrane. However, this is not an ideal mechanism for cellular transport of calcium because the optimal activity of this system requires a $[Ca^{2+}]$ of 10^{-5} M. This is clearly above the physiologic steady-state intracellular $[Ca^{2+}]$ and suggests that mitochondria is not the principal means by which $1,25(OH)_2D$ regulates the movement of calcium through the cell during normal calcium absorption.

$1,25(OH)_2D$ and Transcellular Calcium Absorption: Genomic Pathway

Classical interaction between the hormone–receptor complex and specific genes constitutes the major, long-term (hours to days) mechanism by which $1,25(OH)_2D$ stimulates calcium absorption (Fig. 17.3B). Accumulating evidence suggests that the mechanism of action of $1,25(OH)_2D$ in the enterocytes may involve the induction of more than one protein. At the apical membrane, $1,25(OH)_2D$ may rapidly increase the activity of a channel-mediated calcium influx mechanism discussed previously. Whether this hormone induces the synthesis of such channels or other calcium-translocating proteins at the brush border (Fig. 17.3B, *1*) remains to be explored. A major marker of $1,25(OH)_2D$-mediated gene expression is the synthesis of the calbindin-D. The postulated function of calbindin-D on calcium absorption has been discussed earlier and includes the transcellular calcium buffering and transport (Fig. 17.3B, *2*), as well as a possible role in calcium influx across the brush border membrane (Fig. 17.3B, *1*). It has been further postulated that calbindin-D, and possibly other yet unrecognized proteins, may segregate and accumulate the influxed calcium in lysosomallike vesicles or in Golgi or other intracellular membrane-bound fractions (Fig. 17.3B, *2*). New protein(s) may also function as calmodulinlike proteins, which potentiate calcium exit from mitochondria and deliver it to the Ca^{2+}-ATPase exit pump at the basolateral membrane. The enhancing action of $1,25(OH)_2D$ on the synthesis of Ca^{2+}-ATPase has been mentioned earlier (Fig. 17.3B, *3*).

Altered Vitamin D–Receptor Function

It has been reported that common allelic variants in the gene encoding the vitamin D receptor predicts differences in bone density and can account for up to 75% of the total genetic effect on bone density in healthy individuals. Moreover, the genotype associated with lower bone density was overrepresented in postmenopausal women with a significant reduction in bone density. The mechanism responsible for this association is not clear but has been postulated to be mediated, at least in part, by impaired intestinal calcium absorption. However, several studies could not confirm this association among vitamin D–receptor polymorphism, osteoporosis, and intestinal calcium absorption.

Non–Vitamin D Factors

Convincing evidence for the stimulatory action of $1,25(OH)_2D$ on calcium absorption has eclipsed information on important regulation of calcium absorption by mechanisms not mediated by vitamin D. The participation of vitamin D–independent calcium absorption is mentioned in different sections to this chapter. In addition, the observation that active calcium absorption persists in young, growing rats rigidly deprived of vitamin D and the presence of active calcium secretion in mature rats optimally replete with vitamin D also suggest the participation of factors, other than vitamin D, in the regulation of intestinal calcium absorption. Kinetic analysis of $1,25(OH)_2D$-induced transport mechanism indicates that the transport capacity can be saturated at relatively low levels of luminal $[Ca^{2+}]$, thus raising the question of whether these mechanisms would have major regulatory roles under normal dietary conditions that generate much higher luminal calcium concentrations. There is also suggestive evidence indicating that even under conditions of low dietary calcium intake, the adaptive changes in intestinal absorption of calcium may not be mediated by vitamin D alone. Examples of non–vitamin D agents that may play important roles in calcium absorption include bile salts, lactose, sex hormones such as the prolactin, and other factors that are discussed later.

CALCIUM ABSORPTION: THE CONCEPT OF SEGMENTAL RECRUITMENT

Studies from a number of laboratories have clearly demonstrated that $1,25(OH)_2D$ stimulates active absorption of *both* calcium and phosphate in all segments of the intestine except the colon, where $1,25(OH)_2D$ appears to stimulate calcium absorption only through the transcellular route. Segmental analysis of transport characteristics allows an estimate of the quantitative distribution of these calcium- and phosphate-transporting loci along the length of the intestine (Fig. 17.4). This model is consistent with the observation that the duodenum responds to $1,25(OH)_2D$ with a much greater increase in active calcium absorption than phosphate absorption, whereas the jejunum exhibits a much larger change in active phosphate absorption. Because the total number of calcium- and phosphate-transporting loci are about equal, the model also is consistent with the observation that administration of vitamin D induces equal amount of calcium and phosphate absorption.

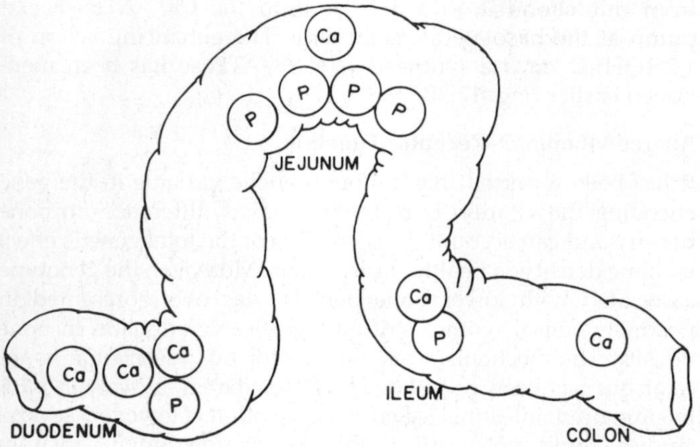

Figure 17.4. Distribution of 1,25(OH)$_2$D-responsive calcium- and phosphate-transporting sites in different segments of the intestine in the rat.

The observation that 1,25(OH)$_2$D is capable of stimulating active calcium absorption in all segments of the intestine raises the question of how this hormone regulates calcium absorption in the intact intestinal tract. Does even minimal Ca-deficit turns on 1,25(OH)$_2$D, which in turn, turns on the entire intestine for active calcium absorption? Based on dose–response studies in the rat, we have demonstrated that low, physiologic doses of 1,25(OH)$_2$D stimulated calcium absorption only in the duodenum. At somewhat higher dosages, the colon also became activated to absorb calcium, but the jejunum and ileum remained unresponsive. Only at clearly pharmacologic dosages of 1,25(OH)$_2$D did the long, midsegments become stimulated, with the jejunum being the least sensitive segment to 1,25(OH)$_2$D stimulation.

Based on these observations, we have proposed the concept of "segmental recruitment" as a mechanism for regulation. In Fig. 17.5, the five columns represent five states of increasing calcium deficits characterized by progressive elevations in endogenous levels of 1,25(OH)$_2$D represented by the solid horizontal line in each column [the normal range of 1,25(OH)$_2$D is depicted by the shaded area]. At the top of each column is a schematized intestinal tract with its four representative segments—D, J, I, C—representing duodenum, jejunum, ileum, and colon, respectively. Shaded segments denote activation by 1,25(OH)$_2$D. The first column represents a state of calcium balance (i.e., no calcium deficit). 1,25(OH)$_2$D level is normal or low-normal, and no intestinal segment is actively absorbing calcium. Of course, calcium is still absorbed passively, and the amount absorbed is excreted in the urine. The second column represents a state of minimal calcium deficit, which increases the level of 1,25(OH)$_2$D toward the upper limit of the normal range. This, in turn, would maximally activate the short but highly efficient duodenum. Once the calcium deficit is repaired, the 1,25(OH)$_2$D level will return to its original level (as in the first column), thus deactivating the duodenum from further active absorption. This level of regulation would most likely be sufficient to maintain calcium balance in virtually all physiologic conditions in adult animals and humans [i.e., by fluctuation in 1,25(OH)$_2$D levels close to or within physiologic range and thus turning "on" and "off" active calcium absorption in the duodenum].

In instances when the need for calcium is greater than usual, 1,25(OH)$_2$D may increase above, but still close to, the upper limit of normal range (Fig. 17.5, third column from left). This would then mobilize the colon for active calcium absorption. On reflection, it appears reasonable to first mobilize the shorter, terminal segment rather than the long midsegments for active calcium absorption. Only under conditions of great physiologic stress (e.g., rapid growth) or during states of vitamin D excess [e.g., administration of large doses of exogenous 1,25(OH)$_2$D] are the long midsegments mobilized into the active calcium absorptive mode. The progressive recruitment of different segments of the intestine for active calcium absorption transforms the otherwise simple, open-ended intestinal tube into an organ capable of both fine and massive adjustment in the regulation of calcium absorption.

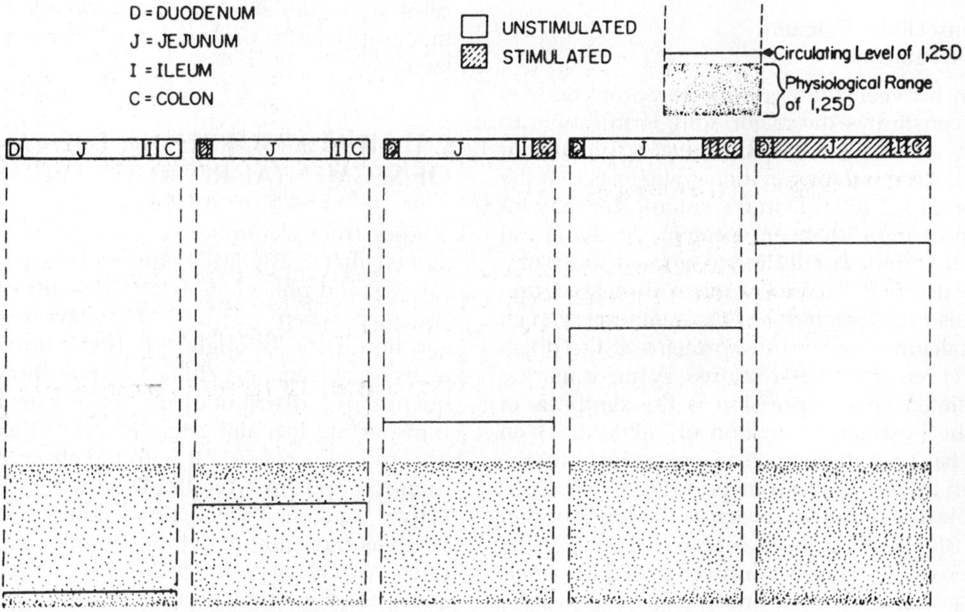

Figure 17.5. "Segmental recruitment" as a mechanism with which 1,25(OH)$_2$D regulates active calcium absorption.

CALCIUM ABSORPTION IN HUMANS AND WHOLE ANIMALS

Importance of Calcium Absorption in the Distal Intestine

Most available information on calcium absorption is based on calcium transport studies in intestinal segments separated from the remainder of the intestinal tract either by actual severance or by other means such as occluding balloons. Such studies, both in animals and in humans, have convincingly demonstrated that the duodenum has the most efficient calcium-absorptive mechanism. Relatively few studies have addressed the quantitative contribution of each segment in the intact intestinal tract in which the functional and structural integrity of the entire intestine is not compromised. Based on observations from such studies, it appears that although the proximal small intestine has the greatest calcium absorptive efficiency, it is the distal small intestine, and in particular the ileum, that accounts for the bulk of calcium absorbed *in vivo*. Using a combination of $^{45}Ca^{2+}$ of a nonabsorbable radionuclide marker, calcium absorption by different segments of the intestine has been estimated in intact rat after an orally administered liquid or solid meal. The proportion of total calcium absorbed by duodenum, jejunum, and ileum were respectively, 15%, 23%, and 62% with liquid meal and 8%, 4%, and 88% with solid meal. The primacy of ileal calcium absorption in intact intestines may be attributed to the very rapid transit of food bolus through the proximal intestine and the long ileal residence time of intestinal content. Using similar techniques, we have demonstrated that within 20 minutes of feeding, 80% of a liquid meal has progressed into the distal intestine and the mean residence time of a meal in ileum is 106 minutes, versus 3 minutes in the duodenum. The importance of the distal intestine, in particular the ileum, in calcium absorption is also evident in patients who had bypass surgery for obesity. Patients who had a better-preserved ileum suffered less from malabsorption or from loss in bone mineral content, or both. In addition to the ileum, it is believed that the large intestine is also important for calcium homeostasis, especially during calcium deprivation or as a consequence of the loss of ileal absorptive function. This is seen in patients who underwent ileostomy after small bowel resection versus those who underwent small bowel resection with ileocecal anastomosis. Calcium absorption was decreased in patients with ileostomy and normal in patients with ileocecal anastomosis.

Net Absorption Versus True Absorption

In the discussion on calcium absorption in humans and whole animals, it is important to distinguish net absorption from true absorption. In a hypothetical normal adult human consuming 1,000 mg of calcium per day, about 350 mg (20% to 40%) is absorbed by the intestine (Table 17.1). In addition, about 200 mg of calcium enters the lumen via intestinal, biliary, and pancreatic secretions, of which 50 mg is absorbed. Total fecal calcium consists of unabsorbed ingested calcium (650 mg) and unabsorbed endogenous calcium (150 mg).

Net calcium absorption (i.e. net gain of calcium to the body) is calculated by subtracting the total fecal calcium from the dietary calcium, that is, 1,000 mg − 800 mg = 200 mg, or 20% of calcium intake. However, the intestine has actually been presented with both dietary and endogenous calcium, totaling 1,200 mg. Hence, true absorption is 1,200 mg − 800 mg, or 400 mg. This represents an absorptive rate of 400/1,200 or 33%. Although the concept of "true absorption" better reflects the overall digestive capacity of the intestine, net calcium absorption is of greater practical importance because it represents the actual transfer of an exogenous source of calcium from the lumen into the body.

TABLE 17.1. Estimates of Dietary and Endogenous Calcium[a]

	Total (mg/day)	Absorbed (mg/day)	In Feces (mg/day)
Dietary calcium	1,000	350	650
Endogenous calcium	200	50	150
Dietary and endogenous calcium	1,200	400	800

[a] Total amount that enters the intestinal lumen (Total), amount absorbed (Absorbed) and amount excreted in feces (In Feces). (See text for discussion on net absorption vs true absorption.)

CALCIUM INTAKE AS A DETERMINATE OF NET ABSORPTION IN HUMANS

The curvilinear relationship between net calcium absorption and dietary calcium intake is illustrated in Fig. 17.6. Net calcium absorption rises steeply as calcium intake increases from 0, and thereafter less steeply as calcium intake exceeds 10 mg/kg per day. At low calcium intake, the active absorptive mechanism most likely predominates. As discussed earlier, for diffusion in the absorptive direction to occur, luminal [Ca^{2+}] has to exceed 2 mM. With low calcium intake, the luminal [Ca^{2+}] may drop below this level, in which case diffusion would occur in the opposite, secretory direction. This, together with the obligatory endogenous secretion associated with digestion, can account for the net negative calcium absorption (i.e., stool calcium exceeds dietary calcium) observed when dietary calcium is below 3 mg/kg per day (Fig. 17.6). At a dietary calcium intake of 3 mg/kg per day, stool calcium equals diet calcium, thereby zero net absorption occurs. Above 3 mg/kg per day, net absorption accelerates rapidly, probably because the luminal [Ca^{2+}] now advances into the range for optimal functioning of the active absorptive mechanism. With further increases in dietary calcium, the slope of the curve becomes less steep. In addition, the curve becomes linear and does not reach a plateau even at the highest calcium intake studied. These observations

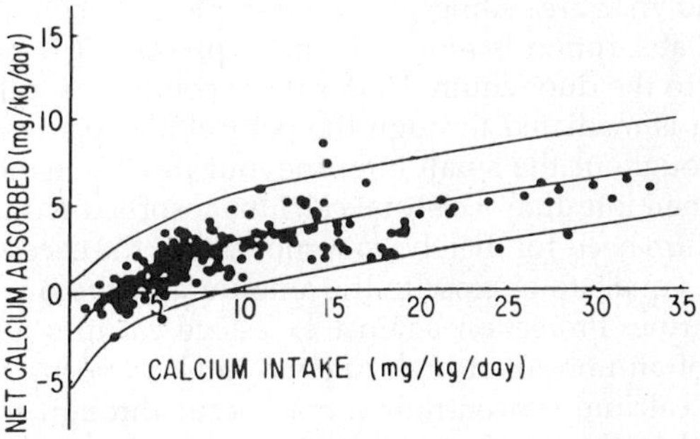

Figure 17.6. Net calcium absorption as a function of dietary calcium. (Reproduced with permission from Wilkinson R. Absorption of calcium, phosphorus and magnesium. In: Nordin BEC, ed. *Calcium phosphate and magnesium metabolism*. Edinburgh and London: Churchill Livingstone, 1976.)

suggest that in face of an ample calcium supply, the passive absorptive mechanism predominates. In any case, reduction or cessation of active calcium absorption is anticipated under the condition of high calcium intake. Closer scrutiny of the curve suggests that a more accurate representation of the data should include an additional change in the slope of the curve as dietary calcium approaches and exceeds 20 mg/kg per day because all the data points above this intake fall below the mean curve. It is possible that at a very high dietary calcium intake, the parallel increase in luminal [Ca^{2+}] could induce local regulation by reducing calcium flux across the paracellular route. An increase in extracellular [Ca^{2+}] is known to increase the "tightness" of the epithelial junction complex, with a consequent reduction in solute traffic across this shunt pathway. In this context, it has been observed that an oral calcium load causes marked and rapid (within 2½ hours) reduction in calcium absorption. It is unlikely that this rapid reduction in absorption is secondary to changes in 1,25$(OH)_2$D synthesis. A more plausible explanation is that the luminal flooding of calcium leads to a reduction in the permeability of the tight junction and thereby an abrupt reduction in the diffusional absorption of calcium.

Although a curvilinear relationship between calcium intake and absorption has been consistently observed, there is considerable variability in net calcium absorption between individuals at any given calcium intake. Both animal and human studies indicate that the habitual calcium intake (calcium status), as well as a variety of other factors discussed next, influence the efficiency of absorption at any level of calcium intake. In woman, even when these factors were held constant or suitably controlled, considerable variation still persisted between individuals. Interestingly though, intraindividual variability was small (i.e., a woman who is a high absorber under one set of conditions is found to be a relatively high absorber under another set of conditions). This suggests that there may be different individual absorptive set points, particularly in women. The relationship between this parameter and vitamin D–receptor gene polymorphism discussed earlier is an interesting speculation.

CALCIUM ABSORPTION: AN INTEGRATED CONCEPT

Integrating available information, we offer the following conceptual framework. Absorption of calcium across the intestinal mucosa is achieved by two parallel processes: a transcellular transport process and a paracellular transport process. In normal adult humans and in grown animals that are in calcium balance and that are eating a calcium-replete diet, transcellular calcium absorption is minimal, and if present, it is mainly restricted to the duodenum. Under these conditions, calcium absorption is mediated through the paracellular pathway occurring throughout the small intestine, but predominantly in the distal small intestine. The total calcium absorbed would satisfy the calcium need for metabolic turnover and the excess calcium (usually equals to or close to the amount absorbed) is excreted in the urine. Protection against excessive calcium absorption in face of an unbridled high calcium intake, and thereby high luminal calcium concentration, may occur through a calcium-mediated "tightening" of the tight junctional complex (which can, in turn, reduce absorptive calcium flux across the paracellular pathway) and through urinary calcium excretion of the excess calcium absorbed. In addition, experimental studies suggest that in face of high calcium availability, transcellular calcium secretion can occur.

When the demand for calcium exceeds the amount of calcium absorbed through this "default" paracellular route, vitamin D–dependent (and vitamin D–independent) transcellular calcium absorption is mobilized by incremental "segmental recruitment" to meet the rising calcium demand. This can occur under normal physiologic conditions when the dietary calcium is unusually low or under conditions of excessive physiologic needs for calcium such as rapid bone turnover states and active growth. Vitamin D under such conditions not only activates transcellular calcium absorption but may also augment intercellular calcium absorption. Despite these adaptive mechanisms, chronic low calcium intake may result in net negative calcium balance and sustained excessive calcium intake can result in unwanted calcium overload.

FACTORS THAT DECREASE CALCIUM ABSORPTION (TABLE 17.2)

In the last section of this chapter, we list factors that have been reported to alter calcium absorption. The validity of these factors as modulators of calcium absorption and the mechanism through which each of these factors may influence calcium absorption are, in most cases, not well established.

Dietary Factors

Phytic Acid and Fiber

It has long been observed that the percentage of dietary calcium absorbed was reduced with the feeding of brown bread instead of white bread. Subsequently, negative calcium balance is observed with the consumption of whole-wheat products, which is attributed to calcium binding (and thereby preventing its absorption) by either the phytate or the uronic acids content in the fiber consumed. It has been calculated that in a typical Western diet, there are 17 g of fiber and 12 mmol of uronic acids, which are capable of binding 152 mg of calcium. A vegetarian diet has sufficient uronic acids to bind 360 mg of dietary calcium. The combination of low calcium intake and high intake of chupaties made from unleavened whole-wheat bread is thought to be a factor in the pathogenesis of late-onset rickets in Asian immigrant children in Great Britain. The interrelationship between fiber consumption and calcium absorption deserves further

TABLE 17.2. Factors That Decrease Calcium Absorption

Dietary factors
Phytic acid and fiber
Low-calcium diet
Excessive phosphorus diet
Fat
Alcohol
Others: fluoride, oxalate, vitamin B_6 deficiency, citrate
Abnormal states of vitamin D metabolism
Chronic renal failure
Aging
Hormonal factors
Parathyroid hormone insufficiency
Glucocorticoids
Other peptide hormones: thyroid hormone, somatostatin
Other conditions
Malabsorption syndrome
Postgastrectomy
Diabetes mellitus
Osteoporosis
Therapeutic agents: colchicine, theophylline, aluminum

scrutiny in susceptible populations, especially in view of the current trend toward increasing fiber intake.

Low Calcium Intake

As mentioned earlier, a low-calcium diet is a known stimulus for transcellular calcium absorption, and this is believed to be mediated through an increase in $1,25(OH)_2D$ synthesis. However, the activation of this mechanism may not translate into a significant increase in net calcium absorption because the low availability of luminal calcium may not provide adequate substrate for transport, even if the transporting mechanism is maximally stimulated. Moreover, the transcellular calcium absorptive process in the rat intestine has an apparent affinity (K_m, the luminal calcium concentration at which active transcellular absorptive process is equal to half its maximal capacity) of 1 mM, and a failure to achieve this calcium concentration would result in the absorptive mechanism functioning at only suboptimal rates. Finally, as already discussed, when luminal calcium concentration drops below 2 mM, the passive calcium flux across the paracellular pathway would be expected to switch from the absorptive into the secretory mode. For all these reasons, low calcium intake may lead to a reduction in net calcium absorption, even in the presence of compensatory stimulation of active, transcellular absorptive mechanism.

Studies in humans have demonstrated that physiologic adaptation to low calcium intake may not be adequate to prevent negative calcium balance (see the discussion relating to Fig. 17.6). In one study, isotopic calcium absorption and calcium balance were carried out in subjects given either 209 or 2,108 mg of calcium/day for 35 days. Subjects receiving the low-calcium diet retained 63.6% of a dose compared with 30.5% in subjects consuming the high-calcium diet. However, calcium balance was −130/day in the low-calcium diet group and +85 mg/day in the high-calcium diet group. In another report, a retrospective survey of calcium-balance studies were collected in 212 adults. Calcium balance was mostly negative in subjects eating a diet containing less than 600 mg of calcium per day. In a third study, two Yugoslavian communities, one with habitual calcium intake of 400 mg/day and the other 900 mg/day, were examined. Both communities were otherwise similar in ethnic background, physical activity, and exposure to sunlight. Both men and women in the low-calcium group demonstrated less skeletal mineralization from age of 30 years and a higher incidence of fractures. These data demonstrate that there is a lower limit of calcium intake, below which adaptive absorption cannot compensate adequately to maintain optimal calcium balance. The critical level appears to be around 400 mg/day.

Many calcium supplements are commercially available in a variety of preparations (liquid and solid). The accompanying anions include carbonate, phosphate, sulphate, acetate, lactate, gluconate, glycerophosphate, citrate, and citrate-malate. The calcium content in these supplements ranges from 10% (calcium gluconate and lactate) to almost 40% (calcium carbonate, oyster shell, hydroxyapatite). Although there is a wide range of solubility of these supplements, the difference in absorbability, by comparison, is small. Furthermore, urinary calcium or calcium balance measurement (both reflect calcium availability for absorption) were not different in subjects given gluconate, carbonate, or citrate. There is disagreement, however, as to the effectiveness of these supplements, particularly when compared with the usual dairy products, in improving bone health.

Excessive Phosphorus Intake

Although phosphorus has been implicated to interfere with calcium absorption (presumably via formation of poorly soluble calcium phosphates), most studies have established that in the presence of adequate dietary calcium and vitamin D, changing the calcium-to-phosphate ratio in the diet over a wide range does not affect calcium absorption in humans and experimental animals. It has been shown that increasing dietary phosphorus from 200 to 2,000 mg/day has no influence on calcium absorption regardless of calcium intake. In low-birth-weight infants, the feeding of formulas with calcium-to-phosphate ratios ranging from 0.6 to 2.4 revealed calcium absorption was dependent on calcium intake and independent of the phosphorus content of the formula.

Fat

In healthy adults, variation in dietary fat from 1% to 32% has no effect on calcium absorption. Calcium absorption is decreased in patients with malabsorption syndrome and increased fecal fat excretion. The complexing of calcium with fatty acids forms insoluble soaps and thereby prevents the absorption of calcium. In contrast to fatty acids, triglycerides may improve the absorption of both fat and calcium. This was shown in preterm infants and in patients with biliary cirrhosis and partial gastrectomies who were supplemented with medium-chain triglycerides.

Alcohol

Calcium absorption may be reduced in chronic alcoholics by a number of factors. Steatorrhea can lead to reduced absorption of both calcium and vitamin D. Liver involvement may cause impairment in 25-hydroxylation of vitamin D. Alcohol has also been shown to cause abnormalities in the microvilli and mitochondria of intestinal mucosal cells. An experimental study in the rat, however, demonstrated that simple feeding of alcohol does not lead to malabsorption of calcium. In healthy young men, the consumption of either 1 L of wine per day or a similar quantity of dealcoholized wine have been reported to improve calcium balance. Because calcium absorption was increased by both forms of treatment, the stimulation of calcium absorption was probably mediated through nonalcoholic components, perhaps through stimulation of gastric acid.

Other Dietary Factors

Fluoride has been shown to reduce calcium absorption in humans and experimental animals. Postulated mechanisms include luminal binding of calcium and interference of calcium transport through inhibition of energy-producing enzymes. Oxalate may bind and precipitate calcium in the intestinal lumen and is often cited as a cause for reduced intestinal calcium absorption. However, definitive evidence for such an association is lacking. Postulated mechanisms include reducing the availability of calcium to its site of transport secondary to calcium-oxalate precipitation or a direct effect of oxalate on calcium transport process. It has been shown that vitamin B_6 deficiency significantly decreases calcium influx and increases calcium efflux in rat enterocytes. These changes induce profound loss of calcium from intestinal epithelial cells manifested by decreased cytosolic free calcium and total cell calcium. Administration of large doses of citrate (5 mmol) significantly depresses calcium absorption (55% compared with 76%), probably as a result of complexation of calcium and citrate in the intestinal lumen.

Abnormal States of Vitamin D Metabolism

Decreased calcium absorption occurs in various disorders of vitamin D metabolism. These disorders include vitamin D–deficiency, vitamin D–dependency, and vitamin D–resistance states. These states as they are related to intestinal phosphate absorption are discussed in Chapter 19, Part 1. Similar comments apply to calcium absorption and are not repeated here.

Chronic Renal Failure

The association between renal failure and reduced calcium absorption has been repeatedly demonstrated in experimental and clinical studies. Reduced 1,25(OH)$_2$D synthesis by the diseased kidney has been incriminated as a major factor in the pathogenesis of calcium malabsorption associated with renal failure. Treatment with 1,25(OH)$_2$D or its analogs restores calcium absorption to normal. It is also possible to restore net calcium absorption to normal by supplementary calcium intake. This is also reflected by the frequent observation of the correction of hypocalcemia or the development of hypercalcemia associated with the use of calcium-containing phosphate binders. The increased oral calcium load would be expected to augment its absorption through the diffusional pathway. Several studies have demonstrated that uremic patients have a habitually lower intake of calcium when compared with nonuremic control subjects, and this may play an important role in aggravating the suboptimal calcium harvest from the intestine. Further discussion of this topic is found in Chapter 77.

Age

Both experimental and clinical studies have supported the notion of an age-related reduction in calcium absorption. Reduction in calcium absorption is particularly apparent in elderly subjects older than 70. Like patients with chronic renal failure, elderly subjects may ingest diets with suboptimal calcium content. Additional factors include an age-related reduction in 1,25(OH)$_2$D synthesis and an age-related intestinal decline in intracellular 1,25(OH)$_2$D-receptor protein resulting in intestinal resistance to 1,25(OH)$_2$D.

Hormonal Factors

Parathyroid Hormone

Numerous reports have documented increased calcium absorption in hyperparathyroid states and diminished calcium absorption in hypoparathyroid states. Many studies have concluded that the action of parathyroid hormone on intestinal calcium absorption is mediated indirectly through its stimulatory action on renal 1,25(OH)$_2$D production.

Glucocorticoids

Although a large number of studies have demonstrated that glucocorticoids suppress intestinal calcium absorption, the precise mechanism through which this action is mediated is unclear. In experimental studies, glucocorticoids may in fact raise circulating levels of 1.25(OH)$_2$D, increase cytosolic 1,25(OH)$_2$D receptors in cultured osteogenic sarcoma cells, and raise calcium-binding protein levels in intestinal mucosa. *In vitro* studies have demonstrated that glucocorticoids may increase calcium absorption in the ileum and colon. These conflicting observations may be explained by work demonstrating a biphasic effect of glucocorticoids on calcium absorption. Low dosages or short treatment periods of glucocorticoids tend to stimulate calcium absorption, and high concentrations or long-term treatment tend to inhibit calcium absorption.

Other studies have shown that dexamethasone administration has differential actions on the jejunum and colon. In the jejunum, dexamethasone increases bidirectional calcium flux (i.e., mucosal-to-serosal, as well as serosal-to-mucosal directions) with more pronounced mucosal-to-serosal calcium flux and abolishes calcium secretion in this segment. Dexamethasone administration increases intestinal fluid absorption. This effect may enhance bidirectional calcium flux via paracellular pathway presumably by the normal and anomalous solvent drag mechanisms. The same effect of dexamethasone on calcium flux has also been observed in the rat ileum and proximal colon. However, in the distal colon, dexamethasone administration resulted in increase unidirectional flux from serosal-to-mucosal surface and net calcium absorption was abolished.

The apparent inhibitory effect of the glucocorticoids on calcium absorption can also be related to their generalized catabolic effect. The catabolic influence of these metabolites on both skeletal and nonskeletal tissue may reduce the demand for intestinal calcium absorption. Clearly, much work is needed to more clearly define the effect of glucocorticoids on calcium absorption.

Other Peptide Hormones

A number of studies have demonstrated that patients with hyperthyroidism have impaired calcium absorption. Whether this effect is mediated indirectly through altered metabolism of vitamin D is unknown. The reduced calcium absorption may be a result of the general catabolic effect of this hormone. Interestingly, studies in chick embryonic intestinal cells indicate that thyroid hormone (10^{-10} M) amplifies the intestinal response to 1,25(OH)$_2$D. Acute infusion of somatostatin decreases intestinal calcium absorption in man. This observation appears to be in accord with the finding that *in vitro* addition of this hormone stimulates the secretory (serosal-to-mucosal) flux of calcium in descending colon and ileum.

Other Factors

Postgastrectomy

Impaired calcium absorption, osteomalacia, osteoporosis, and fractures have been described after gastrectomy. Factors that could lead to postgastrectomy calcium malabsorption include reduced calcium absorption secondary to exclusion of the duodenum and upper jejunum from the intestinal tract, increase in the intestinal transit rate and steatorrhea, and alterations in vitamin D metabolism.

Diabetes Mellitus

Increased incidence of osteoporosis, hip fractures, and reduction in bone mass have been observed in patients with diabetes mellitus. In experimentally induced diabetes mellitus, reduced intestinal calcium absorption and intestinal calbindin-D and low plasma levels of 1,25(OH)$_2$D have been noted. The relevance of these observations to human diabetes remains to be determined.

Osteoporosis

Decreased intestinal calcium absorption and chronic, relative calcium deficiency have been considered important in the pathogenesis of postmenopausal osteoporosis. Because serum 1,25(OH)$_2$D levels decline with menopause and estrogen treatment reverses this trend, 1,25(OH)$_2$D deficiency has been postulated as a cause for calcium malabsorption in postmenopausal osteoporosis. In this context, long-term treatment with low dosages of 1,25(OH)$_2$D has been reported to restore calcium absorption to normal in postmenopausal women. Other studies suggest that estrogen is necessary for preserving normal intestinal responsiveness to 1,25(OH)$_2$D.

Therapeutic Agents and Aluminum

Several therapeutic agents have been reported to reduce intestinal calcium absorption in experimental studies. Perfusing the rat duodenum with 0.1 and 0.5 mM colchicine produced a dose-dependent inhibition in calcium transport without simultaneous changes in water transport. Theophylline has been reported to inhibit active, transcellular calcium transport through a mechanism involving calbindin-D. Aluminum has been reported to inhibit active calcium absorption in duodenal segments but has no effect on calcium absorption in ileal segments, where passive, paracellular calcium absorption predominates. Of more clinical interest, aluminum-containing antacids, even at low dosages (90 ml/day), decrease calcium absorption and increase urinary calcium excretion.

FACTORS THAT INCREASE CALCIUM ABSORPTION (TABLE 17.3)

Dietary Factors

Low-Phosphate Diet

Under rigorous conditions of dietary phosphorus deprivation in humans, both calcium absorption and $1,25(OH)_2D$ production are stimulated. However, calcium balance becomes negative because of a significant increase in urinary calcium loss, which is, at least partly, also caused by increased bone resorption. Similar findings have been noted in experimental studies. However, when protracted phosphorus deprivation results in severe phosphorus deficiency, intestinal calcium absorption may become depressed.

Lactose and Other Sugars

It has been recognized for decades that the feeding of lactose to experimental animals leads to increased calcium absorption. *In vitro* studies have established that calcium absorption is directly stimulated by the presence of lactose in the mucosal compartment, and the effect of this sugar is greatest in the ileum. Under *in vivo* condition, large quantities of ingested lactose is delivered to the ileum because unlike other monosaccharides and disaccharides, lactose is not hydrolyzed in the proximal small intestine. In humans, calcium absorption in infants fed lactose-free formula is significantly reduced when compared with infants fed regular, lactose-containing formula. In healthy adults, calcium absorption, as reflected by the serum appearance of orally ingested calcium, is greater when the isotope is given with regular milk compared with lactose-free milk. The stimulation of calcium absorption by lactose is not vitamin D dependent. The basis for this interesting "lactose effect" is still not fully elucidated, but both paracellular and cellular mechanisms have been proposed. Other sugars, such as mannose and raffinose, have similar stimulatory effect on calcium absorption. Jejunal perfusion studies in humans have confirmed that, like lactose, other sugars (e.g., xylose, sorbitol) also increase calcium absorption. Glucose has also been reported to increase intestinal calcium absorption in both humans and experimental animals. A possible mechanism is that glucose activates the Na-glucose cotransport mechanism, which triggers cytoskeletal contraction and dilation of the "channels" in the tight-junction complex, permitting augmented calcium absorption by solvent drag.

TABLE 17.3. Factors That Increase Calcium Absorption

Dietary factors
Low-phosphorus diet
Lactose and other sugars
Protein and amino acids
Bile salts
Others: small doses of calcium, meal, medium-chain triglycerides, ascorbic acid, antibiotics
Physiologic states of increased calcium demand
Hormonal factors
Parathyroid hormone
Growth hormone
Prolactin
Estrogens
Other factors
Sarcoidosis
Idiopathic hypercalciuria and calcium-stone formers
Milk-alkali syndrome

Protein and Amino Acids

Experimental studies have demonstrated that certain amino acids (e.g., L-lysine and L-arginine) enhance calcium absorption. Of clinical interest is the observation that an increase in purified or semipurified protein consumption is associated with a parallel increase in urinary calcium excretion. This was initially attributed to a protein-induced increase in intestinal calcium absorption. However, subsequent studies failed to substantiate such a postulated relationship. It is now believed that the protein-induced hypercalciuria is a consequence of an insulin-mediated reduction in renal calcium reabsorption. Another theory proposes that high protein intake increases endogenous acid production, which causes skeletal mobilization and urinary excretion of calcium. Controlled human studies, on the other hand, have failed to show that common dietary complex proteins (e.g., meat, dairy products) fed over a long period cause calcium loss in adults. In addition to protein, meat and dairy products contain high levels of phosphorus, which can decrease urinary calcium output, regardless of the calcium intake, thereby counteracting the calciuric effect of the protein.

Bile Salts

Bile salts also enhance calcium absorption in experimental studies through a vitamin D–independent mechanism. These compounds not only increase the solubility of calcium salts but also have a direct enhancing effect on the absorption of calcium from the intestine. The mechanism for this last action has not been fully explored. Bile salts increase transepithelial conductance in rat colon and reversibly increase epithelial permeability to large molecules such as inulin, implicating the shunt pathway as the major locus of action. However, it is also possible that bile salts may affect cellular transport of calcium because they are known to influence active electrolyte transport across the intestine.

Other Dietary Factors

Calcium absorption has been shown to be higher when the daily intake of calcium is divided into smaller doses. This is because the efficiency of calcium absorption varies inversely with the size of the calcium dose fed. Thus 1,000 mg of calcium taken as two doses of 500 mg each resulted in 30% more calcium being absorbed than if it was taken as one dose, and four divided doses resulted in 60% more calcium absorbed. Consuming calcium with a meal also increases calcium absorption compared with calcium ingested on an empty stomach. This may be particularly important for a subset of individuals. Studies indicate that some individuals will substantially malabsorb calcium carbonate when it is given on an empty stomach, even though they absorb the carbonate salt normally when it is taken with a meal. Ascorbic acid, a component of orange juice, has been reported to substantially increase calcium absorption. Antibiotics such as penicillin, chloramphenicol, and neomycin have been shown to increase radiocalcium absorption. The mechanism for this phenomenon is unclear but it has been suggested that these antibiotics may act in a manner similar to lactose.

PHYSIOLOGIC STATES OF INCREASED CALCIUM DEMAND

The two major physiologic states that impose immense demand for calcium are rapid growth and pregnancy and lactation. In both states, increased $1,25(OH)_2D$ synthesis has been demonstrated. Experimental studies also suggest the participation of vitamin D–independent factors. During the neonatal period, the intestine is insensitive to vitamin D and exhibits no saturable process for calcium absorption. Calcium absorption during this period of rapid growth is therefore sustained by the diffusion and solvent drag. Not until weaning (i.e., 3 weeks of age) do rats acquire simultaneously a saturable calcium absorptive process and sensitivity to $1,25(OH)_2D$. Initially, active calcium absorption is observed in both the small and large intestine, but with time, active calcium absorption is limited to the proximal small intestine. Pregnancy and lactation also impose heavy stress on the calcium absorptive system. Experimental studies again have demonstrated that adaptive responses can occur in the absence of vitamin D. It has been found that calcium absorption increased late in pregnancy, peaked during lactation, and fell to control values after weaning in both vitamin D–replete and vitamin D–deficient rats. In pregnant women, both an increase in plasma levels of $1,25(OH)_2D$ and an increase in intestinal calcium absorption have been demonstrated. However, when high dosages of both estrogen and progesterone were given to normal women for 7 weeks, changes similar to those observed in pregnant women could not be duplicated. Thus the mechanisms that stimulate $1,25(OH)_2D$ and intestinal calcium absorption remain incompletely defined.

CALCIUM ABSORPTION IN CLINICAL STATES

Hormonal Abnormalities

The effect of parathyroid hormone excess and deficiency on calcium absorption have been mentioned earlier: excess growth affects calcium absorption; indeed, increased calcium absorption has been reported in patients with acromegaly. The exact incidence and pathogenetic mechanism remain to be defined, but growth hormone–related stimulation in $1,25(OH)_2D$ production has been suspected. Prolactin is another peptide hormone that increases calcium absorption and the generation of $1,25(OH)_2D$. However, a direct vitamin D–independent effect on calcium absorption has also been demonstrated in experimental studies. Cyclical administration of conjugated estrogens has been reported to increase plasma $1,25(OH)_2D$ and intestinal calcium absorption in postmenopausal osteoporotic women.

Other Clinical Conditions

Sarcoidosis increases intestinal calcium absorption through increased production of $1,25(OH)_2D$. The synthesis of this hormone occurs outside the kidney and is accomplished by "sarcoid cells," that is, pulmonary alveolar macrophages and cells from the involved lymph nodes. Increased calcium absorption is also found in patients with hypercalciuria and calcium-stone formation. In some of these patients, increased serum $1,25(OH)_2D$ is demonstrated. This condition is discussed in detail elsewhere in this book. The pathogenetic mechanism of the milk-alkali syndrome is not well understood, but increased intestinal calcium absorption has been considered a contributory factor. The syndrome is characterized by hypercalcemia, reduced renal function, and alkalosis. It is associated with the ingestion of large quantities of milk or calcium carbonate or both.

FACTORS WITH UNCERTAIN EFFECT ON CALCIUM ABSORPTION (TABLE 17.4)

Hypertension

Alterations in calcium absorption in hypertensive patients and experimental animals have been described. Initial surveys in American adults identified a relationship between dietary calcium (dairy products) and blood pressure. The higher the intake of dietary calcium, the lower the blood pressure. However, clinical studies examining the effect of calcium supplementation on blood pressure have been inconclusive. It is possible that only a subset of the population's blood pressure is responsive to dietary calcium therapy. It is also possible that dietary calcium supplementation lowers blood pressure only in subjects with marginal calcium intake and with relative calcium depletion but that it has no effect on blood pressure in subjects with an adequate body calcium store. There is some data showing that hypertensive patients have increased urinary excretion of calcium, which is not caused by an increase in calcium intake. There are some suggestions that the impairment in renal tubular reabsorption of calcium might be secondary to the development of hypertension rather than a primary event.

Reported differences in serum ionized calcium between spontaneously hypertensive rats (SHR) and their genetically matched normotensive control (WKY) have led to the study of intestinal calcium transport in this animal model of hypertension. Although some studies have shown lower intestinal calcium absorption in SHR, no clear understanding of the relationship between rates of calcium absorption and hypertension has emerged from these studies.

Other Factors

The importance of gastric acid for complete absorption of dietary calcium, particularly the absorption of different forms of calcium supplement, remains unclear. Currently, the consensus is that gastric acid is not required for calcium absorption when the calcium source is taken with meals. Luminal pH in the rat small intestine varies from 6.0 in proximal segments to 7.2 in terminal ileum. Because calcium precipitates from solutions when pH is greater than 6.1, it has been postulated that dietary calcium is in a more absorbable form in the duodenum and proximal jejunum. However, the bulk of studies, both clinical and experimental, have failed to demonstrate an association between changes in luminal pH with changes in calcium absorption. The effect of magnesium on calcium absorption is still controversial. Studies have demonstrated stimulatory, inhibitory, and absence of effect of this cation on calcium absorption. Ani-

TABLE 17.4. Factors with Uncertain Effect on Calcium Absorption

Hypertension
Other factors
Gastric acid
Luminal pH
Magnesium
Calcitonin

mal studies using vascularly perfused intestines from vitamin D–replete rats showed an inhibition of calcium absorption at low calcitonin levels and stimulatory effect at high concentrations of the hormone.

Selected Readings

Bronner F. Calcium absorption—a paradigm for mineral absorption. *J Nutrition* 1998;128:917–920.
A recent review on transepithelial calcium transport.

Charles P. Calcium absorption and calcium bioavailability. *J Internal Med* 1992; 231:161–168.
A good discussion of calcium supplements.

Favus W. Factors which influence absorption and secretion of calcium in the small intestine and colon. *Am J Physiol* 1985;248:G147–G157.
A review on 1,25-dihydroxyvitamin D–responsive, transepithelial calcium transport in the small intestine and colon in experimental animals.

Karbach U. Mechanism of intestinal calcium transport and clinical aspects of disturbed calcium absorption. *Dig Dis* 1989;7:1–18.
A comprehensive review of calcium absorption in humans and experimental animals.

Kayne LH, D'Argenio DZ, Meyer JH, et al. Analysis of segmental phosphate absorption in intact rats. A compartmental analysis approach. *J Clin Invest* 1993; 91:915–922.
A new strategy for analyzing segmental phosphate absorption from a spontaneously propelled liquid meal through a structurally and functionally untampered intestinal tract in intact rats. Highlights the importance of transit and dwell time in the overall absorption of phosphate in different segments of the intestine in vivo. This concept is used in the discussion of calcium absorption in this chapter.

Lee DBN, Hardwick LL, Hu MS, Jamgotchian N. Vitamin D-independent regulation of calcium and phosphate absorption. *Miner Electrolyte Metab* 1990;16: 167–173.
A review of vitamin D–independent mechanisms for Ca absorption.

Lee DBN, Walling MW, Levine BS, et al. Intestinal and metabolic effect of 1,25-dihydroxyvitamin D_3 in normal adult rat. *Am J Physiol* 1981;240:G90–G96.
Includes data from which the 'segmental recruitment" theory of Ca absorption regulation is developed.

Nemere I, Norman AW. Transport of calcium. In: Field M, Frizzell RA, eds. *Handbook of physiology*, sect 6, vol 4. Bethesda, MD: American Physiological Society, 1991:337–360.
A good review on the effect and mechanism of action of 1,25-dihydroxy vitamin D on calcium absorption.

Wasserman RH, Fullmer CS. Vitamin D and intestinal calcium transport: facts, speculations and hypotheses. *J Nutrition* 1995;125:1971S–1979S.
A recent review on the role of vitamin D on intestinal calcium transport.

Wood RJ, Fleet JC. The genetics of osteoporosis: vitamin D receptor polymorphisms. *Annu Rev Nutr* 1998;18:233–258.
An update on allelic variations in the vitamin D receptor gene, calcium metabolism, and osteoporosis.

PART 2
Renal Handling of Calcium

Diane Rouse and Wadi N. Suki

Calcium (Ca) is the predominant divalent cation in the body, representing 2% of the total body weight. Approximately 99% of total body Ca is found in the bone and the remaining 1% in the soft tissues and extracellular space. The maintenance of calcium homeostasis is important not only to preserve the integrity of the skeleton but also because Ca is the major ionic intracellular messenger and regulator of many cellular functions. Ca is maintained by the integrated actions of the gut, kidneys, and bone. The following discussion focuses on the mechanisms and control of the renal handling of Ca and the role of the kidneys in the maintenance of body Ca.

EXTRACELLULAR CALCIUM

In the normal human adult, plasma Ca ranges from 8.8 to 10.3 mg/dl or approximately 2.5 mM. The plasma Ca may normally be as high as 11 mg/dl in growing children. Calcium in plasma occurs in three forms: approximately 46% of total Ca is bound to protein, approximately 6% of Ca is complexed with various anions, and approximately 48% is in the form of free Ca ions. The latter two forms, complexed Ca and free Ca ions, together comprise the ultrafiltrable (UF) fraction of plasma Ca, or that portion that is filtered through the glomerulus with the plasma water. The ionic form is thought to be the physiologically important moiety, the form that is transported and is active in cellular functions. The ionized calcium (Ca^{2+}) concentration is normally maintained within a very narrow range; however, changes in total plasma Ca concentration, serum protein concentration and composition, blood pH, and complexing anions may upset this rigid control. These changes may also affect the handling of Ca by the renal tubules.

INTRACELLULAR CALCIUM

Total cellular Ca concentration ranges from 1 to 5 mM; however, most of this is bound to the external surface of the cell membrane. Total intracellular Ca is approximately 0.5 mM and most of this is bound to cytoplasmic proteins and ionic ligands or sequestered in the endoplasmic reticulum and mitochondria. The resting intracellular Ca^{2+} concentration is only 10^{-7} M, four orders of magnitude less than the extracellular concentration. This large chemical gradient, coupled with the negatively charged cell interior, favors Ca entry into the cell. However, the maintenance of intracellular Ca^{2+} at submicromolar levels is crucial for its role as an intracellular messenger and modulator of cellular function. Therefore, to maintain the steep gradient between the extracellular and intracellular compartments and to allow transcellular fluxes of Ca in Ca-transporting cells, movement across the cellular membranes must be regulated (Table 17.5).

Calcium Movement Across the Luminal Membrane

In renal tubular cells, as in most other cells, a small amount of Ca diffuses passively across cell membranes; however, the physicochemical properties of cell membranes are such that they impede the diffusion of highly charged ions such as Ca. Therefore, particularly in cells that transport Ca transcellularly, Ca entry must proceed by a facilitated diffusion transport mechanism, either carrier-mediated or through Ca channels. Carrier-mediated transport mechanisms have not been well described; however, Ca^{2+}-H^+ exchange, coupled to Na^+-H^+ exchange and Ca^{2+}-Cl^- cotransport, have been proposed from functional studies.

The presence of Ca channels in renal tubular cells has been suggested by studies using calcium channel blockers. Several investigators have identified Ca channels from various renal tubule cells by patch clamp analysis. One study identified Ca channels on proximal straight (PST), cortical thick ascending limb (TAL), distal convoluted (DCT), and cortical collecting tubule (CCT) segments. Although conductance and open time measurements varied widely, all channels were voltage regulated, inhibited by nifedipine and verapamil, and stimulated by the Ca channel agonist Bay K 8644. The authors suggested that L-type Ca channels were present throughout the nephron. In a separate study, L-type Ca channels also were demonstrated in

TABLE 17.5. Cellular Proteins Involved in Renal Tubular Transport of Calcium

Protein	Cellular Location	Tubule Segment	Action
Ca channels			
L-type	Luminal membrane	PST, CTAL, DCT, CNT, CCT	Ca influx
Other	Luminal membrane	Proximal tubules, TAL/DCT	Ca influx
Na-Ca Exchanger	Basolateral membrane	DCT/CNT	Ca influx or efflux
Plasma membrane Ca-ATPase	Basolateral membrane	DCT, CCT > PCT, MTAL > PST, CTAL	Ca efflux (Ca^{2+} -H^+ exchange)
Calmodulin	Cytoplasmic	All	↑ Ca-ATPase activity
Regucalcin	? Cytoplasmic	Cortex	↑ Ca-ATPase activity
Extracellular Ca/polyvalent	Luminal membrane	PCT, PST, IMCD	?
ion–sensing receptor	Basolateral membrane	CTAL, MTAL, DCT/CNT	↓ Ca transport (? ↓ Ca influx)

CCT, cortical collecting tubule; CNT, connecting tubule; CTAL, cortical thick ascending limb; DCT, distal convoluted tubule; IMCD, inner medullary collecting duct; MTAL, medullary thick ascending limb; PCT, proximal convoluted tubule; PST, proximal straight tubule; TAL, thick ascending limb.

the connecting tubule (CNT) segment. Other studies have suggested that there are unique Ca channels in cultured proximal tubule and TAL/DCT cells. Both of these channels have a lower conductance than the L-type channel and are activated by hyperpolarization of the cell but not depolarization, which opens L-type channels. The channel in the proximal tubule cells is only active in the presence of PMA (an activator of protein kinase C) and stretch. The channel in the TAL/DCT cells has a long open time and is constitutively active. These studies suggest that multiple channel subtypes are present in the proximal and distal tubule. Molecular studies are just beginning to identify Ca channel proteins in kidney tubules. Using polymerase chain reaction and Northern blot analysis, studies in cultured mouse DCT tubule cells and rat DCT/CNT segments also suggest multiple Ca channel subtypes. Messenger RNA transcripts for at least one of the diagnostic Ca channel proteins have also been demonstrated in PST, cortical TAL, and CCT.

Calcium Movement Across the Basolateral Membrane

The endoplasmic reticulum and mitochondria may act as temporary storage compartments for Ca entering the cell; however, ultimately, the "extra" Ca must be removed. This is especially important in cells that transport Ca transcellularly. Calcium exit at the basolateral membrane of renal tubule cells is against a strong electrochemical gradient; hence, an active or secondary active transport mechanism is required. Two mechanisms exist to facilitate Ca efflux at this membrane, the Na-Ca exchanger and plasma membrane Ca-ATPases (PMCA).

Na-Ca Exchanger

Physiologic studies have suggested an operative Na-Ca exchanger in PCT, DCT, and CNT nephron segments. Other investigations have confirmed the importance of the Na-Ca exchanger in Ca transport in the DCT/CNT segment; however, the existence and role of this protein in proximal tubule Ca transport is controversial. Molecular and immunohistochemical studies have confirmed Na-Ca mRNA and protein in distal nephron segments, primarily the CNT and the putative DCT2 segment, which is a transitional segment between the DCT and CNT in some species, but not in the TAL. The results in the proximal tubule segments are again controversial.

The cardiac Na-Ca (the isoform occurring in most tissues) family of proteins is typically approximately 120 kD; however, Western analysis often reveals three proteins with molecular weights of 160, 120, and 70 kD. The 70-kD protein is thought to be a proteolytic fragment of the 120-kD Na-Ca exchanger protein. One investigator demonstrated Na-Ca exchanger mRNA in proximal tubules isolated by gradient centrifugation and the 70-kD fragment of the Na-Ca exchanger protein in PCT and PST segments isolated from dog and rat kidney. The significance of finding only the proteolytic fragment is not known, especially because other investigators have failed to demonstrate the mRNA transcript or protein in these segments. The discrepancies may be a result of species differences, low abundance of the exchanger protein in these segments, or the presence of an isoform not recognized by the antibodies or nucleotide sequences used to probe for the protein or mRNA, respectively. The intron/exon arrangement of the Na-Ca gene suggests that up to 32 splice variants are possible during transcription. To date, eight different isoforms have been identified and four of these have been demonstrated in the kidney, Na-Ca1, 2, 3, and 7.

Plasma Membrane Ca^{2+}-ATPases

The other transport protein involved in Ca efflux at the basolateral membrane is Ca-ATPase (PMCA). Early studies demonstrated a magnesium (Mg)- and calmodulin-dependent Ca-ATPase in the rabbit nephron. The highest concentration was found in the DCT and CCT, intermediate concentrations in the PCT and medullary TAL, and lower concentrations in the PST and cortical TAL segments. Two calmodulin- and Mg-independent Ca-ATPases with different biochemical profiles were demonstrated in basolateral membrane vesicles prepared from rat kidney cortex. The low-affinity, high-capacity form probably contributes little to intracellular Ca homeostasis under physiologic conditions, whereas the other high-capacity, low-affinity enzyme demonstrates an affinity for Ca close to that of normal intracellular Ca^{2+}.

The first antibody used to identify PMCA protein was directed against the red cell PMCA and detected the protein only on the basolateral membrane of the DCT. However, molecular studies have demonstrated four different isoforms of Ca-ATPase, each with multiple splice variants and each encoding a unique protein. Of the isoforms, PMCA1 and 4 mRNAs are expressed in large quantities in all tissues and are thus thought to be "housekeeping" proteins, that is, responsible for the normal maintenance of intracellular Ca^{2+}. PMCA2 and PMCA3 are generally confined to neural tissue. Expression of the isoforms has been demonstrated to change with development and intracellular Ca^{2+} concentration. In mRNA obtained from whole kidney, PMCA1, PMCA2, and PMCA4 have been demonstrated; however, the isoform distribution in the tubules is controversial. Using isolated tubule segments, one group found only PMCA2 expressed in tubular epithelium derived from the cortex and later demonstrated PMCA1 and 4 in medullary tubular structures and

PMCA3 uniquely expressed in the thin descending limb of Henle's loop. The existence of PMCA3 in the thin descending limb is puzzling because this segment is not known to transport Ca and because PMCA3 is thought to be unique to the nervous system. Using isoform-specific antibodies, only PMCA1 and PMCA4 protein have been demonstrated in human and rat whole kidney preparations and in immortalized mouse proximal tubule cells. The lack of expression of PMCA2 and PMCA3 protein may reflect a low abundance of these proteins in total kidney homogenates or that the mRNA transcripts are not translated to proteins in the kidney under normal conditions.

A protein that may regulate PMCA activity has been described in rat kidney and liver. This protein, named *regucalcin*, has been demonstrated to increase ATP-dependent Ca^{2+} uptake in basolateral membranes isolated from rat kidney cortex. Regucalcin mRNA is upregulated by Ca ingestion. Regucalcin mRNA is downregulated by chronic saline intake and in spontaneously hypertensive rats, conditions associated with increased intracellular Ca^{2+}. ATP-dependent Ca^{2+} uptake is reduced in tissues from the spontaneously hypertensive rats, perhaps due to a decrease in regucalcin. However, ATP-dependent Ca^{2+} uptake is increased in rats after 7 days of saline ingestion. Therefore the role this protein plays in the normal and abnormal renal handling of Ca remains to be determined.

The Extracellular Calcium/Polyvalent Ion–Sensing Receptor

First identified in the parathyroid gland, the Ca/polyvalent ion–sensing receptor (CaSR) has provided a link between the observed effects of extracellular Ca concentrations on various renal transport systems, including Ca and Mg reabsorption and antidiuretic hormone (ADH)–induced water reabsorption. The receptor is coupled to an inhibitory guanosine triphosphate (GTP)–binding protein and when activated by high extracellular Ca, reduces hormone-stimulated cyclic adenosine monophosphate (cAMP) production. The effect of the activated receptor to reduce cAMP production may be secondary to activation of phospholipase A_2 (prostaglandins) or phospholipase C and intracellular Ca release in some cells. The mRNA transcript has been found in the glomerulus, proximal tubule segments, cortical and medullary TAL, DCT/CNT, and collecting ducts. Studies using specific antibodies have demonstrated the CaSR protein in the apical membrane of the PCT, in the PST and inner medullary collecting duct, and in the basolateral membrane of the cortical and medullary TAL and the DCT, but not in the glomerulus. In the CCT, the staining was primarily in the cytoplasm of intercalated cells suggesting that the receptor may be trafficked to either membrane depending on the type of intercalated cell represented. Mutations of this receptor have been implicated in several pathologic conditions, such as familial hypocalciuric hypercalcemia and autosomal-dominant hypocalcemia.

RENAL HANDLING OF CALCIUM

A normal human adult, with a glomerular filtration rate (GFR) of 100 ml/min (or 1440 L/day) and a plasma UF_{Ca} of 60 mg/L, filters 8 to 9 g of Ca per day. However, only 150 to 200 mg/day (the amount of net intestinal absorption) appears in the urine. The remaining 99% of the filtered Ca is reabsorbed by the renal tubules. Alterations in either the filtration or reabsorption of Ca can result in changes in urinary Ca excretion, but the effect of tubular reabsorption plays the predominant role.

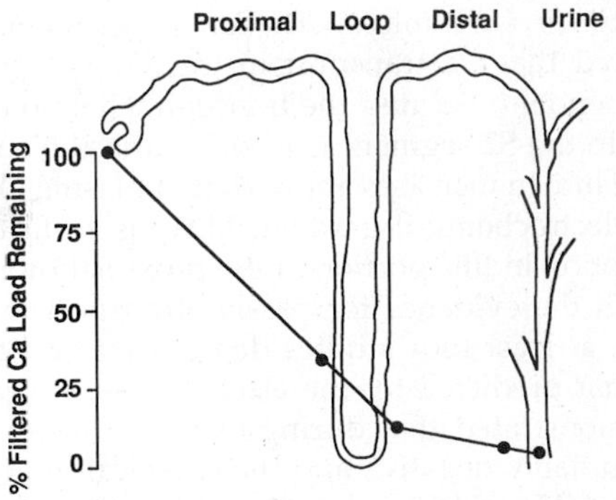

Figure 17.7. Calcium reabsorption along the nephron as demonstrated by micropuncture data. (Reproduced with permission from Rouse D, Suki WN. Renal transport of calcium, magnesium and phosphate. In: Brenner BM, ed. *The kidney,* 5th ed. Philadelphia: WB Saunders, 1996:478.)

In vivo micropuncture data demonstrated that 70% of the filtered Ca is reabsorbed in the proximal tubule segments, 20% in the TAL segments, 5% to 10% in the distal tubule, and less than 5% in the collecting tubule system (Fig. 17.7). The characteristics of Ca handling by individual nephron segments and their contribution to overall Ca homeostasis have been studied using *in vivo* micropuncture and microperfusion and *in vitro* microperfusion techniques.

Calcium Handling by Individual Nephron Segments

Glomerular Filtration

The amount of Ca filtered is dependent on the GFR and plasma UF_{Ca} concentration, although alterations in GFR may or may not result in changes in Ca excretion. Increases in GFR produced by maneuvers such as protein feeding, renal vasodilation, and steroid administration may also enhance tubular reabsorption such that fractional reabsorption and fractional excretion are unchanged (glomerulotubular balance). Maneuvers that disturb glomerulotubular balance, such as volume expansion, usually result in increased Ca excretion. Generally, increases in UF_{Ca} result in an increase in filtered Ca even though high plasma Ca can cause a decrease in GFR. Ca excretion increases as a result of increased filtered load and an inhibition of tubular transport. Some of the effects are mediated through changes in circulating parathyroid hormone (PTH) levels, but others are PTH independent.

Proximal Tubule Segments, S1, S2, and S3

The bulk of filtered Ca is reclaimed in the proximal tubule. Morphologically and functionally, the proximal tubule has been divided into three segments: S1, the first two-thirds of the PCT; S2, the remaining one-third of the PCT and the initial portion of the proximal straight tubule (PST); and S3, the remainder of the PST. Micropuncture studies have demonstrated that the PCT reabsorbs approximately 60% of the filtered load of Ca and the PST reabsorbs approximately 10%.

Transport of Ca in the PCT generally has been considered to be passive; however, evidence for active transport also has been demonstrated. Evidence for passive transport comes from micropuncture studies that demonstrate that sodium (Na), water, and Ca are absorbed in parallel, such that the concentrations of Na and Ca in the tubular fluid (TF) are approximately equal to that in plasma filtrate (PF) at the end of the accessible portion of cortical PCT segments. In addition, *in vivo* and *in vitro* microperfusion studies have demonstrated a large backflux component of Ca transport in this segment indicating a high intrinsic permeability. *In vitro* microperfusion experiments also have demonstrated that Ca transport in the S2 segment is largely voltage-dependent. Because the transepithelial potential difference (PD_t) in the S2 segment is positive and the concentration of Ca in the lumen increases above that of plasma, the small but favorable electrochemical gradient likely is sufficient to drive Ca reabsorption in this portion of the proximal tubule.

Although the evidence for passive transport in the PCT is convincing, at least four studies demonstrate Ca transport in excess of that predicted by the electrochemical gradient. Two studies demonstrated that during osmotic diuresis, when the PD_t is presumably negative and the chemical gradient is zero, the TF/PF for Na and Ca is less than 1.0 at the end of the PCT. Two other *in vivo* micropuncture studies demonstrated an active component for Ca reabsorption under nondiuretic conditions as well. The discrepancy of active versus passive transport may be a result of the experimental design or a function of the puncture site for the micropuncture experiments. The early, S1 portion of the PCT is functionally different from the S2 segment. Reabsorption of many electrolytes is more avid in this segment and the PD_t is generally lumen negative. Thus the electrochemical gradient for transport of positive ions such as Ca is likely unfavorable, and active transport processes may be necessary.

The first portion of the PST segment is morphologically defined as S2 and apparently transports Ca passively, much like the PCT S2 segment. However, the S3 segment of the PST may transport Ca actively. Micropuncture studies have demonstrated a TF/PF for Ca to be less than the TF/PF for Na at the bend of Henle's loop (from juxtamedullary nephrons). Because these values are roughly equal at the end of the cortical PCT, this difference suggests that Ca is reabsorbed in excess of Na in a tubular segment between these two points or that Ca is transported differently in the cortical versus the juxtamedullary PCT. Consistent with the former prediction, two *in vitro* microperfusion studies have demonstrated Ca transport in excess of that predicted by the calculated electrochemical gradient in S3 segments.

The passive movement of Ca in these segments is probably paracellular; however, the translocation is probably not simply solvent drag because the reflection coefficient is 0.9 (the reflection coefficient for water is 0). The active transport component is necessarily transcellular and an active extrusion mechanism at the basolateral membrane is required. Consistent with this requirement, PMCA1 and PMCA4 are thought to be present in these segments and primarily responsible for Ca extrusion at the basolateral membrane. The presence of the Na-Ca exchanger in the PCT is controversial, and physiologic studies suggest that it plays no role or a minor role in Ca extrusion from these cells.

Henle's Loop Segments

The apparent permeability for Ca measured in isolated, perfused segments of thin descending and thin ascending limbs of Henle's loop from the rabbit kidney is very low and net Ca transport is zero even in the presence of an osmotic gradient. The abundance of Ca transporting proteins in these segments is very low or nonexistent, consistent with the finding of no significant net Ca transport in these segments.

The TAL segment of Henle's loop is responsible for the reabsorption of 20% of the filtered load of Ca; however, the mechanism by which this is accomplished is controversial. Three laboratories have shown that Ca transport in isolated, perfused TAL is passive and driven by the PD_t, whereas three other laboratories have demonstrated an active component. The TAL, especially the cortical segment, generally displays a high lumen positive PD_t, which could support the Ca transport observed normally. However, at least one laboratory has demonstrated active Ca transport in the cortical TAL and passive transport in the medullary TAL. This apparent axial heterogeneity may explain in part the discrepancy between the two sets of studies. Another possible explanation is an error in the measurement of PD_t at the perfusion end of the tubule. Because the luminal NaCl concentration decreases axially, increasing the positivity of the luminal PD_t downstream, the voltage used to predict the Ca flux ratio may have been underestimated in some of the studies. However, this cannot explain all of the differences because two studies used perfusion solutions that obviate the increase in PD_t and found opposite results for Ca transport. Another interesting finding is that certain hormones increase Ca transport with no apparent corresponding increase in PD_t. Because Ca transport was found to be passive in the absence of hormones, the explanation given was that the hormones "uncovered" an active Ca transport component. The controversy is yet to be resolved; however, it is agreed that this portion of the nephron plays an important role in Ca reabsorption.

The cellular mechanisms have been partially characterized in the cortical TAL. The transport is saturable at luminal concentrations of 4 mM and above and at high perfusion rates. It is apparently independent of anaerobic metabolism, Na transport, and PMCA activity. These observations are consistent with a primarily passive Ca transport that proceeds through the paracellular route. A transcellular route would necessitate an active or secondary active efflux mechanism at the basolateral membrane. To date, there is no convincing evidence for PMCA or Na-Ca exchanger protein in this part of the nephron, although PMCA2 mRNA was detected in one study. Interestingly, the CaSR is prominent on the basolateral membrane of this segment and suggests that this segment is an important regulatory site for Ca reabsorption.

Distal Tubule Segments

Although the TAL is an important site for Ca transport, the "distal tubule" is considered the site for fine tuning of Ca excretion. Approximately 10% of the filtered Ca is absorbed in this segment; however, this is far below the capacity of the segment for reclaiming luminal Ca. In the absence of complexing anions, which are normally high in concentration at this site, the distal tubule is capable of absorbing 90% of the load delivered to it. Normally, Ca and Na are reabsorbed in parallel in this portion of the nephron; however, Ca transport can be dissociated from Na transport and PD_t under certain conditions. Because the luminal Ca concentration is lower than plasma and the PD_t is negative, Ca transport must be an active process in the distal tubule.

The distal tubule is not a homogeneous structure and has been subdivided into four distinct sections based on morphologic and functional differences. These include an extension of the thick ascending limb segment, a "bright" portion (the distal convoluted tubule), a granular portion, now defined as the connecting tubule (CNT), and a "light" portion that resembles the CCT. In some species, the transition between the DCT and the CNT and the CNT and CCT is abrupt, but in other species it is more gradual and segments with more than one cell type intervene. Portions of the CNT appear at the surface of the kidney and may represent some of the "late" DCT puncture sites defined in early micropuncture studies. Studies of Ca transport in isolated perfused rabbit CNT have demonstrated rates of 0.4 to 4.0 mEq/min/mm. Other studies have shown that this segment is highly responsive to hormones involved in Ca homeostasis. For these reasons, many investigators believe it is here that the primary control of Ca excretion lies.

The machinery for active Ca transport is most abundant in the DCT/CNT. Ca channels are present on the luminal membrane and respond appropriately to hormones involved in Ca homeostasis. In addition, protein and mRNA for both PMCA and the Na-Ca exchanger have been demonstrated in this portion of the nephron as have the vitamin D-stimulated calcium binding proteins, calbindin-D28K and calbindin-D9K. Several studies have suggested that the Na-Ca exchanger is the primary mechanism for Ca extrusion in this segment.

Collecting Duct Segments

The Ca appearing in the final urine is less than that measured by micropuncture at the last accessible portion of the cortical distal tubule. This suggests that Ca is absorbed in the collecting system or that there is greater fractional Ca absorption in the juxtamedullary than in the cortical nephrons. Studies of Ca transport in isolated, perfused CCT segments have yielded results ranging from no transport to a significant and active Ca efflux. The studies demonstrating Ca transport have found that it is unaffected by cAMP and PTH but is abolished in the presence of ADH. *In vivo* microcatheterization studies have suggested that as much as 1.4% of the filtered Ca is absorbed in the medullary collecting duct.

If there is indeed Ca transport in the CCT it is likely active because of the lumen negative PD_t and the low concentration of Ca. Consistent with the idea of Ca transport in this segment is the presence of the calbindins and perhaps significant amounts of PMCA. Transport of Ca in the medullary collecting duct may be passive because the PD_t is lumen positive in this segment.

FACTORS INFLUENCING THE RENAL HANDLING OF CALCIUM

Table 17.6 summarizes commonly encountered conditions and pharmacologic interventions that affect the renal handling of Ca. These conditions and pharmacologic agents may affect Ca excretion by altering the filtered load or the tubular transport of Ca, or both. Generally, the effects on proximal tubule transport are not translated to urinary excretion unless distal tubule transport is also affected.

Plasma Calcium Concentration

Hypercalcemia, in the absence of PTH excess, generally results in an increase in Ca excretion caused by a net increase in the filtered load and a decrease in tubular reabsorption. Hypercalcemia has opposing effects on the two factors that determine the filtration of Ca: the GFR and the concentration of UF_{Ca}. In the presence of intact parathyroid glands, hypercalcemia decreases the ultrafiltration coefficient (K_f) of glomerular membranes causing a decline in GFR; however, the increase in UF_{Ca} usually results in a net increase in the filtered load of Ca. Hypercalcemia also causes a decline in the tubular reabsorption of Ca by PTH-dependent and PTH-independent effects. Hypercalcemia inhibits Ca reabsorption in the proximal tubule segments by inhibiting bulk reabsorption of filtrate, and by inhibiting Ca efflux at the basolateral membrane as a result of the high Ca concentration in the peritubular capillary blood. In addition, the complexed Ca in the filtrate often is increased disproportionately, reducing the transportable Ca pool. These segments also demonstrate the extracellular CaSR on their luminal membranes; however, the role this receptor

TABLE 17.6. Effects on Filtered and Reabsorbed Calcium of Conditions that Increase or Decrease Calcium Excretion

Condition	Filtered Ca	Tubular Transport: Proximal	Tubular Transport: Loop	Tubular Transport: Distal
Associated with Hypercalciuria				
Hypercalcemia:				
Primary hyperparathyroidism	D	I, D, n/c	I	I
Other causes	I	D	D	D(PTH)
Volume Expansion (saline)	I	D	NE	D
Acidosis	I, D, n/c	D	n/c	D
Insulin, glucose	n/c	D	D	D
Phosphate depletion	n/c	D	D(PTH)	D(PTH)
Hypermagnesemia	n/c	D	D	D
Diuretics:				
Osmotic	n/c	D	D	D
Loop-acting	D, n/c	n/c, D	D	D
Associated with Hypocalciuria				
Hypocalcemia:				
Primary hypoparathyroidism	D	NE	I	NE
Other causes	D	I	I	NE
Volume contraction	n/c	I	NE	NE
Alkalosis	n/c	I	NE	NE
Phosphate loading	D, n/c	NE	NE	I
Diuretics:				
Thiazides, amiloride	D, n/c	I	NE	I
Acetazolamide	n/c	D	NE	I

D, decreased; I, increased; n/c, no change; NE, not examined; (PTH), change caused by alterations in circulating PTH.

plays in the modulation of Ca transport in this portion of the nephron is unknown.

Ca transport in the TAL segments also is inhibited by hypercalcemia, largely due to the high Ca concentration in the vasa recta and interstitium. In these segments, the CaSR is located on the basolateral surface and is thought to play a crucial role in limiting Ca transport in these segments. Distal tubule Ca transport also is inhibited without affecting Na transport. This effect is probably caused by the decrease in circulating PTH and probably occurs in both the DCT and CNT segment.

Hypocalcemia causes a reduction in filtered Ca and enhanced tubular reabsorption, which results in a decline in Ca excretion. The increase in circulating PTH results in a decline in GFR and enhanced bulk reabsorption in the proximal tubule. However, Ca reabsorption in the thick ascending limb is also enhanced by PTH-dependent and PTH-independent effects.

Volume Status

Expansion of extracellular fluid volume (ECFV) with saline infusion causes an increase in the excretion of Na and Ca even in the presence of PTH and despite decreased filtered loads of both ions. Conversely, ECFV contraction causes a decrease in the excretion of Na and Ca. Although reabsorption in general is inhibited by volume expansion in the PCT, for hypercalciuria to be observed requires that distal nephron reabsorption be inhibited as well. The distal site is not known; however, it is probably a segment beyond the DCT, perhaps the CNT or early CCT.

Acid–Base Status

In humans, both acute and chronic metabolic acidosis are associated with increased Ca excretion irrespective of changes in filtered Ca load or PTH. Conversely, metabolic alkalosis results in a decrease in Ca excretion. In general, the effects of respiratory acid–base changes parallel those of metabolically induced changes. Acute acidosis has been shown to decrease Ca reabsorption in the proximal tubule. This effect is due in part to a general inhibition of PCT absorption and in part to the decrease in luminal bicarbonate or luminal buffering. There is no known effect of acid–base alterations on Ca transport in the TAL or in the collecting tubules; however, it does affect distal tubule Ca handling. Chronic metabolic acidosis inhibits Ca transport, proportionately more than Na transport, in the distal tubule in the absence of PTH. This effect is reversed by bicarbonate infusion. Conversely, metabolic alkalosis, when induced by potassium salts to avoid a natriuresis, causes an increase in distal Ca reabsorption.

Hormones

PTH and PTH-Related Peptide

PTH is the primary homeostatic regulator of renal Ca excretion. PTH decreases Ca excretion by reducing the filtered load (via reduction of Kf and GFR) and by enhancing tubular reabsorption of Ca. The primary cellular mechanism is thought to be activation of adenylyl cyclase, and the distribution of PTH-sensitive adenylyl cyclase activity along the nephron segments correlates well with the observed actions of this hormone on Ca transport. PTH also may activate the phospholipase C cascade, which, in some studies, appears to be the signal transduction system activated by physiologic concentrations of PTH. In other studies, the activation of both signal transduction mechanisms is necessary to mimic the action of PTH. PTH is a classic hormone secreted by the parathyroid glands; however, another protein, PTH-related peptide (PTHrP), has many of the same actions as PTH but is distributed in many tissues and is thought to play an autocrine/paracrine role. This peptide was first discovered in tumors causing humoral hypercalcemia, but now it is thought to mediate many of the effects previously ascribed to PTH. At least two receptors bind PTH and/or PTHrP: the PTH1 receptor, which binds both peptides, and the PTH2 receptor, which binds only PTH. Two additional receptors have been suggested by functional studies but have not been verified at the molecular level. The primary receptor found in the kidney is the PTH1 receptor; the PTH2 receptor is found only at the vascular pole of the glomerulus in the kidney but is prevalent in brain, lung, pancreas, and vasculature.

No consistent effect of PTH on Ca reabsorption in the PCT has been shown; however, there is a definite effect in Henle's loop. *In vitro* microperfusion experiments have suggested that the cortical, but not the medullary, TAL segment is one site of action for PTH in Henle's loop. PTH also enhances Ca reabsorption along the distal tubule, in portions accessible to micropuncture and beyond. This effect occurs independently of Na reabsorption and alterations in PD_t. This action of PTH may not be mediated solely by cAMP because the administration of cAMP enhances the reabsorption of Na as well as Ca. Studies using cultured mouse distal tubule cells suggest that PTH opens Ca channels on the luminal membrane. In addition, studies using basolateral membranes from rabbit distal tubules demonstrated an increase in Na-Ca exchanger activity. As discussed previously, the distal tubule is a heterogeneous structure, and studies have suggested that the PTH-responsive portion is the CNT.

Vitamin D

Direct tubular effects of vitamin D metabolites have been suggested. Ca reabsorption is decreased in vitamin D–depleted animals with or without PTH; however, the acute administration of active vitamin D metabolites produces no consistent effects. The demonstration of an effect of vitamin D metabolites on proximal tubule Ca transport is lacking. However, there is some evidence for a direct effect of vitamin D metabolites on Ca transport in the distal nephron. Ca uptake has been shown to be decreased in luminal membrane vesicles from distal tubules isolated from vitamin D–depleted rabbits. This study also demonstrated that ATP-dependent Ca transport was inhibited in the basolateral membranes of distal but not proximal tubules from these animals. Other investigators have found no consistent effects of vitamin D on basolateral Ca transport proteins. In cultured distal tubule cells, vitamin D primarily enhanced the effect of PTH to increase Ca transport but had little effect alone. In cultured CNT/CCT cells, the effects of PTH and vitamin D to enhance Ca uptake were mediated via the same pathway in that they were neither additive nor potentiating.

Part of the effect of vitamin D is mediated through the vitamin D–stimulated Ca-binding proteins (calbindin-D28K and calbindin-D9K), which are found in the DCT, CNT, and CCT. These proteins not only sequester Ca and promote further entry but also aid in the translocation of Ca from the luminal to the basolateral membrane. Vitamin D may also increase luminal membrane chloride (Cl) channels and Cl entry. The resulting hyperpolarization of the cell then opens Ca channels enhancing Ca entry, and hence, transcellular Ca transport.

Calcitonin

The effects of calcitonin on the renal handling of Ca are confusing. Superphysiologic doses are hypercalciuric; however, more physiologic doses are hypocalciuric in the absence of PTH. *In vitro* microperfusion studies suggest that calcitonin enhances Ca reabsorption in the medullary TALH via activation of calcitonin-stimulated production of cAMP. In a study using luminal and basolateral membrane vesicles from rabbit distal tubules, calcitonin opened Ca channels in luminal membrane vesicles and stimulated Na-Ca exchange in basolateral membrane vesicles. Both effects were mimicked by cAMP analogs.

Insulin and Glucagon

Insulin administration, hyperinsulinemia, and glucose administration are associated with hypercalciuria. Proximal reabsorption of Na, water, and Ca is reduced; however, only Ca is increased in the urine suggesting an additional distal effect. Studies in diabetic rats have demonstrated a Ca transport defect in Henle's loop and in the terminal nephron beyond the "late" distal tubule. The defects are not corrected by controlling the hyperphagia associated with the diabetes or by PTH infusion. Glucagon also has a natriuretic and calciuretic effect; however, this is probably secondary to increases in renal blood flow and GFR.

Other Hormones

Long-term administration or elevation of growth hormone results in hypercalciuria probably resulting from antagonism of PTH action or from expansion of ECFV. Thyroid hormone and chronic glucocorticoid excess cause increased Ca excretion primarily by increasing bone resorption. Estrogens decrease bone resorption and reduce urinary Ca excretion. Chronic mineralocorticoid administration is hypercalciuric largely mediated by the expansion of ECFV.

Diuretics

Osmotic Diuretics

The osmotic diuresis produced by mannitol, and other osmotic agents, results in a parallel increase in the excretion of both Na and Ca. In the proximal tubule TF/PF Na and TF/PF Ca fall below 1.0 during osmotic diuresis, indicating that these two ions are absorbed in excess of water. Inhibition of proximal tubule absorption increases delivery of fluid to Henle's loop and the distal nephron, overwhelms both Na and Ca reabsorptive mechanisms, and results in a brisk natriuresis and calciuresis.

Thiazide Diuretics

When given acutely, thiazide diuretics produce a small, transient increase in plasma total and ionized Ca, probably through PTH-dependent stimulation of bone resorption. When administered long term, these agents cause a sustained increase in plasma total and ionized Ca resulting from hemoconcentration and decreased urinary excretion of Ca despite the marked natriuresis.

The acute administration of thiazide diuretics results in a marked natriuresis, but there is little or no change in Ca excretion. This effect is due to the direct stimulation of Ca transport in the distal tubule via opening Cl channels and hyperpolarizing the cells, which opens Ca channels. The chronic administration of thiazide diuretics produces frank hypocalciuria, which can be reversed by salt replacement, suggesting that the chronic effect on urinary Ca excretion involves enhanced proximal reabsorption in response to ECFV contraction. This effect, coupled with the direct stimulation of Ca absorption in the DCT, forms the basis for the use of thiazides in the treatment of patients with idiopathic hypercalciuria and those with hypoparathyroidism. With salt restriction and chronic therapy with thiazide agents, luminal Ca is decreased, reducing the potential for hypercalciuria and stone formation, and the plasma Ca can be normalized.

Acetazolamide

The acute administration of acetazolamide is natriuretic, but not calciuretic. Proximal reabsorption is inhibited; however, the distal nephron must reabsorb Ca in excess of Na to produce the urinary findings. The effect on distal tubular reabsorption may be indirect and due to enhanced bicarbonate delivery, which obligates Na and reduces the lumen-negative PD_t in this segment.

Loop-Acting Diuretics

When given acutely, furosemide and related agents produce a large increase in Na and Ca excretion. The primary action is the inhibition of Na and Cl transport in the TAL. This effect of furosemide in the TAL is due to inhibition of the Na^+-K^+-$2Cl^-$ transporter in the luminal membrane, dissipation of the lumen-positive PD_t, and a decline in the driving force for passive Ca transport. With replacement of urinary losses of ions other than Ca, very high Ca excretion rates can be maintained with furosemide treatment. This observation forms the basis for the treatment of severe hypercalcemia with furosemide.

Amiloride, Triamterene, and Spironolactone

Amiloride, triamterene, and spironolactone increase Na and decrease Ca excretion. Amiloride decreases the lumen-negative PD_t in the distal tubule and CCT, which may account for the enhanced Ca reabsorption in this portion of the nephron. Amiloride also exerts a direct effect on Ca reabsorption in the distal tubule at a site distinct from that responsive to thiazides. Amiloride closes Na channels effecting hyperpolarization of the cell, which in turn opens Ca channels. Spironolactone may act primarily by inhibition of the mineralocorticoid effects on the distal nephron.

Other Ions

Phosphate

Phosphate loading causes a decrease in Ca excretion, even in the face of volume expansion. The effect primarily results from an increase in Ca reabsorption in the distal tubule secondary to an increase in PTH secretion, triggered by the initial drop in plasma ionized Ca. Conversely, phosphate depletion is associated with hypercalciuria, which is only partially corrected by the administration of PTH. There may or may not be a reduction in bulk reabsorption in the PCT; however, there is good evidence for a defect in Henle's loop. This defect was corrected by PTH infusion partially in one study and completely in another. The apparent discrepancy may be explained by a difference in plasma PO_4, because the effect of PTH is inhibited by low plasma PO_4. One study also suggests a defect in Ca transport in the distal nephron, beyond the last accessible micropuncture site, which was corrected by phosphate infusion. However, a second study could not demonstrate this defect. Thus although most investigators agree that the hypercalciuria is the consequence of a defect beyond the PCT, the exact site(s) are in dispute.

Magnesium

Hypermagnesemia is associated with hypercalciuria. The mechanism of action appears to be inhibition of basolateral Ca and Mg extrusion in the TALH, similar to that produced by hypercalcemia. The involvement of the CaSR in the inhibition of

Ca transport by high basolateral Mg has not been proven. The receptor does respond to Mg; however, the sensitivity is in the range of 10 mM Mg, an order of magnitude greater than normal plasma Mg. It is possible that the Mg concentration in the interstitium surrounding the TALH, especially the medullary segment, is high enough to activate the receptor and inhibit the transport of both Ca and Mg.

Selected Readings

Carafoli E, Garcia-Martin E, Guerini D. The plasma membrane calcium pump: recent developments and future perspectives. *Experientia* 1996;52:1091–1100.

This is the latest in many reviews of the state-of-the-art in plasma membrane calcium pump physiology and molecular structure. The 41 references include previous review articles and more recent studies.

Chattopadhyay N, Vassilev PM, Brown EM. Calcium-sensing receptor: roles in and beyond systemic calcium homeostasis. *Biol Chem* 1997;378:759–768.

This review article surveys current knowledge of this important receptor in the kidney and other organ systems. The article also suggests areas for further research into the roles this receptor may play in ion homeostasis (55 references).

Freidman PA, Gesek FA. Cellular calcium transport in renal epithelia: measurement, mechanisms, and regulation. *Physiol Rev* 1995;75:429–471.

This article is an extensive review of calcium handling by the renal tubules, including cellular calcium activity and measurement, transport properties, regulation, and mechanisms. A particularly detailed discussion of distal tubule calcium transport is included (418 references).

Hilgemann DW, Philipson KD, Vassort G, eds. Sodium-calcium exchange. Proceedings of the Third International Conference. Annals of the New York Academy of Sciences vol. 779. New York: The New York Academy of Sciences, 1996.

This collection of articles from the international conference on sodium-calcium exchange presents the state-of-the-art knowledge of this important calcium transport protein in several organ systems including the kidney. The topics range from the molecular structure to enzyme kinetics and regulation.

Philbrick WM, Wysolmerski JJ, Galbraith S, et al. Defining the roles of parathyroid hormone-related protein in normal physiology. *Physiol Rev* 1996;76:127–173.

This article reviews the discovery of PTHrP and its gene structure and translation. A detailed discussion of the physiologic functions of this important peptide on various organ systems is then presented (293 references).

Rouse D, Suki WN. Renal transport of calcium, magnesium and phosphate. In: Brenner BM, ed. *The kidney*, 5th ed. Philadelphia: WB Saunders, 1996.

This chapter presents a detailed discussion of the renal handling of calcium as well as magnesium and phosphate (594 references).

PART 3
Dyscalcemias

Shaul G. Massry and Miroslaw Smogorzewski

The regulation of extracellular calcium concentration is a complex process. Three organs, including the skeleton, kidney, and intestine, are involved in this process through their interaction with parathyroid hormone (PTH), parathyroid hormone–related peptide (PTHrP), vitamin D, and calcitonin. PTH protects against hypocalcemia by augmenting calcium mobilization from bone, by increasing renal tubular reabsorption of calcium, and by enhancing intestinal absorption of calcium either directly or indirectly by an effect on vitamin D metabolism. Therefore states with excess PTH may cause hypercalcemia and those with PTH deficiency are associated with hypocalcemia. PTHrP promotes bone resorption, enhances renal reabsorption of calcium, and decreases renal tubular reabsorption of phosphate. Excess of this hormone is responsible for the hypercalcemia of malignancy. Vitamin D and its metabolites increase intestinal absorption of calcium and cause bone resorption; therefore excess vitamin D would induce hypercalcemia. Calcitonin inhibits bone resorption but its physiologic role in the protection against hypercalcemia in humans is not proven.

BODY CONTENT OF CALCIUM AND ITS CONCENTRATION IN SERUM

There are approximately 1.3 kg of calcium ion in a 70-kg man. Approximately 99% of this amount is present in bones and teeth, 1.0% is located in cells of soft tissues, and 0.1% is found in the extracellular fluid. The concentration of ionized calcium in serum is maintained stable despite tremendous fluxes of calcium between skeleton, intestine, and kidney on the one hand and extracellular fluid on the other hand. This is achieved by the regulatory homeostatic processes mentioned above. Approximately 500 mg of calcium leaves the bone daily, and an equal amount is deposited back in the skeleton; the daily urinary losses of calcium are equal to the net amount of calcium absorbed by the gut. Thus calcium balance is maintained, and the level of ionized calcium in serum remains normal.

The concentration of total calcium in serum in normal subjects varies widely and ranges from 4.4 to 5.2 mEq/L (8.8 to 10.4 mg/dl), and this variation results, at least partly, from differences in the concentration of serum albumin among normal individuals (3.9 to 4.8 g/dl), the state of hydration, and the use of a tourniquet during blood sampling.

Total serum calcium consists of two major fractions. The first is the protein-bound fraction, which constitutes 40% ± 5% of total serum calcium concentration, and the second is the non-protein-bound or diffusible fraction, which comprises 60% ± 5% of total calcium levels. Approximately 6% ± 5% of the diffusible moiety of serum calcium exists in the form of calcium complexed with bicarbonate, phosphate, and acetate, and the remaining 94% ± 5% is in the form of calcium ion. Thus the concentration of calcium ion in the serum is approximately 50% of the total serum level, and it is this concentration of calcium ion that is critically controlled by the homeostatic mechanisms.

The relationship between calcium ion and the concentration of protein in the serum is represented by a simple mass action expression: $[Ca^{2+}]$ [proteinate]/calcium, proteinate = K, where [proteinate] equals concentration of serum protein, primarily albumin. Because K is constant, the numerator and denominator must change proportionately in any physiologic or pathologic state. A change in the concentration of total serum calcium will occur after a change in the concentration of serum proteins or alterations in their binding properties and after a primary change in the concentration of calcium ion. A fall in serum albumin reduces the proteinate and the calcium proteinate proportionately, resulting in a fall in total serum calcium level with the free calcium ion concentration remaining normal. Therefore the diffusible fraction will constitute a larger portion of the total serum calcium level. A decrease in the concentration of serum albumin by 1 g/dl is usually associated with a fall of 0.8 to 1.0 mg/dl in the concentration of serum calcium. Such hypocalcemia does not represent a basic disorder in the homeostatic process regulating the concentration of calcium ion in serum.

Because only a small amount of calcium is bound to globulin (1.0 g of globulin binds 0.2 to 0.3 mg of calcium), it is unusual to see a change in the total concentration of serum calcium as a result of alterations in the levels of globulin in blood. However, in instances in which the globulin concentration in serum is extremely high (greater than 8.0 g/dl), such as in multiple myeloma, a mild to moderate hypercalcemia may be seen because of an elevation of the globulin-bound calcium. In addition, certain myeloma proteins (immunoglobulin G [IgG]) may have increased calcium-binding properties, and an elevation in the total level of serum calcium could occur even with a moderate increase in serum levels of globulins. In these circumstances, the concentration of calcium ion in serum is normal, and therefore, this kind of hypercalcemia would not require treatment. Thus in patients with elevations in both total serum calcium and hyperglobulinemia, one should determine the level of the ionized or diffusible fraction of serum calcium to differentiate between true hypercalcemia (elevation of calcium ion concentration) and hypercalcemia secondary to increased binding of calcium by high levels of globulins.

Several factors may alter calcium binding to serum proteins and result either in changes in the total levels of serum calcium or in alterations of the relation between total and ionized levels of calcium. PTH may decrease the binding of calcium to albumin, and patients with excess PTH and normal serum concentration of total calcium may have elevated levels of ionized calcium. This phenomenon has been documented in patients with normocalcemic hyperparathyroidism and in renal transplant recipients with excess serum levels of PTH.

A rise in plasma pH increases binding of calcium to protein, and with each 0.1-unit increment in plasma pH, the concentration of ionized calcium falls by 0.1 mEq/L. This phenomenon has important implications during the treatment of hypocalcemic and acidotic renal failure patients with bicarbonate; the sudden rise of plasma pH may cause seizures because of a fall in the concentration of ionized calcium.

The concentration of sodium in serum may affect the binding of calcium to albumin, resulting in changes in total serum calcium concentration. Severe hyponatremia of less than 120 mEq/L and marked hypernatremia of greater than 155 mEq/L could cause changes in the concentration of total calcium in serum. Hyponatremia causes an increase in protein-bound calcium and therefore slight hypercalcemia, whereas hypernatremia causes a decrease in the protein-bound calcium and hence slight hypocalcemia. In either case, the concentration of calcium ion is not altered.

If a tourniquet is left on the arm for 2 to 3 minutes before obtaining the blood sample, protein-free fluid moves out of the capillary blood, resulting in a higher concentration of blood proteins and consequently a rise in the protein-bound calcium. This phenomenon might cause an elevation of 0.5 to 1.5 mg/dl in the level of total calcium in serum. Therefore every effort should be made to obtain a blood specimen for the measurement of total serum calcium from free-flowing blood.

If, for some physiologic or pathologic reason, the concentration of free calcium ion changes, the calcium proteinate component will also change proportionately; this will result in a proportionate change in levels of total, bound, and diffusible calcium. Therefore, in all hypocalcemic and hypercalcemic disorders resulting from primary changes in the concentration of calcium ion, the ratio of the diffusible to nondiffusible fractions remains constant or normal. This is in contrast to altered ratios between the diffusible and bound fractions of calcium in cases in which the changes in total serum calcium level are due to alteration in the concentration of serum proteins or in their binding properties.

TABLE 17.7. Causes of Hypercalcemia

Malignancy
- With skeletal involvement
- No skeletal involvement
  - PTH-related protein
  - Transforming growth factors (TGF)
  - Interleukin-1 (α and β)
  - Interleukin-6
  - Tumor necrosis factor-β
  - Colony-stimulating factor
  - 1,25-dihydroxyvitamin D

Primary hyperparathyroidism
- Adenoma, hyperplasia, carcinoma
- Multiple endocrine neoplasia type I with pituitary and pancreatic tumors
- Multiple endocrine neoplasia type IIa with medullary carcinoma of the thyroid and pheochromocytoma

Familial hypocalciuric hypercalcemia[a]

Neonatal severe hyperparathyroidism[a]

Other endocrine disorders
- Hyperthyroidism
- Acromegaly
- Pheochromocytoma
- Acute adrenal insufficiency

Granulomatous disorders
- Sarcoidosis
- Tuberculosis
- Berylliosis
- Disseminated coccidioidomycosis or candidiasis
- Histoplasmosis
- Leprosy
- Granulomatous lipoid pneumonia
- Silicone-induced granuloma
- Eosinophilic granuloma
- Farmer's lung

Vitamin overdosages
- Vitamin D
- Vitamin A

Immobilization

Renal failure
- Diuretic phase of acute renal failure, especially due to rhabdomyolysis
- Chronic renal failure
- After renal transplantation

Chlorothiazide diuretics

Lithium ingestion

Theophylline toxicity

Tamoxifin

Estrogen

Vasoactive intestinal polypeptide

Hyperalimentation regimens

Milk-alkali syndrome

Idiopathic hypercalcemia of infancy

Increased serum proteins[b]
- Hemoconcentration
- Hyperglobulinemia due to multiple myeloma

[a] These entities are due to mutation in the calcium receptor gene, resulting in inactivation of the receptor; for details, see text.

[b] Under these circumstances, the levels of ionized calcium in blood may not be elevated despite the elevation in the total concentration of calcium.

PTH, parathyroid hormone.

HYPERCALCEMIA

Etiology

The primary cause of hypercalcemia is an increase in net calcium movement from bone into the extracellular fluid. An augmentation in intestinal calcium absorption and/or a decrease in urinary calcium excretion may contribute to the magnitude of the hypercalcemia. The clinical conditions associated with hypercalcemia are listed in Table 17.7.

Hypercalcemia is commonly found in patients with malignant diseases. It has been estimated that up to 10% to 20% of all patients with carcinoma will have hypercalcemia at some time during their disease, usually in the terminal stages of the illness. Hypercalcemia has been reported in patients with solid tumors and in those with hematologic neoplasms. The most common solid tumor associated with hypercalcemia is lung carcinoma. Approximately 20% of all such patients have hypercalcemia. The cancer in these patients is usually epidermoid (squamous) carcinoma, large cell carcinoma, or adenocarcinoma. Small cell carcinoma of the lung is rarely associated with hypercalcemia. Among patients with carcinoma of the breast, 20% will have hypercalcemia. The latter has been reported in 19% of all cases with squamous carcinoma of the head, neck, esophagus, or the female genital tract, and in 8% of patients with hypernephroma.

Hypercalcemia is common in patients with multiple myeloma, and it has been reported in one-third of these patients. In contrast, hypercalcemia has been encountered in a small fraction of patients (1% to 2%) with lymphoma; it is more common in Burkitt's lymphoma than in Hodgkin's lymphoma, and it is uncommon in leukemia.

Hypercalcemia of malignancy is due to bone metastases and/or the production by the tumor of a bone-resorbing agent(s). The latter mechanism is more important than the former one in the genesis of the hypercalcemia of malignancy. The main humoral factor responsible for the hypercalcemia associated with most solid tumors is the PTHrP. Two observations support this proposition. First, the serum levels of PTHrP are elevated in three-fourths of patients with solid tumor and hypercalcemia and in four-fifths of those with hypercalcemia in the absence of bone metastases; and second, the blood levels of PTHrP are normal in cancer patients without hypercalcemia.

PTHrP has been cloned and synthesized. The human gene of PTHrP is larger than that of human PTH. The gene extends for about 15 kilobase of genomic DNA. The gene has 9 axons and 3 promoters. There are three isoform of PTHrP, which are made of 139, 141, and 173 amino acids and several species of PTHrP messenger RNA. Available data indicate that the hormone is secreted in at least three forms: an amino terminal moiety [PTHrP (1–36)], a midregion fragment that begins with amino acid 36 with undetermined carboxyterminus, and a carboxyterminal species that is recognized by an antibody that detects the 109–138 amino acids region. The carboxyterminal moiety of PTHrP is cleared by the kidney, and therefore its concentration in blood is elevated in chronic renal failure. The PTHrP amino terminal fragment displays homology with that of PTH. Indeed, 8 amino acids of the first 13 in the amino terminus of PTHrP are similar to those of PTH. The PTHrP binds to the PTH–PTHrP receptor, stimulates renal adenylate cyclase, and produces phosphaturia and hypocalciuria. The PTHrP-induced phosphaturia is responsible for the hypophosphatemia that may be seen in patients with hypercalcemia of malignancy. PTHrP induces bone resorption, and this action is mainly responsible for the hypercalcemia; however, the hypocalciuria contributes to the magnitude of the elevation in the plasma calcium levels. It is of interest that the bone resorption induced by PTHrP is not coupled with increased bone formation; indeed, the latter is diminished. This is in contrast to the PTH-stimulated bone resorption that is associated with increased bone formation. The PTHrP may, by itself, cause bone resorption and hypercalcemia, or it may act synergistically with transforming growth factor(s) α (TGF α). The mechanisms for this synergism are complex and not well defined.

Solid tumors may produce other humoral factors that may cause hypercalcemia. These include PTH, $1{,}25(OH)_2D$, prostaglandins, and TGF(s). In a few cases of malignant solid tumors (small cell lung carcinoma, ovarian adenocarcinoma, primitive neuroectodermal cancer) and hypercalcemia, production of PTH by these tumors has been authenticated; in these patients the tumors contained PTH gene transcripts and immunoreactive PTH. Also, the serum levels of PTH were elevated.

Carcinoma of the breast produces PTHrP, and the mRNA of this hormone was detected in cells of breast cancer. The mRNA of the hormone was detected in 70% of tumor metastases in bone, whereas only in 20% of the metastases in other organs. Breast cancer may also produce $1{,}25(OH)_2D$, and this may play a role in the genesis of the hypercalcemia in patients with this cancer. Production of $1{,}25(OH)_2D$ by leiomyoblastoma has also been reported.

Solid tumors, including epidermoid cancer of the tonsils, lung, and penis; carcinoma of the pancreas and kidney; hepatoma; and melanoma, may produce prostaglandins of the E series (PGE_1 and PGE_2). Indeed, some patients with hypercalcemia of malignancy have increased urinary excretion of prostaglandin metabolites and display a fall in the excretion of these metabolites and a fall in their plasma calcium concentration following the administration of prostaglandin synthetase inhibitors. Although these compounds stimulate bone resorption in tissue culture, their role in the genesis of hypercalcemia of malignancy is questionable for several reasons. First, there is a poor correlation between prostaglandin production by the tumors and the levels of serum calcium; second, the blood levels of PGE_2 in these patients are low; and third, inhibitors of prostaglandin synthesis do not control the hypercalcemia of malignancy in most patients.

TGF is present in α and β forms. TGF-α has a molecular weight of 5,000 and consists of 50 amino acids. It is produced by most solid tumors associated with hypercalcemia, and binds to the epidermal growth factor receptors. TGF-α is believed to mediate its action through this receptor binding, and its hypercalcemic effect is due to stimulation of osteoclastic bone resorption. The latter results from an increase in the number of osteoclastlike cells derived from mononuclear cells. TGF-β has a molecular weight of 25,000. It stimulates the release of PTHrP from tumor cells of breast carcinoma, and through this effect contributes to the generation of hypercalcemia.

It has been reported that patients with certain squamous cell carcinoma of the lung and other organs may have hypercalcemia and leukocytosis. A humoral factor with properties similar to colony stimulating factor(s) has been incriminated.

Hematologic neoplasms are often associated with bone involvement, but the hypercalcemia that is encountered in these patients is mediated by cytokines with bone-resorbing activity. These cytokines are released by the tumor cells, and include interleukin-1α, interleukin-1β, tumor necrosis factor-β, and TGF-α. Tumors producing these factors include multiple myeloma, lymphoma, and leukemia. T-cell lympholeukemia may also produce PTHrP. Osteoclastic-activating factor (OAF), which has been implicated in the genesis of hypercalcemia of multiple myeloma, no longer represents one factor but rather a family of cytokines with bone-resorbing activity. Therefore the term *OAF* should not be used as a unique compound responsible for the hypercalcemia of multiple myeloma. In this cancer, the humoral factors responsible for the hypercalcemia include interleukin-1 and interleukin-6 and tumor necrosis factor-β.

High blood levels of $1{,}25(OH)_2D_3$ have been noted in hypercalcemic patients with Hodgkin's disease, and adult T-cell lymphoma. It has been suggested that these tumors produce $1{,}25(OH)_2D_3$. Indeed, cultured lymphoid cells infected with human immunodeficiency virus produce $1{,}25(OH)_2D_3$ from 25-hydroxyvitamin D. Other factors may also be produced by these tumors and contribute to the hypercalcemia.

Primary hyperparathyroidism is second to malignancy as a cause of hypercalcemia. More than 80% of such patients have a single parathyroid adenoma, but some may have multiple adenomas; approximately 15% have primary hyperplasia of all glands, and only a few (4%) may have carcinomas. Familial hyperparathyroidism and hypercalcemia are common among patients with primary parathyroid hyperplasia and occur in up to 50% of these patients. This familial form of primary hyperparathyroidism is autosomal dominant with a high degree of penetrance. It may manifest itself as primary parathyroid hyperplasia alone or as a part of the multiple endocrine neoplasia (MEN) syndromes. In *type I MEN*, primary hyperparathyroidism occurs in 95% of the patients and is associated with pituitary, pancreatic, adrenal, or thyroid adenomas. After surgery, recurrence of hyperplasia in the remaining parathyroid tissue is more common than in the sporadic primary parathyroid hyperplasia. In *type IIa MEN*, primary hyperparathyroidism is present in 20% to 30% of the patients who usually present with medullary carcinoma of the thyroid and pheochromocytoma. In *type IIb MEN*, the incidence of primary hyperparathyroidism is very low, and the patients usually have mucosal neuromas, medullary carcinoma of the thyroid, and pheochromocytoma. Severe *neonatal primary hyperparathyroidism* is rare, and is associated with hyperplasia of the parathyroid glands. It is due to a mutation of the gene of the calcium-sensing receptor resulting in inaction of the receptor. It is seen as sporadic cases in siblings of normocalcemic parents. It is also recognized in few children from families with familial hypocalciuric hypercalcemia; in these cases, there is a homozygous calcium receptor mutation. Similar homozygous or heterozygous mutations have been observed in sporadic cases.

Mortality during the first year of life is very high (more than 50%) in the untreated severe cases. Therefore the early recognition and management of this entity is crucial. These infants display hypotonia, poor feeding, respiratory distress, fractures, and marked hypercalcemia and hypophosphatemia, as well as high PTH levels in the homozygous mutation. The hypercalcemia is severe in these infants, and there is autonomous secretion of PTH. Removal of the hyperplastic parathyroid glands is the treatment of choice.

It is interesting to mention that an increased association between primary hyperparathyroidism and other diseases has been noted. These include goiters, Hashimoto's thyroiditis, hyperthyroidism, Cushing's syndrome, sarcoidosis, medullary sponge kidney, carcinoid tumors, empty sella syndrome, and nonendocrine malignant tumors. Because hyperthyroidism and malignant tumors are also associated with hypercalcemia, the presence of an associated parathyroid adenoma as the underlying cause of the hypercalcemia in these patients should always be considered. Indeed, approximately 30% of patients with primary hyperparathyroidism may develop cancer of other organs before, during, or after the discovery of parathyroid adenoma. Also, in a study of 136 patients with malignancy and hypercalcemia, 4.4% had parathyroid adenoma. Hyperparathyroidism also has been described after low-dose radiation to the head and neck.

Familial hypocalciuric hypercalcemia is an autosomal-dominant disorder with high penetrance at all ages. The biochemical hallmarks of this entity are mild hypercalcemia, hypophosphatemia, hypermagnesemia, hyperchloremic acidosis, hypocalciuria, and hypomagnesiuria. This disorder appears to be due to inherited inactivating mutation of the calcium-sensing receptor in the ascending limb of Henle's loop and distal tubule leading to enhanced reabsorption of both calcium and magnesium in these nephron sites, resulting in hypocalciuria, hypomagnesiuria, hypercalcemia, and hypermagnesemia (see Chapter 18, Part 2). The blood levels of PTH may be normal or mildly elevated but always inappropriately high for the level of serum calcium. The chronic hypercalcemia in these patients is not associated with severe symptoms, and most patients do not require treatment. Peptic ulcer disease and nephrolithiasis have been encountered in 10% of patients with familial hypocalciuric hypercalcemia. In the occasional patient who may require therapy, total parathyroidectomy may be considered because hypercalcemia persists after subtotal parathyroidectomy.

Hypercalcemia may occur in patients with other endocrine diseases. Mild hypercalcemia may be present in up to 20% of the patients with hyperthyroidism, but severe hypercalcemia is uncommon. Thyroid hormones (thyroxine and triiodothyronine) increase bone resorption and lead to hypercalcemia and/or hypercalciuria when bone resorption exceeds bone formation significantly. The effect of thyroid hormones on bone may be a direct one and/or mediated by an increased number of β-adrenergic receptors. The latter notion is indirectly supported by the demonstration of an increased number of β-receptors in other organs in hyperthyroidism and by the ability of propranolol to correct the hypercalcemia of thyrotoxicosis. Because of a possible increased association between hyperthyroidism and parathyroid adenoma, the latter must be ruled out in patients with thyrotoxicosis and hypercalcemia. Furthermore, the hypercalcemia in a patient with thyrotoxicosis could be attributed to this disease only if it resolves after achieving an euthyroid state.

Acromegaly is often (15% to 20% of cases) accompanied by mild hypercalcemia, which results from enhanced intestinal calcium absorption and augmented bone resorption. The blood levels of $1,25(OH)_2D_3$ may be elevated in patients with acromegaly, and this metabolite is probably responsible for the changes in calcium metabolism at the gut and the bone level. The elevation in the blood levels of $1,25(OH)_2D_3$ is most likely caused by an increase in its renal production induced by growth hormone. A second possible mechanism for hypercalcemia in acromegaly is parathyroid hyperplasia. Exogenous growth hormone given to rats produced parathyroid hyperplasia and elevated serum levels of PTH. In acromegalic patients with hypercalcemia, the serum levels of PTH are normal but may be inappropriately high for the levels of serum calcium.

Pheochromocytoma may be associated with hypercalcemia, which disappears after removal of the adrenal tumor. Epinephrine injections can stimulate PTH secretion, but in one report, normocalcemic patients with pheochromocytoma had normal serum concentrations of PTH. In a study of 10 patients with pheochromocytoma, the serum levels of PTHrP were elevated in 7 and became undetectable after resection of the tumor. There was a positive correlation between serum levels of calcium and those of PTHrP. These observations are consistent with the notion that pheochromocytoma may produce PTHrP and that the latter may underlie, at least partly, the hypercalcemia seen in these patients. *Acute adrenal insufficiency* is a rare cause of hypercalcemia. Because these patients may be dehydrated and have hemoconcentration, a rise in serum albumin concentration and increased binding of calcium to serum albumin secondary to hyponatremia may contribute to the increase in serum calcium level. Measurements of ionized calcium have not been made in humans with Addison's disease, but in rats with experimental adrenal insufficiency, the serum levels of calcium ion are elevated.

Patients with a variety of granulomatous diseases may have hypercalcemia. Approximately 17% (1% to 20%) of patients with *sarcoidosis* may have hypercalcemia, which is more common in those with chronic and disseminated disease. Sun exposure may precipitate or worsen the hypercalcemia. The mechanism of the hypercalcemia in sarcoidosis is an increase in both intestinal calcium absorption and bone resorption. These derangements are produced by the elevated blood levels of $1,25(OH)_2D_3$ found in an anephric patient with sarcoidosis, suggesting an extrarenal production of the metabolite, possibly by the sarcoid granuloma. Alveolar macrophages obtained by bronchial lavage from patients with sarcoidosis and hypercalcemia convert $25(OH)D_3$ to $1,25(OH)_2D_3$. The serum levels of PTH are low except in those patients who may have coexisting primary hyperparathyroidism. *Hypercalcemia* has been encountered in patients with *active tuberculosis* before initiation of therapy. It is usually mild, but levels greater than 12 mg/dl have been noted in a few patients. The hypercalcemia may last 1 to 7 months, and it resolves spontaneously with the healing of tuberculosis. The mechanism for this hypercalcemia is most likely similar to that of sarcoidosis. Elevated blood levels of $1,25(OH)_2D_3$ have been reported in patients with tuberculosis and hypercalcemia. Elevated blood levels of $1,25(OH)_2D_3$ were also found in hypercalcemic patients with *leprosy, disseminated candidiasis, silicone-induced granuloma*, and *granulomatous lipoid pneumonia*. Other granulomatous diseases associated with hypercalcemia include *berylliosis, disseminated coccidioidomycosis, histoplasmosis, eosinophilic granuloma*, and *farmer's lung*.

Hypercalcemia caused by *vitamin D intoxication* is seen in patients with hypoparathyroidism or those with chronic renal failure treated with large doses of the vitamin. In the latter patients, the blood levels of $25(OH)D_3$ are elevated, whereas those of $1,25(OH)_2D_3$ may be normal or reduced. This hypercalcemia may persist for weeks to months after the cessation of therapy with vitamin D. The use of $1,25(OH)_2D_3$ for the management of patients with chronic uremia and those treated with dialysis is also associated with hypercalcemia, but the serum levels of calcium return to normal within a few days of discontinuation of therapy (see Chapter 77). The mechanisms responsible for the hypercalcemia associated with the administration of the parent vitamin D, $25(OH)D_3$, or $1,25(OH)_2D_3$ include augmented intestinal calcium absorption and enhanced bone resorption.

Hypercalcemia may be encountered in patients with hypervitaminosis A. It could occur in food faddists and in patients receiving more than 75,000 IU/day of vitamin A for the treatment of acne. The hypercalcemia is due to enhanced bone resorption, and the action of vitamin A may be synergistic with that of vitamin D. Patients with vitamin A intoxication may have periosteal calcification.

Hypercalcemia caused by *immobilization* most often occurs in children or young adults. Among the causes of immobilization are body casts for the management of single or multiple fractures, quadriplegia, and extensive burns. When found in the elderly, the patients usually have polyostotic Paget's disease of the bone. The hypercalcemia usually appears several weeks after the onset of immobilization. The hypercalcemia is more common among patients with an increased rate of bone turnover before immobilization. Impairment of renal function associated with hypocalciuria may accentuate the hypercalcemia.

Hypercalcemia may be observed in patients with acute and chronic renal failure and in renal transplant recipients. The hypercalcemia of *acute renal failure* is discussed in detail in Chapter 49, that of *chronic renal failure* in Chapter 77, and that of *renal transplantation* in Chapter 89, Part 3.

Thiazide diuretics by inducing natriuresis and volume contraction cause hemoconcentration, and a mild rise in the serum levels of total calcium may not occur with the use of other diuretics because thiazides are the only diuretic agents that cause hypocalciuria. Overt hypercalcemia with elevated serum levels of ionized calcium may be encountered during thiazide therapy in patients with conditions associated with increased bone turnover, such as vitamin D therapy, primary and secondary hyperparathyroidism, juvenile osteoporosis, metastases to bone, and phosphate depletion. Thiazide diuretics have a direct effect on bone manifested by increased osteocytic osteolysis, and they potentiate the skeletal actions of PTH as well. The hypocalciuric effect of these diuretics contributes to the magnitude of the hypercalcemia.

Patients receiving long-term therapy with *lithium* may develop mild hypercalcemia and modest elevation in serum levels of PTH. Either intravenous or intragastric *hyperalimentation* regimens may be associated with hypercalcemia. *Milk-alkali syndrome* has been noted in patients with duodenal ulcer receiving therapy with sodium bicarbonate and large amounts of milk. These patients have hypercalcemia, hyperphosphatemia, hypocalciuria, renal insufficiency, and soft tissue calcifications. With the advent of newer therapeutic agents for the management of ulcer disease, the milk-alkali syndrome has become rare. However, with the increased use of calcium supplement in the form of calcium carbonate for the prevention and treatment of osteoporosis, milk-alkali syndrome may be seen more often. Indeed, a substantial number of patients with heart–lung transplantation who were treated with large doses of calcium carbonate for the prevention of glucocorticoid-induced osteoporosis or peptic ulcer developed hypercalcemia, alkalosis, and impaired renal function.

Theophylline toxicity may be associated with hypercalcemia, most likely by stimulation of β-adrenergic receptors in bone. This hypercalcemia is treated successfully by the administration of propranolol (40 mg every 6 hours) or by withdrawal of theophylline therapy.

Idiopathic hypercalcemia of infancy is a rare syndrome of unknown cause. The parathyroid glands of these patients are normal. The hypercalcemia causes constipation, hypotonia, and nephrocalcinosis and may lead to uremia. Other clinical features include abnormal growth and development with hypoplastic mandible, low-set ears, peglike teeth and scoliosis, mental retardation, supravalvular aortic stenosis, and accessory nipples.

Clinical Manifestations

The symptoms and signs of hypercalcemia are listed in Table 17.8. The effects of hypercalcemia on the kidney are discussed in a later part of this chapter. Hypercalcemia adversely affects the function of all organ systems. The severity of

TABLE 17.8. Signs, Symptoms, and Complications of Hypercalcemia

General
Malaise, fatigue, weakness
Neuropsychiatric
Impaired concentration, loss of memory, headache, drowsiness, lethargy, disorientation, confusion, irritability, depression, paranoia, hallucination, ataxia, speech defects, visual disturbances, deafness (calcification of ear drum), pruritus, mental retardation (infants), obtundation, coma
Neuromuscular
Hyporeflexia or absent reflexes, hypotonia, myalgia, muscle weakness, arthralgia, joint effusion, bone pain, dwarfism (infants)
Gastrointestinal
Anorexia, dry mouth, thirst, polydipsia, nausea, vomiting, constipation, abdominal pain, weight loss, acute pancreatitis, ulcer, acute gastric dilation
Genitourinary
Polyuria, nephrocalcinosis, stones, interstitial nephritis, acute and chronic renal failure, see also Table 17.70.
Cardiovascular
Hypertension, bradycardia, first-degree heart block, vascular calcification
Metastatic calcification
Band keratopathy, red eye syndrome, conjunctival calcification, nephrocalcinosis, vascular calcification, pruritus

the signs and symptoms in a given patient is a function of the degree and rapidity of onset of hypercalcemia. As many as 10% of patients with elevated levels of serum calcium are detected by a routine screening test of blood chemistry and are considered to have "asymptomatic hypercalcemia." In the symptomatic patients, the spectrum of the clinical presentation is varied and could be nonspecific. It is not uncommon that many patients with mild chronic hypercalcemia are considered psychoneurotics; malaise, weakness, minor joint pain, and other vague symptoms may mislead the physician until the hypercalcemia is discovered. In patients with severe hypercalcemia, the psychoneurotic pattern may be minimal, and the major symptoms are more likely to be nausea, vomiting, constipation, polyuria, and mental disturbances ranging from headache and lethargy to coma. Recent loss of memory could be prominent and could be a presenting symptom.

The clinical picture of primary hyperparathyroidism is variable, and three clinical presentations may be encountered. In 40% to 45% of these patients, there are minimal or no symptoms and moderate hypercalcemia (11.0 to 13.0 mg/dl) that is usually discovered during a routine examination. Another 40% to 45% of these patients have a chronic course manifested by mild or intermittent hypercalcemia, recurrent renal stones, and complications of nephrolithiasis; in these patients the parathyroid tumor is small (less than 1.0 g) and slowly growing. In another 5% to 10% of these patients, one encounters severe and symptomatic hypercalcemia (more than 13.0 mg/dl) and overt osteitis fibrosa cystica; in these patients the parathyroid tumor is large (greater than 5.0 g). Hypertension is common in patients with primary hyperparathyroidism.

The biochemical hallmarks of primary hyperparathyroidism are hypercalcemia, inappropriately normal or elevated blood levels of PTH, hypophosphatemia, phosphaturia, hypercalciuria, and increased urinary excretion of cyclic adenosine 3',5'-monophosphate (cAMP). Hyperchloremic acidosis may be present, and the ratio of serum chloride to phosphorus is elevated. The serum levels of alkaline phosphatase and of uric acid also may be elevated. The serum concentration of magnesium is usually normal but may be low or high.

In some patients with primary hyperparathyroidism, the concentration of serum calcium may be normal; this entity has been called *normocalcemic primary hyperparathyroidism*. However, we know of no patient in our own experience or in the literature in whom the level of serum calcium found before removal of the adenoma did not fall after surgery. Therefore the normal serum calcium in these patients with so-called normocalcemic primary hyperparathyroidism is in essence elevated in relation to their actual normal concentrations. A significant number of patients with primary hyperparathyroidism may have normal serum phosphorus concentrations. This may be related to the handling of the blood samples. If blood is drawn in the morning, with care to avoid hemolysis, while the patient is in the fasting state, and serum is separated without undue delay, the chances of finding hypophosphatemia are enhanced.

The evaluation of urinary calcium in patients with primary hyperparathyroidism should take into consideration the level of renal function, because renal insufficiency is usually associated with hypocalciuria. PTH also lowers the renal clearance of calcium; therefore, in patients with primary hyperparathyroidism, the degree of hypercalciuria, for any given elevation in serum calcium concentration, is less than that seen in nonparathyroid hypercalcemic disorders. To our knowledge, primary hyperparathyroidism in the presence of normal renal function is the only hypercalcemic disorder in which calcium excretion may be normal or slightly elevated.

Laboratory Findings

Laboratory findings in patients with hypercalcemia include abnormalities related to the underlying disease causing the hypercalcemia, and these are beyond the scope of this chapter. Alterations in the electrocardiogram (ECG) and electroencephalogram (EEG) occur in hypercalcemic patients independent of the cause of the hypercalcemia. The ECG shows a shortened ST segment and therefore a reduced QT interval when corrected for heart rate. In patients with severe hypercalcemia exceeding 16 mg/dl, there is a widening of the T waves, resulting in an increase in the QT interval. Therefore a reduction in interval from the onset of the QRS complex to the beginning of the T wave corrected for the heart rate is a more reliable sign of hypercalcemia. Bradycardia and first-degree heart block may be present in the ECG of patients with acute and severe hypercalcemia. The EEG displays slowing and other nonspecific changes.

Diagnosis

A careful history, physical examination, and routine laboratory tests will, in most patients, lead to the correct diagnosis in hypercalcemia. A flow diagram for the evaluation of hypercalcemia is shown in Fig. 17.8. Hypercalcemia in a patient with cancer may not always be caused by the malignant disorder; in fact, there is an increased association between primary hyperparathyroidism and malignant disorders and especially with carcinoma of the breast. Because both diseases can cause hypercalcemia, one should always consider that the hypercalcemia of malignancy may be due to parathyroid adenoma. Elevated blood levels of PTH provide for the diagnosis. The finding of hypercalcemia with normal or elevated serum levels of PTH should direct attention to primary hyperparathyroidism or familial hypocalciuric hypercalcemia.

The availability of new PTH assay [immunoradiometric assay (IRMA)], which uses two antibodies directed toward epitopes on both ends of the PTH molecule, allows the detection of the intact and biologically active hormone. This assay does not measure cross-reacting substances. Therefore elevated blood levels of PTH by IRMA provide a definite diagnosis of hyperparathyroidism. Although the tests and laboratory evaluation listed in Fig. 17.8 are still helpful for the diagnosis of primary hyperparathyroidism, one can make the definite diagnosis by the accurate measurement of serum levels of PTH by IRMA.

Occasionally, patients with normocalcemic hyperparathyroidism may have borderline elevated blood levels of PTH, and there may be doubt about the diagnosis. In these patients, the thiazide test may be helpful. The administration of 200 mg of hydrochlorothiazide per day for 5 days will cause overt hypercalcemia in these patients. Although this procedure may also produce a mild rise in the serum levels of calcium (0.5 to 0.8 mg/dl) in normal subjects, overt hypercalcemia does not occur.

Localization of the parathyroid adenoma provides valuable information to the surgeon who plans to remove the tumor. However, this is not essential, and an experienced surgeon rarely fails to find the tumor. Computed axial tomography scanning or high resolution ultrasonography of the neck may detect the site of a parathyroid adenoma (1 cm or greater) in 60% to 80% of patients; both false-positive and false-negative results have been noted. Arteriography of the neck also could be helpful but has the disadvantage of being invasive. Selective catheterization of the veins draining the parathyroid glands could be very helpful in localizing the adenoma. This technique is invasive and expensive and is not required before the first

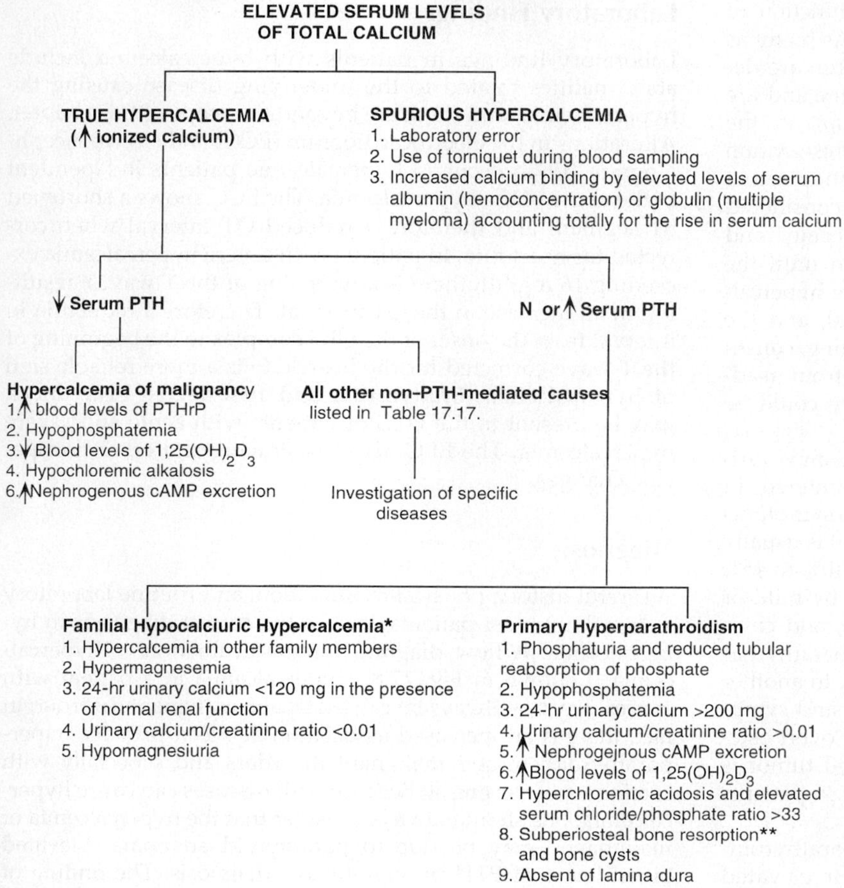

Figure 17.8. A flow diagram for evaluation of hypercalcemia. *Phosphaturia and increased nephrogenous cAMP may be present but are of less magnitude than in primary hyperparathyroidism; **not always present; N, normal.

surgery. The use of this procedure should be reserved for the few patients who need surgical reexploration for the treatment of recurrent hyperparathyroidism or persistent hyperparathyroidism after the initial surgical exploration.

Therapy

Hypercalcemia is managed by treating the underlying cause. However, many patients with marked hypercalcemia (more than 12.0 mg/dl) may require therapy to lower their serum calcium while investigation is being performed to determine the cause of the hypercalcemia. In addition, the nausea, vomiting, and polyuria that may be present in hypercalcemic patients may require fluid volume repletion. In the absence of congestive heart failure, 1 to 3 L of normal saline should be administered over a period of several hours to achieve rehydration.

Theoretically, a decrease in the serum levels of calcium can be achieved by enhancing urinary losses of this ion, augmenting net movement of calcium into bone, inhibiting bone resorption, reducing intestinal absorption of calcium, and/or removing calcium from extracellular fluid by other means. The various therapeutic modalities using these approaches are listed in Table 17.9. The level of serum calcium should not be lowered rapidly and precipitously because such a fall may cause acute hypotension.

Enhance Urinary Excretion of Calcium

All agents that induce sodium diuresis also augment urinary calcium excretion. This phenomenon forms the basis for the use of intravenous infusions of isotonic saline and the administration of a loop diuretic (furosemide) for the management of hyper-

TABLE 17.9. Therapeutic Modalities for the Management of Hypercalcemia

Enhance urinary excretion of calcium
- Intravenous saline-loading with or without loop diuretics
- Intravenous infusion of isotonic sodium sulfate
- Intravenous infusion of EDTA

Increase net movement of calcium into bone[a]
- Intravenous phosphate
- Oral phosphate

Inhibit bone resorption
- Calcitonin
- Mithramycin
- Glucocorticoids[b]
- Biphosphonates
- Indomethacin
- Aspirin
- Propranolol[c]

Reduce intestinal absorption of calcium[d]
- Reduce oral intake of calcium
- Oral ingestion of sodium phytate
- Oral ingestion of cellulose phosphate
- Glucocorticoids[b]

Other methods for calcium removal
- Hemodialysis
- Peritoneal dialysis

[a] Inhibition of bone resorption may also occur during phosphate therapy and partially account for the fall in serum calcium concentration.
[b] Especially in patients with increased sensitivity to vitamin D or in those with vitamin D overdose.
[c] Effective for the therapy of hypercalcemia in patients with hyperthyroidism.
[d] Agents that reduce intestinal absorption of calcium are usually not effective in the treatment of hypercalcemia because augmented intestinal absorption of calcium is not a primary cause of hypercalcemia.

calcemia. Effective lowering of the level of serum calcium requires the infusion of large amounts of isotonic saline (5 to 10 L/day) and the intravenous injection of 100 to 200 mg of furosemide every 2 hours. Ideally, this treatment should be carried out in an intensive care unit with a Swan-Ganz catheter in place to help monitor the amount of fluid administered. If urinary output is maintained at 5 to 10 L/24 hr, urinary calcium excretion may increase to 1 to 2 g, and serum calcium concentration may decrease by 2 to 4 mg/dl. It is absolutely essential that urinary losses of fluid, potassium, and magnesium are quantitatively replaced to prevent dehydration, hypokalemia, and hypomagnesemia. The urinary concentrations of these ions should be measured to guide replacement therapy, and the serum electrolytes should be evaluated at intervals of 2 to 4 hours to detect serious abnormalities. Usually, 20 to 40 mEq of KCl and 15 to 30 mg of magnesium ion per liter of saline infusate are adequate to replenish the urinary losses of these electrolytes. Hypophosphatemia also may develop as a result of increased urinary losses of phosphate; therefore attention should be given to serum phosphate level during this therapy. In some patients, the rate of calcium mobilization from the skeleton may be equal to or exceed the urinary losses, and therapy with saline and diuretics may not lower the levels of serum calcium. The presence of severe cardiovascular disease or congestive heart failure precludes the use of large volumes of saline. Hypercalcemic patients with severe renal failure (creatinine clearance of less than 20 ml/min) may not benefit from this therapy because a marked augmentation in urinary calcium excretion may not be achieved.

Infusion of isotonic solutions of sodium sulfate could be more effective than isotonic saline in lowering serum calcium. This is due to a greater loss of urinary calcium secondary to its complexing with the unabsorbable sulfate ions. The preparation of a sterile solution of sodium sulfate is cumbersome, and in practice, this therapy offers little advantage over the use of saline and diuretics. EDTA chelates serum calcium and forms complexes that are rapidly excreted by the kidney. This therapy is not recommended because it can induce severe renal injury.

Increase Net Movement of Calcium into Bone

Intravenous administration of salts of inorganic phosphate also is effective in acutely reducing the serum calcium levels by causing a shift of calcium out of the extracellular fluid into bone. Inhibition of bone resorption also may occur during phosphate therapy and may partially account for the fall in serum calcium concentration. One gram of elemental phosphorus (33 mmol) infused with saline over 8 to 16 hours is a safe and effective dose. Phosphate therapy is contraindicated if the serum phosphorus level is significantly elevated (above 5.0 to 6.0 mg/dl), and it should be used with caution when renal function is markedly reduced (creatinine clearance below 20% to 30% of normal); in these patients, the dose should be reduced to 0.2 to 0.4 g. It is important to monitor the levels of serum phosphorus, calcium, and creatinine during intravenous phosphate therapy and to adjust additional doses of phosphate according to the therapeutic response given. Intravenous therapy with inorganic phosphorus may be associated with soft tissue calcification. However, this complication can be avoided by the judicious use of this therapy by experienced physicians and by appropriate adjustment of the dose in patients with impaired renal function. This form of therapy is effective in the management of hypercalcemia of any origin and usually has been used in patients with primary hyperparathyroidism and in those with malignant tumors.

Oral phosphate therapy is also effective for the management of hypercalcemia. It is used in patients with primary hyperparathyroidism in whom surgery for the removal of the adenoma is delayed or in those with persistent hypercalcemia after the surgical exploration. The daily dosage is 1 to 3 g of elemental phosphorus given in three divided doses. Monitoring of the serum concentrations of phosphorus, calcium, and creatinine is required. The oral ingestion of phosphate may not be well tolerated because of diarrhea and gastrointestinal upset. Certain patients with primary hyperparathyroidism may display an escape from the effect of oral phosphorus therapy, and hypercalcemia may recur. Such patients will respond to an increase in the dose.

Inhibit Bone Resorption

Calcitonin, a polypeptide hormone that lowers the concentration of serum calcium by decreasing the rate of bone resorption, should theoretically provide an ideal modality for the treatment of hypercalcemia. Intravenous or intramuscular administration of 50 to 100 MRC units of salmon calcitonin or its equivalent every 8 to 12 hours usually produces a decrease in the concentration of serum calcium. However, hypercalcemia recurs within hours after discontinuation of therapy. In addition, many patients escape from the calcium-lowering effect of calcitonin during continued administration. Therefore its use has been disappointing.

Mithramycin is a highly potent cytotoxic antibiotic that blocks bone resorption through an inhibition of RNA synthesis in bone cells. The reduction in serum calcium concentration is accompanied by reduced urinary calcium and hydroxyproline excretion. It is administered by intravenous infusion of a dose of 25 to 50 μg/kg of body weight. A fall in serum calcium may be noted within hours and normocalcemia may persist for days after a single dose. Rapid recurrence has been encountered. Repeated therapy is effective but is limited by the cumulative toxicity of the drug. Side effects include nausea, vomiting, and malaise. The drug may decrease the platelet count and lead to hemorrhage, impair renal function, and cause a transient rise in blood levels of liver enzymes. Although this drug has become quite popular among oncologists in treating hypercalcemia, it is probably most useful in those patients who are resistant to other forms of treatment. The availability of biphosphonates and their approval for clinical use by the Food and Drug Administration have made them the mainstay for the treatment of hypercalcemia of malignancy.

Glucocorticoid may successfully reduce an elevated serum calcium concentration in certain hypercalcemic states such as sarcoidosis and vitamin D intoxication, and dosages as low as 10 mg of prednisone per day for several days are adequate; in these hypercalcemic states, the glucocorticoids reduce intestinal absorption of calcium and inhibit bone resorption as well. The hypercalcemia associated with multiple myeloma, leukemias, lymphomas, and breast cancer is most responsive to glucocorticoid therapy partly as a result of destruction of the tumor. In multiple myeloma, glucocorticoids may block the bone-resorbing effect of a family of cytokines, and they may also interfere with the bone resorption induced by prostaglandin produced by other tumors. The dosage of glucocorticoids for the management of the hypercalcemia of these tumors is 40 to 100 mg/day of prednisone or its equivalent, and most patients respond within 5 to 10 days. Because the prolonged use of high-dose glucocorticoids causes a multitude of side effects, these agents should be discontinued if response is not apparent within 2 weeks. Glucocorticoids are usually ineffective in the treatment of PTH-induced hypercalcemia and are not recommended for the management of the hypercalcemia of primary hyperparathyroidism.

The hypercalcemia associated with malignant tumors that produce prostaglandin may respond to therapy with prostaglandin synthetase inhibitors such as indomethacin or aspirin. The use of these drugs in the treatment of hypercalcemia of malignancy has been disappointing because prostaglandin-induced hypercalcemia is not common. Therefore these drugs are not currently being used for the treatment of hypercalcemia of malignancy.

Biphosphonates are pyrophosphate compounds that localize in the bone and inhibit osteoclastic bone resorption. They are effective in the treatment of hypercalcemia associated with hematologic neoplasias and carcinomas. Etidronate (Didronel) is effective when given intravenously (7.5 mg/kg per day) in combination with saline (3 L/day). Normalization of serum calcium levels may require up to 7 days of such therapy, and the duration of the response may last 1 to 6 weeks. Side effects are usually minimal, although acute renal failure may occur with rapid administration to patients with preexisting renal disease. Oral therapy with these biphates may cause oral ulcers, nausea, esophagitis, and diarrhea. Osteomalacia may follow long-term therapy. Pamidronate disodium is the most potent biphosphonate available. It is usually given as an intravenous infusion over 4 to 24 hours. Available data indicate that the infusion of 90 mg of pamidronate over 4 hours achieved normocalcemia after a mean period of 4 days and the normocalcemia was maintained for a mean period of 28 days. The dosage of pamidronate ranges between 30 to 90 mg depending on the severity of hypercalcemia. An infusion of 60 mg of pamidronate over 4 hours is usually adequate to control moderate hypercalcemia (less than 13.5 mg/dl). Pamidronate also has been used to decrease bone pain in patients with multiple myeloma and in those with breast cancer and bone metastasis. Side effects include fever, leukopenia, myalgia, hypophosphatemia and occasionally hypocalcemia, and hypomagnesemia. Pamidronate does not appear to worsen renal function even in patients with renal insufficiency.

Propranolol when given intravenously (10 mg/hr) may rapidly reverse the hypercalcemia of thyrotoxicosis. Oral therapy with this drug (80 to 100 mg/day) is also effective, and the response becomes apparent within a week. This therapy should not be used in the presence of congestive heart failure or in patients with a history of bronchospasm. The hypercalcemia of thyrotoxicosis is best managed by the restoration of the euthyroid state.

Other Therapeutic Modalities

In postmenopausal women with primary hyperparathyroidism, estrogen therapy may be useful in the management of hypercalcemia. Agents that reduce intestinal absorption of calcium are usually not effective in the treatment of hypercalcemia because augmented intestinal absorption of calcium is not a primary cause of hypercalcemia. Both peritoneal dialysis and hemodialysis with calcium-free dialysate are an effective means for acute lowering of serum calcium concentration. This therapeutic approach is rarely needed, but it may be lifesaving in a patient with multiple complicating problems such as renal failure and congestive heart failure.

Effects of Hypercalcemia on the Kidney

Hypercalcemia produces derangements in the function and structure of the kidneys, and these alterations are grouped together under the name of *hypercalcemic nephropathy*. The disease states that are associated with elevation in serum calcium and may be complicated by hypercalcemic nephropathy are listed in Table 17.7. The functional and structural changes in the kidneys are usually similar regardless of the cause of the hypercalcemia, but the severity of the abnormalities depends on the duration and degree of the hypercalcemia. The various effects of hypercalcemia on renal function and structure are listed in Table 17.10.

TABLE 17.10. Abnormalities in Renal Function and Structure Due to Acute or Chronic Hypercalcemia

Decreased renal plasma flow
Decreased coefficient of filtration, K_f
Reduction in glomerular filtration rate
Inhibition of tubular reabsorption of sodium
Suppression of tubular reabsorption of magnesium
Hypercalciuria
Enhanced tubular reabsorption of phosphate
Reduced tubular reabsorption of phosphate
Enhanced tubular reabsorption of bicarbonate
Impaired acid excretion
Impaired concentrating ability
Prerenal azotemia
Acute renal failure
Chronic renal failure
Hypertension
Nephrocalcinosis
Nephrolithiasis

Renal Hemodynamics

Renal plasma flow and glomerular filtration rate (GFR) may be reduced during acute elevation of the levels of serum calcium, and this effect usually depends on the magnitude of the hypercalcemia and rapidity with which it develops. A rapid and substantial rise in the concentration of serum calcium may cause acute renal failure with oliguria and uremia; occasionally, the urine volume is not scanty and the renal failure is of the nonoliguric type. In states with chronic hypercalcemia, there are proportional reductions in renal plasma flow and GFR without a change in the filtration fraction, and progressive deterioration in renal function resulting in chronic renal failure and uremia may occur.

Concentration and Dilution of Urine

The most common and early abnormality in renal function during hypercalcemia is impairment in concentrating ability. It is usually noted in patients with serum levels of calcium above 13 mg/dl, and many patients with milder degrees of hypercalcemia may retain their ability to concentrate the urine. Clinically, the defect is manifested by polyuria and polydipsia. Urinary osmolality is reduced and may approach isotonicity. The urine is rarely hypotonic, but occasionally the polyuria is marked and the patients excrete large volumes of diluted urine. The effect of hypercalcemia on the concentrating ability of the kidney is most probably due to functional alterations rather than to permanent structural damage because the defect is usually reversible following the control of hypercalcemia.

Inhibition of sodium transport at Henle's loop resulting in reduced sodium content in the renal medulla and lowered medullary tonicity is one possible factor underlying the defect in renal concentration. Hypercalcemia may increase medullary blood flow, leading to washout of medullary tonicity, which may also be a contributory factor. An impairment in the movement of water from the collecting duct into the renal medulla, caused by decreased sensitivity to vasopressin secondary to interference with the action of the hormone on renal adenylate cyclase, is another possible mechanism. Renal prostaglandin production may be stimulated and may antagonize the effect of vasopressin, and as such may contribute to the urinary concentration defect.

It is noteworthy to emphasize that patients with hypercalcemia, but without impairment in renal function, retain their ability to dilute the urine and to excrete water loads normally.

Tubular Transport

Calcium. Acute hypercalcemia produced by calcium infusion causes an increase in both the urinary excretion of calcium and the fraction of filtered calcium excreted. Hypercalcemia per se directly inhibits tubular reabsorption of calcium. This effect occurs throughout the nephron but may be more marked in the ascending limb of Henle's loop. The inhibition of the parathyroid glands by hypercalcemia and consequent fall in the blood levels of PTH contribute to the decreased tubular reabsorption of calcium.

Patients with hypercalcemic disorders have hypercalciuria, and the magnitude of the latter depends on the level of serum calcium, the activity of the parathyroid glands, and the integrity of renal function. PTH enhances tubular reabsorption of calcium, and for any given level of serum calcium and filtered load of this ion, the renal clearance of calcium is lower in states of excess PTH than in those without PTH. This action of PTH would explain (a) the frequent finding of a normal or only slightly elevated renal clearance of calcium in patients with primary hyperparathyroidism; (b) the high clearance of this ion in other disorders with comparable degrees of hypercalcemia but without excess PTH (malignant tumors with osteolytic metastases, sarcoidosis, and vitamin D intoxication); and (c) the hypercalciuria noted in patients with hypoparathyroidism made normocalcemic with vitamin D or calcium supplementation. Hypocalciuria is very common in patients with renal failure and occurs even in those with mild impairment in renal function. Because hypercalcemia may induce renal insufficiency, it is not infrequent to find that such hypercalcemic patients do not have hypercalciuria.

Sodium. Acute hypercalcemia inhibits the renal tubular transport of sodium and produces modest natriuresis. This inhibitory action occurs in the proximal tubules, the ascending limb of Henle's loop, and the distal tubule. Although hypercalcemia is associated with an increase in the excretion of both calcium and sodium, the relationship between their clearances differs from that observed during saline infusion in that calcium clearance significantly exceeds sodium clearance for any degree of sodium diuresis.

Magnesium. The infusion of calcium also causes an increase in the urinary excretion of magnesium, despite maneuvers that acutely reduce GFR and its filtered loads, indicating that the tubular reabsorption of this ion is inhibited during hypercalcemia. This inhibition is mainly located at the ascending limb of Henle's loop. Hypercalcemic states are associated with augmented urinary magnesium, and hence hypomagnesemia may ensue. Patients with primary hyperparathyroidism may have a negative magnesium balance with normal to low levels of magnesium in plasma. After the removal of the parathyroid adenoma, urinary magnesium falls and magnesium balance becomes positive; in some of these patients with severe and generalized bone disease, marked hypomagnesemia may develop after surgery, probably caused by a rapid deposition of magnesium in bone. Hypomagnesemia also has been observed in patients with malignant osteolytic lesions of bone and hypercalcemia.

The inhibition of renal tubular reabsorption of sodium and magnesium could be caused by hypercalcemia per se, but it is also possible that calcium, sodium, and magnesium compete for a common transport mechanism, with the absolute increase in the transport of one ion (calcium) responsible for the reduced reabsorption of the other two (sodium and magnesium). It is of interest that a reduction in the blood concentration of calcium has been associated with enhanced tubular reabsorption of sodium.

Phosphate. After acute infusions of calcium, the urinary excretion of phosphate falls, despite an increase in serum phosphorus. This effect of acute hypercalcemia is caused by an inhibition of secretion of PTH because phosphate excretion is not reduced after an acute elevation of serum calcium in dogs or humans without parathyroid glands. However, changes in the calcium concentration in blood may *directly* affect the renal reabsorption of phosphate. An ipsilateral decrease in urinary phosphate occurs during the acute infusion of calcium into one renal artery. In contrast, an increase in urinary phosphate was noted when the concentration of serum calcium was raised to normal by the prolonged infusion of calcium in patients with untreated hypoparathyroidism. In addition, phosphaturia is present in patients with breast carcinoma and hypercalcemia. This direct effect of calcium on tubular transport of phosphate may be caused by alterations in intracellular calcium concentration.

Bicarbonate. Acute hypercalcemia enhances tubular reabsorption of bicarbonate and acute hypocalcemia decreases transport maximum (T_m) of bicarbonate. Thus alterations in the concentration of serum calcium may affect acid–base homeostasis. Metabolic acidosis has been noticed in patients with hypercalcemia resulting from excess PTH, but patients with hypercalcemia that is not caused by excess PTH may have metabolic alkalosis. It is evident therefore that the effect of hypercalcemia on acid–base homeostasis is modified by the presence or absence of PTH and probably by other factors such as hypophosphatemia.

Potassium. Urinary excretion of potassium is increased during acute hypercalcemia in animals but not in humans, and prolonged hypercalcemia augments urinary output of potassium in humans as well. Patients with chronic hypercalcemia may develop hypokalemia, especially when their potassium intake is not adequate.

Prerenal Azotemia

Acute and severe hypercalcemia (hypercalcemic crisis) is usually associated with nausea, vomiting, abdominal discomfort, and loss of appetite. The loss of fluid with vomiting, the lack of water intake resulting from nausea, and the polyuria secondary to the inability of the kidney to concentrate the urine lead to marked dehydration and prerenal azotemia, which may progress to acute renal failure.

Hypertension

Available data indicate the presence of several interactions between blood pressure and the concentration of serum calcium. Acute and chronic hypercalcemia per se cause hypertension, and correction of the hypercalcemia is often followed by the return of blood pressure to normal levels; chronic hypercalcemia may lead to progressive renal failure, which can cause hypertension. Patients with chronic renal failure are more sensitive to the hypertensive effect of hypercalcemia; and acute hypocalcemia per se is associated with hypotension in humans and in

TABLE 17.11. Clinical States in Which Hypercalcemia Has Been Associated with Hypertension

Primary hyperparathyroidism[a]
Secondary hyperparathyroidism
Chronic renal failure
After renal transplantation
Vitamin D intoxication
Malignant diseases
Prolonged immobilization

[a] 32% to 54% (42% ± 5% SE) of patients with primary hyperparathyroidism and hypercalcemia have hypertension, and the removal of the parathyroid adenoma is followed by normalization of blood pressure in most.

dogs. The clinical states with hypercalcemia and hypertension are listed in Table 17.11.

The mechanisms through which changes in the concentration of serum calcium affect blood pressure are not known. Theoretically, such an effect may be mediated through a primary change in cardiac output and/or peripheral vascular resistance or through altered release and/or action of pressor substances such as renin and catecholamines. The available data indicate that, in humans, the levels of plasma renin activity are not altered during acute hypocalcemia or hypercalcemia, but a modest increase in plasma levels of norepinephrine may occur during acute hypercalcemia. In addition, hypercalcemia appears to interfere with the pressor effect of angiotensin. Thus one may conclude that a change in the plasma levels of pressor agonist or an augmentation in their action does not occur during hypercalcemia. The bulk of evidence suggests that hypercalcemia is associated with increased peripheral vascular resistance, possibly resulting from a direct effect of calcium on the vascular muscle cells.

A role for excess blood levels of PTH in the genesis of hypertension in patients with primary hyperparathyroidism has been suggested. However, PTH is a vasodilator and interferes with the pressor response to norepinephrine and angiotensin II. Despite this, it is possible that PTH interacts with the hypercalcemia and that these together contribute to the hypertension of primary hyperparathyroidism. Studies in rats support this notion. The infusion of calcium in normal rats caused a dose-related rise in serum calcium, and the increment in serum calcium was associated with an increase in mean arterial pressure; the changes in the latter were directly related ($P <.01$) to changes in serum calcium. For a comparable rise in serum calcium, the increments in mean arterial pressure in parathyroidectomized (PTX) rats were significantly ($P <.01$) less than in sham PTX rats (Fig. 17.9). When PTH was given intravenously to PTX rats, the rise in mean arterial pressure in response to calcium infusion was restored. These data suggest that the presence of PTH plays an important permissive role in the hypertensive action of the hypercalcemia. Further support for this concept is provided by the observation that after acute and comparable increments in the concentration of serum calcium produced by calcium infusion in normal subjects and in patients with postsurgical hypoparathyroidism, mean arterial pressure increased significantly only in the normal subjects. These data may explain the increased sensitivity of patients with chronic renal failure and secondary hyperparathyroidism to the hypertensive action of hypercalcemia.

Because PTH has been shown to enhance entry of calcium into cells and to increase the calcium content of many tissues, one might suggest that in the presence of PTH, more calcium may enter the vascular smooth muscle during hypercalcemia, and that such an event augments the hypertensive response to the rise in serum calcium. This action of PTH must be more powerful than its vasodilatory effect, and its full expression is evident only in the presence of hypercalcemia.

Structural Changes: Nephrocalcinosis

Acute hypercalcemia induced by the administration of PTH or vitamin D to animals may cause degenerative and necrotic lesions in the tubular epithelium of the ascending limb of Henle's loop, the distal convoluted tubules, and the collecting ducts; the proximal convoluted tubules are spared. Obstruction of some nephrons by casts and debris leading to dilation of renal tubules also has been noticed. Calcium deposition in the interstitium occurs with hypercalcemia of longer duration.

Clinically, the deposition of calcium salts within the renal parenchymatous tissue is called *nephrocalcinosis.* The localization of the calcium deposition may vary, but it usually involves the medulla and corticomedullary area and occasionally the cortex. Besides hypercalcemia, other disease conditions may also be associated with nephrocalcinosis (Table 17.12). Nephrocalcinosis is detected more often at postmortem examination than by x-ray examination during life.

Nephrocalcinosis per se is usually symptomless; however, the patients may have symptoms and signs produced by the disease causing the nephrocalcinosis. When nephrocalcinosis is associated with renal stones, some or all of the signs, symptoms, and consequences of nephrolithiasis may be present.

The mechanisms of nephrocalcinosis are not clear, may vary from one patient to another, and usually depend on the underlying disease. Prolonged hypercalcemia and/or hypercalciuria,

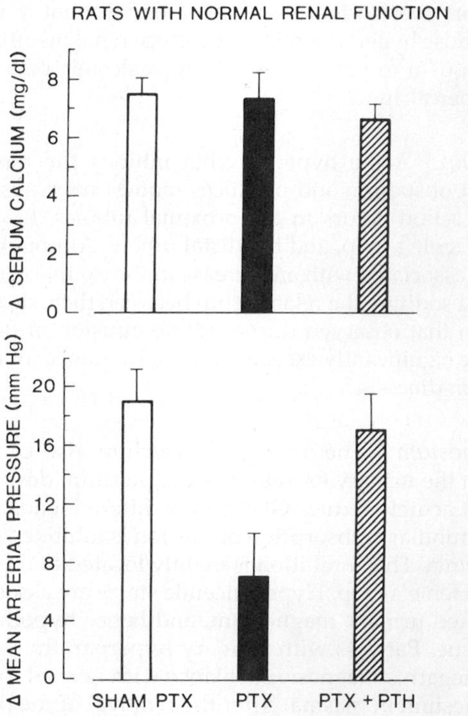

Figure 17.9. Changes in the concentration of serum calcium *(upper panel)* and in mean arterial pressure *(lower panel)* after 2 hours of calcium infusion in parathyroidectomized *(PTX)* and sham PTX rats and in PTX rats receiving parathyroid hormone *(PTH)* (residues 1 to 84) infusion for 2 hours. Each column represents the mean of data, and the bars denote SE. (Reprinted with permission from Iseki K, Massry SG, Campese VM. Effects of hypercalcemia and PTH on blood pressure in normal and renal failure rats. *Am J Physiol* 1986;250:F924–F929.)

TABLE 17.12. Diseases Associated with Nephrocalcinosis

Primary hyperparathyroidism
Milk-alkali syndrome
Vitamin D intoxication
Sarcoidosis
Malignancy with hypercalcemia
Renal tubular acidosis
Chronic renal failure
Primary oxaluria
Oxalosis
Renal cortical necrosis
Renal infarcts
Renal tuberculosis
Medullary sponge kidney
Certain renal tumors
Idiopathic infantile hypercalcemia
Magnesium depletion

excess circulating PTH, impaired urinary acidification, and local injury to renal parenchyma are among the factors that can predispose to nephrocalcinosis.

Renal Function in Patients with Primary Hyperparathyroidism

Patients with primary hyperparathyroidism are hypercalcemic and display various disturbances in renal function, ranging from modest reduction in GFR to advanced renal failure, impaired urinary concentrating ability, hypercalciuria, hypophosphatemia, increased urinary excretion of cAMP, impaired urinary acidification, metabolic acidosis, hypertension, nephrocalcinosis, and nephrolithiasis. These disturbances are due to the hypercalcemia, the elevated blood levels of PTH, and/or the consequences of nephrolithiasis.

Several factors are responsible for the impairment in renal function in patients with primary hyperparathyroidism. Hypercalcemia is an important factor. Chronic excess of PTH causes an elevation in the basal levels of cytosolic calcium in renal cells; this may adversely affect their function. Elevated levels of PTH reduce the coefficient of filtration (K_f) and thus decrease GFR. Available data indicate an interaction between PTH and calcium in the reduction of K_f. Hypercalcemia in normal rats has been associated with a fall in single nephron GFR and whole kidney GFR, and these decrements were mainly due to a reduction in K_f. However, similar hypercalcemia failed to affect K_f or single-nephron GFR in acutely thyroparathyroidectomized rats. In addition, the infusion of PTH to hypercalcemic thyroparathyroidectomized animals produced a marked and significant fall in K_f and single nephron GFR. These data demonstrate that PTH is a critical mediator of the effect of hypercalcemia. This effect of PTH may play a role in the progression of renal failure in patients with renal insufficiency, who usually have secondary hyperparathyroidism. Finally, urinary tract obstruction and infection in those who develop nephrolithiasis contribute to the deterioration in renal function.

Impaired urinary concentrating ability is common in these patients and is most probably related to the hypercalcemia. Urinary tract obstruction caused by renal stones also may contribute to the genesis of this defect. Usually, the abnormality is mild with only slight reduction of maximal urinary specific gravity to 1.010 to 1.020. Occasionally, the defect may be very marked, with the patients excreting as much as 4 to 6 L of hypotonic urine per day. In one series, only 11 of 57 patients had symptoms of polyuria or polydipsia. An inability to elevate urine osmolality above that of plasma could not account for the profound polydipsia and polyuria described above. Increased thirst or a state of acquired nephrogenic diabetes insipidus may exist in unusual cases. In many patients, there is an improvement in maximum urinary concentrating capacity after surgical correction of the hyperparathyroidism.

The hypercalciuria is due to the hypercalcemia, but the magnitude of the hypercalciuria is modified by the degree of elevation in blood levels of PTH because the latter enhances renal tubular reabsorption of calcium. The hyperphosphaturia and increased urinary excretion of cAMP are due to the elevated blood levels of PTH.

Patients with primary or secondary hyperparathyroidism may display abnormalities in acid–base homeostasis and in renal handling of bicarbonate. Many investigators have observed mild acidosis, low levels of serum bicarbonate, and impaired urinary acidification in patients with primary hyperparathyroidism and in those with osteomalacia or malabsorption and secondary hyperparathyroidism. Successful treatment of hyperparathyroidism is usually associated with reversal of these abnormalities. On the other hand, elevated levels of serum bicarbonate were noted in patients with hypercalcemia that was not due to excess PTH and in patients with hypoparathyroidism. In addition, metabolic alkalosis may be present in patients with primary hyperparathyroidism and protracted vomiting.

The presence of hyperchloremic acidosis in patients with parathyroid adenoma is not an all-or-none phenomenon. We noticed this abnormality in 11 of 44 patients with parathyroid adenoma. In another study of 57 patients with primary hyperparathyroidism, it was noted that 24% had blood bicarbonate levels less than 24 mEq/L, and serum chloride levels were above 107 mEq/L in 48% of the patients. In contrast, others reported that only 1 of 13 patients with parathyroid adenoma had hyperchloremic acidosis. These variations in the incidence of hyperchloremic acidosis in patients with hyperparathyroidism stem from the complexity of the mechanisms involved.

It appears that there is an interaction among PTH, body stores of phosphate, and hypercalcemia on the changes in renal tubular bicarbonate reabsorption in patients with hyperparathyroidism, which may be due to a direct action of PTH on the renal tubule and/or to phosphate depletion that develops secondary to the sustained phosphaturic action of excess PTH. On the other hand, the hypercalcemia in these patients may counteract the effect of PTH or phosphate depletion on bicarbonate reabsorption. The net effect on the acid–base status of the patients will depend on the interaction between these factors. Therefore variations in the duration and degree of elevated blood levels of PTH, the magnitude of hypercalcemia, and the severity and the duration of phosphate depletion in patients with hyperparathyroidism may explain the variations in the incidence of metabolic acidosis in these patients. Urinary tract obstruction, if present, may cause impaired urinary acidification and further contribute to the mechanism of the disturbances in acid–base homeostasis.

Other factors may be involved in the genesis of metabolic acidosis in patients with secondary hyperparathyroidism, who are often hypocalcemic and may have vitamin D deficiency. The latter may be associated with renal bicarbonate wasting, and T_m bicarbonate is reduced by hypocalcemia. Thus in patients with secondary hyperparathyroidism, there may be four abnormalities (excess PTH, hypophosphatemia and/or phosphate depletion, hypocalcemia, and vitamin D deficiency) responsible for renal bicarbonate losses and consequently for the metabolic acidosis.

HYPOCALCEMIA

Etiology

The causes of hypocalcemia are listed in Table 17.13. True hypocalcemia is a fall in the level of ionized calcium in serum. A decrease in the concentration of serum albumin is associated with a fall in the total level of serum calcium, but the concentration of ionized calcium is not reduced. It is evident from Table 17.13 that in certain disease conditions multiple factors may underlie the genesis of the hypocalcemia. Detailed discussion of the mechanisms of hypocalcemia in magnesium deficiency is provided in Chapter 18, Part 3; acute renal failure with and without rhabdomyolysis in Chapter 49; chronic renal failure in Chapter 77; and the nephrotic syndrome in Chapter 39, Part 2A. Hypocalcemia of less than 8 mg/dl occurs in 20% to 80% of patients with acute pancreatitis, and levels below 7 mg/dl occur in 10% to 50% of the patients. Several factors contribute to the hypocalcemia in acute pancreatitis including hypoalbuminemia, hypomagnesemia, hypoparathyroidism, skeletal resistance to the calcemic action of PTH, and sequestration of calcium in necrotic tissue (soap formation). Low serum levels of PTH are found in many patients with acute pancreatitis despite the hypocalcemia; the mechanisms for this phenomenon are not fully understood, but temporary damage to the parathyroid glands by pancreatic proteolytic enzymes has been postulated.

TABLE 17.13. Causes of Hypocalcemia

- Diminished protein-bound calcium (hypoalbuminemia)
  - Nephrotic syndrome
  - Cirrhosis
  - Malnutrition
  - Protein-losing enteropathy
  - Acute pancreatitis
- Diminished ionized calcium
  - Parathyroid hormone (PTH) deficiency
    - Hypoparathyroidism
      - Congenital, Di George syndrome (absence of thymus and parathyroid glands)
      - Idiopathic[a]
      - Sporadic
      - Familial
      - Acquired
        - Surgical removal of parathyroid glands
        - Acute pancreatitis
        - Destruction of parathyroid glands by malignant disease of neck (rare)
        - Amyloid of the parathyroid glands
        - Following radioactive iodide therapy of thyroid diseases (rare)
      - Inhibition of release of PTH
        - Magnesium deficiency
      - Following removal of parathyroid adenoma (temporary)
      - Infants of hypercalcemic mothers (temporary)
      - Acute pancreatitis with hypomagnesemia
      - Familial hypercalciuric hypocalcemia[b]
- Resistance of skeleton to the calcemic action of PTH
  - Uremia: acute and chronic renal failure
  - Magnesium deficiency
  - Pseudohypoparathyroidism
  - Acute pancreatitis with renal insufficiency
  - Vitamin D deficiency
    - Nutritional
    - Uremia: acute or chronic renal failure
    - Nephrotic syndrome
    - Intestinal malabsorption
    - Gastrectomy and gastrojejunostomy
    - Biliary cirrhosis
    - Anticonvulsant therapy
    - Vitamin D–dependent rickets (low serum levels of $1,25(OH)_2D_3$)[c]
- Secretion of biologically inactive PTH (Chapter 19, Part 3)
- Hyperphosphatemia
  - Uremia: acute or chronic renal failure
  - Oral or intravenous phosphate administration
  - During treatment of leukemia
- Increased flux of calcium into bone
  - Osteoblastic skeletal metastases in patients with cancer of breast or prostate
  - Healing phase of metabolic bone disease (the hungry bone syndrome) especially after removal of parathyroid adenoma
- Deposition of calcium in necrotic soft tissues
  - Rhabdomyolysis
  - Acute pancreatitis
- Chelation of calcium in blood
  - Citrate administration with blood transfusion
  - EDTA administration
- Miscellaneous[d]
  - Toxic shock syndrome
  - Trauma with fat embolism
  - Sepsis

[a] Idiopathic hypoparathyroidism may have an autoimmune etiology. Idiopathic hypoparathyroidism has also been associated with Kearns-Sayres syndrome (ophthalmoplegia, retinal degeneration, myopathy, and ataxia) and with hereditary nephritis and nerve deafness.

[b] This condition is due to a mutation of a gene of the calcium sensing receptor resulting in its activation. These patients also have hypomagnesiuria. The PTH blood levels are low normal.

[c] In vitamin D–dependent rickets type II, the blood levels of $1,25(OH)_2D_3$ are elevated but the response of the target organs to its action is reduced.

[d] Mechanisms are not defined.

Clinical Manifestations

The signs and symptoms of hypocalcemia depend on the rapidity with which it develops, its magnitude, and its duration but are usually independent of the cause. Chronic and moderate hypocalcemia may not be associated with symptoms, but a precipitous and marked fall in the serum level of ionized calcium is symptomatic. The manifestations of hypocalcemia may include weakness, fatigue, vague ill health, and emotional disturbances such as irritability and emotional lability, impairment of memory, confusion, delusion, hallucination, paranoia, and depression. The decrease in the serum concentration of ionized calcium increases neuromuscular excitability and causes a variety of signs and symptoms related to this phenomenon. A positive Chvostek's or Trousseau's sign may be elicited even in the asymptomatic hypocalcemic patient; many normal subjects may have a positive Chvostek's sign. There may be paresthesias manifested by circumoral tingling and numbness and feeling of pins and needles in the feet and hands, muscle cramps, carpopedal spasms, laryngeal stridor, or frank tetany. Epileptiform and more often Jacksonian seizures may occur but are usually not associated with aura, loss of consciousness, and incontinence.

Patients with chronic hypocalcemia, including those with idiopathic and postsurgical hypoparathyroidism and those with pseudohypoparathyroidism, may have papilledema, elevated cerebrospinal fluid pressure, and neurologic signs simulating a cerebral tumor.

Bilateral cataracts affecting the anterior and posterior subcapsular areas of the cortical portions of the lens may develop after one year of hypocalcemia. Cataracts are encountered more often in pseudohypoparathyroidism and idiopathic hypoparathyroidism than in the postsurgical variety. The cataracts do not resolve after correction of the hypocalcemia.

In patients with idiopathic hypoparathyroidism, the skin could be dry and scaly, eczema and psoriasis may worsen, and moniliasis can occur. The eyelashes and eyebrows may be scanty and axillary and pubic hair may be absent. Because some forms of this disease are caused by an autoimmune etiology, manifestation of other autoimmune diseases such as adrenal, thyroid, and gonadal insufficiency, diabetes mellitus, pernicious anemia, vitiligo, and alopecia areata may be present and should be looked for.

Hypoparathyroidism in children often causes teeth abnormalities such as defective enamel and root formation, dental hypoplasia, or failure of adult teeth to erupt. Severe skeletal mineralization may occur in the fetus of untreated pregnant women with hypoparathyroidism. Severe hypocalcemia in the neonate may cause congestive heart failure. Hypocalcemic patients may have resistance to digitalis therapy.

Laboratory Findings

The alterations in the levels of serum PTH and serum and urinary electrolytes in various hypocalcemic states depend on the mechanisms responsible for the hypocalcemia (Table 17.14), and knowledge of these changes aids in the differential diagnosis of these disorders.

X-ray examination of the skull or computed axial tomography scanning of the brain may reveal intracranial calcifications, especially of the basal ganglia. These have been noted in up to 20% of hypocalcemic patients with idiopathic hypoparathyroidism but are less common in postsurgical hypoparathyroidism unless the disease is longstanding. Such calcifications are also encountered in patients with pseudohypoparathyroidism.

Nonspecific abnormalities in the EEG, particularly an increase in high-voltage slow waves, may be seen in patients with hypocalcemia; these changes reverse with normalization of the level of serum calcium. The ECG shows peaking and inversion of the T waves and prolongation of the heart rate-corrected QT interval.

Therapy

Hypocalcemia associated with neuromuscular disturbances such as carpopedal spasms of tetany requires treatment with intravenous injection of calcium salts. Calcium gluconate is preferred to calcium chloride because the latter may cause necrosis of tissues if it infiltrates outside the vein. This may be given as 10 to 20 ml of 10% calcium gluconate over 10 minutes. The long-term treatment of hypocalcemia is achieved either by oral calcium supplementation or vitamin D administration. Several preparations of calcium salts are available and in prescribing any of them one should take into consideration their content of elemental calcium. The latter constitutes 40% of calcium carbonate, 36% of calcium chloride, 12% of calcium lactate, and 8% of calcium gluconate. A proprietary preparation, Titralac, provides 0.42 g of calcium carbonate and 0.18 g of glycine per tablet (i.e., 160 mg of elemental calcium per tablet). Neo-Calglucon syrup is another preparation well accepted by patients, but it is costly; each 4 ml contains 92 mg of calcium ion. Patients may need 2.0 to 4.0 g of elemental calcium per day. Oral calcium supplementation alone may be adequate to raise serum calcium toward normal.

Hypocalcemia of hypoparathyroidism may be treated with long-term therapy with a thiazide diuretic (chlorthalidone, 50 mg/day) and sodium restriction (50 mEq/day). Such therapy may increase the serum levels of both total and ionized calcium and is associated with hypocalciuria. During such therapy, the patients should be receiving adequate amounts of calcium (800 mg/day).

Parent vitamin D (50,000 to 100,000 units/day) or its potent metabolite 1,25(OH)$_2$D$_3$ (0.5 to 1.5 μg/day) is adequate

TABLE 17.14. Laboratory Findings in Serum and Urine in Disease States Associated with True Hypocalcemia

Serum Phosphorus	
High	Low
Idiopathic or acquired hypoparathyroidism	Malabsorption
Secretion of abnormal PTH	Vitamin D deficiency
Oliguric phase of acute renal failure	Acute pancreatitis
Chronic renal failure	Diuretic phase of acute renal failure
Pseudohypoparathyroidism	
Phosphate administration	
Serum PTH	
High	Low or undetectable
Pseudohypoparathyroidism	Idiopathic or acquired hypoparathyroidism
Vitamin D deficiency	Magnesium deficiency
Malabsorption	Acute pancreatitis
Acute renal failure	
Chronic renal failure	
Secretion of abnormal PTH	
Phosphate administration	
Serum Magnesium	
High	Low
Acute renal failure	Magnesium deficiency
Chronic renal failure	Acute pancreatitis
	Diuretic phase of acute renal failure
Serum Bicarbonate and Blood pH	
High	
Idiopathic and acquired hypoparathyroidism	
Urinary Calcium	
24-hr excretion	
High	Low
During treatment of idiopathic or acquired hypoparathyroidism with Vitamin D	All other hypocalcemic states
Fractional excretion	
High	Low
Idiopathic or acquired hypoparathyroidism	All other hypocalcemic states
Diuretic phase of acute renal failure	
Advanced renal failure	
Urinary Phosphate	
Hypophosphaturia	Hyperphosphaturia
Idiopathic and acquired hypoparathyroidism	Vitamin D deficiency
Pseudohypoparathyroidism	Malabsorption
Magnesium deficiency	Chronic renal failure
	Phosphate administration
Urinary cAMP	
Decreased	Increased
Idiopathic and acquired hypoparathyroidism	Vitamin D deficiency
Pseudohypoparathyroidism	Malabsorption
	Chronic renal failure

PTH, parathyroid hormone.

to maintain normal serum calcium levels between 8.5 and 10.0 mg/dl in most patients with idiopathic or acquired hypoparathyroidism. Hypercalciuria is usually present during this treatment. The required dosage of vitamin D may vary among patients and this therapy requires close monitoring of serum calcium to avoid hypercalcemia and its deleterious effects on renal function. Nephrocalcinosis, renal insufficiency, and uremia have occurred during the chronic management of hypocalcemia with vitamin D. Patients with pseudohypoparathyroidism require larger doses of vitamin D to correct their hypocalcemia. Treatment with vitamin D is not effective in the management of hypocalcemia associated with magnesium deficiency, and magnesium supplementation is the treatment of choice. The hypocalcemia resulting from advanced chronic renal failure and dialysis treatment is best treated with $1,25(OH)_2D_3$ (see Chapter 77).

Selected Readings

Baxter JD, Bandy PK. Hypercalcemia of thyrotoxicosis. *Ann Intern Med* 1966; 65:429–442.

A study of hypercalcemia in a large number of patients with hyperthyroidism.

Caburn JW, Brickman AS, Massry SG. Medical treatment in primary and secondary hyperparathyroidism. *Semin Drug Treat* 1972;2:117–135.

An excellent review and personal experience of the authors in the medical therapy of the hypercalcemia of primary hyperparathyroidism.

Guise TA, Yaneda T, Yates AJ, et al. The combined effect of tumor-produced parathyroid hormone–related protein and transforming growth factor-α enhance hypercalcemia in vivo and bone resorption in vitro. *J Clin Endocrinol Metab* 1993;77:40–45.

A study demonstrating that the hypercalcemic effect of PTHrP is enhanced by TGF-α.

Kaplan L, Katz AD, Ben-Issac C, et al. Malignant neoplasms and parathyroid adenoma. *Cancer* 1971;28:401–407.

The first detailed report on the high incidence of malignant tumors in patients with primary hyperparathyroidism.

Lingrade F, Zetterval O. Hypercalcemia and normal ionized serum calcium in a case of myelomatosis. *Ann Intern Med* 1973;78:396–399.

Documentation of a rise in total level of serum calcium caused by high blood levels of globulins in a patient with multiple myeloma. The patient had normal levels of ionized calcium despite the hypercalcemia.

Masekilde L, Erikson EF, Charles P. Hypercalcemia of malignancy: pathophysiology, diagnosis and treatment. *Crit Rev Oncol Hematol* 1991;11:1–7.

A very good review of the complex issue of hypercalcemia of malignancy.

Mundy GR, Guise TA. Hypercalcemia of malignancy. *Am J Med* 1997;103:134–144.

An excellent review of the pathogenesis of hypercalcemia of malignancy and its management.

Mune T, Katakami H, Kata Y, et al. Production and secretion of parathyroid-related protein in pheochromocytoma: participation of an α-adrenergic mechanism. *J Clin Endocrinol Metab* 1993;76:757–762.

A study of 10 patients with pheochromocytoma, demonstrating production of PTHrP by the tumor.

Pearce SHS, Williamson C, Kifor O, et al. A familial syndrome of hypocalcemia with hypercalciuria due to mutation in the calcium-sensing receptor. *N Engl J Med* 1996;335:1115–1122.

It provides the genetic analysis of this syndrome in 20 affected members of six families and describes the various mutations in the calcium-sensing receptors.

Pollack MR, Brown EM, Chou YWH, et al. Mutation in the human Ca^{2+} sensing receptor gene cause familial hypocalciuric hypercalcemia and neonatal severe hyperparathyroidism. *Cell* 1993;75:1297–1303.

A discussion of the role of Ca^{2+}-sensing receptor gene in the genesis of these calcium disorders.

Porter RH, Cox BG, Heaney D, et al. Treatment of hypoparathyroid patients with chlorthalidone. *N Engl J Med* 1978;298:577–581.

The first report demonstrating the use of chlorthalidone and dietary sodium restriction in the treatment of hypoparathyroidism.

Rodan GA. Mechanisms of action of bisphosphonates. *Annu Rev Pharmacol Toxicol* 1998;38:375–388.

An excellent review of the topic.

Singer FR, Fernandez M. Therapy of hypercalcemia of malignancy. *Am J Med* 1987; 82(2A):34–41.

A good review of the therapeutic modalities for the management of hypercalcemia of malignancy.

Strewler GJ, Nissenson RA. Hypercalcemia of malignancy, *West J Med* 1990;153: 635–640.

A good review of the hypercalcemia of malignancy and a discussion of the role of PTHrP.

Suki WN, Yium JJ, Van Minden M, et al. Acute treatment of hypercalcemia with furosemide. *N Engl J Med* 1970;283:836–840.

A description of the use of diuretics (furosemide) in the treatment of hypercalcemia.

CHAPTER 18

Magnesium Metabolism

PART 1 Intestinal Absorption of Magnesium

Barton S. Levine and Jack W. Coburn

Magnesium is the fourth most abundant metal in living organisms and is the second most prevalent intracellular cation. Many enzymes, involved in key steps of intermediary metabolism and phosphorylation, are activated by magnesium. These enzymes are important in providing energy for transport and in regulating various processes in the cell and at the cell membrane. Magnesium also plays a part in the synthesis of protein and DNA, in DNA and RNA transcription, and in the translation of messenger RNA. Moreover, magnesium may have a critical role in the regulation of mitochondrial function. Disorders of magnesium homeostasis can lead to profound changes in the function and well-being of the organism; the maintenance of normal magnesium metabolism is therefore of vital importance.

The recommended dietary allowance for magnesium is 350 mg/day for a normal adult male and 300 mg/day for an adult female. The average American diet providing 250 to 350 mg of magnesium a day is close to the recommended daily allowance; hence, dietary magnesium intake is actually below dietary requirements for a large percentage of the population. Furthermore, relatively small reductions in dietary magnesium intake and/or increases in dietary magnesium requirement for a prolonged period can alter magnesium balance.

The principal dietary sources of magnesium include cereals, nuts, dairy products, and green leafy vegetables and fats; refined sugars, a major energy source, contain small amounts of magnesium. Dietary sources of magnesium for infants are adequate in most circumstances. The magnesium concentration in human breast milk is 30 mg/L; in infant formulas, 40 to 80 mg/L; and in cow's milk, 130 mg/L. The bioavailability of magnesium varies with different sources. For example, the magnesium from magnesium acetate tablets or from almonds is more bioavailable than magnesium from commercially available enteric-coated magnesium chloride (Slow-Mag).

SITES AND MECHANISMS OF INTESTINAL ABSORPTION

Metabolic balance studies indicate that 25% to 60% of dietary magnesium is absorbed; this percentage may be even higher in low-birth-weight infants ingesting human milk. A small fraction of the magnesium in the feces is derived from endogenous intestinal secretion; this is estimated to be 12 to 24 mg/day or 0.5 to 1.0 mmol/day and is the amount of magnesium found in the stool of a person ingesting a very low magnesium intake.

The data available are somewhat variable with regard to whether the intestine can modify magnesium absorption according to the magnesium content of the diet. Studies using radiolabeled magnesium (^{28}Mg) in animals indicate little variation of the fraction of magnesium absorbed according to the dietary content, and metabolic balance studies reveal an apparent linear increase in the net absorption, because magnesium intake varies from 100 to 500 mg/day. On the other hand, studies of net absorption from a single meal show substantial reductions in the fraction absorbed as the amount of magnesium added to a normal meal is increased substantially from 120 to 950 mg/meal. These data are consistent with a saturable and a nonsaturable component for the absorption of magnesium (Fig. 18.1). The nonsaturable component accounts for absorbing approximately 7% of ingested magnesium. There are no data to suggest that there is intestinal adaptation of magnesium absorption in response to chronic variation to either a high or low magnesium diet.

The localization of magnesium absorption in various segments of the intestine has yielded different results depending on the species studied. Thus magnesium is absorbed in both the small intestine and colon in the rat, but absorption is limited to the small intestine in most other species. In humans, the tem-

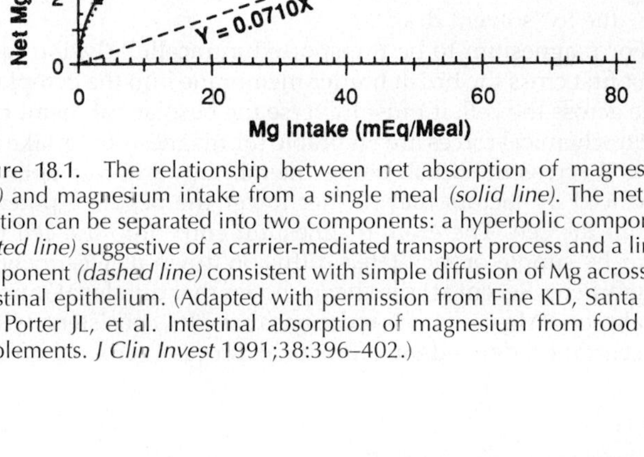

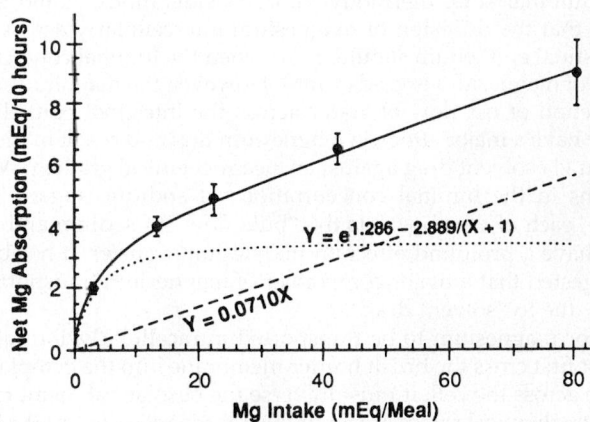

Figure 18.1. The relationship between net absorption of magnesium *(Mg)* and magnesium intake from a single meal *(solid line)*. The net absorption can be separated into two components: a hyperbolic component *(dotted line)* suggestive of a carrier-mediated transport process and a linear component *(dashed line)* consistent with simple diffusion of Mg across the intestinal epithelium. (Adapted with permission from Fine KD, Santa Ana CA, Porter JL, et al. Intestinal absorption of magnesium from food and supplements. *J Clin Invest* 1991;38:396–402.)

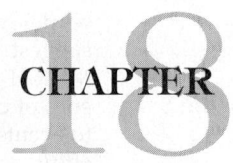

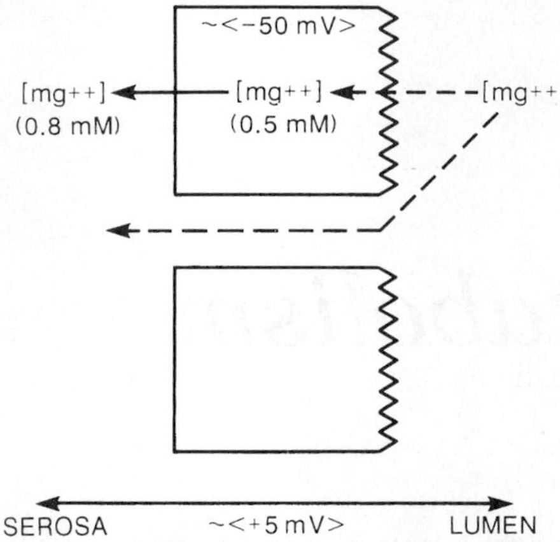

Figure 18.2. Depiction of the transport routes for magnesium across the intestinal mucosa. Magnesium can travel between cells by simple diffusion or solvent drag, or pass through the mucosal cell. Under normal circumstances, electrochemical forces for magnesium would favor both the intercellular movement of magnesium (serosal is +5 mV relative to lumen) and the uptake of magnesium into the cell cytoplasm across the brush border membrane. By contrast, electrochemical forces oppose the movement of magnesium across the basolateral membrane into the extracellular space. *Broken arrows* indicate passive or facilitated diffusion; the *solid arrow* indicates movement of magnesium against an electrochemical gradient. *Numbers in parentheses* indicate the estimated ionic concentration of magnesium.

poral pattern of the appearance of radiolabeled magnesium in the plasma following its ingestion suggests that most absorption occurs in the small intestine. Triple-lumen perfusion studies in humans have demonstrated that magnesium absorption occurs equally well in the ileum and proximal jejunum.

The mechanism of magnesium transport by the intestine has yet to be elucidated. As with calcium, magnesium may move across the intestinal mucosa by both intercellular and intracellular routes (Fig. 18.2). The relative importance of each of these modalities may vary with different intestinal segments and the species studied. For magnesium to cross the intestinal epithelium through an intercellular pathway, it must move against an electrical gradient and, depending on its luminal concentration, against a chemical gradient. Because the serosal side of the intestinal epithelium is approximately 5 mV positive relative to the luminal side, thermodynamic considerations would suggest that the diffusion of magnesium intercellularly across the intestinal epithelium should occur when the luminal concentration of magnesium exceeds 1 mM. However, the magnitude and direction of net flow of water across the intestinal epithelium may have a major effect on magnesium flux and result in movement via solvent drag against an electrochemical gradient. Variations in the luminal concentrations of sodium, sugars, and urea, each of which affects the "bulk flow" of sodium and water, have a profound effect on magnesium transfer. It has been suggested that a major component of magnesium transport occurs due to "solvent drag."

For magnesium to be transported intracellularly, the cation must first cross the brush border membrane into the cytoplasm; once across the cell, it must traverse the basolateral membrane. Electrochemical forces are favorable for magnesium uptake into the cell across the brush border membrane, and this uptake is enhanced by factors that further lower the negative potential within the cell. Therefore magnesium entry into the cell may occur by simple or facilitated diffusion down its electrochemical gradient. Recent studies have shown that duodenal mucosal uptake of ^{28}Mg is linear and nonsaturable, consistent with a concentration-dependent diffusional process across the brush border membrane of this gut segment. In the colon, animal data suggest that magnesium may enter the intestinal cell via a Mg^{2+}-H^+ exchanger whose function is stimulated by the presence of certain volatile fatty acids, such as butyrate. In contrast to events occurring at the brush border membrane, magnesium efflux across the basolateral membrane occurs against a large electrical gradient and presumably is active in nature. An electroneutral Mg^{2+}-anion symporter has been identified in the basolateral membrane of the enterocyte of the tilapia (Oreochromis Mossambicus). Whether this transporter is present in the basolateral membrane of enterocytes from other species is unknown. Various metabolic "poisons" reduce magnesium transport, providing further evidence for the active nature of the transport. The exact nature of this transport process, however, remains to be elucidated. The relative contributions of transcellular and intercellular magnesium transport to intestinal magnesium absorption are unknown and may vary with specific physiologic stimuli and specific pathologic conditions.

Factors that may modify the absorption of magnesium include dietary magnesium, calcium, and phosphorus and hormones, including vitamin D and parathyroid hormone. Variations in normal dietary magnesium intake lead to little if any changes in the fraction of magnesium that is absorbed. Thus the intestine plays a small role in the regulation of body magnesium. This is not surprising considering the low concentration of luminal magnesium required for the intercellular diffusion of magnesium.

Studies of the interrelation between the absorption of calcium and magnesium have yielded conflicting results. Certain observations, which suggest that magnesium absorption decreases as dietary calcium increases and vice versa, have been interpreted to indicate that calcium and magnesium may share and compete for transport pathways. Other data show that the absorption of the two divalent cations changes in the same direction with little evidence for competition. The effect of calcium on magnesium absorption can be modified by several factors. *In vivo* and *in vitro* studies have demonstrated that calcium, in the presence of adequate amounts of phosphorus, reduces the absorption of magnesium, perhaps related to the formation of an insoluble Mg-Ca-P complex. In contrast, calcium gluconate may actually enhance magnesium absorption, perhaps through the formation of volatile fatty acids, which appear to increase magnesium absorption in the gut. Wheat bran blunts the effects of dietary calcium supplementation and enhances the intestinal absorption of magnesium. Thus the interaction between dietary magnesium and calcium is complex, and it is difficult to make conclusions regarding absorptive mechanisms in the intestine from data from dietary studies. Several studies have shown that increasing dietary phosphate alone may inhibit magnesium transport. This effect is magnified by high dietary magnesium intakes.

The overall effect of vitamin D on the intestinal absorption of magnesium is not clearly resolved. Results of studies in vitamin D–deficient animals and in vitamin D–replete pigs indicate a definite effect of vitamin D sterols to augment magnesium absorption. Moreover, perfusion studies of the jejunum of patients with renal failure indicate that 1,25-dihydroxyvitamin D_3 [$1,25(OH)_2D_3$] stimulates magnesium absorption. Other data show no relation between steady-state plasma levels of $1,25(OH)_2D$ and net absorption of magnesium; these findings are in contrast to the close relation between calcium absorption and plasma $1,25(OH)_2D$ levels. Also, when the active vitamin D sterols are given to humans, the effect on net magnesium absorption has been either very small or undetectable.

Available data suggest that parathyroid hormone may have a small effect on magnesium absorption, a process that may be dependent on the action of the hormone on vitamin D metabolism. Growth hormone may increase the intestinal absorption of magnesium slightly, whereas aldosterone and calcitonin have been observed to reduce magnesium absorption slightly. Vitamin B_6 administration has been reported to enhance intestinal absorption of magnesium. High dietary fiber and particularly phytates, which chelate both calcium and magnesium, and an increase in dietary phosphate intake reduce intestinal magnesium absorption. In contrast, a variety of oligosaccharides appear to enhance magnesium absorption via the formation of volatile fatty acids.

CONDITIONS ASSOCIATED WITH ABNORMALITIES IN INTESTINAL ABSORPTION OF MAGNESIUM

Clinical disorders and various conditions associated with altered magnesium absorption are shown in Table 18.1. A reduction in magnesium absorption will accompany a decrease in dietary intake. In a recent diet survey, up to 70% of adults in the United States were found to ingest a diet with a magnesium content below the recommended daily allowance. This is particularly true in the African-American population in which the recent National Health and Nutrition Examination Survey (NHANES) survey, using 24-hour dietary recall, found that African-Americans consume significantly less magnesium than whites, regardless of educational level. Because of their rapid growth, pubertal boys and girls may be more susceptible to magnesium depletion despite ingesting the recommended daily allowance of magnesium; thus a higher magnesium intake may be necessary in this group. A markedly reduced intake most often occurs with the prolonged administration of parenteral fluids or tube feedings that are devoid of magnesium or with prolonged fasting; a reduced intake contributes to the hypomagnesemia of chronic alcoholism. Many disorders reduce the fractional absorption of magnesium, including various malabsorption syndromes, intestinal bypass surgery, and other conditions with shortening or fistulas of the intestinal tract. In addition, malabsorption of magnesium occurs with steatorrhea of various causes and in many diarrheal disorders. The intestinal absorption of magnesium may be reduced in chronic alcoholism, perhaps because of diarrhea. Fecal magnesium concentrations may reach levels as high as 1,000 mg/L in various diarrheal states. Hence, severe diarrhea can cause magnesium deficiency quite rapidly. An inborn error in intestinal absorption of magnesium, which occurs more commonly in males, is manifested by profound hypomagnesemia and hypocalcemia. It is usually detected during infancy or early childhood. The nature of the transport defect is unknown. There is a report of a child with both impaired intestinal magnesium absorption and renal magnesium wasting.

A reduction in urinary magnesium excretion has been described in patients with hypercalciuria and nephrolithiasis. Intestinal perfusion methods that measure magnesium absorption and metabolic balance studies that measure net magnesium absorption indicate that the intestinal magnesium absorption is reduced in such patients. This condition is of particular interest because it is characterized by enhanced intestinal absorption of calcium; thus, this represents a clear dissociation between the transport of calcium and magnesium. However, the administration of magnesium to hyperabsorptive hypercalciurics reduces the enteral absorption of calcium while it increases the net magnesium absorption, both of which may reduce the incidence of stones.

Chronic renal failure is accompanied by altered magnesium metabolism, but data on intestinal absorption of magnesium have provided varying results. Studies of net intestinal absorption of magnesium in patients with uremia have yielded results that are either normal or only slightly decreased (Fig. 18.3). However, data from jejunal perfusion in uremic patients indicate that magnesium absorption is subnormal; this has been attributed to a deficiency of $1,25(OH)_2D_3$. The significance of this finding is unclear because most patients with renal failure exhibit hypermagnesemia and increased body content of magnesium, particularly in bone. In addition, treatment with vitamin D sterols has produced little or no increase in the net absorption of magnesium and no significant increase in serum or urinary magnesium. On the other hand, urinary and serum magnesium levels increase when patients with chronic renal failure are

TABLE 18.1. Conditions Associated with Altered Magnesium Absorption

- Reduced magnesium absorption
  - Reduced intake
  - Parenteral fluids lacking magnesium
  - Tube feeding
  - Prolonged fasting
  - Chronic alcoholism
- Reduced intestinal absorption
  - Malabsorption syndromes
  - Intestinal bypass or fistula
  - Diarrheal disorders
  - Inborn error of intestinal magnesium absorption
  - Nephrolithiasis
  - Chronic alcoholism
  - Chronic renal failure?
- Augmented magnesium absorption
  - Increased oral intake
  - Magnesium-containing laxatives
  - Magnesium-containing antacids
  - Other
  - Magnesium-containing enemas

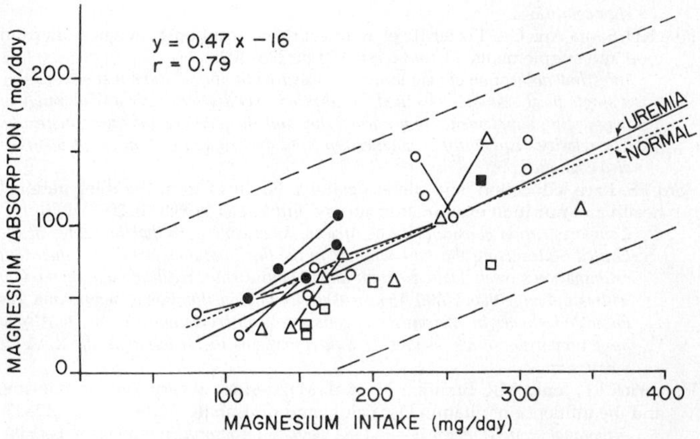

Figure 18.3. The relationship between net magnesium absorption and dietary magnesium intake in patients with chronic renal failure and creatinine clearances below 30 ml/min. The regression line and 95% confidence limits for normal are shown. The lines between symbols connect observations during different levels of magnesium intake in the same patient. The data have been collected from various sources. (Reprinted from Coburn JW, Hartenbower DL, Brickman AS, et al. Intestinal absorption of calcium, magnesium and phosphorus in chronic renal insufficiency. In: David DS, ed. *Calcium metabolism in renal failure and nephrolithiasis.* New York: John Wiley & Sons, 1977:77–109. With permission of John Wiley & Sons.)

given dietary supplements of magnesium; also, hypermagnesemia is common in patients with renal failure who ingest magnesium-containing antacids. If there is a defect in magnesium absorption in uremia, the abnormality must play a quantitatively small role in overall magnesium homeostasis. The component of magnesium absorption that is impaired in uremia may be limited to one or two segments of the intestine, whereas magnesium absorption may be normal or even increased in other segments. The net result is normal or near normal net absorption throughout the entire gut.

Net dietary magnesium absorption is enhanced with increased dietary magnesium intake. An increase in the absorption of magnesium caused by an underlying disease process or pathophysiologic state has not been reported. Although a slight rise in serum magnesium may occur in normal subjects with magnesium supplementation, clinical problems with hypermagnesemia caused by increased magnesium intake arise only when the capacity for renal excretion of magnesium is reduced. A marked increase in net absorption of magnesium can occur with the ingestion of magnesium-containing antacids or magnesium-containing laxatives (Table 18.1). The use of magnesium-containing enemas can cause striking hypermagnesemia in patients with decreased renal function, indicating that magnesium absorption in the colon can be substantial.

Selected Readings

Brannan PG, Vergne-Morini P, Pak CYC, et al. Magnesium absorption in the human small intestine: results in patients with absorptive hypercalciuria. *J Clin Invest* 1976;57:1412–1420.

A study of normal subjects, patients with chronic renal disease, and patients with absorptive hypercalciuria, using a triple-lumen catheter to assess magnesium absorption in the jejunum or ileum. Includes the kinetics of magnesium absorption in both ileum and jejunum, comparison of the absorption of magnesium in patients with renal disease or hypercalciuria with that in normal subjects, and assessment of the interaction of calcium and magnesium.

Fine KD, Santa Ana CA, Fordtran JS. Diagnosis of magnesium-induced diarrhea. *N Engl J Med* 1991;324:1012–1017.

This study evaluates the fecal output of magnesium and the fecal concentration of magnesium under various conditions. Measurements are obtained in normal subjects before and after the induction of diarrhea. Diarrhea is induced either with magnesium-containing compounds or with osmotic agents. Similar measurements are also made in subjects suffering with chronic diarrhea. This study provides a range of fecal magnesium concentrations that may occur under normal and diarrhea conditions.

Fine KD, Santa Ana CA, Porter JL, et al. Intestinal absorption of magnesium from food and supplements. *J Clin Invest* 1991;88:396–402.

Intestinal absorption of magnesium is measured in normal human subjects using a single meal "balance" method. Absorption was assessed over a wide range of magnesium supplements to a normal diet and the data are analyzed kinetically. The relative availability of magnesium from dietary and certain supplements is also evaluated.

Ford ES. Race, education, and dietary cations. Findings from the third national health and nutrition examination survey. *Ethnic Dis* 1998;8:10–20.

Compares cation consumption of African-Americans with that in whites in the United States using the data obtained in the third national health and nutrition examination survey. Data are from the 24-hour dietary recall of more than 6,000 whites and more than 2,000 African-Americans. Consumption of magnesium was found to be lower in African-Americans across all socioeconomic classes. Also, a large proportion of whites and African-Americans ingest less than the RDA for magnesium.

Hardwick LL, Jones MR, Brautbar N, et al. Magnesium absorption: mechanisms and the influence of vitamin D, calcium and phosphate. *J Nutr* 1991;21:13–23.

A thorough, concise review of intestinal magnesium absorption is provided. Both human and animal data are analyzed regarding mechanisms and sites of intestinal magnesium absorption, the possible interaction between calcium, phosphate, and magnesium transport and the effect of vitamin D on intestinal magnesium absorption.

Hodgkinson A, Marshall DH, Nordin BEC. Vitamin D and magnesium absorption in man. *Clin Sci* 1979;57:121–123.

Vitamin D was administered to subjects with osteoporosis, osteomalacia, primary hyperparathyroidism, and hypoparathyroidism, as well as to normal subjects. Vitamin D significantly increased net calcium absorption and to a lesser degree augmented magnesium absorption. However, magnesium balance was not affected.

Marier JR. Magnesium content of the food supply in the modern day world. *Magnesium* 1986;5:1–8.

An article describing several aspects of magnesium metabolism including the results of a large scale survey of dietary magnesium intake in North America and a comparison of the magnesium content of various diets. Also considered are various illnesses that may be improved by magnesium supplementation and various pathophysiologic conditions that may be brought about by magnesium deficiency.

Schmulen AC, Lermon M, Pak CYC, et al. Effect of 1,25 dihydroxyvitamin D_3 therapy on jejunal absorption of magnesium in patients with chronic renal failure. *Am J Physiol* 1980;238:349G–355G.

Evaluation of the effects of administered calcitriol [1,25 $(OH)_2D_3$] on intestinal magnesium absorption in patients with chronic renal failure. Magnesium absorption is assessed using the triple lumen catheter technique.

PART 2
Renal Handling of Magnesium

Gary A. Quamme

In humans, the plasma normally contains magnesium in concentrations of 0.7 to 1.0 mmol/L. Although no single homeostatic control has been demonstrated for magnesium, the cellular availability of this cation is closely regulated by the gastrointestinal tract, kidney, and bone.

The excretory side of magnesium balance involves appropriate changes in renal magnesium handling; indeed, the kidney plays the major role in regulating extracellular magnesium concentration. In humans, with an ultrafiltrable magnesium concentration of 0.5 to 0.7 mmol/L, the filtered load of magnesium amounts to approximately 1,500 mmol/day. Because the normal urinary magnesium excretion rate is approximately 100 mg/day, the urinary output represents about 3% of the filtered load of magnesium. The major portion of filtered magnesium is reabsorbed by the renal tubules. The kidney is able to respond rapidly to changes in concentration of magnesium in the extracellular fluid and to alter tubular reabsorption of magnesium with specific physiologic influences. Thus, in magnesium deficiency, magnesium excretion can approach zero as hypomagnesemia becomes severe. Conversely, with progressive hypermagnesemia, magnesium excretion can attain a value near that filtered at the glomerulus. Present evidence suggests that the renal handling of magnesium is normally a filtration-reabsorption process. Experimental support for secretion remains unconvincing.

Clearance studies over the last two decades have characterized renal magnesium transport as a saturable process or a transport maximum (T_m)-limited system. A maximum reabsorption rate of 58 mmol/min/kg of body weight at a filtered magnesium load of 90 mmol/min was achieved during magnesium infusion in dogs. The titration curve had a considerable splay, and its maximum value (T_m), was appropriately altered by factors that can alter magnesium reabsorption, such as parathyroid hormone (PTH), serum calcium concentration, and extracellular fluid volume expansion.

Renal magnesium reabsorption has distinctive features when compared with reabsorption of sodium and calcium (Fig. 18.4). Approximately 20% to 30% of the filtered magnesium is reabsorbed in the proximal tubule, compared with a fractional absorption of sodium or calcium of 50% to 60%. Although the fractional reabsorption of magnesium is only one-third that of sodium, it changes in parallel with that of sodium in response to changes in extracellular fluid volume. The major portion of filtered magnesium (about 65%) is reabsorbed in Henle's loop. Evidence suggests that magnesium reabsorption in the thick ascending limb (TAL) occurs passively through the paracellular pathway driven by the luminal positive transepithelial

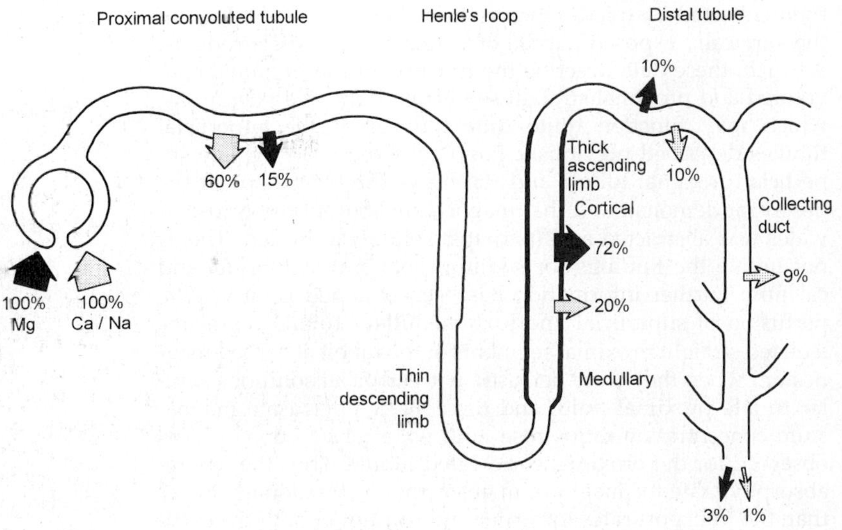

Figure 18.4. Schematic view of segmental reabsorption within the nephron. (Modified from Quamme GA. Renal magnesium handling: new insights in understanding old problems. *Kidney Int* 1997;52:1180–1195.)

voltage. The distal tubule normally reabsorbs about 10% of the magnesium filtered through the glomerulus. Although this seems like a small amount, it represents 70% to 80% of the magnesium delivered to this segment from Henle's loop. Because there is little magnesium reabsorption beyond the distal tubule in the collecting ducts, the segments comprising this portion of the nephron play an important role in determining the final urinary excretion of magnesium. Magnesium reabsorption within the distal tubule is transcellular and active in nature.

TUBULAR REABSORPTION OF MAGNESIUM

Glomerular Filtration

From 70% to 80% of the plasma magnesium is ultrafiltrable as determined by direct sample of fluid from surface glomeruli of Munich-Wistar rats and by the use of artificial membranes. This compares with 60% to 65% for ultrafiltrable plasma calcium. Only 70% to 80% of the filterable magnesium is thought to be in the ionic form (Mg^{2+}), the remainder being largely complexed to anions, particularly phosphate, citrate, and oxalate. The ultrafilterability of plasma magnesium is not affected by magnesium deficiency, magnesium excess, or elevation of plasma calcium concentration. Other factors that may affect glomerular ultrafilterability such as acidosis, alkalosis, and alterations of plasma anion and protein constituents remain to be evaluated. The use of recently developed electrodes for ionized Mg^{2+} will be informative in determining ultrafilterability in these situations.

Proximal Convoluted Tubule

The proximal convoluted tubule reabsorbs approximately 25% of the magnesium filtered at the glomerulus (Fig. 18.4). Luminal magnesium concentration rises with respect to the ultrafiltrable magnesium along the length of the proximal convoluted tubule. The mean tubular fluid:ultrafiltrate (TF/UF) magnesium ratio was found to be 1.7 at a point in the nephron where 50% to 55% of sodium and water had been reabsorbed. This appears to be a common phenomenon in all species studied to date, including primates. The overall fractional magnesium reabsorption in the proximal tubule (20% to 30% of the filtered load) is lower than the fractional reabsorption rate of sodium and calcium (60% to 70%). However, overall magnesium reabsorption in the proximal tubule closely follows changes in sodium and water reabsorption, although at a lower fractional rate. The profile for the TF/UF for magnesium relative to that for inulin remains largely unchanged in a variety of experimental circumstances, including volume expansion, diuretic administration, metabolic acidosis and alkalosis, and changes in plasma levels of calcium and phosphate.

The observation that the tubular fluid magnesium concentration may be about 1.5-fold greater than the plasma concentration suggests that the proximal tubule epithelium possesses a low permeability for magnesium relative to sodium or calcium. A detailed analysis of magnesium transport in the proximal tubule was made using *in vivo* microperfusion techniques. Tubules were perfused with Ringer's solutions containing various amounts of magnesium chloride, and magnesium was measured in the samples collected downstream from the perfusion site. Absolute magnesium concentration increased along the perfused tubule in a linear manner with net water reabsorption, as observed in free-flow micropuncture studies. Moreover, the collected : perfusate magnesium concentration ratio rose whether luminal magnesium concentrations were markedly below or even very significantly (11-fold) above the ultrafiltrable plasma magnesium level, indicating a low permeability of the superficial proximal tubule to magnesium relative to sodium and calcium.

In these *in vivo* perfusion studies, it was demonstrated that magnesium reabsorption is dependent on intraluminal magnesium concentration. Perfusion of rat proximal tubules with solutions containing magnesium in excess of 5 to 7 mM failed to saturate the transport system. Further studies in dogs given magnesium chloride infusions supported these observations. Graded elevations of plasma magnesium resulted in enhanced absolute magnesium reabsorption. This latter observation is possibly the basis for the glomerulotubular balance observed for magnesium. The reabsorptive rate is dependent on the luminal magnesium concentration, which is determined by the concurrent sodium and water transport. In summary, magnesium transport by the superficial proximal tubule is mainly a unidirectional process, is dependent on luminal or filtered magnesium concentration, and is proportional to sodium and water transport but at a fractionally lower rate.

Proximal Straight Tubule and the Descending Limb of Henle's Loop

Present knowledge of magnesium transport by the proximal straight tubule has been gained indirectly by evaluating the fluid collected by micropuncture from the bend of the loop of the surgically exposed papilla of young rats or desert rodents. As such, these data describe the function of the proximal convoluted and proximal straight segments of the deep nephrons, which may function quite differently from the superficial tubules described previously. Fluid collected from the late superficial proximal tubule and the tip of the long loops of the desert rat demonstrated that magnesium concentration rose as water was abstracted and (perhaps) solute was added. This is not unlike the findings for sodium, potassium, chloride, and calcium. Further information has been obtained from *in vitro* perfusion of superficial and juxtamedullary tubule segments. Isolated straight proximal segments of the rabbit absorbed magnesium when they were perfused with artificial solutions similar to late proximal fluid, and the collected:perfusate magnesium concentration ratios rose with water abstraction, as was observed for the proximal convoluted tubule. Thus the real reabsorptive rate for magnesium absorption is fractionally lower than the transport rates for water and sodium in both the cortical and juxtamedullary straight proximal tubules of the rabbit. These observations support the notion that the straight proximal tubule has a low permeability to magnesium and a low reabsorptive rate, which depends on the luminal magnesium concentration, which is influenced by magnesium delivery rate and concurrent sodium transport rate.

Considerable magnesium is reabsorbed within the thin descending limb associated with water absorption. Accordingly, with dehydration magnesium is quantitatively absorbed with water whereas with hydration little water or magnesium is absorbed into the medullary interstitium. It is not known what role magnesium reabsorption in the thin descending limb plays in overall renal magnesium balance.

Thick Ascending Limb of Henle's Loop

Early micropuncture studies indicated that Henle's loop is the major site of magnesium reabsorption. Magnesium concentration in the early distal tubule fluid was found to be distinctly lower than the ultrafiltrable magnesium concentration, with a TF/UF of 0.5 to 0.6. Hence some 50% to 60% of the filtered magnesium was reabsorbed between the last accessible proximal tubule on the surface of the kidney and the early distal tubule (Fig. 18.5). This represents a fractional reabsorption rate greater than that of sodium and calcium, based on the amount filtered at the glomerulus. Other micropuncture studies showed an increase in the mean TF/UF for magnesium at the bend of the descending limb of the loop, indicating that the major site of the marked magnesium reabsorption must be located in the ascending limb of Henle's loop, most likely the thick segment of the ascending limb. Magnesium transport in the thin ascending limb has not been investigated, but a number of studies have been directed at the TAL.

Magnesium is principally reabsorbed within the TAL of Henle's loop. Using microperfusion techniques of isolated mouse TAL segments, researchers have shown that only the cortical thick ascending limb (CTAL) is involved with magnesium reclamation because no transport was observed in the medullary segment (MTAL). They have further demonstrated that magnesium transport is mainly passive in nature, supporting the earlier studies. Net magnesium absorption was entirely dependent on the transepithelial voltage (Fig. 18.5). With luminal positive voltage, magnesium moved from lumen into the bath whereas luminal negative voltage resulted in magnesium secretion into the lumen. No transport was observed at zero voltage consistent with passive transport. It is envisioned that magnesium normally moves across the CTAL epithelium

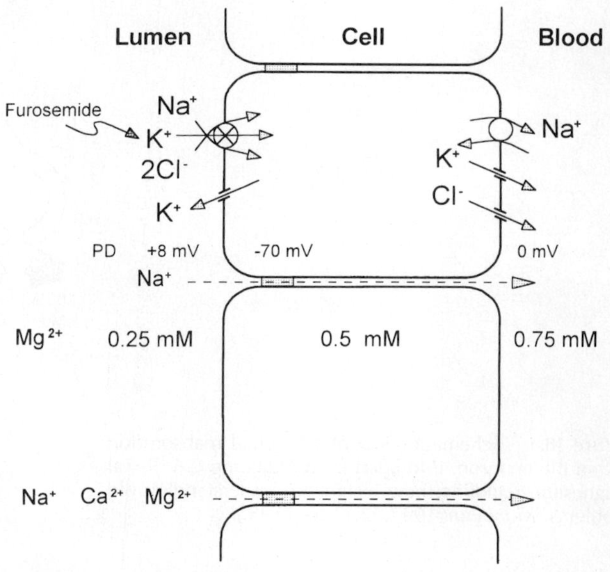

Figure 18.5. Schematic model of magnesium absorption in the thick ascending limb of Henle's loop. (Modified from Quamme GA. Renal magnesium handling: new insights in understanding old problems. *Kidney Int* 1997;52:1180–1195.)

through the paracellular pathway driven by the positive luminal transepithelial voltage. Factors controlling magnesium absorption in this segment act through changes on the voltage and/or the permeability of the paracellular pathway.

Two influences that affect magnesium absorption in the loop have been explained with the use of *in vitro* perfusion experiments. First the loop diuretic furosemide inhibits calcium, magnesium, and sodium chloride absorption in the loop. This would suggest some dependence of calcium and magnesium transport on sodium chloride absorption. Furthermore, the reabsorption of these cations, particularly magnesium, is inhibited to a greater degree than that of sodium chloride. This may indicate that the permeability coefficient for magnesium is lower than that for sodium and that magnesium transport is less for any given sodium chloride absorption. Second, increased flow rates into the thick ascending segment, such as with extracellular volume expansion, may alter the sodium diffusional gradient and the concurrent transmembrane voltage. Extracellular volume expansion leads to a greater fractional excretion of magnesium than sodium; for example, an increase in fractional sodium excretion of 1% to 2% is usually accompanied by a 10% to 15% increment in magnesium excretion. These observations are readily explained if magnesium transport is entirely passive in nature but an active mechanism may also exist within the cells.

Distal Tubule

Most of our early knowledge concerning magnesium transport in the distal tubule has come from micropuncture and microperfusion studies of the superficial nephron. Micropuncture studies showed that significant amounts of magnesium are reabsorbed in the distal tubule. Microperfusion studies indicated that magnesium absorption depended on the luminal magnesium concentration and the flow rate into the distal tubule. More recently, microfluorescence experiments with isolated distal tubule cells have extensively added to our knowledge of how magnesium is absorbed within this segment. Unlike the TAL, magnesium transport in the distal tubule is active and transcellular (Fig. 18.6).

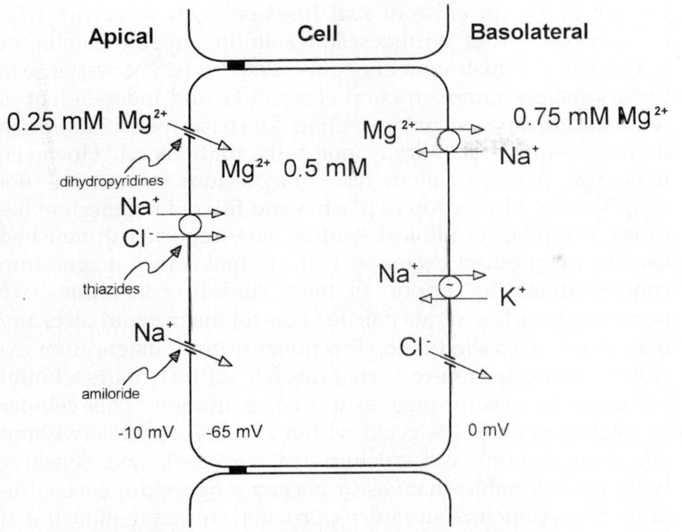

Figure 18.6. Schematic model of magnesium absorption in the distal convoluted tubule. (Modified from Quamme GA. Renal magnesium handling: new insights in understanding old problems. *Kidney Int* 1997;52: 1180–1195.)

FACTORS THAT AFFECT RENAL MAGNESIUM HANDLING (TABLE 18.2)

Renal Plasma Flow and Glomerular Filtration

Like sodium and calcium, magnesium appears to be in glomerulotubular balance. Acute and marked increases in glomerular filtration rate (GFR) and filtered magnesium lead to relatively little change in fractional magnesium excretion. Similar studies evaluating the effects of renal vasodilation with acetylcholine, bradykinin, and other agents have demonstrated only small increases in magnesium excretion, which were proportional to the increase in sodium excretion. The acute administration of atrial natriuretic peptide results in marked increases in urinary magnesium excretion in association with the natriuresis. The tubular sites of these changes have not been systematically studied but are likely related to the marked changes in hemodynamic forces acting within the proximal tubule and the TAL.

Chronic renal failure with its attendant reduction in GFR results in a rise in fractional magnesium excretion proportional to that observed for urinary calcium and sodium excretion. Studies were performed in experimentally induced uremia in dogs, which, like patients with chronic renal failure, have a reduced nephron population and demonstrate marked hyperfiltration per nephron. Micropuncture data demonstrated that the fractional magnesium reabsorption was reduced proportionally with sodium and calcium transport within Henle's loop. Thus an increase in the single-nephron GFR and the filtration fraction increases the peritubular capillary hydrostatic pressure and decreases colloid osmotic pressure, which diminishes proximal sodium and water reabsorption and enhances delivery into Henle's loop. Enhanced distal sodium delivery and putative natriuretic hormones may affect magnesium transport as it affects sodium reabsorption in chronic renal failure. Accordingly, as the nephron population is diminished, each individual nephron adapts by excreting more of the filtered loads, including magnesium, to maintain the fine balance between intake and excretion. These adaptive mechanisms fail only in severe end-stage renal failure, when there are not sufficient numbers of nephrons to excrete the dietary magnesium, resulting in magnesium retention. Additional information on renal handling of magnesium in patients with chronic renal failure is found in Chapter 77.

TABLE 18.2. Factors Affecting Urinary Excretion of Magnesium

Factors that Decrease Urinary Magnesium Excretion
Extracellular volume depletion
Hypomagnesemia and magnesium depletion
Hypocalcemia
Hormones
Parathyroid hormone
Antidiuretic hormone (vasopressin)
Glucagon
Calcitonin
Insulin
Renal innervation
Isoproterenol
Distal diuretics
Amiloride
Triamterene
Factors that Increase Urinary Magnesium Excretion
Extracellular volume expansion
Hemodynamics (renal vasodilation, atrial peptides)
Hypermagnesemia
Hypercalcemia
Loop diuretics
Furosemide
Osmotic diuretics—urea, mannitol, glucose
Chronic thiazide diuretics
Phosphate depletion
Metabolic acidosis—diabetic ketoacidosis
Carbohydrate, protein, alcohol ingestion
Chronic hypermineralocorticoidism

Sodium Balance and Extracellular Fluid Volume

Extracellular volume expansion with saline or Ringer's solution produces an immediate increase in magnesium excretion. The response in magnesium excretion parallels that of sodium and calcium but the fractional excretion rate is approximately twice that of the latter two ions. The high fractional magnesium excretion rate secondary to volume expansion persists despite reduction in renal artery perfusion pressure. The reduction in sodium and water reabsorption occurs principally in the proximal tubule so that fractional reabsorption falls from 30% to 15% when the extracellular volume is expanded to 5% of body weight. The increased amount of magnesium delivered to the loop is largely excreted unchanged in the urine because of the concomitant increase in distal sodium delivery from the proximal tubule.

Hormonal Control of Renal Magnesium Reabsorption

A large number of hormones have been implicated in the control of renal magnesium conservation. PTH, calcitonin, glucagon, vasopressin (AVP), and insulin stimulate magnesium absorption in both the TAL and distal tubule. Renal innervation may also take part in renal conservation because isoproterenol enhances magnesium absorption in both the loop and distal tubule. Finally, steroid hormones influence NaCl and magnesium absorption within the TAL and distal tubule. All of these hormones stimulate magnesium in the TAL and distal tubule cells by very different cellular mechanisms. Using mouse CTAL segments, de Rouffignac and colleagues showed that all of the above hormones enhanced transepithelial voltage and increased magnesium permeability of the paracellular pathway. The cellular mechanisms underlying hormone-induced increase in transepithelial voltage have been clarified. Receptor-mediated activation of basolateral membrane Cl conductance and apical Na-2Cl-K cotransport/K conductance increases the luminal positive voltage (Fig. 18.5). These hormones also increase the paracellular permeability but the mechanisms are not clear. De Rouffignac postulates that hormonal control of paracellular pathway proteins, possibly through phosphorylation, may change the permeability and allow for a greater movement of magnesium across the epithelium from the luminal to the interstitium.

The early micropuncture studies clearly showed that PTH, calcitonin, and glucagon increase magnesium absorption in the distal tubule. More recently, we have shown with microfluorescence studies that these hormones as well as isoproterenol and PGE_2 stimulate Mg^{2+} uptake into isolated distal cells, in part, by the cyclic adenosine monophosphate (cAMP)–dependent mechanisms (Fig. 18.6). The cellular mechanisms whereby hormone-mediated cAMP formation enhances Mg^{2+} entry is unclear, but we speculate that signalling pathways lead to activation of apical membrane channels.

The evidence suggests that steroid hormones augment NaCl absorption and transepithelial voltage in isolated thick descending limb segments. Although there have been no direct studies of the effects of mineralocorticoids on loop magnesium transport, the increment in voltage would be expected to lead to an increase in magnesium absorption. We have studied the effects of aldosterone on Mg^{2+} entry into mouse distal convoluted tubule cells. Incubation of aldosterone, for 16 hours before the determination of magnesium uptake failed to have any effect on basal magnesium transport but potentiated hormone-stimulated magnesium take. Evidence has been given to show that aldosterone may induce protein(s) that control G_s-proteins so that hormonal-mediated cAMP formation is potentiated resulting in an increase in hormone-stimulated magnesium transport. However, chronic hyperaldosteronism leads to extracellular volume expansion and diminished salt absorption in the TAL. This is associated with elevated urinary magnesium excretion. Salt restriction and normalization of the extracellular volume mitigates aldosterone-induced hypermagnesuria. In summary, the effects of steroid hormones within the loop are complex; aldosterone enhances salt retention that leads to volume expansion and in turn leads to increased salt and magnesium excretion.

The aforementioned list of hormones is far from exhaustive and further research will in all likelihood identify others that affect renal magnesium handling. There appears to be no single hormone that alters renal magnesium balance, rather many hormones act in concert to regulate magnesium. Moreover, many of the hormones interact to control magnesium transport in both the TAL and the distal tubule. We postulate that multi-hormonal control of renal magnesium absorption is a more efficient way of maintaining magnesium balance than what would be expected with a dedicated hormone.

Hypomagnesemia and Magnesium Deficiency

Primary magnesium depletion by dietary means is extremely uncommon because the kidney has the remarkable ability to conserve magnesium. When depletion does occur, it is usually caused by gross absorptive abnormalities such as bowel resection or by compromise of real function such as occurs with overzealous use of diuretics, longstanding hypercalcemia, or long-term administration of nephrotoxic drugs. The response to dietary magnesium restriction is sensitive and independent of renal sodium and calcium excretion. The basis for this alteration in magnesium transport is not fully understood. However, it is clear that the fall in renal magnesium excretion is not simply caused by a drop in plasma and filtered magnesium because a number of clinical studies have reported diminished urinary magnesium excretion with normal serum magnesium concentrations. In support of these clinical observations, we performed studies in rats pair-fed control magnesium diets and magnesium-restricted diets. Fractional urinary magnesium excretion of magnesium-restricted rats fell within 8 hours without a change in plasma magnesium concentration. This cellular adaptation is rapid (detected within 2 hours), specific (without effect on sodium and calcium reabsorption), and sensitive (without detectable changes in plasma magnesium concentration). Micropuncture and microperfusion studies demonstrated that the cellular adaptation occurred within the TAL and the distal tubule. This ability to adjust transport appears to be intrinsic to renal cells because we can see an increase in Mg^{2+} uptake in isolated tubule cells growing in hormone-free media deficient in magnesium.

Plasma Magnesium and Calcium Concentration

Elevation of plasma magnesium or calcium concentration inhibits magnesium and calcium reabsorption, leading to hypermagnesuria and hypercalciuria. Inhibition of magnesium transport by elevated extracellular divalent cations occurs in both Henle's loop and the distal tubule but again by different mechanisms. In the TAL, elevation of magnesium or calcium increases the resistance of the paracellular pathway thereby limiting passive absorption of magnesium and calcium. More recently, an extracellular Ca^{2+}-Mg^{2+}–sensing receptor has been cloned and localized to all segments of the nephron, including the TAL, distal tubule, and cortical and medullary collecting ducts. It has been reported that activation of the Ca^{2+}-Mg^{2+}–sensing receptor in the TAL inhibits apical K^+ channels and possibly Na-2Cl-K cotransport in the TAL. This would diminish transepithelial voltage and in turn passive sodium, magnesium, and calcium transport within the TAL leading to increased distal delivery of these electrolytes. We have shown that elevation of extracellular magnesium or calcium activates a Ca^{2+}-Mg^{2+}–sensing receptor in the distal tubule that inhibits hormonal-mediated cAMP formation and active Mg^{2+} transport. Accordingly, hypermagnesemia or hypercalcemia inhibits passive absorption in the loop and active magnesium transport in the distal tubule resulting in elevated urinary magnesium excretion. It has also been shown that elevation of luminal divalent cations in the medullary collecting duct activates the luminal Ca^{2+}-Mg^{2+}–sensing receptor that diminishes water permeability and inhibits volume reabsorption. The net effect is to increase volume flow along with an increase in calcium and magnesium excretion. The notion advanced by these observations is that a concomitant increase in volume flow with inhibition of calcium and magnesium reabsorption would minimize the incidence of stone formation.

Clearance studies have suggested that renal magnesium reabsorption is a T_m-limited process; that is, the kidney possesses a tubular maximum for transport that can be saturated with elevations of plasma magnesium. Determination of the T_m value has been useful in assessment of renal magnesium conservation. Micropuncture studies have shown that this phenomena is due to segmental differences in magnesium absorption. The cellular basis for the T_m is inhibition of magnesium transport within Henle's loop. It is likely that activation of the Ca^{2+}-Mg^{2+}–sensing receptor within the ascending limb plays a role in this T_m phenomenon and as such it is necessary to reassess what a T_m value means in the assessment of renal magnesium balance. These recent observations have given us an additional regulation process of renal magnesium handling. In support of this notion, it has been shown that both inactivating and activating mutations of the Ca^{2+}-Mg^{2+}–sensing receptor are found in clinical medicine. Two rare hypercalcemic disorders, familial hypocalciuric hypercalcemia (FHH) and neonatal severe hyperparathyroidism (NSHPT), result from inactivating mutations when present in the heterozygous or homozygous states, respectively. Renal excretion of both calcium and magnesium is reduced in these patients, leading to hypercalcemia and in some instances to hypermagnesemia. A defective extracellular Ca^{2+}-Mg^{2+} sensing likely results in inappropriate absorption of calcium and magnesium in the loop and distal tubule, leading to diminished excretion and elevated plasma levels of these ions. Supporting this idea, a knockout mouse model has been developed with all of the characteristics of FHH and NSHPT. On the other side, an autosomal-dominant inherited activating mutation has been reported that was associated with hypercalcemia and hypermagnesemia, presumably due to inappropriate renal magnesium wasting, in about half the patients.

Diuretics

Diuretics, acting within the loop, diminish salt absorption by virtue of their ability to inhibit Na-2Cl-K cotransport, leading to a decrease in the luminal positive voltage. These diuretics, such as furosemide, increase urinary magnesium excretion fractionally more than sodium, so they are potent hypermagnesuric agents. Accordingly, inappropriate renal magnesium wasting may occur with chronic use of these diuretics.

Diuretics, acting within the distal convoluted tubule, stimulate magnesium reabsorption. Amiloride, a blocker of Na^+ channels, and chlorothiazide, an inhibitor of NaCl cotransport, hyperpolarize the luminal membrane increasing the driving force for Mg^{2+} entry. It is clear from a large number of clinical studies that amiloride has magnesium-conserving properties in addition to its natriuretic and potassium-sparing effects. On the other hand, the long-term effects of chlorothiazide are equivocal. Some studies have reported that hypermagnesemia may be associated with chronic chlorothiazide use, likely due to renal magnesium wasting. The cellular basis for magnesium wasting is not known but it may be due to hypokalemia, which is often observed with chronic use of chlorothiazide. Hypokalemia and cellular potassium depletion is associated with diminished magnesium absorption within the loop and distal tubule that may lead to increased magnesium excretion. However, there are many instances of hypokalemia without renal magnesium wasting; therefore the relationship between potassium and magnesium balance is unclear at present.

Metabolic Acidosis and Alkalosis

It has long been known that metabolic acidosis is associated with renal magnesium wasting. Some clinicians have reported that 25% of patients with diabetes mellitus have hypomagnesemia. Metabolic alkalosis, on the other hand, consistently leads to a fall in urinary magnesium excretion. Studies with isolated distal tubule cells showed that Mg^{2+} entry may be directly affected by protons so that distal magnesium reabsorption is impaired with acidosis.

Phosphate Depletion

One of the hallmarks of hypophosphatemia and cellular phosphate depletion is the striking increase in urinary excretion of calcium and magnesium. Magnesium excretion may be sufficiently large to lead to overt hypomagnesemia. The increase in divalent ion excretion in both humans and experimental animals occurs within hours after initiation of dietary phosphate restriction. We have shown with isolated distal cells that phosphate depletion decreases magnesium entry, which in turn leads to diminished epithelial magnesium transport. The cellular mechanisms are different to those observed with potassium depletion or acidosis.

Renal Magnesium-Wasting States

Defective magnesium transport or abnormal control of magnesium absorption leads to renal magnesium wasting and hypomagnesemia. Although these diseases are well described, little is known about the cellular mechanisms involved. Familial hypomagnesemia from renal magnesium wasting is an uncommon disease. It is by all accounts an autosomal-recessive disease, but one report provided evidence for dominant penetrance that there may be a spectrum of genetic diseases. Renal magnesium wasting may be caused by defective transport in the TAL or distal tubule, resulting in complex presentation. The intestinal form, which results in diminished dietary absorption, is distinct to the disease in the kidney. Linkage studies have shown that intestinal magnesium malabsorption is on chromosome 9q. Mutation of gene-coding transport proteins are likely to be the basis for these familial diseases. As mentioned previously, mutations of the extracellular Ca^{2+}-Mg^{2+}–sensing receptor have been reported. Inactivating mutations lead to excessive magnesium conservation, whereas activating mutations result in hypomagnesemia due to inappropriate renal magnesium wasting.

Hypomagnesemia is consistently observed in patients with Gitelman's syndrome. This disease is caused by a mutation in the gene coding for the NaCl cotransporter in the distal convoluted tubule. It is not known how this single gene defect results in diminished distal magnesium absorption and renal magnesium wasting. Interestingly, Bartter's syndrome, caused by mutational changes in salt transport in the loop, is associated with renal magnesium wasting in only about 30% of patients.

Other states of magnesium wasting can result from marked volume expansion, systematic hypercalcemia, or prolonged administration of loop diuretics. Smaller degrees of volume expansion, for instance, those associated with primary hyperaldosteronism and inappropriate hypersecretion of antidiuretic hormone, can similarly lead to mild magnesium wasting, but these are not usually of clinical significance. Osmotic diuresis, such as occurs in diabetic ketoacidosis with hyperglycemia and glycosuria or during the rapid infusion of mannitol, can bring about renal magnesium wasting. Finally, hypophosphatemia, hypokalemia, and metabolic acidosis may cause renal magnesium wasting that may be severe enough to lead to hypomagnesemia.

Renal magnesium wasting has been associated with several chemotherapeutic agents, most prominently with *cis*-platin treatment. Patients that become magnesium depleted after *cis*-platin therapy will remain hypomagnesemic, particularly in the presence of a limited dietary magnesium intake. Renal magnesium wasting can be demonstrated in these patients at any level of dietary magnesium intake for a long time after cessation of the *cis*-platin therapy. In most of these patients, the hypomagnesemia is mild and the individuals are asymptomatic, but in some cases, neuromuscular, central nervous system, and cardiovascular symptoms can arise. A detailed investigation of the cause of *cis*-platin toxicity has demonstrated morphologic changes in the straight portion of the proximal tubule but the functional changes are due to diminished magnesium transport in the loop and distal tubule. Aminoglycoside toxicity, especially that caused by gentamicin, may sporadically result in magnesium wasting. Finally, the common immunosuppressive agent cyclosporine has been demonstrated to cause renal magnesium wasting in some patients. Again, the morphologic damage appears to occur within the straight portion of the proximal tubule, but the functional defects are likely to occur more distally in the loop and distal tubule. It is interesting that magnesium wasting induced by cyclosporine, unlike that induced by *cis*-platin, is normally corrected when treatment is terminated. The cellular mechanisms for the cytotoxic effects of these drugs remain to be defined.

Selected Readings

Dail J, Friedman PA, Quamme GA. Mechanisms of amiloride stimulation of Mg^{2+} uptake in immortalized mouse distal convoluted tubule cells. *Am J Physiol* 1997;272:F249–F256.

This study describes the cellular mechanisms of magnesium transport in the distal convoluted tubule and the magnesium conserving properties of amiloride.

Hebert SC. Extracellular calcium-sensing receptor: implications for calcium and magnesium handling in the kidney. *Kidney Int* 1996;50:2129–2139.

This report describes the role of extracellular cation-sensing receptors on magnesium handling within the kidney, which forms the basis for the described T_m for renal magnesium handling.

Massry SG, Coburn JW. The hormonal and nonhormonal control of renal excretion of calcium and magnesium. *Nephron* 1973;10:66–112.

A comprehensive review of the renal handling of calcium and magnesium, with emphasis on the various factors that affect their urinary excretions.

Massry SG, Coburn JW, Kleeman CR. Renal handling of magnesium in the dog. *Am J Physiol* 1969;216:1460–1467.

The first detailed description of the renal handling of magnesium in the mammalian kidney. The studies used clearance techniques and demonstrated the presence of T_m for magnesium in the whole kidney.

Quamme GA. Renal magnesium handling: new insights in understanding old problems. *Kidney Int* 1997;52:1180–1195.

This review highlights some of the new research observations in the field of renal magnesium handling and their significance in understanding disorders of renal magnesium handling.

Rouffignac DE. Multihormonal regulation of nephron epithelia: achieved though combinational mode? *Am J Physiol* 1995;269: R739–R748.

Hormones play an important role in control of renal magnesium conservation; this review details some hormonal actions on magnesium transport.

Rouffignac DE, Quamme GA. Renal magnesium handling and its hormonal control. *Physiol Rev* 1994;74:305–322.

Renal magnesium handling is affected by both hormonal and nonhormonal controls; this report summarizes some of these controls.

PART 3
Dysmagnesemias

Shaul G. Massry and Robert K. Rude

Magnesium is predominantly an intracellular cation, participating in many membrane and enzymatic functions. The adult human body contains about 2,000 mEq of magnesium, with approximately half this amount in the skeleton and the other half in soft tissues. The concentration of magnesium is highest (15 to 20 mEq/kg wet weight) in cells with the highest metabolic activity (i.e., liver, kidney, striated muscle). The extracellular fluid contains only about 1% of the body's magnesium. The normal concentration of magnesium in plasma is maintained within a narrow range of 1.5 to 2.0 mEq/L. Approximately 25% to 35% of magnesium in plasma is bound to proteins (chiefly albumin) and the rest [75% ± 9% (SD)] is present in a diffusible form. The major part of the diffusible fraction is made of free ionized magnesium. The kidneys play an important role in maintaining plasma magnesium within the normal range. Oral or intravenous loads of magnesium are rapidly excreted, and in the magnesium-deficient state or in dietary magnesium restriction, magnesium almost disappears from the urine.

Methods for the determination of total and ionized intracellular magnesium have been developed; however, they are labor intensive and have been applied chiefly as a research tool. Magnesium content or concentration has been determined in a number of tissues, including erythrocytes, lymphocytes, skeletal muscle, and bone. Tissue magnesium does not always correlate well with the plasma magnesium concentration, and an intracellular assessment of magnesium appears to reflect more accurately magnesium status. However, because determination of intracellular magnesium is not available in clinical laboratories, the assessment of magnesium status relies on the plasma magnesium concentration as the index of deficiency. As stated previously, changes in the concentration of magnesium in plasma does not always reflect alteration in total body magnesium. Hypomagnesemia usually indicates some degree of magnesium depletion; however, a normal serum magnesium concentration does not exclude the presence of magnesium deficiency. Intracellular magnesium depletion, along with clinical complications of magnesium deficiency, may exist despite a normal plasma serum magnesium concentration. Diminished magnesium content of muscle has been noted in patients with advanced uremia, despite normal or elevated levels of magnesium in plasma. Alternatively, hypomagnesemia may infrequently develop with normal intracellular magnesium levels such as in extreme hypoalbuminemia or during stress; lipolysis during stress is thought to result in magnesium binding of lipids. Ion-selective electrodes are now available for the determination of serum ionized magnesium concentration that may prove to assess more accurately magnesium status.

HYPOMAGNESEMIA AND MAGNESIUM DEFICIENCY

Definition

Magnesium deficiency is defined as a decrease in total body content of magnesium. Poor dietary intake of this ion is usually not associated with a marked magnesium deficiency. This phenomenon results from the remarkable ability of the normal kidneys to conserve magnesium. It should be emphasized, however, that prolonged and severe dietary restriction of magnesium (less than 1 mEq/day) can produce symptomatic magnesium deficiency in humans. This is caused by the renal and fecal obligatory losses, which may slightly exceed the low intake. Severe hypomagnesemia is usually associated with magnesium deficiency, and a deficiency of 1 to 2 mEq/kg of body weight may exist in patients with significant hypomagnesemia (less than 1 mEq/L).

The prevalence of magnesium depletion may be more common than previously thought. Approximately 10% of patients admitted to a large city hospital are hypomagnesemic. The incidence of hypomagnesemia may be as high as 65% in a medical intensive care unit. These observations do not necessarily mean that all these patients have magnesium depletion, but they certainly indicate that hypomagnesemia is not infrequent.

Etiology

The main factors responsible for the development of hypomagnesemia and magnesium deficiency in disease states are excessive losses of magnesium in urine, feces, or other body fluids, and lack of intestinal absorption. The clinical conditions that could be associated with hypomagnesemia are listed in Table 18.3.

Gastrointestinal Diseases

The decreased intestinal absorption and increased fecal losses of magnesium in patients with disease of the gastrointestinal tract are usually associated with hypomagnesemia and magnesium deficiency. The incidence of hypomagnesemia in patients with malabsorption syndromes, including nontropical sprue, massive resection of the small intestine, and other small bowel disturbances with steatorrhea, is high and in some series approaches 30% to 40%. In the steatorrheic states, fecal excretion of magnesium exceeds magnesium intake because of the formation of magnesium soaps in the stool. Indeed the restriction of dietary intake in fats in patients with massive intestinal resection has caused a decrease in fecal magnesium and the correction of hypomagnesemia. Marked losses of magnesium from the gastrointestinal tract may occur with excessive use of purgatives, in patients with severe diarrhea as in infantile gastroenteritis and ulcerative colitis, and in patients with biliary or intestinal fistulas. The loss of magnesium during nasogastric suction (1 mEq/L) combined with parenteral administration of magnesium-free fluids may cause hypomagnesemia.

TABLE 18.3. Causes of Hypomagnesemia

Decreased intake
Protein-calorie malnutrition
Starvation
Prolonged intravenous therapy without food intake
Decreased intestinal absorption
Malabsorption syndromes including nontropical sprue
Massive surgical resection of small intestine
Neonatal hypomagnesemia with selective malabsorption of magnesium
Excessive losses of body fluids
Prolonged nasogastric suction
Excessive use of purgatives
Intestinal and biliary fistulas
Severe diarrhea as in ulcerative colitis and infantile gastroenteritis
Rarely, prolonged lactation
Excessive urinary losses
Diuretic therapy
Diuretic phase of acute renal failure
Postobstructive diuresis
Posttransplant diuresis
Chronic alcoholism
Prolonged intravenous therapy with excessive sodium administration
Primary aldosteronism
Hypercalcemic states: malignancy, hyperparathyroidism, and vitamin D excess
Metabolic acidosis (starvation, ketoacidosis, renal tubular acidosis)
Diabetes (glucose-induced osmotic diuresis, and during and following treatment of ketoacidosis)
Phosphate depletion (occasionally)
Hyperthyroidism
Idiopathic renal magnesium wasting
Chronic renal failure with renal magnesium wasting
Phosphate depletion
Aminoglycoside toxicity
Amphotericin toxicity
Therapy with *cis*-platinum
Therapy with cyclosporine
Therapy with pentamidine
Miscellaneous
Idiopathic hypomagnesemia
Acute pancreatitis
Bartter's syndrome
Porphyria with inappropriate secretion of antidiuretic hormone
Multiple transfusions or exchange transfusions with citrated blood

Acute Pancreatitis

Moderate hypomagnesemia is encountered in approximately 25% to 35% of patients with acute pancreatitis, and occasionally, the hypomagnesemia in these patients is marked (less than 1 mEq/L). Many patients with acute pancreatitis may have normal levels of serum magnesium at the time of their admission to the hospital but develop a significant hypomagnesemia during the first week of their illness. The hypomagnesemia of acute pancreatitis has been attributed to the formation of magnesium soaps in areas of fat necrosis around the inflamed pancreas. Also, a large number of patients with acute pancreatitis are alcoholics, and chronic alcoholism is associated with hypomagnesemia.

Disorders Associated with Urinary Losses of Magnesium

Excessive urinary losses of magnesium occur in a variety of clinical conditions, and such losses can cause hypomagnesemia and magnesium deficiency even in the face of normal dietary intake.

Diuretics, except acetazolamide and especially those acting at Henle's loop such as furosemide, increase urinary excretion of magnesium. The use of these agents in patients with edematous states can lead to hypomagnesemia and magnesium deficiency. Indeed, low plasma levels of magnesium have been noted in patients with congestive heart failure receiving diuretic therapy. Hypomagnesemia, like hypokalemia, may precipitate digitalis intoxication. Therefore it is important to monitor plasma levels of magnesium in patients with congestive heart failure treated with digitalis and diuretic agents.

Hypercalcemia inhibits the renal tubular reabsorption of magnesium, and patients with hypercalcemic disorders may have hypermagnesuria and hypomagnesemia. Patients with primary hyperparathyroidism may have a negative magnesium balance with normal or low levels of magnesium in plasma. After the surgical removal of the parathyroid adenoma, urinary magnesium falls and magnesium balance becomes positive; in some of these patients who have severe and generalized bone disease, marked hypomagnesemia may develop after surgery, probably due to a rapid deposition of magnesium in bone. Hypomagnesemia is often encountered in patients with hypercalcemia associated with malignancy, especially during the therapy of the hypercalcemia with saline diuresis and loop diuretics.

Patients with hyperthyroidism may have a negative magnesium balance, and their plasma magnesium levels may be low, most probably because of augmented urinary losses of this ion. In myxedema, the blood levels of magnesium tend to be elevated, and magnesium balance is positive. Treatment of thyrotoxicosis or the hypothyroid state restores magnesium homeostasis to normal.

Primary aldosteronism is associated with magnesiuria and hypomagnesemia. Removal of the aldosterone-secreting tumor corrects the abnormality in magnesium metabolism. The magnesiuria in this disease is not due to direct effect of aldosterone on renal magnesium handling but is rather secondary to the action of the hormone on distal tubular reabsorption of sodium. The sodium retention induced by aldosterone produces a modest degree of extracellular fluid volume expansion. This latter effect induces a decrease in the proximal reabsorption of magnesium and sodium and increases delivery of both ions to the distal nephron. In this latter site, aldosterone enhances sodium reabsorption but has no effect on magnesium reabsorption. The net effect would be an increase in urinary magnesium alone.

Both glycosuria and acidosis increase urinary magnesium. It is not surprising therefore that hypomagnesemia and magnesium deficiency develop in patients with poorly controlled diabetes mellitus. During the treatment of severe diabetic ketoacidosis with insulin and fluid therapy, hypomagnesemia may worsen as a result of continued urinary losses and/or insulin-induced secondary shift of magnesium into cells. Approximately 85% of the magnesium administered intravenously to a diabetic patient during the treatment of ketoacidosis is retained, suggesting the presence of magnesium depletion. Although the hypomagnesemia of diabetes mellitus is not symptomatic, tetany may occur during the correction of diabetic ketoacidosis without the supplementation of magnesium.

Hypomagnesemia is often observed in patients with chronic alcoholism, during alcohol withdrawal, and in patients with delirium tremens. The hypomagnesemia of chronic alcoholism is associated with magnesium deficiency. Poor dietary intake and enhanced urinary losses are the main factors responsible for the magnesium-deficient state in these patients. The hypomagnesemia that is seen in some patients with alcoholic cirrhosis is probably related to alcohol ingestion rather than to impaired liver function.

Urinary magnesium losses with subsequent hypomagnesemia is commonly encountered during the administration of a number of drugs such as aminoglycosides, amphotericin B, *cis*-platinum, cyclosporine, and pentamidine. Renal magnesium wasting may also occur during the diuretic phase of acute renal failure, the diuresis following the relief of obstructive uropathy, posttransplant diuresis, and the first two days after various surgical procedures. Phosphate depletion is occasionally associated with hypomagnesemia as a result of increased urinary losses of magnesium. Hypomagnesemia resulting from renal magnesium wasting of unknown cause has been described. A familial disorder characterized by hypokalemia and hypomagnesemia produced by impaired renal conservation of these two ions has also been reported. Hypomagnesemia has been reported in patients with acute intermittent porphyria, most likely because of hemodilution secondary to water retention induced by inappropriate secretion of antidiuretic hormone.

TABLE 18.4. Clinical Manifestations and Laboratory Findings of Magnesium Depletion

Central nervous system
Anorexia, nausea, weakness, and apathy
Muscular fibrillation
Tremors
Ataxia
Vertigo
Carpopedal spasms
Frank tetany
Hyperreflexia, occasionally hyporeflexia
Depression
Irritability
Psychotic behavior
Cardiovascular
Electrocardiographic changes: QT prolongation, shortening of ST segment, broadening of T waves
Increased myocardial irritability; atrial and ventricular arrhythmias
Increased incidence of digitalis intoxication
Reduced myocardial contractility[a]
Hypertension[a]
Musculoskeletal
Abnormal skeletal muscle function
Myopathiclike potentials on electromyogram
Muscle fibrillation
Bone
Resistance to the calcemic action of parathyroid hormone
Increased incidence of osteoporosis
Endocrine
Reduced parathyroid hormone secretion
Resistance to the calcemic action of parathyroid hormone
Increased renin and aldosterone secretion
Reduced lipolytic activity
Cellular[a]
Reduced mitochondrial respiration
Impaired oxidative phosphorylation
Altered cell membrane integrity
Defective Na^+-K^+-ATPase activity
Impaired DNA synthesis
Reduced Krebs cycle activity
Laboratory findings
Hypomagnesemia, hypocalcemia, hypokalemia
Hypophosphatemia, occasionally hyperphosphatemia
Low urinary magnesium and calcium
Low magnesium in cerebrospinal fluid

[a] Experimental observations.

Clinical and Laboratory Manifestations

The signs and symptoms of magnesium depletion are usually mixed with, and sometimes masked by, the clinical manifestations of the basic disorders that caused the magnesium-deficient state. Studies in which experimental magnesium depletion was produced in humans have helped delineate the clinical and laboratory findings of pure magnesium deficiency. The main clinical manifestations of moderate to severe magnesium depletion include neuromuscular hyperexcitability and cardiac arrhythmias. The common biochemical feature of hypokalemia may contribute to the increased myocardial irritability. During magnesium depletion, intracellular potassium falls, and the ability of the kidney to conserve potassium is impaired with the subsequent development of hypokalemia and a total body potassium deficit. Hypocalcemia is also frequently encountered and may contribute to the neuromuscular findings. The mechanism of the hypocalcemia in patients with hypomagnesemia and magnesium deficiency are discussed later in this chapter. The clinical and laboratory findings of magnesium depletion are listed in Table 18.4.

Diagnosis of Magnesium Deficiency

The diagnosis of magnesium deficiency is not easy because blood level of magnesium does not always reflect the state of body magnesium, and it may be a poor guide to the degree of magnesium depletion. Moreover, hypermagnesemia may occur in patients with renal failure, despite cellular magnesium depletion. The concentration of magnesium in erythrocytes or lymphocytes, magnesium content of muscle, body-exchangeable magnesium, and magnesium balance have been used to assist in the diagnosis of magnesium deficiency. These methods either are difficult to perform or do not provide a good index of the state of body magnesium. The fate of an intravenous load of magnesium may help in the diagnosis of magnesium depletion. Normal subjects excrete 85% of the parenterally administered magnesium within 24 hours, whereas subjects with magnesium deficiency may retain more than 20% of the intravenous load of magnesium. Therefore the retention of intravenously administered magnesium is consistent with magnesium deficiency, even in the presence of normal serum magnesium. This test is valid only when renal function is normal and when magnesium depletion is not due to the inability of the kidney to conserve magnesium.

Treatment

Magnesium deficiency is managed by replacement with magnesium salts. Because the magnitude of the deficit is not easy to estimate, the planning of the replacement therapy is usually empirical. A deficit of 1 to 2 mEq/kg body weight may exist in the presence of significant hypomagnesemia. The amount of magnesium required will be twice the estimated deficit because approximately 50% of the administered magnesium will be lost in the urine even when marked deficiency of this ion exists. Magnesium sulfate ($MgSO_4 7H_2O$) is usually used for the parenteral therapy. The molecular weight of this hydrated compound is 246.5, and each gram of the salt contains 8.12 mEq of magnesium. Repletion can be achieved by intramuscular or intravenous administration of magnesium. An effective treatment regimen is the administration of 16 mEq of magnesium every 8 hours intramuscularly. These injections may be painful, and a continuous intravenous infusion of 48 mEq/24 hr may therefore be preferred. The restoration of a normal plasma-magnesium concentration does not indicate repletion, and therapy should be continued for approximately 3 to 7 days. Patients with seizures and/or cardiac arrhythmias may be given 8 to 16 mEq as an intravenous injection over 5 to 10 minutes followed by 48 mEq/day. Patients who have chronic magnesium loss from the intestine or kidney may require continued magnesium supplementation. Oral magnesium may be given in dosages from 25 to 50 mEq/day in divided doses to achieve the desired effect. Oral therapy with magnesium salts may not be tolerated by many patients because of the diarrhea that may complicate such therapy. Frequent measurement of serum magnesium during the parenteral administration of this ion is advised. The dosage of magnesium should be substantially reduced in patients with renal failure, and serial monitoring of serum magnesium is mandatory in these patients.

Finally, attempts should be made to identify the underlying abnormality that has led to the deficient state, and if possible, to treat the underlying cause. In addition, efforts should be undertaken to prevent magnesium depletion in any clinical setting that may predispose to its development. For example, in patients who require gastric suction, or in those who need prolonged intravenous fluid therapy, daily supplement of 10 to 15 mEq of magnesium could prevent magnesium depletion. Magnesium supplementation should also be given to patients with postobstructive diuresis.

HYPERMAGNESEMIA

Etiology

Elevated levels of plasma magnesium are seen in patients with acute (see Chapter 48) and chronic (see Chapter 77) renal failure, during the administration of pharmacologic doses of magnesium, in some infants born to mothers who had been treated with magnesium for eclampsia, and during the use of oral purgatives or rectal enemas containing magnesium. Mild hypermagnesemia also may be present in patients with adrenal insufficiency, acromegaly, or familial hypocalciuric hypercalcemia. Because the kidney is the main organ responsible for the maintenance of plasma magnesium level within the normal range, extreme caution should be exercised with the use of magnesium-containing medications in patients with impaired renal function. Chronic renal failure affects many aspects of magnesium homeostasis, and these are discussed in detail in Chapter 77.

Signs and Symptoms

The signs and symptoms of hypermagnesemia are the result of the pharmacologic effects of this ion on the nervous and cardiovascular systems. Deep tendon reflexes are usually lost when plasma magnesium exceeds 6 mEq/L. Respiratory paralysis, narcosis, hypotension, and abnormal cardiac conduction may occur as plasma levels of magnesium approach 10 mEq/L.

Treatment

Cessation of magnesium administration and the intravenous injection of calcium salts are the initial mandatory steps in the management of symptomatic hypermagnesemia. The administration of 5 to 10 mEq (100 to 200 mg) of calcium ion may be adequate to reverse the manifestation of hypermagnesemia, although greater amounts may be needed. On occasion, peritoneal dialysis or even hemodialysis may be required to control severe hypermagnesemia. In patients who develop respiratory paralysis, artificial respiration should be used until the plasma level of magnesium is lowered.

EFFECT OF HYPERMAGNESEMIA AND MAGNESIUM DEFICIENCY ON THE KIDNEY

Hypermagnesemia

The infusion of magnesium salts with the attendant hypermagnesemia causes an increase in the urinary excretion of sodium and calcium despite significant reduction in their filtered loads, indicating that the natriuresis and calciuria are due to inhibition of the tubular reabsorption of these two ions. Micropuncture studies have shown that hypermagnesemia inhibits the reabsorption of sodium in the proximal tubules. Although the renal excretion of calcium and sodium increases during magnesium infusion, the relationship between the renal clearances of these ions differs from that found during saline infusion. First, the augmented sodium diuresis becomes evident 2 to 3 hours after initiation of magnesium infusion, whereas the increase in calcium excretion occurs almost immediately. Second, there is greater augmentation of calcium clearance, even during periods of the highest sodium excretion. One factor that could play a role in causing the disproportionate increase in calcium clearance over sodium clearance is suppression of the parathyroid glands by hypermagnesemia. Because the renal tubular reabsorption of calcium is enhanced by the parathyroid hormone (PTH), reduction in the level of the hormone would be associated with a rise in calcium clearance without an effect on sodium clearance. The administration of parathyroid extract during magnesium infusion causes a substantial decrease in the clearance of calcium in relation to sodium, but the clearance of calcium still remains significantly above that of sodium. These observations suggest that the preponderance of calcium clearance over sodium clearance is not entirely related to suppression of the parathyroid glands by hypermagnesemia, but it may be that a closer interdependence exists between the renal transport of calcium and magnesium than sodium and magnesium. The effect of hypermagnesemia on renal handling of magnesium is discussed in Chapter 18, part 2.

Acute hypermagnesemia causes a fall in the urinary excretion of phosphate, despite an increase in the concentration of serum phosphorous. The effect of acute hypermagnesemia is due to inhibition of the secretion of PTH, because phosphate excretion is not reduced following an acute elevation in the levels of serum magnesium in thyroparathyroidectomized dogs.

Magnesium Deficiency

Most of the data on the effect of magnesium deficiency on the kidney come from studies of experimental magnesium depletion in the rat. In these animals, magnesium depletion is associated with a fall in the blood level of magnesium, an elevation in the concentration of blood urea nitrogen, a rise in the blood levels of calcium, and a decrease in the potassium content of muscle. There are also abnormalities in renal function and structure. These include reduced glomerular filtration rate (GFR), proteinuria, aminoaciduria, phosphaturia, normal or reduced urinary excretion of calcium, kaliuresis, and renal calcification. Renal concentrating ability may be normal or impaired.

The renal calcification of magnesium depletion deserves a special comment. The earliest lesion is focal medullary calcification and is occasionally seen 4 days after the feeding of a magnesium-deficient diet. Within the second week of magnesium depletion in the rat, microliths containing both calcium and organic matrix may appear within the thin limb of Henle's loop. The accumulation of large numbers of microliths results in the formation of calculus within the lumen of the nephron. Distal to these calculi, cellular debris containing conglomerates of calcareous compounds is present; this material propagates through the thin ascending limb of Henle's loop to its thick part, with the distal convoluted tubule and collecting duct remaining free of such calcareous deposits. Permanent tubular obstruction will follow with consequent nephron destruction and deterioration in renal function. After 5 months of magnesium repletion, scarring of the diseased nephrons occurs, but the calcereous deposits in the inner zone are still present. Calcium deposits may be seen in the cytoplasm or within lysosomelike bodies. The cellular calcification is not seen in the absence of luminal calcification, suggesting that the latter precedes the former. Electron diffraction of these calcium deposits indicates that their structure is similar to that of apatite. Nephrocalcinosis has been observed in humans with magnesium deficiency. The exact mechanisms underlying the renal calcifications of experimental or human magnesium deficiency are not well understood.

MAGNESIUM HOMEOSTASIS, PARATHYROID GLANDS, AND PLASMA CALCIUM

Hypermagnesemia suppresses the activity of the parathyroid glands. The data on the effect of hypomagnesemia are variable. Acute reduction in the concentration of magnesium in blood perfusing the parathyroid glands causes increased release of PTH, and parathyroid gland hyperplasia has been reported in calves with magnesium deficiency. These observations in animals suggest that hypomagnesemia may stimulate the activity of the parathyroid glands. Chronic magnesium deficiency and hypomagnesemia in humans have been associated with low, normal, or elevated plasma levels of PTH. Because these patients are usually hypocalcemic, the blood levels of PTH may represent an inadequate response of the glands to the hypocalcemia, even in those with moderate elevation in their plasma levels of PTH. Convincing data have demonstrated in humans that marked magnesium deficiency and hypomagnesemia inhibit the release of PTH from the parathyroid glands. The intravenous administration of magnesium to hypomagnesemic patients was associated with a marked increase in plasma levels of PTH within 1 minute of magnesium injection. These observations are consistent with *in vitro* studies showing that low magnesium concentration in the incubation medium diminishes the secretion of PTH but not its synthesis by bovine parathyroid glands.

Hypomagnesemia and magnesium depletion is associated with hypocalcemia. The degree of hypocalcemia appears to reflect the severity of the magnesium deficiency because there is a positive correlation between the hypocalcemia and hypomagnesemia. In addition, the fall in serum PTH in experimental human magnesium depletion correlates with the fall in intracellular free magnesium in the erythrocyte. The available data indicate that factors other than inhibition of release of PTH from the parathyroid glands contribute to the genesis of hypocalcemia in patients with magnesium deficiency. These include skeletal and renal resistance to PTH and abnormalities in the equilibrium between bone and extracellular fluid; one or all of these factors may be operative.

Selected Readings

Kreusser WJ, Kurokawa K, Eznar E, et al. Effect of phosphate depletion on magnesium homeostasis. *J Clin Invest* 1978;61:573–581.

Detailed examination of the effects of phosphate depletion on body magnesium homeostasis in rats, with special emphasis on renal handling of magnesium.

Massry SG. Pharmacology of magnesium. *Annu Rev Pharmacol Toxicol* 1977;17:67–82.

A review of magnesium metabolism including renal handling of magnesium.

Massry SG, Seeling MS. Hypomagnesemia and hypermagnesemia. *Clin Nephrol* 1977;7:147–153.

A review of clinical disorders associated with hypomagnesemia and hypermagnesemia.

Mimouni FB. The ion-selective magnesium electrode: a new tool for clinicians and investigators. *J Am College Nutr* 1996;15:4–5.

A review of the use of the ion-selective electrode in the diagnosis of magnesium deficiency.

Rude RK. Magnesium disorders. In: Kokko JP, Tannen RL, eds. *Fluids and electrolytes*, 3rd ed. Philadelphia: WB Saunders, 1996:421–425.

A detailed discussion of magnesium disorders, their etiology, manifestations, and therapy.

Rude RK. Magnesium metabolism. In: Bilesikian JB, Raisz L, Rodan G, et al, eds. *Principles of bone biology*. San Diego: Academic Press, 1996:277–293.

A detailed review of the effect of magnesium deficiency on bone and mineral metabolism.

Whang R, Welt LG. Observations in experimental magnesium depletion. *J Clin Invest* 1963;42:305–313.

An excellent study evaluating the effects of experimental magnesium deficiency on the rat kidney.

CHAPTER 19

Phosphate Metabolism

PART 1
Intestinal Absorption of Phosphate

Laurie H. Kayne, Phuong-Chi T. Pham, Phuong-Thu T. Pham, and David B.N. Lee

TERMS AND NOMENCLATURE

Elemental phosphorus in various biologic samples (e.g., food, plasma, urine, tissue, and feces) is measured and expressed in units of mg/dl. Thus the normal plasma phosphorus concentration is 3.1 mg/dl. However, phosphorus participates in physiologic and biochemical events in the body as phosphate molecules. For example, it is filtered at the glomerulus or transported across the tubule and the intestine as inorganic phosphate, not phosphorus, molecules. For such purposes it is more convenient to use units such as mEq/L or mmol/L. Thus the 3.1 mg/dl phosphorus in plasma is filtered at the glomerulus as 1.0 mmol/L (molecular weight of phosphorus is 31), or 1.6 mEq/L (valence of phosphate at pH 7.4 equals 1.6) of inorganic phosphate. With this understanding in mind, we will use in this chapter the abbreviation *P* interchangeably for either phosphorus or inorganic phosphate.

Under normal conditions, the intestine is the only organ through which environmental P enters the extracellular fluid (ECF), and the kidney is the only organ through which P is excreted from the ECF back into the environment. Although intermediate mechanisms, including P exchange between ECF and the skeleton or the soft tissue, play important roles in the overall metabolism of P, the fundamental process of P balance revolves around intestinal P absorption and the renal excretion of the excess P absorbed by the intestine. Dietary P occurs in both inorganic and organic forms. Most of the P in milk is inorganic, whereas most of the P in meat, vegetables, and other nondairy sources is located intracellularly and is complexed as phosphoproteins, phosphosugars, and phospholipids. Although certain phospholipids may be absorbed in organic forms, the bulk of the P is absorbed as inorganic P, which is released from organic P by hydrolysis within the lumen of the gut.

TRANSEPITHELIAL TRANSPORT OF INORGANIC PHOSPHATE

P Absorption

Overall Concept

Intestinal P absorption represents the net flux of P from the gut lumen, across the intestinal epithelium, and into the bloodstream. This net flux of P (Jnet) represents the difference between two unidirectional fluxes: the absorptive, lumen (mucosal)-to-blood (serosal) flux (Jms) and the opposite, serosal-to-mucosal flux (Jsm), that is, Jnet equals Jms minus Jsm (Fig. 19.1). Each unidirectional flux, in turn, can be resolved into two components; thus, Jms consists of a transcellular flux (J^c_{ms}) and a paracellular flux (J^P_{ms}), and the same is true for Jsm in the opposite direction. The paracellular flux is mediated through solvent drag and diffusional processes, driven by transepithelial chemical and physical (electrical and hydrostatic) gradients, whereas the transcellular flux represents an active, energy-dependent transport process.

Absorption Through the Paracellular Pathway

The flow of water across the paracellular pathway can carry with it solutes such as P. This transport process is known as *convection* or *solvent drag*. Under physiologic conditions, net water flow across the intestinal epithelia is directed in the absorptive

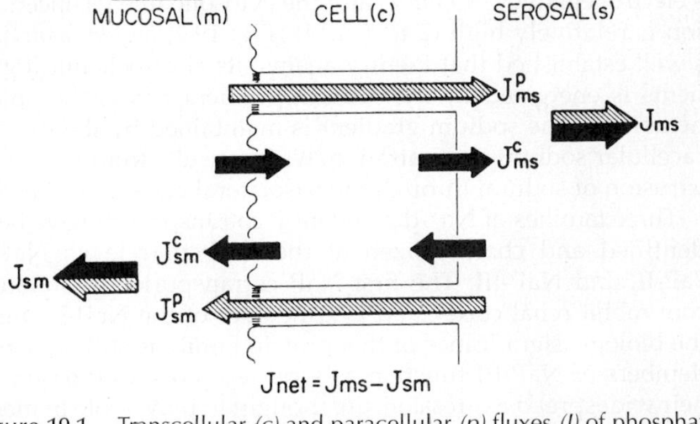

Figure 19.1. Transcellular *(c)* and paracellular *(p)* fluxes *(J)* of phosphate across intestinal epithelium. (Reproduced with permission from Lee DBN. Mechanism and regulation of phosphate transport. *Adv Exp Biol Med* 1986; 208:207–212.)

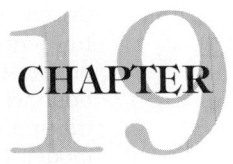

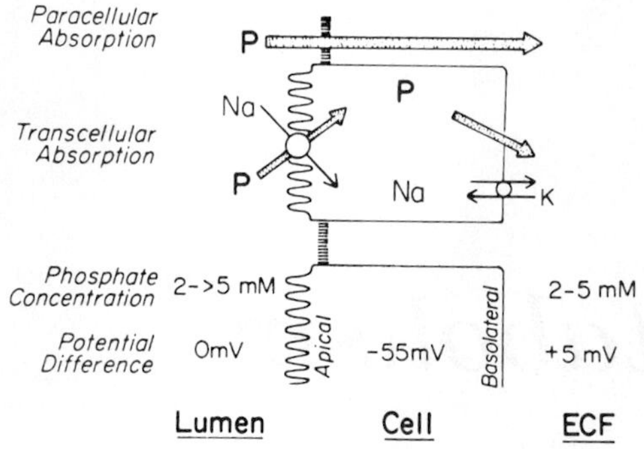

Figure 19.2. Transepithelial electrochemical characteristics in mammalian intestine. (Data compiled from experimental studies.)

direction, thus setting up the condition for net P absorption. Diffusion is another mechanism that can mediate P absorption through the intercellular shunt pathway. The driving force is the electrochemical gradient across the intestinal epithelium. In the rat, for example, a transepithelial potential difference of 5 mV (serosal positive, Fig. 19.2) favors the diffusion of negatively charged P across the paracellular space. Using an average valence of −1.6 for P, and assuming an extracellular P concentration [P] of 2.4 mM (in the rat), it can be predicted from the Ussing equation that net diffusional absorption of P would occur when luminal [P] exceeds 1.8 mM. In humans, diffusion in the absorptive direction would be expected to occur at luminal [P] lower than 1.8 mM, because the average extracellular [P] in humans is lower than 2.4 mM. When measured under fasting conditions, the gut luminal [P] at all levels of the small intestine in humans is approximately 2.0 mM. With feeding, one would clearly expect higher luminal [P]. Indeed, the [P] in human fecal fluid as determined by *in vivo* dialysis was 5.0 mM. Thus, under normal conditions, P absorption through the paracellular conduit could occur throughout the intestinal tract, including the colon. The amount absorbed through this mechanism would be expected to vary directly with luminal [P], which in turn varies with dietary P intake.

Phosphate Absorption Through the Cellular Pathway

Transcellular transport of P across the enterocytes involves at least three steps: transport across the apical membrane, transport through the cytoplasm, and transport across the basolateral membrane (Fig. 19.2, *top panel*).

Energetic considerations would predict that the apical membrane penetration of anionic P, with a calculated valence of −1.6, is an energy-dependent process. This is because the cell interior is electronegative (−55 mV) and the cytosolic free P concentration is relatively high (2 to 5 mM) (Fig. 19.2, *bottom panel*). It is well established that P entry against its electrochemical gradients is energized by the sodium gradient across the apical membrane. The sodium gradient is maintained by the low intracellular sodium concentration, which results from the active extrusion of sodium through the basolateral Na^+-K^+-ATPase.

Three families of Na^+-dependent P cotransporters have been identified and characterized at the molecular level: NaP-I, NaP-II, and NaP-III. The first NaP cotransporter was cloned from rabbit renal cortex and is a member of the NaP-I family. The biologic significance of this protein family is still not clear. Members of NaP-III function as viral receptors and, based on their widespread expression, are thought to play a role in meeting cellular metabolic needs for P. Of the greatest interest to renal physiologists are the members of the NaP-II protein family, which exhibit the functional characteristics of sodium-dependent P transport in the kidney. Surprisingly, neither the transcription nor the expression of this transporter could be demonstrated in the intestine in mammalian models. Cloning of flounder NaP-II, however, demonstrated the presence of these transporters in both the kidney and the intestine of this fish model. The deduced flounder NaP-II protein sequence is highly homologous to the mammalian protein in the hydrophobic, membrane-spanning domains (80% identity, 92% similarity). However, in the hydrophilic portions of the molecule, only minimal similarity is found between the two species (30% identity, 45% similarity). Flounder intestinal NaP-II is, like in mammalian kidney, apical in location. In contrast, flounder kidney NaP-II is located in the basolateral membrane and functions to secrete P. Thus the molecular basis for apical P transport in the intestine remains relatively unexplored.

The mechanism by which P traverses the cytoplasm is not clear. Indirect evidence suggests that the absorbed P mixes with only a small fraction of the total intracellular inorganic P pool, suggesting passage through restricted channels. Thermodynamic considerations at the basolateral membrane are opposite to those at the apical membrane and P exit can be accounted by the electrochemical gradients (Fig. 19.2). Studies using basolateral membrane preparations conflict as to the nature of P transport. Several studies suggest that P transport is accomplished through a sodium-independent, carrier-mediated, electrogenic process, whereas other studies indicate that there is a Na-P transporter that translocates 2 Na^+ to 1 HPO_4^{2-} and is electroneutral.

Studies in young rats indicate the presence of an active, $1,25(OH)_2D$-sensitive, P absorptive mechanism in all segments of the small intestine, but not in the colon. Quantitatively, the jejunum accounts for the bulk of P absorbed through this mechanism. In adult rats, on the other hand, only the duodenum continues to actively absorb P, whereas the jejunum, which during active growth was the major P-absorbing segment, now secretes P. Thus it appears that the transcellular P transport mechanism may act to adjust net P absorption to the need of the body for this mineral. In growing animals with increased demand for P, active P transport is directed in the absorptive direction so that the net P absorption represents the summation of transcellular and paracellular absorptive processes. With aging and decreased need for P, the active P transport (at least in the jejunum) is directed in the secretary direction, and the net P absorption represents the difference between paracellular P absorption and transcellular P secretion.

P Secretion

In addition to transcellular P secretion, net secretion of P also can occur through the paracellular route, particularly when luminal fluid [P] is low. In humans, intestinal lavage using P-free solution leads to diffusion of 4 mg/kg per 30 minutes of P from blood to gut lumen. The quantitative aspects and the physiologic significance of these secretary fluxes of P are not well studied. Under normal conditions, most of the secreted P is assumed to derive from P entering the gut lumen with the digestive juices. This has been estimated to range between 2 to 5 mg/kg per day. The endogenous fecal P excretion represents that portion of the digestive P that is not reabsorbed and is estimated at 0.86 mg/kg per day.

Relative Role of Paracellular and Transcellular P Absorption

In humans, P absorption by the entire intestinal tract is measured by the metabolic balance technique. The difference between dietary and fecal P is termed *net phosphorus absorption*

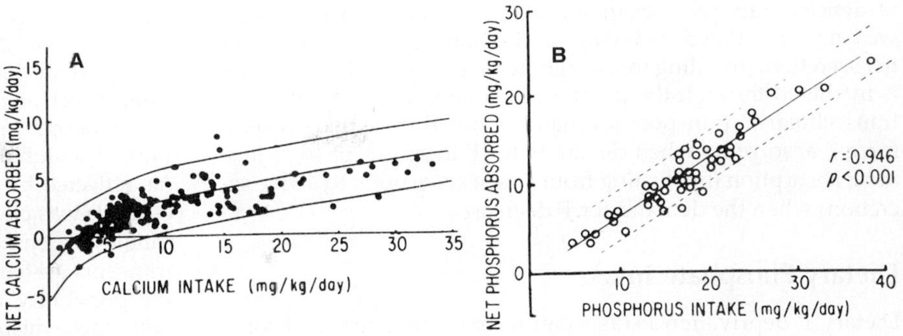

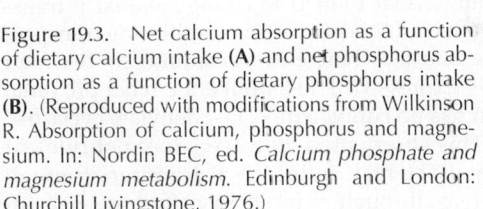

Figure 19.3. Net calcium absorption as a function of dietary calcium intake (**A**) and net phosphorus absorption as a function of dietary phosphorus intake (**B**). (Reproduced with modifications from Wilkinson R. Absorption of calcium, phosphorus and magnesium. In: Nordin BEC, ed. *Calcium phosphate and magnesium metabolism*. Edinburgh and London: Churchill Livingstone, 1976.)

and is expressed either in an absolute amount or as a percentage of P intake. In normal subjects net P absorption is a linear function of dietary P intake. For a dietary P range of 4 to 30 mg/kg/day, the percentage of net P absorption remains constant at 60% to 65% of the P ingested (Fig. 19.3B). These observations indicate that over the customary range of P intake, P absorption varies directly with P intake with no tendency toward saturation and would suggest that convection and diffusional processes account for the bulk of P absorbed under normal conditions.

In contrast to this linear relationship between P absorption and P intake, net calcium absorption is related to calcium intake in a curvilinear way, rising steeply initially as calcium intake rises, and thereafter less steeply and linearly as calcium intake exceeds 10 g/day (Fig. 19.3A). Figure 19.3 also illustrates the point that net fractional absorption of P (60% to 65% of the P intake) is approximately two times higher than that for calcium (20% to 30% of the calcium intake). Although the concentration-dependent P absorption would satisfy P needs under normal conditions, the active cellular absorptive mechanism may become important in metabolic states in which P needs outstrip P supply (e.g., during rapid growth, pregnancy or under circumstances of excessively low dietary P intake), conditions that are also associated with increased synthesis of $1,25(OH)_2D$. In contrast to the paracellular process, the transcellular absorptive process is saturable. The K_m (the concentration of luminal [P] at which active transport is one-half the maximal rate) measured in rat jejunum is about 2 mM. Measurement of jejunal P absorption in humans using the technique of triple lumen perfusion also supports the presence of an active saturable process at low perfusate P concentration (less than 2 to 3 mM/L) and a diffusional process with no tendency toward saturation at higher perfusate P concentrations.

Segmental P Absorption in the Intact Intestine

Based on *in vitro* and *in vivo* studies in isolated segments, the bulk of P absorption occurs in the proximal small intestine. In these studies, however, the transport parameters are measured under conditions quite different from those that an intestinal segment confronts in an untampered intestinal tract *in vivo*. In rats in which segmental absorption was determined from a spontaneously propelled liquid meal, it has been shown that the distal small intestine absorbs as much P as the duodenum. This appears to be attributable to the longer dwell time of the meal in the terminal ileum compared with the proximal small intestine. Other local luminal and dietary factors also may increase the availability of P for absorption and/or activate additional transport mechanisms for P absorption in different regions of the intestine; for example, the presence of bile salts in the distal intestine *in vivo* can increase P transport through increasing tight-junction permeability. This is an important area of P absorption that has been relatively unexplored.

FACTORS REGULATING PHOSPHATE ABSORPTION

Absorptive Surface Area

The effective absorptive surface area of the intestine can be altered by the proliferative activity of the villus and its associated crypts. An increase in absorptive surface would be expected to increase P absorption. Experimental studies indicate that vitamin D increases mucosal cell growth, cell turnover time, villus height, and the number of cells per villus. The duodenal mucosa from patients with renal failure revealed reduced villi and crypt length and ultrastructural abnormalities of the microvilli. In these patients $1,25(OH)_2D$ treatment was associated with normalization of these structural changes. This may be one of the several factors through which $1,25(OH)_2D$ can aggravate hyperphosphatemia in renal failure patients.

Vitamin D

Extensive clinical and experimental studies support the existence of an active, $1,25(OH)_2D$-responsive P transport mechanism in the intestine. This regulatory step appears to be mediated through the apical P entry step discussed previously. Kinetic studies indicate that $1,25(OH)_2D$ increases the maximum number of P transporting sites (V_{max}). In addition to its effect on transcellular P transport, evidence suggests vitamin D can increase paracellular permeability and thereby convective solute transport. The effect of vitamin D on maximizing the intestinal absorptive surface and maintaining its integrity has been mentioned.

Physiologic Need for Phosphate

Under physiologic conditions of increased P demand (e.g., active growth and pregnancy), $1,25(OH)_2D$ synthesis is increased and P absorption stimulated. Experimental studies suggest that physiologic mechanism(s) other than that dependent on vitamin D may also participate in the regulation of intestinal P absorption. For example, in the case of severe vitamin D depletion, continued active P absorption can still be demonstrated in jejunum from young rats. On the other hand, in mature rats, despite normal vitamin D nutritional status, active P secretion (rather than active P absorption) is demonstrated in the same intestinal segment. These observations suggest factors, such as the demand for P to satisfy the stress of growth (as in younger, vitamin D–deficient rats) or the lack of such demand for P when growth reaches a plateau (as in older, vitamin D–replete rats), may modulate net jejunal P absorption and that such factors operate quite independently from the prevailing status of vitamin D nutrition. When exogenous $1,25(OH)_2D$ was given to these rats, active P absorption was further augmented in vitamin

D–deficient rats, whereas in normal adult rats active absorption was also stimulated, reducing or eliminating the pretreatment net secretion. Recalling that a significant portion of P absorption is mediated through the paracellular route, it appears that the transcellular P transport mechanism functions either to reinforce P absorption when demands for P increases or to reduce net P absorption (by turning from active absorption to active secretion) when the demand for P decreases.

Dietary Phosphate Intake

Dietary P deprivation leads to an increase in active P absorption. Increased 1,25(OH)$_2$D production is believed to play a role in the observed increase in P absorption. However, experimental studies both support and refute the need for vitamin D in mediating the P deprivation–induced P absorption.

Luminal Sodium

Both clinical and experimental studies have supported the notion that intestinal P absorption is dependent on the presence of luminal sodium. It is now quite certain that the transcellular absorption of P is initiated by the luminal entry of P into the enterocyte via a Na-P cotransport mechanism. However, there is also evidence suggesting that increasing luminal sodium concentration may increase P absorption through the paracellular pathway. Increased transepithelial absorption of sodium would create greater serosal electropositivity, which in turn could increase diffusional flux of the negatively charged P molecules in the absorptive direction.

Influence of pH

Alterations in pH influences the relative proportion of the monovalent ($H_2PO_4^-$) and divalent (HPO_4^{2-}) P moieties. The monovalent moiety increases proportionately as pH is progressively reduced. Intestinal pH ranges from acidic in the duodenum to alkaline in the jejunum and ileum. An unequilibrated region (about 700 μm thick), however, has been demonstrated in the immediate vicinity of the mucosal surface of the rat jejunum with a pH one to two orders of magnitude lower than the bulk solution pH. Thus the effective pH (approximately 5.4) at the transporting surface would dictate that all P in the immediate ambience would be in the monobasic form. The effect of pH on transcellular P absorption has been examined by studying the effect of varying external pH on P influx across the apical membrane. In rats and rabbits, P influx has been observed to increase with a reduction in medium pH. In chick duodenum and sheep ileum, however, P absorption is similar at acidic and alkaline pH, whereas P transport is twice as high in chick jejunum at higher pHs. Theoretically, in addition to its effect on the dissociation of the P molecule, H^+ ions also may directly affect either the conformation of the cell membrane or the carrier molecules in the membrane. In addition, pH gradients may influence epithelial permeability (both of cell membrane and of tight junction) and generate a diffusion potential, thus causing changes in the membrane potential difference. Finally, changes in transmembrane pH gradients can change Na^+ fluxes through the Na^+-H^+ exchanger. This change in Na^+ flux may in turn affect P influx through the NaP cotransport mechanism already discussed.

Parathyroid Hormone and Adenylate Cyclase

Both clinical and experimental observations suggest a parathyroid hormone (PTH)-stimulatory effect on P absorption. More rigorous analysis has demonstrated that the effect of PTH on intestinal P absorption is mediated through the effect of this hormone on 1,25(OH)$_2$D synthesis. The jejunal adenylate cyclase system does not respond to stimulation by PTH. In addition, direct *in vitro* application of dibutyryl cyclic adenosine 3′,5′-monophosphate (cAMP) failed to change jejunal P transport, although the effect of this nucleotide on chloride transport (as reflected by the marked change in transmural short-circuit current) was clearly expressed. Thus, unlike the renal proximal tubule, the jejunum has no equivalent PTH–adenylate cyclase–P transport system. This observation, however, does not rule out the possibility that PTH may influence P transport through other mechanisms (e.g., through its inhibitory effect on ouabain-sensitive Na^+ pump).

Calcium

Early observations on the reduction of both calcium and P absorption with vitamin D deficiency and their parallel increase following vitamin D treatment has led to the conclusion that vitamin D increases P absorption secondary to its stimulation on calcium absorption, perhaps through vitamin D–mediated stimulation of a cotransport process. It is now clearly established that there are separate calcium and P transport processes in the intestine and that active intestinal P absorption can occur independent of calcium absorption.

Alkaline Phosphatase

Because phosphorylated compounds are not readily absorbed, it has been suggested that intestinal alkaline phosphatase may serve a hydrolytic function to free inorganic P for absorption. This enzyme is clearly increased by vitamin D repletion in vitamin D–deficient animals. It has the highest activity in duodenum and has been localized in both the brush border membrane and the basolateral membrane of the intestine. An apparent paradox is the finding that alkaline phosphatase, with a high optimal pH, is predominantly located in the duodenum, where the pH is usually low. If this enzyme is important in P absorption, one also would expect it to concentrate in the rest of the small intestine, where significant P absorption also occurs. Such difficulty clearly reflects the complexity of this enzyme, which not only exists in several isoenzyme forms in the small intestine but also has an affinity for a large number of substrates, ranging from paranitrophenol phosphate to adenosine 5′-triphosphate (ATP). It can also function as a phosphotransferase. Clearly, the question whether alkaline phosphatase affects intestinal P absorption remains open.

SIMILARITIES AND DIFFERENCES BETWEEN RENAL AND INTESTINAL PHOSPHATE TRANSPORT

In mammalian intestine and kidney, net P transport occurs in the lumen-to-blood direction. In the kidney, the proximal tubule is responsible for reabsorbing the bulk of the P filtered at the glomerulus, whereas in the intestine the entire intestine plays a role in absorbing the dietary P. In both the kidney and the intestine, an active sodium-dependent phosphate absorptive mechanism has been demonstrated although, as discussed previously, NaP cotransporting proteins have been identified in mammalian kidney but not the intestine. The influence of vitamin D on this active absorptive process is well established in the intestine but not in the kidney.

The mammalian renal proximal tubule is capable only of P reabsorption, whereas the jejunum has both active absorptive and secretary mechanisms. Dietary phosphorus deprivation induces active P reabsorption in both the renal tubule and jejunum. The expression of this response in the kidney is vitamin D independent, whereas in the intestine the vitamin D dependency of this response is still an unsettled issue. The pattern of sodium dependency also exhibits interesting differences between the two epithelia. Thus although P influx across the brush border membrane increases with increasing external sodium concentration in both the renal proximal tubule and the jejunum, this direct correlation holds up to [Na^+] of 300 mM in the kidney, whereas in the intestine, the maximal P influx is reached at [Na^+] of 100 mM. Thereafter, further elevation in [Na^+] caused no additional increase in P influx.

As mentioned earlier, an important difference also exists in brush border membrane P influx in relation to changes in pH in the bulk medium. In kidney preparations, phosphate influx increased with increasing extravesicular pH, whereas in intestinal preparations, P influx decreases with increasing external pH. Finally, although diffusional absorptive process plays a major role in intestinal P absorption, it has virtually no role in the reabsorption of P across the renal tubule.

CLINICAL DISORDERS OF PHOSPHATE ABSORPTION (TABLE 19.1)

Decreased Absorption

Dietary Factors

As discussed previously, in human adults who consume the customary range of dietary P (4 to 30 mg/kg per day), the bulk of P appears to be absorbed through a diffusional process, and the fraction of dietary P absorbed remains constant at approximately 60% to 65% of the P intake. Thus the total quantity of P absorbed would vary directly with the amount consumed. However, when the P intake becomes excessively low, the active absorptive component is stimulated. However, the effect of the induction of this active mechanism is not translated into significant increases in net P absorption. This is because the virtually P-free diet would provide little substrate for absorption. Stool P may, in fact, exceed dietary P because of the P loss through obligatory intestinal secretion and shedding. Thus reducing dietary P would reduce diffusional P absorption on the one hand and stimulate active P absorption on the other hand. Because the stimulation of the active absorptive process in the presence of low availability of luminal P contributes little toward increasing the net P absorbed, the overall effect of reducing P intake is one of reducing net P absorbed by the intestine. Reduced P absorption can also result from interaction between dietary P and other ingested material, rendering the intraluminal P unavailable for absorption. For example, phytates, the major organic P in cereals, precipitate with calcium and are not absorbed. The commonly used aluminum- and magnesium-containing antacids also form insoluble salts with P, rendering it nonabsorbable. Sucralfate, a drug for the treatment of peptic ulcer, causes reduction in serum P levels probably through a similar mechanism. It is a polyaluminum hydroxide salt of sucrose sulfate, but its P-binding capacity appears to be greater than that accounted for by its aluminum content. Interest in the search of aluminum-free P binders has rejuvenated the use of oral calcium carbonate as an agent for reducing intestinal P absorption. A new polymer resin that does not contain aluminum and binds P effectively is under development.

TABLE 19.1. Clinical Disorders Affecting Intestinal Phosphate Absorption

Decreased phosphate absorption
Dietary factors
Low phosphate intake
Ingestion of P binders
Vitamin D–related disorders
Deficiency
Dependency
Resistance
Chronic renal failure
Other conditions
Aging
Hypoparathyroidism
Osteoporosis
Cytotoxic drugs
Alcohol abuse
Malabsorption states
Mucosal hypoplasia
Inflammatory disorders
Diarrhea
Increased phosphate absorption
Increase physiologic need for P
Dietary factors
Increased intake
Phosphate-containing laxatives or enemas
Others
Primary hyperparathyroidism
Hypervitaminosis D
Acromegaly
Hereditary hypercalciuric rickets

Vitamin D–Related Disorders

Reduced P absorption can result from a deficiency of vitamin D, the substrate for $1,25(OH)_2D$ synthesis. Vitamin D–dependent rickets (pseudovitamin D–resistant rickets) is an autosomal recessive disorder characterized by dysfunction of 1α-hydroxylase and therefore defective conversion of 25-hydroxyvitamin D to $1,25(OH)_2D$. High dosages of vitamin D fail to influence the course of this disorder in children, whereas $1,25(OH)_2D$ therapy caused restoration of normal growth, healing of rickets, and correction of all biochemical abnormalities. In contrast to vitamin D deficiency and vitamin D dependency, vitamin D–resistant rickets, or osteomalacia, responds only to pharmacologic dosages of vitamin D or to $1,25(OH)_2D$.

X-linked hypophosphatemia is the prototypic vitamin D–resistant rachitic disease. The normal $1,25(OH)_2D$ level found in this disorder has been considered inappropriately low for the prevailing degree of hypophosphatemia. Experimental studies on the murine homologue of this disorder, the hypophosphatemic (Hyp)-mouse, has further demonstrated a generalized defect in the regulation of 25-hydroxyvitamin D-1α-hydroxylase activity in this disorder. In humans, an oral P supplement in association with supraphysiologic dosages of $1,25(OH)_2D$ has been reported to heal vitamin D–resistant osteomalacia in patients with X-linked hypophosphatemia. In all vitamin D–related disorders, reduced intestinal P absorption is considered an important cause for the associated biochemical abnormalities and bone disease. It is possible that the reduced effect of vitamin D in these disorders acts primarily to reduce bone turnover rate and therefore the demand for minerals. Reduced intestinal P absorption may be a secondary effect of this reduction in skeletal demand.

Chronic Renal Failure

In advanced chronic renal failure, the reduction in $1,25(OH)_2D$ synthesis would be expected to affect the active component of P absorption and thus could cause a reduction in net P absorption.

Lower intestinal P absorption in uremic patients has been reported using balance studies and radiophosphate markers. However, in general, a reduction in net P absorption in uremic patients, if and when demonstrated, usually could be accounted for by other factors such as decreased availability of dietary P for absorption (e.g., reduced intake and/or the use of P binders) or as part of a generalized malabsorptive process associated with uremia. A study using a technique that permits measurement of net absorption of dietary constituents after a single meal further confirms that P absorption is not different between hemodialysis patients and normal controls. Because under normal dietary conditions (i.e., with adequate P intake) the bulk of intestinal P absorption is accomplished through diffusion across the paracellular pathway, a uremia-induced loss of the active P absorptive component is not expected to cause perceptible disruption in overall P absorption. The universal practice of prescribing P binders to uremic patients (for reduction of P absorption) attests to the fact that, relative to the body's need, the intestine over-absorbs rather than under-absorbs P.

Other Conditions

Studies in normal subjects of both sexes have demonstrated that P absorption decreases with increasing age. This may be secondary to a reduction in absorptive surface area, because it has been reported that aging is associated with progressive hypoplasia of the intestinal mucosa. Certain studies, however, also demonstrate that there is a significant reduction in Na^+-dependent P transport (resulting from a decrease in V_{max}) and decreased stimulation of P transport by $1,25(OH)_2D$ with age. The changes in P absorption associated with hyperparathyroidism and hypoparathyroidism is probably secondary to the effect of PTH on renal 1α-hydroxylase activities and the synthesis of $1,25(OH)_2D$. Reduced P absorption has been reported in osteoporotic patients with improvement following estrogen treatment. Whether the estrogen affects P absorption directly or indirectly through stimulation of $1,25(OH)_2D$ production is uncertain. Cytotoxic drugs such as cyclophosphamide and adriamycin have been reported to decrease intestinal P absorption. Inhibition of proliferative activity of the intestinal mucosa and damage to the enterocytes are some of the postulated causes.

Reduced intestinal P absorption is one of the many metabolic abnormalities encountered in patients with alcohol abuse. Poor intake, vomiting, diarrhea, and routine intake of antacids are some of the causes that may lead to reduction in P absorption. In experimental studies in which the direct effect of chronic alcohol intake, in the absence of other complications, is tested, no reduction in P absorption was observed.

Other malabsorptive states may reduce P absorption as part of a generalized defective solute absorption, and this may be aggravated by concomitant malabsorption of vitamin D.

Increased Absorption

Clinical conditions that may be associated with increased P absorption include physiologic states of increased P demand. Rapid growth is one example. Increased P intake would lead to increased P absorption. Other than food, the use of P-containing laxatives and enemas could also lead to higher P absorption, sometimes causing dangerous hyperphosphatemia especially in the presence of impaired renal function. Intestinal P hyperabsorption has been described in acromegaly. Whether this is the direct or indirect (e.g., secondary increase in $1,25(OH)_2D$ production) result of growth hormone excess is uncertain. Increased intestinal P absorption has been proposed in the entity called *hereditary hypophosphatemia rickets with hypercalciuria.* This is a disease of early childhood in which renal P leak is considered the primary culprit. This defect in turn leads to the following sequence of events: hypophosphatemia, increased synthesis of $1,25(OH)_2D$, increased calcium and P absorption, suppression of parathyroid glands activity, and hypercalciuria. It has been postulated that this syndrome may represent one end of a spectrum of hereditary absorptive hypercalciurias. Increased intestinal P absorption is inferred from the observation that a standardized oral P load caused greater increments in serum P levels in the patients when compared with normal controls. Long-term P supplementation leads to reversal of all clinical and biochemical abnormalities except the reduced maximal reabsorptive capacity of phosphate (T_mP) per glomerular filtration rate.

ADDITIONAL FACTORS THAT MAY MODIFY INTESTINAL PHOSPHATE ABSORPTION

In addition to the aforementioned clinical disorders, many other agents and factors have been reported to affect P absorption (Table 19.2). In some instances, the same agent or factor may cause increased P absorption in one study and decreased P absorption in another study. It is possible that a given perturbation may affect P absorption directly at the intestinal level or indirectly through altering the need of the body for P. As previously discussed, changes in physiologic need for P can alter intestinal P absorption through both vitamin D–dependent and vitamin D–independent mechanisms. It is thus possible, for example, that thyroxine may, under one set of circumstances, increase P absorption through its action on increasing bone remodeling rate, whereas under a different set of circumstances it may decrease P absorption through its general catabolic effect on tissues.

DIETARY PHOSPHATE, PHOSPHATE ABSORPTION, AND MINERAL METABOLISM

The bone of the skeleton is continually being resorbed and formed, a process referred to as *bone remodeling*. Factors that increase this remodeling rate [e.g., growth, PTH, and $1,25(OH)_2D$] also augment intestinal calcium and P absorption, whereas factors that decrease this remodeling rate [e.g., aging, lack of PTH or $1,25(OH)_2D$] is associated with a reduction in intestinal absorption of these minerals. These observations raise the possibility that skeletal activities may directly regulate intestinal P absorption.

There is also evidence suggesting changes in dietary P, and therefore P absorption, may cause changes in mineral metabolism independent of changes in calcium and PTH. In healthy humans reduction and augmentation in the oral intake of P can cause rapid, sustained and inverse changes in the production rate of $1,25(OH)_2D$. This change in the rate of $1,25(OH)_2D$ synthesis was not associated with significant changes in serum calcium concentrations (both total and ionized fractions) or serum immunoreactive PTH. Serum P was lower with low P intake, but remained unchanged, except for a transient initial rise with high P intake. In both children and adults with moderate renal failure, dietary P restriction is also associated with increases in serum levels of $1,25(OH)_2D$. In contrast, in patients with advanced renal failure and in dogs with 5/6 nephrectomy, reduction in dietary P is not associated with an increase in serum levels of $1,25(OH)_2D$. This is most likely due to the marked reduction in renal mass.

Increased availability of P is known to increase bone formation and mineralization, whether studied *in vitro* or *in vivo.* In clinical practice, chronic P supplementation, generally in association with the treatment of osteoporotic patients, is not

TABLE 19.2. Additional Factors Reported to Modify Phosphate Absorption

Agents	Species	Findings and/or Conclusions[a]
Hormones		
Thyroid	Human	P malabsorption in hypothyroid subjects (balance technique).
		Decreased radioactive P absorption in hypothyroid subjects; reversed by TSH.
		Normal P absorption in hypothyroid subjects, and T_3 treatment did not produce any change (balance technique).
		Thyroxine treatment increased radioactive P influx into intestine.
		P malabsorption in hyperthyroidism by balance technique.
		Normal P absorption in hyperthyroid cases.
		Normal radioactive P absorption in hyperthyroidism.
		Increased net P absorption in thyrotoxic patients.
	Rat	P transfer decreased in duodenum, but no effect on distal segments with thyroxine pretreatment.
		T_4 increased P absorption.
	Chick	Thyroxine and T_3 increased Na^+-dependent P accumulation by cultured embryonic jejunum.
		T_3 increased Na-P cotransport by brush border membrane vesicles (BBMV) from cultured embryonic jejunum.
		T_3 further enhances the stimulatory action of $1,25(OH)_2D_3$ on Na-P uptake by cultured embryonic jejunum.
Calcitonin	Human	Short-term (3 days) administration increased radioactive P absorption in normal subjects; salmon calcitonin decreased P absorption.
	Dog	P transport in perfused jejunal loops was not affected by calcitonin administration.
	Rat	Calcitonin inhibited intestinal P absorption.
Corticosteroids	Human	Dexamethasone increased fecal P; chronic corticosteroid therapy decreased radioactive P absorption.
	Rat	Hydrocortisone pretreatment did not affect *in vivo* P absorption.
		Hydrocortisone inhibits intestinal P absorption.
		Corticosteroids stimulated vitamin D–independent active P uptake; effect of two hormones additive.
		Corticosteroids may stimulate passive P absorption through their effect on passive fluid movement.
	Chick	Corticosteroids stimulated vitamin D–independent active P uptake by embryonic duodenum; effect of two hormones synergistic.
Insulin	Rat	BBMV from streptozotocin diabetic rats exhibited greater Na^+-dependent P accumulation than those from controls.
	Chick	Sustained exposure of cultured small intestine to insulin depressed vitamin D–independent Na^+-P uptake.
		Insulin enhances vitamin D–dependent P uptake in cultured embryonic jejunum.
Dietary items		
Carbohydrates	Rat	Presence of luminal glucose did not affect P absorption (*in vivo* gut loop).
		Glucose required for concentrative P transport (*in vitro* gut sacs).
Lysine	Chick	Inhibited radioactive P absorption from ligated intestinal loops.
L-Phenylalanine	Chick	Decreased radioactive P absorption in *in vivo* loops.
		No effect on radioactive P transport in *in vivo* loops.
	Mouse	Decreased P uptake by intestine *in vitro*.
Cations		
Magnesium (Mg)	Human	Increased Mg intake led to decreased P absorption.
	Rat	Increased P absorption in *in vitro* gut loops from Mg-deficient rats or in normal rats but with Mg removed from ambient medium.
		Increased dietary Mg led to decreased P absorption *in vivo*.
Potassium (K)	Rat	Increased K in bathing medium led to increased concentrative transport of P (everted sacs).
	Sheep	Increased K intake led to decreased fecal P in balance studies.
Ammonium	Chick	Ammonium chloride inhibited radioactive P absorption in ligated duodenal loops.
Drugs		
Antacids	Human	Nonabsorbable aluminum and magnesium compounds increased fecal P.
Diphosphonates	Chick	Decreased radioactive P transport across *in vivo* ileal loops.
Cyclophosphamide	Human	Decreased radioactive P absorption in patients with leukemias and cancers.
Anaerobiosis and cyanide	Rat	Decreased concentrative transport of P in everted gut loops.
Iodoacetate, arsenite,2,4-dinitrophenol	Rat	Decreased P influx and tissue uptake in everted duodenal loops.
Oubain	Chick	Decreased *in vitro* ileal P transport.
Arsenate	Chick	Decreased (^{32}P) P transfer.
Cyanide	Human	Decreased P uptake by small intestinal mucosa *in vitro*.
Tonicity	Rat	Mannitol- or urea-induced changes in perfusing fluid tonicity did not affect P absorption.
	Chick	Urea-induced changes in tonicity had no effect on P absorption.

[a] Each statement represents a finding/conclusion from a different study. *TSH*, thyroid stimulating hormone; *T_3*, 3,5,3′-triodothyronine; *T_4*, thyroxine.
Reproduced with permission from Yanagawa N, Farid N, Kurokawa K, et al. Physiology of phosphorus metabolism. In: Maxwell MH, Kleeman CR, Narins RG, eds. *Clinical Disorders of Fluid and Electrolyte Metabolism.* New York: McGraw-Hill, 1993.

accompanied by an increase in bone mass, possibly because of the induction of secondary hyperparathyroidism neutralizing any potential beneficial effect of P. More encouraging results of increased bone formation have been obtained using brief periods of oral P supplementation, or the ADFR (activate-depress-free-repeat) protocol. P is first given for 3 days to activate bone remodeling units. A second agent, Didronel (a sodium diphosphonate), is then administered for 15 days to depress bone resorption. This is followed by the third phase during which bone formation is free to proceed with no interference from exogenous agents. The cycle is then repeated at regular 90-day intervals.

Selected Readings

Donisi G, Murer H. Inorganic phosphate absorption in the small intestine. In: Field M, Frizzell RA, eds. *Handbook of physiology* Sect. 6, vol. 4. Bethesda, MD: American Physiological Society, 1991:323–336.

A good review on the mechanism and regulation of inorganic phosphate absorption.

Kayne LH, D'Argenio DZ, Meyer JH, et al. Analysis of segmental phosphate absorption in intact rats. A compartmental analysis approach. *J Clin Invest* 1993; 91:915–922.

A new strategy for analyzing segmental phosphate absorption from a spontaneously propelled liquid meal through a structurally and functionally untampered intestinal tract in intact rats.

Hu MS, Kayne LH, Jamgotchian N, et al. Paracellular phosphate absorption in rat colon. A mechanism for enema-induced hyperphosphatemia. *Miner Electro Metab* 1997;23:7–12.

On phosphate absorption through the paracellular pathway.

Werner A, Dehmelt L, Nalbant P. Na^+-dependent phosphate cotransporters: the NaPi protein families. *J Exp Biol* 1998;10:201(Pt 23):3135–3142.

Update on the molecular basis of NaP cotransporters including recent demonstration of the presence of this protein in flounder intestine.

Yanagawa N, Farid N, Kurokawa K, et al. Physiology of phosphorus metabolism. In: Narins RG, ed. *Maxwell and Kleeman's clinical disorders of fluid and electrolyte metabolism*, 5th ed. New York: McGraw-Hill, 1993:307–371.

A summary of important aspects of phosphorus metabolism, including experimental and clinical aspects of phosphate absorption.

PART 2
Renal Handling of Phosphate

Heini Murer, Caroline Slive, Gerard Friedlander, and Jurg Biber

Plasma concentration of inorganic phosphate (Pi) varies with age, sex, dietary intake of Pi and other nutrients, and is regulated by a number of hormones. It also displays a circadian rhythm. Normal concentration of phosphate in humans ranges from 1.1 to 0.77 mmol/L. Inorganic phosphate is ingested via the diet, and Pi is excreted via the kidneys. The kidneys therefore play a central role in the balance of the extracellular concentration of Pi, which is an important prerequisite for normal cellular metabolic activities. Under average steady-state conditions, the amount of phosphate taken up by the small intestine is excreted by the kidneys, and it approximates 20 to 25 mmol/day, which represents approximately 20% of the filtered load. It is of note that other organs, such as the bones and muscles, are also involved in smoothing fluctuations of extracellular Pi and therefore have to be taken into account in the understanding of the various forms of hypophosphatemia and hyperphosphatemia.

Different mammalian sodium-dependent phosphate cotransporters have been identified. This molecular knowledge allows a better understanding of the basic mechanisms involved in renal Pi reabsorption and of the cellular mechanisms determining the net capacity of Pi reabsorption.

GLOMERULAR FILTRATION AND TUBULAR SITES OF RENAL REABSORPTION OF PHOSPHATE

Because 10% to 15% of the inorganic phosphate is bound to proteins and Pi is almost freely filtered, the calculated concentration of Pi in the ultrafiltrate is approximately 90% of that in plasma water. Total urinary excretion of Pi is the result of reabsorptive processes because in mammals no evidence for a secretory pathway has been obtained thus far.

Approximately 80% of Pi is reabsorbed along the proximal tubular segments S1, S2, and S3. Proximal tubular Pi reabsorption exhibits two heterogeneities: (a) more avid reabsorption of Pi is observed in the early convolutions (intranephron heterogeneity) and (b) Pi reabsorption is greater in proximal tubules of juxtamedullary nephrons compared with that of superficial nephrons (internephron heterogeneity). No Pi reabsorption takes place in the thin and thick ascending limb of Henle's loop. However, evidence was obtained that 5% to 10% of the filtered load may be handled beyond the early convoluted distal tubule. The tubular reabsorption of Pi display T_m phenomenon. Several factors affect the urinary excretion of phosphate (Table 19.3).

Cellular Mechanisms

Unidirectional flux of Pi from the lumen (across the apical, brush border membrane) to the peritubular fluid (across the basolateral membrane) requires the presence of sodium on the luminal side and the integrity of the Na^+-K^+-ATPase, which is localized in the basolateral membrane. The basic characteristics of this transepithelial transport of Pi were investigated extensively in *in vivo* and *in vitro* by micropuncture studies, by microperfusions technique, and by using isolated apical and basolateral membranes. These studies have provided a wealth of functional data; however, only by the cloning of some of the sodium-dependent phosphate cotransporters was it possible to understand in more detail single transport steps of proximal Pi reabsorption and the cellular mechanisms involved in the regulation of these transporters.

TABLE 19.3. Factors Affecting Urinary Phosphate Excretion

↑ Increases	↓ Decreases
Parathyroid hormone (PTH)	Phosphate deprivation
High phosphate intake	Vitamin D
↑ P_{CO_2}	Insulin
Dopamine	Growth hormone
Metabolic acidosis	Thyroid hormone
Calcitonin	↓ P_{CO_2}
Extracellular fluid volume expansion	Hypercalcemia
Glucocorticoids	Hypermagnesemia
Diuretics	
Atrial natriuretic factor	
Fasting	
Acute renal denervation	
PTH-related protein	

PTH, parathyroid hormone.

Thus far three nonhomologous mammalian NaPi-cotransporter families have been identified. The three families were named type I, type II, and type III NaPi cotransporters. Whereas type II cotransporters are expressed almost exclusively in the kidneys, type I and type III cotransporters are expressed more ubiquitously.

Type I NaPi cotransporters have been identified in cDNA libraries of rabbit, human, mouse, and rat kidney cortex. In the kidney, expression of type I mRNA and protein is exclusively found in the proximal tubules, and by immunohistochemistry, the type I cotransporter has been localized at the brush border membrane. Type I cotransporter–mediated sodium-dependent Pi transport has been demonstrated after injection of cRNA into oocytes of Xenopus laevis. Interestingly, the type I NaPi cotransporter seems also to operate as a chloride channel and also seems to transport some organic anions, such as benzylpenicillin. Type I–mediated NaPi cotransport is not dependent on extracellular pH. The precise role of type I NaPi cotransporters in renal Pi reabsorption is still unclear. Its activity and/or expression does not appear to be regulated by parathyroid hormone or phosphate in the diet.

Similarly, by expression cloning, *type II NaPi cotransporters* have been identified in cDNA libraries of kidney cortex of various species and in opossum kidney (OK) cells. Depending on the species, type II NaPi cotransporters are of 630 to 650 amino acids in length and are predicted to have eight to ten transmembrane regions. Only few structural features are presently known. For example, *N*-glycosylation has been demonstrated at sites located in an extracellular loop, and by the use of antibodies the N-terminus has been located at the cytoplasmic site. By *in situ* hybridization expression, type II mRNA was observed exclusively in the proximal tubular cells. A congruent pattern was also found for the type II protein, and moreover the type II protein was localized in the apical membrane. Under physiologic conditions, expression of both mRNA and protein was found to be highest in the S1 segments of juxtamedullary nephrons and to gradually decrease toward the end of proximal tubules; this expression, however, in agreement with functional data as described later in this chapter, the expression pattern along the proximal tubules as well as in different nephron generations varies dramatically under certain conditions such phosphate deprivation or hypoparathyroidism. Type II–associated NaPi-cotransport properties have been characterized after transfection in various different cellular systems (MDCK cells, insect Sf9 cells, and oocytes of Xenopus laevis). In all these expression systems, similar transport characteristics were obtained.

The family of *type III NaPi cotransporters* consists of the retroviral receptors of gibbon ape leukemia virus Glvr-1 (Pit1) and mouse amphotropic retrovirus Ram-1 (Pit2). Functional evidence for these receptors being NaPi cotransporters was obtained from transport studies using oocytes of Xenopus laevis. In contrast to type I and type II cotransporters, expression of type III mRNA was found in many tissues suggesting that type III NaPi cotransporters may represent ubiquitously expressed NaPi cotransporters rather than being specifically involved in renal handling of Pi.

Apical Entry Step

Experiments on intact tubules and isolated brush border membrane vesicles demonstrated that Pi entry at the brush border of proximal tubular cells requires the presence of sodium, which guarantees Pi uptake against the electrochemical gradient determined by a membrane potential of approximately −65 mV. From a thermodynamic point of view, which predicts an excess of driving force, one can assume that changes in the net number of NaPi cotransporters within the apical membrane (change in V_{max}) is the major determinant for the overall capacity of proximal Pi reabsorption.

Proximal tubular apical NaPi cotransport is largely performed via the type II cotransporter. The strongest evidences for this role of the type II cotransporter were obtained by type II knockout mice and by the use of antisense oligonucleotides injected intravenously. In both studies it has been shown that either partial (antisense) or complete (knockout) reduction in the type II NaPi cotransporter results in hypophosphatemia. Moreover, after targeted inactivation of the type II NaPi-cotransporter gene (npt2), serum levels of calcium, and $1,25(OH)_2$ vitamin D resembled that observed in hereditary rickets with hypercalciuria. In addition to the aforementioned evidences, studies on the regulation of proximal Pi reabsorption by parathyroid hormone or dietary Pi intake also point toward a key role of the type II NaPi cotransporter. Currently there is no clear picture about the possible roles of the type I and type III NaPi cotransporters in the apical entry step of Pi.

Additional evidence that the type II cotransporter plays a key role in proximal Pi reabsorption stems from transport experiments. Transport characteristics for type II associated NaPi cotransport, as observed in various expression systems (oocytes, MDCK cells, insect Sf9 cells), were in agreement with results obtained in earlier *in vivo* and *in vitro* studies on tubules and isolated brush border membranes. Typically, the apparent $K_m(Pi)$ is approximately 0.1 mM and the apparent $K_m(Na)$ is approximately 50 mM. Strikingly, in all expression systems, type II associated NaPi cotransport was highly dependent on the extracellular pH. Higher rates of transport were observed at alkaline pH consistent with all data obtained in intact tubules and isolated brush border membrane vesicles. Electrophysiologic studies on oocytes revealed that type II associated NaPi cotransport is electrogenic. Detailed analysis of the Pi-induced, inwardly directed current suggested that the stoichiometry for the overall transport reaction is three Na ions per one HPO_4^{2-} ion. Thus each transport cycle involves a net transfer of one positive charge implying that type II related NaPi cotransport is dependent on the membrane potential. Furthermore, the apparent $K_m(Pi)$ increased with depolarizing the membrane potential. Dependence of apical NaPi cotransport on the membrane potential therefore explains decreases in proximal Pi reabsorption as observed in glucose-induced hyperphosphaturia for example.

Besides inorganic phosphate, only arsenate has been described to be transported by the type II NaPi cotransporter and only few inhibitors are known. The best, yet not specific, inhibitors are phosphonic acids, such as phosphonoformic acid.

Because type I cotransporters are expressed in the apical membrane and because they act as NaPi cotransporter, it has to be assumed that the type I NaPi cotransporter contributes to the overall Pi reabsorption as well. However, the fact that the type I cotransporter also acts as a chloride channel and may transport certain organic anions suggests that the role of the type I cotransporter may be more complex than expected. Interestingly, in brush border membranes isolated from type II knockout mice, still approximately 20% of NaPi cotransport compared with that of brush border membranes of normal mice was observed. If the type I or an as yet unidentified NaPi cotransporter accounts for this remaining NaPi-cotransport activity remains to be determined.

The type III cotransporter seems to be expressed uniformly along the entire nephron and evidence was obtained, showing that type III protein is expressed at the basolateral surface. Therefore type III cotransporters may not be of significant importance in the renal handling of Pi but may be regarded as a "housekeeping" NaPi cotransporter.

Basolateral Exit Step

Functional evidence for the existence of both an anion-exchange mechanism and a sodium-dependent Pi transport was obtained from studies on isolated basolateral membranes. Until now, none of these transport pathways have been described at the molecular level. It seems likely that the ubiquitously expressed type III NaPi cotransporter is located at the basolateral membrane but this needs to be firmly established. However, if so, sodium-dependent transport of Pi in the basolateral membrane would be oriented toward the cell interior and would therefore not contribute to the transepithelial Pi transport. It has been suggested that such a mechanism located in the basolateral membrane may provide Pi to the cell under situations of limited luminal uptake.

Regulation of the Capacity of Proximal Pi Reabsorption

Transport of Pi through the apical membrane is the rate-limiting step and determines the overall capacity of proximal Pi reabsorption. In addition to the membrane potential and intraluminal pH, many hormonal and nonhormonal factors have been described to alter the capacity of proximal tubular Pi reabsorption. In the examples analyzed thus far, it has been determined that the type II cotransporter is the key target of these determinants and it seems likely that for every alteration of proximal Pi reabsorption, the possibility of a contribution of type II cotransporters has to be considered.

With respect to the regulation of type II NaPi cotransporter three general statements can be made: First, most, if not all, alterations of proximal apical NaPi cotransport are associated with changes in the number of type II NaPi cotransporters residing within the apical membrane (change of V_{max}); changes in the apparent K_m values for Pi or Na have not yet been described. Although the involvement of other NaPi cotransporters cannot be excluded completely, their contribution to the overall regulatory potential may be minor. Second, most acute changes in proximal NaPi-cotransport activity are due to posttranscriptional events, which include the rate of insertion into the apical membrane and the rate of internalization. The resulting net rate then determines the actual number in the apical membrane (V_{max}). Third, internalized type II cotransporters are routed to the lysosomes and do not enter a recycling compartment as observed in other cases of regulated membrane transports. These statements are summarized in Fig. 19.4.

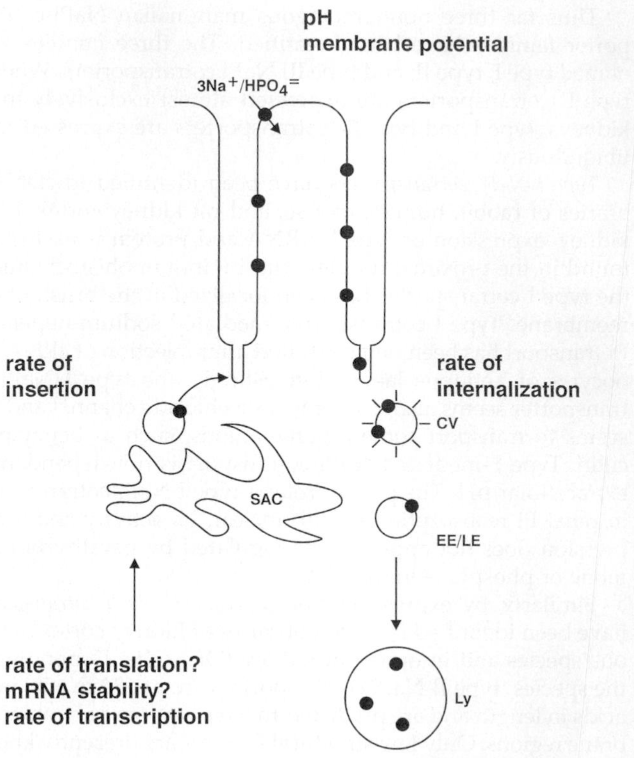

Figure 19.4. Cell parameters determining the rate of proximal tubular reabsorption of phosphate via the type II NaPi cotransporter. Note that the rate is determined by the net number of cotransporter molecules residing in the brush border membrane. CV, coated vesicle; EE, early endosomes; LE, late endosomes; LY, lysosomes; SAC, subapical compartment.

Dietary Content of Phosphate

The amount of inorganic phosphate ingested with the diet is an important regulator of the rate of proximal apical NaPi cotransport. It has been established that most changes of proximal NaPi cotransport observed after changes of the Pi diet can be related to alterations in the number of type II NaPi cotransporters in the brush border membrane. No such changes in the type I NaPi cotransporter (in the rabbit and the mouse) nor in type III NaPi cotransporters (in the mouse) have been observed thus far.

The increase in the rate of NaPi cotransport after the onset of a diet of low Pi content (e.g., 0.1% Pi) is biphasic. The increase in transport and the amount of type II cotransporters is manifested already after a few hours (acute adaptation) and progresses slightly during the following days (chronic adaptation). Stimulated NaPi cotransport is manifested by an increased number of type II cotransporters, and after chronic adaptation a change (up to two-fold) of the type II mRNA also is observed. Interestingly, acute upregulation of NaPi cotransport is insensitive to cycloheximide, suggesting that *de novo* protein synthesis is not involved. The cellular events triggering the acute adaptation are still not known. It also remains to be shown if changes of intracellular concentrations of Pi, adenosine triphosphate (ATP), or calcium (extracellular as well as intracellular) are involved.

After the onset of a high Pi diet (1.2%) given to animals kept chronically (several days) on a low Pi diet, the rate of NaPi cotransport decreases rapidly (within hours) and does not further decrease significantly afterward. Again the decrease of transport matches the decrease in the number of type II cotransporters. This decrease is manifested by an increased rate of internalization at the intermicrovillar clefts via clathrin-coated vesicles. Internalized type II NaPi cotransporters are routed to the lysosomes and degraded.

Parathyroid Hormone

Increased renal excretion of Pi is provoked by parathyroid hormone (PTH) and parathyroidectomy is associated with a decrease in Pi excretion. The main action of PTH on Pi reabsorption is the proximal distal tubule but the hormone inhibits up to 10% of Pi transport in the distal tubule. The acute phosphaturic effect of PTH is accompanied by a selective retrieval of type II NaPi cotransporters from the apical membrane. As in the case of an acute high-Pi diet, PTH leads to an internalization and lysosomal targeting of the cotransporters. In addition, it has been reported that after 2 to 4 days, high PTH concentrations lead to a decrease in type II mRNA content. The reverse situation (decrease of the PTH concentration) has been studied in OK cells. These studies show that recovery of NaPi cotransport upon the removal of PTH requires *de novo* protein synthesis because it was completely blocked by inhibitors of translation. This is in agreement with the notion that internalized type II cotransporters do not enter a recycling compartment but are degraded in the lysosomes. These changes in type II NaPi cotransporters are in agreement with physiologic observations showing that the inhibition of proximal tubular NaPi cotransport by PTH occurs within minutes, whereas recovery may take longer.

Along the proximal tubules, PTH acts via the PTH–PTHrP receptor, PTH R1, which has been localized in both the apical and basolateral membranes. Available data suggest that the receptor PTH R2 is not involved in the regulation of proximal reabsorption of Pi. The action of PTH occurs through the generation of cAMP with a subsequent stimulation of protein kinase A and also through a production of inositol phosphates and stimulation of protein kinase C. Although it seems clear that the activity of either one of these protein kinases is central in determining the actual number of type II cotransporters in the apical membrane, the target of activated kinase activity has not yet been described.

Vitamin D

The effect of 1,25-dihydroxycholecalciferol on proximal absorption of phosphate is rather complex, and results obtained in numerous studies are conflicting because of the possible effects of systemic alterations in calcium and/or phosphate concentrations. Under defined conditions, it seems that low doses lead to an increase, whereas high doses result in a decrease of Pi reabsorption. Furthermore, a role of vitamin D is indicated by the observations that $1,25(OH)_2$vitamin D synthesis is stimulated under low Pi conditions and that $1,25(OH)_2$vitamin D potentiates the stimulatory effect of insulinlike growth factor (IGF)-1 on Pi reabsorption. The mechanisms of these interactions have not been studied in detail and it remains to be shown if the effects of $1,25(OH)_2$vitamin D are on the rates of insertion, on the retrieval of type II cotransporters, and/or on the rate of transcription.

Glucocorticoids

Administration of glucocorticoids to rats leads to a decrease in NaPi cotransport in brush border membrane vesicles, which correlates with a decrease in the abundance of the type II cotransporter as well as its mRNA content. Thus these findings are sufficient to explain the phosphaturic effect observed after chronic administration of pharmacologic doses of glucocorticoids. Parallel changes in the lipid content of the brush border membrane have been described, such as an increase of glycosylceramide and sphingomyelin. However, a direct link between altered lipid content and altered NaPi cotransport remains to be established. Because diacylglycerol is formed during the conversion of the mentioned lipids, a role of a subsequently activated protein kinase C cannot be ruled out.

Dopamine/Serotonin

Dopamine and serotonin exert different paracrine effects. Dopamine (via the receptors DA1 and DA2) is phosphaturic per se, whereas serotonin increases phosphate reabsorption through the binding to 5-HT1B receptors and thereby reduces the phosphaturic effect of PTH. Regarding the abundance of type I and type II cotransporters, no information is available yet.

Growth Factors

Both *in vivo* (such as administration of IGF-1 to hypophysectomized rats) and *in vitro* (in OK cells) studies clearly demonstrate that growth factors increase Pi transport in the proximal tubules. Direct molecular evidence that IGF-1 modulates the abundance of the type II cotransporter has been obtained in studies on OK cells. Similarly, it can be expected that insulin also modulates the transport capacity (increase) via type II cotransporters. The precise mechanism of insulin on proximal NaPi cotransport however may be more complex as may be illustrated by the fact that insulin is required for the renal PTH stimulation of 1α-hydroxylase activity in diabetic rats.

Thyroid Hormone

Thyroid hormone (T_3) stimulates proximal Pi reabsorption. This effect is more pronounced in young compared with adult individuals. Physiologic doses of T_3 resulted in increased contents of type II-cotransporter mRNA and protein. Whether T_3 exerts a direct effect on the transcription of the npt2 gene, or whether T_3 exerts an indirect genomic effect, remains to be established because in known promoter sequences of the npt2/NPT2 genes the presence of known thyroid hormone response elements are not obvious.

Stanniocalcin

Synthesis of stanniocalcin also has been documented in rat and human kidneys and immunohistochemistry provided evidence for the synthesis of stanniocalcin in cells of the distal nephron (thick ascending limb cells and principal cells of distal tubules and collecting ducts). In rat and human, stanniocalcin increases proximal tubular phosphate reabsorption, which in part is related to increased NaPi-cotransport activity in the brush border membrane. Stanniocalcin therefore appears to be a new possible paracrine modulator of proximal Pi reabsorption, however it is not known which of the known cotransporters is affected and how.

Prostaglandins

Prostaglandins were described to antagonize the phosphaturic effect by parathyroid hormone and other phosphaturic stimuli. Evidence was obtained that prostaglandins may act as inhibitors for proximal tubular production of cAMP (e.g., by parathyroid hormone) via inhibition of the adenyl cyclase. However, other phosphaturic stimuli that are not related to the cAMP system are also blunted by prostaglandins.

Volume expansion leads to an increase of phosphaturia; conversely, *volume contraction* reduces phosphaturia. Micropuncture studies and studies with isolated brush border membrane vesicles demonstrated that volume expansion alters reabsorption of Pi in the proximal tubule. This effect of volume expansion may be explained by an indirect hormonal action on the abundance of the type II NaPi cotransporter in the apical membrane.

Diuretics

In general, diuretics lead to a phosphaturia. The extent of the phosphate loss correlates with the degree of the inhibitory action of a diuretic of carbonic anhydrase. Subsequent changes in intracellular and/or extracellular pH might have strong effects on proximal tubular Pi reabsorption by a mechanism such as is known under conditions of acute and chronic acid–base changes (see below).

Calcitonin

Phosphaturia observed after administration of calcitonin can be explained by both indirect (e.g., hypocalcemia) and direct effects. Although calcitonin does not activate proximal tubular adenyl cyclase, a direct action of calcitonin on the proximal cell might be possible such as by transient increases of intracellular calcium.

Plasma Calcium

The most direct phosphaturic influence of altered plasma concentrations of calcium ions is via the parathyroid hormone. A direct effect of calcium on the proximal cell (e.g., on intracellular calcium) presently cannot be excluded entirely.

Acid–Base Status

Part of the fluctuations of phosphatemia observed under altered acid–base status are related to changes in the capacity of the proximal tubules to reabsorb phosphate. However, care has to be taken when interpreting results because the effects of altered pH values on proximal NaPi cotransport are rather complex. NaPi cotransport associated with the type II cotransporter is per se strongly dependent on the extracellular pH (higher rates are observed at more alkaline pH values) in agreement with results obtained in intact tubules and isolated brush border membrane vesicles. This dependence has been explained by a direct interaction of protons with the transport protein, most likely via a competition with sodium-binding sites. However, acute and chronic metabolic acidosis also have been shown to reduce the capacity of proximal apical NaPi cotransport via a reduction in the numbers of cotransporters and under chronic conditions also of type II mRNA.

Aging

Aging is accompanied by a reduced tubular Pi reabsorption. In parallel, the number of type II cotransporters within the apical membrane is reduced resulting in a reduced V_{max} value. In addition, during aging the content of mRNA is reduced by up to a factor of two, indicating changes of the transcriptional rates. The effect of aging may be mediated in part by the elevated blood levels of PTH observed in older individuals.

Heavy Metals

Administration of cadmium to rats for several weeks resulted in reduced proximal NaPi cotransport partly due to a loss of type II cotransporters. This seems to be a specific effect because other apical membrane proteins such as aquaporin-1 or Na-sulfate cotransporter were not affected. In addition, inhibition of NaPi cotransport by direct interactions of heavy metals with the type II NaPi cotransporter have been demonstrated. In most cases, this inhibition is reversible by thiol reagents.

Hypophosphatemias and Hyperphosphatemias

Many forms of acquired or inherited hypophosphatemias and hyperphosphatemias have been described. The acquired forms are rather common in hospitalized patients. Most of the symptoms of acquired hypophosphatemias result from decreased ATP levels caused by many reasons, such as phosphate depletion, alkalosis, or acute intake of glucose. On the other hand, acute and chronic renal failures are common reasons for acquired hyperphosphatemias. Familial hypophosphatemias can be regarded as inherited primary diseases of renal transport of phosphate or inherited complex disorders of metabolic pathways. Familial hyperphosphatemias are rare; for example they may result from a deficiency of PTH secretion.

It is of note that no familial disorder associated with disturbed renal transport of Pi has been directly associated thus far with a primary defect (mutation) in either the type I or the type II NaPi-cotransporter proteins. For example, in X-linked hypophosphatemia (XLH), a case of familial hypophosphatemia leading to an isolated renal phosphate wasting, the basis for altered renal Pi reabsorption, is related to a reduced number of type II cotransporters in the apical membrane but not to a defect in the NPT2 gene. It appears that many of the described forms of hypophosphatemias and hyperphosphatemias will be explained similarly.

In *Hyp* mice, the murine homologue of human X-linked hypophosphatemic rickets, renal Pi wasting is associated with a decreased expression of type II cotransporters but not of the type I cotransporter. In parallel, a reduced content of type II mRNA was observed. Similar findings have been reported for the *Gy* mutant. Yet because in humans, the type II gene (NPT2) is not localized on the X chromosome but on chromosome 5q35, an indirect mechanism of a genetic defect on the X chromosomes has to be assumed. Recently, the gene responsible for XLH has been identified by positional cloning and named *PEX* because the gene product exhibits similarities to endopeptidases. Different mutations in the PEX gene have been identified in families with X-linked hypophosphatemic rickets, suggesting that no hot spot for this disease may exist. In the *Hyp* mouse model, a deletion at the 3′-end was described and in the analogous situation *Gy*, a deletion was mapped at the 5′-end of the PEX gene. The function of the PEX-gene product is not known. The expression pattern of PEX mRNA (bone, lung, ovary) suggests that the product of the PEX gene may act as a humoral factor degrading a putative phosphate-wasting hormone. The identity of such a hormone is still not clear.

CLINICAL DISORDERS ASSOCIATED WITH ABNORMALITIES IN RENAL HANDLING OF PHOSPHATE

Hypoparathyroidism

Patients with hypoparathyroidism exhibit hyperphosphatemia, low phosphate clearance, decreased fraction of filtered phosphate excreted, and increased maximal tubular transport of phosphate per glomerular filtration rate (T_mPi/GFR). However, the amount of phosphate excreted in the urine reflects the dietary intake, and the patients are in phosphate balance but at a higher blood level of phosphate. PTH administration to these patients increases phosphate excretion, and this phenomenon has been used as a test (Ellsworth-Howard test) to differentiate hypoparathyroidism from pseudohypoparathyroidism; the latter patients do not manifest phosphaturia with PTH administration. The low phosphate clearance in patients with hypoparathyroidism is caused by the absence of PTH, but it also may be related to hypocalcemia per se.

Pseudohypoparathyroidism

Patients with pseudohypoparathyroidism have hyperphosphatemia and a decreased phosphate clearance as a result of a defective response of the kidney to PTH. In pseudohypoparathyroidism type I, the administration of PTH does not increase urinary cAMP or cause phosphaturia. In some patients, this abnormality has been attributed to a deficiency of the "N" protein component of the adenylate cyclase, which is essential for the stimulation of the enzyme by PTH. In type II pseudohypoparathyroidism, PTH increases urinary cAMP but does not cause phosphaturia; thus it appears that defects in cellular events beyond the production of cAMP are responsible for the resistance to the phosphaturic action of PTH in patients with this disease.

Primary and Secondary Hyperparathyroidism

Moderate hypophosphatemia due to an increase in both phosphate clearance and fraction of filtered phosphate excretion and reduced T_mPi/GFR are present in patients with primary hyperparathyroidism. Patients with secondary hyperparathyroidism resulting from malabsorption and/or nutritional vitamin D deficiency have similar findings. These patients are usually hypocalcemic, and the hypocalcemia stimulates the activity of the parathyroid glands. The resultant elevation in blood levels of PTH is responsible for the phosphaturia.

Disorders of Tubular Transport of Phosphate

A number of diseases cause decreased tubular reabsorption of phosphate. These conditions include primary hypophosphatemic rickets, vitamin D–dependent rickets, adult hypophosphatemic rickets, hypophosphatemic bone disease without rickets, oncogenous phosphaturic rickets, hypophosphatemia with glycinuria and glycylprolinuria, and Fanconi syndrome. An animal model of X-linked hypophosphatemic mice has been extensively studied. The defect in phosphate reabsorption is not transferred by renal cross transplantation. Numerous studies suggest the existence of a humoral factor, which is not PTH, that contributes to the renal defect. Evidence for a defect in calcitriol metabolism in X-linked hypophosphatemia also has been demonstrated. Detailed discussion of disorders of tubular transport of phosphate is provided in Chapter 23.

Chronic Renal Failure

In patients with chronic renal failure, tubular reabsorption of phosphate is decreased, and this phosphaturia becomes more marked as renal failure progresses. This adaptive response in the renal handling of phosphate is due to several factors, including elevated blood levels of PTH, the decrease in GFR per se, and as yet unidentified factors. These changes in renal handling of phosphate also occur in the absence of PTH in experimental animals with chronic renal failure. Certain studies have shown that early chronic renal failure in rats is associated with increased tubular dopamine synthesis by the residual nephrons and decreased tissue norepinephrine levels. Both of these factors may contribute to the exaggerated phosphate excretion observed in chronic renal failure.

Renal Transplant Recipients

Renal allograft recipients may have reduced tubular reabsorption of phosphate for months or years after renal transplantation despite good function of the graft. This phenomenon may be caused by persistent secondary hyperparathyroidism, administration of glucocorticoids, renal denervation, and primary defect in tubular phosphate transport resulting in renal phospate leak.

Selected Readings

Ambühl PM, Zajicek HK, Wang H, et al. Regulation of renal phosphate transport by acute and chronic metabolic acidosis in the rat. *Kidney Int* 1998;53:1288–1298.

A demonstration that the decrease of proximal Pi reabsorption by acute and chronic metabolic acidosis is associated with a reduced amount of the type II co-transporter. Interestingly this effect was minimal in animals fed a low-Pi diet.

Beck L, Karaplis AC, Amizuka N, et al. Targeted inactivation of Npt2 in mice leads to severe renal phosphate wasting, hypercalcuria and skeletal abnormalities. *Proc Natl Acad Sci* 1998;95:5327–5377.

An important study demonstrating that proximal tubular Pi reabsorption is up to 70% via the type II cotransporter. Biochemical characteristics of this knockout model have similarities with hereditary rickets with hypocalciuria (HHRH).

Custer M, Lötscher M, Biber J, et al. Expression of Na/Pi cotransport in rat kidney: localization by RT-PCR and immunohistochemistry. *Am J Physiol* 1994;266:F767–F774.

By using specific probes, expression of the type II NaPi cotransporter is described in rat kidney. Expression of both the protein and the mRNA was exclusively found in proximal tubules. The protein is located in brush borders only. The findings are consistent with earlier reported sites of renal handling of phosphate.

Forster I, Hernando N, Biber J, et al. The voltage dependence of a cloned mammalian renal type II Na/Pi cotransporter (NaPi 2). *J Gen Physiol* 1998;112:1–18.

A detailed electrophysiologic study of the inwardly directed current provoked by NaPi cotransporter via the type II cotransporter after expression in oocytes of X. laevis. The study was performed under steady-state and pre–steady-state conditions. From obtained data a model was generated describing an ordered kinetic reaction.

Kempson SA, Lötscher M, Kaissling B, et al. Parathyroid hormone action on phosphate transporter mRNA and protein in rat proximal tubules. *J Am Physiol* 1995;268:F784–F791.

The findings demonstrate a direct link between the phosphaturic action of parathyroid hormone and reduced amount of type II Na-Pi cotransporters in the apical membrane of proximal tubular cells.

Keusch I, Traebert M, Lötscher M, et al. Parathyroid hormone and dietary phosphate provoke lysosomal routing of the proximal tubular Na/Pi cotransporter type II. *Kidney Int* 1998;54:1224–1232.

This in vivo study performed with rats demonstrates that both parathyroid hormone and high-Pi diet lead to an internalization of type II cotransporters. Furthermore, evidence is provided that under both conditions internalized cotransporters are routed to the lysosomes. The latter finding likely excludes a recycling of internalized cotransporters.

Kos CH, Tihy F, Murer H, et al. Comparative mapping of Na-phosphate cotransporter genes NPT1 and NPT2 in human and rabbit. *Cytogenet Cell Genet* 1996;75:22–24.

By fluorescence in situ hybridization the human NPT2 gene was mapped to chromosome 5q35.

Magagnin S, Werner A, Markovich D, et al. Expression cloning of human and rat renal cortex NaPi cotransport. *Proc Natl Acad Sci* 1993;90:5979–5983.

The first report describing the cloning of type II NaPi cotransporters. The strategy used was by expression cloning using oocytes of X. laevis. cDNA libraries uses for screening were generated from human and rat kidney cortex tissue.

Pfister MF, Ruf I, Stange G, et al. Lysosomal degradation of renal type II NaPi co-transporter, a novel principle in the regulation of membrane transport. *Proc Natl Acad Sci* 1998;95:1909–1914.

This study demonstrates that in opossum kidney cells, parathyroid hormone leads to the internalization and lysosomal routing of type II cotransporters. As shown by confocal microscopy, lysosomal inhibitors lead to an intracellular accumulation of internalized cotransporters.

Sorribas V, Lötscher M, Loffing J, et al. Cellular mechanisms of the age related decrease in renal phosphate reabsorption. *Kidney Int* 1996;50:855–863.

Aging-associated decrease of renal Pi reabsorption was studied in rats of different ages. Obtained data indicate that aging provokes a reduction of the expression of type II NaPi cotransporters.

Taketani Y, Miyamoto K, Tanaka K, et al. Gene structure and functional analysis of the human Na-phosphate cotransporter. *Biochem J* 1997;324:927–934.

A description of the human NPT2 gene structure including part of the promoter region in which several cis-acting elements are described.

Wagner GF, Vozzolo BL, Jaworski E, et. al. Human stanniocalcin inhibits renal phosphate excretion in the rat. *J Bone Mineral Res* 1997;12:165–171.

Recombinant human stanniocalcin is shown to increase brush border membrane NaPi cotransport. Therefore this study suggests that stanniocalcin may participate in the renal handling of phosphate in mammals.

PART 3
Dysphosphatemias

Shaul G. Massry and Miroslaw Smogorzewski

HYPOPHOSPHATEMIA

Body Stores of Phosphorus

There are 600 to 700 g of phosphorus in the human body, with 85% of it in the skeleton. Only 600 to 700 mg or 1/1,000 of total body phosphorus is found in the extracellular fluid. Approximately 15% of body phosphorus is located in soft tissues, mainly bound to carbohydrates, lipids, and proteins. The amount of inorganic phosphorus in the cell is very small, but this fraction of body phosphorus is important because it provides the source of phosphorus for the resynthesis of adenosine triphosphate (ATP).

Definition

Hypophosphatemia is a decrease in the concentration of plasma phosphorus, and *phosphate depletion* is an absolute reduction in total body phosphorus. For clinical purposes, hypophosphatemia could be divided into moderate or severe. *Moderate hypophosphatemia* may be defined as plasma phosphorus levels between 2.5 to 1.0 mg/dl; it is not uncommon, and it is usually not associated with signs and symptoms. Phosphate depletion may not be present in patients with moderate hypophosphatemia. *Severe hypophosphatemia* denotes plasma phosphorus levels below 1.0 mg/dl. Phosphate depletion is usually present in patients with severe hypophosphatemia. Such patients display signs and symptoms of organ dysfunction.

Hypophosphatemia with and without phosphate depletion is not uncommon. One study showed that 2% of hospital patients had levels of plasma phosphorus below 2.0 mg/dl and that such low levels are noted more frequently among patients with chronic alcoholism. It was reported that plasma levels of phosphorus below 2.0 mg/dl were observed in 10% of patients admitted to the hospital with chronic alcoholism. Also 40% to 80% of patients with septicemia due to a variety of infections, and especially those infected with Gram-negative bacteria, have hypophosphatemia.

Causes

Three categories of disturbances may cause hypophosphatemia and/or phosphate depletion. These include decreased intestinal absorption of phosphorus, increased urinary losses of this ion, a shift of phosphorus from extracellular to intracellular compartments, or a combination of these factors. In addition, hypophosphatemia of variable degrees should be anticipated during administration of nutrients to patients with a wasting illness, starvation, or malnutrition. This is due to the formation of new tissues that requires the incorporation of phosphorus in these tissues. Table 19.4 lists the causes of moderate hypophosphatemia; the conditions that may be associated with severe hypophosphatemia are presented in Table 19.5.

TABLE 19.4. Causes and Mechanisms of Moderate Hypophosphatemia

Cause	Mechanism
Hyperparathyroidism	↑ Urinary losses
Osteomalacia[a]	↓ Intestinal absorption ↑ Urinary losses
Vitamin D deficiency[a]	↓ Intestinal absorption ↑ Urinary losses
Malabsorption[a]	↓ Intestinal absorption ↑ Urinary losses
Renal transplantation	↑ Urinary losses
Renal tubular defects	↑ Urinary losses
Extracellular volume expansion	↑ Urinary losses
Diuretic therapy	↑ Urinary losses
$NaHCO_3$ administration	↑ Urinary losses
Chronic glucocorticoid effect	↑ Urinary losses
Recovery from hypothermia	↑ Urinary losses
Glucagon administration	↑ Urinary losses
Starvation	Lack of intake
Salicylate poisoning[b]	Shift of phosphorus into cells
Acute gout[b]	Shift of phosphorus into cells
Septicemia especially due to infection with gram-negative bacteria[b]	Shift of phosphorus into cells
Insulin administration	Shift of phosphorus into cells
Glucose or fructose administration	Shift of phosphorus into cells
Androgen therapy	Incorporation of phosphorus into cells

[a] In these clinical conditions, the decreased intestinal absorption of phosphorus is due to vitamin D deficiency and the increased urinary losses of phosphorus are due to the associated secondary hyperparathyroidism.
[b] These clinical conditions are associated with hyperventilation and respiratory alkalosis. The latter is associated with movement of phosphorus from extracellular fluid into cells.

TABLE 19.5. Causes of Severe Hypophosphatemia

Prolonged use of phosphate-binding antacid
Diabetes mellitus
Chronic alcoholism
Respiratory alkalosis
Recovery from severe burns
Hyperalimentation
Nutritional recovery syndrome

Pathogenesis of Severe Hypophosphatemia

Prolonged Use of Phosphate-Binding Antacids

Various antacids, such as aluminum hydroxide or carbonate, magnesium hydroxide, or calcium carbonate, bind phosphorus in the intestine and render it unabsorbable. Therefore severe hypophosphatemia and phosphate depletion may develop with the use of these antacids. Indeed, severe hypophosphatemia has been noticed in patients with duodenal ulcer and in those with advanced renal failure who were treated with these compounds.

Diabetes Mellitus

Several mechanisms may underlie the hypophosphatemia in patients with diabetes mellitus. It should be noted that serum phosphorus is usually normal when the disease is adequately controlled. However, hypophosphatemia of varying degrees may develop in patients with untreated diabetes mellitus, and especially when the disease is complicated with ketoacidosis. Osmotic diuresis, metabolic acidosis, and insulin therapy may all be contributory to the genesis of hypophosphatemia (Fig. 19.5). Although hypophosphatemia is common in patients with ketoacidosis, it is usually of short duration and therefore does not cause phosphate depletion. However, in small groups of patients, severe hypophosphatemia may cause resistance to the peripheral action of insulin and result in increased insulin requirement for the treatment of ketoacidosis. In such patients phosphorus supplementation is beneficial.

Chronic Alcoholism

Hypophosphatemia is common in patients with chronic alcoholism. The factors responsible for the fall in serum phosphorus are multiple. They include poor dietary intake, use of

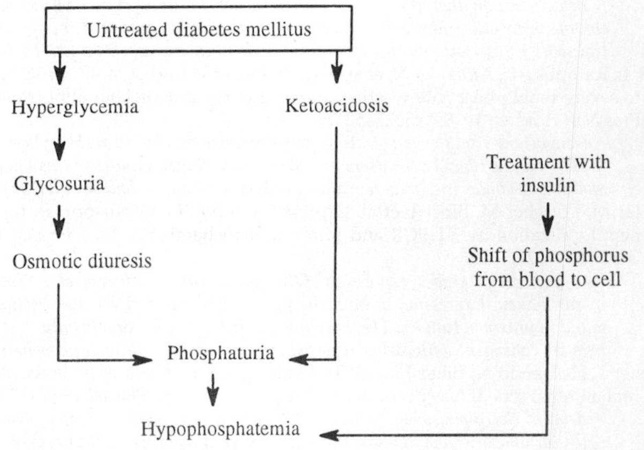

Figure 19.5. Mechanisms of hypophosphatemia in patients with untreated diabetes mellitus and ketoacidosis.

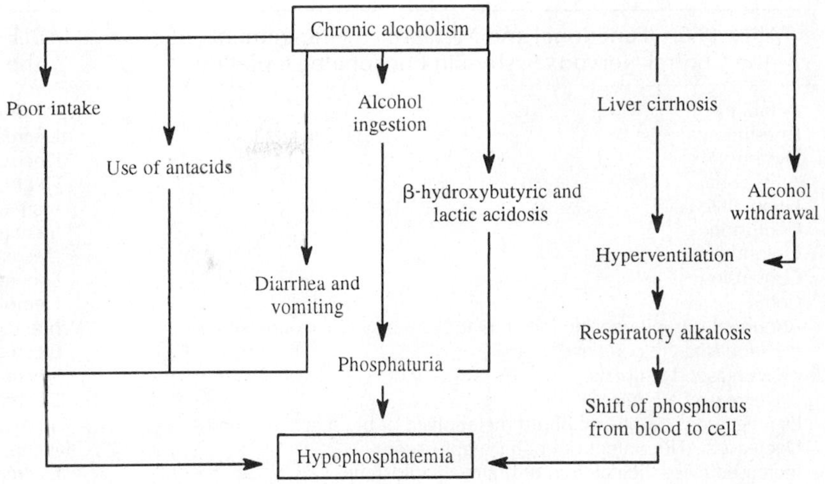

Figure 19.6. Mechanisms of hypophosphatemia in patients with chronic alcoholism.

antacids for the management of gastric disturbances, vomiting and diarrhea, alcohol ingestion per se, metabolic acidosis (β-hydroxybutyric and lactic acidosis), and hyperventilation associated with liver cirrhosis or acute withdrawal syndrome. The interaction between these factors and the pathways through which they may induce hypophosphatemia are depicted in Fig. 19.6. A large number of patients with chronic alcoholism enter the hospital with normal levels of plasma phosphorus and develop hypophosphatemia in the hospital; the fall in plasma levels of phosphorus is most likely due to therapeutic (saline and glucose infusions) and dietary (high carbohydrate diets) regimens given to these patients in the hospital.

Respiratory Alkalosis

Marked hyperventilation causes respiratory alkalosis and profound hypophosphatemia. This is particularly important in clinical conditions associated with prolonged and chronic respiratory alkalosis. The fall in plasma levels of phosphorus during respiratory alkalosis are not due to the rise in blood pH but due to the fall in P_{CO_2}. Indeed, a similar increase in plasma pH without a significant fall in P_{CO_2}, as in metabolic alkalosis, is associated with only a slight fall in plasma phosphorus. In addition,

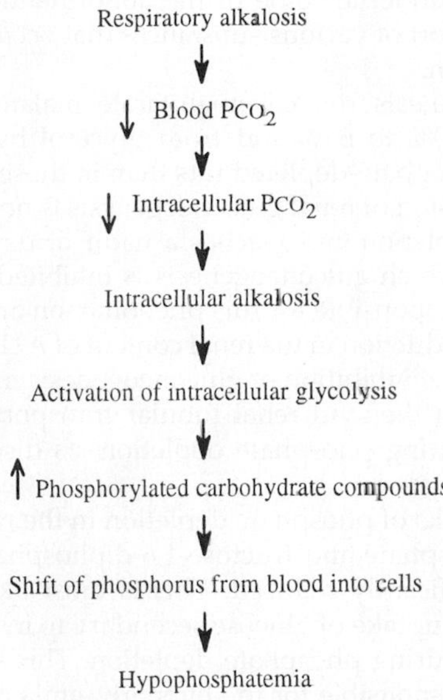

Figure 19.7. Mechanisms of hypophosphatemia during respiratory alkalosis.

phosphorus disappears from the urine in respiratory alkalosis indicating that the hypophosphatemia is due to a shift of phosphorus from the extracellular space into the cells. The sequence of events that leads to hypophosphatemia during respiratory alkalosis are depicted in Fig. 19.7. Respiratory alkalosis is associated with intracellular alkalosis, which in turn activates cellular glycolysis resulting in the generation of carbohydrate intermediary compounds. These compounds are phosphorylated by phosphorus that moves from the extracellular space into the cells. This sequence of events was confirmed in dogs subjected to respiratory alkalosis. It should be emphasized that the effect of respiratory alkalosis on plasma phosphorus occurs only when a small amount of glucose is also given.

Recovery from Severe Burns

The hypophosphatemia in patients recovering from severe and extensive burns is probably due to two factors: (a) augmented urinary losses of phosphorus during the diuresis period that follows the initial salt and water retention and (b) incorporation of phosphorus into newly formed tissues during the period of healing.

Septicemia

Hyperventilation that occurs in this condition causes a shift of phosphorus from the extracellular space into cells. Also septicemia is associated with very high blood levels of tumor necrosis factor-α (TNF-α), interleukin (IL)-6, and soluble IL-2 and IL-6 receptors, especially in those with positive blood cultures. Indeed, the injection of TNF-α or IL-6 into mice caused marked reduction in the plasma levels of phosphorus.

CLINICAL SYNDROME OF PHOSPHATE DEPLETION

Chronic phosphate depletion is associated with multiple organ dysfunction. These derangements are listed in Tables 19.6 through 19.11. It is evident that phosphate depletion adversely affects the function of almost every organ. *Indeed, it has been stated that the complications ascribed to phosphate depletion are only limited by one's imagination.*

Effect on Kidney Function and Plasma Electrolytes

Significant hypophosphatemia and phosphate depletion induce alterations in plasma concentrations of various electrolytes, in cardiovascular function and renal hemodynamics, in renal tubular transport processes, and in renal cell metabolism.

TABLE 19.6. Functional and Metabolic Derangements of the Central Nervous System in Phosphate Depletion

Irritability
Paresthesia
Dysarthria
Anisocoria
Hyperreflexia
Confusion
Obtundation
Convulsion
Coma
Abnormal norepinephrine (NE) metabolism of brain synaptosomes
Decreased NE content
Decreased NE uptake
Decreased NE release
Derangements in phospholipid metabolism of brain synaptosomes
Decreased ATP content of brain synaptosomes
Increased cytosolic calcium of brain synaptosomes
Decreased V_{max} of Ca^{2+}-ATPase and Na^+-K^+-ATPase of brain synaptosomes

ATP, adenosine triphosphate.

TABLE 19.7. Functional and Metabolic Derangements of the Hematopoietic System in Phosphate Depletion

Red blood cells
Decreased ATP content
Decreased hexokinase activity
Decreased 2,3-diphosphoglycerate
Increased affinity of oxygen to hemoglobin
Increased rigidity
Decreased life span
Spherocytosis
Hemolysis
White blood cells
Decreased chemotactic, phagocytic, and bactericidal activity
Decreased oxygen consumption
Decreased ATP content
Increased cytosolic calcium
Platelets
Decreased ATP content
Thrombocytopenia
Shortened platelet survival
Impaired clot retraction
Megakaryocytosis

ATP, adenosine triphosphate.

TABLE 19.8. Functional and Metabolic Derangements of the Musculoskeletal System in Phosphate Depletion

Hypofunction of the parathyroid glands
Bone pain
Pseudofractures
Rickets or osteomalacia
Bone resorption
Marked muscular weakness
Rhabdomyolysis
Increased blood creatine phosphokinase
Increased blood aldolase
Low transmembrane resting potential difference
Impaired bioenergetic processes of muscle
Decreased ATP content
Decreased creatine phosphate
Impaired mitochondrial oxidation
Impaired pulmonary muscle performance

ATP, adenosine triphosphate.

TABLE 19.9. Functional and Metabolic Derangements of the Cardiovascular System in Phosphate Depletion

Decreased myocardial stroke work
Decreased cardiac contractility
Increased left ventricular end diastolic pressure
Congestive heart failure
Impaired bioenergetic and phospholipid metabolism
Decreased ATP content
Decreased mitochondrial oxidation
Impaired fatty acid oxidation
Increased cytosolic calcium of cardiac myocytes
Impaired V_{max} of Ca^{2+}-ATPase and Na^+-K^+-ATPase of cardiac myocytes
Decreased ATP content of peripheral blood vessels
Impaired pressor response to norepinephrine and angiotensin
Hypertension

ATP, adenosine triphosphate.

Glomerular Filtration Rate

In humans and dogs, glomerular filtration rate (GFR) may fall with phosphate depletion and return to control values with phosphate repletion. Although the mechanism of the decrease in GFR is not fully elucidated, it is most likely due to the decrease in cardiac output and tendency toward fall in blood pressure during marked phosphate depletion.

Renal Cell Metabolism

Phosphate depletion may be associated with a fall in the levels of inorganic phosphorus, adenine nucleotides, and phospholipid precursors of the renal cells. The intracellular concentrations of inorganic phosphorus in kidneys of rats begin to fall after 2 weeks of phosphate depletion and remain low thereafter. The levels of ATP and phospholipid precursors (phosphorylcholine, phosphoethanolamine, glycerophosphocholine, and glycerophosphoethanolamine) are significantly reduced by the fourth week of phosphate depletion, but there are no changes in the levels of adenosine diphosphate or adenosine monophosphate. Within 10 to 14 days of phosphate repletion of rats that have been phosphate depleted for 8 weeks, the intracellular levels of inorganic phosphorus and ATP return to normal. These changes may underlie some of the abnormalities in the renal tubular transport of various substances that occur during phosphate depletion.

Gluconeogenesis from α-ketoglutarate, malate, and pyruvate is lower by 50% to 65% and from glycerol by 12% in renal tubules of phosphate-depleted rats than in those of control animals. Suppression of renal gluconeogenesis is noted on day 3 of phosphate depletion and reaches a nadir at day 7. The metabolic step at which gluconeogenesis is inhibited and the exact mechanisms responsible for this phenomenon are not fully elucidated. The reduction in the renal content of ATP may be partly responsible. The inhibition of gluconeogenesis may play an important part in the avid renal tubular transport of phosphate that occurs during phosphate depletion, as discussed later in this chapter.

After 4 weeks of phosphate depletion in the rat, the levels of glucose-6-phosphate and fructose-1,6-diphosphate in the renal cells are significantly reduced. This is most likely due to reduced cellular uptake of glucose secondary to insulin resistance encountered during phosphate depletion. This state of insulin resistance is responsible for the hyperglycemia associated with phosphate depletion.

TABLE 19.10. Carbohydrate Metabolism and Functional and Metabolic Derangements of Pancreatic Islets

Hyperglycemia
Carbohydrate intolerance
Peripheral resistance to the action of insulin
Impaired glucose-induced insulin secretion
Impaired leucine-induced insulin secretion
Decreased ATP content of pancreatic islets
Increased cytosolic calcium of pancreatic islets
Decreased V_{max} of Ca^{2+}-ATPase and Na^{+}-K^{+}-ATPase of pancreatic islets

ATP, adenosine triphosphate.

TABLE 19.11. Effect of Marked Hypophosphatemia and Phosphate Depletion on Renal Function and Fluid and Electrolyte Homeostasis

Serum concentrations
Hypomagnesemia
Elevation in calcium levels and even hypercalcemia
Decrease in bicarbonate levels
Hyperglycemia
Renal hemodynamics
Reduction in GFR in humans and dogs
Renal cell metabolism
Decreased renal content of inorganic phosphorus, ATP, phospholipid precursors, glucose-6-phosphate, and fructose-1,6-diphosphate
Suppression of renal gluconeogenesis
Possible decrease in intracellular hydrogen ion concentration
Reduction in urinary excretion of cAMP
Stimulation of 25-hydroxycholecalciferol-1α-hydroxylase and an increase in the production of 1,25-dihydroxyvitamin D_3
Elevated cytosolic calcium of proximal tubular cells
Down-regulation of the mRNA of the PTHrP receptor
Renal tubular transport and urinary excretions
Enhanced tubular transport of phosphate and hypophosphaturia
Blunted phosphaturic response to acute administration of PTH and calcitonin
Blunted phosphaturic response to acute extracellular volume expansion
Decreased tubular reabsorption of calcium and hypercalciuria
Decreased tubular reabsorption and increased tubular secretion of magnesium and magnesiuria
Decreased proximal reabsorption of sodium without natriuresis
Decreased T_m bicarbonate
Decreased T_m glucose
Decreased tubular reabsorption of amino acids and aminoaciduria
Decreased ammonia excretion
Decreased titratable acid excretion

ATP, adenosine triphosphate; *cAMP*, cyclic adenosine monophosphate; *GFR*, glomerular filtration rate; *mRNA*, messenger ribonucleic acid; *PTH*, parathyroid hormone; *PTHrP*, PTH-related peptide; T_m, maximal tubular transport.

The concentration of hydrogen ions in the renal cell during phosphate depletion has not been measured, but a decrease in hydrogen ion concentration in the muscles of phosphate-depleted dogs has been described. A possible decrease in renal-cell hydrogen ion concentration may also occur and could provide an explanation for the decreased maximal transport capacity (T_m) for bicarbonate during phosphate depletion.

The reduction in urinary cyclic adenosine 3′,5′-monophosphate (cAMP) excretion during phosphate depletion is not due to impaired activity of the renal adenylate cyclase because administration of parathyroid hormone (PTH) to phosphate-depleted animals produces appropriate increases in urinary cAMP excretion. Phosphate depletion is associated with a state of hypoparathyroidism, which in turn is responsible for reduced basal levels of urinary cAMP excretion.

Dietary phosphate restriction could be associated with augmented production of 1,25-dihydroxyvitamin D_3 [1,25$(OH)_2D_3$] secondary to stimulation of the 1-hydroxylase in the renal tubule. In humans, dietary phosphate restriction has been found to result in an increase in the blood levels of 1,25$(OH)_2D_3$ in normal subjects.

Tubular Transport

Calcium, Sodium, and Magnesium. A significant increase in urinary calcium excretion occurs during phosphate depletion in humans, sheep, rats, dogs, and rabbits. The magnitude of the hypercalciuria is related to the severity of the phosphate depletion and the degree of hypophosphatemia (Fig. 19.8). The increase in urinary calcium excretion occurs in hours after reduction of dietary phosphate intake. The hypercalciuria produced by severe phosphate depletion in humans may be marked with urinary calcium reaching values as high as 800 to 1,000 mg/day. The hypercalciuria results from a decrease in the renal tubular reabsorption of calcium. Although a decrease in proximal tubular reabsorption of calcium may occur during phosphate depletion, the bulk of evidence from clearance and micropuncture data indicates that the hypercalciuria is due to a defect in calcium reabsorption at sites distal to the proximal tubule and most likely at Henle's loop. The mechanisms responsible for the reduction in tubular reabsorption of calcium are not evident. Evidence suggests that the blood of phosphate-depleted animals contains a humoral factor capable of producing hypercalciuria in normal kidneys perfused *in vitro* with such blood. The state of relative hypoparathyroidism during phosphate depletion may partially account for the decrease in the tubular reabsorption of calcium. In addition to the decrease in the tubular reabsorption of calcium, a rise in its filtered load secondary to augmented calcium mobilization from the skeleton may contribute to the magnitude of the hypercalciuria. Indeed, studies in healthy subjects have shown that phosphate depletion is associated with negative calcium balance. The administration of thiazides blunts the hypercalciuria of phosphate depletion and induces hypercalcemia.

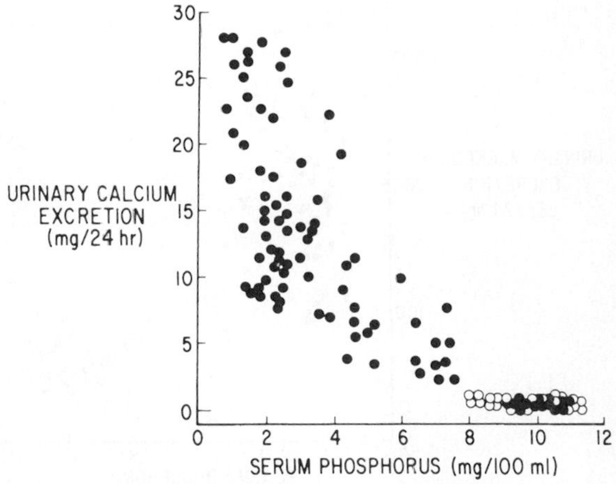

Figure 19.8. The relationship between plasma levels of inorganic phosphorus and urinary excretion of calcium. *Open symbols* denote data before dietary phosphate restriction, and *closed symbols* represent data after dietary phosphate restriction. (Reproduced with permission from Kreusser WJ, Kurowaka K, Eznar E, et al. Phosphate depletion: effect on renal inorganic phosphorus and adenine nucleotides, urinary phosphate and calcium balance. *Miner Electrolyte Metab* 1978;1:30–42.)

Phosphate depletion is associated with a decrease in proximal tubular reabsorption of sodium without natriuresis, indicating that the increased delivery of sodium is completely reabsorbed at sites distal to the proximal tubule. Thus there is no increase in urinary sodium excretion under basal conditions, but a greater fraction of filtered sodium is excreted by phosphate-depleted dogs than by normal animals during both saline infusion or osmotic diuresis.

The renal excretion of magnesium is increased during phosphate depletion. Magnesiuria occurs within hours after reduction of dietary phosphate intake. This increment is modest in humans and dogs but significant in rats. These changes in urinary magnesium are often associated with hypomagnesemia. In the rat, a significant increment in urinary magnesium excretion occurs during the first day of dietary phosphate restriction, and magnesiuria reaches its peak by the third day. The magnitude of the magnesiuria is related to the degree of hypophosphatemia (Fig. 19.9) and is not affected by lowering dietary calcium intake or reducing the hypercalciuria. In the rat, the marked magnesiuria is associated with significant hypomagnesemia. Magnesium balance is negative, and most of the urinary magnesium comes from bone. The magnesiuria of phosphate depletion in the rat is caused by both a decrease in renal tubular reabsorption and an increase in renal tubular secretion (Fig. 19.10) of magnesium.

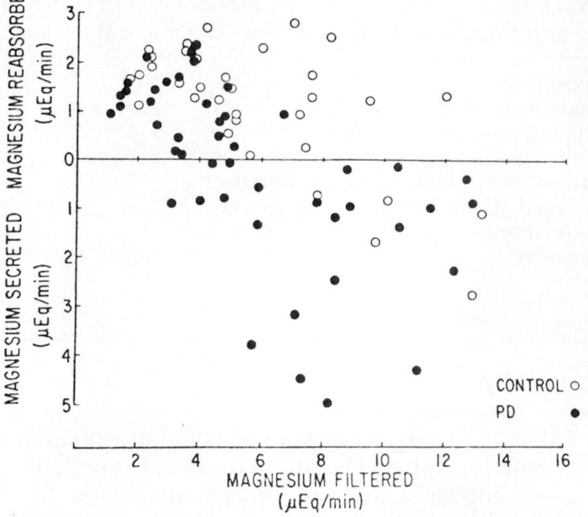

Figure 19.10. The change in the quantity of magnesium reabsorbed or secreted at various levels of filtered magnesium in control and phosphate-depleted *(PD)* states. *Symbols below the line* denote secretion of magnesium. (Reproduced with permission from Sachtjen E, Meyer-Sabellek WA, Massry SG. Evidence for magnesium secretion during phosphate depletion. *Proc Exp Biol Med* 1979;162:416–419.)

Phosphate. Dietary phosphate restriction in humans and experimental animals is associated with enhanced renal tubular reabsorption of phosphate. The urinary excretion of phosphate declines within hours after phosphate reduction in dietary intake, and phosphate virtually disappears from the urine within 1 to 2 days. The changes in renal tubular reabsorption of phosphate and in its urinary excretion may occur before a fall in plasma concentration of phosphorus becomes evident. This renal response to phosphate depletion develops in normal, parathyroidectomized, or vitamin D–deficient animals.

The kidney's ability to conserve phosphate during phosphate depletion can be documented even when phosphaturic stimuli are applied. Thus the phosphaturia produced by extracellular fluid volume expansion or by the acute administration of PTH is markedly blunted or inhibited. It is interesting to note that the lack of phosphaturia during the administration of PTH to phosphate-depleted animals is observed despite a normal increment in urinary cAMP, its generation by renal cortical slices, and normal activation of cAMP-dependent protein kinase; also, the administration of dibutyryl cAMP to phosphate-depleted rats fails to produce phosphaturia. These data suggest that inhibition of cellular metabolic steps beyond the cAMP-dependent protein kinase system is responsible for the lack of effect of PTH on phosphate reabsorption.

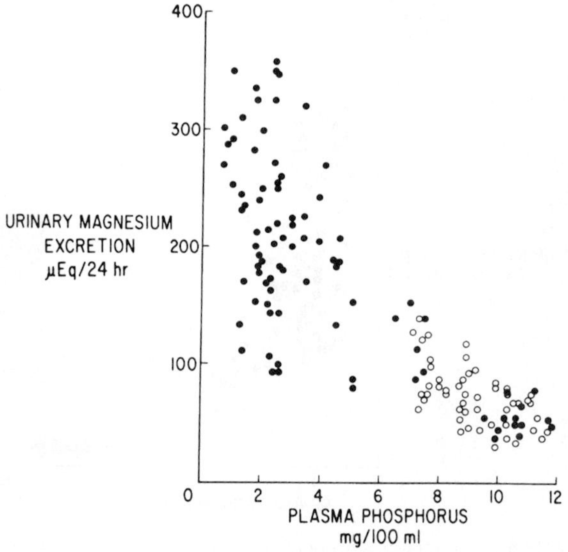

Figure 19.9. The relationship between plasma levels of inorganic phosphorus and urinary excretion of magnesium. *Open symbols* denote data before dietary phosphate restriction, and *closed symbols* represent data after dietary phosphate restriction. (Reproduced with permission from Kreusser WJ, Kurowaka K, Eznar E, et al. Effect of phosphate depletion on magnesium homeostasis. *J Clin Invest* 1978;61:573–581.)

These observations indicate that an additional system for the regulation of renal tubular reabsorption of phosphate exists. This system is independent of PTH and is modulated by dietary intake of phosphate and/or body stores of phosphate. There may be two primary functions for such a system: first, to prevent further depletion of body phosphate stores during low dietary intake of phosphate, and second, to facilitate phosphate repletion when dietary phosphate is increased to correct the state of phosphate depletion.

The PTH-independent adaptive system of renal phosphate transport in response to phosphate supply also responds to the phosphate demands of the body. It has been shown that when the demand of phosphate is reduced, such as in growth arrest, blockage of bone mineralization, pharmacologically induced inhibition of protein synthesis, or starvation, a PTH-independent decrease in tubular reabsorptive capacity for phosphate occurs. The available data are consistent with adaptive mechanism(s) primarily concerned with the maintenance of intracellular pool(s) rather than the concentration of inorganic phosphorus in serum. The controlling factors for this adaptive system are not known but do not include PTH, vitamin D, growth hormone, thyroid hormones, or calcitonin, and an agent(s) as yet unidentified has been suggested.

The proximal tubule is the main segment of the nephron where the adaptation in phosphate reabsorption in response to dietary phosphate intake occurs. The distal tubule and the collecting duct may also participate. The change in the transport of phosphate across the proximal tubule is associated with alterations in the sodium-dependent phosphate transport system located at the luminal membrane. The initial rate of the sodium-dependent phosphate transport by the brush border membrane vesicles is greatly enhanced. A role for the alkaline phosphatase of the brush border membrane in mediating the augmented phosphate reabsorption has been suggested, but the available data indicate that the increase in phosphate transport by brush border membrane vesicles induced by phosphate depletion precedes a demonstrable rise in alkaline-phosphatase activity. The bulk of evidence indicates that the molecular basis of the adaptive mechanism is not related to abnormalities in the adenylate cyclase–cAMP system; the protein kinase system; or the renal cellular content of ATP, adenosine diphosphate (ADP), AMP; or inorganic phosphorus. The suggestion has been made that the suppression of renal gluconeogenesis during dietary phosphate restriction is a possible mechanism for the adaptive augmentation of phosphate transport. During the process of gluconeogenesis, nicotinamide adenine dinucleotide (NAD) is generated in the cytosol resulting in a rise in the $NAD^+/NADH$ ratio. Either NAD^+, a rising $NAD^+/NADH$ ratio, or inhibition of the activity of NAD^+ hydrolyzing enzyme reduces renal tubular transport of phosphate. Suppression of renal gluconeogenesis would thus be associated with a fall in NAD^+ and the $NAD^+/NADH$ ratio, and as a consequence, renal phosphate reabsorption would be enhanced. Indirect evidence exists supporting a role for such a sequence of events in the adaptive mechanism of phosphate transport, although a cause-and-effect relationship between gluconeogenesis and phosphate transport has not been documented. However, it should be mentioned that enhanced phosphate transport during dietary phosphate restriction occurs before the suppression of renal gluconeogenesis becomes evident.

Bicarbonate. Phosphate depletion in dogs is associated with a reduced renal threshold at which bicarbonate appears in the urine, reduced T_m for bicarbonate reabsorption (Fig. 19.11), and a fall in blood bicarbonate concentration with a direct relationship between the blood levels of bicarbonate and phosphate. The parathyroid glands are hypoactive during phosphate depletion, and abnormality in bicarbonate reabsorption noted in phosphate-depleted dogs cannot be attributed to excess PTH but is due to phosphate depletion per se. Micropuncture studies have demonstrated an inverse linear relationship between serum levels of phosphate and the tubular fluid bicarbonate concentrations both in intact and thyroparathyroidectomized dogs. Similar reductions in bicarbonate reabsorption during phosphate depletion have been observed in rats as well. Humans with significant hypophosphatemia may have low blood levels of bicarbonate, suggesting a similar effect of phosphate depletion on bicarbonate reabsorption. The mechanism through which phosphate depletion affects tubular bicarbonate reabsorption may be related to the rise in intracellular pH. A reduction in intracellular hydrogen ion concentration may impair hydrogen ion secretion by the renal tubules and decrease the tubules' ability to reabsorb bicarbonate. Consequently, T_m bicarbonate and serum bicarbonate fall.

The overall effect of the renal losses of bicarbonate during phosphate depletion on acid–base homeostasis is complicated by the finding that phosphate depletion is also associated with release of bicarbonate from bone, which initially may compensate for the renal losses of this ion. Thus a decrease in the serum levels of bicarbonate may become evident after prolonged phosphate depletion or early in its course if bone resorption is inhibited. In addition to its effect on renal bicarbonate reabsorption, phosphate depletion is also associated with a decrease in urinary titratable acid and ammonia excretion. Thus phosphate depletion could cause both proximal and distal renal tubular acidosis.

Glucose. Chronic and prolonged phosphate depletion and marked hypophosphatemia of less than 1.0 mg/dl are associated with a decrease in the tubular reabsorption of glucose.

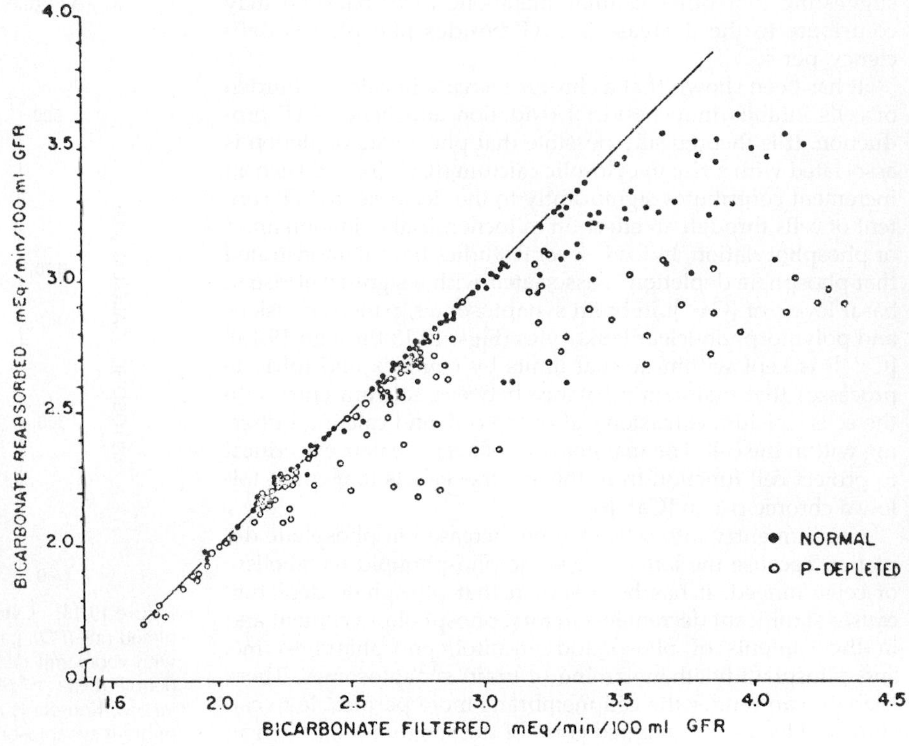

Figure 19.11. The relationship between the quantity of bicarbonate reabsorbed and that filtered for all clearance periods during bicarbonate infusion both before and after phosphate depletion. GFR, glomerular filtration rate. (Reproduced with permission from Gold LW, Massry SG, Arieff AI, et al. Renal bicarbonate wasting during phosphate depletion. A possible cause of altered acid-base homeostasis in hyperparathyroidism. *J Clin Invest* 1973;52:2556–2562.)

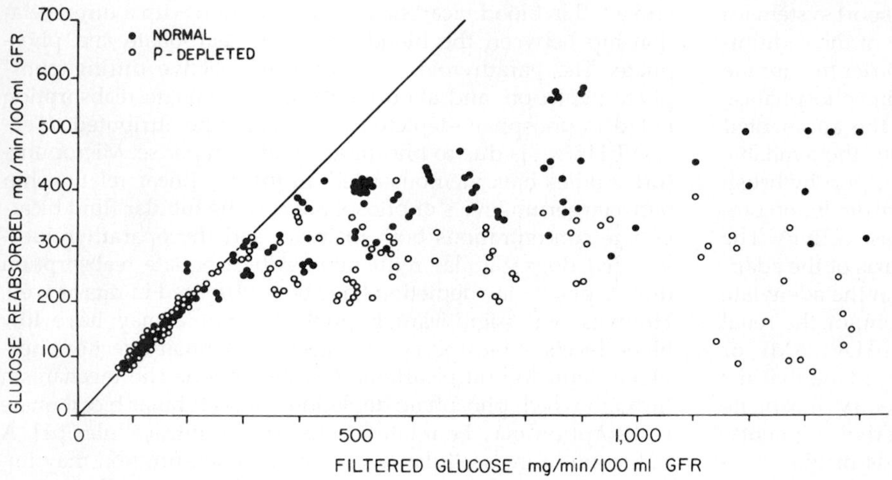

Figure 19.12. The relationship between the quantity of glucose reabsorbed and that filtered for all clearance periods during glucose infusion both before and after phosphate depletion. GFR, glomerular filtration rate. (Reproduced with permission from Gold LW, Massry SG, Friedler RM. Effect of phosphate depletion on renal tubular reabsorption of glucose. *J Lab Clin Med* 1977;89:557–559.)

Both T_m glucose and T_m glucose/GFR (Fig. 19.12) have been shown to fall significantly during phosphate depletion. This change in the renal glucose transport is not due to alteration in GFR but may be related to the fall in levels of cytosolic nucleotides in the renal cells.

Pathogenesis of Organ Dysfunction

Two critical disturbances occur during chronic and marked phosphate depletion, and they have been implicated in the genesis of organ dysfunction associated with phosphate depletion. First, there is a decrease in 2,3-diphosphoglycerate in the red blood cells, and this change is associated with increased affinity for hemoglobin to oxygen resulting in tissue hypoxia. Second, there is also a decrease in tissue content of ATP and therefore a decrease in the availability of energy-rich phosphate compounds that are essential for cell function.

The available data indicate that ATP of cells starts to fall several weeks after a significant decrease in their inorganic phosphorus content and ATP continues to decrease thereafter, suggesting that other cellular metabolic disturbance(s) may contribute to the decrease in ATP besides phosphorus deficiency, per se.

It has been shown that a chronic increase in calcium burden of cells inhibits mitochondrial oxidation and hence ATP production. It is theoretically possible that phosphate depletion is associated with a rise in cytosolic calcium ($[Ca^{2+}]i$), and such an increment contributes significantly to the decrease in ATP content of cells through an effect on mitochondrial oxidation and/or phosphorylation. Indeed, several studies have demonstrated that phosphate depletion is associated with a significant rise in basal levels of $[Ca^{2+}]i$ in brain synaptosomes, pancreatic islets, and polymorphonuclear leukocytes (Figs. 19.13 through 19.15). $[Ca^{2+}]i$ is kept within normal limits by complex and intricate processes that maintain a balance between calcium entry into the cells, calcium extrusion out of the cell, and calcium buffering within the cell. The maintenance of such a balance is critical to protect cell function from the adverse effects that could follow a chronic rise in $[Ca^{2+}]i$.

Calcium entry into cells may be increased in phosphate depletion because the latter affects the phospholipid metabolism of cells. Indeed, it has been shown that phosphate depletion causes significant decrements in total phospholipid content and in the contents of phosphatidylinositol, phosphatidylserine, and phosphatidylethanolamine of brain synaptosomes. These changes can render the cell membrane more permeable to calcium and lead to augmented entry of this ion into cells. Such an event by itself should not increase basal levels of $[Ca^{2+}]i$ because cells are endowed with mechanisms that allow them to pump out excess calcium and/or buffer it by intracellular organelles. Thus the finding of a rise in basal levels of $[Ca^{2+}]i$ in phosphate depletion indicates that the balance between calcium entry into, its extrusion out of, and/or its buffering within the cell is impaired. Calcium extrusion out of cells is accomplished, directly or indirectly, by the intact function of Ca^{2+}-ATPase, Ca^{2+}-Na^+ exchanger, and Na^+-K^+-ATPase. ATP is needed for the functional integrity of these calcium pumps. Therefore an initial fall of ATP secondary to phosphorus deficiency per se, and/or secondary to increased calcium entry into cells, may be followed by a reduction in the activity of these calcium pumps leading to reduced calcium extrusion out of the cells and consequently to a rise in basal levels of $[Ca^{2+}]i$. Also, alterations in phospholipid metabolism of cell membrane adversely affect the activity of Na^+-K^+-ATPase and therefore also contributes to reduced calcium extrusion out of the cell and to rise in $[Ca^{2+}]i$. Indeed, studies in brain synaptosomes, in pancreatic islets, and in cardiac myocytes have shown that the V_{max} of Ca^{2+}-ATPase and Na^+-K^+-ATPase are reduced in phosphate depletion.

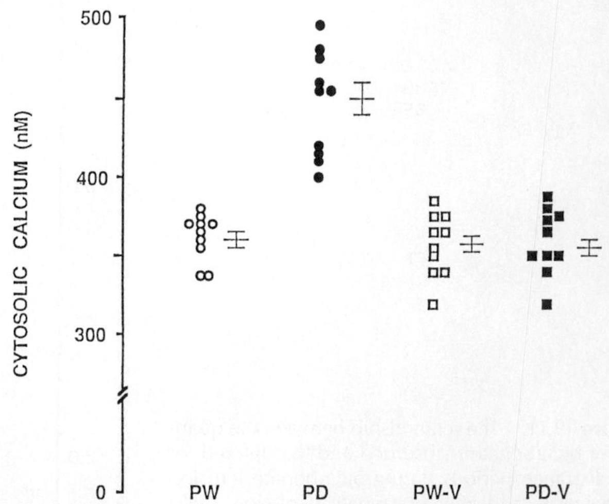

Figure 19.13. Cytosolic calcium of brain synaptosomes of phosphate-depleted rats *(PD)*, pair-weighed animals *(PW)*, and PD and PW rats treated with verapamil *(V)*. Each datum point represents one study and brackets denote mean ±1 SE. (Reproduced with permission from Massry SG, Hajjar SM, Koureta P, et al. Phosphate depletion increases cytosolic calcium of brain synaptosomes. *Am J Physiol* 1991;260:F12–F18.)

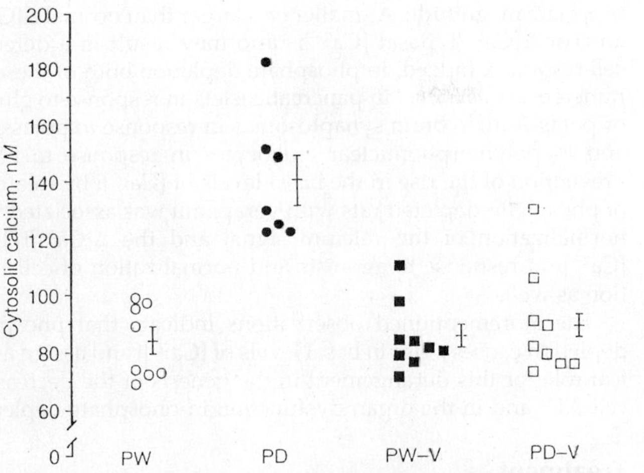

Figure 19.14. Cytosolic calcium of pancreatic islets of phosphate-depleted rats *(PD)*, pair-weighed animals *(PW)*, and PD and PW rats treated with verapamil *(V)*. Each datum point represents one study and brackets denote mean ±1 SE. (Reproduced with permission from Fadda GZ, Thanakitcharu P, Massry SG. Phosphate depletion reduces potassium-induced insulin secretion. *Proc Exp Biol Med* 1991;198:742–746.)

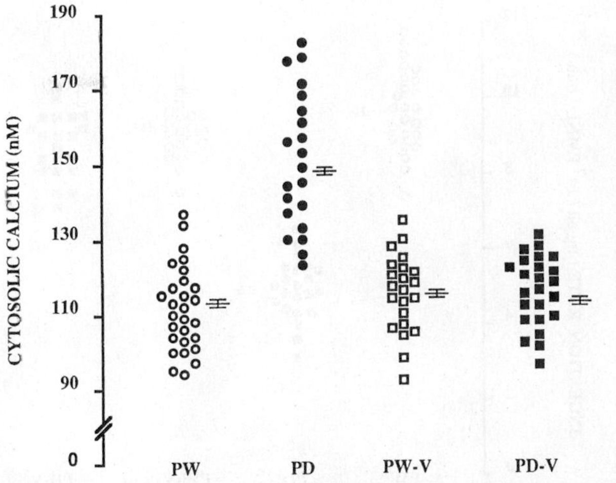

Figure 19.15. Cytosolic calcium of polymorphonuclear leukocytes of phosphate-depleted rats *(PD)*, pair-weighed animals *(PW)*, and PD and PW rats treated with verapamil *(V)*. Each datum point represents one study and brackets denote mean ±1 SE. (Reproduced with permission from Kiersztejn M, Chervu I, Smogorzewski M, et al. One mechanism of impaired phagocytosis in phosphate depletion. *J Am Soc Nephrol* 1992;2:1484–1489.)

Thus the available data are consistent with the notion that calcium entry into cells is increased and calcium extrusion out of the cells is decreased in phosphate depletion. These derangements lead to a rise in $[Ca^{2+}]i$, an event that inhibits mitochondrial oxidation and phosphorylation and hence reduces ATP production. Therefore it seems that the fall in ATP content of cells in phosphate depletion is not only due to the phosphorus deficiency per se, but also to the increase in $[Ca^{2+}]i$. The proposed model for these events is depicted in Fig. 19.16.

If an increase in calcium entry occurs in phosphate depletion and if this plays an important role in the sequence of events described in Fig. 19.16, one should be able to ameliorate or prevent these cellular derangements by blocking calcium entry into the cells. Indeed, the treatment of phosphate-depleted rats with the calcium channel blocker, verapamil, improved or normalized both the metabolic profile and the function of many cells such as ATP content, cytosolic calcium concentration, the activity of Ca^{2+}-ATPase and Na^+-K^+-ATPase, phospholipid profile,

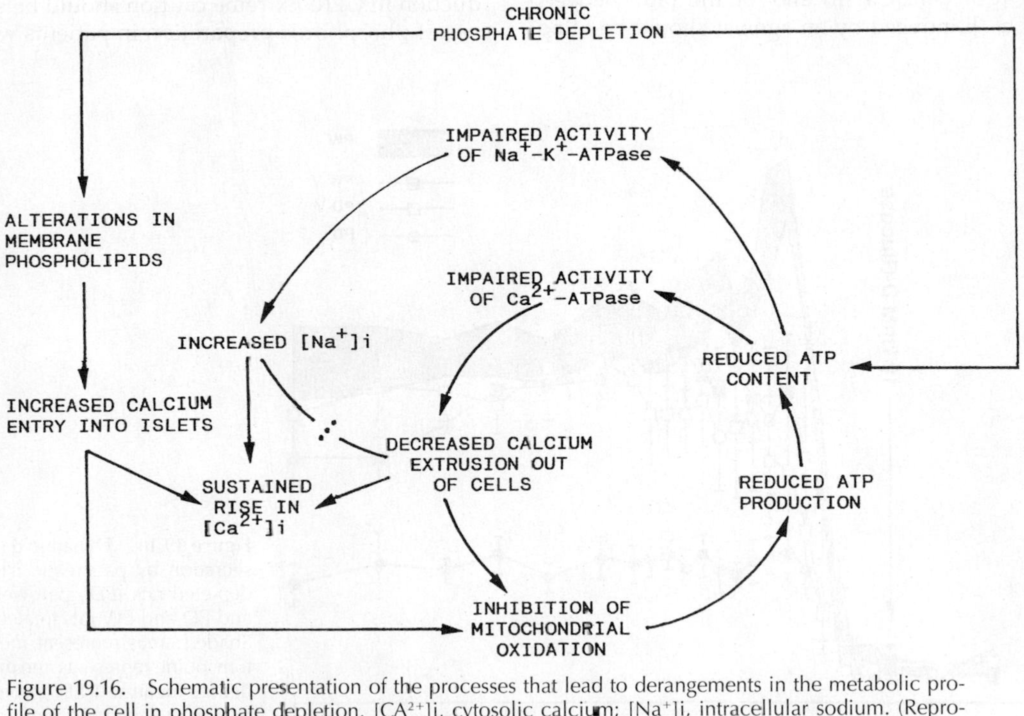

Figure 19.16. Schematic presentation of the processes that lead to derangements in the metabolic profile of the cell in phosphate depletion. $[CA^{2+}]i$, cytosolic calcium; $[Na^+]i$, intracellular sodium. (Reproduced with permission from Massry SG, Fadda GZ, Perna AF, et al. Mechanism of organ dysfunction in phosphate depletion: a critical role for a rise in cytosolic calcium. *Miner Electrolyte Metab* 1992;18:133–140.)

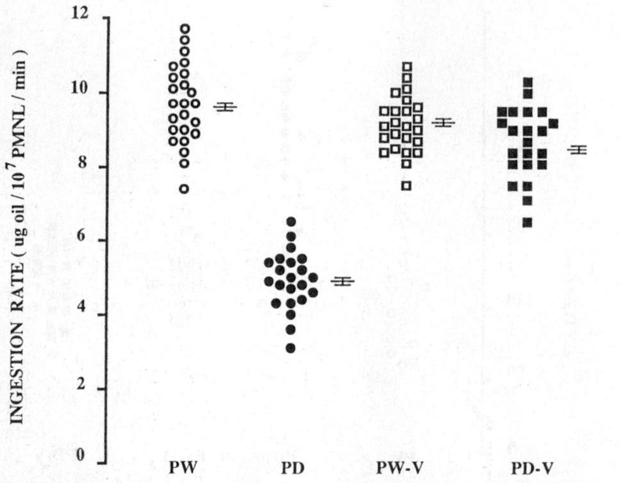

Figure 19.17. Ingestion of oil particles (phagocytosis) by polymorphonuclear leukocytes of phosphate-depleted rats *(PD),* pair-weighed animals *(PW),* and PD and PW rats treated with verapamil *(V).* Each datum point represents one study and brackets denote mean ±1 SE. (Reproduced with permission from Kiersztejn M, Chervu I, Smogorzewski M, et al. On the mechanism of impaired phagocytosis in phosphate depletion. *J Am Soc Nephrol* 1992;2:1484–1489.)

phagocytosis of polymorphonuclear leukocytes (Fig. 19.17), and insulin secretion by pancreatic islets (Fig. 19.18). Of special interest is the observation that despite chronic and marked phosphate depletion, cell ATP was either normal or only modestly reduced when the rise in $[Ca^{2+}]i$ was prevented by verapamil. This again points toward an important role for the rise in $[Ca^{2+}]i$ in the genesis of the decrease in ATP content of cells in phosphate depletion.

The elevation in basal levels of $[Ca^{2+}]i$ in phosphate depletion could also adversely affect cell function. Calcium serves as a second messenger in cell function, and for calcium to act as such, the rise in $[Ca^{2+}]i$ ($\Delta[Ca^{2+}]i$) and/or the ratio between $\Delta[Ca^{2+}]i$/basal $[Ca^{2+}]i$ induced by an agonist should be of appropriate magnitude. A smaller or a larger than normal $\Delta[Ca^{2+}]i$ and/or $\Delta[Ca^{2+}]i$/basal $[Ca^{2+}]i$ ratio may result in a defective cell response. Indeed, in phosphate depletion both of these parameters are *abnormal* in pancreatic islets in response to glucose or potassium, in brain synaptosomes in response to potassium, and in polymorphonuclear leukocytes in response to FMLP. Prevention of the rise in the basal levels of $[Ca^{2+}]i$ by treatment of phosphate-depleted rats with verapamil was associated with normalization of the calcium signal and the $\Delta[Ca^{2+}]i$/basal $[Ca^{2+}]i$ in response to agonists and normalization of cell function as well.

The aforementioned observations indicate that phosphate depletion causes a rise in basal levels of $[Ca^{2+}]i$ and assign a critical role for this derangement in the genesis of the decrease in cell ATP and in the organ dysfunction in phosphate depletion.

Treatment

Hypophosphatemia, per se, usually does not require emergency treatment, and its cause should first be determined. However, severe hypophosphatemia and phosphate depletion should be treated. If oral intake is possible, milk could be used because it is a good source of inorganic phosphorus (1 g or 33 mmol/L of milk). Oral phosphorus preparations (Table 19.12) could also be used. If the patient cannot take phosphorus supplementation by mouth, intravenous administration of phosphorus preparation (Table 19.12) should be used. Phosphorus preparations are not given intramuscularly.

The objective of the treatment of hypophosphatemia and phosphate depletion is to bring plasma phosphorus levels to normal (4.0 to 4.5 mg/dl) and to replenish body stores of phosphorus. Careful monitoring of plasma concentrations of phosphorus and calcium is essential during administration of phosphorus preparation to avoid the development of hyperphosphatemia, hypocalcemia, and soft tissue calcification. The dose of phosphorus given to patients with renal failure should be adjusted in proportion to the magnitude of the reduction in GFR. Extreme caution should be exercised with the use of phosphorus preparation in patients with oliguria.

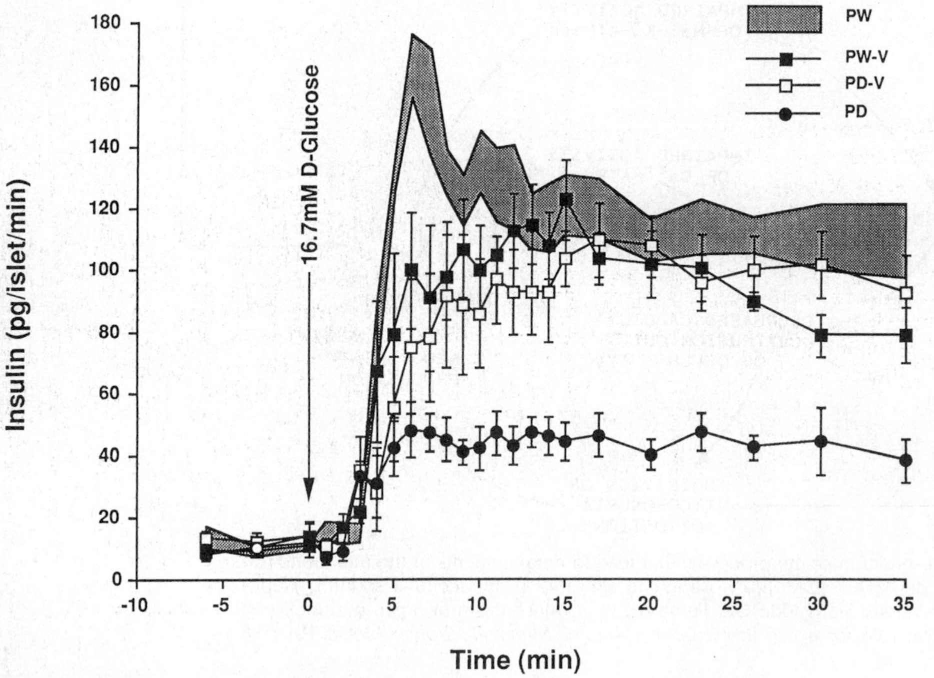

Figure 19.18. Dynamic data on glucose-insulin secretion by pancreatic islets from phosphate-depleted rats *(PD),* pair-weighed animals *(PW),* and PD and PW rats treated with verapamil *(V).* Shaded areas represent mean ±1 SE. Each datum point represents mean value and brackets denote mean ± 1 SE. (Reproduced with permission from Fadda GZ, Hajjar SM, Zhou X-J, et al. Verapamil corrects abnormal metabolism of pancreatic islets and insulin secretion in phosphate depletion. *Endocrinology* 1992;130:193–202.)

TABLE 19.12. Commonly Available Phosphorus-Containing Preparations

	Phosphorus	Sodium	Potassium	Remarks
	mg	*mEq*		
Oral preparations				
K-Phos Neutral tablets (Beach Pharmaceuticals)	250/tab	12/tab	2/tab	4 tablets provide 1,000 mg phosphorus, 48 mEq sodium, 8 mEq potassium
K-Phos tablets (Beach Pharmaceuticals)	114/tab		3.68/tab	9 tablets provide 1,000 mg phosphorus, 33 mEq potassium
Neutra-Phos-K capsules (Willen Drug Co.)	250/cap		14/cap	4 capsules deliver 1,000 mg phosphorus, 57 mEq potassium
Neutra-Phos capsules (Willen Drug Co.)	250/cap	7/cap	7/cap	4 capsules deliver 1,000 mg phosphorus, 28 mEq potassium, 28 mEq sodium
Fleet-Phospho-Soda (C. B. Fleet Co.)	149/ml	6/cap		6.7 ml deliver 1,000 mg phosphorus, 40 mEq potassium
	mg/ml	*mEq/ml*		
Parenteral preparations				
Sodium phosphate (Abbott Pharmaceuticals)	93	4	0	Available in 15-ml vial and 10.75 ml Delivers 1,000 mg phosphorus, 43 mEq sodium
Potassium phosphate (Abbott Pharmaceuticals)	93	0	4	Available in 5- and 15-ml vials and 10.75 ml. Delivers 1,000 mg phosphorus, 43 mEq potassium

In normal subjects, the administration of 1 g of inorganic phosphorus over a 6 hour period distributes in a volume equal to 40% of body weight. Therefore such an amount of phosphorus will increase plasma phosphorus by 3.5 mg/dl. In phosphate depletion, the exact volume of distribution of the administered phosphorus is not known. Therefore the amount of phosphorus required to treat patients with phosphate depletion should be titrated to the need of each individual patient. This is done by frequent monitoring of plasma phosphorus during the therapy, with appropriate adjustment of the phosphorus dose.

It is safe to start oral therapy with 1 g/day of inorganic phosphorus and intravenous therapy with 1 to 2 g of inorganic phosphorus delivered in a liter of fluids over 8 to 12 hours. Additional therapy and adjustment of the dose are dictated by the magnitude of the increment in plasma phosphorus during therapy.

HYPERPHOSPHATEMIA

Causes

Variable degrees of hyperphosphatemia are commonly encountered in clinical medicine. It usually is due to a decrease in urinary excretion of phosphorus with or without increased dietary intake of phosphorus and/or increased intestinal absorption of phosphorus. In addition, an increased shift of phosphorus from cells into extracellular space may cause hyperphosphatemia. The causes of hyperphosphatemia are listed in Table 19.13.

It must be emphasized that acute and chronic renal failure are the most common causes of hyperphosphatemia in clinical medicine. In acute renal failure and other oliguric states, hyperphosphatemia develops as a result of marked reduction in urinary phosphorus excretion. In patients with acute renal failure associated with rhabdomyolysis or other catabolic disorders, the hyperphosphatemia is severe, and plasma phosphorus levels in excess of 10 mg/dl are common. Phosphate homeostasis and the mechanisms of hyperphosphatemia in patients with chronic renal failure are discussed in detail in Chapter 77.

PTH is the major modulator of urinary phosphorus excretion. Therefore patients with hypoparathyroidism and those with resistance to the renal action of PTH (pseudohypoparathyroidism) have reduced urinary phosphorus excretion and hyperphosphatemia. *Growth hormone* enhances tubular reabsorption of phosphorus; in this regard the action of growth hormone is opposite to that of PTH. Patients with acromegaly and elevated blood levels of growth hormone have reduced urinary excretion of phosphorus and hyperphosphatemia.

Hyperphosphatemia, hypocalcemia, tetany, and cataract occurred in few patients with normal or elevated blood levels of PTH. In these patients, there is no resistance to the renal action of PTH, but rather the circulating PTH is ineffective as a result of a defect in conversion of PTH to the active form.

Hyperphosphatemia could follow increased administration of phosphorus salts, administration of vitamin D and its metabolites (which increases intestinal absorption of phosphate), or administration of etidronate to patients with Paget's disease. Indeed, hyperphosphatemia was noted in patients ingesting large amounts of phosphorus-containing laxatives or receiving

TABLE 19.13. Causes of Hyperphosphatemia

- Decreased renal excretion of phosphorus
  - Chronic renal failure
  - Acute renal failure
  - Hypoparathyroidism
  - Pseudohypoparathyroidism type I and type II
  - Abnormal circulating PTH
  - Acromegaly
  - Thyrotoxicosis[a]
  - Tumoral calcinosis
  - Biphosphonates therapy
- Increase in phosphorus release from tissues into the extracellular fluid
  - Therapy of myeloproliferative malignancy
  - Increased catabolism
  - Trauma, extensive burns
- Administration of phosphorus
- Administration of vitamin D and its metabolite
- Miscellaneous
  - Cortical hyperostosis
  - Intermittent hyperphosphatemia
  - Artifacts

[a] The hyperphosphatemia in thyrotoxicosis is mild. It is due to a direct effect of the thyroid hormone in enhancing phosphate reabsorption by the renal proximal tubule and to the suppression of the parathyroid gland secondary to the mild hypercalcemia that is frequently encountered in patients with thyrotoxicosis.
PTH, parathyroid hormone.

enemas containing large amounts of phosphorus salts. In a study of 143 patients who were given a total of 90 ml of Fleet-Phospho-Soda enemas for bowel preparation before elective colonoscopy, a significant rise in plasma phosphorus (mean of 3 mg/dl) was noted. Fatality has been reported in both children and adults as a consequence of severe hyperphosphatemia following the use of large amounts of Fleet-Phospho-Soda. Marked hypocalcemia and metabolic acidosis are consistent findings in severe phosphate intoxication. Risk factors for massive hyperphosphatemia after the use of these phosphate enemas include chronic renal failure and intestinal obstruction. Hyperphosphatemia also has been observed during therapy of the hypercalcemia of malignancy with intravenous phosphorus salts.

Another uncommon disease associated with hyperphosphatemia is *tumoral calcinosis.* This disease occurs in young African-Americans and is manifested by soft tissue calcification around large joints. The blood levels of PTH in these patients are normal, and their phosphaturic response to exogenous PTH is normal as well. The mechanisms of the hyperphosphatemia are not evident, but it has been suggested that these patients have an enhanced renal tubular reabsorption of phosphorus.

Catabolic conditions, trauma, and extensive burns are associated with tissue destruction and increased release of phosphorus from soft tissues into the extracellular space leading to the elevation of the plasma levels of phosphorus. The hyperphosphatemia will be more severe if these patients have impaired renal function as well. A similar phenomenon occurs during therapy of myeloproliferative malignancies. The tumor lysis is associated with increased release of phosphorus from the tumor cells into the extracellular space. Metabolic acidosis, and especially severe ketoacidosis, is associated with hyperphosphatemia. In contrast, hyperphosphatemia is not a feature of chronic respiratory acidosis.

Clinical Effects

Hyperphosphatemia may be associated with hypocalcemia, reduced blood levels of $1,25(OH)_2D$, secondary hyperparathyroidism, and soft tissue calcification. Hyperphosphatemia inhibits the conversion of $25(OH)_2D$ to $1,25(OH)_2D$ by the kidney, leading to a decrease in the blood levels of $1,25(OH)_2D$. Hyperphosphatemia directly, or indirectly through the reduction in the blood levels of $1,25(OH)_2D$, causes hypocalcemia. The latter in combination with the reduction in the blood levels of $1,25(OH)_2D$ induces the stimulation of the parathyroid gland activity leading to secondary hyperparathyroidism.

Persistent and significant hyperphosphatemia increases the calcium–phosphorus product. When this product exceeds 70, soft tissue calcification may develop. This phenomenon assumes significant importance in the genesis of soft tissue calcification in patients with advanced chronic renal failure (see Chapter 77). Severe hyperphosphatemia is frequently associated with metabolic acidosis.

Treatment

Hyperphosphatemia is treated by reduction of dietary intake of phosphorus and by the use of phosphorus-binding drugs that render phosphorus unabsorbable by the intestine. The details of the management of hyperphosphatemia including the various preparations of the phosphorus-binding antacids used for the treatment of hyperphosphatemia are provided in Chapter 77. Medical suppression of the parathyroid gland activity or subtotal parathyroidectomy would correct the hyperphosphatemia in patients with advanced chronic renal failure.

Selected Readings

Barak V, Schwartz A, Kalickman I, et al. Prevalence of hypophosphatemia in sepsis and infection: the role of cytokines. *Am J Med* 1998;104:40–47.

A study of 99 patients with infection. These patients displayed hypophosphatemia and elevated blood levels of cytokines. There was a correlation between the high blood levels of the inflammatory cytokines and hypophosphatemia.

Brautbar N, Baczynski R, Carpenter C, et al. Biochemical alterations in rat myocardium during phosphate depletion. *Am J Physiol* 1982;242:F699–F704.

Studies in rats demonstrating that phosphate depletion causes impaired energy production, shuttle, and utilization by the myocardium. Phosphate depletion causes a fall in myocardial content of inorganic phosphorus, ATP, and creatine phosphate; impaired mitochondrial oxidation; and reduced activity of mitochondrial and myofibrillar creatine phosphokinase.

Brautbar N, Carpenter C, Baczynski R, et al. Impaired energy metabolism in skeletal muscle during phosphate depletion. *Kidney Int* 1983;24:53–57.

Studies in phosphate-depleted rats demonstrating reduced content of inorganic phosphorus, impaired mitochondrial oxidation, and diminished mitochondrial and myofibrillar activity of creatine kinase in skeletal muscle.

Brautbar N, Leibovici H, Massry SG. On the mechanism of hypophosphatemia during acute hyperventilation: evidence for increased muscle glycolysis. *Miner Electrolyte Metab* 1983;9:45–50.

Studies in dogs demonstrating that increased muscle glycolysis and acute hypophosphatemia occur during acute hyperventilation. The study also shows that glucose administration during hyperventilation is required for a marked fall in plasma phosphorus to occur.

Coburn JW, Massry SG. Changes in serum and urinary calcium during phosphate depletion: studies on mechanisms. *J Clin Invest* 1970;49:1073–1087.

A study examining in detail the mechanisms of phosphate depletion–induced hypercalciuria in dogs.

Cohen SM, Waxner SD, Binderow SR, et al. Prospective, randomized, endoscopic-blinded trial comparing precolonoscopy bowel cleansing methods. *Dis Colon Rectum* 1994;37:689–699.

A study demonstrating the frequency of hyperphosphatemia following the use of Fleet-Phospho-Soda for intestinal preparation before rectocolonoscopic examination.

Fadda GZ, Hajjar SM, Zhou X-J, et al. Verapamil corrects abnormal metabolism of pancreatic islets and insulin secretion in phosphate depletion. *Endocrinology* 1992;130:193–202.

A detailed study in rats examining the disturbances in function and metabolism of pancreatic islets in phosphate depletion and the effect of verapamil on these abnormalities.

Gold LW, Massry SG, Arieff AI, et al. Renal bicarbonate wasting during phosphate depletion: a possible cause of altered acid-base homeostasis in hyperparathyroidism. *J Clin Invest* 1973;52:2556–2562.

A study demonstrating impaired renal tubular reabsorption of bicarbonate in phosphate-depleted dogs.

Gold LW, Massry SG, Friedler RM. Effect of phosphate depletion on renal tubular reabsorption of glucose. *J Lab Clin Med* 1977;89:554–559.

A study demonstrating impaired renal tubular reabsorption of glucose in phosphate-depleted dogs. The authors also showed that hyperglycemia developed during phosphate depletion.

Kiersztejn M, Chervu I, Smogorzewski M, et al. On the mechanism of impaired phagocytosis in phosphate depletion. *J Am Soc Nephrol* 1992;2:1484–1489.

A study in rats demonstrating that phosphate depletion is associated with impaired phagocytosis, reduced ATP content, and increased cytosolic calcium of polymorphonuclear leukocytes. Treatment of the phosphate-depleted rats with verapamil normalized phagocytosis and cytosolic calcium and improved ATP content of these cells.

Knochel JP. The pathophysiology and clinical characteristics of severe hypophosphatemia. *Arch Intern Med* 1977;137:203–220.

An excellent review of the pathophysiology, clinical manifestations, and therapy of hypophosphatemia and phosphate depletion.

Lotz M, Ney R, Bartter FC. Osteomalacia and debility resulting from phosphorus depletion. *Trans Assoc Am Physicians* 1964;77:281–295.

The first description of phosphate depletion syndrome in humans.

Marcinkowski W, Smogorzewski M, Zhang G, et al. Renal mRNA of PTH-PTHrP receptor, $[Ca^{2+}]$i and phosphaturic response to PTH in phosphate depletion. *Miner Elect Metab* 1997;23:48–57.

A study demonstrating in phosphate-depleted rats a rise in basal levels of cytosolic calcium in their renal proximal tubule and downregulation of the mRNA of PTH–PTHrP receptor in these cells. Treatment of these rats with verapamil corrected these derangements.

Massry SG, Fadda GZ, Perna AF, et al. Mechanism of organ dysfunction in phosphate depletion: a critical role for a rise in cytosolic calcium. *Miner Electrolyte Metab* 1992;18:133–140.

A detailed discussion of the role of elevated cytosolic calcium in the genesis of organ dysfunction in phosphate depletion.

Massry SG, Hajjar SM, Koureta P, et al. Phosphate depletion increases cytosolic calcium of brain synaptosomes. *Am J Physiol* 1991;260:F12–F18.

The first demonstration that phosphate depletion is associated with an elevation of basal levels of cytosolic calcium. The authors also examined the mechanism underlying the rise in cytosolic calcium. They found that both calcium entry and exit from brain synaptosomes are impaired.

Mitnick PD, Goldfarb S, Slatopolsky E, et al. Calcium and phosphate metabolism in tumoral calcinosis. *Ann Intern Med* 1980;92:482.

A study emphasizing that abnormalities in urinary calcium and phosphorus excretion play an important role in the pathogenesis of tumoral calcinosis.

Saglikes Y, Massry SG, Iseki K, et al. Effect of phosphate depletion on blood pressure and vascular reactivity to norepinephrine and angiotensin. *Am J Physiol* 1985;248:F93–F99.

A study demonstrating low blood pressure and reduced pressor response to norepinephrine and angiotensin II in phosphate-depleted rats.

Slatopolsky E, Rutherford WE, Rosenhaum R, et al. Hyperphosphatemia. *Clin Nephrol* 1977;7:138–146.

An excellent review of hyperphosphatemia, its pathogenesis, and the clinical conditions associated with it.

Smogorzewski M, Islam A, Koureta P, et al. Reduced phospholipid content of brain synaptosomes in phosphate depletion. *Am J Physiol* 1991;261:E742–E747.

A study demonstrating in the rat that the phospholipids of brain synaptosomes are decreased in phosphate depletion.

Travis SF, Sugerman HJ, Ruberg RL, et al. Alterations of red cell glycolytic intermediates and oxygen transport as a consequence of hypophosphatemia in patients receiving intravenous hyperalimentation. *N Engl J Med* 1971;285:763–768.

A study of the changes in red cell metabolism during hypophosphatemia and the effect of these changes on oxygen transport by the red cells.

CHAPTER 20

Acid–Base Metabolism

PART 1

Normal Chemistry and Physiology of Acid–Base Homeostasis

Horacio J. Adrogué

Acid–base homeostasis involves chemical and physiologic processes responsible for the maintenance of the acidity of body fluids at levels that allow optimal function of the whole individual. The chemical processes represent the first line of defense to an acid or alkali load and include the extracellular and intracellular buffers; the physiologic processes modulate acid–base composition by changes in cellular metabolism and by adaptive responses in the excretion of volatile acids by the lungs and fixed acids by the kidneys. The need for the existence of multiple mechanisms involved in acid–base regulation stems from the critical importance of the hydrogen ion (H^+) concentration on the operation of many cellular enzymes and function of vital organs, most prominently the brain and the heart. The task imposed on the mechanisms that maintain acid–base homeostasis is large because metabolic pathways are continuously consuming or producing H^+, and the daily load of waste products for excretion in the form of volatile and fixed acids is substantial. This part of the chapter will examine the determinants of the acidity of body fluids, the mechanisms that maintain normal acid–base composition, and the overall defense to disruption in acid–base equilibrium.

MEASURES OF ACIDITY

Measurement of acid–base balance (and acid excretion) is routinely expressed in millimole (mmol or 10^{-3} mol), whereas that of plasma acidity uses nanomole (nmol or 10^{-9} mol). The strikingly larger unit that quantifies balance in comparison with that of plasma composition is characteristic of H^+ but not of other ions such as sodium, potassium, and chloride. The reason for the use of different units when the concentration of H^+ in body fluids is measured is that although major ions are largely freely dissolved in body fluids, a very small fraction of H^+ is free in solution; the bulk of the acid load produced by tissues is bound to body buffers and/or transported as plasma bicarbonate in the case of volatile acids (carbonic acid). Consequently, the plasma [H^+] is maintained at levels that are approximately 1 million times smaller than those of most anions and cations of extracellular fluid.

Acidity of body fluids may be expressed as a molar concentration such as nanomoles per liter (10^{-9} mol/L) or as a pH value, the latter being the negative logarithm of H^+ activity of a solution in which [H^+] is expressed in mol/L. Yet measurement of acidity is always performed by means of a glass pH electrode. The glass chosen allows protons (H^+) but not other ions to diffuse through it. The glass of the electrode is interposed between the sample to be tested and a known buffer solution. The proton gradient between the sample and the buffer solution creates an electrical potential, which is measured and whose magnitude is proportional to the proton gradient, and that is thus dependent on the [H^+] in the sample to be tested. The pH electrode measures the H^+ "activity" but not the H^+ concentration. In an ideal diluted solution the lack of significant interaction between ions results in a ratio between "activity" and concentration equal to one. Because the [H^+] in most body fluids is very low (i.e., the behavior of H^+ resembles that found in an ideal solution), it is appropriate to equate activity to concentration of H^+.

The major difference between expressing the acidity of a solution in nmol/L and pH units is that the former uses an arithmetic scale, whereas the pH notation is a logarithmic scale. Thus, when acidity is expressed in pH units, due to the logarithmic scale, conceptualization of quantitative changes in acidity can become difficult. For example, a change in pH from 7.40 to 7.10 represents an increase in [H^+] from 40 nmol/L to 80 nmol/L (i.e., 100% increase). Because the first step of a thoughtful approach to reach the correct acid–base diagnosis is to establish the presence of internal consistency of the acid–base data using the Henderson equation, pH values must be converted to [H^+] in nmol/L. Thus any of the three commonly used methods to make this conversion can be applied. The first method, which is the most precise, is as follows: the pH value under study must be first subtracted from 9.00 and its antilog subsequently obtained to convert pH values to [H^+] in nmol/L (nEq/L). The reverse, to convert [H^+] in nmol/L to pH, is accomplished by obtaining first the log of the nmol/L value under study and then subtracting it from 9.00. The rationale for subtracting from 9.00 when expressing acidity in nmol/L is that pH 9.00 represents the start of the scale and amounts to 1 nmol/L (10^{-9} mol/L). For example, the [H^+] for a pH of 7.15 is calculated as follows:

we must first subtract 7.15 from 9.00, which is 1.85; then we should obtain the antilog of 1.85, which is 71; thus a pH of 7.15 is equivalent to a $[H^+]$ of 71 nmol/L. A second method is to apply the rule whereby for each 0.01 pH unit below or above its normal value, 1 nmol/L is respectively added or subtracted. Because a pH of 7.40 is equal to 40 nmol/L (nEq/L) of $[H^+]$, pH values of 7.50 and 7.30 correspond to $[H^+]$ of 30 and 50 nmol/L, respectively. This rule is relatively accurate for a limited range of pH of about 0.2 pH units below and above the normal value (7.20 to 7.60). It must be recognized, however, that this rule is inaccurate for extreme deviations of pH, and therefore should not be used in those circumstances. A third method of converting pH values to $[H^+]$ in nmol/L is the 80% method (or 0.8 method), which is useful for any blood pH value and does not require a calculator with a logarithmic capability. This method requires remembering that a pH of 7.40 and one of 7.00 correspond to $[H^+]$ of 40 nmol/L and 100 nmol/L, respectively. For an increase in pH equal to 0.10 units, one must multiply the $[H^+]$ by 0.8. For example, the $[H^+]$ for a pH of 7.10 and one of 7.20 are 80 nmol/L and 64 nmol/L, respectively. These values are obtained by multiplying 0.8×100 nmol/L ($[H^+]$ for a pH of 7.00) for the former, and $0.8 \times 0.8 \times 100$ nmol/L for the latter. The 80% method is reliable and has practical value.

BODY BUFFERS AS DETERMINANTS OF PLASMA ACIDITY

The relative stability of the pH of body fluids despite the continuous production of sizeable quantities of acid by metabolism in health and disease is fully dependent on the presence of large amounts of body buffers. A buffer is a compound that ameliorates the change in acidity that would otherwise occur in response to the addition of acid or alkali to a solution. A meaningful example of biologic buffering was provided by the classic experiments of Robert Pitts. He compared the addition of identical amounts of HCl to the blood stream of a dog and to a receptacle with distilled water identical in volume to that of the dog's body fluids. Although the pH of the dog's blood decreased only to 7.14, the pH of the distilled water decreased to 1.84. The dramatic fall in the pH of the water contained in the receptacle was due to the fact that water cannot neutralize the hydrogen ions released by the strong acid. The presence of large amounts of buffers, including the bicarbonate and nonbicarbonate body buffer systems, in the dog's fluids ameliorated the change in blood pH. The bicarbonate stores, extracellular and intracellular, were titrated to carbonic acid (H_2CO_3) by the acid load and were subsequently decomposed to CO_2 and water; the excess CO_2 was excreted by the lungs. Thus the following reaction took place:

$$H^+ + HCO_3^- \leftrightarrow H_2CO_3 \leftrightarrow CO_2 + H_2O$$

In addition, the nonbicarbonate buffers such as hemoglobin and other proteins, and intracellular as well as bone phosphate (HPO_4^{2-}) salts, were titrated to their acid forms. This buffer reaction proceeded as follows:

$$A^- + H^+ + Buf^- + Na^+ \text{ (or } K^+ \text{ or } Ca^{2+})^* \leftrightarrow Buf\,H + A^- + Na^+ \text{ (or } K^+ \text{ or } Ca^{2+})$$

These chemical processes of buffering of the acid load depleted the body reserves of buffer base because the level of bicarbonate stores decreased and nonbicarbonate buffers were titrated to their acidic form. Consequently, physiologic processes are recruited, which restore the body reserves of buffer base to their normal level. These physiologic processes, namely the excretion of carbonic acid by the lungs and the excretion of fixed acid/base by the kidneys correct the level and composition of body buffers to their initial state before the acid/base load. It is evident therefore that body buffers are not only the initial line of defense to an acid or alkali load but they are the final line of defense because the action of physiologic processes (i.e., role of the lung and kidney) consist in the restoration of body buffers to their normal state.

The effects of an acid or alkali load derived from any source will alter the composition of the various body buffers, which will subsequently interact with each other according to the isohydric principle. This postulate dictates that the acid–base ratio of all the different buffer pairs present in body fluids (e.g., H_2CO_3-HCO_3^-, $H_2PO_4^-$-HPO_4^{2-}, protein H^+–protein$^-$) is altered in a predictable manner in response to a change in $[H^+]$ of these fluids. The law of mass action is defined by the following formula for the case of $[H^+]$:

$$[H^+] = K_2 \frac{[HA]}{[A^-]}$$

If several buffers are in solution, the relationships among the buffer pairs are as follows:

$$[H^+] = K_{a1} \frac{[H_2CO_3]}{[HCO_3^-]} = \frac{K_{a2}\,[H_2PO_4^-]}{[HPO_4^{2-}]} = K_{a3} \frac{[Protein\ H^+]}{[Protein^-]}$$

where K_{a1}, K_{a2}, and K_{a3} are the respective dissociation constants for each buffer pair. Because the buffer pair quantified in clinical practice to assess acid–base status is the H_2CO_3/HCO_3^-, we use the following formula (Henderson equation):

$$[H^+] = 24 \frac{P_{CO_2}}{[HCO_3^-]}$$

To obtain hydrogen ion activity as pH, the equation is modified by taking the negative logarithm of each side of the equation:

$$pH = 6.1 + \log \frac{[HCO_3^-]}{0.03 \times P_{CO_2}}$$

In the Henderson equation, the $[H^+]$ is expressed in nmol/L, P_{CO_2} in mm Hg, and $[HCO_3^-]$ in mmol/L.

BICARBONATE AND NONBICARBONATE BUFFER SYSTEMS

The physiologic control of $[H^+]$ in humans is not exerted by a direct effect on the pH of body fluids. Instead, acidity is modulated by altering the levels of the components that determine $[H^+]$, namely partial pressure of carbon dioxide (P_{CO_2}) and bicarbonate concentration; whereas P_{CO_2} is regulated by the lungs, the $[HCO_3^-]_p$ is regulated by the kidneys. It must be recognized that the level of P_{CO_2} in body fluids is determined by the relationship between CO_2 production by the tissues and its excretion by the lungs; the latter excrete the CO_2 produced from tissue metabolism that is present in body fluids as dissolved CO_2 and carbonic acid. Thus CO_2 excretion by the lungs maintains a constant P_{CO_2} level in arterial blood and thereby limits the accumulation of carbonic acid. With respect to the concentration of bicarbonate in body fluids, its steady-state value results from ongoing processes that decompose HCO_3^-, counterbalanced by other processes that regenerate it. The major component of bicarbonate decomposition is the release of fixed acids derived from cellular metabolism, whereas regeneration of bicarbonate stores is accomplished by proton consuming metabolic pathways and the excretion of acid by the kidneys.

*Any cation other than H^+.

The relative strength of a buffer system in the defense of pH is quantified by the so-called buffer value. The buffer value of a solution is the amount of acid or alkali required to alter the acidity of a solution by 1 pH unit. It is expressed in units called Slykes (sl) in honor of Donald van Slyke and they are equivalent to mEq/L per pH unit. When the bicarbonate buffer system is compared with the nonbicarbonate buffer system in terms of buffer value, a substantial difference in the strength of buffer action is found. The buffer value of HCO_3^- is 2.3 sl/mmol, whereas that of HPO_4^{2-} is only 0.58 sl/mmol so that the molar buffer value of HCO_3^- is four times that of ordinary buffers like HPO_4^{2-}. The mechanism responsible for the 4-fold enhancement in the buffer value of bicarbonate is the disappearance of the acid (as CO_2 gas), resulting from acid titration of HCO_3^-, which occurs only with the H_2CO_3-HCO_3^- system but not with ordinary buffers, because the acid form of the buffer pair of ordinary buffers remains in solution. To better understand this most valuable characteristic of the H_2CO_3-HCO_3^- system, let us further compare its response with an acid load and that of nonbicarbonate buffers to a similar challenge. We should remember that the $[H^+]$ of body fluids is determined by the ratio of the components of any buffer pair; for example, the ratio of H_2CO_3 to HCO_3^- as dictated by the Henderson equation previously discussed. An acid load typically diminishes the denominator (i.e., A^-, HPO_4^{2-}, protein$^-$) and increases the numerator (i.e., HA, $H_2PO_4^-$, protein H^+) of this ratio to the same degree. Thus with standard buffer systems including the so-called non-HCO_3^- buffers, the ratio is changed by both the decrease in the denominator and the increase in the numerator. Although this concept is true for most buffer systems including the body proteins and HPO_4^{2-}, the H_2CO_3-HCO_3^- system is an exception. Because the numerator is in equilibrium with a gas in an open system and therefore does not accumulate (P_{CO_2}), the change in $[H^+]$ is exclusively the result of a decrease in the denominator ($[HCO_3^-]$). The release of the acid form (carbonic acid) of the buffer pair from the solution substantially increases the buffer value of this system. A second major characteristic that makes the H_2CO_3-HCO_3^- system particularly valuable as a buffer in humans relates to the existence of independent physiologic regulation of the numerator of this ratio by the lungs and that of the denominator by the kidneys. A primary alteration in one component (i.e., decreased HCO_3^- stores due to an acid load) elicits a secondary alteration in the other component (i.e., prompt decrease in P_{CO_2} after an acid load, the so-called respiratory response to acidemia) that would tend to preserve the ratio of the buffer pair, and therefore a more stable pH level. A third major characteristic that makes the H_2CO_3-HCO_3^- system particularly valuable is that the size of this buffer system is large enough to provide approximately 600 mEq of bicarbonate to neutralize an equally large acid load.

A load of fixed acids (as opposed to the volatile carbonic acid) titrates the bicarbonate and the nonbicarbonate buffer systems of all body compartments, including the intracellular and extracellular fluids. Yet as shown in the classic studies of Pitts, two-thirds of an administered load of fixed acids is buffered intracellularly. Although the buffer value of fluids within and outside cells is similar when expressed per liter (approximately 64 slykes), the larger intracellular fluid in comparison with the extracellular fluid (ratio is 2:1) accounts for the greater contribution of the intracellular buffers. It should be recognized that despite the similar buffer value of intracellular fluid and extracellular fluid, the fractional contribution of bicarbonate and nonbicarbonate buffers in each fluid is substantially different. Whereas HCO_3^- accounts for approximately 36% of the intracellular fluid buffer value, the non-HCO_3^- buffers (e.g., proteins, HPO_4^{2-}) account for approximately 64% of this value. The contribution of HCO_3^- to the buffer value of extracellular fluid is very large, amounting to approximately 86%, and the remaining approximate 14% is due to non-HCO_3^- buffers. Thus the fractional contribution of the two buffer systems differs substantially in extracellular fluid with respect to intracellular fluid.

In contrast with the response to a load of fixed acids, which titrates the bicarbonate as well as the nonbicarbonate buffer systems, the volatile carbonic acid challenges exclusively the nonbicarbonate buffer system. Thus the non-HCO_3^- buffer system can be precisely assessed by titration with CO_2 gas as follows:

$$CO_2 + H_2O \leftrightarrow H_2CO_3 \leftrightarrow H^+ + HCO_3^-$$
$$HCO_3^- + H^+ + Buf^- \leftrightarrow HBuf + HCO_3^-$$

In this reaction, the newly generated H^+ resulting from the dissociation of H_2CO_3 is picked up by non-HCO_3^- buffers. The amount of HCO_3^- that is generated during the CO_2 titration is identical to the amount of H^+ removed from the body fluids by the non-HCO_3^- buffers. Therefore the change in plasma $[HCO_3^-]$ per unit change in P_{CO_2} ($\Delta[HCO_3^-]_p$/mm Hg) or per unit change in blood pH ($\Delta[HCO_3^-]_p$/pH) quantifies the buffering response of non-HCO_3^- buffers.

Among the major buffer systems involved in the *in vivo* response to an acid load, in addition to those present in the extracellular and intracellular fluids, are the bone carbonates. This reserve of alkali stored in the skeleton amounts to a total of approximately 35,000 mEq in an adult and contributes significantly to the buffering capacity of the body. It has been estimated that approximately 40% of the buffering of an acute acid load occurs in the bones. The proton acceptance by the skeleton is accompanied by the release of Ca^{2+} or Na^+; alternatively, HPO_4^{2-} uptake by bone tissues from the extracellular fluid may accompany the H^+ acceptance. Patients with chronic metabolic acidosis, especially in the presence of chronic renal failure, develop a major depletion of skeleton mineral content that is partly the result of buffering of H^+ by bone carbonates.

PROTON GENERATION, CONSUMPTION, AND EXCRETION

The equilibrium reaction of water and CO_2, the end product of oxidative metabolism, results in the daily formation of large amounts of carbonic acid. As previously discussed, buffering of carbonic acid is accomplished exclusively by the nonbicarbonate buffer system, hemoglobin being the principal buffer involved in this reaction, whereas other proteins and phosphates play a minor role. Hemoglobin has unique features that facilitate this task, namely its increase in buffer value by deoxygenation and the direct binding of CO_2 forming carbaminohemoglobin. The increased buffer capacity of hemoglobin that occurs with the release of oxygen in peripheral tissues, known as *Haldane effect*, allows the transport of CO_2 to the lungs with only a minimal effect on blood pH. In other terms, due to the Haldane effect, at any given P_{CO_2} more CO_2 can be carried by reduced blood than by oxygenated blood. Conversely, adding carbon dioxide or hydrogen ions to blood decreases the oxygen-binding affinity of hemoglobin, a phenomenon known as the *Bohr effect*. The interactions between the Haldane and Bohr effects promote optimal transport of both oxygen and carbon dioxide, enlarging the difference in oxygen content between arterial and venous blood and reducing the arteriovenous P_{CO_2} gradient. It is estimated that these interactions account for up to 40% of the tissue CO_2 unloading and 20% of tissue O_2 uptake. The acceptance of the H^+ derived from carbonic acid by hemoglobin results in the transformation of carbonic acid into bicarbonate, and this ion transports approximately 80% of the CO_2 added to the blood from the peripheral tissues to the lungs. The higher $[HCO_3^-]$ in venous blood than in arterial blood is precisely due to the CO_2 released from the tissues and added to the blood for its ultimate excretion into the atmosphere. Venous blood $[HCO_3^-]$ is about 2 mEq/L (mmol/L) higher than the arterial value and this arteriovenous difference of $[HCO_3^-]$ may be used to estimate the daily rate of carbonic acid production. The product of the arteriovenous difference of $[HCO_3^-]$/L of blood and the cardiac output in L/min yields the CO_2 production in mmol/L. This value multiplied by 1,440 min provides the daily CO_2 production in mmol. Thus 2 mEq/L × 5 L/min of cardiac output × 1,440 min/day = 14,400 mEq/day (approximately 15,000 mEq/day carbonic acid production). As red cells reach the lungs and oxygen is taken up by hemoglobin, H^+ is released, decomposing bicarbonate into CO_2 that diffuses into the alveoli for final excretion. The presence of carbonic anhydrase in red cells facilitates bicarbonate generation in peripheral tissues and decomposition in the lungs, speeding up the mechanisms of blood CO_2 loading and unloading.

The daily production of fixed acids, commonly referred to as *endogenous acid production*, is approximately 70 to 100 mEq/day (approximately 1.0 to 1.5 mEq of H^+/kg body weight per day) and are removed from body fluids by the kidney according to the classic interpretation. Consequently, the daily production of volatile acid of approximately 15,000 mEq/day is approximately 200-fold that of fixed acids and explains the development of severe acidemia due to CO_2 retention within minutes of a respiratory arrest. It takes days to reach a comparable deviation of acidity as a result of retention of fixed acids in the absence of renal function. The endogenous acid production is mostly composed of waste products and other substances derived from the intermediate metabolism of energy-rich compounds. The relatively small net daily production of acids (70 to 100 mEq/day) in the normal state occurs in the presence of a large proton generation and proton consumption in major metabolic pathways of carbohydrates, lipids, and proteins. Glycolysis is the proton producing pathway from carbohydrates, leading to the synthesis of lactic or pyruvic acids. Conversely, regeneration of glucose from lactic acid or complete oxidation of the latter to CO_2 and water consumes hydrogen ions (Table 20.1). It has been estimated that approximately 1,300 mmol of lactate and H^+ enter the circulation in a resting 70-kg subject every 24 hours and an almost identical amount of this organic acid is removed by the tissues, mostly the liver. A large imbalance between synthesis and consumption of lactic acid is responsible for the development of various forms of lactic acidosis.

Lipolysis in peripheral tissues produces fatty acids, which in turn can undergo partial oxidation leading to the formation of ketoacids. Proton production through these pathways amounts to approximately 300 mmol/day in normal individuals, and an almost identical quantity of these acids is consumed with the synthesis of triglyceride and fatty acids (Table 20.1). However, a large imbalance between degradation and synthesis of body fats is observed in states of diabetic, alcoholic, or starving ketoacidosis.

Disposal of ammonium (NH_4^+) during oxidation of amino acids in an individual with a 100 g of dietary protein intake generates approximately 1,000 mmol/day of H^+ by the liver in the process of urea synthesis. However, an identical H^+ load is consumed in body tissues with complete oxidation of the carbon skeletons of amino acids if the protein entirely consists of neutral amino acids. During oxidation, dicarboxylic amino acids (glutamate and aspartate) generate 2 HCO_3^- for each NH_4^+, whereas basic amino acids (e.g., lysine) generate 2 NH_4^+ for each HCO_3^- (Table 20.1). Excess protons also are produced during degradation of sulfur-containing amino acids by the oxidation of sulfur. In well-fed subjects the type of proteins in the diet largely account for differences in the net daily production of fixed acids. Conversely, in starved subjects the use of endogenous proteins determine the net acid production from this energy source. An imbalance between the proton load generated by urea synthesis and the bicarbonate production from oxidation of the carbon skeletons of amino acids can lead to a deviation of the normal acid–base status. Furthermore, states of abnormal acid–base composition have a major influence on proton generation and consumption in major metabolic pathways, as described later in this chapter.

Acidemia of both metabolic and respiratory origin inhibits glycolysis, whereas alkalemia stimulates it. This effect is mediated, at least in part, by the pH-sensitive enzyme phosphofructokinase, that plays a key rate-limiting role in glycolysis. Acidemia also stimulates renal lactate utilization, but inhibits hepatic lactate utilization. In addition, acid–base balance alters ketoacid metabolism in a comparable manner to that of lactic acid. A low systemic pH inhibits ketoacid production, whereas a high pH stimulates it. Consequently, there is a pH feedback control of endogenous acid production. Under conditions of excessive lactic or ketoacid production, the resultant acidemia feeds back to inhibit the rate of endogenous acid production, thereby serving as a protective mechanism. Similarly, amino acids oxidation is significantly altered in response to changes in systemic acidity. Hepatic urea synthesis and its associated proton generation (two H^+ are generated per molecule of urea synthesized) is inhibited by a low systemic pH. Conversely, alkalemia stimulates urea synthesis and therefore leads to increased proton generation facilitating correction of the altered systemic acidity. Acidemia also has a direct effect on the kidney

TABLE 20.1. Overview of H^+-Producing and H^+-Consuming Pathways in the Metabolism of Carbohydrates, Fats, and Proteins (i.e., amino acids)

	H^+-Producing Pathways	H^+-Consuming Pathways
Carbohydrates	Glucose → 2 Lactate + $2H^+$ Lactate + NAD^+ → Pyruvate + NADH + H^+	2 Lactate + $2H^+$ → Glucose 2 Lactate + $2H^+$ + $6O_2$ → $6CO_2$ + $6H_2O$
Fat stores	Triglyceride → 3 Fatty acid anions + $3H^+$ Palmitate + $6O_2$ → 4 Ketone anions + $3H^+$ + $2H_2O$	3 Fatty acid anions + $3H^+$ → Triglyceride 4 Ketone anions + $3H^+$ + $2H_2O$ → Palmitate Ketone anions + H^+ → CO_2 + H_2O
Proteins	2 NH_4^+ + CO_2 → Urea + $2H^+$ + H_2O (neutral AA: 1NH_4^+; dicarboxylic AA: 1NH_4^+; basic AA: 2NH_4^+)	AA → HCO_3^- (neutral AA: 1HCO_3^-; dicarboxylic AA: 2HCO_3^-; basic AA: 1HCO_3^-)

AA, amino acids.

TABLE 20.2. Effects and Consequences of Acidemia on H^+-Producing Pathways from Oxidation of Protein (i.e., amino acids)

	Direct Effect			Indirect Effect		Consequences
Kidney	Increases urinary NH_4^+ excretion	→	Liver	Reduces supply of NH_4^+ for urea synthesis	→	Alkalinizing effect secondary to decreased H^+ production
Liver	Alters nitrogen disposal pathways:			↑		
	Augments glutamine synthesis delivering substrate to kidney	→	Kidney	Increased urinary NH_4^+ excretion		
	Decreases urea synthesis				→	Alkalizing effect secondary to decreased H^+ production

that increases urinary NH_4^+ excretion, thereby facilitating nitrogen disposal and promoting proton excretion. A synopsis of the direct and indirect effects of acidemia on the liver and kidney is depicted in Table 20.2.

The kidneys are involved in the final disposal of fixed acids produced daily. Because acid production and excretion are identical in a steady state, measurement of urinary acid excretion permits quantification of net acid production. This precise linkage between the tissue production of acids and the renal excretion of acids occurs as follows. The release of fixed acids from the cells generates H^+ and anions. The H^+ will decompose extracellular HCO_3^-, which is excreted as CO_2, and the anion will bind the Na^+ previously bound to the decomposed bicarbonate. The amount of decomposed bicarbonate will be identical to the amount of added fixed acids of both organic and inorganic origin. The sodium salts of the fixed acids released by the tissues will reach the kidney for their final excretion. To maintain acid–base balance, the kidney must fully reclaim the filtered HCO_3^- as a first step in accomplishing its task of excreting the daily acid load. Daily renal HCO_3^- reabsorption is approximately 4,320 mEq/day (180 L/day of glomerular filtration rate $\times$ 24 mEq/L of $[HCO_3^-]$); thus, the magnitude of H^+ secretion required to reclaim all the filtered HCO_3^- is approximately 50 times greater than that required for net daily acid excretion. Complete reabsorption of the filtered HCO_3^-, although of critical importance for the maintenance of acid–base balance, is not responsible for renal excretion of the metabolically produced acids. To accomplish the "net acid excretion" the kidney must regenerate the HCO_3^- decomposed in the tissues by exchanging the cation (usually Na^+) bound to the filtered anion (organic or inorganic, derived from the endogenous acid production) for H^+ secreted by the renal tubules, thus producing the urinary titratable acidity. Excretion of acid by the kidney with simultaneous maintenance of Na^+ and K^+ balance is also accomplished by the production within the kidney of the organic cation NH_4^+ (ammonium), which can be excreted with the filtered anion. To simplify matters we indicated that the H^+ derived from fixed acids generated by cell metabolism decompose exclusively extracellular bicarbonate; but, in fact, these acids titrate all body buffers and the explanation provided also applies for the case of nonbicarbonate buffers. In summary, the role of the kidney in acid–base balance resides on the modulation of $[HCO_3^-]_p$. This is done by adjusting the net acid excretion (sum of titratable acidity and urinary NH_4^+) to a level that will maintain normal acid–base balance. Under most conditions, net acid excretion is precisely adjusted in accordance to "endogenous acid production," dietary intake of acid/alkali, and bicarbonate loss in normal stools of 20 to 40 mmol/day.

The regulation of acid–base equilibrium also includes, as previously explained, changes in cellular metabolism that either accelerate or retard the production of fixed acids in response to changes in systemic pH. Alkalemia stimulates, whereas acidemia inhibits, the production of organic acids such as lactic and β-hydroxybutyric acids. Thus the tissue metabolic response appears as aimed at preserving the normalcy of acid–base equilibrium. In addition, urea production is inhibited by acidemia and this response appears to be homeostatic in nature because ureagenesis consumes bicarbonate ions. Thus changes in cellular metabolism contribute with chemical buffering and acid disposal by emunctories in the maintenance of acid–base balance.

RESPONSE TO AN ALKALI LOAD

Because bicarbonate-rich solutions are frequently prescribed, especially in an intensive care unit (ICU), it is mandatory to properly understand their effects on acid–base status. To determine the expected response to an alkali infusion in terms of the increase in $[HCO_3^-]_p$, it is necessary to express its value in mEq/kg of body weight. This practice allows correction for differences in the size of the fluid compartments among patients. A second reason for expressing the alkali load in milliequivalents per kilogram of body weight is the units in which the change in $[HCO_3^-]_p$ is reported (mEq/L). Remember that 1 kg of body fluid amounts to about 1 liter of fluid, such that the two units will be canceled out when one is divided by the other.

The space of distribution of bicarbonate can be viewed as having two components: an anatomic portion and a nonanatomic one. The anatomic portion corresponds to the extracellular fluid volume in which the infused HCO_3^- is freely dissolved. The nonanatomic portion is a theoretical space large enough to accommodate, at the prevailing $[HCO_3^-]_p$, all of the administered HCO_3^- unaccounted for by the anatomic boundaries. A large fraction of the nonanatomic portion corresponds to the component decomposed by the body buffers.

The major influences on the size of each component of the "bicarbonate space" are as follows. The anatomic portion is increased in patients with substantial edema, featuring a major expansion of extracellular fluid volume. The opposite is true for patients experiencing severe volume depletion (contraction of extracellular fluid volume). The nonanatomic portion is largely modified by two factors: (a) the initial level of $[HCO_3^-]_p$, because low $[HCO_3^-]_p$ expands the HCO_3^- space and high $[HCO_3^-]_p$ contracts it; and (b) the time elapsed from HCO_3^- loading to that of the evaluation of the plasma bicarbonate response. This effect is caused by slow equilibration of tissue buffers and by the effects of endogenous acid production. The impact of the initial $[HCO_3^-]_p$ and time elapsed on the bicarbonate space has been examined in the experimental dog and is depicted in Fig. 20.1.

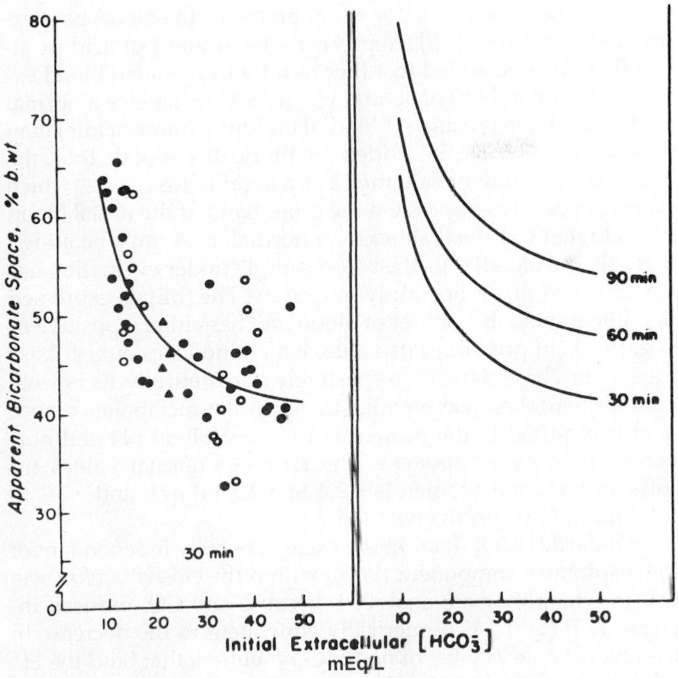

Figure 20.1. Relationship between initial extracellular bicarbonate concentration and apparent bicarbonate space following sodium bicarbonate infusion. The *left-hand panel* depicts the relationship at 30 minutes after infusion. *Filled circles* denote values obtained in dogs with metabolic acid–base disturbances, *open circles,* values in dogs with respiratory acid–base disturbances, and *filled triangles,* values in dogs with normal acid–base status. The *right-hand panel* compares the relationship at 30 minutes with those obtained at 60 and 90 minutes after the infusion. Bicarbonate space is highly correlated with the initial level of extracellular bicarbonate concentration ($[HCO_3]_p$) in dogs with respiratory and metabolic acid–base disturbances but is independent of the initial pH (data not shown). The bicarbonate space increases as a function of time and therefore cannot be assigned a simple value, even at a given bicarbonate concentration. (Reprinted with permission from Adrogué HJ, Brensilver J, Cohen JJ, et al. Influence of steady-state alterations in acid–base equilibrium on the fate of administered bicarbonate in the dog. *J Clin Invest* 1983;71:867–883.)

The empirical equation obtained from those studies, which determines the magnitude of the bicarbonate space as a function of the prevailing plasma bicarbonate is, at the 30-minute mark from the infusion, as follows:

$$\text{Bicarbonate space} = 0.36 + \frac{2.44}{[HCO_3^-]_p}$$

The bicarbonate space of normal subjects, measured at 30 minutes following alkali administration, is approximately 50% body weight. Patients with moderate metabolic acidosis having a $[HCO_3^-]_p$ of 12 to 20 mEq/L feature a bicarbonate space of approximately 60% to 80% of body weight, whereas those with extreme metabolic acidosis (i.e., $[HCO_3^-]_p$ of less than or equal to 5 mEq/L) can exhibit a bicarbonate space that exceeds 100% of body weight. A reduction in the bicarbonate space is observed in metabolic alkalosis, average values being in the range of 30% to 40% body weight. As shown in Fig. 20.1, there is a substantial time-dependent increase of the bicarbonate space, which averages about 10% of body weight at 60 minutes.

Let's now determine the expected increase in $[HCO_3^-]_p$ in response to administering 4 mEq/kg body weight of $NaHCO_3$ to a normal individual whose weight is 50 kg (i.e., 200 mmol of alkali). In the normal state, the apparent space of distribution of the alkali (bicarbonate space) is, as explained previously, approximately 50% body weight; thus the expected increase in $[HCO_3^-]_p$ in our subject is as follows:

$$\Delta[HCO_3^-]_p = \frac{4\ mEq/kg\ (alkali\ load)}{0.5\ (i.e.,\ 50\%,\ bicarbonate\ space)} = 8\ \text{mEq/L}$$

This calculation demonstrates that the expected increase in $[HCO_3^-]_p$ after an alkali load in the presence of a normal bicarbonate space amounts to the alkali load expressed in milliequivalents per kilogram of body weight multiplied by 2. As indicated by the preceding equation, dividing the administered HCO_3^- load by the observed change in $[HCO_3^-]_p$ permits an empiric estimation of the bicarbonate space. For example, if administration of an alkali load of 4 mEq/kg of body weight had resulted in a change in $[HCO_3^-]_p$ of 5 mEq/L, the bicarbonate space, expressed as a percentage of body weight, is as follows:

$$\text{bicarbonate space} = \frac{4\ \text{mEq/kg (alkali load)}}{5\ \text{mEq/L}\ (\Delta[HCO_3^-]_p)} \times 100 = 80\%$$

Administering 1 mEq of sodium bicarbonate (i.e., 1 ml of the usual 1-N preparation) per kilogram of the patient's body weight will increase plasma bicarbonate by 1 or 2 mEq/L for a bicarbonate space of 100% or 50% of body weight, respectively. Being mindful of the possibility of overtreatment, we recommend that bicarbonate requirements be calculated on the basis of a bicarbonate space of 50% of body weight. Thus, to raise plasma bicarbonate from an initial value of 4 mEq/L to a target value of 8 mEq/L, one should administer 2 mEq of sodium bicarbonate per kilogram of the patient's body weight. Except in the case of extreme acidemia, sodium bicarbonate should be dispensed as an infusion (over several minutes to a few hours), rather than as a bolus. Subsequent monitoring of the patient's acid–base status will determine whether additional alkali will need to be administered. In this regard, about 30 minutes must elapse following completion of the infusion before the clinical effect of a bicarbonate load is judged.

RESPONSE TO AN ACID LOAD

Acid infusions are occasionally used in the management of patients with metabolic alkalosis, especially when the pace of correction of the disorder must be accelerated. The distribution of an acute acid load within body fluids is virtually complete within 20 to 30 minutes. Buffering of the hydrogen ions takes place promptly in the extracellular fluid and within cells, and the relative buffering contribution of each of these compartments occurs at a 1:2 ratio. Computation of the amount of acid to be infused is based on a volume of distribution of the acid load equal to a bicarbonate space of 50% of body weight. The solution most commonly used is 0.1 N hydrochloric acid (HCl), thus containing 100 mEq of H^+/L. To reduce plasma bicarbonate concentration, for example, from 50 mEq/L to 40 mEq/L in a 70-kg patient, the amount of H^+ required can be estimated as $10 \times 70 \times 0.5$, or 350 mEq. This amount of H^+ is contained in a 3.5 L of HCl solution. Some clinicians might find it more expedient to base their prescription on the fact that infusion of 5 ml of HCl solution per kilogram of the patient's body weight will decrease plasma bicarbonate concentration by about 1 mEq/L—a proportionality that incorporates the values for the bicarbonate space and the normality of the solution. Although highly effective, infusion of HCl as well as other acidifying agents (e.g., NH_4Cl, arginine monohydrochloride) entails considerable risks.

MEASUREMENT OF ACID–BASE STATUS

To assess a patient's acid–base status, arterial blood pH, partial pressure of carbon dioxide in arterial blood ($PaCO_2$), and plasma bicarbonate concentration are most commonly used. Measurement of arterial blood pH and $PaCO_2$ and calculation of plasma bicarbonate is performed in the blood-gas laboratory, whereas measurement of plasma total CO_2 from a venous blood sample is performed in the chemistry laboratory (plasma bicarbonate makes up approximately 95% of total CO_2, such that plasma total CO_2 and bicarbonate concentrations are used interchangeably). Of course, it is critical to ensure that measurements of acid–base parameters are correct. Unfortunately, certain errors can be introduced during the process of specimen collection or measurement of the individual acid–base parameters. Detection of errors in measurement is facilitated, however, by the fact that the individual components of the bicarbonate-carbonic acid system are always at equilibrium in blood. Thus blood values for pH, $PaCO_2$, and bicarbonate must adhere to the mathematical constraints of the mass-action equation for the bicarbonate-carbonic acid system. Arithmetic rearrangement of this equation yields the Henderson equation, $[H^+] = 24 \times PaCO_2/[HCO_3^-]$, and its logarithmic derivative, the Henderson-Hasselbalch equation, $pH = 6.1 + \log [HCO_3^-]/(0.03 \times PaCO_2)$.

To make sure that the individual acid–base parameters adhere to the expected mathematical relationship, either of these equations can be used. Use of the Henderson-Hasselbalch equation is aided by the wide availability of calculators. Alternatively, application of the Henderson equation to the data, although simple, requires the conversion of the pH obtained from the blood-gas laboratory into hydrogen ion concentration expressed in nanoequivalents per liter, as previously explained. If independently measured values for blood pH, $PaCO_2$, and plasma bicarbonate concentration are available and do not fit into these equations, an error in one or more of the values must be present and repeat determinations should be performed. Because errors are encountered more often in the chemical determination of plasma bicarbonate concentration, it is more suitable to use the derived plasma bicarbonate concentration along with the blood pH and $PaCO_2$ obtained from the blood-gas laboratory to assess acid–base disorders.

It is often assumed that the two determinants of acidity are independent of each other. In actual fact, a major interdependency exists between $PaCO_2$ (the respiratory component) and HCO_3^- (the metabolic component) of the Henderson-Hasselbalch equation. The search for an estimate of the metabolic component that is truly independent of the respiratory component led investigators to derive other parameters, including standard $[HCO_3^-]$ and base excess, which simultaneously quantify changes in bicarbonate and nonbicarbonate buffer systems within a blood sample. Because many laboratories currently use these parameters, it is of importance to properly understand the precise meaning of each of these expressions. Standard $[HCO_3^-]_p$ is the plasma HCO_3^- concentration present in a blood sample that is fully saturated with oxygen and equilibrated *in vitro* at 38° C with PCO_2 equal to 40 mm Hg. The mean normal value is 24 mmol/L, which is identical to the mean normal value of actual plasma $[HCO_3^-]$ in a patient with a normal $PaCO_2$ of 40 mm Hg. Because the level of oxygenation of the hemoglobin alters its buffer value, precise measurement of the metabolic component requires standardization of the blood oxygen level of the sample used for measurement of acid–base composition. When oxygenated hemoglobin releases oxygen, it becomes less acidic and accepts protons more avidly, thus increasing its buffering capacity; the opposite occurs after oxygen is taken up by hemoglobin.

The blood-base excess, or, more precisely, the blood-base excess concentration, $[BE]_b$, represents the amount of acid or alkali that must be added to a liter of fully oxygenated blood exposed *in vitro* to PCO_2 of 40 mm Hg at 38°C to achieve a normal pH (7.40). When the initial blood pH is lower (more acidic) than normal, alkali must be added to titrate the blood, thus the blood sample under evaluation has a *negative base excess*, which is also called a *base deficit*. On the other hand, if the initial blood pH is higher (more alkaline) than normal, acid must be added to titrate the blood, thus the blood sample under evaluation has a *positive base excess* or simply *base excess*. The $[BE]_b$ is expressed in milliequivalents per liter of blood and has either a positive or negative sign preceding its value, which indicates either "base excess" or "base deficit," respectively. Theoretically its normal value is zero, because no adjustment in the metabolic component is required in the presence of normal blood pH and normal respiratory component. The range of normal values for $[BE]_b$ in men and women is −2.4 to +2.2 mEq/L and −3.3 to +1.3 mEq/L, respectively.

Standard $[HCO_3^-]_p$ and base excess are truly independent of the respiratory component (PCO_2) within the closed *in vitro* system in which they are analyzed, because any CO_2-induced increase in $[HCO_3^-]$ is numerically equivalent to the decrease in the anionic equivalency of non-HCO_3^- buffers that bind the H^+ released from the H_2CO_3; the opposite reaction occurs when decreases in blood PCO_2 occur *in vitro* such that the "metabolic component" again remains constant. *In vivo*, however, neither standard $[HCO_3^-]_p$ nor the base excess of plasma or blood are independent of the respiratory component. The reason for this difference is that among the main blood buffers, only HCO_3^- diffuses freely between plasma and interstitial fluid in response to a concentration gradient. The most prevalent non-HCO_3^- blood buffers, which include plasma proteins and hemoglobin, are restricted to the vascular compartment. Therefore the equivalent but reciprocal change in the HCO_3^- and the non-HCO_3^- components of the blood buffers elicited *in vitro* by a change in PCO_2 does not occur *in vivo*.

The relationship between changes in standard $[HCO_3^-]_p$ and in $[BE]_b$ is not entirely linear and varies with the hemoglobin concentration [Hb]; if the [Hb] is abnormally low, as in severe anemia, a change in $[BE]_b$ is equivalent to the change in standard $[HCO_3^-]$, whereas for a normal [Hb] the relationship can be expressed as $\Delta[BE]_b = 1.3 \times \Delta\text{standard } [HCO_3^-]_p$. As misconceptions with respect to the meaning of base excess frequently lead to false interpretations of the acid–base data, let us consider the pathophysiologic correlates of "base excess" and "base deficit." For example, the presence of $[BE]_b$ equal to +10 mEq/L should lead the clinician to consider the presence of conditions characterized by an elevated "metabolic component," such as metabolic alkalosis or chronic respiratory acidosis. In an analogous manner, the presence of $[BE]_b$ equal to −10 mEq/L should lead the clinician to consider the presence of conditions characterized by a diminished "metabolic component," such as metabolic acidosis or chronic respiratory alkalosis. A critique of the use of standard bicarbonate and base excess in the analysis of acid–base disturbances by Schwartz and Relman established that these parameters offer no advantages in the evaluation of the metabolic component of acid–base status as compared with actual plasma bicarbonate concentration. Yet they can be effectively used to assess the acid–base status of the blood.

Blood samples for acid–base measurement should be collected with anticoagulant (i.e., heparin), anaerobically, and should be promptly processed or cooled at 4°C if delays are expected. In addition to arterial blood, venous blood is occasionally sampled to assess the acid–base status. An arterial sample is routinely chosen for evaluation of the acid–base status. The test allows evaluation of pulmonary gas exchange and is assumed to provide an index of acid–base status in the tissues. Yet it is only in the normal state, in which the acid–base values in arterial blood are known to be close to those in mixed venous blood (the aggregate tissue effluent) that firm support for this assumption exists. In fact, an assessment of the acid–base status of the tissues in patients with circulatory failure may be misleading if only arterial blood data are examined (Fig. 20.2). The degree of misrepresentation worsens with the severity of circulatory compromise, and it becomes extreme during cardiac arrest (Fig. 20.3). Therefore information on venous as well as arterial blood gases is required for reliable monitoring of the critically ill patient. In addition, data derived from central and mixed venous blood sampling are practically interchangeable. Because mixed venous blood is obtained through a more risky, technically demanding, and expensive procedure, we recommend sampling of central venous blood. Notably, blood sampling from a peripheral vein may be misleading if regional blood flow is compromised or an occluding tourniquet is applied.

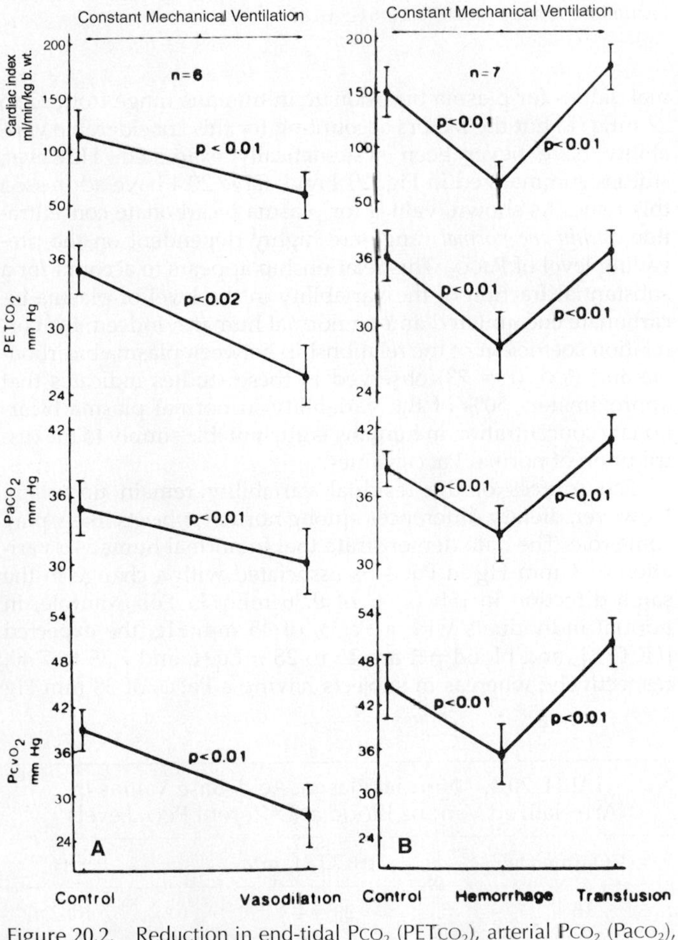

Figure 20.2. Reduction in end-tidal P_{CO_2} (PET_{CO_2}), arterial P_{CO_2} (Pa_{CO_2}), and central venous P_{O_2} (PCV_{O_2}) as a result of diminished cardiac index because of pharmacologic vasodilation **(A)** or hemorrhage **(B)** (changes reversed by transfusion) in the presence of constant pulmonary ventilation. In both cases, arterial hypocapnia occurred in the presence of fixed mechanical ventilation, therefore discounting pulmonary hyperventilation as an obligatory mechanism for its pathogenesis. Moreover, the reduction in arterial P_{CO_2} was in fact associated with a reduction in pulmonary CO_2 excretion, as indicated by the large and significant decrement in PET_{CO_2}. Note also that the reduction in cardiac index led to a significant decrement in venous P_{O_2}. (Reprinted with permission from Adrogué HJ, Rashad MN, Gorin AB, et al. Arteriovenous acid–base disparity in circulatory failure: studies on mechanism. *Am J Physiol* 1989;257:F1087–F1093.)

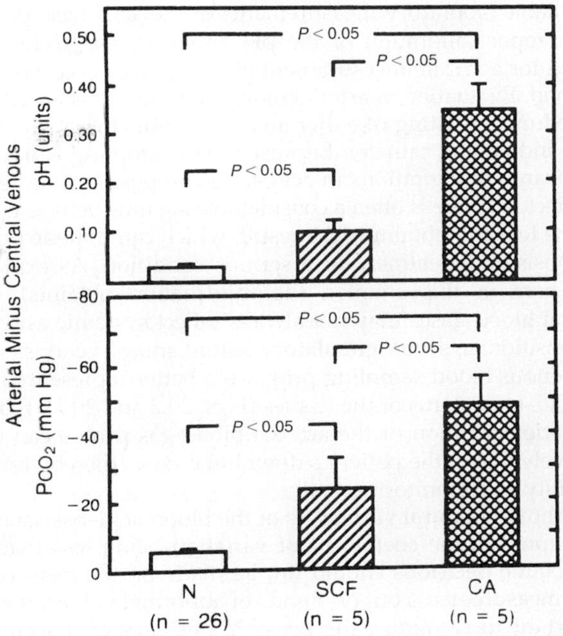

Figure 20.3. Arteriovenous differences in pH and P_{CO_2} in patients with different hemodynamic conditions. Patients with severe circulatory failure or cardiac arrest had a significant widening of the arteriovenous difference in pH and P_{CO_2}. A measure of effective alveolar ventilation is a prerequisite for the widened arteriovenous differences in pH and P_{CO_2} characteristic of circulatory compromise. When severe respiratory failure accompanies circulatory failure, arterial P_{CO_2} keeps pace with the evolving venous hypercapnia, thus preventing an enlargement of the arteriovenous gradients in pH and P_{CO_2}. CA, cardiac arrest in the presence of constant mechanical ventilation; N, normal hemodynamic status; SCF, severe circulatory failure. (Reprinted with permission from Adrogué HJ, Rashad MN, Gorin AB, et al. Assessing acid–base status in circulatory failure. *N Engl J Med* 1989;320:1312–1316.)

The use of venous blood allows measurement of the total CO_2 concentration, which is a reasonable approximation of serum bicarbonate concentration. The value of venous $[HCO_3^-]_p$ is about 2 mEq/L higher than the arterial one because the bulk of the metabolically produced CO_2 that is added to venous blood is carried as HCO_3^-. In addition, venous blood has larger amounts of dissolved CO_2 and carbamino compounds than arterial blood. Detection of acid–base disorders is frequently triggered by the presence of abnormal total CO_2 concentration in venous blood upon examination of serum electrolytes.

Capillary blood is often used, especially in children, for acid–base monitoring after securing proper dilation of the vascular bed by preheating the area. "Arterialized" blood drawn from a vein on the dorsum of the hand also can be used for acid–base measurements after the hand is warmed up to increase blood flow; the values obtained are almost identical to those derived from arterial blood.

LIMITATIONS OF MONITORING ACID–BASE STATUS BY ARTERIAL BLOOD GASES

Measurement of arterial blood gases represents the mainstay of acid–base monitoring and is an indispensable component of a patient's evaluation and follow-up in ICUs. Accurate assessment of the acid–base status requires the use of proper techniques for blood sampling and specimen handling and depends on reliable laboratory measurements of the acid–base parameters. Proper calibration of the pH and P_{CO_2} electrodes is required for accurate measurement of the acid–base composition of blood. Evaluation of arterial blood gases requires an invasive procedure consisting of either an arterial puncture or insertion of an indwelling catheter. Because blood sampling is intermittent, transient alterations in acid–base composition can remain undetected. There is often a considerable lag time between ordering the test and obtaining the result, which can impede prompt diagnosis and treatment of a serious condition. As explained elsewhere in this chapter, the information obtained using arterial blood gases may not always reflect systemic acid–base composition; in severe circulatory failure, mixed venous or central venous blood sampling provides a better representation of the acid–base status of the tissues (Figs. 20.2 and 20.3). Furthermore, deterioration of the arterial blood-gas profile can occur relatively late in the patient's downhill course, thereby limiting its utility as a monitoring tool.

Although natural variability of the blood acid–base status is quite modest, the coefficient of variation being less than 5%, therapeutic decisions should not be made on the basis of isolated measurements but on trends of abnormal values. It is also important to recognize the possible presence of inaccuracies resulting from faulty sampling techniques. Introduction of air bubbles must be avoided. The use of excessive amounts of heparin (more than 0.2 ml) can lead to low Pa_{CO_2} and bicarbonate readings due to a dilutional effect and to artifactually high PaO_2 values. Despite the acidity of the heparin solution, pH is not affected materially because of the excellent buffering capacity of blood. These problems can be minimized by obtaining at least 3 ml of blood, using small needles and minimal amounts of heparin, or using syringes that contain lyophilized heparin. During transport, specimens should be stored on ice to minimize errors resulting from the ongoing metabolism of white blood cells or platelets, especially in patients with leukemia or thrombocytosis.

NORMAL ACID–BASE COMPOSITION

The $[H^+]$ of extracellular fluid is maintained at relatively low levels or, in other words, in the alkaline range by homeostatic mechanisms that result in a ratio of $[HCO_3^-]$ to H_2CO_3 of 20:1, when the values are expressed in mmol/L. The normal blood acid–base composition in adults is shown in Table 20.3. These values are notably stable in each subject. Thus daily variations in resting values for Pa_{CO_2} and $[HCO_3^-]_p$ rarely exceed 2 to 3 mm Hg and 1 to 2 mEq/L, respectively. On the other hand, nor-

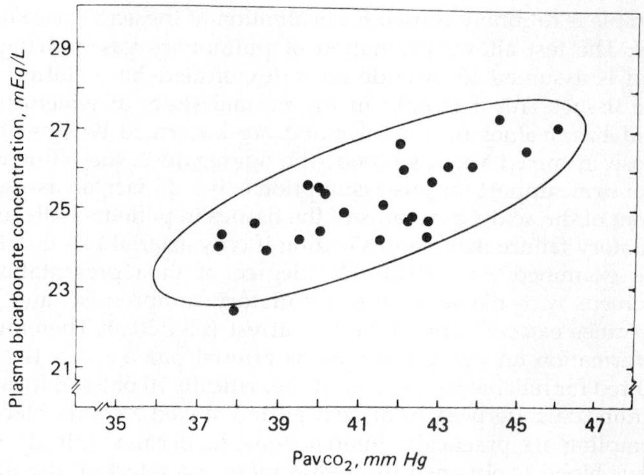

Figure 20.4. Dependency of the bicarbonate concentration on the P_{CO_2} measured in arterialized venous blood ($PavCO_2$) in the normal state. The 90% confidence region depicted as a *solid line* is for a simple blood sample. (Reprinted with permission from Madias NE, Adrogué HJ, Horowitz GL, et al. A redefinition of normal acid–base equilibrium in man: carbon dioxide tension as a key determinant of normal plasma bicarbonate concentration. *Kidney Int* 1979;16:612–618.)

mal values for plasma bicarbonate in humans range from 22 to 27 mEq/L, but the factors accounting for this considerable variability have never been systematically examined. However, studies summarized in Fig. 20.4 and Table 20.4 have addressed this issue. As shown, values for plasma bicarbonate concentration *within the normal* range are highly dependent on the prevailing level of Pa_{CO_2}. This relationship appears to account for a substantial fraction of the variability in the level of plasma bicarbonate encountered among normal humans. Indeed, the correlation coefficient of the relationship between plasma bicarbonate and P_{CO_2} (r = .73) observed in these studies indicates that approximately 50% of the variability in normal plasma bicarbonate concentration in humans is attributable simply to the distribution of normal Pa_{CO_2} values.

The sources of the residual variability remain uncertain. However, dietary differences among normal subjects likely play some role. The data demonstrate that in normal humans a variation of 1 mm Hg in Pa_{CO_2} is associated with a change in the same direction in $[HCO_3^-]_p$ of 0.36 mEq/L. For example, in normal individuals with a Pa_{CO_2} of 45 mm Hg, the expected $[HCO_3^-]_p$ and blood pH are 25 to 28 mEq/L and 7.35 to 7.40, respectively; whereas in subjects having a Pa_{CO_2} of 38 mm Hg

TABLE 20.3. Normal Acid–Base Composition

	Mean	Range
Arterial blood		
pH	7.40	7.36–7.44
$[H^+]$	40 nM	36–44 nM
P_{CO_2}	40 mm Hg	36–44 mm Hg
$[HCO_3^-]$ actual	24 mM	22–26 mM
$[HCO_3^-]$ standard	24 mM	22–26 mM
Base excess	0 mM	−2, +2 mM
Venous blood		
pH	7.38	7.34–7.42
$[H^+]$	42 nM	38–46 nM
P_{CO_2}	46 mm Hg	42–50 mm Hg
CO_2 total	26 mM	23–30 mM

TABLE 20.4. Normal Plasma Acid–Base Values in Arterialized Venous Blood at Different P_{CO_2} Levels[a]

$PavCO_2$ mm Hg	$[HCO_3^-]_p$ mM	pH
38	23.5–24.7	7.40–7.42
39	23.4–25.4	7.38–7.42
40	23.6–25.9	7.38–7.42
41	23.9–26.4	7.37–7.41
42	24.3–26.7	7.37–7.41
43	24.8–26.9	7.37–7.40
44	25.4–27.0	7.37–7.39

[a] The range of $[HCO_3^-]_p$ and pH represent the 90% joint confidence region of the mean steady-state values.

Reprinted with permission from Madias NE, Adrogué HJ, Horowitz GL, et al. A redefinition of normal acid–base equilibrium in man: carbon dioxide tension as a key determinant of normal plasma bicarbonate concentration. *Kidney Int* 1979;16:612–618.

the expected $[HCO_3^-]_p$ and blood pH are in the range of 23 to 25 mEq/L and 7.38 to 7.43, respectively. The difference in acid–base composition between arterial and venous blood from a resting extremity is small; venous blood pH is 0 to 0.03 lower, P_{CO_2} about 6 mm Hg higher, and $[HCO_3^-]$ approximately 2 mEq/L higher than that of arterial blood. The higher P_{CO_2} in venous blood reflects the interposition of peripheral tissues, which add CO_2 to venous blood. As noted previously, venous blood can be "arterialized" *in vivo* by warming up the hand at 45°C for 10 minutes—a procedure that renders the arteriovenous acid–base differences negligible.

Several physiologic factors modify the acid–base status. Compared with the recumbent position, sitting and standing lowers P_{CO_2} by approximately 3 and 4 mm Hg, respectively. Normal women, during the progesterone phase of the menstrual cycle, have Pa_{CO_2} values approximately 2 to 4 mm Hg lower, $[HCO_3^-]_p$ approximately 1 mEq/L lower, and pH approximately 0 to 0.02 higher than in men. Women develop substantial hypocapnia during pregnancy, most notably in the last trimester, with Pa_{CO_2} of 29 to 32, increased alveolar ventilation being driven by the high progesterone levels. Acid–base composition is influenced by age. Whereas normal children have Pa_{CO_2} values of 33 to 37 mm Hg up to age 3, the difference is progressively minimized such that Pa_{CO_2} shifts to 35 to 40 mm Hg by age 15 and becomes identical to adult values by age 17. Diet influences the acid–base status through changes in endogenous acid production. Consequently, a small but detectable decrease in both $[HCO_3^-]_p$ and Pa_{CO_2} is observed when a meat diet is ingested as opposed to a vegetable diet; nonetheless, despite this variation, the acid–base data are generally maintained within the normal range. High-altitude residents or individuals ascending to high altitudes express hypoxemia-induced hyperventilation such that the acid–base values reflect primary hypocapnia (respiratory alkalosis).

SECONDARY RESPONSE TO ALTERATIONS IN ACID–BASE STATUS

When an abnormal acid–base status develops because of a single initial alteration in either the respiratory component (P_{CO_2}) or the metabolic component (measured by actual $[HCO_3^-]_p$, standard $[HCO_3^-]_p$, or base excess), defense mechanisms are recruited that diminish the impact on acidity of the primary insult. These defense mechanisms include buffering (discussed previously) and physiologic processes, the latter involving changes in the rate of excretion of either volatile acid by the lungs or fixed acid by the kidneys. The physiologic processes of acid–base safeguard modify the respiratory component when the initial insult occurs in the metabolic component (i.e., respiratory response to metabolic acidosis and alkalosis) or in the metabolic component when the respiratory one is initially perturbed (i.e., metabolic response to respiratory acidosis and alkalosis). The effect on acidity of this physiologic secondary response is to decrease the deviation in blood pH resulting from the primary insult because the other component of the buffer pair (H_2CO_3 and/or HCO_3^-) changes in the same direction. It should be recognized that the secondary response to a primary disorder affords the best protective effect on blood pH if this "adaptive" response does not alter the acid–base component that was initially perturbed. However, it has been demonstrated that in the chronic phase of acid–base disorders such as metabolic acidosis and alkalosis, the secondary respiratory response further decreases the plasma bicarbonate in the former disturbance and increases the plasma bicarbonate in the latter one as a result of P_{CO_2}-induced changes in renal acidification. Consequently, the benefits of the respiratory adaptation (secondary response) are unmitigated in the initial phase of the acid–base disorder but are diminished or even deleterious when the metabolic disturbance is prolonged. Consequently, the terms *adaptive* or *compensatory response* to primary acid–base disorders should be discarded in favor of the term *secondary response*.

Metabolic Perturbations

Because the metabolic component of acid–base equilibrium may be quantified by actual $[HCO_3^-]_p$, standard $[HCO_3^-]_p$, or base excess, a primary decrease in any of these measured parameters constitutes metabolic acidosis. Conversely, a primary increase in the metabolic component represents metabolic alkalosis. The secondary response to metabolic acidosis consists of hyperventilation and results in hypocapnia, whereas hypoventilation leading to CO_2 retention (hypercapnia) develops when the initial acid–base disorder is metabolic alkalosis. Because acidemia (in metabolic acidosis) and alkalemia (in metabolic alkalosis) are the stimuli for the increased and decreased ventilation, respectively, the secondary physiologic response is never sufficient to restore blood pH to normal in the course of these acid–base disorders. As depicted in Fig. 20.5, significant and highly predictable ventilatory response to chronic metabolic acid–base disturbances have been demonstrated in the experimental animal. Furthermore, the magnitude of the ventilatory response appears to be uniform throughout a wide spectrum of chronic metabolic acid–base disorders extending from severe metabolic acidosis to severe metabolic alkalosis. On average, arterial P_{CO_2} is expected to change by 0.74 mm Hg for a 1-mEq/L chronic change in plasma bicarbonate concentration of metabolic origin. In addition, the data suggest that the ventilatory response to chronic metabolic alkalosis is independent of the particular mode of generation (Fig. 20.5). A comparable rigorous characterization of the respiratory response to metabolic acidosis and alkalosis in humans is not available; however, the

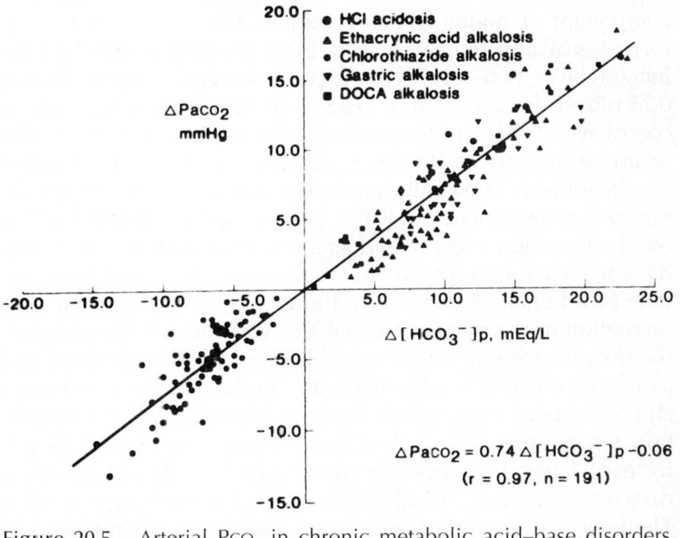

Figure 20.5. Arterial P_{CO_2} in chronic metabolic acid–base disorders. Steady-state relationship between changes (experimental minus control values) in arterial CO_2 tension (Pa_{CO_2}) and plasma bicarbonate concentration ($[HCO_3^-]_p$) in dogs with chronic metabolic acidosis and chronic metabolic alkalosis. Key to symbols is presented. Each point is an average of three observations obtained on consecutive days in a single dog. Regression line drawn through points was calculated from pooled data by method of least squares. (Reprinted with permission from Madias NE, Bossert WH, Adrogué HJ. Ventilatory response to chronic metabolic acidosis and alkalosis in the dog. *J Appl Physiol* 1984;56:1640–1646.)

TABLE 20.5. Secondary Response to Alterations in Acid–Base Status

Condition	Initiating Mechanism	Expected Response	Maximal Level or Response
Respiratory acidosis	↑ $Paco_2$		
Acute		↑ $[HCO_3^-] \approx 0.1\ \Delta Paco_2$	30 mEq/L
Chronic		↑ $[HCO_3^-] \approx 0.3\ \Delta Paco_2$	45 mEq/L
Respiratory alkalosis	↓ $Paco_2$		
Acute		↓ $[HCO_3^-] \approx 0.2\ \Delta Paco_2$	16–18 mEq/L
Chronic		↓ $[HCO_3^-] \approx 0.4\ \Delta Paco_2$	12–15 mEq/L
Metabolic acidosis	↓ $[HCO_3^-]_p$	↓ $Paco_2 \approx 1.2\ \Delta[HCO_3^-]$	10 mm Hg
Metabolic alkalosis	↑ $[HCO_3^-]_p$	↑ $Paco_2 \approx 0.7\ \Delta[HCO_3^-]$	65 mm Hg

response is presumably very similar in these species. The expected secondary response to metabolic alterations in acid–base status based on data collected from human studies is depicted in Table 20.5. The ventilatory response observed in humans and experimental animals is prompt so that a new steady-state Pco_2 is reached within a few hours from the development of the metabolic derangement of acid–base status. The maximum level of adaptation results in an arterial blood Pco_2 as low as approximately 10 mm Hg in metabolic acidosis and as high as approximately 65 mm Hg in metabolic alkalosis.

Respiratory Perturbations

Respiratory acidosis and alkalosis are the acid–base disturbances initiated by an increase and a decrease, respectively, in CO_2 tension of body fluids. Adaptation to acute hypercapnia (respiratory acidosis) elicits an immediate increment in $[HCO_3^-]_p$ produced by titration of nonbicarbonate body buffers. Such buffers generate HCO_3^- by combining with H^+ derived from the dissociation of H_2CO_3, as follows:

$$CO_2 + H_2O \leftrightarrow H_2CO_3 \leftrightarrow HCO_3^- + H^+$$
$$HCO_3^- + H^+ + Buf^- \leftrightarrow HBuf + HCO_3^-$$

where Buf^- refers to the base component and HBuf to the acid component of nonbicarbonate buffers. On average, $[HCO_3^-]_p$ increases by approximately 0.1 mEq/L for each 1-mm Hg acute increment in Pco_2. As a result, $[H^+]_p$ increases approximately 0.75 nEq/L for each 1-mm Hg rise in Pco_2. This adaptation is completed within 5 to 10 minutes of the rise in arterial Pco_2. The adaptive increase in $[HCO_3^-]_p$ observed in the acute phase of hypercapnia is markedly amplified during chronic hypercapnia, as a consequence of HCO_3^- generation by the kidney. This renal adaptation is expressed as a transient increase in net urinary acid excretion (mostly in the form of NH_4^+) that generates new bicarbonate for the body fluids, and as a persistent augmentation in the rate of renal HCO_3^- reabsorption that ensures the maintenance of the increased $[HCO_3^-]_p$. Both proximal and distal acidification mechanisms are involved in the response to chronic hypercapnia, which requires 3 to 5 days for its completion. On average, $[HCO_3^-]_p$ increases approximately 0.3 mEq/L for each 1-mm Hg chronic increment in Pco_2; as a result $[H^+]_p$ rises approximately 0.3 nEq/L for each 1-mm Hg rise in Pco_2. The expected secondary response to respiratory alterations in acid–base status based on data collected from human studies is depicted in Table 20.5.

Respiratory alkalosis, also known as *primary hypocapnia*, results in a prompt fall in $[H^+]$ because of a reduction in the $[H_2CO_3]$ of the body fluids. Adaptation to acute hypocapnia is characterized by an immediate decrement in $[HCO_3^-]_p$ that results from nonrenal mechanisms and is accounted for, principally, by alkaline titration of the non-HCO_3^- body buffers. This adaptation is completed within 5 to 10 minutes after the onset of hypocapnia, and assuming no further changes in arterial Pco_2, no additional, detectable changes in acid–base equilibrium occur for a period of several hours. The $[HCO_3^-]_p$ falls by approximately 0.2 mEq/L for each mm Hg of acute decrement in arterial Pco_2. Consequently, H^+ concentration decreases by approximately 0.75 nEq/L for each mm Hg reduction in arterial Pco_2. A 20 mm Hg reduction in Pco_2 in a subject who initially had a normal acid–base composition ($Paco_2$ 40 mm Hg, $[HCO_3^-]_p$ 24 mEq/L, and $[H^+]$ 40 nEq/L or a pH of 7.40), will result in a $[HCO_3^-]_p$ of 20 mEq/L and a $[H^+]_p$ of 25 nEq/L or a pH equal to 7.60. A larger decrement in $[HCO_3^-]_p$ occurs in chronic hypocapnia, which reflects the renal adaptation to the acid–base disorder. This renal adaptation involves suppression of the mechanisms of urine acidification in both proximal and distal tubules. The body HCO_3^- stores are reduced by a transient decrease in net acid excretion that occurs during the first few days of hypocapnic exposure; the persistent suppression of HCO_3^- reabsorption maintains the hypobicarbonatemia of chronic hypocapnia. Completion of the adaptation requires 2 to 3 days. The $[HCO_3^-]_p$ decreases, generally, by about 0.4 mEq/L for each 1-mm Hg chronic decrement in $Paco_2$ and, as a consequence, $[H^+]$ decreases by approximately 0.5 nEq/L for each 1-mm Hg reduction in $Paco_2$. Chronic adaptation to a $Paco_2$ of 20 mm Hg results in a $[HCO_3^-]_p$ of 16 mEq/L and a $[H^+]_p$ of 30 nEq/L (a pH of 7.52). As previously stated for the secondary respiratory response to metabolic acid–base disorders, the secondary metabolic response to respiratory disturbances also fails to fully restore blood pH to normal levels.

Selected Readings

Adrogué HJ, Brensilver J, Cohen JJ, et al. Influence of steady-state alterations in acid–base equilibrium on the fate of administered bicarbonate in the dog. *J Clin Invest* 1983;71:867–883.

This study describes the determinants of the bicarbonate space based on carefully conducted studies in nonanesthetized animals. The effects of chronic metabolic and respiratory acid–base disorders on the internal distribution of an alkali load are discussed in detail.

Adrogué HJ, Rashad MN, Gorin AB, et al. Arteriovenous acid–base disparity in circulatory failure: studies on mechanism. *Am J Physiol* 1989;257:F1087–F1093.

The importance of central or mixed venous blood sampling in the evaluation of the acid–base status in the presence of an abnormal circulation are studied in experimental animals. The advantages and disadvantages of arterial as compared with venous blood sampling are discussed. The concepts derived from this investigation are relevant in the management of patients admitted in intensive care units.

Adrogué HJ, Wesson DE. *Acid–base. Blackwell's basics of medicine.* Boston: Blackwell Science, 1994.

A text on acid–base that uses simple questions followed by short answers to illustrate the various topics presented. Case discussions help consolidate theoretical principles with practical facts.

Bracket NC Jr, Cohen JJ, Schwartz WB. Carbon dioxide titration curve of normal man. Effect of increasing degrees of acute hypercapnia on acid–base equilibrium. *N Engl J Med* 1965;272:6–12.

This study provides experimental data on the contribution of nonbicarbonate buffers in acid–base homeostasis of normal humans.

Bushinsky DA, Ori Y. Effects of metabolic and respiratory acidosis on bone. *Curr Opin Nephrol Hypertens* 1993;2:588–596.
A review of the effect of metabolic and respiratory acidosis on bone composition. Respiratory acidosis was associated with less calcium loss compared with metabolic acidosis in the rat calvariae.

Cohen JJ, Kassirer JP. *Acid/Base*. Boston: Little, Brown, 1982.
A comprehensive textbook on acid–base chemistry, physiology, and clinical disorders of the acidity of body fluids.

Green J, Kleeman CR. Role of bone in regulation of systemic acid base balance. *Kidney Int* 1991;39:9–26.
The contribution of bone to acid–base balance discussed in detail.

Hills AG. *Acid–base balance: chemistry, physiology, pathophysiology*. Baltimore: Williams & Wilkins, 1973.
This textbook offers a detailed explanation on acid–base theory and buffer systems.

Lennon EJ, Lemann J, Litzow JR. The effects of diet and stool composition on the net external acid balance of normal subjects. *J Clin Invest* 1966;45:1601–1607.
This carefully conducted study describes the effects on acid–base balance of standard diets consumed in North America.

Madias NE, Adrogué HJ, Horowitz GL, et al. A redefinition of normal acid–base equilibrium in man: carbon dioxide tension as a key determinant of normal plasma bicarbonate concentration. *Kidney Int* 1979;16:612–618.
This study demonstrates that acid–base equilibrium in normal humans is characterized by a positive correlation between $[HCO_3^-]_p$ *and* P_{CO_2}. *The independent variable in this relationship is the carbon dioxide tension of body fluids.*

Madias NE, Bossert WH, Adrogué HJ. Ventilatory response to chronic metabolic acidosis and alkalosis in the dog. *J Appl Physiol* 1984;56:1640–1646.
The ventilatory response to chronic metabolic acid–base disorders was quantitated as the slope of the linear regression of the individual changes in P_{CO_2} *as a function of the prevailing changes in plasma bicarbonate concentration. This approach, which is at variance to that used by other investigators that simply correlate the experimental acid–base values, provides a more rigorous definition of the ventilatory response to metabolic acidosis and alkalosis.*

Schwartz WB, Relman AS. A critique of the parameters used in the evaluation of acid–base disorders: "whole-blood buffer base" and "standard bicarbonate" compared with blood pH and plasma bicarbonate concentration. *N Engl J Med* 1963;268:1382–1388.
An intelligent exposition of the various parameters used in the evaluation of acid–base status.

Siggaard-Andersen O. *The acid–base status of the blood*, 4th ed. Baltimore: Williams & Wilkins, 1964.
A complete exposition of the buffer systems of blood and a detailed description of some methods to measure acid–base status are presented. The alignment and curve nomograms of Siggaard-Andersen are explained in great detail.

Tannen RL. Fluid, electrolyte and acid–base disorders. In: Jacobson HR, Striker GE, Klahr S, eds. *The principles and practice of nephrology*. Philadelphia: BC Decker, 1991.
A careful view of relevant aspects of acid–base disorders. Theoretical concepts are presented in harmony with practical applications for the management of patients.

Valtin H, Gennari FJ. *Acid–base disorders. Basic concepts and clinical management*. Boston: Little, Brown, 1987.
Current concepts of acid–base physiology are presented and secondary responses to primary acid–base disturbances are discussed in detail.

PART 2
Renal Handling of Hydrogen and Bicarbonate Ions

Biff F. Palmer and Robert J. Alpern

To maintain acid–base balance, the kidney must excrete net acid at a rate equal to the rate of extrarenal acid production. Extrarenal acid production varies from 0.3 to 1 mEq/kg per day and is markedly dependent on dietary acid intake. Thus, to maintain acid–base balance, the kidney is normally required to excrete 0.3 to 1 mEq/kg of acid per day. In certain settings such as with a patient who is vomiting, the kidney is faced with an extrarenal alkaline load, and thus is forced to excrete net alkali.

The regulation of normal acid–base balance by the kidney requires a number of key features. First, the renal tubules must possess mechanisms for tubular transport of hydrogen and bicarbonate. Second, the kidney must provide mechanisms for provision of buffers. Excretion of 50 mEq of acid in an unbuffered liter of urine would require a urine pH of 1.3. Third, the kidney must regulate rates of H^+ secretion, HCO_3 secretion, and buffer synthesis in an integrated fashion so as to provide precise regulation of renal net acid excretion. Renal net acid excretion (NAE) is calculated using the following formula:

$$NAE = U_{NH_4}V + U_{TA}V - U_{HCO_3}V$$

where NH_4^+ refers to ammonium, *TA* to titratable acidity, and HCO_3 to bicarbonate.

MECHANISMS OF H-HCO_3 TRANSPORT

Glomerulus

The glomerulus is not normally considered to participate in acid–base regulation. However, the glomerulus filters an amount of bicarbonate equivalent to the plasma bicarbonate concentration multiplied by glomerular filtration rate (GFR). This filtered load of bicarbonate is equivalent to HCO_3 secretion. It does not contribute to net acid excretion (NAE), but in fact contributes to alkali excretion. Under normal circumstances, the filtered load of bicarbonate in a human subject is approximately 4,000 mEq/day. Under conditions of metabolic alkalosis, the filtered load may increase significantly. In the presence of metabolic alkalosis, glomerular filtration becomes an important mechanism for excretion of HCO_3 and correction of alkalosis. In this setting, changes in GFR alter the filtered load of HCO_3, and markedly affect HCO_3 excretion. From the standpoint of prevention of or correction of acidosis, glomerular filtration contributes little and places a large load on the tubules. Before the tubules can "regenerate" the HCO_3 consumed by extrarenal metabolism, approximately 30 to 70 mEq/day, they must "reclaim" the filtered load of HCO_3, 4,000 mEq/L.

Proximal Tubule

The proximal tubule reabsorbs approximately 80% to 90% of the filtered load of HCO_3. In addition, by titrating luminal pH from 7.3 down to approximately 6.7, the majority of phosphate, the major titratable buffer, is titrated to its acid form. Lastly, most of ammonia synthesis occurs in the proximal tubule. Ammonia synthesis will be discussed later. Here we discuss the mechanisms responsible for H secretion and HCO_3 absorption.

Figure 20.6 shows a model of the proximal tubule cell. Bicarbonate absorption from the tubular lumen is mediated by H secretion across the apical membrane. This H^+ secretion is active in that the electrochemical gradient favors H^+ movement from lumen to cell. Two mechanisms have been identified that mediate active apical H secretion. Approximately two-thirds of this flux is affected by an apical membrane Na^+-H^+ antiporter. This transporter uses an inward Na gradient to drive the outward secretion of H ions. This process is considered secondary active in that the Na^+-H^+ antiporter does not possess any direct coupling to metabolism. Rather, an Na^+-K^+-ATPase, which is coupled to adenosine triphosphate (ATP), lowers cell Na concentration and provides the driving force for Na entry and secondary H extrusion. The Na^+-H^+ antiporter has been studied extensively. It is almost ubiquitous in vertebrate cells. The Na^+-H^+ exchanger has a 1:1 stoichiometry and is electroneutral. A number of different isoforms of the Na^+-H^+ antiporter

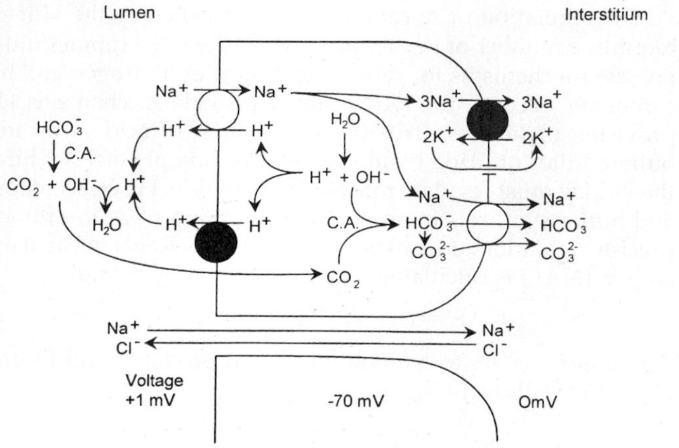

Figure 20.6. Cell model of proximal tubule $NaHCO_3$ reabsorption. H^+ is secreted into the proximal tubule lumen by an Na-H antiporter and an H-ATPase. OH^- generated by apical membrane H^+ secretion reacts with CO_2 to form HCO_3^- and CO_3^{2-}, which exit with an Na^+ on the basolateral membrane Na-HCO_3-CO_3 cotransporter. Na^+ absorbed by the Na^+-H^+ antiporter exits the cell on the basolateral membrane Na^+-K^+-ATPase and the Na-HCO_3-CO_3 cotransporter. K^+, which enters the cell on the Na^+-K^+-ATPase, exits on a basolateral membrane K^+ channel. Carbonic anhydrase catalyzes the conversion of HCO_3^- to CO_2 and OH^- in the lumen, and the reverse reaction in the cell. Electrogenic H^+ secretion generates a small lumen positive voltage, which generates a current flow across the paracellular pathway. •, active transport mechanism; ○, passive transporter; =, channel; CA, carbonic anhydrase.

have been cloned. In general, these isoforms are similar because they possess an N-terminal hydrophobic transmembrane domain and a C-terminal cytoplasmic domain. All Na^+-H^+ antiporters are inhibited by amiloride and amiloride analogs. However, the ubiquitously distributed Na-H antiporter, most likely corresponding to the isoform NHE-1, is exquisitely sensitive to amiloride and its analogs. The Na^+-H^+ antiporter mediating H^+ secretion across the apical membrane of the proximal tubule is less sensitive to amiloride and its analogs and may correspond to the cloned isoform NHE-3.

In parallel with the Na^+-H^+ antiporter, there is an apical membrane H^+ pump. This pump mediates approximately one-third of proximal tubular HCO_3 absorption. The pump is of the vacuolar type, and is similar to the H^+ pump of intracellular vesicles, as well as the collecting duct H^+ pump. There may, however, be some isoform differences among these H^+ pumps.

Both of these H^+ transporters generate base in the cell, which must exit across the basolateral membrane in order to affect transepithelial transport. As previously noted, acid can passively enter the cell, or equivalently, alkali can passively exit the cell. Thus basolateral membrane base exit could be mediated by a simple OH or HCO_3 channel. However, the mechanism that mediates this process is an Na-HCO_3-CO_3 cotransporter. This mechanism carries one Na with one HCO_3 ion and one carbonate ion. It is equivalent to an Na-3HCO_3 cotransporter, and carries two negative charges. Base efflux on this transporter is driven by the cell negative voltage. The transporter is inhibited by disulfonic stilbenes. The net effect of this transporter is that HCO_3 leaves the cell passively, and in addition one Na is carried from the cell, requiring less Na transport on the Na^+-K^+-ATPase, allowing conservation of ATP. The Na-HCO_3-CO_3 cotransporter has been cloned.

Carbonic anhydrase is present in the proximal tubule cytoplasm and on the apical and basolateral membranes. Carbonic anhydrase subserves a number of functions in the proximal tubule. Apical membrane carbonic anhydrase allows secreted H^+ ions, which react with HCO_3 and form H_2CO_3, to then form $CO_2 + H_2O$. This allows the buffering of secreted H^+ ions secondarily causing luminal pH to increase, allowing further H^+ secretion. In addition, OH generated in the cell must react with CO_2 to form HCO_3 and carbonate for efflux across the basolateral membrane. This reaction is catalyzed by either cytoplasmic or basolateral membrane carbonic anhydrase.

Thick Ascending Limb of Henle's Loop

Tubular fluid arriving at the early distal tubule has a pH and HCO_3 concentration similar to that of the late proximal tubule. Because there is significant water extraction in Henle's loop, maintenance of a constant HCO_3 concentration requires reabsorption of HCO_3. The majority of this HCO_3 absorption appears to be accomplished in the thick ascending limb (Fig. 20.7). The thick ascending limb appears in many ways to be similar to the proximal tubule. Bicarbonate absorption is accelerated by carbonic anhydrase. The majority of apical membrane H^+ secretion is mediated by an Na^+-H^+ antiporter. In addition, the cells possess a basolateral membrane Na-HCO_3-CO_3 cotransporter, which likely mediates the majority of base efflux. These cells possess an H^+ pump, but it is not clear what role it plays in acidification.

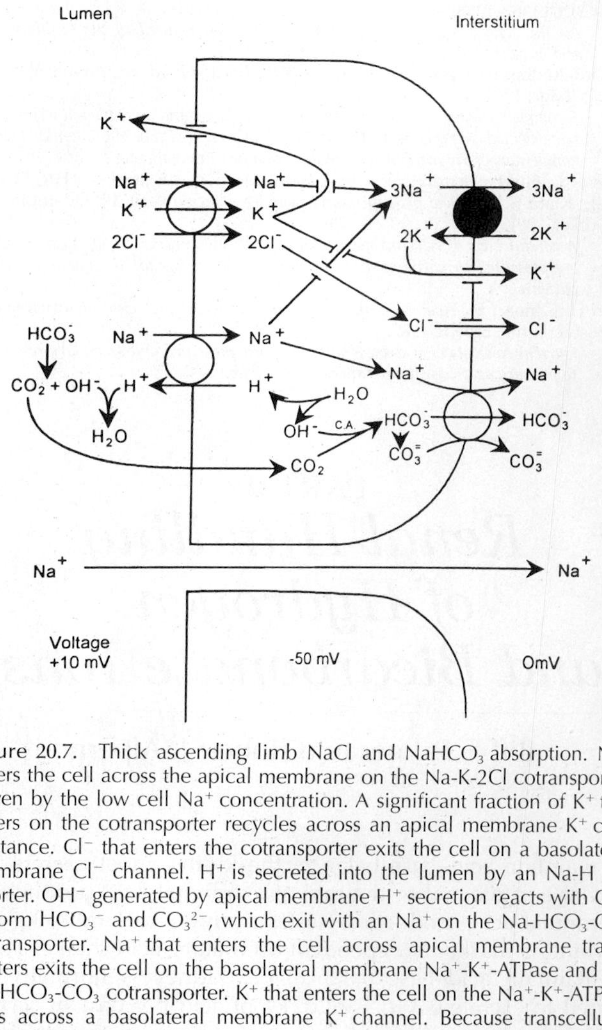

Figure 20.7. Thick ascending limb NaCl and $NaHCO_3$ absorption. Na^+ enters the cell across the apical membrane on the Na-K-2Cl cotransporter, driven by the low cell Na^+ concentration. A significant fraction of K^+ that enters on the cotransporter recycles across an apical membrane K^+ conductance. Cl^- that enters the cotransporter exits the cell on a basolateral membrane Cl^- channel. H^+ is secreted into the lumen by an Na-H antiporter. OH^- generated by apical membrane H^+ secretion reacts with CO_2 to form HCO_3^- and CO_3^{2-}, which exit with an Na^+ on the Na-HCO_3-CO_3 cotransporter. Na^+ that enters the cell across apical membrane transporters exits the cell on the basolateral membrane Na^+-K^+-ATPase and the Na-HCO_3-CO_3 cotransporter. K^+ that enters the cell on the Na^+-K^+-ATPase exits across a basolateral membrane K^+ channel. Because transcellular NaCl absorption is electrogenic, a lumen positive voltage is generated, which drives a paracellular current. •, active transport mechanism; ○, passive transporter; =, channel.

Collecting Duct

From the standpoint of renal acidification, there is much axial and cellular heterogeneity along the collecting duct. The surface distal nephron and the cortical collecting duct are capable of H secretion or HCO_3 secretion, depending on chronic acid–base status. These functions appear to be mediated by distinct cells, acid secreting α-intercalated cells, and base secreting β-intercalated cells. Both types of intercalated cells are rich in carbonic anhydrase.

The α-intercalated cell possesses an apical membrane H^+ pump that is responsible for most of active H transport across the apical membrane (Fig. 20.8). This transporter once again is of the vacuolar type and is inhibited by n-ethylmaleimide and by bafilomycin A. Under certain circumstances, these cells possess an apical membrane H-K pump similar to that present in gastric mucosa. This pump can affect active H secretion and K absorption, and appears to be most prominent functionally in conditions of chronic K deficiency. This pump is inhibited by SCH28080. Alkali generated within the cell exits on the basolateral membrane Cl-HCO_3 exchanger. This Cl-HCO_3 exchanger is inhibited by disulfonic stilbenes and is similar in many respects to the Cl-HCO_3 exchanger of red cells. In fact, molecular studies have demonstrated that the collecting duct basolateral membrane Cl-HCO_3 exchanger is derived from the same gene as the red cell Cl-HCO_3 exchanger, AE1, but is truncated at its amino terminus due to alternative splicing. Chloride ions that enter the cell in exchange for HCO_3^- then exit across the basolateral membrane on a Cl conductance.

The HCO_3 secreting β-intercalated cell is in many respects a mirror image of the α-intercalated cell (Fig. 20.9). It possesses an H^+ pump on the basolateral membrane, which mediates active H^+ ion extrusion. Under certain circumstances, a basolateral membrane H^+-K^+ pump has been suggested to be present. Alkali that is generated within the cell then exits on an apical membrane Cl-HCO_3 exchanger. This Cl-HCO_3 exchanger is more

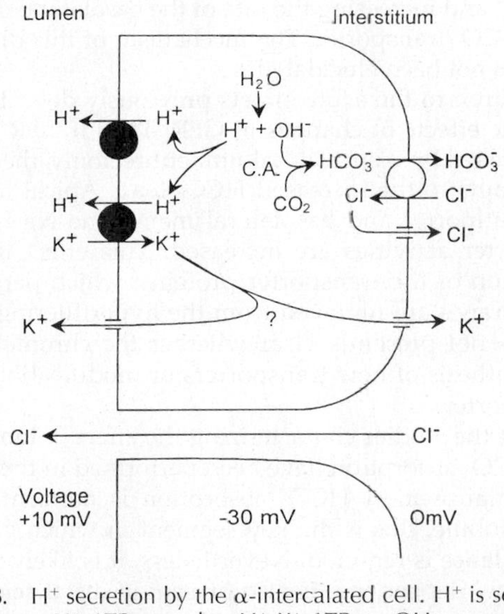

Figure 20.8. H^+ secretion by the α-intercalated cell. H^+ is secreted into the lumen by an H^+-ATPase and an H^+-K^+-ATPase. OH^- generated by apical membrane H^+ secretion reacts with CO_2 to form HCO_3^-, which exits across the basolateral membrane on a Cl-HCO_3 exchanger. Cl^- that enters the cell on the exchanger recycles across a basolateral membrane Cl^- channel. The fate of K^+ that enters the cell on the H^+-K^+-ATPase is not clear. Carbonic anhydrase catalyzes the conversion of CO_2 and OH^- to HCO_3^- in the cell. Electrogenic H^+ secretion generates a lumen positive voltage, which generates a current flow across the paracellular pathway. •, active transport mechanism; ○, passive transporter; =, channel.

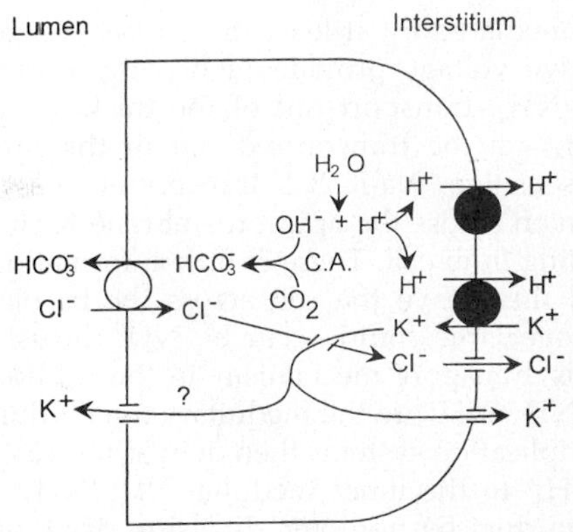

Figure 20.9. HCO_3^- secretion by the β-intercalated cell. H^+ is secreted into the interstitium by an H-ATPase and an H^+-K^+-ATPase. OH^- generated by basolateral membrane H^+ secretion reacts with CO_2 to form HCO_3^-, which exits across the apical membrane on a Cl-HCO_3 exchanger. Cl^- that enters the cell on the exchanger exits across a basolateral membrane Cl^- channel. The fate of K^+ that enters the cell on the H^+-K^+-ATPase is not clear. Carbonic anhydrase catalyzes the conversion of CO_2 and OH^- to HCO_3^- in the cell. •, active transport mechanism; ○, passive transporter; =, channel.

resistant to disulfonic stilbenes than the basolateral membrane Cl-HCO_3 exchanger. The apical membrane Cl-HCO_3 exchanger is not encoded by the AE1 gene. Although a number of different isoforms have been identified for the Cl-HCO_3 exchanger, it is not clear which of these, if any, corresponds to the apical membrane Cl-HCO_3 exchanger. Cl^- that enters the cell in exchange for HCO_3^- then exits across a basolateral membrane conductance.

The medullary collecting duct appears to only possess mechanisms for H^+ secretion. This H^+ secretion is mediated by α-intercalated cells, but also is mediated by cells that morphologically appear distinct from intercalated cells yet functionally appear similar.

AMMONIA SYNTHESIS AND TRANSPORT

Ammonia is synthesized in the proximal tubule. Ammonia synthesis occurs primarily from glutamine, which is actively transported into the proximal tubule cell from both the luminal and peritubular side. Glutamine is then transported into the mitochondria where it is metabolized sequentially to glutamate (phosphate-dependent glutaminase) and to α-ketoglutarate (glutamate dehydrogenase), yielding two ammonias. The α-ketoglutarate can then be metabolized in the tricarboxylic acid cycle to CO_2 and water or can be used in gluconeogenesis. Detailed discussion of ammonia synthesis by the renal tubule is found in Chapter 20, Parts 1 and 3.

Ammonia synthesized in the proximal tubule is preferentially transported into the lumen by two mechanisms. First, NH_3 can diffuse across the apical or basolateral membranes. NH_3 permeability has been found to be equal on these membranes. However, the lower luminal pH serves as a trap for ammonia converting NH_3 to NH_4^+, lowering luminal NH_3 concentration and allowing continued NH_3 diffusion (nonionic diffusion). In addition, NH_4^+ can be transported on the Na-H antiporter. In that this transporter is localized predominantly on the apical membrane, this leads to predominantly luminal secretion.

Most of the ammonia that leaves the surface proximal tubule does not return to the surface distal tubule. Thus there is transport of ammonia out of Henle's loop. This transport appears to occur predominantly in the thick ascending limb of Henle's loop and is mediated by at least three mechanisms. First, the lumen positive voltage provides a driving force for passive paracellular NH_4^+ transport out of the thick ascending limb. Second, NH_4^+ can be transported out of the lumen on the furosemide-sensitive Na-K-2Cl transporter. Last, NH_4^+ can leave the lumen across the apical membrane K channel of the thick ascending limb cell. There is little information as to how NH_4^+ would then leave the cell across the basolateral membrane. However, this could occur by NH_3 diffusion. The net result of this transport mechanism is the addition of large amounts of NH_3/NH_4^+ to the medullary interstitium. Countercurrent multiplication systems then deliver the vast majority of this NH_3/NH_4^+ to the inner medulla. NH_3/NH_4^+ then enters the collecting duct by nonionic diffusion driven by the acid luminal pH.

Thus, based on the preceding discussion, ammonia excretion can be regulated by three mechanisms. First, ammonia synthesis in the proximal tubule can be regulated. Chronic acidosis and chronic K deficiency increase ammonia synthesis, whereas hyperkalemia suppresses ammonia synthesis. Second, ammonia delivery from the proximal tubule to the medullary interstitium can be regulated. Hyperkalemia can inhibit NH_4^+ reabsorption from the thick ascending limb. This may explain the low urinary NH_4^+ concentrations found in hyperkalemic distal renal tubular acidosis (RTA) in addition to decreased synthesis of ammonia by hyperkalemia. In addition, any interstitial renal disease that destroys renal medullary anatomy may decrease medullary interstitial NH_3/NH_4^+ concentration. Last, mechanisms that regulate H^+ secretion can regulate ammonia entry into the collecting duct and excretion.

The only other physiologically significant buffer in the urine is phosphate. This is the major titratable buffer. In general, phosphate excretion is equal to phosphate intake. Thus although the serum phosphate level may be regulated, phosphate excretion is rarely altered in the steady state, and thus is rarely responsible for abnormalities in acid–base balance. One possible exception to this may be the patient with renal failure who is ingesting phosphate binders, which will prevent gastrointestinal phosphate absorption and lower urinary phosphate excretion.

REGULATION OF RENAL ACIDIFICATION

The precise regulation of acid–base balance requires an integrated system that precisely regulates proximal tubular $H\text{-}HCO_3$ transport, distal nephron $H\text{-}HCO_3$ transport, and ammonia synthesis. We review here some of the key determinants.

Luminal Bicarbonate Concentration and pH

Rates of tubular H^+ secretion all along the nephron are exquisitely sensitive to luminal pH and HCO_3 concentration. This can be viewed as analogous to regulation of a reaction by the concentration of the product. Thus the higher the luminal H^+ concentration, the greater the driving force for H^+ movement from lumen to cell and blood, decreasing the net rate of H^+ secretion. In the proximal tubule, luminal pH and HCO_3 concentration regulate the rate of passive paracellular HCO_3 transport. In addition, a lower luminal pH inhibits apical membrane H^+ secretion, lowering cell pH, and secondarily inhibiting basolateral membrane base efflux. In the collecting duct, active transcellular H^+ secretion has been demonstrated to be regulated by luminal pH.

The net result of this form of regulation is that changes in H^+ transport rate early in the nephron will be attenuated along the nephron. Thus for instance, a 50% increase in H^+ secretory rate in the first millimeter of the proximal tubule will lower luminal HCO_3 concentration. This will then lead to inhibition of H^+ secretion in all subsequent segments of the nephron, attenuating the 50% stimulation. This explains why experimental maneuvers known to significantly increase proximal tubular transport may have small effects on total renal H^+ secretion. Thus although the proximal tubule reabsorbs the vast majority of HCO_3, and therefore its regulation would be predicted to be the most important, this may not be the case. Changes in the rate of distal nephron H^+ secretion are less likely to be attenuated, making small changes in distal H^+ secretory rate of possibly great significance.

Luminal Flow Rate

Changes in GFR are associated with proportional changes in the filtered load of HCO_3. This means that in order to maintain acid–base balance, changes in GFR must be accompanied by parallel changes in tubular H^+ secretion rate. This phenomenon is *glomerulotubular balance,* and is similar to the glomerulotubular balance for renal sodium transport. A number of mechanisms are responsible.

First, changes in GFR and luminal flow rate lead to changes in the axial profile for luminal pH and HCO_3 concentration. Thus, in the presence of a higher luminal flow rate, a fixed rate of HCO_3 absorption will lower HCO_3 concentration to a lesser extent. This will cause the HCO_3 concentration and pH in later portions of the nephron to be higher and thus will stimulate H^+ secretion.

When changes in the axial luminal HCO_3 concentration profile are corrected for, studies have demonstrated an additional effect of flow rate. Thus acute increases in luminal flow rate are accompanied by immediate increases in the rate of H^+ secretion that cannot be attributed to changes in measured luminal HCO_3 concentration. Microperfusion studies have shown that increases in luminal flow rate directly increase proximal tubule $Na^+\text{-}H^+$ antiporter activity and rate, secondarily increasing cell pH and increasing the rate of the basolateral membrane $Na\text{-}HCO_3\text{-}CO_3$ transporter. The mechanism of this direct effect of flow has not been elucidated.

In addition to the acute effects previously described, there are chronic effects of changes in GFR. Thus if GFR is chronically increased by contralateral uninephrectomy, the proximal tubule adapts to the increased HCO_3 load. Apical membrane $Na^+\text{-}H^+$ antiporter and basolateral membrane $Na\text{-}HCO_3\text{-}CO_3$ cotransporter activities are increased. This effect involves a modification of the transporter proteins, which persists after the membranes are removed from the hyperfiltering environment. It is not presently clear whether the chronic effect involves synthesis of new transporters or modification of existing transporters.

Most of the studies characterizing the affect of luminal flow rate on HCO_3 absorption have been performed in the proximal tubule. Because most HCO_3 absorption is performed in the proximal tubule, this is the key segment in which glomerulotubular balance is required. Nevertheless, it is likely that some form of flow dependence is also present in distal acidification.

Blood pH

The regulation of acid–base balance requires that in states of acidosis net H^+ excretion increase, and in states of alkalosis net H^+ excretion decrease. This form of regulation involves both acute and chronic mechanisms. In the proximal tubule, acute decreases in blood pH increase the rate of HCO_3 absorption, and acute increases in blood pH inhibit HCO_3 absorption. Both transcellular and paracellular fluxes are regulated. In addition, this type of regulation occurs with changes in P_{CO_2} or HCO_3 concentration. Similarly, in the collecting duct acute changes in peritubular HCO_3 concentration and pH regulate the rate of H^+ secretion. A part of this acute regulation may involve exocytotic insertion of membrane-containing H^+ pumps.

In addition to acute regulation, mechanisms exist for chronic regulation. Chronic acidosis or alkalosis leads to chronic changes in the activities of proximal tubule apical membrane Na^+-H^+ antiporter and basolateral membrane Na-HCO_3-CO_3 cotransporter. The affect of chronic acid–base changes on the H-HCO_3 transporters persists after the transporters are removed from the acidotic environment. Activities appear to change in parallel. In addition, kinetically the effect appears to be a Vmax effect. Changes in Na^+-H^+ antiporter activity are associated with increases in the abundance of mRNA corresponding to the Na^+-H^+ antiporter isoform, NHE-1. When proximal tubule cells are examined in tissue culture, one can also demonstrate that incubation of the cells in acid media leads to an increase in Na^+-H^+ antiporter activity and an increase in NHE-1 mRNA. In addition, chronic acidosis increases proximal tubular ammonia synthesis. Activities of phosphate-dependent glutaminase, phosphoenolpyruvate carboxykinase (PEPCK), and glutamate dehydrogenase have all been shown to be increased. In addition, the abundance of mRNAs corresponding to these proteins has been shown to be increased.

The cortical collecting duct is also modified by chronic acid–base changes. As previously noted, the cortical collecting duct is able to either secrete H^+ ion or secrete HCO_3. If animals are fed an acid-rich diet, cells responsible for H^+ secretion increase their activity, whereas cells responsible for HCO_3 secretion decrease their activity. Conversely, in animals fed an alkali-rich diet, HCO_3 secreting cells increase their activity and H^+ secreting cells decrease their activity. These effects persist *in vitro*. There is some controversy regarding whether this chronic effect involves interconversion between α and β cells or reciprocal atrophy and hypertrophy of the two cell types. In any case, there is no cellular proliferation during these adaptations, indicating that one cell type does not overgrow the collecting duct. Chronic metabolic acidosis also stimulates thick ascending limb HCO_3 absorption, and chronic alkalosis inhibits thick ascending limb HCO_3 absorption. The mechanisms responsible have not been addressed.

Mineralocorticoids, Distal Na Delivery, and Extracellular Fluid Volume

Mineralocorticoid hormones are key in the regulation of distal nephron H^+ secretion. Two mechanisms appear to be involved. First, mineralocorticoid hormone stimulates Na absorption in principal cells of the cortical collecting duct. This leads to a more lumen negative voltage that is able to then stimulate H^+ secretion. This mechanism is indirect in that it requires the presence of Na and the presence of Na transport.

A second mechanism is the direct activation of H^+ secretion by mineralocorticoid hormones. If one perfuses cortical or medullary collecting ducts in the total absence of Na, mineralocorticoid hormones will directly stimulate H^+ secretion. In addition, the outer medullary collecting duct does not transport Na, yet mineralocorticoids stimulate H^+ secretion in this segment. The effect of mineralocorticoids is chronic, requiring long exposure. Mineralocorticoids have been shown to increase the activities of the apical membrane H^+ pump and the basolateral membrane Cl-HCO_3 exchanger in parallel. This effect is most likely transcriptional, as with other steroid hormones.

The relative importance of the direct and indirect mineralocorticoid effects is unclear. Based on the fact that rates of HCO_3 absorption in the outer medullary collecting duct exceed those in the cortical collecting duct, and the fact that the indirect mechanism could not possibly function in the outer medullary collecting duct given the absence of Na transport, it has been concluded that the direct effect of mineralocorticoids is quantitatively more important. However, if one places animals or human subjects on a low dietary Na, a diet expected to decrease distal delivery of Na, there is no effect of mineralocorticoid hormones on H^+ secretion. These studies imply that the indirect mechanism for mineralocorticoid activation is quantitatively the more important. Thus in the absence of Na delivery to the cortical collecting duct, mineralocorticoid hormones cannot stimulate Na absorption, and there will not be a change in voltage. Therefore in this setting there would be no indirect effect on H^+ secretion. Although direct stimulation of H^+ transport is still possible in this setting, no effect on renal acidification is observed.

In this respect, distal Na delivery becomes a regulator of distal acidification. Thus the combination of high mineralocorticoid levels and high distal Na delivery will increase H^+ secretion in the distal nephron and increase renal net acid excretion. This mechanism is responsible for the generation and maintenance of metabolic alkalosis in patients with primary increases in mineralocorticoid levels or in patients on chloruretic diuretics. In volume contracted patients not ingesting a diuretic, high mineralocorticoid levels do not lead to increases in net acid excretion or alkalosis, because there is no distal delivery of Na.

Although volume contraction is not able to increase distal nephron H^+ secretion, volume contraction is known to be the most important factor responsible for maintenance of metabolic alkalosis in many patients. This effect appears to be related to a number of factors. First, volume contraction is associated with a decrease in GFR. This will lower the filtered load of HCO_3 and decreases the load placed on the tubules to maintain net acid excretion. Thus a decrease in GFR can be considered to be equivalent to a decrease in nephron HCO_3 secretion. Volume contraction also has been demonstrated to acutely decrease the paracellular permeability of the proximal tubule. This will tend to decrease HCO_3 backleak around cells, and increase net H^+ secretion in the proximal tubule. Third, chronic volume contraction is associated with an adaptive increase in the activity of the proximal tubule apical membrane Na^+-H^+ antiporter. Because this transporter mediates $NaHCO_3$ and NaCl absorption, both of these capacities will be increased with chronic volume contraction. Lastly, volume contraction limits distal delivery of chloride. In the presence of chronic metabolic alkalosis, the cortical collecting duct is poised for HCO_3 secretion. However, the secretion of HCO_3 requires the presence of luminal Cl (Fig. 20.8), and may be limited by low Cl delivery.

Potassium Deficiency

Potassium deficiency is associated with an increase in renal net acid excretion. This effect is multifactorial. First, potassium deficiency leads to a decrease in GFR, which, as previously discussed, is equivalent to decreasing nephron HCO_3 secretion. Second, chronic K deficiency leads to an adaptive increase in the proximal tubule apical membrane Na^+-H^+ antiporter and basolateral membrane Na-HCO_3-CO_3 cotransporter activities. This effect is similar to that of chronic acidosis and may be due to intracellular acidosis. Chronic K deficiency also increases proximal tubular ammonia production. Activities of phosphate-dependent glutaminase and PEPCK are increased, similar to that seen in chronic acidosis. Once again, these effects may be related to a decrease in intracellular pH. Last, chronic K deficiency leads to an increase in collecting duct H^+ secretion. This appears to be related to an increase in the apical membrane activity of an H^+-K^+ pump. It is not clear whether K deficiency increases the synthesis of these transporters, leads to insertion of a latent pool of transporters into the apical membrane, or merely activates latent transporters in the apical membrane. Such transporters will increase the rate of H^+ secretion, while they also increase the rate of K absorption in the collecting duct. It should be noted that while all of the above mechanisms will increase renal acid excretion and cause alkalosis, K deficiency also decreases aldosterone secretion, which can inhibit distal acidification. Thus in control subjects the effect of K deficiency on acid–base status can be variable. However, in patients in whom mineralocorticoid secretion is nonsuppressible (primary hyperaldosteronism, Cushing's syndrome), K deficiency will markedly stimulate renal acification and cause a profound metabolic alkalosis.

It should be noted that hyperkalemia may have opposite effects on renal acidification. The most notable effect of hyperkalemia is to inhibit ammonia synthesis in the proximal tubule. This contributes to the metabolic acidosis seen in patients with hyperkalemic distal renal tubular acidosis or type IV RTA.

Hormones

In the proximal tubule, the apical membrane Na^+-H^+ antiporter is acutely inhibited by cyclic adenosine monophosphate (cAMP) and stimulated by protein kinase C. A number of hormones regulate the apical membrane Na^+-H^+ antiporter and proximal tubule acidification, possibly working through cAMP and cAMP-dependent protein kinase. Parathyroid hormone (PTH) and dopamine, both capable of increasing cell cAMP levels, inhibit proximal tubule HCO_3 absorption. Conversely, angiotensin II and α-adrenergic catecholamines, both capable of lowering cell cAMP levels, stimulate HCO_3 absorption. There is evidence, however, that these hormones may work by other mechanisms in addition. In this regard, endothelin has been shown to increase the activity of the apical Na^+-H^+ antiporter through a process involving phosphorylation, increased cell calcium, and activation of tyrosine kinase pathways. In Henle's loop, a number of hormones that increase cell cAMP (arginine vasopressin, glucagon, and PTH) inhibit HCO_3 absorption.

In the distal nephron, increases in cAMP stimulate proton secretion, whereas protein kinase C has no effect. Arginine vasopressin, functioning through a V2 receptor was shown to stimulate distal HCO_3 absorption. *In vivo,* PTH also has been shown to stimulate distal HCO_3 absorption, but this effect appears to be secondary to increased distal delivery of phosphate, with phosphate acting as a nonreabsorbable anion and a buffer.

Selected Readings

Alpern RJ. Mechanism of basolateral membrane $H^+/OH^-/HCO_3$ transport in the rat proximal convoluted tubule: a sodium coupled electrogenic process. *J Gen Physiol* 1985;86:613–636.

Demonstration of the mechanism of basolateral membrane HCO_3 transport in the proximal tubule using a fluorescent method to measure cell pH in vivo.

Alpern RJ. Cell mechanisms of proximal tubule acidification. *Physiol Rev* 1990; 70:79–114.

An in-depth review of the cellular mechanisms responsible for proximal tubule acidification.

Alpern RJ, Stone DK, Rector FC Jr. Renal acidification mechanisms. In: Brenner BM, Rector FC Jr, eds. *The kidney.* Philadelphia: WB Saunders, 1991:318–379.

A complete review of mechanisms and regulation of renal tubular acidification.

Hays SR. Mineralocorticoid modulation of apical and basolateral membrane $H^+/OH^-/HCO_3$ transport processes in the rabbit inner stripe of outer medullary collecting duct. *J Clin Invest* 1992;90:180–187.

These studies demonstrate that mineralocorticoid treatment in vivo leads to a parallel increase in the activities of the apical membrane H pump and basolateral membrane Cl-HCO_3 exchanger in the perfused outer medullary collecting duct.

Horie S, Moe O, Tejedor A, et al. Preincubation in acid media increases Na/H antiporter activity in cultured renal proximal tubule cells. *Proc Natl Acad Sci USA* 1990;87:4742–4745.

The first demonstration that chronic incubation of proximal tubule cells in acid media leads to a protein synthesis dependent increase in Na-H antiporter activity.

Knepper MA, Packer R, Good DW. Ammonium transport in the kidney. *Physiol Rev* 1989;69:179–249.

A thorough review of ammonium transport in the kidney.

McKinney TD, Burg MB. Bicarbonate transport by rabbit cortical collecting tubules: effect of acid and alkaline loads in vivo on transport in vitro. *J Clin Invest* 1977;60:766–768.

The first demonstration that the cortical collecting duct was capable of H secretion or HCO_3 secretion, depending on the diet of the animal.

Preisig PA. Luminal flow rate regulates proximal tubule H-HCO_3 transporters. *Am J Physiol* 1992;262(Renal Fluid Electrolyte Physiol 31):F47–F54.

Demonstration that luminal flow rate directly regulates Na-H antiporter activity.

Stone DK, Xie X-S. Proton translocating ATPases: issues in structure and function. *Kidney Int* 1988;33:767–774.

A thorough description of the molecular properties of proton pumps.

PART 3
Metabolic Acidosis

Thomas D. DuBose, Jr.

PATHOPHYSIOLOGY OF ACID–BASE DISORDERS

Definition

Metabolic acidosis occurs as a result of a marked increase in endogenous production of acid (such as lactic acid and ketoacids), loss of HCO_3^- stores (diarrhea or renal tubular acidosis [RTA]), or progressive accumulation of endogenous acids as a result of impaired excretion because of renal insufficiency.

The Anion Gap

The anion gap (AG) serves a useful role in the initial differentiation of metabolic acidoses and should always be calculated. Two broad types of metabolic acidoses are recognized by directing attention to the *AG:* (a) high AG acidoses, and (b) normal AG or hyperchloremic acidoses. The AG is defined (assuming the albumin is 4 g/dl) as follows:

$$AG = Na^+ - (Cl^- + HCO_3^-) = 12 \text{ mEq/L} \quad (1)$$

Metabolic acidosis with a high AG indicates addition of an acid other than hydrochloric acid or its equivalent to the extracellular fluid (ECF). The AG may also be increased as a result of an increase in anionic protein (albumin) or a decrease in non-Na^+ cations (hypocalcemia, hypomagnesemia). Such factitious causes of a high AG are unusual. Most often an elevated AG denotes the presence of a high AG acidosis. If the attendant non-Cl^- acid anion cannot be readily excreted in relationship to the rate of production and is retained after HCO_3^- titration, the anion replaces titrated HCO_3^- without disturbing the Cl^- concentration. Hence, the acidosis is normochloremic and the AG increases. Moreover, in a pure high AG metabolic acidosis the decrement in the serum HCO_3^- (ΔHCO_3^-) will equal numerically the increment in the AG (ΔAG).

A metabolic acidosis with a normal AG (hyperchloremic) suggests that HCO_3^- has been effectively replaced by Cl^- because of one of the following conditions: (a) HCO_3^- loss from the body fluids through gastrointestinal or renal mechanisms, with subsequent Cl^- retention; (b) defective renal acidification with failure to excrete normal quantities of metabolically produced acid—the conjugate base is excreted as the sodium salt, and sodium chloride is retained secondarily; (c) addition of hydrochloric acid (or equivalent) to the body fluids; (d) addition of an acid other than hydrochloric acid, with subsequent titration of HCO_3^- and rapid renal excretion of the accompanying anion and replacement by Cl^-; and (e) rapid dilution of the plasma HCO_3^- by saline.

General Clinical Features

Metabolic acidosis is recognized by the co-occurrence of acidemia (pH less than 7.35) and a low serum bicarbonate concentration (total CO_2 concentration). Metabolic acidosis also be may recognized by an elevated AG, even in the face of normal values for pH and HCO_3^- in plasma. A flow diagram outlining the diagnostic approach to metabolic acidosis, in which the initial consideration is the AG, is displayed in Fig. 20.10.

Respiratory Compensation

When there is a primary decrease in plasma $[HCO_3^-]$ and an increase in alveolar ventilation, a decrease in $Paco_2$ (respiratory compensation) is anticipated because the medullary chemoreceptors are stimulated by acidemia to invoke an increase in ventilation. The ratio of HCO_3^- to $Paco_2$ and the subsequent pH will be returned toward, but not to, normal. This hypocapnic response to acidemia is predictable in simple acid–base disturbances and blunts the magnitude of the decline in blood pH that would occur otherwise. The degree of respiratory compensation expected in a simple form of metabolic acidosis was derived empirically and can be predicted from the following relationship:

$$Paco_2 = (1.5 \times HCO_3^-) + 8 \quad (2)$$

Thus, in a patient with metabolic acidosis and a plasma bicarbonate concentration of 12 mEq/L, a $Paco_2$ between 24 and 28 mm Hg would be anticipated. Values for $Paco_2$ below 24 or greater than 28 mm Hg denote a mixed disturbance (metabolic acidosis and respiratory alkalosis, or metabolic acidosis and respiratory acidosis, respectively). Although this relationship is accurate within 2 mm Hg, the $Paco_2$ also can be estimated more conveniently by adding 15 to the patient's serum $[HCO_3^-]$. Deviations from anticipated values (such as coexistent respiratory acidosis or alkalosis) demand recognition and immediate attention.

Renal Role in Compensation

The kidneys regulate plasma $[HCO_3^-]$ through three processes: (a) "reabsorption" of the filtered HCO_3^-, (b) excretion of titratable acidity, and (c) synthesis and excretion of NH_4^+. *Net acid excretion* is the sum of titratable acid and ammonium, minus any bicarbonate that appears in the urine. Approximately 80%

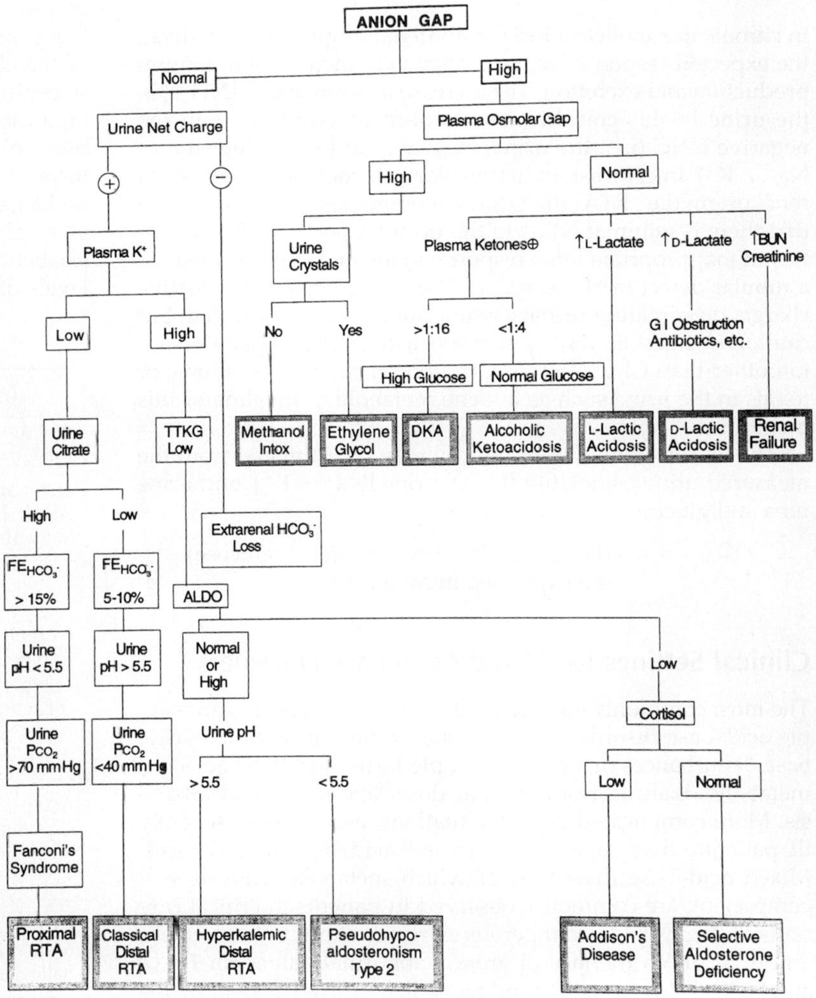

Figure 20.10. Diagnostic approach to metabolic acidosis. The anion gap is the entry point and divides the types of metabolic acidoses into the high anion gap and normal anion gap categories. Final diagnoses are displayed in hatched boxes. Aldo, aldosterone; DKA, diabetic ketoacidosis; RTA, renal tubular acidosis; TTKG, transtubular potassium gradient, which is U_K-P_K/U-P Osm.

to 90% of the filtered HCO_3^- is reabsorbed in the proximal tubule. Under normal conditions, the distal nephron reabsorbs the remainder of the filtered HCO_3^- (approximately 5% to 10%). In addition to the amount of H^+ secreted to absorb the filtered bicarbonate, the collecting duct must secrete a quantity of protons equal to that generated from metabolism and digestion of dietary protein. The quantity of acids produced daily is approximately 40 to 60 mEq. Thus an equal amount of acid must be secreted to prevent the development of chronic positive hydrogen ion balance and metabolic acidosis. Ammonium excretion, the major component of net acid excretion, is regulated by both ammoniagenesis and by ammonium transport.

Estimating Urinary NH_4^+ Excretion: The Urine Net Charge (Anion Gap) and Osmolal Gap

When renal function is normal, the kidney responds to chronic metabolic acidosis by increasing ammonium production and excretion dramatically. Ammonium production and excretion by the kidney may be impaired by chronic renal failure, hyperkalemia, and RTA. Because one of the causes of hyperchloremic metabolic acidosis is RTA, it is important to delineate whether the kidney is responding appropriately to systemic acidosis by increasing ammonium excretion. Ammonium excretion can be estimated from a spot urine sample by consideration of the urine net charge or urinary osmolal gap. The *urine net charge (UNC)* is defined as the difference in the concentration of chloride (Cl^-) and the sum of the urinary cations Na^+ and K^+, as shown in the following equation:

$$UNC = [Na^+ + K^+]_u - [Cl^-]_u \qquad (3)$$

In chronic metabolic acidosis of nonrenal origin (e.g., diarrhea), the expected response by the kidney is to increase ammonium production and excretion. The increase in ammonium $[NH_4^+]$ in the urine in this condition is manifest as an increase in the negative UNC (i.e., the urinary Cl^- would exceed the sum of $Na^+ + K^+$). In contrast, in hyperchloremic metabolic acidosis of renal origin (i.e., RTA) the UNC would be positive, designating that there is minimal NH_4^+ in the urine. A positive UNC signifies an inappropriate renal response to the metabolic acidosis or a tubular defect in H^+ secretion. The utility of the net negative charge in estimating urinary ammonium has been verified, but caution is urged if NH_4^+ is excreted with an accompanying anion other than Cl^-. Ketonuria, the presence of drug anions, or toxins in the urine such as toluene metabolites, invalidates this method.

The urinary ammonium ($U_{NH_4^+}$) may be estimated from the measured urine osmolality (U_{Osm}), urine $[Na^+ + K^+]$, and urine urea and glucose:

$$U_{NH_4^+} = 0.5\,(U_{Osm} - [2(Na^+ + K^+) + \text{urea} + \text{glucose}) \quad \text{(all expressed in mmol/L)} \qquad (4)$$

Clinical Settings for Mixed Acid–Base Disorders

The most commonly encountered clinical disturbances are simple acid–base disorders, that is, one of the four cardinal acid–base disturbances in a pure or simple form: metabolic acidosis, metabolic alkalosis, respiratory acidosis, and respiratory alkalosis. More complicated clinical situations, especially in severely ill patients, may give rise to mixed acid–base disturbances. Mixed acid–base disorders, of which metabolic acidosis is a component, are commonly observed in patients in critical care units and may lead to dangerous extremes of pH, or, conversely, a normal pH in the face of grossly abnormal values for Pa_{CO_2} and HCO_3^-. To appreciate and recognize a mixed acid–base disturbance, it is important to understand the physiologic compensatory responses that occur in the simple acid–base disorders. Mixed metabolic acidosis–respiratory acidosis or mixed metabolic acidosis–respiratory alkalosis can be diagnosed by recognition that the measured Pa_{CO_2} is above, or below, respectively, the predicted value (from equation 2). A mixed high AG metabolic acidosis–metabolic alkalosis is affirmed by appreciation that the increment in the AG exceeds the decrement in the serum HCO_3^- because new HCO_3^- is generated by loss of H^+ and Cl^- in the vomitus. An example of values in a patient with mixed metabolic acidosis–metabolic alkalosis follows: Na^+ 140, Cl^- 95, HCO_3^- 25, AG 20 (i.e., the ΔHCO_3^- is 0 and the ΔAG is +10). In this case, the mixed disorder has reestablished normobicarbonatemia, but in association with retention of the high AG. When the increase in the AG is less than the decrease in serum HCO_3^- concentration, a mixed high AG–normal AG metabolic acidosis is present. This mixed disorder might arise in a patient with both lactic acidosis and diarrhea or ketoacidosis and RTA. A "triple disturbance," which typically includes a high AG metabolic acidosis (usually lactic acidosis), respiratory alkalosis, and metabolic alkalosis, is not uncommon in critically ill patients.

HIGH ANION GAP ACIDOSIS (AG GREATER THAN 12 mEq/L)

There are four major causes of a high AG acidosis: (a) lactic acidosis (usually L-lactic acidosis, rarely, D-lactic acidosis), (b) ketoacidosis, (c) ingested alcohol or toxins, and (d) acute and chronic renal failure (Table 20.6). Identification of the underlying cause of a high AG acidosis is facilitated by consideration of the clinical setting and associated laboratory values. Initial screening to differentiate the high AG acidoses should include (a) a careful history or other evidence for drug or toxin ingestion, (b) arterial blood gas measurement to detect coexistent respiratory alkalosis, (c) oxalate crystals in the urine plus an osmolal gap in the patient with a high AG acidosis suggesting ethylene glycol ingestion, (d) historic evidence of diabetes mellitus (diabetic ketoacidosis), (e) evidence of alcoholism or increased levels of β-hydroxybutyrate (alcoholic ketoacidosis), (f) obser-

TABLE 20.6. Causes of High Anion Gap Acidosis

Ketoacidosis
Diabetic ketoacidosis Alcoholic ketoacidosis Starvation ketoacidosis
Lactic Acidosis

L-Lactic acidosis
  Type A
  Type B
D-Lactic acidosis

Renal Failure
Acute Chronic
Toxins
Ethylene glycol Methyl alcohol Salicylates

vation for clinical signs of uremia and determination of the blood urea nitrogen (BUN) and creatinine (uremic acidosis), (g) the recognition of the numerous settings in which L-lactate levels may be increased (hypotension, cardiac failure, drugs, leukemia, or cancer), and (h) appreciation of the possibility of accumulation of D-lactate in the presence of low gastrointestinal (GI) motility, GI obstruction, G pouches, antibiotic therapy, and bacterial overgrowth.

Ketoacidosis

Diabetic Ketoacidosis

Pathophysiology. Diabetic ketoacidosis (DKA) occurs when insulin deficiency and the relative excess of glucagon leads to increased fatty acid metabolism. An absence of insulin stimulates lipolysis and fatty acid release, and glucagon stimulates the hepatic metabolism of fatty acids to ketoacids.

Clinical Features. DKA, which occurs most often in insulin-dependent diabetes mellitus, is seen clinically in association with an intercurrent illness, particularly infections, which increase insulin requirements temporarily and acutely. The diagnosis is confirmed by the concurrence of a metabolic acidosis, strongly positive plasma ketones in undiluted serum, hyperglycemia, ECF volume depletion, and Kussmaul respiration. Although hyperchloremic acidosis may occur in patients who remain euvolemic, most patients will have an AG acidosis.

Treatment. Two aspects of treatment are universal in DKA: (a) insulin, to inhibit ketoacid production, and (b) intravenous fluids for ECF volume restoration and correction of electrolyte deficits. Low-dose intravenous insulin therapy (0.1 units/kg per hour, after an initial loading dose of the same amount) reduces the plasma glucose, smoothly corrects the ketonemia, lowers the elevated AG, and repairs the acidosis. Although regular insulin also may be administered intramuscularly (0.2 mg/kg initially, then 6 units every hour), it should be noted that intramuscular insulin may not be effective in volume depleted and/or hypotensive patients, as is often the case in ketoacidosis. If hyperglycemia is marked, blood glucose should not be lowered below 300 mg/dl in the first few hours of treatment. Sudden drop of blood glucose below 300 mg/dl may be associated with cerebral edema.

Most, if not all, patients with diabetic ketoacidosis require correction of the ECF volume depletion that almost invariably accompanies the osmotic diuresis and ketonuria. Therapy should be initiated with isotonic saline at a rate of 1,000 ml intravenously per hour. The usual ECF deficit in an adult is in the range of 3 liters of isotonic saline. When the pulse and blood pressure have stabilized and the corrected serum sodium concentration is in the range of 130 to 135 mEq/L, the clinician should switch to 0.45% NaCl. Ringer's lactate should be avoided. If the blood sugar declines below 250 to 300 mg/dl, 0.45% NaCl with 5% dextrose should be administered.

Total body potassium depletion is almost always present, although the plasma potassium on admission is usually elevated, indicating that potassium replacement therapy must be individualized. Potassium depletion occurs as a result of the osmotic diuresis, decreased dietary intake, and vomiting that accompanies DKA. A normal or reduced [K^+] on admission, which is found in certain patients (e.g., in which vomiting was a prominent prodromal symptom), indicates severe potassium depletion. Administration of saline, insulin, and alkali will cause the potassium level to decline further. Frequent monitoring of the plasma potassium is mandatory and a precise recipe is difficult to provide. Caution should be exercised in the presence of hyperkalemia, especially in the patient with renal insufficiency; the clinician should withhold potassium as long as the serum level is greater than 5.0 mEq/L. Nevertheless, when the urine output has been established, 20 mEq KCl should be administered in each liter of fluid as long as the plasma [K^+] is less than 3.5 mEq/L. The plasma [K^+], glucose, HCO_3^-, Na^+, and Cl^- should be monitored and recorded hourly.

The routine administration of phosphate (usually as potassium phosphate) is not advised because of the potential for hyperphosphatemia and hypocalcemia. A significant number of patients with DKA will display hyperphosphatemia before initiation of therapy. In virtually all patients, the elevated phosphorous concentration on admission is followed by a fall in plasma phosphorus levels within 2 to 6 hours after initiation of therapy. In this circumstance, phosphate should be replaced, up to a plasma phosphorus of 4.0 mg/dl. Neutral K-phosphate, 10 to 20 mmol/L of intravenous fluids, should be used unless hyperkalemia coexists, in which case neutral Na-phosphate should be used. Bicarbonate therapy is usually not necessary unless the acidosis is severe (pH less than 7.1, and Pa_{CO_2} is low). In general, the increment in the AG above the normal value represents "potential" bicarbonate, or that bicarbonate that will be realized when circulating ketones are metabolically converted to bicarbonate following primary therapy (insulin). Nevertheless, during therapy, it is difficult to predict to what extent ketones will be converted back to bicarbonate before being lost in the urine when the GFR is normalized. If exogenous bicarbonate is administered, that amount of bicarbonate will be added to that produced endogenously, so an "overshoot alkalosis" may develop. Therefore small amounts of bicarbonate, given initially (45 to 90 mEq intravenous slowly, or 1 to 2 ampules), until the pH reaches approximately 7.2, or the [HCO_3^-] is in the range of 10 to 12 mEq/L, is a prudent goal. With exogenous bicarbonate therapy, additional potassium will be needed.

Alcoholic Ketoacidosis

Pathophysiology. Alcoholic ketoacidosis is a relatively common, but underappreciated, disorder that occurs in alcoholics, particularly in binge drinkers. Ketoacidosis develops when alcohol consumption is abruptly curtailed, usually as a result of vomiting, or abdominal pain. In association with starvation, glycogen depletion, and metabolism of ethanol (which inhibits gluconeogenesis), the glucose concentration is often low or normal. When ECF volume depletion is pronounced and insulin levels are reduced, the acidosis may be severe. The value for the AG is elevated because of elevated ketones, which are predominantly β-hydroxybutyrate. Mild lactic acidosis may coexist because of alteration in the redox state by ETOH in the liver or severe tissue hypoxia because of volume depletion. The nitroprusside ketone reaction (Acetest) can detect acetoacetic acid but not β-hydroxybutyrate, so the initial degree of ketosis and ketonuria may not be appreciated. Typically, insulin levels are low and levels of triglyceride, cortisol, glucagon, and growth hormone are increased, leading to ketoacidosis.

Treatment. The mainstay of therapy is intravenous normal saline to expand the ECF. Insulin is obviously contraindicated, illustrating why the diagnosis of alcoholic ketoacidosis must not be mistaken for DKA. Intravenous replacement of potassium, phosphate, and magnesium deficits, as well as vitamin supplementation (thiamine 100 mg intravenously) are usually necessary and should be given as needed later in the course, particularly in the face of chronic alcoholism and malnutrition. Glucose is necessary if hypoglycemia is present, and it increases the insulin/glucagon ratio, suppressing ketoacid production and permitting resolution of the ketoacidosis. Hypophosphatemia usually emerges several hours after admission; therefore the need for therapy can be overlooked, especially if the serum phosphorus concentration on admission is normal. Profound hypophosphatemia may provoke aspiration, rhabdomyolysis, and coagulopathy. Phosphate should be replaced as either neutral Na^+ or K^+ phosphate, as dictated by the plasma [K^+], at 10 to 20 mmol/L of intravenous fluids. Upper gastrointestinal hemorrhage, pancreatitis, and pneumonia may accompany alcoholic ketoacidosis.

L-Lactic Acidosis

L-Lactic acidosis occurs in a diverse group of disorders that are recognized by an increase in the plasma L-lactate concentration. This disorder is discussed in detail in Chapter 20, Part 4.

DRUG-INDUCED AND TOXIN-INDUCED ACIDOSIS

Salicylates

Aspirin overdose usually gives rise to a complex acid–base disturbance, in which respiratory alkalosis predominates (because of stimulation of respiration by salicylates), and a high AG may occur concomitantly. Only a portion of the increased AG can be attributed to the increased plasma salicylate concentration; for example, a toxic salicylate level of 100 mg/dl can only account for an increase in the AG of 7 mEq/L. Lactic-acid production is also often increased, partly as a direct drug effect and partly as a result of the decrease in P_{CO_2} induced by salicylate.

Treatment

The initial step in therapy should include vigorous gastric lavage followed by activated charcoal administration per nasogastric tube. The mainstay of therapy is afforded by an alkaline diuresis to allow the relatively impermeant anionic form of salicylate to be trapped in tubular fluid and excreted in the urine. To facilitate removal of salicylate, intravenous sodium bicarbonate in amounts adequate to alkalinize the urine (urine pH greater than 7.5) and to maintain urine output is necessary. An alkaline diuresis may be induced by infusion of half isotonic saline plus two ampules of $NaHCO_3$ (45 mEq each). Although this form of therapy is straightforward in acidotic patients, alkalemia from respiratory alkalosis may make this approach hazardous. To avoid serious alkalosis, the arterial pH should be monitored and not allowed to increase above 7.55. Acetazolamide, in small doses (250 mg), is recommended only when an alkaline diuresis cannot be achieved or when the plasma pH exceeds 7.55 because larger doses may result in systemic metabolic acidosis if sodium bicarbonate is not given concomitantly. Moreover, acetazolamide and acetosalicylic acid compete for binding sites on albumin. Coexisting metabolic acidosis greatly impedes salicylate clearance and enhances salicylate entry into the central nervous system and must be avoided. On the other hand, hypokalemia may occur as a result of an alkaline diuresis from either sodium bicarbonate or acetazolamide and should be treated promptly. If renal failure prevents rapid clearance of salicylate or if acetosalicylic acid levels remain in the toxic range (greater than 4 to 5 mM or 40 to 50 mg/dl), hemodialysis against a bicarbonate dialysate (35 mEq/L) should be performed.

Toxin Ingestion (Ethylene Glycol and Methyl Alcohol) and the Osmolal Gap

Pathophysiology

Plasma osmolality (mOsm/kg H_2O) is calculated according to the following expression:

$$P_{Osm} = 2\ Na + Glu/18 + BUN/2.8 \qquad (5)$$

The BUN and glucose are expressed in mg/dl. The calculated and determined osmolality should agree within 10 to 15 mOsm/kg. When the measured osmolality exceeds the calculated osmolality by more than 15 to 20 mOsm/kg, one of two circumstances prevails. First, the serum sodium may be spuriously low, as occurs with hyperlipidemia or hyperproteinemia (pseudohyponatremia), or second, osmolytes other than sodium salts, glucose, or urea have accumulated in plasma. Examples include the accumulation of solutes that can increase the osmolality in plasma, including the alcohols: ethanol, ethylene glycol, and methanol. Less commonly, mannitol or retained radiocontrast agents increase the osmolal gap. In these examples, the difference between the calculated osmolality and the measured osmolality is proportional to the concentration of the unmeasured solute (osmolal gap). With an appropriate clinical history and index of suspicion, the osmolal gap becomes a helpful screening tool in poison-associated AG acidosis.

Clinical Features

Ingestion of ethylene glycol leads to a metabolic acidosis in addition to severe central nervous system, cardiopulmonary, and renal damage. Ethylene glycol (molecular weight = 62 D) increases the osmolar gap (greater than 10 mOsm/kg H_2O), and the increased AG can be attributed to ethylene-glycol metabolites, especially glycolic acid, and other organic acids. L-Lactic acid production also increases owing to a toxic depression in the reaction rates of the citric-acid cycle and altered intracellular redox state. Diagnosis is facilitated by recognizing oxalate crystals in the urine.

Treatment

The principles of treatment of ethylene-glycol intoxication, as with methanol intoxication, is to stop production of toxic metabolites by competitive inhibition of alcohol dehydrogenase through intravenous ethanol administration, coupled with removal of the accumulated toxins. Immediate therapy is necessary to prevent irreversible central nervous system and renal toxicity. Ethanol (10% solution) is given intravenously at a rate of 0.6 g/kg body weight over 30 to 45 minutes followed by a maintenance infusion of 5% ethanol at 110 mg/kg per hour to produce an ethanol serum level of 100 to 150 mg/dl. Thus therapy includes prompt administration of intravenous ethanol; intravenous normal saline to initiate a diuresis; thiamine and pyridoxine supplements (100 mg each, intravenously); and hemodialysis with a high-flux membrane. During dialysis, the rate of ethanol infusion must be increased.

Methanol Ingestion

Methanol ingestion as wood alcohol or in paint thinners causes metabolic acidosis and severe optic nerve and central nervous system manifestations when methanol is metabolized to formaldehyde, then formic acid. More recently, the new alcohol dehydrogenase inhibitor, fomepizole, has been used successfully with or without concomitant hemodialysis.

Clinical Features

This form of toxic acidosis should be considered when an obviously inebriated patient with a high AG metabolic acidosis and visual disturbances is encountered. Nausea, vomiting, and abdominal pain are usually present. Lactic acids and ketoacids as well as other unidentified organic acids may contribute to the acidosis. Due to its high retention and low molecular weight (32 D), an osmolar gap is usually present.

Treatment

The treatment of methanol intoxication is generally similar to that for ethylene-glycol intoxication, including ethanol or fomepizole administration, general supportive measures, volume expansion, and hemodialysis. Initiation of a saline diuresis is less of an issue with methanol than with ethylene-glycol intoxication because renal toxicity is not a direct effect of methanol intoxication and crystals are not present in the urine.

Chronic Renal Failure

Pathophysiology

Progressive renal insufficiency will eventually convert the hyperchloremic acidosis of moderate renal insufficiency to the typical high AG acidosis of advanced renal failure. Low glomerular filtration, continued reabsorption of organic anions, and low ammonium excretion all contribute to the pathogenesis of this metabolic disturbance. As functional renal mass is compromised in the relentless progression of renal disease, the number of functioning nephrons eventually becomes insufficient to maintain NH excretion to the extent necessary to balance net acid production. Thus the HCO_3^- concentration declines, but rarely below 15 mEq/L, and the AG rarely exceeds 20 mEq/L. The acid retained in patients with chronic renal disease is buffered, in part, by alkaline salts derived from bone resulting in loss of bone calcium carbonate, which contributes to the skeletal demineralization with renal acidosis. Metabolic acidosis mobilizes calcium and alkali from bone and also inhibits renal calcium absorption. Thus an additional "trade-off" in chronic renal failure is a decrease in bone mineral content and negative calcium balance as a result of mobilization of bone calcium salts to defend blood pH in the face of chronic metabolic acidosis. Treatment of acidosis with alkali improves calcium balance and bone density.

Treatment

Both severe uremic acidosis and hyperchloremic acidosis of renal insufficiency require oral alkali replacement to maintain the bicarbonate concentration between 20 and 24 mEq/L. This usually can be accomplished with relatively modest amounts of alkali (1.0 to 1.5 mEq/kg per day). Sodium citrate (Shohl's solution) has been shown to enhance the absorption of aluminum from the gastrointestinal tract and should never be administered to patients receiving aluminum-containing antacids because of the risk of aluminum intoxication. If hyperkalemia persists, furosemide (60 to 80 mg/day) should be added.

HYPERCHLOREMIC METABOLIC ACIDOSIS (NORMAL ANION GAP ACIDOSIS)

Pathogenesis and Differential Diagnosis

Alkali may be lost from the gastrointestinal tract (diarrhea) or from the kidneys (RTA). In these disorders (Table 20.7), reciprocal changes in chloride and bicarbonate result in a normal AG. Therefore, in a pure form of simple hyperchloremic acidosis, the increase in chloride above the normal value equals the decrease in bicarbonate. The absence of such a relationship suggests a mixed disturbance. Diarrhea results in the loss of large quantities of HCO_3^- and HCO_3^- decomposed by reaction with organic acids. Instead of an acid urine pH, as is often anticipated with diarrhea, a pH of 6.0 is usually observed because metabolic acidosis and hypokalemia increase renal ammonium synthesis and excretion, thus providing more urinary buffer, which increases urine pH. Metabolic acidosis due to gastrointestinal losses with a high urine pH can be differentiated from RTA because urinary NH_4^+ excretion is low in RTA and high in patients with diarrhea. Urinary NH_4^+ levels can be estimated by calculating the urine net charge (equation 3) or estimating urinary ammonium (equation 4). With extrarenal bicarbonate loss, the Cl^- concentration in urine exceeds the sum of the cations in urine, Na^+ and K^+. If the sum of urine Na^+ and K^+ exceeds the Cl^- concentration, the urine NH_4^+ concentration is low, a finding comparable with RTA. The distinguishing features of the hyperchloremic acidoses are outlined in Table 20.8.

TABLE 20.7. Causes of Hyperchloremic Metabolic Acidosis[a]

Gastrointestinal Bicarbonate Loss
Diarrhea
External pancreatic or small bowel drainage
Ureterosigmoidostomy, jejunal loop
Drugs
Calcium chloride (acidifying agent)
Magnesium sulfate (diarrhea)
Cholestyramine (bile acid diarrhea)
Renal Tubular Acidification Defects
Hypokalemia
Proximal renal tubular acidosis (RTA) (type 2 RTA)
Classical distal RTA (type 1 RTA)
Hyperkalemia
Generalized distal nephron dysfunction (type 4 RTA)
Mineralocorticoid deficiency
Mineralocorticoid resistance
Decreased delivery of Na^+ to the distal nephron
Liver disease
Normokalemia or Hyperkalemia
Early renal failure
Other
Acid loads (ammonium chloride, hyperalimentation with insufficient alkali infusion)
Loss of potential bicarbonate: ketosis with ketone excretion
Expansion acidosis (rapid saline administration)
Posthypocapnic state
Glue sniffing

[a]Must rule out hypoalbuminemia, pseudohyponatremia, pseudohyperchloremia, and paraproteinemia.

TABLE 20.8. Forms of Alkali Replacement

Agent	Alkali Content
Shohl's solution	
Sodium citrate	1 mEq/ml
Citric acid	1 mEq/ml
Sodium bicarbonate	3.9 mEq/tablet (325 mg) or 5.9 mEq/tablet (500 mg)
Baking soda	60 mEq/tsp
K-Lyte	25 or 50 mEq/tablet
Polycitra (K-Shohl)	
Sodium citrate	1 mEq/ml
Potassium citrate	1 mEq/ml
Citric acid	1 mEq/ml

TABLE 20.9. Distinguishing Features of Hyperchloremic Acidoses

	Proximal RTA (Type 2 RTA)	Classical Distal RTA (Type 1 RTA)	Generalized Distal Defect (Type 4 RTA)	Extrarenal HCO_3^- Loss
Anion gap	Normal	Normal	Normal	Normal
Plasma [K^+]	Low (with treatment)	Low	High	Low
Urine anion gap or urine osmolal gap	Low	Low	Very low	High
Urine pH	Low	High	Low or high	Low or high
Urine P_{CO_2}	>70	<40	<40	>70
$FE_{HCO_3^-}$	>15% (with treatment)	5%–10%	10%–15%	<5%
Urine citrate	High	Low	Low	Normal
TTKG	High	High	Low (not high)	Low

RTA, renal tubular acidosis; TTKG, transtubular potassium gradient.

Hyperchloremic Acidosis of Chronic Renal Failure

Pathophysiology

Loss of functioning renal parenchyma by progressive renal failure is commonly associated with metabolic acidosis, which is typically hyperchloremic when the GFR is between 20 and 50 ml/min but may convert to the typical high AG acidosis of uremia with more advanced renal failure (i.e., when the GFR is less than 20 ml/min). Although it is assumed that such a progression is observed more commonly in patients with tubulointerstitial forms of renal disease, it should be emphasized that hyperchloremic metabolic acidosis can occur as frequently with advanced glomerular disease. The major defect in acidification with advanced renal failure is that ammoniagenesis is reduced in proportion to the loss of functional renal mass. In addition, medullary ammonium accumulation and trapping in the medullary collecting duct is impaired. Because of adaptive increases in potassium secretion by the collecting duct and colon, the acidosis of chronic renal insufficiency is typically normokalemic. In the face of hyperkalemia, there is further reduction in ammonium production and excretion because of a direct effect of hyperkalemia to suppress ammoniagenesis, and because of competition between K^+ and NH_4^+ transport in the proximal tubule, Henle's loop, and collecting duct, all of which reduce NH_4^+ excretion, and thus net acid excretion.

DISTAL RENAL TUBULAR ACIDOSIS

This condition is discussed in Chapter 20, Part 5. The various types of distal renal tubular acidosis belong to the category of hyperchloremic metabolic acidosis. The distinguishing features of the various types of hyperchloremic metabolic acidosis are provided in Table 20.9.

Selected Readings

Bidani A, DuBose TD Jr. Cellular and whole-body acid–base regulation. In: Arieff AI, DeFronzo RA, eds. *Fluid, electrolyte, and acid–base disorders.* New York, NY: Churchill Livingstone, 1995.

This review focuses on acid–base biochemistry, cellular and whole body buffering, and regulatory properties. As such the detailed explanation of acid–base balance should be useful to readers interested in fundamental aspects of this process rather than on pathophysiology and disease processes.

Cogan MG. *Fluid and electrolytes.* Norwalk, CT: Appleton & Lange, 1991.

This handbook is an excellent companion for the student or fellow interested in understanding practical aspects of the clinical spectrum of acid–base and electrolyte disorders encountered in the clinical setting.

DuBose TD Jr. Hyperkalemic hyperchloremic metabolic acidosis: pathophysiologic insights. *Kidney Int* 1997;51:591–602.

This review correlates information obtained from animal models of hyperkalemic acidosis to the disorders observed clinically. The role of hyperkalemia in the generation of metabolic acidosis through adverse effects on ammonium production and excretion is emphasized. Tubular abnormalities that commonly lead to hyperkalemia and acidosis are reviewed in detail and a new classification of this large group of disorders is proposed.

DuBose TD Jr. Acid–base disorders. In: Brenner BM, ed. *Brenner and Rector's: The kidney,* 6th ed. Philadelphia: WB Saunders, 2000.

This review by the same author of the attached chapter encompasses more than 1,000 references, has been updated thoroughly, and provides a comprehensive overview of the field of acid–base chemistry, physiology, pathophysiology, and associated clinical disorders. It is suggested that this review serve as a companion reference for more detail on the topics discussed in the previous chapter.

Emmett M, Narins RG. Clinical use of the anion gap. *Medicine* (Baltimore) 1977; 56:38–44.

The anion gap is widely used as a helpful tool in both the understanding of the classification of the metabolic acidoses and in a practical approach to their diagnoses. This now classical paper helped to place this important index into perspective.

Halperin ML, Kamel KS, Narins RG. Use of urine electrolytes and osmolality: bringing physiology to the bedside. In: Narins RG, ed. *Diagnostic techniques in renal disease.* New York, NY: Churchill Livingstone, 1992.

The application of urine electrolytes in the diagnosis of patients with common electrolyte and acid–base disorders is often confusing to the clinician. This practical review is an excellent resource for obtaining the needed "formulas."

Narins RG, Emmett M. Simple and mixed acid–base disorders: a practical approach. *Medicine* (Baltimore) 1980;56:161–168.

Sometimes referred to as son of anion gap (the classic paper cited above), this companion paper was among the first to espouse a practical approach to the recognition of mixed disturbances. The approach described here has withstood the test of time. This and the companion paper above should remain in the collection of any serious student of acid–base disorders.

Narins RG, Kupin W, Faber, MD, et al. Pathophysiology, classification, and therapy of acid–base disturbances. In: Arieff AI, DeFronzo RA, eds. *Fluid, electrolyte, and acid–base disorders.* New York NY: Churchill Livingstone, 1995.

This more detailed and updated approach from the same senior author as above, is an excellent resource. The tables and illustrations are especially informative.

PART 4
Lactic Acidosis

Jeffrey A. Kraut and Nicolaos E. Madias

Lactic acidosis is the acid–base disorder arising from the accumulation of lactic acid in the body fluids as reflected by a serum lactate concentration of 5 mEq/L or greater. It is a common cause of metabolic acidosis in hospitalized adults with a prevalence of approximately 1%. Moreover, more than 45% of adults with severe metabolic acidosis (blood pH less than 7.10) and a large increment in the serum anion gap have lactic acidosis. The diagnosis of lactic acidosis has serious implications because the prognosis of patients with this disorder, particularly when it is caused by compromised tissue perfusion, is very poor. Indeed, survival of adult patients within 30 days of the diagnosis of lactic acidosis was only 17% in one large study. Therefore it is not surprising that considerable effort has been directed at elucidating the pathophysiology of lactic acidosis and developing new modalities of treatment. In this chapter, we summarize normal lactate metabolism, the pathogenesis of lactic acidosis, its causes, the diagnosis and clinical features of this disorder, and its treatment.

NORMAL METABOLISM OF LACTATE AND PATHOGENESIS OF LACTIC ACIDOSIS

The sole reaction that generates or consumes lactate is depicted in equation 1:

$$\text{Pyruvate} + \text{NADH} + H^+ \overset{\text{LDH}}{\leftrightarrow} \text{LACTATE} + \text{NAD}^+ \quad (1)$$

The interconversion of pyruvate and lactate occurs in the cytosol and is catalyzed by the enzyme, lactate dehydrogenase (LDH). Thus lactate is formed through the reduction of pyruvate by reduced nicotinamide adenine dinucleotide (NADH) and is converted back to pyruvate through lactate's oxidation by the oxidized form of the dinucleotide (NAD^+). The equilibrium constant for this reversible reaction favors lactate formation such that the concentration of lactate normally is approximately 10-fold greater than that of pyruvate. Of the two optical isomers, L(+)-lactate is the only natural form in mammals and LDH is stereospecific for the L(+)-lactate reaction. Recasting equation 1 to highlight the equilibrium concentration of lactate yields equation 2:

$$[\text{Lactate}] = \text{Keq} \times [\text{Pyruvate}] \times [\text{NADH}]/[\text{NAD}^+] \times [H^+]_i \quad (2)$$

where *Keq* is the equilibrium constant of the LDH reaction. Consequently, the cytosolic concentration of lactate is determined by the concentration of pyruvate, the $[NADH]/[NAD^+]$ ratio of the cell, otherwise referred to as the *redox state*, and the intracellular hydrogen ion concentration, $[H^+]_i$. The cytosolic concentration of pyruvate depends on the rates of pyruvate production and consumption. The main pathway for pyruvate production is anaerobic (oxygen-independent) glycolysis (Embden-Meyerhof pathway) (Fig. 20.11). The anaerobic glycolysis is regulated by the availability of glucose substrate, the rate of glucose passage through the cell membrane, and the activity of three functionally unidirectional enzymes: hexokinase (HK), 6-phosphofructokinase (PFK), and pyruvate kinase

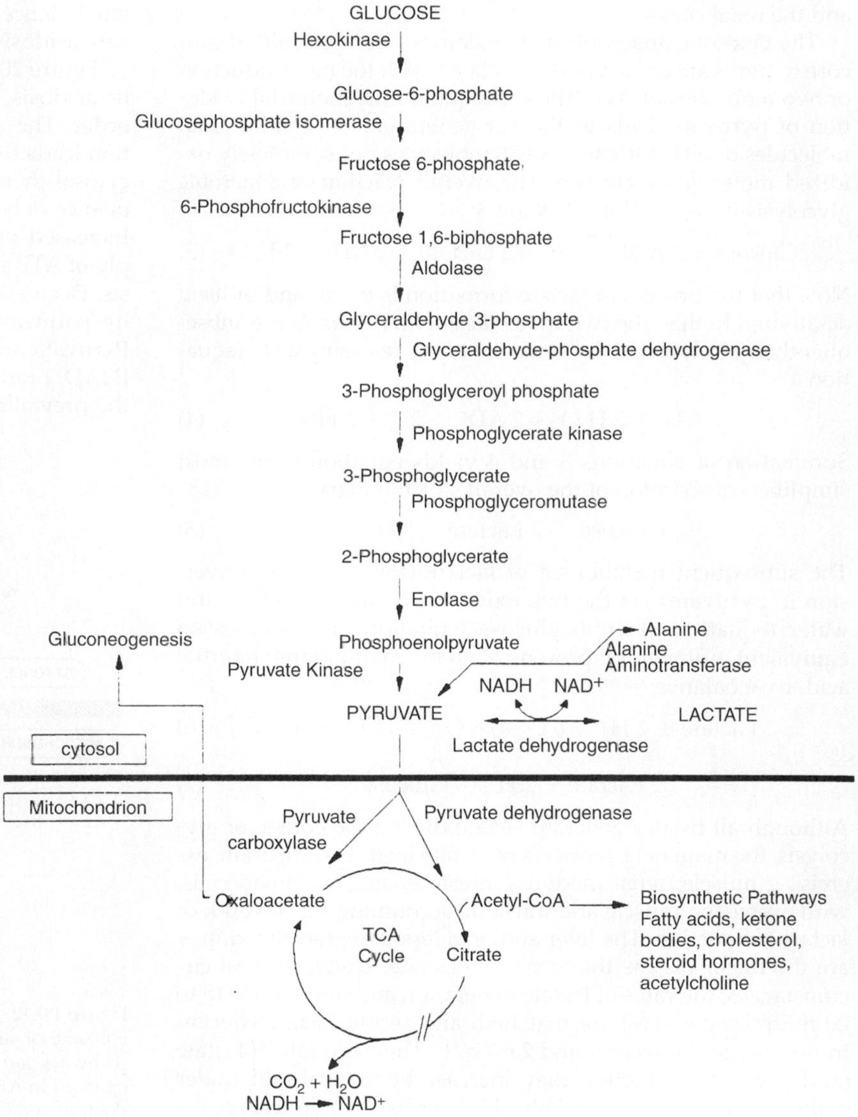

Figure 20.11. Metabolic pathway leading to production of lactic acid from glucose. For sake of simplicity, the reactions are depicted only in the forward direction leading to lactic acid formation. However, only three of the glycolytic reactions (those catalyzed by hexokinase, phosphofructokinase, and pyruvate kinase) are irreversibly catalyzed in the forward direction; thus by circumventing these steps the body can use the same pathway, but in the reverse mode, for gluconeogenesis.

(PK). Adenosine 5′-triphosphate (ATP) is an allosteric inhibitor of the PFK reaction; thus, when ATP stores are reduced, flux through this reaction is augmented and the rate of glycolysis is increased. A key step in glycolysis is the oxidation of glyceraldehyde 3-phosphate during which NAD^+ is consumed and converted to NADH; therefore NAD^+ is essential to the maintenance of glycolysis. Under normal conditions, regeneration of NAD^+ occurs largely via mitochondrial oxidation of NADH. Under hypoxic conditions, however, replenishment of the NAD^+ stores depends on the cytosolic conversion of pyruvate to lactate (equation 1). A small quantity of pyruvate is produced from the transamination of alanine (released from skeletal muscle and gut) and from the metabolism of glutamine during ammoniagenesis. Consumption of pyruvate occurs within the mitochondria via two oxidative pathways (Fig. 20.11). The first of these is oxidative decarboxylation to acetyl-coenzyme A (acetyl CoA), a reaction requiring NAD^+ and catalyzed by a complex of three enzymes collectively referred to as *pyruvate dehydrogenase (PDH).* The resultant acetyl CoA can enter the tricarboxylic acid (TCA) cycle for complete oxidation to CO_2 and water, or it can be used in various biosynthetic pathways (e.g., fatty acids, ketone bodies, cholesterol). The second pathway involves carboxylation of pyruvate to oxaloacetate, a reaction requiring ATP and catalyzed by pyruvate carboxylase (PC); this reaction is the first step to gluconeogenesis, the synthesis of glucose or glycogen that occurs exclusively in the liver and the renal cortex.

The cytosolic anaerobic conversion of one molecule of glucose to pyruvate or lactate is associated with the net production of two molecules of ATP. The subsequent mitochondrial oxidation of pyruvate leads to the net generation of 36 additional molecules of ATP, for a total of 38 molecules per completely oxidized molecule of glucose. The overall reaction of anaerobic glycolysis is depicted in equation 3:

$$\text{Glucose} + 2\ \text{ADP} + 2\ \text{P} \rightarrow 2\ \text{Lactate} + 2\ \text{ATP} + 2\ H_2O \quad (3)$$

Note that the process of lactate formation is not in and of itself acidifying. Rather, the two molecules of ATP formed are subsequently hydrolyzed in the cytosol thereby releasing 2 H^+ (equation 4):

$$2\ \text{ATP} + 2\ H_2O \rightarrow 2\ \text{ADP} + 2\ \text{P} + 2\ H^+ \quad (4)$$

Summation of equations 3 and 4 yields equation 5, the most simplified description of the overall stoichiometry:

$$\text{Glucose} \rightarrow 2\ \text{Lactate} + 2\ H^+ \quad (5)$$

The subsequent metabolism of lactate (following its conversion to pyruvate) via the two oxidative pathways to CO_2 and water (equation 6) or to glucose (equation 7) consumes an equivalent number of protons thereby maintaining internal acid–base balance:

$$2\ \text{Lactate} + 2\ H^+ + 6\ O_2 \rightarrow 6\ O_2 \rightarrow 6\ CO_2 + 6\ H_2O \quad (6)$$

$$2\ \text{Lactate} + 2\ H^+ \rightarrow \text{Glucose} \quad (7)$$

Although all tissues generate lactate during the course of glycolysis, the main net producers of lactate include skin, brain, exercising muscle, renal medulla, intestine, and red blood cells, with exercising muscle and intestine accounting for the bulk of lactate production. The liver and, to a lesser degree, the kidney are the major organs that consume lactate. Under normal circumstances, the rates of lactate generation and utilization (15 to 20 mEq/kg per day) are matched, and serum lactate concentration ranges between 1 and 2 mEq/L. The basal rate of lactate (and proton) production may increase by several-fold under pathologic conditions. Notably, the liver has a large reserve capacity for lactate metabolism that exceeds the basal rate by several-fold. Renal consumption of lactate is augmented in hyperlactatemia, thus contributing to the organism's reserve capacity. Lactate easily crosses cell membranes, including the glomerular barrier. Under normal conditions, filtered lactate is virtually completely reabsorbed in the proximal tubule. Above serum levels of 6 to 7 mEq/L, however, lactate appears in the urine, as the reabsorptive mechanism becomes saturated. Available evidence indicates that in most cases of lactic acidosis both overproduction and underutilization of lactate are implicated. A severe reduction in hepatic perfusion and systemic pH below 7.10 can substantially reduce hepatic lactate use and might even convert the liver into a lactate-producing organ. Similarly, marked renal underperfusion causes a sharp decrease in lactate uptake by the kidney.

Regarding the $[NADH]/[NAD^+]$ term of equation 2, it represents a measure of the redox state of cytosolic pyridine nucleotides. Suppression of mitochondrial function as a result of decreased oxygen availability or other mechanisms reduces the oxidation of NADH. As equation 2 indicates, the resultant increase in the $[NADH]/[NAD^+]$ ratio shifts the equilibrium of the LDH reaction toward lactate formation. Finally, an increase in intracellular $[H^+]_i$ should lead to increased lactate concentration in the cytosol (equation 2). This direct effect is, however, overridden by the property of intracellular acidosis to inhibit the activity of PFK, thereby reducing the rates of glycolysis and lactate production. Nonetheless, the net effect of acidosis on lactate balance can be variable because, as previously noted, severe acidosis can markedly retard hepatic lactate utilization.

Figure 20.12 depicts the mechanism of hypoxia-induced lactic acidosis, by far the most common clinical cause of the disorder. The resultant impaired mitochondrial oxidative function leads to reduced availability of ATP and NAD^+ within the cytosol thereby causing accumulation of pyruvate as a consequence of both increased production and decreased utilization. Increased production occurs because a reduced cytosolic supply of ATP stimulates the PFK reaction and accelerates glycolysis. Decreased utilization of pyruvate reflects the fact that both its pathways depend on mitochondrial oxidative reactions. Pyruvate accumulation coupled with the increased $[NADH]/[NAD^+]$ ratio results in heightened lactate production. Despite the prevailing mitochondrial dysfunction, continuation of gly-

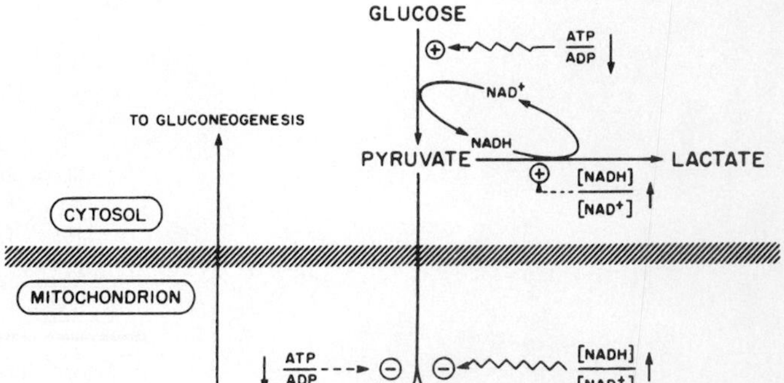

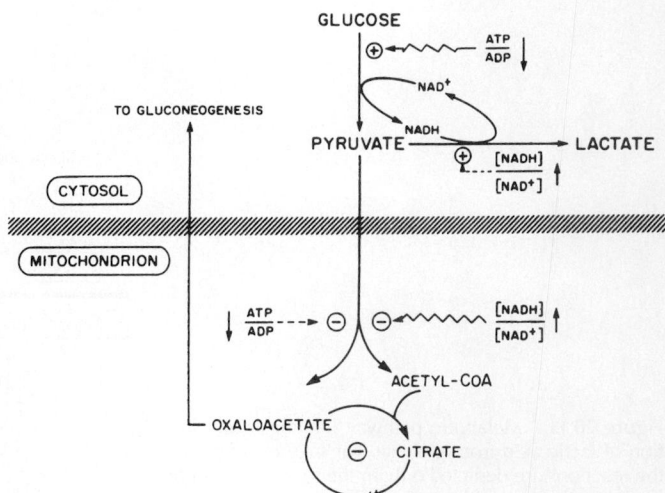

Figure 20.12. Mechanism of hypoxia-induced accumulation of lactate. For sake of simplicity, the individual enzymes involved in the metabolic pathways are omitted. Shown by the − or + signs are the impact of changes in ATP concentration and the $[NADH]/[NAD^+]$ ratio on the production and consumption of pyruvate. (Reproduced with permission from Madias NE. Lactic acidosis. *Kidney Int* 1986;29:752–774.)

colysis is ensured by the cytosolic regeneration of NAD^+ during the conversion of pyruvate to lactate because, as noted, NAD^+ is required for the oxidation of glyceraldehyde 3-phosphate. Thus increased lactate production represents the toll paid by the organism to maintain energy production during anaerobiosis.

CAUSES OF LACTIC ACIDOSIS

The causes of lactic acidosis are shown in Table 20.10. Traditionally, lactic acidosis is divided into two broad categories: type A, in which there is clinical evidence of impaired tissue oxygenation, and type B, in which no clinical evidence of impaired tissue oxygenation is apparent. However, as indicated in the following section, overt clinical signs of inadequate tissue oxygenation are not always present. Therefore the distinction between the two types of lactic acidosis might on occasion be less than obvious.

Type A Lactic Acidosis

Impaired tissue oxygenation might reflect increased oxygen demand as it arises from voluntary exercise, the most common cause of transient lactic acidosis. The quantity of lactic acid produced and the consequent changes in the body's acid–base status depend on several variables, including the intensity, duration, and type of exercise; the continuous versus the intermittent nature of the work; the number of muscle groups involved; and the physical condition of the subject. Training might reduce the quantity of lactate released from exercising muscle. Exertional heat stroke might generate severe lactic acidosis. Substantial hyperlactatemia also occurs with generalized convulsions and hypothermic shivering, clinical equivalents of strenuous voluntary exercise. Lactic acidosis after a single grand mal seizure resolves spontaneously, usually within 1 hour.

TABLE 20.10. Causes of Lactic Acidosis

Type A	Type B
Increased oxygen demand	**Systemic disorders**
Vigorous voluntary exercise	Diabetes mellitus
Generalized convulsions	Liver disease
Hypothermic shivering	Malignancy
Reduced oxygen delivery	Thiamine deficiency
Shock or incipient shock	Pheochromocytoma
Low cardiac output	D(-)-lactic acidosis
Severe hypoxemia	**Drugs and toxins**
Carbon monoxide poisoning	Ethanol
Very severe anemia	Methanol
	Ethylene glycol
	Salicylates
	Biguanides
	Other toxins (e.g., cyanide, acetaminophen, isoniazid, streptozocin, nitroprusside papaverine, paracetamol, nalidixic acid)
	Fructose, sorbitol, and xylitol
	Epinephrine, norepinephrine
	Congenital enzymatic defects
	Glucose-6-phosphatase deficiency (type 1 glycogen storage disease, van Gierke's disease)
	Fructose-1,6-diphosphatase deficiency
	Pyruvate carboxylase deficiency
	Pyruvate dehydrogenase deficiency
	Oxidative phosphorylation defects

By far, the most common cause of clinically significant lactic acidosis is decreased oxygen delivery to the tissues. As already indicated, the pathogenesis of hypoxic lactic acidosis reflects both overproduction and underutilization of lactate (Fig. 20.12). Virtually all tissues might release lactate into the circulation during hypoxia, the main sources being muscle, gut, liver, and kidney. On the other hand, underutilization of lactate stems from hypoxia of the hepatic and renal parenchyma. Overt or incipient shock of any type (cardiogenic, septic, or hypovolemic) is commonly associated with lactic acidosis. Profound hyperlactatemia develops soon after circulatory collapse. However, in slowly evolving circulatory failure, a modest rise in serum lactate might even antedate any substantial reduction in systemic blood pressure, presumably reflecting tissue ischemia from intense peripheral vasoconstriction. The severity of the hyperlactatemia represents a fairly reliable index of the outcome in patients with shock, with survival being rare if baseline serum lactate concentration is greater than 13 mEq/L. The magnitude of the associated acidemia varies widely depending on the direction and degree of change in $Paco_2$. Thus, in many patients with traumatic or septic shock, a coexisting respiratory alkalosis can strikingly limit the decrement in blood pH observed despite profound hyperlactatemia. By contrast, because respiratory arrest often accompanies cardiac arrest, severe acidemia resulting from mixed metabolic and respiratory acidosis is commonly observed.

Patients with depressed cardiac output and pulmonary edema but without frank hypotension often develop a mild to moderate degree of lactic acidosis, reflecting both diminished tissue perfusion and associated hypoxemia. The most severe cases of pulmonary edema have an associated respiratory acidosis and thus feature substantial acidemia.

Clinically, significant tissue hypoxia and lactic acidosis only rarely are produced by acute isolated reduction in arterial oxygen content because hypoxemia elicits a compensatory increase in cardiac output. Nonetheless, asphyxia or severe reduction in Pao_2 to levels below approximately 30 mm Hg will lead to severe lactic acidosis. Profound acidemia resulting from both lactic and respiratory acidosis is characteristic of advanced status asthmaticus, lactic acidosis reflecting the prevailing severe hypoxemia, and the increased work of breathing. Patients with chronic forms of hypoxemia (e.g., chronic obstructive lung disease and congenital heart disease) are less prone to develop significant tissue hypoxia because of adaptive secondary polycythemia and augmented erythrocytic content of 2,3-diphosphoglycerate, which decreases hemoglobin's affinity for oxygen thereby shifting the oxyhemoglobin dissociation curve to the right; both of these mechanisms enhance oxygen delivery to the tissues. By contrast, carbon monoxide poisoning regularly results in lactic acidosis despite reductions in oxyhemoglobin levels of less than 50%. This tendency has been attributed to both absence of a compensatory increase in cardiac output in this setting and impaired efficiency of oxygen release in tissues resulting from a shift of the oxyhemoglobin dissociation curve to the left by carbon monoxide. Last, patients with very severe anemia (hematocrit levels lower than 10%, hemoglobin levels less than 2 g/dl) might suffer sufficient tissue hypoxia to develop lactic acidosis.

Type B Lactic Acidosis

As indicated in Table 20.10, type B lactic acidosis occurs in association with certain clinical disorders, following exposure to certain drugs or toxins, or is congenital in origin.

Diabetes mellitus is widely considered to predispose to lactic acidosis, but the precise relationship between the two entities remains elusive. Insulin promotes the utilization of pyruvate through the oxidative pathway and inhibits the release of alanine (a source of pyruvate) from muscle; thus insulinopenia would tend to facilitate the accumulation of pyruvate and lactate. Notwithstanding, careful observations indicate that no more than 10% to 15% of patients with diabetic ketoacidosis have concomitant lactic acidosis. It is unclear, however, to what extent overt or incipient circulatory failure (caused by hypovolemia, sepsis, or cardiac dysfunction) might have contributed to the development of lactic acidosis in these patients. Only rare reports exist of diabetic, nonketotic patients developing lactic acidosis in the absence of other predisposing conditions (e.g., hepatic failure or treatment with phenformin). Therefore, although diabetes mellitus might predispose to lactic acidosis, development of lactic acidosis is probably rare in the absence of other contributory factors.

Because the liver is the major consumer of lactate, it seems reasonable to anticipate that liver disease would predispose to lactic acidosis. Approximately 30% to 40% of patients with lactic acidosis have evidence of liver disease. However, because of the large reserve capacity of the liver for lactate consumption, it is uncertain whether lactic acidosis can result from defective hepatic utilization of lactate alone, unless the liver disease is of extreme severity. Thus patients with stable hepatic cirrhosis usually have normal serum lactate levels in the basal state, although kinetic studies using lactate infusions have revealed a moderate prolongation in the lactate elimination rate. On the other hand, most patients with fulminant hepatitis have modest elevations in serum lactate levels. Available evidence indicates that in most cases of lactic acidosis in patients with liver disease, overproduction of lactic acid as a result of circulatory impairment or hypoxemia is also a factor. The commonly associated respiratory alkalosis might also contribute to lactate overproduction; intracellular alkalosis stimulates the activity of PFK thereby enhancing the rate of glycolysis.

Lactic acidosis can develop in patients with malignancies in the absence of circulatory failure or hypoxemia. This "paraneoplastic" syndrome can assume a relatively chronic course and is usually associated with acute leukemias or other myeloproliferative disorders, and less commonly with lymphomas or solid tumors. A pathogenic role for overproduction of lactic acid by the neoplastic tissue is supported by the resolution of lactic acidosis following effective treatment of the tumor. Because malignant cells generally have high glycolytic rates, enhanced production of lactate would be expected if the tumor burden were large. Of interest, in some cases, lactic acidosis appears to have been triggered by the administration of total parenteral solutions rich in glucose. Local severe hypoxia resulting from an inadequate blood supply of rapidly proliferating tumors might increase the dependence on anaerobic glycolysis. Hepatic underutilization of lactate might contribute to lactic acidosis in cases of massive invasion of the liver by the tumor. Putative neoplastic factors, which promote lactic-acid production or inhibit its metabolism, have also been proposed. Administration of bicarbonate to patients with malignancy-associated lactic acidosis might increase lactic-acid production, presumably by the malignancy, in all likelihood as a result of intracellular alkalinization (relative or absolute).

Thiamine deficiency, a common occurrence in alcoholic patients, when severe, might cause lactic acidosis. Both underutilization and overproduction of lactic acid appear to contribute. Thiamine pyrophosphate is a coenzyme for PDH and its deficiency results in accumulation of pyruvate and lactate. Moreover, despite an increased cardiac output, patients with thiamine deficiency appear to have regional underperfusion.

Rare cases of lactic acidosis in patients with pheochromocytoma have been described, presumably the result of the vasoconstrictive and metabolic effects of the excess catecholamines released. The presence of pulmonary edema might contribute to the generation of lactic acidosis.

An idiotypic form of lactic acidosis, D(-)-lactic acidosis has been described in patients with the short-bowel syndrome (following small-bowel resection or jejunoileal bypass for treatment of morbid obesity). D(-)-lactic acid, the optical isomer of L(+)-lactic acid, is not normally a product of human intermediary metabolism. The pathogenesis of the disorder relates to delivery of large amounts of undigested carbohydrate to the colon resulting in increased fermentation by colonic bacteria and production of both lactic-acid isomers at rates exceeding the capacity of bacteria for further utilization. The resultant decrease in stool pH favors the overgrowth of acid-resistant, anaerobic species (e.g., *Eubacterium, Lactobacillus*). Both lactic-acid isomers are absorbed from the colonic contents, but the metabolic acidosis is primarily a result of the D(-)-lactic acid because of its slower metabolism by nonspecific dehydrogenases. A special assay must be used for measurement of D(-)-lactate. In addition to metabolic acidosis, patients develop neurologic abnormalities, including confusion, lethargy, bizarre behavior, slurred speech, and ataxic gait. Eradication of the abnormal flora with antibiotics and a marked reduction in carbohydrate intake results in resolution of the syndrome.

Renal failure commonly is found in patients with type A or B lactic acidosis and has been cited as a predisposing factor in the development of lactic acidosis. However, there is no evidence that uremia per se can cause lactic acidosis.

As shown in Table 20.10, a number of drugs and toxins have been associated with the development of lactic acidosis. Ethanol causes a mild increase in serum lactate levels in normal subjects and prolongs the clearance of lactate from the circulation. This phenomenon has been ascribed to underutilization of lactate as a result of inhibition of hepatic gluconeogenesis. This inhibition reflects a marked increase in the hepatic [NADH]/[NAD$^+$] ratio as a result of the oxidation of ethanol. Excessive ethanol intake, especially in chronic alcoholics, can occasionally induce substantial lactic acidosis in the absence of other causative factors (e.g., volume depletion, seizures, severe thiamine deficiency). When lactic acidosis occurs, it usually coexists with alcoholic ketoacidosis. Whether the aforementioned mechanism is sufficient to account for the generation of lactic acidosis in these cases remains uncertain. Methanol and ethylene glycol intoxications commonly result in small rises in serum lactate concentration that contribute by a relatively small measure to the prevailing metabolic acidosis. Hyperlactatemia results from inhibition of mitochondrial oxidation by toxic metabolites of these alcohols. Large doses of salicylates uncouple oxidative phosphorylation, thereby stimulating glycolysis and decreasing lactate consumption. Lactic acid contributes, along with ketoacids and other organic acids, to the metabolic acidosis; a coexisting element of respiratory alkalosis might also enhance lactic-acid production.

The biguanide group of oral hypoglycemic agents, and in particular phenformin, is an established cause of lactic acidosis. The incidence of phenformin-induced lactic acidosis ranged between 0.25 and 14 per 1,000 patient-years, with a mortality of approximately 50%. Consequently, the agent was withdrawn from the U.S. market in 1977 and later from several other markets. Other biguanides, such as metformin and buformin, also cause lactic acidosis but apparently at a substantially lower incidence. Increased plasma levels of phenformin have been found in the bulk of patients with lactic acidosis as a result of decreased renal function or overdosage. The pathogenesis of lactic acidosis reflects both overproduction of lactic acid (stimulation of glycolysis) and its underutilization (inhibition of hepatic and renal gluconeogenesis and decreased lactate oxidation) as a result of toxic suppression of mitochondrial oxidative phosphorylation by phenformin. In addition to renal failure, other predisposing factors to phenformin-induced lactic acidosis include diabetes mellitus, severe liver disease, circulatory failure, advanced age, treatment with tetracycline, and ethanol ingestion. The incidence of lactic acidosis with metformin is very low, 0.03 cases per 1,000 patient-years. As with phenformin, renal insufficiency is the most important factor predisposing to the development of lactic acidosis. Other important predisposing factors include age, presence of severe liver disease, circulatory failure, and ethanol intake.

Among other toxins, cyanide poisoning is regularly associated with lactic acidosis because of its binding to cytochrome C with resultant inhibition of oxidative phosphorylation. A number of other agents have been implicated in causing lactic acidosis including acetaminophen, isoniazid, streptozotocin, nitroprusside, papaverine, paracetamol, and nalidixic acid.

Administration of large amounts of fructose, sorbitol, and xylitol in parenteral solutions can induce lactic acidosis. Metabolism of these substances results in marked depletion of cellular ATP stores with consequent stimulation of glycolysis and inhibition of hepatic utilization of lactate. Ethanol, hypoxemia, severe liver disease, and diabetes mellitus predispose to the generation of lactic acidosis from these substances.

Overdosage of epinephrine or norepinephrine can cause lactic acidosis by producing severe peripheral vasoconstriction and, largely in the case of epinephrine, by direct effects on lactate metabolism (augmentation of glycogenolysis and glycolysis, inhibition of pyruvate oxidation). Administration of pressor doses of norepinephrine to patients with circulatory failure might contribute to the generation of lactic acidosis. Therapeutic doses of the β-adrenergic receptor agonists salbutamol and rimiterol have been shown to produce mild hyperlactatemia.

Congenital lactic acidosis results from a variety of rare enzymatic defects that impair gluconeogenesis or pyruvate oxidation. The diagnosis is usually made in infancy and most patients do not survive childhood; however, the defect is occasionally diagnosed in adults.

Patients with glucose-6-phosphatase deficiency (type 1 glycogen storage disease, von Gierke's disease) and fructose-1,6-diphosphatase deficiency suffer from impaired gluconeogenesis from all precursors. They manifest fasting hypoglycemia and consequent insulinopenia, which enhances mobilization of adipose tissue stores and ketogenesis, and inhibits PDH activity. Thus ketosis and lactic acidosis develop. Treatment consists of sustaining normoglycemia with frequent carbohydrate feedings. Pyruvate carboxylase deficiency also impairs gluconeogenesis and leads to recurrent episodes of lactic acidosis. The associated brain damage causes mental retardation and various types of movement disorders. Some of the cases respond favorably to biotin.

Finally, partial deficiencies in PDH activity or defects in mitochondrial oxidative phosphorylation have been described to cause reduced pyruvate oxidation and thus lactic acidosis. Mental retardation and neurologic defects are also present. Administration of thiamine and lipoic acids and limitation of carbohydrate intake might lessen the severity of the disorder in some cases.

DIAGNOSIS AND CLINICAL FEATURES

As previously noted, serum lactate concentration averages 1.0 ± 0.5 mEq/L in normal individuals. Although the presence of a high anion gap metabolic acidosis in the appropriate clinical setting might strongly suggest lactic acidosis, confirmation of this diagnosis rests on the finding of a serum lactate concentration of 5 mEq/L or greater. Carefully performed studies have demonstrated that the clinical suspicion of lactic acidosis was confirmed in only 43% of cases, thus emphasizing the need to measure serum lactate levels when the diagnosis is being considered. The clinical significance of mildly elevated serum lactate levels in the range of 2 to 4 mEq/L remains uncertain. Although there is some suspicion that these mild degrees of hyperlactatemia might portend the development of more severe lactic acidosis, it is currently unknown how often mild hyperlactatemia progresses to full-blown lactic acidosis. On the other hand, the higher the level of lactate above 5 mEq/L in patients with circulatory failure, the worse the prognosis. Therefore sequential measurements of serum lactate concentrations are extremely useful in evaluating the patient's course and response to treatment.

Traditionally, the diagnosis of lactic acidosis is entertained in patients with circulatory failure and tissue hypoperfusion who also have an elevated serum anion gap, frequently in the company of hypobicarbonatemia and acidemia. However, an elevated serum anion gap might not be observed in a significant percentage of patients with moderate hyperlactatemia (serum lactate 5 to 10 mEq/L). Indeed, in one study almost 50% of patients with these levels of serum lactate concentration had a serum anion gap of less than 12 mEq/L. Moreover, hypobicarbonatemia and acidemia might not be present in many patients because of the frequent coexistence of respiratory alkalosis and metabolic alkalosis, additional acid–base disorders that are often seen in critically ill patients. The diagnosis of lactic acidosis also is considered in patients with a high anion gap metabolic acidosis of unknown origin. The differential diagnosis under such circumstances includes lactic acidosis, uremia, ketoacidosis (both alcoholic and diabetic), and various intoxications such as salicylate, methanol, and ethylene glycol. Mild elevations in serum lactate concentration can be observed in patients with salicylate or methanol intoxication, but the magnitude of the hyperlactatemia in these disorders falls far short of completely accounting for the hypobicarbonatemia and elevation in serum anion gap. Moreover, when the serum anion gap is markedly elevated (anion gap of 30 mEq/L or greater) more than 90% of patients will have either lactic acidosis or ketoacidosis.

The clinical presentation of lactic acidosis is extremely variable and heavily influenced by the manifestations of the underlying disease. Nonetheless, its development is often heralded by the sudden onset of malaise, weakness, anorexia, vomiting, and a deterioration in mental status. Most patients have overt evidence of circulatory shock as manifested by hypotension, tachycardia, and circulatory instability. Myocardial failure, sepsis, severe hemorrhage, and/or multisystem failure are extremely common. Hyperventilation can also be prominent, particularly in the presence of sepsis. These clinical manifestations of lactic acidosis associated with acute hypoperfusion should be distinguished from the more insidious presentation of the rarer forms of chronic lactic acidosis associated with enzyme defects, D-lactic acidosis, and certain drugs.

Certain laboratory derangements frequently have been associated with lactic acidosis. Similar to other forms of organic acidosis, serum potassium concentration is often normal despite significant acidemia. This feature likely reflects the concurrent entry of lactate and protons into cells, thus obviating the necessity of potassium to exit the cells to maintain electroneutrality. On the other hand, if severe renal failure or marked catabolism accompany lactic acidosis, hyperkalemia can be observed. Hypochloremia leading to a rise in the serum anion gap that exceeds the fall in serum bicarbonate concentration has been noted in experimental lactic acidosis in animals. These studies suggest that rather than being an indicator of an antecedent, hidden hyperbicarbonatemic disorder, hypochloremia might be an integral feature of the lactic acidosis. These experimental observations indicate that caution is recommended in diagnosing mixed acid–base disorders in patients with lactic acidosis solely on the basis of an accompanying disproportionate delta anion gap to delta bicarbonate ratio.

Experimental studies indicate that the ventilatory response to lactic acidosis is virtually identical to that observed in mineral acid-induced metabolic acidosis. Nonetheless, in clinical lactic acidosis, the prevailing $PaCO_2$ might vary widely for a given level of hypobicarbonatemia depending on the coexistence of additional processes known to affect alveolar ventilation. As noted previously, respiratory alkalosis is commonly observed in septic patients, whereas respiratory acidosis is frequent in those with cardiopulmonary arrest. Some degree of renal impairment is common in most patients with lactic acidosis and in one study, more than 10% of patients required dialysis within 2 days of diagnosis. Multisystem failure is also common. Respiratory failure necessitating mechanical ventilation is not unusual as is shock liver with marked elevation in liver enzymes. Anemia and a strikingly elevated white blood cell count can be present reflecting the relatively high prevalence of sepsis and decreased margination of leukocytes produced by the accompanying catecholamine surge. Hyperphosphatemia is a common feature of lactic acidosis and likely reflects increased ATP hydrolysis during tissue ischemia and a rise in inorganic phosphate efflux from cells. Hyperuricemia, another manifestation of lactic acidosis, originates both from increased production and decreased excretion of uric acid. The former reflects increased release of adenosine diphosphate (ADP) and adenosine monophosphate (AMP) during the augmented hydrolysis of ATP that accompanies tissue ischemia, whereas the latter represents competitive inhibition of tubular urate secretion by the lactate anion. A modest elevation in the serum osmolal gap (averaging 17.4 ± 5.4 mOsm/kg H_2O in one study) has been described in some patients with lactic acidosis. The explanation for this finding remains uncertain. Of course, alcoholic ketoacidosis and methanol and ethylene glycol intoxications are typically associated with an often substantial elevation in the serum osmolal gap, a feature that represents an important aid in the diagnosis of these entities. Nonetheless, the aforementioned observations indicate that a modest elevation in the serum osmolal gap should not serve to exclude consideration of the diagnosis of lactic acidosis. The salient clinical features of lactic acidosis are summarized in Table 20.11.

TABLE 20.11. Common Clinical Features of Lactic Acidosis

Tachypnea
Respiratory failure
Hypotension
Deteriorating mental status
Hyperlactatemia (serum lactate >5 mEq/L)
Increased serum anion gap
Acidemia and hypobicarbonatemia[a]
Leukocytosis
Renal failure
Anemia
Hyperphosphatemia
Hyperuricemia
Septic, cardiogenic, or hemorrhagic shock[b]
Multisystem failure

[a]Presence of acidemia and/or hypobicarbonatemia is variable and depends on the coexistence of other acid–base disorders such as metabolic alkalosis or respiratory alkalosis.

[b]Circulatory shock secondary to hemorrhage, myocardial disease, and sepsis alone or in combination are present in most patients.

TREATMENT

The treatment of lactic acidosis is centered around the prompt identification and aggressive management of the underlying cause or predisposing disorder whenever possible. Although judicious administration of alkali might be required to lessen the prevailing acidemia, this maneuver should only be regarded as temporizing and adjunctive to cause-specific measures. The need for aggressive treatment of lactic acidosis is emphasized by its dire prognosis: the results of a large prospective study demonstrated that 83% of patients expired within 30 days of the diagnosis.

Tissue hypoxia is the underlying cause in most cases of lactic acidosis. However, the presence of lactic acidosis does not always mean that oxygen delivery to peripheral tissues is markedly reduced, nor does the resolution of lactic acidosis always indicate that tissue oxygenation is improved. Studies using an *in vivo* model of sepsis demonstrated that in some cases overproduction of lactic acid by splanchnic and peripheral tissues can be observed in the absence of marked cellular hypoxia. Be that as it may, therapeutic measures must be directed at augmenting oxygen delivery to the tissues. Cardiovascular collapse, low cardiac output states, hypoxemia, and sepsis should be rapidly evaluated and treated. In general, aggressive monitoring of the patient's hemodynamics, oxygenation, serum lactate concentration, and acid–base status should be used to guide therapy. In addition to arterial blood gases, determination of central venous blood gases might be of special value in managing patients with advanced circulatory failure by providing a better representation of the tissue acidity and oxygenation (see Chapter 20, Part 1). Indeed, arterial blood gases might be close to normal despite significant acidity, hypoxia, and hypercapnia in peripheral tissues. Use of vasoconstrictor agents should be limited in treating low cardiac output states because of their potential for exacerbating ischemia of tissue beds such as skeletal muscle, gut, and liver. Rather, inotropic and afterload reducing agents should be used whenever possible. Although there has been some interest in the use of vasodilators, such as nitroprusside, to improve tissue perfusion, their effectiveness has never been clearly shown. The adequacy of alveolar ventilation should be monitored closely and prompt ventilatory assistance should be given as required. Significant CO_2 retention should be avoided at all costs because it would exacerbate acidemia.

Although restoration of a normal blood pressure and adequate urine output is a valuable sign of improvement, these findings do not ensure that adequate reperfusion of the microcirculation has been attained. Normalization of serum lactate level itself might be the best indicator of restoration of adequate tissue perfusion.

The role of alkali therapy in managing lactic acidosis remains controversial. Proponents have supported the judicious use of base in cases in which severe acidemia is present (arterial blood pH below 7.20, serum bicarbonate concentration below 8 to 10 mEq/L) on grounds that such degrees of acidemia can have potentially catastrophic effects on the cardiovascular system. These include impairment of cardiac contractility, arteriolar dilatation, and peripheral venoconstriction, thereby resulting in reduction of cardiac output, hypotension, decreased hepatic and renal blood flow, and centralization of blood volume with consequent pulmonary congestion, bradycardia, and sensitization to malignant ventricular arrhythmias, and attenuation of the inotropic and chronotropic effects of catecholamines on the heart. It is evident that severe acidemia, per se, can compound the hemodynamic compromise caused by the underlying disease process, and thus enhance lactate production, decrease its metabolism, and impede efforts at restoring tissue perfusion. Also, it has been argued that mortality in patients with lactic acidosis is related primarily to an acidemia-related suppression of ATP generation, leading to an inadequate supply of ATP to vital organs. Base administration in the presence of adequate substrate supply enhances intracellular ATP generation by means of preventing inhibition of PFK by excess hydrogen ion. In this formulation, base administration is a necessary adjunct to treatment along with provision of sufficient glucose to fuel ATP generation. By administering alkali, the clinician aims at achieving the following goals: (a) preventing or reversing the acidemia-related hemodynamic compromise, thereby providing more time to allow control of the underlying disease by cause-specific and general supportive measures; (b) reinstating cardiac responsiveness to endogenous and exogenous catecholamines; and (c) providing a certain measure of safety against the superimposition of additional acidifying stresses: at serum bicarbonate concentrations below 10 mEq/L, a further fall in serum bicarbonate and/or a small increment in Pa_{CO_2} can cause extreme acidemia.

Opponents of alkali administration have cited a number of potential risks of this mode of therapy, including (a) aggravation of systemic and intracellular acidity resulting from an increase in Pa_{CO_2} that results from the decomposition of the alkali in the process of buffering, (b) augmentation of lactate production caused by alkalinization of body fluids, (c) potential deterioration of hemodynamics as manifested by a decrement in cardiac index and blood pressure, (d) overshoot alkalosis secondary to persistent hyperventilation and aggressive increments in serum bicarbonate concentration that reflect inordinately large exogenous alkali loads and regeneration of endogenous alkali from the metabolism of the accumulated lactate, (e) hypertonicity, (f) volume overload, (g) hypokalemia, (h) paradoxical cerebrospinal fluid acidification, and (i) a decrease in oxygen delivery to the tissues as a result of enhancement of hemoglobin's affinity for oxygen. Indeed, observations in animal models of experimental lactic acidosis (e.g., severe hypoxemia coupled with fixed ventilation, or pancreatectomy and phenformin administration) have shown that administration of sodium bicarbonate not only failed to improve the systemic acid–base status, but rather led to deterioration of systemic hemodynamics and unchanged mortality. The abrogation of the potential beneficial effects of alkali in these models of lactic acidosis has been attributed largely to exacerbation of intracellular acidosis resulting from accumulation of CO_2 in tissues. This could in turn decrease hepatic extraction of lactate and impair cardiac contractility. Notwithstanding, a number of well-founded criticisms have been raised against the relevance of these experimental observations to the clinical setting. Moreover, other animal studies of lactic acidosis, including experimentally provoked cardiac arrest in pigs and hypoxia-induced lactic acidosis in dogs, have not confirmed either the exacerbation of intracellular acidosis or the deterioration of hemodynamics following bicarbonate administration. Moreover, a negative effect of bicarbonate on hemodynamics has not been demonstrated in humans. Results of two controlled studies in patients with shock and lactic acidosis have shown no deterioration in hemodynamics or tissue oxygenation after bicarbonate administration. Furthermore, in a large multicenter study, intravenous bicarbonate administration had no appreciable beneficial or detrimental effect on serum lactate, arterial pH, or survival in patients with lactic acidosis.

The limited evidence summarized in the preceding discussion does not indicate that bicarbonate therapy is either deleterious or beneficial in the treatment of lactic acidosis secondary to hypoperfusion. However, given the potentially catastrophic impact of profound acidemia on the circulation and its negative effect on maintaining an adequate supply of ATP for vital organs, the authors believe it is prudent to administer alkali judiciously to treat severe acidemia arising in the context of lactic acidosis. The clinician should aim to restore serum bicarbonate concentration to approximately 8 to 10 mEq/L and blood pH to greater than 7.20. However, the level of serum bicarbonate required to achieve this blood pH can vary substantially depending on the prevailing level of Pa_{CO_2}. In calculating alkali requirements, consideration should be made of the apparent enlargement of the space of distribution for bicarbonate in severe hypobicarbonatemia (serum HCO_3^- less than 5 mEq/ L), which can approach 100% of the body weight (see Chapter 20, Part 1). Every effort should be made to minimize increments in the Pa_{CO_2} of the body fluids while administering alkali. In this regard, alkali should be given as an infusion rather than as a bolus. Moreover, adequate gas exchange should be a prerequisite to alkali administration. If feasible, temporary augmentation of alveolar ventilation during the course of alkali infusion is advisable. In patients with advanced circulatory failure, determination of central venous blood gases will aid in assessing the prevailing P_{CO_2} in the tissues. Although even relative alkalinization of body fluids secondary to alkali administration will tend to increase lactate production, this tendency should be countered by the improved state of tissue perfusion resulting in decreased lactate generation and improved lactate metabolism. This recommended judicious administration of alkali should prevent the transition to an overshoot alkalosis. The complications of hypertonicity and volume overload can be prevented by administering hypotonic fluids and diuretics. If renal failure is present, peritoneal dialysis, hemodialysis, or hemofiltration might be required to remove excess sodium and fluid given to the patient. Moreover, peritoneal dialysis and hemodialysis provide a large source of base. In this regard, if peritoneal dialysis is used, one should use a bicarbonate-based dialysate rather than the more conventional lactate-containing dialysate. Special attention should be paid to the level of serum potassium to prevent hypokalemia during alkali administration, especially in patients receiving digitalis. Finally, concerns that the change in pH induced by cautious alkali administration will produce clinically significant cerebrospinal fluid acidification or a decrease in tissue oxygenation are unfounded. Particular restraint should be exercised in using alkali during cardiopulmonary resuscitation; the markedly reduced pulmonary blood flow can lead to retention of some of the carbon dioxide generated in the process of buffering, potentially exacerbating the prevailing acidosis. Our recommendations for the treatment of lactic acidosis are summarized in Table 20.12.

Given the ominous prognosis of lactic acidosis, clinicians should strive to prevent its development by maintaining adequate fluid balance, optimizing cardiopulmonary function, managing infection, and using cautiously drugs that predispose to the disorder. This is all the more important in patients at special risk for developing lactic acidosis, such as those with diabetes mellitus or advanced cardiac, respiratory, or hepatic disease.

A potentially useful advance in alkali therapy of severe lactic acidosis is the administration of Carbicarb, a solution containing equimolar quantities of sodium bicarbonate and sodium carbonate. By virtue of its pK, sodium carbonate is used in preference to sodium bicarbonate in the process of buffering, thereby obviating the generation of CO_2 (equation 8):

$$\text{Lactate} + H^+ + Na_2CO_3 \rightarrow NaHCO_3 + \text{NaLactate} \quad (8)$$

Promising results have been obtained with the use of Carbicarb in some experimental models of hypoxic lactic acidosis. Arterial pH, myocardial intracellular pH, and cardiac contractility all

TABLE 20.12. Recommendations for Treatment of Lactic Acidosis

Treat cardiovascular collapse, low cardiac output states, hypoxemia, and sepsis vigorously with appropriate measures.
Use inotropic and afterload-reducing agents to maintain cardiac output and blood pressure, as necessary. Limit use of vasoconstrictor agents.
Monitor alveolar ventilation carefully and provide prompt ventilator assistance, as required.
Monitor hemodynamics, oxygenation, serum lactate concentration, arterial acid–base status, and in cases of severe circulatory failure, central venous blood gases.
Institute promptly other course-specific measures, such as operative intervention for trauma or tissue ischemia, dialytic removal of certain toxins (e.g., methanol and ethylene glycol), discontinuation of metformin and nitroprusside, administration of insulin in patients with diabetes mellitus, glucose infusion in those with alcoholism, and correction of thiamine deficiency in cases of ethanol intoxication, short-bowel syndrome, and fulminant beriberi.
Administer bicarbonate judiciously as an isotonic solution. Infuse over several hours to raise and maintain serum bicarbonate concentration at approximately 10 mEq/L and blood pH at approximately 7.20. Estimate bicarbonate requirements based on volume of distribution of 50% of body weight with serum bicarbonate above 10 mEq/L and 100% of body weight with serum bicarbonate below 5 mEq/L. Particular restraint should be exercised in using alkali during cardiopulmonary resuscitation.
If the patient becomes volume overloaded and renal function is severely compromised, consider hemodialysis, peritoneal dialysis with bicarbonate-based dialysate, or hemofiltration.

were improved after Carbicarb administration. Moreover, no rise in the Pa_{CO_2} was noted. The results in humans have been less impressive. In a small study of patients with mild lactic acidosis, Carbicarb improved cardiovascular hemodynamics in only a subset of the patients. Studies in patients with severe lactic acidosis have not been performed, and therefore the role of this compound in the treatment of lactic acidosis remains unclear. At present, Carbicarb is not commercially available.

The conservative approach to administering alkali to patients with hypoxic lactic acidosis advocated previously should also be applied in the treatment of lactic acidosis occurring in association with malignancies. Indeed, massive doses of alkali might not raise plasma bicarbonate concentration substantially because of a direct stoichiometric relationship between alkali administration and acid production, presumably by the tumor itself. In addition to the well-known risks stemming from the administration of large bicarbonate loads, aggravation of the prevailing cachexia might also occur in the patient with cancer and poor dietary intake because the body's glycogen and protein stores might be depleted as a consequence of stimulated lactate production. Consequently, such patients should receive the smallest possible amount of bicarbonate that is sufficient to prevent or treat life-threatening acidemia and always in the company of an adequate nutrient supply.

Considerable excitement had been generated about the therapeutic potential of dichloroacetate (DCA) in the treatment of lactic acidosis. DCA stimulates PDH, thereby accelerating the oxidation of pyruvate to acetyl CoA. Its action has been associated with decreases in the serum and intracellular levels of lactate, decreases in the serum levels of alanine and pyruvate, and elevations in serum and intracellular pH. Moreover, increased ATP content of various tissues including the heart has been observed. Studies in experimental lactic acidosis indicated that DCA improves the disordered lactate metabolism, reduces serum lactate levels, raises plasma bicarbonate, increases blood and intracellular pH, improves systemic hemodynamics, and reduces mortality. Unfortunately, initial promising results in human lactic acidosis have not been borne out. A rigorously controlled study of 252 patients with lactic acidosis demonstrated that DCA caused a mild decrease in plasma lactate levels and small rise in plasma bicarbonate concentration. However, this treatment did not affect systolic blood pressure, cardiac output, and most importantly survival compared with conventional management. Therefore the role of DCA in the treatment of lactic acidosis associated with hypoperfusion remains unproven.

On the other hand, treatment of children with congenital lactic acidosis due to deficiency of PDH with DCA leads to improvement in acid–base status and in some cases improvement in neurologic function. Presently, the drug is available for this purpose through the Food and Drug Administration (FDA) orphan-drug program.

Peritoneal dialysis or hemodialysis using bicarbonate-buffered dialysate has been successfully employed in the management of lactic acidosis, particularly in patients with impaired renal function or congestive heart failure. In addition to preventing or treating volume overload, dialysis provides the needed alkali and removes lactate, thereby lessening the risk of rebound hyperbicarbonatemia. Removal of lactate might confer additional benefit to the extent that hyperlactatemia itself (independent of changes in systemic pH) exerts adverse effects. Indeed, some animal studies have shown that elevated lactate levels reduce oxidative phosphorylation and glucose utilization in myocardial tissue, impair myocardial contractility, and provoke the development of cardiac arrhythmias. Finally, dialysis also can accelerate the removal of drugs or toxins that might contribute to the development of lactic acidosis.

Insulin administration has been suggested as a therapeutic measure in diabetic patients with lactic acidosis, whether or not biguanide agents are involved in the generation of the acidosis. On theoretical grounds, insulin could exert a beneficial effect by stimulating the oxidation of pyruvate through the pyruvate-dehydrogenase pathway and by limiting the flow of gluconeogenic amino acids to the liver. Although the evidence supporting this form of therapy is tenuous, it is probably reasonable to include insulin in the treatment plan in this setting.

Methylene blue, an oxidizing agent, was proposed as treatment of lactic acidosis on the premise that it promotes the conversion of NADH to NAD^+ and thus restores the cellular redox state; however, clinical application of this therapy has not proved successful.

Thiamine and lipoic acids, agents that act as coenzymes for PDH, have been used occasionally in the treatment of patients with lactic acidosis, but experience is limited and therefore their utility remains uncertain. Of course, potentially thiamine-deficient patients such as alcoholics should be given this factor. Thiamine represents remarkably effective specific treatment in patients with lactic acidosis in association with fulminant beriberi.

Treatment of D(-)-lactic acidosis might include, in addition to the administration of base, carbohydrate restriction, avoidance of lactobacillus-containing preparations, and administration of oral antibiotics such as vancomycin or clindamycin.

Selected Readings

Cooper DJ, Walley KR, Wiggs BR, et al. Bicarbonate does not improve hemodynamics in critically ill patients who have lactic acidosis. *Ann Intern Med* 1990; 112:492–498.

A study of the effect of bicarbonate therapy on the hemodynamics of patients with lactic acidosis. Despite improvement in acid–base status, administration of bicarbonate failed to improve the hemodynamics of the patients.

Hindman BJ. Sodium bicarbonate in the treatment of subtypes of acute lactic acidosis: physiological considerations. *Anesthesiology* 1990;72:1064–1076.

An excellent discussion of the pathophysiology of lactic acidosis and the rationale for sodium-bicarbonate administration in certain subtypes of this entity.

Madias NE. Lactic acidosis. *Kidney Int* 1986;29:752–774.

Extensive review of the pathophysiology, causes, and treatment of lactic acidosis.

Mizock BA. Lactic acidosis. *Dis Mon* 1989;35:237–300.

An exhaustive review of the biochemistry, pathophysiology, diagnosis, and therapy of lactic acidosis. One of the best overall reviews of the subject.

Narins RG, Cohen JJ. Bicarbonate therapy for organic acidosis: the case for its continued use. *Ann Intern Med* 1987;106:615–618.

A concise and insightful discussion concerning the benefits of bicarbonate therapy in the treatment of lactic acidosis and other organic acidoses. The article is strongly in favor of the use of bicarbonate.

Stacpoole PW, Wright EC, Baumgartner TG, et al. A controlled trial of dichloroacetate for treatment of lactic acidosis in adults. *N Engl J Med* 1992;327: 1564–1569.

A controlled study of dichloroacetate demonstrating the failure of treatment with this agent to alter the morbidity or mortality of lactic acidosis.

Stacpoole PW. Lactic acidosis. *Endocrinol Metab Clin North Am* 1993;22:221–245.

A excellent exhaustive review of the topic including discussions about pathophysiology and recommendations for diagnosis and treatment.

Stacpoole PW, Wright EC, Baumgartner TG, et al. Natural history and course of acquired lactic acidosis in adults. *Am J Med* 1994;97:47–57.

One of the only long-term prospective studies examining the clinical characteristics and natural history of lactic acidosis in adults. An excellent summary of the salient clinical features and natural history of lactic acidosis.

PART 5
Renal Tubular Acidosis

Sandra Sabatini, Neil A. Kurtzman, and Somchai Eiam-Ong

The renal tubular acidosis (RTA) syndromes are nonuremic defects of urinary acidification. RTA is characterized by a normal anion gap and hyperchloremic metabolic acidosis; plasma potassium may be normal, low, or high depending on the type RTA present. These syndromes differ from uremic acidosis, which is associated with a high anion gap and enhanced proton secretion by each remaining nephron. As new technologies have been applied to biology, we now better understand the basic lesions of these important syndromes. In this chapter, we briefly review the physiology of acid excretion by the kidney. We then discuss the defects of proximal and distal RTA syndromes, including therapy when appropriate.

REVIEW OF ACID–BASE HOMEOSTASIS BY THE KIDNEY

Both volatile acid and nonvolatile acid are produced by normal intermediary metabolism. Approximately 13,000 to 15,000 mmol of CO_2 are formed daily in a normal adult. CO_2 is then transported in the blood to the lungs as hemoglobin-generated bicarbonate and hemoglobin-bound carbamino groups. CO_2 excretion by the lungs responds rapidly to changes in production. Nonvolatile acids account for a smaller quantity of metabolic acid. The high-protein diet, consumed by most persons living in industrialized countries, generates 1.0 to 1.5 mEq/kg body weight of endogenous nonvolatile acid per day. These dietary acids are generated as sulfuric acid from methionine and cysteine and as organic acids from the metabolites of the partial combustion of dietary carbohydrates, fats, proteins, and nucleic acids. Phosphoric acid results from the hydrolysis of phosphate esters in proteins and nucleic acids that are not neutralized by mineral cations. Hydrochloric acid or its equivalent is formed from the metabolism of cationic amino acids. These nonvolatile acids must be excreted by the kidney by a process that is much slower than the lungs' excretion of CO_2 (i.e., hours versus a single breath).

Besides the respiratory and the renal regulatory systems, extracellular and intracellular buffers defend acid–base homeostasis. The bicarbonate–carbonic acid buffer complex is the major extracellular buffer system. Intracellular buffers include hemoglobin, tissue proteins, organophosphate complexes, and bone apatite.

The kidney plays the pivotal role in maintaining acid–base balance by preserving plasma bicarbonate at normal concentrations (i.e., 24 mEq/L). This occurs via two processes, bicarbonate reclamation and bicarbonate regeneration, and both occur by the same mechanism (i.e., hydrogen ion secretion). The proximal tubule reabsorbs about 85% to 90% of the filtered bicarbonate and the distal nephron reabsorbs the remaining 10% to 15%. Proximal bicarbonate reabsorption is mediated by two mechanisms (two-thirds is transported by a luminal Na^+-H^+ antiporter, whereas the other third is controlled by a luminal electrogenic H^+-ATPase). The Na^+-H^+ antiporter is driven by the sodium gradient between luminal and intracellular fluid. This gradient is generated by the basolateral Na^+-K^+-ATPase, which keeps intracellular sodium concentration low (approximately 10 to 12mEq/L). The H^+-ATPase functions independently of sodium; it primarily uses metabolic energy to secrete protons.

Secreted protons combine with filtered bicarbonate to form carbonic acid (H_2CO_3) and under the influence of luminal carbonic anhydrase, dehydrates quickly to CO_2 and water. Some of the CO_2 enters the cell to combine with water, catalyzed by cellular carbonic anhydrase, thus forming H_2CO_3. This breaks down to hydrogen ions and HCO_3. The proton formed is available for secretion while the bicarbonate is returned to the blood with sodium via the basolateral Na-HCO_3 symporter. The pH of the proximal tubular filtrate changes little (i.e., from pH 7.4 to approximately 7.1).

The thick ascending limb also participates in urinary acidification. It reabsorbs HCO_3 by the secretion of proton via a luminal Na^+-H^+ antiporter (NHE-3 isoform) similar to that of the proximal tubule. Avid sodium transport occurs in this segment by the apical Na-K-2Cl cotransporter. As fluid traverses this segment, pH changes little if any.

The distal nephron has the ability to generate a large transtubular gradient despite its small capacity for proton secretion when compared with the proximal tubule. This property enables the kidney to reduce urinary pH to as low as 4.5 and, hence, to maximally titrate the urinary buffers.

The collecting tubule, the final site of urinary acidification, consists of at least two cell types, principal cells and intercalated cells. The intercalated cells are further divided into α and β cells. The α-intercalated cells secrete hydrogen ions through a luminal proton pump, bicarbonate then exits the cell through a basolateral Cl-HCO_3 exchanger. The β-intercalated cells secrete bicarbonate. They resemble the α-intercalated cells except that the Cl-HCO_3 exchanger and proton pump are reversed in polarity. The outer medullary collecting tubule (MCT) has more α-intercalated cells than does the cortical collecting tubule (CCT); β-intercalated cells exist only in the CCT. The CCT can thus secrete either protons or bicarbonate. Furthermore, the CCT actively absorbs sodium, which can secondarily affect acidification by increasing negative transepithelial voltage. No active sodium transport occurs in the MCT where lumen potential difference remains approximately +10 mV, reflecting hydrogen ion (H^+) secretion.

Hydrogen ion secretion in the collecting tubule is mediated by two proton pumps, an H^+-ATPase and an H^+-K^+-ATPase. The H-ATPase is a vacuolar type of proton-translocating ATPase.

It is inhibited by *N*-ethylmaleimide (NEM) and the bafilomycins. It is an electrogenic pump, and its apical charge is balanced by chloride basolaterally.

The H^+-ATPase is distributed along the whole nephron; it is found in greatest amounts biochemically in the proximal convoluted tubule. As a percentage of total measurable ATPase activity, however, the CCT and MCT have the highest H-ATPase activity. H^+-ATPase activity in the collecting duct changes *directly* with the aldosterone level. Serum potassium level has no effect on H^+-ATPase activity. Both metabolic and respiratory acidosis enhance H^+-ATPase activity in the collecting tubule.

An H^+-K^+-ATPase, similar to that of gastric mucosa (and colon), is also found in the kidney with the highest activities detected in the CCT. The H^+-K^+-ATPase belongs to the class of ATPases similar to Na^+-K^+-ATPase. It is inhibited by vanadate, omeprazole, and more specifically by SCH28080. The H^+-K^+-ATPase secretes protons in exchange for potassium, and thus is electrically neutral.

In the collecting duct, H^+-K^+-ATPase activity changes *inversely* with serum potassium concentration. Aldosterone has no effect on H^+-K^+-ATPase activity. In potassium-depleted animals, H^+-K^+-ATPase activity markedly increases and thus appears to play an important role in distal potassium reabsorption. The enzyme also regulates distal acidification in both potassium-depleted and normokalemic conditions, as well as during metabolic acidosis and respiratory acidosis.

In the collecting duct, carbonic anhydrase is also present, but current dogma states that it is thought to reside primarily inside the cell. This is different from the enzyme's location in the proximal tubule where it resides in the cell membrane as well as the cell's interior. This issue is controversial and under intense investigation.

PROXIMAL RENAL TUBULAR ACIDOSIS

Pathogenesis of Proximal Renal Tubular Acidosis

Because the proximal tubule is the major site of bicarbonate reabsorption, a defect at this site results in the delivery of large amounts of bicarbonate out of the proximal tubule. Because the distal tubule has a limited capacity for bicarbonate reabsorption, urinary bicarbonate wastage occurs. The definitive method in diagnosing proximal RTA is to measure the fractional excretion of bicarbonate when the plasma bicarbonate level is near normal. Fractional excretion of bicarbonate is usually greater than 15% in patients with proximal RTA when the plasma bicarbonate concentration is at least 20 mEq/L.

The defect(s) responsible for proximal RTA remain unclear. As can be seen in Fig. 20.13, impaired proximal tubule acidification might result from a defect in any of the following:

1. Apical Na^+-H^+ antiporter (labeled 1)
2. Basolateral Na-HCO_3 symporter (labeled 2)
3. Carbonic anhydrases (labeled 3 and 4)
4. Apical H^+-ATPase
5. Impaired ability to maintain a low intracellular sodium concentration

A defect in numbers 1 through 4 will result in a selective impairment of proximal acidification. The final defect, however, will affect all Na-coupled transport processes, and thus produce Fanconi's syndrome. This abnormality might occur by several mechanisms:

1. Increased cell sodium permeability (labeled 5)
2. Decreased Na^+-K^+-ATPase activity (labeled 6)

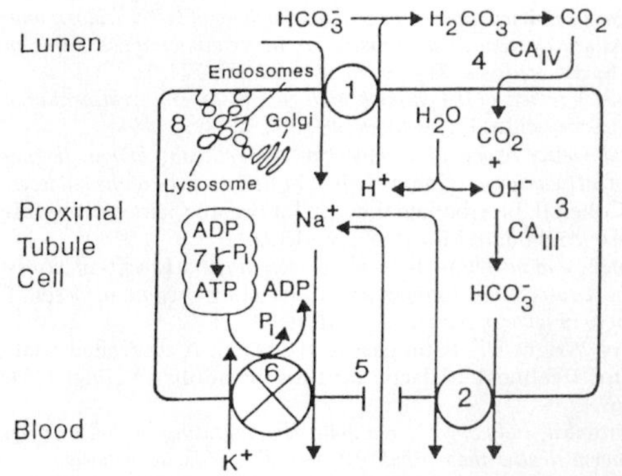

Figure 20.13. Potential cellular mechanisms of proximal (type II) RTA. The possible causes of impaired proximal acidification include defects in the luminal Na-H antiporter *(1)*; the basolateral Na-HCO_3 symporter *(2)*; the intracellular *(3)* or luminal *(4)* carbonic anhydrases (CA); sodium permeability *(5)*; the Na-K-ATPase *(6)*; the intracellular generation of ATP *(7)*; or membrane recycling, metabolism, or trafficking *(8)*. (Reproduced with permission from Cogan MG, Morris RC Jr. In: Massry SG, Glassock RJ, eds. *Textbook of nephrology.* Vol. 1, 2nd ed. Baltimore: Williams & Wilkins, 1988.)

3. Decreased adenosine triphosphate (ATP) generation (labeled 7)
4. Impaired membrane recycling (labeled 8)
5. Impaired vacuolar transport or trafficking (labeled 8)
6. Loss of epithelial mass

An abnormal form or deficient level of red blood cell–carbonic anhydrase (isoform II) has been reported in several families with proximal RTA. This abnormality has been posited as the cause of the syndrome. This is a reasonable supposition, but there are at least five isoforms of carbonic anhydrase. A defect in only one isoform might not compromise proximal acidification completely.

Intravenous administration of fructose to patients with hereditary fructose intolerance (HFI) can induce Fanconi's syndrome. High dosages of maleic acid to animals causes a similar disorder. Maleic acid impairs mitochondrial oxidation and leads to increased glucose uptake. Increased glucose concentration, like fructose administration to patients with HFI, causes increased formation and concentration of phosphorylated glycolytic intermediates, which limit the availability of cellular inorganic phosphate. This impairs mitochondrial oxidative metabolism, increases lactate production, and reduces ATP formation. Obviously, an underproduction of ATP will impair proximal transport. Studies from our laboratory show that this issue is far more complex. The administration of a low dosage of maleic acid that does not impair renal cytosolic ATP concentration also causes Fanconi's syndrome. In these studies, a decrease in proximal tubule (microdissected) Na^+-K^+-ATPase was observed; the compound had no direct effect on proximal collecting tubule H^+-ATPase activity.

Parathyroid hormone (PTH) excess also has been suggested as the cause of bicarbonate wastage in proximal RTA. PTH administration to normal subjects results in bicarbonaturia. Proximal RTA due to intestinal malabsorption is associated with hypocalcemia, vitamin D deficiency, and elevated PTH levels. Vitamin D or calcium therapy in this disorder reduces the hormone levels and decreases the bicarbonaturia. However, chronic PTH excess alone in humans does not cause profound bicarbonate wastage or severe metabolic acidosis, making it unlikely that the hormone plays a primary role in this syndrome.

Clinical Etiologies

Proximal RTA can be divided in two categories, isolated bicarbonate wasting and generalized proximal tubule dysfunction (Fanconi's syndrome). Each type can be further divided by whether or not it is accompanied with systemic or genetic disease (Table 20.13).

Patients with proximal RTA generally maintain a plasma-bicarbonate concentration greater than 15 mEq/L; severe metabolic acidosis rarely develops. In fact, these patients will completely reclaim all the filtered bicarbonate at the reduced plasma bicarbonate level and have normal distal nephron acidification. Thus patients with proximal RTA are able to acidify their urine normally during acidemia. When plasma bicarbonate is raised by exogenous addition of alkali, the reduced proximal capacity to reabsorb bicarbonate leads to bicarbonaturia, as discussed previously. After cessation of alkali administration, urinary bicarbonate wastage continues until the filtered load reaches the level at which the combined reabsorptive capacity of the proximal tubule and the distal tubule is no longer exceeded; urine bicarbonate concentration then becomes very low and urine pH is appropriately acidic.

Isolated defects in proximal tubule bicarbonate reabsorption are rarely identified. Most patients with proximal RTA show multiple defects in proximal tubular function including defective reabsorption of glucose, calcium, phosphate, citrate, uric acid, lysozymes, light-chain immunoglobulins, and amino acids.

Low serum potassium due to distal potassium wasting is a consistent finding in proximal RTA. Kaliuresis is promoted by increased distal delivery of sodium bicarbonate and by hyperaldosteronism resulting from volume contraction. Plasma renin levels are typically elevated. The rate of kaliuresis is therefore proportional to the bicarbonate delivery to the distal nephron and also to the plasma bicarbonate concentration. Administration of alkali to correct acidosis in these patients leads to an exaggeration of the kaliuresis and potassium deficiency.

Patients with proximal RTA may have high urinary calcium excretion; nephrocalcinosis and renal calculi, however, are rare. This may be due to the relatively normal rate of citrate excretion in these patients as compared with most acidotic subjects. Afflicted children are likely to have growth retardation, rickets, osteomalacia, and abnormal vitamin D metabolism. Adults may develop osteopenia but generally without pseudofractures.

Treatment of Proximal Renal Tubular Acidosis

Children and infants with proximal RTA require alkali therapy because of the high incidence of growth retardation secondary to acidemia. In general, 5 to 15 mEq/kg per day of alkali therapy is sufficient to compensate for the urinary bicarbonate losses and the endogenous acid production. Alkali may be given as sodium bicarbonate or its metabolic equivalent (citrate). Potassium supplements are necessary owing to the exacerbation of kaliuresis from high distal-bicarbonate delivery following alkali therapy. Thiazide diuretics, which cause mild volume contraction and hence enhance proximal reabsorption of bicarbonate, can diminish alkali requirements. However, thiazides enhance kaliuresis and worsen hypokalemia, which may require the addition of a potassium-sparing diuretic.

Despite the absence of significant metabolic abnormalities and bone disease, adult patients with proximal RTA may require alkali therapy when plasma bicarbonate is consistently less than 18 mEq/L. Here therapy is to prevent the development of severe acidosis following intercurrent illness.

TABLE 20.13. Clinical Spectrum of Proximal Renal Tubular Acidosis

Selective (Isolated Bicarbonate Wasting)
Primary
Idiopathic or genetic
Transient (Infants)
Carbonic anhydrase deficiency, inhibition, or alteration
Acetazolamide, sulfanilamides
Carbonic anhydrase type II deficiency
Idiopathic
Mafenide acetate
York-Yendt syndrome
Cyanotic congenital heart disease
Generalized (Associated with Fanconi's Syndrome)
Primary (without associated systemic disease)
Genetic
Sporadic
Genetically transmitted systemic diseases
Cystinosis
Dysproteinemic states
Galactosemia
Hereditary fructose intolerance (during fructose ingestion)
Lowe's syndrome
Metachromatic leukodystrophy
Methylmalonic acidemia
Monoclonal gammopathy
Multiple myeloma
Pyruvate carboxylase deficiency
Tyrosinemia
Wilson's disease
Associated with chronic hypocalcemia and secondary hyperparathyroidism
Vitamin D deficiency or resistance
Vitamin D dependency
Drug- or toxin-induced
Arginine
Gentamicin
Glue (toluene)
Lead
Maleic acid
Medullary cystic disease
Mercury
Methyl-3-chromone
Outdated tetracyclines
Renal transplantation
Sjögren's syndrome
Streptozotocin
Tubulointerstitial diseases
Other renal and miscellaneous diseases
Amyloidosis
Bone fibroma
Nephrotic syndrome
Osteopetrosis
Paroxysmal nocturnal hemoglobinurinia
Severe burns

Vitamin D and phosphate are appropriate for patients with rickets and hypophosphatemia and may improve the acidification defect. Patients with fructose intolerance should avoid fructose.

The clinical course of proximal RTA in adults depends largely on the primary disease. Proximal RTA associated with intestinal malabsorption, vitamin D deficiency, secondary hyperparathyroidism, and hypophosphatemia can be cured by vitamin D and calcium therapy. Treatment with alkali, potassium, phosphate, and vitamin D can ameliorate bone disease.

DISTAL RENAL TUBULAR ACIDOSIS

Although described earlier, distal RTA (dRTA) was recognized as a distinct entity by Albright, Burnett, and Parson in 1946. The clinical syndrome described consisted of hypokalemia, hyperchloremic metabolic acidosis, inability to lower the urine pH below 5.5, nephrocalcinosis, and nephrolithiasis. Additional features included osteomalacia or rickets. The syndrome was designated *distal renal tubular acidosis* because the establishment of a large pH gradient between urine and blood is a function of the distal nephron.

Originally, dRTA was thought to have a single pathogenesis. The prevailing view was that the disorder resulted from an inability to generate or maintain a steep hydrogen ion gradient across the distal nephron rather than from failure to secrete protons. This hypothesis was based on the observation that maximal reabsorptive capacity for bicarbonate during bicarbonate loading is either normal or increased in patients with this syndrome. Because proton secretion is thought to be the mechanism responsible for bicarbonate reabsorption, hydrogen ion secretion in the distal nephron was considered to be intact. Furthermore, titratable acid excretion in these patients increased during sodium-phosphate administration also indicating intact distal proton secretory capacity. Accordingly, dRTA often was referred to as *gradient RTA.* However, the expansion of knowledge of the control of distal urinary acidification, new methods to evaluate urinary acidification, and the development of a number of experimental models of dRTA have enlarged and modified our understanding of the pathogenesis of this syndrome.

Pathogenesis of Distal Renal Tubular Acidosis

As stated previously, the distal convoluted tubule and the collecting tubule reclaim approximately 15% of filtered bicarbonate, lower the urine pH to its final value, and titrate most of the nonbicarbonate urinary buffers. In the CCT, acidification is indirectly coupled to sodium transport and is influenced by transepithelial voltage. Active sodium reabsorption in this nephron segment generates a negative electrical potential difference, which facilitates the active secretion of protons. Aldosterone increases this transepithelial voltage and hence CCT acidification. Acidification in the MCT is not influenced by sodium transport and occurs against an electrical gradient. The potential difference in this nephron segment is lumen positive, most likely the result of active proton secretion. The absolute magnitude of proton secretion is greater in the MCT than in the CCT.

Hydrogen ion secretion is mediated by two proton pumps located in the intercalated cells, an H^+-ATPase and an H^+-K^+-ATPase. The H^+-ATPase is regulated by aldosterone, whereas the H^+-K^+-ATPase responds inversely to the serum potassium level. In the lumen, the secreted hydrogen ions combine with ammonia and other buffers and are excreted in urine.

Distal RTA can occur because of the following defects:

1. Impaired proton-pump function (defective H^+-K^+ ATPase, *classical dRTA*; defective H^+-ATPase, *normokalemic* dRTA)
2. Decreased potential difference in CCT (or *voltage-dependent dRTA*)
3. Aldosterone deficiency (or resistance)
4. Decreased capacity to maintain steep pH gradients (or *back-leak dRTA*)
5. Rate-dependent dRTA
6. Abnormal anion exchange
7. Abnormal carbonic anhydrase

Evaluation of Distal Urinary Acidification

Minimal Urine pH During Metabolic Acidosis

Measurement of the urine pH is the first step in assessing the integrity of distal urinary acidification. When systemic pH is below 7.35, the urine pH is usually less than 5.5 in normal individuals. Finding the urine pH below 5.5 suggests, but does not prove, that acidification mechanisms are intact. For example, a urine pH below 5.5 can be found in patients with dRTA due to selective aldosterone deficiency. Moreover, a urine pH below 5.5 can be found in patients with proximal RTA in whom the plasma bicarbonate concentration has fallen to values below the decreased "threshold" for bicarbonate reclamation in the proximal tubule.

The urine pH should be measured on freshly voided urine obtained in the morning and collected under mineral oil to prevent the loss of CO_2. If the patient is acidemic, there is no need to perform an ammonium-chloride (NH_4Cl) loading test because mild acidemia should be sufficient to provoke a maximal decline in urine pH. Urine pH can be influenced by the patient's position and by the rate of urine flow. Because the recumbent position can increase pH, the patient should void, if possible, in the upright position. If systemic acidemia is not present, NH_4Cl should be given orally in a dose of 0.1 g/kg body weight daily for 3 to 5 days. Alternatively, a single dose may be given and the urine collected hourly over the next 2 to 8 hours. We prefer the 3-day test because it seems to give more reliable results and allows time for a maximal increase in ammonium excretion. The urine pH in normal subjects will fall below 5.5 (usually below 5.0) by the first day and will remain below 5.5 for the duration of the test. Ammonium excretion normally increases at least 3-fold by the third day of NH_4Cl administration.

When the urine pH is above 5.5 in the presence of systemic acidemia (and in the absence of urinary tract infection) a diagnosis of dRTA is likely although the type of defect is not elucidated. Some patients with salt-retaining diseases appear to respond abnormally to acidemia because of inadequate distal sodium delivery even though distal acidification is intact. An adequate history and the measurement of sodium concentration in the collected urine can eliminate this possibility. There are a few patients, however, in whom urine pH can fall below 5.5 even though there is a defect in distal acidification. Evidence of such a defect can be disclosed by measuring the urine P_{CO_2} during bicarbonate loading.

Excreted acid appears in the urine either as titratable acid (i.e., mainly phosphate) or ammonium. Because many patients with impaired distal acidification have renal insufficiency, it is important to compare net acid excretion (titratable acid + ammonium bicarbonate) during the loading test or during spontaneous acidemia with values obtained from subjects with renal insufficiency who have similar glomerular filtration rates (GFRs). One should remember that the usual patient with renal insufficiency or renal failure has *increased* acid excretion and *increased* proximal HCO_3 reabsorption when expressed per ml GFR.

Calcium chloride is an alternative acidifying agent that can be used in patients who cannot tolerate NH_4Cl, or in whom its use is contraindicated, as in patients with liver disease. The compound is given in a dose of 2 mEq/kg orally and results in an acidification response almost identical to that observed after the administration of ammonium chloride.

Urine P_{CO_2} as an Index of Distal Acidification

Urine P_{CO_2} During Sodium-Bicarbonate Infusion. After alkalinization of the urine produced by systemic $NaHCO_3$ infusion, the urine P_{CO_2} reaches a value considerably above that of blood. Normally, the urine P_{CO_2} rises above 70 mm Hg after maximal alkalinization of the urine (i.e., pH 7.8 or greater) provided that the urine bicarbonate concentration exceeds 80 mEq/L. Although the factors controlling the generation of urinary P_{CO_2} are still not completely elucidated, renal proton secretion is considered responsible for a major component of the increase.

The rationale for using the urine P_{CO_2} as an index of acidification is that when a proton is secreted into urine containing bicarbonate, the generation of carbonic acid results that, in turn, produces CO_2. The more the hydrogen ion secreted, the higher the urine P_{CO_2}. The test is performed by infusing a solution of $NaHCO_3$ (1M) at a rate of 3 ml/min into a peripheral vein. Timed urine collections over approximately 15 to 30 minutes are obtained by spontaneous voiding in the upright position. Urine is collected (under mineral oil) for measurement of pH and P_{CO_2}. Bicarbonate concentration is calculated using the Henderson-Hasselbalch equation correcting the pKa for ionic strength. Venous blood samples are obtained at the midpoint of every other urine collection for determination of pH and P_{CO_2}. The test is terminated after a pH of 7.8 has been obtained on three consecutive urine collections. An infusion lasting approximately 180 to 260 minutes is usually required. A convenient way of visualizing the results is to plot urine P_{CO_2} against urine bicarbonate concentration.

Urine P_{CO_2} During Neutral Sodium-Phosphate Infusion. A critical dependency of urine P_{CO_2} on urine phosphate concentration exists when the pH of the urine is close to the pKa of a phosphate buffer system (i.e., 6.8).

The test is performed by infusing neutral phosphate (1 mmol/L of total body water dissolved in 180 ml of normal saline) at a rate of 1 ml/min for 3 hours. This procedure usually results in a twofold to threefold increase in plasma phosphate concentration. Urine phosphate concentration must increase to at least 20 mmol/L in two to three successive collections after the beginning of the phosphate infusion. Under these conditions, urine P_{CO_2} is consistently 25 mm Hg above that of blood both in normal individuals and in patients with renal insufficiency.

Sodium-Sulfate Infusion

Normal subjects lower the urine pH below 5.5 provided distal sodium delivery is adequate and sodium reabsorption is avid. The latter requirement can be accomplished by administering 9fludrohydrocortisone, 1 mg orally, 12 hours before the sodium-sulfate test is performed. Urine collections should be continued for 2 to 3 hours after the end of the sodium-sulfate infusion because some subjects have a delayed response. Typically, 500 ml of a 4% solution of sodium sulfate is infused over a 45- to 60-minute period. In addition to a fall in urine pH below 5.5, sodium-sulfate infusion induces a marked increase in potassium and ammonium excretion. The sodium-sulfate test provides the same information as that obtained by infusion of neutral sodium phosphate, the latter being easier to perform.

Furosemide Administration

Although both the sodium-sulfate and sodium-phosphate tests provide much useful information, they are cumbersome, difficult to perform, and seldom performed clinically. A furosemide test has been developed, and it yields the same information much more conveniently. A dose of 40 to 80 mg of furosemide is given orally. Urine is collected 120 to 180 minutes later when the maximum acidification response occurs. Administration of the diuretic furosemide inhibits tubular reabsorption of sodium and chloride in the ascending limb of Henle's loop (via the Na-K-2Cl transporter), resulting in increased delivery of sodium and chloride to the CCT. In normal subjects, this increases voltage-dependent hydrogen ion and potassium secretion in the CCT. Animal data also suggest that furosemide has a direct stimulatory effect on acidification in the MCT.

Bicarbonate Reabsorption

Because patients with dRTA have intact proximal acidification, and because the measurement of maximal bicarbonate reabsorptive capacity during bicarbonate loading is mainly a function of proximal acidification, the T_m for bicarbonate in these patients is not reduced. In fact, it tends to be somewhat increased. This increase probably results from some degree of volume contraction commonly found in these subjects along with their chronic acidemia. Acidemia can stimulate proximal acidification by decreasing intracellular pH. Because patients with dRTA cannot lower urine pH below 5.5, and usually not below 6.0, small amounts of bicarbonate are always present in the urine. Thus a characteristic small leak of bicarbonate is seen during the performance of a bicarbonate titration curve in these patients when the plasma bicarbonate is less than normal. This response contrasts with the bicarbonate-free urine normally elaborated under such circumstances. It is rarely necessary to perform a full titration experiment. A proximal defect in acidification can effectively be excluded by demonstrating a fractional excretion of bicarbonate below 5% when the plasma bicarbonate is above 20 mEq/L.

Urinary Ammonium and the Urine Anion Gap

A normal renal response to acidemia includes an increase in urinary ammonium excretion. If ammonium excretion increases under this circumstance, renal acidification is intact regardless of whether urine pH falls or not. Conversely, urinary acidification is impaired if it does not rise, irrespective of how low the urine pH falls. Urinary ammonium, however, is not usually measured in patients.

In urine, the sum of anions must be equal to the sum of cations. The major ions in bicarbonate-free urine are demonstrated in the following equation:

$$Na^+ + K^+ + Ca^{2+} + Mg^{2+} + NH_4^+ = Cl^- + H2PO_4^- + SO^{2-} + OA^-$$
(organic anion)

Because there are no major changes in phosphate, sulfate, and organic anions when the acid–base status is modified, urine ammonium concentration (NH_4^+) can be estimated from urine anion gap, defined as $(Na^+ + K^+)-Cl^-$. A urine rich in ammonium will have a negative anion gap (n50mEq/L); that is, there will be considerably more chloride present than sodium plus potassium, with the missing cation being ammonium.

The use of the urinary anion gap, as a rough index of urinary ammonium, may be helpful in the initial evaluation of hyperchloremic metabolic acidosis. A negative anion gap suggests gastrointestinal loss of bicarbonate, whereas a positive anion gap reveals the presence of altered distal urinary acidification. Use of the urinary anion gap to estimate ammonium concentration assumes that the difference between the sum of unmeasured cations (e.g., Ca^{2+}, Mg^{2+}, Li^+, drugs) and unmeasured anions (e.g., SO_4^{2-}, $H_2PO_4^-$, organic anions) is relatively constant. This difference is altered in the following circumstances:

1. Increase in bicarbonate excretion
2. Increase of an acid (that is not HCl) with the excretion of its anions (conjugate base—e.g., ketoacids, acetylsalicylic acid, D-lactic acid)
3. Excretion of unusual salts (sodium or potassium salts of certain antibiotics, sodium salicylate, and possibly excessive quantities of lithium salts)

Distal Renal Tubular Acidosis with Hypokalemia

Classical Distal Renal Tubular Acidosis

Basic Pathogenesis. Classical dRTA is a syndrome of hypokalemia, hyperchloremic metabolic acidosis, inability to lower the urine pH below 5.5, nephrocalcinosis and nephrolithiasis, and osteomalacia or renal rickets. The clinical spectrum of classical dRTA is given in Table 20.14. It is apparent from perusing this list that no single pathogenetic mechanism exists. Part of the difficulty also relates to the lack of suitable animal models for study (except for amphotericin-B and possibly toluene), although new insights with transgenic animals and carbonic-anhydrase isoform deficiency appears to be emerging.

A reduced urine P_{CO_2} in patients with classical dRTA indicates that an impairment of proton secretion, rather than increased backleak of protons, is the cause of the defective acidification. In addition, most patients with classical dRTA fail to lower urine pH after sodium sulfate, further supporting the presence of impaired distal hydrogen ion secretion. Studies in amphotericin-treated rats, a model of gradient dRTA, show an intact capacity to generate urinary CO_2.

The discovery of a renal H^+-K^+-ATPase provides new insight into the basic defect of classical dRTA. The failure of H^+-K^+-ATPase leads to both an acidification defect and urinary potassium loss, and hence causes hypokalemic hyperchloremic metabolic acidosis with all the features associated with classical dRTA. Reports from northeastern Thailand showing large numbers of patients with hypokalemic dRTA and achlorhydria suggest that there may be defects in tissue H^+-K^+-ATPases. Victims include not only humans but also water buffaloes, suggesting an environmental inhibitor of the H^+-K^+-ATPase pump as a cause of this syndrome. In animal experiments, chronic administration of sodium orthovanadate to potassium-replete rats caused hypokalemic dRTA with a urine pH of greater than 6 and a low fractional bicarbonate excretion. Collecting tubule H^+-K^+-ATPase activity is markedly decreased in the animals, whereas H^+-ATPase activity appears normal.

An immunocytochemical study of a kidney biopsy from a patient with Sjögren's syndrome who had dRTA showed no H^+-ATPase staining in the collecting tubule intercalated cells (H^+-K^+-ATPase staining was not performed). Current studies are hampered because we are just now identifying which isoforms of the H^+-K^+-ATPase are found in collecting duct tissue. Evidence to date suggests at least two isoforms are present in the distal nephron (one similar to the colonic H^+-K^+-ATPase and one apparently unique to the kidney). Further studies will doubtless be forthcoming to clarify this issue.

Hypokalemia and potassium wasting are consistent findings in classical dRTA, however the underlying mechanisms are not well understood. This may be, in part, a consequence of elevated levels of aldosterone commonly seen during acidosis. Metabolic acidosis results in decreased proximal sodium reabsorption, increased distal delivery of sodium, and hence, increased kaliuresis. The sodium wastage thus causes extracellular volume contraction and secondary hyperaldosteronism. Amelioration of hypokalemia usually occurs following correction of the acidosis with bicarbonate therapy, but the reason for this reduction is not clear. Another explanation for the distal potassium wastage may be that an electrical void is created as a consequence of absent H^+-ATPase proton secretion. Because the positively charged protons would not be secreted into the tubular lumen, a more negative transepithelial potential difference could be generated as Na reabsorption would proceed. Potassium secretion thus would rise passively in response to this steeper electrical gradient.

The inability to secrete protons in the collecting tubule in patients with classical dRTA results in a severe limitation of the titration of nonbicarbonate buffers (i.e., phosphate and ammonia) in the urine, and hence, a marked reduction in net acid excretion (titratable acid + ammonia − bicarbonate). This occurs even when an adequate supply of appropriate luminal buffers is present and ammonia production is normal. In contradistinc-

TABLE 20.14. Clinical Spectrum of "Classical" Distal Renal Tubular Acidosis

Primary (Without Associated Systemic Disease)
Genetic
Idiopathic, sporadic
Genetically Transmitted Systemic Diseases
Ehlers-Danlos syndrome
Glycogenesis type III
Hematologic disorders
Carbonic anhydrase I deficiency (or alteration)
Hereditary elliptocytosis
Sickle cell anemia
Marfan syndrome
Medullary cystic disease (nerve deafness)
Osteopetrosis with carbonic anhydrase type II deficiency
Autoimmune Diseases
Chronic active hepatitis
Hypergammaglobulinemia
Cryoglobulinemia
Familial
Hyperglobulinemic purpura
Primary biliary cirrhosis
Pulmonary fibrosis
Sjögren's syndrome
Systemic lupus erythematosus
Thyroiditis
Vasculitis
Diseases Associated with Nephrocalcinosis
Fabry's disease
Hereditary fructose intolerance (after chronic fructose ingestion)
Hyperoxaluria
Hyperthyroidism
Idiopathic (or hereditary) hypercalciuria
Medullary sponge kidney
Milk-alkali syndrome
Primary hyperparathyroidism
Vitamin D intoxication
Wilson's disease
Drug or Toxic Nephropathies
Amphotericin B
Analgesics
Balkan nephropathy
Cyclamate
Toluene ("glue sniffing")
Tubulointerstitial Diseases
Chronic pyelonephritis (secondary to urolithiasis)
Hyperoxaluria
Leprosy
Myelomonoblastic leukemia
Obstructive uropathy (?)
Renal transplantation (?)
Miscellaneous
Empty sella syndrome
Hepatic cirrhosis

tion to proximal RTA, impaired net acid excretion persists despite severe metabolic acidosis.

Positive hydrogen-ion balance and relentless acid retention inevitably develop and rapidly exhaust extracellular buffers. Blood pH can then be defended only by tapping another source of buffer, the skeleton, which is the only pool big enough to serve this need. Accordingly, basic calcium salts are continually mobilized from bone. Furthermore, metabolic acidosis suppresses proximal and distal calcium reabsorption by decreasing apical calcium entry. The clinical sequelae are hypercalciuria, nephrocalcinosis, and osteomalacia or renal rickets. Nephrocalcinosis can occur in patients with dRTA without hypercalciuria. The simultaneous reduction in urinary citrate levels during metabolic acidosis and the persistently alkaline urine enhance the development of nephrocalcinosis. Growth retardation and failure to thrive are predominant clinical features in infants and children.

Because the ability of proximal tubule to reclaim filtered bicarbonate is intact, only a slight degree of bicarbonaturia (fractional bicarbonate excretion less than 5%) is detected in adult patients with classic dRTA. Infants with dRTA, however, may present with significant bicarbonate wasting, a condition previously known as *type 3 RTA*, now recognized as a variant of classical dRTA.

"Backleak" dRTA

Amphotericin B therapy is the usual cause of this syndrome. It is easily recognized by the history of amphotericin therapy in a patient with hypokalemic dRTA. These patients can be differentiated from other patients with hypokalemic DRTA by their normal U-P pCO_2 gradients. Recently a few patients with this syndrome have been described who never took amphotericin. They appear to have a spontaneous defect in maintaining sharp pH gradients in the distal nephron.

Evaluation and Treatment of Classical Hypokalemic Distal Renal Tubular Acidosis

Because normal anion gap hyperchloremic metabolic acidosis is a feature of patients with classical dRTA, diagnosis begins with a history and physical examination to rule out other conditions (Table 20.15). The laboratory evaluation should be initiated with the examination of the urine. If the acidosis is the result of an extrarenal disorder such as diarrhea, the urine will be rich in ammonium. This can easily be disclosed by measuring the urinary electrolytes. There will be considerably more chloride than sodium (plus potassium), usually greater than 50 mEq/L. In other words, the anion gap will be *minus 50* or more. The missing cation is ammonium. Patients with dRTA or related syndromes typically have more cation than chloride in their urine when they are acidemic, indicating the reduced ammonium excretion and hence defective acidification. Once the diagnosis of an RTA syndrome has been made, the urinary anion gap has no further use because it is abnormal in all RTA syndromes.

The next step is to divide the patients according to the serum potassium, those with a low (or normal) serum potassium and those in whom it is elevated (Fig. 20.14). The first group can be further subdivided into those patients who can lower the urine pH below 5.5 and those who cannot. When proximal RTA has been excluded by measuring fractional bicarbonate excretion, distal RTA can be diagnosed with certainty in those whose urine pH is greater than 5.5. Patients who can lower urine pH below 5.5 and in whom a proximal lesion has been ruled out, can then be given sodium bicarbonate intravenously; if the urine P_{CO_2} fails to rise normally, the diagnosis of rate-dependent dRTA can be made.

Chronic treatment of classical dRTA requires alkali administration equivalent to the sum of endogenous acid production and amount of accompanying bicarbonate wastage. In general, total replacement therapy needed is 1 to 2 mEq/kg per day. Greater amounts are required in children because of the need for base deposition in growing bone and because bicarbonate wastage in children may be greater than in adults. Indefinite maintenance of alkali therapy is necessary. Correction of acidosis will generally ameliorate potassium wasting and hypokalemia. Also, there is an improvement in hypercalciuria; an increase in citrate excretion occurs, which decreases the incidence of nephrocalcinosis and nephrolithiasis.

In children, alkali therapy will allow normal growth and amelioration of hypokalemia, proximal myopathy, polyuria, and listlessness. Alkali administration and glucocorticoid therapy results in improvement in the diminished lacrimal and salivary secretions in Sjögren's syndrome associated with dRTA. Without appropriate therapy, life-threatening systemic acidosis (plasma bicarbonate less than 5 mEq/L) may occur and require emergent intervention, including intravenous bicarbonate and potassium replacement and even respiratory support.

TABLE 20.15. Conditions Associated with Hyperchloremic Metabolic Acidosis

Renal Tubular Acidosis (RTA)[a]
Proximal RTA
Distal RTA
Acid Loads
Ammonium chloride
Arginine or lysine hydrochloride
Methionine sulfate
Hyperalimentation
Sulfur
Ketoacidosis with renal ketone loss
Bicarbonate Losses
Diarrhea
Pancreatic, biliary, or small bowel fistulas or drainage
Ureterosigmoidostomy
Drugs
Calcium chloride
Magnesium sulfate
Cholestyramine
Posthypocapnia

[a] See text for differential diagnosis and evaluation.

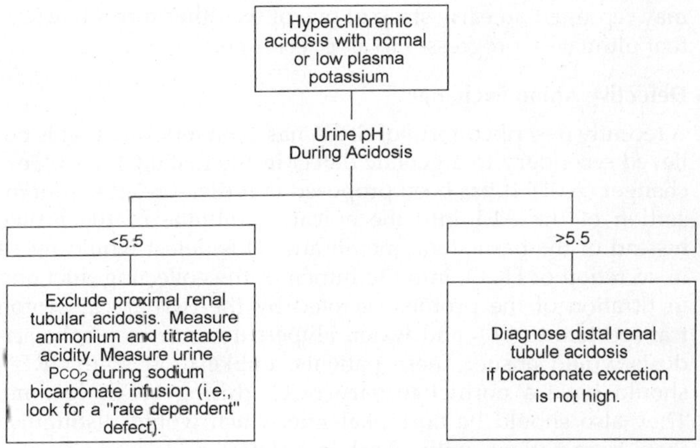

Figure 20.14. Clinical approach to the classification of renal tubular acidosis (RTA) in patients with normal or low plasma potassium; there could be a proximal or distal RTA present.

Distal Renal Tubular Acidosis with Normokalemia

Metabolic acidosis develops during renal failure; this occurs when the GFR has fallen to approximately 20% to 30% of normal. This acidosis is the result of reduced nephron mass, and not the consequence of defective proton secretion. Patients with interstitial renal disease, however, may develop a normokalemic form of dRTA, which we have tentatively ascribed to an isolated failure of the H^+-ATPase. These patients, in contradistinction to those with the acidosis of chronic renal failure, cannot lower the urine pH during acidemia and cannot raise the urine P_{CO_2}. An identical form of normokalemic dRTA is seen in patients with chronic transplant rejection and indeed may be the first sign of rejection.

Rate-Dependent Distal Renal Tubular Acidosis

There is a small subset of patients with decreased renal function who have a subtle defect in distal urinary acidification. These patients cannot raise the urine P_{CO_2} in response to bicarbonate loading, but in all other respects their ability to acidify the urine appears normal. They typically do not have metabolic acidosis. This particular defect is designated as *rate-dependent dRTA*. The definition of "incomplete" dRTA described previously could be broadened to include these patients (i.e., those without overt acidosis who cannot raise the urine P_{CO_2} but who can lower the urine pH). The urine P_{CO_2} reflects the rate of distal acidification; thus a moderate decrease in that rate might be reflected only by decreased urine P_{CO_2}. Only a handful of patients with this disorder have been described and whether the defect is of more than marginal clinical importance is uncertain. The syndrome may represent an early stage of one of the other forms of dRTA that ultimately progresses to an overt state.

Defective Anion Exchange

A recently described form of dRTA has been reported that is believed secondary to a genetic defect in the distal Cl/HCO_3 exchanger (AE1). It has been proposed that dRTA results from insertion of the AE1 into the apical membrane of the tubule instead of the basolateral membrane. This defect would result in secretion of HCO_3 into the lumen of the collecting duct and in titration of the protons secreted by the two apical proton transporters to CO_2 and water. Hyperchloremic metabolic acidosis would ensue. These patients, unlike those with dRTA, should have a normal urinary pCO_2 during HCO_3 loading. They also should be normokalemic which would distinguish them from patients with a back leak defect.

Patients with hereditary ovalocytosis have a mutation of the red blood cell AE1. They typically do not have defective urinary acidification, but occasional patients with the disease have been reported with dRTA. A recent paper described one such patient whose acidosis was associated with a normal U-B pCO_2. This patient, however, was also very hypokalemic. It is not clear whether her defect was secondary to an abnormal AE1 or rather due to a coexisting back leak defect. As mentioned above, back leak defects are usually secondary to amphotericin therapy, but can occur spontaneously.

Abnormal Carbonic Anhydrase

A null mouse has been developed, which lacks the cytoplasmic form of the enzyme [carbonic anhydrase (CA) type II–deficient mouse]. It appears that the other CA isoforms are normally expressed. These animals have dRTA with a low plasma HCO_3, and high urine pH that does not decrease normally with NH_4Cl loading. Other studies showed these animals to have virtually no α- or β-intercalated cells in the collecting duct, but there are many principle cells staining positive for the vasopressin-sensitive water channel, aquaporin (AQP)-2. These animals also have polyuria, an inadequate rise in NH^+_4 excretion with acidemia, but a normal plasma potassium. Many interesting experiments are doubtless forthcoming, and how it should be precisely categorized will soon follow.

Other studies have treated the CA type II–null mouse using genetic techniques that may be soon applicable to humans. Liposomes, containing *human* CA type II–coding sequence driven by a viral promoter, were injected into the renal arteries, and the high urine pH of these animals was noted to decrease from approximately 7.2 to 6.2 pH units. Although the latter number is not that seen in a normal mouse given NH_4Cl (pH approximately 5.7), the fall was highly significant, and in some animals it was maintained for several weeks. Using the polymerase chain reaction (PCR) and reverse transcriptase-PCR (RT-PCR), the injected renal tissue was also found to contain significant amounts of both human CA II cDNA and its corresponding mRNA. Levels were said to peak at 3 days and to remain detectable for approximately 1 month. After 7 days of chronic treatment, intense staining for CA type II was found in the cytoplasm of renal cortex and outer medulla. No staining was observed in the glomerular, vascular, or interstitial structures. If the liposomes were injected unilaterally, no staining was observed in the contralateral kidney. No renal or systemic toxicity was apparent in the mice after gene transfer.

Incomplete Distal Renal Tubular Acidosis

Some patients with classical dRTA can maintain their systemic acid–base parameters at normal levels in the unstressed state. Acid loading in these patients discloses an inability to acidify the urine maximally. These patients have incomplete type of dRTA. These patients often have a normal pH response to sodium-sulfate administration, in contrast to those described in the previous section.

Distal Renal Tubular Acidosis with Hyperkalemia

The CCT actively reabsorbs sodium via an aldosterone-dependent mechanism. Electrogenic sodium reabsorption is accompanied by passive chloride reabsorption and secretion of potassium. The negative intraluminal potential difference generated by sodium reabsorption facilitates active proton secretion by the H^+-ATPase. In both CCT and MCT, aldosterone stimulates this pump directly as well. Impairment of CCT sodium transport suppresses the secretion of potassium and hydrogen; if the H^+-ATPase is also inhibited in MCT, hyperkalemic hyperchloremic metabolic acidosis will ensue. Such disorders include aldosterone deficiency or resistance (known as *type 4 RTA*), and "voltage-dependent" RTA (Table 20.16).

Aldosterone Deficiency

Aldosterone deficiency is the most frequent form of hyperkalemic metabolic acidosis in adults. Although originally described more in the 1960s, the syndrome of isolated aldosterone deficiency (hyporeninemic hypoaldosteronism) has been recognized with regularity since the 1980s. It is much more common than Addison's disease, in which both glucocorticoid and mineralocorticoid deficiency are combined.

Aldosterone deficiency would be expected to cause both voltage-dependent acidosis and proton secretory failure. In humans and experimental animals with aldosterone deficiency, however, the ability to generate pH gradient between blood and urine is relatively normal, but the rate of net acid excretion is reduced. Patients with this syndrome can lower urine pH below 5.5, have a normal urine P_{CO_2} in an alkaline urine, and a normal response to phosphate and sulfate infusion. The rate of titratable acid appears to be normal, whereas urinary ammonium and potassium excretion in response to sodium-sulfate infusion is reduced. The decreased ammonia production and excretion is likely secondary to hyperkalemia. When hyperkalemia is treated

TABLE 20.16. Clinical Spectrum of Distal Renal Tubular Acidosis with Hyperkalemia

Aldosterone Deficiency
Combined deficiency of aldosterone, desoxycorticosterone, and cortisol
Addison's disease
Bilateral adrenalectomy
Bilateral adrenal destruction
Hemorrhage or carcinoma
Congenital enzymatic defects
21-Hydroxylase deficiency
3β-Hydroxysteroid-dehydrogenase deficiency
Desmolase deficiency
AIDS (?)
Isolated aldosterone deficiency
Familial hypoaldosteronism
Corticosterone methyloxidase deficiency, types 1 and 2
Primary zona glomerulosa defect
Transient hypoaldosteronism of infancy
Chronic idiopathic hypoaldosteronism
Heparin administration
Persistent hypotension
Angiotensin-converting enzyme inhibition
Endogenous
Drug therapy (the "prils" and the "sartans"—e.g., captopril and losartan)
Hyporeninemic hypoaldosteronism
Diabetic nephropathy
Tubulointerstitial nephropathies
Nephrosclerosis
Nonsteroidal antiinflammatory agents
AIDS (?)
Aldosterone Resistance
With salt wasting (pseudohypoaldosteronism type I)
Childhood forms
Adult forms with tubulointerstitial nephritis and renal insufficiency
Spironolactone
Without salt wasting (pseudohypoaldosteronism type II)
Combined aldosterone deficiency and resistance
Deficient renin secretion
Cyclosporine nephrotoxicity
Uncertain renin status
Lupus nephritis with deficient renin secretion
Voltage-Mediated Defects
Obstructive uropathy
Amiloride
Lithium
Sickle cell anemia
Triamterene
Lupus nephritis with deficient renin secretion
Uncertain Classification

AIDS, acquired immunodeficiency syndrome.

by cation exchange resins or dietary potassium restriction, ammonia production and excretion rise. Net acid excretion is not completely corrected, however, disclosing a defect in hydrogen ion secretion. In the absence of aldosterone, H^+-ATPase activity should markedly fall and H^+-K^+-ATPase activity should be unaffected. The ensuing hyperkalemia, however, will directly decrease H^+-K^+-ATPase activity. Correcting hyperkalemia without giving aldosterone should only partially correct acidosis.

Diabetes, tubulointerstitial nephropathy, or nephrocalcinosis are common causes of this disorder. Mild to moderate renal insufficiency is generally a persistent finding. Metabolic acidosis and elevation in potassium concentration are disproportionate for the decline in GFR. Decreased renin activity cannot completely explain this syndrome because hyperkalemia, per se, should stimulate aldosterone release. Thus failure of the zona glomerulosa to respond to hyperkalemia appropriately seems to be an integral feature of this disease.

Treatment of this disorder rarely requires mineralocorticoid replacement. Such therapy may, in fact, result in edema formation and even precipitate congestive heart failure. Furosemide administration can lower plasma potassium and enhance distal hydrogen ion secretion provided that salt is not restricted from the diet while the diuretic is administered. Dietary potassium should be reduced and potassium exchange resin given if necessary.

Aldosterone Resistance or Pseudohypoaldosteronism

For every endocrine deficiency disease, there is a corresponding resistance state. The features of the aldosterone resistance are the same as those of aldosterone deficiency except aldosterone levels in the former are normal or increased. Patients with aldosterone deficiency or resistance can lower their urine pH normally, whereas those with voltage-dependent dRTA cannot. There are at least two forms of aldosterone resistance: with or without salt wasting.

Aldosterone resistance in children is associated with profound salt wastage far in excess of that seen in adults. The difference may be attributable, at least in part, to the normal GFR present in children. The disease results from hyporesponsiveness of the distal tubule to aldosterone. Therapy in this group include salt supplement, $NaHCO_3$, and either potassium restriction or ion exchange resins.

Aldosterone resistance without salt wasting occurs in adults and presents with salt retention rather than wastage. These patients usually have chronic renal disease and the acidosis is usually mild. Mineralocorticoid administration fails to increase potassium excretion even when coupled with intravenous infusion of sodium chloride. However, infusion of sodium sulfate results in a normal increase in urinary potassium excretion.

Another form of this disorder results from an inability to generate a negative potential difference in the lumen of the distal nephron as a result of increased permeability of the distal nephron to chloride, that is, a *chloride shunt*. Increased chloride reabsorption causes NaCl retention and suppression of the renin-aldosterone axis. The combination of the low transepithelial potential difference and hypoaldosteronism results in decreased potassium secretion, hyperkalemia, and reduced ammonia production, which leads to decreased net acid excretion, and hence, acidosis. These patients can be effectively treated with salt restriction and thiazide diuretics.

Voltage-Dependent Distal Renal Tubular Acidosis

The defect responsible for voltage-dependent dRTA originally was thought to be the loss of the lumen-negative potential difference in the CCT, which in turn leads to reduced hydrogen and potassium secretion. The features of this syndrome are hyperkalemic hyperchloremic metabolic acidosis, salt wastage (detectable only with marked salt restriction), normal or increased plasma aldosterone, urine pH more than 5.5, low urine P_{CO_2} with bicarbonate loading, and abnormal response to sulfate or furosemide administration. Urinary tract obstruction, amiloride, and lithium are known prototypes of voltage-dependent dRTA. However, there are major differences among these conditions. Urinary tract obstruction and amiloride administration are associated with hyperkalemia and the inability to lower urine pH below 5.5 following sulfate. Lithium administration, however, is not accompanied by hyperkalemia, whereas the ability to lower urine pH below 5.5 following sulfate is preserved. Furthermore, lithium has a greater propensity than amiloride to cause systemic acidosis. Studies of renal ATPase activities provide more insight into the pathogenesis of these syndromes.

After 24 hours of unilateral ureteral obstruction, Na^+-K^{+-}-ATPase activity is depressed along the entire nephron. H^+-ATPase activity is decreased slightly in CCT and markedly in MCT. H^+-K^+-ATPase activity is increased in CCT and decreased in MCT. Chronic administration of amiloride results in decreased Na^+-K^+-ATPase activity in both CCT and MCT, decreased H^+-ATPase activity only in CCT, and unchanged collecting tubule H^+-K^+-ATPase activity. Following chronic lithium therapy, Na^+-K^+-ATPase activity is depressed in both CCT and MCT, and activities of H^+-ATPase and H^+-K^+-ATPase are decreased only in CCT.

Thus it appears that besides the effect on potential difference by inhibiting Na^+-K^+-ATPase activities, these prototypes of voltage-dependent dRTA also influence renal proton pumps. In 24-hour unilateral ureteral obstruction, the enhanced CCT H^+-K^+-ATPase activity likely mitigates the reduced acid secretion caused by decreased H^+-ATPase activity at this site. Thus the overall acidification defect observed in unilateral ureteral obstruction appears due to impaired MCT proton transport. The potassium retention observed in acute unilateral ureteral obstruction is caused by both decreased potassium secretion by reduced Na^+-K^+-ATPase activity and increased potassium reabsorption via the H^+-K^+-ATPase, both in CCT.

With regard to lithium, the inhibitory effect of lithium on both H^+-ATPase and H^+-K^+-ATPase might explain the metabolic acidosis found in this model. The decreased H^+-K^+-ATPase activity likely mitigates reduced potassium excretion caused by decreased Na^+-K^+-ATPase activity and prevents hyperkalemia. Amiloride inhibits H^+-ATPase but not H^+-K^+-ATPase, which likely explains its modest effect on acid–base composition. Intact potassium reabsorption (H^+-K^+-ATPase activity is normal) and the failure of potassium secretion (Na^+-K^+-ATPase activity is decreased) lead to decrease potassium excretion and hence hyperkalemia.

Evaluation and Treatment of Hyperkalemic Distal Renal Tubular Acidosis

Because normal anion gap hyperchloremic metabolic acidosis is also a feature of patients with hyperkalemic dRTA, the diagnosis begins with a history and physical examination and an assessment of the features of the acidosis as outlined in Table 20.15. Because diabetes mellitus with hyporeninemic hypoaldosteronism and urinary tract obstruction are two diseases commonly encountered in medicine, they should be easy to rule out. Addison's disease should also be considered and patients on chronic low-dose heparin (or its analogues) should be tested for isolated aldosterone deficiency or adrenal hemorrhage.

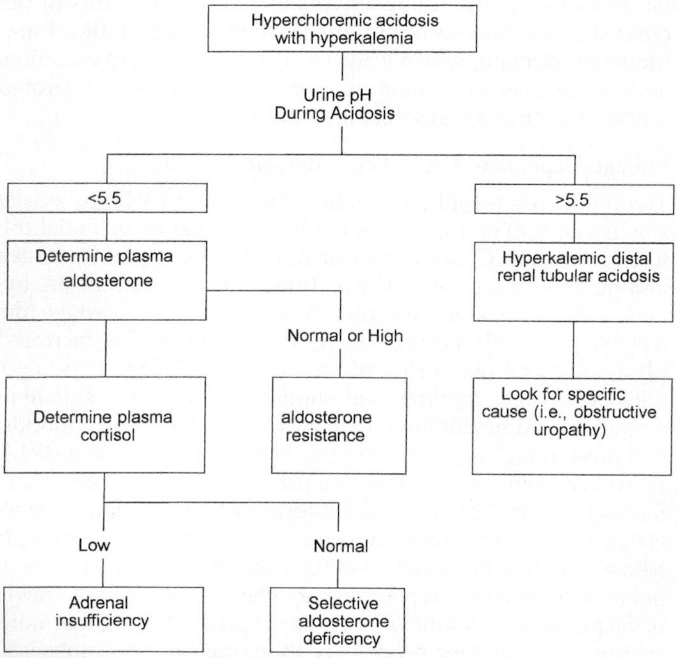

Figure 20.15. Clinical approach to the classification of distal renal tubular acidosis (RTA) in patients with hyperkalemia.

TABLE 20.17. Patterns of Plasma Aldosterone and Urine pH Hyperkalemic dRTA

	Urine pH During Acidemia	Plasma Aldosterone
Aldosterone deficiency	<5.5	Low
Aldosterone resistance	<5.5	Normal or high
Voltage-dependent dRTA	>5.5	Normal or high
Aldosterone deficiency and voltage-dependent dRTA combined	>5.5	Low

dRTA, distal renal tubular acidosis.

Patients with hyperkalemia should also be divided on the basis of urine pH. In those with a pH below 5.5 (Fig. 20.15), a normal plasma cortisol combined with a low aldosterone establishes the diagnosis of selective aldosterone deficiency. Because hyperkalemia stimulates aldosterone release, plasma aldosterone values cannot be interpreted accurately without reference to the serum potassium concentration. When the potassium is elevated, the plasma aldosterone concentration should be at least three times higher. Thus an aldosterone of 15 ng/ml, while ostensibly normal, is low for a patient with a potassium of 6 mEq/L. If both cortisol and aldosterone are low, the patient has Addison's disease. The finding of a normal or high aldosterone suggests aldosterone resistance. In patients with hyperkalemia and a urine pH persistently greater than 5.5, the diagnosis of hyperkalemic or voltage-dependent dRTA is made without further evaluation, but one should look for a specific cause such as obstructive uropathy or a sickle hemoglobinopathy.

Table 20.17 shows the pattern of plasma aldosterone and urine pH seen in patients with aldosterone deficiency, aldosterone resistance, voltage-dependent dRTA, and the combination of aldosterone deficiency and RTA. Note that the patient with the combined disorder is easily distinguished from those with the other disorders. The high urine pH indicates dRTA and the low aldosterone discloses the steroid deficiency.

In summary, the patient with hyperchloremic metabolic acidosis may have a diagnosis as simple as diarrhea (Table 20.15) or one as complex as voltage-dependent dRTA. Unraveling the diagnosis and understanding the pathophysiology is not only a rewarding exercise, it reinforces the basic concepts of acid–base physiology. Appropriate therapy may then be prescribed paying particular attention to the long-term adverse consequences of metabolic acidosis.

Acknowledgements

The research described by the authors was supported in part by a grant from the National Institutes of Health, #R01-DK-36199. The authors thank Betty Lonis for her expert editorial and graphic assistance.

Selected Readings

Battle DC. Hyperkalemic hyperchloremic metabolic acidosis associated with selective aldosterone deficiency and distal renal tubular acidosis. *Semin Nephrol* 1981;1:260–273.

An extensive review of dRTA in aldosterone deficiency.

Caruana RJ, Buckalew VM Jr. The syndrome of distal (type 1) renal tubular acidosis. Clinical and laboratory findings in 58 cases. *Medicine* 1988;67:84–99.

A comprehensive study of clinical and laboratory findings in classical dRTA.

Cogan MG. Disorders of proximal nephron function. *Am J Med* 1982;72:275–288.
A review of the normal physiology and pathophysiology involved in clinical disorders of proximal tubule function.

Dafnis E, Spohn M, Kurtzman NA, et al. Vanadate causes hypokalemic distal renal tubular acidosis. *Am J Physiol* 1992;262:F449–F453.
An experimental study of chronic vanadate administration on fissure levels, renal function and ATPases in microdissected rat nephron segments.

DuBose TD Jr, Caflisch CR. Validation of the difference in urine and blood carbon dioxide tension during bicarbonate loading as an index of distal nephron acidification in experimental models of distal renal tubular acidosis. *J Clin Invest* 1985;75:1116–1123.
An important study using the U-B P_{CO_2} to demonstrate impaired distal nephron proton secretion.

Eiam-Ong S, Kurtzman NA, Spohn M, et al. Insights into the biochemical mechanism of maleic acid-induced Fanconi syndrome. *Kidney Int* 1995;48:1542–1548.
An experimental study of maleic acid on rat nephron segment ATPases.

Garg LC. Respective roles of H-ATPase and H-K-ATPase in ion transport in the kidney. *J Am Soc Nephrol* 1991;2:949–960.
Review of the roles of H-ATPase and H-K-ATPase in acidification along the entire tubule segments.

Gonick HC, Kramer HJ. Pathogenesis of the Fanconi syndrome. In: Gonick HC, Buckalew VM Jr, eds. *Renal tubular disorders.* New York: Marcel Dekker, 1985: 545–607.
A comprehensive review of pathogenesis of Fanconi's syndrome in experimental models.

Kurtzman NA. Disorders of distal acidification. *Kidney Int* 1990;38:720–727.
An article describing new concepts in the pathogenesis of various subtypes of distal RTA and a practical guideline for the approach to renal tubular acidosis.

Pressley T, Sabatini S, Guest Editors. ATPases in biology and medicine. *Miner Electrolyte Metab* 1996;22:1–263.
Several articles on Na-K-ATPase, H-ATPase, and H-K-ATPase as they relate to renal physiology and pathophysiology.

PART 6
Metabolic Alkalosis

John H. Galla and Robert G. Luke

Metabolic alkalosis occurs when a primary stimulus leads to the net accumulation of base within or the net loss of acid from the extracellular fluid (ECF). Unopposed by other primary acid–base disorders, metabolic alkalosis is recognized by elevations in both arterial blood pH (alkalemia) and plasma bicarbonate concentration. This increase in arterial blood pH promptly, normally, and predictably depresses ventilation, resulting in increased Pa_{CO_2} and buffering of the magnitude of the alkalemia. The Pa_{CO_2} increases about 0.5 to 0.7 mmHg for every 1.0-mM increase in plasma HCO_3 concentration. Although a Pa_{CO_2} greater than 55 mmHg is uncommonly encountered, compensatory increases to 60 mmHg have been documented in severe metabolic alkalosis; substantial hypoxia may accompany such marked degrees of hypoventilation. Conversely, failure of an appropriate compensatory increase in Pa_{CO_2} should be interpreted as a mixed acid–base disturbance in which a primary stimulus to hyperventilation (respiratory alkalosis) is superimposed on metabolic alkalosis. Mixed acid–base disturbances are discussed in Part 8 of this chapter.

Metabolic alkalosis is common, and it accounted for half of all acid–base disorders in at least one study. This observation should not be surprising because vomiting and the use of chloruretic diuretics and nasogastric suction are also common among hospitalized patients. The mortality associated with severe metabolic alkalosis is substantial; a morality rate of 45% in patients with an arterial blood pH of 7.55 and of 80% when the pH was greater than 7.65 has been reported. Although this relationship is not necessarily causal, severe alkalosis should be viewed with concern and correction by the appropriate intervention should be undertaken with dispatch when the arterial blood pH exceeds 7.55.

CLASSIFICATION AND DEFINITIONS

A major clinically and pathophysiologically relevant classification can be based on whether the metabolic alkalosis is dependent on chloride depletion. The former is by far more common. The other major grouping, not related to chloride, is that caused by potassium depletion due to mineralocorticoid excess. By definition, chloride-depletion metabolic alkalosis can be corrected without potassium repletion. As noted later, a modest degree of potassium depletion, or at least hypokalemia, is common in chloride-depletion alkalosis because of both the shift of potassium intracellularly in exchange for protons and the usually modest cumulative urinary potassium losses. However, although concomitant potassium repletion is clinically indicated to prevent other potentially harmful effects of potassium depletion, studies have shown that it is not essential to correct the alkalosis. Metabolic alkalosis caused by mixed potassium and chloride depletion also may occur.

Because the normal kidney is so efficient at excreting bicarbonate, base loading, whether exogenous or endogenous (as in bone dissolution), whether patient derived or iatrogenic, is rarely a sole cause of significant *chronic* metabolic alkalosis. *Transient* states of metabolic alkalosis, on the other hand, may occur during and immediately after an oral or intravenous infusion of $NaHCO_3$ or base equivalent (e.g., citrate in transfused blood or fresh-frozen plasma). A state of transient metabolic alkalosis may also occur after the successful treatment of ketoacidosis or lactic acidosis because these organic anions are metabolized to bicarbonate. A third situation for transient metabolic alkalosis is after successful therapy to correct hypercapnia in respiratory acidosis before the kidney can reduce the then inappropriately high plasma bicarbonate concentration, provided that chloride intake is adequate.

In transient states of acute metabolic alkalosis, the urinary pH should be relatively alkaline (greater than 6.2) because the kidney is in the process of excreting the retained bicarbonate. If the urine is relatively acidic, in the face of *chronic* metabolic alkalosis, the diagnostic approach discussed next is recommended.

The course of chronic metabolic alkalosis can be divided into *generation, maintenance,* and *recovery* phases. Generation occurs by loss of protons from the ECF into the external environment or into the cells, or by gain of base by the oral or intravenous route or from the base stored in bone apatite. Important maintenance mechanisms are chloride depletion, mineralocorticoid excess, and potassium depletion, and states of low or absent glomerular filtration rate (GFR) associated with base excess.

Disequilibrium occurs in acute or acute-on-chronic metabolic alkalosis when generation of bicarbonate and resultant elevation of plasma bicarbonate exceeds the capacity of the renal tubule to reabsorb bicarbonate. Transient bicarbonaturia with resulting sodium loss ensues until a new steady state of chronic metabolic alkalosis is achieved and bicarbonate excretion ceases.

PATHOPHYSIOLOGY OF CHLORIDE-DEPLETION ALKALOSES

Generation

Chloride may be lost from the gut, kidney, or skin. The loss of gastric fluid, which contains 60 to 100 mM HCl and lesser variable concentrations of sodium and potassium, results in alkalosis because bicarbonate, generated during the production of gastric acid, returns to the circulation. Although sodium and potassium loss in the gastric fluid varies in amount, the obligate urinary loss of these cations is intensified by bicarbonaturia, which often occurs at the outset of alkalosis and especially with disequilibrium alkalosis. Gastrocystoplasty for bladder augmentation may also result in urinary HCl losses sufficient to produce alkalosis.

Villous adenomas of the colon usually produce a hyperchloremic metabolic acidosis because of the loss of large volumes of colonic fluid, which is rich in potassium and bicarbonate. However, 10% to 20% of these tumors will secrete chloride rather than bicarbonate with potassium and thus result in metabolic alkalosis. Congenital chloridorrhea, a rare disease, has a similar pathogenesis in which Cl-HCO_3 exchange in the ileum is defective, resulting in copious diarrhea with major chloride, potassium, and fluid losses.

Chloruretic agents, such as chlorothiazide, furosemide, and their congeners, all directly produce the loss of chloride, sodium, and fluid in the urine. In turn, these losses promote alkalosis by several possible pathways: (a) diuretic-induced increases in sodium delivery to the late distal convoluted tubule and collecting duct accelerate potassium and proton secretion and excretion; (b) resultant ECF volume contraction stimulates renin and aldosterone secretion, which blunts sodium loss but accelerates the secretion of potassium and protons; (c) as discussed later, potassium depletion independently also accelerates bicarbonate reabsorption in the proximal tubule and stimulates ammonia production, which, in turn, may promote urinary acid excretion; and (d) urinary losses of chloride exceed those for sodium relative to their respective plasma concentrations. The exact mechanisms by which diuretics engender renal proton loss are not yet established.

Respiratory acidosis is compensated by accelerated renal bicarbonate reabsorption with increased urinary chloride excretion. The patient with chronic respiratory acidosis is chloride depleted, and the kidney will maintain this deficit until the hypercapnia is corrected. When respiratory acidosis is corrected, accelerated bicarbonate reabsorption, which is no longer appropriate, will persist if sufficient chloride is not available, and posthypercapneic metabolic alkalosis occurs. The patient with respiratory failure and congestive heart failure who is being managed with NaCl restriction epitomizes this presentation.

Skin losses of chloride may generate alkalosis in cystic fibrosis. Alkalosis may even be the presenting feature in adolescents, with a few of the several hundred mutations in the cystic fibrosis transmembrane regulator (CFTR) gene.

Maintenance

The cessation of events that generate alkalosis is not necessarily accompanied by resolution of the alkalosis, unlike the usual course in metabolic acidosis in which sufficiently increased renal net acid excretion can restore normal acid–base balance. To account for maintained metabolic alkalosis in these instances, the kidney must *a priori* retain bicarbonate either by a decrease in GFR with an accompanying decrease in filtered bicarbonate, by an increase in bicarbonate reabsorption, or by both mechanisms. Because, as we have described, chloride-depletion alkaloses are usually characterized by concurrent deficits of sodium, potassium, and fluid, as well as chloride, controversy has existed regarding which of these deficits is responsible for the maintenance of the alkalosis.

Early studies showed that complete correction of experimental chloride-depletion alkalosis could be effected without potassium or sodium repletion, thus eliminating these deficits as causes of the maintenance in these experimental circumstances. Although these observations led to the conclusion that chloride repletion was pivotal in the correction of the alkalosis, a role for volume repletion per se was not excluded. Subsequently, a widely accepted hypothesis for the pathophysiology of the maintenance and correction of chloride-depletion alkalosis was developed. Volume depletion accompanying alkalosis augments fluid reabsorption in the proximal tubule, and because bicarbonate is preferentially reabsorbed compared with chloride in this segment, alkalosis is maintained. With subsequent ECF volume expansion, fluid reabsorption in the proximal tubule is depressed, delivering more bicarbonate and chloride to the more distal nephron segments, which possess a substantial capacity to reabsorb chloride but a limited capacity for bicarbonate. As a result, chloride is retained, bicarbonate is excreted, and the alkalosis is corrected. In this construct, chloride administration has only a permissive role for volume expansion, which itself is regarded as the extrarenal impetus for correction.

A dominant role for a reduced GFR and the attendant reduction in filtered bicarbonate load in the maintenance of alkalosis and the importance of an primary increase in GFR for its correction has also been propounded and refuted.

The so-called classical hypothesis based on volume has been reappraised in our laboratory in a series of studies of both acute and chronic chloride-depletion alkalosis in humans and rats; the role of GFR has been examined in parallel. In these studies, complete correction of chloride-depletion alkalosis has been effected by the administration of any of several non–sodium chloride salts in the face of persistently low GFR, decreased plasma volume, negative sodium balance, decreasing body weight, continuing urinary potassium loss, persistently high plasma aldosterone concentration, and continued bicarbonate loading, all of which should, if anything, promote alkalosis. Increased bicarbonate delivery out of the proximal tubule, as predicted by the volume hypothesis, was observed during both expansion and contraction of ECF volume but, in either case, without correction of alkalosis in the absence of chloride replacement. Even during sustained volume contraction, however, the administration of chloride promptly induced bicarbonaturia and progressive correction of alkalosis. In human subjects with diuretic-induced alkalosis maintained for 5 days by chloride restriction, alkalosis was corrected as chloride was repleted quantitatively. However, the depression of GFR and renal blood flow and the decreased plasma volume that attended the generation of the alkalosis persisted throughout the correction. Thus we would extend the earlier conclusion to state that chloride is *necessary* and *sufficient* for the correction of chloride-depletion alkalosis. Volume depletion is a commonly associated but not causative or essential factor for the maintenance of alkalosis. Indeed, this relationship is more aptly called *alkalotic contraction* in that sodium and fluid shifts from the extracellular to the intracellular compartment in response to the alkalosis and in the absence of necessary external sodium losses.

We propose that intrarenal mechanisms responsive to chloride depletion can account for the maintenance of alkalosis

TABLE 20.18. Effects of Metabolic Alkalosis on Renal Function

	CDA	KDA
Reduced GFR[a]	X	X
Stimulated renin-aldosterone axis[a]	X	
Enhanced response to mineralocorticoid[a]		X
Accelerated proximal HCO_3 reabsorption[a]		X
Accelerated collecting duct HCO_3 reabsorption[a]	X	X
Decreased HCO_3 secretion (collecting duct)[a]	X	
Increased renal potassium excretion[a]	X	
Reduced urinary concentrating ability	X	X
Chloride wasting (when severe)[a]		X
Renal vasoconstriction		X

[a] May contribute to maintenance of metabolic alkalosis.
CDA, chloride-depletion alkalosis; GFR, glomerular filtration rate; KDA, potassium-depleted alkalosis.

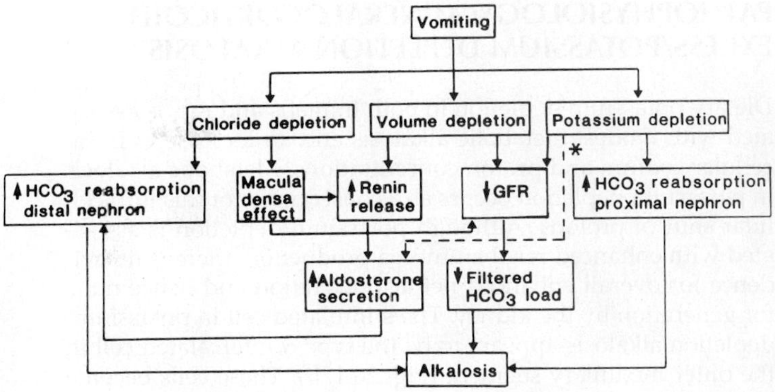

Figure 20.16. Schema for the maintenance of alkalosis during vomiting.

regardless of the status of the ECF volume (Table 20.18; Fig. 20.16). In the absence of volume depletion, chloride depletion may decrease GFR by tubuloglomerular feedback, an intrarenal mechanism for the control of GFR, the afferent signal for which is at the macula densa. In this setting, the signal perceived by the macula densa (chloride concentration or osmolality in tubule fluid at that site) results in a decrease in GFR. Such a protective response by the kidney would blunt the losses of fluid and sodium, which might attend the bicarbonaturia commonly encountered during disequilibrium alkalosis. Chloride depletion also increases renin secretion by a macula densa mechanism, resulting in increased aldosterone secretion, which may be disproportionate to the magnitude of an accompanying hypokalemia and would augment potassium wasting.

A reasonable body of evidence now favors the collecting duct as the major site in the nephron for altered acid–base and electrolyte transport in both maintenance of and recovery from metabolic alkalosis. Additional alterations in renal electrolyte transport occur when the kidney itself is the proximate cause of the defect leading to alkalosis, as in the defect in Henle's loop in Bartter's syndrome. However, the proximal tubule does play an essential permissive role by the appropriate reabsorption of the bicarbonate load (Table 20.19).

The collecting duct is heterogeneous anatomically and functionally throughout its length with regard to both cells and segments. Sodium reabsorption and potassium secretion in the principal cell occurs through electrogenic channels in the luminal membrane. Aldosterone stimulates sodium reabsorption and facilitates potassium secretion by its action on basolateral Na^+-K^+-ATPase and luminal potassium and sodium channel permeability. Overall, potassium depletion would be stimulated by enhanced sodium delivery, increased aldosterone concentrations, increased cellular potassium activity, or diminished availability of chloride in the lumen. All of these factors likely contribute to the kaliuresis seen in chloride-depletion metabolic alkalosis.

The major cell stimulated by chloride-depletion alkalosis is the type B intercalated cell in the cortical segment (Fig. 20.17A). This cell is then poised to secrete bicarbonate when chloride is administered and luminal or cellular chloride concentration or amount increases. During maintenance, bicarbonate secretion does not occur because insufficient chloride is available for bicarbonate exchange and bicarbonate reabsorption is maintained distal to the cortical segment.

TABLE 20.19. Functions of Collecting Duct Cells Relevant to Alkalosis

Segment	Cell	Function
Cortical	Principal	Na^+ and Cl^- reabsorption and K^+ secretion
	α Intercalated	HCO_3^- reabsorption
	β Intercalated	HCO_3^- secretion; Cl^- reabsorption
Outer medullary	α Intercalated	K^+ and HCO_3^- reabsorption[a]
Inner medullary (initial)	α Intercalated	HCO_3^- reabsorption
Inner medullary (terminal)	IMCD	Na^+, Cl^-, HCO_3^- reabsorption

[a] H^+-K^+-ATPase.
IMCD, inner medullary collecting duct.

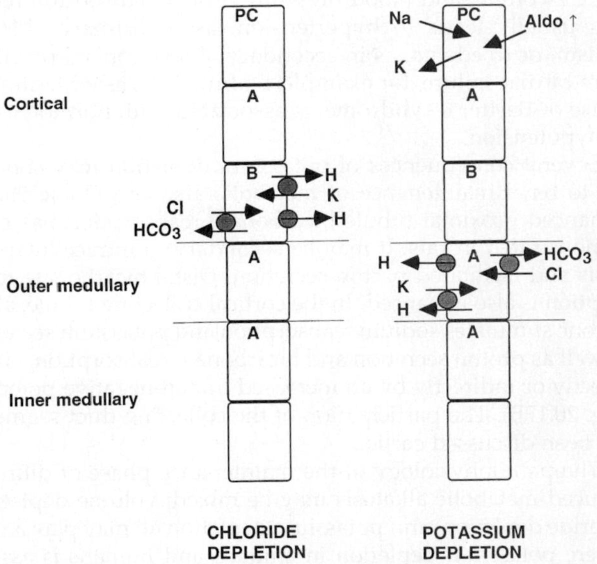

Figure 20.17. Theoretical contributions of transport mechanisms in the collecting duct segments during metabolic alkalosis. In chloride-depletion alkalosis during maintenance, the relative unavailability of Cl in the lumen facilitates HCO_3 reabsorption by an enhanced gradient for Cl secretion in the medullary segment but blunts HCO_3 secretion in the cortical segment because of its requirement for apical Cl-HCO_3 exchange. During correction by Cl, the availability of Cl reverses these effects, HCO_3 secretion becomes the dominant contribution of the collecting duct, and HCO_3 excretion occurs. In potassium-depletion alkalosis caused by primary hyperaldosteronism, for example, aldosterone stimulates K secretion and Na reabsorption in the cortical segment. The resultant K depletion produces an intracellular acidosis and extracellular alkalosis. In the kidney, this accelerates proton secretion primarily in the medullary segment, thereby maintaining the alkalosis. Both H^+-ATPase and H^+-K^+-ATPase may participate in these responses. A, intercalated cell; B, intercalated cell; PC, principal cell.

PATHOPHYSIOLOGY: MINERALOCORTICOID EXCESS/POTASSIUM DEPLETION ALKALOSIS

Dietary potassium depletion in both humans and rats is associated with modest metabolic alkalosis and an increase in intracellular sodium and proton concentrations. Metabolic alkalosis in potassium depletion occurs as a consequence of this intracellular shift of protons. Although potassium depletion is associated with enhanced renal ammonia production, there is no evidence for overall enhanced net acid excretion and hence none for generation by the kidney. The stimulated cell in potassium-depletion alkalosis appears to be the type α intercalated cell in the outer medullary segment (Fig. 20.17B). These cells become increased in size and number in potassium depletion. Intracellular acidosis in renal tubular cells would facilitate luminal proton–potassium exchange with potassium conservation and bicarbonate reabsorption and thus would perpetuate alkalosis. The important role of intracellular acidosis in potassium-depletion alkalosis is supported by correction of the alkalosis by infusion of potassium without any suppression of renal net acid excretion; correction is assumed to occur by the movement of potassium into and of protons out of the cell, which titrates ECF bicarbonate.

Administration of aldosterone causes only a slight degree of metabolic alkalosis if potassium depletion is prevented. Although escape from the sodium-retaining effect of mineralocorticoids occurs at the expense of persistent vascular and ECF volume expansion and resulting hypertension, escape does not occur from potassium-wasting effect, as for example in primary hyperaldosteronism.

The potassium-depletion mineralocorticoid excess classification of metabolic alkalosis can be subdivided by the status of ECF volume and blood pressure. Associated sodium retention usually leads to hypertension, as in primary aldosteronism, or to edema, as in secondary aldosteronism resulting from cardiac failure, for example. Sodium loss, as with diuretic abuse or Bartter's syndrome, is associated with normotension or hypotension.

Several consequences of potassium depletion may contribute to renal maintenance of metabolic alkalosis (Table 20.18). Enhanced proximal tubule bicarbonate reabsorption has been demonstrated in rats. It may be secondary to intracellular acidosis and facilitated proton secretion. Distal bicarbonate reabsorption is also enhanced. In the cortical collecting tubule, aldosterone stimulates sodium reabsorption and potassium secretion as well as proton secretion and bicarbonate reabsorption, either directly or indirectly by an increased lumen-negative potential (Fig. 20.17B). The participation of the collecting duct segments has been discussed earlier.

The pathophysiology of the maintenance phase of diuretic-induced metabolic alkalosis may be mixed; volume depletion, chloride depletion, and potassium depletion all may play a role. Severe potassium depletion in animals and humans is associated with renal chloride wasting, which would intensify metabolic alkalosis caused by chloride depletion. Downregulation of chloride transporters is an early event in potassium depletion.

The pathophysiology of the sometimes severe metabolic alkalosis seen in Bartter's and Gitelman's syndromes and their variants is likely dependent on both potassium depletion and chloride depletion. A primary hereditary defect in coupled Na-K-2Cl reabsorption in the thick ascending limb of Henle's loop explains the tendency toward renal sodium, potassium, and chloride wasting; macula densa and volume depletion–stimulated activation of the renin-aldosterone system; and high renal production of PGE_2 in Bartter's syndrome. Both medullary interstitial PGE_2 excess and severe potassium depletion can further impair Na-K-2Cl reabsorption in the ascending limb. The similarity of the syndrome to that produced by abuse of loop diuretics is evident. In Gitelman's syndrome, a defect in coupled NaCl uptake in the distal convolution has been identified. The association of hypocalciuria in this syndrome is reminiscent of the effect of thiazide diuretics. Bulimia with surreptitious vomiting can produce similar pathophysiologic consequences, but renal conservation of chloride remains normal. Bartter's syndrome and its variants are uncommon, but the pathophysiology is important because they mimic some commonly concealed causes of metabolic alkalosis (Table 20.20).

TABLE 20.20. Conditions Associated with Metabolic Alkalosis That May Mimic Bartter's Syndrome

Diuretic abuse	
	High urinary Cl^- depends on duration of action of recently ingested diuretic
Severe potassium depletion	
	From any cause not associated with HCO_3 wasting
Bulimia with vomiting	
	Urinary Cl low
Magnesium depletion	
	Also may occur in some patients with Bartter's and most patients with Gitelman's syndrome
Laxative abuse	
	Urinary K^+ excretion <30 mEq/day

PATHOPHYSIOLOGY OF MISCELLANEOUS METABOLIC ALKALOSIS

Metabolic alkalosis in the chronic milk-alkali syndrome also has multiple causes, including vomiting, hypercalcemia (which directly increases bicarbonate reabsorption), a reduced GFR (which is secondary to volume depletion), chloride depletion, hypercalcemia, and in some patients, nephrocalcinosis.

Hypoalbuminemia may cause mild metabolic alkalosis because of the diminution of the negative charges that albumin normally contributes to the anion gap and the shift in the buffering curve for plasma.

CLINICAL AND DIAGNOSTIC ASPECTS

The clinical features of metabolic alkalosis per se are difficult to separate from those of depletion of chloride, volume, or potassium. Apathy, confusion, cardiac arrhythmias, and neuromuscular irritability (related in part, perhaps, to a low ionized plasma calcium) are common when alkalosis is severe. Compensatory hypoventilation may cause hypoxia or contribute to pulmonary infection in very ill or immunocompromised patients. The degree of compensation is not influenced by the cause of the alkalosis.

The cause of chronic metabolic alkalosis (Table 20.21) is often evident on the initial assessment of the patient with a careful history and physical examination. In the absence of blood gas measurements, an increase in the anion gap and hypokalemia favor metabolic alkalosis over respiratory acidosis when plasma chloride is low and bicarbonate high. Both increased plasma albumin and lactate concentration may contribute to the increased anion gap. These changes do not usually occur in respiratory acidosis unless there is accompanying severe hypoxia.

Urinary electrolyte measurements before therapy, especially chloride and potassium concentrations, can be of diagnostic

TABLE 20.21. Etiologies of Chronic Metabolic Alkalosis

Chloride Depletion
Gastric losses—vomiting, mechanical drainage, bulimia
Chloruretic drugs
Diarrheal states—villous adenoma, congenital chloridorrhea
Posthypercapneic states
Dietary Cl deprivation and base loading—Cl-deficient infant formulas
Gastrocystoplasty
Cystic fibrosis (high sweat chloride)
Mineralocorticoid Excess
Primary—tumors, hyperplasia
Secondary
Malignant or accelerated hypertension
Adrenal glucocorticosteroid excess, primary, secondary, exogenous
Juxtaglomerular apparatus tumors
Apparent
Drugs—licorice, carbenoxolone
Liddle's syndrome
Excess Intake of HCO_3
Ingestion with renal insufficiency
Acute or chronic milk-alkali syndrome
Other
Bartter's syndrome, Gitelman's syndrome, and their variants
Antibiotics (e.g., carbenicillin)
Laxative abuse
Recovery from starvation
Hypoalbuminemia

value before treatment when the diagnosis is not obvious or the patient is concealing information (Fig. 20.18). A urinary potassium concentration of greater than 30 mEq/L in the presence of hypokalemia indicates renal potassium wasting, often due to diuretics or high aldosterone secretion rates. A urinary potassium concentration of less than 30 mEq/L indicates an extrarenal potassium loss or severe chronic potassium depletion from any cause. When metabolic alkalosis is believed to be primarily caused by potassium depletion, the presence of severe alkalosis should prompt a search for mineralocorticoid excess or additional causative factors, such as chloride depletion or base ingestion. If the cause of the alkalosis is not readily apparent, the urine should be screened for diuretics.

Bulimia is often associated with a metabolic alkalosis of fluctuating severity and with episodes of disequilibrium and recovering alkalosis. The latter is characterized by an "alkaline" urine (pH greater than 6.2) with a urinary sodium greater than 10 mEq/L, urinary potassium greater than 30 mEq/L, and bicarbonaturia; urinary chloride concentration remains low until chloride repletion is nearly complete.

Alkalosis associated with gastric HCl loss is most common. Even in gastric achlorhydria, however, metabolic alkalosis can occur because of relatively high chloride loss with sodium and potassium as the cation. In Zollinger-Ellison syndrome, the alkalosis can be very severe. In pyloric obstruction, significant ECF deficits of both chloride and fluid may exist because of gastric dilation.

Laxative abuse is rarely associated with severe alkalosis. Urinary potassium is always low in laxative abuse and plasma bicarbonate is rarely above 30 to 34 mEq/L. In states of diarrhea, there is a tendency toward loss of base; indeed, in secretory diarrheas such as cholera, hyperchloremic acidosis is the rule. The alkalosis associated with some villous adenomas may result from excessive potassium secretion. Chloridorrhea is associated with persistent watery diarrhea, high stool chloride concentrations, and low urinary chloride and potassium concentrations.

The differential diagnosis of Bartter's and Gitelman's syndromes and their variants is presented in Table 20.21. The genetic causes of these normotensive syndromes associated with hypokalemia and metabolic alkalosis have now been established. Patients with Bartter's syndrome are usually detected in infancy with failure to thrive. In most patients, the mutation is in the Na-K-2Cl cotransporter in the thick ascending limb of Henle's loop; hypercalciuria is prominent, and serum magnesium concentration is usually normal. PGE_2 concentrations in the urine are high, and nonsteroidal antiinflammatory drugs (NSAIDs) may improve the hypokalemia. Hypokalemia is less severe in "variant" Bartter's syndrome, likely because the mutation is in the luminal ROMK channel, which facilitates potassium recycling from the thick ascending limb into the lumen, a step essential for the normal functioning of the Na-K-2Cl cotransporter in that nephron segment. In contrast, Gitelman's syndrome often presents in adults, is less severe, is often heterozygotic, and at least in the United States, is more common than Bartter's syndrome. Gitelman's syndrome is associated with hypocalciuria and hypomagnesemia but not increased urinary prostaglandins. Thus NSAIDs do not help correct the hypokalemia. The genetic defect in this syndrome is in the thiazide-sensitive Na-Cl cotransporter in the distal convoluted tubule. Surreptitious induction of alkalosis can be difficult to differentiate from these syndromes, but certain clues may help establish the diagnosis: (a) the patients are most often female; (b) an underlying psychiatric abnormality may be present; (c) the severity of alkalosis may fluctuate; (d) the patient can easily obtain diuretics; (e) intermittently, alkaline urine can occur with acute-on-chronic vomiting; and (f) patients with surreptitious vomiting may have blackened teeth enamel and scarred knuckles.

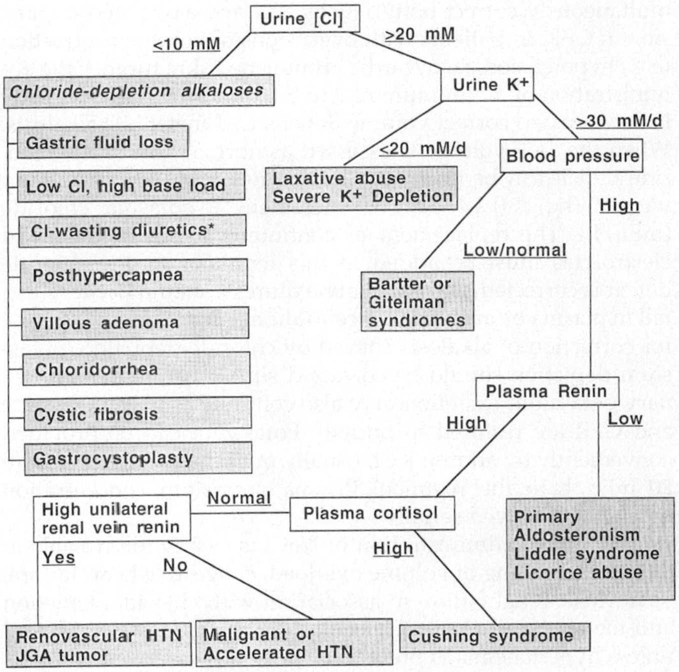

Figure 20.18. Diagnostic algorithm for metabolic alkalosis. This algorithm does not infer any particular prevalence or necessary order in which an evaluation should proceed. It is provided as a framework for the etiologic considerations. Other clinical information will often direct the diagnostic evaluation. *Urine Cl is elevated in diuretic use.

Diuretic abuse usually leads to more severe potassium depletion than vomiting.

Metabolic alkalosis with hypokalemia in patients with mild to moderate hypertension is caused by primary aldosteronism in 40% of such patients. Metabolic alkalosis may accompany hypokalemia and *secondary* hyperaldosteronism (a high renin state in contrast with primary aldosteronism, which is associated with a suppressed plasma renin) in accelerated hypertension and in edematous states, especially during diuretic therapy. Metabolic alkalosis may be severe in ectopic adrenocorticotrophin hormone (ACTH) syndrome even if hypertension is not prominent.

CORRECTION OF METABOLIC ALKALOSIS

Chloride-Responsive Forms

Although replacement of the chloride deficit is central, selection of the accompanying cation—sodium, potassium, or proton—is dependent on assessment of (a) ECF volume status by clinical examination, (b) the presence and degree of associated potassium depletion, and (c) the degree and reversibility of any depression of GFR. If kidney function is normal, bicarbonate and base equivalents will be excreted with sodium or potassium and metabolic alkalosis will be rapidly corrected as chloride is made available. If renal function is severely impaired by acute or chronic renal disease or in the presence of intractable congestive cardiac failure or hyperkalemia, it may be desirable to avoid the administration of sodium or potassium. There are two therapeutic options in such situations: (a) infuse chloride as HCl or (b) provide chloride by dialysis across the peritoneal or hemodialysis membrane so that potassium balance, sodium balance, and plasma volume can be contemporaneously corrected.

If depletion of chloride and ECF volume coexist, as is most common, isotonic NaCl is the appropriate therapy and will simultaneously correct both deficits and any associated depression in GFR. In patients with overt signs of volume contraction (e.g., hypotension, tachycardia, diminished skin turgor), the administration of a minimum of 3 to 5 L of normal saline usually is necessary to correct volume deficits and metabolic alkalosis. When the ECF volume is assessed as normal, total body chloride deficit can be estimated by the following formula: body weight (kg) $\times$ 0.2 $\times$ desired increment in plasma chloride (mEq/L). The replacement of continuing losses of fluid and electrolytes must be added to this regimen. As the chloride deficit is corrected, a brisk alkaline diuresis should occur with a fall in plasma bicarbonate concentration. Although not essential for correction of alkalosis caused by chloride depletion, potassium depletion should be corrected simultaneously. High urinary potassium excretion may also continue as plasma volume and GFR are restored to normal. Potassium can be provided conveniently by adding KCl, usually in a concentration of 10 to 20 mEq/L to the regimen. Plasma potassium concentration should be followed serially.

In contrast, administration of NaCl is clearly inadvisable in the clinical setting of volume overload, congestive heart failure, or intrinsic renal failure in association with chloride depletion and metabolic alkalosis. Chloride should be repleted with KCl unless hyperkalemia is present or the ability to excrete a potassium load is a concern. HCl administration or dialysis with a high-chloride, low-base dialysate should then be considered.

Intravenous HCl is used if NaCl or KCl is contraindicated and immediate correction is required, that is, when the arterial pH is greater than 7.55 and in the presence of hepatic encephalopathy, cardiac arrhythmia, digitalis cardiotoxicity, or altered mental status. The amount of HCl (0.1 or 0.2 M, available in most hospital pharmacies) needed to correct alkalosis is calculated by the following formula: 0.5 $\times$ body weight (kg) $\times$ desired decrement in plasma bicarbonate (mEq/L); continuing losses must also be replaced. The use of 50% of body weight as the volume of distribution of infused protons relates mainly to the prior buffering of alkali, including those in intracellular sites; infused protons must restore these buffers as well as titrating extracellular bicarbonate. Because the goal of such therapy is to rescue the patient from severe alkalosis, it is usually prudent to plan initially to restore the plasma bicarbonate concentration halfway toward normal. HCl must be given through a catheter placed in the vena cava or a large vein draining into it. The placement of the catheter should be confirmed radiographically because leakage of HCl can lead to sloughing of perivascular tissue; in the mediastinum, this could be a catastrophe. Rates of infusion up to 25 mEq/hr have been reported. These patients are best managed in an intensive care unit with frequent measurement of arterial blood gas values and electrolytes.

NH_4Cl, which may be given into a peripheral vein, is an alternative; its rate of infusion should not exceed 300 mEq/24 hr. NH_4Cl is contraindicated in the presence of renal or hepatic insufficiency. In concurrent renal failure, azotemia would be worsened, and in hepatic failure, acute ammonia intoxication with coma could result. Lysine or arginine HCl should be avoided because they have been associated with dangerous hyperkalemia. Although we prefer HCl, we would limit its use to the indications mentioned.

If GFR is adequate (serum creatinine less than 4 mg/dL), the use of acetazolamide (250 to 500 mg/day), which produces a diuresis of primarily $NaHCO_3$ by inhibition of carbonic anhydrase, can be considered. If hyperkalemia is absent, KCl should be administered concurrently because of the high likelihood of developing hypokalemia during the ensuing alkaline diuresis. Acetazolamide can be useful in patients with alkalosis induced by loop diuretics whose high sodium excretion must be maintained or in patients with posthypercapneic alkalosis with cor pulmonale and a high serum potassium. Natriuresis can be sustained while progressive metabolic alkalosis and reductions in GFR induced by tubuloglomerular feedback are avoided.

When the kidney is incapable of responding to chloride repletion or dialysis is necessary for the control of renal failure, exchange of bicarbonate for chloride by hemodialysis or peritoneal dialysis will effectively correct metabolic alkalosis. The usual dialysates for both peritoneal dialysis (including continuous ambulatory peritoneal dialysis) and hemodialysis contain concentrations of bicarbonate or its metabolic precursors, such as acetate, equivalent to 35 mEq; thus the dialysate composition must be modified in the management of metabolic alkalosis. In an emergency, peritoneal dialysis can be performed against sterile solutions of normal saline with appropriate maintenance of plasma potassium, calcium, and magnesium concentration by intravenous infusion.

Additional therapeutic approaches are needed in certain specific clinical situations associated with chloride-depletion metabolic alkalosis. In the presence of pernicious vomiting or when continual removal of gastric secretions is necessary, metabolic alkalosis will continue to be generated and replacement of preexisting deficits will be impeded by these losses. In such circumstances, the administration of a proton pump inhibitor such as omeprazole will blunt gastric acid production. Omeprazole has also been used effectively to blunt the acid loss that occurs with gastrocystoplasty.

Villous adenomas require surgical removal after correction of the sodium, chloride, potassium, and volume deficits. The rare familial disorder of chloridorrhea is responsive to continued repletion of fluid, chloride, and potassium losses by supplementation of the dietary intake; antidiarrheal agents are largely ineffective. Reduction in gastric HCl production by proton pump inhibition has been shown to aid in the maintenance of chloride balance.

Chloride-Resistant Alkaloses

Severe potassium depletion is associated with a mild to moderate metabolic alkalosis in humans unless there is complicating chloride depletion, mineralocorticoid excess, or exogenous base administration, in which case severe metabolic alkalosis may occur. When chloruretic diuretics or laxatives are responsible, these agents should be stopped. Oral KCl (40 to 60 mEq four or five times per day) usually will suffice for correction. However, if a cardiac arrhythmia or generalized weakness is present, intravenous KCl may be given at rates as high as 40 mEq/hr in concentrations not to exceed 60 mEq/L. These very high rates should be used only when life-threatening situations are encountered. The patient should be monitored by electrocardiogram and frequent determinations of plasma potassium concentration because muscle uptake of potassium may initially be diminished by downregulation of muscle Na^+-K^+-ATPase. Glucose should be omitted initially from the solution used to administer potassium because stimulated insulin secretion may cause plasma potassium concentration to decrease even further. However, once potassium repletion is begun, the presence of glucose in the infusion may facilitate cellular potassium repletion. Because nephropathy caused by potassium depletion may impair free-water excretion, plasma sodium should be monitored, particularly if hypotonic fluids are administered.

Because Bartter's and Gitelman's syndromes and their variants probably comprise several disorders with different pathophysiologies, sodium, chloride, magnesium, or potassium deficiencies may be present. Nevertheless, the principal goal of therapy is to prevent urinary potassium loss. In Bartter's syndrome, angiotensin-converting enzyme inhibitors, which reduce angiotensin II production and decrease aldosterone secretion, have been shown to be effective and should be tried first. In Gitelman's syndrome, potassium-sparing diuretics, such as amiloride (5 or 10 mg daily), triamterene (100 mg twice a day), or spironolactone (25 to 50 mg four times a day), will blunt the urinary losses but dietary potassium supplementation may also needed. Because renal prostaglandin production is increased in Bartter's syndrome and may contribute to sodium, chloride, and potassium wasting, prostaglandin synthetase inhibitors, such as indomethacin or ibuprofen, may ameliorate, but usually will not completely correct, the hypokalemic alkalosis. Magnesium depletion, which may also increase urinary potassium wasting, should be corrected. However, the degree to which magnesium repletion corrects alkalosis is uncertain, and magnesium salts often produce an unacceptable degree of gastrointestinal irritation that may compound the patient's problems.

In the group of alkaloses characterized by mineralocorticoid excess, therapy is directed at either removal of the source or mineralocorticoid blockade. Hypertension, occasionally severe, may complicate many of these disorders and require specific therapy. Because mineralocorticoids directly and indirectly stimulate potassium and proton secretion in the distal convoluted tubule and collecting duct (to a great extent in exchange for sodium), the administration of potassium-sparing diuretics, specifically spironolactone in patients with excess aldosterone, will effectively reverse the adverse effects of mineralocorticoid excess on sodium, potassium, and bicarbonate excretion. Restriction of sodium, reduction of potassium loss, and the addition of potassium to the diet will also ameliorate the alkalosis and the hypertension. Correction of the potassium deficit reverses the alkalinizing effects, but reversal of aldosterone excess is essential to permanent correction.

Many primary disorders of mineralocorticoid excess are definitively treated by tumor ablation. ACTH-secreting pituitary tumors may be removed by transsphenoidal resection or irradiation. With adrenal tumors, adrenalectomy, either unilateral or bilateral as appropriate, may be curative. In ectopic ACTH syndrome, the ideal treatment of the secreting tumor can rarely be accomplished. In this instance and in metastatic adrenal tumors, metyrapone, which inhibits the final step in cortisol synthesis, and aminoglutethimide, which inhibits the initial step in steroid biosynthesis, will blunt the myriad manifestations of hypercortisolism. In those disorders in which curative surgery cannot be carried out, mitotane (p,p-DDD), which produces selective destruction of the zona fasciculata and reticularis and leaves aldosterone production intact, has also been used to effectively control many of the manifestations of the disease. However, to the extent that severe fluid and electrolyte disturbances are caused solely by aldosterone production, mitotane may not suffice when hypokalemic alkalosis is present; metyrapone or aminoglutethimide would be better choices. *Cis*-platin has also been used in the treatment of adrenal malignancies, but detailed discussion of the use of these drugs is beyond the scope of this chapter.

Cessation of licorice intake or carbenoxolone allows for potassium retention with resultant correction of alkalosis. When apparent mineralocorticoid excess is caused by constitutive increased activation of the luminal sodium channel in the principal cell of the collecting duct, as in Liddle's syndrome, amiloride is a reasonable treatment.

Among the alkaloses produced by massive exogenous base administration, the milk-alkali syndrome characterized by metabolic alkalosis, hypercalcemia, and renal insufficiency is now rarely seen. Cessation of alkali ingestion and the calcium sources (often milk and calcium carbonate) and chloride and volume repletion for the commonly associated vomiting usually will lead to the prompt resolution of these abnormalities.

Selected Readings

Adrogue HJ, Madias NE. Management of life-threatening acid–base disorders. *N Engl J Med* 1998;338:107–111.

The authors emphasize the need to correct alkalosis when arterial pH is greater than 7.55.

Galla JH, Gifford JD, Luke RG, et al. Adaptations to chloride-depletion alkalosis. *Am J Physiol* 1991;261:R771–R781.

Review of recent studies in acute models of chloride-depletion in humans and rats, supporting the necessary and sufficient role of chloride repletion.

Galla JH, Bonduris DN, Sanders PW, et al. Volume-independent reductions in glomerular filtration rate in acute chloride-depletion alkalosis in the rat. *J Clin Invest* 1984;74:2002–2008.

In alkalosis, GFR was reduced by an intrarenal mechanism, tubuloglomerular feedback, and not by volume contraction.

Javaheri S, Kazemi H. Metabolic alkalosis and hypoventilation in humans. *Am Rev Respir Dis* 1987;136:11011016.

Excellent review of the compensatory respiratory response to metabolic alkalosis.

Jones JW, Sebastian A, Hulter HN, et al. Systemic and renal acid–base effects of chronic dietary potassium depletion in humans. *Kidney Int* 1982;21:402–410.

Unequivocal but mild metabolic alkalosis in response to dietary potassium restriction was shown.

Kassirer JP, Schwartz WB. Correction of metabolic alkalosis in man without repair of potassium deficiency. *Am J Med* 1966;40:19–25.

Despite sustained potassium deficits of 450 mEq, alkalosis was corrected by NaCl in humans.

Rosen RA, Julian BA, Dubovsky EV, et al. On the mechanism by which chloride corrects metabolic alkalosis in man. *Am J Med* 1988;84:449–458.

Despite persistent decreases in GFR and plasma volume, KCl corrected chronic diuretic-induced alkalosis.

Seldin DW, Rector FC Jr. The generation and maintenance of metabolic alkalosis. *Kidney Int* 1972;1:306321.

Seminal review of the course and pathophysiology of metabolic alkalosis.

Simon DB, Lifton RP. The molecular basis of inherited hypokalemic alkalosis: Bartter's and Gitelman's syndromes. *Am J Physiol* 1996;271:F961–F966.
The molecular genetics and pathophysiology of this expanding group of disorders characterized by normotension is updated.
Sojo A, Rodriquez-Soriano J, Vitoria JC, et al. Chloride deficiency as a presentation or complication of cystic fibrosis. *Eur J Pediatr* 1994;153:825–828.
Although cystic fibrosis has often been associated with chloride-depletion alkalosis, it can present with this acid–base disorder mimicking Bartter's syndrome.

PART 7
Respiratory Alkalosis and Acidosis

Eugene Dafnis and Sandra Sabatini

The respiratory acid–base disorders are among the most common abnormalities encountered in clinical medicine. They are characterized by a *primary* change in CO_2 tension in blood with a *secondary* change in blood HCO_3 concentration in the same direction. In this chapter, we first briefly review respiratory function. We then discuss the pathophysiology for the respiratory acid–base disorders, giving treatment when appropriate.

The primary role of the respiratory system is to deliver needed oxygen to the tissues for metabolism and to excrete CO_2 resulting from intermediary metabolism. There is a close regulation between the CO_2 excreted and acid–base homeostasis, and the integrity of the respiratory system is an absolute requirement for this biologic system to function normally. The respiratory system includes the lungs, the chest wall with the diaphragm and intercostal muscles, the pulmonary circulatory system, and the central nervous system. Respiratory function can be divided into four main components: alveolar ventilation, pulmonary gas exchange, the transport of O_2 and CO_2 in the blood to and from the cells, and the regulation of ventilation. These functional components work in concert to achieve normal gas exchange.

REVIEW OF RESPIRATORY FUNCTION

Ventilation

Ventilation is the inflow and outflow of air between the atmosphere and lung alveoli. It is accomplished by expansion and contraction of lungs. Alveolar ventilation is the actual amount of air reaching the alveoli with each breath; it equals the volume of the inspired air with each breath minus the volume of the anatomic dead space. In a "normal" 70-kg subject, the amount of dead space is approximately 1 ml per pound body weight (or approximately 150 ml); the rest of the tidal volume is distributed to the alveoli for gas exchange. Alveolar ventilation in this normal subject at sea level is 4.5 L/min when the respiratory rate is 10 breaths/min.

Pulmonary Gas Exchange

Gas exchange between alveolar air and the pulmonary capillary blood occurs via the alveolar membrane. Oxygen diffuses down its concentration gradient from the alveoli to the pulmonary capillaries while CO_2 crosses the pulmonary membrane in the opposite direction along its concentration gradient. CO_2 diffuses across the respiratory membrane more readily than oxygen and ceases when the alveolar concentration of CO_2 equilibrates with that in the alveolar capillary (i.e., P_{CO_2} = 40 mm Hg).

Transport of Oxygen and Carbon Dioxide in the Blood to and from Cells

Oxygen in the pulmonary blood combines principally with hemoglobin in erythrocytes for subsequent transport to the tissue capillaries, where it is released for metabolism. Oxygen metabolism by tissues results in 13,000 to 15,000 mmol of CO_2 daily; this waste product diffuses from the cells into the tissue capillaries to be immediately buffered within erythrocytes. In the erythrocytes, CO_2 is hydrated in the presence of carbonic anhydrase, producing HCO_3 and protons. The protons are buffered by hemoglobin, and the bicarbonate is exchanged for extracellular chloride (i.e., the chloride shift). The bulk of carboxyhemoglobin (approximately 70%) is transferred to the lungs in combination with HCO_3. In the alveoli, the entire process is reversed; hemoglobin is oxygenated, and the protons are released, combining with HCO_3 to form H_2CO_3, which in the presence of carbonic anhydrase, results in CO_2 and H_2O.

Central Nervous System

Respiratory control is achieved through sensitive and sophisticated mechanisms integrated in the central nervous system (CNS) that are both volitional and involuntary. Modifying signals originate from mechanoreceptors and chemoreceptors to subsequently influence the regulation of respiration. The mechanoreceptors are located in the upper airway, trachea, lungs, and chest wall and are stimulated by physical distortion or irritation occurring in the local environment. The chemoreceptors are slowly adapting receptors, whereas mechanoreceptors are rapidly adapting receptors. Stimulation of the rapidly adapting receptors produces bronchoconstriction and tachypnea, resulting in rapid shallow breathing and tachycardia, which may be clinically significant in the pathogenesis of asthma and reactive airway disease. The chemoreceptors are divided into central and peripheral chemoreceptors.

The central chemoreceptors are located in the ventrolateral surface of medulla, and their goal is to maintain a stable pH and P_{CO_2} within the CNS during systemic acid–base disturbances. The blood–brain barrier, interposed between blood and the cerebrospinal fluid, impedes the free diffusion of HCO_3 and protons but is freely permeable to CO_2. Because hydrogen and bicarbonate are not in electrochemical equilibrium across the blood–brain barrier, the pH of the cerebrospinal fluid can change independently of systemic pH changes. A fall in local extracellular pH (in the CNS) stimulates ventilation; an increase in local CO_2 is the same as a fall in pH.

The peripheral chemoreceptors contribute approximately 15% to 20% to resting ventilation, but it is only when the organism is stressed metabolically that they are activated. There are two groups of peripheral chemoreceptors: the carotid and the aortic bodies. The former are located at the bifurcation of the common carotid artery, and the latter lie along the aortic arch. The carotid bodies transmit their signals to the CNS via the glossopharyngeal nerve (cranial nerve IX), and the aortic bodies transmit their signals through the vagus nerve (cranial nerve X). Signals from the carotid bodies overshadow those from the aortic bodies. Blood flow (1.4 to 2.0 L/min per 100 gram tissue) to these chemoreceptors is extraordinarily high, allowing very small changes in P_{O_2} (or P_{CO_2}) to be detected. Such a high flow is consistent with the organs' critical role as a primary O_2

sensor. When Po_2 falls, there is a significant rise in the rate of afferent firing and a simultaneous release of dopamine. There is minimal responsiveness of these organs to Pco_2 (a rise increases the rate of firing); if denervated, the change in ventilation is less than 20%.

Whereas the peripheral chemoreceptors respond primarily to changes in arterial Po_2, the central chemoreceptors respond to local CO_2 or protons in the CNS and to the change in the respiratory acid–base disturbances that constitutes the common stimuli. Their ventilatory response is additive and is modified to adjust Pco_2 toward normal values. When the two chemoreceptors respond to different stimuli, one or the other predominates. The sensitivity of these chemoreceptors varies from stimulus to stimulus. In acute situations over a range from normal Pco_2 up to moderate hypercapnia (i.e., Pco_2 of approximately 60 mm Hg), the ventilatory response is linear and steep; when the stimulus is hypoxia, the response is hyperbolic. The combined effects of hypoxia and hypercapnia are not simply additive, they are multiplicative. Thus hypoxia lowers the threshold of the chemoreceptors for stimulation to hypercarbia, and hypercapnia lowers the threshold for stimulation to hypoxia. That is, when hypoxia and hypercapnia exist simultaneously, there is a potentiation of the ventilatory response exceeding the sum of the responses of each component. Therefore therapy with oxygen under these circumstances may seriously depress respiratory drive.

Any change in one or more functional components of the respiratory system may alter arterial Pco_2 and, as a consequence, change arterial pH. When primary changes occur in the partial pressure of CO_2 in blood, the term used clinically is a *respiratory acid–base disorder. Respiratory alkalosis* is a primary fall in arterial Pco_2; *respiratory acidosis* is a primary rise in arterial Pco_2. Because the compensatory response of the respiratory acid–base disorders is only fully manifested after several days, these disturbances are further subdivided into *acute* (up to 8 hours) and *chronic* (present for 2 to 3 days longer) disorders. Between the acute and chronic phase, there is a transitional phase that reflects the gradual development of the renal adaptation. Both the acute and chronic forms of the two acid–base disorders are discussed in this chapter, as well as the major pathophysiologic states associated with them.

RESPIRATORY ALKALOSIS

Respiratory alkalosis is a primary decrease in arterial Pco_2 that results in an elevation of arterial pH. The disturbance is usually a consequence alveolar *hyper*ventilation (hypocapnia). Any stimulus increasing ventilation above the levels required to excrete the produced CO_2 lowers the Pco_2 and has the propensity for raising the systemic pH. Table 20.22 illustrates the different causes of respiratory alkalosis, which in hospitalized patients, usually suggests serious underlying disease.

Ventilation can be stimulated by signals from the peripheral receptors (i.e., the mechanoreceptors or the chemoreceptors) as well as by signals from the brainstem or higher centers. Besides hyperventilation, other maneuvers can eliminate excessive CO_2 from the body and lower the Pco_2. These include mechanical ventilation and extracorporeal circulation used during open-heart operations. Increasing minute ventilation by raising the respiratory rate in patients with sufficient alveolar reserve results in hypocapnia. In conditions associated with cerebral edema, respiratory alkalosis is often induced deliberately. Hypocapnia decreases the cerebral blood flow and is thought to reduce brain edema.

TABLE 20.22. Causes of Respiratory Alkalosis

Central Nervous System Stimulation
Neurologic disorders
Cerebrovascular accidents
Trauma
Pontine tumors
Infections (encephalitis, meningitis)
Metabolic factors
Cirrhosis
Pregnancy
Luteal phase of menstrual cycle
Sepsis
Fever
Heat stroke
Overcorrection of metabolic acidosis
Pharmacologic agents
Salicylates and nicotine
Dinitrophenol
Aminophylline
Catecholamines (norepinephrine, dopamine)
Nikethamide
Volitional hyperventilation
Voluntary temporary hyperventilation
Anxiety-induced hyperventilation syndrome
Stimulation of Peripheral Chemoreceptors and Mechanoreceptors
Pneumonia
Pulmonary emboli
Interstitial fibrosis[a]
Asthma[a]
Hemodialysis
High altitude
Carbon monoxide poisoning
Hypotension
Cyanotic congenital heart disease
Severe anemia

[a] May also cause respiratory acidosis if severe.

In hospitalized patients, outcome is correlated to the severity of respiratory alkalosis. Patients with a low Pco_2 (below 15 mm Hg) have a very high mortality rate (approximately 90%). Sudden and unexplained respiratory alkalosis should alert the physician to search for septicemia. Hyperventilation may *precede* the other manifestations of sepsis, occurring before fever, hypotension, or metabolic acidosis. Pulmonary embolism is virtually always associated with hyperventilation; the mechanisms for this are related to the combined effects of hypoxemia and afferent vagal signals from nociceptive receptors in the lung.

Several pharmacologic agents increase ventilation via direct or indirect mechanisms. Aspirin directly stimulates the medullary chemoreceptors. Nicotine can increase the ventilation by stimulation of both peripheral and central chemoreceptors; however, it requires rapid cigarette puffing to induce detectable Pco_2 decrements. Increased production of progesterone, during pregnancy or during the luteal phase of menstrual cycle, increases ventilation by stimulating the brainstem. Decreased degradation of progesterone in the presence of severe liver disease or cirrhosis also increases ventilation by the same mechanism. In cirrhosis, the degree of hypocapnia correlates best with the level of blood ammonia. A low Pco_2 in patients with hepatic failure is an index of poor prognosis.

Acetate hemodialysis often causes hypoxia, hyperventilation, and acute respiratory alkalosis (Fig. 20.19). Whether hypoxia is the primary stimulus for the hyperventilation of hemodialysis

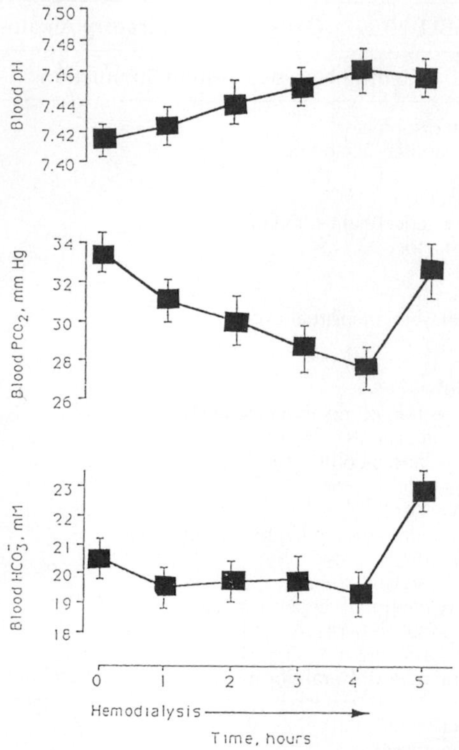

Figure 20.19. Effects of acetate hemodialysis on blood pH, P_{CO_2}, and bicarbonate. During the 4-hour treatment, P_{CO_2} decreases without a significant drop of bicarbonate concentration as respiratory alkalosis develops. (Adapted from Kaiser BA, Potter DE, Bryant RE, et al. acid–base changes and acetate metabolism during routine and high-efficiency hemodialysis in children. *Kidney Int* 1981;19:70.)

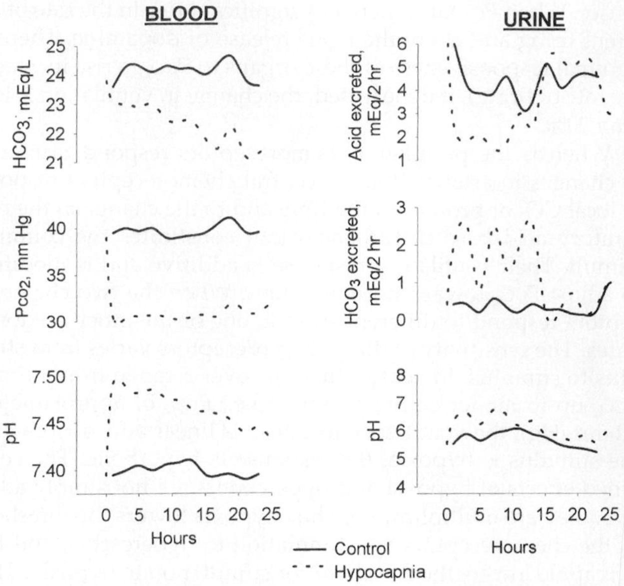

Figure 20.20. Time course for the adaptation to hypocapnia in man. **Left panel:** Early, there is an immediate increase in arterial pH, which gradually returns toward the baseline as serum bicarbonate falls. **Right panel:** Urine acid excretion is significantly reduced until about 12 hours of hypocapnia; urine bicarbonate excretion remains elevated for approximately the same period of time. (Adapted from Gledhill N, Beirne GJ, Dempsey JA. Renal response to short term hypocapnia in man. *Kidney Int* 1975; 8:376.)

is not yet clear because it can be present in patients treated with reuse dialysis or polyacrylonitrile membrane dialyzers, in which case the trapping of circulating leukocytes in pulmonary bed is minimal. The loss of CO_2 across the dialyzer is probably a contributing factor.

Respiratory alkalosis may be either acute or chronic in nature. *Acute respiratory alkalosis* is respiratory alkalosis of less than 24 hours' duration, and arterial pH is always high. It is distinguished from *chronic respiratory alkalosis* by the absence of renal metabolic compensation; arterial pH in this situation may also be high, but of the simple four acid–base disorders, it is the only one that can be completely compensated (i.e., arterial pH can be completely normal).

Between the onset of acute respiratory alkalosis and the establishment of chronic respiratory alkalosis, there is an adaptation phase that reflects the gradual development of the renal compensation. Acute hypocapnia reduces the carbonic acid concentration without significantly changing the plasma bicarbonate concentration (Fig. 20.20, *left panel*). Carbonic acid, however, cannot be reduced by more than a total of about 4 mEq from normal. The acute buffering response is produced exclusively by the tissue nonbicarbonate buffers and by the red cell buffers. The participation of extracellular protein buffer, while it occurs, is trivial. This buffering process is completed within 10 minutes, and despite the early onset of renal adaptation to hypocapnia within 30 minutes, no appreciable changes in acid–base equilibrium are observed for several hours (Fig. 20.20, *right panel*). The protons are derived from intracellular buffers, proteins, phosphate, and hemoglobin. They exit from cells and combine with bicarbonate to form carbonic acid, thus lowering plasma bicarbonate level. There is also substantial evidence that a portion of the fall of plasma bicarbonate results from enhanced organic acid production. Lactic acid generation occurs, resulting in a mild increase in plasma levels (less than 3 mEq/L). Lactic acid generation is likely secondary to stimulation of phosphofructokinase consequent to high intracellular pH.

As part of the renal response to acute respiratory alkalosis, bicarbonate reabsorption and titratable acid excretion decrease and urine pH increases. After 6 hours, acute hypocapnia significantly reduces the activity of H^+-ATPase and Na^+-K^+-ATPase in the proximal tubule, and there is endocytosis of vesicles containing H^+-ATPase. In the distal nephron biochemical activity, all of the acidifying pumps are reduced in both cortical and medullary collecting ducts (i.e., H^+-ATPase, H^+-K^+-ATPase) (Fig. 20.21).

The marked diuresis that occurs during acute respiratory alkalosis is likely the result of decreased activity of renal tubular Na^+-K^+-ATPase and increased atrial natriuretic peptide (ANP). The effect of ANP, however, is blunted by an independent action to stimulate the renal sympathetic nervous system. During acute respiratory alkalosis, there is an increase in plasma chloride that occurs as a result of chloride shift from erythrocytes. A well-designed important study has questioned the traditional view that acute respiratory alkalosis directly causes hypokalemia (Fig. 20.22, *top panel*). Results from normal subjects show a rapid *increase* in plasma potassium of 0.3 mEq/L, presumably the result of increased sympathetic adrenergic activity. The increased level of catecholamines appears to be caused by the fall in plasma bicarbonate and not by alterations in P_{CO_2} or pH. This small hyperkalemic response appears to be secondary to enhanced α-receptor stimulation. It is only after the ventilatory stimulus is reversing does one see a fall in plasma potassium (Fig. 20.22, *top panel*). Acute respiratory alkalosis also decreases serum phosphorus resulting in hypophosphatemia due to the ion's movement into cells. Indeed, urinary

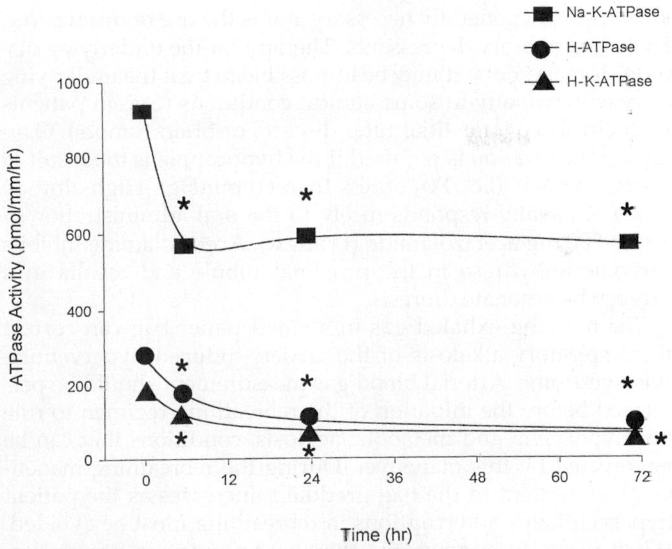

Figure 20.21. Effect of respiratory alkalosis on Na^+-K^+-ATPase, H^+-ATPase, and H^+-K^+-ATPase in microdissected cortical collecting tubule of rats (*$P < .01$). There is a progressive decrement in all enzymes studied in cortical collecting tubule during the kidney adaptation to respiratory alkalosis (similar findings are noted in the medullary collecting duct). In the proximal tubule, Na^+-K^+-ATPase and H^+-ATPase also fell (no significant H^+-K^+-ATPase is found in the proximal tubule). (Adapted from Eiam-Ong S, Laski ME, Kurtzman NA, et al. Effect of respiratory acidosis and alkalosis on renal transport enzymes. *Am J Physiol* 1994;267:F390.)

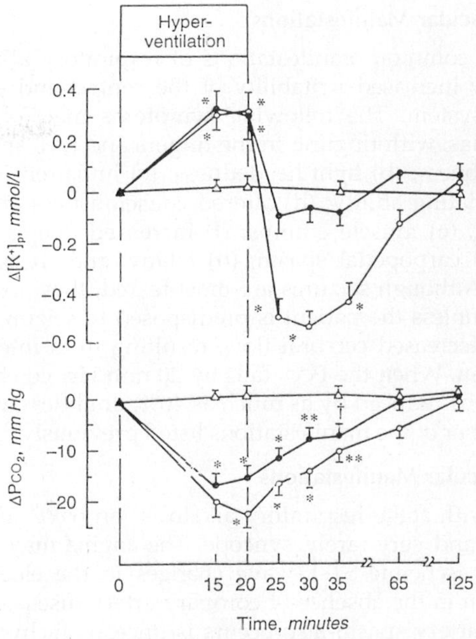

Figure 20.22. Effect of graded degrees of hyperventilation [18 (•) 36 (o) L/min, respectively] compared with controls (Δ), on plasma potassium concentration and blood P_{CO_2}. There is a significant increase of plasma potassium concentration (*$P < .05$) after 15 minutes of hyperventilation, which falls after the cessation of hyperventilation (*$P < .05$). (Reprinted with permission from Krapf P, Caduff P, Wagdi P, et al. Plasma potassium to acute respiratory alkalosis. *Kidney Int* 1995;47:217.)

phosphate falls during respiratory alkalosis. For more details, see Chapter 19, Part 3. There is substantial evidence that renal phosphate handling during acute hypocapnia is modulated by an increase in α-adrenergic activity and is independent of both parathyroid hormone (PTH) and 1,25-dihydroxyD_3 levels.

Chronic respiratory alkalosis decreases the rise in arterial pH that occurs during the acute hypocapnia with a further decrement in plasma bicarbonate. Urinary acidification is inhibited in both the proximal and the distal tubule. Proximal bicarbonate reabsorption falls, acid excretion is decreased, and urine pH rises.

The intracellular alkalosis reduces the availability of hydrogen for exchange with sodium in the proximal tubule. Apical Na^+-H^+ antiporter activity decreases, as does basolateral Na-HCO_3 symporter activity. Natriuresis occurs with bicarbonaturia, not with chloruresis. Volume contraction results, subsequently stimulating proximal sodium and chloride reabsorption. Extracellular volume contraction can be minimized by lowering sodium intake. A decrease in sodium intake will result in a modest impairment of the renal adaptive response, with a smaller reduction in serum bicarbonate. The rise during chronic respiratory alkalosis in plasma chloride is less than the fall in plasma bicarbonate. If arterial P_{CO_2} drops from 40 to 20 mm Hg, the anion gap increases by approximately 3 mEq/L. The factors causing this increase are not known. Lactate generation does not appear to be involved, because in chronic respiratory alkalosis, serum lactate is not increased.

These changes are associated with progressive decrement in H^+-ATPase activity in the proximal tubule compared with that of acute hypocapnia, possibly further contributing to the bicarbonaturia. The collecting tubule further contributes to acid retention. H^+-ATPase and H^+-K^+-ATPase in the collecting tubule continue to fall progressively during the adaptation process over the 72 hours without a further fall in the Na^+-K^+-ATPase activity (Fig. 20.21). The signal(s) for these biochemical changes are not known, but they are independent of aldosterone.

With the development of these compensatory renal mechanisms, plasma bicarbonate falls, bicarbonaturia lessens, and urine pH returns to normal. When the hypocapnia occurs gradually, there is very little bicarbonaturia and the metabolic compensation reducing the plasma bicarbonate results solely from changes in renal acid retention. Sustained respiratory alkalosis (days) in humans results in hyperphosphatemia and a decrease in ionizable calcium. Fractional calcium excretion increases, and phosphate clearance falls. These changes are thought to be a result of a decreased responsiveness of the tubular cells to PTH action because decreased nephrogenous cyclic adenosine 3′,5′-monophosphate (cAMP) excretion has been noted with normal PTH levels. Also, there must be a defect in the secretion of PTH because the blood levels of the hormone fall and then rise in the face of hypocalcemia. Decreased urine magnesium also occurs as a consequence of enhanced tubular reabsorption in the thick ascending limb of Henle's loop.

If the subject has efficiently compensated to chronic respiratory alkalosis and a new hypocapnic stimuli is introduced, the renal response is much less dramatic. The degree of the bicarbonaturia is small, reflecting bicarbonate depletion. It should be noted that patients with chronic renal failure and respiratory alkalosis will manifest severe alkalemia because they cannot excrete bicarbonate normally. More profound alkalemia is predicted in patients receiving peritoneal dialysis, because under normal circumstances, they have already fixed elevated bicarbonate levels in the range of 28 to 30 mEq/L.

Clinical Manifestations

Clinical manifestations of respiratory alkalosis are often overshadowed by the symptoms of the underlying disease. Respiratory alkalosis affects three major organ systems: neuromuscular, cardiovascular, and respiratory.

Neuromuscular Manifestations

The most common manifestations of respiratory alkalosis are caused by increased irritability of the central and peripheral nervous system. The following symptoms may be seen: (a) paresthesias, with tingling in the fingers and toes and circumoral numbness; (b) light-headedness; (c) impaired judgement and calculating ability; (d) altered consciousness and mental confusion; (e) muscle cramps; (f) increased deep tendon reflexes; (g) carpopedal spasm; (h) tetany; and (i) generalized seizures. Although seizures are most feared, they are very uncommon unless the patient is predisposed to seizure disorder. There is decreased cerebral flow, resulting from intense vasoconstriction. When the P_{CO_2} falls by 20 mm Hg, cerebral blood flow may be reduced by as much as 40%, doubtless accounting for a number of the manifestations listed previously.

Cardiovascular Manifestations

Patients with acute respiratory alkalosis can have angina, palpitations, and very rarely, syncope. The angina may be associated with ischemic ST-T–wave changes in the electrocardiogram, even in the absence of coronary artery disease. Whether coronary artery spasm also occurs is unclear. Tachycardia can also be present in these patients, but atrial and ventricular arrhythmias are seen only in those with underlying heart disease. When syncope occurs, it is virtually always precipitated by a ventricular arrhythmia; coexisting cerebral hypoxia has also been documented.

There is a sharp difference in cardiac output and blood pressure when respiratory alkalosis occurs in the awake state as opposed to the effects seen in the anesthetized patient receiving mechanical ventilation. In the awake subject, respiratory alkalosis does *not* significantly alter blood pressure or cardiac output. There are alterations in blood flow to certain beds (e.g., decreased blood flow to the brain, skin, and kidneys and increased blood flow to muscle and liver); however, blood pressure remains normal. Because tachycardia invariably occurs in respiratory alkalosis, a decrease in cardiac contractility may not be seen. By contrast, in anesthetized subjects with respiratory alkalosis caused by mechanical ventilation, a severe reduction of cardiac output and blood pressure is always noted. Systemic vascular resistance subsequently increases, suggesting that some component of acute respiratory alkalosis has a direct depressive effect on the myocardium. Whether it is the increase in arterial pH or the fall in P_{CO_2} tension is unknown, but in the isolated working heart, a rise in perfusate pH (at a constant P_{CO_2}) directly decreases contractile force. In patients on a respirator, the decrease in cardiac output cannot be compensated for because maximal tachycardia already exists and venous return is "fixed" as a result of the effect of mechanical ventilation.

Respiratory Manifestations

Patients with respiratory alkalosis always have some degree of dyspnea; however, it often does not correlate with the degree of coexisting hypoxia. A classic example is the patient with "anxiety-induced" hyperventilation syndrome; virtually all such patients complain of dyspnea but have a high arterial P_{O_2} tension. The absence of increased respiratory rate does not rule out hyperventilation. Increases in tidal volume or frequent "sighs" can rarely increase ventilation. A ventilation-perfusion mismatch has been documented on lung scans; this appears to be pH mediated and not a function of the altered P_{CO_2}.

Treatment

Identification of the cause of respiratory alkalosis usually does not constitute a difficult medical problem. Treatment of the alkalemia is not generally necessary, nor is the use of intravenous HCl or respiratory depressants. Therapy for the underlying disorder is mandatory. It may be impossible to treat the underlying disease maximally in some clinical conditions (e.g., in patients with cirrhosis, interstitial lung disease, or brain tumors). Oxygen administration is required if the hypocapnia is the result of severe hypoxia (i.e., P_{O_2} of less than 60 mmHg). High-altitude sickness usually responds nicely to the oral administration of 250 to 500 mg acetazolamide (Diamox). Acetazolamide inhibits carbonic anhydrase in the proximal tubule and results in a prompt bicarbonate diuresis.

Rebreathing exhaled gas in a small paper bag can correct the respiratory alkalosis of the anxiety-induced hyperventilation syndrome. Arterial blood gas measurement should be performed before the initiation of the rebreathing regimen to rule out hypoxemia and metabolic acidosis, conditions that can be aggravated by this maneuver. During the rebreathing maneuver, CO_2 content in the bag gradually increases as the patient hyperventilates. Interruptions in rebreathing must be avoided. When properly applied, the therapeutic outcome occurs dramatically, usually within a minute or two.

In patients undergoing mechanical ventilation who also develop respiratory alkalosis, decreasing the tidal volume or the respiratory rate usually corrects the abnormality. When this is not feasible, increasing dead space by lengthening the tubing can resolve the problem. Rarely, the dialysis patient with life-threatening alkalemia will require administration of dilute mineral acid via the inferior vena cava.

RESPIRATORY ACIDOSIS

Respiratory acidosis is a primary elevation in arterial P_{CO_2}; it results in a decrease in arterial pH. The elevated P_{CO_2} increases the concentration of carbonic acid, which then dissociates into protons and bicarbonate. Hypercapnia and respiratory acidosis are almost always caused by a decrease in effective ventilation (i.e., alveolar *hypo*ventilation). Because the CO_2 stimulus to ventilation is very potent, any process that interferes with the CNS regulation of the respiratory function or with CO_2 excretion from the lung, as well as any event that increases CO_2 production consequent to metabolism, can result in CO_2 retention. In general, an increase in CO_2 production secondary to metabolism

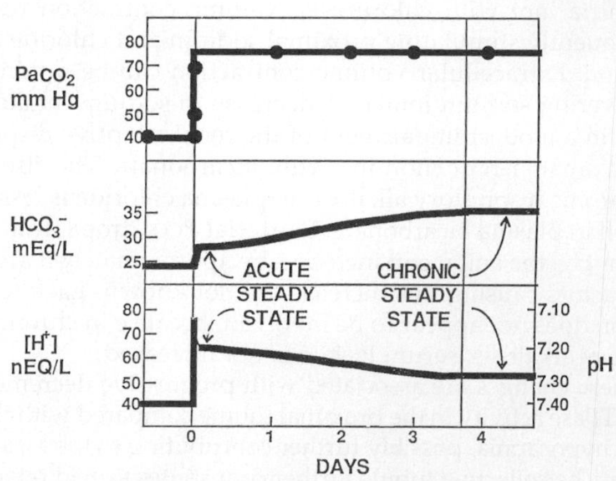

Figure 20.23. Schematic representation of blood HCO_3 and H concentration in acute (<2 days) and chronic (3 to 4 days) respiratory acidosis. P_{CO_2} can be changed in a *single* breath in a patient on mechanical ventilation. (Reprinted with permission from Cohen JJ, Madias NE. acid–base disorders of respiratory origin. In: Brenner BM, Stein JH, eds. *Contemporary issues in nephrology,* vol 2. New York: Churchill Livingstone, 1978:137.)

will not result in appreciable CO_2 retention in subjects with intact respiratory reserve.

There are conditions, however, in which the diminished respiratory reserve, stressed by increased metabolic demands, fails to excrete excess CO_2. Patients with fixed ventilation on a respirator may not be able to excrete the increased CO_2 as a result of excessive use of carbohydrates in enteral or parenteral alimentation. Sorbent-regenerative hemodialysis or high-flux hemodialysis with bicarbonate in mechanically ventilated patients can cause acute respiratory acidosis resulting from diffusion of CO_2 from the dialysate to the blood. A very uncommon cause of respiratory acidosis in the mechanically ventilated patients may be seen during peritoneal dialysis with dialysate containing high glucose concentration.

In *acute respiratory acidosis,* the increase in P_{CO_2} is sudden and usually occurs on the background of previously normal respiratory function (Fig. 20.23). Plasma HCO_3 increases minimally, while arterial pH plummets and arterial hydrogen ion concentration rises. In *chronic respiratory acidosis,* P_{CO_2} rises gradually and remains elevated, but stable, for a prolonged time (Fig. 20.23). Plasma HCO_3 increases (greater than 35 mEq/L), and arterial pH, although low, is somewhat compensated. The causes of respiratory acidosis of clinical importance are virtually always chronic in nature and are listed in Table 20.23.

TABLE 20.23. Causes of Respiratory Acidosis

Acute Respiratory Acidosis	Chronic Respiratory Acidosis
Alveolar hypoventilation	Alveolar hypoventilation
Primary	Primary alveolar hypoventilation
Pharmacologic agents	Primary alveolar hypoventilation
Opiates	Massive obesity ("Pickwickian syndrome")
Barbiturates	Brain tumor
Benzodiazepines	Methadone therapy
Nonbarbiturate sedatives	Chronic sedative abuse on the background of chronic obstructive or restrictive lung disease
Alcohol	Hypothyroidism
Oxygen therapy in chronic hypercapnia	Secondary
Central nervous system lesions	Central nervous system
Head injuries	Chronic bulbar poliomyelitis
Cerebrovascular accidents	Multiple sclerosis
Infections (encephalitis, meningitis)	Peripheral nervous system
Collagen-vascular diseases (systemic lupus erythematosus)	Amyotrophic lateral sclerosis
Secondary	Muscular disease
Central nervous system	Muscular dystrophy
Acute bulbar poliomyelitis	Myositis
Peripheral nervous system	"Permissive" hypercapnia
Guillain-Barré syndrome	Ventilation-perfusion mismatch
Spinal cord injury	Obstructive disease
Bilateral phrenic nerve palsy	Chronic obstructive pulmonary disease
Neuromuscular junction	Restrictive disease
Myasthenia gravis	Kyphoscoliosis
Tetanus	Interstitial fibrosis (sarcoid, silicosis, berylliosis)
Botulism	Fibrothorax
Organophosphate poisoning	Hydrothorax
Curare	Chronic radiation pneumonitis
Succinylcholine	Ascites
Aminoglycosides	Chronic peritoneal dialysis
Muscle	Obesity
Myositis	
Hypokalemia	
Hypophosphatemia	
"Permissive" hypercapnia	
Ventilation-perfusion mismatch	
Acute airway obstruction	
Laryngospasm (laryngitis, chemical irritation)	
Bronchospasm (asthma attack)	
Obstructive sleep apnea	
Aspiration of foreign body	
Bronchoscopy	
Mishaps during mechanical ventilation	
Ventilatory restriction	
Severe pneumonia	
Hemothorax	
Pneumothorax	
Massive pulmonary embolism	
Infant and adult respiratory distress syndromes	
Increased CO_2 production in the presence of fixed ventilation	
Total parenteral nutrition with high carbohydrate content	
Sorbent regenerative hemodialysis	
High flux hemodialysis with bicarbonate	
Peritoneal dialysis with dialysate containing high glucose concentration	
Failure of CO_2 transfer to the lung	
Cardiac arrest	

Suppression of the respiratory center with an overdose of certain medications, including narcotics, benzodiazepines, and barbiturates, decrease minute ventilation, resulting in primary alveolar hypoventilation. Strokes, tumors, or trauma also may produce the same picture. Neuromuscular disorders can cause secondary alveolar hypoventilation as a result of paralysis or spasm of the respiratory muscles. Spinal cord injury above the fifth cervical vertebrae causes varying degrees of paralysis, including acute respiratory arrest if the lesion is above the third vertebrae. Guillain-Barré syndrome, myasthenia gravis, acute botulism, and the acute and severe hypokalemia seen in "familial periodic paralysis" may all result in paralysis of the respiratory muscles and acute respiratory acidosis. (Acute respiratory failure can occur in the presence of intact or even increased ventilatory drive and is due to ventilation-perfusion mismatch. In this situation the degree of hypoxia exceeds the degree of hypercapnia and is usually caused by diseases that directly affect the bronchi or alveoli. Such disorders include acute asthma, severe pulmonary edema, fulminant pneumonia, and chest wall abnormalities such as pneumothorax or fracture of the ribs.)

"Permissive" hypercapnia is a novel strategy for the management of patients requiring mechanical ventilation, and it is done so in an attempt to limit ventilator-induced lung injury. The application of high tidal volumes or normal volumes with high peak airway pressure during conventional mechanical ventilation can cause severe alveolar epithelial and capillary injury from the alveolar overdistention. Permissive hypercapnia involves the deliberate induction of alveolar *hypo*ventilation in an effort to avoid overdistension during mechanical ventilation relegating the normalization of P_{CO_2} to second place. During this novel approach of ventilation, it is recommended that tidal volume be reduced to levels below 7 ml/kg, minute ventilation be decreased to less than 115 ml/kg, and peak airway pressure be maintained below 35 cm H_2O. This mechanical ventilation prescription is thought to ensure efficient alveolar ventilation in the face of high P_{CO_2} levels and respiratory acidosis. The graded hypercapnia is done progressively, in steps not exceeding 10 mm Hg and up to a maximal P_{CO_2} of 80 mm Hg. The accepted levels of pH in this strategy approximates 7.20. Buffering agents are suggested when pH falls below this value.

There is ongoing literature favoring the use of permissive hypercapnia in patients with adult respiratory distress syndrome and some reports show a decrease in mortality. Other advantages of this method are purported to be improved cardiovascular tolerance. Cardiac output increases because the augmented levels of catecholamines overcome the direct suppressive effects of respiratory acidosis on the myocardium. The main disadvantage is related to the vasodilator effect of CO_2 on cerebral vessels and the ensuing increase in intracranial pressure; for this reason, it should be avoided in patients with cerebral trauma or tumors.

Compensation for acute respiratory acidosis is less effective than for acute metabolic acidosis. There are no available extracellular buffers that can buffer the carbonic acid. The buffering capacity of extracellular lactate and plasma proteins is minimal (approximately 3%) and cannot produce appreciable changes in blood hydrogen ion concentration. The nonbicarbonate buffers found inside the cell are the ones that respond to acute hypercapnia. About one-third of the protons appear to be neutralized in the erythrocytes by hemoglobin, and the rest are neutralized by tissue buffers. The buffer capacity of hemoglobin is linear to changes in pH in hypercapnia. For each unit of pH decrease, 1 mmol of hemoglobin produces 3 mEq of new bicarbonate ions. In contrast to acute metabolic acidosis, the bone buffers (i.e., carbonate, bicarbonate, and phosphate) contribute very little to the total tissue buffering capacity in respiratory acidosis. The reasons for this are not understood.

The rise in plasma bicarbonate will not exceed the 3 to 4 mEq/L above normal, even when hypercapnia is extreme. Although during acute hypercapnia chemical processing of the retained CO_2 accounts for the total increase in plasma bicarbonate, there is substantial evidence that renal adaptation begins virtually immediately. Within minutes, the proximal nephron responds and proximal bicarbonate reabsorption increases. This is due to the direct effect of CO_2 (i.e., the fall in arterial pH), which independently stimulates proximal bicarbonate reabsorption, and the decreased effective blood volume due to systemic vasodilation produced by the acute hypercapnia. However, the mechanism is not clear because neither the proximal tubule Na^+-H^+ antiporter nor H^+-ATPase activity is affected. A minimal increase in the plasma sodium occurs, and proximal sodium reabsorption is increased. The chloride shift results in hypochloremia and the slight increase in the potassium concentration is likely due to the exchange of extracellular protons for intracellular potassium. Hyperphosphatemia and hyperphosphaturia occur, but the precise mechanisms for these findings are not completely understood.

The acute phase of respiratory acidosis (up to 8 hours) is followed by the gradual development of the renal response, which develops over 3 to 4 days. With sustained hypercapnia, the kidney plays the major role to raise the blood bicarbonate, and in addition to proximal mechanisms, the distal nephron now responds. During the renal adaptation, there is a transient increase of net acid excretion above the rate of endogenous acid production, leading to the generation of a new bicarbonate. This is coupled with increased proximal bicarbonate reabsorption, which prevents the loss of the new generated bicarbonate, and low urine bicarbonate concentration is seen. The retention of bicarbonate is independent of salt and bicarbonate intake, mineralocorticoid levels, potassium depletion, and oxygen tension.

In chronic hypercapnia, the increased proximal bicarbonate reabsorption presumably is caused by the increased activity of the Na^+-H^+ effect, likely mediated by the stimulated protein kinase C of the renal brush border membrane. This transporter attempts to return renal tubular intracellular pH toward normal values, and its activity is linearly related to the plasma HCO_3 and the proton concentration. There is also a significant rise in the activity of proximal tubule H^+ -ATPase and Na^+-K^+-ATPase 24 hours after the onset of hypercapnia. The H^+-ATPase appears to participate in bicarbonate reabsorption and may be a biochemical marker for proximal acidification.

The increased bicarbonate reabsorption is coupled with decreased chloride reabsorption, increased chloride excretion in the form of ammonium chloride, and an abnormally low serum chloride. Hypercapnia further decreases phosphate reabsorption in the proximal tubule, increasing its delivery to the distal tubule, where it is titrated. The stimulation of distal urinary acidification in chronic hypercapnia is likely mediated by an increased activity of the two proton pumps in cortical and medullary collecting tubules. Both H^+-ATPase and H^+-K^+-ATPase start rising 24 hours after the onset of acute hypercapnia, and at 72 hours, both increase even further (Fig. 20.24). Plasma bicarbonate continues to rise; bicarbonaturia and a high urine pH are noted, both of which are likely caused by the high filtered load of bicarbonate. The precise mechanisms that stimulate H^+-ATPase and H^+-K^+-ATPase in chronic hypercapnia remain unknown. The stimulation of these ATPases as well as the increase in Na^+-K^+-ATPase (Fig. 20.24) is independent of aldosterone and potassium levels as evidenced by their occurrence in adrenalectomized animals. The renal response to respiratory acidosis is usually complete by 72 hours, and a new steady state emerges. The increased ammonium excretion returns to the levels needed to meet daily acid produc-

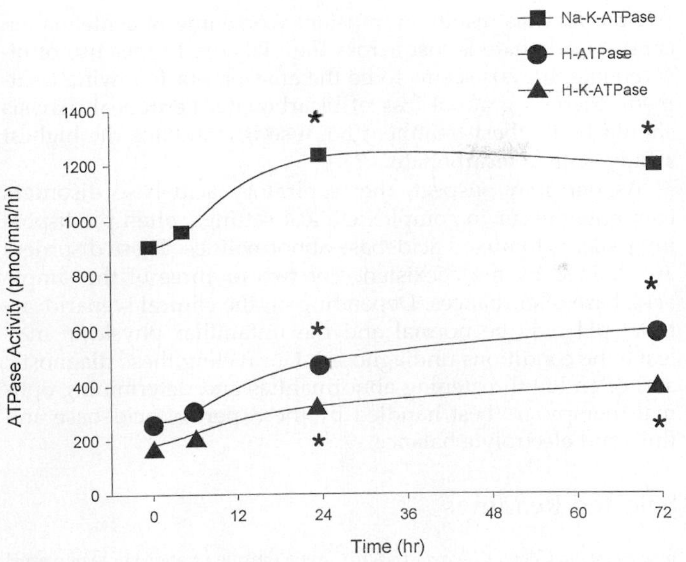

Figure 20.24. Effect of respiratory acidosis on Na^+-K^+-ATPase, H^+-ATPase, and H^+-K^+-ATPase in microdissected cortical collecting tubule after exposure to 72 hours of hypercapnia (*P <0.05). A significant rise in enzymes occurs only after 24 hours of hypercapnia in both the cortical and medullary (data not shown) collecting tubule. Aldosterone levels were high in intact animals, but identical enzyme effects were seen in adrenalectomized animals. (Adapted from Eiam-Ong S, Laski ME, Kurtzman NA, et al. Effect of respiratory acidosis and respiratory alkalosis on renal transport enzymes. *Am J Physiol* 1994;267:F390.)

tion, and the increased filtered load of bicarbonate is precisely balanced by the augmented rate of bicarbonate reabsorption. Chronic respiratory acidosis has a minimal effect in bone metabolism, in sharp contrast to the effect of chronic metabolic acidosis; thus there is little effect on urine calcium excretion.

Clinical Manifestations

Acute respiratory acidosis presents a broad constellation of symptoms that affect the CNS, the cardiovascular system, and the pulmonary system. Severe hypercapnia of short duration is well tolerated and does not present an immediate threat to life, even with a rise in P_{CO_2} at a rate of 3 to 5 mmHg/min. CNS symptoms depend on the degree of the acidemia and the hypercapnia, as well as the rate of their development. In moderate hypercapnia, hyperreflexia and asterixis occur, likely related to the effect of pH on the transmembrane potential of the peripheral nerves. With acute increases of arterial P_{CO_2} (i.e., to more than 60 mm Hg), headache, restlessness, anxiety, disorientation, and coma occur. With severe respiratory acidosis, deep tendon reflexes are decreased and muscle contractility is significantly impaired. This is associated with increased fatigability of skeletal muscle, and if this occurs in the respiratory muscles, respiratory failure will no doubt occur.

Similar degrees of hypercapnia in chronic respiratory acidosis present fewer and less severe symptoms. A fine tremor may be the only manifestation, but when the hypercapnia becomes more severe, confusion, loss of memory, and somnolence occur ("CO_2 narcolepsy"). There is an increase in cerebrospinal fluid pressure because of acidemia-induced vasodilation and increased cerebral flow. The effect of respiratory acidosis on the cardiovascular system is biphasic; first, the cardiac contractile force is acutely depressed, followed by improved ventricular contractility. Respiratory acidosis causes peripheral vasodilation, which is modified by increased sympathetic activity and increased catecholamine secretion.

Treatment

In patients with acute respiratory acidosis, the degree of hypoxemia is probably the single most critical factor determining patient outcome (Fig. 20.25). If the arterial P_{O_2} is less than 60 mmHg, low-flow oxygen administration should be initiated immediately, *regardless* of the potential adverse effects in the patient with chronic obstructive pulmonary disease (COPD). In these patients, the low P_{O_2} is often the only remaining stimulus to the respiratory center. Thus oxygenation may aggravate the hypoventilation and worsen the respiratory acidosis. The decision for the endotracheal intubation is complex and should be based on the entire clinical picture rather than on a single symptom or a single laboratory finding.

The acute decrease of P_{CO_2} with mechanical ventilation without restoration of the extracellular volume contraction due to chloride loss during the adaptation to respiratory acidosis hampers the excretion of the increased serum bicarbonate and results in the so-called posthypercapnic metabolic alkalosis. For this reason, repletion of chloride stores by the administration of NaCl is usually mandatory during the correction of respiratory acidosis.

The administration of alkali for the correction of severe respiratory acidosis has always been controversial. The tolerance to respiratory acidosis is remarkable, and only rarely is administration of alkali required. Nevertheless, in the presence of profound acidosis (i.e., pH less than 7) and when adverse effects of acidosis are anticipated, the administration of alkali is prudent, with the target of pH between 7.15 and 7.20.

The appropriate alkali for the correction of respiratory acidosis remains a matter of debate. There are several concerns regarding the use of bicarbonate. Besides the risk of fluid overload and pulmonary edema, there are several other problems regarding the efficacy of bicarbonate to increase arterial pH. There is substantial excretion of bicarbonate in the urine (i.e., up

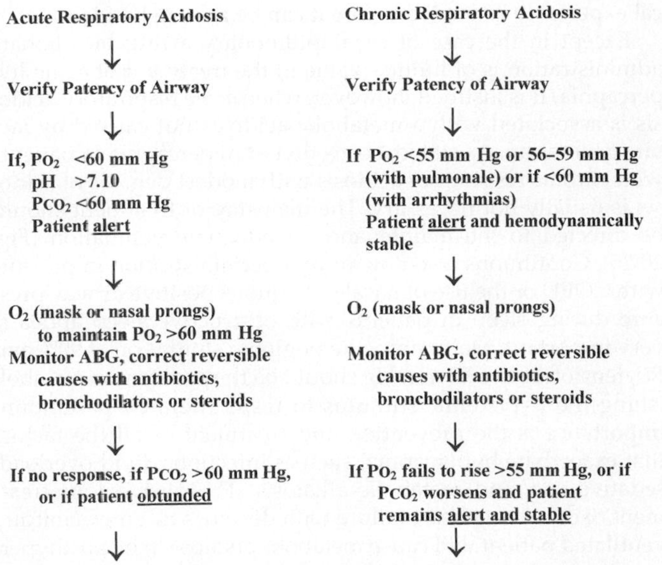

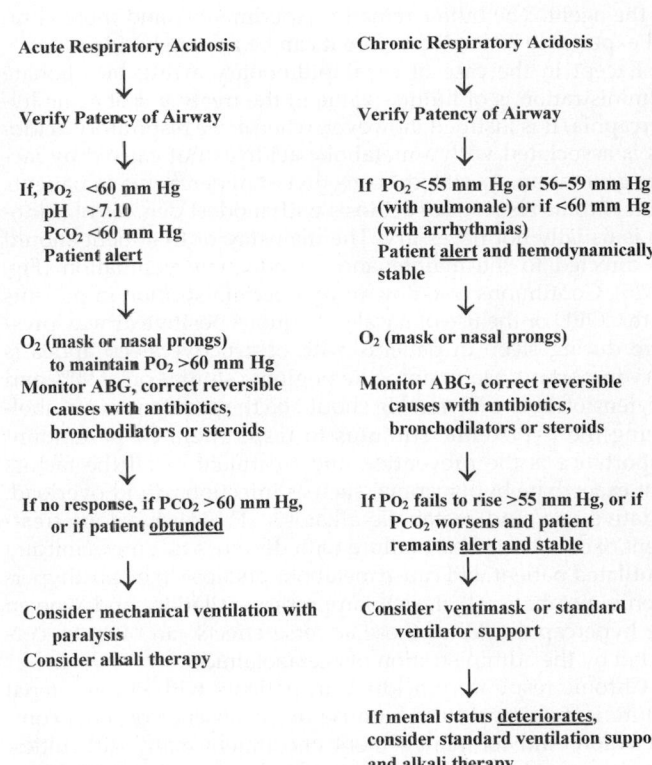

Figure 20.25. Flow diagram for the approach to a patient with respiratory acidosis.

to 40%) after its bolus administration. An appreciable rise of pH in the presence of hypercapnia requires a significant increase in plasma bicarbonate concentration according to the Henderson-Hasselbalch equation (i.e., $pH = 6.10 + \log HCO_3^-/0.03 \times P_{CO_2}$). Bicarbonate has a large volume of distribution, and the amount needed is difficult to calculate precisely. The administration of large doses of bicarbonate transiently worsens the intracellular acidosis. It causes an increase in arterial pH, but the rise of P_{CO_2} will be more pronounced according to the buffering process (i.e., $H^+ + HCO_3^- \rightarrow H_2O + CO_2$). Because CO_2 diffuses readily across cell membranes, intracellular acidosis worsens, the Na^+-H^+ exchanger is further stimulated, and protons are extruded into the extracellular space. (Some suggest that a bicarbonate drip mitigates the paradoxical intracellular acidosis). The generated CO_2 during the buffering process cannot be excreted by the lungs because of reduced alveolar ventilation, and therefore the hypercapnia worsens.

Alternative buffers for the correction of respiratory acidosis have been proposed, but they are considered experimental by most authorities because their safety and efficacy have yet to be established. A mixture of sodium carbonate and bicarbonate (Carbicarb) has been suggested; it has a pKa higher than that of the CO_2–carbonic acid–bicarbonate buffer system. This is apparently the reason that protons are buffered by the carbonate ion *without* CO_2 generation. The avoidance of intracellular acidosis, its lack of detrimental effect on the heart, and its low content of sodium theoretically make it a promising buffer for the correction of respiratory acidosis despite its limited clinical experience. Tris (hydroxymethyl) aminomethane (THAM) is a weak base amine buffer; it is not protein bound and is distributed primarily in the extracellular fluid. The buffer combines with protons, also without generating CO_2. It does not produce fluid overload, and the protonated form is excreted by the kidneys. This latter property precludes its use in patients with impaired renal function. Hypotension, hyperglycemia, and "left shift" of the hemoglobin dissociation curve have been reported. These effects are said to be prevented by a continuous infusion of the agent. The buffer remains experimental, and more clinical experience is needed before it can be adopted widely.

Except in the case of cardiopulmonary arrest, bicarbonate administration is of limited value in the treatment of acute hypercapnia. It is justified, however, when *acute* respiratory acidosis is associated with a metabolic acidosis not caused by lactate generation. As stated, correction of hypercapnia in patients with chronic respiratory acidosis with modest degrees of acidosis is usually not necessary. The mainstay of treatment should be directed to the maintenance of adequate ventilation (Fig. 20.25). Continuous low-flow oxygen administration in patients with COPD or the use of nasal continuous positive airway pressure during sleep in patients with obstructive sleep apnea is very important. Maintaining hemoglobin saturation at 90% and P_{O_2} tension above 60 mm Hg should be the goal to prevent abolishing the hypoxemic stimulus to respiration. Of paramount importance is the prevention and treatment of all the factors that exacerbate hypercapnia, such as infections, fluid overload, sedative use, and metabolic alkalosis. The overzealous treatment of coexisting heart failure with diuretics to a mechanically ventilated patient will cause metabolic alkalosis (i.e., posthypercapnic metabolic alkalosis), suppress ventilation, and worsen the hypercapnia. All of these adverse effects can often be corrected by the administration of acetazolamide.

Chronic respiratory acidosis in patients with chronic renal failure is more profound because of the absence of renal compensation, and its management encounters many difficulties. Bicarbonate administration causes fluid overload and excess intradialytic weight gain, and it is not a good treatment option. Acetate dialysis results in transient worsening of acidemia because bicarbonate is lost across the dialyzer. Proper use of bicarbonate dialysis seems to be the answer, but following treatment, there is gradual loss of bicarbonate. Peritoneal dialysis should be the best treatment because it maintains the highest steady state of bicarbonate.

As one may suspect, the respiratory acid–base disorders commonly occur in complex clinical settings, often predisposing patients to mixed acid–base abnormalities. These disorders are defined by the coexistence of two or three of the simple acid–base disturbances. Depending on the clinical scenario, arterial pH may be normal and the unfamiliar physician may leave the conditions undiagnosed. Unraveling these diagnostic and often life-threatening abnormalities and determining optimal therapy are best handled by the expert of acid–base and fluid and electrolyte balance.

Selected Readings

Bracket NC Jr, Cohen JJ, Schwartz WB. Carbon dioxide titration curve of normal man. Effect of increasing degrees of acute hypercapnia on acid–base equilibrium. *N Engl J Med* 1965;272:6.

Provides an experimental basis for the diagnosis of acute hypercapnia in humans. Includes a description of the acute steady-state plasma acid–base composition in humans with acute respiratory acidosis and an illustration of the relation between P_{CO_2} *and the associated changes of bicarbonate and pH during acute respiratory acidosis.*

Cohen JJ, Madias NE, Wolf CJ, et al. Regulation of acid–base equilibrium in chronic hypocapnia. Evidence that the response of the kidney is not geared to the defence of extracellular [H^+]. *J Clin Invest* 1976;57:1483.

Provides substantial evidence that hypocapnia itself induces the decreased proximal bicarbonate during chronic respiratory alkalosis.

Eiam-Ong S, Laski ME, Kurtzman NA, et al. Effect of respiratory acidosis and respiratory alkalosis on renal transport enzymes. *Am J Physiol* 1994;267:F390.

Examines the changes in H^+*-ATPase,* H^+*-*K^+*-ATPase,* Na^+*-*K^+*-ATPase, and aldosterone in microdissected rat nephron segments in the acute and chronic respiratory acid–base disorders.*

Feihl F, Perret C. Permissive hypercapnia. How permissive should we be? *Am J Respir Crit Care Med* 1994;150:1722.

An in-depth review examining the functional consequences of hypercapnia and respiratory acidosis on organs and integrated systems. Includes a discussion of the tolerance to hypercapnia and a description of permissive hypercapnia giving the indications and contraindications to be expected.

Gennari FJ, Goldstein MB, Schwartz WB. The nature of the renal adaptation to chronic hypocapnia. *J Clin Invest* 1972;51:1722.

Establishes the importance of adequate cation intake for defense of pH and describes the time course of renal response to primary hypocapnia.

Grippi MA. *Pulmonary pathophysiology.* Philadelphia: JB Lippincott, 1995:1–337.

A well-written review of respiratory acid–base physiology and pathophysiology. Selected cases of clinical importance are presented and discussed.

Krapf P, Caduff P, Wagdi P, et al. Plasma potassium to acute respiratory alkalosis. *Kidney Int* 1995;47:217.

Describes the alteration in plasma potassium concentration in acute voluntary hyperventilation in normal subjects. It examines the effect of respiratory alkalosis on sympathoadrenergic activity and documents for the first time that acute respiratory alkalosis results in significant increase in plasma potassium concentration mediated by enhanced α-adrenergic activity.

PART 8
Approach to the Diagnosis of Acid–Base Disorders

Jeffrey A. Kraut and Nicolaos E. Madias

Simple and mixed disturbances of acid–base balance are commonly encountered in clinical practice in stable as well as in critically ill patients. Thus analysis of more than 13,000 arterial blood samples from all patients hospitalized in one medical center revealed that more than 75% had altered acid–base balance. Simple metabolic alkalosis and simple respiratory alkalosis, in that order, were the most prevalent acid–base disturbances. In another series of critically ill patients, respiratory alkalosis was the most common acid–base disorder observed, being seen in 45% of 8,000 patients. On the other hand, mixed acid–base disturbances are also not uncommon. Indeed, the combination of mixed metabolic and respiratory alkalosis was the most common acid–base abnormality noted in an additional large series of seriously ill patients.

Recognizing the precise acid–base disorder(s) present in a patient is extremely important. Certain acid–base disorders can have a substantial impact on the patient's prognosis. In certain situations, disturbances of body acidity might be the sole or primary reason for the patient's illness and their correction can be lifesaving, as with severe diabetic ketoacidosis or renal tubular acidosis. In addition, severe acidemia caused by metabolic or respiratory acidosis, or the combination of the two, can impair cardiovascular function and contribute to the development of life-threatening arrhythmias. Similarly, results of several studies suggest that severe alkalemia, resulting from metabolic or respiratory alkalosis or the combination of the two, can contribute to the morbidity and mortality of hospitalized patients. Furthermore, the finding of a particular acid–base disturbance can provide a clue to an underlying disorder. For example, respiratory alkalosis can precede overt signs of sepsis, and the combination of a high anion gap metabolic acidosis and respiratory alkalosis can suggest the diagnosis of salicylate intoxication.

Proper analysis of acid–base disorders requires a systematic approach, as outlined in Table 20.24. The five critical steps in this process are as follows: (a) assess whether the acid–base parameters are correct using the Henderson equation or the Henderson-Hasselbalch equation, (b) obtain a good history and perform a complete physical examination, (c) calculate the serum anion gap, (d) identify the primary or dominant acid–base disturbance and assess whether a simple or mixed acid–base disturbance is present, and (e) examine the serum electrolytes and other ancillary laboratory data. In certain situations, measurement of urine pH and electrolytes and calculation of the urine anion or osmolal gap can also provide useful information.

TABLE 20.24. Systematic Approach to the Analysis of Acid–Base Disorders

Assess the accuracy of the acid–base parameters using the Henderson equation ($[H^+] = 24 \times PaCO_2/[HCO_3^-]$) or the Henderson-Hasselbalch equation ($pH = 6.1 + \log HCO_3^-/.03 \times PaCO_2$).
Obtain a good history and perform a complete physical examination, looking for clues to a particular acid–base disturbance.
Calculate the serum anion gap: $[Na^+] - ([HCO_3^-] + [Cl^-])$.
Identify the primary acid–base disturbance and assess whether a simple or mixed acid–base disturbance is present.
Examine serum electrolytes and ancillary laboratory data.
Measure urine pH and urine electrolytes, urine urea nitrogen, and glucose to calculate the urine anion gap ($[Na^+] + [K^+] - [Cl^-]$) or urine osmolal gap (measured osmolality − ($2[Na^+ + K^+]$ + urea nitrogen/2.8 + glucose/18).[a]

[a] Measurement of urine Na and Cl and urine pH should be obtained when metabolic alkalosis is present.

Measurement of urine electrolytes, urine glucose and urine pH should be obtained when an element of normal anion gap metabolic acidosis is present.

ASSESSMENT OF THE ACCURACY OF THE ACID–BASE PARAMETERS

The first step in analyzing any acid–base disorder is to ensure that the available measurements of pH, $PaCO_2$, and bicarbonate concentration are correct. The components of the bicarbonate–carbonic acid system are always at equilibrium in the blood; therefore measurements of pH, $PaCO_2$, and bicarbonate must adhere to the mathematical constraints of the Henderson-Hasselbalch equation: $pH = 6.1 + \log [HCO_3^-]/0.03 \times PaCO_2$. Serum bicarbonate is usually determined in the chemistry laboratory using an autoanalyzer technique. In actuality, total CO_2 content is measured, but because serum bicarbonate normally accounts for about 95% of that measurement, total CO_2 content can in practice be taken as equivalent to serum bicarbonate. Routinely, venous blood is used for measurement of total CO_2 content, the resulting value being higher by 2 to 3 mmol/L than that of arterial blood. On the other hand, arterial blood is usually used for measurement of pH and carbon dioxide tension. pH and $PaCO_2$ are measured with a blood gas analyzer using specific electrodes; serum bicarbonate can be derived using the known values for pH and $PaCO_2$. Methodologic errors are somewhat more common with the chemical determination of total CO_2 content. Blood should be collected anaerobically and serum promptly separated from whole blood and stored at 4°C until analyzed to ensure accurate assessment of acid–base equilibrium. The occurrence of spurious hypocapnia and hypobicarbonatemia resulting from the dilutional effect of excessive amounts of sodium heparin solution in the blood sample or failure to completely fill the Vacutainer tube when obtaining blood has been emphasized. Also, an elevation in serum bicarbonate can occur after the blood is obtained if the serum is not immediately separated from the cells because CO_2 continues to be generated by cellular metabolism. More commonly, however, a fall in serum bicarbonate of 3 to 5 mEq/L can be observed because of loss of CO_2 if the serum is left exposed to air for more than 90 to 120 minutes before the determination of CO_2.

When independent measurements of the acid–base parameters are available, the accuracy of the values can be checked using the logarithmic (Henderson-Hasselbalch) or linear (Henderson) form of the mass action equation for the bicarbonate–carbonic acid system. As a matter of convenience, the linear form of the equation is more commonly used at the bedside to evaluate the accuracy of the acid–base parameters: $[H^+] = 24 \times PaCO_2/[HCO_3^-]$, where $[H^+]$ is given in nEq/L, $PaCO_2$ in mm Hg, and $[HCO_3^-]$ in mEq/L. Conversion of pH into $[H^+]$ expressed in nEq/L can be accomplished by solving the equation $[H^+] = \text{antilog}\,(9\text{-pH})$. This interconversion is facilitated by the fact that in the normal arterial blood a pH of 7.40 corresponds to a hydrogen ion concentration of 40 nEq/L. Furthermore, between pH values of 7.2 and 7.5, for every 0.1-unit change in pH, there is a change in hydrogen ion concentration of 10 nEq/L in the opposite direction. Hydrogen ion concentration can also be derived from pH by sequentially multiplying the preceding hydrogen ion concentration by 0.8 when pH rises by 0.1, or by 1.25 when it falls by 0.1. The different methods of translating pH into hydrogen ion concentration are illustrated in Table 20.25. If a calculator is readily available, it is also convenient to use the logarithmic form of the mass action equation (Henderson-Hasselbalch) to accomplish the same purpose. If the independently measured values for pH or hydrogen ion concentration, $PaCO_2$, and bicarbonate concentration do not fit in these equations, repeat determinations should be performed before any analysis of the nature of the acid–base disturbance is made.

TABLE 20.25. Comparison of Methods of Interconversion of pH and Hydrogen Ion Concentration with Actual Values

	Hydrogen Ion Concentration		
	Derived Values		
pH	A	B	Actual Values
	nEq/L		nEq/L
7.80	—	16	16
7.70	—	20	20
7.60	—	26	25
7.50	30	32	32
7.40	40	40	40
7.30	50	50	50
7.20	60	63	63
7.10	—	78	79
7.00	—	98	100
6.90	—	122	126

A, between pH 7.2 and 7.5, with every 0.1-unit change in pH, hydrogen ion concentration changes by 10 nEq/L in the opposite direction; B, with every 0.1-unit rise in pH, multiply preceding hydrogen ion concentration by 0.8; with every 0.1 fall in pH, multiply preceding hydrogen ion concentration by 1.25.

HISTORY AND PHYSICAL EXAMINATION

After the acid–base parameters have been verified, it is necessary to obtain a good history and perform a complete and careful physical examination. These two tasks are often avoided in favor of dissection of the laboratory data. In this regard, it should be emphasized that a given set of acid–base parameters is never diagnostic of a particular acid–base disorder, but rather consistent with a range of acid–base abnormalities. Indeed, what appears to be a straightforward simple acid–base disorder might in actuality reflect the composite of coexisting acid–base disturbances. Clues from the history and physical examination are usually helpful in differentiating among the various possibilities. Thus a patient with severe chronic renal failure or insulin-dependent diabetes mellitus might be expected to have a high anion gap metabolic acidosis, whereas a patient who has a history of vomiting or who is receiving diuretics might be expected to have metabolic alkalosis. Similarly, a patient with a history of a disorder associated with extracellular volume depletion who presents with hypotension and evidence of reduced tissue perfusion might have lactic acidosis, whereas respiratory alkalosis is a likely possibility in a patient in hepatic coma. Physical abnormalities such as optic papillitis detected on funduscopic examination or evidence of severe respiratory distress and obstructive pulmonary disease detected by chest examination might suggest the presence of methanol intoxication or respiratory acidosis, respectively.

CALCULATION OF THE SERUM ANION GAP

The anion gap is the sum of serum [Cl^-] and [HCO_3^-] subtracted from the sum of serum [Na^+] and [K^+]. Many experts ignore potassium in this calculation. Defined in this way, [Na^+] − ([Cl^-] + [HCO_3^-]), the normal anion gap, which reflects primarily the negative charge of circulating proteins, ranges between 8 and 18 mEq/L, with an average of 10 to 12 mEq/L. There might be a spurious increase in the anion gap if the serum sample is left exposed to air: loss of water and CO_2 results in a decrease in bicarbonate and increase in sodium, chloride, and potassium (Δ gap of about 6 mEq/L at 2 hours). Several clinical laboratories have introduced a new method for measuring serum chloride. This new method results in a higher value of serum chloride and therefore a lower serum anion gap (average of 6 to 8 mEq/L). Therefore the clinician should know the normal range of the anion gap in his or her laboratory when evaluating acid–base disorders. Given this variability in the anion gap, if previous electrolyte values are available for the patient when no acid–base or electrolyte disturbance was present, the serum anion gap calculated from these electrolytes should be used as the baseline value.

The anion gap can be modestly elevated with severe metabolic alkalosis; however, an increment in the anion gap of more than 6 mEq/L usually signifies the presence of a high anion gap metabolic acidosis and in fact might be the only clue to the presence of this acid–base disturbance. The rise in the serum anion gap in this type of metabolic acidosis occurs because the addition to the body fluids of any strong acid produces both a fall in serum bicarbonate concentration and a rise in the concentration of the acid anion. If the acid accumulating in the blood is hydrochloric acid (as essentially occurs with bicarbonate loss from the body), the anion gap remains stable because the fall in serum bicarbonate is matched by an equivalent rise in serum chloride concentration. By contrast, if the acid accumulating in the blood is any acid other than hydrochloric acid, for example, lactic acid, the reduction in serum bicarbonate will be matched by a rise in the concentration of the acid anion, in this case lactate. Because chloride and bicarbonate, but not lactate, are the anions considered in the calculation of the serum anion gap, a rise in the serum anion gap will be present. Thus, with a high

TABLE 20.26. Use of the Delta (Δ) Anion Gap in the Diagnosis of Mixed Metabolic Acid–Base Disorders

Blood Chemistries	Normal	High Anion Gap Acidosis	High Anion Gap and Normal Anion Gap Acidosis	Metabolic Alkalosis	High Anion Gap Acidosis and Metabolic Alkalosis
Sodium[a]	140	140	140	140	140
Chloride[a]	106	106	114	94	94
Bicarbonate[a]	24	14	6	34	20
Δ Bicarbonate	—	10	18	10	4
Anion gap[a]	10	20	20	12	26
Δ Anion gap[a]	—	10	10	2	16
pH	7.40	7.29	7.10	7.50	7.38
$Paco_2$[b]	40	30	20	45	35

[a] In mEq/L.
[b] In mm Hg.

anion gap metabolic acidosis, there is usually a close reciprocal stoichiometry between the fall in serum bicarbonate and the rise in the anion gap, termed the *delta* (Δ) *anion gap*. Therefore a reduction in serum bicarbonate of 10 mEq/L is associated with a delta anion gap of 10 mEq/L. Addition of the value for the delta anion gap to the prevailing level of serum bicarbonate allows the derivation of the basal value of bicarbonate existing before the development of the high anion gap metabolic acidosis. Appreciation of this reciprocal relation between the fall in serum bicarbonate (Δ bicarbonate) and the rise in anion gap (Δ anion gap) is important in distinguishing between a pure high anion gap metabolic acidosis and a mixed high and normal anion gap metabolic acidosis, as well as in detecting the presence of a mixed high anion gap metabolic acidosis and metabolic alkalosis. The utility of the delta gap in diagnosing such mixed acid–base disturbances is illustrated in Table 20.26. The magnitude of the anion gap noted with the different causes of metabolic acidosis can vary greatly; however, a level greater than 30 mEq/L is usually observed only with lactic acidosis or ketoacidosis.

IDENTIFICATION OF THE PRIMARY OR DOMINANT ACID–BASE DISORDER AND ASSESSMENT OF WHETHER A SIMPLE OR MIXED ACID–BASE DISORDER IS PRESENT

Each of the cardinal acid–base disorders consists of the primary or initiating event and the secondary or adaptive response. Thus disorders initiated by a change in serum bicarbonate concentration, referred to as *metabolic,* elicit secondary changes in $Paco_2$, whereas those initiated by a change in $Paco_2$, referred to as *respiratory,* elicit secondary changes in the level of serum bicarbonate. These secondary or adaptive responses have a characteristic time course and magnitude and tend to return blood pH toward, but not completely to, normal levels. Thus, with the exception of mild chronic hypocapnia (respiratory alkalosis), some degree of acidemia or alkalemia persists as long as the initiating acidifying or alkalinizing process, respectively, is present.

Accurate assessment of disorders of acid–base equilibrium requires knowledge of both the time necessary for the adaptive responses to reach completion and the magnitude of the anticipated secondary adaptive response to each primary acid–base disorder. The characteristics of the secondary responses to the four cardinal acid–base disturbances are shown in Table 20.27. Analysis of disorders of acid–base equilibrium can also be aided by the use of the acid–base nomogram depicted in Fig. 20.26. This acid–base map schematically presents the limits of compensation for each of the primary acid–base disturbances. Acid–base parameters falling outside the expected range for each simple acid–base disorder denote the presence of a mixed acid–base disturbance. Acid–base data falling within the expected range of a simple acid–base disorder are consistent with, but not diagnostic of, the particular disorder. This is because the range of physiologic response for any simple disturbance is wide enough to allow the superimposition of another primary disturbance without shifting the acid–base equilibrium beyond the expected limits for a simple disorder. Indeed, the simultaneous presence of several acid–base derangements can result in an acid–base profile that is identical to that produced by a simple acid–base disorder. Moreover, the relationship between serum bicarbonate concentration and $Paco_2$ for each of the primary disturbances is derived from data obtained during the steady state. As noted previously, a defined time interval is required for the secondary response to reach completion or to return to normal once the primary disturbance has been corrected. Thus a mixed disturbance might be incorrectly diagnosed when only a simple disturbance is present because insufficient time has elapsed for the secondary response to develop or resolve.

To identify the primary acid–base disorder, it is useful to first examine the serum bicarbonate concentration. A rise in serum bicarbonate represents either metabolic alkalosis or the adaptive response to respiratory acidosis. If blood pH is elevated, metabolic alkalosis is the primary disorder; by contrast, if blood pH is reduced, respiratory acidosis is the primary disorder. Conversely, a reduced serum bicarbonate concentration signifies metabolic acidosis or the adaptive response to respiratory alkalosis. If hypobicarbonatemia is accompanied by a reduced blood pH, metabolic acidosis is the primary disorder, whereas an elevated blood pH in the face of a low serum bicarbonate level indicates the presence of respiratory alkalosis.

After determining which is the primary or dominant acid–base disorder, it is necessary to assess whether a simple or mixed disturbance is present, using the principles delineated earlier. An important clue to the presence of a mixed acid–base disorder is the deviation of serum bicarbonate and $Paco_2$ in opposite directions. An additional clue to the presence of a mixed

TABLE 20.27. Nature of Adaptive Response to Primary Acid–Base Disorders

Primary Acid–Base Disturbance	Initiating Mechanism	Secondary Physiologic Response	Time to Reach Completion	Limits of Compensation
Metabolic acidosis	↓ $[HCO_3^-]_p$	↓ $Paco_2$ of 1–1.3 mm Hg for each mEq/L fall in $[HCO_3^-]_p$ $Paco_2 = 1.5\ [HCO_3^-] + 8 \pm 2$	12–24 hr	$Paco_2$ of 10 mm Hg
Metabolic alkalosis	↑ $[HCO_3^-]_p$	↑ $Paco_2$ of 0.4–0.7 mm Hg for each mEq/L rise in $[HCO_3^-]_p$	24–36 hr	$Paco_2$ of 55 mm Hg[a]
Respiratory acidosis	↑ $Paco_2$	Acute: ↑ $[HCO_3^-]_p$ of 1.0 mEq/L for every 10-mm Hg rise in $Paco_2$	5–10 min	$[HCO_3^-]_p$ of 30 mEq/L
		Chronic: ↑ $[HCO_3^-]_p$ of 3.5 mEq/L for every 10-mm Hg rise in $Paco_2$	72–96 hr	$[HCO_3^-]_p$ of 45 mEq/L
Respiratory alkalosis	↓ $Paco_2$	Acute: ↓ $[HCO_3^-]_p$ of 2 mEq/L for every 10-mm Hg fall in $Paco_2$	5–10 min	$[HCO_3^-]_p$ of 17–18 mEq/L
		Chronic: ↓ $[HCO_3^-]_p$ of 4–5 mEq/L for every 10-mm Hg fall in $Paco_2$	48–72 hr	$[HCO_3^-]_p$ of 12–14 mEq/L

[a] Rare cases with $Paco_2$ values greater than 55 mm Hg have been reported.
p, plasma.

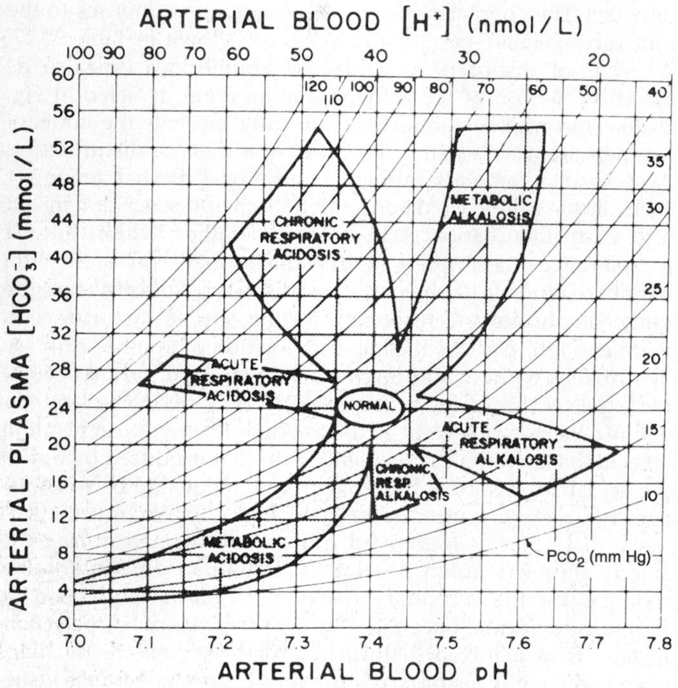

Figure 20.26. Acid–base nomogram. This acid–base map depicts the 95% confidence limits of the normal metabolic and respiratory adaptation to each of the four primary acid–base disorders. (Reprinted with permission from Cogan M, Rector FC. Acid–base disorders. In: Brenner BM, Rector FC, eds. *The kidney*. Philadelphia: WB Saunders, 1986:473.)

disorder is a normal or near-normal blood pH, signifying the coexistence of acid–base disorders with offsetting effects on blood pH. The sole exception to this rule, as noted earlier, is mild respiratory alkalosis: this acid–base disturbance can be present alone when the blood pH is within normal limits.

EXAMINATION OF SERUM ELECTROLYTES AND OTHER ANCILLARY LABORATORY DATA

In addition to the calculation of the serum anion gap, examination of the serum electrolytes, particularly serum potassium, is very helpful in the differential diagnosis of acid–base disorders. The normal anion gap acidoses can be conveniently divided into disorders associated with a high or normal serum potassium concentration and those associated with a low serum potassium concentration. Therefore identification of a normal anion gap metabolic acidosis should be followed by examination of the serum potassium concentration. By contrast, serum potassium concentration can be high or low in the various disorders associated with a high anion gap metabolic acidosis and therefore is of no particular help in the differential diagnosis of this type of metabolic acidosis. Respiratory acid–base disturbances can also cause changes in serum potassium concentration, but the magnitude of these changes is much less than that noted with metabolic acid–base disturbances. Thus significant deviations in serum potassium concentration usually suggest the presence of a metabolic acid–base disturbance.

In patients with high anion gap metabolic acidosis, determination of serum glucose, lactate, and creatinine concentrations; investigation for ketonemia or ketonuria; and screening of blood or urine for certain toxins are very useful. Also, measurement of serum osmolality and comparison of this value with the estimate of serum osmolality derived from consideration of the usual, osmotically active substances in blood can also be of great value. Under normal circumstances, the quantitatively most important moieties contributing to serum osmolality are sodium (and its counterbalancing anions, chloride and bicarbonate), glucose, and urea. Thus serum osmolality can rapidly be estimated using the following formula: $2 \times [Na^+] + [glucose]/18 + [BUN]/2.8$, where [glucose] and [BUN] (blood urea nitrogen) are expressed in mg/dl. An osmolal gap (defined as the difference between the measured and estimated serum osmolality) greater than 10 mOsm/kg H_2O signifies the presence in serum of additional osmotically active particles and supports a number of diagnoses, including alcoholic ketoacidosis and methanol or ethylene glycol intoxication. A mildly increased osmolal gap on the order of 20 mOsm/kg H_2O has been identified in some patients with lactic acidosis or chronic renal failure the explanation for which remains unclear. Thus, in some rare instances, an increased osmolal gap might not indicate toxic alcohol ingestion. On the other hand, methanol or ethylene glycol intoxication can be found in the presence of only a trivial increment in the osmolal gap, particularly if this measurement is obtained many hours after the intoxication, a time when these alcohols might have been largely metabolized to their toxic byproducts.

MEASUREMENT OF URINE ELECTROLYTES AND pH

In addition to the five steps discussed thus far, measurement of urinary electrolytes and pH provides critical information for the differential diagnosis of certain acid–base disorders. Measurement of urinary chloride concentration is a valuable tool in the differential diagnosis of metabolic alkalosis. Based on measurement of urinary chloride, the metabolic alkaloses can be divided into chloride-responsive (low urine chloride concentrations, less than 20/mEq/L) and chloride-resistant (high urine chloride concentration, greater than 20 mEq/L) forms. Moreover, if a measurement of urine chloride concentration is not readily available, measurement of urine Na along with that of urine pH can provide similar information to allow assignment to either one of these categories of metabolic alkalosis. Thus all patients with chloride-responsive forms of metabolic alkalosis will have not only a low urinary chloride concentration but also a low urinary Na concentration, with the exception of those individuals with metabolic alkalosis caused by vomiting or gastric drainage who are observed during the "disequilibrium" phase. In this early phase of vomiting or gastric drainage, urinary Na concentration can be high, but if so, it will be accompanied by an elevated urine pH, reflecting the increased quantities of bicarbonate appearing in the urine. Determination of urine electrolytes can also be helpful in distinguishing among the various causes of normal anion gap metabolic acidosis. Thus low urinary sodium and potassium concentrations are found with diarrhea, high levels of sodium and potassium are found in certain types of renal tubular acidosis, and high sodium and low potassium can be indicative of aldosterone deficiency. Urine electrolytes can also be used to calculate the urine anion gap (defined as $[Na^+] + [K^+] - [Cl^-]$). The urine anion gap can be helpful in grossly estimating urine ammonium excretion in the presence of metabolic acidosis and thereby determining whether a defect in renal acid excretion is contributing to the pathogenesis of the acidosis. Requirements for its use are that the urine does not contain unusual anions (e.g., ketone bodies, carbenicillin) and that bicarbonate excretion is low (urine pH less than 6.5). A negative value for the urine anion gap, that is, $[Cl^-]$ exceeding the sum of $[Na^+]$ and $[K^+]$, indicates that the urine contains substantial quantities of ammonium and is evidence against an impairment in ammonium excretion as the major contributing factor in the pathogenesis of the acidosis. On the other hand, a positive value in the range of 20 to 30 mEq/L indicates that ammonium excretion is low and implicates a reduction in ammonium excretion as an important factor in the production of metabolic acidosis. The accuracy of the urine anion gap in certain situations has been questioned, and the urine osmolal gap has been introduced as an alternative means of assessing ammonium excretion. The urine osmolal gap has the advantage that it can be used to obtain a semiquantitative estimate of ammonium excretion even when bicarbonaturia or organic aciduria is present. The urine osmolal gap is defined as the measured osmolality − (2[Na^+ + K^+] + [urea nitrogen]/2.8 + [glucose]/18), where [urea nitrogen] and [glucose] are measured in mg/dl. An appropriate urine osmolal gap in an acidotic patient is greater than 250 to 300 mOsm/L; in patients with low ammonium excretion, it usually is less than 100 mOsm/L.

Finally, measurement of urine pH in individuals with normal anion gap metabolic acidosis in association with an estimation of urinary ammonium excretion can aid in the detection and/or further characterization of metabolic acidosis resulting from defects in renal acidification. A sample of urine is obtained for measurement of pH and ammonium when the patient is acidemic. If the urine pH is below 5.5, bicarbonate is administered until the urine becomes alkaline or the serum bicarbonate returns to normal. The development of an alkaline urine (pH greater than 6.5) before normalization of serum bicarbonate indicates that proximal renal tubular acidosis is present; if the urine remains acidic, it indicates that other disorders (e.g., diarrhea) might underlie the acidosis. If urine pH is high (greater than 6.0) and remains relatively constant despite bicarbonate administration, distal renal tubular acidosis is present. Measurement of urine pH and determination or estimation of the quantity of urinary ammonium (using the urine anion or osmolal gap) will also help differentiate between nonrenal disorders in which ammonium excretion will be increased and those forms of renal acidoses in which urine pH is appropriately reduced but ammonium excretion is low, such as hyporeninemic hypoaldosteronism.

In summary, using the steps outlined in Table 20.24 and discussed in some detail in the text provides a rational approach to the diagnosis of acid–base disorders. The use of these principles are illustrated in the following case reports. For the purposes of these reports, the following mean normal values for blood acid–base parameters were used: pH, 7.40; hydrogen ion concentration, 40 nEq/L; $PaCO_2$, 40 mm Hg; serum bicarbonate concentration, 24 mEq/L; and serum anion gap, 10 mEq/L.

ILLUSTRATIVE CASES

Case 1

A 60-year-old man with a history of severe osteoarthritis is admitted to the hospital with a 3-day history of confusion and easy bruisability. The patient was taking aspirin for treatment of his arthritis. He had mild hypertension in the past but was presently receiving no medication for this condition. Physical examination on admission reveals a blood pressure of 120/80 mmHg lying. The pulse is 100 beats/min and regular, and respirations are 26 breaths/min and unlabored. Examination of the chest shows it to be clear to auscultation and percussion. Cardiac examination reveals no murmurs or gallops. Examination of the abdomen is negative. Laboratory data obtained on admission reveal the following: Na, 136 mEq/L; K, 3.2 mEq/L; HCO_3^-, 14 mEq/L; Cl, 100 mEq/L; BUN, 22 mg/dl; creatinine, 1.4 mg/dl; pH, 7.35; and $PaCO_2$, 34 mm Hg. Serum osmolality is 285 mOsm/kg H_2O. Urine ketones are trace positive.

At first glance, this patient has a mixed acid–base disturbance: metabolic acidosis and respiratory acidosis. The serum bicarbonate and blood pH were both reduced, indicating the presence of metabolic acidosis. The delta anion gap of 12 mEq/L, when added to the prevailing serum bicarbonate of 14 mEq/L, indicates that serum bicarbonate was 26 mEq/L (within the range of normal values for the laboratory) before the development of metabolic acidosis. Moreover, the $PaCO_2$ is inappropriately high for the degree of hypobicarbonatemia, indicating that an element of respiratory acidosis is also present.

On closer examination, however, the measured serum bicarbonate concentration is substantially lower than the value calculated from the pH and $PaCO_2$ using the Henderson equation: $[H^+] = 24 \times PaCO_2/HCO_3^-$; $45 = 24 \times 34/HCO_3^-$; $HCO_3^- = 24 \times 34/45 = 18$ mEq/L. A repeat measurement of serum HCO_3^- concentration indeed gave a value of 19 mEq/L. Even in the face of the corrected serum bicarbonate value, the patient still had a high anion gap metabolic acidosis. However, the $PaCO_2$ is now appropriately reduced for the degree of hypobicarbonatemia, indicating this patient has a simple metabolic acidosis. Measurement of salicylate levels revealed them to be substantially elevated, and it was concluded that this individual has salicylate intoxication. Although the combined presence of a high anion gap metabolic acidosis and respiratory alkalosis is thought to suggest the diagnosis of salicylate intoxication, in fact, studies have indicated that patients with salicylate intoxication can have pure respiratory alkalosis, pure metabolic acidosis, or mixed metabolic acidosis and respiratory alkalosis.

Case 2

A 30-year-old thin female nurse is seen in the clinic complaining of weakness and fatigue. She denies abdominal pain, nausea, or vomiting. She reports taking no medication. Physical examination reveals a blood pressure of 110/70 mm Hg supine and upright, pulse is 80 beats/min, and respirations are 12 breaths/min and unlabored. The rest of the physical examination is unremarkable. Laboratory data reveal the following: Na, 136 mEq/L; K, 2.8 mEq/L; Cl, 86 mEq/L; HCO_3^-, 36 mEq/L; BUN, 18 mg/dl; creatinine, 0.9 mg/dl; pH, 7.50; and $PaCO_2$, 46 mm Hg. Urine electrolytes are as follows: Na, 40 mEq/L; Cl, 60 mEq/L; and pH, 6.0.

The elevated plasma bicarbonate concentration and blood pH signify the presence of metabolic alkalosis. The $PaCO_2$ is appropriately elevated for this degree of hyperbicarbonatemia, indicating the development of appropriate respiratory adaptation. Although the serum anion gap is slightly elevated (a delta anion gap of 4 mEq/L), this slight increase probably does not reflect a coexisting high anion gap metabolic acidosis. A mild increase in the anion gap (not exceeding 6 mEq/L) is commonly observed in patients with moderate to severe chloride-responsive metabolic alkalosis and reflects the resultant hyperproteinemia and the alkaline titration of plasma proteins. The cause of the metabolic alkalosis is not immediately obvious because the patient denies taking any medication (e.g., diuretics). Urine chloride and sodium are both elevated, excluding surreptitious vomiting or most other forms of chloride-responsive metabolic alkalosis. The elevated urine chloride concentration is consistent with chloride-resistant metabolic alkalosis. The patient does not have an elevated blood pressure, a clinical finding that would appear to exclude most mineralocorticoid excess syndromes. The serum potassium is substantially reduced, but not to the degree to produce metabolic alkalosis by itself. Bartter's or Gitelman's syndrome, two disorders caused by mutations in the Na^+-K^+-$2Cl^-$ and thiazide-sensitive Na^+-Cl^- cotransporter, respectively, could account for this clinical picture. However, a screen of the urine for diuretics was positive, and after further questioning, the patient admitted she was taking diuretics in an attempt to control her weight. Diuretic administration has been classically considered a chloride-responsive form of metabolic alkalosis, and indeed correction of the alkalosis can easily be achieved with administration of sodium or potassium chloride after discontinuation of the diuretic. However, these patients can have low or high urine chloride and sodium concentrations depending on how soon urine electrolytes are measured after diuretic administration. Because this patient was surreptitiously taking diuretics while ingesting a normal salt intake, urine Na and Cl were high. Had the patient withheld the diuretics for many hours before the measurement of urine electrolytes, urine Na and Cl might have been low. This case illustrates the utility and some of the pitfalls of urine electrolyte measurements.

Case 3

A 42-year-old woman with a history of insulin-dependent diabetes mellitus is admitted to the hospital with severe renal failure and cough productive of purulent sputum for 3 to 4 days. The patient has had nephrotic range proteinuria and progressive renal failure for many years. Physical examination on admission reveals the following: blood pressure, 150/100 mm Hg supine and upright; pulse, 100 beats/min; respirations, 22 breaths/min; and temperature, 39.5°C. Her chest is clear to percussion and auscultation. No murmurs or gallops are present. Laboratory data include the following: Na, 135 mEq/L; K, 5.0 mEq/L; HCO_3^-, 15 mEq/L; Cl, 105 mEq/L; pH, 7.24; $Paco_2$, 36 mm Hg; glucose, 200 mg/dl; BUN, 90 mg/dl; creatinine, 9.1 mg/dl; urine and blood ketones were both negative. Microscopic examination of the urine is negative.

The acid–base parameters are consistent with a combination of metabolic and respiratory acidosis. Both the blood pH and serum bicarbonate are reduced, indicating metabolic acidosis. The $Paco_2$ is inappropriately elevated for the magnitude of the hypobicarbonatemia, indicating this patient also has respiratory acidosis. Given a serum bicarbonate concentration of 15 mEq/L, a change of 9 mEq/L, one would anticipate the $Paco_2$ should have fallen by 9 to 13 mm Hg to a level of 27 to 31 mm Hg. In fact, the $Paco_2$ is substantially higher, indicating that some other process was attenuating ventilation, thereby preventing the expression of the appropriate respiratory response to metabolic acidosis. A chest radiograph reveals bilateral pneumonia. Examination of the serum electrolytes and calculation of the ratio of the Δ anion gap to Δ bicarbonate indicate that both a high anion and normal anion gap (hyperchloremic) metabolic acidosis are present. The decrement in serum bicarbonate (9 mEq/L) is greater than the rise in the anion gap (Δ gap, 5 mEq/L). A normal anion gap metabolic acidosis is not uncommon in the early stages of renal failure. As renal failure progresses, the metabolic acidosis can remain a normal anion gap type, evolve into a pure high anion gap metabolic acidosis, or become a mixed high and normal anion gap metabolic acidosis, as in this patient. Patients with diabetic renal disease might be more prone to develop a normal anion gap metabolic acidosis than other patients with renal disease because they often have aldosterone deficiency (hyporeninemic hypoaldosteronism), as did this patient. This type of mixed high and normal anion gap metabolic acidosis can also be observed in patients with diabetic ketoacidosis during their initial presentation or after treatment with saline. However, there was no evidence of ketoacidosis in this patient.

Case 4

A 66-year-old man with a history of chronic obstructive lung disease for many years is seen in the clinic for complaints of increasing shortness of breath and swelling in his feet. Examination of his lungs reveals diminished breath sounds and diffuse wheezing. There is 2 to 3+ pretibial edema. Laboratory data are as follows: Na, 136 mEq/L; HCO_3^-, 30 mEq/L; K, 4.0 mEq/L; Cl, 96 mEq/L; pH, 7.29; Pao_2, 60 mm Hg; and $Paco_2$, 64 mm Hg (on room air).

A diagnosis of acute exacerbation of lung disease and right-sided heart failure is made, and the patient was given a low-salt diet, diuretics, steroids, and antibiotics. He is asked to return to the clinic in 1 to 2 days for reevaluation. Physical examination on the next visit reveals the following: blood pressure, 130/80 mm Hg supine and upright; pulse, 100 beats/min; respirations, 14 breaths/min; and temperature, 37.0°C. Examination of the chest reveals bilateral wheezes. Examination of the heart shows an S_3 gallop at the apex. Examination of the extremities reveals 1+ pretibial and pedal edema. Laboratory data are as follows: Na, 130 mEq/L; HCO_3^-, 34 mEq/L; K, 3.0 mEq/L Cl, 86 mEq/L; pH, 7.40; $Paco_2$, 56 mm Hg; and Pao_2, 72 mm Hg (on room air).

The initial set of acid–base parameters is consistent with either acute superimposed upon chronic respiratory acidosis or the combination of chronic respiratory acidosis and metabolic acidosis. With acute respiratory acidosis, for every acute rise of $Paco_2$ of 10 mm Hg, serum bicarbonate concentration increases, on average, by 1 mEq/L, and hydrogen ion concentration by 7 nEq/L. By contrast, with chronic respiratory acidosis, for every chronic rise of $Paco_2$ of 10 mm Hg, serum bicarbonate concentration is increased by 3 to 4 mEq/L and hydrogen ion concentration by 2 to 3 nEq/L. The rise in serum bicarbonate is caused by both titration of nonbicarbonate buffers and stimulation of net acid excretion by the kidney. The acute adaptation is complete within minutes, whereas the chronic adaptation takes 3 to 5 days before it reaches completion. An individual who chronically maintained a $Paco_2$ level of 64 mm Hg would be expected to have a serum bicarbonate concentration of approximately 31 to 33 mEq/L. In this patient, the rise in serum bicarbonate and hydrogen ion concentration is less than expected for someone with a chronic $Paco_2$ level of 64 mm Hg. The patient has no history to suggest any causes of metabolic acidosis, and other laboratory studies exclude any element of metabolic acidosis. Subsequent review of previous medical records indicate that the patient usually had a chronic $Paco_2$ level of approximately 50 mm Hg.

The second set of acid–base parameters is consistent with the combined presence of chronic respiratory acidosis and metabolic alkalosis. The normal blood pH is an important clue to the coexistence of two primary acid–base disturbances; with the exception of mild respiratory alkalosis, single primary acid–base disturbances are associated with an abnormal blood pH. In this instance, respiratory acidosis and metabolic alkalosis had divergent effects on blood acidity, resulting in a normal blood pH. The level of serum bicarbonate is higher than anticipated for an individual with a $Paco_2$ of 56 mm Hg, indicating the coexistence of metabolic alkalosis. The metabolic alkalosis in this patient was produced largely by the administration of diuretics and a low-salt diet given for the treatment of right-sided heart failure. Although the development of metabolic alkalosis might have been expected to suppress ventilation, thereby resulting in a further rise in $Paco_2$, the treatment of the lung disease with antibiotics and of the congestive heart failure with diuretics actually led to some slight improvement in pulmonary function and therefore a decrement in $Paco_2$.

Case 5

A 36-year-old alcoholic man is admitted to the hospital because of decreased mental status and increasing abdominal girth. Medications on admission include furosemide and spironolactone. Physical examination reveals a cachectic and icteric male who is extremely lethargic. Blood pressure is 100/60 mm Hg supine and 90/50 mm Hg upright. His pulse is 90 beats/min and regular. Respirations are 22 breaths/min. The lungs are clear to auscultation and percussion. Examination of the heart reveals no murmurs or gallops. The abdomen is protuberant, and there is evidence of ascites as manifested by a fluid wave. There is 1+ pretibial edema. Laboratory data on admission reveal the following: Na, 120 mEq/L; K, 3.0 mEq/L; HCO_3^-, 24 mEq/L; Cl, 75 mEq/L; BUN, 10 mg/dl; creatinine, 0.9 mg/dl; bilirubin, 16 mg/dl; albumin, 2.5 mg/dl; SGOT, 150 IU; pH, 7.46; and $PaCO_2$, 35 mm Hg.

At first glance, the acid–base parameters are normal except for mild hypocapnia. However, calculation of the serum anion gap reveals it to be 21 mEq/L. Addition of the delta anion gap of 11 mEq/L to the prevailing serum bicarbonate concentration of 24 mEq/L reveals that the patient's serum bicarbonate had been 35 mEq/L but was presumably reduced to 24 mEq/L by the superimposition of a high anion gap type of metabolic acidosis. The metabolic alkalosis is the consequence of diuretic administration. Thus this patient had metabolic alkalosis and high anion gap metabolic acidosis. Perusal of the serum electrolytes alone without calculating the serum anion gap would have resulted in a failure to detect this complex acid–base disturbance. This case illustrates the importance of calculating the serum anion gap in every acid–base disorder presented to the physician. As noted, the presence of hypocapnia and alkalemia is consistent with a mild respiratory alkalosis. This was presumed to be secondary to decompensated liver disease. This patient had a triple acid–base disturbance. Triple acid–base disturbances are common in seriously ill patients.

Case 6

A 36-year-old male drug addict is admitted to the hospital for the evaluation of mental confusion, unsteady gait, and hypobicarbonatemia. The patient has a long history of drug abuse and has been admitted on several occasions in the past for drug overdose. Physical examination on admission reveals an acutely ill man. Blood pressure is 110/80 mm Hg supine. Pulse is 106 beats/min and regular. Respirations are 34 breaths/min and unlabored. Temperature is 36°C. Examination of the chest is negative. Examination of the heart reveals no murmurs or gallops. Examination of the abdomen reveals no organomegaly. Neurologic examination reveals decreased mental status with a marked decrease in muscle strength. Deep tendon reflexes are normal. Laboratory data on admission reveal the following: Na, 135 mEq/L; K, 2.0 mEq/L; Cl, 113 mEq/L; HCO_3^-, 12 mEq/L; BUN, 20 mg/dl; creatinine, 0.9 mg/dl. pH, 7.26; and $PaCO_2$, 28 mm Hg. Urine electrolytes are as follows: Na^+, 90 mEq/L; K^+, 50 mEq/L; and Cl^-, 100 mEq/L. Urine pH is 6.0.

This patient has a normal anion gap (hyperchloremic) metabolic acidosis. The plasma bicarbonate is depressed, as is the blood pH, signifying the presence of metabolic acidosis. The $PaCO_2$ of 28 mm Hg is appropriately reduced for the degree of hypobicarbonatemia. The serum potassium concentration is significantly reduced, indicating the presence of a form of metabolic acidosis that is associated with large potassium losses. Disorders in this category include gastrointestinal losses of bicarbonate from diarrhea and intestinal fistulae, ureteral diversions, and distal and proximal renal tubular acidosis. The patient has no history of diarrhea, ureteral diversions, or intestinal fistulae. The urine anion gap calculated from urine electrolytes was positive (+40 mEq/L). At first glance, this finding suggests that renal ammonium excretion is reduced, consistent with renal tubular acidosis. However, careful questioning of the friends and relatives of this patient indicated that the patient had sniffed glue "to get high" because he did not have sufficient funds to purchase narcotics. Measurement of urine urea and glucose allowed the calculation of the urine osmolal gap, which was greater than 400 mOsm, consistent with the excretion of large quantities of ammonium in the urine. The urine anion gap was positive (and falsely suggested insufficient excretion of ammonium) because a large quantity of unmeasured anions were being excreted in the urine. Toluene is present in glue and, when inhaled, is metabolized to hippuric acid. The addition of large quantities of hippuric acid to the body leads to metabolic acidosis; although urine ammonium excretion increases strikingly, it is insufficient to generate enough bicarbonate to prevent hypobicarbonatemia. The hippurate anions, which are excreted in the urine swiftly, obligate the excretion of large quantities of sodium and potassium, thereby accounting for the severe hypokalemia and the conversion of the metabolic acidosis from an initial high anion gap form to a hyperchloremic form. This case illustrates the utility of the urine osmolal gap in determining the mechanism underlying the production of normal anion gap metabolic acidosis in certain situations.

Selected Readings

Adrogue HJ, Madias NE. Management of life-threatening acid–base disorders. *N Engl J Med* 1998;338:26–34, 107–111.

A recent review of the management of disorders producing severe acidemia or alkalemia.

Bia M, Thier SO. Mixed acid–base disturbances: a clinical approach. *Med Clin North Am* 1987;65:347–361.

Presentation of an approach to the analysis of mixed acid–base disturbances, emphasizing the integration of clinical and laboratory material.

Gabow PA. Disorders associated with an altered anion gap. *Kidney Int* 1985; 27:472–487.

An exhaustive discussion of disorders associated with deviations in the serum anion gap. Excellent introduction to this important concept in the evaluation of acid–base disorders.

Goodkin PA, Krishna GG, Narins RG. The role of the anion gap in detecting and managing mixed metabolic acid–base disorders. *J Clin Endocrinol Metab* 1984; 13:333–350.

A review of the use of the serum anion gap in dissecting mixed acid–base disturbances. It particularly emphasizes the importance of the serum anion gap in recognizing the coexistence of different types of metabolic acidosis (normal and anion gap varieties) and the presence of both metabolic acidosis and metabolic alkalosis. Frequent clinical examples are used to illustrapte these points. A nice clinical counterpart to the paper by Gabow.

Kamel KS, Ethier JH, Richardson RM, et al. Urine electrolytes and osmolality: when and how to use them. *Am J Nephrol* 1990;10:89–102.

An excellent review of the use of urinary electrolytes and osmolality determinations in the evaluation of patients with disorders of acid–base, fluid, and electrolyte balance. Discusses the benefits and pitfalls of these measurements in the assessment of acid–base disorders.

Laski ME, Kurtzman NA. Acid–base disorders in medicine. *Dis Month* 1996; 42:51–125.

A review of acid–base disorders that updates our knowledge of basic physiology of the kidney and the abnormalities leading to disorders of acid–base balance. An approach to the evaluation of acid–base disorders and basic concepts of treatment is presented. This is a nice complement to the review by Narins.

Narins, RG, Emmett ME. Simple and mixed acid–base disorders: a practical approach. *Medicine* (Baltimore) 1977;59:767–787.

A comprehensive review of acid–base physiology and pathophysiology, stressing practical methods for diagnosing simple and mixed acid–base disturbances. Examples of particular cases and the rationale for therapy are given. Although this paper is more than 20 years old, it still remains an excellent introduction to the careful evaluation of acid–base disorders.

CHAPTER 21

Renal Actions and Use of Diuretics

D. Craig Brater

All diuretics increase renal sodium and water excretion; however, they differ in chemical derivation, efficacy, sites of action, mechanism of action, and the transport pathways they inhibit (Table 21.1). Diuretic choice is dictated by the objective of therapy and the characteristics of the patient's disease. For example, patients with renal insufficiency need loop diuretics because they do not respond to the other agents. Patients with cirrhosis often have secondary hyperaldosteronism as a cause of sodium retention (see Chapters 31 and 55, Part 2); thus diuretic treatment in such patients is initiated with an aldosterone inhibitor, spironolactone. Knowledge of each diuretic agent and an understanding of the patient's disease are essential for effective diuretic use.

Diuretics are used in many clinical conditions (Table 21.2); the most common are the edematous disorders and hypertension. Other uses include treating hypercalcemia with loop diuretics (see Chapter 17, Part 3), treating diabetes insipidus (see Chapter 15, Part 1, and Chapter 26) or hypercalciuria (see Chapter 17, Part 2) with thiazide diuretics, treating glaucoma with carbonic anhydrase inhibitors, and treating cerebral edema with osmotic agents.

When diuretics are used to treat edematous disorders and hypertension, the objective of therapy is to cause a negative sodium balance. Doing so results in decreased vascular volume that stimulates movement of sodium and water from the interstitium into the vascular space, thereby decreasing edema. In hypertensive patients who do not have edema, this effect results in diminished vascular volume and consequent decrease in blood pressure. The ability to attain a negative sodium balance can be offset by sodium intake; effective diuretic use involves counseling patients and their families or caregivers to limit dietary sodium.

In patients with edematous disorders, it is important to assess clinically whether the patient has an expanded or contracted vascular volume. In the former case, patients can tolerate vigorous diuresis. In the latter, overly aggressive diuresis can contract the vascular space enough to result in hypotension. Thus in patients with normal or contracted vascular volumes, as typically occurs in those with nephrotic syndrome or cirrhosis, diuresis should be induced in a slow and controlled fashion, leading one to first use less efficacious diuretics such as the thiazides. On the other hand, patients with expanded volumes, such as those with congestive heart failure (CHF), often are treated with loop diuretics to cause a rapid and extensive diuresis.

TABLE 21.1. Diuretic Characteristics

Type	Site of Action	Chemical Class	Maximum Effect (% of Filtered Sodium Load)
Carbonic anhydrase inhibitors: acetazolamide	Proximal tubule	Sulfonamide derivative	3–5
Osmotic agents: mannitol	Proximal tubule and thick ascending limb of Henle's loop	Sugar	20–25
Loop diuretics: bumetanide, ethacrynic acid, furosemide, torsemide	Thick ascending limb of Henle's loop; Na^+-K^+-$2Cl^-$ cotransporter	Carboxylic acid; sulfonamide derivatives	20–25
Thiazide diuretics: bendroflumethiazide, benzthiazide, chlorothiazide, chlorthalidone, cyclothiazide, hydrochlorothiazide, hydroflumethiazide, indapamide, methyclothiazide, metolazone, polythiazide, quinethazone, trichlormethiazide	Distal tubule; electroneutral NaCl reabsorption	Sulfonamide derivatives	5–8
Potassium-retaining diuretics: amiloride, spironolactone, triamterene	Distal tubule and collecting duct; Na^+, K^+ exchange	Pyrazinoyl-guanidine, 17-spirolactone, and pteridine, respectively	2–3

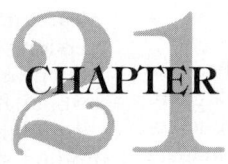

TABLE 21.2. Therapeutic Uses of Diuretic Agents

Type	Uses Diuretic	Uses Nondiuretic
Carbonic anhydrase inhibitors	With loop diuretics in patients with diuretic resistance	Glaucoma, metabolic alkalosis, altitude sickness
Osmotic agents	Acute renal failure	Cerebral edema
Loop diuretics	Edematous disorders, acute renal failure, hypertension in patients with C_{Cr} <40 ml/min or in those with extensive fluid retention	Hypercalcemia, hyponatremia, renal tubular acidosis
Thiazide diuretics	Edematous disorders	Hypertension, hypercalciuria, diabetes insipidus
Potassium-retaining diuretics	Edematous disorders (particularly primary or secondary hyperaldosteronism; e.g., cirrhosis)	Potassium or magnesium loss

C_{Cr}, creatinine clearance.

CHEMISTRY AND HISTORY OF DIURETICS

Carbonic Anhydrase Inhibitors

The structures of clinically used diuretics are presented in Fig. 21.1. The carbonic anhydrase inhibitor acetazolamide (Fig. 21.1A) is a derivative of sulfonamide antibiotics. Its development derived from the observation that the antibiotic sulfanilamide caused a diuresis but with metabolic acidosis as a side effect. Further study showed that sulfanilamide inhibited carbonic anhydrase. Modifying the antibiotic's structure yielded acetazolamide as a drug with more desirable diuretic features. Its ability to inhibit carbonic anhydrase explained its mechanism of action; this knowledge also was used to define the role of carbonic anhydrase in the kidney. This historical precedent is typical of the field of diuretic development, which is inextricably linked to fundamental discoveries in renal physiology.

Osmotic Diuretics

Mannitol is a sugar that remains within the vascular space and is filtered freely at the glomerulus (Fig. 21.1B). After being filtered at the glomerulus, mannitol creates an osmotic force throughout the length of the renal tubule that blunts reabsorption of sodium and water. This same effect occurs with other sugars and results in the volume depletion in patients with uncontrolled diabetes mellitus, in whom renal glucose excretion results in osmotic diuresis.

Loop Diuretics

The first consistently effective diuretics exerted their effects at the thick ascending limb of Henle's loop. These organic mercurials are no longer marketed because better, less toxic agents have been developed.

Ethacrynic acid and furosemide were developed independently and almost simultaneously (Fig. 21.1C). Ethacrynic acid development focused on findings from the era of mercurial diuretics that inhibiting sulfhydryl groups in the kidney would cause diuresis. Screening for such compounds led to the discovery of this agent. At the same time in Germany, screening compounds for diuretic activity resulted in a group of active sulfamylanthranilic acids that were substituted on the amine group of the aromatic ring. Of this group, furosemide and, in later years, bumetanide (Fig. 21.1C), azosemide, piretanide, and torsemide were developed. Other structurally different agents with sites of action at Henle's loop have been studied, but none have been marketed. These loop diuretics were a major breakthrough. Their efficacy made them useful in patients who did not respond to other drugs, including those with severe renal insufficiency and severe heart failure.

Thiazide Diuretics

The discovery of acetazolamide led to the hope that compounds could be discovered that would result in NaCl diuresis rather than the $NaHCO_3$ diuresis caused by carbonic anhydrase inhibitors. Such drugs were predicted to have greater effects but to avoid the undesirable metabolic acidosis of carbonic anhydrase inhibition. Chemical modifications of the sulfa nucleus were explored. One derivative, chlorothiazide, resulted in ring closure that conferred the desired pharmacologic effect. Additional thiazides (Fig. 21.1D) were developed that have different pharmacokinetic features but the same magnitude of effect. These drugs are selected based primarily on their duration of effect and relative cost; their pharmacologic characteristics are the same.

Other modifications of the sulfa nucleus resulted in quinethazone, metolazone, and chlorthalidone, which have pharmacologic effects identical to those of the classic thiazides but represent different chemical categories (Fig. 21.1D). Because their pharmacologic features are identical, these drugs are grouped with thiazides.

Potassium-Retaining Diuretics

Physiologic studies identified the role of aldosterone in stimulating Na^+ reabsorption in the distal tubule and collecting duct in exchange for K^+ and H^+. Derivatives of the steroid nucleus of spirolactone were found to be active in animals with intact adrenal glands and inactive in those with adrenalectomy. Thus it was presumed that these agents acted by blocking aldosterone. As methods for studying steroid receptors and effects became available, these compounds were shown to block the aldosterone receptor competitively. From this series of compounds, spironolactone (Fig. 21.1E) was developed.

Triamterene (Fig. 21.1E) was discovered in studies of the biologic activity of pteridines, some of which were shown to have renal effects. Chemical modification of xanthopterin, a pigment in butterfly wings, resulted in the discovery and development of triamterene. Amiloride (Fig. 21.1E) is chemically similar to triamterene, representing an open-ring version of the pteridines. Like many of the other diuretics, it has been a useful physiologic probe because it specifically blocks the luminal Na^+ channel of the distal tubule.

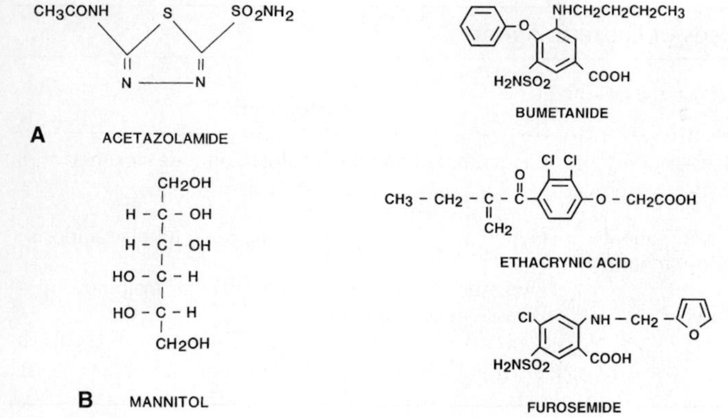

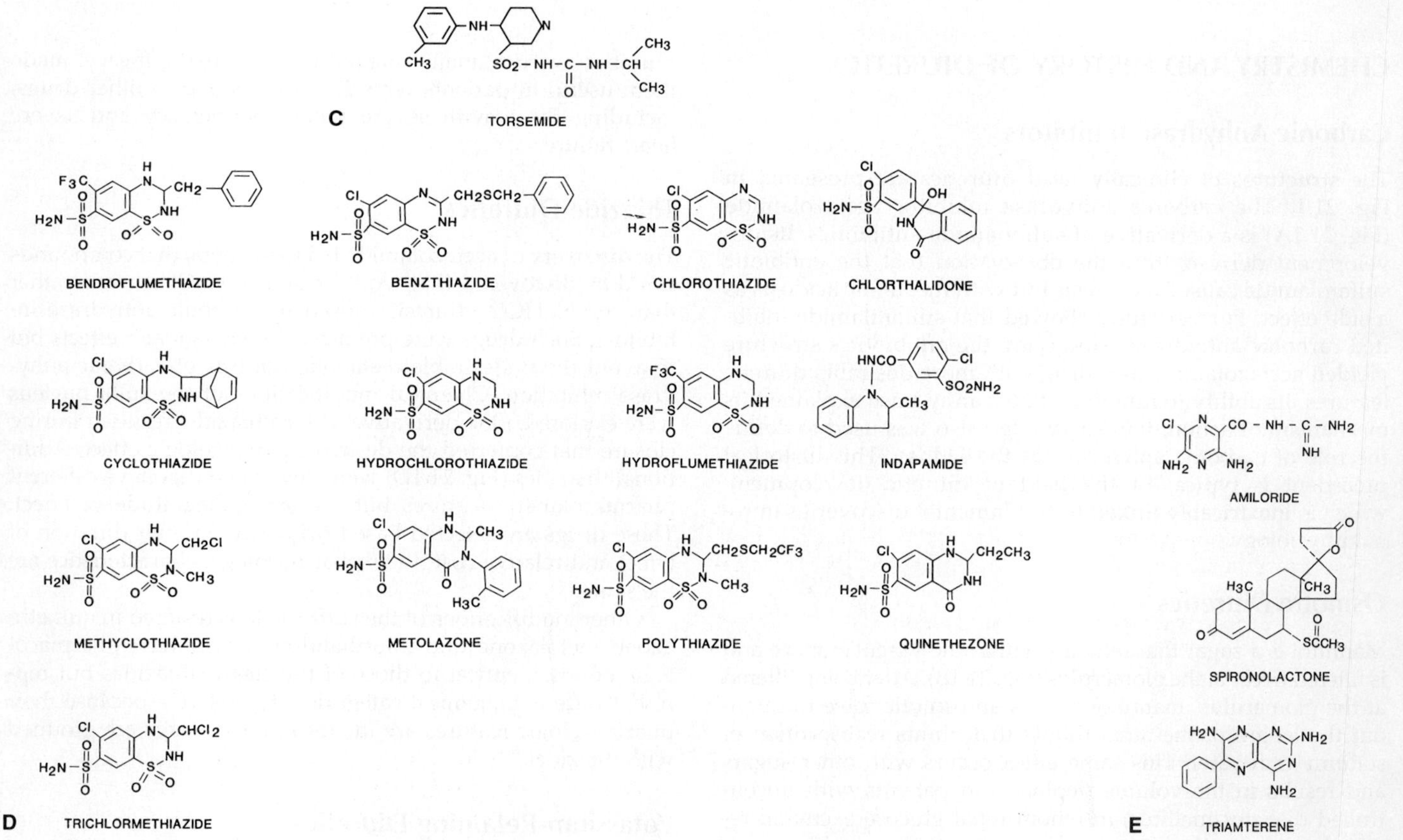

Figure 21.1. Structures of diuretic agents. **A,** Carbonic anhydrase inhibitor. **B,** Osmotic diuretic. **C,** Loop diuretics. **D,** Thiazide diuretics. **E,** Potassium-retaining diuretics.

PHARMACOLOGY OF DIURETICS

General

All diuretics except spironolactone must reach the lumen of the renal tubule to cause an effect. Their primary routes of access are presented in Table 21.3. Their discrete sites of action along the nephron account for the additive effects that occur with combinations of diuretics, or sequential nephron blockade. In addition, the nephron function at these sites of effect accounts for the various responses to different types of diuretics.

Both the organic acid and organic base secretory sites are located in the proximal tubule. Each secretes a variety of different substrates and is subject to competition by a similar group of compounds; thus, other organic acids (e.g., probenecid) can compete for transport of acidic diuretics, and other organic bases (e.g., trimethoprim) can compete for amiloride and triamterene secretion. Such competition can diminish the amounts of these diuretics reaching the tubular lumen and diminish response.

The amount of diuretic reaching its intraluminal site of action can be quantified as its excretion rate in the voided urine. This quantity can be related to the amount of sodium excretion, as illustrated for loop and thiazide diuretics in Fig. 21.2. This relationship is a typical pharmacologic S-shaped (or sigmoidal) curve, a so-called sigmoid E_{max} model wherein critical parame-

TABLE 21.3. Access Routes to Sites of Diuretic Action

Diuretic	Access Route
Carbonic anhydrase inhibitors	Organic acid secretion
Osmotic diuretics	Glomerular filtration
Loop diuretics	Organic acid secretion
Thiazide diuretics	Organic acid secretion
Potassium-retaining diuretics	
Amiloride	Organic base secretion
Spironolactone	Peritubular circulation
Triamterene	Organic base secretion

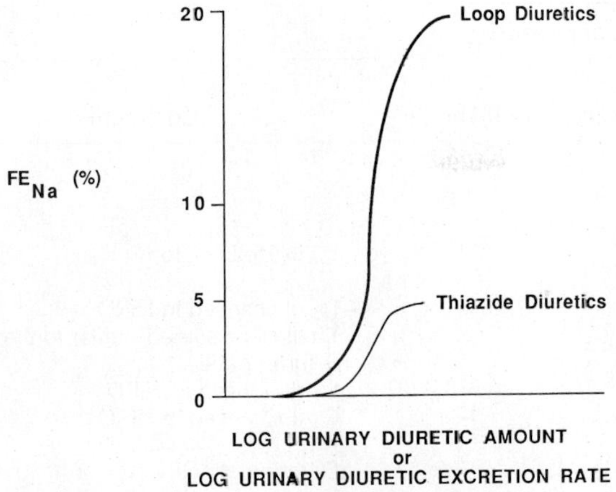

Figure 21.2. Schematized relationship between urinary excretion of loop and thiazide diuretics and sodium excretion.

ters are the basal response, the dosage causing 50% response, an upper asymptote or maximal response, and a slope factor that defines the steepness of the relationship. The maximum dosages of the various diuretics used to treat patients with renal insufficiency, nephrotic syndrome, cirrhosis, and CHF are provided in Table 21.4.

Carbonic Anhydrase Inhibitors

Efficacy

By catalyzing bicarbonate hydration at the proximal tubule, carbonic anhydrase facilitates reabsorption (more accurately regeneration) of nearly all the bicarbonate filtered at the glomerulus. Sodium accompanies this anion to maintain electroneutrality. When the enzyme is inhibited, $NaHCO_3$ is lost in the urine, accompanied by water. This loss of base leads to a metabolic acidosis.

Because the proximal tubule absorbs the majority of filtered sodium, one might expect a proximally acting diuretic to have a large effect. Table 21.1 shows that this is not the case because most but not all of the sodium rejected from the proximal tubule is reabsorbed at the thick ascending limb of Henle's loop. This reclamation diminishes the overall efficacy of proximally acting diuretics. The increased delivery of sodium to the distal nephron and collecting duct results in increased exchange for potassium. In addition, the luminal bicarbonate creates a negative charge that facilitates potassium secretion. The net result is that bicarbonate is excreted with both Na^+ and K^+ and carbonic anhydrase inhibitors, thereby causing potassium depletion.

Pharmacokinetics

Little is known about acetazolamide's disposition (Table 21.5). Its half-life of about 13 hours means that twice-a-day dosing is sufficient and that steady-state concentrations are attained after 2 days of therapy. Presumably, renal acetazolamide elimination is compromised in patients with renal insufficiency.

Therapeutic Uses

As a diuretic, acetazolamide is used infrequently; settings include in combination with loop diuretics to cause sequential nephron blockade and alone to treat metabolic alkalosis that has not responded to other therapies.

In patients refractory to loop diuretics, particularly those with heart failure, proximal tubular sodium reabsorption is elevated. Thus the loop diuretic is limited in its efficacy because less sodium is being delivered to its site of action. Coadministering acetazolamide in this setting occasionally can cause a clinically important diuresis. In this setting, the practice of combining a proximally acting and a loop diuretic is sound. Acetazolamide's adverse effects unfortunately limit its utility. Blocking adenosine receptors at the proximal tubule inhibits sodium reabsorption at this site. Therefore adenosine antagonists are under development.

Because carbonic anhydrase is also important for intraocular fluid formation, inhibitors of this enzyme are effective in decreasing intraocular pressure and are therefore used to treat glaucoma. Acetazolamide, as well as its derivatives, such as methazolamide, are used to treat glaucoma. The latter was developed to have comparable effects on ocular carbonic anhydrase but little systemic effect. Therefore benefit is retained without the degree of diuresis and metabolic acidosis that occur with acetazolamide.

The systemic metabolic acidosis caused by acetazolamide can be used to correct metabolic alkalosis. The typical patient is one with severe chronic obstructive pulmonary disease in whom treatment with other diuretics has resulted in Na^+, Cl^-, and K^+ loss, causing a severe metabolic alkalosis. If sufficiently severe, the alkalosis causes hypoventilation to raise blood CO_2 concentrations to correct systemic pH. However, this hypoventilation can cause further hypoxemia in such patients. Correcting the alkalosis with short-term acetazolamide use can improve oxygenation. Acetazolamide has been proven to be effective in treating and preventing altitude sickness. The mechanism of this effect is not known. This diuretic also is useful as a cotherapy with bicarbonate in treating patients with uric acid stones.

TABLE 21.4. Maximum Loop Diuretic Dosages

Clinical Condition	Dosage (mg)				
	Furosemide		Bumetanide	Ethacrynic Acid	Torsemide
	IV	PO	IV and PO	IV and PO	IV and PO
Renal insufficiency					
C_{Cr} 20–50	80	160	2	100	40
C_{Cr} <20	200	400	8–10	250	100
Nephrotic syndrome with preserved renal function	120	240	4	150	40–60
Cirrhosis with preserved renal function	40	80	1	50	20
Congestive heart failure with preserved renal function	40–80	80–160	1–2	50–100	20–40

C_{Cr}, creatinine clearance.

TABLE 21.5. Diuretic Pharmacokinetics

	Bioavailability (%)	Clearance (ml/min/kg)	Vd (L/kg)	Half-Life (hr)	Comments
Carbonic anhydrase inhibitor					
Acetazolamide				13	
Osmotic agent					
Mannitol		7	0.5	1	$t_{1/2}$ in ESRD = 36 hr
Loop diuretics					
Bumetanide	80–90	2–3.5	0.15	0.3–1.5	$t_{1/2}$ unchanged in ESRD
Ethacrynic acid					Kinetics presumed similar to those of furosemide
Furosemide	10–100	1.5–3	0.15	0.3–3.4	$t_{1/2}$ prolonged in ESRD
Torsemide	80–100			3–4	$t_{1/2}$ unchanged in ESRD
Thiazide diuretics					
Bendroflumethiazide	90	4.3	1–1.5	2.5–5	Duration of action 18–24 hr
Benzthiazide	100			10	Duration of action 12–18 hr
Chlorthalidone	65			24–55	Duration of action 24–72 hr
Chlorothiazide	30–50	4.3	1	15–25	Duration of action 6–12 hr
Clopamide				8–12	Duration of action 18–24 hr
Cyclothiazide					Duration of action 18–24 hr
Hydrochlorothiazide	65–75	4.6	2.5	3–10	Duration of action 6–12 hr
Hydroflumethiazide	75	6.4	5	6–10	Duration of action 18–24 hr
Indapamide	90		1.6	6–15	Duration of action 24–36 hr
Methyclothiazide					Duration of action 24–48 hr
Metolazone					Duration of action 12–24 hr
Polythiazide				25	Duration of action 24–48 hr
Quinethazone					Duration of action 12–24 hr
Trichlormethiazide		3.4		1–4	Duration of action 24 hr
Potassium-retaining diuretics					
Amiloride				17–26	$t_{1/2}$ in ESRD = 100 hr
Spironolactone				1.5	$t_{1/2}$ of active metabolites = 15 hr
Triamterene	83 (55)	14 (0.7)	3.0 (0.14)	3 (3)	Parentheses denote active metabolite; $t_{1/2}$ in ESRD = 10 hr

ESRD, end-stage renal disease; $t_{1/2}$, half-life; Vd, volume of distribution.

One dose at 8 PM keeps the urine alkaline throughout the night.

Toxicity

Metabolic acidosis and potassium depletion are the primary adverse effects of carbonic anhydrase inhibitors; these effects are extensions of the pharmacologic activity of the diuretic. In addition, acetazolamide, particularly in large dosages, can cause central nervous system side effects, including light-headedness, paresthesias (particularly circumoral), weakness, and confusion. The mechanisms of these effects are unknown.

Osmotic Diuretics

Efficacy

Mannitol is freely filtered at the glomerulus. Because it is not reabsorbed in the nephron, it remains in the tubule lumen, where it exerts an osmotic effect, thereby reducing the ability of the proximal tubule and thick ascending limb to reabsorb sodium. The reabsorptive pumps in these nephron segments have a limited ability to counteract the osmotic gradient caused by the intraluminal mannitol.

Although the proximal effect of mannitol causes some bicarbonate excretion, the effect at Henle's loop predominates so that mainly sodium is excreted, along with chloride. In addition, the increased delivery of Na^+ to distal sites allows increased exchange for K^+ so that osmotic agents also enhance potassium excretion. This effect accounts for the potassium deficits commonly encountered in patients with uncontrolled diabetes mellitus and a glucose-mediated osmotic diuresis.

Pharmacokinetics

Mannitol is eliminated quickly, with a half-life of about 1 hour in patients with normal renal function. Thus its effects begin quickly but also dissipate quickly. For this reason, it is often administered as a continuous intravenous infusion. Mannitol elimination is impaired in patients with renal insufficiency (the half-life is 36 hours).

Therapeutic Uses

Since the development of loop diuretics, osmotic diuretics have been relegated to nondiuretic uses. The most common setting of osmotic diuresis is disease related rather than therapeutic, caused by the renal glucose excretion that occurs in uncontrolled diabetes mellitus.

Generating diuresis before potential renal insult (e.g., hypotension, aminoglycoside antibiotics, contrast agents, *cis*-platinum) occurs has been shown to protect renal function in animal models. Mannitol has been explored as prophylaxis in patients likely to suffer ischemic insults to the kidney (as in some types of surgery), and at one time it was used widely before chemotherapy with *cis*-platinum. There is little evidence that osmotic diuresis is better than brisk diuresis caused by parenteral saline administration. In fact, if an osmotic agent causes volume depletion, it could actually worsen the insult. In addition, data in animals suggest that a protective effect is best gained by decreasing renal metabolic demands by blocking Na^+ reabsorptive pump activity at the thick ascending limb. Such an effect can be accomplished with loop but not osmotic diuretics. Overall, rather than using osmotic agents for prophylaxis against renal injury, it is better to ensure adequate volume status in the patient.

Mannitol has also been used in patients with acute renal failure in attempts to "open up" the kidney. There is no evidence that this strategy is effective, and ensuring adequate volume status in the patient probably is the best treatment. This latter strategy is reinforced by the fact that if mannitol is administered to a patient with acute renal failure and the patient's renal function remains suppressed, the mannitol remains in the vascular space, where its osmotic effect expands blood volume and may precipitate heart failure. Under these circumstances, the intracellular K^+ concentration rises as a result of water movement out of the cell, and K^+ leaks out of the cells and aggravates the hyperkalemia of acute renal failure. Therefore mannitol should rarely be used as a diuretic agent.

On the other hand, the osmotic effect of mannitol is highly effective in reducing cerebral edema, and it is used appropriately in neurosurgical procedures and head trauma treatment. This use is associated with a pronounced osmotic diuresis that in this setting is unwanted. Scrupulous attention must be paid to volume repletion in such patients.

Toxicity

The adverse effects of mannitol are a predictable consequence of the pharmacology of this compound. Thus volume depletion and urinary potassium loss are the risks in patients with adequate renal function. Patients with compromised renal function are at risk of volume expansion that can precipitate heart failure. In most patients with renal insufficiency, the risks outweigh any benefits.

Loop Diuretics

Efficacy

Loop diuretics inhibit the Na^+-K^+-$2Cl^-$ reabsorptive pump at the thick ascending limb of Henle's loop, causing a diuresis of NaCl and KCl. At this nephron site, 20% to 30% of filtered sodium is reabsorbed. Because a maximally effective dosage of a loop diuretic can cause excretion of 20% to 25% of filtered sodium, these agents can block nearly all reabsorption by this segment of the nephron.

Because a major component of calcium reabsorption occurs parallel to that of sodium at the thick ascending limb (see Chapter 17, Part 2), use of loop diuretics enhances calcium excretion and can be used to treat hypercalcemia (see Chapter 17, Part 3). However, their use should be withheld until the volume depletion associated with hypercalcemia is corrected with saline infusions. Also, during such therapy attention to the volume status of the patient is essential.

The thick ascending limb is also important for urinary concentrating ability. Forming a concentrated urine requires not only antidiuretic hormone (ADH), which permits water reabsorption across the collecting duct, but also a hypertonic medullary interstitium to act as the osmotic driving force for water absorption (see Chapter 8). In turn, the hypertonicity of the renal medullary interstitium is maintained by solute reabsorption at the thick ascending limb. Thus loop diuretics decrease the driving force for water reabsorption, thereby preventing concentrated urine generation.

Loop diuretics also have a short-lasting venodilating effect when administered intravenously. This effect explains the immediate improvement that often occurs in patients with acute pulmonary edema before any diuresis has occurred. The venodilation results in decreased cardiac preload, a fall in pulmonary artery wedge pressure, and symptomatic relief. However, this effect can also trigger sympathetic nervous system activation, causing increased afterload and diminished cardiac function. Thus this effect is a double-edged sword.

Pharmacokinetics

All loop diuretics are avidly bound to serum albumin (more than 95%) and enter the urine by being secreted actively at the proximal tubule. The high protein binding accounts for the small distribution volumes of these drugs, which are for the most part restricted to the vascular space. In effect, binding to albumin traps the diuretic in the vascular space so that it can be delivered to the kidney and exert its effects. The short half-lives of these agents mean that their duration of action is brief. Thus they cause an intense, short-lived diuresis. When they are given intravenously, response occurs within minutes and is complete within 2 to 3 hours. When they are administered orally, peak response occurs within 30 to 90 minutes and is complete within another 2 to 3 hours. Because of the short duration of action, these drugs must be administered several times a day. Torsemide, the newest loop diuretic, has a longer half-life and duration of action and probably can be administered less frequently.

The bioavailabilities of these three diuretics differ, with that of bumetanide and torsemide being essentially complete (80% or more) and that of furosemide averaging 50%. Therefore, when a patient is switched from intravenous to oral bumetanide or torsemide, dosing is the same; in contrast, the oral furosemide dosage must be twice the intravenous dosage. Unfortunately, absorption of these drugs is not so simple. In particular, furosemide absorption varies greatly, both between patients and within an individual patient from day to day. The range of furosemide absorption is 10% to 100%. In contrast, variability of bumetanide and torsemide absorption is modest. Theoretically, highly variable absorption translates to equally variable response and the potential for a poor long-term outcome. This is indeed the case, as supported by the results of a study in which hospitalized patients with CHF were randomized to either furosemide (variable absorption) or torsemide (predictable absorption) and followed for a year after discharge. Those taking torsemide had significantly fewer hospitalizations for CHF, fewer hospitalizations for any cardiac cause, and better quality of life measures. Thus a predictably absorbed diuretic appears to be better.

In patients with renal disease, less total drug appears in the urine. This accounts for the larger dosages of all three drugs necessary to deliver effective amounts of the diuretic to the site of action. In addition, entry into the urine of furosemide, but not bumetanide and torsemide, is prolonged, so the duration of response is longer than in patients with normal renal function. The explanation for this difference is that nonrenal pathways of bumetanide and torsemide elimination are preserved so that overall clearance and half-life are not affected appreciably when renal function is diminished. In contrast, in patients with hepatic dysfunction, including congestive hepatoathy, elimination of bumetanide and torsemide, but not furosemide, is slowed, resulting in a longer half-life and duration of action.

Therapeutic Uses

Loop diuretics are the most effective diuretics currently available. For this reason and because they are often effective when other diuretics are not, they are also called *high-ceiling diuretics.* Their site of action is the thick ascending limb of Henle's loop. Because loop diuretics can block nearly all reabsorption at this site and only small amounts of sodium are reclaimed at more distal nephron sites, these agents can cause excretion of 20% to 25% of filtered sodium. These agents therefore cause a vigorous diuresis and should not be used when less active diuretics suffice.

Many patients, particularly those with severe heart failure, severe cirrhosis, nephrotic syndrome, and renal insufficiency need loop diuretics to control volume. If creatinine clearance is less than about 40 ml/min, other diuretics as single agents are not likely to be clinically effective, and loop diuretics usually are needed. Patients may need large dosages of these drugs, but small dosages should be tried first, followed by upward titration according to clinical response. Thus 40 mg of furosemide or the equivalent dosage of another agent is given first. If inadequate, the dosage can be doubled sequentially until a response occurs or a maximum dosage is reached. The maximum single dosage that should be tried differs for different clinical conditions and is a function of the pharmacodynamics of loop diuretics in different edematous disorders.

The dose–response relationship of a loop diuretic is expressed by comparing the amount of diuretic at the active site (i.e., the urinary excretion rate of the diuretic) with the response, expressed as the sodium excretion rate or fractional excretion of sodium. When this is done in patients with renal insufficiency (Fig. 21.3), it appears as if remaining nephrons respond normally because the response, expressed as FE_{Na}, is similar to that which occurs in healthy subjects. Because of the impaired delivery of diuretic into the urine in such patients, a higher dosage is needed to maximize the response. For clinical guidance, a dosage can be determined that causes maximal response (Table 21.4). This dosage is the ceiling dosage; larger dosages do not increase the response. Even if a maximum dosage is administered in such patients and remaining nephrons respond adequately, it is clear from the upper-left panel of Fig. 21.3 that response measured as overall sodium excretion is limited by the diminished filtered load of sodium. Response is not increased by dosages higher than the ceiling dosage; it is increased only by administering effective doses on multiple occasions per day.

In patients with CHF, cirrhosis, or nephrotic syndrome, the pharmacodynamics of loop diuretics (and probably others) are altered so that maximal response is lower (Fig. 21.3). The mechanism of this change is unknown and could result from increased proximal or distal sodium reabsorption or a change in the dynamics of the interaction with the Na^+-K^+-$2Cl^-$ transporter. Clinically the most important ramification of this change is that the diminished response to a loop diuretic is not improved by administering large doses of the diuretic. As a consequence, ceiling dosages of loop diuretics in CHF and cirrhosis are modest (Table 21.4). If such dosages do not cause a sufficient overall response, multiple doses should be given rather than larger single doses.

The guidelines in Table 21.4 show that nephrotic syndrome differs from CHF and cirrhosis. This difference is explained by the fact that one-half to two-thirds of the amount of the loop diuretic that reaches the urine in patients with nephrotic syndrome is bound to the urinary albumin consequent to the disease. Thus, higher dosages are needed to attain normal amounts of unbound, active drug in the urine. In addition to this effect is the change in pharmacodynamics shown in Fig. 21.3. The net result in nephrotic syndrome is a need to administer higher dosages; these dosages will not cause the same diuresis as in healthy subjects, and frequent dosing usually is needed.

It is important to emphasize that patients with CHF, cirrhosis, and nephrotic syndrome who have concomitant decreases in renal function need higher dosages than those listed in Table 21.4 to attain effective amounts of diuretic at the site of action.

Once an effective dosage is found, the next decision is its frequency of administration. Dosing frequency must be individualized and depends on the sodium excretion needed, the effectiveness of the drug in the individual patient, and the amount of sodium restriction with which the patient will comply. For example, assume a patient is ingesting 150 mEq sodium/day and the objective is to maintain balance by causing daily excretion of 150 mEq of sodium. If each dose of diuretic causes 75 mEq of sodium to be excreted, twice-daily dosing would be sufficient. If the effective diuretic dosage causes excretion of

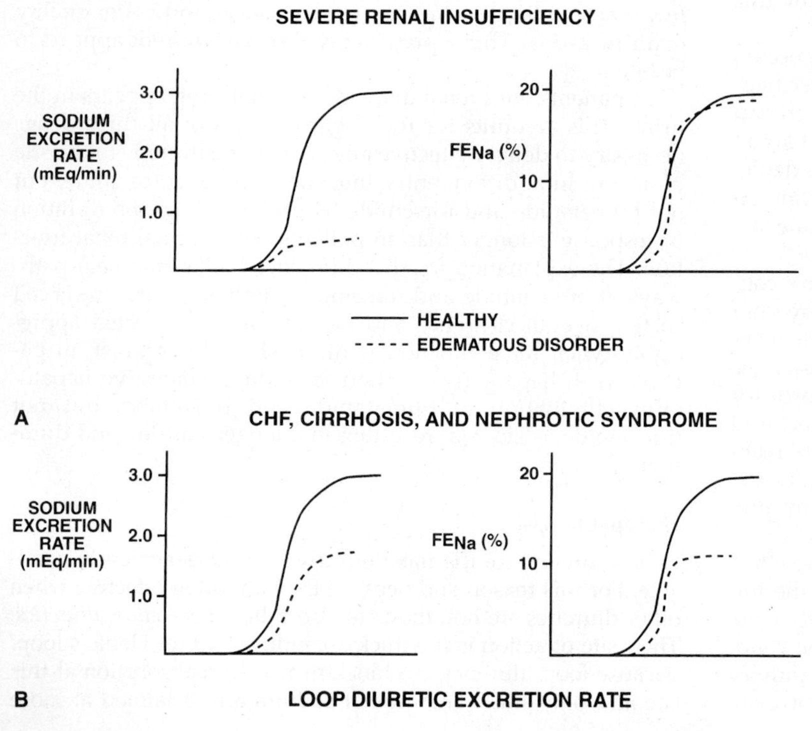

Figure 21.3. Schematized pharmacodynamics of loop diuretics in patients with renal insufficiency **(A)** and with congestive heart failure, cirrhosis, or nephrotic syndrome **(B)**.

TABLE 21.6. Dosages for Continuous Infusion of Loop Diuretics

	Furosemide Loading Dose (mg)	Infusion Rate (mg/hr)	Bumetanide Loading Dose (mg)	Infusion Rate (mg/hr)	Torsemide Loading Dose (mg)	Infusion Rate (mg/hr)
Renal insufficiency						
Moderate	40	20	1	1	20	10
Severe	40	40	1	2	20	20
Congestive heart failure						
Preserved renal function	40	10	1	0.5	20	5
Diminished renal function						
Moderate	40	20	1	1	20	10
Severe	40	40	1	2	20	20

only 50 mEq of sodium, then dosing three times a day would be needed. Alternatively, less frequent dosing would be possible if the patient decreased sodium intake to 100 mEq day. Frequent dosing of loop diuretics also decreases the time during which there is no drug at the site of action. During such times the nephron avidly reabsorbs sodium, causing rebound sodium retention. Unfortunately, noncompliance to sodium restriction is common, necessitating more frequent dosing of these diuretics than would otherwise be necessary.

A continuous intravenous infusion can be used to maximize response to a loop diuretic. Intravenous infusion maintains effective amounts of the diuretic at the site of action, thereby maximizing response and minimizing rebound sodium retention. If this strategy is pursued, dosages indicated in Table 21.6 are suggested. Importantly, a loading dose should be administered at the start of dosing and whenever the infusion rate is increased. If a loading dose is not given, 4 to 20 hours (four times the half-life of the chosen loop diuretic) is needed to reach steady state.

Large dosages of loop diuretics have been tried in patients with acute renal failure to "open up" the kidney, but there is no evidence of efficacy. Therefore there are no data to guide dosing. I prefer to administer no more than 500 mg furosemide intravenously or the equivalent of another loop diuretic. Such a dose should be given as an infusion over 20 to 30 minutes to avoid high peak concentrations that might cause ototoxicity. If this strategy is tried and the patient does not respond, there is no reason to administer a different loop diuretic because the pharmacology of all loop diuretics is the same.

Loop diuretics are also used to treat hypertension. Several studies demonstrate greater efficacy of thiazides than of furosemide in mild hypertension because the thiazides decrease peripheral vascular resistance as well as produce diuresis. On the other hand, low dosages of torsemide (2.5 to 5 mg) are effective as an antihypertensive agent with little or no diuretic effect.

Other renal effects of loop diuretics are used to treat hypercalcemia, hyponatremia, and occasionally renal tubular acidosis. The major site of calcium reabsorption is the thick ascending limb of Henle's loop (see Chapter 17, Part 2). Thus, by inhibiting solute reabsorption at this segment of the nephron, loop diuretics increase calcium excretion and are effective adjunctive therapy of hypercalcemia. Most patients with hypercalcemia are volume depleted, so the first step of therapy is volume replacement with saline. The saline diuresis in itself increases calcium excretion and is sufficient in most patients. If additional therapy is needed, loop diuretics plus replacement of fluid losses to maintain intravascular volume can be helpful.

Loop diuretics cause excretion of water in excess of sodium. Therefore replacement of loop diuretic–induced volume losses with isotonic or hypertonic saline results in a net gain of sodium relative to water, causing the serum sodium concentration to increase. The decision to use this strategy depends on the desired speed of hyponatremia correction.

In some patients with distal renal tubular acidosis who are unable to maintain an adequate systemic pH with conventional therapy, loop diuretics allow excretion of an acid urine and facilitate correction of the metabolic acidosis.

Toxicity

The majority of toxicity from loop diuretics is attributable to their effectiveness. The vigorous diuresis may result in volume depletion or potassium deficits. In addition, loop diuretics can cause both auditory and vestibular toxicity. This usually is associated with high dosages, particularly in patients with renal insufficiency and in those receiving other ototoxic compounds such as aminoglycoside antibiotics. This effect is reversible. Its mechanism is not well understood but is associated with loss of cochlear hair cells. Most clinicians believe that the risk of ototoxicity is greatest with ethacrynic acid, which accounts for its low use compared with other loop diuretics. With the other loop diuretics, it appears that ototoxicity is rare. Large dosages (e.g., 4 to 5 g/day furosemide) have been administered without ototoxic effects.

Allergic interstitial nephritis also occurs with chronic use of loop diuretics. This diagnosis should be entertained in historically stable patients chronically exposed to loop diuretics whose renal function begins to deteriorate. If the diagnosis is made and the patient still needs a loop diuretic, ethacrynic acid is the best alternative because it differs structurally, whereas the chemical structures of other loop diuretics are similar.

Thiazide Diuretics

Efficacy

Thiazide diuretics block electroneutral NaCl reabsorption at the distal convoluted tubule, connecting tubule, and early collecting duct. In sufficient concentrations, all thiazides inhibit carbonic anhydrase, but in clinically used dosages, any effect at the proximal tubule is negligible. Thiazides cause NaCl diuresis, and enhanced distal Na^+ delivery facilitates potassium secretion, so these drugs can also cause potassium depletion. Because the distal tubule reabsorbs only about 5% of filtered sodium, the maximal effect of thiazides is much less than that of loop diuretics. However, these drugs still are sufficient in most patients with mild edematous disorders unless they have concomitant renal dysfunction. In such cases, limited filtered sodium and diminished access of thiazides into the tubular lumen compromise efficacy, and loop diuretics are needed.

The thiazide diuretics have a very flat dose–response curve (Fig. 21.2). This means that there is little difference between the lowest dosage having any effect and the dosage having the greatest effect. Thus the starting dosage of a thiazide is 12.5 mg hydrochlorothiazide, or the equivalent of another agent, and the maximum dosage is 50 mg. Higher dosages result in no greater benefit but increase risks, particularly of potassium depletion and altered glucose and lipoprotein homeostasis.

Pharmacokinetics

Disposition of some of the thiazide diuretics has been defined in detail, whereas that of others has been studied little. Extensive clinical experience with this group of drugs has demonstrated their pharmacologic equivalence. Thus the maximal response to all is the same and they all have flat dose–response curves (Fig. 21.2). Because their potencies differ, different amounts are needed to achieve the same effect.

The major distinguishing features of thiazides are cost and duration of action. Costs vary between pharmacies; patients should be given the option of receiving the thiazide that is least expensive for them. In addition to cost, the duration of effect occasionally is a factor. However, duration of effect and elimination half-life are not always linked, and thiazides with short half-lives often have longer durations of action (Table 21.5). The reasons for this discrepancy are unclear. Thiazides usually are grouped according to short (6 to 12 hours), medium (12 to 24 hours), and long (more than 24 hours) durations of effect. It is best to use the drugs with short and medium half-lives because those with longer duration of effect usually cause more potassium loss.

Therapeutic Uses

Thiazide diuretics are the initial choice for most patients with edematous disorders if renal function is not impaired, but not all patients respond to these agents. If possible, a therapeutic trial of thiazides should be attempted before loop diuretics are used.

The greatest use of thiazide diuretics has been as antihypertensive agents. Initial dosages of a thiazide are associated with diuresis-induced decreases in blood volume and a consequent decrease in blood pressure. However, this decrease in blood volume triggers homeostatic reflexes such as plasma renin-angiotensin-aldosterone and sympathetic nervous system activation, which cause increased proximal tubule sodium reabsorption and restoration of blood volume. However, the antihypertensive effect is maintained because chronic use of these agents results in diminished peripheral vascular resistance. This effect, the mechanism of which is unknown, has made thiazide diuretics a mainstay of antihypertensive therapy. They are effective not only as single agents in patients with mild hypertension but also in multiple-drug therapy for patients with more severe disease. They are particularly useful for blunting the sodium retention that occurs with vasodilators.

The homeostatic reflexes that restore blood volume when thiazides are used to treat hypertension can be helpful in treating hypercalciuria and diabetes insipidus. Some patients with nephrolithiasis have idiopathically elevated urinary calcium excretion. Increased reabsorption of solute (including calcium) proximal to sites at which the thiazides act combined with increased distal reabsorption decreases calcium excretion and prevents renal stone formation. This effect also causes slight increases in serum calcium concentration. Thus although loop diuretics can be used to lower serum calcium, thiazide diuretics can increase it. Importantly, these effects are predictable based on the pharmacology of the drugs and the physiology of calcium homeostasis (see also Chapter 17, Part 2).

The increased proximal solute reabsorption associated with chronic thiazide use is accompanied by increased water reabsorption. In addition, the distal site at which thiazides act is responsible for generating a dilute urine. As a consequence, thiazide diuretics impair the ability to dilute the urine maximally. Patients with central diabetes insipidus generate a maximally dilute urine, which can result in urine volumes of up to 20 L/day. Using thiazides in such patients can diminish urinary output to half its pretreatment value, an effect sufficient to improve the quality of these patients' lives. Thus a diuretic agent in this setting is used to diminish urinary volume, a seemingly paradoxical effect.

Toxicity

As with other diuretics, much thiazide toxicity is predictable based on renal effects of these agents. The same mechanism that decreases urinary calcium excretion increases serum calcium concentrations that can mimic hyperparathyroidism. Similarly, urinary dilution impairment prevents patients who drink large volumes of hypotonic fluids from excreting them. Thus free water is retained and hyponatremia can occur. In fact, thiazide diuretics are the most common drug-induced cause of hyponatremia.

The mild volume depletion caused by thiazide diuretics results in increased proximal tubular reabsorption; thus thiazide administration can affect other cations that are transported in the proximal nephron. The major component of lithium reabsorption occurs at the proximal tubule. Long-term treatment with thiazides increases lithium reabsorption, decreasing its renal excretion and causing accumulation to potentially toxic concentrations. Therefore patients concomitantly treated with thiazides should be given lower dosages of lithium, and dosing should be guided by measured serum concentrations of lithium.

Thiazide diuretics also cause other adverse effects, the mechanisms of which are poorly understood. They disrupt glucose homeostasis. This usually occurs clinically in a patient with borderline blood glucose control who, with thiazide use, becomes sufficiently hyperglycemic to need oral hypoglycemic agents. Alternatively, a patient well maintained on oral agents may deteriorate after thiazide administration and need insulin. Some argue that this adverse effect is linked to potassium depletion and can thereby be prevented by maintaining potassium homeostasis. There seems to be little support for this hypothesis. Thiazides have also been implicated in increasing low-density lipoprotein cholesterol levels. This effect is dose related, and currently recommended antihypertensive dosages of thiazides have negligible effects on low-density lipoprotein cholesterol levels. Low dosages also have negligible effects on glucose, potassium, and magnesium homeostasis.

Potassium-Retaining Diuretics

Efficacy

In the distal nephron and collecting duct, sodium undergoes exchange with K^+ and H^+. This process depends on luminal entry into the cell of Na^+, a pathway blocked by amiloride and triamterene. Exchange of sodium for K^+ and H^+ also is stimulated by aldosterone. There are receptors for aldosterone in the cytoplasm of principal cells in this part of the nephron. Their interaction with aldosterone results in translocation of the hormone–receptor complex to the nucleus of the cell, where protein synthesis, presumably of Na^+ pumps, is stimulated. This entire sequence of events can be blocked by spironolactone, which blocks the receptor for aldosterone.

Thus there are two different mechanisms by which this class of drugs blocks Na^+ reabsorption. That for amiloride and triamterene is independent of aldosterone, whereas that for spironolactone requires the presence of mineralocorticoid. This latter mechanism of action is the rationale for specifically using spironolactone in patients with primary or secondary hyperaldosteronism. It should be apparent that the spironolactone dosage needed depends on the endogenous level of mineralocorticoid in each patient. Thus each patient must undergo titration until an effective dosage is reached. Because the mechanism of action involves protein synthesis blockade, spironolactone's duration of effect is 1 or more days, and plateau effects are not reached until 3 or 4 days of therapy. Therefore, during titration, dosages should not be increased more frequently than every 3 or 4 days. The spironolactone dosage usually used ranges between 25 and 100 mg; occasionally, higher dosages may be used.

The actions of amiloride and triamterene contrast with those of spironolactone. They are effective in the absence of mineralocorticoid and are shorter-acting, making daily dosage adjustments possible. These agents are preferable to spironolactone when a potassium-retaining diuretic is needed in a patient without mineralocorticoid excess. The dosages are 5 to 20 mg/day for amiloride and 100 to 200 mg/day for triamterene.

Because only a small amount of sodium is reabsorbed at the site of action of these agents, they are not sufficiently effective to benefit most patients (excluding those with mineralocorticoid excess). Their use, then, is to correct potassium or magnesium deficiency. The mechanism by which these drugs diminish magnesium excretion has not been fully elucidated.

Pharmacokinetics

Triamterene has a short half-life and duration of effect. Thus it must be dosed multiple times per day. Triamterene itself is not active, and it must be converted to its active metabolite by the liver. This process can be impaired in patients with liver disease, making this drug ineffective in such patients.

Amiloride has a long half-life. In patients with liver disease in whom an alternative to spironolactone is sought, amiloride is preferred over triamterene because metabolic activation is not needed. Amiloride can be administered twice a day, and steady-state effects occur in 2 days.

Although spironolactone has a short half-life, it appears that its activity resides primarily in several metabolites with half-lives of about 15 hours. In addition, the duration of effect is even longer (several days), as discussed earlier.

Therapeutic Uses

Potassium-retaining diuretics are most often used in combination preparations with thiazide diuretics. The rationale for these preparations is that the thiazide component causes renal potassium and magnesium losses, whereas the potassium-retaining agents have the opposite effect. Therefore the combination is presumed to have a neutral effect on potassium and magnesium excretion while lowering blood pressure. However, this rationale for combination products is flawed. First, only about 5% of patients receiving thiazide diuretics alone become potassium depleted. Thus the remaining 95% of patients do not need therapy with potassium-retaining diuretics. Second, potassium-retaining diuretics entail a risk of hyperkalemia, which may be more threatening than potassium depletion. This fact argues against their prophylactic use. Third, patients with a legitimate need for potassium-retaining diuretics often need amounts that are not available in fixed combination preparations. Thus these drugs should be titrated individually.

The most rational approach for using these drugs to maintain potassium and magnesium homeostasis is to use them only in patients who have become hypokalemic or hypomagnesemic. In these patients, potassium-retaining diuretics appear to be more effective at attaining and maintaining homeostasis of these cations than is exogenous replacement with supplements.

Although potassium-retaining diuretics occasionally are used in edematous disorders and hypertension, their weak diuretic effects are insufficient to cause a useful effect in most patients when used as single agents. In patients with excess aldosterone, the specific receptor antagonist spironolactone is the drug of choice. Such patients include those with mineralocorticoid-producing tumors, adrenal hyperplasia, renal artery stenosis, and cirrhosis. It must be titrated to a dosage sufficient to block endogenous aldosterone levels. Therefore the dosage is determined for each individual patient.

Overall, spironolactone is best used in patients with excessive mineralocorticoid effects. The most common clinical setting is the patient with cirrhosis and fluid retention. Spironolactone, amiloride, or triamterene can be used in patients with potassium or magnesium depletion. The long duration of action of spironolactone makes it more difficult to use in this setting, and the other two agents should be used as individual agents rather than in fixed combination with thiazides.

Toxicity

Use of potassium-retaining diuretics entails a predictable risk of hyperkalemia that can be life threatening. As discussed earlier, prophylactic use of these drugs to avoid potassium depletion cannot be justified.

Other settings increase the risk of hyperkalemia with these agents. Coadministering potassium supplements obviously increases the risk. Angiotensin-converting enzyme inhibitors and nonsteroidal antiinflammatory drugs also can cause hyperkalemia, and combined with potassium-retaining diuretics they probably are additive. Finally, patients with renal insufficiency have diminished ability to eliminate potassium; these diuretics are particularly risky in such patients and should be avoided.

Blockade of H^+ exchange for Na^+ by these drugs can cause type IV renal tubular acidosis. Patients may have an acid urine, but they cannot acidify maximally. They characteristically have a hyperchloremic metabolic acidosis with hyperkalemia. Patients with mild renal insufficiency or diabetes mellitus may be particularly susceptible.

Other adverse effects of potassium-retaining diuretics are not extensions of their pharmacologic effects. Rarely, the metabolite of triamterene can precipitate in concentrated urine and act as a nidus for stone formation. High spironolactone dosages have antiandrogenic effects and can cause gynecomastia. This occurs only rarely at conventional dosages.

Other Diuretics

Metolazone is another diuretic that acts on the early distal convoluted tubule. It binds preferentially to thiazide-sensitive receptors that are prominent in the luminal membrane of this segment of the nephron. This drug is very potent when given with a loop diuretic. It is given in a dosage of 2.5 to 20 mg/day. The major side effect of its use is hypokalemia.

Indapamide is an indoline derivative of chlorosulfonamide. It is a mild diuretic but a potent vasodilator. It is used in dosages of 1.25 to 2.5 mg/day to treat hypertension. It is effective in patients with diabetes mellitus, renal insufficiency, and even those treated with hemodialysis. At these dosages, there are almost no substantial effects on potassium, carbohydrate, or lipid metabolism.

DIURETIC COMBINATIONS

The use of potassium-retaining diuretics combined with other diuretics that cause potassium and magnesium losses was discussed earlier. Other diuretic combinations are used to obtain additive or even synergistic effects in patients who respond poorly to single agents. Such patients usually have severe disease (e.g., end-stage heart failure, severe renal insufficiency, severe cirrhosis with persistent ascites, and severe nephrotic syndrome). They have received maximum dosages of loop diuretics, yet sodium excretion is inadequate. If additional sites in the nephron can be blocked, a greater response can be achieved.

The most useful combination of agents for this purpose is that of a loop plus a thiazide diuretic or metolazone. Response to a loop diuretic alone can be blunted by increased reabsorption of sodium at sites distal to the thick ascending limb. In fact, chronic loop diuretic dosing causes hypertrophy of distal tubule cells with an enhanced capacity to reabsorb sodium. Blocking sodium reclamation at these distal sites with thiazide diuretics often increases response to a clinically important degree and can occasionally result in a pronounced diuresis in patients with little or no response to a loop diuretic alone.

Patients should be monitored carefully for volume and potassium status when such combinations are used. If a thiazide or metolazone is combined with loop diuretics in patients with renal insufficiency, it must be given in sufficient dosages to attain effective amounts in the lumen of the nephron. Dosages as high as 200 mg/day of hydrochlorothiazide or the equivalent of other thiazides may be needed. If a thiazide is to be used with a loop diuretic, any thiazide can be selected because their pharmacologies are similar and clinical trials have shown that many of them work similarly in this setting.

Some patients, particularly those with severe heart failure, have elevated proximal tubular reabsorption of sodium, which blunts response to more distally acting agents. Adding an agent with proximal effects such as acetazolamide can be a helpful adjunct to therapy in some patients. It is best to try combinations of thiazides and loop diuretics first and reserve acetazolamide for patients who are still unresponsive.

Distally acting potassium-retaining diuretics also can be used to enhance natriuretic effects. The effects are not as great as those of added thiazides, and this strategy should be used on top of loop diuretics and thiazides. Two studies have shown urinary electrolytes to be useful in predicting which patients will have an additive natriuresis when a distal agent is superimposed. Low Na^+ and K^+ predicts negligible response, whereas low Na^+ and high K^+ predicts response.

SUMMARY

Diuretics are effective for treating edematous disorders and hypertension, and adverse effects are primarily an extension of the pharmacologic characteristics of these agents. All except spironolactone must reach the urine to inhibit sodium reabsorption. Mannitol gains access by filtration at the glomerulus, whereas acetazolamide, loop diuretics, and thiazides are secreted actively by the organic acid transport pump. Amiloride and triamterene are similarly secreted but by the organic base pump.

Diuretics encompass a range of efficacy, with the loop diuretics being the most effective and potassium-retaining diuretics the least effective. Loop diuretics can cause excretion of about 20% of filtered sodium, and they retain their effectiveness in all but the most severe disease states.

Acetazolamide inhibits carbonic anhydrase and blocks sodium reabsorption at the proximal tubule. It causes $NaHCO_3$ diuresis. Mannitol inhibits sodium reabsorption in the proximal tubule and also in the thick ascending limb, causing NaCl diuresis. Loop diuretics block the Na^+-K^+-$2Cl^-$ reabsorptive pump at the thick ascending limb, causing NaCl diuresis and impairing the ability to concentrate the urine. Thiazide diuretics inhibit electroneutral NaCl reabsorption in the distal tubule, causing NaCl diuresis and impairing the ability to dilute the urine. These and all diuretics affecting more proximal sites cause K^+ loss concomitant with Na^+ loss. In contrast, the more distally acting, potassium-retaining diuretics cause K^+ accumulation. Of these diuretics, amiloride and triamterene are independent of aldosterone, whereas spironolactone is a competitive antagonist of this mineralocorticoid.

Most patients initially are treated with thiazide diuretics because they are effective, moderately potent, and inexpensive. Members of this class of drugs differ only in cost and duration of action. They have flat dose-response curves, so little dosage titration is needed. Patients with renal insufficiency and those not responding to thiazide diuretics are treated with loop diuretics, beginning with small dosages and titrating upward according to individual patient needs. Lack of response to ceiling dosages of loop diuretics warrants combining these and thiazide diuretics. Mannitol is used less as a diuretic than as a systemic osmotic agent to treat cerebral edema. Spironolactone is used primarily in patients with liver disease to reverse the secondary hyperaldosteronism associated with this disorder. Amiloride and triamterene are used primarily for patients who become potassium depleted from other more proximally acting diuretics. Knowledge of the pharmacology of diuretics coupled with the physiology of the nephron allows rational and predictable use of these agents.

DIURETIC RESISTANCE

For a variety of reasons, some patients seem to be resistant to the actions of diuretics. They can be divided into two categories: those with apparent (Table 21.7) and those with true resistance. In the former category are patients with poor compliance or those in whom the diuretic dosing intervals are too long. Furthermore, *ad libitum* sodium ingestion can frustrate even the most aggressive diuretic regimen.

The criteria for diuretic effectiveness are listed in Table 21.8. Failing to meet one or more of these criteria leads to true diuretic resistance. The causes of true diuretic resistance are listed in Table 21.9. For each of these causes, one or more of the diuretic effectiveness criteria listed in Table 21.8 has not been met. Diuretics may not reach their tubular sites of action for one or more of the following reasons: When given by mouth, their gastrointestinal absorption is reduced or delayed; their secretion into tubular lumen is reduced; or despite gaining entrance to the tubular lumen, their activity is impaired. Patients with severe CHF often exhibit problems with both absorption and secretion of the drug. The latter circumstance probably is related to circulatory abnormalities. Patients with anasarca can be shown to have gut wall edema and act as if this abnormality impedes drug absorption, often responding dramatically if intravenous diuretic is provided, even in a lower dosage than that

TABLE 21.7. Causes of Apparent Diuretic Resistance

Compliance problems
Patient failure to comply with the drug administration regimen
Patient failure to adhere to or physician failure to instruct the patient in reducing sodium intake
Infrequent diuretic administration, which allows rebound to occur

TABLE 21.8. Criteria for Diuretic Effectiveness

- Glomerular filtration that is not severely compromised
- Diuretic delivery to its site of action within the kidney
- Sodium delivery to the nephron segment at which the diuretic acts
- Responsiveness of the tubular site to the diuretic
- Absence of major reabsorption of rejected sodium ions at nephron sites distal to that of the diuretic's action

TABLE 21.9. Causes of True Diuretic Resistance

I. Failure of the diuretic to reach the tubular site of action in sufficient concentration to effect a natriuresis
  A. Reduced or delayed bioavailability
    1. Decreased or delayed gastrointestinal absorption
      a. Congestive heart failure
      b. Anasarca
    2. Reduced secretion of the diuretic into the tubular lumen
      a. Reduced glomerular filtration rate
        i. Acute or chronic renal failure
        ii. Circulatory compromise or inadequate arterial filling
          (a) Congestive heart failure
          (b) Advanced liver disease
      b. Advanced age
      c. Transplantation
    3. Reduced availability of the diuretic within the tubular lumen
      a. Nephrotic syndrome (protein binding of the drug)
II. Interference by other drugs with diuretic effects
  A. Nonsteroidal antiinflammatory drugs
  B. Captopril
  C. Other antihypertensives
  D. Cimetidine
III. Tubular adaptation to chronic diuretic administration
IV. Failure of the diuretic regimen to block transport at major sodium reabsorption sites

which failed when administered orally. As is the case with many drugs, older adults appear to respond differently to diuretics than do their younger counterparts. A group of patients who received kidney transplants have been reported to respond less well to furosemide than do other transplant recipients, probably because of a decreased ability to secrete the drug into the tubular lumen. In both animals and humans, the presence of large amounts of urinary protein has been found to interfere with the luminal bioavailability of furosemide, limiting the effectiveness of this diuretic in nephrotic syndrome.

Diuretics also are subject to interference from other pharmaceutical agents. The nonsteroidal antiinflammatory drugs reduce natriuresis after furosemide but not hydrochlorothiazide. Cimetidine interferes with the action of amiloride and triamterene, probably by impairing the tubular secretion of these agents. Finally, any antihypertensive agent that lowers renal blood flow and glomerular filtration rate can reduce diuretic effectiveness.

Investigations conducted over the past several years have documented the fact that chronic furosemide or hydrochlorothiazide administration to animals results in a tubular adaptation phenomenon that can manifest itself as resistance to the actions of these drugs when they are given individually. The mechanisms of this phenomenon include hypertrophy of the distal convoluted tubular cells and enhanced transport capacity of this nephron segment. Furthermore, in humans, this phenomenon can be overcome by adding an agent that inhibits sodium reabsorption in the early distal convolution and Henle's loop. This maneuver of sequential nephron blockade also is important in other clinical circumstances. For example, in patients in whom proximal tubular reabsorption appears to have been increased substantially, administering a diuretic that acts proximally in combination with a loop of Henle agent often results in a major natriuresis, whereas neither drug by itself is effective.

There are suggested therapeutic measures for patients in whom noncompliance with medication has been ruled out. First, one must ensure dietary sodium restriction. Usually, patients who begin to manifest diuretic resistance have been receiving drugs orally. If increasingly larger dosages of the drug have been ineffective, administration should be switched to the intravenous route. It is important to reduce the dosage. In patients who have been receiving large oral dosages of furosemide, for example, a brisk natriuresis may result from as little as 40 mg of the drug administered intravenously. On the other hand, there is probably little to be gained by giving a patient with moderately advanced renal failure 40 mg furosemide. Instead, a dosage of 80 mg or more or its equivalent (2 mg bumetanide or 100 mg ethacrynic acid) may be needed. Therapy must be individualized depending on the clinical circumstances and the patient's history of drug responsiveness. Some patients respond to one of the loop of Henle drugs and not others for reasons that are obscure. If no response occurs to the intravenous diuretic in 3 or 4 hours, then the dosage should be increased and the same process repeated in another 3 to 4 hours if necessary. Single bolus doses of furosemide of more than 200 to 240 mg (or their equivalents) are not recommended. Successful natriuresis has been reported with constant furosemide and bumetanide infusion when bolus administration has failed.

Selected Readings

Beermann B, Groschinsky-Grind M. Clinical pharmacokinetics of diuretics. *Clin Pharmacokinet* 1980;5:221–245.

This is a comprehensive compilation of diuretic pharmacokinetics. Although it was published in 1980, only a handful of additional diuretics have been developed since then so the data are still pertinent.

Better OS, Rubinstein I, Winaver JM, et al. Mannitol therapy revisited (1940–1997). *Kidney Int* 1997;51:886–894.

This recent comprehensive article reviews mannitol pharmacology and enumerates studies of its clinical efficacy. The complete reference list includes the primary literature on which the conclusions of this review are based.

Bonvalet JP. Regulation of sodium transport by steroid hormones. *Kidney Int* 1998; 53(Suppl 65):S49–S56.

This review discusses current understanding of the mechanisms of glucocorticoid effects on sodium transport. The mechanism of action of distal-acting potassium-retaining diuretics is discussed.

Brater DC. Resistance to loop diuretics: why it happens and what to do about it. *Drugs* 1985;30:427–443.

This review discusses pharmacokinetic and pharmacodynamic mechanisms of resistance to loop diuretics in edematous disorders. It emphasizes that mechanisms of resistance differ between different clinical conditions; one direct clinical application is in determining the maximum single dosage of a diuretic.

Chennavasin P, Seiwell R, Brater DC, et al. Pharmacodynamic analysis of the furosemide–probenecid interaction in man. *Kidney Int* 1979;16:187–195.

This study shows that it is urinary (or luminal) amounts of loop diuretic that correlate to response and that one feature of this response is the ability to define a dosage that maximizes response.

Dormans TPJ, Gerlag PGG, Russel FGM, et al. Combination diuretic therapy in severe congestive heart failure. *Drugs* 1998;55:165–172.

This brief review discusses the rationale for using combinations of diuretics and offers specific guidelines for drug and dosage selection.

Ellison DH. The physiologic basis of diuretic synergism: its role in treating diuretic resistance. *Ann Intern Med* 1991;114:886–894.

This review discusses the pathophysiology of diuretic resistance. It discusses the distal nephron hypertrophy that probably occurs with chronic use of loop diuretics.

Frelin C, Vigne P, Barbry P, et al. Molecular properties of amiloride action and its Na^+ transporting targets. *Kidney Int* 1987;32:785–793.

This review describes the physiology of the luminal sodium channel that is the site of action of amiloride. It also describes amiloride's mechanism of action.

Ginès P, Arroyo V, Rodés J. Pharmacotherapy of ascites associated with cirrhosis. *Drugs* 1992;43:316–332.

This review discusses the pathophysiology of and therapy for fluid accumulation in cirrhosis. In addition to discussing diuretic use, this article describes large-volume paracentesis and spontaneous bacterial peritonitis.

Martinez-Maldonado M, Cordova HR. Cellular and molecular aspects of the renal effects of diuretic agents. *Kidney Int* 1990;38:632–641.

This review discusses the molecular biology of the solute reabsorptive pathways inhibited by diuretics.

Martinez-Maldonado M, Eknoyan G, Suki WN. Diuretics in nonedematous states. *Arch Intern Med* 1973;131:797–808.

Although this review article is more than 25 years old, it is still relevant in its discussion of uses of diuretics for nondiuretic purposes. Importantly, this article describes these uses in terms of the linkage of renal physiology and pharmacology of different diuretics. These nondiuretic effects are predictable based on renal physiology.

Rose BD. Diuretics. *Kidney Int* 1991;39:336–352.

This article is a comprehensive review of diuretics that is clinically oriented in that it translates pharmacology and pathophysiology into therapeutic strategies.

CHAPTER 22

Idiopathic Edema

Charles R. Kleeman and Victoria L. Szatalowicz

Idiopathic edema is a condition in which a patient manifests edema or excessive weight gain secondary to salt and water retention, with no evidence of cardiac, renal, hepatic, nutritional, allergic, hypoproteinemic, obstructive venous, or lymphatic causes of edema. A mineralocorticoid excess syndrome secondary to bilateral adrenal hyperplasia or an adrenal or extraadrenal tumor should not be present. Likewise, hypothyroidism and hyperthyroidism should be excluded. The patient should not be taking any drugs that can cause sodium retention, such as adrenal glucocorticoids or mineralocorticoids, carbenoxalone, amantadine, indomethacin, methyldopa, estrogens, trimethadione, reserpine, large amounts of licorice or syrup of glycyrrhiza, or diuretics. Diuretic discontinuation can be followed by severe salt and water retention. Finally, cyclic edema of the menstrual period should be excluded.

CLINICAL AND BEHAVIORAL FEATURES

It has been suggested that this syndrome was first described in 1922 by Jungmann but first popularized and delineated in the English literature by Thorn in 1957. In 1968, at the Billing's Lecture before the annual convention of the American Medical Association, Thorn delineated the syndrome in greater detail and outlined what he thought were the pathophysiologic mechanisms underlying it. In this lecture he stated, "In establishing a diagnosis of idiopathic edema or cyclical swelling, three considerations are critical: 1) the demonstration of excessive weight gain or fluid retention; 2) the exclusion or organic disease known to predispose to edema formation; 3) evidence of a substantial psychological or emotional disturbance." The stress Thorn placed on the psychological aspects of the syndrome has been repeated by almost every writer on this subject, and from our own clinical experience with these patients this emphasis certainly is warranted. Various authors have referred to Thorn's calling the syndrome "psychlical" edema. Although we were unable to find this term in Thorn's 1968 article, it does underscore the conclusion many clinicians have made about these patients.

Another outstanding characteristic of the syndrome is the fact that almost all cases occur in women approximately 20 to 50 years old. Fewer than a dozen men have been reported in the medical literature to have had this condition. Idiopathic edema is never seen before menarche and very rarely does it start after the beginning of menopause. These statements can be qualified by the results of Dunnigan, reported in 1990, in which he observed 18 children (15 girls and 3 boys) presenting with clinical features of idiopathic edema starting between birth and 12 years of age, 16 of whom had a family history of idiopathic edema. If the syndrome does begin before menopause, it can continue afterward. Some have stated that idiopathic edema is related to abnormalities of estrogen and progesterone secretion and metabolism; however, it can be seen after total oophorectomy and it is not necessarily related to the far more common and readily treated cyclic edema of the menstrual period.

Further important characteristics generally are not described in the literature but are typical of the syndrome. First, the occurrence of idiopathic edema is related to the patient's socioeconomic status. In a questionnaire study, we found that 76% of the respondents, all of whom were practicing or academic physicians, had seen patients with the process in the preceding year. None of the patients were observed in the clinics serving indigent or low-income populations. Second, the patients almost always have active social or professional lives, often with much contact with the public, and pride themselves on their social and professional achievements. Third, the patients usually are attractive women with an unusual concern about their physical appearance.

History indicates years of going to different doctors with the complaint of "swelling all over," periorbital edema on arising, and increasing tightness of clothes as the day progresses. Patients often describe swelling of the hands, breasts, and abdomen. Their history is replete with years of therapy with diuretics, cathartics, and hormones. Rarely have they been instructed in the proper use of low-salt diets. It is not unusual to note symptoms and signs related to electrolyte disturbances and other complications of long-term excessive diuretic use. A common complaint is, "Every time I try to stop the diuretic, I blow up like a balloon and I feel terrible." This rebound often is called the picket fence effect. This phenomenon has been emphasized as a fundamental part of the syndrome, and great importance has been assigned to diuretic abuse as a cause of the syndrome. Often the patient complains of wide, unexplained weight swings ("Doctor, I can gain 10 pounds from morning to evening" or "Over a weekend, I will gain 20 pounds"). Invariably there is a long history of emotional symptoms, and problems often seem to manifest themselves when the patient is most aware of swelling, edema, and rapid weight gain. However, the same emotional disturbances may be present completely independent of the edema, as emphasized by Thorn.

Therapy must be directed at relieving the underlying emotional difficulties as well as correcting the excessive fluid retention. The resolution of edema cannot be expected to relieve symptoms significantly when the excessive fluid retention resulted from a fundamental psychological disturbance. Loss of edema fluid may improve physical comfort to some extent and may reduce overall irritability, but the physician cannot hope for significant or permanent improvement from this approach alone. Moreover, because the visible signs of the disorder may have enabled the patient to avoid social contacts or responsibilities, their removal without improvement in the basic cause may increase anxiety.

It is believed that the syndrome has not received the proper attention because of the psychological accompaniments. The patient with idiopathic edema apparently needs to overemphasize her symptoms, and this often evokes a negative transference and a degree of hostility on the part of the physician. Often, the patients are so demanding of help that they kindle feelings of aggression in the physician. In our experience, when patients are referred for psychotherapy, they almost invariably resist and often do not accept or improve under this therapy. Finally, they resist a psychophysiologic explanation of the syndrome.

The edema in these patients is worse in those with mild to moderate obesity, and it can be exaggerated by an upright posture. However, it is much more common to find a striking discrepancy between the physical findings of edema and the patient's complaint. Although visible edema, pitting or otherwise, may be lacking, the patient may insist that her eyes and face are puffy, that her breasts and stomach are swollen, and that her thighs and lower legs are stretched and aching. When blood pressure is measured in the lying and standing position, mild orthostatic hypotension may be observed. This is particularly true when diuretic- or cathartic-induced potassium depletion is present. Generally, the patient is sedentary, doing very little regular physical exercise.

On physical examination we usually see an attractive young or middle-aged woman, well groomed in all respects. If an inpatient, she almost never wears the usual unattractive hospital gown but instead wears more attractive garments. There may or may not be moderate pitting or nonpitting brawny tightness of the ankles or lower legs. Although the rest of the physical examination directly related to the syndrome is noncontributory, every effort must be made to look for organic causes of salt and water retention.

PATHOGENESIS

In reviewing the literature on this topic published from 1922 to 1998, we found more than 300 articles, of which nearly one-fourth were published in languages other than English, representing countries all over the world. Of interest, there were no reports of idiopathic edema in undeveloped countries. The English-language publications included single case reports and multipatient studies. To further investigate the demography of this process in a statistically meaningful manner, we chose certain criteria to select articles for more detailed analysis. These criteria included articles reporting more than 10 subjects with idiopathic edema and using any form of statistical analysis to evaluate the reported results. Twenty percent of the English-language articles met these criteria. Further review of these articles revealed that varying hypotheses have been made as to cause, but in only a small percentage of studies do the conclusions follow the findings. Lack of accurate case definition (i.e., alternative causes of edema not ruled out in study patients), lack of appropriate comparison groups, and lack of documented edema, weight gain, or loss in study subjects appear to be the three most common shortcomings in these selected articles. Thus it is no surprise that a clear pathophysiologic schema for the genesis and cause of idiopathic edema remains elusive.

Nonetheless, it appears that some of these patients actually do have true pitting or nonpitting edema and thus an abnormal interstitial accumulation of salt and water in various parts of their bodies. Because rapid weight gains can be observed at times, we must conclude that regardless of whether primary pathophysiologic event is at the capillary and interstitial tissue level (i.e., disturbed Starling equilibrium) or at a more central location (i.e., central nervous system, circulatory system, primary abnormal secretion of an adrenal or ovarian mineralocorticoid), it is clearly causing an inappropriate renal retention of salt and water. However, what is both impressive and frustrating is the striking disparity between the history of intractable edema, body swelling, and weight gains of unbelievable rapidity and magnitude and the minimal degree of objective findings and abnormal changes when the patient is followed closely in the hospital. This latter observation could mean either that the patient has a nonobjective, exaggerated impression of her "abnormalities" or that the hospital setting affords a protective environment in which the nonhomeostatic psychophysiologic reactions do not occur.

In most instances, we admit patients only after a prolonged period of abstinence from diuretics, cathartics, and crash diets and with the stepwise liberalization of sodium intake described later in this chapter. In contrast, when some patients have been studied too soon after discontinuing diuretic use (a few days to a week or so) or the patient has been unable to adhere to the prescribed regimen, we have observed various and inconsistent "defects" in water and salt excretion and often uninterpretable hormone measurements. It is apparent that long-term use of a diuretic, with its salt wasting effects, brings into play a host of physiologic and pathophysiologic consequences such as increased aldosterone and antidiuretic hormone, decreased atrial natriuretic peptide and dopamine, increased epinephrine and norepinephrine with stimulation of the sympathetic nervous system, mild reduction in renal dynamics, and reduction in effective arterial filling volume with peripheral vasodilation. In this setting, discontinuing the diuretic will causes immediate renal retention of salt and proportionate amounts of water, which may last many days. The higher the salt intake when the diuretic is discontinued, the greater the positive salt and water balance and therefore weight gain.

To elucidate the fundamental pathophysiologic mechanisms, we must first eliminate the influences of such iatrogenic factors as diuretics, cathartics, therapeutic agents, and crash diets with variable amounts of carbohydrates. A careful review of the literature on idiopathic edema indicates that few investigators have taken these precautions, which we consider essential prerequisites to careful inpatient or outpatient study of these patients. In fact, proper controls for such patients would be other women without the syndrome who not only have been matched for age, weight, and socioeconomic background but also have agreed to take comparable dosages of diuretics, with and without potassium, for a number of weeks before study when the study patients have a clear history of diuretic use.

Table 22.1 lists the various postulated mechanisms, some of which have not been shown convincingly to be responsible for the syndrome (mechanisms 1 and 2) and some of which have not been investigated (mechanisms 3, 4, and 5). If a given patient, studied under the most rigorous conditions as described earlier, still clearly demonstrates abnormal tissue and renal retention of plasm ultrafiltrate, then it is our intuitive impression

TABLE 22.1. Postulated Mechanisms Responsible for Idiopathic Edema

1. Primary excess secretion of aldosterone or some other undetermined mineralocorticoid.
2. Secondary hyperaldosteronism with elevated renin and angiotensin levels resulting from a reduction of effective arterial filling volumes relative to the degree of arterial tree dilation (capacity).
   a. Plasma albumin abnormality with excessive turnover, decrease in albumin pool, and hypoalbuminemia.
   b. Increased capillary permeability with albumin leak, leading to a fall in plasma and a simultaneous rise in interstitial colloid osmotic pressure.
   c. Circulatory inadequacy with orthostatic blood pooling in the lower extremities, leading to excessive plasma volume reduction followed by inappropriate rise in renin and aldosterone and inappropriate decrease in the glomerular filtration rate and sodium and water retention.
3. Basic abnormality of Starling equilibrium conditions at the capillary level, resulting in a net excess of interstitial volume (pitting and nonpitting edema).
   a. Abnormal regulation of precapillary arteriolar or postcapillary venular sphincters.
   b. Inadequate function of the lymphatics as regulators or interstitial volume.
4. Fundamental defect in tissue prostaglandins; relative balance of a- and b-adrenergic and cholinergic influences at the capillary level; failure of appropriate atrial natriuretic hormone, Na^+-K^+-adenosine triphosphatase inhibitor, or dopamine generation; imbalance of peptide to nonpeptide hormones, affecting renal tubular sodium reabsorption; or excess interleukin production.
5. A basic psychophysiologic disorder in which a primary behavioral problem causes one or more of the preceding physiologic abnormalities.

TABLE 22.2. Drugs Causing Peripheral Edema

Antidepressants
- Monamine oxidase inhibitors

Antihypertensive drugs
- β-Blockers
- Calcium channel blockers
- Clonidine (Catapres)
- Diazoxide (Proglycem)
- Guanethidine (Esimil, Ismelin)
- Hydralazine (Apresoline, Hydra-Zide)
- Methyldopa (Aldoclor, Aldomet)
- Minoxidil (Loniten)
- Reserpine (Diupres, Rogoton, Salutensin)

Hormones
- Corticosteroids
- Estrogen
- Progesterone
- Testosterone

Nonsteroidal antiinflammatory drugs

Adapted from Ciocon JO, Fernandez BB, Ciocon DG. Leg edema: clinical clues to differential diagnosis. *Geriatrics* 1993;48(5):34-40, 45, copyright Advanstar Communications Inc.; and Kraytman M. *The complete patient history.* New York: McGraw-Hill, 1979:49.

that mechanisms 3 and 5 (Table 22.1) will be found to be responsible. Note that we did not include a defect in water excretion per se in our discussions or in Table 22.1. The fact that these patients never have hyponatremia or hyposmolality, unless clearly caused by a diuretic, is a definite indication that free water is handled in an appropriately homeostatic manner.

DIAGNOSTIC EVALUATION

Evaluating the patient with idiopathic edema is best performed in a hospital or clinical research center, if possible. This enables a systematic and rapid search for all other causes of edema, including the drugs listed earlier and in Table 22.2. Although it is simple to rule out the usual causes of edema, other, more unusual or subclinical causes of periodic edema or abnormal salt and water retention may occur. The latter may be observed in subclinical hypothyroidism or low thyroid reserve. Also, on rare occasions a pituitary or ectopic tumor source of adrenocorticotrophic hormone (ACTH) or ACTH-releasing factor may cause a sudden surge of cortisol, deoxycorticosterone, or aldosterone, which leads to acute episodes of salt and water retention and overt edema. These disorders can be confused easily with idiopathic edema.

These patients almost invariably appreciate the admission to the hospital when it is accompanied by the doctor's explanation that a very intense metabolic investigation will be done to search for a hormonal or other organic cause of their condition. However, hospitalization is of no value if the patient is not properly prepared for a number of weeks before admission.

The patient must be instructed very clearly that no proper study can be done as long as she is taking diuretics or the drugs mentioned earlier and in Table 22.2 and that her physician intends to follow her closely for a month to 6 weeks before hospitalization. The patient is told how chronic diuretic use calls into play all the body's mechanisms for sodium and water retention and that these will be unmasked as soon as the diuretic is stopped. In other words, it is explained to the patient that unless diuretic discontinuation is accompanied by rigid dietary sodium restriction, there will invariably be a striking salt and water retention and a very rapid weight gain. The patient has often experienced this phenomenon herself and therefore may argue that she cannot get along without the diuretic. It is best to place the patient on a 1 g/day sodium diet, which is continued for a number of days, and the patient is seen by the physician at the end of this time for physical examination, reassurance, and a spot check of the urine sodium to determine adherence to the diet. After this, there can be a slow and gradual liberalization of the sodium content of the diet up to the time of admission if the latter proves necessary. As mentioned earlier, this regimen may take as long as 6 weeks. If there are any signs, symptoms, or laboratory manifestations of magnesium or potassium depletion or alkalosis, these should be corrected. They usually correct themselves spontaneously when the patient is off diuretics and adhering to the low-sodium regimen. By the time of admission, it is anticipated that the patient will be ingesting a diet that contains at least 3 g/day of sodium, thus approaching a normal sodium intake. In addition to the weighing in the doctor's office, the patient is asked to keep a careful record of morning and evening weights and diary of symptoms. The patient with a true abnormality in salt and water handling usually shows a weight gain from morning to evening of at least 2.0 kg on most days. As noted by Dunnigan, a lesser increase can lead to overdiagnosis. Normal women usually gain no more than 0.6 to 0.8 kg over the same period. Blood and urine electrolytes and creatinine are checked once weekly. The patient is given the maximum encouragement throughout this period and is congratulated for abstaining from diuretics and adhering to the sodium-restricted diet. Assuming that this has been achieved, the patient is admitted into the hospital.

Instead of allowing the patient to spend ad libitum time in bed, she is instructed to spend as many hours a day out of bed as she would on the outside, sitting, walking, exercising in the hospital, and being recumbent only when sleeping in the evening or at specific times ordered by the physician. All the usual causes of edema should be ruled out as quickly as possible. Surreptitious use of diuretics in the hospital should be monitored specifically.

Before and during admission, the patient is weighed twice daily, on arising and before going to bed. On selected days, urine should be collected at 12-hour intervals (i.e., 7 AM to 7 PM and 7 PM to 7 AM) to note any abnormality in the diurnal pattern of water, sodium, chloride, potassium, and creatinine excretion. After a few days of inpatient study, the effect of orthostasis or the upright position on creatinine clearance [glomerular filtration rate (GFR)], electrolyte excretion, and the ability to excrete a standard water load is studied. This is done over a 5-hour period beginning at 8 AM while withholding breakfast. During the first hour (8 AM to 9 AM), a blood sample is taken as painlessly as possible and the first hourly urine is collected. The patient then drinks a liter of water over 10 to 20 minutes and four additional hourly collections of urine are analyzed for volume, for creatinine, sodium, potassium, and chloride concentrations, and for osmolality. On the first day this test is done, the patient reclines in bed or combines this with sitting quietly by the bedside throughout the 5 hours. The next day, the entire procedure is repeated but throughout the 5 hours the patient remains ambulatory, walking around her room or the ward corridor. Thus we have a measure of orthostatic stress on GFR and water and solute excretion in the patient. However, as mentioned earlier, whatever abnormality of water excretion is observed, it is not sustained enough to result in hyposmolality or hyponatremia in these patients. In the blood samples taken on the first and last day of the test, plasma cortisol, aldosterone, and renin also are measured to evaluate the impact of the upright position and ambulation on their concentrations. On selected samples of blood taken during the hospitalization, plasma albumin concentration is measured to rule out any possibility of hypoalbuminemia contributing to the syndrome. If hypoalbuminemia is found, it may be necessary to study the albumin pool and albumin turnover and the rate of albumin loss from the circulation. After these studies, the sodium content of the diet should be doubled to determine the patient's ability to cope with increasing amounts of dietary salt. By the time of discharge, the patient must feel that she has had a complete diagnostic evaluation. This workup should be necessary only in a small group of selected patients.

Many patients, when admitted and evaluated under these circumstances, do not demonstrate any specific abnormality in water and salt metabolism or in the metabolic measurements. In the remaining patients, some tendency toward unusual orthostatic drops in GFR can be observed, and mild defects in handling increasing loads of sodium with the production of mild peripheral edema may be demonstrated. Of the many patients hospitalized and studied in this manner, only a small number demonstrate a serious defect in salt and water excretion and develop exaggerated weight gains and overt peripheral edema. In some, the weight gain from morning to evening exceeds the usual 0.6 to 0.8 kg observed in women of comparable age but without this syndrome.

In summary, we have been more impressed with the absence of any metabolic, cardiovascular, or renal abnormality than with their presence. After performing an in-depth evaluation, we stress to the patient that long-term prevention depends on a permanent change in dietary, weight management, exercise, and drug ingestion habits.

TREATMENT AND LONG-TERM CARE

Treating this difficult syndrome takes great patience, compassion, understanding, and gentle firmness on the part of the physician, and the patient must trust the physician's ability to help her. At the same time, she must be highly motivated to overcome this syndrome with its many distressing symptoms. Because the exact cause of the syndrome is unknown, it is very difficult to formulate specific therapy. However, from our experience and that of others, we believe that success can be achieved with a firm and positive approach that uses few, if any, drugs. A fundamental aspect of management is total abstinence from diuretic use. Of the many publications on idiopathic edema, it is amazing how few are willing to approach therapy without using diuretics. Intermittent edema of unknown cause in most otherwise healthy women seems to result from their use of diuretics, abetted in some patients by self-imposed fluctuations in sodium and carbohydrate intake, and does not appear to be idiopathic. It is clear that recovery cannot be achieved with the continued use of diuretics, although it should be pointed out that cases of idiopathic edema were described before diuretics became widely used.

Some of these patients may benefit from the continued use of such sympathomimetic amines as ephedrine, dextroamphetamine (Dexedrine), and amphetamine sulphate (Benzedrine). Their mechanism of action in this syndrome is unknown. They may have a direct effect on the central nervous system or a peripheral action on the precapillary or postcapillary sphincters. This action might correct a defect in transcapillary fluid exchange, which may be a more fundamental step in salt and water retention. In a study of 16 patients with idiopathic edema, urinary dopamine excretion was lower than in normal subjects. Dopamine generation from the nervous system or the dopaminergic system of the kidney may play an important role in renal sodium excretion and in precapillary and postcapillary sphincter control and the body's ability to eliminate acute and chronic salt loads. Dopamine also negatively modulates adrenal aldosterone secretion. Oral analogs of dopamine may be available for study, and they certainly should be tried in the idiopathic edema syndrome. The dopaminergic agonist bromoergocryptine has been used successfully in a small number of cases, but the gastrointestinal side effects often are prohibitive. In certain cases patients may show hyperreninemic hyperaldosteronism or secondary hyperaldosteronism. The use of angiotensin-converting enzyme inhibitors may result in weight loss and symptomatic improvement.

If the patient is overweight, a reducing diet low in salt should be prescribed. It may be better to use a diet that contains less carbohydrate and therefore has less tendency to cause renal salt and water retention. Crash diets are forbidden. The patient should visit her physician every few weeks. The physician will use this visit for reassurance, brief office psychotherapy, and measurement of urine and serum electrolytes and, in some cases, perform a diuretic screening to determine whether the patient is adhering to the dietary regimen and abstaining from the use of diuretics. Because the patient leaves the hospital or outpatient workup on a diet containing no more than 2 g/day of sodium, the physician outlines a plan for a gradual return to a diet of normal sodium content over approximately 6 months. The patient must be given the opportunity to learn about low-salt cooking. The rate of liberalization of the diet depends on the patient's course from week to week. There must be an aggressive plan of physical activity, physical rehabilitation, and exercise, with special emphasis on developing the leg muscles and conditioning the cardiovascular system. The development of good leg musculature increases pumping action on the veins and lymphatics and thus contributes greatly to the return of excess interstitial fluid to the circulation. The tendency toward orthostatic drops in blood pressure and renal hemodynamics can be minimized by this type of cardiovascular conditioning. The patient continues to weigh herself morning and evening and to keep a diary of these weights. The primary physician continues a psychosocial evaluation and superficial psychotherapy with each visit. The physician can enlist the help of a psychiatrist if the patient is willing. In all, the patient should feel that she and her doctor are partners working toward her rehabilitation.

Selected Readings

Anderson GH Jr, Streeten DH. Effect of posture on plasma atrial natriuretic hormone and renal function during salt loading in patients with and without postural (idiopathic) edema. *J Clin Endocrinol Metab* 1990;71(1):243–246.

The first report of a possible role of atrial natriuretic hormone as a possible etiologic factor in the syndrome. These authors found no association.

Bader KF. Idiopathic edema. In: Brenner BM, Stein JH, eds. *Body fluid homeostasis.* Vol 13. New York: Churchill-Livingstone, 1987:357.

An excellent review of the possible causes of this syndrome. Rather light on clinical description.

Denning DW, Dunnigan MG, et al. The relationship between "normal" fluid retention in women and idiopathic edema. *Postgrad Med J* 1990;66:363–366.

Excellent study in which authors examine the syndrome from an epidemiologic point of view and shed new light on the subject.

Edwards OM, Bayliss RIS. Idiopathic edema of women. A clinical and investigative study. *Q J Med* 1976;45:124–144.

The first careful attempt to delineate postural effects on plasma volume in these patients and to compare the findings with those in matched normal subjects. The authors also give an outstanding description of the clinical syndrome.

Kuchel O, Cuche JL, Buu NP, et al. Catecholamine excretion in "idiopathic" edema: decreased dopamine excretion a pathogenic factor? *J Clin Endocrinol Metab* 1977;44:639.

An interesting investigation of catecholamine metabolism in these patients, with emphasis on dopamine excretion. Idiopathic edema syndrome treatment is discussed.

MacGregor GA, Markander ND, Roulston JE, et al. Is "idiopathic" edema idiopathic? *Lancet* 1979;1:397–400.

The first authors to discuss the possible role of diuretics in this syndrome. Although the authors were too all-inclusive of all cases of idiopathic edema under a diuretic withdrawal etiology, they did emphasize the striking weight gains observed in these patients after diuretic withdrawal.

Paller MS, Ferris TF. Idiopathic edema. In: Dirks JH, Sutton RAL, eds. *Diuretics: physiology, pharmacology, and clinical use.* Vol. 10. Philadelphia: WB Saunders, 1986:192.

An in-depth review of the syndrome and a collation of all laboratory investigations and theories up to the date of its publication.

Rovner DR. The enigma of idiopathic cyclic edema. *Hosp Pract* 1972(April): 103–110.

A detailed study of the behavior of patients with idiopathic edema, including an outline of a systematic approach to workup.

Streeten DHP. Idiopathic edema: pathogenesis, clinical features and treatment. *Metabolism* 1978;27:353–383 and *Curr Ther Endocrinol Metab* 1997;6:203–206.

These reports represent some of the most in-depth investigations of water, electrolytes, and neural and humoral abnormalities in this syndrome, with a recent update.

Thorn GW. Approach to the patient with "idiopathic edema" or "periodic swelling." *JAMA* 1968;206:333–338 and *Am J Med* 1957;23:507–550.

The first authentic descriptions of this disorder. They are classics and should be read by all.

CHAPTER 23

Defects of Renal Tubular Transport

Russell W. Chesney and Antonia C. Novello

All disorders of renal tubular transport reflect a reduction in the net tubular accumulation of ions or organic solutes. Defects in tubular transport can be single or complex and may result from the absence of a specific membrane transport protein or from alterations in tubular epithelium that reduce solute reabsorption. Although most tubular transport disorders have a genetic basis, the transport disorder may be secondary to a particular disease. For example, some metabolite accumulated in the tubule, such as galactose-1-phosphate in galactosemia and fructose-1-phosphate in fructose intolerance, may exert a toxic effect on renal tubular epithelial cells. An alteration caused by a primary net transport defect or a secondary cause will be similar, so hyperexcretion of a particular compound says little about the cause of the disorder.

Renal tubular disorders seem to be diffuse because carbohydrates, amino acids, divalent and monovalent ions, and ketoacids may be lost singly or in groups. Nonetheless, several underlying precepts prevail in these disorders.

- All tubular disorders involve some abnormality of the transport function of the kidney and often of the transport function of the intestine. In general, a transport protein or ion channel is affected.
- Tubular disorders demonstrate the point that the nephron site of the defect defines the alteration of transport function. To know the characteristics of the disease, one must know the function of the nephron site that is impaired.
- Most tubular transport disorders are inherited and involve the loss of a transport protein or an inborn error of metabolism.
- Because many of these transporter proteins and ion channels have been cloned, the precise genetic defect can now be understood in several instances.
- Diseases that perturb energy production of the tubular cell or alter the structural integrity of the nephron result in global or complex transport disorders, such as Fanconi's syndrome, rather than simple disorders.
- The principles of therapy are straightforward and involve replacing the substance lost in the urine, replacing the missing vitamin, or avoiding the toxic substances.
- The replacement therapy dosage relates to the nephron site altered by the disorder. If the site altered is responsible for bulk reabsorption (e.g., the proximal tubule for bicarbonate), then larger dosages are needed than at a site with less reclamation of the lost solute.

Examples of these points are demonstrated for the individual disorders discussed in this chapter.

DISORDERS OF CARBOHYDRATE TRANSPORT

Melituria (glucosuria) results from defective proximal tubule transport or, more commonly, from overflow related to an abnormality of carbohydrate metabolism. Diabetes mellitus is the prime example of the latter type of disorder; the complex prevailing metabolic alterations result in a filtered glucose load that exceeds reabsorptive capacity, leading to an overflow glucosuria.

Pentosuria

The several pentosurias also represent an overflow type of melituria. Essential pentosuria is an inborn error of glucuronic acid metabolism found mainly in Jews, inherited as an autosomal-recessive disorder. About 1 to 4 g L-xylulose appears daily in the urine of affected patients because nicotinamide adenine dinucleotide phosphate–linked xylitol dehydrogenase is reduced and xylulose is not converted to xylitol. Excessive intake of fruit or fruit-flavored candy can result in excessive L-arabinose and L-xylose excretion. D-Ribose hyperexcretion may follow abnormal release of this pentose from muscle in subjects with muscular dystrophy. Finally, the autosomal-recessive disorder essential fructosuria results from reduced activity of fructokinase, the enzyme responsible for phosphorylating fructose at the 1-carbon position. These disorders are detected only by the use of tests for urinary reducing substances, not by glucose oxidase–impregnated test strips. Each of these pentosurias is clinically benign.

Renal Glucosuria

The two autosomal-recessive disorders of hexose transport are unrelated to abnormalities of carbohydrate metabolism. These include primary renal glucosuria, in which a moderate urinary loss of glucose is present, and glucose–galactose malabsorption, with only trivial amounts of glucose lost in the urine. The gene defect in familial glucosuria is in SGLT-2 or the low-affinity, high-capacity glucose transporter. Defective SGLT-1, or the high-affinity glucose–galactose transporter, is defective in glucose–galactose malabsorption.

Primary Renal Glucosuria

Primary renal glucosuria is defined as a state of constant glucosuria without hyperglycemia, ketosis, or other meliturias. It represents a transport defect in either the brush border mem-

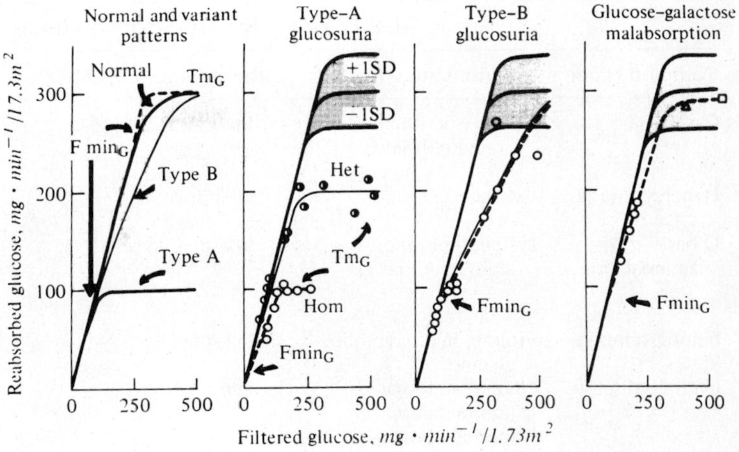

Figure 23.1. Glucose titration curves demonstrating the maximal transport rate (T_{mG}) and the venous plasma threshold (*Fmin*$_G$). The *left panel* depicts both the normal pattern and the pattern in the two variants of renal glucosuria (type A and type B). The *right panel* shows the situation in the inborn errors of hexose transport. *Gray area* represents ±1 standard deviation. Het, heterozygous; Hom, homozygous. (Reprinted with permission from Scriver CR, Chesney RW, McInnes RR. Genetic aspects of renal tubular transport: diversity and topology of carriers. *Kidney Int* 1976;9:149–171.)

brane or the transtubular reabsorptive process for glucose. The glomerular filtration rate (GFR) and intestinal absorption of hexoses are normal in this disorder.

The genetic pattern in renal glucosuria is autosomal-recessive, although glucosuria in heterozygotes has led some investigators to postulate a dominant inheritance. Two forms of this disorder have been described. The type A variant represents a reduction in both the renal threshold for glucose and the maximal rate of glucose reabsorption (T_{mG}). Patients with type B glucosuria have a low renal threshold for glucose but a normal T_{mG}. The principal distinction between types is that patients with type A have massive glucosuria at low plasma glucose concentrations, whereas patients with type B have some glucosuria at low plasma glucose levels, but reabsorption is normal at high levels (Fig. 23.1). A glucose infusion test must be performed to distinguish these types, and clear-cut differences are not always evident, particularly in children.

A possible but unproven pathogenetic mechanism for these two types is that type A glucosuria represents a reduction in the number of membrane transport sites, and type B represents a reduced affinity of the carrier for glucose. Type A glucosuria can be evident as part of the complex tubulopathies, particularly Fanconi's syndrome, whereas type B usually is isolated but may be found in glucoglycinuria or glucosuria with renal hyperphosphaturia. Furthermore, a separation into types A and B may be conjectural because both forms have been found in a single pedigree. An alternative interpretation is that the point mutation of the transporter gene defines the clinical form.

Glucosuria usually is found on routine urinalysis and presumably starts at birth. No clinical manifestations are apparent, and polyuria is not found. The differential diagnosis includes diabetes mellitus and other forms of melituria. A glucose tolerance test proves normal in renal glucosuria, and the glucose oxidase paper strip test can distinguish pentosuria or galactosuria. The glucosuria of uremia is ruled out by normal renal function. No therapy is indicated from this harmless disorder, and dietary restriction of carbohydrates does not alter urinary glucose excretion.

Glucose–Galactose Malabsorption

Glucose–galactose malabsorption is manifested predominantly in the intestine, where jejunal transport is impaired. Renal hexose transport is minimally impaired (Fig. 23.1). A low renal threshold for glucose is found with normal glucose T_{mG} values, as in type B glucosuria, but even less glucose is lost. The high-affinity, low-capacity shared (glucose–galactose) transporter is affected. Galactosuria is not found under usual circumstances because there is no impairment of carbohydrate metabolism. The main symptom is diarrhea after eating carbohydrate-containing foods. Patients with this disorder mimic people with gut disaccharidase deficiency.

DISORDERS OF AMINO ACID TRANSPORT

Amino acids also are reabsorbed in the proximal tubule by at least five major shared transport systems: cyclic and neutral amino acids and glycine, dibasic amino acids, dicarboxylic amino acids, and β-amino acids (Table 23.1). Amino acid reabsorption usually reaches 98% to 99.5% of the filtered load, so aminoaciduria is readily detectable by various chromatographic techniques. Transport defects usually represent an abnormality of one of these shared sites. Nonetheless, specific transport processes for individual amino acids must exist because the isolated hyperexcretion of individual amino acids including threonine, glycine, and cystine has been reported. In addition, an overflow type of aminoaciduria is evident in phenylketonuria, histidinemia, hemocystinuria, maple syrup urine disease, and ketotic hyperglycinemia, in which mutations in amino acid catabolism lead to prerenal hyperaminoacidemia. At least 20 types of overflow aminoaciduria have been described, with evidence of tubular competition between groups seen in such disorders as hyper-β-alaninemia and hyperprolinemia.

Cystinuria

Cystinuria involves a defect in dibasic amino acid transport affecting mainly the epithelial cells of the renal tubule and the gastrointestinal tract. The defective transport is transmitted as an autosomal-recessive trait; it occurs equally in both sexes, but boys are more generally affected and have a higher mortality rate. The heterozygous state may reflect a true recessive or incompletely recessive state in which the affected amino acids are excreted in greater quantities than normal but in lower quantities than in the homozygous state.

Cystinuria is a complex transport disorder in which the sulfur-containing amino acid is excreted in excess quantities, which, because of cystine's relative insolubility, results in stone formation. First described in 1810 by Wollaston, cystinuria usually is characterized by hyperexcretion of cystine and the dibasic amino acids ornithine, arginine, and lysine. At least five forms of this autosomal-recessive inborn error of transport have segregated:

TABLE 23.1. Inborn Errors of Renal Tubular Amino Acid Transport

Common Name	Amino Acids Affected	Other Membranes Affected	Inheritance	Transport Site Altered	Salient Clinical Features
Cystinuria	Cystine, ornithine, arginine, lysine	Intestine, CNS?	AR	Shared cystine–dibasic system	Renal stones, decreased height, renal failure resulting in stones
Hypercystinuria	Cystine	Unknown	AR	Isolated cystine and cysteine system	Renal stones
Dibasic aminoaciduria	Lysine, ornithine, arginine (dibasic)	Intestine, liver?, CNS?	AR or AD	Isolated dibasic group system	Type I hyperammonemia Type II mental retardation with aminoaciduria in heterozygotes
Iminoglycinuria	Proline, hydroxyproline, glycine	Intestine	AR	Shared imino acid and glycine system	Benign trait
Hartnup disease	Neutral amino acids (monoamino-monocarboxylic)	Intestine	AR	Shared system for neutral and aromatic amino acids	Pellagra resulting from tryptophan malabsorption
Dicarboxylic aminoaciduria	Glutamic, aspartic (dicarboxylic)	Intestine	AR	Shared dicarboxylic system	
β-Aminoaciduria	Taurine, β-alanine, β-aminoisobutyric	Unknown	—	Shared α-amino acid system	Not described in humans Inborn error in mice

Adapted from Scriver CR, Chesney RW, McInnes RR. Genetic aspects of renal tubular transport: diversity and topology of carriers. *Kidney Int* 1976;9:149–171.
AD, autosomal dominant; AR, autosomal recessive; CNS, central nervous system.

- Isolated hypercystinuria.
- Type I or classic cystinuria, with absent intestinal cystine, lysine, and arginine transport and normal urinary excretion (silent carriers) of dibasic amino acids by heterozygotes. The gene defect in classic cystinuria involves a single point or deletion mutation of COLA, the dibasic amino acid transporter. This transporter is called *SLC3A1* in humans and its gene is found on chromosome 2.
- Type II, with absent gut lysine transport and dibasic aminoaciduria in heterozygotes.
- Type III, with intact gut transport and urinary hyperexcretion of dibasic amino acid by heterozygotes. This gene is on chromosome 19.
- Cystine–lysinuria, which could represent heterozygotes of types II and III.

The homozygous state has three defined types of cystinuria, which result from allelic mutations. Thus cystinuria is inherited as an autosomal-recessive trait, with at least three different alleles. A variable expression may occur in the first year of life, but the second and third decades are the peak times of its appearance. Detection of cystinuria in the first 6 months of life is difficult because amino acid excretion is increased in infants because of renal tubular immaturity. Screening by DNA analysis recently has been shown to be useful.

The precise membrane location for the defect in cystine and dibasic amino acid transport is unknown. The uptake of these amino acids by renal slices from patients with cystinuria is essentially normal, and both cystine and dibasic amino acids are accumulated by independent transport processes. There is also a shared transport site in the luminal membrane, but a loss of this site could not account for the negative reabsorption of dibasic amino acids (indicative of secretion) found in some patients. It has been speculated that efflux out of the cell at the basolateral membrane is impaired, resulting in backflux of amino acids into urine from the intracellular dibasic amino acid pool. Such a mechanism could account for both decreased reabsorption and net secretion.

Excessive urinary losses of cystine and dibasic amino acids occur with normal or less than normal plasma levels of the affected amino acids. Although the transport mechanism defective in cystinuria has been reported to be shared by cystine and the dibasic amino acids, reports of atypical clinical disorders have questioned this interpretation and indicate that there might be separate systems for cystine and lysine transport by the kidney tubule. In rat renal tubule fragments and isolated brush border membrane vesicles, multiple systems for cystine and lysine transport are evident. Cystine and the dibasic amino acids appear to share the low–Michaelis constant (K_m), high-affinity system that probably is defective in the cystinuric kidney. Studies show that there might be an interaction of cystine and dibasic amino acids at the luminal membrane of the renal tubule. Cysteine, the oxidized form of cystine, shares a cellular efflux system with dibasic amino acids but not an uptake system. An elevation of intracellular cysteine could result from inhibition by lysine of cysteine transport into the peritubular capillary at the basolateral surface.

The only clinical abnormality in cystinuria relates to the insolubility of cystine with stone formation; the loss of the three dibasic amino acids is clinically insignificant. Renal colic is the most common presentation, associated with urinary tract obstruction. Infection, hypertension, and eventual renal failure may occur occasionally and may make the patient seek medical attention.

It was previously thought that cystinuric patients were shorter than the general population and that they had a higher incidence of mental illness. The former has not been substantiated, and in recent studies (testing of a large group of homozygous cystinuric patients for mental deficiency), the latter did not reveal an increased prevalence. Because of the gut transport defect, the bacterial metabolism of arginine and lysine can occur, and the diamines putrescine and cadaverine can be found in stool and urine. A mixed disulfide of cystic and homocystine often is also found in the urine.

The differential diagnosis consists of all causes of renal calculi. The diagnosis is simplified because the cystine stone is yellow-brown with a maple sugar crystal surface, is firm, and is radiopaque. On radiographic examination the stones appear smooth and less dense than other varieties. They tend to occur as staghorn or multiple recurrent stones. The simplest diagnostic procedure is microscopic examination of urinary sediment, which shows the pathognomonic hexagonal shape of the cystine crystals. Similarly, a positive cyanide nitroprusside test, followed by thin-layer chromatography, high-voltage electrophoresis, or quantitative ion-exchange chromatography will establish the diagnosis.

Therapy

Cystine hyperexcretion is a lifelong event. The basic therapy for this disorder is designed to reduce excretion and increase cystine solubility. Thus dietary restriction, increased solubility, and attempts to convert cystine to a more soluble compound have been used.

Dietary Restriction. Because cystine production arises from the essential amino acid methionine, it is probably reasonable to avoid excessive methionine intake, but in reality such a diet is difficult to establish and maintain.

Increased Solubility. Normal subjects excrete less than 60 mg cystine per day per 1.73 m^2 body surface area. By increasing the fluid intake, one can reduce the urinary cystine concentration below 200 mg/L and thus the likelihood of stone formation. Many cystinuric subjects excrete 1 g cystine per day and thus may need an intake of 4 or more liters of fluid every 24 hours. Cystine solubility can also be increased with an alkaline pH (more than 7.5). Although administering bicarbonate, citrate, and carbonic anhydrase inhibitors has been advocated as part of the alkalinizing program to improve solubility, this should be done in conjunction with fluid ingestion. To prevent supersaturation of urine with cystine at night when urine flow is low, some researchers advocate nocturnal hydration therapy (two glasses of water at bedtime and again at 2 AM or 3 AM).

Attempts to Convert Cystine to a More Soluble Compound. The main agent capable of converting cystine to a more soluble mixed disulfide is D-penicillamine (1 to 3 g in a daily divided dose). However, in one-third of patients it may cause rash, fever, bone marrow suppression, lupuslike illness, and proteinuria leading to the nephrotic syndrome. On biopsy these nephrotic patients have membranous nephropathy. Because of these drawbacks of D-penicillamine therapy, this agent should be limited to patients in whom hydration therapy has failed or those who have severe cystine stone disease. A related compound with fewer side effects is *N*-acetyl-D-penicillamine, which is effective in disulfide formation and thus in reducing cystine content. Another drug that should be substituted for penicillamine is mercaptopropionylglycine, which leads to the formation of a mixed disulfide and cysteine. Although not devoid of side effects (e.g., rash, fever, nausea, and soft feces), it does not have the serious hematologic, hepatic, or renal toxicity of D-penicillamine. When these therapeutic approaches do not arrest the cystinuric state, surgical approaches such as catheter irrigation (to dissolve calculi by irrigation), lithotomy (to remove calculi), and transplantation (to replace kidneys destroyed by cystinuria) may be needed. For transplantation, a kidney from a noncystinuric donor usually is effective, with normal amino acid excretion documented as long as 3.5 years after transplantation.

Extracorporeal Shock-Wave Lithotripsy. Extracorporeal shock-wave lithotripsy has been used effectively to fragment large intrapelvic or ureteric stones into smaller pieces that can be passed, obviating surgery. However, lithotripsy may lead to significant morbidity in the form of hematuria, obstruction with stone fragments, infection, and renal parenchymal scarring. Of all stones fragmented, cystine stones are the most resistant to shock-waves.

Hypercystinuria

Hypercystinuria is an autosomal-recessive order with high urinary excretion rates for cystine but normal excretions for lysine, ornithine, and arginine. Cystine clearance is elevated, and tubular reabsorption is decreased. The tubular defect is much less pronounced than in classic cystinuria, and none of the patients described has developed nephrolithiasis. Although the reduction in cystine reabsorption has only minimal clinical importance, it has influenced the theory of the tubular transport system for these amino acids. Originally, it was thought that cystine and the dibasic amino acids were transported by a common carrier. Current evidence indicates that this may not be the only tubular transport system for dibasic amino acids and cystine and that individual systems are present.

Hyperdibasic Aminoaciduria

Clinically and chemically distinguishable from cystinuria, hyperdibasic aminoaciduria is an impairment in transport of dibasic amino acids in the basolateral membrane of intestinal and renal tubular cells. In addition, it is characterized by protein intolerance, leading to hyperammonemia, and slow urea production could be caused by defective hepatic transport of dibasic amino acids. Such a defect could deprive hepatic cells of ornithine, a necessary component for urea production. Hyperdibasic aminoaciduria is inherited as an autosomal trait and it affects girls more than boys by about 2:1. The heterozygous trait may be expressed as a partial impairment in the intestinal elimination of dibasic amino acids after oral loads. Thus, the pattern resembles a recessive trait. Two major clinical patterns are evident. In type I, diamino acid transport is defective in renal tubules and intestine only; in type II, the transport defect is shared by hepatic cells. The characteristic plasma amino acid pattern includes subnormal levels of lysine, arginine, ornithine, leucine, and tyrosine. The diagnosis is based on the findings of dibasic aminoaciduria without cystinuria. Special renal function tests show that GFR is in the lower range of normal, with only 37% of filtered lysine reabsorbed by the tubule on average. Likewise, endogenous reabsorption of arginine and ornithine also is diminished.

Although the mechanism for the hyperammonemia and protein intolerance in these patients remains uncertain, it might reflect arginine or ornithine deficiency at some critical site. This may provide a basis for therapy. Supplementation with arginine, ornithine, or citrulline of an alanine intravenous load abolishes or prevents the hyperammonemic response that occurs after protein. Likewise, citrulline supplementation improves hypolysinemia. An oral supplement of citrulline plus lysine is highly effective in correcting the abnormal amino acid patterns.

Iminoglycinuria

Iminoglycinuria is a benign autosomal-recessive inborn error of membrane transport; heterozygotes may reveal hyperglycinuria without hyperprolinuria. It occurs because of a deletion or alteration of the membrane transport protein of the renal tubule that selectively binds L-proline, hydroxy-L-proline, and glycine during cellular uptake (both imino acids and glycine share a renal transport system). The renal transport of proline, hydroxyproline, and glycine apparently involves several reactive membrane sites, which are under the control of several genes. However, it is the shared group-specific tubular transport system for glycine and the imino acids that is disturbed in iminoglycinuria. In some cases an accompanying defect in intestinal proline absorption is found. Titration studies with L-proline loading in humans demonstrated that net tubular reabsorption undergoes saturation and that a tubular maximum for proline can be achieved. Infusion with one imino acid increases urinary excretion of the other and of glycine, whereas glycine infusion does not increase the rate of excretion of the imino acids. Kinetic analysis of the entry process (in human kidney slices) suggested the existence of two saturable transport systems), one separate and one shared; studies on tubules have shown that both L-proline and glycine are transported by more than one system. The obvious conclusion is that this disorder is accounted for by the loss of the shared carrier but retention of the selective carriers. Several types of iminoglycinuria are evident: Type I has an intestinal defect and heterozygotes have no aminoaciduria; type II shows normal gut transport, again with silent heterozygotes; type III has hyperglycinuria in heterozygotes; and type IV is a K_m mutant for glycine transport in which there is retention of normal imino acid transport (T_m) for proline is normal.

The differential diagnosis includes hyperprolinemia types I and II, which are autosomal-recessive disorders of proline metabolism involving proline oxidase and α-pyrroline-5-carboxylate dehydrogenase, respectively; hydroxyprolinemia, which is an autosomal-recessive deficiency of hydroxyproline oxidase; and glycinuria, seen with deficiencies of propionyl-CoA carboxylase and glycine decarboxylase. In each of these, plasma levels of proline or glycine are elevated. Iminoglycinuria also occurs in Fanconi's syndrome as part of a generalized inhibition of tubular transport. The normal infant has some degree of renal iminoglycinuria up to the third month of postnatal life. Finally, glycinuria without aminoaciduria has also been reported. Glycinuria has also been reported in adults, in adolescents with hypophosphatemic rickets, and in association with type A glucosuria. Hyperprolinemia and hydroxyprolinemia can be ruled out as a cause of iminoglycinuria if the concentration of both imino acids in plasma is normal in iminoglycinuric subjects. Iminoglycinuria is discovered incidentally in most subjects and therefore is a benign condition involving nonessential amino acids for which no treatment is indicated.

Hartnup Disease

Hartnup disease is a complex disturbance in the jejunal and renal epithelial transport of neutral amino acids: alanine, serine, threonine, asparagine, glutamine, valine, leucine, isoleucine, phenylalanine, tyrosine, tryptophan, histidine, and citrulline. It is transmitted as an autosomal-recessive trait. A defect in the neutral amino acid group transporter in gut and renal proximal tubule is presumed. Although first recognized in England, it has been reported to occur in almost all parts of the world. The single recognized constant feature is a massive tubular amino acid defect involving a group of neutral monoamino-monocarboxylic amino acids that are known to share a common renal reabsorption mechanism. This leads to a typical hyperaminoaciduria and intestinal malabsorption with secondary decomposition of amino acids in the stool. This hyperaminoaciduria arises because affected patients have a diminished capacity for the tubular reabsorption of these particular amino acids. This hyperaminoaciduria is remarkably constant and usually massive and correlates with neither the severity of clinical signs nor the therapeutic response. It is also of little clinical importance and has not resulted in any nutritional disturbances. This is not so for the intestinal defect in Hartnup disease. The intestinal bacterial tryptophan decomposition leads to urinary and stool excretion of indican and indoleacetic acid. The malabsorption in the jejunal area, specifically of tryptophan, and its impaired conversion to nicotinamide and kynurenine is responsible for the clinical signs: pellagralike photosensitive rash on exposure to sunlight, attacks of cerebral ataxia, neuropsychiatric symptoms, and delirium. The only disorder in the differential diagnosis is the dietary deficiency pellagra, which has no aminoaciduria or indicanuria, but the North American diet generally precludes the appearance of pellagra. Therapy for Hartnup disease consists of oral nicotinamide, and undue sunlight exposure should be avoided. Temporary reduction of the bacterial decarboxylation of unabsorbed dietary amino acids with neomycin diminishes the absorption of indoles and other amines. Although essential amino acids are lost in the urine and are malabsorbed, intestinal dipeptide and tripeptide absorption remains intact, so these amino acids are absorbed in sufficient quantities.

Hyperdicarboxylic Aminoaciduria

The autosomal-recessive disorder in which glutamic and aspartic acids are not absorbed by the jejunum and undergo urinary hyperexcretion apparently involves the shared dicarboxylic amino acid transport system; infusion of glutamic acid produces a steep increase in aspartic acid excretion. This disorder may represent renal tubular overproduction or a total tubular reabsorption defect resulting in net tubular secretion because in these patients net secretion of glutamate and aspartate was found. Treatment with glutamate and aspartate in one patient seemed to prevent the hypoglycemia found in this disorder. This hypoglycemia is thought to be related to the absence of these key gluconeogenic amino acids.

β-Aminoaciduria

No tubular defect in the β-amino acid (β-alanine, β-aminoisobutyric acid, and taurine) transport system has been described. Isolated β-aminoisobutyric aciduria may occur in normal subjects as a breakdown product of thymine metabolism. This trait is especially common in Asians, Eskimos, and Native Americans, so it can serve as a genetic marker. Thus β-aminoisobutyric acid excretion is a curious laboratory finding.

Two disorders of β-alanine metabolism have been identified in humans. One involves free β-alanine catabolism (hyper-β-alaninemia), the other the degradation of carnosine in serum. In hyper-β-alaninemia, reported in a single child with seizures and coma, increased urinary excretion of β-alanine, β-aminobutyric acid, taurine, and β-aminoisobutyric acid was noted, indicating competition for the β-amino acid renal tubular transport site. A γ-amino component, γ-aminobutyric acid (GABA), was found. The concentrations of β-alanine and GABA also were elevated in the plasma and cerebrospinal fluid.

The selective hyperaminoaciduria involving β-amino acids may be the result of combined overflow and renal mechanisms. β-Aminoaciduria reflects a diminution of β-alanine-Y-ketoglutarate aminotransferase activity. Thus impaired oxidation of β-alanine is the most probable cause of the abnormality. A defective β-amino acid transport system has been found in inbred strains of mice, but not in humans.

Hyperaminoaciduria of Immaturity

In early infancy, urinary amino acid excretion is greater than in later life. Incomplete tubular reabsorption is considered responsible for the physiologic hyperaminoaciduria. When the net excretion rates of individual amino acids are corrected in terms of surface area, only certain amino acids are involved in the physiologic hyperaminoaciduria (threonine, serine, proline, glycine, alanine, and hydroxyproline). The aminoaciduria of infancy is not related to a reduced maximal capacity of tubular reabsorption, but it may be caused by an increased permeability of the tubule cell membrane or by higher intracellular amino acid concentrations permitting a greater fraction of amino acids to backleak out of the cell into the urine.

The precise mechanisms that switch on normal reabsorption of all amino acids in all systems are unknown but may involve the development of new transport (a change in K_m) or the production of more carriers (a change in maximum rate [V_{max}]). There are no known physiologic or clinical consequences of hyperaminoaciduria, but it occurs despite the reduced GFR of the neonatal period. After a varying amount of time, the complete adult pattern of reabsorption emerges.

DISORDERS OF PHOSPHATE TRANSPORT

Phosphate transport disorders can result from the absence of a plasma membrane transport protein as a result of mutation, absence of an effector hormone or failure of the transport process to respond to normal levels of the hormone, exaggerated response to a hormone, absence of or defects in intracellular enzymes important in the transport process, or alteration of energy-producing processes within the tubular epithelium.

Tubular disorders of phosphate transport can result in hypophosphatemia with phosphate hyperexcretion or in hyperphosphatemia caused by decreased phosphate excretion. Both primary hypophosphatemia with rickets and hyperphosphatemia with skeletal abnormalities, which behaved like hypoparathyroidism, were first described by Dr. Fuller Albright. Phosphate hyperexcretion, like disorders of glucose and amino acid transport, can be part of the complex tubulopathy known as *Fanconi's syndrome* (Table 23.2).

Primary Hypophosphatemic Rickets

Hypophosphatemia with hyperphosphaturia, rickets, and short stature is known as *primary hypophosphatemic rickets* and is usually associated with an X-linked mode of inheritance. Other terms used to describe this disorder are *vitamin D–resistant rickets, familial hypophosphatemic rickets,* or *X-linked hypophosphatemic rickets.* Decreased serum phosphate levels lead to a reduction in the mineralization rate of bone matrix, with resultant rickets and short stature. Although X-linked inheritance is the common pattern, autosomal-dominant, autosomal-recessive, and sporadic cases are described. Defects in the phosphate-regulating gene with homologies to endopeptidases on the X chromosome (PEX), found on the X chromosome, account for X-linked hypophosphatemia. PEX produces a protein that presumably regulates the activity of the sodium-dependent phosphate transporter, found on chromosome 5. This transporter is responsible for sodium-dependent phosphate reabsorption in the proximal tubule.

Patients have decreased net tubular phosphate reabsorption even at lower serum phosphate concentrations. The fractional phosphate excretion is further increased by phosphate administrations. Serum parathyroid hormone (PTH) levels in untreated patients are normal or slightly elevated; therefore, secondary hyperparathyroidism is not the cause of hyperphosphaturia unless the renal tubule is supersensitive to the action of PTH, as some have postulated. Nonetheless, even if hypersensitivity to PTH is present in this disorder, this hormone does into evoke decreased reabsorption of amino acids, bicarbonate, and glucose or alter normal cyclic adenosine 3′5′-monophosphate (cAMP) excretion. Hyperphosphaturia may be related to a missing transport protein or binding site in the proximal tubule. In the X-linked hypophosphatemic mouse, which is a comparable animal model of hypophosphatemic rickets, there is a defect in phosphate uptake into brush border membrane vesicles.

Hypophosphatemia is universal with serum phosphorus values of 1.0 to 2.4 mg/dl, which is especially low for children, whose phosphate values are higher than those of adults. Serum calcium is normal or slightly reduced, and alkaline phosphatase activity is less elevated than in nutritional vitamin D–deficiency rickets.

TABLE 23.2. Clinical Disorders of Renal Tubular Phosphate Transport

Disorder	Other Substances Lost	Serum,1,25(OH)$_2$D$_3$ Concentration	Usual Age Detected	Inheritance	Salient Clinical Features
Primary hypophosphatemic rickets	None	Low normal	9–13 mo	Usually X-linked; also AR, AD, or sporadic	Bowing lower segment, short stature?, no myopathy, boys more affected in most common form.
Oncogenous phosphaturic rickets	Glycine?	Low	Birth onward	AD with neurofibromatosis or sporadic	Rickets with fibrous dysplasia, fibromas, or soft tissue tumors; heals with removal of tumor.
Adult hypophosphatemic rickets	Glycine	?	15–50 yr	Sporadic	Bone pain, vertebral flattening, Looser's zones, muscle weakness.
Hypophosphatemic rickets with hypercalciuria	Calcium	Elevated	3 yr to adulthood	AR	Elevated 1,25(OH)$_2$D$_3$ resulting from renal phosphate leak leads to intestinal hyperabsorption of Ca^{2+}.
Hypophosphatemic bone disease without rickets	None	Normal	3 yr to adulthood	AD or X-linked	No rickets; milder short stature may appear in adulthood.
Hypophosphatemia with glycinuria, glucosuria, and glycylprolinuria	Glycine, glucose, glycylproline	?	7 yr	AR?	Muscle weakness, rickets, bone pain, growth failure similar to adult onset?
Fanconi's syndrome	Glucose, amino acids, uric acid, bicarbonate, low-molecular-weight proteins	Normal unless renal function impaired	Any age	AR, AD, X-linked, or sporadic	Osteoporosis, hypokalemia, weakness, acidosis, bone pain from many causes.

1,25(OH)$_2$D$_3$, 1,25-dihydroxyvitamin D; AD, autosomal-dominant; AR, autosomal-recessive.

Patients develop rickets when they begin walking, with rachitic changes involving mainly the legs. Coxa vara, genu valgum, bowing, and pelvic deformities are common. The rickets usually are unresponsive to therapy with vitamin D dosages that are sufficient to cure nutritional vitamin D deficiency. The teeth erupt on time with normal enamel but defective dentin. The patient has a prominent forehead and widened bridge of the nose but none of the myopathy found in other causes of rickets. Patients tend to be very short, but girls are less affected than boys and some may attain normal height with only minimal bowing. Radiographic examination shows rickets without evidence of hyperparathyroidism or Looser-Milkman striae (Fig. 23.2). Classically, patients are said to have smooth bowing of their extremities rather than the sharp, angular bowing of nutritional or vitamin D–deficiency rickets.

In some studies, a transport defect was found in the intestine. A malabsorption of calcium and phosphate is found despite the fact that patients are not hypocalcemic. Because 1,25-dihydroxyvitamin D [$1,25(OH)_2D_3$] synthesis is regulated by these divalent ions, synthesis of this compound is abnormal.

In the differential diagnosis of this disorder, one should consider both vitamin D–deficiency rickets and vitamin D–dependency rickets (Table 23.3), but familial hypophosphatemic rickets can also present as an autosomal-dominant disorder.

Therapy for primary hypophosphatemic rickets consists of oral phosphorus supplementation at 1 to 4 g/day, provided every 4 hours because the phosphate leak is continuous throughout the day. Because oral phosphate impedes calcium absorption, vitamin D must be provided. Massive dosages of this vitamin (20,000 to 100,000 U/day) must be given. The long-term use of $1,25(OH)_2D_3$ (1 mg/day) has been shown to be of benefit in healing the rickets, offsetting phosphate-induced hypocalcemia and reactive hyperparathyroidism, and promoting bone mineralization.

Newer data suggest that treating symptomatic adult subjects with oral phosphate and $1,25(OH)_2D_3$ decreases bone pain in nearly 90% of subjects. Nevertheless, bone biopsies showed evidence of incomplete healing of osteomalacia.

The rare disorder of hypophosphatemic bone disease is described in Tables 23.2 and 23.3.

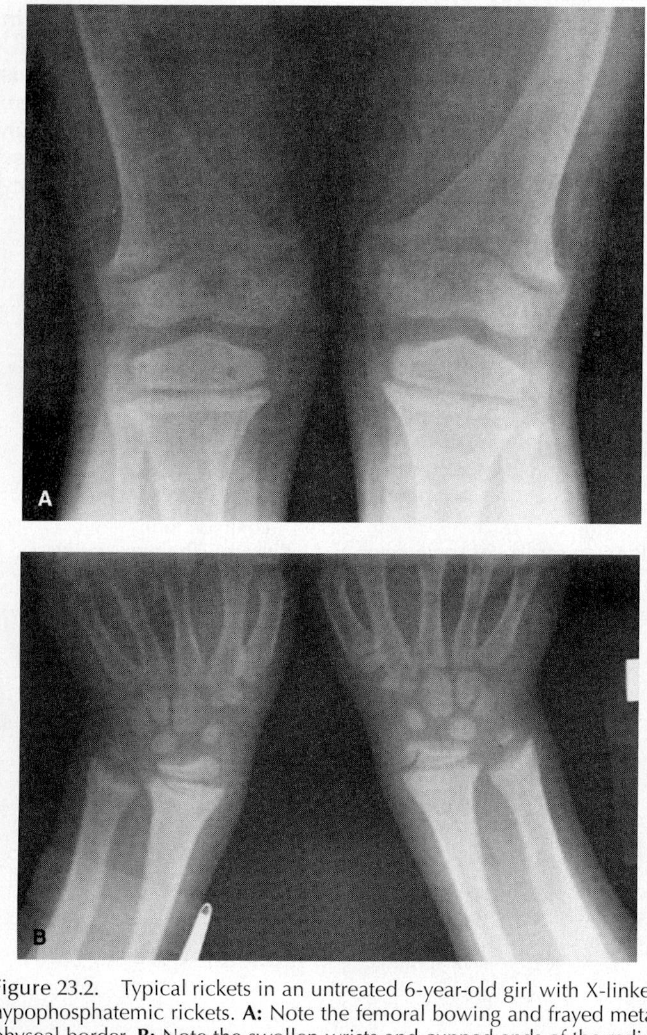

Figure 23.2. Typical rickets in an untreated 6-year-old girl with X-linked hypophosphatemic rickets. **A:** Note the femoral bowing and frayed metaphyseal border. **B:** Note the swollen wrists and cupped ends of the radius and ulna. Diffuse osteopenia also is present.

Vitamin D–Dependent Rickets

Vitamin D–dependent rickets (VDDR) is an autosomal-recessive disorder closely resembling classic vitamin D deficiency, so it may also be called *pseudodeficiency rickets* (Table 23.3). Patients have muscle weakness, enamel hypoplasia, evidence of hyperparathyroidism, aminoaciduria, and hypocalcemia. Disease is apparent at the age of 12 weeks, in contrast to 12 to 18 months in hypophosphatemic rickets. This disorder results from an inherited deficiency of 25-hydroxyvitamin D-1α-hydroxylase activity in which diminished amounts of $1,25(OH)_2D_3$ are produced. Recent cloning of the gene for 25(OH)D-1α-hydroxylase will permit a more complete understanding of this disorder. Several point mutations have been described in affected patients from Japanese families. The hypocalcemia that results from the absence of circulating $1,25(OH)_2D_3$ leads to elevated PTH levels, hyperphosphaturia, aminoaciduria, and rickets with evidence of hyperparathyroid bone disease. The differential diagnosis from other conditions can be seen in Table 23.3. Treatment with 1.0 mg/day of $1,25(OH)_2D_3$ reverses this disorder, whereas 100,000 to 200,000 U/day of ordinary vitamin D may be necessary.

Another group of patients with clinical features of VDDR, elevated blood levels of $1,25(OH)_2D_3$, and decreased target organ responsiveness to $1,25(OH)_2D_3$ (VDDR type II) has been described. These patients often have alopecia totalis and may be the product of first-cousin marriages. Studies in vitro in bone and skin cells demonstrate abnormalities in the nuclear receptor for $1,25(OH)_2D_3$ or the vitamin D receptor. Some patients with this disorder respond to high dosages (6 to 20 mg/day) of $1,25(OH)_2D_3$, and their skin fibroblasts also produce $24,25(OH)_2D_3$ under tissue culture conditions, indicating that their $1,25(OH)_2D_3$ receptors have reduced affinity for this metabolite. Patients who do not respond to $1,25(OH)_2D_3$ presumably lack receptors of this steroid molecule.

Adult Hypophosphatemic Rickets

Patients with adult hypophosphatemic rickets (Table 23.2) develop hypophosphatemic osteomalacia between ages 15 and 60 years. The inheritance is sporadic, and the patients have debilitating bone pains, Looser zones, and a prominent myopathy. They may also have isolated hyperglycinuria and, less often, glucosuria. The pathogenesis of this disorder is unclear, but it involves renal hyperphosphaturia. Blood levels of PTH and $25(OH)D_3$ are normal, although isolated parathyroid adenomas sometimes are found. These patients also have marked angulation of bones, codfish vertebrae, kyphosis, and scoliosis. Calcium levels in serum are normal after phosphate loading. At endogenous phosphate levels (2 to 2.5 mg/day), phosphate reabsorption is normal. Treatment with oral phosphate and high-dose vitamin D is indicated.

TABLE 23.3. Clinical Features of the Forms of Hypophosphatemic Bone Disorders Related to Phosphaturia

	Vitamin D–Deficiency Rickets	Primary Hypophosphatemic Rickets	Hypophosphatemic Rickets with Hypercalciuria	Vitamin D–Dependency Rickets	Hypophosphatemic Bone Disease
Bone disease	Rickets, bowing	Rickets, bowing	Rickets, bowing	Rickets, bowing	Increased trabeculation, no bowing
Muscle weakness	Yes	No	No	Yes	No
Age of onset	9–12 mo	12–18 mo	Infancy	3–6 mo	Variable
Serum calcium level	↓	Normal	Normal	↓	Normal
Serum phosphate level	↓	↓	↑	↓	↓
Serum alkaline phosphatase	↑	↑	↓	↑	↑
Serum immunoreactive PTH level	↑	Normal or minimal ↑	No	↑	Normal
Increased aminoaciduria	Yes	No	↓	Yes	No
T_mP at endogenous levels (phosphate)	↓	↓	↑	↓	Normal
Urinary phosphate at					
Endogenous levels	↑	↑	↑	↑	Normal
Loaded levels	↑	↑	↑	↑	↑
Intestinal calcium absorption	↓	↓	↑↑	↓	?
Genetics	None	X-linked dominant, AD, AR		AR	X-linked, AD
Response to 10 μg/day vitamin D_3	Curative	None	Increased urine Ca^{2+}	None	None
Response to 2 μg/day $1,25(OH)_2D_3$	Curative	None acutely, improvement with chronic use	Increased urine Ca^{2+}	Curative	Possible curative
Response to 1 mg day vitamin D_3	Curative, hypercalcemia	Rickets partially healed, hypophosphatemia persists	Increased urine Ca^{2+}	Curative	Bone disease partially healed, hypophosphatemia
Oral phosphate supplement		Heals rickets, increased growth	Suppresses $1,25(OH)_2D_3$ formation, reduces intestinal Ca^{2+} absorption and heals bone		Increases serum phosphate

Adapted from Chesney RW. Tubular defects in phosphate reabsorption in clinical medicine. In: S Massry, H Fleisch, eds. *Renal handling of phosphate.* New York: Plenum, 1980:321–365.

$1,25(OH)_2D_3$, 1,25-dihydroxyvitamin D_3; AD, autosomal dominant; AR, autosomal recessive; PTH, parathyroid hormone.

Oncogenous Rickets

In some patients, hypophosphatemia may be associated with tumors of soft tissue or bone, fibrous dysplasia or neurofibromatosis, sclerosing hemangioma, cavernous hemangioma, or giant cell tumors. The hypophosphatemia is related to some substance elaborated by the tumor because it disappears when the tumor or fibrous tissue is excised. These tumors appear to produce PEX, the phosphate-regulating protein, in large quantities. Blood PTH levels are normal, aminoaciduria is absent, and calcium levels are normal. When measured, blood levels of $1,25(OH)_2D_3$ are reduced, suggesting that vitamin D metabolism is altered; treatment with vitamin D metabolite has reversed the biochemical and radiologic finding of rickets in two patients. Tumor removal reverses rickets, but for the extensive tumor or metastatic disease, oral phosphate and vitamin D also are needed. Therapy with oral phosphate may cause hypocalcemia, and reactive secondary hyperparathyroidism may ensue. Treatment with vitamin D or one of its metabolites may prevent these complications.

Hypophosphatemic Rickets with Hypercalciuria

Some patients with hypophosphatemic rickets also have evidence of hypercalciuria and stones (Dent disease). In this condition, patients appear to have a primary renal tubular phosphate leak; an increase in $1,25(OH)_2D_3$ synthesis, causing increased intestinal calcium absorption; and augmented urinary calcium excretion. The therapy for this condition consists only of oral phosphate, which reduces $1,25(OH)_2D_3$ synthesis and thereby hypercalciuria. These patients obviously do not need any form of vitamin D in their treatment protocol. The recent recognition of this disorder implies that all hypophosphatemic patients should be monitored to determine urinary calcium excretion values.

Pseudohypoparathyroidism

Pseudohypoparathyroidism is characterized by short stature, a round face and short neck, shortened fourth and fifth metacarpal and metatarsal bones (Fig. 23.3), strabismus, cataracts, subcutaneous calcifications, mental retardation, and hypocalcemic tetany. Blood PTH levels are elevated, and exogenous PTH does not evoke phosphaturia or cAMP excretion, indicating end-organ unresponsiveness to the hormone. The patients have hyperphosphatemia, but hypocalcemia is not universal. Some patients have the same somatic features but normal serum calcium and phosphate levels; this condition is called *pseudo-pseudohypoparathyroidism.* Members of the same family may have both conditions. The genetics of this disorder are confusing but may represent a sex-linked dominant mode of inheritance, with the variable expression dependent on random inactivation of the X chromosome in girls.

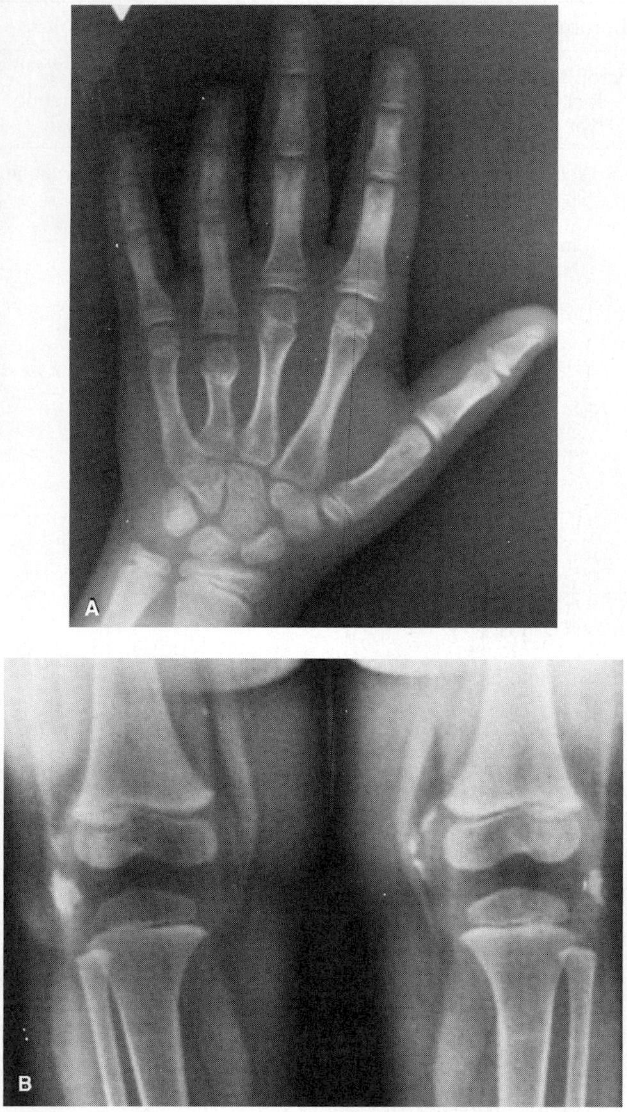

Figure 23.3. **A:** The typical radiologic features of pseudohypoparathyroidism with a shortened fourth metacarpal. **B:** Subcutaneous calcification about the knees in a child with pseudohypoparathyroidism.

Partial or total end-organ unresponsiveness to PTH in kidney and bone accounts for hypocalcemia and hyperphosphatemia. In most cases, there is no PTH-evoked stimulation of tubule adenylate cyclase because of reduced activity of the stimulatory component or N protein in the receptor adenylate cyclase complex. Defective G_5 or the stimulatory component of the G protein is relevant in type I pseudohypoparathyroidism but not type II. High serum phosphate lowers serum calcium and leads to PTH hypersecretion. In some patients, the bone may display an osteoclastic response to PTH, and histologic evidence of osteitis fibrosa cystica is found. Some patients respond to PTH administration with increased urinary excretion of cAMP but without phosphaturia; this form of the disease is called *type II pseudohypoparathyroidism.*

These clinical features fit classic pseudohypoparathyroidism, but patients with normal somatic features, normal height, and hypocalcemia and hyperphosphatemia unresponsive to PTH administration have been described. In addition, prolactin and thyrotropin deficiency with mild hypothyroidism have been reported. Skeletal resistance to PTH with renal responsiveness, with typical somatic features or normal features, also has been described. The various clinical forms of pseudohypoparathyroidism are listed in Table 23.4.

With typical features the diagnosis is not difficult, but it can be confirmed by the absence of urinary cAMP after PTH administration. In contrast, normal subjects and patients with pseudo-pseudohypoparathyroidism have a 10- to 20-fold increase in cAMP excretion after PTH administration. Moreover, the hypocalcemia and hyperphosphatemia are not corrected by PTH administration in pseudohypoparathyroidism.

Tetany and, in part, cataract formation can be prevented with large dosages of vitamin D (50,000 to 150,000 U/day). More recently, therapy with low dosages of $1,25(OH)_2D_3$ (0.5 to 2.0 mg/day) have been found to correct hypocalcemia. This analog with a shorter half-life eliminates the problem of tissue storage that can complicate high dosages of vitamin D_2 or D_3. Long-term $1,25(OH)_2D_3$ therapy ultimately may reduce serum phosphate levels, possibly by the influence of prolonged periods of normocalcemia. Many physicians treating these patients find that hypocalcemia is easier to manage in this condition than in idiopathic hypoparathyroidism.

TABLE 23.4. Clinical Forms of Pseudohypoparathyroidism

Phenotype	End Organ Nonresponsive	Urinary cAMP After PTH	Serum Ca^{2+}	Serum Phosphate	Therapy
Typical somatic features[a]	Bone Kidney	Absent	↓	↑	Vitamin D
Typical somatic features (pseudo-pseudohypoparathyroidism)	None	Normal	N	N	None
Normal features with osteitis fibrosa	Kidney	Absent	↓	↑	Vitamin D
Typical somatic features with osteitis fibrosa	Kidney	Absent	↓	↑	Vitamin D
Normal features with low $1,25(OH)_2D_3$	Bone	Normal	↓	↑	$1,25(OH)_2D_3$
Typical somatic features	Bone	Normal	↓	↑	Vitamin D
Typical somatic features; no phosphaturic response to dibutyryl cAMP infusion	Bone Kidney	Normal	↓	↑	Vitamin D
Normal features; no phosphaturic response to dibutyryl cAMP infusion	Bone Kidney	Normal	↓	↑	Vitamin D
Typical somatic features	Bone Kidney	Absent	N	N	None

[a] Typical somatic features include short neck, round face, short fourth and fifth metacarpals and metatarsals, strabismus, cataracts, subcutaneous and basal ganglia calcification, and mental retardation. $1,25(OH)_2D_3$, 1,25-dihydroxyvitamin D_3; cAMP, cyclic adenosine monophosphate; N, normal.

COMPLEX TUBULAR DEFECTS (FANCONI'S SYNDROME)

The urinary hyperexcretion of amino acids of all classes, phosphate, glucose, bicarbonate, calcium, potassium and other ions, and proteins with molecular weights under 50,000 D, in conjunction with renal tubular acidosis and vasopressin-resistant polyuria, defines the complex tubulopathy called *Fanconi's syndrome.* Other features are rickets, osteoporosis, short stature, and hypokalemia. The fractional reabsorption of nearly all substances transported by the proximal tubule is reduced and the net secretion of *p*-aminohippuric acid also may be impaired.

The numerous causes of Fanconi's syndrome and their accepted modes of inheritance are listed in Table 23.5. The disease is primary or idiopathic when its cause is unknown or when only the genetic mode of inheritance is evident. Idiopathic Fanconi's syndrome may be sporadic, autosomal-dominant, autosomal-recessive, or X-linked. A variety of defective genes are not relevant in this complex disorder, which is truly a syndrome because of its diverse causes.

The clinical features are related directly to tubular dysfunction and its consequences. The onset is in infancy (childhood form) or in the third to fourth decade (adult form), and the diverse symptoms of hypokalemia may be the prominent clinical features. Children have growth failure, anorexia, vomiting, fever muscle weakness, a waddling gait, and paralysis from hypokalemia. Adult patients complain of muscle weakness and bone pain, particularly in the spine position. Uremia may occur in either form.

In most instances, Fanconi's syndrome is related to some systemic disorder. In several of these conditions (Fanconi's syndrome with glycogenosis, galactosemia, hereditary fructose intolerance, tyrosinosis, Wilson's disease, and infantile nephropathic cystinosis), both the liver and the kidney are involved; indeed, the liver disease may be more debilitating. Many patients with Fanconi's syndrome may have progressive renal failure developing well after the features of Fanconi's syndrome are obvious.

The pathogenesis of the syndrome, regardless of its cause, involves one of two basic mechanisms. The first possibility is that renal tubular membranes become leaky, allowing less efficient reabsorption of solutes. The evidence supporting this hypothesis is that glucosuria is of the type A variety, indicating fewer transport sites for glucose reabsorption. Furthermore, phosphate and, to a degree, amino acids are lost at reduced filtered loads. Finally, some patients have negative glucose, amino acid, and phosphate clearance, which suggests secretion through a series of leaky membranes. Nonetheless, conventional transport systems remain partially intact because the infusion of competing hexoses or amino acids increases the excretion of other members of the same transport group.

The second hypothesis suggests that the intracellular metabolism of renal tubule cells does not produce sufficient energy to support transport. Any substance that could be toxic and alter renal tubular metabolism, such as fructose-1-phosphate, galactose-1-phosphate, copper, or other heavy metals, could impair transport processes. Maleic acid, long used to induce Fanconi's syndrome in experimental animals, alters mitochondrial function and causes backflux of amino acids, glucose, and phosphate into urine. These two hypotheses may not be very divergent because cellular energy is needed to maintain the contact between cells and preserve the tubular epithelium.

The clinical presentation depends on the cause. Infantile nephropathic cystinosis, the most common cause of the syndrome, starts with polyuria, polydipsia, constipation, recurrent fevers related to dehydration, rickets, and dwarfism. The disease is symptomatic at age 9 to 14 months, and other features are pale skin and hair, photophobia, and hypokalemia with muscle weakness. Severe rickets is present, related to acidosis, hypophosphatemia, and possibly alterations in vitamin D metabolism. A 100-fold increase in intralysosomal storage of cystine is found in nearly all tissues, but the relationship of these increased levels of cystine to the complex tubulopathy is unclear. However, it is known that the process by which cystine leaves the lysosome (efflux) is impaired in this disorder; the transporter activity is greatly reduced. Although the gene for the lysosomal

TABLE 23.5. Causes of Fanconi's Syndrome with a Demonstrable Inheritance Pattern

Disorder	Inheritance	Glucosuria	Aminoaciduria	Phosphaturia	Bicarbonate Wasting	Polyuria	Rickets or Osteoporosis	Uremia
Cystinosis								
Infantile	AR	Common	Common	Common	Common	Common	Common	Common
Adolescent	AR	Common	Common	Often	Often	Often	Rare	Common
Adult	AR	Absent	Absent	Absent	Absent	Absent	Absent	Absent
Lowe's oculocerebrorenal syndrome	X-linked	Rare	Common	Common	Often	Rare	Common	Often
Tyrosinemia	AR	Common	Common	Common	Often	Often	Common	Absent
Galactosemia	AR	Rare	Common	Rare	Rare	Often	Rare	Absent
Glycogenosis (Fanconi-Bickel syndrome)	AR	Common	Common	Often	Often	Rare	Often	Absent
Wilson's disease	AR	Often	Common	Rare	Often	Rare	Rare	Absent
Fructose intolerance	AR	Rare	Common	Rare	Often	Often	Rare	Absent
Nephrotic syndrome	AR(?)	Common	Common	Often	Common	Often	Often	Often
Idiopathic								
Adult	AR, AD, or X-linked	Common	Common	Common	Common	Common	Common	Often
Childhood		Common	Common	Common	Common	Common	Common	Often

This table represents the findings typical of Fanconi's syndrome when patients with these disorders are symptomatic. If offending metabolites are avoided in tyrosinemia, galactosemia, Wilson's disease, and fructose intolerance, the complex tubulopathy disappears.

AD, autosomal dominant; AR, autosomal recessive.

cystine efflux transporter is not yet cloned, presumably it will be defective in cystinosis. By age 7 to 12 years, uremia develops, heralded by massive proteinuria and a decline in glucose, phosphate, and amino acid excretion, which occurs as the GFR falls. In adolescent cystinosis, the features of Fanconi's syndrome are less prominent, and disease appears between 10 and 20 years of age. Bone disease is less severe and dwarfism is absent. Tissue cystine levels are lower than in the infantile form. Uremia also supervenes in adolescent cystinosis. Adult cystinosis is a benign disorder, with the corneal cystine deposition found in the other forms.

In galactosemia caused by transferase deficiency, hepatomegaly and jaundice are evident at birth. If it is untreated, vomiting, cataracts, inanition, and cirrhosis develop. Fanconi's syndrome disappears after dietary galactose restriction. Refeeding galactose causes hepatic dysfunction in minutes, but renal tubular damage takes several days to become apparent.

In hereditary fructose intolerance caused by fructose aldolase-b deficiency, blocking the conversion of fructose-1-phosphate to glyceraldehyde, the features of the syndrome occur within minutes after exposure to this sugar. Children with fructose intolerance learn early to avoid sweets and fruit sugars, accounting for their notable lack of dental caries.

Tyrosinemia presents in infancy with growth failure, hepatic damage, cataract formation, hypoglycemia related to islet cell hypertrophy, and mental retardation. Liver disease precedes Fanconi's syndrome development. Tyrosinemic patients excrete large amounts of succinyl acetoacetate, and the activity of the hepatic enzyme fumarylacetoacetate hydrolase is impaired. This enzyme is needed to convert fumarylacetoacetic acid and succinylacetoacetic acid to fumarate and succinate, respectively, and acetoacetic acid. Hypophosphatemia and rickets are more prevalent in galactosemia or fructose intolerance than in tyrosinemia. Phosphate is used to phosphorylate these sugars. In some cases, the clinical findings of tyrosinosis have been seen with congenital viral infections of the liver.

In Wilson's disease, cirrhosis and neurologic symptoms predominate, but some patients show Fanconi's syndrome with bicarbonate wasting and nephrocalcinosis with hypercalciuria. Patients with glycogen storage and Fanconi's syndrome (Fanconi–Bickel syndrome) do not have any of the recognizable enzyme defects of glycogen storage disease, but they do have complex abnormalities of carbohydrate metabolism, including glucose intolerance, insulin hyposecretion, ketosis, and a failure to convert galactose to glucose; hyperlipidemia and profound glucose wasting may also be common features. Glycogen deposits are found in renal cells. Mutations in GLUT, the gene for the liver isoform of the facilitative diffusion glucose transporter, are found in patients with the Fanconi–Bickel syndrome. Patients with this variant of Fanconi's syndrome have massive hepatorenal glycogen storage and impaired utilization of glucose and galactose.

Lowe's oculocerebrorenal syndrome is an X-linked disorder characterized by cataracts, glaucoma, high sloping forehead, severe mental retardation, hypotonia, areflexia, and an incomplete form of Fanconi's syndrome. The few females reported (less than 5%) are dependent on random inactivation of the X chromosome or an alternative inheritance pattern. The natural history of the disease has three separate phases. During infancy, central nervous system and ophthalmologic disturbances predominate. During childhood, the features of Fanconi's syndrome are evident, with severe rickets and osteoporosis. In adulthood, the tubulopathy disappears and renal failure, inanition, and pneumonia may lead to death. A peculiar arthritis of the small joints of the hand may be seen.

The Lowe's syndrome gene has been mapped to xq25–q26, and a candidate gene has been proposed. Indeed, Lowe's syndrome appears to encode a protein with a 71% similarity to human inositol polyphosphate-5-phosphatase because this gene codes for a protein that removes 5-phosphate from inositol (1,4,5)-triphosphate. Therefore Lowe's syndrome may be an unborn error of inositol phosphate metabolism.

Fanconi's syndrome with Bence Jones proteinuria can occur with multiple myeloma or with amyloidosis. Clinical features include lassitude, bone pain, muscle weakness, polyuria, osteomalacia, pseudofractures, and cytoplasmic inclusion crystals within tumor cells and renal tubule cells. Bence Jones light chains are of the K type only because l light chains lead to myeloma kidney with acute oliguric renal failure. Polyclonal hyperglobulinemia, sometimes in association with Sjögren's syndrome, results in renal tubular acidosis and, rarely, in Fanconi's syndrome.

Mutations in the mitochondrial genome can present with features of Fanconi's syndrome. Because mitochondrial DNA (M+ DNA) is key in coding for proteins important in cellular energy production, a number of patients have been described who have defective cytochrome oxidase or ATPase or NADH dehydrogenase activity and a diffuse proximal tubulopathy as well as tubulointerstitial disease.

Development of Fanconi's syndrome after renal transplantation, infantile renal vein thrombosis, and antibody-induced interstitial nephritis probably is the result of tubular dysfunction caused by tubular atrophy, scarring, or fibrosis (Table 23.6). In each of these disorders, the syndrome rarely occurs and not all patients have the full-blown syndrome. Tubular scarring and atrophy sometimes are seen in other forms of Fanconi's syndrome including the swan neck lesion, which is narrowing of the proximal tubular epithelium at a site near the glomerulus.

Toxins including outdated tetracycline, dichrome, and heavy metals including lead and cadmium cause Fanconi's syndrome. If tetracycline is stored in a moist, warm environment for a long period of time, the degradation product, anhydro-4-epitetracycline,

TABLE 23.6. Nongenetic Causes of Fanconi's Syndrome (Rare)

Renal allografts
Myeloma of the kidney
Sjögren's syndrome
Hyperparathyroidism
Potassium depletion
Infantile renal vein thrombosis
Amyloidosis with Bence Jones proteinuria
Nephrotic syndrome
Pancreatic carcinoma
Vitamin D deficiency
Interstitial nephritis (with antitubular basement membrane antibodies)
Heavy metals
Cadmium
Mercury
Organomercurials
Lead
Uranium
Copper
Chemical toxins
Lysol
Salicylate
Nitrobenzene
Maleic acid
Methyl-3-chrome
Outdated tetracycline
Ifosfamide

can be formed and this product is responsible for the tubulopathy. The clinical picture is typified by myopathy, dizziness, acidosis, polyuria, and hypokalemia. This disorder was common in nurses' and physicians' families and neighbors who were given outdated professional samples. Recovery is fairly rapid after cessation of the drug but may take up to 2 years. Cadmium-induced disease is found in cadmium battery workers.

Fanconi's syndrome can be found in vitamin D–deficiency or vitamin D–dependency rickets and probably is related to the secondary hyperparathyroidism that follows the hypocalcemia caused by lack of vitamin D. These patients also have metabolic acidosis and severe rickets. This disorder often is described in premature neonates with seemingly mild hepatobiliary disease. Whether disease is from a failure of 25-hydroxylation or vitamin D malabsorption is not established, but PTH levels always are elevated. Children with classic vitamin D deficiency begin to show signs of the disease at age 18 to 36 months. Treatment with the missing vitamin reverses all features of the syndrome, although a failure of ordinary dosages to correct hypocalcemia may indicate vitamin D–dependency rickets.

The laboratory features of Fanconi's syndrome include hypophosphatemia with a phosphate leak even at low endogenous phosphate levels (a low T_m phosphate leak), hypokalemia, hypouricemia, and a proximal renal tubular acidosis with the attainment of an acid urine at low serum bicarbonate levels and defects in urine concentration. Sodium wasting sometimes is present, leading to volume depletion and consequently to metabolic alkalosis, and if patients have large amounts of free water, they may display hyponatremia. Hypocalcemia is uncommon, but intestinal malabsorption and phosphorus can be found in several forms of the syndrome. The relationship of this gut transport defect to abnormalities of vitamin D metabolism is unknown. Proteinuria is of the tubular type, which often can be suspected by its dissolution upon heating after a sulfosalicylic acid precipitation step. Nephrocalcinosis and hypercalciuria are common in Wilson's disease and Lowe's syndrome. Fructose and galactose are found in the urine in fructose intolerance and galactosemia. Tyrosine and methionine plasma levels are elevated in tyrosinosis, but in other disorders plasma amino acid levels are normal. In patients with nephrotic syndrome and Fanconi's syndrome, hypocalcemia is common. Elevations of lactate and pyruvate are described in idiopathic disease and in patients with Fanconi's syndrome associated with cystinosis or glycogenosis.

The differential diagnosis of Fanconi's syndrome is extensive because so many conditions are associated with the disorder. In addition, renal tubular acidosis in children closely resembles infantile forms of Fanconi's syndrome. The muscle weakness and gait disturbances are similar to those found in neuropathies or primary myopathy. Infants with prolonged icterus, hepatomegaly, and growth failure may also have cystic fibrosis, neonatal giant cell hepatitis, extrahepatic biliary atresia, or hypothyroidism. Obstructive uropathy in children, particularly with polyuria and potassium wasting, can mimic Fanconi's syndrome. Adults with osteoporosis or other forms of metabolic bone disease or with myopathies may resemble patients with Fanconi's syndrome. Glucosuria and aminoaciduria may be present in uremia, but hypophosphatemia is uncommon. Movement disorders could also be confused with Wilson's disease. In general, the finding of complex tubular hyperexcretion should lead to a search for an underlying disorder.

Treatment consists of removing the offending metabolite or toxic agent whenever possible. In addition, replacing solutes lost in the urine is indicated. Phosphate and high dosages of vitamin D are used to heal rickets and osteomalacia. Alkalinizing solutions often are needed (bicarbonate, 10 to 15 mEq/kg per day) in children up to 10 years of age to overcome acidosis; potassium citrate is especially useful because it corrects both acidosis and hypokalemia. In adults, therapy corrects both acidosis and hypokalemia. In adults, therapy could be achieved with 30 ml Shohl's solution every 8 hours. Alkali therapy may also improve bone healing because correcting acidosis prevents further use of bone as a buffer. Thiazide diuretics and salt restriction have been useful in some cases. It is not necessary to replace glucose or amino acids.

In cystinosis, transplantation restores renal function but does not prevent further cystine deposition in other tissues. The use of the reducing agent cysteamine appears to offer great promise in preventing uremia in cystinosis. This compound results in breakdown of cystine within the lysosomes and egress from the lysosome of a mixed disulfide consisting of cysteine–cysteamine.

Treatment for Wilson's disease entails removing copper from the body. Although D-penicillamine is the mainstay of therapy aimed at removing copper from various tissue sites, it has many side effects, and its use may result in membranous nephropathy. Some success has been reported with triethylenetetramine dihydrochloride (Triene), which may act by enhancing ceruloplasmin degradation, which in turn would release free copper into plasma and permit excretion of this toxic metal.

DISORDERS OF WATER TRANSPORT

The failure to concentrate the urine despite the presence of high antidiuretic hormone (ADH; arginine vasopressin) levels defines the nephrogenic disorders of water transport and urinary concentration. A partial defect prevails when urine is hypertonic to plasma but not maximally concentrated. A complete defect is denoted by permanent hyposthenuria. Numerous drugs, toxins, and conditions such as hypokalemia or hypercalcemia can result in nephrogenic diabetes insipidus (see Chapter 26). In addition, disorders such as medullary cystic disease, interstitial nephritis, sickle cell anemia, and urinary tract infections that alter the medullary solute concentration are associated with impaired urinary concentration. These disorders are discussed in Chapter 15, Part 1. Our discussion is limited to the X-linked inherited disorder of hereditary nephrogenic diabetes insipidus (NDI). At least two gene defects have been described in NDI; a defect in the vasopressin type II receptor can account for X-linked NDI. Autosomal-recessive or autosomal-dominant disease appears to represent a defect in aquaporin 2, the water channel.

As mentioned in Chapter 15, Part 1, ADH or vasopressin induces increased water permeability in the connecting segment of the distal tubule and in the collecting ducts by first binding to a peritubular membrane receptor and then activating specific adenylate cyclases to form cAMP. This compound leads to phosphorylation of other proteins that alter microtubular structures and permit augmented water permeability. In patients with hereditary NDI, the cAMP generation may be impaired, and administering ADH does not promote antidiuresis as it does in normal subjects. The finding of normal cAMP generation in response to vasopressin administration in some patients with this disorder is similar to the finding of cAMP generation in response to PTH in certain cases of pseudohypoparathyroidism. Rapid inactivation of ADH or production of an inactive molecule by the hypothalamic peptide synthetic system is ruled out by the finding that vasopressin administration leads to belching and abdominal pains, known vascular side effects of the hormone.

Overt disease is always found in boys, but girls may have a partial or complete defect. The hereditary pattern is consistent with X-linked transmission with variable degrees of manifestation of penetration in heterozygous girls. Male patients exhibit complete unresponsiveness to vasopressin. Male-to-male transmission is rare, but incomplete forms of the disease occur in female siblings, female carriers, and female relatives of affected male patients. Several girls have been reported to have as severe a disease as that in affected boys. Different defects in the physiologic sequence from ADH binding to the microtubule changes responsible for water permeability could be of heterogeneous genetic origin. The high prevalence of this disorder in eastern Canada and the northeastern United States has led to the suggestion that most affected patients are descended from Ulster Scottish immigrants who arrived in the New World on a ship called the *Hopewell,* from which most of the "water drinkers" were traced. Of interest, a legend in Nova Scotia attributed the cause of the compulsive "water drinkers" in their midst to the curse of a Gypsy denied water in a pasture. Recently, however, families in Hawaii and an Australian aboriginal kindred with no Caucasian ancestry have been reported with this disorder; thus, a more general distribution is indicated. The disorder is apparent in the first weeks of life with polyuria, severe dehydration, fever, convulsions, hypernatremia, and constipation. Polyhydramnios may be evident at birth. Hypernatremic dehydration is common because the infant cannot indicate thirst. This complication is thought to lead to the high incidence of mental retardation in this disorder. Studies in animals confirm that neurologic damage resulting from brain shrinkage and tearing of veins are the major consequences of the hyperosmolar state. As children grow older, hydronephrosis, dilation of the collecting duct, and nocturia are found. These children are particularly restless in the classroom. Persistent hyposthenuria is a laboratory hallmark. Striking dilation of the urinary tract may develop, progressing to massive hydroureter, hydronephrosis, and enlarged bladder capacity.

The cardinal renal abnormality is the failure of the collecting ducts to increase their water permeability in response to ADH, resulting in hypotonic urine. The concentrating defect is caused by end-organ refractoriness to ADH because dosages of arginine vasopressin (Pitressin) sufficient to cause abdominal cramps and cutaneous blanching have no effect on urine volume and concentration. Four other disturbances in renal function have been apparent: a rise in filtration fraction, the consequence of renal vasoconstriction produced by high circulating ADH concentrations; hyperuricemia, which in adults may be caused by a renal tubular defect in uric acid excretion (in children, however, it may be acquired and possibly related to an elevated filtration fraction or urinary tract dilation); shortening of proximal convoluted tubule segments; and increased NaCl concentrations in sweat, which are not reduced by 9-Y-fluorohydrocortisone administration. In all other aspects, renal function is normal. The differential diagnosis includes central diabetes insipidus, diabetes mellitus, compulsive or psychogenic water drinking, and other vasopressin-resistant disorders such as pyelonephritis, hypokalemia, hypercalcemia, interstitial nephritis, medullary cystic disease, and Fanconi's syndrome.

The treatment consists of massive amounts of water or, more appropriately, dietary salt restriction and the use of thiazide diuretics, which reduce urine flow and increase urine osmolality. This therapy probably reduces solute load and creates a state of extracellular volume depletion, thereby enhancing proximal sodium reabsorption. Neither arginine vasopressin (Pitressin) nor any of its analogs (lysine vasopressin or DDAVP) has any effect in the disease. Inhibitors of prostaglandin synthesis (ibuprofen, indomethacin, aspirin) reduce urine volume, slightly increase urine osmolality, and thus reduce solute delivery to the distal tubule. In one patient, a diet low in NaCl and protein caused a halving of urine volume. Finally, adequate hydration in infancy is mandatory. By diluting infant formula by 25% to 50% with water to reduce the solute load and administering chlorothiazide, the serum osmolality can be maintained within normal range. Glucose polymers can be added to provide adequate calories for normal growth and development.

DISORDERS OF SODIUM, POTASSIUM, AND MAGNESIUM TRANSPORT (TABLE 23.7)

Pseudohypoaldosteronism (Cheek-Perry Syndrome)

In pseudohypoaldosteronism there is salt wasting, failure to thrive, isotonic or hyponatremic dehydration, hyperkalemia, and a failure to respond to deoxycorticosterone acetate or 9-Y-fluorohydrocortisone.

The disease is considered to have an autosomal-recessive mode of inheritance. This disorder occurs as a result of a truncation mutation in subunits of ENaC, the sodium channel in the collecting duct, permitting massive urinary sodium wasting. In several families there might be a persistent disturbance in renal NaCl handling, which might be unmasked by dietary NaCl restriction of or aldosterone antagonist administration. In these families, the disorder appears to be inherited as an autosomal-dominant trait. It is usually recognized in the second week of

TABLE 23.7. Disorders of Sodium, Potassium, and Magnesium Transport

	Serum							Response to	
Disorder	Na^-	K^+	Cl^-	HCO_3^-	Plasma Renin	Plasma Aldosterone	Blood pH	Mineralocorticoids	Therapy
Pseudohypoaldosteronism (Cheek-Perry syndrome)	↓	↑	↓	↑	↑	↑	Alkalotic	None	Oral NaCl to correct NaCl wasting
Tubule secretion defect (Spitzer-Weinstein syndrome)	→	↑	→	↓	↓ or →	→	Acidotic	Normal	Thiazide diuretics and HCO_3^-
Pseudohyperaldosteronism (Liddle's syndrome)	↑ or →	↓	→	↑	↓	↓	Alkalotic	Not indicated	NaCl restriction, potassium supplements, triamterene
Bartter's syndrome	↓	↓	↓	↑	↑↑	↑↑	Alkalotic	Worsens defect	Indomethacin to reduce prostaglandins
Fanconi's syndrome	→	↓	↑	↓	→ or ↑	→ or ↑	Acidotic, rarely	None	Replace NaCl, potassium, HCO_3^-

life, with isotonic or hyponatremic dehydration with hyperkalemia as the presenting findings. Although no other abnormalities are found, urinary aldosterone excretion and aldosterone secretion rates are elevated; similarly, plasma aldosterone concentration and plasma renin activity are high. The defect is caused by a refractoriness of the renal tubules to endogenous mineralocorticoids resulting from the loss of ENaC activity. Generalized glomerular and tubular dysfunction is absent. Although an end-organ unresponsiveness has been suggested, the fact that spironolactone exacerbates the salt loss suggests that the renal tubules are not totally unresponsive to aldosterone. Others have suggested that renal tubule dysfunction results from a deficiency in Na^+-K^+-ATPase. However, the specific activity of renal Na^+-K^+-ATPase is known to be lower whenever there is reduced renal sodium reabsorption. In adrenalectomized animals, net renal sodium reabsorption appears to be a major determinant of specific activity for Na^+-K^+-ATPase.

The pathophysiologic manifestations are consistent with a cellular defect that interferes with the action of aldosterone in the collecting tubules and duct. The main differential diagnostic consideration is congenital adrenal virilizing hyperplasia, particularly 21-hydroxylase or 81-dehydrogenase deficiency. In such cases, aldosterone secretion rates are very low, but corticosterone production increases with age, leading to remissions. The differential diagnosis should also include Fanconi's syndrome, renal tubular acidosis, and occasional cases of salt-losing nephritis. Some low-birth-weight infants may have hyponatremia, hyperkalemia, and inadequate renal conservation of sodium appearing in the second or third week of life. Spontaneous resolution usually occurs by 6 weeks of age as the tubule matures. The high levels of aldosterone encountered in these infants represent a compensatory response to the tendency toward sodium loss.

Cheek-Perry syndrome is treated with 3 to 6 g NaCl supplementation daily, which corrects hyperkalemia and reduces renin and aldosterone levels. Despite clinical improvement, however, elevation of plasma renin activity may persist, so long-term follow-up is justified.

Bartter's Syndrome

Bartter's syndrome is characterized by profound hypokalemic metabolic alkalosis with hypertrophy and hyperplasia of the renal juxtaglomerular apparatus, hyperaldosteronism, hyperrenemia, and diminished blood pressure response to infused angiotensin II. Patients may have polyuria, polydipsia, constipation, poor feeding, vomiting, failure to thrive, weakness, salt craving, dehydration, and hypokalemia with all of its symptoms. Children have salt craving, muscle weakness, and a peculiar facies with a large head, protruding pinnae, and a downturned mouth. This disorder, more common in blacks, has an autosomal-recessive origin. It has occurred in both sexes, with a slight male predominance. The constellation of polyuria, polydipsia, and dehydration is present in about 80% of the reported cases. There is also absence of hypertension and edema. Recent advances have uncovered at least three gene defects responsible for Bartter's syndrome: a loss-of-function mutation in the gene encoding the furosemide- or bumetanide-sensitive Na-K-2Cl cotransporter of the medullary thick ascending limb of Henle's loop, a defect in the chloride channel gene CLCNKB, and mutations of the gene encoding the luminal inwardly rectifying potassium channel Kir 1.1 in the neonatal subtype of Bartter's syndrome.

Abnormalities in erythrocyte and parotid gland sodium transport can be demonstrated. Renomedullary cell hyperplasia with elevated plasma and urinary prostaglandin levels may be present.

Laboratory studies demonstrate hypokalemia, metabolic alkalosis, and low or low normal sodium, and low serum chloride. The GFR is normal. Urinalysis reveals an alkaline pH and hypotonicity and a 30% incidence of proteinuria. Maximal urinary concentration usually is subnormal despite water deprivation, vasopressin administration, and potassium repletion. Urinary acid excretion (after acid loading) generally is inadequate. Sodium transport at the diluting segment is impaired, and normal free-water clearances are found only when massive amounts of filtrate are delivered to the distal nephron. Sodium conservation is abnormal, and more than 50% of patients display elevation in serum potassium during sodium restriction. Plasma renin activity is markedly elevated in all patients. Aldosterone production or excretion is increased, and large angiotensin II infusions (200 ng/kg per minute) are needed to cause an elevation in blood pressure. Hematologic abnormalities are uncommon. A differential diagnosis includes diuretic or laxative abuse, chronic licorice ingestion, or primary hyperaldosteronism, although the latter two are associated with hypertension. Familial chloride diarrhea (Darrow-Gamble syndrome) must be excluded because this disorder also has juxtaglomerular hyperplasia, hyperreninemia, increased aldosterone levels, and hypokalemia. This diagnosis is established by measuring stool volume and electrolyte concentration. Similarly, a presentation of metabolic alkalosis with failure to thrive has been described in infants with cystic fibrosis. The final diagnostic possibility is Fanconi's syndrome with salt wasting and metabolic alkalosis, but other features of tubulopathy help in establishing that diagnosis. The treatment has been symptomatic. Potassium chloride supplements of 5 to 10 mEq/kg per day to children up to age 10 years with normal function have alleviated the symptoms. Indomethacin and aspirin inhibit prostaglandin synthesis and may alleviate or reverse many features of the syndrome. In patients unresponsive to indomethacin, oral KCl and spironolactone or triamterene are beneficial in correcting hypokalemia.

Pseudohypoaldosteronism (Liddle's Syndrome)

Pseudohypoaldosteronism is a potassium-losing disorder characterized by hypertension, hypokalemic alkalosis, and failure of the kidneys to conserve potassium. Aldosterone secretion is low. Urinary electrolyte excretion is unchanged after spironolactone administration. An autosomal-dominant mode of inheritance has been suggested. Symptoms include headaches, paresthesias, epigastric pain, tetany, polyuria, polydipsia, and acute paralysis with weakness. Hypertension is always present and usually is associated with retinopathy.

Liddle's syndrome is a gain of function condition in which the activity of the β and α subunits of ENaC is abnormal, resulting in Na retention and K^+ wasting with metabolic alkalosis.

Laboratory findings show hypokalemic metabolic alkalosis, a normal GFR, and low plasma renin and aldosterone secretion. The basic pathophysiologic mechanism is a renal tubular transport defect characterized by hyperabsorption of sodium and excessive potassium and hydrogen despite low plasma aldosterone levels. The same defect is found in erythrocytes, as indicated by altered sodium transport. Triamterene, which directly alters distal tubule sodium transport, can lead to sodium excretion, potassium retention, and normalization of electrolyte values. The nature of the renal tubule defect has not been elucidated, but its localization distal to the macula densa segments of the distal nephron is in accordance with the known renal actions of triamterene.

The diuretic spironolactone has no effect in this condition, but other agents including amiloride and triamterene can reverse findings and effectively reduce hypertension.

Primary hyperaldosteronism and Bartter's syndrome are in the differential diagnosis, but aldosterone levels are elevated in those disorders. A rare endocrine disorder called *11-β-hydroxysteroid dehydrogenase deficiency* presents with growth failure, hypokalemic alkalosis, and hypertension; in these patients, urinary tetrahydrocortisol is elevated and patients respond to spironolactone. Therapy for Liddle's syndrome consists of sodium restriction, oral potassium supplementation, and triamterene administration.

Renal Tubular Potassium Secretion Defect (Spitzer-Weinstein Syndrome)

Children with Spitzer-Weinstein syndrome have decreased renal tubular secretion of potassium, metabolic acidosis in the absence of GFR reduction, short stature, and in two patients hypertension and weakness. Associated findings are hypoplasia of the upper incisors, urinary tract infections, and calcium oxalate stones.

Laboratory findings show persistent hyperkalemia and metabolic acidosis. Urinalysis is normal, as is GFR. The primary defect appears to be decreased secretion of potassium, with secondary impairment of proximal tubule bicarbonate reabsorption. Decreased aldosterone secretion is in the differential diagnosis, but these patients usually have hyporeninemic hypoaldosteronism in association with diabetes mellitus, pyelonephritis, and impaired renal function with acquired interstitial lesions. Whether a collecting duct K channel is affected is unclear but plausible.

Chlorothiazide usually corrects hyperkalemia and acidosis in these children, presumably by enhancing sodium delivery to the distal tubule, which facilitates potassium secretion, or by affecting the transport of these ions at the distal tubule level. Bicarbonate administration may be needed to correct persistent acidosis. Sodium restriction alone sometimes can be adequate to correct hyperkalemia, acidosis, and hypertension.

Renal Tubular Magnesium Wasting

Hypomagnesemia usually results from an autosomal-recessive disorder in intestinal magnesium absorption. However, hypomagnesemia can be caused by a renal leak. Renal tubular magnesium wasting is found in two groups of patients. The first have renal potassium and magnesium wasting with an autosomal-recessive inheritance pattern; the second have renal hypomagnesemia with aminoaciduria and glucosuria. Hypomagnesemic patients develop tetany, carpopedal spasm, weakness, nausea, and hypocalcemia because of impaired PTH secretion and action. Osteochondrosis cured by magnesium replacement therapy has also been reported. Although magnesium malabsorption should be considered in the differential diagnosis of the hypomagnesemia, renal tubular magnesium wasting is evidenced by greater magnesium excretion than intake or by the failure of parenteral administration of magnesium salts to correct the hypomagnesemia. Some patients with Bartter's syndrome or renal tubular acidosis may also have renal magnesium wasting. This hypocalciuric–hypomagnesiemic variant of Bartter's syndrome was first described by Gitelman and colleagues and appears to be related to a mutation in the distal convoluted tubule thiazide-sensitive NaCl cotransporter. It thus represents a distal tubular disorder. Its clinical features tend to be less severe than those of the neonatal or adult variants of Bartter's syndrome.

Patients with this disorder excrete three to five times more magnesium than control subjects. The patients also have a mild metabolic alkalosis and may show abnormalities in urinary concentration tests. Because about half of the body magnesium is found in bone, bone mineral status may be reduced. Malabsorptive and hormonal disorders such as hyperaldosteronism and hyperparathyroidism must be considered in the differential diagnosis. Treatment with aminoglycosides or cisplatin can also be associated with renal magnesium and potassium wasting, leading to hypomagnesemia and hypokalemia. Therapy for hypomagnesemia consists of oral supplementation of magnesium salts; magnesium oxide is the best tolerated of these. Hypokalemia is treated in a conventional fashion.

Selected Readings

Chesney RW. Noncystic hereditary diseases of the kidney. In: Brady HE, Wilcox CM, eds. *Therapy in nephrology and hypertension: a companion to Brenner and Rector's the kidney.* Philadelphia: WB Saunders, 1998.
A complete review of renal tubular diseases.

Chesney RW. Specific renal tubular disorders. In: Goldman L, Bennett JC, eds. *Cecil textbook of medicine.* 21st ed. Philadelphia: WB Saunders, 1998.
Descriptions of the major renal tubular syndromes.

Econs MJ, Francis F. Positional cloning of the PEX gene: new insights into the pathophysiology of X-linked hypophosphatemic rickets. *Am J Physiol* 1997;273:F489–F498.
The unraveling of the gene defect in X-linked hypophosphatemia in humans and mice.

Saner R, Schneppenheim R, Dombrowski A, et al. Mutations in GLUT 2, the gene for liver-type glucose transporter, in a patient with Fanconi-Bickel syndrome. *Nat Genet* 1997;17:324–327.
A good description of the genetics of this variant of Fanconi's syndrome.

Scriver CR, Beaudet A, Valle D, et al., eds. *The metabolic basis of inherited disease.* 7th ed. New York: McGraw-Hill, 1995.
Includes detailed descriptions of several inborn errors of renal tubular transport, including the molecular basis for these disorders.

Singh PJ, Santella RN, Zawada ET. Mitochondrial genome mutations and kidney disease. *Am J Kidney Dis* 1996;28:140–146.
Defects in mitochondrial DNA can result in Fanconi's syndrome.

Vollmer M, Koehrer M, Topaloghi R, et al. Two novel mutations of the gene of Kir 1.1 (ROMK) in neonatal Bartter syndrome. *Pediatr Nephrol* 1998;12:69–71.
An excellent discussion of the variants and gene defects in Bartter's syndrome.

CHAPTER 24

Fluid and Electrolyte Disorders in Infants and Children

Aaron L. Friedman

Children are at risk for rapid and life-threatening alterations in fluid and electrolyte balance, and the margin for error is smaller than in adults. This chapter presents a practical approach to fluid and electrolyte problems commonly encountered in children. The discussion and tables are focused on assessing and managing fluid and electrolyte disorders in infants and children.

NORMAL FLUID AND ELECTROLYTE PHYSIOLOGY IN CHILDREN

Developmental Physiology and Renal Function

Children are at higher risk than adults for fluid and electrolyte balance disorders because of differences in body composition, metabolism, and regulatory mechanism function. These differences are most marked in the neonate and infant. In early fetal life, the amount of body water is 95% of body mass, in the premature infant it is 80% to 90%, and in the term infant it is 75% to 80%. Body water is primarily extracellular during fetal development. At birth, extracellular water accounts for about 45% of fetal weight and intracellular water about 33%. Total body water content decreases steadily during infancy to reach adult levels of approximately 60% by 1 year of age.

Clamping the umbilical cord not only removes regulation of fluid and electrolytes but also reduces the influx of large amounts of fluid and electrolytes to the fetus. Under normal circumstances the term newborn undergoes weight loss approaching 10% of birth weight during the first 1 to 2 weeks of life.

As the relative distribution in body mass shifts from visceral organs to muscles during the first few months of life, the distribution of water changes from an extracellular to an intracellular locus. This change is associated with a turnover rate of water that is four to five times that of an adult on a per weight basis, underscoring the vulnerability of the infant if water intake is diminished or losses occur. These differences are further exaggerated in premature infants by their higher metabolic rates.

Regulatory organs for fluid and electrolytes, particularly the kidney, are immature at birth. Glomerular filtration rate (GFR) at birth is approximately 20 ml/min/m^2 but doubles within the first week and attains adult values after 6 months. The GFR (creatinine clearance) in infants can be estimated using the following formula:

$$GFR = 0.45\ L/P_{Cr}$$

where L is body length in centimeters and P_{Cr} is plasma creatinine. For children more than 6 months old, the estimated GFR (as creatinine clearance) is as follows:

$$GFR = 0.55\ L/P_{Cr}$$

Despite initial low values, glomerular function exceeds tubular function, so neonates normally exhibit glomerulotubular imbalance. Fractional reabsorption of most filtered solutes is lower in neonates than in infants and older children. Although the glomerular number is complete by 36 weeks' gestation, the newborn has short Henle's loops and is unable to achieve a concentrated urine. Maximum urine osmolality for term infants is 600 to 800 mOsm/kg. This concentrating defect can be reversed by urea infusion, which implies that the relative unavailability of urea to the medullary interstitium plays a major role in the defect. Furthermore, the tubules may be insensitive to antidiuretic hormone (ADH). The capacity of the neonatal kidney to generate a dilute urine is comparable to that of the adult. However, because urinary flow rates are significantly less, the newborn is at risk for water intoxication. Such intoxication may be expected if the volume of intake exceeds 50 ml/kg per hour.

Implications for Treating the Normal Newborn

Maintenance fluid therapy for the first 2 days of life includes a minimum of 75 ml/kg per day to offset insensible losses of 35 ml/kg/day and obligatory urinary losses of 40 ml/kg. Weight loss can be expected from the extracellular loss of fluid in the first few days, with a gradual return to birth weight by 10 days of age. Caloric intake necessary for growth is approximately 100 kcal/kg per day, which can be met by breast milk or formula supplying 150 ml/kg per day. Sodium and potassium needs for growth are approximately 2 to 3 mEq/kg per day and 1 to 2 mEq/kg per day, respectively.

Maintenance Needs of Infants and Children

Pediatricians use several methods for calculating maintenance fluid and electrolyte needs. The caloric method, which is based on fluid intake needed for basal metabolism, is the most physiologic and is the most preferred method (Table 24.1).

TABLE 24.1. Daily Maintenance Fluid and Electrolyte Therapy in Children

Body Weight (kg)	Volume	Sodium (mEq/100 ml)	Potassium (mEq/100 ml)
<10	100 ml/kg	2–3	2
11–20	1,000 ml + 50 ml/kg for each kg >10	2–3	2
>20	1,500 ml + 20 ml/kg for each kg >20	2–3	2

ASSESSMENT FOR ALTERATIONS IN FLUID AND ELECTROLYTE BALANCE

Classic descriptions of dehydration usually differentiate the approach into hypotonic, isotonic, and hypertonic states based on the measurement of serum sodium concentration. The physician should be prepared to manage volume deficits while awaiting results of serum electrolytes so that hypovolemia is treated promptly. Once results of serum electrolytes are obtained, then therapy based on whether the patient has hypotonic, isotonic, or hypertonic dehydration can be initiated.

Recognizing dehydration relies primarily on clinical assessment (Table 24.2). The younger the child, the more critical heart rate becomes for maintaining cardiac output because stroke volume is almost fixed. Any interference with heart rate, such as hypoxia, leads to rapid hypotension. In neonates, signs of extracellular dehydration are subtle even with severe dehydration.

Dehydration is graded into estimated percentages of weight loss. When clinical signs of dehydration just become apparent, weight loss is estimated at 5%; when readily apparent, it is estimated at 10%; and when marked hypotension is present, a 15% weight loss is assumed.

The causes of dehydration (Table 24.3) often can be identified by careful history. Loss of fluid may occur via the skin, gastrointestinal tract, or urinary tract or with hemorrhage. Internal hemorrhage, hypoalbuminemia, or plasma fluid sequestration also can result in dehydration.

TABLE 24.2. Signs and Symptoms of Dehydration in Children

Signs and Symptoms	Hyponatremic and Isotonic Dehydration	Hypernatremic Dehydration
Weight	Decreased	Decreased
Blood pressure	Low	Moderately low to normal
Respirations	Deep, rapid	Marked tachypnea
Apical pulse rate	Marked tachycardia	Mild tachycardia
Peripheral pulse	Weak, thready	Normal
Skin	Tenting	Doughy
Mucous membranes	Dry	Sticky
Eyeballs	Sunken, soft	Slightly sunken
Fontanelle	Depressed	Variable
Mental status	Lethargy	Irritability, convulsions

TABLE 24.3. Causes of Dehydration in Children

Decreased intake
Increased loss
- Gastrointestinal
  - Diarrhea
  - Vomiting
  - Salivary loss from caustic burns
  - Nasogastric suction
  - Ileostomy
- Cutaneous
  - Burns
  - Cystic fibrosis
  - Erythema multiforme bullosa (Stevens-Johnson syndrome)
  - Scaled skin syndrome
  - Heat exposure (ambient, heat shields)
- Urinary
  - Diabetes insipidus (central and nephrogenic)
  - Diabetes mellitus
  - Hypoaldosteronism (adrenogenital syndrome)
  - Pseudohypoaldosteronism
  - Fanconi's syndrome
  - Renal tubular acidosis
  - Sickle cell nephropathy
  - Chronic renal insufficiency (dysplasia/hypoplasia)
  - Obstructive uropathy
  - Postobstructive diuresis
  - Diuretic use
- Distributive
  - Gastrointestinal obstruction
  - Blood loss
  - Nephrotic syndrome
  - Cirrhosis
  - Protein-losing enteropathy (cystic fibrosis, sprue)
  - Septic shock

REHYDRATING INFANTS AND CHILDREN

Conventional Intravenous Therapy

Conventional therapy of the hospitalized child with dehydration in developed countries is with intravenous fluids. The goal is rehydration over 24 hours, except in the case of hypertonic dehydration, in which slower rehydration is safer. Fluid deficits are determined by the actual weight lost, if serial weights are available, or by clinical estimate of dehydration (Table 24.4). Ongoing management consists of serial weights, monitoring of vital signs, frequent clinical assessments, and monitoring of urinary output and its composition. Serum electrolytes are reassessed within 12 hours or more often if the child is not clinically responding.

Oral Rehydration Therapy

The World Health Organization oral rehydration solution (WHO-ORS) was developed because of the need for a practical, cost-effective means of treating children with dehydration secondary to cholera. Children can absorb sodium-containing fluid in the small intestine at rates up to 25 ml/kg per hour. Sodium absorption is facilitated by glucose, with maximal absorption achieved by use of a 2.5% solution. More concentrated glucose may exacerbate diarrhea because of its osmotic effect.

The goal of conventional intravenous therapy is rehydration by 24 to 48 hours, with gradual reintroduction of oral feedings. In contrast, ORT allows rehydration over 6 hours (Table 24.5). During the first 4 hours of rehydration, the WHO-ORS solution is given orally or by nasogastric tube, followed by free water

TABLE 24.4. Intravenous Rehydration Therapy for Isotonic Dehydration

Dehydration (%)	Volume (ml/kg/day)	Sodium (mEq/kg/day)	Potassium (mEq/kg/day)
5	50	6–8	1–3
10	100	8–10	1–3
15	150	10–12	1–3

Example: For a 7.2-kg child who is 10% dehydrated:

	Volume (ml)	Sodium (mEq/kg)	Potassium (mEq/kg)
Maintenance (see Table 24.1)	720	21	21
Replacement	720	72	15[b]
Total for 24 hr	1,440	93	36
Total for first 8 hr[a] (8 hr of maintenance + 50% of replacement)	600	43	14
Total for next 16 hr	840	50	22

For the first 8 hr, the orders should read D5W + 0.45% NaCl + 23 mEq/L KCl to run at 75 ml/hr; for the next 16 hr, the orders should read D5W + 0.33% + 26 mEq/L KCl.

[a] 50% of the deficit is administered over the first 8 hr and the rest over the next 16 hr. Whenever possible, a standard saline solution is used for infusion.

[b] Potassium is added after urinary output is established.

over the remaining 2 hours. Once rehydration is completed, the child is given a maintenance oral solution at a rate of 100 ml/kg per day for the next 18 hours. Continued use of the WHO-ORS beyond the repletion phase is associated with hypernatremia. Dilute formula is reintroduced after the first 24 hours of therapy. Other commercially available solutions that contain a sodium concentration of 75 mEq/L are satisfactory for oral rehydration, but homemade solutions should not be used because of the risk of salt poisoning.

TABLE 24.5. Oral Rehydration Therapy for Infants

Oral Solution	Electrolyte (mEq/L) Concentration: Na^+	K^+	Cl^-	HCO_3^-
Maintenance	50	20	40	30
Replacement (WHO-ORS)	90	20	80	30

Step 1: Volume calculations for rehydration over 6 hr
- Maintenance for 6 hr = 25 ml/kg
- Replacement
  - Dehydration 5% = 50 ml/kg
  - Dehydration 10% = 100 ml/kg
- Provision for ongoing losses = 10 ml/kg

Step 2: Total fluid should be divided into WHO-ORS for first 4 hr and free water for remaining 2 hr.

Step 3: Give maintenance solution for next 18 hr.

Example: A 6.0-kg infant who is 5% dehydrated needs approximately 85 ml/kg (25 ml/kg maintenance, 50 ml/kg replacement, 10 ml/kg ongoing losses), or 510 ml fluid to be given over 6 hr, divided as follows:

First 4 hr	340 ml WHO-ORS
Next 2 hr	170 ml free water
Next 18 hr	450 ml maintenance solution

WHO-ORS, World Health Organization oral rehydration solution.

Success of ORT depends on the child's ability to absorb fluid and on a dedicated provider who will administer the solution. Close supervision by knowledgeable medical personnel is needed. Failure can be expected in children with hypovolemic shock, severe ileus, glucose intolerance, or purge rates greater than 10 ml/kg per hour. Despite these potential obstacles, ORT is successful in more than 75% of children with dehydration secondary to diarrhea. The potential cost savings from such therapy are enormous.

Shock

Shock is a clinical response that occurs when blood flow is insufficient to deliver nutrients needed to maintain tissue metabolism. Shock must be recognized quickly and treated before multiple organ failure ensues and the condition becomes irreversible. Proper management is one of the most challenging fluid problems encountered in pediatrics. Most often, shock is associated with reduced cardiac output secondary to hypovolemia or heart failure. However, cardiac output may be normal or even increased when shock is secondary to sepsis with attendant high metabolic demands. Regardless of cardiac output, regional flow distribution may be irregular and may compromise cellular functions.

Clinical signs include decreased capillary refill, tachycardia, tachypnea that results in respiratory alkalosis, metabolic acidosis, and diminished urinary output. When compensation fails, the child develops obtundation, irregular respirations, hypotension, and severe acidosis as harbingers of cardiopulmonary arrest.

Immediate therapy for the child in shock begins by assessing respiratory status. Supplemental oxygen (100%) should be provided and tapered to provide a Po_2 greater than 80 torr (100% saturation). Intravenous lines should be established. An algorithm for fluid management of hypovolemic shock is provided in Fig. 24.1.

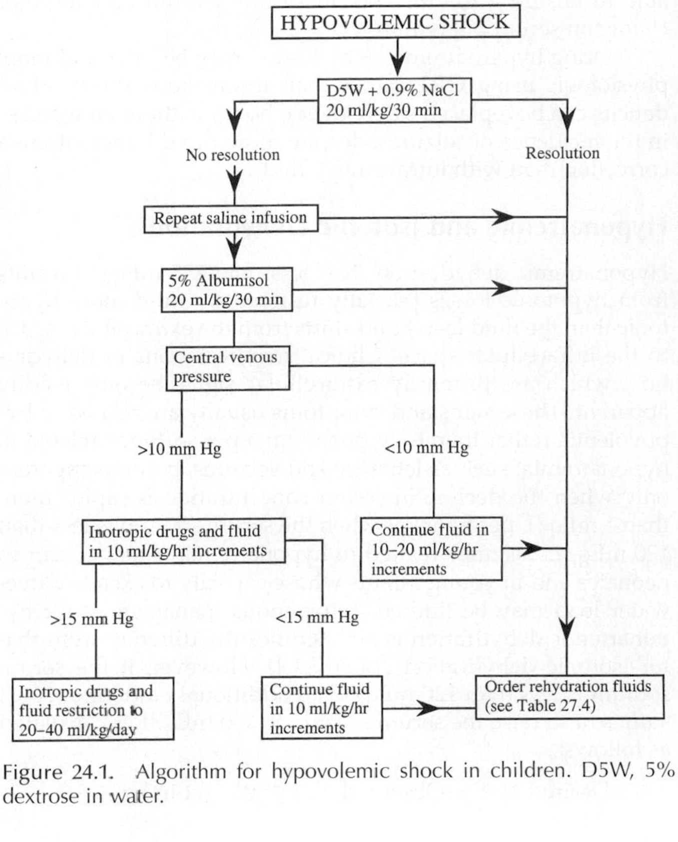

Figure 24.1. Algorithm for hypovolemic shock in children. D5W, 5% dextrose in water.

Hypernatremic Dehydration

Hypernatremic dehydration (Na^+ greater than 150 mEq/L) presents a special problem in children because of its potential for brain damage. Infants are at high risk because of large hypotonic fluid losses associated with diarrhea, inability to express thirst, and dependency on a provider to administer appropriate fluids. The child with hypernatremic dehydration is both water deficient and salt depleted despite an elevated serum sodium concentration. Because of the relative preservation of extracellular fluid volume compared with hyponatremic or isotonic dehydration, classic signs of extracellular dehydration (Table 24.2) may not be present or may be minimal relative to true volume loss. Marked intracellular dehydration may lead to significant central nervous system (CNS) problems, including intracranial hemorrhage. Furthermore, rapid correction of extracellular water deficits (fall in serum sodium greater than 1 mEq/hr) may result in symptomatic cerebral edema.

Children with hypernatremic dehydration often have associated hypocalcemia and hyperglycemia. Hypocalcemia should be corrected so that the seizure threshold is not lowered further. Insulin should not be used to correct hyperglycemia because insulin sensitivity is restored rapidly with volume replacement. Renal failure associated with hypernatremic dehydration may be caused by volume depletion or to associated rhabdomyolysis.

Hypernatremia should be corrected slowly to prevent iatrogenic cerebral edema. Usually it can be avoided if the rate of fall in serum osmolality does not exceed 2 mOsm/kg H_2O per hour. This goal can be accomplished using hypotonic solutions containing 0.45% NaCl in 5% dextrose, administered at a rate that provides maintenance plus replacement of 50% of the calculated deficit in the first 24 hours. Because most children with hypernatremic dehydration also are potassium depleted, the fluid should be supplemented with KCl to provide a potassium level of 3 to 5 mEq/kg per day in patients who are urinating. Frequent measurement of serum sodium and potassium is advisable to ensure a gradual fall in serum sodium and monitor change in serum potassium.

Treating hypernatremic dehydration may be safer and more physiologic using ORT rather than intravenous fluids. Fluid deficits can be replaced safely over 6 hours without an increase in the incidence of seizures, despite more rapid hypernatremia correction than with intravenous fluids.

Hyponatremic and Isotonic Dehydration

Hyponatremic dehydration (Na^+ less than 135 mEq/L) results from hypotonic losses partially restored by fluid more hypotonic than the fluid lost. Fluid shifts from the extracellular space to the intracellular space. Clinical manifestations of dehydration, which are primarily extracellular signs, become readily apparent. These signs and symptoms usually are related to hypovolemia rather than to hyponatremia per se. Signs related to hyponatremia, such as lethargy and seizures, become apparent only when the decline in serum concentration is rapid (more than 1 mEq/L per hour) or when the serum sodium is less than 120 mEq/L. Seizures related to hyponatremia usually occur in neonates and in young infants whose capacity to excrete a free-water load may be limited. Intravenous management for hyponatremic dehydration is not significantly different from that for isotonic dehydration (Table 24.4). However, if the serum sodium is less than 120 mEq/L, an additional amount of NaCl sufficient to raise the serum sodium to 130 mEq/L is calculated as follows:

$$\text{Desired Na}^+ - \text{Observed Na}^+ \times \text{Weight in kg} \times 0.6$$

This can be added to the rehydration solution. Oral rehydration therapy for hyponatremic dehydration is safe, is efficacious, and should be considered.

DISORDERS OF SALT BALANCE

Hypernatremia

Hypernatremia (Na^+ greater than 150 mEq/L) in children usually is associated with gastroenteritis, as previously discussed. However, any condition resulting in hypotonic fluid losses without adequate replacement results in hypernatremic dehydration (Table 24.6). Hypernatremic dehydration without salt loss usually indicates central or nephrogenic diabetes insipidus.

Hypernatremia with excess total body sodium content reflects salt poisoning. Fatal cases of inadvertent poisoning have been associated with excessive salt content of homemade oral rehydration solutions and substituting salt for sugar in preparing infant formulas. Mastitis has been associated with hypernatremia in breast-fed infants as a result of high sodium content and inadequate free water in the milk. Salt poisoning may result also from absorption of salt contained in sodium hypophosphate lavage solutions or enemas, particularly in children with intestinal aganglionosis (Hirschsprung's disease). Iatrogenic salt poisoning has been associated with the use of hypertonic intravenous solutions or dialysate. The physician must also be aware that salt poisoning may reflect child abuse.

Usually, the medical history and physical examination are sufficient to determine the cause of hypernatremia. In addition, the urinary volume and urinary sodium concentration may be helpful. Children with gastroenteritis become oliguric and have low urinary sodium concentrations (less than 10 mEq/L), in contrast with children with nephrogenic diabetes insipidus, who are polyuric with a low urinary sodium concentration. Urinary output is variable in children who are salt poisoned, but urinary sodium concentration usually is high (more than

TABLE 24.6. Causes of Hypernatremia in Children

Salt poisoning
Excessive salt in homemade rehydration solutions
Substitution of salt for sugar in infant formulas
Intravenous hypertonic solutions
Salt-containing enemas
Oral sodium phosphate solutions
Child abuse
Hypotonic losses without sufficient water replacement
Gastrointestinal
Vomiting
Diarrhea
Cutaneous
Heat exposure
Burns
Scalded skin syndrome
Urinary
Diabetes insipidus (central or nephrogenic)
Diabetes mellitus
Hyperalimentation solutions
High solute enteralimination formulas
Renal tubular disease
Decreased water intake
Infants dependent on provider
Comatose patients who cannot express thirst
Inaccessibility of water (lost children)

40 mEq/L). However, in situations of very high serum sodium concentrations (more than 165 mEq/L), urinary sodium concentrations in the dehydrated patient may be greater than 10 mEq/L.

Treating the salt-burdened child entails removing the salt. Volume-induced diuresis usually is an effective means of salt removal. In severe cases (Na^+ greater than 190 mEq/L) peritoneal dialysis is recommended. In children with water deprivation, the free-water replacement is calculated by the following formula:

$$\text{TBW} = \text{Weight in kg} \times 0.60$$

$$\text{Measured sodium} \times \text{TBW}/140 = X, \text{ where } X = \text{TBW}$$

$$X - \text{TBS} = \text{Liters of free water necessary to correct the deficit}$$

where TBW is total body water and TBS is total body salt. Alternatively, the amount of water needed to decrease the serum sodium concentration by 1 mEq is 4 ml/kg body weight.

Hyponatremia

Hyponatremia in children most often is a result of gastrointestinal, renal, or cutaneous salt and water losses in combination with the use of hypotonic replacement fluids (Table 24.7). Rarely is hyponatremia in a child caused by water excess (dilutional hyponatremia). Newborns, especially premature infants, are more susceptible to dilutional hyponatremia because of reduced ability to excrete a water load. Also, the child with renal failure may be unable to excrete a water load in a timely fashion. Edema may not be apparent in the child with water excess, even in one who has had a seizure as a complication of hyponatremia. Other symptoms of hyponatremia include poor feeding and listlessness. Clinical suspicion of dilutional hyponatremia in a child with normal renal function is confirmed by the presence of a low urinary sodium concentration and polyuria.

The cornerstone of treating dilutional hyponatremia in children is fluid restriction to insensible losses of 20 to 40 ml/kg per day or 700 ml/m² per 24 hours. In children with symptomatic hyponatremia, emergency management includes intravenous furosemide (1 mg/kg) and an infusion of hypertonic (3%) saline (1 mEq equals 0.5 ml). The infusion of 6 ml/kg per hour of 3% NaCl should raise the serum sodium concentration by 3 to 5 mEq/L per hour (Table 24.8). The hazards of rapid hyponatremia correction have not been investigated thoroughly in children. Before replacement regimens for hyponatremia are changed, careful clinical investigation is needed.

The syndrome of inappropriate secretion of ADH (SIADH) deserves special mention because it is associated with conditions common to childhood such as meningitis, encephalitis, and head trauma. SIADH may also occur in association with other causes of increased intracranial pressure, such as tumors and hydrocephalus. Bronchopneumonia and asthma in children are associated with SIADH. Regardless of the cause, excessive ADH results in impaired free-water excretion without impairment of sodium excretion. The child develops hyponatremia and low serum osmolality with a high urinary osmolarity. Low uric acid and low blood urea nitrogen are consistent with SIADH and help differentiate SIADH from hyponatremic dehydration where uric acid and blood urea nitrogen values usually are elevated.

The clinical expression of SIADH often is prevented by early water restriction in children at high risk. Total daily fluid intake should be approximately two-thirds of maintenance needs (60 ml/kg per day or 800 to 1,000 ml/m² per 24 hours). SIADH reversal depends on successful treatment of the underlying cause. Chronic SIADH in children is rare.

TABLE 24.7. Causes of Hyponatremia in Children

- Factitious
  - Hyperglycemia
  - Hyperlipidemia (liver disease, nephrotic syndrome)
- Sodium loss
  - Urinary
    - Renal dysplasia or hypoplasia
    - Obstructive uropathy
    - Postobstructive diuresis
    - RTA
    - Pseudohypoaldosteronism (RTA type IV)
    - Nephropathic cystinosis (Fanconi's syndrome)
    - Bartter's syndrome
    - Sickle cell nephropathy
    - Adrenogenital disease
  - Cutaneous
    - Cystic fibrosis
    - Burns
    - Exudative skin lesions
  - Gastrointestinal
    - Vomiting
    - Diarrhea
    - Sequestration, particularly with bowel obstruction
    - Ileostomy
    - Fistulas
    - Peritoneal dialysis in infants
- Water retention
  - Acute renal failure
  - End-stage renal disease
  - Syndrome of inappropriate ADH secretion
  - Congestive heart failure
  - Cirrhosis
  - Hypothyroidism
  - Drugs promoting ADH release
    - Desamino-D-arginine vasopressin
    - Vincristine
    - Barbiturates
  - Drugs interfering with prostaglandin synthesis
    - Salicylates
    - Nonsteroidal antiinflammatory agents

ADH, antidiuretic hormone; RTA, renal tubular acidosis.

TABLE 24.8. Emergency Management of Selected Electrolyte Disorders in Children

	Management	
Problem	Drug	Dosage
Hyponatremia	3% NaCl	6–12 ml/kg/hr
	Furosemide	1 mg/kg
Hyperkalemia[a]	Calcium gluconate (10%)	2 ml/kg slow IV push
	$NaHCO_3$ (7.5%)	1 mg/kg over 30 min
	Glucose (50%)	2 ml/kg slow IV push
	Insulin (regular)	0.1 U/kg IV
	Kayexalate	1 g/kg PO or PR
Hypokalemia	KCl (2 mEq/ml)	1 mEq/kg over 1 hr
Hypocalcemia	Calcium gluconate (10%)	2 ml/kg slow IV push
Hypomagnesemia	Magnesium sulfate (25%)	0.2 mg/kg IM

[a] The drugs are listed in order of priority for the emergency treatment of hyperkalemia.

DISORDERS OF POTASSIUM BALANCE

Hyperkalemia

Hyperkalemia (K^+ greater than 5.5 mEq/L) often is spurious in infants, resulting from hemolysis accompanying phlebotomy by heelsticks. True hyperkalemia occurs almost exclusively in children with renal failure, adrenal insufficiency, or shock. Electrocardiographic changes are rare unless the serum potassium exceeds 7.0 mEq/L. Emergency management of severe hyperkalemia is described in Table 24.8. Shifts of potassium from the intracellular space to extracellular space may accompany acidosis, hemolysis, cellular damage, sodium depletion, glycogenolysis, and glucagon administration. Children with acidosis secondary to gastroenteritis usually are potassium depleted despite hyperkalemia. Inappropriate treatment with bicarbonate for acidosis-related hyperkalemia may result in hypokalemia.

Hypokalemia

Hypokalemia (K^+ less than 3.5 mEq/L) is a common complication in hospitalized children. Investigation entails a systematic review of potassium intake, sources of potassium loss, and conditions that result in a shift of potassium from the extracellular space (Table 24.9). The malnourished child who develops acute gastroenteritis is at particular risk for hypokalemia. Such children may have significant total body depletion and may have serum potassium values of less than 2.5 mEq/L in the face of acidosis. Signs of hypokalemia include ileus, listlessness, and depressed reflexes. It may be difficult to differentiate findings of severe hypokalemia from signs of sepsis in infants.

Hypokalemia treatment entails potassium salt administration. Usually 3 to 5 mEq/kg/day of KCl is needed. Emergency management consists of infusing 1 mEq/kg per hour. Children receiving more than 40 mEq/L by intravenous infusion should be monitored for arrhythmias. Excessive glucose infusion or administration of $NaHCO_3$ exacerbates hypokalemia and should be avoided. Oral KCl salt administration often results in gastritis and vomiting.

TABLE 24.9. Causes of Hypokalemia in Children

- Potassium loss
  - Gastrointestinal
    - Vomiting
    - Nasogastric suction
    - Diarrhea
    - Ileostomies
    - Chloride-losing diarrhea
  - Urinary
    - Renal dysplasia or hypoplasia
    - Obstructive uropathy
    - Cystinosis (Fanconi's syndrome)
    - Bartter's syndrome
    - Renal tubular acidosis types I and II
    - Hyperaldosteronism
    - Diabetes mellitus
    - Renovascular hypertension
    - Hypomagnesemia
    - Drugs
      - Diuretics
      - Aminoglucosides
      - Carbenicillin, ticarcillin
      - Amphotericin B
- Shift from extracellular to intracellular
  - Alkalosis
  - Glucose
  - Insulin
  - Periodic paralysis

DISORDERS OF CALCIUM BALANCE

Hypercalcemia and Hypercalciuria

Hypercalcemia (Ca^{2+} greater than 11.5 mg/dl) is rare in pediatric practice. Hypercalcemia is associated with malignancies (typically osseous), vitamin D excess, hyperparathyroidism, or excessive calcium supplementation in patients with renal insufficiency. The combination of failure to thrive, mental retardation, valvular heart disease, and elfin facies constitutes the syndrome of idiopathic hypercalcemia in infancy (Williams syndrome). Clinical features include headache, nausea, anorexia, weakness, and hypertension. Treatment of hypercalcemia involves withdrawing vitamin D preparations and supplemental calcium, forcing diuresis with volume, furosemide, and in selected cases (serum calcium greater than 14 mg/dl) calcitonin or biphosphonates. Experience with biphosphonates in children is limited.

Hypercalciuria (greater than 4 mg/kg/day) associated with a normal to slightly elevated serum calcium often occurs in adolescents who undergo prolonged immobilization. Gross hematuria and hypertension can complicate immobilization hypercalciuria. Idiopathic renal hypercalciuria often is associated with microhematuria in children. Therapy is primarily preventive, ensuring adequate hydration and high urinary flow. Adjunctive use of thiazide diuretics decreases urinary calcium losses.

TABLE 24.10. Causes of Hypocalcemia in Children

- Hypoproteinemia
- Decreased intake or absorption
  - Inadequate exposure to sunlight
  - Dietary deficiency of calcium or vitamin D
  - Malabsorption
    - Cystic fibrosis
    - Sprue
    - Regional enteritis
    - Pancreatitis
- Hypoparathyroidism
  - Idiopathic
  - Pseudohypoparathyroidism
  - Maternal hyperparathyroidism
  - Neonatal tetany
  - DiGeorge's syndrome
  - Neonatal disorders
    - Sepsis
    - Tetany
    - Prematurity
    - Infant of a diabetic mother
  - Infiltration of parathyroid with iron
    - Transfusion therapy for thalassemia, sickle cell disease, Diamond-Backfan syndrome
- Renal disease
  - Acute renal failure
  - Chronic renal failure
  - Renal tubular acidosis
- Drugs
  - Phenobarbital
  - Dilantin
  - Furosemide
  - High-dose corticosteroids
  - Laxatives
  - Aminoglycosides
- Other
  - Liver failure
  - Nephrotic syndrome
  - Sepsis
  - Rhabdomyolysis
  - Hypernatremic dehydration
  - Hypomagnesemia
  - Acute lymphoblastic leukemia

Hypocalcemia

Hypocalcemia (Ca^{2+} less than 8.5 mg/dl) is a common laboratory finding in children but infrequently produces symptoms. The causes of hypocalcemia are listed in Table 24.10. Hypocalcemia in normal newborns develops in association with the absorption of high-phosphorus formulas at a time when the GFR is low. Functional hypoparathyroidism probably plays a minor role in normal newborns but may be important in the development of hypocalcemia in premature infants.

Cardinal clinical signs of hypocalcemia indicative of neonatal tetany are poor feeding, abdominal distension, jitteriness, seizures, and apnea. Infants and older children may develop similar manifestations along with weakness, inspiratory stridor, and tingling of the extremities. Chvostek's and Trousseau's signs are not necessarily present.

Acute treatment of symptomatic hypocalcemia (Table 24.8) entails infusing 1 to 2 ml/kg 10% calcium gluconate. The dose can be infused at a rate of 1 ml/min, up to 20 ml/hr. Longer-term infusions may be necessary (4 to 6 ml 10% calcium gluconate/kg per 24 hours). For oral replacement, in nonemergent situations one can use different calcium preparations delivering 20 to 30 mg/kg per 24 hours of elemental calcium. Continuous electrocardiographic (ECG) monitoring for bradyarrhythmias must be done during infusion, and extreme care must be taken to avoid infiltration because calcium extravasation may cause tissue necrosis.

DISORDERS OF MAGNESIUM BALANCE

Hypermagnesemia

Clinically significant abnormalities in magnesium metabolism are rare in childhood. Hypermagnesemia (Mg^{2+} greater than 3 mg/dl) has been reported in newborns as a result of magnesium sulfate administration during labor. Affected newborns are lethargic and may have respiratory depression. Management is supportive. Hypermagnesemia in infants and children has occurred with accidental massive ingestion of magnesium-containing antacids and in association with acute and chronic renal failure. In children on dialysis, hypermagnesemia without apparent clinical symptoms has been associated with the use of conventional dialysate solutions containing 1.5 mEq/L magnesium. Most infants now undergo dialysis with a 0.75 mEq/L magnesium solution.

Hypomagnesemia

Hypomagnesemia in childhood is most common in newborns with neonatal tetany, usually in association with hypocalcemia but without hyperphosphatemia. Hypomagnesemia in older children is seen most often with intestinal malabsorption associated with cystic fibrosis, sprue, or inflammatory bowel disease; inherited tubulopathies such as cystinosis and type I renal tubular acidosis (RTA); Gitelman's syndrome; and severe malnutrition. Children with hypomagnesemia (less than 1.0 mEq/L) may be asymptomatic or may show signs of irritability, confusion, and seizures.

DISORDERS OF ACID–BASE BALANCE

Alkalosis

Metabolic alkalosis in children most often is caused by vomiting. Pyloric stenosis is a special situation in young infants. Other causes include diuretic use, inadvertent administration of alkali or of chloride-deficient formulas, cystic fibrosis, Bartter's syndrome, and compensation for respiratory acidosis. Management entails correcting the underlying disorder, if possible, and replacing lost chloride as NaCl and KCl along with appropriate volume to correct dehydration.

Acidosis

Metabolic acidosis should not be viewed as a specific disease (except in the case of RTA) but rather as a failure to compensate for a net increase in acid production. Acidosis develops quickly in the sick neonate, whose capacity for buffering is less than that of the older child. Regardless of the child's age, the physician should focus immediately on the possibility of hypoperfusion, sepsis, or toxic ingestion (e.g., salicylate) as the three most common causes of acidosis in children.

Children may tolerate lower blood pH levels than adults. The best therapy is to treat the underlying disorder. The tendency to provide bolus bicarbonate in children should be avoided. In neonates, bolus bicarbonate use may lead to hypokalemia, intracranial bleeding, an unwanted shift to the left in the oxyhemoglobin dissociation curve, and paradoxical CNS acidosis if the CO_2 generated from buffering cannot be eliminated. Intravenous infusion of bicarbonate should be limited to children with a serum pH of less than 7.2 or a serum bicarbonate of less than 10 mEq/L and only after adequate ventilation is established and potassium deficiencies have been corrected.

TUBULAR DISORDERS OF CHILDHOOD

Bartter's Syndrome

Bartter's syndrome is a set of abnormalities involving renal electrolyte transport. Recent molecular genetic techniques have shown that Bartter's syndrome involves the Na-K-2Cl cotransporter on chromosome 15 (neonatal Bartter's syndrome), the renal chloride channel on chromosome 13 (classic Bartter's syndrome), and the Na-Cl cotransporter on chromosome 16 (Gitelman's syndrome). All appear to be autosomal-recessive traits. Neonatal and classic Bartter's syndrome are similar in that patients typically have polyuria and polydipsia, salt craving, and growth retardation with dehydration. Metabolic alkalosis and hypokalemia usually are seen and urinary sodium chloride and calcium excretion are high. Hyperreninemia, hyperaldosteronemia, and hypertrophy of juxtaglomerular apparatus also are noted. By definition, neonatal Bartter's syndrome presents in the first few weeks of life, whereas classic Bartter's syndrome has a later onset. Gitelman's syndrome is more subtle, presenting in childhood or adulthood without salt craving or dehydration but with metabolic alkalosis and hypokalemia. Sodium chloride excretion may be high, but magnesium excretion is high and calcium excretion low. Hyperreninemia and hyperaldosteronemia often are present. In general, therapy is supportive and aimed at replacing lost electrolytes or fluids. No therapy to date specifically addresses the transporter or channel defects noted earlier.

Pseudohypoaldosteronism

Children with pseudohypoaldosteronism have a relative unresponsiveness of the renal tubule to aldosterone. Other aldosterone receptor sites may likewise be unresponsive; for example, sweat glands may produce a false-positive sweat chloride test for cystic fibrosis. Serum aldosterone levels in the euhydrated

TABLE 24.11. Laboratory Diagnosis of Selected Salt-Losing Disorders of Childhood

	Serum Electrolytes			Urinary Electrolytes	
Disorder	Na^+	K^+	HCO_3^-	Na^+	K^+
Bartter's syndrome	↓	↓	↑	↑	↑
Pseudohypo-aldosteronism	↓	↑	↓	↑	↓
Renal tubular acidosis type I	↓	↓	↓	↑	↑
Cystinosis	↓	↓	↓	↑	↑
Adrenogenital syndrome	↓	↑	↓	↑	↓
Pyloric stenosis	↓	↓	↑	↓	↑

state are elevated, yet serum sodium is low and serum potassium is elevated with a metabolic acidosis (Table 24.11). The children are polyuric, with high concentrations of urinary sodium and low urinary potassium. It is unusual for the serum potassium to exceed 7.0 mEq/L without significant ECG changes.

Treatment involves maintaining normal hydration and salt supplementation. The fluid needed may exceed 200 ml/kg/day, and the amount of sodium may exceed 30 mEq/kg/day. Forced feeding by nasogastric tube may be necessary to maintain adequate hydration and electrolyte balance. Most affected children acquire sufficient responsiveness to endogenous aldosterone by 2 years of age, so supplementation may be minimal or unnecessary. However, under stress the defect may become clinically significant.

Nephrogenic Diabetes Insipidus

Predominantly an X-linked recessive disease, nephrogenic diabetes insipidus is characterized by unresponsiveness to ADH, leading to urinary water loss. Affected patients often have hypernatremic dehydration in infancy, often without antecedent gastroenteritis. Repeated episodes of dehydration may be associated with seizures and may result in mental retardation. Other clinical manifestations include short stature, malnutrition, polydipsia, and polyuria. High urinary output often leads to hydronephrosis, hydroureter, and megacystis. Once these infants are identified, management is oriented toward maintaining hydration and providing calories as close to the Recommended Daily Allowance as possible. Urinary solute load is reduced by using low-solute formulas and hydrochlorothiazide (1 to 3 mg/kg per day). This diuretic reduces free-water clearance by enhancing proximal sodium and water reabsorption, but hypokalemia should be anticipated.

Renal Tubular Acidosis

RTA is characterized by hyperchloremic (normal anion gap) acidosis. The three most common types are proximal RTA (type II), distal RTA (type I), and hyperkalemic RTA (type IV). In type II, bicarbonate reabsorption is defective. In type I, bicarbonate generation is defective because of the inability of the distal tubule to generate a hydrogen ion gradient for excreting titratable acid and ammonium chloride. Hypercalciuria leading to renal lithiasis is common. Children with type IV RTA either are aldosterone deficient or are unresponsive to the hormone. Further discussion of RTA is provided in Chapter 20, Part 5.

Regardless of type, children characteristically experience severe failure to thrive, and polyuria with type I RTA nephrocalcinosis is common. Also seen are acidosis, hypokalemia (except in type IV RTA), and hyponatremia, especially in type II RTA. Urinary pH is high, almost always above 5.5.

Type I RTA is treated with 2 to 3 mEq/kg/day $NaHCO_3$. In addition, 2 to 4 mEq/kg/day KCl may be necessary. For types II and IV, 4 to 10 mEq/kg/day $NaHCO_3$ may be necessary. Prognosis for preservation of renal function is excellent in children if therapy is initiated before they develop severe nephrocalcinosis.

Fanconi's Syndrome or Cystinosis

Fanconi's syndrome is a generalized proximal tubulopathy. Manifestations in infancy include dehydration from polyuria, polydipsia, failure to thrive, and rickets. Laboratory features include hypokalemia, hypophosphatemia, hypouricemia, low serum bicarbonate, and sometimes hyponatremia. Urinary findings include glycosuria, aminoaciduria, high urine pH (bicarbonate loss), and phosphaturia.

The most common cause of Fanconi's syndrome in children is cystinosis. Cystinosis is a defect in cystine transport out of lysosomes. Cystine accumulates in lysosomes and eventually in intracellular space, leading to cellular injury. Patients present with Fanconi's syndrome and growth failure. The renal disease is related to tubular injury. Growth failure persists despite treatment for the Fanconi's syndrome and rickets. Photophobia may be reported and is caused by cystine deposition in the cornea. Eventually other organs become involved (leading to hypothyroidism, diabetes mellitus, myopathy, and peripheral neuropathy).

Treatment includes replacement therapy with potassium (2 to 4 mEq/kg per day), bicarbonate offered as citrate (2 to 6 mEq/kg per day), phosphate as Neutra-Phos (500 mg to 2 to 3 g/day given in 4 or 5 divided doses), and ready access to sodium and water. Vitamin D replacement as dihydrotachysterol (0.125 mg to 0.25 mg/day) or calcitriol (0.25 mg to 0.5 mEq three times/week to daily). Therapy directed at cystinosis includes phosphocysteamine to enhance solubility and allow transport of cystine–cysteine moiety from lysosome into intracellular space.

Management includes cysteamine and meticulous attention to nutrition and fluid and electrolyte alterations. Polycitra (550 mg potassium citrate, 500 mg sodium citrate, 334 mg citric acid; 2 mEq base equals 1 ml) is given in three or four divided doses and adjusted to maintain a serum bicarbonate level of 18 to 20 mEq/L. Oral neutral phosphate (1 to 3 g/day) in four divided doses is used to control hypophosphatemia. Total fluid intake in infancy should be at least 150 ml/kg per day.

SPECIAL FLUID AND ELECTROLYTE DISORDERS OF CHILDHOOD

Pyloric Stenosis

Pyloric stenosis is the most common cause of metabolic alkalosis in infants younger than 2 months of age. Hypertrophy of the pyloric muscle results in partial gastric outlet obstruction, causing vomiting. Infants exhibit projectile vomiting within minutes of feeding. Oral intake usually remains normal or even high because of relative starvation. Constipation and dehydration are common. Physical examination often reveals a cachectic infant who is near or below birth weight. In addition to signs of dehydration and malnutrition, the infant may have visible peristaltic waves and a palpable mass (commonly called an olive), usually in the epigastric area just to the right of the midline. Often, the olive is detected only after vomiting or after aspiration of stomach contents.

The major fluid and electrolyte abnormalities result from gastric chloride loss and the apparent paradoxical renal response of acidic urine in the face of metabolic alkalosis (see Chapter 20, Part 6).

Management is aimed at restoring volume and replacing chloride deficits with NaCl-KCl–containing solutions. Replacement for at least 10% dehydration typically is needed. The dextrose solution should contain at least 0.45% NaCl and 3 to 5 mEq/kg per day of KCl. Deficits usually can be restored within 24 to 48 hours with such a prescription. Surgery, which usually is curative, should be postponed until alkalemia and hypovolemia are corrected.

Cystic Fibrosis

Cystic fibrosis is an autosomal-recessive disease with an incidence of 1 : 2,000 in Caucasian children. Major clinical manifestations include repeated episodes of bronchopneumonia, leading to chronic lung diseases and cor pulmonale and fat malabsorption, leading to chronic diarrhea and malnutrition. Other manifestations include cirrhosis, diabetes mellitus, and intestinal obstruction, particularly in neonates who develop meconium ileus.

The hallmark of the disease is a positive sweat chloride test. Normal sweat chloride content is less than 20 mEq/L, whereas children with cystic fibrosis have more than 60 mEq/L. Sweat chloride losses lead to hypochloremic, hypokalemic metabolic alkalosis. Hyponatremia and dehydration usually are present. Treating the electrolyte deficiency entails both NaCl and KCl supplementation, especially in climates or conditions where sweat losses are high.

Adrenogenital Syndrome

Of the many varieties of adrenogenital syndrome, the most common and the most clinically significant is 21-hydroxylase deficiency. Affected girls have masculine features at birth because 17-hydroxyprogesterone cannot be converted to 11-deoxycortisol, resulting in testosterone overproduction. Boys with this syndrome may be overlooked because no phenotypic abnormality is apparent except for a slightly enlarged phallus. In this syndrome, aldosterone production is blocked so that affected infants have urinary sodium losses and potassium retention, resulting in hyponatremia, hyperkalemia, and acidosis. A rare infant may need emergency peritoneal dialysis to treat hyperkalemia. Hypoglycemia is also common. Affected newborns usually present with vomiting and dehydration. Shock may be present secondary to hypovolemia or hypoglycemia. In addition to normal saline, affected infants need mineralocorticoid (fluorohydrocortisone, 0.01 to 0.15 mg/day) and glucocorticoid (hydrocortisone, 10 to 30 mg/day) substitution therapy.

Sickle Cell Nephropathy

Sickle cell nephropathy, characterized by hyposthenuria, hematuria, proteinuria, nephrotic syndrome, and renal insufficiency, has its origins in childhood but often is not fully expressed until adolescence. The earliest recognized manifestation is an inability to concentrate the urine. This condition is improved with aggressive sickle cell disease management before 15 years of age but is irreversible thereafter. Affected children are at high risk for rapid dehydration because of high obligatory urinary volume. Dehydration, in turn, leads to increased sickling and further tubular function impairment. Prevention and crisis treatment include fluid intakes of more than 150 ml/kg/day.

Tumor Lysis Syndrome

Tumor lysis syndrome is secondary to rapid breakdown of tumor mass by chemotherapeutic agents or radiation. One should expect this syndrome with non-Hodgkin's lymphoma, particularly Burkitt's lymphoma, and in children with leukemias in whom initial peripheral white counts exceed 100,000 cells/mm^3. As a consequence of rapid lysis of tumor cells, intracellular electrolytes and water are released into the extracellular environment. Affected children rapidly develop renal dysfunction with hyperkalemia, hyperphosphatemia, severe hypocalcemia, and hyperuricemia. Such children may have laboratory evidence of acute renal failure before chemotherapy and are at very high risk for fatal arrhythmias once tumor lysis begins.

Therapy is primarily preventive. If renal function is normal, the child should be given fluids to maintain a forced diuresis with administration of 1.5 to 2.0 times maintenance fluids. Alkalinization of urine reduces urine acid deposition in the kidney and allopurinol reduces serum uric acid and uric acid delivery to the kidney. Continuous mannitol infusion (0.25 g/kg per hour) after a loading dose of 1 g/kg over 20 minutes may facilitate diuresis and may prevent acute renal failure. Frequent monitoring of serum osmolarity and electrolytes is necessary with mannitol use. Diuresis also facilitates phosphorus excretion. However, for children with severe renal failure, hemodialysis or peritoneal dialysis should be initiated before therapy and continued as needed during induction.

Nephrotic Syndrome

In contrast to adults, children with nephrotic syndrome often are intravascularly volume depleted despite having total body fluid and salt overload. Tachycardia and orthostatic hypotension may be present. Poor peripheral perfusion in combination with elevated fibrinogen levels and thrombocytosis puts the child at risk for thromboembolism.

Initial treatment of clinically ill children must be directed at restoring intravascular volume with the use of 10 to 20 ml/kg per hour 0.9% NaCl or 5% albumin until vital signs are normal. Diuretics should not be used in the initial management phase. Once the child is clinically stable, fluid and electrolyte intake can be reduced to maintenance needs. Diuretics and albumin can then be used to mobilize edema fluid.

Selected Readings

Fuller PJ, Lim-Tio S. Aldosterone action, sodium channels and inherited disease. *J Endocrinol* 1996;148:387–390.

Excellent overview of aldosterone excess and deficiency, inherited defects of sodium channels, and associated hypertension.

Holliday MA. The evolution of therapy for dehydration: should deficit therapy still be taught? *Pediatrics* 1996;98:171–177.

A reconsideration of deficit therapy and a reevaluation of acute bolus therapy for dehydration.

Holliday MA, Segar WE. The maintenance need for water parenteral fluid therapy. *Pediatrics* 1957;19:823–832.

The manuscript that describes the method used by most practitioners to determine maintenance therapy for children. A classic.

Perkin RM, Levin DL. Shock in the pediatric patient. Part 1. *J Pediatr* 1982;101:163–169.

Perkin RM, Levin DL. Shock in the pediatric patient. Part 2. *J Pediatr* 1982;101:319–332.

Both articles are useful compendia for pathophysiology and guides to fluid volume, electrolytes, and inotropic therapy in the patient with shock.

Rodriguez-Soriano J. Bartter and related syndromes: the puzzle is almost solved. *Pediatr Nephrol* 1998;12:315–327.

Excellent review of up-to-date information on neonatal and classic Bartter's syndrome and Gitelman's syndrome.

Schneider JA, Clark KF, Greene AA, et al. Recent advances in the treatment of cystinosis. *J Inherit Metab Dis* 1995;18:387–397.

Update on cystinosis and Fanconi's syndrome treatment with information on progression of renal disease in patients with cystinosis receiving cysteamine and phosphocysteamine therapy.

Schwartz GJ, Feld LG, Langford DL. A simple estimate of glomerular filtration in infants in the first year of life. *J Pediatr* 1984;104:849–854.

A simple formula to estimate creatinine clearance and GFR

Infants: GFR = 0.45 L/P_{Cr}

Children: GFR = 0.55 L/P_{Cr}

where L is length in centimeters and P_{Cr} is plasma creatinine in milligrams per deciliter.

Snyder JD. Use and misuse of oral therapy for diarrhea: comparisons of U.S. practices with American Academy of Pediatrics recommendations. *Pediatrics* 1991;87:28–33.

Very interesting analysis of the failure of U.S. physicians to incorporate oral rehydration into widespread use.

SECTION IV

Cardinal Manifestations of Renal Diseases

CHAPTER 25

Oligurıa and Anuria

Bruce A. Molitoris

Oliguria and anuria are common and important indicators of renal dysfunction, especially in the acute setting. *Oliguria* is defined as urine output of less than 400 ml/24 hr or less than 20 ml/hr. The reasoning behind this definition comes from the kidney's restricted ability to concentrate urine. Because maximal urinary concentrating ability is 1,200 mOsm and the average daily intake of solute is 600 mOsm, 500 ml of maximally concentrated urine every 24 hours is needed to maintain solute equilibrium. The use of 20 ml/hr comes from the setting in which urinary output is monitored with the use of a bladder catheter to determine whether a patient is oliguric. In children, oliguria is defined as a urine output of less than 0.8 ml/kg/hr. The inability to maintain solute equilibrium results in the accumulation of creatinine, blood urea nitrogen (BUN), Na^+, K^+, H^+, and water, leading to hypervolemia, hyperkalemia, and acidosis. Anuria is the total cessation of urine output. Although both oliguria and anuria require rapid medical attention, anuria represents the severe end of the spectrum and is a true medical emergency. Anuria results from a total lack of glomerular filtration rate (GFR) from either complete occlusion of arterial or venous blood flow or complete obstruction of urine flow bilaterally or from a solitary kidney. The characteristics of oliguria, which result from a decrease in GFR, are listed in Table 25.1. The differential diagnosis is functionally divided into prerenal, intrarenal, and postrenal etiologies.

PRERENAL CAUSES OF OLIGURIA

Oliguria occurs in conditions leading to prerenal azotemia. This is a rapidly reversible process if the underlying cause can be corrected because cellular injury has not yet occurred. Therefore its morbidity and mortality rates are low if the condition is diagnosed and treated rapidly. Prerenal azotemia, also called

TABLE 25.1. Characteristics of Oliguria

Functional	Pathophysiology	Etiology	Examples*
Localization			
Prerenal	Mild to Moderate ↓ RBF	↓ Effective arterial volume	Congestive heart failure, ECFV depletion
		Bilateral renal artery or venous stenosis or partial thrombosis	Bilateral renal artery stenosis
		Loss of renal autoregulation	Angiotensin-converting enzyme inhibitors
Intrarenal	Cell injury	Moderate to severe ↓ RBF (ischemia)	Shock, sepsis, bypass surgery, NSAIDs
		Nephrotoxins	Aminoglycosides, *cis*-platin, heme pigments, radiocontrast agents
		Small vessel vasculitis	Pauci immune glomerulonephritis, hemolytic uremic syndrome
		Acute glomerulonephritis	Rapidly progressive glomerulonephritis, endocarditis
		Interstitial nephritis	Methicillin, any drug
		Intratubular crystals	Uric acid, sulfonamides, methotrexate, acyclovir
Postrenal	Obstruction of urine flow	Bilateral ureteral obstruction	Ovarian cancer, nephrolithiasis, retroperitoneal fibrosis
		Lower urinary tract obstruction	Benign prostatic hypertrophy

*The list of examples is not intended to include all potential clinical situations. ECFV, extracellular fluid volume; NSAIDs, nonsteroidal antiinflammatory analgesics; RBF, renal blood flow.

TABLE 25.2. Reduced Effective Arterial Volume as a Cause of Prerenal Azotemia

Extracellular Fluid Volume Reduced
Hemorrhage, burns, surgery, dehydration, diuretics third spacing of fluids, gastrointestinal losses (including diarrhea, vomiting, and nasogastric suctioning), pancreatitis
Extracellular Fluid Volume Normal
Sepsis, cirrhosis, anaphylaxis, vasodilatory drugs, and anesthetic agents
Extracellular Fluid Volume Increased
Congestive heart failure, cardiac tamponade, aortic stenosis, reduced serum albumin, cor pulmonale, ascites, and venocaval syndromes

TABLE 25.3. Indexes Useful in Differentiating Prerenal Azotemia and Causes of Ischemic or Nephrotoxic Acute Renal Failure

	Prerenal Causes	Renal Causes
Urinary Na^+	<20	>40
Urinary $FENa^+$ (%)	<1	>2
Ratio of urinary to plasma creatinine	>40	<20
Ratio of urinary to plasma osmolality	>1.5	<1.1
Plasma BUN-to-creatinine ratio	>20	<20
Fractional excretion of lithium (%)	<7	>20

BUN, blood urea nitrogen; $FENa^+$, fractional excretion of sodium.

functional renal failure, results from mild to moderate reductions in renal blood flow (RBF), primarily as a result of a reduction in the effective arterial blood flow (Table 25.2). *Effective arterial blood flow* is the amount of arterial blood effectively perfusing vital organs. It represents the functional component of extracellular fluid (ECF) volume. The ECF compartment can be divided into intravascular volume, consisting of venous and arterial components, and interstitial volume. Venous and interstitial volumes serve to support arterial volume. The ECF volume may have no relationship to effective arterial volume because the ECF volume can be either reduced, normal, or increased with a decreased effective arterial volume (Table 25.2). Furthermore, arterial volume and cardiac output can be either normal or increased and effective arterial volume reduced in cases of systemic vasodilation and selective renal vasoconstriction such as septic shock or cirrhosis. Therefore the determinants of effective arterial volume include the actual arterial volume, cardiac output, and vascular resistance. Although venous and interstitial volumes can be estimated by careful physical examination, effective arterial volume cannot. However, two useful estimates of the effective arterial volume include invasive cardiac monitoring and determination of the fractional excretion of Na^+ ($FENa^+$).

A low urinary Na^+ (<20) or $FENa^+$ (less than 1%) is generally indicative of prerenal azotemia as the cause of oliguria (Table 25.3). In prerenal azotemia, the proximal tubule functions appropriately to avidly reabsorb Na^+ and water. This results from reduced tubular flow and increased proximal tubule affinity secondary to increased angiotensin II– and adrenergic-mediated vasoconstriction. Increased proximal Na^+ reabsorption reduces distal Na^+ delivery, resulting in increased renin secretion. This in turn mediates enhanced aldosterone production, which leads to increased distal Na^+ reabsorption. The result is a low $FENa^+$. Exceptions to this rule include the use of diuretics within the previous 24 hours, chronic renal insufficiency with a high baseline urinary Na^+ excretion, glucosuria, an alkaline urine, and in the early stages of obstruction, acute glomerular nephritis, pigment nephropathy, and intrinsic acute renal failure (ARF) induced by radiographic contrast agents. A reduced effective arterial volume state also stimulates antidiuretic hormone (ADH) release. This results in increased distal water and BUN reabsorption. Some investigators have used a low fractional excretion of BUN as a diagnostic indicator of prerenal azotemia, although specific guidelines are not available. This can be especially advantageous in states of high urinary output prerenal azotemia, as occurs in cases of high solute administration, such as in burn and trauma patients. Other useful indicators of prerenal azotemia are listed in Table 25.3. As the tubule retains its ability to reabsorb water, measurements of concentrating ability are appropriate with high ratios of urinary to serum creatinine and osmolarity. The serum BUN-to-creatinine ratio also increases as urinary BUN is retained and creatinine is excreted. Finally, the FE of lithium has been used in experimental situations because lithium is specifically reabsorbed by the proximal tubule. Therefore lithium reabsorption can be used to selectively evaluate proximal tubule function. Another indicator of prerenal azotemia in oliguric patients is significant elevation in blood levels of uric acid.

INTRARENAL CAUSES OF OLIGURIA

A wide spectrum of renal disease processes causes oliguria (Table 25.1). Ischemia and nephrotoxins are responsible for most cases, but consideration must be given to all potential causes. When RBF is reduced to an extent that intracellular adenosine triphosphate (ATP) falls below the threshold necessary to maintain vital cellular processes, cell injury occurs and prerenal azotemia becomes ischemic ARF. Therefore prerenal azotemia and ischemic ARF represent a spectrum of renal perfusion with the extent and duration of decreases in RBF determining the pathologic outcome. This is why it is essential to rapidly diagnose and treat prerenal azotemia as the clinical outcome of ischemic ARF remains poor. ARF resulting from hyperfusion or nephrotoxins has been termed acute tubular necrosis, based on the occasional occurrence of mild patchy sites of necrosis on pathologic evaluation. More appropriate terms include *ischemic* or *nephrotoxic ARF* or *acute tubular dysfunction* (ATD). ATD accurately describes the pathophysiologic state of the kidney as this represents a reversible process dependent primarily of tubular cell injury. Tubular cell dysfunction is responsible for the high $FENa^+$, limited ability to excrete H^+, and the reduced concentrating ability. Recovery of tubular function mirrors the return in GFR as tubular cells undergo repair and differentiation.

Nephrotoxins induce tubular cell injury by four primary mechanisms. Nephrotoxins such as aminoglycosides, amphotericin, heavy metals, foscarnet, pentamidine, and *cis*-platin cause direct tubular cell injury. Other toxins such as nonsteroidal antiinflammatory drugs (NSAIDs) cause vasoconstriction and induce injury through reductions in RBF. Many nephrotoxins cause both vasoconstriction and direct cellular toxicity. These include radiographic contrast agents, cyclosporine, and heme pigments. Efferent vasodilation by angiotensin II–receptor antagonists or angiotensin-converting enzyme inhibitors can also lead to a reduced GFR secondary to a reduced filtration fraction with near-normal RBF. This is characteristically rapidly reversible if detected early and the offending agent withdrawn.

The third mechanism is crystal-induced tubular obstruction; compounds known to do this include uric acid, acyclovir, sulfonamides, methotrexate, triamterene, and ethylene glycol. Finally, any drug can induce interstitial nephritis by an idiosyncratic immune-mediated mechanism and results in ARF. Methicillin is the classic example.

Although we try to limit our diagnosis to one specific cause of oliguria or ARF, it is often the case that two or more factors combine in a synergistic fashion to induce renal injury and oliguria. When this occurs, it is termed multifactorial ARF. This is particularly true for interactions between nephrotoxins and reduced RBF or ischemia to induce ARF. Examples include aminoglycosides, radiographic contrast agents, cyclosporine, *cis*-platin, uric acid, and heme pigments. For aminoglycosides, renal hypoperfusion increases the incidence of ARF from approximately 7% to 30% to 50%. Therefore it is essential to ensure adequate renal perfusion by correcting any deficit in volume status and maximizing RBF before administering potential nephrotoxic agents. This is also true in the treatment of endogenous nephrotoxic compounds, such as heme pigments and uric acid.

Diagnosing small-vessel vasculitis, acute glomerulonephritis (GN), nephrotic syndrome, crystal-induced nephropathy, or acute interstitial nephritis as a cause of oliguria in large part depends on the urine analysis. For the characteristics specific for each of this diagnosis, see Chapters 39–42.

POSTRENAL CAUSES OF OLIGURIA

Obstruction of the urinary tract is a common problem, especially in elderly men, in whom the primary cause is benign prostatic hypertrophy (BPH). Prostatic carcinoma can also present in a similar fashion. Retroperitoneal fibrosis commonly presents as alternating oliguria and polyuria, which often makes the diagnosis difficult. Retroperitoneal lymphoma and metastatic carcinoma, especially breast carcinoma, can cause ureteral obstruction. Blood clots within the urinary tract can also present with obstruction. Nephrolithiasis is also in the differential diagnosis for this condition; however, pain will usually be a presenting symptom with this situation. The ability to evaluate for obstruction using ultrasonographic techniques has virtually eliminated the use of tests that require a contrast medium. A high index of suspicion for obstruction should be present in all cases of ARF, especially in older patients and patients in whom the cause of ARF remains unknown after routine evaluation. Obstructive neuropathy is discussed in Chapter 50.

ANURIA

Anuria is the absolute lack of urine production. Diagnosis requires placement of a urinary catheter to drain previously formed urine and to document the lack of new urine production. Although there are several potential causes (Table 25.4), the primary cause is total urinary obstruction. This could occur at the level of the ureters, as with retroperitoneal fibrosis, or at the level of the urethra. Total occlusion of the renal arteries or the renal venous system bilaterally by thrombosis or an embolism can also result in total lack of urine flow. Finally, severe forms of hypoperfusion resulting in cortical necrosis or severe, rapidly progressive glomerulonephritis can also produce this syndrome. Whatever the cause, the diagnostic and therapeutic approaches must be fast and efficient. Because occlusion of either the urinary tract or the renal vascular system are potentially reversible conditions, each may need to be ruled out.

TABLE 25.4. Etiologic Factors in Anuria

Bilateral renal artery occlusion
Bilateral renal vein occlusion
Complete obstruction of both ureters
Complete obstruction of the urethra
Cortical necrosis secondary to severe ischemia (rare)
Rapidly progressive GN (rare)

GN, glomerulonephritis.

APPROACH TO THE OLIGURIC PATIENT

Because ARF results from a wide range of clinical insults, the approach involves meticulous history taking, a complete physical examination, and the efficient and cost-effective use of the laboratory to establish the diagnosis and to direct therapy. It is of paramount importance to differentiate prerenal azotemia from ischemic ARF rapidly; failure to do this can result in the development of ischemic ARF in patients presenting with prerenal azotemia. It is vital to pay close attention during history taking and physical examination to the patient's volume status and any recent exposure to potential nephrotoxins. It is essential to review the patient's hospital pharmacologic records and anesthesia notes. In all patients, a careful urinalysis should be conducted. Critical information narrowing the diagnosis down will be forthcoming, especially in intrarenal causes of ARF. For example, in ischemia or nephrotoxin-induced ARF, the urinalysis will show mild proteinuria and pigmented granular casts. However, in acute RPGN there will be high protein content, white and red cell counts, and cellular casts. In interstitial nephritis, there will be moderate proteinuria, white and red cell counts, and eosinophils. Urinary diagnostic indices should be sent for evaluation in any case in which prerenal azotemia is in the differential diagnosis. A very high serum creatinine level does not preclude a diagnosis of prerenal azotemia. I have seen one patient recently with a creatinine level of 13 who had prerenal azotemia. Renal ultrasonography should be performed if the potential of obstruction exists. Ultrasonography is the preferred way to evaluate for obstruction because the use of radiocontrast agents could be potentially harmful and further worsen the clinical situation. Besides evaluating for obstruction, ultrasonographic examination can give valuable information regarding kidney size as well as the size, quality, and quantity of renal cortical parenchyma. This may also give information regarding the chronic nature of the disease process. If the clinical situation dictates evaluation of the renal vasculature, isotopic scans, Doppler flow studies, or angiography should be used, depending on the clinical situation and urgency of diagnosis. In general, angiography should be avoided because of the potential for contrast-induced nephrotoxicity. However, there are instances such as renal artery thrombosis in which angiography is essential.

Selected Readings

Anderson RJ, Linas SL, Berns AS, et al. Non-oliguric acute renal failure. *N Engl J Med* 1977;296:1134–1138.

Analysis of clinical outcomes of patients with either oliguric or nonoliguric acute renal failure.

Blantz RC. Pathophysiology of pre-renal azotemia. *Kidney Int* 1998;53:512–523.

Extensive review of the pathophysiology and clinical significance of prerenal azotemia.

DuBose TD Jr, Warnock DG, Mehta RL, et al. Acute renal failure in the 21st century: recommendations for management and outcomes assessment. *Am J Kidney Dis* 1997;29:793–799.

Overview of what is known and what needs to be evaluated in ARF in the clinical and laboratory setting.

Klahr S, Miller SB. Acute oliguria. *N Engl J Med* 1998;38:671–675.
Review of clinical approach to acute renal failure.

Lieberthal W. Biology of acute renal failure: therapeutic implications. *Kidney Int* 1997;52:1102–1115.
Review of the biology of ARF, interrelating potential therapies to the underlying pathophysiology.

Miller TR, Anderson RJ, Linas SL, et al. Urinary diagnostic indices in acute renal failure. *Ann Intern Med* 1978;89:47–50.
Evaluation of use of urinary diagnostic indices in prerenal azotemia and ARF.

Molitoris BA. Cell biology of aminoglycoside nephrotoxicity: newer aspects. *Curr Opin Nephrol Hypertens* 1987;6:384–388.
A review detailing the synergistic interactions of nephrotoxins and ischemia to induce ARF.

Nolan CR, Anderson RJ. Hospital-acquired acute renal failure. *J Am Soc Nephrol* 1998;9:710–718.
Overview of the causes, diagnosis, prevention, and management of hospital-acquired ARF.

Sutton TA, Molitoris BA. Mechanisms of cellular injury in ischemic ARF. *Semin Nephrol* 1998;18:490–497.
Overview of the role of proximal tubular cell injury in the pathophysiology of a reduced granular filtration rate in ischemic ARF.

Thadhani R, Pascual M, Bonventre JV. Acute renal failure. *N Engl J Med* 1996; 334:1448–1460.
Extensive review detailing clinical findings of acute renal failure and the cell biology of tubular cell injury.

CHAPTER 26

Polyuria and Nocturia

Eric E. Simon and Jules B. Puschett

Based on data that are available in the literature as well as consensus opinion, *polyuria* is said to be present when the 24-hour urine volume exceeds approximately 3 L. However, *nocturia* is a more qualitative term; it refers to the frequency of urination during the nighttime hours. In young individuals, the amount of urine excreted during the day often approaches twice that excreted at night, whereas in elderly persons, day and night urine volumes are often equivalent. Total urinary volume in healthy subjects, both young and old, averages about 1.5 L/day.

PHYSIOLOGY OF WATER AND SOLUTE DIURESIS

In the hydrated subject, urine may be considered to be excreted in two (theoretical) portions. The solute or osmolal clearance (C_{Osm}) is that portion of the urine containing all of the solute excreted over a 24-hour period dissolved in enough water such that this "packet" is isotonic with plasma (roughly 290 mOsm/kg). The other portion of the urine, which contains no solute (the "solute-free water") is the water that remains once the requirement for fluid in the isotonic solute–containing portion has been satisfied. In mathematical terms, therefore, urine flow rate (V; milliliters per minute) is equal to solute clearance, C_{Osm} in milliliters per minute, plus solute-free water clearance (denoted C_{H2O}), and also expressed as milliliters per minute. Thus:

$$V = C_{Osm} + C_{H_2O}$$

As with any other solute (e.g., sodium) excreted by the kidney, solute clearance can be calculated as the product of urinary flow rate and urinary osmolality divided by the value for the plasma osmolality.

$$C_{Osm} = \frac{U_{Osm}V}{P_{Osm}}$$

Therefore, if one solves the equation for C_{H_2O}, it becomes:

$$C_{H_2O} = V - C_{Osm}$$

Substituting for C_{Osm}, the expression becomes:

$$C_{H_2O} = V - \frac{U_{Osm}\ V,}{P_{Osm}}$$

or

$$C_{H_2O} = V\left(\frac{1 - U_{Osm}}{P_{Osm}}\right)$$

Based on these relationships, several matters become clear. First, urine flow may increase *either* because solute-free water excretion or solute excretion increases, or both. Second, according to the convention that has been adopted to express the relationship between urine flow rate, solute clearance and solute-free water excretion, free water cannot be cleared when urinary osmolality is either equivalent to or exceeds plasma osmolality. Thus, when the latter situation obtains, not only is there no free water generation, but "negative free water formation" occurs. In this circumstance, water is abstracted from the tubular lumen, resulting in solute-free water reabsorption, or T^cH_2O. Third, a free water diuresis is characterized by an increase in V and a low urinary osmolality; therefore the larger the water diuresis, the greater the urine flow rate and the lower the urinary osmolality. Young normal subjects can achieve a urinary osmolality in the ranges of 50 to 70 mOsm/kg while older persons usually demonstrate a minimal urinary osmolality of from 100 to 110 mOsm/kg during water diuresis. Fourth, it is obvious from the previous formula presented that at any given urinary flow rate, solute clearance is at its highest when free water formation is minimal ($C_{Osm} = V - C_{H_2O}$). Finally, an increase in urinary flow rate can be a consequence of either an increase in free water clearance or an increase in osmolal (solute) clearance or both.

Figure 26.1 depicts the relationship between the urine-to-plasma osmolality ratio and either V or solute clearance. Notice that whether the patient is contracted (Fig. 26.1, *A*) or hydrated (Fig. 26.1, *B*), an increase in solute excretion or V leads to an alteration in urinary osmolality, so that it approaches (but does not reach) the osmolality of plasma. The causes of solute diuresis are provided next.

Water diuresis is accomplished by changes that occur predominantly in the midbrain, hypothalamus, and posterior pituitary, as well as in the kidney. Free-water diuresis is initiated, under physiologic circumstances, by a fall in plasma osmolality. This change is sensed by the paraventricular and supraoptic nuclei on the basis of the activity of osmoregulators present in the midbrain. As a consequence, the elaboration and secretion of antidiuretic hormone (ADH; arginine vasopressin) is suppressed. (For further discussion of the interaction of blood osmolality and ADH secretion, see Chapter 15, Part 1.) Thus the excretion of urine containing increased amounts of solute-free water ultimately represents an interaction between hormonal, hemodynamic, and tubular transport factors that take place in the kidney.

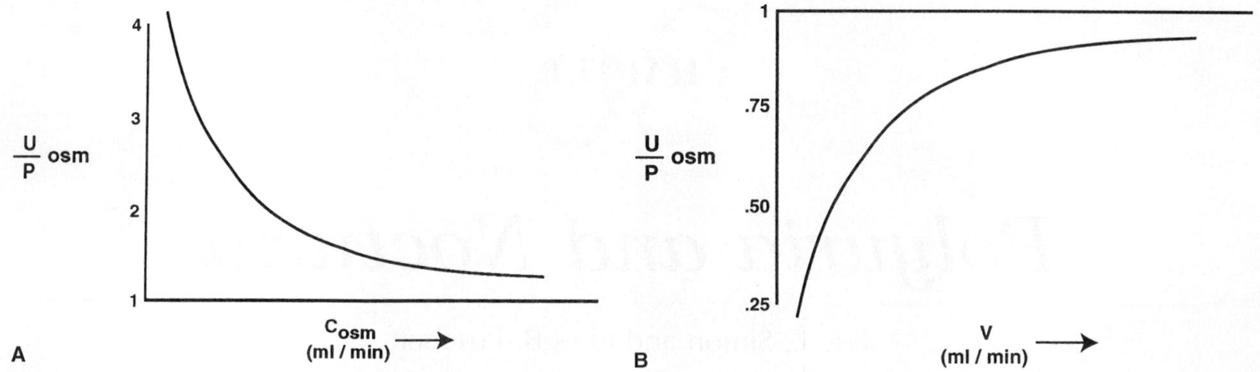

Figure 26.1. Diagrammatic representation of the relationship between the urine-to-plasma osmolal ratio (U/P_{Osm}) and osmolal clearance (c_{Osm}) during solute diuresis in the volume contracted subject **(A)** and between U/P_{Osm} and urine flow rate (V) during water plus solute diuresis in a hydrated subject **(B)**.

Figure 26.2 shows the electrolyte and water transport sites of the various nephron segments. In the proximal nephron (site 1), it has been estimated that 60% to 70% of the filtered sodium and attendant anions is reabsorbed. Furthermore, this process occurs in an isotonic manner; that is, equivalent amounts of water and solute are transported by the proximal tubular epithelium. Thus the fluid that enters the descending limb of Henle's loop is isotonic to plasma. In the process of traversing Henle's loop, major changes in tubular fluid osmolality occur. First, as the fluid passes through the descending limb, the osmolality rises related both to an abstraction of fluid and the addition of solute. As a result, as the tubular fluid enters the thick or outer medullary portion of the ascending limb of Henle's loop (site 2), it is significantly hypertonic to plasma. This nephron segment is the major site of urinary dilation within the kidney. This function of the ascending limb is based on two properties: (a) the epithelium of this nephron segment behaves as if it is essentially impermeant to water, and (b) located at this nephron site is an electroneutral cotransporter that simultaneously reabsorbs one sodium and one potassium ion in association with two chloride ions. In this segment of the nephron, approximately 15% to 25% of the filtered load of sodium is transported.

Because solute is reabsorbed and water is retained in the tubular lumen, the tubular contents are "freed" of solute and solute-free water is generated. Thus the fluid that issues from the ascending limb is hypotonic to plasma. Labeled "site 3" in Fig. 26.2, is the distal convoluted tubule which has a sodium chloride transporter that accounts for the reabsorption of between 5% and 8% of filtered sodium. Fluid exiting this segment remains hypotonic. However, whether the urine that is excreted will be isotonic, hypotonic, or hypertonic to plasma crucially depends on the functioning of the most distal nephron segment—the collecting duct (site 4). This nephron segment is responsive to ADH, whereas the sites in the kidney previously discussed are not. When ADH is absent, this site likewise serves as a diluting segment because solute is transported from the tubular contents, but in the absence of ADH, the tubular epithelium is impermeant to water. Because the collecting duct is also sensitive to the action of ADH, suppression of the release of this hormone likewise prevents the flow of water from the tubular contents into the medullary interstitium, resulting in the elaboration of a hypotonic urine. In this manner, urinary dilution occurs and solute-free water is generated or "cleared" by the kidneys.

If, on the other hand, ADH had been present, the tubular epithelium of the most distal nephron segments would have been rendered permeant to water. Under these circumstances, tubular water would have crossed the tubular epithelium into the hypertonic medullary interstitium of the kidney. Thus ADH permits fluid to flow from an area of lower osmolality to an area of higher osmolality down a concentration gradient. The renal medulla is hypertonic because of the transport of solute (sodium, associated anions, and urea, principally) that has occurred along the nephron, from the tubular contents. Defects in urinary concentrating ability, may thus be a result of abnormalities in the generation of the medullary osmotic gradient or defects in the utilization of the gradient. Defects in the generation

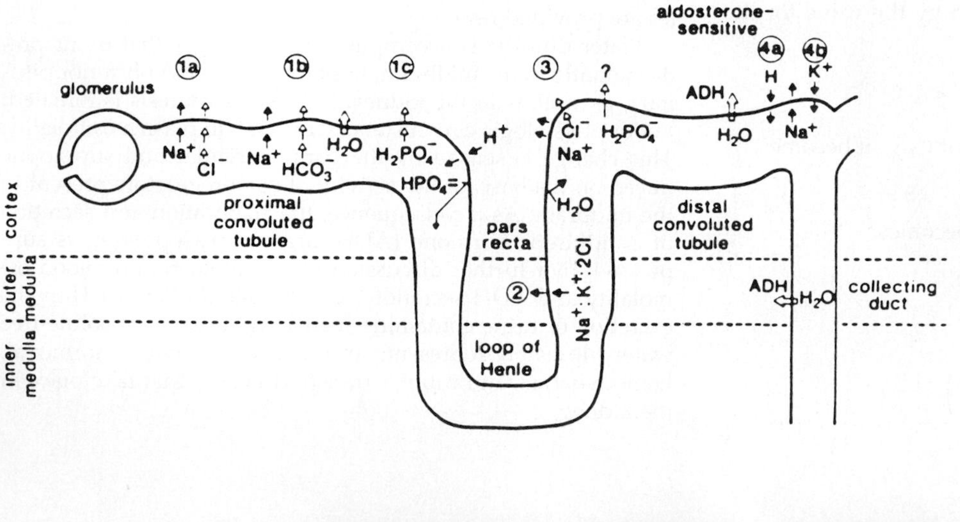

Figure 26.2. Nephron sites of electrolyte and water transport.

of the osmotic gradient include decreased delivery of sodium to the thick ascending limb, decreased sodium reabsorption by the thick ascending limb, and decreased urea delivery. The gradient may be disrupted by increased medullary blood flow. Decreased gradient utilization occurs because of defects in ADH secretion or action. Solute diuresis is characterized by multiple defects, including decreased proximal tubule sodium reabsorption, inadequate sodium capture from Henle's loop (relative to the increased delivery), increased medullary blood flow, and incomplete osmotic equilibration in the collecting duct.

A group of tubular proteins called aquaporins have been identified that represent water channels and have been determined to play an important role in the reabsorption of water from the tubular contents. The major aquaporin involved in the collecting duct transport of water is aquaporin 2 (AQP2). When inserted into the apical membrane of the renal tubular cell, AQP2 permits the selective passage of water. It appears that the expression of this protein is mediated by the action of ADH. Evidence has accumulated that abnormalities in the expression of these proteins may serve as the basis for some forms of nephrogenic diabetes insipidus (DI), as discussed in the following section. In other cases, disorders of the vasopressin receptor (V_2) may be involved.

TABLE 26.1. Some Causes of Solute Diuresis

Electrolyte
Sodium chloride
Saline loading
Furosemide
Sodium bicarbonate
Sodium bicarbonate loading
Nonelectrolyte
Glucose
Uncontrolled diabetes
Mannitol
Radiocontrast agents
Urea
Renal insufficiency
Protein loading
Mixed Electrolyte and Nonelectrolyte
Electrolyte and urea
Posturinary obstruction
Recovery from acute tubular necrosis

POLYURIA

Polyuria may be the consequence of water diuresis, solute diuresis, or a combination. Thus the first issue in the care of the patient with polyuria is to categorize the urine output into solute or water diuresis. This distinction can generally be made based on the urinary osmolality. A hypotonic urine (osmolality less than 150 mOsm/kg) indicates that the urine is largely driven by urinary water losses. On the other hand, a urine osmolality higher than 300 signifies that there is a significant solute diuresis. Intermediate values suggest that there is a mixed water and solute diuresis.

Solute Diuresis

As described previously, the presence of solutes in the urine obligates fluid losses and, when excessive, impairs urinary concentrating ability. During solute diuresis the urine osmolality usually approaches that of plasma (Fig. 26.1). The list of abnormalities causing solute diuresis is limited (Table 26.1); often the cause is obvious. In a hospitalized patient, solute diuresis is much more common than DI.

The most common offending solute is glucose from uncontrolled diabetes mellitus. The administration of large amounts of mannitol or radiocontrast agents will usually be obvious. Other causes of solute diuresis include diuretics, relief of urinary obstruction and recovery from acute renal failure. Polyuria may be driven by excessive intake of sodium chloride, such as with the intravenous infusion of saline solution. Less obvious, but also commonly seen in a hospitalized patient, is a diuresis driven by urea as a result of amino acid infusions or in patients with renal insufficiency.

If it is established that the patient has a solute diuresis or a mixed solute and water diuresis but the cause is not clear, it is useful to measure the contribution of the urinary electrolytes and urea to the solute load. A 24-hour urine electrolyte excretion of more than 600 mOsm/24 hr confirms that the solute excretion is driven by electrolytes. The measurement of the usual electrolytes (sodium, potassium, and chloride) along with measurement of urinary pH will allow the determination of whether the diuresis is from sodium chloride, sodium bicarbonate, or a more unusual cause. If the electrolyte excretion is less than 600 mOsm/24 hr, a nonelectrolyte osmotic diuresis is present. If the patient does not have glycosuria or another obvious cause, measurement of urine urea excretion may be helpful to confirm the diagnosis. A random urine sample can also be used to extrapolate the daily excretion of electrolytes and urea, but a 24-hour collection is more accurate.

In estimating fluid losses and the propensity for hypernatremia, it should be recognized that it is the electrolyte-free water clearance and not the free-water clearance (as classically calculated using total urine osmolality) that is critical. Thus, if a patient were to excrete a urine that was virtually electrolyte free but isotonic because of the presence of large amounts of urea, the patient would still eventually develop hypernatremia if the water losses were not replaced. Therefore patients with solute diuresis may be prone to hypernatremia, depending on the nature of the solutes.

Water Diuresis

A diuresis of hypotonic urine signifies a water diuresis. Having established that the patient has a water diuresis, one of four etiologic types may be present (Table 26.2): (a) inadequate ADH (central DI), (b) inadequate response to ADH (nephrogenic DI), (c) excessive water intake, and (d) gestational DI. The clinical features and management are discussed later.

The causes of DI are often obvious. Clues to the diagnosis include the clinical history and laboratory examination. Central DI is usually abrupt in onset; the patient may be able to indicate the exact time of onset. These patients prefer ice-cold fluids to drink. The serum osmolality may help distinguish between true DI and polydipsia driven by water intake. In true DI, either central or nephrogenic, the serum sodium and osmolality tend to be in the high normal range; the polyuria leads to inappropriate urinary water losses, which then tends to drive up serum osmolality, which then drives thirst. On the other hand, when the problem is excessive water intake, the inappropriate water intake tends to lower serum osmolality, which in turn causes appropriate water diuresis. Unfortunately, there is much overlap among patients. Thus it may be necessary to

TABLE 26.2. Some Causes of Water Diuresis

Central DI
Head trauma*
Surgery*
Following benign brain tumor resection
Posthypophysectomy
Idiopathic*
Congenital
Abnormal vasopressin-neurophysin
Tumors
Craniopharyngioma
Metastatic breast cancer
Vascular
Cerebrovascular accidents
Aneurysm
Diffuse hypoxemia encephalopathy
Granulomatous disease
Sarcoidosis
Tuberculosis
Infections
Encephalitis
Nephrogenic DI
Hereditary
Vasopressin V_2 receptor abnormality
Aquaporin 2 abnormality
Drugs
Lithium carbonate*
Demeclocycline
Amphotericin B
Methoxyflurane
Electrolyte abnormalities
Severe potassium deficiency
Hypercalcemia*
Renal interstitial and structural diseases
Sickle cell disease or trait
Amyloidosis
Sjögren's syndrome
Polycystic and medullary cystic kidney diseases
Functional disorders of urinary concentrating ability
Postobstruction*
Post-ATN*
Primary polydipsia
Primary polydipsia*
Psychogenic polydipsia
Dipsogenic polydipsia
Idiopathic
Hyperreninemia
Thirst center lesions
Hypokalemia
Gestational DI

*Most common causes.
ATN, acute tubular necrosis; DI, diabetes insipidus.

resort to more sophisticated maneuvers to distinguish among the possibilities. A standard water deprivation test may be helpful. This is performed as follows: after initial voiding, the patient is deprived of water and urine is collected, along with a blood sample for osmolality. The patient is then weighed hourly, urine specimens are collected hourly, and plasma osmolality is obtained very 4 to 6 hours. When several consecutive urine specimens are collected with no further increase in osmolality (no increase in hourly urine osmolality greater than 30 mOsm/kg), or if the plasma osmolality reaches 295 mOsm/kg, or if the patient loses 3% to 4% of body weight, exogenous ADH is given. In a patient with complete nephrogenic DI, the urine osmolality remains low and there is no response to ADH. In complete central DI, the urine osmolality remains low until ADH is given, which then produces a significant rise in urine osmolality. In incomplete nephrogenic DI, the urine osmolality rises but is never completely concentrated. Again, ADH administration produces no further rise in urine osmolality. In incomplete central DI, urine osmolality rises but rises further after the administration of ADH. Unfortunately, primary polydipsia will often behave like incomplete nephrogenic DI. These patients will generally be unable to maximally concentrate their urine because of "medullary washout" of solute from chronic high water intake.

It is important to monitor patients for surreptitious water intake during the water deprivation test; preferably, this test should be done where there will be no access to water. Second, monitoring the patient is critical because the patient with true DI may become profoundly volume depleted when deprived of water. Third, if the patient is already hypernatremic, water deprivation is unnecessary and dangerous. ADH can be given and the response should establish whether the patient has central or nephrogenic DI. Finally, the simple water deprivation test described here illustrates the pathophysiology of the conditions and is adequate to establish the diagnosis in cases of complete DI whether central or nephrogenic but in partial DI there is a significant (up to 25%) rate of erroneous categorization.

In partial DI, further diagnostic precision can be gained from measurements of ADH and concomitant plasma and urine osmolalities during the water deprivation test. Patients with nephrogenic DI have ADH levels that are higher than normal for the degree of plasma osmolality, yet their urine osmolalities are below normal for the concomitant plasma ADH level. Patients with central DI have ADH levels that are below normal; in primary polydipsia, the ADH levels are normal. However, one must compare the ADH levels with the plasma and urine osmolalities using published nomograms. Furthermore, for adequate discrimination, the plasma osmolality at the end of the water deprivation test should be in the frankly hyperosmolal range (greater than 295 mOsm/kg) to provide an unequivocal stimulus to endogenous ADH release. If it is not, hypertonic saline solution may be infused. When the water deprivation test is combined with ADH measurements, more than 95% of patients will be correctly classified. However, certain precautions for the assay of ADH are critical, including handling of the blood specimen, and a good assay may not be available to all clinicians. Furthermore, these are not available in an emergency situation.

Another diagnostic maneuver that may be helpful is the administration of an ADH analog such as DDAVP (1-desamino-8-D-arginine vasopressin) for several days. If DDAVP decreases polydipsia and urine volume without producing hyponatremia, the patient most likely has central DI. If there is no response, the patient most likely has nephrogenic DI. If the polyuria improves but polydipsia does not, leading to hyponatremia, the patient very likely has primary polydipsia. This diagnostic and therapeutic trial must be done in the hospital under supervised conditions.

Central Diabetes Insipidus

Central (also called neurogenic) DI may be congenital or acquired, partial or complete. The most common forms of central DI result from trauma or pituitary surgery. Trauma causing DI is generally severe, with more than 95% having loss of consciousness and with a high frequency of skull fractures. Temporary DI has been observed in patients with moderate head trauma. When the upper infundibular stalk sustains damage, usually the DI is permanent, whereas if the lower stalk or neurohypophysis is damaged, the DI is usually transient. After transsphenoidal hypophysectomy, about 25% of patients will have DI, but most of these are transient. After trauma or surgery, the DI usually appears within the first 24 hours. In many patients, this resolves after several days. However, a classic triphasic response may be seen in 5% to 10% of cases. The initial diuresis (phase 1), lasting 1 to 8 days, is followed by a period of antidiuresis (phase 2), lasting 5 to 6 days, which may be mistakenly taken for recovery. However, in this case, the antidiuresis is due to release of ADH from dying cells. Later, permanent DI ensues (phase 3). It is important to recognize the potential for the second phase of increased ADH release, because in this case, unregulated ADH release in the face of continued hypotonic fluid infusion may lead to significant hyponatremia.

Various other CNS insults affecting the hypothalamus or posterior pituitary may cause central DI (Table 26.2). The congenital form is caused by a defect in neurophysin, the ADH precursor, which prevents proper folding and ultimately leads to the death of the magnocellular neurons. Because of the neuronal destruction that prevents the expression of normal ADH from the other allele, the inheritance is autosomal dominant. The syndrome is rare in neonates, manifesting itself in individuals between a few months of age and adolescence. Various primary brain tumors such as craniopharyngioma may cause (either at the time of diagnosis of DI or as a postoperative complication). Metastatic cancer as a cause of DI is less common but has been reported in patients with breast cancer. Granulomatous diseases, such as sarcoid or tuberculosis, may rarely destroy the magnocellular neurons. Cerebrovascular accidents or Sheehan's syndrome may cause DI. Diffuse hypoxemic encephalopathy may be the result of various insults, including cardiac arrest and has an extremely poor prognosis. Many agents inhibit ADH secretion, notably ethanol, and may contribute to polyuria although they rarely alone cause polyuria.

In approximately 25% of patients with central DI, no cause is found and the DI is called idiopathic. There is an associated high incidence of autoimmune disorders and antibodies to the ADH-secreting neurons, suggesting an autoimmune pathogenesis of DI in at least some of these patients. Idiopathic central DI can start at any age but has a median age of onset of 16 years. It has no hereditary predisposition and is usually permanent.

When the defect in ADH secretion is only partial, increased ADH secretion, driven by increases in plasma osmolality, increases urine osmolality. This is the basis for the partial ability to concentrate the urine. Even when the DI is severe, patients generally do not present overt dehydration and hypernatremia as long as they are allowed free access to water. Infants are at particular risk of becoming dehydrated because they may not have access to the required water. Similarly, adults with complete central DI are at risk from dehydration if an intercurrent illness limits their water intake because they are unable to concentrate their urine at all. Some patients with central DI have concomitant damage to the thirst center, and in these cases, the potential for dehydration is a constant concern.

Patients with DI who present with hypernatremia and volume depletion should be resuscitated with saline solution. Once they are euvolemic, hypotonic fluids should be given to correct hypernatremia. Treatment of central DI is generally via hormone replacement. In the setting of acute central DI, it is generally preferable to use a short-acting parenteral preparation such as aqueous vasopressin, so that if hyponatremia should develop, vasopressin can be held and hormone levels will quickly fall. In this regard, as noted earlier, patients with traumatic central DI are at particular risk because of the potential for changing levels of endogenous ADH. The starting dose is 2 to 5 U of aqueous vasopressin, administered subcutaneously or intramuscularly. Subsequent doses and frequency will depend on the urine output desired. The goal should be to reduce urine flow to a reasonable range (such as 100 ml/hr) and subsequent doses should be given when the urine output starts to exceed this level which will usually mean dosing every 4 to 6 hours. Intravenous boluses of ADH should be avoided because of the potential pressor effect. In some cases of hemodynamic instability or when a precise regulation of hourly urine output is needed, ADH can be given as a continuous infusion starting at 2.5 U/hr. The duration of action is short (the half-life is approximately 20 minutes), and thus if hyponatremia develops, it can be rapidly reversed. In the setting of acute posttraumatic DI, patients should be supplemented with glucocorticoids until impairment in glucocorticoid secretion has been ruled out.

Treatment of chronic central DI is accomplished by the administration of the synthetic ADH analog, DDAVP. For long-term use, a nasal spray is available with a usual dosage of 5 to 20 μg every 12 hours. Patients generally tolerate DDAVP even with constant levels because they generally regulate their water intake by thirst. However, it is preferable to undertreat to avoid overhydration. To further limit the potential for overhydration, at least once a week, the DDAVP should be withheld to allow a diuresis. DDAVP is also available for parenteral use (intravenous or subcutaneous) in hospitalized patients with chronic DI who cannot use the intranasal preparation. The dose is about one-tenth the intranasal dose.

Chlorpropamide has also been used for long-term treatment of patients with incomplete DI. Chlorpropamide probably enhances the effect of endogenous ADH at the level of the collecting duct. Most patients tolerate this therapy but they should be observed for hypoglycemia, especially in the presence of concomitant anterior pituitary abnormalities (glucocorticoid and growth hormone). Chlorpropamide is especially useful when costs are a consideration because DDAVP replacement generally costs at least $1,000 per year.

Nephrogenic DI

Impairment of urinary concentrating ability is characteristic of many forms of renal disease. In most cases, however, patients do not experience true polyuria because the defect is not severe, and furthermore, the decrease in glomerular filtration rate (GFR) limits the diuresis. Nephrogenic DI is usually the consequence of a more limited list of diseases (Table 26.2) than the large number of diseases that cause defects in urinary concentrating ability. These diseases primarily affect the medullary portion of the kidney.

Like central DI, nephrogenic DI may be congenital or acquired, partial or complete; most commonly, nephrogenic DI is acquired and incomplete. One of the most common causes is lithium carbonate: about half of patients receiving chronic lithium therapy show impaired urinary concentrating ability and about 20% show frank polyuria. Demeclocycline causes a dose-related impairment in urinary concentrating ability that may be exploited to treat the syndrome of inappropriate ADH secretion. Both lithium and demeclocycline inhibit cellular cyclic adenosine monophosphate (cAMP) production in response to ADH. Another drug that may cause nephrogenic DI is the anesthetic methoxyfluthrane. In most cases of drug-induced DI, the disorder abates when the offending agent is withdrawn, but in the case of lithium, polyuria may persist. Electrolyte disturbances, including hypercalcemia and hypokalemia, may cause DI, although the case will usually be mild.

Several intrinsic renal diseases are noteworthy for their ability to produce polyuria. Chronic partial urinary tract obstruction may lead to structural changes in the medulla and collecting duct that impair responsiveness to ADH and maintenance of medullary hypertonicity. Polyuria is common after release of bilateral ureteral obstruction. The diuresis is partially a solute diuresis from urea and sodium chloride retention and partially a water diuresis from

ADH resistance. The diuresis may be perpetuated by continued fluid replacement of urinary losses. Sickle cell disease or trait may also occasionally produce nephrogenic DI as a result of its propensity for destroying medullary structures.

There are two general varieties of congenital or genetic forms of DI. The more common variety is the X-linked recessive form, characterized by a defect in the AVP V_2 receptor. Many mutations in the receptor have now been identified in various kindreds. Most of the mutations apparently block the insertion of the protein into the plasma membrane although some of the defects are only partial. The second variety is autosomal recessive and is caused by defects in the water channel of the collecting duct, aquaporin 2. The defects described prevent the protein from inserting into the plasma membrane. Heterozygotes are unaffected. In contrast to hereditary central DI, the congenital forms of nephrogenic DI are manifest from birth. Consequently, these infants are more prone to dehydration and hypernatremia with attendant problems such as mental retardation. Furthermore, the increase in urinary volumes may lead to dilation of the collecting duct system.

The polyuria of nephrogenic DI can be blunted by the use of a low-salt diet plus a thiazide diuretic. The low-salt diet limits the obligate urine loss from the osmotic component as well as promoting volume depletion in the face of the diuretic. The volume depletion limits diuresis by enhancing proximal tubule fluid reabsorption. Thiazide diuretics do not impair urinary concentrating ability and thus are useful in the treatment of DI. Loop diuretics, although producing volume depletion, impair maximal urinary concentrating ability and should be avoided. Furthermore, hypokalemia should be avoided in the thiazide diuretic–treated patients as this may impair urinary concentrating ability. Amiloride may be used both for its diuretic and potassium-sparing effects, usually in combination with thiazides. Nonsteroidal antiinflammatory drugs (NSAIDs) may also be useful probably because of their ability to inhibit medullary prostaglandin synthesis. Because PGE_1 normally antagonizes the effect of ADH, prostaglandin inhibition would be expected to enhance the effect of ADH. A combination of thiazide and NSAIDs may also be used if the effect of the thiazide alone is not adequate. Some patients with partial nephrogenic DI will respond to DDAVP therapy with some decrease in polyuria, but usually its cost will not justify its use in this situation.

In patients receiving lithium, serum levels should be monitored and if they are elevated, the dosage should be reduced. Administration of a single daily dose may also be used to limit toxicity. Amiloride is particularly useful in the treatment of polyuria associated with lithium. In addition to its diuretic and potassium-sparing effects, it may block lithium uptake into collecting duct cells.

Primary Polydipsia

The excessive urinary output of dilute urine seen in primary polydipsia strictly defines DI, although some investigators would exclude primary polydipsia from DI. Excessive water intake can be the result of two types of abnormalities. In classic *psychogenic polydipsia,* the patient's water intake is not strictly tied to osmolality; hence thirst is often not the primary driving force for fluid ingestion. Water intake may continue despite significant hypoosmolality, and these patients generally have plasma osmolalities ranging from the low end of normal to the frankly hyposmolal level. These patients may have an overt psychiatric illness, such as schizophrenia. They are also prone to developing episodes of inappropriate ADH secretion, which may lead to symptomatic hyponatremia. A second group of patients has an apparent decrease in the osmotic thirst threshold. These patients have what is termed *dipsogenic DI* and are otherwise normal. Although they are stimulated to drink fluids at a lower osmotic threshold than normal, as their plasma osmolality falls, ADH is suppressed and a maximally dilute urine is formed. These patients tend to have plasma osmolalities in the normal range. In some patients, no cause of the increase in thirst will be found, although diverse causes of increased thirst include hyperreninemic states, hypokalemia, and structural lesions of the thirst center.

Because of the high urine output, ultimately primary water drinkers may generate a form of nephrogenic DI. These patients have decreased solute in the medulla from "medullary washout," and consequently are unable to maximally concentrate their urine. As discussed previously, this often presents problems in differential diagnosis, making it sometimes difficult to separate this group from partial nephrogenic DI of other causes.

Distinguishing primary polydipsia from DI is critical if one contemplates treatment with DDAVP. The use of DDAVP or other ADH analogs may have disastrous consequences in patients who continue to ingest fluid when ADH levels are normal or high. However, some of these patients can be given DDAVP at night to eliminate troublesome nocturia. If it is given only at night, usually significant hyponatremia does not develop.

Gestational Diabetes Insipidus

DI starting in pregnancy is rare. It is caused by increased blood levels of vasopressinase synthesized in the placenta. The levels of this enzyme increase during normal pregnancy but increase even more in patients with DI. Partial central DI may also be exacerbated by pregnancy. The disease remits soon after delivery of the placenta. Measuring ADH levels is generally not helpful because ADH is rapidly degraded by the vasopressinase in the tube in which the blood sample is collected unless the vasopressinase is inhibited. The treatment during pregnancy is DDAVP, which is relatively resistant to the vasopressinase.

NOCTURIA

A number of factors affect nocturnal urination; these include age, structural components of the urinary tract from the kidney to urethra, psychologic factors, and daytime fluid retention (if any). Nocturia may be associated with polyuria, as defined earlier (i.e., water and osmotic diuresis). However, nocturia may also occur as the consequence of an edema-forming state such as congestive heart failure, nephrotic syndrome, and cirrhosis, in which total urine output may be normal or decreased but the normal diurnal pattern is disrupted. The supine position during sleep promotes reabsorption of dependent edema with subsequent urine production.

ADH levels normally rise at night, which limits nocturia. The achievement of the normal diurnal variation in ADH levels is usually seen by 7 years of age. Some children with persistent enuresis have deficient nocturnal ADH release (without frank DI). The loss of diurnal variation in urine output also becomes increasingly common with advancing age. As a consequence the incidence of nocturia increases with age, with more than 80% of patients experiencing nocturia by 80 years of age. Many factors could contribute to nocturia in elderly persons, including decreased bladder compliance or size, increased bladder contractions, decreased renal concentrating ability because of intrinsic renal disease, and urologic disease. However, in many patients, bladder capacity is normal, and a careful measurement of urine volumes shows a loss of diurnal variation. Plasma

ADH levels are variable in elderly persons, but some studies suggest that in those with nocturia, levels are lower than normal. The role of daytime fluid retention in elderly patients with nocturia but without congestive heart failure is not clear.

It should also be emphasized that significant nocturia disrupts sleep, and in elderly persons, it is a significant risk factor for hip fractures. Patients should limit fluid intake before bedtime and should avoid ethanol. However, some elderly patients will become dehydrated in their attempt to avoid nocturia. A definite role for DDAVP has not been established in the treatment of these patients; however, low dosages of DDAVP have been used successfully to control troublesome nocturia in some patients with neurologic disease, such as multiple sclerosis.

Selected Readings

Batlle DC, von Riotte AB, Gaviria M, et al. Amelioration of polyuria by amiloride in patients receiving long-term lithium therapy. *N Engl J Med* 1985; 312:408–414.

This study shows the beneficial effects of amiloride on lithium-induced diabetes insipidus.

Blevins LS, Wand GS. Diabetes insipidus. *Crit Care Med* 1992;20:69–79.

This review emphasizes the diagnosis and treatment of diabetes insipidus in the critical care setting.

Donahue JL, Lowenthal DT. Nocturnal polyuria in the elderly person. *Am J Med Sci* 1997;314:232–238.

Comprehensive review of mechanisms of nocturia in patients without overt edema-forming states. Treatment options are discussed.

Durr JA, Hoggard JG, Hunt JM, et al. Diabetes insipidus in pregnancy associated with abnormally high circulating vasopressinase activity. *N Engl J Med* 1987; 316:1070–1074.

Vasopressinase levels were measured in the plasma of pregnant women and were found to be significantly elevated.

Gennari FJ, Kassirer JP. Osmotic diuresis. *N Engl J Med* 1974;291:714–720.

This comprehensive review of the mechanisms of osmotic diuresis still remains pertinent.

Greenberg, A. Disorders of body water metabolism. In: Puschett JB, ed. *Disorders of fluid and electrolyte balance.* New York: Churchill Livingstone, 1985.

This brief review includes discussions of urinary concentrating defects and hypernatremia.

Kirkland J, Lye M, Levy DW, et al. Patterns of urine flow and electrolyte excretion in health elderly. *Br Med J* 1983;287:1665–1667.

This study shows that the proportion of urine passed at night increases in elderly patients.

Narins RG, Riley LJ Jr. Polyuria: simple and mixed disorders. *Am J Kidney Dis* 1991;17:237–241.

This review of solute diuresis emphasizes the importance of nonelectrolyte water excretion in the production of hypernatremia.

Knoers NV, van Os CH. Molecular and cellular defects in nephrogenic diabetes insipidus. *Curr Opin Nephrol Hypertens* 1996;5:353–358.

Current, brief review of the genetic disorders associated with nephrogenic diabetes insipidus.

Oster JR, Singer I, Thatte L, et al. The polyuria of solute diuresis. *Arch Intern Med* 1997;157:721–729.

The causes of solute diuresis are reviewed. A detailed algorithm aids in the categorization of patients into water, solute, or mixed disturbances and then, when solute diuresis is present, will help to identify the type (or types) of contributing solute.

Robertson, GL. Diabetes insipidus. *Endocrinol Metab Clin North Am* 1995;24: 549–572.

This comprehensive review of diabetes insipidus gives nomograms for relating the plasma and urine osmolalities to plasma ADH levels for the diagnosis of diabetes insipidus as well as covering pathogenesis and treatment.

Seckl JR, Dunger DB. Diabetes insipidus. Current treatment recommendations. *Drugs* 1992;44:216–224.

This review contains a particularly useful discussion on the use of DDAVP, specifically, the different types of administration methods for intranasal use with their potential problems.

Zerbe RL, Robertson GL. A comparison of plasma vasopressin measurements with a standard indirect test in the differential diagnosis of polyuria. *N Engl J Med* 1981;305:1539–1546.

This study directly compares the accuracy of determining the causes of diabetes insipidus using the traditional water deprivation test to the water deprivation test combined with measurement of plasma ADH levels. Approximately 25% of patients were misclassified when ADH levels were not used. None of the patients with complete DI were incorrectly classified.

CHAPTER 27

Dysuria and Frequency

Richard J. Glassock

The symptom complex of difficult and painful passage of urine (dysuria) accompanied by a pattern of repetitive voiding of relatively small amounts of urine (frequency; pollakiuria) and a sense of an imperative need to void (urgency) is quite familiar to all clinicians. Although bacterial cystitis or urethritis is the most common cause of these complaints, many nonbacterial, infection-associated conditions can yield similar symptoms. Polyuria (discussed in Chapter 26) can lead to frequent voiding, usually of large rather than small amounts of urine. Dysuria should not be present unless the polyuric state is complicated by another condition. Partial obstruction of the flow of urine in the lower urinary tract or a neurogenic bladder can also give rise to frequency (e.g., overflow incontinence), with or without dysuria.

The dysuria–frequency complex is seen far more frequently in women than in men. Table 27.1 lists the causes of dysuria and frequency in both sexes. Because there are distinct gender differences in causation, the approaches to diagnosis of dysuria in women and men will be discussed separately.

DYSURIA IN WOMEN

Infectious Causes

Pyelonephritis, Cystitis, and Urethritis

Upper urinary tract bacterial infection (pyelonephritis) is often accompanied by fever, costovertebral angle tenderness (unilateral or bilateral), frequency of urination, and dysuria. Such renal infections may also be asymptomatic. When dysuria is not accompanied by upper urinary tract symptoms or signs, one must distinguish symptoms arising from bladder or urethral pain from pain associated with urination across inflamed external genitalia (labia and vagina).

Quantitative urine cultures of spontaneously voided (midstream) urine has long been used as a standard for the definition of urinary tract infection (upper or lower). When properly collected, urine containing greater than 100,000 colonies (10^5) per milliliter of urine can be assumed to represent an "infection" of the urinary tract, regardless of the presence or absence of symptoms (symptomatic or asymptomatic bacteruria). The false-positive rate of quantitative bacteruria will vary according to the adequacy of the collection. With one specimen, a false-positive rate of 10% to 14% can be expected. Two or more consecutive specimens showing high colony counts with the same organism yields a false-positive rate of less than 5%. However, women with the dysuria/frequency symptom complex commonly (at least 50% of the time) excrete far fewer organisms (10^2 to 10^4, usually coliform bacilli), despite higher counts from aspirated bladder urine. Pyuria (increased excretion of leukocytes; greater than 200,000/ml urine) combined with low urinary colony counts (10^2 to 10^4) strongly suggests a bacterial origin for the symptom complex. Gram-stain evaluation of unspun urine may be helpful if colony counts are high, but it is not very useful if colony counts are low. Nitrite dipstick tests to detect bacterial degradation and tests to detect polymorphonuclear leukocyte enzymes may be useful adjunctive procedures, but because of a high frequency of false-negative results, they should not be used as a substitute for careful examination of the urinary sediment in patients with the symptom complex. The presence of dysuria and pyuria despite negative test results for bacterial infection are characteristic of a *Chlamydia trachomatis* urinary tract infection, urinary tuberculosis, and occasionally a chemically induced cystitis.

Chlamydia, a common cause of urethritis or cystitis in young, sexually active women, is an intracellular gram-negative bacterial organism that requires special isolation techniques for detection (cell culture, monoclonal antibodies). Symptoms of chlamydial infection are similar to those of other bacterial infections of the urinary tract, except for a more insidious onset and less hematuria. Treatment with 100 mg doxycycline twice a day for 7 days or 1 g macrolide (azithromycin) by mouth is effective.

Genitourinary tuberculosis (further discussed in Chapter 41, Part 2) is a bloodstream-derived infection that often (but not necessarily) originates from the lungs. Sterile pyuria with or without hematuria is common. A positive tuberculin skin test is expected and a diagnosis can be established by a series of first-voided specimens cultured for mycobacterium tuberculosis. Smears for acid-fast bacilli are not useful because of potential contamination with other nontubercular acid-fast organisms. In endemic areas, *Schistosoma hematobium* bladder infection may also be a cause of sterile pyuria and terminal (end of voiding) hematuria. In this infection, the urine will ordinarily contain the characteristic ova, but occasionally biopsy at the time of cystoscopy will be required for accurate and definitive diagnosis.

Vaginitis can also produce dysuria and is often associated with vaginal discharge, vulvar pruritus, and painful intercourse. Several organisms may be implicated in the infectious

TABLE 27.1. Causes of Dysuria

Urinary tract infection
Enterobacteriaceae
Gram-positive organisms
Chlamydia trachomatis
Mycobacterium tuberculosis
Viruses: adenovirus II, cytomegalovirus
Parasites: *Schistosoma haematobium*
Vaginitis
Fungal: *Candida albicans*
Bacterial:
Bacterial vaginosis (*Gardnerella vaginalis*)
Neisseria gonorrhoeae
Treponema pallidum (endourethral chancre)
Chlamydia trachomatis
Protozoa: *Trichomonas vaginalis*
Genital infection
Herpes simplex (genitalis)
Condyloma acuminatum
Paraurethral glands
Estrogen deficiency
Interstitial cystitis (Hunner's ulcers)
Chemical irritants
Douches, deodorant aerosols
Contraceptive jellies
Bubble bath
Medications: cyclophosphamide
Impedance to flow
Urethral caruncle or diverticula
Meatal stenosis or stricture
Transient urethral edema
Chronic fibrosis after trauma
Impaired synergy: bladder contraction and sphincter relaxation
Pregnancy
Systemic or regional disease
Reiter's syndrome
Behçet's syndrome
Crohn's disease
Diverticulitis
Cervical radium implant
Bladder tumor

process, including *Candida albicans, Trichomonas vaginalis, Gardnerella, Neisseria gonorrhea,* and *Herpes simplex*.

Candida vaginitis is characterized by a thick, white, adherent, curd-forming discharge. Hyperglycemia, high estrogen levels, and pregnancy promote this infection. Diagnosis is established by detecting the *Candida* spherules in fresh wet-mounted specimens of the discharge. Topical treatment with clotrimazole or miconazole generally yields satisfactory results. *Trichomonas vaginitis* produces a profuse, frothy, malodorous discharge. Wet-mount specimens of the discharge will confirm the diagnosis in more than 70% of cases. The treatment is oral metronidazole 500 mg twice daily for 5 days or 2 g metronidazole given in a single dose. The patient's sexual partners should be treated concomitantly. *Gardnerella vaginitis* is characterized by overgrowth of the normal endogenous lactobacillus with anaerobic bacteria and mycoplasma. It is characterized by a thin, yellow, malodorous discharge with a low pH. The addition of 10% potassium hydroxide to the discharge produces a fishy odor that is caused by the release of polyamines. "Clue cells," or vaginal epithelial cells covered with adherent coccobacilli, are frequently found. Treatment with metronidazole 500 mg twice daily for 5 days is very effective. *N. gonorrhea* is becoming a more common cause of vaginitis in sexually active women. This infection is characterized by a purulent discharge, sometimes with fever and vaginismus resembling an acute urinary tract infection. Pelvic examinations may reveal tender adnexa. A Thayer-Martin culture will establish the diagnosis in a high percentage of cases. Treatment in uncomplicated cases consists of intramuscular single-dose administration of ceftriaxone 200 mg, followed by a week-long course of doxycycline or azithromycin for possible associated chlamydial disease. Spectinomycin 2 g given intramuscularly can also be used. *H. simplex* vaginitis can be diagnosed by inspection and responds to oral or topical antiviral therapy (acyclovir) but recurrences are frequent.

Noninfectious Causes

Atrophic Vaginitis

Atrophic vaginitis results from estrogen deficiency in postmenopausal women. It leads to dysuria, perineal irritation, pruritus, and vaginal discharge accompanied by painful intercourse. It may be complicated by infections (e.g., with *Trichomonas*). A wet smear of exfoliated cells will demonstrate low estrogen effect. This disorder responds satisfactorily to topical estrogen replacement.

Chronic Interstitial Cystitis

Chronic interstitial cystitis is a difficult and aggravating disorder of uncertain cause and pathogenesis. Affected women complain of severe urinary frequency, marked urgency, and dysuria. Pyuria and hematuria may also occur, but bacteruria is usually absent. The diagnosis can only be established through cystoscopy, where multiple petechiae are seen with bladder distention. The bladder capacity is reduced and superficial stellate ulcers (Hunner's ulcers) are observed. Biopsy also shows inflammation, edema, vasodilation, and fibrosis. Most therapies are not successful in eradicating symptoms, except transiently. Many surgical approaches, including bladder denervation, neocystoplasty, and urinary diversion, have been used in seriously affected patients with variable results.

Chemical and Physical Injuries

Chemical or physical injury to the bladder may also cause severe dysuria. High-dose intravenous or oral administration of cyclophosphamide can induce dysuria as a result of excretion of toxic metabolites such as acrolein. Ifosfamide also may induce hemorrhagic cystitis and dysuria. Forced diuresis and the use of mesna can reduce this complication. X-ray irradiation of the bladder area can produce radiation cystitis. Rarely, an intentional self-induced trauma to the urethra (malingering) is the cause of dysuria.

Occasionally, dysuria can be caused by other noninfectious bladder lesions, such as bladder cancer or renal parenchymal diseases. Irritative symptoms are likely to occur in the presence of gross hematuria. Cystoscopy may become necessary to elucidate the underlying cause.

Urethral Syndrome

Urinary frequency, dysuria, and urgency in women in whom a urinary tract infection cannot be documented by culture of voided urine is a common problem. Some of these patients have true infection with positive bladder aspiration cultures and low but abnormal voided urinary bacterial colony counts (10^2 to 10^4). These patients will respond, at least temporarily, to conventional antimicrobial therapy. Others may have infections with *Chlamydia, Mycoplasma,* or *Mycobacterium tuberculosis.* For the remainder of symptomatic patients, antimicrobial therapy is ineffective and ill advised because of the effect on intestinal and vaginal flora. If bladder irritation and incontinence is present, an antispasmodic agent such as oxybutynin may be used. Diazepam can also be used and has shown varying degrees of success. A careful history should be obtained to determine any bladder–urethral trauma, local irritant factors, excessive douching, or use of bubble baths. During the physical examination, the physician should search for urethral caruncle and meatal stenosis. Systemic diseases such as Behçet's syndrome, Crohn's disease, ileocolitis, and Reiter's syndrome should be considered, as should an infiltrating bladder carcinoma. Voiding mechanisms should be evaluated in refractory cases to assess dyssynergy between bladder contraction and sphincter relaxation.

DYSURIA IN MEN

The most common causes of dysuria and frequency in men are urinary tract infections (urethritis, cystitis, and pyelonephritis) and prostatic disease (including acute and chronic prostatitis). Prostatic infection is particularly common in older individuals in association with benign prostatic hypertrophy or prior bladder instrumentation. The site of localization is suggested by terminal dysuria, perineal discomfort, and a purulent appearance in expressed prostatic fluid (by postprostatic massage). Because of poor antimicrobial penetration into prostatic fluid, many antibiotics are unsuitable for the management of prostatic infection. Current recommendations include trimethoprim-sulfamethoxazole. Prolonged therapy (6 to 12 weeks) may be required to fully eradicate infection and lower the likelihood of relapse. *N. gonorrhea, C. trachomatis,* and *Mycoplasma* also cause urethritis or cystitis in men and can be diagnosed and treated by procedures identical to those described for women. *Trichomonas* infection can cause dysuria in males engaging in unprotected intercourse with infected partners. Urethritis can also accompany Behçet's syndrome and Reiter's syndrome and can be accompanied by balanitis. The manifestations of genitourinary tuberculosis and schistosomal infection are similar in men and women.

APPROACH TO PATIENTS WITH DYSURIA AND FREQUENCY

A history of prior urinary tract infection, previous antimicrobial therapy, urinary instrumentation, passage of stone, gross hematuria, fever, flank pain, diabetes, exposure to x-ray or alkylating agent therapy, and travel to endemic areas for tuberculosis and schistosomiasis should be elicited in all cases. Information on menstrual history, vaginal discharge, use of contraceptives, sexual activity, bathing, douching practices, and pregnancy should be obtained for women. The temporal relationship of dysuria to the act of voiding should be carefully analyzed.

The physical examination should include careful inspection of the external genitalia, including a pelvic examination and inspection of the cervix and palpation of the adnexa in women. Vaginal or urethral discharge in women and urethral discharge in men should be inspected with careful attention to consistency, odor, and color. Costovertebral angle or bladder tenderness should be assessed. Prostatic massage in men may be a valuable adjunct to diagnosis. Urinalysis, with examination of a freshly voided urine sediment, should be performed in every case. Quantitative urine culture should be obtained in patients suspected of having a bacterial infection. Radiologic or ultrasonographic evaluation may be required to assess obstruction, stone, or urogenital anomalies. Cystoscopy is required when chronic interstitial cystitis or malignancy is considered possible.

Selected Readings

Fairley KF, Birch DF. Detection of bladder bacteriuria in patients with acute urinary symptoms. *J Infect Dis* 1989;159:226–231.

One of a number of reports demonstrating a high yield of low numbers of conventional uropathogens and fastidious bacteria on bladder urine aspiration in symptomatic adults with equivocal findings on conventional culture studies. Thirty-one percent of 1,817 women and 12% of 300 men were found to be culture positive, primarily with fastidious bacteria (70%). Bacterial counts were below 10^5 colony-forming units in 67% of samples. Fifty percent of the culture-positive patients had pyuria.

Koziol JA, Clark DC, Gittes RF, et al. The natural history of interstitial cystitis: a survey of 374 patients. *J Urol* 1993;149:465–469.

This survey of a large population of patients with well-documented interstitial cystitis provides information on the demography, risk factors, symptoms, psychosocial determinants, and alleviating and aggravating factors. Despite the wide variety of therapeutic agents attempted, fewer than half the patients reported relief from medication. An apparent plateau in symptoms of frequency and urgency was observed after approximately 5 years.

Norrby SR. Short-term treatment of uncomplicated lower urinary tract infection in women. *Rev Infect Dis* 1990;12:458–467.

This meta-analysis of 28 trials of various antibiotics and treatment intervals conducted on women with uncomplicated cystitis found single-dose therapy was less effective than a 3- or 5-day course in eradicating bacteriuria. Considerable differences were found among various antibiotics. Optimal treatment time with trimethoprim-sulfamethoxazole appeared to be 3 days, whereas β-lactams should be administered for 5 days or more.

Sobel JD. Vaginal infections in adult women. *Med Clin North Am* 1990;74:1573–1602.

A well-referenced review of the differential diagnoses and approaches to women with symptomatic and asymptomatic vaginitis. The epidemiology, pathogenesis, clinical features, diagnosis, and treatment of infectious causes are thoroughly and critically considered.

Stapleton A, Latham RH, Johnson C, et al. Postcoital antimicrobial prophylaxis for recurrent urinary tract infection. A randomized, double-blind, placebo-controlled trial. *JAMA* 1990;264:703–706.

Postcoital single-dose trimethoprim-sulfamethoxazole was found to be a safe, effective, and inexpensive means to prevent recurrent urinary tract infections in infection-prone young women with both low and high intercourse frequencies.

CHAPTER 28

Hematuria and Pigmenturia

Richard J. Glassock

Hematuria is the excretion of abnormal quantities of erythrocytes in the urine. When present, hematuria should be regarded as a sign of disease originating in the kidneys, of lesions present anywhere along the urinary tract from the renal pelvis to the distal urethra, or as a consequence of a systemic disturbance that as only secondarily affected the kidneys and urinary system. *Pigmenturia,* on the other hand, seldom arises solely as a result of a disease originating in the urinary system but is a manifestation, displayed in the urine, of some extrarenal disturbance.

HEMATURIA

Detection and Quantification

The detection of erythrocytes in urine is relatively simple, but the clear separation of normal from abnormal rates of excretion may be more difficult, especially when using semiquantitative methodology. Examination of a freshly voided, concentrated urine specimen by microscopic techniques after centrifugal sedimentation is a widely used method. Preparation of the urinary specimen for microscopic examination is discussed in detail in Chapter 100. With careful rather than casual examination, as little as one erythrocyte per 10 to 20 high-powered fields (hpf) can be detected. The orthotolidine-impregnated paper strips (Hemastix, Ames) will give a positive result in a urine specimen that contains as few as five erythrocytes per hpf of resuspended centrifuged urinary sediment. The orthotolidine test also will be positive in hemoglobinuria and myoglobinuria. In the latter instances, the paper strip usually gives a diffuse positive reaction rather than a speckled one, as is seen in the case of hematuria alone. False-negative test results may be seen in patients who take large amounts of ascorbic acid (vitamin C). If the urine specimen is hypotonic or has been allowed to stand for some time, free hemoglobin may be released and only erythrocyte ghosts remain, giving rise to confusion. Microscopic examination can mistakenly identify *Candida* spherules, calcium oxalate crystals, starch granules, and air bubbles as erythrocytes, under which circumstances the orthotolidine test will be negative. *Candida* spherules are larger than red cells and frequently may be seen to bud, especially in urine that has been allowed to stand at room temperature.

Hematuria may be quantified in one of two ways. When gross bleeding is present, a simple urocrit assessment may be obtained in the same fashion as one determines hematocrit. This may be useful in the follow-up of hematuria occurring in patients with severe bleeding in the urinary tract. When lesser degrees of hematuria are present (microscopic or macroscopic), timed overnight specimens of urine are necessary for quantification of hematuria (Addis counts). Counting the number of erythrocytes in *uncentrifuged,* freshly voided urine by use of a hemocytometer chamber and a calibrated pipette followed by calculation of the number of erythrocytes per milliliter of urine has proved useful and may be helpful in longitudinal studies of individual patients.

Normal Values of Erythrocyte Excretion

Normal individuals excrete small numbers of erythrocytes in the urine. Fewer than 4% of normal male subjects excrete more than three erythrocytes per hpf. This value commonly is accepted as the upper limit of normal. The urine sediment cannot be interpreted safely using voided specimens from menstruating females or urine samples obtained by urethral catheterization. Under both circumstances, the red cell count in the urine may be spuriously elevated. When quantitative tests (Addis counts) are used, normal individuals usually excrete 10^7 erythrocytes per day. When direct counting of erythrocytes in freshly voided urine is done, an upper limit of normal of 8,000 erythrocytes per milliliter (using centrifuged urine) or 13,000/ml (using uncentrifuged urine) is commonly accepted. Most of the erythrocytes in normal urine are *dysmorphic,* indicating a glomerular source. After vigorous exercise, normal individuals increase erythrocyte excretion to between 50,000 and 100,000/ml. Such exercise-induced erythrocyturia is associated with persistence of the dysmorphic appearance of the red cells. Dilute urine (specific activity below 1.005) can cause erythrocyte hemolysis and a considerable decline (30% to 70%) in the number of intact erythrocytes.

Localization of Hematuria

Several clues may help differentiate between hematuria arising from the renal parenchyma and that arising from the renal pelvis, ureters, bladder, or urethra because of local lesions, such as infection, tumors, stones, or arteriovenous malformations.

The presence of concomitant erythrocyte casts (red cell casts) always indicates a renal parenchymal origin, mainly glomerulonephritis or interstitial nephritis.

The concomitant presence of heavy proteinuria nearly always signifies a glomerular origin for hematuria. This can be illustrated by a few simple calculations. The entry of sufficient whole blood at a venous hematocrit of 40% into the bladder from a bleeding tumor or trauma of sufficient degree to result in a urocrit value of 0.5% would yield a urine specimen with a grossly hemorrhagic appearance to visual inspection. If one assumes that the prevailing plasma protein concentration is 7.0 g/dl (70 mg/ml) and the total daily urine volume is 1,500 ml, then 7.5 ml of packed erythrocytes derived from 18.7 ml of whole blood, and 11.2 ml of plasma (i.e., hematocrit of 40%) have been added to the urine. This 11.2 ml of plasma contains approximately 785 mg of plasma proteins. Therefore the concentration of protein in the final urine should be equal to the normal urinary protein concentration (10 mg/dl or less) plus that added to the urine by virtue of the entry of the plasma protein fraction of whole blood (e.g., 785 mg/1,500 ml or approximately 52 mg/dl). Thus the total urinary protein concentration would not exceed 62 mg/dl unless, of course, hemolysis had occurred, releasing additional hemoglobin into the supernatant, which would be measured by certain techniques as protein. This value would give a semiquantitative estimate of proteinuria (Dipstix method) of about 2+ and not more than 1 g of protein per day on quantitation using timed urinary specimen. A lower venous hematocrit or higher plasma protein concentration would require adjustments to this somewhat oversimplified analysis. Hemolysis of red cells is more likely to occur in a hypotonic urine (U_{Osm} below 280 mOsm/kg H_2O) that has been allowed to sit at room temperature for several hours. The contribution of released hemoglobin to the measured value of urine protein can be significant but seldom results in protein levels exceeding 1.0 g/day unless bleeding is very severe. Such contribution can be assessed by urinary protein electrophoresis because hemoglobin migrates as a β-globulin. The principal message is that rather massive bleeding into the urinary tract is required to elevate the protein concentration in the 100 to 300 mg/dl range and to the values of greater than 1.0 g/24 hr commonly observed in patients with glomerular disorders. Milder degrees of macroscopic or microscopic hematuria accompanied by heavy qualitative proteinuria (3+ to 4+) should always be assumed to have a glomerular or interstitial cause.

Red blood cells emanating from lesions confined to the renal pelvis, ureter, bladder, or urethra usually retain their uniform biconcave shape in isotonic or hypertonic urine (isomorphic or normomorphic erythrocyturia), whereas red blood cells arising in the urine consequent to a glomerular (and probably also tubulointerstitial) disease are commonly disfigured as they traverse the nephron and appear in the final urine as fragmented, distorted erythrocytes (dysmorphic erthyrocyturia). Such dysmorphic cells are best recognized with phase contrast microscopy. However, both a supravital stain with eosin-Y or Sternheimer-Malbin stain (Sedi-Stain) and standard light microscopy and a Wright's stain of a smear prepared from a drop of centrifuged sediment mixed with a drop of 5% albumin in normal saline solution are accurate methods for the assessment of erythrocyte shape and hemoglobin content. Because the dysmorphic cells are smaller than the isomorphic cells, Coulter Counter analysis (flow cytometry) of freshly voided urine with estimation of mean corpuscular diameters and the dispersion of these values also can be used as a rapid and automated method to detect and quantify the dysmorphism of urinary erythrocytes. The red cells in normal urine are nearly all dysmorphic, suggesting a renal parenchymal origin. Normomorphic erythrocytes in urine, even within the normal range, suggest an abnormality distal to the ducts of Bellini. Large numbers of dysmorphic erythrocytes (greater than 10^6/ml) suggest underlying glomerular disease.

Abnormally increased erythrocyte excretion that accompanies vigorous exercise is nearly always of the normomorphic variety (i.e., bladder origin). If dysmorphic hematuria follows exercise, it suggests an underlying renal parenchymal disease.

Dysmorphic red cells characterized by knoblike projections (acanthocytes) may be more specific in glomerular diseases. The degree of dysmorphism may be influenced by urine concentration and time from passage of urine. A drug-induced diuresis may transiently convert dysmorphic hematuria to normorphic one.

Because the analysis of urinary erythrocyte dysmorphism is observer dependent and influenced by many non–disease-related factors, it should be carried out under well-standardized conditions and by experienced personnel to optimize its value.

Of course, there may be other clinical clues that permit one to make more than an educated guess as to the site of origin of hematuria. These include the presence of suprapubic pain (bladder disease), loin pain (kidney disease), or the passage of clots, the last usually indicating bleeding from renal tumors or lesions in the ureter, pelvis, or bladder. Passage of clots should not be encountered in patients with glomerular disease.

Pattern of Hematuria

Three basic terms are used to describe the patterns of hematuria. These are related to the color and appearance of the urine, the timing of hematuria, and the presence or absence of associated urinary tract symptoms. First, in relation to the color or appearance of the urine, the terms *gross* and *macroscopic* are used to designate urine that is obviously discolored with blood. Only 5 ml of blood in 1 L of urine will give rise to visible hematuria (25×10^9 erythrocytes/L or 25×10^6 cells/ml). Gross hematuria is a more extreme degree of macroscopic hematuria. The appearance in acid urine may be brown to brownish red, smoky, or coffee- or tea-colored. When bleeding is brisk and active or in highly alkaline urine, the appearance may be bright red. *Covert* or *microscopic* hematuria refers to urine not distinguishable from normal in gross appearance but that has abnormal quantities of erythrocytes on microscopic examination. Second, the pattern of hematuria with respect to time is described by the use of the self-explanatory terms *persistent* or *constant* and *intermittent* or *recurrent*. Finally, the coexistence of other findings referable to the urinary tract is designated by the use of the terms *symptomatic* or *asymptomatic* (painless) hematuria. These descriptive terms are useful because certain disorders are more likely than others to result in particular patterns of color and appearance, timing, and associated symptoms.

Causes of Hematuria

The causes of hematuria are multiple and have been categorized into renal parenchymal, urinary tract, and systemic coagulation disturbances (Table 28.1). The precise origin of the erythrocytes in the urine in instances of glomerular or tubulointerstitial renal parenchymal disease is unknown. Localized rents or tears in glomerular capillary walls, rupture of tubular basement membrane, and invasion of blood vessels and tubules by tumors may be augmented by locally impaired thrombus generation and excessive thrombolysis. Entry of erythrocytes into tubular lumina proximal to the site of Tamm-Horsfall mucoprotein synthesis and excretion (i.e., the medullary and cortical ascending limb) may give rise to their incorporation into casts (red cell casts), especially in the presence of heavy proteinuria. When accompanied by glomerular hematuria, these casts contain plasma immunoglobulins (IgG) in addition to Tamm-Horsfall protein.

The major causes of asymptomatic hematuria, either gross or microscopic, in the absence of degrees of proteinuria that definitely indicate the presence of underlying glomerular disease

TABLE 28.1. Causes of Hematuria

Renal Parenchymal Diseases	Urinary Tract Diseases
Glomerular disease	Renal pelvis
Primary	Transitional cell carcinoma
Mesangial IgA nephropathy (Berger's disease)	Varices
Mesangial proliferative glomerulonephritis with IgM and/or C3 deposits	Calculi
Membranoproliferative glomerulonephritis	Trauma
Crescentic glomerulonephritis	Severe hydronephrosis
Focal glomerulosclerosis	Nevi
Membranous glomerulopathy (<20%)	Ureter
Minimal change disease (<20%)	Calculi (uric acid, calcium oxalate, calcium phosphate, struvite, cystine, adenine, xanthine)
Fibrillary glomerulonephritis	Transitional cell carcinoma
Multisystem	Periureteritis (appendicitis, ileocolitis, abscess)
Systemic lupus erythematosus nephritis	Retroperitoneal fibrosis
Microscopic polyangiitis	Ureterocele
Wegener's granulomatosis	Varices
Henoch-Schönlein purpura	Endometriosis
Goodpasture's disease	Tuberculosis
Infection	Bladder
Poststreptococcal glomerulonephritis	Carcinoma of the bladder
Infective endocarditis	Cystitis (bacterial, viral, parasitic, fungal)
Shunt nephritis	Chronic interstitial cystitis (Hunner's ulcers)
Other postinfectious glomerulonephritis	*Schistosoma haematobium*
Hereditary disease	Radiation cystitis
Alport's syndrome	Nitrogen mustard or cyclophosphamide cystitis
Nail–patella syndrome	Hypersensitivity (allergic) cystitis
Fabry's disease	Bladder calculi
Thin basement membrane nephropathy	Sudden decompression of severe overdistention
Other	Foreign bodies
Primary idiopathic renal hematuria with or without hypercalciuria	Vascular anomalies
Vascular and tubulointerstitial diseases	Amyloidosis
Hypersensitivity	Trauma
Acute hypersensitivity interstitial nephritis	Jogger's or marathon runner's hematuria
Tubulointerstitial nephritis with uveitis	Tuberculosis
Neoplastic	Prostate
Tumors (renal cell carcinoma, Wilms' tumor, leukemic infiltrates, angiomyolipoma)	Benign prostatic hypertrophy
Metastatic tumors (uncommon)	Carcinoma of the prostate
Hereditary	Acute or chronic prostatitis
Polycystic kidney disease (autosomal dominant variety)	Urethra
Medullary sponge kidney	Meatal ulcers
Vascular	Urethral prolapse
Malignant hypertension	Urethral caruncle
Renal arterial emboli or thrombosis	Acute or chronic urethritis
Loin pain–hematuria syndrome	Carcinoma of the urethra or penis
Arteriovenous malformations	Vascular anomalies
Thrombotic microangiopathy	Trauma
Chemolytic-uremic syndrome, thrombocytopenic purpura	Foreign body
Papillary necrosis	Condyloma acuminatum
Analgesic abuse nephropathy	Other (endometriosis)
Sickle cell trait	In association with a systemic coagulation disturbance (with or without diseases previously listed)
Diabetes mellitus	Platelet defect
Alcoholism	Idiopathic or drug-induced
Ankylosing spondylitis	Thrombocytopenic purpura
Obstructive uropathy	Thrombasthenia
Trauma	Bone marrow diseases
Acute bacterial pyelonephritis	Coagulation protein deficiency
Acquired cystic disease of renal failure and dialysis	Hemophilia A or B
	Heparin therapy
	Warfarin therapy
	Other congenital and acquired defect in coagulation
	Other
	Scurvy
	Hereditary telangiectasia
	Surreptitious (malingering)

(e.g., less than 1.0 g/day) include tumors of the kidney, renal pelvis, ureter, bladder, prostate, and urethra; hypercalciuric states; vascular anomalies; papillary necrosis from analgesic abuse or sickle cell trait and coagulation abnormalities; and certain primary, secondary, and hereditary glomerular diseases. The last category includes mesangial proliferative glomerulonephritis with deposits of IgA (Berger's disease), IgM, and/or C3; primary renal hematuria with thin basement membranes (possibly a variant of Alport's syndrome); polycystic kidney disease; and medullary sponge kidney. The character of systemic symptomatology or the presence of recognizable underlying disease may be very helpful in elucidating the cause, site, and origin of hematuria. For example, a recent streptococcal infection of the skin or throat may point to a resolving acute poststreptococcal glomerulonephritis; the presence of rash or arthritis may point to systemic lupus erythematosus, vasculitis, or Henoch-Schönlein purpura; hemoptysis and microcytic hypochromic anemia may indicate the presence of Goodpasture's syndrome; deafness in a clear-cut X-linked family history of renal disease may be a clue to the presence of Alport's syndrome; acroparesthesias and cutaneous angiokeratomas may indicate Fabry's disease; chronic atrial fibrillation or a recent acute myocardial infarction may be a clue to underlying embolic disease; loin pain in young women on birth control pills may indicate the presence of the loin pain—hematuria syndrome; dysuria, frequency, and suprapubic pain may point to the presence of hemorrhagic cystitis; the development of acute renal colic may indicate renal calculi; hypercalciuria may be associated with idiopathic hematuria or medullary sponge kidney; and episodes of hematuria following long-distance running may indicate marathon runner's hematuria. The specific details regarding the characteristics of each of the disorders in which hematuria is found are described in other sections of this book and need not be examined in detail here. However, two clinical entities are reviewed briefly because hematuria is their chief mode of presentation.

Loin Pain–Hematuria Syndrome

Loin pain–hematuria syndrome is often, but not exclusively, found in young women receiving estrogen-containing birth control medication. It occurs with recurrent bouts of gross or microscopic hematuria with or without dysuria but almost always with unilateral or bilateral loin pain. It often is misdiagnosed initially as "acute pyelonephritis," although leukocyturia usually is not observed. Low-grade fever may be present. Blood pressure and renal function are normal. Proteinuria is mild (less than 1 g/day). Urine sediment evaluation usually reveals only erythrocytes. Renal arteriograms may demonstrate narrowing and tortuosity of terminal branches and segmental ischemia. Technetium-99m dimercaptosuccinic acid (DMSA) or diethylenetriamine pentaacetic acid (DTPA) scans may show zones of segmental ischemia during episodes of pain. Renal biopsies may reveal normal glomeruli and arteriolar thickening by light microscopy and C3 deposits in arterioles by immunofluorescence microscopy. Treatment, in general, is not very satisfactory, but discontinuance of oral contraceptives may result in some relief of loin pain and disappearance of hematuria. If symptoms persist, some improvement has been observed with the administration of oral anticoagulants. Autotransplantation of the kidney has been successful in eradicating pain, but recurrences may develop. Renal failure does not occur.

Marathon Runner's Hematuria

This form of gross hematuria occurs after prolonged running (usually more than 15 km a week), predominantly but not exclusively in males. The hematuria may be associated with the passage of clots and suprapubic and perineal discomfort, but usually not with loin pain. It may develop repetitively but usually disappears quickly when the patient rests. Urinalysis reveals minimal or no proteinuria, but hyaline casts may be seen. The excreted red cells are usually normomorphic. Blood pressure and renal function are normal. Cystoscopy during episodes of hematuria may show ecchymosis and capillary congestion of the posterior bladder and interureteric ridge. This finding is presumed to be caused by the to-and-fro motion of a partially filled bladder traumatizing the posterior bladder base. No treatment is required other than reassurance and reduction of running intensity. Running with a completely empty bladder may help.

Evaluation of Hematuria

Above all, the evaluation must include a very careful microscopic examination of the urinary sediment done by the physician to confirm the presence or absence of true hematuria and to differentiate other causes of brownish, coffee-colored, or red urine. This urinalysis also will provide invaluable clues, reviewed previously as to the presence or absence of features indicative of a renal parenchymal source. Having such data in hand at the outset of the evaluation will often direct one's attention into specific areas and will avoid unnecessary, costly, and potentially hazardous investigations, such as retrograde pyelograms, arteriography, and renal biopsy.

The history must be thorough and complete, emphasizing the pattern of hematuria with respect to time, the presence of associated symptoms, such as dysuria, frequency, colic, and loin pain, and the appearance of the urine. The relation of episodes to exercise, medication, and voiding also is helpful. Careful attention should be paid to elucidating a history of weight loss (malignant tumors or tuberculosis) or gain (nephritis or nephrotic syndrome), fever (infection), abdominal pain, loin pain, colic (stones), frequency and dysuria (infection), paresthesias (Fabry's disease), joint pain (systemic lupus erythematosus), skin rashes (systemic lupus erythematosus, Henoch-Schönlein syndrome, drug hypersensitivity), hearing loss (Alport's syndrome), bleeding tendency, hemoptysis (Goodpasture's disease), tinnitus (vasculitis), recent throat or skin infections (poststreptococcal glomerulonephritis), tooth extractions (infective endocarditis), previous heart murmur (endocarditis), irregular heartbeat (renal emboli), and previous renal calculi (hypercalciuria).

A history of drug ingestion and/or self-medication with proprietary preparations is important. These include compound analgesics (papillary necrosis), birth control pills (loin pain–hematuria syndrome), antimicrobials (interstitial nephritis), anticoagulants, and cyclophosphamide or nitrogen mustard (chemical cystitis). Excessive consumption of alcohol (papillary necrosis) and/or cigarettes (bladder cancer) should be noted.

A family history of renal disease, hematuria, deafness, sickle cell disease, bleeding tendency, or polycystic kidney disease is especially relevant. Foreign travel, especially in areas in which *Schistosoma haematobium* is endemic, should be documented.

Through physical examination blood pressure and cardiac rhythm should be determined, and a careful search should be made for ecchymosis, petechiae, skin rashes, pigmentation, telangiectasia, angiomas, and other nodular cutaneous infiltrates. The heart and lung examination for murmurs and rales is equally essential. Corneal and lens abnormalities and sensorineural hearing loss should be routinely searched for. The abdominal examination must be particularly thorough, searching for masses, renal enlargement, or tenderness. The bladder should be palpated and percussed, and a rectal examination should assess prostatic size, consistency, and contour. The pelvic examination should carefully assess the external urethral meatus.

Many clues to the correct diagnosis often will be obtained as a result of the initial history, physical examination, and carefully done urinalysis, thus allowing the physician to move confidently into more specific diagnostic procedures. Heavy proteinuria, dysmorphic erythrocyturia, or red cell casts should always direct one's attention to a renal parenchymal source. However, most patients should receive a minimal set of laboratory studies. These should include a hemogram (hematocrit, hemoglobin, erythrocyte count with calculation of red blood cell indices, white blood cell count, differential, platelet estimation, and assessment of leukocyte and erythrocyte morphologic structure), erythrocyte sedimentation rate, serum creatinine or blood urea nitrogen test, chest x-ray evaluation, and screening blood chemistries (SMA 12 or equivalent). If any history or physical examination finding suggests a coagulation disturbance, a prothrombin time, partial thromboplastin time, and bleeding time should be added to this list. Among the population of patients with African ancestry, hemoglobin electrophoresis should be performed.

In the presence of qualitative proteinuria of 1+ or greater in a concentrated urine specimen, an estimate of 24-hour urinary protein levels should be obtained. Urinary protein electrophoresis can be helpful when massive hematuria is present. When the symptoms or urinalysis findings suggest active urinary tract infection, a urine culture with antimicrobial sensitivities is appropriate. If the results of prior tuberculin skin tests are unknown or negative in a patient with unexplainable hematuria, a 5-TU tuberculin skin test should be undertaken. A positive result or a known conversion from negative to positive may require evaluation for renal tuberculosis. This could be done by obtaining concentrated morning urine cultures for *Mycobacterium tuberculosis* on 3 separate days. A search for the ova of *S. haematobium* is usually unnecessary, unless travel through endemic areas is documented.

The presence of macroscopic hematuria without features suggestive of a glomerular or renal parenchymal source (normomorphic erythrocyturia) could next be evaluated with a three-glass test. Predominance of hematuria in only the first 10 to 15 ml of voided urine indicates a urethral site, bleeding in only the final 10 to 30 ml (terminal hematuria) suggests a bladder origin, and hematuria in all three samples suggests upper urinary tract bleeding. Bleeding at the very end of urination is suggestive of *S. haematobium* infestation, or bladder lesion at the trigone.

Patients with normal renal function and without significant proteinuria, dysmorphic erythrocytes, and/or red cell casts require intravenous urography (IVU), or a computed tomography (CT) scan with contrast when a renal tumor is suspected. Providing that the IVU does not give an unequivocal diagnosis and no features indicative of glomerular disease are present, gross bladder infection is absent, polycystic kidney disease is not suspected, and gross bleeding continues, one could proceed directly to cystoscopy. Patients older than 40 years of age who have or continue to smoke *must* be suspected of having bladder cancer, and urinary cytology and cystoscopy are mandatory procedures. In patients who are at high risk of developing acute renal failure (ARF) as a result of contrast media-induced nephrotoxicity (see Chapter 49, Part 7) and who are suspected of having hematuria resulting from obstructive uropathy, ultrasonographic or CT studies without contrast compound are helpful and could precede IVU. If cystoscopy is performed in addition to careful inspection of the bladder for foreign bodies, vascular anomalies, tumors, and ulcers, one should attempt to collect urine as atraumatically as possible from each ureter to determine whether hematuria is originating in one or both ureters. Urinary cytologic evaluation is a particularly useful tool in the diagnosis of hematuria in patients suspected of having a neoplasm involving the bladder, ureter, or renal pelvis (transitional cell carcinoma). A urine calcium measurement should be performed in patients with otherwise unexplained normomorphic hematuria.

Although in many patients the cause of hematuria will be evident after a thorough history and physical examination, an initial screening test as a stepwise systematic approach is useful in those instances when a diagnosis is still uncertain. Such a schema is outlined in Tables 28.2 and 28.3. The use of this approach will often permit one to arrive at a final diagnosis with

TABLE 28.2. Approach to the Evaluation of Hematuria

- Group A (glomerular and tubulointerstitial disease)
  - Characteristics
    - Initial history, examination, and screening laboratory nondiagnostic; RBC casts, dysmorphic erythrocytes in sediment, and/or proteinuria in excess of that expected for degree of hematuria
  - Approach (depending on clinical findings [see also Table 28.3])
    - Laboratory group
      - Fluorescent antinuclear antibody
      - Antinative DNA
      - Antistreptolysin O
      - Antihyaluronidase
      - Anti-DNAse
      - Antiglomerular basement or tubular basement membrane antibody
      - Antineutrophil cytoplasmic antibody
      - C3, C4, C3 nephritic factor
      - Cryoglobulins
      - Immunoglobulin levels
      - IgA-fibronectin complexes
      - IgA rheumatoid factor
      - Urinary interleukin-6
      - Urinary platelet factor 4
      - C-reactive protein
      - Serum and urine immunoelectrophoresis
      - Blood cultures
      - Urinary eosinophils
      - Audiogram
    - Then,
      - Renal biopsy with light, immunofluorescence, and electron microscopy
    - Then,
      - If all negative or nondiagnostic, idiopathic renal hematuria
- Group B (nonglomerular hematuria)
  - Characteristics
    - Initial history, examination, and screening nondiagnostic; no RBC casts or dysmorphic cells in sediment, protein excretion less than or equal to that predicted by degree of hematuria
  - Approach (perform IVU and/or CT scan and renal ultrasound)
    - Parenchymal renal mass; ultrasound and/or CT scan; then arteriogram for solid mass or cyst puncture for cystic mass
    - Bilateral enlarged kidneys; ultrasound; radionuclide or CT scan; no cystoscopy
    - Filling defect in pelvis or ureter: cystoscopy, retrograde pyelogram, urine cytology
    - Papillary necrosis: hemoglobin electrophoresis (if of African ancestry) urine cytology, review drug exposure
    - Ectasia of collecting tubules: urinary calcium, urine culture, and sensitivity
    - Ureteral stricture and/or dilation: repeat tuberculin test, fresh urine for *Mycobacterium tuberculosis*
    - Urinary calculus: nonopaque—evaluate uric acid excretion, xanthine, adenine, urine pH; opaque—evaluate for cystine, calcium, oxalate; urine culture and sensitivity; serum calcium, phosphorus and intact parathyroid hormone
    - Medial or lateral deviation of ureter: evaluate for lymphoma, aortic aneurysm; abdominal CT scan, methysergide administration
- Group C (indeterminant hematuria)
  - Characteristics
    - History, examination, and screening laboratory nondiagnostic; IVU, CT scan or renal ultrasonography normal or nondiagnostic; RBC casts or dysmorphic cells absent; proteinuria less than or equal to that expected for degree of hematuria
  - Approach
    - Proceed to cystoscopy (with or without retrograde pyelogram)
      - Hematuria confined to bladder: diagnosis made by inspection, biopsy, culture, or cytology
      - Hematuria from one ureter only: proceed to retrograde pyelogram, CT scan, renal ultrasound, radionuclide scan, arteriogram, and/or urine cytology
      - Hematuria from both ureters *or* no bladder or urethral lesion: proceed as in group A

CT, computed tomography; IVU, intravenous urogram; RBC, red blood cells.

TABLE 28.3. Glomerular Hematuria: Common Causes and Suggested Laboratory Evaluation

Suspected Disease	Laboratory Tests
Systemic lupus erythematosus	Fluorescent antinuclear antibody (FANA), anti-double-stranded DNA antibody (anti-ds DNA), C3, C4, anti-neutrophil cytoplasmic antibody (ANCA), anti-Clq antibody
Vasculitis	ANCA, FANA, antiglomerular basement membrane antibody (anti-GBM), cryoimmunoglobulin (cryo-Ig), C3, C4, sedimentation rate, C-reactive protein (CRP), rheumatoid factor, blood cultures
Goodpasture's disease	Anti-GBM, ANCA (IgG and IgM), cryo-Ig, C3, C4, single breath carbon monoxide lung uptake
Idiopathic pauci-immune crescentic glomerulonephritis	Anti-GBM, ANCA, C3, C4, cryo-Ig, FANA
Henoch-Schönlein purpura	Serum IgA level, IgA-fibronectin complexes, IgA-rheumatoid factor, urinary IL-6, skin biopsy for IgA
Poststreptococcal glomerulonephritis	Anti-streptolysin O, anti-hyaluronidase, anti-DNA-ase, C3, C4, C3 nephritic factor (C3 Nef)
Infective endocarditis	Blood cultures, C3, C4, rheumatoid factor
Shunt nephritis	Rheumatoid factor, cultures
Acute interstitial nephritis	Urinary and blood eosinophils, CRP
Fibrillary glomerulonephritis	Serum and urinary immunoelectrophoresis, C3, C4, quantitative Ig
Membranoproliferative glomerulonephritis	C3, C4, C3 Nef, cryoglobulins, anti-hepatitis C hepatitis B surface antigen
IgA nephropathy	Serum IgA levels, IgA-rheumatoid factor, urinary platelet factor 4 (PF-4), urinary IL-6, IgA-fibrinectin aggregates
Thin basement membrane nephropathy	Audiogram, urinary PF-4, urinary IL-6, skin biopsy for IgA
Alport's syndrome	Audiogram, slit-lamp examination

TABLE 28.4. Causes of Pigmenturia

Source of Pigment	Color of Urine	Compound Responsible
Exogenous	Pink-red or red-orange	Analgesics: phenazopyridine, antipyrine
		Anticoagulants: phenindione, warfarin
		Anticonvulsants: phenytoin, phensuximide
		Laxatives: phenolphthalein, danthron senna, cascara (in alkaline urine)
		Foods: beets, blackberries, rhubarb, paprika
		Sedatives: sulfonal
		Antibiotics: rifampicin, thiazolsulfone, azosulfisoxazole
		Tranquilizer: phenothiazine
		Other: azathioprine, deferoxamine mesylate, doxorubicin
	Brown-black	Antibiotics: nitrofurantoin, metronidazole, sulfas, chloroquine
		Antihypertensives: methyldopa
		Analgesics: phenacetin, salicylates
		Antiparkinsonian: levodopa
		Muscle relaxants: methocarbamol
		Other: cresol, phenol, iron sorbitol citrate
	Blue-green	Dyes: methylene blue, Evans blue, indigo blue
		Diuretics: triamterene
		Vitamins: riboflavin
		Tranquilizers: amitriptyline
Endogenous	Red to red-brown	Myoglobin
		Hemoglobin
		Porphyrins (porphyria, hepatitis, lead poisoning, pellagra)
		Serratia marcescens infection
		Amorphous urates (brick red)
	Golden brown	Bilirubin
	Green-blue	*Pseudomonas* infection: bilirubin + infection → biliverdin
	Brown-black	Melanin (melanoma)
		Homogentisic acid (alkaptonuria)
	White, milky	Chyluria (traumatic, neoplastic, pregnancy)

a minimum of risk, cost, and inconvenience. However, it should be recognized that in 10% to 15% of patients, no satisfactory explanation for hematuria will ever be found. Hematuria in many of these patients may be caused by subtle glomerular or tubulointerstitial disease or by small arteriovenous malformations that are very difficult to localize. *The exclusion of treatable tumors of bladder or renal origin and infections should be foremost in the mind of physicians approaching patients with otherwise unexplained hematuria.* Gross, painless normorphic hematuria always requires a systematic urologic evaluation of the urinary tract, especially the bladder in older individuals.

PIGMENTURIA

Pigmenturia may be defined as the presence of any soluble or insoluble colored substance in the urine that imparts a distinct alteration in the normal straw-yellow color of the urine. Pigmenturia could be produced by endogenous or exogenous compounds excreted into the urine. These compounds are listed in Table 28.4 according to the color changes they impart. The causes of pigmenturia ordinarily can be differentiated by a careful history of food or drug intake or by adjustment of the urinary pH. For example, the red color of phenolsulfonphthalein will disappear with acidification of the urine, and porphyrins may be extracted in chloroform. On occasion, specific chemical assays may be required for accurate diagnosis.

One of the most important classes of pigments found in the urine arises as a result of breakdown of muscle (myoglobin) or red blood cells (hemoglobin). Both myoglobinuria and hemoglobinuria may result in specific abnormalities in renal function (ARF) and may be confused with true hematuria. A method of differentiating true hematuria and the endogenous pigmenturias that impart a reddish or reddish brown color to urine is given in Table 28.5.

Myoglobinuria

Myoglobin is an iron-containing, oxygen-binding respiratory protein present in skeletal and smooth muscle. It is a single-chain protein with a molecular weight of approximately 16,800 (effective molecular radius, 19 Å) and is loosely bound to a

TABLE 28.5. Differentiation of Hematuria and Pigmenturia

Disorder	Color of Urine	Orthotolidine Test Strip	Albumin Test Strip	Heat and Acetic Acid Test	Color of Spun Serum	Microscopic Examination of Unspun Urine	Color of Spun Urine
Hematuria	Red, red-brown, brown	4+, diffuse or speckled	0–4+*	0–4+	Normal clear	Red blood cells	Clear (unless hemolyzed)
Hemoglobinuria	Same	4+, diffuse	0–1+	0	Pink	Negative	Red, red-brown
Myoglobinuria	Same	4+, diffuse	0–1+	0	Normal clear	Negative	Orange-red, brown
Porphyrins	Red	Negative	0 0	0	Normal clear	Negative	Red (chloroform extractable)
Exogenous pigments	Red, red-orange	Negative		0	Normal clear	Negative	Red (may change with adjustment in pH)

*Depending on whether glomerular disease is responsible.

plasma α_2-globulin (not haptoglobin). The maximum myoglobin-binding capacity of this plasma protein is about 20 mg/dl of plasma. Myoglobin normally is present in very small amounts in the plasma, detectable only by sensitive radioimmunoassays. Small amounts are present in normal urine. The renal threshold for myoglobin is approximately 21 mg/dl of plasma or just above the maximum binding of myoglobin to plasma protein. Once this threshold plasma concentration is exceeded, the fractional clearance of myoglobin is about 75% of the prevailing level of the glomerular filtration rate (GFR). At a lower plasma myoglobin concentration, only about 50% of the myoglobin is plasma protein bound. Therefore the fractional clearance of myoglobin is reduced well below the value of 75%. Plasma concentrations of myoglobin above 100 mg/dl are required to impart a distinct, visible pinkish color to plasma. Myoglobin in the urine is initially pink but is rapidly converted to a brown or brownish black pigment, metmyoglobin. Myoglobin and hemoglobin are both soluble in dilute acetic acid after heating. Plasma proteins usually are quite insoluble following such treatment. Myoglobin is soluble in 3.2 M ammonium sulfate, but hemoglobin is not. This latter property serves as a basis for chemical tests differentiating there two endogenous pigments. The isoelectric point of myoglobin is approximately 6.9. Thus, in acid urine, the molecule is cationic. Cationic protein molecules may interact or polymerize with anionic mucoproteins, such as Tamm-Horsfall protein. Furthermore, at a pH level of less than 5.4, myoglobin and hemoglobin dissociate to globin and ferrihemate. The latter may be directly nephrotoxic.

Because of the high renal clearance of myoglobin at plasma concentrations above plasma protein-binding capacity, it is difficult to achieve plasma concentrations of myoglobin that would impart a pinkish hue to plasma (levels above 100 mg/dl) unless GFR is significantly reduced or myonecrosis is very severe. The space of distribution of myoglobin is approximately 40% of body weight, and skeletal muscle contains myoglobin levels of approximately 4 mg/g. Assuming negligible renal excretion, it would require total dissolution of over 7 kg of muscle mass in a 70-kg individual to achieve myoglobin concentrations exceeding 100 mg/dl. Myoglobinuria ordinarily is not detectable until plasma levels exceed 1.5 mg/dl, an amount equivalent to the dissolution of about 100 g of skeletal muscle. Radioimmunoassays can detect much smaller quantities of myoglobin and therefore can detect dissolution of even smaller quantities of skeletal or smooth muscle. For example, detectable myoglobinuria occurs quite often after myocardial infarction. Physical training can greatly increase the myoglobin content of skeletal muscle. Thus more myoglobinuria can be expected with equivalent degrees of muscle destruction in well-trained athletes than in sedentary individuals. The magnitude of urinary myoglobin concentration expected for any given degree of myonecrosis, therefore, is conditioned by the muscle myoglobin content, plasma protein binding, plasma myoglobin concentration, prevailing GFR, and urine flow rate.

The causes of myonecrosis and myoglobinuria are outlined in Table 28.6. They may be divided into several fundamental categories, namely, an imbalance between muscle energy consumption and production (the latter of which can be genetically based or acquired), primary muscle injury, decreased muscle oxygenation, infections, and toxins.

Myoglobin may be released from muscle as a result of frank cell destruction or alterations in cell membrane integrity, causing leakage of intracellular contents without cell death. During muscle injury, release of certain other intracellular contents is concomitant with release of myoglobin; these include creatine kinase (MM type), creatine phosphate, aldolase, purine precursors, adenine nucleotides, and neutral proteases. This may lead to the increased concentration of these compounds in plasma, urine, or both. The most common causes of rhabdomyolysis encountered in clinical medicine are related to abuse of alcohol, heroin, and other drugs; severe exercise in unconditioned individuals; trauma; and prolonged coma with immobilization. In many of these patients, ARF may ensue. The rhabdomyolysis of heroin abuse is discussed in Chapter 47, Part 6.

The mechanisms of ARF in myoglobinuric states are not known, but any one or more of the following could be involved: (a) intranephronal obstruction resulting from precipitation of myoglobin (as a polymer with Tamm-Horsfall protein) in the ascending limb, (b) precipitation of uric acid crystals with resultant intranephronal obstruction, (c) renal ischemia resulting from concomitant release of potent vasoconstrictor substances or their conversion to active compounds from inactive precursors under the influences of proteolytic enzymes released from damaged muscles, and (d) direct nephrotoxicity of myoglobin or its breakdown products (e.g., ferrihemate) with tubular necrosis and intranephronal obstruction or backleak of filtrate. Whatever the mechanism, rhabdomyolysis should be suspected when ARF supervenes in any of the clinical situations described in Table 28.6 and when pigmenturia is documented. Other biochemical features that are common accompaniments of acute rhabdomyolysis include elevated serum creatine kinase (often above 100,000 units/ml) and serum aldolase. No correlation exists between the magnitude of the elevation in serum levels of these enzymes and the risk of ARF. However, impaired renal function is seldom seen with creatine kinase levels below 2,000 units/ml. Marked hyperuricemia out of proportion to azotemia (often higher than 20 mg/dl) and early and severe hypocalcemia and hyperphosphatemia are usually associated with oliguria. The serum calcium may be profoundly depressed (below 6 mg/dl), most likely because of the combined effects of hyperphosphatemia (above 10 to 15 mg/dl) and an acquired state of 1,25-dihydroxyvitamin D deficiency. Metastatic calcification (as calcium phosphate or calcium carbonate) in damaged muscle

TABLE 28.6. Causes of Rhabdomyolysis and Myoglobinuria

- Increased energy consumption
  - Severe exercise
  - Amphetamine, phencyclidine, cocaine, and lysergic acid diethylamide intoxication
    - Delirium tremens
  - Status epilepticus
  - High voltage shock
  - Tetanus
  - Succinylcholine administration
  - Hyperthermia, malignant neuroleptic syndrome
  - Heat stroke and cramps
  - Muscular dystrophies
- Decreased energy production: genetic, congenital affecting carbohydrate metabolism
  - Myophosphorylase deficiency
  - α-Glucosidase deficiency
  - Amyloglucosidase deficiency
  - Phosphohexosisomerase deficiency
  - Phosphofructokinase deficiency
  - Diabetic ketoacidosis
  - Nonketotic hyperosmolar coma
  - Adenine deaminase deficiency
  - Carnitine deficiency
  - Carnitine palmitoyltransferase deficiency
- Decreased energy production: acquired
  - Potassium depletion (severe)
  - Phosphate depletion
  - Ethanol
  - Myxedema
  - Hypothermia
  - Diabetic ketoacidosis
- Primary muscle injury
  - Polymyositis
  - Dermatomyositis
  - Trauma, crush injury
  - Severe burns
  - Vasculitis
- Decreased muscle oxygenation
  - McCardle's syndrome
  - Decreased muscle blood flow
    - Potassium depletion
    - Compressive vascular occlusion
    - Arterial thrombosis or embolism
  - Prolonged cardiac surgery
  - Carbon monoxide poisoning
  - Shock
  - Trauma
  - Sickle cell trait
- Infections
  - Gas gangrene
  - Tetanus
  - Leptospirosis
  - Viral influenza
  - Coxsackie infections
  - Shigellosis
  - Reye's syndrome
  - Myxomavirus
  - Legionnaires' disease
  - Infectious hepatitis
- Miscellaneous toxins
  - Venoms
    - Snake bite
    - Hornet bite
    - Brown recluse spider bite
  - Drugs
    - Ethanol
    - Cocaine
    - Heroin
    - Barbiturates
    - Propoxyphene
    - Methadone, codeine
    - Glutethimide
    - Amphetamines
    - Plasmacid
    - Licorice, carbenoxolone (potassium deficiency)
    - Amphotericin B
    - Diazepam
    - ϵ-Aminocaproic acid
    - Peanut oil (arachidonic acid)
    - Phencyclidine (angel dust)
  - Others
    - Quail ingestion
    - Isopropyl alcohol
    - Ethylene glycol
    - Haff disease
    - Hypernatremia
    - 2,4-Dichlorophenoxyacetic acid

mitochondria also may participate. During the early phases of rhabdomyolysis with ARF, serum parathyroid hormone levels are often greatly increased. The serum creatinine concentration is disproportionately elevated in relation to the blood urea nitrogen concentration, and marked creatininuria will be present if renal function remains relatively intact. A portion of the elevation of total serum creatinine is owing to an increase of noncreatinine chromogen production. Because of the non–steady-state conditions and the often very high rates of creatinine excretion, calculation of the true fractional excretion of sodium may be difficult and provide erroneous data. However, a low fractional excretion rate of sodium may be seen in ARF associated with rhabdomyolysis. Disseminated intravascular coagulation commonly may supervene, especially in patients with heat stroke and septic shock.

Because of local swelling and entrapment of tissues and vessels in fascial compartments, a second wave of rhabdomyolysis may occur after the initial injury as viable muscle is further compromised by the steadily increasing fascial compartment pressure impairing local blood flow. Urgent fasciotomies may be required.

Prevention and treatment of rhabdomyolysis are directed at recognition of individuals at high risk (e.g., poorly conditioned athletes undergoing vigorous exercise under conditions of volume depletion, potassium depletion, and exercise-induced lactic acidosis). A starved, volume-depleted, potassium-depleted, phosphate-depleted alcoholic patient is at particular risk for the development of rhabdomyolysis. Once myoglobinuria has developed, urine flow should be maintained at 100 to 200 ml/hr with isotonic or hypertonic mannitol. The urine should be alkalinized to a pH of 7.0 or greater with intravenous sodium bicarbonate. Fluid deficits, if any are present, should be promptly corrected. Hypocalcemia and hyperphosphatemia, if mild, require no therapy, although the infusion of large amounts of alkali in an attempt to alkalinize the urine may result in tetany in profoundly hypocalcemic patients. Parenteral furosemide may convert patients from oliguric to nonoliguric ARF. Intravenous calcium salts should be avoided, especially in the face of marked hyperphosphatemia and oliguria. Severe metastatic calcification may appear in patients given excessive quantities of intravenous calcium in this setting. Early hemodialysis usually will be required for the treatment of ARF because patients tend to be severely hypercatabolic. During recovery from ARF, which usually occurs in 7 to 14 days after the initial injury, some patients develop hypercalcemia. This hypercalcemia is most often of a mild and asymptomatic nature and requires no specific therapy. However, occasionally it is severe and if phosphate levels have not fallen concomitantly, the hypercalcemia may lead to extraskeletal calcifications. The mechanism of the development of hypercalcemia in the diuretic phase is thought to be a rapid return of 1,25-dihydroxyvitamin D biosynthesis in the kidney under the influence of persisting high parathyroid hormone levels. The hypercalcemia may be augmented by the dissolution of extraskeletal (primarily muscle) calcifications. In the absence of serious extrarenal disease, such as might occur from a severe crush injury, the prognosis for ultimate recovery in patients with rhabdomyolysis and myoglobinuria is good. Mortality rates of 5 to 10% have been commonly observed.

Hemoglobinuria

Hemoglobin is an iron-containing, oxygen-binding respiratory protein present exclusively in the erythrocyte. It is a protein composed of four chains (2 α, 2 β) with a molecular weight of 68,000. It has an isoelectric point of 6.99, and in plasma it is tightly and irreversibly bound to a plasma α_2-globulin (haptoglobin). The α chain of the tetrameric haptoglobin molecule binds to the β chain of oxyhemoglobin, forming a large macromolecular complex that is taken up by the hepatic Kupffer cells. Plasma haptoglobin levels fall precipitously with the development of intravascular hemolysis and hemoglobinemia. At normal plasma haptoglobin levels of 50 to 150 mg/dl, the maximum binding capacity for hemoglobin varies between 40 and 200 mg/dl, depending on the haptoglobin phenotype.

Hemoglobin is present in only trace quantities in nonhemolyzed plasma (below 1 mg/dl), and because of its high molecular weight and haptoglobin-binding properties, it is not present in normal urine unless hematuria is present or unless the capacity for haptoglobin binding is impaired or exceeded. The fractional renal clearance of hemoglobin at plasma levels above the maximum binding capacity of haptoglobin is only about 3% that of the prevailing level of GFR. The threshold for urinary excretion of hemoglobin is approximately 150 mg/dl. Plasma may acquire a distinct pinkish hue at plasma levels of hemoglobin above 50 mg/dl. Hemoglobin in urine is bright red at alkaline pH but in acid urine is converted to brownish black pigmented methemoglobin. Hemoglobin is insoluble in 3.2 M ammonium sulfate, which aids in its differentiation from myoglobin. Electrophoresis, immunoassays, and absorption spectra are other more accurate methods of differentiating myoglobin from hemoglobin.

Because of the low renal clearance of hemoglobin, plasma concentrations sufficient to result in pinkish discoloration are quickly achieved with only modest amounts of intravascular hemolysis. Hemoglobin once filtered at the glomerulus is partially reabsorbed in the proximal tubule, where the heme iron is reincorporated into ferritin and hemosiderin. Hemosiderinuria and increased urinary iron occur in the course of chronic hemoglobinemic states.

The causes of hemoglobinemia and hemoglobinuria are listed in Table 28.7. Fundamentally, destruction of autologous or homologous erythrocytes is responsible. Hemoglobinuria ensues if the rate of destruction exceeds the capacity for complexing with haptoglobin. Thus most very-low-grade chronic hemolytic anemias are not associated with significant degrees of hemoglobinuria.

As with myoglobinuria, clinical conditions associated with brisk hemoglobinuria may be associated with the development of ARF. The mechanism of ARF in hemoglobinuric states is not known, but the following could be involved: (a) intranephronal obstruction resulting from precipitation or polymerization of the globin portion of the hemoglobin molecule with acidic mucoproteins (e.g., Tamm-Horsfall protein), (b) renal ischemia resulting from concomitant release of potent vasoconstrictor substances, and (c) direct nephrotoxicity of breakdown products (ferrihemate) with resultant tubular necrosis and/or backleak of filtrate. Regardless of the mechanism, hemoglobinuria should be suspected when ARF supervenes in any of the clinical situations described in Table 28.7 and when pigmenturia can be documented.

Other biochemical features that are common accompaniments of hemoglobinuria include severe anemia, elevated reticulocyte count, elevated serum lactic dehydrogenase, significant reduction in serum haptoglobin concentration, abnormalities in the red cell morphologic picture on peripheral smear, and the presence of abnormal immunoproteins, especially antibodies to erythrocyte cell wall antigens. Profound hyperuricemia, hyperphosphatemia, and hypocalcemia, as seen in myoglobinuric states, usually are not observed in conditions associated with hemoglobinuric ARF.

The prevention and treatment of hemoglobinuria are, as in rhabdomyolysis, directed at the recognition of individuals at high risk (e.g., mismatched blood transfusions, hemoglobinopathies, congenital erythrocyte enzyme deficiencies). The coexistence of volume depletion, acidosis, and dehydration

TABLE 28.7. Causes of Hemoglobinuria

Inherited (congenital) hemolytic disorders
- Defects in erythrocyte membrane or erythrocyte glycolytic enzymes (e.g., hereditary spherocytosis, pyruvate kinase deficiency)*
- Deficiencies in pentose phosphate pathway and glutathione metabolism
- Glucose-6-phosphate dehydrogenase deficiency and exposure to oxidant drugs (sulfa, *p*-aminosalicylic acid, phenacetin, aniline dyes, chlorates, phenol, fava beans)*
- Defects in globin structure and synthesis
  - Unstable hemoglobin diseases*
  - Sickle cell disease*
  - Thalassemia*
  - Other*

Acquired hemolytic disorders
- Immunohemolytic disorders
  - Transfusion of incompatible blood*
  - Autoimmune hemolytic anemia resulting from warm-reactive antibody*
  - Autoimmune hemolytic anemia resulting from cold-reactive antibody (cold agglutinin disease, paroxysmal cold hemoglobinemia)
- Traumatic/microangiopathic
  - Prosthetic valves
  - Disseminated intravascular coagulation
  - March hemoglobinuria
- Infectious
  - Malaria (falciparum, blackwater fever)
  - Clostridial infection
- Chemicals
  - Oxidant drugs and glucose-6-phosphate dehydrogenase deficiency*
  - Nonoxidant chemical (arsine, distilled water or hypotonic fluids, hemodialysis, abortifacients)
  - Quinine
- Physical agents
  - Thermal injury
- Other
  - Severe hypophosphatemia
  - Paroxysmal nocturnal hemoglobinuria
  - Rapid infusion of hypotonic fluids (e.g., dialysis with erroneous diluted dialysate)

*Most common causes.

may aggravate the susceptibility to hemoglobinuric ARF. Once hemoglobinuria has been documented, the urine flow should be maintained at 100 to 200 ml/hr with the infusion of isotonic saline solution or isotonic or hypertonic mannitol. There may be value in alkalinizing the urine to a pH of 7.0 or greater with intravenous sodium bicarbonate. Peritoneal dialysis or hemodialysis may be required for those patients developing prolonged oliguria from ARF. Administration of furosemide in 40- to 200-mg doses may be protective, provided it is not given to patients who are already volume depleted. During recovery from ARF resulting from hemoglobinuria, which usually occurs 7 to 14 days after the initial injury, patients may develop a tendency to polyuria and renal salt wastage. Provided extrarenal disease is mild and not life threatening, the immediate mortality rate of ARF in hemoglobinuric conditions is low (below 10%).

Selected Readings

Abuelo GJ. The diagnosis of hematuria. *Arch Intern Med* 1983;143:961–970.

An excellent simple analysis of the causes of and approach to hematuria.

Alento BG, Stock JA, Kaplan B. Hematuria in children. A practical approach. *Urol Clin North Am* 1995;22:43–55.

An excellent overview of hematuria.

Cameron JS. The patient with proteinuria and hematuria. In: Davison AM, Cameron JS, Greenfield J-P, eds. *Oxford Textbook of clinical nephrology,* 2nd ed. Oxford, England: Winearls, 1998:444–455.

An excellent overview.

Fairley KF, Birch DF. Hematuria: a simple method for identifying glomerular hematuria. *Kidney Int* 1982;21:105–108.

A detailed description of the use of phase contrast microscopy in the detection of dysmorphic hematuria.

Knochel JP. Rhabdomyolysis and myoglobinuria. *Semin Nephrol* 1981;1:75–85.

A review of the mechanisms and consequences of muscle injury.

Mariani AJ, Mariani MC, Macchioni C, et al. The significance of adult hematuria: 1000 hematuria evaluation including a risk-benefit and cost-effectiveness analysis. *J Urol* 1989;141:350–355.

A comprehensive study.

CHAPTER 29

Renal Colic and Flank Pain

Fredric L. Coe

RENAL COLIC

Renal colic is the term for the pain syndromes that may occur when the urinary tract is acutely dilated because of obstruction. The pain is proportional to the rate at which dilation of the renal pelvis or the ureters occurs, so passage of a kidney stone, a blood clot, a sloughed renal papilla, or other obstructing body can be extremely painful, whereas chronic dilation from an intraluminal or extraluminal cause is often painless, even when it is severe enough to produce renal failure. Colic usually follows a typical pattern that is easy to recognize, but atypical or variant forms can present important diagnostic challenges.

Typical Renal Colic

Onset

Discomfort or pain, often described as an ache or scratchy feeling, appears suddenly and can be so mild that it is almost unnoticeable at first. The sensation begins in one flank or loin, the side of the body, or along a broad band, about the width of the palm, extending from the side downward, across the abdomen to the groin. Within 20 to 30 minutes, the discomfort advances to pain of indescribable severity.

Plateau Phase

Like the pain that arises from distension of an obstructed portion of the intestine, renal colic seems to come from inside the body and localize on the body surface only vaguely. The victim of colic usually moves about in bed or by walking, hoping to find a comfortable position but mainly as a distraction from the pain, which, of course, is unaffected by posture or any other external maneuver or voluntary action. Although the kidneys and urinary tract are retroperitoneal, nausea and vomiting that is associated with reduced bowel sounds or even paralytic ileus may be prominent consequences. When these symptoms accompany colic that happens to radiate strongly along the upper abdominal wall, an intraperitoneal disease may be suspected. This is especially true when colic arises from ureteropelvic junction obstruction of the right kidney because the pain, and even muscle spasm, localize to the right upper quadrant of the abdomen, as in acute cholecystitis.

As for the intensity of the pain, one must turn to the artist because no description in our workaday can convey its horror. Richard Selzer, a surgeon and deft writer, has captured what I believe is a good likeness of its appalling nature. He wrote*:

> Whom the stone grips is transformed in one instant from man to shark; and like the shark that must remain in perpetual motion, fins and tail moving restlessly lest it, helpless, sink to terrible black depths of pressure, so the harborer of stone writhes and twists, bending and unbending in ceaseless turmoil. Now he straightens, stretches his limbs, only to draw them upon his trunk the next moment and fling his body from one side to another, finding ease in neither. From between his teeth come sounds so primitive and elemental as to trigger the skin to rise and creep. He shudders and vomits as though to cast forth the rock that grinds within.

In corroboration of Selzer's description, I have been assured by many women that the pain of stone passage greatly exceeds that of childbirth in severity.

Disappearance

Most of the time, we cannot observe the natural resolution of colic because pain medication has been given. However, in an untreated patient, sudden disappearance of pain follows the relief of the acute obstruction that occurs, for example, after the passage of the stone or blood clot through the ureter. Sudden resolution of pain helps distinguish renal colic from other urinary symptoms, none of which have this characteristic.

Location of Colic

In general, the area of the body from which the pain of colic seems to arise is determined by the site of obstruction, but there are so many exceptions to the rule that predictions made on the basis of symptoms in any given patient often are wrong. Colic from a stone or clot at the ureteropelvic junction or in the proximal ureter localizes in the flank and may radiate from there to the upper abdominal quadrant or the loin, or even into the lower abdomen or groin. Obstruction at the midureter may cause pain to appear first in the flank or loin or along a band coursing downward, laterally and inferiorly, across the abdomen. Pain from stones that have traversed the upper ureter without causing obstruction but lodge in and obstruct the lower third of the ureter usually begins in the anterior-lateral

* Selzer R. Mortal lessons: notes on the art of surgery. New York: Simon & Schuster, 1976:83.

abdomen, the groin, or ipsilateral testicle or vulva, but it also may begin in the flank. Stones or blood clots that obstruct at the ureterovesical junction produce symptoms of trigone irritation: frequency, urgency, urethral pain, and dysuria. Renal colic itself may not occur at all, so infection of the bladder is suspected. From time to time, a stone that lodges at the end of the ureter may cause chronic pain in the scrotum, penis, or the labia, on one side. Frequency and urgency may or may not occur, and diagnostic studies may be directed to a region that harbors no pathologic process.

Variant or Atypical Colic

The same process that causes typical colic, acute obstruction by stone, clot, or tissue can cause a group of less severe pain syndromes that may be designated variant or atypical colic. Lesions that intermittently obstruct the infundibulum draining a calyx and never enter the renal pelvis cause flank pain that has the visceral quality of colic but is milder and comes in episodes, when obstruction occurs. There may be hematuria. An object free in the renal pelvis may occlude the ureteropelvic junction like a ball valve and give rise to brief episodes that begin like typical colic but remit quickly or at irregular intervals and cause incomplete cycles of pain. Chronic biliary disease can be suspected if the right kidney is involved. Obstructing lesions at the ureterovesical junction or in the intramural segment of the ureter typically cause urinary frequency and urgency, dysuria, and pain that radiates upward along the usual path of renal colic or downward into the penis, scrotum, or labia. If the object remains in place, urinary infection or diseases of the genital system often are suspected. Finally, renal colic may occur with severe vomiting, nausea, and diarrhea that may mimic intestinal disease or with unusually mild pain that, although typical in onset, location, radiation, character, and speed of remission, is not at first thought of as renal colic because it is not severe.

Differentiation of Renal Colic from Other Pains (Fig. 29.1)

Renal colic is not a great mimic because its character, location, pattern of radiation, and course are distinctive and not like those of most other intraabdominal or retroperitoneal diseases. A patient who has had authentic colic can usually be trusted to identify it correctly if it ever recurs and to distinguish it reliably from other pains. Therefore one must be attentive to the opinion of an experienced patient concerning the likelihood of recurrent colic. Conditions that can be confused with renal colic and pose diagnostic problems are listed in Table 29.1.

Biliary Colic

Right upper quadrant abdominal pain, persistent nausea and vomiting, and abdominal tenderness can be caused by an acute obstruction of the right ureteropelvic junction. If the kidney is infected, there may be fever, leukocytosis, and even slight jaundice from sepsis, and a mistaken diagnosis of acute cholecystitis might easily be made. Renal outflow obstruction usually causes more flank than anterior tenderness, and the pain is more severe than biliary colic. Hematuria and leukocyturia are not features of acute cholecystitis. Radiation of the pain to the right shoulder or subscapular region occurs in acute cholecystitis but not with renal outflow obstruction.

Appendicitis

The initial pain of appendiceal dilation is a visceral colic, centered vaguely near the umbilicus and not at all like renal colic. After 4 to 6 hours, however, the pain tends to localize in the right lower quadrant as periappendiceal inflammation creates localized peritonitis, and at this stage, the location of the pain is like that of a lower ureteral stone. Usually, the differential diagnosis is not difficult. A patient with appendicitis prefers to lie quietly and has rebound and direct abdominal tenderness; renal colic provokes a patient to move, and the pain is not altered by

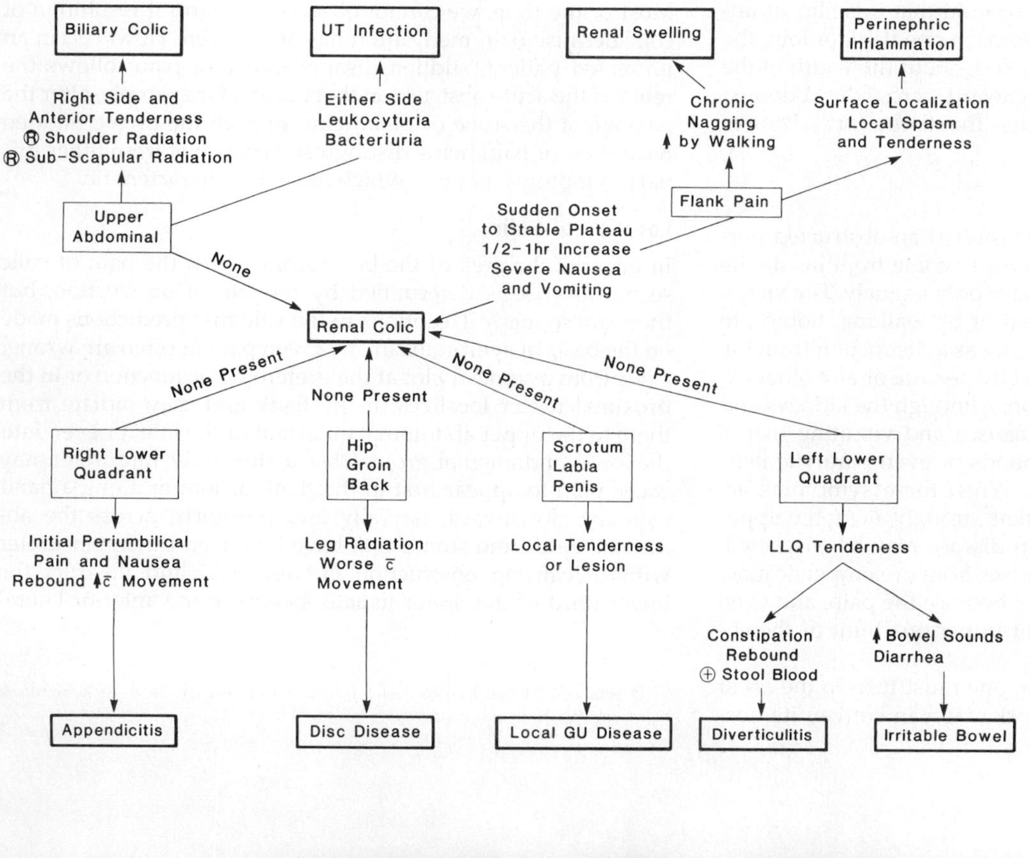

Figure 29.1. Characteristics of states that can cause renal colic and those that could be confused with renal colic. *UT,* urinary tract; *R,* right; *LLQ,* left lower quadrant; *GU,* genitourinary.

TABLE 29.1. Differential Diagnosis of Renal Colic

Biliary colic
Appendicitis
Diverticulitis
Diverticulosis
Irritable colon syndrome
Musculoskeletal pain
Urinary tract infection
Testicular, scrotal, or labial disease
Systemic and metabolic disease
Acute intermittent porphyria
Familial Mediterranean fever
Lead poisoning

abdominal palpation. Hematuria and leukocyturia can occur when an inflamed appendix lies near the right ureter or the bladder, but there are at most a few red and white cells compared with the marked hematuria that is usual in stone passage. Fever and leukocytosis, typical of appendicitis, are not present in uncomplicated colic. Most of all, the severity of the pain and the time course differ in these two conditions. In appendicitis, pain shifts from the periumbilical region to the right lower quadrant over a period of hours, whereas renal colic tends to stay in one place or move from the flank downward. Also, the pain of renal colic is usually much more severe than that of early appendicitis.

Diverticulitis, Diverticulosis, and Irritable Colon Syndrome

Left-sided colic from lower ureteral obstruction, if not too severe, may raise the possibility of diverticulitis in the descending colon when pain localizes in the left lower quadrant. Colic from a low ureteral stone sometimes causes a sense of rectal fullness that increases the suspicion of colon disease. However, diverticulitis is much less painful than renal colic, and often there are localized abdominal tenderness, direct and rebound muscle spasm, and guarding. The stool is positive for occult blood in 25% of diverticulitis cases, constipation, not usual in renal colic, is a common finding, and hematuria is uncommon. Acute colicky pain also can arise from diverticulosis in the absence of diverticulitis and produce a brief acute pain syndrome with no abdominal physical findings except tenderness of the sigmoid colon. Hematuria is absent. Irritable colon syndrome, especially in its most severe forms, can pose a serious diagnostic problem. Abdominal distension is marked, and the pain is severe and associated with low backache. Furthermore, it tends to occur in people who are abnormally preoccupied with their health and therefore are less likely to describe their symptoms precisely. I have observed some patients with this disorder who have also suffered from stone disease, and it has not always been easy for the patient to distinguish left-sided renal colic and recrudescence of colon symptoms. As a rule, diarrhea is severe during an acute attack of pain from irritable colon syndrome, and bowel sounds are hyperactive rather than hypoactive, as in renal colic. There may be abdominal tenderness and spasm and tenderness of the colon itself.

Musculoskeletal Pain

Protrusion of a lumbar intervertebral disk causes unilateral backache with radiation into the hip, groin, or thigh, symptoms that can resemble those of a low ureteral stone. The two most common sites of protrusion are at the L4-5 and L5-S1 interspaces. Complete rupture of a disc is not likely to be confused with stone because the pain radiates prominently to the leg, and there usually are neurologic defects, such as reduced reflexes or sensation. However, L4-5 disc degeneration can produce unilateral lumbar back pain radiating into the hip, groin, and thigh, not accompanied by neurologic abnormalities. Strain or trauma can produce an acute attack of severe pain. Usually, the differentiation from renal colic is easy because the pain is aggravated by certain postures and relieved by immobility, and vomiting and anterior abdominal radiation are absent, as are urinary symptoms and hematuria.

From time to time, patients who have formed stones also have chronic back pain, not colic, and there arises the question of what relation the chronic pain may have to stone disease. In general, chronic back pain does not result from obstructing lesions of the urinary tract, especially a pain that is worsened by particular postures or exercise and relieved by rest. For this reason, the cause of the pain should be sought as if a urinary lesion were not present. The exceptions to this dictum are (a) chronic pelvic pain that radiates into the sacral region and is clearly unilateral and (b) chronic flank pain. Pelvic pain may arise from obstructing lesions at the ureterovesical junction or from inflammatory, infective, or neoplastic lesions in the bladder, prostate, or genital structures. Chronic flank pain can arise from intrarenal obstructing lesions of the type that can also produce colic, such as stones or clots.

Lesions obstructing the ureterovesical junction may produce symptoms resembling urinary tract infection. Stones lodging in the intramural segment of the ureter may cause urinary frequency and dysuria, with or without unilateral mild pain in the groin, testicle, labia, or low back, and often without an antecedent attack of typical colic. In this situation, hematuria is usually present, but leukocyturia is minimal and urine culture is sterile. Even if it is a radiopaque stone, the lesion may not be recognized as such by plain abdominal x-ray evaluation because of overlying bony and soft tissue shadows and the high frequency of small pelvic calcifications caused by phleboliths.

Scrotal, Penile, or Labial Disease

A variant form colic also arises from chronic lodgment of an object at the ureterovesical junction. The presence of frequency, dysuria, and sacral or low lumbar back pain may help to differentiate the scrotal, penile, or labial pain caused by variant renal colic from that caused by localized disease of these areas.

Causes of Renal Colic

Passage of kidney stones is by far the most common reason for renal colic—so much so that the two are often wrongly taken as synonymous. The pain of colic comes from the acute obstruction and consequent dilation of a ureter or the renal pelvis, not from the hardness or abrasive qualities of a stone, so blood clots or tissue fragments may cause the symptoms just as well. Colic from blood clots is not rare in sickling disorders that predispose to renal papillary bleeding, hereditary, or acquired disorders of blood clotting, trauma, bleeding after percutaneous renal biopsy, benign and malignant neoplasms of the kidney or urinary tract, renal cysts, polycystic renal disease, renal vascular malformation, invasion of the urinary tract by adjacent neoplasm, papillary necrosis, tuberculosis, and infarction of a portion of one kidney from arterial or venous occlusion. Papillary necrosis occurs in sickle cell disease and trait, analgesic abuse, diabetes mellitus, chronic alcoholism, and severe pyelonephritis in the presence of obstruction. Neoplasms of a benign and malignant nature can cause colic by sloughing off of some tissue. This usually results from malignant tumors of the urothelium in the renal pelvis or in the ureter. Polypoid tumors, benign or malignant, may produce colic by acting as a ball valve obstruction, as well as by bleeding or sloughing tissue. Finally, true colic, but brief, occurring only during micturition, can occur when vesicoureteral reflux is present. This transient pain can be a valuable clue to reflux.

Approach to the Patient with Renal Colic (Fig. 29.1)

Once it is clear that renal colic is present, in contrast to another pain syndrome, urinalysis and abdominal flat plate evaluation are the most important studies. The most common findings to be anticipated are a radiopaque calculus in the region of the renal pelvis, along the ureter, or at the ureterovesical junction on the side of the pain, accompanied by microscopic hematuria. Calcium oxalate or phosphate stones, cystine stones, and struvite ($MgNH_4PO_4$) stones are all radiopaque. Uric acid stones, blood clots, and sloughed tissue, including renal papillae, usually are radiolucent, however, and may not be accompanied by hematuria. The kidney on the side of the colic may be larger than the other one because of obstruction, but I rarely have found this sign helpful, because the two kidneys may differ in length normally.

Unless there is a contraindication, such as allergy to contrast material, intravenous pyelography should be performed to assess the extent of urinary obstruction that may be present and to verify or define the cause of the colic. In many instances, the stone or other obstructing object may have passed by the time of the pyelogram, leaving only mild unilateral dilation of the ureter, renal pelvis, or calyces in its wake. In the presence of severe azotemia, intravenous pyelography may not provide adequate visualization of the excretory system. If intravenous pyelography cannot be performed or visualization is unsatisfactory, retrograde pyelography may be indicated instead. However, the latter procedure is unpleasant and carries a small but real risk of morbidity from infection and ureteral damage.

Patients with renal colic should have all their urine filtered through gauze in the hope of capturing stones, clots, or tissue that can provide important clues to the cause of the colic. Straining the urine is worthwhile, even weeks after colic, because a stone or tissue can reside in the bladder for a very long time without producing symptoms. Any discrete object must be studied to determine its nature and never be discarded until its composition is fully understood.

If renal colic is clearly present, the patient must receive adequate analgesic medications promptly. One cannot exaggerate the pain of renal colic, and it is pointless to withhold medication during diagnostic studies unless there is a serious question about the presence of an intraabdominal disease whose evaluation could be hampered if the patient were given medications for pain. In general, narcotic drugs are needed to control colic, and they must be used at full therapeutic dosage.

FLANK PAIN

The flanks are those regions of the back bounded above by the ribcage, below by the crest of the ilium, medially by the spine, and laterally by the sides of the body. As a rule, the flanks are not the site of the common backaches and pains that afflict most of us at one time or another, so significant flank pain must always raise considerable concern, even if it is not very severe. It is natural to suspect a renal origin for flank pain, and in most cases, this is a reasonable suspicion.

Flank Pain of Renal Origin (Table 29.2)

TABLE 29.2. Causes of Flank Pain

Pain of renal origin
Renal swelling
Acute nephritis
Nephrotic syndrome
Renal vein thrombosis
Urinary obstruction
Pyelonephritis
Renal cysts
Renal cell carcinoma
Perinephritic inflammation
Renal infarction
Embolic arterial occlusion
Atherosclerotic arterial occlusion
Polyarteritis
Venous occlusion
Infection
Cyst rupture
Tumor
Trauma
Pain of nonrenal origin
Musculoskeletal
Malignant neoplasm
Pancreatitis
Aortic aneurysm

Renal Swelling

Stretching the capsule of the kidneys gives rise to pain that is localized to the flank because the renal capsule and flank both receive their sensory innervation from T10 to T12 spinal cord segments. The pain is an aching or heavy inward sensation that is not felt directly on the body surface and is unlike renal colic in that it is less severe and is nagging and persistent rather than explosive and unbearable. It often is worse with standing or at the end of the day and is unassociated with nausea or vomiting.

In several disease processes, the kidneys swell, but the mechanisms for pain may be different. In acute glomerulonephritis, nephrotic syndrome, renal vein thrombosis, and acute interstitial nephritis, the swelling reflects interstitial edema that could result from inflammation (acute glomerulonephritis and interstitial nephritis) or from abnormal transcapillary Starling forces (renal vein thrombosis and nephrotic syndrome). Acute urinary obstruction causes tubular dilation, with consequent renal enlargement. Narrowing of the ureteropelvic junction can cause swelling and pain after a high fluid intake as the urine flow rises through a narrowed passage. Renal cysts, isolated or as a part of polycystic renal disease, can enlarge rapidly and cause capsular distention. Finally, rapidly growing renal cell carcinoma may cause swelling and pain.

Perinephric Inflammation

If a disease process causes inflammation outside the renal capsule, a new kind of pain syndrome results. The kidneys, their vessels, and the urinary tract lie in the retroperitoneal space, essentially just inside the posterior body wall. Inflammation of the body wall interior causes highly localized flank pain and local muscle spasm and tenderness. Unlike renal colic, which is unaffected by posture, and the aching produced by renal swelling, the pain of perinephric inflammation is worsened by movement of the flank and by jarring of the body surface, and the patient usually prefers to lie quietly. A common cause of perinephric inflammation is acute bacterial interstitial nephritis (pyelonephritis), especially when it is severe and extends beyond the confines of the renal capsule. Infarction of the kidney by extrinsic mechanical, embolic, or atheromatous vascular occlusion, aneurysm, or classic polyarteritis nodosa may be associated with perinephric inflammation and flank pain. A useful clue to infarction is a very high serum level of glutamic-oxaloacetic transaminase, released from the damaged kidney. Rupture of a renal cyst, hemorrhage or necrosis of a tumor mass in the kidney or urinary collecting system, and urine extravasation or renal hemorrhage incident to trauma are other causes of perinephric inflammation.

Unlike the kidneys themselves, the perinephric space has no natural drainage path, so infection or necrotic tissue can create a need for surgery. In the common situation of pyelonephritis, perinephric inflammation is mainly in the region of the renal capsular surface and tends to resolve if treatment is given. However, if infection extends deeply into the space because of diabetes mellitus, urinary tract obstruction, or other cause of reduced resistance to infection, a perinephric abscess can form. Such an abscess usually will require surgical drainage. A clue to perinephric abscess is loss of the clear renal outlines on abdominal flat plate or of the lateral border of the psoas muscle. Another is the development of an unexplained pleural effusion on the affected side.

Flank Pain of Extrarenal Origin

Because it is contiguous with the retroperitoneal space, the flank area can share in inflammatory processes that arise from the large blood vessels, the pancreas, or retroperitoneal malignancies. The local picture produced is like that of perinephric inflammation. Acute pancreatitis releases proteolytic and lipolytic enzymes into the flanks, and severe hemorrhage and inflammation can result. Rupture of an aortic aneurysm also may cause flank pain if hemorrhage happens to occur at that level. Any retroperitoneal sarcoma or lymphatic malignancy can produce pain in one flank, although this is an uncommon occurrence. Pelvic infections in the uterus or fallopian tubes or malignant tumors at either site can spread upward into the flanks.

Finally, there are musculoskeletal causes of flank pain. Like any portion of the back, the flanks can be painful if intervertebral disk disease is present and causes irritation to sensory nerve roots. This situation is less common in the thoracic than in the lumbar or cervical spine, perhaps because the mobility of the thoracic spine is limited, and it is not subjected to the torsion forces that occur elsewhere. T11–12 or T12-L1 disk disease, however, or degenerative osteoarthritis at these sites can produce pain, muscle spasm, and tenderness in the flank that resembles perinephric inflammation of renal or extrarenal origin. Clues to a neuromuscular origin include an onset related to back strain, sensory deficits in the areas of pain, and radiographic evidence of intervertebral disk space narrowing or osteoarthritis. Systemic evidence of tissue inflammation, such as fever and leukocytosis, is absent.

Selected Readings

Bretland PM. *Acute ureteric obstruction.* New York: Appleton-Century-Crofts, 1972.

A charming, short book that describes the experience of a consulting radiologist and summarizes the colic syndromes, their differential diagnosis, and relevant clinical investigation.

Cordell WH, Larson TA, Lingeman JE, et al. Indomethacin suppositories versus intravenously titrated morphine for the treatment of ureteric colic. *Ann Emerg Med* 1994;23:262–269.

Randomized, double-blind, double-dummy, two-period crossover study to compare the analgesic efficacy and side effect profiles of two types of analgesics. The conclusion of this study was that patients treated with intravenous morphine had significantly greater pain relief at 10 minutes than patients treated with indomethacin suppositories. At 20 and 30 minutes there was no difference, and at no time was there any difference in vital sign data or the numbers of side effects.

Erwin BC, Carroll BA, Sommer FG. Renal colic: the role of ultrasound in initial evaluation. *Radiology* 1984;152:147–150.

A prospective comparison of sonography and intravenous pyelogram in the detection of renal calculi. Sonography had no false-negative and only one false-positive result and can be used as a screening tool before x-ray evaluation.

Grenabo L, Holmlund D. Indomethacin as prophylaxis against recurrent ureteral colic. *Scand J Urol Nephrol* 1984;118:325–327.

One hundred patients with retained stones were treated with indomethacin or placebo in a prospective controlled trial to determine whether indomethacin reduces the severity of recurrent colic as such stones pass. Compared with control subjects, patients who took indomethacin had fewer episodes of recurrent pain, and their pain was of shorter duration, even though passage of retained stones that are in the midst of passing may be best treated with indomethacin to avoid severe pain episodes as the stones traverse the ureter.

Lehtonen T, Kellokumpu I, Permi J, et al. Intravenous indomethacin in the treatment of ureteric colic. *Ann Clin Res* 1983;15:197–199.

A prospective randomized trial of indomethacin compared with pethidine and metamizol. Indomethacin was as effective as pethidine, a centrally acting analgesic, and metamizol, a peripheral antagonist of prostaglandin synthesis. Intravenous administration of indomethacin may be a reasonable substitute for narcotic agents in control of acute colic.

Lundstam S, Whihed A, Suurkula M, et al. Acute radiorenography during attacks of renal colic. *J Urol* 1983;130:855–857.

The hippuran renogram was compared with the intravenous pyelogram in 22 patients with clinical signs suggesting renal colic. The renogram successfully detected all of the 16 patients who had stones producing urinary obstruction but was normal in 2 patients with nonobstructing stones causing only hematuria. The renogram is a sensitive test for detecting obstruction from stones, and a negative result may indicate that an abdominal x-ray evaluation without dye infusion may be sufficient for a complete evaluation.

Oosterlinck W, Philp NH, Charig C, et al. A double-blind single dose comparison of intramuscular ketorolac tromethamine and pethidine in the treatment of renal colic. *J Clin Pharmacol* 1990;30:336–341.

Ten milligrams of ketorolac tromethamine, a nonsteroidal antiinflammatory drug, was substituted for narcotics in the management of renal colic. This constitutes a new approach to the treatment of such pain.

Sacks M, Fajardo LL, Hillman BJ, et al. Prospective comparison of plain abdominal radiography with conventional and digital renal tomography in assessing renal extracorporeal shockwave lithotripsy patients. *J Urol* 1990;144:1341–1346.

Finding stones by flat plate evaluation can pose a problem and send us searching for other tests. Here, modern methods seem precise and much more sensitive. Although the title concerns shockwave lithotripsy, the materials concern finding stones for any purpose, such as evaluating a patient with pain.

CHAPTER 30

The Renal Mass

Thomas G. Cangiano and Jean B. deKernion

MASSES IN CHILDREN

It is extremely important to diagnose a renal mass in children. The diagnostic dilemma of a palpable renal mass deserves expeditious attention because damage to renal function and other systemic sequelae can be lethal. With the routine use of prenatal ultrasonographic screening, many genitourinary anomalies, including renal masses, are being detected and diagnosed *in utero.* This has led to the development of innovative forms of fetal intervention. Furthermore, from the emerging field of genetics we have seen new techniques in gene sequencing that have linked congenitally detected renal masses. The implications of all this are still not known, but we are entering the twenty-first century armed with the knowledge to begin to recognize and understand diseases that were previously beyond our comprehension.

Multicystic Dysplastic Kidney

The most common cause of an abdominal mass found in the first 48 hours of life is a multicystic dysplastic kidney (MCDK). Most of these are detected on routine prenatal ultrasonographic screening, although it can be difficult to distinguish MCDK from hydronephrosis by ultrasound imaging. Hydronephrosis caused by obstruction or reflux is less common in the first 2 days of life because of immature renal function and low urine output. As the neonatal kidney takes over filtration from the maternal placenta, urine output increases dramatically and hydronephrosis can manifest.

MCDK is most commonly seen on the left side and is unilateral. Bilateral MCDK is incompatible with life. Only if the cysts are large is the mass palpable in neonates. Again, MCDK can usually be diagnosed by ultrasonography, but the condition can also resemble a ureteropelvic junction obstruction. Ultrasonography may show noncommunicating cysts of varying sizes, with no one predominant cyst. Although the diagnosis can be suspected by reviewing the sonogram, this should be confirmed by a renal scan with technetium-99m diethylenetriamine-pentaacetic acid (DTPA) or mercaptoacetyltriglycerine (MAG-3) imaging. This is usually performed at 2 to 4 weeks of age. With MCDK, a photopenic defect will confirm no function. On histologic analysis, primitive tubules are seen; therefore no radiotracer agent is excreted. Imaging of the contralateral kidney is recommended because 18% of these can have an associated anomaly. One-third of these patients have vesicoureteral reflux; therefore a voiding cystourethrogram (VCUG) should be part of the workup for these patients.

The treatment approach is controversial, unless the MCDK is large, causing symptoms or signs, or there are suspicious findings, such as hypertension, associated nephroblastoma, malignancy, and renal blastema (precursor of Wilms' tumor). If the cysts are small, they can be followed conservatively. Follow-up with serial 1-year ultrasonography and physical examination is prudent. If the cysts grow significantly in size or malignancy is suspected, the kidney can be removed by cyst puncture though a small incision. The long-term potential for malignancy is controversial, but this possibility must be discussed with the family before deciding any course of action. It seems the risk is too low to recommend routine nephrectomy in these patients, and each must be treated individually.

Hydronephrosis

Congenital ureteropelvic junction (UPJ) obstruction has an incidence of about 1 in 1,000 children. Approximately 40% of patients are diagnosed prenatally by ultrasonography. Fewer than 15% of neonates with UPJ obstruction present with an abdominal or renal mass. Approximately two of three patients with UPJ obstruction are boys. In 60% of patients, the left side is involved. The cause of a UPJ obstruction may be anatomic or functional. Twenty percent of patients have a crossing vessel, and these are considered anatomic obstructions. The other 80% may be obstructed by a maldevelopment of the ureter at the UPJ: collagen and circular muscle fibers replace the usual longitudinal fibers, preventing adequate propulsion of urine. The pelvis then expands and drapes over this segment, exacerbating the obstruction.

The diagnosis of hydronephrosis caused by UPJ obstruction is made by ultrasonography. On a sonogram, cysts may be found; a medial cyst predominates, and the cysts are seen to communicate. The pelvis is usually dilated but the ureter is not, as is found in reflux. If bilateral hydronephrosis is present, if there is a solitary kidney with hydronephrosis, or an abdominal mass is detected, a more prompt diagnosis must be made. If the sonogram exhibits no hydronephrosis in the first 2 weeks of life, ultrasonography should be repeated at 1 month. Fifteen percent of patients with UPJ obstruction have reflux; therefore a VCUG must be obtained. In neonates, at least 5% function must be documented to distinguish this from an MCDK that has less than 5% function. An intravenous pyelogram (IVP) is generally not performed in neonates because it is difficult to concentrate the contrast agent and the prominent overlying bowel gas obscures the collecting systems. IVPs are generally reserved for use in infants or older children. A DTPA scan or MAG-3 scan with a furosemide washout phase is important not only to assess function but also may be critical in the diagnosis of a potential obstruction. The time for half the radiotracer to be excreted ($T_{1/2}$) is used as an indication of potential obstruction, but controversy exists as to the true definition of obstruction. Usually, a $T_{1/2}$ of less than 10 minutes is considered to be normal; 10 to 20 minutes is intermediate. A $T_{1/2}$ greater than 20 minutes is thought to represent significant delay in contrast excretion and is defined as potential obstruction. Not all researchers agree on what constitutes obstruction, and this will be important when discussing therapy.

Nephrogenesis is complete during the first 36 weeks of gestation, and the glomerular filtration rate (GFR) increases dramatically during the first 6 months of life. Obstruction can decrease the filtration rate and renal blood flow. With progressive obstruction, the GFR may be decreased indefinitely. Furthermore, compensatory hypertrophy and hyperfiltration may affect the contralateral kidney. With long-term hyperfiltration, nephrosclerosis can occur. The congenitally obstructed kidney has a great potential to return to normal function when the obstruction is removed; blood flow may be reestablished to the cortical nephrons that were obstructed. Thus it seems logical that treatment be considered, but in addition to controversy among pediatric urologists as to the true definition of obstruction, some investigators question whether pyeloplasty really reduces renal injury. Recent evidence suggests that many patients with UPJ obstruction may be followed conservatively. If this approach is used, the parents must be reassured that further damage may not be imminent.

Nevertheless, the mainstay of treatment is still surgery. Controversy exists whether a percutaneous nephrostomy tube should be placed; however, sepsis and bilateral UPJ obstruction mandate tube placement. Timing is a consideration: proponents for intervention recommend repair when severe hydronephrosis is present (grades IV and V). Grades I through III can be managed conservatively if the contralateral kidney is normal and renal function is greater than 40%. If there is deterioration of renal function or function is decreased in the washout curve on the DTPA scan, pyeloplasty should be considered and discussed with the parents. Proponents of intervention have also recommended that patients with a solitary kidney and an abdominal mass undergo repair. If such repair is undertaken, the dysfunctional segment of ureter at the UPJ must be excised.

Renal Vein Thrombosis

Renal vein thrombosis, more commonly seen in neonates, results from dehydration, which may cause sludging and subsequent clotting in the small renal venules. The classic features are a palpable renal mass (60%), gross hematuria (70%), thrombocytopenia (90%, below 75,000/μL), consumptive coagulopathy (elevated clotting time; fibrin split products), leukocytosis, proteinuria, and anemia (32%). Patients with bilateral renal vein thrombosis will have elevated blood urea nitrogen and serum creatinine levels. The prognosis for a patient with bilateral renal vein thrombosis is poor, as it is for a patient with vena caval thrombosis. For patients in whom renal vein thrombosis is suspected, ultrasonography is the diagnostic procedure of choice. Usually, an enlarged kidney is seen, and Doppler scanning will show minimal flow in the renal vein and inferior vena cava (IVC). A DTPA scan may also be useful to assess renal function.

Initial management consists of intravenous hydration and correction of electrolyte abnormalities. This can usually prevent new clot formation. Investigators have not yet reached consensus on the efficacy of heparinization in this situation. Because of the potential for side effects, the use of thrombolytic agents such as urokinase and streptokinase should be reserved for cases of bilateral renal vein thrombosis. If concomitant IVC occlusion is present, thrombectomy is controversial because collateral circulation tends to develop. Long-term sequelae include renin-mediated hypertension resulting from an atrophic kidney, but this only occasionally occurs. In these cases, a nephrectomy may be curative.

Mesoblastic Nephroma

Mesoblastic nephroma was first reported in 1967. It is the most common solid tumor in infants; the mean age at diagnosis is 3.5 months. It occurs more commonly in boys and also may be associated with polyhydramnios; 14% of patients may have other associated anomalies. There has been a trend to detect these tumors prenatally. Imaging cannot reliably distinguish this from other solid tumors, but the age of presentation provides the best clue for diagnosis.

Pathologically, the tumor is dense, is firm, and appears as a leiomyoma. The cell count is dense, and 25% of patients have a high mitotic index. Treatment is complete excision of the tumor. The completeness of resection will predict relapse. Metastases are rare and warrant chemotherapy and/or radiotherapy.

Multilocular Cyst

Multilocular cyst is also known as *multilocular cystic nephroma*. The most common feature is an abdominal or renal mass. There are two age peaks: pediatric, with blastema in septa of cysts; and adult, which usually has fibrous tissue in the septa. Usually, the tumor is well circumscribed, filled with cysts of varying size. These are best managed by nephrectomy or partial nephrectomy. No distant metastases or tumor recurrence has been reported.

Autosomal Recessive Polycystic Kidney Disease

Autosomal-recessive polycystic kidney disease (ARPKD) occurs in approximately 1 in 10,000 births. It is characterized by kidneys that are enlarged because of bilateral cystic disease. ARPKD is caused by a genetic defect on chromosome 6. Seventy-five percent of patients present in the neonatal period with an abdominal or flank mass. These may be associated with pulmonary hypoplasia and renal failure in the first year of life. In these patients, the cause of death is pulmonary hypoplasia and respiratory failure, not renal failure. If the infant survives the newborn period, he or she will eventually develop renal insufficiency and hypertension. Seventy-nine percent of infants born with ARPKD are alive at 12 months. As these children age, an increased percentage will develop renal insufficiency and hepatic fibrosis. The latter involves fibrosis of the portal spaces, and portal hypertension ensues.

ARPKD is always bilateral. The pathogenesis is unknown, except for the mode of transmission (autosomal recessive), but there is a spectrum of phenotypic expression. The cysts are usually small but pepper the kidney in a radial arrangement. Microscopically, these are dilated collecting ducts and tubules from the medulla to the cortex. Oligohydramnios is not always present.

On ultrasonography, the kidneys are both seen to be enlarged. Numerous fine cysts are found throughout the medulla and cortex. There is increased echogenicity, reflecting the cysts within the tubules; this gives the characteristic pattern of medullary echoes. Ultrasonography of the liver will show dilated bile ducts and increased echogenicity.

Two systems need to be treated: the renal and the hepatic. These patients may need bilateral nephrectomy and renal transplantation if the kidneys are large. The sequelae of congenital hepatic fibrosis are best treated with a portocaval shunt.

The prognosis for these patients is poor. It is of the utmost importance that parents of an affected child receive genetic counseling because there is no cure. Siblings of an affected child have a 25% chance of being affected, and the parents have a 50% chance of carrying the heterozygous allele.

Wilms' Tumor

Wilms' tumor is the most common malignant solid tumor of the urinary tract in children; 80% of genitourinary tumors in children younger than 15 years are Wilms' tumors. The peak incidence at diagnosis is 3.5 years of age. This tumor has also been diagnosed in utero by fetal sonography. The cause is thought to be a loss of a tumor suppressor gene (WT1) at 11p13. There is a 5% to 10% incidence of bilateral Wilms' tumor.

Wilms' tumor is diagnosed as an abdominal or renal mass in 75% of affected children. Microhematuria is seen in about 25% of patients with this tumor; gross hematuria is relatively uncommon. On physical examination, an abdominal or renal mass may be palpated but rarely crosses the midline. Hypertension, seen in 65% of patients, is caused by compression of renal tissue, leading to renal ischemia with subsequent renin release. Fifteen percent of children have other congenital anomalies and 6% have other genitourinary anomalies. These include aniridia, WAGR syndrome [*W*ilms' tumor, *a*niridia, *g*enitourinary anomaly of fusion (hypospadias, cryptorchidism), and mental *r*etardation], hemihypertrophy, and Beckwith-Wiedemann syndrome (visceromegaly, hemihypertrophy, omphalocele, microcephaly, mental retardation, and macroglossia).

Intravenous pyelography may demonstrate a mass in the kidney splaying the collecting system. Ultrasonography will show a solid mass in the kidney with or without calcifications. The computed tomography (CT) scan is the radiologic imaging test of choice once a solid mass is documented. This will show a solid renal mass with a sharp demarcation from the normal parenchyma. Calcifications on the rim may be seen on CT scan, and the contralateral kidney can be assessed for tumor and relative function. The CT scan gives some information on staging, but it does not supplant exploration to confirm pathologic stage and contralateral involvement. Because the lungs are the most common site of metastases, a chest x-ray evaluation is performed.

Pathologically, most Wilms' tumors are well demarcated and encapsulated. Microscopically, they contain blastemal, epithelial, and stromal cells. The histopathologic features can be divided into favorable and unfavorable findings. The histologic studies will be important in predicting the patient's prognosis and clinical course. An unfavorable histologic finding would include an anaplastic Wilms' tumor, which is relatively chemoresistant and represents 4.8% of cases. This is usually seen in older children, and histologically there is an increase in nuclear size, hyperchromatic nuclei, and abnormal and frequent mitotic figures. Planning for the intensity of chemotherapy will be guided by the histologic picture (Table 30.1).

Complete nephrectomy with contralateral exploration is the standard of treatment. Tumor spillage must be avoided. Chemotherapy and radiotherapy should be considered in cases in which the tumor is bilateral, intracaval (extensive), or considered unresectable. There is no evidence that preoperative chemotherapy or radiotherapy improves long-term survival. The mainstay of chemotherapeutic agents for Wilms' tumor includes actinomycin D, vincristine and Adriamycin. The National Wilms' Tumor Study Group IV found that survival rates were higher with combination chemotherapy than with monotherapy. Patients with stage III and IV tumors and unfavorable histologic findings receive the aforementioned chemotherapeutic agents. In the same stage patients with unfavorable histologic findings, a more intensive chemotherapeutic regimen is given. In patients with stage V disease, a biopsy of the tumor is initially performed and preoperative chemotherapy is given, followed by surgical restaging and nephron-sparing surgery. Stage V tumors can be understaged in many patients; therefore exploration of the contralateral side in any patient with a Wilms' tumor is necessary.

The prognosis for patients with Wilms' tumor depends heavily on histologic findings. All stages with a favorable histologic picture have a better prognosis than any stage with unfavorable histologic evidence. Patients must be followed with serial chest x-ray evaluation because this is the most common site of recurrence. Patients with renal failure who have survived Wilms' tumor can safely undergo transplantation if they are found to be free of disease at 24 months. Table 30.2 provides currently available data on postnephrectomy survival in patients with Wilms' tumors.

Nephroblastomatosis or nephrogenic rests are thought to be a precursor to Wilms' tumor. Nephrogenic rests are abnormally present nephrogenic cells that can be secondarily induced to form Wilms' tumor. This is found in 30% to 44% of patients with Wilms' tumor.

Nephroblastomatosis is the diffuse or multifocal presence of nephrogenic rests. Nephrogenic rests can change over time and can undergo transformation to form Wilms' tumor. These rests can be indistinguishable from Wilms' tumor and should be followed serially with CT scan. Any increase of growth may be a sign of Wilms' tumor, and appropriate therapy must be instituted.

TABLE 30.1. Staging of Wilms' Tumor as Determined by the National Wilms' Tumor Study Group IV

Stage I	Tumor confined to the capsule, completely resected without rupture
Stage II	Tumor outside of capsule (by direct invasion of capsule, extrarenal vascular extension or tumor spillage), completely resected (includes biopsied tumor)
Stage III	Incomplete surgical resection with residual tumor remaining within the abdomen (includes nodal metastases, tumor spillage or peritoneal seeding)
Stage IV	Any local stage with hematogenous metastasis
Stage V	Bilateral renal involvement at time of diagnosis

TABLE 30.2. Four-Year Postnephrectomy Survival in Patients with Wilms' Tumor

	FH	UH
Stage I	97%	68%
Stage II	92%	68%
Stage III	84%	68%
Stage IV	83%	55%
Stage V	46% (3 yr)	—

FH, Favorable histology; UH, unfavorable histology.

MASSES IN ADULTS

Renal masses in adults are approached differently from those found in children. Most renal masses found in adults are "guilty until proven innocent"; that is, they are carcinoma until definitely proven benign. Although in some cases this is clear cut, many cases still exist that challenge the physician's ability to make a diagnosis using currently available diagnostic modalities. The history plays an extremely important role when evaluating the renal mass in adults because symptoms and signs can develop that will give clues to the diagnosis.

We have categorized renal masses in adults into benign and malignant categories. This is not to say that one may not be associated with the other but that diagnostic evaluation and management in each category may be similar. An algorithm for the diagnosis of a renal mass in the adult is given in Fig. 30.1.

Benign Lesions

Inflammatory Lesions

Xanthogranulomatous pyelonephritis (XGP) is an uncommon inflammatory process of the kidney. It is usually associated with obstruction of part of the kidney and is often caused by calculous disease. This lesion is one of the great mimickers of neoplastic disease because it forms a heterogeneous mass that may be indistinguishable from renal cell carcinoma. A staghorn or large obstructing calculus will give a clue to the diagnosis. There is also a tendency for XGP to spread, which may lead to a diagnostic dilemma. Clinically, the patient may have nonspecific symptoms or symptoms or signs of infection, including flank pain, low-grade fever, chills, and malaise. XGP most commonly occurs in middle-aged women. The urinalysis will often reveal leukocytosis without white cell casts. Bacteriuria may be seen in 50% of the cases, indicating the association with urinary tract infection (UTI).

Sonography may reveal nephrolithiasis and perinephric extension of the inflammatory process. If the lesion is focal, it will appear isoechoic to parenchyma. A CT scan is a helpful diagnostic tool. Usually on CT scan a stone will be seen along with nephromegaly and a perinephric reaction on the noncontrast phase. This reaction will often involve Gerota's fascia and even the psoas muscle. The CT density numbers are called *Hounsfield units* (HU) and will vary between −15 and +10 HU. They may be lower than normal parenchyma because of the lipid-laden macrophages, or "foam cells," that are contained within the reaction to infection. When an intravenous contrast medium is administered, only the compressed surrounding parenchyma will be enhanced because obstruction of the XGP is usually seen. Although one faces a diagnostic dilemma in distinguishing XGP from renal cell carcinoma, both are treated with nephrectomy; therefore the importance of knowing this ahead of time is less imperative.

Renal Abscess

Renal abscesses usually occur as a complication of acute pyelonephritis. Ascending infection associated with tubular obstruction appears to be the primary pathway for development of gram-negative abscesses. Gram-positive abscesses are associated with hematogenous spread and have rarely been seen in the era of antibiotics. Microabscesses can form from areas of necrosis in small parts of the kidney. These microabscesses may enlarge and coalesce to form a full-blown abscess.

The clinical hallmarks are persistent fever, chills, abdominal or flank pain, malaise, and leukocytosis despite appropriate antibiotic therapy for suspected pyelonephritis. Complicated UTIs associated with stones or obstruction, as well as diabetes, will predispose a patient to formation of abscesses. Bacteruria and

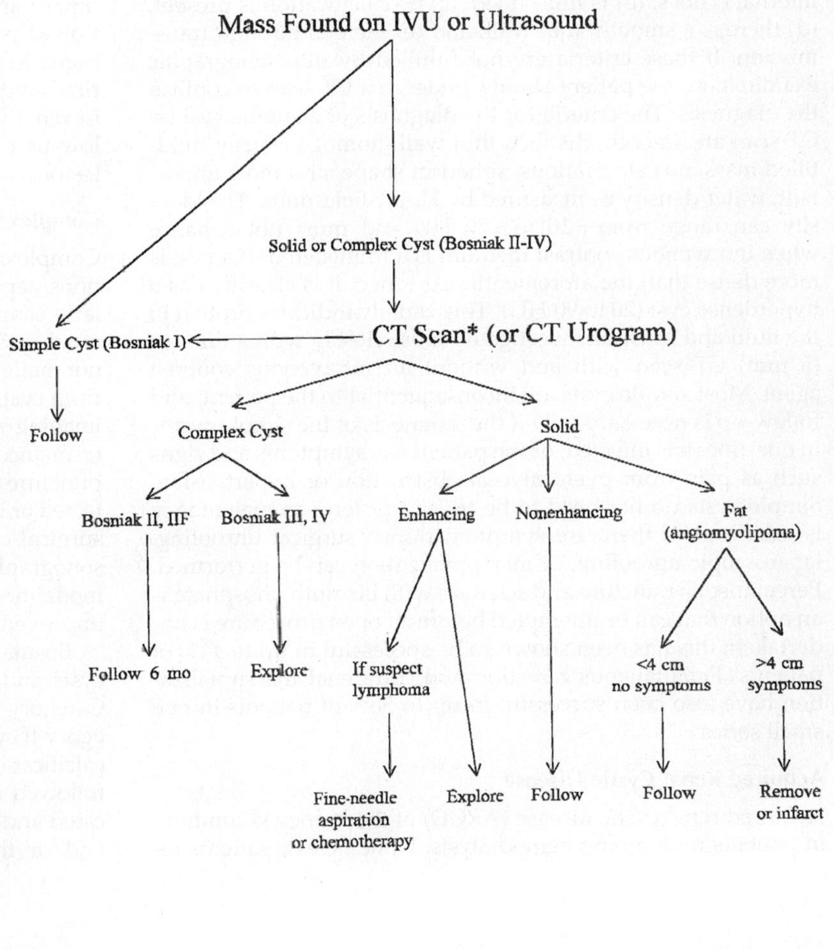

Figure 30.1. A schema for the diagnosis of a renal mass in an adult patient. IVU, intravenous urogram.

pyuria may not be present because the abscess usually does not connect to the collecting system.

Ultrasonography will identify a focal, fluid-filled, space-occupying lesion with through transmission; it may contain low-level echogenic debris. On contrast-enhanced CT scan, there will be a focal, sharply demarcated area that does not enhance with intravenous contrast medium. A thick wall distinguishable from the renal parenchyma will usually surround the area of liquefaction. The center may be hyperdense secondary to the protein content of the fluid. If the abscess is identified early, treatment is with empiric antimicrobial agents and careful observation. Percutaneous drainage may obviate open surgical management if the abscess is not loculated. If the lesion does not resolve, it can be drained in an open surgical procedure. Any obstruction must be relieved with a stent or percutaneous nephrostomy tube.

Simple Cysts

Renal cystic disease is quite common. The incidence of simple renal cysts increases with age: from birth to age 18, incidence is 0.22%; at age 40, incidence is 20%; at age 60, 33%. These cysts can also be part of an inherited disorder. Simple cysts do not connect to any part of the nephron. Typically, they are fluid filled, lined with cuboidal epithelium, and usually are thin walled and smooth. Most cysts are discovered incidentally with intravenous pyelogram, ultrasonography, or CT scan performed for reasons other than renal disease. Very rarely, cysts can produce pain or cause hematuria if they rupture into the collecting system. Cysts may grow over time and can obstruct the collecting system, causing pain and, rarely, hypertension. It is thought that the mass effect of the cysts on the parenchyma or renal vessels may cause local ischemia and subsequent renin-dependent hypertension.

Ultrasonography can reliably aid in making a diagnosis of a simple cyst if the mass fulfills the following criteria: (a) has no internal echoes, (b) is fluid filled, (c) no calcification is present, (d) there is a smooth, thin wall, and (e) there is through transmission. If these criteria are not fulfilled by ultrasonographic examination, the patient should undergo a CT scan to confirm the diagnosis. The criteria for the diagnosis of a simple cyst by CT scan are smooth, distinct, thin wall, homogeneously fluid-filled mass, no calcifications, spherical shape, and most important, water density as measured by Hounsfield units. This density can range from −10 to +20 HU and must not enhance when intravenous contrast medium is administered. If a cyst is more dense than the aforementioned range, it is classified as a hyperdense cyst (20 to 90 HU). This usually indicates protein in the fluid and must be investigated more closely with a fine-cut (5 mm) CT scan with and without an intravenous contrast agent. Most simple cysts are inconsequential to the patient, and follow-up is necessary only if the diagnosis of the simple cyst is in question, it is infected, or the patient has symptoms and signs such as pain from pyelocalyceal obstruction or hypertension. Simple cysts do not need to be treated as long as malignancy is ruled out. If there are symptoms, open surgical unroofing, laparoscopic unroofing, or marsupialization can be performed. Percutaneous puncture and sclerosis with bismuth phosphate is an option that can be attempted before an open procedure is undertaken; this has been shown to be successful in up to 44% of patients. Percutaneous resection and intrarenal marsupialization have also been successful in up to 50% of patients in one small series.

Acquired Renal Cystic Disease

Acquired renal cystic disease (ARCD) of the kidney is common in patients undergoing hemodialysis. Nonetheless, patients receiving peritoneal dialysis and those with chronic renal failure may develop renal cysts. The mechanisms responsible for these cyst formations are not well understood. The incidence of ARCD rises with time in patients who have end-stage renal disease (ESRD). The incidence at 3 years is as high as 44%, and at 10 years it rises to 90%. There is also a higher incidence of ARCD with increased age, male gender, and patients with end-stage kidney disease. The significance of ARCD is twofold: first, the cysts can bleed and produce pain and hematuria; second, there is increased incidence of benign and malignant renal lesions in these renal cysts in patients with renal failure. (For further discussion on ARCD in patients with renal failure, see Chapter 46, Part 3.)

Most patients with ARCD who have symptoms present with loin pain or hematuria. Infection of these lesions in ESRD patients with an unexplained fever should be entertained. Most cysts do not communicate with the collecting system of the kidney and are located in the cortex. They are generally bilateral and average 0.5 to 1.0 cm. Adenomas and renal cell carcinomas may develop in these cysts. The adenomas are usually multiple, bilateral, and small in diameter. In these patients, tumors smaller than 1 cm are likely to be adenomas, whereas tumors 1 to 3 cm are indeterminate, and tumors larger than 3 cm are more likely to be carcinomas. CT scanning is the modality of choice for detecting these small renal lesions, and if the patient is receiving hemodialysis, an intravenous contrast agent can be given safely.

The cysts of patients with ARCD tend to regress after renal transplantation. The malignant potential in the lining of the cysts still remains the same. It is therefore important that these cysts not be ignored when a patient undergoes renal transplantation and begins to receive immunosuppressive therapy. The native kidneys account for 4.5% of malignancies in renal transplant patients. In general, renal transplant recipients should have their native kidneys screened yearly. On the other hand, it is not cost-effective to screen the entire population of patients with ESRD. The incidence of renal cell carcinoma in patients with end-stage renal disease is three to six times higher than the general population. Treatment of ARCD in renal failure patients or transplant recipient is careful follow-up of cysts or adenomas and removal of suspicious renal lesions.

Complex Cysts

Complex cysts take a variety of forms. If a cyst has calcifications, septations, proteinaceous fluid, or is thick-walled, irregularly shaped, or hyperdense, then it is not considered a simple renal cyst. It is of the utmost importance to define the cyst as nonmalignant. Cystic neoplasms can be difficult to distinguish from cysts with one or more of the above features. With newer imaging modalities such as spiral CT scanning and magnetic resonance imaging (MRI), a clearer diagnosis can be made. Cyst puncture and aspiration are rarely indicated, but if the cyst is infected or if it is of borderline character in a patient who is a poor surgical candidate, aspiration may be considered. With better sonography and CT scanning and careful follow-up using these modalities, the safety margin for following these lesions will be improved.

Bosniak has developed a classification system for complex cysts and has divided these into four categories (Table 30.3). Category I lesions fulfill all of the criteria for simple cysts. Category II cystic lesions that may have fine sepatations, fine, small calcifications and/or, of high density. Most of these cysts can be followed radiographically. Category III cysts are more complicated and include several thick-walled septae, a thick cyst wall, and/or thick, extensive calcification. These lesions must be

TABLE 30.3. Bosniak Classification for Complex Renal Cysts

Category	Features	Treatment
I	Simple cyst, thin smooth wall, no enhancement	None
II	Pencil-thin septation, fine calcific; can be hyperdense, minimal internal echoes	Follow with US or CT
III	Extensive, thin calcification; thin multiple septae, thick wall; no enhancement	Explore
IV	Cystic enhancing mass, thick wall, numerous thick calcifications	Explore/radical nephrectomy

CT, Computed tomography; US, ultrasonography.

treated on an individual basis based on patient health status, but for the most part they must be explored for fear of malignancy, because up to 46% of category III lesions have been found to be malignant. Category IV lesions are cystic malignancies that have a solid component; these must be excised surgically with a partial nephrectomy or radical nephrectomy, depending on size and location. A CT scan of a complex cyst of Bosniak category IV is shown in Fig. 30.2.

The major disagreement among radiologists is in distinguishing category II and III lesions. A fifth classification has emerged to help clinicians manage patients with category II lesions that are questionable with regard to wall thickness, extent of calcifications and number and thickness of septae. This category has been named *IIF*. This indicates patients who should be followed with interval CT scans and explored if growth occurs or there is a change characteristics that would resemble category III lesions.

Autosomal-Dominant Polycystic Kidney Disease

The pathogenesis, genetics, clinical presentation, diagnosis, and treatment of autosomal-dominant polycystic kidney disease (APCKD) are discussed in detail in Chapter 46, Part 1. The most sensitive radiographic modality for detecting APCKD is the CT scan, but ultrasonography can also be useful. In patients at risk for APCKD, early screening with ultrasonography will detect about 7% of patients with the disease. In patients 30 years or older, ultrasound sensitivity approaches 100%. If patients are thought to have bleeding into a cyst or have a cyst associated with infection, a CT scan with and without an intravenous contrast medium will be useful to make the diagnosis. With infected cysts, Indium-111–labeled leukocyte scanning may also be useful for detecting infection associated with cysts, especially in those with compromised renal function.

Angiomyolipoma

Renal angiomyolipoma (AML) is a benign tumor of the kidney. As the name implies, AML is a tumor that contains fat, smooth muscle, and thick-walled vessels. The incidence in the general population is between 0.07% and 0.3%. Patients with AML may present with flank pain, hematuria, or rarely, a flank mass and vascular collapse associated with an acute bleeding episode. Increasingly, these lesions are being diagnosed during routine imaging studies. They occur much more commonly in women. Tuberous sclerosis is a hereditary and familial condition of mental retardation, adenoma sebaceum (tubers), and epilepsy. Approximately 80% of patients with tuberous sclerosis have an AML, whereas 50% of patients with AML have some stigmata of tuberous sclerosis. Patients with tuberous sclerosis may have AMLs of the brain, eye, heart, and lung. Ultrasonography may give a clue to the diagnosis, because it will show hyperechogenicity of the fat. CT scan is the diagnostic method of choice. A radiolucent area within the mass indicates fat and is pathognomonic for AML. Since these tumors have large vessels, they will enhance with intravenous contrast. At times, AMLs with low fat content are difficult to distinguish from renal cell carcinoma. The fat may not be appreciated on CT scan, and there have been several reports of AML associated with renal cell carcinoma. If the margin of tumor and kidney are indistinct or there is calcification within the mass, renal cell carcinoma should be suspected. Treatment of AML depends on size and symptoms. If flank pain or hemorrhage is present, selective embolization of the tumor should be considered. If this is unsuccessful, a partial or total nephrectomy should be performed. Asymptomatic tumors are treated based on size because the size may indicate their potential to bleed.

Asymptomatic patients with tumors less than 4 cm can be observed with yearly or semiannual follow-up; asymptomatic

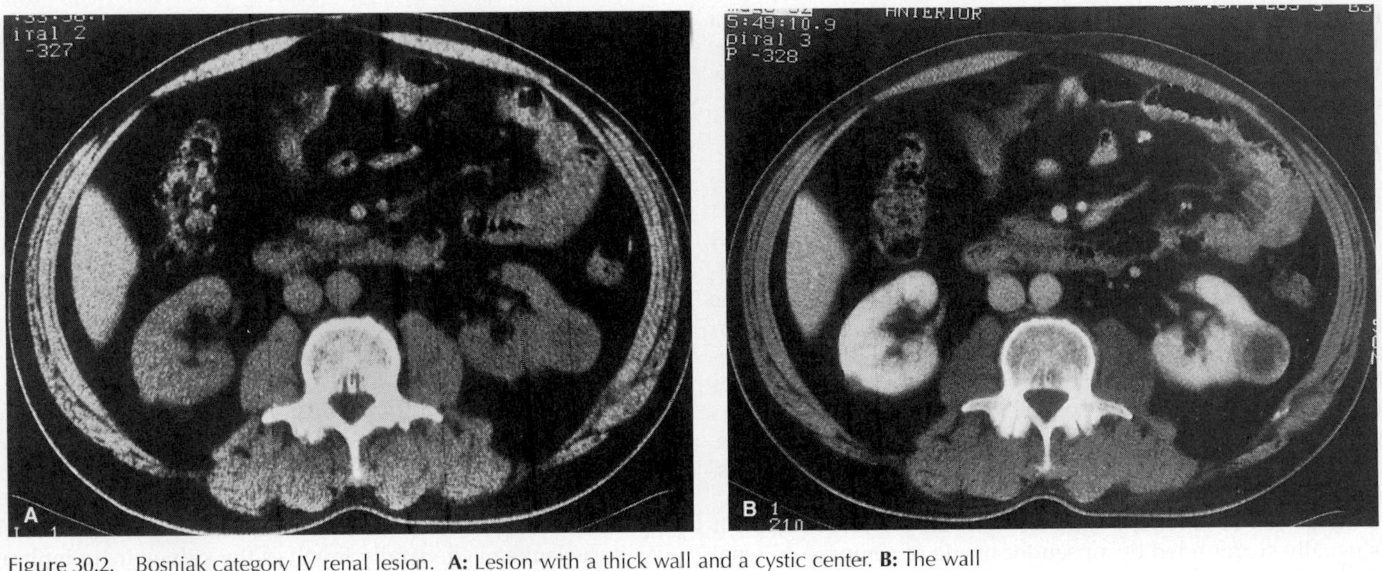

Figure 30.2. Bosniak category IV renal lesion. **A:** Lesion with a thick wall and a cystic center. **B:** The wall enhances with intravenous contrast medium; note cystic nonenhanced center. A radical nephrectomy was performed that on final pathologic analysis was grade 1 renal cell carcinoma.

patients with tumors larger than 4 cm have an increased risk of bleeding. The latter patients should have their tumors selectively embolized or removed with partial or total nephrectomy.

Cortical Adenoma

Controversy exists among pathologists regarding the diagnosis of cortical adenomas. Some believe that renal adenomas are benign tumors, and others believe that these simply represent early stage of renal cell carcinoma. Renal adenomas are less than 3 cm in size and have no clear cells, mitotic activity, nuclear polymorphism, cell stratification, or necrosis. These lesions are well circumscribed but not encapsulated, merging into the adjacent renal parenchyma. Symptoms are rare unless there is growth into the collecting system. Usually renal adenomas are detected on routine imaging studies as an incidental finding. A CT scan will not distinguish this from a small renal cell carcinoma. For this reason, most of these tumors are treated with radical nephrectomy or partial excision, depending on the size and location within in the kidney, because our preoperative diagnostic abilities are presently inadequate to rule out cancer.

Oncocytoma

Renal oncocytoma has an incidence of 3% to 7% of solid renal cortical tumors. They are more common in men than in women. Most commonly, they are unilateral, but 6% of patients may have bilateral tumors. Oncocytomas are usually asymptomatic and are diagnosed incidentally during abdominal imaging for various unrelated conditions. There is no specific finding on CT scan or sonogram, but occasionally a CT scan shows a central scar. On angiography, the typical pattern of appearance is that of a spoke-wheel or stellate pattern on the arterial phase, with associated venous pooling and arteriovenous malformations. Oncocytomas are usually indistinguishable from a hypovascular renal cell carcinoma because many oncocytomas will contain vessels that enhance with an intravenous contrast medium on CT scans. Histologically, the tumors have typical oncocytic features, including large eosinophilic cells with uniform nuclei, granular cytoplasm, and a characteristic polygonal form. On high-power examination, a typical granular cystoplasm is seen, indicating the presence of numerous mitochondria. Histologically, it can be difficult to distinguish renal cell carcinoma with oncocytic features from an oncocytoma. Because of the difficulty in identifying these tumors preoperatively, most lesions need to be explored surgically and excised with a partial nephrectomy or radical nephrectomy. Even if a patient has a synchronous or metachronous lesion, current radiographic techniques are unreliable, and these lesions should be treated as a renal cell carcinoma and be removed.

Malignant Lesions

Renal Cell Carcinoma

Patients with renal cell carcinoma (RCC) are being diagnosed with smaller, lower grades of the tumor because more incidental tumors are being discovered during routine imaging studies for various abdominal symptoms. RCC affects men more often than women, in a ratio of 2:1. There are no racial differences between African-Americans and whites. There are certain groups with an increased risk of renal cell carcinoma, such as patients with a familial form of RCC and von Hippel-Lindau disease. These are also characterized with bilateral and multiple tumors. The incidence of bilaterality is 2% in sporadic RCC.

Renal cell carcinoma originates from the proximal tubule. It is usually surrounded by a pseudocapsule of compressed renal tissue. Grossly, the tumors are yellow or brown with a soft consistency. Usually, hemorrhage and necrosis occur, especially in larger tumors. Eighty percent of RCCs are of the clear cell variety, with large clear cells containing glycogen, cholesterol, and phospholipids. Other types of RCC include the chromophobe type, which carries an excellent prognosis, and the sarcomatoid variant, which is aggressive and carries a poor prognosis.

Presentation of RCC is highly variable. Only 10% of patients will present with the classic triad of flank pain, hematuria, and a palpable mass. Other findings include weight loss, fever, night sweats, and sudden development of varicocele in a male patient (from venous obstruction). Paraneoplastic syndromes include hypercalcemia, erythrocytosis, and abnormal liver function tests. Hypercalcemia has been reported in up to 10% of patients. It is thought to be caused by a parathyroid hormone–like protein. Removal of the primary tumor will usually allow the calcium to return to normal, unless bony metastases are present. Nonmetastatic hepatic dysfunction associated with RCC is known as *Stauffer's syndrome.* Patients manifest elevated liver function test results, white blood cell loss, fever, and areas of hepatic necrosis without evidence of hepatic metastases. In most patients with this syndrome, hepatic function returns to normal once the primary tumor is removed. Erythrocytosis is thought to be caused by erythropoietin release by the kidney under hypoxic insult from the tumor or be released by the tumor itself. Hypertension can be caused by various factors, including elevated renin, arteriovenous fistula formation, hypercalcemia, ureteral obstruction, cerebral metastases, or polycythemia.

With the increased use of ultrasonography and CT and MRI scanning, more renal tumors are diagnosed at earlier stages. Classically, urography played a role in the diagnosis of a suspicious mass on the nephrotomograms. Ultrasound has the advantage of being less invasive and can distinguish between solid and cystic lesion of the kidney. Any lesion that is not clearly identified as a simple renal cyst must be investigated further using CT scanning, which is the modality of choice for detecting and staging RCC. Therefore, in any patient suspected of having a solid renal mass, CT scanning should be performed because it is the most cost-effective and reliable test for the diagnosis. Currently, with spiral CT scanning, the scans can be performed with a single 20-second breath-hold. The CT scan usually displays a spherical, solid, heterogeneous mass that may or may not have necrosis and hemorrhage. With intravenous contrast, there will be enhancement secondary to neovascularity of the tumor. Hounsfield units can range from −1,000 (air) to zero (water) to +1,000 (cortical bone). Soft tissue such as renal parenchyma or tumor will be greater than 35 HU. If after intravenous contrast there is an increase of 15 to 20 HU, which is considered enhancement, the diagnosis is RCC until proven otherwise. The CT scan will also give an indication of stage, especially when referring to lymphadenopathy, abdominal metastases, and an associated tumor thrombus in the renal vein or inferior vena cava. If there is vena caval involvement, an MRI may be useful to define the proximal extent of the thrombus, especially on the coronal images. Otherwise, the role of MRI in routine imaging and staging of RCC is still under investigation and currently not cost-effective. The use of routine fine needle aspiration cytology of suspicious lesions in the kidney is controversial because there is a false-negative rate between 8% and 25% and a false positive rate of 5%. Moreover, the puncture site can lead to metastatic spread in the puncture tract, tumor pseudocapsule disruption or hemorrhage.

Renal Lymphoma

Whereas leukemia generally involves the kidney in an infiltrative pattern, lymphoma involves the kidney in an infiltrative pattern early in its course but then expands and grows into a lymphomatous mass. Of patients with lymphoma, 34% have renal involvement. CT scan is the diagnostic method of choice and shows four different patterns of renal involvement. There can be multiple intraparenchymal nodules, direct contiguous lymph node masses, solitary renal nodule, and diffuse infiltration. These lesions, when nodular, can mimic the appearance of renal cell carcinoma since there is enhancement of the lesion. Nonetheless, the usual pattern of enhancement is peripheral with a less enhancing center. Also, multiple and bilateral masses with associated retroperitoneal adenopathy will almost always be seen. If the situation dictates and question exists, an aspiration biopsy may aid in the diagnosis between RCC and lymphoma and can be accurate in up to 80% of cases. We believe that when lymphoma is suspected and diagnosis is difficult, this is one of the few indications for fine-needle aspiration.

Renal Metastases

Because of its high blood supply, the kidney is a common site of metastases and are seen in 12% of patients with solid cancers. Metastatic lesions are usually small, multifocal, and bilateral. They are seldom associated with any symptoms but hematuria and flank pain can exist. They are usually noted on routine staging examinations for the primary tumors. Tumors that most commonly metastasize to the kidneys are lung, breast, ovarian, bowel, or any other solid malignancy. CT scan is the method of choice for diagnosis. Usually, the mass (masses) will be isodense on the noncontrast phase of the CT scan and will enhance slightly on the postcontrast scan. These lesions are usually inconsequential and are rarely removed because of the nature and course of metastatic disease.

Selected Readings

Bosniak MA. Diagnosis and management of patients with complicated cystic lesions of the kidney. *Am J Radiol* 1997;169:819–821.

Describes the Bosniak classification of renal cysts. Clarifies and discusses controversies in management of each category.

Bosniak MA, Birnbaum BA, Krinsky GA, et al. Small renal parenchymal neoplasms: further observations on growth. *Radiology* 1995;197:589–597.

Describes the results of patients followed with small incidentally discovered lesions. Discusses pitfalls of current techniques in the diagnosis of small renal lesions.

Goethys H, Van Poppel H, Oyen R, et al. The case against fine-needle aspiration cytology for small solid kidney tumors. *Eur Urol* 1996;29:284–287.

Outlines reasons not to use fine-needle aspiration cytology in the routine evaluation and management of a renal mass.

Kaplan DM, Rosenfield A, Smith RC. Advances in the imaging of renal infection. *Infect Dis North Am* 1997;11(3):681–705.

Shows how helical CT has revolutionized the imaging of renal infections. Many radiographs to familiarize the reader with the appearance of renal infections on CT. Other imaging modalities are also described.

Sampaio CA, McLain D, Klein E, et al. Renal masses simulating primary renal cell carcinoma in patients with advanced malignancies. *J Urol* 1994;151:1505–1508, 1994.

Review of masses that simulate renal cell carcinoma. Outcome of evaluation and treatment of seven of such patients.

Weiner JS, Coppes MJ, Ritchey ML. Current concepts in the biology and management of Wilms' tumor. *J Urol* 1998;159:1316–1325.

The most current review on Wilms' tumor genetics, biology, and management.

Wolf JS. Evaluation and management of solid and cystic renal masses. 1998; *J Urol* 159:1120–1133.

Current literature review of management of cystic masses and solid renal lesions. Results of nephron-sparing surgery are compared.

CHAPTER 31

Edema

Hervé Favre, Eric Féraille, and Pierre-Yves Martin

Edema is a clinical term that defines an increase of the interstitial component of the extracellular fluid (ECF) volume. In this context, the intravascular volume (or blood volume) could be either increased, normal, or decreased. The distribution of body fluid between the intravascular and interstitial compartments of the ECF is regulated by the equilibrium linking the net transcapillary flux driving the fluid from the intravascular compartment to the interstitial compartment and the lymph flux returning the fluid from the interstitial compartment to the intravascular compartment. The net transcapillary flux is described by the Starling equation (Net transcapillary flux = Kf $[(\pi i - \pi c) + (Pc - Pi)]$), taking into account the coefficient of ultrafiltration (Kf), the capillary oncotic pressure (πc), the interstitial oncotic pressure (πi), the capillary hydrostatic pressure (Pc), and the interstitial hydrostatic pressure (Pi). At equilibrium, both fluxes are equal. (The regulation of transcapillary fluid exchange in normal and pathological states is discussed in detail in Chapter 14, Part 2.)

Disequilibrium between these two fluxes resulting from a local pathologic condition leads to localized edema. Examples include ankle edema from vein insufficiency, edema from obstruction of lymphatic vessels of tumoral origin, or edema associated with inflammatory processes. Localized edema expresses a pathologic event that, in a well-limited part of the body, promotes a redistribution of the ECF at the expense of the interstitial compartment without interfering with the total body sodium balance. Conversely, generalized edema is the manifestation of an increase in ECF volume, which is determined by its total sodium content. Thus a positive sodium balance resulting from increased renal sodium retention is a common characteristic of generalized edema. For a 70-kg patient, edema becomes apparent after 4 to 6 L of isotonic solution accumulate in the ECF volume. Under these circumstances, edema is observed in the parts of the body subjected to the highest hydrostatic pressure, resulting in a net transcapillary flux greater than the lymphatic flux and creating the driving forces required to expand the interstitial compartment of the ECF.

Thus the localization of edema depends on the patient's position. In a standing person, edema will appear at the ankle and legs, whereas in a supine person, edema will be localized to the sacral area. In addition to the typical interstitial space expansion, edema can also be found in the peritoneal cavity (as ascites) or pleural cavity (as pleural effusion) in relation to specific changes in the microcirculation. The generalized edema associated with nephrotic syndrome, hepatic cirrhosis, and congestive heart failure is called *pitting edema.* This term refers to the fact that an indentation will remain after pressure has been applied and then released on a given area.

REGULATION OF SODIUM BALANCE

Schematically, the mechanisms controlling body fluid's homeostasis include three component systems: sensor, integrator, and effector. The integrator system receives signals from the receptors, which are sensitive to variations of specific parameters, such as blood pressure (BP), atrial and vascular intramural tension, osmolality, and sodium concentration. This information is translated into hormonal messages that induce the changes in the effector system that are necessary to maintain homeostasis. Applied to the regulation of ECF volume, changes in the function of the effector system promoted by activation or inhibition of the sensor systems have to be appropriate to correct any alteration made to this body fluid compartment. Because sodium is the most important cation in the ECF, sodium balance is the key determinant of the regulation of the ECF volume. Under physiologic conditions, any sodium added (with its associated anion) to the ECF, either intravenously or orally, will cause an increase in ECF volume, leading to a modification of the sensor activities and a subsequent adaptation of the effector systems. For instance, sodium reabsorbed from the gastrointestinal tract enters the ECF volume, creating a transient hyperosmotic state. To return the ECF osmolality to normal, the organism can do two things: transfer water from the intracellular to the extracellular space or increase arginine vasopressin (AVP) release in response to the activation of the osmoreceptors to enhance renal water reabsorption. The result is an increase in ECF volume, which is sensed by the baroreceptors. Subsequent adjustment in renal sodium and water handling will depend on the integration of these signals in the body's homeostasis. The multiple control systems and their components, from the sensors to the effectors, are shown in Table 31.1 and Fig. 31.1.

Sensors detect ECF volume either by responding to the actual blood volume or by reacting to the *effective blood volume.* Effective blood volume consists of the blood volume itself, the cardiac output, and the peripheral systemic resistance. Sensors located in the vascular system determine the ECF volume by taking into account each of these three components.

The kidney has four regulating pathways for controlling sodium excretion. First is the glomerular filtration rate (GFR):

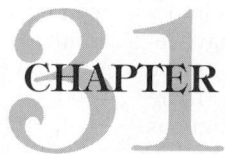

TABLE 31.1. Components of the Control Systems Responsible for the Maintenance of Sodium and Water Homeostasis

Sensor	Afferent Pathway	Integrator	Efferent Pathway
Low-pressure baroreceptors (volume receptors)			
Atria/pulmonary vessels	Glossopharyngeal/ vagus nerves	Solitary tract nucleus of the medulla oblongata	AVP SNS (Brain: ANP, OLS)
Atria	Direct pathway: heart to heart		ANP
High-pressure baroreceptors (pressure receptors)			
Carotid sinus/aortic arch	Glossopharyngeal/ vagus nerves	Solitary tract nucleus of the medulla oblongata	AVP SNS (Brain: ANP, OLS)
Juxta-glomerular apparatus	Direct pathway: kidney to kidney		Renin-angiotensin II (Brain: angiotensin II →, AVP↑, OLS↑)
*Hepatic**			
Pressure receptors: hepatic vasculature	Hepatic nerves	Solitary tract nucleus of the medulla oblongata	SNS
[Na] receptors: portal vein	Hepatic nerves	Solitary tract nucleus of the medulla oblongata	SNS
*Central nervous system**			
[Na] receptors: hypothalamus?	Direct pathway: brain to brain		SNS OLS?

*The roles of hepatic and central nervous system receptors have not been completely determined.
ANP, atrial natriuretic peptide; AVP, arginine vasopressin; OLS, ouabainlike substance; SNS, sympathetic nervous system.

an increase in GFR increases the filtered sodium load, an appropriate response to an increased ECF volume. Conversely, a diminished GFR helps maintain the sodium balance when ECF volume is reduced. This mechanism plays only a minor role in the kidney's regulation of sodium balance. It has been demonstrated that the natriuretic response to a perfusion of isotonic saline solution occurs even in the presence of a reduced GFR, produced by clamping the renal artery. Evidence from micropuncture studies performed in physiologic and pathophysiologic conditions indicates that changes in the sodium filtered load can be completely blunted by the subsequent tubular sodium reabsorption occurring at different segments of the nephron.

Second are the antinatriuretic hormones. The renin-angiotensin-aldosterone system is the most important and the best studied. It is a good example wherein the kidney is the sensor and the integrator, thus producing the effector. When the ECF volume diminishes, plasma concentrations of renin, angiotensin, and aldosterone increase; the reverse occurs when ECF volume increases. The sympathetic nervous system and the nonosmotic release of arginine vasopressin are the other neurohormonal systems.

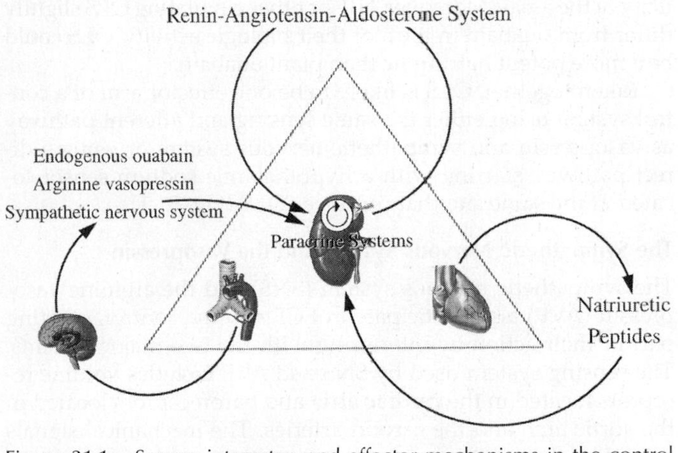

Figure 31.1. Sensor, integrator, and effector mechanisms in the control of extracellular fluid homeostasis.

The third pathway involves the natriuretic hormones—a family of natriuretic peptides that are now well defined both in chemical and in physiologic activity terms, and the endogenous ouabainlike substances that inhibit the Na^+-K^+-ATPase activity.

The fourth pathway, the paracrine systems, includes the prostaglandins, nitric oxide (NO), and the endothelins, to mention the most important systems. (The renal handling of sodium is discussed in detail in Chapter 15, Part 2.)

Control Systems with Sensor and Effector Localized in the Same Site

The Renin-Angiotensin-Aldosterone System

The sensing system, which stimulates the release of renin, is located in the afferent arteriole at the juxtaglomerular apparatus. This baroreceptor is sensitive to arterial pressure and pulse pressure. Its activation directly stimulates the release of renin by the juxtaglomerular apparatus, a structure that includes sensor and effector. At the renal level, angiotensin II is a factor in the control of the glomerular hemodynamic when the systemic perfusion pressure decreases. Angiotensin II has two types of G-protein–coupled receptors: type 1 (AT_1) and type 2 (AT_2). Binding of angiotensin II to these receptors triggers a complex cascade of signal transduction events, resulting principally in a decrease in cyclic adenosine monophosphate (cAMP) generation through inhibition of adenyl cyclases, an increase in intracellular Ca^{2+} through generation of inositol triphosphate (IP_3), and activation of protein kinase C and tyrosine kinases. The vascular effects of angiotensin II are transmitted through AT_1 receptors located in afferent and efferent arterioles as well as in the glomerular mesangium. The vasoconstrictor effect of angiotensin II is stronger in the efferent arteriole than in the afferent vessel; this promotes an increase in filtration pressure, permitting maintenance of the GFR when renal perfusion pressure drops below 70 mm Hg. In addition, angiotensin II stimulates sodium reabsorption by the proximal convoluted tubule, where

AT_1 receptors have also been found to enhance Na^+-H^+ exchange at the luminal domain of the cellular plasma membrane. Aldosterone adjusts the rate of sodium reabsorption across the collecting duct, the key segment of the nephron for the final regulation of the sodium balance. In this segment, aldosterone stimulates both the apical and basolateral steps of sodium reabsorption through an amiloride-sensitive epithelial sodium channel and the Na^+-K^+-ATPase, respectively. Finally, the renin-angiotensin-aldosterone system (RAAS) is modulated by several hormones and neurotransmitters that have a role in ECF volume regulation, moderating or enhancing the renal-mediated response. (The physiology of the renin-angiotensin system and its effects on the kidney are discussed in Chapter 13, Part 3.)

The Natriuretic Peptides

During the mid-1970s, it was demonstrated that extracts from cardiac atria injected in rats evoked a 40-fold increase in natriuresis. These results stimulated a search for an atrial natriuretic factor, which was first isolated and synthesized in 1983. The first substance recognized was a polypeptide hormone of 28 amino acids called *atrial natriuretic peptide* (ANP). ANP is the first member of a family of natriuretic peptides that share a conserved central core but exhibit variable N and C terminal sequences. Subsequently described peptides are brain natriuretic peptide synthesized in atria and ventricle; C natriuretic peptide synthesized in brain and endothelial cells, where it exerts a paracrine activity; and urodilatin, found only in the distal tubule cells and urine. The biologic roles of these peptides are very similar, but the best-investigated peptide is ANP, which is the only member of this family to circulate in the blood at levels compatible with physiologic activity. The activation of the low-pressure baroreceptors located in the atria induced by atrial stretch or pressure is the stimulus for the release of ANP. There are two classes of natriuretic peptide receptors (NPR): those transmitting the function (NPR-A and NPR-B) and those responsible for clearance of the hormone (NPR-C). Functional receptors are particulate guanylyl cyclases, which are composed of an extracellular binding site, a single membrane-spanning domain, and an intracytoplasmic catalytic domain containing the guanylyl cyclase domain. ANP binding activates the guanylyl cyclase moiety, leading to the conversion of guanosine triphosphate to cyclic guanosine monophosphate (cGMP), which is the sole messenger of all the actions of ANP. When converted, the intracellular amount of cGMP is then regulated by the activity of cGMP phosphodiesterases, which control cGMP degradation. Clearance receptors are responsible for the very short half-life (1 to 3 minutes) of ANP. They work as an endocytosis-mediated receptor, bringing ANP from the cell surface to the lysosomes, where it is hydrolyzed. In addition, natriuretic peptides are cleared by neutral endopeptidases.

ANP exerts three types of action: vasomotor, natriuretic, and inhibition of the RAAS. The hypotension induced by ANP is secondary to multiple effects on cardiovascular hemodynamics. ANP diminishes cardiac output by decreasing the plasma volume and central venous pressure. Decreased plasma volume results, at least in part, from a change in capillary permeability, allowing a shift of fluid from the plasma to the interstitial compartment. In addition, ANP stimulates vagal activity, which contributes to the hypotension. This mechanism permits a normal BP to be maintained and protects the cardiac function in the presence of an increase in ECF volume. When hypertension is caused by an augmented vascular peripheral resistance induced by angiotensin II or catecholamines, ANP acts as a vasodilator to reduce the BP and increase cardiac output by diminishing the afterload. The vasodilatory effect of ANP results principally from its antagonism of angiotensin II and catecholamines.

The natriuretic activity of ANP is related to its effect on renal hemodynamics, tubular sodium transport, and RAAS. There is no important natriuretic response to ANP without an increase in GFR and sodium filtered load, which results from the combined effect of vasodilation of the afferent arteriole and vasoconstriction of the efferent arteriole. This produces an increase in sodium delivery to Henle's loop and the inner medullary collecting duct, which, combined with an increase in medullary interstitial pressure and an inhibition of apical sodium entry, leads to natriuresis. In addition to these mechanisms, the ANP natriuretic effect also depends on its antagonist action to the RAAS. ANP blocks the synthesis and release of renin and of aldosterone. Decreased renin secretion induced by ANP results from increased sodium delivery to the macula densa and is mediated by NO as ANP fails to blunt renin secretion when the increased sodium load arriving at the macula densa is impeded or the NO synthesis blocked by specific inhibitor. Inhibition of aldosterone secretion results both from the reduced renin secretion and from a direct action of ANP on aldosterone synthesis in the adrenal zona glomerulosa. (Natriuretic peptides are discussed in more detail in Chapter 13, Part 8.)

Other Systemic Control Systems

Endogenous Ouabainlike Substances (OLS)

There is now evidence that an isomer of ouabain is present in the bovine hypothalamus as well as in the adrenal gland, and there is evidence that an isomer of ouabain is circulating in the human blood, from which it has been isolated. However, there are some differences in the biologic activity of the hypothalamic inhibitor factor (HIF) and ouabain. Elevated circulating concentration of OLS has been reported by several groups in primary hyperaldosteronism, congestive cardiac failure, chronic renal failure, high dietary sodium intake, pregnancy, preeclampsia, and hypertension. All these reports support the theory that OLS has a role in controlling ECF volume and in the genesis of hypertension. Even if there is no doubt about the existence of circulating OLS in the blood of mammals, including humans, there is still speculation on their natriuretic role along two lines of argument: (a) not all of the studies reach the same conclusion concerning the concentration of OLS in comparable physiologic or pathophysiologic situations, and (b) perfusion of ouabain or use of digoxin does not promote natriuresis. However, OLS is often estimated by using the cross-reactivity of an immunoassay of ouabain, digoxin, or other cardiac glycosides but not validated for OLS itself; therefore the chance of detecting OLS depends largely on the specificity of the assay. Moreover, HIF or other circulating OLS slightly differ from ouabain in term of their biologic activity. OLS could be a more potent natriuretic than plant ouabain.

Taken together, OLS is likely to be one effector arm of a control system using either the same sensing and afferent pathway as vasopressin and sympathetic nervous system or using a direct pathway starting with a hypothalamic sodium sensor located at the same site that produces OLS (Fig. 31.1).

The Sympathetic Nervous System and the Vasopressin

The sympathetic nervous system (SNS) and the arginine vasopressin (AVP) also participate in ECF volume control, exerting part of their action by interfering with the two major systems. The sensing system used by SNS and AVP includes volume receptors located in the cardiac atria and baroreceptors located in the aortic arch and the carotid arteries. The mechanical signals sensed by these receptors are translated in neural messages that reach the hypothalamus through parasympathetic pathways (glossopharyngeal and vagus nerves). The downloading of these receptors, either by a decrease in intrathoracic filling volume or hypotension, will stimulate the nonosmotic release of AVP and the sympathetic nervous system. Conversely, an increase in intrathoracic filling volume or hypertension will inhibit the SNS and the AVP release. These two systems exert a direct effect on the kidney, through which they control ECF volume. Another important part of their effect results from their interaction with the RAAS and the natriuretic peptides.

Sympathetic Nervous System. The kidney is rich in noradrenergic fibers that innervate the afferent and efferent arterioles, the juxtaglomerular apparatus, and the nephron itself. Stimulation of the SNS reduces the renal blood flow (RBF) through α_1-adrenergic receptors, inducing vasoconstriction of both afferent and efferent arterioles. Catecholamines also increase the tubular sodium reabsorption in the proximal tubule through α_1-adrenergic receptors by enhancing the luminal Na^+-H^+ exchange, the basolateral Na^+-K^+-ATPase activities, and the renin release through the α_2-adrenergic receptors. For instance, in animal models of sodium retention, renal denervation increases sodium excretion without altering renal hemodynamics.

Arginine Vasopressin. The major factor known to influence AVP secretion in normal circumstances is plasma osmolality. Neurons called *osmoreceptors* are located in the anterior hypothalamus close to the supraoptic nuclei. These osmoreceptors are very sensitive to changes in effective plasma osmolality, which are sensed through changes in their intracellular water content. At plasma osmolalities below a certain level (average, 280 mOsm/kg), AVP secretion is undetectable. Above this threshold level, plasma AVP concentrations are directly related, in normal circumstances, to plasma osmolality.

In addition to these hypothalamic osmoreceptors, AVP secretion is also controlled by an anatomically separate pathway that is responsive to nonosmotic stimuli. The major nonosmotic pathway for vasopressin involves the autonomic nervous system. The input from these pathways appears to be inhibitory under basal conditions because interrupting them results in a sharp rise in plasma vasopressin and arterial pressure. Changes in systemic hemodynamics may therefore influence AVP secretion. A decrease of 10% or more in arterial pressure or a fall in blood volume of more than 8% can stimulate AVP secretion.

This minimal effect of changes in blood volume and pressure on vasopressin contrasts with the remarkable sensitivity of the osmoreceptors. Osmoregulation is not inhibited by modifications in systemic hemodynamics, but there is a shift in the relationship between plasma osmolality and plasma AVP. For instance, in the presence of hypotension, the plasma AVP level can also be suppressed by a decrease in plasma osmolality, but this effect occurs at a lower plasma osmolality than in normal conditions. This hemodynamically mediated secretion of AVP is the most important cause of AVP hypersecretion in pathophysiologic states such as cirrhosis or cardiac failure.

AVP has a vasoconstrictor effect through V_1 receptors located on the vascular smooth muscle cells and an antidiuretic effect through the V_2 receptors, located on the basolateral membranes of the principal cells of the collecting duct. Stimulation of the V_2 receptors activates aquaporin-2, the water channels located on the apical membrane, thus increasing water permeability. In addition, AVP exerts a variable action on the tubular sodium transport, depending on the sodium balance of the subject and the species. AVP appears to be natriuretic when the sodium balance is positive and antinatriuretic when the sodium balance is negative.

Renal Paracrine Systems

Prostaglandins

Prostaglandins are locally active substances (autocoids) originating from arachidonic acid and synthesized by several structures of the kidney (blood vessels and tubules). Their synthesis depends on two cyclooxygenases isoforms: COX-1 and COX-2, both detected within the kidney and inhibited by nonsteroidal antiinflammatory drugs (NSAIDs). When synthesized, prostaglandins act on specific receptors that either stimulate adenylate cyclase and increase intracellular cAMP or increase intracellular Ca^{2+} and activate protein kinase C (PKC), the messengers responsible for their biologic effects. Prostaglandin synthesis is stimulated by vasoconstrictive substances such as endothelins, angiotensin II, and AVP; prostaglandins are considered protective substances from renal ischemia because they antagonize the effects of all the vasoconstrictive hormones acting on the kidney. Although their role in the control of the basal vascular tone is minor, they maintain GFR by promoting an increase in the filtration pressure by vasodilating the afferent arteriole in activated vasoconstrictor systems. At the tubular level, they antagonize the antidiuretic action of AVP. All these effects can be suppressed by the use of NSAIDs, which inhibit the cyclooxygenases. Prostaglandins counterbalance the renal effect of the systemic regulating factors participating in the ECF volume control without altering their extrarenal function but may be facilitating or limiting factors for their final renal effects. (For a detailed discussion of the physiology of prostaglandins and their effects on the kidney, see Chapter 13, Part 1.)

Nitric Oxide

NO is synthesized from L-arginine by three isoforms of the enzyme nitric oxide synthase (NOS), which are all present within the kidney. The biologic effects of NO are principally mediated by cGMP and protein kinase G. NO plays a major role in the control of systemic BP as well as renal BP regulation. Chronic systemic inhibition of NO synthesis increases BP and leads to an increase in renal vascular resistance (RVR), a fall in renal plasma flow (RPF), and a smaller fall in GFR. Within the kidney, administration of endothelium-dependent vasodilators produces renal vasodilation and natriuresis that are mediated by both NO and prostaglandins. The systemic infusion of low doses of NOS inhibitors does not affect BP but increases RVR and decreases RBF, thus demonstrating an enhanced sensitivity of the renal circulation to NOS inhibitors in physiological condition. The vasoconstrictor effect of NOS inhibition predominates on the afferent glomerular arterioles which decreases the glomerular plasma flow. The role of NO in regulating renin release has yielded conflicting conclusions; some authors have concluded that NO suppresses renin release, whereas others have concluded that NO stimulates renin release. These contrasting results could be caused by the different function of NOS isoforms with respect to the control of renin release.

In addition to being a potent vasodilator in the renal vasculature, NO appears to be essential in coupling an increase in renal perfusion pressure with a decrease in tubular sodium reabsorption by mechanisms that are independent of glomerular events. NO regulates medullary blood flow and inhibition of NO in the interstitial medullary interstitial space, decreased renal medullary blood flow without changing cortical blood flow, and decreased sodium and water excretion without modifying GFR or BP. Finally, NO may have a tubular effect, either directly through an increase in cGMP or indirectly through antagonizing such substances as angiotensin II. (For additional discussion on NO and its interaction with the kidneys, see Chapter 13, Part 6.)

Endothelins

Endothelins (ETs) are members of a family of three highly related peptides (ET1, ET2, and ET3). Both ET1 and ET3 are synthesized by the kidney. Endothelins bind to either ETA or ETB receptors that are expressed in a tissue-specific manner. ETA receptors are found on vascular structures and preferentially bind ET1, whereas ETB receptors are the predominant form expressed by kidney epithelial cells and bind all three ETs equally. ET1, the most potent vasoconstrictor known, exerts its effect through ETA receptors; by contrast, activation of vascular ETB receptors has a vasodilatory effect, most likely through stimulation of NO generation. The effects of ETs on sodium and water excretion are very complex and depend on the actions of ETs on systemic hemodynamics, renal microcirculation, and transport properties of the renal tubule epithelial cells. Schematically, at low dosages, exogenous ET1 is diuretic and natriuretic, whereas at high dosages, ET1 induces renal vasoconstriction and sodium and water retention. (For a more detailed discussion of ETs and their interaction with the kidneys, see Chapter 13, Part 5.)

EDEMA FORMATION

In most circumstances leading to sodium retention, the systemic control systems respond adequately to ECF volume status. The different systems [RAAS, ANP, and endogenous ouabain (OLS), AVP, SNS, and the paracrine systems] interact to adapt the response of the kidneys to the ECF volume situation to provide the most appropriate compensation. Thus these multiple systems are not redundant but are necessary for the fine-tuning of ECF volume regulation (Table 31.2). Under physiologic conditions, the blood concentrations of the neurohormonal substances involved in systemic control of ECF volume are at the level expected for the ECF volume size because it correlates fairly well with the effective blood volume. In edematous states, however, this is not the case and the equilibrium between the different effector systems is altered because the effector systems are not efficient in restoring a normal "effective blood volume," as sensed by the different baroreceptors. The disruption of this equilibrium can be caused either by alteration of the parameters determining the effective blood volume, such as decreased cardiac output or increased vasodilation, or by alterations of the kidney's responses, or both. In addition, the kidneys may respond poorly to an adequate action of the systemic regulators because of renal hypoperfusion, dysfunction of the paracrine systems (i.e., prostaglandins, NO, endothelins), or primary or secondary intrinsic functional alterations of the tubular cells at different levels of the nephron, and more specifically, the collecting duct. Specific alterations of these mechanisms in the major edematous states encountered in clinical practice are now discussed.

TABLE 31.2 Neurohormonal Responses to Decreases or Increases in ECF Volume Role of the Paracrine Systems and Their Interactions

ECF volume	Decreased	Increased
Neurohormonal systems		
RAAS	Activated	Suppressed
Atrial natriuretic peptide (ANP)	Suppressed	Activated
Endogenous ouabain (Ouabainlike substances (OLS))	Suppressed	Activated
Arginine-vasopressin (AVP)	Stimulated	Suppressed
Sympathetic nervous system (SNS)	Stimulated	Suppressed
Renal target	Increased sodium and water reabsorption	Increased sodium and water excretion
Paracrine systems		
Prostaglandins	Vasodilator: antagonize the effects of AVP, endothelins, angiotensin II, and SNS	
Nitric oxide	Vasodilator: antagonizes the effects of AVP, angiotensin II, endothelins, and SNS; stimulates renin release	
Endothelins	Vasoconstrictor: stimulate release of prostaglandins and NO	
Interactions		
ANP	Decreases synthesis renin/aldosterone Antagonizes all the known functions of angiotensin ii Antagonizes the vasoconstrictor effects induced by humoral or autonomic systems (SNS, AVP)	
Angiotensin II	Increases NO and prostaglandins Increases ANP Increases Aldosterone Increases OLS (feed back mechanism)	
OLS	Decreases renin release and SNS Potentiates the vasoconstrictor effects induced by humoral or autonomic systems	
SNS	Increases renin	
AVP	Increases ANP Increases OLS Increases prostaglandins	

ECF, extracellular fluid; NO, nitric oxide; RAAS, renin-angiotensin-aldosterone system.

NEPHROTIC EDEMA

Two biologic alterations, massive proteinuria and hypoalbuminemia, define nephrotic syndrome, while generalized edema is its clinical expression. Nephrotic syndrome usually accompanies glomerulopathies of different histologic categories but may occasionally occurs in tubulointerstitial diseases. In nephrotic edema, fluid accumulates as a result of avid sodium and water reclamation by the kidney into the interstitial component of the extracellular volume. This location implies a rupture of the equilibrium existing between the intravascular and the interstitial components of the extracellular compartment. (For further discussion of the transcapillary fluid exchange in nephrotic syndrome, see Chapter 14, Part 2.)

Although renal sodium and water retention are recognized as the key event in the development of edema in nephrotic syndrome, there is no consensus concerning the pathogenic mechanisms. Two opposite pathogenic concepts have been proposed (Fig. 31.2). First, the classic *underfilling hypothesis* assumes that the initiating event for sodium and water retention is the fall in plasma protein concentration originated from the renal protein leak. This reduction in capillary oncotic pressure produces extravasation of a large amount of fluid from the intravascular to the interstitial compartment, generating edema and secondary intravascular hypovolemia. According to this model, this hypovolemia initiates sodium and water retention by the kidneys through the activation of the homeostatic mechanisms in an attempt to restore the blood volume. In contrast, the *overflow hypothesis* assumes that a primary intrarenal defect drives sodium and water retention. In this model, vascular hypervolemia develops during the initial phase of sodium and water retention; edema formation represents an adaptive process that prevents intravascular fluid volume from overload. The relative roles in nephrotic edema formation of the body fluid homeostasis regulators on the kidney, as contrasted with an primary intrinsic renal defect leading to sodium retention, are discussed next.

Role of Decreased Plasma Oncotic Pressure in Nephrotic Edema

Edema in nephrotic syndrome results from disturbed body fluid homeostasis with increased ECF volume. The net transcapillary flow is initially increased by the diminution in plasma oncotic pressure in nephrotic syndrome; however, the rapid decrease in interstitial protein concentration from the diluting effect of the protein-free plasma ultrafiltrate and removal of proteins from the interstitial compartment by an enhanced lymph flow that returns albumin from the interstitial to the intravascular compartment normalizes the difference between plasmatic and interstitial oncotic pressures.

Several lines of evidence argue against a key role for hypoalbuminemia in the pathogenesis of nephrotic edema: (a) in nephrotic syndrome, the difference between plasmatic and interstitial oncotic pressures is preserved despite severe hypoproteinemia; (b) in analbuminemic humans, sodium balance is normal and edema is usually absent; (c) in analbuminemic rats, blood and interstitial fluid volumes are normal and the difference between plasmatic and interstitial oncotic pressures is preserved; (d) in dogs, hypoproteinemia induced by plasmapheresis has not been shown to result in a significant fall in plasma volume or in sodium retention until plasma protein concentration has been decreased by more than 50%; and (e) in rats with Heymann's nephritis (a model of glomerulonephritis induced by injection of antitubular basement membrane antibody), despite the presence of hypoproteinemia, sodium retention does not occur in the absence of plasma volume expansion that is produced by creating a renal failure by subtotal nephrectomy. Therefore decreased plasma oncotic pressure caused by hypoalbuminemia cannot account for the production of large interstitial fluid accumulation, which requires massive sodium and water retention by the kidney.

Role of Decreased Intravascular Volume in Nephrotic Edema

The role of blood volume in the pathogenesis of the renal sodium and water retention characteristic of nephrotic syndrome has been debated. According to the underfilling hypothesis, the decrease in plasma or blood volume initiates renal sodium and water retention through activation of the homeostasis control system and hormonal mediators (Fig. 31.2).

The concept of hypovolemia is supported by occasional observations of circulatory collapse and acute renal failure, which may occur in the course of nephrotic syndrome. However, measurement of plasma volume and blood volume using the distribution volume of iodine-125 (^{125}I) albumin and chromium-51 (^{51}Cr) red cells, respectively, did not permit generalization of these observations. In most instances, patients with nephrotic syndrome exhibit a blood volume within the normal range; in one-third of these patients, this volume is even increased. Similarly, in rat models of nephrotic syndrome, plasma volume is either normal or increased. Preservation of blood volume in the absence of a rise in albuminemia during diuretic- or steroid-induced natriuresis is additional evidence against a vascular volume decrease in nephrotic syndrome. In nephrotic syndrome, plasma volume remains stable despite large variations in interstitial fluid volume—in contrast with chronic renal failure or acute glomerulonephritis, two conditions in which the plasma volume is proportional to the interstitial volume. These findings demonstrate that the relationship between plasma and interstitial fluid volume is flattened in nephrotic syndrome and that the excess of ECF stored in the interstitial compartment preserves the integrity of the intravascular compartment, even

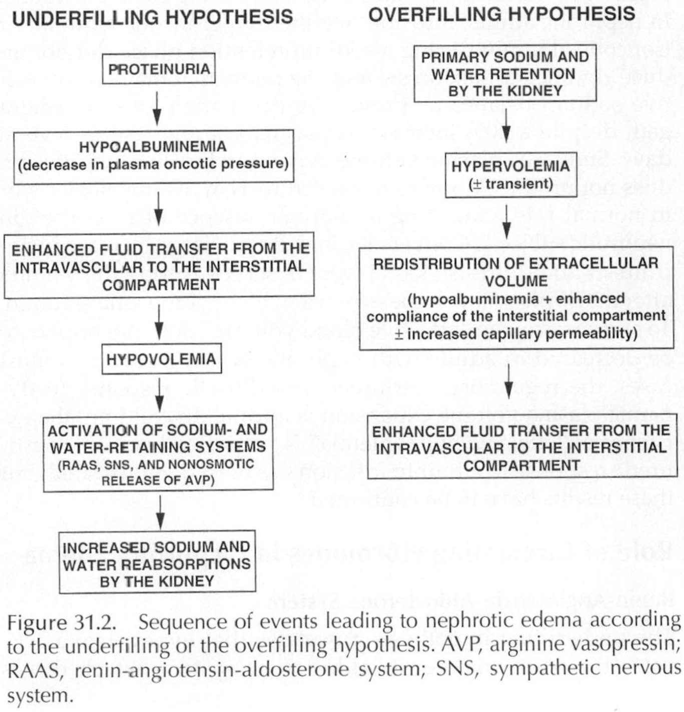

Figure 31.2. Sequence of events leading to nephrotic edema according to the underfilling or the overfilling hypothesis. AVP, arginine vasopressin; RAAS, renin-angiotensin-aldosterone system; SNS, sympathetic nervous system.

during an active phase of ECF depletion. Increased compliance of the interstitium, combined with low plasma oncotic pressure and a possible increase in capillary permeability, may explain this observation (Fig. 31.2). Although hypovolemia has been reported in some cases of nephrotic syndrome, and more often in children than in adults, it is not a common presentation. Globally, the studies of intravascular volume do not support the underfilling hypothesis and propose other mechanisms to explain the renal water and sodium retention consistently found in nephrotic syndrome.

Although decreased total blood volume was not found in most cases of nephrotic syndrome using static measurement techniques, the possibility of a decreased "effective blood volume" exists. The role of this effective blood volume was assessed by studies measuring the functional response to a dynamic increase in blood volume either by head-out water immersion or by albumin infusion. Water immersion increases central vascular volume to a similar extent in normal and in nephrotic individuals. This procedure causes an increase in natriuresis and diuresis by 150% to 170% in nephrotic patients, except for one case-control study demonstrating that the natriuretic and diuretic effects of this procedure were blunted in nephrotic syndrome. However, it should be mentioned that (a) in most studies, nephrotic subjects were either in an equilibrated or in a negative sodium balance, as indicated by the high basal sodium excretion rate (60 to 150 mmol/24 hr) that exceeded the sodium intake by two to three times; (b) no control group was studied under the same conditions except for one study reporting a blunted response in nephrotic subjects; and (c) most patients had received diuretics or steroids, or both, before the study. Thus, in these studies, most patients exhibited a normal regulatory response to an acute increase in central plasma volume, but none of them was in a sodium-retaining phase.

Relevance of basal natriuresis to the natriuretic response to water immersion was demonstrated in one study showing that the diuretic and natriuretic response to water immersion was blunted in nephrotic subjects with a low basal urinary sodium excretion rate (less than 50 mmol/24 hr) but preserved in patients with a high basal urinary sodium excretion rate (more than 50 mmol/24 hr). Studies of plasma and blood volume expansion by albumin infusion have led to more constant results. In nephrotic adults, infusion of either hyperoncotic-albumin or isoncotic-albumin during a sodium retention phase did not induce significant natriuresis and the patients remained in positive sodium balance as proved by calculation and by weight gain despite a 20% increase in plasma volume lasting several days. Similarly, plasma volume expansion by albumin infusion does not produce diuresis nor natriuresis in healthy subjects or in normal rats, indicating a "normal absence of response" in nephrotic subjects. Conversely, in children, large increase in natriuresis and diuresis (400%) were observed during the 6 hours after a 20% plasma volume expansion by hyperoncotic albumin. To summarize, the "effective blood volume" does not appear to be decreased in adults with nephrotic syndrome, and in most cases, the regulatory natriuretic and diuretic response to dynamic plasma volume expansion is normal. In children, the existence of "effective hypovolemia" is suggested because a natriuretic response to albumin infusion has been demonstrated, but these results have to be confirmed.

Role of Circulating Hormones in Nephrotic Edema

Renin-Angiotensin-Aldosterone System

The underfilling hypothesis postulates that hypovolemia activates the renin-angiotensin-aldosterone system, which drives renal sodium retention to restore the "effective plasma flow." However, a large body of evidence strongly argues against a determinant role of the RASS in the pathogenesis of the sodium retention characteristic of the nephrotic syndrome: (a) in nephrotic patients, basal plasma renin activity (PRA) and plasma aldosterone concentrations do not correlate with blood volume, BP, or natriuresis; (b) during intravascular volume expansion, PRA and plasma aldosterone concentrations fall, but these changes do not correlate with the amount of natriuresis; (c) during remission of nephrotic syndrome, PRA and plasma aldosterone concentrations decrease at the beginning of the natriuretic phase, to return to their previous levels by the end of this period, without changes in plasma protein concentration; (d) in human puromycin-aminonucleoside (PAN)–induced nephrotic syndrome, inhibitors of the angiotensin-converting enzyme (ACE) or angiotensin II antagonists have no effect on natriuresis despite a large fall in plasma aldosterone concentration; and (e) in the PAN-induced nephrotic syndrome in rats, the total suppression of aldosterone secretion by surgical adrenalectomy increases sodium excretion in both control and nephrotic rats, but nephrotic rats remain in a positive sodium balance. Therefore activation of the RAAS is not the causal mechanism of sodium retention in nephrotic syndrome.

Atrial Natriuretic Peptide

Because ANP is the major hormone that increases excretion of renal sodium and water, a defect in ANP secretion or efficacy may participate in the pathogenesis of nephrotic edema. In human nephrotic syndrome, basal plasma concentration of ANP is unchanged or decreased. By contrast, in rats with the adriamycin (ADR)-induced nephrotic syndrome, ANP levels are elevated. During intravascular volume expansion, the rise in plasma level of ANP is similar in nephrotic patients and in control subjects, demonstrating that regulation of ANP release by changes in intravascular volume is preserved in nephrotic syndrome. In nephrotic patients, in contrast to control subjects, the increase in diuresis and natriuresis induced by a bolus of ANP is diminished in absolute terms but unchanged in relative terms. In ADR-induced nephrotic syndrome in rats, the diuretic and natriuretic response to ANP infusion is blunted despite an increase in GFR, indicating a dissociation between the hemodynamic and the tubular effects of ANP. Similarly, the natriuretic and diuretic effects of ANP (at a dosage that does not modify the GFR) was decreased in the PAN-induced nephrotic syndrome in rats. This blunted excretory response to ANP is not related to a decrease in number or in affinity of renal ANP receptors. Therefore the tubular insensitivity to ANP should take place after the binding step. ANP receptors are coupled to guanylate-cyclase, and ANP binding raises intracellular cGMP concentrations. The effect of ANP on the generation of cGMP was investigated in ADR-induced nephrotic syndrome. Urinary cGMP excretion, taken as an index of intracellular cGMP generation, was found either normal or decreased in nephrotic rats. In isolated glomeruli or inner medullary collecting ducts from nephrotic rats, intracellular cGMP accumulation in response to ANP was decreased in both structures, whereas in the presence of inhibitors of phosphodiesterases, intracellular cGMP accumulation in glomeruli and inner medullary collecting ducts was similar in nephrotic and in control rats. These results indicate that the reduced intracellular cGMP accumulation found in nephrotic rats is secondary to an enhanced phosphodiesterase activity. However, it should be stressed that the decrease in intracellular cGMP accumulation was similar in both glomerulus and inner medullary collecting duct, although the effect of ANP on GFR is preserved in this model of nephrotic syndrome.

Therefore additional "tubule-specific" mechanisms of "ANP resistance" have to be speculated.

Vasopressin

In nephrotic patients, excretion of an oral water load (20 ml/kg) is delayed and the maximal power of diluting the urine is lowered. Therefore the role of AVP in these alterations in water excretion has been investigated. In nephrotic syndrome, basal plasma concentration of AVP is increased. After an oral water load or an intravenous plasma volume expansion, plasma AVP levels decrease less in nephrotic patients than in control subjects. However, in nephrotic subjects, the plasma concentration of AVP was no longer correlated with the plasma osmolality or the capacity of excreting a water load. In addition, plasma AVP concentration remains elevated after remission of the nephrotic syndrome. Finally, the delayed excretion of water and the decrease in the diluting capacity of the urine are not related to the elevated blood concentration of AVP but are correlated to the GFR, suggesting an intrarenal consequence of the functional adaptation of the residual nephrons rather than a dysregulation of the hormonal control of the tubular water transport. This conclusion is further supported by observations that rats without circulating AVP (Brattleboro rats) and normal rats retain sodium and water to the same extent in PAN-induced nephrotic syndrome.

Functional Alterations of the Kidney in Nephrotic Edema

Because in most humans with nephrotic syndrome hemodynamic or circulating hormone alterations cannot explain the renal sodium and water retention, a primary renal defect has been hypothesized. The most convincing evidence for the existence of such an intrarenal defect comes from unilateral drug-induced nephrotic syndrome studies in which salt retention and proteinuria occur only in the injected kidney.

Renal Hemodynamics

In the absence of change in the total number of functional nephrons, a fall in GFR can result from a decrease in RBF, which may drive a sustained sodium and water retention and a change in glomerular hemodynamics, as expressed by a low filtration fraction (FF). In human nephrotic syndrome, GFR decrease corresponds to a low FF with a normal or increased RBF. In drug-induced experimental nephrotic syndrome, the decrease in single-nephron GFR is also accompanied by a decreased FF. Furthermore, neither the increase in RBF accompanying plasma volume expansion nor the pharmacologic increase of RBF produced by ACE inhibitors (which increases RBF without a parallel increase in GFR) had any effect on sodium and water excretion in nephrotic humans. Therefore alteration in RBF is not involved in the pathogenesis of nephrotic edema.

Renal Nerves

The role of sympathetic nerves has been investigated in both humans and experimental models with nephrotic syndrome. Basal plasma norepinephrine concentration, taken as an index of the overall activity of sympathetic innervation, was either normal or increased in nephrotic subjects. However, plasma norepinephrine concentration reduction induced by plasma volume expansion did not correlate with the changes in diuresis and natriuresis among these subjects. In ADR-induced nephrotic syndrome, restoration of the kidney's ability to excrete a sodium load was taken as an evidence for a contribution of the renal nerves to the sodium retention. However, this observation should be interpreted with caution because (a) the day-to-day sodium balance was not different between sham-operated and denervated nephrotic rats and (b) renal denervation by itself impairs the normal growth of rats, and cumulative sodium balance, when normalized for growth, becomes positive in denervated control subjects and identical between denervated and nondenervated nephrotic rats. Therefore it is unlikely that sodium retention is mediated by increased SNS activity in nephrotic syndrome.

Kidney Tubules

Considering the sodium and water retention characteristic of the nephrotic syndrome as a consequence of a primary tubular dysfunction, several investigators have made efforts to localize the segment(s) of the nephron responsible for the sodium retention using clinical approaches or experimental nephrotic syndrome models.

In humans, results obtained using the so-called technique of distal tubular blockade by ethacrynic acid and thiazide diuretics indicated that the "proximal" tubular fractional reabsorption of sodium was decreased in nephrotic subjects; therefore sodium retention should occur beyond the proximal convoluted tubule. In rats, micropuncture studies performed either in immune or in drug-induced nephrotic syndrome models have demonstrated that (a) absolute proximal sodium reabsorption is decreased and the sodium delivery to Henle's loop is normal, (b) sodium reabsorption by Henle's loop and by the distal tubule is normal, and (c) sodium retention occurs in the collecting duct. In nephrotic syndrome, the proximal tubular function is adapted to the decreased filtered sodium load to provide a physiologic distal sodium delivery; thus enhanced sodium and water reabsorption occurs in the collecting duct, which is the site of the final adaptation of urine composition.

Among the possible mechanisms of sodium retention by the collecting duct, the role of an increased Na^+-K^+-ATPase activity in the collecting duct was investigated in rats with PAN-induced nephrotic syndrome. Na^+-K^+-ATPase is localized at the basolateral border of the tubular epithelium, and it drives tubular sodium reabsorption through the active exchange of intracellular sodium against extracellular potassium. In isolated collecting ducts from PAN-induced nephrotic rats, the activity of Na^+-K^+-ATPase was increased twofold, whereas the activity of the enzyme was normal in the proximal convoluted tubule and in the thick ascending limb of Henle. In this model of nephrotic syndrome, the sodium retention and the increase in Na^+-K^+-ATPase activity exhibit a similar time course and are significantly correlated. In addition, nephrotic mice with spontaneous lupuslike glomerulonephritis also exhibit an increased Na^+-K^+-ATPase activity specifically localized in the collecting duct. Therefore increased Na^+-K^+-ATPase activity, which promotes an enhanced sodium reabsorption though an increase in the driving force for transepithelial sodium transport in the collecting duct, might be the molecular basis of sodium retention during nephrotic syndrome (Fig. 31.3).

In nephrotic syndrome, the isotonicity of ECF is preserved, implying isotonic sodium and water retention by the kidney. It should be noted that regulated water reabsorption also takes place in the collecting duct. Studies performed in PAN- or ADR-induced nephrotic syndrome have shown that expression of aquaporin-2, the apical water channel, as well as aquaporin-3 are decreased in this setting. This finding can explain, at least in part, the decrease in maximal concentrating power of the kidney in nephrotic syndrome. However, in both experimental models of nephrotic syndrome, the aquaporin-2 ratio of the plasma membrane to intracellular vesicles is increased. Therefore the collecting duct in a nephrotic rat most likely exhibits a significant level of basal water permeability, allowing isoos-

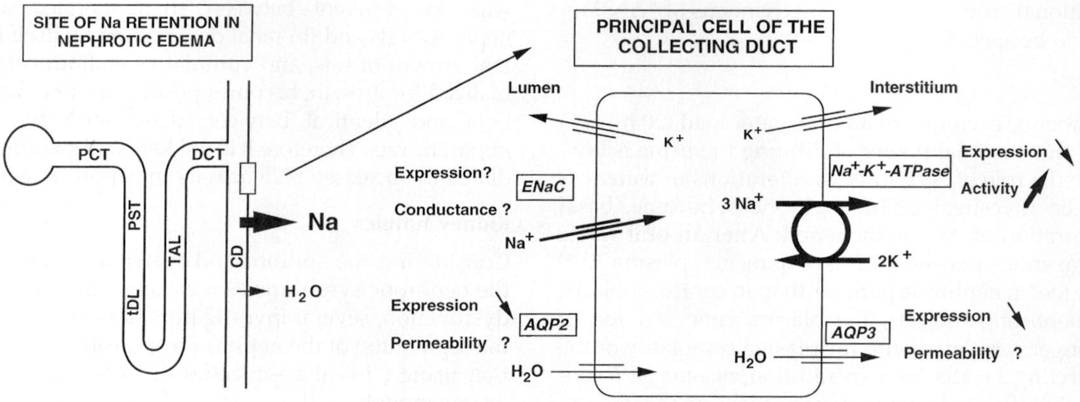

Figure 31.3. Sites of increased sodium and water reabsorption in experimental nephrotic syndrome and summary of the documented alterations in expression and activity of Na^+ and water transporters. AQP2; aquaporin-2; AQP3; aquaporin-3; CD, collecting duct; DCT, distal convoluted tubule; EnaC, epithelial sodium channel; PCT, proximal convoluted tubule; PST, proximal straight tubule; TAL, thick ascending limb of Henle's loop; tDL, thin descending limb of Henle's loop.

motic water reabsorption along with sodium reabsorption in the collecting duct (Fig. 31.3).

Conclusion

Rather than a hemodynamic disease, edema of nephrotic syndrome appears to be more like a glomerulotubular disease. According to this point of view, the following simplified model can be proposed: (a) glomerular defect with loss of anionic charges is responsible for massive proteinuria which results in hypoproteinemia; (b) a tubular defect that originates in the collecting duct drives sodium and water retention through enhanced Na^+-K^+-ATPase activity; and (c) hypoproteinemia in association with enhanced compliance of the interstitium protects from intravascular volume overload, facilitating accumulation of the excess of extracellular fluid in the interstitial space. The precise mechanism of Na^+-K^+-ATPase activation in nephrotic syndrome remains an open question.

NEPHRITIC EDEMA

Nephritic syndrome, typically caused by poststreptococcal glomerulonephritis, is another primary renal disorder associated with edema. In contrast with nephrotic syndrome, hypoproteinemia is absent and hypertension is almost always present. In addition, edema of nephritic syndrome is smaller than edema of nephrotic syndrome and develops more rapidly. In nephritic syndrome, plasma and blood volume are increased and this increase in intravascular volume is responsible for the salt-dependent hypertension of the syndrome. The presence of hypertension in nephritic syndrome may reflect the absence of peripheral adaptation protecting intravascular volume from rising, such as the increased compliance of the interstitium observed in nephrotic syndrome. Similar to the findings in investigations of nephrotic syndrome, human studies and animal-model micropuncture experiments in subjects with immune glomerulonephritis have shown that in acute glomerulonephritis, sodium retention originates from an increase in sodium reabsorption in the collecting ducts. These observations taken with the specific increase in cortical collecting duct Na^+-K^+-ATPase activity found in a mouse model of immune glomerulonephritis, suggest a common mechanism for the sodium retention of glomerular diseases leading to either nephrotic or nephritic syndrome.

CARDIAC EDEMA

Cardiac edema is present in patients with advanced heart failure and results from avid sodium and water retention by the kidneys. In this setting, ECF volume, plasma volume, and blood volume are all expanded. Edema results from an increased transcapillary hydraulic pressure, leading to an enhanced net transcapillary flux that overcomes the capacity of fluid removal from the interstitial compartment by lymph flow. The current pathogenic concept assumes that sodium and water retention is initiated by the decrease in cardiac output. This decrease is sensed as an underfilling of the effective blood volume, subsequently activating homeostatic mechanisms that promote arterial vasoconstriction and sodium and water retention to restore adequate fullness of the arterial compartment. In contrast to the physiologic response, the resulting increased ECF volume is not followed by an efficient counterregulatory diuretic response. Thus the maintenance of expanded ECF compartment implies an imbalance between factors promoting renal sodium and water retention or excretion. In this section, the mechanisms leading to this imbalance in cardiac edema are discussed.

Renal Functional Alterations in Cardiac Edema

In chronic heart failure (CHF), RPF is reduced as a result of decreased cardiac output and systemic vasoconstriction. This decrement is more important in renal cortical blood flow, whereas medullary blood flow appears to be less affected. However, GFR is relatively preserved by an increased filtration fraction until cardiac function is severely altered. In the rat model of ischemic heart failure, it has been shown that the increased filtration fraction is accounted for by a striking rise in the efferent arteriolar resistance, leading to an increased glomerular capillary hydraulic pressure, thus preserving the GFR. A decrease in GFR by itself is not the primary cause of the sodium and water retention since sodium retention is observed in patients and animals with CHF not associated with a decreased GFR.

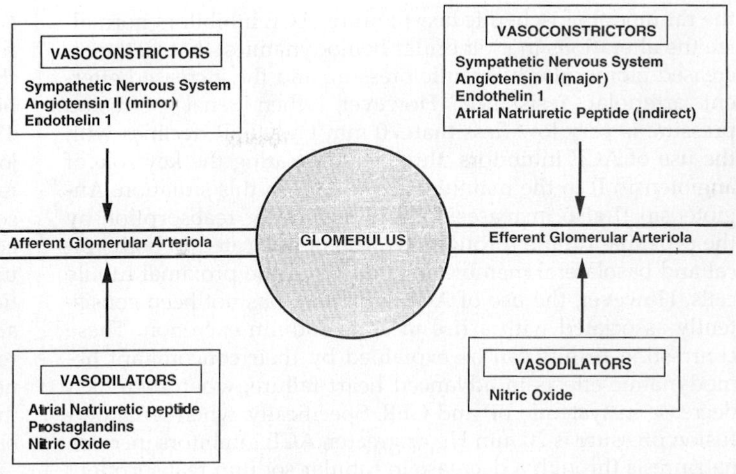

Figure 31.4. Vasoactive factors controlling glomerular hemodynamics.

However, the adaptive mechanisms that modify glomerular hemodynamics (Fig. 31.4) also control tubular sodium and water reabsorption, which play a key role in the development of abnormal renal sodium and water handling. Indeed, the most important cause is increased renal tubular sodium reabsorption. Homeostatic mechanisms activated in CHF, such as RAAS and SNS, are antinatriuretic through their hemodynamic effects and through direct tubular action. These mechanisms have been demonstrated in the rat model of ischemic heart failure (i.e., low cardiac output), in which fluid reabsorption is enhanced in the proximal tubule (Fig. 31.5). The rise in filtration fraction might participate in this process through an increased oncotic pressure in peritubular capillaries, thus enhancing the driving force for passive fluid transfer from the proximal tubule. By contrast, in one human study and in the aortocaval fistula rat model of heart failure (i.e., high cardiac output), proximal tubule reabsorption was normal but was increased in Henle's loop through a yet undefined mechanism (Fig. 31.5). Interestingly, in rats with high-output heart failure, the activity of Na^+-K^+-ATPase, which provides the driving force for vectorial sodium transport in the kidney tubule, is increased in the thick ascending limb of the Henle's loop in compensated heart failure but is increased in both proximal tubule and thick ascending limb in decompensated heart failure.

Role of Increased Activity of Antidiuretic Factors in Cardiac Edema

Renin-Angiotensin-Aldosterone System

The RAAS plays a key role in the hemodynamic and sodium handling alterations of heart failure. Activation of the RAAS has an unfavorable effect on the outcome of heart failure, and ACE inhibitors reduce the symptoms and increase the survival rate of CHF patients. Decreased RBF is a strong stimulus for renin release by the myoepithelial cells of the afferent glomerular arteriole, leading to the generation of angiotensin II. In addition to its systemic vasoconstrictor effect, angiotensin II preferentially constricts the efferent glomerular arteriole and therefore participates in the preservation of the GFR. In patients with mild to moderate heart failure, ACE inhibitors increase RPF and decrease filtration fraction without altering GFR. Similarly, in

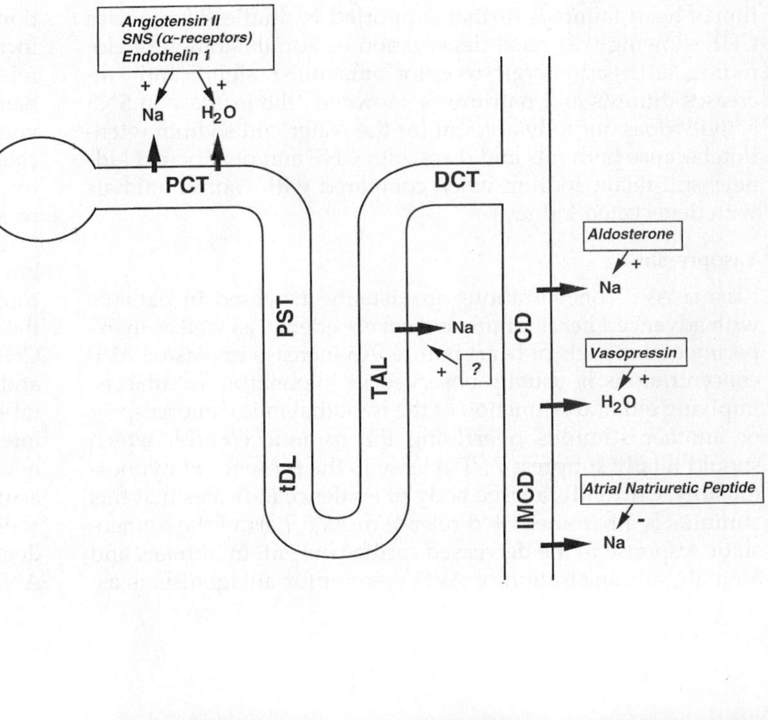

Figure 31.5. Sites of increased sodium and water reabsorption in chronic heart failure. CD, collecting duct; DCT, distal convoluted tubule; IMCD, inner medullary collecting duct; PCT, proximal convoluted tubule; PST, proximal straight tubule; TAL, thick ascending limb of Henle's loop; TDL, thin descending limb of Henle's loop.

the rat model of ischemic heart failure, ACE inhibitors normalize the alterations in glomerular hemodynamics, that is, the increased glomerular hydraulic pressure and the increased efferent arteriolar resistance. However, when renal perfusion pressure is very low (less than 70 mm Hg), GFR declines with the use of ACE inhibitors, thus demonstrating the key role of angiotensin II in the maintenance of GFR in this situation. Angiotensin II also increases sodium and water reabsorption by the proximal tubule through AT_1 receptors located in both apical and basolateral membrane domains of the proximal tubule cells. However, the use of ACE inhibitors has not been consistently associated with a rise in renal sodium excretion. These contrasting results can be explained by their concomitant hemodynamic effects in advanced heart failure, when there is a decrease in systemic BP and GFR. Specifically, when renal perfusion pressure is 70 mm Hg or greater, ACE inhibitors increase natriuresis through a decrease in tubular sodium reabsorption, as indicated by a rise in the fractional sodium excretion. In addition, in a rat model of high-output heart failure induced by an aortocaval fistula, losartan, an inhibitor of AT_1 receptors, increases natriuresis. Finally, angiotensin II also stimulates synthesis of aldosterone, the major hormone that stimulates sodium reabsorption in the collecting duct. ACE inhibitors as well as AT_1 antagonists decrease plasma aldosterone concentration in heart failure. Aldosterone also participates in the sodium retention of heart failure, as indicated by the natriuretic response to the administration of a large dose of spironolactone, an antagonist of aldosterone, in patients with heart failure.

Sympathetic Nervous System

The SNS is strongly activated in heart failure, as indicated by increased plasma norepinephrine concentration. The extent of SNS activation correlates with the severity of cardiac failure. SNS may contribute to the renal sodium and water retention of heart failure indirectly through stimulation of renin secretion and directly through stimulation of tubular fluid reabsorption, or both. Studies in animal models of cardiac failure have shown that renal sympathetic nerve activity is increased and is associated with impaired arterial and cardiac baroreceptor reflexes. This increase in SNS activity is, at least in part, responsible for the decreased RPF observed in CHF. In the rat model of ischemic heart failure, renal denervation decreases both afferent and efferent arteriolar resistance partially through decreased angiotensin II generation. The role of SNS in the sodium retention of heart failure is further supported by studies in rats with CHF showing that renal denervation or administration of clonidine, an α_2-adrenergic receptor antagonist, significantly increases diuresis and natriuresis. However, the increase in SNS activity does not fully account for the water and sodium retention because both rats and dogs with CHF and denervated kidneys still retain sodium when compared with control animals with denervated kidneys.

Vasopressin

Plasma AVP concentrations are usually increased in patients with advanced heart failure and severe edema, as well as in experimental models of heart failure. An increase in plasma AVP concentrations is usually observed in hyponatremic subjects, implying either dysfunction of the hypothalamic osmoreceptor or another stimulus overriding the osmotic control, which should totally suppress AVP release in the presence of hypoosmolality. Currently, a large body of evidence indicates that this stimulus is a baromediated release of AVP, part of the homeostatic response to the decreased cardiac output. In humans and animals, administration of AVP-V_1–receptor antagonists is associated with a decrease in BP, thus supporting a vasopressor role for AVP in CHF through activation of the V_1 receptors. In the rat model of ischemic heart failure, AVP hypothalamic biosynthesis is increased as a result of nonosmotic stimulation. The resulting increase in plasma AVP concentration is the major cause of renal water retention in CHF. Specifically, in CHF rats, aquaporin-2 water channels—the molecular target of vasopressin in collecting ducts—are significantly upregulated; administration of AVP-V_2–receptor antagonists abolishes this upregulation and induces a marked diuresis. Moreover, in patients with severe heart failure, AVP-V_2–receptor antagonists administration induces solute-free water diuresis and downregulation of the urinary excretion of aquaporin-2 water channel. The urinary excretion of aquaporin-2 is an estimation of the expression of this water channel onto the luminal membranes of collecting duct cells.

Endothelins

Plasma concentrations of ET1 are usually elevated and play a role in the vasoconstricted state characteristic of CHF patients. Acute administration of the ETA/ETB-receptor antagonist bosentan improves systemic hemodynamic in CHF patients, decreasing systemic vascular resistance (SVR) and increasing cardiac output. Like angiotensin II, ET_1 may also participate in the progressive deterioration of cardiac function as suggested by the improvement in long-term survival of CHF rats treated with bosentan. A role for ET1 in abnormal renal homeostasis of heart failure has also been demonstrated. Administration of ETA-receptor antagonists in dog and rat models of CHF increases RPF, GFR, and sodium and water excretion. By contrast, ETB-receptor antagonists have opposite effects, further decreasing GFR and sodium and water excretion. Whether the renal effects of ETA-receptor antagonists are due to the associated improvement in cardiac output and the decrease in systemic arterial resistance or to the antagonism of the effects of ET1 on renal microcirculation and tubular function still needs to be determined.

Role of Decreased Activity of Natriuretic Factors in Cardiac Edema

Atrial Natriuretic Peptide

The baroreceptor-mediated neurohumoral response (RAAS, AVP, SNS) triggered by CHF induces sodium and water retention, resulting in increased total blood volume. The subsequent increase in atrial pressure caused by hypervolemia induces the release of ANP, which should, in physiologic conditions, enhance diuresis and natriuresis and thus restore normal blood volume. The persistence of hypervolemia in heart failure indicates that this compensatory mechanism is somewhat inoperative. Many investigations have been undertaken to elucidate the reasons for ANP "failure" in CHF.

In human and experimental heart failure, plasma ANP and brain natriuretic peptide (structurally similar to ANP) concentrations are elevated. The increase correlates significantly with the severity of CHF, and these hormones are used to evaluate CHF patients. In addition to the increase in ANP release, cardiac and extracardiac ANP biosynthesis is augmented in experimental heart failure. Taken together, these results demonstrate the integrity of the sensor mechanisms in CHF. This ANP response nevertheless has some benefits in CHF: (a) in CHF rats, the acute administration of an ANP antagonist decreased RPF, GFR, sodium excretion rate, and fractional sodium excretion; (b) in dogs with rapid ventricular pacing–induced heart failure, chronic ANP suppression by bilateral atrial appendectomies was associated with a rise in plasma renin activity and aldosterone as well as a decrease in sodium excretion; and (c) in patients with heart failure, the increase in plasma ANP concentration is associated and strongly correlated with urinary cGMP excretion, the intracellular second messenger of ANP. Taken together, these results demonstrate that ANP has biologic activity at the kidney level and participates in the maintenance of sodium balance in CHF. However, in patients with heart failure and in CHF animals, the natriuretic effect of ANP is reduced, thus suggesting a renal resistance to the effects of the peptide. Indeed, a decrease in intracellular cGMP accumulation in response to ANP has been documented in both glomeruli and inner medullary collecting ducts from CHF rats. This decrease in cGMP accumulation is accounted for by a decrease in the number of biologically active ANP receptors (NPR-A receptors) and an increase in cGMP phosphodiesterase activity. Improvement of the natriuretic response to ANP by an inhibitor of cGMP phosphodiesterases in CHF rats suggests that increased cGMP degradation is an important mechanism of renal ANP resistance. This renal resistance to ANP appears to be at least partly dependent on angiotensin II because losartan, an AT_1-receptor antagonist, improves the intrarenal generation of cGMP and the natriuresis in response to ANP.

Other Natriuretic Systems

Fewer investigations have been conducted concerning the role of other local or systemic natriuretic systems in the sodium and water retention associated with heart failure. Among these factors, NO can increase renal sodium and water excretion through both general and regional hemodynamic effects as well as direct tubular effects. Decreased NO production has been documented in patients with heart failure and may participate in systemic and renal vasoconstriction. However, a study in CHF rats has shown that intrarenal NO production is preserved and that the decreased renal vasodilatory response to NO is related to angiotensin II–mediated vasoconstriction. Adrenomedullin is another factor controlling renal sodium handling. Plasma adrenomedullin concentrations are increased in dogs with experimentally induced heart failure and might counterbalance the sodium-retaining effects of the RAAS and SNS. Finally, renal prostaglandins have an important role in counteracting the influence of sodium-retaining factors and preserving the GFR in heart failure. Indeed, inhibition of prostaglandin synthesis by indomethacin decreases RPF, GFR, and sodium excretion in heart failure.

EDEMA IN HEPATIC CIRRHOSIS

Abnormalities in renal excretion of sodium and water are commonly found in cirrhosis in humans as well as in animal models. These abnormalities eventually lead to ascites, a common complication of cirrhosis and a cause of morbidity and mortality.

The pathogenesis of renal water and sodium retention in cirrhosis is not related to an intrinsic abnormality of the kidney but to extrarenal mechanisms. Specifically, when kidneys from cirrhotic patients are transplanted into persons with normal liver function, renal sodium and water retention no longer occur. Similarly, liver transplantation in patients with hepatorenal syndrome (HRS) allows recovery of renal function. Several hypotheses have been proposed to explain ascites formation in patients with chronic liver disease. It is generally agreed that the initial event is the onset of hepatic dysfunction and increased sinusoidal pressure, but the mechanism by which the diseased liver affects renal function is not completely elucidated.

The Underfilling Theory

The underfilling theory considers that portal hypertension disrupts the Starling equilibrium within the hepatic sinusoids and splanchnic capillaries, leading to an increase in fluid first in the interstitium, then, when the lymphatic system is saturated, in the peritoneal cavity. The subsequent decrease in plasma volume is compensated by enhanced renal sodium and water retention. Although local factors contribute to the maintenance of ascites, the underfilling theory of ascites formation does not fit with the hemodynamic abnormalities. Most important is that plasma volume has been found to be increased, not decreased, in cirrhosis.

The Overflow Theory

The overflow theory proposes that renal sodium and water retention is the primary event, resulting in expansion of plasma volume and adaptive circulatory changes. Multiple observations suggest the existence of a link between the liver and the kidney; among them, a glucagon-induced increase in water and sodium excretion depends on a prior action of glucagon on the liver, and plasma cAMP could be this link. Glomerulopressin, a low-molecular-weight hepatic hormone, was also proposed a few years ago. Finally, a neuronal link through the parasympathetic system has been suggested. Because liver is the diseased organ in cirrhosis, an alteration of this hepatorenal link through the activation of intrahepatic receptors and a decreased hepatic clearance of sodium-retaining substances and a decreased hepatic synthesis of a liver-borne diuretic has been suggested. For instance, it has been demonstrated that extracellular circulating cAMP was diminished in cirrhotic patients. Similarly, alterations in eicosanoid regulation by the cytochrome P450 liver system may lead to increased production of hydroxyeicosatetraenoic acid (HETE) metabolites, which are vasoactive and affect transport in several nephron segments. Finally, downregulation of hepatic and renal 11β-hydroxysteroid dehydrogenases has been demonstrated in rats with cirrhosis. These enzymes are responsible for the interconversion of active to inactive glucocorticosteroids on the mineralocorticoid receptors, acting as a glucocorticoid-receptor protector. The downregulation may contribute to the enhanced sodium retention in distal and collecting tubular cells. Although all these proposed mechanisms are very appealing, the available data do not yet permit direct implication in cirrhosis-related renal dysfunction. More important, a primary renal defect does not explain the neurohumoral reflexes that are activated in cirrhosis, thus suggesting arterial underfilling rather than overfilling, which should abolish these reflexes, as the primary mechanism of sodium and water retention.

The Peripheral Arterial Vasodilation Hypothesis

The peripheral arterial vasodilation hypothesis has been proposed to explain the mechanism of ascites formation and renal dysfunction because many features characterizing cirrhotic patients with ascites could not be explained on the basis of the two previous theories. This theory is based principally on the systemic hemodynamic abnormalities observed in cirrhosis.

Systemic Abnormalities in Cirrhosis: Peripheral Arterial Vasodilation

A hyperdynamic circulation characterized by low arterial BP, high cardiac output, and low SVR was first described in cir-

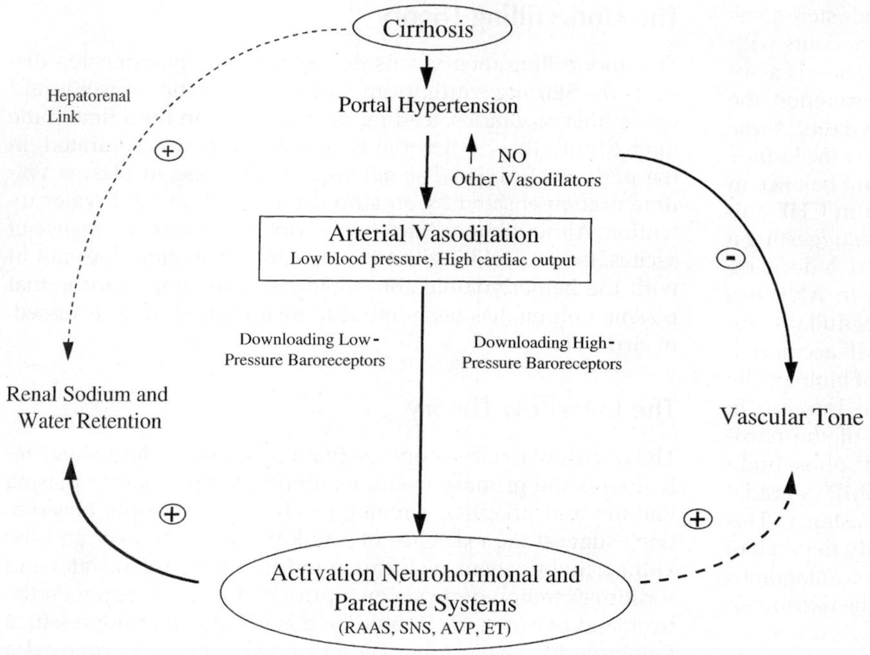

Figure 31.6. Potential mechanisms involved in the pathogenesis of sodium and water retention in cirrhosis. Primary arterial vasodilation is considered the principal event that leads to a baroreceptor-mediated neurohumoral response. This response has two major consequences: increased vascular tone and enhanced renal sodium and water retention. When this response is sufficient to counterbalance the primary vasodilation, baroreceptors stimulation decreases and a new equilibrium is reached at the expense of an increased extracellular fluid (ECF): compensated cirrhosis. When this response is insufficient to counterbalance the primary vasodilation, baroreceptor stimulation further increases, leading to further renal sodium and water retention and ascites formation: decompensated cirrhosis. In addition, it is possible that a direct stimulation toward renal sodium and water retention occurs directly from the liver (hepatorenal link).

rhotic patients more than four decades ago. In animal models and patients with advanced cirrhosis, cardiac output may increase twofold to threefold and SVR can be extremely low, almost comparable to patients with septic shock. Thus chronic liver disease has been classified with states that are characterized by high cardiac output, such as thiamin deficiency (beriberi), thyrotoxicosis, arteriovenous fistulas, septic shock, anemia, and pregnancy, all of which have in common a low peripheral vascular resistance. It has been proposed that this low peripheral vascular resistance, principally in the splanchnic circulation, is the primary mechanism leading to a relative underfilling of the arterial circulation and a hyperdynamic circulation in cirrhosis. This arterial underfilling unloads the high pressure baroreceptors, which activate the renin-angiotensin-aldosterone axis, SNS, the nonosmotic release of AVP, and the ETs. This sequence of events results in enhanced renal water and sodium retention in an attempt to compensate the relatively underfilled arterial circulation (Fig. 31.6). Initially, these compensatory mechanisms succeed at the expense of increased plasma volume, which attenuates the signals activating the antinatriuretic and vasoconstrictor systems. At this time, renal sodium and water balance is reestablished, a state called *compensated cirrhosis.* When the liver disease progresses and the splanchnic arteriolar vasodilation further increases, these mechanisms can no longer compensate for the underfilled arterial circulation and are therefore continuously stimulated; this results in ascites and edema formation: the state of *decompensated cirrhosis.*

There is now a strong body of evidence supporting this hypothesis. Blockade of the vascular effect of angiotensin II or AVP is associated respectively with a fall in BP and SVR in cirrhotic patients and rats with ascites, whereas this blockade does not change the systemic hemodynamics in normal subjects. These studies demonstrate that these neurohormones have a compensatory role in maintaining the systemic hemodynamics. In animal models, there is a close chronologic relationship between onset of sodium retention and a decrease in BP. In rats with partial portal vein ligation, a model of presinusoidal hypertension, the fall in SVR occurs before there is a detectable increase in total body sodium (Fig. 31.7).

Induction of cirrhosis by carbon tetrachloride in spontaneously hypertensive rats has been undertaken to better detect an early fall in BP than in nonhypertensive rats. The authors found a direct correlation between the onset of a decrease in arterial pressure and renal sodium retention.

In cirrhotic patients, there is an abnormal distribution of the blood volume and a decreased central blood volume when care-

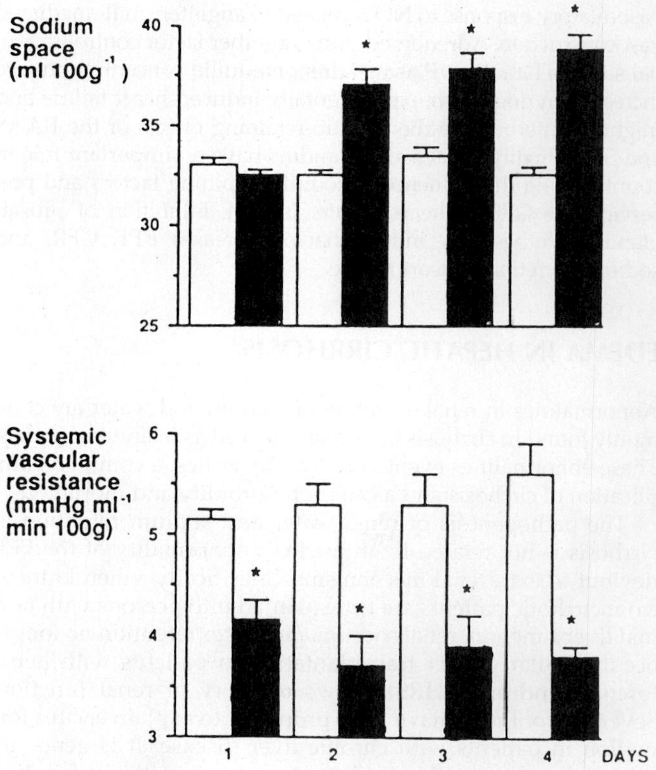

Figure 31.7. Temporal relationship between decreased peripheral vascular resistance and increased sodium space in rats with prehepatic portal hypertension *(black bars)* versus control rats *(white bars)*. $P < .05$. (Reprinted from Albillos A, Colombato L, Groszmann R. Vasodilation and sodium retention in prehepatic portal hypertension. *Gastroenterology* 1992;102:931–935.)

fully estimated by magnetic resonance imaging. Head-out water immersion, a maneuver that increases the central blood volume corrects the abnormal renal sodium and water retention in cirrhotic patients with ascites only when associated with concomitant maintenance of SVR with exogenous norepinephrine. The results of this latter study demonstrate the major role of the peripheral arterial vasodilation in the pathogenesis of ascites. Finally, portal hypertension is known to be associated with splanchnic arterial vasodilation that may play a critical role in initiating the hemodynamic alterations and also contribute to the formation of ascites by perturbing the local microvascular pressures. It has been demonstrated in cirrhotic patients that superior mesenteric artery blood flow, as estimated by Doppler ultrasonography, significantly correlates with SVR index and parallels the degree of liver dysfunction.

Pathogenesis of Peripheral Arterial Vasodilation in Cirrhosis

Nitric Oxide

Since the discovery of the major role of the endothelium in the control of the vascular tone, several endothelial vasoactive factors have been implicated in the pathogenesis of the hemodynamic abnormalities of cirrhosis. It has been known since 1965 that responsiveness to endogenous vasoconstrictors was impaired in patients with cirrhosis. The endothelium appears to play a major role in this abnormal vascular resistance because removal of the vascular endothelium abolishes the difference in vascular reactivity between cirrhotic and control vessels. There is now considerable evidence that the endothelial vasodilator NO is produced in excess by the vasculature of cirrhotic animals and patients. In rat models of cirrhosis or portal hypertension, evidence for increased production of NO can be detected early in the course of the disease. Similarly, several studies in cirrhotic patients have shown increased NO production. Normalization of NO production in cirrhotic rats with ascites to the level of the NO production of the controls corrected the hyperdynamic circulation of cirrhosis, thus supporting a major role for NO in the pathogenesis of the arterial vasodilation associated with cirrhosis. Moreover, normalization of NO production is accompanied by a significant increase in urinary sodium and water excretion, with a concomitant decrease of ascites in cirrhotic rats (Fig. 31.8). These effects of NO inhibition and reversal of the hyperdynamic circulation were associated with a decrease in plasma renin activity and in aldosterone and vasopressin concentrations. It should be stressed that the mechanisms leading to increased NO vascular production are not yet elucidated. Among them, increased shear stress, a circulating factor, and a liver-borne substance have to be considered as potential stimulators of NO production.

Other Causes

Although increased vascular NO production is the most reported abnormality, other derangements of the cirrhotic vessels have been described. The potassium channels that influence the vasodilatory state of the vessels by regulating the membrane potential have a blunted response when stimulated by potassium channel activators in cirrhosis. In addition, impairment of the G-protein transduction pathway has been reported in vessels from portal-hypertensive animals. It has been hypothesized that increased activity of adenosine participates in the hemodynamic abnormalities associated with cirrhosis. Adenosine is an endogenous nucleoside derived mainly from intracellular catabolism of ATP, which is a vasodilator in most vascular territories but not in the kidneys, where it induces marked vasoconstriction and reduces GFR by increasing the responsiveness of afferent arterioles to angiotensin II. Finally, the plasma levels of several substances that have a vasodilatory effect mainly mediated by NO are elevated in cirrhotic patients; these include substance P, calcitonin gene–related peptide, and insulin. Adrenomedullin, a vasodilator peptide that is biosynthesized by several tissues, including endothelium and kidneys, has also been shown to be elevated in human cirrhosis, and this elevation does not seem to be a homeostatic response to counteract the effects of vasoconstrictors. Whether these increased plasma concentrations of adrenomedullin contribute significantly to arterial vasodilation in cirrhosis remains to be established.

Mechanisms of Sodium Retention in Cirrhosis

Sodium retention is the earliest and most common renal abnormality in cirrhosis. It has been established that sodium retention precedes ascites. In compensated cirrhosis without ascites, patients do not have overt sodium retention because most of them

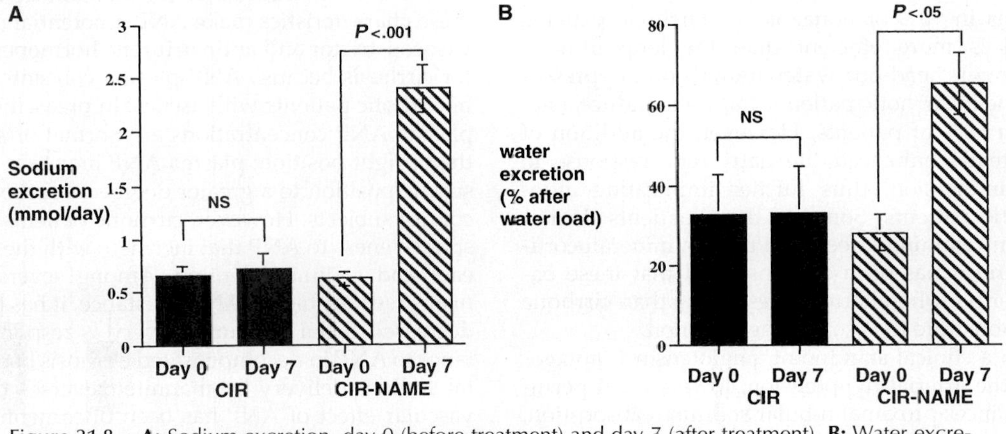

Figure 31.8. **A:** Sodium excretion, day 0 (before treatment) and day 7 (after treatment). **B:** Water excretion, day 0 and day 7 in cirrhotic rats with ascites either untreated *(black bars)* or treated with N^G-nitro-L-arginine methyl ester (L-NAME) 0.5 mg/kg/day *(hatched bars)* for 1 week. Mean values are given from 10 rats in each group. (Adapted from Martin PY, Ohara M, Gines P, et al. Nitric oxide synthase (NOS) inhibition for one week improves renal sodium and water excretion in cirrhotic rats with ascites. *J Clin Invest* 1998;101:235–242.)

are in sodium balance, although with an increased plasma volume. However, they are often unable to handle a sodium load and demonstrate abnormal sodium handling when they are in the upright position. In patients with ascites, baseline urinary sodium levels can be variable, and this has been shown to be of prognostic value. Alterations in GFR, RBF, and renal perfusion pressure could contribute to sodium retention, but in many instances, they have been reported to be unchanged during active sodium retention. When present, reduced renal perfusion is usually accompanied by more marked sodium retention. Reduced renal perfusion has been attributed predominantly to cortical vasoconstriction, with relative maintenance of medullary blood flow. However, in one study, a decrease in papillary blood flow was demonstrated in experimental cirrhosis coexisting with reduced water and sodium excretion. This study further demonstrated that volume expansion induced a smaller increase in papillary blood flow and renal interstitial hydrostatic pressure (RIHP) in cirrhotic animals than in control rats and was accompanied by a blunted natriuresis. An important role of RIHP has emerged in the control of salt and water reabsorption by the proximal tubule and Henle's loop, and it is possible that a decreased RIHP could facilitate sodium and water tubular reabsorption in cirrhosis. Finally, micropuncture studies in animals have demonstrated increased sodium resorption in proximal and thick ascending limb of Henle's loop in liver cirrhosis. Taken together with the known elevation of plasma aldosterone leading to an increase in distal and collecting tubule sodium resorption, it is fair to say that sodium retention is enhanced in all nephrons' segments. The factors involved in the imbalance between natriuretic and antinatriuretic mechanisms characterizing the edematous state of cirrhosis are now reviewed.

Renin-Angiotensin-Aldosterone System

Stimulation of the renin-angiotensin-aldosterone axis has antinatriuretic effects and has been shown to be activated in cirrhosis. First, in a situation of decreased renal perfusion pressure, angiotensin II increases glomerular efferent arteriole resistance and thus provides preservation of the GFR by enhancing filtration fraction. However, the resulting decrease in hydraulic and colloidal pressures within the peritubular capillaries enhances proximal tubular sodium reabsorption. Angiotensin II also has a direct effect to enhance sodium reabsorption in the proximal tubule. In addition, aldosterone promotes sodium reabsorption in the cortical collecting duct. Competitive antagonism of the tubular action of aldosterone with high dosages of spironolactone (200 to 400 mg/day) results in natriuresis in 90% of nonazotemic cirrhotic patients with ascites and is more efficient than the loop diuretic furosemide. Although head-out water immersion suppresses plasma aldosterone in cirrhotic patients, failure to induce a natriuresis occurs in 50% of patients. However, the addition of spironolactone greatly enhanced the natriuretic response to head-out water immersion, thus further implicating aldosterone in cirrhotic patients. Some of these patients do not escape the sodium-retaining effect of synthetic mineralocorticoid hormones, and it has been demonstrated that these patients have a lower peripheral arterial resistance than cirrhotic patients who demonstrate the escape phenomenon.

However, from a clinical standpoint, angiotensin II antagonism aggravates the arterial hypotension, lowers renal perfusion pressure, enhances proximal tubular sodium reabsorption, and decreases distal sodium delivery. Similarly, aldosterone antagonism may worsen the hypotension of cirrhosis. These findings suggest that activation of the angiotensin-aldosterone axis in cirrhosis is a compensatory response.

Sympathetic Nervous System

Activation of the SNS can decrease RBF and GFR through the α-adrenoreceptors on the afferent and efferent glomerular arterioles. In addition, α_1-adrenoreceptors can directly enhance proximal tubular sodium reabsorption and β-adrenoreceptors on the afferent arterioles mediate renin release. Circulating norepinephrine (NE) and epinephrine are elevated in cirrhotic patients; a positive correlation between plasma NE and urinary sodium excretion has been documented in cirrhotic patients with ascites. When NE samples have been collected from the renal vein to quantify the sympathetic tone in cirrhotic patients, a significant inverse relationship has been found between NE concentration and RBF. Finally, renal denervation increases sodium excretion in experimental cirrhosis, particularly in cirrhotic animals on a low-sodium diet.

Endothelin System

The endothelin system is a potent vasopressive and antinatriuretic regulatory system. This system appears to be activated in cirrhotic patients, at least in decompensated cirrhosis, but the pathophysiologic importance of the ET system in cirrhosis is not yet delineated. Compared with the other systems implicated in the pathogenesis of sodium and water retention of cirrhosis, the predominant paracrine action of the endothelin system makes investigation of its role in cirrhosis more difficult. Molecular studies and use of ET antagonists have demonstrated that activation of the ET system contributes significantly to the hepatic pathogenesis of portal hypertension. Concerning its role in renal abnormalities, there are no convincing studies that demonstrate that the ET system plays a major role in sodium and water retention. Further use of more specific ET antagonists should bring a better answer to this question.

Atrial Natriuretic Peptides

ANP is the most studied natriuretic peptide in cirrhosis, although a role for brain natriuretic peptide (BNP) and urodilatin is also probable but less well defined. ANP is a potent natriuretic peptide secreted in response to atrial wall stretch; however, in conditions such as cirrhosis, in which central blood volume is low, increased secretion of ANP comes primarily from the ventricles where ANP mRNA levels from cirrhotic rats are fourfold higher than in controls. ANP promotes vasodilation of afferent arterioles and vasoconstriction of efferent arterioles and inhibits sodium reabsorption in medullary collecting tubules. In addition, ANP inhibits renin and aldosterone secretion. All these characteristics make ANP a potential counterregulator of vasoconstrictor and antinatriuretic hormones with implications for cirrhosis because ANP plasma concentrations are elevated in cirrhotic patients with ascites. In preascitic cirrhotic patients, plasma ANP concentrations are normal or slightly elevated in the upright position; plasma ANP increases significantly in the supine position to a greater degree in cirrhotic patients than in control subjects. However, cirrhotic patients develop a hyporesponsiveness to ANP that increases with the severity of the disease and sodium retention. Among several possible mechanisms responsible for ANP resistance, it has been proposed that decreased distal sodium delivery is responsible for the resistance to ANP in decompensated cirrhosis because increased distal sodium delivery by mannitol reverses this resistance. The vascular effect of ANP has been documented in experimental cirrhosis. Administration of HS-142-1, a receptor antagonist of ANP, to cirrhotic rats with ascites leads to a dramatic fall in RBF and GFR, as well as a significant increase in plasma renin activity and aldosterone. Thus endogenous ANP appears to play a critical role in the maintenance of renal function and regulation of the renin-aldosterone axis in cirrhosis.

Prostaglandin System

Renal prostaglandins are important to the preservation of renal function in situations with elevated plasma concentrations of angiotensin II, NE, or vasopressin. Urinary excretion of E_2 (PGE_2) and prostacyclin metabolites (6-oxo-PGF1α) are increased in cirrhosis. Administration of NSAIDs in this setting is accompanied by a fall in GFR and an increase in sodium and water retention. Moreover, comparison of the effects of NOS inhibitors and NSAIDs (either given separately or together) in experimental cirrhosis has nicely demonstrated that the predominant role of NO was on the systemic hemodynamics, whereas prostaglandin integrity was essential for maintenance of renal function in cirrhosis.

Mechanism of Water Retention in Cirrhosis: The Role of Vasopressin

In some patients with advanced cirrhosis, the severity of the urinary diluting disorder is such that they retain most of the water ingested and develop hyponatremia and hypoosmolality. In a multivariate analysis of 39 variables in a large cohort of cirrhotic patients, hyponatremia (less than 133 mmol/L) was the strongest independent predictor of the occurrence of hepatorenal syndrome.

Studies in human and experimental animals have provided strong evidence that AVP plays a major role in the pathogenesis of water retention in cirrhosis with ascites. Plasma NE, renin activity, aldosterone, and AVP are significantly higher in cirrhotic patients with impaired water excretion, and there is a strong positive correlation between concentrations of plasma norepinephrine and AVP concentrations after water loading in these patients. The role of vasopressin in impaired water secretion of cirrhosis has been further confirmed by animal studies. There is a clear temporal dissociation between sodium retention and the defect in water excretion—sodium retention preceding the impairment in water excretion by 2 weeks. Administration of a V_2-AVP–receptor antagonist normalizes water excretion in cirrhotic rats. This hypersecretion of AVP is caused by an increased synthesis because the hypothalamic AVP mRNA content is increased in cirrhotic rats. Finally, the collecting duct water channel, aquaporin-2 (AQP2), which is regulated by AVP, has been shown to be increased in cirrhotic rats with ascites.

The most likely explanation for the hypersecretion of AVP in cirrhosis is a nonosmotic stimulation because cirrhotic patients have a degree of hyponatremia and hypoosmolality that would suppress AVP release in normal subjects. Head-out water immersion has been shown to consistently improve sodium and water excretion and suppress plasma norepinephrine, renin activity, aldosterone, and AVP in decompensated cirrhotic patients. However, a complete normalization of water and sodium excretion was obtained only when this maneuver was concomitant with an NE infusion. Thus increased central blood volume with simultaneous maintenance of SVR normalizes renal sodium and water excretion in decompensated cirrhotic patients. The importance of the hemodynamic stimuli for AVP hypersecretion in cirrhotic rats with ascites has been demonstrated by using a V_1-AVP–receptor antagonist and an angiotensin II inhibitor. These drugs did not have any hemodynamic effect in control subjects, whereas both further reduced the mean arterial pressure in cirrhotic rats and were additive. These findings further support a role for hypersecretion of AVP as a compensatory mechanism to the peripheral arterial vasodilation.

As noted earlier, chronic NOS inhibition decreases plasma AVP in cirrhotic rats with ascites and improves their renal ability to excrete water. Decreased renal production of prostaglandins in cirrhosis has been demonstrated to enhance the tubular effect of AVP in cirrhosis in addition to the hormone's hemodynamic effect.

Consequences of Sodium and Water Retention

The development of ascites in cirrhotic patients results in a significant increase in morbidity and mortality; 5-year survival has been estimated at 50% after the first appearance of ascites. When cirrhotic patients have to be hospitalized for the treatment of ascites, the 1-year survival rate has been reported to be 56%. Development of ascites is a marker of the severity of the liver disease and portal hypertension, both of which account for the high mortality rate. Moreover, ascites also contributes directly to the increased morbidity and mortality because it predisposes to spontaneous bacterial peritonitis. Diuretic-induced renal failure has been estimated to be as high as 20% in cirrhotic patients. In addition, about 10% of cirrhotic patients with ascites develop refractory ascites, which necessitate more invasive therapies, including therapeutic paracentesis, peritoneovenous shunting, or placement of percutaneous transjugular intrahepatic portosystemic shunt. Finally, hepatorenal syndrome is a common complication: the probability of developing this syndrome is 20% at 1 year and 40% at 5 years in cirrhotic patients with ascites.

Conclusion

Primary peripheral arterial vasodilation is the major initiating event of water and sodium retention in cirrhosis. Increased NO production by the endothelial cells plays a major role in the pathogenesis of the peripheral arterial vasodilation. Sodium retention is the first renal abnormality in cirrhosis and there is evidence that sodium retention starts after the hemodynamic abnormalities. Activation of the renin-angiotensin-aldosterone axis and the SNS, both vasoconstrictor and antinatriuretic neurohormones, constitutes the major mechanism contributing to sodium retention. Impaired water excretion and dilutional hyponatremia related to nonosmotic release of vasopressin is a marker of the severity of the disease and the accompanying hemodynamic abnormalities. Ascites is associated with multiple complications, including subacute bacterial peritonitis, esophageal varices, and hepatorenal syndrome. Thus, when ascites in cirrhotic patients occurs, morbidity and mortality are significantly increased.

APPROACH TO THE PATIENT WITH EDEMA

The most important principle is that the underlying pathologic condition responsible for the edema must be identified quickly. Ordinarily, this is not difficult: symptoms of fatigue, breathlessness, and a history of cardiac disease direct attention to congestive heart failure. Enlarged heart, gallop rhythm, murmurs, distended neck veins, pulmonary rales, and hepatomegaly with hepatojugular reflux confirm the cardiac origin of the edema.

Jaundice, spider angiomas, hepatomegaly, ascites, and abnormal liver function test results point to cirrhosis of the liver as the cause of edema.

Pallor, heavy proteinuremia, hypoalbuminemia, and hyperlipidemia coupled with normal liver and cardiac function would indicate that the edema is caused by nephrotic syndrome.

Rare causes of generalized edema, such as protein-losing enteropathy, capillary leak syndrome, and inferior vena cava obstruction, can be suspected from the characteristic clinical and laboratory findings. (For more information on idiopathic edema, see Chapter 22.)

MANAGEMENT OF EDEMA

Indications for Treatment of Edema

The presence of edema is not in itself an indication for vigorous treatment, and in an otherwise asymptomatic patient, a mild degree of edema does not need to become the primary focus of attention. Rather, specific indications must be present to warrant treatment. The side effects and possible complications of treatment—in particular those associated with severe salt restriction and diuretic administration—must be weighed carefully against the possible benefits of correcting the edema. On the other hand, the decision as to how vigorously to treat the edema will be significantly influenced by the presence of complications attributable to edema or ascites. Some of these complications are listed in Table 31.3. They include local complications, such as discomfort from swelling of extremities and digits, as well as stasis dermatitis and skin ulceration. More general complications consist of the psychologic impact of altered physical appearance and any limitations in physical activity imposed by the edema and the underlying condition that led to its formation. Specific organ systems are affected by accumulation of the fluids of edema. In addition to the respiratory difficulties associated with pulmonary vascular congestion, pleural effusions and impaired diaphragmatic excursion from large collections of ascites may further compromise respiratory function. Expanded plasma volume leads to hypertension and increased cardiac workload, which will aggravate heart failure. Passive congestion of the liver is associated with anorexia, nausea, and vomiting (cardiac cachexia).

If the congestion persists chronically, cardiac cirrhosis with disordered liver function may develop. Engorgement of the splanchnic vasculature may lead to protein-losing enteropathy and intestinal malabsorption. Other complications of ascites include spontaneous bacterial peritonitis, esophageal reflux, and formation of umbilical and inguinal hernias. Scrotal and penile edema may be particularly disabling, and urinary obstruction may develop from this complication. The presence of one or more of these complications of fluid retention and edema formation may demand specific treatment.

TABLE 31.3. Complications of Edema and Ascites

Peripheral edema
Cellulitis
Venous thrombosis
Impaired vision from periorbital edema
Pain
Unacceptable cosmetic impact
Scrotal and penile edema
Limitation of physical activity
Pleural effusions
Ascites
Impaired intestinal absorption
Esophageal reflux
Dyspnea from impaired diaphragmatic excursion
Umbilical, inguinal hernias
Spontaneous bacterial peritonitis

General Measures in the Management of Edema

The treatment of edema can be considered as consisting of *general measures*, which are effective in all edema-forming states, and *specific* additional *measures*, which can be employed in certain settings. The available treatments are summarized in Table 31.4.

Treatment of the Underlying Disease

In all cases of edema formation, treatment of the underlying disease process should be the primary focus of attention. Thus therapeutic measures directed at the failing myocardium in patients with congestive heart failure or at altered glomerular permeability in patients with nephrotic syndrome will, if successful, treat the edema as well.

A full discussion of the therapeutic approach to the organ dysfunctions leading to accumulation of edema fluid is beyond the scope of this chapter. However, from a practical viewpoint, this principle has only limited applicability; treatment of chronic liver disease and many forms of nephrotic syndrome may only stabilize but not correct the primary disease, and many forms of heart disease will progress despite optimal medical therapy. Thus management of edema in these settings must of necessity rely on other measures.

Bed Rest. Bed rest with elevation of the edematous extremities is usually helpful in mobilizing the edema. If the supine position is maintained for several hours, there is an augmentation of blood volume in the central circulation as a result of diminution of peripheral venous pooling. This results in increased cardiac output and perhaps, in the edematous state, in augmented renal perfusion and sodium excretion. In addition, recumbency is associated with diminished plasma levels of AVP and aldosterone, which may facilitate increased water and sodium excretion, respectively. The diuretic response to bed rest may be better in heart failure than in either cirrhosis or nephrosis, primarily through diminished cardiac work rather than through any differences in volume redistribution among the three disorders.

Outpatients whose edema is refractory to diuretics may become more responsive to diuretic therapy on enforced hospital bed rest. Whether this is a result of hemodynamic changes or of more reliable patient compliance in taking prescribed medications and diet is unclear. The use of supportive stockings tends to increase the velocity and volume of limb venous blood flow and minimizes venous stasis, helping to mobilize edema,

TABLE 31.4. Treatment of Edema

General measures
Treatment of the primary disease
Bed rest
Sodium restriction
Diuretic administration
Specific measures
Fluid removal
Pleurocentesis (heart failure, cirrhosis, nephrosis)
Paracentesis (heart failure, cirrhosis, nephrosis)
Plasma volume expansion
Infusion of plasma or hyperoncotic albumin solutions (cirrhosis, nephrosis)
Ascitic fluid reinfusion (cirrhosis)
Peritoneovenous shunt (cirrhosis)
Headout water immersion (cirrhosis, nephrosis)
Pharmacologic therapy
Vasodilators (heart failure)
Angiotensin-converting enzyme inhibitors (heart failure)
Continuous arteriovenous hemofiltration (heart failure)

whether such stockings are used alone or are combined with bed rest.

Sodium Restriction. In most edematous patients not receiving diuretic therapy, the rate of urinary sodium excretion is very low (often below 10 mEq/day). The exception to this rule is in patients with chronic renal insufficiency, in whom sodium excretion usually resembles dietary sodium intake. To create a negative sodium balance (i.e., daily sodium excretion in excess of daily sodium intake) would require rigid dietary sodium restriction, which necessitates an intake of less than 20 mEq/day. Such a diet is unpalatable, and patient acceptance is low. For these reasons, salt restriction is more important in limiting the development of *further* edema than in causing resolution of preexisting edema. Sodium restriction is also useful because it allows moderation of the dose of diuretic required to induce a negative sodium balance, thus diminishing the likelihood of diuretic toxicity.

Diuretics. In all but the mildest cases of edema, diuretics are one of the mainstays of management. The various classes of diuretics, their site and mechanism of action, and their use and dosage in various edematous states are discussed in Chapter 21.

Specific Measures for Treatment of Edema

The plethora of treatments in addition to those outlined in the previous section is testimony to the fact that general measures are not always effective in treating edema. Some of these additional treatments are listed in Table 31.4. *Pleurocentesis* and *paracentesis* can be used for direct removal of edema fluid accumulated in thoracic and abdominal cavities. If no other treatment is provided concomitantly, the fluid usually reaccumulates. The indications for these procedures relate to symptoms caused by them, although small volumes may be removed for diagnostic purposes. Pleurocentesis should be undertaken when the pleural effusion is large and compromises respiration either through the sense of dyspnea or through impairment of gas exchange by compression of lung parenchyma.

Recent experience has shown that large-volume paracentesis (4 to 6 L or even the total removal of ascitic fluid) can be safely carried out in patients with cirrhosis if a plasma expander is given during a procedure or within a few hours afterward. The removal of ascitic fluid without concomitant plasma expansion causes a constant reduction of intravascular volume that may be associated with the development of renal failure (hepatorenal syndrome) or hyponatremia in a significant proportion of patients. The optimal plasma expander seems to be albumin (6 to 8 g/L of ascitic fluid removed), but synthetic molecules (polymerized gelatin, dextran-70) may also be used. Several recent studies comparing large-volume paracentesis with plasma volume expansion versus administration of diuretics have shown that paracentesis is more rapid and effective and is associated with a lower incidence of complications (renal failure, electrolyte disorders, and encephalopathy) than conventional diuretic therapy, thus offering a new approach to treatment of ascites in cirrhosis.

Many plasma volume expansion maneuvers have been recommended for the treatment of cirrhotic and nephrotic edema in an effort to correct the renal hypoperfusion state that characterizes these conditions. Plasma and hyperoncotic albumin infusions preferentially expand the plasma compartment while maintaining or increasing plasma oncotic pressure. These may transiently improve renal function, even to the point of increasing sodium excretion. In liver disease, fresh-frozen plasma infusions may supplement depleted clotting factors. However, this approach has limited utility in the management of edema. The infusions are expensive, and the effects on renal function are at best transient. Moreover, they have no effect on the underlying disease process. In addition, gastrointestinal bleeding in cirrhotic patients is increased after volume expansion, and the infused protein is rapidly excreted into the urine in nephrotic patients. For these reasons, alternative approaches to volume expansion therapy have been advocated. In cirrhotic patients, ascites fluid reinfusion reduces the volume of ascites and restores it to the plasma compartment. This technique, when carried out in an acutely ill patient, has improved renal function and promoted natriuresis, particularly if it is accompanied by administration of high-ceiling diuretics. However, because it is a cumbersome procedure with a high risk of infection and sepsis, air embolus, and activation of the clotting system, is no longer carried out.

A method of chronic ascitic fluid infusion is achieved with the surgical insertion of a peritoneovenous (LeVeen) shunt. Tubing containing a one-way valve is placed with one end in the peritoneal cavity. It is tunneled subcutaneously, and the other end is inserted into the right atrium through the internal jugular vein. Whenever intraabdominal pressure exceeds right atrial pressure, ascites is delivered by this route into the bloodstream. Although initial uncontrolled experience with this technique yielded favorable results in the management of intractable ascites, data from controlled studies have not indicated clear-cut advantages to the use of the technique, particularly in view of its high percentage of shunt failures, sepsis, and activation of the clotting cascade. As a consequence, it too is used only rarely.

One other form of central blood volume expansion has been used in the treatment of cirrhotic and nephrotic edema. This is the technique of head-out water immersion, in which the patient is immersed to the neck in a tub of thermoindifferent water for 4 or 5 hours. The water pressure redistributes blood volume from the periphery to the great veins of the thorax, which then corrects sensed underfilling and by reflexive response acts on the kidneys to lead to natriuresis. Although the increase in sodium excretion during immersion is impressive, patients revert to their avid sodium-retaining state after they come out of the immersion tub. The benefit is thus only transitory, and no published report comments on its use in the long-term management of edema. Rather, its utility lies in the ability to explore some of the pathophysiologic mechanisms that lead to sodium retention and edema formation in these conditions.

The technique of continuous arteriovenous hemofiltration affords a means of fluid removal over the short term in patients with congestive heart failure. Using an extracorporeal circulation, arterial BP provides the force for ultrafiltration of plasma water through a semipermeable membrane contained in a small cartridge. Ultrafiltration rates can be extremely high with this system. Its major drawback is the requirement for an extracorporeal circuit, but it can be used to assist volume control until other measures improve cardiac function sufficiently to allow the native kidneys to resume their homeostatic function. (This technique is discussed in detail in Chapter 84, Part 3.)

Selected Readings

Albillos A, Colombato L, Groszmann R. Vasodilation and sodium retention in prehepatic portal hypertension. *Gastroenterology* 1992;102:931–935.

Very convincing experiments demonstrating the early onset of vasodilation in cirrhosis.

Angeli P, Jimenez W, Arroyo V, et al. Renal effects of natriuretic peptide receptor blockade in cirrhotic rats with ascites. *Hepatology* 1994;20:948–954.

This study emphasizes the counterregulatory role of ANP in cirrhosis, especially for the maintenance of renal function.

Arroyo V, Bosch J, Gaya-Beltran J, et al. Plasma renin activity and urinary sodium excretion as prognostic indicators in nonazotemic cirrhosis with ascites. 1981;94:198–201.

First demonstration of the prognostic role of activation of the RAAS and renal sodium retention in cirrhotic patients.

Bennhold H, Klaus D, Scheurlen PG. Volume regulation and renal function in analbuminaemia. *Lancet* 1960;2:1169–1170.

A study showing that analbuminemia does not alter renal sodium handling, nor does it produce edema.

Brown EA, Markandu ND, Sagnella G, et al. Evidence that some mechanism other than the renin system causes sodium retention in nephrotic syndrome. *Lancet* 1982;2:1237–1240.

A study showing that inhibitors of the angiotensin-converting enzyme does not increase natriuresis despite a fall in plasma aldosterone in subjects with nephrotic syndrome.

Féraille E, Vogt B, Rousselot M, et al. Mechanism of enhanced Na-K-ATPase activity in cortical collecting duct from rats with nephrotic syndrome. *J Clin Invest* 1993;91:1295–1300.

A demonstration of the functional increase in collecting duct Na^+-K^+-ATPase activity of rats with puromycinaminonucleoside-induced nephrotic syndrome.

Geers AB, Koomans HA, Roos JC, et al. Preservation of blood volume during edema removal in nephrotic subjects. *Kidney Int* 1985;28:652–657.

A study showing that blood volume does not decrease with diuretic treatment of nephrotic edema.

Hamlyn JM, Hamilton BP, Manunta P. Endogenous ouabain, sodium balance and blood pressure: a review and a hypothesis. *J Hypertens* 1996;14:151-167.

Review discussing the evidence in favor of the existence of endogenous ouabain in humans as well as the correlation between the blood level of the substance and the size of ECF volume in different pathologic conditions.

Ichikawa I, Pfeffer JM, Pfeffer MA, et al. Role of angiotensin II in the altered renal function of congestive heart failure. *Circ Res* 1984;55:669–675.

A study demonstrating the role of angiotensin II in the alterations of glomerular hemodynamics and proximal tubule fluid reabsorption in chronic heart failure.

Lüscher TF. Endothelin, endothelin receptors, and endothelin antagonists. *Curr Opin Nephrol Hypertens* 1994;3:92–98.

Review describing in detail the endothelin system and its physiologic role.

Maack T. Role of atrial natriuretic factor in volume control. *Kidney Int* 1996;49: 1732–1737.

Review updating our knowledge on the natriuretic peptides.

Martin PY, Ohara M, Gines P, et al. Nitric oxide synthase (NOS) inhibition for one week improves renal sodium and water excretion in cirrhotic rats with ascites. *J Clin Invest* 1998;101:235–242.

This study demonstrates that NO is an important factor not only in the pathogenesis of the hemodynamic abnormalities of cirrhosis but also in the pathogenesis of renal sodium and water retention.

Moller S, Sondergaard L, Mogelvang J, et al. Decreased right heart blood volume determined by magnetic resonance imaging: evidence of central underfilling in cirrhosis. *Hepatology* 1995;22:472–478.

This article gives good evidence for a central underfilling in cirrhosis.

Richards AM. The renin-angiotensin-aldosterone system and the cardiac natriuretic peptides. *Heart* 1996;76 (Suppl 3):36–44.

Article briefly presenting the two systems and outlining their interactions.

Schrier RW, Arroyo V, Bernardi M, et al. Peripheral arterial vasodilation hypothesis: a proposal for the initiation of renal sodium and water retention in cirrhosis. *Hepatology* 1988;8:1151–1157.

The original paper in which a group of experts elaborated the peripheral arterial vasodilation hypothesis to better explain the pathogenesis of ascites in cirrhosis.

Volpe M, Tritto C, DeLuca N, et al. Abnormalities of sodium handling and of cardiovascular adaptations during high salt diet in patients with mild heart failure. *Circulation* 1993;88:1620–1627.

A study showing that sodium avidity of the kidneys is observed early in the course of chronic heart failure.

Wada A, Tsutamoto T, Fukai D, et al. Comparison of the effects of selective endothelin ETA and ETB receptor antagonists in congestive heart failure. *J Am Coll Cardiol* 1997;30:1385–1392.

A demonstration of the role of ETs in the sodium and water retention of chronic heart failure and showing the cardiovascular and renal effects of ETA- and ETB-receptors antagonists.

Xu DL, Martin PY, Ohara M, et al. Upregulation of aquaporin-2 water channel expression in chronic heart failure rat. *J Clin Invest* 1997;99:1500–1505.

A study suggesting that increased aquaporin-2 expression in the collecting duct is the molecular basis for enhanced water reabsorption in chronic heart failure.

Zhang PL, Mackenzie HS, Totsune K, et al. Renal effects of high-dose natriuretic peptide receptor blockade in rats with congestive heart failure. *Circ Res* 1995; 77:1240–1245.

A study showing the role of endogenous ANP in antagonizing the sodium and water retention promoted by vasoconstrictors in heart failure.

CHAPTER 32

Proteinuria

Richard J. Glassock

The abnormal excretion of protein into the urine is one of the most important pathophysiologic disturbances accompanying renal diseases. However, it is worthwhile to emphasize that such proteinuria may arise under diverse circumstances, not related to any underlying renal disorder. Thus the evaluation of a patient with proteinuria requires a sound understanding of the principles of glomerular permeability to protein macromolecules, the tubular reabsorption of filtered protein, and the various methods for detection, analysis, and quantification of proteins in the urine. These subjects are also discussed in Chapters 4, 7, Part 5, and 101.

The recognition that proteinuria plays an important role in the progression of certain types of renal diseases has increased the importance of its early recognition, classification and quantitation.

NORMAL VALUES FOR PROTEIN EXCRETION

The normal rate of protein excretion into the urine in healthy adults is 80 ± 24 mg/24 hours (1 SD). Thus more than 95% of normal adults excrete less than 150 mg of protein per day. Protein excretion is somewhat higher in healthy children and adolescents, and a value of 250 mg/day often is used as the upper limit of normal in these individuals. Urinary protein excretion rises modestly in normal pregnancy. Normally, 70% to 80% of urine protein is excreted during quiet, upright ambulation. The excretion of an abnormal amount of protein in a 24-hour period, coupled with an exaggeration of the protein excretion pattern with respect to posture, is found in patients who have fixed and reproducible orthostatic proteinuria. Fever, severe exercise, congestive heart failure, and acute infusions of hyperoncotic albumin, or many pressor agents (e.g., angiotensin II, norepinephrine) may also transiently increase protein excretion in otherwise normal individuals.

DETECTION OF PROTEINURIA

The detection of abnormal proteinuria is discussed in detail in Chapter 101. Various methods can be used. The simplest and least expensive is the use of dye-impregnated paper strips (e.g., Multistix, Ames), which depend on a color change of a pH-sensitive dye (tetrabromophenol blue buffered to pH 3). These strips detect protein, chiefly albumin, down to a concentration of 20 mg/dl and provide a semiquantitative estimate up to 300 mg/dl. The strips are relatively insensitive to globulins (e.g., Bence Jones protein) and may give false-positive reactions in highly buffered alkaline urine. Reagent strips that detect lower concentrations of protein (albumin) have also been developed. These maybe useful in the evaluation of microalbuminuria (exertion rates of albumin of 15 μg/min to 150 μg/min or 20 mg/day to 200 mg/day) below the level of overt proteinuria.

The evaluation of low but abnormal excretion rates of albumin aids in early detection of diabetic glomerulopathy and in assessment of risk for complications of cardiovascular and cerebrovascular disease. Variations in the concentration of urine (as determined by specific gravity or osmolality) greatly influence the ability of these strips to detect abnormal proteinuria. For example, a patient excreting 1,000 mg of protein per day (a clearly abnormal value) in a total urine volume of 5,000 ml/day with a specific gravity of 1.006 (a water diuresis) would have a urinary protein concentration of only 20 mg/dl, a value barely detectable as abnormal by the conventional dye-impregnated paper strip method. However, an individual excreting 150 mg/day in a urine volume of 500 ml/day with a specific gravity of 1.030 (a severe antidiuresis) would have a urine protein concentration of 30 mg/dl, a value that would be considered suspiciously abnormal by the conventional dye-impregnated strip technique. Similar caveats apply to the more quantitative colorimetric and turbidimetric methods. However, these latter techniques have increased sensitivity (down to 5 to 10 mg/dl) and react more equally to a broader class of proteins. Thus they are preferred when low levels of proteinuria are expected, quantitative results are desired, or abnormal proteins other than albumin (e.g., globulins) are being investigated.

Hematuria, hemoglobinuria, or myoglobinuria could confound the interpretation of proteinuria (see Chapter 101), but these can be accounted for by examination of the urine sediment and/or plasma color and by the performance of cellulose acetate electrophoresis of urine if needed.

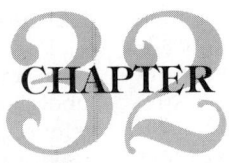

Urine samples for evaluation of proteinuria should be collected early in the morning when the patient arises and again after several hours of upright ambulation. In this fashion, the orthostatic component of proteinuria will be manifest. Because vigorous exercise and high fever produce proteinuria in otherwise healthy individuals, it is best to avoid collecting urine under these circumstances or to repeat values at a later time if abnormal proteinuria is detected under these conditions. Similar caveats apply to other patients with acute illnesses, such as acute myocardial infarction. It is important to know of the situations that may produce a false positive test for proteinuria (see Chapter 101) lest unnecessary investigations be initiated.

When heavy proteinuria (e.g., more than 100 mg/dl) is detected in screening by the conventional dye-impregnated paper strip method, it is useful to quantitate urinary protein by timed urine samples (e.g., 24 hours) or by comparing the concentration of protein (in mg/dl) with a filtration marker, such as creatinine (in mg/dl).

COMPOSITION OF URINARY PROTEIN

Urinary protein is derived from three sources: (a) plasma proteins filtered by the glomerulus and escaping reabsorption by the proximal tubule, (b) renal tissue proteins secreted by tubular cells or leaking into the urine by virtue of tubular cell damage, and (c) urinary tract proteins, secreted by the urinary bladder, urethra, or accessory glands or leaking into the urine as a result of tissue injury or inflammation. The proteins in normal urine consist of about 50% plasma protein and 50% renal and urinary tract protein. Albumin is the principal plasma protein in normal urine (Table 32.1). The rest of the plasma protein in urine consists chiefly of low-molecular-weight proteins: immunoglobulin, principally IgG and IgA, and the κ and λ light chains of immunoglobulin. Tamm-Horsfall mucoprotein is the principal renal tissue protein in the urine and accounts for about 40 mg/day. This mucoprotein is synthesized by the cells of the ascending limb of Henle's loop and is the major constituent of urinary casts.

Inflammation in the urinary tract may increase the fraction of tissue proteins and immunoglobulin in urine, and exercise increases the plasma protein fraction in urine. Specific disease states affect the profile and composition of urinary protein.

CLASSIFICATION OF ABNORMAL PROTEINURIA

Abnormal proteinuria generally is classified according to the underlying pathophysiologic disturbance responsible for proteinuria. However, other approaches to classification may be used, such as pattern with respect to quantity (e.g., nephrotic versus nonnephrotic), time and posture (constant versus orthostatic), or associated urinary abnormality (isolated proteinuria versus proteinuria with hematuria).

Pathophysiologic Types of Proteinuria

There are four principal pathophysiologic types of abnormal proteinuria: (a) glomerular, (b) tubular, (c) overflow, and (d) tissue proteinuria. Glomerular proteinuria results from a perturbation of the mechanisms responsible for maintenance of normal glomerular permselectivity to plasma proteins (see Chapter 4). Plasma proteins, chiefly albumin and globulins, are found in the urine. The quantity of abnormal proteinuria may range from slightly above normal (200 mg/day) to massive (more than 20 g/day). Proteinuria above 3.5 g/day/1.73 m^2 of body surface area (in an adult) is often referred to as *nephrotic proteinuria.* In a child, urine protein excretion rates above 40 mg/m^2/day are regarded as in the nephrotic range. Protein excretion below 3.5 g/day/1.73 m^2 of body surface area is referred to as *nonnephrotic proteinuria.* If the ratio of urinary protein (in milligrams) to urinary creatinine (in milligrams) in a random voided urine is greater than 3.0, the proteinuria generally can be considered as falling within the nephrotic range.

Tubular proteinuria results from inadequate reabsorption of normally filtered proteins, although glomerular and tubular proteinuria can coexist (see Chapter 7.5). Tubular proteinuria usually consists of low-molecular-weight proteins (e.g., as β_2-microglobulin), which migrate in the α and β regions by electrophoresis. The quantity of protein excretion can vary widely

TABLE 32.1. Protein Composition of Normal Urine

	Urinary Protein		
	Excretion Rate		Percentage of Total
	μg/min	*mg/day*	*%*
Plasma proteins			
Albumin	8 (4–15)	12 (5–25)	15
IgC	2 (1–3)	3 (2–7)	
IgA (secretory)	0.7 (0.2–2.0)	1 (0.4–3.0)	5.4
IgM	0.2	0.3	
Light chains	2.6	3.7	4.6
κ		2.3	
λ		1.4	
β_2-Microglobulin	0.8	0.12	<0.2
Other plasma proteins and enzymes (total)	13.8	≈20	25
Subtotal of all plasma proteins	27.5 μg/min	40 mg/day	50%
Nonplasma proteins			
Tamm-Horsfall protein	28	40	50
Other renal-derived proteins	<0.7	<1	<1
Subtotal of nonplasma proteins	28 μg/min	40 mg/day	50%
Total protein	55 ±17 μg/min (1SD)	80 ± 24 mg/day (1SD)	100%

but is generally in the range of 200 mg to 2.0 g/day. The ratio of urinary protein to urinary creatinine in random samples is generally below 3.0.

Overflow proteinuria is caused by the filtration across the glomerular capillaries and incomplete tubular reabsorption of a plasma protein that, by virtue of its molecular dimensions (size, shape, and flexibility) is readily filtered across the capillary wall. Urinary protein excretion increases because of an increase in the plasma concentration of the protein and/or a biochemical change in a plasma protein that results in enhanced glomerular permeability across a normal glomerular capillary wall. Examples of overflow proteinuria include hemoglobinuria, myoglobinuria, and the excretion of monoclonal light-chain fragments of immunoglobulin. The abnormal protein can be readily detected by electrophoresis, immunodiffusion, or immunoprecipitation. The amount of abnormal protein in urine may vary widely from trace amounts to massive quantities.

Tissue proteinuria is generally associated with some structural, inflammatory, or neoplastic abnormality in the urinary tract. It seldom gives rise to heavy proteinuria and usually is found in amounts less than 500 mg/day.

Patterns of Proteinuria

As stated previously, proteinuria may be nephrotic or nonnephrotic based on whether protein excretion rates fall above or below an arbitrary value of 3.5 g/day/1.73 m^2 of body surface area. It should be emphasized that protein excretion rates that are above the threshold value of 3.5 g/day (or 40 mg/m^2/hr in children) have little diagnostic value. However, massive proteinuria (more than 20 g/day) is more likely to be associated with glomerular disease of amyloidosis, focal and segmental glomerulosclerosis (including the collapsing variant), and membranous glomerulonephritis. Nevertheless, prognosis in terms of risk of progressive renal failure is directly related to the quantity of protein excreted in the urine, over a broad range of values. The pattern of proteinuria with respect to time and posture, although of little diagnostic value, does have some prognostic significance. Transient proteinuria, generally appearing in connection with an acute illness, is a reversible phenomenon and by definition seldom indicates a serious, underlying renal lesion. Intermittent proteinuria is a condition that waxes and wanes on serial observation and may have greater pathologic significance, particularly when the episodes of abnormal proteinuria are heavy. Persistent proteinuria, a repeatedly documentable form of proteinuria, is often a feature of a more serious disease. Constant proteinuria occurs when abnormal proteinuria is detected both during overnight recumbency and during quiet upright ambulation. Constant proteinuria has greater pathologic significance than orthostatic proteinuria, in which abnormal qualitative proteinuria occurs only during upright ambulation. Orthostatic proteinuria, when fixed and reproducible, has a benign, long-term prognosis even though renal biopsies reveal various nonspecific abnormalities in 10% to 60% of patients. When orthostatic proteinuria is accompanied by definite abnormalities in the urinary sediment (e.g., hematuria or hypertension), the prognosis is less certainly benign. A high percentage, perhaps 70% to 80%, of patients with fixed and reproducible orthostatic proteinuria will gradually return to normal over many years. Persistence of orthostatic proteinuria for well over 20 years with a benign outcome has often been documented. However, an evolution of orthostatic proteinuria into constant proteinuria signifies a transition into more progressive disease.

Isolated proteinuria is the term applied when an abnormal rate of excretion of protein is the *only* abnormal finding in the urine. The excretion of erythrocytes and other cells is normal. Hyaline and granular casts may be found but are usually not in abundance. Isolated proteinuria may be of glomerular, tubular, overflow, or tissue origin. Asymptomatic proteinuria is said to occur when the patient has no other abnormal history, physical examination, or laboratory findings pointing to disease of the kidney or urinary tract. The patterns of proteinuria described do not necessarily remain fixed in an individual but may evolve from one type to another over time or under the influence of treatment.

When the composition of urine protein is studied in patients with nephrotic range proteinuria, several patterns emerge. Selective proteinuria is present when albumin (and other proteins of similar molecular dimensions) are the principle proteins detected. Nonselective proteinuria is present when proteins of large molecular dimension (e.g., globulins) are present along with albumin. The relative urinary clearance of IgG to transferrin is a convenient way of measuring selectively. An IgG-to-transferrin clearance ratio of less than 0.1 indicates highly selective proteinuria, whereas a ratio greater than 0.2 indicate poorly selective proteinuria.

Minimal changes disease, at least in children, is characterized by highly selective proteinuria, whereas other structural glomerular diseases, such as focal and segmental glomerulosclerosis, are associated with poorly selective proteinuria.

DIFFERENTIAL DIAGNOSIS OF ABNORMAL PROTEINURIA

The causes of abnormal proteinuria are many and varied and are best considered according to the underlying pathophysiologic disturbance. Table 32.2 provides a list of disease entities, or pathologic states, that may cause one or more of the various pathophysiologic types of abnormal proteinuria. These entities are discussed in greater detail in other chapters.

APPROACH TO EVALUATION OF ABNORMAL PROTEINURIA

When abnormal proteinuria has been detected by a conventional qualitative test on a random urine specimen, the following three-phase approach is taken: (a) initial confirmation and screening studies, (b) preliminary investigation, and (c) definitive evaluation.

Initial Confirmation and Screening of Abnormal Proteinuria

In addition to a thorough history and physical examination regarding the kidney and urinary tract, the first approach to a patient with an abnormal test result for qualitative proteinuria is to assess the likelihood of a false positive result (e.g., excessively concentrated urine, specific gravity 1.026 and above, and highly buffered alkaline urine) and to determine whether the urine specimen was collected following vigorous exercise or if it accompanies a high fever. The urinary sediment should be examined carefully, preferably using phase contrast microscopy or supravital staining. If the likelihood of a false positive test is low, if the degree of abnormality is great (e.g., protein more than 300 mg/dl), or if the urinary sediment is abnormal, further preliminary investigations should be undertaken without delay. If the qualitatively abnormal proteinuria has been detected by dye-impregnated paper strips, it should be confirmed with another test based on a different principle, such as precipitation

TABLE 32.2. Differential Diagnosis of Proteinuria Based on Pathophysiologic Mechanism

- Glomerular proteinuria
  - Primary glomerular disease
    - Minimal change lesion
    - Mesangial proliferative GN (including IgA and IgM nephropathy)
    - Focal and segmental glomerulosclerosis
    - Membranous GN
    - Mesangiocapillary GN
    - Fibrillary glomerulonephritis
    - Crescentic glomerulonephritis
  - Secondary glomerular disease
    - Medications (mercurials, gold compounds, heroin, penicillamine, probenecid, captopril, lithium, NSAID)
    - Allergens (bee sting, pollen, milk)
    - Infectious (bacterial, viral, protozoal, fungal, helminthic)
    - Neoplastic (solid tumors, leukemia)
    - Multisystem (SLE, Henoch-Schönlein purpura, amyloidosis)
    - Heredofamilial (diabetes mellitus, congenital nephrotic syndrome, Fabry's disease, Alport's syndrome)
    - Other (transplant rejection, reflux nephropathy, toxemia of pregnancy)
    - Other glomerular proteinuria
      - Postexercise proteinuria
      - Benign orthostatic proteinuria
      - Febrile proteinuria
- Tubular proteinuria
  - Toxins and drugs
    - Endogenous
      - Light-chain damage to proximal tubule
      - Lysozyme (myelomonocytic leukemia)
    - Exogenous
      - Mercury
      - Lead
      - Cadmium
      - Outdated tetracycline
      - Arginine or lysine infusions
  - Tubulointerstitial disease (chiefly and predominantly involving proximal nephron)
    - Lupus erythematosus
    - Acute hypersensitivity interstitial nephritis
    - Acute bacterial pyelonephritis
    - Obstructive uropathy
    - Chronic interstitial nephritis (e.g., Sjögren's syndrome, Balkan endemic nephropathy, tubulointerstitial nephritis with uveitis)
    - Fanconi syndrome
- Overflow proteinuria
  - Multiple myeloma
  - Light chain disease
  - Amyloidosis (see also Glomerular proteinuria)
  - Hemoglobinuria
  - Myoglobinuria
  - Certain pancreatic or colon carcinomas (rare)
- Tissue proteinuria
  - Acute inflammation of urinary tract
  - Uroepithelial tumors

NSAID, nonsteroidal antiinflammatory drugs; SLE, systemic lupus erythematosus.

with sulfosalicylic acid or heat and acetic acid and the results compared. If a false-positive or transient proteinuria is suspected, repeat qualitative observations should be made before initiating a series of preliminary investigations designed to establish the most likely pathophysiologic abnormality responsible for the proteinuria.

Preliminary Investigations

The extent and nature of preliminary investigations that should be undertaken in patients with confirmed abnormal proteinuria are most appropriately guided by three critical observations made during the initial approach, including the history and physical examination. These observations are (a) the findings in the urinary sediment (especially hematuria), (b) the patient's age and the coexistence of abnormal findings in the history and physical examination that would suggest the presence of renal disease (e.g., diabetes mellitus) or a specific cause of proteinuria (e.g., carpal tunnel syndrome, anemia, bone pain, or hypertension), and (c) the extent of the qualitative abnormality and the magnitude of proteinuria as assessed by the dye-impregnated paper strip method compared with other methods.

If proteinuria is accompanied by hematuria, two questions must be answered (see Chapter 28): (a) Is the degree of proteinuria out of proportion to the degree of hematuria? and (b) Is the hematuria dysmorphic or normomorphic? Heavy or mild proteinuria in the presence of microscopic dysmorphic hematuria indicates a glomerular source (Table 32.2). Proteinuria without hematuria may be of the glomerular, tubular, or overflow type. Red cell casts in the urinary sediment have the same significance as dysmorphic erythrocytes. Severe pyuria, bacteriuria, and proteinuria may all develop in connection with infection-induced inflammation.

Patients older than 40, especially those with concomitant unexplained renal failure, anemia, hypercalcemia, neuropathy, weight loss, or bone pain, should be suspected of having an overflow type of proteinuria owing to the excessive production of monoclonal light-chain fragments of immunoglobulin. All such individuals should be assessed using immunodiffusion or immunoprecipitation analysis of urine for monoclonal light chains. Qualitative tests for Bence Jones proteins are relatively insensitive and may give false-positive results in tubular proteinuria, in which abnormal excretion of polyclonal light chains is common. In addition, when results from the dye-impregnated paper strip method is less positive than other precipitation tests, there is the possibility of abnormal light chain excretion because the dye-impregnated paper strips are less sensitive than precipitation methods to abnormal amounts of excreted globulins. Younger patients should be studied for orthostatic proteinuria by testing urine specimens after overnight recumbency and after 4 to 6 hours of quiet upright ambulation. Other clinical or urinalysis findings also will dictate the specifics of the approach to preliminary investigation. For example, glycosuria may direct an investigation for diabetes mellitus or other manifestations of a proximal tubular reabsorptive defect. With retinopathy, one would investigate diabetic glomerulosclerosis. A thorough history for toxin exposure (especially lead, cadmium, mercury, or gold) and drugs (especially analgesics, nonsteroidal antiinflammatory drugs, or penicillamine) must be undertaken in every case. The specific symptoms or signs associated with disease (Table 32.2) should be sought where appropriate.

All patients with confirmed, qualitatively abnormal proteinuria should have the following tests performed, in addition to a complete urinalysis and urinary sediment examination: (a) complete blood count, including differential; (b) serum creatinine and blood urea nitrogen; (c) serum albumin and total protein; and (d) serum electrolytes and calculation of the anion gap (multiple myeloma may reduce anion gap). As indicated previously, tests for light chain excretion should be conducted in patients older than 40, and tests for orthostatic proteinuria should be done in patients younger than 40.

Additional tests included in a biochemical profile (e.g., calcium, phosphate, uric acid, bilirubin, alkaline phosphatase, transaminases, cholesterol, lactic dehydrogenase) are optional. However, such complete biochemical screening should be done if any of the required tests results are abnormal.

Quantitation of the magnitude of proteinuria by 24-hour collections or by calculation of the urinary protein-to-creatinine ratio on random urine specimens should be conducted as a routine part of the preliminary investigations. If nephrotic-range proteinuria is found, especially with a depressed serum albumin concentration, increased cholesterol, or edema, further investigation should be directed to glomerular proteinuria and nephrotic syndrome if abnormal monoclonal light-chain excretion has been excluded.

Evaluation of the urinary tract is probably not needed initially unless there is a history of recurrent urolithiasis or urinary tract infection or if renal masses are noted in the physical examination. Ultrasound examination is preferred as the initial step, especially if the serum creatinine concentration is elevated, because intravenous urography using radiocontrast media may exacerbate renal disease. In younger patients with recurrent urinary tract infection, one should consider an investigation of the urinary tract for vesicoureteral reflux, such as a cystourethrogram.

Definitive Evaluation

The subsequent evaluation of patients with abnormal proteinuria to determine the precise cause and mechanism will depend on the results from the initial and preliminary investigations.

If abnormal proteinuria is less than 3 g/day, monoclonal light-chain excretion can be excluded, and the serum albumin is normal, an evaluation for tubular proteinuria is in order. This is especially true if preliminary investigations reveal findings suggestive of Fanconi syndrome, such as lysozymuria, glucosuria, hypophosphatemia, hypouricemia, and non–anion gap acidosis. This evaluation is best accomplished using urinary protein electrophoresis and/or comparing the concentrations of albumin and β_2-microglobulin in urine samples. A low ratio of albumin to β_2-microglobulin indicates defective tubular reabsorption, and the disorders listed under tubular proteinuria in Table 32.2 should be considered. Normal values for the ratio of albumin to β_2-microglobulin are 50 to 200 (average is 100). Patients with tubular proteinuria show values ranging from 1 to 14, whereas patients with glomerular disorders show values ranging from 1,000 to 14,000. Both albumin and β_2-microglobulin can be measured using immunoprecipitation, immunodiffusion, or radioimmunoassay methods. The combination of glomerular and tubular proteinuria (e.g., nephrotic-range proteinuria, elevated β_2- microglobulin excretion) usually implies tubulointerstitial damage accompanying glomerular disease and suggests a worse prognosis.

A reduced anion gap (more than 8 mmol/L), elevated globulin concentration, abnormal monoclonal light-chain excretion (κ or λ), or a greatly elevated erythrocyte sedimentation rate demands an investigation for multiple myeloma or amyloidosis. This would include bone marrow aspiration and biopsy, plasma protein electrophoresis, serum immunoglobulin quantitation, metabolic bone survey, and perhaps an abdominal fat pad or rectal biopsy for amyloidosis.

If nephrotic-range proteinuria is present, particularly when the serum albumin concentration is decreased and serum total cholesterol concentration is increased, a renal biopsy should be considered unless the nature of the disease provoking the nephrotic syndrome is obvious from the clinical examination and compatible with the known natural history of the disease (e.g., diabetic nephropathy). When no useful information is expected to be obtained from an examination of renal biopsy tissue, the performance of renal biopsy should be considered investigational (see Chapter 99).

If nonnephrotic constant proteinuria is present and all of the studies point to a glomerular origin (e.g., hematuria in the urinary sediment, elevated ratio of albumin to β_2-macroglobulin, negative test results for monoclonal light chains), it is more difficult to decide whether to perform a renal biopsy. A renal biopsy can be deferred if proteinuria is between 200 and 1,000 mg/day, the urinary sediment is benign, renal function is completely normal, and hypertension is absent. All other situations occurring with nonnephrotic proteinuria of glomerular origin are probably best assessed by renal biopsy unless contraindications to the performance of this procedure exist (see Chapter 96), the disease causing the proteinuria is evident on clinical examination, or the diagnosis can be established by other means (e.g., rectal biopsy for amyloidosis).

Pure, fixed, and reproducible orthostatic proteinuria accompanied by normal serum creatinine, blood pressure, and urinary sediment need not be further evaluated but should be followed at 6-month to 1-year intervals to ensure that evolution to a constant proteinuria has not occurred.

Selected Readings

Cameron JS. The patient with proteinuria and hematuria. In: Davison AM, Cameron JS, Gruenfeld JP, et al, eds. *Oxford Textbook of Clinical Nephrology*, 2nd ed. Oxford: Oxford Medical Publications, 1998:444–445.

An excellent overview.

Cameron JS, Glassock RJ, eds. *The Nephrotic Syndrome*. New York: Marcel Dekker, 1988.

A definitive treatise on proteinuria and nephrotic syndrome.

Mallick NP, Short CD. The clinical approach to hematuria and proteinuria. In: Cameron JS, Davison AM, Grunfeld JP, et al, eds. *Oxford Textbook of Clinical Nephrology*. Oxford: Oxford Medical Publications, 1992:227–239.

An excellent overview with algorithms.

CHAPTER 33

Hypertension

Unini Odama, Nauman Tarif, and George L. Bakris

The detailed definition of hypertension, its accurate measurement, the clinical and laboratory evaluation of a patient with hypertension, and the identifiable causes of hypertension are discussed in Chapter 61. Hypertension is defined by the Joint National Committee Report VI (JNC VI) as an arterial pressure of 140/90 mm Hg or greater. Both unilateral and bilateral renal parenchymal disease can cause this problem. Chronic renal parenchymal disease from various etiologies is the most common secondary form of arterial hypertension. In fact, it accounts for about 50% to 60% of all secondary causes of hypertension. It is a major etiologic risk factor among individuals with renal parenchymal disease; indeed, hypertension and especially poorly controlled hypertension in such individuals can hasten the decline of renal function.

Hypertension as an etiology for end-stage renal disease (ESRD) development has been questioned, and many authors do not believe that essential hypertension per se causes renal failure. Among African-Americans, hypertension may cause renal failure, but these patients may have other concomitant, unidentified, renal diseases such as glomerulonephritides to account for their renal failure. However, this does not preclude hypertension as being a contributing factor to ESRD development because in many cases it accompanies renal failure and, if uncontrolled, leads to a quicker decline in renal function. This latter observation is exemplified in an analysis of the Modification of Dietary Protein in Renal Disease trial (MDRD). In this trial, more than 80% of patients with renal failure had hypertension, an association that correlated positively with the degree of preexisting renal insufficiency.

Hypertension resulting from renal parenchymal disease is usually seen in the presence of bilateral rather than unilateral kidney disease. The mechanisms that generate elevation in blood pressure in most of these cases relate to volume overload and altered sodium homeostasis. In addition, areas of intrarenal ischemia lead to activation of neurohumoral systems (i.e., renin-angiotensin-aldosterone system and sympathetic nervous system) that also contribute to increases in blood pressure.

However, in certain cases unilateral renal disease such as cystic diseases, tumors, obstructive uropathy, hydronephrosis, tuberculosis, and unilateral vesicoureteral reflux (VUR) may lead to hypertension, as evident by its elimination after nephrectomy. The etiology of hypertension in unilateral VUR is unclear. In a study of 86 nephrectomy specimens from patients with unilateral VUR, focal segmental glomerulosclerosis (FSGS) was found in 18 (21%) of the specimens; FSGS was further associated with proteinuria and hypertension in these patients. In a separate study that followed 294 patients with unilateral and bilateral VUR, hypertension was found in the patients with unilateral disease but was more frequent in patients with bilateral VUR and severe parenchymal disease.

Regardless of the etiology, it is clear that reducing blood pressure to levels below 140/90 mm Hg in healthy patients and below 130/85 mm Hg in those with renal disease or diabetes reduces cardiovascular disease risk and renal disease progression. However, only 27% of all nonelderly people with a diagnosis of hypertension are adequately controlled; that is, their blood pressure is less than 140/90 mm Hg. Moreover, if you include those older than 65 and those at high risk (patients with diabetes and renal insufficiency) who require blood pressure reduction to less than 130/85 mm Hg, fewer than 3% of the cases would be controlled. These sobering facts have resulted in a flattening of the previously declining mortality rates from cardiovascular events associated with hypertension treatment. Moreover, this degree of blood pressure reduction has never had an effect on the incidence of renal failure in the United States.

Other studies indicate that blood pressure needs to be reduced to lower levels to maximally protect against declines in renal function. In the first renal trial to randomize and assess the impact of different levels of blood pressure, the MDRD trial, patients with renal insufficiency and proteinuria who were randomized to a mean arterial pressure of less than 92 mm Hg manifested significantly slower rates of decline in renal function when compared with those randomized to mean pressures between 102 and 106 mm Hg. Moreover, the subgroup of African-Americans randomized to the lower blood pressure in this trial also had better renal outcomes. The observation that lower levels of blood pressure are required to maximally slow renal disease progression is also seen in a *post hoc* analysis of the Multiple Risk Factor Intervention Trial (MRFIT). In this trial of more than 330,000 people with hypertension, the relative risk for development of ESRD started to climb significantly when the average blood pressure rose above 127/82 mm Hg. However, the question of whether further reductions in blood pressure to lower levels will optimally slow or stop progression of renal disease will be definitively answered by the results of the ongoing African-American Study of Kidney Disease (AASK) trial due to be completed in 2002.

A new lower level of blood pressure control is also recommended for those with diabetic renal disease. Evidence from

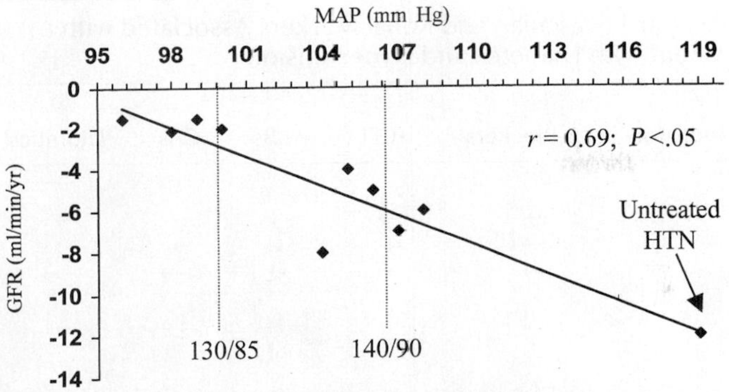

Figure 33.1. A summary of clinical trials, each 3 years' or more duration in diabetic and nondiabetic persons with renal insufficiency, that demonstrate the importance of the degree of blood pressure reduction. Each datum point represents one trial. (Adapted from Bakris GL. *Diabetes Res Clin Pract* 1998;39(Suppl):35–42.)

post hoc analyses of prospective studies in diabetic nephropathy as well as meta-analyses of available data supports the notion that arterial pressure must be reduced to 130/85 mm Hg or less to maximally slow or prevent progression of nephropathy (Fig. 33.1).

Last, no discussion about blood pressure level would be complete without a discussion of the J curve. Since its inception in 1979, the concept that reducing diastolic blood pressure to levels below 85 mm Hg results in a paradoxical increase in cardiovascular mortality has been controversial. However, a J curve exists among patients with established symptomatic coronary artery disease or unstable angina, as well as those who are in the immediate postmyocardial infarction period. A *post hoc* analysis of the only clinical trial to date to randomize to two levels of blood pressure, the MDRD trial, demonstrates no significant increase in cardiovascular events among those with renal insufficiency, proteinuria, and diastolic blood pressures of less than 85 mm Hg. Further evidence to support the absence of a J curve in the general population comes from the Hypertension Optimal Treatment (HOT) trial. This trial did not have a higher cardiovascular event rate in the group randomized to a diastolic blood pressure of 80 mm Hg. Moreover, in the high-risk group of diabetics, a higher cardiovascular event rate at a diastolic blood pressure goal of less than 85 mm Hg was not seen in the United Kingdom Prospective Diabetes Study (UKPDS) trial. Thus each patient needs to be treated in the context of these observations. In the absence of any clear evidence of coronary disease or unstable angina, high-risk patients such as African-Americans and those with diabetes or renal insufficiency should have their blood pressures aggressively reduced to less than 130/85 mm Hg.

Given this background it is important that a physician have a logical and methodical approach to the treatment of hypertension. This chapter presents an approach to the treatment of hypertension predicated on the JNC VI. This chapter focuses on the level to which blood pressure should be reduced as well as how to achieve these lower blood pressure levels and still maximize risk reduction.

Detailed discussion on the pathophysiology of blood pressure control is found in Chapter 59, on genetics of hypertension in Chapter 60, on clinical aspects of essential hypertension and its management in Chapter 61, on renovascular hypertension in Chapter 62, on endocrine hypertension in Chapter 63, on pediatric hypertension in Chapter 64, on geriatric hypertension in Chapter 65, and on hypertension in African-Americans in Chapter 66.

TREATMENT OF THE HYPERTENSIVE PATIENT

The goal of treatment and management of hypertension in the general population is to reduce morbidity and mortality by the least intrusive means possible. All mortality trials to date demonstrate that a reduction of pressure to less than 140/90 mm Hg will greatly reduce the incidence of strokes and other cardiovascular events, including myocardial infarction and heart failure, and somewhat slow the progression of renal disease. Lifestyle modification and/or pharmacologic therapy achieve this goal.

Adequate assessment and management of the hypertensive patient begins by obtaining a concise medical history and by properly measuring blood pressure (see Chapter 61). Evaluating patients with hypertension has three objectives: (a) to identify known causes of high blood pressure; (b) to assess the presence or absence of target organ damage and cardiovascular disease, the extent of the disease, and the response to therapy; and (c) to identify other cardiovascular risk factors or concomitant disorders that may define prognosis and guide treatment.

SELECTION OF INITIAL DRUG THERAPY

Selection of an initial antihypertensive agent and add-on antihypertensive medications for a given patient depends on many factors, including a risk factor profile (e.g., smoking, obesity) and presence of comorbid conditions (e.g., asthma, gout). Thus patients may be grouped as uncomplicated and complicated. The remainder of this discussion is based on these terms.

Uncomplicated Patients

An uncomplicated patient is one with an absence of comorbid conditions, such as being from a particular race, or presence of dyslipidemia, obesity or surrogate markers of target organ disease such as left ventricular hypertrophy (LVH) or microalbuminuria. Many trials have been carried out in such patients. A review of all long-term, randomized, double-blind controlled trials reveal that diuretics and to a lesser extent β-blockers are the classes of medications shown to reduce mortality from vascular events (strokes) and to a lesser extent coronary events in persons with uncomplicated hypertension.

Complicated Patients

A complicated patient has the presence of comorbid conditions, such as older age, particular race, smoking, dyslipidemia, obesity, or surrogate markers of end-organ disease such as LVH or microalbuminuria. These comorbid conditions in a persons with hypertension mandate tailoring antihypertensive therapy to reduce cardiovascular risk and renal disease progression. Four prominent risk factors associated with a high cardiovascular mortality are LVH, microalbuminuria, dyslipidemia, and renal dysfunction. Presence of these risk factors must be considered when choosing antihypertensive medications. A summary of the effects of various antihypertensive agents is summarized in Table 33.1.

Left Ventricular Hypertrophy

LVH results from chronic elevations in arterial pressure causing cardiac myocyte hypertrophy and remodeling of the coronary resistance vessels. LVH is an independent risk factor for predicting an adverse cardiovascular event. In the Framingham study, there was a significant relationship between the presence of LVH and a high cardiovascular morbidity and mortality. In

TABLE 33.1. Effects of Antihypertensive Therapy on Metabolic, Cardiovascular, and Renal Markers Associated with Increased Morbidity and/or Mortality in the Patient with Diabetes and Hypertension

	Central Agonists	α-Blockers	α,β-Blocker	Vasodilator	β-Blockers	ACEI	ARBs	CAs	Diuretics
Metabolic									
Cholesterol (LDL)	→	→	→	→	→*↑	→	→	→	→↑
Insulin resistance	→	↓	→↑	→↑	→↑	↓	↓	→	→↑
Glucose control	→	→	→	→	→↑	→↑	→	*↑→	→↓
Cardiovascular									
Left ventricular hypertrophy	↓	↓	↓	→↑	↓	↓	↓	↓	→↑
Renal									
Microalbuminuria	→	→	→↓	→	→↓	↓	↓	†↓→	→↓

*Only β-blockers with intrinsic sympathomimetic activity; only when used at high dosages (e.g., 480 mg/day diliazem, 480 mg/day verapamil, 90 mg/day nifedipine.
†Only nondihydropyridine calcium antagonists (CAs, verapamil, diltiazem).
Note: This table summarizes the general trends in the literature.
HDL, high-density lipoprotein; LDL, low-density lipoprotein; ACEI, angiotensin-converting enzyme inhibitor; ARB, angiotensin II–receptor antagonist; CA, calcium antagonist; →, no effect; ↑, increase; ↓, decrease.

the Treatment of Mild Hypertension Study (TOMHS) nutritional hygienic measures such as weight loss, reduced salt and alcohol, intake and exercise were effective by themselves to regress LVH. However, the presence of a diuretic added to the benefit.

There are pharmacologic differences in the effects of various drugs on the degree of LVH regression. A meta-analysis of randomized controlled trials revealed that angiotensin-converting enzyme (ACE) inhibitors were the most successful for regressing LVH followed by calcium antagonists, diuretics and β-blockers in that order. The most important factor responsible for this beneficial effect was the prolonged reduction of systolic blood pressure. In contrast, direct vasodilators such as minoxidil and hydralazine, which work through opening [K^+] channels, do not reduce LVH. This is thought to result from profound sympathetic stimulation and subsequent increase in cardiac workload. Thus if these agents are used to lower arterial pressure, they should always be used in the presence of a β-blocker to reduce sympathetic activity and a diuretic to counteract their effect on sodium retention.

Microalbuminuria

Microalbuminuria is a predictor of cardiovascular and renal death in diabetic patients. However, it is weaker as a predictor of renal disease progression in nondiabetic, hypertensive patients. Frank albuminuria is a risk factor for cardiovascular disease and progression of renal failure. In fact, in the presence of albuminuria, more aggressive control of hypertension is required.

Hypertension is commonly present in patients with type 2 diabetes. Importantly, a large number of these patients have cardiovascular events before progressing to ESRD. Reduction of hypertension has proven beneficial not only for reducing renal disease progression but also for reducing cardiovascular morbidity and microangiopathic complications in such patients. A blunted rise or reduction in microalbuminuria is associated with a slowed progression of renal disease. The class of antihypertensive medications known to have the most potent effects on microalbuminuria reduction is the ACE inhibitors. These agents reduce albuminuria by reducing intraglomerular pressure as well as decreasing glomerular size selectivity. The effects of different classes of antihypertensive agents on microalbuminuria, as well as related metabolic parameters, are summarized in Table 33.1.

It should be clear that any agent or group of agents that adequately lowers arterial pressure to levels less than 130/85 mm Hg will slow progression of nephropathy. From the available clinical data, both ACE inhibitors and nondihydropyridine calcium antagonists reduce albuminuria and together have additive antialbuminuric effects independent of further reductions in blood pressure. In addition, these agents are generally well tolerated. Therefore ACE inhibitors should be first-line treatment of hypertension in diabetes and included in all "antihypertensive cocktails."

The role of angiotensin-receptor blockers for treatment of diabetic nephropathy is unclear at this time. However, all animal studies suggest that these agents will be as good as ACE inhibitors in slowing the progression of renal disease. This class has a significantly lower incidence of cough and hyperkalemia compared with an ACE inhibitor.

Renal Dysfunction

From the available data, it is clear that aggressive blood pressure reduction (less than 130/85 mm Hg) is needed to maximally slow progression of renal disease, especially among patients with elevated serum creatinine (1.4 mg/dl or greater). As previously stated, ACE inhibitors slow the progression of diabetic nephropathy more than other antihypertensive agents, assuming blood pressure is reduced to around 140/90 mm Hg. Their effect on the progression of nondiabetic renal disease is also excellent, although it is more a function of the level to which blood pressure is reduced. Moreover, ACE inhibitors tend to reverse endothelial dysfunction in the coronary bed.

Despite this evidence from many long-term clinical trials, there is a general fear by clinicians to use ACE inhibitors in such patients. This stems from a potential rise in serum creatinine following the use of these drugs. Although this may be a concern, it should be worrisome only if the serum potassium rises or if the creatinine continues to climb after a month of therapy. The time sequence and causes of this rise in serum creatinine following ACE inhibitor administration are shown and explained in Fig. 33.2. It is common to see reductions of 5% to 10% in the glomerular filtration rate (GFR) within 1 to 4 weeks of ACE inhibitor initiation. Long-term clinical trials have confirmed that this reduction in renal function plateaus within a month. Moreover, after ACE inhibitors were discontinued following 10 years of therapy, GFR returned to baseline.

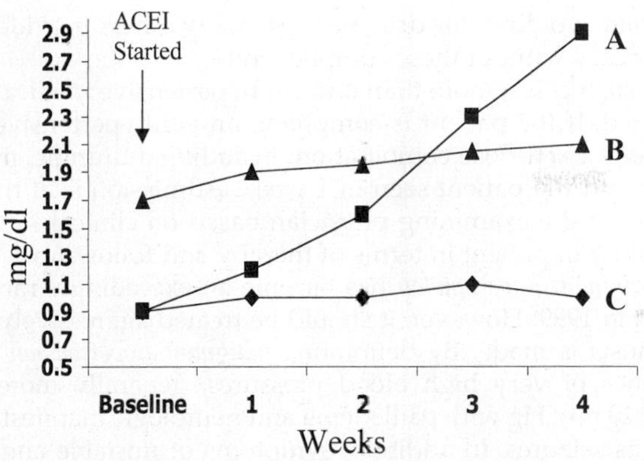

Figure 33.2. The potential effects of an ACE inhibitor on serum creatinine (shown on the ordinate) under three separate scenarios: **A:** person who is either volume depleted or has heart failure with volume depletion or has bilateral renal artery stenosis. **B:** Person with renal insufficiency who is euvolemic. **C;** Normal renal function with euvolemia.

This return to baseline GFR has not been reported with the other class of antihypertensive agent studied.

Thus, although any class of antihypertensive agent may be used to achieve this new recommended lower blood pressure to preserve renal function, the following should be kept in mind. First, blood pressure may not be adequately controlled in patients with renal insufficiency without the use of a diuretic, usually a loop diuretic. Second, various combinations of medications will be needed to reduce blood pressure. One of these combinations should contain an ACE inhibitor. If side effects are noted with the ACE inhibitor, an angiotensin II–receptor blocker may be substituted to ensure renal protection and reduce blood pressure reduction.

Dyslipidemia

Many hypertensive patients are obese and have the presence of diabetes with associated dyslipidemia. A spectrum of metabolic derangements usually accompany essential hypertension and contribute to the development of atherosclerosis. It is clear that reduction of low-density lipoprotein cholesterol reduces mortality. Moreover, low-density lipoprotein cholesterol has been implicated in the genesis of renal injury. Certain classes of antihypertensive agents, such as β-blockers and moderate-dose diuretics, may have an adverse effect on the lipid profile and should not be given for therapy unless absolutely required (Table 33.2). All such patients should be treated for elevated cholesterol, especially if antihypertensive agents are used that worsen the lipid profile.

COMBINATION ANTIHYPERTENSIVE THERAPY

It is well known that an agent from a single antihypertensive drug class will reduce blood pressure to less than 140/90 mm Hg in only 45% to 50% of individuals with hypertension. This percentage is much lower in patients with renal insufficiency or diabetic nephropathy, especially because the target blood pressure in these patients is less than 130/85 mm Hg. Moreover, data from clinical trials show that between 3.5 and 4.2 different antihypertensive medications are required to lower blood pressure to less than 130/85 mm Hg in patients with renal insufficiency. Thus combination therapy using fixed-dose combination drugs provides a way to potentially improve compliance because a person can take the same number of medications in half the pills.

In the early 1960s, fixed-dose combination antihypertensive therapy was introduced with a reserpine–thiazide diuretic combination. Since then, many new fixed-dose combinations have been introduced. Because of their convenient dosing schedule (once daily), these agents are of particular use in high-risk populations that require aggressive reduction of blood pressure.

An ideal way to halt the progression of renal disease and better control arterial pressure is to combine two complementary groups of medications. Lower-than-therapeutic doses of two different drugs are combined in a single pill to reduce arterial pressure to the same level as a higher dosage of an individual component. In this way, they not only are additive for blood pressure reduction, but also have fewer side effects. Moreover, many fixed-dose combinations act to counteract each other's side effects. For example, ACE inhibitors significantly reduce pedal edema associated with dihydropyridine calcium antagonists. In addition, ACE inhibitors mitigate against the adverse lipid effects seen with diuretics. Thus the physician may now select agents with complementary modes of action that minimize side effects and maximize compliance in order to achieve better rates of blood pressure control.

REFRACTORY HYPERTENSION

There are many problems that account for refractory hypertension. Noncompliance with medication is very common. However, this problem primarily results from related side effects of

TABLE 33.2. Factors to Consider before Selection of Antihypertensive Therapy in the Hypertensive Patient

Factor	Useful	Not Useful or Unsafe
Hyperkalemia	Non-DHPCAs, diuretic, α-blocker	ACEI, β-blockers
Renal failure* (GFR <30)	Non-DHPCAs, loop-active diuretic, ? ACEI, ? ARB	High-dose ACEI
Nephrotic syndrome	ACEI with or without non-DHPCAs, ? loop-active diuretic, ? ARB	Minoxidil, hydralazine, ? α-blockers
Coronary artery disease	ACEI, non-DHPCAs, β-blockers	Minoxidil, hydralazine
Autonomic neuropathy	Central α-agonists, ? β-blockers	α-Blockers, hydralazine, minoxidil
Microalbuminuria	ARBs, ACEI, non-DHPCAs	DHPCAs, minoxidil, hydralazine
Side effect profile	ARB, ACEI, CAs	β-Blocker, diuretic, central α-agonists, minoxidil, hydralazine, β-blockers
Peripheral vascular disease	ARBs, ACEI, non-DHPCAs, α-blockers	

*This population usually needs diuretic therapy in addition to other antihypertensive therapy for edema control. All CAs increase renal blood flow in early diabetes, which may not be of benefit. Non-DHPCAs are only subclass of CAs shown to consistently decrease albuminuria.

GFR, glomerular filtration rate; ACEI, angiotensin-converting enzyme inhibitor; CA, calcium antagonist; non-DHPCAs, nondihydropyridine calcium antagonists; ARBs, angiotensin-receptor blockers; central α-agonists, (clonidine, methyldopa).

the medication or cost. A 5-year retrospective chart review of more than 500 patients in a university hypertension clinic demonstrated that more than 88% of the patients referred for refractory hypertension had intolerance of the medications as the most common etiology for not taking the medication as prescribed. Use of fixed-dose combination therapy was able to achieve target blood pressure in more than 90% of these patients with improved tolerability. The most common combinations used were ACE inhibitor/calcium antagonists with or without angiotensin-receptor blocker/diuretics.

Other conditions that contribute to refractory hypertension include use of concomitant medications that interfere with blood pressure control as well as noncompliance because of sexual dysfunction. These are discussed in greater detail.

Concomitant Medications

Failure to adequately reduce blood pressure may be a result of multiple factors, including secondary causes of hypertension and noncompliance. However, a common cause of uncontrolled blood pressure is related to concomitant over-the-counter medications. The two most prevalent types being nonsteroidal antiinflammatory agents, such as ibuprofen, and sympathomimetics, such a pseudoephedrine, in cold preparations. In addition, oral contraceptive and steroid medications will blunt the antihypertensive effect of most agents. In prospective studies, calcium antagonists and to a lesser degree diuretics maintain their antihypertensive effects in the presence of all these medications.

Sexual Dysfunction

A common cause of refractory hypertension in males is noncompliance because of the development of impotence. Almost all medications have been implicated in causing impotence, but the incidence is highest for the central α_2-agonists, diuretics, and β-blockers. Yet in most cases, with the exception of the central α_2-agonists and possibly β-blockers, the drug is only an indirect cause of the problem.

The primary problem of impotence relates to abnormal vascular homeostasis within the penile circulation that results from a large delta change in blood pressure. When blood pressure is dramatically reduced and maintained at lower levels, there is a period of readjustment. In many cases, impotence resolves on its own but may take as long as 4 to 6 months. Thus all patients, including diabetics without neuropathy, should be encouraged to continue taking their medications if arterial pressure is controlled because the problem should resolve.

SITUATIONS THAT REQUIRE IMMEDIATE REDUCTION OF HYPERTENSION

It is important to differentiate between hypertensive urgency and emergency (malignant hypertension). The dosages of the proposed medications are provided in Chapter 61.

Hypertensive urgency is defined as an elevation in arterial pressure in the range of stage III hypertension (diastolic pressure of 110 mm Hg or higher) with either mild or no acute end organ damage and no clinical symptoms. In these situations, it is desirable to reduce blood pressure to 140/90 mm Hg within a few days to a week. This can generally be done in an outpatient setting. Medications routinely used for this include clonidine and labetalol. Use of sublingual nifedipine is absolutely contraindicated for acute pressure reduction. Major complications can result when used in this setting. There should not be a problem avoiding this drug because many others provide similar efficacy without these complications.

In such cases, more than one antihypertensive medication is required. If the patient is compliant, an antihypertensive regimen of a fixed-dose combination, including a diuretic, may be given and the patient seen in 1 week. Admission is at the discretion of the examining physician based on clinical state and reliability of patient in terms of therapy and follow-up.

Malignant hypertension has become an exceedingly rare condition in 1999. However, it should be treated aggressively if the diagnosis is made. By definition, *malignant hypertension* is the presence of very high blood pressures, generally more than 180/120 mm Hg with pailledema and neurologic manifestations such as seizures. In addition, symptoms of unstable angina or impending aortic aneurysm rupture may be present. Treatment of this condition should include intravenous rather than oral medication to reduce the pressure to levels between 140/90 and 160/95 mm Hg. Intravenous nitroprusside, fenoldopam (selective dopamine-1-receptor agonist) or labetalol should be considered as first-line agents. It is desirable to reduce blood pressure by 20% in the first 1 to 2 hours, then slowly over the next 48 hours to between 140/190 and 150/95 mm Hg to avoid cerebral complications such as a hypoperfusion. The selected intravenous medication should be titrated to reduce pressure to the aforementioned goal with the patient monitored. If the patient remains stable, oral antihypertensive agents should then be started and the patient evaluation begun.

SUMMARY

The target blood pressure reduction for the general population is less than 140/90 mm Hg, and for those with renal disease or diabetes, it is less than 130/85 mm Hg. Patients with uncomplicated hypertension should begin therapy with either a diuretic or a β-blocker unless there are compelling or specific reasons to use another class of medications. The reason for this choice is that these agents have been shown to reduce cardiovascular associated mortality in hypertensive patients.

For those with complicated hypertension that require multiple medications to achieve the aforementioned blood pressure targets, use of an ACE inhibitor/diuretic, angiotensin-receptor blocker/diuretic, or ACE inhibitor/calcium antagonist should be strongly considered. The data from clinical trials show that these agents reduce cardiovascular mortality and renal disease progression with minimal side effects, if blood pressure is lowered to less than 130/85 mm Hg. Table 33.2 lists the factors to be considered before drug selection for the therapy of hypertension patient.

Selected Readings

Bakris GL. Treatment of hypertension in diabetes. In: Izzo J, Black H, eds. *Hypertension Primer.* Philadelphia: Lippincott Williams & Wilkins, 1999:421–423.

Discusses the treatment approach to lowering blood pressure among patients with diabetes with and without renal disease.

Sobel B, Bakris GL. *Hypertension: A Clinician's Guide to Diagnosis and Treatment*, 2nd ed. Philadelphia: Hanley and Belfus, 2000:1–137.

A book written for practicing clinicians that presents an in-depth approach to the treatment and diagnosis of hypertension in any person with high blood pressure.

Tarif N, Bakris GL. Renal components of the hypertension syndrome. *J Cardiovasc Risk* 1997;4:271–278.

An overview of the mechanisms involved in the genesis of hypertension along with a treatment approach to optimally reduce blood pressure in a hypertensive person.

The Sixth Report of the Joint National Committee on Prevention, Detection, Evaluation, and Treatment of High Blood Pressure. (JNCVI) *Arch Intern Med* 1997;2413–2446.

Presents the most recent recommendations for the evaluation and treatment of hypertension in a variety of clinical settings.

CHAPTER 34

Uremia

Richard Amerling and Nathan W. Levin

Uremia is a syndrome that affects all body systems. It profoundly influences the way afflicted individuals function. It is striking how ill a uremic patient can appear. In advanced uremia, patients look and, in fact, are moribund. It is equally striking how much better they get with proper treatment. The reversal of uremia is one of the most dramatic events in medicine. For this reason, life-and-death decisions in patients with end-stage renal failure are not made until there has been an adequate trial of dialysis. This chapter discusses the pathophysiology, diagnosis, and clinical manifestations of uremic syndrome.

PATHOPHYSIOLOGY

Uremic syndrome cannot be explained simply by the retention of nitrogenous and other dialyzable solutes. If this were true, dialysis alone would resolve all symptoms and there would be even less need for nephrologists. Many uremic manifestations are direct consequences of the failure of various kidney functions. Chronic anemia and hyperparathyroidism alone account for considerable uremic morbidity. Inadequate catabolism of peptides and globulins results in toxicity, much of which is not cured by dialysis due to the size of the toxins. The pathophysiology and treatment of the various components of the uremic syndrome is covered in detail elsewhere in this book. This chapter provides an overview that is useful in guiding therapy (Table 34.1).

Sodium Balance

Patients with chronic renal failure have abnormalities in sodium handling. The majority retain sodium and are chronically volume overloaded. Some, particularly those with tubulointerstitial and postobstructive nephropathies, lose sodium and may become volume depleted on a sodium-restricted diet. Patients with the nephrotic syndrome often become edematous long before they develop significant azotemia.

Sodium toxicity in uremic syndrome is important because it aggravates hypertension and heart failure. Hypertension speeds the progression of chronic renal failure, and its detection and control should always be given high priority. Depending on local mechanical factors, there may be pleural effusions, pulmonary congestion, ascites, and/or peripheral edema. Severe anasarca may worsen renal function by distorting intrarenal architecture. In some patients with severe congestive heart failure, anasarca from nephrotic syndrome, or refractory ascites, sodium overload dominates the clinical picture and may force the issue of dialysis at levels of creatinine and urea clearance that would otherwise be acceptable.

Water Metabolism

Urinary concentration and dilution require adequate glomerular filtration and an intact countercurrent multiplier mechanism, formed by Henle's loops and the vasa recta. Because the desired effect is tied to precise juxtaposition of these structures, it is not surprising that the ability to concentrate and dilute the urine is an early casualty in the progression of chronic renal disease. Hence, a precocious and ubiquitous symptom of chronic renal failure is nocturia. The osmolality of the urine approaches that of plasma (isosthenuria), even with moderate dehydration. With an average solute load, most individuals can drink 2 to 4 L of water per day without danger of hypotonicity. Therefore water or fluid restriction is not indicated until very low levels of glomerular filtration are attained. Some may be at risk of developing hypernatremia when fluid deprived. Symptomatic hyponatremia and hypernatremia are rare in conscious, uremic patients because an intact thirst mechanism will automatically adjust water intake to produce isotonicity.

Potassium Balance

The kidney's ability to excrete potassium is usually well preserved until the glomerular filtration rate (GFR) falls to 10 to 15 ml/min. Because potassium is secreted down an electrochemical gradient, potassium clearance can exceed the GFR. There is also an increase in intestinal potassium excretion as filtration diminishes. When hyperkalemia is observed at more moderate levels of renal insufficiency, there is often a tubular defect of potassium secretion. A hyperchloremic metabolic acidosis often coexists, as a result of inadequate ammoniagenesis, and the ensemble is labeled *type IV RTA*. Patients most likely to develop this complication are those with tubulointerstitial, postobstructive, and diabetic nephropathies.

Potassium need not be routinely restricted in all patients with chronic renal failure. Some may actually be hypokalemic and require supplementation.* Caution must be used when prescribing potassium to patients with chronic renal failure, especially if

* The presence of hypokalemia in a patient with moderate to advanced chronic renal failure, without obvious gastrointestinal losses, usually indicates poor nutritional status.

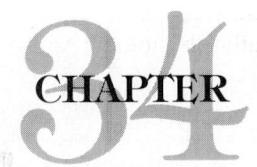

TABLE 34.1. Pathophysiologic Approach to Uremia

Normal Function	Loss of Function	Clinical Manifestation
Sodium balance	Na-retention; salt-wasting (rare)	Edema, HTN, CHF, ascites, pleural effusion
Water balance	Water retention or loss	Hyponatremia; hypernatremia (rare)
Potassium balance	Inability to excrete K load	Hyperkalemia, arrhythmias, muscle weakness, paralysis
Acid-base regulation	Inability to excrete acid load; retention of acid, loss of tissue buffers	Metabolic acidosis → bone disease, ↑ protein catabolism, myopathy, insulin resistance
Calcium, phosphorus, magnesium, and vitamin D metabolism	↓ PO_4, ↓ Ca, ↓ 1,25vitD, ↑ PTH, ↑ magnesium, ↑ aluminum	Osteitis fibrosa, osteomalacia, pruritus, soft-tissue calcification, neuropathy, myopathy, bone marrow fibrosis, anemia, dementia, cardiomyopathy
Erythropoietin production	↓ RBC production, ↓ platelet–endothelium interaction, ↓ platelet function, ↑ pituitary hormones, aldosterone, gastrin, glucagon	Anemia, fatigue, poor exercise tolerance, heart failure, impotence, cognitive impairment, prolonged bleeding time
Catabolism of peptides, β_2-microglobulin, light chains	↑ Insulin, glucagon, GH, ACTH β_2-microglobulin, prolactin, calcitonin, GIF, DIP, light chains	Hypoglycemia/hyperglycemia, impotence, infertility, ? anorexia, amyloidosis, ? ↑ catabolism, ↓ immunity
Excretion of dialyzable solutes	Retention of urea, uric acid, purines, p-cresol, indoxyl sulfate, guanidines, polyamines	Anorexia, ↓ protein intake and catabolism; CNS toxicity, ↓ immunity, glomerular sclerosis
Excretion of drugs and metabolites	Accumulation of drugs and metabolites	Drug toxicity

ACTH, adrenocorticotropic hormone; CHF, congestive heart failure; CNS, central nervous system; DIP, degranulation–inhibiting proteins; GH, growth hormone; GIP, granulocyte-inhibiting proteins; HTN, hypertension; PTH, parathyroid hormone; RBC, red blood cell.

there is a tendency toward hyperkalemia. Likewise, potassium-sparing diuretics and agents that inhibit the renin-angiotensin system, such as angiotensin-converting enzyme (ACE) inhibitors, should be used with extreme care. β-Blocking agents may inhibit potassium entry into cells, but hyperkalemia caused solely by this is not observed clinically. Hyperkalemia and hypokalemia can cause muscle weakness and cramping and precipitate cardiac arrhythmias. Hyperkalemia may require dialysis.

Acid-Base Regulation

It is the kidney's responsibility to not only reclaim all the filtered bicarbonate but also regenerate the bicarbonate consumed titrating daily acid production. This important function is impaired early in the course of chronic renal failure, especially in patients with tubulointerstitial disease. Metabolic acidosis is a common finding in patients with chronic renal failure. The absence of metabolic acidosis (or the appearance of a metabolic alkalosis) in advanced renal failure is a clue to vomiting or poor protein intake.

Acidosis plays a prominent role in the malnutrition of advanced renal failure. It causes accelerated bone loss by consumption of bone buffers and increases muscle catabolism. Acidosis stimulates protein catabolism by increasing branched-chain amino acid oxidation and cortisol secretion. It contributes to insulin resistance and may also promote synthesis of proteolytic enzymes and depress the response of insulinlike growth factor to growth hormone. For these reasons, treatment of chronic metabolic acidosis in the uremic patient with alkali is recommended. The toxicity of acidosis in uremia is further discussed in Chapter 68, Part 6.

Calcium, Phosphorous, Magnesium, and Vitamin D Metabolism

The kidney is a major player in calcium, phosphorous, and magnesium homeostasis. It is an effector organ for parathyroid hormone (PTH) and indirectly controls its level by controlling the rate of synthesis of 1,25$(OH)_2D_3$. It is the principal route of excretion of phosphorous, and hyperphosphatemia appears as the GFR declines to 20 to 30 mL/min. This, along with low levels of 1,25$(OH)_2D_3$, causes hypocalcemia and hyperparathyroidism. The uremic state is characterized by end-organ resistance to calcitriol. This is most likely because of downregulation of vitamin D receptors, the inhibition of the interaction between vitamin D and its receptors by unidentified toxins, and intranuclear, vitamin D response elements. There is also well-documented skeletal resistance to PTH, which contributes to hyperparathyroidism. Sustained hyperparathyroidism causes osteitis fibrosa and low levels of 1,25 $(OH)_2D_3$. 1,25 vitamin D (and/or end-organ resistance) may produce osteomalacia. Bone biopsy evidence of both diseases is seen in most patients at the time of entry into dialysis programs. Chronic elevation of phosphorous and calcium predisposes the patient to soft-tissue calcification, which can affect the brain, eyes, heart, lungs, viscera, skin, muscle, and blood vessels. Calcification in the microcirculation may produce local ischemia. Hyperparathyroidism also has been linked to neuropathy, myopathy, and insulin resistance. It may also cause worsened anemia and resistance to erythropoietin due to marrow fibrosis. There is evidence in animals and humans of a causative role for PTH (or a fragment) in the pathogenesis of uremic encephalopathy. The toxicity of excess PTH in uremia is discussed in Chapter 68, Part 1.

Aplastic bone disease is a recognized uremic manifestation. It is characterized by low rates of osteoid formation and bone mineralization with concomitant increase in soft-tissue calcification. The etiology is probably complex: relative hypoparathyroidism, subtle aluminum poisoning, and protein malnutrition may all be involved.

Aluminum is excreted by the kidney and may accumulate in patients with chronic renal failure, even in the predialysis setting. Aluminum not only is present in certain phosphate binders but also can be ingested with food, particularly if prepared in aluminum containers. It is an abundant metal and may contaminate water supplies. Oral citrate greatly enhances aluminum absorption in the gut. Aluminum is a uremic toxin that causes bone disease, refractory anemia, dementia, myopathy, neuropathy, and cardiomyopathy. Severe intoxication is unusual in the nondialyzed chronic renal failure population, but they are not routinely screened for aluminum. Chapter 68, Part 2 provides detailed information on aluminum toxicity in uremia. Symptomatic hypermagnesemia is rare in chronic renal failure but may result from the injudicious prescription of magnesium-containing antacids, laxatives, and enemas.

Erythropoietin Production

The anemia of chronic renal failure, mainly caused by inadequate erythropoietin production, is a major cause of morbidity and mortality. Other factors, such as shortened red blood cell survival time and bone marrow fibrosis, also contribute to the anemia of uremia. Anemia unquestionably causes uremic symptoms, such as fatigue, impotence, pruritus, decreased exercise tolerance, cognitive dysfunction, congestive heart failure, and a general impairment in the quality of life. Treatment with recombinant human erythropoietin ameliorates these symptoms and has greatly improved the quality of life for patients with chronic renal failure. It is routinely prescribed once the hematocrit falls below 30%. This has helped elucidate some nonerythropoietic effects of erythropoietin. In dialysis patients, increasing hematocrit may be associated with elevations in blood pressure. The mechanism of this effect involves increasing blood volume and viscosity, improving cardiac contractility, and eliminating anemia-induced peripheral vasodilatation. Elevated levels of the endogenous vasopressor endothelin-1 have been noted in dialysis patients receiving intravenous erythropoietin. Erythropoietin mRNA has been detected in the brain, spleen, testes, and lung. Treatment with rHuEpo is associated with significant decreases in the levels of somatotropin, luteinizing hormone, follicular-stimulating hormone, adrenocorticotrophic hormone (ACTH), cortisol, aldosterone, glucagon, and gastrin, and increases in the levels of insulin, estradiol, testosterone, atrial natriuretic peptide, and thyroxine. These changes return to baseline after 6 months to a year, although anemia remains corrected, which suggests an effect of erythropoietin independent of anemia correction.

Erythropoietin also increases intracellular calcium in platelets, which improves platelet function before restoration of the hematocrit. The prolonged bleeding time seen in uremia is largely a function of anemia, resulting from decreased platelet–endothelial interaction, and commonly improves when the hematocrit is raised above 30%.

Catabolism of Peptides

The kidney plays an important role in protein catabolism. Many small peptide hormones and fragments, immunoglobulin light chains, and other small proteins are filtered, reabsorbed, and digested in the proximal tubules. The loss of this catabolic function causes diverse metabolic derangements, which contribute heavily to the uremic syndrome. As many of these substances are poorly cleared by dialysis, their toxic effects often persist after initiation of dialysis.

β_2-Microglobulin amyloidosis, which presents itself as carpal tunnel syndrome, bone cysts, fractures, arthropathies, and occasional visceral problems, is the first clear example of uremic pathology linked to the accumulation of an abnormal substance of middle molecular weight. Although there is build-up of β_2-microglobulin before end-stage disease is reached, its contribution to the uremic syndrome is unknown.

Other peptides have been identified in the ultrafiltrate and peritoneal effluent of dialyzed uremic patients that impair polymorphonuclear leucocyte (PMNL) function *in vitro*. Granulocyte inhibiting proteins I and II are analogs of immunoglobulin light chains and β_2-microglobulin, respectively. Free light chains have also been found to inhibit PMNL function, and their level may be five times higher in chronic renal failure. Two other proteins that block PMNL degranulation are called, appropriately, degranulation inhibitory proteins (DIP I and II). DIP I was found to be identical to angiogenin, a tumor-derived protein found in normal plasma and in higher concentrations in uremic plasma. DIP II turned out to be a complement factor. Together, these peptides can be considered uremic toxins that contribute to an impairment of host defenses.

Insulin is a filtrable peptide that is largely catabolized by the proximal tubules. Its half-life is prolonged in advanced chronic renal failure, an effect due also to impaired hepatic uptake and metabolism. Insulin resistance occurs in renal failure; the mechanism of this resistance is unknown but may be related to metabolic acidosis. Hypoglycemia is noted in patients with advanced chronic renal failure receiving exogenous insulin or oral hypoglycemic medications and may occur spontaneously.

Insulin resistance and elevated blood levels of insulin seen in some uremic patients may play an important role in the dyslipidemia of uremia and is potentially of importance for long-term morbidity. Cardiovascular mortality is excessive in these patients, and hyperlipidemia may be a factor in the progression to end-stage disease. Lipid abnormalities develop in early chronic renal failure and are not corrected by dialysis. In general, triglycerides are increased, high-density lipoprotein (HDL) is reduced, and low-density lipoprotein (LDL), intermediate-density lipoprotein (IDL), and very-low-density lipoprotein (VLDL) are all increased. Insulin resistance and hyperparathyroidism are associated with hypertriglyceridemia. Both insulin and parathyroid hormone affect the metabolism of hepatic (HL) and lipoprotein lipase (LPL). LPL and HL activity are decreased in chronic renal failure. Lipoprotein catabolic rate is decreased and VLDL synthesis is enhanced. Synthesis of HDL-associated apolipoproteins, apoA-I and apoA-II, are decreased. Lecithin cholesterol acyl transferase, a required enzyme for HDL synthesis, is reduced. Apo(a), associated with increased cardiovascular risk in the general population, is increased in chronic renal failure. It is unknown whether specific therapy of dyslipidemia will improve mortality or slow the progression of chronic renal failure. Low total cholesterol, probably as a marker of poor nutritional status, is associated with increased mortality in the chronic renal failure population. The hyperlipidemia of chronic renal failure is discussed in detail in Chapter 74, Part 2, and the role of excess PTH in this abnormality is discussed in Chapter 68, Part 1.

Glucagon and the biologically inert proglucagon are metabolized by the kidney. A threefold increase in biologically active glucagon is observed in uremic individuals as a result of decreased clearance. High glucagon levels cause glucose intolerance in animals, as well as anorexia, ketosis, and hypoaminoacidemia. Whether hyperglucagonemia contributes to excessive protein catabolism in uremia remains to be established.

Cortisol and its metabolites are excreted by the kidney, and its half-life is prolonged in chronic renal failure. Diurnal variation and ACTH responsiveness is generally normal. Tests of suppression produce variable results, making the diagnosis of Cushing syndrome problematic. It may be that hypercortisolism is present in some patients with renal failure and could contribute to insulin resistance as well as the tendency toward a negative protein balance.

Prolactin levels are elevated in uremia, likely as a result of inadequate renal filtration and catabolism. This results in female infertility and male impotence.

Iodide is cleared by glomerular filtration and accumulates in chronic renal failure, ultimately resulting in decreased uptake of radiolabeled iodide. T_3 levels are often low, a product of decreased peripheral conversion of T_4 and of diminished protein binding. The latter may be due to competition for binding sites by retained creatinine, indoles, and phenols. The peptide hormones thyroid-stimulating hormone (TSH) and thyroid-releasing hormone (TRH) are cleared by the kidney. This may explain why the TSH response to exogenous TRH is often blunted and delayed. TSH does respond normally to changes in T_3/T_4 and is reliably increased in hypothyroidism. This is fortunate because the symptoms of hypothyroidism mimic those of the uremic syndrome (fatigability, edema, constipation, lethargy, and dry skin).

Calcitonin is another peptide metabolized by the kidney. In addition to its modest role in calcium homeostasis, it acts in the central nervous system to suppress appetite. Levels are elevated in uremia and may contribute to anorexia.

Advanced glycosylation end products (AGE) are substances of middle molecular weight that are metabolized by the kidney and accumulate in chronic renal failure. They are breakdown products of glycosylated proteins, released by macrophages into the circulation, where they may exert biologic activity. Levels of AGE are highest in diabetic patients with renal failure but are also elevated in nondiabetic patients with renal failure; in fact, they are higher than in diabetic patients without renal failure. Their properties make them potential uremic toxins. They are reactive, able to cross-link large and small proteins, such as β_2-microglobulin, are chemotactic for monocytes and macrophages, and stimulate cytokines. They seem to increase vascular permeability and enhance coagulation.

Endothelin-1, a potent endogenous vasoconstrictor peptide, accumulates in renal failure and may contribute to hypertension. A digitalislike substance, probably ouabain, has been detected in uremic plasma. It also may be a factor in hypertension because inhibition of Na^+-K^+-ATPase causes increased intracellular calcium and enhanced vascular tone.

Cytokine levels are increased in uremia, presumably as a result of impaired catabolism. In patients dialyzed with bioincompatible membranes, cytokine production may be stimulated, leading to even higher levels. Tumor necrosis factor-α may be an important mediator of protein wasting in uremic patients.

Resistance to insulinlike growth factor-1 may be caused by decreased renal breakdown of insulinlike growth factor binding proteins, as well as smaller, unidentified dialyzable solutes.

Excretion of Dialyzable Solutes

Loss of glomerular filtration causes retention of those substances normally cleared by filtration. Many small, dialyzable compounds have been studied as possible uremic toxins (Table 34.2). None have consistently been shown to cause toxicity at levels found in uremic patients. Interaction between numerous retained solutes very likely occurs and may be responsible for some uremic toxicity *in vivo*. Urea is a soluble end product of protein catabolism. Its rate of excretion correlates well with protein catabolic rate, which in the steady state is determined by protein intake. Urea clearance, normalized to total body water volume, correlates with mortality in dialyzed (and very likely nondialyzed) uremic patients. For this reason, urea has been used as a marker solute for kinetic modeling analyses of dialysis adequacy and protein catabolic rate. Level of blood urea nitrogen is proportional to the protein catabolic rate and inversely proportional to total urea clearance. Urea is considered non-toxic, but headache, fatigue, nausea, and vomiting were noted in a study of normal volunteers dialyzed against a high-urea dialysate.

Two dialyzable products of amino acid catabolism have been added to the list of potential uremic toxins. Indoxyl sulphate is formed in the liver from indole, which is derived from colonic bacterial degradation of the amino acid tryptophan. It accumulates in chronic renal failure and inhibits albumin binding and lymphocyte blast formation. It may also contribute to glomerular scarring via stimulation of transforming growth factor-β and collagen production. The toxicity of indoxyl sul-

TABLE 34.2. Dialyzable Solutes Retained in Uremia

Solute	Possible Toxicity
Urea	Headache, vomiting, fatigue; carbamylation of hemoglobin and/or other proteins via isocyanate
Creatinine	No known toxic effects; clearance overestimates GFR
Purines: uric acid, xanthine, hypoxanthine, hippuric acid(s)	Anorexia, weight loss; interference with protein binding; resistance to calcitriol (uric acid)
Guanidines: methylguanidine, guanidinosuccinic acid	GI symptoms, polyneuropathy, ↓ seizure threshold, immune suppression
Polyamines: spermidine, spermine, putrescine, cadaverine	Cellular poisons: affect messenger systems, protein synthesis, membrane function; may cause anorexia, CNS toxicity, immune depression, inhibit erythropoiesis
Amino acid metabolites: p-cresol, indoxyl sulfate, asymmetric dimethyl arginine, homocysteine	Inhibits PMNL glucose oxidation; inhibits protein binding, erythroid colony formation, lymphocyte blast formation, thyroxine hepatocyte transport; may stimulate glomerular sclerosis; competitive inhibitor NOS: ↑ BP; accelerate atherosclerosis

BP, blood pressure; CNS, central nervous system; GFR, glomerular filtration rate; GI, gastrointestinal; PMNL, polymorphonuclear leukocyte.

phate is discussed in detail in Chapter 68, Part 5. P-cresol, a byproduct of gut metabolism of phenylalanine and tyrosine, has been shown to inhibit PMNL glucose consumption in response to various stimuli and may contribute to impaired immune defense in uremia.

Another altered amino acid, asymmetric dimethyl arginine, has been demonstrated in uremic plasma. This compound is a naturally occurring antagonist of nitric oxide synthase and may cause or worsen hypertension by inhibiting synthesis of nitric oxide.

Homocysteine is a metabolite formed in the conversion of methionine to cysteine. Hyperhomocystinemia is observed in chronic renal failure and may contribute to accelerated atherosclerosis. The toxicity of homocysteine in uremia is discussed in detail in Chapter 68, Part 3.

Excretion of Drugs and Metabolites

The kidney is a principal organ of drug elimination. Many drugs, such as digoxin and aminoglycosides, depend wholly on renal excretion for their elimination. Others are first processed in the liver then excreted renally. When the hepatic metabolite is pharmacologically active, as in *N*-acetyl procainamide, or morphine-6-glucuronide, the renal excretory pathway assumes major importance in their elimination. In addition, protein binding of drugs may be altered in uremia. An example is phenytoin, which is less protein bound in chronic renal failure, resulting in increased free drug level.

DIAGNOSIS AND CLINICAL MANIFESTATIONS

The diagnosis of uremia is straightforward when an azotemic patient has classical symptoms and signs (Table 34.3). In patients with slowly progressive chronic renal failure, deciding when a symptom can be attributed to uremia can be vexing. Paradoxically, uremia is often most difficult to diagnose today in patients already undergoing renal replacement therapy. This is because uremia can masquerade as a host of other disease entities. However, it reflects the notion that uremia is a diagnosis of exclusion and our reluctance to believe that a dialyzed patient might be uremic. Inadequate dialysis is all too common, and seemingly obvious uremic manifestations are routinely present and may be misdiagnosed in dialysis patients. Although one should have a broad differential diagnosis for any symptoms or signs, when a patient with known renal failure has a complaint, uremia should be considered above all other explanations. In other words, the most likely explanation for the appearance of any of the uremia symptoms listed in Table 34.3 in a patient with renal failure is uremia. In a nondialyzed patient, treatment should be instituted and the response observed. In a patient already undergoing dialysis, an assessment of dialysis adequacy and perhaps an increase in the prescribed dosage is in order. If the patient fails to improve, further investigation is necessary. This approach will spare many patients morbidity and mortality and will promote cost-effective use of diagnostic testing.

The diagnosis of volume overload in chronic renal failure patients may be difficult when the jugular venous pressure is hard to ascertain, arterial pressures are normal, and there is no peripheral edema. A useful rule is to assume volume overload unless there is clear evidence of volume depletion (i.e., reduced central venous pressure, orthostatic hypotension). This is helpful when a patient with renal failure exhibits pulmonary infiltrates. Most of these patients can readily be managed with diuretics or ultrafiltration.

In contrast, salt-wasting patients may become volume depleted and show acute worsening of renal failure. A high index of suspicion is required to accurately diagnose these patients, usually in the presence of orthostasis or low central venous pressure. A saline challenge is then of diagnostic import.

Clinical Manifestations of Uremia

It is beyond the scope of this chapter to discuss each uremic symptom in detail. These manifestations are discussed in detail in other chapters of this book. Many of the manifestations listed in Table 34.3 are readily diagnosed and easily attributable to

TABLE 34.3. Clinical Manifestations of Uremia

Neurologic manifestations	**Cardiovascular manifestations**	**Muscoloskeletal manifestations**
Behavioral changes	Congestive heart failure	Bone disease: osteitis fibrosa; osteomalacia; amyloid
Memory dysfunction	Hypertension	Arthralgias, arthropathies
Inability to concentrate	Ascites, edema, pleural effusion	Proximal myopathy
Sleep pattern disorder (reversal)	Arrhythmia	Periarticular (and other soft tissue) calcification
Mood disorders	Pericarditis, +/− effusion	Carpal tunnel syndrome
Neuromuscular irritability	Conduction abnormality	Muscle wasting
Peripheral neuropathy	Cardiomegaly	**Fluid and electrolyte disorders**
Psychosis	**Pulmonary manifestations**	Hyperkalemia
Convulsions	Infiltrate on x-ray	Hyponatremia
Coma	Pleuritis	Metabolic acidosis
Headache	Dyspnea, orthopnea	Hypermagnesemia
Irritability	Cough	Hypocalcemia/hypercalcemia
Akathisia	Hemoptysis	Hyperphosphatemia
Gastrointestinal (GI) manifestations	Abnormal breathing	**Endocrine disorders**
Anorexia	Sleep apnea syndrome	Sexual dysfunction
Dysgeusia	**Dermatologic disorders**	Growth retardation (children)
Nausea, vomiting	Xerosis	Hyperprolactinemia
Diarrhea, constipation	Pruritis	Insulin resistance/sensitivity
GI bleeding	Prurigo nodularis	Hyperglycemia/hypoglycemia
Hiccough	Frost	
Stomatitis, parotitis	**Hematologic manifestations**	
Weight loss	Anemia	
	Platelet functional disorder	
	Immunodeficiency	

uremia. Neurologic, gastrointestinal, and certain other manifestations are less obvious. Some clinical examples will be used to highlight more difficult diagnostic issues.

Neurologic Manifestations

As can be seen from Table 34.3, neurologic manifestations of uremia run the gamut from subtle behavioral changes to "coma, convulsions, and death," the infamous endpoints of most systemic poisonings. Uremic encephalopathy describes a nonspecific and variable disorder of psychomotor function, consciousness, cognition, speech, memory, perception, and emotion, commonly observed in advanced chronic or acute renal failure, and generally reversible with dialysis. Symptoms include sleep pattern reversal, inability to concentrate, emotional lability, restlessness, difficulty with abstract concepts, memory lapses, bizarre behavior, hallucinations, akathisia, painful extremities, withdrawal from friends and family, and loss of libido. Symptoms are often subtle, elicited only through careful questioning of patient and family, who are often unaware because of the gradual nature of the change. The differential diagnosis encompasses other organic encephalopathies including portosystemic, hypoxic, HIV-associated, myxedematous, and syphilitic. Senile and presenile dementia, alcoholic brain syndrome, vitamin B_{12} deficiency, chronic subdural hematoma, frontal lobe tumor, lupus cerebritis, chronic fatigue syndrome, and endogenous depression may all present with similar symptomatology. When a patient with renal failure develops a neurologic or behavioral symptom, a B_{12} level, VDRL, blood ammonia level, HIV antibodies, head computed tomographic (CT) scan, and neurology and nephrology consults may be needed. Psychiatric diagnoses should not be given to patients with renal failure until uremia has been unequivocally eliminated.

Several cases demonstrate this point: (a) A 53-year-old woman with renal failure and systemic lupus, receiving peritoneal dialysis for more than a year, suddenly began hallucinating, had severe memory lapses, and had frequent spontaneous crying episodes. She was hospitalized and underwent a workup for lupus cerebritis, including lumbar puncture. Her dialysis prescription was empirically increased, and over a 2-week period, her neuropsychiatric symptoms vanished. (b) A 60-year-old man started hemodialysis after undergoing bilateral nephrectomies for urothelial cancer. He was readmitted several months later with an altered mental status. He had become completely withdrawn and had stopped eating. Formerly a robust, gregarious person, he was observed on rounds curled in a fetal position; the only sounds he made were occasional hiccoughs. The house staff diagnosed severe depression and prescribed tricyclics. A psychiatrist was consulted for possible electroconvulsive therapy. Although the blood urea nitrogen was 30 mg/dl, he was given daily hemodialysis treatments. Within 7 days his symptoms completely resolved. Study of his arteriovenous fistula revealed a significant venous stenosis which compromised the efficiency of the dialysis treatments he had been receiving. (c) In a similar scenario, a 46-year-old former professor with a history of endogenous depression developed chronic renal failure, requiring dialysis. He experienced an exacerbation of depression with insomnia, anorexia, and suicidal ideation that led to hospitalization and electroconvulsive therapy. He was found to have a venous stenosis of the AV graft, which was dilated successfully. Whether resulting from enhanced dialysis or psychiatric manipulations, his condition improved greatly and he was discharged. Subsequent bouts of acute depression were temporally linked with recurrence of the venous stenosis. (d) A 77-year-old man with chronic renal insufficiency from obstruction was admitted with a hypertensive intracerebral bleed. He survived but was left with an expressive aphasia. During the hospitalization, he became severely demented. This was associated with worsening renal failure. Although the creatinine clearance was in the 10 to 15 ml/min range, he was given a trial of dialysis. After 2 weeks, his dementia cleared. He remains aphasic on thrice-weekly hemodialysis.

Gastrointestinal Manifestations

Uremia may be associated with any acute or chronic inflammation of the gastrointestinal tract. This can cause dyspepsia, anorexia, nausea and vomiting, ulcerlike pain, diarrhea, constipation, and bleeding. Anorexia is commonly encountered and is a nonspecific symptom of many disease states. It tends to have a central component in uremia and is generally reversible with dialysis. This can be of diagnostic utility. (a) A 72-year-old man with nephrotic syndrome and chronic renal failure of unknown etiology presented with severe anorexia and weight loss. The blood urea nitrogen was 100 mg/dl, and the creatinine was 4 mg/dl. He was dialyzed several times with no improvement in appetite or general condition. A saline infusion improved renal function to a blood urea nitrogen of 63 mg/dl and a creatinine of 2.6 mg/dl. Over the next few days, he developed a left pleural effusion, which was tapped. Cytologic examination was positive for adenocarcinoma. This case illustrates the diagnostic value of a trial of dialysis, as well as the common exacerbation of chronic renal failure by volume depletion in a patient with poor oral intake.

Other Manifestations

It is increasingly accepted that decreased immunity is part of the uremic syndrome. The diagnosis of "failure to thrive" in a patient with renal failure is usually synonymous with uremia. However, once this is ruled out, chronic infection or cancer must be considered in such cases. (a) A 76-year-old man receiving chronic hemodialysis complained of dyspepsia and weight loss. His dialysis dosage was excellent by conventional standards of urea kinetics, but his treatment time was empirically increased. No improvement was noted, and he was referred for gastrointestinal evaluation. Upper endoscopy revealed severe esophageal reflux. He was treated with H_2-blockers and metoclopramide, and his symptoms gradually improved. However, 6 months later, he again began to lose weight. Repeat endoscopy with biopsy demonstrated adenocarcinoma of the lower esophagus. (b) A 53-year-old man with hypertensive renal disease was stable receiving dialysis for 9 years. He began to lose weight and feel poorly. Access recirculation was 17%, and a fistula angiogram revealed significant anatomical problems. As corrective surgery was planned, dialysis time was extended, but there was no relief. Hematuria was noted, and renal sonography demonstrated bilateral solid masses, confirmed by contrast CT as probable hypernephromas. Bilateral nephrectomies were followed by clinical improvement.

Confusion may arise when patients with renal failure and systemic inflammatory diseases, such as lupus erythematosus, develop signs of inflammation. It has long been observed that nonrenal manifestations of lupus diminish once the renal failure progresses to the point of requiring dialysis. This observation lends support to the concept of uremia as an immunocompromised state. This is exemplified by the following case: A 45-year-old woman with chronic renal failure and systemic lupus was treated with peritoneal dialysis. After about a year, renal function improved and her dialysis prescription was decreased. She came in one day with severe left-sided pleuritic chest and shoulder pain. Electrocardiogram and echocardiogram were unchanged, and the chest radiograph was unremarkable. She was given a diagnosis of pleuritis. Because her dialysis indices were recently measured and within the acceptable range and she had no other uremic manifestations, she was treated with oral steroids and improved after a few days.

Selected Readings

Bergstrom J. Anorexia in dialysis patients. *Semin Nephrol* 1996;16(3):222–229.

Very comprehensive review of all aspects of malnutrition in uremia with 88 references.

Felsenfeld AJ, Llach F. Parathyroid gland function in chronic renal failure. *Kidney Int* 1993;43:771.

A detailed review, extensively referenced.

Niwa T, Ringoir SM, Massry SG, eds. Uremic toxicity. *Kidney Int* 1997;62:S1–S92.

Proceedings of the Third International Symposium on Uremic Toxicity. A superb compilation of original articles by international experts.

Sherrard DJ, Hercz G, Pei Y, et al. The spectrum of bone disease in end-stage renal failure—an evolving disorder. *Kidney Int* 1993;43(2):436–442.

An excellent histology-based study of a large number of renal failure patients with comprehensive analysis of results.

Vanholder R, Ringoir S. Infectious morbidity and defects of phagocytic function in end-stage renal disease: a review [Editorial]. *J Am Soc Nephrol* 1993;3(9): 1541–1554.

Erudite review of a complex topic.

SECTION V

Renal Immunopathology

CHAPTER 35

General Concepts of Immunopathology

Richard J. Glassock

It is clear that a majority of glomerulonephritic renal diseases and a growing number of tubulointerstitial and vascular diseases of the kidney result from abnormal immunologic processes. These processes may directly injure renal structures, such as glomerular capillaries, or participate in the evolution and progression of diseases initiated by other, nonimmune mechanisms. However, the evolution of immune-mediated renal diseases may, at least in part, depend on the superimposition of other nonimmune events (see Chapter 67, Part 2).

Our understanding of the immunopathogenesis of renal disease continues to evolve as new insights are gained into a wider variety of experimental models and a greater array of immunologic interactions. Fundamentally, immune-mediated renal disease can be categorized according to the character of the immune response (humoral or cellular), the nature of the antigen(s) involved (native or nonnative, exogenous or endogenous, circulating or planted, soluble or insoluble, and renewable or nonrenewable), and the source of the effector (exogenous or endogenous). In addition, the ability of an immune mechanism to result in tissue injury and the extent and character of the tissue injury observed are conditioned or modulated to a significant degree by soluble (complement components, coagulation proteins, cytokines chemokines, peptide hormones, and eicosanoids) and cellular (leukocytes, platelets) mediators of inflammation. Table 35.1 provides a classification of the immune mechanisms of renal disease.

MECHANISMS INVOLVING CIRCULATING ANTIBODY

Renal diseases that result from the reaction of a circulating antibody with its corresponding antigen are the best studied of the categories of immune-mediated renal disease. The antibody can arise endogenously as a result of antigenic stimulation and proliferation of B cells, with a resultant secretion of immunoglobulins (IgG, IgM, IgA, and IgE) with specificity for defined epitopes on the antigen. On the other hand, the antibody can be administered artificially from an exogenous source after another animal develops it by antigenic stimulation.

The antibody can then react with the epitopes on antigens. These antigens may be native to the organ or tissue that is injured. If the antibody is endogenous and the antigen is native to the kidney, one usually refers to this process as organ-specific autoimmunity, and the antibody is described as an autoantibody. Nonnative antigens are those that are extrinsic to the organ or tissue that is injured. Nonnative antigens can be exogenous (i.e., derived from another animal), such as bovine serum albumin (BSA), or endogenous, such as deoxyribonucleic acid (DNA) or thyroglobulin. Antigens are further characterized according to their solubility. Many native antigens, particularly basement membrane or extracellular matrix antigens, are quite insoluble. Thus the reaction with the antibody tends to be confined to the site of the antigen rather than in the circulation (see Chapter 36, Part 1). Other antigens, because of their solubility, tend to diffuse into the vascular compartment and, as a result, are found in the circulation as well as in the vicinity of the site of synthesis. In the circulation these antigens form soluble or insoluble circulating immune complexes upon interaction with a circulating antibody. Once formed, these immune complexes can localize in various renal structures (glomerular capillaries or mesangium) because of their physical properties and/or the local hemodynamic milieu (see Chapter 36, Part 3).

The mononuclear phagocyte system removes circulating immune complexes in the liver and spleen. The erythrocyte may play an important role in transporting immune complexes to the hepatic Kupffer cells by binding immune complexes that have incorporated C3b via the complement receptors located on the erythrocyte surface. Complement components may play a critical role in dissolving those immune complexes that have formed an insoluble lattice, thus minimizing their deposition in tissues. Once deposited in the tissue, immune complexes are in a constant state of dynamic equilibrium with both the circulating antigen and circulating antibody.

Certain antigens have an affinity for glomerular capillary walls as a result of antibody reactivity, electrostatic charge, or a biochemical reaction. These antigens, although not normally native or intrinsic to the capillary wall, may be planted at this site and serve as a focus for an *in situ* antigen-antibody reaction with a circulating antibody. An IgG antibody bound to a native antigen by virtue of an immune reaction may act as a planted antigen on subsequent reactions with a circulating antiimmunoglobulin antibody, such as rheumatoid factor or antiidiotypic antibody (see Chapter 36, Part 2).

TABLE 35.1. Classification of the Immunologic Mechanisms of Glomerular, Vascular, and Tubulointerstitial Diseases of the Kidney

I. Mechanisms involving the synthesis of circulating, endogenous antibody
   A. Reacting with a native, insoluble, endogenous, nonrenewable antigen
      1. Anti-GBM antibody-induced nephritis (including Goodpasture's disease)
      2. Antitubular basement membrane antibody nephritis
      3. Mercuric chloride-induced nephritis in Brown-Norway rats
      4. Lupus nephritis (?)
   B. Reacting with a native, soluble, endogenous, renewable antigen (in situ immune complex disease)
      1. Active Heymann's nephritis (gp 330)
      2. Idiopathic membranous glomerulonephritis (?)
      3. Microscopic polyangiitis (myeloperoxidase) (?)
   C. Reacting with a nonnative, soluble, exogenous or endogenous, nonrenewable antigen planted at the site of injury (in situ immune complex disease)
      1. Cationized bovine serum albumin or ferritin
      2. Viruses (?)
      3. Histone, DNA (?)
      4. Bacterial products (?): poststreptococcal glomerulonephritis
      5. IgG (autologous phase of nephrotoxic serum nephritis)
      6. Idiotypes on IgG, IgM, or IgA
   D. Reacting with nonnative, soluble, exogenous, nonrenewable, circulating antigen (circulating immune complex disease)
      1. Acute serum sickness (serum protein antigens)
      2. Acute postinfectious glomerulonephritis
   E. Reacting with nonnative, soluble, endogenous, renewable, circulating antigen
      1. Normal tissue antigens (thyroglobulin, HLA antigens, erythrocyte membrane antigens, DNA)
      2. Abnormal tissue antigen (tumor-associated antigens, drug-tissue antigen copolymer, altered DNA)
   F. Reacting with a nonnative, soluble, exogenous, renewable, circulating antigen
      1. Bacterial endocarditis
      2. Viruses
II. Mechanisms involving the administration of exogenous antibody
   A. Reacting with a native, insoluble, endogenous, nonrenewable antigen
      1. Classic nephrotoxic serum nephritis (NTN, Masugi's nephritis)
   B. Reacting with a native, soluble, endogenous, renewable antigen (in situ immune complex disease)
      1. Passive Heymann's nephritis (gp 330)
      2. Mesangiopathic nephritis (anti-Thy1.1)
   C. Reacting with a nonnative, soluble, exogenous or endogenous, nonrenewable antigen planted at the site of injury
      1. Passively augmented NTN
      2. Concanavalin A nephritis
   D. Reacting with nonnative, soluble, exogenous, nonrenewable, circulating antigen
      1. Passive serum sickness
III. Mechanisms involving cell-mediated immunity
   A. Reacting with native, insoluble, endogenous, nonrenewable antigen
      1. Anti-GBM antibody disease (cellular component)
      2. Antitubular basement membrane
   B. Reacting with nonnative, soluble, exogenous or endogenous, nonrenewable antigen planted at the sites of injury
      1. IgG (autologous phase of NTN)
      2. Viruses?
      3. Bacterial antigens?

GBM, glomerular basement membrane; HLA, human lymphocyte antigen; NTN, nephrotoxic nephritis.

Finally, antigens can be categorized in terms of their ability to be continuously renewed. Antigens such as exogenously administered BSA would be regarded as nonrenewable antigens unless administered continuously over a long period. On the other hand, a replicating bacterium or virus could provide a continuing source of exogenous antigen. Native antigens are renewable or nonrenewable. Antigens of the extracellular matrix are nonrenewable or only slowly renewable, whereas cell surface antigens, such as those associated with the epithelial or endothelial cells, can be resynthesized and reexpressed even after they have been shed from the cell surface and interacted with an antibody to form an *in situ* immune complex.

Theoretically, any of the immunoglobulin isotypes could participate in the renal injury induced by this type of immunologic reaction, but IgG is the most common. In the case of the native and planted antigens, the distribution of antibody deposits can be uniform or nonuniform or can be localized to discrete segments or structural components of the nephron. Thus, when a circulating antibody reacts with an antigen *in situ*, a variety of patterns of IgG deposits, as recognized by immunofluorescent studies of renal biopsy material, may be seen. Linear deposits of IgG along the capillary wall imply a reaction of an antibody with a native or planted antigen that is uniformly and continuously expressed within the basement membrane (anti-basement membrane antibody disease). A granular or irregular deposition of IgG along the capillary wall suggests that the antibody has reacted *in situ* in one of three scenarios: (a) with a native or planted antigen that is discontinuously distributed along the capillary wall, (b) with an antigen that is associated with the cell surface or epithelial or endothelial cell and then aggregates into discrete deposits after being shed from the cell surface as an immune complex, or (c) that antigen-antibody complexes have deposited from the circulation. Granular or irregular immune deposits confined to the luminal aspect of the capillary wall or mesangium suggest that immune complexes (soluble or insoluble) have been deposited from the circulation or that circulating antibody has reacted *in situ* with a fixed and native or planted antigen at these sites. Thus the pattern of deposition of immunoglobulins does not strictly relate to a unique or specific immunopathogenetic mechanism. Differences in location and distribution of the immunologic reaction may indicate a spectrum of histologic and functional manifestations ranging from a pure capillary wall abnormality to structural lesions involving the mesangium or the tubulointerstitial region. Occasionally, Ig (IgG, IgM) and/or complement (C3) deposits may be present in glomerular or tubular structures unrelated to an immune pathogenesis as a result of nonspecific trapping or binding by altered glomerular or tubular structures. Thus some caution should be exercised in interpreting patterns of Ig and/or C3 deposits in terms of underlying immunopathogenesis.

The binding of extrinsic antigenic compounds to the glomerulus represents an intriguing mechanism. Such a binding would permit the development of a renal disease in which neither circulating antibodies to renal structures nor circulating immune complexes would be detectable and the variety and sources of putative antigenic compounds would be extremely wide.

The reaction of a circulating antibody with a nonrenal exogenous or endogenous antigen within the circulation, thereby producing a circulating immune complex, has long been presumed to be a major cause for human renal disease. Although the formation of circulating immune complexes is a relatively common event, deposition within glomeruli is not observed in all instances. Thus the deposition of circulating immune complexes in the renal structures is best viewed as a breakdown in the normal mechanism of removal and disposal. The complement system and the mononuclear phagocytic systems of the spleen, liver, circulating blood, and glomerular mesangium play important roles in this process. The hemodynamic profile that prevails in the glomerular and peritubular capillary circulation also participates in the uptake and removal of immune aggregates.

Although a great deal is understood about the interaction of antigens and antibodies in renal diseases, little is known about how the antibody develops in the first place, especially when it is an autoantibody. The mechanisms of autoantibody formation are complex but fundamentally involve a breakdown in the body's ability to distinguish self from nonself.

MECHANISMS INVOLVING CELL-MEDIATED IMMUNITY

For many years, it was believed that sensitized cells, derived from T cell lineage, had little to do with the development of glomerular or tubulointerstitial diseases in humans. With the emergence of new tools for the study of lymphoid cells and their constituent subsets and biological products (cytokines), a better understanding of the genetic control of immune responses, and the recognition of important interactions between T cells (i.e., T helper cells, T suppressor cells, and T inducer cells) and B cells, it is apparent that cell-mediated factors are active participants in many immunologic disorders of the kidney.

It seems reasonable to assume that the native renal tissue antigen, either modified or unmodified, could also be the target of a cell-mediated, autoimmune response. Such instances have been described in experimental models. A simple demonstration of an *in vitro* correlate of cell-mediated immunity using a modified or unmodified native tissue antigen is insufficient to prove the necessary involvement of cell-mediated immunity in renal disease. Clearly, both humoral antibody formation and cell-mediated immunity coexist, each under separate genetic control, yet one or both may be required for the full expression of the disease.

MEDIATORS OF IMMUNOLOGIC RENAL INJURY

The pathogenetic mechanisms of immunologic forms of renal disease noted previously result in tissue injury by activation of a variety of mediator systems (Table 35.2). These mediator systems may be described as soluble or cellular. The former are represented by a series of serum products, peptides, fatty acids, or amines that may be activated from some precursor forms, secreted from storage sites, or synthesized *de novo* in response to some immunologic or phlogogenic stimulus. C3 is among the better known and studied of these factors. The individual components of the C3 cascade participate in tissue injury in several ways, including (a) direct, by promoting cell lysis, alteration of membrane permeability, and/or solubilization or precipitation of immune complex, and (b) indirect, by calling forth the participation of polymorphonuclear and mononuclear cells. Fibrinogen and the coagulant proteins participate in renal injury by formation of localized thrombi and generation of biologically active peptide fragments that interact with complement or cells. The prostaglandins, thromboxanes, and leukotrienes can be synthesized *de novo* during immune-induced inflammation and participate in local vasomotor changes and vascular permeability. Kinin formation, histamine release, and angiotensin production also participate in local vasomotor phenomena and altered permeability. These changes may be vital determinants of the morphologic and clinical manifestations of renal injury.

Cellular factors participate as mediators by virtue of the local release of enzymes, procoagulant factors, mitogens, and lymphokines or monokines. These cellular factors require the presence and expression of accessory proteins called adhesion molecules so that cells can be mobilized and directed to sites of lesions. Cellular proliferation and differentiation accompanies local damage by digestion of structural proteins or thrombosis.

TABLE 35.2. Mediators of Immunologic Renal Injury

Mediators	Effect
Soluble	
Complement (C3, C5–9, membrane attack complex)	Chemoattractant for polymorphonuclear and mononuclear cells Alters glomerular permeability Solubilizes immune complexes Directs cytolysis
Fibrinogen	Localized coagulation Mitogenic for monocytes (?)
Prostaglandins (thromboxanes)	Vasomotor changes Alter permeability
Leukotrienes and lipoxins	Chemoattractant Vasomotor effects
Kinins	Vasomotor effects
Histamine	Alters permeability Vasomotor effects
Angiotensin II	Vasomotor effects, growth factor
Platelet-activating factor (PAF)	Mitogenic for mesangial cells
Interleukins (IL-1, IL-4, IL-6, IL-10)	Activate cells, induce proliferation
Tumor necrosis factor (TNF)	Promotes interleukin release
Transforming growth factor (TGF)	Promotes collagen deposition
Chemokines	Promote inflammation
Cellular	
Polymorphonuclear cells	Local release of lysosomal enzymes with digestion of structural proteins Toxic oxygen radicals Procoagulant factors
Mononuclear cells	Local release of lysosomal enzymes with digestion of structural proteins Monokine (IL-1) release Procoagulant factors Mitogenic and/or growth factor release Toxic oxygen radical
Platelets	Procoagulant factors Mitogenic and/or growth factor release (PDGF) Vasomotor effects
Lymphocytes	Direct cytolysis (killer cells) Lymphokine release

Some of the synthetic products of the infiltrating cells or the fixed cells driven to hyperplasia and/or terminal differentiation may be important components of the reparative process (e.g., transforming growth factor). Examples include collagen synthesis, organization of the fibrin thrombus, and mesangial and/or smooth muscle proliferation. The damage induced by such mediators may release new antigens or modify existing ones, thereby permitting secondary humoral or cellular responses to the damage-related neoantigen. This may serve to perpetuate a progressive form of immune injury.

Selected Readings

Betani T, Remuzzi G, eds. *Glomerular Injury 300 Years After Morgagni.* Milan: Wichtig Editore, 1983.

An excellent monograph dealing with many facets of immune-mediated glomerular injury.

Wilson CB, ed. *Immunological Mechanisms of Renal Disease, Contemporary Issues in Nephrology,* Vol 3. New York: Churchill Livingstone, 1979.

An excellent and comprehensive monograph dealing with fundamental principles.

Wilson CB, Dixon FJ. *The Kidney,* 3rd ed. Philadelphia: WB Saunders, 1986.

A comprehensive review.

CHAPTER 36

Immune Mechanisms of Glomerular and Vascular Diseases

PART 1

Nephritogenic Immune Reactions Involving Native Renal Antigens

David C. Kluth and Andrew Rees

Autoimmune diseases are a leading cause of acute and chronic renal failure involving both glomerular and interstitial injury. Over the last 10 to 15 years there has been a dramatic increase in our understanding of the cellular and molecular mechanisms that underlie the immune response in autoimmune diseases with implications for their treatment. This chapter examines the potential role of renal autoantigens in the pathogenesis of glomerular and interstitial disease, discusses which antigens have been shown to be the target of the immune response, and analyzes the cellular and molecular events involved in the production of injury.

In antiglomerular basement membrane (anti-GBM) disease, the target of autoimmunity has been clearly characterised. This chapter highlights the mechanisms involved in the production of pathogenic antibodies and the molecular and cellular events involved in the effector phase of glomerular inflammation. Anti-GBM is the clearest example where the renal autoantigen has been identified; however, there are a number of glomerulonephritides where putative antigenic targets have been proposed (Table 36.1). This chapter also outlines the potential antigens in membranous nephropathy and analyzes the mechanisms by which the immune deposits in this disease can lead to glomerular injury. Last, this chapter outlines the potential for the involvement of other renal antigens in other inflammatory renal disease, including antineutrophil cytoplasmic antigen (ANCA) associated vasculitis and postinfectious glomerulonephritis.

ANTIGLOMERULAR BASEMENT MEMBRANE DISEASE

Anti-GBM disease is characterised by the production of autoantibodies directed principally at the glomerular and pulmonary basement membranes, resulting in severe inflammatory disease. The classic clinical pattern of the disease is for the patients to develop progressive renal failure secondary to glomerulonephritis and develop pulmonary hemorrhage, particularly in smokers. This clinical pattern is often referred to as Goodpasture's syndrome, after an original description of a patient by Ernest Goodpasture in 1919. However, the term is applied to clinical conditions presenting with glomerulonephritis and pulmonary hemorrhage with systemic vasculitis being the predominant cause. Goodpasture's disease is synonymous with anti-GBM disease and is one of the causes of Goodpasture's syndrome. (For clarity Goodpasture's disease will be referred to as anti-GBM disease in this chapter.) This disease is caused by antibodies directed at a specific part of the α3 chain

TABLE 36.1. Human Glomerular Diseases and Their Causative Renal Autoantigens

Disease	Renal Antigen
Anti-GBM disease	NC1 domain of α3 chain of type IV collagen
Anti-GBM disease in renal transplant in Alport's patients	Mainly α5 chain of type IV collagen; minority have antibodies to α3 chain
Membranous nephropathy	Component of glomerular epithelial cell
ANCA-associated vasculitis	Glycoprotein on glomerular endothelium
Postinfectious glomerulonephritis*	Streptococcal antibodies may cross-react with type IV collagen, heparan sulfate, and laminin in GBM
IgA nephropathy	Antigens identified from glomeruli that react with IgG antibodies from patients; characterized only by molecular weights of 185, 160, and 30–40 kD

Note: For the majority of glomerular diseases, the pathogenic antigen or antigens are not clearly defined. For anti-GBM disease, the target of autoimmunity has been shown to be the NCI domain of on the α3 chain of type IV collagen. For the remainder of diseases listed, there is experimental evidence to identify renal antigens as potentially involved.

ANCA, antineutrophil cytoplasmic antigen; GBM, glomerular basement membrane.

*The most important antigens involved in poststreptococcal glomerulonephritis appear to be derived from the streptococcal organism itself. These antigens bind to the glomerular capillary wall. Although an immune response to glomerular autoantigens does occur, the role of these autoantibodies in the pathogenesis of the disease remains uncertain (see text).

of type IV collagen, which is present in the glomerular basement membrane and other specialised basement membranes, including the lung, cochlear membrane, and retinal capillaries. The clinical entity of Goodpasture's disease is described in detail in Chapter 42, Part 6.

Glomerular Basement Membrane and the Goodpasture Antigen

The glomerulus is a highly specialised structure designed for the formation of filtrate from plasma, which excludes macromolecules on the basis of their size, shape, and charge. This filtration barrier is composed of three layers: (a) the endothelium, which has large, open pores unlike most other endothelium, (b) the glomerular basement membrane, and (c) the podocytes (Fig. 36.1A). The glomerular basement membrane forms the backbone of this structure with the endothelial cells adherent to the inner side and the podocytes attached to the outer surface. It is composed of an organized meshwork of glycoproteins whose major components are type IV collagen, laminin, heparan sulfate glycoproteins, and chondroitin sulfate glycoproteins. Each chain of type IV collagen consists of a central, long collagenous domain, a collagenous N-terminus (called the 7S domain, and the noncollagenous C-terminal (NC1 domain). Three α-chains self assemble to form a monomer, and these monomers are linked at their NC1 domains by disulphide bridges producing a fixed hexamer. The monomers are also linked at the 7S domains thereby stabilizing this complex meshwork (Fig. 36.1B).

α1 and α2 chains of type IV collagen are the major components, but α3, α4, and α5 are also present and are probably responsible for some of the special qualities of this basement membrane because their absence leads to disease as in Alport's syndrome (see Chapter 43, Part 2). The glomerular basement membrane is exposed to circulating blood by virtue of the fact that the endothelium has fenestrae not found in other organs, enabling circulating anti-GBM antibodies to bind readily to the GBM. These antibodies are directed at the Goodpasture antigen, which is located on the C-terminal NC1 domain of the α3 chain of type IV collagen. The pathogenicity of these antibodies has been confirmed by eluting the antibodies from human kidney fixed tissue and injecting these antibodies into monkeys. The antibodies bound to the monkey GBM and elicited characteristic glomerular inflammation.

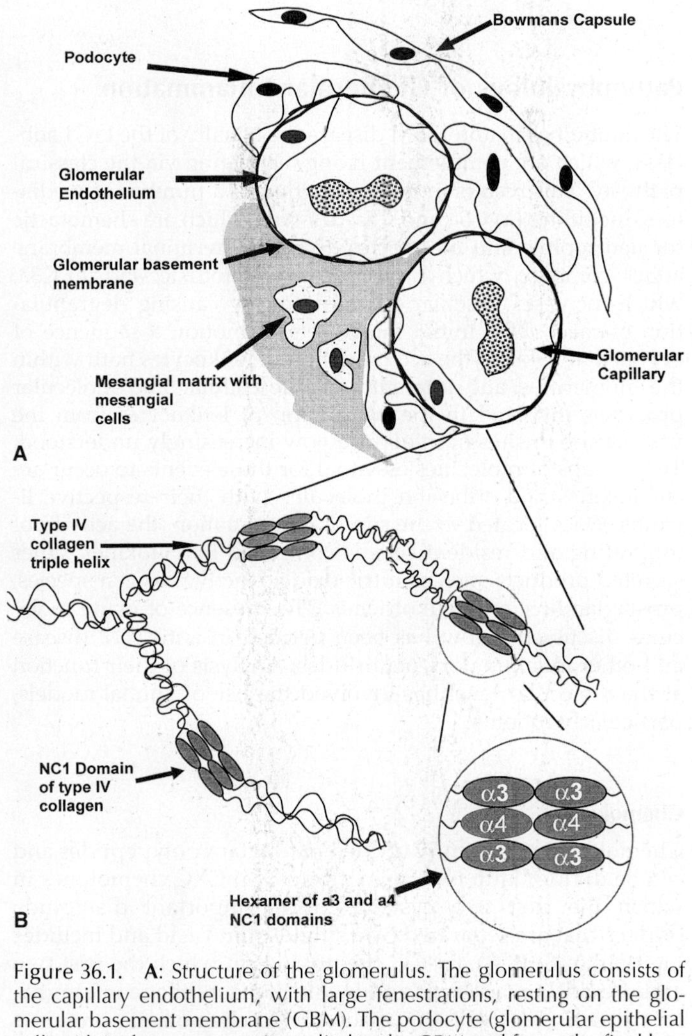

Figure 36.1. **A**: Structure of the glomerulus. The glomerulus consists of the capillary endothelium, with large fenestrations, resting on the glomerular basement membrane (GBM). The podocyte (glomerular epithelial cell) with its foot processes is applied to the GBM and forms the final barrier before the filtrate reaches the urinary space. **B**: Structure of the collagen network in the GBM. The GBM contains a meshwork of type IV collagen linked by both their NC1 domains, which forms hexamers, and disulphide bonds at their amino terminus. The target for autoimmunity in anti-GBM disease is the NC1 domain of the α3 chain of type IV collagen.

Pathology

The most characteristic pathologic finding is linear binding of IgG to the GBM, which is visualized by direct immunofluorescence. The histologic pattern of the disease starts with mesangial expansion and hypercellularity and progresses to focal and segmental glomerulonephritis with infiltration by leukocytes. Later, glomeruli develop extensive crescent formation composed of parietal epithelial cells and macrophages (Fig. 36.2), destroying the GBM. Interstitial inflammation is usually present and may relate to the binding of the antibody to the basement membrane of distal convoluted tubules.

In addition to linear IgG along the basement membrane, approximately 30% of GBM have linear IgM and/or IgA as well, and 60% have linear C3, which can be seen with immunofluorescence. There are also case reports of linear IgM alone, IgA alone, and C3 alone.

Etiology

Anti-GBM disease is relatively rare, accounting for about 5% of glomerulonephritis and 2% of end-stage renal failure. However, it provides valuable insights into the mechanisms of autoimmunity and in the particular the role of human leukocyte antigens (HLA) class II molecules in predisposing patients to the disease.

Antigen Presentation

The first stage in the production of antibodies is the uptake and processing of an antigen. A number of cells can preform this function, including macrophages, B cells, and specialist antigen presenting cells called dendritic cells. The antigen is digested within the endosomal compartments into peptides, and some of these peptides bind with newly synthesized major histocompatibility complex class II molecules. The complex of class II molecules with peptide is directed to the cell surface and presented to CD4 positive T cells along with costimulatory signals such as B7-1 and B7-2 (Fig. 36.2). CD4 positive T cells activated by this complex provide specific help to B cell, which leads to their differentiation, division, and production of antibodies directed at the original antigen. In the case of anti-GBM disease, the original antigen is the NC1 domain of the α3 chain of type IV collagen.

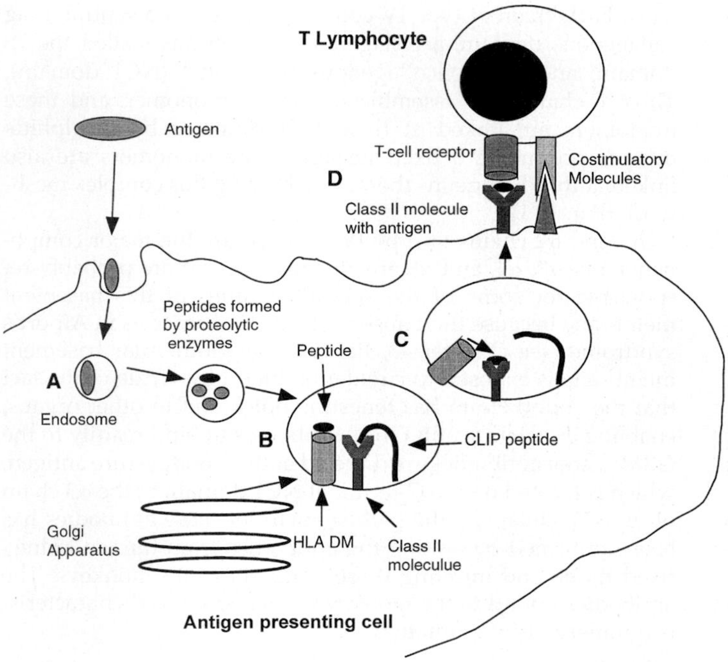

Figure 36.2. Antigen processing and presentation. **A**: Antigen is taken up by an antigen-presenting cell, such as a macrophage or dendritic cell, into the endosomal compartment. The antigen is digested by proteolytic enzymes, such as cathepsins, into peptides. **B**: These endosomes fuse with compartments containing newly synthesized class II molecules. These consist of a DR molecule with its binding groove protected by a CLIP peptide derived from invariant chain, and adjacent to the DR is a DM molecule, which initially binds the peptides. **C**: DM delivers the peptide to the DR molecule, and as this occurs the CLIP protein is removed exposing the antigen-binding groove. **D**: Peptide bound to class II molecules is then delivered to the surface for presentation to T lymphocytes. This complex along with costimulatory molecules activates the T cell, which then initiates the adaptive immune response.

HLA Complex

The importance of the class II molecules from the HLA-DR, DQ, and DP gene complex in antigen presentation is evident, and most autoimmune diseases have associations with specific alleles from this region. Positive associations have been identified with HLA-DR2 and HLA-DR4, whereas negative associations have been found with HLA-DR7 and HLA-DR1 for anti-GBM disease. Class II HLA molecules are heterodimers composed of an α chain that is encoded by single functional genes (DRA, DPA1, and DQαA) and a β chain that shows greater polymorphism. There are at least 18 DRβ alleles, and HLA-DR2 has been split into DR15 (comprising the alleles DRB1*1501 through 1505) and DR16 (comprising the alleles DRB1*1601 through 1606). Analysis of these subsets in anti-GBM disease has shown that the disease is associated with DRB1*1501 and 1502 but not with any of the DRB1*16 alleles.

Peptides derived from exogenous antigens bind to a groove formed on the Class II molecule that holds about 12 amino acids. Side chains projecting from the peptide are accommodated in pockets in the groove that occur at positions 1, 4, 6, 7, and 9 within the groove. Comparison of the DR2 alleles that predispose to disease (DRB1*1501 and 1502) with those that do not (DRB1*16) shows that they differ in pockets at positions 4 and 7 of the peptide groove. Therefore binding of Goodpasture's antigen–derived peptides to specific DR15 alleles increases disease susceptibility. It is not understood how the binding interaction of specific DR molecules with the Goodpasture antigen promotes disease. It is possible that DR15 binds the Goodpasture's-derived peptides with a high affinity to present to T cell receptors with unique efficiency. It is also possible that DR15 binds α3(IV)NC1 peptides with reduced affinity so failing to tolerise autoreactive T cells, which are later activated under specific circumstances leading to autoimmunity.

These are not the only mechanisms involved because DR 15 is common in the general population and anti-GBM disease is rare. There are clearly other genes important in allowing disease expression, and environmental triggers such as infections, exposure to hydrocarbons, and renal trauma induced by lithotripsy, have all been implicated in the onset of disease.

Pathophysiology of Glomerular Inflammation

The antibodies in anti-GBM disease are usually of the IgG1 subclass, which are complement fixing/activating via the classical pathway. This results in the production of a number of mediators, including (a) C5a and C5a-des-Arg, which are chemotactic for neutrophils and monocytes; (b) C5b-9 terminal membrane attack complex, which can be directly cytotoxic; and (c) C3a, which increases vascular permeability by causing degranulation of mast cells. Initial injury sets in motion a sequence of events that leads to the accumulation of leukocytes both within the glomerulus and interstitium. The cellular and molecular processes involved in the emigration of leukocytes from the vasculature to sites of injury are now increasingly understood. Two groups of molecules essential for these events to occur are chemokines and adhesion molecules with their respective ligands. Once located to the site of inflammation, the activity of infiltrating and resident cells is controlled by cytokines, other secreted products such as nitric oxide, reactive oxygen species, prostaglandins, and leukotrienes. The presence of many molecules discussed below has been verified in anti-GBM disease and other inflammatory nephritides. Analysis of their function at the molecular level has involved the use of animal models, particularly rodents.

Chemokines

Chemokines are a family of chemoattractant polypeptides and can be divided into two main groups: (a) CXC chemokines in which the first two cysteines form important disulphide bridges that are separated by a single amino acid and includes interleukin-8 (IL-8); (b) CC chemokines in which the first two amino acids are adjacent and includes macrophage inflammatory protein-1α (MIP-1α), macrophage chemotactic protein-1 (MCP-1), and regulated or activated T-cells expressed and secreted. Two other chemokine families have also been identified with a different structure: lymphotactin and fractalkine. The latter can act both as a chemoattractant and as an adhesion molecule. The binding of chemokines to their receptor on

TABLE 36.2. Cytokines and Their Effects on Inflammation

Cytokine	Source	Main Functions
Proinflammatory Cytokines		
Interleukin-1	Macrophages, PMN, and most other cell types	Fever, synthesis of acute-phase proteins, promotes leucocyte adhesion to endothelium, stimulates secretion of other cytokines (including IL-8, TNF, IL-1, IL-6, IL-1ra, IL-4 and GM-CSF), increases collagen synthesis, and promotes proliferation of fibroblasts.
Tumor necrosis factor	Mainly macrophages, but also synthesised by PMN and lymphocytes	Activates macrophages and neutrophils, stimulates secretion of cytokines, increases NO and reactive oxygen species synthesis, triggers cell death, and promotes differentiation of macrophages to cytotoxic cells
Interferon-γ	Lymphocytes	Promotes Th1 cell development, activates macrophages
Interleukin-8	Macrophages, PMN, most other cells	PMN chemotaxis and adhesion
Interleukin-12	Macrophages, B cells	Promotes Th1 cells, inhibits Th2 cell development
GM-CSF	Macrophages, endothelium	Differentiation and activation of PMN and macrophages
Antiinflammatory Cytokines		
Interleukin-4	T cells	Induces Th2 cells, deactivates macrophages
Interleukin-6	Macrophages, most cells	Stimulates synthesis of acute-phase proteins and cortisol, inhibits synthesis of IL-1 and TNF, promotes B cell development
Interleukin-10	Macrophages, T cells	Deactivates macrophages, inhibits Th1 cell development
Interleukin-13	Macrophages, T cells	Deactivates macrophages
Interleukin-1 receptor antagonist	Macrophages, PMN	Inhibits actions of IL-1
TGF-β	Macrophages, platelets	Deactivates macrophages, stimulates matrix synthesis

GM-CSF, granulocyte mocrophage colony stimulating factor; IL, interleukin; NO, nitric oxide; PMN, neutrophils; TBF-β, transforming growth factor-β; Th1, immune response characterized by cell-mediated immunity; Th2, immune response characterized by humoral immunity; TNF, tumor necrosis factor.

leukocyte cell surfaces alters the cell shape and increases expression of molecules involved in adhesion to the endothelial surface. This topic is covered in detail in Chapter 37, Part 2.

Adhesion

Adhesion molecules are known to play a vital role in cell-to-cell and cell-to-matrix interactions, which are important in glomerulonephritis. They include the immunoglobulin superfamily (ICAM-1, VCAM-1, and PECAM 1) and their ligands the β1 (Mac1 and LFA1) and β2 integrins (VLA-4), the selectin family, and the recently described chemotactic adhesin, fractalkine. Selectins are believed to mediate early "rolling" interactions between leukocytes and endothelium, which is later followed by tight adhesion mediated by integrins and migration across the endothelium. The expression of these adhesion molecules has been shown to be upregulated in a number of human glomerulonephritides. Both ICAM-1 and VCAM-1 expression is increased on endothelial cells of glomeruli with crescentic glomerulonephritis, IgA nephropathy, lupus nephritis, and tubulointerstitial nephritis. In addition, there is increased expression of ICAM-1 on the luminal surface of proximal and distal tubules, whereas VCAM-1 expression is increased on proximal tubule cells in acute glomerulonephritis. These molecules play a pivotal role in directing inflammatory cells to the focus of injury. In experimental models of glomerulonephritis, blocking their function can reduce the degree of inflammation. This topic is discussed in detail in Chapter 37, Part 6.

Cytokines

In anti-GBM disease the glomerulus and interstitium are infiltrated by macrophages, neutrophils, and lymphocytes. Cytokines produced by these cells are important in the propagation and control of inflammation. There are a large number of cytokines, which can be broadly divided into those with principally proinflammatory effects and those with antiinflammatory effects, that include chemokines mentioned above (Table 36.2).

The expression of many of the cytokines and chemokines discussed here has been verified in acute glomerular inflammation, including anti-GBM disease. The detail of the regulatory network has been demonstrated in *in vivo* models and is beginning to provide more specific approaches to control acute glomerular inflammation.

Proinflammatory Cytokines. The principal cytokines in this group, produced at sites of inflammation, include interleukin-1β (IL-1β) and tumor necrosis factor (TNF), are largely produced by infiltrating macrophages and interferon-γ, which is produced by activated T-helper cells. These cytokines activate other inflammatory cells and alter the endothelium to enhance the localization of leukocytes to the site of injury. The effects of IL-1β and TNF are regulated by a number of naturally synthesized antagonists. IL-1 receptor antagonist (IL-1ra) is produced by macrophages and neutrophils and executes its antiinflammatory effect by binding to the IL-1 receptor on the cell surface without activating the receptor. The activity of IL-1β is also controlled by the characteristics of the two sorts of IL-1 receptor, type I and type II. The type I receptor mediates the biologic effects of IL-1β, whereas the type II receptor binds IL-1β but does not generate a signal, in effect acting as a decoy receptor. In addition, the type II receptor is found in a soluble form that binds IL-1β and decreases the concentration of the cytokine. Similarly for TNF there are naturally occurring soluble forms of the receptors that bind and inhibit the biologic effect of TNF. The net effect on inflammation is a balance between the proinflammatory cytokines and their antagonists.

Antiinflammatory Cytokines. Several cytokines act to reduce inflammatory activity of infiltrating cells. Some of these such as IL-4, IL-10, and IL-13 are produced by regulatory T-helper cells, whereas others, such as transforming growth factor-β, IL-6, and IL-13, are produced by resident glomerular cells and macrophages. An outline of their influences on inflammation is provided in Table 36.2. Broadly, this group of molecules reduces the synthesis of proinflammatory cytokines IL-1 and TNF, increases production of their antagonists IL-1ra and soluble TNF receptors, decreases production of inflammatory mediators such as reactive oxygen intermediates, nitric oxide, and certain prostaglandins, and increases synthesis of other antiinflammatory cytokines (i.e., IL-4 increases IL-10 synthesis by macrophages). The topic of cytokines is discussed in detail in Chapter 47, Part 2.

ANTI-GBM DISEASE AFTER TRANSPLANTATION IN PATIENTS WITH ALPORT'S SYNDROME

The molecular defect in Alport's syndrome is most commonly a mutation in the gene for α5 chain of type IV collagen on the X chromosome. Failure of expression of the α5 chain also leads to the absence of α3 and α4 type IV collagen in the specialized GBM. This leads to hematuria and subsequently renal failure. When such patients receive a renal transplantation, they are in theory exposed to novel antigens in the form of α3, α4, and α5 chains of type IV collagen, which could be identified as foreign by the recipient's immune system. The majority of such patients have a routine posttransplant course, however; a minority develop anti-GBM disease with associated inflammation within the allograft. In most cases of such posttransplant anti-GBM, the antibody appears to be directed at the α5 chain and leads to a crescentic glomerulonephritis similar to that seen with anti-GBM. This topic is also discussed in Chapter 43, Part 2.

MEMBRANOUS NEPHROPATHY

Membranous nephropathy is a glomerular disease characterised by subepithelial deposition of immune deposits leading to diffuse thickening of the glomerular capillary wall in the absence of inflammatory or proliferative changes. It is the most common cause of nephrotic syndrome in adults and is associated with a large number of diseases, including hepatitis B, solid tumors (colon, lung, breast, and kidney), lymphomas, systemic lupus erythematosus, and drug reactions (captopril, gold, and penicillamine). Most cases are idiopathic and the antigen to which the IgG antibodies are directed is most likely a component of the glomerular epithelial cell pedicel.

Pathogenesis

Immunogenetics

Idiopathic membranous nephropathy (IMN) shows a strong link to the major histocompatability complex. Between 55% and 78% of north European Caucasians with membranous nephropathy have HLA-DR3 compared with 20% to 25% of control subjects whereas only 33% of Greek patients were DR3 positive compared with 15% of control subjects. These findings are similar to the findings of a study in North American patients. There have also been reports of associations with HLA-B8 and HLA-B18 in Caucasian patients with IMN as well. In Japanese patients there is a strong association with HLA-DR2 (B1*1501) with approximately 80% possessing this allele versus 30% to 39% of control subjects. The mechanisms explaining how both DR2 and DR3 predispose to IMN are not certain but could include the following: (a) Both DR molecules have the required properties to confer disease susceptibility, (b) The DR molecules are in linkage disequilibrium with the true susceptibility gene(s), or (c) Pathogenesis of IMN is different in different populations.

Evidence from both European and Japanese studies point to the second of these mechanisms where the true susceptibility gene is a DQ allele. In a study of British patients, the primary association was with DQA1, which is inherited with HLA-DR3 and DR5, whereas a Japanese study showed DQA was present in 86% with IMN versus 14% of control subjects.

Formation of Deposits and Mechanism of Injury

The characteristic feature of membranous nephropathy is the formation of subepithelial immune deposits. There are three mechanisms that could explain this phenomenon. First, preformed immune complexes could become trapped in the glomerulus. This has been demonstrated experimentally in rabbits induced with serum sickness by injection of bovine serum albumin; however, there is little evidence of circulating immune complexes in patients with IMN. Second, immune deposits could form on an exogenous antigen trapped in the glomerulus. Such a mechanism may be more likely in secondary causes of membranous nephropathy such as those associated with autoimmune disease or malignancy. Third, the antibody in IMN could be directed at an antigen expressed in the subepithelial space, such as a component of the glomerular epithelial cell. This represents the most likely explanation according to experimental models.

Heymann nephritis represents a useful model for the third possibility. This model was originally induced in rats by immunizing them with a mixture of antigens purified from the brush border of proximal tubules (Fx1A). Over the span of a few weeks, the rats develop subepithelial deposits containing IgG and complement, accompanied by proteinuria and then nephrotic syndrome. The main antigen against which the IgG is directed has been identified as megalin, a glycoprotein found in the clathrin coated pits of podocytes. However, antibodies to megalin are not sufficient to cause proteinuria and antibodies to other membrane glycolipids appear to be important to induce proteinuria. Antibodies to megalin have not yet been identified in human disease, and in human IMN the target may be a different component expressed on podocytes.

Subepithelial immune deposits probably mediate their injury through a number of mechanisms, including activation of complement and generation of oxygen radicals. This has been most clearly demonstrated in Heymann nephritis where it appears to be the formation of the C5b-9 membrane attack complex that allows the development of proteinuria. C5b-9 inserts into the cell membrane of the podocyte and is taken up into endosomes and then exocytosed from the podocyte into the urinary space, eventually appearing in the urine. In humans with IMN, a number of groups have found increased levels of urinary C5b-9, which has also been associated with disease activity.

Both mesangial and glomerular epithelial cells produce inflammatory mediators in response to C5b-9, including TNF, IL-1, reactive oxygen species, and extracellular matrix components, which could mediate changes in both cell function and glomerular basement membrane structure. Sublytic attack by C5b-9 on the glomerular epithelial cell results in increased cell surface expression of NADPH oxidoreductase enzyme complex. This results in increased generation of reactive oxygen species that interact with the GBM matrix and result in lipid peroxidation (LPO) adducts on monomeric and dimerized NC1 domains of type IV collagen. These structural changes in the GBM could have functional consequences. Interestingly, treatment with probucol, an LPO antagonist, reduces proteinuria in Heymann nephritis. A potential source of the polyunsaturated lipids required for LPO production could be lipoproteins, which have been shown to accumulate in immune deposits. There is evidence for increased protease activity in Heymann nephritis, which could damage the GBM leading to increased protein leak. Also, the presence of large subepithelial immune deposits could cause a mechanical disruption to the function of the podocyte.

Another epithelial antigen that may serve as a target for autoantibodies is the glomerular enzyme dipeptidyl peptidase type IV (gp90/DPP IV). Autoantibodies directed against this molecule were discovered in mice suffering from chronic graft-versus-host disease, an inducible model of autoimmune-mediated glomerulonephritis. A chronic graft-versus-host reaction can be induced by using congenic mouse strains in selected parent–parent or parent–hybrid combinations. The recipient mice develop a variety of pathologic changes, including a lupus type of nephritis, associated with a positive Coombs' test and the formation of autoantibodies directed against components of the GBM and against DPP IV. Binding of anti-DPP IV autoantibodies leads to a rearrangement of this molecule on the glomerular epithelial cell surface. DPP IV functions as an adhesion molecule on the glomerular epithelial cell surface, and its rearrangement may be related to an altered function of these cells and increased permeability of the glomerular capillary wall.

ANCA-ASSOCIATED VASCULITIS

Antibodies to ANCA are found in vasculitides affecting small vessels, including Wegener's granulomatosis, Churg-Strauss syndrome, and microscopic polyarteritis, diseases in which focal necrotizing glomerulonephritis may be the primary pathology. These conditions present with rapidly progressive glomerulonephritis, and renal biopsies often show extensive crescent formation and capillary thrombosis.

These antibodies were initially defined by their pattern of staining on neutrophils. Cytoplasmic pattern of antineutrophil cytoplasmic antibody (c-ANCA) shows a diffuse, granular pattern of staining in the neutrophil cytoplasm, and the main antigen associated with this antibody is proteinase-3 (PR3). The second staining pattern is perinuclear (p-ANCA), and the principal antigen associated with this is myeloperoxidase (MPO). The strong association of ANCA with glomerulonephritis has led to the hypothesis that these antibodies are pathogenic. Potential mechanisms include the following:

1. ANCAs bind to neutrophils, resulting in their activation. Because the antigens are normally intracellular, they need to be expressed on the cell surface to bind the antibody. TNF-stimulated neutrophils demonstrate ANCA antigens on the cell surface. It is presumed that neutrophils activated in this way would then release proteolytic enzymes, reactive oxygen metabolites, and proinflammatory cytokines, which further propagate the acute inflammation. There is also evidence that once neutrophils are bound by ANCA, they lose their ability to transmigrate across the endothelium and remain immobilized within the capillary/small vessel where they continue to elicit injury.
2. Neutrophils release ANCA antigens, which are then bound to the endothelial cell surface. This planted antigen could then become a target for ANCAs, resulting in endothelial activation, injury, and acute inflammation. Also ANCA could prevent PR3 from being inactivated by its natural inhibitor α_1-antitrypsin, thereby allowing prolonged extracellular proteolytic activity.
3. The third possible role for ANCA could be direct binding of these antibodies to the glomerular endothelium. Cytokine-treated endothelial cells in culture have been shown to express PR3. In addition, membrane protein fractions from human glomeruli contain an antigen that binds cANCA. This glomerular glycoprotein was called gp130. A monoclonal antibody raised to gp130 bound to glomerular endothelial cells and also to human neutrophils in a pattern similar to that seen with cANCA. The antigen within the neutrophils to which this antibody bound was isolated as human lysosome associated protein membrane-2 (H-lamp-2). This raises the possibility that ANCAs could bind to glomerular endothelial antigens, and then binding of neutrophils and macrophages via Fc receptors or activation of complement could initiate inflammation. Or, ANCA could cross link neutrophil to endothelium, leading to activation of both cells.

Once injury is initiated, the neutrophils, macrophages, and T cells will infiltrate the glomerulus and interstitium using adhesion pathways and following chemotactic signals as already outlined. The activity of these inflammatory cells leads to the characteristic focal necrotizing glomerulonephritis and progressive renal failure. The clinical entity of membranous glomerulonephritis is discussed in detail in Chapter 39, Part 6.

POSTSTREPTOCOCCAL GLOMERULONEPHRITIS

Poststreptococcal glomerulonephritis (PSGN) is caused by infection with group A β-hemolytic streptococci of the nephritogenic M type. The incidence of this disease has decreased in most developed nations over the last 20 years. Histologically, PSGN appears as a diffuse proliferative glomerulonephritis with proliferation of endothelial and mesangial cells and infiltration by neutrophils and macrophages. A number of streptococcal antigens have been identified as being potentially nephritogenic, including endostreptosin, streptokinase, and streptococcal cationic proteinase or its precursor zymogen.

The antigens involved are a matter of speculation as is the mechanism of immune injury. One possibility is that glomerulonephritis is a result of immune complex deposition. In immune complex–mediated experimental models of nephritis, the immune complexes are deposited in a subendothelial location because they are unable to cross the GBM. In PSGN the immune deposits are both subepithelial and subendothelial. For the antigen, antibody, or immune complex to locate them requires a net positive because the GBM has a net negative charge. Cationic immune complexes have not been identified in patients with PSGN. Another possibility is that the causative streptococcal antigen is deposited within the glomerulus and then preformed antibodies bind to it, resulting in local immune complex formation and injury. Evidence exists in support of the latter possibility.

A third possibility is that antibodies formed against streptococcal antigens cross-react with native glomerular antigens, leading to antibody deposition and acute inflammation. One group of researchers observed that antibodies reactive with streptococcal cell wall also bound to glomeruli, and other researchers have identified antibodies to type IV collagen, heparan sulfate, and laminin in the serum of PSGN patients.

A fourth possibility is that streptococcal infection induces an autoimmune reaction. In a number of patients with PSGN, rheumatoid factor can be found with IgG rheumatoid factor being more common. Neuraminidase (sialidase) is produced by streptococci and can deplete IgG of sialic acid. This modified IgG can induce the formation of anti-IgG rheumatoid factor in rabbits, and in patients these antibodies could lead to the formation of cryoglobulins. Neuraminidase has also been shown to affect activity of neutrophils and monocytes. Treatment of these cells with neuraminidase promotes their localization to glomeruli and interstitium. The clinical entity of poststreptococcal glomerulonephritis is discussed in Chapter 39, Part 3A.

ANTIMESANGIAL ANTIBODY DISEASES

Little is known about the role of antigens located in the glomerular mesangium as specific targets for immune reactions. Primary IgA nephropathy is a common form of glomerulonephritis with a diverse range of clinical presentations, leading to slowly progressive renal failure in a substantial proportion of the patients. Characteristically, deposits of IgA1, derived from the bloodstream, are found in the glomerular mesangium. Increased plasma levels of IgA1 and IgA1-containing immune complexes are believed to be of pathogenic importance, although the mechanism of the mesangial deposition remains unclear. Several studies suggest that the binding of immunoglobulins to the mesangium in IgA nephropathy may be mediated through either a fibronectin–collagen interaction or through autoantibodies directed at glomerular molecules. In patients with IgA nephropathy, antibodies directed against laminin and a collagenase-sensitive antigen present in type IV collagen α-chains have been found. These antibodies are believed to bind to the mesangial extracellular matrix and may be responsible for the induction of glomerular inflammation. In an experimental model in rats, antibodies directed against the mesangial cell surface glycoprotein Thy1.1 induce mesangiolysis and inflammation by mechanisms discussed below.

In anti-Thy1.1–mediated glomerulonephritis in rats, increased synthesis of mesangial matrix components is preceded by cell proliferation and increases of steady-state mRNA levels for these molecules. The evolution of glomerular injury in this model of immune complex–mediated glomerulonephritis is accompanied by an extensive matrix remodeling process, reflected by the upregulation of not only basement membrane molecules themselves but also basement membrane degrading enzymes, such as type IV collagenase. Complement depletion prevents the histologic abnormalities, as well as the increased expression of matrix proteins. These studies indicate that antibody-mediated immunologic injury involving structural renal antigens present in the mesangium may result in overproduction of mesangial matrix components. In this model, recent studies have strongly implicated a role for TGF-β, which may be released by monocytes-macrophages, platelets, or the mesangial cells themselves. TGF-β probably is involved in the regulation of both the mesangial cell proliferative response and the altered extracellular matrix homeostasis. Based on such observations, the concept has emerged that growth factor–mediated cell proliferation in glomerulonephritis should be regarded as part of a repair process that may either be successful or lead to the development of glomerulosclerosis.

Selected Readings

Brainwood D, Kashtan C, Gubler MC, et al. Targets of alloantibodies in Alport antiglomerular basement membrane disease after renal transplantation. *Kidney Int* 1988;53:762–766.

Assesses the antibody binding of serum from Alport's patients who developed anti-GBM disease post renal transplant to recombinant α3, α4, and α5 NC1 domains of type IV collagen. They show that the antibodies are principally directed against α5 NC1 domain rather than α3.

Cockwell P, Tse WY, Savage CO. Activation of endothelial cells in thrombosis and vasculitis [Review]. *Scan J Rheum* 1997;26:145–150.

Reviews the interaction between neutrophils and endothelium in ANCA-positive vasculitis and, in particular, how inhibition of migration by ANCA antibodies could promote inflammation and endothelial damage.

Kain R, Matsui K, Exner M, et al. A novel class of autoantigens of antineutrophil cytoplasmic antibodies in necrotizing and crescentic glomerulonephritis: the lysosomal membrane glycoprotein h-lamp-2 in neutrophil granulocytes and a related membrane protein in glomerular endothelial cells. *J Exp Med* 1995; 181:585–597.

Assesses possible cell surface targets for ANCA antibodies in both neutrophils and glomeruli. The paper shows that ANCA cross reacts with glycoprotein human lysosomal-associated membrane protein 2 (H-lamp-2) on neutrophils and with a 130-kDa glycoprotein on endothelial cell surfaces. This raises the possibility that ANCA antibodies directly bind to endothelium to initiate disease.

Kerjaschki D, Neale TJ. Molecular mechanisms of glomerular injury in rat experimental membranous nephropathy (Heymann nephritis) [Review]. *J Am Soc Nephrol* 1996;7:2518–2526.

This review summarizes current molecular aspects of the formation of characteristic subepithelial immune deposits in the glomerular basement membrane and describes the development of glomerular capillary wall damage resulting in proteinuria in both Heymann's nephritis and membranous nephropathy. It discusses the mechanism of formation of C5-9 membrane attack complex associated with the antigen megalin and how prevention of lipid peroxidation using probucol may be valuable in reducing proteinuria.

Kluth DC, Rees AJ. Inhibiting inflammatory cytokines [Review]. *Semin Nephrol* 1996;16:576–582.

Reviews the role of proinflammatory and antiinflammatory cytokines in regulating glomerular inflammation. It discusses the role of IL-4, IL-6, IL-10, and IL-13 in downmodulating the acute inflammatory response.

Phelps RG, Rees AJ. The HLA complex in Goodpasture's disease: a model for analysing mechanisms of genetic susceptibility to autoimmunity. *Kidney Int* 1999;56:163–1653.

Reviews the evidence for the association of Goodpasture's disease to the HLA complex and analyzes the biology of antigen presentation of Goodpasture's-derived peptides to T cells.

Takano T, Brady HR. The endothelium in glomerular inflammation [Review]. *Curr Opin Nephrol Hyperten* 1995;4:277–286.

Reviews the molecules involved in adhesion of inflammatory leukocytes to glomerular endothelium and the potential for inhibiting these processes in modulating renal inflammation.

Turner N, Forstova J, Rees A, et al. Production and characterization of recombinant Goodpasture antigen in insect cells. *J Biol Chem* 1994;269:17141–17145.

Describes the characterization of Goodpasture antigen as the NC1 domain of the α3 chain of type IV collagen and describes the production of recombinant antigen, which has proved valuable in the study of this disease.

PART 2
Nephritogenic Immune Reactions Involving Planted Renal Antigens

Richard J. Glassock

Antigenic substances not normally native to the kidney may bind to or localize in renal structures by virtue of an immunologic, biochemical, or biophysical (charge or size) interactions. In the presence of a humoral or cellular reaction to the bound or planted antigen, a local or *in situ* immune complex may be formed and subsequently a cascade of immunopathologic events elicited, leading to glomerular injury.

This category of immune reactions also participates in the pathogenesis of antibody-mediated renal disease, in which the antibody is directed to native renal antigens, or in renal diseases involving the deposition of circulating immune complexes. In these circumstances the deposited immune reactants also serve as planted antigens (see Chapter 36, Parts 1 and 3).

BINDING OR LOCALIZATION OF NONNATIVE ANTIGENS TO RENAL STRUCTURES

Table 36.3 outlines the various mechanisms by which nonnative antigenic substances can bind or localize in renal structures, including immune reactions, biochemical interactions, and biophysical interactions (including charge and/or size).

TABLE 36.3. Mechanisms Involved in Binding of Nonnative Antigenic Substances to Renal Structures

Immune Interactions	Biochemical Interactions
Autologous phase of nephrotoxic serum nephritis or passive Heymann nephritis	Concanavalin A, SLE nephritis, poststreptococcal glomerulonephritis, IgA nephropathy and gelatin-induced nephritis
Biophysical Interactions	
(Charge/Size) Cationized ferritin, histones, cationic cell wall proteins, DNA-histone, aggregated cationic IgG, cryoimmunoglobulins, and IgA-fibronectin	

SLE, systemic lupus erythematosus.

Immune Interactions

Antibodies directed to constituents of glomerular basement membrane (GBM) may evoke antiantibody responses (e.g., antiidiopathic antibody). These antibodies may react with the bound (planted) antibody to evoke or perpetuate disease. A cell-mediated response to the bound antibody may also occur. When the planted antibody is from another species, the response is to the heterologous determinants on the bound foreign protein. When the planted antibody is host-derived, the response is to cryptic or neo-neo-epitopes (e.g., idiotypes) on the autologous protein. Examples of the former include the autologous phase of nephrotoxic serum nephritis and the autologous phase of passive Heymann nephritis. Examples of the latter include rheumatoid factor and antiidiotypic antibody interactions in autoimmune diseases of the kidney.

Circulating immune complexes deposited in the kidney may also be the site of a planted antigen interaction; therefore DNA bound locally may react with anti-DNA from the circulation and form an immune complex *in situ* that can then react with rheumatoid factor or antiidiotypic antibody.

Biochemical Interactions

Theoretically, any chemical substance having a strong infinity for constituents of the glomerular capillary wall, mesangium, or the tubular basement membrane and which is capable of eliciting a cellular and/or humoral response can participate in the pathogenesis of renal disease due to planted renal antigen mechanisms.

The capillary wall, mesangium, and basement membranes of glomeruli and tubules are composed of glycoproteins, exogenous substances may have strong affinity. Concanavalin A is a plant protein that has an affinity for carbohydrate residues of glycoproteins (e.g., lectin activity). This glycoprotein can elicit glomerulonephritis when administered to rats preimmunized to concanavalin A. Bacteria (e.g., group A streptococci) also contain similar lectin-like substances that could bind to renal structures and evoke nephritis. The collagenous component of GBM may bind DNA-histone molecules, and the presence of anti-DNA antibody may produce nephritis. Certain bacterial antigens also have an affinity for fibronectin, a normal constituent of the mesangial matrix, and may thereby plant in glomeruli and serve as a focus for an immune reaction. Abnormally glycosylated proteins, such as galactose-deficient IgA_1 may acquire properties of binding to mesangial structures (or alternatively, to form molecular aggregates through IGA_1–IGA_1 interactions).

Biophysical Interactions

The physical attributes of charge and size of macromolecules may confer renal binding or localizing properties. The GBM is normally anionic due to the presence of sulfated glycoproteins such as sialic acid and heparan sulfate (Fig. 36.3). These negative charges are concentrated particularly at the surface of the podocyte, in the laminarara interna and externa, and on the endothelial surface. Cationized antigens (e.g., ferritin, IgG, bovine serum albumin) readily bind to these antionic sites in an electrostatic fashion, particularly in the subendothelial and subepithelial spaces. The binding of these cationic molecules form large aggregates, which, when they subsequently react with circulating antibodies, lead to the formation of subepithelial or subendothelial immune deposits. Anionic molecules, on the other hand, preferentially localize in the mesangium. Cationic antibodies (e.g., those with isoelectric points greater than 8.0) preferentially and initially bind electrostatically to anionic sites and then co-localize antigens to which the cationic antibody is directed. Cationic anti-DNA forms glomerular immune complex deposits with anionic DNA in this fashion. Anionic molecules can also localize in the GBM when the negative charges of the GBM have been neutralized as with the systemic administration of low molecular weight polycations (polyethual imine). The endogenous release of cationic proteins such as platelet factor 4 (polyethylenimine) lysozyme, beta thromboglobulin, or cathepsin (from leukocytes or platelets) may cause a similar neutralization of the normal glomerular anionic charge and alter the affinity of cationic or anionic immunogenic proteins for renal structures.

Histones are highly cationic proteins, normally a constituent of a nuclear chromatin, that bind to GBM with high affinity. Glomerular-bound histone may bind circulating single-stranded DNA, which can then react with circulating anti-DNA to form *in situ* immune complexes.

Finally, large aggregated molecules (e.g., heated IgG) or polymers of native proteins (e.g., IgA_1 polymers) can be trapped in the glomerular structures, particularly in the mesangium, by exceeding the capacity for removal or phagocytosis. Once trapped in this site, these molecules serve as a nidus for reaction with circulating antibodies or sensitized cells.

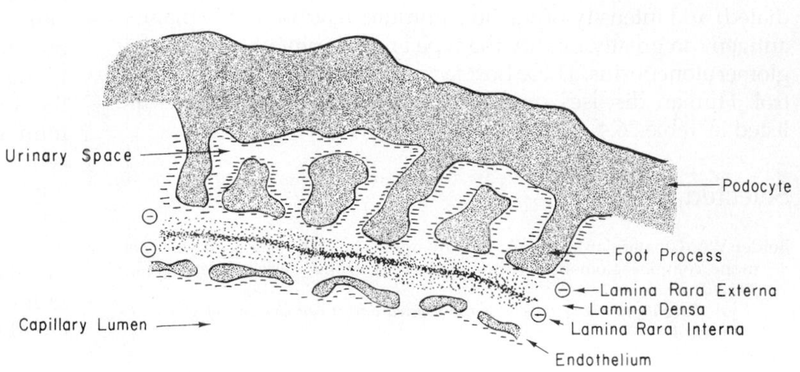

Figure 36.3. Distribution of charges in the glomerular capillary wall.

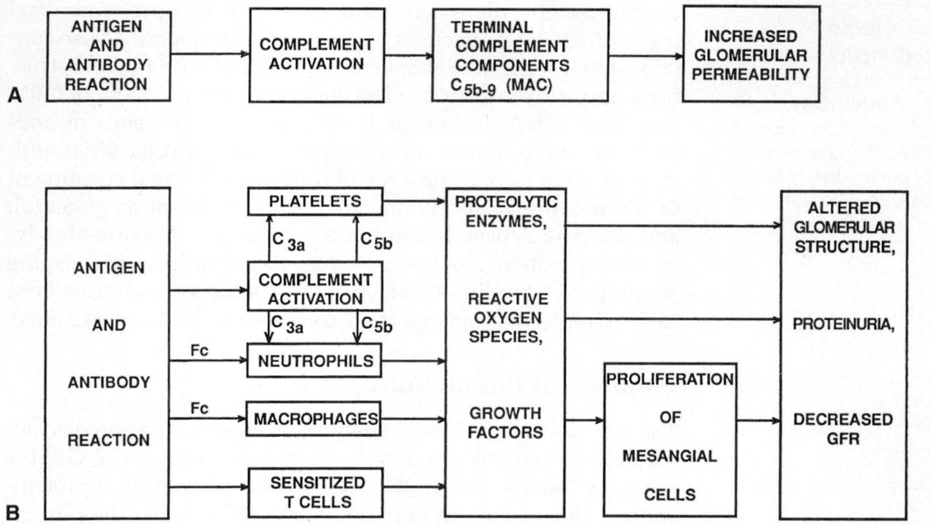

Figure 36.4. Patterns of mediation of glomerular injury according to the site of localization of immune reactions. **A**: Subepithelial localization. **B:** Subendothelial/mesangial localization.

TABLE 36.4. Human Renal Diseases Possibly Involving Planted Antigens

Disease	Planted Antigen
SLE	Histone/DNA
IgA nephropathy	Galactose-deficient polymeric IgA_1
Postinfectious glomerulonephritis (e.g., poststreptococcal GN, hepatitis B)	Cationic bacterial or viral proteins (streptococcal zymogen)
Neoplasia-associated GN	Cationic oncofetal neoantigens
Membranous glomerulonephritis	Idiotypic determinants on IgG
Serum sickness	Heterologous IgG (horse Ig)

GN, glomerulonephritis; SLE, systemic lupus erythematosus.

CONSEQUENCES OF PLANTED ANTIGEN INTERACTIONS

The site of the deposits of planted antigens and their subsequent reaction with antibodies or sensitized cells play crucial roles in the pathologic consequences of the immune reaction. For example, antigens planted predominantly in a subepithelial site evoke a membranous-type nephropathy with minimal proliferative response. The proteinuria in this circumstance is complement dependent and leukocyte independent (Fig. 36.4). On the other hand, antigens planted primarily in a subendothelial or mesangial location tend to produce proliferative or exudative responses in a leukocyte-dependent and complement-independent fashion. This pattern is similar to that of immune interactions involving native renal antigens. Of course, the nature (humoral or cell mediated) and intensity of the host immune reaction to the planted antigen can greatly modify the type and severity of the resulting glomerulonephritis. These host factors may be under genetic control. Human diseases possibly involving planted antigens are listed in Table 36.4.

Selected Readings

Border WA. Glomerular acceptors: new thoughts about the pathogenesis of immune complex glomerulonephritis. *Plasma Ther Transfusion Technol* 1984;5:395–401.

A thought-provoking review of the planted antigen mechanism of glomerulonephritis.

Chan TM. Different mechanisms by which monoclonal anti-DNA antibodies bind to human endothelial cells and glomerular mesangial cells. *Clin Exp Immunol* 1992;88:68–74.

Describes new mechanisms for binding DNA to the glomerulus.

Comussi G, Tetto C, Segonoli G, et al. Platelet activating factor-induced loss of glomerular anionic charges. *Kidney Int* 1984;25:73–81.

Demonstration that endogenous cationic proteins neutralizes glomerular anionic charge.

Rodriguez-Ikube B. Post-infectious glomerulonephritis. *Am J Dis* 2000;35:xlvi–xlviii.

An excellent review, including interpretation of data, of the role of planted antigens in poststreptococcal glomerulonephritis.

Schmiedke TMJ, Stoeckl FW, Weber R, et al. Histones have high affinity for the glomerular basement membrane. *J Exp Med* 1989;169:1879–1894.

Examination of the potential role of histones in the pathogenesis of lupus nephritis through in situ immune complex formation.

Vogt A. New aspects of the pathogenesis of immune complex glomerulonephritis: formation of subepithelial deposits. *Clin Nephrol* 1984;21:15–20.

An analysis of charge and size factors in subepithelial immune deposit formation.

Zanetti M, Wilson CB. A role for antiidiotypic antibodies in immunologically mediated nephritis. *Am J Kidney Dis* 1986;7:445–449.

A thorough review of the idiotype-antiidiotypic network in the pathogenesis of nephritis.

PART 3
Immune Complex Diseases

Christine Abrass

Immune complexes form when antibodies combine with antigens. An immune complex disease is a state in which organ dysfunction results from injury caused by deposition of immune complexes rather than the agent or event that initiated the immune complex formation. Granular deposits of immunoglobulin and complement, detected by immunofluorescence microscopy, are frequent findings in immune complex–mediated glomerulonephritis. In many cases, the nature of the antigen(s) is not known, and therefore the etiology of the disease cannot be established. Significant progress has been made in this area in the past 5 years. With technical advances, immune complex isolation is possible, and the antigen content of circulating immune complexes has been established in some

TABLE 36.5. Diseases in Which Immune Complexes Participate in Pathogenesis of Glomerulonephritis

Definite role[a]
Lupus erythematosus
Poststreptococcal glomerulonephritis
Bacterial endocarditis
Visceral abscess
Infected atrioventricular shunts
Thyroiditis
Specific infections (e.g., hepatitis B and C and syphilis)
Membranoproliferative glomerulonephritis, type I
IgA nephropathy
Uncertain role
Idiopathic rapidly progressive glomerulonephritis
Idiopathic membranous glomerulonephritis
IgM mesangial glomerulonephritis
Henoch-Schönlein purpura

[a] These diseases are sometimes associated with hypocomplementemia (see Chapter 37, Part 5).

diseases. For practical purposes, it is useful to categorize the various forms of human glomerulonephritis into those that have an immune complex pathogenesis and those for which, although immune deposits are present, the pathogenic mechanism(s) is unknown (Table 36.5).

BIOLOGIC BASIS OF IMMUNE COMPLEX DISEASE

The immune system is divided into a cellular and a humoral arm. The humoral component functions through the production of antibody molecules that recognize and bind to specific target antigens. The latter may be present on a cell membrane or may be free in a body fluid. In either case, the result of the union of antigen and antibody is the formation of an antigen–antibody (immune) complex. When immune complexes are formed in the circulation, they can be delivered to organs containing large numbers of mononuclear phagocytes (e.g., liver, spleen), which remove them. This forms the basis of immune elimination, which also occurs when opsonized bacteria are effectively removed to protect the host from infection and its consequences. In some cases circulating immune complexes are formed in such large amounts that they overwhelm the clearance mechanisms. In other cases, unique biochemical characteristics of the circulating immune complexes allow them to escape removal by phagocytes. In this situation, circulating immune complexes persist and can deposit in capillary beds, where they initiate an inflammatory reaction and tissue injury.

Antigens present in the circulation can arise from exogenous sources (e.g., bacterial, viral, drug-related antigens) (Table 36.6) or from endogenous sources (e.g., DNA, histones, thyroid antigens) (Table 36.7). If the immune system functions effectively, most exogenous antigens are eliminated from the circulation after binding to an antibody because specific antibody synthesis decreases and circulating immune-complex formation ends. In this case, the resulting tissue injury may heal if significant scarring has not already occurred. When antibodies are formed to endogenous antigens (autoantibody), it is usually the consequence of abnormal regulation of the immune response. The constant supply of endogenous antigen can lead to more chronic forms of immune complex–mediated tissue injury. Similarly, in some cases of infection (e.g., hepatitis C virus, HIV), antibody formation occurs, but the antibodies and/or cellular immune response are ineffective at eliminating the source of the antigen.

TABLE 36.6. Exogenous Antigens Implicated in Human Immune Complex Glomerulonephritis

Nonreplicating antigens
Foreign serum proteins
Tetanus antitoxin
Antisnake venom
Antilymphocyte globulin
Drugs and chemicals
Penicillin
Sulfonamide
Captopril
Penicillamine
Heavy metals
Food allergens
Milk
Replicating antigens
Bacterial
Coliforms
Streptococcus
Staphylococcus
Pneumococcus
Meningococcus
Salmonella
Treponema
Mycobacterium
Viral
Hepatitis B virus
Hepatitis C virus
Epstein-Barr virus
Cytomegalovirus
Varicella-zoster virus
Human immunodeficiency virus (HIV)
Fungal
Coccidioidomycosis
Aspergilla
Protozoal
Malaria
Toxoplasmosis
Helminthic
Filariasis
Schistosomiasis

TABLE 36.7. Endogenous Antigens Implicated in Human Immune Complex Glomerulonephritis

Nuclear and cytoplasmic constituents
Cytoskeletal proteins
Deoxyribonucleic acid (DNA)
Histones
Ribonucleic acid (RNA)
Saline extractable nuclear antigen (e.g., Smith antigen)
Tumor-specific antigens
Carcinoembryonic antigen (CEA)
Melanoma-specific antigen
Organ-specific proteins
Renal tubular antigens
Thyroglobulin
Structural proteins
Collagen
Fibronectin
Laminin
Cell membrane proteins
Red blood cell membrane antigen
Receptors (e.g., acetylcholine receptor)
Serum proteins
α_1-Antitrypsin
Clq
Hormones (e.g., insulin)
Immunoglobulins
Rheumatoid factors
Antiidiotypic antibodies

Persisting infection can lead to chronic tissue deposition of circulating immune complexes and progressive injury as occurs in autoimmune diseases.

Recent studies indicate that the specificity of antibodies produced to target antigens is genetically determined. Features unique to the antibody can determine its ability to efficiently eliminate antigen, cross-react with self-antigens, and participate in controlled regulation of the intensity and duration of the immune response to a given antigen. Thus the host immune response, as well as features unique to the antigen, can influence the propensity to develop immune complex–mediated disease. Once formed in the circulation, immune complexes may deposit in vascular beds throughout the body. The most susceptible site for such deposition appears to be the renal glomerulus, where accumulation of immune complexes can produce a spectrum of structural and functional alterations.

Experimental Immune Complex Disease

Clinical and pathologic data indicate that 50% to 80% of human glomerular diseases are immunologically mediated and are characterized by granular deposits of immunoglobulin and complement within the glomerulus. To better understand why only some circulating immune complexes result in tissue injury and to define the mechanisms whereby injury occurs, a number of animal models were developed. These have been studied extensively and have made major contributions to our understanding of glomerular diseases. Early in these studies, it was recognized that immune complexes can be formed when antibodies are made to either exogenous or endogenous antigens. Given the potential differences in pathogenesis and outcome of these two forms of immune complex diseases, animal models of both types were studied.

Acute serum sickness in the rabbit is induced by immunization with bovine serum albumin (BSA). Antibodies are made to this exogenous protein. At the time of immune elimination of the antigen from the circulation, some circulating immune complexes are cleared by the mononuclear phagocyte system, and others deposit in the kidney. A self-limited glomerulonephritis occurs, characterized by a proliferative reaction, hematuria, and proteinuria. This model is analogous to poststreptococcal glomerulonephritis in humans. In contrast to the self-limited disease that develops with a single injection of BSA, a chronic, scarring form of glomerulonephritis is induced by repeated injections of BSA. Although most rabbits in these experiments develop capillary wall deposits of antigen and antibody with diffuse cellular proliferation, some animals develop mesangial forms of glomerulonephritis or membranous glomerulonephritis. Thus a spectrum of histopathologic lesions analogous to various human diseases can be induced with the same antigen. This observation suggests that the nature of the host's immune response influences the type of glomerular disease that develops. Also the complexity and genetic determination of the immune response likely explain why some individuals exposed to particular infections develop an associated glomerulonephritis and others do not.

Immune complex diseases in which the antigen is endogenous are similar to those in which an exogenous antigen replicates *in vivo* or repeated doses of an antigen are administered experimentally. In all these cases chronic antigen exposure leads to persistent immune complex formation and tissue injury. The best-studied autoimmune model of renal disease is the mouse model of systemic lupus erythematosus (SLE). The Fl hybrid of the New Zealand black and New Zealand white mouse strains develops a severe autoimmune disorder with many features and a course similar to human SLE. Antinuclear antibodies, circulating immune complexes, and Coombs-positive hemolytic anemia are early findings. Nephritis is apparent in the majority of animals by six months of age, and many animals die of renal failure by one year. Immunofluorescence studies have shown that glomeruli contain IgG, C3, DNA, and other nuclear constituents. If immunoglobulin is eluted from the glomeruli, it can be shown to contain antinuclear antibodies. In addition, these animals are chronically infected with a variety of viruses. Glycoproteins related to the viral envelope and antibodies to these proteins are found in circulating immune complexes and in glomerular deposits. Some anti-DNA antibodies from several different mouse models of SLE are cross-reactive with laminin. Direct binding of these antibodies to laminin in the glomerulus can lead to injury. All of this offers strong evidence that the renal disease of this hybrid mouse is a result of immune complex deposition involving antibodies reactive with both endogenous nuclear antigens, glomerular antigens, and viral antigens. Many endogenous antigens have been implicated in human immune complex diseases. In these instances, the antibody may be considered an autoantibody (Table 36.7).

IMMUNE COMPLEX FORMATION

The size and composition of immune complexes formed in the circulation will depend on many factors, including the affinity and valence of antibodies, the molecular size and structure of the antigens, and the absolute and relative concentrations of each. These factors govern the relative ease with which antibodies react with antigenic sites to cross-link antigens and form a lattice structure. Thus antigens with multiple antigenic sites, antibodies with high affinities, and increased concentrations of both reactants will all increase the tendency to form larger complexes.

The most important factor influencing the composition of soluble immune complexes is the relative concentration of antigen and antibody. Antigen excess results in the covering of available antibody sites so that cross-linking is prevented and only simple immune complexes are formed (Fig. 36.5). This effect occurs regardless of antigen valence and accounts for the classic observation that precipitated immune complexes can be resolubilized by the further addition of antigen.

Cross-linking of antigen is maximized at combining ratios near equivalence because the number of antigenic sites equals the number of antibody binding sites by definition, and competition for available reactive sites is minimized. The size of immune complexes formed at equivalence will greatly depend on the valence of the antigen. Univalent and oligovalent antigens will have limited opportunities for cross-linking and will, therefore, form smaller soluble immune complexes or precipitates (Fig. 36.5).

The composition and size of circulating immune complexes are important for two reasons. First, the molecular composition of immune complexes can affect their detection by assays. Second, and of more pathogenic significance, the fate of circulating immune complexes in the host is affected by size. Large soluble immune complexes with sedimentation rates in excess of 30S are rapidly removed from the circulation within seconds of being injected into experimental animals. Intermediate-size immune complexes of 11S to 30S persist in the circulation for minutes to hours, but ultimately most immune complexes of this size are selectively removed. Very small immune complexes (less than 11S) persist in the circulation for longer periods and may have disappearance times that do not differ from the normal catabolism of other plasma proteins.

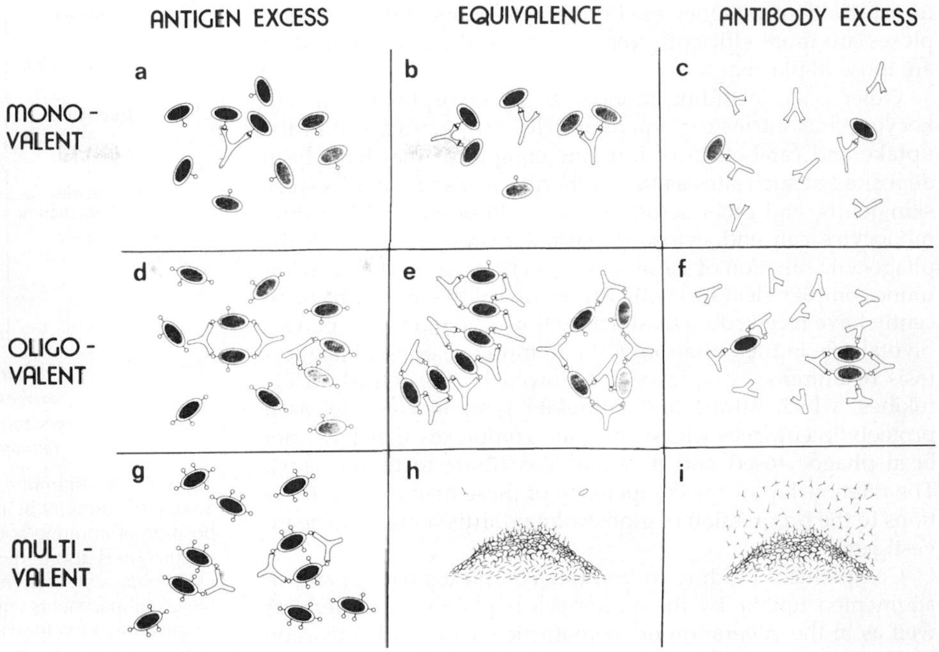

Figure 36.5. The effects of valence of antigen and the antigen-to-antibody ratio on the size and composition of immune complexes. Valency of antigens is shown on the left. A monovalent antigen has only one antigenic site per molecule; an oligovalent antigen has a few antigenic sites per molecule; a multivalent antigen has many antigenic sites per molecule. Antigen excess, equivalence, and antibody excess refer to the molar ratio between antigen and antibody in a given state. *Black dots*, antigen; ♀, the antigenic site; Y, antibody of the IgG class. Section *a* shows a small soluble complex composed of one antibody molecule and two monovalent antigen molecules formed in a state of antigen excess. In contrast, *i* shows the formation of an insoluble and large immune complex composed of many antibody molecules and many multivalent antigen molecules formed in a state of antibody excess. The other sections (*b* to *h*) represent various combinations of immune complex formation.

Features critical to the nature of the antigen, the character of the antibody response, and the relative concentration of each in the circulation determine immune complex formation. The initial steps in antibody synthesis depend on antigen processing and presentation of selected epitopes to T cells. Target antigens are phagocytosed and cleaved into fragments by proteolytic processes. A subset of these fragments will associate with the host's major histocompatibility complex class II antigens, which are polymorphic and genetically determined. The class II molecule–antigen fragment complex will be expressed on the surface of antigen-presenting cells, where it can bind to a T cell–antigen receptor and initiate an epitope-specific immune response. Production of specific antibodies is usually geared to eliminate exogenous antigens. However, selection for antibody production of a foreign antigen fragment that shares structure with an endogenous protein can lead to autoimmune reactions. Other abnormalities in the regulation of antibody synthesis also can lead to the production of autoantibodies. In addition to the epitope specificity of primary antibodies, other aspects of antibody structure are important to the biologic activity of the immune complex. Genetic influences will determine the class (IgM, IgG, or IgA), subclass (e.g., IgG1-4), and affinity of antibodies that are synthesized, as well as the antigen epitope to which the antibody binds. The type of antibody determines its half-life in plasma, its valence, its ability to bind and activate complement, and its efficiency of removal by the mononuclear phagocyte system.

When antibodies combine with antigens, a new macromolecule is formed. Conformational changes in antigens and antibodies expose new regions that can activate complement and interact with tissue proteins through charge, receptor–ligand binding, or other protein–protein interactions. After the binding of the primary antibody to the antigen, Clq binds to the Fc region of IgG. Clq is a collagenlike molecule that can bind fibronectin in plasma, as well as that within basement membranes. In turn, Clq and fibronectin in the immune complex can bind to receptors on monocytes, lymphocytes, and possibly intrinsic glomerular cells. These interactions may facilitate immune complex deposition in the glomeruli.

The initial conformational changes that occur in the circulating immune complex may expose new epitopes in the Fc and Fab regions of the primary antibody. Rheumatoid factors (antibodies to IgG) are often synthesized during the immune response that can bind to the Fc region of the primary antibody. Antiidiotypic antibodies can bind to regions of the Fab portion of immunoglobulin adjacent to the antigen-combining site, or they can mimic the antigen and compete for antigen binding to the primary antibody. When conformational changes in the structure of antigen and antibody occur as a consequence of these binding reactions, adjacent molecules are brought into close proximity such that Fc-Fc and other molecular interactions can further alter the size and compactness of the macromolecule. As these complex reactions occur, the ability to bind complement, clearance properties, and nephritogenic potential of circulating immune complexes are altered further. Although our knowledge of the biochemistry of some of these reactions has grown, we still have little understanding of why some circulating immune complexes deposit in the kidney and initiate local injury and others do not.

DISAPPEARANCE FROM THE CIRCULATION

Mononuclear phagocytes are quantitatively the most important cells for the removal of soluble immune complexes from the circulation. Kupffer cells in the liver clear 60% to 80% of an injected test dose of soluble immune complexes. Macrophages in the spleen and lymph nodes also play an important role. They have specific cell surface receptors for the Fc portion of immunoglobulin molecules and for the activated third component of complement and its degradation products. Such cells can attach individual immune complexes at multiple sites and thereby selectively remove soluble immune complexes from the circulation. Once bound, immune complexes are endocytosed in vacuoles. Lysosomes then fuse and release their proteolytic enzymes into the vacuoles, and the immune complexes are degraded. Erythrocytes also play an important role in immune complex removal. Erythrocytes express C3b receptors, which bind immune complexes and pull them out of solution. As erythrocytes pass through the liver and spleen, the immune complexes are removed from the erythrocyte surface and taken up by resident phagocytes. Erythrocyte-bound immune complexes are more efficiently removed from the circulation than are those in plasma.

Other cells, including monocytes, polymorphonuclear leukocytes, and intrinsic glomerular cells, may participate in the uptake and catabolism of immune complexes that have been deposited at such sites as the glomeruli, walls of blood vessels, skin, joints, and other serosal surfaces. Resident and invading monocytes can endocytose deposited material. Although the phagocytic function of these cells is of critical importance to immune complex clearance, other functions of the macrophage recently have received increased attention. The monocyte plays a pivotal role in the initiation of the immune response. Phagocytosis of immune complexes is followed by the release of cytokines, which attract and stimulate lymphocytes. Released proteolytic enzymes digest immune complexes that have not been phagocytosed and may also contribute to tissue injury. The relationship of the competency of these macrophage functions to the progression of glomerulonephritis remains to be investigated.

Complement binding to immune complexes participates in augmented uptake by the mononuclear phagocyte system, as well as in the generation of chemotactic factors and activation of the terminal complement components. Recently, complement attachment has been shown to solubilize immune complexes. Once solubilized with complement, the immune complexes are inactivated and do not appear capable of further initiation of inflammation. These solubilized complexes contain C3bi, a degradation product of C3b, which binds to a receptor for C3bi on the surface of macrophages. Complement deficiency has been postulated to contribute to impaired clearance of circulating immune complexes and persistence of tissue deposits in SLE. Further discussion of the complement system in immune complex disease is found in Chapter 39, Part 7.

It is important to recognize that immune complex formation, deposition, and catabolism are in a continual state of flux. Antigens and antibodies are entering the circulation at rates that vary independently. Immune complexes are in equilibrium with their component parts and with each other. Complement components are being bound and activated. Complexes are being deposited in tissues and removed from the circulation by the mononuclear phagocyte system. Immune complexes deposited in tissues are in a similar dynamic state (Fig. 36.6), where available sites can bind free antigens or antibodies from the circulation and, thereby, augment lattice growth. In part, this dynamic equilibrium contributes to clinical relapses and remissions of glomerular disease.

Although mononuclear phagocytes clearly play the major role in catabolism of immune complexes, it is unclear whether a failure of these cells accounts for pathologic tissue deposition of immune complexes. Defective clearance of soluble immune complexes from the circulation might result in their increased availability for deposition in the kidney. Alternatively, impaired removal of already deposited immune complexes could lead to their accumulation in tissues to levels capable of eliciting an inflammatory reaction. Such defects might be qualitative, in that certain potentially pathogenic complexes might escape removal, or quantitative, in that removal mechanisms might simply be saturated. The fact that many conditions are associated with abnormal levels of immune complexes in the blood shows that the mechanisms for their removal from the circulation can fail. What is less clear is whether this failure accounts for the pathologic deposition of immune complexes because many patients with high levels of circulating immune complexes do not appear to suffer any adverse effects from these soluble immune

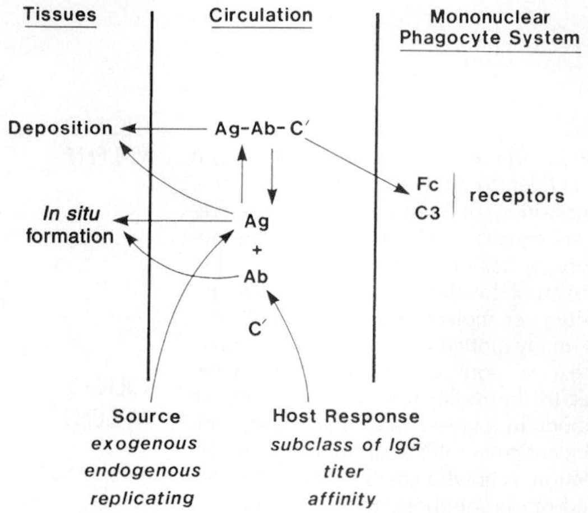

Figure 36.6. Immune complex disease. A dynamic equilibrium exists among the amount of antigen, production of antibody, and rate and composition of immune complexes formed. Each of these components in the circulation is also in dynamic equilibrium with clearance by the mononuclear phagocyte system and tissue deposition. An alteration in one of these compartments will have an effect on each of the others. Sampling a single compartment (tissue biopsy or circulating immune complex detection) is unlikely to provide adequate information for understanding the delicate balance that exists *in vivo*.

complexes. The relationship of defective phagocytic clearance to accelerated immune complex–mediated injury is well established in animal models of nephritis, but the difficulty of evaluating the function of tissue macrophages has left this observation unsupported in humans.

MECHANISMS OF TISSUE DEPOSITION

The glomerular capillary filter is particularly susceptible to immune complex deposition. Several characteristics make it different from other capillary systems. First, the blood flow to the kidney is 25% of the cardiac output, and therefore the glomerulus receives material suspended in plasma at a very high rate of delivery. Second, the endothelial cell of the glomerulus is fenestrated and thus has large pores through which protein may pass into the basement membrane region. Third, as the protein-free ultrafiltrate of plasma is formed, serum proteins are sequentially inhibited from passage into the urinary space by the complex sieving properties of the glomerular capillary wall. The permselectivity of the glomerulus is discussed in detail in Chapter 4. Fourth, as the ultrafiltrate moves into Bowman's space, proteins trapped in the capillary lumen become progressively more concentrated. This local accumulation could favor the formation of complexes between antigen and antibody existing in monomeric form in low concentration in the circulation. The direction of solute flow, pressures within the glomerulus, and integrity of the sieving properties of the glomerular capillary wall influence the site of localization of immune deposits within the glomerulus (Fig. 36.7). The multitude of factors that can influence glomerular deposition of circulating immune complexes is summarized in Table 36.8.

The glomerular basement membrane is composed of type IV collagen and glycosaminoglycans and other proteins that are attached to it. The basement membrane is rich in heparan sulfate, a negatively charged proteoglycan, which contributes a net negative charge to the basement membrane. This serves to repel the movement of negatively charged particles through the glo-

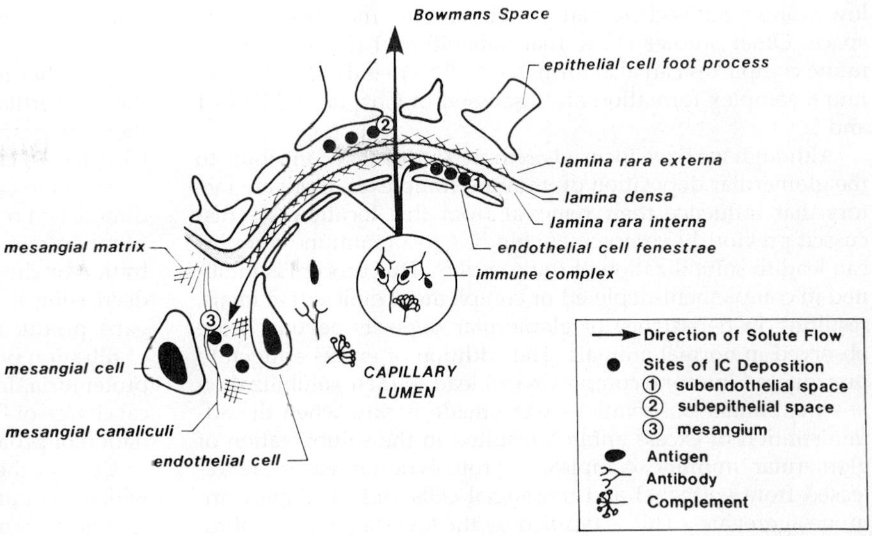

Figure 36.7. Immune complex deposition in the glomerulus. As the ultrafiltrate of plasma moves through the subendothelial space into the mesangial canaliculi and across the capillary wall into Bowman's space, immune complexes *(IC)* and free antigens and antibodies are carried to sites where they can accumulate. Their enhanced local concentration leads to lattice formation and growth in size of the immune deposits.

TABLE 36.8. Factors That Influence Glomerular Deposition of Immune Complexes

Factors related to the immune complex
Quantity
Rate of formation
Size
Antigen-to-antibody ratio
Antigen
Exogenous/endogenous/replicating
Valence
Sialic acid content
Polysaccharide content
Antibody
Class
Subclass
Affinity
Antiidiotypic antibodies
Molecular charge
Antigen
Antibody
Complex
Complement content
Factors related to the kidney
Structural integrity
Blood flow
Intraglomerular pressure
Charge of the glomerular capillary wall
Kidney receptors (Fc, C3, ? others)
Urinary tract obstruction
Systemic factors
Mononuclear phagocyte system
Systemic
Local
Hemodynamic
Blood pressure
Turbulence
Prostaglandins
Vascular permeability
Steroids
Vasoactive amines
Nutritional status
Protein intake
Fatty acid content of the diet
Hormonal status
Catecholamines (stress)
Diabetes mellitus (glucose and insulin)

merular capillary wall. However, it also serves to attract positively charged molecules, which are therefore more freely filtered. This charge-selective property of the glomerular capillary wall has been shown to influence the type and amount of immune complexes that become trapped in the glomerulus.

The specialized chemical composition and structure of many molecules determine their activities *in vivo*. Many molecules participate in molecular activation after binding to another molecule. Molecular charge, hydrophobicity, polysaccharide content, and tertiary structure are some of the known characteristics of molecules that influence their binding to each other. Positive selectivity of interaction between two molecules by each of these mechanisms has been postulated to contribute to immune complex localizaton within the glomerulus. The presence of C3b and Fc receptors has been thought to extract immune complexes from the circulation. Lectins, such as concanavalin A, which bind to polysaccharides, can also bind to similar constituents in the glomerulus and may thereby plant monomeric antigens or antibodies, as well as those already bound in an immune complex. Thus special chemical characteristics of molecules may influence their propensity to deposit in the glomerulus.

Immune complexes can deposit in the glomerular capillary wall or mesangium in four different ways: (a) filtration or mesangial trapping of intact immune complexes formed in the circulation, (b) binding of circulating antibody to a glomerular or glomerular-fixed antigen, (c) interaction of free antigen and antibody when their local concentrations reach critical levels to produce lattice formation, and (d) reaction of free antigen and/or antibody with previously deposited or formed immune complexes. Evidence from experimental animal models indicates that all of these mechanisms can occur. It is also likely that more than one of these mechanisms may be operative in the evolution and progression of human glomerulonephritis. Demonstration of circulating immune complexes of a specific composition with coincident tissue accumulation of complexes of an identical composition strongly supports the concept of tissue deposition of preformed material. Other animal data generated by passive administration of preformed immune complexes and immune aggregates clearly show that this is a feasible mechanism, especially for subendothelial and mesangial deposits. Small immune complexes, particularly those containing low-affinity antibodies, can penetrate into the subepithelial space. Other studies show that subepithelial deposits of immune complexes can also form *in situ*. The details of *in situ* immune complex formation are discussed in Chapter 39, Parts 1 and 2.

Although we have focused on those factors that contribute to the glomerular deposition of immune complexes, there are factors that influence their removal from this location. As discussed previously, complement binding to an immune complex can lead to solubilization of the complex. This process is inhibited in complement-depleted or complement-deficient animals, resulting in persistence of glomerular deposits beyond those observed in normal animals. The addition of excess antigen to precipitated immune complexes can lead to their solubilization *in vitro*. Similar observations were made *in vivo* when the administration of excess antigen resulted in the solubilization of glomerular immune complexes. Proteolytic enzymes are released from epithelial and mesangial cells and can digest immune aggregates. This is typified by the late stages of membranous nephropathy when the deposits become rarefied and may even disappear. Exogenous administration of proteolytic enzymes can remove immune complexes. Local infiltration by phagocytic cells also contributes to the removal of immune deposits, and mesangial cells that express Fc receptors may slowly clear deposited immune complexes. This accumulation and persistence of glomerular immune deposits is a balance between their rate of formation and deposition and their local removal (Fig. 36.6).

MECHANISMS OF RENAL INJURY

Tissue-deposited immune complexes that are not removed may stimulate an inflammatory response. Such immune complexes fix and activate complement, which results in local generation of chemotactic factors. These factors cause an infiltration of polymorphonuclear leukocytes and monocytes that liberate proteolytic enzymes and oxygen radicals that damage glomerular capillary walls. Also, immune complexes bind to surface receptors on mast cells, and this binding initiates the release of vasoactive amines (e.g., histamine), which can contribute to changes in local blood flow and vascular permeability. Release of platelet-activating factor also greatly augments capillary permeability. Immune complex binding to platelets and the release of tissue thromboplastin initiate coagulation and alter glomerular blood flow. Immune complex glomerulonephritis is associated with changes in the rate of synthesis of several components of arachidonic acid metabolism. These eicosanoids may locally mediate changes in glomerular blood flow and filtration rate, as well as the magnitude of the inflammatory reaction produced. Immune complex interaction with monocytes leads to the release of cytokines (interleukin-1), which can stimulate proliferation of mesangial cells and increase production of the mesangial matrix. In most forms of immune complex–mediated glomerulonephritis, there is some increase in glomerular basement membrane and mesangial matrix material. Proliferation of epithelial and mesangial cells and the infiltration of circulating phagocytes contribute to the glomerular hypercellularity that is often observed.

In addition to the generation of chemotactic factors and the consequent secondary inflammation, complement activation can lead to the generation of the membrane attack complex (MAC). The MAC of complement has been demonstrated in immune deposits in both animal models and human diseases. This complex causes the immune lysis of erythrocytes that is characteristic of complement activation *in vitro*. When the MAC is assembled on the surface of nucleated cells, it leads to alterations in membrane permeability and the release of cytokines, which may further mediate inflammation. Attachment of the MAC to the glomerular epithelial cell might contribute to the development of proteinuria in membranous glomerulonephritis (see Chapter 39, Part 7).

Immune complex–mediated glomerular injury may lead to diminished renal plasma flow and thus decrease the glomerular filtration rate. Immune complex deposition also may impair filtration by diminishing the available capillary surface area or by decreasing its permeability. Membrane damage may result in gaps, producing a leaky filter or disrupting the normal integrity of filtration pores, and thus lead to altered permselectivity and proteinuria. Immune complex deposition may alter the electrical charge of the glomerular capillary wall and result in transudation of protein, particularly albumin, into the urinary space.

Cells of the MPS express receptors for the Fc portions of Ig which facilitate phagocytosis. In this capacity FcR plays a critical role in immune elimination. Recently, new functions for FcR have been described that indicate they are required for initiation of immune complex–mediated inflammation. This may also be relevant to the kidney where mesangial and visceral epithelial cells express FcR. When immune complexes bind to these FcR, immunomodulatory cytokines are released and extracellular matrix synthesis is increased. Recently, it has been shown that mice lacking FcR fail to develop glomerular injury or sclerosis despite immune complex deposition and complement activation.

In addition to the humoral factors discussed, T cells sensitized to the deposited antigen can infiltrate the glomerulus and contribute to chronic inflammation and renal dysfunction. This mechanism of renal injury is well documented in animal models of glomerular and tubular disease (see Chapter 39, Part 1, and Chapter 40). The presence of activated lymphocytes in human renal biopsies supports a role for this mechanism of injury in human nephritis.

DETECTION AND QUANTITATION OF CIRCULATING IMMUNE COMPLEXES

The widely accepted importance of circulating immune complexes in the pathogenesis of glomerulonephritis prompted the development of assays for their detection in blood samples. More than 50 assays for the detection of circulating immune complexes have been published, and it is beyond the scope of this chapter to discuss them in detail. In general, all assays are based on similar properties. Large immune complexes are separable from serum based on their size and enhanced precipitation in the cold. These large macromolecules are detected by their Ig content and/or ability to bind and activate complement.

With the development of assays for circulating immune complexes, it was hoped that (a) their detection would be specific for those diseases in which immune complexes caused the tissue injury and thus would aid in the definition of the pathogenesis of various forms of glomerulonephritis, (b) their detection would correlate with disease activity and thus be clinically useful for the management of patients, and (c) their detection would lead to methodology for their isolation. This would provide the tools to identify their mysterious antigen content and, thereby, to discover the etiology of the immune complex–mediated glomerular diseases. Not all of these hopes have been realized.

Application of immune complex testing to various diseases has generated some surprising findings. Circulating immune complexes have been detected in many diseases, such as acute myocardial infarction, cystic fibrosis, and halothane anesthesia, which are not associated with evidence of immune complex injury. In patients with nephritis, elevated serum levels of immune complexes do not consistently predict an active disease course and therefore cannot be used as a guide in therapeutic management.

Experience with immune complex detection has often failed to show a correlation between assay techniques. Because different assays are based on different physical and immunologic properties of immune complexes *in vitro*, it is not surprising that their ability to detect complexes differs. The quantity and character of *in vivo*–formed immune complexes may vary independently, resulting in a heterogeneous population of immune complexes within a particular disease or patient, as well as among different diseases or patients. In addition, the immune complexes that remain in the circulation (and are, therefore, detected by the assays) are not those that have deposited in the glomerulus. Thus detection of circulating immune complexes after a disease has developed may not provide the information of greatest relevance to the definition of disease pathogenesis.

Immune complex detection has greatly facilitated subsequent isolation of the immune complexes. Recent advances in biochemical analysis have provided important insights into the antigens and unique properties of antibodies. The mixed cryoglobulins that are common to hepatitis C infection have been extensively characterized. They contain HCV material, polyclonal IgG with anti-HCV activity, and a monoclonal IgM with a unique epitope that is cross-reactive with other rheumatoid factors. Immune complexes from patients infected with HIV and hepatitis B contain viral material from both agents as well as their respective antibodies. When antigen binds to antibody, C1q binding is initiated. Tertiary rearrangement of bound C1q initiates anti-C1q synthesis. The anti-C1q antibodies are common in SLE and IgA nephropathy. Antigens from immune complexes isolated from patients with SLE contain DNA, cytoskeletal proteins, and laminin. The presence of complexes containing antibodies to laminin is often associated with lupus nephritis. As our knowledge of the nature of antigens in immune complexes grows, it is likely that we will realize the goal to identify the etiology of many forms of glomerulonephritis. Hepatitis C is just the first example (see Chapter 39.3A). Immune complex assays continue to have a role in the investigation of glomerulonephritis, but they are of uncertain and very limited use in the diagnosis and treatment of patients with immune-mediated renal diseases.

Selected Readings

Abrass CK. Autologous immune complex nephritis in rats: influence of modification of mononuclear phagocyte system function. *Lab Invest* 1984;51:162–171.

Demonstration that alterations in activity of the mononuclear phagocyte system can influence the load of circulating immune complexes delivered to the tissues and thereby influence the severity of glomerulonephritis.

Clynes R, Dumitru C, Ravetch JV. Uncoupling of immune complex formation and kidney damage in autoimmune glomerulonephritis. *Science* 1998;279:1052–1054.

An elegant study demonstrating the role of the Fc receptor in mediating glomerular injury following immune complex deposition.

Gauthier VJ, Abrass CK. Circulating immune complexes in renal injury. *Semin Nephrol* 1992;12:379–394.

Includes a detailed review of the biochemical features of antigens, genetic regulation of antibody synthesis, and nephritogenic properties of immune complexes.

Glotz D, Druet P. Immune mechanisms of glomerular damage that affect the kidney. In: Cameron S, Davison A, Grunfeld JP, et al, eds. *Oxford Textbook of Clinical Nephrology*. Oxford: Oxford Medical Publication, 1992:240–261.

Excellent contemporary review of immune pathogenesis of glomerular injury.

Iskandar SS, Jennette JCN. Influence of antibody avidity on glomerular immune complex localization. *Am J Pathol* 1983;112:155–159.

This study confirms the influence of antibody avidity on the site of localization of glomerular immune complex deposits.

Mannik M. Pathophysiology of circulating immune complexes. Arthritis Rheum 1982;25:783–787.

A review of the pathogenic significance of immune complexes to glomerular and rheumatologic diseases.

Mannik M. Mechanisms of tissue deposition of immune complexes. *J Rheumatol* 1987;14:35–42.

Summarizes in detail the reactions of immune complex components with capillary beds and the rearrangements and lattice formations within the macromolecular complex that contribute to immune complex deposition and persistence.

Mannik M, Agodoa LYC, David KA. Rearrangement of immune complexes in glomeruli leads to persistence and development of electron-dense deposits. *J Exp Med* 1983;157:1516–1527.

Explains that the persistence of glomerular immune deposits, which subsequently determines the risk for disease, requires lattice formation and growth of the immune precipitate in the tissue after the complex has deposited from the circulation.

Ravetch JV. Fc receptors. *Curr Opin Immunol* 1997;9:121–125.

A comprehensive review of the multiple functions of Fc receptors.

Sansonno D, Iacobelli AR, Cornacchiulo V, et al. Immunochemical and biomolecular studies of circulating immune complexes isolated from patients with acute and chronic hepatitis C virus infections. *Eur J Clin Invest* 1996;26: 465–475.

Demonstrates that antigen composition and antibody specificity can be determined in some immune complex diseases.

Wilson CB. The renal response to immunologic injury. In: Brenner B, Rector F, eds. The Kidney. Philadelphia: WB Saunders, 1991:1062–1181.

A comprehensive and encyclopedic review with more than 2,000 references.

PART 4
Cell-Mediated Immunity

W. Kline Bolton

The immune system consists of T cells, B cells, natural killer cells, macrophages, and dendritic cells. Most antibody responses require T cells, but classically cell-mediated immunity (CMI) is considered the arm of the immune system comprised of cells rather than antibodies. In truth, there is a large degree of overlap. The emerging knowledge about cells of the immune system, their interaction with each other and with cells not of the immune system, and the elaborate network of interactive factors suggests that classic paradigms of CMI will evolve rapidly. Indeed, recruitment of CMI by non–T cell mechanisms requires a reassessment of the concept of CMI.

Over the years, cells of the immune system have been observed in the kidney in many types of renal diseases. The significance and importance of these cells and the understanding of their role in the pathogenesis and prognosis of disease has evolved as better tools have been developed. Different types of cells of the immune system are involved in various kidney diseases. Generally, diseases can be divided into those that are immune mediated and those not mediated by classic immune mechanisms. Most immune-mediated processes in the kidney appear to be autoimmune in nature.

Renal diseases in which cellular immune processes are prominent include glomerulonephritis (GN), tubulointerstitial nephritis, renal allograft rejection, inflammation of other structures in the kidney such as vasculitis, and cells associated with reparative and structural processes. The emphasis of the present chapter is on CMI in GN.

HISTORICAL PERSPECTIVE

For decades, it was thought that antibodies alone mediated autoimmune processes in the kidney. As recently as 1970, sensitized cells present in GN were considered a natural consequence of the autoimmune process which had no pathogenic role. Since then, it has become increasingly clear that CMI in concert with humoral immunity, and with a host of accompanying effectors, is actually involved in the process of autoimmune nephritis. Evidence for CMI in GN was obtained from the observation that lymphocytes were present around and in glomeruli in certain diseases; that macrophages were a prominent feature both within glomerular crescents and the interstitium; that multinucleated giant cells characteristic of delayed type hypersensitivity (DTH) could be observed in certain types of nephritis; and the cellular infiltrate and histologic appearance were similar in various types of GN regardless of whether there was antibody deposited as apparent immune complexes or as antibody to the glomerular basement membrane (GBM). In addition, the intense interstitial disease of both glomerular and nonglomerular injury was very similar to acute cellular rejection, clearly a CMI event.

In the 1970s and 1980s, with few tools available for analysis of pathogenetic events, several investigators suggested that T cells and macrophages were intimately involved in the pathogenesis of GN and interstitial nephritis. T cells could be documented to occur in various models of anti-GBM antibody disease. In nephrotoxic nephritis (NTN), lymphocytoid cells were seen within glomerular capillary lumens within 15 minutes of administration of nephrotoxic serum (NTS) and could be abrogated by irradiation and antilymphocyte globulin. Transfer of T cells specifically sensitized to heterologous serum resulted in GN in rats that were given heterologous serum as subnephritic anti-GBM antibody or immune complexes, whereas rats that were given control lymphocytes showed no alterations. In these studies, specifically sensitized lymphocytes were required to produce nephritis under the experimental conditions. The influx of T cells in the various experimental forms of GN appears to be relatively transient and can be detected only when there are significant T-cell infiltrates. This probably led to earlier claims that T cells were not present within glomeruli in GN. When T cells are observed within glomeruli, various activation antigens, including interleukin-2 (IL-2) receptor, can be identified, indicating that these cells are not only present but are also in an activated state.

Investigators demonstrated a role for macrophages in the lesion both in anti-GBM and immune complex disease by treating animals with antimacrophage antiserum. A decrease in the number of macrophages within glomeruli and interstitium was associated with a significant reduction in proteinuria and proliferative nephritis. It was later shown that the macrophages in these experimental models were of bone marrow origin. Infiltration of the glomeruli by lymphocytes in the models previously noted caused endogenous cells within the glomerulus to proliferate. The proliferating cells were both endothelial and mesangial in origin.

Assessment of certain human renal diseases suggested that there was frequent disparity between the degree of lymphocyte and mononuclear cell infiltration in patients with GN and the presence or absence of antibodies within the glomerulus. Some patients later were found to have microscopic vasculitis. However, many without vasculitis or glomerular antibody had GN with interstitial infiltrates, which were phenotypically indistinguishable from those with antibodies deposited on the basement membrane or present as immune complexes. Phenotypic analysis showed that the cells found in the interstitium, crescents, and glomeruli consisted of CD4+ cells with a few CD8+ cells and B cells and a large number of activated macrophages. Thus animal models and human renal biopsies provided evidence for a role of CMI in the development of GN.

Experimental models provided early evidence that T cells were pivotally involved in the pathogenesis of certain types of GN. Nude mice lacking functional T cells did not develop GN

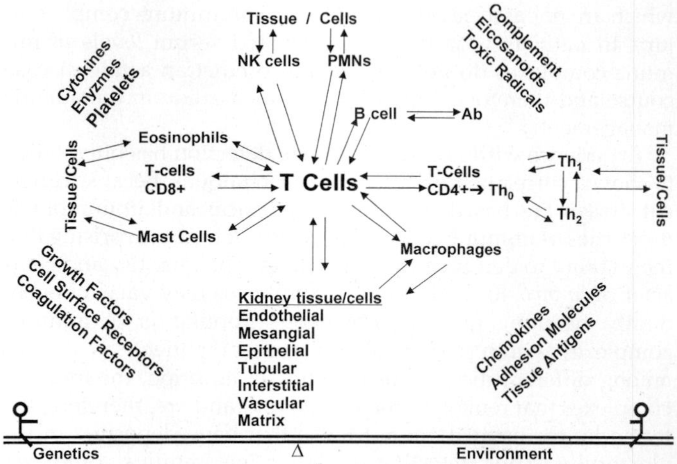

Figure 36.8. The various cells and soluble factors that interact with T cells in cell-mediated immunity are shown. This cascade operates within a balance of genetics and the environment.

and antilymphocyte globulin-aborted GN. Chickens rendered incapable of producing antibodies to GBM still developed proliferative GN upon immunization with GBM antigen indistinguishable from that seen in birds with antibody present on the basement membrane. This latter disease could be transferred with sensitized T cells.

Since these early observations, the complexity of the relationship of CMI to renal disease has greatly increased. It is now obvious that multiple regulatory and counterregulatory systems are involved in pathogenesis, that there is a dynamic interaction between infiltrating and resident cells within the kidney, and that various cells involved in the pathogenesis of immune renal disease can undergo transdifferentiation and change their identity. These relationships are illustrated in Figure 36.8, some of the components of which will be discussed below. It is no longer possible to think of CMI in renal disease as an isolated event dependent only on cells without considering the wide array of dynamic interactions with other cells of the immune system, with resident renal cells, and a variety of other confounding factors. The balance of these various factors, strongly influenced by genetics and the environment, result in an ever-changing balance that will affect the pathogenic process, histologic appearance, clinical course, and prognosis for any given disease.

DEVELOPMENT OF CELL-MEDIATED IMMUNE RENAL DISEASE

Development of GN requires initiation of an immune response to either endogenous or exogenous antigens that become planted within the kidney. Much work has been done with experimental animal models, and some of these pertain more clearly to human diseases than others. Some types of renal disease result from systemic autoimmune diseases that may result from either errors in central or peripheral tolerance at the T- or B-cell level with consequent multisystem autoimmune disease, polyclonal activation of B and/or T cells, or disturbances in the immunoregulatory systems. In these situations, multiple organs are involved, of which the kidney is one.

In terms of organ-specific disease, various theories of pathogenesis have been proposed. The first is release of anatomically sequestered or cryptic antigen. This has been considered a major factor in Goodpasture's disease because the Goodpasture's antigen is revealed by dissociation of type IV collagen chains with exposure of the epitope responsible for the disease (see Chapter 42, Part 6). The second organ-specific mechanism is self-ignorance. This hypothesis suggests that mature resting T cells, specific for extrathymic antigen, are anergic. Under circumstances where appropriate costimulatory factors are present, they can become activated and cause tissue-specific damage. The third mechanism, molecular mimicry, depends on cross-reactive determinants on exogenous sources, such as bacteria and food particles. that would have enough homology to self-antigen and yet enough difference to elicit an immune response involving the self-antigen. The fourth mechanism, or modified self-mechanism, suggests that self-determinants to which the immune system is tolerant may become modified so that they are no longer recognized as self. These neoantigens can result in the initiation of an immune response with consequent damage. Once a response against a self-determinant has been initiated, consequent waves of responses against other determinants can occur through the process of epitope spreading, either by release of epitopes on the same protein or on a close neighbor. The initial autoimmune response to one or a few epitopes can then spread to other epitopes leading to disease expression. In other words, an antigen that causes or triggers a cellular and antibody response can then be followed by an immune response to epitopes that were not present in the immunizing antigen. This can occur by actual damage to the kidney with release of antigens and the initiation of autoimmune disease, or T cells may respond to new linear peptides resulting in the development of B-cell help, which allows unreactive B cells primed to elaborate autoantibodies to begin making these antibodies. This process has been demonstrated in many autoimmune diseases, including oophoritis, diabetes, gastritis, encephalomyelitis, thyroiditis, and interstitial nephritis. The pivotal cell in this process appears to be the T cell, necessary for both the development of DTH as well as the antibody repertoire.

Figure 36.8 depicts the author's view of CMI in renal diseases. CMI damage is related to a very complex interaction with multiple cells of the immune system as well as resident renal cells. This occurs through cell–cell interaction as well as via the influence of various soluble mediator and effector systems addressed in detail in Chapter 37, Part 2, 3, and 4. The cascade of events involves multiple interdigitating loops of upregulation and downregulation of cells, as well as similar modulation of numerous soluble mediators. The balance of these various factors, including genetic predisposition and environmental factors, direct the final phenotypic presentation. Essential for autoimmune disease are T cells that can differentiate into CD4+ cells that further differentiate from Th_0 cells into Th_1 and Th_2 subsets defined by their cytokine profiles. Th_1 cells produce IL-2, tumor necrosis factor (TNF), and interferon gamma (IFN-γ) in addition to mediating DTH-type responses. Th_2 cells produce IL-4, IL-5, IL-6, IL-10, and IL-13, and induce immunoglobulin synthesis. Th_1 cells are inhibited by IL-4 and IL-10, and INF-γ inhibits the Th_2 response. Thus there is reciprocal inhibition of Th_1 and Th_2. Strains of mice have been developed that have a predominant Th_1 phenotype whereas others have a Th_2 phenotype in response to antigens. C57BL/6 mice, which have a predominant Th_1 phenotype, develop severe crescentic GN after NTS with glomerular T cell and macrophage influx with fibrin crescents. This is reduced by monoclonal antibody to IFN-γ and CD4+ cells. BALB/c mice, a Th_2 strain, after the same NTS challenge, develop intense deposits of glomerular IgG and complement with significant attenuation of crescent formation, greatly diminished glomerular infiltration with macrophage and T cells, GN, and fibrin deposition. CD4+ cell depletion does not affect proteinuria or polymorphonuclear leukocytes infiltrates in these BALB/c mice. CD4-deficient mice have abrogation of the GN, whereas CD8-deficient mice develop severe crescentic GN with NTS. This nephritic effect of CD4+ cells is present even in the absence of glomerular bound antibodies. Genetically IL-4 deficit mice with enhanced Th_1 function have exaggerated GN, though administration of the Th_2 cytokines, IL-4, and IL-10 attenuate the GN. These findings suggest that in the mouse model of NTS, GN is a CD4-dependent and CD8-independent DTH reaction within the glomerulus. Similar studies in WKY rats have demonstrated an opposite effect suggesting that CD8+ cells play a pivotal role in crescent formation in rats. Depletion of CD8+ cells decreases macrophage infiltration and proteinuria and ameliorates the GN. IL-4 alone has been shown to ameliorate NTS in rats, but IL-4 alone without IL-10 was not protective in the mouse NTS model. Indeed, IL-10 has been reported to aggravate GN in MRL/lpr lupus-prone mice. In a murine model of autoimmune GN (Steblay model), T cells alone have been reported to transfer disease but only in susceptible strains with associated transfer of antibody production to GBM. These studies provide further evidence of the pivotal role of T cells and CMI in the pathogenesis of GN with and without glomerular-bound antibodies. However, the strain of animal and species influence the experimental model significantly. Thus extrapolation directly to human disease must be made with caution.

Fc Receptors

Classically antibodies have been considered as the arm of the immune system responsible for autoimmune glomerular disease. This was based on early studies of immune complex GN, NTS, and Steblay nephritis referred to above. Multiple studies of decomplementation and IgG isotype association with disease provided support for this concept. However, it is now becoming increasingly clear that antibodies can fix within the glomerulus and be demonstrable as anti-GBM antibodies without nephritis and that complement is present only in certain patients and animal models with anti-GBM disease. Indeed complement-deficient mice can develop anti-GBM–mediated GN, and complement is not present in autoimmune–anti-GBM nephritis in rats. The presence of Fc receptors on multiple members of the cellular immune system provides an alternate method by which CMI can be involved in autoimmune GN. Fc receptors are present on multiple cells and are classically responsible for phagocytosis by macrophages and neutrophils, antibody dependent cellular cytotoxicity, release of mediators by cells, and feedback inhibition of antibody production. In addition, a number of functions are associated with Fc receptors on lymphocytes, including inhibition of antigen-induced activation of B cells, enhanced IgM production by B cells, antigen processing and presentation by B cells, and interaction between T cells, B cells and other functions. In one model of rabbit nephrotoxic nephritis, it was shown that the Fc receptor on macrophages alone was capable of inducing GN with abrogation of nephritis in animals that received NTS consisting only of $F(ab')_2$. Furthermore, the generation of autoantibodies and glomerular deposition of immune complexes in a model of murine systemic lupus erythematosus can be completely abrogated by disruption of a single gene which encodes the γ chain of the Fc receptor. Despite comparable amounts of immune reactants, Fcγ-deficient mice had significantly attenuated disease compared with their wild-type controls. Thus antibody–Fc receptor interaction between various members of the cellular immune system may play a pivotal role in immune damage in the glomerulus.

Macrophages

Throughout the history of nephrology, both in humans and in experimental animal models, macrophages have been identified as a major component of interstitial, periglomerular, glomerular, and crescentic proliferation. Macrophages bearing activation antigens, including tissue factor, appear to be involved in the rupture of Bowman's capsule and consequent formation of fibrous crescents. Macrophages are present in all immune processes as well as most nonimmune processes associated with a mononuclear cell infiltrate in the kidney. The number of macrophages present within glomeruli correlates with proteinuria and renal function. As noted previously, maneuvers to deplete macrophages, such as treatment with antimacrophage antiserum or toxins to decrease circulating macrophages, cause diminution in the histologic abnormalities. Not only may circulating monocytes migrate to inflamed areas to assume their macrophage role, but cells within the glomerulus, the podocyte, may detach from basement membranes, express macrophage-associated antigens, and presumably function as bonafide macrophages. Macrophages appear capable of migrating in and out of the glomerulus, can undergo cell division and proliferate, and can move down the luminal side of tubules, which can express monocyte chemoattractant protein (MCP-1). This chemokine attracts macrophages, which attach to tubular epithelial cells and cause damage from both sides of the basement membrane. Interference with the ability of macrophages to be attracted to renal sites of injury ameliorates damage. Antibody to MCP-1 ameliorates nephrotoxic nephritis when given at day 4 but not if delayed to day 8. Administration of antibodies to adhesion molecules markedly attenuates autoimmune GN in various rat models.

As is described in the following, the attraction of macrophages into the kidney, especially the glomerulus and the consequent dynamic interaction between the macrophage and cells within the glomerulus appear to be a major factor in the phenotypic expression of disease and course.

Other Migratory Cells

Recent attention focused on T cells, histologic analysis of human biopsies, and some experimental models suggest that other cells beside macrophages may also be involved in GN. Certain models of NTS in mice are PMN and complement independent. In the active model of NTS, the first cell that generally arrives is the polymorphonuclear leucocyte as opposed to the presensitization model. Natural killer and antibody dependent cellular cytotoxicity cells have been shown to be responsible for hapten mediated cell transfer of GN in a WKY rat model which is independent of antibodies. In addition, the prominent infiltration within the interstitium and occasionally the glomerulus with eosinophils in certain diseases in humans, including vasculitis, allograft rejection, acute allergic interstitial nephritis, and diabetes, as well as some types of crescentic and other GN, suggest that these cells likewise may play more than an innocent bystander role. The chemokines, cytokines, and growth factors elaborated in the kidney during the course of inflammation are all known to induce migration and activation of these other cells into the injured area. In addition, expression of the products of the cells in immune renal disease has been demonstrated. Further study is needed to determine their roles in the phenotype expression, pathogenesis and progression of associated lesions.

Recruitment of Cells

In the last 10 years, a great deal has been learned about the manner in which cells within the intravascular compartment are recruited into areas of immune and nonimmune damage. As described earlier, specifically sensitized lymphocytes migrate into areas containing their target antigen within minutes of implantation. It is now known that T cells elaborate various chemokines and cytokines (see Chapter 37, Part 2) responsible for recruiting multiple cells into areas of damage. These include importantly IL-2 and RANTES (regulated upon activation normal T cell expressed presumed secreted). Macrophages, the key cells recruited then elaborate multiple chemokines and cytokines for amplification. Leukocyte adhesion molecules play a major role in providing lymphocytes and macrophages access to areas of injury (see Chapter 37, Part 6). These are molecules on the surface of endothelial and other cells that allow leukocytes to adhere, become immobilized, change shape, and transmigrate through the endothelial layer into areas containing either antibodies or antigens to which the cells are attracted. A variety of adhesion molecules are involved in a ligand–receptor interaction specific for different types of cells. Blocking of adhesion molecules with antibodies can significantly ameliorate GN in rats and markedly decrease the macrophage accumulation associated with GN. These various adhesion molecules are dependent upon conditions of local inflammation and chemokines, which are expressed locally. Antibodies to various adhesion molecules appear to be most efficacious when given in close proximity to the immune insult, raising questions as to the degree of efficacy in patients who may already have established GN.

A host of different chemokines are involved in the attraction of macrophages into areas of inflammation. These include MCP-1, RANTES, and macrophage inflammatory protein (MIP). Both RANTES and MCP-1 are chemoattractant for T cells as well as macrophages. Blocking MCP-1 and RANTES decreases cellular infiltration and ameliorates disease. RANTES and MCP-1 are upregulated in various autoimmune renal diseases, providing evidence that chemokines may be involved in human disease. This cascade of chemokines, cytokines, and growth factors continues to recruit macrophages and nonsensitized T cells into areas of inflammation until feedback controls begin to occur. Under ideal conditions, order is restored, recruitment of CMI components is curtailed, and normalcy returns. However, once initiated these processes develop a course of their own that is difficult to control and associated with histologic and functional sequelae that are well known.

RESIDENT RENAL CELLS

In various experimental models of GN and in humans, proliferation of endothelial, mesangial, and epithelial cells have been observed. In early studies, this was shown by histologic examination of cells and observation of mitotic figures as well as ultrastructural characteristics. Trafficking studies demonstrated that the hypercellularity observed in GN and other diseases of the kidney is accompanied not only by an influx of cells into the various compartments of the kidney but also by an increase in the number and extracellular matrix substances of cells already residing in the kidney. An experiment of nature in which kidneys were transplanted from females to males showed that recurrent membranoproliferative GN with mesangial hyperplasia was not associated with Y body–positive nuclei. Crescents present in several of these patients did have Y body–positive cells, and interstitial infiltrates contained Y body–positive cells, indicating both endogenous proliferation and infiltration with cells of exogenous donor origin. Although the mechanisms for these proliferative events were poorly understood at the time, the dynamic interaction between growth factors, chemokines, cytokines, and various cell types noted in this chapter and de-

TABLE 36.9. Products and Activities of Activated Resident Renal Cells

Adhesion molecules		
Antigen presentation molecules		
Complement proteins		
Fc receptor expression		
Growth factors and chemokines		
PDGF	GM-CSF	IL-2
IL-1	IGF-1	Osteopontin
IL-6	TGF-β	IL-1 receptor antagonists
TNF-α	MCP-1	γIP-10
RANTES	MIP-2	IL-8
Matrix components		
Collagen (I, III, IV, and V)		
Laminin		
Fibronectin		
Thrombospondin		
Heparan sulfate proteoglycans		
Phospholipase products		
PAF		
12 HETE		
Eicosanoids		
Proteinase/inhibitors		
Collagenase		
Gelatinase		
TIMP		
Reactive oxygen species		
Transdifferentiated macrophages		
Upregulated MHC class I and II		

bFGF, basic fibroblast growth factor; GM-CFS, granulocyte/monocyte colony stimulating factor; IFN, interferon; IGF, insulinlike growth factor; IL, interleukin; γIP-10, interferon inducible protein 10; MCP, monocyte chemoattractant protein; MIP, macrophage inflammatory protein; PAF, platelet activating factor; PDGF, platelet derived growth factors; RANTES, regulated upon activation normal T cell expressed presumed secreted; TGF, transforming growth factor; TIMP, tissue inhibitor of metalloproteinase; TNF, tumor necrosis factor.

TABLE 36.10. Cellular Mediation of Renal Damage

CMI Product	Mechanism
IL-1	Protein activation of multiple cell surface receptors, expression of ligands elaboration of multiple cytokines, and other soluble products
TNF-α	Protean manifestations similar to IL-1
IL-6	Mesangial cell proliferation
PAF	Depress GFR, blood flow
PDGF	Mesangial, endothelial, fibroblast proliferation
bFGF	Cellular proliferation and matrix elaboration
TBF-β	Matrix elaboration, macrophage accumulation
Eicosanoids	Hemodynamic effects, cellular proliferation
Procoagulant activity	Coagulation initiation, fibrin in crescents
Proteolytic enzymes	Matrix deposition and remodeling, tissue damage
Nitric oxide	Hemodynamic changes, cellular toxicity
Reactive oxygen species	Tissue damage
IFN-γ	Involved in most immune/inflammatory reactors. Regulation of growth and differentiation, activation of various immune cells and most cells of the kidney
Cytokines, chemokines,	Amplification of injurious processes and growth factors

bFGF, basic fibroblast growth factor; GM-CFS, granulocyte/monocyte colony stimulating factor; IFN, interferon; IGF, insulinlike growth factor; IL, interleukin; γIP-10, interferon inducible protein 10; MCP, monocyte chemoattractant protein; MIP, macrophage inflammatory protein; PAF, platelet activating factor; PDGF, platelet derived growth factors; RANTES, regulated upon activation normal T cell expressed presumed secreted; TGF, transforming growth factor; TIMP, tissue inhibitor of metalloproteinase; TNF, tumor necrosis factor.

tailed in Chapter 37, Parts 2 and 3) clearly provide a mechanism for these observations. Table 36.9 provides a partial list of the products and activities of activated resident renal cells. These broad categories clearly illustrate how various soluble and nonsoluble factors can have an impact on both endogenous and exogenous infiltrating cells from a morphologic and functional perspective.

CELLULAR MEDIATION OF RENAL DAMAGE

Injury from CMI may take the form of damage due to direct cell-to-cell contact with the induction of apoptosis, cell lysis with perforins, and injury mediated by a host of soluble mediators (Fig. 36.8). In simplified schema of earlier investigations, complement-mediated immune damage and participation of the coagulation system were considered key factors in the phenotypic expression of GN. With the development of molecular biologic tools, an increasing array of monoclonal antibodies, and the rapid expansion in the number of soluble mediators, it became clear that cell-mediated immune damage as an isolated event is extremely rare and probably nonexistent. As described earlier, transfer of GN by sensitized lymphocytes, participation of macrophages, and even damage by antibody-dependent cellular cytotoxicity appear to be operative. GN develops in the absence of antibodies both in experimental animal models and in humans, but the consequent renal injury most likely results from soluble mediator products of immune system cells and resident renal cells. The latter respond to CMI mediators by elaboration of their own set of soluble substances and by transdifferentiation. Table 36.10 provides a listing of various products related to CMI and the manner in which renal damage can ensue. These mediators and mechanisms of damage are examined in detail in Chapter 37, Part 1 and 7.

CELL-MEDIATED INTERSTITIAL NEPHRITIS

Most forms of GN are associated with an interstitial inflammatory response, and there is persuasive evidence for the communication between various kidney compartments by soluble mediators to account for this. The ultimate functional abnormalities of GN are more closely matched with the degree of interstitial disease than glomerular process. Interstitial nephritis with normal glomerular architecture and an infiltrate of CMI components is associated with impaired renal function, progressive fibrosis, scarring, and development of endstage renal disease in both animals and humans. This occurs as a result of autoimmune processes directed to various components of the nonglomerular compartments, such as acute and chronic cellular rejection in renal transplantation and nonimmune-mediated renal disease. These are addressed in relationship to autoimmune interstitial renal disease in Chapters 38 and 86.

OTHER CELL-MEDIATED RENAL DISEASES

For decades, renal pathologists and clinicians have observed the histologic picture of progressive renal damage of multiple etiologies with its associated interstitial infiltrates and declining renal function. Multiple nonimmune, noninflammatory animal models have an associated infiltration of various renal compartments with components of the CMI. Examples include analgesic nephropathy in humans, focal segmental glomerular sclerosis, and practically any progressive renal disease with proteinuria and decreased renal function. Experimental animal models illustrate this point even more strikingly. Ureteral obstruction models, adriamycin, partial ablation models, experimental diabetes, puromycin aminonucleoside nephrosis, and protein overload nephropathy, are a few examples of progressive renal diseases in humans and animals. These progressive renal diseases are associated histologically with the presence of CMI components that can be ameliorated with maneuvers to alter the CMI system. These various diseases are subtypes of CMI-mediated damage, but stress or damage to any of the resident renal cells can induce elaboration of the cytokine/chemokine/growth factor cascades outlined above and described in detail in Chapter 37, Parts 2 and 3. While these processes do not include specific antigen sensitized T cells, they do include macrophages and other components of the CMI system as effectors of damage recruited by the same mechanisms involved in sensitized T cell–mediated. Some of these can evolve into autoimmune, renal damaging processes with the development of sensitization to antigens of the kidney. Examples include the development of anti-GBM disease after renal damage with cortical necrosis, acute tubular necrosis, and various forms of GN.

Correction of the lesion that is inducing the nonimmune damage does not necessarily result in the cessation of the immune process because the cascade of events associated with CMI, once set in motion, are difficult to abort.

TREATMENT OF CMI RENAL DISEASE

When we thought that CMI renal disease consisted of sensitized T cells and macrophages responding in an orderly fashion to specific antigens in the kidney, efforts at intervention seemed straightforward (i.e., impact the T cells or impact the macrophages). Early studies in humans and experimental animals focused on treatment with broad spectrum immunosuppressives such as prednisone or cyclosporine, cyclophosphamide, azathioprine, and other agents. As we have learned more about the intricate, complex, and redundant systems actually involved in the production of CMI injury, we know these early approaches were inadequate. Emerging knowledge has led to more specific and rational approaches to therapy with monoclonal antibodies to various mediators and cell surface proteins, utilization of soluble receptors or receptor antagonists to attempt to control the inflammatory process by natural negative feedback, and by use of peptides or proteins that might mimic epitopes responsible for consequent autoimmune disease. These approaches have been limited by the necessity for starting them early either prior to the insult or shortly thereafter. This situation is not feasible in most human diseases because of the emergence of host antibodies to various interventive measures and the development of redundant systems to replace those that have been impaired or deleted by molecular techniques. Nevertheless, the explosion in knowledge regarding the CMI, soluble mediators that are their product, and the dynamic interaction between members of the CMI and resident renal cells brings us increasingly closer to rational and specific therapy of various immune diseases in the kidney. Increasing knowledge regarding genetic susceptibility to different diseases has the potential to help identify patients likely to develop various immune mediated renal diseases and provide the possibility of preemptive intervention.

It is clear that sensitized cells are involved in GN. There is persuasive evidence that members of the cellular immune system, both sensitized and nonsensitized, play a pivotal role in a wide variety of disease entities involving all compartments of the kidney. They play a role as members of the inflammatory response to antigen-specific stimuli and as active participants in non–antigen-evoked damage.

The challenge for the 21st century is to further elaborate and clarify mechanisms by which these cells are recruited and induce renal damage. We must develop strategies that can anticipate and prevent consequent damage and intervene to arrest or even reverse the phenotypic and functional alterations that result from CMI in the kidney. Continued study of *in vivo* and *in vitro* models of disease with judicious extrapolation to human disease should continue to clarify the role of CMI in GN and renal disease. This should lead to more specific and less toxic intervention of these disease entities.

Selected Readings

Bolton WK. Mechanisms of glomerular injury: injury mediated by sensitized lymphocytes. *Semin Nephrol* 1991;11:285.

Review of mechanisms of glomerular injury and evidence for the role of specifically sensitized lymphocytes and other members of the cellular immune system in the pathogenesis of GN.

Bolton WK, Benton FR, Lobo PI. Requirement of functional T cells in the production of autoimmune glomerulotubular nephropathy in mice. *Clin Exp Immunol* 1978;33:474.

Experimental model documenting the need for T cells in the production of autoimmune GN.

Bolton WK, Innes DJ, Sturgill BC, et al. T cells and macrophages in rapidly progressive glomerulonephritis: clinicopathologic correlations. *Kidney Int* 1987; 32:869.

Phenotypic analysis of renal biopsies in patients with severe GN showing participation of components of the cellular immune system in human GN.

Bolton WK, Tucker FL, Sturgill BC. New avian model of experimental glomerulonephritis consistent with mediation by cellular immunity. *J Clin Invest* 1984; 73:1263.

Paper describing antibody-deficient chickens (induced by bursectomy) with intact delayed hypersensitivity able to develop GN comparable to GN mediated by antibodies.

Kelly CJ, Frishberg Y, Gold DP. An appraisal of T cell subsets and the potential for autoimmune injury. *Kidney Int* 1998;53:1574.

Review of T-cell subsets and the role of subsets in murine models of autoimmune disease.

Li S, Holdsworth SR, Tipping PG. Antibody independent crescentic glomerulonephritis in μ chain deficient mice. *Kidney Int* 1997;51:672.

One of several papers by this group showing the ability to induce GN in the absence of antibody in specific strains of mice and detailing the role of CD4+ and CD8+ cells and genetic background in disease susceptibility.

Lynch RG. The biology and pathology of lymphocytes Fc receptors. *Am J Pathol* 1998;152:631.

Review of Fc receptors on lymphocytes and the role of Fc receptors in disease

Nikolic-Paterson DJ, Lan HY, Atkins R. Macrophages in immune renal injury. In: Neilson EG, Couser WG, eds. *Immunologic Renal Diseases*. Philadelphia: Lippincott–Raven, 1997:575.

Review of the role of macrophages in GN, including mechanisms involved in recruitment and damage associated with macrophage infiltration.

Stilmant MM, Bolton WK, Sturgill BC, et al. Crescentic glomerulonephritis without immune deposits: clinicopathologic features. *Kidney Int* 1979;15:184.

One of the earliest references to demonstrate GN in the absence of deposits of immune reactants in humans.

Tung KS, Lou YH, Garza KM, et al. Autoimmune ovarian disease: mechanism of disease function and prevention. *Curr Opin Immunol* 1997;9:839.

Review of factors involved in antigen recognition, molecular mimicry and epitope spreading in induction of autoimmune disease.

CHAPTER 37

Role of Mediator Systems in Glomerular and Vascular Diseases

PART 1
Role of Coagulation in Glomerular and Vascular Diseases

Carla Zoja, Piero Ruggenenti, and Giuseppe Remuzzi

Studies performed over many years have provided evidence for accumulation of fibrin within the glomerular tuft in several forms of renal disease, which likely reflects an impaired balance between coagulation and fibrinolytic systems. Glomerular fibrin deposits may form within vessels as well as develop in Bowman's space in association with extracapillary crescents.

In the early 1960s, Vassalli and McCluskey were the first to suggest the importance of glomerular fibrin deposition in glomerulonephritis on the basis of the observation of conspicuous accumulation of fibrin both in patients with acute glomerulonephritis and in experimental crescentic anti-glomerular basement membrane (GBM) glomerulonephritis. The autologous phase of this model was extensively employed in the following years contributing greatly to the understanding of the mechanisms of glomerular fibrin deposition in glomerulonephritis. The accumulation of fibrin seems to implicate activation of the intrinsic pathway of coagulation (Fig. 37.1), as indicated by the presence in the deposits of factor VIII and factor XII (Hageman factor). The extrinsic pathway triggered by activation of the tissue factor procoagulant (factor III, thromboplastin) is also involved. Activation of factor X through both pathways leads to the formation of thrombin that converts fibrinogen to fibrin. Tissue factor is a transmembrane glycoprotein that can be expressed in many cells, including macrophages, endothelial cells, and glomerular cells. Some observations support a central role for activated macrophages as producers of the procoagulant signal essential to initiating the formation of glomerular fibrin. Thus, in experimental anti-GBM nephritis, glomerular infiltration by macrophages and enhanced glomerular synthesis of tissue factor coincided with fibrin deposition and crescent formation. On the other hand, depletion of macrophages by mustine hydrochloride treatment reduced glomerular procoagulant activity and abrogated fibrin deposits. Similarly, in human crescentic glomerulonephritis glomerular damage is associated with macrophage accumulation, enhanced glomerular procoagulant activity, and fibrin deposition. Activated macrophages while producing tissue factor themselves, secrete proinflammatory cytokines such as interleukin-1 (IL-1) and tumor necrosis factor (TNF) that convert endothelial cells from an antithrombotic to a procoagulant phenotype. Thus cytokine-stimulated endothelial cells express tissue factorlike procoagulant activity, acquire the capacity to bind factor VII/VIIa and trigger the extrinsic pathway of the coagulation cascade, and release von Willebrand factor and plasminogen activator inhibitor, with a concomitant

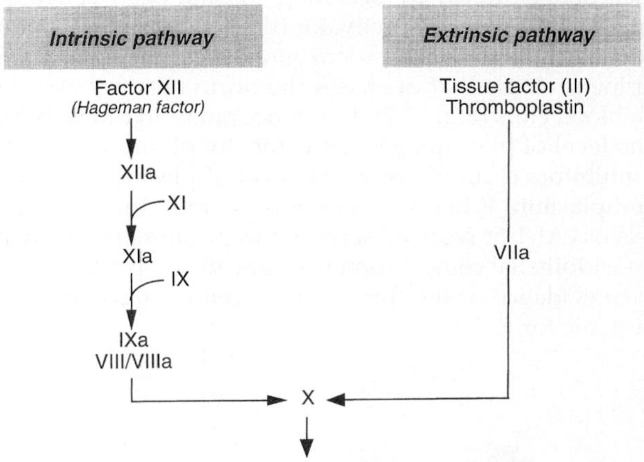

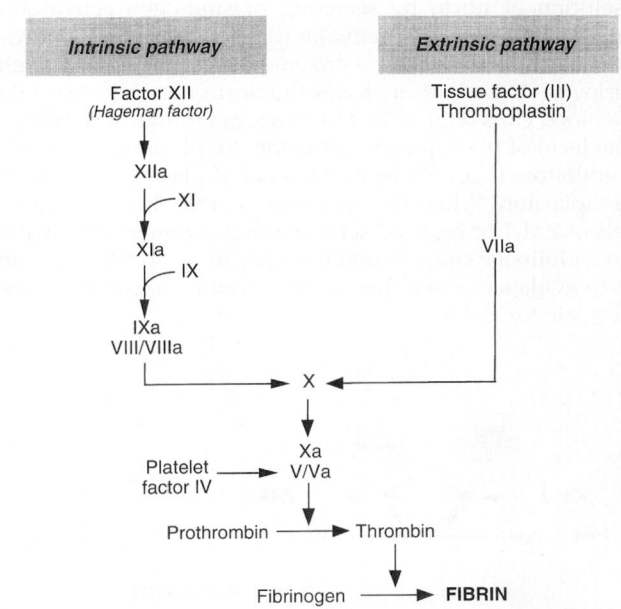

Figure 37.1. A summary of coagulation cascade. Intrinsic and extrinsic pathways of coagulation are both responsible for initiation of fibrin deposition in glomerulonephritis. Platelet factor 3 released by platelets also participates in the coagulation system.

suppression of the protein C anticoagulant activity. The relevance of these *in vitro* findings to the prothrombotic changes promoted by IL-1 in endothelial cells *in vivo*, manifests with fibrin strands associated with the luminal surface of arteries in rabbits infused with IL-1, as shown by scanning electron microscopy.

PARTICIPATION OF ENDOTHELIAL CELLS TO THE FORMATION OF INTRAVASCULAR THROMBI

When endothelial cells are altered by vascular injury or inflammation, platelets respond rapidly by attaching firmly to the site of lesion, where exposure of subendothelial matrix may have occurred. Von Willebrand factor (vWF) is an adhesive protein that in the presence of shear forces becomes essential in the initiation of platelet adhesion and thrombus formation by binding the glycoprotein (GP)Ib and IIb–IIIa complex on platelet surface. At high shear stress, vWF is the only molecule that can bind to the exposed subendothelium and to platelets via GPIb. Molecular conformational changes produced by shear forces favor this process. vWF interaction with GPIb promotes platelet activation with the subsequent formation of GPIIb–IIIa complex that binds the Arg-Gly-Asp (RGD) sequence of both vWF and fibrinogen leading to thrombus formation. Following a series of platelet–platelet interactions, a platelet mass accumulates with thrombus formation. Concomitant deposition of fibrin, arising from blood coagulation, contributes to strengthen platelet aggregates by providing additional fibrous links between individual platelets.

Thrombin and fibrin are the major products of the coagulation cascade. Thrombin, a serine protease generated at sites of vascular damage, proteolytically converts fibrinogen to insoluble fibrin and is, together with collagen, the most potent activator of platelets responsible for thrombus formation at sites of vascular damage. Thrombin exerts procoagulant effects on endothelial cells, stimulating tissue factor and vWF and platelet activating factor. It also affects the fibrinolysis system, inducing endothelial production of plasminogen activator inhibitor (PAI)-1. Endothelial cells normally participate in the dissolution of fibrin by secreting plasminogen activators—tissue-type plasminogen activator (tPA) and urokinase (uPA)—that convert the inactive proenzyme plasminogen to plasmin, a serine protease that degrades the fibrin network associated with blood clots (Fig. 37.2). Fibrin degradation can be blocked at the level of plasminogen activators by plasminogen activator inhibitors (1 and 2) or at the level of plasmin, mainly via α_2-antiplasmin. When the system is altered, due to increased levels of PAI-1 or reduced secretion of plasminogen activators from endothelial cells, thrombosis may develop. Of note is the *in vivo* evidence of the formation of venous thrombi in mice transgenic for PAI-1.

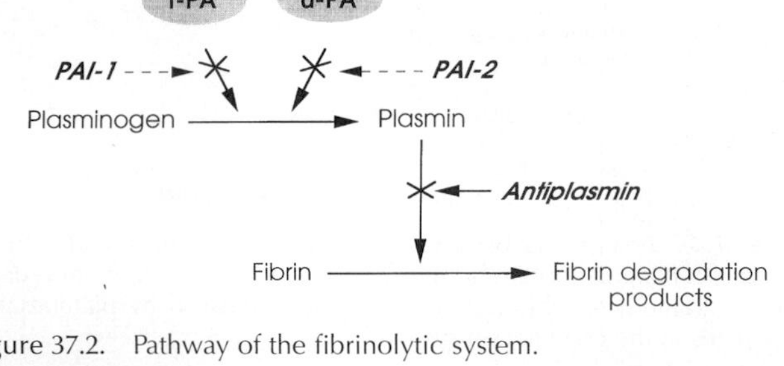

Figure 37.2. Pathway of the fibrinolytic system.

GLOMERULAR CELLS HAVE BOTH PROCOAGULANT AND FIBRINOLYTIC PROPERTIES

Glomerular cells have the potential to modulate local coagulation processes by producing tissue factor-procoagulant activity as well as plasminogen activator and its inhibitor PAI-1. In 1985, De Prost and Kanfer reported that isolated rat glomeruli contained a procoagulant activity with the characteristics of thromboplastin/tissue factor and Wiggins and colleagues measured procoagulant activity in glomeruli and urine of rabbits with nephrotoxic nephritis. A few years later it was documented that rat glomerular mesangial cells in culture released tissue factor in small amounts when in resting conditions, but at a great extent after stimulation with cytokines or endotoxin, thus implying a direct involvement of mesangial cells in fibrin formation during glomerular injury or inflammation. On the other hand, human mesangial cells in culture constitutively express tPA and PAI-1, which are both upregulated by thrombin, especially PAI-1 that is formed in more amounts than tPA. Thus thrombin, besides favoring fibrin formation by virtue of its procoagulant potential, also inhibits fibrin degradation by enhancing mesangial PAI-1 production. Thrombin and cytokines modulate the release of uPA, tPA, and PAI-1 by glomerular epithelial cells, which indicates that glomerular epithelial cells also participate actively in the regulation of extracapillary fibrinolysis in the glomeruli during local inflammatory and immune processes.

INTRAVASCULAR GLOMERULAR FIBRIN DEPOSITION

Intravascular thrombosis is a common feature of hemolytic uremic syndrome (HUS), thrombotic thrombocytopenic purpura (TTP), and other thrombotic microangiopathies that may complicate the course of pregnancy and of several systemic diseases, including systemic sclerosis (Table 37.1). These syndromes of microangiopathic hemolytic anemia and thrombocytopenia share the same histologic lesion—widening of the subendothelial space and intraluminal platelet and fibrin thrombi—and a similar pathophysiologic process that, through platelet consumption and erythrocyte disruption in the injured microcirculation, leads to thrombocytopenia and hemolytic anemia. These entities are discussed in detail in Chapter 42, Part 9.

Endothelial dysfunction appears to be an important factor in the sequence of events leading to microvascular thrombosis. Consistent with this interpretation are data indicating that most agents associated with the disease are toxic to endothelial cells. Thus bacterial endotoxins and verotoxins may trigger the microangiopathic process in some cases of *Escherichia coli* and *Shigella dysenteriae* infection, antibodies and immunocomplexes in systemic lupus erythematosus, cancer, or kidney transplant; and barotrauma in malignant hypertension or scleroderma crises. Even radiation and certain drugs, including mitomycin and cyclosporine, may directly damage the endothelium and trigger the disease. On the contrary, the role of estrogens in mediating the microangiopathic process occasionally associated with pregnancy or birth control pills is controversial.

Hemolytic Uremic Syndrome and Thrombotic Thrombocytopenic Purpura

The role of activated coagulation in formation of vascular thrombi has been extensively investigated in diarrhea-associated HUS (D+HUS). Infection with verotoxin-producing *E. coli* (VTEC) is

TABLE 37.1. Classification of Thrombotic Microangiopathies

Hemolytic Uremic Syndrome
Typical, verotoxin-associated Atypical Plasma resistant
Thrombotic Thrombocytopenic Purpura
Acute Chronic relapsing Plasma resistant
Familial Forms
Secondary Forms

Pregnancy-associated
  TTP
  Severe preeclampsia/HELLP syndrome
  Postpartum HUS
HIV infection-associated
Systemic disease-associated
  Systemic lupus erythematosus, systemic sclerosis
  Antiphospholipid syndrome
  Malignant hypertension
Cancer- and chemotherapy-associated
Transplant- and cyclosporine-associated

HELLP, hemolysis, elevated liver enzymes, and low platelet count; HUS, hemolytic uremic syndrome; TTP, thrombotic thrombocytopenic purpura.

the most common cause of D+HUS. After the ingestion of contaminated food or water, *E. coli* binds to specific receptors on the colonic mucosa, multiplies, and causes cell death. This process usually leads to diarrhea, and strains of the bacteria capable of producing verotoxins, such as *E. coli* O157:H7, can damage the mucosal vasculature causing hemorrhagic colitis. Once the toxin has gained access to the systemic circulation, it may bind specific receptors in the microcirculation of target organs and trigger the microangiopathic process. It has been suggested that verotoxin binding to vascular endothelium may cause endothelial cell activation with consequent prothrombotic changes, including upregulation of tissue factor that in turn may lead to activation of the extrinsic pathway and consequent thrombin formation. Preliminary studies, however, failed to document any change in levels of coagulation factors and soluble circulating fibrin and found only slight increases in fibrinogen turnover following radio-labelled fibrinogen injection. On the other hand, evidence of increased levels of fibrin degradation products in urine and plasma, and raised levels of fibrinopeptide A in children with HUS suggested a role for activated coagulation in the genesis of microvascular thrombi in HUS. The availability of more precise markers of activity of the coagulation system, including thrombin-antithrombin III (TAT) and prothrombin fragment 1+2 (F1+2), allowed an activation of coagulation either in HUS or TTP to be demonstrated. In particular, enhanced TAT and F1+2 levels were taken to indicate activation of coagulation in 25 children with severe VTEC associated D+HUS requiring dialytic treatment. Increased D-dimer and tPA antigen levels documented an increased fibrinolytic turnover that, however, was at least in part inhibited by a parallel net increase in PAI-1 activity. Reduced plasma fibrinolytic potential in the setting of an activated coagulation system was therefore suggested to contribute to stabilization of glomerular and arteriolar thrombi in D+HUS. On the other hand, different mechanisms must be advocated for persistency of fibrin deposits in non–diarrhea-associated HUS and in adult forms of HUS, where PAI-1 activity is not significantly increased and inhibited fibrinolysis is unlikely to play an important role. Whatever the role of the coagulation system, treatment with antithrombotic or fibrinolytic agents was ineffective in childhood D+HUS, in D-HUS, and in adult HUS, and may increase the risk of severe hemorrhage.

At variance with HUS, the microvascular thrombi of TTP are composed predominantly of aggregated platelets combined to large amounts of vWF, with little or no fibrinogen/fibrin. This led some authors to hypothesize that the intrusion in the circulation of one or more platelet-aggregating agents—such as a protein of 59kD, or a 37-kD protein capable of binding to platelet GPIV and inducing clumping—may play a pivotal role in the process of microvascular thrombosis in TTP. Others have reported that in TTP patients, endothelial cells have a reduced capacity to form the potent platelet-aggregation inhibitor prostacyclin (PGI_2), which may reflect underlying endothelial dysfunction and account for decreased endothelial thromboresistance. In acute TTP, Ca^{2+}-dependent cysteine proteinases (calpain) or lysosomal-derived non–Ca^{2+}-dependent cathepsin-type cysteine proteinase (likely expression of tissue injury), may bind to platelet GPIX and GPIIb-IIIa sites on platelets and platelet microparticles, and may cleave vWF multimers into fragments capable of clumping platelets. Abnormal vWF fragmentation is also common in condition of enhanced shear stress (Fig. 37.3). Following endothelial cell injury, subendothelial expansion and myointimal swelling and proliferation may cause narrowing or obliteration of vascular lumina. Vascular narrowing, by increasing resistances, enhances fluid shear stress (i.e., the tractive force produced by blood flowing over the endothelial cell surface), which in turn alters the normal processing of vWF and the interaction of platelets with the endothelium (Fig. 37.3). The attachment of vWF to platelet surface may occur initially to the shear-altered GPIb component of platelet GPIb-IX-V receptors and subsequently to activated platelet GPIIb-IIIa. This process is dependent on vWF binding to activated platelets and may account for the vWF-rich, fibrin-poor platelet thrombi documented in the microcirculation of TTP patients. In turn, the formation of thrombi in the microcirculation may further increase shear stress and perpetuate the phenomenon. Besides vWF, shear stress also influences endothelial nitric oxide (NO) synthesis and release. NO, by inducing TNF-α and IL-1 release from inflammatory cells, promotes leukocyte activation and further amplifies the vascular damage. Shear stress may sustain the microangiopathic process even in some cases of HUS characterized by severe preglomerular arteriolar narrowing and secondary glomerular ischemia. In four dramatic cases, in which persistent thrombocytopenia, refractory hypertension, and hypertensive encephalopathy put the patient in imminent danger of death, bilateral nephrectomy was followed within 2 weeks by complete hematologic and clinical remission. The rationale of the procedure rests on evidence that removing the kidneys eliminates a major site of vWF fragmentation, which would limit platelet activation and protect patients from the further spreading of microvascular lesions. On the other hand, it must be emphasized that bilateral nephrectomy is a rescue therapy for extremely rare and selected cases. The infusion or exchange of fresh-frozen plasma is the first line therapy for all cases of TTP and adult HUS, and for the atypical forms of HUS with signs of neurologic involvement. The procedure is likely effective by providing plasma components—conceivably defective in HUS/TTP patients—involved in vWF processing. It must be continued up to complete remission of the neurologic symptoms, normalization of platelet count, and signs of hemolysis.

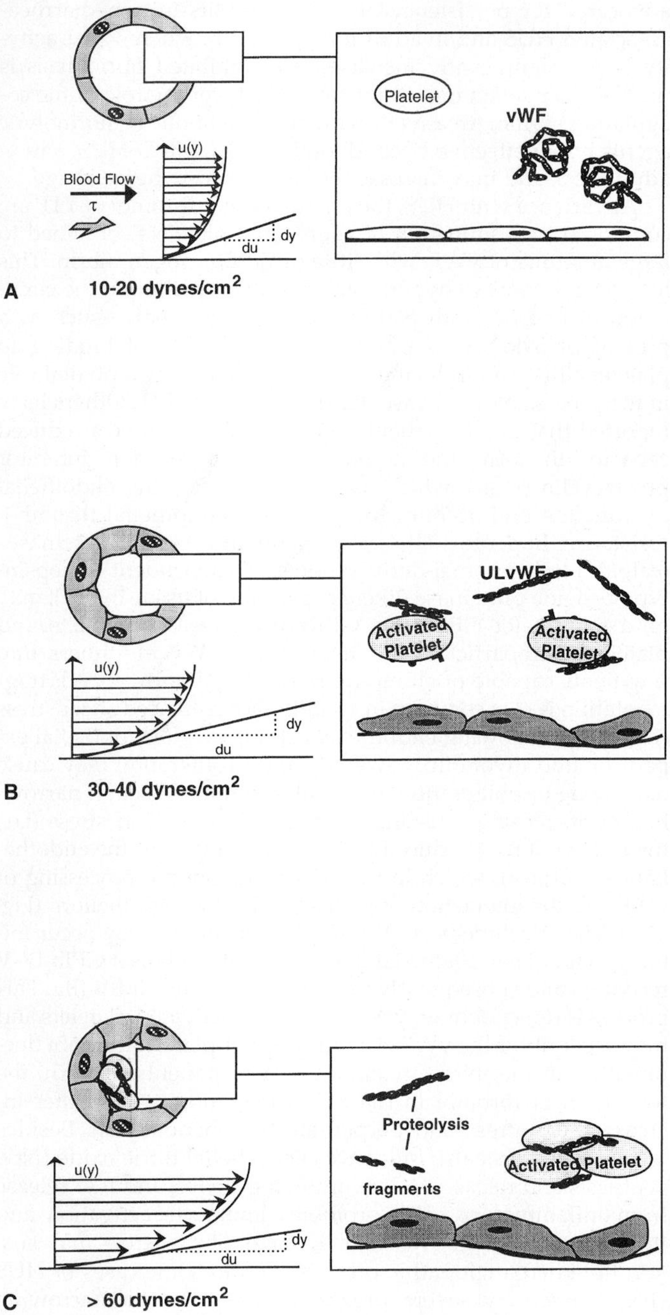

Figure 37.3. A hypothetical sequence of events leading to vascular thrombosis through endothelial cell injury and enhanced shear stress. In normal conditions, blood flow is laminar and vWF multimers circulate in a coiled form *(panel A)*. Upon endothelial cell injury and swelling, blood flow in narrowed vascular lumina becomes turbulent. The consequent increase in shear stress induces platelet activation and vWF multimers uncoiling *(panel B)*. Uncoiled vWF multimers become exposed to the activity of circulating proteases with consequent abnormal fragmentation. vWF fragments bind activated platelets and contribute to platelet aggregation and thrombi formation *(panel C)*.

PREECLAMPSIA AND THE HELLP SYNDROME*

Pregnancy is considered a "hypercoagulable state" characterized by increased plasma levels of several coagulation factors and enhanced risk of thromboembolic complications. Twofold to threefold increases in factor VIII and fibrinogen may occur in normal pregnancy, which are only partially counterbalanced by concomitant increases in α_2-macroglobulin, heparin cofactor II, and tissue-factor pathway inhibitor. Furthermore, plasma levels of protein C and antithrombin III (AT-III) do not change, protein S activity may fall by approximately 50%, and resistance to activated protein C may develop, especially during the third trimester. On the other hand, tPA and uPA, as well as PAI types 1 and 2, increase in parallel, so net plasminogen activator activity is unaffected. These changes reflect enhanced thrombin production and secondary fibrinolysis, which occur even in normal pregnancy, as documented by increased plasma levels of thrombin–antithrombin complexes, fibrin degradation products, and D-dimers. The consequent hypercoagulable state is likely designed to limit the risk of maternal bleeding at the time of delivery, but also may predispose to microvascular thrombosis when endothelial cell injury or platelet activation are superimposed. This is the case of preeclampsia, a syndrome of hypertension, proteinuria, and edema—occasionally complicated by generalized convulsions (eclampsia)—that manifests during the third trimester in 5% to 10% of pregnancies, most commonly in nulliparas, in particular teenagers and women older than 30 years. The disease is triggered by a congenital or acquired defect of placentation resulting in abnormal uterine spiral arteries remodeling and consequent fetoplacental ischemia. Then uncharacterized factors released into the maternal circulation by the ischemic fetoplacental unit would trigger endothelial dysfunction with consequent vascular hyperreactivity, proteinuria, and platelet activation. Loss of the physiologic refractoriness to angiotensin II may account for the "high resistance state" of preeclampsia as compared with normal pregnancy, with further impairment of the placental blood flow and increase in systemic blood pressure. An imbalance between vasodilator and vasoconstrictor eicosanoids could account for platelet activation in preeclampsia and increased responsiveness to pressor peptides. An altered placental PGI_2/thromboxane (TxA_2) ratio may favor local platelet activation and vasoconstriction contributing to placental insufficiency and fetal distress. According to this hypothesis, the restricted flow in the umbilical side of the placental circulation would result in reduced uterine blood flow; fetal hypoxia; and in genetically susceptible patients, a secondary increase in blood pressure. Interestingly, in pregnancies characterized by high placental resistances, mean platelet count in the umbilical blood at time of delivery is significantly lower than in normal pregnancies and is associated with a reduced platelet life span and increased platelet turnover. Thrombocytopenia and increased platelet activity and consumption occur in 10% to 15% of cases of preeclampsia in parallel with an activation of coagulation manifested by depressed AT-III and protein C levels and modest increases in thrombin–antithrombin III complexes and fibrin D-dimers. However, routine coagulation studies, including the prothrombin time (PT), activated partial thromboplastin time (aPTT), and fibrin split products, are usually in normal ranges. A fulminant consumptive coagulopathy may complicate the course of the hemolysis, elevated liver enzymes, and low platelet count (HELLP) syndrome, a form of severe preeclampsia in which, besides hypertension and renal dysfunction, there is evidence of microangiopathic hemolysis and liver involvement. The syndrome is most common in white multiparous women with a history of poor pregnancy outcome. It arises in the antepartum period in 70% of cases. Postpartum symptoms usually arise within 24 to 48 hours from delivery, occasionally after an uncomplicated pregnancy. Diagnosis is based on (a) hemolysis (defined as fragmented erythrocytes in the circulation and lactic dehydrogenase 600 U/L or greater), (b) elevated liver enzymes (serum glutamic oxaloacetic transaminase greater than 70 U/L), and

*HELLP denotes hemolysis, elevated liver enzymes, and low platelet count.

(c) low platelets (platelet count less than 100,000/μl). Overt disseminated intravascular coagulation (DIC) is reported in 25% of cases. Biochemical evidence of secondary fibrinolysis is common, but bleeding or an abnormal PT, aPTT, or fibrinogen are rare in the absence of abruptio placenta. Intrahepatic hemorrhage, subcapsular liver hematoma, and liver rupture are rare, life-threatening complications. The maternal and perinatal mortality rates range from 0% to 24% and from 7.7% to 60%, respectively. Most of the perinatal deaths are related to abruptio placentae, intrauterine asphyxia, and extreme prematurity. As many as 44% of the infants are growth retarded.

Termination of pregnancy is the only definitive therapy of preeclampsia and HELLP syndrome. Antihypertensive therapy may limit the risks of cerebrovascular complications and heart failure. Magnesium sulphate is the treatment of choice to prevent and treat convulsions. Plasma exchange may help recovery in patients with persistent hemolysis and platelet consumption 72 hours or more after delivery. Platelet transfusions are needed only for clinical bleeding or severe thrombocytopenia (platelet count less than 20,000/μl).

Systemic Sclerosis

Systemic sclerosis is a generalized disorder classified among connective tissue diseases and characterized by widespread fibrosis and proliferative and occlusive vascular changes involving the skin, joints and tendon sheaths, muscles, and viscera, including the gastrointestinal tract, lungs, heart, and kidneys. In 5% to 15% of cases, renal function rapidly deteriorates in parallel with a sudden increase in arterial blood pressure. This "renal crisis," often complicated by malignant hypertension and thrombotic microangiopathy, is the most common cause of death in virtually all series reported. Endothelial dysfunction is likely the primary event that may result in vasoconstriction, vascular ischemia, intravascular coagulation, and pulmonary hypertension. Antiendothelial antibodies; a heat-stable, nondialyzable protease with esterolytic activity; and high hydraulic pressure placed on the vessel wall by severe hypertension in the setting of renal crises have been implicated as potential triggers of vascular damage. Then enhanced fluid shear stress in vascular lumina narrowed by swollen endothelial cells may interfere with the complex process of platelet interaction with the endothelium, leading to vascular thrombosis. Increased plasma levels of vWF antigen, increased rates of fibrinogen breakdown, and fibrin deposition in tissues are the expression of an activated coagulation. Autoantibodies to fibrin-bound tPA, found in the circulation of patients at increased risk of pulmonary hypertension, have been suggested to indicate a concomitant abnormal fibrinolysis. Activated platelets adhered to injured vessel surface are a source of growth factors, such as fibroblast-activating factors and transforming growth factor-β that promote the expansion of a subset of fibroblasts capable of inducing the synthesis of type I and type III collagen, proteoglycans, hyaluronic acid, and fibronectin. Further vascular narrowing exacerbates renal ischemia, activation of the renin-angiotensin system, and the release of factors that sustain systemic hypertension in a vicious circle leading to further vascular injury, platelet activation, and intravascular thrombosis. Control of severe hypertension by vasodilators, by angiotensin-converting enzyme inhibitors, and in most severe cases, by ultrafiltration is the only effective therapy in scleroderma renal crisis. Plasma exchange can be attempted in cases complicated by thrombotic microangiopathy, and bilateral nephrectomy may be the last available approach in patients in imminent danger of death because of refractory, malignant hypertension. The role of fibrinolytic therapy is still under investigation. The clinical entity of systemic sclerosis is discussed in Chapter 42, Part 8.

EXTRACAPILLARY FIBRIN DEPOSITION

Crescentic Glomerulonephritis

The autologous phase of crescentic glomerulonephritis in rabbits is the most commonly investigated model of glomerular fibrin deposition with extracapillary crescent formation. The disease is induced by injection of heterologous anti-GBM antibodies that bind to rabbit GBM and lead to glomerular injury. This early phase (heterologous phase) is characterized by a mild proliferative glomerulonephritis. The autologous phase develops several days after injection of nephrotoxic serum and results from the production of host antibodies and cellular sensitivity against the heterologous antibodies fixed to the GBM. In this phase a severe glomerulonephritis manifests with proliferation of glomerular cells, neutrophil and macrophage infiltration, intracapillary and extracapillary fibrin deposits, and crescent formation. Studies consistently indicated that fibrin formation in the Bowman's space is essential for the development of crescents that consist mainly of macrophage infiltrates and proliferating cells from the parietal epithelium of Bowman's capsule (Fig. 37.4). Crescents may also be invaded by fibroblastlike cells associated with extracapillary matrix deposition leading to irreversible nephron loss. Macrophages appear to be crucial for glomerular fibrin deposits and crescent formation. They accumulate early in glomerular capillary and sometimes in periglomerular infiltrates in the rabbit anti-GBM nephritis or in some forms of human glomerulonephritis. Later, increasing numbers of macrophages accumulate in crescents. The signals for macrophage recruitment into the glomerulus are only partially known. Chemotactic factors in the fibrin deposits, such as thrombin or fibronectin fragments, may attract monocytes into the Bowman's space, an event that is facilitated by breaks in the glomerular capillary wall or Bowman's capsule. Immunoglobulins have also been reported to favor monocyte accumulation in some forms of glomerulonephritis. Monocytes and macrophages may contribute to crescent formation through increasing fibrin deposition by the release of tissue factor or by producing

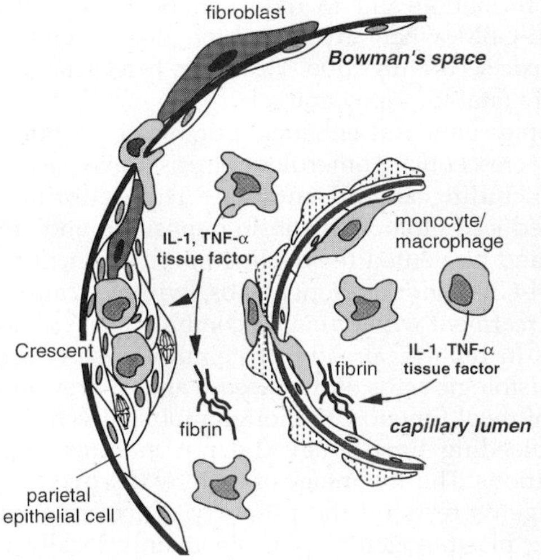

Figure 37.4. Representation of mechanisms possibly involved in fibrin and crescent formation in crescentic glomerulonephritis. Macrophages participate in crescent formation through increasing fibrin deposition by the release of tissue factor or by producing cytokines with procoagulant activity. Cytokines in turn stimulate proliferation of fibroblasts and parietal epithelial cells, which consolidate the crescent structure.

cytokines with procoagulant activity. A procoagulant factor is clearly essential to initiate fibrin deposition. This has been directly documented by a study showing that administration of antibodies to tissue factor in rabbits with crescentic glomerulonephritis inhibited glomerular tissue factor activity, significantly reduced fibrin deposits in Bowman's space and crescent formation, and protected from renal function impairment. A significant reduction in proteinuria was also observed. Of interest, this study also provided evidence that the tissue factor has other functions in addition to its role in activation of coagulation that may contribute to glomerular injury, as demonstrated by decreased major histocompatibility complex class II expression in glomeruli and tubulointerstitial areas in the animals treated with the antitissue factor antibodies.

Besides factors that promote coagulation, an impairment in the fibrinolytic system may also account for glomerular fibrin accumulation. Dysregulation of the plasminogen/plasmin system with decreased glomerular fibrinolytic activity associated with decreased tPA and increased PAI-1 expression has been demonstrated at the peak of the disease in experimental crescentic glomerulonephritis and in human glomerulonephritis.

The recent demonstration of a protective role for plasminogen and plasminogen activators against inflammatory renal injury in crescentic glomerulonephritis was documented by inducing glomerulonephritis in mice with genetic deficiencies of plasminogen or plasminogen activators. Thus deficiency of plasminogen or combined deficiency of tPA and uPA was associated with enhanced glomerular hypercellularity, macrophage infiltration, fibrin accumulation, and crescent formation.

Treatments that interfere with coagulation have been employed, with the aim of limiting fibrin deposition and the consequent glomerular obsolescence and progression of the disease. Results were variable. Some authors showed that high doses of heparin prevented fibrin deposition, reduced glomerular hypercellularity, and limited crescent formation in rabbits with anti-GBM. At variance, other authors did not find any beneficial effect of heparin in a model of severe anti-GBM glomerulonephritis in the rabbit or in nephrotoxic serum nephritis in rats. Differences in severity of the models, difficulty in their standardization, or differences in secondary mediators of injury have been taken as possible explanations for the conflicting results. Another anticoagulant, warfarin, was found to protect against crescent formation and to reduce hypercellularity in rabbits with anti-GBM when given at high doses before and after nephrotoxic serum injection. However, hemorrhagic complications were fatal for many animals.

Therapies aimed at enhancing or replacing fibrinolytic activity in crescentic glomerulonephritis have also been proposed, including ancrod and tPA. The defibrinating agent ancrod reduced glomerular fibrin deposition and crescent formation, and prevented the decline in renal function in rabbits with anti-GBM glomerulonephritis, without causing hemorrhages. Treatment with human recombinant tPA of nephrotoxic nephritis in rabbits, already proteinuric, was effective in reducing histologic signs of the disease and in preventing deterioration of renal function. Although rabbits given tPA had prolonged bleeding times, they did not manifest hemorrhagic complications. The advantage offered by tPA over other thrombolytic agents rests on the property of exerting its effect of activating plasminogen to plasmin mainly locally within the fibrin clot, without degradation of fibrinogen. However, as highlighted by McCluskey, there are serious difficulties in the use and evaluation of the effectiveness of agents that either prevent or dissolve glomerular fibrin deposits in humans with crescentic glomerulonephritis, as indicated by previous studies using heparin, warfarin, and antithrombotic agents combined with steroids and immunosuppressants or ancrod. This is essentially due to the fact that crescentic glomerulonephritis is not a homogeneous entity but it comprises various forms with different underlying causes and pathogenic mechanisms that may differ in severity and progression. Moreover, the major forms of crescentic glomerulonephritis, anti-GBM nephritis, Wegener's granulomatosis and idiopathic necrotizing, and crescentic glomerulonephritis are quite uncommon, which makes it difficult to perform controlled trials in patients with a given type of crescentic glomerulonephritis. Another problem is that these diseases can progress very quickly and severe glomerular injury has often developed by the time diagnosis is provided. Finally, lung hemorrhage sometimes occurs in patients with crescentic glomerulonephritis, which may be a contraindication for anticoagulant and fibrinolytic therapy. Nevertheless, it is conceivable that in some cases, these therapies combined with immunosuppression, and started early after diagnosis, might have a place in the treatment of human crescentic glomerulonephritis. Crescentic glomerulonephritis is further discussed in Chapter 39, Part 9.

Selected Readings

Fritzel MJ, Hart DA, Wilson D, et al. Antibodies to fibrin bound tissue type plasminogen activator in systemic sclerosis. *J Rheumatol* 1995;22:1688–1693.

An important work investigating the role of activation of coagulation and discussing the potential effectiveness of fibrinolytic therapy in systemic sclerosis.

Kitching AR, Holdsworth SR, Ploplis VA, et al. Plasminogen and plasminogen activators protect against renal injury in crescentic glomerulonephritis. *J Exp Med* 1997;185:963–968.

An elegant study on the role of plasminogen and plasminogen activators in the development of inflammatory glomerular injury in crescentic glomerulonephritis that employs mice with genetic deficiencies of plasminogen and plasminogen activators.

McCluskey RT. Tissue factor in crescentic glomerulonephritis. *Am J Pathol* 1997; 150:787–792.

The author provides a commentary on the role of tissue factor in glomerular fibrin deposition and crescent formation and discusses the anticoagulant and fibrinolytic therapies so far employed for treatment of experimental and human crescentic glomerulonephritis.

McCrae KR, Cines DB. Thrombotic microangiopathy during pregnancy. *Semin Hematol* 1997;34:148–158.

An important review of the changes in the coagulation system during normal pregnancy and in the several forms of thrombotic microangiopathy that may occur during pregnancy, with particular focus on preeclampsia and the HELLP syndrome.

Moake JL. Studies on the pathophysiology of thrombotic thrombocytopenic purpura. *Semin Hematol* 1997;34:83–89.

An updated and provocative review of the mechanisms underlying intravascular platelet aggregation and endothelial cell-platelet interaction in normal conditions and in thrombotic thrombocytopenic purpura.

Nevard CHF, Jurd KM, Lane DA, et al. Activation of coagulation and fibrinolysis in childhood diarrhea-associated haemolytic uraemic syndrome. *Thromb Haemost* 1997;78:1450–1455.

An important study documenting the role of activated coagulation in the pathogenesis of intravascular thrombi in D+HUS.

Remuzzi G, Ruggenenti P, Bertani T. Thrombotic microangiopathies. In: Tisher CC, Brenner BM, eds. *Renal pathology,* 2nd ed. Philadelphia: JB Lippincott, 1994:1154–1184.

An in-depth review of primary and secondary forms of thrombotic microangiopathy with particular focus on the main pathologic changes and underlying pathogenetic mechanisms.

Ruggeri ZM. The role of von Willebrand factor and fibrinogen in the initiation of platelet adhesion to thrombogenic surfaces. *Thromb Haemost* 1995;74: 460–463.

A review on the mechanisms of platelet function that allow thrombus propagation initiated and mediated by adhesive components at the site of vessel injury.

Wiggins RC, Glatfelter A, Brukman J. Procoagulant activity in glomeruli and urine of rabbits with nephrotoxic nephritis. *Lab Invest* 1985;53:156–165.

This study demonstrates increased procoagulant activity in glomeruli and urine during fibrin formation in Bowman's space of rabbits with crescentic glomerulonephritis.

Zoja C, Corna D, Macconi D, et al. Tissue plasminogen activator therapy of rabbit nephrotoxic nephritis. *Lab Invest* 1990;62:34–40.

Demonstration that the fibrinolytic agent tPA can reduce glomerular fibrin deposition and crescent formation in experimental anti-GBM glomerulonephritis.

PART 2
Role of Cytokines and Chemokines in Glomerular, Tubular, and Vascular Injury

David J. Nikolic-Paterson and Robert C. Atkins

The infiltration and subsequent activation of leukocytes within the kidney plays an important role in the induction and progression of renal injury. Regardless of the nature of the initial insult, renal leukocytic infiltration is prominent in most forms of kidney disease. Infiltrating leukocytes can cause renal damage through a wide variety of mechanisms ranging from cell-mediated immunity (Chapter 36, Part 4) to the production of cytokines, growth factors (Chapter 37, Part 3), metalloproteinases, eicosanoids (Chapter 37, Part 4), coagulation factors (Chapter 37, Part 1), and oxygen radicals (Chapter 37, Part 7). Cytokines and chemokines regulate the entry of leukocytes into the kidney and their subsequent activation. This chapter discusses the role of cytokines and chemokines in leukocyte-mediated renal injury with an emphasis on experimental blocking studies and the potential for therapeutic intervention in human kidney disease.

OVERVIEW OF CYTOKINES AND CHEMOKINES IN RENAL INJURY

Cytokines and chemokines are small secreted proteins that bind to target cells via cell surface receptors, eliciting either a proinflammatory or antiinflammatory response. A generalized scheme of how cytokines and chemokines participate in renal injury is shown in Fig. 37.5. A renal insult induces production of the major proinflammatory cytokines including interleukin-1 (IL-1), tumor necrosis factor-α (TNF-α), and macrophage migration inhibitory factor (MIF). These cytokines upregulate expression of leukocyte-adhesion molecules, chemokines, colony-stimulating factors, and proinflammatory lipids causing the recruitment and activation of blood leukocytes, resulting in renal damage. Persistent leukocyte-mediated damage leads to renal fibrosis, which is the final common pathway of irreversible kidney destruction.

Leukocytes can cause renal damage through innate and/or cellular immunity. These two responses are regulated by cytokines. In innate immunity, macrophages are activated to function as effector cells via engagement of Fc receptors, engagement of complement receptors, or by stimulation with cytokines such as IL-1, TNF-α, and MIF. The antigen-specific cellular immune response is based on CD8+ cytotoxic T cells and the Th_1 subset of CD4+ T cells (Chapter 36, Part 4). The Th_1 cells, through production of cytokines such as MIF, interferon-γ (IFN-γ), and TNF-α, recruit and activate macrophages as effector cells in a delayed-type hypersensitivity (DTH) response. In contrast, the Th_2 subset of CD4+ T cells produce cytokines IL-4 and IL-10, which promote B-cell proliferation and antibody secretion.

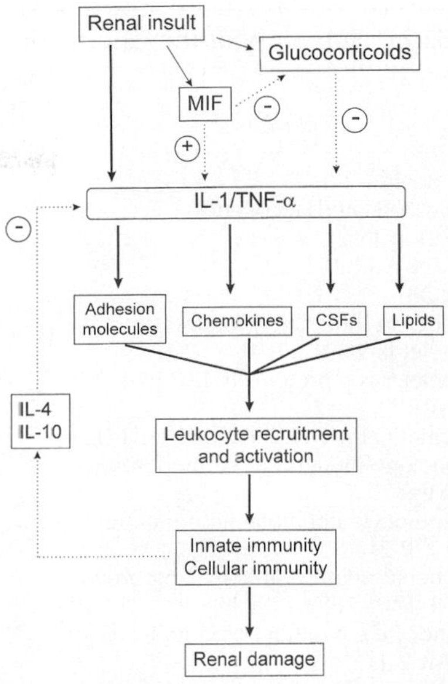

Figure 37.5. Schematic diagram showing the role of cytokines and chemokines in the development of leukocyte-mediated renal damage. Both proinflammatory and antiinflammatory actions are indicated (+ or −). CSFs, colony-stimulating factors; MIF, macrophage migration inhibitory factor.

The accumulation of leukocytes within the kidney is a dynamic process, with infiltrating leukocytes turning over in a matter of days rather than weeks or months. There is constant recruitment, local proliferation (in some cases), and rapid removal of infiltrating cells. Recruitment depends on chemokines and adhesion molecules for the attachment of blood leukocytes to endothelium and subsequent migration into the kidney. Local macrophage proliferation, probably driven by macrophage colony-stimulating factor (M-CSF), is a feature of severe forms of human and experimental kidney disease and is thought to be a mechanism for amplifying macrophage accumulation and effector functions. Although most macrophages die within the inflamed kidney through apoptosis, both T cells and macrophages can leave the kidney via the lymphatic drainage. Indeed, it is the dynamic state of leukocyte recruitment, proliferation, and removal that makes it feasible to inhibit leukocyte accumulation in established disease by blocking the actions of cytokines and adhesion molecules. It is also worth noting that intrinsic renal cells, particularly tubular epithelial cells, are an important source of the cytokines, chemokines, and adhesion molecules, which maintain this dynamic process of leukocyte recruitment, proliferation, and activation.

Chemokines

Chemokines are low-molecular-weight (8 to 10 kD), secreted proteins whose principal function is to induce leukocyte chemotaxis. A wide range of leukocyte and nonleukocytic cell types, including endothelium, mesangial cells, and tubular epithelial cells, can be induced to express chemokines. More than 40 structurally distinct chemokines have been described thus far, the best characterized of which are summarized in Table 37.2. They have been divided into four subgroups based on amino acid sequence. The α, or CXC, subgroup has one amino acid between the first two cysteine residues in the molecule. The β, or CC, subgroup has no amino acid between these two cysteine residues and, more recently, the CX_3C and C subgroups have been described. The structural basis for subgrouping

TABLE 37.2. Summary of the Chemokine Family

Family	Members	Upregulated in Kidney Disease
α (CXC)	Interleukin-8 (IL-8)	Yes[a]
	Growth-related oncogenes	
	(GROα/CINC)	Yes[a]
	(GROβ/MIP-2)	Yes[a]
	(GROγ)	ND
	Interferon-inducible protein-10 (IP-10)	Yes
	Platelet factor-4 (PF-4)	Yes
	Platelet basic proteins (CTAP III, β-TG, NAP-2)	ND
	Stromal cell-derived factor-1 (SDF-1)	ND
	Monokine induced by γ-interferon (Mig)	ND
	Granulocyte chemotactic protein-2 (GCP-2)	ND
	Epithelial neutrophil-activating protein 78 (ENA-78)	ND
β (CC)	Monocyte chemotactic protein-1 (MCP-1)	Yes[a]
	MCP-2,3,4,5	Yes (MCP-3)
	Macrophage inflammatory protein-1	
	(MIP-1α)	Yes[a]
	(MIP-1β)	Yes
	Regulated on activated T-cell expressed and secreted (RANTES)	Yes[a]
	1309 (TCA3)	Yes
	Eotaxin	ND
(CX_3C)	Fractalkine	ND
(C)	Lymphotactin	ND

[a] Blocking these chemokines inhibits leukocyte infiltration in experimental kidney disease. Note, this is not an exhaustive list of all known chemokines.
ND, not determined.

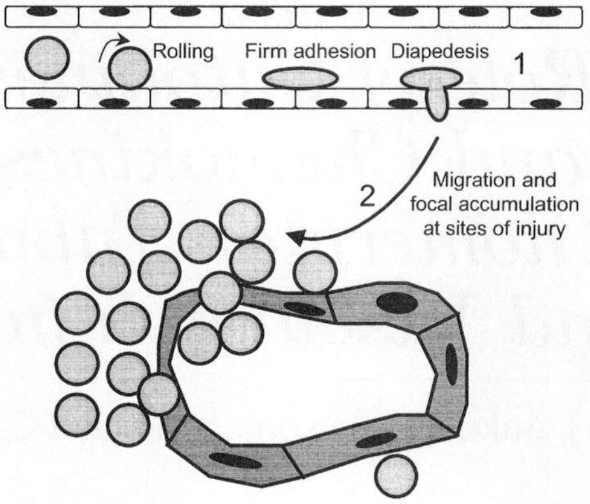

Figure 37.6. Diagram illustrating the two major steps involved in leukocyte accumulation leading to renal damage. Step 1 is the recruitment of blood leukocytes into the kidney, a process called *diapedesis*. Step 2 is the migration of focal accumulation of leukocytes within the glomerulus and interstitium. See text for details.

chemokines also carries biologic relevance in that α (CXC) chemokines act predominantly on neutrophils, whereas the β (CC) chemokines act on other leukocytes including monocytes, T cells, and eosinophils. However, there can be considerable variation in chemokine function within the α and β subgroups. Fractalkine (CX_3C) is chemoattractant for T cells and monocytes, whereas lymphotactin[3] (C) is chemoattractant for T cells only.

Chemokines stimulate cells though binding to G-protein–coupled cell-surface receptors, which contain seven transmembrane-spanning domains. An interesting feature of these receptors is that they can be monogamous (such as the IL-8 receptor A), or permissive (allowing binding by many members within the same subgroup). It has also been proposed that the nonfunctional chemokine receptor present on red blood cells, called the *Duffy antigen receptor complex,* acts as a sink to remove chemokines from the circulation.

There are two stages at which chemokines play a critical role in the development of leukocyte-mediated renal damage; the entry of blood leukocytes into the kidney (see Chapter 37, Part 6), and the subsequent migration and focal accumulation of leukocytes at sites of injury (Fig. 37.6). Following an injury, there is rapid synthesis and release of chemokines by endothelium, platelets, and cells in the underlying extravascular space. Chemokine molecules become attached to the endothelial surface through electrostatic binding to glucosaminoglycans or presentation by distinct membrane-bound structures. Leukocytes rolling along the activated endothelium under the influence of selectin molecules encounter chemokines such as MCP-1 or MIP-1α, which cause an extremely rapid (within seconds) increase in the affinity of integrin molecules on the leukocyte surface for their ligands (ICAM-1, VCAM-1) on the surface of the activated endothelium. This results in firm adhesion of leukocytes to the endothelium—an essential step in diapedesis. Chemokines may also induce polarization of adherent leukocytes resulting in the formation of the characteristic pseudopod-like projection required for leukocyte migration through the endothelial cell junction. In addition, chemokines can induce leukocyte secretion of proteinases, which is necessary for migration through the endothelial basement membrane and into the extravascular space.

Once leukocytes have left the blood and entered the kidney, chemokine production by intrinsic glomerular and tubular cells is thought to promote focal leukocyte accumulation. This is supported by the ability of a wide range of stimuli, including IL-1 and TNF-α, to induce chemokine synthesis and secretion by mesangial cells, podocytes, and tubular epithelial cells.

Chemokines in Experimental Kidney Disease

Based on the known functions of chemokines, it has been postulated that α (CXC) chemokines promote glomerular neutrophil infiltration, whereas β (CC) chemokines promote monocyte and T-cell infiltration. The role of chemokines has been best studied in the acute heterologous phase of rat anti–glomerular basement membrane (GBM) glomerulonephritis. The injection of anti-GBM serum leads to a rapid deposition of foreign immunoglobulin on the GBM causing complement activation and a transient glomerular neutrophil infiltration, peaking 3 to 4 hours later, followed by monocyte infiltration, which is maximal by 24 hours. There is a rapid induction of glomerular gene expression of the α (CXC) chemokines GROα (CINC), GROβ (MIP-2), PF4, and IP-10 in this model, which peaks at 3 hours, concurrent with maximal neutrophil infiltration. The functional significance of these observations was confirmed by the ability of neutralizing antibodies against CINC or MIP-2 to cause a 40% reduction in glomerular neutrophil influx and the accompanying proteinuria. The pattern of glomerular gene expression of the β (CC) chemokines is more diverse, with MIP-1α being induced within 30 minutes of anti-GBM serum injection, whereas MCP-1 mRNA peaks at 15 hours and RANTES is not upregulated for several days. Another α (CXC) chemokine, IL-8, has been examined in rat immunocomplex-induced glomerulonephritis in which anti–IL-8 antibody treatment caused a 40% reduction in glomerular neutrophils and completely prevented any increase in urinary protein excretion.

Given that leukocyte infiltration is prominent in most forms of kidney disease, we would predict that chemokine gene expression also is upregulated in these diseases. This is indeed the case. The best studied chemokine, MCP-1, is upregulated in animal models of anti-GBM disease, immunocomplex glomerulonephritis, tubulointerstitial nephritis, mesangial proliferative nephritis, murine lupus nephritis, puromycin aminonucleoside nephrosis, remnant kidney, lipid-induced glomerular injury, and hydronephrosis. Localization studies using *in situ* hybridization and immunohistochemistry staining have shown that little or no MCP-1 is expressed in the normal kidney, but that glomerular endothelial cells, podocytes, mesangial cells, and tubular epithelial cells can be stimulated to produce MCP-1 in disease. Administration of a neutralizing anti–MCP-1 antibody has been shown to significantly reduce glomerular macrophage accumulation in rat anti-Thy1 mesangial proliferative nephritis and in the acute phase of rat anti-GBM disease. In a recent study, anti–MCP-1 antibody treatment of mouse anti-GBM glomerulonephritis caused a 35% to 50% inhibition of renal T-cell and macrophage accumulation, a 50% reduction in proteinuria, suppression of glomerular crescent formation (55% to 10%), and an inhibition of renal fibrosis (collagen deposition). The inhibition of glomerular crescent formation is consistent with a functional role for MCP-1 in the skin DTH response and in glycan-induced granuloma formation in the rat. Interestingly, administration of a RANTES antagonist caused a similar degree of inhibition of renal leukocyte infiltration in this disease model, but failed to reduce crescent formation or collagen deposition, indicating important pathologic differences in the roles of these two β (CC) chemokines in renal disease.

The clear importance of MCP-1 in renal macrophage and T-cell infiltration has prompted many investigators to examine the factors regulating the expression of this chemokine. There are multiple binding sites for the nuclear factor-kappa B (NF-κB) in the promoter region of the MCP-1 gene, and activation of this transcription factor is crucial for the induction of MCP-1 mRNA synthesis. It is therefore no surprise that IL-1 and TNF-α, cytokines that are known to cause activation of NF-κB, are the best characterized inducers of MCP-1 production in mesangial cells, podocytes, and tubular epithelial cells. Many other stimuli have been described that can induce MCP-1 gene expression, including bacterial endotoxin, interferon-α, leukemia inhibitory factor, IL-6, platelet-derived growth factor, thrombin, oxidized lipoprotein, high concentrations of albumin, and the binding of IgA to Fc-α receptors. In contrast, TGF-β1 has been shown to inhibit lipopolysaccharide (LPS)-induced MCP-1 production by macrophages.

CHEMOKINES IN HUMAN KIDNEY DISEASE

The study of chemokines in human kidney disease has largely focused on MCP-1. The reported pattern of MCP-1 expression in human kidney disease varies significantly, except for the consistent observation that MCP-1 is produced by tubular epithelial cells. However, a general picture has emerged in which MCP-1 is expressed by infiltrating leukocytes, glomerular endothelium, mesangial cells, podocytes, and tubular epithelial cells in the more severe forms of human glomerulonephritis (such as idiopathic or crescentic glomerulonephritis, Wegener's granulomatosis, and active lupus nephritis), with levels of MCP-1 expression associated with marked glomerular and interstitial macrophage accumulation. In contrast, less severe forms of human glomerulonephritis have little or no glomerular MCP-1 expression, although tubular MCP-1 expression is increased, which is associated with interstitial macrophage accumulation.

An alternative approach to investigating the role of MCP-1 in leukocyte infiltration is to measure chemokine levels in serum and urine by using the enzyme-linked immunosorbent assay (ELISA). Low levels of MCP-1 can be detected in both serum (101 ± 24 pg/ml) and urine (130 ± 30pg/mg creatinine) of healthy volunteers. In a study of 37 patients with a wide variety of glomerulonephritides, a positive correlation was found between urinary MCP-1 levels and glomerular macrophage accumulation. Studies focusing on lupus nephritis have shown that patients with active disease have a 10- to 20-fold higher level of urinary MCP-1 compared with patients with inactive disease, whose levels are essentially normal. A significant correlation was found between urinary MCP-1 levels and leukocyte infiltration in patients with active disease. Steroid treatment of active disease caused a rapid reduction in urinary MCP-1 levels, and relapse during treatment was predicted by a marked rise in urinary MCP-1.

PROINFLAMMATORY CYTOKINES IN KIDNEY DISEASE

Interleukin-1 (IL-1) is a classical proinflammatory cytokine that causes fever when administered to healthy volunteers. IL-1 stimulation of immune and nonimmune cells causes activation of NF-κB, which upregulates expression of a wide variety of proinflammatory molecules including TNF-α, leukocyte adhesion molecules, chemokines, and CSFs, resulting in leukocyte infiltration. IL-1 is a potent activator of macrophages causing production of a wide range of mediators of tissue injury, such as thrombin, reactive oxygen species, metalloproteinases, complement components, and growth factors. In addition, IL-1 is a mesangial cell-growth factor.

The site(s) of IL-1 production within the injured kidney is controversial. Although *in vitro* studies have demonstrated that many cell types, including glomerular endothelial cells, podocytes, mesangial cells, tubular epithelial cells, and renal fibroblasts can synthesize IL-1, it is not clear whether such expression occurs *in vivo*. Studies of acute rat anti-GBM disease and puromycin aminonucleoside nephrosis have attributed renal IL-1β production to infiltrating macrophages. However, a study of severe crescentic anti-GBM glomerulonephritis in the rat showed high levels of renal IL-1β mRNA by Northern blotting. This was confirmed by *in situ* hybridization and two color immunohistochemistry staining, which showed a dramatic upregulation of IL-1β production by infiltrating macrophages and by intrinsic renal cells (glomerular endothelium, mesangial cells, podocytes, and tubular epithelial cells). IL-1β production by glomerular mesangial cells has also been demonstrated in rat anti-Thy1 mesangial proliferative nephritis. Studies of human glomerulonephritis have shown glomerular IL-1β expression by infiltrating macrophages, by mesangial cells, and most prominently by podocytes. Tubular IL-1β expression also has been described in several studies of human glomerulonephritis. Urinary IL-1β, although detectable in patients with various forms of glomerulonephritis, has not proven to be a particularly useful marker in terms of diagnosis or in predicting disease progression.

A number of strategies have been used to block IL-1 function *in vivo*, including neutralizing antibodies, the IL-1 receptor antagonist (IL-1ra), and soluble IL-1 receptors. Blockade of IL-1 in the acute phase of rat anti-GBM disease has produced variable results, with some studies showing a partial inhibition of macrophage infiltration and proteinuria, and others failing to show any effect. This apparent discrepancy has been attributed to differences in the models and IL-1 blocking strategies employed. IL-1ra treatment during the first 14 days of rat anti-GBM disease was shown to suppress leukocyte infiltration and proteinuria and to prevent glomerular crescent formation and a loss of renal function. More importantly, a subsequent study showed that delaying IL-1ra treatment until crescentic disease was already established was able to halt disease progression in terms of preventing further leukocyte accumulation, partially reversing glomerular crescent formation, stabilizing proteinuria, and returning renal function to normal. The success of IL-1ra treatment has been attributed to the inhibition of leukocyte adhesion molecules ICAM-1, VCAM-1, osteopontin, and CD44, resulting in the suppression of leukocyte accumulation. In addition, the reduction in local macrophage proliferation seen in IL-1ra treatment animals was associated with a reduction in renal M-CSF expression.

The importance of IL-1 in different types of kidney disease has been demonstrated in a number of studies. Anti–IL-1β antibody treatment was shown to suppress renal injury in puromycin aminonucleoside nephrosis, whereas administration of the IL-1ra suppressed the development of spontaneous IgA nephropathy in *ddY* mice. Furthermore, IL-1ra treatment of rat anti-Thy1 nephritis reduced mesangial proliferation by 25%, demonstrating a pathologic role for IL-1 in mesangial cell proliferation.

Tumor necrosis factor-α (TNF-α) is the second classical proinflammatory cytokine. TNF-α has many functions in common with IL-1, including activation of NF-κB. One interesting difference between the two cytokines is that TNF-α can directly induce apoptosis of target cells. Localization of TNF-α production in tissue sections has proved easier than for IL-1β, with broad agreement that TNF-α is constitutively expressed by tubules in normal kidney with marked upregulation of TNF-α expression by infiltrating macrophages, glomerular mesangial cells, and tubular epithelial cells in both experimental and human glomerulonephritis. A correlation between renal TNF-α expression and upregulation of the adhesion molecule ICAM-1 has been described in various forms of human glomerulonephritis.

Treatment of acute rat anti-GBM disease with anti–TNF-α antibodies or a soluble TNF receptor (TNFbp) produced a significant reduction in glomerular macrophage accumulation and proteinuria. In longer term studies, anti–TNF-α antibody treatment was found to reduce proteinuria by 50% on day 8 of anti-GBM disease. In a separate study, TNFbp treatment of rat crescentic anti-GBM disease over days 0 to 14 produced a 55% to 70% inhibition in macrophage accumulation, a 34% reduction in proteinuria, prevented a loss of renal function, and abrogated glomerular crescent formation.

Because IL-1 and TNF-α share many proinflammatory functions, two studies have addressed the question of whether added benefit can be drawn from combined treatment. In rat crescentic anti-GBM disease, it was found that IL-1ra or TNFbp treatment alone provided a similar degree of protection from renal injury, whereas a combination of IL-1ra plus TNFbp treatment produced no additional benefit over that seen with each treatment alone. This suggests that IL-1 and TNF-α act through the same pathway in mediating renal damage, with activation of NF-κB a logical point at which the actions of two cytokines converge. However, a study of puromycin aminonucleoside nephrosis found that treatment with anti–IL-1β plus anti–TNF-α antibodies gave a greater degree of inhibition of proteinuria compared with either antibody used alone. The apparent discrepancy in these two studies may reflect the different disease models employed or the use of suboptimal doses of neutralizing antibodies.

Macrophage migration inhibitory factor (MIF) is a proinflammatory cytokine that has a number of unique characteristics. In contrast to IL-1 and TNF-α, whose secretion is tightly regulated, MIF is constitutively expressed by most tissues in the body and is readily detectable in the circulation of healthy individuals. MIF plays a key role in macrophage accumulation in the skin DTH response, is a potent activator of macrophage effector functions, and is a costimulator of the primary immune response. A unique aspect of MIF is its ability to override glucocorticoid-mediated immunosuppression. Administration of recombinant MIF overcomes glucocorticoid protection from lethal endotoxemia in mice, while MIF overrides glucocorticoid-mediated inhibition of LPS-induced IL-1 and TNF-α production by macrophages. This places MIF in a unique position in the inflammatory cascade (Fig. 37.6).

MIF is constitutively expressed by tubular epithelial cells and occasional podocytes in normal rat kidney. Following the induction of anti-GBM disease, there is marked upregulation of MIF expression by intrinsic renal cells, including glomerular endothelium, podocytes, parietal epithelial cells, and tubules; infiltrating macrophages and T cells express MIF and serum MIF levels increase. Using *in situ* hybridization and immunohistochemistry, a similar pattern of upregulation of MIF production by intrinsic renal cells and infiltrating leukocytes has been described in human proliferative glomerulonephritis.

Treatment of rat crescentic anti-GBM glomerulonephritis with a neutralizing antibody over days 0 to 14 reduced glomerular macrophage accumulation by 60% and virtually abrogated interstitial leukocyte infiltration and activation. This was associated with a 65% reduction in proteinuria, maintenance of normal renal function, and almost complete prevention of crescent formation (32% reduced to 3%). These effects were attributed to a marked inhibition of renal expression of IL-1β, ICAM-1 and VCAM-1. In a second study, anti-MIF treatment was delayed until day 7 at which time animals had developed crescentic disease. Compared with the rapidly progressive disease apparent in control animals by day 21, anti-MIF antibody treatment partially reversed the disease in terms of restoring normal renal function and significantly reducing crescent formation compared with that seen on day 7. An examination of serum corticosterone levels found that anti-MIF antibody treatment caused a significant increase in endogenous glucocorticoid levels, which correlated with reversal of the disease. Thus MIF can promote renal damage by enhancing innate and cellular immunity and by suppressing the endogenous antiinflammatory glucocorticoid response.

Macrophage colony-stimulating factor (M-CSF) is a potent macrophage growth factor, being the main hematopoietic cytokine responsible for monocyte production in the bone marrow. M-CSF is chemotactic for monocytes, can stimulate monocyte proliferation and survival, and can prime macrophages for activation. Increased renal M-CSF production is evident in lupus-prone mice before the development of macrophage infiltration and renal injury, with tubules being an important source of M-CSF within the kidney. A pathologic role for M-CSF in amplifying macrophage-mediated renal injury comes from studies in which implantation of tubular epithelial cells, genetically engineered to secrete bioactive M-CSF, under the kidney capsule induces macrophage and T-cell infiltration and renal damage in lupus-prone mice, but not in normal mice. Upregulation of renal M-CSF production by glomerular and tubular epithelial cells has also been described in rat crescentic anti-GBM disease, in which it correlates with macrophage proliferation. These proliferating macrophages show high levels of M-CSF receptor expression. However, M-CSF also can be associated with glomerular macrophage infiltration in the absence of local proliferation, such as in lipid-induced glomerular injury in genetically susceptible rats.

Interferon-γ (IFN-γ) is a cytokine produced by T cells, macrophages, and tubular epithelial cells. IFN-γ is a potent activator of macrophage effector functions and stimulates antigen-specific immunity through upregulation of major histocompatibility complex (MHC) molecule expression and by promoting a Th_1 immune response. Although IFN-γ is known to play an important role in a number of immune-mediated diseases, relatively little is known of this cytokine in kidney disease. A pathologic role for IFN-γ in the development of murine lupus nephritis has been demonstrated by a strategy in which IFN-γ gene knockout mice were backcrossed onto the lupus prone *lpr* genetic background. The resulting mice had significantly reduced lymphadenopathy, reduced titres of IgG2a and IgG2b serum immunoglobulins and autoantibodies, and substantially decreased renal disease.

Interleukin-12 (IL-12) is a cytokine produced by T cells, macrophages, and tubular epithelial cells. IL-12 plays a pivotal role in determining the Th_1/Th_2 balance of the immune response such that CD4+ T cells, which maintain expression of the IL-12 receptor, develop a Th_1 response, whereas loss of the receptor switches the cell toward a Th_2 response. Administration of IL-12 has been shown to suppress immunologic disease in Th_2-biased mice, whereas anti–IL-12 antibodies can inhibit immunologic disease in Th_1-biased mice. These findings have been extended in a study of accelerated anti-GBM disease in Th_1-biased mice. Treatment with an anti–IL-12 antibody from the time of immunization suppressed renal injury and crescent formation. In a separate study, IL-12 treatment of murine lupus nephritis reduced the production IgG1 autoantibodies, but did not affect immunoglobulin deposition within the kidney.

Antiinflammatory Cytokines in Glomerular Injury

An alternative approach to the treatment of inflammatory renal injury is to make use of the antiinflammatory properties of some members of the cytokine family. Both IL-4 and IL-10 have been shown to suppress a number of immunologic diseases in Th_1-biased mice. In addition, they can inhibit some macrophage functions, suggesting that these cytokines may have some benefit for the treatment of cellular immune renal damage.

Interleukin-4 (IL-4) is a cytokine that promotes the Th_2 immune response, stimulates immunoglobulin production, and suppress the Th_1 immune response. In addition, IL-4 can inhibit macrophage IL-1 production and promote secretion of the IL-1ra. Examination of normal human kidney by *in situ* hybridization revealed low levels of IL-4 mRNA expression. There is marked upregulation of IL-4 mRNA expression in mesangial cells, podocytes, and parietal epithelial cells in IgA nephropathy, proliferative glomerulonephritis, lupus nephritis, and membranous nephropathy. Glomerular IL-4 mRNA expression correlated with the degree of mesangial hypercellularity and matrix expansion in IgA nephropathy and non-IgA proliferative glomerulonephritis, whereas glomerular IL-4 mRNA expression correlated negatively with renal function in lupus nephritis. However, it is unclear from these studies whether endogenous IL-4 production acts to limit renal injury or whether it is actually causing injury.

This issue has been addressed in experimental disease models. Administration of recombinant IL-4 caused a small (24%), though significant, reduction in glomerular macrophage accumulation and a marked (73%) reduction in albuminuria on day 4 of rat-accelerated anti-GBM disease. This was associated with marked upregulated glomerular mRNA for the IL-1 receptor type II (the so-called decoy receptor, which is thought to 'mop-up' secreted IL-1), which may account for the apparent ability of IL-4 treatment to inhibit glomerular macrophage activation. In a study of anti-GBM disease in Th_1-biased mice, IL-4 treatment from the time of immunization with normal sheep IgG caused a 70% reduction in glomerular macrophage accumulation and complete abrogation of crescent formation. This was associated with 57% reduction in proteinuria, but inexplicably failed to prevent a loss of renal function. In a second set of experiments, IL-4 treatment of established disease (days 3 to 10) caused a modest reduction in glomerular T-cell and macrophage accumulation, but there was no effect on crescent formation, proteinuria, or loss of renal function. To examine the role of IL-4 in murine lupus nephritis, IL-4 gene knockout mice were backcrossed onto the lupus-prone *lpr* genetic background. This significantly reduced lymphadenopathy, reduced titres of serum IgG1 and IgE immunoglobulins and autoantibodies, and substantially decreased renal disease, consistent with the known role for IL-4 in promoting antibody production.

Interleukin-10 (IL-10) is a pleiotropic cytokine produced by activated macrophages and T lymphocytes that promotes the Th_2 immune response and immunoglobulin production. IL-10 can inhibit a number of diseases in Th_1-biased mice, including the skin DTH response, through inhibiting MHC class II expression and antigen presentation. In addition, IL-10 can suppress macrophage production of effector molecules, including IL-1β and reactive oxygen species. On the other hand, IL-10 can also promote monocyte differentiation into CD16+ (FcγRIII+) macrophages with enhanced phagocytic and cytolytic capacity, and IL-10 can induce recruitment and activation of CD8+ T cells and NK cells. Thus IL-10 administration has potentially both beneficial and detrimental effects on kidney disease.

IL-10 treatment of accelerated anti-GBM disease in Th_1-biased mice from the time of immunization with normal heterologous immunoglobulin significantly inhibited glomerular macrophage accumulation, crescent formation, proteinuria, and loss of renal function. Delaying IL-10 treatment until disease was established produced a trend toward disease suppression, but no significant effects were observed. As seen with IL-4, treatment with IL-10 had a more profound effect on the primary rather than secondary Th_1 immune response. It was interesting, however, that combined IL-4 and IL-10 treatment gave some added benefit in suppressing renal injury in this disease model.

In a separate study of accelerated anti-GBM disease in Sprague-Dawley rats, which have no Th_1 or Th_2 bias and therefore are more relevant to human disease, IL-10 administration over days 0 to 14 provided no benefit in terms of proteinuria, loss of renal function, or histologic damage. This lack of renal protection was in spite of a significant inhibition of the skin DTH response to the immunizing antigen. Further examination found that IL-10 treatment partially reduced renal IL-1β mRNA levels and MHC class II expression by infiltrating macrophages. However, IL-10 treatment augmented the humoral response, as evidenced by increased titres of antigen-specific IgG and increased glomerular deposition of C3, and caused an increase in glomerular macrophage accumulation and proliferation. The latter finding was associated with a 3-fold increase in the number of macrophages expressing the M-CSF receptor.

The role of IL-10 has also been examined in lupus nephritis. Peripheral B-cells from patients with lupus exhibit IL-10-dependent production of autoantibodies. It was not surprising therefore that IL-10 treatment of (NZBxNZW)F1 mice increased autoantibody production and accelerated death from glomerulonephritis. Conversely, treatment with anti–IL-10 antibodies or the IL-10 inhibitor drug, AS101, suppressed autoantibody production and inhibited nephritis. In this context, it is interesting that a clinical trial of IL-10 as in inhibitor of the "cytokine-release phenomenon" accompanying OKT3 therapy in renal transplant recipients suffering acute allograft rejection was abandoned because IL-10 treatment stimulated the development of neutralizing antibodies against OKT3.

An unexpected function of IL-10 is that it is a mesangial cell growth factor. The addition of IL-10 directly induces proliferation of growth-arrested mesangial cells *in vitro*. Furthermore, administration of IL-10 to normal rats results in glomerular hypercellularity with evidence of mesangial cell proliferation. Although it is clear from studies of IL-10 gene knockout mice that IL-10 is not essential for normal mesangial and glomerular development, endogenous IL-10 production following renal injury could promote mesangial proliferation. There is upregulation of IL-10 mRNA expression in rat anti-GBM disease as shown by semiquantitative polymerise chain reaction. Localization of IL-10 mRNA expression by *in situ* hybridization found IL-10 production by both glomerular and tubular epithelial cells. In rat anti-Thy1 mesangial proliferative nephritis, *in situ* hybridization found upregulation of IL-10 mRNA expression within mesangial proliferative lesions. However, definitive proof that IL-10 promotes pathologic mesangial proliferation awaits the results of blocking studies.

Leukemia inhibitory factor (LIF) is a member of the neuropoietic cytokine family that exerts a wide range of effects on immune and nonimmune cell types. The question of whether this cytokine has an antiinflammatory action is controversial. Conflicting results have been obtained on the ability of LIF to suppress experimental models of endotoxemia. Glomerular expression of LIF mRNA is increased during the acute phase of rat anti-GBM disease and LIF has been reported to induce MCP-1 production by glomerular mesangial cells. To determine whether LIF plays a protective or injurious role in this acute disease model, rats were continuously infused with recombinant LIF for 24 hours. This caused a 60% reduction in glomerular macrophage infiltration and an 85% reduction in proteinuria. Longer-term studies are required to determine whether LIF can suppress renal inflammation in progressive disease and to assess possible adverse effects of LIF in the nephrotic state.

Interleukin-6 (IL-6) is a pleiotropic cytokine that has both proinflammatory and antiinflammatory actions. It is best known as a *B-cell growth factor*. Great interest was generated when IL-6 was identified as a growth factor for rat mesangial cells and a significant correlation was found between the severity of mesangial proliferative IgA nephropathy and glomerular IL-6 immunostaining and urinary IL-6 levels. This conclusion was supported by the development of mesangial proliferative nephropathy in transgenic mice producing elevated levels of IL-6. However, subsequent studies have produced conflicting results. Some studies have failed to find a relationship between urinary IL-6 levels and mesangial proliferative glomerulonephritis, whereas other studies have shown that urinary IL-6 levels are dependent on tubular function. The role of IL-6 in mesangial proliferation has also been questioned. Two studies failed to show IL-6 stimulation of mesangial cell proliferation *in vitro*, and another study found that IL-6 actually inhibits proliferation of cultured mesangial cells. Indeed, IL-6 gene knockout mice develop a normal glomerular architecture and show the same degree of mesangial proliferative nephritis induced by Habu snake venom as normal litter-mate controls. In addition, constant infusion of IL-6 does not effect mesangial cell proliferation in suboptimal rat anti-Thy1 mesangial proliferative nephritis. Indeed, administration of recombinant IL-6 in the acute phase of rat anti-GBM disease caused a 25% reduction in proteinuria, although no effect was seen on glomerular macrophage infiltration or the loss of renal function.

SYNTHESIS

It is clear from the many successful blocking/treatment studies in experimental kidney disease that chemokines and cytokines play a crucial role in the development of leukocyte-mediated renal damage. This raises the question, which of these strategies has the best therapeutic potential?

The chemokine family is very large, suggesting substantial redundancy. Indeed, the permissive nature of some of the chemokine receptors support this concept. However, the ability to suppress experimental anti-GBM glomerulonephritis with anti–MCP-1 antibodies demonstrates that targeting a single chemokine can be effective. There has been rapid progress in developing chemokine receptor antagonists following the discovery that HIV uses these receptors as docking molecules during infection of leukocytes. Antagonists of permissive receptors have the potential to block the action of many individual chemokines. Such reagents may be effective in blocking leukocyte recruitment in inflammatory kidney disease. In addition, there is significant early promise in the use of urinary MCP-1 levels as a means to monitor inflammation within the kidney. This could provide a more rapid and sensitive index of patient response to treatment compared with changes in renal function.

The cytokine family is extremely diverse (Table 37.3), but these molecules exert a powerful influence on the development of leukocyte-mediated injury. The most logical strategy is to block the action of the cytokines that act at the start of the inflammatory cascade (e.g., MIF, IL-1 and TNF-α) to prevent the production of downstream mediators. The IL-1ra is an attractive therapeutic drug because it is naturally occurring, is extremely well tolerated, and has proven clinical efficacy in phase III clinical trial of rheumatoid arthritis. The ability of IL-1ra to halt established rat crescentic anti-GBM glomerulonephritis argues for the development of a clinical trial of this drug in rapidly progressive glomerulonephritis. Blocking TNF-α provides equal benefit to that obtained with blocking IL-1 in experimental studies. Therefore drugs such as soluble TNF-α receptors are a good alternative to the IL-1ra. Indeed, a humanized anti–TNF-α monoclonal antibody has produced good results in clinical trials of rheumatoid arthritis.

The ability of MIF to not only induce the inflammatory cascade, but also to override the antiinflammatory effects of glucocorticoids, makes this cytokine a most attractive therapeutic target. Indeed, the ability of anti-MIF antibody treatment to suppress, and even partially reverse, crescentic glomerulonephritis in the rat was associated with virtually complete inhibition of the upregulation of renal IL-1β production together with an increase in endogenous glucocorticoid levels. The high levels of MIF in kidney disease may be a crucial factor in limiting the efficacy of high dose glucocorticoid therapy. Therefore it will be important to determine whether a combination of anti-MIF antibody plus glucocorticoid treatment can provide a greater degree of benefit compared with either treatment alone. If so, a combination of anti-MIF treatment with low dose glucocorticoids would be a most attractive therapeutic strategy.

The use of IL-4 and IL-10 treatment has shown promise in Th_1-biased models of experimental anti-GBM disease. How-

TABLE 37.3. Summary of Cytokine Blockade and Cytokine Treatment of Experimental Kidney Disease

Cytokine	General Properties	Effect of Cytokine Blockade/Cytokine Treatment
Interleukin-1 (IL-1)	Proinflammatory	Anti-IL-1 Ab, IL-1ra, and soluble IL-1 receptor inhibit acute glomerular injury in rat anti-GBM disease IL-1ra inhibits development of crescentic anti-GBM disease IL-1ra halts progression of established rat crescentic anti-GBM disease IL-1ra suppresses IgA nephropathy in the *ddY* mouse Anti-IL-1β Ab inhibits rat puromycin aminonucleoside nephrosis IL-1ra inhibits mesangial proliferation in rat anti-Thy1 nephritis
Tumor necrosis factor-α (TNF-α)	Proinflammatory	Anti-TNF-α Ab and soluble TNF-α receptor inhibit acute injury and crescent development in rat anti-GBM disease Anti-TNF-α Ab inhibits rat puromycin aminonucleoside nephrosis
Macrophage migration inhibitory factor (MIF)	Proinflammatory	Anti-MIF Ab suppresses development of crescentic anti-GBM disease in the rat and partially reverses established crescentic disease
Macrophage colony-stimulating factor (M-CSF)	Macrophage chemoattractant and growth factor	Local administration of M-CSF promotes tissue injury in lupus prone, but not in normal, mice
IL-12	Promotes Th_1 and inhibits Th_2 response	Anti-IL-12 Ab inhibits crescentic anti-GBM disease in Th_1-biased mice IL-12 treatment did not affect immunoglobulin deposition in lupus-prone mice
Interferon-γ (IFN-γ)	Promotes Th_1 response	IFN-γ promotes autoantibody production and nephritis in lupus-prone mice
IL-4	Promotes Th_2 response and inhibits Th_1 response; some antimacrophage activity	IL-4 treatment suppresses crescentic anti-GBM disease in Th_1-biased mice Promotes autoantibody production and nephritis in lupus-prone mice
IL-10	Promotes Th_2 response and inhibits Th_1 response; some antimacrophage activity	IL-10 treatment suppresses crescentic anti-GBM disease in Th_1-biased mice IL-10 treatment has no effect on rat crescentic anti-GBM disease (no Th_1/Th_2 bias) IL-10 treatment exacerbates murine lupus nephritis Anti-IL-10 Ab inhibits autoantibody production and nephritis in lupus-prone mice
IL-6	Has both proinflammatory and antiinflammatory actions	IL-6 treatment inhibits glomerular injury in the acute phase of rat anti-GBM disease
Leukemia inhibitory factor (LIF)	Has both proinflammatory and antiinflammatory actions	LIF treatment inhibits glomerular injury in the acute phase of rat anti-GBM disease

Ab, antibody.

ever, the ability of these cytokines to promote the humoral response, including autoantibody production such as in lupus nephritis, together with possible stimulatory actions on macrophage recruitment and Fc-receptor expression would appear to rule out their use in the treatment of human kidney disease—with the possible exception of pauci-immune glomerulonephritis, although even in this case the potential for stimulating the humoral immune response must be considered.

One striking feature of kidney disease that is often overlooked is the ability of tubular epithelial cells to produce many different chemokines and cytokines such as MCP-1, IL-8, IL-1β, TNF-α, MIF, M-CSF, IL-6, and IL-12. Indeed, tubular cells may play a crucial role in promoting focal leukocyte accumulation and, in leukocyte activation, in the development of renal damage. Therefore a novel approach would be to target chemokine and cytokine production by tubular cells. Although no drug delivery systems are currently available that specifically target tubular epithelial cells, the ability to block activation of NF-κB or the IL-1 signal transduction pathway could in theory inhibit renal damage without causing a generalized state of immunosuppression in the patient.

Selected Readings

Adams DH, Lloyd AR. Chemokines: leucocyte recruitment and activation cytokines. *N Engl J Med* 1997;349:490–495.

This is an informative and clearly presented review of chemokine structure, function pertaining to areas of leukocyte recruitment, leukocyte activation, angiogenesis, inflammatory disease, human immunodeficiency virus (HIV) infection, and therapy.

Calandra T, Bucala R. Macrophage migration inhibitory factor (MIF): a glucocorticoid counter-regulator within the immune system. *Crit Rev Immunol* 1997;17:77–88.

This review discusses what is known of the role of MIF in the immune response and the ability to MIF to counterregulate glucocorticoid action, providing a synthesis of an emerging and exciting new area.

Ishida H, Muchamuel T, Sakaguchi S, et al. Continuous administration of anti-interleukin-10 antibodies delays onset of autoimmunity in NZB/W F1 mice. *J Exp Med* 1994;179:305–310.

This paper uses treatment with IL-10 or anti–IL-10 antibodies to demonstrate the crucial role the IL-10 plays in promoting autoantibody production and subsequent nephritis in lupus-prone mice.

Lan HY, Bacher M, Yang N, et al. The pathogenic role of macrophage migration inhibitory factor in immunologically induced kidney disease in the rat. *J Exp Med* 1997;185:1455–1465.

This study uses a neutralizing anti-MIF antibody to inhibit leukocyte infiltration and renal injury and to abrogate crescent formation in rat anti-GBM disease. This treatment is associated with a marked reduction in renal expression of IL-1β, ICAM-1, VCAM-1, and iNOS expression.

Lloyd CM, Minto AW, Dorf ME, et al. RANTES and monocyte chemoattractant protein-1 (MCP-1) play an important role in the inflammatory phase of crescentic nephritis, but only MCP-1 is involved in crescent formation and interstitial fibrosis. *J Exp Med* 1997;185:1371–1380.

This study shows that administration of an anti-MCP-1 antibody can suppress leukocyte infiltration, crescent formation, collagen deposition, and renal injury in a mouse model of anti-GBM glomerulonephritis. In contrast, administration of a RANTES antagonist had little effect on renal injury or crescent formation.

Nikolic-Paterson DJ, Lan HY, Atkins RC. IL-1 receptor antagonism. *Semin Nephrol* 1996;16:583–590.

This review discusses the IL-1 gene family, IL-1 receptors, regulation of IL-1 activity, blockade of IL-1 in experimental glomerulonephritis, mechanisms of IL-1 mediated injury, and potential therapy.

Schlöndorf D, Nelson PJ, Luckow B, et al. Chemokines and renal disease. *Kidney Int* 1997;51:610–621.

This comprehensive review covers chemokine structure and receptors, chemokine production by renal cells, expression of chemokines in experimental and human renal disease, and discusses directions for future studies.

PART 3
Role of Growth Factors in Glomerular, Tubular, and Vascular Injury
A: Transforming Growth Factor-β Superfamily

Kumar Sharma and Fuad N. Ziyadeh

The transforming growth factor-β (TGF-β) superfamily is made up of more than 40 related proteins, with the three mammalian isoforms of TGF-β (-β1, -β2, and -β3) and the bone morphogenetic proteins (BMPs) being the best characterized. Although these factors have pleiotropic effects, a common characteristic is that they limit cell proliferation in a variety of cell types, including endothelial, epithelial, and hematopoietic cells. This is in contradistinction to other cytokines that trigger mitogenic pathways. In the 1990s, there has been extensive literature supporting important roles for the TGF-β superfamily in several types of kidney diseases. In particular, the renal TGF-β system plays a central role in cell growth and differentiation, in chemotaxis (of fibroblasts, monocytes, and neutrophils), and in stimulation of synthesis of various extracellular matrix molecules. In this section, we summarize the salient features of the TGF-βs and BMPs and review their role in normal kidney development and what has been learned about their involvement in various renal disorders.

GENERAL PROPERTIES

The TGF-β1 System

Members of the TGF-β superfamily are unique in that they all use serine–threonine kinase transmembrane receptors rather than the tyrosine–kinase receptors that mediate signaling from a variety of mitogenic growth factors. TGF-β1 is the prototype of the superfamily and the best studied with respect to its gene regulation, cell biology, and *in vivo* pathophysiology. Unless otherwise specified, the discussion here focuses on TGF-β1 because it is also the most ubiquitously expressed in different renal and extrarenal cell types. In the adult kidney, TGF-β1 expression has been described in tubular epithelial cells (both proximal and distal), interstitial cells, and to lesser extent in glomerular mesangial, endothelial, and epithelial cells. TGF-β3 follows a similar pattern of expression but in quantitatively lower amounts. The TGF-β2 protein is largely restricted to the juxtaglomerular apparatus, where it may play an important role in renin metabolism. Of relevance to renal homeostasis, TGF-β1 activity in the kidney can be contributed by platelets, macrophages, and vascular smooth muscle cells.

Bioactivation of TGF-β1

Regulation of TGF-β1 expression occurs at multiple levels, including transcriptional and posttranslational, and its effects are mediated by a complex signaling cascade. The promoter of TGF-β1 does not contain the classic CAAT or TATA boxes, either of which is usually present in constitutively active genes; instead, there are sites that bind early-response genes such as c-*jun*, c-*fos*, and a variety of oncogenes, including *ras* and *src*. These promoter sites allow a rapid stimulation of TGF-β1 gene expression during tissue injury and cell turnover.

In its mature, active form, TGF-β1 is a homodimer of two cysteine-rich 12.5-kD polypeptide subunits derived from the C-terminal end of the gene product and linked by a single disulfide bond. The active form is capable of binding to the signaling receptor and propagating a signal. TGF-β1 is secreted from cells or released from platelets in an inactive form linked noncovalently to the N-terminal precursor molecule called *the latency-associated peptide (LAP)*, which blocks binding to the signaling receptor. TGF-β may also exist in a large latent complex wherein LAP is covalently bound to latent TGF-β–binding protein (LTBP). Proteolytic processing by furin endoprotease plays a role in correct folding and dimerization of the latent complex (Fig. 37.7). Plasmin-mediated activation of TGF-β1 involves binding of the latent form to the mannose-6-phosphate receptor on the cell surface and the concerted action of transglutaminase and plasmin to remove LAP. A protease-independent conformational change of the latent complex also can occur when thrombospondin, derived from the α-granules of platelets, allows the active TGF-β moiety to bind to its cell-surface receptor. Another mechanism of activation of latent TGF-β, which may be important in autoimmune diseases, involves internalization of immunoglobulin–TGF-β complexes through cell-surface Fc-receptors and the subsequent release of active TGF-β. *In vitro* activation of TGF-β1 can be achieved by treatment with acid (pH 4), alkali, heat (80°C), or detergents.

Local activation of secreted TGF-β1 often involves several cell types. It has been demonstrated that latent TGF-β1 secreted by smooth muscle cells or pericytes requires adjacent vascular endothelial cells to convert it to the active form. Locally released TGF-βs act in an autocrine or paracrine fashion, but there is also a circulating pool of TGF-β1 (possibly bone marrow derived), associated noncovalently with α_2-macroglobulin, IgG, or thrombospondin, that may have important endocrine effects in pathophysiologic states. In contrast, TGF-β2 and TGF-β3 are released locally and are not detectable in the circulation.

Signal Transduction

The three TGF-β isoforms share a common receptor system and have similar biologic activities. The actions of these iso-

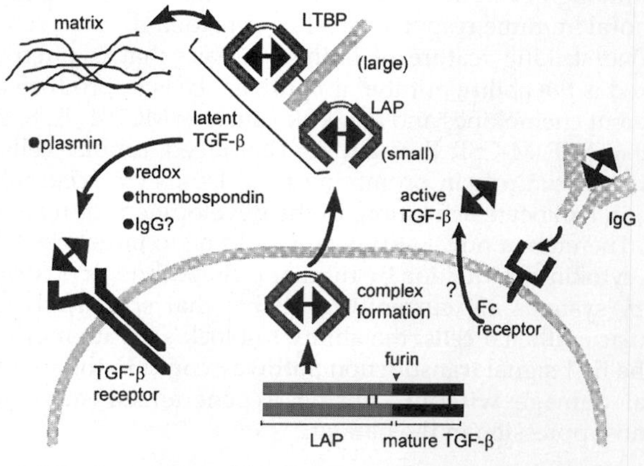

Figure 37.7. Secretion and bioactivation of TGF-β. Latent TGF-β is secreted from cells in the form of a precursor molecule, which is then either sequestered by extracellular matrix or activated by a variety of mechanisms, described in the text. The latent form is either a small complex that contains the latency-associated peptide *(LAP)* or a larger complex that also contains the TGF-β-binding protein *(LTBP)*. The mature form is a homodimer that is cleaved off by a variety of mechanisms (e.g., by plasmin or furin) and is available to bind the receptor and propagate a signal. (Reproduced with permission from Roberts AB. Molecular and cell biology of TGF-β. *Miner Electrolyte Metab* 1998;24: 111–119.)

forms on target cells involves a complex cascade of receptors and intracellular signaling molecules. Virtually all cell types produce one or more isoforms of TGF-β and also express TGF-β receptors. Three major types of TGF-β receptors have been identified: type I, type II, and type III. Type III (also called *betaglycan*) lacks an identifiable cytoplasmic signaling domain and is thought to act as a reservoir of TGF-β on the cell surface. A similar molecule found on endothelial cells is called *endoglin.* Types I and II receptors are the signaling receptors that belong to the transmembrane serine/threonine-kinase receptor family. The type II receptor is also called the *primary receptor* because it directly binds ligand. The ligand–type II receptor complex is then recognized and bound by the type I receptor. Upon cross-phosphorylation of the type I receptor at a "GS site" by the constitutively active type II receptor, the type I receptor's serine-threonine kinase becomes catalytically active. The type I receptor then transiently interacts with a member of the Smad family of intracellular proteins (Fig. 37.8). Receptor-activated Smad 2 and Smad 3 are specific for the TGF-β isoforms, whereas Smad 1 and Smad 5 are specific for BMP. Smad 2 or Smad 3 are phosphorylated by the type I receptor at MH-domains, which allows the interaction of Smad 2 or Smad 3 with Smad 4 (also called *DPC4*), a member of the Smad family that does not get phosphorylated by the type I receptor. The Smad 2–Smad 4 complex translocates into the nucleus and interacts with other transcription factors, including FAST-1, CBP (cyclic AMP–response element–binding protein), and AP-1, allowing for a coordinated transcriptional response. In addition to the receptor-activated Smad proteins, there are specific Smad molecules that are inhibitory, such as Smad 6 and Smad 7, which may inhibit the binding of Smad 2 or Smad 3 to the type I receptor. The BMP-7 system of signal transduction employs homologous but not identical pathways. Experimental evidence indicates that the Smad pathway is directly involved in mediating cell-cycle regulation by TGF-β; however, mediation of other

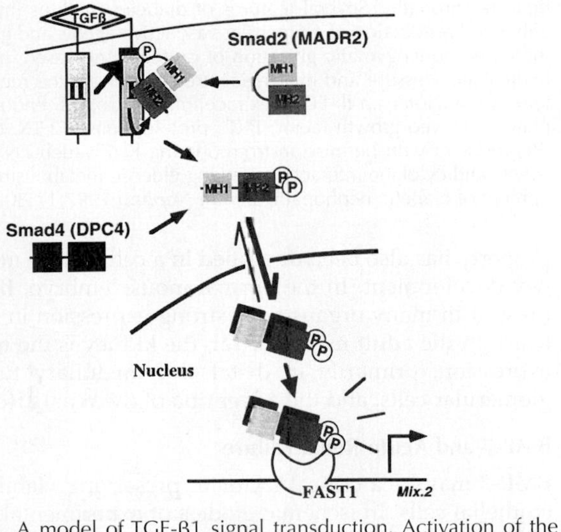

Figure 37.8. A model of TGF-β1 signal transduction. Activation of the serine-threonine kinase receptors begins with binding of TGF-β1 to the type II receptor. The ligand–type II receptor complex then binds the type I receptor. The type I receptor is phosphorylated by the constitutively active type II receptor. The type I receptor recruits Smad 2 and phosphorylates it at MH-2 domains. This leads to dissociation of phosphorylated Smad 2 from the receptor complex, followed by association with Smad 4 and nuclear accumulation. In the nucleus, heteromeric complexes of Smad 2 and Smad 4 then associate with DNA-binding proteins, such as FAST-1, to activate transcription of target genes. (Reproduced with permission from Wrana JL. TGF-beta receptors and signalling mechanisms. *Miner Electrolyte Metab* 1998;24:120–130.)

characteristic functions of TGF-β such as extracellular matrix molecule synthesis is not well defined.

Role of TGF-β in Kidney Development

Basal levels of TGF-β activity may be necessary for normal development of the organism because lack of expression of the TGF-β receptors leads to intrauterine mortality from lack of yolk-sac development. The type II receptor knockout mouse dies of defective yolk-sac vasculogenesis. The TGF-β isoforms themselves do not appear to play a crucial role in guiding renal development. The TGF-β1 knockout mouse has no malformation of renal architecture. However, due to a fatal, multiorgan autoimmunelike disease there is deposition of autoantibodies in glomeruli and a mild glomerulonephritis. The TGF-β2 and TGF-β3 knockout mice also develop normal kidneys although the mice die of craniofacial, lung, or cardiac abnormalities resulting from impaired mesenchyme–epithelial interactions. In contrast, the factor BMP-7, initially described as osteogenic protein-1, plays a dominant role in renal development and tubular epithelial cell differentiation because mice lacking BMP-7 have rudimentary kidneys.

Cellular Effects of TGF-β

Understanding the cellular distribution of the components of the TGF-β system in the kidney (Table 37.4) and the major properties of the TGF-β family is instructive in predicting the response to renal injury. TGF-β1 characteristically stimulates extracellular matrix accumulation, suppresses inflammation, induces chemotaxis, and inhibits epithelial and endothelial cell proliferation. The matrix-stimulating effects are primarily via the stimulation of gene expression of matrix molecules such as fibronectin, proteoglycans, and several collagen isotypes. Importantly, TGF-β also inhibits matrix degradation via a dual-pronged pathway of suppressing the expression and activity of serine, thiol, and metalloproteinases (e.g., plasminogen activator, collagenase, elastase, stromelysin), as well as through its effects to stimulate the tissue inhibitors of metalloproteinases (TIMPs) and plasminogen activator inhibitor-1 (PAI-1). TGF-β1 also regulates expression of integrins and thereby enhances the ability of cells to interact with specific matrix proteins. Excess TGF-β1 activity is important also in mediating fibroproliferative disorders because of its potent chemotactic properties for macrophages and fibroblasts and its ability to stimulate proliferation of fibroblasts under certain conditions.

TGF-β1 exerts a major effect on cell turnover. Inhibition of proliferation has been documented in tissue culture in epithelial and endothelial cells. The effects of TGF-β1 on mesenchymal cell growth can be biphasic. Mesangial cell proliferation can be either stimulated or inhibited by TGF-β1 depending on dosage, cell density, and other tissue-culture conditions. Similarly, renal fibroblasts from the NRK strain demonstrate inhibition of cell proliferation in response to TGF-β1 alone, but they respond by stimulation when TGF-β1 plus epidermal growth factor are added together. In general, the inhibition of cellular proliferation involves activation of the Smad pathway by TGF-β1 and consequent arrest of the cell in the G1 phase of the cell cycle. Specifically, TGF-β1 appears to downregulate phosphorylation of the retinoblastoma protein Rb and increase the activity of p27 and p21, which are proteins that inhibit many cyclin-dependent kinases. The effects of TGF-β1 to suppress inflammation are poorly understood but likely involve growth-inhibitory activities on T and B cells and possibly its ability to inhibit synthesis of the inducible nitric oxide synthase (iNOS) pathway. Under certain conditions, high levels of TGF-β can also induce apoptosis in some cell types.

TABLE 37.4. Expression of TGF-β Isoforms, TGF-β Receptors (R), and the TGF-β–Binding Protein (LTBP-1) in the Adult Mammalian Kidney

	TBF-β1	TGF-β2	TGF-β3	LTBP-1	Type I R	Type II R	Type III R/ Endoglin
Glomerulus	+	+		+	+	+	+
Mesangium	+			+	+	+	+
Epithelial cells	+			+	+	+	
Endothelial cells							+
Juxtaglomerular apparatus		+					
Tubules	+	+	+	−	+	+	+
Proximal tubule	+			−		+	
Distal tubule/collecting duct	+			−		+	
Arterioles	+	+		+		+	
Interstitium	+			+			

Reproduced with permission from Ando T, Okuda S, Yanagida T, et al. Localization of TGF-beta and its receptors in the kidney *Miner Electrolyte Metab* 1998;24:149–153.

+, respective protein expressed; −, respective protein not expressed; blank field, no data available.

Interactions of TGF-β1 with Other Factors

TGF-β1 production is stimulated by a host of cytokines and growth factors such as the mitogen platelet-derived growth factor (PDGF) and the vasoactive agents angiotensin II, thromboxane, and endothelin. In addition, TGF-β1 inhibits the production of nitric oxide, a potent vasodilator. Thus it would appear that TGF-β1 expression may be stimulated in states of mesangial cell proliferation because this is usually driven by PDGF. In addition, conditions that are associated with upregulation of the renin-angiotensin system would be expected to upregulate TGF-β1 expression. The effects of TGF-β1 to suppress inflammation would suggest that this factor plays a role in the healing response after an inflammatory insult. Because TGF-β1 inhibits cell proliferation, it can dampen the mitogenic effects of PDGF and possibly angiotensin II on mesangial cells while at the same time markedly stimulating extracellular matrix accumulation. Dysregulation of the TGF-β system in profibrotic states often represents an unregulated degree of tissue repair that swings the balance toward excess scar deposition. A peculiar property of TGF-β1 is its ability to induce its own production, thereby amplifying in a positive-feedback fashion the fibroproliferative response. High intraglomerular hydrostatic pressure can induce mesangial cell stretching and stimulation of production of TGF-β isoforms. Interestingly, renal production of TGF-β1 is increased in diabetes mellitus, and this is mainly due to metabolic factors, most notably high ambient glucose concentration and nonenzymatically glycated proteins, which can aggravate the profibrotic response (Fig. 37.9). This issue is further discussed in Chapter 45.

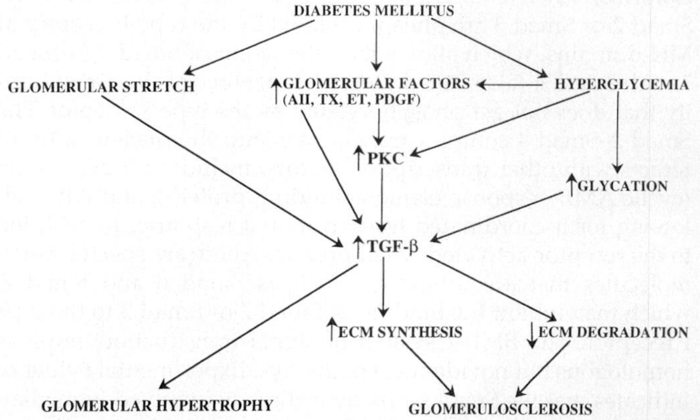

Figure 37.9. Interactions of TGF with other factors in diabetic nephropathy. Note the central role that TGF-β overproduction and activation may play in mediating glomerular hypertrophy and glomerulosclerosis in diabetic nephropathy. Several features of diabetes mellitus (hyperglycemia, enhanced production of glomerular vasoactive agents and growth factors, increased nonenzymatic glycation of proteins, increased intraglomerular hydrostatic pressure and mesangial stretch) activate the renal TGF-β system. AII, angiotensin II; ECM, extracellular matrix; ET, endothelin; PDGF, platelet-derived growth factor; PKC, protein kinase C; TX, thromboxane. (Reproduced with permission from Sharma K, Ziyadeh FN. Biochemical events and cytokine interactions linking glucose metabolism to the development of diabetic nephopathy *Semin Nephrol* 1997;17:80–92.)

Actions of BMP-7

BMP-7 is much less studied than TGF-β; however, it appears to promote cell differentiation and improve vascular and cell integrity by opposing apoptosis. In addition, BMP-7 inhibits expression of intracellular adhesion molecule-1 (ICAM-1) and interleukin-6 (IL-6). In cell culture, BMP-7 enhances differentiation of tubular epithelial cells as reflected by inducing expression of alkaline phosphatase and parathyroid hormone-mediated cyclic adenosine monophosphate (AMP) production in the proximal tubule. During renal organogenesis, BMP-7 is expressed in the ureteric bud tips, in the comma- and S-shaped bodies, and in developing glomeruli. Gene knockout of BMP-7 in mice leads to marked renal agenesis and absent nephrons leading to a uremic death shortly after birth. Thus BMP-7 is required for induction of the metanephric mesenchyme by the ureteric bud. This property has also been described in a cell culture model of kidney development. In the normal mouse embryo, BMP-7 is expressed in many organs with strong expression in kidney and heart. In the adult mouse or rat, the kidney is the major site of expression, primarily in distal and medullary tubular cells, glomerular cells, and the adventitia of the renal arteries.

BMP-7 and Acute Renal Failure

BMP-7 may be a critical factor in preserving viability of renal epithelial cells. In ischemic models of experimental acute renal failure in rats, the major injury-provoking events appear to be during warm ischemia and during reperfusion. The former phase is likely due to anaerobic damage and cell apoptosis and necrosis, whereas the latter is largely due to generation of oxygen radicals. Inflammatory cells are recruited during reperfusion, and there is elaboration of inflammatory cytokines (e.g., IL-1, IL-6, IL-8, tumor necrosis factor-α) and enhanced production of ICAM-1. Interestingly, shortly after the ischemic insult there is a marked downregulation of BMP-7, primarily in the medulla. If BMP-7 is administered systemically to the rat before, or even after, the ischemic insult, there is significant preservation of renal function. This is consistent with the known actions of BMP-7 to promote cell differentiation, improve vascular integrity, and inhibit ICAM-1 and IL-6 expression. Thus it appears that BMP-7 is a critical factor in preserving viability of renal epithelial cells, whereas its downregulation may be harmful for cell survival.

TGF-β1 expression has been found to be quite variable following renal ischemia and likely does not play a critical role. However, there may be important effects of TGF-β1 because it has been shown that systemic administration of TGF-β1 to septic mice improves blood pressure and decreases mortality. This is likely due to the effect of TGF-β1 to inhibit iNOS expression and function. However, it should be noted that inhibition of iNOS via a nonspecific inhibitor of NOS may enhance glomerular thrombosis.

ROLE OF TGF-β IN RENAL DISEASES

Glomerulonephritis

In human glomerular diseases characterized by progressive glomerulosclerosis, all three isoforms of TGF-β are upregulated in the glomerular compartment, whereas there is no such upregulation in glomerular disorders that are not progressive (e.g., minimal-change disease, thin basement membrane disease). Relevance to human kidney disease has been ascertained by immunohistochemical and *in situ* studies of renal biopsies. Increased renal and urinary TGF-β1 levels have been reported in adults and children with a variety of glomerular diseases, including IgA nephropathy, Henoch-Schönlein purpura, idiopathic mesangial proliferative glomerulonephritis, focal glomerulosclerosis, membranous nephropathy, lupus nephritis, anti–glomerular basement membrane (GBM) disease, and human immunodeficiency virus–associated nephropathy. In these diseases, TGF-β1 overexpression can be demonstrated in glomeruli as well as in the interstitium.

In the resolution phase of the anti-Thy1 antibody-induced model of glomerulonephritis in the rat, there is upregulation of TGF-β1 and the type II receptor in the glomeruli. Studies in this model of mesangioproliferative glomerulonephritis have demonstrated that blocking the activity of TGF-β by administering neutralizing anti–TGF-β antibodies or the proteoglycan decorin decreases the glomerular scarring following the inflammatory phase. In general, increased expression of TGF-β1 correlates with mesangial matrix expansion. However, in the Heymann model of membranous nephropathy in the rat (in which there is no mesangial matrix expansion), there is increased expression of the isoforms TGF-β2 and TGF-β3 in the visceral epithelial cells of the glomerulus, as well as increased expression of the type I and type II receptors.

Another model in which overproduction of TGF-β1 has been demonstrated is the anti-GBM–induced glomerulonephritis in the rabbit. This model gives rise initially to proliferative crescentic glomerulonephritis followed by glomerulosclerosis and tubulointerstitial fibrosis. TGF-β1 protein and bioactivity are increased in glomeruli from affected kidneys, and levels of urinary TGF-β also correlate with the time course of the development of fibrosis.

Although TGF-β1 continues to be overexpressed in chronic models of glomerulonephritis, its role in mediating the development of progressive kidney fibrosis and renal insufficiency remains unproven, because specific anti–TGF-β therapy for long-term periods have not yet been attempted. It should be noted that although it is evident that TGF-β promotes renal fibrosis, it is possible that there may be beneficial effects of TGF-β to suppress inflammatory cytokines and halt cellular proliferation. In this regard, it is important to note that the TGF-β1 knockout mouse has increased MHC classes I and II expression in the kidney and accumulation of antibodies in glomeruli.

A well-established model of chronic glomerular disease is the 1 5/6 nephrectomy model in the rat. TGF-β1 has been shown to be upregulated in the remnant glomeruli in this model. Furthermore, reduction of protein intake appears to decrease glomerular expression of TGF-β1, and this property may partly explain the renoprotective effects of protein restriction. One of the beneficial effects of angiotensin-converting enzyme (ACE) inhibitors in delaying the progression of renal failure and the development of tubulointerstitial fibrosis may relate to the inhibition of angiotensin II production, a potent stimulus for TGF-β1 production.

Diabetic Nephropathy

There is now a convincing body of experimental evidence supporting a crucial role for TGF-β1 in the pathogenesis of early and late stages of diabetic kidney disease (see also Chapter 45). In fact, Koch's postulates regarding the involvement of a cytokine in a given kidney disease have all been fulfilled with regards to the TGF-β system and diabetic nephropathy: (a) High ambient glucose and recombinant TGF-β1 exert similar actions on renal cells (i.e., cell hypertrophy and increased extracellular matrix synthesis). (b) Increased amounts of TGF-β1 are produced in renal cells when grown in high glucose (e.g., mesangial, proximal tubular, and renal interstitial cells). (c) Increased renal production and urinary levels of TGF-β1 are observed in diabetic animals and humans. (d) Upregulation of TGF-β receptors is observed in the glomerular and tubular compartments of experimental diabetic animals. (e) Genetic manipulation to overexpress TGF-β1 leads to glomerulosclerosis and tubulointerstitial fibrosis. (f) Many vasoactive agents in the glomerulus (thromboxane, angiotensin II, and endothelin), and increased levels of nonenzymatically glycated proteins and intraglomerular hypertension, which are features of the diabetic state, can all increase glomerular TGF-β1 production. (g) Inhibition of TGF-β bioactivity using neutralizing anti–TGF-β antibodies leads to reversal of the glucose-induced stimulation of matrix production in cultured renal cells. (h) Systemic treatment with neutralizing pan-selective anti–TGF-β antibody or antisense TGF-β1 oligodeoxynucleotides prevents the early manifestations of diabetic renal disease in streptozotocin-diabetic mice. In fact, long-term (8 weeks) anti–TGF-β antibody therapy *in vivo* is efficacious in preventing renal insufficiency and mesangial matrix expansion in diabetic db/db mice, a model of type II diabetes. (i) Finally, patients with type II diabetes have increased renal production of TGF-β1 before established overt nephropathy (Fig. 37.10), and the increased glomerular expression of TGF-β1 correlates with glycemic control. A recent study suggests that part of the renoprotective effects of captopril in patients with diabetic nephropathy is correlated with reduction of TGF-β1 production.

Tubulointerstitial Disease

In models of primary interstitial disease, there is increased expression of TGF-β isoforms, likely as a consequence of the initial inflammation. Increased TGF-β expression is also a hallmark of tubulointerstitial fibrosis that characterizes many renal

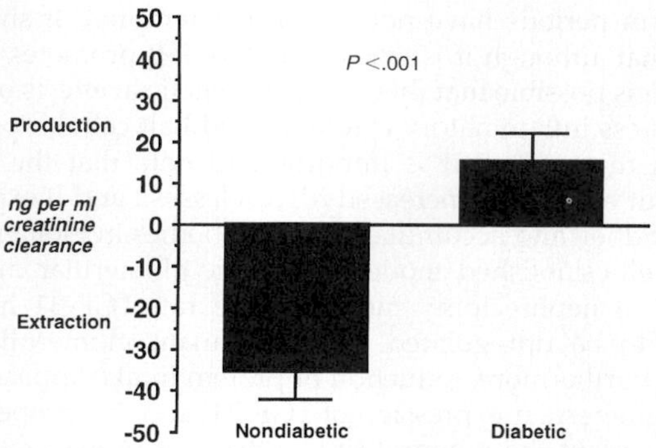

Figure 37.10. Increased renal production of TGF-β1 in diabetic patients. Aortic and renal vein plasma levels of TGF-β1 were measured in 14 type II diabetic patients and 11 nondiabetic control patients who were undergoing elective cardiac catheterization for coronary artery disease. Renal blood flow was also measured in order to calculate the TGF-β1 mass per minute of plasma flow across the renal vascular bed. Values of TGF-β1 mass were factored per milliliter of creatinine clearance. Diabetic patients demonstrated net renal production of immunoreactive TGF-β1, whereas nondiabetic patients demonstrated net renal extraction of circulating TGF-β1. Not shown, urinary levels of bioassayable TGF-β were also significantly increased in diabetic patients. (Reproduced with permission from Sharma K, Ziyadeh FN, Alzahabi B, et al. Increased renal production of transforming growth factor-B1 in patients with type II diabetes mellitus *Diabetes* 1997;46:854–859.)

diseases including primary glomerular and vascular diseases. In all these situations, decreased renal function is correlated with the degree of tubulointerstitial fibrosis and tubular atrophy as well as the expression of interstitial TGF-β. A possible scenario to explain the relationship between the degree of proteinuria in primary glomerular diseases and progressive renal insufficiency may be related to tubular uptake of protein and upregulation of chemoattractant proteins (e.g., MCP-1) with consequent interstitial infiltration of macrophages. The latter are a rich source of TGF-β1 and many proinflammatory molecules, and they promote the switch of fibroblasts to activated myofibroblasts. Synthesis and deposition of fibrillary collagens types I and III are stimulated. Therefore the greater the degree of proteinuria, the greater is the degree of tubulointerstitial fibrosis, which is produced by increased levels of TGF-β1. Treatment with ACE inhibitors reduces TGF-β1 production and delays the progression of renal failure and the development of tubulointerstitial fibrosis.

Obstructive Nephropathy

In animal models of unilateral ureteral obstruction, TGF-β expression is increased in obstructed kidneys compared with the contralateral (control) kidneys. Tissue injury and fibrosis are mediated by macrophage infiltration followed by excessive matrix accumulation. TGF-β1 appears to play a major role in these events following obstructive disease. Pilot studies in human subjects have shown significantly elevated urine levels of TGF-β1 in children with ureteropelvic junction obstruction and posterior urethral valves. Urinary TGF-β1 expression correlates with the severity of interstitial fibrosis and intrarenal TGF-β1 production. ACE inhibitor therapy inhibits production of angiotensin II, and thus of TGF-β1 production. In fact, treatment regimens with enalapril halts tubulointerstitial fibrosis in rats with obstructive nephropathy.

Kidney Allograft Dysfunction

The TGF-β isoforms are important in the early phase of acute rejection, during chronic rejection, and as a mediator of cyclosporine-induced nephrotoxicity. In patients with acute rejection, all three isoforms of TGF-β are increased in the tubulointerstitium. TGF-β is produced by resident cells and inflammatory cells. The role of TGF-β in suppressing inflammation by inhibiting B- and T-cell proliferation may be beneficial, but it may also contribute to the inflammation by recruiting leukocytes. In chronic rejection it is likely that TGF-β contributes to tubulointerstitial scarring. Several studies employing human biopsies of chronic rejection have demonstrated increased TGF-β isoforms in the tubulointerstitium, vascular walls, and glomeruli. Studies that failed to demonstrate upregulation of TGF-β may reflect the heterogeneity of chronic rejection and the varying stages of scarring from the analyzed samples.

Much of the harmful effects of cyclosporine on the kidney have been attributed to TGF-β1. Cyclosporine stimulates endothelin, which may contribute to the renal vasoconstrictive effects and to TGF-β1 stimulation, thus promoting chronic fibrosis in tubulointerstitial areas and vascular hyalinosis.

Selected Readings

Border WA, Noble NA. Transforming growth factor-β in tissue fibrosis. *N Engl J Med* 1994;331:1286–1292.

The authors have performed ground-breaking studies in identifying TGF-β as a critical cytokine in mediating the fibrotic effects that may occur in inflammatory injury to the glomerulus. The review profiles the role of TGF-β in various diseases characterized by tissue fibrosis.

Diamond JR, Ricardo SD, Klahr S. Mechanisms of interstitial fibrosis in obstructive nephropathy. *Semin Nephrol* 1998;18:594–602.

The interactive roles of angiotensin II and TGF-β in the fibrosis that develops in obstructive nephropathy is highlighted in this review article.

Dudley AT, Lyons KM, Robertson E. A requirement for bone morphogenetic protein-7 during development of the mammalian kidney and eye. *Genes Dev* 1995;9:2795–2807.

This original article shows that knockout of BMP-7 leads to severe renal dysplasia and supports an important role for BMP-7 in states of renal regeneration.

Khanna A, Li B, Sharma VK, et al. Immunoregulatory and fibrogenic activities of cyclosporine: a unifying hypothesis based on transforming growth factor-beta expression. *Transplant Proc* 1996;28:2015–2018.

The authors demonstrate stimulation of TGF-β by cyclosporine and provide evidence supporting a role for TGF-β in mediating the immunosuppressant and profibrotic effects of cyclosporine.

Letterio JJ, Bottinger EP. TGF-β knockout and dominant—negative receptor transgenic mice. *Miner Electrolyte Metab* 1998;24:161–167.

The authors review the lessons learned from knocking out the genes encoding the three mammalian TGF-β isoforms and their receptors in transgenic mice. The autoimmune manifestations of the TGF-β1 knockout mice clearly demonstrate a critical role for TGF-β1 in curbing the activity of the immune system.

Roberts A. Molecular and cell biology of TGF-β. *Miner Electrolyte Metab* 1998; 24:111–119.

This is an authoritative and up-to-date review by one of the leading investigators who identified the basic biology of the TGF-β system and explores its role in pathophysiology. The review highlights several concepts related to stimulation of the TGF-β promoter and regulation of the latent molecule to its biologically active form.

Sharma K, Ziyadeh FN. Hyperglycemia and diabetic kidney disease: the case for transforming growth factor-beta as a key mediator. *Diabetes* 1995;44:1139–1146.

This review highlights the seminal observations of various investigators implicating TGF-β as an important growth factor in mediating many of the effects of high ambient glucose in cell-culture models and the effects of hyperglycemia in animal models of diabetic kidney disease. Emerging clinical data appear to support the importance of TGF-β in playing a role in the pathogenesis of human diabetic nephropathy.

Sharma K, Guo J, Jin Y, et al. Neutralization of TGF-β by anti-TGF-β antibody attenuates kidney hypertrophy and the enhanced extracellular matrix gene expression in STZ-induced diabetic mice. *Diabetes* 1996;45:522–530.

This is the first interventional study using anti–TGF-β antibodies in a murine model of type I diabetes mellitus showing that the early upregulation of renal TGF-β1 system precedes the development of renal hypertrophy, and it implicates the increase in renal TGF-β activity as an important etiologic agent in mediating diabetes-induced renal extracellular matrix upregulation and glomerular hypertrophy.

Vukicevic S, Basic V, Rogic D, et al. Osteogenic protein-1 (bone morphogenetic protein-7) reduces severity of injury after ischemic acute renal failure in rat. *J Clin Invest* 1998;102:202–214.

This study demonstrated that administration of BMP-7 before and after ischemic injury in rats was protective of renal function and overall survival. This study, in concert with other studies that found suppression of BMP-7 expression in the kidney following acute ischemic renal injury, suggests that BMP-7 plays an impor-

tant role in renal tubular epithelial cytoprotection and recovery from ischemic insult.

Yamamoto T, Noble NA, Cohen AH, et al. Expression of transforming growth factor-β isoforms in human glomerular diseases. *Kidney Int* 1996;49:461–469.
Interesting correlative studies derived from biopsy samples from various progressive glomerulopathic disorders demonstrating increased expression of all TGF-β isoforms in both glomerular and tubulointerstitial compartments, whereas nonprogressive renal disorders do not show similar changes.

B: Platelet Derived and Fibroblast Growth Factors

J. Ashley Jefferson, Leah A. Haseley, and Richard J. Johnson

The renal response to injury is mediated by a complex interaction between a wide variety of proteins, including proinflammatory cytokines, vasoactive mediators, growth factors, matrix proteins, and proteases. Many of these proteins have been identified, and among these, platelet-derived growth factor (PDGF) and basic fibroblast growth factor (bFGF) have been studied extensively and found to play central roles.

PLATELET-DERIVED GROWTH FACTOR

PDGF was initially discovered in 1974 within the α granules of platelets and was found to stimulate the proliferation of vascular smooth muscle cells. Since then, it has been identified in various cell types, including macrophages, endothelial cells, smooth muscle cells, and mesangial cell. One of its principal roles appears to be the stimulation of growth of cells of mesenchymal origin (fibroblasts, vascular smooth muscle cells, and mesangial cells), but it is also involved in many other processes, including chemotaxis, atherosclerosis, organogenesis, malignant transformation, wound healing, and various fibrotic disorders.

Biology of Platelet-Derived Growth Factor

PDGF is a 28- to 32-kD basic glycoprotein composed of two peptide chains linked by disulfide bonds. These peptide chains have been named *PDGF-A* (14 kD) and *PDGF-B* (16 kD) and exhibit 60% homology in amino-acid sequence. PDGF-B is encoded by the c-sis proto-oncogene localized to the long arm of chromosome 22 and is highly homologous to the v-sis viral-oncogene partly responsible for the cell proliferation seen with simian sarcoma virus infection. The PDGF molecule exists as a homodimer or heterodimer with three isoforms (PDGF-AA, PDGF-AB, PDGF-BB), which may have differing biologic effects on different tissues.

The PDGF receptor (PDGF-R) is a G-protein–coupled cell membrane receptor consisting of a dimer of two subunits (α and β) again forming one of three isoforms (PDGF-Rαα, PDGF-Rαβ, PDGF-Rββ). PDGF-Rαα will bind all three PDGF isoforms, whereas PDGF-Rββ will only bind PDGF-BB. Following ligand binding, the two subunits of the PDGF-R are brought together resulting in rapid activation of a tyrosine kinase located in the intracellular domain and autophosphorylation. Signal transduction through a series of protein–tyrosine kinases results in the generation of second messengers [inositol-(1,4,5)-triphosphate (IP_3) and diacylglycerol (DAG)] that induce an increase in intracellular calcium concentration and activate protein kinase C. The PDGF signaling cascade induces the production of various proto-oncogenes and immediate early response genes (including c-fos, c-myc, egr-1) within the nucleus and eventually leads to new DNA synthesis.

Role of Platelet-Derived Growth Factor in Glomerular Development

Embryologically, the kidney develops through a series of three successive excretory systems: the pronephros, mesonephros, and metanephros—all derived from primitive mesoderm. PDGF-A expression has been demonstrated in the developing metanephric kidney predominantly localized to visceral epithelial cells, collecting duct structures, and the smooth muscle cells of the arterial vasculature. PDGF-B expression has also been found in primitive nephronal epithelial structures, and as glomerular differentiation proceeds, both PDGF-B and PDGF-Rβ are expressed in the developing mesangium.

Knockout studies in mice have demonstrated the critical role that PDGF plays in glomerular development. Both PDGF-B and PDGF-Rβ mice homozygous for null mutations die *in utero* with heart dilation, hematologic abnormalities, and hemorrhages. Examination of their kidneys reveals malformed glomeruli with a virtually absent mesangium resembling mesangiolysis (Fig. 37.11). Approximately 50% of PDGF-A knockout mice survive to birth, but die postnatally from weight loss and lung emphysema. They do not show any of the phenotypic features of the PDGF-B knockout mice, in particular, they have morphologically normal glomeruli at both prenatal and postnatal stages. A strong analogy can be made between the effect of PDGF-B on mesangial cell development and that of PDGF-A on alveolar myofibroblast cell development. Both cell types are induced to express α-smooth muscle actin and have a phenotype intermediate between smooth muscle cells and fibroblasts. PDGF-Rα knockouts die *in utero* from severe mesenchymal defects.

Role of Platelet-Derived Growth Factor in the Glomerulus

In the glomerulus, PDGF expression has been identified in both resident (epithelial, mesangial, and endothelial cells) and nonresident cells (platelets and activated macrophages). Mesangial cells can express PDGF-A and PDGF-B transcripts and are known to release PDGF. Glomerular epithelial cells have been shown to produce PDGF *in vitro* and in models of glomerular disease (passive Heymann nephritis), but only parietal and not visceral epithelial cells have been shown to express PDGF-Rβ. Endothelial cells have been shown to produce PDGF *in vitro*, but not in disease models. The expression of PDGF-A and PDGF-B by these cells can be induced by a variety of cytokines including epidermal growth factor (EGF), tumor necrosis factor-α (TNF-α), transforming growth factor-β (TGF-β), bFGF, and PDGF itself. Other stimuli that induce PDGF expression *in vitro* include angiotensin II, endothelin, thrombin, lipoproteins, phospholipids, and mechanical stress.

Mesangial Cell Proliferation

The mesangial cell is a smooth muscle–like cell that provides structural support to the glomerulus and characteristically proliferates in a variety of glomerular diseases, such as IgA nephropathy, membranoproliferative glomerulonephritis, and lupus

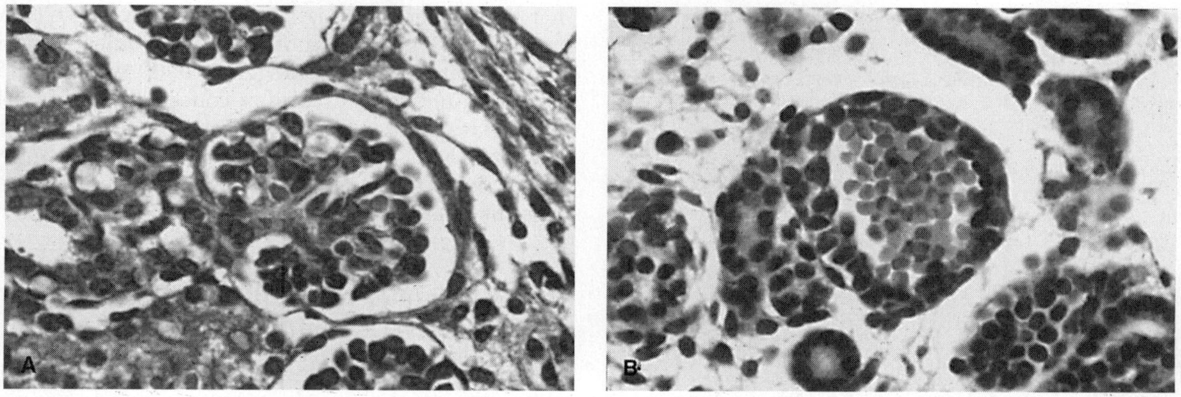

Figure 37.11. PDGF-B chain knockout mice have abnormal glomerular development. Normal embryonic glomerulus **(A)**. Malformed glomerulus from PDGF-B chain knockout mouse demonstrating the complete absence of mesangial development **(B)**. (Reproduced with permission from Belsholtz C, Raines EW. Platelet derived growth factor: a key regulator of connective tissue cells in embryogenesis and pathogenesis. *Kidney Int* 1997;51:1361–1369.)

nephritis. In disease states, the mesangial cell also changes its phenotype to that of a myofibroblast, expressing contractile proteins and interstitial collagens. This may be followed by mesangial extracellular matrix deposition, which may contribute to progressive glomerulosclerosis and the deterioration of renal function.

In Vitro Studies. Early studies demonstrated that cultured mesangial cells could synthesize both PDGF-A and PDGF-B and that PDGF was an important mitogen for these cells. The proliferative response to the PDGF-BB and PDGF-AB isoforms was greater than with PDGF-AA and implied the presence of both PDGF-Rα and PDGF-Rβ receptors on the cells. This was subsequently confirmed by expression studies. In some studies PDGF had only minor mitogenic effects on mesangial cells unless other cytokines such as interleukin-1 (IL-1) or insulinlike growth factor 1 (IGF-1) were present, suggesting under certain circumstances it may act as a competence factor.

Descriptive In Vivo Studies. The anti-Thy1.1 model is probably the best studied model of mesangial proliferative glomerulonephritis. Following injection of the antibody to the Thy1 antigen on the mesangial cell surface, an acute complement-dependent loss of mesangial cells (mesangiolysis) occurs associated with an influx of platelets and macrophages, which peaks at 24 hours. A massive proliferation of mesangial cells and an alteration in mesangial cell phenotype to myofibroblast occurs, followed by increased synthesis and deposition of extracellular matrix. This is followed by the resolution phase during which mesangial cell and macrophage cell numbers return to normal, excess extracellular matrix (ECM) is removed, and normal glomerular architecture is restored.

In this model, there is a marked increase in expression of PDGF-A and PDGF-B localized to mesangial cells, which correlates with the degree of mesangial cell proliferation. There is also upregulation of PDGF-Rβ mRNA and protein in these cells (Fig. 37.12), but not PDGF-Rα, suggesting that the proliferative effect is primarily modulated by PDGF-BB and PDGF-Rβ receptors acting in an autocrine fashion.

Enhanced PDGF expression has also been demonstrated in nonimmunologically mediated renal disease. The remnant kidney model of progressive glomerulosclerosis is induced by unilateral nephrectomy and ligation of two of three branches of the contralateral renal artery. Mesangial cell proliferation is seen during the first week, and its intensity correlates with PDGF-B mRNA and protein expression by the mesangial cell. Correlation of PDGF expression with mesangial cell proliferation has also been demonstrated in other models of glomerular disease (aminonucleoside nephrosis, Habu snake venom–induced nephritis, streptozotocin-induced diabetes).

The expression of mesangial PDGF and PDGF-R in human glomerulonephritis has recently been investigated. Both PDGF-B chain and PDGF-Rβ protein and mRNA have been demonstrated in the mesangium of patients with a variety of proliferative nephritides including IgA nephropathy and lupus nephritis. PDGF expression has also been shown to correlate with the histologic severity of disease, albeit an exact relationship with mesangial cell proliferation has yet to be demonstrated.

Functional Studies In Vivo. The demonstration of a temporal association of PDGF expression with mesangial cell proliferation is suggestive evidence of a direct mitogenic role for this growth factor. By amplifying or antagonizing the activity of PDGF, we can more accurately assess its functional significance. When normal rats were treated with an infusion of human recombinant PDGF, they developed only mild mesangial cell proliferation. However, when these rats were pretreated with a

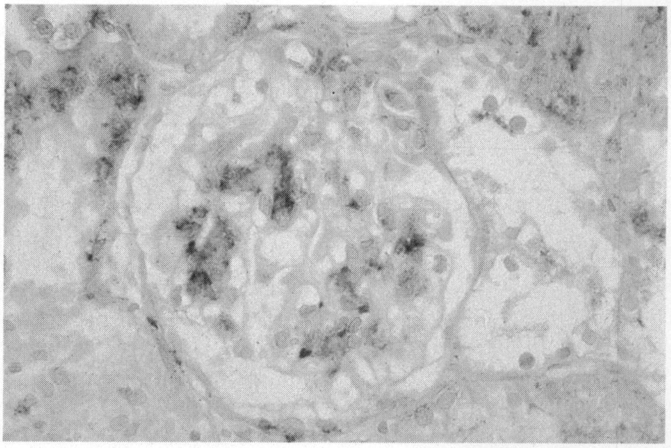

Figure 37.12. PDGF is expressed in experimental mesangial proliferation glomerulonephritis. Mesangial expression of PDGF-B chain mRNA is increased in the anti-Thy1.1 model of mesangial proliferative glomerulonephritis. (*In situ* hybridization × 400; PDGF expression marked by brown staining.)

subnephritogenic dose of anti-Thy1 serum the mesangial cells were rendered more responsive to the action of PDGF and developed massive mesangial cell proliferation. It was possible that the PDGF infusion affected mesangial cell proliferation by its hemodynamic action (PDGF is known to be a potent vasoconstrictor). However, when the human PDGF gene was selectively transfected into one rat kidney by a liposomal system with the contralateral kidney acting as control, a similar markedly proliferative lesion was found.

Antagonizing the action of the cytokine with antibody or antagonists showed the converse with a reduction in mesangial cell proliferation. In the anti-Thy1.1 model, treatment with polyclonal anti-PDGF immunoglobulin for 4 days following induction of the disease resulted in a 50% reduction in mesangial cell proliferation at day 4 and a reduction in ECM accumulation (Fig. 37.13). Trapidil, an antiplatelet agent, has been shown to act as a PDGF-receptor antagonist, and also reduces mesangial cell proliferation in this model.

The evidence, derived from both descriptive and functional studies is therefore convincing that PDGF plays a major role in mesangial cell proliferation

Extracellular Matrix Accumulation

There is a very close relationship between mesangial cell proliferation and the accumulation of extracellular matrix. PDGF may stimulate the production of ECM proteins in addition to its role in mesangial cell proliferation. Mesangial cells have been shown both *in vitro* and *in vivo* to produce matrix proteins such as laminin, fibronectin, and type IV collagen in response to exposure to advanced glycosylation end-products. This effect is abolished by anti-PDGF antibodies (as well as anti–TGF-β antibodies). The ECM accumulation in the anti-Thy1.1 model can also be reduced by anti-PDGF antibodies.

It remains unclear whether the action of PDGF on ECM accumulation is a direct effect or whether it is mediated by other cytokines. TGF-β is well established as the predominant growth factor determining ECM accumulation, and PDGF has been shown to induce TGF-β production in mesangial cells *in vitro*. The stimulation of TGF-β expression by PDGF may be partly mediated by the glycoprotein SPARC. SPARC has been shown to increase TGF-β mRNA and protein both in cultured mesangial cells and in the anti-Thy1.1 model of mesangial proliferative glomerulonephritis. The expression of SPARC is increased in cultured mesangial cells by PDGF. Another protein that may play a role in this process is thrombospondin 1 (TSP1). TSP1 is known to have a direct mitogenic effect on mesangial cells; however, it is also capable of activating latent TGF-β. The expression of TSP1 is increased by PDGF in the anti-Thy1.1 model. The finding that both SPARC and TSP1 are induced in mesangial cells by PDGF may partly explain the well-known association of mesangial cell proliferation with matrix expansion.

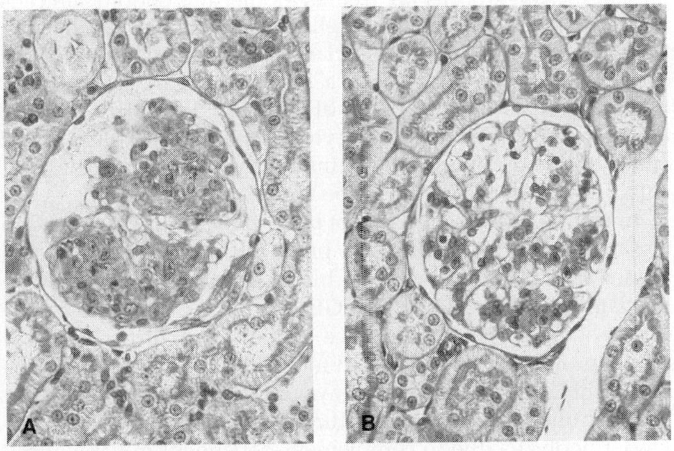

Figure 37.13. Inhibition of PDGF with neutralizing antibody reduces mesangial cell proliferation in the anti-Thy1.1 model. A marked glomerular hypercellularity develops in rats with anti-Thy1.1 nephritis at day 5 administered control IgG **(A)**. In contrast, the hypercellularity is markedly reduced in rats with anti-Thy1.1 nephritis that are treated with anti-PDGF neutralizing antibody **(B)**.

Crescentic Glomerulonephritis

A role for PDGF in crescent development is suggested by recent descriptive and functional studies. Using *in situ* hybridization, PDGF-B chain mRNA has been demonstrated in the crescents of human biopsy tissue from patients with idiopathic RPGN. Both PDGF-B chain and PDGF-βR transcripts have been detected in crescents from patients with lupus nephritis. When a murine model of crescentic nephritis was created in transgenic mice expressing the soluble external domain of the PDGF-β receptor, crescent thickness was significantly reduced, suggesting a protective effect of the soluble receptor, and an active role for PDGF in crescent growth.

Other Biologic Roles in Glomerulus

Chemotaxis. PDGF has been shown to act as a chemoattractant for smooth muscle cells and cultured mesangial cells that migrate in the direction of a PDGF gradient. This fact may play an important role in the repopulation of the mesangium following mesangial cell injury. In the anti-Thy1.1 model, early mesangiolysis is followed by a directional influx of a small number of mesangial progenitor cells from the juxtaglomerular apparatus and hilar area, which divide to repopulate the entire mesangium. PDGF is also known to induce the expression of monocyte chemoattractant protein-1 on vascular smooth muscle cells, but may also act as a direct leukocyte chemoattractant.

Renal Hemodynamics. PDGF induces contraction of mesangial cells both *in vitro* and *in vivo*. Infusion of PDGF into the rat kidney has been reported to produce a reduction in renal blood flow and glomerular filtration rate consistent with a contractile effect of PDGF on smooth muscle and mesangial cells.

Low-Density Lipoprotein Uptake. PDGF has been shown to increase the uptake of low-density lipoprotein (LDL) by vascular endothelial cells and mesangial cells. There are many similarities between focal segmental glomerulosclerosis and atherosclerosis and the uptake of lipid into resident glomerular cells may be important. Hyperlipidemia is also a known risk factor for progression of renal disease and in animal models HMG-CoA reductase inhibitors have been shown to slow the progression of some diseases. Although this may be related to non-PDGF effects, such as inhibition of the mevalonate pathway, lovastatin has been shown to decrease the expression of both PDGF-B and PDGF-Rβ in cultured mesangial cells, and simvastatin has been shown to inhibit PDGF-induced DNA synthesis both in cultured human glomerular mesangial cells and in the anti-Thy1.1 model.

Role of Platelet-Derived Growth Factor in Interstitial Disease

Morphologic studies have revealed a strong correlation between the extent of tubulointerstitial disease and the decline in renal function in a variety of renal diseases. Analogous to the mesangial cell, fibroblasts proliferate and elaborate ECM in response to injury leading to interstitial fibrosis. As in the glomerulus, PDGF in the interstitium may be derived both from infiltrating leukocytes as well as resident epithelial cells and fibroblasts. Vascular endothelial cells are also a potential source of PDGF.

Most studies of PDGF in the interstitium have focused on its role as a mitogen. Proximal tubular cells have been shown be unresponsive to the mitogenic action of PDGF; however, renal interstitial fibroblasts express PDGF-Rβ and proliferate in response to PDGF *in vitro*. Infusion of PDGF-BB into normal rats induced renal tubulointerstitial fibroblast proliferation and alteration of cell phenotype to that of a myofibroblast. These features were also associated with an increase in tubulointerstitial matrix accumulation. In models of interstitial disease caused by cyclosporine or angiotensin II infusion, the development of interstitial fibrosis is associated with increased expression of PDGF.

Therapeutic Possibilities

We have shown that PDGF plays a key role in the glomerular response to injury. If it were possible to block the effects of this cytokine, there may be beneficial effects in reducing the amount of mesangial cell proliferation and the accompanying extracellular matrix accumulation. However, PDGF plays a vital role in development and appears to be important in repopulating the mesangium following mesangiolysis in the anti-Thy1.1 model. Blocking the regenerative effects of PDGF in these situations may be detrimental.

Anti-PDGF antibodies have been shown to decrease PDGF-induced mesangial cell proliferation in models of glomerular disease; however, these would not be practical to administer on a long-term basis given the rapid development of an immune response against foreign immunoglobulin. Antisense oligonucleotide therapy may be an alternative method of decreasing available PDGF. At the level of the PDGF receptor, trapidil, an antiplatelet agent that acts as a PDGF-receptor antagonist, has been shown to reduce mesangial cell proliferation in cell culture and in models of mesangial proliferative glomerulonephritis. Another approach used transfection of a chimeric gene encoding the extracellular domain of PDGF-Rβ fused to the Fc portion of an IgG heavy chain. This acted as a competitive inhibitor of PDGF and was shown to decrease mesangial cell proliferation in the anti-Thy1.1 model.

Agents that interfere with PDGF-receptor signaling (receptor–tyrosine kinase inhibitors, phosphodiesterase inhibitors, bone morphogenic protein 2) or interfere with cell proliferation at the level of the cell cycle (cyclin–kinase inhibitors) have also been investigated. It is also interesting to note that agents that are used commonly in these settings for other reasons may also exhibit anti-PDGF activity. Ramipril, an angiotensin-converting enzyme (ACE) inhibitor, has been reported to decrease the expression of PDGF-A and PDGF-B in fetal calf serum (FCS)-activated human mesangial cells in culture. Simvastatin, an HMG-CoA reductase inhibitor, decreased the expression of both PDGF-B and PDGF-Rβ in FCS-activated murine mesangial cells.

BASIC FIBROBLAST GROWTH FACTOR

Basic fibroblast growth factor (bFGF, also known as *FGF-2*) is the second member of a family of fibroblast growth factors that are known to be potent mitogens for a variety of mesoderm and neuroectoderm-derived cell types, and play a major role in many functions, including development, wound healing, hematopoiesis, and tumorigenesis.

Biology

bFGF is an 18-kD single-chain cationic polypeptide that, along with FGF-1, is unique among the FGFs in being translated without a signal peptide sequence. Although the exact mode of cellular bFGF release is unclear, it is thought to be primarily liberated from cytosolic storage sites following cell injury.

The high-affinity FGF receptors (FGF-R1 to FGF-R4) are transmembrane glycoproteins with intrinsic tyrosine–kinase activity encoded by four different genes. They each have multiple splice variants that generate numerous isoforms of each receptor type. In addition, there are low-affinity glycosaminoglycan receptors that are known to bind FGF directly but also facilitate the binding of bFGF to its high-affinity receptors.

bFGF is constitutively expressed in rat glomeruli by mesangial cells, podocytes, and parietal epithelial cells. All four FGF receptors are expressed in rat glomeruli; however, they are expressed only in specific isoforms of each, raising the possibility that FGF action may be partly regulated in the glomeruli by selective expression of FGF-R isoforms.

Role in Kidney Development

In early kidney development, an epithelial tubule called the *ureteric bud* invades a mass of mesenchymal cells called the *metanephrogenic mesenchyme*. The ureteric bud rescues the mesenchymal cells from apoptosis and induces epithelialization. Certain signaling molecules are released from the ureteric bud, many of which remain to be identified. In cell-culture experiments of transformed ureteric bud cells, bFGF has been identified as a survival factor for metanephrogenic mesenchyme, rescuing these cells from apoptosis. bFGF expression has also been demonstrated *in vivo* in the ureteric bud at the time of its invasion of the mesenchyme. However, bFGF knockout mice have morphologically normal kidneys and the subsequent maturation and epithelialization of the mesonephric mesenchyme appears to be mediated by factors other than bFGF.

Role in Glomerular Disease

Mesangial Cell

In cell culture, bFGF is known to be mitogenic for both rat and human mesangial cells (as well as glomerular endothelial cells and podocytes). In mesangial cells at the level of the cell cycle, this has been shown to be associated with reduced levels of the cyclin-kinase inhibitor $p27^{Kip1}$, a nuclear protein, which negatively regulates the cell cycle. bFGF may also partly mediate the mitogenic effect of other cytokines, such as PDGF, IL-1α and IL-1β, as the effect of these mitogens is reduced in the presence of bFGF neutralizing antibodies.

In animal models, infusion of bFGF by itself does not lead to mesangial cell proliferation. A prior cell injury is required to render the cells responsive to bFGF, a response that may be mediated by upregulation of FGF receptors. In the anti-Thy1.1 model of mesangial-proliferative glomerulonephritis, glomerular cell proliferation is increased fourfold by bFGF infusion. The role of bFGF in this model, however, is complex. bFGF is released from mesangial cells during the early phase of anti-Thy1.1 nephritis due to complement-dependent mesangial cell injury. This phase is also associated with increased levels of nitric oxide (NO) and blocking this NO production with the NO-synthase inhibitor L-NMMA has been shown to reduce mesangial cell lysis by 90%. bFGF is known to induce NO production in mesangial cells and may therefore contribute to the early mesangiolysis seen in this model. In support of this, antagonizing the action of bFGF in the anti-Thy1.1 model with anti-bFGF antibodies ameliorates the initial mesangiolysis and reduces the subsequent mesangial cell proliferation and ECM accumulation.

Glomerular Epithelial Cell

The visceral glomerular epithelial cell proliferates in cell culture in response to bFGF; however, *in vivo*, the cell is highly differentiated and does not proliferate under normal conditions. Treatment of rats with a prolonged infusion of bFGF, without prior cell injury, does however lead to structural changes in the podocyte such as cell hypertrophy, the presence of mitotic figures, and widespread cell vacuolation. The podocytes enter the cell cycle but cannot complete cell division and terminate in binucleated cells, which may be susceptible to mechanical stress. Long-term administration of bFGF leads to progressive podocyte injury resulting in a pattern similar to focal segmental glomerulosclerosis (FSGS) and it is noteworthy that binucleated podocytes are also described in human FSGS.

Passive Heymann nephritis (PHN) is a model of membranous glomerulonephritis induced in rats by an antibody to a glomerular epithelial cell antigen. It is typified by heavy proteinuria with minor degrees of glomerulosclerosis and minimal renal insufficiency. Daily intravenous boluses of bFGF in this model markedly enhanced glomerular injury, resulting in increased proteinuria and the development of glomerulosclerosis and interstitial fibrosis. The podocytes demonstrated *de novo* expression of FGF-R1 accompanied by marked structural changes with increased numbers of mitoses, pseudocyst formation, and increased desmin expression, a marker of podocyte injury. Similarly, administration of bFGF-neutralizing antibody to rats with puromycin aminonucleoside nephropathy, a rodent model resembling minimal-change disease, ameliorated histologic markers of podocyte injury and reduced proteinuria. bFGF-induced podocyte injury may be a common mechanism of disease progression in diseases such as membranous glomerulonephritis and FSGS.

Role in Interstitial Disease

bFGF has been shown to induce cell growth in skin fibroblasts; however, it has not been shown to be mitogenic to renal fibroblast cell lines. Despite this, bFGF plays an important role in the development of interstitial fibrosis. TGF-β is a growth factor that is known to promote the accumulation of extracellular matrix. In cultured human proximal tubular cells, bFGF induces the secretion of latent TGF-β1 from intracellular stores (without altering mRNA levels) and in bovine aortic endothelial cells, bFGF has been shown to activate latent TGF-β by the induction of plasminogen activator. TGF-β also has been shown to increase the expression of bFGF mRNA and protein in human proximal tubular cells, which may promote a positive feedback loop.

In a rat model of human immunodeficiency virus (HIV) nephropathy, mice made transgenic for a subgenomic proviral HIV-1 construct develop progressive renal disease characterized by glomerulosclerosis with severe podocyte lesions and microcystic distortion of the renal interstitium similar to patients infected with HIV. In this model, the extensive interstitial changes were associated with increased expression of low-affinity bFGF binding sites and increased bFGF expression by immunohistochemistry, suggesting an important role for this growth factor in HIV nephropathy.

Therapeutic Options

The antagonism of the effects of bFGF has not been investigated to the same extent as anti-PDGF therapy. Anti-bFGF neutralizing antibodies have been shown to ameliorate the early mesangiolysis and the subsequent cell proliferation and ECM accumulation in the anti-Thy1.1 model. This effect has also been shown using antagonistic bFGF peptides corresponding to partial amino-acid sequences of the protein. Anti-bFGF antibody also reduces renal injury in rats with puromycin aminonucleoside nephropathy. Future studies will no doubt address blockade of bFGF actions at receptor, receptor-signaling, and cell-cycle levels.

Selected Readings

Abboud H, Bhandari B, Ghosh Choudhury G. Cell biology of platelet-derived growth factor. In: Bonventre J, Schlondorf D, eds. *Molecular nephrology: kidney function in health and disease.* New York: Marcell Dekker, 1995:573–590.
Review of the biology of PDGF.

Floege J, Eng E, Lindner V, et al. Rat glomerular mesangial cells synthesize basic fibroblast growth factor. Release, upregulated synthesis, and mitogenicity in mesangial proliferative glomerulonephritis. *J Clin Invest* 1992;90(6):2362–2369.
In vivo study that first showed the important role of bFGF in a model of mesangial proliferative glomerulonephritis.

Floege J, Eng E, Young BA, et al. Infusion of platelet-derived growth factor or basic fibroblast growth factor induces selective glomerular mesangial cell proliferation and matrix accumulation in rats. *J Clin Invest* 1993;92(6):2952–2962.
In vivo study demonstrating mitogenic effects of PDGF and bFGF infusion in normal rats and increased effects in those with subclinical mesangial cell injury.

Isaka Y, Fujiwara Y, Ueda N, et al. Glomerulosclerosis induced by *in vivo* transfection of transforming growth factor-beta or platelet-derived growth factor gene into the rat kidney. *J Clin Invest* 1993;92(6):2597–2601.
Selective overexpression of PDGF-B demonstrates a direct role for PDGF in the pathogenesis of glomerulosclerosis.

Johnson RJ, Raines EW, Floege J, et al. Inhibition of mesangial cell proliferation and matrix expansion in glomerulonephritis in the rat by antibody to platelet-derived growth factor. *J Exp Med* 1992;175(5):1413–1416.
In vivo study demonstrating inhibition of mesangial cell proliferation by blocking the actions of PDGF.

Kunz D, Walker G, Eberhardt W, et al. Platelet-derived growth factor and fibroblast growth factor differentially regulate interleukin 1beta- and cAMP-induced nitric oxide synthase expression in rat renal mesangial cells. *J Clin Invest* 1997; 100(11):2800–2809.
In vivo study demonstrating effects of PDGF and bFGF on NO production, which may play a role in apoptosis and mesangiolysis.

Leveen P, Pekny M, Gebre-Medhin S, et al. Mice deficient for PDGF B show renal, cardiovascular, and hematological abnormalities. *Genes Dev* 1994;8(16):1875–1887.
In vivo study of PDGF-B chain knockout mice that show abnormal glomerular architecture with failure of mesangial development.

Ray PE, Bruggeman LA, Weeks B, et al. bFGF and its low affinity receptors in the pathogenesis of HIV-associated nephropathy in transgenic mice. *Kidney Int* 1994;46(3):759–772.
In vivo study demonstrating a central role for bFGF in a model of HIV nephropathy.

Stein-Oakley AN, Maguire JA, Dowling J, et al. Altered expression of fibrogenic growth factors in IgA nephropathy and focal and segmental glomerulosclerosis. *Kidney Int* 1997;51(1):195–204.
Demonstration of PDGF expression in human disease from renal biopsy specimens.

Tang WW, Ulich TR, Lacey DL, et al. Platelet-derived growth factor-BB induces renal tubulointerstitial myofibroblast formation and tubulointerstitial fibrosis. *Am J Pathol* 1996;148(4):1169–1180.
In vivo study demonstrating interstitial fibroblast proliferation, alteration of cell phenotype, and increased matrix formation in normal rats in response to PDGF-BB infusion.

PART 4
Role of Eicosanoids in Glomerular, Tubular, and Vascular Injury

Prasun K. Datta and Elias A. Lianos

Injury to renal tissue is initiated and mediated by a complex array of biologically active molecules and cells. Antibodies, coagulation factors, complement proteins, immunocompetent cells, leukocytes, and platelets represent factors that commonly participate in renal tissue injury. In this chapter, we discuss a cohort of biologic mediators collectively known as *eicosanoids* that originate from the polyunsaturated fatty acid, arachidonic acid. The eicosanoids are recognized as short-range regulatory molecules that act in a paracrine or autocrine manner to regulate responses to injury and tissue remodeling. The pathways of synthesis of eicosanoids from arachidonic acid via the cyclooxygenase and lipoxygenase pathways and their biologic effects are reviewed in detail in Chapter 13, Part 1.

CELLULAR SOURCES OF EICOSANOIDS IN GLOMERULAR AND VASCULAR INJURY

The most commonly encountered forms of microvascular injury that target the glomerular capillary are hemodynamic (i.e., systemic hypertension), metabolic (i.e., diabetes mellitus and hyperlipidemia), immune (i.e., glomerulonephritides), and inflammatory (i.e., vasculitides). Following initiation of these forms of injury, the cellular sources of eicosanoids become multiple and include blood-borne leukocytes and platelets that are recruited and become activated at the site of injury, and intrinsic glomerular cells (endothelial, epithelial, and mesangial) as a result of activation of these cells by immunologic or inflammatory reactants (i.e., antibody and complement components and leukocyte-derived cytokines). Adhesion of recruited leukocytes to the endothelium also results in release of specific eicosanoids and can be regulated by them.

To distinguish between intrinsic glomerular versus blood-borne cellular sources of eicosanoids in various forms of glomerular injury, investigators have used two approaches: (a) culture of individual cell populations (endothelial, epithelial, mesangial) and assessment of eicosanoid synthesis in response to defined agonists that are deposited or released in the glomerular microvasculature in various glomerulopathies, and (b) measurement of specific eicosanoids in glomeruli isolated from animals with experimental glomerulopathies.

Eicosanoids that originate from cultured mesangial and epithelial cells in response to stimulation with various agonists or from glomeruli isolated following immune or inflammatory injury are: prostaglandin (PG)E_2, $PGF_{2\alpha}$, PGI_2; thromboxane (Tx)A_2; 12- and 15-hydroxyeicosatatraenoic acids (HETE); the leukotrienes (LT)B_4 and C_4; and lipoxin (Lx)A_4. The above eicosanoids may also originate from blood-borne platelets and leukocytes recruited to the glomerular microvasculature following initiation of injury and can act on intrinsic glomerular cells in a paracrine manner to elicit an array of biologic effects.

BIOLOGIC EFFECTS OF EICOSANOIDS ON GLOMERULAR CELLS

Investigators have assessed responses of cultured glomerular endothelial, mesangial, and epithelial cells to individual eicosanoids. The responses most extensively studied were vasoconstriction, proliferation of glomerular cells and extracellular matrix synthesis, changes in expression of endothelial and mesangial cell adhesion molecules that promote adherence of inflammatory cells, and changes in the expression of immunomodulatory molecules (i.e., major histocompatibility antigens).

Table 37.5 correlates these responses with specific eicosanoids in cultured glomerular cells. It can be appreciated that each response can be induced by more than one structurally different eicosanoid and that each eicosanoid can elicit multiple responses, an observation that makes it difficult to conclude which particular eicosanoid induces a given response *in vivo* or whether different eicosanoids act individually or synergistically to elicit the response. Of the various eicosanoids with proinflammatory effects, those implicated in mediating the renal vasoconstriction and progression of glomerular injury are thromboxane A_2 and the leukotrienes. Receptors for TxA_2 have been identified *in vivo* and shown to be localized mainly in glomerular endothelial cells. Receptors for LTD_4 have been identified in cultured mesangial cells. Binding of TxA_2 and LTD_4 to these receptors elicits signaling events, such as phospholipase C activation and hydrolysis of phosphatidylinositol, resulting in generation of phosphoinositide messenger molecules, contraction of mesangial cells, and proliferation. In addition, TxA_2 induces synthesis of extracellular matrix components (collagen type IV, laminin, and fibronectin) by mesangial cells. The contractile effect of TxA_2 and LTD_4 on mesangial cells has been proposed to account for changes in plasma filtration by the glomerular capillary as a result of changes in the ultrafiltration coefficient K_f. Indeed, when LTD_4 is infused systemically, decrements in single nephron glomerular filtration rate (GFR) occur and are mainly due to reductions in K_f. In addition to their vasoactive effects, TxA_2 and the leukotrienes are well-established proinflammatory eicosanoids. Thus TxA_2 aggregates platelets and has chemotactic activity for leukocytes. LTB_4 is a potent chemotactic eicosanoid for neutrophils and eosinophils; it enhances expression of C3b and IgG receptors; expression of cell adhesion molecules, thereby facilitating adherence of leukocytes recruited to the site of vascular injury; and expression of immunomodulatory molecules such as the major histocompatibility complex (MHC) class II antigens.

TABLE 37.5. Responses Induced by Eicosanoids on Glomerular Cells

Proliferation (mesangial endothelial)	$PGF_{2\alpha}$, TxA_2, 12-HETE, 15-HETE, LTC_4, LTD_4
Extracellular matrix synthesis (mesangial)	TxA_2
Changes in structural organization/ contraction (mesangial, epithelial, endothelial)	TxA_2, $PGF_{2\alpha}$, LTC_4, LTD_4
Expression of adhesion molecules (endothelial, mesangial)	TxA_2, leukotrienes
Expression of MHC class II antigens	Leukotrienes

HETE, hydroxyeicosatetraenoic acid; LT, leukotriene; PG, prostaglandin; Tx, thromboxane.

ROLE OF EICOSANOIDS IN GLOMERULAR INJURY

Table 37.6 correlates specific eicosanoids of the arachidonic acid cyclooxygenase and lipoxygenase pathway with various forms of glomerular injury in which a definitive role of these eicosanoids in the pathophysiologic expression of the disease was demonstrated. Of the various eicosanoids, TxA_2 and the leukotrienes have been linked most convincingly with vasoactive and proinflammatory events occurring in various forms of glomerular and vascular injury. In most forms of immune-mediated injury, enhanced synthesis of TxA_2 and LTB_4 in isolated glomeruli or in kidney cortical tissue has been demonstrated, and these eicosanoids may originate from infiltrating platelets and leukocytes or from intrinsic glomerular cells such as resident glomerular macrophages as shown for LTB_4.

TABLE 37.6. Forms of Renal Immune Injury Associated with Enhanced Eicosanoid Synthesis

Disorders	Eicosanoids
Experimental anti-GBM disease	TxA_2, PGE_2, $PGF_{2\alpha}$, 5- and 12-HETE
Experimental membranous nephropathy	TxA_2, PGE_2, LTB_4
Experimental mesangioproliferative nephritis	TxA_2, LTB_4, 12-HETE
Experimental immune complex GN	TxA_2, LTB_4
IgA nephropathy	TxA_2
Lupus nephropathy	TxA_2, LTB_4, LTC_4
Renal allograft rejection	TxA_2, LTB_4, LTC_4
Diabetic nephropathy	TxA_2

GBM, glomerular basement membrane; GN, glomerulonephritis; HETE, hydroxyeicosatetraenoic acid; LT, leukotriene; PG, prostaglandin; Tx, thromboxane.

Role of Prostaglandins

Early studies using nonsteroidal anti-inflammatory drugs (indomethacin) in dosages that inhibit renal arachidonate cyclooxygenation to prostaglandins (PGs) found that these drugs decrease urinary protein excretion and GFR in patients with chronic glomerulopathies and the nephrotic syndrome. To dissect the two effects, studies assessed the immediate and longer-term (5-day) effects of indomethacin on urinary protein excretion and on GFR in patients with the nephrotic syndrome caused by membranous nephropathy and focal glomerulosclerosis with GFR levels ranging from near normal to moderately impaired. When indomethacin (a single oral dose of 75 mg followed by a daily dose of 50 mg) was given in volume-depleted patients, protein excretion was reduced by 45%. This decrement in proteinuria was more than two times greater than the fall in creatinine clearance and it was observed both acutely (1 hour following the 75-mg oral dose) and over a 5-day period. These studies concluded that mechanisms involving inhibition of eicosanoids of the cyclooxygenase pathway may account for decrements in urinary protein excretion.

The effect of arachidonate cyclooxygenase inhibition on renal function was also assessed in patients with active lupus nephritis. In these patients, the urinary excretion of immunoreactive PGE was significantly higher compared with that found in normal subjects. Aspirin administration (4.8 g daily) decreased urinary immunoreactive PGE_2 excretion as well as GFR and effective renal blood flow. These changes were reversible. In another clinical study, the effect of cyclooxygenase inhibition was assessed in 20 women hospitalized with chronic immune-mediated glomerular disease, in 18 of whom the clinical diagnosis was confirmed by renal biopsy. Two patients had the nephrotic syndrome and five patients fulfilled the criteria for the diagnosis of systemic lupus erythematosus. It was found that the urinary excretion of the 6-keto-$PGF_{1\alpha}$ metabolite of prostacyclin was significantly reduced, whereas the excretion of urinary PGE_2 was unchanged. One-week treatment with ibuprofen (1.2 g daily) markedly reduced the urinary excretion of both eicosanoids, and this was associated with decrements of GFR and renal blood flow (RBF) by 28% and 35%, respectively. The reduction of both hemodynamic parameters was inversely related to the urinary excretion of 6-keto-$PGF_{1\alpha}$ but not to that of PGE_2. No changes were observed in healthy women in response to ibuprofen administration despite similar suppression of renal prostacyclin synthesis. In contrast to indomethacin, administration of Sulindac for 1 week (0.4 g daily) had no effect on renal prostacyclin synthesis or renal function despite a marked inhibition of extrarenal cyclooxygenase activity. It was concluded that Sulindac may be a safe substitute for other nonsteroidal antiinflammatory drugs in patient with chronic immune glomerulopathies.

The aforementioned studies provide suggestive evidence for a role of arachidonate cyclooxygenation products in altering glomerular permeability to protein in immune-mediated glomerulopathies. They also point to a critical dependence of renal hemodynamics on these eicosanoids in these glomerulopathies. This dependence makes use of nonsteroidal antiinflammatory drugs unwarranted. A notable exception is the use of low-dose aspirin, which selectively inhibits platelet-derived thromboxane.

Role of Thromboxane

The rationale for assessing the effect of thromboxane synthesis in glomerular immune injury is based on observations of enhanced glomerular synthesis or urinary excretion of this vasoconstrictor and proinflammatory eicosanoid in clinical and experimental forms of glomerular injury, and on the demonstration of thromboxane receptors in glomeruli and in cultured glomerular cells. The development of pharmacologic inhibitors of thromboxane synthesis and of antagonists of the thromboxane receptor led investigators to make important observations on the role of this eicosanoid in the pathophysiology of glomerular injury. Thromboxane synthase inhibition, using the pyridyl methyl phenyl-methylacrylate compound, OKY-1581, or the imidazole methyl-indolepropanoic acid compound, UK-38485, ameliorates decrements in GFR at the early stages of anti–glomerular basement membrane (GBM) antibody-mediated glomerular injury. Thromboxane A receptor antagonism, using the 7-oxabicyclo heptane compound, SQ-29,548, ameliorates antimesangial cell (Thy1.1) antibody-mediated acute decrements of GFR and RBF, and of the ultrafiltration coefficient, K_f, that occur following mesangial cell injury. At later stages of glomerular immune injury, GFR may not be reduced despite significant increments in glomerular thromboxane levels, and thromboxane synthase inhibition may have no protective effect. The mechanism of this apparent hyporesponsiveness or unresponsiveness of the glomerular microvasculature to the vasoconstrictor effect of TxA_2 is unknown and may involve downregulation of glomerular TxA_2 receptors in the course of glomerular immune injury as has been shown in anti-GBM disease and in autoimmune murine lupus nephritis. Theoretically, incremental changes in vasodilatory PGE_2 production could also be involved.

The role of thromboxane in mediating impairment of renal function was also investigated in acutely rejecting renal allografts in rats. Kidneys transplanted from Lewis rats to Brown-Norway recipients, then undergoing acute rejection, show marked decrements in the clearances of inulin and *para*-aminohippuric acid (PAH). As renal function deteriorates, TxB_2 production by *ex vivo*-perfused renal allografts increases progressively, whereas PGE_2 and 6-keto-$PGF_{1\alpha}$ production remained unchanged. There is a significant inverse correlation between the *in vivo* clearance of inulin and the log of *ex vivo* TxB_2 production. Infusion of the thromboxane synthetase inhibitor, UK-37248 (imidazole ethoxy benzoic acid, Dazoxiben) into the renal artery of 3-day allografts significantly decreases urinary TxB_2 excretion and partially but significantly increases RBF and GFR. In the same disease model, the effect of long-term administration of the thromboxane synthase inhibitor, OKY-046, was evaluated. In animals receiving 75 mg/kg/day of OKY-046 by intermittent intraperitoneal injections, allograft function was not improved, nor was thromboxane production inhibited. In contrast, animals receiving an equivalent dose of OKY-046 by continuous intraarterial infusion for 4 days maintained GFR and RBF at levels no different from those of nonrejecting isografts. In these animals, OKY-046 significantly reduced renal allograft TxB_2 production as well as urinary TxB_2 excretion. Despite the beneficial effects on allograft function, OKY-046 did not alter the morphologic appearance of the cellular infiltrate nor the systemic proliferative and cytotoxic cellular immune responses. The effects of long-term administration of the thromboxane synthase inhibitor, OKY-046, were also evaluated on the alloimmune effector cell function in rejecting rat renal allografts. Following transplantation of fully allogeneic kidneys, spleen cells and inflammatory cells eluted from the graft were assessed. It was found that the frequency of antidonor precursor cytotoxic T cells was consistently lower in the allografts from OKY-046–treated animals compared with those receiving vehicle treatment. In short-term cultures (10 to 15 days), lymphocytes from treated and control allografts were equally proficient in specifically lysing donor targets. Proliferative response to donor stimulators, measured by mixed lymphocyte reaction assays, were consistently greater in spleen cells than in allograft eluate cells, but there were no significant differences between OKY-046–treated and vehicle-treated groups in terms of either splenocyte or allograft eluate proliferative responses. These studies on experimental models of renal allograft rejection implicate thromboxane as a hemodynamic mediator of renal impairment during the early stages of acute renal allograft rejection and also point to a role of this eicosanoid in regulating cytotoxic and immunoregulatory T-cell function.

In clinical studies involving patients with kidney allografts undergoing rejection, enhanced urinary excretion of immunoreactive TxB_2 was found. Studies also assessed the correlation between TxA_2 formation and the cytologic inflammatory cell score of fine-needle renal parenchymal aspirates. It was shown that the score correlated significantly with TxB_2 formation originating from cells in the aspirate. A significant correlation was also shown to exist between the percentage of monocytes and macrophages in the aspirates and TxB_2 formation from these cells. These data support the contention that the enhanced urinary TxB_2 excretion in these patients is a useful marker of renal allograft rejection.

Clinical studies also assessed the role of thromboxane in mediating renal functional impairment in patients with active lupus nephropathy. In a randomized, double-blind, crossover study, 10 patients with biopsy-proven lupus nephritis were given a 48-hour continuous infusion of the selective thromboxane receptor antagonist, BM13,177 (a sulfonamide phenyl carboxylic acid). These patients had markedly elevated baseline urinary TxB_2. Infusion of the TxA_2 receptor antagonist increased the inulin and PAH clearances significantly and induced increments in urinary sodium excretion. The bleeding time in these patients doubled, indicating occupancy of platelet thromboxane receptors. In a group of patients studied in parallel, low-dose aspirin (20 mg twice daily for 4 weeks) produced a selective cumulative inhibition of platelet cyclooxygenase activity and a doubling of bleeding time. Yet, it had no effect on inulin clearance or on the urinary levels of TXB_2 or 6-keto-$PGF_{1\alpha}$ excretion. These studies provide evidence that impairment of renal function in active lupus nephritis is at least partially mediated by enhanced thromboxane synthesis and that infiltrating platelets are not a major source of TxA_2 synthesis and action within the kidney.

The effects of enhanced glomerular thromboxane synthesis on glomerular permeability to protein were investigated in various models of glomerular immune injury. The results of these studies have been contradictory. In anti-GBM antibody-mediated glomerular injury in rats, long-term administration of a thromboxane synthase inhibitor, OKY-1581, had no effects on urinary protein excretion. In a rat model of unilateral glomerulonephritis induced by *in situ* formation of cationic immune complexes, the thromboxane synthase inhibitor, UK-38,485, did not ameliorate proteinuria or glomerular hypercellularity at 24 hours after induction of glomerular injury, despite inhibition of both glomerular and systemic thromboxane synthesis. In contrast, in a variant model of passive Heymann nephritis (the experimental equivalent of membranous nephropathy), thromboxane synthase inhibition using OKY-046 significantly reduced proteinuria at the early stages of injury (2 hours) and this effect was independent of changes in renal hemodynamics. At late stages of glomerular injury in passive Heymann nephritis, thromboxane synthase inhibition using the UK-3845 inhibitor had no effect.

In nonimmunologic forms of glomerular injury, it was demonstrated that thromboxane plays a role in the progression of glomerulosclerosis secondary to subtotal nephrectomy and ureteral obstruction and in diabetic glomerulopathy.

In summary, pharmacologic inhibition of thromboxane synthesis or antagonism of its receptor attenuates the impairment in GFR and RBF occurring at early or active stages of renal immune injury (e.g., anti-GBM disease, lupus nephritis, transplant rejection). At later stages of injury, inhibition of thromboxane synthesis may not have a significant effect on impaired renal hemodynamics, despite sustained increments in the synthesis of this eicosanoid. Enhanced thromboxane synthesis may also have an immunoregulatory effect on immunocompetent cells involved in mediating renal immune injury. Finally, most experimental evidence indicates that in glomerular immune injury, the enhanced glomerular thromboxane synthesis does not specifically mediate alterations in glomerular permselectivity to protein.

Role of the Leukotrienes

Although there have been no definitive reports showing enhanced LTD_4 synthesis in experimental glomerular immune injury, systemic administration of the LTD_4 receptor antagonist, SKF104353, was shown to prevent the acute decrements in glomerular ultrafiltration coefficient and in single nephron GFR in anti-GBM antibody-induced glomerular injury in the rat and to attenuate proteinuria in experimental membranous nephropathy. In rat anti-GBM disease, arachidonate 5-lipoxygenase (LO) inhibition using the 5-LO activating protein inhibitor, MK-886, ameliorates the proliferative response of glomerular cells to injury. In the same disease model, 5-LO inhibition using the 5-LO inhibitor, U-66858, ameliorates decrements in GFR. The LTB_4 receptor antagonist, U-75302, has no protective effect, indicating that leukotrienes other than LTB_4 mediate decrements in GFR following immune injury. Finally, the 12-LO inhibitor, Baicalein, partially but significantly protects GFR, implicating 12-HETE as an additional mediator of renal hemodynamic impairment following anti-GBM antibody-induced glomerular injury. In anti-Thy1 antibody-mediated mesangial nephritis, inhibition of arachidonate 5-LO using the inhibitor MK-886 attenuates the acute decrements in GFR and RBF, apparently by inhibiting leukocyte-derived leukotrienes. The beneficial effect on GFR was found to be due to preservation of the glomerular capillary ultrafiltration coefficient, K_f, and to normalization of the increment in resistance of the afferent glomerular arteriole, both assessed by micropuncture techniques. In the same disease model, the extent of mesangial cell proliferation in response to anti-Thy1.1 antibody-induced injury is reduced in rats treated with the arachidonate 5-LO inhibitor, MK-886. Treatment with the thromboxane synthase inhibitor, Furegrelate, or the 12-LO inhibitor, Baicalein, has no effect.

Enhanced renal cortical synthesis of leukotriene B_4 and C_4 was shown in acutely rejecting renal allografts in the rat and in murine lupus nephritis. In this model, a significant inverse correlation was found between GFR and renal cortical production of LTB_4 and LTC_4. Moreover, the specific peptido-leukotriene receptor antagonist, SKF 104353, significantly improved GFR and RBF.

In a clinical study assessing levels of gene expression of 5-LO and 5-lipoxygenase-activing protein (FLAP) in kidney tissue of patients with IgA nephropathy associated with mesangioproliferative changes, 40% of the patients expressed both genes. Expression of the FLAP gene was higher than that of the 5-LO gene. Patients whose kidney tissues expressed 5-LO and FLAP had a lower GFR and an increased level of blood urea nitrogen, serum creatinine, and proteinuria, indicating that augmented arachidonic acid metabolism via the 5-LO pathway may play an important role in human forms of glomerulonephritis, as was established in experimental forms.

EFFECT OF DIETARY MANIPULATION OF EICOSANOID SYNTHESIS

In addition to the availability of pharmacologic inhibitors of the synthesis or action of vasoactive and proinflammatory eicosanoids, it is also possible to alter their synthesis by dietary means. This is accomplished by the administration of marine diets rich in eicosapentaenoic acid rather than eicosatetraenoic (arachidonic) acid. Prolonged feeding with these diets results in a replacement of arachidonic acid in cell membranes by eicosapentaenoic acid, which, when metabolized via cyclooxygenases and lipoxygenases, results in the synthesis of eicosanoids (i.e., TxA_3 or LTB_5) that lack the vasoactive, proaggregatory, or proinflammatory effects mediated by the arachidonic acid-derived eicosanoids (TxA_2, LTB_4). Using this approach, it was demonstrated that eicosapentaenoic acid-rich diets ameliorate the clinicopathologic expression and prolong the survival of animals with experimental lupus nephritis or anti-GBM disease. A large multicenter trial has demonstrated the beneficial role of eicosapentaenoic acid-rich diet in IgA nephropathy (i.e., showing the progression of renal insufficiency).

In addition to the beneficial effect of marine diets, essential fatty acid-deficient diets were also shown to inhibit glomerular synthesis of vasoactive and proinflammatory eicosanoids such as TxA_2 and LTB_4. This effect was shown to be due to depletion of glomeruli of resident immunocompetent macrophages capable of producing these eicosanoids. This potentially beneficial effect of essential fatty acid-deficient diets was assessed in experimental kidney allograft rejection, in which it was demonstrated that kidneys from rats fed essential fatty acid-deficient diets and depleted of resident glomerular macrophages survived and functioned when transplanted across an MHC-antigen barrier and in the absence of immunosuppression of the recipient.

EFFECT OF EICOSANOID ADMINISTRATION

Systemic administration of the stable prostaglandin PGE_1 was shown to ameliorate glomerular hypercellularity, antibody deposition, and proteinuria and to prolong survival of NZBxNZW F_1-hybrid and of MRL/1 mice with murine lupus-associated nephritis. Beneficial effects of PGE_2 treatment have been shown in a murine model of apoferritin-induced immune complex glomerulonephritis and were associated with reduced production of antiapoferritin antibody. Similar effects also were described in rats with anti-GBM disease treated with the stable compound, (S)-15-methyl-PGE_1. Glomerular hypercellularity and proteinuria were reduced. PGE_1 was also shown to suppress glomerular macrophage infiltration and to ameliorate proteinuria and glomerular hypercellularity in rats with a macrophage-dependent form of glomerulonephritis (the accelerated form of nephrotoxic serum nephritis). The beneficial effects of these eicosanoids on the expression and course of renal immune injury have been attributed to their suppressive effect on mitogenesis or on function of immunocompetent cells.

In conclusion, most investigations on the role of eicosanoids in modulating the hemodynamic and histopathologic severity of renal immune injury point to specific endogenous eicosanoids as mediators of at least two of the manifestations of injury: impaired glomerular capillary plasma filtration and proliferation of intrinsic glomerular cells. These eicosanoids are TxA_2, the leukotrienes, primarily LTD_4, and 12-HETE. Moreover, strong evidence points to a beneficial effect of PGE_1 administration on the histopathologic severity and proteinuria in various forms of nephritis. Further investigation is needed to determine whether selective inhibition of TxA_2, the leukotrienes, and 12-HETE, or administration of PGE_1 can retard progression of renal immune injury to end-stage disease. Demonstration that this indeed occurs will result in novel therapeutic strategies in the management of patients with various forms of immune-mediated glomerulopathies.

ROLE OF EICOSANOIDS IN TUBULAR INJURY

Compared with the wealth of information that has been compiled on the role of eicosanoids in glomerular injury, far less is well established regarding their role in renal tubular injury. Investigations have explored the role of eicosanoids in models of ischemic tubular injury, immune-mediated interstitial nephritis, kidney transplant rejection–associated interstitial nephritis, and pyelonephritis.

In acute and chronic animal models of tubular injury induced by total renal ischemia followed by reperfusion, administration of the vasodilatory prostaglandin PGE_1 at reperfusion attenuates the extent of tubular injury (acute tubular necrosis), whereas delayed treatment with PGE_1 is ineffective. This beneficial effect was attributed to the observation that renal vascular resistance does not increase in PGE_1-treated animals compared with those that do not receive PGE_1, in which vascular resistance is increased by 2-fold in response to ischemia. Arachidonic acid itself was also shown to have a cytoprotective effect in isolated rat proximal tubules subjected to hypoxia. This cytoprotection was not specific for arachidonic acid because other unsaturated free fatty acids (e.g., linoleic acid) had a similar effect. The protective effect of arachidonic acid was postulated to be due to inhibition of phospholipase A_2.

In addition to being a vasodilatory eicosanoid, PGE_1 has also immunosuppressive effects as shown in *in vitro* assays of immune responsiveness and in autoimmune diseases. This effect was investigated in a model of autoimmune interstitial nephritis in mice. Mice given PGE_1 treatment do not develop interstitial nephritis, nor do they display delayed-type hypersensitivity to the immunizing renal tubular antigen preparation that induces the interstitial nephritis. This immunosuppressive effect of PGE_1 was shown to be critically dependent on its administration during the period of effector T-cell induction. It was further shown that PGE_1 inhibits T-cell induction and that this effect is indirect and mediated via nonspecific suppressor lymphokines, in particular interleukin-1 (IL-1). In a different model of autoimmune tubulointerstitial nephritis in the rat, a PGE_1 analog [(15S)-15-methyl prostaglandin E_1] given as daily subcutaneous injections (1 mg/kg per day) markedly inhibited or completely abrogated the development of both the acute polymorphonuclear and the subsequent mononuclear interstitial infiltrates.

Leukotriene (LT)B_4 and peptidoleukotrienes (LTC_4, LTD_4, LTE_4) have been convincingly shown to play distinct roles in the pathogenesis of tubulointerstitial nephritis that characterizes renal allograft rejection. In animal models of kidney transplant rejection, there is enhanced renal synthesis of these leukotrienes. Suppression of LT production by a specific 5-LO inhibitor (compound MK 886) results in improved renal function and reduced severity of vascular, interstitial, and endothelial injury that accompany the rejection process. A profound inhibition of expression of donor MHC class II antigens of kidney cells is also observed. A peptido-leukotriene receptor antagonist (compound SKF 106206) also has a beneficial effect albeit of lesser magnitude that that seen with the 5-LO inhibitor.

REGULATORY INTERACTIONS BETWEEN EICOSANOIDS AND OTHER PROINFLAMMATORY MEDIATORS

In their capacity as short-range regulatory molecules, eicosanoids can modulate synthesis of other mediators of inflammatory injury, in particular cytokines and nitric oxide (NO). On the other hand, these mediators can regulate production of eicosanoids. Such interactions have been explored in cultured glomerular cells and in models of glomerular immune injury and renal allograft rejection.

Interactions with Cytokines

In mesangial cells, potent proinflammatory cytokines such as IL-1 and tumor necrosis factor-α (TNF-α) stimulate synthesis and secretion of phospholipase (PL)A_2, a key enzyme that cleaves arachidonic acid from cell membrane phospholipids to be converted to prostaglandins, mainly PGE_2. The secreted PLA_2 can stimulate arachidonic acid release and PGE_2 synthesis by adjacent endothelial and epithelial cells. Thus PLA_2 expression and secretion triggered by proinflammatory cytokines may crucially participate in the pathogenesis of inflammatory injury within the glomerulus. In mesangial cells, IL-1 and TNF-α also induce expression and activity of the inducible cyclooxygenase isoform known as *prostaglandin endoperoxide synthase-II* or *cyclooxygenase (COX)-II* resulting in PGE_2 synthesis. Cyclosporine effectively inhibits this effect of IL-1 and TNF-α indicating that this well-established immunosuppressive agent targets the inducible cyclooxygenase isoform thereby interfering with synthesis of vasodilatory prostaglandins (PGE_2). This may partially explain the vasoconstrictor effects of cyclosporine on the renal vasculature in kidney transplant recipients who develop cyclosporine nephrotoxicity. Available data suggest that endothelium release is the more likely mediator of the cyclosporine-induced vasoconstriction.

Evidence that eicosanoids regulate cytokine expression and production was shown mainly in macrophages. PGE_2 and PGI_2 suppress IL-1 production by murine resident peritoneal macrophage in response to stimulation with lipopolysaccharide (LPS). Leukotriene (LT)B_4 enhances IL-1 production by LPS-stimulated human peripheral blood monocytes. LTD_4 has a similar but less potent effect. PGE_2 suppresses TNF-α gene expression and production in LPS-stimulated macrophages.

Evidence that eicosanoids can regulate cytokine expression in renal immune injury was shown in a mouse model of lupus nephritis. A strain of mice known as *MRL-lpr/lpr* spontaneously develops an autoimmune disease including nephritis that histopathologically resembles human lupus nephritis. In these animals, treatment with E-series prostaglandins ameliorates renal disease and prolongs survival. Administration of the prostaglandin E_1 (PGE_1) analog, misoprostol, by twice daily subcutaneous injection for 2 days attenuates renal cortical IL-1β expression (mRNA levels) without a significant change in the extent of interstitial inflammatory cell infiltration. This points to a direct regulatory effect of PGE_1 on IL-1β expression.

Interactions with Nitric Oxide

In its capacity as a reactive radical gas, NO binds avidly to iron and iron-containing enzymes. A multitude of effects mediated by NO has been attributed to its high affinity for iron-containing substrates. Arachidonate cyclooxygenase may become a target for NO because it contains an iron-heme center at the site that confirms its hydroperoxidase function. Binding of NO to this center may enhance cyclooxygenase activity. Evidence that this may indeed occur has emerged recently. The initial observations pointing to upregulation of cyclooxygenase activity by NO were based on macrophages stimulated with endotoxin. In these cells, endotoxin stimulated the inducible form of nitric oxide synthase (iNOS) as well as the inducible isoform of cyclooxygenase (COX-II) resulting in large production of NO and of prostaglandins, respectively. Pharmacologic inhibition of iNOS not only reduced the release of NO but also the release of prostaglandins. In these studies the iNOS inhibitors employed were specific in that they did not have an effect on COX activity, nor did they alter the level of induction of COX-II. To further explore the role of NO in upregulating COX-II activity, interleukin (IL-1β)-stimulated human fibroblast cells that did not possess an endogenous L-arginine–NO pathway were exposed to exogenous NO. Exposure of IL-1β–stimulated fibroblasts to either NO or to two NO donors, sodium nitroprusside and glyceryltrinitrite, increased COX activity by at least fourfold and increased production of prostaglandins. This was independent of an effect of NO on the soluble guanylate cyclase. A likely mechanism by which NO activates COX is direct stimulation of the enzyme. Indeed, NO directly increases COX activity of microsomal sheep seminal vesicle as well as the activity of murine recombinant COX-I and COX-II. The exact molecular mechanism by which NO activates COX remains to be identified.

In vivo studies supporting regulatory interactions between the arachidonic acid and the L-arginine–NO pathways are also emerging. In endotoxin-induced septic shock in rats, inhibition of NOS using aminoguanidine reduces the release of prostacyclin (PGI_2) by approximately 85% in plasma and urine. Rat islet cells or vascular smooth muscle cells stimulated with IL-1β release NO and prostaglandins; inhibition of NO production blocks PGE_2 release. In bovine coronary microvascular endothelial cells, NO activates constitutive cyclooxygenase leading to increased production of prostacyclin. In a rat model of experimental glomerulonephritis resembling human forms of rapidly progressive crescentic nephritis, iNOS inhibition using a relatively selective pharmacologic inhibitor results in reduced synthesis of the arachidonate cyclooxygenation products, PGE_2 and PGI_2, in isolated glomeruli without an effect on TxA_2.

Arachidonate lipoxygenases may also become NO targets because they contain nonheme iron. Indeed, bond formation between NO and the nonheme iron of lipoxygenase was demonstrated using purified soybean 15-LO and methods of electron spin resonance spectroscopy. Whether this binding results in upregulation or downregulation of lipoxygenase activity is of apparent importance in forms of glomerulonephritis characterized by enhanced arachidonate lipoxygenation to HETE and leukotrienes and by enhanced generation of iNOS-derived NO. In this regard, it was shown that in experimental rapidly progressive nephritis, pharmacologic inhibition of iNOS results in reduced synthesis of 5-HETE, 15-HETE and LTB_4.

Evidence that eicosanoids may regulate generation of NO is also emerging. Arachidonic acid and the leukotrienes (LTB_4) stimulate generation of NO in neutrophils and platelets in amounts sufficient to inhibit platelet aggregation. On the other hand, eicosanoids can modulate NOS expression. In this regard, PGE_2 negatively modulates iNOS induction in glomerular mesangial cells in response to IL-1. In experimental rapidly progressive glomerulonephritis, inhibition of cyclooxygenase or of 5-LO enhance expression of iNOS in isolated glomeruli.

It becomes clear from the evidence reviewed previously that regulatory interactions between arachidonate cyclooxygenation or lipoxygenation pathways and the L-arginine–NO pathway may develop in the glomerular milieu in the course of glomerulonephritis. Such interactions may potentiate adverse hemodynamic and cytotoxic effects thereby amplifying the extent of renal hemodynamic impairment and glomerular cell injury. For example, NO-driven stimulation of proinflammatory eicosanoids (TxA_2 and leukotrienes) would promote platelet aggregation (TxA_2), leukocyte adhesion to the glomerular capillary endothelium via increased expression of adhesion molecules (TxA_2 and leukotrienes), and constriction of the glomerular arterioles (TxA_2, LTD_4). On the other hand, regulation of iNOS by eicosanoids would modulate NO generation.

NOVEL EICOSANOIDS

Epoxyeicosatrienoic Acids

Recently, a new route for the metabolism of arachidonic acid has been described. This pathway is known as the *cytochrome P450 (cP450) monooxygenase system.* It involves chemical reactions, including epoxidation of unsaturated double bonds of arachidonic acid to generate epoxyeicosatrienoic acids (EETs), hydroxylation of arachidonic acid to generate hydroxyeicosatetraenoic acids (HETEs), and allylic oxidation of arachidonic acid to generate regioisomeric hydroxyeicosatetraenoic acids (HETEs).

Microsomal preparations of renal cortex produce primarily 14,15- and 11,12-EETs; their corresponding diHETEs; and products of ω- and ω-1 oxidation; and 19- and 20-HETE and 20-carboxy-arachidonic acid. The proximal tubule and cortical collecting duct are the major source of epoxygenase activity, whereas the thick ascending limb and proximal tubule contain ω- and ω-1 cP450 enzyme activities that produce 19- and 20-HETE.

A brief outline of the biologic actions of the cP450 metabolites of arachidonic acid under normal physiologic and pathophysiologic conditions in the kidney follows.

20-HETE, the primary cP450 metabolite of amino acids in the renal cortex, acts as a potent vasoconstrictor of aortic rings and renal arteries *in vitro*. However, infusion of 20-HETE into the renal artery has no effect on RBF and GFR. In isolated perfused rabbit kidneys preconstricted with phenylephrine, 5,6-EET is a vasodilator. However, infusion of 5,6- and 8,9-EETs into the renal artery of rat lowers RBF and GFR. In a study assessing actions of epoxygenase metabolites on the preglomerular vasculature, it was demonstrated that 11,12-EET and 14,15-EET vasodilates, whereas 5,6-EET vasoconstricts interlobular and afferent arterioles. 14,15-EET has been reported to inhibit renin release in the kidney *in vitro*. EETs affect renal epithelial cell ion transport and cell proliferation. They inhibit sodium reabsorption and potassium secretion by inhibiting Na^+-K^+-ATPase. EETs stimulate proliferation of cultured glomerular mesangial cells. Inhibition of proximal tubule epithelial cell epoxygenase with ketoconazole or clotrimazole inhibits epidermal growth factor-stimulated cell proliferation. Inhibition of epoxygenase activity by ketoconazole also results in increased glomerular filtration and plasma flow in uninephrectomized rats. The production of EETs (11,12-, 14,15-, and 8,9-EET) in the kidney is enhanced by high-salt diet. In spontaneously hypertensive rats (SHR) there is enhanced renal cortical cP450 enzyme activity and gene expression suggesting an involvement of cP450 metabolites of arachidonic acid in the development of hypertension.

Isoprostanes

Isoprostanes (IsoPs) are PGF_2-like compounds produced in abundance *in vivo* by a free radical mechanism independent of the cyclooxygenase enzyme. Because these compounds are isomeric to cyclooxygenase-derived $PGF_{2\alpha}$, they were termed *F_2-isoprostanes* (F_2-IsoPs). Subsequently, it was also demonstrated that PGD_2-like compounds (D_2-IsoPs) and PGE_2-like compounds (E_2-IsoPs) are also produced *in vivo* via a cyclooxygenase-independent, free radical-mediated mechanism. Four different regioisomers of each of these classes of IsoPs are formed, each of which can be comprised of eight racemic diastereomers. Thus 64 different F_2-IsoPs, E_2-IsoPs, and D_2-IsoPs can be formed. Interest in these molecules stems not only from the fact that quantification of IsoPs can provide a valuable index of free radical-induced lipid peroxidation *in vivo* but also from the observation that these compounds are capable of exerting potent biologic activities.

Two of the IsoPs documented to be formed *in vivo*, 15-F_{2t}-IsoP (8-iso-$PGF_{2\alpha}$) and 15-E_{2t}-IsoP (8-iso-$PGE_{2\alpha}$) are potent vasoconstrictors of the renal vascular bed. 15-F_{2t}-IsoP (8-iso-$PGF_{2\alpha}$) has been shown to induce the release of endothelin and induce mitogenesis in rat aortic vascular smooth muscle cells. Renal ischemia-reperfusion injury increases urinary excretion of 8-epi-prostaglandin $F_{2\alpha}$ (8-epi-$PGF_{2\alpha}$) and related compounds by 300% over baseline level. Intrarenal arterial infusion of 8-epi-$PGF_{2\alpha}$ induces dose-dependent reduction in GFR and renal plasma flow, with renal function ceasing at 2 mg/kg per minute infusion rate. Micropuncture measurements reveal a predominant increase in afferent arteriolar resistance, resulting in a decrease in transcapillary hydraulic pressure difference and leading to reductions in single nephron GFR and plasma flow.

In *cis*-platin–induced tubular cell injury it was shown that production of F_2-isoprostanes is increased, and it is hypothesized that these arachidonic acid peroxidation products may be partially responsible for the *cis*-platin–induced renal vasoconstriction.

In a study performed in an animal model of rhabdomyolysis, it was shown that urinary excretion of F_2-isoprostanes increases by 7.3-fold compared with controls. Administration of alkali, a treatment for rhabdomyolysis, improves renal function and significantly reduces the urinary excretion of F_2-isoprostanes by approximately 80%.

Lipoxins

Lipoxins (LX) are another potent product of lipoxygenase pathway (e.g., LxA_4, LxB_4). These compounds have antiinflammatory and vasodilatory effects. They also inhibit cell adhesion and proliferation. The production, metabolism, and biologic effects of these compounds are discussed in Chapter 13, Part 1.

Selected Readings

Davies P, MacIntyre DE. Prostaglandins and inflammation. In: Gallins JI, Goldstein IM, Synderman R, eds. *Inflammation: basic principles and clinical correlates.* 2nd ed. New York: Raven Press, 1992:123–138.

A review of the nomenclature of prostaglandins and thromboxanes, their biosynthesis by cells responding to inflammatory stimuli, and their role in mediating the various manifestations of inflammation.

Fan PY, Ruiz P, Pisetsky DS, et al. The effects of short-term treatment with the prostaglandin E_1 analog misoprostol on inflammatory mediator production in murine lupus nephritis. *Clin Immunol Immunopathol* 1995;75:125–130.

An experimental study that demonstrates that administration of PGE_1 analog misoprostol in a mouse model of lupus nephritis ameliorates renal disease and prolongs survival by modulating IL-1β expression, thus implicating a direct regulatory effect of PGE_1 on cytokine gene expression.

Imig JD. Epoxyeicosatrienoic acids. In: Lianos EA, ed. *Methods in molecular biology,* vol. 120. Totowa, NJ: Humana Press, 1999:175–192.

This chapter focuses on the localization of cytochrome P450 enzymes that generate EETs, the regulation of cytochrome P450 enzymes and EETs formation, and the biologic actions of EETs.

Lianos EA. Activation and potential interactions between the arachidonic acid and L-arginine–nitric oxide pathways in glomerulonephritis. *Kidney Int* 1998;53: 540–547.

This review emphasizes the regulatory interactions that may occur between eicosanoids and NO in glomerulonephritis, and addresses issues regarding the cytotoxic potential of such interactions.

Morrow JD, Roberts LJ II. The isoprostanes: current knowledge and directions for future research. *Biochem Pharmacol* 1996;51:1–9.

This review discusses the novel aspects of the biochemistry of isoprostane formation and their biologic activities. The authors describe in-depth the utility of measuring isoprostanes as markers of oxidant injury both in vitro and in vivo.

Rifai A, Sakai H, Yagame M. Expression of 5-lipoxygenase and 5-lipoxygenase activating protein in glomerulonephritis. *Kidney Int* 1993;43:595–599.

A clinical study that demonstrates how the use of modern methods of molecular biology in kidney biopsy material from patients with IgA nephropathy and mesangioproliferative glomerulonephritis allow assessment of the expression of the genes encoding for the arachidonate 5-lipoxygenase enzyme and the gene encoding the synthesis of 5-lipoxygenase–activating protein. The study also demonstrates that the enhanced intraglomerular levels of transcription of these genes may correlate with clinical parameters of disease activity, such as reduced glomerular filtration rate, increased serum creatinine, and proteinuria.

Roman RJ, Harder DR. Cytochrome P450 metabolites of arachidonic acid in control of vascular tone. In: Rubanyi GM, ed. *Mechanoreception by the vascular wall.* New York: Futura, 1993:155–172.

This article discusses the cellular sources, biologic activities, and role of cytochrome P450 metabolites of arachidonic acid in regulation of vascular tone and local regulation of blood flow under a variety of physiologic and pathophysiologic conditions.

PART 5
Role of Complement in Glomerular and Vascular Injury

Lee A. Hebert, Fernando G. Cosio, and Daniel J. Birmingham

The complement system evolved as part of the innate (natural, nonspecific) immune system, which also includes monocytes, macrophages, and natural killer (NK) cells. The innate immune system is characterized by its ability to "recognize" and disable invading microorganisms, even though there may have been no previous contact with the microorganisms. This recognition of invading microorganisms by the innate immune system is mediated by proteins encoded in germ-line (inherited) DNA. Thus the innate immune system is "hard wired" to interact with specific molecules, in particular the carbohydrates and lipopolysaccharides of bacteria and certain components of immunoglobulins.

The innate immune system is more than 400 million years old and predates the acquired (adaptive, specific) immune system, which consists of B and T lymphocytes. The innate immune system is present in virtually all multicellular organisms. The acquired immune system is present only in higher species beginning with cartilaginous fishes.

The evolutionary interaction of the innate and acquired immune systems represents a true synergism with respect to protection against invasion by microorganisms. For example, complement opsonization of antigens strengthens the response of the acquired immune system, and enhances its power to kill microorganisms, as discussed later in this chapter. Ironically, this evolutionary intersection of the innate and acquired immune systems also renders the host vulnerable to immune complex (IC)–mediated diseases.[1] For example, if antigen–antibody immune complexes accumulate in glomeruli faster they can be cleared, severe glomerulonephritis may develop as the ICs of the acquired immune system interact with the complement and cellular components of the innate immune system.

It is rare, however, that the kidney or other organs fall victim to the generally "friendly fire" that emanates from the innate and acquired immune systems. Indeed, the overarching role of these systems is to protect the individual against disease, including IC disease. In this chapter, we particularly examine the complement system and its role in renal protection and renal injury. Also included is a discussion of the clinical and diagnostic significance of measuring complement components, and how manipulation of the complement system might favorably influence the outcome of certain diseases.

ACTIVATION OF THE COMPLEMENT SYSTEM

The complement system consists of (a) 14 plasma proteins (C1q, C1r, C1s, C2–C9, factors B and D, and properdin) that participate in the activation of the system, (b) 5 plasma proteins (C1 inhibitor, C4 binding protein, factors H and I, and protein S) that regulate the activation of the system (the mechanism of action and biologic effects of these proteins are listed in Table 37.7), and (c) 5 cell-associated proteins (DAF, MCP, CR1, C8 binding protein, and CD59), which also regulate the activation of the system (their mechanism of action and their biologic effects are listed in Table 37.8.

Activation of the complement system occurs via two separate and distinct pathways: the *classical pathway* and the *alternative pathway.* Figure 37.14 provides a general overview of these pathways, and Fig. 37.15 details the various steps involved in the activation of the complement system.

The *classical pathway* activation is initiated by the interactions between C1 proteins (C1q, C1r, and C1s) and IgG or IgM antibodies that have interacted previously with their respective antigen (panel 1, Fig. 37.15). Activated C1s cleaves C4 into C4a and C4b, which binds to an acceptor surface (panel 2, Fig. 37.15). C2 then binds to C4b, and the former is cleaved by C1s to release C2a, leaving activated C4b and C2b attached to the acceptor surface (panel 3, Fig. 37.15). *C4b2b is the classical pathway C3 convertase.* It cleaves C3 into C3a and C3b; the latter binds to an acceptor surface (panel 4, Fig. 37.15). C5 binds to

[1] The term *IC disease* refers to disease in which there is tissue injury associated with substantial accumulation of electron-dense deposits in the affected tissues. These deposits contain immunoglobulin and are associated with complement components indicative of activation of the classical and/or alternative complement pathways.

TABLE 37.7. Plasma Proteins That Are Regulators of Complement Activation

Plasma Protein	Mechanism of Action	Biologic Effects
C1 inhibitor	Binds to activated C1 and dissociates C1q from C1r + C1s	Inhibits activated C1 Inhibits classical pathway activation
C4 binding protein	Binds to C4b and C3b Cofactor for factor I Accelerates C4b2b dissociation	Inhibits classical pathway C4, C3, and C5 activation
Factor H	Cofactor for factor I Binds to C3b Accelerates C3bBb dissociation Inhibits the binding of C5 to C3b	Inhibits classical and alternative pathway activation of C3 and C5
Factor I	Serine protease that degrades C4 and C3 in the presence of cofactors	Inhibits classical and alternative pathway activation of C3 and C5 Generates biologically active C3 fragments
Protein S (vitronectin)	Binds to C5b-7 and inhibits its insertion into cell membranes	Inhibits the generation of membrane attack complex on cell membranes

TABLE 37.8. Complement Regulatory Proteins Expressed on Cell Membranes

Membrane Protein	Mechanism of Action	Biologic Effects
DAF (decay accelerating factor)	Prevents formation of C4bC2b and C3bBb Accelerates the decay of C3 and C5 convertases	Inhibits classical and alternative pathway activation of C3 and C5 Inhibits complement-mediated lysis
MCP (membrane cofactor protein)	Binds to C3b and C4b Cofactor for factor I	Inhibits activation of C3 and C5 Contributes to the generation of C3b degradation products Inhibits complement-mediated lysis
CR1 (complement receptor type 1)	Binds C3b and C4b Cofactor for factor I Accelerates decay of C3 convertases Inhibits binding of C5 to C3b	Inhibits activation of C3 and C5 With factor I, generates biologically active C3b degradation products Mediates binding of C3b coated particles to cells Inhibits complement-mediated lysis
C8 binding protein (C8bp)	Binds to C8	Inhibits binding of C8 to C5b-7 and thus the formation of the membrane attack complex Inhibits complement-mediated cell lysis
CD59	Binds homologous C8	Inhibits binding of C8 to C5b-7 and thus the formation of the membrane attack complex Inhibits complement-mediated cell lysis

C3b on the acceptor surface and is cleaved by the adjacent C4b2b convertase to release C5a. C5b remains bound to C3b, forming a complex C3b5b (panel 5, Fig. 37.15), which activates the common terminal pathway.

The *alternative pathway* is initiated by the reaction of C3 with water ($C3H_2O$) to form a confirmationally altered molecule that

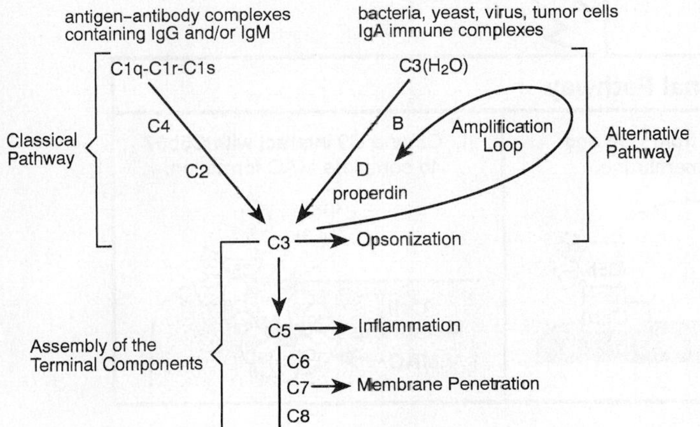

Figure 37.14. A general overview of the classical, alternative, and terminal pathways of complement activation.

is capable of binding factor B. This binding renders factor B susceptible to cleavage by factor D, releasing Ba (panel a, Fig. 37.15). $C3H_2OBb$ is capable of cleaving native C3, releasing C3a, and producing C3b, which binds covalently to an activating surface (panel b, Fig. 37.15). These two steps are catalyzed by aggregated IgA, carbohydrate molecules, and other particulate materials (e.g., yeast). In the next step of the activation process, factor B binds to C3b and is cleaved by factor D, releasing Ba and forming C3bBb. This is the *alternative pathway convertase* (panel c, Fig. 37.15). The C3bBb cleaves additional C3b (panel d, Fig. 37.15), which would interact with more factor B, producing additional C3bBb convertase. This process can be further amplified by the binding of properdin with C3bBb, forming a more stable form of the convertase (C3bBbP). This phenomenon produces an *amplification loop,* leading to a positive feedback effect. Next, C5 binds to C3b and is cleaved by an adjacent Bb, releasing C5a and forming C3b5b, which activates the common terminal pathway (panel e, Fig. 37.15) in a fashion similar to that of the classical pathway.

There are three steps in the *common terminal pathway* First, C6 and C7 associate with C5b (panel i, Fig. 37.15). Next C5b67 is released and inserts into a cell membrane, for example, an erythrocyte. Finally, C8 and multiple C9 molecules interact with C5b67 to form the membrane attack complex (MAC), C5b-9. This complex results in an alteration of the cell membrane, with consequent lysis of nonnucleated cells or in activation of nucleated cells.

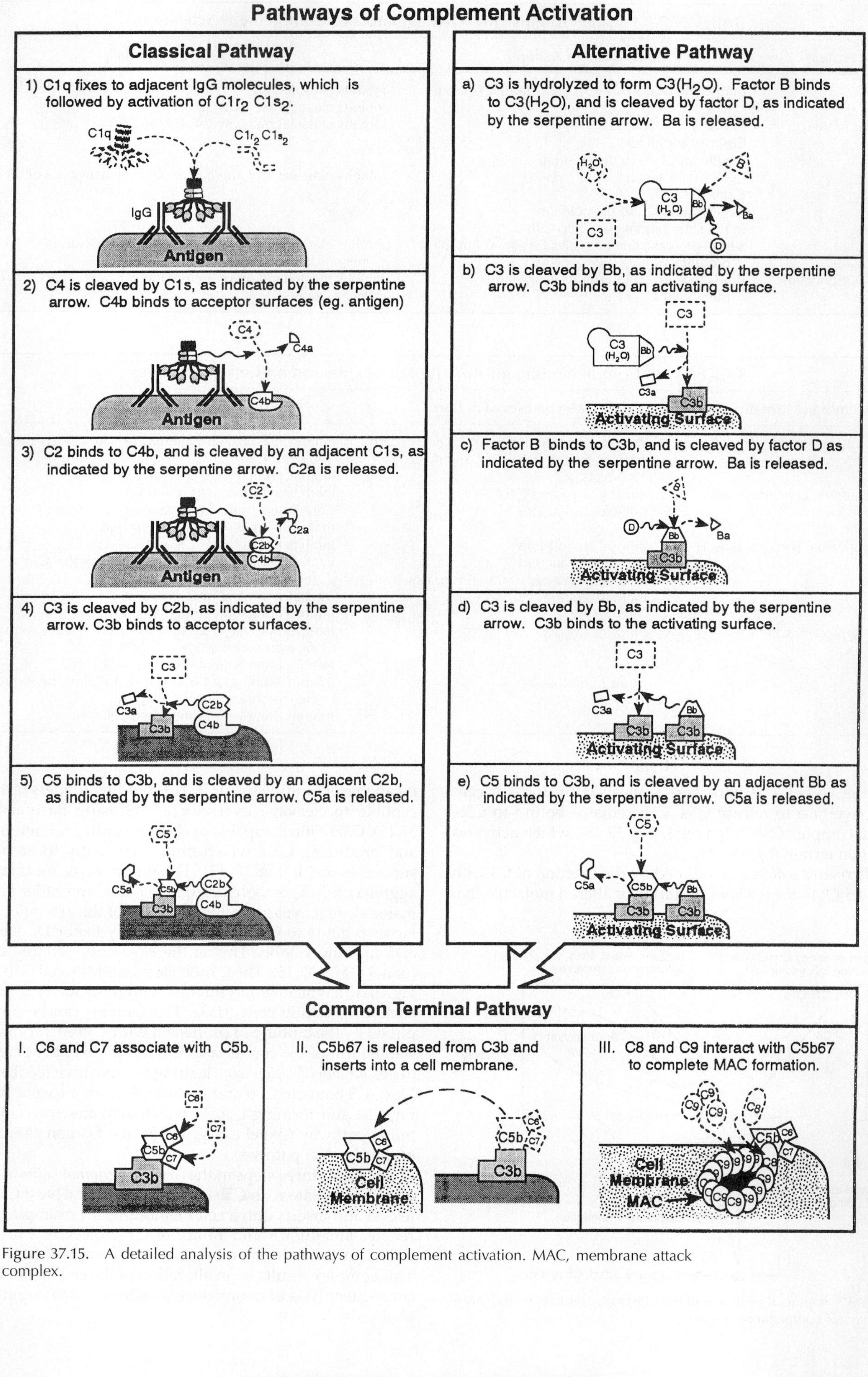
Pathways of Complement Activation
Classical Pathway
1) C1q fixes to adjacent IgG molecules, which is followed by activation of C1r2 C1s2.
C1q
C1r2 C1s2
IgG
Antigen
2) C4 is cleaved by C1s, as indicated by the serpentine arrow. C4b binds to acceptor surfaces (eg. antigen)
C4
C4a
C4b
Antigen
3) C2 binds to C4b, and is cleaved by an adjacent C1s, as indicated by the serpentine arrow. C2a is released.
C2
C2a
C2b
C4b
Antigen
4) C3 is cleaved by C2b, as indicated by the serpentine arrow. C3b binds to acceptor surfaces.
C3
C3a
C2b
C4b
C3b
5) C5 binds to C3b, and is cleaved by an adjacent C2b, as indicated by the serpentine arrow. C5a is released.
C5
C5a
C5b
C2b
C4b
C3b
Alternative Pathway
a) C3 is hydrolyzed to form C3(H2O). Factor B binds to C3(H2O), and is cleaved by factor D, as indicated by the serpentine arrow. Ba is released.
H2O
B
C3 (H2O)
Bb
Ba
C3
D
b) C3 is cleaved by Bb, as indicated by the serpentine arrow. C3b binds to an activating surface.
C3
C3 (H2O)
Bb
C3a
C3b
Activating Surface
c) Factor B binds to C3b, and is cleaved by factor D as indicated by the serpentine arrow. Ba is released.
B
D
Bb
Ba
C3b
Activating Surface
d) C3 is cleaved by Bb, as indicated by the serpentine arrow. C3b binds to the activating surface.
C3
C3a
Bb
C3b
C3b
Activating Surface
e) C5 binds to C3b, and is cleaved by an adjacent Bb as indicated by the serpentine arrow. C5a is released.
C5
C5a
C5b
Bb
C3b
C3b
Activating Surface
Common Terminal Pathway
I. C6 and C7 associate with C5b.
C6
C7
C5b
C3b
II. C5b67 is released from C3b and inserts into a cell membrane.
C5b
C6
C7
Cell Membrane
C3b
III. C8 and C9 interact with C5b67 to complete MAC formation.
C9
C8
C5b
C6
C7
Cell Membrane
MAC

Figure 37.15. A detailed analysis of the pathways of complement activation. MAC, membrane attack complex.

Vitronectin (protein S) binds to C5b-9 released into the fluid phase, rendering the complex hydrophilic. This inhibits its insertion into the cell membrane lipid bilayer. Vitronectin deposits are present in glomeruli in patients with immune complex nephritis suggesting that these ICs were deposited from the circulation, rather than formed *in situ*. Clusterin, a large plasma glycoprotein, may function in a manner similar to that of vitronectin. Clusterin expressed on cell surfaces may also limit complement-mediated injury.

Control of complement activation requires a complex system of regulatory factors. Control of complement activation serves to (a) limit the amount of complement components activated (consumed) by a given stimulus, (b) protect normal bystander cells (self-protection) while allowing sufficient complement activation to damage the intended targets of complement activation (e.g., bacteria, abnormal cells), and (c) control the generation of biologically active complement fragments that can modify both inflammatory and immunologic responses. The control of complement activation is exercised by a variety of plasma proteins and by proteins expressed on cell membranes.

The *plasma proteins* that regulate complement activation are listed in Table 37.7. The cofactor function of factor H and C4 binding protein, referred to in Table 37.7 is the ability of these proteins to bind C4b or C3b in such a way that the ability of factor I to cleave C3b and C4b is markedly increased. The sites in the pathways of complement activation at which each of these inhibitory proteins acts can be visualized by applying the descriptions of Table 37.7 to the depictions in Fig. 37.15.

The *cell-associated* complement regulatory proteins are listed in Table 37.8. These regulatory proteins are needed because when complement is activated, C3b binds indiscriminately to both self and nonself. If it were not for self-protection, complement activation would lead to undesired self-injury. Thus, mechanisms evolved that protect self, but not the intended targets of complement, from the adverse effects of complement activation.

Evidence that DAF and CD59 provide renal protection has been shown in experimental models of immune-mediated renal disease in which administration of antibodies to these molecules worsen the glomerulonephritis. Clinical evidence that these cell-associated complement regulatory proteins are involved in renal protection is suggested by upregulation of DAF in human glomerulonephritis. Also, CR1 is lost from glomerular podocytes in severe glomerulonephritis suggesting that the severity of the glomerulonephritis may be related to loss of CR1.

THE RENOPROTECTIVE ROLE OF THE COMPLEMENT SYSTEM

Protection Against Renal Disease Caused by Infection

The complement system is a key component of our defense against bacterial infections, particularly those with pyogenic organisms, such as *Staphylococcus*, *Streptococcus*, and *Neisseria*. Bacterial infections can damage the kidney directly by invasion, and indirectly in the following ways: (a) certain acute or chronic infections can give rise to IC deposition and/or *in situ* formation that damages the kidney, (b) severe sepsis can result in hypotension and causes renal ischemia, (c) infections can trigger diffuse intravascular coagulation that results in intrarenal thrombosis, and (d) certain bacterial infections can precipitate the hemolytic uremic syndrome (HUS).

If the antigen shown in Fig. 37.15, panel 1, was a microorganism, binding of specific IgG antibody to the microorganism would activate the classical pathway to completion, with insertion of the C5b-9 complex in the bacterial cell wall resulting in lysis of the microorganism. Also, the C3b and C4b deposited on the microorganism would facilitate its phagocytosis by neutrophils and macrophages that express receptors for C3b and C4b (complement receptor type 1, CR1). The alternative pathway also protects against infection because bacterial cell walls, particularly those of Gram-negative organisms, serve as an activating surface for the alternative pathway (Fig. 37.15, panel b). As a consequence, the alternative pathway C3 convertase (C3bBb) can be formed, leading to the generation of more C3 deposits on the bacterial cell wall (Fig. 37.15, panels b, c, and d). Some of these C3b deposits result in formation of the alternative pathway C5 convertase (C3bBbC3b, Fig. 37.15, panel e), which initiates activation of the terminal complement pathway. This results in lysis of the microorganism.

Protection Against Renal Diseases Caused by Immune Complexes

The clearest evidence that the complement system protects against IC-mediated diseases is provided by examining the clinical course of patients with genetic deficiency of specific complement components or deficiency of the regulators of complement activation that can lead to complement deficiency. Almost all instances of inherited complement deficiency involve only a single complement component or regulator. Inherited deficiency of virtually all of the complement components and regulators has been identified. Thus it is possible to provide a comprehensive analysis of the influence of a deficiency of each complement component or regulator on the development of IC-mediated renal disease.

If deficiency of certain complement components or regulators predisposes to IC-mediated diseases, it should be possible to show an increased incidence of these diseases. Furthermore, patients with homozygous deficiencies for the given complement component or regulator should show a greater tendency to IC disease than those with heterozygous deficiencies because the homozygous-deficient patient will produce no gene product, whereas the heterozygous-deficient patient will produce at least some gene product. As shown in Table 37.9 the expectations

TABLE 37.9. Relationship Between an Inherited Deficiency of an Individual Complement Component or Complement Control Protein and Development of SLE or Other Immune Complex–Mediated Disease

Deficient Complement Component	Frequency of SLE or Other Immune Complex Disease[a]	
	Complete Deficiency	Partial Deficiency
C1q, C1r, or C1s	+++	?
C1 inhibitor	+	None reported
C4 (A or B)	++++ (for A and B)	+ (for A only)
C2	+++	+
C3	+++	?
Factor H or I	+	?
C5, 6, 7, 8, or 9	±	?

[a] Frequency of SLE/IC disease is based on a composite of the reviewed literature (see text).

++++, approximately 90% or more; +++, approximately 50% to 90%; +, above levels in the general population but less than 25%; ±, probably above levels in the general population; ?, data insufficient for analysis; SLE, systemic lupus erythematosus.

discussed are fulfilled. Deficiency of complement components required for classical pathway activation or deficiency of those control proteins that inhibit activation of C3 strongly predisposes to the development of IC-mediated diseases. If complete deficiency of the relevant complement components or regulators is present, virtually all of those patients develop IC-mediated diseases. Furthermore, those with partial deficiency of the relevant complement components or regulators show an increased incidence of IC-mediated disease. The mechanism by which specific complement components or regulator deficiencies predispose to IC-mediated renal disease are discussed in the following section.

Complement Deficiencies Predispose to Development of Infections

The types of infections seem most commonly in patients with deficiency of a classical pathway component or regulator or deficiency of an alternative pathway regulator are infections with pyogenic organisms, such as *Staphylococcus* and *Streptococcus*. Patients with deficiency of a terminal pathway component are particularly susceptible to *Neisseria* infections. Acute infection with certain pyogenic organisms, most notably nephritogenic strains of *Streptococcus* group A, can give rise to an acute, postinfectious IC-mediated glomerulonephritis (GN). Chronic infection with a wide variety of bacteria, both gram positive and gram negative, can give rise to a chronic IC-mediated GN. However, predisposition to infection can only partly explain the high incidence of IC-mediated renal disease in patients with deficiency of a complement component or regulator. That is, in many of these patients, chronic or recurring infections are not a problem, yet IC-mediated GN is nearly universal, particularly in those with a total deficiency of specific complement component or regulator (Table 37.9).

Complement Deficiency Affects the Formation, Clearance, and Solubilization of Immune Complexes

The mechanisms and significance of these effects of complement deficiency are discussed in the succeeding paragraphs.

Inhibition of Immune Precipitation by Complement. An intact classical pathway prevents the formation of insoluble ICs in the circulation. The formation of the latter appears to be highly pathogenic at least in part because of the greater ability of large insoluble ICs to cause activation of the complement system, compared with smaller more soluble ones. Large ICs composed of IgG or IgM activate the classical pathway. In addition, their large size permits sustained activation of the alternative pathway, apparently by providing protected sites for C3b deposition within the IC lattice. Thus when ICs form in the circulation, as they do normally, patients with defects in classical pathway activation or regulation are at risk to form large, insoluble, pathogenic ICs in the circulation.

Classical pathway activation inhibits immune precipitation by the binding of C1 to the Fc regions of the antibodies of the IC (Fig. 37.15, panel 1). The presence of C1 prevents Fc–Fc interactions among ICs, which is required for the rapid formation of large insoluble ICs. In addition, the binding of C1 to the IC leads to formation of the classical pathway C3 convertase, resulting in the deposition of numerous C3b and C4b molecules on the antigen and antibody of the IC. C3b and C4b deposited on the antibody of the IC interfere with Fc–Fc interactions and therefore with the formation of large insoluble ICs. Moreover, the C3b molecules deposited on the antibody weaken the bond between antigen and antibody, thereby disrupting the ICs. This reduces the size of the IC and increases its solubility. The alternative pathway also plays a role in inhibition of immune precipitation. The alternative pathway C3 convertase (C3bBb) can be formed from C3b deposited by classical pathway activation. Thus, the alternative pathway can provide additional deposited C3b to disrupt the IC.

The types of antibodies involved in the IC also appear to be important in complement-mediated inhibition of immune precipitation. For example, the presence of IgM rheumatoid factor interferes with complement-mediated inhibition of precipitation. Similarly, the presence of IgG4 antibodies, which do not activate the classical complement pathway, interferes with the ability of IgG1 antibodies to activate complement and promote inhibition of immune precipitation. Because IgG4 antibodies tend to increase in titer with prolonged immunization, the admixture of IgG4 antibodies with IgG1 and IgG3 antibodies, which are good complement activators, could increase the pathogenicity of the ICs that form chronically.

However, the site of IC deposition within the glomerulus is altered by conditions that can influence complement-mediated inhibition of immune precipitation. This was shown when acute IC-mediated GN was induced in rats acutely depleted of C3 by cobra venom factor (CVF) or studied when complement replete. When complement depleted, larger amounts of ICs were deposited in the glomeruli, particularly in the subendothelial space. When complement replete, lesser amounts of ICs were deposited in the glomeruli, and the immune deposits tended to localize in the subepithelial space. The latter observation is consistent with previous studies showing that subepithelial immune deposits may be the result, at least in part, of deposition of circulating ICs in the subendothelial space, with disassembly of the subendothelial ICs and subsequent reassembly of the ICs in the subepithelial space. Although complement activation interferes with the formation of large ICs that form in the fluid phase (i.e., circulating ICs), complement activation does not interfere with ICs that form *in situ*.

Complement-Mediated Solubilization of Precipitated Immune Complexes. ICs that have formed insoluble aggregates can be solubilized by the effects of complement activation. This mechanism could protect against IC-mediated renal disease by promoting the mobilization of ICs from the glomerulus before the complexes can assemble into larger aggregates that could further activate the complement system and/or disrupt glomerular function by virtue of the bulk of the deposit.

Complement-mediated solubilization of immune precipitates has an absolute requirement for an intact alternative pathway. The mechanism appears to involve intercalation of C3b into the IC lattice. This disrupts Fc–Fc interactions and the binding of antibody to antigen. The result is a decrease in IC size and an increase in IC solubility.

Studies in the rat show that complement depletion delays the removal of immune deposit in glomerular capillaries and peritubular capillaries. However, it has been pointed out that complement is 10 times more efficient at inhibiting immune precipitation than in inducing solubilization of an IC. In addition, the process of solubilizing immune deposits by complement is itself injurious because of the local effects of complement activation and because of release of anaphylotoxins during complement activation. Thus complement-mediated inhibition of immune precipitation would appear to be biologically more important than complement-mediated solubilization of deposited ICs.

Complement-Mediated Clearance of Immune Complexes from the Circulation. The presence of C4b and/or C3b on an IC permits the complex to bind to CR1. ICs bound to erythrocyte CR1 are prevented from depositing in vulnerable organs, such as the kidney. Instead, the ICs remain bound to erythrocytes until the erythrocytes traverse liver or spleen, where the ICs are stripped from the erythrocytes and taken up by the macrophages of liver and spleen. The transfer of IC from the erythrocyte to the macrophage involves the binding of the Fc regions of the IC to macrophage Fc receptors. After transfer of the IC from the erythrocyte to the macrophage, which occurs quickly, the erythrocyte returns to the circulation, once again able to participate in what we have termed the *erythrocyte–immune complex clearing mechanism*. If ICs in the circulation are unable to bond to erythrocyte CR1, the ICs will be trapped in increased amounts in vulnerable organs, such as the kidney. Thus based on acute experimental studies in humans and nonhuman primates, the complement-mediated binding of circulating ICs to erythrocytes may be an important means of protection against IC-mediated renal disease. Erythrocyte CR1 are decreased in systemic lupus erythematosus (SLE). This may impair the safe clearance of ICs from the circulation.

The erythrocyte CR1 system and complement also may play a role in the regulation of antibody production. ICs bound to erythrocyte CR1 via C3b are rapidly cleaved by factor I, with degradation of the C3b sites to C3dg, then to C3d. ICs expressing C3d are then able to bind to the CR2/CD19 complex of B cells. Depending on the circumstances of ligation, the B cells may either be activated or suppressed. C3d bearing antigens also enhance T-cell immunity.

Nonprimates do not express CR1 on erythrocytes but do express CR1 on platelets. In nonprimates, the platelet CR1 system may be involved in IC clearance with a manner analogous to that of the erythrocyte CR1 mechanism. However, the biologic value of the platelet IC-clearing mechanism of the nonprimate is not clear.

Infusion of recombinant CR1 (rCR1) into the circulation of rodents results in substantial reduction in complement-mediated immune and nonimmune (ischemic) injury. In humans and other primates, the CR1 expressed on erythrocytes may play an anti-inflammatory role similar to that shown when rCR1 is infused into rodents with various forms of experimental immune and nonimmune injury.

THE RENOINJURIOUS ROLE OF THE COMPLEMENT SYSTEM

Conditions in which activation of the complement system is thought to be detrimental to the kidney are listed in Tables 37.10 and 37.11.

Immune Disorders that Cause Injury Associated with Complement Activation

Excessive Formation of Circulating Immune Complexes

When pathogenic ICs form in the circulation at a rate that exceeds the body's capacity to safely clear them, the complexes will deposit in vulnerable locations, such as the glomerulus. The ICs initiate complement activation while they are forming

TABLE 37.10. Immune Disorders in Which Activation of the Complement System May Be Detrimental to the Kidney

Condition	Specific Examples
Formation of pathogenic circulating immune complexes at an excessive rate	SLE, postinfectious glomerulonephritis, the glomerulopathy of chronic infections, models of experimental immune complex glomerulonephritis
Production of antibodies directed at endogenous glomerular antigens	Goodpasture's syndrome, some form of idiopathic membranous nephropathy? Heymann, Thy1.1, and nephrotoxic serum glomerulonephritis
Production of antibodies against planted antigens in the glomerulus	Some forms of idiopathic membranous nephropathy models of experimental glomerulonephritis, such as cationic BSA, and concanavalin A
Renal transplant rejection	Rejection of xenografts or allografts

BSA, bovine serum albumin; SLE, systemic lupus erythematosus.

TABLE 37.11. Nonimmune Conditions in Which Activation of the Complement System May Be Detrimental to the Kidney

Condition	Specific Examples
Nonselective proteinuria	Severe forms of nephrotic syndrome, such as severe diabetic glomerulosclerosis, result in glomerular filtration of complement and its activation on tubular brush border
Ischemic/toxic renal injury	Hemodialysis with nonbiocompatible (complement-activating dialysis membranes) in nonoliguric acute renal failure may delay or prevent recovery of renal function
Atheroembolic disease	Atheromata activate the complement system This may mediate some of the renal injury in atheroembolism
Renal ammonia production by diseased kidneys	In ablative nephropathy, renal ammonia production results in increased deposition of C5b-9 in renal tissue
Hypertension	Hypertension-induced glomerular injury is less in C5-deficient versus C5-sufficient mice
Tumor necrosis factor (TNF) + lipopolysaccharide (LPS) administration	TNF + LPS administration (mimicking sepsis) result in complement-mediated tissue injury in rats
Aging, chronic diabetes mellitus	C5b-9 deposits are present in glomerulus, interstitium, and vessels in diabetic renal disease and with aging
Factor-H deficiency or other abnormality that permits unregulated alternative pathway activation	Some instances of type II MPGN (dense deposit disease)

in the circulation. After deposition of the ICs, complement activation continues, as shown by the fact that C5b-9 is also deposited at the sites of IC deposition.

The amount of IC formation in the circulation that will result in net accumulation of IC in glomeruli appears to be relatively large. For example, in an experimental model of IC glomerulonephritis in the nonhuman primate, antigen in amounts sufficient to consume all of the circulating precipitating antibody to that antigen must be infused daily for approximately 3 to 4 weeks before glomerular ICs are readily detectable by electron microscopy. This amount of IC formation must be considered large because it is virtually all of the insoluble IC that the animal is capable of forming to that antigen over a 3- to 4-week period.

If the bulk of the antibody in the circulating IC is IgA, rather than IgG, it is possible that excessive amounts of IC may form at a lower total amount of circulating IC. This is suggested by the fact that IgA ICs, which do not activate the classical pathway, will not be influenced by classical pathway inhibition of immune precipitation. In addition, IgA ICs bind poorly to the erythrocyte CR1 when compared with IgG ICs, perhaps because IgA fixes C3 inefficiently. This would increase the pathogenicity of IgA IC by decreasing the ability of the erythrocyte-IC clearing mechanism to efficiently clear IgA ICs from the circulation.

Production or Infusion of Antibodies Directed at Endogenous Glomerular Antigens

The classic example of this disorder in humans is Goodpasture's syndrome. In this disorder, the antibodies, almost always IgG, are directed at the noncollagenous domain of the type IV collagen of glomerular basement membrane (GBM). Some forms of idiopathic membranous nephropathy in humans also may be the result of antibodies directed at endogenous antigens expressed on glomerular epithelial cells. The forms of experimental GN that are the result of antibodies directed at endogenous glomerular antigens include Heymann nephritis, Thy1 GN, and nephrotoxic serum nephritis.

Production or Infusion of Antibodies Against Antigens That Are Planted in the Glomerulus

The membranous nephropathy that is seen with therapy with gold salts or captopril may be an example of GN in which drugs are the planted antigen. In experimental animals, cationic bovine serum albumin (BSA) and concanavalin A are examples of antigens that can be planted in the glomerulus and then reacted with specific antibody to induce GN.

Experimental Renal Transplant Rejection, Either Xenografts or Allografts

At least part of the injurious aspect of the rejection process in these models is mediated by antibody and complement.

Known Immune Disorders That Cause Tissue Injury Associated with Complement Activation

Nonselective Proteinuria

In glomerular disorders in which large amounts of protein are lost in the urine nonselectively (i.e., both large and small molecules are filtered at the glomerulus), all of the components necessary for activation of the alternative complement pathway can be present in tubular fluid. In such patients, C3b deposits are present on proximal tubular brush border. Complement degradation products and MAC are present in urine. Studies in rats with experimental nonselective proteinuria show that complement activation by the proteinuria on the renal tubules is a major contributor to the tubulointerstitial injury seen in this model.

Ischemic/Toxic Renal Injury

Exposure of ischemically injured kidneys to products of complement activation (for example, infusing zymosan into rats with experimentally induced ischemic acute renal failure) results in generation of C5a, which upregulates adhesion molecules on neutrophils. These become lodged in the microcirculation of the injured kidney and contribute to the renal injury. The clinical counterpart to this situation appears to be patients with ischemic/toxic acute renal failure who receive hemodialysis with bioincompatible membranes (membranes that activate the complement system). Such patients showed delayed or insufficient recovery of kidney function, compared with similar patients but who received dialysis with biocompatible membranes.

Atheroembolic Disease

Atheromata are known to activate both the classical and alternative complement pathways *in vitro.* Humans experiencing spontaneous or catheter-induced atheromatous embolization develop hypocomplementemia (decreases in C4 and/or C3 levels). C5b-9 is seen in areas of atheromata formation.

Renal Ammonia Production by Diseases Kidneys

In animals with reduced numbers of functioning nephrons, the amount of ammonia produced per nephron is increased. Because ammonia can cause a nucleophilic attack on C3, thereby activating C3, it is possible that some of the damage in ablative nephropathy is the result of alternative complement pathway injury of renal tissue induced by renal ammonia production.

Hypertension-Induced Renal Injury

C5b-9 deposits are present in renal arterioles in hypertensive nephrosclerosis, suggesting that complement activation could play an injurious role in hypertension-induced injury.

Intravenous Infusion of Tumor Necrosis Factor and Lipopolysaccharide

Infusion of tumor necrosis factor (TNF) and lipopolysaccharide (LPS) mimics the effects of bacterial sepsis. The ability of bacterial sepsis to promote shock and tissue injury in mice is related to activation of the terminal complement pathway because C5-deficient mice infused with TNF and LPS are protected against shock and tissue injury, whereas C5-sufficient mice are not.

Aging of Tissues

Natural aging and aging accelerated by long-standing diabetes mellitus are associated with C5b-9 deposits in areas of renal sclerosis, which include the glomerulus, arterioles, and renal interstitium.

Factor-H Deficiency or Other Abnormality That Permits Unregulated Alternative Pathway Activation

Inherited factor-H deficiency in pigs results in dense deposit disease that is indistinguishable from type II *membranoproliferative glomerulonephritis* (MPGN) of humans. It is thought that chronic unregulated generation of C3 damages the renal glomerulus and causes the intramembranous dense deposits characteristic of MPGN type II. Most patients with MPGN type II do not have factor-H deficiency although they usually have evidence of increased alternative complement pathway activation.

MECHANISMS BY WHICH COMPLEMENT ACTIVATION PROMOTES RENAL INJURY

To assess the role of complement, most previous studies induced transient (up to 3 days) complement depletion by intravenous infusion of CVF. More recently mice with genetic C3, C4, or C5 deficiency, and rabbits or rats with genetic C6 deficiency have also been studied. The discussion that follows is based on an analysis of these models of complement depletion.

From the studies of complement depletion in the various models of immune-mediated GN, a reasonably clear picture has emerged suggesting the following.

1. In the heterologous (acute) phase of nephrotoxic serum or anti-GBM nephritis, the Thy1 model, or the concanavalin A model, complement activation has been regarded as the cause of the proteinuria and glomerular hypercellularity. However, studies using genetically altered mice ("knock-out" of C3 or C4) show that C3 activation via the classical pathway determines glomerular neutrophil accumulation but only partially determines proteinuria.
2. In the autologous phase of nephrotoxic serum nephritis or anti-GBM nephritis (i.e., after the host animal has mounted an immune response to the heterologous antibodies deposited in the glomerulus), complement activation does not play a major role in the pathogenesis of the glomerulonephritis. Instead, monocyte infiltration of the kidney appears to be more important.
3. In Heymann nephritis, complement activation apparently mediates the proteinuria in the acute (passive) model but may not in the chronic (active) model of this disorder. The latter is suggested by studies of active Heymann nephritis in the C6 deficient rat, which developed proteinuria despite evidence of inability to form C5b-9.
4. In the IC-mediated GN of acute serum sickness in the rabbit, terminal pathway complement activation is not needed to induce glomerular injury but does play a role in mediating proteinuria. In models of acute serum sickness in the mouse, complement activation appears to be essential to the development of proteinuria. Models of glomerulonephritis in rodents involving acute deposition of negatively charged antigens also requires C5b-9 deposition in glomeruli to fully express proteinuria. The mechanisms by which complement activation exerts its effects in GN are discussed in the following section.

Site of Immune Complex Localization in the Glomerulus as a Determinant of Complement Effects

A key aspect of how complement activation affects the evolution of the GN is whether the complement activation is occurring primarily in the subepithelial space (Heymann nephritis, some models of chronic infusion of heterologous proteins) or whether the complement activation is occurring primarily in or near the glomerular capillary lumen (nephrotoxic serum nephritis, Concanavalin A model, Thy1 model). ICs that form in the glomerular subepithelial space appear to be less able to induce infiltration of the glomerulus by circulating leukocytes, compared with models in which the ICs form in the subendothelial or mesangial space, or on GBM. Apparently, C5a generated by complement activation acts more effectively as a chemoattractant for neutrophils and monocytes when the complement activation occurs within the glomerular subendothelial space or mesangium. However, this distinction appears not to be absolute. Complement-mediated localization of monocytes to the kidney contributes to the induction of proteinuria in Heymann nephritis, even though the ICs form in the subepithelial space.

Effects of Glomerular Subepithelial Immune Complex Formation

When ICs form in the glomerular subepithelial space, the classical pathway is activated because the antibodies are virtually always IgG. Complement activation results in deposition of C5b-9 on the glomerular epithelial cell membrane. The amount of C5b-9 deposited may be greater if the antibodies bind to epitopes expressed on the glomerular epithelial cells (GEC), rather than to planted antigens in the glomerular subepithelial space. If the amount of C5b-9 deposited on the GEC membrane is sublytic (i.e., does not result in lysis of the GEC), the cell can become activated to produce collagen and products of arachidonic acid metabolism (increased thromboxane, $PGF_{2\alpha}$, and PGE production). The products of arachidonic acid metabolism appear to play a protective role as suggested by worsening of nephrotoxic serum nephritis by cyclooxygenase inhibition.

Sublytic doses of C5b-9 can also stimulate the production of oxidants and proteinases by GEC. This could promote proteinuria and impaired kidney function by the following mechanisms: (a) damage to the GEC results in separation of the GEC from GBM. This leads to increased ultrafiltration at that site and increased proteinuria, apparently by bulk flow through the site of increased hydraulic conductivity. (b) loss of GBM anionic charge, which promotes albuminuria, and (c) damage to GBM with the development of shunt pathways that permit nonselective proteinuria.

A key role for glomerular C5b-9 deposition in causing proteinuria in membranous nephropathy is indicated by studies of C6 depletion in the Sprague-Dawley rat with glomerular subepithelial deposits induced by infusion of cationized human IgG, and in studies involving complement depletion in the media of isolated glomeruli of Sprague-Dawley rats treated with anti-Fx1A antibody. Nevertheless, heavy proteinuria can occur in active Heymann nephritis in the absence of C5b-9 formation as shown in studies in genetically C6-deficient rats, which are unable to form C5b-9. In these studies the size of the glomerular subepithelial electron-dense deposits correlated with the magnitude of the pronteinuria. Taken together these studies suggest that the proteinuria induced by glomerular subepithelial IC formation is influenced both by the ability to generate C5b-9 and the mechanical effects of the subepithelial deposits.

Effects of Glomerular Subendothelial or Mesangial Immune Complex Formation

When ICs form in the subendothelial space or when complement activation is a result of antibodies binding to GBM, the resulting C3b deposition on GBM can itself alter glomerular function and induce proteinuria. In addition, C3b on glomerular structures permits immune adherence of neutrophils and monocytes via CR1 expressed on those cells. Complement activation also promotes adherence of neutrophils and monocytes by inducing upregulation of adhesion molecules on endothelial cells. Moreover, activated neutrophils can initiate complement activation by release of H_2O_2, creating a "vicious cycle." Infiltrating neutrophils and monocytes release proteases, which may be important causes of glomerular injury. Neutrophils also release oxidants (which have been shown to induce glomerular injury and proteinuria) and eicosanoids (which may be protective). The accumulation of neutrophils and monocytes in glomeruli is chiefly the result of the chemotactic effects of C5a. C5a can also directly cause renal vasoconstriction and decrease GFR.

Studies in the genetically C6-deficient rat have shown that C5b-9 generation in the glomerulus is necessary to fully express the lesions of the anti-Thy1.1 model of nephritis: mesangial necrosis, glomerular platelet accumulation, mesangial cell proliferation, and proteinuria. Nitric oxide, induced by complement activation in anti-Thy1.1 nephritis, may play an important role in the glomerular injury of this model.

Interaction of complement with complexed antibody and antigen in the vicinity of endothelial cells increases endothelial cell permeability, perhaps as a direct result of insertion of C5b67 into endothelial cells. This results in the formation of gaps between endothelial cells but does not result in endothelial cell death or necrosis. This complement-mediated increase in capillary permeability would contribute to the inflammatory process.

Complement and Platelets in Glomerulonephritis

In nonprimates (e.g., rodents), platelets may aggregate at sites of glomerular injury via adherence of the platelet C3b receptors to deposited C3b. Primate platelets, including those of humans, lack C3b receptors and may be less likely than nonprimate platelets to localize at sites of complement-mediated injury. This could be an important difference between the responses of the primate kidney and the nonprimate kidney to complement-induced injury. Indeed, there is impressive evidence that in nonprimates, complement-dependent platelet accumulation mediates many of the adverse effects of glomerular IC formation including impaired GFR, proteinuria, and proliferation of resident cells of the glomerulus. It remains to be determined whether the platelets or their products (e.g., PDGF) in humans and other primates can play a similar role.

Production of Complement Components Within the Kidney

Production of complement components C2,3,4 and factor B by resident kidney cells (glomerular and tubular) has been demonstrated under various *in vivo* and *in vitro* circumstances. The role of local synthesis of complement components is not clear. However, they could participate in the inflammatory process or serve paracrine or autocrine roles. Of note is that C3 may act as a growth factor. Thus it is possible that local C3 generation is part of normal defense/repair/growth processes, which are intensified under conditions of biologic stress.

Other events that promote glomerular injury in immune nephritis, but are not directly the result of complement activation, include the adherence of neutrophils and monocytes via their Fc receptors to the glomerular immune deposits, the adherence of neutrophils and monocytes to endothelium via adhesion molecules expressed on their surfaces, and the recruitment of sensitized T cells to the glomerulus.

DIAGNOSTIC SIGNIFICANCE OF SERUM COMPLEMENT LEVELS

The measurement of serum or plasma complement levels, particularly C3, C4, and CH50, commonly are used to assess for the presence of IC-mediated disease or, in patients with a known IC-mediated disorder, to assess for disease activity. Table 37.12 shows the principal IC-mediated disorders that are associated with hypocomplementemia.

For patients whose complement status is being evaluated for the first time, we recommend the measurement of serum C3 and C4 levels and CH50 levels generally from ethylenediaminetetraacetic acid (EDTA) treated plasma. The CH50 assay assesses the overall function of the classical and terminal complement pathway components C1 to C8 (C9 is not required for hemolysis in the CH50 assay). Thus, the measurement of CH50 is useful as a screening test for hypocomplementemic states that would be missed if only C3 and C4 levels were measured. The CH50 assay is less useful as a monitor of serial changes in serum complement levels because, for example, C3 and C4 levels may be abnormally low, yet the capacity of the patient's serum to hemolyze the sensitized sheep erythrocytes, the basis for the CH50 assay, may remain within the normal range. In addition, results of the CH50 assay may be more variable because it is more difficult to standardize than immunoassayable serum C3 and C4 levels.

In patients with classical complement pathway activation, C3 and C4 levels are changed proportionately (Fig. 37.16). In patients with primarily alternative complement activation, C4 levels are preserved but C3 levels are decreased. Some reports have suggested that in certain IC-mediated disorders (e.g., type II cryoglobulinemia or SLE), C4 levels are disproportionately low compared with C3 levels. This has led to the suggestion that in these disorders there may be increased consumption of C4 as compared with C3. However, it is more likely that the low C4 levels relative to C3 levels in these disorders represent the effects of C4 null genes in the affected individuals. C4 null genes occur commonly in the general population and with increased frequency in IC-mediated diseases such as SLE.

When serum complement levels are measured serially to assess activity of SLE, it is sufficient to measure only C3 levels. Although changes in serum C3 and C4 levels are highly correlated in SLE because the normal range for C4 levels is relatively much greater than that of C3 levels (an effect of the presence of C4 null genes in the general population), serum C3 levels are more likely to change from normal to abnormal during SLE activity than are serum C4 levels.

TABLE 37.12. Immune Complex–Mediated Diseases Associated with Hypocomplementemia

Disease	Patterns of Hypocomplementemia
SLE	C3, C4, decreased proportionately
MPGN type 1	C3 decreased more than C4 (effect of C3 Nef)
Cryoglobulinemia	
types I, III	C3, C4 decreased proportionately
type II	C4 may be decreased more than C3
GN of chronic infection (e.g., endocarditis)	C3, C4 decreased proportionately
Postinfectious GN (e.g., poststreptococcal GN)	C3 decreased much more than C4
Other conditions: Rheumatoid vasculitis, idiopathic vasculitis, repeated injection of foreign proteins, drug-induced SLE, hypersensitivity to drugs, chemotherapy for malignancy with IC formation, thyroid disease and GN, jejunoileal bypass with vasculitis, B cell lymphoproliferative disorder with IC formation	Generally, C3, C4 decreased proportionately

C3 Nef, C3 nephritic factor (an antibody that stabilizes C3bBb); GN, glomerulonephritis; MPGN, membranoproliferative glomerulonephritis; SLE, systemic lupus erythematosus.

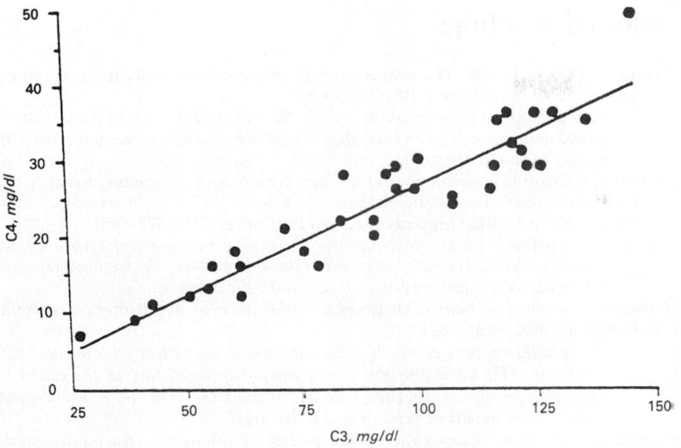

Figure 37.16. Relationship between serum C3 and C4 levels in a typical patient with SLE and glomerulonephritis. The correlation coefficient of this relationship is 0.93 ($p < .001$). The complement levels in this patient were measured by nephelometry.

The role of measurement of products of complement activation (such as C3a des Arg, C3bi, C3dg, Bb, C5b-9) in assessing clinical activity of IC diseases has not been determined.

Although hypocomplementemia often predicts or is evidence of active IC-mediated disease, there are numerous nonimmunologic conditions that also can cause hypocomplementemia. It is important to be aware of these conditions because some of them can induce a systemic disorder that can be easily confused with a IC-mediated vasculitis. These conditions are shown in Table 37.13. In addition, a nonimmunologic condition that causes hypocomplementemia can develop in a patient with an IC-mediated disorder that is inactive. If the physician does not recognize that the hypocomplementemia is the result of the nonimunologic condition, this could lead to incorrect treatment of the patient. The nonimmunologic conditions that could spuriously suggest activity of an IC-mediated disorder, when the nonimmunologic condition develops in a patient with a known IC-mediated disorder, are listed in Table 37.14.

TABLE 37.13. Common Nonimmunologic Diseases That Can Mimic an IC-Mediated Vasculitis Because They Cause Multisystem Disorders and Hypocomplementemia

Disease	Complement Levels	Comment
Atheroembolism	↓ C3, ± ↓ C4	Hypocomplementemia is transient, occurring mainly during active embolization[a]
Severe sepsis	↓ C3, ↓ C4	Development of shock increases likelihood of sepsis causing hypocomplementemia
HUS/TTP	↓ C3, ± ↓ C4	Hypocomplementemia occurs in about 1/2 of cases
Acute pancreatitis	↓ C3, ↓ C4	Hypocomplementemia clears in a few days[a]

[a] By contrast, the hypocomplementemia of active SLE usually requires weeks to return to normal, with successful therapy.

HUS, hemolytic-uremic syndrome; IC, immune complex; TTP, thrombotic thrombocytopenic purpura.

TABLE 37.14. Common Nonimmunologic Conditions That Can Cause Hypocomplementemia and, Should They Be Present in a Patient with Inactive IC-Mediated Disease, Could Spuriously Suggest Activity of the IC-Mediated Disease

Disease	Complement Levels	Comment
The conditions listed in Table 37.13	See Table 37.13	See Table 37.13
Severe malnutrition[a]	↓ C3, ± ↓ N C4	C1q is also low
Severe liver disease	↓ C3, ↓ C4	C1q levels are normal
Inherited C4 deficiency	N1 C3, ± ↓ C4	20% to 40% of normals have 1 or 2 C4 null genes; SLE patients have a higher incidence of this genetic defect

[a] The protein depletion of uncomplicated nephrotic syndrome does not cause low C3 or C4 levels.

↓, decreased; IC, immune complex; N, normal; SLE, systemic lupus erythematosus.

Not all IC-mediated disorders, or disorders mediated by specific binding of antibody to tissues, are associated with hypocomplementemia. The absence of hypocomplementemia in these disorders is probably related to a lesser mass of antibodies involved in these processes. The IC-mediated renal diseases that are rarely or never associated with hypocomplementemia are membranous GN, Henoch-Schönlein purpura, IgA nephropathy, Goodpasture's syndrome, Wegener's granulomatosis, immunotactoid and fibrillary GN, and C1q glomerulopathy.

Certain conditions can raise serum complement levels and therefore could offset the effect of an IC-mediated disease to lower serum complement levels. Of particular relevance in this regard are pregnancy, systemic infections, and noninfectious chronic inflammatory states such as rheumatoid arthritis and idiopathic vasculitis. If these conditions coexist with an active IC-mediated disorder, it is possible that hypocomplementemia might not develop, even though the IC-mediated disease is active. The interaction between a condition that can raise complement levels and a condition that can lower serum complement levels has been particularly well described in SLE patients who become pregnant. In normal pregnancy, serum complement levels often increase to above normal values. Thus a normal complement level in a pregnant SLE patient could indicate activity of her SLE.

PHARMACOLOGIC APPROACHES TO CONTROL COMPLEMENT-MEDIATED RENAL DISEASE

If ICs accumulate within the glomerulus or if complement-activating antibodies bind to endogenous or planted glomerular antigens, the complement system becomes the enemy. Under such conditions, it seems likely that patients would be benefited if complement activation could be attenuated, at least temporarily.

There are four basic approaches to diminish the biologic effects of the complement system: (a) activate the complement system to deplete key component(s), (b) administer an inhibitor of complement activation, (c) administer substances that can absorb activated complement components thereby sparing normal tissue, or (d) physically remove complement components from the circulation.

Approach a has been used extensively in experimental models when CVF is administered to induce C3 depletion. Animals with experimental complement-mediated diseases are usually benefited by CVF treatment. Unfortunately, worsening of tissue injury may occur initially as C3 is depleted by activation of the complement system. As discussed previously, the worsening involves neutrophil activation by complement causing these inflammatory cells to adhere to sites of tissue injury.

In light of the aforementioned concerns, approach b (inhibition of complement activation) may be more desirable than approach a (depletion of complement by activating complement). Presently, heparin is the only inhibitor of complement activation that is available clinically. Unfortunately, the use of heparin for this purpose is not clinically feasible because it must be administered in amounts much greater than that needed to achieve anticoagulation.

The experimental complement inhibitor, soluble recombinant CR1 (sCR1), has been shown to be effective in reducing the acute complement-mediated injury associated with experimental myocardial ischemia, xenografts, gut ischemia, thermal and other forms of skin and lung injury, experimental allergic encephalomyelitis, and experimental nephritis (Con A, Thy1.1, and passive Heymann nephritis). sCR1 can also inhibit complement activation by bioincompatible dialysis membranes.

The results of sCR1 in experimental models of complement injury are encouraging. However, the clinical utility of sCR1 remains to be established. Of interest is that CR1 is normally shed into the plasma, mainly by cleavage of CR1 from neutrophils. Thus plasma CR1 might be a natural mechanism for control of complement activation. Other inhibitors of complement activation, soluble recombinant MCP (sMCP) and DAF (sDAF), have recently been developed. sMCP inhibits complement activation in human and primate systems, but not in rodents. sCR1, sMCP, and sDAF are large proteins that are immunogenic. Thus if these inhibitors are found to be clinically useful it will probably be for the acute, not chronic, treatment of complement-mediated disorders.

Approach c (control of complement activation by infusion of a substance that absorbs activated complement components before they can bind to tissue and initiate further complement activation) is currently being used when high doses of intravenous immunoglobulins (IVIg) are administered. The Fc portion of Ig absorbs C3b and C4b, and dimers of IgG (up to 10% of total IgG in IVIg) bind C1q. These effects of IVIg could explain some of the benefits attributed to IVIg in the treatment of acute immune disorders such as Wegener's granulomatosus.

Approach d (removal of complement) occurs during plasmapheresis, which also removes other plasma components including antibodies and coagulation factors. Plasmapheresis is reported to be of value in the management of a number of immune-mediated disorders. However, the portion of the benefit of plasmapheresis that is attributable to complement removal is not clear. In a controlled prospective randomized trial in SLE patients with severe glomerulonephritis, an 8-week course of plasmapheresis, which had little effect on C3 and C4 levels, did not improve patient outcomes.

In summary, there is considerable evidence that the ability to acutely attenuate the effects of complement activation would be beneficial to patients with certain immune-mediated disorders. At present, there is no entirely satisfactory means to achieve this goal. However, the development of specific inhibitors of complement activation offer hope that this goal may be achieved in the not-too-distant future.

Selected Readings

Fearon DT, Locksley RM. The instructive role of innate immunity in the acquired immune response. *Science* 1996;272:50–54.

This work provides an insightful view of the respective roles of the innate and acquired immune systems and how their interaction produces a true synergism with respect to immune protection.

Hebert LA, Cosio FG, Birmingham DJ. Complement and complement regulatory proteins in renal disease. In: Neilson EG, Couser WG, eds. *Immunologic Renal Disease.* Philadelphia: Lippincott-Raven Publishers, 1997:377–395.

The renoprotective and renoinjurious effects of the complement system are reviewed in detail. The new insights into the mechanism of the immunoprotective role of the complement system in renal disease are examined.

Hebert LA, Cosio FG, Neff J. Diagnostic significance of hypocomplementemia. *Kidney Int* 1991;39:811–821.

A clinically relevant approach to the analysis of the patient with hypocomplementemia. This work also provides a comprehensive listing of the causes of hypocomplementemia, both immune and nonimmune. The use of complement measurement in patient management is discussed.

Morita Y, Nomura A, Yuzawa Y, et al. The role of complement in the pathogenesis of tubulointerstitial lesions in rat mesangial proliferative glomerulonephritis. *J Am Soc Nephrol* 1997;8:1363–1372.

This work shows for the first time the important effect of nonspecific proteinuria to cause tubulointerstitial injury from activation of complement. This work provides a strong rationale regarding the beneficial effects of reductions of proteinuria on progression of proteinuric renal diseases.

Ross GD. *Immunobiology of the complement system.* Boston: Harcourt Brace Jovanovich, 1986.

This textbook is a concise yet detailed discussion of all aspects of the complement system. The many clear figures and tables facilitate understanding of the complexities of the complement system. This work is intended to help those who are not expert in complementology.

PART 6
Role of Leukocytes and Leukocyte Adhesion Molecules in Glomerular, Tubular and Vascular Diseases

Hamid Rabb, Kulwant Modi, and Michael O'Donnell

In many forms of renal disease, white blood cells are found to invade parts of the kidney that are normally sparse in leukocytes. Other forms of renal disease not characterized by obvious leukocyte infiltration may nonetheless respond to immunosuppressive treatment directed against leukocytes. Thus leukocytes have been frequently invoked in the pathogenesis of these kidney diseases. Over the last two decades, advances in immunology and molecular biology have shed light on numerous leukocyte functions and novel ways in which such functions can be studied and regulated.

Movement of leukocytes from the circulation to a site of inflammation is driven by local production of cytokines and chemoattractant substances. Leukocyte infiltration requires that leukocytes first adhere to the vascular endothelium before emigrating across the endothelium and basement membrane to reach the tissue site of inflammation. Adherence of leukocytes to the endothelium involves cell surface molecules known as *leukocyte adhesion molecules* (LAMs) present on both endothelial cells and leukocytes. Once leukocytes have traversed blood vessel walls and reached the site of inflammation, they can release cytokines and chemoattractants to enhance the process of leukocyte infiltration, then release lysosomal enzymes and reactive oxygen molecules that cause tissue injury characteristic of the inflammatory process. In addition, leukocytes attach to parenchymal cells (e.g., glomerular mesangial cells or tubular epithelial cells in the kidney) through specific adhesion molecules, and alter cell function. Of clinical significance, manipulation of LAMs offers the potential for novel therapies in the treatment of leukocyte-mediated kidney diseases. In this chapter, we review some basic features of LAMs, discuss the clinical context of leukocyte involvement in kidney diseases, review experimental data on LAM modulation to treat renal diseases, and propose some future directions in this field.

BIOLOGY OF LEUKOCYTE ADHESION MOLECULES

LAMs were first discovered when parallel studies revealed that children with rare childhood immunodeficiency characterized by recurrent bacterial infections were deficient in a leukocyte cell-surface receptor, CD11/CD18. This receptor was found to regulate numerous leukocyte functions, including adhesion to endothelium, phagocytosis, and antigen recognition. Molecular cloning revealed that the CD11/CD18 molecule belonged to a larger family of cell-adhesion receptors called *integrins,* which span cell membranes to facilitate communication between the extracellular environment and the cell interior.

To date, 10 major subfamilies of integrins have been discovered. The integrins are heterodimeric transmembrane proteins that each contain an α and β subunit. Integrin subfamilies (e.g., β_1, β_2) are defined by the presence of a common β subunit that interacts with different α subunits. Chemoattractants, such as complement (C) fragment C5a and leukotriene (LT)B_4, and chemokines such as interleukin (IL)-8, can augment the cell-surface expression of integrins as well as integrin affinity for endothelial cell counterreceptors. The intracellular domains of integrins associate with cytoskeleton proteins, such as talin and vinculin. Integrins demonstrate selectivity of cell expression and bind to a variety of different ligands. The reader is referred to Table 37.15 to assist with understanding of the current nomenclature of integrins and other LAMs.

At least three integrin subfamilies are of known importance to the nephrologist. β_1 integrins have been identified on cell membranes of lymphocytes and glomerular endothelial, epithelial, and mesangial cells, and are involved in both cell–cell and cell–matrix interactions. β_1 integrins are also referred to as the *very late activation* (VLA) family because these antigens were first discovered to be expressed 2 to 4 weeks after leukocyte stimulation. The β_1 integrin VLA-4 ($\alpha_4\beta_1$) is expressed by lymphocytes, basophils, and eosinophils, but usually not on neutrophils, and binds to an inducible adhesion-molecule receptor on endothelial cells known as *vascular cell adhesion molecule-1* (VCAM-1). Epithelial and mesangial cells also express VCAM-1, facilitating these cells to interact with leukocytes bearing VLA-4. β_1 integrins also serve as receptors for the extracellular matrix proteins collagen, laminin, and fibronectin. Ligands for β_1 integrins include arginine–glycine–aspartic acid (RGD) sequences of fibronectin and laminin, as well as the fibronectin sequence CS-1.

The β_2 integrins include several CD11/CD18 subtypes expressed exclusively on leukocytes. CD11a/CD18 (LFA-1) is found on the outer cell membranes of all leukocytes, and binds primarily to the inducible receptor *intercellular adhesion molecule-1* (ICAM-1) on endothelial cells, epithelial cells, glomerular mesangial cells, and leukocytes themselves. CD11a/CD18 also binds to the constitutive receptor ICAM-2 on endothelial cells, as well as to ICAM-3 on leukocytes. Expression of CD11b/CD18 and CD11c/CD18 appears to occur only in monocytes/macrophages, neutrophils, natural killer cells, and some B cells. CD11b/CD18 binds to ICAM-1 on endothelial cells, and both CD11b/CD18 and CD11c/CD18 bind

TABLE 37.15. Major Families and Examples of Leukocyte Adhesion Molecules

Family	Adhesion Molecule	Alternate Name(s)	Distribution	Ligand(s)
Selectins	E-selectin	ELAM-1	Endothelium	sLe^x, GlyCAM-1
	L-selectin	LAM-1, Mel-14	Leukocytes	sLe^x, GlyCAM-1
	P-selectin	CD62P	Platelets, endothelium	sLe^x, PSGL-1
Integrins				
β1 integrins (VLA proteins)	VLA-4	$\alpha_4\beta_1$	Leukocytes	VCAM-1, CS-1
β2 integrins	CD11a/CD18	LFA-1, $\alpha_L\beta_2$	Leukoctyes	ICAM-1, -2, -3
	CD11b/CD18	Mac-1, Mo-1, $\alpha_M\beta_2$	Monocytes, neutrophils	ICAM-1, iC3b
	CD11c/CD18	p150, 95	Monocytes, neutrophils	iC3b, fibrinogen
	CD11d/CD18	$\alpha_d\beta_2$	Leukocytes	ICAM-3
β7 integrins	$\alpha_4\beta_7$	LPAM-1	B and T cells	VCAM-1, fibronectin
Ig superfamily	ICAM-1	CD54	Leukoctyes, endothelium, epithelium, mesangium	CD11a/CD18, CD11b/CD18
	ICAM-2		Endothelium	CD11a/CD18
	ICAM-3		Lymphocytes	CD11a/CD18
	VCAM-1	INCAM 110	Endothelium, epithelium, mesangial cells Glomerular parietal cells	VLA-4, $\alpha_4\beta_7$
	LFA-2	CD2	T cells	LFA-3
	LFA-3	CD58	Erythrocytes	LFA-2
Cadherins	E-cadherin	L-CAM	Adult epithelial cells	
	N-cadherin	A-CAM	Adult nerve and muscle	
	P-cadherin		Adult placenta and epithelial cells	

Modified from Rabb H, O'Meara YM, Maderna P, et al. Leukocytes, cell adhesion molecules and ischemic acute renal failure. *Kidney Int* 1997;51:1463–1468.

complement fragment iC3b and fibrinogen. CD11d/CD18 is less well understood but may be involved in macrophage adhesion.

The β_3 integrin subfamily contains the important platelet receptor GPIIb/IIIa (CD41/CD61), which binds fibrinogen and von Willebrand's factor. Enhanced adhesion of platelets through IIb/IIIa is a major factor in the pathogenesis of clot formation. Naturally occurring mutations in this receptor predispose to coronary ischemia in humans, and recombinant antagonists of IIb/IIIa are in clinical use for the treatment of myocardial ischemia. This integrin is a potential target to modulate platelet-mediated renal diseases.

Adhesion molecules that serve as ligands for integrins include immunoglobulin supergene family members (Table 37.15). ICAM-1 is found on many cell types and binds leukocyte CD11/CD18. Pathogens such as malaria, rhinovirus, and respiratory syncytial virus also bind ICAM-1 during host invasion. VCAM-1 binds the β_1 integrin VLA-4. Other adhesion molecules now classified in this family include CD4 and CD8 molecules on T cells and the tumor marker, carcinoembryonic antigen (CEA).

Adhesion molecules termed *selectins* are expressed on the cell membranes of endothelial cells (E-selectin, P-selectin), platelets (P-selectin), and leukocytes (L-selectin), and are responsible for initial leukocyte tethering and rolling on endothelium before emigration into inflamed tissue (Table 37.15). The selectins are referred to as such because they are members of the group of carbohydrate-containing binding proteins known as *lectins*. E-selectin is not expressed by normal, inactivated endothelium, but rather expression is induced by local production of proinflammatory cytokines, including IL-1β, tumor necrosis factor-α (TNF-α), and interferon-γ. L-selectin is constitutively expressed by neutrophils, monocytes, and some lymphocytes. Selectin ligands are only beginning to be characterized, but many appear to require fucosylation to be active. The requirement of sugars for selectin function is of potential clinical significance because of the possibility of developing sugar-based therapy to interrupt selectin function.

Addressins are a family of adhesion molecules that appear to mediate selective leukocyte recruitment to specific organ sites, or "addresses." Leukocyte homing to inflamed gut is known to be mediated by specific addressins. As yet, kidney-specific addressins have not been reported.

It should be noted that the number of adhesion molecules and their known functions is growing steadily. The avidity of adhesion molecule binding to ligand, the quantity of adhesion molecule expression, and other features of adhesion molecule function can be regulated by many different substances. In this regard, certain cytokines (e.g., TNF-α, IL-1β) have been found to stimulate expression of ICAM-1, VCAM-1, and L-selectin ligands. Chemokines such as cytokine-induced neutrophil chemoattractant (CINC) and macrophage inflammatory protein-2 (MIP-2) may also modulate LAM expression. Recently, a family of soluble and cell-surface molecules dubbed *disintegrins* has been discovered. These molecules may inhibit competitively integrin binding to ligand, and may be important in the regulation of cell-matrix interactions.

ROLE OF LEUKOCYTES AND LEUKOCYTE ADHESION MOLECULES IN GLOMERULAR DISEASES

Glomerular leukocyte infiltration is a common feature of many types of glomerulonephritis (GN), including diffuse proliferative GN, rapidly progressive GN, membranoproliferative GN, and focal mesangial or focal necrotizing GN. In some cases, deterioration in renal function and ultimate outcome appear to be related to leukocytic infiltration. This is exemplified in lupus nephritis, in which the diffuse proliferative subtype has a much poorer outcome than the subtype with membranous changes and a paucity of leukocytes. Investigators have also used special stains to identify infiltrating leukocytes that are not readily detected by routine light microscopy. These studies have indicated that, in addition to diseases in which leukocyte infiltration has been obvious using conventional techniques, other human renal diseases are also characterized by pronounced leukocyte infiltration. Indeed, pauci-immune glomerulonephritis has been shown recently to have prominent T-cell infiltration.

In an effort to understand how leukocytes infiltrate the glomerulus, numerous studies have searched for altered glomerular expression of LAMs in human biopsies, as well as in experimental models of GN. Increased glomerular and tubular ICAM-1 expression has been found in most human GN specimens. Interestingly, increased ICAM-1 expression may also occur in glomerular diseases that are not characterized by leukocyte infiltration, such as minimal-change disease and membranous nephropathy. Glomerular and tubular expression of VCAM-1 is prominent in many cases of lupus nephritis, crescentic GN, and IgA nephritis. It is important to note that LAM function may be related more to receptor activation state than to actual receptor levels. Thus it is possible that increased glomerular adhesion of leukocytes might occur without a detectable increase in levels of LAMs. Conversely, decreased leukocyte infiltration can occur in the setting of persistent LAM expression.

In experimental models of GN, glomerular localization of circulating leukocytes has long been recognized. The model of anti–glomerular basement membrane (GBM) nephritis has been extensively studied regarding the role of leukocytes and LAMs in the pathogenesis of glomerular injury. Acute anti-GBM nephritis is characterized by glomerular neutrophil infiltration, whereas the chronic phase is characterized primarily by monocyte/macrophage infiltration. Leukocyte infiltration in this model is necessary for glomerular injury, as manifested by proteinuria, and for the subsequent development of glomerulosclerosis.

Because glomerular neutrophil infiltration is a hallmark of acute anti-GBM nephritis, several studies have investigated the possible role of selectins in the pathogenesis of this glomerular disease. In rats with anti-GBM nephritis, glomerular E-selectin was found to be upregulated, but neither anti-E–selectin antibody nor anti-P–selectin antibody reduced polymorphonuclear leukocyte (PMN) infiltration or proteinuria. Platelet P-selectin can facilitate leukocyte–leukocyte and leukocyte–endothelial adhesion, which in turn creates microvascular ischemia (Fig. 37.17). In mice with anti-GBM nephritis, glomerular endothelial expression of P-selectin was found just before PMN infiltration, and anti-P–selectin antibody reduced PMN infiltration and proteinuria. By contrast, in a different study, P-selectin–deficient mice with anti-GBM nephritis had increased PMN infiltration and *worse* proteinuria than P-selectin–replete mice.

The role of L-selectin in glomerular PMN infiltration is also not clear. L-selectin has been found to mediate PMN adhesion to glomerular endothelial cells *in vitro*, and cytokine activation of endothelial cells induced the expression of L-selectin ligand. Collectively, the aforementioned studies indicate that the role of selectins in glomerular neutrophil influx characteristic of immune-mediated GN is equivocal. Indeed, it has been suggested that selectins may be relatively unimportant for endothelial adhesion of neutrophils in anti-GBM nephritis because glomerular capillary blood flow may be slow as a result of intracapillary coagulation or thrombosis. Rather, β_2 integrins may be much more important for leukocyte adhesion and emigration in such a setting.

Several lines of evidence support a role for interactions between CD11/CD18 and ICAM adhesion molecules in the patho-

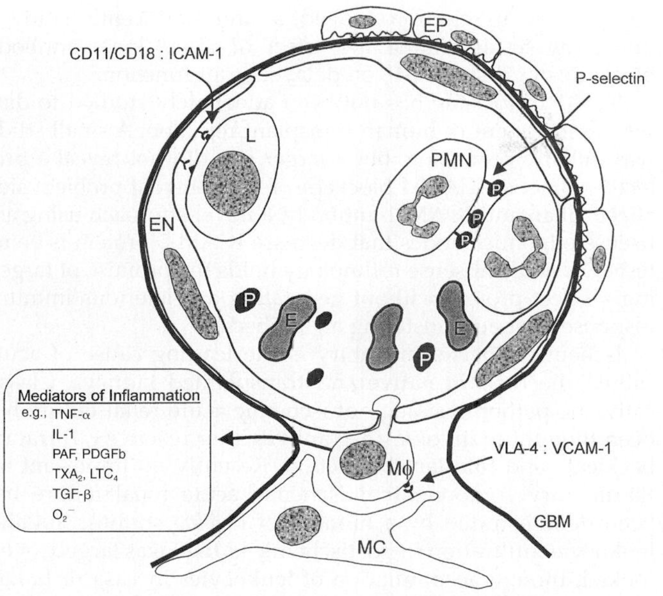

Figure 37.17. Leukocytes and adhesion molecules in glomerular inflammation. Neutrophils, macrophages, and T cells can adhere to activated glomerular endothelium via selectins, CD11/CD18–ICAM-1 and VLA-4–VCAM-1 interactions. Transmigration between endothelial cells occurs, followed by infiltration into the mesangial space. Leukocytes are recruited by numerous cytokines and chemokines, and upon invasion into mesangium, serve to further upregulate inflammation and to contribute to fibrosis. In addition, platelets, via P-selectin, can form bridges between leukocytes in the glomerular capillary, contributing to thrombosis and facilitating extravasation of cells. E, erythrocyte; EN, endothelial cell; EP, epithelial cell; GBM, glomerular basement membrane; L, lymphocyte; MC, mesangial cell; Mϕ, macrophage; P, platelet; PMN, polymorphonuclear leukocyte.

genesis of experimental GN. In rats with anti-GBM nephritis, ICAM-1 is upregulated on the glomerular endothelium and mesangium, and ICAM-1 upregulation is dependent on local production of TNF-α and IL-1β. Both anti-CD11/CD18 and anti–ICAM-1 antibodies have been found to reduce PMN influx in rats with acute anti-GBM nephritis, and to inhibit PMN adhesion to glomerular endothelial and mesangial cells *in vitro*. Evidence suggests that CD11b/CD18 may be of particular importance for PMN infiltration. In addition, PMNs may infiltrate the glomerulus through interactions between CD11/CD18 and ICAM-2, which is constitutively expressed on glomerular endothelial cells.

Studies have also indicated CD11/CD18-independent mechanisms of glomerular neutrophil infiltration and activation. In this regard, platelets appear to augment glomerular neutrophil influx in rats with acute anti-GBM nephritis. Indeed, platelets and neutrophils comigrate into the glomerulus, with platelets expressing the β_3 integrin, IIb/IIIa. Coactivation of neutrophils and platelets then occurs via interaction of IIb/IIIa with fibrinogen, and appears to be important for development of glomerular injury.

β_1 integrins may also be important for glomerular neutrophil influx. Studies have shown that neutrophils can express VLA-4, and that anti–VLA-4 antibody blocks glomerular neutrophil influx and reduces proteinuria in rats with anti-GBM nephritis. A major ligand for VLA-4, VCAM-1, is upregulated in glomerular endothelium and mesangium of rats with anti-GBM nephritis.

Glomerular macrophage infiltration appears to be important for glomerular structural and functional changes that characterize chronic glomerular disease. Monocytes can migrate into the mesangium, where they are transformed into macrophages that persist throughout the chronic phase of many lesions. Macrophages are also particularly prominent in crescentic glomerular lesions, and are believed to play an important role in the process of progressive glomerular scarring through the release of fibrogenic cytokines such as transforming growth factor-β (TGF-β).

Several studies of experimental anti-GBM nephritis suggest that LAMs such as selectins and integrins are important for glomerular monocyte/macrophage infiltration. In rats with anti-GBM nephritis, an anti–P-selectin antibody inhibited glomerular macrophage accumulation and reduced proteinuria. In addition, L-selectin was found to mediate adhesion of monocytes to glomerular endothelial cells *in vitro*.

Monocyte infiltration of inflamed glomeruli appears also to depend on interaction between integrins and ICAM-1. In one study of rats with anti-GBM nephritis, anti-CD11a/CD18 and anti-ICAM-1 antibodies were found to inhibit glomerular monocyte infiltration. Anti-CD11a/CD18 antibody also prevented the development of crescents. In a different study, administration of anti-CD11/CD18 antibody together with anti–VLA-4 antibody reduced monocyte infiltration and proteinuria in nephritic rats although neither antibody alone had an effect. Evidence also suggests that VLA-4 plays a role in glomerular monocyte infiltration. In rats with anti-GBM nephritis, anti–VLA-4 antibody partially reduced monocyte infiltration, but only when preceding neutrophil infiltration was prevented. As previously mentioned, the ligand for VLA-4, VCAM-1, is upregulated in glomeruli of rats with anti-GBM nephritis.

ROLE OF LEUKOCYTES AND LEUKOCYTE ADHESION MOLECULES IN RENAL TUBULAR AND VASCULAR DISEASES

Many renal diseases are characterized by leukocyte infiltration in the interstitium. Acute transplant rejection and acute interstitial nephritis are prominent examples of peritubular leukocyte infiltration. In these acute diseases, leukocytes are felt to directly mediate renal dysfunction (Fig. 37.18). By contrast, in chronic transplant rejection ("chronic allograft nephropathy") and chronic GN, mononuclear leukocytes are usually observed in the interstitium, but their role in disease progression is unclear. In acute tubular necrosis, leukocytes have not classically been associated with disease, but use of special stains has clearly demonstrated leukocyte infiltration in the vulnerable outer medulla of the kidney. Obstructive nephropathy also has been shown to be associated with interstitial leukocyte infiltration, which correlates with renal dysfunction.

Acute allograft rejection is characterized by vascular injury and peritubular leukocyte infiltration. Most current antirejection therapies, including steroids, antibodies against leukocytes, and the immunophilin-binding agents cyclosporine and tacrolimus, are directed against leukocytes. Resolution of an episode of acute rejection is often associated with diminishment of leukocyte infiltration, supporting a role for leukocytes in rejection. It should be noted, however, that leukocyte infiltration is sometimes seen in cases in which acute rejection is not clinically overt. Moreover, renal graft dysfunction may sometimes respond to immunosuppression even in the absence of obvious leukocyte infiltration.

Despite these inconsistencies, acute rejection is accompanied by an upregulation of graft ICAM-1, VCAM-1, and E- and P-selectins. In addition, levels of soluble ICAM-1, VCAM-1, and E-, P-, and L-selectins can be found in the circulation. Unfortunately, infections as well as renal dysfunction itself (by decreasing clearance) can cause an increase in soluble adhesion molecules, limiting the usefulness of monitoring soluble LAMs in detecting rejection. Evaluation of graft LAMs to diagnose rejection is also constrained by findings that ischemia

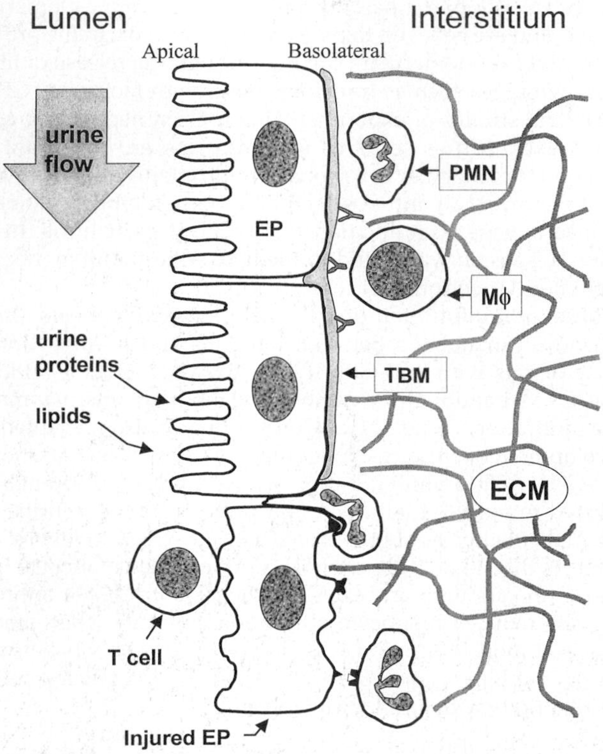

Figure 37.18. Leukocytes and adhesion molecules in tubular injury. Leukocytes are found in the interstitium during interstitial nephritis, allograft rejection, ischemic injury, obstruction, chronic renal failure, and many other diseases. Extravasation occurs at postcapillary venules followed by diapedesis through matrix that includes collagen, laminin, and fibronectin. Leukocytes adhere to tubular epithelial cells and transmigrate between cells. Lipids and protein in urine can recruit inflammatory cells to the interstitium. Epithelial cells, which are injured, are particularly susceptible to both de-adherence from basement membrane and increased adherence to leukocytes. ECM, extracellular matrix; EP, epithelial cell; TBM, tubular basement membrane.

and medications, including cyclosporine, can lead to increased LAM levels in the graft and in the circulation.

Despite the current limits on measurement of LAMs to monitor rejection, upregulation of LAMs during acute rejection has provided the impetus to evaluate LAM blockade as potential therapy for rejection. Blockade of ICAM-1 has been shown to attenuate acute rejection in animal models of renal and heart transplantation. Early blockade of ICAM-1 along with CD11/CD18 during experimental organ transplantation has led to long-term graft tolerance in some studies. Blockade of the VLA-4/VCAM-1 pathway has been less studied, but encouraging data exist to justify further study of the effects of modulating this pathway on both acute and chronic transplant rejection. The VLA-4/VCAM-1 pathway is important in T-cell costimulation, mononuclear cell adhesion, and smooth muscle growth, all of which are potential targets in treating chronic rejection. Selectin blockade is also being evaluated for treatment of acute and chronic transplant rejection. To date, however, experimental studies targeting selectins in transplant rejection have not been as promising as studies targeting integrins or integrin ligands, perhaps, in part, because effective reagents for selectin blockade have not been widely available for testing.

Limited studies in humans with renal allografts have demonstrated that blockade of CD11a/CD18 decreases the incidence of delayed graft function. However, when this pathway was targeted in an attempt to treat acute rejection, minimal protection was seen. Thus modulation of CD11a/CD18 might be more efficacious in treating allograft ischemia-reperfusion injury than acute rejection. Indeed, a large multicenter study is underway to determine the effect of monoclonal antibody blockade of CD11a/CD18 on delayed graft function.

ICAM-1 blockade has not been adequately studied to date for the treatment of human transplant rejection. A small study was initially promising, but a larger one did not reveal a protective effect of ICAM-1 blockade. To circumvent problem side effects of an anti-ICAM-1 antibody, a novel approach using antisense oligonucleotides that decrease ICAM-1 protein is being tested. Use of antisense technology holds the promise of targeting a select protein without generating a deleterious immune response after administering an antibody.

Ischemic reperfusion injury is the leading cause of acute tubular necrosis in native and transplanted kidneys. Classically, the pathophysiology of ischemic acute renal failure has been thought to involve aberrant vascular reactivity, filtration backleak, and tubular obstruction. Recently, an important inflammatory component of ischemic acute renal failure has been demonstrated by a number of *in vivo* studies. Initially, leukocyte infiltration in postischemic kidney was largely overlooked, though accumulation of leukocytes in vasa recta had been recognized for some time. Subsequently, using specific staining, neutrophils, macrophages, and lymphocytes have been shown to infiltrate into postischemic kidney in a number of different species. Leukocytes could potentially worsen postischemic intravascular stasis and release enzymes and oxygen-free radicals (O_2^-) that lead to tubular cell damage.

In an attempt to delineate the role of leukocytes in acute renal failure, the neutrophil was initially targeted because of the large numbers of these cells that infiltrate into postischemic kidney in experimental models, as well as strong evidence for a role of neutrophils in ischemic cardiac injury. However, experimental studies using different neutrophil-depletion techniques have yielded conflicting results, suggesting either a prominent role or no role of neutrophils in the pathogenesis of renal ischemia-reperfusion injury. Interpretation of these studies is complicated also by the clinical observation that neutropenic patients can develop ischemic acute renal failure. Thus the role of neutrophils in the pathogenesis of acute renal failure is still unclear.

Despite conflicting results regarding the role of neutrophils in acute renal failure, the availability of reagents targeting LAMs has led to studies evaluating the effects of LAM blockade on acute renal failure. Studies in rats have consistently shown an important role for ICAM-1 and CD11/CD18 in the pathogenesis of acute renal failure. It also appears that P-selectin is an important mediator of acute renal failure in rats. Studies in mice also support an important role for ICAM-1 and selectins in acute renal failure. Conversely, the few studies in rabbit models of acute renal failure have not shown a role for LAMs in mediating kidney dysfunction.

One might question why blocking LAMs reduces injury in acute renal failure, whereas neutrophil depletion has variable effects. One possible interpretation is that other cell types are involved in the development of ischemia-reperfusion injury, and that LAMs are responsible for more than just mediating neutrophil infiltration to postischemic kidney. Thus LAM blockade could affect other cell types, such as T cells, macrophages, and even resident kidney cells. The results of human studies investigating the effects of LAM blockade on delayed graft function are anticipated eagerly, but with some caution in view of previous failures to date to demonstrate any specific therapy for acute renal failure.

A current clinical controversy that relates to the role of leukocytes and LAMs is the choice of dialysis modality during acute renal failure. Conventional cellulose-based dialysis membranes activate complement, which leads to systemic leukocyte activation and increased avidity of LAMs. This could theoretically facilitate further kidney injury and retard the improvement of acute renal failure. Some clinical trials have demonstrated that use of biocompatible dialysis membranes that cause less complement activation are superior to cellulose membranes with regard to resolution of acute renal failure. This appears to be particularly important when patients are nonoliguric. It appears that delayed graft function in the early transplant period also may be exacerbated by the use of a bioincompatible membrane. However, this issue is not resolved, because some studies have failed to show any beneficial effect of dialysis membrane choice on patient outcome. Another important question is the role of continuous dialysis in the treatment of acute renal failure. Continuous dialysis may be more effective in clearing the deleterious inflammatory mediators that perpetuate acute renal failure. At this time, however, there is no clear answer as to which dialysis membrane or modality best minimizes further kidney injury in acute renal failure.

The incidence of atheroembolic renal disease is increasing, in part due to increased vascular procedures in the aging population. Clear evidence exists for a role of the immune system in the pathogenesis of this disorder. Indeed, organ dysfunction may occur from abnormal tissue inflammatory response to microemboli. Although limited studies evaluating steroid treatment have not shown clear benefit, mononuclear cell infiltration surrounding and close to cholesterol clefts in the kidney suggest that attempts to target these cells, potentially with LAM blockade, could prove fruitful.

Leukocyte infiltration is a common feature of tubulointerstitial nephritis, antitubular basement membrane disease, and obstructive nephropathy. The mechanisms of leukocyte migration into interstitium, their effects on matrix and tubular epithelial cells, and movement into urinary space are essentially unknown. LAMs are upregulated in tubulointerstitial nephritis and reduction of macrophage influx in experimental models of ureteral obstruction is associated with improvement of renal function. However, the role of LAMs in these diseases remains to be investigated.

SUMMARY

LAMs are cell-surface proteins expressed on leukocytes and endothelium, and, in the kidney, on tubular epithelial and mesangial cells. LAMs mediate leukocyte adhesion to endothelial cells, an event that precedes leukocyte migration across the endothelium. LAMs also mediate leukocyte adhesion to parenchymal cells such as epithelial and mesangial cells, and facilitate communication between cells and extracellular matrix proteins. The major families of LAMs include the integrins, selectins, and certain immunoglobulin superfamily members that serve as ligands for integrins.

LAMs play an important role in a variety of normal physiologic processes of the kidney, including cell anchorage, epithelial cell polarity, membrane ion transport, extracellular matrix assembly, and cell differentiation. In addition, an abundance of experimental and clinical evidence indicates that LAMs play a critical role in mediating inflammatory disease processes characterized by tissue leukocyte infiltration. In the kidney, leukocyte infiltration is seen in glomerulonephritis, acute interstitial nephritis, acute and chronic allograft rejection, and postischemic acute renal failure.

Administration of antibodies against specific LAMs has significantly reduced renal injury in animals with experimental glomerulonephritis, acute transplant rejection, and postischemic acute renal failure (Table 37.16). Alternatively, antisense oligonucleotides, which reduce LAM proteins, have reduced renal injury in some animal models of leukocyte-mediated renal disease. Limited studies suggest that anti-LAM antibodies may also ameliorate acute renal failure in human allografts. Of potential clinical significance would be the use of similar therapy to treat native kidney acute renal failure, which at this time has no specific effective therapy. Increasing experimental evidence demonstrates that functional effects of LAM blockade can be dissociated from effects on leukocyte infiltration into kidney. The study of LAMs has revealed much insight into normal and diseased kidney, and holds promise for targeted therapy for immune-mediated renal diseases.

TABLE 37.16. LAM Involvement and Potential Therapies in Select Renal Diseases to Date

Disease	LAM Potentially Involved	Comments and Potential Therapies
Glomerulonephritis		
PMN infiltration	Selectins	Role is equivocal; many experimental studies suggest selectins are not essential for glomerular PMN infiltration
	CD11/CD18–ICAM-1 interactions	Anti-CD18 and anti–ICAM-1 antibodies reduce injury in rats with experimental GN
	VLA-4–VCAM-1 interactions	Anti–VLA-4 antibody reduces PMN influx and proteinuria in rats with experimental GN
Monocyte/Macrophage infiltration	Selectins	Anti–P-selectin antibody reduces MØ accumulation and proteinuria in rats with experimental GN
	CD11/CD18–ICAM interactions	Anti–LFA-1 and anti–ICAM-1 antibodies inhibit glomerular monocyte infiltration in rats with experimental GN; anti–VLA-4 and anti–CD18 antibodies together reduce injury in nephritic rats
Acute allograft rejection	ICAM-1	Blockade attenuates acute rejection in animal models, but has minimal effects in humans; antisense oligonucleotides to reduce ICAM-1 protein are being tried in humans
	VCAM-1	Blockade of VLA-4–VCAM-1 interactions appears to reduce rejection in animal models
	Selectins	Selectin blockade has not been promising in animal models; effective reagents still need to be developed
	CD11a/CD18	Early studies in humans suggest that blockade does not protect against acute rejection but may ameliorate delayed graft function
Acute renal failure	P-selectin	Anti–P-selectin antibody and soluble P-selectin ligand ameliorate ischemic acute renal failure in rats
	ICAM-1 CD11/CD18	Anti-CD11/CD18 and ICAM-1 antibodies ameliorate ischemic ARF in rats and mice; ICAM-1 antisense oligonucleotides reduce postischemic injury in rats

GN, glomerulonephritis; PMN, polymorphonuclear leukocytes.

Selected Readings

Arnaout MA. Leukocyte adhesion molecule deficiency: its structural basis, pathophysiology and implications for modulating the inflammatory response. *Immunol Rev* 1990;114:145–180.

An in-depth review that lays a framework for investigation into both molecular aspects of leukocyte adhesion molecules and clinical studies.

Chiao H, Kohda Y, Craig L, et al. Alpha-melanocyte-stimulating hormone protects against renal injury after ischemia in mice and rats. *J Clin Invest* 1997;99: 1165–1172.

An article that demonstrates that targeting renal inflammation conducted by different mediators, including cytokines and LAMs, is feasible by the use of a single immune-regulating hormone.

Cosio FG, Zager RA, Sharma HM. Atheroembolic renal disease causes hypocomplementaemia. *Lancet* 1985;ii:118–121.

Evidence for mononuclear cell infiltration during experimental cholesterol emboli syndrome.

Gauer S, Yao J, Schoecklmann HO, et al. Adhesion molecules in the glomerular mesangium. *Kidney Int* 1997;51:1447–1453.

An in-depth review focusing on adhesion in the mesangium, a critical area in the pathogenesis of glomerulonephritis. Interactions with matrix and cross talk between cells are highlighted.

Lefkowith JB. Leukocyte migration in immune complex glomerulonephritis: role of adhesion receptors. *Kidney Int* 1997;51:1469–1475.

A review that demonstrates the nuances of LAM involvement in experimental glomerulonephritis. Macrophage migration is contrasted with neutrophils, and underlying mechanisms are discussed.

Mulligan MS, Johnson KJ, Todd RF, et al. Requirements for leukocyte adhesion molecules in nephrotoxic nephritis. *J Clin Invest* 1993;91:577–587.

A comprehensive study that demonstrates a role for different LAMs in an experimental glomerulonephritis model.

Rabb H, Martin JG. An emerging paradigm shift on the role of leukocyte adhesion molecules. *J Clin Invest* 1997;100:2937–2938.

A new hypothesis, based on experimental data, that much of the tissue effects of LAMs during inflammation may actually be independent of mediating leukocyte infiltration into the affected organ. This challenges the conventional rationale for using LAMs to block inflammation.

Rabb H, Mendiola CC, Dietz J, et al. Role of CD11a and CD11b in ischemic acute renal failure in rats. *Am J Physiol* 1994;267:F1052–F1058.

A study that demonstrates by using a rat model of ischemic reperfusion injury that blockade of CD11/CD18 can decrease renal structural and functional damage. Antibodies are used that also block skin responses to bacterial toxin and allergen-induced asthma, demonstrating that diverse diseases may rely on the same effector LAMs.

Rabb H, O'Meara YM, Maderna P, et al. Leukocytes, cell adhesion molecules and ischemic acute renal failure. *Kidney Int* 1997;51:1463–1468.

A review of the conflicting literature on the role of the leukocyte in ischemic acute renal failure, and evidence supporting the role of LAMs. A joint effort to balance the information in this field by two groups of authors who have observed divergent effects of LAMs on acute renal failure.

Springer TA. Traffic signals for lymphocyte recirculation and leukocyte emigration: the multistep paradigm. *Cell* 1994;76:301–314.

A thorough review integrating the complexity of leukocyte emigration from microvasculature that integrates existing knowledge of LAMs and molecules that regulate them.

PART 7
Role of Toxic Oxygen Radicals in Glomerular Injury

Philip R. Mayeux, Norishi Ueda, and Sudhir V. Shah

Treatment of glomerular diseases is empiric because underlying mechanisms that cause glomerular injury are not well known. Thus glucocorticoids and/or immunosuppressive drugs are often used to treat different forms of glomerulonephritides. A better understanding of the mechanisms of glomerular diseases may lead to treatment that is not associated with the complications of glucocorticoids and immunosuppressive drugs.

Oxygen normally accepts four electrons and is converted directly to water. However, partial reduction of oxygen can and does occur in biologic systems leading to the generation of partially reduced and potentially toxic reactive oxygen. Thus sequential reduction of oxygen along the univalent pathway leads to the generation of superoxide anion, hydrogen peroxide, hydroxyl radical, and water. Superoxide and hydrogen peroxide appear to be the primary species generated (Fig. 37.19). These may then play a role in the generation of additional and more reactive oxidants, including the highly reactive hydroxyl radical (or a related highly oxidizing species). Iron salts play a catalytic role in a reaction, commonly referred to as the *metal-catalyzed Haber-Weiss (Fenton) reaction.* In this reaction, superoxide serves as the reductant for Fe^{3+} to generate Fe^{2+}. Fe^{2+} reduces hydrogen peroxide to generate hydroxyl radical. The protective effect of iron chelators, specifically deferoxamine, in numerous model of oxidant injury in the kidney may be explained by its ability to prevent iron from participating in these reactions. However, recent studies suggest that deferoxamine may have other effects unrelated to iron chelation.

Additional reactive oxygen metabolites can be formed as a result of the metabolism of hydrogen peroxide, by neutrophil-derived myeloperoxidase (MPO, the enzyme responsible for the green color of pus), to produce highly reactive toxic products including hypochlorous acid (HOCl, the active ingredient in Clorox Bleach). These oxygen metabolites, including the free radical species, superoxide and hydroxyl radical, and other metabolites such as hydrogen peroxide and hypohalous acids, are often collectively referred to as *reactive oxygen metabolites* (ROM). Recent studies have begun to delineate the importance of a new class of nitric oxide (NO)–derived oxidants that augment the toxicity of ROM.

NO is a relatively stable free radical gas generated from the amino acid L-arginine. The enzyme nitric oxide synthase (NOS) performs a five electron oxidation of L-arginine to yield NO and citrulline. NO is an extremely important cell-signaling molecule. In normal physiology NO generated by vascular endothelial cells plays a key role in regulating systemic vascular tone through its activation of soluble guanylyl cyclase and the formation of the vasodilator cyclic guanosine monophosphate (cGMP). This function is essential for the regulation of medullary and glomerular capillary blood flow. Activated inflammatory cells acquire the ability to generate large amounts of NO through induction of NOS. The induction of NOS is triggered by cytokines in these cells and in glomerular mesangial cells.

NO itself is relatively benign. However, in the presence of superoxide, NO and superoxide react rapidly in a metal-independent manner to form peroxynitrite ($ONOO^-$) (Fig. 37.20). Neither NO nor superoxide are strong oxidants toward most types of organic compounds. However, peroxynitrite is a potent oxidant and nitrating species that can attack a range of biologic

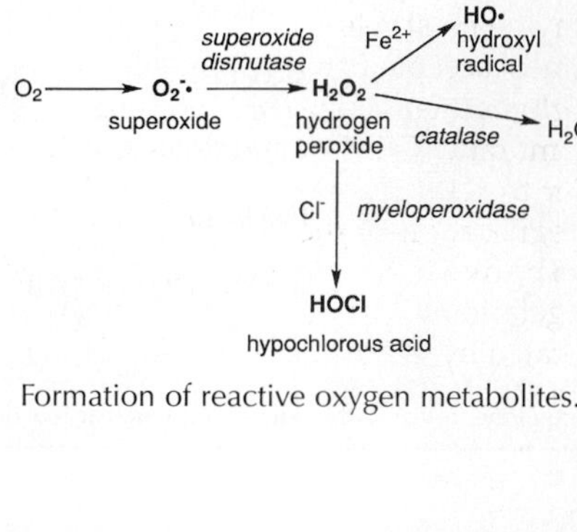

Figure 37.19. Formation of reactive oxygen metabolites.

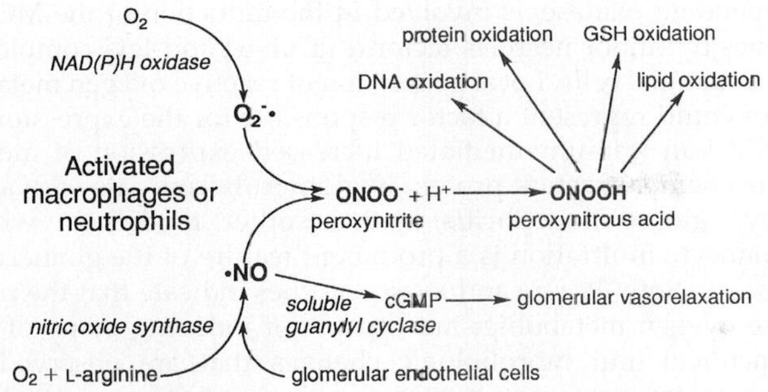

Figure 37.20. Formation of nitric oxide (NO)–derived oxidants.

targets. In the anionic form, it is relatively stable, allowing it to deliver a range of reactivities over a relatively long distance. In the protonated form, it exhibits hydroxyl radical–like activity and can carry out oxidation reactions involving 1- or 2-electron processes. Oxidation of lipid, proteins, and DNA have been reported. The major cellular defense against peroxynitrite is oxidation of cysteine or glutathione.

Although the generation of NO is critical to normal physiology, the generation of peroxynitrite is considered pathologic. Only within the last few years has the importance of peroxynitrite as an oxidant been realized. Hydroxyl radical-scavenging antioxidants, shown to be protective in numerous models of glomerular injury, also scavenge peroxynitrite. In addition, the iron chelator, deferoxamine, is also a potent selective scavenger of peroxynitrite. Thus the importance of Fenton chemistry in the generation of hydroxyl radical in models of glomerular injury in which deferoxamine is protective may need to be reevaluated. It is particularly important to consider the role of NO and peroxynitrite because the rate of reaction between superoxide and NO is three times faster than that between superoxide and detoxifying superoxide dismutase (SOD). Under conditions of infiltrating activated macrophages and neutrophils, the glomerular microenvironment is primed for the generation of both superoxide and NO and thus peroxynitrite.

In the 1990s, numerous studies have examined the role of oxidants in leukocyte- dependent and leukocyte-independent models, and some of the biologic effects of oxidants relevant to glomerular pathophysiology. In this chapter, we present the available evidence in support of the role of oxidants in experimental glomerular disease.

EFFECTS OF REACTIVE OXYGEN METABOLITES RELEVANT TO GLOMERULAR DISEASE

The major manifestations of glomerular disease are proteinuria, altered glomerular filtration rate (GFR), and depending on the type of glomerular disease, some morphologic changes. We have divided the biologic effects of reactive oxygen metabolites into those that may be most relevant to the occurrence of proteinuria, those that may be most relevant to altered GFR, and those that may be most relevant to the morphologic changes.

It is generally accepted that leukocytes cause proteinuria (a hallmark of glomerular diseases) by damaging the glomerular basement membrane (GBM), which serves as the major ultrafiltration barrier to restrict the entry of proteins into the urinary space. The degradation of the GBM by stimulated neutrophils was shown to be due to the activation of a latent metalloenzyme (most likely gelatinase), by hypochlorous acid, or by a similar oxidant generated by the myeloperoxidase–hydrogen peroxide–halide system (Table 37.17).

TABLE 37.17. Effects of Reactive Oxygen Metabolites Relevant in Glomerular Pathophysiology

Relevant to the Occurrence of Proteinuria
ROM participate in GBM degradation
Lipid peroxide induces enhanced generation of gelatinase by mesangial cells.
ROM decrease *de novo* synthesis of glomerular proteoglycans.
ROM increases albumin permeability in freshly isolated glomeruli *in vitro*.
Infusion of phorbol myristate acetate, an activator of neutrophils, results in proteinuria and a fall in GFR; these effects are prevented by catalase.
Hydrogen peroxide infused directly into the renal artery causes massive transient proteinuria by inducing a molecular-size selectivity defect.
Infusion of myeloperoxidase–hydrogen peroxide induces proteinuria.
Relevant to Altered GFR
Reactive oxygen metabolites generated enzymatically or by stimulated neutrophils:
Increase glomerular eicosanoid synthesis.
Increase glomerular cAMP content.
Induce a reduction in glomerular and mesangial cell planar surface and myosin light-chain phosphorylation; these effects appear to be mediated by PAF.
ROM have an effect on release and inactivation of TNF-α.
Relevant to Morphologic Changes
Infusion of myeloperoxidase–hydrogen peroxide causes significant proteinuria, marked influx of platelets, endothelial cell swelling, and epithelial cell foot process effacement; 4–10 days later a marked proliferative glomerular lesion develops.
Scavengers of ROM prevent the reduction in glomerular ADPase activity and increase in platelet aggregation in anti-Thy1 and anti-GBM antibody disease models.
Rats immunized with myeloperoxidase and perfused with lysosomal enzyme extract and hydrogen peroxide developed a proliferative glomerulonephritis.

cAMP, cyclic adenosine monophosphate; GBM, glomerular basement membrane; GFR, glomerular filtration rate; PAF, platelet-activating factor; ROM, reactive oxygen metabolites; TNF, tumor necrosis factor.

Several other studies have shown that oxidants could contribute to GBM damage by increasing its susceptibility to proteolytic damage and by inactivating the α1-proteinase inhibitor (the primary regulator of neutrophil elastase), thus allowing the released elastase to more readily inflict damage to the extracellular matrix. Oxidants also can impair the synthesis of glomerular heparan sulfate proteoglycans. The nascent core peptide appears to be highly susceptible to "selective" direct damage from reactive oxygen metabolites during *de novo* synthesis of heparan sulfate proteoglycans. These molecules are needed to maintain integrity of the GBM and normal glomerular ultrafiltration. The direct *in vivo* effects of reactive oxygen metabolites on glomerular function have been examined in several studies. For example, hydrogen peroxide infused directly into the renal artery caused massive transient proteinuria with no effect on GFR and renal plasma flow. Fractional clearances of graded-sized neutral dextrans of larger molecular radii, an index of glomerular size selectivity, was significantly and substantially elevated after hydrogen peroxide infusion.

These studies indicate that hydrogen peroxide and/or its metabolites generated by neutrophils can cause proteinuria. It can be reasoned that hydrogen peroxide-mediated injury may involve the myeloperoxidase–hydrogen peroxide–halide system. The postulate is particularly attractive in view of the high cationic nature of myeloperoxidase with an isoelectric point of greater than 10. Infusion of myeloperoxidase followed by hydrogen peroxide in a chloride-containing solution into the renal artery in rats results in significant proteinuria followed in 4 to 10 days by the development of a marked proliferative glomerular lesion. These studies indicate that the myeloperoxidase–hydrogen peroxide–halide system is capable of inducing glomerular injury that results in proteinuria.

The effects of ROM that potentially contribute to altered GFR are summarized in Table 37.17. ROM reduce glomerular and mesangial cell planar surface and increase myosin light chain phosphorylation, a biochemical marker of contraction. This suggests that they could modulate the surface area of mesangial cells thus modifying ultrafiltration coefficient and leading to a decrease in the GFR. Generation of NO could also modulate glomerular filtration through cGMP-mediated changes in glomerular hemodynamics. Increased production of prostaglandins and thromboxane have been implicated as important mediators causing proteinuria and/or a fall in the GFR in various experimental models of glomerular disease, including anti-GBM antibody disease, Adriamycin-induced nephrotic syndrome in rats, and complement-mediated glomerular injury. Both reactive oxygen metabolites and NO can increase the synthesis of prostaglandins and thromboxane by activating or inducing cyclooxygenase. Thus some of the observed effects of reactive oxygen metabolites and NO may be mediated through their effect on prostaglandin and thromboxane synthesis. These autocoids may in turn play an important role in the regulation of GFR and in the alterations in renal plasma flow that have been described.

Several studies suggest that reactive oxygen metabolites have several effects that may contribute to the morphologic changes observed in various glomerular diseases (Table 37.17). As mentioned previously, infusion of myeloperoxidase and hydrogen peroxide causes a marked influx of platelets, endothelial cell swelling, and epithelial cell–foot process effacement followed later by a marked proliferative glomerular lesion. In addition, it has been shown that low doses of hydrogen peroxide stimulate the proliferation of cultured rat mesangial cells.

It has been suggested that glomerular adenosine diphosphatase (ADPase) is of major importance in preventing intraglomerular thrombus formation triggered by ADP in experimental glomerulonephritis. Membrane-associated enzymes are apparently highly susceptible to reactive oxygen metabolites. There is a marked decrease in the activity of these enzymes in two models of glomerulonephritis (anti-GBB and anti-thymocyte serum 1 [anti-Thy1]), which are characterized by influx of polymorphonuclear neutrophils. Scavengers of oxygen metabolites prevented the decrease in glomerular ADPase, suggesting a role of reactive oxygen metabolites in the reduction in the glomerular ADPase activity.

Necrotizing crescentic glomerulonephritis associated with anti-MPO antibodies are part of the antineutrophil cytoplasmic autoantibodies (ANCA)–associated glomerulonephritis and is characterized by segmental fibrinoid necrosis of the GBM and marked infiltration of neutrophils and mononuclear cells. The close association of pauci-immune necrotizing glomerulonephritis and anti-MPO antibodies suggests a pathogenic role for anti-MPO–directed immune response. In rats immunized with MPO and perfused with lysosomal enzyme extract and hydrogen peroxide, glomerular intracapillary thromboses developed followed by a proliferative glomerulonephritis characterized by glomerular capillary wall necrosis, extracapillary cell proliferation, infiltration of neutrophils and monocytes, and vasculitis.

A number of monocyte-specific cytokines have been described and include the monocyte colony-stimulating factor (CSF-1), and the monocyte chemoattractant protein (MCP-1). Generation of reactive oxygen species, possibly by NADPH-dependent oxidase, is involved in the induction of the MCP-1 genes by tumor necrosis factor-α (TNF-α) and IgG complexes in mesangial cells. Local generation of reactive oxygen metabolites could represent a factor responsible for the expression of MCP-1 in immune-mediated increased expression of monocyte chemoattractant protein in glomeruli from rats with anti-Thy1 glomerulonephritis, and in other models in which monocyte infiltration is a prominent feature of the glomerular disease. Both *in vitro* and *in vivo* studies indicate that the reactive oxygen metabolites are capable of inducing many of the functional and morphologic changes that are observed in glomerular diseases.

Reactive oxygen metabolites have usually been regarded as toxic metabolites with cytotoxic properties. As mentioned previously, at low concentrations reactive oxygen metabolites seem to play a significant regulatory role without inducing cell death. The effects of reactive oxygen metabolites in altering the cAMP levels and MCP-1 and the CSF-1 genes have been described previously. In addition, regulated generation of low concentrations of reactive oxygen metabolites may serve as intracellular signals for gene activation involving specific transcription factors such as NF-kB in mesangial cells. It is important to note that NOS is also induced by peroxide. Thus the generation of ROM can initiate a cascade of cellular signaling that may augment injury. There are likely to be important interactions between reactive oxygen species and other mediators yet to be described.

ROLE OF OXIDANTS IN LEUKOCYTE-DEPENDENT GLOMERULONEPHRITIS

Several studies have shown that depletion of neutrophils by antineutrophil antibody prevents proteinuria during the heterologous phase of anti-GBM–induced glomerulonephritis and in anti-ConA–induced glomerulonephritis. Furthermore, depletion of monocytes by antimonocyte antibody prevents proteinuria during the autologous phase of anti-GBM–induced glomerulonephritis. Thus these studies strongly support the view that leukocytes mediate glomerular injury that results in proteinuria (Table 37.18).

In neutrophil-dependent glomerulonephritis, circulating PMNs are recruited at the site of immune deposits at subendothelial and mesangial areas by a series of events that involve initial adherence and subsequent migration across the endothelium. Following adherence to the immune site, a wide variety of soluble and particulate stimuli can activate neutrophils and monocytes, resulting in the release of enormous amounts of oxygen-derived and NO-derived oxidants. Of particular interest is the demonstration that several immune reactants, such as serum-treated zymosan (a C3b receptor stimulus), heat aggregated IgG (an Fc receptor stimulus), immune complexes, and complement components, have all been shown to trigger the oxidative burst. Oxygen-derived oxidants are products of a number of enzymes such as oxidases. However, it is important to note that NOS can produce superoxide and hydrogen peroxide in addition to NO. Antineutrophil cytoplasmic autoantibodies present in the circulation of patients with pauci-immune necrotizing vasculitis and pauci-immune crescentic glomerulonephritis have been shown to significantly increase the generation of superoxide by neutrophils. Thus stimulated neutrophils or monocytes are potential sources of oxidants in leukocyte-dependent glomerular injury.

Anti-GBM Antibody Disease

One of the best-characterized models of complement- and neutrophil-dependent glomerular injury is the heterologous

TABLE 37.18. Oxidants in Leukocyte-Dependent Glomerular Disease

In Vitro Studies
A wide variety of soluble and particulate stimuli, including immune complexes, complement components, and ANCA, enhance generation of oxidants by leukocytes.
In Vivo Studies
Cytochemical detection of the presence of superoxide- and hydrogen peroxide–generating leukocytes in anti-GBM–induced and anti-Thy1–induced glomerulonephritis
Enhanced superoxide and hydroxyl radical generated by macrophages isolated from glomeruli of rabbits with anti-GBM antibody disease or glomeruli from the anti-Thy1 model
Induction of nitric oxide synthase in infiltrating leukocytes from human renal biopsy tissue of proliferative glomerulonephritis and in the anti-GBM model
Enhanced generation of nitric oxide by glomeruli isolated from the anti-Thy1 model
Significant reduction in proteinuria by catalase, a hydroxyl radical scavenger, and an iron chelator in complement- and neutrophil-dependent heterologous phase of anti-GBM antibody disease
Protective effect of inhibitors of nitric oxide synthase or an L-arginine–restricted diet in the anti-Thy1 model of proliferative glomerulonephritis

Modified with permission from Shah SV. The role of reactive oxygen metabolites in glomerular disease. *Ann Rev Physiol* 1995;57:245-262.

ANCA, antineutrophil cytoplasmic autoantibodies; GBM, glomerular basement membrane; anti-Thy1, anti-thymocyte serum 1.

phase of anti-GBM antibody disease. Infiltrating neutrophils and macrophages generate large amounts of superoxide anion, hydrogen peroxide, and NO in this model of glomerulonephritis. Treatment with catalase markedly reduces the proteinuria as does dimethylthiourea, a potent hydroxyl radical scavenger, and deferoxamine. Although the role of iron is not completely understood, the protective effect of iron chelators generally has been taken as evidence for the participation of hydroxyl radical in tissue injury because iron is critical in the generation of hydroxyl radical. However, deferoxamine is now known to be an effect scavenger of peroxynitrite. Support for the role of NO in this animal model comes from the ability of the NOS inhibitor, *N*-monomethyl–L-arginine, to protect against the development of proteinuria.

The anti-Thy1 model of glomerulonephritis is also dependent on infiltrating neutrophils and macrophages and their ability to generate oxygen- and NO-derived oxidants. As in the anti-GBM model, *N*-monomethyl–L-arginine protects against the development of proteinuria and mesangial cell injury. Furthermore, a diet low in L-arginine (the substrate for NOS) is also protective. It is clear that stimulated neutrophils or monocytes may serve as sources of ROM and NO in proliferative and exudative glomerulonephritides.

ROLE OF OXIDANTS IN LEUKOCYTE-INDEPENDENT GLOMERULONEPHRITIS

Puromycin Aminonucleoside Model of Minimal-Change Disease in Humans

A single intravenous injection of puromycin aminonucleoside results in marked proteinuria and glomerular morphologic changes that are similar to minimal-change disease in humans. It is clear that ROM play an important role the development of this model (Table 37.19). Puromycin aminonucleoside enhances the generation of superoxide anion, hydrogen peroxide, and hydroxyl radical when added to freshly isolated glomeruli. Glomerular epithelial cells have been shown to be the target of injury in many of the noninflammatory forms of glomerular disease including the nephrotic syndrome induced by the injection of puromycin aminonucleoside. In response to puromycin aminonucleoside, cultured glomerular epithelial cells have been shown to enhance the generation of hydrogen peroxide.

Evidence for the role of superoxide in this model of minimal-change disease comes from the ability of allopurinol (an inhibitor of xanthine oxidase) and superoxide dismutase to protect against puromycin aminonucleoside–induced nephrotic syndrome. Furthermore, proteinuria was significantly reduced in rats receiving polyethylene glycol/catalase suggesting a role for both hydrogen peroxide and superoxide anion in this model of glomerular disease. Several studies have, in fact, shown that enhanced generation of hydrogen peroxide and superoxide anion is accompanied by enhanced generation of hydroxyl radical (or a similar highly oxidizing species). Both hydroxyl radical scavengers and the iron chelator deferoxamine are protective in puromycin aminonucleoside–induced nephrotic syndrome. Although this suggests an iron-catalyzed generation of hydroxyl radical, the role of NO in this model has not yet been investigated.

Several studies indicate a role of reactive oxygen metabolites in glomerular diseases; however, there is no information of whether iron capable of catalyzing free radical reactions is increased in models of glomerular diseases. The role of "catalytic" iron in a model of minimal-change nephrotic syndrome induced by injection of puromycin aminonucleoside to rats was evaluated using deferoxamine. Bleomycin-detectable iron (iron capable of catalyzing free radical reactions) was markedly increased in glomeruli from nephrotic rats when compared with controls. Deferoxamine prevented the increase in the bleomycin-detectable iron in glomeruli and provided complete protection against proteinuria suggesting an important pathogenic role for glomerular catalytic iron in the puromycin aminonucleoside–induced minimal-change nephrotic syndrome.

Several other lines of evidence support a role for reactive oxygen metabolites in puromycin aminonucleoside–induced nephrotic syndrome (Table 37.19). Glucocorticoid administration results in an increase in the activity of superoxide dismutase, an enzyme that scavenges superoxide anion. This is accompanied by protection against both puromycin aminonucleoside–induced and hydrogen peroxide–induced proteinuria. Glutathione peroxidase is a seleno-enzyme that catalyzes the reduction of hydrogen peroxide to water. Feeding rats a selenium-deficient diet results in marked diminution of glutathione peroxidase and is accompanied by a marked increase in urinary protein following puromycin aminonucleoside injection, suggesting an important role of glutathione peroxidase in this model of glomerular disease. Similarly, inhibition of superoxide dismutase

TABLE 37.19. Evidence for the Role of Reactive Oxygen Metabolites in Puromycin Aminonucleoside Model of Minimal-Change Disease

In vitro, cultured glomerular epithelial cells and glomeruli have enhanced generation of hydrogen peroxide.
Scavengers of reactive oxygen metabolites and antioxidants results in reduction in proteinuria in this model of minimal-change disease.
A selenium-deficient diet results in marked diminution of glutathione peroxidase and an increase in proteinuria.
Induction of antioxidant enzymes by glucocorticoids protects against puromycin aminonucleoside-induced proteinuria.
Catalytic iron is increased in glomeruli.

From Baliga R, Ueda N, Shah SV. Oxidant mechanisms in glomerular disease. *Curr Nephrol* 1997;20:135–151..

augments puromycin aminonucleoside–induced proteinuria. These studies not only demonstrate the importance of endogenous antioxidant defenses, but also provide additional support for the role of reactive oxygen metabolites in these models of glomerular injury.

Passive Heymann Nephritis Model of Membranous Nephropathy

Passive Heymann nephritis, induced by a single intravenous injection of anti-Fx1A, is a complement-dependent and neutrophil-independent model of glomerular disease that resembles membranous nephropathy in humans.

Numerous studies suggest that ROM play an important role in this model of membranous nephropathy (Table 37.20). However, the nature of the oxidant is still unclear. Although administration of scavengers of hydroxyl radical or deferoxamine markedly reduce proteinuria, superoxide dismutase or catalase (native or polyethylene glycol-coupled) does not. The protective effects of both the hydroxyl radical scavengers and deferoxamine suggest a role of the hydroxyl radical in passive Heymann nephritis. Similarly, hydroxyl radical scavengers significantly reduced the proteinuria in the cationized gamma globulin–induced immune complex glomerulonephritis, a complement and neutrophil-independent model of membranous nephropathy. Glutathione peroxidase is also an important defense enzyme in this model. Rats on a selenium-deficient diet have decreased glutathione peroxidase activity and a worsening of proteinuria. Taken together these studies suggest an important role for hydroxyl radical in animal models of membranous nephropathy. Initiation of lipid peroxidation by hydroxyl radical may be a key factor in the development of proteinuria in passive Heymann nephritis. Malondialdehyde adducts (a marker of lipid peroxidation) are localized to the GBM, and type IV collagen is modified by malondialdehyde adducts. This site of injury may explain alterations of glomerular permselectivity that results in proteinuria.

TABLE 37.20. Evidence for the Role of Reactive Oxygen Metabolites in an Animal Model of Membranous Nephropathy

In the Passive Heymann Nephritis Model of Membranous Nephropathy
Glomeruli demonstrate the presence of hydrogen peroxide.
Hydroxyl radical scavengers and an iron chelator and probucol reduced proteinuria.
Feeding selenium-deficient diet results in marked diminution of glutathione peroxidase and worsening of proteinuria.
Feeding iron-deficient diet results in a reduction in proteinuria.

From Baliga R, Ueda N, Shah SV. Oxidant mechanisms in glomerular disease. *Curr Nephrol* 1997;20:135–151.

CONCLUSIONS

A sufficient body of *in vitro* and *in vivo* information exists to postulate that reactive oxygen metabolites and NO appear to be important mediators in glomerular pathophysiology. Nonetheless the multifaceted nature of tissue injury makes it almost a certainty that the cooperative and sometimes complex interaction between different injurious mechanisms are important in the final expression of injury. In addition, there are many differences between animal models of glomerular diseases and glomerular diseases in humans. For example, the animal model of minimal-change disease is a toxic model, whereas the mechanism of minimal-change disease in humans is not known. Similarly, the anti-Fx1A antibody that is used for the animal model of membranous nephropathy has been difficult to demonstrate in human membranous nephropathy. Furthermore, the beneficial effects of scavengers of reactive oxygen metabolites or modulators of NO synthesis after the onset of proteinuria have not been demonstrated. Future studies will hopefully provide the answer to the question of the relevance of these studies in animal models to human disease.

Selected Readings

Crow JP, Beckman JS. The importance of superoxide in nitric oxide-dependent toxicity: evidence for peroxynitrite-mediated injury. In: Snyder R, ed. *Biological reactive intermediates V.* New York: Plenum Press, 1996:147–161.

This review presents evidence for the biologically relevant interactions between superoxide and NO and proposes that peroxynitrite is primarily responsible for nitric oxide-mediated pathology in a number of inflammatory conditions.

Diamond JR. The role of reactive oxygen species in animal models of glomerular disease. *Am J Kidney Dis* 1990;19:292–300.

Includes a section on the role of oxidants in progressive renal disease.

Halliwell B, Gutteridge JMC. Role of free radicals and catalytic metal ions in human disease: an overview. *Meth Enzymol* 1990;186:1–85.

Excellent review of free radical biochemistry and detailed explanation of the importance of catalytic iron.

Kaushal GP, Shah SV. Proteases and oxidants in glomerular injury. In: Couser WG, Neilson EG, eds. *Immunologic renal diseases.* Philadelphia: Lippincott-Raven, 1997:397, 415.

Extensive reference list with more than 200 references.

Nath KA, Fischereder M, Hostetter TH. The role of oxidants in progressive renal injury. *Kidney Int* 1994;45(Suppl 45):S111–S115.

Excellent review on the role of oxidants in tubulointerstitial injury and its link with progressive renal disease.

Shah SV. The role of reactive oxygen metabolites in glomerular disease. *Ann Rev Physiol* 1995;57:245–262.

This review provides a comprehensive review of the literature and includes a section on antioxidant defenses.

CHAPTER 38

Immunopathogenesis of Tubulointerstitial Diseases

Catherine M. Meyers

Primary tubulointerstitial nephritis has emerged as an important and distinct clinicopathological entity that accounts for approximately 20% to 40% of chronic renal failure cases and 10% to 25% of acute renal failure cases. Moreover, clinical studies have demonstrated that even in primary glomerular diseases, the extent and severity of tubulointerstitial involvement correlates closely with glomerular filtration rate and the ultimate prognosis for renal function. These observations have therefore stimulated a growing interest in understanding the mechanisms of tubulointerstitial injury.

Concomitant with recognizing the importance of tubulointerstitial damage in renal disease, many observations have also suggested that, like glomerulonephritis, many forms of tubulointerstitial injury are immune-mediated (Table 38.1). For example, primary tubulointerstitial nephritis typically occurs with a dense mononuclear cell infiltrate, is frequently seen as a sequelae to an allergic drug reaction, and is occasionally associated with granular or linear IgG and/or (C3) deposition along the tubular basement membrane (TBM). The earliest models employed to study these phenomena focused primarily on the antibody or immune complex deposition along the TBM and within the tubulointerstitium. In view of the propensity for mononuclear cell infiltrates in most forms of human tubulointerstitial disease, newer studies have evaluated the cell-mediated responses within the tubulointerstitium. These experimental systems have provided useful reagents to further investigate effector mechanisms of deleterious tubulointerstitial immune processes.

To understand events leading to tubulointerstitial injury, the nephritogenic immune response may be dissected into three distinct processes (Table 38.2). The first comprises the immune recognition of the tubulointerstitium, which includes expression, processing, and presentation of a relevant antigen, as well as the genetically determined ability of the organism to respond to that antigen. Regulatory events that modulate quantitative and qualitative expression of an immune response may either amplify or dampen these responses at their initiation or after the immune response is established. Such regulatory responses may be mediated by endogenous regulatory T cells, or cytokines derived from them, and by α-idiotypic antibodies. Administration of exogenous immunosuppressive agents such as cyclosporine and cyclophosphamide has also been successful in abrogating tubulointerstitial injury. The third limb of this nephritogenic immune response involves effector pathways of tubulointerstitial injury. This process may include antibody-mediated damage through immune complex deposition and *in situ* formation, cell-mediated events with antigen-specific T cells, activated macrophages, and natural killer cells, or damage mediated by soluble factors.

This review uses this framework of the nephritogenic immune response to examine experimental models of tubulointerstitial nephritis and their relevance to human disease. The first section evaluates requirements for immune recognition and response to the tubulointerstitium. The second section discusses studies that have characterized tubulointerstitial cell-mediated events. The third section considers humorally mediated responses, including immune deposit–mediated and αTBM antibody–mediated disease. The final section examines regulation of tubulointerstitial immune responses, discussing experimental manipulations that downregulate expression of disease, as well as factors that affect progression of interstitial damage.

TABLE 38.1. Human Tubulointerstitial Disease

Cell-mediated responses
Primary tubulointerstitial nephritis
drug-induced tubulointerstitial nephritis (β-lactams, nonsteroidal antiinflammatory drugs, sulfa drugs)
Infection-related tubulointerstitial nephritis
Medullary cystic disease
Chronic obstructive pyelonephritis
Hydronephrosis
Idiopathic tubulointerstitial nephritis
Progressive glomerulonephritis
Renal transplant rejection
Humorally mediated responses
Associated with αTBM antibodies
Renal transplantation
Drug-induced tubulointerstitial nephritis (methicillin, phenytoin, rifampin)
Primary αTBM disease
αGBM disease
Associated with immune complexes
Systemic lupus erythematosus
Sjögren's syndrome
Essential mixed cryoglobulinemia
Idiopathic tubulointerstitial nephritis
Progressive glomerulonephritis

TABLE 38.2. Nephritogenic Immune Response

Immune Recognition	Regulatory Mechanisms	Effector Pathways
Genetic susceptibility (Ir genes)	Antigen-specific	Humorally mediated
Abrogation of self tolerance	Regulatory T-cell subsets:	Immune complex deposition
Antigen expression	Th, Ts, Tcs	*In situ* formation
Antigen processing and presentation	Antiidiotypic reactions	T cell–mediated
Antigen recognition by Th and B cells	Antigen-nonspecific	Cytotoxicity (perforin, serine esterases)
	Cyclophosphamide	Delayed-type hypersensitivity
	PGE_1	Activated macrophages, natural killer cells
	Nitric oxide	Proinflammatory/fibrotic events
	Antiinflammatory cytokines	Chemoattractant release (chemokines)
	AII	Complement, oxygen radical release
		Cytokines (IL-1, IL-6, TGF-β, TNF-α)
		Nitric oxide
		AII
		Proteinuria

AII, angiotensin II; PGE, prostaglandin E.

INDUCTION OF THE NEPHRITOGENIC IMMUNE RESPONSE

To initiate an immune response, the target antigen must be expressed within the tubulointerstitium and may subsequently elicit either humoral or cellular immune responses. TBM-associated antigens have been extensively studied, but experimental models have suggested that other renal tubular cell components, such as the proximal tubular brush border, Tamm-Horsfall protein, and nonnative soluble and trapped antigens, may also induce nephritogenic immune responses within the tubulointerstitium. Disease susceptibility may also depend on genetic expression of relevant antigens. For example, genes encoding the relevant antigen in αTBM disease are polymorphic and not expressed in all mammals. Therefore experimental animals that do not express this target antigen are protected from immune responses directed against this antigen. Such genetic variations in TBM antigens have also been observed in humans who either lack these determinants or, as observed in nephronophthisis, express genetically altered antigens.

In addition to target antigen expression as an initial requirement for susceptibility, the target antigen must also be immunologically visible to circulating lymphocytes. Such visibility requires that the antigen not be sequestered in an immunologically privileged site. This sequestration may be an important mechanism for maintaining tolerance to many tissue-specific antigens that become exposed to circulating immune cells only after structural tissue damage. Another hypothesis for immune recognition of the tubulointerstitium suggests that a component of an infectious particle or drug may possess a cross-reactive epitope that is expressed within the tubulointerstitium. Therefore an immune response directed against the inciting agent would theoretically also target the tubulointerstitium. The nephritogenic potential of such a response has not been tested within an experimental system.

Visibility also requires that the target epitope of an antigen be expressed with major histocompatibility complex (MHC) determinants, class II MHC for presentation to CD4+ T cells and class I MHC for CD8+ T cells. Experimental evidence both *in vitro* and *in vivo* have demonstrated that renal tubular epithelial cells can process and present antigens to T cells. For example, in αTBM disease murine proximal tubular cells express the target antigen and can present it to syngeneic CD4+ T cells, an interaction blocked by αCD4 or αclass II MHC antibodies. Class II MHC expression on parenchymal cells is generally low, but its expression can be significantly upregulated by proinflammatory cytokines such as interferon-γ (IFN-γ) and tumor necrosis factor-α (TNF-α). Although a clearly defined role for antigen presentation by tubular cells in tubulointerstitial disease has not been established, cytokine-induced class II MHC expression on tubular cells *in vivo* may be important in amplifying or maintaining an autoimmune response targeting the tubulointerstitium.

The target antigen of αTBM-associated interstitial nephritis, called 3M-1, has been isolated from collagenase-solubilized TBM preparations. Murine 3M-1 is a 48-kD glycoprotein that is synthesized by proximal tubular cells and expressed on the lateral border of the TBM. It does not appear to be an integral basement membrane component. 3M-l demonstrates conserved antigenicity across a number of mammalian species (rabbit, rat, guinea pig, and human) although there is some molecular weight variation. Sequencing data obtained from screening of a murine cDNA library made from tubular epithelial cells suggest that 3M-1 is a unique, complex protein containing five distinct amino acid termini, all sharing a common framework domain. This framework domain encodes a protein that shares a 37% nonrepetitive structural similarity with some intermediate filament–associated proteins.

CELL-MEDIATED NEPHRITOGENIC RESPONSES

The role of cell-mediated immunity in tubulointerstitial nephritis has been extensively characterized in the murine model of αTBM disease. Experimental αTBM disease is induced by immunizing susceptible rodents with heterologous renal tubular antigen in complete Freund's adjuvant. Circulating and deposited αTBM antibodies are apparent in all species 1 to 2 weeks after immunization. However, the time course of interstitial disease varies among species. Interstitial mononuclear cell infiltration is observed in guinea pigs and rats 2 to 3 weeks following immunization, whereas immunized mice generally require 6 to 8 weeks to develop such lesions. Dense mononuclear cell infiltrates are composed of a heterogeneous population of T cells, B cells, plasma cells, natural killer cells, and macrophages, and are typically associated with evidence of tubular dilatation and destruction. This progressive inflammatory lesion is eventually replaced by interstitial fibrosis, which ultimately results in end-stage renal disease. A prominent pathogenic role for T cells in

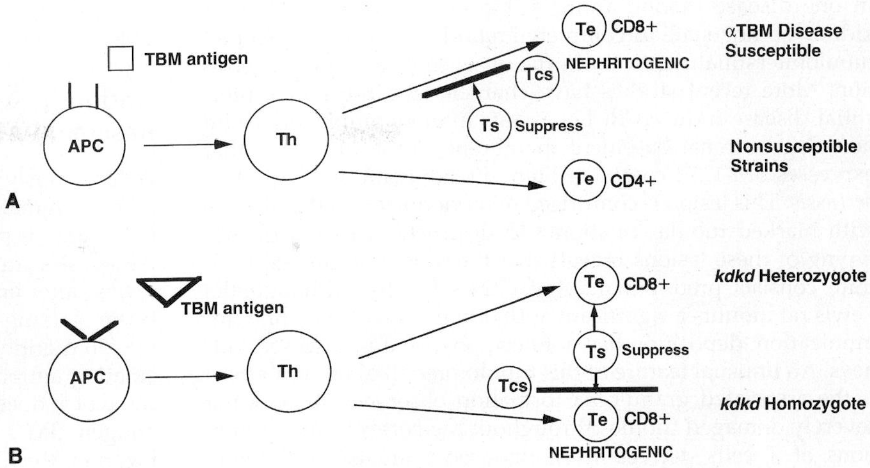

Figure 38.1. T-cell networks in experimental models of tubulointerstitial nephritis. In each model system there is an antigen-presenting cell that presents relevant TBM antigen to the Th cell repertoire, and a peripheral selection process (Ts and Tcs cells) that regulates the phenotype of emerging Te cells. **A:** In αTBM disease nonsusceptible mice develop CD4+ Te cells, class II MHC-restricted, while disease-susceptible strains develop a CD8+ Te cell repertoire, class I MHC-restricted. **B:** In kdkd disease the homozygous mouse develops a CD8+ T cell nephritogenic repertoire that is not seen in heterozygous progeny. (Modified from Meyers CM. T-cell regulation of renal immune responses. *Curr Opin Nephrol* 1995;4:270-276, with permission.)

murine αTBM disease has been demonstrated by the ability of sensitized T cells from diseased animals to adoptively transfer tubulointerstitial nephritis to naive syngeneic recipients. Moreover, no significant differences in humoral responses are apparent between immunized susceptible and nonsusceptible strains of mice. Unlike other rodent models of αTBM disease, murine αTBM antibodies do not transfer tubulointerstitial disease, further supporting a central role for T cells in mediating this lesion.

Susceptibility to murine αTBM disease is an autosomal dominant trait that maps to the class I MHC locus ($H\text{-}2k^{s,d}$). Within several days following immunization with renal tubular antigen, or the relevant target antigen, 3M-1, CD4+ helper T (Th) cells proliferate in lymph nodes of both susceptible and nonsusceptible mice (Fig. 38.1). The Th from susceptible mice do not directly induce tubulointerstitial injury but are required for differentiation of the class I MHC-restricted nephritogenic CD8+ effector T (Te) cells.

In nonsusceptible mice, 3M-1–specific CD4+ Te cells differentiate, which mediate delayed-type hypersensitivity (DTH) responses to the target antigen but do not typically induce tubulointerstitial injury. However, under some experimental conditions 3M-1–specific CD4+ Te cells can induce disease. For example, if class II MHC expression is first upregulated by IFN-γ administration, these CD4+ Te cells will infiltrate the kidney and produce tubulointerstitial nephritis in otherwise nonsusceptible strains. Therefore the presence of antigen-sensitized Te cells that can adequately recognize 3M-1 in association with appropriate (class I) MHC determinants defines susceptibility (Fig. 38.1).

Class I MHC–restricted 3M-1–specific CD8+ Te cells that differentiate in susceptible mice also bear idiotypes cross-reactive with those found on antibodies eluted from nephritic kidneys. Following adoptive transfer they acutely induce interstitial lesions in naive syngeneic mice within 5 to 7 days. These CD8+ Te cells also mediate DTH and cytotoxic responses to the target antigen 3M-l. Previous histologic evidence suggests that both of these activities may be relevant to tubulointerstitial immune injury. The inflammatory tubulointerstitial lesion observed in αTBM disease is strikingly similar to a cutaneous DTH response, with a mononuclear infiltrate of T cells, B cells, plasma cells, natural killer cells, and macrophages. With disease progression there is concurrent evidence for cytotoxicity, suggested by tubular cell atrophy, dilatation, and subsequent scarring.

Analysis of the Te cell response in susceptible animals has revealed clones of distinct function, either DTH-reactive or cytotoxic. *In vitro* study of relevant cytokine mRNA also reveals differential expression of cytokines such as interleukin-2 (IL-2), transforming growth-factor-β (TGF-β), and perforin (a mediator of cytotoxicity) between DTH-reactive and cytotoxic Te clones. As previously stated, progressive inflammation is also associated with TBM thickening, tubular atrophy, and interstitial fibrosis. Relevant soluble factors such as TGF-β, nitric oxide, or angiotensin II (AII), may play an integral role in altering tubular epithelial cell function, synthesizing of basement membrane constituents, or stimulating fibroblast proliferation, which collectively could affect the characteristic histologic changes of tubulointerstitial nephritis. Further definition of the role of T cell–derived cytokines in tubulointerstitial disease remains an area of intense investigation.

The effector T cell response in a spontaneous model of tubulointerstitial nephritis in kdkd mice, a mutant subline of the CBA/Ca strain, has also been extensively evaluated (Fig. 38.1). This disease exhibits an autosomal recessive inheritance pattern with 100% penetrance. Animals are normal at birth but develop progressive renal disease, characterized histologically by peritubular mononuclear cell infiltrates and tubular dilatation, with eventual irreversible damage and tubulointerstitial fibrosis. Cell-mediated immunity has been implicated in the pathogenesis of this disease largely because of the preponderance of tubulointerstitial mononuclear cell infiltrates and also the ability to transfer disease through radiation bone marrow chimeras. In addition, disease expression can be suppressed following thymectomy or protein-calorie restriction. The lack of renal-specific antibodies in the serum or kidney throughout the course of the disease further supports the primary role of cellular immunity in this spontaneous form of tubulointerstitial nephritis. As observed in murine αTBM disease, this interstitial lesion can be acutely transferred by adoptive transfer of tubular antigen–reactive CD8+ Te cells isolated from peripheral lymph nodes and kidneys of diseased kdkd mice. In addition, these CD8+ Te cells will mediate tubular antigen–specific DTH-reactivity to renal tubular antigen preparations. Although the relevant antigen of this disease has not been purified, it appears to be distinct from the 3M-1 antigen of αTBM disease.

Cell-mediated events have also been studied in rat models of tubulointerstitial nephritis. Early studies demonstrated mononuclear cell inflammation in the absence of antibody deposition following intrarenal injection of aggregated proteins. Subsequent studies have examined tubulointerstitial lesions induced in Lewis rats following immunization with renal antigen preparations. The Lewis rat is an interesting host to study because it does not express the relevant antigen, 3M-1, of αTBM disease.

In one disease model, animals immunized with autologous kidney homogenate in complete Freund's adjuvant developed tubulointerstitial nephritis in the absence of antibody deposition. More recent studies have characterized the tubulointerstitial disease induced in Lewis rats after immunization with homologous renal basement membrane, from an animal that expresses 3M-1, in complete Freund's adjuvant and *Bordetella pertussis*. This lesion is comprised of mononuclear cell infiltrates with marked tubular dilation and destruction. *In situ* phenotyping of these lesions reveals that the mononuclear cell infiltrate consists predominantly of CD4+ T cells. Although the Lewis rat mounts a significant antibody response following immunization, deposition has not been observed in diseased kidneys. An unusual feature of this tubulointerstitial injury pattern is the associated granuloma formation observed surrounding severely damaged tubules throughout the cortex. Bulk populations of T cells derived from diseased animals will acutely transfer this granulomatous tubulointerstitial disease to naive animals.

Cell-mediated immunity is the predominant effector mechanism implicated in human tubulointerstitial nephritis. This hypothesis is supported by histologic evidence from various tubulointerstitial diseases that demonstrates polymorphonuclear and mononuclear cell interstitial infiltrates without demonstrable antibody deposition. However, αTBM antibodies and immune complexes are occasionally seen in some forms of tubulointerstitial nephritis. The role of cellular immunity is further supported in human disease by reports of *in vivo* (cutaneous DTH responses) and *in vitro* (lymphoblast transformation) evidence of hypersensitivity to specific inciting antigens. Phenotypic evaluation of interstitial infiltrates has been conducted by a number of investigators. T cells constitute a large portion of the mononuclear cells detected within tubulointerstitial lesions. Both CD4+ and CD8+ T cell subsets have been identified within interstitial infiltrates, although a single subset has not been uniformly associated with interstitial injury. The predominant subset may vary depending on the underlying cause, the time course of the disease, and the therapeutic modalities, particularly immunosuppressive therapy, undertaken to alter disease activity.

Understanding the role of cell-mediated immunity in human interstitial disease remains an investigative challenge as our knowledge of distinct renal antigens that initiate T cell–mediated responses is quite limited. Tamm-Horsfall protein has been implicated in a few human diseases because it has been detected within interstitial infiltrates in a number of patients with chronic obstructive pyelonephritis, hydronephrosis, chronic idiopathic tubulointerstitial nephritis, and medullary cystic disease. As discussed in the previous section, it is tempting to speculate that drugs or infection-related agents may crossreact with or alter endogenous renal antigens and, in effect, induce an immune response targeting the tubulointerstitium. Further examination of this hypothesis awaits an appropriate experimental model.

HUMORALLY MEDIATED NEPHRITOGENIC RESPONSES

Antibodies may participate in the production of tubular cell damage either by direct toxicity or through the formation of tubulointerstitial immune complexes. However, in the setting of tubulointerstitial disease, deposition of antibody or immune complexes is generally associated with tubulointerstitial mononuclear cell infiltration. Nephritogenic antigens that incite such responses may be directed against basement membrane antigens, renal tubular cell products, surface antigens, or other soluble antigens.

Antibody Recognition of the Tubular Basement Membrane

As previously described, αTBM antibody responses in experimental animals are typically induced after immunization with heterologous preparations of renal tubular antigen in adjuvant. All species studied predictably develop an αTBM antibody response after immunization, as evidenced by antibody titers and linear staining of the TBM with IgG antibody. Renal deposition of αTBM antibody is generally observed in the presence of circulating antibodies. An exception is again found in the Lewis rat, which does not express the relevant tubular epithelial target antigen, 3M-1, recognized by αTBM antibodies. After immunization, the Lewis rat develops circulating αTBM antibodies, but they do not deposit within the kidney.

αTBM antibodies will adoptively transfer tubulointerstitial nephritis in guinea pigs and rats. Studies in guinea pigs demonstrate that either IgG1 or IgG2 antibodies will transfer disease. Full expression of disease appears to be C3-dependent, as C3 depletion with cobra venom factor prior to transfer is disease protective. Adoptive transfer of tubulointerstitial nephritis to Brown Norway rats with αTBM antisera results in progressive renal IgG deposition, which is detected within 24 hours after transfer. Evaluation of tubulointerstitial lesions reveals polymorphonuclear cells, mononuclear cells, and giant cells, as well as C3 deposition. Tubulointerstitial lesions in rats that are C3-depleted with cobra venom before αTBM antibody transfer express the usual pattern of αTBM antibody deposition. However, the associated mononuclear cell infiltration is significantly diminished. These findings suggest that activation of complement may be an important effector pathway for antibody-mediated interstitial damage, which potentiates mononuclear cell infiltration. Previous investigations have also demonstrated that αTBM antibodies can act as an informational bridge between the humoral and cellular immune response via antibody-dependent cell-mediated cytotoxicity reactions.

B-cell responses in αTBM disease in rats have been characterized through the study of a library of monoclonal αTBM antibodies, all of which are specific for the 3M-1 TBM antigen. These studies suggest that there may be some limited, biased use of immunoglobulin variable region heavy chain genes to form these αTBM antibodies. Similar epitopic specificity of the 3M-1 antigen and a shared cross-reactive idiotype were also apparent on these monoclonal antibodies. However, the paratope assembled to represent these antibodies is more dependent on recombinatorial diversity than somatic mutation. Therapeutic intervention with rabbit α-idiotypic antisera directed at this shared variable region inhibited disease induction in naive rats and was also effective in preventing progression of tubulointerstitial disease in previously immunized animals.

A number of studies have also characterized the B cell response in various strains of immunized mice. As previously stated, αTBM antisera does not transfer disease in mice. Susceptible and nonsusceptible strains cannot be distinguished on the basis of antibody titers, expression of cross-reactive idiotype, or αTBM-antibody epitope specificity. Moreover, αTBM antibodies may provide a protective function in immunized mice, as they decrease class II MHC expression by tubular epithelial cells. In nonsusceptible mice, αTBM antibody deposits can be detected within the tubulointerstitium following immunization, but they are not pathologic and are not associated with tubulointerstitial infiltration.

αTBM antibody deposition is observed in a number of human renal diseases, but its pathogenic significance has not been formally established. Primary αTBM disease occurs occasionally in humans and, as observed in experimental animals, the immune response appears to be directed at the tubular antigen 3M-l. Linear deposition of IgG along the TBM associated with mononuclear cell infiltrates has been reported in several cases of drug-associated interstitial nephritis (particularly related to methicillin therapy), and is also a frequently observed complication of αGBM disease. αTBM antibody deposits are reported most commonly following renal transplantation. In this setting antibody deposition may reflect the polymorphic expression of human tubulointerstitial antigens and is generally not of functional significance to the allograft.

Immune Deposit–Mediated Tubulointerstitial Nephritis

The Heymann brush border antigen and Tamm-Horsfall protein in the thick, ascending limb and distal convoluted tubule have been implicated in local immune complex formation within the tubulointerstitium. Animals immunized to produce Heymann's nephritis develop tubular IgG and C3 deposits, often associated with marked tubulointerstitial mononuclear cell infiltrates. The characteristic glomerular proteinuria of this disease appears to facilitate antibody deposition because it provides filtered antibodies access to the tubular lumen. If animals with serum sickness–induced proteinuria are administered αFx1A antibodies, these antibodies induce a complement-independent tubular epithelial cell lysis. Similar findings have been observed in experimental animals with proteinuria treated with antibodies to the Tamm-Horsfall protein. Immunizing rats or mice with Tamm-Horsfall protein results in basilar immune deposits on ascending limb tubular cells. However, rabbits immunized in a similar fashion develop interstitial inflammation without immune deposits. Tamm-Horsfall protein deposition with antibodies in human tubulointerstitial lesions in the setting of urinary tract obstruction or reflux nephropathy further suggests its potential as a nephritogenic target antigen in previously diseased kidneys.

Tubulointerstitial immune complex disease has been reported in humans, although it is generally not an isolated finding. Immune complex and complement deposition along the TBM is seen in systemic diseases that involve the kidney, such as systemic lupus erythematosus, particularly in those patients afflicted with predominantly tubulointerstitial pathology. It has also been observed in Sjögren's syndrome, essential mixed cryoglobulinemia, and cutaneous vasculitis. These deposits may be accompanied by tubulointerstitial infiltrates, and are almost always associated with glomerular immune complex deposits and glomerular damage. Primary glomerular lesions such as proliferative glomerulonephritis and membranous nephropathy have also been associated with interstitial immune complex deposition.

REGULATION OF THE NEPHRITOGENIC IMMUNE RESPONSE

A number of studies in murine αTBM disease have examined the regulation of nephritogenic Te cell differentiation (Fig. 38.1). Early observations noted the preferential selection of CD4+ Te cells in nonsusceptible strains of mice and CD8+ Te cells in susceptible strains. This phenotypic selection appears dependent on antigen-specific regulatory T cells, which are differentially expressed in susceptible and nonsusceptible strains. Suppressor T (Ts) cells inhibit CD8+ Te cell expansion in nonsusceptible strains. However, in susceptible strains these Ts cells are abrogated by Vicia Villosa lectin-adherent contrasuppressor T (Tcs) cells, which facilitate the maturation of injurious nephritogenic CD8+ Te cells. A similar analysis of Te cell regulation has been conducted in the kdkd model of spontaneous tubulointerstitial nephritis (Fig. 38.1). T cells derived from the ancestral nondisease prone CBA/Ca strain will suppress disease activity in kdkd mice. Similar disease-suppressing Ts cells are also detected in kdkd mice prior to the onset of disease. Therefore expression of tubulointerstitial nephritis is not a result of Ts cell deletion from the T cell repertoire in kdkd mice but rather occurs with the emergence of antigen-specific Tcs cells that negate the function of Ts cells and permit differentiation of nephritogenic Te cells. These findings suggest that endogenous regulation of Te cell differentiation is critical in defining host susceptibility to disease.

Newer studies in αTBM disease have demonstrated that a number of different experimental manipulations can inhibit expression of CD8+ Te cells and tubulointerstitial inflammation. Antigen-nonspecific modalities that inhibit αTBM disease include treatment with cyclophosphamide, cyclosporine, PGE1, and protein-calorie restriction. In addition, a variety of antigen-specific modalities have successfully suppressed the nephritogenic immune response in αTBM disease. These experimental maneuvers in susceptible animals have included immunizing with renal tubular antigen in incomplete Freund's adjuvant, injecting tubular antigen-reactive T lymphoblasts that bear cross-reactive idiotypes, injecting α-idiotypic antisera, and inducing Ts cell networks. Ts cells are induced following intravenous injection of splenocytes to which tubular antigens have been chemically coupled with 1-ethyl-3-(3-dimethylaminopropyl) carbodiimide. In αTBM disease this Ts network consists of two phenotypically and functionally distinct populations. Suppressor-inducer, or Ts1 cells, are CD4+ T cells that inhibit an early stage in the differentiation of CD8+ Te cells and also induce a population of suppressor-effector, or Ts2 cells. These CD8+ Ts2 cells directly inhibit the function of nephritogenic CD8+ Te cells via a noncytotoxic mechanism. The suppressive effects of both Ts1 and Ts2 cells, which require new mRNA and protein synthesis, are mediated by soluble protein factors synthesized by these cells and present in their lysates (TsF1 and TsF2).

Both TsF1 and TsF2 inhibit αTBM disease. TsF2 will downregulate disease expression even if transferred to an animal after disease onset. Examination of the effects of TsF2 on nephritogenic Te clones has revealed that this antigen-specific protein factor inhibits DTH reactivity and cytotoxicity, in addition to its suppressing adoptive transfer of tubulointerstitial nephritis. Further analysis of TsF2-induced changes in cytokine expression in suppressed Te clones demonstrates changes in transcription of IL-2, IFN-γ, and TGF-β. The close temporal association of these cytokine changes with loss of functional activity in these antigen-specific Te suggests that they are relevant to disease suppression.

Studies of αTBM disease in rodents have also demonstrated that oral administration of crude renal tubular antigen preparations prior to immunization alters the intensity of both interstitial nephritis and renal insufficiency produced by immunization with renal tubular antigen. Moreover, prevention of interstitial disease with oral antigen feeding is dose-dependent. Interestingly, inhibition of renal disease is not dependent on uniform alteration of all renal tubular antigen–specific immune responses, as DTH reactivity and antibody responses are not similarly modulated. However, mechanisms that induce tolerance to oral antigens have not been delineated. Investigations in other models of oral tolerance reveal that antigen feeding changes T cell cytokine profiles, inducing antiinflammatory cytokine production (IL-4 and TGF-β) in susceptible hosts. These studies in interstitial nephritis may be noteworthy because oral tolerance induced by crude renal antigen preparations may have potential therapeutic impact on human interstitial disease, either primary or in the setting of initial glomerular inflammation.

In general, the role of TGF-β in renal disease has been considered one of inducing glomerulosclerosis and enhancing extracellular matrix production and tubulointerstitial fibrosis. However, investigations of nephritogenic T-cell subsets indicate an immunosuppressive and disease-protective effect of this endogenous peptide growth factor. Previous experiments in αTBM disease demonstrate that TGF-β1 inhibits antigen-specific nephritogenic T-cell cytotoxicity and proliferation and blocks their ability to adoptively transfer interstitial disease to naive recipients. Furthermore, analysis of cell-surface markers that are critical for T cell activation, such as CD4, IL-2R, LFA-1, and transferrin receptor, are diminished after exposure to TGF-β1.

Proinflammatory chemotactic mediators, or chemokines, have been studied in a number of renal disease models associated with marked tubulointerstitial infiltration. Molecules such as RANTES and monocyte chemotactic peptide-1 (MCP-1), chemoattractants for CD4+ T cells and monocytes, have been characterized best. Both RANTES and MCP-1 are expressed *in vitro* by cytokine-stimulated tubular epithelial cells and are apparent in renal biopsies obtained in the setting of allograft rejection and glomerulonephritis. However, *in situ* phenotyping of interstitial lesions induced by distinct chemokines appear to differ in various experimental animals studied. Such analyses suggest that chemoattractants may promote interstitial injury *in vivo* by complementary recruitment of distinct populations of mononuclear cells.

FACTORS THAT INFLUENCE PROGRESSION OF INTERSTITIAL DAMAGE

As most forms of chronic renal disease are associated with progressive interstitial injury, the nephritogenic role of a number of nonimmune host factors have been studied in experimental models of chronic renal injury. Although interstitial lesions are typically comprised of mononuclear cells (T cells, B cells, and monocytes/macrophages), the exact phenotypic composition of reported interstitial lesions in experimentally induced disease varies, depending on the disease model. Interstitial lesions observed in primary forms of interstitial nephritis may differ considerably from those seen in secondary forms of interstitial disease (Table 38.3). Infiltrates induced by nonspecific immune cells, such as macrophages, are likely quite different from those induced by T-cell lymphocytes. In addition, interstitial chemoattractant stimuli in settings of proteinuria, lipiduria, or ischemia may induce interstitial inflammation via distinct signaling pathways. Tubular epithelial cell expression of extracellular matrix proteins, such as osteopontin and thrombospondin-1, has been studied in a number of models of glomerular disease. Upregulated expression of such markers at sites of interstitial inflammation and injury in various models suggests a pathogenic role of these glycoproteins in inducing progressive interstitial damage in settings of glomerular disease.

As previously stated, early observations that detected Tamm-Horsfall proteins in human interstitial lesions initially implied a nephrotoxic role for endogenous proteins in chronic renal disease. One hypothesis suggests that protein overload of tubular cells, as a result of glomerular pathology, may be an important initiating factor of interstitial inflammation in early phases of parenchymal injury. Analysis of protein accumulation and interstitial cellular infiltration in progressive renal disease in two different models of proteinuric nephropathies, remnant kidney following 5/6 renal ablation, and passive Heymann nephritis, reveals similar patterns of proximal tubular cell accumulation of albumin and IgG in early stages of disease prior to evidence of interstitial infiltration. In both models, osteopontin is apparent in proximal tubular cells congested with protein at sites of interstitial infiltration. In light of its chemoattractant properties, osteopontin may represent one of the primary regulators of tubulointerstitial inflammation in significant proteinuria.

TABLE 38.3. Experimental Models of Interstitial Injury

Primary	Secondary
αTBM disease	Glomerular diseases with proteinuria
Spontaneous interstitial nephritis (kdkd mice)	Systemic autoimmune diseases
Cyclosporine-associated nephritis (high-dose)	Puromycin aminonucleoside nephrosis
	αThyl nephritis
	Heymann nephritis
	Unilateral ureteral obstruction
	Remnant kidney after renal ablation

In the experimental setting, protein overloading of proximal tubular epithelial cells, with albumin and other proteins, clearly upregulates transcription of a number of genes encoding vasoactive and inflammatory molecules, including endothelin-1, RANTES, and MCP-1. In view of their chemotactic activities, tubulointerstitial release of these molecules could recruit monocytes/macrophages and T-cell lymphocytes and propagate interstitial inflammation and renal disease progression. Proximal tubular cell protein overload may provide a distinct signal that induces interstitial inflammation in the setting of significant proteinuria. Understanding mechanisms of protein-associated damage in glomerulonephritis may have therapeutic implications for most forms of chronic, progressive renal disease in humans.

Activation of the nitric oxide synthase (NOS) pathway is an important mediator of organ damage in inflammatory and ischemic models of renal injury. These effects may be related to the ability of nitric oxide to act as a cytotoxic mediator and oxidant in diseases characterized by macrophage infiltration and activation. In contrast to these injurious effects of nitric oxide, iNOS activation can have immunosuppressive effects on T-cell lymphocytes. In mice immunized to produce αTBM disease, exposure to L-NAME and L-NIL, a highly selective inhibitor of iNOS, develop more severe tubulointerstitial disease than untreated control mice. Evaluation of cytokine profiles reveals that L-NIL–treated animals shift their cellular immune response toward a Th1-like response, with augmented IFN-γ/IL-4 and IL-2/IL-4 ratios. These observations indicate that generation of nitric oxide through the iNOS pathway can have host-protective effects on T cell–mediated renal immune responses. Similar observations of the protective effects of nitric oxide production on renal injury have also been reported in a rat model of cyclosporine-associated nephropathy.

Experimental models of chronic interstitial injury, both primary and secondary, have facilitated studying mechanisms of fibrosis. Interstitial fibrosis is particularly relevant because it constitutes a common final pathway of most forms of progressive renal injury. Recent observations in a model of cyclosporine-associated nephropathy, as well as experimental unilateral ureteral obstruction, demonstrate that progressive interstitial damage is associated with significant increases in tubulointerstitial cell apoptosis. Moreover, levels of such apoptosis correlate with the development of interstitial fibrosis. Chronic interstitial changes in these models appears to be mediated, at least in part, by AII, as experimental animals treated with AII type 1 receptor blockade have significantly less disease than untreated controls. These observations indicate that AII may play an important role in progressive interstitial fibrosis in some settings, and that renal ischemia may perhaps be a critical event in this process.

Selected Readings

Bannister KM, Ulich TR, Wilson CB. Immunological mechanisms in experimental models of tubulointerstitial nephritis. In: Davison AM, ed. *Nephrology*. London: Balliere Tindall, 1988:618–635.

A detailed review of the relative roles of antibody and cell-mediated mechanisms in tubulointerstitial nephritis in the rat.

D'Amico G. Tubulo-interstitial damage in glomerular diseases: its role in the progression of the renal damage. *Nephrol Dial Trans* 1998;1:80–85.

A comprehensive review that discusses studies of interstitial inflammation observed in the context of glomerular damage.

Gabbai FB, Boggiano C, Peter T, et al. Inhibition of inducible nitric oxide synthase intensifies injury and functional deterioration in autoimmune interstitial nephritis. *J Immunol* 1997;159:6266–6275.

Important observations that describe disease-protective effects of nitric oxide in autoimmune interstitial nephritis.

Kelly CJ. T cell regulation of autoimmune interstitial nephritis. *J Am Soc Nephrol* 1990;1:140–149.

A concise and well-written summary of observations derived from multiple studies of T cell–mediated tubulointerstitial disease in rodents.

Kelly CJ, Roth DA, Meyers CM. Immune recognition and response to the renal interstitium. *Kid Int* 1991;39:518–530.

A summary of immune mechanisms of interstitial injury derived from experimental models of tubulointerstitial nephritis.

Lehman DH, Wilson CB, Dixon FJ. Extraglomerular immunoglobulin deposits in human nephritis. *Am J Med* 1975;58:765–786.

An important examination of the occurrence of extraglomerular deposits in immune-mediated nephritis.

Meyers CM. T-cell regulation of renal immune responses. *Curr Opin Nephrol* 1995; 4:270–276.

A review that focuses on T cell–mediated events that induce tubulointerstitial nephritis in the experimental setting.

Meyers CM, Kelly CJ. Effector mechanisms in organ-specific autoimmunity. I. Characterization of a CD8+ T cell line that mediates murine interstitial nephritis. *J Clin Invest* 1991;88:408–416.

Characterization of a unique tubular antigen-specific T-cell line, derived from animals with αTBM disease, that adoptively transfers tubulointerstitial nephritis to naive recipients.

Meyers CM, Kelly CJ. Inhibition of murine nephritogenic effector T cells by a clone-specific suppressor factor. *J Clin Invest* 1994;94:2093–2104.

Characterization of nephritogenic T cells rendered unresponsive by a soluble clone-specific suppressor factor.

Meyers CM, Tomaszweski JE, Glass JD, et al. The nephritogenic T cell response in murine chronic graft-vs.-host disease. *J Immunol* 1998;161:5321–5330.

A recent characterization of nephritogenic T cell clones, derived from kidneys of animals with autoimmune glomerulonephritis, that induce interstitial inflammation and damage.

Neilson EG, Gasser DL, McCafferty E, et al. Polymorphism of genes involved in anti-tubular basement membrane disease in rats. *Immunogenetics* 1983;17: 55–65.

An analysis of the genetic determinants of susceptibility to αTBM disease in rodents.

Neilson EG, McCafferty E, Mann R, et al. Murine interstitial nephritis III. The selection of phenotypic (Lyt and L3T4) and idiotypic T cell preferences by genes in Igh-1 and H2-K characterized the cell-mediated potential for disease expression: susceptible mice provide a unique effector T cell repertoire in the response to tubular antigen. *J Immunol* 1985;134:2375–2382.

A characterization of the T-cell repertoire producing murine αTBM disease.

Neilson EG, Sun MJ, Kelly CJ, et al. Molecular characterization of a major nephritogenic domain in the autoantigen of anti-tubular basement membrane disease. *Proc Natl Acad Sci USA* 1991;88:2006–2011.

Sequence analysis and isolation of an immunodominant region of the target antigen of αTBM disease.

Pham K, Smoyer WE, Archer DC, et al. Oral feeding of renal tubular antigen abrogates interstitial nephritis and renal failure in Brown Norway rats. *Kidney Int* 1997;52:725–732.

An important study describing the disease-protective effects of antigen feeding on autoimmune T cell–mediated interstitial disease.

Wilson CB. Nephritogenic tubulointerstitial antigens. *Kid Int* 1991;39:501–517.

A comprehensive review of nephritogenic antigens in experimental models of tubulointerstitial nephritis.

SECTION VI

Diseases of the Kidney and Urinary Tract

CHAPTER 39

Glomerular Diseases

PART 1
Syndromes of Glomerular Diseases

Richard J. Glassock

Disorders that adversely affect the functional and morphologic integrity of the glomeruli can manifest themselves clinically in only a limited number of ways. The clinical and biochemical disturbances that accompany the *glomerulopathies* are the direct or indirect result of a few fundamental disturbances, namely (a) alteration of the permselectivity of the glomerular capillary wall, leading to the passage of abnormal quantities of plasma proteins into Bowman's space and hence into the urine, which is recognized as *proteinuria* (see Chapters 4 and 32); (b) alteration in the filtering surface area and/or intrinsic hydraulic conductivity of the capillary wall of many or most glomeruli or loss of entire nephron units in a focal manner, with either or both leading to reduction in total kidney *glomerular filtration rate* (GFR) (see Chapter 3); (c) disturbances in the regulation of NaCl and H_2O excretion, leading to expansion of the extracellular fluid volume as modified by the state of Starling's forces in the peripheral capillary circulation; the NaCl and H_2O retention may manifest as edema and/or hypertension (see Chapters 31 and 33); and (d) facilitated migration of circulating cellular elements of blood into the lumen of individual nephrons manifested as increased urinary excretion of formed elements, such as erythrocytes, leukocytes, casts, and tubular epithelial cells. Various presentations of proteinuria, reduced GFR, edema and hypertension, and abnormal urinary sediment result in the *major clinical syndromes of the glomerulopathies* (Table 39.1).

TABLE 39.1. The Major Clinical Syndromes of the Glomerulopathies

Acute glomerulonephritis
Rapidly progressive glomerulonephritis
Chronic glomerulonephritis
Nephrotic syndrome
Asymptomatic hematuria and/or proteinuria

ACUTE GLOMERULONEPHRITIS

Acute glomerulonephritis may be defined as the abrupt onset of hematuria, often accompanied by proteinuria, edema, hypertension, and reduced GFR and sometimes associated with oliguria. The term connotes the appearance of fresh clinical manifestations of previously absent disease and must be distinguished from an exacerbation of a chronic underlying but not previously diagnosed illness. Also implicit in the term is the notion of reversibility and self-limited behavior, although clearly some cases may subsequently evolve into other syndromes of rapidly progressive glomerulonephritis, chronic glomerulonephritis, or nephrotic syndrome. With resolution of the acute process, many cases may evolve into the picture of asymptomatic proteinuria and hematuria. The causative factors that underlie the syndrome of acute glomerulonephritis can be broadly divided into infectious and noninfectious groups (Table 39.2).

TABLE 39.2. Causative Factors of the Syndrome of Acute Glomerulonephritis

Infectious
Acute poststreptococcal glomerulonephritis (group A, β-hemolytic streptococcal infection)
Nonpoststreptococcal glomerulonephritis
Infective endocarditis
Staphylococcal bacteremia
Pneumococcal pneumonia
Meningococcemia
Typhoid fever
Secondary syphilis
Acute viral infection (cytomegalovirus, varicella, Epstein-Barr, hepatitis B, coxsackie)
Mycoplasma (rare)
Trichinosis
Toxoplasmosis
Falciparum malaria
Noninfectious
Multisystem diseases
Systemic lupus erythematosus
Henoch-Schönlein purpura
Necrotizing vasculitis
Goodpasture's disease
Alport's syndrome
Primary glomerular disease
IgA nephropathy (Berger's disease)
Mesangial proliferative glomerulonephritis
Membranoproliferative glomerulonephritis

Each of the entities listed is discussed in detail in other sections of this book. Among the infectious causes, a diffuse endocapillary proliferative glomerulonephritis is the most commonly encountered histologic lesion. Conditions that may mimic acute glomerulonephritis include acute hypersensitivity interstitial nephritis, IgA nephropathy, thromboembolic renal disease, thrombotic thrombocytopenic purpura, and hemolytic uremic syndrome.

RAPIDLY PROGRESSIVE GLOMERULONEPHRITIS

The syndrome of rapidly progressive glomerulonephritis (RPGN) resembles that of acute glomerulonephritis except for the dramatic tendency for progressive deterioration of GFR, often leading to oliguria and end-stage renal disease in a matter of weeks or months. Proteinuria is often only modest, perhaps because of the severe loss of GFR. The multiple causative factors involved in the syndrome of RPGN are listed in Table 39.3. The individual entities are discussed in other sections of this book. The glomerular lesion that is found most frequently to underlie RPGN is extracapillary proliferative (crescentic) glomerulonephritis. Conditions that may clinically mimic RPGN include malignant hypertension, scleroderma, thromboembolic renal disease, thrombotic thrombocytopenic purpura, hemolytic uremic syndrome, and acute hypersensitivity interstitial nephritis.

TABLE 39.3. Causative Factors of the Syndrome of Rapidly Progressive Glomerulonephritis

Infectious diseases
- Poststreptococcal glomerulonephritis
- Infectious endocarditis
- Visceral sepsis
- Hepatitis B or hepatitis C infection with vasculitis and/or cryoimmunoglobulinemia

Drugs and toxic agents
- Allopurinol
- D-Penicillamine
- Hydralazine
- Rifampin

Multisystem diseases
- Systemic lupus erythematosis
- Goodpasture's disease
- Henoch-Schönlein purpura
- Necrotizing vasculitis (including Wegener's granulomatosis)
- Cryoimmunoglobulinemia (hepatitis B or C related)
- Neoplasia (colon, lung)
- Relapsing polychondritis
- Behçet's disease

Superimposed on primary glomerular disease
- Membranoproliferative glomerulonephritis (type I, II)
- Membranous glomerulonephritis
- IgA nephropathy (Berger's disease)

Primary disease
- Type I: antiglomerular basement membrane antibody disease
- Type II: immune complex-mediated disease
- Type III: pauciimmune (often antineutrophil cytoplasmic antibody associated)
- Type IV: mixed antiglomerular basement membrane antibody and antineutrophil cytoplasmic antibody associated disease
- Type V: idiopathic

CHRONIC GLOMERULONEPHRITIS

The term *chronic glomerulonephritis* encompasses a broad array of glomerular diseases. It is best viewed as the expression of the persistence and/or progression of the initiating underlying pathologic process. The syndrome of chronic glomerulonephritis is characterized by abnormal proteinuria, often in the so-called nonnephrotic range (less than 3.5 g/1.73 m^2/day), and accompanied by varying degrees of abnormal urinary sediment, hypertension, and reduced GFR. The time period over which chronic glomerulonephritis evolves is measured in years or decades. Ultimately, the process will lead to contracted granular kidney and irreversible end-stage renal failure. The glomerular lesions that underlie chronic glomerulonephritis vary widely and are best discussed under the heading of the syndromes from which chronic glomerulonephritis evolves. It is often presumed that the evolution to chronic renal insufficiency represents the continuation of the processes that initiated the disorder. However, such factors as complicating systemic hypertension, microvascular sclerosis secondary to intrarenal hemodynamic adjustments, damaging hyperfiltration in less affected residual nephrons, dietary regimens, and hormonal disturbances of renal insufficiency may contribute to the gradual loss of the renal functioning nephron mass.

NEPHROTIC SYNDROME

Nephrotic syndrome is principally defined on the basis of the presence of heavy proteinuria (greater than 3.5 g/1.73 m^2/day), often accompanied by hypoalbuminemia, hyperlipidemia, lipiduria, and edema. It must be emphasized that the selection of a single value for the separation of nephrotic and nonnephrotic-range proteinuria is quite arbitrary. However, it is useful in that disorders that principally affect the extraglomerular vasculature and/or tubulointerstitial areas do not commonly evoke proteinuria of nephrotic magnitude. Although nephrotic-range proteinuria is often a concomitant of glomerular lesions, many glomerular diseases seldom produce heavy proteinuria. The disorders that cause nephrotic syndrome are listed in Table 39.4. It should be emphasized that nephrotic syndrome may have early features of acute glomerulonephritis and may progress to chronic glomerulonephritis.

Nephrotic-range proteinuria, when persistent, often results in a number of biochemical and circulatory disturbances, largely the consequence of the loss of a variety of plasma proteins into the urine (Chapter 4). Thus hypoalbuminemia contributes to the development of edema, hyperlipidemia as manifested by increased cholesterol and/or triglycerides may conceivably alter the risk of cardiovascular disease, the loss of anticoagulant or antithrombotic factors may predispose to thrombosis, and other deficiency states may ensue. The metabolic and endocrine disturbances of the nephrotic syndrome are discussed in Chapter 39, Part 2.

The mechanisms that underlie the alteration in glomerular permeability are reviewed in Chapter 4. Fundamentally, two functional barriers to transglomerular passage of plasma proteins may be breached: (a) a *size-selective barrier* preventing passage of large protein molecules (molecular weight greater than 150,000), such as IgM, α_2-macroglobulin, fibrinogen, and high-density lipoprotein; and (b) a *charge-selective barrier* preventing passage of lower-molecular-weight proteins (70,000 to 150,000) bearing a net negative charge at physiologic pH (albumin). Some indirect evidence of the relative importance of defects in these barriers can be obtained by examining the fractional clearance of neutral dextran or polyvinylpyrrolidone relative to inulin (size-selective barrier) or by evaluating albumin excretion relative to other neutral molecules or to larger protein molecules (charge-selective barrier). Although of considerable fundamental interest, such measurements do not have great clini-

TABLE 39.4. Causative Factors of Nephrotic Syndrome

- Infectious diseases
  - Bacterial
    - Poststreptococcal glomerulonephritis
    - Infective endocarditis
    - "Shunt nephritis"
    - Syphilis, leprosy, tuberculosis
  - Viral
    - Hepatitis B or C infection
    - Cytomegalovirus
    - Epstein-Barr virus
    - Human immunodeficiency virus (HIV)
  - Protozoal
    - Quartan malaria, toxoplasmosis
  - Helminthic
    - Schistosomiasis, filariasis
- Neoplastic
  - Carcinoma of colon, lung, stomach, breast, kidney, thyroid, ovary, cervix, prostate, pancreas
  - Wilms' tumor
  - Malignant melanoma
  - Mesothelioma
  - Leukemia
  - Hodgkin's disease
  - Non-Hodgkin's lymphoma
  - Multiple myeloma (amyloidosis)
- Multisystem disease
  - Systemic lupus erythematosus
  - Mixed connective tissue disease
  - Rheumatoid arthritis
  - Henoch-Schönlein purpura
  - Wegener's granulomatosis
  - Necrotizing vasculitis
  - Sjögren's syndrome
  - Dermatomyositis
  - Amyloidosis (primary and secondary)
  - Sarcoidosis
- Metabolic diseases
  - Diabetes mellitus
  - Myxedema
- Heredofamilial diseases
  - Alport's syndrome
  - Fabry's disease
  - Nail-patella syndrome
  - Sickle cell disease
  - Congenital nephrotic syndrome (Finnish type)
  - α_1-Antitrypsin deficiency
- Heredofamilial diseases *(continued)*
  - Jeune's syndrome
  - Cystinosis
- Drugs, toxins, allergies
  - Organic or inorganic, elemental mercury
  - Organic gold
  - Penicillamine
  - "Street" heroin
  - Probenicid
  - Paradione, trimethadione
  - Captopril
  - Bee sting
  - Pollens
  - Poison ivy and poison oak
  - Antitoxins
  - Vaccines
  - Lithium
  - Nonsteroidal antiinflammatory drugs
  - Tolbutamide
  - Phenindione
  - Silver
  - Insect repellant
- Miscellaneous
  - Pregnancy-associated (toxemia of pregnancy)
  - Chronic renal allograft rejection
  - Malignant nephrosclerosis (essential)
  - Vesicoureteric reflux
  - Renal arterial stenosis
  - Chronic ulcerative colitis
  - Partial lipodystrophy with type II membranoproliferative glomerulonephritis
- Primary glomerular diseases
  - Minimal change disease
  - Mesangial proliferative glomerulonephritis with IgA deposits (Berger's disease), IgM deposits, or other
  - Focal and segmental glomerulosclerosis
  - Membranous glomerulopathy
  - Membranoproliferative glomerulonephritis
    - Type I (subendothelial deposits)
    - Type II (dense deposit disease)
    - Other types
  - Crescentic glomerulonephritis (rare)
  - Fibrillary (immunotactoid glomerulonephritis)
  - Collagen III glomerulopathy
  - Lipoprotein glomerulopathy

cal usefulness because of overlapping values, probably representing mixed defects in both size and charge-selective barriers.

Although the quantitation of total urinary protein excretion rates serves as the basis for defining nephrotic-range proteinuria, it should be emphasized that a striking reduction in plasma albumin concentration and/or GFR may place limits on urinary protein excretion. Thus expressing the defect in permeability in nephrotic states as a clearance value relative to a marker, such as inulin or creatinine, may provide a more accurate reflection of the magnitude of the permselectivity defect. The nature of the permeability defect also conditions to some extent the character of the protein deficiency state that is an integral part of the biochemical consequences of nephrotic syndrome.

Although the causes of the nephrotic syndrome are many and varied (Table 39.4), only a relatively small number of disorders constitute the bulk of the conditions encountered in clinical practice. These include nephrotic syndrome resulting from primary glomerular diseases (Chapters 39, Parts 4 to 14) and the secondary forms of nephrotic syndrome. The primary glomerular lesions of minimal change disease (Chapter 39, Part 4), mesangial proliferative glomerulonephritis (Chapter 39, Part 8), focal sclerosis (Chapter 39, Part 5), membranous nephropathy (Chapter 39, Part 6), membranoproliferative glomerulonephritis (Chapter 39, Part 7), and uncommonly, crescentic glomerulonephritis (Chapter 39, Part 9) constitute the group known as *idiopathic nephrotic syndrome.* Among the common secondary forms of nephrotic syndrome are diabetes mellitus with nephropathy (Chapter 45), amyloidosis (Chapter 42, Part 10), multisystem diseases (systemic lupus erythematosus; Chapter 42, Part 1), neoplasia (Chapter 55, Part 3), and exposure to various drugs and infectious agents. Only after thorough and careful consideration that rules out a possible secondary cause should the diagnosis of idiopathic nephrotic syndrome be entertained. This may prove extraordinarily difficult because some of the underlying diseases may be difficult to detect in their early stages (hepatitis B, systemic lupus erythematosus, or neoplasia) and a history of an exposure to a drug or other agent may not be readily obtainable. Renal biopsy is indicated in the evaluation of nephrotic syndrome of unknown cause (idiopathic nephrotic syndrome in adults) but often can be deferred in children because of the high likelihood of minimal-change disease (a steroid-responsive lesion).

ASYMPTOMATIC HEMATURIA AND/OR PROTEINURIA

Asymptomatic hematuria and/or proteinuria may be defined as including the appearance of varying degrees of hematuria (microscopic or macroscopic, persistent or recurrent) with or without abnormal but nonnephrotic-range proteinuria or the occurrence of nonnephrotic-range proteinuria as an isolated finding. In both instances, renal function is normal and hypertension is absent or rare. As such, the definition excludes those multisystem, hereditary, biochemical disorders that may evoke glomerular disease and be clinically associated with hematuria and/or proteinuria. The onset of hematuria may be abrupt and thus resemble acute glomerulonephritis, and the degree of proteinuria, although initially minimal, may progress to a full-blown nephrotic syndrome. Finally, substantial numbers of patients initially experiencing asymptomatic hematuria and/or proteinuria may evolve, over time, to classic glomerulonephritis, or patients with end-stage renal disease may provide a history of bouts of hematuria or incidentally discovered proteinuria many years or decades earlier.

The use of the term *asymptomatic* may be misleading because many of the patients at the time of discovery of the hematuria or proteinuria do have specific complaints, such as fever or myalgia, but in most instances, such clinical symptoms are not specifically referable to the urinary tract.

The causes of the syndrome of asymptomatic hematuria with or without proteinuria are delineated in Chapter 2, Part 8. The primary glomerular diseases that are associated with this syndrome are given in Table 39.5. The discovery of isolated, nonnephrotic proteinuria incidentally during a preemployment or insurance physical examination (chance proteinuria) is a common occurrence and worthy of brief discussion. Such a finding may be the first indication of an underlying structural glomerular, vascular, or tubulointerstitial disease, such as diabetes mellitus, amyloidosis, focal sclerosis, membranous nephropathy, hypertensive nephrosclerosis, or chronic tubulointerstitial nephritis, or on occasion, it may represent overflow of an abnormal paraprotein into the urine as a multiple myeloma or light-chain disease. Determination of the biochemical, antigenic, and electrophoretic character of the excreted protein (Chapters 32 and 101) provides useful clues for the diagnosis. Comparison of the excretion rates of β_2-macroglobulin and albumin aids in the separation of glomerular from tubulointerstitial proteinuria. Some patients excrete abnormal quantities of protein in the urine only during quiet upright posture (orthostatic proteinuria). Such patients are not likely to have serious underlying structural glomerular disease. Constant proteinuria, on the other hand, often indicates a structural disease of the nephron (Chapter 32). Renal biopsy may be indicated in the evaluation of hematuria and/or proteinuria.

TABLE 39.5. Primary Glomerular Diseases Associated with Asymptomatic Hematuria with or without Proteinuria

Mesangial proliferative glomerulonephritis
With IgA mesangial deposits (Berger's disease, IgA nephropathy)
With IgM mesangial deposits (IgM nephropathy)
With IgG mesangial deposits
With C3 mesangial deposits (? resolving postinfectious glomerulonephritis)
Without Ig or C3 deposits
Membranoproliferative glomerulonephritis
Thin basement membrane nephropathy

Selected Readings

Cameron JS. A clinician's view of the classification of glomerulonephritis. In: Kincaid-Smith P, Mathew TH, Becker EL, eds. *Glomerulonephritis: morphology, natural history and treatment*. New York: Wiley, 1973:63–72.

An excellent overview of the classification of glomerular diseases from the perspective of an experienced clinician.

Glassock RJ, Adler S, Ward H, et al. Primary glomerular diseases: secondary glomerular diseases. In: Brenner B, Rector F, eds. *The kidney*. Philadelphia: WB Saunders, 1986:792–1086.

A comprehensive review of the clinical features, pathologic findings, prognosis, and treatment of glomerular diseases. An excellent source of references.

PART 2
Metabolic and Endocrine Complications of the Endocrine System
A: Calcium and Vitamin D

Shaul G. Massry

Abnormalities in calcium metabolism in patients with nephrotic syndrome are not uncommon. Although many patients with nephrotic syndrome may have renal insufficiency, which may contribute to or be responsible for the derangements in calcium metabolism, it should be emphasized that these disorders are encountered in patients with nephrotic syndrome and normal renal function (Table 39.6). With the better understanding of the metabolism of vitamin D and the availability of reliable assays for its various metabolites, it became apparent that patients with nephrotic syndrome and normal renal function may have

TABLE 39.6. Abnormalities in Calcium and Vitamin D Metabolism in Patients with Nephrotic Syndrome and Normal Renal Function

Serum level of total calcium	↓
Serum level of ionized calcium	↓ or normal
Serum level of parathyroid hormone	↑ or normal
Serum level of vitamin D–binding protein	↓ or normal
Serum level of 25(OH)D	↓
Serum level of $1,25(OH)_2D$	↓ or normal
Serum level of $24,25(OH)_2D$	↓ or normal
Calcemic response to parathyroid hormone	↓
Intestinal absorption of calcium	↓ or normal
Urinary excretion of vitamin D–binding protein	↑
Urinary excretion of calcium	Marked hypocalciuria
Bone histology	Evidence of osteomalacia Evidence of enhanced bone resorption Normal histology
Growth in children	Could be retarded

a deficiency of one or more of the vitamin D metabolites. This potential vitamin D–deficient state is responsible for many of the derangements that may occur in calcium homeostasis in these patients.

VITAMIN D METABOLISM

The metabolite 25-hydroxyvitamin D [25(OH)D] circulates in the blood bound to an inter-α-globulin called *vitamin D–binding protein.* It has a smaller molecular weight (58,000) than albumin (69,000). Therefore both vitamin D–binding protein and 25(OH)D are lost in the urine in patients with nephrotic syndrome and heavy proteinuria. The serum levels of 25(OH)D are low in these patients (Fig. 39.1), and there is an inverse and significant relationship between the serum levels of this metabolite and the magnitude of the proteinuria (Fig. 39.2). Spontaneous decrease in the proteinuria or its improvement after treatment with glucocorticoids is associated with a rapid rise in the serum levels of 25(OH)D toward normal. Intestinal absorption of vitamin D is not reduced in nephrotic syndrome.

The serum levels of total 1,25$(OH)_2$D and 24,25$(OH)_2$D may be low or normal. Several reasons may account for the variability in the total levels of the dihydroxylated metabolites of vitamin D in the serum of patients with nephrotic syndrome. These include the magnitude of the decrease in the serum levels of their precursor 25(OH)D, the degree of their possible loss in the urine, and the presence or absence of impaired production secondary to renal tubular damage by the heavy proteinuria. Indeed, a reduced renal capacity to convert 25(OH)D to 1,25$(OH)_2$D has been documented in experimental animals with renal tubular damage without reduction in the glomerular filtration rate (GFR). The measurement of free 1,25$(OH)_2D_3$ showed that the level of this free metabolite is usually normal despite a reduction in its total levels.

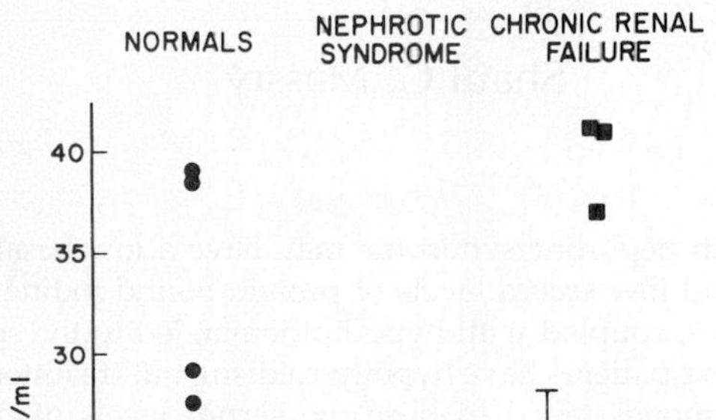

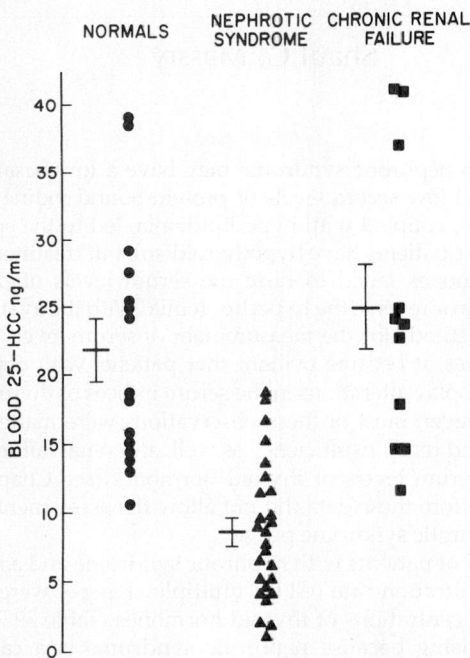

Figure 39.1. Blood levels of 25-hyroxyvitamin D (*25-HCC*) in normal subjects, patients with nephrotic syndrome, and those with renal failure but without proteinuria. *Bars* indicate means ± SE. (Reprinted with permission from Goldstein DA, Oda Y, Kurokawa K, et al. Blood levels of 25-hydroxyvitamin D in nephrotic syndrome. *Ann Intern Med* 1977;87: 664–677.)

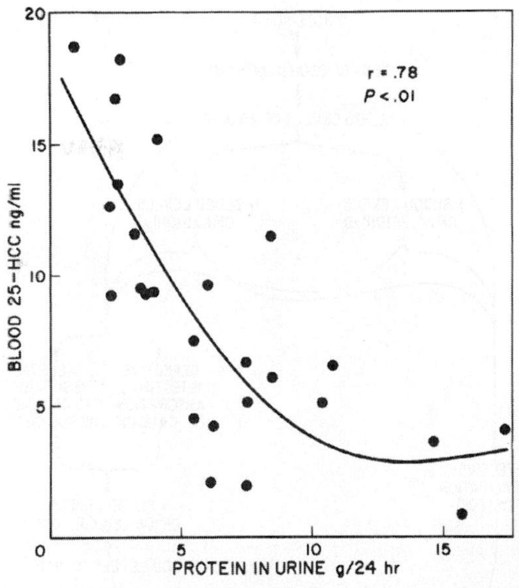

Figure 39.2. The relationship between the blood levels of 25-hydroxyvitamin D (*25-HCC*) and the degree of proteinuria in 26 patients with nephrotic syndrome. The *line* represents the best fit obtained with computer analysis of the data using polynomial equations. (Reprinted with permission from Goldstein DA, Oda Y, Kurokawa K, et al. Blood levels of 25-hydroxyvitamin D in nephrotic syndrome. *Ann Intern Med* 1977; 87:664–677.)

CALCIUM HOMEOSTASIS (FIGS. 39.3 AND 39.4)

Patients with nephrotic syndrome display skeletal resistance to the calcemic action of parathyroid hormone (PTH). Intestinal absorption of calcium may be normal or impaired. Both of these defects result from the vitamin D–deficient state, and both are

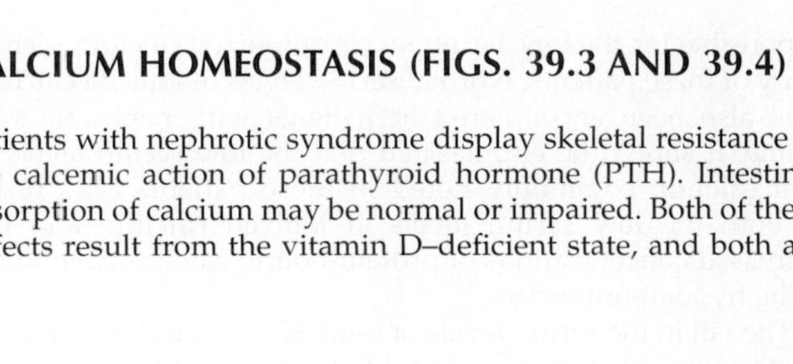

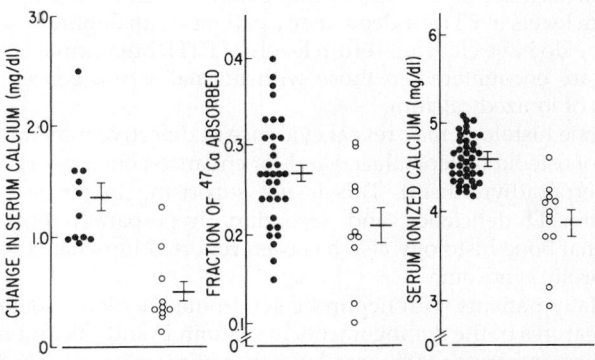

Figure 39.3. The calcemic reaction to the infusion of the parathyroid hormone, intestinal absorption of calcium, and serum levels of ionized calcium in patients with nephrotic syndrome and normal renal function (*open circles*) and in normal subjects (*solid circles*). *Bars* indicated means ± SE. (Reprinted with permission from Goldstein DA, Haldiman B, Sherman D, et al. Vitamin D metabolites and calcium metabolism in patients with nephrotic syndrome and normal renal function. *J Clin Endocrinol Metab* 1981;25:116–121.)

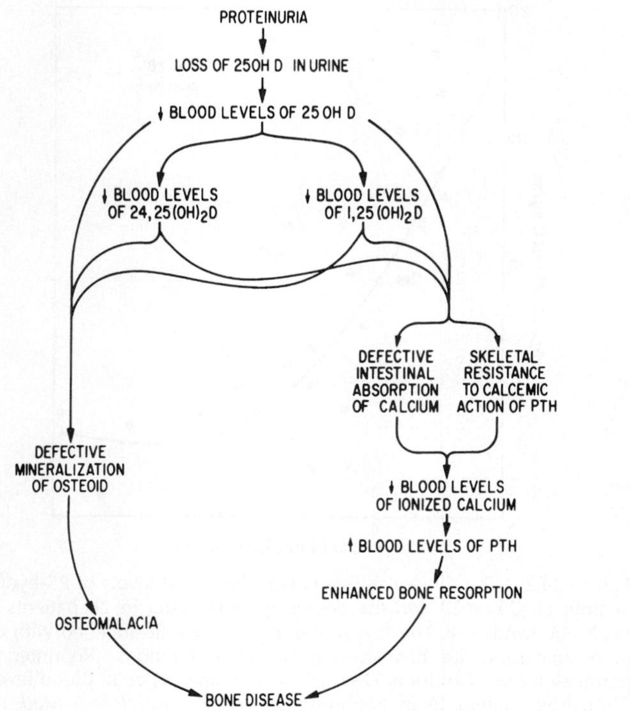

Figure 39.4. A schematic presentation of the pathogenesis of altered vitamin D metabolism and calcium homeostasis in patients with nephrotic syndrome and normal renal function. PTH, parathyroid hormone. (Reprinted with permission from Goldstein DA, Haldiman B, Sherman D, et al. Vitamin D metabolites and calcium metabolism in patients with nephrotic syndrome and normal renal function. *J Clin Endocrinol Metab* 1981;25:116–121.)

responsible for the low serum levels of ionized calcium seen in many of these patients. Normal serum levels of ionized calcium have also been encountered in patients with nephrotic syndrome. It should be emphasized that the low serum levels of total calcium commonly noted in these patients are caused by both the low serum levels of ionized calcium and the decreased concentrations of protein-bound calcium secondary to the hypoalbuminemia.

The fall in the serum levels of ionized calcium should stimulate the activity of the parathyroid glands, resulting in elevated serum levels of PTH. Indeed, many patients with nephrotic syndrome do have elevated serum levels of PTH, but normal levels also are encountered in those with normal serum concentrations of ionized calcium.

Bone histology may reveal evidence of defective mineralization of osteoid (osteomalacia) and/or enhanced bone resorption (hyperparathyroidism). This is not surprising in the face of vitamin D deficiency and secondary hyperparathyroidism. Normal bone histology also has been reported in patients with nephrotic syndrome.

Many patients with nephrotic syndrome may have some of the features of the derangements in vitamin D and calcium metabolism, whereas others may have the entire scope of these disorders. Figure 39.4 is a schematic presentation of the possible pathogenetic processes responsible for the various features of the abnormalities in vitamin D and calcium metabolism in patients with nephrotic syndrome.

Oral supplementation with vitamin D or $25(OH)D_3$ corrects the low serum levels of 25(OH)D in patients with nephrotic syndrome irrespective of the level of the GFR and also causes a rise in serum levels of $1,25(OH)_2D$ in those with normal renal function. A dosage of 20 to 40 μg/day of $25(OH)D_3$ is adequate. Management with $25(OH)D_3$ should be considered when the patients have clear-cut evidence of disturbances in calcium homeostasis and bone disease, especially when nephrotic syndrome is chronic and is not responsive to therapy.

Selected Readings

Goldstein DA, Haldiman B, Sherman D, et al. Vitamin D metabolites and calcium metabolism in patients with nephrotic syndrome and normal renal function. *J Clin Endocrinol Metab* 1981;25:116–121.

Studies of intestinal calcium absorption, calcemic response to PTH, plasma levels of ionized calcium, and serum levels of $1,25(OH)_2D$ and $24,25(OH)_2D$ in patients with nephrotic syndrome and normal renal function.

Goldstein DA, Oda Y, Kurokawa K, et al. Blood levels of 25-hydroxyvitamin D in nephrotic syndrome. *Ann Intern Med* 1977;87:664–667.

The first demonstration of reduced blood levels of 25(OH)D in patients with nephrotic syndrome.

Malluche HH, Goldstein DA, Massry SG. Osteomalacia and hyperparathyroid bone disease in patients with nephrotic syndrome. *J Clin Invest* 1979;63: 494–500.

Static and dynamic evaluation of bone histology in patients with nephrotic syndrome and normal renal function.

Mizokuchi M, Kubota M, Tomino Y, et al. Possible mechanism of impaired calcium and vitamin D metabolism in nephrotic rats. *Kidney Int* 1992;42:335–340.

A study examining the mechanisms of the abnormalities in calcium and vitamin D metabolism in experimental nephrotic syndrome in rats.

Shimotsuji T, Hiejima T, Seino Y, et al. A specific competitive protein binding assay for serum 24,25-dihydroxyvitamin D in normal children and patients with nephrotic syndrome. *Clin Chim Acta* 1980;106:145–154.

A study evaluating the serum levels of 24,25-dihyroxyvitamin D in normal and nephrotic children. The latter had low serum levels of this vitamin D metabolic.

Vaziri ND. Endocrinological consequences of the nephrotic syndrome. *Am J Nephrol* 1993;13:360–364.

A succinct review of the various abnormalities in the endocrine system in nephrotic syndrome.

B: Thyroid Hormone Indices

Shaul G. Massry

Patients with nephrotic syndrome may have a low basal metabolic rate and low serum levels of protein-bound iodine. These abnormalities, coupled with hyperlipidemia, led to the speculation that these patients have hypothyroidism, but treatment with thyroid hormones failed to raise the serum levels of protein-bound iodine or reverse the hyperlipidemia. With the availability of reliable methods for the measurement of serum levels of thyroid hormones, it became evident that patients with nephrotic syndrome display alterations in the serum indices of thyroid hormones. However, most of these observations were made in patients who had renal insufficiency as well, and renal failure by itself affects serum levels of thyroid hormones (see Chapter 74, Part 4). Therefore these data did not allow the assessment of the effect of nephrotic syndrome per se.

In a study of patients with nephrotic syndrome and a normal glomerular filtration rate (GFR), multiple changes were noted in serum concentrations of thyroid hormones (Table 39.7). This is not surprising because nephrotic syndrome is a catabolic condition and represents a state of an acute or chronic illness, conditions known to alter the serum indices of thyroid hormones. The low serum levels of total thyroxine (T_4) and triiodothyronine (T_3) primarily result from decreased binding of these hormones to thyroxine-binding globulin (TBG). A decrease in the levels of TBG secondary to its loss in the urine may contribute to the magnitude of the decrease in the serum levels

TABLE 39.7. Alterations in Serum Thyroid Hormone Indices in Patients with Nephrotic Syndrome and Normal Glomerular Filtration Rate

Total thyroxine	↓ or normal
Free T_4 index	↓ or normal
Free T_4 by dialysis	Normal
Total triiodothyronine	↓ or normal
T_3/T_4 ratio	Normal
Total reverse T_3 (rT_3)	↓
Free rT_3	↓
Thyroxine-binding globulin	↓ or normal
Thyroid-stimulating hormone	Normal
TSH response to thyrotropin-releasing hormone	Normal and prolonged

T_4, thyroxine; T_3, triiodothyronine; TSH, thyroid-stimulating hormone.

of T_4 or T_3. The mechanism for the decreased binding of T_4 and T_3 to TBG is not known, but it most likely is caused by inhibitors known to be present in serum of patients with nonthyroidal illnesses. If one accepts the magnitude of the hypoalbuminemia as an index of the severity of nephrotic syndrome, and hence reflects the magnitude of the loss of TBG in the urine, one might expect a good correlation between the levels of total T_4 and T_3 and those of serum albumin levels. Indeed, available data show that a significant direct correlation exists between the serum levels of both T_4 and T_3 and serum albumin in patients with nephrotic syndrome.

The finding that the T_3/T_4 ratio is normal is consistent with normal conversation of T_4 to T_3, making decreased production of T_3 as a cause of the low serum level of total T_3 less likely. The serum levels of free T_4 and of thyrotropin (TSH) are normal. Earlier studies found that the serum levels of total and free reverse T_3 (rT_3) are normal in patients with nephrotic syndrome who have a normal GFR. However, with the use of a more sensitive and specific assay for rT_3, it was found that both total and free rT_3 levels in serum of nephrotic syndrome and normal renal function are decreased. The reduction in the level of both these thyroid hormones occurred in the face of normal serum levels of free T_4, suggesting that the conversion of T_4 to rT_3 is impaired in these patients.

Despite all the serum alterations in the thyroid hormone indices, patients with nephrotic syndrome, as with other nonthyroidal illnesses, do not have hypothyroidism and do not require thyroid hormone therapy. However, it was reported that some patients with nephrotic syndrome may have true hypothyroidism, which is reversed after the remission of nephrotic syndrome. This situation is not common.

Children with congenital nephrotic syndrome may have low serum levels of free T_4 and elevated levels of TSH, indicating that these children have true hypothyroidism and may require thyroxine therapy.

Selected Readings

Feinstein EI, Kaptein EM, Nicoloff JT, et al. Thyroid hormone in patients with nephrotic syndrome and normal renal function. *Am J Nephrol* 1982;2:70–76.

A detailed study of thyroid hormone function in 15 patients with nephrotic syndrome and normal glomerular filtration rate.

Fosenca V, Thomas M, Sweny P. Can urinary hormone loss cause hypothyroidism? Lancet 1991;338:475–476.

A report of true hypothyroidism in nephrotic syndrome. With the remission of nephrotic syndrome, the hypothyroidism was reversed.

Kaptein EM, Hoopes MT, Parise M, et al. rT_3 metabolism in patients with nephrotic syndrome and normal GFR compared with normal subjects. *Am J Physiol* 1991;260(Endocrinol Metab 23):E641–E650.

A detailed study of rT_3 metabolism in 10 patients with nephrotic syndrome and normal glomerular filtration rate. The investigator evaluated serum rT_3 kinetics utilizing a three-model pool.

Holmberg C, Laine J, Ronnholm K, et al. Congenital nephrotic syndrome. *Kidney Int* 1996;49:S51–S56.

A study of children with congenital nephrotic syndrome in whom true hypothyroidism as evidenced by low serum levels of thyroxine and levels of TSH.

C: Hyperlipidemia

George A. Kaysen

PATTERNS OF HYPERLIPIDEMIA

Hyperlipidemia is a prominent manifestation of nephrotic syndrome. It is usually observed when the serum albumin level is below 2.0 gm/dl. Defects in metabolism of plasma lipoproteins in nephrotic syndrome affect all classes of lipoproteins, altering their concentration in plasma, their composition, and their metabolic rate. Hypercholesterolemia is almost always present. Abnormalities in lipoprotein composition include an increase in the ratio of cholesterol to triglycerides (TG) and of lipids to apolipoproteins (apo). The relative abundance of apolipoproteins in each lipoprotein fraction is changed. The cholesterol-rich low-density lipoproteins (LDLs) and intermediate-density lipoproteins (IDLs) are increased, and high-density lipoproteins (HDLs) may be normal or even decreased. The LDL/HDL ratio is increased. Within the HDLs, the lower molecular weight (200 kD) HDL3 variety remains unaffected while the larger (400 kD) HDL2 is decreased. This change is important because it is believed that it is the HDL2 rather than HDL3 that constitutes the negative cardiovascular risk factor. The triglyceride-rich very-low-density lipoprotein (VLDL) levels in plasma are increased. Although changes in plasma concentrations of apolipoprotein A-I (apoA-I) and A-II (apoA-II) are variable, apolipoprotein B (apoB) is increased consistently. On rare occasions, nephrotic syndrome may not be accompanied by hypercholesterolemia. Lipid levels decrease as renal function fails despite persistence of proteinuria.

Lipoprotein(a) [Lp(a)] has been identified as a prominent risk factor in atherogenesis. Generally, the quantity of this lipoprotein in plasma is genetically determined and is not affected by diet. Lp(a) consists of a molecule to LDL fused via a disulfide bridge to the protein apo(a). Apo(a) consists of amino acid domains called *kringles*. Apo(a) contains one kringle 5 domain and a genetically determined variable number of kringle 4 repeats. The molecular weight of Lp(a) thus increases as the number of kringle 4 repeats increases. Those individuals having the largest apo(a) isoforms have the lowest concentration of Lp(a) in plasma, especially in the Caucasian population.

Lp(a) levels are increased in patients with nephrotic syndrome, and they decrease during remission from nephrotic syndrome. Thus increased Lp(a) in nephrotic patients represents an acquired disorder in lipid levels resulting from the nephrotic state and is not a consequence of a "nephrotogenic" effect of an inherited increase in Lp(a) levels. The mechanism of increased Lp(a) in nephrotic patients is an increase in the rate of its synthesis. Unlike inherited increases in plasma Lp(a) levels, acquired increases in Lp(a) are not associated with increased size of apo(a). Whether an acquired increase in Lp(a) has the same implications for the development of cardiovascular disease is unknown.

PATHOGENESIS

The normal metabolism of VLDLs is shown in Fig. 39.5. Hyperlipidemia in nephrotic syndrome is a consequence both of increased synthesis and decreased catabolism of lipoproteins. The clearance of both chylomicrons (CMs) and VLDLs is reduced. Decreased catabolism of lipoproteins appears to be the predominant cause of hyperlipidemia both in humans and in experimental models of nephrotic syndrome. Increased synthesis of LDLs also contributes to hyperlipidemia. Increased Lp(a) levels are entirely a consequence of increased synthesis.

Increased Synthesis

Hepatic synthesis and secretion of lipoproteins are increased in nephrotic syndrome in the rat as evidenced by direct measurement of lipoprotein synthesis and secretion and by kinetic analysis of the turnover rate of ^{125}I-labeled apolipoproteins. Apolipoprotein synthesis and secretion are also increased. In nephrotic syndrome, the gene encoding apoA-I is regulated at the transcriptional level, whereas apoE and apoB are regulated posttranscriptionally. Similar changes both in apolipoprotein levels and in hepatic gene expression occur in the condition of hereditary analbuminemia in the rat, suggesting that reduced plasma albumin concentration or the reduced oncotic pressure (π) in someway is responsible for establishing the increased concentration of these apolipoproteins in plasma, as well as altering hepatic gene expression.

Conflicting data on lipoprotein synthesis in patients with the nephrotic syndrome have been reported. Triglyceride synthesis was reported to be increased or unchanged. Measurement of the disappearance of ^{125}I apoB showed that its rate of synthesis was increased in nephrotic subjects and that this change correlated with proteinuria in those patients in whom urinary protein loss exceeded 9 g/day. ApoB synthesis was not increased in patients with less proteinuria. We measured synthesis of both VLDL apoB 100 and LDL apoB 100 directly using ^{13}C valine and found that although synthesis tended to be increased, the controlling factor determining VLDL apoB levels in these patients was a decrease in the fractional clearance rate (Fig. 39.6). LDL synthesis, however, was increased, and in some patients, LDL apoB 100 synthesis was greater than the of VLDL apoB 100, consistent with evidence of direct LDL production by the liver in nephrotic syndrome bypassing the normal delipidation pathway requiring LDL to arise from VLDL and IDL (Fig. 39.5).

Mechanism of Increased Hepatic Synthesis of Lipoproteins

Most evidence suggests that the principal organ responsible for increased synthesis both of lipids and of apolipoproteins in nephrotic syndrome is the liver. Furthermore, evidence suggests that reduced extracellular albumin concentration and/or reduced extracellular π in some way regulates apolipoprotein synthesis and lipogenesis by the hepatocyte.

It has been suggested that lipoprotein synthesis was increased in parallel with that of albumin in nephrotic syndrome because all share a common secretory pathway. Although synthesis of some proteins parallels that of albumin in both nephrotic humans and rats, this is not the case for apoB 100. Instead, if increased synthesis of this latter protein does occur, it is not related to that of albumin. Although albumin specifically regulates secretion of apoB by HepG2 cells, it has not been established that this is the mechanism whereby hypoalbuminemia stimulates lipogenesis *in vivo,* and this mechanism cannot explain the effect of nonalbumin macromolecules (dextran and polyvinyl pyrrolidone) on hyperlipidemia or the effect of nonprotein solutes on lipoprotein secretions by cultured hepatocytes. Therefore, although changing the albumin concentration might modulate synthesis of some apolipoproteins, this cannot be the entire effect of albumin on blood lipid levels, but the effect of albumin may be mediated by changes on π. HDL arises initially as a cholesterol, phospholipid bilayer called *nascent HDL* (Fig. 39.5). The cholesterol on the surface of this bilayer is esterified by the action of lecithin cholesterol ester transferase (LCAT) forming lysolecithin and cholesterol esters. The latter sink into the core of the nascent HLD, forming a spherical particle, HLD3. Further action of this same enzyme matures HLD3 to the larger HDL2, a particle whose core is now rich with cholesterol esters. The transfer of this cholesterol ester–rich core of HLD2 to VLDL remnant particles is catalyzed by cholesterol ester transfer protein (CETP), creating LDL. As a result, plasma LDL cholesterol is increased at the expense of HDL cholesterol. Also, CETP plays a significant role in the enrichment of VLDL with cholesterol esters and may also contribute to increased concentrations of apoB lipoproteins. CETP is increased in the

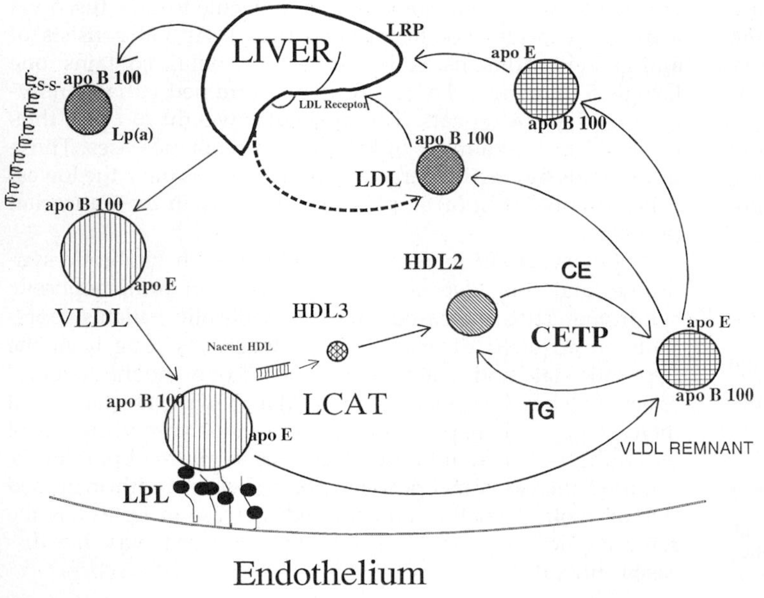

Figure 39.5. Metabolism of VLDL. Very-low-density lipoprotein *(VLDL)* is secreted by the liver and is hydrolyzed on the vascular endothelium by lipoprotein lipase *(LPL).* LPL (the small filled circles), is bound electrostatically to heparan sulfate and, in the presence of apoC-II, hydrolyzes triglycerides *(TG),* releasing free fatty acids, monoglycerides, and diglycerides for cellular uptake. Other surface constituents of VLDL, free cholesterol, and phospholipids participate in the formation of nascent HDL. The free cholesterol on the surface of nascent HDL is esterified by the action of lecithin cholesterol ester transferase *(LCAT)* to produce cholesterol esters. These sink into the core of nascent HDL, which is metabolized to the small, dense HDL3, and finally into the cholesterol ester *(CE)*–rich HDL2. The relatively TG-depleted VLDL remnant particle is released from the endothelial surface and is then either taken up by the liver directly via the remnant receptor or interacts with CE-rich HDL2. In that interaction, catalyzed by cholesterol ester transfer protein (CETP), the CE-rich core of HDL2 is exchanged for the TG-rich core of the VLDL remnant, yielding a TG-rich HDL molecule (not shown) and LDL. The later is then taken up by liver through the LDL receptor, and the former is processed by lipases to HDL3 to continue the cycle. LDL arises both from delipidation of VLDL and by direct synthesis because the rate of synthesis of apoB 100 in LDL may be greater than that of apoB 100 in VLDL. Lp(a) is also synthesized and secreted directly. Plasma concentration is proportional to its rate of synthesis.

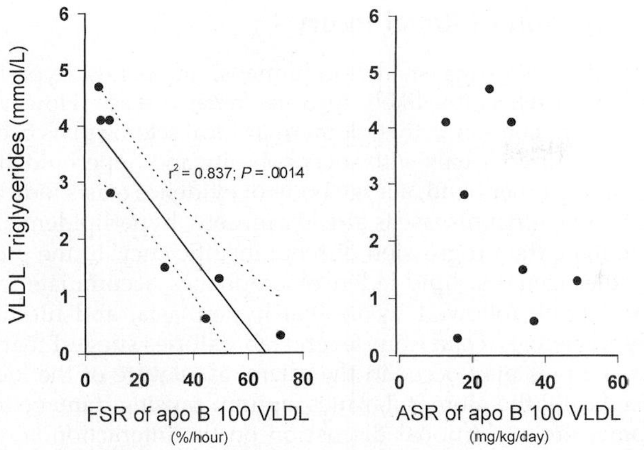

Figure 39.6. The concentration of very-low-density lipoprotein (VLDL) triglycerides is inversely correlated with VLDL fractional synthesis rate *(FSR)*, which at steady state **(left panel)**, is equal to its rate of catabolism. Although VLDL absolute synthesis rate *(ASR)* may be elevated in some patients **(right panel)**, there is no relationship between VLDL ASR and lipid levels in nephrotic patients. (Reproduced with permission from De Sain-van der Velden MG, Kaysen GA, Barrett HA, et al. Increased VLDL in nephrotic syndrome results from a decreased catabolism while increased LDL results from increased synthesis. *Kidney Int* 1998;53:994–1001.)

plasma of nephrotic patients and correlates positively with VLDL cholesterol and negatively with HDL cholesterol. CETP levels decreases significantly following reduction of proteinuria after treatment with an angiotensin-converting enzyme (ACE) inhibitor, in conjunction with a reduction in VLDL and LDL. The mechanism responsible for increased plasma CETP levels in nephrotic patients is unknown.

Plasma LCAT activity increased in the plasma of both patients and rats with the nephrotic syndrome when measured in assays using excess exogenous substrate. The treatment with ACE inhibition and the consequent 40% reduction of proteinuria was associated with a partial normalization of LCAT activity and a decrease in VLDL and LDL cholesterol. LCAT catalyzes two separate reactions: (a) the transfer of an acyl group, usually arachidonic acid, to free cholesterol, increasing the cholesterol ester content of HDLs, and (b) the lysolecithin acyltransferase (LAT) reaction, which takes place on LDLs. Although esterified cholesterol correlated positively with LCAT activity in normal rats, it correlated negatively in nephrotic animals, suggesting that increases of the enzyme *in vivo* may increase the LAT reaction rather than the LCAT reaction.

The observation that HDL3 is preserved in plasma in nephrotic patients at the apparent expense of HDL2 suggests that the LCAT reaction is reduced in nephrotic patients. However, increased activity of CETP could also explain this pattern of HDL distribution by rapidly cycling the core of HDL2 to VLDL remnant particles, thus increasing the flux of cholesterol from the surface of nascent HDL into the core of LDL by increased activities of both LCAT and CETP (Fig. 39.5).

Decreased Lipoprotein Catabolism

Chylomicrons are synthesized in the gut and VLDL in the liver. Both are catabolized on the vascular endothelium by lipoprotein lipase (LPL). The nascent CMs and VLDLs are decorated with a series of apolipoproteins by interacting with HDLs. Of these apolipoproteins, apoC-II is a necessary cofactor for LPL activity and apoC-III a competitive inhibitor. Thus the interaction between properly functioning HDLs and both CMs and VLDLs and the relative amounts of apoC-II and apoC-III are critically important determinants of the rate of lipolysis of these lipoproteins on the vascular endothelium in the presence of LPL.

Once the action of LPL is completed, remnant particles enriched in cholesterol and apolipoproteins are released. The chylomicron remnant particles are immediately catabolized by the liver; this process is impaired in the livers of nephrotic rats, but the mechanism for this defect has not been clarified. VLDL remnants may also be taken up immediately and may also be further processed to LDLs by the enzymatic action of CETP through interaction with HDLs. These processes are also impaired in nephrotic syndrome. Therefore the rate of catabolism of TG-laden lipoproteins, CMs, and VLDLs is greatly reduced in nephrotic syndrome, and their clearance is delayed.

Chylomicron metabolism has not been studied in human nephrotic syndrome. However, the fractional catabolic rate (FCR) of Intralipid, a surrogate for CMs administered intravenously, is lower in nephrotic patients than in healthy control subjects.

Although the delayed catabolism of TGs and the TG-rich lipoproteins has been very well established, much less is known about the catabolism of cholesterol and cholesterol-rich lipoproteins. LDL catabolism has been reported to be either normal or reduced in patients with nephrotic syndrome and only marginally reduced in nephrotic rats. LDL is not the principal cholesterol bearing lipoprotein in rats, however. That function is carried out by HDLs. The catabolism of the protein moieties, apoA-I, and apoC is reduced in HDLs by 50% in nephrotic rats irrespective of whether the HDL is derived from normal or nephrotic rats. However, nothing is known about the fate of cholesterol in HDLs in nephrotic syndrome.

Mechanism of Decreased Catabolism

The impaired catabolism of lipoproteins in nephrotic syndrome is in major part caused by the reduction in the activity LPL. It appears that reduction of the LPL, which is attached to the vascular endothelium, is the critical moiety responsible for the reduced catabolism of VLDLs and CMs in nephrotic syndrome. Indeed, we found that whereas catabolism of CMs by hearts isolated from nephrotic rats is decreased *in vitro* and the LPL pool bound to the vascular endothelium is reduced by approximately 90%, in contrast LPL activity of the heart, which is not bound to the vascular endothelium and hence unable to interact with large lipoproteins, was normal.

The relationship between reduced endothelial-bound LPL activity and decreased catabolism of CMs and VLDLs may not be the only mechanism responsible for the impaired catabolism of lipoproteins in nephrotic syndrome. It was found that HDL isolated from normal animals corrects defective catabolism of VLDL isolated from nephrotic rats by LPL *in vitro*, whereas HDL isolated from nephrotic rats did not. Furthermore, VLDL and CM catabolism by analbuminemic rats was normal despite a significant reduction in heparin-releasable LPL activity. Thus multiple separate defects in the peripheral catabolism of triglyceride-rich lipoproteins may be responsible for the delayed clearance of these particles from the circulation.

In humans with nephrotic syndrome, as in nephrotic rats, the fractional turnover rates of TGs is reduced and the $t_{1/2}$ of TG is prolonged from 4 to 11 hours in VLDLs. The delay in lipolysis in humans with nephrotic syndrome is also caused by a decrease in LPL activity. LPL activity is reduced in children with nephrotic syndrome, and the activity of the enzyme increases after remission of the nephrosis. Furthermore, there is a tight inverse correlation between LPL activity and the concentration of TGs in the VLDL fraction.

At steady state, the FCR and fractional synthesis rate (FSR) of a protein are the same. In nephrotic syndrome, the serum TG levels correlated with the FSR of apoB 100 in VLDLs, but there was no correlation between either VLDL cholesterol or triglyceride levels and the absolute synthesis rates of VLDL apoB 100. These findings are consistent with the notion that it is the FCR of VLDL and not its absolute synthesis rate that established its level in plasma in nephrotic patients (Fig. 39.5).

Total plasma apoC-II is elevated in nephrotic patients; however, the amount of this LPL cofactor per unit of VLDL is reduced by more than 50% because the total amount of VLDL is increased more than the rise in total apoC-II. These findings are similar to those described in rats. This derangement may play a role in the impaired activity of LPL.

The decrease in activity of this biologically active pool of LPL may be important in the defective lipolysis in nephrotic syndrome, but it is probably not the sole defect in this disorder because rats with hereditary analbuminemia also have reduced LPL activity but catabolize both CMs and VLDLs normally. When proteinuria is induced in rats with hereditary analbuminemia, a severe defect in both CM and VLDL clearance becomes apparent. Therefore it appears that neither hyperlipidemia nor defective removal of lipoproteins from the circulation is linked to albumin synthesis or serum albumin concentration but results, at least in part, from proteinuria.

CONSEQUENCE OF LIPID DISORDERS

There are two potential adverse effects of the lipid disorders in nephrotic syndrome. The first is increased risk for atherosclerotic cardiovascular diseases, and the second is the role of hyperlipidemia in mediating progression of renal injury.

Cardiovascular Risk

The relationship between hyperlipidemia, especially hypercholesterolemia, and atherosclerotic disease is generally well established, although no definitive epidemiologic studies have proven clearly that increased risk of atherogenesis occurs in nephrotic patients. However, accelerated atherosclerosis has been reported in patients with proteinuria and hyperlipidemia and in some studies has been associated with a sharply increased incidence of cardiovascular disease and stroke. One study reported an 85-fold increase in the incidence of ischemic heart disease in such patients. In another retrospective analysis of 142 patients with proteinuria greater than 3.5 g/day, the relative risk of myocardial infarction was found to be 5.5 and the risk of cardiac death 2.8 compared with age- and sex-matched controls.

Hyperlipidemia of the nephrotic syndrome may be severe and is characterized by a high LDL/HDL cholesterol ratio. This pattern is associated with accelerated atherosclerosis in other clinical situations, and there is no reason to believe that hyperlipidemia of the nephrotic syndrome would not have similar consequences should this metabolic disorder persist. These abnormalities are further complicated by the increase in plasma Lp(a) levels, increased platelet aggregability, increased plasma viscosity, and increased concentration of highly atherogenic remnants of VLDL and CM catabolism in plasma. It would be surprising indeed if hyperlipidemic patients with nephrotic syndrome did not have considerable risk for development of serious atherosclerotic disease. For this reason, there is no rationale for leaving pronounced hyperlipidemia for prolonged periods in a patient with nephrotic syndrome without treatment.

Progression of Renal Injury

Available data suggests that in humans, unlike rats, hyperlipidemia by itself is not likely to cause renal disease. However, it should be mentioned that glomerular focal sclerosis has been reported in individuals with severe obesity and hyperlipidemia.

On the other hand, a large body of evidence exists indicating that when renal disease is already present, hyperlipidemia may potentiate the progression of renal insufficiency. In the process of atherogenesis, lipid-laden macrophages accumulate in the vessel wall, followed by intimal hyperplasia, and ultimately atherosclerosis. Data from several laboratories suggest that similar changes may occur in the microvasculature of the kidney, specifically the glomerular mesangium, causing damage to the glomerulus. Additional discussion on the interaction between lipids and the kidney is found in Chapter 56, Part 1.

MANAGEMENT

Treatment of the hyperlipidemia of nephrotic syndrome should primarily be directed at (a) treating the primary renal disease if possible and (b) using nonspecific treatments to reduce proteinuria. If the primary mechanism causing the nephrotic syndrome can be directly treated, such as with the use of glucocorticoids for the management of minimal-change nephrotic syndrome, then treatment of hyperlipidemia is of limited clinical utility. If the primary disease process causing the nephrotic syndrome is untreatable and proteinuria is anticipated to be prolonged, specific therapy should be directed at reducing significantly elevated blood lipid levels.

Proteinuria predicts a bad renal outcome in many diseases that cause nephrotic syndrome. Microalbuminuria predicts progression of renal disease in diabetic patients, and the combination of microalbuminuria and hypercholesterolemia predicts the development of atherosclerosis. Although treatment of microalbuminuria would not be anticipated to alter blood lipid levels, if a component of the dyslipidemia of nephrotic syndrome is a consequence of either a liporegulatory substance lost in the urine or of the synthesis of an inhibitor of lipid metabolism by the proteinuric kidney, then a significant reduction in urinary protein excretion should result in decreased blood lipid levels. Indeed, this is the case.

Treatment of nephrotic patients with either ACE inhibitors or cyclooxygenase inhibitors results in a decline in both proteinuria and blood lipid levels, even if plasma albumin concentration does not increase or increases only slightly. The decline in blood lipid levels includes a decrease in total cholesterol, Lp(a), and VLDL and LDL cholesterol; in addition, the activities of CETP and LCAT are decreased. The effect of ACE inhibitors is a class effect and appears to be shared by all drugs within this class.

As with ACE inhibitors, treatment with cyclooxygenase inhibitors may cause hyperkalemia, especially in patients with diabetic renal disease and in patients with underlying hyperkalemia. The decrease in GFR caused by these agents may also limit their utility. Unlike ACE inhibitors, cyclooxygenase inhibitors are likely to increase renal sodium retention, potentially worsening edema formation or increasing the need for diuretic therapy. Other potential risks of cyclooxygenase inhibition include acute renal failure and interstitial nephritis, in addition to gastrointestinal disturbances, including bleeding. For these reasons, cyclooxygenase inhibitors are not the agent of choice.

ACE inhibitors should be started with a small dose (e.g., 6.25 to 12.5 mg of captopril or 2.5 to 5 mg of enalapril). Blood pressure should be checked within 24 hours to make certain that the decline in pressure is not clinically unacceptable, such as might occur with renal artery stenosis. It should be mentioned that normotensive patients do not exhibit a significant fall in blood pressure during therapy with ACE inhibitors. Renal function and serum potassium should be evaluated within a week of initiation of therapy and white blood cells should be checked within a month. If renal function remains stable, one may increase the ACE inhibitor dosage.

Urinary protein excretion declines gradually, even if the fall in blood pressure is abrupt. Urinary protein excretion should be evaluated at the end of the first month of therapy. If urinary protein excretion has not decreased or if there has been no effect on blood pressure in the hypertensive patients, reduction in proteinuria may be elicited by either restricting dietary sodium or adding a diuretic. If high dosages of ACE inhibitors have no effect on either blood pressure or proteinuria, even after sodium restriction and/or the use of loop diuretics, therapy with the ACE inhibitor should be discontinued. Angiotensin II–receptor inhibitors are also effective in lowering the proteinuria of nephrotic syndrome.

Dietary Treatment

Dietary Proteins

High-protein diets should not be prescribed for adults patients with nephrotic syndrome in an attempt to repair depleted albumin stores. Dietary protein augmentation causes an increase in urinary albumin excretion and albumin synthesis rate and may actually cause a decrease in serum albumin concentration. Therefore diets that provide more than the recommended daily allowance for protein of 0.8 g/kg are probably not helpful. The composition of the diet, specifically the type of protein provided by the diet, may also be of significance. The ability of high-protein diets to increase urinary albumin excretion in the rat is a consequence of only a few of the amino acids. The branch-chain amino acids proline, arginine/aspartate and glutamine are without effect on proteinuria. The increase in proteinuria during high protein intake may worsen the hyperlipidemia.

On the other hand, diets consisting essentially of vegetable proteins cause a reduction in urinary protein excretion when compared with isonitrogenous diets consisting of a mixture of foods, including animal protein. Patients receiving the soy-protein diet also exhibited a decrease in total serum cholesterol, LDL cholesterol, and apoB. It is unclear whether the reduction in blood lipids was a consequence of a reduction in dietary lipid intake or a consequence of reduced urinary protein excretion.

Dietary Fat

It is probably prudent to restrict dietary cholesterol and saturated lipids in patients with nephrotic syndrome. It is indeed possible that the changes in lipoprotein levels that follow consumption of a soy-protein diet are a consequence of the lipid composition of the diet, rather than of the amino acid composition. Several uncontrolled studies have demonstrated a reduction in urinary protein excretion in patients treated with lipid lowering agents. Knowing whether this effect is indeed a result of reduction in plasma lipids alone will require a double-blind prospective trial.

Fish Oils

Lipids derived from marine sources are enriched with omega-3 polyunsaturated fatty acids (PUFA) [eicosapentaenoic acid (EPA)], whereas those derived from vegetable oils are enriched with omega-6 PUFA [arachidonic acids (AA)]. The effect of dietary supplementation with PUFA, particularly fish oil, has been studied in a variety of experimental models of renal disease, including nephrotic syndrome.

In adriamycin-induced nephrosis in the rat, plasma levels of cholesterol and triglycerides, proteinuria, and serum creatinine were significantly lower in animals fed fish oil than in those fed beef tallow. Glomerular hyalinosis and endothelial swelling were also less in the rats fed fish oil, and these changes correlated with the changes in plasma concentration of triglyceride and cholesterol. However, the effect of fish oil on the kidney depends on the disease model. For example, fish oil actually accelerates renal damage when fed to rats after partial renal ablation.

The effects of fish oil on either renal disease or the lipid disorders in patients with nephrotic syndrome are less clear-cut than are the data from experimental animals. Although fish oil supplementation lowered serum triglycerides and VLDL cholesterol in patients with systemic lupus, there was no effect on proteinuria or GFR. The addition of fish oil to a soy-protein diet had no further effect on proteinuria or on serum triglycerides. The long-term effect of dietary supplementation with fish oil in human nephrotic syndrome are as yet unknown and cannot be recommended for treatment of nephrotic syndrome except within the context of a controlled investigative trial.

Lipid-Lowering Agents

If specific therapy for the disease causing nephrotic syndrome is not available and if hyperlipidemia does not remit after dietary intervention and reduction in proteinuria with an ACE inhibitor, the hyperlipidemia can be treated with a variety of specific lipid-lowering agents.

The 3-hydroxy-3-methylglutaryl coenzyme A reductase (HMG CoA reductase) inhibitors have proved especially useful. Treatment with pravastatin caused an approximately 28% reduction in cholesterol and 31% reduction in triglycerides in a group of 11 severely hyperlipidemic patients with nephrotic syndrome. The decrease in cholesterol was essentially entirely due to a decrease in LDL cholesterol, resulting in an increase in the HDL/LDL cholesterol ratio. Similar results have been obtained with simvastatin and lovastatin. The use of these agents may engender some morbidity such as rhabdomyolysis with lovastatin, especially when given in combination with gemfibrozil. Serum lipid levels should be monitored, and patients should also be followed for evidence of rhabdomyolysis.

Antioxidants such as probucol have proved useful in lowering serum cholesterol and ameliorating the progression of renal diseases in the rat. This agent also reduced both LDL and total serum cholesterol in nephrotic patients. Probucol also tends to lower HDL levels. Reduction in cholesterol level is less than that reported with HMG CoA reductase inhibitors. Gemfibrozil have been reported to reduce triglycerides by as much as 50% when used in conjunction with colestipol. Although the drug lowers triglyceride levels in nephrotic patients, it is not effective in lowering cholesterol levels. Clofibrate (Atromid) may be toxic in usual doses in nephrotic patients. This drug is tightly bound to albumin, and in hypoalbuminemic states, higher plasma levels of free drug develop, with the usual doses leading to muscle damage manifested by muscle pain and elevated plasma levels of muscle enzymes. Other side effects include gallbladder stones, skin rash, and interference with warfarin therapy. Decreasing the dose of clofibrate to one-third of the usual dose will minimize the side effects.

Nicotinic acid (niacin) but not nicotinamide will lower cholesterol and is particularly useful when combined with gemfibrozil. Flushing and hyperuricemia are undesirable side effects.

Exchange resins, such as cholestyramine (Questran) and colestipol (Colestid), are effective in lowering both total cholesterol and LDL. A major disadvantage of these agents in patients with nephrotic syndrome is their effect on intestinal absorption of vitamin D, which aggravates the vitamin D–deficient state of nephrotic syndrome. Because these medications carry the potential for serious side effects, there is clearly no indication to use them to reduce blood lipids in nephrotic patients who do not have significant hyperlipidemia.

Selected Readings

Davies RW, Staprans I, Hutchinson FN, et al. Proteinuria, not altered albumin metabolism, affects hyperlipidemia in the nephrotic rat. *J Clin Invest* 1990;86:600–605.

Metabolism of both CMs and VLDLs were the same in normal rats with hereditary analbuminemia (HA), even though HA rats were hyperlipidemic and had no detectable albumin in plasma. The hyperlipidemia in HA rats is most likely caused by increased synthesis and not by decreased clearance of lipids. When proteinuria was induced in HA or normal rats, a severe and identical defect in both CM and VLDL clearance was acquired in both groups, and blood lipid levels were increased to a similar degree in both groups. Neither hyperlipidemia nor defective removal of lipoproteins from the circulation is linked to albumin synthesis or serum albumin concentration but result, at least in part, from proteinuria.

De Sain-van der Velden MG, Kaysen GA, Barrett HA, et al. Increased VLDL in nephrotic patients results from a decreased catabolism while increased LDL results from increased synthesis. *Kidney Int* 1998;53:994–1001.

Increased VLDL in nephrotic patients results from a decreased catabolism, whereas increased LDL results from increased synthesis. Although VLDL synthesis is increased in nephrotic patients, the predominant determinant of serum triglyceride levels and VLDL levels is decreased clearance. Serum levels of both triglycerides and VLDLs are independent of their rates of synthesis. LDL synthesis is increased, and the rate of synthesis of LDL apoB 100 is greater than that of VLDL apoB 100 in some patients, suggesting the LDL is synthesized directly by passing the normal delipidation pathway, where VLDL serves as the analog for LDL. Synthesis of apoB 100 does not correlate with that of albumin, suggesting the augmentation of synthesis of albumin and of apoB 100 are regulated separately in nephrotic syndrome.

De Sain-van der Velden MGM, Reijngoud DJ, Kaysen GA, et al. Evidence for increased synthesis of lipoprotein (a) in the nephrotic syndrome. *J Am Soc Nephrol* 1998;9:1474–1481.

The sole mechanism of increased Lp(a) levels in nephrotic syndrome is an increased rate of synthesis. Plasma levels directly correlate with the rate of synthesis of this protein, and no change in Lp(a) clearance occurs. Alteration in synthesis of this lipoprotein differs from that of LDL and VLDL.

Furukawa S, Kirano T, Mamo JCL, et al. Catabolic defect of triglyceride is associated with abnormal very-low-density lipoprotein in experimental nephrosis. *Metabolism* 1990;39:101–107.

Hydrolysis of triglyceride from VLDL by LPL in vitro was significantly less in the presence of HDL from nephrotic rats compared with HDL from normal rats.

Liang K, Vaziri, ND. Acquired VLDL receptor deficiency in experimental nephrosis. *Kidney Int* 1997;51:1761–1765.

The VLDL receptor plays a role in binding to and internalizing VLDL in heart, skeletal muscle, brain, and adipose tissue. The VLDL receptor and mRNA encoding this protein is reduced in heart and skeletal muscle of rats with puromycin-induced nephrotic syndrome, suggesting one mechanism for defective clearance of VLDL in nephrotic syndrome.

Liang K, Vaziri ND. Gene expression of lipoprotein lipase in experimental nephrosis. *J Lab Clin Med* 1997;130:387–394.

Reduced levels of LPL may play a role in decreased catabolism of VLDLs and CMs in nephrotic syndrome. LPL activity and the mRNA encoding this protein are shown to be reduced in muscle and fat of rats with puromycin-induced nephrotic syndrome. This finding suggested that reduced synthesis of LPL may play a role in the reduced levels of LPL in tissues and provide a mechanism for reduced lipid catabolism.

Moberly JB, Cole TG, Alpers DH, et al. Oleic acid stimulation of apolipoprotein B secretion from HepG2 and Caco-2 cells occurs post-transcriptionally. *Biochim Biophys Acta* 1990;1042:70–80.

Incubation of hepatocytes of intestinal cells in culture with fatty acids stimulated apoB synthesis. Binding of fatty acids by albumin prevented this stimulation.

Sun X, Jones H Jr, Joles JA, et al. Apolipoprotein gene expression in analbuminemic rats and in rats with Heymann nephritis. *Am J Physiol* 1992;262:F755–F761.

The concentration of apoA-I, apoB, and apoE are all increased in rats with nephrotic syndrome. ApoA-I is increased by mechanisms involving increased gene transcription, whereas apoE and apoB are posttranscriptionally modulated.

Takegoshi T, Kitoh C, Haba T, et al. A study of the clinical significance of lipoprotein (a) in nephrotic syndrome. *Jpn J Med* 1991;30:21–25.

Lp(a) concentrations were found to be elevated in eight nephrotic patients but decreased after treatment with prednisolone. Lp(a) did not correlate with serum albumin and other lipoprotein or lipid levels.

Warwick GL, Caslake MJ, Bouillon-Jones JM, et al. Low density lipoprotein metabolism in the nephrotic syndrome. *Metabolism* 1990;39:187–192.

In subjects with less than 10 g of urinary protein loss per day, hypercholesterolemia was a result of reduced LDL receptor–mediated clearance. Heavier proteinuria caused increased VLDL and increased LDL synthesis.

D: Thromboembolic Complications

Shaul G. Massry and Nosratola D. Vaziri

Increased predisposition to thromboembolic complications in nephrotic syndrome was first noted by Addis, who reported in 1949 a high incidence of leg vein thrombosis during the "degenerative state" of glomerulonephritis. Since then, numerous reports have described thromboembolic complications involving various arteries and veins in nephrotic patients (Table 39.8). Based on these observations, nephrotic syndrome is considered a hypercoagulable state. Patients with nephrotic syndrome also have deficiencies of various clotting factors and therefore may also manifest bleeding complications.

THE COAGULATION SYSTEM IN NEPHROTIC SYNDROME (TABLE 39.9)

Deficiency of several procoagulant factors may be encountered in patients with nephrotic syndrome. A deficiency of *factor XII (Hageman factor)*, which is at the crossroads of several important proteolytic pathways, has been noted in patients with nephrotic syndrome. Excessive urinary losses, abnormal extravascular distribution, and *in vivo* activation may each (or all) be responsible for low plasma levels of Hageman factor. This deficiency is associated with prolonged partial thromboplastin time (PTT). Nephrotic patients with isolated factor XII deficiency are hemostatically competent and can undergo renal biopsy without added risk of bleeding despite their *in vitro* defect. In fact, acquired factor XII deficiency may paradoxically contribute to thrombotic diathesis, as has been demonstrated in inherited factor XII deficiency. *Factor XI* activity is normal in most patients with nephrotic syndrome, but a deficiency of this factor occasionally may be noted.

Factor IX procoagulant activity is often elevated in nephrotic syndrome. However, moderate to severe deficiency of *factor IX*

TABLE 39.8. Reported Thromboembolic Complications in Nephrotic Syndrome[a]

Pulmonary thromboembolism
Mesenteric artery thrombosis with small bowel and omental necrosis
Inferior vena cava thrombosis
Sagital sinus thrombosis
Axillary artery thrombosis
Iliac vein thrombosis
Splenic vein thrombosis
Right ventricular mural thrombosis with massive pulmonary embolism
Coronary artery thrombosis
Peripheral artery thrombosis with ischemic necrosis of the foot
Renal vein thrombosis

[a] The most common thrombotic complication among those listed in the table is renal vein thrombosis.

TABLE 39.9. Alterations in Plasma Levels of Various Components of the Coagulation System in Patients with Nephrotic Syndrome

Component	Plasma Level
Factor XII (Hageman factor)	↓
Factor XI	Normal
Factor IX[a]	↓ or ↑
Factor VIII	↑
Factor X	Normal
Factor V	↑
Factor VII[a]	↓ or ↑
Prothrombin	Normal or ↓
Fibrinogen	↑
Fibronectin	↑
Factor XIII	↑
Antithrombin III	↓
Protein C[b]	↑
Protein S[b]	↑
Platelets	↑
Plasminogen	↓
Tissue plasminogen activator	Normal
α_2-Antiplasmin	↑
Fibrinogen degradation production (FDP)	↑

[a] Elevated levels are more common than reduced ones.
[b] Reduced functional levels despite increased total levels may occur.

may exist in children and adults with nephrotic syndrome due to various histologic lesions. This deficiency causes prolonged thromboplastin generation time and prolonged PTT. The deficiency of this factor is most likely a result of urinary losses. Because plasma factor IX activity rarely falls below 10% of normal level, spontaneous hemorrhagic complications because of deficiency of this factor are quite uncommon. However, surgical procedures or renal biopsy may be complicated by severe bleeding when performed in the presence of very low activity of factor IX. Prothrombin complex and/or fresh-frozen plasma may be administered in preparation for renal biopsy. The plasma disappearance rate of factor IX may be so fast in some patients that a satisfactory level cannot be sustained for a reasonable period of time. In such patients, the renal biopsy may have to be postponed.

Plasma levels of *factor VIII* (antihemophilic globulin) are significantly elevated in most patients with nephrotic syndrome. This derangement leads to shortening of PTT and may therefore mask the effect of possible deficiency of other coagulation factors evaluated by this screening test. Increased synthesis of this factor by endothelial cells is responsible for its elevated levels, but contracted intravascular distribution may also be contributory.

Factor X levels usually are normal in patients with nephrotic syndrome, but a rapid disappearance rate of this factor has been noted in some patients. *Factor V* levels are elevated in most patients with nephrotic syndrome. Increased synthesis and contracted intravascular distribution are thought to be responsible for this abnormality.

The *extrinsic coagulation pathway* leads to production of prothrombinase, which is functionally identical with that produced during activation of the intrinsic pathway. However, the extrinsic pathway bypasses the steps initiated by contact activation involving factors XII, XI, IX, and VIII. Instead, it requires only tissue thromboplastin and *factor VII.* The latter is a protein synthesized by the liver and requires vitamin K. Factor VII is the main factor involved in the extrinsic pathway. Both increased and decreased plasma levels of factor VII have been noted in patients with nephrotic syndrome. Deficiency of factor VII in nephrotic patients is a result of urinary losses. Isolated factor VII deficiency is associated with prolonged prothrombin time, normal PTT, and normal thrombin time. Severe factor VII deficiency is rare but, when present, may result in spontaneous bleeding. Renal biopsy or other surgical procedures may be associated with bleeding complications in patients with severe deficiency of factor VII. The deficiency state of factor VII and the associated bleeding tendency resolve in parallel with the resolution of the proteinuria. Elevated levels of factor VII are more commonly seen in patients with nephrotic syndrome because of increased hepatic synthesis. Plasma prothrombin *(factor II)* activity and concentration usually are normal despite the demonstrated urinary losses in nephrotic syndrome. However, mild prothrombin deficiency has been reported to occur in some patients.

Hyperfibrinogenemia and elevated plasma fibronectin concentration are common in patients with nephrotic syndrome. The plasma concentration of fibrinogen displays an inverse correlation with those of serum albumin and a direct correlation with serum levels of cholesterol. The elevation in the plasma levels of fibrinogen results from increased hepatic synthesis and contracted intravascular distribution. The fibrinogen degradation rate is normal. In addition to quantitative changes, the fibrinogen molecule may be abnormal in some patients, as evidenced by prolonged thrombin time reported in nephrotic syndrome caused by membranous nephropathy. Hyperfibrinogenemia can significantly increase red blood cell aggregation and thus increase blood viscosity and cause disturbances in blood flow. The latter two changes can contribute to thrombogenesis. Indeed, studies in patients with nephrotic syndrome have shown a significant increase in red blood cell aggregation. Elevation of plasma fibrinogen concentration recently has been identified as an independent risk factor for ischemic cardiovascular disease in the general population. Accordingly, hyperfibrinogenemia can potentially contribute to morbidity from cardiovascular disease in patients with chronic or intermittent nephrosis, compounding the effects of the associated hyperlipidemia.

Plasma *factor XIII* (fibrin-stabilizing factor) activity is increased in most patients with nephrotic syndrome, although normal or subnormal values may be seen in some patients. Increased synthesis combined with negligible urinary losses of this relatively large-molecular-weight protein (160,000 to 320,000) account for the elevation of factor XIII concentration, which seems to be unrelated to the underlying etiology of nephrotic syndrome or histopathologic changes. Interestingly, depressed plasma factor XIII levels have been shown to signify severity and progression of certain active glomerulonephritides characterized by glomerular fibrin deposition. Likewise, a fall in factor XIII activity may occur with acute thrombotic processes because of the active consumption of this protein. Accordingly, a marked fall in plasma factor XIII activity may indicate either progression of the underlying glomerular lesion or occurrence of thrombotic complications in nephrotic syndrome.

A deficiency of *antithrombin III,* which is an α_2-globulin and is the main inhibitor of thrombin, is present in patients with nephrotic syndrome. This abnormality in plasma levels of antithrombin III results from urinary losses. In one study of nephrotic patients, a significant correlation between the degree of antithrombin III deficiency and thromboembolic phenomena was found.

Protein C is an important naturally occurring anticoagulant and fibrinolytic agent whose deficiency is associated with a thrombotic diathesis. This compound is markedly increased in plasma of patients with nephrotic syndrome. Likewise, the level of plasma *protein S,* a compound necessary for activation of protein C by thrombin, is also elevated in nephrotic syndrome. The elevation of protein C and protein S in the plasma of patients with nephrotic syndrome probably reflects increased synthesis of these proteins. Although the clinical significance of elevated plasma protein C and S levels is not known, they may afford some measures of protection in the hypercoagulable state of the nephrotic syndrome. However, reduced plasma level of functionally active free protein S has been reported in some patients with nephrotic syndrome.

Thrombocytosis is common in patients with nephrotic syndrome. Occasionally, thrombocytopenia may be observed, and it should suggest the presence of an underlying disease or associated systemic conditions capable of causing thrombocytopenia, such as systemic lupus erythematosus or disseminated intravascular coagulation. Platelet function is also altered in nephrotic syndrome. Adenosine diphosphate (ADP)-induced and collagen-induced platelet aggregation is increased in children and adults with nephrotic syndrome and significantly correlates with the degree of proteinuria. The observed hyperaggregability is, in part, a result of the associated hypercholesterolemia, which alters platelet membrane composition and resembles that seen in familial type II hyperlipidemia. In addition, hypoalbuminemia, which is known to influence the conversion of arachidonic acid into its platelet aggregating metabolites, may play a role in the genesis of platelet hyperaggregability in nephrotic syndrome.

The fibrinolytic system often is altered in nephrotic syndrome. Blood plasminogen concentration usually is reduced in nephrotic patients because of renal losses. The degree of the plasminogen deficiency correlates with the extent of the proteinuria. Among the several known inhibitors of plasmin, α_1-antitrypsin levels usually are reduce and α_2-macroglobulin and α_2-antiplasmin levels may be reduced or increased in nephrotic syndrome. α_2-Antiplasmin is the most potent plasmin inhibitor, and its plasma levels are particularly elevated in nephrotic patients with renal vein thrombosis. Accordingly, an increased α_2-antiplasmin level may signify a predisposition to thromboembolism in such patients. Likewise, increased plasma concentrations of fibrinopeptide A, fibrin monomer, and its soluble complexes with fibrinogen, fibrin degradation products, or other monomers may denote active thrombus formation. In contrast, an increased level of urinary fibrin/fibrinogen degradation products generally is of little significance in nephrotic syndrome because it usually represents proteolysis of filtered fibrinogen in the urine and enhanced filtration of fibrinogen degradation products through leaky glomeruli.

Several of these abnormalities may be responsible for the increased incidence of thromboembolic phenomena in patients with nephrotic syndrome. These include elevated plasma levels of factors V, VIII, and VII; hyperfibrinogenemia; antithrombin III deficiency; free protein S deficiency; fibrinolytic abnormalities; platelet hyperactivity; and thrombocytosis. In addition, the presence of lupus anticoagulants and/or antiphospholipid antibodies in patients with lupus erythematosus or other autoimmune disorders can result in a thrombophilic state. The use of diuretic agents and the consequent volume contraction may play a contributory role in the genesis of thrombotic complications in nephrotic patients.

RENAL VEIN THROMBOSIS

Renal vein thrombosis may be encountered in a variety of clinical conditions (Table 39.10). Our discussion focuses on renal vein thrombosis in patients with nephrotic syndrome.

TABLE 39.10. Clinical Conditions Associated with Renal Vein Thrombosis

Extension of clots in the vena cava
Invasion of renal veins by tumors
Severe dehydration in children
Renal amyloidosis (rare)
Glomerular diseases associated with nephrotic syndrome
After renal transplantation (rare)

Renal Vein Thrombosis: Cause or Consequence of Nephrotic Syndrome?

For many years, various investigators believed that renal vein thrombosis was the primary event in the association between renal vein thrombosis and the nephrotic syndrome, and most textbooks include renal vein thrombosis among the causes of nephrotic syndrome. The available data, however, strongly support the contention that renal vein thrombosis is a consequence rather than a cause of nephrotic syndrome. The evidence includes the following: (a) obstruction of the vena cava above the renal vein or even renal vein thrombosis may not be associated with nephrotic syndrome, (b) patients with nephrotic syndrome and patent renal veins may develop renal vein thrombosis in the course of their disease, (c) nephrotic syndrome is a hypercoagulable state, and thrombotic events occur in various arteries and veins (Table 39.9) and are not limited to the renal veins, (d) there are no differences in renal pathology in patients with nephrotic syndrome with or without renal vein thrombosis, (e) patients with nephrotic syndrome and unilateral renal vein thrombosis have bilateral proteinuria, and (f) renal vein thrombosis occurs with high frequency in patients with nephrotic syndrome caused by membranous glomerulonephritis and is rare in those with nephrotic syndrome from other causes.

Incidence

It is difficult to assess the incidence of renal vein thrombosis in patients with nephrotic syndrome because selective renal venography has not been performed in all patients. In three series in which such studies were performed, renal vein thrombosis was noted in 1 of 54 patients (1.8%), 33 of 151 patients (21%), and 6 of 21 patients (28%). Thus the overall incidence in this population of 226 patients was 17.7%. The incidence of renal vein thrombosis appears to be much higher (more than 30%) in patients with nephrotic syndrome caused by membranous glomerulonephritis. There may also be a higher incidence in those having membranoproliferative glomerulonephritis. Renal vein thrombosis is not common among patients with nephrotic syndrome from other causes.

Clinical and Laboratory Manifestations

Acute renal vein thrombosis may occur without a specific clinical presentation or may be associated with certain signs and symptoms. These include acute flank pain, marked costovertebral angle tenderness, hematuria, and a rise in the serum concentration of creatinine. When such symptoms occur in a patient with nephrotic syndrome, the diagnosis of acute renal vein thrombosis should be entertained. Intravenous pyelography (IVP) may disclose enlargement of the kidney and pelvocalyceal irregularities on the affected side. Renal biopsy obtained at the time of the acute episode may reveal, in addition to the disease causing the nephrotic syndrome, interstitial edema and margination of polymorphonuclear leukocytes in the glomerular capillaries.

Longstanding renal vein thrombosis in patients with nephrotic syndrome is usually asymptomatic. There are no significant differences in the magnitude of proteinuria, hypoalbuminemia, and hyperlipidemia or in renal function or renal pathology among patients with nephrotic syndrome resulting from membranous or membranoproliferative glomerulonephritis with or without renal vein thrombosis. The kidney on the affected side usually is not enlarged, and occasionally, ureteral notching because of extensive venous collateral circulation may be seen on IVP.

Patients with acute or longstanding renal vein thrombosis may display clinical manifestations due to other thromboembolic events (Table 39.8). The most serious among these complications is pulmonary embolism. In patients with nephrotic syndrome who have a clinical picture suspected to be pulmonary embolism, an aggressive diagnostic approach should be used. If the diagnosis of pulmonary embolism is confirmed, appropriate treatment should be initiated.

Diagnosis

The diagnosis of renal vein thrombosis can be made only by selective renal venography. This test should be performed when the nephrotic patient displays signs and symptoms consistent with renal vein thrombosis. These include (a) sudden onset of flank pain, (b) appearance of hematuria, (c) unexplained rapid deterioration in renal function, and (d) occurrence of other thromboembolic phenomena. Controversy exists as to whether nephrotic patients should undergo a routine venography for the diagnosis of a possible but clinically unsuspected renal vein thrombosis. Because of the high incidence of this abnormality in patients with nephrotic syndrome caused by membranous glomerulonephritis, it is our opinion that venography should be performed routinely at the initial workup of these patients. This approach is not generally accepted, and others may prefer to perform venography only when suspicion of renal vein thrombosis is justified by clinical presentation.

In view of the potential nephrotoxicity of radiocontrast material, use of other sensitive imaging modalities is recommended. In this regard, magnetic resonance imaging (MRI), computed tomography (CT), radioisotope scanning, and Doppler ultrasonography can provide valuable functional and anatomic clues as to the presence of renal vein thrombosis.

Treatment

Data from controlled studies on the use of anticoagulation therapy in patients with renal vein thrombosis are limited. Treatment with anticoagulant agents should be initiated in patients with renal vein thrombosis and proven current thromboembolic phenomena and should be strongly considered in those who have evidence of a previous thromboembolic event. The length of the therapy has not been defined, but the treatment should be continued for at least 3 to 6 months. Long-term therapy is indicated in those with recurrent thromboembolic events. The role of prophylaxis with anticoagulant agents in patients with nephrotic syndrome and without renal vein thrombosis or other thromboembolic complications is not established. Surgical removal of the clot from the renal vein is not advisable or helpful because thrombosis of the venous intrarenal tributaries is most likely present.

Several reports have demonstrated successful use of various fibrinolytic agents in the treatment of new-onset renal vein thrombosis. In addition, subcutaneous administration of low-molecular-weight heparin has been reported in a limited number of patients as a safer and more effective substitute for oral anticoagulants.

Selected Readings

Llach F. *Renal vein thrombosis.* Mount Kisco, NY: Futura, 1983.

An excellent monograph on all aspects of renal vein thrombosis, including abnormalities in the clotting system in the nephrotic syndrome. This book is highly recommended for the reader interested in the topic.

Llach F. Hypercoagulability, renal vein thrombosis, and other thromboembolic complications of nephrotic syndrome. *Kidney Int* 1985;28:429–439.

This review article provides an excellent summary of renal vein thrombosis and coagulation abnormalities in nephrotic syndrome as they were known at the time of its publication.

Llach F, Arieff AI, Massry SG. Renal vein thrombosis and nephrotic syndrome: a prospective study of 36 adults. *Ann Intern Med* 1974;83:8–14.

The first prospective study on the prevalence of renal vein thrombosis in 36 patients with membranous or membranoproliferative glomerulonephritis and the nephrotic syndrome. A high incidence (33%) of renal vein thrombosis was found. There were no clinical, laboratory, histologic, or immunopathologic findings diagnostic of renal vein thrombosis.

Llach F, Papper S, Massry SG. The clinical spectrum of renal vein thrombosis: acute and chronic. *Am J Med* 1980;69:819–827.

A prospective study evaluating the spectrum of renal vein thrombosis in 151 patients with nephrotic syndrome. The incidence of renal vein thrombosis was 27% in patients with membranous or membranoproliferative glomerulonephritis but 9% in patients with other causes of the nephrotic syndrome.

Vaziri ND. Renal vein thrombosis. In: Glassock R, ed. *Current therapy in nephrology and hypertension.* St Louis: Mosby, 1992:286–291.

This review article provides a summary of causes of renal vein thrombosis and its treatment.

Vaziri, ND, Barton CH. Renal vein thrombosis. In: Glassock RJ, ed. *Current therapy in nephrology and hypertension.* St Louis: Mosby, 1998:269–274.

In this review article, the authors describe the use of various laboratory and imaging modalities in the diagnosis of renal vein thrombosis. In addition, the approach to treatment, including use of conventional and more novel agents such as low-molecular-weight heparin and various fibrinolytic agents, are presented in detail.

Vaziri ND, Gonzales EV, Barton CH, et al. Factor XIII and its substrates fibronectin, fibrinogen, and α_2-antiplasmin in plasma and urine of patients with nephrosis. *J Lab Clin Med* 1991;117:152–156.

This study demonstrated marked elevation of plasma factor XIII, fibrinogen, and fibronectin in patients with nephrotic syndrome. In addition, the study revealed urinary excretion and mild but significant reduction in plasma α_2-antiplasmin in a group of nephrotic patients compared with normal controls. Other coagulation and related abnormalities previously reported in nephrotic syndrome have been noted and well referenced in this article.

Vaziri ND, Toohey JA, Paule P, et al. Urinary excretion and deficiency of prothrombin in nephrotic syndrome. *Am J Med* 1984;77:434–436.

This study demonstrates urinary excretion of prothrombin in a group of nephrotic patients, some of whom showed low plasma prothrombin levels, whereas others had normal or elevated values.

E: Sodium Homeostasis and Edema

Robert W. Schrier and Robert G. Fassett

Patients with nephrotic syndrome often demonstrate sodium retention and edema; however, there has been recent controversy over the distribution of the fluid. Some believe there is plasma volume expansion in most patients (overfill mechanism) for the genesis of sodium retention and edema formation, and others believe there is a broad range of intravascular volume states with a significant number of patients demonstrating intravascular volume depletion (underfill mechanism) for the genesis of edema. The underlying events leading

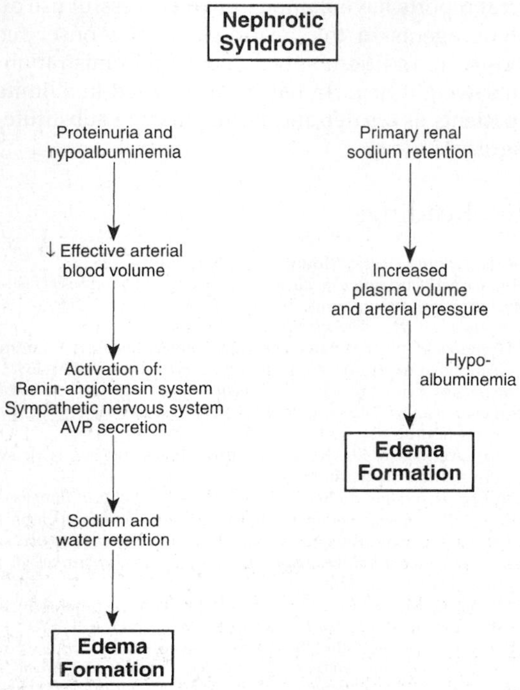

Figure 39.7. Pathogenesis of edema formation in nephrotic syndrome. The proteinuria and decrease in plasma oncotic pressure may induce arterial underfilling with sodium and water retention in nephrotic syndrome (*left:* hypovolemic patients). Primary renal sodium retention may also exist in some patients with nephrotic syndrome and lead to hypervolemia (*right:* hypervolemia patients). AVP, arginine vasopressin.

to sodium retention and edema in nephrotic syndrome are presented in Fig. 39.7.

Clearly, patients with nephrotic syndrome associated with renal failure become volume expanded and hypertensive; in addition, they have a suppressed renin-angiotensin-aldosterone system. Nephrotic patients with normal renal function, however, do not usually demonstrate clinical signs of intravascular volume expansion, nor the low plasma renin activity and high atrial natriuretic peptide (ANP) states seen in acute glomerulonephritis. However, some authors suggest that patients with nephrotic syndrome have an intrarenal defect associated with enhanced tubular sodium reabsorption, predominantly in the distal tubule. This defect is believed to override extrarenal volume regulatory mechanisms. In this setting, nephrotic patients become plasma volume expanded (overfilled) in the presence of normal renal function.

Plasma volume measurements have been assessed in many studies of patients with the nephrotic syndrome over the last 18 years and have produced conflicting results. Some studies in nephrotic patients have shown plasma volume to be expanded; however, a large report analyzing 217 patients from 10 studies found only 25% of nephrotic patients were plasma volume expanded. In fact, the results of this review supported a Gaussian distribution of plasma volume measurements, with 25% having plasma volume expansion, 42% having a normal plasma volume, and 33% having a reduced plasma volume. Thus an issue to be considered is whether the sensitivity of plasma volume measurements is adequate to distinguish between the overfill and underfill mechanisms for the genesis of edema in nephrotic patients. The reproducibility of plasma volume measurement techniques can vary ±10%, which is a range within which renal sodium excretion is regulated by extrarenal mechanisms. Plasma volume measurements may also vary according to the method used to present the data. For example, a particular plasma volume measurement in an edematous nephrotic patient may be increased if adjusted for dry weight or decreased if adjusted for wet weight. In addition, the posture of the patient can influence plasma volume measurement. Patients with nephrotic syndrome who have a normal plasma volume measurement when in the supine position have been demonstrated to have an exaggerated fall in plasma volume in the orthostatic position as compared with the recumbent position.

If plasma volume expansion occurred in most patients with nephrotic syndrome, it would be expected that there would be a consistent suppression of the renin-angiotensin-aldosterone system (RAAS). In a review of nine studies, however, 50% of patients with nephrotic syndrome had elevated plasma renin concentrations. In addition, the posture of the patient also should be considered when assessing plasma renin concentrations because an increase in RAAS activity may only be demonstrable when the patient is upright. Initial studies using an angiotensin-converting enzyme (ACE) inhibitor in nephrotic patients demonstrated a significant reduction in plasma aldosterone concentrations without a natriuresis. Therefore the authors concluded that aldosterone was not an important factor in the genesis of sodium retention in nephrotic syndrome. In this study, however, the ACE inhibitor also reduced blood pressure by a mean of 10 mm Hg, and this hemodynamic effect could in itself be antinatriuretic and thereby override any natriuretic response secondary to the fall in plasma aldosterone concentration. In a subsequent study in patients with nephrotic syndrome, large doses (200 mg orally twice daily) of the competitive aldosterone antagonist spironolactone were used. When compared with a control group of six normal subjects receiving the same constant sodium intake, a natriuretic response to spironolactone was seen only in the nephrotic subjects. These findings led to the conclusion that aldosterone was contributing to the sodium retention in this group of nephrotic patients. An earlier study demonstrated that adrenalectomy in experimental animals with nephrotic syndrome reduced sodium retention. Taken together, these studies support the underfill rather than the overfill hypothesis of edema formation in nephrotic syndrome.

The activity of the sympathetic nervous system also provides indirect evidence for diminished intravascular volume in some patients with nephrotic syndrome. Increased plasma and urinary catecholamine concentrations have been found in nephrotic patients, and in addition, recent investigations assessing catecholamine kinetics have shown increased norepinephrine turnover, suggesting increased production rather than decreased clearance in nephrotic patients. Renal denervation has also been shown to decrease the sodium and water retention in experimental nephrotic syndrome, thus providing additional support for a role of the sympathetic nervous system in edema formation. Renal denervation in nephrotic rats has also been shown to reverse the resistance to ANP. Taken together, these features of increased sympathetic activity in nephrotic animals and humans are also supportive of underfilling of the circulation.

Nonosmotic arginine vasopressin (AVP) release normally occurs with plasma volume depletion (approximately 8% to 10%), and several studies have suggested an involvement of AVP in the water retention in nephrotic syndrome. In this regard, a direct correlation between the decrement in plasma volume and the increase in plasma AVP concentrations has been demonstrated in nephrotic patients.

Plasma volume expansion with saline, hyperoncotic or isoncotic albumin, or head-out water immersion (HWI) improves, but does not normalize, sodium excretion in patients with nephrotic syndrome. Thus, it has been argued that if underfilling is present in nephrotic syndrome, correcting the plasma volume depletion should correct the renal sodium and water retention. However, because prior sodium restriction has been shown to impair and prior sodium excess to enhance the natriuretic response to volume expansion, an impaired response to volume expansion would be expected in underfilled nephrotic patients. Alternatively, patients with nephrotic syndrome who are overfilled may fail to excrete a sodium load because of the presence of a primary intrarenal defect. Such a defect has been demonstrated in a rat model of toxic experimental nephrotic syndrome. Micropuncture techniques have localized this lesion to the collecting duct in superficial nephrons. As noted, studies in patients with nephrotic syndrome have demonstrated that spironolactone decreases sodium reabsorption in the collecting duct.

Hypoalbuminemia does not necessarily result in interstitial edema because compensatory mechanisms can develop. The increase in transcapillary transport of fluid secondary to a decrease in plasma oncotic pressure is initially counterbalanced by a rise in interstitial pressure and increased lymphatic flow, thus minimizing or avoiding edema formation. Moreover, the fluid transport into the interstitium reduces interstitial oncotic pressure, which creates a new steady state with maintenance of the normal transcapillary oncotic gradient. Capillary permeability to protein may also decrease as a result of hypoalbuminemia, which can help maintain plasma oncotic pressure. Patients with analbuminemia do not generally develop severe edema, further supporting a role for these compensatory mechanisms. However, some conditions associated with hypoalbuminemia (e.g., Kwashiorkor, protein-losing gastroenteropathy, and dermopathy) may be associated with significant edema. In clinical states such as these, the compensatory responses to lowered capillary oncotic pressure must be insufficient to prevent interstitial edema.

Last, the debate regarding whether patients with nephrotic syndrome are underfilled or overfilled has important clinical implications. If most nephrotic syndrome patients are underfilled, then diuretic administration may aggravate the underfilling and even precipitate acute renal failure. On the other hand, if most nephrotic syndrome patients are overfilled, diuretic administration is appropriate and safe. It is most likely that a spectrum of arterial circulatory filling states occurs in association with nephrotic syndrome, depending on the degree of renal function impairment, severity of hypoalbuminemia, stage of the disease, and treatment. A clinical assessment of the volume state in the individual patient with nephrotic syndrome is therefore essential when deciding whether it is safe to aggressively administer diuretics.

Selected Readings

Palmer BF, Alpern RJ. Pathogenesis of edema formation in the nephrotic syndrome. *Kidney Int* 1997;51(Suppl 59): S21–S27.

A comprehensive review of edema formation in nephrotic syndrome, with an emphasis on overfilling as the predominant mechanism.

Schrier RW. Pathogenesis of sodium and water retention in high output and low-output cardiac failure, nephrotic syndrome, cirrhosis and pregnancy. *N Engl J Med* 1988;319:1065–1072, 1127–1134.

Review of the pathogenesis of edema formation in conditions without intrinsic renal disease.

Schrier RW, Fassett RG. A critique of the overfill hypothesis of sodium and water retention in the nephrotic syndrome. *Kidney Int* 1998;53:1111–1117.

A review of potential underfill and overfill mechanisms in edema formation in nephrotic syndrome.

F: Other Complications

Richard J. Glassock and Shaul G. Massry

In addition to the complications of nephrotic syndrome discussed in parts A through E of this chapter, there are other disturbances that occur either less frequently or have uncertain clinical consequences. These include (a) orthostatic hypotension; (b) acute renal failure; (c) fluid, electrolyte, and acid–base disturbances; (d) alteration in metabolism of proteins; (e) immune system abnormalities; (f) alterations in erythropoietin metabolism; and (g) derangement in the pituitary-gonadal axis.

ORTHOSTATIC HYPOTENSION

It is uncommon for patients with nephrotic syndrome who have not been treated with diuretics to manifest clinical signs of frank *hypocalcemia* (e.g., orthostatic hypotension or acute renal insufficiency). On rare occasions, however, especially with very massive proteinuria and profound hypoalbuminemia, this can occur. When orthostatic symptoms appear in nephrotic syndrome in association with milder degrees of proteinuria, other processes should be suspected, such as autonomic neuropathy secondary to amyloidosis or diabetes or complicating, acute blood loss.

ACUTE RENAL FAILURE

Acute renal failure may supervene in nephrotic syndrome unrelated to hypovolemia. The cause of this phenomenon is uncertain, but several factors are suspected to play a role: (a) interstitial renal edema, (b) tubular obstruction secondary to intratubular protein aggregation, and (c) widespread epithelial foot process effacement and slit-pore obliteration causing pronounced reduction in glomerular filtering surface area. This complication is predominantly seen in older patients (rare in children) who have minimal-change disease. Recovery of acute renal failure under these circumstance is delayed and is associated with increased risk of mortality.

Sometimes, patients with such acute renal failure will respond to infusion of loop-acting diuretics (furosemide) or, in the case of minimal-change disease, to intravenous methylprednisolone. It should be recalled that patients with nephrotic syndrome are at increased risk for the development of hypersensitivity interstitial nephritis secondary to drugs, renal vein thrombosis, and crescentic glomerulonephritis, any one of which could cause an acute and sustained reduction in glomerular filtration rate (GFR).

Aggressive use of diuretic in patients with nephrotic syndrome and very low serum albumin (less than 2.0 gm/dl) may cause severe intravascular volume contraction and lead to acute renal failure.

FLUID, ELECTROLYTE, AND ACID–BASE DISTURBANCES

Although the vasopressin system is activated in nephrotic syndrome, *hyponatremia* is uncommon in patients who have not received diuretics. Nevertheless, with diuresis, especially when thiazide or thiazidelike drugs are used, hyponatremia may develop, in part as a result of the specific renal effects of the drug to reduce free-water clearance but also because of aggravation of the enhanced vasopressin release related to the effects of hypovolemia on receptors in the arterial and venous circulations, which monitor the degree of vascular filling.

Despite the presence of secondary hyperaldosteronism in many patients with nephrotic syndrome, *hypokalemia* is not commonly seen, except in patients concomitantly receiving diuretics, especially metolazone. *Metabolic alkalosis* is a complication of continued diuretic therapy, although in hypoalbuminemic states, the plasma bicarbonate may be elevated with relatively normal chloride concentrations (hypoproteinemic metabolic alkalosis). The plasma anion gap (sodium − chloride + bicarbonate) is usually reduced in nephrotic syndrome in proportion to the degree of hypoalbuminemia. The anion gap is reduced by 3 to 4 mEq/L for each 1.0 g of albumin less than normal.

Some patients, particularly those with underlying focal and segmental glomerulosclerosis, may have features of *Fanconi's syndrome,* with phosphaturia, glycosuria, hypouricemia, hypophosphatemia, and proximal renal tubular acidosis. Such patients often have massive proteinuria. Conversely, a mild form of hyperkalemic, hyperchloremic *metabolic acidosis* (type IV renal tubular acidosis), may be seen in association with membranoproliferative glomerulonephritis, acute poststreptococcal glomerulonephritis, and lupus nephritis, as well as in association with underlying renal vein thrombosis. Prolonged administration of glucocorticoids can aggravate the tendency toward sodium retention and facilitate the development of hypokalemic metabolic alkalosis. This is particularly true when formulations of glucocorticoids that have significant mineralocorticoid effects are used.

TABLE 39.11. Protein Deficiency States in Nephrotic Syndrome

Protein	Possible Effect
Albumin	Edema, ascites Pleural effusion Hyperlipidemia (? atherosclerosis)
Transferrin	Microcytic anemia (iron-resistant)
Ceruloplasmin	Copper deficiency
Thyroxine-binding globulin	Reduced total T_4, T_3
Cortisol-binding protein	Increased free cortisol Altered cortisol metabolism
Antithrombin III and other inhibitors of coagulation (protein C)	Thrombosis?
Factor B of alternative complement system	Impaired opsonization of bacteria Increased susceptibility to infection
Immunoglobulin G	Increased incidence of bacterial infection (especially encapsulated organisms)
25-Hydroxycholecalciferol–binding protein	Hypocalcemia Intestinal calcium malabsorption Osteomalacia Secondary hyperparathyroidism
Prostaglandin-binding protein	Altered prostaglandin metabolism Thrombosis?
Zinc-binding protein	Hypozincemia Dysgeusia Impotence? Poor wound healing?
Lipoprotein lipase	Altered very-low-density and low-density lipoprotein metabolism
Lecithin-cholesterol acyltransferase	Hyperlipidemia

T_3, triiodothyronine; T_4, thyroxine.

METABOLISM OF PROTEINS

Enhanced glomerular permeability to plasma proteins is a fundamental abnormality in nephrotic syndrome. The bases of these changes in permeability are defects in the charge- and/or size-selective barrier functions. Thus the escape of plasma proteins into the urine depends on the size and charge of the protein, as well as on the nature of the glomerular permselectivity defect. Albumin is a negatively charged protein at physiologic pH and is predominantly lost into the urine in disorders associated with defects in the charge-selective barrier, such as minimal-change disease. In disorders associated with structural abnormalities of the glomeruli and defects in the size-selective barrier, albumin and other protein molecules of similar or larger size (e.g., IgG) are lost in the urine (Table 39.11). Through poorly understood mechanisms, the urinary albumin loss causes a stimulation of hepatic albumin synthesis, thus partially compensating for the escape of albumin into the urine and into the interstitial compartment. A reduction in the plasma oncotic pressure mediated primarily by hypoalbuminemia in the hepatic sinusoids is thought to be the stimulus for this effect. High-protein diets do not correct hypoalbuminemia because they augment urinary protein loss. On the other hand, low-protein diets accompanied by administration of angiotensin-converting enzyme (ACE) inhibitors reduce protein excretion and tend to increase serum albumin levels and total albumin pools.

The effects of the ACE inhibitors is probably due to a direct effect on the glomerular capillary circulation and/or on glomerular permeability.

IgG levels in the serum are commonly reduced in nephrotic syndrome. The degree of reduction does not correlate with the magnitude of urinary losses. For example, IgG levels are decreased in minimal-change disease despite the paucity of IgG losses in the urine. Other mechanisms appear to be involved, such as inhibition of synthesis or increased extrarenal fractional catabolism (e.g., gastrointestinal loss of protein). IgM and IgA levels may be increased in some patients with nephrotic syndrome. For example, IgM levels in minimal-change disease tend to be increased even after remission. As previously discussed, the loss of hormone-binding proteins (e.g., cholecalciferol-binding protein, thyroxin-binding protein) may greatly influence the relationship of free to bound hormone in the plasma and thus alter space of distribution and whole body clearance rates. *Cortisol-binding protein* is reduced in nephrotic syndrome, thus altering the distribution and fate of exogenously administered glucocorticoids. Such alterations could be responsible for the suggestion that nephrotic patients develop clinical Cushing's syndrome more rapidly and at lower dosages than do nonnephrotic patients. In patients not receiving exogenous glucocorticoids, these changes in cortisol metabolism are of little clinical significance.

Loss of *transferrin, ceruloplasmin,* and *zinc-binding proteins* in the urine may contribute to the development of deficiencies of the essential metallic elements iron, copper, and zinc. These deficiencies may interfere with red cell production or the function of critical enzymes. Severe transferrin deficiency rarely occurs in nephrotic syndrome but, when present, can be associated with a microcytic hypochromic anemia unresponsive to oral or parenteral iron therapy.

Copper deficiency usually is asymptomatic, but we have encountered a few patients with nephrotic syndrome who developed "kinky hair" and severe muscular cramps that were responsive to exogenous copper administration. Zinc deficiency is relatively common in nephrotic syndrome but usually of little clinical significance. Nevertheless, zinc deficiency theoretically could contribute to poor wound healing, dysgeusia, impotence, or abnormalities of cell-mediated immunity. Patients with clinical symptoms possibly attributable to zinc deficiency should probably be given a trial of zinc replacement. It is possible that other trace element deficiencies may occur in nephrotic syndrome, particularly in situations in which trace elements are bound to plasma proteins of a molecular size and charge characteristics leading to their excessive urinary loss in patients with nephrotic syndrome.

IMMUNE SYSTEM ABNORMALITIES

To a certain extent, the abnormalities of cellular or humoral immunity found in nephrotic syndrome are a part of the underlying disturbances responsible for the glomerular disease or occur as a consequence of its therapy. Nevertheless, the nephrotic state per se, in all likelihood, also produces changes in the function of the immune system. For example, extensive loss of IgG in the urine may produce a state of partial acquired hypogammaglobulinemia and thus contribute to enhanced susceptibility to bacterial infection, especially with those bacteria with carbohydrate-containing capsules, such as *Streptococcus pneumoniae.*

Enhanced excretion of complement components could contribute to deficiencies in the opsonic activity of serum. Vitamin D deficiency and secondary hyperparathyroidism also could contribute to defects in cell-mediated or humoral immunity. The accumulation of immunoregulatory lipids (low-density lipoprotein, intermediate-density lipoprotein) may participate in defects of cell-mediated immunity, such as reduced delayed cutaneous hypersensitivity or the capacity of T cells from nephrotic patients to respond to mitogens or antigens *in vitro.* Defects of macrophage function and variation in the phenotypic distribution of T and B cells in blood have been described in nephrotic syndrome. However, it is difficult to know how many of these alterations are the consequence of nephrotic syndrome per se or are events associated with the underlying disease pathogenesis. The superimposition of impaired renal function in some patients only confounds interpretation of the results because chronic renal failure causes disturbances in the immune system.

Whatever the case may be, patients with nephrotic syndrome do not appear to be at greatly increased risk for the development of opportunistic viral, fungal, or mycobacterial infection if they are not receiving prolonged therapy with glucocorticoids, cytotoxic agents, or cyclosporine. Nevertheless, patients with nephrotic syndrome do have some increased risk of bacterial infection, particularly with encapsulated organisms. Spontaneous bacterial peritonitis was a greatly feared complication of nephrotic syndrome in the past but is now seldom observed. Infections observed in patients with nephrotic syndrome are more commonly the consequence of immunosuppressive therapy.

ALTERATIONS IN ERYTHROPOIETIN METABOLISM

Patients with nephrotic syndrome may display reduced plasma concentration of erythropoietin and marked excretion of the hormone in the urine. This phenomenon was noticed in nephrotic patients with normal glomerular filtration rate. These observations were confirmed in rats with puromycin-induced nephrotic syndrome. The animals had increased urinary excretion of erythropoietin and marked attenuation in the rise in plasma erythropoietin in response to graded anemia or hypoxia.

Kinetic studies in nephrotic rats demonstrated that the endogenous rate of erythropoietin production is reduced, its disappearance rate is increased, and its volume of distribution is expanded. Thus it appears that these nephrotic animals have relative deficiency of erythropoietin, with the augmented urinary losses of the hormone playing an important role in this phenomenon.

The clinical significance of such relative deficiency of erythropoietin has not been carefully evaluated. Most patients with nephrotic syndrome and normal renal function do not have anemia. However, it is conceivable that this abnormality may interfere with the patients' ability to maintain a normal rate of erythropoiesis when challenged by conditions that may cause anemia.

PITUITARY-GONADAL AXIS

Urinary losses of sex hormone–binding globulin is increased in patients with nephrotic syndrome, and this can result in increased elimination of these hormones. In rats with puromycin-induced renal failure, there were significant reductions in the plasma levels of testosterone, a significant elevation in plasma levels of luteinizing hormone, and marked urinary losses of testosterone. Although the latter contributes in major part to the low plasma levels of testosterone, it appears that there may also be impaired gonadal steroidogenesis. This phenomenon may be related to the catabolic state of nephrotic syndrome. The response of the pituitary to gonadotropin-releasing hormone is not altered in nephrotic syndrome.

Selected Readings

Elias AN, Carreon G, Vaziri ND, et al. the pituitary-gonadal axis in experimental nephrotic syndrome in male rats. *J Lab Clin Med* 1992;120:949–954.
A study evaluating the function of the pituitary-gonadal axis in rats with puromycin-induced nephrotic syndrome.

Glassock RJ, Adler S, Ward H, et al. Primary glomerular disease. In: Brenner B, Rector F, eds. *The kidney*. Philadelphia: WB Saunders, 1991:1182–1279.
An encyclopedic overview of syndromes of glomerular disease.

Vaziri ND, Kaupke CJ, Barton CH, et al. Plasma concentration and urinary excretion of erythropoietin in adult nephrotic syndrome. *Am J Med* 1992;92:35–40.
A study demonstrating a significant increase in urinary excretion of erythropoietin and a decrease in the blood levels of the hormone in patients with nephrotic syndrome.

Zhou XJ, Vaziri ND. Erythropoietin metabolism and pharmacokinetics in experimental nephrosis. *Am J Physiol* 1992;263:F812–F815.
A study examining the metabolism and kinetics of erythropoietin in rats with puromycin-induced nephrotic syndrome.

PART 3

Glomerulonephritis Associated with Infection

A: Poststreptococcal Glomerulonephritis

Bernardo Rodríguez-Iturbe and Gustavo Parra

Poststreptococcal glomerulonephritis (PSGN) is the best known of a variety of nephritides associated with infections. Two centuries ago, it was noted that dark and scanty urine were the hallmarks of a feared complication of the convalescence of scarlet fever. The first pathologic description of the renal lesion and Bela Schick's suggestion that the disease resulted from allergic reactivity appeared in the first decade of the twentieth century. Shortly afterwards, it was recognized that β-hemolytic streptococcus is the etiologic agent of scarlet fever. As a consequence, the terms *acute glomerulonephritis* (pathologic characteristics), *nephritic syndrome* (typical clinical presentation), and *poststreptococcal glomerulonephritis* (etiologic definition) have been used interchangeably in the past.

EPIDEMIOLOGY

The incidence of PSGN is decreasing in the United States and Central Europe, but sporadic cases of the disease continue to be reported from all over the world. Epidemics appear recurrently in certain regions of the world for reasons that remain elusive; most of these areas share the characteristic of crowded housing with poor hygienic conditions.

Acute PSGN typically affects children between the ages of 2 and 14 years, but in most large series, 5% are younger than 2 years and 10% are older than 40 years. The clinical cases of PSGN are twice as common in males as in females, but subclinical disease occurs in both sexes with equal frequency. Familial incidence of PSGN is almost 40%; however, the search for a genetic marker of the disease has been unsuccessful.

The skin and the throat are the usual sites of the preceding infection. In the southern United States and in the tropics, PSGN follows pyodermitis with streptococci of M types 47, 49, 55, and 57. Other M types, particularly types 1, 2, 4, and 12, are isolated more frequently from throat infections associated with nephritis. The risk of nephritis after infection varies considerably in different studies but overall is about 15%. Interestingly, skin infections with M type 49 have a 25% nephritis risk, but only a 5% risk if the site of infection is the upper respiratory tract.

PATHOGENESIS

PSGN is an immunologically mediated disease. Many investigators have attempted to clarify the nature of the antigen(s) involved, the site of their interaction, and the role played by autoimmune reactivity, yet these issues are still incompletely defined.

Streptococcal Antigens

Over the years, many streptococcal fractions have been proposed as the putative nephritogen, but most of them have failed the test of time. M protein was the first and most extensively studied, but it has not been convincingly shown in biopsies, and with the ever-increasing number of M types isolated from patients with PSGN, is difficult to reconcile with the idea of a limited number of nephritis-inducing antigenic fractions.

At present, two antigens are actively investigated: the "preabsorbing antigen" (endostreptosin) and streptococcal zymogen. In an effort to study the preabsorbing antigen, it was found that fluorescein-labeled convalescent sera stain biopsies taken in the first week of PSGN, presumably identifying the relevant nephritogen localized in the glomeruli. Additional studies resulted in the isolation of a protein (molecular weight of 50,000) that preabsorbs the staining capacity of convalescent sera (presumably reacting with the specific antibody). The antigen directly activates the alternative complement cascade and subsequently induces specific antibody response

Other investigators directed their studies to cationic fractions because their charge would make them attracted to the glomerular basement membrane (GBM). Early work identified a cationic proteinase in cultures of nephritogenic streptococci. Subsequent studies have shown that this fraction is zymogen, a precursor of the streptococcal exotoxin B. Zymogen is present in renal biopsies of acute PSGN, and a multicenter study has demonstrated that high antizymogen serum titers are the best marker of streptococcal infection associated to acute glomerulonephritis.

Autoimmunity

Autoimmune reactivity is present in PSGN. Anti-Ig reactivity is indicated by the following findings: (a) 32% to 43% of patients have positive rheumatoid factor in the first week of the disease; IgG-rheumatoid factor is twice as common as IgM-rheumatoid factor; (b) anti-Ig deposits are found in 30% of the renal biopsies; (c) the antibody eluted from the kidney in a fatal case was predominantly IgG with significant anti-IgG reactivity; and (d) IgG anti-IgG antibodies with the capacity to activate the alternate complement pathway (C3Nef) have been demonstrated.

The mechanism of induction of anti-Igs is controversial. Streptococcal neuraminidase (sialidase) could produce loss of sialic acid from autologous Ig, a modification capable of inducing anti-Ig reactivity and nephritis. Neuraminidase has been isolated from nephritogenic streptococcal strains and neuraminidase activity, and free sialic acid have been found in the sera of patients with acute PSGN. In other studies, lectins have been used to identify in kidney biopsies carbohydrate radicals that could have been exposed by sialic acid depletion. Specifically, peanut agglutinin reactive sites have been found in deposits and in infiltrating leukocytes.

Loss of sialic acid is not the only mechanism capable of generating anti-IgG reactivity. Similar autoantigenicity may result from the binding of the Fc fragment of IgG to type II receptors in the streptococcal wall.

Anti-IgG is not the only manifestation of autoimmunity in PSGN: DNA–anti-DNA complexes and ANCA antibodies have also been reported. It is undefined whether autoimmune reactivity is an epiphenomena or if it plays an important role in the pathogenesis of PSGN.

Site of Immune Reactivity and Charge-Dependent Effects

Traditionally, acute PSGN has been considered a disease caused by the deposition of circulating immune complexes, the human counterpart of acute, one-shot, experimental serum sickness. Yet, there is increasing circumstantial evidence in favor of *in situ* antigen–antibody reactivity in many glomerulonephritides, and acute PSGN is no exception. The cationic charge of the zymogen/proteinase described previously would make it an attractive candidate to induce subepithelial deposition because cationic antigens easily fix and readily penetrate the GBM. Antibody charge could also be important: sialic acid-depleted and naturally occurring cationic immunoglobulins may get planted in the anionic basement membrane and act as targets for the antigen.

Participation of Complement

Reduction of the serum complement levels and renal deposition of C3 and other components of the C cascade are well-known characteristics of PSGN. The participation of complement stimulates chemotaxis (C5a), increases capillary permeability, and induces the release of cytokines and platelet-derived inflammatory mediators. Important as it is, the participation of the complement system is not indispensable for the development of experimental models of nephritis that have similitude with human PSGN, such as acute serum sickness.

Cellular Immunity

In addition to the antibody-dependent mechanisms, cellular immunity may also play an important pathogenetic role in PSGN. In the experimental model of acute serum sickness, proteinuria has a temporal correlation with the infiltration of monocytes, and it can be abrogated with antimacrophage serum as well as with cyclosporine treatment. Macrophage migration inhibition factor (MIF) is secreted by infiltrating lymphocytes. In acute PSGN, the participation of immunocompetent cells is suggested by the early infiltration of CD4+ lymphocytes and monocytes. This infiltration is favored by overexpression of adhesion molecules CD54 (ICAM-1) and CD18 (LFA-1) and by the release of cytokines by these cells. Other studies indicate that the loss of sialic acid in the peripheral blood leukocytes favors their accumulation in the kidney, suggesting yet another potential pathogenetic role for neuraminidase.

Cytokines

Cytokines, with the potential to participate and amplify the damage and the immune reactivity, are liberated in PSGN. Interleukin-6 (IL-6) and tumor necrosis factor-α (TNF-α) are increased in serum and in renal biopsies. It is likely that IL-6 stimulates mesangial hypercellularity in PSGN, as it does in lupus nephritis and IgA nephropathy. Platelet-aggregating factor (PAF) is increased in the serum of PSGN patients and, interestingly, is unchanged in uncomplicated streptococcal throat infection.

CLINICAL MANIFESTATIONS

Streptococcal Infection and Antistreptococcal Antibodies

Streptococcal impetigo is a common complication of scabies in the tropics and usually is manifested by small vesicles that break easily and leave a thick crust. Regional lymphadenopathy is present in 80% to 90% of patients with active infection. Postimpetigo nephritis has an incubation period of 3 to 6 weeks. Streptococcal pharyngitis may cause only sore throat or may be associated with fever, cervical adenopathy, and purulent exudate. If the last three manifestations are present, the likelihood of a streptococcal etiology is very high, and antibiotic treatment should be given irrespective of the culture results. In contrast, fewer than 3% of the sore throats in which all three manifestations are absent are streptococcal. The latent period of PSGN after upper respiratory infections is 1 to 3 weeks. During the latent period, one-third of patients have microscopic hematuria and mild albuminuria.

Success in culturing group A streptococci from the site of infection is variable. During epidemics, positive cultures are obtained in 10% to 70% of the cases. The diagnosis of streptococcal infection is usually confirmed by serologic evidence of

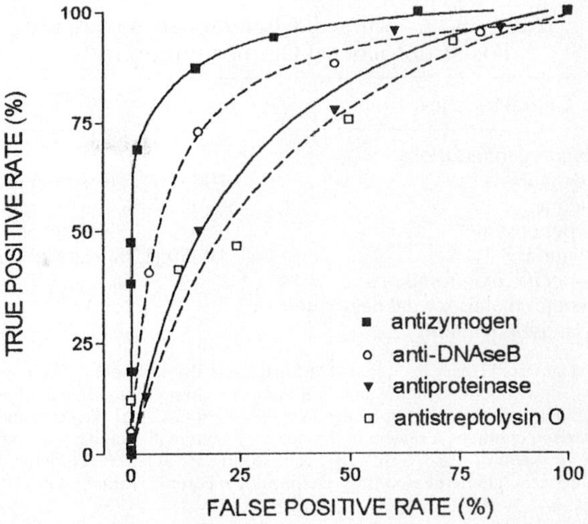

Figure 39.8. Receiver operating characteristics (ROC) curves for antibody tests in the diagnosis of streptococcal infection associated with glomerulonephritis. Antizymogen and antiproteinase curves are drawn with uninterrupted lines. Antizymogen titers are superior to the rest at all levels of the curve. (Reproduced with permission from Parra G, Rodríguez-Iturbe B, Batsford S, et al. Antibody to streptococcal zymogen in the serum of patients with acute glomerulonephritis. A multicentric study. *Kidney Int* 1998; 54:509–517.)

recent infection in serial testing, but not all antistreptococcal antibody determinations are equally helpful. In a large series of cases, antizymogen titers are the best available marker of streptococcal infection in patients with nephritis (Fig. 39.8). In fact, a titer 1:1600 or greater, representing two dilutions above the mean found in controls, has a sensitivity of 88% and a specificity of 85% in the detection of streptococcal infections in patients with nephritis. Antizymogen titers decrease in the following weeks but are still elevated 3 months after the infection. Unfortunately, antizymogen determinations are not widely available. Increased anti-DNAse B, antihyaluronidase, ASO, and antistreptokinase titers have been found in 73%, 38%, 33%, and 7% of patients with PSGN, respectively. Antibodies directed against streptococcal M protein are type specific, appear 4 to 6 weeks after infection, and last for years; this characteristic makes them useful in retrospective analysis of epidemics.

Nephritis

Microscopic hematuria and a fall in serum complement characterize *subclinical PSGN*. Hypertension may or may not be present. These patients have endocapillary glomerulonephritis, but the short- and long-term prognosis is invariably good and renal biopsy is not indicated. A wide variation in the incidence of subclinical disease has been reported (subclinical/clinical ratios ranging from 0.5 to 19), but the best estimates come from prospective studies in which repeated testing was done in families and contacts of index cases. In these studies, subclinical disease is four to five times more common that clinical nephritis. *Acute nephritic syndrome* (hematuria, edema, and hypertension, with or without oliguria) is the most common clinical presentation of PSGN. Fewer than 5% of the children and 20% of adults have proteinuria of more than 3 g/day, and this "*nephrotic*" presentation is associated with a worse long-term prognosis. Fewer than 1% of the patients develop a *rapidly progressive glomerulonephritis*,

TABLE 39.12. Clinical Characteristics of Acute Poststreptococcal Glomerulonephritis

Characteristics	%
Cardinal manifestations	
Hematuria	100 (30% gross hematuria)
Edema	80–90 (60% chief complaint)
Hypertension	60–80 (50% severe)
Oliguria	10–50 (15% <200 ml/day)
Nonspecific manifestations	
General malaise, weakness, anorexia	50
Nausea, vomiting	15

Data from Lewry JE, Salinas-Madrigal L, Herdson PB, et al. Clinicopathological correlations in acute poststreptococcal glomerulonephritis. *Medicine* 1971;50:453–501; Travis LB, Dodge WH, Beathard GA, et al. Acute glomerulonephritis in children. A review of the natural history with emphasis on prognosis. *Clin Nephrol* 1973;1:169–181; and Rodríguez-Iturbe B. Epidemic poststreptococcal glomerulonephritis (Nephrology Forum). *Kidney Int* 1984;25: 129–136.

associated with extensive extracapillary glomerular crescent formation.

The relative frequencies of the various clinical manifestations of are shown in Table 39.12. Microscopic hematuria with red blood cell casts is invariably present. Edema is the chief complaint in most patients. In fact, Well's masterful report of the disease in the early nineteenth century dealt with "the dropsy which succeeds scarlet fever." Generalized edema is more common in infants. Hypertension is very common, and in half of the patients, it is severe; yet, hypertensive encephalopathy is very unusual. Hemodynamic studies demonstrate increased plasma volume and cardiac output in practically all patients, and the severity of hypertension and the degree of fluid retention are directly correlated. The volume-sensitive hormonal systems are responding appropriately to a primary fluid overload: plasma renin activity and aldosterone levels are decreased and atrial natriuretic factor is stimulated. The clinical manifestations of acute PSGN usually resolve in less than 2 weeks, although microscopic hematuria and/or proteinuria may persist for many months. As shown in Table 39.13, the complications, and consequently, the early mortality, are much more common in elderly patients than in children.

TABLE 39.13. Complications of Acute Poststreptococcal Glomerulonephritis

	Children[a] (%)	Elderly Patients[b] (%)
Congestive heart failure	<5	43
Massive proteinuria (>3 g/day)	4–10	20
Azotemia	25–40	83
Early mortality	<1	25

[a] Data from Lewry JE, Saliner-Madrigal L, Herdson PB, et al. Clinicopathological correlations in acute poststreptococcal glomerulonephritis. *Medicine* 1971;50:453–501; Travis LB, Dodge WG, Beathard GA, et al. Acute glomerulonephritis in children. A review of the natural history with emphasis on prognosis. *Clin Nephrol* 1973;1:169–181; and Rodríguez-Iturbe B. Epidemic poststreptococcal glomerulonephritis (Nephrology Forum). *Kidney Int* 1984;25:129–136.

[b] Data reviewed by Melby PC, Musick WD, Luger AM, et al. Poststreptococcal glomerulonephritis in the elderly: report of a case and review of the literature. *Am J Nephrol* 1987;7:235–240.

SEROLOGIC FINDINGS

In the first week of symptoms, serum hemolytic complement activity (CH_{50}) and C3 levels are depressed in 90% of the patients; properdin, C2, and C4 also may be low, suggesting that the alternative as well as the classical pathways of complement are activated. C5b-C9 plasma levels are elevated and decrease with the time. After 2 months, patients with uncomplicated PSGN have normal complement levels.

Serum IgG and IgM are increased in 80% of patients and return to normal after 1 to 2 months. Serum IgA levels are normal in PSGN, in contrast with the findings in rheumatic fever in which serum IgA is frequently high.

Positive rheumatoid factor is present in 32% to 42% of the patients in the first week of nephritis. Cryoglobulins and circulating immune complexes (measured by the C1q binding activity) are found in two-thirds of the patients in the first week of the illness. ANCA antibodies have been found in 9% of the patients and they seem to associate with a more severe disease.

DIAGNOSIS

Many renal diseases may present with edema, hematuria, and hypertension. Systemic lupus erythematosus, IgA nephropathy, anti-GBM disease, essential cryoglobulinemia, bacterial endocarditis, and microscopic polyarteritis, among others, may appear at onset as glomerulonephritis without systemic manifestations. Serum complement levels and the urinary protein excretion are helpful in the initial evaluation of patients with the acute nephritic syndrome of PGSN. A normal serum complement would be against the diagnosis of PSGN, lupus nephritis, membranoproliferative glomerulonephritis types I and II, cryoglobulinemia, and bacterial endocarditis because 90% or more of the patients with these entities have hypocomplementemia. In contrast, a low serum complement would argue against IgA nephropathy, microscopic polyarteritis, and anti-GBM disease. Proteinuria in the nephrotic range is very common (70% to 90% of cases) in nephritis caused by visceral abscesses, membranoproliferative nephritis, lupus nephritis, shunt nephritis, and focal segmental glomerulosclerosis, yet is rare (fewer than 5% of the cases) in acute PSGN, IgA nephropathy, and microscopic polyarteritis.

INDICATIONS FOR RENAL BIOPSY

Because of the excellent prognosis of PGSN, renal biopsy is justified only if unusual features raise the possibility of a different diagnosis. Renal biopsy is worthwhile in patients with normal serum complement in the acute phase, as well as in those in whom the complement remains low after 2 months. Persistence of hypertension after 3 to 4 weeks and proteinuria of more than 3 g/day are also potential indications for biopsy. Increasing azotemia suggests a rapidly progressive course, and renal biopsy is important to document crescentic glomerulonephritis.

PATHOLOGY

Acute PSGN is the prototype of acute endocapillary glomerulonephritis. Proliferating mesangial and endothelial cells are mostly responsible for the hypercellularity of the glomerular tuft. Mesangial expansion is at times important and associated with increased transforming growth factor-β (TGF-β) expression. Cells from the circulation infiltrate the glomeruli; among them, polymorphonuclear leukocytes may predominate in some early biopsies, a characteristic that defines so-called exudative glomerulonephritis, in which there is intense glomerular expression of IL-8. Monocytes and CD4+ lymphocytes are also present. Interstitial infiltration with neutrophils, monocytes, and T lymphocytes, barely mentioned in early descriptions, has been emphasized recently. Tubules are normal.

Granular immune deposits of IgG, IgM, C3, C4, properdin, and the terminal membrane attack complex C5b-C9 are found in the mesangium and capillary loops. Anti-IgG reactivity has mainly a mesangial localization. Three patterns of glomerular immune deposition have been described: mesangial, starry-sky, and garland. In the *mesangial pattern*, the deposits are irregular and granular and are confined to the mesangium. In the *starry-sky* variety, the deposits are scattered randomly throughout mesangial and capillary wall locations. In the *garland* form, gross, irregular deposits are present in the capillary loops. The mesangial and starry-sky patterns are associated with a favorable prognosis, whereas the garland type of deposition is associated with massive proteinuria, unusually prominent subepithelial electrodense deposits, and a higher incidence of chronic renal damage.

Ultrastructural studies show electron-dense deposits in subepithelial, subendothelial, and intramembranous areas. The subepithelial deposits (humps) are typical but not exclusive of PSGN.

The acute proliferative changes improve progressively after a few weeks, but some degree of hypercellularity may persist for months. After several years, focal glomerulosclerosis and mesangial matrix expansion, in association with immune deposits, may be demonstrated in some biopsies, even in the absence of any clinical evidence of renal disease. The clinical significance of these findings remains undetermined.

Evidence indicates that apoptosis is increased in PSGN. Because apoptosis and proliferation are directly correlated, it is probable that apoptosis represents a physiologic form of resolution of the disease.

PROGNOSIS

Early death is extremely rare in children, but not in elderly patients (Table 39.13). There is no demonstrable correlation between the severity of hypertension, oliguria, or edema in the acute phase and the prognosis of PSGN. Patients with proteinuria in the nephrotic range deserve a close follow-up because they are more likely to show late renal damage.

Clinical series reported between 1930 and 1940 indicated excellent prognosis, but the follow-up was relatively short. Since 1970, several studies, comprising more than 900 patients followed for 10 to 15 years, have been published. Taken collectively, these studies indicate that chronic renal insufficiency occurs in fewer than 1% of patients. Proteinuria occurs in 8% to 13% of the individuals in most studies, but the range is very wide (1.4% to 46%). The incidence of hypertension varies from 42% to low values, similar to the frequency expected in the general population. Our own data in children with epidemic and sporadic PSGN (Table 39.14) indicate that after 15 years of follow-up, the incidence of hypertension, proteinuria, and microscopic hematuria is similar to that encountered in our control population.

TABLE 39.14. Abnormal Findings After 15 Years of Follow-Up in Children with PSGN

	Epidemic and Sporadic PSGN		Controls	
	Positive/Total	%	Positive/Total	%
Hypertension	2/98	2.0	1/60	1.6
Proteinuria	8/110	7.2	3/60	5.0
Hematuria	6/110	5.4	2/60	3.3
Azotemia	1/100	0.9	0/60	0.0
C_{cr} <70 ml/min	6/60	10	6/60	10.0

Data shown correspond to abnormalities present in at least two determinations done with an interval of week.
C_{cr}, creatinine clearance.

TREATMENT

All patients should be treated as if they had active streptococcal infection. Appropriate treatments are a single intramuscular injection of 1.2 million units of benzathine penicillin (half this amount in small children) or, alternatively, oral benzyl penicillin 200,000 units every 6 hours for 7 to 10 days. Erythromycin (250 mg every 6 hours for 7 to 10 days) could be used in patients allergic to penicillin. Preventive antibiotic treatment may be given to the siblings of index cases because the familial incidence of PSGN is almost 40%.

Restriction of salt and water intake is beneficial to all patients with the acute nephritic syndrome. Loop diuretics may increase urine output several-fold and, consequently, improve cardiovascular congestion and hypertension. Antihypertensive medication is required in about half of the patients, and sublingual nifedipine, parenteral Apresoline, diazoxide, and very rarely, nitroprusside may be needed. Occasionally, pulmonary edema is present, and morphine, oxygen, loop diuretics, and rotating tourniquets are required. Digitalis is not effective, and digitalis intoxication is likely. Dialysis should be used early if life-threatening hyperkalemia occurs or if there are clinical manifestations of uremia. Enforced bed rest is of no demonstrable value in the treatment of PSGN.

Selected Readings

Baldwin S, Gluck MC, Schacht RG, et al. The long-term course of poststreptococcal glomerulonephritis. *Ann Intern Med* 1974; 80:342–358.

Clinicopathologic follow-up studies in 126 patients showing a high incidence of glomerulosclerosis, proteinuria, and hypertension. This study was the first and most important in raising concern about the late prognosis of acute PSGN.

Marin C, Mosquera J, Rodríguez-Iturbe B. Histological evidence of neuraminidase involvement in acute nephritis: desialized leukocytes infiltrate the kidney in acute post-streptococcal glomerulonephritis. *Clin Nephrol* 1997;47:217–221.

Histopathologic study demonstrating desialized leukocytes infiltrating the glomeruli in PSGN and suggesting a role of neuraminidase in the infiltration observed in PSGN.

Mezzano S, Burgos ME, Olavarría F, et al. Immunohistochemical localization of interleukin-8 and transforming growth factor-β in streptococcal glomerulonephritis. *J Am Soc Nephrol* 1997;8:234–241.

Immunohistochemical study in biopsies of patients with PSGN describing an association between immunostaining of IL-8 and TNF-β with neutrophil infiltration and mesangial matrix expansion.

Odi T, Yoshizawa N, Takeuchi A, et al. Glomerular proliferating cell kinetics in acute poststreptococcal glomerulonephritis (APSGN). *J Pathol* 1997;183:359–368.

Demonstration that proliferating glomerular cells in acute PSGN are mainly endothelial cells in the early phase, followed by proliferation in mesangial cells. Proliferation was found also in macrophages.

Parra G, Rodríguez-Iturbe B, Batsford S, et al. Antibody to streptococcal zymogen in the serum of patients with acute glomerulonephritis. A multicentric study. *Kidney Int* 1998;54:509–517.

Multicentric international study demonstrating that high antizymogen titers are the best available marker to diagnose streptococcal infection associated with nephritis.
Poon-King R, Bannan J, Viteri A, et al. Identification of an extracellular plasma binding protein from nephritogenic streptococci. *J Exp Med* 1993;178:759–763.
Demonstration that nephritogenic streptococcal strains produce zymogen (streptococcal proteinase precursor).
Rodríguez-Iturbe B. Epidemic poststreptococcal glomerulonephritis. *Nephrol Forum* 1984;25:129–136.
Review article. Covers etiopathogenesis, participation of autoimmunity and mechanisms responsible for immune injury, clinical picture of a large series of patients, and pathophysiology of the acute nephritic syndrome.
Sorger K. Postinfectious glomerulonephritis: subtypes, clinicopathological correlations, and follow-up studies. *Veroff Pathol* 1986;125:1–110.
Extensive clinicopathologic studies describing three patterns of glomerular immune deposits, with correlation with ultrastructural findings and urinary abnormalities in follow-up.
Soto H, Mosquera J, Rodríguez-Iturbe, et al. Apoptosis in proliferative glomerulonephritis: decreased apoptosis expression in lupus nephritis. *Nephrol Dial Transplant* 1997;12:273–280.
Pathologic study in human renal biopsies describing a linear correlation between apoptosis and proliferation in PSGN, in contrast with the lack of correlation in lupus nephritis.
Yoshizawa N, Oshima S, Sagel I, et al. Role of a streptococcal antigen in the pathogenesis of acute poststreptococcal glomerulonephritis. *J Immunol* 1992;148: 3110–3118.
Update of a series of papers indicating characteristics, biopsy localization, and complement reactivity of the "preabsorbing" antigen.

B: Viral Hepatitis

Shaul G. Massry and Miroslaw Smogorzewski

Six species of hepatitis virus are known. They include hepatitis A (HAV), B (HBV), C (HCV), D (HDV), E (HEV), and G (HGV). HAV and HEV do not possess a lipid-containing outer viral envelope. They are secreted into the bile, reach the intestine through this route, and are excreted in the feces. Therefore their spread is by fecal–oral transmission. In contrast, HBV, HCV, and HDV do possess a lipid-containing envelope and therefore are inactivated when they are secreted into the bile. Therefore their mode of transmission is through blood in individuals practicing intravenous drug abuse, transfusion of infected blood, sexual intercourse, anal penetration in homosexual and/or sheds from mucosal surfaces.

Renal abnormalities are encountered in patients with HAV, HBV, and HCV infection. The nature, type, and scope of the manifestation of the renal involvement associated with these infections vary. The renal involvement in HCV infection is discussed in detail in Chapter 42, Part 11; the issues related to viral hepatitis in dialysis patients are provided in Chapter 73, Part 2; and related issues in renal transplant recipients are discussed in Chapter 89, Part 5.

HAV INFECTION

HAV causes acute hepatitis but rarely chronic infection. It occurs worldwide and especially in regions where the standard of sanitation is inadequate, a situation that promotes the spread of the disease.

After intravenous inoculation of marmoset with HAV, the virus antigen was detected in the glomeruli and appeared to be distributed along the basement membrane in a pattern suggestive of immune complex deposition. In another study, such inoculation with HAV produced proliferative glomerulonephritis and renal vasculitides.

Sporadic cases of glomerulonephritis in association with HAV infection have been reported. In one patient with HAV, microscopic hematuria, red blood cell casts, and proteinuria were present. Biopsy-proven mesangial proliferative glomerulonephritis was reported in patients with HAV; this entity is mediated by immune complexes. Indeed, IgM and C_3 deposits were prominent. Cytoplasmic tubuloreticular particles were also demonstrated, the structure of which was suggestive of a vial derivative. The outcome of HAV-associated glomerulonephritis is not known.

Although acute renal failure can develop in more than 80% of cases of fulminant viral hepatitis with massive hepatic necrosis, acute renal failure complicating acute nonfulminant HAV infection is exceedingly rare. When acute renal failure occurs, it could be the result of acute glomerulonephritis, acute tubular necrosis, or hepatorenal syndrome. The patients with HAV acute renal failure usually have oliguria and occasionally anuria. Of 28 reported patients in the world literature, renal biopsy was performed in 13. Different histologic changes were described in these biopsies. There were degenerative changes of tubular epithelium, interstitial nephritis, minor tubular necrosis, mild lymphocytic infiltrate with focal tubular atrophy, moderate interstitial edema with generalized vacuolization of tubular epithelium and focal disruption of proximal tubules consistent with acute tubular necrosis, recovery stage of acute tubular necrosis, normal glomeruli on light microscopy but heavy mesangial deposits of IgG on immunofluorescence microscopy, mild membranoproliferative glomerulonephritis with mesangial hypercellularity and capillary wall thickening but no deposits on immunofluorescence, mesangial proliferative glomerulonephritis with immunofluorescence demonstrating focal granular immune complex deposits predominantly of IgM and C_3, dilation of Bowman's capsule, tubular degeneration and cellular infiltration in interstitium, intraglomerular deposition of fibrinogen, and acute tubular necrosis with and normal glomeruli. Of the 28 patients, 27 recovered renal function; 21 patients required dialysis therapy, 18 with hemodialysis and 2 with peritoneal dialysis; 2 patients were treated with plasma therapy, and 5 patients recovered without treatment. One patient died as a result of sepsis.

HBV INFECTION

During acute infection with HBV, renal disease is rare. However, typical proliferative infective–associated glomerulonephritis has been reported. On the other hand, chronic HBV infection is associated with two major forms of renal involvement: polyarteritis nodosa and various types of glomerulonephritis (the most common of which is membranous and membranoproliferative). IgA nephropathy may also be encountered in patients with HBV infection. The glomerulonephritides associated with HBV are common in areas of high endemicity, such as China, Taiwan, Korea, Hong Kong, and some parts of Africa.

Polyarteritis Nodosa

Polyarteritis nodosa (PAN) is discussed in detail in Chapter 42, Part 4, which deals with the overall topic of vasculitis. PAN caused by HBV infection is seen almost exclusively in adults, but it could rarely occur in children. PAN has been reported weeks to months after mild acute infection with HBV, occasionally may develop in patients with chronic infection, and rarely may precede the clinical presentation of the HBV infection. The clinical presentation is that of vasculitis affecting many organs.

The renal involvement may be manifested with microhematuria, nonnephrotic or nephrotic proteinuria, renin-dependent hypertension, and on occasion, renal failure. Hypocomplementemia may be encountered in about 20% of patients with reductions in blood levels of C_3, C_4, and CH_{50}. ANCA is negative. HBsAg and anti-HBc are present, but anti-HBs is absent.

Membranous Glomerulonephritis

The association of an HBV carrier state with membranous glomerulonephritis (MGN) is well established, particularly in children, in whom the frequency of the carrier state in MGN correlates with that in the general population. Adults also can be affected. Children with HBV-MGN usually experience a nephrotic syndrome between the ages of 2 and 12 years. Hypertension is present in fewer than 25% of patients, and renal insufficiency is very unusual. More than 80% of patients are males. The viral infection is acquired both by vertical transmission from mothers and by horizontal transmission from siblings. There is usually no clinical or laboratory evidence of liver disease in children, whereas adults are much more likely to have a history of acute hepatitis, abnormal transaminase, and chronic active hepatitis on liver biopsy. Children may have spontaneous remission, but adults may have a relentless progressive course. HBsAg and anti-HBc usually can be demonstrated in the circulation. About 60% to 80% also have circulating HBe antigen. Serum C_3 and C_4 levels may be reduced or normal. Circulating immune complexes are present in up to 80% of patients.

The pathogenesis of HBV-MGN involves *in situ* formation of immune complexes, with planting of HBV antigen in the glomeruli. Circulating immune complexes may be trapped by the glomeruli and contribute to the development of MGN as well.

The diagnosis of HBV-MGN is confirmed by demonstrating one or more of hepatitis B antigens, such as HBsAg, HBeAg, and HBcAg or their antibodies in the glomerular immune deposits. However, HBeAg is the major antigen in these immune deposits.

The light microscopic findings in the renal biopsy often are indistinguishable from findings in idiopathic membranous nephropathy. Electron microscopy reveals viral-like particles in the subepithelial and subendothelial areas and within glomerular cells. Besides subepithelial immune deposits, there may be subendothelial and mesangial deposits. On immunofluorescence, IgG and C_3 are present along the capillary walls. IgM and IgA are seen less commonly.

Membranoproliferative Glomerulonephritis

In adults with HBV infection, membranoproliferative glomerulonephritis (MPGN) is the most common glomerular lesion. Patients often have nephrotic syndrome and microhematuria. Hypertension is seen in 45% and renal insufficiency in 20% of patients. Hypocomplementemia with a reduction in C_3 and C_4 levels is often observed. Liver biopsy usually shows chronic active or persistent hepatitis. Renal histology is similar to that of MPGN type I or may sometimes resemble type III. ABsAg is localized to the glomerular capillary wall. HBsAg and HBcAg are also found in the mesangium. HBeAg was found in the capillary wall in one patient.

Other Renal Lesions

Other histologic lesions seen in association with HBV infection are mesangial proliferative glomerulonephritis with IgG/IgM deposits or with IgA deposits (resembling IgA nephropathy) and, rarely, a combination of IgA and membranous nephropathy.

Management

No controlled studies on the effects of glucocorticoids in HBV-MGN have been reported. Uncontrolled studies in children suggest that spontaneous remission rates are the same as in children with idiopathic MGN. As many as two-thirds of children with HBV-MGN are in remission at 3 years after diagnosis, and glucocorticoids do not appear to provide any additional benefit. In fact, they may be deleterious because they may retard the ability of the host to eradicate HBV injection and may increase the risk of progression of liver disease to chronic active hepatitis. The initial results of the treatment with interferon-γ (IFN-γ) were encouraging in a few patients. An open randomized study conducted in 40 patients evaluated the effect of INF-γ on MGN of HBV infection. The INF-γ was given by subcutaneous injection three times a week for 12 months. The patients receiving INF-γ were free of proteinuria by the end of 3 months. HBeAg seroconversion after 4 to 6 months of therapy and HBsAg seroconversion after 10 to 12 months treatment occurred in 40% of the patients. Lamivudine at a dosage of 100 mg/day given for 6 months induced sustained HBV DNA suppression during the treatment. No report on a beneficial effect of this drug on the renal lesions associated with HBV is available.

Selected Readings

Jamil SM, Massry SG. Acute anuric renal failure in nonfulminant hepatitis A infection. *Am J Nephrol* 1998;18:329–332.

A report of a patients with anuric acute renal failure in HAV infection and a review of the renal pathology in HAV infection.

Johnson RJ, Couser WG. Hepatitis B infection and renal disease: clinical, immunopathogenetic and therapeutic consideration. *Kidney Int* 1990;37:663–676.

An exhaustive review of the renal lesions associated with hepatitis B infection, their pathogenesis, and management.

Lai KN, Ho RTH, Tam JS, et al. Detection of hepatitis B virus DNA and RNA in kidney of HBV-related glomerulonephritis. *Kidney Int* 1996;50:1965–1977.

An original study demonstrating the presence of viral transcription in glomerular cells and renal tubular epithelia. Also, discusses the pathogenesis of HBV-related glomerulonephritis.

Lin C-Y. Treatment of hepatitis B virus-associated membranous nephropathy with recombinant alpha-interferon. *Kidney Int* 1995;47:225–230.

An open randomized study of 40 patients with MGN caused by HBV infection that evaluates the efficacy of INF-γ in the management of this disease.

Nevens F, Main J, Honkoop P, et al. Lamivudine therapy for chronic hepatitis B: a six-month randomized dose-ranging study. *Gastroenterology* 1997;113:1258–1263.

A randomized trial in 51 patients with HBV infection that evaluates the effect of 6 months of monotherapy with lamivudine.

C: Renal Syndromes Associated With Human Immunodeficiency Virus Infection

Paul L. Kimmel

Patients with human immunodeficiency virus (HIV) infection develop several renal syndromes, including fluid, electrolyte, and urinary abnormalities; renal tubular disorders; acute renal failure; and chronic renal failure (Table 39.15). The different presentations of renal disease may vary among different susceptible populations, providing initial clues to diagnoses. Host factors and responses, as well as viral and environmental differences,

TABLE 39.15. Renal Syndromes Associated with HIV Infection

Fluid and electrolyte disorders
Urinary abnormalities
Isolated hematuria
Isolated proteinuria
Isolated pyuria
Combinations
Disorders of renal tubular function
Nephrolithiasis
Acute renal failure
Prerenal azotemia
Urinary tract obstruction
Acute tubular necrosis
Interstitial nephritis
Glomerulonephritis
Vasculitis
Cryoglobulinemia
Chronic renal failure
HIV-associated nephropathy (HIVAN)
HIV-associated focal glomerulosclerosis
HIV-associated focal glomerulosclerosis—collapsing variant
Mesangial abnormalities
HIV-associated immune-complex glomerulonephritis
Lupuslike lesions
Sclerotic lesions
Mixed picture
HIV-peptides
Cryoglobulinemia
Viral hepatitis related
Other complexes—postinfectious
HIV-associated IgA nephropathy
HIV-associated thrombotic microangiopathies

are probably critical in determining both the presence and the type of renal disease that may develop in an individual patient. Diagnosis can be facilitated by using a syndrome analysis approach. Results of the history and physical examination, review of the urinalysis, and tests of renal function and serologies allow the clinician to make provisional diagnoses. Renal biopsy may be indicated in selected patients if the diagnosis is unclear or to guide specific therapies.

FLUID, ELECTROLYTE, AND URINARY ABNORMALITIES

Common fluid and electrolyte abnormalities in HIV-infected patients include the occurrence of volume depletion secondary to diarrhea, hyponatremia, and disorders of potassium metabolism. Hyponatremia is present in HIV-infected patients for the same reasons it occurs in the general population, conceptually characterized by ingestion of water in quantities that exceed the limited ability of its renal excretion. The clinician must be aware, however, that there exists a high prevalence of disorders of the hypothalamic-pituitary-adrenal axis in such patients and that the presence of pulmonary and central nervous system disease may be associated with the common occurrence of the syndrome of inappropriate secretion of antidiuretic hormone (SIADH). In addition to decrements in glomerular filtration rate (GFR), HIV-infected patients are prescribed numerous medications that potentiate antidiuretic hormone (ADH) action or interfere with renal water excretion. Hypokalemia may be associated with poor nutritional intake or gastrointestinal losses secondary to diarrhea, but it is often exacerbated by abnormally increased urinary potassium excretion. The latter occurs in HIV patients with metabolic alkalosis or magnesium deficiency; during the polyuric phase of acute tubular necrosis (ATN); with therapy with amphotericin, aminoglycoside antibiotics, and rifampin; and less commonly with therapy with pentamidine or foscarnet. Use of didanosine and itraconazole has also been associated with the development of hypokalemia in HIV-infected patients. Hyperkalemia is often the result of abnormal limitations in renal potassium excretory capacity, typically because of a disorder in mineralocorticoid production or action, renal tubular disease, or drug effects. Patients prescribed trimethoprim, at the high dosages used for treatment of *Pneumocystis carinii* infection, may develop hyperkalemia as a result of its amiloridelike effects on the distal tubule. Dapsone can amplify the hyperkalemia. Hyperkalemia may also be encountered in HIV patients with acute renal failure.

Urinary abnormalities are common in patients with HIV infection. Bacterial, mycobacterial, fungal, protozoal, and viral pathogens may involve the renal parenchyma and cause urinary tract infections, which should be evaluated in patients with hematuria and/or pyuria. Perinephric abscesses, renal lymphoma, amyloidosis, and Kaposi's sarcoma and other tumors, as well as nephrocalcinosis, may also be associated with the development of urinary abnormalities and decrements in GFR, reflected clinically in increased levels of blood urea nitrogen (BUN) and creatinine concentrations. The treatment of these diseases is focused on an approach to the complicating infection or tumor, as well as continued therapy for the HIV infection. Renal imaging may be useful in delineating parenchymal abnormalities. Hematuria may be caused by coagulopathies or may be a sign of thrombotic microangiopathy. Patients treated with indinavir, acyclovir, or sulfadiazine may have renal colic as a result of crystalluria and nephrolithiasis. These abnormalities may be complicated by urinary tract infection and/or obstruction in the presence of urinary abnormalities.

Proteinuria may be common in HIV-infected patients, in the presence and absence of renal disease. Its prevalence may vary in specific patient populations and different regions, along with the stage of viral illness. Abnormal glomerular and tubular proteinuria may be present in up to one-third of outpatients with HIV infection, in the absence of other signs of renal dysfunction, and may be related to the pathogenesis of "febrile proteinuria," perhaps related to the viral illness or its superinfections. Urinary protein excretion greater than 1 g/24 hr, the coexistence of hematuria and proteinuria, or the finding of red blood cell casts should prompt an investigation into whether the patient has a disorder consistent with the presence of nephritic or nephrotic syndromes.

ACUTE RENAL FAILURE

Acute renal failure is common in HIV-infected patients, variously reported as having a 3% to 24% prevalence in hospitalized patients. Different populations are affected by this complication at approximately equal rates. The same causes underlie the development of acute renal failure in patients with HIV infection as in uninfected patients, primarily prerenal azotemia, usually secondary to volume depletion. Nonsteroidal antiinflammatory drugs (NSAIDs) may exacerbate renal vasoconstriction, resulting in azotemia. Trimethoprim and cimetidine may falsely mimic changes in GFR by diminishing renal tubular creatinine secretion, in which case the BUN should not be elevated. A bland microscopic urinalysis will be key to establishing such diagnoses.

Urinary tract obstruction should be suspected and ruled out, particularly in HIV-infected patients with lymphoma or other abdominal tumors, retroperitoneal adenopathy, or fibrosis. Therapy with indinavir, sulfadiazine, acyclovir, and foscarnet may also be associated with the development of crystalluria and intrarenal tubular obstruction. Recently, tubular interstitial disease has also been reported in patients treated with indinavir.

ATN often develops in patients with HIV infection, secondary to volume depletion, sepsis, and the administration of nephrotoxic drugs such as aminoglycoside antibiotics, amphotericin B, pentamidine, and radiocontrast agents. Mortality has been reported between 70% in patients with hemodynamic instability and 50% in patients with aminoglycoside nephrotoxicity, probably reflecting the severity of the underlying illnesses in this population. Overall mortality in a recent report was 60%. In the remainder, most recovered renal function, although the need for dialysis is common. Interestingly, mortality rates appear to be similar to those of patients with ATN without HIV infection. Acute interstitial nephritis may be seen in patients treated with antibiotics, including penicillins, cephalosporins, and trimethoprim-sulfamethoxazole combinations, rifampin, phenytoin, interferon-α, allopurinol, and NSAIDs. Recently, the protease inhibitors have been associated with the development of reversible decrements in GFR. Such complications have been reported with ritonavir and indinavir, although the underlying pathogenic mechanisms remain unclear. Hemodialysis, as well as peritoneal dialysis and continuous arteriovenous and continuous venovenous hemofiltration, have all been used successfully in HIV-infected patients with acute renal failure when specific complications occur.

In an HIV-infected patient, nephritic syndrome may represent an HIV-associated renal disease, or the renal disease may be associated with another infection (e.g., syphilis, hepatitis B or C virus infection) or may be caused by an immunologic reaction to a drug the patient is receiving. These syndromes, including cryoglobulinemia and vasculitis, are discussed in the following sections.

CHRONIC RENAL FAILURE

Various renal diseases have been pathogenically closely associated with HIV infection. Such chronic renal diseases include the spectrum of HIV-associated nephropathies, immune-mediated renal diseases associated with the host's response to HIV, and the thrombotic microangiopathies. The pathologic outcome likely depends on several intercurrent factors, including the patient's genetic background, the type and chronicity of the patients' immune response, and factors intrinsically related to the virus.

HIV-ASSOCIATED NEPHROPATHY

HIV-associated nephropathy (HIVAN) continues to be the most common renal pathologic finding in biopsy and autopsy studies of patients with HIV infection and renal disease. This may relate to the tendency to defer biopsies in patients with HIV infection who do not have nephrotic syndrome or who have only mild renal abnormalities. Although it is usually encountered in patients who have nephrotic-range proteinuria, the disease may be present in patients who excrete less than 3.5 g of proteinuria per day. HIVAN comprises a spectrum of abnormalities (Fig. 109.55). HIVAN has been characterized as a "pan nephropathy" because typical pathologic findings include abnormalities of glomeruli, tubules, and the interstitium. The most common finding is a form of focal segmental glomerulosclerosis (FGS). In reports of some populations, a collapsing variant of FGS may be more common. Mesangial abnormalities, such as diffuse hypercellularity, hyperplasia, expansion, and proliferation have also been noted in HIV-infected patients with renal disease and are perhaps most commonly seen in populations including Caucasians and children. The role of variation in geographic location, patient ethnic makeup, or age in determining pathologic outcomes is unclear. Glomerular epithelial cell abnormalities are a typical finding regardless of the pathologic diagnosis. Features such as tubular simplification, loss of the brush border, and microcystic dilation and atrophy are all common. Apoptosis of cells in several compartments may be appreciated in special studies. Interstitial edema, fibrosis, and an inflammatory immune cell infiltration composed primarily of T cells are also usually present. At the electron microscopic level, tubular reticular inclusions are commonly found in renal endothelial cells by electron microscopy.

The disease affects up to 10% of HIV-infected patients, but the overwhelming majority are men of African descent. The nephropathy can occur at any stage of HIV infection, but newer data regarding the natural history of the infection and studies using quantification of CD4 counts and viral burden suggest that the disease is a relatively late manifestation of the viral illness. Patients with HIVAN typically present with nephrotic-range proteinuria and hypoalbuminemia. Hypertension, edema, and hyperlipidemia are reported to be less common in HIV-infected patients than other patients with nephrotic-range proteinuria. In the past, this has been attributed to nutritional abnormalities, the wasting syndrome seen in HIV infection, or presentation at a late stage of viral illness; however, because of advances in diagnosis and in antiretroviral therapies, the patients are living longer, and therefore contemporary patients may exhibit hypertension, if this is an underlying, separate disease. Renal ultrasound shows large echogenic kidneys. Patients may have rapidly progressive renal insufficiency or may present with advanced renal failure. Early studies, before the availability of potent antiretroviral therapies or other interventions, suggested that the disease progresses to end-stage renal disease (ESRD) within weeks to months. It is uncertain whether this bleak prognosis still applies in the era of highly active antiretroviral therapy.

The pathogenesis of the disease is unknown, but studies in children and animal models suggest it is definitely related to HIV infection, rather than primarily to behavioral responses. However, viral characteristics, immune responses, and other host responses may play paramount roles. The finding of nephrotic-range proteinuria and/or renal insufficiency in an HIV-infected patient should not be considered diagnostic of HIVAN because other entities (e.g., HIV-associated immune complex renal diseases, diseases related to other viral infections, minimal-change disease, amyloidosis, diabetic nephropathy) have all been found in such patients. The lack of specificity of these signs and symptoms of renal disease suggests a renal biopsy is important if the clinician is in doubt about aspects of diagnosis and therapy.

Many uncontrolled, observational, and retrospective studies before the advent of protease inhibitors suggested a lower incidence or improved outcome of renal disease in HIV-infected patients treated with zidovudine, compared with untreated patients. The role of antiretroviral therapy has not been studied in well-designed, contemporary controlled trials of patients with HIVAN. Remission of nephrotic syndrome was reported in an uncontrolled trial of three children with HIVAN treated with cyclosporine. Uncontrolled studies have also suggested that glucocorticoids might ameliorate renal insufficiency in patients with HIVAN. Improvement in urinary protein excretion and renal function was noted in 20 patients with HIV infection and renal disease who were treated with a high-dose, tapered prednisone regimen. Opportunistic infections, steroid-induced psychosis, upper gastrointestinal bleeding, and relapses of renal dysfunction and progression to ESRD occurred commonly during and after therapy with steroids, but the study design hampers valid interpretation. The role of glucocorticoid therapy in children is even more unclear.

Treatment of patients with HIVAN with angiotensin-converting enzyme (ACE) inhibitors has been studied. In a nonrandomized, case-control study, patients with renal biopsy-determined HIVAN were treated with captopril (6.25 to 25 mg orally three times daily as tolerated). Survival time to the onset of ESRD or death in patients treated with captopril was significantly longer than that of patients with HIVAN in the control group. Only treatment with captopril and antiretroviral medications, but not demographic characteristics, CD4 count, and level of renal function, were associated with outcome. Two of the study patients have survived with serum creatinine concentrations of less than 2 mg/dl for more than several years. Similar findings were noted in patients with HIVAN who were treated with fosinopril. Patients with HIVAN who are treated with ACE inhibitors should be monitored for onset of hyperkalemia and loss of renal function.

Large, randomized, double-blinded, placebo-controlled trials, controlling for variation in level of renal dysfunction, histologic parameters, stage of viral illness, and medications administered, must be undertaken to determine whether treatment with antiretroviral drugs, cyclosporine, glucocorticoids, or ACE inhibitors are effective and safe therapeutic regimens for forestalling progression to ESRD for patients with HIVAN.

HIV-ASSOCIATED IMMUNE-COMPLEX RENAL DISEASES

There have been continued reports of HIV-infected patients whose renal biopsies demonstrated membranoproliferative and diffuse proliferative glomerulonephritis, as well as IgA and membranous nephropathy since the beginning of the epidemic. These findings suggest an immune-mediated etiology, and circulating HIV peptide antigen–antibody complexes are commonly present in HIV-infected patients at all stages of infection. European reports documented a high prevalence of glomerulonephritis in patients with renal disease, in Caucasian compared with HIV-infected patients of African descent with renal abnormalities. A French multicenter study confirmed that most Caucasian patients with HIV infection and renal disease had glomerulonephritis, but a substantial minority of patients from North Africa had a form of immune-complex renal disease as well. In this study, classic HIVAN was present in most of the patients of African descent with HIV infection and renal disease and in some of the Caucasian patients as well. A relatively high proportion of Caucasian patients with HIV infection and renal disease evaluated by renal biopsy in the United Kingdom had a form of glomerulonephritis consistent with immune-mediated mechanisms, in contrast to patients with classic HIVAN, most of whom were of African descent. In an Italian multicenter study of Caucasian HIV-infected patients, most of whom were intravenous drug users, a spectrum of different glomerulonephritides was noted, including diffuse proliferative glomerulonephritis, mesangial proliferative glomerulonephritis, membranoproliferative glomerulonephritis, membranous and IgA nephropathy, and minimal-change disease; however, no patient had HIVAN. Other studies have demonstrated that one-fourth to one-third of patients in the United States may have immune-mediated glomerulonephritis in the setting of HIV infection, even in populations of African-American patients. The renal disease has been shown by immunochemical methods to be immune-mediated glomerulonephritis caused by immune complexes composed of HIV gp120 or p24 and reactive antibodies.

However, other newer studies have suggested that glomerulonephritis in HIV-infected patients may not be directly related to the HIV infection, but rather to superinfections with hepatitis B or C virus, associated cryoglobulinemia, or postinfectious glomerulonephritis. A range of different glomerular histologic findings was present in African-American and Hispanic intravenous drug users with dual HIV and hepatitis C virus (HCV) infections, including membranoproliferative and mesangial proliferative glomerulonephritis as well as membranous nephropathy. In patients with cryoglobulinemia and HIV infection, HCV infection should be suspected as a cause of any renal disease. Immunochemical analysis, however, may determine that the cryoglobulinemia is an immunologic response to HIV peptides or a result of the immune dysregulation seen in HIV infection. Vasculitic renal disease is uncommon in HIV-infected patients. It is uncertain in the absence of immunochemical studies whether such renal disease is associated with the HIV or hepatitis virus infections, and the role of disordered immune regulation secondary to HIV infection plays in the pathogenesis and progression of the disease remains to be elucidated.

Such immune-mediated glomerulonephritis has been categorized as a lupuslike type, a sclerotic variety, and a mixed (sclerotic-inflammatory) type. Microscopic hematuria and nephrotic-range proteinuria, renal insufficiency, and hypoalbuminemia are common findings. There are limited data regarding outcome, but progression to ESRD appears common, while some patients have stable renal function or die before needing dialysis.

In addition, HIV-associated IgA nephropathy has been reported from centers in North America and Europe, typically in Caucasian or Hispanic men, but at least one case was documented in a black American patient. The disease may be a result of renal deposition of circulating idiotypic IgA molecules directed against HIV peptide–immunoglobulin complexes. Patients usually also have proteinuria and may have renal insufficiency, but hematuria is typically the presenting complaint. These features are consistent with current concepts regarding IgA nephropathy in patients in the absence of HIV infection.

The prognosis for patients with HIV-associated IgA nephropathy, a typically slowly progressive or stable course, appears to be better than that of patients with other HIV-associated renal diseases. Patients with HIV-associated IgA nephropathy and rapidly progressive glomerulonephritis have been treated with glucocorticoids, but as in the case of patients with other HIV-associated immune-mediated renal diseases, the absence of randomized, controlled treatment trials precludes the elaboration of evidence-based recommendations.

HIV-ASSOCIATED THROMBOTIC MICROANGIOPATHIES

Patients with HIV-related hemolytic uremic syndrome or thrombotic thrombocytopenic purpura can present with acute or chronic renal disease. The diagnosis usually requires the presence of renal and central nervous system disease, and thrombocytopenia is often accompanied by the presence of anemia and is confirmed by the demonstration of microangiopathic hemolytic anemia on the peripheral smear and in biochemical studies. Hemolytic uremic syndrome is generally characterized by more prominent renal insufficiency and evidence of hemolysis, whereas thrombotic thrombocytopenic purpura is thought to be associated with greater thrombocytopenia and mild renal disease, but these distinctions may be somewhat arbitrary. The pathogenesis of HIV-associated thrombotic microangiopathies is not known, but the role of endothelial cell responses to HIV infection is likely to be critical.

Patients with HIV-associated thrombotic microangiopathies have been treated with a variety of approaches, including use of plasmapheresis and/or plasma exchange and, in more refractory cases, vincristine, corticosteroids, aspirin, dipyramidole, and immunoglobulin infusions, with variable success. Splenectomy is generally reserved as a last resort in refractory patients.

There are no well-designed, randomized controlled trials to guide therapy in such patients.

RENAL REPLACEMENT THERAPY FOR HIV-INFECTED PATIENTS

HIV infection is the third leading cause of ESRD in African-American men in the United States, although the prevalence of HIV infection in the U.S. ESRD program appears to have plateaued. The prevalence of HIV infection in ESRD centers is highest on the east coast of the United States and may vary from 7% to 39% of patients in hemodialysis units in cities in this region. The incidence of HIV infected patients in the U.S. ESRD program was 0.8% in 1993. However, HIV infection was present in 5.0% of men and 1.8% of women between 25 and 44 years of age beginning ESRD therapy, and in 11.8% of black men and almost 5% of black women between 25 and 44 years of age.

Early surveys of survival in patients with AIDS and ESRD who were treated with dialysis, performed before identification of HIV as its causative agent, suggested a dismal prognosis, as compared with patients who developed acute renal failure and needed renal replacement therapy. Newer studies have suggested that the outcome is much improved for contemporary HIV-infected patients with ESRD. This disparity probably stems from at least two developments. Surveillance for HIV infection and consequently diagnostic accuracy are improved, and patients are currently often placed on dialysis before an AIDS-defining illness is present. In addition, there has been a generalized improvement in survival in HIV-infected patients after the development of antiretroviral medications and combination therapeutic strategies. It should be noted that confidentiality requirements for HIV testing in dialysis patients differ among the states, and surveillance may therefore be variable, leading to difficulties in epidemiologic surveys. Therefore the need for universal precautions to be strictly followed is an imperative in the dialytic setting, to prevent both nosocomial transmission and staff infection. However, isolation of HIV-infected patients is not required. Patient survival varies in different studies as a result of different population variables, including variation in case mix (intravenous drug users versus other risk factors), demographic factors, and antiretroviral and dialytic treatments. The patient's age, stage of viral illness, extent of hypertension, functional status, and presence of antiretroviral therapy have been proposed as the important survival predictors in HIV-infected ESRD patients. The few studies that are extant suggest survival is comparable in patients treated with hemodialysis and continuous ambulatory peritoneal dialysis (CAPD). Although controversial, some studies suggest increased susceptibility to peritonitis, often with opportunistic organisms, in HIV-infected patients. Such findings, however, may be the result of differential case mix in the populations studied, and center effects may be important in determining outcome. Spent peritoneal dialysate must be disposed of with caution because viable virus may be present.

Renal transplantation is usually not recommended as a renal replacement therapy for HIV-infected patients with ESRD. In part, this is because of the perception that immunosuppressive therapy may enhance progression of the viral illness, although there are some tantalizing reports to the contrary, and that the life span of recipients may be limited. In any event, management of prescription and surveillance of immunosuppression in such patients may be difficult, in part because of the lack of proper studies to guide therapy in this setting.

Counseling is perhaps the most important part of initiation of renal replacement therapy in HIV-infected patients. Prognosis and the risks of therapy must be balanced against any expected benefits. Therefore the patients' stage of illness and functional status must be paramount considerations. Counseling regarding physician and patient expectations should include family members and significant others. It is wise to let patients and others know that foregoing initiation of therapy where little benefit is to be expected and that withdrawal from therapy if quality of life is not acceptable are commonly chosen options and may be considered throughout the course of treatment.

Few studies on the pharmacokinetics of antiretroviral medications in HIV-infected patients with renal insufficiency and especially ESRD who are treated with different modalities are available, but renal excretion is the route of elimination for many of them. Zidovudine has been safely used in this population, but dosages must be reduced for patients with extensive renal insufficiency or ESRD. Therapy with didanosine, zalcitabine, stavudine, and lamivudine, as well as, in partial listing, acyclovir, ethambutol, fluconazole, ganciclovir, and pyrazinamide, must also be adjusted in patients with renal insufficiency and ESRD. Delavirdine and a major metabolite of nevirapine as well are primarily excreted through the kidneys. The protease inhibitors are for the most part not subject to elimination through renal routes, and changes in dosage according to renal function is not generally recommended. It may be especially important, however, to monitor patients with renal insufficiency treated with ritonavir or indinavir for unexpected progression of renal disease. In the absence of the availability of convenient measurement of drug levels, signs of incipient clinical toxicity from each individual medication must be monitored.

Selected Readings

Berns JS. Hemolytic uremic syndrome and thrombotic thrombocytopenic purpura associated with HIV infection. In: Kimmel PL, Berns JS, Stein JH, eds. *Renal and urologic aspects of HIV infection.* New York: Churchill Livingstone,1995: 111–133.

A comprehensive review of the possible pathogenesis of thrombotic microangiopathies in patients with HIV infection, and results of therapy.

Chertow GM, Rennke HG, Brady HR. Renal vasculitis with HIV seropositivity: potential manifestation of cytomegalovirus infection. *Am J Kidney Dis* 1997; 30:428–432.

The authors describe a patient with pauci-immune necrotizing renal vasculitis, adding to the spectrum of renal diseases encountered in HIV infected patients. The pathogenesis of the disorder, however, remains incompletely understood.

Clayman RV. Crystalluria and urinary tract abnormalities associated with indinavir. *J Urol* 1998;160:633.

This report documents the increasingly important spectrum of complications associated with the crystalluria seen in patients treated with indinavir.

Cohen AH. HIV-associated nephropathy. *Nephrol Dial Transplant* 1998;13:540–542.

A short but comprehensive recent review of the clinical and pathologic aspects of HIV-associated nephropathy, with emphasis on current notions of possible pathogenic mechanisms.

D'Agati V, Appel GB. HIV infection and the kidney. *J Am Soc Nephrol* 1997;8:138–152.

A comprehensive overview of the types of renal disease associated with HIV infection, and a review of currently accepted therapeutic options.

D'Agati V, Appel GB. Renal pathology of human immunodeficiency virus infection. *Semin Nephrol* 1998;18:378–395.

A state of the art review of the pathologic kidney findings in patients with HIV infection, focussing on HIV-associated nephropathy.

Gurtman A, Borrego F, Klotman ME. Management of antiretroviral therapy. *Semin Nephrol* 1998;18:459–480.

A state of the art review of the antiretroviral therapies available for patients with HIV infection, and their possible implications for patients with renal disease.

Humphreys MH. Human immunodeficiency virus-associated glomerulosclerosis. *Kidney Int* 1995;48:311–320.

A review focussing on possible pathogenic mechanisms underlying the development of classic HIV-associated nephropathy.

Ifudu O, Mayers JD, Matthew JJ, et al. Uremia therapy in patients with end-stage renal disease and human immunodeficiency virus infection: Has the outcome changed in the 1990s? *Am J Kidney Dis* 1997;29:549–552.

A study suggesting the survival of HIV-infected patients treated with end-stage renal disease with various renal replacement therapies has improved dramatically over the past decade.

Kimmel PL. Renal diseases in HIV infected patients: pathogenesis, diagnosis and treatment. *AIDS Patient Care STDs* 1996;10:342–348.

A review of the pathogenesis and treatment of the four types of HIV-associated renal diseases focussing on a syndrome approach to diagnosis.

Kimmel PL. Treatment of HIV nephropathies. In: Glassock RJ, ed. *Current therapy in nephrology and hypertension.* St Louis: Mosby, 1998:146–151.
A comprehensive, up-to-date review of the treatment of the HIV-associated renal diseases.

Kimmel PL, Bosch JP, Vassalotti JA. Treatment of human immunodeficiency virus-associated nephropathy. *Semin Nephrol* 1998;18:446–458.
A state of the art critical review of the treatments available for HIV-infected patients with various kidney diseases, focussing on HIV-associated nephropathy and the treatment of patients with end-stage renal disease.

Kimmel PL, Ferreira-Centeno A, Farkas-Szallasi T, et al. Viral DNA in microdissected renal biopsies of HIV infected patients with nephrotic syndrome. *Kidney Int* 1993;43:1347–1352.
A review of the findings on renal biopsies in HIV-infected patients with the nephrotic syndrome, showing that a large proportion have glomerulonephritis, and that a few patients have renal disease unrelated to the HIV infection. These findings underscore the need for renal biopsy, if clinicians want to make a precise diagnosis of the underlying renal disease in patients with HIV infection.

Kimmel PL, Phillips TM, Ferreira-Centeno A, et al. HIV-associated immune mediated renal disease. *Kidney Int* 1993;44:1327–1340.
A study definitively demonstrating the existence of an immune complex renal disease related to the patients' immune response to HIV infection.

Kimmel PL, Phillips TM. Immune complex glomerulonephritis associated with HIV infection. In: Kimmel PL, Berns JS, Stein JH, eds. *Renal and urologic aspects of HIV infection.* New York: Churchill Livingstone, 1995:77–110.
A review of the pathogenesis and findings of the various inflammatory renal diseases associated with HIV infection.

Kopp JB, Miller KD, Mican JAM, et al. Crystalluria and urinary tract abnormalities associated with indinavir. *Ann Intern Med* 1997;128:118–125.
A landmark paper illustrating the clinical spectrum of renal and urologic syndromes associated with the use of indinavir, accompanied by superb illustrations of indinavir crystalluria.

Navarro JF, Quereda C, Quereda C, et al. Nephrogenic diabetes insipidus and renal tubular acidosis secondary to foscarnet therapy. *Am J Kidney Dis* 1996;27:431–444.
A case report illustrating distal renal tubular complications of therapy with foscarnet—renal resistance to the action of vasopressin and hydrogen ion secretory defects, resulting in the reversible development of hypernatremia and metabolic acidosis.

Martinez F, Moomeja-Marin H, Estepa-Maurice L, et al. Indinavir crystal deposits associated with tubulointerstitial nephropathy. *Nephrol Dial Transplant* 1998; 13:750–753.
Two cases of patients with HIV infection, treated with indinavir, who developed renal insufficiency. Both patients had urinary protein excretion rates of less than 1 g/d, and had renal biopsies showing interstitial inflammatory infiltration and fibrosis, and crystals within tubules. Both patients responded with improvement in renal function after discontinuation of the drug.

Perinbasekar S, Brod-Miller C, Mattana J. Absence of edema in HIV-infected patients with end-stage renal disease. *J AIDS Hum Retrovirol* 1996;13:368–373.
This paper provides evidence confirming earlier findings demonstrating that edema is relatively uncommon in patients with HIV-associated nephropathy. Studies suggesting prior weight loss, diarrhea, hypotension and advanced stage of the viral illness may be associated with the absence of edema in HIV-infected patients with severe hypoalbuminemia (and nephrotic range proteinuria) are presented.

Perinbasekar S, Brod-Miller C, Pal S, et al. Predictors of survival in HIV-infected patients on hemodialysis. *Am J Nephrol* 1996;16:280–286.
A study documented better long term survival of HIV-infected patients with ESRD treated with hemodialysis, confirming earlier data suggesting that higher CD4 counts (and antiretroviral therapy) are associated with improved survival.

Rao TKS. Acute renal failure in human immunodeficiency virus infection. *Semin Nephrol* 1998;18:378–395.
A comprehensive review illustrating the spectrum of causes of acute renal failure in patients with HIV infection, and suggesting that outcomes are improving, but are related to the stage of the viral illness.

Stokes MB, Chawla H, Brody RI, et al. Immune complex glomerulonephritis in patients co-infected with HIV and hepatitis C virus. *Am J Kidney Dis* 1997;29:514.
Various kinds of glomerulonephritides were documented in twelve patients with coexisting HIV and hepatitis C infection, illustrating the range of disease that may be encountered in this population.

D: Malarial Nephropathy

Visith Sitprija and Raja Sinniah

Malaria remains a world problem. It has been estimated that the incidence of malaria in the world is about 300 to 500 million clinical cases each year, with countries in tropical Africa accounting for more than 90%. Mortality varies from 1.5 to 2.7 million per year. The disease primarily affects erythrocytes, with effects on microcirculation and the immune system. As a highly vascularized organ, the kidney is therefore commonly involved. The disease is determined by certain characteristics inherent for each malarial parasite. *Plasmodium vivax* and *Plasmodium ovale* infect young erythrocytes. *Plasmodium malariae* infects aging cells, whereas *Plasmodium falciparum* infects erythrocytes of all ages. Heavy parasitemia is thus common in *P. falciparum* malaria. Among the four species of malarial parasites, which include *P. falciparum, P. vivax, P. malariae,* and *P. ovale,* nephropathy is commonly caused by *P. falciparum* and *P. malariae. P. falciparum* infection usually causes mild glomerular lesion, and reversible renal failure can occur in severe infection. *Quartan* malaria due to *P. malariae* infection may be associated with transient glomerular lesion, nephrotic syndrome, or chronic progressive glomerulonephritis leading to chronic renal failure.

PATHOPHYSIOLOGY

Parasitized erythrocytes play a central role in the disease pathogenesis through decreased erythrocytes deformability, cytoadherence between the knobs on parasitized erythrocytes and the vascular endothelium, rosette formation, erythrocyte sequestration, and hemolysis. Adhesion molecules, including ICAM-1, ELAM-1, VCAM-1, thrombospondins, and CD36, are important in causing cytoadherence. This is true for *falciparum* malaria. The number of knobs increases as the parasite becomes more mature. There is no cytoadherence between *P. malariae–* and *P. vivax*–infected erythrocytes and vascular endothelium. Microcirculation is therefore less compromised. As in other parasitic infections, circulating malarial antigens can trigger immune reactions, monocytes, and complement activation. Glycosylphosphatidylinositol (GPI) moieties covalently linked to the surface antigens of malarial parasite can activate a receptor on the monocyte (CD14) and induce tumor necrosis factor (TNF) and interleukin (IL) release. Many cytokines, especially TNF, IL-1, IL-6, IL-8, and interferon-γ, play a very important role in the acute-phase reaction, expression of adhesion molecules, and release of vasoactive mediators, causing plasma leakage from the intravascular compartment. Catecholamines, kinins, prostaglandins, leukotrienes, histamine, serotonin, nitric oxide, endothelin, complements, and reactive-oxygen species are among inflammatory mediators involved. Because of heavy parasitemia, cytoadherence, sequestration, and the effects of cytokines and mediators, hemodynamic alterations are an integral part in pathophysiology of *falciparum* malaria. Similar to sepsis, there is peripheral vasodilation; the cardiac output is increased, but the renal blood flow is decreased. Initially, there is hypervolemia, but in severe cases or at the later stage, blood volume is decreased because of increased vascular permeability induced by mediators and cytokines. Various nonspecific factors integral to infection, including blood hyperviscosity, hemolysis, rhabdomyolysis, jaundice, intravascular coagulation, high fever, reactive-oxygen species, and complement activation, further contribute to decreased renal perfusion and can lead to renal failure (Fig. 39.9). Renal failure is therefore ischemic in type. Because heavy parasitemia and cytoadherence between parasitized erythrocytes are unique for *falciparum* malaria, acute renal failure is common in *falciparum* malaria but is uncommon in *vivax* and *quartan* malaria.

Immune response to malarial antigens is responsible for the pathogenesis of glomerulonephritis. This is facilitated by Th_2 cells, which are essential for humoral immunity. Glomerulonephritis in malaria is immune complex in type, and the present evidence indicates that the immune complexes are mediated through the implanted malarial antigens. Deposition of immune complexes leads to infiltration of inflammatory cells and mesangial proliferation, which in turn modulates local cellular immune response.

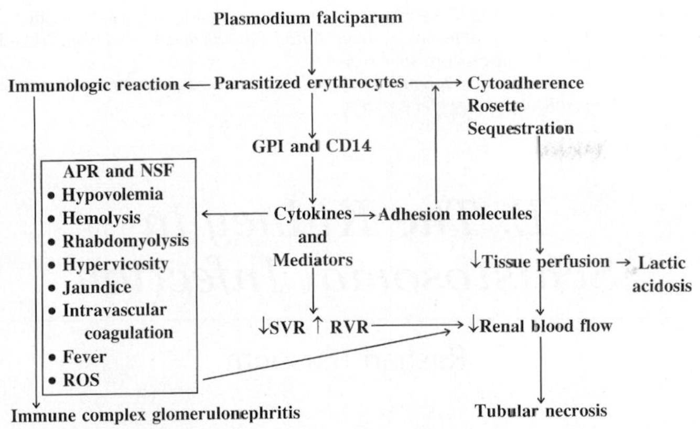

Figure 39.9. Pathogenesis of nephropathy in *falciparum* malaria. APR, acute-phase response; CD_{14}, receptor on monocyte; GPI, glycosylphosphatidylinositol; NSF, nonspecific factors; ROS, reactive-oxygen species; RVR, renal vascular resistance; SVR, systemic vascular resistance. (Reproduced with permission from Eiam-Ong S, Sitprija V. Falciparum malaria and the kidney: a model of inflammation. *Am J Kidney Dis* 1998;32:361–375.)

FALCIPARUM MALARIA NEPHROPATHY

Although renal manifestation may not be apparent in the benign form of *falciparum* malaria, mild proteinuria and urine sediment changes with few erythrocytes, leukocytes, and granular casts are common. These changes resolve quickly when the disease is under control. Nephritic syndrome and nephrotic syndrome are unusual in *falciparum* malaria.

Fluid and Electrolyte Abnormalities

Fluid and electrolyte changes in malaria are interesting. Hyponatremia is noted in 67% of the patients and is usually asymptomatic. The causes are multiple, including reset of osmoreceptor, increased antidiuretic hormone, and volume depletion resulting from low sodium intake and sodium loss. Hypernatremia may be observed in malarial patients with severe brain damage and diabetes insipidus. This is rare and has a poor prognosis. As in many febrile diseases, hypokalemia attributed to respiratory alkalosis due to fever is common in malaria. Hyperkalemia is usually associated with intravascular hemolysis, rhabdomyolysis, or renal failure. Lactic acidosis is observed in severe infection. Hypocalcemia and hypophosphatemia can be found in severe malaria without renal failure. Hypocalcemia is attributed to decreased parathyroid hormone and the effect of IL-1. Hypophosphatemia is caused by respiratory alkalosis with phosphate shift into the cells.

Decreased response to water load can occur in moderate to severe malaria. This is associated with hypervolemia, decreased peripheral vascular resistance, and increased cardiac output. In such patients, there are elevated plasma renin activity, increased plasma norepinephrine, high plasma arginine vasopressin, and increased renal vascular resistance. Low serum sodium is an important clinical marker of these patients. Of the hyponatremic patients, 20% have decreased response to water load. In severe malaria, renal vascular resistance is significantly increased, resulting in renal ischemia and acute renal failure (Fig. 39.9). A positive correlation between the plasma levels of cytokines and the severity of malaria including renal failure has been observed.

Acute Renal Failure

Acute renal failure, usually associated with heavy parasitemia (more than 5% of erythrocytes are infected) or intravascular hemolysis is observed in 1% to 4% of cases of *falciparum* malaria. In 60% of the patients, renal failure is catabolic, with rapid rises in blood urea nitrogen and serum creatinine and high blood urea nitrogen:serum creatinine ratio. Cholestatic jaundice is common in severe cases. Hemoglobinuria is observed in the patients with intravascular hemolysis, usually associated with glucose-6-phosphate dehydrogenase deficiency. Myoglobinuria may also occur. The duration of renal failure varies from a few days in mild cases to several weeks in severe ones.

Quinine is the drug of choice. The initial dose during the first 24 hours need not be modified despite impaired renal function. The following doses, however, should be judged by renal function. Exchange blood transfusion is an effective treatment for reducing the parasite count and jaundice in patients with heavy parasitemia and hyperbilirubinemia. Artemisinin derivatives have been used with promising result in decreasing parasitemia. Fluid administration should be done cautiously in patients with moderate and severe malaria, especially in patients with hyponatremia as a result of decreased response to water load. Fluid overload and pulmonary edema may occur. In patients with decreased response to fluid load, furosemide is helpful. In mild renal failure, the combination of dopamine and furosemide may attenuate the progress of renal failure. When dialysis is needed, it should be performed frequently because of hypercatabolism. Hemodialysis is preferred. However, peritoneal dialysis can also be used. Fortunately, transport through the peritoneal membrane is improved after treatment.

Pathology

Mesangial proliferation is commonly observed. Parasitized erythrocytes are rarely seen. Pigment-laden macrophages can be found in the glomerular capillaries during the acute phase of the disease. Subendothelial and mesangial electron-dense deposits are seen by electron microscopy. Various degrees of tubular degeneration and necrosis are evident in patients with acute renal failure. All levels of the nephron are affected, but the changes are prominent in the distal convoluted tubules and the collecting tubules. Heme and granular casts are often seen in Henle's loop and the collecting tubules. In severe infection, peritubular capillaries are congested with parasitized erythrocytes, malarial pigmented-laden macrophages, lymphocytes, and plasma cells. Fibrin deposition may be seen. Interstitial edema and inflammatory cell infiltration are often observed. By immunofluorescence, there is granular deposition of IgM and C_3 in the mesangial area and along the capillary walls. IgG deposition may also be noted. Malarial antigens can be seen along the mesangium, glomerular endothelium, and medullary capillaries. Major histocompatibility complex (MHC) class I and II antigens are present in the glomerular mesangium, capillary endothelium, and interstitium. Immune cells positive for CD4+ and CD8+ markers are seen around small arteries and interstitium. In *P. berghei* infection, which corresponds to *falciparum* malaria in human, enhanced expression of ICAM-1 is observed in the glomerular mesangium, endothelia of blood vessels, and proximal tubular epithelial cells. The tubules and endothelia of blood vessels show enhanced expression of TNF-α, IL-1, IL-6, and granulocyte monocyte-colony stimulating factor (GM-CSF). Positive staining for ligand leukocyte function antigen-1 and complement receptor type 1 is seen in the glomerular infiltrating inflammatory cells and mesangium.

QUARTAN MALARIA NEPHROPATHY

Most patients are children, with a mean age of 5 years. The common renal manifestations include proteinuria and microhematuria. Transient glomerulonephritis can occur and resolve when the infection is controlled. In these cases, serum complement levels, serum cholesterol value, renal function, and blood pressure are usually normal. However, the infection can cause persistent glomerulonephritis with nephrotic syndrome, which can eventually progress to chronic renal failure. The onset of nephrotic syndrome is usually insidious. Progression of renal failure occurs over 3 to 5 years. Renal manifestations in these patients include nonselective proteinuria, hematuria, hypoproteinemia, edema, and urinary loss of large quantities of malarial antibody. The serum complement is normal but may be decreased in the early stage. Slow progression is associated with azotemia and hypertension.

Spontaneous remission has been reported but is rare. Antimalarial treatment fails to resolve proteinuria. Prednisolone is usually ineffective, but response may occur in patients with highly selective proteinuria and mild glomerular lesion. Fewer than 50% of patients with highly selective proteinuria respond to prednisolone. Cyclophosphamide may reduce proteinuria and occasionally cause remission.

The basic pathologic lesion in *quartan* malaria with persistent glomerular lesion includes thickening of the glomerular capillary walls due to subendothelial deposits of immune complexes. Segmental sclerosis of the glomerular tufts may be noted. By immunofluorescence, the deposits can be either coarsely granular or finely granular or mixed. The coarsely granular deposits contain IgG_3, IgM, and C3, whereas in the diffuse finely granular deposits, IgG is present in the form of IgG2. *Plasmodium* antigens are detected in 25% to 33% of the patients. Electron microscopy reveals subendothelial deposits of electron-dense or basement membrane–like material, accompanied by the formation of intramembranous lacunae. A mesangial proliferative lesion is often noted in adults. Crescents are rare. The extent of tubular involvement depends on the severity of glomerular lesions. In most patients, the renal pathology is diffuse and progressive, leading to end-stage renal disease with total glomerulosclerosis. Glomerulonephritis in *quartan* malaria is immune mediated. Continued renal injury can occur in the absence of antigens due to production of autoantibodies at the initial tissue damage. Several factors are incriminated in the pathogenesis of chronic persistent glomerular lesions. These factors include associated bacterial and viral infections, especially Ebstein-Barr virus infection; malnutrition; autoimmunity; and genetic predisposition.

P. VIVAX AND *P. OVALE* INFECTION

Mild mesangial proliferative glomerulonephritis with IgM and C_3 deposition can be seen in infection by *P. vivax* and *P. ovale*. Benign urinary sediment changes may be observed. Acute renal failure is uncommon.

Selected Readings

Adeniyi A, Hendrickse RG, Soothill JF. A controlled trial of cyclophosphamide and azathioprine in Nigerian children with nephrotic syndrome and poorly selective proteinuria. *Arch Dis Child* 1979;54:204–207.

A controlled trial of the use of cyclophosphamide or azathioprine in the treatment of nephrotic syndrome caused by quartan malaria in Nigerian children.

Eiam-Ong S, Sitprija V. Falciparum malaria and the kidney: a model of inflammation. *Am J Kidney Dis* 1998;32:361–375.

This is a review of pathophysiology of falciparum malarial nephropathy, with emphasis on renal hemodynamics and the role of cytokines and mediators.

Rui-Mei L, Kara AU, Sinniah R. Dysregulation of cytokine expression in tubulointerstitial nephritis associated with murine malaria. *Kidney Int* 1998;53:845–852.

An interesting study of the role of proinflammatory cytokines in the pathogenesis of renal lesions, especially tubulointerstitial changes in murine malaria.

Sitprija V, Boonpucknavig V. Renal involvement in parasitic disease. In: Tisher C, Brenner BM, eds. *Renal pathology: with clinical and functional correlation.* 2nd ed. Philadelphia: JB Lippincott, 1994:626–657.

A comprehensive description of renal pathologic changes in malaria with emphasis on pathophysiology of the disease.

E: The Kidney in Schistosomal Infection

Rashad Barsoum

Schistosomiasis is a parasitic disease that is known to affect more than 300 million people in five continents. In addition, 400 million people are at risk of infection. The disease is responsible for considerable, although widely variable, morbidity primarily involving the urinary and gastrointestinal tracts, with secondary involvement of the lungs, brain, genital tract, skin, eyes, and other organs.

Seven species affect humans, the most widely spread being *Schistosoma hematobium* mainly in Africa, *Schistosoma mansoni* in Africa and South America, and *Schistosoma japonicum* in the Far East. Within each species, there are many strains, which may influence the virulence of infection. Coinfection with certain bacteria (e.g., salmonella) or viruses (e.g., hepatitis B or C) may have a significant impact on pathogenicity. Morbidity is often amplified by associated parasitic infestations or nutritional deficiency.

Infection is acquired by contact with fresh water in the rivers and canals. The "cercariae," the infective agents, penetrate through the skin and migrate through the lymphatics to reach the bloodstream, already grown up into small worms called *schistosomulae*. The latter ultimately find their way into the portal venous system, where they are trapped upstream in the hepatic sinusoids. According to the infective species, the schistosomulae either stay in the portal vein (*S. mansoni* and *S. japonicum*) or further migrate through venous collaterals into the perivesical plexus (*S. hematobium*). Upon reaching their final destination, the schistosomulae mature into adult worms, which are distinguished into males and females. Only one or two couples survive the host's defense and may persist for two or three decades. The couple remains in almost constant copulation; the female leaves only to migrate toward a mucosal surface to lay eggs. This can be the colon and rectum with *S. mansoni* and *S. japonicum*, or the bladder and lower ureters with *S. hematobium*.

The eggs penetrate through the mucosal surface, thanks to their spikes, which are located terminally *(S. hematobium)* or laterally (*S. mansoni* and *S. japonicum*). They pass to the exterior with the respective excreta. Upon reaching fresh water, they hatch, liberating the "miracidia," which infect certain snails, which are specific for each species, hence defining the endemicity of infection in a particular geographic location. The life cycle is completed asexually in the snail, eventually releasing the cercariae, thereby completing the life cycle.

PATHOGENICITY

Morbidity is the outcome of the host's immune response against the parasitic infection. Two patterns of such response are known: (a) a T-cell mediated, delayed hypersensitivity reaction, usually against the ova trapped in the gut or bladder mu-

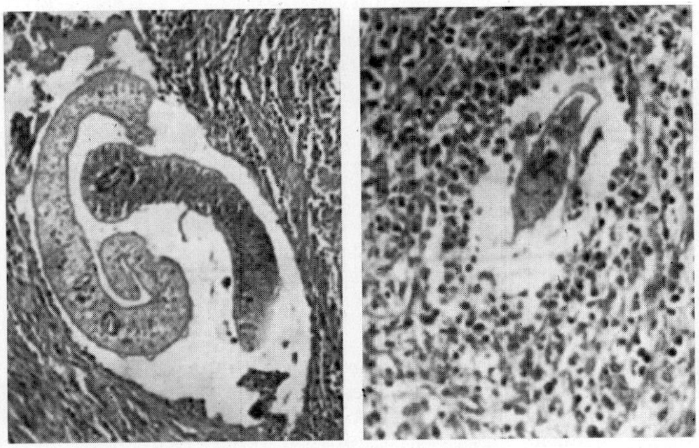

Figure 39.10. Schistosomal granulomas. *Left panel:* A pair of worms trapped in the bladder submucosa surrounded by a mononuclear cellular infiltrate and dense fibrosis. *Right panel: S. hematobium* ovum (note the terminal spike) surrounded by mononuclear cells, a few eosinophils and neutrophils.

cosa, and (b) an immune complex–mediated reaction, usually against worm antigens.

T-Cell Response

Soluble egg antigens (SEA) are released from the trapped ova through shell micropores. These are taken up by antigen-presenting cells, usually the local macrophages, and expressed along with class II major histocompatibility complex (MHC) antigens. Perturbation of the macrophages initially leads to the release of interleukins (IL) 1, 6, and 12, which lead to the proliferation of T-helper 1 (Th_1) cells, which subsequently release tumor necrosis factor-α (TNF-α), which further amplifies the macrophage response. Other cells, mainly the eosinophils, basophils, and fibroblasts, are activated through the subsequent release of IL-2, IL-13, and other cytokines from activated Th_1 cells. All these cells surround single or clusters of ova-forming granulomata, which constitute the characteristic pathologic unit in schistosomiasis (Fig. 39.10).

Macrophages subsequently change their cytokine profile, with predominance of Th_2-activating mediators, particularly IL-4. The predominance of Th_2 cells in late schistosomal granulomata results in the release of such cytokines as IL-5 in small animals, IL-10 in humans, and transforming growth factor-β (TGF-β) in both. These have been shown to have a pivotal role in downregulating the macrophages, thereby modulating the schistosomal granuloma, which tends to shrink, becomes increasingly fibrotic, and ultimately becomes calcified.

Antibody Response

B cells participate in the immune response to schistosomiasis, both by acting as antigen-presenting cells and as targets of late cytokines released by Th_2 cells. The result is the secretion of antibodies, expectedly starting with IgM, and subsequently switching to IgG and IgA. IgE has a pivotal role throughout the evolution of infection, being required for the antibody-dependent cell-mediated cytotoxicity (ADCC) of eosinophils. Switching reflects the pattern of cytokine predominance through the effect of these mediators on the C-gene for the heavy chain in chromosome 14. Whereas IL-2 favors IgG synthesis, IL-4, IL-5, and IL-10 favor IgA.

Antibodies have been identified against more than 100 antigens in schistosomiasis. Those against SEA are useful indicators of infection and are indeed used as diagnostic tools. Antibodies against worm tegument antigens are important in limiting the intensity of infection and conferring immunity against reinfection. The latter are the basis of several vaccines that are currently being developed in different laboratories.

Antibodies against the worm's gut antigens tend to form immune complexes, which are able to activate complement and induce clinical disease. The latter may be acute, presenting as "Katayama fever," which affects foreigners acquiring fresh infection in endemic areas. More often, however, immune complex–mediated disease in schistosomiasis is chronic, affects natives, and presents as glomerulonephritis.

SCHISTOSOMIASIS OF THE LOWER URINARY TRACT

The lower urinary tract is the target of *S. hematobium*, although *S. mansoni* may be the causative parasite when both species coexist in the same locality. The lesions start in the bladder mucosa, mostly in the trigone, and extend centrifugally to involve the rest of the bladder wall, the ureters, urethra, seminal vesicles, and vagina. The initial lesion is an aggregate of granulomata, which appear as small tubercles surrounded by a hyperemic halo. With heavy infection, these coalesce to form sessile or pedunculated masses. The lesions soon ulcerate, leading to terminal hematuria, the typical presentation of the disease. The ulcers eventually heal by fibrosis and calcification, which gives the bladder mucosa the appearance of "sandy patches." Areas of healthy bladder mucosa may be entrapped within the fibrotic strands leading, to a glandular appearance called *cystitis glandularis;* the epithelium soon become atrophic, leading to a cystic appearance, *cystitis cystica.*

Although the acute lesions are responsible for the major clinical presentation of urinary schistosomiasis, they seldom lead to any significant morbidity. On the other hand, chronic fibrotic lesions are the cause of serious, often life-threatening complications. These are generally classified into three categories:

1. Chronic cystitis with ulceration and secondary infection. This may lead to primary bladder stone formation, particularly in children. Ultimate fibrosis may interfere with the bladder capacity and motor function.
2. Development of bladder malignancy (Fig. 39.11), usually a squamous cell carcinoma, which is often circumscribed owing to the surrounding fibrosis. This has been attributed to a variety of carcinogens generated by the parasite, its associated infections, and/or the metabolic consequences of its effect on the hepatocytes. On the basis of experimental evidence, these toxins seem to lead to oxidative breakage of chromosome 11. Mutation of the p53 tumor suppressor gene has also been suggested as a potential mechanism of carcinogenicity of urinary schistosomiasis.
3. Interference with the internal vesical sphincter, leading to bladder neck obstruction, which amplifies the motor disorder of the bladder. The fibrotic process also distorts the ureterovesical junctions, leading to obstruction and/or reflux. The latter may lead to back pressure, which often results in hydronephrosis and chronic pyelonephritis. Disorders of tubular function, including distal tubular acidosis and sodium wastage, have been attributed to schistosomal obstruction. Hypertension, associated with reflux-induced focal sclerosis, has been recognized for many decades. These complications are often mixed, eventually leading to renal failure. About one-fifth of all patients on regular dialysis in Egypt are attributed to complicated lower urinary tract schistosomiasis.

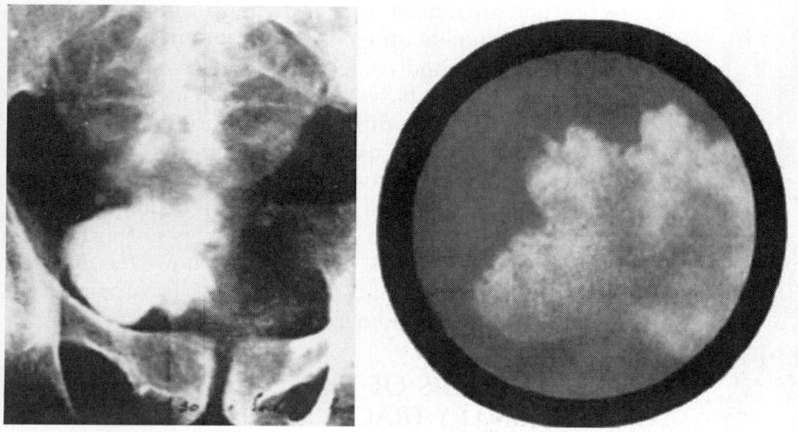

Figure 39.11. Schistosomal bladder cancer. *Left*: Plain radiogram showing irregular erosion by the tumor mass of densely calcified bladder wall. *Right*: Cystoscopic appearance of the growth.

Following a few case reports from Brazil and Egypt by the late 1960s and early 1970s, it was soon realized that immune complexes containing schistosomal antigens are able to induce different forms of glomerulonephritis in humans as well as many experimental animals.

All three major human-pathogenic species of schistosomiasis have been incriminated. However, whereas *S. japonicum* has been the most widely used species in experimental models, its epidemiologic impact in humans is negligible. Conversely, *S. hematobium* is hardly able to induce experimental glomerulonephritis, while its role in initiating glomerular lesions in humans is quite evident. It remains for *S. mansoni* to constitute the most impressive schistosomal species that leads to significant and progressive glomerular disease both in experimental animals and in humans.

Several antigens originating from the worm's gut have been blamed. Of these, a glycoprotein that migrates to the cathode in an electrical field (cathodal antigen) and a proteoglycan (anodal antigen) are most often detected in the glomerular deposits. Both have been found in the circulation as free antigens or immune complexes with almost all known classes of immunoglobulins. Immune deposits are detected mainly in the glomerular mesangium. Subendothelial, intramembranous, and subepithelial deposits have also been described.

A variety of glomerular lesions have been described. The different histopathologic patterns seem to reflect certain pathogenetic differences and to predict deviant prognosis. Accordingly, they may be classified into five "classes" (African Association of Nephrology "AFRAN" Classification) (Table 39.16, Fig. 39.12).

The mild glomerular lesions, usually categorized as class I, are encountered with all schistosomal species. They may be entirely asymptomatic and associated with microalbuminuria, microhematuria, or overt proteinuria that seldom reaches the nephrotic range. Hypertension is unusual, and renal failure does not occur.

Exudative glomerulonephritis (class II) is usually associated with heavy proteinuria, together with manifestations of salmonella-related toxemia. The latter is expressed by pyrexia, a vasculitic skin eruption on the abdomen and flexor surfaces of the extremities, secondary anemia, splenomegaly, and hair changes. The increased catabolism amplifies the hypoproteinemia, leading to gross anasarca. Renal function is usually preserved, but mild impairment may be caused by shrinkage of the blood volume facing a decreased filtration fraction. Hypertension is exceptional. Plasma lipids are reduced despite severe hypoproteinemia because of decreased hepatic synthesis.

Mesangiocapillary glomerulonephritis (class III) and focal segmental sclerosis (class IV) are most often associated with ad-

TABLE 39.16. Classification of Schistosomal Glomerulopathies

Class	Histologic Lesion	Glomerular Deposits	Causative Agent(s)	Clinical Features
I	Mesangioproliferative	Schistosomal gut antigens IgM, IgG C_3	*S. hematobium* *S. mansoni* *S. japonicum*	Microalbuminuria Microhematuria Overt proteinuria
II	Exudative	C_3 Salmonella antigens	*S. hematobium* or *mansoni* *plus* *Salmonella typhi* or paratyphi A	Rapidly developing nephrotic syndrome *plus* Infective toxemia
III	Mesangiocapillary	IgG, IgA, IgM, C_3 Schistosomal antigens (occasionally)	*S. mansoni* ? *S. hematobium*	Hepatosplenomegaly Overt proteinuria Nephrotic syndrome Hypertension Renal failure
IV	Focal and segmental glomerulosclerosis	IgG, IgA, IgM, C_3	*S. mansoni*	Hepatosplenomegaly Overt proteinuria Nephrotic syndrome Hypertension Renal failure
V	Amyloidosis	AA protein	*S. mansoni* *S. hematobium*	Hepatosplenomegaly Overt proteinuria Nephrotic syndrome Hypertension Renal failure

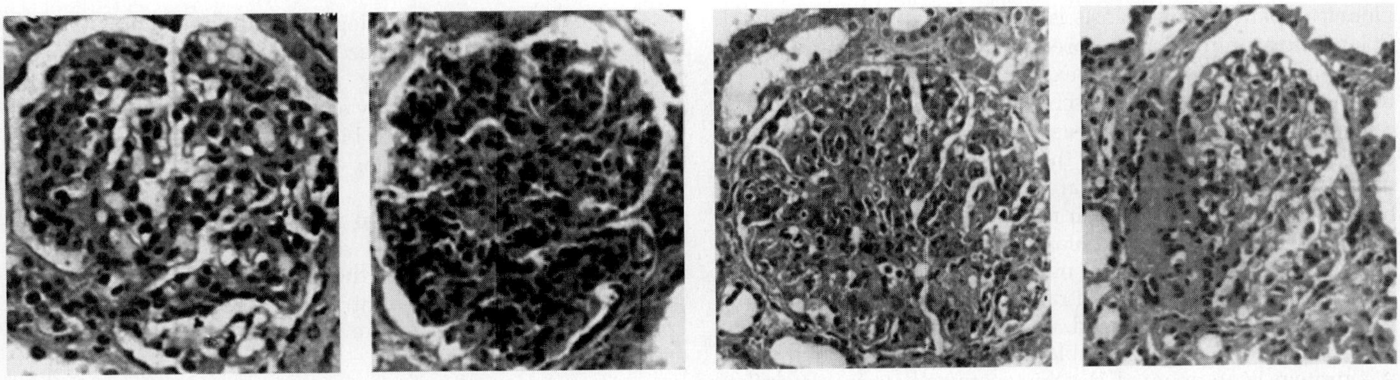

Figure 39.12. Classes I-IV schistosomal glomerulopathy. *Left to right*: Axial mesangial proliferation; exudative glomerulonephritis; mesangiocapillary glomerulonephritis; focal segmental sclerosis.

vanced hepatic fibrosis. For unclear reasons, there seems to be some bias of class III to South America and of class IV to Africa. However, the incidence of both types is remarkably similar in both continents, being encountered in 15% to 20% of patients with schistosomal hepatic fibrosis.

In addition to having fibrotic livers and enlarged spleens, all patients present with proteinuria and often microhematuria. Nephrotic syndrome is common, but its precise incidence is not clearly documented. Hypertension was present in about 50% of patients in different clinical series. Longitudinal studies have substantiated the progressive nature of these classes to end-stage renal disease, being responsible for about 9% of patients on renal replacement therapy in Egypt.

The importance of hepatic fibrosis in the pathogenesis of these classes is based on many experimental and clinical observations. This is classically attributed to the shunting of schistosomal antigens from the portal blood, thereby escaping hepatic clearance mechanisms. Available evidence suggests that impaired clearance of mucosal IgA may play an important role in the progression of glomerular pathology, which shows an almost linear correlation with mesangial deposition of this immunoglobulin.

There is also evidence that the augmented mucosal synthesis of IgA may be crucial in progression of the lesions, as shown by the significant increase of serum antigliadin IgA antibodies. In fact, this seems to be part of a widely spread B-lymphocyte switching favoring IgA at the expense of IgM secretion. It is presumable that switching is initiated in a mucosal B-cell clone exposed to the high IL-10 concentration that supervenes in late schistosomal granulomata. Migration of those lymphocytes via the thoracic duct may disseminate the message to distant aggregations.

On the other hand, several studies have documented the development and progression of classes III and IV without IgA deposits. It has been suggested that some of these cases may be attributed to persistence of schistosomal antigens that continue to fire immune complexes into the glomeruli for many decades. However, this mechanism is unlikely in most patients in whom the chances of detecting schistosomal antigens in the glomeruli decline with disease progression. Autoimmunity is an attractive alternative explanation, supported by many associated clinical and serologic features such as bronchial asthma, cutaneous vasculitis, positive rheumatoid factors, anti-DNA, and antiphospholipid antibodies.

Amyloid deposits (class V) are seen in about one-sixth of patients with schistosomal glomerular disease (Fig. 39.13). They are also encountered in some patients with *S. hematobium*–associated interstitial nephropathy without immune-mediated

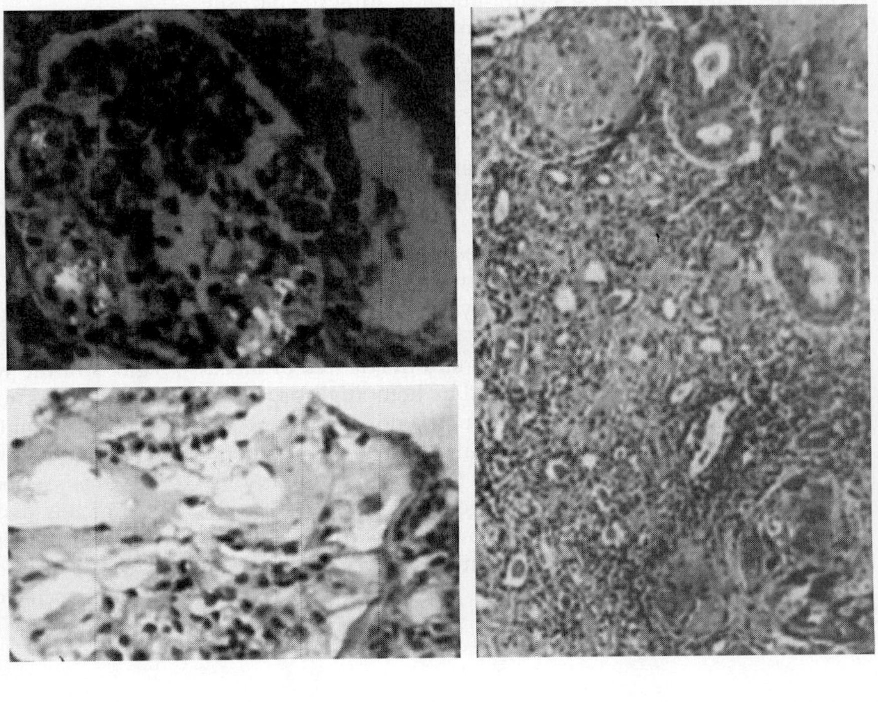

Figure 39.13. Class V schistosomal glomerulopathy (amyloidosis). *Top left:* Amyloid deposits seen as (green) birefringence under polarized light (Congo red stain). *Bottom left*: Amyloid infiltration of a glomerulus amidst mild mesangial proliferation. *Right*: Two glomeruli heavily infiltrated with amyloid amidst dense interstitial round cell infiltration and fibrosis. A schistosomal granuloma is seen in the lower-right corner of the section.

glomerulopathy. Amyloidosis is even more often encountered in laboratory animals, being predominantly seen in mice, hamsters, and rabbits exposed to experimental infection by any of the three human-pathogenic schistosomes.

Patients with schistosoma-associated amyloidosis are clinically indistinguishable from those with other forms of glomerular involvement. They are usually nephrotic and often hypertensive; in addition, their renal function progressively deteriorates. The kidneys are enlarged in only 25% of cases. The liver and spleen are enlarged in most cases, but this is usually an expression of schistosomal rather than amyloid infiltration. Serum AA is usually elevated, and the amyloid deposits contain AA protein. It is presumable that the hepatic generation of AA protein is augmented in schistosomiasis under the influence of IL-1 and IL-6, facing downregulated monocyte uptake by IL-10.

Thanks to the newer antiparasitic drugs, it is now possible to cure the majority of schistosomal infections within a few days. Praziquantel, a pyrazinoisoquinoline derivative, is the first drug of choice against all species of human-pathogenic schistosomes, with a cure rate of 80%. The recommended dose is 40 mg/kg body weight as a single morning dose for *S. hematobium* and *S. mansoni.* In *S. japonicum,* the dose should be increased to 60 mg/kg-body weight given in two divided doses on the same day. The drug is safe, but a few side effects have been reported, including abdominal pains, headaches, dizziness, and skin rash.

Other antischistosomal drugs, of more or less historic interest, include niridazole and metrifonate, which are effective only against *S. hematobium* infections, and oxamniquine, which is effective only against *S. mansoni.* Besides their narrow spectrum, the cure rate with these agents is much lower that with praziquantel.

Unfortunately, parasitologic cure can only be meaningful during the early phases of infection because most clinical problems in schistosomiasis occur late, along with the healing of granulomata. Among the lesions that respond very well to antischistosomal treatment are the acute intestinal and lower urinary, the back pressure induced by trigonal edema and acute vesicoureteric reflux, and possibly the acute glomerular lesions categorized as class I. Exudative glomerulonephritis (class II) also responds well to combined antiparasitic and antisalmonella treatment. Indeed, it is impossible to cure the bacterial infection in those cases without eradicating the parasite.

On the other hand, the chronic glomerular lesions (classes III through V) are progressive despite successful parasiticidal therapy, reflecting the associated copathogenetic mechanisms. Glucocorticoids and immunosuppressive agents do not offer any additional advantage. Patients with extensive lower urinary pathology often need surgical treatment, including the relief of obstruction, correction of reflux, removal of stones, and excision of masses.

Those with end-stage renal disease associated with hepatosplenic schistosomiasis constitute a considerable challenge for renal replacement therapy. Many patients cannot stand any peritoneal dialysis owing to the high protein content of their ascitic fluid. Others are at a major risk of bleeding from esophageal varices if treated by hemodialysis, unless subjected to sclerotherapy and regular endoscopic surveillance. Many patients have an associated infection with hepatitis B and/or C virus, constituting a significant risk for long-term renal replacement therapy in general. Impaired hepatic function often constitutes a clinical problem with the metabolism of immunosuppressive agents in patients subjected to renal transplantation.

Lower urinary tract pathology is an additional problem with renal transplantation. Increased incidence of urinary leaks has been reported, necessitating the resort to nonconventional methods of urinary continuity as ureteroureteric anastomosis to avoid cutting into the fibrotic bladder wall. Yet, the ureter, by its own right, may be equally or even more severely involved in some cases.

Recurrence of schistosomal glomerulopathy was reported in a few patients in whom live worms have been overlooked before transplantation. Despite the rarity of this event, it is recommended to perform a relevant serologic assessment during the pretransplant workout. Active infection must be treated before the transplant surgery.

Selected Readings

Abdel-Wahab MF. *Schistosomiasis in Egypt.* 4th Ed. Florida: CRC Press, 1982.

A comprehensive monograph on the fundamentals of schistosomiasis, including parasitologic and clinicopathologic features of the disease.

Badr MM. Surgical management of urinary Bilharziasis. In: Dudley H, Pories WJ, Carter DC, et al, eds. *Rob and Smith's operative surgery.* London: Butterworth, 1986.

A very well-written chapter on the urologic aspects of schistosomias. It describes the time-honored experience of Egyptian surgeons dealing with the disease since pharaonic ages.

Barsoum RS. Schistosomal glomerulopathies. *Kidney Int* 1993;44:1–12.

A review of the current concepts about renal schistosomiasis, with emphasis on the glomerular involvement, explaining the potential underlying pathogenetic mechanisms.

Houba V. Experimental renal disease due to schistosomiasis. *Kidney Int* 1979; 16:30–43.

An excellent review of the experimental data on schistosomal glomerulopathies. It gives all the necessary details about different animal models and provides insight into pathogenesis.

Wahl SM, Frazier-Jessen M, Jin WW, et al. Cytokine regulation of schistosome-induced granuloma and fibrosis. *Kidney Int* 1997;51:1370–1375.

A very good review of the cytokine profiles in schistosomal granulomata, explaining the essence of the immune response and subsequent fibrosis.

F: Other Bacterial, Viral, Parasitic, and Fungal Infections

Karpal S. Chugh and Vivekanand Jha

Glomerular involvement can occur in a number of infections, of which poststreptococcal glomerulonephritis is the best known. Other bacterial, viral, fungal, and parasitic infections that can cause glomerulonephritis are discussed here (Table 39.17).

Differences in the socioeconomic and environmental conditions appear to be responsible for a significant variation in the profile of infection-related glomerular diseases in different regions of the world. For example, poststreptococcal glomerulonephritis is now extremely uncommon in developed countries. The availability of potent antibiotics and aggressive surgical intervention have led to a decline in the incidence of glomerulonephritis associated with occult infections such as infective endocarditis and infected ventriculoatrial shunts. On the other hand, two new entities that have emerged over the last two decades include hepatitis virus–related glomerular disease and HIV-associated nephropathy.

TABLE 39.17. Nonpoststreptococcal Infective Glomerulonephritis

Bacterial
Streptococcus viridans
Staphylococcus albus and *Staphylococcus epidermidis*
Gram-negative bacilli (*Pseudomonas aeruginosa, Escherichia coli, Proteus vulgaris)*
Salmonella typhosa
Leptospira species
Treponema pallidum
Mycobacterium leprae
Yersinia enterocolitica
Neisseria meningitidis, Neisseria gonorrhoeae
Corynebacterium diphtheriae
Coxiella burnetii
Brucella abortus
Listeria monocytogenes
Viral
Hepatitis B
Epstein-Barr (infectious mononucleosis)
Coxsackie B
ECHO virus
Cytomegalovirus
Varicella-zoster
Mumps
Rubella
Retrovirus (HIV)
Influenza
Fungal
Histoplasma capsulatum
Candida
Coccidiodes immitis
Protozoal
Plasmodium falciparum and *Plasmodium malariae*
Toxoplasma gondii
Trypanosoma
Helminthic
Schistosoma mansoni and *Schistosoma haematobium*
Wuchereria bancrofti
Brugia malayi
Loa loa
Onchocerca volvulus
Trichinella spiralis

The cause-and-effect relationship between infections and glomerulonephritis has been established mainly by epidemiologic studies. The evidence includes the demonstration of specific glomerular abnormalities following certain infections and their resolution following specific treatment. However, there are a few caveats in this approach. The pattern of glomerular disease is not uniform, and the same organism has been shown to produce different morphologic appearances in different patients or in different geographic areas. Even in epidemics, not every infected person develops a glomerular disease. For example, hepatitis B infection has been reported to lead to different histologic types of glomerulonephritides in different age groups and in different geographic areas. In contrast, different infections may have an identical histologic picture. Thus the patient factors as well as the characteristics of the microbe appear to be important. The type of the lesion depends on the nature of the antigen, the duration of exposure, the host immune response, and finally, the glomerular response to injury.

Glomerular lesions similar to those found in humans have been induced in animal models using bacterial, viral, fungal, or parasitic antigens. In most instances, the lesions of infection-associated glomerulonephritis have been thought to be immune complex mediated. A direct causal link can be proved only by identification of either a specific antigen within the glomerulus or by eluting an immunoglobulin that reacts specifically with the antigen. Although the association between some of these infections and glomerulonephritis appears to be very strong in these studies, confirmation of this link may not always be possible because of nonavailability of specific antisera. In these situations, epidemiologic studies remain the cornerstone of the diagnostic association. The availability of highly sophisticated techniques such as reverse transcriptase polymerase chain reaction and *in situ* hybridization has now made identification of these antigens possible with almost 100% sensitivity and specificity. Chronic antigenic stimulation resulting from certain infections can lead to glomerular involvement due to amyloidosis. On the other hand, infections such as measles may induce a remission in the nephrotic state associated with minimal-change disease, possibly by reduction in interleukin production due to inhibitory effect on T cells. Similar effects have rarely been reported following varicella-zoster, *Salmonella typhi,* and pneumococcal infections. Only the commonly encountered nonstreptotoccal infection-related glomerulopathies are discussed here. Glomerulonephritides caused by HIV and hepatitis virus, schistosoma, and malaria are discussed in other sections.

BACTERIAL INFECTION

Infective Endocarditis

Renal involvement in infective endocarditis was recognized as early as 1910 by Lohlein, who described the lesions as an "embolic non-suppurative glomerulonephritis." Subsequently, the embolic nature of the lesions was questioned, and an immunologic mechanism was suggested. This was supported by the demonstration of hypocomplementemia, presence of immune complexes in the glomeruli as well as in the circulation and elution of specific antibodies from the involved kidneys.

Endocarditis most commonly affects heart valves that are either congenitally abnormal or have been damaged as a result of rheumatic or degenerative diseases. With almost complete eradication of rheumatic heart disease in the developed countries and availability of effective antibiotic therapy, the clinical presentation of infective endocarditis has shown a dramatic change. On the other hand, three new groups of patients with infective endocarditis have emerged: habitual parenteral drug abusers, patients with prosthetic cardiac valves, and patients with prolonged central lines. In the last group, the diagnosis of endocarditis may not be obvious, and symptoms related to involvement of other organs may dominate the clinical picture.

The clinical presentation depends on the virulence of the infecting organism and the underlying cardiac disease. Low-virulence organisms, such as *Streptococcus viridans,* commonly infect previously damaged valves and produce a subacute form of endocarditis. In contrast, the newer generation of patients mentioned previously are often affected by virulent organisms such as *Staphylococcus aureus*, gram-negative bacilli, and fungi. In particular, the incidence of *S. aureus* endocarditis has increased in the last decade especially in intravenous drug abusers. Other organisms, isolated particularly from immunosuppressed individuals with infective endocarditis, include α- and β-hemolytic streptococci, *S. mitis, S. mutans, S. epidermidis,* enterococci, gonococcus, *Pseudomonas aeruginosa, Coxiella burnetii, Chlamydia psittaci, Hemophilus aphrophilus,* and *Salmonella* species.

Patients often present with fever, malaise, arthralgias, anemia, and purpura. Some of the signs, such as splinter hemorrhages, Osler's nodes, and Janeway lesions, which were regarded as classical at one time, are seldom seen. The fundus examination may reveal Roth's spots.

The frequency with which glomerulonephritis occurs in infective endocarditis is not well documented. In one autopsy study, 22% of patients showed glomerular lesions, with the majority having right-sided endocarditis. Renal lesions are seen with equal frequency in acute as well as subacute endocarditis. The frequency of renal involvement is higher among those who remain untreated for a long time, have negative blood cultures, and have involvement of the right side of the heart. In most such patients, the classical presentation with peripheral signs of endocarditis is unusual. The blood culture is positive in about 60% to 70% of cases. Exhibition of prior antibiotic therapy may alter the clinical picture as well as the culture positivity rate. Therefore a high index of suspicion is necessary to confirm or exclude this diagnosis. Infective endocarditis should be considered in the differential diagnosis of all patients who show signs of renal involvement in the setting of systemic vasculitis disorders, especially if they exhibit one of the risk factors mentioned earlier.

Renal involvement may manifest with gross or microscopic hematuria and mild proteinuria. Mild to moderate azotemia may be present. Occasionally, patients may present with rapidly progressive glomerulonephritis with crescent formation. Advanced renal failure indicates the presence of diffuse glomerular alterations and failure of antibiotic therapy to eradicate infection. Nephrotic syndrome is distinctly unusual. Laboratory finding include a normocytic normochromic anemia, leukocytosis, increased erythrocyte sedimentation rate, and C-reactive protein. Activation of the immune system may be evident from the high titres of circulating rheumatoid factor, type III cryoglobulins, and the presence of immune complexes. Serum C3, C4, C2, and C1q levels are often decreased in the acute phase. Antineutrophil cytoplasmic antibodies with cytoplasmic pattern (cANCA) and proteinase-3 specificity have been demonstrated in patients with subacute bacterial endocarditis and glomerulonephritis. The clinical and serologic abnormalities are known to disappear after antibiotic therapy.

Pathology

Externally, the kidneys are enlarged and smooth, with small subcapsular hemorrhages (flea-bitten kidneys). Light microscopy reveals two distinct patterns of glomerular damage. In so-called acute endocarditis, the most common finding is diffuse cellular proliferation with or without foci of necrosis. An irregular thickening of the glomerular capillary wall with duplication may also be seen. Less commonly, membranous nephropathy and mesangiocapillary glomerulonephritis type I are observed. Immunofluorescence reveals widespread deposits of IgG, IgM, and C3 in the glomeruli. Ultrastructurally, dense subendothelial, subepithelial, and mesangial deposits are observed.

In the subacute form, focal segmental proliferative lesions with fibrinoid necrosis or capillary thrombi are more common. Immunofluorescence studies reveal diffuse immune deposits limited to the mesangium, and the subendothelial region is usually spared. Occasionally, a crescentic form of glomerulonephritis is observed. In one autopsy study of patients with infective endocarditis dying of renal failure, extracapillary crescents involving more than 50% glomeruli were seen in all patients. Rarely, patients with longstanding, unrecognized infective endocarditis have been reported to develop amyloidosis.

In addition to the glomerular changes, tubulointerstitial infiltration with mononuclear cells and tubular atrophy and fibrosis may be seen. Presence of large number of eosinophils in the infiltrate suggests the superimposition of drug-induced acute interstitial nephritis (AIN), most commonly caused by one of the antibiotics used for treatment.

The other renal lesions encountered in these patients include embolic infarcts and pyemic abscesses, especially in those with *S. aureus* endocarditis. The presenting symptoms in both these conditions include flank pain, oliguria, hematuria, and pyuria. Renal failure may be seen if the involvement is bilateral and extensive. Occasionally, acute tubular necrosis may result from septicemia and/or antibiotic use.

Pathogenesis

The pathogenetic mechanism involves immune complex formation leading to complement activation through direct pathway. Higher levels of circulating immune complexes have been detected in patients with renal involvement compared with those without it. The increase is particularly marked in the subacute form of infective endocarditis. The levels usually decline with successful treatment, but the fall is less marked in patients with glomerular involvement. In an experimental study, immune complexes were detected in 13 of 18 rabbits with infective endocarditis and glomerulonephritis. Gel filtration studies showed the complexes of the size ranging from Ca 4.10 to 3.10 D. Direct immunofluorescence showed IgM to be the predominant immunoglobulin in the glomerular deposits. The role of immune complexes has also been confirmed by elution of antibodies specific to the infecting organism from the glomeruli and the demonstration of streptococcal and staphylococcal antigens *in situ. S. aureus* can also activate the alternative pathway due to nonimmune interaction of staphylococcal cell wall protein A with immunoglobulin complement components and platelets.

Treatment and Prognosis

The course and prognosis are variable. Successful treatment of endocarditis results in resolution of the inflammatory phase of glomerulonephritis. Antibiotics must be given for 4 to 6 weeks to ensure complete eradication of endocarditis. The dosage should be modified in accordance with renal function. All patients who have recovered from an episode of endocarditis must be advised to take prophylactic antibiotics in situations in which bacteremia is likely to occur, such as tooth extraction or instrumentation of urinary tract.

No specific therapy is required for the renal lesions. High-dose prednisolone and plasmapheresis have not been shown to be useful. The use of intravenous methyl prednisolone pulses followed by oral prednisolone has been advocated for treatment of adults with rapidly progressive (crescentic) glomerulonephritis due to infective endocarditis. Some patients may be left with varying degrees of renal insufficiency, hypertension, or proteinuria depending on the severity of initial involvement, more so in those with crescentic disease.

Shunt Nephritis

Ventriculoatrial and ventriculoperitoneal shunts are inserted for decompression of dilated cerebral ventricles. In 1965, Black was the first to describe lobular proliferative glomerulonephritis in two children with a Spitz-Holter ventriculoatrial shunt. Nearly 30% of these shunts have been observed to become infected after insertion. Glomerulonephritis has been reported to complicate 0.7% to 2.25% of all infected shunts. Although more than two-thirds of the colonization occurs within the first 3 months, glomerular involvement has been reported as early as 2 weeks and as late as 21 years after shunt insertion. In most studies, renal lesions have been seen primarily in association with ventriculoatrial shunts. Ventriculoperitoneal shunts are rarely complicated by the development of nephritis. In one series of 212 patients with ventriculoperitoneal shunts, 14 got infected and only one had developed nephritis. The decreasing incidence of this complication can be explained by the increasing use of extravascular ventriculoperitoneal devices.

More than 100 cases have been described in the world literature so far. The causal organism is *Staphylococcus albus* in 70% of patients and *S. aureus* in about 20%. The remainder are caused by *Pseudomonas species, Bacillus cereus* and *subtilis, Listeria monocytogenes, Moraxella nonliquefaciens, Acinetobacter Lwoffi, Propionibacterium acnes, Serratia, Peptostreptococcus,* and diphtheroids.

Clinical Features

The clinical presentation is nonspecific and includes prolonged fever, arthralgias, malaise, weight loss, anemia, signs of increased intracranial pressure, skin rash, and hepatosplenomegaly. The onset is often insidious and may not be recognized for weeks or months. In one series, the diagnosis was delayed up to 1.5 years after the onset of clinical manifestations. Development of palpable purpura sometimes provides a clue to the diagnosis. Hypertension is a common feature, and malignant hypertension is seen occasionally. The blood culture is positive in untreated cases. Varying degrees of azotemia may be seen. Because of the nonspecific nature of symptoms and serologic findings, the infection may be overlooked until the renal failure becomes irreversible. Microscopic hematuria is a constant finding, but gross hematuria is uncommon. Varying degrees of proteinuria may be noted, and nephrotic syndrome is seen in about 25% of cases. Presence of infection may be indicated by leukocytosis and a raised erythrocyte sedimentation rate. Reduced levels of C3 and C4 and elevated levels of C-reactive proteins, rheumatoid factor, antinuclear antibodies, and cryoglobulins may be seen.

Pathology

On histology, the renal lesions resemble mesangiocapillary glomerulonephritis type I, with endocapillary proliferation, lobular accentuation, and double contouring of the basement membrane. Other lesions include segmental or diffuse proliferative glomerulonephritis with or without crescent formation. Electron microscopy reveals subendothelial and mesangial electron-dense deposits, and immunofluorescence reveals granular deposits of IgM, IgG, and C3. Antigens specific to *S. albus* and other bacteria have also been demonstrated within the glomerular deposits.

Pathogenesis

Like most infection-associated glomerulonephritides, the renal lesions are immune complex mediated. The prolonged antigenemia leads to antibody production and immune complex formation, which is indicated by the demonstration of rheumatoid factor and cryoglobulins. In one study, the shunt was found to be infected in more than 85% of patients who showed increase in the levels of circulating immune complexes. *S. albus* antigen and specific antibody have been demonstrated in these immune complexes. The antigen contains glycerol teichoic acid and staphylococcal nuclease during the acute phase. Evidence of classical complement pathway activation is provided by depression of C3 levels. The alternative pathway of complement activation may also be involved. A role for intracellular adhesion molecules such as ICAM-1 and E-selectin has also been postulated. Rarely, shunt nephritis may be seen without the demonstration of a pathogenic organism (sterile shunt nephritis). In such cases, induction of antibodies by silicone elastomers such as polydimethylsiloxane may lead to immune complex formation and complement activation. In a follow-up study, C3 rose to normal within 1 week and urinary abnormalities resolved after a few months. However, there was only a moderate improvement in glomerular histology on repeat biopsy after 2 years. The immune complexes may persist for months despite shunt removal and appropriate antibiotic therapy.

Treatment and Prognosis

Treatment mandates a prompt removal of the infected shunt because antibiotic therapy alone is usually inadequate. The current practice is to replace the shunt with a ventriculoperitoneal shunt. Prognosis depends on the speed with which the diagnosis is made and shunt removed. Although the abnormalities resolve in most cases, renal dysfunction of varying severity may persist in cases in which there is a delay in the diagnosis and/or in removal of the shunt. The dysfunction may ultimately progress to end-stage renal failure. In contrast to ventriculoatrial shunt, the low incidence of nephritis following ventriculoperitoneal shunt placement makes the latter modality preferable for treatment of hydrocephalus. Because colonization of ventriculoatrial shunt is thought to occur in the intraoperative period, the necessity of perioperative antibiotic prophylaxis during insertion of ventriculoatrial shunts has been emphasized. If renal replacement therapy is required, whether continuous ambulatory peritoneal dialysis (CAPD) can be started with a ventriculoperitoneal shunt *in situ* remains controversial because of the risk of peritonitis and meningitis.

Visceral Sepsis

Glomerulonephritis has been reported to follow pulmonary, intraabdominal, pelvic, and cutaneous infections, and also is seen in individuals with infected vascular prostheses. A common feature is severe infection present for many months. A variety of microorganisms have been isolated. The clinical presentation is variable and ranges from mild urinary abnormalities to severe fulminant renal failure. Some patients may develop nephrotic syndrome. Serum levels of complement may be low. No single specific renal histologic entity has been described in association with these infections. The most commonly reported lesions are of diffuse proliferative or mesangial proliferative glomerulonephritis. Occasionally, mesangiocapillary, membranous, or focal proliferative glomerulonephritis has been observed. A varying number of epithelial crescents may be noted, and crescentic glomerulonephritis is seen in 30% of cases. The duration of infection is important in determining the type of glomerular lesion. When infection antedates renal involvement by less than 2 months, mesangial and endothelial cell proliferation occur more commonly, and if the interval is longer, crescentic glomerulonephritis is observed more frequently.

Management is primarily directed at treating the underlying infection. Identification of the offending organism on culture helps in instituting proper antibiotic therapy. The drug dosage has to be modified according to the renal function, and the duration must be long enough to ensure a complete eradication of the infection. Plasmapheresis has been used in some cases with varying success. Recovery of renal function is unpredictable. Complete recovery can be expected only if the treatment is started early. A proportion of patients show an insidious progression to chronic renal failure after initial improvement. Neither the severity of the presenting illness nor the presence of hypertension or the degree of endocapillary proliferation correlates with the eventual outcome. However, crescentic change in the glomeruli is indicative of a poor prognosis.

Typhoid

Typhoid fever is common in the tropical and subtropical regions and is known for its varied manifestations. The clinical picture is dominated by intermittent fever, splenomegaly, and gastrointestinal symptoms. Complications involving the urinary tract include cystitis, pyelitis, and acute renal failure. Although overt glomerular involvement is rare and is seen in fewer than 2% of all cases, hematuria and mild to moderate proteinuria can be detected in 25% to 40% of cases. In a series of children with typhoid fever reported from South Africa, edema of more than 1 month's duration was detected in more than 50% of cases. In a report from Israel, a familial clustering of typhoid nephritis was described, although no HLA haploid-type link could be demonstrated. Renal involvement may also occur as a part of the syndrome of disseminated intravascular coagulation or hemolytic uremic syndrome. The diagnosis is made by demonstrating *S. typhi* or paratyphi in blood, stool, or urine culture, or rising titers in the Widal test. C3 levels are often depressed. Serum IgA levels may be elevated, probably secondary to the intestinal mucosal involvement.

In addition to a direct glomerular involvement, typhoid bacteremia has been implicated in the genesis of nephrotic syndrome in patients with hepatosplenic schistosomiasis in Egypt, Brazil, and Sudan. The proof for etiologic role of this infection has been provided by disappearance of urinary abnormalities following effective treatment of salmonellosis in patients who were demonstrated to have salmonella bacteremia and persistence of abnormalities in those without the bacteremia. This suggests that salmonella leads to aggravation of preexisting subclinical schistosomal glomerulopathy by causing additional lesions directly related to bacteremia.

Pathology

Various histologic lesions have been described. These include diffuse exudative proliferative glomerulonephritis, mesangial proliferative glomerulonephritis, and IgA nephropathy. Variable number of crescents may be observed. The capillary walls are usually normal. The interstitium usually shows localized small cell infiltration. Electron microscopy reveals electron-dense deposits in the paramesangial areas, with occasional thickening of the lamina rara interna. Immunofluorescence microscopy reveals deposition of IgM, IgG, and C3 in the mesangium and along the capillary walls. A small number of cases show dense granular deposits of IgA in the mesangium, along with small amounts of IgM and C3. Salmonella Vi antigen has been demonstrated in the affected glomeruli.

Treatment and Prognosis

The prognosis usually depends upon the extent of systemic involvement due to typhoid. The renal involvement is usually transient and does not require any specific therapy. In some series, however, glomerular involvement has been associated with an increase in mortality from 8% to 30%.

Pneumococcal Infections

Streptococcus pneumoniae (pneumococcus) is a common cause of community acquired pneumonia, especially in developing countries. The clinical and pathologic evidence of nephritis following this infection was well documented in the preantibiotic era, but the incidence decreased drastically following the widespread availability of effective antibiotics. Clinical manifestations include microhematuria and moderate proteinuria. Renal failure is seen in an occasional case.

Sporadic reports have documented mesangiocapillary or mesangioproliferative lesions. Ultrastructural studies reveal electron-dense deposits in the subepithelial, mesangial, and intramembranous regions, and immunofluorescence shows immunoglobulin and complement components corresponding to these deposits. The demonstration of pneumococcal antigen (especially type 14) in the deposits provides the proof for immune complex nature of the disease. The polysaccharide capsular antigen activates the alternative complement pathway as in the case of poststreptococcal glomerulonephritis. A limited activation of classical pathway has also been demonstrated. The course of glomerulonephritis is self-limiting, and the urinary findings disappear after successful treatment of infection.

Leprosy

Leprosy is a chronic granulomatous disorder caused by the acid-fast bacillus *Mycobacterium leprae.* The clinical manifestations of leprosy form a continuum dictated largely by the degree of cell-mediated immunity in the patient. The usual mode of presentation is with anaesthetic skin lesions, peripheral neuropathy, and palpable enlargement of peripheral nerves. This disease continues to be prevalent in most parts of Asia, Africa, and Latin America. The global number of leprosy cases was estimated around 10 to 12 million in the 1970s and 1980s, but according to newer estimates (World Health Organization, 1991), the number has decreased to about 5.5 million.

The occurrence of nephritis in leprosy was first reported by Hansen and Looft in 1894. In the first half of the twentieth century, renal failure was an important cause of death in leprosy. Glomerulonephritis and secondary amyloidosis are the commonest renal lesions seen in leprosy. Other abnormalities include acute tubular necrosis, acute and chronic interstitial nephritis, and tubular function defects without histologic lesions.

Glomerulonephritis

Although fewer than 2% of patients are suspected to have glomerulonephritis on clinical evaluation, renal biopsies have revealed glomerulonephritis in 13% to 71% of cases in different studies. Much of this variability is related to differences in the patient selection. The lower figures come from studies that evaluated unscreened patients, whereas biopsies from patients selected on the basis of urinary abnormalities reveal a higher incidence. Glomerulonephritis is equally common in both lepromatous and nonlepromatous disease. In the former, the glomerulonephritis often occurs during episodes of erythema nodosum leprosum.

In a study of 64 cases from India, a significant relationship was found between the renal involvement and duration of leprosy. Renal involvement could be demonstrated in 2% of nonlepromatous and 63% of lepromatous leprosy, with 100% of patients with lepra reaction showing urinary abnormalities.

Most patients with leprosy-associated glomerulonephritis present with asymptomatic urinary abnormalities, but some may develop nephrotic syndrome. A few patients may present with acute nephritic syndrome and, rarely, with rapidly progressive renal failure. Hypertension is uncommon. In one study, all patients with lepra reaction exhibited urinary abnormalities and a decline in glomerular filtration rate (GFR). Hypocomplementemia is seen often in these patients, especially those showing a picture of mesangiocapillary glomerulonephritis on biopsy. Defects in urinary acidification and concentration may be demonstrated in some cases.

The most common histologic lesions are mesangial proliferative and diffuse proliferative glomerulonephritis, although virtually all morphologic lesions, including crescentic glomerulonephritis, have been reported. Acid-fast bacilli can be demonstrated rarely. Electron microscopy reveals electron-dense deposits in the mesangial and subendothelial regions. Intramembranous and subepithelial deposits are found less frequently. Other findings include focal foot process widening, areas of glomerular capillary basement membrane reduplication with mesangial interposition, and endothelial swelling with cytoplasmic vacuolation. On immunofluorescence, granular deposits of IgG, C3, and less frequently, IgM, IgA, and fibrin are seen in the mesangium and along the capillary walls. Vascular changes resembling microscopic polyarteritis have been reported in Japanese patients dying of leprosy. The significance of these findings, however, is not clear.

The abnormalities observed on electron microscopy and immunofluorescence indicate that the varied glomerular lesions are manifestations of immune complex glomerulonephritis. This hypothesis is further supported by the observation that glomerulonephritis occurs more frequently in lepromatous leprosy complicated by erythema nodosum leprosum (ENL), another immune complex–mediated process. Immune complexes can be detected in circulation in more than 75% of patients with active ENL compared with only one-third in those with lepromatous disease without ENL.

The exact nature of the antigen in the immune complexes is not yet known but is suspected to be a product of *M. leprae.* The observation of glomerulonephritis in nonlepromatous forms of the disease has raised the possibility of involvement of a nonmycobacterial antigen in the generation of glomerulonephritis. The postulated antigens include those derived from microorganisms that coinfect these individuals and dapsone–antidapsone antibodies. In one autopsy study of 133 cases, renal lesions were thought to be secondary to infections in other organs in more than 40% of patients.

Circulating cryoglobulins have been demonstrated in patients with leprosy and also have been identified in the glomerular deposits. Complement activation occurs primarily by the alternative pathway, triggered by the immunoglobulins present in the cryoprecipitates. Cell-mediated immune injury is a possible, but not yet proven, cause of glomerular damage.

Amyloidosis

The incidence of renal amyloidosis in the earlier studies ranged from 2% to 55%, but newer studies put the figure between 2% and 8%. This variability is largely related to geographic differences. Whereas about 55% cases were reported to have amyloid in both autopsy and biopsy studies from the United States, similar studies from Mexico, Africa, and India found the incidence to be less than 10%. The reason for this variability has been thought to be related to genetic differences, frequency of lepra reactions, nutritional status, and different standards of management of leprosy. Amyloidosis is far more common in lepromatous than in tuberculoid leprosy. The occurrence of repeated episodes of erythema nodosum leprosum in lepromatous leprosy may predispose these patients to the development of amyloidosis because each episode is associated with a marked and persistent elevation of serum amyloid A protein. Chemical analysis of the amyloid deposits in these patients has demonstrated the fibrils to be primarily composed of AA protein. Amyloidosis is seen rarely in the tuberculoid form of the disease, and these patients typically have longstanding trophic ulcers preceding the development of this complication.

Management

The treatment of leprosy entails the use of a combination of dapsone, rifampicin, and clofazimine. Glucocorticoids and thalidomide are effective in controlling the systemic manifestations of ENL. Although earlier studies had failed to demonstrate any beneficial effect of steroids or antileprosy drugs on the course of glomerular disease, more recently, prednisolone has been shown to reverse renal failure in some patients during episodes of ENL. Early and aggressive treatment of leprosy with particular attention to preventing recurrent episodes of ENL may be helpful in preventing renal amyloidosis. In patients undergoing renal transplantation, there is an enhanced risk of recrudescence of leprosy as a result of immunosuppressive therapy.

Tuberculosis

Tuberculosis is a common chronic bacterial infection encountered in developing countries. Renal involvement is characterized by chronic caseous destruction and fibrosis and, less commonly, by diffuse interstitial nephritis and granuloma formation. Studies reported in the preantibiotic era frequently associated glomerulonephritis with tuberculosis. In the recent times, only stray reports have described the occurrence of immune complex glomerulonephritis in tuberculosis. Renal lesions of dense-deposit disease have also been reported in isolated instances, but the cause-and-effect relationship has not been proved and chance associations cannot be excluded. A well-known complication, however, is amyloidosis, which is still seen in a significant proportion of patients in economically poor countries where the disease often remains untreated for long periods. Renal tuberculosis is further discussed in Chapter 41, Part 2.

Miscellaneous Bacterial Infections

There are reports of glomerulonephritis occurring in patients with some other bacterial infections. In some of these, the bacterial antigen has been demonstrated in the deposits, confirming the etiologic association. These include *Escherichia coli* and *Klebsiella pneumoniae* infections, meningococcal meningitis, *Yersinia gastroenteritis,* and infection with *Mycoplasma pneumoniae.* The histology shows varying degrees of endocapillary, mesangial, and extracapillary proliferation and at times membrane thickening. Immunofluorescence confirms the immune complex nature of the lesions. IgA deposits may predominate in some patients. The renal disease often resolves after treatment of the infection. Relative rarity of reports of glomerular disease in such infections, which are otherwise not so uncommon, casts a doubt on the causal relationship.

VIRAL INFECTION

Cytomegalovirus

Cytomegalovirus (CMV) is the most frequent pathogen encountered in immunosuppressed patients, including renal transplant recipients. The latter develop this infection either through reactivation of latent infection, reinfection, or a primary infection in a seronegative recipient receiving an organ from a seropositive donor. Clinical CMV syndrome presents most commonly with a febrile illness, along with leukopenia, pneumonia, hepatitis, and gastrointestinal ulcers. It also increases the risk of infections with other opportunistic organisms. There is little agreement on the renal manifestations with this organism. CMV nephropathy has been reported rarely in children with severe congenital disease. Although granular deposits of IgG and C3 have been demonstrated in glomerular capillary walls, no viral antigen has been shown. A distinct glomerulopathy was first reported in a patient with fatal CMV disease in 1979. The kidneys showed mesangial deposits of immunoglobulins, complement components, and most importantly, CMV antigen in the glomeruli. Elution studies revealed the presence of specific antibodies. In a biopsy study conducted among renal transplant recipients with graft dysfunction, four of seven patients with CMV viremia showed a unique lesion that was characterized by hypertrophy and necrosis of endothelial cells, narrowing or obliteration of capillary lumina, fibrillar deposits in the glomerular capillaries, mesangial hypercellularity, and mononuclear cell infiltration. Immunofluorescence showed IgG, IgM, and C3 deposits along the glomerular basement membrane and within the mesangium. In another study in which characterization of glomerular infiltrate was attempted, the lesions contained a large number of CD8+ T lymphocytes. Others have cast a doubt on the etiologic relationship between CMV infection and the glomerular lesions. In three large studies on immunosuppressed patients, including renal allograft recipients with CMV infection who showed glomerular pathology similar to that described in other reports, neither an anti-CMV antibody nor the antigen or DNA could be detected by immunohistochemistry and *in situ* hybridization.

One case of immunotactoid glomerulopathy has been reported in a renal transplant recipient with CMV infection that resolved after ganciclovir therapy and withdrawal of immunosuppression. Intracytoplasmic CMV inclusions have been demonstrated in glomerular epithelial and capillary endothelial cells by light and electron microscopy, and they have been confirmed by immunohistochemistry and *in situ* hybridization. Similar inclusions have been noted in the tubular epithelial cells in renal biopsies from transplant recipients with CMV infection in the absence of any glomerular lesions. In all these cases, however, the characteristic glomerular lesions of CMV were not seen. Thus it seems unlikely that CMV-associated glomerulopathy results from a direct cytopathic effect of the virus. It has been speculated that the glomerular injury could be the result of an increased expression of both class I and II MHC antigens on the renal parenchymal cells. The infiltrating CD8+ lymphocyte may act as the primary effector cell in this process. Why only a minority of viremic individuals develop CMV-associated glomerulopathy is not clear and may be related to differences in the individual host tissue responses and varying degrees of immunosuppression.

Influenza

Influenza is a common viral illness occurring in all parts of the world. The illness primarily affects the respiratory tract and may be accompanied by systemic symptoms. Goodpasture was the first to report the syndrome of glomerulonephritis and pulmonary hemorrhage in an 18-year-old patient with typical influenza during the 1918–1919 pandemic. Similar cases were reported during the influenza pandemic of 1957–1958. The association between the two has since been documented by several workers. The cause-and-effect relationship, however, remains unproven because virologic studies were not performed in these cases. It has been speculated that the pulmonary insult exposes and alters the alveolar basement membrane antigens and elicits the formation of an antibody that cross-reacts with the basement membranes of the lung and kidney. Various reports have documented the deposition of IgG and C3 deposits in linear fashion in the glomerular and renal tubular basement membranes as well as the alveolar septal membrane. In rare instances, properdin deposition has also been shown, suggesting activation of the alternative complement pathway. Most patients develop the typical syndrome of rapidly progressive renal failure. Histopathologic examination reveals focal or diffuse proliferative glomerulonephritis with exuberant crescent formation, and immunofluorescence reveals linear deposition of immunoglobulins along the glomerular and tubular basement membranes. Rarely, the renal function may be normal or minimally altered despite the presence of proliferative glomerulonephritis and linear immunoglobulin deposits in the glomerular basement membrane, suggesting a spectrum that may range from subclinical alterations to rapidly progressive glomerulonephritis. Further discussion on Goodpasture's syndrome is found in Chapter 42, Part 7.

Hemolytic uremic syndrome has also been reported in some patients after influenza A virus infection. Histologic examination showed typical subendothelial deposition in the glomerular capillaries.

Measles

Measles is a common viral exanthematous illness with a worldwide distribution. Measles virus can often be cultured from the kidneys obtained at autopsies of patients dying of this infection, and the antigen has been demonstrated by immunofluorescent antibody technique in the urinary epithelial cells. In one autopsy study, renal histology in patients dying of measles revealed mild hyperplastic and degenerative changes of parietal epithelium of Bowman's capsule, but no change was noted in the glomerular tufts.

Clinical renal involvement has not been reported frequently. A case of acute endocapillary proliferative glomerulonephritis 4 days after onset of measles has been reported from Taiwan during one of the epidemics. Electron microscopy revealed discrete electron-dense deposits within and in the subepithelial region of glomerular basement membrane. Measles virus antigen could be demonstrated along the capillary loops and in the mesangium. The urinary abnormalities resolved completely within 6 weeks. Measles antigen has been demonstrated in the glomeruli of a patient with subacute sclerosing panencephalitis, which is also caused by the measles virus.

Measles infection is reputed to induce a remission of nephrotic syndrome in patients with minimal-change disease. Primary measles vaccination has been used for therapeutic purposes.

Parvovirus

Parvovirus B-19 has been implicated in the development of aplastic crisis in patients with sickle cell disease. A link between this virus and renal disease was first suspected when nephrotic syndrome was noted in two siblings with sickle cell disease and hypoplastic crises. This association has been confirmed subsequently. Nephrotic syndrome may appear as early as 3 days and as late as 7 weeks after the aplastic crisis. Renal involvement without marrow hypoplasia has been reported but is less common. Patients in whom biopsies were performed during the acute phase show a focal or diffuse proliferative glomerulonephritis or membranoproliferative glomerulonephritis. Varying degrees of interstitial disease are also seen. Rarely, rapidly progressive glomerulonephritis with crescent formation has also been observed. In late stages, the histologic picture is consistent with focal and segmental glomerulosclerosis. Steroid therapy may be helpful in halting the decline of renal function in patients with rapidly progressive course. Attempts to demonstrate the viral antigen within the glomerular lesions have so far been unsuccessful.

Mumps

Mumps is an acute communicable disease of viral etiology characterized by painful parotidomegaly and occasional involvement of gonads and pancreas. Renal involvement was reported during an outbreak of mumps in Taiwan in 1990. Of 124 children, 36 had microhematuria and 8 had proteinuria. Renal biopsy in a patient with persistent hematuria showed mesangial proliferative glomerulonephritis. The demonstration of immunoglobulins, complement, and mumps virus antigen on immunofluorescence clearly proved the causal link between the infection and glomerular disease. The urinary abnormalities disappeared in most cases after resolution of the infection.

Epstein-Barr Virus

Epstein-Barr virus, a DNA virus, is the causative agent of infectious mononucleosis and several malignancies, including Burkitt's lymphoma. About 15% of patients with infectious mononucleosis develop proteinuria, and hematuria develops in about 11%. A decline in renal function, however, is seen much less commonly, and only some patients show severe impairment. Renal histology reveals various lesions, including mesangiocapillary glomerulonephritis, diffuse proliferative glomerulonephritis, and IgA nephropathy. The urinary abnormalities disappear with resolution of the infection.

Dengue Hemorrhagic Fever

Endemic in Southeast Asia, the Western Pacific, and the Caribbean, dengue hemorrhagic fever (a severe febrile illness) is caused by four dengue serotypes of the family Flaviviridae. The infection is transmitted to humans by the bite of *Aedes aegypti* mosquito. The clinical features reflect increased vascular permeability and include severe muscular pains, gastrointestinal symptoms, bleeding manifestations, and shock. Renal involvement is manifested by microhematuria and mild to moderate proteinuria. Acute renal failure is seen in patients with severe shock. Light microscopy of the kidney reveals features of endocapillary proliferative glomerulonephritis with mononuclear cells in glomerular capillaries. Mild mesangial proliferation, an increase in mesangial matrix, and irregular thickening of capillary walls may also be seen. Electron microscopy shows electron-dense particles between endothelial cytofolds and paramesangial area. Focal splitting of the capillary basement membrane is also noted where the monocytes come in contact with the membrane. Immunofluorescence during the third week of the disease reveals dense deposits of IgM, IgG, and C3 in the glomeruli, mainly in mesangial areas, and occasionally along the capillary walls. However, the antigen has not been demonstrated.

Coxsackie Viruses

Coxsackie A1-24 and B1-6 are common viruses of the enterovirus family and spread mainly by the fecal–oral route. Most patients develop mild upper respiratory symptoms, but myositis and myocarditis may rarely be noted. Renal involvement is seen after infections with B-5 and A-4 strains. B-5 antigen has been isolated in exfoliated cells in the urine sediment. The usual manifestations are transient microhematuria and mild proteinuria without any permanent sequelae. A full-blown acute nephritic syndrome may be seen in children. A decline in renal function has been recorded in fatal cases. Histologic examination reveals focal or diffuse proliferative glomerulonephritis. The glomeruli are swollen and hypercellular and exhibit proliferation of endothelial and mesangial cells. Interstitial nephritis also may be noted. Electron microscopy shows focal widening of endothelial fenestrae, edema of lamina rara interna, and obliteration of podocytes. Immunofluorescence reveals Coxsackie B-4 antigen within the glomeruli and interstitium.

SPIROCHETES

Syphilis

Syphilis, caused by *Treponema pallidum,* used to be a common cause of nephrotic syndrome in developing countries. Because of the mass treatment campaigns, the infection has been eradicated from a large part of the world, although it still occurs in parts of Africa, Asia, and Oceania.

Nephropathy has been observed both in congenital and in acquired forms of the disease. In congenital syphilis, evidence of renal disease may be apparent at birth or may appear in the first few months of life. Two clinical forms have been recognized. The most common is nephrotic syndrome, but some patients present with an acute nephritic illness, with hematuria, oliguria, and varying degrees of renal dysfunction. Fewer than 60 cases of both forms of glomerulonephritis have been reported in the literature. In one report, urinary abnormalities were detected in 45% of patients with congenital syphilis. On histologic examination, the most common renal lesion is that of membranous nephropathy with mild mesangial proliferation. Endocapillary and extracapillary proliferative glomerulonephritis and membranoproliferative lesions with or without crescents have also been documented. Electron microscopy reveals subepithelial-dense deposits, and immunofluorescence shows IgG, C3, and C1q along the basement membrane. *Treponema* antigen has been identified in these deposits, and elution studies have yielded antitreponemal antibodies. Tubulointerstitial nephritis is often observed along with the glomerular lesions. The lesion is considered to be immune complex mediated, and circulating immune complexes have been demonstrated. Treatment with penicillin is followed by a prompt and complete disappearance of all abnormalities. In some cases, however, proteinuria may persist and may require repeated courses of penicillin. Immunologic studies show increased T-helper cells (CD4+) and low levels of T-suppressor cells. The T. *pallidum* hemagglutination titer is usually very high.

In acquired syphilis, nephropathy is seen in approximately 0.3% of all patients. Renal involvement becomes clinically manifest in the secondary phase of the disease but may also be seen during the latent phase. Rarely, glomerulonephritis may occur in association with syphilitic hepatitis. Nephrotic syndrome is the most common presentation, but microhematuria, azotemia, and hypertension may be observed rarely. The most common light microscopic abnormality is a membranous nephropathy, although mesangial, endocapillary proliferative, minimal-change disease, and crescentic glomerulonephritis have also been reported. The lesion differs from the usual membranous nephropathy in that distinctive segmental lesions are present at the tubular poles and the glomeruli exhibit mild mesangial cell proliferation. Electron microscopy shows subepithelial electron-dense deposits, which consist of IgG and C3 IgG on immunofluorescence. The treponemal antigen and antitreponemal antibody have been demonstrated in these deposits. Nephrotic syndrome and renal histologic abnormalities resolve after penicillin therapy, but some patients have entered spontaneous remission. Methylprednisolone and plasmapheresis produce a favorable response in rapidly progressive glomerulonephritis.

Glomerulopathy following syphilitic infection is presumed to be immune complex mediated. An increase in the levels of circulating immune complexes has been demonstrated both in humans and in animal models. There is a dramatic disappearance of circulating immune complexes after penicillin therapy.

LEPTOSPIROSIS

Leptospirosis is caused by infection with *Leptospira interrogans.* This disease is encountered worldwide but is seen more often in the tropics. Sporadic cases have also been reported. The organism gains access to humans through contact with the urine of infected animals (e.g., rats, wild mice, dogs, foxes) during occupational or recreational activities. In the tropics, an increase in *Leptospira* infection was noted during heavy rains.

The clinical manifestations may be mild to severe. The spectrum of the disease may vary from fever and an influenzalike syndrome to a fulminant illness with jaundice, meningitis, acute renal failure, and hemorrhagic diathesis (Weil disease). Leptospirosis may be associated with mesangioproliferative glomerulonephritis most likely mediated by immune complexes, interstitial nephritis, or acute renal failure resulting from acute tubular necrosis. Acute renal failure is more common in those with severe jaundice; it is nonoliguric in more than 50% of the cases, and it is associated with normokalemia or hypokalemia. Hydration and the use of furosemide have been found to be helpful in this setting. The outcome of the acute renal failure is usually favorable.

Leptospirosis responds to treatment with antibiotics. In mild cases, doxycycline (200 mg/day) given orally for 5 to 7 days is adequate. In severe cases, penicillin (1.5 million units every 6 hours) given for 7 days is preferred. The various renal lesions are reversible after treatment of the infection.

PARASITIC INFESTATIONS

Toxoplasmosis

Toxoplasma gondii is an intracellular parasite that specifically involves reticuloendothelial and nervous systems. Infection may be congenital or may develop later in life. Congenital toxoplasmosis may present with asymptomatic infection or severe disease with hydrocephalus, neonatal hypoglycemia, increased intracranial pressure, and visual impairment. In adults, the most common presentation is with infectious mononucleosislike illness, but immunocompromised patients may develop severe systemic involvement.

Renal involvement is rare, and only a few cases have been reported. Congenital toxoplasmosis generally presents with nephrotic syndrome, and renal biopsy shows a mesangial proliferative glomerulonephritis. *Toxoplasma* antigen and IgM can be demonstrated on immunofluorescence. Disappearance of the antigen has been documented in renal biopsy material after clinical remission. Renal involvement is equally rare in acquired toxoplasmosis. In one study, 150 consecutive renal biopsies were tested by immunofluorescence for reactivity with anti-*toxoplasma* conjugate, but only 1 was positive. Subsequent serologic evaluation revealed anti-*Toxoplasma* antibodies. The light microscopic picture is consistent with mesangiocapillary glomerulonephritis, and immunofluorescence shows IgG, IgA, IgM, C3, and fibrinogen along the glomerular capillary walls and in the mesangial region. Most patients present with nephrotic syndrome and moderate renal failure. The histologic abnormalities are known to reverse after treatment with pyrimethamine and sulphafurazole along with prednisolone.

Kala-Azar

Leishmaniasis is seen in various parts of the world in endemic, epidemic, or sporadic forms. The cutaneous form, caused by *L. tropica,* is seen mostly in the Middle East and Mediterranean regions, and the visceral from (caused by *L. donovani*) is reported mostly from India and East Africa. The usual features include prolonged fever, weight loss, anemia, and splenomegaly. Mild to moderate proteinuria and/or microscopic hematuria are observed in more than 50% of patients. Renal dysfunction, however, is exceptional. Renal histology reveals acute diffuse proliferative, mesangial proliferative, or membranous glomerulonephritis. The glomeruli are slightly enlarged with moderate increase in mesangial cellularity along with varying degrees of sclerosis. Basement membrane thickening has been seen in a few patients dying of this disease. Tubulointerstitial lesions and amyloid deposits in the glomeruli have also been reported. Electron microscopy shows paramesangial and subepithelial electron-dense deposits, as well as thickening and irregularities of lamina densa of the basement membrane. Experimental studies have documented similar lesions in dogs and hamsters infected with *Leishmania.* On immunofluorescence, immunoglobulin deposits are seen mainly in the mesangium. *Leishmania* antigen has been demonstrated in the glomeruli of hamsters infected with *L. donovani* but not in patients with kala-azar. The cause-and-effect relationship has not been proved beyond doubt, and it has been suggested that the renal lesions could be due to concomitant malnutrition and other infections. Indirect proof, however, comes from complete disappearance of urinary abnormalities after successful treatment of kala-azar.

Trypanosomiasis

Trypanosoma is a hemoflagellate parasite that is transmitted to humans through insects bites. Two forms of trypanosomiasis are known. The American form (Chagas' disease), seen in the southern United States and Latin American countries, is caused by *T. cruzei,* which is transmitted by the feces of reduviid bugs. Clinical manifestations may appear years to decades after the initial infection and consist of cardiac rhythm disturbances and gut dysmotility leading to megaesophagus and megacolon. The African form is caused by *T. brucei,* which is transmitted through bites of tsetse flies. The symptoms are mainly related to the nervous system (sleeping sickness). The disease is seen typically in the nonimmune tourists upon their return home after a brief sojourn to an endemic area. The association between either form of trypanosomiasis and a nephropathy has not been confirmed in humans. However, ample evidence is available from animal experiments that mice, especially those of the BALB/C variety, develop a moderate to severe proliferative or mesangiocapillary glomerulonephritis after infection with either *T. brucei* or *T. cruzei.* The lesions typically are seen 4 to 6 months after the infection. Immunoglobulin and complement deposits are observed in the mesangial, subendothelial, and subepithelial regions. Although the trypanosomal antigen has not been demonstrated in the deposits, specific antitrypanosoma antibodies have been found in the eluates. In addition, antibodies against glomerular basement membrane, laminin, and gp-330 have been demonstrated both in circulation and in glomerular eluates. It has been suggested that the immune complexes lead to molecular rearrangement of the basement membrane components after *in situ* binding.

NEMATODES

Filariasis and Related Infections

Filarial worms are nematodes that dwell in the subcutaneous tissues and lymphatics. Of the eight filarial species that infect humans, renal involvement has been reported with *Onchocerca volvulus, Wucheria bancrofti, Brugia malayi,* and *Loa loa* infections. These are transmitted to humans through arthropod bites and produce symptoms depending on the location of microfilariae and adult worms in the tissues. An association between filariasis and glomerular disease has been reported from India, Cameroon, and some other areas.

Loiasis is prevalent in west and central Africa and characteristically manifests with localized areas of allergic inflammation and Calabar swellings. Subconjunctival presence of adult worms may result in pain and intense lacrimation. Onchocerciasis (river blindness) is characterized by subcutaneous nodules, pruritic skin rash, sclerosing lymphadenitis, and ocular lesions. *Bancroftian* and *Brugia* infections cause febrile episodes associated with acute lymphangitis and lymphadenitis. In advanced cases, hydrocele and elephantiasis may be the predominant clinical manifestations. This form of filariasis is endemic in Africa and Southeast Asia.

The prevalence of renal involvement in loiasis is difficult to estimate. The clinical features suggesting glomerular disease include hematuria, proteinuria, and nephrotic syndrome. In one study, 25% patients were shown to have hematuria and 5% had nephrotic-range proteinuria. Renal function may occasionally be impaired. Renal histology reveals diffuse basement membrane thickening with a mild increase in the number of endocapillary cells. Other glomerular lesions, including mesangioproliferative, membranoproliferative, chronic sclerosing glomerulonephritis, and collapsing variant of focal segmental glomerulosclerosis, have also been reported. Mononuclear interstitial infiltration and microinfarcts around blood vessels have also been demonstrated. Microfilariae of *Loa loa* may be found in the glomerular capillary lumina. Electron microscopy shows widely spaced subepithelial or intramembranous deposits and spikes. Sheaths and cuticular ridges of *Loa loa* may also be seen. Although Loa antigen has not been demonstrated in the glomeruli, reactivity with hyperimmune anti-*Onchocerca* serum has been observed, raising the possibility of antigenic cross-reactivity.

The prevalence of proteinuria is 5.5 times greater in populations hyperendemic for onchocerciasis compared with control populations. In one population study, greater than 2+ Albustix proteinuria was demonstrated in 11% patients and nephrotic syndrome in 2.7% patients. A creatinine clearance of less than 65 ml/min was observed in 23% cases. Histologic examination shows a gamut of lesions, including mesangial proliferative, mesangiocapillary, minimal-change and, chronic sclerosing glomerulonephritis. Immunofluorescence reveals deposits of IgM, IgG, and IgA along with *O. volvulus* antigen. Microfilariae can be demonstrated in glomeruli, tubules, and interstitium. The natural history of glomerulonephritis is not known, but a transition from mild to more advanced disease has been shown.

The frequency of renal involvement in *W. bancrofti* and *B. malayi* infections (lymphatic filariasis) is not known. A significantly increased incidence of proteinuria has been noted in patients infected with *B. malayi* compared with control subjects. No difference has been observed in the incidence between asymptomatic patients and those with filarial fever or obstructive filariasis. Other presenting features include microscopic hematuria and hypertension. Renal histology shows mesangioproliferative, membranoproliferative, or diffuse proliferative forms of glomerulonephritis. There are large numbers of eosinophils among the infiltrating cells. A small number of crescents may also be noted. Immunofluorescence reveals immunoglobulin deposits in the mesangium and along the capillary walls. *B. malayi* antigen has been demonstrated in a few cases.

Pathogenesis

Glomerulonephritis associated with various forms of filariasis appears to the immune complex mediated. This is corroborated by the demonstration of immune complexes in the glomeruli and increased levels of IgG and IgM rheumatoid factors in the peripheral blood. Circulating immune complex levels are increased and correlate with the adult worm burden, and not with circulating microfilariae. Studies in dogs infected with *Dirofilaria immitis* have shown development of glomerular lesions similar to those seen in human filariasis. In one experimental study, where one renal artery was selectively catheterized and infused with *D. immitis* after immunization, glomerular lesions developed in the infused kidneys of all the eight animals. Milder lesions were noted in the contralateral kidneys in three dogs. This observation supports the hypothesis of *in situ* immune complex formation. In some cases, the administration of diethylcarbamazine (DEC) antedates the development of proteinuria, suggesting that the latter could be the result of immune response related to the release of antigens into circulation from the dead parasite.

Treatment

In patients with nonnephrotic proteinuria and/or hematuria, treatment with DEC results in complete resolution of renal manifestations. However, the response is inconsistent in those with nephrotic syndrome, and renal function deterioration may continue despite clearance of microfilariae with treatment.

Trichinosis

Trichinella spiralis and *paraspiralis* are the causative nematodes of human trichinosis. The clinical features are secondary to the successive phases of parasitic enteric invasion leading to abdominal pain and diarrhea. Larval migration may lead to hypersensitivity reactions and muscle encystment manifested by myalgias, muscle edema, and weakness involving the extraocular muscles, biceps, back, and diaphragm. Renal involvement is rare and can affect both glomerular and tubulointerstitial components. The glomerular involvement manifests as nonnephrotic-range proteinuria and microscopic hematuria. Hypertension and renal insufficiency have not been reported. C3 levels are low. Histology shows mesangial proliferative glomerulonephritis, and electron microscopy reveals electron-dense deposits in the paramesangial areas. On immunofluorescence, IgM is seen evenly distributed in mesangium and along the capillary walls, with IgA and IgG in weaker intensity. Pronounced deposits of C3 are seen along the arteriolar walls. The glomerular involvement is thought to be immune complex mediated, although a specific antigen has not been demonstrated in the involved glomeruli. Urinary abnormalities disappear within 2 weeks of successful treatment with thiabendazole. Acute renal failure may develop secondary to volume depletion and rhabdomyolysis.

FUNGAL INFECTIONS

Out of the large number of fungi that cause human disease, glomerulonephritis has been documented in association with only a few. About one-third of all patients with disseminated histoplasmosis exhibit urinary abnormalities, but histologic abnormalities have been shown in one patient only. Similarly, a mesangial proliferative glomerulonephritis has been documented in one patient with mucocutaneous candidiasis. The candidal antigen was demonstrated in the glomeruli, and the abnormalities improved with therapy. Given the rarity with which renal involvement has been noted, the etiologic relationship remains speculative.

Selected Readings

Beaufils M, Morel-Maroger L, Sraer JD, et al. Acute renal failure of glomerular origin during visceral abscesses. *N Engl J Med* 1976;295:185–189.
An extensive clinical and pathologic experience, comprehensively reviewed.

Chugh KS, Sakhuja V. Glomerular disease in the tropics. *Am J Nephrol* 1990; 10:437–450.
A comprehensive account of primary and secondary glomerular diseases in the tropics, emphasizing the differences between disease prevalent in the tropics and other geographic regions.

Haffner D, Schindera F, Aschoff A, et al. The clinical spectrum of shunt nephritis. *Nephrol Dial Transplant* 1997;12:1143–1148.
A comprehensive account of this rare entity.

Hunte W, al-Ghraoui F, Cohen RJ. Secondary syphilis and nephrotic syndrome. *J Am Soc Nephrol* 1993;3:1351–1355.
An excellent description of clinical and histologic characteristics of syphilitic nephropathy.

Neugarten J, Gallo GR, Baldwin DS. Glomerulonephritis in bacterial endocarditis. *Am J Kidney Dis* 1984;3:371–379.
A detailed review of glomerular lesions in infective endocarditis.

Ngu JL, Chatelanat F, Luke R, et al. Nephropathy in Cameroon: evidence for filarial derived immune complex pathogenesis in some cases. *Clin Nephrol* 1985; 24:128–134.
The first demonstration of filarial antigen in glomerulonephritis associated with filariasis.

Ponce P, Ramos A, Ferreira ML, et al. Renal involvement in leprosy. *Nephrol Dial Transplant* 1989;4:81–84.
Comprehensive review of renal abnormalities in patients with leprosy.

Schoenfeld MR, Edis GT. Trichinosis and glomerulonephritis. *Arch Pathol* 1967; 84:625–626.
The first description of glomerular involvement in trichinosis.

Sinniah R, Churg J, Sobin LH. *Renal disease: classification and atlas of infectious and tropical diseases.* Chicago: ASCP Press, 1988.
An invaluable pictorial collection of gross and histologic renal abnormalities seen in various infectious and tropical diseases.

PART 4
Minimal-Change Disease

Amir Tejani and Lea Emmett

The entity minimal-change disease (MCD) is not a glomerular disease but a histologic lesion that is noted in many patients with nephrotic syndrome. Prior multicenter studies have clearly identified the lesion as being the most common in young children who develop nephrotic syndrome. Because nephrotic syndrome with this lesion is predominantly seen in the pediatric population, most of our information regarding the clinical data and therapy is derived from pediatric renal literature. Because no registries are devoted to enrolling patients with nephrotic syndrome per se, it is difficult to determine the incidence either in children or in adults. However, the lesion of MCD is found to underlie nephrotic syndrome in about 80% of children and about 20% of adults undergoing renal biopsy for this indication. Nephrotic syndrome can be seen in various clinical settings. It can occur secondary to lupus nephritis, Henoch-Schönlein purpura, diabetic nephropathy, sickle cell disease, AIDS, hepatitis infection, and a host of other diseases. When nephrotic syndrome occurs as a primary renal disorder, a renal biopsy in a child is likely to reveal one of the following histologic lesions: MCD, IgM nephropathy, IgA nephropathy, membranoproliferative lesion, membranous nephropathy, or focal segmental glomerulosclerosis (FSGS). In the case of an adult patient with nephrotic syndrome, a biopsy is often required to determine whether the syndrome is caused by a primary glomerular disease.

DEFINITION AND CLINICAL FINDINGS

The definition was set in an era when other tools such as a renal biopsy were not available. In the present day context, a strict separation of nephrotic- and nonnephrotic-range proteinuria may not be meaningful. Protein excretion in excess of 3.5 g/day is considered in the nephrotic range for adults, and for children, the definition is proteinuria in excess of 40 mg/m^2 per hour (more than 1 g/m^2 per day). Collecting a 24-hour sample of urine in a small child is often difficult, and the definition simply uses a 10-fold increase (4 mg/m^2 per hour being normal excretion). Additional definitions often used in children are hypoalbuminemia less than 2.5 g/dl and hypercholesterolemia.

The hallmark of idiopathic nephrotic syndrome is edema. In a child, edema is usually the first symptom to be noticed, often following an upper respiratory tract infection. This edema is often explosive and generalized in contrast to the edema of glomerulonephritis, which is mostly seen as puffiness around the eyelids. The edema is pitting on pressure, and whereas in an adult patient it tends to localize in the limbs, in young children, the eyes and the abdominal wall bear the brunt. In addition, a large number of infants with nephrotic syndrome develop ascites as a result of fluid accumulation in the peritoneal cavity. Pleural fluid collections are rare but do occur in children. Pericardial fluid collection is unlikely to occur in uncomplicated nephrotic syndrome. In addition to the viral upper respiratory infection often preceding nephrotic syndrome, there is a higher incidence of allergic and atopic diathesis in children who develop MCD, and an association with HLA-B12 has also been demonstrated in children who develop the disease.

In MCD, hypertension is seen in 5% to 7% of the children but may be seen more often in adults. Gross hematuria is rare in all age groups, and its presence should lead to a reconsideration of the diagnosis of MCD. However, persistent microscopic hematuria occurs in up to 25% of patients. Elevation of serum urea nitrogen is commonly seen in both adults and children, but a rise in serum creatinine is seen in fewer than 5% of pediatric patients. Patients who are older than 45 years of age may present with acute renal failure resulting from a minimal change lesion. The mechanism is not well understood but is thought to be related to the development of intrarenal edema.

LABORATORY ABNORMALITIES

Urinalyses shows heavy proteinuria. Timed collections in children will show the nephrotic-range proteinuria to be in excess of 40 mg/m^2 per hour and more than 3.5 g/24 hr in adults. Serum albumin concentration is significantly diminished, and when associated with nephrotic-range proteinuria, the albumin level will be below 2.5 g/dl. In children, there is often marked hypoalbuminemia to levels as low as 1 g/dl. Serum calcium levels are also depressed, partly because of the lowering of protein-bound calcium and partly because of an actual decrease in the ionized portion. In most children, serum creatinine values will be normal or transiently decreased with MCD; however, one-third of adult patients may show a slight increase in serum creatinine at presentation. Severe depression of renal function may be seen in association with marked hypovolemia. Total cholesterol and triglyceride levels are elevated, and fractionation of the lipids will reveal elevation in low-density lipoprotein (LDL) and very-low-density lipoprotein (VLDL) fractions. The plasma volume of patients with MCD may be normal, elevated, or occasionally, decreased. In general, when there is massive proteinuria and marked depletion of the serum albumin level, the plasma volume tends to be low; however, even in MCD, the plasma volume can be elevated because of increased plasma aldosterone secretion, and the extent of the edema does not correlate to the degree of change in plasma volume. The primary concern is the exhibition of powerful loop diuretics in infants with a reduced plasma volume precipitating a vascular collapse. Other abnormalities in the serum consist of a decrease in plasma sodium concentration (pseudohyponatremia) as a result of the hyperlipidemia, and a rise in the hematocrit and the hemoglobin if the plasma volume is depleted. The platelet count and the sedimentation rate, as well as the plasma viscosity, are elevated. This, together with the rise in plasma fibrinogen, tends to promote thrombosis.

PATHOGENESIS

The tendency of nephrotic syndrome to manifest and relapse after viral infections or an allergic diathesis, the association with HLA antigens, and the therapeutic response to steroids and immunosuppressives such as cyclosporine suggest a possible immunologic role in its pathogenesis. Neither circulating nor *in situ* complexes have been consistently demonstrated in patients with nephrotic syndrome, but evidence of intrarenal T-cell infiltration has been shown. Lymphocyte-mediated immune mechanisms have been implicated in the genesis of nephrotic syndrome since Shalhoub's hypothesis in 1974, following which Oii observed a circulating factor designated as lymphocytotoxin in the blood of patients with nephrotic syndrome. Next, in 1975, Lagrue identified the presence of a lymphokine in the supernatant of serum of patients with nephrotic syndrome. In 1984, Schnaper identified a factor in the serum labeled soluble immune response suppressor. More recently, elevated levels of circulating cytokines have been observed in patients with both MCD and FSGS. In 1988, we observed that in patients with nephrotic syndrome (both MCD and FSGS), there was an increase in the interleukin-2 (IL-2) level in the supernatant obtained from patients after incubation with PHA, and patients with elevated levels showed a better response to cyclosporine. Because the half-life of IL-2 in the plasma is brief, studies have focused on the soluble receptor IL-2r, and a correlation of IL-2r with disease activity has been shown. Soluble IL-2r binds IL-2 effectively, and IL-2r is shed into the serum after lymphocyte stimulation. When activated, T cells not only produce IL-2 but also express IL-2r on their cell surface and release a soluble form of the receptor into the plasma. Human IL-2r is a glycoprotein composed of both an α and a β chain. The soluble form of IL-2r is about 45 kD and is similar to the α portion of the membrane-bound form. The elevation of circulating IL-2r levels is thought to indicate T-cell activation and has been shown to correlate with disease activity in systemic lupus erythematosus, rheumatoid arthritis, T-cell leukemia, and acute allograft rejection. The function of soluble IL-2r is not clear, but it is thought that by binding free IL-2, soluble IL-2r either down-regulates IL-2–dependent processes or prolongs the half-life of IL-2.

We have prospectively studied IL-2r in 70 children during active disease using an enzyme-linked immunosorbent assay. IL-2r levels were elevated in 32 of the 70 patients (range, 227 to 919 U/ml). Nonwhite patients had a higher mean IL-2r level of 1,042 $\pm$ 22 U/ml, compared with white patients who had a mean level of 737 $\pm$ 23 U/ml ($P = .034$). Repeat IL-2r levels measured in 14 patients after treatment with cyclosporine demonstrated a decrease in their IL-2r level from a mean of 1,583 $\pm$ 44 to a mean of 8,904 $\pm$ 36 U/ ml ($P = .002$). More interestingly, there was a significant decrease in the individual IL-2r levels in 13 of the 14 patients, and the only patient who did not show a drop in the level after cyclosporine administration had a relapse of the disease a week later.

Similar data of the rise of IL-2 levels with the onset of the disease and fall with cyclosporine-induced remission have been described. Others have shown that raised levels of circulating IL-2r are seen in patients with MCD in established relapse, as well as in focal segmental sclerosis. The mechanism of cytokine-induced injury is obscure. It has been suggested that IL-2 induces a vascular leak syndrome by altering the permselectivity of the glomerular basement membrane. In the animal model, injected recombinant IL-2 has been shown to reduce the number and density of anionic sites of the glomerular basement membrane, which is associated histologically with fusion of epithelial foot processes and massive proteinuria. In the rat model, administration of recombinant IL-2 induces proteinuria in a dose-dependant manner, and the administration of human IL-2 for cancer chemotherapy has led to the development of nephrotic-range proteinuria, which resolves after the treatment is discontinued. The studies presented so far indicate a role for IL-2 in the pathogenesis of nephrotic syndrome in patients with MCD but do not establish a role as an effector, suppressor, or mediator of the altered glomerular permeability. To assign a role to the cytokine IL-2 in the induction of proteinuria necessitates determining its presence in the renal parenchyma during an episode of relapse.

To ascertain whether IL-2 is present intrarenally, we studied renal biopsy tissue from children with a variety of histologic lesions, all of which manifest with nephrotic-range proteinuria. IL-2r mRNA was detected in 14 of 20 patients with FSGS, in 5 of 7 MCD patients, and in 5 of 7 IgM nephropathy patients. The presence of IL-2R mRNA in renal tissue of nephrotic patients with a variety of histologic lesions suggests that it may have a role in the pathogenesis of the disorder; however, it is more likely that its action in the proliferation and differentiation of T lymphocytes to release other cytokines and growth factors may be more relevant. IL-2 mRNA was not detected in any of the biopsy specimens. The role of the newly described protein nephrin, which is localized to the epithelial cell slit-pore membrane, remains to be elucidated.

Current postulates are that a cytokine-induced permeability factor or factors are involved in altering the charge-selective glomerular capillary barrier that normally prevents a protein leak. In patients with MCD as well as in patients with focal segmental sclerosis, such circulating permeability factors have been identified; however, the factors are not universally observed. The selective proteinuria, which in MCD consists mostly of albumin, leads to a marked reduction in the capillary oncotic pressure, setting up the edema that is so characteristic of this disease. The reduced plasma oncotic pressure from hypoalbuminemia induces increased hepatic lipoprotein production. The mechanisms that underlie the marked alterations seen in the lipid profile of patients with nephrotic syndrome have not been clearly elucidated, but a clear lowering of the plasma lipids occurs when hyperoncotic albumin is infused in nephrotic patients, suggesting that the drop in the colloid osmotic pressure is involved in the genesis of lipid abnormalities.

RENAL PATHOLOGY

There is a marked predilection for MCD to affect young children. The peak incidence is seen between the ages of 2 and 4 years. Whereas in the past it was assumed that the lesion is MCD in almost all children, in recent years, renal biopsy in children older than 12 years of age has shown the minimal-change lesion to be present in only a quarter of the population. Particularly in African-American adolescent children, the lesion is more likely to be focal segmental sclerosis. As noted previously, MCD is found in about 20% of adults undergoing renal biopsy of the evaluation of nephrotic syndrome.

Light Microscopy

The glomerular volume is normal in MCD, the capillary walls are thin, and the parietal epithelial cells are normal. Save for a mild increase in mesangial cell number, the glomerulus is essentially normal. Increased cellularity of the mesangium (more than three mesangial cells per high-power field) makes distinction from mesangial proliferative glomerulonephritis necessary because the prognosis of the latter condition is different from that of MCD. Mesangial proliferative lesions are usually associated with an increase in the mesangial matrix, whereas MCD will not exhibit matrix increase. The tubular architecture in MCD is normal as well, particularly in children, although in adult patients, occasional focal areas of tubular atrophy may be seen. The presence of tubular atrophy with interstitial fibrosis should raise the suspicion of a superimposed focal sclerotic lesion, particularly in the absence of juxtaglomerular region. Because focal sclerosis is a more severe lesion, the diagnosis to exclude it can be made only with an adequate sample and fewer than 10 glomeruli in the sample should give pause to the clinician.

Electron Microscopy

Unlike the paucity of changes seen in light microscopy, electron microscopy will consistently reveal abnormalities of the visceral epithelial cells of all or most of the glomerular capillaries. Effacement of the foot processes of the podocytes and obliteration of the slit–pore membrane complex in varying degrees is seen in all nephrotic patients and is more striking when the proteinuria is massive. Occasionally, epithelial cell vacuolization and detachment from the underlying basement membrane may also be seen, but a collapse of the basement membrane is rare and should raise the suspicion of focal sclerosis. Some pathologists have suggested that ultrastructural lesions such as glomerular enlargement, diffuse epithelial cell vacuolization, and capillary wall collapse are sufficient to make the diagnosis of focal sclerosis even in the absence of light microscopic evidence of focal sclerotic glomeruli.

Immunofluorescence

Most of our knowledge on the renal morphology in childhood nephrotic syndrome is based on studies by the International Study of Kidney Disease in Children (ISKDC), which evaluated light and electron microscopic data. Unfortunately, the study did not include immunofluorescence data, and the presence of immune deposits in a MCD renal biopsy is controversial. In most uncomplicated MCD biopsies, there is absence of immunoglobulin and complement deposition. However, several investigators have described diffuse mesangial deposits of IgM and corresponding electron-dense deposits in the mesangium and the paramesangial areas. This entity has been called *IgM nephropathy,* and whereas some investigators consider the presence of these deposits to be an epiphenomenon, others have considered them to be nephritogenic. Whether IgM nephropathy is a distinct entity is irrelevant, what is germane is the response of these patients to corticosteroid therapy, and the outcome of patients with IgM deposits appears to not be as benign as that seen in MCD, particularly when mesangial cells hypercellularity is present. There is also a transition from benign disease such as MCD to a severe form of disease such as focal segmental sclerosis, with IgM nephropathy being an intermediate stage as discussed in the following section.

Morphologic Transition in Minimal-Change Disease

From the foregoing discussion of the renal pathology in MCD it becomes obvious that the diagnosis of the lesion is one of exclusion. In children, both IgM nephropathy and focal segmental sclerosis may mimic the clinical and early histologic picture, whereas in adult patients, the early light microscopic picture and the clinical findings resemble focal sclerosis or membranous nephropathy. It is therefore necessary to obtain both immunofluorescence and electron microscopic confirmation before making a definitive diagnosis. The problem is more acute in children because many pediatric renal centers will not perform a renal biopsy in children up to 12 or 14 years of age, presuming the diagnosis to be MCD, initiating a course of corticosteroid therapy, and resorting to a renal biopsy only if the patient is nonresponsive. MCD has an excellent prognosis, but whether the lesion remains unaltered in patients who become frequent relapsers is another controversial area. As discussed in the section on therapy, frequent relapse is defined as two or more relapses in a given 6-month period, and there is sparse information regarding the persistence of MCD in these patients. The initial description of morphologic transition in MCD was described by McGovern in 1964, who noted that of his 39 patients, 9 showed focal segmental sclerosis on repeat biopsy. Since then, numerous authors have drawn attention to this phenomenon, both in adults and children. On the other hand, pediatric nephrologists dealing with a homogenous population have shown that the outcome of Caucasian children diagnosed as having MCD remains excellent despite numerous relapses because their lesion presumably continues to be minimal change.

Over a number of years, we have adopted a policy of performing a repeat biopsy in all children with a frequently relapsing course. In a previous study, we noted that of 33 children who underwent a repeat biopsy, 45% converted to focal segmental sclerosis from the original diagnosis of MCD and 27% converted to the diagnosis of IgM nephropathy from their original diagnosis of MCD. In nine children, the lesion remained the same; however, on a third biopsy, five of these nine patients showed focal segmental sclerosis, and one exhibited IgM nephropathy. We have evaluated more than 50 children with repeat biopsies. Again, we have noted that of 25 children who initially were diagnosed as MCD, the lesion evolved into IgM nephropathy in 7 patients and into focal sclerosis in 14 patients. There were 12 patients whose initial biopsy diagnosis was IgM nephropathy; of these, 50% exhibited focal segmental sclerosis on the repeat biopsy. The patient population studied in both instances was mixed, with non-Caucasian children forming a majority. These observations lead us to think that the three histologic lesions commonly found in pediatric patients with idiopathic nephrotic syndrome may constitute a single disease entity rather than an expression of heterogeneity of pathogenesis. Our speculation cannot be further advanced without additional knowledge of etiology and pathogenesis; however, we believe that with the armamentarium of drugs available for the treatment of frequent relapsers, a judicious choice would be to tailor therapy to the lesion and that continuing to administer corticosteroids to all patients with frequent relapses without confirmation of the histology may not be in the best interest of the patient.

COURSE AND THERAPY

MCD is exquisitely sensitive to glucocorticoid therapy; however, despite the sensitivity, the pattern is one of relapses and remissions. Presumably spontaneous remissions of this disorder do occur, although the frequency of spontaneous remissions, particularly in children, is impossible to judge because all children are treated and rarely is steroid therapy intentionally withheld from an adult patient. In the preglucocorticoid era, spontaneous remissions eventually occurred in as many as 30-% to 40% of patients. Anecdotal reports of a remission following an attack of measles in a child are often quoted; however, measles vaccination has failed to induce a remission.

Because the disorder is most commonly observed in very young children, a waxing and waning course with relapses and remissions can be seen for several years. Relapses tend to diminish and occasionally disappear after puberty, although a relapse can be noted even after 10 years of freedom from disease. The overall prognosis is extremely favorable in Caucasian children, with fewer than 5% of children who are steroid sensitive developing end-stage renal disease. The prognosis in not so sanguine in the frequently relapsing group, particularly among African-American and Hispanic children, in whom the lesion begins as minimal change and over the course of time converts into a more ominous lesion of focal segmental sclerosis. Because MCD comprises only about 20% of all the adult patients with nephrotic syndrome, it is extremely difficult to ascertain the long-term prognosis in adult patients; those who respond early to steroid therapy and remain in remission would obviously have an excellent prognosis. Adult patients who develop acute renal failure in the course of their disease have poorer prognoses. Prolonged oliguria may be present.

The dosing scheme for glucocorticoids therapy is not standardized. Different regimens are required for optimal results in adults and children. Many pediatric nephrology centers follow the ISKDC regimen for the initial episode of the nephrotic syndrome in children. Prednisone 60 mg/m^2 (not to exceed 80 mg/day) is given in one or two divided doses daily. This dose is maintained for 4 weeks irrespective of response. At the end of 4 weeks, the dose is reduced to 40 mg/m^2 given every other day and continued for 4 more weeks, at the end of which steroid therapy is abruptly discontinued.

When treated in this format, the following responses at 8 weeks and beyond may be seen in a pediatric patient:

1. *Primary response* wherein the patient has complete remission of the proteinuria and remains in lasting remission after a single course of therapy. Approximately 10% to 20% of pediatric patients will be fortunate enough to fall into this category.
2. *Infrequent relapser* wherein the patient has a remission but develops a relapse separated by more than 6 months and sometimes years. About 40% of the pediatric patients will fall into this category.
3. *Frequent relapser* wherein the patient has a remission and develops two or more relapses in the ensuing 6 months or four or more relapses in the ensuing 12 months. Most pediatric patients will fall into this category. This is the controversial group because many nephrologists believe that these patients have an excellent prognosis and should continue to be treated with steroid therapy, whereas others believe that these are the patients who may undergo a morphologic transition and should have a renal biopsy before further treatment.
4. *Primary nonresponder* wherein the patient does not respond to the initial course of steroid therapy. This group makes up 5% to 7% of the pediatric patients, and almost all centers would perform a renal biopsy to determine the lesion. In some instances, there is an initial biopsy before starting therapy and the question arises whether the original diagnosis could be a sampling error. Because other effective drugs are now available, most pediatric nephrologists would not push further steroid therapy in either higher dosage or for prolonged periods in patients who fail to respond to the initial course of steroids.

Thus 90% to 95% of children with MCD will develop a complete remission of proteinuria within 8 weeks of commencing glucocorticoid therapy. On the other hand, adults with MCD respond more slowly and less completely to glucocorticoid therapy compared with children. Using dosing schedules (60 to 80 mg/day or 1 mg/kg per day of prednisone), only about 50% of adult patients will experience a complete remission by 8 weeks, but this increases to about 80% to 85% after 20 to 24 weeks of therapy. Many adult nephrologists would consider an adult patient to be more responsive only after 16 to 20 weeks of daily or alternate-day glucocorticoid therapy. Following a complete remission, relapses occur less often in adults than in children.

Prognostic Signs of Glucocorticoid Responsiveness

In MCD, the proteinuria consists of low-molecular-weight proteins such as serum albumin and transferrin, with large protein molecules such as IgG and IgM less frequently seen. It has been suggested that measuring the selectivity of the proteinuria by using the ratio of observed clearances of IgG and transferrin can help determine response to steroid therapy. The greater the selectivity of the proteinuria, the better the potential for steroid response. Additional information regarding steroid response can be obtained from the biopsy. In patients with large glomeruli, in patients with mesangial and paramesangial deposits, and in patients with any degree of loss of tubular architecture, the response to steroid therapy is likely to be less than optimal. When steroids are used for treatment, the proteinuria in most children will respond within 4 weeks, and those whose response is delayed into the second month of therapy will often become frequent relapsers. Also ominous is the inability of the initial remission to last longer than 6 months. Children who develop their first relapse within fewer than 6 months after discontinuation of steroid therapy are invariably destined to become frequent relapsers.

Treatment of Relapses

A relapse is considered to have occurred when proteinuria reappears in the urine. The patient does not necessarily become edematous and nephrotic at the onset of a relapse, but an untreated relapse will eventually render the patient edematous. Most pediatric nephrologists will consider the presence of 2+ protein in the urine for three consecutive examinations as evidence of relapse and reinitiate steroid therapy. The ISKDC regimen recommends reinitiating steroids at 60 mg/m^2 daily until the proteinuria disappears, at which time the dosage should be reduced to 40 mg/m^2 and administered every other day for a total of 8 weeks. This is designed to minimize the exposure to steroids; however, some centers would administer steroids for a relapse at the same dosage and schedule as that used for the initial episode.

Steroid-Dependent Patients

In the group designated as frequent relapsers, there is a subset of patients who will relapse immediately or very soon after a course of steroid therapy or during the tapering phase of treatment. Such patients need continuous steroid therapy. A good regimen in patients whose lesion continues to be minimal change would be to give an 8-week course of therapy at the end of which, rather than to withdraw the steroids completely, a slow taper is used over another 4 weeks to the lowest alternate-day dose that keeps the patient free of proteinuria. This approach should not be taken lightly because in many instances, the mother, who is taught to check the urine daily, will increase the steroid dosage on her own upon observing proteinuria. Covert steroid toxicity such as posterior subcapsular cataracts and osteoporotic lesions can be easily missed in such steroid-dependent patients. It is our policy not to continue to administer steroids to patients who are steroid dependent, but instead to use other drug therapy that would provide respite from continuous steroid use. In all patients who are treated with repeated courses of steroids or who are steroid dependent, there is always the potential for the physical disabilities manifested by acne, moon facies, and growth retardation. In addition, the clinician must be alert for the development of peptic ulceration, aseptic necrosis of the femoral head, and other osteoporotic lesions.

Alternative Therapy for Frequent Relapses and Steroid-Dependent Patients

The use of alkylating agents such as cyclophosphamide and chlorambucil has been effective in these patients. The dosage for cyclophosphamide is 3 mg/kg per day administered daily for 60 days, and many centers will use the drug together with 5 or 10 mg of prednisone daily. The rationale for a 60-day cutoff is to avoid the gonadal toxicity of the drug, which is likely to occur at cumulative doses exceeding 300 mg/kg for females and 500 mg/kg for males. A 60-day course of therapy will have the cumulative dose of 180 mg/kg. The concomitant use of a small amount of prednisone is to prevent the myelosuppression usually associated with the use of cyclophosphamide. Chlorambucil is used at the dosage of 0.15 to 0.2 mg/kg per day for 60 days. A major advantage of both these drugs is that patients will respond, and about 60% to 75% will remain in remission for at least a year. Dosages for adults are similar, and a 12-week course of cyclophosphamide has been shown to provide better results. There is no superiority of chlorambucil over cyclophosphamide—both seem to work equally well; however, there seems to more familiarity with cyclophosphamide in the United States and a greater use of chlorambucil in Europe. The gonadal toxicity and the myelotoxicity of both drugs is similar, although chlorambucil has a greater tendency to induce seizures in children. A common concern with both drugs is loss of hair, which is dose related but tends to stop with drug discontinuation. Hemorrhagic cystitis is not commonly seen at the recommended dosages, particularly if the patient is well hydrated. Second courses of cyclophosphamide when a patient relapses after the initial course tend to produce a similar remission; however, the long-term oncogenic potential of these drugs together with the gonadal toxicity makes their use hazardous beyond a single course of therapy, and this is now unnecessary because cyclosporine can be used for such patients.

Therapy For Steroid-Nonresponsive Patients and for Those Who Relapse After a Course of Alkylating Agents

Studies have shown the futility of using cyclophosphamide or chlorambucil for patients who are not responsive to the initial course of steroid therapy. Cyclosporine, a fungal decapeptide, is a calcineurin inhibitor first used in the treatment of steroid-nonresponsive patients in 1985. Since then, considerable literature has developed regarding its efficacy in such patients, whether the lesion is minimal change or focal segmental sclerosis. Controlled trials in both adults and children have demonstrated that the drug is more effective in inducing a remission in children than in adults. The mechanism of action of cyclosporine in inducing a remission of nephrotic syndrome is postulated to be an alteration in the permeability of the filtration barrier, although this will remain unelucidated until the pathogenesis of the disease is established.

Cyclosporine therapy is initiated at 5 to 6 mg/kg per day in pediatric patients; somewhat lower dosages (4 to 5 mg/kg per day) may be adequate in adult patients. There is no magic to this dosage; it is simply an extrapolation of the maintenance dose of cyclosporine used in solid organ transplantation. Higher dosages may be required at initiation in patients who exhibit very high levels of serum cholesterol (greater than 400 mg/dl). A response to cyclosporine therapy is slow in most cases, requiring 4 to 6 weeks before the proteinuria begins to diminish. The drug is much more effective in patients who are steroid responsive frequent relapsers. Almost all such patients will undergo a remission within 8 weeks, at which time the dosage can be reduced to 4 mg/kg per day. After 4 more weeks of therapy, the dosage can be further reduced to 3 mg/kg per day, held there for 2 more weeks, and then reduced to 2 mg/kg per day. It has been our observation that more than 60% of the patients will require a 2-mg/kg maintenance dose for an additional 4 months. Discontinuation of the 2-mg/kg dose earlier will result in a relapse, which will necessitate higher dosages. About 30% of the patients can discontinue the 2-mg/kg dose after a month of therapy and remain in a remission for at least a year. It is difficult to determine which patients will tolerate early drug withdrawal, but in general, Caucasian patients and younger children fall into this category. Failure to respond to cyclosporine after 4 consecutive months of therapy at dosages of 5 to 6 mg/kg per day should dictate a discontinuation of the drug.

The management of steroid-nonresponsive MCD patients with cyclosporine is similar to that used for steroid-resistant focal segmental glomerulosclerosis, although some believe that it is easier to induce a remission in MCD patients then in FSGS patients. It is our observation that the lesion of MCD in steroid-resistant patients evolves into FSGS, so we treat them in the same manner. A major distinction between children and adults is that benign neglect or symptomatic therapy is extremely difficult to practice in children, so strenuous efforts are often made to obtain a remission. The mode of therapy described is not for the fainthearted, but diligently pursued, it will induce a remission in at least 60% to 70% of steroid-resistant patients. Similar responses have occurred in adult patients with MCD, but information on this issue is limited because of the lower frequency of MCD in adults.

Therapy for Steroid-Resistant Nephrotic Syndrome with Intractable Edema

This management can be carried out only in an inpatient setting. Simultaneous attempts to induce a diuresis are made by using pulse methylprednisolone, albumin infusions, intravenous furosemide, and high-dose cyclosporine therapy. Methylprednisolone is administered in bolus doses of 100 mg twice daily, and albumin infusion of 0.5 g/kg of salt-poor albumin is given twice daily, followed by intravenous furosemide 3 to 5 mg/kg (not to exceed 100 mg/dose) twice daily. Cyclosporine is started at 10 mg/kg per day, and in the presence of severe hypercholesterolemia, the cyclosporine dosage is increased by 2 mg/kg every 4 days. A diuresis with reduction in the edema and proteinuria is usually observed within 7 to 10 days of therapy. If no response is observed within 2 weeks of therapy, the administration of high-dose cyclosporine is abandoned. During this regimen, a very close watch on the serum electrolytes must be maintained. Patients are likely to develop hypokalemia and metabolic alkalosis, and the use of a potassium-sparing diuretic, such as amiloride 2.5 to 5 mg twice daily, may be necessary. With the high-dose cyclosporine therapy, there will be a rise in serum creatinine, which may not be acceptable and may require abandonment of cyclosporine therapy. Generally, the rise in serum creatinine is not greater than 0.4 mg/dl in most children; elevations greater than 0.6 or 0.7 mg/dl will necessitate lowering the cyclosporine dosage. The elevation in serum creatinine will diminish as the cyclosporine dosage is reduced. This should be done as the proteinuria diminishes.

Duration of Therapy

Steroid-resistant patients who respond to cyclosporine will require prolonged therapy with this drug. In children, we generally use maintenance doses of 7 of 8 mg/kg per day for up to 6 months together with 10 to 20 mg of prednisone daily, depending on the weight of the child. The cyclosporine dosage should be reduced to 5 to 6 mg/kg per day in the second 6 months of therapy. The duration of cyclosporine therapy in these refractory patients has to be individualized, but with careful observation and dosage titration, we have maintained remissions (proteinuria of less than 500 mg/day) with long-term cyclosporine therapy in many such patients. These dosages may not be tolerated in adults in whom the maintenance dose is 4 to 5 mg/kg per day combined with 10 to 20 mg of prednisone daily. However, all patients who receive cyclosporine for more than 12 months are at risk for long-term nephrotoxicity, and renal biopsy may be considered every 12 to 18 months to look for tubular atrophy and interstitial stripe fibrosis, which would require discontinuation of the drug.

Selected Readings

Baqi N, Singh A, Balachandra S, et al. The paucity of minimal change disease in adolescents with primary nephrotic syndrome. *Pediatr Nephrol* 1998;12:105–107.

Demonstrates that beyond the childhood years (1 to 11), the frequency of MCD is significantly reduced.

Hulton SA, Shah V, Byrne MR, et al. Lymphocyte subpopulations, interleukin-2 and interleukin-2 receptor expression in childhood nephrotic syndrome. *Pediatr Nephrol* 1994;8:135–139.

Establishes the role of IL-2r in MCD pathogenesis by measuring it in patients and controls.

Ingulli E, Harmon WE, Arbus GS, et al. Alterations in interleukins during the active phase of idiopathic nephrotic syndrome [Abstract]. *Pediatr Res* 1993; 33:358A.

Measures IL-2r levels in the largest number of nephrotic patients during relapse and remission. Correlates the rise and fall of IL-2r levels with specific immunosuppressive therapy.

Ingulli E, Tejani A. Severe hypercholesterolemia inhibits cyclosporin efficacy in a dose dependent manner in children with nephrotic syndrome. *J Am Soc Nephrol* 1992;3:254–259.

Cyclosporine enters the cell via receptor-mediated endocytosis. The receptor is downregulated in the presence of high serum cholesterol levels, which are always seen in patients with nephrotic syndrome. This study provides evidence of inhibition of cyclosporine efficacy in the face of hypercholesterolemia and suggests a novel method to overcome this inhibition.

Lagrue G, Branellec A, Blac C. A vascular permeability factor in lymphocyte culture supernatants from patients with nephrotic syndrome. Pharmacological and physiochemical properties. *Biomedicine* 1975;23:73–75.

Demonstrates for the first time the presence of a factor in the supernatant of serum of nephrotic patients. This factor is shown to alter glomerular capillary permeability.

Oii BS, Orlina AR, Masmitis L. Lymphocytotoxins in primary renal disease. *Lancet* 1974;ii:1348–1350.

Extends the hypothesis of T-cell dysfunction by observing the role of lymphocytotoxins, a precursor of cytokines in the pathogenesis of nephrotic syndrome.

Schnaper HW, Pierce CW, Aune RM. Identification and initial characterization of concanavalin-A and interferon-induced human suppressor factors: evidence for a human equivalent of murine soluble immune response suppressor (SIRS). *J Immunol* 1984;132:2429–2435.

Identifies a suppressor factor in the serum of nephrotic patients. The authors claim that this factor suppresses the immune response of the patient, thereby leading to the induction of the nephrotic state.

Shalhoub RJ. Pathogenesis of lipoid nephrosis: a disorder of T-cell function. *Lancet* 1974;ii:556–559.

Provides the first enunciated hypothesis of the pathogenesis of nephrotic syndrome.

Tejani A. Morphological transition in minimal change nephrotic syndrome. *Nephron* 1985;39:157–159.

With the use of repeat renal biopsies, all performed percutaneously, shows that MCD in frequently relapsing patients is not a static lesion but a progressive disorder.

Tejani A, Butt KMH, Trachtman H, et al. Cyclosporine induced remission of childhood nephrotic syndrome. *Kidney Int* 1988;33:729–734.

Measures T-cell growth factors and cytokines in the serum of patients with nephrotic syndrome and demonstrates the role of IL-2 in the genesis of childhood nephrotic syndrome that is refractory to corticosteroid therapy.

Tejani A, Strehlau J, Pavalakis M, et al. IL-4, IL-2, IL-2r expression in renal biopsy tissue in children with nephrotic syndrome [Abstract]. *J Am Soc Nephrol* 1996; 7:1782.

This is a pivotal study, which for the first time, measures various cytokines in the renal biopsy tissue of patients with nephrotic syndrome, and by using reverse transcription polymerase chain reaction, quantitates the actual cytokine levels.

Tejani A, Tejani C, Adamson O, et al. Efficacy of cyclophosphamide (CY) in steroid-responsive relapsing nephrotic syndrome of children with different morphological lesions. *Nephron* 1985;41:170–173.

Demonstrates the lack of efficacy of cyclophosphamide in the treatment of steroid-responsive relapsing nephrotic syndrome patients in whom the histologic lesion has evolved into FSGS.

PART 5
Focal and Segmental Glomerulosclerosis

Stephen M. Korbet

Primary focal segmental glomerulosclerosis (FSGS) is a clinicopathologic entity defined by the presence of proteinuria, commonly nephrotic in range, and by segmental glomerular scars involving some glomeruli. First described by Rich in 1957, FSGS is distinguished clinically from minimal-change disease (MCD) by hematuria, hypertension, and renal insufficiency at presentation;

TABLE 39.18. Classification of Focal Segmental Glomerulosclerosis (FSGS)

I. Primary (Idiopathic) FSGS
II. Secondary FSGS
  A. Secondary to reduced nephron mass/glomerular adaptations
    1. Reflux nephropathy
    2. Renal dysplasia
    3. Oligomeganephronia
    4. Morbid obesity
    5. Sickle cell disease
    6. Primary glomerular diseases
  B. Secondary to hereditary nephropathies
  C. Secondary to focal proliferative glomerulonephritis
  D. HIV-associated nephropathy
  E. Heroin-associated FSGS
III. Super-imposed on another primary glomerular disease (e.g., membranous glomerulonephritis)

FSGS, focal segmental glomerulosclerosis.

TABLE 39.19. Prevalence of Glomerular Lesions in Nephrotic Adults

	African-American	White
MCD	10%	20%
FSGS	65%	20%
MGN	20%	40%
MPGN	2%	5%
Other	3%	15%

FSGS, focal segmental glomerulosclerosis; MCD, minimal-change disease; MGN, membranous glomerulonephritis; MPGN, membranoproliferative glomerulonephritis; Others, IgA nephropathy, fibrulary GN, crescentic GN, amyloidosis.

by significantly poorer response to steroid therapy; and by progression to uremia. A lesion morphologically similar to FSGS occurs in a number of clinical settings (Table 39.18), with a presentation indistinguishable from primary FSGS. Because the pathogenesis and treatment of these disorders may differ significantly, secondary conditions associated with FSGS must be excluded before making the diagnosis of primary FSGS.

Primary FSGS accounts for 7% to 20% of glomerular lesions in children and adults presenting with proteinuria, most often the nephrotic syndrome. Recently it has been recognized that the prevalence of primary FSGS in black patients is 2 to 4 times that in white patients, accounting for 65% of cases as compared with 20% of cases, respectively (Table 39.19). Over the last 20 years, a marked increase in the incidence of this lesion has been observed. From 1974 to 1993, the yearly incidence of primary FSGS has risen by twofold to threefold from 10% to 25%. This has been attributed, in part, to an increase in the identification of histologic "variants" of FSGS.

PATHOLOGY

Because of the focal nature of FSGS, the biopsy sample size becomes critical in diagnosing this glomerular lesion. If the prevalence of segmentally scarred glomeruli is 10%, there is a 35% probability that *no* abnormal glomeruli will be found in a biopsy sample that contains only 10 glomeruli, resulting in the misdiagnosis of minimal-change disease. The probability of missing the glomerular lesion drops to 12% or less when 20 or more glomeruli are present in the biopsy sample. Furthermore, because the lesion initially affects the juxtamedullary glomeruli, it is important that a deep enough sample (corticomedullary junction) be obtained. (For further discussion, see Chapter 109.)

Light Microscopy

The histologic diagnosis of focal segmental glomerulosclerosis requires the presence of scarring in a portion (segment) of some (focal) glomeruli. The glomeruli in FSGS (primary or secondary) are hypertrophic as compared with glomeruli of normal patients or those with minimal-change disease, and this may be of pathophysiologic importance. The scar comprises collapsed glomerular capillaries, adhesions between the tuft and Bowman's capsule, and hyaline deposits. Uninvolved areas of the glomerulus are otherwise normal in appearance. The glomerular scarring in primary FSGS may be accompanied by other features such as segmental or global mesangial hypercellularity (which may be diffuse in some cases), endocapillary foam cells, and tubulointerstitial disease.

In addition to segmental glomerular scars, other morphologic features or variants have been included under the diagnosis of primary FSGS. The most recent lesions to attract interest are those involving segmental or global collapse of glomerular capillaries. The areas of collapse contain foam cells and are associated with hypertrophy and hyperplasia of the surrounding glomerular epithelial cells (GEC). This finding has been referred to as the *cellular lesion* of FSGS. When the cellular lesion is confined to the take-off of the proximal tubule, it has been called the *tip lesion*. The pathogenetic significance of the cellular lesion is controversial but we believe that it represents an early, active stage of FSGS that heals to form a segmental scar. Others interpret this finding as a discrete entity with different prognostic and therapeutic implications from classic FSGS and call it *collapsing glomerulopathy*.

The best evidence supporting the pathogenetic evolution from the cellular lesion to glomerular scarring is seen in serial biopsies from allograft recipients who develop recurrent FSGS in which the early onset of massive proteinuria is seen with minimal light microscopic signs of glomerular disease and with ultrastructural pathology limited to foot-process effacement. With time, cellular lesions develop, and segmental scars are seen even later in the course.

Immunofluorescence Microscopy

Immunofluorescence microscopy may be negative. However, some glomeruli may demonstrate segmental deposits of IgM and C3 in the areas of scarring. The significance of these findings is unknown and may merely represent trapping of immunoglobulins and complement in the damaged areas.

Electron Microscopy

Ultrastructural features of primary FSGS mirror those seen by light and immunofluorescence microscopy with capillary collapse, mesangial expansion and hypercellularity, and occasional mesangial electron-dense deposits. Glomerular epithelial foot-process effacement is usually widespread or diffuse but may occasionally be focal, especially in those cases with nonnephrotic proteinuria and in secondary forms of FSGS. In scarred portions of the glomerulus, the glomerular epithelial cell is often separated from the basal lamina by multiple thin layers of basement membranelike material, suggesting an attempt at repair.

PATHOGENESIS

Primary Focal Segmental Glomerulosclerosis

The pathogenesis of primary FSGS, like MCD, is unknown but may be the result of a T-cell mediated disorder that results in the production of a circulating "permeability factor(s)," possibly a lymphokine or cytokine. The permeability factor leads to visceral GEC injury, altering charge and function, and resulting in proteinuria and hypoalbuminemia. Alterations in intraglomerular hemodynamics, due in part to a decrease in oncotic pressure from hypoalbuminemia, result in an increase in transcapillary hydrostatic pressure and hyperfiltration. These hemodynamic changes along with the primary GEC injury lead to the subsequent formation of segmental scars, and ultimately glomerular obsolescence.

Trafficking of macromolecules through the mesangium and reabsorption of filtered proteins by the tubules may also result in the activation of cytokines such as transforming growth factor-β (TGF-β), which stimulate cell proliferation and matrix synthesis. TGF-β increases matrix synthesis by interstitial fibroblasts, and decreases matrix degradation by downregulating the production of matrix degradation proteins, and promoting the generation of proteinase inhibitors. This results in increased interstitial fibrosis and further reduction in nephron mass. The reduction in nephron mass results in further alterations in intraglomerular hemodynamics, which contribute to progressive renal disease.

Evidence for the presence of a circulating permeability factor in FSGS comes from transplant patients with recurrent FSGS. A 50- to 100-kD molecule has been isolated from these patients' serum, which leads to increased glomerular permeability *in vitro*. Furthermore, removal of this factor by plasmapheresis or immunoadsorption has lead to both clinical and histologic remission. The pathogenesis of primary FSGS in nephrotic patients may well differ because some patients are clearly steroid-sensitive with stable renal function and others are steroid-resistant progressing to end-stage renal disease (ESRD). Furthermore, not all patients with primary FSGS are nephrotic. Nonnephrotic patients with FSGS have a more indolent course, progressing to ESRD rarely and only after 10 to 15 years, most often associated with poorly controlled hypertension. Thus in these patients hypertensive or hyperfiltration injury rather than a circulating factor may be the primary mode of injury.

Secondary Focal Segmental Glomerulosclerosis

The etiology of segmental sclerosis in secondary forms of FSGS varies and depends on the underlying condition (Table 39.18). Glomerular epithelial cell injury is thought to be the primary mechanism for FSGS in heroin-associated nephropathy and HIV-associated nephropathy (due to viral infection of GEC with HIV). In segmental necrotizing or proliferative forms of glomerulonephritis, such as microscopic polyarteritis or IgA nephropathy, segmental scars may be a result of the healing process. Obesity and conditions associated with a reduced nephron mass (Table 39.18) lead to FSGS as a result of functional adaptations in the glomeruli, leading to intraglomerular and hyperfiltration hypertension associated with glomerular hypertrophy. In addition, as in primary FSGS, promoters of glomerular growth such as angiotensin II, platelet-derived growth factor, insulinlike growth factor, TGF-β, and tumor necrosis factor are felt to be important in the progression of renal disease in secondary forms of FSGS.

CLINICAL PRESENTATION

The presenting feature in all patients with primary FSGS is proteinuria, often resulting in the nephrotic syndrome; however, a nonnephrotic presentation (proteinuria less than 3.0 g/24 hr without hypoalbuminemia) is not unusual, particularly in adults (Table 39.20). In addition, microscopic hematuria, hypertension, and renal insufficiency are common presenting features. Although some have found adults with FSGS are more likely than children to have hypertension and renal insufficiency at presentation, others report the occurrence of hematuria, hypertension, and level of renal function do not significantly differ between these two groups. However, adults do present with the nephrotic syndrome less frequently than children. The clinical presentation of patients with nonnephrotic FSGS is remarkably similar to that of nephrotic patients with the exception that African-American patients are more often nephrotic (Table 39.21).

In secondary forms of FSGS, patients are less often hypoalbuminemic as compared with patients with primary FSGS, despite having the same level of massive proteinuria and similar levels of renal function. This is commonly seen in conditions associated with secondary FSGS that result from hyperfiltration such as obesity, reflux nephropathy, and reduced nephron mass. It is speculated that hypoalbuminemia fails to develop in these patients due to decreased catabolism of filtered proteins by the proximal tubules as compared with primary FSGS. Thus the actual protein loss in patients with secondary FSGS is less than in patients with primary FSGS and apparently similar levels of proteinuria.

TABLE 39.20. Primary Focal and Segmental Glomerulosclerosis: Clinical Features at Presentation

	Children	Adults
Nephrotic[a]	90%	70%
Male	55%	60%
Hypertensive	30%	45%
Hematuria	55%	45%
Renal insufficiency[b]	20%	30%

[a] Urinary protein excretion >3.5 gm/l accompanied by hypoalbuminemia.
[b] Serum creatinine more than 1.3 mg/dl.

TABLE 39.21. Primary Focal and Segmental Glomerulosclerosis in Adults: Clinical Features at Presentation

	Nephrotic	Nonnephrotic
African-American	65%	25%[b]
Male	60%	50%
Renal insufficiency[a]	65%	60%
Hypertension	45%	65%
Hematuria	40%	25%
Proteinuria median (g/d)	8	2[b]

[a] Serum creatinine more than 1.3 mg/dl.
[b] Significantly different.
From Rydel JJ, Korbet SM, Borok RZ, et al. Focal segmental glomerular sclerosis in adults: presentation, course and response to treatment. *Am J Kidney Dis* 1995;25:534–542.

CLINICAL COURSE

Based on Clinical Features at Presentation

The relevance of any clinical or pathologic feature of primary FSGS is dependent on its prognostic significance. The clinical feature most often used to predict the clinical course in FSGS is the degree of proteinuria at presentation. The presence of nephrotic range proteinuria (greater than 3 to 3.5 g/24 hr) has consistently been associated with a poor outcome in primary FSGS with 50% of patients reaching ESRD over 6 to 8 years. Massive proteinuria (more than 10 g/24 hr), portends an even more "malignant" course with ESRD occurring by 3 years in most patients. This is contrasted by the more favorable prognosis in patients with nonnephrotic proteinuria in which a renal survival of more than 80% is observed after 10 years and subsequent development of the nephrotic syndrome is unusual. In our experience, nonnephrotic patients progressing to ESRD are usually those with therapeutically unresponsive hypertension.

An additional clinical feature of prognostic significance is the presenting serum creatinine. A serum creatinine greater than 1.3 mg/dl is associated with a significantly poorer renal survival than those 1.3 mg/dl or less, irrespective of the level of proteinuria (10 year renal survival of 27% versus 100%).

Racial differences in the course of primary FSGS have been suggested by some. In nephrotic children with FSGS, progression to ESRD is significantly greater for African-American patients as compared with white patients over a 9 year follow-up (80% versus 30%). In adults, African-American patients tend to present less often with nonnephrotic range proteinuria than white patients, and in this respect may have a poorer prognosis. However, when evaluating only nephrotic FSGS patients, there is no significant racial difference in the rate of decline of renal function or renal survival (10-year renal survival: 64% for African-American patients and 55% for white patients).

The progression of FSGS has shown no significant correlation with age, sex, or the presence of hematuria. Even hypertension at presentation has not been found to be of prognostic significance. One could speculate that this may be the result of aggressive blood pressure control in these patients.

Given the poor prognosis of nephrotic patients with primary FSGS, it is of note that multivariate analysis has more often demonstrated the level of serum creatinine at presentation, rather than proteinuria, to be an independent, positive predictor of progression to ESRD. Although some have found the degree of proteinuria to be independently predictive, others have been unable confirm this observation. This discrepancy may be explained on the basis of the unusually high rate of remission in the nephrotic patients reported in the later studies, all of whom had excellent long-term renal survival. When patients entering a remission were eliminated from the analysis, proteinuria along with serum creatinine became independently predictive.

Based on Pathologic Features

The prognostic significance of histologic features of FSGS has also been extensively assessed. Neither the percentage of glomeruli with segmental scars nor the percentage of glomeruli with global sclerosis are predictive of outcome. The extent (20% or more) of interstitial fibrosis has been shown to consistently predict a poor prognosis.

The presence of diffuse mesangial hypercellularity has been associated with a more rapid loss in renal function. However, several large studies have failed to support any relationship between the presence of this finding and the prognosis of primary FSGS. The significance of the location of the segmental scar within the glomerulus has been controversial. Initial studies suggested that patients with the tip lesion (peripheral lesion) were distinguished from patients with primary FSGS because of a better response to therapy and a more benign clinical course. However, a number of investigators were unable to reproduce these observations, concluding the response to treatment and renal survival was not significantly different from that of patients with FSGS without the tip lesion.

The cellular lesion is thought to be the precursor of the glomerular scar in FSGS, representing the initial sign of glomerular damage in primary FSGS. Overall, patients with the cellular lesion have more severe proteinuria at biopsy and progress to ESRD more rapidly than those patients with the classic FSGS. However, achievement of a remission is associated with excellent renal survival in both groups of patients. The response to treatment is equally good in patients with classic and cellular lesions, the exception being patients with biopsies having extensive involvement with cellular lesions (20% or more of glomeruli).

Recently, patients demonstrating extensive segmental and global glomerular capillary collapse with severe tubulointerstitial disease that is out of proportion to the glomerular process have been described. Although similar in appearance to the cellular lesion, these patients are characterized by a black racial predominance, massive proteinuria, advanced renal insufficiency at presentation (serum creatinine 3.5 mg/dl or more), and are unresponsive to therapy with a malignant course, progressing to ESRD over 12 to 18 months. It has therefore been suggested that these patients represent a distinct entity that should be distinguished from primary FSGS and should be referred to as *collapsing glomerulopathy*.

The morphologic features now accepted under the diagnosis of primary FSGS have evolved significantly from that of the classic description. Our ability to further define the prognostic significance of these variants will require careful evaluation and long-term follow-up of larger numbers of patients.

Remission

Of all the clinical and histologic characteristics evaluated in primary FSGS, the only significant *negative* predictor of progression to ESRD has been the presence of a remission in proteinuria. The clinical course for nephrotic patients is significantly improved for those patients fortunate enough to enter and maintain a remission. Patients in remission demonstrate a significant decrease in the rate of decline in renal function and a prolonged renal survival as compared with those not in remission. In nephrotic adults and children alike, less than 15% of patients entering a complete remission (most often defined as proteinuria of less than 300 mg/24 hr) progress to ESRD, whereas up to 50% of persistently nephrotic patients progress to ESRD over 5 years. Even a partial remission (variably defined as proteinuria of less than 2.0 to 3.0 g/24 hr but greater than 0.3 to 0.5 g/24 hr, or by a 50% or more decrease in proteinuria from baseline) is associated with a better renal survival than patients in whom the nephrotic syndrome persists. Thus achieving a remission significantly improves the prognosis of nephrotic patients with FSGS.

Because spontaneous remissions are rare, occurring in fewer than 6% of nephrotic patients, it is in nephrotic FSGS patients that a trial of therapy is recommended. Unfortunately, there are no reliable clinical or histologic features at presentation that allow the nephrologist to determine which patients will enter a remission, and "treatment" is the only factor that predicts remission. Thus the best clinical indicator of outcome is the response to therapy.

TREATMENT OF PRIMARY FOCAL SEGMENTAL GLOMERULOSCLEROSIS

It must be recognized that any recommendations on the treatment of primary FSGS are limited by the fact that our understanding of the response to therapy in adults, and with few exceptions, in children, is based almost entirely on retrospective analyses. From this experience, encouraging insights have emerged, but prospective controlled trials are still required to better define the therapeutic approach to patients with primary FSGS.

Nephrotic Patients

Initial Treatment

Glucocorticoids. The initial treatment of FSGS in nephrotic children consists of prednisone 60 mg/m^2 per day (up to 80 mg/day) given in divided doses for 4 weeks followed by 40 mg/m^2 per day (up to 60 mg/day) given in divided doses 3 consecutive days out of 7, or on alternate days, for 4 weeks and then tapered off over 4 more weeks. The complete remission rate for children with primary FSGS using this treatment protocol is between 20% to 25%. When a more prolonged course of prednisone therapy (up to 6 months) has been used in children, complete remission rates of up to 50% have been achieved.

In nephrotic adults, the experience with steroid treatment in primary FSGS published before 1980 was extremely disappointing, with complete remission rates of less than 20% observed in most studies. In at least half of the reports, no patient attained a complete remission with the course of steroid treatment provided. Thus it is not surprising that nephrologists had become reluctant to subject adults with primary FSGS to a course of steroid or immunosuppressive therapy.

Since 1980, however, a more optimistic picture has evolved. In more than 80% of studies (none of which have been prospective controlled trials, unfortunately), complete remission rates in excess of 30% have been reported (Table 39.22). The improvement in response appears to be associated with a more prolonged duration of steroid therapy because the initial dose of prednisone used has been similar among these studies (ranging from 0.3 to 2 mg/kg per day). The total duration of prednisone therapy in those studies with complete remission rates of less than 30% was 2 months or less as compared with 6 to 9 months in studies achieving complete remissions in 30% or more patients (Table 39.23). It should be noted that in the studies reporting better remission rates, the initial dose of prednisone (often 1 mg/kg per day, up to 80 mg) was generally maintained for 2 to 3 months and then tapered over the remaining treatment duration.

TABLE 39.22. Primary Focal and Segmental Glomerulosclerosis: Response to Treatment with Glucocorticoids/Cytotoxic Agents in Adults

Reference	*n*	Complete Remission	Partial Remission	No Response
Miyata et al.	32	44%	12%	44%
Pei et al.	18	39%	0	61%
Banfi et al.	59	61%	0	39%
Agarwal et al.	38	32%	26%	42%
Rydel et al.	30	33%	17%	50%
TOTAL	177	45%	10%	45%

Reproduced with permission from Korbet SM. Primary focal segmental glomerulosclerosis [disease of the month]. *J Am Soc Nephrol* 1998;9:1333–1340.

TABLE 39.23. Primary Focal and Segmental Glomerulosclerosis: Remission in Relationship to Initial Steroid Treatment Duration in Adults

Response	Dose (mg/kg/day)	High-dose Duration (months)	Total Duration (months)
>30% Remissions	0.5–1.5	2–3	6–9
<30% Remissions	0.5–1.5	1	2

Less than one-third of adults who ultimately achieve a complete remission do so by 8 weeks of therapy. The median time to complete remission is 3 to 4 months, with the majority of patients reaching a complete remission by 5 to 9 months from the beginning of treatment. As a result, it is now proposed that steroid resistance in adults be defined as the persistence of the nephrotic syndrome after a 4-month trial of therapy with prednisone at a dose of 1 mg/kg per day.

Because of concerns about complications related to daily steroid use, particularly in older adults, the potential value of alternate-day steroid therapy has been explored. In young adults, the response to alternate-day regimens has been disappointing. However, in the elderly (60 years of age or older), a complete remission rate of more than 40% has been observed using 1.0 to 1.6 mg/kg (up to 100 mg) of prednisone every other day for 3 to 5 months, and is well tolerated without complication. The excellent response to alternate-day steroid therapy in these patients (comparable to that in younger adults on daily steroid therapy) may be due to the decrease in clearance of steroids with increasing age resulting in a more sustained steroid effect.

Cytotoxic Agents. The combination of cytotoxic agents along with steroids as initial therapy has been evaluated and appears to confer no added benefit in attaining a complete remission when compared with steroids alone. However, their use has been associated with fewer relapses and more sustained remissions than that observed with steroids alone.

Based on the information to date, a trial of steroid therapy in primary FSGS is warranted in nephrotic patients with reasonably well-preserved renal function (serum creatinine 3 mg/dl or less) in whom it is not otherwise contraindicated. Unfortunately, the optimal dose and duration of steroid therapy is unknown. An initial course of treatment for adults should consist of prednisone given at a dose of 1 mg/kg per day (up to 80 mg) for 3 to 4 months. In patients demonstrating a response to treatment (a complete or partial remission), the dosage of prednisone can be reduced to 0.5 mg/kg per day (or 60 mg every other day) and treatment continued for 6 to 8 weeks and then tapered off over 4 to 6 weeks. Patients unresponsive to the initial course of therapy should be tapered off prednisone more rapidly, over 4 to 6 weeks. In the elderly, the use of an alternate-day regimen of prednisone (1 to 2 mg/kg, up to 120 mg) for 4 to 5 months seems prudent.

Relapsing Patients

The improved outcome associated with a remission in primary FSGS depends on that remission being sustained because recurrence of the nephrotic syndrome portends a prognosis similar to primary nonresponders. Fortunately, of those patients who relapse, the majority (more than 75%) are able to reachieve a remission when treated.

Glucocorticoids. The therapeutic approach to the patient who relapses depends on the frequency with which relapses occur. In the patient relapsing after a prolonged remission off steroids (6 months or more), a second course of steroid therapy may be sufficient. For frequent relapsers (two relapses or more within 6 months, or three to four relapses within 12 months), steroid-dependent patients (two relapses occurring with steroid taper or a relapse within 1 month of ending treatment), or those patients in whom a more steroid-conservative approach may be desired, the use of cytotoxic agents or cyclosporine has been beneficial (Table 39.24).

Cytotoxic Agents. A course of cytotoxic therapy (commonly cyclophosphamide 2 mg/kg per day) for 2 to 3 months, often in combination with a short course of prednisone (1 mg/kg per day, up to 80 mg, for up to 1 month, then tapered off over a month) leads to the reestablishment of a remission in more than 70% of children and adults.

Cyclosporine. Cyclosporine (5 to 6 mg/kg per day in two divided doses) is also highly successful in reestablishing a remission in steroid-responsive patients with primary FSGS who have gone on to relapse. Response is seen within the first month of cyclosporine treatment in the majority of patients. However, the remission is generally maintained only with continuous cyclosporine therapy because more than 75% of patients relapse upon taper or discontinuation of the drug. In this setting, the trade off for steroid dependence (and toxicity) becomes that of cyclosporine dependence and the potential risk of cyclosporine nephrotoxicity.

Thus, for the frequently relapsing or steroid-dependent patient with FSGS, the use of cyclophosphamide appears most beneficial in achieving a more sustained remission. To minimize the toxicity (see succeeding section) associated with this agent, a course of treatment should be limited to 3 months.

Steroid-Resistant Patients

The treatment of steroid-resistant FSGS poses one of the most perplexing and frustrating problems for the nephrologist. The therapeutic options most used are the same as those for relapsing patients (cyclophosphamide or cyclosporine). Unfortunately, the response to these agents in steroid-resistant FSGS has been quite disappointing when compared with that of patients who were initially steroid-responsive (Table 39.24).

Cytotoxic Agents. In children, 3 months of cyclophosphamide in combination with a 12-month course of alternate-day prednisone has achieved no better response than prednisone alone. In steroid-resistant adults, the duration of treatment with cyclophosphamide is usually 2 to 3 months but has been as long as 18 months or more. Irrespective, the complete remission rates achieved are disappointingly low at less than 20% in most cases. The rates may not be different than prednisone-only treatment.

Cyclosporine. Cyclosporine has also resulted in complete remission rates of less than 25% in patients with steroid-resistant FSGS. The combined use of low-dose prednisone with cyclosporine may enhance the likelihood of remission; however, if a response to cyclosporine is not observed by 4 to 6 months, it is unlikely to occur. Several prospective, randomized, controlled trials of cyclosporine have been conducted in adults and children with steroid-resistant FSGS (Table 39.25). Cyclosporine, 3.5 to 6 mg/kg per day, is given in two divided doses for 6 months, adjusting the dosage to maintain 10- to 12-hour trough levels of 100 to 200 ng/ml (whole-blood monoclonal immunoassay). The complete remission rate with cyclosporine was low (less than 20%) in most of these studies; however, the overall remission rate (complete plus partial) was significantly better than that observed in the control groups. As expected, relapse rates were high after discontinuation of cyclosporine; however, progression to ESRD in the cyclosporine-treated patients was one-third that of patients on placebo.

In the treatment of steroid-resistant FSGS, even though none of the present options generate much cause for optimism, cyclosporine appears to demonstrate an advantage over that of cytotoxic agents. In either case, the trial of therapy should be limited to reduce the risk of complications. For cytotoxic agents, this should be limited to 3 months (irrespective of the final response) and for cyclosporine, 4 to 6 months. In patients responding to cyclosporine treatment, a more prolonged course may be required to maintain the remission. Recent evidence suggests that patients remaining in remission on cyclosporine for more than 12 months may be slowly tapered off cyclosporine without subsequent relapse. Thus an attempt at taper-

TABLE 39.24. Primary Focal and Segmental Glomerulosclerosis: Response to Cytotoxic and Cyclosporine Therapy in Relationship to Initial Response to Steroid Therapy

	Complete Remission	Partial Remission	No Response
Cytotoxic Therapy			
Steroid responsive	52%	24%	24%
Steroid resistant	15%	10%	75%
Cyclosporine Therapy			
Steroid responsive	69%	8%	23%
Steroid resistant	22%	25%	53%

Reproduced with permission from Korbet SM. Primary focal segmental glomerulosclerosis [disease of the month]. *J Am Soc Nephrol* 1998;9:1333–1340.

TABLE 39.25. Randomized Controlled Trials of Cyclosporine in Steroid-Resistant Patients with Primary Focal Segmental Glomerulosclerosis

	Complete Remission	Partial Remission	*P*
Ponticelli[a]			
Cyclosporine	20%	40%	<0.001
Control	0	33%	
Cattran[b]			
Cyclosporine	12%	57%	<0.001
Placebo	0	20%	
Liebman[c]			
Cyclosporine	33%	66%	<0.05
Placebo	0	17%	

[a]Ponticelli C, Rizzoni G, Edefonti A, et al. A randomized trial of cyclosporine in steroid resistant idiopathic nephrotic syndrome. *Kidney Int* 1993;43:1377–1384.

[b]Cattran DC, Appel GB, Hebert LA, et al. A randomized trial of cyclosporine in patients with steroid-resistant focal segmental glomerulosclerosis. *Kidney Int* 1999;56:2220–2226.

[c]Lieberman KV, Tejani A. A randomized double-blind placebo-controlled trial of cyclosporine in steroid-resistant idiopathic focal segmental glomerulosclerosis in children. *J Am Soc Nephrol* 1996;7:56–63.

Reproduced with permission from Korbet SM. Primary focal segmental glomerulosclerosis [disease of the month]. *J Am Soc Nephrol* 1998;9:1333–1340.

ing cyclosporine in patients with prolonged remissions should be made to minimize possible nephrotoxicity.

Nonnephrotic Patients

At this time, the comparatively favorable prognosis of nonnephrotic patients with FSGS does not support the use of steroids or other immunosuppressive agents. Nonetheless, the progressive renal failure observed in some patients, many of whom are hypertensive, underscores the importance of close follow-up and good blood pressure control. To this end, the use of angiotensin-converting enzyme (ACE) inhibitors in nonnephrotic FSGS patients would appear to be particularly beneficial given their additional renoprotective effects (see the following discussion).

COMPLICATIONS OF IMMUNOSUPPRESSIVE THERAPY

Glucocorticoids

The potential for adverse effects of steroid use can be substantial. At present, significant side effects from the doses and prolonged courses of steroid therapy used in primary FSGS have not been routinely encountered, even in studies with average treatment durations of up to 9 months. However, more experience and longer follow-up is needed to establish the actual risk in these patients.

Cytotoxic Agents

Reports of adverse events from the use of cytotoxic agents are rare. Most patients receive cytotoxic therapy for up to 3 months; however, in some cases, the course of treatment has been significantly longer. Concern of gonadal dysfunction or acute leukemia is particularly appropriate with prolonged use of alkylating agents. The cumulative dose of a 3-month course of 2 mg/kg per day of cyclophosphamide (180 mg/kg, or 12.6 g in a 70-kg patient) is below that which has generally been associated with gonadal dysfunction (greater than 250 mg/kg) or the development of acute leukemia (greater than 25 g). In assessing for acute leukemia, it must be recognized that a substantial lag time (2 to 4 years or more) between the drug exposure and development of leukemia exists. Thus we must remain cognizant of the importance of limiting the exposure of our patients to these agents.

Cyclosporine

The potential nephrotoxicity of long-term cyclosporine therapy is another area of concern because it one that is difficult to evaluate. Continuous cyclosporine use over 12 to 38 months is associated with significant increases in tubular atrophy and interstitial fibrosis. The development of nephrotoxicity may not be apparent clinically because there is a lack of correlation between the structural damage and renal function. The severity of the tubulointerstitial disease in follow-up biopsies of patients taking cyclosporine has a positive and significant correlation with the percentage of segmental scars on the initial biopsy, the serum creatinine at the time of the initial biopsy, and a cyclosporine dosage of greater than 5.5 mg/kg per day. Thus cyclosporine should be used cautiously in FSGS patients with preexisting renal insufficiency and tubulointerstitial disease. In addition, cyclosporine may actually accelerate the progression of FSGS despite remission of proteinuria. A significant increase in glomeruli with segmental scars, obsolescent glomeruli, and interstitial fibrosis/infiltrates as compared with precyclosporine biopsies has been demonstrated, even in FSGS patients in remission. Unfortunately, a major dilemma remains in deciding whether any progressive damage is the result of cyclosporine, the underlying disease, or both. Limiting the cyclosporine dosage to less than 5.5 mg/kg per day and duration of therapy to 12 months in responsive patients should help minimize the potential for nephrotoxicity.

ALTERNATIVE TREATMENT CONSIDERATIONS

Nonsteroidal antiinflammatory drugs (NSAIDs) have been used in severely nephrotic patients unresponsive to the more conventional therapies. In a few cases, complete remissions have been attained in steroid-resistant FSGS. The mechanism(s) by which NSAIDs work is unknown but is more complex than can be explained on the basis of alterations in intrarenal hemodynamics alone because the decrease in proteinuria is often disproportional to the modest reduction in renal function observed in most responsive patients. We rarely use NSAIDs as a specific treatment for FSGS. An issue to recognize is the potential for hyperkalemia when NSAIDs are used in combination with an ACE inhibitor, a drug we do commonly use.

During the past several years, the renoprotective effects of ACE inhibitors in the treatment of glomerular disease have been increasingly appreciated. The beneficial effects afforded by ACE inhibitors result from a combination of systemic blood pressure control, normalization of intraglomerular hemodynamics, and a reduction in proteinuria. In addition, ACE inhibitors act through nonhemodynamic mechanisms to reduce progression of renal disease by decreasing the production of various growth factors that lead to fibrosis such as TGF-β.

Several studies in patients with primary glomerulopathies, including FSGS, have shown that ACE inhibitors not only reduced proteinuria by up to 45% but were also renoprotective. An overall reduction in risk of progressive renal insufficiency (doubling of serum creatinine) of greater than 50% for patients with initial proteinuria of more than 1 to less than 3 g/24 hr, and more than 65% for those patients with greater than 3 g/24 hr, has been observed with the use of ACE inhibitors in patients with nondiabetic renal disease. These findings suggest that ACE inhibitor portends a significantly better prognosis not only for patients who are at greatest risk for progressive renal disease (those with nephrotic-range proteinuria), but may further improve the prognosis for patients with nonnephrotic proteinuria as well. Presently, the addition of ACE inhibitors (or possibly angiotensin II–receptor antagonists) to the treatment regimen of either nephrotic or nonnephrotic patients with FSGS would appear to be prudent.

TREATMENT OF SECONDARY FOCAL SEGMENTAL GLOMERULOSCLEROSIS

The treatment of secondary FSGS is directed at the underlying cause. HIV-associated nephropathy has responded to treatment with retroviral agents as well as to steroid therapy and the use of ACE inhibitors (see Chapter 39, Part 3). In obese patients, weight loss has led to a decrease in proteinuria and a decrease in the progression of renal insufficiency. A beneficial effect from the use of ACE inhibitors has been observed in patients with secondary FSGS due to a reduced nephron mass. An argument can be made for the use of ACE inhibitors or angiotensin II–receptor antagonists in essentially all forms of FSGS attributed to hyperfiltration and intraglomerular hypertension.

RENAL TRANSPLANTATION IN FOCAL SEGMENTAL GLOMERULOSCLEROSIS

It is well known that FSGS recurs in approximately 25% to 40% of renal transplants, leading to graft loss in half of these cases. Recurrence has been reported to occur within hours of transplantation but is more often seen within 3 months. In patients with "malignant" FSGS, the risk of recurrence is reported to be more than 50% and the likelihood for a second recurrence in an individual losing the initial graft to recurrent FSGS is reported to be as high as 85%. Thus not only the initial course, but even the posttransplant course for patients with primary FSGS pose a number of dilemmas with which the nephrologist must contend. Fortunately, a remission in proteinuria has also been associated with an improved prognosis for patients with recurrent FSGS.

The use of plasmapheresis or a protein adsorption device in the treatment of FSGS has been proposed based on the premise that the circulating "permeability factor(s)" responsible for FSGS will be removed. Trials of this approach in the treatment of transplant patients with recurrent FSGS have been encouraging because lasting remissions associated with marked histologic improvement in glomerular abnormalities have been achieved in some patients, providing that treatment with plasmapheresis is initiated early in the course of recurrent disease, before sclerotic lesions have developed in the transplanted kidney. Unfortunately, the use of plasmapheresis in steroid-resistant patients with primary FSGS has failed to produce the same beneficial results.

Selected Readings

Agarwal S, Dash S, Tiwari S, et al. Idiopathic adult focal segmental glomerulosclerosis: a clinicopathological study and response to steroid. *Nephron* 1993;63:168–171.

A retrospective study of 65 adults with idiopathic FSGS. Nephrotic syndrome was present in 38 patients, all of whom were treated with high-dose steroids for up to 12 weeks, after which they were tapered slowly for a total duration of therapy of up to 6 months.

Artero ML, Sharma R, Savin V, et al. Plasmapheresis reduces proteinuria and serum capacity to injure glomeruli in patients with recurrent focal glomerulosclerosis. *Am J Kidney Dis* 1994;23:574–581.

An uncontrolled trial demonstrating a beneficial effect of plasmapheresis in recurrent FSGS. The likelihood of remission with plasmapheresis was greatest in those patients identified and treated early in the course of the recurrence of proteinuria (within 1 week).

Banfi G, Moriggi M, Sabadini E, et al. The impact of prolonged immunosuppression on the outcome of idiopathic focal-segmental glomerulosclerosis with nephrotic syndrome in adults: a collaborative retrospective study. *Clin Nephrol* 1991;36:53–59.

A retrospective study of 59 adults with FSGS who were treated with prolonged courses of immunosuppressive agents. The therapeutic approach fell into three groups: (a) high-dose steroids alone, (b) high-dose steroids combined with cytotoxic agents (chlorambucil, cyclophosphamide, or azathioprine), and (c) cytotoxic agents with low-dose prednisone. These therapies were used from a median of 5 to 19 months. The therapeutic response was more than 60% with improved renal survival in those patients attaining a remission. The only feature predictive of a poor renal outcome was the presence of interstitial fibrosis on the renal biopsy.

Cameron JS. The enigma of focal segmental glomerulosclerosis. *Kidney Int* 1996; 50(Suppl 57):S119–S131.

This is an excellent in-depth review of FSGS.

Cattran DC, Appel GB, Hebert LA, et al. for the North American Nephrotic Syndrome Study Group. A randomized trial of cyclosporine in patients with steroid-resistant focal segmental glomerulosclerosis. *Kidney Int* 2000;56: 2220–2226.

This randomized prospective trial demonstrates the benefit of a 6 month course of cyclosporine in patients with steroid-resistant FSGS. Seventy percent of the treatment group versus only 4% of the placebo group had a partial or complete remission in proteinuria by 26 weeks. Relapse of proteinuria occurred by 78 weeks in 60% of the patients initially remitting. However, only 25% in the treatment group compared with 52% of controls had a 50% decrease in baseline creatinine clearance over 4 years of follow-up.

Cattran DC, Panduranga R. Long-term outcome in children and adults with classic focal segmental glomerulosclerosis. *Am J Kidney Dis* 1998;32:72–79.

This retrospective study of 55 adults and 38 children with FSGS is an ongoing follow-up of the original report by Pei et al. (reference follows). The 10-year renal survival in adults and children with remission was 100% compared with 62% in adults and 58% in children who did not attain a complete remission.

Korbet SM. Primary focal segmental glomerulosclerosis. In: Brady HR, Wilcox CS, eds. *Therapy in nephrology and hypertension: a companion to Brenner and Rector's the kidney.* Philadelphia: WB Saunders, 1998:178–188.

This is an extensive, in-depth review of the clinical presentation, treatment, and course of primary FSGS.

Korbet SM. Primary focal segmental glomerulosclerosis [disease of the month]. *J Am Soc Nephrol* 1998;9:1333–1340.

This is a review of primary FSGS.

Meyrier A, Noel LH, Auriche P, et al. Long-term renal tolerance of cyclosporin A treatment in adult idiopathic nephrotic syndrome. *Kidney Int* 1994;45: 1446–1456.

This is a prospective study of the use of cyclosporine in nephrotic adults with minimal-change disease and FSGS. All patients were biopsied before the initiation of therapy and after 19 months of cyclosporine therapy. Factors predictive of cyclosporine nephrotoxicity included a dose greater than 5.5 mg/kg per day, the presence of renal insufficiency before treatment, and the percentage of glomeruli with lesions of FSGS on the initial biopsy. It was recommended that a repeat biopsy be performed after 1 year of treatment with cyclosporine to determine whether treatment can be continued safely. Patients in remission for a year or more on cyclosporine were able to be tapered off without relapse.

Miyata J, Takebayashi S, Taguchi T, et al. Evaluation and correlation of clinical and histological features of focal segmental glomerulosclerosis. *Nephron* 1986;44: 115–120.

Patients were divided into two groups based on the presence or absence of mesangial hypercellularity. Those patients with mesangial hypercellularity were less steroid responsive, less likely to have permanent remissions, and more likely to have progressive renal insufficiency.

Pei Y, Cattran D, Delmore T, et al. Evidence suggesting under-treatment in adults with idiopathic focal segmental glomerulosclerosis. *Am J Med* 1987;82: 938–944.

This is an in-depth retrospective study of 55 adults and 38 children with a prolonged course of steroid therapy (the median duration was 6 months). The 5-year renal survival (absence of creatinine clearance of less than 15 ml/min) was 96% in patients attaining a complete remission compared with 55% in those patients without a complete remission.

Rydel JJ, Korbet SM, Borok RZ, et al. Focal segmental glomerular sclerosis in adults: presentation, course and response to treatment. *Am J Kidney Dis* 1995; 25:534–542.

This retrospective study evaluates the clinical presentation, response to therapy, and course in 81 adult patients with primary FSGS. Seventy-four percent of patients presented with nephrotic syndrome. The 10-year survival for nephrotic patients was 57% compared with 92% for nonnephrotic patients. Thirty nephrotic patients received a prolonged course of therapy with steroids (up to 6 months on average). Fifty percent of patients achieved a remission by 3.7 months. The 10-year renal survival for patients in remission was 100% compared with 41% for patients not achieving a remission.

Savin VJ, Sharma R, Sharma M, et al. Circulating factor associated with increased glomerular permeability to albumin in recurrent focal segmental glomerulosclerosis. *N Engl J Med* 1996;334:878–883.

This prospective study in 33 patients with recurrent FSGS tries to evaluate and better define the circulating factor responsible for glomerular injury in primary FSGS. Based on an in vitro assay, they found that recurrence of FSGS occurred in only 17% of patients, with a pretransplant permeability activity of less than 0.5 compared with recurrence in 86% of patients with an activity of 0.5 or more. Furthermore, they demonstrate the benefit of plasmapheresis in reducing the level of the permeability factor and significantly reducing the level of proteinuria.

Schwartz MM, Korbet SM. Primary focal segmental glomerulosclerosis: pathology, histologic variants, and pathogenesis. *Am J Kidney Dis* 1993;22:874–883.

This is an in-depth review of the significance of various histologic features associated with primary FSGS.

Schwartz MM, Korbet SM. The cellular lesion of focal segmental glomerulosclerosis: therapeutic response and prognosis. American Society of Nephrology 30th Annual Meeting [Abstract]. *J Am Soc Nephrol* 1997;8:98.

This is a retrospective study in 100 patients (75 nephrotic, 25 nonnephrotic) with FSGS. The study compares 36 nephrotic patients with classic lesions of FSGS with 39 nephrotic patients with cellular lesions (collapsing lesions). Progression to ESRD occurred in 44% of nephrotic patients with the cellular lesion compared with only 14% of patients with classic segmental scars. The rate of remission in treated nephrotic patients with cellular or classic segmental scars was essentially the same (53% versus 52%) and the 5-year survival of both groups was 100% for patients entering in a remission compared with 16% in patients with cellular lesions and 69% for patients with classic scars who did not enter a remission with therapy.

PART 6
Membranous Glomerulonephritis

Claudio Ponticelli and Patrizia Passerini

Membranous glomerulonephritis (MG) is a pathologic term that defines a glomerular disease characterized by diffuse and uniform thickening of the glomerular basement membranes (GBMs) due to the deposition of subepithelial immune complexes. Clinically, MG is usually associated with nephrotic syndrome. The disease may slowly progress to renal failure, but a number of patients maintain normal renal function and may even have spontaneous remission of proteinuria.

MG typically occurs in adults, accounting for approximately 30% to 40% of cases of nephrotic syndrome; it is rare in childhood. It is difficult to estimate the prevalence of MG in the elderly because many nephrologists were reluctant to perform renal biopsy until recently. However, the general impression is that MG represents by far the most common cause of idiopathic nephrotic syndrome in the elderly; it is even more common in people older than 60 years of age than in the younger population. Overall, MG is predominant in males, with a 2:1 ratio.

ETIOLOGY

In most cases of MG, no etiologic factor can be identified and the disease is classified as idiopathic. However, in approximately one-fourth to one-third of cases, MG is associated with infection, neoplasia, and rheumatologic disorders other diseases, or with exposure to drugs or toxins resulting in secondary MG (Table 39.26). The association may merely reflect a chance finding, but in most cases, there is a genuine association, which is confirmed by the resolution of MG if the primary condition is removed or successfully treated. The overall prevalence of secondary MG seems to be higher in children than in adults. Malaria, schistosomias, and hepatitis B and C are the most common causes of secondary MG, particularly in endemic areas. MG can also be associated with systemic lupus erythematosus (SLE) and may sometimes precede the typical serologic abnormalities of lupus even by years. In approximately 10% of cases, MG may be associated with malignant neoplasias; it is important to note that in 40% to 45% of cases, renal disease may antedate the initial manifestations of the underlying cancer by months. Among drugs causing MG, penicillamine and gold salts are two well-recognized agents. However, nonsteroidal antiinflammatory drugs are probably the most common agents responsible for secondary MG, particularly in elderly patients.

In idiopathic disease, an immunogenetic diathesis is likely. An association between MG and HLA-DR3 has been well documented in Caucasian patients, whereas in Japanese patients, there is an association of the disease with HLA-DR2. The gene encoding the complement component Bf may also be involved. Two alleles have been found with increased incidence in patients with MG, BfF1, and BfS. Rarely, MG may affect siblings or other members of the same family.

TABLE 39.26. Possible Causes of Secondary Membranous Glomerulonephritis

Infections	
Enterococcal endocarditis	Quartan malaria
Filariasis	Schistosomiasis
Hepatitis B or C	Streptococcal infection
Hydatid disease	Syphilis (congenital or secondary)
Leprosy	
Neoplasia	
Benign tumors	Mesothelioma
Carcinomas	Non-Hodgkin's lymphoma
Hodgkin's disease	Pheochromocytoma
Melanoma	Retroperitoneal sarcoma
Rheumatologic Disorders	
Ankylosing spondylitis	Rheumatoid arthritis
Dermatomyositis	Systemic lupus erythematosus
Mixed connective tissue disease	Systemic sclerosis
Drugs or Toxic Agents	
Captopril	Lithium
Diclofenac	Mercury compounds
Fenoprofen	Penicillamine
Formaldehyde	Probenecid
Gold	Sulindac
Hydrocarbons	Thiola
Ketoprofen	Trimethadione
Miscellaneous Conditions	
Adult polycystic kidney disease	Periaortic fibrosis
α_1-Antitrypsin deficiency	Primary biliary cirrhosis
Crohn's disease	Renal transplantation
Dermatitis herpetiformis	Sarcoidosis
Diabetes mellitus	Sickle cell disease
Guillan-Barré syndrome	Sjögren's syndrome
Hemolytic uremic syndrome	Systemic mastocytosis
Kimura's disease	Temporal arteritis
Miller Fisher syndrome	Thyroid disease
Multiple sclerosis	Urticarial vasculitis
Myasthenia gravis	Weber-Christian disease
Myelodysplasia	

PATHOGENESIS

The pathogenesis of human MG is not completely understood. However, there is general agreement that MG is an immunologically mediated disorder, as demonstrated by the finding of immune complexes deposition along the GBM. Moreover, experimental models, in which a histologic lesion virtually identical to that found in humans can be produced, provided clear evidence that MG is an immune mediated disease.

For many years, it was thought that MG resulted from the trapping within glomeruli of circulating immune complexes of appropriate size, formed by a specific endogenous antibody reacting with either endogenous or environmental antigen(s). Further studies showed that this mechanism might be operating in some cases of secondary MG but probably not in the idiopathic form. Circulating immune complexes have been detected in MG associated with SLE, hepatitis B, or neoplasia. In some of these cases of secondary MG, the antigen was eluted from glomeruli. On the contrary, immune complexes were found rarely in the sera of patients with idiopathic MG. No study could show that the circulating immune complexes material was the same as that deposited in the glomeruli. Rather, experimental studies support the hypothesis that in idiopathic MG there is an *in situ* formation of immune complexes as a consequence of a reaction between an antibody and either an intrinsic glomerular antigen or an antigen "planted" in the subepithelial position.

Heymann nephritis represents the paradigm of the *in situ* formation of immune complexes in the glomeruli. It is an autoimmune-mediated glomerulonephritis that closely mimics the functional and morphologic features of human MG. There are two models of Heymann nephritis. In the first model, or *active* Heymann nephritis, the renal damage is induced by immunizing a rat with crude proximal tubular brush border extract. In the *passive* model, Heymann nephritis is induced by injecting preformed antibodies against this extract into a normal animal. With both models, subepithelial glomerular immune deposits form, followed by proteinuria 5 or 6 days later. Several attempts have been made to identify the pathogenetic antigen(s) involved in Heymann nephritis. Initially, the pathogenetic activity was recovered in a lipoprotein fraction named *FX1A* and its subfraction named *RTEα5*. Later gp330, a major component of FX1A, was identified as the target antigen. Gp330, now named *megalin*, is a 515-kD glycoprotein present in clathrin-coated pits located at both the base of the microvilli in the proximal tubular brush border and along the sides and the base of the podocyte foot processes. This double location explains why a glomerular disease can develop after the injection of crude proximal tubular brush border extract. More recently a second protein (44 kD) that binds to gp330/megalin, was also shown to be a target antigen. This protein was called *receptor-associated protein*, or *RAP*. Both gp330/megalin and RAP have been cloned and sequenced, and their role in normal epithelial cells has been explored. Gp330/megalin is a member of the low-density lipoprotein-receptor gene family and functions as a multiligand endocytic receptor for the uptake of a variety of macromolecules such as plasminogen, plasminogen activator, lactoferrin, Ca^{2+}, and the like. RAP associates with gp330/megalin and appears to function as its intracellular chaperon, assisting in the folding of gp330/megalin in the endoplasmic reticulum and its transport to the cell surface. For the pathogenesis of immune-deposit formation it is relevant that gp330/megalin is an endogenous renal antigen, present on the bases of foot processes of podocytes where initial immune complexes are formed. Figure 39.14 summarizes the early events in the formation of an immune deposit in passive Heymann nephritis. Circulating anti-gp330/megalin IgG crosses the GBM and approaches gp330/megalin located in clathrin-coated pits of glomerular epithelia (Fig. 39.14A). Then anti-gp330/megalin IgG binds specific "pathogenetic epitopes" of its antigen gp330/megalin in the coated pits, forming an initial immune complex (Fig. 39.14B). The initial immune complex is detached from the cell surface and becomes attached to the GBM as early as 15 minutes after injection of the antibody (Fig. 39.14C). The immune deposit then grows by repeated cycles of *in situ* immune-complex formation and shedding into the lamina rara externa of the GBM, until it eventually encroaches on the area of the slit diaphragm. The glomerular epithelial cells respond by increasing the rate of synthesis of gp330/megalin. Vesicular transport of these new molecules of gp330/megalins exposes them in the membranes of coated pits adjacent to immune deposits. By repeated cycles of this process, more immune complexes can accumulate at the same spot, and eventually the immune deposits become morphologically apparent.

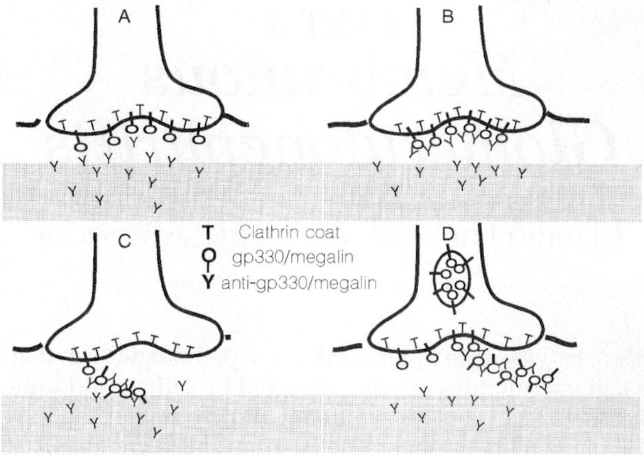

Figure 39.14. Formation of immune deposits in passive Heymann nephritis (see text for further explanation). Circulating anti-gp330/megalin IgG crosses GBM and approaches gp330/megalin located in clathrin-coated pits of glomerular epithelia **(A).** Then anti-gp330/megalin IgG binds specific "pathogenetic epitopes" of its antigen gp330/megalin in the coated pits, forming an initial immune complex **(B).** The initial immune complex is detached from the cell surface and becomes attached to the GBM as early as 15 minutes after injection of the antibody **(C).** (Modified from Kerajaschki D. Molecular pathogenesis of membranous nephropathy. *Kidney Int* 1992;41:1090–1105.)

Another important topic to examine is how proteinuria develops. In experimental models, depletion of complement by cobra venom factor inhibits the occurrence of proteinuria and does not interfere with the formation of immune deposits. Soon after the identification of gp330/megalin as the antigen responsible for inducing immune deposits, it became apparent that antimegalin antibodies were unable to produce proteinuria. In passive Heymann nephritis, proteinuria was demonstrated to depend on activation of complement and formation of the membrane attack complex C5b-9. It has been discovered that within anti-FX1A and antimicrovillar sera, there are at least two IgG fractions of relevance for the development of passive Heymann nephritis: one directed against gp330/megalin, which is responsible for the development of immune deposits, and a second specific glycolipid antigen(s), which activate(s) the complement cascade. C5b-9 causes upregulation of expression of the nicotinamide adenine–dinucleotide phosphate–oxidoreductase enzyme complex by glomerular cells. Subsequently, there is a local production of reactive oxygen species, which flood the entire GBM and its matrix proteins. Here, the formation of lipid peroxidation adducts triggers structural changes within the GBM matrix proteins, thus causing proteinuria.

This sequence of pathogenetic events of Heymann nephritis is thought to be operating also in human MG, although there are still some unanswered questions. The target antigen in human MG, for example, has yet to be identified. There is a gp330-related glycoprotein present in human proximal tubules, but it is absent in normal glomeruli and is not detectable in immune deposits from renal biopsies of patients with MG. Moreover, it is not clear whether a single antigen provides the target for all cases of human MG or whether different antigens are involved in different circumstances. These data raise the possibility that the term *idiopathic* will remain unchanged for the majority of cases of MG.

PATHOLOGY (SEE CHAPTER 109)

The typical lesions of MG can be easily recognized at light microscopy. They consist of a uniform thickening of the peripheral capillary loop basement membrane without any significant increase in the cellular components of the glomerular tuft. Immunofluorescence shows diffuse granular deposits of IgG and C3 along the capillary walls, with IgG deposits being more prominent. Electron microscopy may show electron-dense deposits in subepithelial position.

Different stages of glomerular lesions have been described. In *stage I*, the glomeruli appear almost normal at light microscopy, but granular deposits of IgG and C3 can be seen at immunofluorescence. At electron microscopy there are small subepithelial electron-dense deposits and diffuse foot process fusion. In *stage II*, at light microscopy there is a diffuse, uniform thickening of the GBMs with characteristic spikes on silver stain. Electron microscopy shows that these spikes are due to projections of the GBM. The deposits are larger and more numerous than in stage I. In *stage III*, the deposits are incorporated within the GBM, which appears thickened at light microscopy. The increased thickness might be caused by deposition of novel chains of type IV collagen ($\alpha3$ and $\alpha4$), laminin, and nidogen as a response to the deposition of large immune aggregates. In *stage IV*, the GBM is markedly but irregularly thickened. By electron microscopy electron-lucent areas replace the electron-dense deposits. The intensity of immunofluorescence may be rather low. A *stage V* has also been described with more than 10% of glomeruli showing global sclerosis, particularly in the juxtamedullary area. Not all the authors, however, accept the existence of stage V.

The clinical relevance of staging remains uncertain. Some authorities believe that the different stages develop sequentially with time and that patients with stages I and II are more likely to go into remission, either spontaneously or after treatment. However, other investigators did not find any correlation between the glomerular stage and renal outcome. An unfavorable prognostic role has been attributed to the finding of a focal and segmental glomerulosclerosis superimposed to the typical glomerular lesions of MG. Rarely an extracapillary proliferation can also superimpose on the other glomerular lesions, leading to a rapidly progressive course. If the significance of glomerular stages is still unclear, there is a general agreement that tubulointerstitial changes are of utmost importance in assessing the prognosis. A number of multivariate analyses outlined that the degree of interstitial fibrosis and tubular atrophy, rather than glomerular changes, is the histologic finding more strictly associated with the renal outcome of MG.

CLINICAL PRESENTATION AND NATURAL COURSE

Approximately 70% to 80% of patients with an underlying MG have nephrotic syndrome at presentation. The remaining patients have asymptomatic proteinuria, which is usually nonselective. Macroscopic hematuria is rare, whereas microscopic hematuria can be seen in approximately half of patients. Red blood cell casts are rare. Arterial hypertension and renal dysfunction may be present at clinical onset in several cases. In some patients, however, renal insufficiency simply reflects a condition of hypovolemia either caused by severe hypoalbuminemia or induced by diuretic therapy.

Idiopathic MG may have a variable course. Spontaneous remission of the nephrotic syndrome may occur, and approximately 20% of patients may even show complete disappearance of proteinuria. Remission usually develops after 3 years or more and can be followed by further relapses of the nephrotic syndrome. Other patients show persisting nephrotic syndrome but

TABLE 39.27. Factors That May Influence the Prognosis of Membranous Glomerulonephritis

Prognostic Factor	Good	Bad
Age	Children	Adults
Sex	Female	Male
Serum albumin	Normal-low	Very low
Renal function	Normal	Impaired
Hypertension	Absent	Present
Proteinuria	Nonnephrotic	Profuse and persistent
Remission	Yes	No
Glomerular staging	1–2	3–4
Focal sclerosis	Absent	Present
Mesangial sclerosis	Present	Absent
Tubulointerstitial changes	−/+	++/+++
HLA	DR2	DR3, DR5, B37

HLA, human leukocyte antigens.

maintain normal renal function over time, whereas a number of patients show progression to renal failure or die from complications caused by their nephrotic status. Although the better management of hyperlipidemia, hypertension, thrombosis, and edemas has probably improved the prognosis of MG in the last few years, recent reviews reported that in the Caucasian population 40% to 50% of untreated nephrotic patients either died or had to be submitted to dialysis within 10 years from clinical onset. The prognosis is better in Japanese patients.

Several factors seem to influence the renal prognosis (Table 39.27). Female sex, younger age, asymptomatic proteinuria, normal blood pressure, normal renal function, and glomerular stages I and II at renal biopsy have been found to be associated with a fair prognosis, whereas patients with HLA-DR3-DR5 and B37 have been reported to have a greater likelihood of developing renal failure. However, when multivariate analyses were performed, the presence of severe tubulointerstitial lesions at renal biopsy had the most reliable predictive value, being significantly associated with an increased risk of renal failure. Two dynamic variables are important in assessing the renal prognosis. One is the persistence of elevated proteinuria for months (more than 8 g for 6 months, or more than 4 g for 18 months), which usually indicates a poor prognosis. On the other hand, complete remission of proteinuria, whether spontaneous or induced by treatment, is a strong predictor of a favorable outcome. In our experience, plasma creatinine remained stable in 33 patients with complete remission who were followed for at least 10 years after the disappearance of proteinuria. Moreover, by reviewing the literature, we found that only 1 of 157 patients who had attained complete remission eventually progressed to end-stage renal failure.

Apart from renal function deterioration, MG may expose the patient to the clinical complications of the nephrotic syndrome. Patients with MG are particularly exposed to the risk of thrombotic events. An overall incidence of approximately 30% of renal vein thrombosis, 20% of pulmonary embolism, and 10% of deep venous thrombosis may occur in nephrotic patients with MG. The thrombotic complications are probably the consequence of the typical coagulation abnormalities caused by the nephrotic syndrome. An imbalance between increased procoagulant factors (e.g., fibrinogen, platelet adhesiveness, plasma viscosity, plasminogen activator inhibitor) and decreased anticoagulant factors (e.g., decreased active proteins C and S, decreased levels of antithrombin III) leads to a hypercoagulable state that promotes thrombosis. Intravascular thrombosis is particularly frequent and severe in older patients. The risk of coronary heart disease and arterial occlusion is also increased. Several factors such as older age, hypertension, hypoalbuminemia, hyperfibrinogenemia, the hypercoagulable state, hypercholesterolemia, and increased levels of lipoprotein(a) may contribute to these complications. Moreover, nephrotic patients may show higher incidence of infection, malnutrition, hydro-electrolyte disorders, peritonitis, or pulmonary or cerebral edema.

In the long term, approximately 40% of patients who maintain normal renal function may reach a partial remission (i.e., proteinuria between 0.2 and 3.5 g/day). Relapse of nephrotic syndrome can occur within 10 years in about half of patients who do not develop renal failure. However, only a minority of these patients achieve a complete disappearance of proteinuria. In our experience, only 5% of untreated patients who presented with a nephrotic syndrome were without proteinuria at 10 years. It is difficult to predict which patient may have spontaneous remission of proteinuria. In some series it was found that women and patients with glomerular stages I or II had better chances of spontaneous remission. Instead, the presence of mesangial sclerosis at renal biopsy was associated with an extremely low rate of spontaneous remission.

TABLE 39.28. List of the Most Common Cancers Responsible for Secondary Membranous Glomerulonephritis

Lung
Colon
Rectum
Kidney
Breast
Stomach

TABLE 39.29. Causes of Rapid Deterioration of Membranous Glomerulonephritis

Cause	Diagnostic Approach	Therapy
Acute renal vein thrombosis	Echo-color Doppler scan Renal venography Magnetic resonance imaging	Fibrinolytic agents
Interstitial nephritis	Renal biopsy Blood smear	High-dose corticosteroids
Extracapillary GN	Renal biopsy Urinary sediment	High-dose corticosteroids Cyclophosphamide
Hypovolemia	Central vein pressure Bioimpedance	Plasma expanders Rehydration

GN, glomerulonephritis.

DIAGNOSIS

Although the diagnosis of MG may be suspected on clinical grounds, it requires renal biopsy to be confirmed because other primary or secondary glomerular diseases may present with a similar clinical pattern. After the histologic diagnosis has been obtained, it is important to recognize whether the disease is idiopathic or secondary to other causes. At renal biopsy, subendothelial deposits and mesangial proliferation may be seen in secondary MG; they are generally absent in the idiopathic form. The finding of IgA and/or C1q deposits by immunofluorescence also suggests a secondary MG. In many instances, thorough history and clinical examination are sufficient to identify the cause in secondary MG. Some laboratory investigations may help in recognizing a possible underlying cause. These include a serologic screening for viruses B and C, anti-DNA antibodies, and serum levels of C3 and C4 (which may be low in lupus MG and normal in idiopathic MG) and appropriate tests for malaria, filariasis, and schistosomiasis in endemic areas. Two underlying diseases may pose difficult diagnostic problems: SLE and malignant neoplasia. MG may be the first manifestation of lupus and may precede the typical serologic abnormalities of lupus even by years. The presence of subendothelial and mesangial deposits and especially C1q deposits at immunofluorescence strongly suggest a diagnosis of lupus nephritis but only the presence of viruslike particles (tubuloreticluar inclusions) or tubular basement deposits seen with electron microscopy are considered to indicate the presence of lupus nephritis. Also in the case of MG secondary to malignancy, the renal signs may antedate the initial manifestations of cancer by months or even years. Many clinicians do not carry out exhaustive tests for neoplasia. Considering which are the most common causes of underlying cancer in patients with MG (Table 39.28), we believe that it is appropriate to recommend at least a stool guaiac examination, renal ultrasonography, chest x-ray examination, and prostatic antigen. Mammography and colonoscopy should be considered in patients older than 50 years. Aged patients should be closely followed because cancer is more common in the elderly and may be undetectable on initial screening.

In patients who develop renal insufficiency, the progression is usually slow and the decrease in creatinine clearance is often linear. Rarely, however, an abrupt deterioration of renal function can occur favored by diuretics by hypovolemia related to severe hypoalbuminemia or caused by an acute dehydration. Hypovolemia is easy to recognize and may be treated with plasma volume expanders with rapid restoration of renal function. Acute renal dysfunction may be caused also by renal vein thrombosis, by a superimposed interstitial nephritis, or by extracapillary glomerulonephritis (Table 39.29). Chronic renal vein thrombosis usually does not affect renal function but an acute renal vein thrombosis can precipitate a sudden fall in renal function. The diagnosis can be suspected by the onset of a flank pain and macrohematuria and can be confirmed by echo-color Doppler scan, renal venography, or magnetic resonance imaging. An early administration of fibrinolytic agents can obtain recovery of renal function. Interstitial nephritis can be suspected by a rapidly progressive renal failure associated with fever, rash, or eosinophilia in a patient taking diuretics, allopurinol nonsteroidal antiinflammatory agents, or other drugs. Renal biopsy is often necessary to confirm the diagnosis. Stopping the causal drug and an early course of high-dose corticosteroids may reverse renal insufficiency completely. Missing the diagnosis may favor the development of irreversible interstitial fibrosis with progression to end-stage renal failure. An extracapillary glomerulonephritis can be heralded by an increase in erythrocytes and leukocytes in the urine sediment followed by a rapid deterioration of renal function; however, the final diagnosis can be performed only with renal biopsy. Prognosis and treatment of these latter cases does not differ from that of rapidly progressive pauci-immune glomerulonephritis (Table 39.29).

THERAPY (FIG. 39.15)

Symptomatic Therapy

Before considering the so-called specific therapy of MG, the importance of a well-planned symptomatic therapy, which includes treatment of edema, hypertension, hyperlipidemia, and

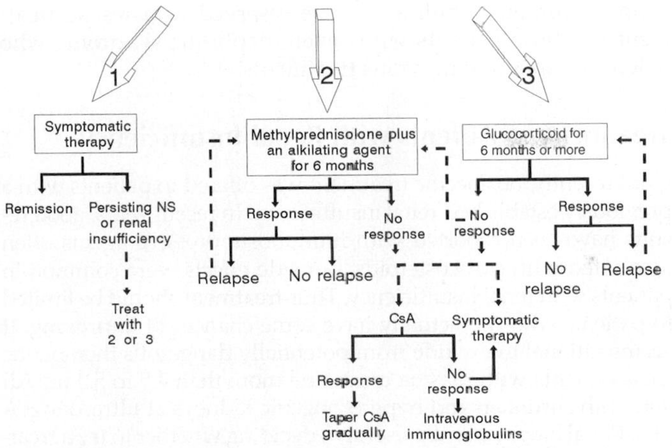

Figure 39.15. Suggested algorithm for treatment of patients with membranous glomerulonephritis and nephrotic syndrome.

hypercoagulability, must be noted. The combination of low-salt diet, diuretics, angiotensin inhibitors, and hypolipidemic drug may maintain many patients with nephrotic proteinuria in an almost asymptomatic state. The use of angiotensin-converting enzyme (ACE) inhibitors and/or antagonists of angiotensin receptors is particularly useful because these agents not only reduce systemic and intraglomerular hypertension but may also diminish urine protein excretion. In order to maximize the antiproteinuric effect, these drugs should be given at the highest-tolerated doses together with a low-salt intake or with diuretics. HMG-CoA reductase inhibitors are the preferred agents for handling hyperlipidemia. These drugs are usually well tolerated and may obtain a dose-dependent reduction of serum cholesterol. The development of myopathy is rare but may occur when high dosages are given. It is recommended to regularly check creatine phosphokinase levels, particularly in the first period of therapy, to catch early the signs of myopathy. Whether nephrotic patients should also receive anticoagulant therapy is still under discussion, although decision analyses concluded that in nephrotic patients with MG the benefits of anticoagulation are superior to the risks. At any rate, there is consensus that bedridden patients and those with more severe nephrotic syndrome (serum albumin lower than 2.5 g/dl, proteinuria more than 10 g/day), and/or antithrombin III levels lower than 75% should be given appropriate anticoagulation.

Specific Therapy

The few patients with nonnephrotic proteinuria do not need a specific therapy because they are asymptomatic and run a minimal risk of renal failure. These patients should be followed regularly, however, to recognize a possible increase in proteinuria. Whether a specific therapy should be used in patients with a nephrotic syndrome is still a matter of controversy. Some clinicians think that no effective treatment for MG is available and prefer not to expose their patients to potentially toxic drugs. Others believe that therapeutic trials should be reserved only for patients at higher risk (i.e., those with proteinuria more than 10 g/day and/or initial renal insufficiency) because in the other cases, MG may run an indolent course. A number of other nephrologists, including ourselves, think that an adequate treatment may favor remission of the nephrotic syndrome and may protect from renal function deterioration and also believe that the earlier the treatment the higher the potential benefit of therapy.

Glucocorticoids and cytotoxic drugs are the agents most commonly used in the treatment of MG. Randomized studies gave conflicting results with the use of corticosteroids. A schedule based on the administration of high-dose alternate-day prednisone (in mean 120 mg every other day) given for 8 weeks was able to reduce proteinuria and to prevent renal insufficiency in a randomized U.S. study but did not show any benefit in a double-blind, placebo-controlled trial carried out in the United Kingdom. Other trials based on short-term administration of corticosteroids or on longer treatment with low-dose prednisone failed to show any benefit. However, a high rate of remissions was reported by some retrospective studies when corticosteroids were given at high dosages for 6 months or more. Therefore it seems that corticosteroids given at high dosages for a short time or at moderate dosages for longer periods are generally ineffective. The use of high dosages for several months might favor remission but clearly exposes the patient to iatrogenic morbidity. Should corticosteroids be chosen for treating patients with MG, one might use a schedule with alternate-day oral prednisone (1 mg/kg per day every 48 hours, given in a single morning dose) for about 6 months. Another possible schedule consists of intravenous methylprednisolone pulses (1 g each) every 24 hours for 3 consecutive days followed by alternate-day oral prednisone (0.5 mg/kg every 48 hours) for 2 months. The cycle is repeated three times for a cumulative period of 6 months. A similar schedule may obtain complete or partial remission of the nephrotic syndrome in approximately 40% of patients, with little risk of side effects.

Some controlled studies showed that a prolonged treatment with chlorambucil or with cyclophosphamide may reduce proteinuria, but the effects on renal function were difficult to assess because of the short follow-ups. There is concern that a prolonged administration of a cytotoxic agent may expose to infectious and oncogenic complications in the long term. Thus alkylating agents should be given for no longer than 6 months. To give an effective treatment while reducing the side effects, we proposed a 6-month course of steroids alternated with a cytotoxic agent. Treatment consisted in 1 month of methylprednisolone (1 g for 3 days intravenously, then 0.4 mg/kg per day orally for 1 month) followed by 1 month with chlorambucil (0.2 mg/kg per day). This 2-month course was repeated three times. Three multicenter randomized trials performed in Italy showed that this therapy may favorably alter the outcome of MG. In a first study, patients with MG and a nephrotic syndrome were randomly assigned to receive supportive therapy or a 6-month treatment with methylprednisolone and chlorambucil. At 10-year follow-up, 92% of treated patients versus 60% of controls were alive without dialysis. The reciprocal of plasma creatinine was reduced by 20% at 10-year follow-up in treated patients and by 50% in untreated patients: 61% of treated patients did not have nephrotic syndrome at 10-year follow-up (of these, 40% were without proteinuria at all) versus 33% of controls (only 5% without proteinuria). In a second study, the aforementioned regimen with methylprednisolone-chlorambucil was compared with methylprednisolone alone at the same cumulative dosage used in the other arm. After a mean follow-up of 54 months, 64% of patients given the combined therapy versus 38% of patients treated with steroids alone were without nephrotic syndrome. There was a trend toward a better slope of the reciprocal of plasma creatinine in patients who received the combined therapy but the difference with the group given steroids alone was not significant because of the small number of patients followed for 4 or more years. In a third study, treatment with methylprednisolone and chlorambucil was compared with methylprednisolone at the same doses alternated every other month with cyclophosphamide (2.5 mg/kg per day). The probability of remission of nephrotic syndrome (82% versus 93% as a first event), the time to remission, and the risk of relapse were similar in the two arms.

These studies show that when compared with the natural course in untreated patients, a 6-month course of steroids alternated with an alkylating agent can prevent, in the long term, death or dialysis in approximately one-third of patients; can obtain remission of nephrotic syndrome in a high number of patients; and is more effective than steroids alone. It is important to point out that the response to treatment tends to occur toward the end of the treatment or even months later. Severe side effects, including leukopenia, infections, diabetes, or gastric intolerance, may develop in approximately 10% of treated patients. These side effects are usually reversible. However, the use of cytotoxic agents may also expose to the risk of irreversible azoospermia. The risk of malignancy seems to be low. In the cumulative experience of the three Italian studies among patients given chlorambucil, 3 cases of malignancy of 662 patient/years or 4.5/1,000 patient/years were observed, a rate similar to that of 4.3/1,000 found in the general, white, male population.

Cyclosporine and intravenous immunoglobulins may be used as alternative therapeutic options. Cyclosporine may reduce proteinuria to a nonnephrotic range in approximately two-thirds of patients. The response may occur after 2 or more months. Unfortunately, proteinuria generally increases after cyclosporine is stopped; however, a few patients may maintain without nephrotic syndrome, particularly if cyclosporine is tapered off very gradually. With cyclosporine use, the renal function should be monitored carefully. If plasma creatinine increases more than 30%, cyclosporine should be stopped and should be reassumed only after plasma creatinine returns to the baseline levels. Some small series reported that intravenous immunoglobulins (0.4 g/kg per day for 3 days repeated every 3 weeks for three times; then a single bolus repeated every 3 weeks for 10 months) can obtain substantial reduction and even the disappearance of proteinuria in a number of patients with initially normal renal function. However, this treatment is quite expensive and is not devoid of side effects. Apart from the risk of viral contamination and allergic reactions, some cases of acute renal failure have been reported.

In summary, approximately 80% of patients treated with methylprednisolone and an alkylating agent may attain remission of the nephrotic syndrome as a first event. Among responders, 20% to 30% of patients may have relapse of nephrotic syndrome. A re-treatment usually obtains the same type of response observed with the first treatment. It must be noted that patients who achieved remission tend to maintain stable renal function over time, independent of whether relapses of the nephrotic syndrome occur. Cyclosporine may obtain remission in approximately 60% of cases, but relapses are frequent if the drug is stopped or the dosage is reduced. On the basis of the available results, we suggest the following algorithm for nephrotic patients with MG. According to the clinical conditions of the patient and his or her own conviction, the physician can start with either symptomatic therapy alone or with corticosteroids for 6 months or more or with methylprednisolone alternated with a cytotoxic agent for 6 months. For patients who attained remission and then had relapse of nephrotic syndrome, the original treatment can be repeated because the probability of response to re-treatment is similar to that observed after the first course. If a patient was not treated and shows prolonged and severe nephrotic syndrome or progression to renal insufficiency, a trial with corticosteroids or with methylprednisolone plus chlorambucil or cyclophosphamide may be offered later. In the case of persisting severe nephrotic syndrome 6 to 12 months after the end of the therapeutic cycle (the response can be delayed in many cases), a trial with cyclosporine may be offered. Intravenous immunoglobulins may be reserved as a rescue treatment for those patients with severe nephrotic syndrome who failed to respond to previous treatments.

Treatment of Patients with Renal Insufficiency

Until recently, no specific treatment was offered to patients with a previously established renal insufficiency. In recent years, good results have been reported with immunosuppressive agents often associated with corticosteroids, but side effects were common in patients with renal insufficiency. Thus treatment should be limited to patients who can actually have some chances of improving. It seems rational to exclude from potentially dangerous therapeutic trials patients with plasma creatinine more than 4.5 to 5.0 mg/dl and with shrunken and hyperechogenic kidneys at ultrasonography. Renal biopsy may be useful in deciding whether to try a treatment in patients with declining renal function. Severe tubulointerstitial changes and diffuse glomerular sclerosis clearly represent a contraindication to aggressive therapies, whereas moderate tubulointerstitial lesions, moderate mesangial sclerosis, and the presence of fresh immune deposits at immunofluorescence may justify a therapeutic trial. It is difficult to recommend a specific regimen for patients with renal insufficiency. Reduction of proteinuria and improvement of renal function have been reported by several investigators with a 6-month treatment alternating methylprednisolone and chlorambucil. To reduce the risk of side effects, the dosages of methylprednisolone pulses may be reduced to 0.5 g and the dosages of oral chlorambucil may be reduced to 0.1 mg/kg per day. Good results have also been reported with prolonged administration of oral cyclophosphamide (1 to 2 years).

Treatment of Elderly Patients

Whether and how to treat older patients with MG is also controversial. Most physicians do not give any specific treatment because of the increased risk of side effects in older patients. On the other hand, elderly patients are particularly exposed to the thrombotic and cardiovascular complications of the nephrotic syndrome. Moreover, the reduced nephron mass makes the elderly kidney more susceptible to the risk of renal failure. The therapeutic decisions should be based mainly on the clinical characteristics of the patients. Corticosteroids alternated with alkylating agents may obtain the same rate of response in older and in younger adults but the frequency and the severity of side effects are increased in elderly patients. As for patients with renal insufficiency, we now also recommended that in older patients the doses of methylprednisolone pulses should not exceed 0.5 g and those of chlorambucil 0.1 mg/kg per day. In the case of contraindication to the use of corticosteroids, a 6-month treatment with cyclophosphamide (1.5 to 2.0 mg/kg per day) or chlorambucil (0.1 mg/kg) might be tried, paying particular attention that white blood cells do not fall below 3,000/cmn.

Selected Readings

Cameron JS, Healy MJR, Adu D. The Medical Research Council Trial of short-term high-dose alternate day prednisolone in idiopathic membranous nephropathy with nephrotic syndrome in adults. *Q J Med* 1990;274:133–156.

A double-blind controlled trial showing the inefficacy of an 8-week treatment with prednisone both on proteinuria and on renal function.

Cattran DC, Pai Y, Greenwood CMT, et al. Validation of a predictive model of idiopathic membranous nephropathy: its clinical and research implications. *Kidney Int* 1997;51:901–907.

A mathematic model based on the amount and duration of proteinuria for predicting the risk of renal insufficiency in patients with membranous nephropathy.

Collaborative study of the adult idiopathic nephrotic syndrome. A controlled study of short-term prednisone treatment in adults with membranous nephropathy. *N Engl J Med* 1979;301:1301–1306.

A randomized trial showing that an 8-week treatment of high-dose alternate-day prednisone can favor a transient remission of the nephrotic syndrome.

Kerjaschki D. Molecular pathogenesis of membranous nephropathy. *Kidney Int* 1992;41:1090–1105.

A study showing the main steps in the formation of immune deposits in passive model of Heymann nephritis.

Kerjaschki D, Farquhar MG. The pathogenic antigen of Heymann nephritis is a membrane glycoprotein of the renal proximal tubule brush border. *Proc Natl Acad Sci USA* 1982;79:5557–5561.

An experimental study that allowed identification in gp330 of the major antigen in Heymann nephritis.

Mathieson PW, Turner AN, Maidment CGH, et al. Prednisolone and chlorambucil treatment in idiopathic membranous nephropathy with deteriorating renal function. *Lancet* 1988;2:869–872.

A study showing that immunosuppression may reduce proteinuria and improve renal function in patients with established renal insufficiency. However, the risk of iatrogenic side effects was increased in these patients.

Ponticelli C, Altieri P, Scolari F, et al. A randomized study comparing methylprednisolone plus chlorambucil versus methylprednisolone plus cyclophosphamide in idiopathic membranous nephropathy. *J Am Soc Nephrol* 1998;9: 444–450.

A multicenter, randomized controlled trial showing the equivalent efficacy of chlorambucil and cyclophosphamide in the treatment of patients with membranous nephropathy.

Ponticelli C, Passerini P. Membranous nephropathy. In: Ponticelli C, Glassock RJ, eds. *Treatment of primary glomerulonephritis.* Oxford: Oxford Medical Publications, 1997:146–186.

A review of factors influencing the prognosis of membranous nephropathy and a critical assessment of the controlled and uncontrolled therapeutic trials attempted in this disease.

Ponticelli C, Passerini P, Altieri O, et al. Remission and relapses in idiopathic membranous nephropathy. *Nephrol Dial Transplant* 1992;7(Suppl 1):85–90.

Complete remission of proteinuria, either spontaneous or after treatment, predicts a fair renal outcome even in the long term.

Ponticelli C, Zucchelli P, Passerini P, et al. A 10-year follow-up of a randomized study with methylprednisolone and chlorambucil in membranous nephropathy. *Kidney Int* 1995;48:1600–1604.

A randomized study showing that patients assigned to receive a 6-month treatment with steroids and chlorambucil had significantly better probabilities than untreated patients of being alive with their kidneys functioning at 10 years. The number of patients with remission of the nephrotic syndrome was also significantly higher in the treated group.

Reichert CJM, Koene KAP, Wetzels JFM, et al. Preserving renal function in patients with membranous nephropathy: daily oral chlorambucil compared with intermittent monthly pulses of cyclophosphamide. *Ann Intern Med* 1994;121: 328–333.

A randomized study showing that methylprednisolone-chlorambucil can obtain better results than monthly intravenous pulses of cyclophosphamide in patients with membranous nephropathy and renal insufficiency.

Rostoker G, Belghiti D, Ben Maadi AB, et al. Long-term cyclosporin A therapy for severe idiopathic membranous nephropathy. *Nephron* 1993;63::335–341.

A study showing that cyclosporine may obtain a good rate of remission in membranous nephropathy.

Sacks SH, Warner C, Campbell RD, et al. Molecular mapping of the HLA class II region in HLA-DR3-associated idiopathic membranous nephropathy. *Kidney Int* 1993;43(S39):S13–S19.

A good review of the genetics of membranous nephropathy.

Sarasin FR, Schifferli JA. Prophylactic oral coagulation in nephrotic patients with idiopathic membranous nephropathy. *Kidney Int* 1994;45:578–585.

A decision analysis showing that the benefits of anticoagulation overcome the potential side effects in patients with membranous nephropathy and nephrotic syndrome.

Susani M, Schulze M, Exner M, et al. Antibodies to glycolipids activate complement and promote protein in passive Heymann nephritis. *Am J Pathol* 1994; 144(4):807–819.

An experimental study showing that specific antibodies for glycolipid antigen(s) activate the complement cascade and promote proteinuria in passive Heymann nephritis.

PART 7
Membranoproliferative Glomerulonephritis

C. Frederic Strife and Clark D. West

Membranoproliferative glomerulonephritis (MPGN) is the term first used by Habib in 1968 to define the pathologic appearance of a chronic and usually progressive form of glomerulonephritis, an appearance that, a few years earlier, had been described in association with persistent hypocomplementemia. Following this earlier description, it was learned that hypocomplementemia was present initially in only 70% of the patients with this glomerular morphology and as a result, the glomerular alterations became the basis for the diagnosis. This form of MPGN, which is often associated with electron-dense subendothelial deposits, became known as *type I MPGN.* Habib also classified as type II MPGN a form of nephritis described in the early 1960s in which the lamina densa of the glomerular basement membrane is replaced by electron-dense ribbonlike material, a form also called *dense deposit disease.* In the mid-1970s, use of the methenamine silver stain on biopsies to differentiate nonargyrophilic capillary loop deposits from argyrophilic basement membrane resulted in recognition of a third type of MPGN. Type III MPGN was characterized by segments of glomerular basement membrane that contained deposits and that had a laminated, fenestrated appearance. Because type III MPGN is reliably distinguished from type I only by electron microscopy of silver impregnated material, a stain not widely used, and by a detailed complement profile, most studies have not distinguished between patients with these two types. This chapter describes these types as separate and distinguishable nephritides.

Whereas MPGN type I can be both idiopathic and secondary to several systemic diseases, types II and III are idiopathic only. MPGN type II has been associated with partial lipodystrophy, suggesting a common pathogenesis. These associations have led to the classification shown in Table 39.30. The common association of type I MPGN with chronic hepatitis C infection (with or without cryoglobulinemia) is discussed in Chapter 39, Part 3B, and in Chapter 42, Part 11.

TABLE 39.30. Classification of Membranoproliferative Glomerulonephritis (MPGN)

- I. MPGN type I
  - A. Idiopathic
  - B. Secondary
    - 1. Chronic infections:
      - Bacterial: endocarditis, visceral abscesses, infected intravascular shunts, osteomyelitis
      - Viral: hepatitis B and C, HIV
      - Protozoal: malaria, schistosomiasis
      - Other: mycoplasma, fungal
    - 2. Immunologic (autoimmune) diseases
      - Systemic lupus erythematosus
      - Chronic active hepatitis
    - 3. Paraprotein deposition diseases
      - Cryoglobulinemia
      - Light-chain disease
    - 4. Neoplastic diseases
      - Leukemia/lymphoma
      - Nephroblastoma
    - 5. Miscellaneous
      - Chronic liver disease
- II. MPGN type II
  - A. Idiopathic with or without partial lipodystrophy
- III. MPGN III
  - A. Idiopathic

PATHOLOGY (SEE CHAPTER 109)

Membranoproliferative Glomerulonephritis Type I

By light microscopy, MPGN type I is the most proliferative of the three types. The proliferation is almost entirely of mesangial cells. It results in a paucity of open capillary lumens and often enlarges the glomerulus. Neutrophils may be present as in acute nephritis. Viewing methenamine silver–stained sections by light microscopy, mesangial interposition into the capillary wall can be identified by double contours of the basement membrane, considered a hallmark of this type. With time, the mesangial proliferation may be replaced by centrolobular hyaline zones with functioning capillaries festooned at the periphery of the lobules, an appearance known as *lobular glomerulonephritis.* By electron microscopy with both uranyl-lead and methenamine silver staining, the basement membrane appears intact. Subendothelial deposits are always present if the level of C3 is low at biopsy and are present in approximately 50% of the biopsies obtained when the C3 level is normal (Table 39.31). Isolated and scanty subepithelial deposits on the loops may accompany the subendothelial deposits. Differing from type III, subepithelial deposits on the paramesangial portion of the basement membrane, so-called paramesangial deposits, are very rare (Table 39.31). By immunofluorescence, the pattern of type I is distinctive; first, in that C4 is usually present as compared with its usual absence in types II and III and second, that C3, C4, and IgG are concordant in their distribution and usually confined to the periphery of the lobules, a distribution suggesting that only the peripheral capillaries are being perfused.

TABLE 39.31. Percentage of Biopsies Obtained at Low and Normal Levels of Serum C3 in Which Subendothelial and Subepithelial Paramesangial Deposits Were Found

	Subendothelial		Subepithelial Paramesangial	
	Normal C3	Low C3	Normal C3	Low C3
Type I	47(17)	100(17)	0(17)	12(17)
Type II	0(11)	0(14)	0(11)	86(14)
Type III	0(18)	54(26)	44(18)[a]	96(26)

[a] Of the total 44 type III biopsies, 33 were obtained when the C3 level was low or had been low in the preceding year. Of these 33, 31 (94%) had paramesangial deposits, whereas of 11 obtained after long-standing normocomplementemia, 2 (18%) had paramesangial deposits.

Number of biopsies examined given in parentheses.

Membranoproliferative Glomerulonephritis Type II

MPGN type II is less proliferative than type I. Viewed by light microscopy, the capillary walls in methenamine silver–stained preparations appear thickened and in some areas may be nonargyrophilic. This basement membrane abnormality, which constitutes the hallmark of the disease, is seen by electron microscopy to consist of a widening and increased density of the lamina densa, best appreciated in uranyl-lead–stained preparations. The increased density may be continuous and have a ribbonlike appearance. By methenamine silver stain, the thickened membrane is homogeneously black and the densification cannot be appreciated. Although this form is often designated dense deposit disease, the densification appears to be the result of an intrinsic change in basement membrane structure—the nature and origin of which is not understood—rather than a deposit. In addition, by electron microscopy, paramesangial deposits will be found in a high percentage of biopsies obtained during hypocomplementemia but are not seen in those obtained from normocomplementemic patients (Table 39.31). Subepithelial deposits on the loops, resembling the humps seen in acute nephritis, are present in less than half the biopsies and appear unrelated to the C3 level. Submesangial deposits are rare and subendothelial deposits are absent. By immunofluorescence with labeled antibody to C3c, three structures have been described. The margins of the abnormal glomerular basement membrane may fluoresce, giving an appearance described as railroad tracks; small rings of fluorescence may be seen in the mesangium; and, in biopsies obtained during hypocomplementemia, brightly fluorescing granules may be seen in the mesangium, which are the counterpart of the paramesangial deposits. Although these granules may appear abundant by immunofluorescence, considerable searching may be required to find paramesangial deposits in the ultrastructure. Usually immunoglobulins and C4 are not present.

Membranoproliferative Glomerulonephritis Type III

By light microscopy, the usual case of MPGN type III is distinctly less proliferative than is type I and the proliferation present is often focal in distribution. Mesangial interposition with double contours is rare. By electron microscopy, paramesangial, subendothelial, and submesangial deposits may be present, as well as subepithelial deposits on the capillary loops. A feature distinguishing type III from type I is the so-called type III lesion. In methenamine silver–stained material, widened segments of the basement membrane appear laminated, fenestrated, and disrupted, an appearance apparently produced by several generations of subepithelial and subendothelial deposits forming in conjunction with multiple interruptions of the lamina densa so that the deposits appear confluent. The laminations result from the covering of each generation of deposit by new lamina densa. By uranyl-lead stain, the type III lesion manifests as a thickened basement membrane containing discontinuous intramembranous deposits, an appearance that can lead to the mistaken diagnosis of type II. The type III lesion persists for long periods after the C3 level has come into the normal range. Recently, other means of differentiating types I and III have been described. In type I, paramesangial deposits are rarely found but are present with high frequency (94%) in patients with type III who are hypocomplementemic at biopsy or were hypocomplementemic in the year preceding biopsy (Table 39.31). Additional differentiation may be afforded by subendothelial deposits. Their absence with a low C3 level at biopsy is evidence for type III and their presence with a normal C3 level is evidence for type I. The reverse could be seen with either type. By immunofluorescence using labeled antibody to C3c, fluorescing structures are abundant, particularly if the biopsy was obtained during hypocomplementemia. Mesangial granules corresponding to paramesangial deposits are difficult to identify among the fluorescing subepithelial and subendothelial deposits. C4 is rarely found. IgG may be present in about half the biopsies but its distribution is usually not concordant with that of C3, evidence that immune complexes are not present. On follow-up biopsies, an evolution from type I to type III has been described rarely.

CLINICAL AND LABORATORY MANIFESTATIONS

Clinical Features

The three types of idiopathic MPGN have no specific geographic distribution, but are uncommon in African-Americans, suggesting a genetic predisposition. A slight preponderance of females has been inconsistently reported. The onset of all types is usually in late childhood or young adulthood.

The presenting clinical features of the three types of idiopathic MPGN are similar and generally fall into three groups

TABLE 39.32. Clinical Features of MPGN at Initial Presentation

	MPGN		
	Type I	Type II	Type III
Major Presenting Features			
Edema	20%	40%–60%	20%
Gross hematuria	25%	20%–40%	65%
Hematuria/proteinuria, no renal symptoms	30%	35%	20%
Associated Clinical Features			
Hypertension	30%–40%	30%–50%	30%
Renal insufficiency	30%–60%	10%–40%	10%–20%
Low serum C3 level	68%	92%	84%
Partial lipodystrophy	—	6%–14%	Reported
Acute infection preceding abnormal urine	40%	50%–80%	?

(Table 39.32). Approximately one-third of patients present because of edema and are found to have hematuria with red blood cell and granular casts, heavy proteinuria, and mild to moderate hypoalbuminemia. In addition, there may be constitutional complaints including lassitude, malaise, and weight loss. In our experience, constitutional symptoms are most common in children with type I MPGN. Approximately 25% of patients present with an acute nephritic syndrome with gross hematuria; mild hypoalbuminemia and hypertension; and, especially in children with this presentation, the initial working diagnosis is often acute poststreptococcal glomerulonephritis (APSGN). Indications for biopsy to distinguish MPGN from APSGN are a normal initial serum C3 level, found in approximately 30% of MPGN and 10% of APSGN patients, and failure of an initially reduced C3 level to become normal 6 to 8 weeks after presentation. An occasional patient with MPGN, especially type II, will have an acute nephritic syndrome with rapid deterioration of renal function. The course could be consistent with a rapidly progressive glomerulonephritis or with APSGN and is again an indication for biopsy. The remaining cases are discovered by investigation of the chance finding of microscopic hematuria and proteinuria in an otherwise healthy individual. This is a frequent presentation in children with type III. Hypertension is present initially in about one-third of all patients with MPGN. Interestingly, an elevation of serum creatinine at initial evaluation is less common in type III MPGN, presumably because of less mesangial proliferation.

Laboratory Findings

The frequency at diagnosis of hypocomplementemia, defined as a low serum level of C3, is approximately 78% in children. It is somewhat lower in adults and in patients with type I (Table 39.32). The hypocomplementemia is multifactorial. In MPGN types II and III, it is produced by autoantibodies known as *nephritic factors.* The nephritic factor in type II was originally designated C3NeF but was subsequently named the nephritic factor of the amplification loop, NF_a. It is directed against the activated factor B component (Bb) of the alternative pathway C3 convertase, C3b, Bb. This convertase is always circulating but in low concentration because it is both unstable and highly susceptible to dissociation by factors H and I. However, when in the form C3b, Bb, NF_a, its half life is extended from 90 seconds to 50 minutes.

The nephritic factor in MPGN type III is the more recently described NF_t, or nephritic factor of the terminal pathway. Whereas NF_a activates only the amplification loop of the complement system, NF_t activates this loop and the terminal pathway. Also NF_t is properdin dependent, whereas NF_a is not. Because of its properdin dependence and the fact that several C3b molecules in close proximity are necessary for terminal pathway activation, its composition is thought to be $C3b_n$,Bb,P,NF_t.

In mixtures of normal and nephritic serum, C3 conversion by NF_a is complete after 30 minutes of incubation, whereas the maximum effect of NF_t is found only after 3 to 4 hours. Because NF_t perturbs the terminal pathway and the amplification loop, the complement profile produced by it is very different from that produced by NF_a. Thus, with abundant NF_a in type II, only the level of C3 is markedly depressed and levels of properdin and terminal components are normal or minimally depressed. In type III, on the other hand, levels of properdin and C5, as well as C3, are depressed and one or more of the other terminal components may also be in low concentration.

In MPGN type I, glomerular morphology, immunohistology, and the complement profile are compatible with a pathogenesis based on circulating immune complexes. The complement profile may give evidence of classical pathway activation; approximately half of hypocomplementemic patients will have a low serum level of C4 and in many of these, the C2 level will be depressed also. However, approximately one-third will have minimal evidence of classical pathway activation and serum levels of C6, C7, and/or C9 will be reduced, indicating the presence of NF_t. However, other aspects of the nephritis in these patients will be compatible with type I. Why some have circulating NF_t is not known.

In addition to the complement abnormalities, a few patients with MPGN will have a normochromic, normocytic anemia out of proportion to the degree of renal insufficiency. The origin of this anemia is unclear. Some authors have suggested "innocent bystander" lysis of erythrocytes by activated complement components. Obviously, in addition, many will have the usual laboratory abnormalities associated with renal failure and nephrotic syndrome.

PATHOGENESIS

MPGN type I is presumably a response to the glomerular deposition of circulating immune complexes or their *in situ* formation. This origin is evident from the glomerular ultrastructure, the immunohistology, the complement profile, and from the fact that a similar glomerular morphology can be seen with the nephritides associated with chronic antigenemia. Although a variety of antigens of infectious, immunologic, and oncotic neoplastic origin have been associated with the secondary forms of MPGN type I (Table 39.30), the origin and nature of the antigen in idiopathic type I MPGN is not known.

In type II MPGN, the frequent recurrence of dense intramembranous alterations in cadaver renal transplant recipients is evidence that this disorder has its origin in a systemic process. The altered lamina densa can be present for a very long time without clinical evidence for glomerulonephritis. Thus it may be necessary for a second, undefined process to occur to induce clinical glomerulonephritis.

There is evidence that some of the glomerular abnormalities of MPGN types II and III are related to C3 convertase stabilized by nephritic factor. First, as seen in Table 39.31, paramesangial deposits in MPGN types II and III and subendothelial deposits in type III are closely associated with the presence, or the presence over the previous year, of nephritic factor. Second, in certain "experiments of nature" in which native, unstabilized convertase circulates in excess such as factor H deficiency, the main glomerular deposits are paramesangial. Although convertase circulating in excess seems to be a common denominator in these nephritides, there is no evidence that it is a component of the deposits, and the nature of the association between circulating convertase and the deposits is not clear. It should be noted that the dense intramembranous deposits in MPGN type II do not demonstrably relate to the presence of nephritic factor stabilized convertase.

There is also compelling evidence for a genetic predisposition to idiopathic MPGN. MPGN of all types is rare in African-Americans and the disease has been reported in siblings. In patients with MPGN types I and III the extended haplotype, HLA-B8, DR3, SC01, GLO2, on the short arm of chromosome 6 was noted in 13% compared with 1% in controls. The association of this haplotype with other diseases of autoimmune origin (type 1 diabetes mellitus, gluten sensitive enteropathy, systemic lupus erythematosus) suggests the possibility of autoimmune phenomena in MPGN. Patients with MPGN types I or III also have a significantly higher incidence of inherited defects of the complement system than do controls (23% versus 6.7%). Although these observations give evidence that factors basic to the pathogenesis of types I and III are similar, their many differences warrant considering them as different entities.

NATURAL HISTORY AND PROGNOSIS

The natural history of MPGN is such that in the absence of effective treatment, irrespective of type, 50% develop end-stage renal disease by 10 years after diagnosis and 90% have renal insufficiency by 20 years. Untreated patients with proteinuria initially in the nephrotic range and/or renal insufficiency and/or hypertension progress more rapidly. According to a recent observation, seven initially nonnephrotic, untreated children with MPGN had normal renal function and a serum albumin greater than 3.0 g/dl after a median follow-up of 9.8 years. Presentation with gross hematuria may also correlate with poorer outcome. As might be expected, the presence of crescents in the initial biopsy is a poor prognostic indicator, and some series have found patients with type II, a type with a high incidence of crescents, to deteriorate more rapidly.

TREATMENT

The progressive nature of MPGN has led to numerous treatment regimens, many not tested by controlled trials. The benefit suggested by early uncontrolled studies using a combination of Coumadin and dipyridamole and, in some, cyclophosphamide could not be substantiated in subsequent controlled prospective trials. Likewise, early enthusiasm for inhibition of platelet function with aspirin and dipyridamole, although associated with short-term stabilization of renal function, was found to be as ineffective as placebo in long-term trials.

There have been several reports of uncontrolled trials of an alternate-day prednisone regimen used either alone or in combination with immunosuppressive agents and/or dipyridamole. Although they have employed a variety of dosage schedules, the reports have all indicated improvement in renal function, glomerular morphology, urinalysis, and patient survival in comparison with historic controls. Two placebo-controlled trials support the uncontrolled observations. In one trial conducted by the International Study of Kidney Diseases in Children, 80 children with MPGN, irrespective of type, who had heavy proteinuria and a glomerular filtration rate in excess of 70 ml/min/m^2 body surface area were randomized to receive prednisone, 40 mg/m^2 per dose on alternate days versus placebo for 5 years. The two groups were compared for *treatment failure,* defined as an increase from baseline of serum creatinine of at least 30%, or more than 35 μmol/L (0.4 mg/dl). Treatment failure occurred in 55% of the placebo-treated and 40% of the prednisone-treated patients. Renal function remained unchanged (i.e., increase in serum creatinine less than 30% or less than 35 μmol/ml from baseline) after 130 months in 61% of the treated patients versus 12% of the placebo group. When types I and III patients were analyzed separately from the type II patients, treatment failed in 33% of the prednisone-treated patients compared with 58% of patients receiving placebo. The efficacy of prednisone could not be assessed in the small number of type II patients. In a smaller study, after an average follow-up of 6 years, 8 prednisone-treated patients had stable or improved renal function, whereas 4 of 10 placebo-treated patients had progressed to end-stage renal failure. The improvements in glomerular morphology seen after 2 years of the alternate-day prednisone regimen include an increase in the number of open capillary lumens, reductions in capillary wall thickening, and mesangial proliferation. However, often associated with this improvement are "chronic" changes including increased glomerulosclerosis and tubular atrophy. The development of these changes appears confined to the 1 or 2 years after institution of the alternate-day regimen and may be responsible for persistence of proteinuria despite evidence that the disease is in remission.

There have been no published studies comparing the response to the alternate-day regimen in the three types of MPGN. It is our experience, however, that children with type I are the most responsive. Within 1 year, preexisting nephrotic syndrome disappears in 80%, serum C3 level returns to normal in most (Fig. 39.16), renal function improves or is stabilized, and microscopic hematuria and often proteinuria are no longer present. A repeat biopsy shows less mesangial proliferation and more open capillary lumens. In contrast, patients with type III, although often with a less severe nephritis initially, improve more slowly. After 2 or 3 years, the serum C3 level may still be low (Fig. 39.16) and the improvement in urinalysis and glomerular morphology is less marked than in patients with type I.

Although accumulated data indicate long-term benefit from steroid treatment of all three types of idiopathic MPGN, the optimal dose, dosage schedule, and duration of treatment needs continuing investigation. Some have advocated postponing treatment until there is evidence of deterioration in an effort to avoid or minimize adverse steroid effects. On the other hand, our data indicate that the outcome of children started on alternate-day prednisone within 1 year of onset is significantly better than that of patients in whom treatment is delayed. Thus with the possible exception of patients with very mild proteinuria or the unusual patient with mild "focal" MPGN, delaying therapy may compromise outcome. The value of initiating treatment with a short course of intravenous methylprednisolone or with daily prednisone before starting the alternate-day regimen has not been determined. The doses of prednisone given at one time on alternate days reported to be effective range from 40 to 60 mg/m^2, with a maximum dosage of 60 to 80 mg. In patients with type I, the dose may be reduced by stepwise reductions of one-fourth of the initial dose so that the regimen is stopped after 2 to 4 years, but our experience would indicate that the dose should be lowered more slowly in patients with types II and III. Reduction in dosage depends on the clinical response, especially with respect to improvement in the urinalysis, normalization of the serum C3 level, and the degree of improvement in the follow-up renal biopsy

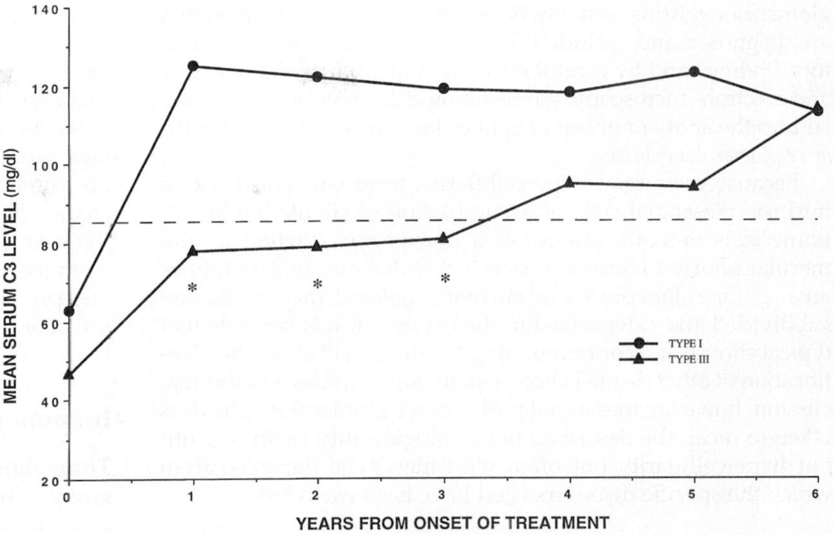

Figure 39.16. The yearly mean serum C3 concentrations from 28 patients with MPGN type I are compared with those from 32 patients with type III for 6 years following onset of the alternate-day prednisone regimen. A significant difference ($P < .05$) between the yearly mean values is indicated by an asterisk. The lower limit of normal C3 concentration is indicated by the dashed horizontal line.

obtained after 2 years of treatment. An important clinical criterion of improvement is reduction and disappearance of hematuria. Hypertension, often present at diagnosis and aggravated by the alternate-day regimen, should be aggressively treated and its presence is not an indication to discontinue the prednisone or reduce the dose. As the steroid dose is reduced and discontinued, continued monitoring is necessary to detect disease relapse, most often seen with types II and III. It has been manifested by recurrence of hematuria and/or an increase in proteinuria, often with a reduction in the serum C3 level. Relapses usually respond to an increase in the dose of prednisone given on alternate days.

Selected Readings

Cameron JS, Turner DR, Heaton J, et al. Idiopathic mesangiocapillary glomerulonephritis: comparison of types I and II in children and adults and long-term prognosis. *Am J Med* 1983;74:175–192.

An overview of the clinical features and prognosis of MPGN with respect to age and disease type.

Droz D, Nabarra B, Noel L-H, et al. The recurrence of dense deposits in transplanted kidneys: I. Sequential survey of the lesions. *Kidney Int* 1979;15:386–395.

Details of the clinical course and glomerular morphology of 11 patients with MPGN type II who underwent renal transplantation. The emphasis is on recurrence of dense intramembranous deposits in the transplanted kidney.

Habib R, Gubler M-C, Loirat C, et al. Dense deposit disease: a variant of membranoproliferative glomerulonephritis. *Kidney Int* 1975;7:204–215.

A detailed study of the clinical onset, renal pathology and long-term outcome of 44 patients with MPGN type II. The results include complement measurements over many years and outcome of renal function (kidney survival).

Habib R, Kleinknecht C, Gubler MC, et al. Idiopathic membranoproliferative glomerulonephritis in children. Report of 105 cases. *Clin Nephrol* 1973;1:194–214.

A detailed analysis of clinical and pathologic presentation of a large cohort of patients with MPGN. Long-term follow-up enables an understanding of the natural history of MPGN.

Jackson EC, McAdams AJ, Strife CF, et al. Differences between membranoproliferative glomerulonephritis types I and III in clinical presentation, glomerular morphology, and complement perturbation. *Am J Kidney Dis* 1987;9:115–120.

Patients with type III MPGN more often presented with chance proteinuria and hematuria and had more open capillary lumens on initial biopsy than patients with type I. Activation of the classical pathway of complement was evidenced in type I by lower serum C4 levels and greater frequency of C4 and IgG in the glomerular deposits than in type III.

Lamb V, Tisher CC, McCoy RC, et al. Membranoproliferative glomerulonephritis with dense intramembranous alterations: a clinicopathological study. *Lab Invest* 1977;36:607–617.

A detailed description of the glomerular morphology and clinical course of 10 patients with MPGN type II before and after renal transplantation.

McEnery PT, McAdams AJ, West CD. The effect of prednisone in a high-dose, alternate day regimen on the natural history of idiopathic membranoproliferative glomerulonephritis. *Medicine* (Baltimore) 1985;64:401–424.

A single-center uncontrolled evaluation of the long-term outcome of patients with MPGN treated with an alternate-day prednisone regime compared with historic controls.

Strife CF, McEnery PT, McAdams AJ, et al. Membranoproliferative glomerulonephritis with disruption of the glomerular basement membrane. *Clin Nephrol* 1977;7:65–72.

A description of the lesion of the glomerular basement membrane that characterizes MPGN type III (the so-called type III lesion) and a comparison of type III with type I with respect to immunohistology and other aspects of the ultrastructure.

Tarshish P, Bernstein J, Tobin JN, et al. Treatment of mesangiocapillary glomerulonephritis with alternate-day prednisone—a report of The International Study of Kidney Disease in Children. *Pediatr Nephrol* 1992;6:123–130.

A prospective, randomized, controlled trial of alternate-day prednisone versus placebo in children with MPGN. This study suggests that patients treated with alternate-day prednisone had improved outcome when compared with placebo-treated patients.

West CD, McAdams AJ. Membranoproliferative glomerulonephritis type III: the association of glomerular deposits with circulating nephritic factor stabilized convertase. *Am J Kidney Dis* 1998;32:1–9.

Glomerular deposits present in MPGN types I and III as found in biopsies obtained at low and normal C3 levels are compared.

PART 8
Mesangial Proliferative Glomerulonephritis

Arthur H. Cohen and Sharon G. Adler

Mesangial proliferative glomerulonephritis is a morphologic entity that is defined by light microscopy and, in its complete form, is characterized by glomerular mesangial hypercellularity usually affecting all lobules to a more or less equal degree. Capillary walls are thin and single contoured, and initially, there are no complicating abnormalities such as adhesions or segments of sclerosis. This lesion may be manifested by near-normal glomeruli with only mild expansion and no hypercellularity of mesangial regions (termed *mesangial injury glomerulonephritis*). Immune deposits in mesangial regions, however, may be detected by both immunofluorescence and electron microscopic examinations. This pattern of glomerular injury is associated with varying degrees of proteinuria, often with hematuria. It should be appreciated that this morphologic definition includes many well-characterized glomerulonephritides, including mesangial lupus glomerulonephritis, IgA nephropathy (Berger's disease), Henoch-Schönlein purpura nephritis, resolving postinfectious glomerulonephritis, and others. When these well-defined entities are diagnosed and excluded on the basis of clinical and laboratory findings and by careful evaluation by immunofluorescence and electron microscopy, the resulting collection of lesions constitutes the entity or group of entities known as *mesangial proliferative glomerulonephritis.*

Because mesangial hypercellularity, from either increase in intrinsic mesangial cells or accumulation of circulating blood-borne cells or both, represents a nonspecific reaction to glomerular injury, it is entirely conceivable that mesangial proliferative glomerulonephritis as currently defined may be further subdivided and categorized in the future, for it is possible that typical clinical and/or immunologic features will allow the identification of other distinct clinical–pathologic entities. For this discussion, however, mesangial proliferative glomerulonephritis is taken to mean the described morphologic entity (with or without hypercellularity but often with mesangial deposits) from which the specific disorders cited have been excluded.

CLINICAL AND LABORATORY FEATURES

The incidence of mesangial proliferative glomerulonephritis is unknown, but this entity accounts for between 5% and 10% of renal biopsies performed for low-grade proteinuria, nephrotic syndrome, hematuria with or without proteinuria, and azotemia. Most often, patients with this lesion have asymptomatic proteinuria, microscopic hematuria, or heavy (nephrotic-range) proteinuria with or without microhematuria. Red blood cell casts or gross hematuria occasionally may be seen. Mild hypertension may be evident at onset in up to one-third of affected patients. At the time of diagnosis, mild to moderate azotemia is present in roughly 25% to 50% of patients. Because these clinical features may be observed in many other glomerulopathies, the diagnosis is made by examination of renal tissue at biopsy. Results of laboratory studies, such as serum complement, immunoglobulin levels, and antinuclear and antistreptococcal antibodies, are normal or negative. As with other forms of glomerular injury with nephrotic-range proteinuria, serum albumin may be low and lipids elevated. Circulating immune complexes are present in 50% to 70% of the patients onset, although their significance is not known. Genetic determinants have not been identified, although familial forms of this disorder with mesangial IgM deposits have been described. It is of interest to note that other glomerulopathies, including IgA nephropathy, were present in other family members.

PATHOLOGY

Light Microscopy (Fig. 109.10A)

The hallmark of this glomerulopathy is, as expected, in mesangial regions of glomeruli. They are expanded and have varying degrees of increased cellularity, characteristically affecting all lobules of all glomeruli to an equal degree, often with a concomitant increase in mesangial matrix. Deposits may be identified in mesangial or paramesangial regions when appropriate histochemical techniques, such as Masson's trichrome stain, are performed. This finding is present in up to 50% of biopsies. Typically, capillaries are patent, and basement membranes are thin and single contoured. Early in the course of the disease, tubular and interstitial lesions are absent, although with heavy proteinuria, protein reabsorption droplets may be seen in tubular epithelial cell cytoplasm. Arteriolar sclerosis (insudative lesion) is present in up to 50% of patients.

As the lesion progresses both clinically and pathologically, the basic glomerular abnormalities may be complicated by focal and segmental sclerosis, the morphology of which is identical to that occurring in idiopathic focal and segmental glomerulosclerosis. As will be discussed, the morphologic lesions, both with and without segmental sclerosis, and the clinical presentations are sometimes considered part of the spectrum of minimal-change disease–focal and segmental glomerulosclerosis. Under these circumstances, the morphologic overlap with both lesions is understandable. On the other hand, if one considers mesangial proliferative glomerulonephritis a distinct entity, it is not unusual to expect segmental glomerulosclerosis as a complication, as in many other diverse glomerulopathies.

Immunofluorescence Microscopy (Fig. 109.10B)

Throughout the years, many series of mesangial proliferative glomerulonephritis have not included regular immunofluorescence microscopic examination of biopsies. As a result, it was and is difficult to assess the occurrence of some of the more specifically named glomerulopathies in the groups of patients with this morphologic lesion. This is especially true for excluding cases of IgA nephropathy, the morphology of which may be identical to that of mesangial proliferative glomerulonephritis at both light and electron microscopic levels of examination. Once IgA nephropathy is excluded, however, there is a relatively limited number of combinations of protein deposits found by immunofluorescence. Most commonly, IgM is the predominant immunoglobulin, deposited in all mesangial regions in a granular pattern. There also may be isolated granular capillary wall deposits. IgM is accompanied often by C3 and less often by C1q in a similar distribution. Some investigators have delineated this as a distinct clinical and pathologic entity known as *IgM nephropathy.* When IgM is present, other immunoglobulins are almost always absent. Other patterns have been described and, based on the predominant protein deposit, have given rise to the names of different and, perhaps, distinct nephropathies. For C1q nephropathy (see Chapter 39, Part 11), in addition to C1q (which is in greatest intensity), variable IgG, IgA, IgM, and C3 are in mesangial regions in all glomeruli. IgG, with or without C3, is known as *IgG nephropathy*, whereas C3 alone is known as *C3 nephropathy.* Perhaps no more than 5% of biopsies in which mesangial hypercellularity occurs in the clinical setting described have negative immunofluorescence.

Electron Microscopy (Fig. 109.10C)

The ultrastructural abnormalities affect both the mesangium and the glomerular capillary walls. Increased numbers or size of existing mesangial cells may be observed. In the latter instance, enlargement of the cytoplasm and prominence of organelles are found. There is also increased matrix. In roughly 50% of the biopsies, typically when immunofluorescence is positive, electron-dense deposits are noted in the mesangium. The deposits are usually smaller and less conspicuous than in IgA nephropathy. Perhaps 25% of the biopsies with positive fluorescence will have ill-defined electron densities occurring within the mesangial matrix. In the remaining biopsies, no electron-dense deposits of any type are noted. In patients with heavy proteinuria, the foot processes of epithelial cells are effaced. Basement membranes are of normal thickness and appearance. Capillary wall electron-dense deposits are absent. When the glomerular lesion is complicated by segments of sclerosis, the ultrastructural features of that lesion are also present.

PATHOGENESIS

The presence of granular immune and electron-dense deposits suggests that the lesion results from immune-complex deposition and complement fixation. However, it is also possible that altered mesangial function may result in nonspecific trapping of these proteins and that the deposits may well represent an epiphenomenon. As with other forms of glomerular injury with mesangial deposits, the existence of deposits does not always elicit a cellular response. Hence, the alternative terms *mesangial injury* or *mesangiopathic* rather than proliferative glomerulonephritis are used to indicate the lack of hypercellularity but not the lack of injury or damage to the mesangium. Nevertheless, regardless of the manner in which the proteins accumulate in the mesangium, the precise relation between the mesangial injury and the manifestations of proteinuria and/or hematuria is unknown.

DIFFERENTIAL DIAGNOSIS

Because few clinical or laboratory features permit differentiation of mesangial proliferative glomerulonephritis from other entities associated with the clinical manifestations, this entity may be confused with any glomerulopathy with proteinuria and/or hematuria. By definition, systemic signs or serologic evidence pointing to a specific disease (secondary glomerulonephritis) are not present in this disorder. Therefore the differential diagnosis includes all of the primary glomerulopathies responsible for the urine abnormalities described. Patients with heavy proteinuria need to be distinguished from those with membranous glomerulonephritis, minimal-change disease, focal and segmental glomerulosclerosis, IgA nephropathy, or membranoproliferative (mesangiocapillary) glomerulonephritis. This last entity may be excluded by the absence of hypocomplementemia and circulating C3 nephritic factor. Although it is possible to make a correct diagnosis among the former choices by using such data as the presence or absence of azotemia, hypertension, episodes of hematuria, degree of selectivity of proteinuria, patient age, responsiveness to glucocorticoid therapy, and serum IgM and IgA levels, no combination of clinical or serologic data permits the establishment of a definitive diagnosis. Causes of low-grade proteinuria include the entire gamut of glomerular, tubular, urologic, and systemic disorders that can manifest themselves in a similar fashion. Patients whose major clinical presentation is hematuria must be distinguished from those affected with IgA nephropathy or with renal infections, such as tuberculosis, renal and urinary tract neoplasms, various forms of cystic disease, arteriovenous malformations, loin pain–hematuria syndrome, thin basement membrane nephropathy, heredofamilial nephritis, and toxic nephropathies.

TREATMENT

Therapy for mesangial proliferative glomerulonephritis has not been well defined. In most instances, patients with microhematuria with or without mild proteinuria are untreated, primarily because the long-term prognosis is good and specific therapies are thought to be ineffective. When present, hypertension should be treated rigorously. On the other hand, a more aggressive approach has been advocated for patients with nephrotic-range proteinuria. To some extent, the rationale for the use of glucocorticoids in this group is derived from the belief that mesangial proliferative glomerulonephritis, especially with IgM deposits, may be an intermediate form in the spectrum of disorders that includes minimal-change disease at the more benign end and focal and segmental glomerulosclerosis at the more malignant end. Consequently, many investigators have modeled therapy of mesangial proliferative glomerulonephritis with nephrotic syndrome on that used for patients with minimal-change disease. With high-dose oral prednisone (60 mg/day or 120 mg every other day in adults), remissions have been reported in as many as 65% of patients. However, frequent relapses, steroid dependence, and partial remissions are common. Nephrotic patients without hematuria are more likely to be steroid responsive than are those with hematuria. In children who are initially unresponsive to glucocorticoids, late remission of nephrotic syndrome is common.

Therapy with cytotoxic agents is somewhat controversial. However, in small groups of patients, cyclophosphamide and chlorambucil appear to be useful adjuncts to glucocorticoids in treating steroid-unresponsive, steroid-dependent, or frequently relapsing nephrotic syndrome. Cytotoxic agents occasionally have been reported to induce remission of nephrotic syndrome in a small number of steroid-unresponsive patients. Although cyclosporine has been employed in a few patients with minimal-change disease or focal and segmental glomerulosclerosis who are either steroid resistant, steroid dependent, or frequent relapsers, the usefulness of this agent in mesangial proliferative glomerulonephritis remains to be determined. A single patient treated with FK506 did not respond to therapy. The efficacy of other therapies, such as nonsteroidal antiinflammatory drugs, angiotensin-converting enzyme inhibitors, and in inducing remission or diminishing proteinuria has not been specifically studied in this lesion. Renal transplantation has been reported in relatively few patients with mesangial proliferative glomerulonephritis, especially with IgM deposits. Isolated instances of recurrence of clinical and pathologic lesions have appeared, but the exact incidence of this feature is unknown.

COURSE AND PROGNOSIS

The clinical course may be as variable as the major presenting manifestations and, to some degree, is linked to the initial manifestation. Most reports suggest that patients with isolated hematuria usually maintain normal renal function for a prolonged period of time, although microscopic hematuria persists and, as with IgA nephropathy, may be punctuated by episodes of gross hematuria. Patients with low-grade proteinuria with or without accompanying microscopic hematuria also have a favorable long-term prognosis. On the other hand, patients with heavy proteinuria are most likely to develop more progressive renal insufficiency, culminating in end-stage renal disease, often within several years of onset. Multivariate analysis of clinical, histologic, and immunopathologic variables indicated that the duration of time from diagnosis to end-stage renal disease is adversely influenced by the following factors identified at the time of biopsy: elevated serum creatinine, heavy proteinuria, microscopic hematuria, complete glomerulosclerosis affecting more than 10% of the glomeruli, segmental glomerulosclerosis, increased mesangial matrix, and pronounced mesangial hypercellularity. The loss of renal function is heralded by the appearance of worsening of hypertension and heavier proteinuria. Progressive azotemia is more likely in nephrotic patients who are steroid dependent or steroid resistant. At this stage of the illness, repeat biopsies will show focal and segmental sclerosing lesions of glomeruli and tubular atrophy and interstitial fibrosis. These latter patients are uniformly unresponsive to glucocorticoids.

Selected Readings

Border WA. Distinguishing minimal change disease from mesangial disorders. *Kidney Int* 1988;34:419–434.

A thoughtful overview of minimal-change disease and mesangial injury glomerulonephritis with IgM deposits, providing a rational basis for separating these entities from one another.

Ginesta JC, Almirall J, Torras A, et al. Long-term evolution of patients with isolated C3 mesangial glomerulonephritis. *Clin Nephrol* 1995;43:221–225.

Review of clinical manifestations and course in a series of 11 patients from one institution.

Habib R, Churg J, Bernstein J, et al. Minimal change disease, mesangial proliferative glomerulonephritis and focal sclerosis: individual entities or a spectrum of disease? In: Robinson RR, ed. *Nephrology*. New York: Springer-Verlag, 1984: 634–644.

A thorough analysis of the controversy surrounding the interrelation of minimal-change disease, mesangial proliferative glomerulonephritis, and focal sclerosis.

Iskander SS, Browning MC, Lorentz WB. C1q nephropathy; a pediatric clinicopathologic study. *Am J Kidney Dis* 1991;18:456–465.

A series of children with C1q nephropathy with poor response to oral prednisone.

Yoshikawa N, Iijima I, Shimomura M, et al. IgG-associated primary glomerulonephritis in children. *Clin Nephrol* 1994;42:281–287.

A case made for IgG mesangial proliferative glomerulonephritis as a distinct entity.

PART 9
Crescentic Glomerulonephritis

Roger C. Wiggins and David B. Kershaw

Crescentic glomerulonephritis is the nonspecific response of the glomerulus to severe inflammation. The major structural feature is that Bowman's space, which is normally a protected area for the collection of glomerular filtrate, becomes occupied by fibrin, cells, and matrix materials that lead to obliterative scar formation and permanent loss of that nephron. Crescentic nephritis is a treatable condition in its early phases, but if not treated urgently may lead to permanent loss of renal function. The clinical syndrome associated with extensive glomerular crescent formation is called *rapidly progressive glomerulonephritis (RPGN).* The diagnosis and treatment of RPGN is a medical emergency.

PATHOGENESIS AND PATHOLOGY

Glomerular inflammation leading to crescent formation is associated with a variety of different underlying pathogenic processes as shown in Fig. 39.17. Although antibody-driven mechanisms are thought to play a role in several forms of crescentic nephritis, it is very likely that T-cell–driven processes are important elements in initiation and progression to scar formation. T-cell–dependent (Th_1 or Th_2 predominant) pathways may determine outcome.

Severe inflammation rapidly forces the glomerulus through a series of recognizable structural "stages" that can be recognized readily on the renal biopsy (Fig. 39.18). These stages include accumulation of cells in glomerular capillaries (stage 1), fibrin formation in Bowman's space (stage 2), the accumulation of cells in Bowman's space to form a cellular "crescent" (stage 3), the accumulation of matrix materials to replace damaged intrinsic glomerular cells and structures (stage 4), and the subsequent permanent replacement of the glomerulus by scar (stage 5). The stages before stage 4 are potentially reversible. It is scar formation that causes permanent loss of structure and function thereby sealing the fate of the glomerulus. Minor or segmental crescent

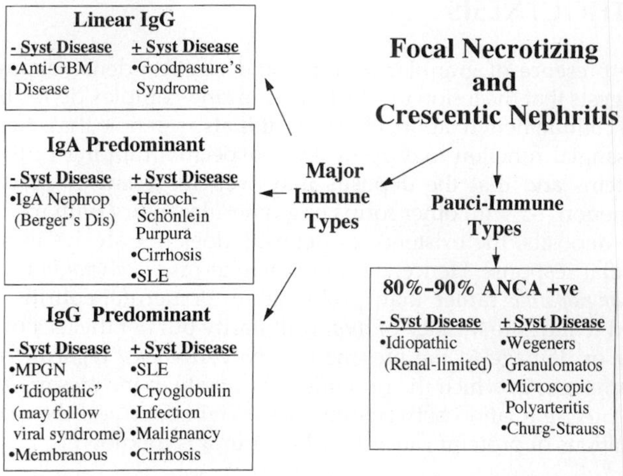

Figure 39.17. Major potential mechanisms driving glomerular inflammation as assessed by an immunofluorescent analysis of the renal biopsy. Immunofluorescent analysis of the renal biopsy taken in conjunction with the clinical picture (± systemic disease) provides helpful information about the likely underlying mechanisms responsible for glomerular inflammation and injury. General categories only are given. SLE, systemic lupus erythematosus.

formation is common in many forms of glomerular inflammation. The pathologist usually counts only those glomeruli containing large circumferential crescents (more than 50% of glomerular circumference) because these are most closely associated with poor outcome. Severe crescent formation is also commonly accompanied by inflammation, edema, and scarring in the interstitial (periglomerular) compartment, which itself contributes significantly to progression of injury and dysfunction.

Factors other than circulating antibodies or immune complexes may be necessary to trigger acute severe glomerular inflammation and injury. Thus individuals may have circulating antibodies [e.g., anti–glomerular basement membrane (GBM) antibodies or anti–neutrophil cytoplasmic antibodies (ANCA)] but not have active disease. Intercurrent infection or other immune stimulation may activate the immune/inflammatory systems nonspecifically, thereby allowing the presence of circulating antibodies or immune complexes to target the glomerulus and initiate the sequence of events leading to crescent formation. Hypertension may also be a factor in promoting enhanced glomerular injury in the face of circulating immune complexes. Similar triggering processes probably also occur in IgA nephropathy, lupus nephritis, and infection-associated glomerular injury. Whether the lung is involved in anti-GBM disease appears to be determined in part by whether an individual smokes or inhales fumes that are toxic to pulmonary tissue (e.g., cocaine). This is an example of local factors helping to target the immune attack, which in turn determines the shape of the clinical syndrome in an individual patient. Thus these "autoimmune diseases" are multifactorial with more than a single motivating force causing the disease process and the particular presenting clinical syndrome. This concept helps explain the protean nature of many of the disease processes that have glomerular inflammation as one component of their potential constellation of features.

The complete cycle of glomerular inflammation from initial immune attack through to obliterative scarring in crescentic nephritis takes approximately 30 days. Figure 39.18 shows the time course for an individual glomerulus. Not all glomeruli are in the same phase of injury at any one time. Thus the proportion of glomeruli involved and the synchronicity of glomerular injury will help to determine both the acuteness of presentation as well as the potential for recovery. This time course is similar to other wound healing–like processes, whether the damage is caused by the immune system or by other processes. As is illus-

A. Pathology and Time Course

Normal Glomerulus	Inflammation Necrosis in Glom Tuft	Fibrin in Bowmans Space	Cells in Bowmans Space	Collagen Synthesis Accumulation	Scarred Glomerulus

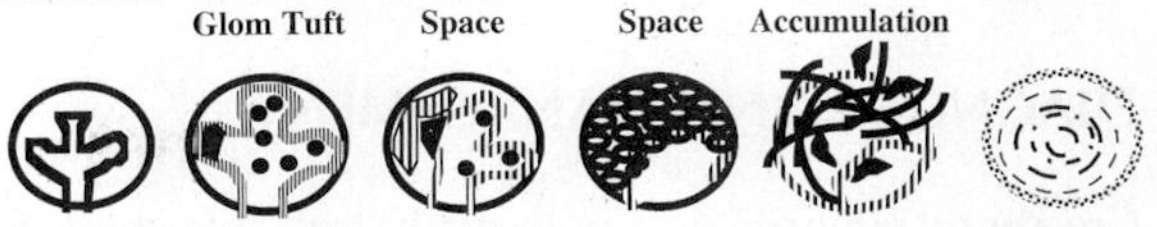

Stage 0	Stage 1	Stage 2	Stage 3	Stage 4	Stage 5
Day 0	Day 3	Day 7	Day 14	Day 21	Day 30

B. Clinical Parameters

Hematuria	-	+	+	+	+	
RBC Casts	-	+	+	+	+	
Proteinuria	-	+	+	+	+	
Decreased Function	No	No	Maybe	Yes	Marked	Absent

C. Reversibility		Yes	Yes	Probable	Unlikely	No

Figure 39.18. Diagrammatic illustration of a crescent's progress with time and in relation to clinical parameters and the potential for reversibility. *Top panel:* Pathologic stages of progression from initial inflammation to obliterative scarring of the glomerulus together with the time course in days for a single glomerulus passing through these stages based on experimental models. *Middle panel:* The associated clinical implications in terms of urine sediment and renal function. *Lower panel:* The potential for reversibility of the lesion back to normal structure and function. The major point to be made from this analysis is that by the time renal function is measurably abnormal, major pathologic changes have taken place and the glomerulus is well on its way toward scarring and permanent loss of normal structure and function. On the other hand, an active urinary sediment including red blood cell casts is an early and sensitive indication of glomerular inflammation.

trated in Fig. 39.18, from the time the injury is established and is detectable to the clinician, scar formation in an individual glomerulus takes approximately 10 to 14 days. Thus it is logical to conclude that the diagnosis and treatment to attempt to prevent progression and preserve useful renal function in RPGN should be approached as a medical emergency. Having made the previous statement, it is important to point out that there is no controlled trial data to show that delay in diagnosis and treatment is associated with worse outcome, although it is not likely that such a trial will be conducted in the future.

Not every condition associated with crescent formation is associated with rapid loss of renal function. For example, the glomerulonephritis associated with systemic vasculitis or infective endocarditis may progress in a more indolent fashion with crescent formation occurring in only a few glomeruli at a time. The result may be progression to end-stage renal disease (ESRD) over months or years. Similarly, in IgA nephropathy at the time of macroscopic hematuria, small crescents may be widespread on renal biopsy, but more than 30 days later when macroscopic hematuria has resolved, the crescents have spontaneously regressed. Factors determining the potential reversibility of crescent formation for an individual glomerulus include the underlying process driving crescent formation (e.g., anti-GBM antibody–associated crescents rarely regress, whereas those associated with IgA nephropathy or ANCA may commonly regress), the severity of injury to the glomerulus (the size of the crescents), the degree of interstitial inflammation and scarring, and whether treatment is instituted early in the sequence of events. The urgency of diagnosis requires knowledge about the rate of progression of the disease process as judged by the rate and degree of rise of the serum creatinine. An indolent process requires a less urgent diagnosis than does a rapidly evolving process. A rapidly evolving crescentic glomerulonephritis requires a diagnosis and treatment within hours rather than days, if this can be done safely.

CLINICAL SYNDROMES ASSOCIATED WITH CRESCENT FORMATION

The Syndrome of Rapidly Progressive Glomerulonephritis

The presenting features of RPGN are the consequence of acute injury to the glomerulus. These include a rapid and progressive decrease in renal function causing a rise in the serum creatinine over days or weeks. RPGN is commonly associated with signs and symptoms of renal dysfunction, such as decreased urine formation and edema, which may be associated with hypertension. The urine may show evidence of inflammation of the glomerulus as manifest by the presence of red blood cell (RBC) casts, leukocytes, protein, dysmorphic RBCs, and other types of casts. The urine may be frankly bloody, a sign that will make the patient seek medical attention urgently, when there is often still time to prevent progression to ESRD. Constitutional symptoms including malaise and fever may also be associated with flank pain or tenderness that give rise to a constellation of symptoms that is commonly mistaken for pyelonephritis.

Indolent Progressive Loss of Renal Function

Crescent formation may involve only a small proportion of glomeruli at any one time resulting in a more indolent progressive scarring process. This occurs in infective endocarditis, in some individuals with ANCA-positive clinical syndromes, in membranoproliferative glomerulonephritis (MPGN), in cryoglobulinemia, and in IgA nephropathy. The actual incidence of this mechanism of progression may be underestimated because renal biopsies are often not performed in these patients, and if a renal biopsy is done, then crescents would be unlikely to be seen in the few glomeruli sectioned in a single biopsy.

Episodic Apparently Reversible Renal Dysfunction

Individuals with chronic and recurrent glomerular inflammation of any cause, such as MPGN or IgA nephropathy, may have episodes of renal dysfunction associated with macroscopic hematuria. We know that renal biopsy at the time of macroscopic hematuria is associated with the presence of crescents in Bowman's space, but if biopsy is delayed for several weeks, crescents are rarely seen. These individuals may have associated decrease in renal function at the time of macroscopic hematuria, which appears to resolve with disappearance of the macroscopic hematuria. Thus crescent formation must be spontaneously reversible in this situation, although presumably each time glomerular inflammation with crescent formation occurs, some glomeruli are at risk for scarring so that progressive loss of renal function occurs over time. Interstitial inflammation, profuse RBC aggregation in renal tubular lumina, and tubular necrosis are common accompaniments of this syndrome, especially in IgA nephropathy. Crescentic glomerular involvement is typically less than 50%. The nonglomerular alterations may account for the reduced renal function.

DIAGNOSIS AND MANAGEMENT

Crescentic nephritis is a potentially treatable condition regardless of the underlying mechanism driving the process. However, as noted previously, the scarring process is rapid. Thus in order to prevent glomerular scarring associated with crescent formation, the diagnosis by renal biopsy and institution of appropriate treatment must be done urgently.

The three major steps in the diagnosis and management of crescentic nephritis are as follows:

Step 1: Detect, diagnose, and treat the crescentic process. Make the diagnosis (usually by urgent/emergent renal biopsy) and institute treatment to control the immune and inflammatory process as an urgent/emergent matter. The immediate goal is to preserve the greatest amount of renal structure and function possible in the short term by intensive early intervention.

Step 2: Control and monitor the underlying process. Gain long-term control of the underlying disease process by induction of disease remission. Institute an effective monitoring program for recurrence of the underlying disease process.

Step 3: Preserve residual renal function. Preserve the residual renal function by using general strategies that minimize hyperfiltration, systemic hypertension, proteinuria, hyperlipidemia, hyperphosphatemia, and other damaging influences.

Diagnostic Strategy

The steps toward making the diagnosis in RPGN are as follows: (a) consider the diagnosis based on a progressive rise of the serum creatinine and other evidence of decreasing renal function (see Table 39.33 for differential diagnosis); (b) detect blood, protein, and leukocytes in the urine, and proceed to identify red cell casts by urine microscopy; and (c) perform a renal biopsy to confirm the diagnosis and determine the immunofluorescent pattern in the biopsy. Serologic studies such as anti-GBM antibody and ANCA also play a critical role in the differential diagnosis. Armed with this information, it is usually straight forward to develop an appropriate treatment strategy and to implement it. Without this information, treatment is often delayed and tentative.

TABLE 39.33. Differential Diagnosis of Rapid Progressive Deterioration of Renal Function with an Active Urine Sediment

Crescentic glomerulonephritis with or without vasculitis
Acute glomerulonephritis ± crescents
Acute interstitial nephritis
Acute tubular necrosis
Malignant hypertension
HUS/TTP
Atheroembolic disease
Thromboembolic disease
Renal vein thrombosis
Scleroderma
Myeloma-associated ARF
Cryoglobulinemia
Others

ARF, acute renal failure; HUS, hemolytic uremic syndrome; TTP, thrombotic thrombocytopenic purpura.

TABLE 39.34. Information Available from the Renal Biopsy

Confirmation of the presence and extent of crescent formation.
Identification of the underlying pathologic process from immunofluorescent analysis (see also Fig. 39.17).
Determination of the degree of fibrosis and potential for reversibility.

The renal biopsy is often helpful in decision making in crescentic nephritis. Table 39.34 lists the three major pieces of information available from the renal biopsy in this setting. This information should be available to the clinician within 4 to 24 hours of performing the biopsy. The confirmation of a diagnosis of crescentic nephritis is a key step in management. Table 39.33 provides a list of some of the many other pathologic processes that can present with a similar picture.

A renal biopsy is useful in most cases of RPGN unless there are contraindications to performing the biopsy such as a low platelet count, abnormal coagulation, or uncontrolled severe hypertension. The risks of performing a biopsy must be weighed against not performing the renal biopsy, with consequent lack of certainty about the diagnosis and optimal treatment strategy that commonly leads to tentative treatment. Serologic studies may be very useful in directing the initial diagnostic and therapeutic approach to RPGN.

Treatment Strategy

The first step in the treatment strategy of crescentic nephritis is to exclude underlying infection as a cause. If present, infection should be treated by removal of the source of infection if possible (e.g., an intravenous line or shunt) and by use of antibiotics. Immunosuppressive agents are rarely needed because they are likely to reduce the rate of removal of the infectious agent.

Having excluded infection as an underlying cause, the available immunosuppressive agents are very effective if used early in the sequence of events. The major options include (a) glucocorticoids to suppress inflammation and scar formation, (b) cyclophosphamide to reduce further immune activation and prevent scar formation, and (c) plasma exchange to remove circulating factors that might prolong and extend the degree of injury, such as anti-GBM antibody and occasionally ANCA. The specific combination of these approaches depends on the underlying diagnosis and the degree of established injury and potential reversibility. These strategies are outlined in brief in the following sections. The reader is directed to chapters dealing with the specific conditions identified in this text.

Infection-Associated Crescentic Nephritis

A wide variety of infections can cause an immune-complex disease resulting in severe acute glomerulonephritis (RPGN) and leading to chronic indolent glomerulonephritis leading to ESRD. These include bacterial, viral, fungal, and parasitic infections. The best recognized infection-associated glomerulonephritis is *postinfective glomerulonephritis* caused commonly by streptococcal infection of the throat or skin. Crescents associated with this condition are not uncommon, although they are often small; rapidly progressive glomerulonephritis requiring urgent renal biopsy is rarely associated with postinfective glomerulonephritis. However, infections involving intravenous lines of various types, shunts, infections of cardiac valves, and other sites and abscesses are all potential causes of glomerulonephritis. Less pathogenic infectious agents can also be responsible, particularly in immunocompromised or immunosuppressed individuals, and in intravenous drug users. Idiopathic crescentic nephritis with immune deposits is probably associated with viral infection that remains unidentified.

If present, the first priority is to treat the infection quickly and effectively using appropriate means. This may include surgery, drainage, removal of the infected foreign body, and antibiotics as appropriate. Immunosuppressive agents are rarely used in this setting.

Anti-GBM Antibody–Associated Diseases

RPGN associated with antibody directed at the C-terminal part of one of the basement membrane–collagen molecules (the $\alpha3$ chain of the type IV collagen) is often rapid, severe, and irreversible. Goodpasture's syndrome, the combination of alveolar hemorrhage and crescentic nephritis, most commonly occurs in individuals with circulating anti-GBM antibodies who also smoke tobacco. Only a single, small, controlled trial on the treatment of anti-GBM disease has been published, therefore available information is limited. It is likely that early diagnosis and treatment does result in preservation of renal function, but this has not been unequivocally proven by a large, prospective, clinical trial.

For anti-GBM disease, the available data support the following conclusions and general approaches to treatment, which are determined in part by the level of renal function at presentation: (a) If the serum creatinine is only moderately elevated at presentation (less than 2 mg/dl), then the combination of glucocorticoids and cyclophosphamide alone are a reasonable therapeutic option. There is no evidence that the addition of plasma exchange is helpful under these conditions. (b) For nonoliguric patients with serum creatinine values between 2 and 6 mg/dl at presentation, plasma exchange in addition to immunosuppressive strategies outlined previously are generally used. (c) If the serum creatinine is more than 6 mg/dl, and particularly if the patient is oligoanuric, it is unlikely that useful renal function will be recoverable despite triple therapy with steroids, cytotoxic agents, and plasma exchange. Thus the intensive use of immunosuppressive agents should be tempered in this setting.

The aforementioned guidelines should be taken in association with the potential for recovery as determined from the renal biopsy. For example, acute tubular necrosis induced by intravenous use of contrast material or other factors may be superimposed on the glomerulonephritis and thereby obscure potential for recovery as assessed from functional studies alone. Thus a biopsy with relatively few involved glomeruli or glomeruli at early stages of crescent formation would lead to a more intensive strategy designed to preserve useful renal function, whereas a biopsy showing widespread and severe glomerular and interstitial scarring would lead to the opposite conclusion. Individuals who have a combination of anti-GBM antibodies and ANCA (30% to 40% of patients with anti-GBM disease) have a better prognosis than do those with anti-GBM antibodies alone. Approximately 30% of the double-positive group can be expected not to require long-term dialysis, compared with the need for permanent dialysis in patients with the anti-GBM antibody alone in the setting of oligoanuric renal disease. Finally, associated alveolar hemorrhage, which may be life-threatening and require intensive pulmonary support including artificial ventilation, appears to be improved by addition of plasma exchange to intensive immunosuppressive therapy.

The absence of detectable circulating anti-GBM antibody by the enzyme-linked immunosorbent assay (ELISA) does not rule out anti-GBM antibody–associated glomerulonephritis, probably because high-affinity antibodies are rapidly removed from the circulation. However, the assay itself is reliable with a low false positive and negative rates for measuring the presence and absence of these antibodies (less than 5%). Although titers of anti-GBM antibody do not closely parallel the disease intensity, plasma levels can be used as a general measure of plasma exchange efficacy. Plasma exchange should continue until the anti-GBM antibody titer is reduced to close to baseline and/or the patient's condition is improving and stabilized. At this time plasma exchange can be stopped and immunosuppression continued for 3 to 6 months. The anti-GBM titer can be monitored. Intercurrent infection may trigger recurrence of anti-GBM glomerulonephritis.

Antineutrophil Cytoplasmic Antibody–Positive Crescentic Nephritis

ANCA appears to be an enhancing factor that helps to target and amplify the immune response to the glomerulus and cause crescent formation. It is most often associated with glomerulonephritis without significant immune deposits *(pauci-immune glomerulonephritis).* If immunoglobulins are detected, they are usually in small amounts and of the IgM and/or C3 variety.

The following associations with ANCA have been defined: (a) Wegener's granulomatosis and pauci-immune crescentic nephritis are 90% ANCA positive (mostly C-ANCA directed at proteinase-3); (b) microscopic polyarteritis syndrome and/or pauci-immune glomerulonephritis as renal-limited diseases are 80% ANCA positive (mostly P-ANCA directed at myeloperoxidase); (c) pauci-immune noncrescentic glomerulonephritis are 20% ANCA positive (mostly P-ANCA); and (d) anti-GBM disease are 35% ANCA positive (mostly P-ANCA). Treatment and improved clinical outcome is often associated with a reduction in titer of circulating ANCA, and recurrence of disease is often associated with a reappearance or a rise in the ANCA titer.

In ANCA-positive RPGN, unlike anti-GBM disease as outlined previously, even if renal function is severely abnormal and the patient is oligoanuric before treatment is initiated, useful renal function may be recovered for the long term in up to 50% of cases. Thus oligoanuria is not a contraindication to intensive treatment in ANCA-associated RPGN. Like anti-GBM disease, ANCA-positive syndromes may present as a pulmonary–renal syndrome that requires ventilation and plasma exchange in association with glucocorticoids and cyclophosphamide therapies.

ANCA-Negative Pauci-Immune Crescentic Nephritis

Pauci-immune crescentic nephritis, which is ANCA negative, is generally treated using the same guidelines as the ANCA-positive pauci-immune group.

IgA-Associated Crescentic Nephritis

Henoch-Schönlein purpura presents in severe cases with acute progressive loss of renal function associated with vasculitis involving the skin, joints, and gastrointestinal tract. Renal biopsy shows IgA immune deposits commonly associated with crescent formation. Glucocorticoids alone are usually used in this circumstance. However, the addition of immunosuppression and plasma exchange may provide additional benefit, but no controlled trial exists. As noted previously, IgA nephropathy (Berger's disease) commonly has small crescents present if the biopsy is performed at the time of macroscopic hematuria. These crescents presumably spontaneously regress. There is no data to support the use of long-term glucocorticoids in this setting. Anecdotal data have supported the use of high-dose intravenous immunoglobulin. Lupus and cirrhosis-associated–immune-complex disease can also present with IgA-predominant–immune-complex disease in the glomerulus.

Lupus Nephritis in Association with Crescents

Diffuse proliferative and focal proliferative glomerulonephritis of lupus are often associated with crescent formation. The general approach should be as outlined in Chapter 42. Part 1. However, if crescents are present in association with a high-chronicity index (established scarring), this signals a worse prognosis and may require more intensive therapy to preserve renal function.

Other Conditions Associated with Crescent Formation

The strategy of treating most widespread crescentic nephritis associated with the RPGN syndromes (not caused by infection) with steroids with or without cyclophosphamide in the short term is a reasonable one, given the risks and costs of allowing a person to progress to ESRD. However, it must be stated that there is no controlled trial information available to support the treatment of these conditions intensively.

Specific Therapeutic Strategies Used to Treat Crescentic Nephritis in the Short Term

There are two immediate goals of therapeutic intervention. The first goal is to halt the inflammatory process causing crescent formation and to prevent fibrosis of the glomerulus and interstitial compartment. The initial intervention is to use high-dose glucocorticoid usually accompanied by cyclophosphamide to halt inflammation and the scarring process as quickly as possible. Once control of the glomerular inflammation is established, the secondary goal is to substitute a regimen that will maintain control of the underlying immune process (disease remission) so that recurrence of glomerular inflammation is prevented and glomerular structure and function is allowed to recover to the optimal extent.

Glucocorticoids

High-dose pulse glucocorticoid use is the first line treatment. The high dose is justified by the concept that severe inflammation and edema in the kidney reduces blood flow. Thus in order to get effective amounts of glucocorticoid to sites of inflammation, high doses are required. Methylprednisolone (1 g given intravenously over 20 minutes each day for 3 days) is frequently used. This is followed by prednisone 1 to 2 mg/kg daily orally for 2 to 4 weeks until inflammation is reduced as assessed by renal function and urine sediment [white blood cell (WBC) and granular casts]. The glucocorticoid dose is then reduced to a maintenance level for up to 6 months or until the underlying disease process has been controlled and the disease is in remission as judged by renal function measurements and the disappearance of the driving mechanism (e.g., anti-GBM or ANCA). Steps to minimize the effect of glucocorticoids on the gastrointestinal tract should be routinely used. Lower dosages of methylprednisolone or prednisone can be used if renal function is relatively normal. Long-term, high-dose glucocorticoid must be avoided by use of steroid-sparing agents such as cyclophosphamide, azathioprine, or mycophenolate mofetil if necessary.

Cyclophosphamide

In severe crescentic nephritis, cyclophosphamide is commonly used as an adjunct to glucocorticoids in anti-GBM disease, in pauci-immune crescentic nephritis including the ANCA-positive group, and in some case of severe lupus nephritis. The data supporting this strategy are not buttressed by prospective, controlled, clinical trials with long-term follow-up.

Cyclophosphamide is converted to the active metabolite in the liver. It is used as either an intravenous pulse starting at 0.5 g/m^2 and being adjusted to achieve a WBC count of 3,000 to 5,000/mm^3, reaching a nadir approximately 2 weeks after injection, or as oral cyclophosphamide at 1 to 2 mg/kg per day to achieve and maintain a WBC count of approximately 5,000/mm^3.

Most published series using cyclophosphamide report deaths from complications of cyclophosphamide treatment. Thus it is imperative to carefully monitor the WBC count initially twice per week so that the trends of the decline of WBCs can be anticipated and the dosage modified before severe leukopenia develops. Once a dose has been established, a weekly WBC count should be monitored. In taking the responsibility to use cyclophosphamide, some important caveats must be kept in mind: (a) The effect of a dose of cyclophosphamide on the bone marrow takes 2 weeks to be seen in the peripheral WBC count. Therefore a change in dosage will not be reflected by a change in peripheral WBC until 2 weeks later. Thus a falling WBC count can be used to anticipate a change in requirement for cyclophosphamide and the dosage modified before severe leukopenia is present. (b) Glucocorticoids are marrow protective against cyclophosphamide. Therefore as the dosage of glucocorticoid is reduced, the dosage of cyclophosphamide required to maintain the WBC count at 5,000/mm^3 will need to be reduced. (c) Over time the marrow appears to become more sensitive to cyclophosphamide so that a dose required to maintain a WBC count at 2 months may be more than is required at 6 months. (d) Renal failure may affect the disposal of toxic metabolites of cyclophosphamide, thus dosage reduction in the presence of renal failure is a prudent step.

The length of time of treatment depends on the level of clinical disease activity and measurement of serologic parameters of activity. In general, treatment is maintained for at least 6 months, and may be continued for 1 to 2 years if evidence of disease activity remains or recurrence of disease occurs. Because side effects are dose related, the sooner cyclophosphamide treatment can be reduced or stopped, the less likely it is to cause side effects. Intravenous pulse treatment is less likely to cause bladder injury (inflammation/malignancy) because of the shorter time of interaction between urine metabolites and the bladder wall. Similarly, encouraging high fluid intake reduces the local concentration of cyclophosphamide metabolites in the bladder. These effects can also probably be reduced by mesna.

Because both the effects and side effects of cyclophosphamide are dose related, it may be possible to gain control of the disease by use of oral cyclophosphamide when control cannot be achieved by monthly intravenous cyclophosphamide. This may be because approximately twice the amount of cyclophosphamide is used with oral therapy as with intravenous therapy.

Dose-related side effects include leukopenia leading to infection and death, induction of malignancy, loss of hair, ovarian failure (age-related) and azoospermia, and fibrotic and hemorrhagic cystitis. The total cyclophosphamide dose should be less than 0.5 g/kg if possible. Higher total doses appear to be associated with an increase in the incidence of malignancy (mainly skin, bladder, and lymphoma).

Plasma Exchange

Most plasma exchange regimens use albumin in exchange for plasma in four liter exchanges. Plasma exchange is usually performed daily for 5 to 7 days and then every other day for a total of 10 to 14 exchanges to achieve and maintain removal of pathogenic circulating antibodies. The clinical severity of disease, particularly lung hemorrhage, as well as anti-GBM antibody or other serologic parameters, can be monitored as a guide to the need for further exchanges. Plasma exchange will also remove creatinine resulting in artificial lowering of this and other parameters of renal function as well as drugs used to treat the underlying condition. The techniques and the side effects of plasma pheresis are discussed in detail in Chapter 95.

Other Immunosuppressive Agents

The reader is referred to chapters dealing with specific diseases, including systemic lupus erythematosus (SLE), systemic vasculitis, and IgA nephropathy, for guidance in long-term management of these diseases and the use of other agents to achieve maintenance suppression of the disease process. This includes the use of mycophenolate; azathioprine and its analogs; cyclosporine; and T-cell, endothelial-cell, and inflammatory-cell modulation by antibodies directed against cell-surface receptors. Azathioprine or mycophenolate may be useful agents to consolidate a remission induced by cyclophosphamide but may be weaker agents for the induction of remission.

Maintaining Remission of the Underlying Disease

Many of the conditions that are associated with crescent formation may recur. This includes SLE, ANCA-positive syndromes, Henoch-Schönlein purpura, and other conditions. Relapse is common in C-ANCA–associated crescentic nephritis (approximately 30%). Anti-GBM disease does not usually recur as long as the anti-GBM titer has returned to baseline. However, a recurrence can be provoked by intercurrent infection. The reader is directed to chapters dealing with these conditions for information on maintaining disease remission.

Preserving Renal Function in the Long Term

It is common to succeed in preserving renal function in the short term only to lose it in the longer term through poor control of hypertension and other noninflammatory mechanisms.

The damaged glomerulus is particularly susceptible to further damage by glomerular hypertension either in isolation or associated with systemic hypertension (Fig. 39.19). Furthermore, angiotensin II itself may play a part in driving the scarring process in association with TGF-β and related mediators. Thus long-term follow-up with a focus on the following factors is important to maintain renal function: (a) education of the patient to measure his or her own blood pressure at home and to understand the principles of prevention of progression; (b) the use of angiotensin-converting enzyme (ACE) inhibition and/or angiotensin II antagonists whenever possible, compatible with maintenance of renal function and potassium status; (c) treatment of systemic hypertension to the 120/80 level; (d) minimization of proteinuria by use of ACE inhibitors and/or angiotensin II antagonists; (e) control of lipid levels; and (f) moderate protein-restricted diet (1 g/kg per day).

Long-term monitoring to detect and prevent recurrence and to preserve residual renal function is essential. Many individuals successfully retain useful renal function in the short term only to become lost to follow-up and lose their remaining renal function through associated hypertension and proteinuria in the long term.

Risks and Costs of Biopsy and Treatment Versus Progression to End-Stage Renal Disease

We know the approximate risks and costs of allowing a patient to progress to ESRD. This risk depends on age and other factors, but mortality is 10% to 15% for the first year for the average patient on dialysis. For individuals with crescentic nephritis it may be higher. In the United States, the cost is $50,000 per year for a stable dialysis patient not including lost earnings and other costs to the family. The life of the patient is often transformed for the worse by loss of employment and other changes associated with established ESRD.

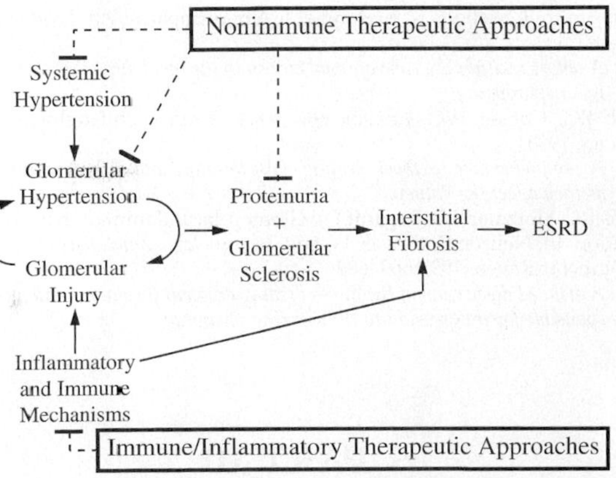

Figure 39.19. Preservation of renal function after established injury. Diagrammatic representation of pathways to preserve renal function. Following injury the glomerulus may be exposed to intraglomerular hypertension and/or systemic hypertension, which themselves cause further injury to the glomerulus resulting in proteinuria and glomerulosclerosis. These changes, along with the inflammatory process, lead to interstitial fibrosis. The combination of these factors results in ESRD. The specific antiimmune and antiinflammatory approaches outlined previously are designed to deal with underlying causative mechanisms. However, "nonimmune" approaches including the use of angiotensin-converting enzyme inhibitors/angiotensin II antagonists to reduce intraglomerular hypertension and proteinuria are indicated in the long-term management to preserve useful renal function.

What are the risks and costs associated with diagnosis and treatment of crescentic nephritis? We know the cost of a renal biopsy and its analysis is approximately $3,000 in the United States and the risk of death from a percutaneous renal biopsy is approximately 0.2%. The risks are not increased in the elderly. These risks may be somewhat higher in an acutely ill patient. We know that the increased incidence of malignancy from receiving cyclophosphamide for 1 year is approximately 8% after a 12-year follow-up (less than 30 g total dose). This malignancy is limited primarily to the skin, and is usually treatable.

Considering the aforementioned discussion, we can therefore conclude that a renal biopsy performed under carefully monitored conditions followed by supervised treatment with cyclophosphamide (if appropriate) for 6 to 12 months carries significantly less risk and cost than allowing a patient to progress to ESRD. If intensive diagnosis and treatment in an individual patient might save renal function, then the risk and cost of such a strategy are usually on the positive side.

Selected Readings

Bolton WK. Goodpasture's syndrome. *Kidney Int* 1996;50:1753–1766.
A current review of anti-GBM Disease and its management.

Bolton WK. Rapidly progressive glomerulonephritis. *Semin Nephrol* 1996;16: 517–526.
A perspective for the diagnosis and treatment of rapidly progressive glomerulonephritis.

Couser W. Rapidly progressive glomerulonephritis: classification, pathogenetic mechanisms and therapy. *Am J Kidney Dis* 1988;9:449–464.
An in-depth review of mechanisms and therapy in rapidly progressive glomerulonephritis.

Falk RJ, Jeanette JC. ANCA small-vessel vasculitis. *J Am Soc Nephrol* 1997;8: 314–322.
A review of the relationship between ANCA and the various clinical syndromes associated with ANCA.

Kincaid-Smith P, Nicholls K. Mesangial IgA nephropathy. *Am J Kidney Dis* 1983;2: 90–102.

A report relating the time of renal biopsy to the incidence of crescent formation in IgA nephropathy.

Neilson EG, Couser WG. *Immunologic renal diseases.* Philadelphia: Lippincott-Raven, 1996.

A comprehensive textbook dealing with immune and inflammatory mechanisms as they affect the kidney.

Wiggins RC, Holzman LB, Legault DJ. Glomerular inflammation and crescent formation. In: Neilsen E, Couser W, eds. *Immunologic renal diseases.* Philadelphia: Lippincott-Raven, 1997:669–682.

A detailed discussion of the forces driving crescent formation and mechanisms responsible for progression to the scarring phenotype.

PART 10 *Fibrillary Glomerulonephritis and Immunotactoid Glomerulopathy*

Agnes B. Fogo and Robert G. Horn

Glomerulopathies of many and various forms are a consequence of the deposition in glomeruli, in a multitude of patterns and with highly variable functional consequences, of material containing immunoglobulin molecules or derivatives thereof. Most commonly, the deposited material is in the form of immune complexes with associated complement components, and in these cases of immune complex–mediated glomerulonephritis (GN), antigenic target material is assumed to be present but rarely demonstrated. Numerous other patterns of glomerulopathy are now recognized to be present as a consequence of deposition of material derived from immunoglobulins or immunoglobulin fragments, occurring as a result of neoplastic or otherwise unregulated overproduction of monoclonal paraproteins.

This large category of immunoglobulin deposit–mediated glomerulopathies is analyzed and classified (a) by defining the retained antigenic characteristics of the deposited immunoglobulin molecules, and if possible, other associated material by immunofluorescence microscopy (IF); (b) by defining with electron microscopy (EM) the pattern of distribution of the deposited material, either in the mesangial region and/or along the glomerular basement membranes (either subendothelial, subepithelial, and in some cases, by the appearance of a structured or ordered pattern to the deposited material); and (c) by considering these EM and IF findings in the light of accompanying pathologic changes produced in glomeruli and aberrations of renal function associated with those structural alterations.

The material deposited in glomeruli is ordinarily easily identified by EM as "exogenous" material because it is of substantially greater density than ordinary extracellular tissue constituents in the electron optical image. At the degree of resolution and magnification ordinarily used in clinical EM, the deposited dense material is usually rather homogeneous in image texture, although at the higher levels of magnification, a "granular" or "reticular" quality is evident, similar to the pattern that might be observed by the close-up macroscopic examination of a bowl of "granulated" sugar or a spoonful of table salt. In a minority of cases, EM will reveal irregularly distributed areas of increased density in various patterns (e.g., irregularly curving "wormlike" lines are commonly seen, particularly in lesions which appear to be quite chronic); however, no particular significance or helpful predictability of associations with such vague patterns has been appreciated. On the other hand, in a smaller minority of cases, EM examination discloses much more regular patterns of density variation, patterns in which the consistency and orderliness in the substructure of the deposits suggest some coherent principle underlying the nonrandom pattern that is produced.

Early on, as information was accumulated on the ultrastructural alterations seen in the various forms of GN, occasional cases were seen in which deposits in the glomeruli were composed of or contained dense material arrayed in a pattern indicating that the dense material existed in the form of elongated linear structures. In many of these cases, the linear structures appeared to be straight, unbranched, randomly disposed in relation to each other, and without further resolvable substructure (think of "a handful of toothpicks tossed on the table") (Fig. 39.20A). In perhaps the first published report describing such a case, the substantial similarity of the deposits to the fibrillar deposits of amyloid was observed, and the point was emphasized that in the reported case the deposited fibrillar material resembled the fibrils of amyloid by EM examination, but the material did not stain with Congo red and therefore appeared to be something other than a β-pleated sheet of amyloid.

Other cases were also studied in which material deposited in glomeruli contained elongated linear structures of a clearly different morphologic form from the fibrils described in the preceding paragraph and pictured in Fig. 39.20B. Such cases contained deposited material that, while elongated and straight, also showed at high resolution a distinctly tubular or cylindrical structure. An early description of a case of this type, with strikingly depicted deposits, was published by Schwartz and Lewis in 1980. In this carefully studied, dramatically depicted, and compellingly analyzed case, numerous important points were made. The patient had, as evidence of an underlying paraproteinemia, free κ light chains in the urine, and deposited material in the glomeruli appeared to contain a monoclonal immunoglobulin (IgG heavy chain and κ light chain staining by IF). The authors postulated that the organized tubular deposits were probably analogous to crystallike aggregates of monoclonal protein, similar to the so-called tactoids of HbS hemoglobin observed in sickled erythrocytes. Based on this assumption, the authors proposed to utilize the term *immunotactoid* to describe structures of this form and presumed origin. In the same seminal case, Schwartz and Lewis also described and more forcefully depicted that the microtubular deposits tend to be disposed, not in an entirely random array, but rather as evenly spaced structures, often oriented in parallel arrays resembling "a box of soda straws, half-full". Finally, in this case, Schwartz and Lewis noted the patient's microtubular immunotactoid deposits were "similar in size and shape to microtubular aggregates described in the serum and glomeruli of certain patients with cryoglobulinemia" (although in this index case, cryoglobulinemia was never demonstrated), and they noted that a number of other patterns of ultrastructural organization had been observed in a variety of different situations.

In the two or three decades during which these such cases, with fibrillary and/or immunotactoid deposits have been observed, described, commented upon, and reported, most who have written on the subject have concluded that most of these cases can be fairly assigned to one or the other of the aforemen-

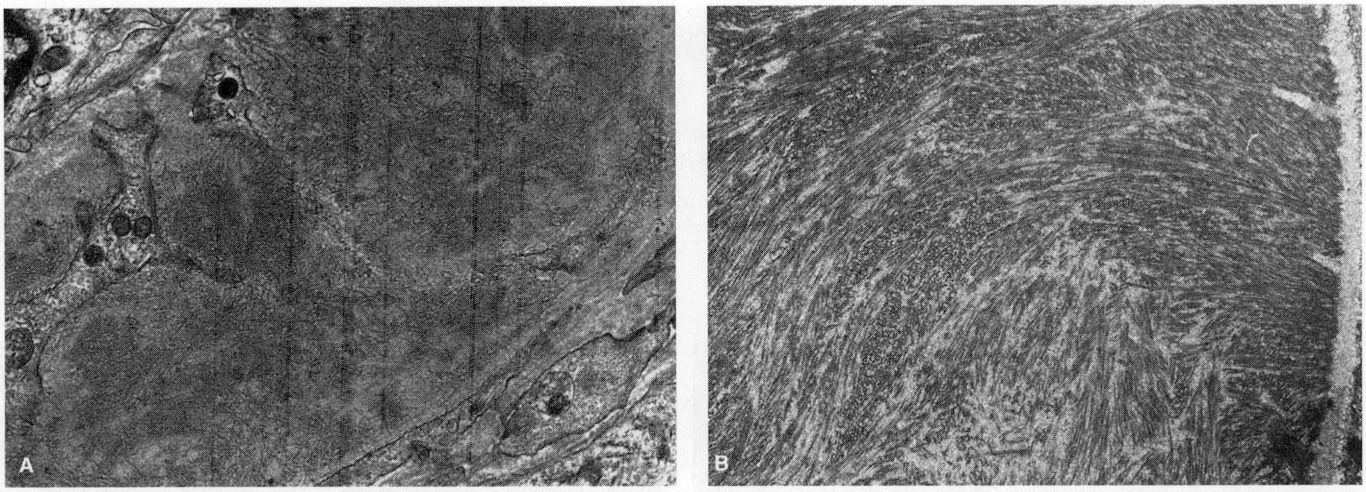

Figure 39.20. Randomly oriented fibrils are characteristic of fibrillary glomerulonephritis **(A)**, whereas microtubular deposits in organized, parallel arrays are typical of microtubular immunotactoid glomerulopathy **(B)** (transmission electron microscopy, × 26,250).

tioned two categories. That is, such a case, with morphologically ordered elongated deposits, will have deposits composed of or containing either (a) amyloidlike (but Congo red negative) delicate (15 to 25 nm), straight, unbranched, apparently nontubular "fibrils," the "toothpicks," randomly arrayed and not aligned with each other in regular array or proximity; or (b) larger (greater than 30 nm), microtubular (i.e., cylindrical) structures, the "soda straws," often with a suggestion of some orderly nearly visible substructure, and often regularly disposed in parallel arrays of very evenly spaced structures, individual arrays being arranged in interlacing bundles.

Although most observers would appear to agree that most of these cases contain either amyloidlike fibrils or larger microtubular structured deposits, there has been much disagreement on the preferred terminology for these cases, and perhaps more importantly, there has been substantial disagreement as to whether the character of the deposits was predictive of the likelihood of an associated underlying disease that had led to the generation of the deposits. Current use appears to favor applying the term *fibrillary* exclusively to those cases with delicate amyloidlike fibrils, using such terminology as *fibrillary glomerulopathy* or *glomerulonephritis with fibrillary deposits.* The earlier frequent use of the descriptive *nonamyloid* adjective now seems redundant, although in earlier discourse the use of this term indicated that the fibrils resembled but differed from amyloid, a then (and occasionally still) quite useful distinction.

Selection of a term to describe the cases with larger, highly ordered, microtubular deposits is more complex and less settled. Some writers, ourselves included, have used the term *immunotactoid* to define these cases with microtubular deposits. This is based largely on the elegant description of the seminal case of Schwartz and Lewis described previously and their creation and use of that term to describe the highly ordered microtubular deposits in that case. It is also based on their suggestion that such deposits were composed of crystallike arrays of proteinaceous material of immunoglobulin origin. In later work, Schwartz, Lewis, and others have used the term *immunotactoid* to include not only the cases with microtubular deposits but also the larger set of cases with fibrillary deposits as defined earlier and perhaps cases with less well-defined orderly substructure in the deposits. It is etymologically justified to use the term *immunotactoid* to encompass both the fibrillary and the microtubular deposits because it seems quite likely that the smaller fibrillary deposits are also ordered structures of immunoglobulin origin. On the other hand, use of the term *immunotactoid,* without other modifiers, to describe the two groups of cases may obscure meaningful differences between the two (or more) groups of cases encompassed by the term. In this chapter, we hereafter use the term *fibrillary glomerulonephritis* to describe the cases with smaller amyloidlike fibrils, and the term *microtubular immunotactoid glomerulopathy* to encompass the cases with ultrastructurally defined clearly microtubular cylindrical deposits.

PATHOLOGY

The characteristic feature in this group of disorders is the presence of deposits with ultrastructural features of either fibrillary, randomly oriented deposits, or microtubular deposits with varying degrees of organization. These deposits stain with immunoglobulin and complement, but by definition, they do not stain with the Congo red stain. Other systemic disorders may have ultrastructural findings that overlap or are indistinguishable from the EM findings in fibrillary glomerulonephritis or immunotactoid glomerulopathy. These include amyloidosis, paraproteinemia-associated diseases, and occasionally, lupus nephritis. The organized nature of deposits in cryoglobulin-related renal disease, including those related to chronic hepatitis C viral infection, has long been recognized. Thus the presence of substructure with microtubular or short, curvilinear fibrils should suggest the possibility of cryoglobulin-related disease. Of note, cryoglobulin-related glomerulonephritis can manifest with varying morphologic changes, few of which are pathognomonic. Deposits can range from frank, diagnostic cryoglobulin plugs in capillary lumina or may have only vague, wormy substructure or frank microtubular immunotactoid morphology. Thus cryoglobulinemic glomerulonephritis is most often a clinicopathologic diagnosis, whereas immunotactoid glomerulopathy is a diagnosis based primarily on morphologic appearance. Therefore distinction between these two diagnostic possibilities may be difficult and somewhat artificial because it relies largely on imprecise additional clinical tests.

The light microscopic appearance of this group of disorders is not specific (Table 39.35). Most cases show varying

TABLE 39.35. Pathologic Features of Fibrillary Glomerulonephritis and Microtubular Immunotactoid Glomerulopathy

	Fibrillary GN	Microtubular Immunotactoid GP
Light microscopy	Varying mesangial or membranoproliferative pattern	Occasional proliferation
Immunofluorescence	Mesangial > capillary, IgG_4 predominant, polyclonal	Capillary > mesangial, IgG predominant, polyclonal or monoclonal
Electron microscopy	Randomly oriented fibrils (14–25 nm)	Organized microtubules (>30 nm)

GN, glomerulonephritis; GP, glomerulopathy.

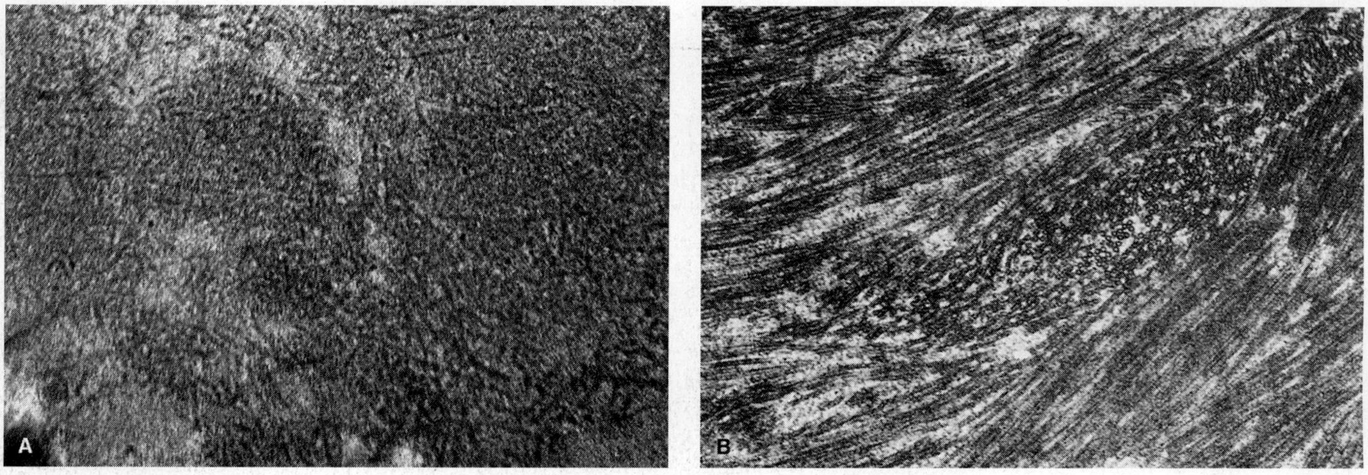

Figure 39.21. Deposits in fibrillary glomerulonephritis **(A)** and microtubular immunotactoid glomerulopathy **(B)** (transmission electron microscopy, ×55,000).

degrees of mesangial proliferation, some with proliferation extending to capillary loops. The overall pattern may be one of a mesangioproliferative glomerulonephritis or, in nearly half of the cases, a membranoproliferative or focal or diffuse proliferative lesion. Occasionally, the appearance may be that of a membranous-type glomerulopathy. Crescents are found in approximately one-fourth to one-third of patients with fibrillary glomerulonephritis but are seen much less commonly with microtubular immunotactoid glomerulopathy. Extensive glomerulosclerosis is typical at presentation in fibrillary glomerulonephritis, involving approximately 20% to 30% of glomeruli, with proportional interstitial inflammation and fibrosis as well as tubular atrophy. Mild to moderate hyalinization of vessels and arteriolosclerosis and arteriosclerosis are often present. Congo red stains are uniformly negative.

IF findings are characteristic in fibrillary glomerulonephritis, with moderate to intense, predominantly mesangial IgG staining with weaker, granular, and sometimes irregular glomerular basement membrane staining. Trace staining for IgA and/or IgM in the same pattern may be present in a minority of cases. In some cases of fibrillary glomerulonephritis, a distinctly "linear" pattern of IgG staining along the glomerular basement membranes may be seen. This pattern of linear staining is seen in glomeruli where abundant fibrillary material permeates the basement membrane, and this appearance may lead to diagnostic confusion with nephritis induced by anti–glomerular basement membrane antibody if seen in a case with crescentic lesions. In fibrillary glomerulonephritis, IgG_4 is the dominant subclass, with weak IgG_1 and absent IgG_2 and IgG_3. However, the deposits are polyclonal, with both κ and λ light chains in more than 80% of patients. In immunotactoid glomerulopathy, IgG4 subclass is not dominant. Deposits are typically polyclonal, and in our cases, mostly IgG with capillary wall deposits more prominent than mesangial deposits.

EM is the cornerstone of diagnosis of these disorders. In fibrillary glomerulonephritis, randomly arranged microfibrils, on average 14 to 25 nm wide, are present (Figs. 39.20A and 39.21A). This is slightly larger than typical amyloid fibrils (7.3 nm). Fibrils are abundant in mesangial areas and may extend to subendothelial areas or subepithelial areas, or they may be transmembranous. These fibrils are scattered in a background of loose, amorphous matrix. Usual type immune complexes with typical dense appearance may be interspersed. In contrast, microtubular immunotactoid glomerulopathy has larger, microtubular structures (usually more than 30 nm wide) that are focally organized with parallel bundles (Figs. 39.20B and 39.21B). Foot-process effacement is diffuse in most biopsies with either morphologic appearance.

PATHOGENESIS

Several studies have suggested an association of the immunotactoid glomerulopathy type with paraproteinemia. In one study, this group of disorders with organized deposits was subdivided into those with fibrillary deposits with negative Congo red stain, and compared with those with distinct tubular appearance or with organized arrays. Patients with cryoglobulinemia, which is a known underlying disease associated with hepatitis C viral infection, that can manifest as organized, immunotactoidal deposits in the glomerulus, were not included in the second group to avoid bias. Differences emerged based on this morphologic classification. The patients with immunotac-

TABLE 39.36. Clinical Presentation

	Fibrillary GN	Microtubular Immunotactoid GP
Age (yr; average and range)	50 ± 12[a] 9–81	62 ± 2[a] 10–68
Gender	Female > male[b] 1.3:1	Male > female[b] 2.6:1
Race	Caucasian > African-American[b] 9:1	Not known
Proteinuria	Invariable, most with nephrotic syndrome	Invariable, most with nephrotic syndrome
Hematuria	>70%	>70%

[a] From case series in Fogo A, Qureshi N, Horn RG. *Am J Kidney Dis* 1993;22:367–377.
[b] From review in Brady HR. *Kidney Int* 1998;53:1421–1429.
GN, glomerulonephritis; GP, glomerulopathy.

toid morphology were older, 62 ± 2 years versus 50 ± 12 years in the fibrillary glomerulonephritis group.

Of patients with fibrillary lesions, 44% had developed end-stage renal disease after an average 23 months of follow-up. In contrast, renal function appeared stable in patients with immunotactoid morphology. There were also associated hematopoietic abnormalities in four of the six patients with immunotactoid morphology, with either monoclonal proteins and/or abnormal plasma cell proliferation present in three. One patient in the fibrillary glomerulonephritis group developed multiple myeloma, but the deposits did not show monoclonality. These findings were echoed in a large review based on reported cases in the literature in which 186 patients with either fibrillary glomerulonephritis or immunotactoid glomerulopathy were evaluated for association with malignancy. From 33% to 41% (depending on whether fibril size or arrangement was used for classification) of patients with immunotactoid glomerulopathy had malignancy, compared with 7% with fibrillary glomerulonephritis. This difference appeared largely due to malignancy associated with a paraprotein in immunotactoid glomerulopathy because the incidence of malignancy in the two diseases was the same when patients with paraprotein were excluded.

In addition to increased hematopoietic abnormalities in immunotactoid glomerulopathy, a variety of other systemic disorders, including Sjögren syndrome, leukocytoclastic vasculitis, mixed connective tissue disease, gastric or liver adenocarcinoma, hepatitis C, and tuberculosis infection, have also been reported in patients with fibrillary glomerulonephritis or microtubular immunotactoid glomerulopathy. However, many of these associations are based on individual case reports.

Mechanisms of Fibrillogenesis

The prominence of IgG and C3 staining of the areas with deposits suggests an immunologic origin. Ultrastructural immunohistochemical studies have shown that IgG and C3 indeed colocalize with the fibrils in fibrillary glomerulonephritis, and amyloid-P component is associated with the fibrils. These studies suggest that IgG, C3, and amyloid-P might all play a role in fibrillogenesis, although clearly a β-pleated sheet does not result (i.e., Congo red negative). An interesting report shows a serum fibrillar cryoprecipitate in a patient with fibrillary glomerulonephritis, with the fibrils consisting of IgG and IgM heavy chain, κ and λ high chains, and fibronectin.

A newly described rare familial form of non–immune complex glomerulonephritis, so-called fibronectin glomerulopathy, is characterized by prominent, fibrillar deposits containing large amounts of fibronectin and scant, if any, immunoglobulin. Studies have failed to show any mutation in the fibronectin gene in these kindreds. Animal models point to the possibility of a primary abnormality in uteroglobulin in this disease. Uteroglobin is a ubiquitously expressed protein that modulates fibronectin homeostasis, resulting in large fibronectin-containing deposits, which are fibrillar by EM. These findings point to a novel pathway of fibrillogenesis involving uteroglobin-mediated abnormalities in handling of and binding of plasma-derived fibronectin. That plasma-derived proteins play a role in fibrillogenesis is also supported by the recurrence of fibrillary deposits in renal transplants in patients with fibrillary glomerulonephritis.

Thus varying pathogenic mechanisms and types of molecules may give rise to fibrillogenesis. The presence of immunotactoid-type deposits (i.e., microtubular immunotactoid glomerulopathy) should prompt the search for associated paraprotein and/or malignancy, whereas no such distinct association has been shown for fibrillary glomerulonephritis. It is anticipated that new molecular studies will further elucidate various mechanisms of fibrillogenesis.

CLINICAL PRESENTATION

Fibrillary glomerulonephritis was present in 1% of biopsies in two large series of native kidney biopsies, primarily in adults. This incidence is similar to that of anti–glomerular basement membrane antibody disease and myeloma cast nephropathy in those series. The age range of patients with this disorder is wide, from 9 years old to as old as 81 years, with a slight female preponderance among the fibrillary glomerulonephritis group and a slight male preponderance in the microtubular immunotactoid glomerulopathy group (Table 39.36). There is a preponderance of Caucasians, with a 9:1 ratio of Caucasians to African-Americans. Patients typically present with proteinuria, often nephrotic range (in 71%), and more than half have renal insufficiency at presentation. There is often associated hematuria (71%). Serologic investigation of patients typically shows normal complement and negative antinuclear antibodies, anti–neutrophil cytoplasmic antibodies and anti–glomerular basement membrane antibodies. Antibodies to hepatitis C virus may be found in those patients who are chronically infected with this virus.

PROGNOSIS AND TREATMENT

End-stage renal disease occurs commonly in fibrillary glomerulonephritis, in 40% to 50% of patients over 2 to 4 years of follow-up (Table 39.37). Older age and elevated serum creatinine at diagnosis were associated with a higher incidence of end-stage

TABLE 39.37. Clinical Course

	Fibrillary GN	Microtubular Immunotactoid GP
Progression to ESRD	~40%	Less frequent?[a]
Association with paraprotein	4%[b]	~36%[b]
Recurrence in transplant	>50%, slower progression in transplant than in native kidney	Case report

[a] From case series in Fogo A, Qureshi N, Horn RG. *Am J Kidney Dis* 22:367–377.
[b] Calculated from review in Brady HR. *Kidney Int* 1998;53:1421–1429.
ESRD, end-stage renal disease; GN, glomerulonephritis; GP, glomerulopathy.

renal disease in one large series. Only 3 of the 28 patients younger than 40 years of age at time of diagnosis of either fibrillary glomerulonephritis or immunotactoid glomerulopathy reported in the literature developed end-stage renal disease, compared with 21 of 37 patients with either lesion who was older than 40 years. The presence of crescents in fibrillary glomerulonephritis did not uniformly correlate with a poor prognosis. Thus, in one series, only four of seven patients with crescents in fibrillary glomerulonephritis developed end-stage renal disease. The percentage of obsolescent glomeruli at diagnosis was also not different between crescentic and noncrescentic cases. In our small series of six cases with immunotactoid glomerulopathy, renal function remained stable over the follow-up period, suggesting that prognosis may be somewhat better than in fibrillary glomerulonephritis.

Treatment has generally yielded disappointing results. No controlled trials have been conducted, and none are expected because of the rarity of the condition. Not surprisingly, combinations of glucocorticoids and immunosuppressive agents have been most commonly used, with only an occasional patient showing a "response." Those with underlying neoplasia and/or monoclonal gammopathies have received cytotoxic agents with varying results.

Selected Readings

Alpers CE. Immunotactoid (microtubular) glomerulopathy: an entity distinct from fibrillary glomerulonephritis? *Am J Kidney Dis* 1992;19:185–191.
Presents a case of immunotactoid glomerulopathy as it was first described. Also discusses how to separate fibrillary GN and immunotactoid glomerulopathy on morphologic grounds.

Brady HR. Fibrillary glomerulopathy. *Kidney Int* 1998;53:1421–1429.
A review of reported cases with either randomly arranged fibrils or microtubular deposits, including the author's own series. This review shows that overall incidence of malignancy was ~33% in patients with immunotactoid type versus ~7% with the fibrillary-type deposits, but if cases with a paraprotein were excluded, both groups has similar incidence of malignancy (~7%).

Fogo A, Quereshi N, Horn RG. Morphological and clinical features of fibrillary glomerulonephritis versus immunotactoid glomerulopathy. *Am J Kidney Dis* 1993;22:367–377.
A large series of cases with fibrillary, randomly arranged deposits were compared with cases with microtubular, organized deposits, indicating hematopoietic diseases were associated with the latter morphology more frequently than the former. Clinical characteristics and prognosis were also compared, showing worse prognosis in fibrillary deposits patients despite their younger age.

Iskandar SS, Falk RJ, Jennette JC. Clinical and pathologic features of fibrillary glomerulonephritis. *Kidney Int* 1992;42:1401–1407.
Detailed description of a large series of fibrillary glomerulonephritis cases with randomly arranged fibrils, showing polyclonal IgG_4 in the deposits and detailing clinical characteristics and prognosis. At 24 months follow-up, there was 48% renal survival.

Korbet SM, Rosenberg BF, Schwartz MM, et al. Course of renal transplantation in immunotactoid glomerulopathy. *Am J Med* 1990;89:91–95.
Report of recurrence of disease in one of two renal transplant recipients. Autopsy performed in the patient without recurrence showed no systemic evidence of immunotactoid deposits.

Markowitz GS, Cheng JT, Colvin RB, et al. Hepatitis C viral infection is associated with fibrillary glomerulonephritis and immunotactoid glomerulopathy. *J Am Soc Nephrol* 1998;9:2244–2252.
Report of four cases of fibrillary glomerulonephritis and two cases of immunotactoid glomerulopathy in association with hepatitis C infection, with cryoglobulin detected in one case.

Pronovost PH, Brady HR, Gunning ME, et al. Clinical features, predictors of disease progression and results of renal transplantation in fibrillary immunotactoid glomerulopathy. *Nephrol Dial Transplant* 1996;11:837–842.
A review of 161 previously reported cases and 25 cases from the authors' institutions. Recurrence of disease occurred in three of five allografts, but with slower deterioration of renal function than in the native kidney.

Rosenmann E, Eliakim M. Nephrotic syndrome associated with amyloid-like glomerular deposits. *Nephron* 1977;18:301–308.
Original description of nonamyloid fibrillary deposits.

Rostagno A, Vidal R, Kumar A, et al. Fibrillary glomerulonephritis related to serum fibrillar immunoglobulin-fibronectin complexes. *Am J Kidney Dis* 1996;28:676–684.
Case report of cryoprecipitable fibronectin-polyclonal immunoglobulin in serum of a patient with fibrillary glomerulonephritis.

Schwartz MM, Lewis EJ. The quarterly case: nephrotic syndrome in a middle-aged man. *Ultrastruct Pathol* 1980;1:575–582.
Discussion of a case with deposits with microtubular substructure, with coinage of the term immunoglobulin tactoids.

Ström EH, Banfi G, Krapf R, et al. Glomerulopathy associated with predominant fibronectin deposits: a newly recognized hereditary disease. *Kidney Int* 1995;48:163–170.
Report of a familial disease with fibronectin deposits, a condition in which deposits also have substructure.

Yang GCH, Nieto R, Stachura I, et al. Ultrastructural immunohistochemical localization of polyclonal IgG, C3, and amyloid P component on the congo red-negative amyloid-like fibrils of fibrillary glomerulopathy. *Am J Pathol* 1992;141:409–419.
Association of fibrils with amyloid-P component and the polyclonal nature of deposits are demonstrated by immunoelectron microscopy.

Zhang Z, Kundu GC, Yuan C-J, et al. Severe fibronectin-deposit renal glomerular disease in mice lacking uteroglobin. *Science* 1997;276:1408–1412.
Mice lacking uteroglobin develop a glomerular disease with fibronectin deposits, suggesting uteroglobin is necessary to prevent fibronectin dimerization and deposits.

PART 11
C1q Nephropathy

J. Charles Jennette and Ronald J. Falk

C1q nephropathy is an uncommon glomerular disease that usually manifests as steroid-resistant asymptomatic proteinuria or nephrotic syndrome. The disease has a predilection for older children and young adults and is most common in African-Americans. In an analysis of 3,914 consecutive nontransplant renal biopsies evaluated in the University of North Carolina (UNC) Nephropathology Laboratory, C1q nephropathy was diagnosed in 2.5% of the specimens obtained from patients with proteinuria greater than 3g/24 hr. In an analysis of renal biopsy specimens obtained from children with nephrotic syndrome, persistent proteinuria, or persistent nephritis, C1q nephropathy was diagnosed in 16% of the children.

The light microscopic appearance of C1q nephropathy can mimic minimal-change glomerulopathy, mesangioproliferative glomerulonephritis, or focal segmental glomerulosclerosis, but the conspicuous C1q-containing immune deposits demonstrable by immunohistology and electron microscopy rule out these diseases. The major diagnostic differential consideration is lupus nephritis.

PATHOLOGY

The *sine qua non* of C1q nephropathy is the presence of mesangial C1q-containing immune complexes (Fig. 39.22, Table 39.38). To identify a category of patients with distinctive clinical features of renal disease, C1q nephropathy should be defined as 2+ or greater (out of 0–4+), predominantly mesangial immune complex immunostaining for C1q. This mesangial C1q is almost always accompanied by IgG and IgM, which may be less intense, equally intense, or more intense. Table 39.38 details the pathologic features in the last 113 renal biopsy specimens given a diagnosis of C1q nephropathy in the UNC Nephropathology Laboratory. Note that approximately 90% of the specimens have staining for IgG and IgM along with the C1q staining, and about half of the specimens have low-intensity IgA staining.

By light microscopy, C1q nephropathy can have no glomerular changes, focal mesangial hypercellularity, or focal segmental glomerular sclerosis, and thus can mimic minimal-change glomerulopathy, focal segmental glomerulosclerosis, or other proliferative glomerulonephritides. Table 39.38 demonstrates a high frequency of both glomerular hypercellularity and sclerosis in our specimens. In pediatric series, 8 of 15 specimens had no glomerular lesions by light microscopy, 3 had mesangial hypercellularity, and 4 had focal segmental glomerular sclerosis. This suggests that the pathologic changes may be less severe in younger patients.

TABLE 39.38. Pathologic Features in the Last 113 Renal Biopsy Specimens Given a Diagnosis of C1q Nephropathy in the UNC Nephropathology Laboratory

Immunofluorescence Microscopy

Antigen	% Positive	Mean Intensity When Positive[a]
C1q	100%	2.6+
C3	88%	1.0+
IgG	95%	1.5+
IgM	90%	1.1+
IgA	50%	0.8+
κ Light chain	96%	1.2+
λ Light chain	94%	1.1+

Light Microscopy

Feature	Frequency
Glomerular sclerosis	80%
Glomerular hypercellularity	70%
Glomerular crescents	5%
Glomerular necrosis	3%
Tubular atrophy	89%
Interstitial fibrosis	88%
Interstitial leukocytes	85%
Arteriosclerosis	44%

Electron Microscopy

Feature	Frequency
Mesangial deposits	94%
Subendothelial deposits	16%
Subepithelial deposits	15%
Tubuloreticular inclusions	3%

[a] On a scale of 0.5+ = trace to 4+ = maximum immunofluorescence staining.

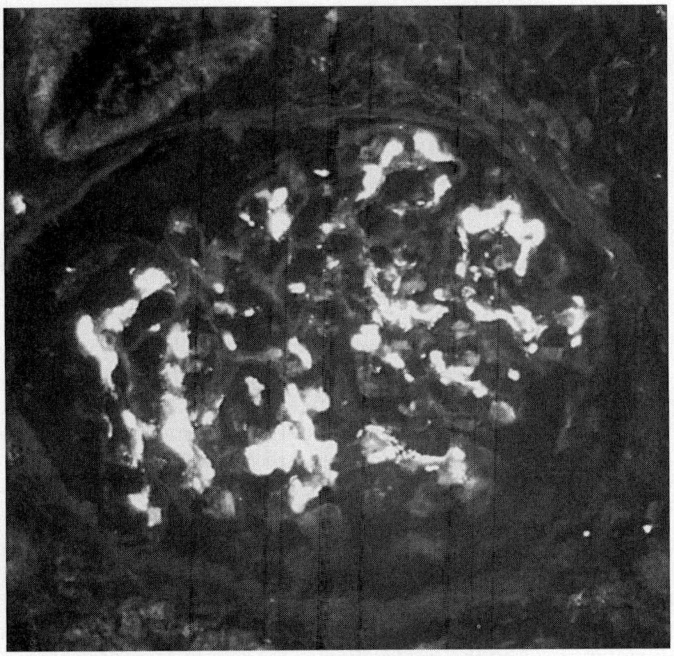

Figure 39.22. Intense mesangial immunostaining for C1q in a glomerulus from a patient with C1q nephropathy (magnification, × 400). (Reproduced with permission from Jennette JC, Hipp CG. C1q nephropathy: a distinct pathologic entity usually causing nephrotic syndrome. *Am J Kidney Dis* 1985;6:103–110.)

Electron microscopy usually demonstrates well-defined mesangial electron-dense deposits (Fig. 39.23, Table 39.38). Fewer than one-fifth of the specimens will have capillary wall–dense deposits, which usually are few and scattered. Endothelial tubuloreticular inclusions are rare, which contrasts with their frequency in lupus nephritis, and thus is a useful diagnostic feature.

DIFFERENTIAL DIAGNOSIS

When no glomerular changes are present by light microscopy, the differential diagnosis includes minimal-change glomerulopathy, but this is readily excluded once immunofluorescence microscopy and electron microscopy demonstrate immune complex–type deposits. Likewise, in specimens with segmental sclerosis, the immune complex–type deposits exclude focal segmental glomerulosclerosis. The sclerotic lesions of focal segmental glomerulosclerosis often contain trapped C1q, which should not be confused with C1q within immune complex–type deposits.

In patients with mesangial immune deposits with intense C1q staining and mesangial hypercellularity, the pathologic differential consideration is mesangioproliferative lupus nephritis (i.e., class II lupus nephritis). The major pathologic difference between these diseases is the high frequency of endothelial tubuloreticular inclusions in lupus nephritis and their usual absence in C1q nephropathy. The differentiation between C1q nephropathy and lupus nephritis, however, can be done with confidence only by

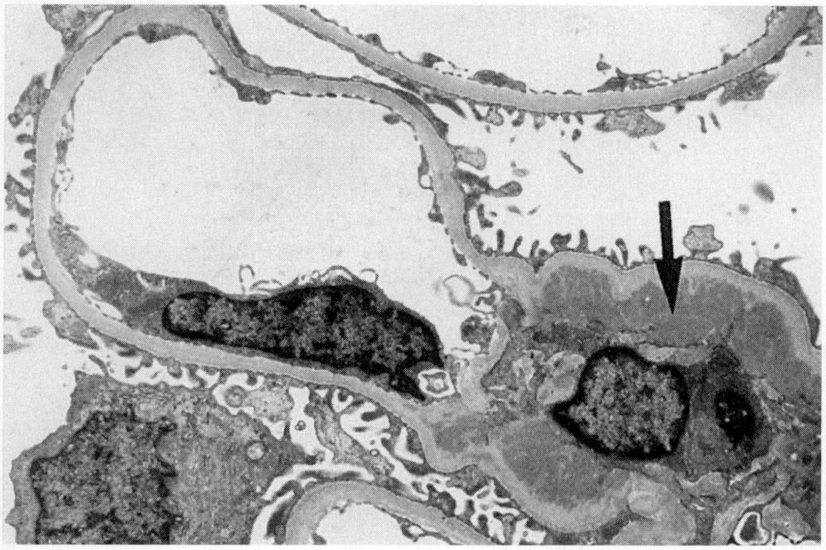

Figure 39.23. Mesangial electron-dense deposits *(arrow)* in a glomerulus from a patient with C1q nephropathy (magnification, × 4,000). (Reproduced with permission from Jennette JC, Hipp CG. C1q nephropathy: a distinct pathologic entity usually causing nephrotic syndrome. *Am J Kidney Dis* 1985;6:103–110.)

careful serologic and clinical exclusion of systemic lupus erythematosus. In a careful evaluation of 34 patients with a diagnosis of C1q nephropathy, no patients developed serologic or clinical evidence for lupus after a mean follow-up of 31 months.

Type I membranoproliferative glomerulonephritis often has intense immunostaining for C1q. This phenotype of glomerular disease, however, can be readily differentiated from C1q nephropathy by its distinctive light microscopic and ultrastructural features.

CLINICAL MANIFESTATIONS

Unless the pathologic criteria for C1q nephropathy define a category of disease that is distinctive with respect to clinical manifestations, natural history, and response to treatment, this pathologic category of disease is not worth recognizing. In fact, patients with the C1q nephropathy pathologic phenotype have a very characteristic clinical profile.

In a clinical analysis by The Glomerular Disease Collaborative Network of 34 patients with C1q nephropathy, a distinctive age distribution, racial predilection, clinical presentation, and natural history were observed. As shown in Table 39.39, there is a slight male predominance and a marked racial predilection for African-Americans compared with whites. Although C1q nephropathy occurs in all age groups, approximately 90% of patients are between 15 and 30 years of age when diagnosed. There is one report of neonatal C1q nephropathy, and we are aware of several possible familial instances of C1q nephropathy.

Virtually all patients have proteinuria at the time of diagnosis, but most are asymptomatic, including some patients with nephrotic-range proteinuria. Approximately 45% have edema, 40% have hypertension, and 30% have microscopic hematuria. Proteinuria caused by C1q nephropathy is most often first detected during a physical examination required for participation in sports, induction into the military, or obtaining insurance.

In our experience, no patient diagnosed as having C1q nephropathy after clinical and serologic exclusion of systemic lupus erythematosus has subsequently developed evidence for lupus. Because patients with evidence for lupus are excluded, no C1q nephropathy patients have antinuclear or anti-DNA antibodies. Unlike patients with lupus nephritis, patients with C1q nephropathy rarely have hypocomplementemia.

TABLE 39.39. Clinical Features of 34 patients with C1q Nephropathy at the Time of Renal Biopsy

Male:female ratio	1.8:1	
African-American:white ratio	4.7:1[a]	
Edema	44%	
Hypertension	41%	
	Mean	**Range**
Age	23.4 ± 11.7 yr	2–66[b]
Proteinuria	5.9 ± 4.3 g/day	0.6–19.8
Creatinine	1.5 ± 0.9 mg/dl	0.4–5.9
Albumin	3.3 ± 0.8 g/dl	1.9–4.7
Cholesterol	294 ± 105 mg/dl	159–567

[a]The expected ratio of African-Americans to whites in this renal biopsy population is 0.3:1.

[b]Of 34 patients, 31 (91%) were from 14 to 31 years old.

Derived from data in Jennette JC, Wilkman AS, Hogan SL, et al. Clinical and pathologic features of C1q nephropathy (C1qN). *J Am Soc Nephrol* 1993;4:681.

NATURAL HISTORY AND MANAGEMENT

The natural history of C1q nephropathy is characterized by persistent proteinuria that typically does not respond completely to steroid treatment. Approximately 90% of patients with C1q nephropathy continue to have proteinuria after a mean follow-up of 2.5 years.

An analysis by The Glomerular Disease Collaborative Network of 12 untreated and 21 prednisone-treated patients is summarized in Table 39.40. Patients treated with prednisone had no statistically significant improvement in proteinuria or preservation of renal function compared with untreated patients; however, of the treated group, three had complete remission of proteinuria and one had end-stage renal failure, compared with no complete remission of proteinuria and three cases of end-stage renal failure in the untreated group. The three cases of remission in the treated group, however, occurred months to years after cessation of steroid treatment and therefore may not have been induced by the treatment.

Others have also observed a poor response of C1q nephropathy to corticosteroid treatment but have suggested that patients with no glomerular abnormalities by light microscopy

TABLE 39.40. Changes in Laboratory Values After a Mean Follow-Up of 31 Months in 34 Patients with C1q Nephropathy Who Received No Specific Treatment Compared with Those Who Received Prednisone

	At Time of Biopsy	After Follow-Up
Untreated Patients (n = 12)		
Proteinuria (g/24 hr)	5.2	2.4
Creatinine (mg/dl)	1.7	3.0
Albumin (g/dl)	3.6	3.7
Cholesterol (mg/dl)	269	210
Complete remission		0%
ESRD		25%
Treated Patients (n = 21)		
Proteinuria (g/24 hr)	7.0	3.9
Creatinine (mg/dl)	1.2	1.3
Albumin (g/dl)	2.9	3.5
Cholesterol (mg/dl)	338	232
Complete remission		14%
ESRD		5%

ESRD, end-stage renal disease.

may have a better response than those with glomerular sclerosis or hypercellularity.

Life table analysis has demonstrated renal survival of 84% at 3 years. Elevated serum creatinine at the time of diagnosis is the clinical parameter that correlates best with progressive renal failure.

PATHOGENESIS

The etiology and pathogenesis of C1q nephropathy are unknown; however, the immunohistologic and ultrastructural features incriminate *in situ* formation or deposition of immune complexes as the cause. The conspicuous C1q in the immune complexes could be (a) bound to the Fc region of immune-complexed IgG or IgM, (b) bound to the Fab region of anti-C1q antibodies, or (c) bound to the antigen component of the complexes.

C1q binds to IgG and IgM during classical pathway complement activation. This does not necessarily result in conspicuous immunostaining for C1q in immune deposits, as evidenced by specimens with extensive immune complex deposits containing intensely staining IgG and IgM but no or scant C1q (e.g., idiopathic membranous glomerulopathy). C1q in immune complex may facilitate localization in the glomerular mesangium because mesangial cells have specific receptors for C1q.

Anti-C1q antibodies are known to occur in some patients with glomerulonephritis, such as lupus nephritis and the nephritis associated with hypocomplementemic vasculitis. Anti-C1q antibodies have not been reported in patients with C1q nephropathy.

Because C1q is a very basic molecule, it binds to many polyanionic substances, such as DNA, RNA, polynucleotides, and lipopolysaccharides. One explanation for the intense C1q immunostaining observed in most lupus nephritis specimens is that the C1q is binding to the anionic nucleic acids comprising the immune complexes. Similarly, C1q nephropathy may be caused by immune complexes that contain polyanionic antigens, such as microbial cell wall lipopolysaccharides, that electrostatically bind large amounts of C1q.

Selected Readings

Iskandar SS, Browning MC, Lorentz WB. C1q nephropathy: a pediatric clinicopathologic study. *Am J Kidney Dis* 1991;18:459–465.

An analysis of C1q nephropathy in 15 children. Noted that even patients with no lesions by light microscopy responded poorly to steroid treatment.

Jennette JC, Hipp CG. C1q nephropathy: a distinct pathologic entity usually causing nephrotic syndrome. *Am J Kidney Dis* 1985;6:103–110.

First published description of C1q nephropathy. The 15 patients ranged in age from 14 to 27 and had steroid-resistant proteinuria.

Jennette JC, Hipp CG. Immunohistopathologic evaluation of C1q in 800 renal biopsy specimens. *Am J Clin Pathol* 1985;83:415–420.

Pathologic analysis demonstrating that C1q nephropathy, lupus nephritis, and type I membranoproliferative glomerulonephritis are the only glomerular diseases that frequently have conspicuous C1q within immune deposits.

Kuwano M, Ito Y, Amamoto Y, et al. A case report of congenital nephrotic syndrome associated with positive C1q immunofluorescence. *Pediatr Nephrol* 1993;7:452–454.

A report of typical C1q nephropathy in a 1-month-old infant with nephrotic syndrome.

Shappell SB, Myrthil G, Fogo A. An adolescent with relapsing nephrotic syndrome: minimal-change disease versus focal segmental glomerulosclerosis versus C1q nephropathy. *Am J Kidney Dis* 1997;29:955–970.

A review of the pathologic, clinical, and prognostic differences between C1q nephropathy, focal segmental glomerulosclerosis, and minimal-change glomerulopathy.

van den Dobbelsteen ME, van der Wouda FJ, Schroeijers WE, et al. Both IgG- and C1q-receptors play a role in the enhanced binding of IgG complexes to human mesangial cells. *J Am Soc Nephrol* 1996;7:573–581.

Report of an in vitro study that demonstrated the presence of receptors for C1q on mesangial cells that were capable of binding immune complexes that contain C1q.

PART 12
IgA Nephropathy

L.A. van Es

IgA nephropathy is the most common type of primary glomerulonephritis in many parts of the world. It is characterized by the predominant deposition of IgA in the mesangial area of the glomeruli. The histology may vary from mild mesangial proliferation to severe crescentic glomerulonephritis. Clinically, the disease begins with episodes of hematuria, followed frequently several years later by proteinuria, hypertension, and progressive reduction of the glomerular filtration rate (GFR). Deposits of IgA in the walls of extrarenal vessels may occur, but the presence of cutaneous leukocytoclastic vasculitis is more suggestive of anaphylactoid purpura or Henoch-Schöenlein purpura. A full understanding of the etiology and pathogenesis remains illusive after decades of clinical and laboratory investigations. Although prognosis is better understood, effective treatment regimens are only now emerging for selected groups of patients.

IgA nephropathy was first described by Berger in 1969, years after the introduction of the immunofluorescence technique in the mid 1950s. The disease was discovered relatively late because hematuria without any other renal manifestations was not considered a major clinical problem, and therefore renal biopsies were not regularly performed. The disease received more attention in the early 1980s, when long-term follow-up data illustrated that a considerable number of patients with IgA nephropathy have a slow indolent course to end-stage renal failure. It subsequently became clear that the low prevalence of IgA nephropathy in certain parts of the world could be attributed to a restrictive policy with regard to renal biopsies in this disease. Because therapy is not yet fully understood, most clinicians in the United States believe that taking a renal biopsy of a patient with isolated hematuria represents an

TABLE 39.41. Diseases Reported in Association with IgA Mesangial Deposits

Rheumatic diseases
- Ankylosing spondylitis
- Rheumatoid arthritis
- Reiter's syndrome

Gastrointestinal diseases
- Celiac disease
- Ulcerative colitis
- Crohn's disease

Hepatic diseases
- Hepatic cirrhosis
- Alcoholic liver disease

Dermatologic diseases
- Dermatitis herpetiformis
- Psoriasis

Neoplastic diseases
- Mycosis fungoides
- Sézary syndrome
- Bronchial carcinoma
- Laryngeal carcinoma
- IgA monoclonal gammopathy (IgA myeloma)

Unclassified
- Idiopathic pulmonary hemosiderosis
- Retroperitoneal fibrosis
- Sarcoidosis
- Properdin deficiency
- AIDS
- Episcleritis

invasive diagnostic procedure without therapeutic consequences. For this reason, studies on IgA nephropathy often appear from Europe and Asia, where renal biopsies are performed more regularly. When it was realized that IgA nephropathy is a relatively common type of glomerulonephritis, at least in the developed part of the world, scientific interest in IgA nephropathy gained considerable momentum. The progress made in the 1990s not only has given more insight in the pathogenesis of the disease but also has led to a better understanding of natural history and treatment.

IgA mesangial deposits have been reported to be associated with other diseases such as liver cirrhosis, ankylosing spondylitis, celiac disease, dermatitis herpetiformis, malignancy, and many other conditions (Table 39.41). The common denominator that could explain the development of IgA mesangial deposits in these diseases is unknown. When no other diseases are present, the diagnosis of primary IgA nephropathy or Berger's disease is established when glomerular mesangial deposits of IgA predominate. Henoch-Schönlein purpura, which is also characterized by mesangial deposits of IgA, can be regarded as a multisystem form of IgA nephropathy.

PATHOLOGY

The glomerular lesions described in renal biopsies of patients with IgA nephropathy can vary from mild mesangial or focal and segmental intracapillary proliferation, or mesangioproliferative glomerulonephritis to moderate or severe intracapillary and extracapillary proliferative lesions, including crescent formation (see Chapter 109). If present, the crescents are usually not circumferential. Biopsies with mild mesangial lesions show very few polymorphonuclear leukocytes (PMNs) and mononuclear cells in the glomeruli. However, when the glomerular lesions are more severe, numerous mononuclear cells are found in the mesangium and in Bowman's space. The number of macrophages in the glomeruli correlate with the severity of proteinuria and presence of crescents. In crescentic IgA nephropathy, not only macrophages but also T cells can be detected in the glomeruli. On the basis of the increased expression of the receptor for interleukin-2 (IL-2), it is assumed that these lymphocytes are activated. Biopsies from patients with crescentic IgA nephropathy show more activated T lymphocytes than in noncrescentic biopsies. Some patients may present with minimal glomerular lesions similar to minimal-change disease.

When IgA nephropathy progresses, tubulointerstitial changes develop. Mononuclear cells appear in the interstitium. These cells consist of macrophages and CD4- or CD8-positive lymphocytes. In more advanced stages of the disease, mononuclear cells and tubular atrophy are found together with interstitial fibrosis, leading to widening of the interstitial space. The size of the cortical interstitial space correlates with the serum creatinine level. Patients with acute reversible renal failure observed in association with episodes of macroscopic hematuria frequently demonstrate many large red cell casts in tubules, acute tubular necrosis, and interstitial nephritis.

The mesangial deposits of IgA are often accompanied by IgG and C3. Biopsies with moderate to severe glomerular lesions do not show a higher percentage of IgG deposition than biopsies showing mild or minimal glomerular changes. IgM can also be present but is less common than IgG. C3 is often accompanied by properdin, whereas components of the classical pathway (C1q) are rarely seen. The IgA_1 subclass predominates in the mesangial deposits often accompanied by the λ light chain. Although J-chain may also be associated with IgM, the presence of J-chain strongly suggest that at least part of the IgA deposits, if not all, consist of polymeric IgA_1. These deposits are often accompanied by components of the alternative pathway and the terminal sequence of the membrane attack complex complement. Secretory piece of IgA is absent.

By immunoelectronmicroscopy, IgA, IgG, IgM, and C3 can be detected between mesangial cells. Occasionally, smaller masses of IgA and C3 can be observed along the glomerular capillary loops. The IgA deposits found in the capillary loops are usually localized in a subendothelial position, but they can also be intramembranous or subepithelial. Electron microscopy usually demonstrates large mesangial or paramesangial dense deposits.

CLINICAL PRESENTATION AND NATURAL HISTORY

Clinical Presentation

Patients with IgA nephropathy are usually young to early middle-age individuals, often male, who have asymptomatic microscopic hematuria (Table 39.42). The usual age range at the time of diagnosis is between 10 and 40 years. About 40% of patients have recurrent macroscopic hematuria, often preceded 1 or 2 days earlier by infections ("synpharyngitic nephritis"). Upper airway infections have been observed most frequently, but other infections have also been implicated, including urinary tract infections and mastitis. In about 30% of cases, unilateral or bilateral loin pain can be present, giving rise to confusion with a urinary tract infection or passage of a stone. A family history of glomerulonephritis or IgA nephropathy occurs in a minority of cases. Mild proteinuria is not uncommon, whereas heavy proteinuria and the nephrotic syndrome are present in only a few cases. Proteinuria often antedates hypertension and the insidious but progressive loss of renal function. Some patients may present with acute reversible renal failure following

TABLE 39.42. Clinical Features of IgA Nephropathy at Presentation

Clinical Feature	Prevalence (%) Mean	Range
Age	30.4 yr	19–42 yr
Male:female ratio	2.16	1.1–10.3
Loin pain	31%	7%–37%
Family history	11%	3%–20%
Microscopic hematuria	87.5%	53%–100%
Macroscopic hematuria	42.7%	5%–87%
Infection-related exacerbations	40.7%	10%–69%
Proteinuria 1–3 g/24 hr	46.8%	18%–81%
>3 g/24 hr	10.8%	0%–38%
Hypertension	25.2%	7%–52%
Reduced glomerular filtration rate	20.7%	5%–38%

Modified with permission from Ibels LS, Györy AZ. IgA nephropathy: analysis of the natural history, important factors in the progression of renal disease, and a review of the literature. *Medicine* 1994;73:79–102.

TABLE 39.43. Clinical and Histologic Features That Predicts a Higher Likelihood of Future Progression of IgA Nephropathy

Clinical Features
Persistent proteinuria (>1–2 g/24 hr)
Hypertension
Reduced glomerular filtration rate at presentation (elevated serum creatinine ≥1.5 mg/dl)
Persistent microscopic hematuria
Persistence of hyaline casts
Histologic Features
The extent of glomerulosclerosis
Crescent formation
Capsular adhesions
Tubular atrophy
Interstitial inflammation
Interstitial fibrosis
Blood vessel thickening
Immunologic Features
Density and mesangiocapillary pattern of IgA and C3 deposits

an upper respiratory infection and macroscopic hematuria. Malignant hypertension is rarely the initial clinical finding.

Natural History

Spontaneous remission has been documented in children and in adults. Of the 38% of Japanese children who went in clinical remission, very few histologic lesions were seen in the repeat biopsy. Clinical remission may also occur in 6% to 12% of adults with IgA nephropathy, however, without histologic improvement.

Patients with recurrent attacks of macroscopic hematuria following an upper airway infection may have leucocyturia with a negative urine culture. Macroscopic hematuria occurs more often in children than in adults. Its prevalence varies with geographic areas, being lower in Asia and Northern Europe and higher in Southern Europe and Australia. The long-term prognosis of patients with infection-related and recurrent macroscopic hematuria is more favorable. Patients with gross hematuria and a significant rise of their serum creatinine frequently have intracapillary and extracapillary lesions with crescent formation in their biopsies, as well as tubular interstitial lesions. Patients can even develop acute renal failure either on the basis of crescentic glomerulonephritis, on the basis of renal tubular obstruction by red blood cell casts, or on the basis of the inflammatory effects of hemoglobin in tubular lumina.

The disease has an indolent course in most patients with chronic or intermittent microscopic hematuria. Because the disease may remain undetected for many years, it is difficult to establish the onset of the disease. It has been detected by periodic screening of Japanese school children at a young age, but in European studies, it is usually detected in adults in their twenties or thirties. When biopsies of adults are compared with biopsies of children, the prevalence of tubulointerstitial changes is not higher, suggesting that not all cases of IgA nephropathy start at an early age.

Attacks of macroscopic hematuria become less frequent over the course of IgA nephropathy. The level of proteinuria, the severity of hypertension, and the degree of microscopic hematuria are indicators of progression of the disease, manifested by a steady loss of GFR (Table 39.43). It is obvious that when GFR is reduced at presentation, end-stage renal failure may develop sooner. The persistence of hyaline casts was also reported as a prognostic indicator. The initially mild proteinuria may progress to heavy proteinuria in the nephrotic range. Worsening of proteinuria is usually considered an indication of poor prognosis.

The extent of segmental and global sclerosis together with capsular adhesions are prognostic indicators (Table 39.43). Biopsies of children going into remission or going into a progressive course did not differ in their clinical presentation or the severity of the renal lesions in their initial biopsies. The two groups did not differ in the frequency of crescents or the degree of mesangial hypercellularity. However, an increase of mesangial matrix was usually seen in the follow-up biopsy of patients with persistent hematuria and proteinuria and not in biopsies of patients in clinical remission. Other studies have found a correlation between crescent formation and an adverse outcome. The progression in IgA nephropathy correlates with the severity of tubulointerstitial damage, such as tubular atrophy, interstitial infiltration by macrophages and T lymphocytes, and interstitial fibrosis.

Hyperplasia of the wall of intrarenal arteries and arterioles, together with hyalinosis, has been observed in the absence of hypertension. These observations suggest the possibility that the vascular changes are not caused by hypertension but that systemic hypertension may be the consequence of these vascular changes. Studies have shown that low dosages of angiotensin-converting enzyme (ACE) inhibitors can reduce the proteinuria, the tubulointerstitial changes, and the vascular changes without influencing the level of the systemic blood pressure, suggesting that angiotensin II may play a role in the pathogenesis of tubulointerstitial and vascular damage.

Several studies have shown that both the intensity of deposition of IgA and C3 in the mesangium as well as the extension of these deposits in the glomerular capillary walls correlate with a progressive course of the disease. Children in clinical and histologic remission have a significant diminution of IgA deposition. Multivariate analysis showed an independent unfavorable effect of combined mesangial and capillary deposition of IgM on renal outcome. However, the presence of IgM and C3 could also be explained by its association with sclerotic lesions in the glomeruli.

TABLE 39.44. Actuarial Renal Survival in Patients with IgA Nephropathy

	Renal Survival (%)[a]	
	Mean	Range
5 yr	94	83–100
10 yr	86.4	78–94
15 yr	77.4	71–88
20 yr	70	50–83

[a]Percentage of renal survival as defined by freedom from the need for chronic dialysis or renal transplantation, obtained from 22 reports and reviewed in Ibels LS, Györy AZ. IgA nephropathy: analysis of the natural history, important factors in the progression of renal disease, and a review of the literature. *Medicine* 1994;73:79–102.

IgA nephropathy was initially considered a benign disease. When 20-year follow-up data became available, it was realized that each year, a consistent percentage of this population develops end-stage renal failure. About 7% to 10% of patients receiving chronic hemodialysis have IgA nephropathy as their original renal disease. Calculated from the first renal symptom, about 1.5% of patients reach the need for chronic dialysis each year. When calculated from the time of biopsy, about 1.3% of patients develop end-stage renal failure each year (Table 39.44). While these figures can be applied to groups of patients with IgA nephropathy, they cannot be applied to individual patients. Some patients have a very rapid course and others do not progress at all. Prognostication at the level of the individual patients is fraught with inaccuracies, but individual patients with a worse-than-average or a better-than-average prognosis can be identified by a simulation of clinical (e.g., serum creatinine level, urinary protein excretion) and histologic features (glomerulosclerosis and interstitial fibrosis) at the time of diagnosis.

GEOGRAPHIC DIFFERENCES

The geographic differences in incidence and prevalence of IgA nephropathy are heavily influenced by the accessibility to medical care and the policy for performing renal biopsy. Despite these confounding factors, some striking differences have been reported. The incidence and prevalence of IgA nephropathy in Japan and probably other Asian countries is high compared with the estimated incidence and prevalence in Europe. The incidence in American Indians is the highest reported. The factors responsible for these geographic and racial differences are not known. They could be environmental, genetic, or both.

GENETIC PREDISPOSITION

In an extensive family study in the United States, 60% of patients from eastern Kentucky were related to at least one other patient. Environmental factors such as occupation, types of residence, or food were excluded. This may suggest a genetic predisposition in the members of this pedigree. Several studies have reported the occurrence of IgA nephropathy in first-degree relatives. However, in about 90% of the cases, IgA nephropathy is a sporadic disease. The development of IgA nephropathy has been linked to various polymorphic genetic systems encodecd within the HLA major histocompatibility complex (MHC), such as the class I and class II HLA molecules; the complement components C2, C4, and factor B (class III); and tumor necrosis factor. The disease has been associated with several phenotypes of the HLA MHC. However, these associations may differ widely among geographic areas. Disease association with HLA-B12 has been reported in the United States, whereas the association with HLA-B35 has been reported in France, Australia, and the United States. The association with HLA-DR4 was found in France and Japan and for HLA-DR1 in England. Other studies from Germany, The Netherlands, Japan, France, Italy, The United States, England, Finland, and Hungary were unable to find associations with HLA allotypes. HLA-B35 and HLA-DR4 have also been implicated in a more rapid progression of the disease.

The complement components C4 and factor B (Bf) are encoded within the MHC locus. An association of IgA nephropathy was found with a homozygous C4 null phenotype and the Bf FF phenotype. A significant excess of the C3FF phenotype was found in a German and Dutch population. The disease has also been associated with the polymorphism of the heavy chain switch region. A significant increase in the 7.4 kb $S_{\alpha 1}$ phenotype was observed in patients with IgA nephropathy. A very interesting association was found between a more rapid decline of renal function and the DD genotype of angiotensin converting enzyme, but an association between the prevalence of IgA nephropathy and ACE polymorphism remains controversial.

ETIOLOGY

The onset or exacerbation of IgA nephropathy is often preceded by a respiratory tract infection or infections at other locations a few days earlier. The association with *Campylobacter jejuni, Yersinia enterocolitica,* and *Mycoplasma pneumoniae* has been reported. Except in individual cases, no specific bacterial infection has been detected to be associated with the development of IgA nephropathy. Several viruses have been implicated in the etiology of this disease. Extensive virologic investigation for adenovirus, Coxsackie virus, varicella-zoster virus, cytomegalovirus, or Epstein-Barr virus in tonsils, renal tissue, and mouth washings did not reveal any positive results. Hepatitis B and C do not seem to play any role.

IgA nephropathy has also been associated with hypersensitivity to specific food components such as gluten. Withdrawal of gluten from the diet of these selected patients resulted in both immunologic and clinical improvement. In a large series of Italian patients, antigliadin antibodies occurred in only 3% of patients. Antigliadin antibody–positive patients had small intestinal mucosal atrophy and reacted favorably on a gluten-free diet also with respect to their IgA nephropathy. These data suggest that IgA nephropathy may occur as a complication of celiac disease, but in most patients with IgA nephropathy, hypersensitivity to gluten does not seem to play a pathogenetic role. The IgA antibody titer directed against bovine γ-globulin, β-lactoglobulin, chicken γ-globulin, ovalbumin, pig γ-globulin, soy flour extract or surface protein of streptococcus mutans does not differ between patients and controls, whereas deposits of soy bean and casein antigens could not be demonstrated in the glomeruli of Japanese patients. These studies suggest that IgA nephropathy may not be just one disease, but rather a complication due to an abnormal response of the mucosal immune system to various antigens. Thus it appears that genetic as well as environmental factors may play a role in the causation of IgA nephropathy in some patients, but as yet a unifying hypothesis involving a single gene locus or a specific environmental factor is lacking.

PATHOGENESIS

The predominance of IgA in the mesangium strongly suggests, but does not prove, that these deposits are the consequence of an immune response initiated at the mucosal level. The association of recurrent macroscopic hematuria with infections of the upper respiratory tract suggests further that microbial antigens may be involved in the IgA immune response. However, no specific microbial antigen has until now been implicated. Interestingly, the IgA deposited in the mesangium belongs almost exclusively to the IgA_1 subclass. Several explanations could be given for the selective mesangial deposition of IgA_1. First, the B lymphocytes stimulated at a particular mucosal site could have a predilection to produce IgA_1 antibodies. The IgA subclass distribution varies with different mucosal locations. Second, the responsible antigen could induce preferentially an IgA_1 response as is known for proteins, whereas carbohydrates induce preferentially an IgA_1 response as is known for proteins, whereas carbohydrates induce preferentially an IgA_2 response. However, after vaccination of patients with viral antigens, both IgA_1 and IgA_2 responses can be observed. Third, IgA nephropathy patients could also have a selective hyperresponsiveness for IgA_1. Fourth, the molecular characteristics of IgA_1 in patients with IgA nephropathy could favor self-aggregation and mesangial deposition or promote an autoantibody response to autologous IgA_1, resulting in the formation of immune complexes. The recognition of defective galactosylation of a subset of IgA_1 molecules supports this explanation.

Macromolecular IgA in the Circulation

A pivotal observation with regard to the pathogenesis of IgA nephropathy is the high recurrence rate of mesangial IgA deposits in kidneys transplanted into recipients who had IgA nephropathy as their original disease. On the other hand, kidneys from patients with IgA nephropathy unintentionally transplanted into recipients who did not originally have IgA nephropathy show spontaneous recovery. These clinical observations indicate that a circulating factor in IgA nephropathy patients is responsible for mesangial deposition of IgA. This factor has not been clearly identified. It could be circulating IgA_1-containing immune complexes or aggregates of IgA_1 (polymeric IgA). The finding of extrarenal IgA deposits are consistent with such a mechanism. Another possibility would be that circulating IgA antibodies react with antigens, receptors, or any other molecules on the surface of the mesangial cell, including native as well as "planted" antigens. It is even conceivable that the hypothetical binding structure on the mesangial cell surface is more easily induced in IgA nephropathy patients than in healthy individuals. It should be noted that the IgA deposits frequently recur, but clinical manifestations of IgA nephropathy in renal allografts are uncommon. It is assumed that the immunosuppressive regimen in transplant recipients prevents the full development of an inflammatory reaction after deposition of IgA has occurred in the mesangium.

The presence of macromolecular IgA in the circulation of patients with IgA nephropathy was first documented by sucrose density gradient ultracentrifugation of sera from patients with this disease. The macromolecular IgA was varied in size between 300 and 1000 kD. Because this IgA was capable of binding to secretory component (SC), it probably represents polymeric IgA (pIgA) or complexes of IgA and antigen. Control subjects and IgA nephropathy patients with mucosal infections both respond with increases in serum concentrations of pIgA, but in patients the pIgA, levels rise higher and persist longer. Episodes of macroscopic hematuria are associated in children with elevated levels of pIgA and IgA-containing immune complexes. During infection-related relapses of macroscopic hematuria, children have more IgA-bearing B lymphocytes in their circulation that produce more pIgA than is seen in control children with infections. The presence of elevated serum levels of pIgA during relapses does not exclude the simultaneous presence of IgA immune complexes in the circulation. Because the antigen putatively involved in the pathogenesis of IgA nephropathy is not known, the distinction between pIgA and pIgA-containing immune complexes cannot easily be made. Several antigen-independent techniques have been developed to demonstrate the presence of IgA complexes in sera of patients with IgA nephropathy. In contrast to the IgA complexes found in patients with anaphylactoid purpura, the macromolecular IgA in sera of IgA nephropathy patients is not easily precipitated in 3% polyethylene glycol, suggesting a smaller size than is found in anaphylactoid purpura.

Elevated Levels of Serum IgA

Concentrations of serum IgA are elevated in about half of the patients with IgA nephropathy. Increased levels of serum IgA in diseases associated with IgA mesangial deposits, such as ankylosing spondylitis, are well known. The increase in serum IgA levels is only significant for the IgA_1 subclass. Whether the serum concentrations of polymeric IgA or IgA_1 are higher than in controls is still controversial. The controversy could be explained by the clinical condition of the patient. Half of the patients with an episode of macroscopic hematuria have elevated polymeric IgA, whereas none of the patients had this during a quiescent phase of the disease.

The increase in serum IgA could be the result of either decreased degradation or increased production. Studies on the elimination of IgA in rodents have little relevance to humans because rodents have predominantly polymeric IgA in their circulation and SC receptors on the sinusoidal side of their hepatocytes. In humans, IgA is also eliminated by the liver, but humans have no or very few SC receptors on their hepatocytes. Human hepatocytes have asialoglyprotein receptors, which bind to desialylated galactosyl residues of the olgiosaccharide side chains of the IgA molecule. After endocytosis, the receptor–ligand is dissociated and IgA is degraded in the lysosomal compartment of the hepatocyte. Few studies have been performed in human IgA nephropathy. Using radiolabeled IgA–IgG aggregates, a slower clearance rate was found in IgA nephropathy patients than in controls.

Increased synthesis of IgA in patients was found after parenteral immunization. Following subcutaneous vaccination with tetanus toxoid, significantly higher IgA antibody titers were found than in controls. In another study, specific IgA responses against tetanus toxoid were found to be similar in patients and controls, but patients produced more polymeric IgA antibodies and the polymeric IgA response lasted longer. Higher IgA antibody responses were also found after intramuscular vaccination with inactivated influenza virus. These antigens probably represent recall antigens. The increased production of influenza-specific IgA antibodies was significantly higher only for IgA_1 antibodies and not for IgA_2, IgG, or IgM. Elevated production of monomeric and polymeric IgA was found in the bone marrow of IgA nephropathy patients. The connection between the mucosal immune system and the bone marrow, the so-called mucosa–bone marrow axis, is not based on the overflow of IgA antibodies from the mucosa into the vascular compartment, but it is probably based on traffic of either antigen presenting cells or antigen-specific lymphocytes from the mucosa to the bone marrow. After intranasal challenge with a neoantigen [cholera toxin B (CTB), patients with IgA nephropathy do not develop a specific mucosal immune response and have significantly lower IgA responses by their peripheral blood mononuclear cells, lower IgA anti-CTB plasma levels, and a lower IgA anti-CTB response in their bone marrow compared with healthy controls. Apparently, these patients have a defective mucosal response after intranasal challenge with a neoantigen and they may need a more frequent and/or prolonged antigen exposure before they can develop an effective mucosal (memory) response. As a consequence of the repetitive mucosal exposure to ubiquitous antigens, the IgA production in the bone marrow and the IgA plasma levels are elevated when the mucosal response is adequate enough to protect against recurrent nasal infections.

Formation of Mesangial Deposits

It has been suggested that the high levels of serum IgA in themselves could be responsible for mesangial IgA deposition. Although serum IgA levels are often elevated in IgA nephropathy, it does not occur in all patients. The rare occurrence of IgA mesangial deposits in AIDS patients strongly argues against high serum IgA levels as a pathogenetic factor because these levels are significantly higher in AIDS patients than in IgA nephropathy patients.

Because circulating macromolecular IgA cannot be detected in all patients with IgA nephropathy, other hypotheses have been proposed than the deposition of circulating IgA immune complexes or IgA in the mesangium. In one theory, circulating IgA antibodies react with antigens either planted on the surface of the mesangial cell or intrinsically expressed by the mesangial cell. Sera of patients with IgA nephropathy have been tested by immunofluorescence microscopy and by fluorescence-activated cell sorting. No IgA antimesangial antibodies were detected. Antibodies directed against umbilical vein endothelium were found in sera of some patients. The prevalence of specific IgA and IgG antibodies in these patients varies between 15% and 35%. Autoantibodies directed against nuclear antigens, histone, and myeloperoxidase occur in a minority of patients. False-positive results due to the presence of IgA rheumatoid factor have not been sufficiently excluded. The involvement of microbial and dietary antigens has been suggested in case reports, but such involvement has not been demonstrated in larger series. Another theory has suggested that IgA is not bound to the mesangium by its antigenic specificity but by its carbohydrate composition, giving it an affinity to the fibronectin matrix in the mesangium. This hypothesis has not been supported by experimental studies. Research on the carbohydrate composition of IgA_1, in sera of IgA nephropathy patients, suggest that the O-linked carbohydrates in the hinge region contain less terminal galactose. Such defective galactosylation appears to be due to a deficiency of $\beta_{1,3}$-galactosyltransferase in IgA-secreting B cells. Reduced galactosylation of IgA_1 could lead to poor hepatic clearance. The abnormal galactosylated IgA_1 has a tendency to self-aggregate and bind to mesangium. These abnormal IgA_1 molecules could also provoke autoantibody formation, leading to the development of immune complexes. Another possibility could be that mesangial cells in IgA nephropathy patients have a high affinity for pIgA via specific Fc_α receptors ($Fc_{\alpha R}$). Whether such receptors are present in human the mesangium remains controversial.

The Inflammatory Reaction in the Glomerulus

The acute initial phase of the disease is characterized by mesangial proliferation. Few monocytes are present unless the intracapillary and extracapillary inflammation is severe enough to lead to crescent formation. Crescents are often found during relapses characterized by macroscopic hematuria and reduction of GFR. Biopsies taken during relapses show more monocytes and T cells than biopsies of IgA nephropathy patients without crescents. During relapse, these mononuclear cells express IL-2 receptors as a sign of activation. PMNs occur at very low numbers.

Several mediator systems have been implicated in the inflammatory process in the glomeruli. In analogy to models of experimental nephritis, complement activation has been studied in human biopsies. C3 and properdin are found at the same location as the IgA deposits in 75% to 100% of the cases. The presence of the membrane attack complex in the deposits correlates with disease activity. On the other hand, C9 does not seem to be essential because IgA nephropathy occurs also in patients with congenital C9 deficiency. Components of the classical pathway (C1q) are found in fewer than 10% of cases, suggesting that C3 and the membrane attack complex are activated by the alternative pathway.

THE PROLIFERATIVE RESPONSE IN THE GLOMERULUS

This stage of the disease is characterized by proliferation of renal cells. Studies on the induction of cytokine production by mesangial cells raise the possibility that the proliferative response of the mesangium might be the result of local cytokine production. IgA immune complexes and pIgA induce the activation of rat mesangial cells. In contrast to monomeric IgA, polymeric IgA binds efficiently to mesangial cells. This binding is not influenced by fibronectin or asialofetuin. IgA immune complexes as well as pIgA induce IL-6 production by mesangial cells in a dose dependent fashion.

Activated mesangial cells produce monocyte chemotactic protein-1 (MCP-1), which attracts monocytes and T lymphocytes but not polymorphonuclear leucocytes. The influx of monocytes can be responsible for the release of IL-1, and TNF-α. These cytokines are capable of inducing the expression of adhesion molecules in endothelial cells. The expression of ICAM-1 in the glomerular capillaries of IgA nephropathy patients correlates with the severity of the glomerular lesions. Once mesangial cells are activated by these cytokines, they start to produce IL-1, IL-6, platelet-derived growth factor (PDGF), and transforming growth factor-B (TGF-β). These and other cytokines have a proliferative effect on mesangial cells *in vitro.*

In renal biopsies of IgA nephropathy patients, mRNA for IL-1, IL-6, TNF-α, and PDGF B chain can readily be demonstrated in monocytes and macrophages by *in situ* hybridisation. Weaker staining can be observed in mesangial, tubular, and endothelial cells. IL-1 and IL-6 stimulates the proliferation of mesangial cells *in vitro.* It is unclear whether IL-6 has the same effect *in vivo.* The correlation that was observed between the level of IL-6 excretion in the urine and the severity of the glomerular lesions in IgA nephropathy suggests that IL-6 may also play an important role *in vivo.* Mesangial cells express mRNA for both the A and the B chain of PDGF. In IgA nephropathy, the glomeruli show increased expression of PDGF and PDGF receptors. PDGF released by platelets, monocytes and mesangial cells may stimulate mesangial cells to proliferate. These observations strongly suggest that the mesangial proliferation seen in the chronic stage of IgA nephropathy is the result of local production of cytokines by monocytes/macrophages, T lymphocytes, and mesangial cells.

The Development of Glomerulosclerosis and Interstitial Fibrosis

Repeat biopsies in IgA nephropathy patients have shown a high correlation of interstitial infiltrate with progression to end-stage renal failure. A positive correlation of glomerulosclerosis with progression of the disease would be expected but is less well established. It has been puzzling to most investigators how glomerular abnormalities would lead to tubular atrophy, interstitial infiltrate, and fibrosis. For many years, these changes were explained by glomerular ischemia and obsolescence resulting in functional deterioration of the downstream nephron. With the discovery of cytokine production by mesangial, tubular, and endothelial cells of the kidneys, new concepts have been evolved to explain the tubulointerstitial abnormalities that develop as a result of glomerular pathology. Cytokines produced by recruited cells like monocytes and T lymphocytes or produced by intrinsic cells in the glomeruli could reach the tubulointerstititum either by glomerular filtration or by transportation via the postglomerular capillaries. These cytokines may exert not only their effector functions in the tubulointerstitium but also may stimulate the production of cytokines by renal tubules. Proximal renal tubular epithelial cells produce MCP-1, IL-1, IL-6, TNF-α, and TGF-β in the presence of increased tubular traffic of proteins. The intensity of macrophage infiltration in the interstitium correlates with the tubular staining of MCP-1 in biopsies of IgA nephropathy patients. MCP-1 is not the only chemotactic factor produced by renal tubules. Osteopontin, IL-6, and RANTES are also chemoattractants that are produced by renal tubules. Cytokines produced by infiltrating macrophages may also stimulate cytokine production by tubular epithelial cells. Another important stimulant of cytokine production is angiotensin II. It is a growth factor not only for smooth muscle cells but also for mesangial cells and tubular epithelial cells. Mesangial cells have AT_1 receptors for angiotensin II. *In vitro* angiotensin II stimulates the proliferation of mesangial cells, which is inhibited by prostaglandin E_1 and atrial natriuretic peptide. Angiotensin II also induces the synthesis of collagen type I by mesangial cells. ACE inhibitors prevent the development of glomerulosclerosis and interstitial fibrosis in several animal models. This effect is independent of the hemodynamic effects of ACE inhibitors.

Angiotensin II is an autocrine as well as a paracrine cytokine. Renal tubular epithelial cells express the mRNA and protein of components of the renin-angiotensin system, including angiotensinogen, converting enzyme, and the AT_1 and AT_2 receptors. Tubular epithelial cells contain more angiotensin II than is present in the circulation, suggesting its intracellular production. Angiotensin II stimulates the production of TGF-β by tubular epithelial cells. PDGF and TGF-β, together with basic fibroblast growth factor (bFGF), strongly stimulate matrix production by fibroblasts. Activated fibroblast in renal biopsies of IgA nephropathy patients have been implicated as predictors of progression. However, it is not clear which cells are responsible for the process of fibrosis. The matrix components deposited in the interstitium can be produced not only by fibroblasts but also by renal tubular epithelial cells. These cells are of mesenchymal origin and may transdifferentiate into matrix-producing cells. After matrix components such as collagen type I, III, IV, and V; laminin; and fibronectin have been secreted, they are deposited and rearranged to form fibrils, which ultimately may lead to fibrosis and shrinkage of the renal cortex.

TREATMENT

The therapeutic approach to IgA nephropathy is undergoing a transition from the nihilistic belief that it is a disorder not fundamentally influenced by therapeutic interventions to the more optimistic view that some patients would be benefited by available therapy. For example, it has been recognized for many years that a small subset of patients presenting with nephrotic syndrome and minimal glomerular changes on renal biopsy responds to glucocorticoids in a fashion similar to that described for patients with minimal-change disease unassociated with IgA deposits in the mesangium. In addition, the exceptional patients with extensive crescents and rapidly progressive renal failure often responds to an aggressive regimen of glucocorticoids and cyclophosphamide combined with plasma exchange. On the other hand, patients with IgA nephropathy who have mild histologic abnormalities, normal renal function, and minimal proteinuria (less than 1 g/24 hr) tend to have a benign long-term prognosis and are best managed conservatively by nonspecific measures such as blood pressure control. Nevertheless, these patients will require careful follow-up because subsequent evolution to heavy proteinuria and/or the development of poorly controlled hypertension may presage subsequent renal functional deterioration. Early and aggressive management of hypertension and agents that reduce urinary protein excretion, such as ACE inhibitors or angiotensin II–receptor blockers, may be indicated.

The issue of specific therapeutic intervention mainly concerns those patients with more severe histologic abnormalities, initially abnormal renal function (e.g., serum creatinine concentration greater than 1.4 mg/dl), and/or heavy proteinuria (greater than 1 g/24 hr). A wide variety of approaches have been tried in such patients, and reported studies have included both uncontrolled and controlled observations. Although from the perspective of the indolent nature of the disease, follow-up in these studies are relatively short (usually less than 7 years), collectively indicate promising advances in therapeutic intervention.

Glucocorticoids

Glucocorticoids, given orally (on a daily or alternative-day basis) over short-term periods (less than 3 months) do not seem to have a clear beneficial effect in IgA nephropathy. However, when glucocorticoids are administered over longer periods (usually 6 months to 2 years) in moderate dosages, the risk of development of progressive renal failure can be reduced, especially in those with initially well-preserved renal function (serum creatinine less than 1.5 mg/dl, creatinine clearance greater than 70 ml/min), even when initial proteinuria is moderate to heavy (greater than 1 to 2 g/24 hr). Such treatments seem to be particularly effective in patients with diffuse proliferative glomerulonephritic lesions. Initial oral dosage is usually 0.8 to 1.0 mg/kg per day for 30 to 60 days, followed by slow tapering of the dose to 10 to 20 mg/day and subsequent conversion to an alternate-day regimen of 20 to 40 mg/day. Some regimens include a course of 1 g intravenous methylprednisolone every other month accompanied by oral prednisone 0.5 mg/kg body weight every other day for a total of 6 months, at which time the treatment is stopped. Patients with more advanced renal disease (e.g., serum creatinine greater than 1.5 mg/dl, creatinine clearance less than 70 ml/min) are much less responsive to such a glucocorticoid regimen. These findings indicate that glucocorticoids have their primary beneficial effects when used early in the course of disease.

Fish Oils

High dosages of fish oils [omega-3 fatty acids; mixtures of eicosapentanoic (EPA) and doxosohexanoic acid (DHA)] given over 6 months to 2 years has been shown to confer beneficial effects measured in terms of reducing future progression to end-stage renal disease in patients with moderately impaired renal function and with heavy proteinuria. Unfortunately, this finding has not been consistently observed, although the single largest study conducted at the Mayo Clinic has shown beneficial effects with long-term follow-up. Fish oils have a low profile of adverse side effects, although they do result in an unpleasant "fishy odor," and they must be taken in large doses of up to 3 g/day (1.8 g of EPA and 1.2 g of DHA daily) for 2 years. Fish oils may be well suited to the treatment of patients who have heavy proteinuria and have advanced to a stage of their disease when glucocorticoids alone are not likely to be effective.

Azathioprine

In a single retrospective study, patients with IgA nephropathy associated with moderately impaired renal function (serum creatinine greater than 1.5 mg/dl) had a better long-term outcome when treated with oral azathioprine (1.5 to 2.0 mg/kg per day), often accompanied by low-dose glucocorticoids. All of these patients had moderate proteinuria, greater than 1 g/24 hr. The beneficial effects of azathioprine have not yet been confirmed in a prospective controlled trial.

Warfarin and Dipyridamole

Anticoagulant and antithrombotic agents, often given as combined therapy, have been studied in small series of controlled observations. The combination of warfarin (international normalized ratio (INR) of 1.3 to 1.5 prothrombin time relative to control) and dipyridamole (75 mg three times daily) given for 3 years has been associated with an improved outcome among patients with increased proteinuria and modestly reduced renal function. Repeat biopsy observations have shown no beneficial effects on the histologic changes. The controlled studies were generally performed in small numbers of patients followed over relatively short periods; therefore the benefit of these agents over the long term remains uncertain. Dipyridamole alone has not been shown to have beneficial effects in IgA nephropathy in controlled trials.

Intravenous Immunoglobulins

Several uncontrolled observations suggest that high-dose (2 g/kg body weight per month) intravenous immunoglobulin given for 3 successive months, followed by 0.35 ml of pooled immunoglobulins every 3 months for another 6 months may be associated with improved renal function in patients with "severe" IgA nephropathy and Henoch-Schönlein purpura. Such therapy might be reserved for patients with a particularly poor prognosis with very "active" lesions on renal biopsy.

Combined Immunosuppression

Combinations of oral glucocorticoids, azathioprine, or cyclophosphamide anticoagulant and antithrombotics have been used to treat "severe" forms of IgA nephropathy, including crescentic glomerulonephritis with rapidly progressive renal failure. These studies, which include some prospective observations, strongly suggest that an aggressive approach to treatment of the "severe" forms of IgA nephropathy may be associated with an improved outcome. This may be particularly true in younger age populations. Combinations of fish oil, azathioprine, and low-dose glucocorticoids would be an attractive option because of an expected low incidence of undesired side effects, but this approach has not yet been tested in clinical trials.

Antimicrobials

Antimicrobial agents, including tetracycline (250 mg/day) and minocycline (100 mg/day) given for 6 months have been studied for possible beneficial effects. They do not appear to alter the natural history of the disease in terms of slowing progression to renal failure; however, they may be associated with a reduction in the frequency of episodes of gross hematuria.

Tonsillectomy

Tonsillectomy has been performed to treat IgA nephropathy for many years, particularly in Europe and Japan. The results have been inconsistent and inconclusive. Occasionally, patients subjected to this procedure experience acute exacerbations of macroscopic hematuria and reduced renal function. Some uncontrolled studies have shown increased clinical remission rates following tonsillectomy.

Other Therapies

The effects of alkylating agents (chlorambucil or cyclophosphamide) have been examined in only a limited number of trials. They have often been used in combination with other agents, most notably dipyridamole, warfarin, heparin, or prednisone. Most of the trials have involved small numbers of patients with relatively short-term follow-up and the beneficial effects have been modest, chiefly reduced proteinuria. Because of the multiplicity of combinations used, it is difficult to ascertain whether the results are due to the alkylating agent itself or to the other components of the regimen. Patients with the rare variant rapidly progressive glomerulonephritis due to extensive crescentic lesions may respond to a combination of intravenous or oral glucocorticoids, oral alkylating agents, and plasma exchange.

Limited trials of cyclosporine have been reported. Short-term (4 months) therapy with cyclosporine at dosages of 5 mg/kg per day have been associated with modest, transient reductions in proteinuria, unfortunately, often accompanied by deterioration of renal function. Interestingly, the prevalence of recurring IgA nephropathy in renal allografts has not been appreciably reduced in the cyclosporine era as compared with the azathioprine era, further implying lack of efficacy of this agent in IgA nephropathy.

Mycophenolate mofetil is a new immunosuppressive agent that acts by impairing *de novo* purine synthesis (see Chapter 88, Part 2C). Anecdotal reports have suggested that it may be effective at dosages of 1 to 2 g/day in severe forms of IgA nephropathy, including that associated with extensive crescentic disease. In addition, anecdotal reports have suggested efficacy in severe recurrent disease in renal allografts. Randomized trials are under way in patients with moderately severe forms of IgA nephropathy. Mizoribine is a new imidazole nucleoside immunosuppressive agent capable of directly inhibiting B-cell function. It is still an experimental agent in the United States, but short-term uncontrolled trials in patients with IgA nephropathy have shown reduced proteinuria and improved creatinine clearance. Further studies are needed to more fully evaluate the role of this agent in IgA nephropathy.

Numerous other approaches to the therapy of IgA nephropathy have been described. Most have been discarded because of a lack of proven efficacy or undesirable side effects, while others remain incompletely evaluated. Phenytoin will reduce serum IgA levels, but other than a decrease in episodes of macrohematuria, no beneficial effects have consistently been found in two randomized, prospective trials. Danazol, a compound capable of solubilizing immune complexes, has been associated with a reduction in proteinuria, but this effect has not been confirmed by further evaluations. Sodium cromoglycate and 5-aminosalicylic acids have been evaluated in limited controlled and uncontrolled trials. Sodium cromoglycate lowers IgA levels but has no other beneficial effects. 5-Aminosalicylic acid also lowered proteinuria but had no other beneficial effects.

ACE Inhibitors and Angiotensin II–Receptor Antagonists

Based on extensive experimentation in animals with laboratory-induced disease and on clinical trials in humans with progressive disease of diverse etiology, there seems little doubt that inhibition of the angiotensin system by converting enzyme inhibitors or angiotensin II–receptor antagonist, have salutory effects on the progression of renal disease, particularly when such therapy is accompanied by a reduction in proteinuria. Although many clinical trials demonstrating such beneficial effects have included large numbers of patients with IgA nephropathy, relatively few prospective randomized trials that have specifically addressed the effects of inhibition of the angiotensin system in patients with IgA nephropathy have been reported. Nevertheless, these trials, which have relatively short-term follow-up, suggest that patients with IgA nephropathy who have initially heavy proteinuria (particularly those with 3 g/day) or who demonstrate progressive disease can be benefited by administration of ACE inhibitors or angiotensin II antagonist, providing that urinary protein excretion declines significantly (greater than 30% to 40% from baseline values). Maximum benefit on progression of renal failure is seen in patients with proteinuria greater than 3.0 g/24 hr and the beneficial effects appear to be largely independent of the blood pressure–lowering effects. Other agents, such as β-blockers and nondihydropyridine (diltiazem, verapamil) calcium channel antagonists also have antiproteinuric effects, but these appear to correlate with the magnitude of decline in blood pressure. Some investigators have suggested that the deletion (DD) ACE genotype is associated with more rapid progression and that the beneficial effect of angiotensin antagonism is limited to those with the DD genotype. This is not yet consistently confirmed. In summary, it would appear that patients with IgA nephropathy who have moderate to significant proteinuria (e.g., greater than 1 to 2 g/24 hr) would be benefited by treatment with either an ACE inhibitor or an angiotensin II–receptor antagonist, in terms of a decrease in risk of future progression to end-stage renal disease. These effects are dependent on the magnitude of reduction in urinary protein excretion. Because the effects on proteinuria of these agents are dependent both on dosage and may be on the prevailing status of the extracellular fluid volume, it may be necessary to use maximal doses, in conjunction with sodium restriction or diuretics in order to obtain the desired results. Caution should be exercised with these in patients with advanced renal failure.

Irrespective of concomitant therapy, all patients with IgA nephropathy and significant proteinuria are candidates for treatment with an ACE inhibitor or an angiotensin II–receptor antagonist.

Selected Readings

Cattran DC, Greenwood C, Ritchie S. Long-term benefits of angiotensin-converting enzyme inhibitor therapy in patients with severe immunoglobulin a nephropathy: a comparison to patients receiving treatment with other antihypertensive agents and to patients receiving no therapy. *Am J Kidney Dis* 1994;23:247–254.

A retrospective study that strongly supports the concept that ACE inhibitors slow the progression of renal disease in patients with IgA nephropathy.

Clarkson AR, Woodroffe AJ, Bannister KM, et al. The syndrome of IgA nephropathy. *Clin Nephrol* 1984;21:7–14.

A comprehensive review of the varied clinical manifestations of IgA nephropathy.

D'Amico G. The commonest glomerulonephritis in the world: IgA Nephropathy. *Q J Med* 1987;245:709–727.

A review that includes an analysis of the geographical variation in prevalence of IgA nephropathy.

Feehally J. Immune mechanisms in glomerular IgA deposition. *Nephrol Dial Transplant* 1988;3:361–378.

An excellent review of immunologic disturbances in IgA nephropathy.

Feehally J, Allen AC. Structural features of IgA molecules which contribute to IgA nephropathy. *J Nephrol* 1999;12:59–65.

An excellent review of the abnormalities in glycosylation of the IgA_1 molecule in IgA nephropathy.

Glassock RJ. The treatment of IgA nephropathy: status at the end of the millenium. *J Nephrol* 1999;12:288–296.

A comprehensive review of the treatment of IgA nephropathy.

Ibels LS, Györy AZ. IgA nephropathy: analysis of the natural history, important factors in the progression of renal disease, and a review of the literature. *Medicine* 1994;73:79–102.

A comprehensive and detailed analysis of IgA nephropathy with particular emphasis on prognostic factors.

Lévy M, Lesavre P. Genetic factors in IgA nephropathy (Berger's disease). *Adv Nephrol* 1992;21:23–49.

This is a review and analysis of various genetic loci and their impact on susceptibility of IgA nephropathy.

Van Es LA. Pathogenesis of IgA nephropathy. *Kidney Int* 1992;41:1720–1729.

This provides a review of the various mechanisms involved in IgA mesangial deposition.

PART 13
Thin Basement Membrane Disease

Fernando G. Cosio

Thin basement membrane disease (TBMD) is a common familial disorder characterized by abnormal narrowing of the glomerular basement membrane (GBM). The disease most often presents clinically as isolated microscopic hematuria. TBMD was initially described in 1973 by the demonstration of abnormal GBM thinning in kidney biopsies from several members of a large family who presented with microscopic hematuria and had a benign renal prognosis. TBMD is now recognized as a unique entity, separate from other forms of familial nephritis. The diagnosis of TBMD is hampered by several issues: (a) the diagnosis requires electron microscopy studies of renal biopsies, including measurements of GBM thickness in several capillary loops; (b) there is considerable variation on the width of GBM that is considered to be diagnostic of TBMD; (c) thinning of GBM has been described in patients with Alport's syndrome and in the glomeruli of some patients with acquired nephropathies, suggesting the possibility that in some patients, GBM thinning may be acquired; and (d) the clinical presentation of TBMD is indistinguishable from that of some other glomerulopathies such as IgA nephropathy. On occasion, the terms *TBMD* and *benign familial hematuria* are used interchangeably. However, we believe this is not appropriate because not all patients with benign familial hematuria have thinning of the GBM and not all patients with TBMD have a benign course and the disease may be of a sporadic nature. For example, recent studies have shown associations between TBMD and other nephropathies, suggesting that patients with this disorder may be at risk of developing other forms of renal disease and/or hypertension.

CLINICAL PRESENTATION

Patients with TBMD most commonly present with persistent microscopic hematuria. TBMD is the second most common cause, after IgA nephropathy, of microscopic hematuria in both adults and children. Episodic gross hematuria is rare and occurs in fewer than 10% of patients with TBMD. Proteinuria of greater than 500 mg/24 hr occurs in 30% of patients, and nephrotic-range proteinuria can occur but is quite rare. It is difficult to ascertain the prevalence of renal insufficiency at the time of diagnosis of TBMD because most published studies excluded patients with azotemia. However, long-term follow-up of patients with TBMD and a normal serum creatinine level indicate that most of these patients will maintain normal renal function. Although most patients with TBMD are asymptomatic, at least two previous studies have suggested an association between TBMD and the syndrome of loin pain hematuria (LPH). The latter is a poorly understood condition characterized clinically by episodes of severe flank pain, microscopic or macroscopic hematuria, and generally, normal renal function. Renal biopsies in patients with LPH most often are normal, except for the deposition of complement components, mainly C3, in the walls of arterioles. Some patients with LPH also demonstrate abnormal thinning of the GBM, and it has been hypothesized that this structural abnormality allows the escape of erythrocytes through the glomerular filter, resulting in intratubular red blood cell (RBC) cast formation, obstruction of tubular flow, and increased intrarenal pressure that may cause flank pain. This hypothesis is supported by the observation that in some patients with TBMD and LPH, flank pain is associated with increases in the concentration of RBCs in the urine, which sometimes results in macroscopic hematuria. Further discussion on LPH is found in Chapter 28.

PATHOLOGY

In patients with uncomplicated TBMD, examination of the kidneys by light microscopy demonstrates normal glomeruli or very mild degrees of mesangial cell proliferation. One study has suggested that, compared with normal individuals, patients with TBMD may have an increased number of globally sclerotic glomeruli. This observation has not been confirmed. The tubulointerstitial compartment of the kidney is also normal, although one often can observe erythrocytes inside tubular lumens, supporting the postulate that the hematuria is of glomerular origin.

By immunofluorescence microscopy there is no accumulation of immunoglobulins or complement components in glomeruli. However, there occasionally is deposition of C3 in the wall of renal arterioles. The significance of this latter finding is unclear, but vascular C3 deposition appears to be a rather nonspecific finding that can be demonstrated in several other forms of glomerular disease, such as diabetic glomerulosclerosis and IgA nephropathy.

The characteristic findings of TBMD are demonstrated by electron microscopy, where the overall width of the GBM and, in particular, the lamina densa is strikingly thin. Illustrations of the renal histologic finding are provided in Chapter 109. This finding can be diffuse, affecting all glomerular capillaries. However, in our experience, it is more common to observe segmental thinning of the GBM, affecting portions of capillary loops. It is of historical interest that the first family of patients with TBMD included patients with segmental GBM thinning. Neither the degree of thinning nor the extent of the abnormality (diffuse versus segmental) correlate with the patient's clinical presentation or prognosis. GBM thickness is greater in normal males (373 ± 42 nanometers) than in normal females (326 ± 45 nm). Most authors agree that an average GBM thickness of less than 264 nm, that is, two standard deviations below the mean of normal adult values, should be considered abnormal and suggestive of TBMD. In children, the GBM is thinner than in adults, and the criteria to be used to diagnose TBMD in children have not been clearly established. Multiple measurements of orthogonal (perpendicular) cuts of the GBM in several glomerular capillaries should be made, particularly in patients with segmental thinning of the GBM. When GBM thinning is diffuse, the pathologic diagnosis is not difficult. However, in patients with segmental GBM thinning, the pathologic diagnosis can be more uncertain, particularly if only a limited number of glomeruli are available for observation. In previous studies, we have used the following pathologic criteria to make the diagnosis of TBMD in patients with segmental thinning of the GBM: (a) the segments of GBM that are abnormally thin involve at least 50% of the length of the capillaries examined, (b) the thinning affects more than one glomerular capillary loop, and (c) specimens that also demonstrate splitting of the GBM and/or the presence of intramembrane dense bodies should be excluded because those findings are characteristic of Alport's syndrome and are not present in TBMD. The reliability of these pathologic criteria is supported by the observation that 92% of the patients diagnosed with TBMD using this method had familial microscopic hematuria.

DIAGNOSIS, FREQUENCY, AND MODE OF INHERITANCE

TBMD is quite common; for example, it has been shown that between 5% and 10% of transplant kidney donors have abnormal thinning of the GBM. It is unknown whether all of these individuals also have microscopic hematuria. In patients with hematuria of renal origin (i.e., patients with negative urologic workup) and normal kidney function, the prevalence of TBMD is similar to that of IgA nephropathy (both approximately 30% of cases) and frequency is similar in adults and in children. Ideally, the diagnosis of TBMD should be made only in patients who meet all of the following criteria: (a) characteristic clinical presentation; (b) positive family history of persistent hematuria; (c) lack of family history of deafness, ocular abnormalities, or renal failure; and (d) characteristic renal pathologic findings by electron microscopy. The presence of a family history of hematuria is a critical component of the diagnosis as illustrated by previous studies in which we showed that more than 90% of patients with TBMD have one or more relatives with microscopic hematuria. Furthermore, 46% of the relatives examined had microscopic hematuria. It should be emphasized that in our experience, most relatives of patients with TBMD are not aware that they have hematuria. Thus the determination of whether the patient has familial hematuria should be based on examination of urine samples from the patient's relatives. In addition, it is clearly advantageous to obtain urine sediment from as many family members as possible because one would expect that approximately half of those relatives will have hematuria.

Eighty-two percent of patients with isolated microscopic hematuria, normal renal function, minor proteinuria (less than 2 g/24 hr), and a positive family history of hematuria, but no deafness, have TBMD. Thus we believe that it is unnecessary to do a renal biopsy in these patients to establish the diagnosis of TBMD. However, in the absence of a positive family history, the odds that the patient has TBMD are reduced to approximately 30%, and in those patients, a kidney biopsy may be necessary to confirm the diagnosis. Patients with a benign clinical presentation, as described earlier, should be followed periodically with reassessment of their clinical status.

Previous studies suggested that TBMD is inherited as an autosomal-dominant trait, and the data discussed previously are consistent with that postulate.

DIFFERENTIAL DIAGNOSIS

It is important to differentiate TBMD from other forms of familial nephritis, such as Alport's syndrome, and from other glomerulopathies, such as IgA nephropathy, for at least two reasons: (a) there are significant differences in the prognosis of these diseases, and (b) the correct diagnosis will determine the risk of renal disease in other family members.

The differentiation between Alport's syndrome and TBMD may be difficult, but the following clinical and pathologic criteria are often useful in making that distinction: (a) in contrast to patients with Alport's syndrome, patients with TBMD have no family history of deafness or ocular abnormalities and rarely have a family history of azotemia; (b) pathologically, sclerotic glomeruli and interstitial fibrosis are more commonly found in Alport's syndrome, although it can be present in TBMD; (c) by electron microscopy, segmental thinning of the GBM is often observed in the glomeruli of patients with Alport's syndrome; however, most often these glomeruli demonstrate other GBM changes, including splitting of the lamina densa and the presence of intra-GBM small dense bodies (these latter changes are not observed in patients with TBMD); and (d) it has been suggested that the presence or absence of the Goodpasture's antigen (i.e., the noncollagenous portion of collagen type IV) in the GBM can be used to differentiate between Alport's syndrome and TBMD. Several studies have shown that Goodpasture's antigen is present in the GBM of patients with TBMD but is often absent, or its expression is decreased, in the GBM of patients with Alport's syndrome. Data from several studies that have addressed this issue led to the following conclusion: the absence of Goodpasture's antigen in GBM argues strongly against the diagnosis of TBMD and in favor of the diagnosis of Alport's syndrome. However, decreased intensity of staining for Goodpasture's antigen can be seen in both Alport's syndrome and TBMD. Thus this latter finding is not useful to differentiate between these two conditions. Other studies described a linkage between TBMD and alterations in the collagen IV gene that can also be found in Alport's syndrome. These studies concluded that alterations in the collagen IV gene can result in either Alport's syndrome or TBMD.

TBMD and IgA nephropathy cannot be differentiated reliably on clinical grounds alone. However, the presence of familial hematuria is the rule in TBMD and the exception in patients with IgA nephropathy. In general, pathologic examination of kidney biopsy tissue will differentiate conclusively these two diseases. However, some biopsies demonstrate both TBMD and IgA nephropathy, that is, positive immunofluorescence for mesangial IgA and mesangial electron-dense deposits. When this observation was initially made, it was suggested that thinning of the GBM can be acquired in patients with other forms of glomerular pathology. However, those studies did not exclude the presence of familial hematuria in these patients. In contrast, the results of other studies suggest that the presence of TBMD together with IgA nephropathy most likely represents the occurrence of a *de novo* glomerulopathy in a patient with TBMD. This conclusion is based on the observation that patients with IgA nephropathy and TBMD have a positive family history of hematuria significantly more often than patients with IgA nephropathy but without TBMD. The concurrence of these two diseases may not be surprising considering that TBMD is present in 5% to 10% of the general population.

PROGNOSIS

The large majority of patients with TBMD will have persistent microscopic hematuria but will maintain normal renal function throughout their lives. However, several studies suggest that this "benign" course may not apply to all patients with TBMD. For example, some studies indicate that patients with TBMD have an increased prevalence of systemic hypertension during follow-up; in addition, rare cases of TBMD and progressive azotemia have been described. We noted before that patients with TBMD may have significant proteinuria, even in the nephrotic range, and those patients should be monitored closely for evidence of progressive azotemia. Finally, in patients who have TBMD and an additional acquired glomerulopathy, the renal prognosis is most likely dictated by the severity of the secondary glomerular disease, and it is likely that these patients will have a worse prognosis than patients who have only TBMD.

The discovery of patients with TBMD and an acquired glomerulopathy raises the possibility that TBMD may predispose to another glomerulopathy. For example, among a large group of renal biopsies obtained in patients with a variety of renal disease, the prevalence of TBMD was 5%. However, among patients with IgA nephropathy, TBMD was significantly more common (12%). Recalculation of these data using an updated database that now contains 1,948 biopsy specimens showed similar results. Thus 143 of these biopsies (7%) showed TBMD, but a significantly greater number of patients with IgA nephropathy (30 of 184, or 16%) had TBMD. In contrast, TBMD was present in 7% of patients with focal glomerulosclerosis (7%), a prevalence similar to the general population.

We should reemphasize that most patients with TBMD have an excellent renal prognosis. However, the studies mentioned earlier led to the suggestion that these patients should be monitored periodically for evidence of disease progression by measuring serum creatinine, urine protein excretion, and blood pressure.

TBMD AND RENAL TRANSPLANTATION

The diagnosis of TBMD is sometimes made during the evaluation of an individual who wants to donate one of his or her kidneys to a relative with renal failure. This clinical situation prompts at least three important questions: (a) Do patients with TBMD and/or their relatives have an increased prevalence of renal failure? We discussed this issue previously. (b) Should kidney biopsies be done in individuals with microscopic hematuria discovered during a donor workup for a relative with renal failure? In our opinion, a kidney biopsy in these patients will achieve two important goals: to rule out the presence of significant structural damage in a kidney with TBMD and to rule out a diagnosis other than TBMD. Furthermore, a kidney biopsy should be considered in these patients even if they are not going to be donors because the association of microscopic hematuria with a family history of renal failure suggests diagnoses other than TBMD (e.g., Alport's syndrome), and establishing those diagnoses may be of benefit to the potential donor. (c) Is kidney donation safe in patients with TBMD? In patients with TBMD, isolated microscopic hematuria without proteinuria, and normal renal histology by light and immunofluorescence microscopy, kidney donation appears to be quite safe and is routinely practiced in most transplant centers.

Selected Readings

Cosio FG, Falkenhain ME, Sedmak DD. Association of thin glomerular basement membrane with other glomerulopathies. *Kidney Int* 1994;46:471–474.

Review of cases of TBMD with particular emphasis on the association of TBMD with other pathologic abnormalities in the biopsy. Original description of the association between TBMD and IgA nephropathy. Examination of urine sediment in family members proves the familial nature of these cases.

Dische FE, Anderson VER, Keane SJ, et al. Incidence of thin membrane nephropathy: morphometric investigation of a population sample. *J Clin Pathol* 1990; 43:457–460.

Careful morphometric assessment of GBM thickness in 76 kidney biopsies obtained from normal transplant donors. TBMD is found in 9% of the healthy population in England.

Hebert LA, Betts JA, Sedmak DD, et al. Loin pain-hematuria syndrome associated with thin glomerular basement membrane disease and hemorrhage into renal tubules. *Kidney Int* 1996;49:168–173.

Description of the association between TBMD and the syndrome of loin pain hematuria. Description of kidney biopsies in these individuals that demonstrate a high number of renal tubules occluded by RBC casts.

Rogers PW, Kurtzman NA, Bunn SM Jr, et al. Familial benign essential hematuria. *Arch Int Med* 1973;131:257–261.

Original description of TBMD. Description of clinical presentation, familial clustering of findings, and histopathology.

Steffes MW, Barbosa J, Basgen JM, et al. Quantitative glomerular morphology of the normal human kidney. *Lab Invest* 1983;49:82–86.

Normal values for morphometric parameters in normal human kidney biopsies. Variations with age and gender.

Tiebosch ATMG, Frederick PM, van Breda Vriesman PJC. Thin-basement membrane nephropathy in adults with persistent hematuria. *N Engl J Med* 1989; 320:14–18.

Examination of a large cohort of patients from The Netherlands presenting with microscopic hematuria and no familial evidence of Alport's syndrome. The article highlights the high prevalence of TBMD that is similar to that of IgA nephropathy. Striking similarities in the clinical presentation of these two entities.

Trachtman H, Weiss RA, Bennett B, et al. Isolated hematuria in children: indications for renal biopsy. *Kidney Int* 1993;25:94–99.

This is one of the few studies that has evaluated the prevalence of TBMD in children presenting with isolated hematuria. The authors also correlate the prevalence of TBMD versus other findings with the patient's clinical presentation.

Yoshikawa N, Matsuyama S, Iijima K, et al. Benign familial hematuria. *Arch Pathol Lab Med* 1988;112:794–797.

Prevalence of TBMD according to the patient's clinical presentation. These data can be used to justify not performing a kidney biopsy in patients presenting with isolated microscopic hematuria, normal renal function, and absence of family history consistent with Alport's syndrome.

PART 14
Collagenofibrotic and Lipoprotein Glomerulopathies

Arthur H. Cohen

Over the past decade or so, new and uncommon glomerular diseases have been described and established as distinct clinicopathologic entities. Among them are lipoprotein glomerulopathy and collagen type III or collagenofibrotic or glomerulopathy. Both are characterized by accumulation of material either produced by or trapped in glomeruli. Both may occur in families. Interestingly, both are most commonly reported in Japanese patients, although they appear to have a worldwide distribution.

COLLAGENOFIBROTIC GLOMERULOPATHY (COLLAGEN TYPE III GLOMERULOPATHY)

A small group of patients has been described with a glomerulopathy seemingly structurally similar to that occurring in nail-patella syndrome; the patients, however, did not have either skeletal or cutaneous manifestations. First thought to represent a forme fruste of nail-patella syndrome, it has become apparent that the glomerulopathy is clearly a distinct clinical and pathologic entity.

Collagenofibrotic glomerulopathy has been reported from many countries, although most patients are from Japan. This disorder occurs in both children and adults; the youngest child was 3 months of age. It is slightly more common in males and is inherited in an autosomal-recessive pattern; many sibling pairs, both children and adults, are reported. Parental consanguinity has also been described. The usual presenting manifestation is proteinuria, commonly with hematuria and infrequently with nephrotic range or hematuria alone. Nephrotic syndrome, hypertension, and slowly progressive renal insufficiency develop during the course of the disease, usually after many years. End-stage renal disease has been described in few patients. Associated disorders are reported in some patients. One child developed hemolytic uremic syndrome, and siblings of two unrelated patients died with hemolytic uremic syndrome, one after several years of proteinuria. Another patient had complete deficiency of factor H and persistent hypocomplementemia. One patient had hepatic perisinusoidal fibrosis with collagen III deposition.

Although no laboratory tests are diagnostic of this disorder, it is of interest that in the patients evaluated, serum concentrations of procollagen III peptide are elevated. This peptide is the N-terminal sequence of the precursor procollagen molecule, which is cleaved in the serum. This finding is not specific because serum procollagen III peptide is increased in patients with renal dysfunction and in many nonrenal disorders with increased collagen synthesis. However, in contrast to other conditions, this peptide is greatly elevated in collagenofibrotic glomerulopathy, a feature that makes this finding presumptive evidence of the glomerulopathy. It has been suggested that this may be a systemic disease because of the occasional extrarenal manifestations.

The illustrations of the renal pathology are provided in Chapter 109. The glomerular structural features are distinctive. Capillary walls are thickened, and mesangial regions are widened without accompanying increased cellularity; there is lobular architecture in adults but not in children. Mesangial regions and subendothelial aspects of capillary walls are infiltrated by pale staining material. Capillary walls often have double contours. Capillary lumina are narrowed. Ultrastructure indicates the abnormal material in capillary walls and mesangium to consist of collagen fibrils with periodicity of approximately 60 nm. The fibrils are typically in the subendothelial zone and not within the basement membrane proper (lamina densa); this distinguishes collagenofibrotic glomerulopathy from nail-patella syndrome, in which collagen type III is in multiple foci within the basement membranes. In both disorders, staining of ultrathin sections with phosphotungstic acid may be necessary to demonstrate the fibrils. Peripheral mesangial migration is present in some capillary walls. Immunofluorescence for immune deposits is negative. Immunohistochemical evaluation documents collagen III in mesangial regions and capillary walls.

There is no specific treatment. The possibility of recurrence in transplants is not known.

LIPOPROTEIN GLOMERULOPATHY

First described in 1987, lipoprotein glomerulopathy affects both children and adults; most have been sporadic cases, although a few familial clusters are described. Approximately 25 cases have been reported; the vast majority are from Asia, with most from Japan. The usual presentation is proteinuria, often in or progressing to nephrotic syndrome. Microscopic hematuria is uncommon. Advanced renal insufficiency or end-stage renal disease occurs over a variable period.

The glomerular morphology is distinctive and initially provided the basis for delineating important metabolic abnormalities (see Chapter 109). The capillaries are dilated and filled with pale-staining, slightly tan amorphous material occasionally with a meshlike appearance. Oil red-0 stain on frozen tissue is positive. Alterations of the tufts include segmental capillary wall thickening with double contours, mild mesangial widening, and segmental glomerulosclerosis. The ultrastructure of the luminal "thrombi" is distinctive; there are stratified layers of pale granular extracellular material with lipid droplets and occasional entrapped platelets. Red blood cells are often deformed and displaced to peripheral aspects of the capillary lumina. Thrombi are not in all capillaries. Immunohistochemical stains indicate the thrombi to be composed of apolipoproteins E and B. Presence of thrombi in vessels other than glomerular capillaries is not reported.

Patients with this disorder characteristically have features of type III hyperlipidemia; intermediate-density lipoproteins (IDLs) and very-low-density lipoproteins (VLDLs) are elevated, as are cholesterol, triglycerides, and apolipoprotein E. Apolipoprotein E, important in lipid metabolism, is polymorphic with three main variants, termed *apoE2*, *apoE3*, and *apoE4*; apoE3 is most common. Six genotypes are possible; all have been reported in lipoprotein glomerulopathy, although apoE2/3 is most frequently found. One study using DNA sequence analysis documented a substitution of proline for arginine at amino acid 145 of apoE in three Japanese patients, two of whom were related. Although other patients with lipoprotein glomerulopathy have not been similarly evaluated, it is possible that this mutation, termed *apoE-Sendai*, is responsible for many additional cases.

Some patients have progressed to end-stage renal disease; the lesion has recurred in the transplant in at least two reported patients. Corticosteroids and cyclophosphamide have not affected the course of the disease or proteinuria. An occasional patient has responded to probucol with diminished proteinuria and hyperlipoproteinuria and with improvement in glomerular lesions on repeat biopsy. Lipid-lowering agents have not altered the course of the disease.

Selected Readings

Abt AB, Cohen AH. Newer glomerular diseases. *Semin Nephrol* 1996;16:501–510.
A comprehensive review of all reports of lipoprotein glomerulopathy, collagen type III glomerulopathy, and fibronectin glomerulopathy, all newly described and rare entities.

Gubler MC, Dommergues JP, Foulard M, et al. Collagen type III glomerulopathy: a new type of hereditary nephropathy. *Pediatr Nephrol* 1993;7:354–360.
The largest series of collagen type III glomerulopathy; also describes possible association with thrombotic microangiopathy.

Oikawa S, Matsunaga A, Saito T, et al. Apolipoprotein E Sendai (Arginine 145 → proline): a new variant associated with lipoprotein glomerulopathy. *J Am Soc Nephrol* 1997;8:820–823.

Saito T, Oikawa S, Sato H, Chiba J. Lipoprotein glomerulopathy and its pathogenesis. *Contrib Nephrol* 1997;120:30–38.

Yang AH, Ng YY, Tarng DC, et al. Association of apolipoprotein E polymorphism with lipoprotein glomerulopathy. *Nephron* 1998;78:266–270.
Suggested molecular/genetic pathogenesis of lipoprotein glomerulopathy proposed in all three papers.

CHAPTER 40

Tubulointerstitial Nephropathies

Garabed Eknoyan

The renal lesions that develop in a motley group of unrelated diseases affect mainly the interstitium and tubules while sparing the glomeruli and vasculature of the kidney. The distinct clinicopathologic entity that results accounts for some 10% to 25% of cases of acute renal failure and, in its primary form, 20% to 40% of cases of chronic renal failure. Initially referred to as *interstitial nephritis,* the more descriptive nomenclature of *tubulointerstitial disease, tubulointerstitial nephritis,* and *tubulointerstitial nephropathy* are now the preferred terms used to identify this entity, in which the dominant structural changes are restricted to the interstitium and tubules of the kidney and whose hallmark of disordered pathophysiology is abnormalities of tubular function. The preferential use of the term *tubulointerstitial* in describing these lesions is not meant to belittle the role of the interstitium in the pathogenesis of these disorders. It is in the interstitium that the initial morphologic changes are often most evident and may well account for much of the tubular dysfunction that ensues. However, in most cases, the tubular structural changes become ultimately more evident, and being functionally more important, they always account for much of the clinical and functional manifestations that characterize the interstitial nephritides. In addition, there is increasing experimental evidence for a role of the tubular epithelial cells in the immunopathogenesis and progression of the renal involvement. This is not to imply that glomerular dysfunction does not occur in tubulointerstitial nephropathies (TIN), most of which will ultimately develop functional and structural changes of the glomeruli and vasculature. These relatively late changes, the structural hallmark of which is glomerulosclerosis and arteriolosclerosis, manifest themselves by a progressive decline in glomerular filtration, the development of glomerular proteinuria, and volume-dependent hypertension. These late manifestations notwithstanding, the characteristic and differentiating features of TIN are an insidious onset in which tubular dysfunction is the dominant feature and, even in the presence of glomerular dysfunction, out of proportion to any increment in blood urea nitrogen (BUN) and serum creatinine (Cr) levels.

Although diseases that affect primarily the glomeruli and vasculature are excluded by definition from the primary forms of TIN, interstitial alterations can be an important component of glomerular and vascular diseases. The extent and severity of concurrent tubulointerstitial changes that develop in such cases contribute significantly to their clinical course. In fact, the presence and severity of tubulointerstitial lesions in the initial kidney biopsy of different primary glomerular and vascular diseases has come to be recognized as a significant and more important determinant of the rate of progression to renal failure than that of the glomerular or vascular lesions. Although this form of secondary TIN may develop in any primary glomerular disease, it is more evident in cases of membranoproliferative glomerulonephritis (MPGN), membranous nephropathy (MGN), focal and segmental glomerulosclerosis (FSGS), lupus nephritis, and IgA nephropathy. A common feature of all such cases is persistent proteinuria, with a demonstrated correlation between the magnitude of the proteinuria and the severity of the secondary TIN that develops. As such, tubulointerstitial nephritis is the final common pathway of all forms of progressive renal failure, independent of the original site of renal disease.

STRUCTURAL AND FUNCTIONAL FEATURES

The portion of normal renal tissue occupied by the interstitium increases from the cortex to the papilla. In the cortex, the peritubular capillaries occupy most of the space between the tubules, and the interstitium constitutes only about 7% of the relative cortical volume. Approximately half of the cortical interstitial space is occupied by rather inconspicuous interstitial mononuclear cells, and the remainder by extracellular space made up of a fibrillar net of collagen filled with a glycosaminoglycan-rich ground substance and interstitial fluid. The interstitial cells consist either of type I cells, which participate in maintenance of the interstitial matrix, or type II cells with macrophage-like capacity for phagocytosis and antigen processing and presentation.

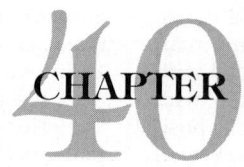

In the medulla, the relative portion of interstitium increases in increments that gradually become larger toward the tip of the papilla. The increase in interstitial volume begins in the inner zone of the outer medulla, where the interstitial spaces are meager in the region of vascular bundles but occupy some 10% to 20% of the volume in the interbundle regions occupied by the tubules. In the inner medulla, the differentiation into vascular bundles and interbundle regions becomes gradually less obvious and the relative volume of interstitial space continues to increase, such that at the papillary tip, it occupies 30% to 40% of the relative volume. There are three kinds of cells in the medullary interstitium. The majority consist of the interstitial cells that contain lipid droplets and have characteristic transverse appositions to their adjoining structures, specifically to the limbs of Henle's loop and the capillaries but not to the collecting ducts. In addition to providing structural support, one of the principal functions of these cells is prostaglandin production. The two other types of medullary interstitial cells are pericytes and mononuclear cells, which have the same features and functions as those in the cortex. Detailed discussion of the renal interstitium is found in Chapter 1, Part 2.

Independent of the initiating pathogenetic process, the principal morphologic feature of TIN is an increase in interstitial volume, resulting from edema in its acute form and fibrosis in its chronic form. This increase is accompanied by varying degrees of infiltration by inflammatory cells, most of which are mononuclear. The cortical and medullary interstitial mononuclear cells are presumed to be precursors of some of these cellular infiltrates, most of which are infiltrative cells recruited from the circulation. The cellular infiltrate is always dominated by T lymphocytes with only a modest number of B cells, monocytes, macrophages, and only rarely, polymorphonuclear leukocytes. Differential characterization of the infiltrating lymphocytes reveals a near equal number of CD4 and CD8 lymphocytes, with a slight preponderance of CD4. Wherever examined, these cells express surface markers of antigenic activation (HLA II), intercellular adhesion molecules (ICAM-1), and interleukin-2 (IL-2) receptors.

Although the normal structural and functional correlates of the interstitial spaces are still poorly defined, the changes in the interstitial composition and structure that characterize TIN, by altering normal exchange and equilibration processes, are reflected in changes in tubular function, apart from those resulting from direct tubular injury. The severity of tubular dysfunction that results will be determined by the extent of injury that has occurred. The type of insult responsible for the TIN will determine the location of the injury to either the cortex or the medulla. Because of the focal nature of the lesions and the segmental nature of normal tubular function, the pattern of tubular dysfunction that develops will vary depending on the principal site of injury. Cortical lesions will affect either the proximal or the distal tubule, whereas medullary lesions will affect Henle's loop or the collecting duct. The deviation from normal function of each of these segments will then determine the altered tubular function that is encountered clinically (Table 40.1). Lesions affecting mainly the proximal tubule will result in aminoaciduria, glucosuria, phosphaturia, uricosuria, β_2-microglobulinuria, and bicarbonaturia [proximal renal tubular acidosis (RTA)]. Lesions affecting the distal tubule will result in inability to acidify the urine (distal RTA), secrete potassium, and regulate sodium balance. Lesions that affect the medulla and papilla will result in the inability to concentrate the urine maximally and nephrogenic diabetes insipidus, which are manifested by polyuria and nocturia. Despite the usefulness of this general framework in localizing the site of injury, some degree of overlap is often encountered clinically, with varying degrees of proximal, distal, or medullary tubular dysfunction being present in the same patient.

As a rule, the magnitude of the decline in glomerular filtration rate (GFR) appears to correlate with the severity and extent of interstitial fibrosis in chronic TIN, whereas the increase in interstitial space and cellular infiltrate seems to have a limited bearing on the GFR. This is in contrast to acute TIN, in which it is the extent of the cellular infiltrate that shows a better correlation with the degree of reduction in GFR and consequent azotemia. In cases of chronic TIN that present late in the course of their disease with renal insufficiency, abnormalities of tubular function, unless specifically sought, may remain undetected. However, early in the course of the illness, the hallmarks of glomerular disease (i.e., salt retention, edema, and hypertension) are absent, and tubular dysfunction is almost always out of proportion to any coexistent glomerular dysfunction. At this stage, serial sections through the kidney indicate that severe tubular atrophy due to chronic TIN is associated with otherwise histologically normal appearing but atubular glomeruli (i.e., functionless glomeruli). Later in the course of the disease, when the glomerular lesions (glomerulosclerosis and periglomerular fibrosis) are prominent and azotemia is quite severe, the morphology may be difficult to differentiate from that of end-stage kidney disease of any etiology. Differential features in favor of a diagnosis of TIN would be the smaller size of the end-stage kidneys, because the bulk (80%) of the renal volume is composed of tubules, and their higher echogenicity on ultrasonography, because the amount of interstitial fibrosis is quite severe.

TABLE 40.1. Principal Sites and Causes of Tubular Injury in Acute and Chronic Tubulointerstitial Nephropathy (TIN)

Site of Injury	Acute TIN	Chronic TIN	Tubular Dysfunction
Cortex Proximal tubule	Antibiotics Multiple myeloma Lymphoproliferative disorders	Heavy metals Immunologic disorders Cystinosis Multiple myeloma	↓ Reabsorption of amino acids, bicarbonate, glucose, protein (β_2-microglobulin), phosphate uric acid, sodium
Distal tubule	Antibiotics Immunologic disorders Analgesics Nonsteroidal antiinflammatory drugs	Hypercalcemia Obstructive uropathy Amyloidosis Granulomatous diseases Immunologic diseases Sickle hemoglobinopathy	↓ Reabsorption of sodium ↓ Secretion of potassium, hydrogen
Medulla	Analgesics Metabolic disorders Infection Immunologic diseases Sickle hemoglobinopathy Sulfonamides Multiple myeloma	Analgesic nephropathy Metabolic disorders Infection Obstructive uropathy Sickle hemoglobinopathy Granulomatous diseases Hereditary diseases Amyloidosis	Impaired urine concentrating ability ↓ Reabsorption of sodium
Papilla	Infections Sickle hemoglobinopathy	Analgesic nephropathy Diabetes mellitus Obstructive uropathy Transplanted kidney Sickle hemoglobinopathy Infection	Impaired urine concentrating ability ↓ Reabsorption of sodium

PATHOGENESIS AND MECHANISMS OF INJURY

As initially deduced from the morphologic features of TIN, in which mononuclear cell infiltrates are an invariable feature, a local inflammatory process is the principal pathogenetic pathway of tubulointerstitial diseases. The demonstration that the infiltrating cells are antigenically activated lymphocytes implicates a cell-mediated immune mechanism of injury. Considerable laboratory evidence accrued over the past decade has unravelled the mechanism of recruitment of inflammatory cells and provided compelling support for an immune mechanism of TIN. The process entails a three-phase response of antigen recognition or expression, integration and regulation of the immunopathogenic response, and an effector or mediator phase. In the kidney, this entails a complex integrative operation between tubular epithelial cells, resident interstitial cells, and infiltrating inflammatory cells (Fig. 40.1). The interaction depends on messages transmitted by a host of cytokines released by these cells at various stages of the process and of the increased expression of specific surface receptors by the cells. A large and increasing number of identified stimulatory signals with different, often overlapping, functions modulate, interact, and amplify the inflammatory reaction that accounts for the tubulointerstitial lesions. Some of these are cell surface markers, which have *antigenic* [major histocompatibility complex (MHC), HLA class II, secreted protein acidic and rich in cysteine (SPARC)] or *adhesive* (intercellular or vascular adhesion molecule-1, ICAM-1, VCAM-1; integrins; selectins) properties. Others are cytokines, which are *chemoattractants* [monocyte chemoattractant protein-1 (MCP-1), osteopontin, regulated on activation, normal T-cell expressed and secreted, (RANTES), macrophage inflammatory protein-1 (MIP-1)]; *proinflammatory* [IL-6 and IL-8, platelet-derived growth factor-β (PDGF-β), granulocyte monocyte-colony stimulating factor (GM-CSF), tumor necrosis factor-α (TNF-α), transforming growth factor-α (TGF-α)]; *vasoactive* [nitrous oxide (NO), endothelin-1 (ET-1), adenosine]; *cytotoxic* [metalloproteinases (MP), and their tissue inhibitors TIMP-1; reactive-oxygen radicals (O), ferric ion]; or *fibrogenic* [TGF-β, PDGF, IL-1, IL-6, TNF, and plasminogen activator inhibitor (PAI)].

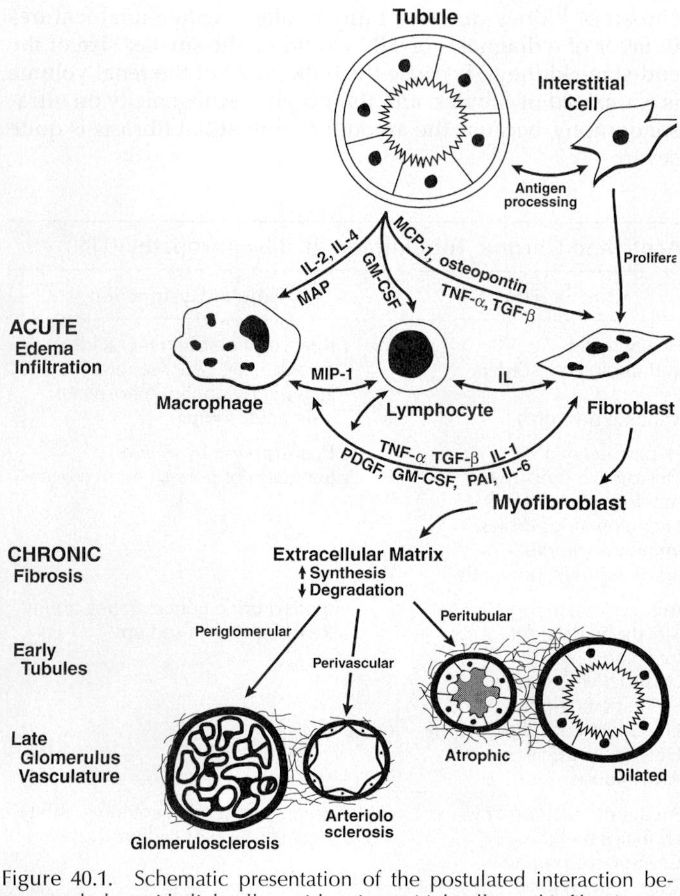

Figure 40.1. Schematic presentation of the postulated interaction between tubular epithelial cells, resident interstitial cells, and infiltrating inflammatory cells and the implicated cytokines that initiate and perpetuate tubulointerstitial lesions.

The initiating cell injury may be a drug, an infectious agent, a filtered protein (albumin, transferrin, lipoprotein, complement, immunoglobulin), mechanical (obstruction), or ischemic (vasculitis). The process begins by antigen recognition, uptake and processing, or expression by the tubular epithelial cells and resident interstitial cells, followed by recruitment of inflammatory cells (Fig. 40.2). The course of events during this subsequent integrative or regulatory phase will either suppress the effector phase (as in arrest or reversal of the transient injury in mild forms of acute TIN) or intensify it (as in progressive injury in severe forms of acute TIN). In acute TIN, feedback mechanisms restore the initial orchestrated response to injury to its baseline dormant state. In chronic TIN, either persistent injury or dysregulation of normal feedback results in perpetuation of the effector phase, which results in differing rates of progressive and permanent tubulointerstitial damage. An integral component of this progressive stage is activation of the interstitial fibroblasts, which undergo upregulation and increased expression of new or constitutive receptors for the fibrogenetic cytokines released by the tubular epithelial and infiltrating cells (TGF-β1, PDGF, TNF-α, IL-1, IL6, PAI) and begin to undergo phenotypic changes, including acquisition of smooth muscle (actin) and mesenchymal (vimentin, desmin) cell markers. Their subsequent evolution into myofibroblasts results in the increased desposition of extracellular matrix (collagen I, III, IV; fibronectin; laminin). In addition to their evolution from resident fibroblasts, myofibroblasts can be derived from the transdifferentiation into fibroblasts of the renal tubular epithelial cells, vascular pericytes, and recruited macrophages. While the initial result is that of increased peritubular and interstitial fibrosis, there is also varying degrees of progressive perivascular and periglomerular fibrosis (Figs. 40.1 and 40.2). The latter is always a feature of severe and late stages of chronic TIN and account for the progression to end-stage renal disease (ESRD) and the onset of hypertension. The vascular changes may assume a gradually increasing role in the pathogenesis of TIN. Microvascular constriction due to edema or released vasoactive agents in the acute phase and obliteration due to perivascular fibrosis in the chronic phase would induce ischemia, which itself is a cause of TIN; increase intraglomerular capillary pressure, a known cause of progressive glomerular injury; and increase production of angiotensin, which magnifies ischemic injury and is a known direct stimulant of several cytokines (e.g., MCP-1).

It is now evident that the tubular epithelial cells play a central role and actively participate at all phases of the development and progression of tubulointerstitial disease by acting as antigen-processing and presenting cells; secreting cytokines, which recruit inflammatory cells; upregulating their surface markers (ICAM, VCAM) to interact with interstitial infiltrates; and transforming into activated fibroblasts, which contribute directly to the irreversible fibrosis that results. As such, continuous exposure of the epithelial cells to the initiating injury is an implicated and conceivable cause of progression and chronic TIN. Of the various stimuli that have been incriminated as a cause of chronic epithelial cell injury, the most convincing evidence ascribes a role to proteinuria and angiotensin.

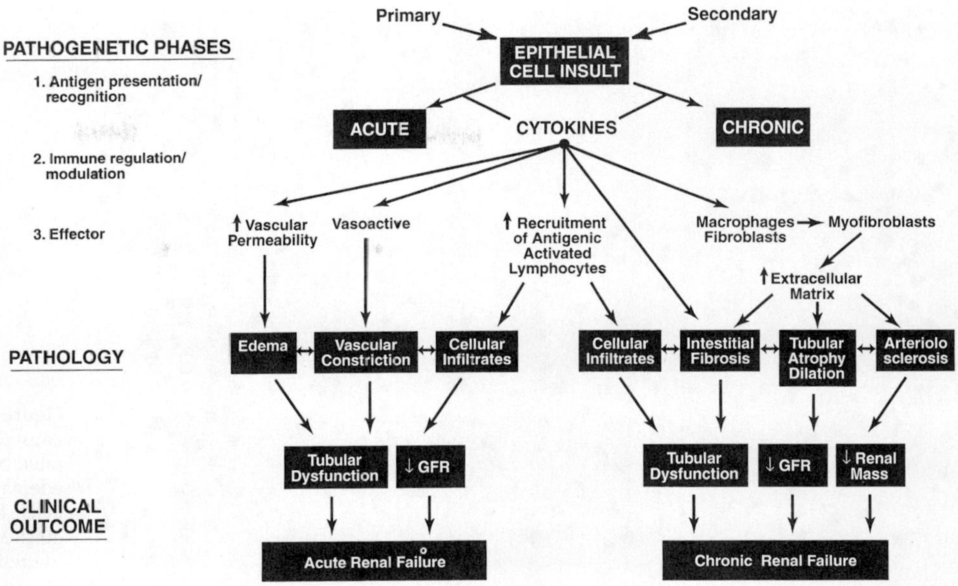

Figure 40.2. Pathogenetic pathways implicated in primary and secondary forms of acute and chronic tubulointerstitial nephritis.

Proteinuria resulting from glomerular disease has a direct role in activating the cascade initiated by epithelial cell injury that perpetuates the interstitial disease. Clinical studies in a host of glomerular diseases (FSGS, MGN, IgA, MPGN) show a direct correlation between the degree of proteinuria and the rate of progression of renal failure and of the extent of TIN. The detrimental role of proteinuria in the progression of diabetic nephropathy, which had long been recognized, has now been substantiated and shown to relate to the severity of TIN. In addition, the results of the Modification of Diet in Renal Disease (MDRD) study have clearly established that a higher baseline level of proteinuria is directly associated with a more rapid decline of GFR and progression to ESRD. The role of proteinuria in the pathogenesis of progression of renal failure is discussed in more detail in Chapter 67, Part 2.

Another injurious agent that has been documented is angiotensin II. Although circulating levels of angiotensin II are not elevated, there is evidence that its local autacoid activity is increased and TIN can be induced by the infusion of angiotensin II. Moreover, in various experimental models of TIN, the renal lesions can be ameliorated by angiotensin-converting enzyme (ACE) inhibitors. Thus the renoprotective effects of ACE inhibitors are not limited to their hemodynamic effect on glomerular intracapillary pressure, but just as importantly to their ability to favorably affect the lesions of TIN.

Increased ammonia generation due to proteinuria or caused by the remaining intact tubules has also been implicated as a cause of chronic injury. Ammonia possesses the capability to Amidate C_3, which acts as C_3/C_5 convertase and activates the alternative complement pathway C5b-9. Experimentally, the administration of bicarbonate to correct acidosis and reduce renal ammonia generation, in a partial remnant model of renal disease, has been shown to reduce TIN and ameliorate the course of renal failure.

Many of these pathogenetic mechanisms have been marshalled from experimental laboratory models and confirmed to be operative in humans from *in situ* hybridization and histochemical studies of kidney biopsies. Although still difficult to use routinely, the human studies provide not only confirmation but also the potential for diagnostic and clinical application. Thus the urinary excretion of antigenically active inflammatory cells and ET-1 has been shown to be increased and, when examined, to correlate with the extent of tubulointerstitial injury. Also, fine-needle aspiration biopsy has been shown to allow for quantification, characterization, and chemokine expression of infiltrating cells. More importantly, the implicated pathogenetic mechanisms provide a basis for the therapy of TIN. The early inflammatory cell-mediated immune response is amenable to steroid therapy in acute TIN. Experimental evidence also supports a role of other forms of cell directed therapy with cyclosporine or cyclophosphamide. The renoprotective effect of ACE inhibitors on TIN processes, coupled with their ability to reduce proteinuria, makes them the logical agent of choice in the management of such cases, even in the absence of hypertension. Correction of acidosis with bicarbonate deserves equal consideration. Finally, accrued evidence for a balanced extracellular matrix biosynthesis and degradation processes provides hope for the identification of components of the matricial degrading enzymes and their potential therapeutic role in reversing renal fibrosis, at least in its early stages. Detailed discussion of the immunopathogenesis of tubulointerstitial diseases are provided in Chapter 38.

ACUTE TUBULOINTERSTITIAL NEPHROPATHY

The acute form of TIN is characterized by a rapid deterioration of renal function, the constant pathologic features of which are edema and inflammatory cell infiltration of the interstitium, in the absence of suppuration or interstitial fibrosis, and the sparing of the glomeruli and vasculature (Fig. 40.3). As a rule, the infiltrates are focal, most evident at the corticomedullary junction; are peritubular in distribution; and consist primarily of mononuclear cells that have been identified as activated lymphocytes. Polymorphonuclear cells and macrophages are rare; their presence reflects prolonged exposure to the inciting antigen and poorer prognosis of recovery, especially when granulomas are formed.

Varying degrees of tubular injury may be present, but there is no tubular atrophy. In contrast to cases of acute tubular necrosis, the tubular injury generally affects the basement membrane and the basilar surface of the cells, whereas the luminal side of the cells is relatively preserved. The distinguishing features of the so-called tubulitis, which results from focal infiltrating mononuclear cell disrupting the tubular basement membrane (TBM) and its lining epithelial cells, is considered characteristic of

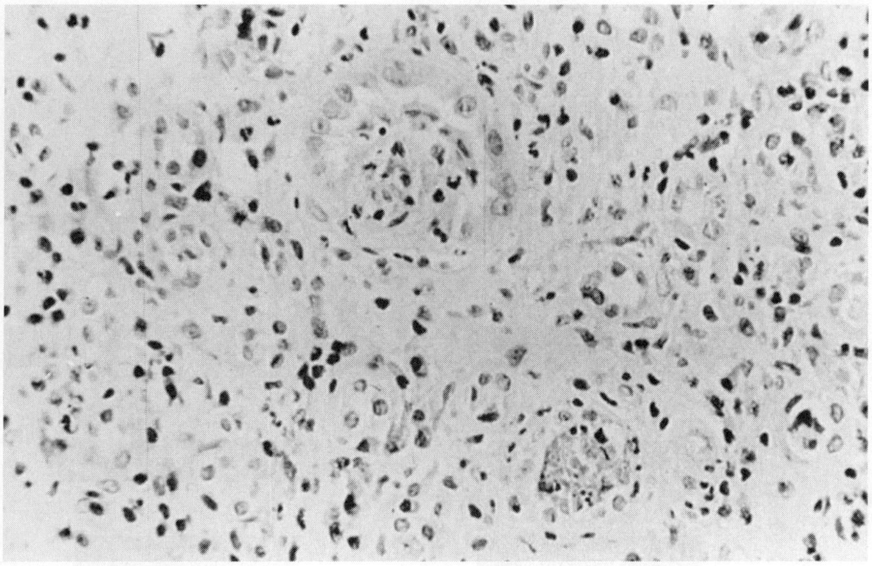

Figure 40.3. Acute tubulointerstitial nephropathy caused by methicillin. The tubules are widely separated because of the considerable degree of interstitial edema. Most of the infiltrate consists of mononuclear cells. Bilobed eosinophilic leukocytes can be distinguished in the *center* of the figure. The tubules appear injured and filled with debris.

TABLE 40.2. Conditions Associated with Acute Tubulointerstitial Nephropathy

Drugs (Table 40.3)
Antibiotics
Sulfonamides
Nonsteroidal antiinflammatory drugs
Others
Infections
Direct—invasion of renal parenchyma
Indirect—systemic infections
Systemic diseases
Metabolic disturbances: urate, oxalate, calcium, potassium
Heavy metals: cadmium, lead
Immunologic diseases: systemic lupus, sarcoidosis
Hematopoietic infiltrative disorders: lymphoproliferative diseases, plasma cell dyscrasias
Idiopathic

acute TIN. In such cases, increased epithelial cell mitotic activity and pleomorphic nuclei are often present, but extensive necrosis of the epithelial cells is absent. Although acute TIN may be suspected clinically, its diagnosis can be confirmed only by the presence of the characteristic morphologic changes noted on a biopsy specimen or at postmortem examination of the kidney. The adjective *acute,* used in referring to this entity, reflects the sudden onset of the clinical syndrome rather than the pathologic features observed, which are notable for their mononuclear cell infiltrate rather than the polymorphonuclear leukocytes associated with acute inflammatory and suppurative reactions.

The two most common causes of acute TIN are drugs and infections. Less commonly, it may occur in a number of systemic diseases or in the absence of any identifiable cause (Table 40.2).

Drugs (Fig. 109.15)

A hypersensitivity reaction to a variety of unrelated drugs is the most common cause of acute TIN encountered clinically. The reaction is not dose related, occurs only in a small number of patients who are exposed to the causative agent, and recurs upon reexposure to the same drug. The renal changes that develop are usually associated with systemic manifestations of hypersensitivity and, less commonly, with circulating antibodies to the responsible drug and laboratory evidence of altered immune mechanisms.

The most commonly incriminated agents are the penicillin congeners, especially methicillin, ciprofloxacin, other β-lactam derivatives, sulfonamides, and rifampin. Deposits of a methicillin metabolite, dimethoxyphenyl penicilloyl, have been implicated as the cause of methicillin-induced acute TIN, but they are also detected in the kidneys of asymptomatic individuals who do not have any functional or structural changes. Acute TIN resulting from sulfonamides appears to be more common in the setting of preexisting reduced renal function. The predisposition to an adverse reaction to sulfonamides has been attributed to differences in metabolism, the idiosyncratic reaction being more common in slow acetylators of sulfonamide, presumably because of the accumulation of metabolites, which are responsible for the reaction. Its occurrence in patients with renal failure has been attributed to their inability to excrete these metabolites. Most cases of rifampin-induced TIN have been noted during intermittent therapy or upon readministration after a hiatus in its daily uneventful use. However, cases of acute TIN during continuous rifampin therapy have been noted. Circulating antibodies to rifampin have been detected in most cases of rifampin-induced TIN but are probably nonspecific because they are also detected in the serum of patients without any adverse drug reactions.

Nonsteroidal antiinflammatory drugs (NSAIDs) whose principal detrimental effect on the kidney is hemodynamic, due to inhibition of prostaglandin synthesis, may also cause an acute deterioration of renal function by causing a distinctive form of TIN. NSAID-induced TIN, unlike other drug-induced TINs, is often associated with the insidious onset of massive proteinuria, which precedes the development of renal failure. In some 15% of cases, renal failure occurs without massive proteinuria, whereas in another 10% of cases, nephrotic syndrome occurs without renal failure. About three-fourths of the reported cases have been associated with the propionic acid derivatives, such as fenoprofen, ibuprofen, and naproxen. Another unique feature of NSAID-induced TIN is the rarity (20% of cases) of associated symptoms of hypersensitivity reaction. Their absence may actually reflect the beneficial effect of NSAIDs on the symptoms of hypersensitivity reactions in general, rather than being a unique feature of this type of TIN. Further discussion of NSAID-induced TIN is found in Chapter 47, Part 3.

Another agent that was a relatively common incriminated cause of TIN, phenindione, is now rarely encountered since cessation of its manufacture in the United States, where it is available only as an investigational drug. Relatively fewer cases of TIN have been reported in association with allopurinol cimetidine, phenytoin, and diuretics. The list of drugs that have been implicated in causing acute TIN continues to expand (Table 40.3) and includes occasional cases attributed to nonprescribed, self-administered herbal remedies. However, the association of TIN with several of these drugs is rare and based on isolated, often single, case reports. The evidence for a causative role of the implicated agents is less than convincing, especially in reports in which more than one agent was being administered and no kidney biopsy was obtained. An *in vitro* lymphocyte stimulation test of the various drugs ingested by an individual patient can be useful in identifying the agent responsible for the acute TIN.

The archetypical prototypes in which acute TIN has been best studied are those associated with methicillin and, to some extent, penicillin and its derivatives. The following clinical features, which are commonly encountered in such cases, have a variable occurrence in other forms of drug-induced acute TIN, the more notable differences being the absence of systemic manifestations and presence of nephrotic-range proteinuria with NSAIDs. The impairment of renal function that develops is preceded and accompanied by a characteristic but nonspecific triad of fever, skin rash, and eosinophilia. The fever, which is present in 70% to 100% of cases, usually appears after the subsidence of the febrile reaction due to the original infection or disease for which antibiotic therapy had been instituted. The skin rash is less common (30% to 50% of cases); consists of erythematous maculopapular lesions, which are often pruritic and generally fleeting; and affects the trunk and proximal portion of the extremities. The eosinophilia is transient and unless specifically sought may go undetected. Skin rash with eosinophilia is uncommon in patients with acute TIN caused by NSAIDs. A nonspecific arthralgia is present in some 15% to 20% of cases. There is a history of preceding flank pain in most cases, and one-third of cases have a history of gross hematuria.

Microscopic hematuria, pyuria, and/or proteinuria are present in almost all cases. The pyuria is nonspecific, except when eosinophils are detected in a carefully examined sediment that has been appropriately stained with Hansel's stain, which improves the detection of urinary eosinophils compared with that of conventional stains. Eosinophiluria is not a unique marker of drug-induced TIN. It can be detected in any infection of the urinary tract or inflammatory disease of the kidney. Only when more than 5% of the urinary white cells are eosinophils in clinically suspected cases can the eosinophiluria be considered as corroborative evidence of acute TIN. It can occur in cases that on kidney biopsy have no eosinophilic infiltrates, or conversely, it can be absent in those with infiltrating eosinophils. The proteinuria is mild and generally of tubular origin, but it may be glomerular and in the nephrotic range, especially in NSAID-induced TIN. β_2-Microglobulinuria may be a prominent feature. The serum level of IgE, an acute serum reactant, is elevated in as many as 50% of cases, and IgE-containing plasma cells have been demonstrated in the renal infiltrate. Coombs' test may be positive in some cases. Ultrasonography generally reveals enlarged kidneys with no evidence of increased echogenicity. A gallium scan may reveal increased uptake by the kidneys but is nonspecific and is positive in all cases of interstitial inflammatory reaction.

The kidney biopsy is diagnostic. In most cases, the diagnosis can be established from light microscopic examination. Electron microscopic and immunofluorescent studies are negative in most cases, except in rare instances in which immunoglobulins, complement, and electron-dense deposits are detected along the TBM. Diffuse interstitial edema and focal cellular infiltrates are the most common findings. Tubular epithelial cell injury varies in severity from vacuolization, decreased height, and simplification in mild cases, to detachment from the basement membrane and necrosis in severe cases. The presence of eosinophils, although of some diagnostic import, is variable. The severity of renal failure correlates with the diffuseness of the cellular infiltrates, the presence of a granulomatous reaction, infiltration with polymorphonuclear leukocytes, and the presence of focal segments of tubular epithelial cell injury or necrosis. Most of the infiltrating mononuclear cells are activated T lymphocytes, with a preponderance of T_4 cells. In general, the lymphocytes that invade the tubules and present the features of "tubulitis," are of the T_8 variety, which are cytotoxic and reflect the severity of the lesions.

The impairment in renal function is variable, ranging from discrete changes of tubular function to an acute reduction in GFR with frank azotemia. The renal failure is nonoliguric in two-thirds of the cases and oliguric in the remainder. Oliguria, which almost always follows a period of polyuria reflecting tubular injury, is more likely to develop in older patients and in those in whom the initial azotemia goes undetected and the administration of the causative agent is continued. Following proper therapy, reversal of renal failure and return to baseline function is the rule. Persistent renal failure can occur in patients

TABLE 40.3. Drugs Associated with Acute Tubulointerstitial Nephropathy

Antibiotics
Penicillins
Methicillin,[a] ampicillin,[a] penicillin,[a] cloxacillin,[a] carbenicillin, oxacillin, nafcillin, amoxicillin
Cephalosporins
Cephalothin,[a] cephradine, cephalexin, cefoxitin, cefazolin, cefaclor
Others
Rifampin,[a] minocycline, doxycycline, gentamicin, vancomycin, lincomycin, mezlocillin, chloramphenicol
Sulfonamides
Cotrimoxazole,[a] sulfamethoxazole,[a] sulfisoxazole, sulfamerazine
Nonsteroidal antiinflammatory drugs
Fenoprofen,[a] ibuprofen,[a] naproxen,[a] glafenenin,[a] tolmetin, zomepirac, indomethacin, diflunisal, phenylbutazone, sulindac, phenazone, sulfinpyrazone, aminopyrine
Anticonvulsive agents
Phenytoin,[a] phenobarbital, carbamazepine
Anticoagulant agents
Phenindione,[a] warfarin
Diuretics
Thiazides,[a] furosemide, triamterene, chlorthalidone
Immunosuppressive agents
Azathioprine, cyclosporine
Miscellaneous
Allopurinol, cimetidine, captopril, clofibrate, amphetamine, *p*-aminosalicylic acid

[a] More commonly incriminated agents.
The drugs in each group are listed in descending order of frequency of associated acute TIN.

in whom the diagnosis is delayed, interstitial fibrosis has set in, or kidney biopsies reveal a granulomatous reaction.

Infection (Fig. 109.14)

Acute TIN may result from direct invasion of the renal parenchyma by an infective organism or may complicate a systemic infection in the absence of bacteremia and renal parenchymal invasion. Before the antibiotic era, acute TIN was a relatively common complication noted at autopsy in cases of β-hemolytic streptococcal infections, particularly in fatal cases of scarlet fever and diphtheria, about one-fourth of which demonstrated an acute TIN. In fact, the term *acute interstitial nephritis* was coined at the turn of the 19th century to describe the renal lesions associated with systemic streptococcal infections. The availability of specific vaccines and antibiotics has ameliorated the severity and frequency of streptococcal infections, such that although TIN continues to complicate their course occasionally, the clinical outcome is now more favorable. Actually, it is now increasingly difficult to establish infection as the cause of TIN because of the concomitant use of antibiotics and other therapeutic agents in their management, most of which have come to be implicated as a cause of acute TIN. Contrary to the glomerular lesions of postinfectious glomerulonephritis that develop 2 to 3 weeks after these infections, the lesions of acute TIN occurs early in the course of the infection, generally during its first few days and rarely after 10 to 12 days. These lesions always appear in the absence of the morphologic features of glomerulonephritis.

The more classic, and certainly more common (at least morphologically), cause of TIN is direct bacterial invasion of the renal parenchyma. Although generally caused by bacterial organisms, it may also be caused by fungal, viral, and parasitic infections. The clinical features of the acute pyelonephritis that results are quite characteristic and consist of the sudden onset of fever, chills, costovertebral pain and tenderness, dysuria, leukocytosis, pyuria, bacteriuria, and urinary casts. The urine culture is almost always positive. The renal lesions are lobular in distribution, and the inflammatory foci, which are arranged radially, are equally prominent in the cortex and the medulla. Numerous polymorphonuclear leukocytes are found in the interstitium and in the walls and lumens of tubules, with evidence of suppuration in severe cases. This is in sharp contrast to the lesions of acute TIN caused by systemic streptococcal infections, in which the infiltrates are focal, form circular bands around the tubules, are more prominent at the corticomedullary region, and rarely contain polymorphonuclear leukocytes. Acute bacterial pyelonephritis does not usually result in a decline of renal function, except when it occurs with urinary tract obstruction or in diabetic patients. In fact, renal function is well preserved, except for an impairment in urine concentrating and acidifying ability, which is reversible when the infection is controlled. Although generally rare in cases that are bacterial in origin, acute deterioration in renal function does occur in TIN due to leptospirosis, brucellosis, and candidiasis. In most of these conditions, the renal changes subside after resolution of the infection, although instances of progression to chronic TIN with interstitial fibrosis, tubular atrophy, and residual impairment of renal function can occur in chronic forms of the disease.

Systemic Diseases

An acute deterioration of renal function in which the structural changes of the kidney are those of TIN occurs in a variety of systemic diseases. The renal involvement may be due to metabolic disturbances, the infiltrative nature of the primary disease, or the immunologic basis of the systemic disease process.

The metabolic disturbances in which acute TIN develops are those due to an abnormality in the metabolism of urate, oxalate, calcium, potassium, or heavy metals. The two principal conditions in which an immune mechanism may cause acute TIN, with only limited glomerular involvement, are systemic lupus erythematosus and kidney transplantation. They have also been noted, but only rarely, in Sjögren's syndrome, mixed cryoglobulinemia, IgA nephropathy, and Wegener's granulomatosis. The infiltrative disorders are in general the neoplastic diseases but, in fact, occur mostly with lymphoproliferative disorders and plasma cell dyscrasias. These entities are discussed in their respective appropriate chapters and are not considered further here, other than to note their association with acute TIN.

Idiopathic Acute Tubulointerstitial Nephritis

Despite exhaustive investigation no evidence of drug exposure, infection or systemic disease can be substantiated in some 10% to 20% of cases of reversible acute renal failure with the finding on kidney biopsy of interstitial edema and mononuclear cell infiltration. The systemic manifestations of a hypersensitivity reaction are generally absent in most of these cases. Uveitis has been a feature of a small subset of these cases, which have been termed *renal-ocular syndrome* or *tubulointerstitial nephritis and uveitis (TINU) syndrome.* Bone marrow granulomas may be another common feature that has been noted in a few of the reported cases. Both the renal and ocular changes often respond favorably to a brief course of steroid therapy.

Therapy of Acute TIN

In drug-induced cases, the cornerstone of therapy is early recognition of renal injury and elimination of the agent responsible for the hypersensitivity reaction. This is not always easy. Early recognition depends on careful monitoring for any increments in BUN and serum Cr, even when the reported levels are within normal limits, particularly in the presence of any evidence of tubular dysfunction, such as polyuria, glycosuria, hypouricemia, elevated urine pH, and eosinophiluria. Even when suspected, patients are usually taking multiple drugs and the decision of which agent to eliminate is empiric. Although it is natural to eliminate those agents that are commonly a cause of acute TIN (Table 40.2), the choice is not always a correct one because any of the unsuspected other drugs could be the inciting agent.

Close monitoring of renal function is essential after discontinuation of the suspected offending agent. If the concentrations of BUN and Cr are only modestly elevated and there are no further increments, it will suffice to provide symptomatic treatment consisting of maintaining adequate hydration; monitoring for volume depletion or overload; adjusting the dosage of other drugs to the level of renal function; avoiding drugs that compromise renal function, such as NSAIDs and ACE inhibitors; and instituting specific therapy for any coexistent infection. If renal insufficiency persists and progresses after elimination of the suspected drugs, consideration should be given for a renal biopsy to establish the diagnosis. If renal function continues to deteriorate and the biopsy is diagnostic, the institution of steroid therapy should be considered. A short course of steroids (60 mg prednisone per day for 10 to 14 days) can shorten the course of renal insufficiency and hospitalization. The duration of steroid therapy will depend on the clinical response but is not indicated for longer than 2 to 4 weeks. In patients with severe renal failure or those who are poor candidates for renal biopsy and unable to be medicated orally, intravenous pulse steroids (1 g methylprednisolone per day for 3 days) can be used. Steroids have not proven to be effective in cases caused by NSAIDs, in which recovery is protracted (months) after withdrawal and return to baseline renal function relatively less common.

In oliguric patients or those with progressive renal failure, dialysis should be initiated early, using biocompatible high-flux membrane dialyzers. Dialysis may be required in about one-third of patients and for the duration of the oliguria, which varies from a few days to several weeks. The outcome with supportive dialytic therapy is favorable in 90% of patients after withdrawal of the inciting agent. Actually, independent of the severity of renal failure, recovery of normal renal function is the rule after the incriminated agent has been discontinued. Instances of persistent reduction of renal function after recovery from the acute renal failure episodes have been reported. It is especially in these patients that a brief course of high-dose steroids can expedite the recovery period and is of particular value when renal failure is protracted. It is important that the patient be informed of the cause of TIN and that future exposure to the same agent be avoided. Reexposure can result in the rapid, precipitous onset of severe renal failure.

Because of the cell-mediated immune basis of acute TIN, the use of cyclophosphamide or cyclosporine has also been suggested. This is primarily based on experimental studies with very limited clinical evidence of their effectiveness. In cases that fail to respond to steroids, a limited course of cyclophosphamide (2 mg/kg per body weight daily) may be tried. Therapy for longer than 4 to 6 weeks is not indicated. Plasmapheresis has been used in occasional cases with demonstrated circulating anti-TBM antibodies and complement consumption.

In cases of acute TIN caused by infection, early diagnosis and proper antibiotic therapy will reverse the renal changes. In fact, in such cases, the tubular dysfunction and modest increments in the levels of BUN and Cr may go undetected. It is when the infection is protracted or in difficult cases when the diagnosis is unsuspected (e.g., in psittacosis) or delayed (e.g., in Hanta virus) that acute renal failure becomes evident. Supportive therapy, including early dialysis, is important in preventing uremic syndrome, which otherwise would aggravate the infection. Because of the difficulty in differential diagnosis, a common error is to attribute the deterioration of renal function to acute tubular necrosis (ATN). The urinary indices are not helpful because both are associated with increased fractional excretion of sodium, and eosinophiluria is neither sensitive nor always present. A biopsy is indicated when acute TIN is highly suspected. Although the supportive therapy for both ATN and acute TIN is the same, proper diagnosis is essential when consideration is given to the use of steroids in cases due to acute TIN. Actually, until the infective agent is identified and specific antibiotic therapy is instituted, the use of steroids is fraught with the risk of aggravating the infection. Under any circumstance, steroids should be reserved for patients with severe and protracted renal failure that persists after proper therapy for the infection is instituted and in whom the diagnosis of acute TIN is established on kidney biopsy.

In patients with acute TIN due to systemic diseases, therapy of the primary disease process will reverse the renal lesion. To the extent that most of these are immune-mediated processes that require steroid therapy (lupus, allograft rejection), the decision to use steroids is easier to make than in those due to infection.

The response of idiopathic forms of acute TIN to a short course of steroids is dramatic and should be initiated immediately after the diagnosis is established to prevent persistent injury that would otherwise compromise return of baseline renal function.

CHRONIC TUBULOINTERSTITIAL NEPHROPATHY

The diseases implicated as a cause of chronic TIN are quite diverse (Table 40.4), having in common only the predominant morphologic features of the kidney in this entity and the course of the renal disease that develops.

The principal morphologic features of chronic TIN are interstitial fibrosis, proliferating fibroblasts, inflammatory mononuclear cell infiltration, and varying degrees of tubular dilation, degeneration, and atrophy (Fig. 40.4). Some degree of thickening of the tubular basement is almost always present, whereas that of the vascular walls and Bowman's capsule is variable and a late occurrence. The lesions may be diffuse but are generally patchy in distribution. Intimal fibrosis, medial hypertrophy, microvascular obliteration, and glomerular changes of sclerosis, atrophy, and periglomerular fibrosis, although not present, will ultimately become a dominant feature (Fig. 40.5). By this late stage, tubular changes are more severe and a cross-section of patent tubules contain hyalinized casts that mimic thyroid follicles, hence the term *thyroidization.*

Renal insufficiency is slow to develop, and the early manifestations of renal involvement are those of tubular dysfunction. The pattern of tubular dysfunction that develops will vary depending on the responsible etiologic agent and the principal site of tubular injury associated with it (Table 40.1). Continued exposure to the causative agent will result in progressive injury, and the severity of tubular dysfunction noted clinically will depend on the extent of tubular damage caused. With progressive injury, reduction in GFR will occur. Early during the course of the disease, the characteristic clinical features of glomerular dysfunction (peripheral edema, significant proteinuria, and hy-

TABLE 40.4. Conditions Associated with Chronic Tubulointerstitial Nephropathies

Immunologic diseases
Systemic lupus erythematosus, allograft rejection, cryoglobinemia, Sjögren's syndrome, IgA nephropathy, Goodpasture's syndrome
Drugs
Analgesics, nonsteroidal antiinflammatory drugs, cyclosporine, *cis*-platinum, nitrosureas, lithium
Infection
Bacterial, viral, fungal, mycobacterial
Obstructive uropathy
Vesicoureteral reflux, mechanical
Hematopoietic diseases
Sickle hemoglobinopathies, plasma cell dyscrasias, lymphoproliferative disorders
Heavy metals
Cadmium, lead
Metabolic disorders
Urate, oxalate, cystinosis, hypercalcemia, potassium depletion
Granulomatous diseases
Sarcoidosis, tuberculosis, Wegener's granulomatosis, candidiasis, drug addiction nephropathy
Vascular diseases
Inflammatory, sclerotic, emboli
Hereditary diseases
Hereditary nephritis, medullary sponge kidney, medullary cystic disease, polycystic kidney disease
Endemic diseases
Balkan nephropathy, nephropathia epidemica
Idiopathic

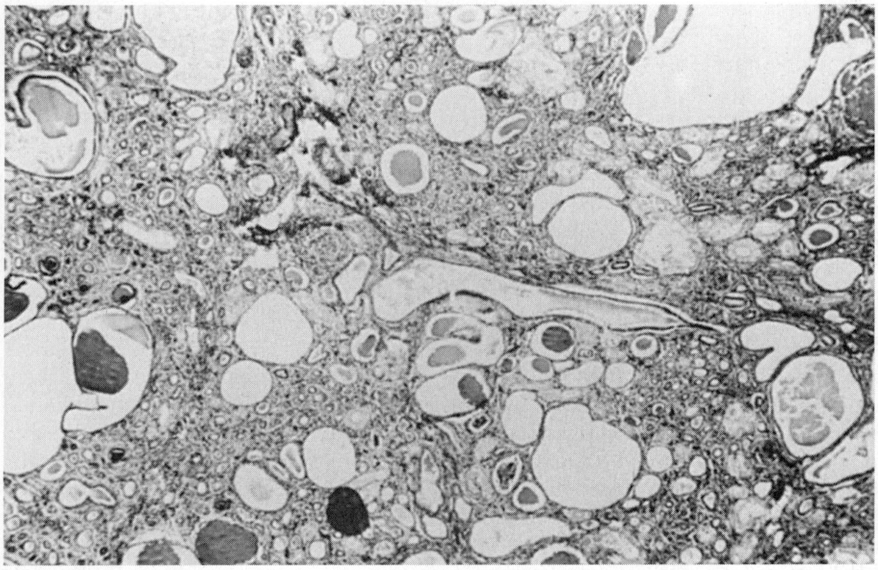

Figure 40.4. Chronic tubulointerstitial nephropathy of undetermined etiology. There is diffuse tubular atrophy, degeneration, and dilation. The interstitium is fibrotic with scanty mononuclear cell infiltration.

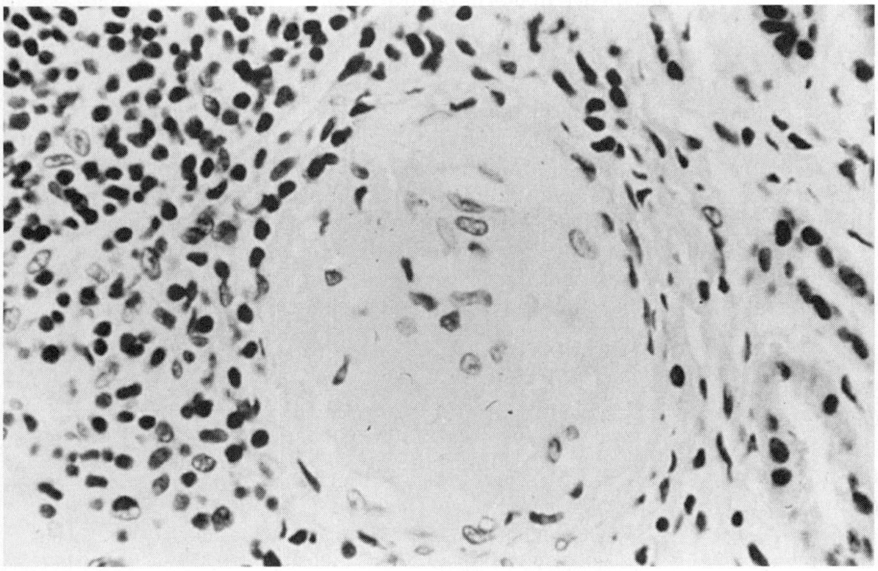

Figure 40.5. Sclerotic glomerulus from a patient with chronic tubulointerstitial nephropathy. Note the periglomerular fibrosis and mononuclear cell infiltration.

pertension) are absent, and tubular dysfunction is almost always out of proportion to any coexistent glomerular dysfunction. The magnitude of reduction in glomerular filtration shows a direct correlation with the extent and severity of the interstitial fibrosis and, to a much lesser degree, with the extent of tubular atrophy. Later in the course of the disease, when the glomerular sclerotic lesions are advanced, massive proteinuria, edema, and hypertension will develop; it may then be difficult to differentiate them from end-stage disease of any etiology.

Because of the insidious onset of renal failure, the renal injury of tubulointerstitial nephropathy may go unrecognized until significant renal damage has occurred. It is therefore very important to maintain a high index of suspicion of this entity whenever any tubular dysfunction is noted clinically because in some one-third of patients with ESRD, the primary cause of renal failure is chronic TIN. In at least two-thirds of these cases, the cause of TIN is a known drug or toxin and the condition is therefore potentially preventable or treatable if recognized early enough, before progression to irreversible renal failure.

Immune Diseases

Although the mechanism of interstitial injury remains to be fully elucidated, considerable experimental and clinical evidence exists for a cell-mediated immune mechanism of tubulointerstitial injury. Primary TIN mediated by humoral immune complexes is rare in humans. It is most commonly encountered clinically in lupus nephritis, in which evidence for an immune complex–mediated injury has been adduced from the demonstration of DNA in the deposits seen along or within the TBM and around the peritubular capillaries and the interstitium. Tubulointerstitial electron-dense deposits have also been described in Sjögren's syndrome, IgA nephropathy, renal allografts, and mixed cryoglobulinemia. However, aside from lupus nephritis, in which the antigen has been demonstrated, and mixed cryoglobulinemia, in which IgG and anti-IgG antibodies have been identified in the deposits, there is only limited evidence for an immune complex–mediated mechanism in other diseases, including chronic allograft rejection whose classic morphologic feature is that of chronic TIN. A potential role of Tamm-Horsfall protein, a surface membrane glycoprotein of the ascending limb of Henle's loop and the distal tubule, has been implicated in certain forms of human TIN. Antibodies to this protein have been detected in the sera of patients with vesicoureteral reflux and pyelonephritis and have been demonstrated in the interstitium of patients with hereditary nephritis, hydronephrosis, and medullary cystic disease. However, antibodies are not regularly associated with the Tamm-Horsfall deposits that have been noted in these patients. The clinical evidence for anti-TBM antibodies as a cause of TIN is even less convincing but has been demonstrated in cases of Goodpasture's syndrome, in renal allograft rejection, and rarely, in otherwise idiopathic forms of the disease.

In contrast to the rarity and variability with which immune complex deposits and anti-TBM antibodies are noted in chronic TIN, some degree of interstitial cell infiltration is an almost invariable and essential component of the lesion. Most cells constituting the infiltrate are T cells, some of which have been further characterized as activated lymphocytes. The T cells may be of the helper/inducer or cytotoxic/suppressor subset, although there generally seems to be a slight preponderance of the former. B cells, which may also be present, constitute less than 20% of the cellular interstitial infiltrate. As a rule, infiltration with T cells is more diffuse, whereas those of B cells are more focal in their distribution. This profile of immunocompetent cells supports the role for cell-mediated immune injury in most cases of chronic TIN. Fibroblasts constitute a significant number of the interstitial cells in severe cases, and in isolated culture, they synthesize four to five times more total collagen per cell as compared with fibroblasts isolated from normal kidneys.

Drugs

The prolonged and excessive consumption of drugs is a leading cause of chronic TIN. This is best exemplified by analgesic nephropathy, which represents one of the most common causes of end-stage kidney disease in some geographic areas (see Chapter 47). In fact, it is to a great extent the appreciation of the role of analgesic mixtures in the causation of "chronic interstitial nephritis" that corrected the erroneous attribution of all interstitial lesions to pyelonephritis and led to the identification of TIN as the uniform renal response to various other disorders (Table 40.4). The association between the ingestion of analgesic compounds and the development of chronic TIN with papillary necrosis is now well established. Other implicated drugs include cyclosporine, nitrosurea compounds, *cis*-platinum, lithium, and NSAIDs. The risk of developing chronic TIN with these agents is quite small, often preventable, and generally reversible on reduction of the dosage administered. Of interest are reports of chronic TIN resulting from the use of herbal medications that in the course of storage had become contaminated with a fungus.

The most common deleterious effect of these agents is in the distal tubule, with impairment of urine concentrating ability, polyuria, and nocturia as the earliest detectable derangements of renal function. Other defects of distal tubular function, specifically hydrogen and potassium secretion, if not evident clinically, can be documented on appropriate testing.

Infection

Contrary to earlier notions, the role of recurrent renal infection as a cause of chronic TIN in the absence of urinary tract obstruction is doubtful. Chronic "atrophic pyelonephritis" with the classic lesions of chronic TIN is a disease of childhood that manifests itself as renal failure in adults. It is children younger than 6 years of age in whom the chronic urinary tract infection is coexistent with severe vesicoureteral reflux and pyelotubular back flow who seem to be at risk of developing chronic TIN.

There is also limited but unsubstantiated clinical evidence for an immune-mediated response to bacterial antigens as the cause of renal parenchymal injury in the absence of obstruction. The experimental data for such a mechanism are more convincing. Acute bacterial infection of experimental animals is accompanied, during the active phase of the infection, by an active immune response by B lymphocytes, a depression of T-lymphocyte suppressor/cytotoxic cells, and an increased local production of IgG, IgM, and IgA by the infiltrating cells of the infected kidney. Whether these reactions persist and contribute to the perpetuation of renal parenchymal injury is a possibility that remains to be documented.

Obstruction and Reflux

Urinary outflow obstruction is characterized by the classic morphologic features of chronic TIN (see Chapter 50). In a carefully studied rat model of unilateral ureteral obstruction, it has been shown that the sequence of events in the development of these lesions is identical to that of the development of interstitial disease in other forms of glomerular proteinuria or tubular epithelial cell injury. Of special interest is the important pathogenetic role of local production of angiotensin and the ability of ACE inhibitors to attenuate the infiltrative and fibrotic processes of urinary obstruction. On the other hand, angiotensin II–receptor blockade decreases the fibrosis but does not appear to affect the influx of mononuclear infiltrating cells.

Clinically, urinary tract obstruction and vesicoureteral reflux result in tubulointerstitial injury in the absence of complicating infections. However, as noted, it is mainly children in whom infection and vesicoureteral reflux persist despite treatment who are at risk of developing chronic TIN. The extent of renal injury depends on the magnitude of the pressure that develops, the degree of incompetence of the vesicoureteral valves, and the length of time that either of these two defects persists before it is corrected. A role for the extravasation of Tamm-Horsfall protein in causing an immune-mediated injury in the absence of infection has been demonstrated experimentally and suggested to be operative in humans. Figure 109.17 (Chapter 109) provides the findings in renal biopsy of the chronic interstitial nephropathy in reflux nephropathy.

Hematopoietic Disorders

The hematopoietic disorders associated with TIN are the sickle hemoglobinopathies, plasma cell dyscrasias, and lymphoproliferative disorders.

Sickle Cell Hemoglobinopathies

The lesions are most common in sickle cell disease but are also encountered in patients with sickle cell trait, sickle cell hemoglobin C disease, and sickle cell thalassemia. The propensity of hemoglobin S to polymerize in an environment of low oxygen tension, hypertonicity, and reduced pH, all of which characterize the renal medulla, is conducive to the intraerythrocytic polymerization of hemoglobin S and consequent sickling in the medullary vessels. The initiating event is an occlusive lesion that affects the medullary vasculature. As a result, the TIN lesions involve mainly the renal medulla, and renal papillary necrosis is common in sickle hemoglobinopathies (see Chapters 43, Part 1 and 51). Inability to concentrate the urine and impaired distal tubular secretion of hydrogen and potassium are the principal disorders encountered early in the course of renal involvement, before the onset of azotemia.

Plasma Cell Dyscrasias

The pathogenesis of renal involvement in plasma cell dyscrasias is of varied etiology. The characteristic lesions that result directly from excessive production of light-chain proteins are due to their precipitation in the distal tubule. The affected tubules become surrounded by chronic inflammatory cells, interstitial fibrosis, and multinucleated giant cells—the classic appearance of myeloma cast nephropathy. The initiation of this series of events depends on (a) the physical properties of the light chains, which are probably why λ light chains are more injurious than κ light chains; (b) the quantity of light chains produced and therefore delivered to the tubules; and (c) the pH of the tubule fluid, which is why the lesions are more common in the distal acid fluid. Increasing the rate of urine flow and alkalinization of the urine will prevent or reverse cast formation, whereas treatment of the plasma cell dyscrasia will reduce the load of light chains presented to the kidney. Plasmapheresis, to reduce the load of abnormal proteins, may be useful in severe cases.

Direct tubular toxicity of the reabsorbed light chains may also contribute to renal dysfunction. The myeloma cast nephropathy, localized in the distal tubule, accounts for the distal tubule dysfunction, whereas the reabsorption of the light chains, which is a function of the proximal tubules, accounts for the proximal tubule dysfunction in these patients.

The interstitial and perivascular deposition of paraproteins, either as amyloid fibrils or as fragments of light chains, is another reason that TIN develops in patients with plasma cell disorders. Finally, metabolic disorders (hyperuricemia or hypercalcemia), which occur in some patients, can cause or contribute to TIN.

Lymphoproliferative Disorders

Infiltrates of the kidney by malignant cells are localized to the interstitium and result in tubular atrophy while sparing the glomeruli and, as such, mimic the classic morphologic features of TIN. They are most common in lymphoproliferative disorders, especially in non-Hodgkin's lymphomas and lymphoblastic leukemias. Chemotherapy of the lymphoproliferative disorder will reverse the renal lesions.

Heavy Metals

Environmental exposure to cadmium and lead are the two most common sources of heavy metals associated with chronic TIN. Occasional cases of TIN have also been reported after exposure to arsenic, barium, bismuth, chromium, copper, iron, mercury, platinum, silicon, and uranium.

Cadmium is preferentially concentrated in the proximal tubule as a cadmium–metallothionein complex, which has a biologic half-life of 10 years. It results in a slowly developing form of chronic TIN, the major manifestations of which are those of proximal tubule dysfunction. Renal calculi develop in one-fourth of these cases.

Focal lesions of TIN occur in half of the cases exposed to lead, in the absence of the classic findings of systemic lead intoxication. This subclinical total body lead overload has been implicated in the causation of hyperuricemia, hypertension, and renal failure. The infusion of calcium EDTA to mobilize excessive stores of lead has been shown to be a useful diagnostic tool for the detection and ultimate treatment of this condition. More discussion on the effects of heavy metals on the kidneys is found in Chapter 47, Part 4.

Metabolic Disorders

Changes in the metabolism of urate, oxalate, cystine calcium, and potassium have been implicated as causes of TIN. The effects of each of these on the kidney are discussed elsewhere and are discussed only briefly in this chapter.

Urate

Depending on the load of urate presented to the kidney, one of three forms of disorders will result: (a) acute urate nephropathy, which occurs during episodes of sudden massive overproduction of uric acid; (b) uric acid nephrolithiasis, which occurs in chronic overproducers and overexcretors of uric acid; and (c) chronic urate nephropathy, which occurs in chronic hyperuricemics who excrete normal amounts of uric acid.

The principal renal lesion of chronic hyperuricemia is the deposition in the interstitium of amorphous urate crystals, which elicits a surrounding giant cell reaction. An earlier and coexistent change in these cases is the precipitation of birefringent uric acid crystals in the acid environment of the collecting tubules, with consequent tubular obstruction, dilation, atrophy, and interstitial fibrosis. The earlier notion that these lesions account for the occurrence of renal disease in patients with hyperuricemia has been questioned in the light of prolonged follow-up studies. Renal dysfunction could be documented only when the serum urate was persistently greater than 13 mg/dl in men and 10 mg/dl in women. The deterioration of renal function in those with lower levels of hyperuricemia has been attributed to coexistent hypertension, diabetes mellitus, and arteriosclerosis. Treatment with allopurinol of isolated asymptomatic hyperuricemia that is below these deleterious levels would be of questionable merit, particularly because the drug itself is not an innocuous agent. Evidence has been advanced for an association between hyperuricemia, hypertension, and renal dysfunction in individuals with a history of exposure to lead who had only subclinical lead toxicity. The adverse effects of urate on the kidney are discussed in detail in Chapter 44.

Oxalate

The increased renal excretion of oxalate, whether due to its overproduction or overabsorption, results in the intratubular precipitation of calcium oxalate. Atrophy of the affected tubules with surrounding inflammatory cell infiltration and fibrosis result in the classic morphologic features of chronic TIN. The lesions first occur in the proximal tubules, where oxalate is secreted, but are more severe in the renal medulla, where the increasing concentration of tubular fluid fosters the further precipitation of calcium oxalate. Recurrent calcium oxalate stones in these patients can contribute to the development of TIN by causing obstruction.

Cystinosis

This rare autosomal inherited disorder of amino acid metabolism is characterized by the deposition of cystine crystals throughout the body. In the kidney, the early lesions are those of proximal tubular injury and characteristic rhomboid crystal deposits in the adjacent interstitium. Progressive interstitial fibrosis, tubular atrophy, and interstitial inflammatory reaction eventuate in end-stage renal failure due to chronic TIN.

Hypercalcemia

Focal degeneration and necrosis of the tubular epithelium, primarily affecting the medulla, where calcium is concentrated in an acid tubular medium, develop shortly after persistent hypercalcemia. The affected tubules atrophy and become obstructed, with consequent dilation and pressure injury to the proximal segments of the tubule. The subsequent calcification and destruction of the TBM result in an infiltrative and proliferative cellular reaction in the adjacent interstitium. The deposition of calcium in the injured areas results in nephrocalcinosis. The ultimate lesion of focal scarred areas of tubular atrophy interstitial fibrosis and mononuclear cell infiltration is a classic example of chronic TIN.

Potassium Depletion

The several functional changes associated with potassium depletion notwithstanding, the characteristic structural changes that develop are limited to the proximal tubule and consist of vacuolization of the epithelial cells due to the dilated cisternae of their endoplasmic reticulum and basal infoldings. In protracted cases, microcystic dilation of the affected tubules occurs. Whether these changes can progress to chronic TIN in humans is uncertain, although in severe persistent experimental potassium depletion, interstitial fibrosis and scarring have been demonstrated in the rat kidney.

Granulomatous Diseases

Interstitial granulomatous reaction is a rare but singular feature of certain forms of chronic TINs that occur in sarcoidosis, tuberculosis, xanthogranulomatous pyelonephritis, Wegener's granulomatosis, berrylliosis candidiasis, oxalosis, phenytoin hypersensitivity, and drug-addiction (heroin) nephropathy.

Noncaseating granulomatous infiltrates of the renal interstitium may be detected in most of patients with sarcoidosis. As a rule, they are few in number, with no clinical evidence of renal involvement. It is when they are more widely distributed that renal dysfunction becomes apparent. The deterioration of renal function due to acute granulomatous reaction is responsive to steroid therapy. Regression of the acute granulomatous reaction, following steroid therapy, can result in residual interstitial fibrosis and progressive renal failure in the more diffuse forms of the disease. The characteristic increased intestinal calcium absorption due to the high levels of circulating 1, $25(OH)_2$ vitamin D_3 and consequent hypercalcemia and hypercalciuria contribute to the progression of the TIN and possibly account for the TIN that is encountered in some cases in the absence of granulomatous lesions.

The pathogenetic sequence of events is similar in tuberculosis of the kidney. The granulomatous reaction due to the infective mycobacteria responds to antituberculous treatment, but the residual fibrosis results in TIN even in the absence of caseating lesions. More common is obstructive uropathy, which develops after ureteral scarring due to urinary tract seeding by mycobacteria, which can cause chronic TIN due to urinary outflow obstruction. The renal lesions in tuberculosis are discussed in Chapter 41, Part 2.

Vascular Diseases

Tubular atrophy, interstitial fibrosis, and cellular infiltration develop wherever there is ischemia due to intrarenal vascular involvement by any vascular disease. This accounts for the TIN of nephrosclerosis caused by hypertension and contributes to the renal interstitial lesions of diabetes mellitus, sickle hemoglobinopathies, and radiation nephritis. In addition, the vascular obliterative lesions of severe TIN play an important role in the progressive nature of these lesions.

Mechanical obstruction of the intrarenal vasculature by emboli, be they atheromatous or thrombotic, results in patchy infarction and an adjacent tissue reaction of classic TIN.

Hereditary Diseases of the Kidney

Tubulointerstitial lesions are a prominent component of the structural changes occurring in a number of hereditary diseases, such as medullary cystic disease, familial juvenile nephrophthisis, polycystic kidney disease, medullary sponge kidneys, and hereditary nephritis.

Endemic Diseases

Balkan nephropathy and nephropathia epidemica are two endemic diseases in which the characteristic renal lesions are those of TIN. The former is truly an endemic disease; it is restricted to the geographic regions bordering the Danube River, and its etiology remains elusive. The latter, although initially thought to be restricted to the Scandinavian countries, has since been shown to have a more universal occurrence and termed *hemorrhagic fever with renal syndrome*, the causative agent of which has been shown to be a rodent-transmitted virus of the genus *Bunyavirus*.

Idiopathic Disease

Despite extensive workup, it is not possible to determine the etiology of chronic TIN noted on biopsy in some 15% to 20% of patients who present with renal insufficiency of undetermined etiology.

Selected Readings

Bohle A, Muller GA, Wehrmann M, et al. Pathogenesis of chronic renal failure in the primary glomerulopathies, renal vasculopathies, and chronic interstitial nephritides. *Kidney Int* 1996;49(Suppl):54.

An analysis of more than 2,000 kidney biopsies from cases of glomerular and vascular disease. Illustrates that impaired renal function most closely relates to the severity of tubulointerstitial disease regardless of the primary disease.

D'Amico G. Influence of clinical and histological features on actuarial renal survival in adult patients with idiopathic IgA nephropathy, membranous nephropathy and membranoproliferative glomerulonephritis: survey of the recent literature. *Am J Kidney Dis* 1992;20:315–323.

The title says it all. It is not glomerular damage but the extent of interstitial inflammatory infiltrates and fibrosis that determine the outcome of kidney disease.

Ditlove J, Weidman P, Bernstein M, et al. Methicillin nephritis. *Medicine* (Baltimore) 1977;56:483–491.

A thorough review of the clinical and morphologic features of a common cause and prototype of drug-induced acute tubulointerstitial nephropathy.

Eddy AA. Experimental insights into the tubulointerstitial disease accompanying primary glomerular lesions. *J Am Soc Nephrol* 1994;5:1273–1287.

Review of the demonstrated processes that account for the development of tubulointerstitial lesions in experimental models of primary glomerular injury.

Eknoyan G, McDonald MA, Appel D, et al. Chronic tubulo-interstitial nephritis: correlation between structural and functional findings. *Kidney Int* 1990;38: 736–743.

A study of the functional and structural changes in 46 cases of primary chronic tubulointerstitial nephritis.

Kelly CJ. T cell regulation of autoimmune interstitial nephritis. *J Am Soc Nephrol* 1990;1:140–149.

A review of autoimmune effector mechanisms and the renal antigens implicated in the immunopathogenesis of tubulointerstitial nephritis.

Klahr S, Levey AS, Beck GJ, et al. The effects of dietary protein restriction and blood pressure control on the progression of chronic renal disease. *N Engl J Med* 1994;330:877–884.

Results of a national study demonstrating that baseline urinary protein excretion is directly associated with a more rapid decline of GFR and progression to ESRD. Course favorably modified by control of the blood pressure and possibly by dietary protein restriction, an amelioration that correlates with the reduction in proteinuria by these interventions.

Kleinknecht D, Vanhille PH, Morel-Maroger L, et al. Acute interstitial nephritis due to drug hypersensitivity. An up-to-date review with a report of 19 cases. *Adv Nephrol* 1983;12:277–308.

A well-referenced review of the topic.

Kliem V, Johnson RJ, Alpers CE, et al. Mechanisms involved in the pathogenesis of tubulointerstitial fibrosis in 5/6-nephrectomized rats. *Kidney Int* 1996;49: 666–678.

Evidence for the role of chronic inflammatory cell infiltrates on the course of renal failure in the experimental model of renal ablation.

Laberke HG, Bohle A. Acute interstitial nephritis: correlations between clinical and morphologic findings. *Clin Nephrol* 1980;14:263–273.

A correlation of the structural and functional features in 30 cases of acute tubulointerstitial nephropathy.

Michel DM, Kelly CJ. Acute interstitial nephritis. *J Am Soc Nephrol* 1998;9:506–515.
A personal view of the topic based on the authors experience, coupled with a selective review of the literature on experimental models of acute tubulointerstitial nephritis.

Nath KA. Tubulointerstitial damage as a major determinant in the progression of renal damage. *Am J Kidney Dis* 1992;20:1–17.
An in-depth review of the mechanisms and role of tubulointerstitial lesions that contribute to the progressive nature of renal diseases.

Palmer BF. The renal tubule in the progression of chronic renal failure. *J Invest Med* 1997;45:346–361.
A thorough and well-referenced review of the experimental and clinical evidence in support of the central role of epithelial cells in the tubulointerstitial injury that mediate progressive renal disease.

Rastegar A, Kashgarian M. The clinical spectrum of tubulointerstitial nephritis. *Kidney Int* 1998;54:313–327.
An overview of tubulointerstitial nephritis that focuses on analgesic nephropathy, sarcoidosis, lead nephropathy, and drug-induced hypersensitivity interstitial nephritis.

Ruffing KA, Hoppes P, Blend D, et al. Eosinophils in urine revisited. *Clin Nephrol* 1994;41:163–166.
A study of some 200 cases of pyuria in which the sensitivity of eosinophiluria was 40%, specificity 72%, and positive predictive value 38% in establishing a diagnosis of acute tubulointerstitial nephritis.

Sutton JM. Urinary eosinophils. *Arch Intern Med* 1986;146:2243–2244.
A review and discussion of sensitivity and specificity of urinary eosinophils in the diagnosis of acute tubulointerstitial nephropathy.

Toto RD. Acute tubulointerstitial nephritis. *Am J Med Sci* 1990;299:392–410.
A well-referenced review of the subject.

CHAPTER 41

Renal Infections

PART 1
Urinary Tract Infections

Martina Franz, Sabine Schmaldienst, and Walter H. Hörl

Urinary tract infection (UTI) accounts for one of the most common diseases in the population, occurring from the neonate up to geriatric individuals. Of adult women, 40% to 50% have a history of at least one UTI. In hospitalized patients and in patients after kidney transplantation, UTI is a major cause of gram-negative sepsis.

UTI defines a condition in which the urinary tract is infected with a pathogen causing inflammation. In females, most uropathogenic microorganisms such as *Escherichia coli* colonize the colon, the perianal region, the introitus vaginae, and the periurethral region and may further ascend to the bladder and/or to the kidneys. UTI results from the encounter of a uropathogen and the host. The microorganisms may have particular uropathogenic properties, explaining infection in an otherwise normal urinary tract. Usually, nonuropathogenic strains can induce acute infection in cases of urologic abnormalities or when the host's defense mechanisms are impaired, for example, in children and elderly people, during pregnancy, in diabetic patients, and in immunocompromised patients including patients after renal transplantation.

HOW URINARY TRACT INFECTIONS DEVELOP: THE MICROBE AND THE HOST

The Pathogen: The Commensal Flora

The role and composition of the commensal flora of the distal urethra should be considered to understand that UTI is often caused by organisms that are normal commensals in adjacent sites. The most common route of infection is ascending. The well-recognized gender difference in the prevalence of UTI is clearly related to the short length of the urethra in females. Most uropathogens are part of the fecal flora. These bacteria colonize the perianal region and then ascend to the introitus vaginae, which is a reservoir of several uropathogens, particularly if vaginal flora and vaginal pH are not intact. The process of colonization proceeds to the periurethral area, to the urethra, and into the bladder depending on sexual practices. It is believed that females whose introitus vaginae are colonized by uropathogens develop UTI depending on sexual activities, whereas other females do not. During voiding, there is sufficient turbulence in the female urethra to allow backflow of organisms that may enter the bladder. The role of normal vaginal flora in the defense against genital colonization with potentially pathogenic adhering *E. coli* has been demonstrated. The reported vaginal colonization rate of *E. coli* varies from 6% to 26%. Defensive properties of the commensal flora against invasion by bowel organisms include production of inhibitors against potential pathogens, aggregate formation of commensal species with microbes of the same specimen or with potential pathogens, colonization of epithelial surfaces, and competition with potential pathogens for site of adhesion. The quantitative relationship of vaginal *E. coli* with phases of the menstrual cycle delineates hormonal determinants in vaginal colonization with *E. coli*. Local trauma such as sexual intercourse or urethral massage may promote invasion of microorganisms into the urinary tract. Therefore, in the presence of colonization of the introitus vaginae by uropathogens, women may suffer from recurrent UTI, whereas in the absence of colonization, UTI is rare in sexually active women. Repeated or prolonged administration of antibiotics may inhibit growth of *Lactobacillus* usually colonizing the vagina and may result in change of the urethral and vaginal colonization by uropathogenic bacteria and predispose for UTI. A vaginal pH of 4 or less can protect against vaginal and urogenital infections. *Lactobacillus* generates this acidic vaginal pH and interferes with the adhesion of *E. coli*, one of the most common uropathogens in otherwise normal women. It has been demonstrated that weekly vaginal instillation of *Lactobacillus casei* as a suppositorium for 1 year in premenopausal women reduces the rate of UTI by approximately 80%. It is also likely that soaps for cleaning the genitals may impair the milieu and balance of the respective flora. In addition, the use of diaphragm, cervical cap, or spermicides for contraception is associated with a higher incidence of UTI in women when compared with other contraceptive methods. Other possible risk factors for UTI are certain practices such as the use of diapers and bubble baths (Table 41.1).

In females with recurrent UTI, it is supposed that also hormonal factors influence epithelial cell receptivity for bacterial attachment. Variable adherence has been observed at different

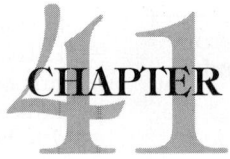

TABLE 41.1. Asymptomatic Bacteriuria and Recurrent Urinary Tract Infections in Females: Preventive and Prophylactic Measures

High fluid intake
Frequent voiding
Voiding at bedtime
Voiding after coitus
Avoidance of diaphragm use
Avoidance of spermicidal agents
Avoidance of bubble bath
Avoidance of chemical additives in bath water
Intravaginal application of *Lactobacillus*
Intravaginal estrogen application
Drinking of cranberry juice
Administration of antimicrobial drugs

times during the menstrual cycle in particular, and adherence appeared maximal in cells obtained during peak estrogen stimulation *in vivo*. Administration of estrogens may cause change in the quality and quantity of the mucopolysaccharide layer of the bladder and urethra. Estrogens also increase visceral smooth muscle tone and contractility of lower urinary tract. The presence of estrogen receptors supports the possible role of estrogens in directly influencing the bacterial receptivity of genitourinary mucosal cells. Experimental studies and clinical observations suggest that ovarian hormones may contribute to UTI in premenopausal women. On the other hand, estrogen deficiency in postmenopausal women is associated with higher risk for UTI because *Lactobacillus* disappears from the vaginal flora due to the atrophic mucosa. In consequence, vaginal pH increases and the vagina is predominantly colonized by Enterobacteriaceae, especially *E. coli*. In a controlled trial, the intravaginal administration of estriol significantly reduced the incidence of UTI in postmenopausal women with recurrent UTI. *Lactobacillus* reappeared after 1 month in 61% and mean vaginal pH declined from 5.5 to 3.8. Thus topically applied vaginal estriol can prevent recurrent UTI in postmenopausal women, probably by modifying vaginal flora (Table 41.1).

In summary, preservation or restoration of intact vaginal milieu is a major factor in the prevention and treatment of UTI in females—a factor that is often underestimated or neglected.

The Inflammation: The Host–Pathogen Reaction

Frequency and severity of UTI are determined by both local defense mechanisms of the urinary tract and the pathogenicity (virulence factors) of uropathogenic microorganisms. Specific virulence factors allow bacteria to survive and to replicate in the host. Virulence factors of several uropathogens such as *E. coli* or *Proteus mirabilis* are well established and include synthesis of aerobactin and enterobactin (iron-binding proteins with extremely high affinity to iron, which is necessary for replication of uropathogens) as well as production of hemolysin and expression of fimbriae. Mannose-sensitive fimbriae (type 1-fimbriae) have been found on pathogenic and nonpathogenic *E. coli* species, whereas mannose-resistant fimbriae (P-fimbriae) have been detected on uropathogenic *E. coli* species only. P-fimbriae are called *pyelonephritis-associated pili* because they can attach specifically to epithelial receptors of the urogenital tract and can further ascend from the bladder up to the kidneys. Abnormalities of the urinary tract such as vesicoureteral reflux or diagnostic procedures (cystoscopy, micturition urography, bladder lavage) favor ascendance of pathogens.

Pyelonephritic *E. coli* species have P-fimbriae in more than 90%. These virulent properties are not essential for lower UTI in girls and women, whereas virulent pathogens are necessary to induce lower UTI in the male urinary tract, which is considered to be relatively resistant to infections (most likely due to longer urethra in males, presence of bacteriostatic secretions of the prostate). Another important uropathogen is *Staphylococcus saprophyticus*. This microorganism can cause acute cystitis or pyelonephritis predominately in young women. Compared with *S. aureus* and *S. epidermidis, S. saprophyticus* displays not only the strongest attachment to uroepithelial cells but also has additional invasive properties resulting in penetration into the respective cells. Bacterial attachment is mediated by α-1-microglobulin.

Investigations on virulence factors of uropathogens have found that P-fimbriae and/or F-adhesins are present in 50% to 65% of *E. coli* strains in patients with cystitis and in 75% to 90% of isolates from patients with pyelonephritis, whereas they are present in only 10% to 15% of fecal *E. coli* from patients without UTI. Women with recurrent UTI have frequent and persistent vaginal *E. coli* colonization. An increased attachment of *E. coli* to vaginal epithelial cells has been demonstrated. It is also of interest that nonsecretors of blood group antigens, easily determined in the saliva, are prone to recurrent UTI.

E. coli and other gram-negative bacilli can be classified by the somatic antigens (O antigens) present in the lipopolysaccharide component of the cell wall. Approximately 150 serotypes have been identified and a limited number have been implicated as urinary pathogens. However, correlation between particular serotypes and parenchymal invasion has not been established. Other somatic antigen markers include the K antigens of capsular origin, overlying the O antigens of the cell wall. A correlation between K-rich strains and evidence of renal parenchymal involvement was found in pregnant women with bacteriuria. K-rich *E. coli* may be relatively resistant to phagocytosis and to destruction by complement.

During UTI, cytokines are released as a result of local and/or systemic reactions. A considerable proportion of women with bacteriuria have increased urinary interleukin (IL)-6 levels independent of accompanying symptoms. However, serum IL-6 levels are elevated only in women with acute pyelonephritis. In contrast, pregnant women with acute pyelonephritis have decreased urinary and serum IL-6 production. Decreased cytokine and immunoglobulin production during pregnancy may explain, at least in part, enhanced susceptibility in these patients. Women and men of advanced age and with bacteriuria have increased IL-1α and IL-6. The latter is synthesized by epithelial cells of the bladder and kidney, and by peripheral mononuclear blood cells after contact with attached *E. coli*. Determination of urinary IL-6 may differentiate between asymptomatic bacteriuria and contamination. However, in other clinical studies, urinary IL-6 levels did not correlate with the degree of pyuria and with urinary IL-8 concentrations, whereas urinary IL-8 concentrations significantly correlated with the amount of pyuria. Recruitment of polymorphonuclear leukocytes (PMNL) into the urine seems to be associated with local production of IL-8, whereby both uroepithelial cells and PMNL produce IL-8. It has been demonstrated that 4 hours after intravesical instillation of lipopolysaccharide, neutrophils infiltrate into the bladder and mRNA for inducible nitric oxide synthase (iNOS) and the cytokines IL-6 and IL-10 are detected in the rat bladder but not in the kidney. This localized inflammatory response demonstrates the importance of lipopolysaccharide as a mediator of the host response in UTI and supports the use of urinary measurements of nitrate and cyclic guanosine3′,5′-monophosphate (cGMP) in humans as indicative of the localized induction of iNOS in UTI. IL-1α is detectable in urine samples of patients with either asymptomatic or symptomatic UTI, but IL-1β, tumor necrosis factor (TNF)-α, or TNF-β are not found.

Mechanisms leading to chronic UTI are not yet clarified. Predisposing factors include urinary tract obstruction, vesicoureteral reflux, neurogenic bladder, stone disease, diabetes, and immunosuppressive treatment. Uroepithelial cells and red blood cells carry specific receptor components (glycosphingolipids) for P-fimbriae, which are also determined by the P-blood group system. The presence of P1-antigens is associated with an individual's risk for UTI. P1-antigens have been found more frequently in patients with symptomatic infections or with renal scar formation. The latter may be induced by phagocytotic inactivation of uropathogenic microorganisms due to release of superoxide, oxygen radicals, or proteinases.

Host-specific factors associated with UTI include immunoresistance of local mucosa, production of secretory immunoglobulin A and the presence of Tamm-Horsfall mucoprotein (THP), as well as urodynamic factors or bactericidal properties of the serum. THP has specific receptors for several uropathogens and the bound bacteria are excreted into the urine.

THE SPECTRUM OF URINARY TRACT INFECTION

Definitions

Significant Bacteriuria

Traditionally, the concept of significant bacteriuria (Fig. 41.1) for the diagnosis of UTI was based on the notion that the quantitative bacterial count could help distinguish between infection and contamination. The utility and consistency of the criterion of at least 10^5 colony-forming units per milliliter (cfu/ml) of clean-catch urine for the diagnosis of UTI has been validated repeatedly. In children, rapid and reliable diagnosis of UTI is mandatory due to the higher risk for severe illness and complications (e.g., irreversible renal damage). Here, UTI is defined as bacterial count in excess of 10^4 cfu/ml urine, obtained by microscopic examination because contamination frequently results in false-positive culture tests.

Low-Count Bacteriuria

Only half of women with symptoms of acute lower UTI meet the criterion of at least 10^5 cfu/ml. It is suggested that low-count bacteriuria might be an early phase of UTI (Fig. 41.1). Most patients with bacterial counts between 10^2 and 10^4 cfu/ml shows microorganisms typical for UTI. Symptoms may arise from a transitional phase of UTI in which the urethra is the primary site of colonization and inflammation. According to this concept bacteria may enter the bladder transiently but, because of urodynamic and other host defense mechanisms, they are not able to grow sufficiently to achieve the high densities that are observed in well-established UTI. The phenomenon of low-count bacteriuria may be explained as follows: First, it is likely that symptomatic bacteriuria of less than 10^5 cfu/ml reflects ongoing UTI, and therefore microbiologic criterion should be reduced to more than 10^2 cfu/ml in symptomatic patients. Second, a low number of bacteria in the urine may be the result of increased urine output due to high fluid intake. Third, low-count bacteriuria may be produced by slow growth of some uropathogens such as *S. saprophyticus*. Thus one major common error in the diagnosis of UTI is to underestimate low-count bacteriuria.

Asymptomatic Bacteriuria

Asymptomatic bacteriuria is frequently detected in routine investigations. Bacterial counts in excess of 10^5 cfu/ml in two consecutive clean-catch urine samples, however, differentiate between asymptomatic UTI and contamination (Fig. 41.1). For infections with *S. saprophyticus* and *Candida* species, the cutoff level is defined as 10^4 cfu/ml or more.

Asymptomatic bacteriuria is extremely rare in the early childhood period in the absence of anatomic abnormalities (prevalence in males 0.001% between the ages of 0 and 5 years). In females asymptomatic bacteriuria increases up to 10% until

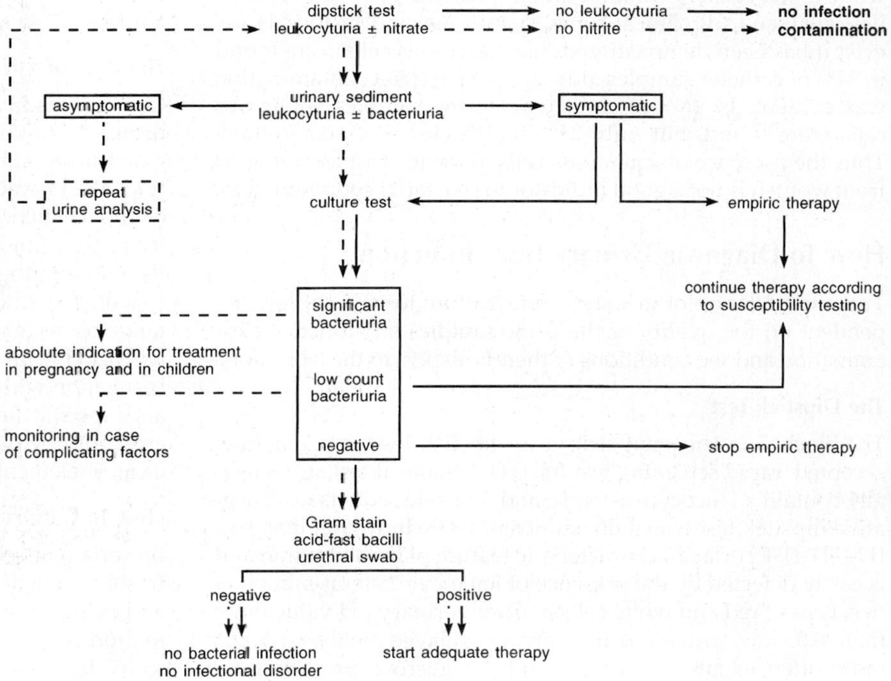

Figure 41.1. Urine analysis and management of urinary tract infections.

an age of 65 years. In elderly males, the percentage is even higher if there is retention of urine due to hyperplasia of prostate. Asymptomatic bacteriuria and leukocyturia exist in up to one-third of hemodialysis patients. The reason for this is the decrease of urine output and therefore the lack of adequate rinsing, which allows the bacteria to grow.

A further common error in the diagnosis and treatment of UTI is the underestimation or overestimation of asymptomatic bacteriuria. The information about the presence or absence of bacteriuria in asymptomatic patients is a prerequisite to decide who should be treated and who should be monitored. Asymptomatic bacteriuria should not be treated except in pregnancy (Fig. 41.1). The dilation of the urinary tract during pregnancy allows bacteria to ascend easily to the kidneys. Acute pyelonephritis during pregnancy is associated with a high frequency of abortion.

Patients with asymptomatic bacteriuria, such as hemodialysis patients evaluated for kidney transplantation, should be treated concomitantly with undergoing invasive urologic diagnostics in order to prevent severe septic complications. Whether diabetic or immunosuppressed patients with asymptomatic bacteriuria should receive antibiotic therapy is currently under debate.

Contamination

Contamination is likely if small numbers of bacteria or mixed growths are recovered. *Lactobacilli, Corynebacteria* species, *Gardnerella*, α-hemolytic streptococci, and aerobes are considered urethral and vaginal contaminants that may be passed into the voided urine. Infection may be confirmed by urine samples obtained by urethral catheterization or, better, by suprapubic aspiration. True polymicrobic infection is rare, except in patients with ileal conduit, neurogenic bladder, or vesicocolic fistula, and in patients with complicated UTI due to stones, chronic renal abscesses or long-term indwelling urinary catheters. The isolation of more than one organism from a single specimen of urine must be always be interpreted in the light of (a) whether one organism is dominant, (b) the type of the specimen (chronic catheterization versus midstream specimen), (c) the presence of other features suggesting either true infection (presence of white blood cells) or contamination (presence of vaginal epithelial cells), and (d) clinical signs, symptoms, and history. However, it has been demonstrated that squamous cells were found in 94% of catheter samples although no bacterial contamination was evident. In 96% of midstream urine samples squamous cells were found, but only 21% had bacterial contamination. Thus the presence of squamous cells in urine samples obtained from women is not a good indicator for bacterial contamination.

How To Diagnose Urinary Tract Infection

The interpretation of urinalysis and culture tests is entirely dependent on the quality of the urine samples submitted for examination and the conditions of their transport to the laboratory.

The Dipstick Test

The biochemical reagent strip test (dipstick test) is a generally accepted, rapid screening test for UTI. Chemical test strips usually contain a leucocyte esterase and a nitrate reductase. A negative dipstick test is usually sufficient to exclude true infection (Fig. 41.1). Pyuria is a characteristic feature of inflammation and is easily detected by the presence of leukocyte esterase. In practice, lysis of red and white cells in urine (urinary pH value more than 6.0, low urinary osmolality or delayed analysis) leads more often to false-negative results in microscopy than false positives by the dipstick method. The presence of leukocyturia does not always correlate with bacteriuria. The source may be from sites of inflammation other than the urinary tract, such as the female genital tract. Leukocyturia is also present in acute glomerulonephritides. Moreover, leukocyturia may continue even if bacteriuria has cleared spontaneously or after treatment. The nitrite test depends on the detection of nitrite in the urine formed from nitrate by many uropathogens. The nitrite field is highly specific for bacteria, but several uropathogens do not reduce nitrate to nitrite and therefore its utility is restricted to *Enterobacteriaceae*, which give a positive test result (Fig. 41.1). In addition, some foodstuff contains nitrate/nitrite and can therefore influence the urinary nitrite test giving positive test results although UTI is not evident. A urine pH in excess of 7.5 suggests UTI.

The Clean-Catch Urine Specimen

In general, patients with symptoms suggesting UTI should have a clean-catch specimen sent for urinalysis and culture test. Because the bacterial count of early morning specimens is usually greater than at other times, it has become conventional to collect the first urine of the day. This sample is the most concentrated, and bacteria in the bladder have had time to multiply overnight. When samples are obtained later in the day, as in routine practice, a more dilute urine and a partial bacterial washout due to multiple voids may markedly lower the colony counts. Because initial urine flushes out urethral contaminants, collection of midstream specimens is the standard means for diagnosis. In women, collection of midstream specimens requires far greater care and cooperation than in men. Spreading the labia, the introitus vaginae should be cleaned with water- or saline-soaked swabs. Soaps or antiseptics should never be used because they may result in misleading low bacterial counts. Obviously, a suitable sterile container for urine collection is mandatory. In uncircumcised men, the foreskin should be pulled back due to possible colonization of the preputial sac. Problems occur in the interpretation of urinalysis particularly in the elderly and adipose women because of technical difficulties of sample collection. Elderly female patients are reported to have a high false-positive test rate. Therefore in those incapable of providing midstream clean-catch urine specimens the procedure should be assisted by a nurse.

The Role of Microscopic Examination of Urine

UTI can readily be diagnosed by microscopic examination of urine. A standardized, centrifuged urinary sediment investigated under a coverslip is recommended as a routine method (Fig. 41.1) because it is cheap and the differentiation of formed elements such as red and white blood cells or bacteria is easier in thin fluid layers than in traditional (e.g., Bürker, Fuchs-Rosenthal) glass chambers. Centrifugation always introduces a loss of particles and may produce inaccurate results in quantitative terms. On the other hand, with unspun samples a number of relevant elements can be missed. Thus the use of centrifugation with a standardized procedure gives more sensitive and specific findings. When compared with bright-field microscopy, the phase contrast technique allows a better detection of most elements, but especially bacteria.

How to Culture Urine

Bacteria will continue to multiply in the warm medium of freshly voided urine. It is therefore mandatory that urinalysis and culture tests be performed without delay. If bacterial examination is delayed beyond 2 hours, specimens must be stored at 4°C for no longer than 48 hours to ensure growth on the culture medium. Dip-slide culture or a similar semiquantitative method of culture is generally preferable. These methods offer the advantage of reflecting the true approximate concentration of bacteria at the time the sample is taken, making storage at low temperature unnecessary. Results from a test-strip measurement or microscopic counts of elements should be used for correct interpretation of bacterial cultures. The correct procedure and interpretation of the antibiotic sensitivity of urinary pathogens is also highly relevant to best patient care (Fig. 41.1).

Occasionally, unusual or fastidious bacteria may induce UTI. These bacteria may be difficult to detect without examining the urine by Gram stain. For example, *Haemophilus influenzae* and *H. parainfluenza* do not grow well in culture media commonly used for enteric bacteria and as a result may go undetected. Other unusual organisms include *Pneumococcus, Campylobacter, Legionella pneumophila, Salmonella, Shigella, Corynebacterium* group D2, acid-fast bacilli (including *Mycobacterium tuberculosis* and atypical mycobacteria), and fungi (e.g., *Blastomyces* and *Coccidioides*). Gram and acid-fast stains should be performed for patients with urinary symptoms and significant pyuria for whom routine cultures are reported to be negative (Fig. 41.1).

THE DIFFERENT CLINICAL PRESENTATION OF URINARY TRACT INFECTION

The clinical presentation of a patient with UTI ranges from asymptomatic bacteriuria up to acute pyelonephritis (bacterial interstitial nephritis) or urosepsis depending on the localization and the severity of the infection. Additional differentiation between uncomplicated and complicated UTI is another essential issue to ensure adequate therapy strategies, which includes evaluation for complicating factors in the latter (Table 41.2).

Lower Versus Upper Urinary Tract Infection

The clinical presentation of a patient gives some evidence to distinguish lower and upper UTI. Usually, lower UTI displays no alterations of acute-phase reactants and body temperature is below 38°C. Upper UTI causes elevation of inflammatory parameters such as C-reactive protein or leukocytosis and high fever. Diagnostic procedures for an accurate localization of the infection are pretentious and are not without risk due to bladder and/or ureteral catheterization. A variety of methods have been proposed to distinguish between lower (urethra, bladder) and upper (kidney) UTI, emphasizing contributions of renal nuclear medicine. In clinical practice, symptoms and monitoring of bacteruria may help differentiate between lower and upper UTI, retrospectively. For example, if bacteriuria diminished after 1 day or short-term (3 days) treatment, one may assume the presence of a lower UTI. Urinary excretion of *N*-acetyl-β-glucosaminidase (NAG), a lysosomal enzyme present in the proximal convoluted tubule, has been used for differentiation of UTI. Urinary NAG excretion was significantly higher in patients with upper UTI than in patients with lower UTI or in healthy adults.

TABLE 41.2. Initial Evaluation of the Patient Presenting with Urinary Tract Infection and Detailed Medical History for Evidence of Complications

Patient Evaluation
Male or female
Neonate, child, adolescent, or adult
Asymptomatic or symptomatic
Mild or severe illness
Sporadic or recurrent episodes of UTI
Presence or absence of complicating factors
Complicating Factors
Anatomic abnormalities of the urinary tract
Neurogenic disorders of urine transport
Polycystic kidney disease
Analgetic abuse
Sickle cell anemia
Impaired immunologic defense mechanisms
Transplantation
Immunosuppression
Diabetes mellitus
Pregnancy
Indwelling urinary catheter
Prostatitis
Treatment failure

Symptomatic Versus Asymptomatic Urinary Tract Infection

Based on clinical signs and symptoms we have to distinguish between asymptomatic (asymptomatic bacteriuria) and symptomatic (dysuria, frequent voiding, flank pain, fever) UTI. In case of "symptomatic abacteriuria," bacterial infection with low counts of uropathogens may cause the so-called urethral syndrome. Other causes for symptomatic abacteriuria include infection with chlamydia, mycoplasma, trichomonas, gonococci, *Candida,* or mycobacteria. Similar symptoms can also arise from bladder stones or tumors. Renal abscess without connection to the urinary tract, complete ureteral obstruction, antimicrobial treatment, or antiseptics (incorrectly obtained urine sample) can also be associated with symptomatic abacteriuria.

Complicated Versus Uncomplicated Urinary Tract Infection

It has been demonstrated that persistent or recurrent infection in adults with anatomically and functionally normal urinary tracts rarely, if ever, leads to renal damage. Therefore emphasis has been placed on distinguishing between complicated and uncomplicated UTI (Table 41.2). Complicated UTI includes all infections of the urinary tract, which is anatomically or functionally altered (uropathy), with the consequence of relevant changes in the urodynamic properties. The attribution "complicated" is related to complicating factors along the urinary tract, and encompasses all abnormalities of the urinary tract that alter urinary flow or influence voiding mechanism. Except UTI in uropathies, UTI is also termed complicated in case of nephropathies (e.g., single- or double-sided renal damage) or in association with other relevant disorders that favor the development of UTI (Table 41.2). Uncomplicated infections occur mainly in otherwise healthy females with structurally normal urinary tract and intact voiding mechanisms. In contrast, complicating factors put individuals of both genders at a higher risk to develop severe renal damage, bacteremia, and urosepsis.

Complicated UTI is caused by gram-negative and gram-positive microbes. It could be demonstrated that the incidence of certain uropathogens correlated with complicating factors of the urinary tract. Furthermore, for accurate treatment of UTI it is important that the complicating factor be eliminated during therapy (e.g., removal of stones), if possible.

DIAGNOSTIC RADIOLOGIC IMAGING PROCEDURES

Radiologic imaging is recommended in patients with suspected complicated UTI to identify abnormalities predisposing to infection and to define the presence of abnormalities that may affect management or predispose to renal damage (Table 41.3). A rational diagnostic strategy is the cornerstone for both optimal clarification of UTI and saving of costs.

Conventional Radiologic Techniques

Ultrasound and plain abdominal radiography are the imaging methods of choice, especially for emergency imaging in patients with severe loin pain and fever. Ultrasound alone does not allow reassurance that the urinary tract is normal. It gives little anatomic detail of the pelvocalyceal system and cannot identify minor degrees of ureteral dilation. Sonographically detected, upper urinary tract wall thickening is reported to occur in UTI, urinary tract stone disease, and vesicoureteral reflux (VUR). Therefore voiding cystourethrography seems to be justified in all cases of upper urinary tract wall thickening. Nonrefluxing systems should be further evaluated with intravenous urography for exclusion of urinary tract obstruction.

Plain abdominal radiographs are of value in monitoring renal stone disease. However, intravenous urography seems to remain the investigation of choice because it provides a broad range of information on anatomic details of the calyces, pelvis, and ureter, and additional adequacy of bladder emptying. Routine performance of intravenous urography generally is not accepted. There is also little indication during acute infection because the results are of poor quality and additional nephrotoxicity is encountered. This investigation is indicated when complicating factors such as obstruction, stones, papillary necrosis, or renal scars are supposed. These conditions are associated with increased risk for renal damage if further infection occurs, and with a more difficult eradication of the infection. Intravenous urography should not be performed during pregnancy because of radiation hazard, and it is useless in renal impairment.

TABLE 41.3. Indications and Impact of Diagnostic Imaging Procedures in Patients with Urinary Tract Infection

Indications for Diagnostic Imaging Procedures
Neonates and young children with first febrile UTI
Men with recurrent UTI
Women with frequent and severe reinfection
Persistent infection after 48 to 72 hours of adequate therapy
Renal transplant recipients with recurrent UTI
Imaging Methods
Ultrasound
Hydronephrosis
Abscess
Plain abdominal radiography
Renal stone disease
Intravenous pyelography
Urinary tract obstruction
DMSA scanning
Renal damage
Reflux
Voiding cystoureterography
Reflux
Bladder emptying disorders
Computed tomography
Microabscesses
Perinephritic abscess

DMSA, dimercaptosuccinic acid; UTI, urinary tract infection.

Dimercaptosuccinic Acid Scanning

Renal cortical scintigraphy with Technetium-99m (^{99m}Tc)-dimercaptosuccinic acid (DMSA) represents a relatively new technique that provides an excellent imaging modality for the assessment of cortical damage secondary to UTI. Renal cortical scanning for the diagnosis of acute pyelonephritis is presented as an example of an existing nuclear medicine method that is accurate and cost effective, and should be the primary imaging tool for children presenting with acute urinary infection (Table 41.3). Cortical scintigraphy should be added to the initial examination of children with their first acute febrile UTI, and this could be supplemented by voiding cystourethrography alone, with ultrasonography having a second role. DMSA scan detects renal changes 10-fold more than does ultrasonography. Children older than 2 years of age and those with reinfection have a significantly higher incidence of renal lesions than do younger children. Among those kidneys that presented abnormal cortical scintigraphy, VUR is present in about 75%.

Comparing planar scintigraphy with single-photon emission computed tomography (SPECT) using a triple-head gamma camera in children with UTI, SPECT scanning was superior in detecting kidney lesions (positive findings in 36 kidneys versus 18 kidneys). Moreover, uncorrected metabolic acidosis may be associated with an unusual pattern of isotope uptake, noteworthy because patients referred for imaging with renal disease may also have abnormalities of acid–base balance.

Voiding Cystourethrography

Voiding cystourethrogram is the method of choice to establish VUR (Table 41.3). VUR is a major risk factor for childhood infections and has been identified in up to 40% of children with recurrent UTI. However, ultrasonography and DMSA scan, where available, should be considered the first step for accurate diagnosis and follow-up of children with UTI. This more aggressive workup is recommended for patients at greater risk for pyelonephritis and renal scarring, including infants younger than 1 year of age and all children who have systemic signs of infection concomitant with UTI. In contrast to voiding cystourethrogram, cystosonography with echocontrast using galactose suspension as an echogenic contrast media seems a promising imaging technique for detecting and grading VUR with a sensitivity of 100% and without exposing patients to ionizing radiation. Voiding cystourethrography is rarely carried out in adults with UTI, but it is suggested that VUR is more common in adults than was previously suspected. The renal transplant recipient with recurrent or chronic UTI should undergo a voiding cystourethrogram for identification of VUR into the renal transplant and/or native kidneys, which may affect graft function and maintain chronic infection.

Computed Tomography

Although computed tomography (CT) scanning is the most precise method to identify infection involving the kidney (Table 41.3), the exposure to contrast media with respect to its increased nephrotoxicity in patients with renal infection has to be considered. CT without contrast shows only a large kidney in case of acute bacterial interstitial nephritis and is of limited diagnostic value. In the broad spectrum of UTI, CT scanning is rarely employed in routine practice, but can help to delineate and identify microabscesses within the kidney and extension or rupture of the infection into the perinephritic space. CT provides greater sensitivity because sonography may not detect lesions smaller than 2 cm wide. CT scanning also may be helpful to identify infection of cysts in patients with polycystic disease, which usually occurs as a complication of ascending UTI. However, differentiation between infected cyst(s) and bleeding into a cyst may be impossible.

Cystoscopy

Cystoscopy is not indicated in isolated UTI. In patients with recurrent UTI, particularly in older patients with hematuria, cystoscopy should always be performed because bladder cancer may be suspected. In addition, the renal transplant recipient with recurrent UTI and hematuria should undergo this procedure because of the relatively high incidence of nephrogenic adenoma. It is obvious that cystoscopy is performed only when the urine obtained previously is sterile. Additional prophylaxis with single-dose antimicrobial therapy is associated with a low risk for iatrogen infection.

TREATMENT

Management of Uncomplicated Urinary Tract Infection

In general, antimicrobial therapy should be started in all symptomatic patients with UTI (Fig. 41.1). However, duration of therapy is unclear. Short-term treatment (once dosing, 1-day or 3-day therapy) of a limited number of patients suffering from lower UTI is possible. Treatment trials indicate that 3-day therapy for uncomplicated lower UTI provides an optimal balance between efficacy and adverse effects when compared with single-dose therapy or treatment for 7 to 10 days. However, one has to keep in mind that the recurrence of UTI is significantly enhanced after short-term compared with long-term treatment. The cure rate is also influenced by the uropathogen. Single-dose therapy is ineffective for *S. saprophyticus*, but effective for *E. coli* infection. Approximately 80% of women suffering from UTI can be cured after a 7- to 10-day antibiotic regimen, with up to 100% cured after 3 weeks. The choice of antibiotics must be based on its probable effectiveness against uropathogenic bacteria, lack of side effects, acceptability to the patient, and cost. Trimethoprim and cotrimoxazole [trimethoprim-sulfamethoxazole (TMP-SMX)] are among the most widely used antibiotics. These drugs have remained popular because they are mostly well tolerated and are relatively inexpensive. Side effects are more likely linked to the sulfonamide component in TMP-SMX. Several studies have indicated superiority of this drug to ampicillin, possibly because it is more effective in reducing fecal, vaginal, and periurethral colonization. Arguments for sulfonamides as part of therapy include the lower risk for developing drug resistance. Arguments against sulfonamides include allergic reactions that resulted in trimethoprim monotherapy in many centers. Trimethoprim alone is considered by many as the drug of first choice.

In case of treatment failure, or also as first-line therapy in community-acquired infections, administration of fluoroquinolones is indicated. The most commonly used substances are ciprofloxacin and ofloxacin. The latter undergoes very low metabolism with the consequent risk for accumulation in impaired renal function. Therefore the elderly patient population is particularly prone for adverse side effects such as central nervous system symptoms. Norfloxacin 800 mg once daily is as effective and safe as norfloxacin 400 mg twice daily for a 7- to 10-day treatment period, but norfloxacin carries the disadvantage of low penetration rates into interstitial tissue. The new quinolone antibiotics, levofloxacin and sparfloxacin, have improved action against gram-positive microbes compared with that of older fluoroquinolones, and are usually administered once daily. Fosfomycin may be a useful alternative for single-dose therapy of uncomplicated UTI. Its activity is higher than that of the rest of the antimicrobials commonly used for therapy of uncomplicated UTI. It has been shown that single-dose treatment with fosfomycin is at least as effective as 3- to 7-day treatment; however, *Pseudomonas aeruginosa* and *Acinetobacter* species were more resistant to this drug compared with fluoroquinolones.

Oral cephalosporin therapy represents an alternative proposal if fluoroquinolones cannot be used (e.g., because of drug resistance or side effects). Cephalosporins of the third generation are highly effective against enterobacteria, but their efficacy against *S. aureus* is insufficient, and both *Pseudomonas* and *Enterococci* are not sensitive at all. Aminopenicillins without or with β-lactamase inhibitor (e.g., ampicillin/amoxicillin, amoxicillin-clavulanic acid, ampicillin-sulbactam) have lower sensibility than fluoroquinolones or oral cephalosporins in UTI with enterobacteria, and often lead to selection of *Klebsiella*. Aminopenicillins therefore are not recommended as first-line therapy in uncomplicated UTI.

Management of Asymptomatic Bacteriuria

The significance of asymptomatic bacteriuria (presence in excess of 10^5 cfu/ml of the same bacterial species in two consecutive midstream urine samples) and indications for treatment remain controversial. It has been proposed that transient bacteriuria merely reflects colonization of the bladder without tissue invasion, which clears spontaneously and returns, or probably turns into true infection with pyuria over the time. With advancing age, asymptomatic bacteriuria increases in both prevalence and incidence. Postmenopausal estrogen deficit and decrease in lactobacilli colonization with lower vaginal pH results in increased vaginal colonization with possible uropathogenic and gastrointestinal bacteria that, in part, may account for the generally higher incidence of bacteriuria in elderly women as opposed to elderly men. In general there is little evidence that routine treatment of positive cultures are required, except during pregnancy and in children. Treatment of asymptomatic bacteriuria in elderly patients is disputed. No difference in the overall mortality rate has been observed whether the patients have been treated or not. However, in the morbid and bedridden elderly patient, antibiotic treatment should be considered because of the possible acceleration to life-threatening urosepsis.

RECURRENT URINARY TRACT INFECTION: RELAPSE AND REINFECTION

A major problem of treating UTI is to manage recurrent infections. Recurrent UTI is defined as more than four events every year, but each patient appears to have a unique pattern of recurrence, such as sporadic or multiple episodes, related to sexual intercourse. Therefore the usefulness of the concepts of relapse and reinfection is undergoing reevaluation. These two types of recurrent infection can be distinguished only by properly timed, sequential urine cultures. Relapsing infection is defined as prompt recurrence with the same organism following treatment. Relapse implies that there has been a failure to eradicate the infection, but rather, relapses occur in association with urologic abnormalities or other complicating factors. Treatment has to be prolonged to 2 to 6 weeks, respectively, because relapses with the same organism are mainly due to an inadequate duration of therapy. Particularly in patients receiving single-dose therapy, persistent vaginal and periurethral colonization may lead to rapid recurrent infection with the same organism.

Reinfection occurs much more commonly (80% of recurrent infections) and is defined as eradication of bacteriuria by appropriate treatment, followed by infection with a mostly different organism at variable time intervals. In young women, recurrent infections are mostly reinfections. Reinfection is due to persistence of factors predisposing to reinvasion of the urinary tract; therefore prophylactic measures should replace urologic evaluation, which is not routinely indicated because of the rarity of urologic abnormalities. One of the most likely risk factors for UTI is recent sexual intercourse, two others are diaphragm and spermicide use.

The major problem in women with recurrent UTI is the vaginal colonization with uropathogens and their establishment within the bladder. Supportive measures against recurrent UTI include modification of behavioral factors such as high fluid intake and frequent voiding to maintain bacterial clearance by day (Table 41.1). Healthy women who drink less and void infrequently at work have a 2.2-fold higher risk of UTI. The beneficial effect of drinking and frequent voiding is lost overnight therefore low-dose prophylaxis with antimicrobials should be prescribed at bedtime. Trimethoprim, cotrimoxazole, and nitrofurantoin are the most commonly used drugs because side effects and resistant strains are unusual. For prophylaxis only, prescription of nitrofurantoin represents an accepted and safe strategy because a relatively low and nontoxic dosage (one-eighth of the original therapeutic dosage) is administered. For long-term prophylaxis, oral cephalosporins and fluoroquinolones are cost prohibitive. Recurrence rates are significantly greater after shorter periods of prophylaxis, therefore treatment should be maintained for 6 to 12 months, particularly in patients with very frequent symptomatic recurrences.

Estrogen deficiency, particularly when prolonged, is associated with a wide range of urogenital complaints including frequency, nocturia, incontinence, UTI, and the "urge syndrome." These may coexist with vaginal symptoms of dryness, itching, and burning. Of women ages 55 to 85 years, approximately 48% are affected with these urogenital complaints. The intravaginal administration of estriol can significantly reduce the incidence of UTI in postmenopausal women with recurrent UTI. Thus topically applied vaginal estriol can prevent recurrent UTI in postmenopausal women, probably by modifying vaginal flora.

Ovarian hormones may contribute to UTI also in premenopausal females. A vaginal pH of 4 or less can protect against vaginal and urogenital infections. Weekly vaginal instillation of *Lactobacillus casei* for one year in premenopausal women can lower the rate of UTI by approximately 80% but does not prevent all urogenital infections. It is also likely that soaps for cleaning the genital tract may impair the milieu and balance of the respective flora. Other possible risk factors for invasion are certain practices, such as the use of diapers and bubble baths.

Experimental studies have demonstrated that cranberry juice inhibits the expression of P-fimbriae of *E. coli.* Fully inhibited bacteria had a 100% reduction in expression of fimbriae. There is evidence that cranberry juice acts on the cell wall, preventing proper attachment of the fimbrial subunits or as a genetic control preventing the expression of normal fimbrial subunits or both. Because bacterial adherence to epithelial cells is mediated by lectin–sugar interactions, consumption of food containing lectins or carbohydrates might affect the infection process. The underlying mode of action of cranberry juice *in vitro* may be explained by at least two inhibitors of lectin-mediated adherence of uropathogens to eucaryotic cells. One of these constituents is the fructose that is also present in orange juice and pineapple juice, and that inhibits the adherence of type 1 fimbriated *E. coli.* The other is a substance (or substances) that inhibits binding of P-fimbriated *E. coli.* However, the orange and pineapple juices did not inhibit the P-fimbriated bacteria.

MANAGEMENT OF COMPLICATED URINARY TRACT INFECTION

According to the underlying complicating factor and the diversity of anatomic and functional abnormalities of the urinary tract, patients with complicating UTI display a pronounced heterogeneity. In addition, recurrent infections are frequently observed in this patient population. Their incidences mostly correlate with the ability to restore normal urodynamics. In the case of incomplete restitution, effective treatment remains questionable. Therefore therapy strategies should focus on the individual problem.

After thorough evaluation of the clinical situation and respective initiation of antimicrobial drugs, urologic procedures should follow targeting restoration of the urinary tract. Antimicrobial treatment has to be continued until urodynamics are normal. In contrast, antimicrobial treatment is not effective in some disorders such as renal stones, neurogenic bladder, or permanent indwelling catheter.

Complicated infections encompass a broad spectrum of clinical conditions for which it is difficult to make all-inclusive recommendations for empiric treatment. Widespread resistance is present to ampicillin, amoxicillin, sulfonamides, and first-generation cephalosporins, which makes these drugs less attractive for empiric therapy of most types of complicated UTI. In general, regimens for such infections should be broad spectrum, with fluoroquinolones being especially useful in the outpatient management of complicated infections. However, increased resistance has emerged against this relatively new class of drugs, probably once again explained by the indiscriminate and excessive use of these antimicrobials. Quinolones have a broad antimicrobial spectrum and a high potency and, so far, are associated with a low incidence of microbial resistance. Some quinolones are available as both parenteral and oral formulations, making possible an early switch from parenteral to oral therapy. Other favorable characteristics include a high oral bioavailability, extensive tissue penetration, and in the case of some of the newer quinolones, long elimination half-lives. According to their *in vitro* activity, all fluoroquinolones tested other than rufloxacin showed similar rates of resistance (approximately 15%) against uropathogens. However, the increased use of fluoroquinolones is associated with the emergence of ciprofloxacin-resistant *E. coli* from urinary tract sources.

There is a high suspicion for complicated UTI, including treatment failure, if bacteriuria does not resolve or if clinical signs and symptoms persist after a 48-hour period of antibiotic drug therapy. Careful patient monitoring and repeated culture tests (including blood cultures) during and after treatment should be performed. There is now strong indication for performing kidney and urinary tract imaging by ultrasonography, plain abdominal radiography, CT, or intravenous urogram to establish possible complicating factors like renal stones and other urologic disorders or abscesses (Table 41.3).

URINARY TRACT INFECTIONS AFTER RENAL TRANSPLANTATION

One of the major problems for successful organ transplantation is the reaction of the recipient's immune system against the donor organ. This could lead to acute and chronic rejection and, in case of unsuccessful treatment, to the loss of the transplant. The immunosuppressive therapy used today is relatively unspecific and targets many immunologic functions. The net state of immunosuppression is a complex function determined by the interaction of a number of factors, the most important of these are the dose, duration, and temporal sequence in which immunosuppressive drugs are used. Regarding this, it is obvious that any kind of immunosuppressive protocol is associated with an increased risk for infection.

By far the most common form of bacterial infection in the renal transplant recipient is UTI. The incidence varies widely in the literature. There are reports from 6.1% to 85% following renal transplantation, and up to 84% following simultaneous kidney and pancreas transplantation. This wide range of values may be explained by differences in the definition of UTI, in urine sampling, and in the use or absence of perioperative and postoperative antibiotic prophylaxis. Further discussion on infections in the renal transplant recipient is found in Chapter 89, Part 1.

Bacterial Invasion

Bacteria are introduced mainly via the bladder catheter, particularly in the early period after kidney transplantation. As a consequence, there is a high risk for bacterial invasion of the kidney because of initial immunosuppressive regimen such as induction therapy using monoclonal or polyclonal antibodies, and the vulnerability of the graft following surgical manipulation. Once a Foley catheter is in place, an incidence of bacteriemia of 5% to 10% per day is reported. The early postoperative removal of the bladder catheter (within 36 hours) is associated with a low rate of UTIs, and without an increase in urologic complications.

The possible impact of UTIs lies in two areas: the direct morbidity and mortality due to the infection itself, and the possible effect of the infection in activating the rejection. Early UTIs after kidney transplantation are associated with increased parenchymal invasion of the organ.

Risk Factors

Some factors are associated with an increased risk for bacterial invasion, such as female gender, histories of UTIs before kidney transplantation, vesicoureteral reflux, polycystic kidney disease with a history of recurrent upper UTIs without binephrectomy performed before renal transplantation, diabetes mellitus, chronic viral infections, and increased urinary aluminium excretion in patients with previous aluminium overload. The contamination of cadaver donor renal allografts before transplantation due to UTIs or septic complications of the donor, or due to contamination of the perfusate, is remarkable. The risk of urinary catheters has been mentioned previously. Furthermore, there is a significant correlation between the cumulative dose of antirejection treatment (monoclonal and polyclonal antibodies), chronic uremia, and incidence of infections (Table 41.4).

Bacterial Spectrum (Table 41.5)

The bacteria causing UTI in renal transplant recipients are similar to those causing UTIs in the nonimmunocompromised population; *E. coli* is the leading microorganism. UTIs are caused by *E. coli* in 80% of the normal population. In kidney transplant recipients, this organism is involved only in 29% to 61%. *Proteus mirabilis* and *Klebsiella pneumoniae* were positive in 30% and gram-positive cocci in 20% of the urine cultures. Other uropathogens are *Enterobacter* species, enterococci, *Serratia, Acinetobacter, Citrobacter,* and *P. aeruginosa. P. mirabilis* can cause stone formation as an uncommon complication in renal allograft recipients. However, stone formation due to urease-forming microorganisms such as *P. mirabilis, Proteus vulgaris, P. aeruginosa, Klebsiella,* or *S. saprophyticus* is common in nontransplanted individuals suffering from UTI.

As discussed previously, UTIs are very common in the early posttransplant period. The mean time for acquisition is 7 days (range, 3 to 11). Occurrence of UTI leads to a prolongation of hospitalization. In addition, in pediatric patients UTIs were most common in the first 6 months after renal transplantation. Eighty percent of the infections were located in the lower urinary tract, mostly without clinical symptoms.

UTIs during the first month after kidney transplantation are more often associated with pyelonephritis, bacteriemia, and a high rate of relapses when treated with a conventional course of antibiotics. It has been shown that the urinary tract is the source of septicemia in 40% to 60% of transplant recipients, and 7% of UTIs are complicated by septicemia. Recurrence of UTIs was found in 40.1% of the patients, equally distributed in males and females (which is markedly different from the nonimmunosuppressed patient population). Sixty-one percent of UTIs in the transplant patients were reinfections by different microorganisms.

Asymptomatic bacteriuria is frequently observed in kidney transplant recipients. There is a direct correlation between bacterial concentration and diuresis. Therefore by increasing the urinary output, urinary bacterial counts can be diminished. On

TABLE 41.4. Risk Factors for Urinary Tract Infections After Renal Transplantation

Female sex
Histories of UTIs before kidney transplantation
Vesicoureteral reflux
Polycystic kidney disease
Diabetes mellitus
Chronic viral infections
Increased urinary aluminium excretion
Urinary catheters
Antirejection therapy (monoclonal and polyclonal antibodies)
Vulnerability of the graft following surgical manipulation
Contamination of the perfusate

UTIs, urinary tract infections.

TABLE 41.5. Main Bacilli Causing Urinary Tract Infection in Renal Transplant Recipients

Escherichia coli (29% to 61%)
Proteus mirabilis (up to 30%)
Klebsiella pneumoniae (up to 30%)
Gram-positive cocci (20%)
Enterobacter species
Enterococci
Serratia
Acinetobacter
Citrobacter
Pseudomonas aeruginosa

the other hand, one also has to consider that some bacteria, such as *S. saprophyticus,* have long generation times. It is therefore rare to find high colony-forming units per milliliter (cfu/ml), although lower bacterial counts are pathogenic under these conditions. In evaluating bacteriuria, urine production, type of uropathogens, and generation time of bacteria have to be considered when deciding about the necessity and modality of antibiotic treatment.

UTIs that occur in a later period after kidney transplantation are normally benign and are seldom associated with structural abnormalities of the urinary tract. They are easy to handle with a conventional course of antibiotic treatment. Positive urine cultures were mainly observed in combination with urologic complications, such as vesicoureteral reflux.

Comparison of Immunosuppressive Protocols

After transplantation of solid organs, various immunosuppressive protocols are established, depending on the source of the donor kidney, human leukocyte antigen (HLA) match, and sensibilization of the host. The individual cumulative immunosuppression depends on rejection episodes, but may have a direct correlation on the incidence of infectious complications.

The comparison of conventional immunosuppressive therapy (azathioprine and prednisone) with dual therapy (cyclosporine and prednisone) revealed no influence of the immunosuppressive regimens on the rate of infections observed.

Steroids are often accused of provoking an increased risk for bacterial infections in the transplant recipient. Patients treated with intravenous methylprednisolone for acute rejection are more likely to develop septicemia and wound infections than patients treated with oral steroid pulse therapy. Immunosuppressive protocols using mycophenolate mofetil instead of azathioprine cause fewer UTIs in renal transplant patients probably due to lower rejection rates.

An increasing number of transplantation centers are using tacrolimus (FK506) instead of cyclosporine in their immunosuppressive protocols, mainly in liver allograft recipients. These patients seem to have a slightly lower risk of developing bacterial infections (30% versus 40%) compared with cyclosporine. In kidney transplant recipients, a lower infection rate among patients treated with FK506 was observed, compared to patients who received cyclosporine. However, in a prospective randomized trial of FK506 after kidney transplantation, no lowered risk regarding infections was found. Also, a higher frequency of bacterial infections, mainly UTIs and pyelonephritis, was reported in patients treated with FK506 compared with those who were treated with cyclosporine A. Therefore the impact of FK506 on the incidence of UTIs is not clear.

An important factor is the cumulative dose of immunosuppressive agents. The reexposure to OKT3 is associated with an increasing number of bacterial infections. However, when a low-dose regimen of OKT3 was compared with a standard-dose regimen of OKT3, no significant difference with respect to infectious complications could be found. Regarding these findings it is proposed that not a single dose of antirejection therapy, but the maximal immunosuppression after repeated courses of treatment for acute rejection, which is often necessary in multitransplanted patients, is of great importance. When OKT3 was used in a prophylactic manner the incidence of infections was 16% compared with 100% after third use.

Comparing antilymphocyte globulin (ATG) and the monoclonal antibody OKT3 as part of an induction protocol, there is no great difference in the incidence of bacterial infections. The development of life-threatening infections after the therapy for acute rejection is more frequent in transplant recipients being treated by OKT3 than by conventional antirejection therapy, such as steroids or ATG. Patients with ATG (29%), OKT3 (48%), or both antibodies sequentially (50%), show a significantly higher incidence of bacterial infections.

There are a few new antibodies available, such as T10B9.1A-31, a monoclonal antibody that detects an epitope on the α and β chains of the T-cell–antigen receptor. T10B9.1A-31 was employed to treat biopsy-proven acute cellular allograft rejection compared with OKT3. The overall incidence of infections was less in the group receiving the new antibody. Another agent is the anti–IL-2 receptor monoclonal antibody, which has been administered during the first 10 days postgrafting. Bacterial infections seemed to appear in the same rate compared with the ATG group.

PROPHYLACTIC ANTIBIOTIC TREATMENT

Three different modes of antimicrobial treatment are described: (a) a therapeutic mode, (b) a prophylactic mode, and (c) a preemptive mode, in which antimicrobial agents are administered to a subgroup of patients before the appearance of clinical disease. Because of the risk of transplanted infections and the surgical manipulations, a perioperative antibiotic prophylaxis is indicated.

Summarizing the literature, many antimicrobial protocols are shown to be effective: oxacillin in combination with streptomycin, mezlocillin, cloxacillin, amoxicillin, piperacillin, and also different cephalosporins. Cefazolin, cefamandole, or ampicillin should be emphasized preoperatively because they are effective against most uropathogens and staphylococci.

As mentioned previously, the urinary tract is a common site of bacterial infections, both in the normal population and in renal transplant recipients. In nonimmunosuppressed, high-risk women, prophylaxis with TMP-SMX is an effective regimen to prevent urinary tract infections. A beneficial influence of TMP-SMX prophylaxis in the first months following kidney transplantation could be demonstrated as well. A decreasing incidence of infections due to gram-negative bacilli, enterococci, and *S. aureus* is observed. The incidence of bacterial infections, mainly UTIs, was significantly lowered (up to a 2-fold reduction after removal of the Foley catheter) in patients receiving prophylactic treatment. These patients needed 50% fewer hospitalization days due to less complications. UTIs occurring without TMP-SMX prophylaxis were commonly symptomatic (fever, tenderness of the graft), whereas transplant recipients receiving 160 mg TMP and 800 mg SMX once daily at bedtime often have an asymptomatic bacteriuria easily treated by a conventional course of antibiotics over 10 to 14 days. TMP-SMX prophylaxis is effective even in maximally immunosuppressed patients receiving OKT3. Furthermore, opportunistic infections seem to be effectively inhibited by TMP-SMX.

In renal transplant recipients on TMP-SMX prophylaxis, a greater incidence of oral candidiasis was observed, promptly responding to oral Mycostatin therapy. There is a tendency that infections caused by *P. aeruginosa* are more frequent in the prophylaxis group, but these pathogens were sensitive to various antibiotics. During hospitalization, a higher dosage of TMP-SMX is recommended because of unexpectedly low blood levels, particularly in transplant patients who need dialysis for oliguria or in posttransplant acute renal failure. Worth mentioning is a 15% higher serum creatinine in individuals receiving TMP-SMX and cyclosporine, which may be caused by inhibition of the creatinine excretion by TMP-SMX in the presence of cyclosporine. When prophylaxis is stopped, creatinine decreases to normal baseline levels. No case of TMP-SMX–associated interstitial nephritis could be demonstrated in biopsies of immunosuppressed renal transplant patients. There is also no statistically relevant effect of TMP-SMX on cyclosporine pharmacokinetics. TMP-SMX alone and in combination with azathioprine may cause hematologic disorders, but the risk of granulocytopenia is very low.

NEW DIAGNOSTIC PARAMETERS

In the early posttransplant period, fever is often seen in these patients. Sometimes it is hard to decide if fever occurred due to acute rejection or viral or bacterial infection. Fever in the first 16 days is more likely to be due to rejection than to infection. Therefore fever is an unspecific parameter that does not allow differentiation between infection and rejection.

Serum and urinary proteins may be helpful for diagnostic purposes. An increase of C-reactive protein (CRP) in the urine can be induced by both acute rejection and UTI. An extreme increase of urinary CRP in the case of vascular rejection might be caused by endothelial damage. A ratio of CRP (serum) to CRP(urine) of less than one is associated with an acute rejection episode, whereas a CRP(serum):CRP(urine) ratio of more than one is a sign of bacterial infection. α_2-Macroglobulin in the urine is a parameter of postglomerular origin because of the high molecular weight (720 kD). In renal transplant patients, α_2-macroglobulin is extremely increased during rejection crises (vascular more than interstitial). An elevation, but to a lower extent, is observed during episodes of UTIs and urosepsis. When CRP in the serum is increased, as mentioned previously, the diagnosis of bacterial UTI can be made, whereas the combination of negative α_2-macroglobulin and elevated CRP(serum) is compatible with an extrarenal bacterial infection. In the diagnostic cascade, a third urinary protein has been evaluated. Myeloperoxidase could be detected in all cases of UTI, but was within the normal range in the case of vascular or interstitial rejection. In association with fever, an FE(urea) of less than 35% [FE(urea) = U(urea)/P(urea) × P(creatinine)/U(creatinine) × 100%] is due to viral infection, whereas FE(urea) of more than 35% is a sign of bacterial infection in the kidney transplant recipient.

A noninvasive method to distinguish between urinary infection caused by the renal allograft or by native polycystic kidneys is gallium-67 scintigraphy. The scan can also localize which of the kidneys (native or transplant) may be the site of persistent infection. However, it should be stressed that all of these noninvasive diagnostic procedures do not have enough sensitivity and specificity in order to replace biopsy if rejection has been considered.

Why the Risk for Bacterial Infections Is Increased in the Immunosuppressed Host

Usually, there are many immunologic defense mechanisms to combat bacterial invasion. Both the humoral system and the cellular system are involved in bacterial killing. Cellular host defense includes neutrophil chemotaxis, degranulation, phagocytosis, and killing mechanisms due to reactive oxygen intermediates. However, immunosuppressive therapy affects multiple functions of PMNL.

Kidney transplant recipients suffering from recurrent bacterial infections and with low IgG levels improved with parenteral gamma-globulin therapy. In patients after renal transplantation, low levels of one or more immunoglobulin fractions are found in 35.5%. FK506 is proven to be a potent inhibitor of IgG and IgM production by mononuclear cells via a T-cell–dependent mechanism. In the case of cyclosporine A, a direct inhibitory effect on the response of B cells can be observed. FK506 inhibits B-cell activation in a T-cell–dependent manner via the cytokine network. FK506 and rapamycin inhibit B-cell activation caused by stimuli that induce a rise in intracellular calcium. Therefore secretion of IL-1β is decreased in T cells by the aforementioned agents. When mononuclear cells from transplant recipients are incubated with *S. aureus*, both proliferation and immunoglobulin production are lower compared with controls. This may be due to suppressed IL-2 production in T cells affected by cyclosporine. Thus B-cell abnormality in transplant patients could be caused by a lack of T-cell lymphokines and additionally by an intrinsic B-cell defect. Altered receptors may occur in patients on azathioprine therapy because this drug inhibits DNA and RNA synthesis and thus may alter protein synthesis. When mononuclear cells are incubated with activated neutrophils, they display a marked decrease in both natural killer activity and mitogen-dependent–DNA synthesis. This effect seems to be due to reactive oxygen metabolites. Myeloperoxidase from neutrophils is thought to interact with the glucose oxidase system of mononuclear cells. These findings may explain the increased risk of infection associated with the administration of OKT3. When neutrophils are incubated with this monoclonal antibody, both degranulation and oxidative burst are increased in a dose-dependent manner.

A lower release for lactoferrin and elastase as parameters for degranulation is observed under the influence of cyclosporine and/or azathioprine. A further major neutrophil defect is depressed granulocyte adherence early postoperatively at the time of rejection crisis, when prednisone dosage is maximal. Chemotactic activity improves progressively after transplantation despite large doses of prednisone and azathioprine. Phagocytosis is enhanced early postoperatively and also at the time of rejection crisis. Bactericidal activity is unaffected by renal transplantation and immunosuppressive therapy in recipients of living related donors, but is depressed in recipients of cadaveric kidneys. Impaired oxidative metabolism due to immunosuppressive agents is described. A slight but significant negative correlation between cyclosporine blood levels and values of neutrophil chemiluminescence is found, suggesting that cyclosporine causes a dose-dependent inhibition of neutrophil function. Cyclosporine-mediated alteration of granulocyte function is only partial and restricted to phagocytosis. Renal transplant recipients treated with a combination of azathioprine and prednisolone also have lower levels for zymosan-stimulated chemiluminescence. Oxidative burst from polymorphonuclear cells measured as chemiluminescence was equally inhibited by methylprednisolone, prednisolone, and dexamethasone. The impaired oxidative burst by leukocytes may contribute, at least in part, to impaired microbial killing and may explain, at least in part, the increased morbidity and mortality from infection in renal transplantation. Summarizing these findings, the higher risk for bacterial infectious complications in renal transplant recipients compared with the normal population may result from the coincidence of impaired humoral and cellular host-defense mechanisms.

SUMMARY OF URINARY TRACT INFECTION IN RENAL TRANSPLANT RECIPIENTS

Bacterial infections are common after kidney transplantation, particularly UTIs. In the posttransplant period, UTIs occur in an average of 50% and are associated with acute rejection triggered by the infection itself (in up to 90% of the cases). The most severe complication of UTI is septicemia/bacteriemia. Antibiotic prophylaxis reduces the risk of UTI and shortens hospitalization.

However, in this case approximately half of the transplant recipients receive antibiotic therapy without any evidence for UTI. The spectrum of bacilli causing UTIs in renal transplant patients is nearly identical to that in nonimmunosuppressed individuals. The incidence of the different microorganisms is changing dramatically. Furthermore, immunosuppressive protocols may also contribute to the high risk of bacterial infections because they not only effect T and B cells, but also neutrophil counts and specific granulocyte functions.

REFLUX NEPHROPATHY

Reflux nephropathy is the end result of severe VUR, which may be associated with UTI, hypertension, proteinuria, or renal failure. Primary VUR is a common congenital abnormality of the urinary tract and the most frequent clinical presentation in early life is as a complicating UTI. However, the role of bacterial infection in the pathogenesis of renal damage in reflux nephropathy is still under debate. Whether sterile reflux can cause renal scarring is also uncertain, but it is obvious that VUR, particularly intrarenal reflux, promotes rapid entry of uropathogens into renal parenchyma. Potentially damaging to renal parenchyma is high-pressure VUR and intrarenal reflux in infants due to urodynamic factors, such as bladder and sphincter dysfunction. It is supposed that the increased pelvic pressure could exceed filtration pressure and efferent arteriolar pressure, causing ischemia and papillary atrophy. The risk of developing reflux nephropathy is related to the grade of the reflux. Other mechanisms that may contribute to renal damage in association with VUR is extravasation of urine into the renal parenchyme with the result of developing tubulointerstitial nephritis. Thereby, Tamm-Horsfall glycoprotein is the most interesting urinary constituent investigated. However, it is uncertain whether tubulointerstitial nephritis in patients with reflux nephropathy occurs due to autoimmune response directed against this protein.

The defect of primary VUR is a shortness of the submucosal segment due to congenital lateral ectopia of the ureteric orifice. With increasing age, the intravesical ureter lengthens and VUR tends to improve toward puberty and may resolve completely. Hereditary VUR seems to be a disorder with Mendelian-dominant inheritance. When VUR is discovered in symptomatic siblings, it is usually high grade and associated with a higher incidence of reflux nephropathy. Family screening programs offer the prospect of detecting VUR before scars develop with UTI. Analysis of families demonstrated phenotypic variation and the regular detection of both sterile reflux and reflux nephropathy. Secondary VUR may occur with several conditions, such as inflammatory disorders of the vesicoureteric junction (tuberculosis, bilharziasis), bladder neck obstructions, irradiation of the bladder, or in association with other congenital abnormalities or with neurogenic bladder defects.

Voiding cystourethrography is still the most precise method available for demonstration and classification of grades of VUR. At present, the most widely favored classification is that used by the International Reflux Study Committee. VUR without dilation of the urinary tract may be restricted to the ureter only (grade I) or may compromise ureter, pelvis, and calyces (grade II). Mild, moderate, or severe dilation of the ureter and the pelvis as well as tortuosity of the ureter are seen in higher grades of VUR. Grade III reflux is associated with normal or slightly blunted fornices, grade IV reflux with complete obliteration of the sharp angles of the fornices (Fig. 41.2), and in grade V reflux papillary impressions of calyces is diminished. Intrarenal reflux may occur in association with either grades IV or V reflux. Ultrasonography may provide a 92% sensitivity in the detection of reflux grade III and above when dynamic aspects of real-time studies are performed by experts. However, its nonvoiding nature is a limiting factor. Radionuclide micturition cystography is also considered a method that is at least as sensitive as the conventional voiding cystourethrogram and comparable in the radiation exposure. This technique is preferred for follow-up of patients with VUR treated either by surgery or conservative measures. Voiding ultrasonography of the bladder with echo enhancement also seems to be as good as voiding cystourethrography in the detection or exclusion of VUR, and thus will make it possible to reduce the number of children having to be exposed to ionizing radiation.

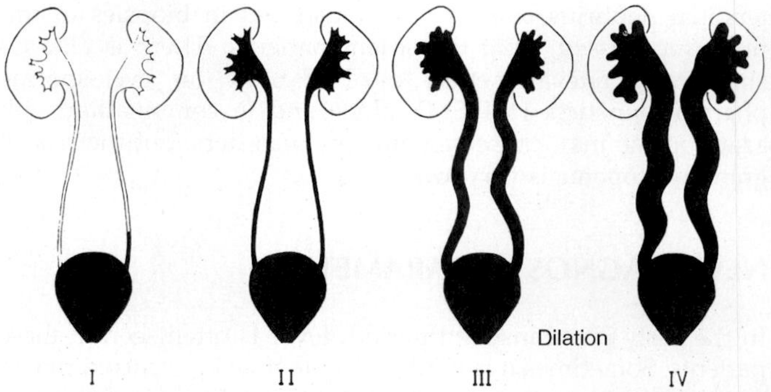

Figure 41.2. Diagrammatic representation of the various grades of vesicoureteral reflux seen with voiding cystoureterography. *I*, mild reflux in one ureter; *II*, reflux in both ureters into the pelvis, without dilation; *III*, reflux in both ureters reaching the pelvocalyceal system, with dilation; *IV*, severe reflux in both ureters reaching the pelvocalyceal system, with marked dilation of ureters and pelvis. (Reproduced with permission from Winberg J, Larson H, Bergstrom T. Comparison of the natural history of urinary infection in children with and without vesicoureteric reflux. In: Kincaid-Smith P, Farley NF, eds. *Renal infection and renal scarring*. Melbourne, Australia: Mercedes Publishing Services, 1970:293–302.)

Reflux nephropathy (i.e., renal scarring) with VUR and UTI is primarily a diagnosis on renal imaging. ^{99m}Tc-DMSA scanning appears to be the preferred method for the detection of renal cortical scarring. DMSA scanning more accurately identifies scarring with a higher sensitivity (76% versus 29%) and specificity (98% versus 92%) than does ultrasound. On the ^{99m}Tc-DMSA study, pinhole imaging had the highest accuracy (92%) when compared with planar (90%) and SPECT (87%) data. It has been demonstrated that levels of serum soluble IL-2 receptor were significantly higher in children with reflux nephropathy who had total uptake of DMSA than in those with normal total uptake. Serum levels of soluble IL-2 receptor correlated significantly with levels of creatinine, suggesting a useful predictor of progression of renal injury in these patients. Other findings suggest that circulating endothelial leukocyte adhesion molecule-1 (ELAM-1) levels reflect increased tissue damage in children with VUR and reflux nephropathy, probably as a result of progressive, localized inflammatory responses.

Approximately 40% of children with UTI demonstrate VUR. There is evidence that infancy and early childhood are the critical periods for renal scarring associated with reflux. In some infants renal damage clearly occurred *in utero*. Renal parenchymal damage may occur in those kidneys subjected to severe degrees of reflux (grades III to IV), whereas lesser degrees of reflux (grades I and II) usually are not associated with renal damage. Gross VUR (grade V) is the only degree of reflux associated with progressive renal damage. Clinically and radiologically, long-term follow-up of patients however demonstrated that serial long-term renal imaging studies do not provide additional information that will alter clinical management in children with damaged kidneys, who no longer have VUR after successful surgical correction. Complicating UTIs are the most common manifestations of VUR or reflux nephropathy in children. The reasons for the predisposition to these infections are not clear, but they are certainly multifactorial in origin. In neonates and young infants, UTIs are more common in boys than in girls, and in both there is a high incidence for abnormalities of the urinary tract, the most common being VUR. The natural history of VUR first detected in adulthood has shown a high incidence of UTI. In adult patients with VUR combined with reflux nephropathy, 95% had upper with or without lower UTI. Symptoms and findings associated with the urinary tract preceded the diagnosis of VUR by median 14 years. Hypertension was present in 34% of the patients, and five times more frequent in patients with bilateral reflux nephropathy than in those with unilateral reflux nephropathy.

Reflux nephropathy is associated with hypertension. Hypertension in reflux nephropathy contributes significantly to morbidity including deterioration of renal function. The mechanism of onset of hypertension is not clear, although abnormalities of the renin-angiotensin system and in sodium–potassium adenosine triphosphatase (ATPase) activity has been described in some cases. Treatment with angiotensin-converting enzyme inhibitors in patients with reflux nephropathy was reported to be useful in reducing microalbuminuria and may have slowed the progression of renal damage.

Besides patients with severe bilateral reflux nephropathy who may develop renal failure, there is another group of patients who also show deterioration of renal function despite surgically corrected or spontaneously ceased VUR, and despite the absence of UTI or hypertension. These patients present with persistent proteinuria due to focal or segmental glomerulosclerosis with hyalinosis in unscarred segments of the kidney. It is suggested that the loss of renal mass produces maladaptive hemodynamic changes in the glomeruli, which has been termed the *hyperfiltration theory.* Glomerulopathy may induce hypertension, and hypertension may accelerate glomerulosclerosis, with the result of developing chronic renal failure. Reflux nephropathy is an important cause of end-stage renal disease and still seems to be underdiagnosed in many centers. Reflux nephropathy should be excluded in any patient presenting with renal insufficiency and proteinuria, with or without hypertension or UTI.

Selected Readings

Franz M, Hörl WH. Common errors in diagnosis and management of urinary tract infections. I: Pathophysiology and diagnostic techniques. *Nephrol Dial Transplant* 1999;14(11):2746–2753.

The interaction of virulence factors of uropathogens and the host-defense mechanisms are reviewed. Correct procedures for an accurate diagnosis of urinary tract infections are discussed and the broad spectrum of clinical conditions are overviewed.

Kim ED, Schaeffer AJ. Antimicrobial therapy for urinary tract infections. *Semin Nephrol* 1994;14:551–569.

The selection of an antimicrobial agent for urinary tract infection (UTI) is dependent on host, organism, and drug pharmacologic factors. This review presents an overview of antimicrobial therapies for commonly seen UTIs such as acute uncomplicated cystitis or pyelonephritis in women, complicated UTI, or recurrent UTI. Treatment strategies for UTI occurring during pregnancy and management of bacterial prostatitis, fungal infections, and catheter-associated UTI are also discussed.

Kunin CM. Urinary tract infections in females. (State-of-the-art). *Clin Infect Dis* 1994;18:1–12.

Definition and classification of urinary tract infections (UTI) is important to ensure optimal clinical management. Low-count bacteriuria should not be neglected because it may reflect ongoing infection. The only indication for treatment of asymptomatic bacteriuria is during pregnancy. The broad spectrum of clinical conditions of UTI and its pathogenesis is the subject of this article, with recommendations for diagnostic methods and treatment.

Schmaldienst S, Hörl WH. Bacterial infections after renal transplantation. *Nephrol* 1997;75:140–153.

An overview of the time course and the risk factors for urinary tract infections in renal transplant recipients.

Stamm WE, Hooton TM. Management of urinary tract infections in adults. *N Engl J Med* 1993;329:1328–1334.

Management strategies designed for specific groups of patients with urinary tract infections (UTIs) can maximize therapeutic benefits while reducing costs and the incidence of adverse reactions. Choice of antimicrobial drugs, duration of therapy, and indication for urologic evaluation depends on the clinical setting of the patient and the presence or absence of complicating factors. Clinical management and therapeutic strategies in the field of UTI are discussed.

Stapleton A. Prevention of urinary tract infections in women. *Lancet* 1999;353:7–8.

Strategies to enhance the effect of prophylactic antimicrobial therapy.

Stapleton A, Stamm WE. Prevention of urinary tract infection. *Infect Dis Clin North Am* 1997;11:719–733.

Increased susceptibility to recurrent UTIs among otherwise healthy women is an exceedingly common clinical problem. Intrinsic host factors and exogenous exposures or behaviors are illuminated, and effective prophylactic measures against recurrent UTI are summarized.

PART 2
Renal Mycobacterial Diseases

John B. Eastwood, Susan A. Dilly, and John M. Grange

The human mycobacterial diseases include tuberculosis, leprosy, and less specific opportunist infections caused by mycobacteria normally found in the environment. Tuberculosis is usually caused by *Mycobacterium tuberculosis,* but a minority of cases are caused by *M. bovis* (the bovine tubercle bacillus) and *M. africanum.* On the basis of DNA homology, these are really variants of a single species. The genus *Mycobacterium* contains approximately 80 other species, including rapid growers, slow growers, and the leprosy bacillus (*M. leprae*), which has never been cultivated *in vitro.* Most of these other species are free-living environmental saprophytes but some, listed in Table 41.6, cause human disease, particularly in immunosuppressed persons including recipients of renal transplants. They are often present in the lower urethra and on the external genitalia and are thus often isolated from urine, but they are extremely rare causes of disease of the genitourinary tract. The kidney may be involved as part of multiorgan disease, usually due to the *M. avium* complex, in patients with AIDS.

Globally, tuberculosis is a common disease, with 8 to 10 million new cases annually and a rising incidence, particularly in regions with a high incidence of HIV infection. Most often the lung is affected, but after lymphadenopathy, the most common form of nonpulmonary tuberculosis is genitourinary disease, which accounts for 20% to 27% of nonpulmonary cases in the United States and United Kingdom. Within developed countries, various forms of nonpulmonary tuberculosis are relatively more common in patients from ethnic minority groups, except for genitourinary tuberculosis, which is uncommon in these groups. In the United Kingdom, genitourinary tuberculosis accounts for 5% of nonpulmonary tuberculosis cases in ethnic minorities, compared with 27% in the general population.

Tuberculosis due to *M. bovis* is now rare in industrially developed nations, accounting for fewer than 1% of all cases of tuberculosis, and is usually due to reactivation of old, dormant, disease. In approximately 25% of such cases the genitourinary system is involved.

TABLE 41.6. The Principal Causes of Mycobacterial Disease in Humans[a]

Obligate Pathogens	
The *M. tuberculosis* complex: *M. tuberculosis (M. bovis, M. africanum)*	Tuberculosis (*M. bovis* principally causes tuberculosis of cattle)
M. leprae	Leprosy
Causes of Other Named Mycobacterial Diseases	
M. marinum	Swimming pool granuloma
M. ulcerans	Buruli ulcer (an uncommon tropical skin disease)
Slowly Growing Mycobacteria Causing Nonspecific Tuberculosis-Like Disease	
M. avium complex[b]	*M. kansasii*
M. malmoense	*M. scrofulaceum*
M. xenopi	*(M. asiaticum)*
(M. celatum)	*(M. gordonae)*
(M. haemophilum)[c]	*(M. simiae)*
(M. szulgai)	
Rapidly Growing Pathogens	
M. chelonae	*M. fortuitum*
(M. flavescens)	
Slowly Growing Mycobacteria Causing HIV-Associated Disseminated Disease	
M. avium complex	*(M. genavense)*

[a] Less common causes are in parentheses.
[b] Contains the closely related species *M. avium* and *M. intracellulare.*
[c] An uncommon cause of skin lesions in renal transplant recipients and other immunosuppressed patients.

PATHOGENESIS OF TUBERCULOSIS

Infection with the tubercle bacillus principally occurs via the respiratory tract. If the bacilli overcome local defence mechanisms and replicate, a primary focus of disease develops in the lung. Bacilli are transported from the primary focus to the local lymph nodes from which dissemination to other organs occurs via the bloodstream. Overt primary tuberculosis occurs in approximately 5% of infected people as a result of progression of the primary complex or development of disease in a distant organ (e.g., meninges, bone, kidney). Primary renal tuberculosis tends to present 3 to 8 years after initial infection, which is later than primary disease in other nonpulmonary sites.

In most infected persons the primary complex resolves, but bacilli may persist in a dormant state for long periods of time. Postprimary tuberculosis develops, as a result of either endogenous reactivation of latent infection or exogenous reinfection, in approximately 5% of those who overcome the primary infection. Postprimary tuberculosis is characterized by excessive tissue destruction as a result of necrotizing delayed-type hypersensitivity reactions. This necrosis generates pulmonary cavities that communicate with the bronchi and thereby enable the bacilli to enter the bronchial secretions and be spread to other persons. Likewise, organisms enter the urine when cavities in the kidney erode into the renal pelvis. Renal involvement in postprimary tuberculosis is probably underestimated because, unless there are definite symptoms, the genitourinary tract is usually not examined in patients with pulmonary tuberculosis. Destructive lesions of the genitourinary system develop in an estimated 4% to 8% of such patients.

Renal granulomas, resulting from the implantation of small numbers of tubercle bacilli during early hematogenous spread, usually appear first in association with glomeruli, probably because of the high blood flow and favorable oxygen tension. At this stage, cortical granulomas are typically bilateral but remain dormant until other, poorly understood, factors permit the bacilli to proliferate. The enlarging granulomas may rupture into the proximal tubule enabling bacilli to reach Henle's loop, a site where they appear to survive well, possibly because phagocytosis is impaired in the hypertonic environment. Bacillary proliferation leads to granuloma formation in the medulla and the disease process may be destructive enough to cause papillary necrosis and rupture through the calyceal wall. Bacilli can then reach the renal pelvis, ureters, bladder, prostate, and epididymis. There may also be spread to these organs via the local lymphatics or by direct hematogenous spread from the primary focus (usually pulmonary), which explains why there can occasionally be genital involvement without the urinary tract being affected. Chronic tuberculosis commonly gives rise to amyloidosis, and in India, is a common cause of renal amyloid, but in contrast to leprosy, glomerulonephritis is an uncommon complication.

CLINICAL MANIFESTATIONS OF TUBERCULOSIS

Classical Genitourinary Tuberculosis

Tuberculosis of the urinary tract is easily overlooked, and it is not uncommon for the diagnosis to be made either at operation or on postmortem examination. One report refers to 25 patients with renal tuberculosis, 18 of whom presented only after advanced cavitating disease had developed. In practice, most patients present with lower urinary tract symptoms typical of "conventional" bacterial cystitis and suspicions are aroused only when the patient fails to respond to the usual antibacterial agents or when urine examination reveals pyuria in the absence of a positive culture on routine media. Other symptoms of urinary tract tuberculosis, such as dysuria; back, flank, or suprapubic pain; hematuria; frequency; and nocturia, might also suggest conventional bacterial urinary tract infection. Renal colic is unusual, occurring in up to 10% of patients, and constitutional symptoms such as fever, weight loss, and night sweats are also unusual. Only one-third of the patients have abnormal chest radiographs.

Generalized parenchymal destruction in advanced bilateral renal tuberculosis may lead to a reduction of glomerular filtration rate (GFR) and eventually to end-stage renal failure. A more common cause of reduced GFR is ureteric and bladder involvement due to seeding of *M. tuberculosis* into the urine. Such seeding can lead to ureteric scarring with distortion and urinary tract obstruction and to considerable fibrosis and contraction of the bladder.

In the male, genital tuberculosis usually results from seeding from infected urine and the most common manifestation is epididymoorchitis. Tuberculous prostatitis also occurs. The urinary tract should be investigated in men with genital tuberculosis because 75% of those with epididymoorchitis have evidence of urinary tract involvement. Tuberculosis of the urethra and penis is uncommon but can present with papulonecrotic skin lesions, fistulae, and genital ulceration. Although usually resulting from direct seeding of infected urine, penile tuberculosis can be acquired by direct inoculation from contaminated surgical instruments (e.g., in circumcision) or clothing. By contrast, tuberculosis of the genital tract in the female is accompanied by urinary tract tuberculosis in fewer than 5% of cases, probably because tuberculosis of the female genital tract is almost always the result of direct hematogenous spread.

Tuberculous Interstitial Nephritis

A more insidious form of renal tuberculosis also occurs. In one report, three patients presented with advanced renal failure in whom imaging had revealed equal-sized smooth kidneys without evidence of calcification or gross anatomic distortion. Tubercle bacilli were not found in the urine but renal biopsies revealed acid-fast bacilli in two cases, caseation in two cases, and interstitial infiltrates with chronic inflammatory cells and granulomas in all three patients. Two patients had radiologic evidence of pulmonary tuberculosis and one patient had tuberculous peritonitis. In another report, a renal biopsy from a patient with reduced GFR and equal-sized smooth kidneys on intravenous urography showed interstitial fibrosis with epithelioid and giant cell granulomas, one of which showed caseation. Acid-fast bacilli were not seen in the biopsy nor grown from biopsy material or urine but a Mantoux test was strongly positive. The patient received a 12-month course of antituberculosis therapy and the GFR improved over the next 3 years. Tuberculosis had not been considered before the biopsy because there was no other evidence of this disease and five of the six urine specimens were free of leukocytes. These cases show that there may be tuberculous involvement of the kidneys, sufficient to cause renal failure, in the absence of either the typical renal destruction with calcification and fibrosis or urinary tract obstruction.

Tuberculosis as a Cause of End-Stage Renal Failure

Tuberculosis is an important cause of progressive renal failure, but unlike most other causes, it is preventable and treatable. In 1991, the European Dialysis and Transplant Association (EDTA) registry reported that, among the 35 countries submitting returns, 195 (0.65%) of 30,064 new patients assigned a diagnosis had renal failure due to renal tuberculosis, an incidence similar to that in earlier years. Greece had the highest incidence (4.51% of new patients) and it was also common in Portugal, Belgium, Spain, Italy, and Yugoslavia. In Portugal, there were local areas of high incidence: over a 10-year period in the Algarve, tuberculosis was the cause of renal failure in as many as 12 of 345 patients starting hemodialysis. In some instances, patients presented terminally but with no previous symptoms of tuberculosis. Among other populations it is less common; for example, only 2 of 1,786 patients accepted for dialysis/transplantation in Australasia in 1997 were found to have renal tuberculosis. Unfortunately, data is generally lacking in regions of the world where there is a high prevalence of tuberculosis.

It is probable that the reported number of patients with tuberculosis as a cause of end-stage renal disease is an underestimate because, although most individuals with classical urinary tract tuberculosis will be identified, the interstitial form can easily be overlooked. It is important to consider tuberculosis in all patients with equal-sized smooth kidneys without a clear-cut diagnosis, especially in high-risk groups, and in such patients, renal biopsy should be seriously considered.

TUBERCULOSIS IN DIALYSIS AND TRANSPLANT PATIENTS

Tuberculosis is a problem in dialysis and transplant patients. In the former, it often presents insidiously with anorexia, low-grade fever, and weight loss. Most cases have been extrapulmonary or, less often, miliary. Tuberculosis appears to be much more common among hemodialysis patients than in the general population, and the type of presentation suggests that dialysis is associated with reactivation of quiescent disease. In developed nations there may be a significant excess of persons with renal failure from ethnic minorities groups who may also have a higher incidence of tuberculosis. There are fewer reports of tuberculosis in patients undergoing continuous ambulatory peritoneal dialysis (CAPD) but there is no reason to suspect that reactivation of tuberculosis is any less likely to occur in these patients. Several cases of tuberculous peritonitis have been reported and one study suggests that, provided that adequate antituberculosis treatment is given, CAPD can be continued successfully.

Tuberculosis has always been a worrisome clinical challenge in renal transplant patients but has received less attention than opportunist infections such as *Pneumocystis carinii* and cytomegalovirus. A literature search of the first 30 years of renal transplantation revealed only 42 cases of tuberculosis in transplanted patients. In a subsequent report, 14 cases occurred among 403 renal transplant patients, an incidence 50 times greater than in the general population, and a high proportion of patients had miliary disease. The risk of developing tuberculosis was unrelated to tuberculin test reactivity. In a few cases tuberculosis followed transplantation of an infected kidney.

Chemoprophylaxis is effective in preventing tuberculosis in transplant patients. In one series there were no cases of tuberculosis among patients receiving chemoprophylaxis, but there were 6 cases among 27 high-risk patients who did not receive chemoprophylaxis. It has been suggested that isoniazid 300 mg daily with pyridoxine 25 to 50 mg daily should be given for 1 year to transplant patients with any of the following: a history of inadequately treated tuberculosis, an abnormal chest radiograph, a tuberculin test more than 10 mm wide, and contact with a case of active tuberculosis; this treatment should also be given to tuberculin-negative patients who receive a kidney from a tuberculin-positive donor. Our practice is to give isoniazid 100 mg daily with pyridoxine for 6 months to patients originating from countries where there is a high incidence of tuberculosis.

LABORATORY DIAGNOSIS OF RENAL TUBERCULOSIS

Urine samples, preferably early-morning midstream specimens collected on 3 successive days in sterile containers, are examined by microscopy and culture. Specimens should be delivered to the laboratory without delay to prevent replication of contaminating bacteria but if delays are unavoidable, specimens should be refrigerated but not frozen. Microscopy may reveal leukocytes, erythrocytes, and keratinous debris. Acid-fast bacilli are seen in a minority of cases; small numbers should be interpreted with caution because they may be environmental mycobacteria derived from the lower urethra or external genitalia.

Biopsies are cultured after homogenization. Best results are obtained with tissue surrounding necrotic lesions, rather than the necrotic material itself.

Growth of tubercle bacilli on traditional culture media is slow and there is a delay of 2 to 6 weeks before growth is visible. Automated radiometric techniques and some newer nonradiometric techniques based on the activation or quenching of dyes permit a more rapid detection of growth, and various molecular techniques such as the polymerase chain reaction, some available in kit form, provide even more rapid results. However, they have not yet been extensively evaluated in the diagnosis of renal tuberculosis.

HISTOPATHOLOGY OF TUBERCULOSIS

Tuberculosis of the renal tract may take the form of miliary disease, in which the kidney is speckled with firm, white, small nodules, or cavitating or "caseous" tuberculosis, in which there is destruction of the parenchyma. In both forms of the disease, the classical microscopic finding is the granuloma, which may caseate with the center becoming necrotic.

The initial lesions are bilateral. In the miliary form small granulomas develop in the renal cortex adjacent to glomerular capillaries; in the cavitating form the medulla is the site primarily involved. It is this form that can progress to focal papillary damage with erosion into the urinary tract. These areas may coalesce to destroy a large amount of renal parenchyma.

Bacteria may spread throughout the renal pelvis and down the ureter to the bladder. The resulting tissue destruction and attempts at healing may lead to fibrosis that produces strictures and obstructive damage. The most common sites for obstruction are the neck of a calyx, the pelvoureteric junction, the midureter, the ureterovesical junction, and, in females, the point where the ureter passes under the broad ligament. Involvement of the urethra is uncommon and difficult to diagnose but may present with unusual fistulae involving the perineum, rectum, and anus or as long strictures that are difficult to treat. In the bladder, tuberculosis may present as persistent cystitis because of ulceration of the mucosa and may eventually reduce the bladder capacity as a result of fibrosis of the wall. Tuberculous epididymoorchitis generally presents with swelling, abscesses, or sinuses.

Calcification is common in renal tuberculosis, occurring in approximately one-fourth of cases, and appears to have increased in incidence with the advent of effective chemotherapy, possibly because more patients survive long enough to develop calcification. It may take the form of staghorn calculi, ureteric stones, bladder stones, renal parenchymal calcification, or calcification in the wall of the urinary tract. In the end-stage kidney this dystrophic calcification produces a so-called cement kidney and a "cumulus cloud" appearance on radiology.

Effective chemotherapy can promote healing of active lesions without the development of damaging fibrosis or calcification but areas of established fibrosis do not improve. Before antituberculosis therapy became available, chronic inflammation led to leukoplakia of the renal pelvis and caused normal transitional epithelium to become squamous, with associated hyperplasia and keratinization. The large amounts of keratin formed could cause local obstruction and, sometimes, repeated episodes of renal colic.

Tissue Changes in Tuberculosis (Fig. 109.21)

The tissue reaction in tuberculosis is a spectrum ranging from classical caseating granulomas to multibacillary histiocytosis and depends on the stage of the disease and the immune status of the patient. The classical tuberculoid granuloma consists of macrophages, many of which are modified to be epithelioid cells and Langhans' giant cells. Necrosis may be present and may appear bland and eosinophilic (caseous necrosis). Alternatively, necrotic areas may contain nuclear debris and polymorphonuclear leukocytes or be more fibrinoid or granular in appearance. Acid-fast bacilli are few in number or not seen in the tissue sections. Different stages of development may be present within the kidney, so the appearance is often a mixture of noncaseating granulomas and areas of caseous necrosis, with the effects of attempts at healing and repair leading to fibrosis.

The picture may be altered if the patient is immunosuppressed, in which case the characteristic appearance is that of immature macrophages containing numerous bacilli so that the cytoplasm has a foamy appearance. Necrosis, giant cells, granulomas, and epithelioid cells are generally not seen. Mycobacterial infection is not the only cause of granulomas, although those associated with other diseases rarely caseate. Other granulomatous conditions include sarcoidosis, Wegener's granulomatosis, reaction to foreign/abnormal material (e.g., myeloma protein, ruptured tubules, crystals), brucellosis, and certain fungal infections.

IMAGING

Intravenous urography (IVU) is very useful in the detection of urinary tract tuberculosis because of its ability to detect calcification (which is seen in approximately 30% of cases), to provide a detailed image of anatomy, and to show the multiple lesions that commonly occur. Renal tuberculosis may be unilateral or bilateral and may present a variety of calcific patterns—punctate, speckled, or hazy. In advanced tuberculosis, the whole pelvocalyceal system and ureter may be outlined by calcification, the so-called tuberculous autonephrectomy.

Early tuberculosis is seen on IVU as irregularity of the papillae. Cavities, either smooth or irregular, then develop and communicate with the pelvocalyceal system. As destruction progresses there is associated parenchymal loss. Fibrosis leads to strictures, and when these affect the calyceal infundibula, there is no calyceal filling at urography and the infundibulum shows a typical "pinched off" appearance. Fibrosis at the pelvoureteric junction causes obstruction at this level. Local granuloma formation or dilated obstructed calyces that do not fill with contrast medium may produce a mass effect. Extension of infection into the perinephric space with abscess formation may occur. Fistulae may develop, particularly to the skin and gut, and retrograde ureterography or sinography may be required to show them fully.

Tuberculosis of the ureter and bladder is usually secondary to renal tuberculosis therefore the kidneys usually show radiologic abnormalities. The earliest ureteric change is ulceration but this is rarely demonstrated radiologically. Strictures then develop and there may be associated filling defects if there is florid granuloma formation. As fibrosis progresses the ureter shortens and the wall thickens. Involvement of the vesicoureteric junction may result in vesicoureteric reflux. The bladder wall thickens and granulomas may cause filling defects. With generalized involvement, bladder capacity is reduced. Calcification in the ureter and bladder occur only with fairly advanced disease. Calcification may also occur in the seminal vesicles, vas, and prostate if these are involved.

Ultrasonography shows many of the changes of advanced disease such as pelvocalyceal dilation, large localized lesions, and calcification although it is a less sensitive detector than urography even of advanced disease. Computed tomography is a good method for demonstrating the many changes in advanced disease: calcification, pelvocalyceal dilation, scars, strictures, and extrarenal spread. Its sensitivity in early disease has not been assessed but is likely to be less than urography because it shows less detailed pelvocalyceal anatomy.

Follow-up studies of patients on chemotherapy reveal that ureteric strictures may develop during treatment. They may occur at sites apparently normal on the IVU obtained at presentation, presumably because mucosal ulceration at the affected site was not visualized. A limited IVU is the best method for detecting new ureteric strictures and their effects on the upper tracts.

TREATMENT OF TUBERCULOSIS

Although most clinical trials of antituberculosis drug regimens have involved pulmonary disease, modern short-course regimens appear effective in all forms of tuberculosis, including those involving the genitourinary system. These regimens are based on an intensive phase of treatment lasting 2 months, during which almost all tubercle bacilli are killed, and a continuation phase lasting 4 months, during which the few remaining persisters are eliminated. In the most frequently used regimen, four drugs [rifampicin, isoniazid, pyrazinamide, and ethambutol (or streptomycin)] are given in the intensive phase and two drugs (rifampicin and isoniazid) are given in the continuation phase. Strict adherence to the drug regimen should be ensured by direct supervision of all doses. To facilitate this, drugs may be given two or three times weekly during the continuation phase.

Multidrug-resistant tuberculosis (i.e., resistance to rifampicin and isoniazid with or without resistance to other drugs) requires the use of at least four drugs selected, on the basis of drug susceptibility tests, from ethionamide, prothionamide, quinolones (e.g., ofloxacin), newer macrolides (e.g., clarithromycin), cycloserine, kanamycin, viomycin, capreomycin, thiacetazone, and *para*-aminosalicylic acid (PAS). These are less effective and often more toxic and/or costly than the first-line drugs. Duration of therapy is based on bacteriologic response but may be 18 months or longer. Daily doses of the principal antituberculosis agents are shown in Table 41.7.

Because rifampicin, isoniazid, pyrazinamide, ethionamide, and prothionamide are either eliminated in the bile or metabolized they may be given in normal dosages to patients with impaired renal function. Considerable care must be taken when using streptomycin (and other aminoglycosides) and ethambutol because both are wholly excreted via the kidney; both have major adverse side effects—ototoxicity and optic neuritis—respectively. Reduced dosages of ethambutol should be given according to GFR (i.e., 25 mg three times weekly if the GFR is between 50 and 100 ml/min and twice weekly if it is between 30 and 50 ml/min). Streptomycin and other aminoglycosides are nephrotoxic and should be avoided, if possible, if there is impairment of renal function. They are contraindicated in patients on cyclosporine because they enhance the risk of nephrotoxicity.

Encephalopathy is a rare complication of isoniazid therapy and its incidence is reduced by prescription of pyridoxine (25 to 50 mg/day). A few cases of isoniazid-induced encephalopathy that failed to respond to pyridoxine have been reported in patients on hemodialysis but the condition resolved when isoniazid was withdrawn. Care must also be taken with rifampicin in renal transplant patients because it increases the rate of metabolism of corticosteroids, cyclosporine, and tacrolimus, all of which are often given to transplant patients. Blood concentrations of cyclosporine and tacrolimus should be regularly monitored in patients receiving rifampicin.

Surgical intervention is indicated in cases of urinary obstruction, in advanced unilateral disease complicated by pain or hemorrhage, and for bladder augmentation. Surgical excision of nonfunctioning kidneys or extensive lesions in partly functioning kidneys is controversial.

OTHER MYCOBACTERIAL DISEASES

Although direct invasion of the kidney by *M. leprae* is unusual, renal damage is an important cause of morbidity and mortality in leprosy patients in whom many different renal diseases, including most histologic forms of glomerulonephritis, interstitial nephritis, and secondary amyloidosis occur. Between 11% and 38% of leprosy patients die of renal failure, but percutaneous renal biopsy shows that the incidence of renal disease is much more common. Glomerulonephritis, due to the deposition of

TABLE 41.7. Daily Doses of the Antituberculosis Agents[a]

Agent	Daily Dose: Adults	Daily Dose: Children
Rifampicin	450 mg if body wt < 50 kg 600 mg if body wt ≥ 50 kg	10 mg/kg to maximum of 600 mg
Isoniazid	200–300 mg	5 mg/kg
Pyrazinamide	1.5 g if body wt < 50 kg 2.0 g if body wt ≥ 50 kg	25 mg/kg
Ethambutol	15 mg/kg	As for adult
Streptomycin	750 mg if body wt < 50 kg 1 g if body wt ≥ 50 kg 750 mg if age ≥ 40 yr 500 mg if age ≥ 60 yr	15 mg/kg to maximum of 750 mg
Thiacetazone	150 mg	50 mg
Para-aminosalicylic acid	10–12 g	300 mg/kg
Ethionamide and Prothionamide	500 mg if body wt < 50 kg 750 mg if body wt ≥ 50 kg	15–20 mg/kg
Ofloxacin	800 mg	Avoid

[a] See text for dose modifications needed in patients with renal failure.

immune complexes, and amyloidosis are most frequent in patients with multibacillary leprosy.

Disease of the kidney and other parts of the genitourinary tract (epididymis and prostate) due to environmental mycobacteria (EM) is extremely rare and diagnosis is not easy because these bacteria are often present as contaminants in urine. A firm diagnosis usually requires isolation of EM from granulomas demonstrable in biopsies. In HIV-positive and other immunosuppressed patients, renal involvement by EM is a manifestation of disseminated disease.

The iatrogenic immunosuppression in renal transplant patients predisposes to mycobacterial disease, either tuberculosis itself or disease due to EM. The latter may manifest as pulmonary or disseminated disease or as skin lesions. Because the symptoms are often masked by the immunosuppression, diagnosis may be delayed and the mortality is high (approximately 30%). Some infections have occurred in patients on hemodialysis and in some cases were the result of contamination of the dialysis machine by EM. Peritonitis resulting from EM has occurred in patients on intermittent or ambulatory peritoneal dialysis and requires drainage of the dialysis fluid, removal of the catheter, and transfer of the patient to hemodialysis. The treatment of disease due to EM depends on the *in vitro* drug susceptibility of the organism. Expert guidance should be sought.

Selected Readings

Ahsan N, Wheeler DE, Palmer BP. Leprosy associated renal disease: case report and review of the literature. *J Am Soc Nephrol* 1995;5:1546–1552.

A review of renal disease associated with leprosy.

Carl P, Stark L. Indications for surgical management of genitourinary tuberculosis. *World J Surg* 1997;21:505–510.

A review of the surgical treatment of genitourinary tuberculosis.

Collins CH, Grange JM, Yates MD. *Tuberculosis bacteriology: organisation and practice*, 2nd ed. Oxford: Butterworth Heinemann, 1997.

A description of the mycobacteria causing human disease and a detailed account of diagnostic laboratory procedures, including collection of specimens.

Eastwood JB, Dilly SA, Grange JM. Tuberculosis, leprosy and other mycobacterial diseases. In: Cattell WR, ed. *Infections of the kidney and urinary tract*. Oxford: Oxford University Press, 1996:291–318.

A detailed and extensively referenced account of mycobacterial disease of the kidney and urinary tract.

Heptinstall RH. Renal manifestations of various infective conditions. In: Heptinstall RH, ed. *Pathology of the kidney*, 4th ed. Boston: Little, Brown, 1992:1936–1939.

Includes an account of the pathologic manifestations of renal tuberculosis.

Hussain MM, Baker N, Roujouleh H. Tuberculosis in patients undergoing maintenance dialysis. *Nephrol Dial Transplant* 1990;5:584–587.

Tuberculosis as an important complication of dialysis for renal failure.

Morgan SH, Eastwood JB, Baker LRI. Tuberculous interstitial nephritis—the tip of the iceberg. *Tubercle* 1990;71:5–6.

Tuberculosis as an often overlooked cause of renal failure.

Qunibi WY, Al-Sibai MB, Taher S, et al. Mycobacterial infection after renal transplantation: a report of 14 cases and review of the literature. *Q J Med* 1990; 77:1039–1060.

Disease due to mycobacteria other than tubercle bacilli in recipients of renal transplants.

CHAPTER 42

Renal Involvement in Multisystem Diseases

PART 1
Lupus Nephritis

Gerald B. Appel and Vivette D'Agati

Renal disease is a common manifestation of systemic lupus erythematosus (SLE). Although the multiple immunologic abnormalities of lupus can affect virtually any organ system, involvement of the kidneys is often a major source of patient morbidity and mortality. Renal involvement in SLE is extremely diverse, ranging from asymptomatic urinary findings to fulminant renal failure or florid nephrotic syndrome.

Pathologic alterations may affect the glomerular, tubulointerstitial, and vascular compartments. The diagnosis of SLE often can be established by the presence of certain clinical and laboratory features defined by the 1982 modified American Rheumatism Association (ARA) criteria (Table 42.1). Renal involvement is defined for these purposes as persistent proteinuria exceeding 500 mg/day (or 3+ on the dipstick) or the presence of cellular casts (consisting either of erythrocyte, hemoglobin, granular, tubular, or mixed casts). The development of any 4 of the 11 ARA criteria during a patient's course confers a 96% sensitivity and specificity for SLE. At presentation, an individual patient may display fewer than four of these criteria, only to fulfill the ARA criteria at a later time. It is rare, however, for patients with severe proliferative lupus nephritis to present before fulfilling the ARA criteria for SLE. On the other hand, patients with purely mesangial or membranous lesions may present with renal involvement as an initial manifestation, even before serologic tests for SLE are positive.

Both the terms *lupus nephritis* and *lupus glomerulonephritis* are commonly applied to the many patterns of glomerular involvement in SLE. This includes mesangial lesions, formerly designated as *lupus glomerulitis,* and membranous patterns, sometimes termed *membranous lupus nephropathy* rather than *true nephritis* because of the lack of a glomerular inflammatory component. Likewise, those occasional patients with predominant involvement of the blood vessels (e.g., vasculopathy or thrombotic microangiopathy) and the tubulointerstitial compartment with little or no glomerular disease are still considered within the disease spectrum of lupus nephritis.

In the United States, the incidence and prevalence of SLE, and hence of lupus nephritis, vary considerably among different studies. The reported incidence ranges from 1.8 to 7.6 cases per 100,000 per year with a prevalence of 14.6 to 50.8 cases per 100,000. SLE is most common among young females, with the highest reported incidence in African-American females. Although severe renal involvement can affect lupus patients regardless of age, race, or sex, a number of studies have found more severe renal involvement in African-Americans. The roles of socioeconomic and biologic-genetic factors remain to be clarified in this population.

TABLE 42.1 Revised American Rheumatism Association Criteria for Systemic Lupus Erythematosus

Malar rash
Discoid rash
Photosensitivity
Oral ulcers
Nondeforming arthritis
Serositis—pleuritis or pericarditis
Renal disease—persistent proteinuria, casts
Central nervous system disease—seizures or psychoses
Hematologic disorder—anemia, leukopenia, lymphopenia, thrombocytopenia
Immunologic disorder—+ LE prep, + anti-DNA, + anti-Sm, + false-positive VDRL
Positive antinuclear antibody

Modified from Tan EM, Cohen AS, Fries JF, et al. The 1982 revised criteria for the classification of systemic lupus erythematosus. *Arthritis Rheum* 1982;25:1271–1277.

A number of factors have been documented to influence the incidence of SLE and its renal manifestations. The importance of genetic factors is supported by the reported African-American racial predominance, the increased frequency of certain HLA haplotypes, familial clustering, common serologic abnormalities [e.g., positive antinuclear antibodies (ANA)] in relatives of patients with SLE, and the increased susceptibility to lupus among patients with deficiencies of early complement components. Exposure to sunlight or ultraviolet radiation can trigger a flare of systemic disease including lupus nephritis. Certain drugs, such as hydralazine, procainamide, isoniazid, and methyldopa, may precipitate a lupus-like syndrome manifesting many of the serologic and clinical features of SLE. In general, however, renal involvement is rare in drug-induced SLE. The influence of estrogens and sex hormones on the pathogenesis of lupus nephritis can be inferred from the strong female predominance, the unfavorable effect of female sex hormones on the course of experimental lupus nephritis, and the exacerbations of systemic or renal disease with the use of oral contraceptives or pregnancy.

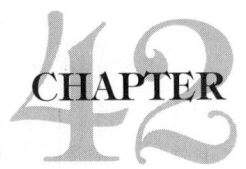

PATHOGENESIS

Glomerular involvement in SLE is considered a human prototype of the classic schema of immune complex–induced renal damage as defined in experimental models. In SLE, there is a loss of self-tolerance with B-cell hyperactivity and the overproduction of autoantibodies reacting against subcellular nuclear and cytoplasmic constituents. B-cell hyperactivity may be caused by altered T-cell regulatory function, including decreased numbers of cytotoxic and suppressor T cells, increased helper CD4+ T cells, and dysfunctional T-cell signaling. It may also be due to autogenous B-cell activation or more complex defects in immune regulation. The autoantibodies produced include antibodies to single-stranded and double-stranded DNA, ribonucleoproteins and histones, and in some circumstances, extracellular matrix proteins such as laminin. The chronic deposition of circulating immune complexes formed by autoantibodies and "self" antigens may play a major role in the mesangial and endocapillary proliferative patterns of lupus nephritis. The glomerular localization of circulating immune complexes is influenced by many factors, including the size, charge, and avidity of the complexes; the clearing ability of the mesangium; and local hemodynamic factors. The involvement of the factors in the deposition of immune complexes in the glomeruli are discussed in detail in Chapter 36, Part 3. Once immune complexes are deposited, activation of the complement cascade leads to complement-mediated damage, activation of procoagulant factors, leukocyte infiltration, release of cytokines and proteolytic enzymes, and induction of glomerular cellular proliferation and matrix synthesis. Cross-reactivity of circulating autoantibodies with intrinsic basement membrane antigens such as laminin, collagen IV, or heparan sulfate proteoglycans may also be operant. In some cases, particularly in membranous glomerulopathy, the initiating event may be the local binding of nucleosomes, histones, or other autoantigens to glomerular subepithelial sites, causing *in situ* immune complex formation. Histones and nucleosomes, which are cationic, have particular affinity for the intrinsic negative-charge sites in the glomerular capillary wall, promoting planting of autoantigens; this process is covered in detail in Chapter 36, Part 2. Glomerular and vascular damage may be exacerbated by hypertension and intravascular coagulation. The presence of antiphospholipid antibodies and their attendant alterations in endothelial and platelet function may lead to intravascular coagulation, producing thrombotic glomerular and vascular lesions.

PATHOLOGY

Both morphologically and clinically, lupus nephritis is an extremely pleomorphic disease with the capacity to transform over time. This tremendous diversity of disease expression is evident whether one is comparing renal biopsy findings from different patients or adjacent glomeruli in an individual biopsy. This morphologic heterogeneity posed problems in formulating a pathologic classification of lupus nephritis that was accurate, reproducible, and able to provide information about the disease course and prognosis. Early classifications relied predominantly on glomerular histologic changes, distinguishing between glomerulitis and glomerulonephritis, whereas later schema integrated histologic findings with quantification and location of immune deposits as detected by fluorescence and electron microscopy. The World Health Organization Classification (WHO) and its modified and expanded system developed by the International Study of Kidney Disease of Childhood is currently the formulation most widely accepted by pathologists and clinicians (Tables 42.2 and 42.3). This has markedly improved the uniformity and reproducibility of renal biopsy interpretation. It has also enhanced the development of important clinical pathologic correlations and prognostic correlations, as well as served as a guideline for treatment of lupus nephritis. A limitation of the WHO schema is that it uses only glomerular changes to classify lupus nephritis and does not integrate potentially important information about vascular or tubulointerstitial disease.

TABLE 42.2 Original WHO Classification of Lupus Nephritis

Class I	Normal glomeruli (by LM, IF, EM)
Class II	Purely mesangial disease
	a) Normocellular mesangium by LM but mesangial deposits by IF and/or EM.
	b) Mesangial hypercellularity with mesangial deposits by IF and/or EM.
Class III	Focal segmental proliferative glomerulonephritis
Class IV	Diffuse proliferative glomerulonephritis
Class V	Membranous glomerulonephritis

EM, electron microscopy; IF, immunofluorescence; LM, light microscopy.

TABLE 42.3 Modified WHO Classification of Lupus Nephritis

I. Normal glomeruli (by LM, IF, EM)
II. Pure mesangial alterations
   a) Normal by LM, mesangial deposits by IF and/or EM
   b) Mesangial hypercellularity and deposits by IF and/or EM
III. Focal segmental glomerulonephritis
   a) Active necrotizing lesions
   b) Active and sclerosing lesions
   c) Sclerosing lesions
IV. Diffuse glomerulonephritis (severe mesangial, endocapillary or mesangiocapillary proliferation and/or extensive subendothelial deposits)
   a) Without segmental lesions
   b) With active necrotizing lesions
   c) With active and sclerosing lesions
   d) With sclerosing lesions
V. Diffuse membranous glomerulonephritis
   a) Pure membranous glomerulonephritis
   b) Associated with lesions of category II (a or b)
   c) Associated with focal segmental proliferative lesions (category III)
   d) Associated with diffuse proliferative lesions (category IV)
VI. Advanced sclerosing glomerulonephritis

EM, electron microscopy; IF, immunofluorescence; LM, light microscopy.

Histologic Classes of SLE Nephropathy (See Chapter 109, Atlas of Renal Pathology)

Class I: Normal Biopsies

In class I, the kidneys are entirely normal by light microscopy (LM), immunofluorescence (IF), and electron microscopy (EM). In the literature and in clinical practice, true class I biopsies are rarely observed, because even SLE patients with no detectable clinical renal disease often have evidence of mesangial immune deposits when studied carefully by the more sensitive techniques of IF and EM. The low incidence of class I biopsies is likely also explained by referral bias, because few SLE patients lacking clinically evident renal disease are referred for renal biopsy.

Class II: Pure Mesangial Lesions

Patients with class II biopsies have lesions confined to the mesangium. Class IIa is defined by glomeruli that are normal by LM but have mesangial immune deposits detectable by IF and/or EM. Class IIb biopsies have mild to moderate mesangial hypercellularity with immune deposits limited to the mesangium. Mesangial hypercellularity is generally defined in 3 micron sections as greater than three cells in mesangial regions distant from the vascular pole. All other changes seen in patients with classes III, IV, and V lesions are usually superimposed on a substrate of these mesangial alterations. In the past, some patients with moderate mesangial hypercellularity in a diffuse and global distribution were at times misclassified as diffuse proliferative lupus nephritis (WHO class IV). However, the absence of subendothelial deposits along the peripheral capillary walls as detected by IF and EM distinguishes true class IIb lupus nephritis from class IV lupus nephritis.

Class III: Focal Proliferative Glomerulonephritis

Biopsies from patients with class III lupus nephritis are characterized by predominantly focal and segmental endocapillary proliferation. Mesangial cells, endothelial cells, and infiltrating mononuclear and polymorphonuclear leukocytes may contribute to the glomerular hypercellularity. The glomerular proliferation is arbitrarily defined as involving less than 50% of the total glomerular capillaries. The lesions may be focal and segmental, diffuse and segmental, or focal and global as long as the percentage of total glomerular area involved is less than 50%. Active glomerular lesions in class III lupus nephritis often display fibrinoid necrosis, nuclear pyknosis or karyorrhexis, rupture of the glomerular basement membrane, and leukocyte infiltration. Monoclonal antibody studies have demonstrated infiltration of the tuft by monocytes and T lymphocytes, as well as neutrophils. Crescents may accompany the more active lesions. Hematoxylin bodies consisting of swollen basophilic nuclear material acted upon by antinuclear antibodies, the *in vivo* tissue equivalent of the LE body, may rarely be seen in areas of necrosis. Subendothelial immune deposits are often identifiable histologically as "wire loop" lesions or large intraluminal masses, so-called hyaline thrombi. Glomerular immune deposits are typically present in a focal and segmental subendothelial distribution as well as in the mesangium. By IF, subendothelial wire loop deposits are usually semilinear to granular and at times confluent. Positivity for fibrin-related antigen is common in areas of segmental necrosis and in association with crescents. Less involved neighboring glomeruli may show only mesangial alterations by LM. Chronic lesions are typically characterized by progression to focal segmental and global glomerulosclerosis. Segmental crescents may scar as synechiae between the tuft and Bowman's capsule.

Class IV: Diffuse Proliferative Glomerulonephritis

Patients with diffuse proliferative lupus nephritis have glomerular endocapillary proliferation that is qualitatively similar to that seen in class III biopsies. However, the lesions involve more than 50% of the glomerular capillary surface area in a predominantly diffuse and global distribution. Active lesions may include the histologic features of fibrinoid necrosis, infiltrating leukocytes, wire loop–type subendothelial deposits, hematoxylin bodies, and crescents. In general, the severity of the glomerular changes is greater and the distribution more diffuse than in class III lupus nephritis. By IF and EM, subendothelial immune deposits are found more extensively along the glomerular capillary walls, sometimes associated with positivity for fibrin-related antigens. There are several morphologic variants of class IV lupus nephritis as outlined by the modified WHO classification (Table 42.3) that deserve special mention because they may pose diagnostic problems. These include biopsies with severe mesangial proliferation associated with diffuse subendothelial immune deposits. Another variant of class IV lupus nephritis is characterized by minimal glomerular hypercellularity but extensive subendothelial immune deposits. A third variant manifests prominent membranoproliferative (i.e., mesangiocapillary, which is discussed in Chapter 39, Part 7) features with widespread mesangial interposition and glomerular basement membrane (GBM) double contours resembling idiopathic membranoproliferative glomerulonephritis.

Virtually all the changes found on biopsies of patients with class IV lesions can be found to a lesser extent in biopsies of patients with class III lesions. Therefore many investigators believe that these two classes represent quantitative differences in the same qualitative lesion. In this way, they can be considered closely related entities along a disease continuum. Other workers have suggested that patients with class III biopsies have a different pathogenesis and much more benign prognosis compared with patients who have class IV lesions, especially when the proliferative lesions involve a minority of the glomeruli, are discretely segmental, lack necrotizing features, and have few subendothelial deposits.

Class V: Membranous Nephropathy

Class V lupus nephritis is characterized by numerous subepithelial glomerular immune deposits. In the early stages, there may be no abnormalities detected by LM, but subepithelial deposits can be demonstrated by IF and EM. Well-developed lesions demonstrate thickening of glomerular capillary walls and "spike" formation between the subepithelial deposits. Because most biopsies of patients with membranous lupus have coexistent mesangial hypercellularity and mesangial immune deposits, it is unnecessary and redundant to classify these as a class V and class II combined lesion. The presence of scattered small subendothelial deposits in addition to the membranous changes is not inconsistent with a diagnosis of class V lupus nephritis. However, if there is endocapillary hypercellularity or more widespread subendothelial deposition in addition to the membranous component, a combined diagnosis of classes V and III or classes V and IV is appropriate (classes Vc and Vd, respectively, according to the Modified WHO Classification). It is also not uncommon for occasional scattered subepithelial deposits to occur in other classes of lupus nephritis. Therefore a designation of class V (membranous) lupus nephritis should be reserved only for those patients in which the membranous pattern predominates.

Class VI: Sclerosing Glomerulonephritis

Some biopsies, especially from patients with prior severe renal disease but who are currently inactive, have glomerulonephritis that is predominantly in an extremely advanced, sclerosing phase. In such cases, IF and EM are usually required to establish a diagnosis of SLE by demonstrating residual immune deposits. The modified WHO classification (Table 42.3) has added class VI to categorize these lesions and distinguish them from those with persistent activity.

Immunofluorescence Microscopy

By IF, renal immune deposits typically contain a variety of immunoglobulin and complement components. IgG, the most frequently detected immunoglobulin, is often accompanied by

IgM and IgA. Complement components C3, C1q, and C4, as well as properdin, are also commonly found, indicating both classical and alternative pathway complement activation. Deposits that are often granular in texture may be observed in the glomeruli (in a mesangial, subendothelial, and/or subepithelial location), in the interstitium, along the tubular basement membranes, or in vessel walls. Immune deposits in the tubulointerstitial compartment may consist of immunoglobulin and complement or of complement alone. Active necrotizing lesions and crescents often display strong reactivity for fibrin/fibrinogen. Nuclear staining is commonly observed in renal specimens due to ANA activity of the patient serum binding *in vitro* to nuclei exposed in the course of cryostat sectioning of the frozen tissue sample.

Ultrastructural Features

Renal biopsies of SLE patients from any histologic class may show certain characteristic features by EM in addition to glomerular electron-dense deposits in the locations outlined previously. Numerous intracytoplasmic tubuloreticular inclusions (TRIs) are commonly observed within the cytoplasm of glomerular and vascular endothelial cells. These 24-nm branching tubular structures are located within dilated cisternae of the endoplasmic reticulum. They are not specific for SLE but are inducible upon exposure to α-interferon (so-called interferon footprints) and can be seen in biopsies of patients with human immunodeficiency virus (HIV) and other viral infections. Electron-dense deposits in lupus nephritis sometimes demonstrate a characteristic fingerprint substructure composed of curvilinear parallel arrays measuring 10 to 15 nm in diameter. Subendothelial or intracapillary fibrin tactoids may be seen in cases of active necrotizing glomerulonephritis.

Tubulointerstitial Disease

Although information about tubulointerstitial disease is not used in formulating the WHO classification, tubulointerstitial lesions may be prominent in some biopsies and often correlate well with the degree of renal functional impairment. Active lesions include interstitial edema and inflammatory infiltrates that contain T lymphocytes (including CD4- and CD8-positive cells), monocytes, and plasma cells. Chronic changes include interstitial fibrosis and tubular atrophy. Immune deposits may be seen by IF and/or EM along the tubular basement membranes, along the basement membranes of interstitial capillaries, or in the interstitial connective tissue. Severe acute interstitial changes and tubulointerstitial immune deposits are most commonly found in patients with active class IV lupus nephritis and to a lesser extent in classes III and V. However, there is not a good correlation between the presence of interstitial inflammatory changes and the presence of tubulointerstitial immune deposits. Indeed, some biopsies with severe interstitial inflammation lack any identifiable tubulointerstitial immune deposits.

Vascular Lesions

The vascular lesions of SLE are not factored into either the WHO classification or the activity and chronicity indices, yet they may contribute significantly to renal dysfunction and may influence overall renal survival. Uncomplicated vascular immune deposits are the most common vascular lesion, particularly in patients with active class III and IV lupus nephritis. They are detected by IF and EM as granular immune deposits in the media and intima of small arteries and arterioles, which usually appear normal by LM. A less common vascular lesion consists of a noninflammatory necrotizing vasculopathy that primarily affects arterioles, especially in active class IV lupus nephritis. Involved arterioles are severely narrowed or occluded by fibrinoid deposits without an inflammatory component. A true necrotizing inflammatory arteritis resembling polyarteritis has only rarely been described in biopsies from lupus patients, and it may be systemic or limited to the kidneys. Finally, some patients with SLE may have evidence of a thrombotic microangiopathy involving the interlobular arteries, arterioles, and glomerular capillaries. Some have a thrombocytopenic purpuralike syndrome or evidence of circulating antiphospholipid antibodies.

Activity and Chronicity Indices

Many centers have used a semiquantitative scoring system to grade the renal biopsy's features of activity (i.e., predominantly potentially reversible lesions) and features of chronicity (i.e., those lesions that are irreversible and hence untreatable). The most widely used system computes the sum of scores 0 to 3+ for each of six histologic features of activity, including endocapillary proliferation, glomerular leukocyte infiltration, wire loop deposits, fibrinoid necrosis and karyorrhexis, cellular crescents, and interstitial inflammation (Table 42.4). The individual scores (0 to 3+) for the severe lesions of crescents and fibrinoid necrosis are accorded double weight (i.e., multiplied by 2), giving a total possible Activity Index score of 0 to 24. Features of irreversible renal damage, including glomerulosclerosis, fibrous crescents, tubular atrophy, and interstitial fibrosis, are also graded from 0 to 3+, giving a total possible Chronicity Index of 0 to 12. Workers at the NIH have correlated a high Activity Index (greater than 12) and especially a high Chronicity Index (greater than 4) with a poor long-term renal survival. Others have not been able to confirm the prognostic value of these scoring systems in either large populations of lupus patients representing all WHO classes or even in series limited to WHO class IV. Nevertheless, in the individual patient, these indices may be of value, especially when comparing sequential biopsies. Thus the findings of persistent or worsening activity despite ongoing therapy may favor a change in treatment. Likewise, a major decline in activity on repeat biopsy is reassuring if discontinuation of vigorous treatment is being considered. Finally, increasing chronicity on repeat biopsy can document progressive renal damage not reflected in measurements of serum creatinine or even the creatinine clearance. Additional studies at the NIH suggest the combination of elevated Activity Index

TABLE 42.4 Activity and Chronicity Index

Indices of Activity
Endocapillary hypercellularity Leukocyte Infiltration Subendothelial hyaline deposits Necrosis/karyorrhexis Cellular crescents Interstitial inflammation
Indices of Chronicity
Sclerotic glomeruli Fibrous crescents Tubular atrophy Interstitial fibrosis

Modified from Austin HA, Muenz LR, Joyce KM, et al. Diffuse proliferative lupus nephritis: identification of specific pathologic features affecting renal outcome. *Kidney Int* 1984;25:689–695.
EM, electron microscopy; IF, immunofluorescence; LM, light microscopy.

(greater than 7) and an elevated Chronicity Index (greater than 3) or the combination of cellular crescents and interstitial fibrosis on renal biopsy predicts a poor long-term prognosis in patients with severe lupus nephritis.

LABORATORY FINDINGS

The clinical laboratory tests play an important role in SLE in three areas: (a) initial diagnosis of SLE, (b) initial evaluation of renal disease, and (c) follow-up evaluation of remission, relapse, and response to therapy.

As mentioned, 4 of the 11 criteria used in the diagnosis of SLE are laboratory findings: (a) abnormal urinalysis, (b) abnormal blood counts, (c) positive lupus erythematosus (LE) cell tests or antinative DNA antibody or anti-Sm antibody or false-positive serologic tests for syphilis, and (d) positive antinuclear antibody. Indeed, a diagnosis of SLE can be made with a reasonable degree of certainty by clinical laboratory testing in a patient with overt renal disease even in the absence of extrarenal symptoms or signs of SLE. Patients with lupus nephritis may initially present with only abnormal urinalysis and abnormal serologic test results. On the other hand, as many as 10% of patients who fulfill the clinical criteria for the diagnosis of SLE may fail to display abnormal serologic findings (ANA-negative SLE).

In the usual patient with SLE, the fluorescent antinuclear antibody (FANA) test is positive with a titer exceeding 1:80. Unfortunately, the low specificity of the FANA (60% to 70%) for SLE often requires additional confirmatory tests, especially in patients with atypical manifestations and/or a prior history of ingestion of drugs known to provoke false-positive FANA results. The most useful confirmatory test is the assay for circulating antibodies to native or double-stranded (ds) DNA. Such antibodies are found in about 70% of untreated patients with SLE. Anti-Sm antibody is more specific for SLE, but it has low sensitivity and therefore is of limited diagnostic value. Testing for antibodies to single-stranded (ss) DNA or to ribonuclear antigens (anti-Ro/SSA, anti-La/SSB, anti-RNP) may be of value in patients with negative FANA findings or those with atypical or overlap syndrome (i.e., mixed connective tissue disease; Part 2 of this chapter) or those with a history of drug ingestion that can cause false-positive FANA findings. Patients with overt renal disease who have both a high titer of FANA and anti-ds DNA antibody can be regarded as having SLE until proven otherwise.

Abnormalities in serum complement values are often observed in patients with SLE, especially in those with active lupus nephritis, dermatitis, or cerebral involvement. These abnormalities may be either congenital or acquired. The most common pattern of these acquired changes is reduced levels of C3, C4, and CH50; however, in patients with congenital complement deficiency, CH50 level may be reduced while C3 and C4 values remain normal. Testing for complement abnormalities has only limited diagnostic usefulness because of its low sensitivity and specificity.

Other serologic abnormalities, such as antiphospholipid antibodies, rheumatoid factor, cryoglobulins, and circulating immune complexes, have limited diagnostic usefulness because of their variable sensitivity and specificity for SLE. Antibodies to C1q are highly correlated with active lupus nephritis.

Urinalysis is the most important test for the initial evaluation of renal involvement in a patient known to have SLE or suspected of having the disease. The abnormalities in urinalysis vary widely, from isolated hematuria to heavy proteinuria accompanied by florid nephritic urinary sediment (i.e., hematuria, leukocyturia, and cellular and erythrocyte casts). Abnormal urinalysis may be found even in a patient who has mild renal involvement. Quantitation of urinary protein excretion is a valuable initial step in assessing renal disease, because the presence of nephrotic-range proteinuria (greater than 3.5 g/24 hr) points toward an underlying membranous or proliferative glomerulonephritis. The selectivity of proteinuria is poor, with large amounts of IgG and other high-molecular-weight proteins present in the urine.

Measurement of renal function by serum creatinine levels or by creatinine clearance is useful. However, a normal result may still be accompanied by significant underlying renal disease.

CLINICAL MANIFESTATIONS

The clinical manifestations of kidney involvement in SLE are as varied as the corresponding renal pathologic lesions. It is rare for patients to present with severe lupus nephritis as the initial manifestation of SLE. Renal involvement typically develops concurrently with or following other systemic manifestations of the disease. It most often follows a chronic course with periods of remission and recrudescence. Although some patients will have prominent tubulointerstitial or vascular lesions of lupus nephritis, there is usually a good correlation between the clinical renal involvement and the degree of glomerular involvement in SLE.

It is unusual to find a patient who fulfills the ARA criteria for SLE and who has a totally normal renal biopsy by LM, IF, and EM (WHO class I). Such patients will have no evidence of clinical renal disease. It is likely that most SLE patients with mild or no clinical renal disease and who never undergo renal biopsy and certainly most of those who have renal biopsy would display mesangial glomerular lesions (WHO class II). Patients with class II lupus nephritis may have active serologic tests for SLE (e.g., a high anti-DNA antibody titer and low serum complement) but typically have mild clinical renal involvement. They usually have inactive urinary sediment, mild proteinuria (usually less than 1 g/24 hr), and a normal serum creatinine and glomerular filtration rate (GFR). It is rare for class II patients to have a significantly elevated serum creatinine, and nephrotic-range proteinuria (more than 3 g/24 hr) is virtually never found. Hypertension occurs in a minority of cases and is usually easily controlled.

Patients with class III, focal and segmental proliferative, lupus nephritis often present with active lupus serology, active urinary sediment, and proteinuria. One-fourth to one-third will have nephrotic syndrome at presentation. Hypertension is not uncommon, and a reduced GFR and elevated serum creatinine are present in up to one-fourth of patients at the time of renal biopsy. The degree of clinical renal involvement usually parallels the extent and severity of the glomerular involvement. However, the degree of serologic activity does not necessarily correlate with the severity or activity of the glomerulonephritis.

Patients with WHO class IV, diffuse proliferative, lupus nephritis comprise the largest group of biopsied patients with SLE in most series. They present with the most active clinical nephritis and positive lupus serologies, with high anti-DNA antibody titers and low serum complement levels. They typically have very active urinary sediment, with erythrocytes, red cell casts, and other casts present on urinalysis, as well as proteinuria that is often in the nephrotic range. Hypertension is found in more than half of these patients, and a decreased GFR is usually present even when the serum creatinine appears normal for the laboratory standards.

Although patients with membranous lupus nephropathy (WHO class V) comprise from 10% to 25% of biopsied lupus patients, until recently they have been underrepresented in the literature. Patients with membranous lupus nephropathy typically have proteinuria, and about 60% will present with nephrotic syndrome as their major clinical manifestation. Although active urine sediment, hypertension, and renal dysfunction may occur, these features are often overshadowed by the degree of proteinuria and its manifestations. Lupus serologies may or may not be positive. The clinical presentation of lupus membranous nephropathy often has distinctive features. Some patients are considerably older than the average patient presenting with other WHO classes of lupus nephritis. Membranous lupus patients may also have heavy proteinuria and nephrotic syndrome *before* developing other manifestations of SLE. In such cases, the renal biopsy findings of mesangial immune deposits, endothelial tubuloreticular inclusions, and in some cases, tubulointerstitial or small subendothelial deposits are helpful in differentiating lupus from idiopathic membranous glomerulopathy. Some patients with membranous lupus nephritis develop pulmonary emboli as a consequence of renal vein thrombosis with symptoms of cough, hemoptysis, and shortness of breath as an initial manifestation of their disease. Lupus patients may have mixed lesions consisting of a membranous component combined with a focal or diffuse proliferative glomerulonephritis. In general, their symptoms will reflect the presence of both lesions, with heavy proteinuria as well as active clinical renal disease.

Patients with class VI sclerosing glomerulonephritis usually have had a prolonged course of treatment spanning many years, with repeated lupus flare-ups, punctuated by periods of inactivity. They may continue to manifest microhematuria and proteinuria, usually less than 3 g/24 hr, despite the absence of active lesions on biopsy. Hypertension and a decreased GFR are common, but lupus serologies are usually negative.

Monitoring Clinical Disease

The course of lupus nephritis is typically characterized by flares of activity, remissions, and relapses. It is important in the management of lupus patients to be able to predict clinical and renal relapses and minimize their injurious effect through the judicious use of immunosuppressive agents. Although measurement of many laboratory tests for clinical activity (including anti-ds DNA, complement components, erythrocyte sedimentation rate, C-reactive protein, circulating immune complexes, and levels of cytokines and interleukins) have been followed in the course of the disease, the levels of anti-DNA antibody and the total serum complement (CH_{50}) remain the two most useful measures of disease activity. Circulating serum levels of DNA antibody typically rise as the clinical activity of SLE increases and usually before there is a clinical renal deterioration. Likewise, serum CH_{50} total hemolytic complement levels typically decline preceding or concurrent with the onset of active clinical disease. Increases in the activity of the urine sediment may be helpful if the urine is examined by an experienced clinician and if baseline values are available for comparison. An increase in proteinuria from levels of less than 1 g/24 hr to more than this amount and certainly from low to nephrotic levels is a clear indication of either increased activity or a change in renal histologic class.

Silent Lupus Nephritis

Rarely, patients will have no clinical evidence of renal involvement despite the findings of severe glomerular lesions on renal biopsy. Although so-called silent lupus nephritis has been described in several series of patients, many investigators have been unable to document a single case of biopsy-proven diffuse proliferative lupus nephritis that meets the criteria for true silent renal disease: inactive urinary sediment, absence of proteinuria, and normal GFR. Cases of silent lupus nephritis with negative lupus serologies are even less commonly described. Thus, although silent lupus nephritis may exist, biopsies of lupus patients without clinical renal findings will usually show mesangial or very mild focal proliferative lesions and only extremely rarely more active and severe diffuse proliferative lesions.

Transformations

During the course of lupus nephritis, the histologic pattern on renal biopsy may transform from one WHO class to another. This occurs in 15% to 40% of rebiopsied patients. Clearly, if all patients were rebiopsied, the incidence would be much higher. Some patients with mesangial or mild focal proliferative lesions may develop increased renal activity over time, heralded by increased activity of the urinary sediment, worsening proteinuria (often reaching nephrotic levels), and hypertension. On rebiopsy, such patients may display class IV lesions. Patients with membranous lupus may also develop clinical activity and on rebiopsy transform to a superimposed class III plus V or a predominant class IV lesion. Cases of diffuse proliferative or severe focal proliferative lupus nephritis may respond to therapy, with subsequent resolution of endocapillary proliferation and subendothelial deposits. Lesions of glomerular endocapillary proliferation, interstitial inflammation, and edema may resolve while areas of glomerular necrosis and crescents inevitably scar, producing foci of glomerulosclerosis and fibrous crescents. Some cases of class IV lupus nephritis develop inactive mesangial proliferative and sclerosing lesions after treatment. Other patients with an initial biopsy described as class III or IV but showing both subendothelial and subepithelial deposits may transform from an active proliferative lesion (class III or IV) into a membranous pattern (class V) after treatment. This transformation is consistent with the observation that subepithelial deposits tend to resorb less readily than subendothelial deposits. Thus lupus nephritis may undergo both transformations in class as well as alterations in activity and chronicity, which may occur spontaneously or subsequent to treatment. It is unusual for these morphologic transformations to occur very rapidly; therefore renal biopsies need only rarely be repeated at less than 6-month intervals.

Pregnancy and SLE

Pregnancy in an SLE patient poses unique problems for both mother and fetus. Some problems are independent of renal involvement, such as the frequent miscarriages seen in patients with antiphospholipid antibodies. The offspring of lupus mothers with high titer of anti-Ro antibodies may be born with heart block. Data are conflicting regarding the risks that pregnancy will initiate flares of SLE, especially in the third trimester or postpartum period. In general, for patients with SLE that has been quiescent for at least a year and who have a normal GFR and are normotensive, the chances are excellent for a healthy child and mother. If proteinuria has been present before pregnancy, it is likely to worsen during pregnancy, often associated with edema. Hypertension, when present, is also likely to be exacerbated by pregnancy. Worsening of hypertension should be treated aggressively. Although there are conflicting data in the literature, patients with clinical and serologic activity at the time they become pregnant or early in the pregnancy have the worst fetal outcomes. Moreover, this population and those with a significantly elevated serum creatinine are most likely to develop maternal renal damage. Although high-dose glucocorticoids and azathioprine have been used during pregnancy, cyclophosphamide is relatively contraindicated, making the management of some patients with very active renal involvement even more difficult.

Pregnancy should not be prohibited in women with lupus nephritis, but risks to the mother and fetus should be discussed thoroughly with the patients. In general, termination of pregnancy is not indicated in lupus patients unless the disease poses a life-threatening situation to the mother that does not respond to appropriate therapy.

Many believe that intensification of glucocorticoid therapy in the immediate postpartum period is advisable to prevent exacerbation of the disease.

Vascular Lesions

Involvement of the renal vasculature in SLE is not uncommon and may take a number of different patterns. Evidence for immune complex deposition in the walls of vessels of the arterial and venous tree are common and usually lack clinical manifestations. A noninflammatory necrotizing vasculopathy involving arteries and arterioles (i.e., "lupus vasculopathy") is a lesion that typically occurs in the setting of active class IV lupus nephritis and is often complicated by severe hypertension and renal insufficiency. True inflammatory necrotizing vasculitis like that seen in microscopic polyarteritis (polyangiitis) rarely occurs in SLE patients and is usually associated with severe hypertension and progressive renal functional deterioration. An important and not uncommon vascular lesion in lupus nephritis is thrombotic microangiopathy, which may involve glomerular capillaries as well as arterioles and small arteries. Although intravascular coagulation at the level of the glomerular capillaries is commonly observed in active necrotizing glomerulonephritis, this feature of severe diffuse or focal proliferative lupus nephritis must be distinguished from cases of thrombotic microangiopathy lacking clinical or histologic evidence of active lupus nephritis. Some such patients will fulfill the criteria for thrombotic thrombocytopenic purpura or a hemolytic uremic syndrome complicating SLE. They will have the presence of microthrombotic renal involvement (often without evidence of severe proliferation or subendothelial immune deposits), central nervous system (CNS) disease, fever, microangiopathic hemolytic anemia, and thrombocytopenia in the presence of normal coagulation studies and absence of antiphospholipid antibodies. Another subset of patients with thrombotic microangiopathy prove to have circulating antiphospholipid antibodies. Although 40% to 75% of all SLE patients have evidence of antiphospholipid antibodies, most of these never develop clinically evident thrombotic complications. Antiphospholipid antibodies may be detected by a variety of assays [anticardiolipin antibodies by enzyme-linked immunosorbent assay (ELISA) or (RIA)], by biologic false positive tests for syphilis, and by interference with standard coagulation tests leading to a high activated partial thromboplastin time (i.e., the lupus anticoagulant). Some patients with high titers of these antibodies will develop the full antiphospholipid syndrome, with livedo reticularis, spontaneous abortions, neurologic symptoms ranging from memory loss to strokes and seizures, thrombocytopenia, and a predisposition to major arterial and venous thromboses. Thrombotic microangiopathy involving interlobular arteries, arterioles, and glomerular capillaries in the absence of active lupus nephritis (WHO class III or IV) has been described in this population.

TREATMENT

Despite numerous controlled and uncontrolled treatment trials, the therapy of lupus nephritis remains controversial. In part, this is because of the variable nature of the renal histopathology, the chronic course of the disease with periods of exacerbation and remissions, and the myriad conflicting studies dealing with treatment issues. Therapy can be simplified if the WHO classification is used as a treatment guide as shown in Table 42.5.

TABLE 42.5 Treatment of Lupus Nephritis by WHO Class

Class I:	Treat extrarenal manifestations.
Class II:	Treat extrarenal manifestations. If increased clinical activity, rebiopsy and treat appropriately for change in class.
Class III:	For mild lesions, initiate therapy with glucocorticoids. For severe lesions, treat as class IV.
Class IV:	Initiate vigorous immunosuppressive therapy.
Class V:	Initially, use glucocorticoid therapy to obtain serologic remission and remission of nephrotic syndrome, especially in those with heavy proteinuria and progressive renal failure. If no response, either no further treatment or use other agents depending on clinical situation.[a]

[a] Some believe that class V lupus nephritis does not require an aggressive immunosuppressive therapy. Treatment of extrarenal manifestation and hypertension may suffice.

In general, those rare patients with normal renal biopsies (class I) and those with mesangial lesions (class II) need be treated only for extrarenal manifestations of SLE. If a patient develops greater renal involvement with increasing proteinuria or more active urinary sediment, a repeat biopsy can be performed and the patient treated appropriately. Patients with class III lesions may respond to a brief trial of high-dose glucocorticoids (vide infra), especially if the active lesions are limited to small segments of few glomeruli and the glomeruli do not contain necrotizing features, cellular crescents, or extensive subendothelial deposits. Most clinicians would advocate treating class III patients with more active lesions in the same way as class IV patients. There is universal agreement that patients with diffuse proliferative lesions warrant the most vigorous treatment efforts to prevent irreversible renal damage. For patients with membranous lupus nephropathy, there have been conflicting data regarding the course, prognosis, and response to treatment. Many patients with class V lupus nephritis will have a prolonged course of heavy proteinuria and nephrotic syndrome, and some will progress to end-stage renal disease. Patients with severe unremitting nephrotic syndrome and renal insufficiency are at particular risk for progression. Certainly, for patients at high risk for progressive renal damage, therapy designed to induce a remission of nephrotic syndrome and stabilize renal function is warranted. For patients with a benign prognosis, some investigators use only a brief trial of steroids alone. However, in several series, membranous patients with superimposed proliferative disease developed progressive renal failure over the long term and therefore deserve vigorous treatment modalities (e.g., cyclophosphamide, cyclosporine). Trials at the NIH have randomized patients with membranous lupus nephropathy to intravenous cyclophosphamide, corticosteroids, or cyclosporine therapy. All study arms have appeared effective in inducing remissions of nephrotic syndrome, but the relapse rate when the drugs are discontinued in this preliminary study appears highest with cyclosporine.

Therapy for active class IV diffuse proliferative nephritis has included a vast array of immunosuppressive and antiinflammatory medications such as high-dose daily or alternate-day glucocorticoids, azathioprine, nitrogen mustard, intravenous pulse methylprednisolone, plasmapheresis, oral or intravenous cyclophosphamide, cyclosporine, and other less well-studied treatment modalities such as ancrod, total lymphoid irradiation, thromboxane inhibitors, and intravenous gammaglobulin

TABLE 42.6 Vigorous Therapy of Lupus Nephritis
Daily glucocorticoids
Alternate-day high-dose glucocorticoids
Azathioprine
Plasmapheresis
Nitrogen mustard
Oral cyclophosphamide
Intravenous pulse glucocorticoids
Intravenous cyclophosphamide
Cyclosporine
Ancrod, thromboxane antagonists, intravenous gammaglobulin
Mycophenolate mofetil, LJP 394, Bindarit, anti-CD40 ligand
Bone marrow transplant

(Table 42.6). Few modalities have been shown to be effective in well-controlled trials; none is without major potential side effects, and no modality is uniformly effective. Newer therapeutic agents, including mycophenolate mofetil, LJP 394, Bindarit, and monoclonal antibodies such as anti-CD40 ligand, are currently under study.

Despite the consensus that high-dose glucocorticoids (prednisone 1 mg/kg per day initially, followed after 4 to 6 weeks by 2 mg/kg given on alternate days) is effective therapy for severe lupus nephritis, there are no controlled trials documenting its efficacy. In early trials in the 1950s and 1960s, low-dose therapy was not effective in halting the progression of active severe lupus nephritis, and when compared with retrospective controls, high-dose treatment proved more efficacious. Some clinicians still use initial glucocorticoid treatment for severe lupus nephritis, reserving other immunosuppressives for patients who fail to respond to several months of therapy or who have evidence of rapid clinical progression of renal disease. Others initiate therapy immediately with the alternative agents described next, either because they believe them to be more effective in preventing renal failure or because they wish to avoid the side effects of chronic glucocorticoid therapy. High-dose oral alternate-day glucocorticoids (in doses up to 250 mg every other day) have been used to provide effective treatment without the side effects of high-dose daily glucocorticoids. Controlled trials, however, have not been performed with this regimen. The use of a second immunosuppressive agents such as azathioprine or nitrogen mustard in conjunction with glucocorticoids has proved an effective steroid-sparing regimen in many patients. However, newer data suggest, but do not prove, that glucocorticoids or steroids plus azathioprine may not be an optimal therapy for severe lupus nephritis (vide infra).

Plasmapheresis in combination with a number of other treatments has enjoyed anecdotal success in severe lupus nephritis. Some patients have experienced correction of active serology and remissions of severe clinical and histologic renal disease. However, a large, controlled trial of more than 80 patients randomized to standard therapy with steroids and cytotoxics or standard therapy plus plasmapheresis showed no benefit for the plasmapheresis group with respect to clinical activity, renal survival, or patient survival. Although this study was criticized for less vigorous "standard" therapy than is given currently by many clinicians and although the patient population appears to have had worse initial renal function than many other study groups, the results nonetheless suggest that plasmapheresis should not be used as routine therapy for severe lupus nephritis. Whether there is a role for plasmapheresis in certain patients (e.g., those who failed other treatment modalities, patients with a thrombocytopenic purpuralike syndrome) remains to be proven.

Pulse methylprednisolone was first used in lupus nephritis in the 1970s. Adapting a regimen that was effective for acute transplant rejection, three consecutive daily intravenous doses of 1 g of methylprednisolone were given over 30 to 60 minutes to patients with diffuse proliferative disease and deteriorating renal function. Renal parameters markedly improved, with GFRs returning toward normal in a matter of days. In patients with persistently active glomerulonephritis, the initial pulse therapy may be followed by a single dose given monthly for 6 to 12 months. Subsequent reports used a variety of pulse glucocorticoid regimens with or without other immunosuppressive agents with favorable but anecdotal results. A large, retrospective analysis of 34 patients treated with pulse glucocorticoids plus other agents showed that fewer than one-third had a favorable course, with a 20% decrease in plasma creatinine within 2 months. Patients who responded to treatment included those with more active proliferative lesions on biopsy, those with recent deterioration of their GFR, and those with the most positive lupus serologies. A controlled, randomized trial at the NIH showed that pulse steroids were not as effective as monthly intravenous cyclophosphamide in preventing a doubling of the serum creatinine over 5 years in patients with severe proliferative disease. Monthly pulse intravenous methylprednisolone has proven effective when used with intravenous cyclophosphamide, but there is a higher incidence of side effects with such combination regimens.

Several early studies on the use of oral cyclophosphamide could not prove that it was more effective than high-dose glucocorticoids in preventing renal failure. Nevertheless, in one well-performed study of 50 patients with diffuse proliferative disease, the group receiving cyclophosphamide experienced fewer flares of renal activity over the course of 4 years, suggesting the potential for improved long-term renal survival. Subsequent studies at the NIH examined five treatment regimens in severe lupus nephritis: high-dose oral glucocorticoids for 6 months, oral cyclophosphamide, oral azathioprine, combined oral azathioprine plus oral cyclophosphamide, and intravenous cyclophosphamide (up to 1 g/m^2 every third month), all given with low-dose glucocorticoids. After 120 months of follow-up, there was a significant improvement in renal survival in the intravenous cyclophosphamide–treated group compared with the steroid only–treated group. Moreover, side effects of treatment seemed least severe and troublesome in the intravenous cyclophosphamide–treated group. At 200 months of follow-up of the same population, the azathioprine-treated patients were now statistically no better in terms of renal survival than the glucocorticoid only–treated group. However, overall patient survival was not measurably improved by the more aggressive immunosuppressive regimens. Another study at the NIH recently compared three treatment regimens in diffuse proliferative lupus nephritis patients: monthly pulse methylprednisolone, monthly intravenous cyclophosphamide for 6 months, and monthly intravenous cyclophosphamide for 6 months followed by every third month continued treatment. At more than 5 years of follow-up, almost half of the pulse steroid–treated patients doubled their serum creatinine in comparison to only about one-fourth of the cyclophosphamide-treated groups. Relapses were less common in the group receiving long-term cyclophosphamide therapy. We and others have achieved similar favorable long-term results with monthly intravenous cyclophosphamide in conjunction with a high-dose tapering regimen of glucocorticoids in similar populations of severe lupus nephritis patients followed long term. Moreover, noting a high incidence of relapses at 6 to 12 months after therapy, we also have followed the initial six monthly pulses with an every third month follow-up dose for three or more doses.

Current pulse cyclophosphamide therapy includes a single dose of 0.5 to 1.0 g/m^2 given monthly for 6 to 12 months to be followed by a single dose every 3 months until remission has been achieved for about 12 months. Some investigators replace cyclophosphamide with another immunosuppressive, such as oral azathioprine or mycophenolate mofetil, after six monthly intravenous cyclophosphamide doses to avoid potential toxic side effects. In our population of more than 75 patients treated with monthly pulse cyclophosphamide and in other reported series, hemorrhagic cystitis has not been a complication of this regimen of intravenous cyclophosphamide, and so far, no tumors have been noted. Complications such as infections, alopecia, and infertility are usually transient, but permanent premature menopause in older females treated with this regimen may limit its usefulness. An additional study from the NIH examined issues of efficacy and potential side effects in severe lupus nephritis. Patients were randomized to either monthly pulses of intravenous methylprednisolone versus monthly intravenous cyclophosphamide, versus a combination of both therapies. The remission rate was highest in the combination therapy group but so were the infectious and overall side effects. Thus many clinicians still favor pulse intravenous cyclophosphamide as first-line therapy for severe lupus nephritis, reserving the combination therapy for resistant cases or those at lowest risk from the potential complications of treatment.

Not all investigators believe the promising results obtained with intravenous cyclophosphamide can be attributed to the immunosuppression alone, but should also be attributed to improved medical management of hypertension, hyperlipidemia, and the metabolic and infectious complications of SLE.

Other therapies used in patients with lupus nephritis include cyclosporine, total lymphoid irradiation, ancrod, thromboxane antagonists, and intravenous gammaglobulin. None has been proven effective in controlled trials or been used in large numbers of patients. Low-dose cyclosporine (4 to 6 mg/kg per day) administered with a variety of other immunosuppressive agents has been used in uncontrolled trials in more than 100 SLE patients. One most promising report describes 26 patients with lupus nephritis resistant to other forms of treatment. The response to 2 years of cyclosporine plus tapering glucocorticoids was dramatic in terms of improvements in lupus serology, clinical activity, proteinuria, and renal histology. Moreover, there was no increase in serum creatinine after 2 years of treatment with this potentially nephrotoxic medication. We have had similar favorable results in a 2-year trial of cyclosporine therapy in patients with membranous lupus nephropathy. Ancrod, pit-viper venom, used in one series of patients with severe lupus nephritis did not appear to give impressive results when compared with other therapies available today. Total lymphoid irradiation has also been used in one series of patients, but more data about the long-term course of the patients are needed before further trials should be undertaken. Intravenous thromboxane antagonists have resulted in a transient improvement in GFR and renal blood flow in a small group of lupus patients. Whether this can be sustained by oral therapy and whether complete blockade of thromboxane synthesis is feasible with oral treatment remains to be proven. Although intravenous gammaglobulin has been used in SLE patients to treat thrombocytopenia and other lupus manifestations, more data about the effects of this therapy on renal function and histology are needed.

Mycophenolate mofetil, an inhibitor of *de novo* purine synthesis, is widely used in transplantation as a potentially more effective immunosuppressant than azathioprine. It has been used in several small series of patients with SLE who either failed standard therapy or were developing intolerable side effects of standard therapy. At dosages lower than used in transplantation (e.g., 250 to 1,000 mg twice daily), it led to decreased proteinuria and remission of clinical renal disease in these small uncontrolled trials. In humans with SLE, active renal lesions correlate with high levels of the beta chemokine, monocyte chemoattractant protein 1. Bindarit, a novel immunosuppressant that selectively inhibits this chemokine, has led to remission of clinical and histologic disease in animal models of SLE. Likewise, LJP 394, an intravenous agent that prevents anti-DNA antibody production, and anti-CD40 ligand, a potent immunosuppressant that interferes with B cell–T cell communication, have both proven useful in experimental animal models of lupus nephritis. All three of these agents are undergoing clinical trials in lupus nephritis patients. Preliminary results of LJP 394 study have been encouraging.

Preliminary results using high-dose chemotherapy and bone marrow transplantation in patients with severe, therapy-resistant lupus nephritis are very encouraging, but further trials are needed to fully evaluate this risky and expensive modality.

Antiphospholipid antibodies are present in 40% to 75% of lupus patients. Because most patients do not experience thrombotic complications, it is clear that many require no prophylaxis against large vessel and microvascular thromboses. In patients who experience a thrombotic event, most investigators favor chronic anticoagulation with warfarin as long as antiphospholipid antibody titers remain high. In patients with high titers of antiphospholipid antibody without a documented thrombotic event, some still favor full anticoagulation, whereas others use one aspirin daily or no specific therapy. The titer of the antiphospholipid antibody often does not correlate with other lupus serologic activity (anti-DNA antibody titer and serum complement) and therefore must be monitored individually.

COURSE AND OUTCOME

The course of patients with lupus nephritis is complicated by episodic exacerbations and remissions, transitions in histology, modification by treatment, and intercurrent illnesses. Patients with mesangial lesions (whether class IIa or IIb) have generally had a very favorable long-term renal prognosis. Progression to renal failure is extremely uncommon unless they transform to a more active class of lupus nephritis.

Patients with WHO class III focal proliferative lupus nephritis have a variable course. Those patients with small areas of mild segmental involvement without necrosis, crescents, or large amounts of subendothelial immune deposits have a benign long-term prognosis. Those with numerous necrotizing lesions and focal crescent formation have a prognosis akin to patients with diffuse proliferative lesions. In virtually all series, patients with class IV lesions have the most unfavorable renal and patient survival. In part, the poorer patient survival reflects the severe complications that may occur in this ill population subjected to vigorous immunosuppression. The 5-year renal survival for this groups still varies from 60% with older regimens to more than 90% with newer treatment modalities and better supportive care. Data from the NIH and other investigators suggests that approximately one-fourth of patients with class IV lesions will double their serum creatinine at 5 years. This is the population at highest risk for renal failure at longer follow-up. It is also clear that many patients with nephrotic syndrome, renal insufficiency, and severe active lesions on biopsy may go into remission with a variety of therapies and remain free of active disease long after major immunosuppressive treatment has been discontinued.

Several studies have clarified those factors in severe proliferative lupus nephritis that correlate with long-term renal outcome. Factors correlating with a poor prognosis include African-American race, elevated serum creatinine, increased proteinuria, anemia, increased combined Activity Index (greater than 7) and Chronicity Index (greater than 3), and the combination of cellular crescents and interstitial fibrosis on renal biopsy. The presence of renal flares of activity during the course of SLE in one study led to a sevenfold increase in long-term renal failure, while "nephritic" flares with an acute rise in serum creatinine led to a 27-fold increase in renal failure.

Patients with class V lesions have not been studied extensively in comparative treatment trials. Five-year renal survival is 85% to 95% and is most favorable in those patients who experience a remission of nephrotic syndrome. Without vigorous immunosuppressive regimens, some investigators have found lower survival rates, especially among patients with persistent nephrotic syndrome. Others have reported far more favorable results with 90% 10-year survival rates in patients treated with vigorous immunosuppression. When treated with short-term anticoagulation, the presence of renal vein thrombosis does not appear to adversely affect the long-term course of membranous lupus patients. African-American race, increased levels of proteinuria, elevated serum creatinine, and superimposed proliferative lupus lesions have all been associated with a poor prognosis. Transition to a pattern with superimposed proliferative lesions (classes V and III or classes V and IV) clearly adversely influences prognosis.

Vascular lesions are common in lupus patients and the influence of these lesions on the outcome of lupus nephritis has also been studied. A study of more than 200 lupus patients found that patients without vascular lesions had a 90% 5-year survival, whereas patients with vascular lesions had only a 68% to 80% survival. Patients with fibrinoid necrotizing vasculopathy and true vasculitis had the most unfavorable outcomes. Involvement of the tubulointerstitial compartment also correlates with outcome and renal survival. Patients with more severe interstitial inflammation and fibrosis are more likely to have elevated serum creatinines and hypertension and experience progressive renal insufficiency over time. The presence of interstitial and tubular immune deposits, however, does not correlate with renal function or renal outcome.

END-STAGE RENAL DISEASE IN LUPUS PATIENTS

Whether due to noncompliance with treatment, intercurrent infections requiring interruption of treatment, or treatment failures, some patient with lupus nephritis will develop end-stage renal disease. Some patients, when maintained on hemodialysis or peritoneal dialysis, may become clinically and serologically inactive. A small group of patients will retain serologic activity despite the absence of clinical symptoms of SLE; they require no treatment for their laboratory abnormalities. Finally, occasional patients will have serologic activity and clinical signs of active SLE despite prolonged dialysis. These patients rarely have major organ involvement, and symptoms usually resolve with low dosages of glucocorticoids or other immunosuppressives. There are reports of lupus patients with end-stage renal disease who when treated with dialysis therapy recover adequate renal function after several months to permit their survival without dialysis. In the end-stage renal disease population with lupus, mortality is greatest during the first 3 months of dialysis and can be attributed largely to infectious complications. The prognosis for survival beyond this point is no different from that for other dialysis populations. Renal allograft survival in SLE patients is comparable to the general transplant population. Lupus nephritis rarely recurs in the allograft (less than 2%), with fewer than two dozen documented recurrences. Most clinicians allow 6 to 12 months of clinical and serologic inactivity before proceeding to transplantation in patients with lupus nephritis.

Selected Readings

Appel GB, Pirani CL, D'Agati VD. Renal vascular involvement in systemic lupus. *J Am Soc Nephrol* 1994;4:1499–1515.

An in-depth review of the pathology and clinicopathologic correlations of the vascular lesions found in lupus patients. Includes review of coagulation abnormalities and the antiphospholipid syndrome.

Appel GB, Valeri A. The course and treatment of lupus nephritis. *Adv Intern Med* 1994;45:525–537.

An analysis of the clinical features and clinicopathologic correlations and course of lupus patients using the WHO classification.

Austin HA, Balow J. Natural history and treatment of lupus nephritis. *Semin Nephrol* 1999;19:2–11.

A review of treatment approaches and prognostic features in lupus nephritis.

Austin HA, Boumpas DT, Vaughan EM, et al. Predicting renal outcomes in severe lupus nephritis: contributions of clinical and histologic data. *Kidney Int* 1994;43:544–550.

An analysis of prognostic clinical and histologic features predicting renal outcome in 65 patients with severe lupus nephritis all receiving therapy with either intravenous methylprednisolone or cyclophosphamide.

Balow JE, Boumpas DT, Fessler BJ, et al. Management of lupus nephritis. *Kidney Int* 1996;49(Suppl):S88–S92.

A review of the therapy of lupus nephritis.

Bansal VK, Beto JA. Treatment of Lupus nephritis: a meta-analysis of clinical trials. *Am J Kidney Dis* 1997;29:193–199.

A meta-analysis of 19 prospective controlled trials of severe lupus nephritis showing the advantages of immunosuppressive agents over glucocorticoids.

Boumpas DT, Austin HA, Vaughn EM, et al. Controlled trial of pulse methylprednisolone versus two regimens of cyclophosphamide in severe lupus nephritis. *Lancet* 1992;340:741–745.

A randomized controlled trial of monthly high-dose intravenous methylprednisolone versus monthly intravenous cyclophosphamide treatment of two different durations.

Cheigh JS, Stenzel KH. End-stage renal disease in systemic lupus erythematosus. *Am J Kidney Dis* 1993;21:2–8.

An in-depth review of lupus patients who have developed end-stage renal disease, including their course on dialysis and with renal transplantation.

D'Agati VD. Renal disease in systemic lupus erythematosus, mixed connective tissue disease, Sjogren's syndrome and rheumatoid arthritis. In: Jennette JC, Olson JL, Schwartz MM, et al, eds. *Heptinstall's pathology of the kidney,* 5th ed. Philadelphia: Lippincott-Raven, 1998:541–624.

A detailed review of the morphologic features of lupus nephritis with clinicopathologic correlations.

Donadio JV, Glassock RJ. Immunosuppressive drug therapy in lupus nephritis. *Am J Kidney Dis* 1993;21:239–250.

A review of immunosuppressive regimens used in SLE with emphasis on their influence on the course of lupus nephritis.

Dooley MA, Hogan S, Jennette C, et al. Cyclophosphamide therapy for lupus nephritis: poor renal survival in black Americans. *Kidney Int* 1997;51: 1188–1195.

An analysis of the clinical and histologic features of 89 patients with diffuse proliferative lupus nephritis that influence prognosis showing that African-American race is a major determinant of adverse outcome.

Gourley MF, Austin HA, Scott D, et al. Methylprednisolone and cyclophosphamide, alone or in combination, in patients with lupus nephritis. *Ann Intern Med* 1996;125:549–557.

A randomized, controlled trial of 82 patients with severe lupus nephritis treated with three different treatment regimens looking at efficacy and complications of therapy.

Kashgarian M. Lupus nephritis: lessons from the path lab. *Kidney Int* 1994;45: 928–938.

A review of lupus nephritis viewed from the histopathologic standpoint.

Lewis EJ, Hunsicker LG, Lan SP, et al. For the lupus collaboration study group. A controlled trial of plasmapheresis therapy in severe lupus nephritis. *N Engl J Med* 1992;326:1373–1379.

A randomized, controlled trial of plasmapheresis in patients with diffuse proliferative lupus nephritis.

Madaio M. The role of autoantibodies in the pathogenesis of lupus nephritis. *Semin Nephrol* 1999;19:48–56.

A review and update on the pathomechanisms of glomerular immune complex formation in lupus nephritis.

Magil AB, Puterman ML, Ballon HS, et al. Prognostic factors in diffuse proliferative lupus glomerulonephritis. *Kidney Int* 1988;34:511–517.

Analysis of features associated with an adverse outcome in lupus patients with diffuse proliferative disease.

Moroni G, Qualini S, Maccario M, et al. "Nephritic flares" are predictors of bad long-term renal outcome in lupus nephritis. *Kidney Int* 1996;50:2047–2053.

Retrospective analysis of 70 SLE patients followed for up to 30 years showing the significance of renal flares and especially "nephritic" renal flares along their course.

Park MH, D'Agati VD, Appel GB, et al. Tubulointerstitial disease in lupus nephritis: relationship to immune deposits, interstitial inflammation, glomerular changes, renal function, and prognosis. *Nephron* 1986;44:309–319.
A study of more than 100 biopsied lupus patients analyzing tubulointerstitial immune deposits and inflammatory lesions and correlating these to glomerular lesions, clinical features, and course of the patients.
Pasquali S, Banfi G, Zucchelli A, et al. Lupus membranous nephropathy: long-term outcome. *Clin Nephrol* 1993;39:175–182.
A long-term analysis of the outcome of patients with membranous lupus nephropathy including a comparison to patients with diffuse proliferative disease.
Ponticelli C, Zucchelli P, Moroni G, et al. Long-term prognosis of diffuse lupus nephritis. *Clin Nephrol* 1987;28:263.
Favorable results in a large population of patients with diffuse proliferative disease treated with immunosuppressive regimens.
Radhakrishnan J, Valeri A, Kunis C, et al. Use of cyclosporine in systemic lupus. In: Tejani A, ed. *Contributions in nephrology.* Basel: Karger, 1995;114:59–72.
Review of published animal and human trials with cyclosporine in SLE.
Seliger S, Barr RG, Zuniga R, et al. Prognosis in proliferative lupus nephritis: role of race and socioeconomic status. *J Am Soc Nephrol* 1998;9:99A.
Analysis of 129 patients with either severe focal or diffuse proliferative lupus nephritis analyzing racial, socioeconomic, and clinical features predictive of a poor prognosis.
Sloan RP, Schwartz MM, Korbet SM, et al. Long-term outcome in SLE membranous glomerulonephritis. *J Am Soc Nephrol* 1996;7:299–305.
A retrospective analysis of 73 membranous lupus patients, of whom 30 had pure membranous lupus, analyzing the effect of histologic and clinical features on long-term outcome.
Steinberg AD, Steinberg SC. Long-term preservation of renal function in patients with lupus nephritis receiving treatment that includes cyclophosphamide versus those treated with prednisone only. *Arthritis Rheum* 1991;34:945–950.
A 20-year follow-up by life-table analysis of the course of patients with severe lupus nephritis treated in a controlled trial at the NIH with a variety of immunosuppressive regimens.

PART 2
Mixed Connective Tissue Disease

Robert W. Hoffman

Mixed connective tissue disease (MCTD) was first described by Sharp and colleagues in 1972 when they reported on a group of patients with overlapping clinical manifestations consisting of features of systemic lupus erythematosus (SLE), polymyositis (PM), and progressive systemic sclerosis (SSc), and the presence of a distinctive antibody profile. These patients designated as having MCTD were found to have antibodies against a crude antigenic extract called *extractable nuclear antigen* (ENA). Antibodies from patients with MCTD were later defined more precisely as reacting with nuclear ribonucleoprotein (RNP), which is now known to consist of a complex of uridylic acid–rich RNAs and a series of discrete, small nuclear ribonucleoproteins (snRNP). These snRNP normally aggregate in the nucleus of cells, where they participate in the splicing and assembly of messenger RNA. Since that original description, the concept has become more refined, and substantial evidence has been published supporting the idea that MCTD is a distinct rheumatic disease. Advances in characterizing the genetics of MCTD and in characterizing the autoantibodies found in MCTD have added further evidence supporting the concept of MCTD as being distinct.

Classification criteria for MCTD have been published by investigators from several countries. The criteria of Alarcón-Segovia and Cardiel is regarded by many as the best presently available for classification of patients with MCTD (Table 42.7). Clinically, the features that predominate in MCTD are the constellation of swollen hands, arthralgia/arthritis, sclerodactyly, Raynaud's phenomenon, esophageal dysmotility with frequent symptoms of gastroesophageal reflux, and myositis, which is often mild.

TABLE 42.7. Criteria for Classification of Mixed Connective Tissue Disease (MCTD)

A. Criteria used for classification of MCTD are as follows:
   1. Serologic: positive RNP antibodies present in high titer
   2. Clinical:
      a. Edema of the hands
      b. Synovitis
      c. Myositis
      d. Raynaud's phenomenon
      e. Acrosclerosis

B. Application of the above criteria for the classification of a patient as having MCTD are as follows:
   1. Serologic finding of anti-RNP antibodies at moderate to high levels in patients' sera
   2. At least three of the clinical findings listed above
   3. The association of edema of the hands, Raynaud's phenomenon, and acrosclerosis requires the addition of at least one of the other two clinical criteria (i.e., b. synovitis or c. myositis)

Modified from Alarcón-Segovia D, Cardiel MH. Comparison between 3 diagnostic criteria for mixed connective tissue disease. Study of 593 patients. *J Rheumatol* 1989;16:328–334.

PATHOGENESIS

One of the first hallmarks of MCTD recognized was the presence of very high levels of anti-ENA antibodies typical of the IgG isotype in patients' sera. In some cases, these antibodies have been demonstrated to account for one-third of total serum immunoglobulin. Biochemical studies have shown that the crude ENA antigen contains both the RNP and Sm antigens. High serum levels of anti-RNP antibodies are strongly associated with MCTD, whereas anti-Sm antibodies are highly specific for SLE. The RNP and Sm antigens have been biochemically characterized to be components of uridylic acid–rich RNA (U) snRNP complexes. The RNP antigen consists of the 70-kD, A, and C snRNP polypeptides associated with U1 RNA, whereas the Sm antigen consists of the B1-2, D1-3, E, F, and G snRNP polypeptides associated with U1, U2, U4/U6, and U5 RNA. U snRNP are part of the spliceosome complex involved in the excising of introns during the processing of the larger pre-mRNA to final mature mRNA. Although U snRNP complexes normally reside and function intracellularly, B- and T-cell immune reactivity against this complex exist in the immune repertoire of MCTD patients. Although it is not known why this immune reactivity exists or how activation of the anti-RNP immune repertoire occurs, it has been proposed that it may occur as cells undergo apoptosis or necrosis. During apoptosis, the normally intracellular RNP antigens are potentially exposed to and could stimulate the immune system of an individual possessing the appropriate genetic background that confers susceptibility to disease (see the following section). Alternatively, immune activation may occur through molecular mimicry with microbial pathogenesis or with other cross-reactive self-antigens and is then misdirected at self-antigens.

Genetic studies from several countries have demonstrated that susceptibility to produce anti-RNP antibodies and to develop MCTD per se is associated with major histocompatibility complex class II genes. The strongest and most consistently found association has been with HLA-DR4. Studies have also found an association with a specific genotype of HLA-DR2, which is labeled HLA-DRB1*1501. Molecular genetic studies have shown that the specific genotypes of HLA-DR4 and HLA-DR2 that are associated with anti-RNP antibody production and MCTD all share common amino acids at positions 26, 28, 30-32, 70, and 73 on the HLA-DR β chain. These studies suggest that this common HLA structural motif, or so-called shared epitope, may be important in disease susceptibility.

One model that has been proposed, for the preferential association of certain HLA genes with the production of high levels of anti-RNP autoantibodies, is that MCTD is driven by an immune response against the RNP autoantigen or some component of the RNP complex. In such a model, the RNP complex could bind preferentially to select HLA-DR4/DR2 alleles, and this RNP-HLA complex then stimulate autoreactive T cells to expand and produce cytokines. Cytokines released could assist in the expansion of autoreactive T and B cells in an exocrine or paracrine fashion and could also directly mediate tissue damage. In support of this model of disease pathogenesis, it has been found that MCTD patients have circulating T cells that are reactive with RNP and that the presence of such cells parallel the presence of anti-RNP antibodies found in their sera. In addition, these RNP-reactive T cells have a T-helper cell phenotype and have been shown to produce cytokines, which are known to be important in B-cell help and differentiation.

CLINICAL FEATURES

Clinical features that predominate in MCTD are the constellation of Raynaud's phenomenon, arthralgia, arthritis, swollen hands, sclerodactyly, abnormal esophageal motility, and myositis. It has also been appreciated that pulmonary disease may frequently be present in MCTD. The development of pulmonary hypertension occurs in a minority of patients but is often a very serious clinical event. Pulmonary hypertension and subsequent heart failure are the most common causes of disease-related death in MCTD.

Raynaud's phenomenon is the most prevalent clinical finding in MCTD, being present in more than 90% of patients. Arthralgias occur in most patients, with objective synovitis occurring in three-fourths of patients during their disease course. The arthritis is typically nonerosive and nondeforming. Rheumatoid factor is commonly detected in MCTD, occurring in more than half of all patients. In some patients, deforming arthritis may develop, which resembles rheumatoid arthritis with associated ulnar deviations, swan neck, and boutonniere deformities.

Swollen hands and/or sclerodactyly occur in three-fourths of MCTD patients and is typical early in disease. The swelling of the digits may result in diffuse swelling or so-called sausage-shaped appearance of the digits. Such swelling may remain fixed or may progress to a tapering of the digits or so-called sclerodactyly. In some patients, the diffuse swelling of the fingers appears to be associated with synovitis. In some patients, it may resolve without leaving residual abnormalities over a period of several months to years.

Esophageal involvement is found to be present in three-fourths of patients with MCTD when it is sought, such as in clinical research studies using manometrics and radiologic evaluation of patients prospectively. Clinically symptomatic dysphagia and heartburn are also very prevalent in MCTD. Other regions of the gastrointestinal tract can less frequently be involved. This can result in intestinal hypomotility, bacterial overgrowth, pseudoobstruction, vasculitis, small and large bowel perforation, secretory diarrhea, acute pancreatitis, pancreatic pseudocyst formation, Budd-Chiari syndrome, chronic active hepatitis, and pneumatosis intestinalis.

Myositis is a prominent feature of MCTD. In most patients, the myositis is mild, often occurring without proximal weakness. Severe PM or dermatomyositis can less commonly be present. A longitudinal study comparing MCTD patients with myositis to PM and dermatomyositis without anti-RNP antibodies found that the MCTD group has less severe disease on biopsy and a more rapid response to treatment with glucocorticoids.

Pulmonary involvement in MCTD is common. Longitudinal studies have demonstrated its occurrence in 85% of patients studied. Pulmonary hypertension is the most serious pulmonary manifestation of MCTD. The histopathologic basis for pulmonary hypertension in MCTD is a progressive proliferative vasculopathy, rather than interstitial pulmonary fibrosis.

Cardiac disease is common in MCTD. Pericarditis has been reported to occur in 10% to 43% of patients. Myocarditis can occur, and the proliferative vasculopathy of MCTD may involve epicardial and intramural coronary arteries. Cardiac failure can complicate advanced pulmonary hypertension.

Neurologic involvement occurs in approximately 10% of patients with MCTD. Trigeminal neuralgia is the most commonly recognized problem, followed by vascular headaches. Cognitive abnormalities, aseptic meningitis, cerebral vasculitis, organic mental syndromes, seizures, and other neurologic abnormalities have been reported in MCTD, but these appear to be much less common than in SLE.

RENAL DISEASE

Renal disease occurs overall in approximately 25% of MCTD patients and may be more severe and more common in children. Renal findings in MCTD are summarized in Table 42.8. It has been reported to occur in almost half of all children with MCTD. Often, renal disease in MCTD is asymptomatic and is found only on routine laboratory testing or when specifically sought, such as in clinical research studies. Focal proliferative glomerulonephritis appears more common than diffuse proliferative glomerulonephritis, which is rare. Proliferative vascular lesions, similar to those occurring in the lungs and other tissues, may be found in the kidneys in MCTD. Proliferative vascular lesions in MCTD have been associated with renovascular hypertension. Although overall renal disease occurs much less commonly in MCTD than in SLE, it has been reported that MCTD patients possessing the HLA-DR2 phenotype and antibodies directed against the D polypeptide of the Sm antigen are more likely to have severe renal disease.

The precise prevalence of renal disease in MCTD is difficult to ascertain with certainty from the literature because of differ-

TABLE 42.8. Renal Disease in Mixed Connective Tissue Disease (MCTD)

Renal involvement reported to occur in approximately 10%–25% of MCTD patients.
Renal involvement may be clinically silent or mild, consisting of proteinuria or hematuria.
Serious renal disease reported to be more common in children with MCTD.
HLA-DR2 phenotype, anti-Sm-D peptide antibodies, and anti-double-stranded DNA antibodies are associated with severe renal disease.
Membranous or focal disease are the most common lesions; membranoproliferative glomerulonephritis is uncommon.
Proliferative vascular lesions were found in the kidneys and may be associated with the development of malignant hypertension in a small number of patients.
Secondary Sjögren's syndrome can lead to interstitial nephritis and associated renal tubular dysfunction, such as renal tubular acidosis.

ences in criteria used to classify patients as MCTD in different published series. Among patients classified using the classification criteria, such as those of Alarcón-Segovia and Cardiel (Table 42.7), it would appear that the incidence of serious renal disease is very low. In series of MCTD patients that exclude patients with antibodies against the Sm antigen or antibodies to double-stranded DNA, glomerulonephritis is rare. A published longitudinal 29-year study, which used the criteria of Alarcón-Segovia and Cardiel for MCTD classification, found that among the 47 patients studied, there was an 11% cumulative incidence of renal disease.

Malignant hypertension associated with a proliferative vasculopathy, similar to that seen in SSc, has been reported in MCTD and may result in hypertensive renal crisis and end-stage renal disease. Adverse reactions to nonsteroidal antiinflammatory drugs (NSAIDs) occur and may cause drug-associated renal disease (see Chapter 47, Part 3) in patients with MCTD. Patients with MCTD and secondary Sjogren's syndrome may have interstitial renal disease with associated clinical findings, such as renal tubular acidosis.

LABORATORY FINDINGS

Virtually all MCTD patients have antinuclear antibodies, which typically give a speckled pattern on indirect immunofluorescence using HEp2 cells as a substrate in so-called antinuclear antibody (ANA) or fluorescent antinuclear antibody (FANA) testing. These antibodies are primarily reactive against ENA and RNP, which can be demonstrated by more specific testing. MCTD patients typically will not have persistent or high levels of antibodies reactive with the Sm antigen or double-stranded DNA.

Many assays can detect antibodies to ENA; however, sensitivity and specificity vary significantly, as does the ability of the assay to distinguish between the individual antigens. More commonly used assays for detecting ENA include the FANA, immunodiffusion, and hemagglutination. Highly specific but less widely used assays for detecting ENAs include immunoblotting and enzyme-linked immunosorbent assay (ELISA). The presence of specific antibodies, such as those against RNP, can currently be detected using a variety of techniques. The methods most commonly used to detect anti-RNP antibodies are double immunodiffusion, immunoelectrophoresis, or ELISA.

Although FANA testing may detect both anti-RNP antibodies and anti-Sm antibodies, it cannot distinguish between the two. Immunodiffusion can differentially detect both anti-RNP and anti-Sm antibodies. In some instances, however, such as when anti-RNP or anti-Sm antibodies are present in low titer by hemagglutination or ELISA, immunodiffusion may fail to detect these antibodies. To detect antibodies against the individual snRNP polypeptides, such as U1-70kD or Sm-D, immunoblotting or an ELISA must be used.

Other antibodies that are distinctive in MCTD are those against U1 RNA and heteronuclear RNP-A2/RA33. Antibodies against U1 RNA are detected exclusively in patients with antibodies against RNP. Unlike antibodies to RNP, where serum levels fluctuate slowly over time, the serum levels of antibodies to U1 RNA can change very quickly and may correlate directly with disease activity in some patients.

Antiphospholipid (aPL) antibodies, such as those detected as lupus anticoagulants, anticardiolipin antibodies, and false-positive test results for syphilis, have been reported to occur in patients with MCTD at a similar frequency to that found among patients with SLE. Unlike in SLE, the presence of aPL antibodies in MCTD has not been found to correlate with an increased risk of venous or arterial clotting events. In MCTD, however, aPL antibodies are associated with pulmonary hypertension.

Hypergammaglobulinemia is common in MCTD, and rheumatoid factor occurs in more than half of all patients. Complement components C3, C4 are typically normal in MCTD, although they may be reduced in patients with renal disease or severe MCTD.

Anemia or leukopenia occurs in approximately one-third of MCTD patients. The anemia is typically an anemia of chronic inflammation, although autoimmune hemolytic anemia has been described. Leukopenia is typically mild, but abnormalities of granulocyte chemotaxis and host defense can result in significant risk of serious or event fatal infections in MCTD. Infections remain one of the leading causes of disease-related death in MCTD. Immune-mediated thrombocytopenia appears more common in children and may be severe. Thrombotic thrombocytopenia and red cell aplasia have been reported to occur in MCTD.

Histopathology in MCTD shows that salivary glands, muscle, and other tissues may be massively infiltrated with lymphocytes and plasma cells. There also may be massive lymphoproliferation in MCTD. Histopathology is characterized by proliferative vascular lesions, including intimal thickening and medial hyperplasia, which may resemble vascular lesions in SSc. In the lungs in MCTD, however, there is vasculopathy with the absence of interstitial pulmonary fibrosis and selective increase of type III collagen in contrast to SSc.

TREATMENT AND PROGNOSIS

Controlled clinical trials have not been done to examine therapy in MCTD; therefore current treatment guidelines are based on retrospective analyses and clinical experience. In mild MCTD without serious end-organ involvement, patients' symptoms can often be managed with combinations of NSAIDs and the antimalarial, hydroxychloroquine, without the use of corticosteroids. The NSAID ibuprofen and sulindac have been associated with a hypersensitivity meningitis in MCTD, so the clinician should be alert to this rare possibility with the use of an NSAID. Patients should be encouraged to avoid cold exposure, and calcium channel blockers can be used to control Raynaud's phenomenon when it is severe. Esophageal symptoms appear to respond favorably to proton pump inhibitors.

For patients with RA-like joint involvement, hydroxychloroquine, low-dose glucocorticoid (e.g., 5 to 15 mg/day in a single morning dose) or low-dose methotrexate (e.g., 7.5 to 15 mg/wk) may be used in addition to an NSAID. Mild SLE-like symptoms, including pleuritis, rash, anemia, and leukopenia, typically respond to low- to moderate-dose (e.g., 0.5 mg/kg per day of prednisone in single or divided doses) glucocorticoid and hydroxychloroquine therapy.

Major organ involvement such as myocarditis, polymyositis, thrombocytopenia, glomerulonephritis, or central nervous system involvement requires moderate to high dosages (e.g., 1 to 2 mg/kg per day of prednisone in divided doses) of glucocorticoid therapy. The addition of a cytotoxic drug may be needed for patients requiring continued high-dose glucocorticoids to control their disease or in patients in whom disease remains active despite high-dose glucocorticoid therapy. Early intervention with cytotoxic drugs may also be considered for patients with severe or potentially life-threatening MCTD. Based on favorable experience in controlled trials treating lupus nephritis and more limited uncontrolled data in MCTD, many clinicians now favor the use of intermittent pulse cyclophosphamide as the cytotoxic agent of choice in severe MCTD. Azathioprine, cyclosporine, and other immunosuppressants have also been used to successfully treat MCTD.

Pulmonary hypertension appears to be the most common disease-related cause of death in MCTD. Patients with asymptomatic pulmonary hypertension, suggested by findings on physical examination, pulmonary function testing (decreased diffusion capacity for carbon monoxide), or echocardiography, should undergo cardiac catheterization for right-sided heart pressure measurements and definitive diagnosis. Although optimal treatment for such patients is uncertain, many would treat patients found to have elevated right-sided heart pressure documented by right-sided heart catheterization. Patients with symptomatic pulmonary hypertension have a much poorer prognosis. Although the efficacy of intervention in such patients remains unproven, some patients have been reported to respond to therapy. Treatment of pulmonary hypertension has included careful administration of a high dosage of a vasodilator, such as calcium channel blocking agents, oxygen therapy, and anticoagulation. Other agents that have been used to treat pulmonary hypertension in MCTD include angiotensin-converting enzyme inhibitors, prostaglandins, cyclosporine, and hydralazine. Sustained improvement of pulmonary hypertension in MCTD has been described in case reports with treatment of the disease using high-dose corticosteroids and the cytotoxic agent cyclophosphamide.

The prognosis of MCTD has been the subject of a longitudinal study that examined 47 patients followed for as long as 29 years. It was found that patients rarely evolved into SLE or SSc and that most had a favorable outcome, with pulmonary hypertension the most common disease-related cause of death. Outcome studies in children with MCTD have been less favorable, with excess early death occurring in as many as one-third of children with MCTD, especially in those patients with renal disease.

Selected Readings

Alarcón-Segovia D, Cardiel MH. Comparison between 3 diagnostic criteria for mixed connective tissue disease. Study of 593 patients. *J Rheumatol* 1989;16:328–334.

A comparative analysis of three published criteria for the classification of MCTD among 593 connective tissue disease patients from Mexico. The authors present classification criteria that are straightforward and easily applied. These criteria appear to have sensitivity and specificity equal to or superior to other published classification criteria for MCTD.

Burdt M, Hoffman RW, Deutscher SL, et al. Long-term outcome in mixed connective tissue disease: longitudinal clinical and serologic findings. *Arthritis Rheum* 1999;42:899–909.

A longitudinal study of 47 MCTD patients from one center followed over 29 years. This is the largest published long-term outcome study of patients from North America to date. It reports that patients classified as having MCTD, using the criteria such as that described by Alarcón-Segovia and Cardiel, rarely evolved into SLE or PSS and that most had a favorable outcome, with pulmonary hypertension being the most common disease-related cause of death.

Hamaeenkorpi R, Ruuska P, Forsberg S, et al. More evidence of distinctive features of mixed connective tissue disease. *Scand J Rheumatol* 1993;22:63–68.

*An immunogenetics study of Finish MCTD patients that demonstrates that disease susceptibility is associated with the HLA-DR4/Dw4 (HLA-DRB1*0401) genotype. This work adds to earlier studies of others (see Kaneoka et al. and references therein) that demonstrated association of anti-RNP (anti-U1-70kD) antibody production with HLA-DR4.*

Holyst M-M, Hill DL, Hoch SO, et al. Analysis of human T cell and B cell responses against U-small nuclear ribonucleoprotein 70kD, B and D polypeptides among patients with systemic lupus erythematosus and mixed connective tissue disease. *Arthritis Rheum* 1997;40:1493–1503.

This study found that MCTD patients have circulating T cells, which can be isolated from their peripheral blood and are reactive with RNP, and that the presence of such cells parallel the presence of anti-RNP antibodies found in their sera. In addition, these RNP-reactive T cells have a T-helper cell phenotype and have been shown to produced cytokines, which are known to be important in B-cell help and differentiation, suggesting that they have an important role in disease pathogenesis.

Kaneoka H, Hsu KC, Takeda Y, et al. Molecular genetic analysis o HLA-DR and HLA-DQ genes among anti-U1-70kD autoantibody-positive connective tissue disease patients. *Arthritis Rheum* 1992;35:83–94.

*A comprehensive molecular genetic analysis of the contribution of major histocompatibility genes to susceptibility to MCTD. The work extends the earlier studies of Genth et al., Hoffman et al., and Black et al. (cited herein) showing association of HLA-DR4 with the production of anti-RNP/U1-70-kD polypeptide antibodies. The study of Kaneoka et al. identifies the association of disease susceptibility to select genotypes of HLA-DR4, including HLA-DRB1*0401, and to the HLA-DRB1*1501 genotype of HLA-DR2.The study identifies a so-called shared epitope of HLA, which may be important in peptide selection and binding and which is common to all HLA-DRB1 genotypes associated with anti-RNP/U1-70kD autoantibody production.*

Smolen JS, Steiner G. Mixed connective tissue disease: to be or not to be? *Arthritis Rheum* 1998;41:768–777.

A critical review of the evidence that MCTD is a distinct entity. This review examines recent data, which demonstrate that the patterns of specific autoantibodies produced by patients with MCTD and genetics of the disease are distinct, and supports the concept of MCTD as being a unique rheumatic disease.

PART 3
Rheumatoid Arthritis and Rheumatic Fever

Arthur H. Cohen

Abnormalities of the kidneys in rheumatoid arthritis may be direct manifestations of the disease and/or the results of treatment directed at its control (Table 42.9). Indeed, a consideration of the various therapies indicates virtually the entire spectrum of iatrogenic forms of renal damage in rheumatoid arthritis (RA). Similarly, the clinical features are those of most renal syndromes and include mild and severe urinary abnormalities, acute and chronic renal failure, and less often, rapidly progressive glomerulonephritis. Those lesions that are "intrinsic" to or a direct complication of RA are described first, followed by lesions that are associated with therapy.

The incidence of any type of kidney abnormality in RA is not precisely known and depends, in part, on the patient pop-

TABLE 42.9. Abnormalities of the Kidneys in Rheumatoid Arthritis

Changes resulting from rheumatoid arthritis per se
Membranous glomerulonephritis
Mesangial proliferative glomerulonephritis
Diffuse proliferative glomerulonephritis
Necrotizing and crescentic glomerulonephritis
Necrotizing vasculitis
Changes resulting from chronic inflammatory state
Renal amyloidosis (AA type)
Changes resulting from therapeutic agents
Gold
Membranous glomerulonephritis
Minimal-change disease
Acute tubular necrosis
Penicillamine
Membranous glomerulonephritis
Crescentic glomerulonephritis
Minimal-change disease
Nonsteroidal antiinflammatory agents
Acute tubular necrosis
Acute interstitial nephritis
Minimal-change disease
Analgesic drugs
Papillary necrosis
Chronic interstitial nephritis
Azathioprine
Acute interstitial nephritis
Bucillamine
Membranous glomerulonephritis
Cyclosporine
Chronic ischemic changes
Miscellaneous
Renal calculi

ulation studied and the sources of data. For example, most reports on glomerular involvement are derived from renal biopsy studies and files, thereby emphasizing a type of lesion without necessarily indicating the pool of RA patients from which those selected for biopsy were gathered. Alternatively, it is not known whether significant renal pathologic findings can be clinically silent or trivial, thereby possibly making clinical studies nonrepresentative or underestimating the true frequency of any renal damage. Nevertheless, as many as 50% of patients with RA, irrespective of treatment, are estimated to have renal involvement in the form of either abnormal urine findings or decreased glomerular filtration or both. It should be noted that renal involvement in juvenile rheumatoid arthritis and ankylosing spondylitis also occurs, although it is less frequently reported.

Virtually all immune-mediated renal abnormalities in RA were long thought to be consequent to therapeutic agents. However, it has become apparent that several forms of immune complex–mediated glomerulonephritis, including membranous glomerulonephritis, may occur in the absence of therapy. For membranous glomerulonephritis, the clinical manifestations of low-grade or nephrotic-range proteinuria with or without hematuria are largely the same as those of the idiopathic form of the disease. As is well known, there is a high association of RA with HLA-DR4. However, patients who develop membranous glomerulonephritis during gold or penicillamine therapy are often positive for DRw2 or w3 antigens, and those who develop membranous glomerulonephritis unrelated to treatment generally are DRw4 positive. This suggests that there might be a genetic predisposition for gold- or penicillamine-induced renal complications, whereas in the DRw4-positive, DRw2- or DRw3-negative patient, membranous glomerulonephritis, which occurs without a predisposing factor or therapy, may be an integral part of the rheumatoid disease.

Some debate persists as to whether mesangial proliferative (or mesangial injury) glomerulonephritis occurs as an integral part of RA. Reports appear to support the contention that patients with RA and generally mild hematuria or proteinuria may have, on renal biopsy, a lesion of mesangial injury or proliferative glomerulonephritis. Indeed, some investigators consider it to be a common extraarticular manifestations or RA. IgM is most commonly found; fewer biopsies have predominant IgA in the mesangium. Some investigators have suggested that mesangial clearance of circulating rheumatoid factor may account for the mesangial abnormalities. Although more than 25% of RA patients undergoing renal biopsy for urinary abnormalities have been found to have this form of glomerular damage, it is still uncertain whether the lesions are integral to or merely coexisting with RA. For example, a large study from Finland comparing patients with RA with age- and sex-matched controls found no difference in the prevalence of isolated microscopic hematuria in the two groups.

In one study, patients with isolated hematuria had normal renal function and hematuria at follow-up. Proteinuria, whether alone or in association with hematuria, was temporally related to administration of gold or penicillamine; in these patients, renal function remained stable, although proteinuria often persisted after discontinuation of the drugs.

Other forms of proliferative glomerulonephritis, often with greater and more widespread hypercellularity than those just described, have been infrequently reported. Glomeruli have more extensive and widespread immune complex deposits in both mesangium and capillary walls and are characterized by numerous leukocytes within the capillaries and substance of the glomerulus, as well as by increased intrinsic glomerular cells. Patients with this form of injury have heavy proteinuria, hematuria, and progressive renal failure. It is possible that some of these patients also have or ultimately develop systemic lupus erythematosus.

An additional form of glomerulonephritis has been emphasized to belong to the spectrum of glomerular lesions in RA, including juvenile rheumatoid arthritis. A necrotizing glomerulonephritis with or, more frequently, without immune deposits but with crescent formation may occur in the absence of a systemic rheumatoid vasculitis. It may also be associated with antineutrophil cytoplasmic antibodies (ANCA) and systemic vasculitis. It has been reported in the absence of penicillamine therapy, although penicillamine is known to be associated with this form of glomerular injury. As with other forms of crescentic and destructive glomerulonephritis, it may eventuate in a short time in end-stage renal disease. This form of glomerulonephritis may also respond to cyclophosphamide or azathioprine and prednisone therapy. As with pauci-immune crescentic glomerulonephritis in other settings, renal and patient death are not uncommon.

Patients with longstanding deforming RA with subcutaneous nodules and high levels of rheumatoid factor, often with depressed serum complement (C3), develop a systemic necrotizing vasculitis. Approximately 15% of affected patients have renal abnormalities, most commonly proteinuria and/or hematuria, often becoming manifest at the time that the cutaneous vasculitic lesions appear. There may be severe hypertension and progressive irreversible loss of renal function. Microscopically, the medium-sized arteries are most affected by necrosis and inflammation in varying stages of evolution, similar to the classical form of polyarteritis nodosa. Glomerular necrosis and crescents, variably associated with immune deposits, represent the major renal structural lesion. It should be noted that this glomerular lesion is virtually identical to the crescentic and destructive glomerulonephritis described previously; the relationship between the two is not known.

Amyloidosis is estimated to occur in approximately 20% of individuals with longstanding RA. Renal involvement is usually in the form of glomerular infiltrates of AA amyloid, although it has been suggested that interstitial amyloid, even in the absence of glomerular amyloid, may be more common in RA patients than in others with AA amyloidosis. The clinical manifestations and course of renal amyloid in RA are the same as in patients with amyloid associated with other disease processes (see Chapter 42, Part 10).

With more prevalent use of cyclosporine in treating RA, features of chronic cyclosporine toxicity have been noted. With lower dosages, both functional and morphologic adverse effects are lessened; biopsy studies have disclosed minimal or no significant chronic tubulointerstitial lesions in patients treated with no more than 5 mg/kg per day. Renal lesions caused by other therapeutic agents are quite varied and include membranous glomerulonephritis in patients treated with gold, especially parenterally administered (see Chapter 47, Part 4); penicillamine; and a related agent, bucillamine. Penicillamine may also induce a necrotizing and crescentic form of glomerulonephritis. Nonsteroidal antiinflammatory drugs may be responsible for a variety of lesions, which include acute renal failure resulting from acute tubular necrosis, acute interstitial nephritis, heavy proteinuria with minimal-change disease as the glomerular lesion, or a combination of these manifestations (see Chapter 47, Part 3). Finally, long-term use of analgesics at high dosages may cause chronic interstitial nephritis and renal papillary necrosis (see Chapter 47, Part 5). Acute tubular necrosis may also result from administration of gold salts.

The types and incidence of renal lesions in patients with acute rheumatic fever are less impressive than those of RA. Because both acute rheumatic fever and acute glomerulonephritis are consequences of streptococcal infections, the possibility of coexistence of cardiac and renal abnormalities in the same patient has intrigued investigators for many years and has led to a number of morphologic studies in an attempt to document such concurrence. Studies conducted between 1932 and 1962 showed a widely varying prevalence of glomerular abnormalities, ranging from 1.3% to 38.6% in patients with acute rheumatic carditis or rheumatic heart disease. The lesions encountered were most often mild, but on occasion, typical diffuse glomerulonephritis was noted. Although these and other studies show wide variation in renal, especially glomerular, involvement in rheumatic fever, a number of points make interpretation of the data difficult in the light of modern concepts of glomerular injury. It is most probable that the instances of glomerular changes in chronic valvular disease, especially with mitral valve involvement and pulmonary hypertension, actually represent the spectrum of glomerular alterations that have been described in patients with pulmonary hypertension, cor pulmonale, chronic lung disease, polycythemia, or cyanotic heart disease. These abnormalities consist of glomerular enlargement, often with varying degrees of mesangial hypercellularity. Although instances of active bacterial endocarditis were excluded from most of the aforementioned studies, some cases of prior infective endocarditis with associated glomerulonephritis in a "healed" state were probably included. It is also possible that forms of glomerulonephritis not associated with streptococcal infections were also included; for example, some of the patients with "focal glomerulonephritis" could easily have had independently occurring IgA nephropathy. Last, most of the aforementioned observations were made on tissues studied primarily with thick hematoxylin and eosin-stained sections, enhancing the opportunity for overinterpretation of the findings. The more modern approach toward evaluation of the kidneys in acute rheumatic fever was first undertaken in a study in 1967. Renal biopsies were performed on 22 patients with acute rheumatic fever. Proteinuria and/or hematuria was present in 18 patients, although heavy proteinuria and an active urinary sediment occurred in only three. The remainder had only slight (trace to 1+) proteinuria. Glomerular abnormalities, detected by either light or electron microscopy, were described in 17 cases; in only seven patients were electron-dense deposits documented. The light microscopic changes were generally those of segmental and/or mesangial hypercellularity. As emphasized earlier, some of the glomerular lesions indicated are probably not directly related either to streptococcal infections or to acute rheumatic fever or cardiac manifestations, and they may be examples of well-defined glomerulopathies occurring coincidentally in affected patients.

Although isolated reports continue to emphasize the coexistence of glomerulonephritis and acute rheumatic fever, careful review of these indicates that approximately half of the patients actually had a poststreptococcal glomerulonephritis at the time of acute rheumatic carditis. The renal structural findings and clinical courses of these patients appear to be identical to those of others of the same age with acute poststreptococcal glomerulonephritis.

The infrequent concurrence of acute rheumatic fever and acute poststreptococcal glomerulonephritis is a poorly understood phenomenon. It should be recalled that acute rheumatic fever may follow pharyngeal infection with any group A hemolytic *Streptococcus* infection, whereas glomerulonephritis may follow pharyngeal or cutaneous infections with only a limited number of serotypes of group A streptococci. Thus it is likely that "rheumatogenic" as well as "nephritogenic" strains of streptococci exist, but these two properties seldom occur simultaneously. Elevated levels of circulating immune complexes have been detected in patients with rheumatic fever or poststreptococcal glomerulonephritis.

Selected Readings

Harper L, Cockwell P, Howie AJ, et al. Focal segmental necrotizing glomerulonephritis in rheumatoid arthritis. *QJM* 1997;90:125–132.
Series of patients with crescentic glomerulonephritis with clinicopathologic correlations and therapeutic results.

Helin HJ, Korpela MM, Mustonen JT, et al. Renal biopsy and clinicopathologic correlations in rheumatoid arthritis. *Arthritis Rheum* 1995;38:242–247.
Retrospective analysis of and correlations in a large series (110 patients) indicating mesangial proliferative glomerulonephritis to be most common renal lesion, followed by amyloidosis.

Ito S, Nozawa S, Ishikawa H, et al. Renal stones in patients with rheumatoid arthritis. *J Rheumatol* 1997;24:2123–2128.
Study suggesting renal stones often with hematuria are more common in patients with RA than in controls.

Korpela M, Mustonen J, Heikkinen A, et al. Isolated microscopic hematuria in patients with rheumatoid arthritis compared with age and sex matched controls. A population based study. *J Rheumatol* 1995;22:427–431.
Description of hematuria of diverse origins in patients with and without RA.

Korpela M, Mustonen J, Teppo AM, et al. Mesangial glomerulonephritis as an extra-articular manifestation of rheumatoid arthritis. *Br J Rheumatol* 1997;36:1189–1195.
Detailed description of immunopathology of glomerular mesangium and an assertion that this form of glomerulonephritis is integral to RA.

Landewe RB, Dikhmans BA, van der Woude FJ, et al. Long-term low dose cyclosporine in patients with rheumatoid arthritis; renal function loss without structural nephropathy. *J Rheumatol* 1996;23:61–64.
Effects of low-dose cyclosporine on kidney function and structure.

Rodriguez F, Krayenbuhl JC, Harrison WB, et al. Renal biopsy findings and follow-up of renal function in rheumatoid arthritis patients treated with cyclosporine A. *Arthritis Rheum* 1996;39:1491–1498.
Study of the renal effects and dosage correlations of cyclosporine therapy.

PART 4
Vasculitis

Gill Gaskin and Charles D. Pusey

The primary systemic vasculitides are a group of disorders characterized by necrotizing inflammation of blood vessels. The clinical manifestations of systemic vasculitis depend on the size of vessels affected, whether there is associated granuloma formation, and which organ systems are involved. Those forms of vasculitis affecting small blood vessels may cause a focal necrotizing glomerulonephritis, often with crescent formation, which presents as the clinical syndrome of rapidly progressive glomerulonephritis (RPGN). Vasculitis of larger blood vessels may also affect the kidney, often by causing regional ischemia or infarction. This chapter deals principally with vasculitis affecting small vessels, including Wegener's granulomatosis, microscopic polyangiitis, and Churg-Strauss syndrome. It is also increasingly recognized that pauci-immune crescentic glomerulonephritis represents a renal limited form of small vessel vasculitis.

CLASSIFICATION OF VASCULITIS SYNDROMES

The original description of many forms of vasculitis was based on postmortem findings. Kussmaul and Maier first reported "periarteritis nodosa" in a patient with nodular swellings of medium-sized arteries in several organ systems. The term *polyarteritis nodosa* was used by Rose and Spencer in 1957 when it was realized that the arterial wall itself was the target of inflammation. Davson and co-workers, in 1948, first used the term *microscopic polyarteritis* when describing patients with systemic vasculitis accompanied by patchy fibrinoid necrosis of glomerular tufts. Subsequently, in recognition of the involve-

TABLE 42.10. Classification of Vasculitis, According to Chapel Hill Consensus Nomenclature (Jennette et al, 1994)

Syndromes Affecting Small Vessels (Capillaries, Venules, and Arterioles)	
Wegener's granulomatosis	Granulomatous inflammation in the respiratory tract/necrotizing vasculitis affecting small- to medium-sized vessels
Churg-Strauss syndrome	Eosinophil-rich and granulomatous inflammation in the respiratory tract; necrotizing vasculitis affecting small- and medium-sized vessels; asthma and eosinophilia
Microscopic polyangiitis	Necrotizing vasculitis, with few or no immune deposits, affecting small vessels
Henoch-Schönlein purpura	Vasculitis, with IgA-dominant immune deposits, affecting small vessels
Essential cryoglobulinaemic vasculitis	Vasculitis, with cryoglobulin deposits, affecting small vessels, and associated with circulating cryoglobulins
Cutaneous leukocytoclastic angiitis	Isolated cutaneous leuocytoclastic angiitis without systemic vasculitis or glomerulonephritis
Syndromes Affecting Medium-Sized Vessels	
Polyarteritis nodosa	Necrotizing inflammation of medium-sized or small arteries without glomerulonephritis or vasculitis in arterioles, capillaries, or venules
Kawasaki disease	Arteritis involving large, medium-sized, and small arteries; associated with mucocutaneous lymph node syndrome
Syndromes Affecting Large Vessels	
Giant cell arteritis	Granulomatous arteritis of the aorta and its major branches, with a predilection for the extracranial branches of the carotid artery
Takayasu arteritis	Granulomatous inflammation of the aorta and its major branches

ment of capillaries and venules in this condition, the term *microscopic polyangiitis* was introduced.

Wegener's granulomatosis, defined by a triad of respiratory tract lesions, granulomata, and glomerulonephritis, was initially described by Klinger but fully characterized by Wegener in 1936. This condition was comprehensively described by Godman and Churg in 1954, and limited forms of the disease, sparing the kidneys, were subsequently recognized by Carrington and Liebow and others. Churg and Strauss in 1951 described a granulomatous form of vasculitis, characterized by asthma, eosinophilia, and multisystem disease (Churg-Strauss syndrome). Segmental glomerular lesions were commonly seen but were rarely severe.

Following these early descriptions, it was appreciated that there was a spectrum of systemic vasculitis, with both distinct and overlapping features. Several simple classifications were proposed based on the size of vessel principally involved and the presence or absence of granulomata. However, it is only in the last 10 years that more systematic classification systems have been developed. In 1990, the American College of Rheumatologists identified clinical features most commonly associated with certain vasculitic syndromes and proposed combinations of features that would identify patients with each of the syndromes concerned. Unfortunately, the list of diagnoses did not include microscopic polyarteritis (a condition seen more frequently by nephrologists), resulting in some confusion. In particular, patients with small vessel vasculitis affecting internal organs, but without granulomata or ENT (ear, nose, and throat) symptoms, could not readily be classified.

The situation improved after a multidisciplinary international consensus conference at Chapel Hill, North Carolina, in 1994. This conference was concerned with standardizing the nomenclature of systemic vasculitis and not with developing diagnostic criteria. The distinction between the different syndromes was based chiefly on the size of the vessel affected, together with the presence of other specific features (Table 42.10). Each syndrome is classified according to the smallest vessel affected, such that Wegener's granulomatosis (a small vessel vasculitis) can be diagnosed in the presence of involvement of muscular arteries, but polyarteritis nodosa may not be diagnosed in the presence of necrotizing glomerulonephritis. The Chapel Hill classification did not include renal-limited vasculitis, although this is now frequently regarded as a form of microscopic polyangiitis. In fact, cases of apparently renal-limited vasculitis may be found at autopsy to have more widespread disease or may in time develop clinical features characteristic of Wegener's granulomatosis or microscopic polyangiitis.

ANTINEUTROPHIL CYTOPLASM ANTIBODIES

The discovery that autoantibodies directed against cytoplasmic components of neutrophils and monocytes were associated with various vasculitic syndromes has made a great impact on the diagnosis and management of these conditions. The association of antineutrophil cytoplasm antibodies (ANCAs) with Wegener's granulomatosis was first described in 1985 and was closely followed by the recognition that ANCAs were also associated with microscopic polyangiitis and isolated focal necrotizing glomerulonephritis. Patients with Churg-Strauss syndrome are frequently reported to have ANCAs, whereas patients with vasculitis of medium-sized and large vessels generally do not. Thus the presence of ANCAs appears to identify those forms of systemic vasculitis that principally affect small vessels and that may lead to focal necrotizing glomerulonephritis. They are commonly grouped together as ANCA-associated vasculitis.

Two neutrophil primary granule enzymes are the targets of the majority of ANCAs in systemic vasculitis (Fig. 42.1). ANCAs directed against proteinase 3 produce a granular cytoplasmic staining pattern (C-ANCA) by indirect immunofluorescence on ethanol-fixed neutrophils. C-ANCAs are particularly associated with Wegener's granulomatosis and generally account for around 90% of ANCA in this condition. However, they are also found in up to 50% of cases of microscopic polyangiitis. ANCAs directed against myeloperoxidase produce a perinuclear staining pattern (P-ANCA) on ethanol-fixed neutrophils. However, they produce a cytoplasmic staining pattern on formalin-fixed neutrophils, suggesting that the perinuclear distribution of MPO is a consequence of ethanol fixation. P-ANCAs are particularly associated with microscopic polyangiitis, accounting for more than 50% of ANCAs in this condition and are also by far the most common type in isolated focal necrotizing glomerulonephritis. A detailed description of other types of ANCA is outside the scope of this chapter. However, it is worth noting that ANCAs in vasculitis may occasionally be directed against other neutrophil proteins, including elastase,

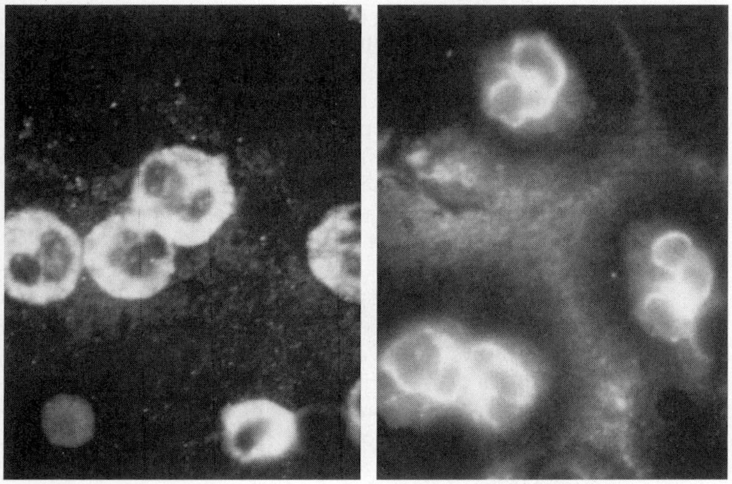

Figure 42.1. Anti-neutrophil cytoplasm antibodies detected by an immunofluorescence assay on ethanol-fixed neutrophils. A cytoplasmic pattern (C-ANCA) is shown on the left and a perinuclear pattern (P-ANCA) on the right.

alpha-enolase, lactoferrin, and bactericidal/permeability-inducing protein (BPI). ANCAs to proteinase 3 or myeloperoxidase are rarely found in diseases other than vasculitis, in which ANCAs of other specificities are more common. The diseases concerned include inflammatory bowel disease (particularly ulcerative colitis), primary sclerosing cholangitis, rheumatoid arthritis, and a variety of infections.

EPIDEMIOLOGY OF SYSTEMIC VASCULITIS

Small vessel vasculitides are uncommon, but their incidence appears to be increasing. In the United Kingdom, the incidence was reported as around 5 cases per 1 million population per year in the early 1980s and this had risen to around 15 per 1 million per year by the mid-1990s. Current estimates suggest that this has now risen to 20 per 1 million per year, with a prevalence of around 150 per 1 million of the population. At least part of this increase may be related to greater ease of diagnosis following the introduction of testing for ANCAs. Small vessel vasculitis is most commonly a disease of adult life. The median age in most published series is in the sixth decade, although population studies demonstrate the highest age-specific incidence between the ages of 64 and 75. Wegener's granulomatosis and microscopic polyangiitis are both rare in children, and such patients often show atypical features. There is a slight male predominance reported in most series of Wegener's granulomatosis and microscopic polyangiitis. There is a striking racial distribution, with the majority of cases being European Caucasoids. The disease appears to be exceptionally rare in African-Americans, but we have seen several cases in Indian Asians.

Genetic Predisposition

The literature contains several reports of familial vasculitis, although these are rare. Most reports involve siblings, some of whom had lived apart for many years, suggesting that genetic, rather than environmental factors, were important. We have, however, studied monozygotic twins discordant for vasculitis. As in other autoimmune diseases, it might be suspected that there would be associations with HLA genes. A number of reports over the years have identified weak associations, but these have generally used serologic typing methods and diagnostic criteria were not always clear. Studies using more accurate genotyping methods have generally failed to demonstrate a consistent HLA association. Perhaps the larger studies now in progress will do so. There are reported associations with polymorphisms of the C3 component of complement and, in particular, an increased frequency of the C3f allele in patients with vasculitis. There are also consistently reported associations with polymorphisms of α_1-antitrypsin, the major physiologic inhibitor of proteinase 3. In particular, the frequency of deficient Z alleles appears to be increased in Wegener's granulomatosis.

Environmental Factors

Several reports suggest a link between small vessel vasculitis and various infections. The first reports of ANCA were made in patients with vasculitis associated with Ross River virus infection. Small numbers of cases have been associated with human immunodeficiency virus and parvovirus B19. There is an established link between hepatitis B and polyarteritis nodosa (but not small vessel vasculitis). An infectious etiology or precipitant is also suggested by reports of a seasonal variation in presentation. In Wegener's granulomatosis, the frequency of relapse is higher in nasal carriers of *Staphylococcus aureus*. In these cases, it is possible that local infection may provoke disease. Small vessel vasculitis may also be precipitated by a variety of drugs. The most commonly implicated are D-penicillamine, propylthiouracil, and hydralazine and less commonly allopurinol and rifampicin. There are also suggestions of an association between ANCA-associated vasculitis and silica exposure and aminoguanidine therapy.

CLINICAL FEATURES

Because small vessel vasculitis may affect blood vessels anywhere in the body, the range of clinical features is very broad. However, some organs are consistently affected more often than others, for reasons that are not clear. The main clinical features in patients with Wegener's granulomatosis and microscopic polyangiitis, seen at the Hammersmith Hospital, are summarized in Fig. 42.2. It should be remembered that the frequency of clinical features reported in the literature depends in part on the interest of the center concerned, for example, nephrologists see a different spectrum of disease to rheumatologists.

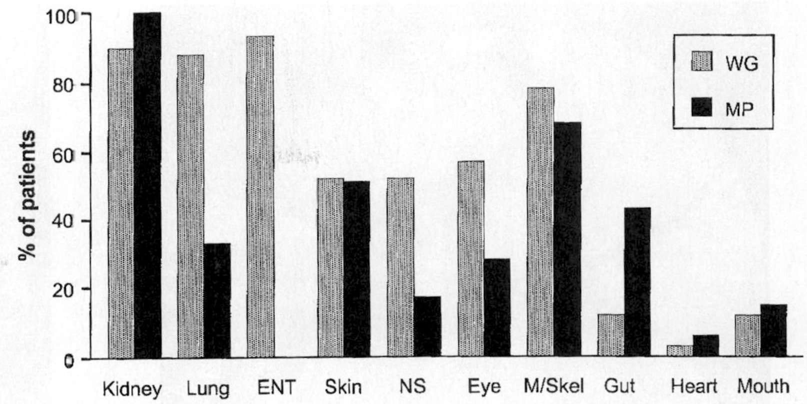

Figure 42.2. Clinical features in patients with Wegener's granulomatosis (WG) and microscopic polyangiitis (MP) treated at Hammersmith Hospital. (ENT, ear, nose, and throat; NS, nervous system; M/Skel, musculoskeletal)

Constitutional Symptoms

Many patients with small vessel vasculitis report malaise, weakness, fever, weight loss, or flulike symptoms at presentation. These are present in more than 50% of patients in most series. Arthralgia and myalgia are common, but true arthritis is rare.

Renal Disease

The characteristic renal lesion in small vessel vasculitis is a focal and segmental necrotizing glomerulonephritis, which becomes more diffuse and crescentic as the disease progresses. Microscopic hematuria, granular and red cell casts, and proteinuria suggest glomerular involvement. Macroscopic hematuria and nephrotic-range proteinuria are relatively uncommon. Hypertension is found in fewer than half of the patients at presentation but becomes more common as renal failure progresses. Without treatment, renal function often declines rapidly, such that end-stage renal failure is reached within a few weeks or months. However, the rate of progression is variable, and occasional patients may have mild renal disease for years.

Pulmonary Disease

In Wegener's granulomatosis, granulomatous inflammation in the lung is apparent in up to 90% of patients. Symptoms include dyspnea, cough, hemoptysis, and chest pain. Chest radiography reveals rounded lesions, often with central cavitation. Granulomata may also be present in the bronchi and can cause bronchial stenosis. All three of the small vessel vasculitides may present with alveolar haemorrhage. This was a common finding in our series of patients with microscopic polyangiitis (Fig. 42.2). Small vessel vasculitis is now the most common cause of Goodpasture's syndrome, the combination of rapidly progressive glomerulonephritis and lung hemorrhage. Diagnosis of alveolar hemorrhage is made by the combination of hemoptysis, dyspnea, anemia, and hypoxia, accompanied by diffuse alveolar shadowing on chest radiography. A sensitive test for lung hemorrhage is elevation of the corrected transfer factor for carbon monoxide (KCO). Some patients with small vessel vasculitis, particularly those with microscopic polyangiitis, may develop features suggestive of pulmonary fibrosis. It is thought that this may reflect scarring from persistent alveolar capillaritis.

Upper Airways Disease

In Wegener's granulomatosis, the upper airways are affected in more than 90% of patients. Symptoms include epistaxis, rhinorrhea, nasal pain, sinus involvement, tinnitus, conductive deafness, and hoarseness. Destruction of the nasal cartilage leads to the characteristic saddle nose deformity (Fig. 42.3), but gross destruction of bone or skin is unusual. Subglottic stenosis is a serious complication and may be diagnosed by analysis of the flow-volume loop. Nasal polyps are common in Churg-Strauss syndrome, but the upper respiratory tract is rarely involved in microscopic polyangiitis.

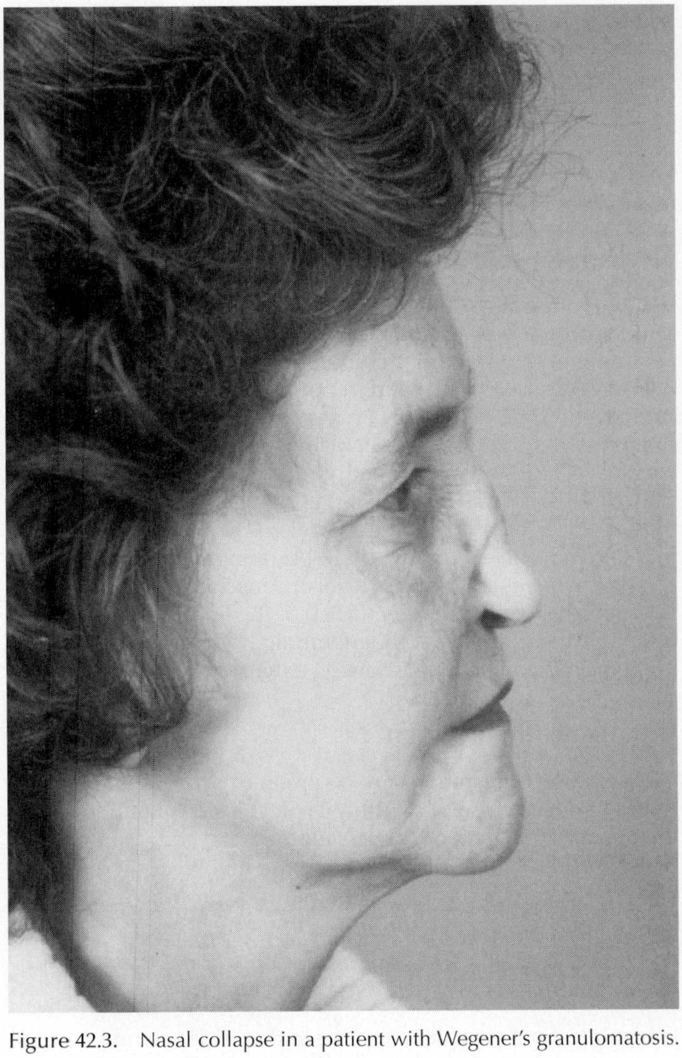

Figure 42.3. Nasal collapse in a patient with Wegener's granulomatosis.

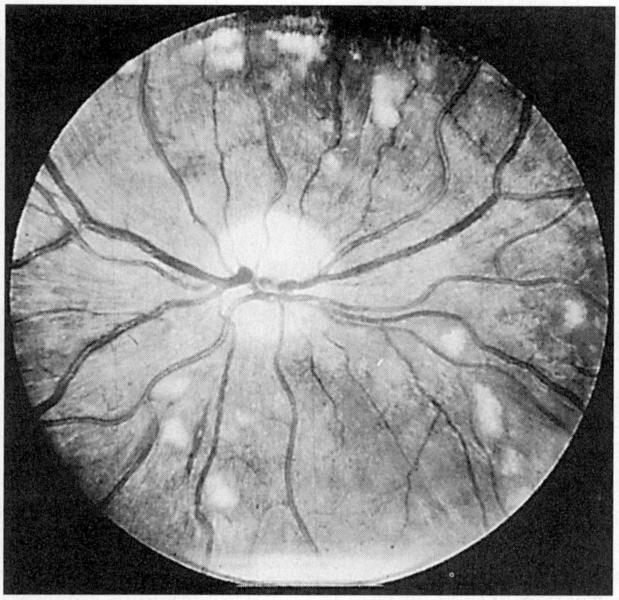

Figure 42.4. The appearance of the ocular fundus in a patient with microscopic polyangiitis. Note the multiple exudates.

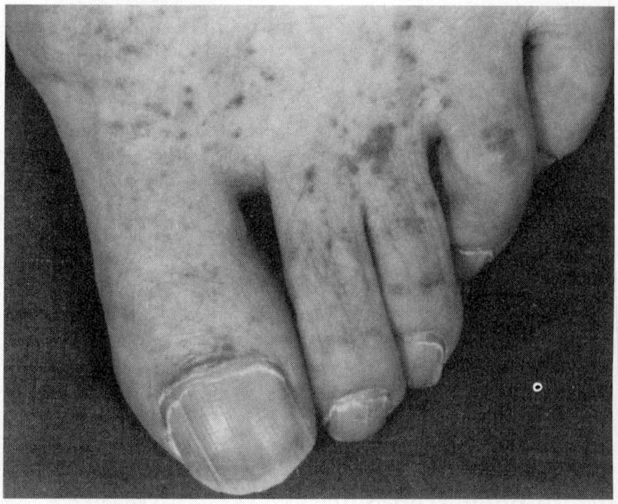

Figure 42.5. Purpuric rash in a patient with microscopic polyangiitis.

Eye Involvement

Eye involvement is most serious in Wegener's granulomatosis and may affect up to 50% of patients. There may be episcleritis, corneal ulceration, uveitis, retinal vasculitis, and optic neuropathy. Proptosis results from orbital involvement, and obstruction of nasolacrimal duct is common. Episcleritis is the most common ocular manifestation of microscopic polyangiitis, but exudates may occasionally be seen in the retina (Fig. 42.4).

Nervous System Involvement

The nervous system may be involved in up to 50% of patients with Wegener's granulomatosis, but this appears to be less common in those with microscopic polyangiitis. Peripheral nerve involvement is often reported in Churg-Strauss syndrome. Peripheral lesions typically cause an asymmetric mononeuritis multiplex or, occasionally, a distal sensory neuropathy. Peripheral neuropathy may be more common in polyarteritis nodosa. Cranial nerves may be affected either individually or in combination. Cerebral vasculitis may lead to major neurologic defects or to more subtle abnormalities, such as alteration in behavior, reduced level of consciousness, or seizures. Magnetic resonance imaging (MRI) of the brain is often helpful, although there are no pathognomonic changes. We have seen good recovery in patients showing extensive lesions on MRI.

Cutaneous Involvement

Cutaneous manifestations are common (up to 50%) in all three forms of small vessel vasculitis. Typical lesions include palpable purpura, nail bed or finger pulp infarcts, and splinter hemorrhages (Fig. 42.5). If larger vessels are involved, there may be ischemia or infarction of the extremities, producing ulcers or gangrene.

Gastrointestinal Tract Disease

Gastrointestinal vasculitis appears rather more common in microscopic polyangiitis than in Wegener's granulomatosis. It may present with abdominal pain, diarrhea, or gastrointestinal bleeding. Occasionally, there may be life-threatening major bleeding or bowel perforation. Severe ulceration of the oral mucosa occurs in some patients, and gingival hypertrophy is a feature of Wegener's granulomatosis. It should be remembered that some patients with inflammatory bowel disease may have positive tests for ANCA. Ischemia or infarction of various visceral organs (gallbladder, small intestine, spleen, or kidney) may be seen in polyarteritis nodosa.

Cardiac Involvement

Cardiac disease is relatively uncommon, except in Churg-Strauss syndrome. Arrhythmias, cardiac failure, cardiomyopathy, and pericarditis have all been reported. Coronary artery lesions, including myocardial infarction, can be seen in polyarteritis nodosa.

PATHOLOGY

The pathologic features of small vessel vasculitis are considered only briefly here. Glomerular pathology is discussed in Chapter 109 and is illustrated in the Atlas of Renal Pathology. Light microscopy of the renal biopsy reveals a focal and segmental necrotizing glomerulonephritis. There is evidence of crescent formation affecting a variable proportion of glomeruli in the great majority of patients (Fig. 42.6). Severely affected glomeruli may be seen adjacent to virtually normal glomeruli, and it is not clear why the disease process is so patchy. Fresh necrotizing lesions may be seen in the same sample as fibrocellular crescents or sclerosed glomeruli. This probably represents consecutive waves of disease activity and is rather unlike anti–glomerular basement membrane (GBM) disease in which most lesions are of a similar age. There is often interstitial infiltration by inflammatory cells, including T lymphocytes and macrophages. In a small number of patients, acute interstitial nephritis, sometimes accompanied by granulomata, may occur in the presence of normal glomeruli. Vasculitis of intrarenal arteries and arterioles is observed in only 20% to 30% of cases.

Direct immunofluorescence of the renal biopsy may be negative or may show scanty deposits of immunoglobulin and complement—hence the term *pauci-immune* crescentic glomerulonephritis. It is clear, however, that there is a spectrum of intensity of immune deposits, although these do not appear to correlate with the clinical features. Electron microscopy may re-

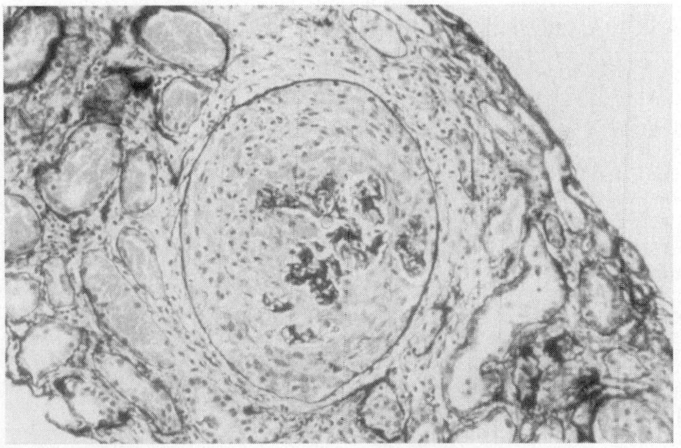

Figure 42.6. Renal biopsy in a patient with Wegener's granulomatosis showing severe crescentic glomerulonephritis.

veal breaks in Bowman's capsule or the GBM, confirm the presence of cellular crescents, and exclude the presence of electron-dense immune deposits.

The diagnosis of small vessel vasculitis is often suggested or confirmed by biopsies from other affected organs, particularly the skin, nose, and lung. Biopsy of the upper airways is relatively easy but unfortunately does not often produce diagnostic material. Similarly, transbronchial lung biopsies often produce samples that are too small and fragmented for accurate diagnosis. Open-lung biopsy is more reliable but also more invasive. Cutaneous biopsy provides a relatively easy way of confirming the presence of vasculitis, although findings are not specific and should be considered in association with the clinical picture.

DIFFERENTIAL DIAGNOSIS

It is extremely important to distinguish primary systemic vasculitis from other causes of crescentic nephritis, and from RPGN in association with other systemic diseases. In general, the diagnosis of systemic vasculitis will be made on the basis of clinical features, the presence of a positive test for ANCA, and when possible, consistent histologic findings. Anti-GBM disease (Goodpasture's disease) is one of the most important differential diagnoses of pulmonary renal syndrome. It should be distinguished by a lack of other systemic features and by the presence of circulating and deposited anti-GBM antibodies. Other causes of pulmonary renal syndrome include systemic lupus erythematosus, mixed cryoglobulinemia, and Henoch-Schönlein purpura (Table 42.11). In many of the diseases causing pulmonary renal syndrome, there are distinctive serologic features or characteristic immunofluorescence findings on renal biopsy.

TABLE 42.11. Immune-Mediated Pulmonary Renal Syndromes

More common	Microscopic polyangiitis
	Wegener's granulomatosis
	Anti-GBM disease (Goodpasture's disease)
	Systemic lupus erythematosus
Less common	Churg-Strauss syndrome
	Henoch-Schönlein purpura
	Hemolytic uremic syndrome
	Behçet's disease
	Essential mixed cryoglobulinemia
	Rheumatoid vasculitis
	Penicillamine therapy

GBM, glomerular basement membrane.

Other systemic conditions associated with renal failure (but not necessarily crescentic nephritis) include cholesterol emboli, infective endocarditis, and a variety of infections (including leptospirosis, Hanta virus, and meningococcus). In the absence of systemic disease, crescentic glomerulonephritis on a background of primary glomerulopathy should be considered, together with acute interstitial nephritis. Renal biopsy should be diagnostic in these situations.

It is increasingly recognized that ANCA-positive systemic vasculitis may coexist with anti-GBM disease. ANCAs may be detected in 20% to 30% of patients with anti-GBM disease, whereas anti-GBM antibodies may be found in 5% to 10% of patients with ANCAs. There are anecdotal reports that these "double positive" patients behave more like those with systemic vasculitis.

INVESTIGATIONS

Hematological investigations typically reveal anemia, usually with a normochromic, normocytic pattern; neutrophil leucocytosis; and thrombocythemia. Marked eosinophilia is a particular feature of the Churg-Strauss syndrome. Slight eosinophilia is often reported in other forms of vasculitis. Markers of the acute-phase response, including erythrocyte sedimentation rate and C-reactive protein, are usually increased in active disease. The latter is more specific in renal failure and more sensitive to changes in disease activity. Biochemical findings include an elevated blood urea nitrogen and creatinine, although values in the normal range do not exclude nephritis. There is often a low serum albumin (even in the absence of severe proteinuria), a raised alkaline phosphatase, and diffuse hyperglobulinemia.

Immunoassays for ANCA are positive in most patients with active disease. The titer of ANCA by immunofluorescence (IF) correlates broadly with the activity and extent of the vasculitis. ANCA is less often positive (in around 60%) in limited forms of Wegener's granulomatosis. As discussed, the ANCA pattern may be cytoplasmic or perinuclear; C-ANCAs are more strongly associated with Wegener's granulomatosis, and P-ANCAs with microscopic polyangiitis or isolated renal vasculitis. It should be remembered that P-ANCAs may be mimicked by ANAs, and the presence of ANAs by standard methods should be excluded. The specificity of ANCA testing in vasculitis is increased to more than 90%, by combining the IF assay with solid-phase immunoassays for antibodies to proteinase 3 and myeloperoxidase, although with some loss of sensitivity. It is recommended that enzyme-linked immunosorbent assays (ELISAs) for ANCA are performed in all suspected cases of vasculitis, and at a minimum, they should be performed on any sample positive for ANCA by IF. Table 42.12 summarizes the performance of standardized assays for ANCA in a large European study. Vasculitis patients presenting to a range of specialists were included; not all had active glomerulonephritis.

Most ANCA assays detect either all immunoglobulins or IgG. Some authors suggest that IgM ANCAs are particularly associated with pulmonary renal syndrome, although others have detected coexisting IgG ANCAs or have not been able to confirm this association. The presence of IgA ANCAs has been reported in patients with Henoch-Schönlein purpura, but these findings have not been widely confirmed. Antiendothelial cell antibodies have been described in some reports but are not invariably detected, and this test does not currently have a clinical role. Rheumatoid factor may be weakly positive but has no specificity for vasculitis. Complement levels are usually normal or slightly raised, as part of the acute-phase response.

TABLE 42.12. Performance of Standardized ANCA Assays in a Large European Study

	C-ANCA or P-ANCA	C-ANCA and anti-Pr3	P-ANCA and anti-MPO	C-ANCA/anti-Pr3 or P-ANCA/anti-MPO
Sensitivity in Newly Diagnosed Patients				
Wegener's granulomatosis	85%	57%	16%	73%
Microscopic polyangiitis	81%	15%	49%	67%
Renal-limited vasculitis	81%	36%	46%	82%
Churg-Strauss syndrome	66%	22%	33%	56%
Classical polyarteritis nodosa	40%	10%	10%	20%
Specificity in Control Patients				
Disease controls	76%	99%	99%	98%
Healthy controls	94%	100%	100%	100%

Reproduced with permission from Hagen EC, Daha MR, Hermans J, et al. Diagnostic value of standardized assays for anti-neutrophil cytoplasmic antibodies in idiopathic vasculitis, EC/BCR project for ANCA assay standardization. *Kidney Int* 1998;53:743–753.

Radiologic investigations may assist in diagnosis as described previously. Chest radiography may reveal the typical rounded lesions of Wegener's granulomatosis, although computed tomography is more sensitive (Fig. 42.7). Chest radiographs may show the diffuse alveolar shadowing suggestive of alveolar hemorrhage, although this may be difficult to differentiate from infection or pulmonary edema. The KCO is of particular value in such cases. Upper airways involvement, such as sinus abnormalities, may be revealed on plain radiography. However, MRI of the upper airways, sinuses, and orbit is more sensitive and better suited to repeated investigation. For renal involvement, the ultrasound appearances are not diagnostic, although there may be increased cortical echogenicity. This investigation is of most value in excluding other causes of renal dysfunction and in guiding renal biopsy. Arteriography is not routinely performed in suspected cases of small vessel vasculitis but may be of particular value when involvement of medium-sized arteries is suspected. In the latter, angiography may show the presence of aneurysms, arterial occlusions, or more widespread irregularities in vessel caliber. Radiolabeled white cell scans may identify the presence of vasculitis in various organ systems, including the respiratory tract and gut. Cerebral vasculitis is best detected by MRI.

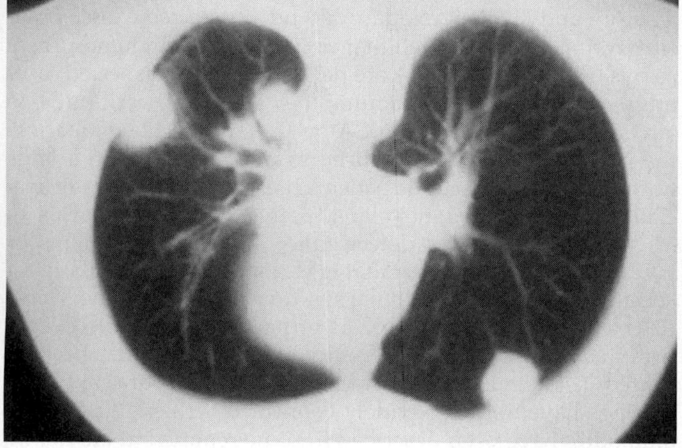

Figure 42.7. CT scan of the chest in a patient with Wegener's granulomatosis, showing discrete rounded lesions.

PATHOGENESIS

The pathogenesis of primary systemic vasculitis remains unclear. As discussed earlier, there is increasing evidence that various genetic factors underlie susceptibility to the disease. However, we are not yet in a position to assess the relative importance of these factors, and we do not know how they predispose to the development of vasculitis. It is disappointing that no clear HLA associations have emerged because this would strengthen the case that small vessel vasculitis is a distinct T-cell–mediated autoimmune disorder. Nonetheless, it seems likely that T cells are involved, both in providing help for the production of antigen-specific, class-switched antibodies (ANCAs) and also perhaps in mediating tissue injury. Several groups have reported specific proliferation of T cells from patients with vasculitis, in response to the antigens proteinase 3 and myeloperoxidase. There is a prominent T-cell infiltrate in biopsies from patients with vasculitis, although their specificity remains unknown. However, study of T cells from biopsies of giant cell arteritis reveals expansion of selected Vβ families of the T-cell receptor (TCR), suggesting an oligoclonal antigen-driven response. In addition, cytokines suggestive of a Th_1-like response have been identified in biopsy specimens. There are also reports of expansion of certain TCRs in the peripheral blood of patients with microscopic polyangiitis and Wegener's granulomatosis. A further suggestion, based on the association of vasculitis with various infections, is that T-cell stimulation may be caused by superantigens derived from microbial pathogens. So far, there is little evidence for this phenomenon in small vessel vasculitis.

More interest has been focused on the role of ANCA in pathogenesis. As described previously, ANCA titers generally correlate with disease activity and several studies have shown a rise in ANCA titer preceding disease relapse. It should be noted, however, that other reports have failed to confirm this observation. Numerous experiments have demonstrated important biologic effects of ANCAs in cell culture systems. ANCAs are capable of activating polymorphs and monocytes to undergo a respiratory burst and to secrete proinflammatory mediators, such as reactive oxygen species, cytokines, and various enzymes. There is controversy as to whether the effects of ANCAs on neutrophils are mediated via Fc receptors. In some studies, intact antibody has been required, but in others, $F(ab)_2$ fragments appear to mediate similar effects. Overall, it seems likely that the effects of ANCA are at least partly Fc receptor dependent, but the reasons for the different experimental results remain unexplained.

Coculture experiments have shown that ANCA-activated neutrophils are capable of damaging endothelial cells. It is also possible that ANCAs may directly damage endothelial cells, which have bound-released ANCA antigens on their cell surface. There is considerable debate as to whether endothelial cells themselves can synthesize and express proteinase 3 at the cell membrane. If so, this would provide an alternative source of antigen to act as a target for ANCAs. The potential for ANCAs to stimulate neutrophil-mediated endothelial damage is supported by experiments demonstrating ANCA-induced neutrophil adherence to endothelial cells and reduced deformability of neutrophils (making their passage through capillaries more difficult). ANCAs could also lead to endothelial injury by increasing the potential toxicity of locally released proteinase 3 or myeloperoxidase by blocking the binding to these enzymes of their specific inhibitors. For example, it has consistently been observed that proteinase 3–specific ANCA block the binding of α_1-antitrypsin to proteinase 3.

Unfortunately, there are no good animal models of ANCA-associated vasculitis. Detailed consideration of current models is outside the scope of this chapter. However, several different *in vivo* models do provide some support for the potential pathogenic role of ANCAs. For example, rats preimmunized with myeloperoxidase developed glomerulonephritis when their kidneys were perfused, *ex vivo,* with products of activated neutrophils. In another model, preimmunized rats developed glomerulonephritis when injected parenterally with subnephritogenic doses of anti-GBM antibodies, suggesting that anti-MPO antibodies can enhance glomerular inflammation.

There are several reports of the presence of antiendothelial cell antibodies (AECAs) in small vessel vasculitis. In a small number of studies, these antibodies have been shown to cause endothelial cell damage *in vitro.* However, AECAs are not a consistent finding in vasculitis, and their role remains far from clear.

NATURAL HISTORY

The bleak prognosis of untreated vasculitis was clearly demonstrated in historical studies in Wegener's granulomatosis; mean survival was only 5 months, with renal failure and extensive respiratory disease the main killers. The first drugs to make a significant impact were glucocorticoids, but escalating doses were often required until the disease became resistant to therapy. The empirical addition of alkylating agents—initially nitrogen mustard, and subsequently cyclophosphamide—by investigators of the National Institutes of Health (NIH) was a major advance in the treatment of Wegener's granulomatosis, and combined steroid–cyclophosphamide regimens have been the cornerstone of therapy since the 1970s. Similar regimens have been used in the treatment of microscopic polyangiitis and polyarteritis nodosa since the reporting of better outcomes in patients treated with combination therapy than with steroids alone. The NIH steroid and cyclophosphamide regimen, summarized in Table 42.13, was accepted as the gold standard and

TABLE 42.13. NIH Prednisolone and Cyclophosphamide Regimen for Wegener's Granulomatosis

	Starting Dose	Tapering Schedule
Prednisolone (oral)	1 mg/kg daily	Converted to 60 mg alternate days over 1–2 mo Reduced to 20 mg alternate days by 6–12 mo Subsequently tailed off if no disease activity
Cyclophosphamide (oral)	2 mg/kg	Maintained until in remission for 1 yr Tapered by 25 mg every 2–3 mo if no disease activity White blood cell count maintained at > 3,000–3,500/mm^3

widely used. Data on its efficacy and drawbacks have added greatly to our understanding of long-term problems in vasculitis therapy and shaped our current approaches.

OUTCOMES WITH IMMUNOSUPPRESSIVE THERAPY

Initial Disease Control

A response to first-line therapy is seen in around 90% of patients. Complete suppression of disease activity is not invariable, and some patients continue to have "grumbling" or "smoldering" extrarenal disease. Up to 10% of patients presenting with severe generalized vasculitis die in the early stages of treatment, typically from diffuse alveolar hemorrhage, which may be compounded by superimposed infection.

Resolution of Glomerulonephritis

Recovery of renal function, with subsequent stability, is usual when renal impairment is not severe at presentation. Recovery from advanced renal impairment is also common, although the rate varies substantially between series. Oliguria, severe renal impairment, and an initial need for dialysis have been identified as risk factors for permanent renal failure. This may reflect the contribution of irreversible renal damage, as indicated by interstitial scarring and tubular atrophy, because these independently predict a poorer prognosis. A low percentage of normal glomeruli also suggests a poorer outlook, but this is not simply a function of the extent of the involvement of the glomeruli by crescents (crescent score), which alone is not prognostic. In general, histologic parameters are an unreliable predictor of outcome in individual patients and should not be used to decide whether to withhold immunosuppressive therapy. Patients who make a good response to initial therapy and who remain in remission tend to maintain stable renal function long term.

Relapse

Between one-third and one-half of patients with small vessel vasculitis will relapse during follow-up. Relapse occurs in both Wegener's granulomatosis and microscopic polyangiitis, although the risk appears to be highest in those with proteinase 3–specific ANCA. The consequences may be severe, including progression to end-stage renal failure and death, particularly if recognition of disease activity is delayed. Relapse can occur at any time during follow-up and remains a risk even after the onset of permanent renal failure requiring replacement therapy. In the NIH series, the first relapse occurred after 16 years of remission in one patient; we have treated a similar case. In our experience, most relapses occur in patients no longer receiving combined steroid and cytotoxic therapy, and this accords with other reports of relapse after reduction or discontinuation of immunosuppressive therapy. Consequently, withdrawal of immunosuppressive treatment should be gradual, performed only when there is no sign of disease activity and accompanied by close monitoring for early signs of relapse. Unfortunately, a minority of patients relapse despite continuing therapy, at comparable doses to those who remain in remission and with no other explanation apparent.

Infection is also a recognized precipitant of relapse. Furthermore, data suggest that patients with Wegener's granulomatosis who are nasal carriers of *S. aureus* have a sevenfold higher relapse rate than those who are not; staphylococcal exotoxins with superantigen activity have been implicated.

Organ Damage Due to Disease

Many patients give a history of several months of symptoms before a diagnosis of vasculitis is finally made, and treatment may not be immediately or totally effective in suppressing inflammation. Therefore it is hardly surprising that irreversible organ damage is common. In the NIH series of patients with Wegener's granulomatosis, irreversible organ damage from vasculitis affected 86% of the patients. Table 42.14 summarizes some of the recognized patterns of organ damage.

Renal scarring is of particular concern in vasculitis patients presenting to the nephrologist. A proportion of the patients who are dialysis independent after initial therapy later progress to end-stage renal failure. This was particularly notable in a series from North Carolina, in which the probability of independent renal function at 5 years from diagnosis was close to zero in patients presenting with a creatinine of 10 mg/dl. Many of these patients have an incomplete response to initial therapy, either because of extensive glomerular sclerosis and interstitial damage at presentation or because of insufficiently aggressive initial therapy; in the North Carolina series, a poorer renal outcome was noted in patients treated with steroids alone. Other patients sustain further renal damage during relapse, against a background of limited renal reserve, and this triggers an inexorable decline to end-stage renal failure.

TABLE 42.14. Patterns of Organ Damage in ANCA-Associated Vasculitis

Organs Affected	Consequence
Kidney	Glomerular and interstitial scarring leading to irreversible renal impairment or end-stage renal failure
Lung	Interstitial fibrosis (particularly associated with anti-MPO–associated microscopic polyangiitis); bronchial stenoses (in Wegener's granulomatosis)
Ear, nose, and throat	Subglottic stenosis, tinnitus, deafness, nasal bridge collapse, sinus drainage problems
Eyes	Visual loss following orbital inflammation (in Wegener's granulomatosis), retinitis
Peripheral nerves	Residual sensory and motor deficits following mononeuritis multiplex

Fortunately, the prognosis for vasculitis patients receiving renal replacement therapy (RRT) is comparable to patients treated with RRT as a whole. The optimal modality of RRT is debated; one series did not identify particular problems with either hemodialysis or peritoneal dialysis, while data from Guy's Hospital, London, suggest that immunosuppressed patients receiving continuous ambulatory peritoneal dialysis (CAPD), including patients with vasculitis, have a higher incidence of infectious complications than nonimmunosuppressed patients. Renal transplantation is also an acceptable option in the absence of other contraindications, and conventional drug therapy may be used. ANCA positivity should not preclude transplantation, but there remains a risk of disease relapse, affecting 17% of transplanted vasculitis patients in one analysis. Necrotizing glomerulonephritis may recur in the graft.

The emphasis of care in vasculitis patients receiving RRT often shifts to their renal failure management, and there is a risk that the diagnosis of relapse may be delayed or misdiagnosed as a complication of RRT. We have seen pulmonary hemorrhage misdiagnosed as fluid overload and intestinal vasculitis with perforation treated as CAPD peritonitis; the true diagnoses were revealed at autopsy.

Complications of Therapy

Of Wegener's granulomatosis patients in the NIH series, 42% suffered adverse effects from their treatment (Fig. 42.8). Cyclophosphamide therapy was associated with a 33-fold increase in risk of bladder cancer and an 11-fold increase in risk of lymphoma. Increased susceptibility to these malignancies was confirmed in a Swedish series in which the cancer incidence was compared with a regional database. Substitution of azathioprine added instead to the risk of skin carcinoma, which was also increased in patients receiving steroid therapy for more than 4 years.

Significant infections occurred during follow-up in 46% of the NIH patients, especially in the early stages of treatment; half of the serious infections occurred during the period of daily steroid therapy. A study from our own unit confirmed the importance of steroids in predisposition to infection; the dosage of steroids was the most important factor in a cohort of patients

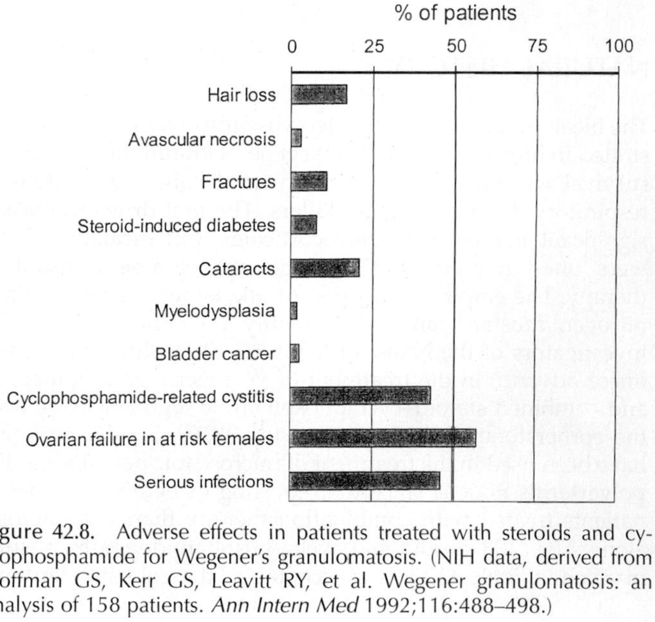

Figure 42.8. Adverse effects in patients treated with steroids and cyclophosphamide for Wegener's granulomatosis. (NIH data, derived from Hoffman GS, Kerr GS, Leavitt RY, et al. Wegener granulomatosis: an analysis of 158 patients. *Ann Intern Med* 1992;116:488–498.)

treated for immune-mediated renal diseases. The variety of infecting organisms reflects the range of precipitating factors: drug effects on humoral and cell-mediated immunity, disease-induced organ damage, hospitalization, and invasive procedures. Bacterial infections are common: sinus and nasal damage are associated with *S. aureus* infections, and dialysis access sites may become infected; respiratory infections are also common. Other infections that are widely recognized include *Pneumocystis carinii* (particularly in the presence of drug-induced lymphopenia) and *Herpes zoster;* other opportunist organisms such as *Nocardia* and *Aspergillus* have also been reported. Fatal infections are most common in the first year of treatment, and elderly patients appear to be particularly susceptible.

Infection can progress rapidly in immunocompromised patients, particularly in the presence of drug-induced leukopenia, and empirical treatment is often warranted. The differential diagnosis may also include manifestations of vasculitis, and a two-pronged approach to investigation, and even to treatment, may be required.

Overall Survival

Around 10% of patients with generalized vasculitis and renal involvement die in the first few weeks of treatment; early deaths are typically the result of uncontrolled disease, and often result from pulmonary hemorrhage. A small number of deaths occur later in the first year, with a significant contribution from opportunist infections. One-year survival rates are generally around 80%. Causes of late deaths include relapse and the adverse effects of therapy. The remainder are attributable to unrelated causes in a predominantly elderly population. Happily, prognosis has improved with early recognition of relapse and the more judicious use of immunosuppression: 5-year survival rates of 55% to 75% are the norm even when many of the patients present with advanced renal impairment.

There are certain subgroups in whom mortality is increased, including those with advanced renal failure at presentation. Indeed, probability of survival is generally lower in patients with renal disease than in those without. Failure to achieve independent renal function with initial therapy also carries an increased mortality, although this is no higher than that of patients with end-stage renal failure due to other causes. Older patients fare less well in many series, with a higher incidence of fatal infections.

CURRENT APPROACHES TO THERAPY

Strategies to Minimize Cyclophosphamide Toxicity

Most strategies retain cyclophosphamide and corticosteroids to induce remission, particularly in the presence of renal involvement, but aim to avoid the long-term risks of cyclophosphamide by using lower total doses.

For the last 20 years, we have favored a regimen in which the duration of cyclophosphamide has been limited to 2 to 3 months, with a switch to azathioprine for maintenance therapy. A comparison of this approach with the use of one year's oral cyclophosphamide has been undertaken by the European Vasculitis Study Group; preliminary results indicate equal efficacy. Substitution of mycophenolate mofetil for cyclophosphamide at 3 months has been tested in a small open study, but there are as yet no controlled trial data to indicate that it is preferable to azathioprine in this setting.

An alternative strategy, based on protocols used successfully in systemic lupus erythematosus, is to administer cyclophosphamide as intermittent pulses, with two potential advantages: a reduction in the total dose administered (provided the course of therapy is not unusually long) and the easy concomitant use of mesna to prevent bladder toxicity. Pulsed cyclophosphamide has now been tested in both open and randomized studies in Wegener's granulomatosis and other syndromes of ANCA-associated glomerulonephritis and vasculitis. It has been used most frequently, and most effectively, in first-line therapy. Dose intervals in the published reports varied from 2 weekly (initially) to 2 monthly; typical pulse size varied from 0.5 to 0.75 g/m^2, with adjustments for renal failure, age, and leukopenia; and pulses were usually, but not invariably, given intravenously. The open studies reported mixed results, which were to some extent repeated in the three published randomized, controlled trials, summarized in Table 42.15. Pulsed cyclophosphamide appeared to induce remission effectively and was associated with a lower infection risk than conventional oral dosing. However, one should be cautious in extrapolating the results of the study reported by Guillevin and co-workers, because the overall incidence of fatal infection, and the incidence of *P. carinii* in particular, was unusually high; the high dosages of steroids used and the policy of deliberate suppression of the neutrophil count may have contributed. The principal drawback of pulsed administration of cyclophosphamide is that disease control may not be sustained; circumventing this problem by prolonging the course of pulses abolishes the total dose advantage, which confers the reduction in certain adverse events.

It is worth noting that few patients with severe renal impairment have been included in published trials of pulsed therapy. Haubitz and colleagues reported on 10 dialysis-requiring patients in each limb of their study. At the end of the study, 2 of 10 in the pulse treatment limb and 5 of 10 in the continuous treatment limb were dialysis independent; 2 of 10 of the continuous limb had died of severe infection. Larger studies, with greater power, are still needed to define the place and optimal duration of pulsed therapy in the treatment of vasculitis with significant renal involvement.

Weekly methotrexate has recently been tested as an alternative to cyclophosphamide in patients with Wegener's granulomatosis, using a comparable regimen to that used for rheumatoid arthritis. It was used in combination with oral steroids and given orally at a starting dose of 0.3 mg/kg per week, increasing gradually until a mean stable weekly dose of 20 mg was reached, and continuing until patients had been in remission for 1 year. Remission was achieved in 73% of the 41 patients studied, at a median of 4.2 months, but was complicated by relapse during therapy in just under a quarter. Side effects included abnormal liver enzymes, necessitating a dosage reduction (in 25%) and reversible methotrexate-induced pneumonitis (in 7%). The overall incidence of opportunist infections was 9.5%, and included two fatal cases of *Pneumocystis* in patients also taking high-dose steroids; no prophylaxis was used. The likely role of methotrexate is as an induction agent for patients with non–life-threatening Wegener's granulomatosis or as a maintenance therapy in those who relapse on, or are tolerant of, azathioprine. It is unlikely to have a place in the routine treatment of patients with moderate or severe renal impairment because of the increased risk of toxicity.

Prophylaxis Against Adverse Effects

Prophylactic regimens for patients with vasculitis have not been subjected to rigorous study. Nonetheless, the pattern of adverse effects in patients treated for vasculitis and experience in other diseases suggest that a number of measures should be considered, including the use of proton pump inhibitors for gastric protection and the use of selected antimicrobial agents to pre-

TABLE 42.15. Three Published Randomized, Controlled Trials of Pulsed Cyclophosphamide in ANCA-Associated Vasculitis

	Adu et al, 1997	Guillevin et al, 1997	Haubitz et al, 1998
Diagnoses	WG, MP, PAN	WG	WG, MP
No. of patients	54	50	47
Common steroid regimen	(differed in 2 limbs)	Methylprednisolone 15 mg/kg days 1–3, followed by Prednisolone 1 mg/kg tapered from 6 wk	Methylprednisolone 0.5 g days 1–3, followed by Prednisolone 1 mg/kg tapered from 2 wk
Pulse Cyc schedule	15 mg/kg Increasing intervals (2–3–4–5–6 wk) to 76 wk (total of 18 pulses). With: Methylprednisolone 10 mg/kg with Cyc pulses (all pulses split into three oral doses on consecutive days from wk 7) Prednisolone 0.15 mg/kg on alternate days	0.7 g/m² 3-week intervals until remission, then at increasing intervals (4–5–6) to 2 yr	0.75 g/m² 4-week intervals to 1 yr
Continuous Cyc schedule	Cyc 2 mg/kg daily until remission (at median 3 mos); then azathioprine 1.5 mg/kg until 52 wk With: Prednisolone 0.85 mg/kg tapered from 2 wk	Cyc 0.7 g/m² at presentation, then Cyc 2 mg/kg daily from day 10, tapering from 1 yr	Cyc 2 mg/kg daily until 1 yr
Cyc dose adjustments	For renal impairment and cytopenia (both limbs)	For renal impairment (pulse limb only) For cytopenia (in both limbs) To suppress PMN count (aim nadir 1,500–3,000/mm³ in both limbs)	For renal impairment and cytopenia (both limbs)
Significant differences	None	Higher relapse rate in pulse limb Fewer severe infections (including PCP) in pulse limb	Fewer episodes of leukopenia and severe infections in pulse limb

Cyc, cyclophosphamide; MP, microscopic polyangiitis; PAN, polyarteritis nodosa; PCP, *Pneumocystitis carinii* pneumonia; PMN, neutrophils; WG, Wegener's granulomatosis.

vent infection. These include low-dose cotrimoxazole prophylaxis against *P. carinii,* isoniazid prophylaxis against reactivation of previous tuberculosis in susceptible patients, and oral antifungal therapy to prevent mucosal candidiasis. Cyclophosphamide dosage adjustments should be built into protocols to prevent severe neutropenia; our practice is to temporarily discontinue the drug if the total leukocyte count is less than 4,000/mm³ and to reintroduce it at a lower dosage once the level has risen again.

The significant risk of steroid-induced osteoporosis must also be considered. Many patients with vasculitis are elderly and have reduced bone density before therapy, and baseline bone densitometry is useful to guide management. Unfortunately, the use of biphosphonates is commonly precluded by severe renal dysfunction, so bone protection depends chiefly on calcium supplementation and appropriate formulations of vitamin D. Hormone replacement may be considered in postmenopausal women, although the increased thrombotic tendency associated with active vasculitis should be borne in mind.

Cyclophosphamide treatment should be combined with a high fluid intake (renal function permitting) to minimize bladder toxicity from its metabolite, acrolein. Mesna should be administered when high-dose, pulsed, therapy is used. Finally, because immunosuppressive drugs increase the risk of skin cancer, it is prudent to advise all patients on measures to reduce sun exposure.

Strategies to Minimize Organ Damage

The key issue for the nephrologist is how to avoid residual renal damage. Early diagnosis and prompt treatment are critical but are unlikely to prevent patients from presenting with severe renal impairment. In particular, patients with renal-limited disease are likely to present late, in the absence of extrarenal symptoms to alert them and their physicians to the problem. Two therapies, used in addition to conventional drugs, have gained considerable acceptance as adjunctive measures for patients with severe renal impairment. They are pulsed intravenous methylprednisolone and plasma exchange. There are many reports of benefit attributed to these therapies in uncontrolled studies. Proponents of the two strategies also report beneficial effects on other manifestations of severe vasculitis, including lung hemorrhage and neurologic involvement, although these aspects have not been studied in randomized trials.

Pulsed intravenous methylprednisolone is widely used in vasculitis with renal involvement, although there are no controlled trials. The doses reported in uncontrolled studies vary from 250 to 30 mg/kg per pulse, although most clinicians adopt doses of 0.5 to 1 g. Published outcomes also vary, with 50% to 75% of patients recovering renal function after initial dialysis dependence.

Plasma exchange has been tested in several controlled trials that included patients with vasculitis-associated glomerulonephritis. Two early European studies did not demonstrate a convincing effect, but neither study rigidly separated those who received plasma exchange from those who did not, and both included patients with rapidly progressive glomerulonephritis associated with a variety of systemic diseases. Two more recent trials (one from our unit) suggested benefit in the patient subgroups with advanced renal failure but no benefit in patients with lesser degrees of renal impairment at presentation. Pusey and colleagues in 1991 randomized patients to receive at least five 4-L exchanges in addition to oral steroids, cyclophosphamide, and azathioprine; 10 of 11 dialysis-dependent patients treated with plasma exchange discontinued dialysis, whereas only 3 of 8 patients in the control group did so. Cole and colleagues in 1992 randomized patients to receive 10 exchanges, each of one plasma volume, in addition to a regimen of intravenous methylprednisolone, prednisone, and azathioprine. Three of four dialysis-dependent patients treated with plasma exchange discontinued dialysis; only two of seven in the control group did so.

We now have data on 73 patients presenting with a creatinine greater than 500 μmol/L treated with a combination of oral steroids, cyclophosphamide, and five or more plasma exchanges. At 2 months, 74% were alive with independent, improved renal function; 16% were dialysis dependent, and 10% had died. Renal recovery was maintained long term in most responders.

A randomized, controlled comparison of plasma exchange and methylprednisolone is in progress by the European Vasculitis Study Group. Published uncontrolled comparisons have suggested similar efficacy. Both treatments have disadvantages and risks. Plasma exchange requires specialized equipment and expertise; it carries the risks of bleeding due to depletion of clotting factors and anticoagulation and the risks of allergic reactions and blood-borne infections associated with replacement solutions. Routine exchange for fresh-frozen plasma is inadvisable; albumin solutions are to be preferred, although clotting factor replacement may be required in patients at particular risk of bleeding. Methylprednisolone is cheaper than plasma exchange and widely available, but it may be associated with an increased infection risk and with increased corticosteroid toxicity, including avascular necrosis of bone. The two strategies have been used together successfully by some authors, but others have drawn attention to the risk of sepsis in patients in whom multiple immunosuppressive strategies are combined.

Strategies to Reduce Relapse Risk

There are wide variations in the policies adopted to maintain a remission induced with corticosteroids and cyclophosphamide. The European Vasculitis Study Group conducted a survey of 15 European centers and identified eight different drug combinations used in the first year. There was even greater variability in the second year, and by this time, patients in four centers were off therapy completely. In our unit, treatment duration has progressively lengthened since the 1970s, with a corresponding fall in relapse rate. Other groups concur that early discontinuation of therapy is associated with recurrence of disease, but controlled data are not yet available to confirm that the ratio of benefit (in preventing relapse and consequent organ damage) to risk (of adverse effects of therapy) is favorable. Our maintenance regimen comprises prednisolone and azathioprine, with azathioprine substituted dose for dose for oral cyclophosphamide once remission is achieved, typically at about 3 months. Our experience suggests that relapse in patients receiving treatment is rarely severe, and if diagnosed promptly, permanent renal damage is unusual. The optimal duration of therapy is unknown. Although relapse can occur years after diagnosis, a policy of lifelong treatment in all patients would subject many of them to unacceptable toxicity. Our current impression is that patients with persisting ANCA, irrespective of specificity, and patients whose disease was initially associated with proteinase 3–specific ANCA are at greatest risk of relapse and merit continuing low-dose immunosuppression.

An alternative approach to maintenance of remission without undue treatment risk is to use a nonimmunosuppressive therapy. A randomized, placebo-controlled trial in Wegener's granulomatosis has confirmed the value of cotrimoxazole; a significant reduction in relapses was achieved in the treated group, predominantly due to a reduction in relapse affecting the respiratory tract. However, 20% of the patients discontinued cotrimoxazole because of its adverse effects. Patients who are nasal carriers of *S. aureus* appear to be at particular risk of relapse and it is possible that the beneficial effect of cotrimoxazole is mediated through the eradication of this organism.

To apply preventive strategies that may themselves carry risks, tools to identify patients at risk from relapse are critically important. Many reports suggest that useful information can be gained from serial estimations of ANCAs, whether specific for proteinase 3 or myeloperoxidase. Immunofluorescence titers correlate in general with disease activity, although some authors find the association too weak to be prognostically useful. Persisting ANCAs point to risk of relapse, and rising titers may precede relapse. The interval is typically 1 to 3 months, but occasionally, it is much greater; ANCAs sometimes persist for long periods at high titer without evidence of relapse. Few clinicians escalate drug therapy on the basis of rising ANCA levels alone, but many will increase their vigilance and maintain existing therapy.

Other markers of relapse risk include nasal carriage of *S. aureus* (in Wegener's granulomatosis), which confers a sevenfold risk, and ANCA specificity for proteinase 3, which carries a roughly fourfold higher relapse risk than ANCA specificity for myeloperoxidase. The relapse rate is lower after transplantation than in dialysed patients, although this is likely to reflect the routine use of immunosuppressive drugs.

Management of Relapse

Confirmation of suspected relapse follows the same general principles as investigation of the presenting illness. However, the clinical picture may be less clear, with infectious complications of therapy an important differential. The clinical manifestations of relapse may differ from the presenting illness: features of extrarenal vasculitis may develop in patients who initially have isolated renal disease, and the characteristic features of Wegener's granulomatosis may occasionally emerge in a patient with an initial diagnosis of microscopic polyangiitis. The erythrocyte sedimentation rate is slow to reflect changes in disease activity, and estimations of C-reactive protein are more reliable. Nonetheless, these markers are not specific and sometimes reflect the presence of infection rather than active vasculitis. Objective assessment of disease activity, which is essential for clinical trials, is difficult. Scoring systems have been designed to assign a numerical value to disease activity, but they have not been widely adopted.

Minor relapses can often be managed by a short course of steroids or by a temporary increase in maintenance immunosuppression; however, relapses affecting the function of vital organs are usually treated with higher-dose steroids and cyclophosphamide. Adjunctive therapy may occasionally be required for severe renal or neurologic relapse or alveolar hemorrhage. A minority of patients with vasculitis will show relentless progression of disease despite aggressive therapy or will continue to show disease activity for such prolonged periods that toxicity of conventional treatment becomes limiting. Therapeutic agents that have been used in this situation include both monoclonal and polyclonal anti–T-lymphocyte antibodies, following meticulous exclusion of infection as an alternative diagnosis.

Some patients have multiple relapses and risk the adverse effects of high cumulative doses of cytotoxic agents. One agent that has been used to improve disease control in this setting is intravenous immunoglobulin. A typical schedule comprises 2 g/kg given in divided doses over 5 days, and there are anecdotal reports of successful remission maintenance using follow-up doses of 0.5 to 1 g/kg at intervals of 1 to 3 months. The principal risk is nephrotoxicity in patients with abnormal renal function before therapy. Another approach that may be considered in frequently relapsing patients is the addition of co-trimoxazole (in patients with Wegener's granulomatosis). Cyclosporine appears to be useful in selected cases.

FUTURE CHALLENGES

The goal of the physician is to steer a careful path between disease morbidity and treatment toxicity, which presents a particular challenge in the increasing number of elderly patients with vasculitis. Current efforts to optimize the use of existing therapies in multicenter studies should bear fruit soon, and data on the value of "biologic" therapies in vasculitis are likely to be available in the next few years. Anti–tumor necrosis factor strategies, which have proved successful in rheumatoid arthritis and Crohn's disease, are promising, and other antiinflammatory and immunomodulatory agents are likely to be tested; new drugs, designed initially for organ transplantation or rheumatic diseases, are also emerging. It remains to be seen whether they will deliver the desired efficacy and the safety of more selective immunosuppression.

Selected Readings

Adu D, Pall A, Luqmani RA, et al. Controlled trial of pulse versus continuous prednisolone and cyclophosphamide in the treatment of systemic vasculitis. *QJM* 1997;90(6):401–409.
A randomized, controlled trial of pulsed cyclophosphamide.

Allen AR, Pusey CD, Gaskin G. Outcome of renal replacement therapy in ANCA-associated systemic vasculitis. *J Am Soc Nephrol* 1998;9:1258–1263.
A study of the outcome of vasculitis patients on RRT.

Bajema IM, Hagen EC, Hermans J, et al. Kidney biopsy as a predictor for renal outcome in ANCA-associated necrotizing glomerulonephritis. *Kidney Int* 1999;56(5):1751–1758.
A study of renal biopsy findings predictive of renal prognosis.

Cole E, Cattran D, Magil A, et al. A prospective randomized trial of plasma exchange as additive therapy in idiopathic crescentic glomerulonephritis. *Am J Kidney Dis* 1992;20:261–269.
A controlled trial of plasma exchange in RPGN.

Guillevin L, Cordier J-F, Lhote F, et al. A prospective, multicenter, randomized trial comparing steroids and pulse cyclophosphamide versus steroids and oral cyclophosphamide in the treatment of generalized Wegener's granulomatosis. *Arthritis Rheum* 1997;40(12):2187–2198.
A randomized, controlled trial of pulsed cyclophosphamide.

Hagen EC, Daha MR, Hermans J, et al. Diagnostic value of standardized assays for anti-neutrophil cytoplasmic antibodies in idiopathic systemic vasculitis. EC/BCR project for ANCA assay standardization. *Kidney Int* 1998;53:743–753.
Performance of standardized ANCA assays in a large European study.

Haubitz M, Schellong S, Gobel U, et al. Intravenous pulse administration of cyclophosphamide versus daily oral treatment in patients with antineutrophil cytoplasmic antibody-associated vasculitis and renal involvement: a prospective randomized study. *Arthritis Rheum* 1998;41(10):1835–1844.
A randomized, controlled trial of pulsed cyclophosphamide.

Hewins P, Cohen Tervaert JW, Savage COS, et al. Is Wegener's granulomatosis an auto-immune disease? *Curr Opin Rheumatol* 2000;12:3–10.
A review of the possible pathogenic role of ANCA.

Hoffman GS, Kerr GS, Leavitt RY, et al. Wegener granulomatosis: an analysis of 158 patients. *Ann Intern Med* 1992;116:488–498.
A detailed study of outcome, including adverse effects, in patients treated with steroids and cyclophosphamide.

Hogan SL, Nachman PH, Wilkman AS, et al, and The Glomerular Disease Collaborative Network. Prognostic markers in patients with anti-neutrophil cytoplasmic autoantibody-associated microscopic polyangiitis and glomerulonephritis. *J Am Soc Nephrol* 1996;7:23–32.
A study demonstrating the low probability of long-term renal survival in patients presenting with severely impaired renal function.

Jennette JC, Falk RJ, Andrassy K, et al. Nomenclature of systemic vasculitides. Proposal of an international consensus conference. *Arthritis Rheum* 1994;37:187–192.
Consensus nomenclature of systemic vasculitis.

Jennette JC, Wilkman AS, Falk RJ. Anti-neutrophil cytoplasmic autoantibody-associated glomerulonephritis and vasculitis. *Am J Pathol* 1989;135:921–930.
An overview of the pathologic findings in ANCA-associated vasculitis.

Nachman P, Segelmark M, Westman K, et al. Recurrent ANCA-associated small vessel vasculitis after transplantation: a pooled analysis. *Kidney Int* 1999;56:1544–1550.
An analysis of the outcome of kidney transplantation in patients with ANCA-associated vasculitis.

Pusey CD, Rees AJ, Evans DJ, et al. Plasma exchange in focal necrotizing glomerulonephritis without anti-GBM antibodies. *Kidney Int* 1991;40:757–763.
A randomized, controlled trial of adjunctive plasma exchange in vasculitis-associated glomerulonephritis.

Savige J, Davies D, Falk RJ, et al. Anti-neutrophil cytoplasmic antibodies and associated diseases: a review of the clinical and laboratory features. *Kidney Int* 2000;57:846–862.
A review of the clinical and serologic features of small vessel vasculitis.

Sneller MC. Evaluation, treatment, and prophylaxis of infections complicating systemic vasculitis. *Curr Opin Rheumatol* 1998;10(1):38–44.
A review of the infectious complications of vasculitis.

Sneller MC, Hoffman GS, Talar-Williams C, et al. An analysis of forty-two Wegener's granulomatosis patients treated with methotrexate and prednisone. *Arthritis Rheum* 1995;38(5):608–613.
An open study of methotrexate in Wegener's granulomatosis.

Stegeman CA, Cohen Tervaert JW, de Jong PE, et al. Trimethoprim-sulphamethoxazole (Co-trimoxazole) for the prevention of relapses of Wegener's granulomatosis. Dutch Co-Trimoxazole Wegener study group. *N Engl J Med* 1996;335:16–20.
A randomized, controlled trial of cotrimoxazole for remission maintenance in Wegener's granulomatosis.

Watts RA, Lane SE, Bentham G, et al. Epidemiology of systemic vasculitis. *Arthritis Rheum* 2000;43(2):414–19.
A population-based study of the incidence and prevalence of vasculitis.

Westman KW, Bygren PG, Olsson H, et al. Relapse rate, renal survival, and cancer morbidity in patients with Wegener's granulomatosis or microscopic polyangiitis with renal involvement. *J Am Soc Nephrol* 1998;9(5):842–852.
A long-term follow-up study containing a systematic analysis of cancer risk in vasculitis patients treated with immunosuppression..

PART 5
Henoch-Schönlein Purpura

George B. Haycock

Henoch-Schönlein (anaphylactoid) purpura is a form of vasculitis affecting skin and other organs, especially joints, the gut, and kidneys. It is the most common vasculitis of childhood. A purpuric rash is essential to the diagnosis and is occasionally the only manifestation, but other systems just named are usually involved. The diagnosis is clinical: there is no specific confirmatory test, although the presence of IgA in biopsies of affected skin or renal tissue is strongly supportive of the diagnosis.

CLINICAL FEATURES

The disease may occur at any age, but most patients are children younger than 10 years of age. It is rare in infancy and uncommon in adult life. There is a 2:1 male predominance. It is most common in the winter months, and there is often a recent history of infection, usually respiratory. It is more common in Caucasians than in those of African descent, at least in Europe and North America. It is mainly a disease of the world's temperate climatic zones. The rash may precede or follow involvement of other organs; the skin should be inspected carefully for early signs of purpura in children with unexplained abdominal or joint pain or in those with urinary abnormalities or other evidence of nephritis. Recurrent crops of palpable purpura may occur over a few weeks, usually diminishing in severity with time. Signs and symptoms generally resolve within 3 months of onset, except for the nephritis, which may be chronic and progressive. Occasional patients, usually adults and older children, run a chronic, relapsing course for years. Urinary abnormalities may appear during recurrences of purpura even when they were not present at the time of the first attack.

Skin

The rash of Henoch-Schönlein purpura mainly affects the extensor surfaces of the limbs, being especially prominent over the ankles, calves, and buttocks and to a lesser extent the elbows. The trunk is usually spared anteriorly and above a line joining the iliac crests posteriorly. The head and scalp are occasionally involved, particularly in very young patients (younger than 4 years). The rash begins as slightly raised, pink, nonitchy, urticarialike papules. Erythema multiforme–like lesions may be seen. Within hours or a day or two, purpura develops within and between the lesions, which in severe cases may become confluent. The fully developed eruption is maculopapular, is purple in color, and does not blanch on pressure (palpable purpura). The purple fades to brown and then to yellow before disappearing. In severe cases, the rash may be bullous. Desquamation may occur.

Joints

Two-thirds of patients experience joint pain: it is the presenting symptom in up to a fourth of patients. The large limb joints (knees, ankles, wrists, and elbows) are mainly affected. The tissues around involved joints may be diffusely swollen and tender, often with a bruised appearance. In other cases, there may be pain without obvious swelling. Synovial effusions are absent, differentiating Henoch-Schönlein purpura arthropathy from other childhood arthritides. The arthritis is self-limiting and leaves no permanent damage but may be very painful. Opiate analgesics may be required.

Gastrointestinal Tract

Colicky, often severe abdominal pain affects most children with Henoch-Schönlein purpura. Gastrointestinal bleeding occurs in 80% of cases, ranging from a positive stool test for occult blood to major hemorrhage. Intussusception may occur, secondary to edema and intramural hemorrhage of the intestine, and can be difficult to differentiate from the colicky pain and melena that occur much more commonly. Bowel infarction may rarely occur. When abdominal pain is present before the rash, diagnosis can be difficult and children are occasionally operated on for a suspected abdominal emergency before the correct diagnosis is established. Careful inspection of the skin is an important part of the examination of the child with acute abdominal pain of unknown cause. Scrotal involvement may mimic torsion of the testis in boys, particularly if it precedes other manifestations of the disease (idiopathic scrotal edema).

Kidney

The renal disease of Henoch-Schönlein purpura presents with the usual features of glomerulonephritis: dysmorphic hematuria, proteinuria, casts, oliguria with fluid retention, edema and hypertension, and reduced glomerular filtration rate with azotemia. Nephrotic syndrome occurs in some patients. Hematuria, with or without proteinuria, is usually the first sign of significant renal involvement. The proportion of patients with Henoch-Schönlein purpura that show evidence of renal disease varies greatly according to the criteria used to define it and the way in which patients are selected, but most reports that describe unselected patients from general pediatric units give figures of 25% to 50% for urinary abnormalities but only 1% to 2% with evidence of long-term progression. The clinical syndromes that may be seen range from transient urinary abnormalities to rapidly progressive glomerulonephritis with early development of chronic renal failure (weeks to months).

Other Organs

Almost every organ has been described anecdotally as being involved in Henoch-Schönlein purpura, mostly very rarely. Seizures are observed from time to time, of which some at least result from hypertension, but cerebral damage with permanent neurologic sequelae is fortunately very rare. Occasional case reports have appeared of Henoch-Schönlein purpura affecting the heart, lungs, pancreas, and ureters. Hemoptysis may rarely occur.

Edema

As previously mentioned, localized edema can often be seen around joints affected by Henoch-Schönlein purpura. Generalized edema occurs less commonly. It may be due to nephrotic syndrome, but it can also develop in patients who have no proteinuria. In some of these, with severe gastrointestinal disease and low plasma albumin concentration, the cause is protein-losing enteropathy. Others have edema with normal plasma albumin: it is likely that the cause is a change in capillary permeability caused by generalized vasculitis. These possibilities should be borne in mind when the diagnosis of nephrotic syndrome is entertained.

ETIOLOGY AND PATHOGENESIS

Most patients with Henoch-Schönlein purpura give a history of a recent intercurrent infection, usually of the respiratory tract. Numerous pathogens have been implicated, including β-hemolytic streptococci; bacteria of the genera *Staphylococcus, Mycobacterium, Haemophilus,* and *Yersinia;* and numerous viruses. Less commonly, attacks have followed exposure to a variety of drugs and ingestion of foods of many different kinds. Post hoc is not propter hoc, and in many of these reported cases, the association between the putative agent and Henoch-Schönlein purpura may be casual rather than causal.

Documented cases of food or drug allergy in which administration of the suspected antigen is repeatedly followed by relapse of the disease are rare. Organisms, drugs, and foods that have been claimed to precipitate Henoch-Schönlein purpura are listed in Table 42.16.

Clinical and laboratory evidence strongly favor an immunologic basis for Henoch-Schönlein purpura. The history of exposure to an organism, food, or drug has already been mentioned. Immunoglobulins and complement components are consistently found in skin and glomeruli from affected patients. An increase in the concentration of IgA in the serum, as well as changes in its composition (polymeric, as opposed to monomeric in normal subjects), have been described. Both IgA_1 and IgA_2 subclasses may be increased. Immune complexes and rheumatoid factors containing IgA have been found in the blood by several groups. In one observation, so far unconfirmed, the presence of IgG as well as IgA in the complexes was a predictor of significant renal involvement. An increased num-

TABLE 42.16. Microorganisms, Drugs, and Foods That Have Been Implicated in the Causation of Henoch-Schönlein Purpura

Microorganisms	Drugs	Foods
Bacteria	Aspirin	Nuts
β-hemolytic streptococcus	Erythromycin	Blackberries
Mycobacterium tuberculosis	Griseofulvin	Egg
Hemophilus parainfluenzae	Iodide	Milk
Streptococcus pneumoniae	Penicillin	Potato
Mycoplasma pneumoniae	Phenacetin	Wheat
Yersinia enterocolitica	Phenothiazines	Meat (various)
Staphylococcus spp.	Quinidine	Fish
Legionella spp.	Sulfonamides	Chocolate
Salmonella hirschfeldii	Tetracycline	Chicken
Campylobacter jejuni	Thiazides	Tomato
	Chlorpromazine	Alcohol
Viruses	Acetaminophen	
Varicella zoster	Dihydrocodeine	
Vaccinia	Thiram	
Measles	Carbamazepine	
Human parvovirus	Streptokinase	
Human immunodeficiency virus	Enalapril	
Influenza vaccine	Lisinopril	
	Fluoroquinolones	

ber of IgA-secreting B lymphocytes and alterations in T-cell regulation of antibody synthesis have been reported. A consistent and satisfactory explanation of the immunopathogenesis of Henoch-Schönlein purpura, and in particular of the associated glomerulonephritis, is not yet available. Many consider Henoch-Schönlein purpura to be a multisystem form of IgA nephropathy or, conversely, that IgA nephropathy is a monosymptomatic form of Henoch-Schönlein purpura. For further information on this issue, see Chapter 39, Part 12. Because the etiology of neither disease is adequately understood, the argument is sterile and akin to debating the number of angels that can dance on the head of a pin.

LABORATORY FINDINGS

Urine

Hematuria is the most common urinary abnormality in Henoch-Schönlein purpura and usually the first to appear. As in other forms of glomerulonephritis in children, hematuria in the absence of proteinuria is generally a benign finding. However, it is an indicator that the kidney is definitely involved in the disease process and the patient should be monitored carefully for other evidence of renal disease as long as hematuria persists. Proteinuria is a more significant finding, particularly if heavy and persistent. Proteinuria in the nephrotic range (more than 40 to 50 $mg/m^2 \cdot hr^{-1}$) for more than a few days, or if accompanied by reduced glomerular filtration rate, may portend progressive disease and is an indication for renal biopsy. Dysmorphic erythrocytes and hyaline, granular, and red cell casts may be present as in any proliferative glomerulonephritis.

Blood

The blood count, including the platelet count, is usually normal: the purpura is nonthrombocytopenic. The erythrocyte sedimentation rate and C-reactive protein may be nonspecifically raised. Plasma concentrations of electrolytes, urea, and creatinine reflect renal function. The plasma albumin concentration is usually normal but may be reduced if the disease is complicated by nephrotic syndrome, protein-losing enteropathy, or (perhaps) a generalized increase in capillary permeability to albumin. Serum IgA and IgM concentrations are often raised; the IgG is usually normal. An increase in the proportion of total serum IgA in multimeric form has been found by several groups; whether this finding represents molecular aggregates of IgA alone or immune complexes is disputed. Serum C3 and C4 complement proteins are usually normal, but evidence of activation of the alternative complement pathway is sometimes present (low CH_{50} and properdin).

PATHOLOGY

Skin

Biopsies of affected skin show leukocytoclastic vasculitis, with accumulation of inflammatory cells and red cells around the capillaries and postcapillary venules. Fragmented nuclear material is present in the infiltrate. Fibrinoid necrosis and small vessel thrombosis are seen in the more aggressive lesions. IgA, C3, fibrinogen, and fibrin are demonstrable by immunofluorescent or immunoperoxidase staining techniques in vessels and connective tissue in clinically involved skin and in vessels alone in clinically noninvolved skin.

The Kidney

The renal pathologic findings in Henoch-Schönlein purpura are indistinguishable from those of idiopathic IgA nephropathy (Berger's disease). They are described in Chapter 109 (Atlas of Renal Pathology).

Light Microscopy

The basic renal lesion of Henoch-Schönlein purpura is a focal and segmental mesangial proliferative glomerulonephritis. Infiltration with polymorphonuclear leukocytes and other inflammatory cells is seen in some biopsies. In the more severe cases, extracapillary (epithelial) proliferation occurs with variable crescent formation: as in other forms of proliferative glomerulonephritis, the presence of numerous crescents is an important adverse prognostic factor. The severity of the lesion can be classified according to criteria agreed upon by pathologists of the International Study of Kidney Disease in Childhood (ISKDC), as shown in Table 42.17.

Immunofluorescent and Immunoperoxidase Staining

The immunopathologic hallmark of Henoch-Schönlein purpura is deposition of IgA and C3 in the glomerular mesangium and, to a lesser extent, in the capillary walls. Less intense deposits of IgG are seen in a majority, and IgM in a minority, of cases. Properdin and fibrin are detectable in about two-thirds of biopsies. C4 and C1q are seldom present.

Electron Microscopy

Typical findings on electron microscopy include moderate expansion of mesangial matrix and electron-dense deposits in the mesangium in most cases, subendothelially in about half, and subepithelially rarely. Immunoelectron microscopic studies confirm that these deposits contain IgA and C3 and may therefore be immune complexes.

TABLE 42.17. Classification of the Histologic Appearance of Henoch-Schönlein Purpura Glomerulonephritis, Agreed upon by Pathologists of the International Study of Kidney Disease in Childhood

I. Minimal changes
II. Pure mesangial proliferation
  a) Focal
  b) Diffuse
III. Mesangial proliferative glomerulonephritis with < 50% crescents
  a) Focal
  b) Diffuse
IV. Mesangial proliferative glomerulonephritis with 50%–75% crescents
  a) Focal
  b) Diffuse
V. Mesangial proliferative glomerulonephritis with >75% crescents
  a) Focal
  b) Diffuse
VI. Membranoproliferative (mesangiocapillary) glomerulonephritis

Modified from Heaton JM, Turner DR, Cameron JS. Localization of glomerular 'deposits' in Henoch-Schönlein nephritis. *Histopathology* 1977;1:93–104.

NATURAL HISTORY

The nonrenal aspects of Henoch-Schönlein purpura are self-limiting, although there may be several crops of purpura after the initial attack, with or without abdominal and articular involvement. With the exception of the rare relapsing variant referred to previously, the disease has usually run its course in 6 weeks and almost always within 3 months. In contrast, in cases with evidence of more than minimal renal involvement, it is common for the urinary abnormalities to persist for months or years, often with temporary exacerbations of hematuria during intercurrent infections. A very small number of patients develop rapidly progressive glomerulonephritis with rapid deterioration to renal failure; the renal biopsy in such cases typically shows extensive crescent formation.

Some patients with persisting urinary abnormalities undergo progressive deterioration of renal function with eventual slow decline into renal failure; the majority do not. Attempts have been made to identify patients at high risk for progression of renal disease according to both clinical and histologic criteria. Four broad categories of clinical outcome are recognized, and these are listed in Table 42.18. The clinical and histologic predictors of long-term outcome are summarized in Fig. 42.9. It will be seen that patients with combined nephritic and nephrotic features are at high risk for poor outcome, as are those with renal biopsy appearances in ISKDC categories 4 to 6 (especially category 5) (Table 42.18). Histology is a better predictor than clinical features alone, and it is recommended that a renal biopsy be performed in patients whose clinical features suggest a significant risk of poor outcome.

TABLE 42.18. Classification of Clinical Status at Follow-Up of Patients with Henoch-Schönlein Purpura Glomerulonephritis

	Outcome Group
A Normal	Normal physical examination, no urinary abnormality, normal renal function
B Minor urinary abnormality	Normal physical examination; hematuria (microscopic ± intermittent macroscopic) and/or proteinuria (<1 g/24 hr); normal renal function
C Active renal disease	Proteinuria (≥1 g/24 hr) ± hypertension; normal renal function
D Renal insufficiency	Glomerular filtration rate <60 ml/min/1.73 m²; death or renal replacement therapy

Reproduced with permission from Haycock GB. The treatment of glomerulonephritis in children. *Pediatr Nephrol* 1988;2:247–255.

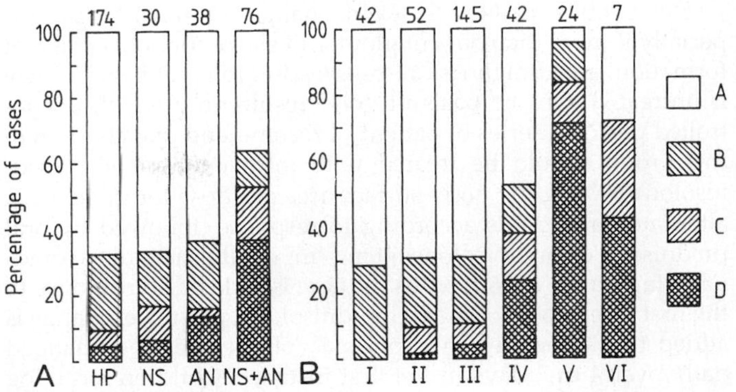

Figure 42.9. The influence of clinical **(A)** and histologic **(B)** features at presentation on eventual outcome in patients with Henoch-Schönlein purpura nephritis. AN, acute nephritic syndrome; HP, hematuria proteinuria; NS, nephrotic syndrome. Histologic categories I to VI as in Table 42.17; outcome categories A through D as in Table 42.18.

MANAGEMENT

The extrarenal manifestations of the disease require symptomatic treatment only and are not discussed here. Hypertension, if present, should be controlled with antihypertensive drugs. Patients without evidence of renal involvement need no treatment, but they should be observed with regular monitoring of urinalysis and blood pressure until all clinical evidence of disease has disappeared.

The great majority of children with Henoch-Schönlein purpura nephritis recover without evidence of permanent renal damage or loss of renal function; clearly, these patients need no treatment. Because the pathologic findings are more accurate predictors of prognosis than the clinical features alone, a renal biopsy should be performed in children with more than transient evidence of reduced renal function (low glomerular filtration rate or high plasma creatinine) and those with persistent nephrotic syndrome, especially if accompanied by "nephritic" features such as hypertension and circulatory volume expansion. It is also advisable to perform a renal biopsy when patients exhibit extrarenal disease activity that persists beyond the usual few weeks or with other atypical features because the absence of the characteristic immunohistologic findings of Henoch-Schönlein purpura nephritis raises the possibility of systemic vasculitis of non–Henoch-Schönlein type.

No treatment has ever been shown in controlled trials to be of benefit in the management of Henoch-Schönlein purpura nephritis of any degree of severity. Treatments tried and found wanting include glucocorticoids, immunosuppressive and cytotoxic agents given alone and in combination, anticoagulants and antiplatelet drugs, and rifampicin. Claims have been made for efficacy of high-dose intravenous immunoglobulin therapy in severe Henoch-Schönlein purpura. In the absence of a prospective controlled trial, this claim cannot be regarded as conclusive.

However, patients with severe changes on renal biopsy, especially if more than 50% of glomeruli show epithelial crescent formation, are at high risk of progression to renal insufficiency if untreated. On the basis of good results in a small, uncontrolled personal series of patients, I recommend that children in this group should be treated with intravenous methylprednisolone 600 mg/m^2 body surface area per dose for three to six alternate daily doses according to response, followed by oral prednisone or prednisolone 60 mg/m^2 on alternate days, gradually tapering over 6 months. If there is little or no response to the first three doses of methylprednisolone, plasma exchange is added to the regimen, two plasma volumes being exchanged daily over 4 to 7 days in the first instance. Children receiving plasma exchange are also treated with cyclophosphamide 2.5 to 3 mg/kg per day for 8 weeks. It is recognized that this regimen is toxic and potentially dangerous, but the prognosis without treatment is so bad that it is justified if it prevents a significant number of patients from developing end-stage renal failure, which carries its own morbidity. Of 12 children treated in this way at Guy's Hospital over a 17-year period, 2 are in end-stage renal failure, 6 have urinary abnormalities with normal glomerular filtration rate, and 3 are clinically and biochemically normal. Comparison with historical controls suggests that this outcome is probably better than that to be expected without treatment, despite the admitted weakness of the evidence base for this assertion. Whether this regimen is effective and safe in adult patients with similarly severe disease is unknown.

TRANSPLANTATION

There are published reports, mostly from France and Japan, of about 30 patients with end-stage renal disease resulting from Henoch-Schönlein purpura nephritis treated by renal transplantation. Recurrent glomerulonephritis has been seen in some cases, but so far, curiously, only in living-related donor grafts, in whom the risk appears to be about 30%. No case of clinical recurrence has been described in a cadaveric graft. Admittedly, the numbers are small, but it seems prudent to recommend cadaveric grafting in the first instance until further data either confirm or refute this suspicion.

Selected Readings

Allen DM, Diamond LK, Howell DA. Anaphylactoid purpura in children (Schönlein-Henoch syndrome). *Am J Dis Child* 1960;99:833–854.

A comprehensive description of the major clinical features of Henoch-Schönlein purpura based on a personal series of 131 patients.

Coppo R, Mazzucco G, Cagnoli L, et al. Long-term prognosis of Henoch-Schönlein nephritis in adults and children. *Nephrol Dial Transplant* 1997;12:2277–2283.

Follow-up of 95 adults and 57 children with Henoch-Schonlein purpura nephritis for up to 20 years.

Gairdner D. The Schönlein-Henoch syndrome (anaphylactoid purpura). *Q J Med* 1948;17:95–122.

The first modern classic account of the clinical features of the disease.

Goldstein AR, White RHR, Akuse R, et al. Long-term follow-up of childhood Henoch-Schönlein nephritis. *Lancet* 1992;339:280–282.

Follow-up of a large series of children with Henoch-Schonlein purpura originally described by Meadow et al. in 1972.

Haycock GB. The treatment of glomerulonephritis in children. *Pediatr Nephrol* 1988;2:247–255.

A review of the literature with some original data on the management of aggressive Henoch-Schönlein nephritis, among other glomerulopathies.

Haycock GB. The nephritis of Henoch-Schönlein purpura. In: Cameron JS, Davison AM, Grufeld J-P, et al, eds. *Oxford textbook of clinical nephrology,* 2nd ed. Oxford, 1998:858–877.

A more detailed and fully referenced version of the clinical features, histopathology, and management of Henoch-Schönlein nephritis.

Heaton JM, Turner DR, Cameron JS. Localization of glomerular "deposits" in Henoch-Schönlein nephritis. *Histopathology* 1977;1:93–104.

An immunohistologic and electron microscopic study of the renal lesion of Henoch-Schönlein purpura, providing support for the hypothesis that the disease is caused by immune complex deposition.

Knight JF. The rheumatic poison: a survey of some published investigations of the immunopathogenesis of Henoch-Schönlein purpura. *Pediatr Nephrol* 1990;4:533–541.

A review of current knowledge of the immunologic findings in Henoch-Schönlein purpura and their possible role in its causation.

Meadow SR, Glasgow EF, White RHR, et al. Schönlein-Henoch nephritis. *Q J Med* (New Series) 1972;41:241–258.

Clinical and laboratory features of 88 children and adolescents with Henoch-Schönlein purpura and renal involvement.

Oner A, Tinaztepe K, Erdogan Ö. The effect of triple therapy on rapidly progressive type of Henoch-Schönlein nephritis. *Pediatr Nephrol* 1995;9:6–10.

An uncontrolled but interesting study suggesting that immunosuppressive therapy, including high-dose intravenous steroids, can favorably influence the outcome of rapidly progressive Henoch-Schönlein purpura nephritis.

PART 6
Goodpasture's Disease

Richard J. Glassock

In 1919, during the influenza pandemic, Ernest Goodpasture described a patient with hemorrhagic pneumonitis who also showed evidence of glomerulonephritis at autopsy. Later, his name was applied as an eponym for a syndrome consisting of pulmonary (alveolar) hemorrhage, chiefly manifested by hemoptysis, and glomerulonephritis, often of a rapidly progressive (crescentic) variety. Coexistence of these two clinical findings is now well recognized to result from a variety of disease states (Table 42.19). Thus, in the broadest sense, the term *Goodpasture syndrome* might be used to refer to any instance in which both pulmonary hemorrhage and glomerulonephritis are encountered, regardless of underlying cause. However, with the recognition of an important role for anti–glomerular basement membrane (GBM) antibody production in the pathogenesis of many cases exhibiting these clinical manifestations, a more strict definition that incorporates the pathogenetic mechanism, thus delineating a triad of *pulmonary hemorrhage, glomerulonephritis,* and *anti-GBM antibody production,* has been advanced. Anti-GBM an-

TABLE 42.19. Disorders in Which Renal Diseases Are Accompanied by Pulmonary Hemorrhage (Goodpasture's Syndrome)

Anti-GBM antibody–mediated disease (Goodpasture's disease)
Systemic lupus erythematosus
Systemic necrotizing vasculitis (microscopic polyangiitis)[a]
Wegener's granulomatosis[a]
Henoch-Schönlein purpura
D-Penicillamine hypersensitivity
Mixed IgG/IgM cryoimmunoglobulinemia
Thrombotic thrombocytopenic purpura
Legionnaire's disease[b]
Advanced uremia secondary to renal parenchymal disease with superimposed congestive heart failure
Pulmonary embolism (with infarction) resulting from renal vein thrombosis secondary to membranous or membranoproliferative glomerulonephritis, or amyloidosis

[a] These disorders are often accompanied by antineutrophil cytoplasmic antibody.
[b] The usual renal disease is tubulointerstitial nephritis.
GBM, glomerular basement membrane.

tibody disease has been discussed in detail in Chapter 36, Part 1. This constellation of findings can be used to define a unique entity, here called *Goodpasture's disease,* to distinguish it from the disorder having a more heterogeneous basis, called *Goodpasture syndrome.* Patients with this disease may have fulminating pulmonary hemorrhage associated with very mild renal disease, only recognized by renal biopsy; may have both mild renal disease and relatively inconsequential pulmonary bleeding; or may have severe and fulminant glomerulonephritis coexisting with a wide range of severity of pulmonary manifestations. *Goodpasture's disease* should be viewed as resulting from glomerular and pulmonary injury fundamentally resulting from anti-GBM antibody production, the latter reactive with glomerular, tubular, or alveolar basement membrane antigens.

Goodpasture's disease is rare. Based on finding autoantibodies to GBM antigens, it occurs in about 0.5 cases per 1 million per year, although seasonal outbreaks may be associated with much higher incidence. Depending on series and referrals, it accounts for about 2% to 5% of all primary glomerulonephritis, and about 10% to 30% of crescentic glomerulonephritis. It is more common in Caucasians than in African-Americans or Asians.

Goodpasture syndrome is more common, with most cases resulting from an underlying vasculitis, most often of the antineutrophil cytoplasmic antibody (ANCA)–positive variety. This chapter deals with the clinical and pathologic aspects of Goodpasture's disease as contrasted to Goodpasture syndrome.

CLINICAL AND LABORATORY FEATURES

Renal

The clinical features of renal involvement are varied, but most cases initially evidence or subsequently develop a picture of rapidly progressive renal functional impairment resulting from glomerulonephritis. Blood pressure is often normal or only mildly increased. Urinalysis reveals dysmorphic microhematuria and proteinuria often associated with erythrocyte casts. The proteinuria is only occasionally massive and rarely evokes the biochemical features of nephrotic syndrome. On rare occasions, the urinalysis and renal function may be entirely normal; nonetheless, renal biopsies may reveal typical immunologic features of anti-GBM antibody disease outlined in the following. When recurrent hemoptysis is the dominant clinical feature, such patients may be diagnosed as having *idiopathic pulmonary hemosiderosis.*

Pulmonary

Hemoptysis and pulmonary infiltrates are usually the presenting features of pulmonary involvement. The pulmonary manifestations usually precede the nephritis by days or weeks or even longer periods of time. Episodes of hemoptysis may have been present for several years before the development of overt renal disease, but this is not common. On occasion, hemoptysis may not be present initially but appears later as the disease progresses. The presence of pulmonary hemorrhage in anti-GBM antibody disease is highly correlated with concomitant exposure to pulmonary irritants, especially cigarette smoke. Cocaine inhalation may also provoke bouts of pulmonary bleeding. Nonsmokers with anti-GBM antibody disease seldom develop pulmonary hemorrhage. Because advanced uremia with congestive heart failure can, at times, produce blood-streaked or frankly bloody sputum, confusion may be present regarding the true nature of disease when the patient is seen clinically with already far-advanced renal failure. From time to time, intrapulmonary bleeding occurs without any overt hemoptysis and is discovered only as the result of a chest x-ray examination, concomitant iron deficiency anemia, the presence of macrophages in the sputum, or a reduced arterial oxygen saturation. Arterial Po_2 levels may be quite low and fail to rise with 100% oxygen delivery in cases of extensive hemorrhage. Cough and shortness of breath are common symptoms, but pleuritic chest pain is rare and when present should give rise to the suspicion of systemic lupus erythematosus, vasculitis, or pulmonary emboli.

Chest x-ray examination reveals bilateral perihilar alveolar infiltrates often without air bronchograms. In severe disease, generalized pulmonary involvement may be present. Pleural effusions are rare except when advanced renal failure has ensued. Lobular consolidation or cavitation should suggest an underlying infectious illness, pulmonary emboli, or a vasculitis such as Wegener's granulomatosis. ^{59}Fe scanning of the lung may reveal extensive iron sequestration in the form of hemosiderin. $C^{15}O$ scans may reveal increased uptake and/or delayed disappearance of carbon monoxide resulting from binding to the intraalveolar hemoglobin. The single-breath carbon monoxide uptake is *increased,* and this test is a useful way of evaluating the presence and progress of underlying intrapulmonary bleeding. Patients with congestive heart failure and uremia with pulmonary edema often have reduced pulmonary carbon monoxide uptake. Hemosiderin-laden macrophages are found in sputum samples, but this is not a specific finding and reflects only chronic or intermittent intrapulmonary bleeding. As stated previously, the degree of intrapulmonary bleeding may vary from a clinically silent process detected only by careful laboratory examination, including arterial Po_2, carbon monoxide uptake, and chest x-ray examination, to a fulminant, immediately life-threatening pulmonary hemorrhage associated with profound hypoxemia and a picture resembling the adult respiratory distress syndrome.

General Features

A preceding, vague, influenzalike illness with fever and myalgias is not uncommon, and a few patients have had well-documented influenza A disease. Some series have suggested a common environmental exposure to volatile hydrocarbons, although this is not always present in the history. Mini-"epidemics" of Goodpasture's disease have been described, suggesting an infectious etiology. The disorder may be seen with a seasonal peak in the spring months. Affected individuals are usually young men between the ages of 20 and 30 years, although this disorder may affect nearly any age or either sex. Patients between 50 and 60 years of age, particularly females, are being increasingly recognized. Arthritic complaints and occasional central nervous system abnormalities may be seen, but frank arthritis, palpable purpura, and lymphadenopathy should make one more suspicious of an underlying systemic lupus erythematosus or vasculitis. Severe anemia of a microcytic, hypochromic, iron deficiency type may be present if intrapulmonary bleeding has been severe and protracted. A microangiopathic hemolytic anemia is not seen, and Coombs' tests are uniformly negative. Fever is usually absent at the time the patient is seen clinically unless there is a complicating infectious process. Rarely, the disorder may be associated with other diseases such as Hodgkin's lymphoma, celiac disease, myasthenia gravis, Hashimoto thyroiditis, partial lipodystrophy, nail-patella syndrome, or Alport's syndrome (postrenal transplant), as well as following lithotripsy.

Laboratory Findings

The general laboratory examination often is rather unrewarding. The serum complement components C3 and C4 are nearly always normal. Immunoglobulin levels are not consistently altered. Rheumatoid factor, antinuclear antibody, and circulating immune complexes are absent. The most regular finding, present in more than 90% of the patients, is a circulating IgG autoantibody to a basement membrane antigen, commonly detected by indirect immunofluorescence, enzyme-linked immunosorbent assay (ELISA), or radioimmunoassay (RIA). The latter test uses a solubilized collagenase-extracted antigen from pooled human GBM and will detect IgG antibodies with a high degree of sensitivity and specificity. The antibody reacts with the NC-1 domain of the $\alpha 3$ chain of type IV collagen. The reactive epitope is normally sequestered within this globular domain and consists of a 27- to 54-kD glycoprotein (see Chapter 36, Part 1). A negative ELISA or RIA test for circulating anti-GBM antibody, properly done, in a patient with pulmonary hemorrhage and evidence of glomerulonephritis, reduces the probability of Goodpasture's disease (as defined earlier) to less than 5%. The indirect immunofluorescence assay for anti-GBM antibody is less sensitive, with about a 15% to 20% false-negative rate. However, the indirect immunofluorescence assay and the RIA have approximately equal specificity, with only 1% or less false-positive results. False-negative results are more likely to be seen in patients beginning treatment late in the course of the disease or in sera collected after treatment. An occasional patient may develop an IgA anti-GBM antibody, which will not be detected in a conventional ELISA or RIA, which detect only IgG autoantibodies. The titer or level of anti-GBM antibody correlates poorly with the severity of the pulmonary and renal manifestations. The circulating antibody, as well as renal eluates, will react with normal renal, alveolar, and choroid plexus basement membrane antigens and sometimes with other GBM constituent (e.g., laminin, 7S collagen). Patients with pulmonary hemorrhage and glomerulonephritis resulting from other causes often have other serologic markers of their underlying disease, such as depressed complement components, positive antinuclear antibody, elevated circulating immune complexes, positive rheumatoid factor, positive antineutrophil cytoplasmic antibodies, or elevated cryoimmunoglobulins. Fibrin-reactive antigens are increased in the urine, although this is not a specific finding because similar changes are found in many patients with diffuse proliferative glomerulonephritis. Antistreptolysin O and other antibodies to streptococcal exoenzymes are usually normal. In 20% to 30% of patients with anti-GBM antibody disease, there may be coexistence of ANCA and systemic polyangiitis. The prevalence of HLA-DR2 antigen is greatly increased in patients with Goodpasture's disease. Approximately 85% to 90% of patients with Goodpasture's disease are positive for HLA-DR2, whereas this antigen is found in only 25% to 30% of the normal population (relative risk equals 13). Additional association with HLA-DR4, HLA-DQR, and Gm haplotype 1, 2, 21 (oxg) have been described. Coexistence of the HLA-DR2 and HLA-B7 antigens confers a worse prognosis because of more severe glomerular crescentic disease. Cases in identical twins have been reported. Chapter 36, Part 1 provides a detailed description of genetic susceptibility.

PATHOLOGY (SEE CHAPTER 109, ATLAS OF RENAL PATHOLOGY)

The renal pathology is quite varied. Patients displaying a course of rapidly progressive renal failure most often have the features of crescentic glomerulonephritis identical in all respects with that found in patients with crescentic glomerulonephritis caused by anti-GBM antibodies but without pulmonary hemorrhage. The only finding that serves to differentiate Goodpasture's disease from this form of rapidly progressive (crescentic) glomerulonephritis is the presence of covert or overt pulmonary hemorrhage in the former. Glomerular involvement with crescents is often very severe, involving 80% to 100% of the glomeruli in the renal biopsy sample. The glomerular crescents are often circumferential, occasionally contain giant cells and stainable fibrin, and are associated with segmental glomerular necrosis and extensive periglomerular cellular reaction. The glomerular tufts may appear "compressed" by the circumferential crescent. In patients with milder disease, a focal and segmental proliferative and/or necrotizing glomerulonephritis may be seen. On occasion, light microscopic analysis of renal biopsy tissue is not greatly different from normal; however, in all cases, the typical immunopathologic features described next should be present. Varying degrees of tubulointerstitial nephritis are commonly observed. Severe tubulointerstitial nephritis may be seen in the group of patients that develops, in addition to anti-GBM antibody, high levels of an antibody reacting with tubular basement membrane antigens. With progression of disease, the glomeruli undergo obsolescent changes as the crescents undergo fibrous organization. Intrarenal vasculitis is usually not observed.

The pulmonary pathology is that of extensive alveolar hemorrhage with focal loss of endothelial and capillary wall integrity. Polymorphonuclear leukocyte infiltration of the alveolar wall is common. Extensive hemosiderin-laden macrophages may be seen if bleeding has been protracted and severe. Necrotizing vasculitis and granuloma formation are not seen in classic Goodpasture's disease. In rare cases, inflammatory changes in the choroid plexus have been observed.

Immunofluorescence studies of renal tissue reveal typical and characteristic abnormalities. The glomeruli reveal *diffuse, ultralinear deposits of IgG*, indicating binding of anti-GBM antibodies with their respective antigens in the GBM. When advanced glomerular disease is present, there may be extensive distortion of the capillary wall, making recognition of the linear pattern difficult. On rare occasions in patients with mild, nonprogressive disease, serial biopsies have revealed the transformation of the deposit from a linear pattern to a combination linear-granular pattern, indicating the superimposition of an immune complex–mediated disease. Deposition of complement components is less regularly observed, and the pattern is more of an interrupted linear deposit. Fibrin and fibrinogen are regularly seen among the crescents in patients with advanced crescentic disease. Some cases reveal extensive linear deposits of IgG along some, but not all, tubular basement membranes and/or Bowman's capsule. A rare case will have predominantly IgA rather than IgG linear deposits. Table 42.20 lists diseases with linear IgG deposits in glomeruli. Eluates of renal tissue have revealed that the deposited IgG is capable of binding to normal basement membrane antigens of the glomeruli, tubules, and alveoli. Such eluted antibody is also capable of transferring the disease to subhuman primates. The antibody eluted from the glomeruli is similar in composition to the circulating antibody.

Lung biopsies have revealed linear deposits of IgG along the alveolar basement membrane; however, the distribution of the deposits is irregular, and lung biopsies may be negative for IgG deposition. Eluates of these tissues have likewise revealed that the deposited antibody will react with both glomerular and alveolar basement membrane. Because assays for circulating anti-GBM antibody have been developed using principally GBM antigens, it is not certain that the antibodies detected in these as-

TABLE 42.20. Renal Disorders Associated with Linear Deposits of IgG Along the Glomerular and/or Tubular Basement Membrane

Antibasement membrane antibody disease
Goodpasture's disease
Crescentic glomerulonephritis due to anti-GBM antibody
Membranous glomerulonephritis complicated by anti-GBM disease
Nonantibasement membrane antibody disease
Diabetic nephropathy
Following *ex vivo* perfusion of renal allograft
Polyarteritis (rare)
Minimal change disease (rare)
Systemic lupus erythematosus (rare)

GBM, glomerular basement membrane.

says are identical with those that have deposited *in vivo* in the alveolar capillary wall. It is possible that there are several species of antibodies, each directed to a specific but similar antigen in glomerular, tubular, and alveolar basement membranes. Linear deposits of IgG are not found in skin or other tissues.

Electron microscopic findings are quite similar in Goodpasture's disease and idiopathic crescent glomerulonephritis due to anti-GBM antibodies. Glomeruli revealing extensive crescent formation often display focal discontinuities or gaps in the GBM. Monocytic cells and polymerized fibrin may be seen in the glomerular crescent. A fluffy, inhomogeneous, electron-lucent deposit may be seen in the subendothelial zone of the glomerular capillary wall, occasionally lifting the endothelial cell away from the underlying basement membrane. Electron-dense deposits are not observed, except when slowly progressive disease has been associated with the emergence of an immune complex–mediated lesion. A rare patient with idiopathic membranous nephropathy may develop superimposed anti-GBM antibody–mediated glomerulonephritis. In these instances, electron-dense subepithelial deposits may be found and pulmonary hemorrhage does not occur.

PATHOGENESIS

The pathogenesis of Goodpasture's disease is reasonably well understood, although the etiologic factors that induce the disease are by and large unknown. The mechanisms that underlie anti-GBM antibody disease are discussed in Chapter 36, Part 1.

COURSE AND TREATMENT

The wide spectrum of clinical behavior in Goodpasture's disease is to be emphasized. At one extreme are those patients who develop minor and inconsequential episodes of pulmonary hemorrhage, manifested as recurring bouts of hemoptysis over many years, eventually associated with the development of minor abnormalities in the urinary sediment such as hematuria or nonnephrotic proteinuria. These cases may be labeled *idiopathic pulmonary hemosiderosis,* and only after measurement of circulating anti-GBM antibody levels does the true nature of the disease become apparent. Some of these patients, after many years of an apparently benign clinical course, may develop rapidly progressive glomerulonephritis of an explosive nature or develop serious pulmonary hemorrhage in association with a seemingly minor infectious disease. At the other end of the spectrum are those patients who are seen clinically for the first time with either fulminant and life-threatening pulmonary hemorrhage or rapidly progressive glomerulonephritis or both. Such patients may initially be confused with those with other multisystem diseases, such as systemic lupus erythematosus or vasculitis; however, again, the measurement of anti-GBM antibodies in the circulation readily provides an accurate diagnosis. In between these two extremes are those patients with overt manifestations of renal disease who have mild and non–life-threatening pulmonary hemorrhage or to rapidly progressive renal failure or both. On rare occasions, patients with mild renal disease have apparently undergone spontaneous remissions. Bouts of pulmonary hemorrhage may disappear inexplicably even in the absence of treatment and may be precipitated by associated infectious disease, not necessarily associated with pulmonary involvement.

The introduction of various treatment modalities has significantly altered the natural history of Goodpasture's disease, which previously was a lethal disease in most instances. Although few large-scale randomized, controlled, and prospective trials have yet been conducted because of the relative rarity of this condition, anecdotal data have strongly suggested a positive and beneficial effect of several forms of treatment. First, it seems clear that large doses of glucocorticoids administered intravenously as "pulses" of methylprednisolone (1 to 2 g/pulse per day for 2 to 3 days) are effective in reducing the severity of pulmonary hemorrhage and terminating serious life-threatening hemoptysis. Unfortunately, a beneficial effect of such therapy on the renal component of Goodpasture's disease has not been conclusively demonstrated. Conventional oral doses of prednisone (1 mg/kg of body weight per day) have, on occasion, been reported to result in a reduction in the "activity of disease" as assessed by the frequency of bouts of hemoptysis and/or the rate of change of renal functional parameters. Because this form of therapy has most often been administered to patients with relatively mild disease, it is not clear whether similar degrees of improvement might have occurred spontaneously.

For patients with Goodpasture's disease associated with rapidly progressive (crescentic) nephritis, the use of *intensive plasma exchange combined with conventional immunosuppression* has resulted in often dramatic recovery of renal function, provided this form of therapy was instituted *before* the development of oligoanuria or the requirement for hemodialysis or peritoneal dialysis. Such plasma exchange treatments involve the removal of up to 4 L of plasma per day initially, with replacement fluid consisting of 5% albumin or purified protein fractions. Early, daily, and intensive plasma exchange therapy combined with conventional oral doses of prednisone (60 mg/day) and an alkylating agent (cyclophosphamide 1 to 2 mg/kg per day) have been associated with significant improvement in renal function in more than 80% of patients, provided the therapy was begun before the serum creatinine rose to greater than 6.8 mg/dl. Patients who have already evolved to end-stage renal disease, who have serum creatinines of more than 6.8 mg/dl, or who require hemodialysis therapy frequently do not respond with improvement in renal function following plasma exchange (Table 42.21). Monitoring of anti-GBM antibody levels may be helpful in determining the intensity of plasma exchange therapy because the goal would be to reduce the levels of circulating antibody to low or undetectable levels as quickly as possible and then to maintain these levels by intermittent plasma exchange or by continuation of the immunosuppressive components of the therapy. The cyclophosphamide component of the regimen is usually discontinued after 8 weeks, and glucocorticoids are tapered providing no relapse of pulmonary hemorrhage occurs; relapses may be retreated by reinstitution of therapy. Plasma exchange may be discontinued after 10 to 14 treatments unless high levels of anti-GBM antibody persist. It does seem clear that such intensive

TABLE 42.21. Effect of Plasma Exchange and Immunosuppression on Outcome of Patients with Goodpasture's Disease

Treatment with Plasma Exchange + Immunosuppression Begun When:	Percent of Patients Not Requiring Dialysis Treatment at 1 Year	Total Patient Number
Serum creatinine <600 μM/L (<6.8 mg/dl)	73%	66
Serum creatinine >600 μM/L (>6.8 mg/dl)	11%	56

Adapted with permission from Turner N, Rees AJ. Antiglomerular basement membrane antibody disease. In: Cameron JS, Davison J, Grünfeld JP, et al, eds. *Oxford textbook of clinical nephrology.* Oxford: Oxford Medical Publications, 1992:438–455.

plasma exchange therapy reduces the levels of circulating anti-GBM antibody more rapidly than would have occurred spontaneously. Patients with combined anti-GBM antibody and ANCA-associated disease are unusually refractory to therapy. Antineutrophil antibody–associated vasculitis may develop subsequent to the initial presentation. Serial levels should be assessed in most cases.

Pulmonary hemorrhage that has been refractory to pulse methylprednisolone therapy often resolves during such intensive plasma exchange, and the improvement in pulmonary hemorrhage occurs irrespective of the effect of plasma exchange on renal function.

Anticoagulants are contraindicated because of the possibility of exacerbating serious pulmonary bleeding. Episodes of pulmonary hemorrhage and/or recrudescence of renal functional impairment may develop in connection with either pulmonary or nonpulmonary infectious complications, exposure to pulmonary irritants, or too rapid tapering of the intensity of plasma exchange and immunosuppression. Such relapses may not be associated with a change in the levels of circulating anti-GBM antibodies. Spontaneous relapses in patients who have been successfully treated for pulmonary hemorrhage and/or renal disease with intensive plasma exchange are relatively uncommon.

Patients with very severe initial disease with extensive crescentic involvement in glomeruli who do obtain an improvement in renal function after plasma exchange may later develop progressive renal failure associated with heavy proteinuria that is refractory to renewal of therapy. The precise mechanism for this later development of progressive renal disease is not at all clear but may be similar to that in other conditions associated with marked reduction in nephron population. A low-protein diet and the use of angiotensin-converting enzyme inhibitors may slow the progression of the disease.

Patients who fail to respond to therapy or who begin treatment at a late stage of their disease and therefore are placed on a regimen of chronic maintenance dialysis therapy without treatment directed to their renal disease are often candidates for renal transplantation. Recurrences of glomerulonephritis undoubtedly occur in the renal allograft. The precise prevalence of such recurrent disease is difficult to determine with certainty but may be as high as 30%. Fortunately, most instances of recurrence are mild and chiefly manifested by the immunopathologic findings of linear deposits of IgG along the GBM of the renal allograft. However, on occasion, fulminant crescentic nephritis may redevelop in the renal allograft. Such clinically significant recurrences are more likely to develop if transplantation is carried out at a time when high levels of circulating anti-GBM antibodies are present. Thus all patients who are considered candidates for renal transplantation should be monitored serially for circulating levels of anti-GBM antibody and should receive transplants only when such levels have fallen to low or undetectable quantities. Patients receiving renal grafts from identical twins should continue immunosuppression in both the pretransplant and posttransplant period to prevent a recrudescence of anti-GBM antibody activity. The role of "prophylactic" plasma exchange in patients with known Goodpasture's disease who are subjected to renal allotransplantation is unknown. The added risk of recurrence of glomerulonephritis in Goodpasture's disease may be a factor in the choice between a cadaveric organ donor versus a living-related donor.

Among those patients who have reached end-stage renal disease, bilateral nephrectomy has often been suggested as a means of treatment for serious pulmonary hemorrhage and has been advocated as a preliminary step in preparation of patients for renal transplantation. Although there are undoubted instances of termination of pulmonary hemorrhage promptly following bilateral nephrectomy, most patients can now be treated effectively with pulse methylprednisolone and/or intense plasma exchange. Thus bilateral nephrectomy should be reserved for patients with undoubted Goodpasture's disease who have biopsy-proven disease of an irreversible nature and whose pulmonary hemorrhage has failed to respond to high dosages of pulse methylprednisolone and intensive plasma exchange with immunosuppression. It is rarely necessary to resort to bilateral nephrectomy.

There is no convincing evidence that bilateral nephrectomy before renal transplantation will reduce the prevalence of recurring disease in the renal allograft, other than the fact that such a procedure often delays the performance of renal allotransplantation until such time as the anti-GBM antibody has fallen to low or undetectable levels. In fact, several instances of recurring disease have been described in patients who have undergone preliminary bilateral nephrectomy. Thus, at the present state of our knowledge, elective prophylactic bilateral nephrectomy should rarely be performed.

Recurrences of pulmonary hemorrhage may occur in patients with renal transplantation. Patients with Alport's syndrome receiving cadaveric renal allografts may, at times, develop circulating anti-GBM antibodies after transplantation and have rarely developed a Goodpasture-like disease. This topic is discussed in Chapter 43, Part 2. Presumably, underlying this occurrence is the fact that patients with Alport's syndrome are congenitally deficient in the relevant GBM antigen and thus are quite capable of making a primary immune response to the GBM antigens provided by the donor renal allograft. Such antibodies will be reactive only with the renal antigens of the allograft and not with the patient's native kidneys. However, it is conceivable that the patient with Alport syndrome will not be deficient in the basement membrane antigens of the pulmonary alveoli, and thus will be susceptible to the development of a Goodpasture-like disease.

Selected Readings

Cohen AH, Glassock RJ. Anti-GBM glomerulonephritis Goodpasture disease. In: Tisher CC, Brenner BM, eds. *Renal pathology,* 2nd ed. Philadelphia: JB Lippincott, 1994:524–552.

An excellent contemporary review with emphasis on pathology and pathogenesis.

Glassock RJ. Intensive plasma exchange. Help or no help? *Am J Kidney Dis* 1992;20:270–275.

A review of therapy of anti-GBM and non–anti-GBM rapidly progressive glomerulonephritis.

Hudson BG, Wieslander J, Wisdom BJ, et al. Goodpasture's syndrome. Molecular architecture and function of basement membrane antigen. *Lab Invest* 1990;61:256–269.
An excellent overview of biochemistry of the Goodpasture antigen.
Jayne DRW, Marshall PD, Jones SJ, et al. Antibodies to GBM and neutrophil cytoplasm in rapidly progressive glomerulonephritis. *Kidney Int* 1990;37: 1390–1992.
Description of the coexistence of anti-GBM and ANCAs.
Johnson JP, Moore J Jr, Austin H, et al. Therapy of anti-glomerular basement membrane antibody disease: analysis of prognostic significance of clinical, pathologic and treatment factors. *Medicine (Baltimore)* 1985;64:219–227.
A study of 17 patients showing that pathologic features in addition to treatment determine prognosis.
Salant D. Immunopathogenesis of crescentic glomerulonephritis and lung purpura. *Kidney Int* 1987;32:408–425.
An excellent review of basic mechanisms, diagnosis, and therapy.
Savage CO, Pusey CD, Bowman C, et al. Antiglomerular basement membrane antibody disease in the British Isles. *Br Med J* 1986;292:302–304.
A summary of the extensive experience at Hammersmith Hospital with Goodpasture's syndrome.
Turner AN, Rees AJ. Anti-glomerular basement membrane disease. In: Pusey C, Rees A, eds. *Rapidly progressive glomerulonephritis.* Oxford: Oxford Medical Publisher, 1998:108–124.
A definitive review of the immunology and clinical findings.
Wilson CB, Dixon FJ. Anti-glomerular basement membrane antibody induced glomerulonephritis. *Kidney Int* 1973;3:74–84.
A classic article, worth reading in the original.

PART 7
Sjögren Syndrome

Robert L. Winer

Sjögren syndrome (SS) is a chronic inflammatory disorder characterized by lymphocyte and plasma cell infiltration of lacrimal and salivary glands, with the resultant functional derangements of xerophthalmia and xerostomia (sicca complex). On occasion, other organs, such as the lungs and kidneys, may be involved. Conceptually, SS includes a primary form (sicca complex alone) and a secondary form (sicca complex plus rheumatoid arthritis (RA) or other connective tissue disease). There also is a stage characterized predominantly by lymphocyte aggressive behavior (lymphocytic infiltration, pseudolymphoma, or malignant lymphoma). The diagnosis of SS requires two of the following three major criteria: (a) xerophthalmia, (b) xerostomia, or (c) associated autoimmune disorder. Approximately 50% of patients with SS have RA, 5% to 8% have progressive systemic sclerosis, and 5% have systemic lupus erythematosus (SLE). Interestingly, 10% to 20% of patients with RA and 30% with SLE have features suggestive of SS. Also, about 40% of patients with xerophthalmia have either primary or secondary SS. Some other disorders that have been associated with SS include polymyositis, polyarteritis nodosa, mixed connective tissue disease, fibrosing alveolitis, partial and complete lipodystrophy, thrombotic thrombocytopenic purpura (TTP), Crohn's disease, psoriasis, and certain hepatic conditions such as primary biliary cirrhosis and chronic active hepatitis.

CLINICAL AND LABORATORY FEATURES

Sjögren syndrome is an uncommon disease complex primarily affecting females (90% of cases), with an average age of onset between 44 and 54 years of age (range, 5 to 70 years). In general, the clinical and laboratory manifestations are determined by which form of SS is present. Patients with the secondary form will have the sicca complex plus features of their associated connective tissue disease, usually RA. Those with the primary form have, in addition to the sicca complex, a high prevalence of extraglandular involvement, such as peripheral and cranial neuropathy, myopathy, Raynaud's phenomenon, nonthrombocytopenic purpura, interstitial pneumonitis, and renal disease. A European classification system of SS has emphasized the exocrine (glandular) and nonexocrine (extraglandular) clinical manifestations of the disease, with further subdivision of these two groups based on pathogenetic mechanisms and clinical expression.

Laboratory findings include a mild normochromic normocytic anemia (25%), leukopenia (30%), elevated erythrocyte sedimentation rate (90%), positive direct Coombs' test (25%), rheumatoid factor (75% to 90%), antinuclear antibodies (homogeneous or speckled pattern, 70%), and positive lupus erythematosus cell preparation (10%). Eosinophilia may be present, and this is most marked when there is extraglandular disease activity. Multiple organ-specific antibodies have been noted, including those directed against smooth muscle, gastric parietal cells, salivary and pancreatic duct epithelium, thyroid microsomes, and thyroglobulin. Polyclonal hyperglobulinemia is frequent (50% to 70%). Free monoclonal light chains ($\lambda > \kappa$) also have been found in the serum and urine, especially in patients with extraglandular involvement or pseudolymphoma. Cryoglobulins, often of the mixed IgG-IgM type, and hyperviscosity due to IgG-IgG or IgG-IgM intermediate complexes have been noted. About 85% of patients have circulating immune complexes, many of which contain IgA. Even though complement levels usually are normal, except when SLE or cryoglobulinemia with nephritis is present, increased fluid phase levels of C5b-9 have been detected. Serum levels of β_2-microglobulin may be elevated in patients with renal dysfunction.

A spectrum of renal disorders occurs in SS (Table 42.22), with the most common ones being primarily related to tubular dysfunction. Distal renal tubular acidosis (RTA), either overt or latent, occurs in 20% to 25% of patients. Fanconi's syndrome with proximal RTA has rarely been reported. However, isolated proximal tubular defects have been observed, such as altered uric acid transport and abnormal renal phosphorus handling, the latter of which occurred without any alterations in calcium or parathyroid hormone metabolism. Increased urinary excretion of β_2-microglobulin and other markers of tubular proteinuria are frequent (25% to 50%) as is enzymuria (30%), again indicating proximal tubular dysfunction. Of note, some of these patients with altered proximal tubular function also have impaired urinary concentrating ability or distal RTA, suggesting heterogeneity of nephron segment involvement in SS.

Urinary titratable acidity is usually decreased, and neither titratable acid nor ammonium excretion increases appropriately with an ammonium chloride acid load. Although failure to

TABLE 42.22. Renal Manifestations of Sjögren's Syndrome

Renal tubular acidosis
Distal > proximal
Impaired concentrating ability
Interstitial nephritis
Acute, chronic, pseudolymphoma
Hypercalciuria, nephrocalcinosis, nephrolithiasis
Urinary tract infection
Glomerular disease
Secondary > primary
Necrotizing vasculitis

acidify the urine is characteristic of distal RTA, an occasional patient with RTA can lower urinary pH in the presence of acidosis. Some patients with SS and distal RTA have nonthrombocytopenic purpura and hyperglobulinemia, and reviews of hyperglobulinemic patients with distal RTA have revealed a high prevalence of SS. The globulin levels per se appear to be unrelated pathogenetically to RTA, because in one large series of hyperglobulinemic patients, there were no differences between those with and without RTA, except for the presence of intense renal interstitial infiltrates in the former. Hypokalemia may be present in these patients with SS and distal RTA, and up to one-third of them may have hypercalciuria, nephrocalcinosis, and a slight decrease in creatinine clearance. Evidence of osteomalacia has been detected in about 20% of patients. Hypocitraturia and reduced renal tubular reabsorption of phosphate have been observed in 75% and 67% of patients with primary SS. Clinical nephrolithiasis has been reported, although its occurrence appears to be uncommon.

A variable degree of nephrogenic diabetes insipidus may be present in 40% to 50% of patients with SS, and it is often associated with RTA. The patients are hyporesponsive to vasopressin administration or overnight fluid deprivation. Clinical manifestations are mild, and the patients usually do not have proteinuria, azotemia, abnormal urinary sediment, or electrolyte disorders.

There appears to be an increased incidence of urinary tract infections in SS. Women with RA accompanied by SS have an eightfold greater risk of recurrent lower urinary tract infections than do women with RA alone. The incidence was particularly high in that subset of patients with vaginal sicca symptoms. Furthermore, 58% of these SS patients had chronic or recurrent pyuria. It has been suggested that there may be defective mucosal and local immunologic barriers, which may be partly explained by the generalized alterations in exocrine and immunologic function. Urinary tract obstruction with functional sequelae may also occur. Although it is rare, pseudolymphomatous involvement of the ureter has been reported.

Heavy proteinuria is distinctly uncommon, with urine protein excretion of more than 500 mg/day being found in fewer than 3% of patients in one large series. Glomerular disease as a primary event in SS is unusual, and its occurrence suggests an associated disease process such as SLE or mixed cryoglobulinemia. Glomerular alterations have been observed in SS patients with associated TTP or lipodystrophy. Three patients with the primary form of SS and circulating immune complexes had membranoproliferative glomerulonephritis or membranous nephropathy. Progressive glomerular sclerosis with renal functional insufficiency has been observed.

Some patients with SS may have progressive deterioration in renal function related to interstitial fibrosis, glomerular obsolescence, or more frequently, extensive renal interstitial infiltration by lymphocytes and plasma cells. Acute renal failure secondary to extensive pseudolymphomatous involvement of the renal interstitium has been reported. Such patients usually have evidence of lymphocyte aggressive behavior in other organ systems as well.

PATHOLOGY

The major pathologic alteration in SS is a chronic inflammatory infiltrate consisting of lymphocytes and plasma cells, which may be extensive enough to form epimyoepithelial islets. Occasionally, the infiltrates are pleomorphic with primitive or invasive features, evolving to actual malignancy. Renal changes are those of a moderate to severe interstitial nephritis with lymphocyte and plasma cell infiltration, loss of tubular definition, tubular atrophy, epithelial cell degeneration, and hyaline cast formation. In one large series of patients with primary SS, renal biopsy revealed variable degrees of tubulointerstitial alteration in approximately 50% of the cases. Mild and nonspecific glomerular changes consisting of segmental mesangial cell proliferation, increase in mesangial matrix, periglomerular fibrosis, or occasional glomerular obsolescence may occur in half to two-thirds of patients with primary SS. These changes usually are secondary to the tubular alterations. The presence of more significant glomerular lesions, often with clinical manifestations, usually is related to an associated autoimmune or connective tissue disease, especially SLE. Membranous, focal and segmental proliferative, diffuse endocapillary and extracapillary proliferative, and membranoproliferative glomerulonephritis have been described. Necrotizing arteritis and arteriolitis have also been noted. Hyaline thrombosis of glomerular capillaries and arterioles has been observed in patients with SS and TTP.

There are limited reports of immunofluorescence findings in SS. IgG has been noted in the cells of the interstitial infiltrates and in tubular cell cytoplasm, the latter probably representing protein reabsorption droplets. Focal tubular basement membrane deposits of IgG, IgM, and C3 in the absence of glomerular involvement have also been observed. Glomerular immunoglobulin and complement deposits are uncommon; when they are present, one should suspect another disease process, for example, SLE or mixed cryoglobulinemia.

There are very few electron microscopic studies of renal lesions in SS. The occasional patient with overt glomerulopathy may have the ultrastructural features characteristic of a specific lesion (e.g., membranous and focal or diffuse proliferative glomerulonephritis and thrombotic microangiopathy). However, in most patients, glomerular alterations are usually nonspecific, consisting of irregular thickening and wrinkling of basement membranes. Focal tubular basement membrane deposits have also been observed.

PATHOGENESIS

SS is an autoimmune disorder with immunoregulatory alterations manifest primarily by impaired suppressor T-cell function and B-cell hyperactivity. Functional alterations and expression are at the epithelial cell level, giving rise to the concept of an autoimmune epithelitis. Fox has summarized some of the key pathogenetic features of SS. There is a failure at the thymic level to delete autoimmune T cells, and these lymphocytes then hone in on and clonally expand in salivary and epithelial glands. There also is an inappropriate and selective expression by the glandular epithelial cells of HLA class II molecules, the proto-oncogene c-myc and adhesion molecules, along with secretion of proinflammatory cytokines [e.g., interleukin (IL)-1 and IL-6] by the epithelial cells and infiltrating lymphocytes. The glands have decreased neural innervation, and the residual glandular tissue fails to appropriately express secretory function. There appears to be a failure of the normal mechanisms of apoptosis to remove the autoimmune lymphocytes, which may be related, in part, to defects in a Fas antigen gene and expression of the Fas antigen on cell surfaces. It is reasonable to presume that similar pathogenetic phenomena may be operative in nonglandular tissues, including the kidney.

There are a variety of clinical laboratory markers of T-cell dysfunction and B-cell hyperactivity. The latter is suggested by polyclonal hyperglobulinemia, occasional monoclonal gammopathy, along with multiple organ and non–organ-specific autoantibodies, including precipitin systems peculiar to the different forms of SS [anti-Ro (SS-A), anti-La (SS-B), RA precipitin].

The production of and response to B-cell growth factor are normal; however, there is an exaggerated response to B-cell stimulatory factors. Circulating immune complexes and rheumatoid factors are often present, and there is abnormal Fc receptor–mediated clearance of IgG-sensitized autologous erythrocytes, implying defective clearance of immune complexes by the phagocytic mononuclear system. However, the presence of circulating immune complexes does not correlate with disease activity. Salivary gland infiltrates can synthesize immunoglobulin, and along with the epithelial cells, they can produce a variety of proinflammatory cytokines. Studies of salivary gland T cells using monoclonal antibodies have revealed a preponderance of helper cells expressing activation antigens. The cells infiltrating the renal interstitium are of the T-helper variety, but there also are variable foci of B cells. It is possible that the renal infiltrates may be functionally similar to the salivary gland infiltrates, particularly with respect to immunoglobulin and cytokine production. Interestingly, Fas is expressed on tubular epithelial cells and Fas-ligand on infiltrating cells of patients with SS and interstitial nephritis, but not in controls; suggesting a possible role for the Fas-Fas ligand apoptosis system in the interstitial nephritis of SS.

SS is a disease that seems to have a phasic evolutionary pattern, with the immunologic and clinical features paralleling each other. The disease is initially characterized by polyclonal B-cell hyperactivity and isolated glandular involvement. There may then be an intermediate stage of poly-oligo-monoclonal B-cell hyperactivity with systemic extraglandular manifestations; finally, some patients may progress to a stage of monoclonal B-cell hyperactivity and B-cell lymphoma.

There appears to be a genetic predisposition to SS, illustrated by an increased frequency (21%) of autoimmune diseases, including SS itself, in family members of patients with SS, while 12% of patients with SS have one or more relatives with the same disease. Segregation analysis has indicated a Mendelian-dominant genetic defect. There also are definite associations of the disease with HLA-D locus antigens. The DRw52 specificity seems to be a primary genetic marker for all patients with SS. HLA-DR3 and/or DR2 are associated with autoantibodies to the oligoribonucleoproteins SS-A (Ro) and SS-B (La), which are present in patients with the most severe disease. That different immune response genes might be operative is suggested by different HLA specificities for the primary and secondary forms of SS. The primary form is associated with HLA-B8 and HLA-DR3 and is characterized by a high prevalence of antibodies to SS-A and SS-B and frequent extraglandular involvement, including renal disease. Patients with secondary SS, especially that associated with RA, have a high prevalence of HLA-DR4 with clinical manifestations of the sicca complex and their connective tissue disease.

Viruses probably play a role in many of the autoimmune diseases, and there are data indicating that they may be operative in the pathogenesis of SS as well. Some circumstantial evidence includes the finding of Epstein-Barr viral protein and DNA in salivary gland infiltrates and renal proximal tubular cells and circulating antibodies to the retroviral antigens p24 and p19. That retroviruses may act in a genetically susceptible host is an attractive hypothesis. Chronic infection with hepatitis C virus has also been implicated in the pathogenesis of SS.

There is a large body of evidence supporting a role for sex steroids in the pathogenesis and modulation of autoimmune diseases, especially in women. SS, like many of the other autoimmune disorders, is predominantly a disease of women, which is consistent with a sex steroid–immune system interaction.

The tubulointerstitial disease in SS may be immunologically mediated. Tubular basement membrane deposits suggest an immune complex mechanism, probably as a result of *in situ* formation, as has been proposed for the autologous immune complex interstitial nephritis model in rabbits. Also, immune complexes might initiate the interstitial infiltrates, with subsequent tissue damage related to cell-mediated immunity and/or cytotoxic antibody. Alternatively, cell-mediated mechanisms may play a primary role, with secondary formation of localized immune complexes.

As indicated previously, renal tubular dysfunction correlates best with the presence of interstitial inflammatory cells. Immunocytochemical analysis of renal tissue from several patients with SS and distal RTA has shown a complete absence of vacuolar H^+-ATPase in the collecting duct as the functional basis for impaired hydrogen ion transport. That tubulotoxic humoral factors may be important is suggested by several recent observations. Transient RTA and polyuria were noted in the neonate of a mother with SS, and tubular dysfunction in the child was temporally associated with the presence of an IgG antibody reactive with distal tubular cell antigens and Tamm-Horsfall protein. This antibody was also present in the maternal circulation. A patient with SS and pseudohypoparathyroidism had a circulating autoantibody that reacted *in vitro* with renal tubular plasma membranes. Functional significance for this factor was suggested by the observation that it blocked parathyroid hormone–induced phosphaturia in the rat.

DIFFERENTIAL DIAGNOSIS

Clinically, symptoms of the sicca complex may be caused by a variety of diseases and conditions that may simulate SS. Examples include amyloidosis, lipoprotein abnormalities, sarcoidosis, chronic graft-versus-host disease following bone marrow transplantation, some persistent viral infections, neoplasia, fibromyalgia, autonomic dysfunction, and certain medications such as the anticholinergic drugs. This may be quite problematic, especially if less stringent diagnostic criteria for SS are used. Of particular concern is the complex of clinical and pathologic findings in patients with either human immunodeficiency virus (HIV) or hepatitis C infection. In addition to the clinical history, slit-lamp examination of the cornea after rose bengal staining, stimulated parotid flow rate, and salivary gland scintigraphy have been useful diagnostic adjuncts. In view of disease mimicry, the diagnosis of SS may depend on the demonstration of autoimmunity and focal tissue lymphocytic infiltrates. However, certain serologic markers, such as antibodies to SS-A and SS-B, as well as characterization of circulating lymphocytes and the immunohistochemical and cytochemical evaluation of salivary gland or other tissue biopsies may be helpful in establishing the diagnosis. For example, the infiltrating T cells in the interstitial nephritis of SS are primarily of the CD4 variety, whereas CD8 T cells predominate in other forms of interstitial nephritis, including that seen in the diffuse infiltrative lymphocytosis syndrome associated with HIV infection.

Distal RTA and nephrogenic diabetes insipidus may occur under a variety of conditions, and patients with evidence of such tubular dysfunction should be evaluated for other features of SS. Similarly, SS should be considered in patients with tubular defects and unexplained progressive renal functional insufficiency. Patients with the secondary form of SS may have renal abnormalities related to the associated disease process (e.g., SLE). The presence of extensive lymphocyte and plasma cell infiltration without evidence of infection or other suggestive history is more supportive of SS. The multiple immunologic abnormalities seen in SS should also help in this differentiation. On immunofluorescence microscopy, positive staining of interstitial inflammatory cells for immunoglobulin suggests SS. The demonstration of isolated tubular basement membrane immune complexes in the presence of interstitial infiltrates might also lead to the diagnosis of SS, although rare patients with SLE may have isolated tubular basement membrane deposits.

MANAGEMENT

In general, the management of SS is supportive and includes such measures as the use of methylcellulose ophthalmic preparations (artificial tears), proper attention to oral hygiene, maintenance of adequate fluid intake, and use of humidifiers. Phosphodiesterase inhibitors, oral pilocarpine, hydroxychloroquine, and especially cyclosporine eyedrops have shown some promise in either experimental or clinical studies. For most patients, the renal manifestations are fairly mild. Although muscle paralysis secondary to severe hypokalemia has been reported, RTA usually does not have to be treated; if necessary, only small amounts of supplemental sodium citrate and potassium are required. The urinary concentrating defect usually requires no specific form of therapy, except for awareness of the condition and possible situations in which volume depletion and dehydration may occur. Systemic glucocorticoids are indicated only when there is evidence of active muscle disease, progressive pulmonary fibrosis, hemolytic anemia, or severe renal involvement. Distinction should be made between primary glomerular disease and that related to an associated disease process, such as SLE. Steroids have been used to successfully treat membranous and membranoproliferative glomerulonephritis, with improvement in renal function and proteinuria. If hyperviscosity syndrome or cryoglobulinemic acute renal failure with proliferative glomerulonephritis are present, then glucocorticoids, cytotoxic agents, D-penicillamine, or plasmapheresis may be in order. If renal function is markedly impaired and extensive interstitial inflammatory infiltrates are present, glucocorticoids and immunosuppressive therapy may be tried. Cytotoxic therapy should be considered for patients with lymphomatous transformation. Future therapeutic modalities may include the use of monoclonal antibodies directed toward some of the elements in the immunologic system, particularly proinflammatory cytokines.

COURSE AND PROGNOSIS

For most patients with SS, longevity is not determined by the mild renal involvement that is usually seen. An occasional patient may have progressive renal insufficiency related to (a) primary or secondary glomerulopathy, (b) interstitial fibrosis and vascular changes, or (c) nephrocalcinosis. Extraglandular lymphoproliferation may progress to a malignancy such as non-Hodgkin's lymphoma or Waldenström's macroglobulinemia. In one large series of patients followed for 8 years, there was a 44-fold increase over the expected incidence for non-Hodgkin's lymphoma. One should carefully monitor SS patients for the development of lymphoma because early therapy may be curative.

Selected Readings

Fox RI, ed. Sjögren's syndrome. *Rheumatic Disease Clin North Am* 1992;18:507–717.
A multiauthored monograph covering the pathogenesis, immunology, genetics, diagnosis, nonrenal clinical manifestations, and treatment of SS. There also is a section on the clinical similarities between SS and the diffuse infiltrative lymphocytosis syndrome associated with HIV-1 infection.

Fox RI. Sjögren's syndrome. Pathogenesis and new approaches to therapy. *Adv Exp Med Biol* 1998;438:891–902.
A review of current concepts in pathogenesis, especially molecular biologic phenomena. Controversies in classification of SS, with implications for therapy are summarized.

Parke AL, ed. VIth International Symposium on Sjögren's Syndrome. *J Rheumatol* 1997;24(Suppl 50):1–52.
A recent presentation of current observations, including controversies, on the diagnosis, pathogenesis, immunology, and treatment of SS. Abstracts of current research are included.

Pavlidis NA, Karsh J, Moutsopoulos HM. The clinical picture of primary Sjögren's syndrome: a retrospective study. *J Rheumatol* 1982;9:685–690.
An analysis of 47 patients referred to the National Institutes of Health between 1967 and 1979. Extraglandular manifestations were most frequently characterized by renal involvement and vasculitis. Of the 10 patients who had renal biopsy, 7 had interstitial nephritis and 4 had focal glomerulonephritis.

Talal N, Zisman E, Schur PH. Renal tubular acidosis, glomerulonephritis and immunologic factors in Sjögren's syndrome. *Arthritis Rheum* 1968;11:774–786.
A description of 12 patients with SS, 6 of whom had impaired urinary acidification. Renal biopsy showed interstitial nephritis, tubular atrophy, and mononuclear cell infiltration; one patient had focal proliferative glomerulonephritis, and two had necrotizing arteritis and arteriolitis.

Winer RL, Cohen AH, Sawhney AS, et al. Sjögren's syndrome with immune-complex tubulointerstitial renal disease. *Clin Immunol Immunopathol* 1977;8:494–503.
A description of the clinical course and renal histology of a patient with primary SS and renal insufficiency. Intense interstitial nephritis associated with IgG, C3, and electron-dense tubular basement membrane deposits, without significant glomerular alterations, was observed. Possible pathogenetic mechanisms of this renal disease are discussed.

PART 8
Progressive Systemic Sclerosis

Richard J. Glassock

Progressive systemic sclerosis (PSS), also known as *scleroderma*, is a multisystem disease of uncertain origin, which is characterized by the accumulation of excessive amounts of connective tissue in many organs and tissues, as well as in blood vessels. Cutaneous involvement (scleroderma) leads to progressive thickening of the subcutaneous tissue, and visceral involvement is associated with organ dysfunction, morbidity, and mortality. The principal target organs are the skin, kidneys, gastrointestinal tract, lungs, and heart, but blood vessel involvement may be quite widespread. The pathogenesis of PSS is not well understood, but autoimmune reactions are likely candidates, especially because of serologic findings and the association of PSS with other disorders such as systemic lupus erythematosus, mixed connective tissue disease, rheumatoid arthritis, dermatomyositis, and polymyositis.

CLINICAL FEATURES

Progressive systemic sclerosis is seen in all geographic areas, has a marked female preponderance, and has an increased prevalence in African-Americans. The average age of onset of PSS is between 30 and 50 years. It is a somewhat rare condition, with an estimated incidence of about 20 cases per 1 million population per year in the United States. A genetic predisposition to the disease exists and an association with HLA DR3, DR5, and C4 null genes has been noted.

Early clinical manifestations are mild and include nonpitting edema of the face and hands, telangiectasia, and nail bed capillary changes. The latter can be best visualized by use of the ophthalmoscope and a small drop of immersion oil placed over the nail bed. Corkscrewing and capillary dropout are characteristic. Serologic features, such as a positive fluorescent antinuclear antibody (speckled pattern), positive anti-Scl-70 (anti-DNA topoisomerase I), anticollagen, and anticentromere antibodies may be present even at this early stage. On occasion, patients may be seen clinically with predominant visceral involvement and a paucity of cutaneous findings. Alternatively, progressive cutaneous sclerosis may develop with little or no visceral involvement. Limited cutaneous forms (morphea) also exist. However, in most patients, the skin edema gives way to a progressive thickening of the skin, leading to firm, taut integument proximal to the metacarpophalangeal joints (sclerodactyly) and of the face. At this time, the diagnosis can usually be made clinically with relative ease. Skin biopsies are often unnecessary. Raynaud's phenomenon may often be a prominent feature. Overlaps with other diseases are common, and PSS is a frequent late feature of mixed connective tissue disease (see Chapter 42, Part 3). These latter patients frequently demonstrate very high titers of antiribonucleoprotein (anti-RNP) autoantibodies.

Gastrointestinal involvement leads to dysphagia, esophageal and intestinal hypomotility, and malabsorption. Pulmonary fibrosis may lead to hypoxia and respiratory failure. Severe pulmonary hypertension may also be observed. Cardiac involvement causes diastolic dysfunction and congestive heart failure, often aggravated by concomitant hypertension and increased left ventricular afterload. A variant of PSS called the *CREST syndrome* is associated with calcinosis, Raynaud's phenomenon, esophageal hypomotility, sclerodactylia, and telangiectasia. Anticentromere autoantibodies, anti-Scl4, and anti-Scl6 are particularly common in this disorder, especially with Raynaud's phenomenon. As mentioned, autoantibodies to nucleolar constituents (giving rise to a speckled pattern on fluorescent antinuclear antibody) and to Scl70 (anti-DNA topoisomerase) are particularly common in PSS.

Sclerodermalike syndromes may be seen after exposure to rapeseed oil, vinyl chloride monomer, silicone or paraffin breast implants, bleomycin, carbidopa, and L-tryptophan. Systemic graft-versus-host disease can also induce a PSS-like disorder.

RENAL INVOLVEMENT

Renal disease is the most common cause of death in PSS and is found clinically in 40% to 70% of cases. Upon pathologic examination, the frequency of involvement of the kidney in PSS is even higher.

A decrease in renal plasma flow and/or glomerular filtration rate is found in 50%, proteinuria in 35%, and hypertension in 25% of patients with PSS. Malignant hypertension is seen in almost half of the patients with elevated blood pressure. Renal involvement usually occurs in one of two forms. The first, and most common, is slowly progressive renal insufficiency accompanied by hypertension and moderate proteinuria. Nephrotic syndrome is uncommon. A second and less common form manifests as acute renal failure with or without malignant hypertension *(scleroderma renal crisis).* This latter form of renal involvement often occurs abruptly and constitutes a true medical emergency because without intervention permanent renal failure or even death may ensue. Scleroderma renal crisis usually develops early in the course of PSS, is more often seen in the winter months, and may be preceded by rapid progression of skin involvement. The onset is heralded by features of severe hypertension, including headaches, visual blurring, and confusion. Rarely, acute renal failure may ensue in the absence of hypertension. Congestive heart failure, seizures, and microangiopathic hemolytic anemia may be encountered. The plasma renin activity is extremely elevated. Kidney size is usually normal, renal function profoundly is depressed, and oliguria may be present. Circulating immune complexes, rheumatoid factor, and cryoimmunoglobulins are usually normal, and complement components are not abnormal.

RENAL PATHOLOGY

The histologic changes in renal blood vessels are nearly always seen in PSS. In moderately advanced disease, tubulointerstitial fibrosis and tubular atrophy is also observed. Types I, III, and V collagen are increased in blood vessels and in the tubulointerstitial areas. The arcuate, interlobular, and small arteries and arterioles are principally affected. Marked intimal thickening with a mucinous appearance to the subintimal tissue is characteristic. Staining for acid mucopolysaccharides may be strongly positive. Intimal cell proliferation and edema are seen early with fibrosis, particularly of the adventitia, and periadventitial tissue is a common later consequence. Such perivascular fibrosis is more characteristic of PSS than hypertensive arteriolonephrosclerosis. Fibrinoid necrosis indistinguishable from malignant hypertension may be found, especially in association with scleroderma renal crisis. The glomerular changes are usually secondary to ischemia. The juxtaglomerular apparatus may be quite prominent, consistent with the profound elevations in plasma renin activity. Immunofluorescence studies are nonspecific with occasional glomerular and vascular deposits of IgM, C3, and/or fibrin. Electron-dense deposits are not seen.

PATHOGENESIS

The etiology and pathogenesis of PSS are unknown, but an immunologic disorder resulting in overproduction of collagen is suspected. Activation of fibroblasts and endothelial cells by unknown factors, perhaps growth factors (transforming growth factor-β), cytokines (interleukin[IL]-2), or a regulator of collagen gene activation, are prime candidates. Vasospasm and microvasculature abnormalities underlie some of the clinical manifestations of PSS (e.g., Raynaud's phenomenon). The role of autoantibodies to collagen and/or nuclear constituents is unknown, but these autoantibodies are useful markers of the disease process. The Scl-70 antigen is a basic chromosomal nonhistone protein immunologically related to DNA topoisomerase I. Antibodies to Scl-70 are found in 20% to 30% of patients with PSS and are rarely found in other diseases. Anti-Scl-70 may also be found when lung carcinoma is associated with PSS. Antibodies to other nucleolar constituents (RNA polymerase I, fibrillarin, KV, PM-Scl) may also be found in PSS. An antibody that mediates endothelial cell injury via antibody-dependent cell-mediated cytotoxicity is found in some patients. Plasma endothelin levels may be elevated. Some studies have suggested that the transplacental passage of immunocompetent lymphoid cells from the fetus to the mother may induce a graft-versus-host disease, leading to the late onset of PSS in the mother. This mechanism is also postulated to explain the development of PSS in the recipients of bone marrow allograft.

MANAGEMENT

The therapy of cutaneous and nonrenal visceral involvement is difficult and generally unsatisfactory. Physical exercise, joint protection, skin care, and avoidance from cold are all useful. Glucocorticoids are without benefit and can precipitate scleroderma renal crisis. Renal vasoconstriction may initiate a vicious cycle of renal ischemia, excessive renin or endothelin production, and further vasoconstriction leading to impairment of renal blood flow and glomerular filtration rate, as well as to intimal proliferation, intravascular thrombosis, and fibrinoid necrosis of vessel walls. Interruption of this cycle is best achieved by the use of angiotensin-converting enzyme (ACE) inhibitors or angiotensin II–receptor antagonists. Use of these agents have been associated with a marked improvement in survival from 18% to more than 75% at 1 year.

Therefore blood pressure and renal function should be monitored carefully, particularly in patients with rapidly advancing skin manifestations. Captopril or other ACE inhibitors (e.g., enalapril, ramipril, benazepril, lisinopril) are probably of equal efficacy but have different side effect profiles. Vigorous therapy, even using intravenous enalaprilat or nitroprusside, is indicated in patients with scleroderma renal crisis or in patients with severe hypertension and markedly elevated plasma renin activity. Other vasodilators, such as minoxidil or hydralazine, can be used if patients are intolerant of ACE inhibitors. Calcium channel blockers and diuretics may be of added benefit, particularly in the presence of Raynaud's phenomenon. Initiation of ACE inhibitors should be cautious if patients appear to be fluid volume depleted. Blood pressure can be controlled in nearly every instance, but rarely, refractory hypertension may be present and this may respond dramatically to bilateral nephrectomy. Nevertheless, recurrence of hypertension after bilateral nephrectomy has been reported. Dialysis therapy may be required in scleroderma renal crisis, but with adequate therapy, renal function will often return at sometime only after several months of treatment. Slowly progressive renal failure is seldom reversible unless it is accompanied by malignant hypertension. Maintenance of vascular access for hemodialysis may be difficult. Peritoneal dialysis is a usually well-tolerated and effective form of maintenance therapy, but some patients will develop progressive peritoneal fibrosis.

Kidney transplantation may be performed in patients with end-stage renal failure, but in patients with scleroderma renal crisis, this should be delayed to allow the patient opportunity for spontaneous complete or partial recovery. Extrarenal organ involvement (particularly cardiomyopathy) may limit survival. Recurrent disease in the renal allograft has been observed, but relatively infrequently. The vascular and pathologic changes of recurrent PSS may resemble chronic allograft rejection. Overall, the extent of cutaneous and nonrenal visceral involvement determines the eventual outcome and potential benefits of renal transplantation in PSS. Patients with PSS may be more susceptible to the vascular toxicity of cyclosporin. The overall outcome of patients with PSS and renal involvement has greatly improved in recent years, with a 60% cumulative 10-year survival in current reports.

Selected Readings

D'Agati V, Cannon P. Scleroderma (systemic sclerosis). In: Tisher CC, Brenner B, eds. *Renal pathology*, 2nd ed. Philadelphia: JB Lippincott, 1994:1058–1086.
An excellent up-to-date review.

Maricq H, Weinberger A, LeRoy E. Early detection of scleroderma spectrum disorders by in-vivo capillary microscopy. *J Rheumatol* 1982;9:289–291.
An excellent description of the method of nailfold microscopy and its diagnostic utility.

Merino G, Sutherland D, Kjellstrand C, et al. Renal transplantation for progressive systemic sclerosis and renal transplantation. *Am J Surg* 1977;133:745–749.
A compilation of extensive experience in renal transplantation.

Reimer G. Auto-antibodies against nuclear, nucleolar and mitochondrial antigens in systemic sclerosis. *Rheum Dis Clin North Am* 1990;16:169–183.
A good review of the serologic abnormalities in systemic sclerosis.

Steen V, Costantino J, Shapiro A, et al. Outcome of renal crisis in systemic sclerosis relative to availability of angiotensin converting enzyme inhibitors. *Ann Intern Med* 1990;113:352–357.
A good review of results of converting enzyme therapy in scleroderma renal crisis.

Traub YM, Shapero AP, Rodnan G, et al. Hypertension and renal failure in progressive systemic sclerosis: review of a 25 year experience in 68 cases. *Medicine* 1983;62:335–354.
A definitive account of scleroderma renal crisis.

PART 9
Hemolytic Uremic Syndrome and Thrombotic Thrombocytopenic Purpura

Bernard S. Kaplan

There is a distinctive form of hemolytic uremic syndrome (HUS) and a distinctive form of thrombotic thrombocytopenic purpura (TTP). The designation TTP-HUS is no longer helpful because the causes, pathogenesis, treatment, and prognosis of HUS and TTP differ. A new, less confusing terminology for the Shiga-like toxin family is shown in Table 42.23, and a more log-

TABLE 42.23. New Nomenclature for the Shiga-Like Toxin (Verotoxin) Family

Current Names	Proposed Gene Name	Proposed Protein Name
Shiga toxin (Stx)	**stx**	**Stx**
Shiga-like toxin 1 (SLT-I) Verotoxin I (VT1)	stx1	Stx1
Shiga-like toxin II (SLT-II) or Verotoxin II (VT2)	stx2	Stx2
Shiga-like toxin IIc (SLT-IIc) or Verotoxin IIc (VT2c)	stx2c	Stx2c
Shiga-like toxin IIe (SLT-IIe) or Verotoxin IIe (VT2e)	stx2e	Stx2e

Reproduced with permission from Kaplan BS, Meyers KW, Schulman SL. The pathogenesis and treatment of the hemolytic uremic syndromes. *J Am Soc Nephrol* 1998;9:1126–1133.

TABLE 42.24. A Proposed New Terminology for Hemolytic Uremic Syndromes

Current	Proposed	Abbreviation
Hemolytic uremic syndrome		HUS
Classical, typical, sporadic, epidemic, diarrhea-associated, D+ HUS	Shiga toxin–associated HUS	Stx HUS
Atypical D− HUS	Idiopathic HUS	

Reproduced with permission from Kaplan BS, Meyers KW, Schulman SL. The pathogenesis and treatment of the hemolytic uremic syndromes. *J Am Soc Nephrol* 1998;9:1126–1133.

ical nomenclature for the types of HUS is shown in Table 42.24. The term *Shiga toxin–associated HUS* (Stx HUS) is used for cases caused by, or presumed to be caused by, Stx-producing bacteria that include *Escherichia coli* and *Shigella dysenteriae* type 1. The broad classification of HUS into typical D+ (diarrhea associated) and atypical D− (nondiarrhea associated) forms is helpful, but an etiologic classification is more appropriate (Table 42.25). In this context, the term *idiopathic HUS* is preferable to that of *atypical D− HUS*. However, *D+ HUS* and *Stx HUS* are used interchangeably as are *atypical D− HUS* and *idiopathic HUS*. It is also classified clinically into mildly affected and severely affected cases on the basis of the presence and duration of anuria and histopathologically into the predominant type of renal injury, which may be glomerular, arteriolar, or cortical necrosis.

Stx HUS is the typical D+ form of HUS, is usually caused by Stx-producing *E. coli*, occurs mainly in childhood, is uncommon in African-Americans, and follows a prodromal illness of acute gastroenteritis. Bloody diarrhea is a common finding. There is rapid onset of acute hemolytic anemia, thrombocytopenia, and acute renal injury. Renal failure almost always predominates over brain involvement.

The onset of ***idiopathic HUS*** (atypical D− HUS) is often insidious without a recognizable prodrome, all age and racial groups are affected, prognosis is often poor, and relapses may occur before and/or after renal transplantation. Patients who initially have what appears to be idiopathic (atypical D− HUS) may have HUS inherited by an autosomal-recessive or autosomal-dominant mode.

Fever, thrombocytopenia, hemolysis, jaundice, neurologic involvement, and renal manifestations in various combinations, often at different times, define the typical form of TTP. TTP occurs mainly in adults, African-Americans and whites are affected with equal frequency, the onset is often insidious, bloody diarrhea is uncommon, and brain involvement predominates over renal disease.

Thrombotic microangiopathy (TMA) is a term often used to encompass the spectrum of TTP and HUS. However, not all cases of Stx HUS have evidence of TMA. *TMA* is a descriptive histopathologic term that may be useful in patients who develop features of HUS or TTP after bone marrow transplantation or in association with malignancy, human immunodeficiency virus (HIV) infection, systemic lupus erythematosus, and systemic sclerosis. TMA is a pathologic observation and is used best when tissue examination has confirmed the presence of renal arteriolar and glomerular thrombi.

TABLE 42.25. Etiologic Classification of Hemolytic Uremic Syndromes

Infections
- *Escherichia coli* O157:H7 and other serotypes, *Shigella dysenteriae* type 1, *pneumoniae, Aeromonas,* HIV

Hereditary HUS
- Autosomal recessive, autosomal dominant, inborn error of cobalamin metabolism

Drug- and treatment-associated HUS
- Cyclosporine, tacrolimus, mitomycin-C, oral contraceptives, quinine, ticlopidine hydrochloride, irradiation, OKT3, crack cocaine, gencytobine

HUS associations
- Pregnancy, solid organ transplant, bone marrow transplant, malignancy, systemic lupus, systemic sclerosis, Sjögren syndrome, poststreptococcal glomerulonephritis, membranoproliferative glomerulonephritis

Idiopathic HUS (atypical D- HUS)
- With recurrent episodes, without recurrent episodes
- With complement deficiency, without complement deficiency

From Kaplan BS, Meyers KW, Schulman SL. The pathogenesis and treatment of the hemolytic uremic syndromes. *J Am Soc Nephrol* 1998;9:1126–1133.

HEMOLYTIC UREMIC SYNDROME

Stx HUS (Typical D+ HUS)

Etiology and Pathogenesis

To cause HUS, an agent must be able to injure endothelial cells. The Stx-producing bacteria that most frequently are incriminated are various serotypes of *E. coli*, especially O157:H7 and *Shigella dysenteriae* type 1. Shiga toxin and Stx1 are almost identical, whereas Stx2 is more antigenically distinct. The β subunits of Stx bind the holotoxin to a glycolipid receptor galactotriosylceramide (Gb3) on the surface of human kidney endothelial and proximal tubule epithelial cells. The α subunit is the toxic moiety of the Stx. The holotoxin enters the cell by receptor-mediated endocytosis. The α subunit is separated from the β subunits and, after "activation," inhibits protein synthesis and injures the cell (Table 42.26).

Lipopolysaccharides (LPS) and tumor necrosis factor-α independently sensitize cells to Stx. Circulating LPSs are detected in Shigella-associated HUS, and elevated titers of agglutinins and IgM antibodies against *E. coli* O157:H7 derived LPS are found in Stx HUS. LPS is not directly cytotoxic but acts in synergism with cytokines and leukocytes. Activated neutrophils participate in the pathogenesis of Stx HUS. There is a leukocytosis, serum neutrophil elastase levels are increased, α_1-antitrypsin levels are increased, circulating neutrophils are degranulated, and neutrophils from HUS patients adhere to endothelial cells.

Although fibrin thrombi may be seen in glomerular capillaries and arterioles, coagulation factors, fibrinogen levels, and fibrinogen turnover are usually normal. Serum and urine levels of fibrin breakdown products are increased. Most patients have increased serum levels of plasminogen activator inhibitor-1 (PAI-1), an inhibitor of glomerular fibrinolysis. The role of the fibrinolytic system is discussed in more detail in Chapter 37, Part 1. Von Willebrand factor (vWF) antigens are elevated acutely, and large multimeric forms of vWF are decreased. No consistent changes are found in prostacyclin activity, but Stx inhibits prostacyclin synthesis *in vitro*. Plasma levels of vWF cleaving protease are uniformly normal. This finding clearly differentiates HUS from TTP.

Epidemiology

Stx HUS occurs mainly in children between 6 months and 4 years of age, but infants and adults can be affected. More than 90% of children with HUS have the D+ form compared with

TABLE 42.26. Pathogenesis of Stx HUS: A Theoretical Succession of Interrelated, Overlapping, Synchronous, and Asynchronous Events

1. Stx-producing *Escherichia coli* infection
   - Colonic injury
   - Entry of Stx into circulation
   - Stx attachment to Gb3 receptors on glomerular endothelial cells
   - Stx attachment to Gb3 receptors on renal tubular epithelial cells
   - Inhibition of cell protein synthesis
   - Cell injury and death—necrosis and apoptosis
2. Access of lipopolysaccharide (LPS)
   - LPS stimulates production of cytokines, TNF-a, and IL-1
   - Stx, LPS, and cytokines synergistically injure endothelial and tubular epithelial cells
3. Neutrophil leukocytosis
   - LPS activate leukocytes
   - Leukocytes release TNF-a, IA-1, elastase, free radicals
   - Transient leukocyte infiltration in glomeruli
   - Stx stimulates leukocyte adhesion
   - Stx upregulates adhesive proteins on endothelial cells
4. Activation of platelets
   - Local procoagulant state
   - Early, transient thrombi in glomeruli, afferent arterioles
   - Removal of platelets by spleen and liver
5. Endothelial cell injury
   - Perturbed endothelial cell functions—prostacyclin, von Willebrand factor, endothelin, nitric oxide, PAI-1
   - Collagen exposure
   - Endothelial cell swelling, injury, detachment
   - Narrow lumen, reduced glomerular filtration rate
6. Acute renal tubular injury
   - Stx attachment to Gb3 receptors on renal tubular epithelial cells
   - Inhibition of cell protein synthesis
   - Cell injury and death—necrosis and apoptosis
   - Tubular obstruction, acute renal failure
7. Hemolysis, thrombocytopenia
   - Secondary to vascular injury
   - Secondary to peroxidative damage

From Kaplan BS, Meyers KW, Schulman SL. The pathogenesis and treatment of the hemolytic uremic syndromes. *J Am Soc Nephrol* 1998;9:1126–1133.
IL, interleukin; TNF-α, tumor necrosis factor-α.

fewer than 50% of adults. Slightly more females are affected, there is a seasonal incidence (mainly summer), and there is almost a worldwide distribution. Clusters of cases occur, and affected siblings have HUS at about the same time. Large epidemics have occurred in the northwestern states of America, Japan, Scotland, and Southern Africa. The epidemic that occurred in Seattle, Washington, followed the ingestion of undercooked ground meat contaminated with *E. coli* O157:H7. Ground meat should be cooked to a temperature of not less than 68°C (155°F). HUS has also resulted after ingestion of contaminated fruit, vegetables, water, apple cider, milk-containing products, and many different kinds of undercooked and ground meats. Patients are usually healthy before the onset of acute gastroenteritis. Precise diagnosis in adults may be more difficult, but adults who have acute renal injury, acute hemolytic anemia, and thrombocytopenia, after a prodrome of bloody diarrhea, have the D+ form of HUS whether or not there is central nervous system involvement. Recurrent episodes after recovery from D+ HUS are extremely rare.

Clinical Findings

Sudden onset of pallor usually begins a few days after cessation or improvement of gastrointestinal symptoms. This is often followed by increasing edema and, occasionally, mild jaundice, petechiae or seizures. Hypertension, with or without congestive heart failure and pulmonary venous congestion, may result in part from excessive fluid administration before recognition of oliguria.

Gastrointestinal. Initial gastrointestinal symptoms are abdominal pain, vomiting, and diarrhea, usually with bloody and/or mucoid stools. Stx HUS can occur in the absence of diarrhea and may even be associated with a urinary tract infection. The prodrome lasts from 1 to 14 days and may improve before onset of the triad of features that define HUS. The colon is the focus of the gastrointestinal injury, and the symptoms resemble those of ulcerative colitis, appendicitis, intussusception, rectal prolapse, gastroenteritis, or acute bacterial enterocolitis. Examination by sigmoidoscopy (which is rarely indicated) shows combinations of mucosal friability, petechiae, ulcer, edema, bowel wall thickening, and nodularity. The acute colitis is usually transient, but complications include rectal prolapse, toxic megacolon, and bowel wall necrosis. Hepatomegaly is common. An abdominal plain film may show gas accumulation in the colon and bowel wall thickening. The findings on barium enema (which is rarely indicated) may be normal, or there may be thumbprinting, pseudotumor, and transverse ridging. Serum transaminase levels may be elevated because of anoxic injury to the liver or hepatitis. High lactic dehydrogenase levels usually reflect hemolysis. Hypoalbuminemia is a common finding and may be caused by a protein-losing enteropathy. Pancreatic dysfunction causes marked elevation of serum amylase and lipase levels, and islet cell necrosis results in hyperglycemia with low insulin levels. Thrombosis of submucosal and intramural vessels with mucosal ulceration, hemorrhagic mucositis, and pseudomembrane formation occur in severe cases. Widespread thromboses can cause colonic gangrene.

Renal. Renal failure is universal in the patients. Oligoanuria occurs in about half the cases, and some patients have nonoliguric renal failure. Microscopic hematuria occurs more often than macroscopic hematuria. Blood pressure is usually normal at the onset of the illness but often increases after a blood transfusion. Signs of fluid overload are edema, hypertension, and cardiac failure. Urinalysis reveals red blood cells and various casts. Every patient has at a minimum microscopic hematuria and proteinuria. Biochemical changes of renal dysfunction include elevated serum levels of creatinine, potassium, phosphorus, hydrogen ion, uric acid, and blood urea nitrogen (BUN). The serum potassium concentration may be low initially as a result of potassium loss secondary to diarrhea and gastroenteritis. Hyperkalemia may develop as a result of reduced glomerular filtration rate, hemolysis, and transcellular shifts caused by acidosis. Serum concentrations of sodium, calcium, bicarbonate, and albumin are low, especially in severely ill patients. Serum levels of cholesterol, triglycerides, and phospholipids may be elevated. Doppler ultrasound studies of renal blood flow reveal reduced diastolic flow and can be a useful way of predicting return of renal function. Endothelial cell injury results in local intravascular coagulation and mechanical destruction of erythrocytes and platelets by fibrin strands in narrowed vessels. Platelet adherence contributes to formation of microthrombi.

Histopathologic findings include combinations of glomerular, arteriolar, and arterial lesions in varying degrees of severity. The characteristic glomerular lesion is often focal and consists of endothelial cell swelling and a widened subendothelial space, which results in a thickened capillary wall and reduced capillary lumen. Fibrinlike substances and lipids accumulate in the subendothelial space. The glomerular basement membrane is intact. Thrombi may occlude capillary lumens. The mesangium is expanded. Leukocytes are noted in specimens obtained soon after the onset of HUS. Occasionally, there may be crescents and signs of necrosis. The glomeruli often have a lobulated appearance. There is a patchy distribution of arterial and arteriolar lesions with intimal cell proliferation, thickening and necrosis of the wall, thrombi, and narrowed lumens. There may be evidence of acute tubular necrosis and tubulointerstitial disease. In some cases, there is patchy necrosis, and in others, widespread cortical necrosis is present. Deposits of fibrin, fibronectin, IgM, and C3 can be demonstrated along capillary walls, in the mesangium, and in the subendothelial spaces of capillaries and arterioles by immunofluorescent microscopy. Ultrastructural changes include swollen endothelial cells with prominent nuclei and damaged membrana fenestrata; detachment of endothelial cells and formation of a subendothelial space with deposition in this space of fibrin, cellular fragments, lipids, and occasional platelets; and swollen epithelial cells with effacement of foot processes. In D+ HUS, the lesions are predominantly glomerular, but some patients have cortical necrosis and the evidence for direct Stx-mediated renal tubular injury is increasing. A renal biopsy is rarely indicated in patients with D+ HUS.

Hematologic. The severity of the microangiopathic hemolytic anemia varies from slight decreases in hemoglobin concentration to levels as low as 3 g/dl. There is often no correlation between the severity of hemolysis and that of renal failure. Repeated episodes of hemolysis may occur during the first few weeks. The erythrocytes are fragmented as a result of a microangiopathic injury and/or peroxidative damage. Other findings of hemolysis are increased serum levels of lactic dehydrogenase, unconjugated bilirubin, and an increased reticulocyte count. Haptoglobin levels are decreased and the Coombs' test results are usually negative. A leukocytosis occurs during the first week of D+ HUS. Thrombocytopenia lasts for up to 2 weeks and has no relationship to the course of the renal disease. Increased numbers of immature platelets are seen on peripheral blood smears. Evidence of peripheral platelet destruction includes a reduced half-life of radiolabeled infused autologous platelets and their increased uptake by the spleen and liver. Platelet aggregation in response to agonists is impaired, and levels of intraplatelet β-thromboglobulin, platelet factor 4, and serotonin are reduced. Serum concentrations of β-thromboglobulin, platelet factor 4, and serotonin are increased. The coagulation profiles (e.g., prothrombin time and partial thromboplastin time) are usually normal. However, an inhibitor of glomerular fibrinolysis, PAI-1, which can be removed by peritoneal dialysis, is detected in most patients with HUS.

Neurologic. Many patients have neurologic symptoms such as irritability, somnolence, behavioral changes, restlessness, ataxia, dizziness, tremors, and twitching. Major neurologic dysfunction occurs in one-third of the cases, can be the presenting feature, and may determine the outcome. Seizures may be focal or generalized. Less often, there are combinations of hemiparesis, decerebrate or dystonic posturing, cortical blindness, or brainstem involvement with stupor and coma. Central nervous system injury may be caused by the Stx and hyponatremia, hypocalcemia, markedly increased BUN, and accelerated hypertension may be additional inciting or aggravating factors. Neurologic involvement occasionally occurs during convalescence. Computed tomography scans may be normal in cases with focal findings, but scans that first show hypodense areas may later demonstrate hemorrhage into the same areas. Magnetic resonance imaging may be more sensitive for early detection of structural lesions. Brain edema and microthrombi are found in some cases at autopsy.

Cardiopulmonary. The cardiovascular abnormalities usually result from volume overload, but some patients have myocarditis or cardiogenic shock caused by microthrombi, cardiomyopathy, or aneurysms. Some patients have adult respiratory distress syndrome.

Treatment

Electrolyte and fluid balance should be managed carefully. Dehydrated patients must receive appropriate fluid repletion, and if oliguria does not respond to a fluid challenge, care must be taken to avoid volume overload. Hyponatremia, hyperkalemia, hyperphosphatemia, and metabolic acidosis are managed conservatively as needed. If this fails, dialysis or hemodiafiltration are used. Dialysis is generally started once it is apparent that the patient manifests clinical symptoms of uremia or is anuric. There are no apparent advantages for peritoneal dialysis over hemodialysis. Continuous hemodiafiltration can be used in patients who have a precarious hemodynamic status or colonic gangrene. Packed red blood cells are transfused when the hemoglobin concentration falls below 6 g/dl. Blood is given slowly because of the danger of severe hypertension. Platelet transfusions are indicated if there is active bleeding or if surgery is needed. Hypertension is treated by fluid removal and, if this is unsuccessful, by vasodilators. Adequate nutrition should be maintained because of a high catabolic rate.

There is no specific treatment for colitis, and antibiotic treatment is not recommended. Commercial immune globulin preparations are ineffective in eliminating organisms from the bowel and lack anti-Stx2 antibodies. Surgery is indicated if ischemic bowel lesions are suspected. Diabetes mellitus and seizures are treated by established methods. There is no evidence to support the use of antithrombotic, fibrinolytic, or antiplatelet agents; fresh-frozen plasma; or plasmapheresis. Posttransplant recurrences are uncommon in these patients regardless of the source of the donor kidney or the use of cyclosporine.

Outcome

In general, the longer and more severe the diarrheal phase, the worse the outcome. The longer the period of anuria, the less likely the return of normal renal function. A very high initial neutrophil count is associated with a poorer outcome. Patients with severe neurologic impairment have a poorer prognosis, but there is the potential for improvement and recovery. There are no consistent correlations between age at onset and outcome in childhood. Older patients may have a poorer outcome in part because of comorbid conditions. Mild, nonoliguric cases of D+ HUS that have patchy cortical necrosis or mainly glomerular involvement have a favorable outcome. The renal outcome is worse in patients with diffuse cortical necrosis. The acute mortality rate is less than 5% in Stx HUS caused by *E. coli* and is up to 60% in Stx caused by *Shigella dysenteriae* type 1. This difference may be due in part to the more frequent occurrence of the latter in impoverished patients living in underdeveloped countries.

The long-term prognosis based on data from Western European series show the following: acute mortality 9%, complete recovery 64%, chronic renal insufficiency with hypertension 4%, late sequelae 12%, and end-stage renal disease 9%.

Idiopathic HUS (Atypical D− HUS)

Idiopathic HUS excludes patients who have a cause of HUS or a prodromal illness of bloody diarrhea. In the remaining group of heterogeneous patients, there is by definition no causal agent or seasonal pattern. Onset is usually insidious, the course is often progressive, and features of nephrotic syndrome may precede HUS. The outcome is more often serious than with Stx HUS: a higher mortality rate and more sequelae of proteinuria, severe hypertension, and chronic renal failure. Recurrences may occur before and/or after renal transplantation. The pathogenesis is not known. The renal histopathologic findings include collapsed ischemic glomeruli, intimal hyperplasia of afferent arterioles, and thrombi that appear to originate in the efferent arterioles with extensions into glomeruli.

Other Forms of HUS

Streptococcus pneumoniae

Features of HUS may occur in patients infected with *Streptococcus pneumoniae*. The organism produces a neuraminidase, which removes sialic acid from erythrocytes, platelets, and glomeruli and thereby exposes the T-cryptantigen (Thomsen-Freidenreich antigen). Preexisting serum IgM directed against this antigen causes agglutination and glomerular injury. There are widespread microthrombi. *The diagnosis must be made in this uncommon variant of HUS because treatment with blood products may aggravate agglutination. S. pneumoniae*–associated HUS is suspected when one or more of the following occurs in the context of HUS: a toxic patient, pneumonia, a positive Coombs' test, a hemolytic anemia without a reticulocyte response, difficulties in ABO cross-matching, or a positive minor cross-match. These patients should be treated with penicillin. Plasma should not be given until the results of blood cultures, Gram stains, and pneumococcal antigen tests are known because of the danger of providing additional anti–T-antigen IgM. The prognosis, which has been poor, is improving.

Human Immunodeficiency Virus

HUS, TTP, and TMA occur in patients with HIV infection. The incidence of this association has increased 16-fold over the past 20 years. The male:female ratio is 9:1 compared with female predominance in adults with typical TTP. Most of the patients are homosexual men or intravenous drug users. Microthrombi are found in many organs. There is no specific treatment, and the prognosis is extremely poor.

Oral Contraceptives

There is circumstantial evidence that oral contraceptives cause HUS or TTP. In most reports of an apparent association between oral contraception and HUS, there is evidence of preexisting disease, nonspecific viral prodromal illness, family history of HUS, or recurrent episodes of HUS with and without oral contraception use.

HUS in Families

Patients with autosomal-recessive or autosomal-dominant inheritance of HUS have similar clinical and renal histopathologic features to idiopathic HUS (atypical D− HUS). A diagnosis of inherited HUS cannot be made without an informative family history. The onset of both types of inherited HUS is usually insidious.

Autosomal-Recessive HUS. The interval between onset in affected siblings is often more than a year, adults are occasionally affected, and the ages of affected siblings is often similar. There is no seasonal incidence or typical prodrome. The renal lesion is predominantly arteriolar, and the mortality rate is greater than 65%. Some patients have a TTP-like phenotype.

Autosomal-Dominant HUS. There is a family history of HUS in a parent or grandparent, and adults are usually affected. There is no specific prodrome, although some females with the dominant form develop HUS in association with pregnancy or use of an oral contraceptive. The renal lesion is mainly arteriolar, relapses are uncommon, and the mortality rate is greater than 90%. Most survivors have chronic renal failure.

The pathogenesis of inherited HUS is unknown. There may be linkage in some kindreds with dominantly inherited HUS to the factor H locus on chromosome 1. There is no specific treatment for inherited HUS, and the prognosis is poor. In some cases, HUS may recur before and/or after renal transplantation. Treatment with fresh-frozen plasma and/or plasmapheresis is advocated without definitive data to demonstrate their value.

Transplantation, Cyclosporine, and Tacrolimus

Recurrent or *de novo* HUS after transplantation are uncommon. Patients who may be at risk for a recurrence usually have idiopathic HUS (atypical D− HUS), inherited HUS, or a history of a recurrence before transplant. Recurrences may occur after transplantation without a prior history of recurrent episodes. The possibility of a recurrence cannot be predicted unless the patient has had one or has a family history of HUS. Recurrences may occur after transplantation with living-related or cadaver allografts, in one of two allografts in the same patient, or in more than two allografts. HUS has recurred whether or not cyclosporine or tacrolimus was used. However, there is evidence that cyclosporine and tacrolimus can cause *de novo* HUS after renal, liver, or heart transplantation.

HUS with TMA can occur after heterologous or autologous bone marrow transplantation (BMT). These patients have been treated with total body irradiation and some have received cyclosporine. There is no effective treatment, and the prognosis is poor.

Pregnancy

Severe acute renal failure is a prominent feature in intrapartum and postpartum HUS. In postpartum HUS, pregnancy and delivery are usually normal, and the onset of HUS occurs after a symptom-free interval of 2 days to a month. Many patients have a nonspecific influenzalike illness before onset. The outcome is poor, with a 55% mortality rate. Although treatment with fresh-frozen plasma and/or plasmapheresis is advocated, there are no data that prove their value.

Cancer-Associated TMA

HUS with TMA may occur in patients with neoplasms whether or not chemotherapeutic agents are used. Microangiopathic hemolytic anemia predominates in HUS associated with mucin-secreting carcinoma. Gastric carcinoma accounts for half the cases. Most patients with cancer-associated TMA have metastatic disease. There is no specific treatment, and the prognosis is poor.

Chemotherapy-Associated HUS

The clinical features in patients with chemotherapy-associated HUS resemble HUS more than TTP, and renal involvement is characteristic. HUS associated with mitomycin-C is uncommon in patients given less than 30 mg/m^2 or fewer than two cycles of treatment. HUS can occur after treatment with combinations of *cis*-platinum and bleomycin. The fatality rate of HUS induced by mitomycin-C is 60% to 70%. Chemotherapy-associated HUS is reported in association with other chemotherapeutic agents, but a causal relationship is unproven. Encouraging results have been obtained using protein A immunoadsorption of plasma.

THROMBOTIC THROMBOCYTOPENIC PURPURA

TTP is a syndrome, not a disease (Table 42.27). There is an overlap between TTP and the secondary forms of HUS. A precise cause for TTP has not been found. The heterogeneous nature of TTP is shown by the fact that many patients with TTP have other disorders such as systemic lupus or progressive systemic sclerosis (scleroderma). TTP is less common than HUS, and the prevalence is from 1 in 45,000 to 1 in 1 million. TTP occurs mainly in adults and is uncommon in infants and children. Females are affected more often than males, and 20% to 30% of patients are African-American. There is no seasonal incidence, and epidemics have not been reported.

Hemolytic anemia, thrombocytopenic purpura, and waxing and waning neurologic signs are present in 74% of all cases; these features together with fever and renal disease occur in 40% of patients. Onset is often insidious, and the manifestations may be asynchronous. Presenting manifestations in order of frequency are neurologic, hemorrhagic, malaise, weakness, fatigue, nausea, vomiting, fever, pallor, abdominal pain, jaundice, arthralgia, and myalgia. Brain injury is more prominent than nephropathy. Occult blood is occasionally detected in stools, but bloody diarrhea is rare. Although renal involvement is common, gross hematuria occurs in only 15% of cases, proteinuria and microscopic hematuria are often detected, but oliguria, acute renal failure, and uremia are uncommon. Inheritance of TTP is uncommon. Relapses occur in some cases.

The pathogenesis of TTP has been greatly clarified by studies of the processing of vWF multimeres. Patients with chronic relapsing forms of idiopathic TTP have been shown to have greatly reduced plasma levels of a methyl-containing vWF cleaving protease. This protease normally degrades large multimeres of vWF, thereby preventing the proplatelet aggregating effects of large vWF multimeres. Such patients cannot be shown to have a circulating inhibitor of the vWF cleaving protease; therefore the deficiency is due to an abnormality in the production, survival, or function of this protease. In contrast, patients with acute nonrelapsing TTP, a more common entity, have reduced plasma vWF cleaving protease activity due to the presence of an IgG inhibitor. These findings account for the frequent occurrence of elevated vWF multimeres in plasma of patients with TTP.

TABLE 42.27 Classification of Thrombotic Thrombocytopenic Purpura (TTP)

Idiopathic TTP
Chronic relapsing (due to congenital or acquired vWF protease deficiency)
Acute nonrelapsing (due to an IgG auto antibody inhibitor of vWF protease)
Secondary TTP
Systemic lupus erythematosus
Progressive systemic sclerosis
Cancer associated
HIV associated
Drug induced (ticlopidine, crack cocaine, quinidine)
Heredofamilial (rare)

HIV, human immunodeficiency virus; vWF, von Willebrand factor.

Very importantly, the vWF protease deficiency is not found in HUS (D+ or D−). This critical finding also differentiates these superficially similar entities. These observations also explain the efficacy of plasma exchange and plasma infusion in TTP. Plasma exchange presumably removes the IgG autoantibody inhibitor, and fresh-frozen plasma infusion replaces the deficient protease. Plasma exchange alone would be ineffective in cases due to protease deficiency without the IgG inhibitor antibody, whereas plasma exchange and plasma infusion would be effective in cases with an IgG inhibitor.

The hematologic findings in TTP are similar to those in HUS. Coagulation studies are usually normal. Abnormally large factor VIII:vWF multimers are detected in the sera of patients with relapsing TTP during remission; these are undetectable during relapses. Serial measurement of serum levels of lactic dehydrogenase (LDH) may provide useful information on the activity of the disease. Falling serum levels of LDH may indicate subsiding disease activity.

Widespread arteriolar and capillary microthrombi, of different stages or organization, are seen in postmortem specimens. The characteristic lesion is a nonobliterative, finely granular hyaline thrombus, composed of fibrin and platelets. The thrombus is composed of aggregated platelets and vWF multimers and is covered by proliferating endothelial cells.

The therapy of TTP is controversial because few controlled trials have been performed. Nevertheless, many experienced clinicians favor the use of daily administration of 3 to 4 units of fresh-frozen plasma, often combined with one or more inhibitors of platelet aggregation such as dipyridamole (300 to 400 mg/day) in divided doses. Intensive daily plasma exchange has improved the survival of TTP patients, and many believe that it is the preferred initial therapeutic approach, whereas others reserve plasma exchange for patients failing to respond to plasma infusion plus antiplatelet aggregation therapy. Studies of vWF protease activity and its inhibition by IgG autoantibody should clarify treatment decision making in TTP. Patients with vWF protease deficiency without IgG autoantibody inhibition should respond to plasma infusion alone. Those with vWF protease deficiency due to IgG autoantibody inhibition will require plasma exchange and plasma infusion. Whether the addition of glucocorticoids is of further benefit is unknown. Splenectomy or vincristine therapy may be of value in some patients with a chronic or relapsing course primarily manifested by thrombocytopenia or hemolysis. Platelet infusions should be scrupulously avoided because they may be associated with a wave of *in vivo* platelet aggregation and sudden deterioration of central nervous system function.

The outcome of TTP is often poor, with high morbidity and mortality rates, but the prognosis has improved recently from a mortality rate of 90% to less than 20%. Relapses occur is some patients.

Selected Readings

Boyce TG, Swerdlow DL, Griffin PM. Escherichia coli 0157:H7 and the hemolytic-uremic syndrome. *N Engl J Med* 1995;333:364–368.

This is an important review of the epidemiology of what may ultimately be a preventable disease.

Hughes AK, Stricklett PK, Kohan DE. Cytotoxic effect of Shiga toxin-1 on human proximal tubule cells. *Kidney Int* 1998;54:426–437.

New insights are provided into the pathogenesis of Stx HUS. The demonstration of direct Stx-induced tubule injury further differentiates Stx HUS from TTP.

Hymes KB, Karpatkin S. Human immunodeficiency virus infection and thrombotic microangiopathy. *Semin Hematol* 1997;34:117–125.

This is a superb review of all aspects of this association.

Kaplan BS, Meyers KW, Schulman SL. The pathogenesis and treatment of the hemolytic uremic syndromes. *J Am Soc Nephrol* 1998;9:1126–1133.

A review of the pathogenesis of Stx HUS and its treatment with a careful attempt to focus as precisely as possible on several specific types of HUS.

Melnyk AMS, Solez K, Kjellstrand CM. Adult hemolytic-uremic syndrome. A review of 37 cases. *Arch Intern Med* 1995;155:2077–2084.

A retrospective analysis of HUS in adults in which HUS is not confused with TTP. Treatments and outcomes are evaluated on the basis of the causes of the HUS.

Moake JL. Moschcowitz, multimeres and metalloprotease. *N Engl J Med* 1998;339:1629-1631.

This is an excellent summary of the seminal findings that demonstrate two different mechanisms for abnormal von Willebrand factor (vWF) in TTP: autoantibodies to metalloproteinase and deficiency in the metalloproteinase.

Moake JL. Studies on the pathophysiology of thrombotic thrombocytopenic purpura. *Semin Hematol* 1997;34:83–89.

The pathogenesis of TTP is reviewed in relation to the formation of the platelet thrombi in TTP a result of platelet–endothelial cell interactions.

Rock G, Shumak K, Kelton J, et al. Thrombotic thrombocytopenic purpura: outcome in 24 patients with renal impairment treated with plasma exchange. Canadian Apheresis Study Group. *Transfusion* 1992;32:710–714.

Fifteen of 25 patients who responded fully or partially to this regimen (acetylsalicylic acid, dipyridamole and plasma exchange) by the end of the first cycle survived.

Snyder HW Jr, Mittelman A, Oral A, et al. Treatment of cancer chemotherapy-associated thrombotic thrombocytopenic purpura/hemolytic uremic syndrome by protein A immunoadsorption of plasma. *Cancer* 1993;71:1882–1892.

The 1-year survival rate for patients with cancer chemotherapy-associated TTP in complete or partial remission was 74% compared with 22% for case controls.

Tsai HM, Rice L, Sarode R, et al. Antibody inhibitors to von Willebrand factor metalloproteinase and increased binding of von Willebrand factor to platelets in ticlopidine-associated thrombotic thrombocytopenic purpura. *Ann Intern Med* 2000;132:794–799.

von Willebrand factor (vWF) is involved in the pathogenesis of ticlopidine-associated TTP with development of autoantibodies to the vWF metalloproteinase.

PART 10
Amyloidosis

Mark S. Kindy and Frederick C. De Beer

Amyloid is a general term used to define deposition of extracellular proteinaceous material that is associated with a number of disease states. Karl Rokitansky described a lardaceous substance in 1842, first identifying these deposits, and in 1854, Rudolf Virchow coined the term *amyloid* because of its iodine staining properties similar to starch and cellulose. Amyloidosis is characterized by the tissue deposition of insoluble protein fibrils—a process resulting in organ dysfunction and death. The typical fibrillar deposits are common to all amyloid diseases and define this pathologic entity even though a group of diverse precursor proteins can form fibrils. Fibrils are 7 to 10 nm wide and form antiparallel cross β-pleated sheets. This structural arrangement rarely occurs in nature except for silk and keratin and is particularly resistant to enzymatic digestion and clearance.

Other common features of amyloid deposits are the presence of serum amyloid P component (SAP), apolipoprotein E (apoE), and glycosaminoglycans, in particular the basement membrane form heparan sulfate proteoglycan (HSPG). The structural commonality of amyloidoses and the relative importance of subcomponents in fibrillogenesis have been studied extensively. Systemic amyloids such as amyloid A protein (AA) amyloid, amyloid L (AL) amyloid, transthyretin (TTR) amyloid, and islet amyloid polypeptide (IAPP) amyloid, as well as cerebral amyloids such as prion protein (PrP) amyloids and β-amyloid (Aβ) of Alzheimer's disease (AD) are included in this group of fibrillar diseases. The amyloid associated with chronic dialysis therapy, β_2-microglobulin (β_2M) amyloid, is discussed is Chapter 84, Part 1E.

BIOCHEMICAL AND PATHOLOGIC PROPERTIES OF AMYLOID

As described, the fibrils associated with various forms of amyloid are comprised of monoclonal light chains (κ and λ), heavy chains (IgG_1), serum amyloid A protein, β_2M, transthyretin (prealbumin), β-peptide, and polypeptide hormones, among others (Table 42.28). The fibrils are 7 to 10 nm wide and variable lengths, depending on the type of fibril and the tissue in which the fibrils are deposited. These fibrils are highly insoluble and resistant to proteolysis. The amorphous configuration of amyloid deposits appears extracellularly and can lead to cell death and disruption of tissue structure. The characteristics are determined by the cross β-pleated sheet conformational structure of the fibrils as determined by circular dichroism (CD), nuclear magnetic resonance (NMR), and x-ray diffraction studies. Fibril formation and deposition depend on the existence of a precursor protein, which can have an altered protein structure or concentration or both. In most cases, the proteolytic processing of the fibrils is important in the generation of an amyloidogenic protein or peptide required for fibrillogenesis. However, it is possible for the precursor protein itself to exist as a full-length entity such as in transthyretin or β_2M fibrils.

The initiation of amyloidogenesis requires the generation or synthesis of a precursor protein in sufficient quantities to allow for deposition. In AA amyloid, a continuous inflammatory response results in a sustained increase in serum amyloid A (SAA) levels. This 103–amino acid precursor is proteolytically cleaved to a 76–amino acid amyloid A peptide that deposits as fibrils. The presence of myeloid or plasma cells producing high levels of a monoclonal light-chain protein results in deposition of AL fibrils. β_2M is usually catabolized in the kidneys. Hemodialysis is incapable of removing the β_2M protein. Therefore high plasma concentrations in patients with renal failure who are receiving dialysis result in amyloid deposition after 6 to 8 years of dialysis. The continuous maintenance of high levels of the precursor seems to be required to generate a nidus for more rapid amyloid deposition. Activation of macrophages (or microglia in the brain) by cytokines appears to be important for the processing and progression of the disease (particularly for AA, Aβ, and PrP amyloids). Finally, altered clearance of the amyloid proteins (turnover) is needed to allow for increased deposition of the amyloidogenic proteins. The combination of these factors serves as the mechanism by which amyloid depositions occur and are potential targets for therapeutic approaches.

Several other components are found associated with all amyloid fibrils; these are SAP component, apoE, and proteoglycans. These factors form complexes with the amyloid fibrils and appear to play a role in the formation and/or maintenance of the fibrillar deposits. Inactivation of both the SAP and apoE genes in mice showed a delay and reduction in the deposition of amyloid in the mouse model of AA amyloidosis. The apoE gene knockout animals also demonstrate a reduction in development of Aβ plaques when crossed with Alzheimer's precursor protein (APP) transgenic mice. In addition, the administration of small-molecule anionic sulfates and sulfonates blocked the deposition of systemic amyloid and did allow for increased resorption of the amyloid fibrils. These molecules interfere with the amyloidogenic protein–heparan sulfate interactions and alter amyloid deposition. These studies suggest that these com-

TABLE 42.28. Classification of Amyloidoses

Type[a]	Precursor	Clinical Manifestation
AA[b]	Serum amyloid A (apoSAA)	Reactive systemic amyloidosis associated with rheumatoid arthritis, chronic inflammatory diseases, familial Mediterranean fever, Muckle-Wells syndrome. Referred to as *secondary amyloidosis*
AL	Monoclonal immunoglobulins light chain (κ, λ)	Primary amyloidosis, systemic amyloidosis associated with multiple myeloma and monoclonal gammopathy, also can have single organ localization without systemic involvement
AH	Heavy chain (IgG_1, γ1)	
ATTR	Transthyretin (prealbumin)	Systemic senile amyloidosis (TTR-normal protein) Familial amyloid polyneuropathy (FAP) Portuguese (Met30)[c] Familial amyloid polyneuropathy II (Indiana/Swiss) (Ser84) Familial amyloid cardiomyopathy (Danish) (Met111)
AApoAI	Apolipoprotein AI	Familial amyloid polyneuropathy (Iowa) (Arg26), normal AI protein in amyloid Systemic senile amyloidosis (TTR)
Agel	Gelsolin	Familial amyloidosis (Finnish)
ACys	Cystatin C	Hereditary cerebral hemorrhage with amyloid, Icelandic (Gln68)
Aβ	β-protein precursor (βPP)	Alzheimer's disease, Down's syndrome, hereditary cerebral hemorrhage with amyloid, Dutch (Gln618 and other mutations)
$A\beta_2M$	β_2-microglobulin	Chronic dialysis
Acal	Pro-calcitonin	Medullary carcinoma of the thyroid
Alac	Pro-lactin	Pituitary amyloid
AFibAα	Fibrinogen	Nephropathy
Alys	Lysozyme	Renal and hepatic amyloid
AScr (PrP)	Prion protein (Scrapie)	Creutzfeldt-Jakob disease (Scrapie protein 27-30) Gertsmann-Straüssler-Scheinker syndrome (Leu 102)
AANF	Atrial natriuretic factor	Isolated atrial amyloid
AIAPP	Islet amyloid polypeptide	Type II diabetes, insulinoma, islets of Langerhans (Ser20Gly mutation)
AApoAII	Apolipoprotein AII (murine)	Senescence accelerated amyloid in the mouse
AIns	Insulin (rodent)	Islet amyloid in the degu

[a] Nomenclature as determined by Husby G, Araki S, Benditt EP, et al. The 1990 guidelines for nomenclature and classification of amyloid and amyloidosis. In: Natvig JB, Forre O, Husby G, et al, eds. *Amyloid and amyloidosis 1990.* Dordrecht: Kluwer Academic Publishers, 1991:7–11; and the WHO-IUIS Nomenclature Sub-Committee. Nomenclature of amyloid and amyloidosis. *Bull WHO* 1993;71:105–108.
[b] AA, amyloid A amyloidosis.

ponents are involved in the process of amyloidogenesis and may provide targets for therapeutic intervention.

In primary amyloidosis (AL), the fibrils are comprised of the amino terminal portion of the variable or hypervariable region of the light chain of a monoclonal antibody. The process involves the κ and λ light-chain fragments, which are deposited into amyloid fibrils. Light-chain amyloid can occur with no apparent coexisting disease or can be associated with multiple myeloma. Both processes are a result of the proliferation of plasma or B cells that gives rise to increased levels of the light-chain fragment. Studies have shown that injection of mice with Bence Jones proteins (an amyloidogenic light chain) resulted in the deposition of light-chain amyloid in these animals. Deposition is similar to that seen in humans, in that fibrils are detected in the kidneys, spleen, liver, and heart. In addition, the amyloid fibrils are associated with SAP. Injection of a nonamyloidogenic light-chain protein did not results in amyloid deposition.

AA amyloid is associated with chronic inflammatory disease, amyloidosis, familial Mediterranean fever (FMF), and familial amyloid nephropathy (FAP). The amyloid fibrils are derived from the SAA proteins, which are acute-phase proteins, normally produced in the liver. The SAA proteins are induced several hundred-fold by interleukin (IL)-1, IL-6, and tumor necrosis factor (TNF) in response to an inflammatory stimuli. The SAA precursor is a 12.5-kD protein associated with the high-density lipoprotein (HDL) particles. The AA fibrils are usually a result of cleavage from the SAA proteins and consist of 40 to 103 (full-length precursor) amino acids. The role of cleavage in the generation of amyloid fibrils is not clear. Varying lengths of AA fibrils are detected in different tissues, suggesting that the cleavage may occur after deposition and that the length depends on the types of proteases in the particular tissue. In addition, because full-length precursor can be found in the amyloid tissue and can be used for *in vitro* fibril formation, this suggests that cleavage is not essential. It is more likely that the precursor concentrations and sustained levels of precursor are important in fibril formation.

Animal models of AA amyloid have proven useful in understanding the process of amyloid formation. Animals given chronic inflammatory stimuli with a modified casein suspension have sustained levels of SAA production and develop systemic AA amyloid. This process can be shortened to 3 days with the injection of amyloid-enhancing factor (AEF) and silver nitrate. AEF appears to be preformed amyloid fibrils that act as a nidus to stimulate deposition. As in humans, extensive deposition is detected in the spleen, liver, heart, lungs, kidneys, and intestine. These animals are being used to study the role of factors such as SAP and apoE in fibrillogenesis. Studies of SAA transgenic mice have shown selective deposition of AA amyloid in the presence and absence of inflammatory response.

NOMENCLATURE AND CLASSIFICATION OF AMYLOIDOSES

The pathologic features usually determine the classification of the diseases. The nomenclature and classification of amyloid diseases is confounded by similarities between the different types of amyloidoses. All amyloidoses stain with Congo red to give an apple-green birefringence under polarized light (Fig. 42.10), and in light and electron microscopic analysis, amyloid fibrils are almost identical (Fig. 42.11). In several different amy-

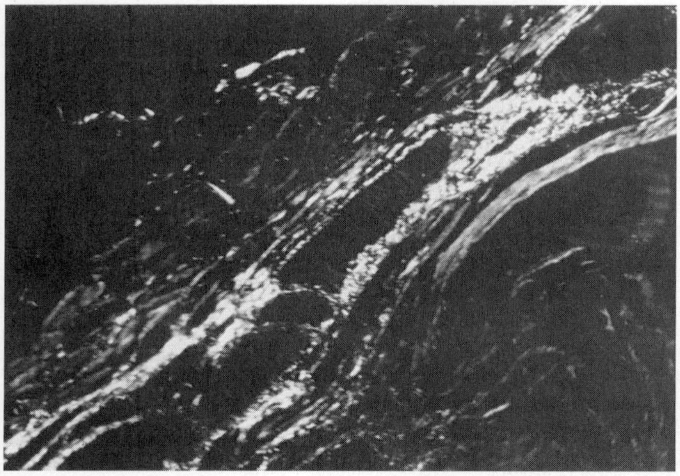

Figure 42.10. Light microscopic appearance of glomerular amyloidosis. A patient with diagnosed renal insufficiency and kidney failure demonstrated amyloid in the glomeruli of the kidney. Congo red stained glomeruli visualized with polarized light shows the characteristic birefringent material of primary (AL) amyloidosis. (Magnification × 40.)

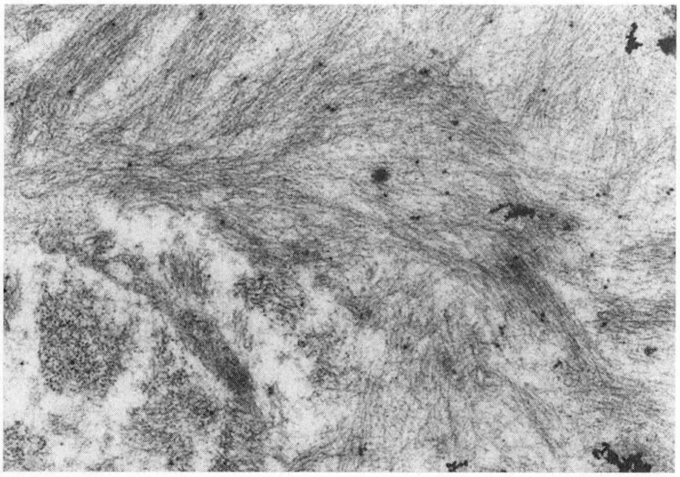

Figure 42.11. Electron microscopic analysis of AA amyloidosis. Negatively stained amyloidotic kidney showing evidence of 7- to 10-nm fibrils with nonspecific arrangement. Fibrils appear extracellular in nature. (Magnification × 25,000.)

loid diseases, there are overlapping sites of localization. In AA amyloidosis (secondary), the spleen, liver, kidney, heart, and gut are involved in the disease, whereas AL amyloidosis (primary) can involve the kidney, heart, lung, peripheral nerves, and blood vessels. The current classification is determined by the protein component that is associated with the amyloid deposits. This can be achieved by isolation and characterization of the amyloid fibrils or by immunocytochemical analysis of amyloid biopsies. Several studies have demonstrated the coexistence of different types of amyloidogenic proteins in a single deposit, complicating identification.

DISEASE DIAGNOSIS

The key to diagnosing amyloid is histopathologic analysis of diseased tissue and immunohistochemical analysis to determine the type of amyloid. These results are limited because of the amount of the tissue obtained for analysis. In addition, the extent of the disease cannot be assessed adequately. A technique for the assessment of the extent of disease was developed based on the properties of the SAP protein to specifically and reversibly bind to amyloid fibrils. Purified SAP can be radiolabeled with the short half-life, moderate-range γ emitter, ^{123}I and used *in vivo* to determine the degree of amyloid deposition. Injection of labeled SAP and whole body imaging can be used to detect amyloid in specific organs. In addition, regression of amyloid after treatment can be assessed. Although this is a very sensitive and noninvasive technique to measure organ involvement and the extent of amyloid deposition, the short half-life and limited availability of the ^{123}I limits its use. ^{99m}Tc (technetium) scanning has been used but has low sensitivity. Abdominal fat biopsy may be a helpful first diagnostic step in patients suspected of having amyloidosis.

PRIMARY AMYLOIDOSIS (AL, MONOCLONAL IMMUNOGLOBULIN AMYLOID)

AL amyloid is a progressive disease resulting from deposition of fragments of monoclonal immunoglobulin light chains, which are produced by abnormal plasma or B cells. AL can occur as a result of monoclonal gammopathy, Waldenström's macroglobulinemia, or multiple myeloma. Diagnosis of the AL amyloid depends on several characteristics of the disease. Characteristic is the presence of light-chain protein (M-protein) in the urine or serum that is associated with congestive heart failure, peripheral neuropathy, carpal tunnel syndrome, orthostatic hypotension, and nephrotic syndrome or renal insufficiency. Urine M-protein is detected by immunoelectrophoresis in 73% of the patients, and monoclonal λ type is twice as frequent as κ type light chains. Patients also present with fatigue, weight loss, and organ enlargement, particularly of the liver and spleen. Many other organs, such as the tongue, intestine, and bronchus, can be involved.

A large Mayo Clinic study of 229 patients in 1983 demonstrated the overall outcome of individuals with AL amyloid. The average age of presentation of the disease was 59 to 64 years depending on the sex of the individual (women or men, respectively), and the median survival time was 12 to 24 months. The median life expectancy for patients with myeloma was shown to be 5 months. Patients with congestive heart failure had a median life expectancy of 6 months, and in orthostatic hypotension, 9 months. Individuals with nephrotic syndrome or carpal tunnel syndrome due to AL amyloidosis had a median survival time of 17 months and 31 months, respectively. Amyloid involvement of cardiac tissue resulting in congestive heart failure and arrhythmias was related to 40% of the deaths in this disease.

Multiple organ involvement is common, with the kidney affected approximately 50% of the time. Patients with nephrotic syndrome account for more than 30% of individuals with AL amyloidosis. These patients almost always develop renal failure. Amyloid deposition in the kidney leads to renal enlargement in 45% of patients; however, this is not specific for diagnosis. The proteinuria resulting from the disease is nondiscriminative and may be massive, reaching more than 2 g/24 hr in some patients. Tubular dysfunction has been documented and can lead to acidosis or nephrogenic diabetes insipidus. Renal biopsy can be done safely in patients with renal amyloidosis. About 10% of patients older than 60 years of age with nephrotic syndrome are found to have AL amyloidosis, which was not suspected clinically.

SECONDARY AMYLOIDOSIS (AA, REACTIVE SYSTEMIC AMYLOID)

AA amyloidosis is associated with rheumatic diseases, certain chronic inflammatory diseases, chronic infections, and some malignant disorders (Table 42.29). Ulcerative colitis and systemic lupus erythematosus (SLE) are rarely complicated by amyloidosis. This contrasts with Crohn's disease and rheumatoid arthritis (particularly juvenile rheumatoid arthritis) in which amyloidosis is a well-known complication. The basis for this difference is possibly a deficiency in the cytokine-mediated increase in the precursor serum amyloid A production in patients with SLE. Renal carcinoma and Hodgkin's disease are known to be associated with fevers and systemic inflammatory features leading to serum amyloid A induction. It is not clear whether amyloid complicating advanced carcinoma of the cervix is the result of concomitant chronic inflammation or derived from the tumor per se. The overall incidence of AA amyloid has decreased significantly over the last 20 to 30 years as a result of therapeutic modalities that control chronic inflammation. However, the ability to sustain patients suffering from trauma, particularly spinal cord injuries, contributes to an increase in systemic AA amyloidosis due to chronic urinary tract infections. Also, the inability of physicians to recognize the syndrome and test for amyloid deposits demonstrates an underestimation of this disease in the population. Idiopathic inflammatory disease (rheumatoid arthritis, juvenile rheumatoid arthritis, and chronic infections) is the leading cause of AA amyloidosis in the Western hemisphere. Generally, 50% of patients with amyloidosis succumb to the disease within the first 5 years after diagnosis, and an additional 25% succumb between 5 and 15 years.

Deposition of AA fibrils involves multiple organs initially without any symptomatic manifestation. Approximately 25% of individuals with amyloidosis ultimately present with renal or glomerular involvement. The typical clinical presentation is proteinuria due to glomerular deposition of amyloid fibrils. This results in a nephrotic syndrome, which leads to renal insufficiency or end-stage renal failure, the most common cause of death in these patients. Deposits can usually be detected in the spleen, with some involvement of the liver, adrenals, and to a lesser degree, the heart, gut, and other tissues. Remarkably, it has been reported that dialysis and renal transplantation can exacerbate deposition in other tissues.

TABLE 42.29. Diseases Complicated with Secondary Amyloidosis

Inflammatory Diseases
Ankylosing spondylitis
Behçet's syndrome
Juvenile rheumatoid arthritis
Polymyositis
Psoriatic arthritis
Reiter's syndrome
Rheumatoid arthritis
Sjögren's syndrome
Takayasu arteritis
Third-degree burns
Whipple's disease
Infectious Diseases
Bronchiectasis
Chronic infection due to burns
Chronic lung and pleural infections
Chronic pyelonephritis
Cystic fibrosis
Drug abuse
HIV infection
Leprosy
Parasitic infections
Paraplegia (recurrent urinary tract infection)
Syphilis
Tuberculosis
Neoplastic Diseases
Cervical cancer
Hodgkin's disease
Lymphoma
Medullary carcinoma
Multiple myeloma
Renal cell carcinoma
Solid tumors
Waldenström's macroglobulinemia
Familial Diseases
Familial Mediterranean fever (recessive)
Glycogen storage disease, type Ib

β_2-MICROGLOBULIN AMYLOIDOSIS (AMYLOID ASSOCIATED WITH CHRONIC DIALYSIS)

Patients who are maintained on long-term hemodialysis therapy (i.e., more than 7 years' duration) develop dialysis-related amyloidosis (DRA). This is the result of deposition of β_2M in the synovium and carpal ligaments, resulting in arthropathy, carpal tunnel syndrome, and deposits in soft tissue. In addition, cases of β_2M amyloidosis have been reported in nondialyzed patients with chronic renal failure.

β_2M is a protein of 11.8 kD is produced by a number of different cell types, including lymphoid cells. The plasma levels of β_2M protein are 1 to 2 mg/L, which are selectively cleared by the kidneys. β_2M, produced by lymphoid cells, is involved in the stabilization of the major histocompatibility complex (MHC) class I antigen. During end-stage renal failure, concentrations can increase to 70 mg/L due to the inability of dialysis to remove the β_2M protein, and these elevated, sustained levels of protein result in the deposition of amyloid. Increased duration of dialysis can result in an increase in deposits in patients, and most patients subject to dialysis for more than 20 years have amyloid deposits. Treatment revolves around the use of nonsteroidal antiinflammatory drugs and/or corticosteroids, indicating a role of inflammation in the disease. In addition, high-flux dialysis can be used to reduce the levels of β_2M, with variable results. High-flux dialysis in combination with cellulose column absorption resulted in a slight improvement in patients. Renal transplantation will prevent the progression of the disease. This issue is discussed in detail in Chapter 84, Part 1E.

FAMILIAL AMYLOIDOSES

Familial amyloidoses are divided into several specific groups. The two most prevalent are familial amyloid polyneuropathy (FAP) and familial Mediterranean fever (FMF). FAP is an autosomal-dominant disorder that involves the transthyretin or prealbumin (TTR) protein. The most common mutation is the Met30, a substitution of methionine for valine at position 30 in the mature protein. At least 60 other mutations have been identified, some of which result in amyloid deposition while others do not. This disorder is mainly neuropathic in nature; however, renal involvement can occur. The disease is characterized as a progressive peripheral and autonomic neuropathy that can result in death as early as 10 years after diagnosis. Because TTR is mainly produced in the liver, hepatic transplantation has become standard therapy for amelioration.

FMF (autosomal-recessive inheritance) involves AA amyloid deposition in the kidneys of Sephardic Jews. It also occurs in Ashkenazi Jews, Druse, Kurds, Turks, and Armenians, with sporadic cases being reported in many other nationalities. The clinical presentation is febrile attacks and polyserositis (sporadic abdominal pains resembling acute abdomen, arthritis, and high fever). Initiation of febrile attacks starts during childhood, followed by amyloid deposition later in life. These attacks result in increased levels of SAA protein that result in AA fibril formation. The gene responsible for this disorder has been identified as the pyrin gene (MEFV) on chromosome 16p13.3. Missense mutations in this apparent transcription factor gene may lead to altered inflammatory response and eventually to amyloid deposition. Amyloidosis occurs as a result of glomerular AA fibril deposition and is complicated by nephrotic syndrome often leading to renal insufficiency. This disease can be controlled by prophylactic treatment with colchicine doses of at least 1.5 mg/day. Colchicine reduces the acute polyserostitic attacks and prevents the deposition of amyloid. Colchicine treatment is effective in symptom prevention in 60% to 70% of patients with FMF. In 25% to 30%, only partial protection is provided, but amyloid deposition is still prevented.

Other less common forms of hereditary amyloidoses are amyloidosis of the Ostertag type (mutant lysozyme protein amyloid), Muckle-Wells syndrome (AA amyloid), and apolipoprotein A-I (mutant A-I protein amyloid and normal A-I protein). In addition, other forms of hereditary amyloidoses have proteins of unknown origin. These forms of amyloid are also discussed in Chapter 43, Part 6.

TREATMENT OF AMYLOIDOSES

There are no specific effective treatments for amyloid diseases. Current opinion is that reduction or elimination of increased levels of the amyloidogenic precursor proteins would slow the development of the disease and potentially reverse the effects. Treatment of AA amyloid has focused on the reduction of the inflammatory response using antiinflammatory agents and immunosuppression in rheumatoid arthritis and inflammatory diseases to decrease the synthesis of SAA protein. Several studies have shown that treatment of patients with AA amyloidosis complicating rheumatoid arthritis (or juvenile rheumatoid arthritis) with chlorambucil or cyclophosphamide reduced proteinuria. Subsequently, the process of amyloidosis is suspended and reversed, and patients demonstrate a regression of amyloid. In addition, renal function is maintained in individuals receiving therapy.

AL amyloid is the result of increased immunoglobulin light-chain synthesis from a monoclonal generation of plasma cells. Therapeutic approaches are targeted at suppression of light-chain synthesis or removal of overexpressing plasma cells. Chemotherapeutic regimens using a combination of melphalan and prednisone have been used to treat the amyloidosis associated with multiple myeloma and monoclonal gammopathy with limited success. Other cytotoxic therapies have been reported to be beneficial to individuals with AL amyloid [treatment with VAD (vincristine, doxorubicin, and dexamethasone)]. However, bone marrow transplantation has not been successful. Some patients treated for plasma cell dyscrasia demonstrated a resolution of nephrotic syndrome, reduction in light-chain synthesis, normalization of hepatic enzymes, and a reduction in spleen and liver size indicative of amyloid resorption. Analyses of liver biopsies indicated that there was an abatement of amyloid deposits.

Other types of amyloidoses, such as hereditary (transthyretin, TTR) and hemodialysis (β_2M), require more invasive procedures for eradication of the disease. For hereditary amyloidosis (FAP), some mutations in the TTR gene can result in an amyloidogenic variant. To eliminate the source of the variant protein, orthotopic liver transplantation is required. Once the synthesis of the variant protein has been removed, regression of amyloid in other tissues can occur. For hemodialysis amyloidosis, the inability to properly clear the β_2M during kidney failure results in elevated levels of the protein, which could reach 20 to 70 times the normal levels. Dialysis to remove the protein is usually insufficient, and ultimately treatment requires renal transplantation to prevent amyloid deposition. Successful renal transplantation will decrease β_2M levels and allow for regression of the amyloid deposits.

POTENTIAL THERAPEUTIC APPROACHES TO AMYLOID DISEASES

New therapeutic strategies have been developed in animal models, and clinical trials have been initiated to slow or to reverse the process of amyloidosis. As described earlier, it was predicted that the interaction between amyloid fibrils and HSPG were important interactions, and disruption of these contacts may prevent amyloid deposition. Oral administration of low-molecular-weight anionic sulfates or sulfonates reduced amyloid development in the mouse model. In addition, they interfered with Aβ fibril formation *in vitro*, suggesting that they may have application to other amyloid diseases. Another compound, methyl 4,6-*O*-[(R)-1-carboxyethylidene] β-D-galactopyranoside (MOβDG), which interferes with SAP interaction with fibrils, has been shown to reduce amyloid fibrillogenesis *in vitro* and *in vivo* in the mouse. Finally, 4′-iodo-4′-deoxydoxorubicin (I-DOX, which may interfere with fibril deposition) was originally introduced as a chemotherapeutic agent. I-DOX was tested on a small group of individuals with AL amyloid and demonstrated a slight improvement in patient outcome as well as some regression of amyloid deposits.

Selected Readings

Gertz MA, Kyle RA. Response of primary hepatic amyloidosis to melphalan and prednisone: a case report and review of the literature. *Mayo Clin Proc* 1986;61:218–223.

This is a case report of one patient with AL amyloid treated with melphalan and prednisone demonstrating a reduction in amyloidosis after treatment. This is one in a series of articles that demonstrates the utility of melphalan and prednisone in the elimination of AL amyloid deposits and maintenance of the disease.

Gertz MA, Kyle RA. Secondary amyloidosis: response and survival in 64 patients. *Medicine (Baltimore)* 1991;70:246–256.

A study of 64 patients with AA amyloidosis secondary to rheumatoid arthritis seen at the Mayo Clinic. Renal involvement was detected in more than 90% of the individuals in the study.

Hawkins PN, Lavender JP, Pepys M. Evaluation of systemic amyloidosis by scintigraphy with ^{123}I-labeled serum amyloid P component. *N Engl J Med* 1990;323:508–513.

Method of detection, diagnosis, location, and monitoring of amyloid fibrils in patients with systemic amyloidosis.

Holmgren G, Ericzon BG, Groth CG, et al. Clinical improvement and amyloid regression after liver transplantation in hereditary transthyretin amyloidosis. *Lancet* 1993;341:1113–1116.

Description of clinical outcome of patients with a long history of FAP having received liver transplantation to remove the amyloidogenic TTR protein. Follow-up after transplantation demonstrates improvement of patients and regression of amyloid deposits.

Kindy MS, Rader DL. Reduction in amyloid A amyloid formation in apolipoprotein-E-deficient mice. *Am J Pathol* 1998;152:1387–1395.

This paper demonstrates the applicability of the mouse AA model to study amyloid formation. This study describes the reduction in amyloid formation in mice deficient in apoE. In addition, comments on SAP inactivation mice and common elements are provided.

Kisilevsky R. Anti-amyloid drugs: potential in the treatment of disease associated with aging. *Drugs Aging* 1996;2:75–83.

Description of potential therapeutic treatments for amyloid diseases from AA amyloid to Alzheimer's disease.

Koch KM. Dialysis-related amyloidosis. *Kidney Int* 1992;41:1416–1429.

Case study of individual placed on dialysis after presentation of end-stage renal disease due to mesangioproliferative glomerulonephritis. Indication of extreme β_2M amyloid deposition associated with 19 years of hemodialysis. Treatment paradigms and therapeutic considerations are discussed.

Pras M. Familial Mediterranean fever: from the clinical syndrome to the cloning of the pyrin gene. *Scand J Rheumatol* 1998;27:92–97.

Editorial review of FMF, clinical presentation, treatment with colchicine, and the eventual cloning of the gene that is potentially responsible for the disease. Identification of the missense mutations responsible for the altered function of the protein.

Tan S-Y, Irish A, Winearls CG, et al. Long term effect of renal transplantation on dialysis-related amyloid deposits and symptomatology. *Kidney Int* 1996;50: 282–289.

Exacerbation of dialysis-related amyloid in patient with renal transplantation and potential long-term effects after transplantation.

Tan S-Y, Pepys MB, Hawkins PN. Treatment of amyloidosis. *Am J Kidney Dis* 1995;26:267–285.

In-depth review of amyloidosis. This review examines the development, diagnosis, management, and treatment of amyloid diseases as they relate to kidney involvement. Describes a number of therapeutic approaches in the maintenance of amyloid disease and potential outcomes.

PART 11
Mixed Cryoglobulinemia

Giuseppe D'Amico and Alessandro Fornasieri

Cryoglobulinemia is a pathologic condition in which the blood contains immunoglobulins that reversibly precipitate in the cold. According to the most widely used classification, based on the chemistry of the cryoglobulins involved, proposed by Brouet in 1974 and still accepted, there are three types of cryoglobulinemia. In type I cryoglobulinemia, the cryoprecipitable immunoglobulin is a single monoclonal immunoglobulin, usually a myeloma protein or a macroglobulin. Types II and III cryoglobulinemias are both mixed cryoglobulinemias (MCs), composed of at least two immunoglobulins. In both, a polyclonal IgG is bound to another immunoglobulin, acting as an anti-IgG rheumatoid factor. The important difference between these two types of MCs is that in type II, the antiglobulin component, which is usually of the IgM class, is monoclonal, whereas in type III, it is polyclonal.

MCs constitute 60% to 75% of all cryoglobulinemias, and a high proportion are found in connective tissue diseases, infectious or lymphoproliferative disorders, hepatobiliary diseases, or immune glomerular diseases; these are called *secondary mixed cryoglobulinemias*. For 30% of all MCs, the etiology was unclear and cryoglobulinemia was referred to as essential until new serologic markers of hepatitis C virus (HCV) infection revealed that nearly all of these patients have antibodies against viral antigens and also HCV RNA, proving active viral replication.

The clinical syndrome of MC was first described by Meltzer and co-workers in 1966. It was characterized by purpura, weakness, arthralgia, and in some of the patients, glomerular lesions. Many subsequent reports have more fully characterized this syndrome. They also indicate that the incidence of MC varies in different geographic areas, the majority of cases having been reported in the Mediterranean countries, namely Italy, France, Spain, and Israel, where HCV infection is endemic. They have confirmed that the syndrome can be associated with either type II and type III cryoglobulins. In the rheumatologic surveys, patients with type III MC outnumbered those with type II MC. On the contrary, surveys based on renal involvement indicated a large prevalence of type II MC, the monoclonal component being nearly always an IgM kappa. Although the glomerular lesions were variable in the few cases of type III MC with renal involvement, a well-characterized pattern of glomerular disease (cryoglobulinemic nephropathy) has been described in type II MC, in which IgM kappa was the monoclonal component.

MANIFESTATIONS OF GLOMERULONEPHRITIS ASSOCIATED WITH TYPE II MIXED CRYOGLOBULINEMIA

Pathology

At light microscopy, a particular type of membranoproliferative glomerulonephritis is found in the majority of patients, especially in the acute stages. The pattern of the glomerular involvement differs from that of the idiopathic type of membranoproliferative glomerulonephritis and from that of the diffuse proliferative glomerulonephritis of systemic lupus erythematosus (SLE) in the following characteristic features: (a) the presence of a massive infiltration of leukocytes, mainly monocytes, that is the major constituent of endocapillary proliferation; (b) the frequent presence of the so-called intraluminal thrombi (amorphous, eosinophilic, PAS-positive deposits of variable size and diffusion, lying against the inner side of the glomerular capillary wall and sometimes filling the capillary lumen completely); and (c) thickening of glomerular basement membrane (GBM), with a double-contoured appearance, that is more diffuse and evident than in lupus nephritis and in idiopathic membranoproliferative glomerulonephritis. Electron microscopy shows that monocytes are in close contact with the subendothelial and intraluminal deposits, involved in their degradation, and can often be found in the double-contoured capillary wall, between the basement membrane and the endothelial cells or the newly formed basement membrane–like material. In this area, peripheral interposition of mesangial matrix and cells is not as marked as in idiopathic membranoproliferative glomerulonephritis. Mesangial sclerosis is found in late stages in the central area of the glomerular lobules (lobular glomerulonephritis) in a minority of patients. In all other cases, mesangial sclerosis is a late and usually mild feature. Another peculiar feature that can be found in at least one-third of patients biopsied in the acute stages, especially when signs of systemic vasculitis coexist, and in a larger percentage of postmortem specimens is a vasculitis of small and medium renal arteries. Perivascular infiltrating cells are mainly monocytes. In biopsies taken in later stages, perivascular infiltration appears to be replaced by perivascular fibrosis. The pattern found by immunofluorescence microscopy in specimens taken when an acute nephritic syndrome is present and massive intraluminal deposits can be seen by light microscopy is characterized by intense staining of such deposits, usually associated with faint irregular segmental parietal staining of some peripheral loops in a subendothelial position. In more chronic stages, when intraluminal thrombi are absent, the pattern is that of intense granular diffuse staining of peripheral loops, very similar to that of type I idiopathic membranoproliferative glomerulonephritis. IgM and IgG are the prevailing immunoreactants, suggesting that the deposits are locally trapped or precipitated cryoglobulins. This identity is further confirmed by the finding that the intracapillary electron-dense deposits, which are usually amorphous by electron microscopy, may have in some patients a peculiar crystalloid structure (cylinders with a hollow axis), which is identical to that seen in the *in vitro* cryoprecipitate of serum of the same patients.

Clinical Features

Type II MC manifests itself usually from the fourth to fifth decade of life, although first presentation has been reported for younger patients. Women outnumber men in nonselected populations.

Renal symptoms are usually a late manifestation of type II MC. They appear a few years after the extrarenal signs, which are mainly purpura, arthralgias, leg ulcers, systemic vasculitis, Raynaud's syndrome, hepatic involvement, and peripheral neuropathy. However, the concomitant appearance of renal and systemic signs of the disease is rather common. In some patients, renal involvement may be the main manifestation of the disease, before the appearance of the more evocative purpura.

An acute nephrotic syndrome, characterized by macroscopic hematuria, severe proteinuria, hypertension, and sudden increase in blood urea, is present at the onset of renal disease in 25% of cases and is complicated by an acute oliguric renal failure in 5%. At this acute stage, biopsy shows the typical cryoglobulinemic glomerulonephritis, that is, a severe membranoproliferative exudative glomerulonephritis characterized by intense monocyte infiltration and massive intraluminal deposits, which obliterate many capillary lumens.

However, the most common renal syndrome is an isolated proteinuria with microscopic hematuria, sometimes associated with signs of moderate chronic renal failure or, less frequently, nephrotic-range proteinuria. The corresponding histologic picture is that of a membranoproliferative glomerulonephritis characterized by less conspicuous intraluminal deposits and monocyte infiltration, sometimes with a lobular pattern, while immunofluorescence usually reveals subendothelial deposits, sometimes segmental, of IgM, IgG, and C3. In a few patients with isolated urinary abnormalities, a rather unspecific picture of mild segmental mesangial proliferation may be observed, without significant monocyte infiltration and capillary wall alterations.

Hypertension is very common at the apparent onset of renal disease, even in patients without nephritic syndrome. The renal disease has a variable course. In nearly one-third of patients, a remission of renal symptoms, partial or complete, has been described, even if at presentation, an acute nephritic syndrome or a severe nephrotic syndrome was present. Remission after acute nephritic syndrome may occur before any treatment is started and is associated with the disappearance of the massive intraluminal deposits that characterize such acute events. In one-third of patients, renal disease has a rather indolent course and does not progress to renal failure for several years, despite the persistence of urinary abnormalities. In as many as 20% of patients, reversible clinical exacerbations, such as nephritic or nephrotic syndrome, occur in the course of the disease, sometimes associated with flare-ups of the systemic signs of the disease. The new episodes of nephritic syndrome are often associated with the recurrence of massive intraluminal thrombi and intense monocyte infiltration. Several exacerbation episodes may occur in a single patient at variable intervals.

A moderate degree of renal failure, if not already present at clinical onset, is often found at later stages. However, progression to end-stage renal failure is less common than was believed in the past, even in patients with multiple relapses of renal disease. Chronic uremia developed in only 14% of the patients after 10 years of long-term follow up. The survival rate was 49% at 15 years, the most common causes of death being cardiovascular diseases, infections, liver failure, and neoplasia.

Laboratory Findings

Two laboratory findings are specific for MC: the presence of circulating cryoglobulins and a typical pattern of hypocomplementemia. The amounts of circulating cryoglobulins may vary from one patient to the other, and in the same patients at different times. The thermal instability of cryoglobulins may vary from one patient to another. Some cryoglobulins will precipitate at room temperature (20°C), whereas others require more prolonged incubation at lower temperatures (4°C). We found cryocrits ranging between 2% and 70%, with large variations during the course of the disease. There is no correlation between these laboratory parameters and the degree of activity of the disease, but high cryoglobulin concentration was correlated with a bad prognosis in our experience. The serum complement pattern is specific in cryoglobulinemic nephritis. Early complement components (C1q, C4) and CH_{50} are usually very low, C3 is slightly but significantly low, and later components tend to be higher than in normal controls. The complement pattern does not change very much with changes in clinical activity of the disease. In fact, early complement components tend to remain low, whatever the degree of activity of the systemic and renal disease.

Pathogenesis

While the polyclonal anti-IgG immunoglobulins involved in type III MC derive from the disruption and amplification of the physiologic immunoregulating mechanism of antiglobulin production and are probably antigen driven, the monoclonal anti-IgG immunoglobulins of type II MC may derive from the abnormal proliferation of a special clone of B lymphocytes and probably represent the consequence of a lymphoproliferative disorder, even though patients with type II MC show (with rare exceptions of late progression to lymphoma) very little evidence of lymphoid malignancy, and their dominant manifestation results from the tissue deposition of IgM-IgG immune complexes.

Many groups of investigators from Europe and the United States, using an enzyme-linked immunoabsorbent assay (ELISA) and an even more sensitive recombinant immunoblot assay (RIBA), demonstrated a very high rate of positivity of anti-HCV antibodies in the sera of patients with all types of MC (essential and secondary), but not type I cryoglobulinemia.

In type II MC, several groups of investigators, using reverse transcription and DNA amplification, have documented an even greater prevalence of HCV RNA. Finally, HCV antibodies have been detected, at an higher concentration, even in the cryoprecipitate.

These findings suggest a direct role of the viral infection in the development of all types of MC. It is possible that HCV could promote the underlying lymphoproliferative disorder in patients with this disease by triggering the emergence of B cell clones, producing a monoclonal or polyclonal IgM rheumatoid factor. This hypothesis is consistent with the fact that the HCV virus can infects peripheral blood mononuclear cells and particularly B lymphocytes, even though the presence active viral replication in lymphocytes is still controversial.

It can be postulated that there is a subgroup of patients with chronic HCV infection in whom possible direct active viral replication in B lymphocytes induces type III MC by triggering B-cell clone activation to hyperproduce polyclonal IgM rheumatoid factors. This situation is not associated with a specific glomerular disease. Some additional event, still unknown, might induce abnormal proliferation of a specific B cell clone that produces the monoclonal rheumatoid factor characterizing type II MC and cryoglobulinemic glomerulonephritis in only part of the total population.

Because evidence of HCV infections has been found in all types of MC, the presence of the virus in the precipitable cryoglobulins is probably not relevant to the determination of their preferential deposition in the glomerulus that characterize cryoglobulinemic glomerulonephritis. Cryoglobulinemic membranoproliferative glomerulonephritis occurs only when a monoclonal rheumatoid factor (usually an IgM kappa) is produced, as a consequence of the HCV infection even though the possibility that HCV can induce an immune complex–mediated membranoproliferative glomerulonephritis independently of type II MC induction cannot be totally excluded. The presence in the serum of an IgM kappa rheumatoid factor with specific affinity for glomerular structures like cellular fibronectin seems to be essential to the development of the glomerular damage associated with HCV infection.

Treatment

In the past 15 years, glucocorticoids and/or cyclophosphamide have been used by the majority of investigators to treat cryoglobulinemic glomerulonephritis. Methylprednisolone pulses and plasmapheresis have been added to oral glucocorticoids and cyclophosphamide for the more acute stages of the renal or systemic disease, especially when there is an acute nephritic syndrome and/or signs of vasculitis. This therapeutic approach is probably responsible for the reduced evolution to end-stage renal failure in patients with type II MC and renal involvement. The outcomes of this disease in patients with or without renal complication are now comparable.

The beneficial effects of interferon-alpha therapy on the clinical and biochemical manifestations of type II MC in some uncontrolled studies and in two randomized, controlled studies have been reported. Before the demonstration of the pathogenetic role of HCV infection in the pathogenesis of this disease, the response to this drug had been supposed to be related to its antiproliferative and immunomodulating effect. The controlled trial in 53 patients with HCV-associated type II MCs documented that the clinical effect of interferon-alpha, accompanied by a reduction in serum cryoglobulin concentration, was limited to patients in whom HCV RNA disappeared from the serum and was therefore due to its antiviral action. The study also showed that the virus reappears in the majority of treated patients after discontinuation of the drug, suggesting the advisability of using high dosages for long periods. It was proposed that dosages of 4.5 to 6.0 mU interferon-alpha-2a thrice weekly for 6 months be used and continued at a dosage of 3 mU thrice weekly for 6 additional months if there is a beneficial effect and HCV RNA disappears from the serum. Although three-fourths of the patients studied in this manner had renal damage and displayed a small improvement of their renal disease (a small significant reduction in serum creatinine, but not of the urinary protein-creatinine index), the majority of the large studies have not focused on evaluation of the specific effect of this antiviral drug, given as a single agent, in patients with cryoglobulinemic glomerulonephritis and HCV infection. Specific favorable responses of the signs of the renal disease in very small numbers of patients have been reported. A large controlled trial in patients with cryoglobulinemic glomerulonephritis and HCV infection is definitely necessary to define the precise role of interferon-alpha in the management of this disease entity. Until the results of such a trial become available, our policy is to use this antiviral agent as the sole therapeutic tool during the chronic stage of the renal disease. In some cases, we have obtained reduction of proteinuria and serum creatinine levels and probably prevented acute flare-ups. However, when a patient presents with an acute nephritic syndrome and/or signs of acute renal and systemic vasculitis, we still prefer to combine glucocorticoids (starting with intravenous pulses of 1.0 g of methylprednisolone each given on 3 consecutive days). This is followed with oral administration of 0.5 to 0.7 mg/kg of body weight per day of prednisone; this therapy should be tapered over several weeks to a small maintenance dose. This therapy should be combined with 2 to 3 mg/kg body weight per day for at least 3 months. In the most severe cases of acute renal insufficiency, the aforementioned therapy should be combined with plasmapheresis. The combined therapeutic approach has been well tolerated even when there was concomitant hepatic damage.

Selected Readings

Agnello V, Chung RT, Kaplan LM. A role for hepatitis C virus infection in type II cryoglobulinemia. *N Engl J Med* 1992;327:1490–1495.
One of the first study suggesting a close relation between MC and chronic HCV infection.

Brouet JC, Clauvel JP, Danon F, et al. Biological and clinical significance of cryoglobulins. A report of 86 cases. *Am J Med* 1974;57:775–778.
The most complete description of cryoglobulins, with the most valid classification.

Cacoub P, Lunel Fabiani F, et al. Mixed cryoglobulinemia and hepatitis C virus. *Am J Med* 1994;96:124–132.
A recent study demonstrating a close relation between MC and HCV infection.

Cordonnier D, Renversez JC, Vialtel P, et al. The kidney in mixed cryoglobulinemias. *Springer Semin Immunopathol* 1987;9:395–415.
An excellent overview of the kidney involvement in MC.

D'Amico G, Colasanti G, Ferrario F, et al. Renal involvement in essential mixed cryoglobulinemia. *Kidney Int* 1989;35:1004–1014.
A comprehensive overview of the pathogenetic and clinical aspects of cryoglobulinemic glomerulonephritis and vasculitis.

D'Amico G, Fornasieri A. Cryoglobulinemic glomerulonephritis: a membranoproliferative glomerulonephritis induced by hepatitis C virus. *Am J Kidney Dis* 1995;25:361–368.
A recent overview on clinical, pathologic, and pathogenetic mechanisms of glomerulonephritis associated with MC.

D'Amico G, Madias NE, Fornasieri A, et al. Renal involvement in hepatitis C infection: cryoglobulinemic glomerulonephritis-discussion. *Kidney Int* 1998;54:650–671.
A stimulating discussion on many aspects of cryoglobulinemic glomerulonephritis made by experts in the field.

Gorevic PD, Kassab HJ, Levo Y, et al. Mixed cryoglobulinemia: clinical aspects and long-term follow-up of 40 patients. *Am J Med* 1980;69:287–308.
The first exhaustive report on the clinical course of patients with MC.

Johnson RJ, Gretch DR, Yamabe H, et al. Membranoproliferative glomerulonephritis associated with hepatitis C virus infection. *N Engl J Med* 1993;328:465–470.
A study in which HCV infection is found to be associated to membranoproliferative glomerulonephritis.

Tarantino A, Campise M, Banfi G. Long-term predictors of survival in essential mixed cryoglobulinemic nephritis. *Kidney Int* 1995;47:618–623.
A good long-term study of patient with MC.

PART 12
Paraproteinemic Disorders

Manuel Martínez-Maldonado and Julio E. Benabe

MULTIPLE MYELOMA

Multiple myeloma is a neoplastic transformation of plasma cells with an incidence of about 2 to 4 per 100,000 population; there are nearly 15,000 new cases each year in the United States. It mostly affects patients older than 60 and reaches its peak incidence in the eighth decade in men; fewer than 1% of patients have been diagnosed before age 40. For unclear reasons, the incidence is higher in African-Americans. The disease is incurable and has a median survival of approximately 3 years. In 99% of patients, an abnormal production and secretion of a clone of unique immunoglobulin proteins or immunoglobulin light or heavy chains (paraproteins) is detected. Plasmacytoma or myeloma develops in hematopoietically active bone marrow or, occasionally, at extramedullary sites. Although initially local, plasma cell neoplasia soon become generalized.

Clinical Manifestations

Presenting symptoms are predominantly related to bone disease and include skeletal pain, pathologic fractures, and diffuse osteoporosis. When multiple myeloma coexists with renal tubular dysfunction, osteomalacia and pseudofractures are prominent. Areas of osteolysis without osteoblastic reaction are characteristic. Normochromic, normocytic anemia is usually related to a tumor mass of more than 10^{12} cells. A hemoglobin value less than 8 g/dl carries a poor prognosis. Renal dysfunction, malnutrition, and cachexia also worsen anemia. Leukopenia, thrombocytopenia, hemolysis, and a high sedimentation rate can also be present. In the presence of renal failure, the degree of anemia in multiple myeloma is greater than that due to the degree of renal failure.

The prevalence of hypogammaglobulinemia varies with the type of abnormal protein produced, being most marked when only the light chain unattached to the heavy chain of the immunoglobulin molecule is secreted ("light-chain disease"). In these cases, the erythrocyte sedimentation rate can be normal. Serum levels of normal polyclonal immunoglobulins can be reduced because of an increase in fractional catabolism or expansion of the plasma volume. Also, some patients develop circulating mononuclear phagocytes that can impair the capacity of normal B cells to secrete or produce normal immunoglobulins. Hypogammaglobulinemia, together with malnutrition, cachexia, and renal failure have made infections a common cause of death in these patients. Early use of nonnephrotoxic antibiotics at the first sign of infections is essential.

Acute or chronic renal failure occurs in plasma cell disorders as shown in Table 42.30. The development of sensitive techniques that detect monotypical light-chain deposition in kidney tissue has often uncovered plasma cell dyscrasia after a renal biopsy is performed to diagnose the nature of the renal disease. Progressive renal failure, nephrotic syndrome, nephrotic-range proteinuria, acute renal failure, and mild proteinuria with or without hematuria can be presenting manifestations of multiple myeloma.

Electrolyte Abnormalities

Abnormal gamma globulins can lead to electrolyte abnormalities in serum and provide a clue to the diagnosis of multiple myeloma. Pseudohyponatremia, as measured by flame photometry but not by ion-selective electrodes, occurs because in the presence of large quantities of circulating protein, the total water per volume of serum is reduced. Correction for the portion of serum from which water has been displaced by protein usually reveals the values of serum sodium concentration to be normal. In these pseudohyponatremia patients, plasma osmolality and serum sodium measured by ion-selective electrodes are normal. The difference between measured osmolality and calculated osmolality [(Serum sodium × 2) + (Serum urea nitrogen, mg/dl, ÷ 2.8) + (Blood glucose, mg/dl, ÷ 18)] is referred to as the *osmolal gap*, and its presence is helpful in the diagnosis of pseudohyponatremia.

TABLE 42.30. Plasma Cell Disorders

	Prevalence[a] (%)	Associated Light Chain	Bence Jones Proteinuria[b] (%)	Renal Failure[b] (%)	Clinical Findings
IgG myeloma (γ)	50	κ>λ	60	40	Circulating aggregates of IgG_3; most common; best prognosis
IgA myeloma (α)	20	κ>λ	70	60	Circulating polymers; hypercalcemia; associated with extramedullary plasmacytomas
IgM myeloma (μ) Waldenström's macroglobulinemia	12	κ>λ	70	20	Hyperviscosity syndrome; multiple organ infiltration; plasmacytoid lymphocytes in marrow
IgD myeloma (δ)	4	κ>λ	90	90	Frequently normal serum protein electrophoresis; detected by immunoelectrophoresis; organ infiltration
IgE myeloma (ϵ)	1	κ>λ	70		Circulating plasma cells (plasma cell leukemia)
Light-chain myeloma	10	κ>λ	100	80	Severe bone disease; polyclonal hypogammaglobulinemia; rouleaux formation absent; Bence Jones proteinemia detected with onset of renal failure
Heavy-chain disease (μ, α, γ)	<1	κ?	Only μ-chain disease	Rare	Large vacuolated plasma cells in marrow; lymphomalike presentation
Primary (AL type) amyloidosis	<1	λ>κ	30	40	Evolving plasma cell neoplasm; less renal failure than secondary type
Monoclonal gammopathy of undetermined significance	3 (> 70)	κ>λ	10	Rare	24% develop some type of neoplastic process or amyloidosis on follow-up

[a] Approximate values, relative to all plasma cell disorders.
[b] Approximate values, occurence among patents with specific plasma cell disorder.

A low anion gap may be found in multiple myeloma because large amounts of immunoglobulin possessing net positive electrostatic charges tend to reduce the normal anion gap by increasing the amount of neutralizing anions in the serum. The result may be an anion gap of less than 5 mEq/L (normal is about 12 mEq/L). In 42% of patients with multiple myeloma, particularly those of the IgG type, the anion gap is lower than in normal subjects. In contrast, patients with IgA myeloma do not have a low anion gap because the abnormal proteins are negatively charged at the physiologic pH; therefore cations are attracted, leading to an increase in the anion gap. However, the anion gap is usually maintained at or near normal values because of concomitant hypoalbuminemia.

Hypercalcemia is the most common electrolyte disturbance in this disease. Rarely, the myeloma protein can bind calcium and produce a syndrome of pseudohypercalcemia, with normal ionized calcium concentration despite elevated total serum calcium concentration. *Hyperphosphatemia* can result from a similar mechanism when some myeloma proteins bind phosphate and spuriously raise serum values. *Hypophosphatemia* has also been described in patients with multiple myeloma and proximal tubule abnormalities leading to Fanconi's syndrome. In addition, asymptomatic, prolonged hypophosphatemia resulting from spurious reductions in phosphate as a result of interference of large amounts of abnormal IgG with the Beckman CX7 autoanalyzer assay for phosphate determination has been described. Use of other automated or manual methods that precipitate plasma proteins with trichloroacetic acid demonstrate normal phosphate levels in the same samples. It is of interest that spurious hyperphosphatemia has also been reported in hypergammaglobulinemic patients when an automated autoanalyzer similar to the Beckman was used for the measurement. *Hypercupremia* occasionally resulting in Kayser-Fleischer–like rings has been described. Serum copper concentration rises as a result of increased binding of copper to anomalous proteins in the blood. *Hyperkalemia* associated with hyporeninemic hypoaldosteronism has been described in multiple myeloma.

Diagnosis

Diagnosis and classification of multiple myeloma rest on the identification and quantification by electrophoretic analysis of serum and urine of the abnormal immunoglobulin molecule produced by the neoplastic clone. In more than two-thirds of patients, a monoclonal gammopathy is detected in the serum. Quantitative assay of the abnormal immunoglobulin ("M" component) is one of the best indices to follow the progression of the disease and the response to treatment.

Examination of the urine can reveal the presence of light chains, also known as Bence Jones proteins, which provides further support for the diagnosis (Table 42.31). The approximate concentration of light-chain proteins in the urine of normal individuals is 2.5 mg/ml. Patients with monoclonal gammopathies of undetermined significance or with hepatitis C virus–related chronic liver disease can have urinary light-chain concentrations from 0.02 to 0.5 mg/ml. This is usually much higher (range, 0.02 to 11.5 mg/ml) in patients with multiple myeloma or Waldenström's macroglobulinemia. The amount of light chain excreted is often insufficient for detection using turbidimetric and heat tests (Bence Jones assay); diagnosis therefore rests with antibody detection assays, which confirm the presence and monoclonal nature of the light chain (Table 42.30). Immunofixation electrophoresis, which is very sensitive, detects light chains even in very low concentrations. However, the presence of a small amount of monoclonal light chain can be masked by coexistent tubulointerstitial disease that produces significant proximal tubule damage and therefore results in increased excretion of low-molecular-weight proteins that include polyclonal light chains. The diagnostic hallmark of plasma cell dyscrasias is Bence Jones proteinuria. The causes of monoclonal light-chain proteinuria are listed in Table 42.32. Rifampin can induce Bence Jones proteinuria and renal failure from cast nephropathy. Light-chain overproduction resolves by stopping the administration of the drug.

Renal monoclonal light-chain deposition may be found by kidney biopsy in the absence of detectable serum or urine paraproteins by immunoelectrophoresis in 30% to 50% of patients with documented glomerular light-chain deposition. Immunophenotyping of bone marrow biopsy can document a monoclonal population of plasma cells when other tests are ambiguous. Plasma cells in excess of 20% of nonerythroid cells, especially if they are vacuolated, bizarre, and multinucleated,

TABLE 42.31. Detection of Bence Jones Proteinuria

Test	Specification
Colorimetric Tetrabromophenol blue reagent (Dipstix, Ames)	Typically will not detect Bence Jones protein. Sensitivity to protein concentrations > 20 mg/dl.
Turbidimetric Nitric acid reagent Sulfosalicylic acid Toluene sulfonic acid Trichloroacetic acid	Will detect Bence Jones protein, but also other proteins. Sensitive to ≥ 10 mg/dl.
Heat test Appearance of urine precipitate at 40°-60°C, dissolve at 100°C and reprecipitate on cooling at 40°C	False-positive resluts can be seen in the presence of polyclonal light chains (e.g., tubular proteinuria). The test requires at least 200 mg/dl of light chains. False-negative results can occur with very high amounts of Bence Jones proteinuria (600 mg/dl).
Electrophoresis Cellulose acetate	Single peak with β or γ mobility representing monoclonal light chains. Two peaks with β and γ mobility representing monomers and dimer of light chains; or two peaks representing intact immunoglobulin and free light chain.
Immunoelectrophoresis—1% agar or agarose gel with use of monospecific antibodies to κ or λ	Used for final identification of monoclonal or polyclonal light chains and immunoglobulins in serum or urine.
Immunodiffusion (Ouchterlony)—uses monspecific antibodies to κ or λ	More sensitive than immunoelectrophoresis. Can be used as screening test. To identify monoclonality, immunoelectrophoresis is still needed.
Immunofixation electrophoresis—uses monospecific antibodies to κ or λ	Very sensitive test; widely used. Presence of tubulointerstitial damage can mask monoclonal light chain.

TABLE 42.32. Causes of Bence Jones Proteinuria

Multiple myeloma
Amyloidosis, type AL
Systemic light chain deposition disease
Waldenström's macroglobulinemia
Heavy-chain disease (μ)
Monoclonal gammopathy of undetermined significance (unusual)
Chronic lymphoproliferative disease (rare)
Rifampin therapy (rare)

support a diagnosis of multiple myeloma. A negative bone marrow biopsy does not rule out the existence of a population of bone marrow cells producing abnormal light chains that deposit in the kidney and cause renal failure. Patients with renal failure from documented light-chain deposition and no evidence of plasma cell dyscrasia on routine evaluation of the bone marrow may develop overt multiple myeloma over time. Patients with monoclonal gammopathy of undetermined significance without evidence of renal dysfunction should be followed closely because over time, as many as 25% will develop overt multiple myeloma, amyloidosis, macroglobulinemia, or a malignant lymphoproliferative disorder.

Renal Involvement

Virtually all areas of the kidney parenchyma can be damaged by monoclonal light-chain deposition (Table 42.33). Immunoglobulin light chains undergo glomerular filtration and are reabsorbed by the proximal tubule, where they are ordinarily catabolized and the amino acid components are returned to the circulation. Saturation of the reabsorptive process will permit light chains to reach the distal nephron fluid and the urine. Parenteral administration of certain human light chains into mice reproduces the glomerular, tubular, and vascular lesions found in humans. In humans, simultaneous occurrence of two or more of these lesions is unusual, and some patients may excrete large amounts of monoclonal light chains and have no clinically evident renal dysfunction. The type of renal lesion induced by light chains may depend on the physicochemical properties of the excreted protein. Although structurally similar, each light chain is a distinct and unique molecule. The characteristics or mechanisms that render these molecules nephrotoxic properties have yet to be identified but may include isoelectric points above 5.1, interference with sodium-dependent transport, and inhibition of Na^+-K^+-ATPase activity. Also, light chains may compete for endocytosis of other low-molecular-weight proteins and disrupt molecular cell trafficking. Evidence for inhibition of DNA synthesis by light chains has also been advanced.

Glomerulopathies

Light chains may polymerize to form AL amyloid, or they can be deposited unaltered as granular, punctate, electron-dense material (granular light-chain deposition disease). Electron microscopy characterizes amyloid as randomly oriented, nonbranching fibrils 8 to 10 nm wide and localized primarily in mesangial and/or subepithelial glomerular areas. For amyloid deposition to occur in glomeruli, amyloid P glycoprotein must also be present. The amyloid P component is not a part of the amyloid fibrils, but it binds them. This glycoprotein is a constituent of normal human glomerular basement membrane and elastic fibrils. In contrast to AL amyloid, granular light-chain deposits are punctuate and electron dense and are identified in the mesangium and/or subendothelial space. These deposits contain both intact and fragmented light chains. Amyloid P component is absent in the granular, nonamyloid deposits of light chains. Amyloid is also known for its peculiar tinctorial properties and classically stains with Congo red, producing an apple-green birefringence when the tissue section is examined under polarized light and also if stained with thioflavin T and S; these special stains do not identify granular light-chain deposits. Another difference between AL amyloid and light chain deposits is the tendency for the granular deposits to be composed of κ light chains, whereas amyloid is typically composed of λ light chains. The λVI class is particularly amyloidogenic. Amyloid and granular nonamyloid deposits have been demonstrated in the same patient. Both diseases can involve organs other than the kidney, such as the heart, liver, nerves, and blood vessels. Amyloid more commonly involves the gastrointestinal tract and lungs, whereas granular light-chain deposition disease more commonly involves the liver.

Glomerular involvement from both amyloid and granular light-chain deposition leads to a nodular glomerulopathy reminiscent of diabetic nephropathy, although glomerular morphology can vary (Table 42.32). Early amyloid and granular light-chain deposition can be subtle and difficult to distinguish from minimal-change nephropathy. When a morphologic renal lesion, such as minimal-change nephropathy, does not follow the expected clinical course, a light chain–related renal lesion should be considered. Advanced amyloid and granular light-chain deposition diseases typically produce a nonproliferative, noninflammatory glomerulopathy. Unlike amyloid, however, a proliferative lesion often occurs early in the course of granular (nonamyloid) light-chain deposition. Mesangial proliferation varies from mild to fairly intense. A proliferative glomerulonephritis may represent an early manifestation of granular light-chain deposition disease; progression from membranoproliferative glomerulonephritis to nodular glomerulopathy has been documented. Heavy chains may also participate in some of these lesions. Concomitant deposition of heavy chains occurs in some monoclonal light chain–related glomerulopathies, and some authors have suggested the term *monoclonal light- and heavy-chain deposition disease.* In those specimens, the punctate electron-dense deposits appear larger and more extensive than those deposits that contain only light chains, but it is unclear whether the clinical course of these patients differs from the course of isolated light-chain deposition alone. On rare occasions, systemic (liver and renal) amyloidosis may be composed primarily of an atypical heavy-chain protein. These findings suggest that overproduction of this protein can also result in amyloidosis and subsequent organ failure.

Tubulointerstitial Lesions

Proximal tubule injury leading to Fanconi's syndrome is associated with Bence Jones proteinuria. A plasma cell dyscrasia should be considered present in any adult with this syndrome. In patients with glomerular lesions associated with light chains, severe damage to proximal tubule epithelium occurs rather consistently. On occasion, isolated proximal tubule damage from light-chain deposition can produce clinical renal failure. Experimental studies have shown that certain human Bence

TABLE 42.33. Renal Lesions of Multiple Myeloma

I. Glomerulopathies
- A. Amyloid, type AL
- B. Granular light-chain deposition disease
- C. Fibrillary (monotypical membranous) glomerulonephritis

II. Tubulointerstitial lesions
- A. Fanconi's syndrome
- B. Proximal tubule necrosis (acute tubular necrosis, or "tubulopathy")
- C. Cast neuropathy ("myeloma kidney")
- D. Tubulointerstitial nephritis

III. Vascular lesions

IV. Asymptomatic Bence Jones proteinuria

V. Hypercalcemic nephropathy

VI. Hyperviscosity syndrome

VII. Pyelonephritis

VIII. Neoplastic cell infiltration

IX. Obstructive nephropathy

Jones proteins produce morphologic and functional defects in the proximal tubule after endocytosis. The same morphologic lesions occurred in human proximal tubule epithelium exposed to certain Bence Jones proteins. The mechanism of damage to the proximal epithelium appears to develop with accumulation of toxic Bence Jones proteins in the endolysosomal system. The atypical appearance of the lysosomes in proximal tubule epithelium suggests the presence of Bence Jones proteinuria. A few patients have been found to have an acute tubulopathy (acute tubular necrosis) associated with polymerization of light chains in the cytoplasm of proximal tubule cells.

Cast nephropathy, or "myeloma kidney," is another common tubulointerstitial lesion resulting from light-chain deposition. This noninflammatory tubulointerstitial nephropathy develops with formation of light-chain casts in the distal nephron, a site that provides an optimal environment for precipitation of light chains. Casts occur in part because light chains coaggregate with Tamm-Horsfall glycoprotein, which is synthesized exclusively by cells of the thick ascending limb of Henle's loop. In normal individuals, the majority of urinary protein is Tamm-Horsfall glycoprotein. This glycoprotein is the major constituent of urinary casts and is also an important component of intranephronal casts formed by light chains. Cast-forming Bence Jones proteins bind to a common portion of the peptide backbone of Tamm-Horsfall glycoprotein; binding results in coaggregation of these proteins and subsequent occlusion of the tubule lumen from precipitated protein complexes. Intranephronal obstruction and renal failure ensue. The carbohydrate moiety of Tamm-Horsfall glycoprotein also appears to be critical for coprecipitation of these proteins because deglycosylated Tamm-Horsfall glycoprotein does not coprecipitate with light chains. Colchicine prevents cast formation by light chains *in vivo* in the rat by removing the carbohydrate component of Tamm-Horsfall glycoprotein. Coaggregation of Tamm-Horsfall glycoprotein with light chains also depends on the ionic environment and the physicochemical properties of the light chain because not all light chains are cast forming. Increasing concentrations of sodium chloride or calcium, but not magnesium, facilitate coaggregation. Interestingly, furosemide augments coaggregation and accelerates intraluminal obstruction *in vivo* in the rat. Finally, the lower tubule fluid flow rates of the distal nephron allow more time for Bence Jones proteins to interact with Tamm-Horsfall glycoprotein and subsequently obstruct the lumen. Situations in which flow rates are further reduced, such as volume depletion, can accelerate tubule obstruction or convert nontoxic light chains into cast-forming proteins.

Light-chain deposition can cause an unusual lesion that contains inflammatory infiltrates, often including eosinophils, associated with active tubular damage. A careful search usually detects subtle light-chain deposits along the tubular basement membranes almost exclusively in the areas of interstitial inflammation. This interstitial inflammatory pattern is sometimes associated with glomerular involvement; cast formation is rare. Failure to detect the deposits of light chains along the basement membrane may lead to the erroneous interpretation that the lesions are a hypersensitivity reaction to drugs, most notably nonsteroidal antiinflammatory agents, which can also produce a combined lesion consisting of minimal-change glomerulopathy and tubulointerstitial nephritis. An underlying plasma cell dyscrasia may therefore be missed.

Vascular Lesions

Glomeruli and other vessels are concomitantly affected by light-chain deposition; thus isolated involvement of the renal vasculature is unusual. Amyloid or granular (nonamyloid) light-chain deposits can be found. Light-chain deposits are generally localized to the walls of arterioles and small and medium arteries. Both proliferative and nonproliferative vasculopathies can occur. Vascular lesions can be prominent and contribute to progressive loss of renal function in some patients.

Hypercalcemia and Hypercalcemic Nephropathy

Mild hypercalcemia (11 to 13 mg/dl) occurs in more than 25% of patients; marked hypercalcemia (more than 13 mg/dl) may also be encountered. The hypercalcemia is secondary to enhanced bone resorption mediated by osteoclast-activating factors (OAF), a family of cytokines [including lymphotoxin, interleukin (IL)-1β, parathyroid related protein (PTHrP), and IL-6] produced by the neoplastic cells or by marrow stromal cells. The demonstration of OAF produced by myeloma cells has been inconstant. Nevertheless, PTHrP mRNA has been demonstrated in myeloma cells and the protein identified in the marrow and the plasma of some patients, suggesting that PTHrP plays an important role in the skeletal lesions and in the hypercalcemia of the disease. In some patients with markedly elevated serum levels of abnormal immunoglobulins, the total concentration of serum calcium is elevated because of binding to globulins, but the ionized fraction remains normal. This pseudohypercalcemia does not require treatment. In some patients, despite mild hypercalcemia (11 to 13 mg/dl), severe systemic manifestations may be present. Nausea, vomiting, renal salt wasting, and polyuria cause dehydration and volume depletion, resulting in increasing degrees of azotemia and renal failure. In most cases, treatment of volume contraction with the infusion of saline and correction of hypercalcemia will reverse the process. Renal histology in patients with multiple myeloma, renal failure, and hypercalcemia at times shows extensive proteinaceous cast formation, calcium deposits, and associated epithelial necrosis. This indicates that the tubular dysfunction caused by Bence Jones proteins and calcium deposition, and dehydration and volume depletion, may lead to tubular necrosis and acute renal failure. Saline administration usually reverses hypercalcemia, provided renal function is not irreversibly severely impaired. Loop diuretics also increase calcium excretion, but furosemide, because it may facilitate nephrotoxicity from light chains, *should not be administered until the patient is clinically euvolemic.* Generally, most patients respond to volume repletion and chemotherapy. Glucocorticoid therapy (prednisone 60 mg/day) is helpful for the management of multiple myeloma and hypercalcemia; nevertheless, it rarely corrects the calcium elevation. Rarely, more aggressive management is necessary. Mithramycin (25 mg/kg) lowers serum calcium levels to normal within 24 to 36 hours, and normocalcemia persists for almost 1 week without additional therapy. Because of the availability of other agents, mithramycin probably should be used only with life-threatening hypercalcemia (serum calcium concentration greater than 16 mg/dl). Hypercalcemia of malignancy also responds to gallium nitrate and the bisphosphonates. Both agents are nephrotoxic and should be administered only to euvolemic patients. Gallium nitrate appears to be more nephrotoxic and should not be given to patients with renal insufficiency. Bisphosphonates are now used to treat hypercalcemia (serum calcium greater than 13 mg/dl) unresponsive to other measures. Currently available bisphosphonates include etidronate and pamidronate. Although these agents may prove effective when administered orally, intravenous infusion of the agent over 3 to 7 days is recommended. Because bisphosphonates may chelate calcium and cause symptomatic acute hypocalcemia, intravenous infusion rates should be slow. Response occurs within the first several days of treatment: interrupting therapy is indicated as the calcium level normalizes. The effect of these agents is transient but often allows time for chemotherapy and hydration to prevent recurrence of hypercalcemia. Second-generation bisphosphonates, such as pamidronate, are efficacious in the treatment of symptomatic bone disease in myeloma. Further discussion of the treatment of hypercalcemia is found in Chapter 20, Part 3.

Dehydration and Contrast Media–Induced Renal Failure

Acute renal failure has been reported after intravenous pyelography in patients with multiple myeloma. This was originally attributed to the formation of aggregates of contrast media and the abnormal immunoglobulins. Several investigators have demonstrated that contrast media in large doses decrease renal blood flow and glomerular filtration rate transiently. Precipitates of Tamm-Horsfall glycoprotein in the presence of contrast media have also been demonstrated. Some contrast materials are uricosuric and may result in urate precipitation in the kidney. Hypercalcemia and Bence Jones proteinuria have been present in most patients who developed this syndrome. Dehydration and volume depletion potentiate all of the aforementioned factors in the development of acute renal failure. Thus intravenous pyelography is contraindicated in patients with multiple myeloma.

Acute Uric Acid Nephropathy

Hyperuricemia in patients with multiple myeloma results from the increased nucleic acid turnover, either spontaneously or as a result of chemotherapy. Patients with lymphomas and leukemias may have marked hyperuricemia and acute uric acid nephropathy, but these complications are rare in patients with multiple myeloma. However, if such complications are expected, the induction of water and solute diuresis together with alkalinization of the urine should be considered. Treatment with allopurinol may also be helpful.

Pyelonephritis

Infections and sepsis are among the most common causes of death in multiple myeloma, and the most frequent portal of entry is the urinary tract. Causes that predispose to infection are age (older than 60 years), hypogammaglobulinemia, neurogenic bladder, prostatic hypertrophy with obstructive uropathy, and the use of indwelling catheters. Instrumentation of the lower urinary tract should be avoided. If institution of antibiotic therapy is necessary, avoidance of nephrotoxic drugs must be considered when possible.

Obstructive Nephropathy

Obstructive nephropathy directly related to myelomatosis can occur secondary to (a) ureteral amyloid deposits, (b) nephrolithiasis, (c) papillary necrosis, (d) huge proteinaceous renal pelvic cast formation, and (e) neurogenic bladder secondary to spinal cord or nerve injury resulting from vertebral collapse.

Other renal involvement that may occur in multiple myeloma or in Waldenström's macroglobulinemia, such as lymphocytoid infiltration, hyperviscosity syndrome, and immunologically mediated glomerulopathy, are discussed in a following section.

Clinical Course, Management, and Prognosis

The clinical course of patients with monoclonal light chain–related renal diseases varies. If untreated, however, virtually all of the renal lesions cause progressive loss of renal function. A peculiar course of some patients with granular light-chain deposition disease resembles rapidly progressive glomerulonephritis with irreversible relentless reduction of renal function over weeks to months. In general, granular light-chain deposition disease that shows a nodular glomerulopathic morphologic pattern has a poor prognosis, with most patients progressing to end-stage renal failure. Progressive renal failure is common in patients with AL amyloidosis. These patients have a poor prognosis, with a median survival of 12 months, although prolonged survival is possible in some patients. The proximal tubule lesion (acute tubulopathy) contributes to progressive loss of renal function in patients also exhibiting monoclonal light chain–related glomerulopathies. With adequate control of light-chain proteinuria, however, proximal tubule lesions may improve.

The mainstay of therapy of these disorders is to abolish production of immunoglobulin light chains, the pathogenic feature of all of these renal lesions. As a group, the renal lesions responsible for renal failure, which occurs in more than half of patients with multiple myeloma, belong to an unusual class of potentially reversible renal diseases. The standard chemotherapeutic regimen that includes melphalan and prednisone ameliorates renal failure in more than half of patients who have renal failure and multiple myeloma.

Although successful chemotherapy decreases the bone marrow biosynthesis of abnormal monoclonal light chains in patients with glomerular lesions from monoclonal light-chain deposition, light chain–related lesions associated with glomerulopathy are particularly resistant to chemotherapy. Alkylating agents and prednisone decrease proteinuria, ameliorate nephrotic syndrome, and improve renal dysfunction in some patients with AL amyloidosis. Chemotherapy appears to prolong survival, although the overall response rate to chemotherapy approaches only 20%. Generally, however, progressive amyloid deposition continues, and progressive renal failure is the rule. Unlike amyloidosis in familial Mediterranean fever, treatment of AL amyloidosis with colchicine (0.6 mg/dl twice daily) has been disappointing. Uncontrolled trials of chemotherapy in granular light-chain deposition disease have suggested benefit in some patients by preventing progression of renal failure and occasionally improving renal function. Most studies examining the role of chemotherapy in the management of glomerular lesions from light-chain deposition are flawed or uncontrolled. Nevertheless, given the inexorable progression of these glomerular lesions when untreated and the proven pathogenic role of monoclonal light chains in these glomerulopathies, a trial of chemotherapy should be considered, especially if the initial serum creatinine concentration is less than 2 mg/dl. To identify these early lesions, however, a careful and comprehensive pathologic evaluation of kidney tissue must be performed early in the course of the disease.

Unlike glomerular lesions resulting from light-chain deposition, reducing plasma light-chain concentration has been shown to improve renal function in cast nephropathy. However, progressive loss of renal function subsequently occurs in many of these patients. Less attention has been given to potential treatments designed to disrupt coprecipitation of Tamm-Horsfall glycoprotein with cast-forming light chains. Hypercalcemia, an acidic urine, furosemide, and radiocontrast materials may aggravate nephrotoxicity of light chains by facilitating its coprecipitation with Tamm-Horsfall glycoprotein. Correction of hypercalcemia usually improves renal function. Alkalinization of the urine prevents renal failure from Bence Jones proteins in rats. In one inadequately controlled trial in humans, however, alkalinization of the urine by itself has not been beneficial. Thus alkalinization should be used only in conjunction with other measures, especially those aimed at enhancing hydration and keeping the urine flow rate high and the sodium chloride concentration in the distal nephron low. It is prudent to recommend a daily intake of 2 to 3 L of dilute fluids as long as a significant defect in excreting free water does not coexist. Clinicians have long recognized the detrimental effect of radiocontrast agents on renal function, and these should be avoided or not used at all in patients with multiple myeloma. Use of nonsteroidal antiinflammatory agents in myeloma has been associated with a significant incidence of renal failure in some studies and should therefore be avoided if possible. Because furosemide aggravates cast formation in experimental animals *in vivo*, this loop diuretic should be used with caution, especially when extracellular volume depletion is present.

With current management, median survival of patients with mild renal failure and multiple myeloma is 20 months. For all patients with myeloma, median survival approaches 25 months; for significant renal failure (creatinine concentration 180 mmol/L or greater, or 2 mg/dl), median survival decreases to 4.3 months. Patients with renal insufficiency are also predisposed to infection, which represents the major cause of death in myeloma. Mortality and morbidity from renal failure in this patient population should therefore decrease as diagnosis is made earlier in the course by use of a comprehensive diagnostic approach and with the emergence of new treatment modalities that result from improved understanding of the pathophysiology of light chain–mediated renal damage. These treatment strategies will not only attack the production of nephrotoxic light chains, but also will act to prevent binding and deposition of these proteins in various structures of the nephron.

Renal replacement therapy in the form of hemodialysis or peritoneal dialysis is generally recommended in patients with renal failure from monoclonal light chain–related renal diseases, especially if the renal failure is of recent onset. Recovery of renal function sufficient to survive without dialysis occurs in as many as 5% of patients with multiple myeloma, but in some patients, recovery requires months. In addition, although multisystem involvement and advanced age at the time of diagnosis of myeloma shorten life span with death occurring early in the course of treatment, some patients, particularly those with disease limited mostly to the kidney, may achieve functional rehabilitation and survive more than 2 years.

In contrast to dialysis as a form of therapy for end-stage renal failure, the role of renal transplantation is less clear cut. Generally, for patients with myeloma, extrarenal manifestations of the disease should be absent for more than 1 year before renal transplantation is considered. Suitable patients may then undergo successful transplantation. Similarly, extrarenal manifestations should be controlled in patients who do not have documented multiple myeloma but who have systemic light-chain deposition (AL amyloidosis or light-chain deposition disease). Renal transplantation in these individuals may be particularly beneficial if the disease has remained limited to the kidney. In one large study of 62 patients, 15 of whom had AL amyloidosis, 65% of patients were alive 5 years after renal allograft implantation. Whereas amyloid was found to involve the graft in 10%, in only 3% was the graft lost as a result of this involvement. Transplant experience in patients with granular light-chain deposition disease is even more limited, but the disease may also recur in the allograft and cause renal failure. Renal transplantation, however, remains a potential therapy in selected patients.

WALDENSTRÖM'S MACROGLOBULINEMIA

Macroglobulinemia is distinct from multiple myeloma; it is rare and has a variable clinical course. It represents a different neoplastic transformation, probably of a more immature B cell. The condition behaves more like a lymphoma, and many of its manifestations can be attributed to organ infiltration and hyperviscosity of blood. Cytopenia, serum IgM level, splenomegaly, and lymphadenopathy correlate with poor prognosis. The neoplastic cell, a large plasmacytoid lymphocyte, has the capacity to produce and secrete monoclonal IgM (macroglobulin). Some of the immunoglobulins behave as cryoglobulins and cause cryopathic signs and symptoms.

The most dramatic symptoms and signs are attributed to the circulating abnormal macroglobulin. Symptoms of increased blood viscosity and hypervolemia are usually the presenting manifestation and include a bleeding diathesis, neurologic disturbances, or cardiac dysfunction. Usually, there are no osteolytic lesions, and renal impairment can occur in up to 30% of cases. Although Bence Jones proteinuria can be detected by immunologic methods in more than 90% of patients, cast formation and myeloma kidney are rarely seen. Renal dysfunction is usually the consequence of (a) lymphocytoid cell infiltration of the kidney, (b) hyperviscosity syndrome, (c) amyloidosis, (d) immunologically mediated glomerulonephritis, or (e) nonspecific IgM glomerular deposits.

Lymphocytoid Cell Infiltration

Neoplastic infiltration of the kidneys occurs in fewer than 30% of patients with IgG multiple myeloma. By contrast, neoplastic involvement of kidneys is found in 50% to 60% of patients with macroglobulinemia. On some occasions, especially when associated with amyloidosis, the kidneys may attain a huge size and become palpable by abdominal examination. The appearance of IgM in the urine usually provides the diagnosis. Plasmacytoid cells have been recovered from urine sediment in patients with massive cell infiltration.

Hyperviscosity Syndrome

Symptoms and signs attributable to hyperviscosity and hypervolemia are present in 100% of patients with macroglobulinemia at some time during the course of the illness. In contrast, only 4.2% of patients with IgG multiple myeloma show symptoms attributable to increased serum viscosity. This striking difference probably relates to the predominantly intravascular localization of the IgM globulin, whereas only 40% of IgG is intravascular in multiple myeloma, and to the abnormal shape and structure of multimeric IgM. IgG_3 and IgA multiple myeloma may sometimes be evidenced by hyperviscosity syndrome, the former by causing circulating aggregates and the latter by forming covalently linked polymers. The characteristics of this syndrome are attributed to the increased blood viscosity and hypervolemia with resultant stasis, sluggish blood flow, distension of capillary beds, and interference with normal coagulation. It is usually manifested by impaired urine concentration, azotemia, and occasionally hematuria. Very rarely, it can cause acute renal failure or permanent renal damage.

The diagnosis of hyperviscosity syndrome rests on the typical clinical findings, which may also include bleeding diathesis, neurologic disturbances, or cardiac dysfunction, and on measurement of "relative" serum viscosity, but this parameter does not correlate linearly with serum concentration of abnormal immunoglobulins. This discrepancy may be due to aggregatability, polymerization, cryoprecipitability, and euglobulin formation *in vitro.* These factors must be kept in mind when faced with a slightly augmented relative serum viscosity and a picture of the full-blown syndrome. A relative serum viscosity of more than 4 and serum concentration of abnormal immunoglobulin of more than 5 g/dl are usually encountered when symptoms of hyperviscosity are present. On some occasions, a whole blood viscosity determination is needed for correlation with the clinical findings. A positive Sia water test (euglobulin formation) may be a clue to the diagnosis in patients with monoclonal IgM.

Under emergency situations, plasmapheresis with the removal of large amounts of macroglobulins can be accomplished by the following methods: (a) removal of 500 ml of blood and centrifugation for 5 minutes at 5,000 rpm and (b) use of a cell separator, always maintaining an adequate hemoglobin concentration (9 g/dl). Plasmapheresis should be continued until viscosity is lowered to acceptable levels and symptoms improve. Exchange transfusions may be done, but the risk of viral hepatitis is present. On some occasions, peritoneal dialysis is helpful. Chemotherapy in the form of alkylating agents and prednisone will help maintain a stable serum viscosity.

Immunologically Mediated Glomerulopathy

Glomerular disease is not a common finding in multiple myeloma, except in patients with amyloidosis or light-chain nephropathy. However, glomerular lesions are common in patients with macroglobulinemia; in some patients, a cryoglobulin associated with immune complex nephritis can be detected. Massive subendothelial deposits of IgM can be found in up to 40% of patients with macroglobulinemia. These deposits must be differentiated from amyloid by Congo red staining, electron microscopy, and immunofluorescence studies. Other immunoglobulins and complement are usually absent. A new entity, atypical membranous glomerulonephritis with organized monoclonal IgG deposits, has been described.

Amyloidosis

Amyloidosis (AL type) develops in about 10% of patients with multiple myeloma but less frequently in those with macroglobulinemia. There is no difference in organ infiltration between primary or myeloma-associated amyloidosis. Overall, patients with myeloma and amyloidosis have a poor prognosis, with a median survival of less than 12 months; but in patients with remissions induced by chemotherapeutic agents, survival time can be prolonged and amyloid deposits can be shown to regress.

MONOCLONAL GAMMOPATHY OF UNDETERMINED SIGNIFICANCE

Approximately 3% of patients older than 70 years of age may have a serum monoclonal (M) spike by electrophoresis without initial overt evidence of plasma cell neoplasm or other malignancy. On follow-up, almost 25% of these patients manifest an increase in M component concentration or the appearance of overt plasma cell neoplasm or amyloidosis. It has been emphasized that if the initial M component concentration is greater than 2 g/dl, a malignancy may be present. Bone marrow and radiographic studies, as well as blood cell counts, have failed to identify those patients in whom overt malignancy will develop. Serum and urine protein analyses are the best indices for the follow-up of the clinical course. The appearance of significant Bence Jones proteinuria or a progressive increase in M component concentration should alert the physician to the potential presence of a plasma cell neoplasm or other associated diseases such as lymphoma, amyloidosis, or pancreatic cancer.

Renal disease in association with monoclonal gammopathy of undetermined significance usually manifests clinically as endothelial and mesangial proliferative glomerulonephritis. Electron microscopy has shown intramembranous, endothelial, and subepithelial electron-dense deposits. Immunofluorescence studies demonstrate monoclonal immunoglobulin deposits in the glomeruli; specific antisera have shown them to be the circulating M component. Although this renal involvement resembles immune complex nephritis, elution studies have failed to reveal a specific antigen. There are two possible explanations for the presence of M component in the glomerulus: (a) passive glomerular adsorption takes place and (b) the glomerular lesions result from circulating immune complexes and/or cryoglobulins. A distinct choice between these two possibilities cannot be made with the information available at present.

Selected Readings

Buxbaum JN, Chuba JV, Hellman GC, et al. Monoclonal immunoglobulin deposition disease: light chain and heavy chain deposition diseases and their relation to light chain amyloidosis. *Ann Intern Med* 1990;112:455–464.

Excellent description of biopsy-proven monoclonal light chain–related glomerular lesions, including analysis of glomerular lesions related to light- and heavy-chain deposition.

Ganeval D, Rabian C, Guérin V, et al. Treatment of multiple myeloma with renal involvement. *Adv Nephrol* 1992; 21:347–370.

Excellent summary of 80 patients with multiple myeloma treated at the Necker Hospital. Focuses on renal failure in myeloma and the response to treatment.

Henick K, Vescio RA, Berenson JR. Recent advances in the treatment of multiple myeloma. *Curr Opin Hematol* 1998;5:254–258.

A recent review of available therapies.

Kyle RA. "Benign" monoclonal gammopathy: after 20 and 35 years of followup. *Mayo Clin Proc* 1993;68:26–36.

A classic article dealing with the renal complications in multiple myeloma. Special emphasis is placed on pathophysiologic features of myeloma cast nephropathy.

Kyle RA, Greipp PR. Amyloidosis (AL): clinical and laboratory features of 229 cases. *Mayo Clin Proc* 1983;58:665–683.

Describes the Mayo Clinic experience with primary amyloidosis, including clinical manifestations, treatment, and survival.

Malpas JS, Bergsagel DE, Kyle RA, eds. *Myeloma: biology and management.* Oxford: Oxford Medical Publications, 1995.

A compendium of excellent chapters on the biology and complications of myeloma, including kidney disease, hypercalcemia, and amyloidosis.

Sanders PW, Booker BB, Bishop JB, et al. Mechanisms of intranephronal proteinaceous cast formation by low molecular weight proteins. *J Clin Invest* 1990;85:570–576.

Demonstration that accumulation of tubulotoxic light chains in the proximal tubule produce cellular injury or form tubule lumen casts when light chains coprecipitate in vitro with Tamm-Horsfall glycoprotein, a protein made by cells of the thick ascending limb of Henle's loop.

Sanders PW, Herrera GA, Kirk KA, et al. Spectrum of glomerular and tubulointerstitial renal lesions associated with monotypical immunoglobulin light chain deposition. *Lab Invest* 1991;64:527–537.

Comprehensive description of the extensive renal manifestations associated with deposition of monoclonal immunoglobulin light chains.

Sanders PW, Martinez-Maldonado M. Paraproteinemic disorders. In: Massry GS, Glassock RA, eds. *Textbook of nephrology.* Baltimore: Williams & Wilkins, 1995.

Summarizes the effects of serum and urine protein abnormalities in multiple myeloma and correlates these with the changes in renal function and renal histology.

Tsujimura H, Nagamura F, Iseki T, et al. Significance of parathyroid-related protein as a factors stimulating bone resorption and causing hypercalcemia in myeloma. *Am J Hematol* 1998;59:168–170.

A study demonstrating that PTHrP may be a cause of hypercalcemia in myeloma.

PART 13
Sarcoidosis

Richard J. Glassock

Sarcoidosis is a disseminated noncaseating granulomatous disease of unknown cause. The granulomas consist of epithelioid and multinucleated giant cells surrounded by lymphocytes (predominantly CD8+) and macrophages. The organs most commonly affected include the lungs, skin, liver, eyes, nerves, heart, lymph nodes, parotid glands, joints, bone, and kidneys. Disordered renal structure or function occurs commonly in association with sarcoidosis and may be the result of direct granulomatous involvement of the tubulointerstitial regions of the kidney, the development of a glomerulopathy, longstanding hypercalcemia, or hypercalciuria with nephrocalcinosis or secondary to hyperglobulinemia.

RENAL MANIFESTATIONS

Granulomatous Disease of the Tubulointerstitial Region

Widespread involvement of the renal parenchyma by noncaseating granulomata occasionally may produce renal failure. The urinary sediment changes are nonspecific, but sterile pyuria is common. Proteinuria is most often mild and of a "tubular" character. Concentrating and acidifying capacity may be markedly diminished. The kidneys may be enlarged or of normal size. Gallium scans often show a generalized but irregular increase in uptake. Technetium-DMSA (dimercaptosuccinic acid) scans reveal irregular isotope uptake.

Renal biopsies demonstrate typical noncaseating epithelioid granulomata that do not contain acid-fast organisms, as demonstrated by special stains. Giant cells are present, but necrotizing vasculitis is absent. Similar lesions have been described in cases of diphenylhydantoin or allopurinol hypersensitivity. The lesion is responsive to glucocorticoid therapy, although a prolonged course may be required, and chronic fibrosing lesions may ultimately develop.

Nephrocalcinosis and/or Nephrolithiasis

Acquired disorders of calcium metabolism are among the most common abnormalities observed in sarcoidosis. These disorders may lead to hypercalcemia, hypercalciuria, nephrocalcinosis, nephrolithiasis, obstructive uropathy, urinary tract infection, and chronic progressive renal failure. The fundamental defect appears to be either increased sensitivity to vitamin D by its target organs or enhanced synthesis of 1,25-dihydroxyvitamin D [1,25$(OH)_2$D] by the sarcoid granulomata. Evidence in support of the latter includes elevated blood levels of 1,25$(OH)_2$D in sarcoid patients and even in an anephric patient with sarcoidosis. It is worthy of note that other granulomatous diseases, such as tuberculosis and berylliosis, have also been associated with hypercalcemia and/or hypercalciuria. Consequent to the elevated levels of 1,25$(OH)_2$D, enhanced gastrointestinal absorption of calcium occurs, leading to suppression of endogenous parathyroid hormone production (even in the face of mild to moderate impairment of the glomerular filtration rate) and to hypercalciuria. Because there seems to be an increase in the prevalence of parathyroid adenoma in sarcoidosis, an elevated serum parathyroid hormone level in a patient with sarcoidosis and hypercalcemia should suggest the possibility of an underlying parathyroid adenoma. The hypercalcemia and hypercalciuria of sarcoidosis are extraordinarily sensitive to the suppressive effects of oral glucocorticoids in modest dosage (as little as 10 mg of prednisone per day). These doses of glucocorticoid will not treat hypercalcemia in a patient with parathyroid adenoma. Excessive exposure to sunlight or ultraviolet irradiation may promote 25(OH)D synthesis and aggravate the hypercalcemia.

When severe hypercalcemia develops (serum calcium greater than 14 mg/dl), impairment of the glomerular filtration rate may occur via a direct effect on the contractile proteins of the mesangium. Polyuria may also result from marked impairment of concentrating ability. Mild hypercalcemia and hypercalciuria predispose to the development of nephrocalcinosis, which in turn may lead to chronic interstitial nephritis, urinary tract infection, and eventually, chronic renal failure. The effects of acute or chronic hypercalcemia on renal function and structure are discussed in detail in Chapter 17, Part 3. Early recognition and treatment of disorders of calcium metabolism in patients with sarcoidosis can, by and large, prevent these complications.

Hyperglobulinemia and Impaired Acidification

Many patients with sarcoidosis develop severe polyclonal gammopathy with marked hyperglobulinemia. On occasion, and for poorly understood reasons, the hyperglobulinemia may be associated with a form of distal renal tubular acidosis in which the maximal acidification of urine is impaired. Whether this abnormality is the direct result of increased globulin levels or secondary to tubulointerstitial disease is unknown. Impaired acidification of urine and reduced citrate excretion may also predispose to calcium phosphate or calcium oxalate crystallization and to nephrolithiasis.

Sarcoid Glomerulopathy

The association of glomerulonephritis and sarcoidosis is reasonably well established but is relatively uncommon. The clinical manifestations of glomerular involvement in sarcoidosis are varied but principally are those of nephrotic syndrome. The serum levels of C3 component of complement are usually normal or increased. The underlying glomerular lesions responsible for the clinical syndrome are varied. Membranous glomerulopathy, diffuse endocapillary proliferative glomerulonephritis, focal and segmental glomerulosclerosis, minimal-change disease, amyloidosis, and crescentic glomerulonephritis all have been observed. There are no morphologic features that distinguish the sarcoid form of glomerulopathy from the primary forms of glomerular disease. Immunofluorescent observations have usually revealed extensive capillary wall or mesangial glomerular deposits of IgG, IgM, and C3. Electron microscopy has most often revealed electron-dense deposits in the mesangium or capillary walls. These findings suggest an immune complex–mediated lesion, although the antigen and antibody systems involved are unknown. Patients with sarcoidosis often have evidence of a hyperactive humoral immune system (hyperglobulinemia, cryoglobulinemia, increased antiglobulins, various autoantibodies, and circulating immune complexes) while at the same time they have evidence of defective T-cell immunity (anergy to common microbial antigens, depressed response to phytohemagglutinin, abnormal mixed lymphocyte reactivity, and T-lymphocytopenia). The role of these immunologic abnormalities in the production of renal disease, specifically glomerulopathy, is poorly understood.

EXTRARENAL MANIFESTATIONS

The extrarenal manifestations of sarcoidosis are protean in nature. Pulmonary involvement may take the form of diffuse interstitial infiltrates, pulmonary fibrosis with the development of cysts, bullae, and airway obstruction resembling pulmonary emphysema. Such patients most frequently demonstrate a reduction in total lung capacity with only a slight increase in residual volume. Early disease may be associated only with a reduction in diffusion capacity. The forced expiratory volume in 1 second is decreased relative to the functional vital capacity. Severe lung involvement may be associated with hypoxemia. Gallium scanning of the lungs is often diffusely positive. Enlargement of the hilar lymph nodes may be especially prominent and is useful in differentiating sarcoidosis from other forms of diffuse interstitial lung disease. Rarely, periaortic lymph node enlargement has produced obstructive nephropathy and renal artery compression with hypertension.

Uveitis, parotid enlargement, fever, and lymphadenopathy are commonly present. Iridocyclitis and chorioretinitis are common eye findings. Skin involvement may consist of the development of firm papulonodular lesions representing the cutaneous development of typical noncaseating granulomata. Erythema nodosum may be the presenting feature in some patients (Lofgren's syndrome), especially in those with isolated hilar adenopathy. Lupus pernio represents a violaceous discoloration and thickening of the skin of the ear, nose, and cheek and may also be a cutaneous manifestation.

Hepatic involvement may produce liver enlargement and abnormalities in liver function tests, chiefly rising serum levels of alkaline phosphatase. Parenchymal cell injury with marked jaundice or a rise in serum levels of glutamic-oxaloacetate transaminase is unusual. Splenomegaly and generalized lymphadenopathy may develop. Pituitary and/or hypothalamic involvement may lead to diabetes insipidus or other deficiency syndromes. Involvement of the cardiac conduction system may lead to heart block and arrhythmias. Involvement of the salivary, lacrimal, and parotid glands may cause marked enlargement of these organs. Cranial nerve palsies, especially of the facial nerves, may be the presenting feature. Osseous involvement is particularly evident in the distal phalanges, with osteolytic lesions representing localized granulomatous involvement of bone. An acute multiarticular arthritis may also be a presenting feature. Hypercalcemia and disorders of calcium metabolism are discussed earlier in this chapter. Hyperglobulinemia indicative of polyclonal B-cell activation is very common and, if severe, could be partially responsible for elevation of total serum calcium. Anergy to common microbial antigens and defective delayed hypersensitivity to chemical agents such as dinitrochlorobenzene are almost always present during active disease. Interestingly, amyloidosis almost never occurs as a consequence of this disease, even after many years of activity.

DIAGNOSIS AND DIFFERENTIAL DIAGNOSIS

Sarcoidosis is more common in African-Americans and individuals of Swedish, German, or Danish descent. Approximately two-thirds of patients are younger than 40 years of age at the time of diagnosis. Females are slightly more affected than males. There is no evidence of linkage to the human leukocyte antigen (HLA) system.

In typical cases seen clinically with pulmonary lesions, hilar adenopathy, uveal or parotid involvement accompanied by hyperglobulinemia, anergy, and hypercalcemia or hypercalciuria, the diagnosis is not difficult. In atypical cases seen clinically with fever, arthritis, renal failure, hepatic disease or adenopathy, biopsy of suspicious skin lesions, liver, lymph nodes, or kidney may be indicated. Unfortunately, the finding of noncaseating granulomata in these tissues is not specific for sarcoidosis; these lesions are also found in berylliosis, Wegener's granulomatosis, hypersensitivity disease (especially diphenylhydantoin or allopurinol), and other chronic inflammatory disorders. The Kveim test—in which sterile extract of splenic or lymph node tissue from a patient with known sarcoidosis is injected intradermally, followed to 6 weeks later by biopsy of the area searching for noncaseating granuloma—is diagnostic of the disease but seldom performed because of the limited availability of well-standardized test material. Approximately 60% to 85% of patient with active sarcoidosis have a positive Kveim test. Serum levels of angiotensin-converting enzyme are often greatly elevated in active sarcoidosis, but false-positive test results do occur, and the test is mainly of value as a confirmatory tool. Marked elevation of angiotensin-converting enzyme activity also occurs in patients with leprosy and Gaucher's disease. Gallium scanning of the lungs or kidneys must be useful in assessing the extent and/or activity of visceral involvement.

The differential diagnosis includes disseminated tuberculosis, human immunodeficiency virus (HIV), other infectious granulomatous diseases, lymphoma Wegener's granulomatosis, drug hypersensitivity, berylliosis, and systemic lupus erythematosus. Cases with prominent hypercalcemia or hypercalciuria may be confused with primary hyperparathyroidism, chronic vitamin D intoxication, milk-alkali syndrome, idiopathic hypercalciuria, or primary renal tubular acidosis.

COURSE AND THERAPY

The therapy of sarcoidosis is largely predicated on the site and severity of organ involvements. Severe uveitis, marked pulmonary involvement, severe cardiac or central nervous system involvement, hypercalcemia, hyperciuria, and renal failure secondary to renal parenchymal granulomatous disease are indications for an aggressive approach to treatment. Mild pulmonary disease, isolated hilar adenopathy, cutaneous involvement, or mild hepatic disease need not necessarily be treated unless one or more of the severe organ involvements listed previously supervene. Excessive exposure to sunlight might aggravate hypercalcemia or hypercalciuria and is to be avoided. The disorder may wax and wane in its activity over many years. Chloroquine seems to be effective for the treatment of clinically active skin lesions and may diminish the severity of polyarthritis. Nonsteroidal antiinflammatory agents may at times result in dramatic symptomatic relief. Treatment with oral glucocorticoids at modest dosages (10 to 20 mg/day) is very effective in treating hypercalcemia. If hypercalcemia persists despite therapy with glucocorticoids, other causes of hypercalcemia should be considered. The use of thiazide diuretics should be avoided because they may induce hypercalcemia. High dosages of glucocorticoids are required for the management of proven renal parenchymal granulomatous involvement such as interstitial nephritis or glomerulonephritis.

The aim of therapy is to prevent irreversible complications such as pulmonary fibrosis, blindness, renal failure, and renal calculi without exposing the patient to the potential hazards of longstanding glucocorticoid therapy. Thus maintenance of patients with sarcoidosis on the lowest dosage of glucocorticoids consistent with the desired effect is a reasonable goal. More aggressive therapy, including the use of immunosuppressive agents, may be indicated in those cases with very serious life-threatening disease such as crescentic glomerulonephritis.

Selected Readings

Barbour GL, Coburn JW, Slatopolsky E, et al. Hypercalcemia in an anephric patient with sarcoidosis: evidence for extrarenal generation of 1,25-dihydroxyvitamin D. *N Engl J Med* 1982;305:440–443.

The demonstration of extrarenal production of 1,25-dihydroxyvitamin D in a patient with granulomatous disease.
Bell NH, Stern PH, Pantzer E, et al. Evidence that increased circulating 1,25-dihydroxyvitamin D is the probable cause for abnormal calcium metabolism in sarcoidosis. *J Clin Invest* 1979;64:218–225.
A study demonstrating abnormal vitamin D metabolism in sarcoidosis.
Hannedouche T, Grateaw G, Noel L, et al. Renal granulomatous sarcoidosis: a clinical and pathologic study. *Nephrol Dial Transplant* 1990;5:18–24.
An excellent clinical description.
James DG, ed. *Sarcoidosis and other granulomatous disorders.* New York: Marcel Dekker, 1994.
A comprehensive treatise on sarcoidosis.
McCoy RC, Tisher CC. Glomerulonephritis associated with sarcoidosis. *Am J Pathol* 1972;68:339–353.
A well-written and complete description of glomerular disease in sarcoidosis.
McCurley T, Salter J, Glich X. Renal insufficiency in sarcoidosis. A clinical and pathological study. *Arch Path Lab Med* 1990;114:488–492.
A good review of cases illustrating the effects of sarcoidosis on renal function.

PART 14
Cutaneous Diseases

Richard J. Glassock

Abnormalities of the integument may occur in connection with renal diseases in one of two clinical circumstances. First, the cutaneous lesions occur as a part of multisystem, heredofamilial, or infectious diseases, or as a component of adverse reactions to drugs. Cutaneous involvement may be an integral part of a syndrome in which the renal lesion is also a dominant feature (Table 42.34).

TABLE 42.34. Cutaneous Manifestations of Multisystem, Heredofamilial, or Infectious Disorders Associated with Renal Diseases

Disorder	Principal Cutaneous Manifestations
Multisystem disease	
Henoch-Schönlein purpura	Palpable purpura (leukocytoclastic angiitis)
Polyangiitis	Palpable purpura; ischemic necrosis, urticaria
Behçet's disease	Mucosal ulcers
Rheumatoid arthritis	Subcutaneous nodules, ischemic necrosis
Rheumatic fever	Erythema marginatum
Scleroderma	Dermal thickening, Raynaud's phenomenon; telangiectasia
Mixed connective tissue disease	Dermal thickening, Raynaud's phenomenon
Systemic lupus erythematosus	Highly variable; macular, maculopapular, purpuric, bullous, "butterfly" malar rashes; atrophic lesions, alopecia, and photosensitivity are common; mucosal ulcers
Cryoglobulinemia	Purpura, skin necrosis
Amyloidosis	Papules or nodules, purpura with mild trauma
Sarcoidosis	Lupus pernio, papular or plaque sarcoid, erythema nodosum
Gout	Tophi
Diabetes mellitus	Necrobiosis lipoidica, eruptive xanthoma
Thrombotic thrombocytopenic purpura	Purpura
Sjögren's syndrome	Palpable purpura
Relapsing polychondritis[a]	Saddle nose, tracheal collapse, thickened ear cartilage
Mycosis fungoides (cutaneous lymphoma)	Skin infiltration, skin erythema
Kimura's disease	Subcutaneous nodules
Heredofamilial diseases	
Fabry's disease	Angiokeratomas of scrotum, trunks, and buttocks, anhydrosis
Nail-patella syndrome	Onychodysplasia
Cystinosis	Hypopigmentation
Partial lipodystrophy	Acanthosis nigricans
Tuberous sclerosis	Adenoma sebaceum
Alport's syndrome	Ichthyosis, eczematoid dermatitis
Sickle cell disease	Ischemic ulcer
Neurofibromatosis (pheochromocytoma)	Café-au-lait, cutaneous fibromata
Infectious diseases	
Poststreptococcal glomerulonephritis	Impetigo, scabies, erysipelas, purpura
Infective endocarditis	Osler's nodes, Janeway lesions, splinter hemorrhages, petechiae, palpable purpura
Viral diseases (measles, varicella)	Maculopapular rash
Hepatitis B	Jaundice, maculopapular rash
Staphylococcal bacteremia	Skin abscesses, epidermal necrolysis, diffuse erythema
Leprosy	Dermal thickening, hypoalgesia, autoamputation, erythema nodosum
E. coli	Hemolytic uremic syndrome (jaundice and purpura)
Secondary syphilis	Maculopapular rash
Human immunodeficiency virus	Kaposi's sarcoma
Drug-related diseases	
Acute hypersensitivity interstitial nephritis (methicillin)	Maculopapular rash
Halogenated hydrocarbons	Jaundice
Paracetamol poisoning	Jaundice
Mercury poisoning	Acrodynia, dyshidrosis
Organic gold therapy	Maculopapular rash
Penicillamine therapy	Maculopapular rash

[a] Relapsing polychondritis is a rare inflammatory disorder principally affecting the cartilaginous structures of the ears, nose, and trachea. Destruction of cartilage may lead to deformities of the nose, thickening of the ears, and tracheal collapse. Conjunctivitis, aortic aneurysms, and deafness may also be seen. Patients with concomitant crescentic glomerulonephritis have been described.

TABLE 42.35. Cutaneous Disorders with Renal Involvement

Psoriasis
Erythema multiforme
Toxic epidermal necrolysis
Atopic dermatitis
Gardner-Diamond syndrome
Mycosis fungoides
Kimura's disease
Behçet's disease

These disorders are discussed in detail in various chapters of this book. Second, the skin lesions are the primary and dominant clinical feature, and the signs of the renal involvement are often, but not necessarily, minor or are found only incidentally (Table 42.35). These disorders are discussed in the following sections.

PSORIASIS

Psoriasis is a chronic skin condition of unknown cause that is characterized by an enormous increase in the rate of turnover of epidermal cells. This process leads to the development of plaques covered with silvery scales, mostly involving the scalp, elbows, and knees. On occasion, a more generalized lesion may occur. In some patients, the lesion of psoriasis may coexist with an atypical form of rheumatoid arthritis (psoriatic arthritis) or ankylosing spondylitis.

In severe disease, uric acid production is increased, and both serum uric acid concentration and uric acid excretion may rise, predisposing the patient to gout or nephrolithiasis.

Renal disease is uncommon, but when arthritis or spondylitis is severe, it may be associated with amyloidosis. Rarely, focal glomerulosclerosis and IgA nephropathy have been observed. It is not known whether this is a chance association or a part of the clinical spectrum of psoriasis.

ERYTHEMA MULTIFORME

Erythema multiforme is a disorder in which uncommon self-limited eruptions occur on the skin and mucous membranes. The typical lesion appears in localized areas and resembles a target or iris. More severe disease may involve wide areas of the skin and oral and vaginal mucous membranes (Stevens-Johnson syndrome). The disorder may follow a wide variety of bacterial, viral, fungal, or protozoal infections; may develop as cutaneous manifestations of malignancy or collagen-vascular disease (systemic lupus erythematosus); may appear consequent to an allergic reaction to a drug (sulfonamides); or may be idiopathic. Skin biopsy reveals lymphocytic vasculitis with IgG, IgM, and C3 deposits in the dermal vessels.

Renal involvement is uncommon when the lesion occurs in the absence of an underlying infection or collagen-vascular disease. When present, the renal lesion is most often mild and manifested by hematuria and mild proteinuria. On rare occasions, a proliferative glomerulonephritis has been observed. Acute renal failure secondary to acute tubular necrosis has been described in Stevens-Johnson syndrome.

TOXIC EPIDERMAL NECROLYSIS

Toxic epidermal necrolysis (scalded skin syndrome, Lyell's disease) is uncommon and characterized by widespread erythema and detachment of the epidermis. This process leads to the scalded skin appearance typical of the disorder. In many instances, it resembles severe cases of erythema multiforme. The disease may occur secondary to bacterial or viral infection, drug allergy, or underlying neoplastic disease. Staphylococcal infection may be associated with toxic shock syndrome, which in turn may produce diffuse erythema, bullae, and acute renal failure.

Renal involvement is found in about 15% of patients. It is usually mild, manifested by only hematuria or proteinuria. On occasion, nephrotic syndrome and/or renal failure have been observed secondary to membranous or proliferative glomerulonephritis.

ATOPIC DERMATITIS

Atopic dermatitis is a chronic, intensely pruritic condition that often occurs in association with a history of allergic rhinitis, hay fever, or asthma. The lesion is usually found in flexor creases of the arms and legs but may become generalized. There may be a hereditary background. Papules and lichenification are often seen.

The renal lesion most often associated with atopic dermatitis is minimal-change disease with steroid-sensitive nephrotic syndrome. Such patients have a higher prevalence of HLA-B12. Allergy to milk proteins may be the underlying cause in some patients. Both the dermatitis and the nephrotic syndrome may resolve on the introduction of a dairy food–free diet.

GARDNER-DIAMOND SYNDROME

Gardner-Diamond syndrome is a rare disorder in which recurrent crops of painful pruritic lesions appear. The affected patients are usually young women, often under psychologic stress. Some patients have been observed to have positive skin tests to autologous erythrocytes, and the disorder is thought to be due to autoerythrocyte sensitization. Circulating immune complexes have been found, and in one patient, membranous nephropathy with glomerular deposition of erythrocyte antigen–antibody complexes was documented.

MYCOSIS FUNGOIDES

Mycosis fungoides is a neoplastic process with cutaneous infiltration by malignant T lymphocytes. It is associated with generalized erythema and firm papules and nodules. IgA nephropathy or minimal-change disease may be found to coexist in some patients.

KIMURA'S DISEASE (ANGIOLYMPHOID HYPERPLASIA WITH EOSINOPHILIA)

Angiolymphoid hyperplasia is a rare condition associated with subcutaneous nodules, usually around the head and neck, and blood eosinophilia. Most patients are Asian males usually between the ages of 20 and 40. The subcutaneous lesions reveal lymphoid hyperplasia, angioid proliferation, and tissue eosinophilia. Proteinuria and nephrotic syndrome due to a variety of renal lesions have also been found, including minimal-change disease, membranous glomerulonephritis, mesangial proliferative glomerulonephritis, and focal segmental glomerulosclerosis.

BEHÇET'S DISEASE

Behçet's disease is a multisystem disorder predominantly associated with painful mucocutaneous ulcerations of mouth, gastrointestinal tract, and genital areas. Panuveitis, retinal vasculitis, transient neurologic involvement (resembling strokes or meningoencephalitis) erythema nodosum, seronegative arthritis, venous and arterial occlusive disease, and purpura are also seen. Renal disease, principally proliferative and/or crescentic glomerulonephritis, may occasionally arise.

Selected Readings

Gilchrest B, Rowe J. Cutaneous aspect of renal disease. In: Fitzpatrick TB, Eisen AZ, Wolff K, et al, eds. *Dermatology in general medicine,* 3rd ed. New York: McGraw-Hill, 1987:1977–1980.

A review of the clinical manifestations of cutaneous diseases that may be associated with renal diseases.

James GD. Behçet's disease. In: Fitzpatrick TB, Eisen AZ, Wolff K, et al, eds. *Dermatology in general medicine,* 3rd ed. New York McGraw-Hill, 1987:1239–1244.

An excellent review of Behçet's disease.

Krumlovsky FA, Del Greco F, Herdson PB, et al. Renal disease associated with toxic epidermal necrolysis (Lyell's disease). *Am J Med* 1974;57:817–824.

A case report and a review of the literature on toxic epidermal necrolysis associated with renal disease.

Yamada A. Membranous glomerulonephritis associated with eosinophilic lymphofolliculosis of the skin (Kimura's disease). A report of a case and review of the literature. *Clin Nephrol* 1982;18:211–215.

An excellent review article on a rare disease.

CHAPTER 43

Renal Involvement in Heredofamilial and Congenital Disease

PART 1
Kidney in Sickle Cell Hemoglobinopathy

Antonio Guasch

The sickle hemoglobinopathies are caused by a mutation in a single base pair of DNA encoding the β-globin molecule, which results in the substitution of valine for glutamic acid at the sixth position of the hemoglobin β chain and the formation of an abnormal hemoglobin tetramer, hemoglobin S ($\alpha_2\beta^s_2$). Normal individuals inherit two β-globin genes and four α-globin genes, so, following classic mendelian genetics, patients may be heterozygous for hemoglobin S (AS genotype, sickle cell trait) or homozygous (Hb SS, sickle cell disease). Other hemoglobin variants (e.g., hemoglobin C, E) and α- and β-thalassemia may coexist with hemoglobin S, producing double heterozygous states (hemoglobin SC disease, Sβ+ thalassemia, Sβo thalassemia, or Hb SS with α-thalassemia). Sickle hemoglobinopathies affect mostly individuals of African, Asian, or Mediterranean origin, where the sickle cell mutation is thought to confer survival advantage against malaria, a disease endemic in those geographical areas. In the United States, about 8% of African-Americans are heterozygous for Hb S (sickle cell trait), and sickle cell disease occurs in about 1 in 500 African-American newborns.

The β-globin gene cluster consists of a long segment of DNA containing the β-globin and other globin genes. There are genetic polymorphisms in the β-globin gene cluster that can be defined as haplotypes, using site-specific restriction endonuclease DNA cleavage. In Africa and India, specific haplotypes are associated with ethnic groups from different geographic areas (probably a reflection of the multiplicity of times the sickle mutation originated) and define an individual's origin from Benin, Central African Republic, Senegal, Saudi Arabia, Cameroon, or India. Patients with the Central African Republic or Benin haplotype have more severe clinical manifestations, whereas individuals with the Senegal haplotype have a less protracted course. Other genetic or phenotypic factors like the coexistence of α-thalassemia and/or the persistence of higher levels of fetal hemoglobin are associated with a more benign prognosis.

The pathologic manifestations of sickle cell anemia (SCA) arise from the intracellular polymerization of hemoglobin S and the formation of sickle red blood cells. This phenomenon is enhanced by increased intracellular Hb S concentration (intracellular dehydration), acidosis, increased erythrocyte 2,3-biphosphoglycerate or a low oxygen tension (hypoxia). Polymerized Hb S distorts the erythrocyte membrane, promoting calcium entry into the cell and stimulation of the Ca^{2+}-activated K^+ channel. This leads to K^+ efflux, water loss, and intracellular dehydration, and favors further sickling. Acidosis promotes sickling by activating the erythrocyte potassium–chloride cotransport, leading to K^+ and Cl^- efflux, water loss, and erythrocyte dehydration.

The clinical manifestations of SCA result from chronic hemolysis and the development of vasoocclusive events. Sickle erythrocytes are much less deformable and have a much shorter life span than normal erythrocytes, resulting in chronic hemolysis. Vasoocclusive events are a very dynamic process involving complex interactions between SS erythrocytes and vascular endothelial cells, and not the result of simple mechanical obstruction. Polymerization of SS hemoglobin alone is not enough to cause vasoocclusive events as emphasized by kinetic measurements of the rate of hemoglobin polymerization that exceeds the microcirculation transit time. Oxygenated SS erythrocytes have increased stickiness to the vascular endothelium under both static and dynamic flow conditions, and this enhanced adhesiveness correlates with disease severity. This process is mediated by the interaction between erythrocyte membrane molecules (sulfated glycoglycans, CD36, and $\alpha_4\beta_1$ integrin) and endothelial membrane receptors (VCAM1, CD36, and $\alpha_v\beta_3$ integrin). Other molecules, such as thrombospondin, high-molecular-weight von Willebrand factor, and other products of platelet activation, could promote erythrocyte adhesion to endothelial cells by bridging together erythrocyte and endothelial membrane receptors. A similar effect in facilitating adhesion could result from the release of proinflammatory cytokines [interleukin (IL-1), interferon (IFN), tumor necrosis factor-α (TNFα)], which upregulate endothelial VCAM1 expression and favor erythrocyte adhesion. Once initial adhesion of SS

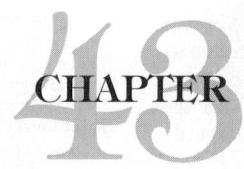

TABLE 43.1. Clinical Abnormalities in Patients with Sickle Cell Anemia

Glomerular
Sickle cell glomerulopathy
Albuminuria
Renal insufficiency
Postinfectious glomerulonephritis
Membranoproliferative glomerulonephritis
Acute renal failure
Tubulointerstitial
Concentrating defects
Hematuria
Renal papillary necrosis
Incomplete renal tubular acidosis
Distal renal tubular acidosis
Hyperkalemia
Hyperuricemia
Hyperphosphatemia
Malignancy
? Medullary renal cell carcinoma

erythrocytes to the endothelium has occurred, other SS erythrocytes could adhere via cell–cell interaction, reduce vascular lumen, and promote the entrapment of poorly deformable sickle erythrocytes. In summary, a dynamic microvascular process occurs in SCA, mediated in part by an intrinsic enhanced stickiness of the erythrocyte to the endothelial cell, which, in turn, is modulated by inflammatory conditions and prothrombotic mediators. This favors the entrapment of other erythrocytes, slows down microvascular flow, promotes sickling, and ultimately results in vascular occlusion.

BLOOD PRESSURE ABNORMALITIES

Patients with SCA have a hyperdynamic circulation, resulting from a decrease in systemic vascular resistance and a high cardiac output, probably the result of adaptations to a chronic anemic state. Systolic and diastolic blood pressure values in patients with SS disease are 5 to 15 mm Hg lower, on average, than age-, gender- and race-matched controls. In patients with SC disease, blood pressure levels tend to be lower than in healthy individuals but not as low as in SS individuals. Because of the lower systemic blood pressure levels in the SCA population, the definition of hypertension based on epidemiologic studies in nonanemic individuals may not apply to SCA patients. The National Cooperative Study of Sickle Cell Disease demonstrated a higher mortality, due mostly to vascular events, in both male and female SCA patients with systolic and diastolic blood pressure values above the 90th percentile of the blood pressure distribution for the SCA population. In patients with SS disease, this corresponds to systolic blood pressure values higher than 128 to 132 mm Hg and diastolic values higher than 80 to 84 mm Hg. Relative hypertension in SCA individuals should be properly identified and aggressively treated.

RENAL ABNORMALITIES

Renal abnormalities are common in patients with SCA, probably because of the highly vascular nature of the kidney. Table 43.1 lists the most common renal clinical findings in patients with SCA.

Renal Hemodynamics (Table 43.2)

Children with SCA have very high renal blood and plasma flows (hyperperfusion), increased glomerular filtration rate (GFR) (hyperfiltration), and a low filtration fraction. These abnormalities are not corrected by multiple transfusions to replace transiently Hb S by normal hemoglobin and correct the anemia, indicating that they are not related to adaptations to anemia. The elevated GFR decreases with age, so by the third decade, the GFR is similar to that of healthy adults; nevertheless, a relative hyperperfusion (consequence of renal vasodilation) persists and the filtration fraction remains lower than that in normal individuals. The mechanisms mediating renal vasodilation are not known, but involvement of vasodilatory prostaglandins and/or the nitric oxide system has been postulated.

Glomerular Damage in Sickle Cell Anemia

Two large series from the southeastern United States have emphasized that proteinuria is a very common finding in SCA and can be detected by urinary dipstick in 25% to 30% of adults. The proteinuria is of glomerular origin, as indicated by the presence of abnormally high albumin excretion rates (AER). In a series from our institution (Table 43.3), macroalbuminuria (AER greater than 300 mg/g creatinine) occurred in 27% of adult patients with SS disease, and microalbuminuria (AER between 30 and 300 mg/g creatinine) was present in 41% of them, with a combined prevalence of albuminuria of 68%. Only about one-third of adults with Hb SS disease have normoalbuminuria. As

TABLE 43.2. Glomerular Function in Patients with Sickle Cell Anemia

	SBP (mm Hg)	DBP (mm Hg)	Serum Creatinine (mg/dl)	GFR	RPF (ml/min/1.73m²)	FF	Renovascular Resistance (mm Hg) (ml/min/1.73)	Ultrafiltration Coefficient (ml/min). mmHg⁻¹ × 1.73mm²	AER (μg/min)
Healthy individuals	116 ± 3	75 ± 2	0.8 ± 0.1	98 ± 4	498 ± 26	0.20 ± 0.01	0.19 ± 0.01	16 ± 2	5 ± 1
SCA controls	118 ± 5	66 ± 5	0.7 ± 0.1	108 ± 7	699 ± 66[a]	0.16 ± 0.01[a]	0.13 ± 0.01[a]	12 ± 2	15 ± 4
SCA-CRF	125 ± 4	69 ± 4	1.6 ± 0.3[b]	41 ± 5[a,b]	356 ± 56[a,b]	0.13 ± 0.01[a,b]	0.37 ± 0.07[a,b]	4 ± 1[a,b]	973 ± 219[a,b]

[a] $P < .05$ versus healthy controls.
[b] $P < .05$ versus SCA controls.
Adapted from Guasch A, Cua M, You W, et al. Sickle cell anemia causes a distinct pattern of glomerular dysfunction. *Kidney Int* 1997;51:826–833.
AER, albumin excretion rate; DBP, diastolic blood pressure; FF, filtration fraction; SBP, systolic blood pressure; SCA, sickle cell anemia.

TABLE 43.3. Prevalence of Albuminuria in Adult Patients with Sickle Cell Anemia

	Hb SS Disease (n = 146)	Other Sickle Hemoglobinopathies (Hb SC, Sβ Thalassemia, n = 87)
Normoalbuminuria	32%	58%
Microalbuminuria	41%	36%
Macroalbuminuria	27%	6%

Normoalbuminuria: albumin excretion rate, AER <30 mg/g creatinine. Microalbuminuria: AER between 30–300 mg/g creatinine. Macroalbuminuria: AER >300 mg/g creatinine.

patients with SS live longer due to better care, renal insufficiency in SS patients could become a major clinical problem in this population. Glomerular damage is less common in patients with non-SS sickle hemoglobinopathies (Hb SC and Sβ thalassemia). In our series, macroalbuminuria, microalbuminuria, and normoalbuminuria was present in 6%, 36% and 58%, respectively, of adult patients with non-SS sickle hemoglobinopathies (Table 43.3).

Pathophysiology of Sickle Glomerulopathy

The pathogenesis of sickle glomerulopathy is not well understood (Fig. 43.1). In the early stages of the disease, there is glomerular hyperperfusion and hyperfiltration. Renal histology in patients with SCA but without clinical renal dysfunction is remarkable for glomerular hypertrophy and open, dilated glomerular capillary loops. Later, the GFR returns toward normal values, despite the persistence of a high renal blood flow. At this preclinical stage, physiologic studies using dextran sieving analysis have revealed an increased glomerular permeability to macromolecules, resulting from an increase in the glomerular pore size. This increased glomerular permeability and enhanced transglomerular protein trafficking does not result in clinical albuminuria, presumably because of increased proximal tubular protein reabsorption. Subsequently, some patients will develop clinical proteinuria, with enhanced excretion of albumin and other high-molecular-weight proteins such as IgG, the result of a glomerular size-selective defect. At this albuminuric stage, the GFR is still preserved, but a reduction in the glomerular ultrafiltration coefficient can already be demonstrated. A further reduction in the glomerular ultrafiltration coefficient results in the development of renal insufficiency. This is accompanied by worsening proteinuria. In summary, a glomerulopathy occurs in SCA that is manifested initially as albuminuria and progresses to clinical renal insufficiency and end-stage renal disease (ESRD).

The findings of early glomerular hyperfiltration and hyperperfusion with glomerular hypertrophy, followed by late proteinuria, renal insufficiency, and focal glomerulosclerosis (see Pathology), are suggestive of a glomerulopathy mediated by increased flows and enhanced intraglomerular pressure. This is also supported by the reduction in proteinuria in SCA patients with renal insufficiency when receiving angiotensin-converting enzyme (ACE) inhibitors. However, the early pattern of glomerular dysfunction with renal vasodilation and a generalized increased permeability to macromolecules is unlike that described in other hemodynamically mediated glomerulopathies. In experimental animals, acute isovolemic anemia does not result in intraglomerular hypertension, and the latter is unlikely to occur in the early stages of glomerular dysfunction in SCA. It is possible that the massive glomerular hypertrophy that occurs in SCA as described by Bhathena or that the increased transglomerular macromolecular trafficking as a consequence of increase glomerular permeability could result in late glomerulosclerosis. Alternatively, focal glomerulosclerosis could result from the interaction between the sickle erythrocyte and the glomerular vasculature. Once renal insufficiency occurs, common mechanisms to all glomerular diseases could operate to promote further glomerular injury (Fig. 43.1).

Prevalence of Renal Insufficiency

In a retrospective analysis of 725 SS and 209 SC patients in southern California, Powars and co-workers found a preva-

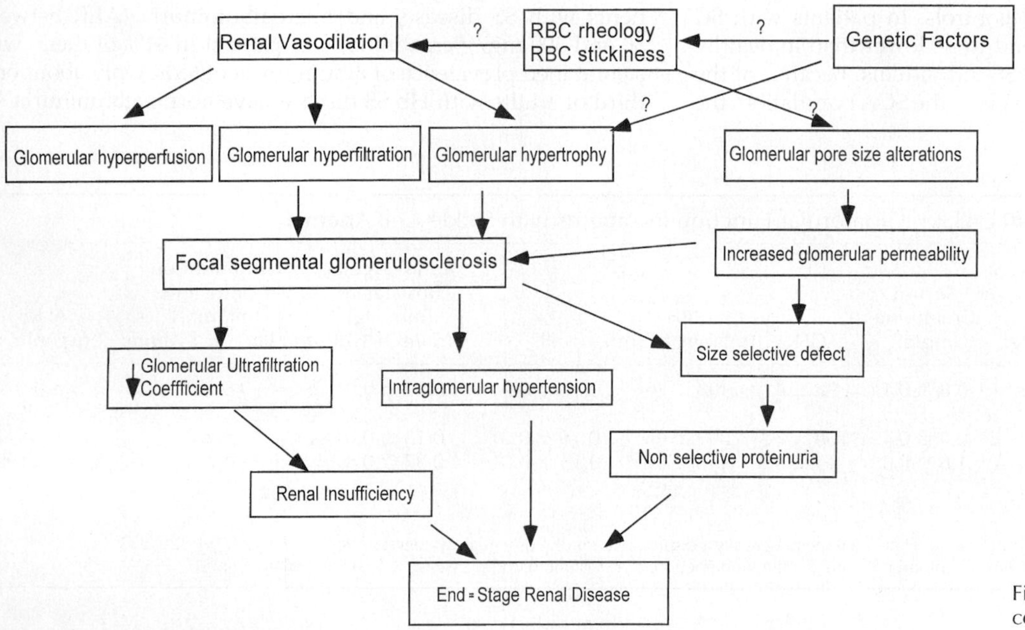

Figure 43.1. Pathogenesis of sickle cell glomerulopathy.

lence of renal insufficiency (defined as serum creatinine higher than 1.5 mg/dl) of 4.2% and 2.4% in SS and SC patients, respectively. The median age at presentation was 23 years in SS disease and 50 years in patients with SC disease. Clinical factors associated with renal insufficiency were ineffective erythropoiesis, hypertension, proteinuria, and hematuria. The relative low prevalence of renal insufficiency in Powars' study probably represents an underestimation of the true prevalence of renal insufficiency in SCA. Serum creatinine values in SCA patients are lower than those in healthy individuals, probably a reflection of lower muscle mass in SCA patients. At our institution, we found that only 41% of individuals with SCA who had an abnormally low GFR had elevated serum creatinine values (1.4 mg/dl or greater in males and 1.2 mg/dl or greater in females). Conversely 100% of those with elevated serum creatinine values also had abnormally low GFR. Renal insufficiency is a strong predictor of mortality in SCA patients. The life expectancy of SCA patients with renal insufficiency is 10 years lower than that of SCA patients without renal insufficiency. Moreover, the frequency of hospitalizations, episodes of acute chest pain syndrome, and other major organ failure is increased in SCA patients with renal insufficiency.

Genetic Influences on Sickle Glomerulopathy

Genetic studies have shown that the coinheritance of α-thalassemia and SCA (Hb SS) is associated with a lower prevalence of sickle glomerulopathy than in SCA patients with normal α-globin genes, indicating that the coinheritance of α-thalassemia confers renal protection. The mechanisms of renoprotection are not known, but are not related to differences in the degree of anemia or the severity of hemolysis between SCA patients with and without α-thalassemia. This provides further support to the hypothesis that the hemodynamic adaptations to a chronic anemic state are not enough for the development of sickle glomerulopathy. Individuals with α-thalassemia have a lower mean corpuscular hemoglobin concentration than non-thalassemic SCA individuals. Moreover, SS erythrocytes with α-thalassemia have a lower transmembrane Na^+-K^+ flux, indicating improved intracellular hydration, and are more deformable than nonthalassemic sickle erythrocytes. This suggests that intraerythrocyte factors are important in the development of sickle glomerulopathy. In the same study, there was no association between the geographic origin of the sickle cell mutation (β-globin haplotypes) and the development of sickle cell glomerulopathy.

Clinical Presentation of Glomerulopathy

Sickle cell glomerulopathy typically presents in early adulthood or in middle-aged adult patients, and it occurs more commonly in patients with Hb SS disease. Males and females are affected equally. The presentation is usually insidious, with proteinuria being discovered at the time of a routine urinalysis. Most patients present with subnephrotic-range proteinuria, typically 1 to 2 g of protein per day, and a minority may present with nephrotic syndrome. Urinalysis is typically bland. Urine protein electrophoresis, when performed, reveals nonselective proteinuria, indicating a glomerular origin. The presence of hematuria or red blood cell casts should alert the clinician to other forms of glomerulonephritis. Serum creatinine is typically normal in the early stages of the disease. As the disease progresses, renal insufficiency ensues, leading to ESRD. Blood pressure is usually not elevated, although it may be inappropriately high for the population. Because SCA patients have been exposed in their lifetime to multiple blood transfusions, infection-associated glomerulonephritis (hepatitis or HIV-associated) should be ruled out. Acute glomerulonephritis has also been described in association with parvovirus infection and aplastic crises.

Pathology of Glomerulopathy

In patients with nephrotic syndrome, two patterns of glomerular lesions have been described. In the mid-1970s, Pardo and coworkers reported on five patients with nephrotic syndrome resulting from an immune-complex proliferative glomerulonephritis resembling membranoproliferative glomerulonephritis. There was glomerular hypertrophy and mesangial cell proliferation and matrix expansion, along with glomerular capillary mesangial interposition, producing a double-contour of the peripheral capillary walls. Immunofluorescence revealed staining for IgG, IgM, C1q, C3, C4, and C2 in a granular, mesangial, and glomerular capillary wall pattern that corresponded to mesangial and subendothelial electron-dense deposits seen on electron microscopy. An additional report described 13 children with proteinuria (6 with nephrotic syndrome) and SCA. Eight had focal segmental glomerulosclerosis and five had mesangial proliferation. The prognosis was worse in children with focal glomerulosclerosis, with six of them developing ESRD or deterioration of renal function, as compared with only one patient with mesangial proliferation who developed progressive renal insufficiency.

Others have described the pathologic features in 10 adult patients with SCA (Hb SS) and proteinuria. The majority, 9 of 10 patients, had proteinuria between 1 to 2 g/24 hr, and only 1 patient had nephrotic syndrome. Histologically, there was glomerular hypertrophy and focal segmental glomerulosclerosis in 8 of 10 patients. In the other two patients, only global sclerosis could be identified. In the sclerosed glomeruli, there was adhesion to Bowman's capsule and focal hyalinosis. Immunofluorescence in the nonsclerosed glomeruli was either negative or revealed only trace mesangial amounts of IgM or C3. By electron microscopy, there was focal effacement of epithelial podocytes and no electron-dense deposits.

In summary, early reports emphasized the occurrence of mesangioproliferative glomerulonephritis, probably a reflection of undiagnosed infection-associated glomerulonephritis. More recently, the pathologic findings of sickle cell glomerulopathy are those of glomerular hypertrophy, mild mesangial proliferation (a feature seen mostly in younger children), and the occurrence of focal segmental glomerulosclerosis in older children and adults.

Treatment of Glomerulopathy

The findings of glomerular hypertrophy, proteinuria, and focal segmental glomerulosclerosis have prompted the use of angiotensin converting enzyme (ACE) inhibitors in proteinuric patients with sickle cell glomerulopathy. To date, only short-term studies have been reported. In one study enalapril was administered at 5 to 10 mg/day over a 2-week period in patients with mild to moderate renal insufficiency. Proteinuria was reduced in all patients, on average by 57% (range 23% to 79%), without lowering systemic blood pressure levels or decreasing GFR. Although no long-term studies have been reported, ACE inhibitors are a reasonable therapeutic choice in patients with sickle cell glomerulopathy. In patients with more advanced renal insufficiency, ACE inhibitors should be used cautiously because they could exacerbate the tendency to hyperkalemia.

End-Stage Renal Disease (ESRD)

Dialysis and/or transplantation can be offered to SCA patients who reach ESRD. Early reports indicated a dismal survival on dialysis, with a median survival of only 2 years. However, here is the clinical impression that survival on dialysis has improved in the last decade. Based on reports from the United States Renal Data System, most patients with ESRD and SCA are treated in the United States with center hemodialysis. Unfortunately, there is a paucity of information regarding the clinical course of the disease in the dialysis population. Studies comparing hemodialysis and peritoneal dialysis outcomes in SCA individuals with ESRD are also needed, because acute volume shifts, rapid changes in acid–base status, and so forth, could have a major impact on the clinical manifestations of the disease. Erythropoietin, which is routinely used in SCA patients with ESRD; it decreases transfusion dependency in SCA patients and may improve anemia. In contrast to other ESRD patients, SCA patients require significantly higher doses of erythropoietin.

Renal transplantation has also been performed successfully in SCA patients with ESRD. After renal transplantation, however, a higher incidence of vasoocclusive episodes has been reported in SCA, and sickle cell glomerulopathy can recur in the transplanted kidney. Moreover, antilymphocyte preparations could precipitate vasoocclusive crises and the acute chest pain syndrome and should be used with caution. For these reasons, there are differences among transplantation centers in their acceptance of SCA patients as transplant candidates. Agodoa and colleagues reviewed the outcome of renal transplantation in African-American patients with ESRD due to sickle glomerulopathy versus other causes of ESRD. The incidence of delayed graft function and 1-year renal allograft survival was similar in SCA versus non-SCA recipients (78% versus 77%, respectively). However, the 3-year cadaveric graft survival was lower in the SCA group (48% versus 60%, in SCA versus non-SCA, respectively) because of an increased risk of graft loss in SCA individuals. Despite a slightly worse outcome in transplanted SCA patients, there was a trend toward increased patient survival in SCA recipients versus SCA patients on a waiting list and being treated with dialysis. These findings may prompt a reevaluation of current transplant policies for SCA patients. However, even with a more open policy toward renal transplantation for SCA patients, difficulties in finding compatible organs for SCA patients will persist because of their highly immunized status and a relative lack of suitable living donors due to the familial occurrence of SCA.

Renal Medullary Defects

An inability to maximally concentrate the urine has been well documented in homozygous and heterozygous patients with SCA (Table 43.4). This concentrating defect is more pronounced in patients with Hb SS and Hb SC disease than in patients with sickle cell trait and worsens with age (Table 43.4). In individuals with sickle cell trait, maximal urinary concentration in older children and young adults is rarely above 800 mOsm/kg, and older individuals do not concentrate more than 450 mOsm/kg. In patients with SS disease, maximal urinary concentration is about 400 mOsm/Kg after the age of 10 years. Initially, in young children, the concentrating defect is of a functional nature, as indicated by the restoration of normal concentrating ability by multiple transfusions. However, in children older than 10 years of age and in adults, the concentrating defect cannot be reversed with transfusions, with the administration of vasopressin or indomethacin, or with the ingestion of high-protein diets, indicating permanent medullary damage. Microangiographic studies have revealed obliteration of vasa recta and near absence of vessels in the renal medulla and papillae as a consequence of vascular occlusion. Such alterations in the medullary circulation may disrupt the formation of urea and sodium gradients in the medullary interstitium, reduce medullary tonicity, and interfere with concentrating ability. In contrast to the concentrating defect, the ability to generate free water and dilute the urine is unimpaired in patients with SCA. The impairment in the concentrating ability is not of major clinical significance under normal conditions because the obligatory water losses of 1.5 to 2 L of urine per day can easily be maintained with normal fluid intake. However, in febrile states, excessive heat, and so forth, patients could easily become volume depleted and precipitate a vasoocclusive episode. SCA patients are advised to drink enough water to maintain urinary volumes of 2 to 3 L/day.

TABLE 43.4. Renal Hemodynamics and Concentrating Ability in Sickle Cell Hemoglobinopathies[a]

	Hb AA (n = 9)	Hb AS (n = 9)	Hb SS (n = 10)
Age (yr)	30 ± 4 (21-51)	33 ± 3 (23-53)	27 ± 3 (18-42)
Hematocrit (%)	39 ± 1	40 ± 1	27 ± 1[b]
Inulin clearance (C_{in}) (ml/min/1.73 m^2)	97 ± 5 (71-118)	95 ± 9 (62-136)	124 ± 11[c] (78-186)
Paraaminohippurate clearance (C_{PAH}) (ml/min/1.73 m^2)	440 ± 29 (301-575)	514 ± 59 (282-875)	837 ± 34[b,c] (495-1145)
Filtration fraction (C_{in}/C_{PAH} [%])	22 ± 1 (19-25)	19 ± 1[d] (14-22)	15 ± 1[d] (13-21)
U_{osm} max (mOsm/kg H_2O)	995 ± 56 (764-1260)	593 ± 35[e] (469-779)	407 ± 10[b] (400-493)

[a] Values are mean ± SE; ranges are in parentheses.
[b] $P<.025$ versus Hb AA and Hb AS.
[c] Three of 10 patients with Hb SS had supranormal C_{in} (>3 SD above the mean of controls); eight of 10 patients with Hb SS had supranormal C_{PAH}; all were 32 years old or younger.
[d] $P<.05$ versus Hb AA.
[e] $P<.001$ versus Hb AA.
Adapted from Oster JR, Lespier LE, Lee SM, et al. Renal acidification in sickle cell disease. *J Lab Clin Med* 1976;88:389–401.

ACIDIFICATION DEFECT

Under normal conditions, patients with SS disease have normal acid–base balance or a mild chronic respiratory alkalosis. A large number of patients, however, have an incomplete form of distal renal tubular acidosis and are unable to lower the urine pH to less than 5.3 when exposed to an acute acid load (normal response is less than 5.0). This is due to a reduction in titratable acid and not in ammonium excretion. Proximal bicarbonate reabsorption is normal. Patients with sickle cell trait have no acidification abnormalities.

HYPERKALEMIC HYPERCHLOREMIC METABOLIC ACIDOSIS

Six patients with SCA (three with SS disease, two with sickle cell trait, and one with Hb SC disease) with a hyperkalemic hyperchloremic form of metabolic acidosis and moderate renal insufficiency have been described. All patients had a decreased fractional potassium excretion. Some patients had a selective aldosterone deficiency (hyporeninemic hypoaldosteronism or type IV renal tubular acidosis [RTA]), whereas others had a voltage-dependent form of distal renal tubular acidosis with an inability to generate a normal transepithelial electrical gradient. Further discussion on distal renal tubular acidosis is found in Chapter 20.5.

Proximal Tubular Function

Proximal tubular transport processes are generally increased in sickle cell anemia. An increase in the maximal reabsorption of phosphate per GFR (TmP/GFR) has been demonstrated in patients with SCA and may account for the hyperphosphatemia observed in some patients. Similarly, proximal tubular sodium and β_2-microglobulin reabsorption are also increased. Some excretory functions are also increased. An enhanced secretion of uric acid has been observed and may partially mask the tendency to hyperuricemia in SCA patients, which results from an increased erythrocyte turnover and overproduction of uric acid. Despite the increased uric acid production, gout is uncommon in SCA.

Hematuria

Gross hematuria, sometimes accompanied by renal colic, is a relatively common manifestation of SCA and usually very disturbing for the patient. Hematuria may occur in both Hb SS and sickle cell trait and is more common in males than in females. The left kidney is affected four times more frequently than the right kidney and is bilateral in about 10% of cases. The pathogenesis is not completely understood but is thought to result from microinfarctions or severe stasis in peritubular capillaries associated with the obliterative vasculopathy. Pathologic examination of nephrectomy specimens reveals minimal gross pathologic alterations with only stasis in peritubular capillaries with extravasation of blood into the collecting tubules. Patients with SCA may have a higher incidence of renal cell carcinoma, and all first episodes of hematuria should be evaluated thoroughly.

In general, with the first episode of hematuria the patient should be admitted to the hospital to identify the cause and to institute intravenous hydration. Patients with mild episodes with a previous negative workup may be managed as outpatient, but periodic reevaluation may be needed, especially in the elderly, to rule out malignancies. Treatment includes vigorous hydration with hypotonic fluids, diuretics, urine alkalinization, and bed rest. In persistent cases, epsilon aminocaproic acid (EACA) may be administered at a dosage of 4 to 12 g/day in four divided doses after adequate diuresis has been initiated. Chronic relapsing hematuria can be treated with exchange transfusion, EACA, iron supplementation, and the avoidance of intense physical activities. Severe cases may need selective embolization, but nephrectomy is not indicated unless life-threatening hemorrhage is present, because it could recur in the contralateral kidney.

Renal Papillary Necrosis

Renal papillary necrosis is a relatively common occurrence in patients with SCA and results from localized ischemic necrosis of the medullary tip. In the largest series reported in 1984, renal papillary necrosis was present in 39% of patients with Hb SS disease, being asymptomatic in the majority of instances or presenting with microscopic hematuria or a urinary tract infection. Occasionally, it may present as a renal colic or obstruction due to the sloughing of the renal papillae. Diagnosis can be made with intravenous pyelography, or ultrasonography or computed tomography (CT) scan. Initial radiographic findings are irregular, fuzzy calyces. As the disease progresses, a sinus tract forms along the papillae, producing the radiographic "arc sign." In late stages, there is complete sequestration of the necrotic area or "ring sign," and "clubbing" of the papillae due to sloughing or reabsorption of the renal papillae. Ultrasonographically, there is increased echogenicity in the inner medulla and medullary tips as a consequence of fibrosis and calcification. Sloughed papillae may give the ultrasonographic appearance of a renal filling defect. Computed tomography scan is not as sensitive as ultrasound to detect renal papillary necrosis. In contrast to other forms of renal papillary necrosis, renal function is relatively preserved and the long-term prognosis is good. The treatment involves maintaining adequate hydration and aggressive treating superimposed urinary tract infections.

Malignancy

The overall incidence of cancer in the SCA population is comparable to that of the African-American population. A retrospective study suggests that there is an increased incidence of renal cell carcinoma of the medullary type in patients with SCA. In a series of 33 SCA patients with medullary carcinoma, the presentation was gross hematuria and abdominal pain, and less frequently, weight loss and flank pain. The right kidney was involved in 23 of the 33 patients, and because of the aggressive nature of the tumor, survival was only 15 weeks. Sickle erythrocytes were identified microscopically in all patients, but clinical information was limited. Nine patients had sickle cell trait and one had SC disease. The significance of these findings is unclear at this time, but until additional information is available, a careful urologic evaluation should be performed in SCA patients with hematuria and/or flank pain.

Selected Readings

Allon M, Lawson L, Eckman JR, et al. Effects of nonsteroidal antiinflammatory drugs on renal function in sickle cell anemia. *Kidney Int* 1988;34:500–506.

Glomerular function and tubular solute and water handling was studied before and after nonsteroidal antiinflammatory administration in SCA patients without renal insufficiency. Both drugs reduced GFR by about 15% in SCA individuals, but not in healthy controls. Nonsteroidal drug administration in SCA patients caused a higher increase in urinary osmolality and a decrease in the fractional sodium excretion in the medullary thick ascending limb of Henle's loop than in healthy controls, suggesting that prostaglandins mediate these effects. However, the overall renal effect of nonsteroidal drugs in SCA is antinatriuretic due to enhanced proximal tubular sodium reabsorption.

Batlle DC, Itsarayoungyuen K, Arruda JAL, et al. Hyperkalemic hyperchloremic metabolic acidosis in sickle cell hemoglobinopathies. *Am J Med* 1982;72: 188–192.

Six patients (three with Hb SS, one Hb SC, and two with sickle cell trait) with mild to moderate renal insufficiency and hyperkalemic hyperchloremic metabolic acidosis were reported. All patients had decreased ability to excrete potassium as compared with GFR-matched non-SCA individuals. Two patterns of impaired urinary acidification were observed. Four patients had distal renal tubular acidosis based on a urinary pH more than 5.5 despite systemic acidosis. Two other patients hyporeninemic hypoaldosteronism with low rates of ammonium excretion but were able to lower urinary pH to less than 5.3.

Bhathena DB, Sondheimer JH. The glomerulopathy of homozygous sickle hemoglobin (SS) disease: morphology and pathogenesis. *J Am Soc Nephrol* 1991;1: 1241–1252.

Histomorphometric analysis of kidney biopsy specimens from six Hb SS patients that revealed focal sclerosis in maximally hypertrophied glomeruli. It proposes that glomerulosclerosis results as consequence of hemodynamic injury in a susceptible subset of maximally hypertrophied glomerular.

Davis CJ, Mostofi FK, Sesterhenn IA. Renal medullary carcinoma. The seventh sickle cell nephropathy. *Am J Surg Pathol* 1995;19:1–11.

Retrospective analysis of the cases of renal medullary carcinoma from one institution that suggests that this type of malignancy occurs preferentially in individuals with either sickle cell trait or disease. Extent of clinical information was limited in some patients.

Falk RJ, Scheinman J, Phillips G, et al. Prevalence and pathologic features of sickle cell nephropathy and response to inhibition of angiotensin-converting enzyme. *N Engl J Med* 1992;326:910–915.

Landmark study that describes a high prevalence of clinical proteinuria in SCA and emphasizes the pathologic findings of glomerular hypertrophy and focal segmental glomerulosclerosis in proteinuric patients with renal insufficiency. Provides the first evidence that ACE inhibitors acutely reduce proteinuria in sickle glomerulonephropathy.

Guasch A, Cua M, Mitch WE. Extent and the course of glomerular injury in patients with sickle cell anemia. *Kidney Int* 1996;49:786–791.

Glomerular function was measured in 34 adult patients with SCA to determine the mechanisms of renal insufficiency. Renal insufficiency results from a glomerulopathy, characterized by an enhanced excretion of albumin and IgG and a loss of glomerular ultrafiltration capacity. Albuminuria is the earliest clinically detectable marker of sickle glomerulopathy and is accompanied by a reduction in the ultrafiltration coefficient even when the GFR is still normal. Determination of albuminuria should be used clinically to detect early sickle glomerulopathy.

Guasch A, Cua M, You W, et al. Sickle cell anemia causes a distinct pattern of glomerular dysfunction. *Kidney Int* 1997;51:826–833.

Glomerular function and dextran sieving analysis were studied in 27 patients with SCA. In patients with preserved glomerular function and no proteinuria, there was renal vasodilation and a generalized increased in dextran permeability, which resulted from an increase in glomerular pore size. Patients with renal insufficiency had a defect in glomerular size-selectivity and a reduction in the total number of glomerular pores, which accounted for the proteinuria and the renal insufficiency, respectively. Because the pattern of glomerular dysfunction is different from that found in other hemodynamically mediated glomerulopathies, it is postulated that unique mechanisms mediate sickle cell glomerulopathy.

Guasch A, Zayas CF, Eckman JR, et al. Evidence that microdeletions in the a globin gene protect against the development of sickle cell glomerulopathy. *J Am Soc Nephrol* 1999;10:1014–1019.

Genetic analysis was performed in a cohort of patients with Hb SS to define genetic markers associated with sickle glomerulopathy. Deletions in one or more of the α-globin genes were associated with a lower prevalence of sickle glomerulopathy. In contrast, β-globin haplotypes were not associated with sickle glomerulopathy.

Ojo AO, Govaerts TC, Schmouder RL, et al. Renal transplantation in end-stage sickle cell nephropathy. *Transplantation* 1999;67:291–295.

Largest series reported to date on the outcome of renal transplantation in SCA patients with ESRD. Emphasizes that early transplant outcomes are similar to those of non-SCA African-Americans, but allograft survival at 3 years is lower in than in other conditions.

Oster JR, Lespier LE, Lee SM, et al. Renal acidification in sickle-cell disease. *J Lab Clin Med* 1976;88:389–401.

Renal acidification study in patients with sickle cell trait and SS disease showing that an incomplete distal renal tubular acidosis occurs frequently in SCA despite the lack of systemic acidosis.

Pegelow CH, Colangelo L, Steinberg M, et al. Natural history of blood pressure in sickle cell disease: risks for stroke and death associated with relative hypertension in sickle cell anemia. *Am J Med* 1997;102:171–177.

Data from the Cooperative Study of Sickle Cell Disease was analyzed regarding blood pressure values and its relationship to stroke. Blood pressure was lower in SCA patients than in healthy individuals matched for age, sex, and race, and it was directly correlated to mortality and risk for stroke. Individuals with high values relative to the population were at an increased risk for stroke and death.

Powars DR, Elliott-Mills DD, Chan L, et al. Chronic renal failure in sickle cell disease: risk factors, clinical course, and mortality. *Ann Intern Med* 1991;115:614–620.

Large, retrospective study of nearly 1,000 patients with sickle hemoglobinopathies followed in southern California. Renal failure was associated with early death despite the availability of dialysis. Hypertension, hematuria, proteinuria, progressive anemia, and the CAR β-globin haplotype were associated with a higher risk for renal failure.

Tejani A, Phadke K, Admason O, et al. Renal lesions in sickle cell nephropathy in children. *Nephron* 1985;39:352–355.

Review of the clinical course of 13 children with proteinuria and sickle cell disease seen between 1968 and 1982. Presentation was isolated proteinuria or nephrotic syndrome with or without hematuria. Renal biopsy revealed mesangial proliferation in five, and focal segmental glomerulosclerosis in eight. Children with focal segmental glomerulosclerosis tended to be older and had a more aggressive course, requiring dialysis in four cases. Children with mesangial proliferation had less proteinuria, relatively preserved renal function and none of them required dialysis over the observation period.

Vaamonde CA. Renal papillary necrosis in sickle cell hemoglobinopathies. *Semin Nephrol* 1984;4:48–64.

Comprehensive review of the clinical, pathogenetic, radiographic, and therapeutic aspects of renal papillary necrosis in SCA. Renal papillary necrosis occurs often in asymptomatic SCA patients with microscopic hematuria, but in contrast to other forms of renal papillary necrosis, rarely progresses to end-stage renal failure.

Zayas CF, Platt J, Eckman JR, et al. Prevalence and predictors of glomerular involvement in sickle cell anemia [Abstract]. *J Am Soc Nephrol* 1996;7:1401.

The authors screened 233 adult patient with SCA (146 Hb SS, 54 Hb SC, and 33 Sb-thalassemia) for the presence of glomerular injury as evidenced by increased albumin excretion rate. Albuminuria was present in 68% of SS individuals: 27% had macroalbuminuria and 41% microalbuminuria. Albuminuria was somewhat less prevalent in non-SS sickle hemoglobinopathies, occurring in 42% of individuals and only 6% had macroalbuminuria. In contrast to other glomerulopathies, hypertension was uncommon in albuminuric SCA individuals.

PART 2
Alport Syndrome

Clifford E. Kashtan

Alport syndrome is a genetic disorder of type IV (basement membrane) collagen characterized clinically by the onset of hematuria in early childhood and ultimate progression to renal failure, predominantly in males. In many, but not all, families with Alport syndrome, affected individuals exhibit sensorineural deafness as well as a variety of ocular lesions. The first report of the entity now known as *Alport syndrome* is credited to Guthrie, who in 1902 described a family in which multiple individuals displayed hematuria. In 1927, Alport observed that many members of this family exhibited deafness and that affected males developed uremia while affected females survived into old age. Several hundred unrelated kindreds with progressive hereditary nephritis (with or without deafness) have been reported in the medical literature, representing all geographic and ethnic groups. Alport syndrome accounts for about 2% of children with end-stage renal disease (ESRD) in the United States and about 0.2% of adults with ESRD.

CLINICAL FEATURES (TABLE 43.5)

Hematuria is the key clinical feature of Alport syndrome. Affected males have persistent microscopic hematuria. Many also have episodic gross hematuria, precipitated by upper respira-

TABLE 43.5. Clinical Features of Alport Syndrome by Organ System

Renal
Hematuria
Persistent microhematuria is present from early childhood in XLAS males and both sexes with ARAS.
XLAS females may have persistent or intermittent microhematuria; 5%–10% of obligate carriers have no hematuria.
Episodic gross hematuria is not unusual in childhood and adolescence.
Proteinuria
Usually detectable by late childhood or early adolescence; may increase into nephrotic-range; substantial proteinuria is typical of XLAS males and both sexes with ARAS, but uncommon in XLAS females.
Hypertension
Usually detectable by late childhood or early adolescence.
Significant hypertension is typical of XLAS males and both sexes with ARAS but uncommon in XLAS females.
Renal insufficiency
All XLAS males and both sexes with ARAS eventually develop end-stage renal disease.
The rate of progression among XLAS males varies between families but is fairly constant within families.
Chronic renal failure occurs in 10%–15% of XLAS females.
Ocular
Perimacular flecks are the most common lesion (30%–35%).
Anterior lenticonus is pathognomonic; occurs in about 20% to XLAS males.
Other lesions: posterior polymorphous dystrophy, recurrent corneal erosions.
Cochlear
High-frequency sensorineural deafness occurs in 80% of XLAS males, and virtually all ARAS patients.
It is never congenital, always bilateral.
Leiomyomatosis
Occurs in a small number of XLAS families.
Smooth muscle tumors of the esophagus, tracheobronchial tree, and female external genitalia are seen.
Esophageal tumors present as dysphagia.

ARAS, autosomal-recessive Alport syndrome; XLAS, X-linked Alport syndrome.

tory infections, during the first two decades of life. Hematuria has been discovered in the first year of life in affected boys, in whom it is probably present from birth. Boys who are free of hematuria during the first 10 years of life are unlikely to be affected. Affected females with XLAS may have persistent or intermittent hematuria; some obligate female heterozygotes never manifest hematuria.

Proteinuria, usually absent in the first few years of life, appears eventually in affected males. Initially mild, proteinuria increases progressively with age, and development of nephrotic syndrome is not unusual in affected males. Similarly, hypertension is a finding that increases in incidence and severity with age and, like proteinuria, occurs more frequently in affected males.

End-stage renal disease develops inevitably in affected males. The rate of progression to renal failure is fairly constant among affected males within a particular family. In contrast, there is significant interkindred variability in the rate of progression to renal failure.

The prognosis in affected females is generally benign, with most surviving into old age with minimal renal disease. Gross hematuria in childhood, nephrotic syndrome, sensorineural deafness, anterior lenticonus, and diffuse glomerular basement membrane (GBM) thickening by electron microscopy are features predictive of progressive nephritis in affected females. As in women with other chronic nephritides, pregnancy does not appear to adversely affect renal function in those with mild disease but may be associated with accelerated loss of function in those with more severe disease.

In those Alport kindreds in which deafness is a component of the syndrome, hearing loss is never congenital, usually develops by age 15 in affected boys, and is always accompanied by evidence of renal involvement. In its early stages, the hearing deficit is detectable only by audiometry, with bilateral reduction in sensitivity to tones in the range of 2,000 to 8,000 Hz. In affected males, the deficit is progressive and eventually extends to other frequencies, including those of conversational speech. In affected females, hearing loss is less common and tends to occur later in life. Brainstem auditory evoked responses implicate the cochlea as the site of the aural lesion in Alport syndrome. Families with progressive hereditary nephritis but lacking sensorineural hearing loss have been reported. In some of these families, affected members have exhibited ultrastructural GBM lesions diagnostic of Alport syndrome. In addition, such families exhibit biochemical alterations of basement membranes pathognomonic of Alport syndrome and have mutations in the same gene (i.e., COL4A5) involved in kindreds with the Alport nephropathy and deafness. Thus the presence of sensorineural deafness is not required for the diagnosis of Alport syndrome.

Ocular defects are not unusual in patients with Alport syndrome, occurring in 15% to 30% of patients. Anterior lenticonus, the conical protrusion of the central portion of the lens into the anterior capsule, is virtually pathognomonic of Alport syndrome and is restricted to kindreds with rapid progression to end-stage renal disease (i.e., before age 30) and deafness. The lesion is bilateral in about 75% of patients. Anterior lenticonus is absent at birth, usually appearing during the second to third decade of life, and occurs more frequently in affected males. Progressive distortion of the lens may occur, accompanied by increasing myopia. Lens opacities may be seen in conjunction with lenticonus, occasionally resulting from rupture of the anterior lens capsule. A variety of other ocular lesions has been reported in patients with Alport syndrome. Perhaps the most commonly occurring abnormalities are pigmentary changes in the perimacular region, consisting of whitish or yellowish granulations surrounding the foveal area. These lesions are often accompanied by anterior lenticonus but may also occur in the absence of lenticonus. Corneal endothelial vesicles (posterior polymorphous dystrophy) and recurrent corneal erosion have also been observed in Alport patients.

In 1972, Epstein and co-workers described two families in which hereditary nephritis and deafness were associated with megathrombocytopenia. Affected members of these families usually manifested a bleeding tendency early in life, often diagnosed as idiopathic thrombocytopenic purpura, with later development of hematuria, albuminuria, and sensorineural hearing loss. The nephropathy was progressive, with light microscopic features similar to those characteristic of Alport syndrome. Several other kindreds with hereditary nephritis, deafness, and megathrombocytopenia have been described since Epstein's initial report. Ichthyosis may also be seen in Epstein's syndrome. The molecular relationship of Epstein's syndrome to Alport syndrome is uncertain.

The association of Alport syndrome with leiomyomatosis of the upper gastrointestinal tract and tracheobronchial tree has been reported as both a familial and sporadic disorder. Affected females in these kindreds typically exhibit genital leiomyomas as well, with clitoral hypertrophy and variable involvement of the labia majora and uterus. Bilateral, posterior subcapsular cataracts also occur frequently in affected individuals in these kindreds.

GENETICS (TABLE 43.6)

For many years, it had been the prevailing view that Alport syndrome was an autosomal-dominant disorder, and a variety of models were proposed to explain the rarity of father-to-son transmission of the disease and the greater severity of involvement in affected males compared with affected females. By refining the criteria used to identify affected individuals in large Alport pedigrees, O'Neill and colleagues were able to present a persuasive argument in favor of X-linked dominant inheritance. Atkin and colleagues in 1988 mapped the Alport locus to the long arm of the X chromosome (Xq22) by analysis of linkage to restriction fragment length polymorphisms. In 1990, Hostikka and co-workers cloned a gene (COL4A5) for a basement membrane collagen chain (the α5 chain of type IV collagen) and mapped this gene to Xq22. Barker and colleagues identified this gene as a locus for X-linked dominant Alport syndrome by detecting mutations in COL4A5 in three Alport kindreds. Since then, a variety of mutations in COL4A5 have been described in families with Alport syndrome. Most of these mutations are single base-pair substitutions, and many of these convert a glycine residue in the collagenous portion of the α5(IV) chain to an amino acid with a bulkier side chain. Other mutations alter messenger RNA splice sites. Deletions of all or a portion of the COL4A5 gene appear to account for approximately 10% of mutations in Alport kindreds. The association of Alport syndrome and diffuse leiomyomatosis represents a contiguous gene disorder, involving the COL4A5 and COL4A6 genes, which are adjacent to each other in a head-to-head (i.e., 5 end-to-5 end) arrangement on the X chromosome. Deletion of part or all of the COL4A5 gene and deletion of the first two exons of COL4A6 are found in all patients with this disease complex.

In addition to the X-linked dominant form of Alport syndrome, which accounts for about 80% of families with the disease, autosomal varieties of Alport syndrome are well documented. Autosomal-recessive Alport syndrome arises from mutations in either COL4A3, which encodes the α3 chain of type IV collagen, or COL4A4, which codes for the α4(IV) chain. COL4A3 and COL4A4 are located adjacent to each other on chromosome 2. An autosomal-dominant form of Alport syndrome has been mapped to chromosome 2 in the region of COL4A3 and COL4A4, but specific mutations have yet to be described.

TABLE 43.6. Inheritance of Alport Syndrome

Locus	Affected Gene Product	Chromosome	Inheritance
COL4A5	α5(IV)	X	X-linked dominant Alport syndrome
COL4A5 + COL4A6[a]	α5(IV) + α6(IV)	X	X-linked Alport syndrome + leiomyomatosis
COL4A3	α3(IV)	2	Autosomal-recessive Alport syndrome
COL4A4	α4(IV)	2	Autosomal-recessive Alport syndrome
COL4A3?[b]	α3(IV)?	2	Autosomal-dominant Alport syndrome
COL4A4?[b]	α4(IV)?	2	Autosomal-dominant Alport syndrome

[a] The Alport syndrome–diffuse leiomyomatosis complex results from deletion mutations involving both COL4A5 and COL4A6. The breakpoint of the deletion within the COL4A6 gene must fall within its second intron to produce leiomyomatosis; if the deletion breakpoint occurs more distally within COL4A6, leiomyomatosis will not result.

[b] Autosomal-dominant Alport syndrome has been mapped to region of chromosome 2 in which the COL4A3 and COL4A4 genes are located (Jefferson JA et al. *Nephrol Dial Transplant* 1997;12:1595–1599), but specific mutations have yet to be described. Benign familial hematuria due to a mutation in one allele of COL4A4 has been reported (Lemmink HH et al. *J Clin Invest* 1996;98:1114–1118).

PATHOLOGY

There are no pathognomonic light microscopic lesions in Alport syndrome. The histologic features are similar in patients with and without hearing loss or ophthalmologic abnormalities. Most specimens have both glomerular and tubulointerstitial lesions. Although at one time Alport syndrome was believed to be a primary chronic tubulointerstitial nephritis, the advent of transmission electron microscopy allowed recognition of unique glomerular lesions.

Renal biopsy early in the course of the disease, usually before the age of 5 years, reveals normal or nearly normal nephrons and vessels by light microscopy. The tubules and interstitium are usually normal during early childhood. The kidney in the older child (5 to 10 years old) may also demonstrate only minor abnormalities, but definite mesangial and capillary wall lesions, consisting of segmental to diffuse mesangial cell proliferation and matrix increase along with thickened capillary walls, are usually visible. Tubulointerstitial damage, characterized by focal tubular basement membrane thickening, interstitial fibrosis, tubular ectasia, and tubular atrophy, is often present, and interstitial foam cells are commonly found. Although renal failure may develop in the first decade of life, it is commonly during the second through the fifth decades of life that the glomerular and tubulointerstitial lesions progress to end-stage renal disease. Declining renal function is accompanied by the appearance of segmental sclerosis and hyalinosis, which develop at or near the vascular pole. The capillary walls become diffusely thickened, and double contours are more apparent. The focal tubulointerstitial lesions progress to diffuse tubular atrophy, irregular interstitial fibrosis, and chronic inflammation, and in approximately 40% of biopsies, sparse to abundant and diffuse interstitial foam cells are seen.

Routine immunofluorescence microscopic studies of renal biopsy specimens from patients with Alport syndrome show nonspecific changes. Many specimens are entirely negative, but granular deposits of C3 and IgM within the mesangium and vascular pole and along the glomerular capillary walls in segmental or diffuse distribution may be seen. As segmental sclerosis/hyalinosis appears, subendothelial deposits of IgM, C3, properdin, and C4 can be found.

The GBM of males with Alport syndrome frequently lacks reactivity with human anti-GBM autoantibodies and with monospecific antibodies directed against the α3, α4, or α5 chains of type IV collagen (Table 43.7). Such abnormalities are unique to Alport syndrome and can be diagnostic in cases in which electron microscopy of the glomerulus yields equivocal findings. It should be noted that GBM reactivity with anti-GBM sera or anti-α3(IV)–α5(IV) antibodies is preserved in some Alport kindreds, so a normal result when such an assay is used does not exclude the diagnosis.

Ultrastructural examination of the kidneys of patients with Alport syndrome reveals diagnostic morphologic changes. The cardinal fine structural feature is the variable thickening, thin-

TABLE 43.7. Immunostaining for Type IV Collagen α3–α6 Chains in Alport Basement Membranes[a]

	GBM	BC	dTBM	EBM
X-Linked				
Males				
α3(IV)	Absent	Absent	Absent	Normally absent
α4(IV)	Absent	Absent	Absent	Normally absent
α5(IV)	Absent	Absent	Absent	Absent
α6(IV)	Absent	Absent	Absent	Absent
Female[b]				
α3(IV)	Mosaic			Normally absent
α4(IV)	Mosaic			Normally absent
α5(IV)	Mosaic			Mosaic
α6(IV)	Mosaic			Mosaic
Autosomal Recessive (Males and Females)				
α3(IV)	Absent	Absent	Absent	Normally absent
α4(IV)	Absent	Absent	Absent	Normally absent
α5(IV)	Absent	Present	Present	Present
α6(IV)	Absent	Present	Present	Present

[a] In some AS kindreds, staining of basement membranes for type IV collagen chains is entirely normal. Therefore a normal result does not exclude a diagnosis of X-linked or autosomal-recessive AS.

[b] Some obligate carriers have normal basement membrane immunoreactivity for type IV collagen chains. Thus a normal result does not exclude the carrier state.

BC, Bowman's capsule; dTBM, distal tubular basement membrane; EBM, epidermal basement membrane; GBM, glomerular basement membrane.

ning, basket-weaving, and lamellation of the GBM, which is identified in many affected members of kindreds with Alport syndrome. The thick segments measure up to 1,200 nm, usually have irregular outer and inner contours, and are found more commonly in males than in females. The lamina densa is transformed into a heterogeneous network of membranous strands, which enclose clear electron-lucent areas. The electron-lucent zones may be entirely clear or contain round granules of variable density 20 to 90 nm wide. The origin of these granules is unknown, but it has been hypothesized that they represent degenerating islands of visceral epithelial cell cytoplasm. The altered capillary walls typically demonstrate epithelial foot process fusion, which may be extensive even in the absence of significant proteinuria. Young children and females, and adult males on occasion, may have diffusely attenuated segments of GBM measuring as little as 100 nm or less.

The specificity of the GBM changes has been questioned. Foci of lamina densa splitting and lamellation have been observed in 6% to 15% of specimens in two large series of unselected renal biopsies. These foci of splitting occur most commonly in postinfectious glomerulonephritis, focal segmental glomerulosclerosis and hyalinosis, IgA nephropathy, and mesangioproliferative glomerulonephritis associated with nephrotic syndrome. For this reason, clinical correlation and immunofluorescence microscopic examination of all biopsies are necessary when Alport syndrome is the suspected diagnosis. Diffuse thickening and splitting of GBM is strongly suggestive, if not pathognomonic, of Alport syndrome.

Not all Alport kindreds demonstrate these characteristic ultrastructural features. Thick, thin, normal, and nonspecifically altered GBM have all been described. Although diffuse attenuation of GBM has been considered the hallmark of benign familial hematuria (see Chapter 39, Part 13), some patients with this abnormality are members of kindreds with a history of progression to renal failure, and other patients have isolated microscopic hematuria and no family history of renal disease, ophthalmologic lesions, or hearing impairment. Thus a careful family history, along with follow-up examinations for proteinuria, hearing loss, ophthalmologic abnormalities, and azotemia, are warranted when thin lamina densae are found in a renal biopsy.

PATHOGENESIS

Type IV collagen is present ubiquitously in human basement membranes, where it is the major collagenous constituent. At least six genetically distinct chains of type IV collagen exist. The six genes are arranged in pairs on three chromosomes: COL4A1 and COL4A2 on chromosome 13, COL4A3 and COL4A4 on chromosome 2, and COL4A5 and COL4A6 on the X chromosome.

Collagen IV chains consist of a major collagenous domain containing the repetitive triplet sequence glycine(Gly)-X-Y, in which *X* and *Y* represent a variety of other amino acids, and a carboxyterminal noncollagenous domain. Individual type IV collagen chains associate intracellularly to form triple helical molecules, which are secreted and incorporated into the extracellular matrix. Formation of triple helices of type IV collagen is initiated by the establishment of disulfide bonds between the carboxyterminal noncollagenous domains of associating chains. Folding of the chains a triple helix then proceeds toward their aminotermini, a process that has been likened to the zipping of a zipper.

Unlike the interstitial collagens, which lose their carboxyterminal noncollagenous domains after secretion through proteolytic cleavage, type IV collagen triple helices retain their carboxyterminal domains. Numerous interruptions are present in the repetitive Gly-X-Y sequence of the collagenous domain, enhancing the flexibility of the triple helix. Type IV collagen triple helices form networks through several types of intermolecular associations. These include end-to-end linkages involving the carboxyterminal domains of two type IV collagen triple helices, covalent interactions between four triple helices at their aminoterminal ends, and lateral associations between triple helices via binding of the carboxyterminal domains to sites along the collagenous region of the triple helix. These interactions result in a flexible, nonfibrillar polygonal assembly that serves as a scaffolding for the deposition of other matrix glycoproteins and for the attachment of cells.

Evidence from a variety of sources indicates the probable existence of several separate collagen networks in basement membranes. The α1 and α2 chains of type IV collagen are present in all human basement membranes and are always codistributed. The distribution of the α3–α6(IV) chains is comparatively restricted. One network probably consists of the α1 and α2(IV) chains, while another is composed of the α3, α4, and α5(IV) chains, and a third is comprised by the α5 and α6(IV) chains. These networks may serve distinct functions in basement membranes and similarly may have different effects on the cells with which they make contact.

The α5 chain of type IV collagen is composed of 1,685 amino acids, including a signal peptide of 26 residues, a collagenous domain of 1,430 residues with 22 interruptions of the Gly-X-Y repetitive sequence, and a carboxyterminal noncollagenous domain of 229 residues. The carboxyterminal noncollagenous domain is encoded by five exons at the 3′ end of the COL4A5 gene. The amino acid sequence of the noncollagenous domain includes 12 highly conserved cysteine residues, which participate in intrachain disulfide bonds that establish its globular conformation.

With this background in mind, the consequences of some of the mutations found in COL4A5 in patients with Alport syndrome can be predicted. Deletion or splicing mutations of COL4A5 could result in a truncated translational product, a product with nonsense sequence downstream of the deletion, or no product at all, depending on the site of the deletion and whether the transcriptional reading frame is preserved. Mutations resulting in loss of the carboxyterminal noncollagenous domain would prohibit the formation of triple helices involving the α5(IV) chain, because formation of type IV collagen triple helices is initiated by disulfide bonding between the carboxyterminal noncollagenous domains of associating chains. Similarly, a point mutation eliminating a conserved cysteine residue in the carboxyterminal noncollagenous domain would result in loss of an intrachain disulfide bond and a change in the conformation of this domain, which could interfere with normal chain associations.

Many COL4A5 mutations result in replacement of a glycine residue in the collagenous domain by another amino acid. In this regard, it is worth noting that most of the mutations found in COL1A1, the gene for the α1 chain of type I collagen, in patients with osteogenesis imperfecta (OI) convert a glycine residue to another amino acid. The formation of collagen triple helices requires glycines at every third position in the associating chains, as glycines lack side chains and are the only amino acids so small that three of them can fit into the interior of the tightly wound triple helix. The impact of a glycine substitution in OI, and most probably in Alport syndrome as well, is influenced by the position of the glycine residue in the collagen chain. Some glycine substitutions completely prohibit folding into a triple helix, whereas others may have little or no effect on folding. The abnormally folded triple helices resulting from OI mutations are excessively vulnerable to extracellular proteases, undergoing degradation following secretion. In this way, the mutant collagen chain facilitates the destruction of the normal chains with which it has associated, amplifying the effect of the mutation.

Immunohistologic and immunochemical studies of GBM from males with X-linked Alport syndrome indicate that these basement membranes lack the α3 and α4(IV) chains (Table 43.7). Mutations in the α5(IV) chain might prevent the formation of triple helices involving the α3, α4, and α5(IV) chains or increase the susceptibility of such triple helices to degradation so that none of these chains appear in basement membranes. Alternatively, COL4A5 mutations might in some way affect transcription of the genes encoding the α3(IV) and α4(IV) chains. Similar events may occur in autosomal-recessive Alport syndrome, although the primary abnormality affects the α3(IV) or α4(IV) chain. Regardless of the precise mechanism, COL4A3, COL4A4, and COL4A5 mutations result in basement membranes lacking an apparently vital component—the collagenous network formed by the α3, α4, and α5 chains of type IV collagen. The process by which loss of this network eventuates in glomerulosclerosis has yet to be delineated. The glomeruli in Alport syndrome exhibit overexpression and ectopic distribution of the α1 and α2(IV) chains, type V collagen, and type VI collagen. Accumulation of these and/or other matrix proteins may contribute to glomerulosclerosis in Alport syndrome.

TREATMENT

There are currently no treatments of proven benefit for Alport syndrome. Experimental studies of gene therapy approaches and angiotensin-converting enzyme inhibition, using spontaneous canine models of Alport syndrome, are under way. However, it seems prudent to treat hypertension and proteinuria as is recommended for these abnormalities in other renal diseases.

RENAL TRANSPLANTATION

Because Alport syndrome is a familial disorder, potential living-related kidney donors for Alport patients with ESRD must be selected with care. Hematuria will serve to exclude all related affected males and most affected females. Because some female heterozygotes are asymptomatic carriers of mutations at the COL4A5 locus, a normal urinalysis does not guarantee that a female member of an Alport kindred is not a carrier. Molecular genetic studies will make it possible to precisely identify asymptomatic carriers in many Alport families.

Anti-GBM nephritis involving the renal allograft is a rare, but dramatic, manifestation of Alport syndrome. Data from several transplant centers indicates an incidence of 3% to 4% of anti-GBM nephritis in transplanted Alport patients. It is important that Alport patients who suffer allograft dysfunction undergo evaluation for anti-GBM nephritis for several reasons. First, anti-GBM nephritis may respond to appropriate therapy. Second, Alport patients who develop allograft anti-GBM nephritis are very likely to have recurrent anti-GBM nephritis in subsequent allografts. Finally, allograft anti-GBM nephritis may occur in more than one member of an Alport kindred.

Alport patients who develop posttransplant anti-GBM nephritis are usually male, always deaf, and are likely to have reached end-stage renal disease before the age of 30. Because this profile describes the majority of Alport patients presenting for renal transplantation, its predictive value is limited. Alport females are at little risk for posttransplant anti-GBM nephritis, unless they have autosomal-recessive disease.

Most cases of posttransplant anti-GBM nephritis are diagnosed within the first year after transplantation. Three-fourths of affected allografts have been lost. Anti-GBM nephritis has recurred in most retransplanted patients. Allograft anti-GBM nephritis may recur despite an interval of many years between transplants and in the absence of detectable circulating anti-GBM antibodies before retransplantation.

Anti-GBM antibodies from patients with X-linked Alport syndrome usually identify the noncollagenous domain of the α5(IV) chain, whereas the target antigen in patients with autosomal-recessive disease is the α3(IV) chain. Susceptibility to the development of posttransplant anti-GBM nephritis is probably determined by at least two factors: (a) the nature of the patient's mutation (mutations preventing the synthesis of immunogenic protein would prevent establishment of immunologic tolerance) and (b) the strength of the host's immune response.

Because posttransplant anti-GBM nephritis is rare, Alport patients facing a first transplant can be offered organs from living or cadaveric donors. Transplanted Alport males should be monitored regularly for circulating anti-GBM antibodies during the first year after transplantation. Allograft biopsy is indicated if circulating anti-GBM antibodies are detected or in the event that hematuria or allograft dysfunction develops. Patients with posttransplant anti-GBM nephritis may benefit from treatment with plasmapheresis and cyclophosphamide in the absence of superior therapies. Some patients may have circulating anti-GBM antibodies but no histologic evidence of glomerulonephritis; close observation is appropriate in these cases. Given the high likelihood of recurrence of anti-GBM nephritis in subsequent allografts, the advisability of retransplantation should be considered carefully.

Selected Readings

Barker DF, Hostikka SL, Zhou J, et al. Identification of mutations in the COL4A5 collagen gene in Alport syndrome. *Science* 1990;248:1224–1227.
A seminal paper that identifies the COL4A5 gene as the Alport locus.

Brainwood D, Kashtan C, Gubler MC, et al. Targets of alloantibodies in Alport anti-glomerular basement membrane disease after renal transplantation. *Kidney Int* 1998;53:762–766.
An analysis of anti-GBM antibodies from transplanted Alport patients.

Hostikka SL, Eddy RL, Byers MG, et al. Identification of a distinct type IV collagen chain with restricted kidney distribution and assignment of its gene to the locus of X chromosome-linked Alport syndrome. *Proc Natl Acad Sci USA* 1990;87:1606–1610.
A paper describing the cloning of the COL4A5 gene and the discovery of the α5 chain of type IV collagen.

Kalluri R, Shield CF, Todd P, et al. Isoform switching of type IV collagen is developmentally arrested in X-linked Alport syndrome leading to increased susceptibility of renal basement membranes to endoproteolysis. *J Clin Invest* 1997;99:2470–2478.
A description of a study suggesting that Alport GBM has an increased susceptibility to proteolysis.

Kashtan CE, Kim Y. Distribution of the α1 and α2 chains of collagen IV and of collagens V and VI in Alport syndrome. *Kidney Int* 1992;42:115–126.
A paper describing overexpression and ectopic distribution of several collagen types in Alport GBM.

Kashtan CE, Michael AF. Perspectives in clinical nephrology: Alport syndrome. *Kidney Int* 1996;50:1445–1463.
An extensive review of clinical, pathologic, and molecular aspects of Alport syndrome.

Kleppel MM, Fan WW, Cheong HI, et al. Evidence for separate networks of classical and novel basement membrane collagen. Characterization of 3(IV)-Alport antigen heterodimers. *J Biol Chem* 1992;267:4137–4142.
A study supporting the existence of two distinct collagenous networks in basement membranes.

Kleppel MM, Kashtan CE, Butkowski RJ, et al. Alport familial nephritis. Absence of 28 kilodalton non-collagenous monomers of type IV collagen in glomerular basement membrane. *J Clin Invest* 1987;80:263–266.
A paper documenting the absence of the α3 and α4 chains of type IV collagen from Alport GBM.

Lemmink HH, Nillesen WN, Mochizuki T, et al. Benign familial hematuria due to mutation of the type IV collagen α4 gene. *J Clin Invest* 1996;98:1114–1118.
A paper showing that at least some families with benign familial hematuria have type IV collagen mutations.

Lemmink HH, Schröder CH, Monnens LAH, et al. The clinical spectrum of type IV collagen mutations. *Hum Mutat* 1997;9:477–499.
An excellent review of type IV collagen mutations in Alport syndrome.
Mochizuki T, Lemmink HH, Mariyama M, et al. Identification of mutations in the α3(IV) and α4(IV) collagen genes in autosomal recessive Alport syndrome. *Nat Genet* 1994;8:77–82.
The first paper to identify mutations in patients with autosomal-recessive Alport syndrome.
Thorner PS, Zheng K, Kalluri R, et al. Coordinate gene expression of the α3, α4 and α5 chains of collagen type IV: evidence from a canine model of X-linked nephritis with a COL4A5 gene mutation. *J Biol Chem* 1996;271:13821–13828.
A study suggesting that a COL4A5 mutation may suppress transcription of the COL4A3 and COL4A4 genes.
Tryggvason K, Heikkila P, Pettersson E, et al. Can Alport syndrome be treated by gene therapy? *Kidney Int* 1997;52:1493–1499.
A discussion of issues related to gene therapy for Alport syndrome.
Zhou J, Mochizuki T, Smeets H, et al. Deletion of the paired α5(IV) and α6(IV) collagen genes in inherited smooth muscle tumors. *Science* 1993;261:1167–1169.
A molecular genetic analysis of kindreds expressing Alport syndrome and leiomyomatosis.

PART 3
Fabry's Disease

Richard J. Glassock

Angiokeratoma corporis diffusum universale, known commonly as *Fabry's disease,* is an X-linked hereditary disorder of glycosphingolipid metabolism. The deficiency of a specific α-galactosidase. A leads to the accumulation of ceramide trihexoside [galactosyl]-(α4)-galactosyl(β4)-glycosyl-(β1) ceramide] in many organs. The vessel wall, kidneys, and nerves are favorite sites of deposition. The cutaneous manifestations of this disorder, which were first recognized by Fabry in 1898, consist of multiple angiokeratomas distributed particularly on the scrotum, back, hips, and buttocks. These skin lesions may at times be entirely absent in patients with otherwise typical Fabry's disease.

EXTRARENAL MANIFESTATIONS

The *cutaneous* manifestations include the presence of reddish purple papules distributed over the midtrunk (bathing suit area) chiefly involving the scrotum, buttock, upper thighs, umbilicus, and oral mucous membrane. The lesions are shown to be typical angiokeratomas on histologic examination. These lesions usually become evident at the time of puberty. The skin findings may be lacking in females or in African-Americans. *Peripheral nerve involvement* is classically manifested by the development of burning pain in the distal extremities (acroparesthesias), which appears early in the course of the disease, waxes and wanes in severity, and usually declines in intensity with the appearance of renal disease. *Autonomic nervous system involvement* may produce hypohidrosis or postural hypotension. Postprandial is common. Involvement of the central nervous system does not occur, except for vascular disease. *Corneal opacities* are often found, especially in females with the disease (cornea verticillata), similar to chloroquine or amiodarone toxicity. *Tortuosity of the conjunctival or retinal vessels* and *cataracts* are also often seen. *Visceral involvement* usually takes the form of vascular disease with ischemia. Thus coronary arterial disease with angina pectoris and/or myocardial infarction or cerebral arterial insufficiency with strokes or transient ischemic episodes may develop. Mitral insufficiency and a short PR interval may be seen. Periorbital puffiness and pedal edema may appear even in the absence of cardiac or renal involvement.

RENAL MANIFESTATIONS

The initial clinical manifestations of renal involvement are mild and subtle, consisting primarily of asymptomatic nonnephrotic proteinuria occasionally accompanied by hematuria. Nephrotic syndrome is quite unusual. Occasionally, patients may develop more severe renal tubular functional abnormalities such as nephrogenic diabetes insipidus or distal renal tubular acidosis. Hypertension is usually mild. Renal involvement seldom appears before the age of 20 years and is usually slowly progressive, leading to end-stage renal failure by the age of 40 years. Rarely, patients with very indolent disease have survived into the sixth decade of life. The renal findings are most often nonspecific, and the diagnosis is usually suspected on the basis of the extrarenal manifestations. However, careful examination of the urinary sediment by light or electron microscopy may reveal characteristic foamy epithelial cells containing birefringent lipid and "myelin figures." Complement levels are normal.

GENETICS AND BIOCHEMISTRY

The disorder is X-linked and is usually fully expressed in hemizygous males. However, in heterozygous females, according to the Lyon hypothesis, early inactivation of one of the X chromosomes leads to a heterogeneous population of cells in females, some affected with the mutant gene, whereas others are spared. Thus the manifestations of the disease are more variable in females; some have only mild atypical nonprogressive disease, whereas other cases resemble the hemizygous males in severity. The gene defect is localized on X chromosome between Xg 21 and Xg 24.

The biochemical lesion is the result of a single gene defect leading to reduced or absent α-galactosidase A. The gene has been cloned and the disorder is due to multiple point mutations or deletions. This enzyme is essential for the catabolism of ceramide trihexoside, a glycosphingolipid. Thus this glycosphingolipid accumulates in many organs, including the vascular wall, nerves, and kidneys.

α-Galactosidase A activity is reduced in serum, urine, leukocytes, hair follicle roots, and amniotic fluid. Levels of α-galactosidase A in hemizygous males are most often less than 10% of normal, and the levels in females vary widely from undetectable to normal. Ceramide trihexoside levels are increased in plasma and urine only in severely affected hemizygous males. Other data have suggested the presence of inhibitors of α-galactosidase in some patients. Asymptomatic female carriers can be detected by slit-lamp examination for corneal deposits or by restriction fragment length polymorphisms.

PATHOLOGY

The most characteristic finding in the kidney by light microscopy is the presence of finely vacuolated, lipid-laden visceral glomerular epithelial cells. The glomerular endothelial cells, parietal epithelial cells, and distal tubular cells may also be involved. The vacuoles stain with Sudan black and oil red O but not with periodic acid–Schiff. Immunofluorescence microscopy is negative or reveals nonspecific deposits of immunoglobulins in sclerotic glomeruli. By electron microscopy, a very characteristic, but not necessarily pathognomonic, lesion is observed. The visceral epithelial cells of the glomerulus contain numerous, dense, osmophilic, round or ovoid, laminated and whorled bodies. These bodies, called *myelin figures* or *zebra bodies,* represent the storage sites of ceramide trihexoside. Similar deposits may also be seen in endothelial cells and distal tubular cells. Extrarenal involvement with deposits may be seen in arterial endothelium, the vascular wall, and neural tissue. Deposits of a similar character can also be seen in asymptomatic heterozygous females. Deposits with similar electron microscopic features may also occasionally be seen in patients with longstanding heavy proteinuria from other causes. Foamy, lipid-laden cells may also be seen by light microscopy in the kidney in Alport syndrome, Gaucher's disease, Niemann-Pick disease, carnitine deficiency, severe hyperlipidemia, and lecithin-cholesterol acyltransferase deficiency. The urinary sediment may contain desquamated epithelial cells having the distinctive morphologic features, thus permitting the diagnosis of Fabry's disease without renal biopsy. As the renal disease progresses, the glomeruli undergo segmental and global sclerosis. Variable degrees of tubular atrophy and interstitial fibrosis invariably are seen in advanced cases.

DIAGNOSIS AND DIFFERENTIAL DIAGNOSIS

Fabry's disease should be suspected in any individual, male or female, initially seen clinically with unexplained nonnephrotic proteinuria and renal failure in early adult life. A careful search for angiokeratomas, conjunctival or retinal vascular tortuosity, corneal opacities, and coronary arterial disease should be undertaken, and the history should attempt to elicit features of prior or current acroparesthesias. The diagnosis can be confirmed by finding reduced levels of α-galactosidase A in urine or serum or by the finding of elevated ceramide trihexoside in serum. Electron microscopy of urinary sediment can also be useful as stated previously. Occasionally, renal biopsy will be required or the diagnosis will be made by such biopsies in patients not previously suspected to have Fabry's disease. Once having found the typical morphologic lesions in such circumstances, the diagnosis should be confirmed by appropriate enzyme or glycosphingolipid measurements, especially if typical extrarenal findings are lacking. Direct molecular diagnosis in asymptomatic carriers is possible by examining the α-galactosidase A gene for mutations. Prenatal diagnosis is possible in female carriers by chorionic villus sampling before the 9th week on by amniocentesis by the 16th week of pregnancy. The differential diagnosis of Fabry's disease includes other causes of nonnephrotic proteinuria and renal failure that may be associated with acroparesthesias and corneal opacities. These diseases include amyloidosis, adult-onset cystinosis, lecithin-cholesterol acyltransferase deficiency, and congenital syphilis.

COURSE AND TREATMENT

The course of renal involvement in Fabry's disease is usually relentlessly progressive, although at variable rates. The neural manifestations are often mild or absent by the time renal failure has developed. No form of therapy has been efficacious in preventing the evolution of disease to end-stage renal failure. Theoretically, replacement of deficient α-galactosidase A by transplantation of tissues capable of continued production of the enzyme or by recombinant gene therapy might be of benefit. A trial approved by the Food and Drug Administration approved using human recombinant α-galactosidase A is currently in progress. Painful acroparesthesias will respond to carbamazepine (Tegretol), and gastrointestinal hypomotility can be reduced by metoclopramide.

Although chronic dialysis may alleviate some of the symptoms related to glycosphingolipid deposition, renal allotransplantation remains the treatment of choice. Interestingly, despite the widespread nature of the enzymatic defect, recurrence of disease in the allograft has been observed only rarely. It is possible that the transplanted kidney itself may provide a source of the defective or missing α-galactosidase A. Clinical improvement of extrarenal manifestations of Fabry's disease is frequently observed following allotransplantation; however, the levels of α-galactosidase A do not regularly increase following such grafting. Indeed, transplantation of a kidney from an asymptomatic heterozygous female to an unaffected daughter with end-stage renal disease resulting from other causes has revealed that the characteristic dense bodies of the glomerular visceral epithelial cells remain unchanged. Besides renal failure, coronary artery and cerebral vascular disease remain major causes of death.

Selected Readings

Cohen AH, Adler SG. Nail patella syndrome, lipodystrophy, Fabry's disease and familial lecithin cholesterol acyl transferase deficiency. In: Tisher CC, Brenner BM, eds: *Renal pathology,* 2nd ed. Philadelphia: JB Lippincott, 1994:1267–1290.

An excellent overview with an emphasis on pathology.

Desnick RJ, Sweeley C. Fabry's disease: α-alactosidase A deficiency (angiokeratoma corporis diffusum universale). In: Fitzpatrick TB, Eisen AZ, Wolff K, et al, eds: *Dermatology in general medicine,* 3rd ed. New York: McGraw-Hill, 1987:1739–1760.

A summary and description of the cutaneous manifestations of Fabry's disease.

Eng CM, Resnick-Silverman LA, Niehaus DJ. Nature and frequency of mutations in the *alpha*-galactosidase gene that cause Fabry disease. *Am J Hum Genet* 1993;53:1186–1197.

A description of the molecular defect underlying Fabry's disease.

Meroni M, Sessa A, Battini G, et al. *Vol. 122: Hereditary kidney diseases.* In: Sessa A, Conte F, Meroni M, et al, eds. *Contributions to nephrology.* Basel: S. Karger AG, 1997:178–184.

A comprehensive treatise proving clinical details of Fabry's disease.

Sakuraba H, Oshima A, Fujukara Y, et al. Identification of point mutation in the α-galactosidase gene in classical and atypical hemizygotes with Fabry's disease. *Am J Hum Genet* 1990;47:784–789.

Description of the genetic bases of Fabry's disease.

PART 4
Nail-Patella Syndrome

Richard J. Glassock

The nail-patella syndrome, also known as *hereditary osteoonychodysplasia,* is a rare genetic disease associated with osseus and renal abnormalities. The latter include asymptomatic proteinuria, nephrotic syndrome, and renal failure. The disorder is transmitted as an autosomal-dominant trait closely linked to the ABO erythrocyte antigens, and the gene is assigned to the distal end of the long arm of chromosome 9 (9 q 34). The responsible gene may be a transcription factor related limb development in vertebrate (LMX1B). Two allelic mutations of the gene may occur; one is associated with nephropathy while the other is not. Both sexes are equally affected. The biochemical lesion responsible for the bone and renal abnormalities is unknown. It is a rare disease, affecting 221 million population.

The typical clinical findings are dysplastic or hypoplastic nails of the fingers and toes, with the thumbs and great toes most severely involved. The patellae are reduced in size and, on occasion, are entirely absent. Abnormalities of the elbow joint may prevent full extension of the forearm. Osseus spurs projecting posteriorly from the iliac wings are seen in most cases.

Heterochromia of the irises may be present. No defects in the central nervous system function are present.

The most common renal manifestation of nail-patella syndrome is mild nonnephrotic proteinuria commonly associated with microhematuria. About 30% to 40% of patients with this disorder will develop proteinuria, sometimes with nephrotic syndrome, usually first discovered during childhood or adolescence.

Progressive renal failure occurs in about 30% of cases and usually appears during adulthood. The proteinuria is nonselective and hypertension is mild. Serum levels of complement are normal. Associated diseases include anti–basement membrane antibody nephritis, membranous nephropathy, IgA nephropathy, and vasculitis.

By light microscopy, renal biopsies reveal nonspecific findings consisting of focal and segmental glomerulosclerosis, focal thickening of the capillary wall, and mesangial hypercellularity. By immunofluorescence, focal and segmental nonspecific glomerular deposits of IgM and C3 have been described. Electron microscopy reveals a characteristic lesion consisting of localized areas of rarefraction of the glomerular basement membrane with intramembranous deposits having the appearance and periodicity of mature collagen (Fig. 105.39). Types I, III, and VI collagen have been detected in lesions by immunohistochemical methods. Sometimes, the basement membrane is deficient in normal structural antigens.

In many patients, the disease pursues a benign course with only persistent asymptomatic proteinuria. Those with more severe degrees of proteinuria, including nephrotic syndrome, may eventually develop renal insufficiency. No treatment is known to be effective. Patients with nail-patella syndrome should be regarded as good candidates for renal transplantation, because no cases of recurrent renal disease or posttransplant anti–glomerular basement membrane antibody disease have yet been recorded.

Selected Readings

Bennett WM, Musgrave JE, Campbell R, et al. The nephropathy of nail-patella syndrome. A clinical-pathologic analysis of 11 kindreds. *Am J Med* 1973;54:304–311.
A good analysis of the inheritance and clinical features of nail-patella syndrome.

Cohen AH, Adler SG. Nail-patella syndrome, lipodystrophy, Fabry disease and familial lecithin cholesterol acyl transferase deficiency. In: Tisher CC, Brenner BM, eds. *Renal pathology,* 2nd ed. Philadelphia: JB Lippincott, 1994:1267–1290.
An excellent overview with an emphasis on pathology.

Hoyer JR, Michael AF, Vernier RL, et al. Renal disease in nail-patella syndrome: clinical and morphologic studies. *Kidney Int* 1972;2:231–238.
A review of the clinical and pathologic features of well-documented patients with nail-patella syndrome.

Sabris S, Antonovych T, Argy WP, et al. Nail-patella syndrome. *Clin Nephrol* 1980;14:148–153.
An excellent clinical review of the topic.

Vollrath D, Jaramillo-Babb VL, Clough MV. Loss-of-function mutations in the LIM-homeodomain gene, LMX1B, in nail-patella syndrome. *Hum Mol Genet* 1998;7:1091.
A description of the gene defect possibly responsible for nail-patella syndrome.

PART 5
Congenital Nephrotic Syndrome

Niilo-Pekka Huttunen and Juhani Rapola

Nephrotic syndrome (NS) manifested soon after birth is rare, but it comprises several diseases with different etiologies. NS is arbitrarily called *congenital* when it is observed before the age of 3 months. The causes of nephrotic syndrome seen within the first few months of life are presented in Table 43.8.

TABLE 43.8. The Causes of Nephrotic Syndrome Manifested at Birth or in Early Infancy

Congenital nephrotic syndrome of the Finnish type (CNF)
Diffuse mesangial sclerosis (DMS)
Malformation syndromes
Denys-Drash syndrome (DDS)
Galloway-Mowat syndrome
Frasier syndrome
Hereditary onycho-osteodysplasia (nail-patella syndrome)
Secondary nephrotic syndromes
Syphilis
Cytomegalovirus
Toxoplasmosis
Human immunodeficiency virus (HIV)
Hepatitis B
Systemic lupus erythematosus (SLE)
Idiopathic nephrotic syndromes
Minimal-change nephrotic syndrome (MCNS)
Focal segmental glomerulosclerosis (FSGS)
Diffuse mesangial proliferation
Membranous glomerulonephritis

CONGENITAL NEPHROTIC SYNDROME OF THE FINNISH TYPE

Genetics

Congenital nephrotic syndrome of the Finnish type (CNF) is a distinct disease entity with an autosomal-recessive inheritance. Although CNF has a worldwide distribution, it is more common in Finland than elsewhere. The incidence of CNF pregnancies in Finland during 1975 to 1988 was 14.2 per 100,000 births, but the birth prevalence is now lower due to antenatal diagnosis and termination of CNF pregnancies during the early weeks of gestation. It is calculated that the frequency of heterozygotes among the Finnish population is about 1:200, but in certain areas, it may be up to 1:20. The disease causing NPHS1 gene is located in the q13.1 region of chromosome 19. Two mutations have been identified in the Finnish families. The first is *Fin major,* which is a 2 bp deletion in exon 2 consisting 78% of the Finnish CNF chromosomes. The second, called *Fin minor,* is a nonsense mutation CGA to TGA in exon 26 consisting 16% of Finnish CNF chromosomes. The remaining portion of 6% consists of unknown mutations. The CNF families outside of Finland seem to have different mutations in NPHS1 gene. The product of NPHS1 gene is nephrin, which is constitutively expressed only in glomerular epithelial cells.

Clinical Picture

The onset of CNF takes place already *in utero* and the signs of the disease are recognizable at birth. A large placenta is a firm hallmark of the disease. The placental/fetal weight ratio is 0.43 on average and always it is more than 0.25. These children tend to be born prematurely. They are small for the gestational age. The retardation of the intrauterine growth seems to occur during the last 2 months of gestation. As a sign of fetal stress, the amniotic fluid is often meconium stained and the low Apgar score is a common finding. Fetal death just before birth is not rare. Breech presentation is more common among CNF fetuses than among average ones. Edema is usually seen during the first week and invariably during the first month of life. Postural deformities, such as pes calcaneovalgus, are seen in CNF children more often than in other children. The sutures of the skull are often broad. In ultrasonographic examination, the kidneys are large and hyperechogenic. In the past when there was no active supportive treatment, the CNF children later had a marked growth retardation and muscular wasting. Frank edema often disappeared, and marked abdominal distension was a dominant feature. Because of the abdominal distension, the children lied in an opisthotonic position and umbilical hernias were common. Their psychomotor development was very poor. Life-threatening bacterial infections and severe thrombotic complications were common and often the cause of death. Without renal transplantation, CNF is definitely a fatal disease. Before the active treatment had been established, half of the Finnish CNF children died before the age of 6 months and fewer than every 20th child reached the age of 2 years; none has known to reach the age of 5 years. The active treatment with albumin substitution, nephrectomy, and renal transplantation has dramatically changed the prognosis of CNF children. Serious physical and mental retardation have been overcome, and most of the transplanted CNF children are capable of going to a normal school.

Laboratory Findings

Massive proteinuria is always seen already in the first urine sample. The 24-hour urinary protein excretion varies from 1 to 6 g without treatment, but during the albumin infusions, it may rise up to 20 g. Urinary proteins are mainly albumin, but small but significant amounts of transferrin, apoproteins, IgG, lipoprotein lipase, antithrombin III, and thyroid-binding globulin (TBG) are also lost into urine. Proteinuria is mainly highly selective, thus comparable with minimal-change nephrotic syndrome (MCNS), but in some CNF children with advanced renal pathology, the proteinuria is less selective. The tubular component of proteinuria increases with advancing tubular atrophy. Microscopic hematuria and mild glucosuria are not rare. Protein leakage into urine decreases with declining renal function. Hypoproteinemia is detectable already in the cord blood. Without any albumin substitution, total serum protein content is between 30 and 40 g/L, but even lower concentrations have been seen. Serum albumin is usually less than 7 g/L. On the other hand, the concentration of high-molecular-weight serum proteins such as α_2-macroglobulin, fibrinogen, and IgM are increased. Due to urinary loss of apoproteins and lipoprotein lipase, the serum concentrations of cholesterol and triglyceride-rich lipoproteins are increased. After nephrectomy, triglyceride and cholesterol levels in serum decrease but still remain at higher levels than in healthy children. Urinary loss of TBG leads to low concentrations of thyroxine and tri-iodothyronine in the serum. The concentration of thyroid-stimulating hormone (TSH) may be in the normal range soon after birth but usually rises in older age. Blood urea concentration is usually normal before nephrectomy. Before the era of active treatment, the serum creatinine concentration was abnormally low during the first year of life because of muscular wasting, but the creatinine clearance had a declining tendency after the fourth month of life (Fig. 43.2).

Renal Pathology (See Chapter 109, Atlas of Renal Pathology)

The CNF kidneys appear macroscopically large, smooth surfaced, pale, and soft. The renal cortex relative to medulla is somewhat broader than normal. The histologic changes are present in the renal cortex, and the medulla is spared. The cortical lesions are progressive with age. Fetal kidneys in the third trimester of pregnancy show occasional dilated tubules with low cuboidal epithelium containing bright eosinophilic and colloidlike material. These tubules are usually located close to the medullary border. The glomeruli of the fetal kidneys appear normal in light microscopy, but the most mature glomeruli show a loss of the foot processes in electron microscopy. In the first month after birth, the histologic changes are usually slight. A moderate increase of mesangial cells is present in otherwise normal glomeruli. Fetal glomeruli are present, but they are also seen in normal kidneys at this age. A few dilated proximal tubules located in the deep renal cortex can be found. In electron microscopy, the loss of foot processes is evident in all glomeruli and morphometric measurement shows a thin glomerular basement membrane (GBM). The light microscopic changes at this age are so focal and subtle that a needle biopsy sample may be interpreted as consistent with the MCNS. The characteristic pathologic changes appear usually from the age of 2 months on. Radial dilations of the tubules are present. The proximal tubules are the most dilated, but with advancing age, the distal ones are also affected. Most glomeruli show mesangial hypercellularity, but collapse of the glomerular tuft and glomerular sclerosis with fibrotic thickening of the glomerular capsule increase with age. Interstitial fibrosis and interstitial chronic inflammation appear in some kidneys. In autopsy and nephrectomy specimens of the children older than 8 months of age, sclerotic glomeruli, wide cystic dilations of the tubules, and interstitial fibrosis with inflammation govern the histologic picture, but the individual variation is great in this age group. The CNF kidneys show neither immunodeposits in immunofluorescence studies nor dense deposits in electron microscopy.

Pathogenesis

The basic defect in CNF is a leaky glomerular barrier for vital serum proteins. As a consequence of this genetically determined defect, massive proteinuria begins as soon as the glomerular filtration starts in the fetal kidneys. A sign of this fetal protein leakage is the high α-fetoprotein (AFP) content in the amniotic fluid of mothers bearing CNF fetuses. The content of type IV collagen, laminin, nidogen, and fibronectin, which are the important components of the structure of GBM, has shown to be normal in CNF. The amount of anionic proteoglycans are also within in the normal limits in the GBM of CNF children. The mutant NPHS1 gene codes nephrin, which is a transmem-

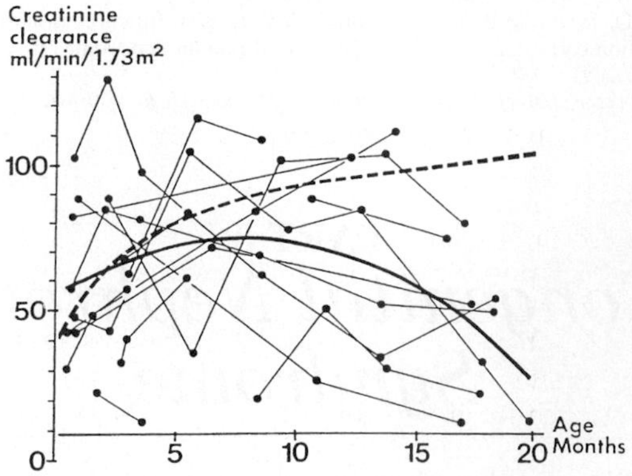

Figure 43.2. The early increase and later decline of glomerular filtration rate of nonnephrectomized CNF infants. The *closed circles* connected by *solid lines* represent individual patients. The *dotted curve* shows the development of creatinine clearance in healthy infants, and the *solid one* is the regression curve of the repeated measurements of creatinine clearance in 15 CNF infants.

brane protein of the immunoglobulin superfamily. Nephrin is expressed only in glomerular epithelial cells. It is presumed that the zipperlike structure of the slit membrane between podocyte foot processes is formed by nephrin. When the building of the slit membrane is defective, albumin and other serum proteins are leaked into urine.

Treatment

Steroids and other immunosuppressive drugs are ineffective in CNF. The results of trials with indomethacin and captopril in reducing the protein leakage are controversial. Intravenous albumin substitution since birth, a high-protein diet, hyperalimentation, bilateral nephrectomy at weight of about 10 kg, peritoneal dialysis, and renal transplantation are the cornerstones of the treatment. Albumin (3 to 4 g/kg per day) as 20% solution divided in one to four doses with fursemide 0.5 mg/kg is given through a deep indwelling catheter. The target level of serum albumin is 15 g/L. The recommended daily energy supply is 130 kcal/kg, and the amount of protein in the diet should be at least 4 g/kg per day. Thyroxin substitution is started immediately after birth, and the dosage is adjusted according to the TSH level. To avoid thromboembolic complications, warfarin medication is started at the age of 1 month and the target level of plasma prothrombin time is 20% to 30% of normal. When surgical interventions are necessary, warfarin is stopped and the operations are performed under protection of antithrombin III infusion with a dose of 50 IU/kg. Although the CNF children in the nephrotic phase are prone to serious bacterial infections, no prophylactic use of antibiotics or immunoglobulins are recommended; however, every proven infection should be treated aggressively. Bilateral nephrectomy should be performed when the child has reached the weight of 7 to 10 kg. Before nephrectomy, a peritoneal dialysis catheter is placed and possible hernias are corrected. Dialysis is started with increasing volumes of dialysate. If there are no problems in dialysis, nephrectomy is performed about 2 weeks after the placement of the catheter. After nephrectomy, continuous cyclic peritoneal dialysis (CCPD) is started. Eight to ten exchanges with a filling volume of 30 to 40 ml/kg are performed during the night and one to two manual exchanges during daytime. Heparin 200 to 500 IU should be added in every dialysate batch. Treatment of erythropoietin should be started with a dosage of 50 IU/kg three times per week, later adjusting the dosage according to response. If necessary, alfacalcidol pulse therapy by mouth is started to prevent hyperparathyroidism. Episodes of bacterial peritonitis are treated with intraperitoneal vancomycin and netilmycin for a few days. Renal transplantation should not be performed until the child has been receiving dialysis at least for 2 months. Standard immunosuppressive treatment with three drugs should be started already before and during the operation with azathioprine, methylprednisolone, and cyclosporine. Anti-CMV (cytomegalovirus) immunoglobulin is given for 4 months for those who have received a graft from a CMV-positive donor. Trimethoprim-sulfamethoxazole prophylaxis is given through the first year after transplantation. The 5-year patient survival of Finnish CNF patients has been 98%, and graft survival has been 82%. Most children have had a distinct catch-up growth after transplantation. Of 43 children, 7 have needed growth hormone therapy. Of 43 Finnish CNF children, 9 have developed posttransplant NS, which is clearly a higher proportion than seen in children transplanted for reasons other than CNF. In no case did the pathologic findings in the graft include typical features of CNF. Therefore this NS after transplantation cannot be regarded as a recurrence of the original disease. In most Finnish CNF patients, infection with CMV or Epstein-Barr virus (EBV) has preceded the development of posttransplantation NS. The histopathologic findings in the diseased graft have been comparable with those seen in adult transplantation patients with previous CMV infection. The best results in the treatment of posttransplantation nephrotic syndrome have been achieved with combination therapy with methylprednisolone and cyclophosphamide.

Antenatal Diagnosis

In CNF pregnancies, AFP content is invariably increased in the amniotic fluid since the early weeks of gestation. Thus determination of amniotic fluid AFP is found be a useful tool in prediction of CNF fetus in risk families. Also, maternal serum AFP content is usually high when the mother is bearing a CNF fetus. Screening of maternal serum AFP has been performed in some areas in Finland, where the prevalence of CNF is high. When maternal serum AFP is higher than normal, the amniocentesis has been done to confirm the high content of AFP in the amniotic fluid. However, maternal serum AFP is not elevated in all CNF pregnancies, and it may also be high when a mother is bearing a healthy heterozygous CNF fetus. Because the AFP based method is an indirect indication of fetal CNF and carries a risk of both false-negative and false-positive results, it seems obvious that methods of molecular genetics will soon replace the determination AFP in maternal serum and amniotic fluid in the prenatal diagnosis of CNF in Finland. However, in the families with unknown mutations of NPHS1, the identification of the possible CNF fetus is still based on the determination AFP content in the amniotic fluid.

DIFFUSE MESANGIAL SCLEROSIS

Diffuse mesangial sclerosis (DMS) is a clinicopathologic entity with typical renal histology, early appearance of NS, and rapid progression to end-stage renal failure (ESRF). Autosomal-recessive inheritance is suspected because familial occurrence of DMS is not infrequent and it is equally seen in both sexes. NS is sometimes already seen at birth or a few months later. However, the great majority of the children with DMS have had the onset of their disease after the first year of life. Usually, the first sign of nephropathy is proteinuria often associated with hematuria. Full-blown NS develops later and is not seen in every patient with DMS. The protein leakage into urine is usually less than that seen in CNF. Soon after onset of proteinuria, the glomerular filtration rate (GFR) decreases rapidly, leading to ESRF within a few weeks to some years. Arterial hypertension is almost a constant finding. DMS children may have miscellaneous additional signs such as nystagmus, cataract, myopia, mental retardation, muscular dystrophy, cardiac arrhythmia, or dysmorphic facies. Renal pathology is characteristic in DMS, but it appears that the pathologic lesions of DMS cover a wider spectrum of congenital renal diseases than the solitary form of DMS. In the early phase, the glomerular mesangium is expanded by an increase of fibrillary matrix, and podocytes show hypertrophy. In the more advanced, diagnostic phase, the GBM is thickened and the mesangial cells are embedded in the abundant PAS-positive fibrillar matrix. The capillary lumens disappear due to mesangial expansion, and the glomeruli look like solidified globules within slightly dilated urinary space. There is no cellular proliferation in the DMS glomeruli, but a single layer of large podocytes looks like a corona around the shrunken tufts. There is often a corticomedullary gradient of the sclerotic glomeruli, the deepest glomeruli being the least affected. In electron microscopy, the

GBM is multilayered, wavy, and thickened. The mesangial matrix contains filaments and collagenlike fibrils. In immunofluorescence studies, deposits of IgM, C1q, and C3 in the glomeruli have been seen occasionally, but most authors agree that DMS is not a immune complex–mediated disease. Tubulointerstitial lesions include atrophic and dilated tubules and interstitial fibrosis with inflammation. The tubular dilation is not as extensive as that in CNF. DMS is resistant to steroids and other immunosuppressive agents. Thus the treatment of DMS is principally the same as for CNF. Because the proteinuria is not so heavy as seen in CNF, the need of albumin substitution may be less. Most patients need antihypertensive treatment. Nephrectomy is not mandatory if the urinary protein leakage is not heavy and the blood pressure is under control.

MALFORMATION SYNDROMES

Denys-Drash syndrome (DDS) is characterized by a triad of ambiguous genitals, progressive nephropathy, and Wilms' tumor. It is caused by a mutation in the WT1 gene, which is a tumor suppressor gene located in p13 of chromosome 11. DDS children carry a single germline mutation of the zinc finger domain of the WT1 gene. A great majority of children have ambiguous external genitals or female phenotype, but most of them have male genotype. True hermaphroditism is rare. The average age of the appearance of nephropathy is 1.4 years, with a range of 0.01 to 17 years. The first sign of nephropathy is proteinuria, which does not always lead to NS. Hypertension is common. Nephropathy leads to ESRF at the age of 2 years on average. Among those DDS children who have died of renal failure, the age at death has ranged from 1 month to 7 years. Usually, Wilms' tumor is found before the age of 2 years, but it may be manifested as late as in the second decade of life. Not all DDS children have developed Wilms' tumor during the observation time. The pathologic changes in DDS kidneys are similar to those of DMS. It has been speculated that some DMS children without Wilms' tumor may present an abortive form of DDS. The therapy of DDS consists control of hypertension, bilateral nephrectomy, dialysis, and renal transplantation.

Galloway-Mowat syndrome (GMS) consists of congenital microcephaly, mental retardation, and NS. It is fatal within the first 3 years of life. It is regarded to be inherited in autosomal-recessive trait. Renal histopathology is identical with that of DMS.

SECONDARY NEPHROTIC SYNDROMES

Early-onset NS secondary to perinatal infection is rare. It has been described in connection with congenital syphilis, toxoplasmosis, rubella, and CMV infection. The clinical picture has varied from proteinuria to full-blown NS. Congenital syphilis is often associated with membranous glomerulonephritis combined with interstitial nephritis, showing lymphocytes and plasma cells. It is a rare example of immune complex–mediated glomerulonephritis in the newborn. Congenital syphilis is successfully treated with penicillin. The pathologic changes in congenital CMV, toxoplasmosis, and rubella are variable. Showing the presence of the typical inclusion bodies in the renal biopsy sample confirms the diagnosis of CMV infection. Nephropathy associated with human immunodeficiency virus (HIV) or hepatitis B infection is rarely manifested in early infancy, but some occasional cases have been reported. Lupus nephritis is usually seen in older children and adults, but some cases of lupus nephritis have been seen at the age of few months.

IDIOPATHIC NEPHROTIC SYNDROME

Idiopathic NS rarely manifests in early infancy. It is a group with variable renal pathology and clinical course. MCNS has been reported to appear under the age of 1 year and even in newborns. Some patients with MCNS respond to steroids and cytotoxic agents, whereas others do not, having a less favorable prognosis than seen in MCNS appearing in later age. Patients with focal segmental glomerular sclerosis (FSGS) may have the onset of their disease under the age of 1 year. About half of the described cases have responded to immunosuppressive treatment, whereas others have developed ESRF during the first or second decade of life. Infantile NS with diffuse mesangial proliferation is not a homogenous group. Some have mesangial deposits of immunoglobulin, and the response to steroid therapy is variable.

DIFFERENTIAL DIAGNOSIS OF THE EARLY-ONSET NEPHROTIC SYNDROME

If NS is manifested at birth and a child has large placenta, normal genitals, and head circumference, there is a strong suspicion of CNF. However, large placenta is a sign of intrauterine onset of the disease and is not exclusively seen in CNF, but it has reported to occur also in connection with intrauterine infection and in congenital forms of DMS and FSGS. If the methods of molecular genetics are available, the presence of a mutation in NPHS1 gene in the DNA sample of the child with congenital NS confirms the diagnosis of CNF. Renal biopsy has not been used for many years in Finland to establish the diagnosis, but elsewhere the renal biopsy may be reasonable if NS is observed in a newborn infant without gross anomalies. If a child has ambiguous genitals and proteinuria DDS is suspected. If the first urine sample is negative for protein, repeated urine samples are necessary in a child with ambiguous genitalia, because the nephropathy in DDS may appear later in life. Galloway-Mowat syndrome is suspected if an infant, in addition to proteinuria, has congenital microcephaly and poor mental development. If NS is observed after birth and a child has no obvious anomalies, DMS, systemic lupus erythematosus, MCNS, or other forms of idiopathic NS are the possibilities. The main difference between CNF and DMS is that in the latter disease, urine contains less protein and the deterioration of renal function is more rapid. Diagnostic renal biopsy is mandatory in NS manifested in infants after the neonatal period.

Selected Readings

Cooperstone BG, Fredman A, Kaplan BS. Galloway-Mowat syndrome of abnormal gyral patterns and glomerulopathy. *Am J Med Genet* 1993;47:250–254.

A report of three patients with GMS and a comprehensive review of findings and associated anomalies in GMS.

Habib R. Nephrotic syndrome in the first year of life. *Pediatr Nephrol* 1993;7:347–353.

A concise overview of congenital and infantile NS with an emphasis on DMS.

Heinonen S, Ryynänen M, Kirkinen P, et al. Prenatal screening for congenital nephrosis in East Finland: Results and impact on the birth prevalence of the disease. *Prenat Diagn* 1996;16:207–213.

The results of a large population based screening for CNF with determination of AFP in maternal serum.

Holmberg C, Antikainen M, Rönnholm K, et al. Management of congenital nephrotic syndrome the Finnish type. *Pediatr Nephrol* 1995;9:87–93.

A comprehensive review of the modern treatment of congenital NS.

Huttunen N-P. Congenital nephrotic syndrome of Finnish type: a study of 75 patients. *Arch Dis Child* 1976;51:344–348.

A report of clinical features and outcome of 75 Finnish CNF patients before the time of modern treatment.

Kestilä M, Lenkkeri U, Männikkö M, et al. Positionally cloned gene for novel glomerular protein-nephrin is mutated in congenital nephrotic syndrome. *Molecular Cell* 1998;1:575–582.

The first report of the cloning of NPHS1 gene and definition of the gene product—nephrin—which is expressed only in glomerular epithelial cells. Two mutations of NPHS1 gene are found in Finnish CNF families.

Laine J, Jalanko H, Holthöfer H, et al. Post-transplantation nephrosis in congenital nephrotic syndrome of Finnish type. *Kidney Int* 1993;44:867–874.

A report of the high frequency of posttransplantation nephrosis in CNF children with a comment of the possible viral etiology of posttransplantation syndrome.

Ljungberg P, Holmberg C, Jalanko H. Infections in infants with congenital nephrosis of the Finnish type. *Pediatr Nephrol* 1997;11:148–152.

A detailed analysis of bacterial and viral infections in CNF children with guidelines to prophylaxis and treatment.

Männikkö M, Kestilä M, Lenkkeri U, et al. Improved prenatal diagnosis of the Finnish type based on DNA analysis. *Kidney Int* 1997;51: 868–872.

A good report on how to confirm the diagnosis of homozygous CNF fetus or healthy heterozygous CNF fetus in the case of elevated amniotic fluid AFP.

Mueller RF. The Denys-Drash syndrome. *J Med Genet* 1994;31:471–477.

A good review of clinical features, karyotypes, and genetics in DDS.

Rapola J, Sariola H, Ekblom P. Pathology of fetal congenital nephrosis: immunohistochemical and ultrastructural studies. *Kidney Int* 1984;25:701–707.

The results of this study confirms that CNF has an intrauterine onset.

Ruotsalainen V, Ljungberg P, Wortiovaara J, et al. Nephrin is specially located at the slit membrane of glomerular podocytes. *Proc Natl Acad Sci USA* 1999;96:7962–7967.

This study shows that the product of NPHS1 gene is located at the slit membrane between the foot processes of glomerular podocytes.

PART 6
Other Heredofamilial Diseases

Richard J. Glassock

A multitude of hereditary or familial disorders may be associated with glomerular lesions, tubular dysfunction, or derangements in the structure of the renal parenchyma manifested as cysts, dysplasia, or hypoplasia. The disorders of tubular function are discussed in Chapter 23, the cystic diseases of the kidney in Chapter 46, and many of the glomerular disorders in various other chapters of this book. This discussion deals with those heredofamilial diseases with major or predominant glomerular involvement that have not been discussed elsewhere in this book. Table 43.9 provides a comprehensive list of the heredofamilial diseases associated with glomerular lesions.

DISEASES WITH AUTOSOMAL-DOMINANT INHERITANCE

Diseases with autosomal-dominant inheritance include Alport syndrome (Part 2 of this chapter), nail-patella syndrome (Part 4), Muckle-Wells syndrome of systemic amyloidosis, Ostertag amyloid nephropathy, neuropathic forms of systemic amyloidosis, hereditary osteolysis with glomerulonephritis, and some forms of benign hematuria with thin glomerular basement membrane.

Hereditary Amyloidosis

Muckle-Wells Syndrome

The clinical manifestations of Muckle-Wells syndrome appear in early adolescence or adulthood. The patients display a recurring urticarial eruption accompanied by a fever, malaise, and limb pains. They all have sensory neural deafness. Deposition of amyloid in the basement membranes of glomeruli and tubules is regularly seen and leads to proteinuria, nephrotic syndrome, and chronic renal failure.

Ostertag Amyloid Nephropathy

Ostertag amyloid nephropathy is characterized by the development of hematuria, proteinuria, and hepatosplenomegaly in early adult life. The clinical course is progressive, leading to uremia in the fourth to sixth decade of life. Extensive glomerular, hepatic, splenic, and adrenal amyloid deposits are found. Some of the deposits are associated with foam cells and giant cells.

Neuropathic Forms of Familial Amyloidosis

Neuropathic forms of familial amyloidosis may also be characterized by significant renal involvement. The *Portuguese type* is seen in the third and fourth decade of life and is associated with a sensory neuropathy beginning in the lower extremities leading to loss of sensation of pain, temperature, and position. Autonomic dysfunction with impotence, orthostatic hypotension, hypohidrosis, and disordered gastrointestinal motility may occur. Amyloid deposition is more predominant in the interstitium and tubules than in the glomeruli. The patients may have proteinuria. Nephrotic syndrome and uremia do not occur. In the *Swedish variety,* the neurologic manifestations are similar to those described for the Portuguese type except that genitourinary abnormalities are more frequent. Urinary retention and hematuria may develop secondary to bladder involvement. Proteinuria secondary to glomerular amyloidosis occurs, but renal failure is rare. In the *Finnish type,* lattice dystrophy of the cornea, cranial neuropathy, and thickening of the skin occur. Mild proteinuria may be present, but nephrotic syndrome and renal failure are distinctly unusual. *Amyloid neuropathy with peptic ulcer (Iowa variety)* is evidenced by shooting pains and weakness of the lower extremities. Later, the disease progresses to involve the upper extremities and autonomic nervous system. Duodenal ulcer is frequently found. Deafness and cataracts may also develop. Renal failure is common. Urinalysis reveals moderate proteinuria, hematuria, and leukocyturia. Nephrotic syndrome does not occur.

Hereditary Osteolysis with Nephropathy

Hereditary osteolysis with glomerulonephritis is characterized by the development of acute inflammation of the wrist and ankles in childhood. Later, progressive sclerosis and lysis of the involved bones lead to severe joint deformities. Hypertension, chronic progressive glomerulonephritis with nephrotic syndrome, and amyloidosis may ensue.

Familial, Recurrent, Benign Hematuria

Some patients with familial, recurrent, benign hematuria may have extensive attenuation ("thinning") of the glomerular basement membranes demonstrated by ultrastructural analysis of renal biopsy material, that is, thin basement membrane nephropathy (see Chapter 39, Part 11). It is possible that these patients represent variants of Alport syndrome, because identical or very similar lesions have been described in patients with the typical extrarenal manifestations of Alport syndrome. Both autosomal-dominant and autosomal-recessive modes of inheritance have been suggested for this disorder.

Diseases with Autosomal-Recessive Inheritance

Diseases with autosomal-recessive inheritance include familial Mediterranean fever, congenital nephrotic syndrome, diffuse mesangial sclerosis, lecithin-cholesterol acyltransferase

TABLE 43.9. Heredofamilial Diseases with Predominant Glomerular Involvement[a]

Disease	Mode of Inheritance	Major Manifestations: Renal	Major Manifestations: Extrarenal
Alport syndrome (Chapter 43, Part 2)	X-Linked or autosomal dominant with variable penetrance	Hematuria, chronic renal failure	Deafness, lenticonus, thrombocytopenia, leiomyomata
Fabry's disease (Chapter 43, Part 3)	X-linked	Hematuria, proteinuria, chronic renal failure	Angiokeratoma, acroparesthesia, corneal opacities, coronary artery disease
Nail-patella syndrome (Chapter 43, Part 4)	Autosomal dominant, ABO-linked	Proteinuria, chronic renal failure	Onychodysplasia, iliac horns, absence of patella
Amyloidosis (Chapter 42, Part 10)			
Familial Mediterranean fever	Autosomal recessive[b]	Nephrotic syndrome, chronic renal failure	Periodic fever, serositis, arthritis, rash
Muckle-Wells syndrome	Autosomal dominant	Proteinuria, chronic renal failure	Deafness, urticaria, fever acroparesthesias
Neuropathic forms (Portuguese, Swedish, Finnish, with ulcer)	Autosomal dominant	Proteinuria, chronic renal failure	Peripheral neuropathy, peptic ulcer
Congenital nephrotic syndrome (Chapter 43, Part 5)	Autosomal recessive	Nephrotic syndrome, chronic renal failure	Polycythemia, enlarged placenta
Diabetes mellitus types I and II	Polygenic type I linked to HLA, type II not linked to HLA	Nephrotic syndrome, hypertension, chronic renal failure	Retinopathy, neuropathy, peripheral vascular disease
Sickle cell disease	Autosomal, intermediate	Proteinuria, chronic renal failure, nephrogenic diabetes insipidus, renal tubular acidosis, hyperkalemia	Painful crisis, hemolytic anemia, bilirubin gallbladder stones
Lecithin-cholesterol acyltransferase deficiency	Autosomal recessive	Hematuria, proteinuria	Deafness, corneal opacities, splenomegaly, absent serum α-lipoprotein, hypertriglyceridemia
Partial lipodystrophy (Barraquer-Simons disease)	Autosomal recessive or sporadic	Nephrotic syndrome, chronic renal failure	Loss of subcutaneous fat in face and limbs only, diabetes mellitus, hirsutism
Benign hematuria with thin glomerular basement membrane	Autosomal dominant or recessive	Recurrent hematuria	None
Hereditary osteolysis	Autosomal dominant	Hematuria, proteinuria	Acute arthralgias, wrist and ankle deformities
Imerslund's syndrome (selective malabsorption of vitamin B_{12})	Autosomal recessive	Proteinuria	Megaloblastic anemia
Charcot-Marie-Tooth disease	Autosomal recessive	Proteinuria, nephrotic syndrome	Peripheral neuropathy with atrophy of muscle of feet, deafness
α_1-Antitrypsin deficiency	Autosomal, intermediate	Hematuria, proteinuria	Emphysema
Laurence-Moon-Bardet-Biedl syndrome	Autosomal recessive	Proteinuria, nephrotic syndrome, chronic renal failure	Retinitis pigmentosa, obesity, mental retardation, hypogonadism, polydactyly
Jeune's syndrome	Autosomal recessive	Proteinuria, chronic renal failure, proximal tubular dysfunction	Constriction of thorax, short limbs
Cystinosis	Autosomal recessive	Proteinuria, chronic renal failure, Fanconi syndrome	Growth retardation, rickets, photophobia, decreased skin pigmentation, blood hair
Von Gierke's disease	Autosomal recessive	Proteinuria, chronic renal failure	Hepatomegaly, hypoglycemia, hyperuricemia, lactic acidosis

[a] Only the major and extrarenal manifestations are listed. For further details, refer to the appropriate part of this chapter (in parentheses).
[b] Common in Sephardic Jews, Armenians, and other inhabitants of the Mediterranean basin.

deficiency, partial lipodystrophy, Imerslund's syndrome, Charcot-Marie-Tooth disease, Laurence-Moon-Bardet-Biedl syndrome, Jeune's syndrome, and cystinosis.

Familial Mediterranean Fever

Familial Mediterranean fever is characterized by recurring episodes of serosal inflammation and is inherited as a single gene recessive trait. The responsible gene, MEFV, is located on the short arm of chromosome 16. It encodes a 781–amino acid protein called *pyrin* or *marenostin,* which is expressed exclusively on neutrophils. The gene product regulates transcription of peptides involved in inflammation. Multiple missense mutations of the gene are responsible for informational changes in the protein. The M694V mutation affects mainly North African Jews. Ashkenazi Jews, Druze, and Arminicius predominantly have the V72A mutation associated with mild disease. A C52/IL-8 deficiency may be present in some patients.

Familial Mediterranean fever is commonly associated with systemic amyloidosis. Renal involvement with extensive amyloid deposits in glomeruli and arterioles contributes in a major way to the morbidity and mortality of this disorder. It occurs predominantly in inhabitants of the Mediterranean basin, including Sephardic Jews, Armenians, and Arabs. Renal amyloidosis is very common in Sephardic Jews but uncommon in Armenians. The principal clinical manifestations are recurring, self-limited, unpredictable episodes of fever, serositis, arthritis, and an erysipeloid rash. Pericarditis is uncommon, but peritonitis and pleuritis are frequent. Hepatosplenomegaly, macroglossia, neuropathy, and cutaneous and cardiac involvement are rare. Gastrointestinal involvement may lead to malabsorption. Nephrotic syndrome and progressive renal failure are the usual clinical manifestations of the renal involvement. Most patients develop uremia before the age of 40 years. Colchicine (0.6 mg two or three times per day) definitely decreases the frequency of the episodes but is of little value in the treatment of an attack. Prophylactic use of colchicine also impedes the development of amyloidosis. Institution of dialysis treatment for the management of uremia in these patients is associated with a reduction in the frequency of the attacks.

Lecithin-Cholesterol Acyltransferase Deficiency

This autosomal-recessive disorder is caused by a genetic defect on the long arm of chromosome 16 causing a deficiency of the enzyme lecithin-cholesterol acetyltransferase. The enzyme catalyzes the conversion of lecithin and cholesterol to lysolecithin and cholesterol esters. Thus patients with deficiency of this enzyme have decreased plasma levels of cholesterol esters and lysolecithin and elevated plasma levels of unesterified cholesterol and lecithin. Hypertriglyceridemia is found, and the pre- and pre-1 bands in lipoprotein electrophoresis are greatly reduced or absent. Differences in the size and in apoprotein and lipid composition of very-low-, low-, and high-density lipoproteins are also observed. Clinical features include corneal deposits of lipids, normocytic, normochromic anemia with target cells, and occasionally splenomegaly. The anemia is due to hemolysis and inadequate erythropoiesis. "Sea blue" histiocytes are found in the bone marrow. Premature atherosclerosis and hyperuricemia are other features. Some patients have very high antistreptolysin O titers (greater than 50,000 Todd units/ml) when sheep erythrocytes are used but normal values with rabbit erythrocytes. The renal manifestations include hematuria, proteinuria, and slowly progressive renal failure. The renal lesion consists of foamy endothelial cells in glomeruli and progressive fibrosis and hyalinization of glomerular capillaries (see Atlas of Renal Pathology, Chapter 109). Plasma infusions may transiently correct the enzymatic defect; a low dietary fat intake is recommended. Renal transplantation has no effect on the enzyme deficiency but provides satisfactory treatment for the renal failure.

Partial Lipodystrophy

Also known as the *Barraquer-Simons disease,* partial lipodystrophy is characterized by the loss of subcutaneous fat of the face, upper arms, and trunk but normal fat distribution elsewhere in the body. Females are affected more than males. The onset of the disease is usually in childhood or adolescence. The disorder may appear after an infectious illness. Some patients may develop insulin-dependent or insulin-resistant diabetes mellitus, hepatomegaly, hyperpigmentation, hyperlipidemia, hirsutism, or acanthosis nigricans. The predominant finding of nephrologic interest is the association of this disorder with membranoproliferative glomerulonephritis and hypocomplementemia. Many patients with partial lipodystrophy have diminished serum C3 component of complement levels but normal C1q, C4, and C2. These patients also have a circulating IgG autoantibody to the C3-converting enzyme of the alternative pathway of complement activation. The glomerular lesion most frequently encountered is membranoproliferative glomerulonephritis type II or dense deposit disease (see Chapter 39, Part 7). A few patients have type I membranoproliferative glomerulonephritis. Several patients have been described in whom the hypocomplementemia has been present without overt clinical manifestation of glomerulonephritis. Renal biopsy in a few of the latter groups of patients has revealed pathologic lesions of dense deposit disease. The nature of the association between lipodystrophy and hypocomplementemia is not known. However, the hypocomplementemia may predispose to glomerulonephritis by altering the defense mechanism for the control of chronic infections or by interfering with normal clearance mechanisms of immune complexes.

Cystinosis

Cystinosis is the result of a generalized storage of cystine throughout the body tissues. The biochemical defect underlying this abnormality is unknown but is associated with an abnormality in transporting cystine out of liposomes. In the *infantile* form of the disease, the predominant clinical manifestations are growth retardation, rickets, metabolic acidosis, Fanconi's syndrome, and polyuria secondary to an acquired defect in urinary concentrating ability. Most patients have blond hair, fair complexion, and photophobia. The erythrocyte sedimentation rate is markedly elevated. Hypothyroidism may be present. Crystals of cystine in the cornea can be found by slit-lamp examination. Crystals of cystine may also be found in the circulating leukocytes and bone marrow cells. Cystinuria and renal cystine stones do not occur. Although tubular abnormalities dominate the early clinical picture, glomerular disease eventually ensues, causing proteinuria and progressive renal failure. Some patients may have the clinical manifestations delayed until adolescent or adult life. In the *adult form* of the disease, tubular abnormalities may be mild, whereas glomerular lesions may dominate the renal involvement. The renal pathology consists of cystine deposition in tubules, interstitium, and glomerular epithelial cells. Atrophy of the proximal tubule may be found (swan neck deformity). Epithelial alterations in the glomeruli may be associated with focal and segmental glomerulosclerosis and giant cell formation. Nephrotic syndrome may ensue. Infantile forms are treated with fluids, alkali, phosphate, and vitamin D replacement. Cysteamine may be useful. Favorable results have been obtained by renal transplantations for patients with cystinosis who developed uremia. Cystine crystals have been found in the mesangium and interstitium of the transplanted kidney.

Other Disorders

Imerslund's syndrome consists of selective malabsorption of vitamin B_{12} leading to the development of megaloblastic anemia in infancy. Nonnephrotic proteinuria is the principal renal abnormality. The underlying renal lesion is not well defined. Treatment is with parenteral administration of vitamin B_{12}.

Charcot-Marie-Tooth disease is a slowly progressive peripheral neuropathy involving the feet and hands. Glomerular disease may evoke proteinuria and nephrotic syndrome. The presence of deafness suggests a relation to Alport syndrome. The glomerular tubulointerstitial pathology is not distinctive and consists of tubular atrophy, interstitial fibrosis, and thickening of the glomerular capillary wall.

Laurence-Moon-Bardet-Biedl syndrome is characterized by retinitis pigmentosa, obesity, hypogonadism, mental retardation, and polydactyly. A variety of renal abnormalities occur, including medullary cystic disease, renal hypoplasia, nephrosclerosis, and glomerulonephritis. The latter chiefly consists of focal segmental glomerulosclerosis. Proteinuria with progressive renal failure is common.

Jeune's syndrome consists of severe deformities of the thorax, leading to marked and progressive respiratory distress, short limbs, and developmental abnormalities of the pelvis. Defects of proximal tubular dysfunction may lead to Fanconi's syndrome. Glomerular involvement has varied in severity, but several patients have developed lesions similar to focal segmental glomerulosclerosis with nephrotic syndrome. In other patients, the disease has resembled medullary cystic disease or infantile polycystic disease.

Von Gierke's disease (glycogen storage disease type I) is a disorder characterized by a deficiency of glucose-6-phosphate dehydrogenase. It may be associated with chronic renal failure caused by progressive focal segmental glomerulosclerosis. Patients demonstrate hepatomegaly, hypoglycemia, hyperuricemia, short stature, lactic acidosis, platelet dysfunction, xanthomas, and perimacular retinal lesions. It is inherited in autosomal-recessive fashion. Renal lesions are consistent with glycogen storage in renal tubules, renal and glomerular enlargement, and focal sclerosis. A form of "hyperfiltration" injury is thought to be responsible for renal disease. Overproduction of urate may lead to hyperuricemic nephropathy. *Gaucher's disease, Refsum's disease,* and other rare sphingolipidoses may very uncommonly be associated with renal abnormalities presumably due to lipid accumulation in renal tissue.

DISEASES WITH OTHER FORMS OF INHERITANCE

Other forms of inherited diseases include those that are transmitted with X-linked, autosomal intermediate or polygenic modes of inheritance. Among those with X-linked inheritance are Alport syndrome (Chapter 43, Part 2) and Fabry's disease (Chapter 43, Part 3); sickle cell disease (Chapter 43, Part 4) and α_1-antitrypsin deficiency are examples of autosomal intermediate modes of inheritance. Diabetes mellitus has a polygenic basis of inheritance. Concordance in identical twins for type I diabetes mellitus is approximately 50%, whereas for type II diabetes mellitus concordance is nearly complete.

α_1-Antitrypsin deficiency is present in patients who are homozygous for the Pi^z allele of the α_1-antitrypsin protein. This deficiency leads to an imbalance in the protease-antiprotease activity in the body. In the lungs, this deficiency leads to emphysema. Also, for poorly understood reasons, this deficiency may cause cirrhosis of the liver. In several patients, necrotizing vasculitis or membranoproliferative glomerulonephritis have been associated with the Pi^z allele.

ASSOCIATION OF GLOMERULAR DISEASES WITH THE MAJOR HISTOCOMPATIBILITY COMPLEX

The major histocompatibility complex contains genetic loci that determine the synthesis of discrete antigenic glycoproteins on the surface of mammalian nucleated cells (see Chapter 86). Some of the genes at this locus play a central role in the immune response to environmental agents and to normal or altered autologous tissue antigens. It is not surprising, therefore, that associations should exist between immunologically mediated glomerular diseases and antigens determined by genes of the major histocompatibility complex, namely the human leukocyte antigens (HLA). Table 43.10 lists the reported associations between HLA and human glomerular diseases. In many circumstances, the relative risk of developing a glomerular disease

TABLE 43-10. Glomerulopathies Associated with Human Leukocyte Antigens

Disorder	HLA	Relative Risk[a]
Systemic lupus	DR2	3
erythematosus	DR3	3 to 6
(Caucasian)	B8	2.1
	B5	1.7
Systemic lupus	A10, A25,	
erythematosus	B18, DR2	
with C2 deficiency	haplotype	
Goodpasture's disease	DR2	13.1
	B18, B7	
Henoch-Schönlein purpura	Bw35	4.9
Rheumatoid arthritis	B27	1.7
	DR4	
Ankylosing spondylitis	B27	
Caucasian		87.4
Jewish		109.5
Japanese		324.5
Sjögren's syndrome	DR3	9.7
	B8	3.2
Sarcoidosis with arthritis	B8	13.5
Penicillamine- or gold-		
induced nephropathy	DR3	32.0
Diabetes mellitus, type I	DR3	5.7
(insulin-dependent)	DR4	2.8
Acute streptococcal	B12	3.4
glomerulonephritis		
Minimal change disease,		
steroid-responsive		
With atopy	B12	27.7
	DR4	2.9
Without atopy	B8, B7	2.9
Membranous glomerulopathy	DR3 (Caucasian)	12.0
	DR2 (Oriental)	3.0
	B18, BfF1	
Focal sclerosis	DR4	3.0
IgA nephropathy	Bw35	4.3
	DR4	4.0
Membranoproliferative	"B cell antigen"	
glomerulonephritis	B7	

[a] Relative risk higher than 1 indicates that the frequency of the antigen is increased in patients with the disease. The value of the relative risk indicates how many times more frequently the disease occurs in a group of individuals carrying the antigen relative to a group lacking the antigen.

in an individual positive for a given HLA is increased by a factor of two to five. An example of an exception to this generalization is the HLA-DR2–positive individual, who has a 13.1 times greater chance of developing Goodpasture's disease than an HLA-DR2–negative individual.

Selected Readings

Cohen AH, Adler SG. Nail patella syndrome, lipodystrophy, Fabry disease and familial lecithin cholesterol acyl transferase deficiency. In: Tisher CC, Brenner BM, eds. *Renal pathology,* 2nd ed. Philadelphia: JB Lippincott, 1994:1267–1291.
An excellent overview with an emphasis on pathology.

Hors J, Gony J. HLA and disease. *Adv Nephrol* 1986;15:329–351.
A compendium of information on the association of HLA antigens with disease.

Rees AJ. The HLA complex and susceptibility to glomerulonephritis. *Plasma Ther Transf Tech* 1984;5:455–570.
A discussion of the association between various glomerulonephritides and HLA complex.

Samuels J, Aksentijevich I, Torosyan Y. Familial Mediterranean fever at the millennium. Clinical spectrum, ancient mutations, and a survey of 100 American referrals to the National Institutes of Health. *Medicine* 1998;77:268–288.
A comprehensive review of the genetics and the clinical findings of familial Mediterranean fever.

Schneider J, Lovell H, Calhoun F. Update on nephropathic cystinosis. *Pediatr Nephrol* 1990;4:645–653.
A good review of renal involvement in cystinosis.

PART 7
Other Congenital Disorders

Richard J. Glassock and Shaul G. Massry

Congenital abnormalities of the kidney and urinary tract arise as a consequence of maldevelopment during embryogenesis. They occur either in association with other developmental derangements or as an isolated defect. Certain clinical features may suggest the presence of a congenital urogenital abnormality; examples are a single umbilical artery, a transverse palmar crease, and abnormal facial features (Potter facies) consisting of hypertelorism, curved nose, receding chin, and low-set ears.

Although all hereditary abnormalities may also be regarded as congenital, rarely are the congenital defects hereditary. The various congenital abnormalities of the kidney and the urinary tract are listed in Table 43.11. There are also genetic and heredofamilial disorders associated with malformations involving the kidney and urinary tract, as listed in Table 43.12.

KIDNEY ABNORMALITIES

Agenesis

Bilateral agenesis of the kidneys is incompatible with life, although infants born at term with this abnormality may survive for a brief period. Potter facies and pulmonary hypoplasia are frequently found. The ureters and a portion of the bladder also fail to develop. *Unilateral agenesis* of the kidney often escapes detection in childhood and is most often discovered accidentally during adulthood. The normal kidney shows hypertrophy. Some reports have suggested that the longstanding hyperperfusion of the normal kidney may evoke proteinuria, hypertension, and progressive focal segmental glomerulosclerosis. The ureter and a portion of normal, but the volumes of the individual glomeruli are 7 to 10 times normal. A diffuse form of interstitial fibrosis is also present. The urogenital system is normal. This congenital abnormality is more common in boys than in girls. Renal insufficiency is usually present at birth and progresses to end-stage renal failure by the end of the first decade of life (age 10 to 12 years). Polyuria, polydipsia, and episodes of dehydration may be the first clinical features that bring these individuals to medical attention. The signs and symptoms may include failure to thrive, vomiting, hypothermia, azotemia, metabolic acidosis, salt wasting, growth retardation, and osteodystrophy. Hypertension and proteinuria are present, and hematuria is usually absent.

Segmental Hypoplasia (Ask-Upmark Kidney)

Segmental hypoplasia was first described by Ask-Upmark in 1929 in six young children with severe hypertension. Since then, numerous reports have confirmed the initial observations and emphasized the importance of this congenital abnormality as a cause of hypertension in children and adolescents. Girls are affected more than boys.

The disorder is usually recognized during an investigation for the cause of hypertension and/or renal insufficiency. Intravenous urography reveals unilateral hypoplasia affecting both the cortex and medulla of a segment of the kidney at either pole or between the poles, and the calyces draining the involved area appear abnormal (swallow tail abnormality). Computed axial tomography or radionuclide imaging confirms the presence of segmental renal hypoplasia. The renal angiogram shows normal and patent renal arteries with size and luminal diameter proportional to the renal mass. Increased renin production from the hypoplastic segments may be documented by selective renal venous sampling in some cases. The degree of renal insufficiency correlates with the extent of the renal tissue involved.

Pathologically, the hypoplastic areas appear as notches or cavities at the outer border of the kidney. The hypoplastic area of the kidney is clearly demarcated from the normal renal tissue. The glomeruli in the hypoplastic segment are small, poorly

TABLE 43.11. Congenital Abnormalities of Kidney and Urinary Tract

Kidney abnormalities
Agenesis
Bilateral
Unilateral
Hypoplasia
Oligomeganephronia
Segmental hypoplasia (Ask-Upmark kidney)
Ectopia
Simple
Crossed
Horseshoe kidney
Urinary tract abnormalities
Ureteric
Atresia and agenesis
Duplication
Ectopic
Ureterocele
Vesicoureteral reflux
Bladder
Urachus
Exstrophy
Urethra
Valves
Hypospadias

TABLE 43.12. Genetic and Heredofamilial Disorders with Malformations Involving the Kidney and Urinary Tract

Condition/Syndrome[a]	Major Extrarenal Manifestations	Major Renal/Urogenital Anomalies
Chromosomal abnormalities		
Trisomy 18	Multiple congenital anomalies	Horseshoe kidney Renal agenesis Ectopic kidney
Trisomy 21	Down's syndrome	Renal dysplasia
Trisomy 13	Multiple congenital anomalies	Adult polycystic kidney Glomerular cysts
Trisomy 8 (Warkany syndrome)	Mental retardation Destructive facies Vertebral anomalies Destructive toes	Obstructive uropathy
Trisomy 9	Multiple congenital anomalies	Microcystic disease
Sex-chromosome (Ullrich-Turner) syndrome	Ovarian dysplasia Webbed neck	Duplication of ureters Malrotation Horseshoe kidney
Syndromes of cerebral malformations and renal dysplasia (genetic transmission)		
Goldston syndrome (autosomal recessive)	Defect in vermis Dandy-Walker malformation	Cystic dysplasia
Miranda syndrome (autosomal recessive)	Severe CNS abnormalities Intrahepatic fibroductal proliferation	Cystic dysplasia
Ivemark's syndrome (autosomal recessive)	Hepatic and pancreatic dysplasia Central nervous system abnormalities	Cystic dysplasia
Tuberous sclerosis (autosomal dominant)	Epilepsy Mental retardation Angiofibroma Intracerebral calcifications	Hamartoma of kidney Adult polycystic kidney disease
Von Hippel-Lindau disease (autosomal dominant)	Reticial angiomata Cerebellar tumors Pancreatic cysts	Renal cysts resembling adult polycystic kidney disease Hypernephroma
Meckel's syndrome (autosomal recessive)	Central nervous system malformation Cleft palate Heart disease Adrenal hypoplasia Pseudohermaphroditism	Renal hypoplasia or dysplasia with cysts
Lissencephaly syndrome	Smooth brain surface Microcephaly Polydactyly Corneal clouding	Renal agenesis Cystic dysplasia
Zellweger's cerebrohepatorenal syndrome (autosomal recessive)	Central nervous system abnormalities Pear-shaped head Severe hypotonia Liver disease Hemisclerosis	Multicystic kidney
Smith-Lemli-Opitz syndrome (autosomal recessive)	Microcephaly Mental retardation Incomplete development of external genitalia	Cystic dysplasia and renal hypoplasia
Syndromes of musculoskeletal and connective tissue abnormalities and mental dysplasia		
Ehlers-Danlos syndrome (autosomal dominant, recessive, and X-linked locus)	Multiple cutaneous hyperelasticity	Multiple cysts
Schwartz-Jampel syndrome (autosomal recessive)	Myotonia Blepharophimosis	Micromulticystic kidney
Jeune's syndrome (asphyxiating thoracic dystrophy)	Constricted thorax Short limbs	Fanconi syndrome Cystic dysplasia Focal glomerulosclerosis
Orodigitofacial syndrome (X-linked)	Cleft tongue and palate	Polycystic kidney disease
Chondrodysplasia punctata, rhizomelic type (autosomal recessive)	Severe symmetric shortness of humerus and femora Microcephaly	Micromulticystic kidney
Short-rib polydactyly syndrome (SRP), *Majewski* type (autosomal recessive)	Lethal dwarfism Polydactyly Short ribs	Cystic dysplasia
SRP syndrome, *Saldino-Noonan* type (autosomal recessive)	Thoracic dystrophy Polydactyly Metaphyseal dysplasia	Cystic dysplastic kidney
Elejade syndrome (autosomal recessive)	Gigantism Hexadactyly Acrocephaly Thick skin	Bilateral cystic dysplasia

TABLE 43.12. Genetic and Heredofamilial Disorders with Malformations Involving the Kidney and Urinary Tract—*cont'd.*

Condition/Syndromea	Major Extrarenal Manifestations	Major Renal/Urogenital Anomalies
Other syndromes		
Kallmann syndrome (autosomal recessive)	Anosmia Hypogonadotrophic hypogonadism	Renal agenesis
Renal-retinal dysplasia (autosomal recessive)	Retinal blindness Hepatic fibrosis Iminoglycemia	Cystic dysplasia Medullary cystic disease
Laurence-Moon-Bardet-Biedl syndrome (autosomal recessive)	Retinitis pigmentosa Obesity Mental retardation Hypogonadism Polydactyly	Focal glomerulosclerosis Medullary cysts Renal hypoplasia
Torticollis, keloids, and cryptorchidism (autosomal recessive)	Torticollis Keloids Sterility Cutaneous nevi	Renal dysplasia
Peutz-Jegher syndrome (autosomal dominant)	Pigmentation of buccal mucosa Intestinal polyposis	Polycystic kidney disease
Prune belly syndrome (unknown)	Absent abdominal musculature Megaloureter	Urethral and bladder dilation
Wiedemann-Beckwith syndrome (sporadic)	Exomphalos Macroglossia Hydronephrosis Gigantism Hypoglycemia Wilms' tumor	Renomegaly
Liban-Kozenitsky syndrome (autosomal recessive?)	Similar to Wiedemann-Beckwith syndrome	Nephroblastomatosis
G-syndrome (autosomal dominant)	Micrognathia Short trachea Hypospadias Pulmonary abnormalities	Bifid ureter Vesicoureteral reflux
Goldenhar's syndrome (sporadic)	Multiple abnormalities of viscera and aortic arch	Unilateral cystic kidney Renal pelvis abnormality
Kaufman syndrome (autosomal recessive?)	Multiple vertebral anomalies Heart disease	Ureteral ectases Bifurcation of pelvis
VATER syndrome (autosomal dominant)	Vertebral anomalies Anal atresia Tracheoesophageal fistula Esophageal atresia Radial dysplasia	Renal dysplasia Renal agenesis Renal ectopia Hypospadias
Drash syndrome (sporadic)	Male pseudohermaphroditism Wilms' tumor	Diffuse mesangial sclerosis Congenital nephrotic syndrome

[a] Inheritance, if known, is given in parentheses.
Adapted from Gilbert E, Optiz J. Renal involvement in genetic-hereditary malformation syndromes. In: Hamburger J, Crosnier J, Grunfeld J-P, eds. *Nephrology.* New York: Wiley-Flammarion, 1979:909–944.

developed, and show ischemic changes. The tubules are randomly scattered within a fibrous matrix; they may be dilated and filled with colloid casts or they may be atrophic and collapsed. The arteries are tortuous and show obliterative fibroelastic endarteritis. Normal kidney tissue may display arteriolonephrosclerosis if hypertension is severe and longstanding.

Early diagnosis is important because surgical removal of a unilaterally involved kidney or excision of a hypoplastic segment often cures the hypertension. Bilateral disease cannot be managed surgically, and rigorous treatment of the hypertension with angiotensin-converting enzyme inhibitors or β-blockers is indicated. Rarely, when both kidneys are involved but the degree of the hypoplasia is not uniform, excision of the more severely involved segments may ameliorate the hypertension. For patients with progressive renal failure and uncontrolled hypertension, nephrectomy followed by dialysis therapy and transplantation may be the treatment of choice.

Ectopia

Simple Ectopia

In simple ectopia, the kidney ascends abnormally but does not cross the midline. It must be distinguished from a ptotic kidney, a condition in which the kidney descends secondarily from its normal position, usually in association with a large renal artery. In nephroptosis, the right kidney is more frequently involved than the left. The ectopic kidney may be found anywhere from the thorax to the pelvis, but the latter position is more common. An ectopic kidney in the pelvis could be differentiated from a ptotic kidney by its shorter ureter and a renal artery originating from the pelvic artery. Fetal lobulations are often present, and because of malrotation, the pelvis faces anteriorly. Occasionally, a simple ectopic kidney is associated with agenesis of the opposite kidney; removal of the ectopic kidney mistaken for a mass has led to renal failure in such patients.

Crossed Ectopia

Crossed ectopia occurs when one kidney ascends abnormally and crosses the midline. The ectopic kidney often fuses with the normally placed opposite kidney but may also be located in the pelvis. Crossed ectopia is more common in males, and left-to-right ectopia is more common than right-to-left. Malrotation invariably accompanies ectopia. The ureter may join the bladder in an abnormal location.

Horseshoe Kidney

In horseshoe kidney, a relatively common condition (1 in 400 of the population), the two kidneys fuse across the midline, most commonly at the lower poles. Malrotation is almost always found, and the ureters emerge anteriorly and pass in front of the isthmus. This may occasionally result in ureteric obstruction, which is then complicated by infection and stone formation. Horseshoe kidney may be found with other developmental abnormalities such as Turner's syndrome. Multiple renal arteries may be present.

URINARY TRACT ABNORMALITIES

Ureters

Atresia and Agenesis

Bilateral ureteral agenesis is incompatible with life, because without a normal ureteric bud, the kidney will not develop. If unilateral, the ipsilateral kidney and the trigone are absent, and the opposite kidney is hypertrophic. In ureteral atresia, the kidneys are dysplastic and connected to the bladder by a fibrous band. Bilateral atresia is not compatible with life.

Duplications

Various forms of ureteral duplication are common (1 in 125 autopsies) and are usually incidental findings. A *bifid ureter* is bifurcated in the upper two-thirds, the two limbs joining together before they enter the bladder. Urine may oscillate between the two limbs because of asynchronous peristalsis (the yo-yo phenomenon) and thus leads to stasis or dilation. A *double ureter* is made up of a normal and an ectopic ureter. Both drain a single kidney. The ectopic ureteral orifice is below and medial to the orifice of the normal ureter.

Ureterocele

A ureterocele is a cystic dilation of the distal end of the ureter that projects into the bladder. It may provoke ureteric obstruction or be associated with hematuria or infection.

Vesicoureteral Reflux

Incompetence of the vesicoureteric valvular mechanism may be congenital or acquired; the latter may result from bladder infection and/or ureteral obstruction with decompensation of the bladder. The proper function of the vesicoureteric valves depends on the normal development of ureteric and bladder (trigone) musculature, the length and course of the intramural ureter, and the size and shape of the ureteral orifice. Thus ectopic ureters that are laterally displaced are likely to display reflux. Primary reflux may occur *in utero* and could result in dilation of the upper urinary tract before birth. The development of urinary tract infection in the early postnatal period may be an indicator of congenital vesicoureteral reflux. Cortical scarring from intrarenal reflux, especially in association with infection, may result. Bilateral vesicoureteral reflux, or unilateral reflux with contralateral renal hypoplasia or agenesis, may produce renal failure and heavy proteinuria. Reimplantation of the ureter may correct the reflux, but if heavy proteinuria has already developed, progression of renal failure will continue. The diagnosis of vesicoureteral reflux may be established by voiding cystourethrogram, cystogram, or cystoscopy.

Unlike many congenital abnormalities, vesicoureteral reflux may also be familial and hereditary. A family study has shown that the prevalence of vesicoureteral reflux in siblings is 10 times higher than that expected in a normal population. Thus, if vesicoureteral reflux is diagnosed, screening studies for urinary tract infection and reflux should be conducted in all siblings.

Bladder

Persistent Urachus and Urachal Cyst

In embryonic life, the vesicoureteric canal extends to the umbilicus. As the bladder descends, this canal is replaced by the urachus, which then becomes progressively obliterated. Persistence of the lumen of the urachus provides a blind-ended channel extending from the bladder. Dilation and cyst formation may result in abdominal pain and/or infection.

Exstrophy

Exstrophy is a rare condition that results in the interior of the bladder being exposed to the abdominal wall. The pubic symphysis fails to develop. Bilateral ureteric diversion with an ileal bladder is required for treatment.

Urethra

Urethral Valves

Urethral valves are caused by reduplication of the urethral mucous membrane. They often cause lumen obstruction. Two types are recognized. In one type, the obstruction is unidirectional and only the forward passage of urine is impaired, but an instrument or sound can be easily introduced in a retrograde fashion. In the other type, a bidirectional obstruction is present. If unrecognized, urethral valves can cause severe renal damage in young children.

Epispadias and Hypospadias

In *epispadias,* a groove on the upper surface of the penis leads to a cleft in the proximal urethra that connects to a defect in the bladder wall. Thus incontinence is present. In *hypospadias,* a more common condition than epispadias, the urethra terminates in the undersurface of the penis. Hypospadias may be classified depending on the site of the abnormal opening: glandular, penile, periscrotal, scrotal, perineal, or pseudovaginal. Hypospadias is due to a congenital defect in the production of testosterone by the fetal testis. It may be associated with other developmental anomalies, most commonly undescended testes.

Selected Readings

Bernstein J, Gilbert-Barness E. Congenital malformations of the kidney. In: Tisher CC, Brenner BM, eds. *Renal pathology,* 2nd ed. Philadelphia: JB Lippincott, 1944:1355–1386.

An excellent overview with an emphasis on pathology.

Lyundquist A, Lagergren C. The Ask-Upmark kidney. *Acta Pathol Microbiol Scand* 1962;56:277–282.

Description of the pathology of segmental hypoplasia of Ask-Upmark kidney.

Moffat DB. Development abnormalities of the urogenital systems. In: Chisholm GD, Williams DI, eds. *Scientific foundations of urology.* Chicago: Year Book, 1982:357–374.

An excellent overview of the developmental abnormalities of the urinary tract.

Royer P. Malformations of the kidney. In: Royer P, Habib R, Mathiue R, et al, eds. *Pediatric nephrology.* Philadelphia: WB Saunders, 1974:9–27.

A concise review of congenital malformations of the kidney seen in pediatric age populations.

Scheinman JL, Abelson HJ. Bilateral renal hypoplasia with oligonephronia. *J Pediatr* 1970;76:389–397.

A clinical and pathologic description of oligomeganephronia.

CHAPTER 44

Gout and Renal Disease

Bryan T. Emmerson

In any understanding of the relationship between gout and renal disease, it is essential to appreciate that two distinct syndromes exist: one in which kidney disease is the primary phenomenon and gouty arthritis a secondary development, and the other in which gouty arthritis is the primary process and renal disease supervenes as a sequel to the gout. When a patient is seen with both gout and renal disease, it is sometimes difficult to determine whether the gout or the renal disease came first, and this difficulty has caused confusion in the concept of there being two distinct clinical syndromes. An unequivocal distinguishing feature would be a clear history of the development of gout at a time when renal disease was not present or the presence of renal disease before the patient suffered any acute gout. A comparison of two such groups indicated that although there was some variation between individuals, a patient with gout had usually suffered between 20 and 30 attacks of gouty arthritis over a 10-year period and had developed tophi before renal disease was detected. By contrast, in a patient with primary renal disease, the renal disease had usually been known for about 10 years before the development of gout and was usually of the tubulointerstitial type (Table 44.1).

TABLE 44.1. Patients with Both Renal Disease and Gout

	Gout Antedating Renal Disease	Renal Disease Antedating Gout
Males (%)	75	35
Age at onset of gout (yr)	40	40
Age at onset of renal disease (yr)	50	30
Duration of gout before renal disease (yr)	10 (20 attacks)	
Duration of renal disease before gout (yr)	—	10
Number of attacks of gout	50+	3
Gout affecting upper limbs (%)	75	10
Presence of tophi (%)	50	5-10

GOUT SECONDARY TO RENAL DISEASE

Gout or gouty arthritis is a clinical syndrome characterized by recurrent acute attacks of arthritis that is predominantly monarticular and is caused by an inflammatory response to the deposition of monosodium urate monohydrate (urate) crystals. The formation of these crystals occurs from supersaturated body fluids, and the risk of crystallization appears to be proportional to the degree and duration of the hyperuricemia. Urate solubility in a particular body fluid depends on its electrolyte composition, pH, temperature, protein content, and the presence or absence of substances such as proteoglycans that maintain urate in solution.

Although hyperuricemia implies an elevated concentration of urate in plasma, it is difficult to define precisely the upper limit of the normal or optimal concentration. Reference ranges vary between populations and even in one population with time. Solubility limits *in vitro* often cannot be extrapolated to the *in vivo* situation. A pragmatic approach suggests an upper limit of normal as the value above which urate crystallization is frequent and below which urate crystallization is infrequent. Such a dividing line is usually accepted as being at plasma urate concentrations of 7 mg/dl (0.42 mmol/L).

Body urate is a balance between urate production and urate elimination. Urate is chiefly produced by degradation of purine nucleotides, either from nucleic acid catabolism or from degradation of dietary purines. Urate elimination occurs principally by the kidney. However, one-third is excreted into the alimentary tract by processes that appear to be passive and dependent on the plasma urate concentration.

Urate is only minimally bound to plasma protein at body temperature and is almost entirely filterable at the glomerulus. Within the tubules, it is extensively reabsorbed, particularly in the proximal tubule, and most of the excreted urate enters the lumen by active tubular secretion. Although the urate clearance is approximately one-tenth the glomerular filtration rate (GFR), there is a wide normal range of 8.7 ± 2.5 (SD) ml/min. Accordingly, some normal subjects can have a urate clearance as low as 4 ml/min, whereas other normal subjects may have a urate clearance as high as 14 ml/min. Those with a high urate clearance have a greater facility for excreting urate than those with a low urate clearance and have a proportionately lower risk of hyperuricemia. In healthy subjects, between 60% and 80% of the urate clearance is determined by genetic factors. The renal handling of uric acid is discussed in detail in Chapter 7, Part 3.

Renal Causes of Hyperuricemia

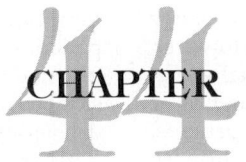

Hyperuricemia of renal origin may thus be caused by a reduced ability to excrete urate by a kidney that is completely normal in every other regard. Families with a low renal excretory capacity for urate may develop primary gout of renal origin. However, there are also many reversible factors that impair renal excretion of urate, principally drugs such as the oral diuretics or metabolites such as lactate or ketone bodies. In such patients, the hyperuricemia is associated with a relatively low urinary urate excretion.

Effect of Kidney Disease on Urate Homeostasis

As renal disease develops, even before there is a fall in the GFR, the urate clearance becomes impaired and the serum urate tends to rise. Whether this rise moves the urate concentration into the hyperuricemic range or keeps it within the normal range depends on the previous value of the serum urate and the extent of urate production, particularly from dietary purines. As the GFR falls further, the urate clearance continues to fall and there is a greater tendency to hyperuricemia. Moreover, the absolute excretion of urate in the urine falls, and there is an increased elimination of urate into the alimentary tract. Despite the global fall in urinary urate elimination, urate excretion per nephron actually increases.

The rise in the plasma urate concentration is not progressive in renal failure because of these adaptive mechanisms, and the urate concentration rarely exceeds 10 mg/dl (0.6 mmol/L) in stable chronic renal failure. Concentrations greater than this in chronic renal failure suggest that an additional mechanism is contributing. This could be either an agent such as a drug or metabolite which is further reducing renal excretion of urate or (b) an increase in urate production or (c) an acute process interfering with urate elimination. Nonetheless, hyperuricemia is disproportionately great for a particular GFR in certain varieties of chronic renal disease, and those in which disproportionate hyperuricemia is persistent tend to be associated with gout. Marked hyperuricemia may occur in patients with acute renal failure resulting from rhabdomyolysis or acute pancreatitis and in patients with severe prerenal azotemia resulting from profound dehydration.

Types of Kidney Disease Predisposing to Gout

Several specific varieties of renal disease have been documented as having an association with disproportionate hyperuricemia and gout. These tend to be tubulointerstitial rather than the glomerulonephritic variety, which is much less commonly associated with the development of secondary gout.

Particular varieties include chronic lead nephropathy, polycystic disease of the kidneys, renal amyloidosis, medullary cystic disease, analgesic nephropathy, obstructive nephropathies, and many varieties of familial renal disease. Studies of urate metabolism in such patients have shown that urate production remains within normal limits in the presence of increasing renal dysfunction but that renal elimination steadily decreases to about one-third of urate production. As the renal disease progresses, extrarenal excretion of urate becomes increasingly important and ultimately becomes the major route of excretion.

Most of the types of renal disease associated with secondary gout have a long duration and a slow intrinsic rate of progression. Gout has also been reported as an important complication of medullary cystic disease, and hyperuricemia has been demonstrated before any other evidence of renal insufficiency in patients with histologic evidence of this condition. Gout has also been reported in one-third to one-fourth of patients with polycystic disease of the kidney, although the significance of these reports has been questioned by studies that failed to confirm any increased impairment of urate excretion in this condition. Gout is well documented in cases of renal amyloidosis, in patients with analgesic nephropathy (usually a chronic nonprogressive type of renal disease in those patients who have stopped taking analgesics), and in patients with bilateral hydronephrosis resulting from an obstructive nephropathy.

There is also an increasing number of reports of patients with a familial nephropathy who develop gout at a young age (usually younger than 20 years of age). Although the renal disease is clearly primary, its precise nature and form of inheritance seem to vary and may represent several different types, rather than a homogeneous form, of familial nephropathy. Some may be a variety of medullary cystic disease, although the nature of the renal disease has been difficult to define in life. The major feature of all of these is disproportionate hyperuricemia with a reduced fractional excretion of urate and the early onset of gout.

Chronic Lead Nephropathy

Lead poisoning has long been believed to aggravate the development of gout, and even Garrod in 1876 noted the frequency of lead intoxication in his gouty subjects. It is estimated that 50% of patients with chronic lead nephropathy have suffered from gout. Much of the evidence relating to this has come from three sources: chronic renal disease following childhood lead poisoning in Queensland, Australia; the nephropathy of "moonshine" drinkers in the southern states of the United States; and the study of renal disease in lead workers in Paris and the United States.

Toward the end of the nineteenth century, many young children in Queensland developed lead poisoning because of the chronic and persistent ingestion of lead paint from weathered verandah railings. Careful epidemiologic studies in several hundred of these patients established a clear relation between childhood lead poisoning and the subsequent development of renal disease. In such cases, the kidneys were uniformly and severely contracted with granular surfaces, and there was an increased concentration of lead in bone. This elevated bone lead was uniformly associated with a characteristic, although not pathognomonic, renal pathology, whereas the other varieties of chronic renal disease were associated with a normal bone lead content. In these lead-intoxicated patients, a standardized infusion of calcium EDTA produced an increase in urinary lead excretion that was significantly greater than in normal subjects or in subjects with renal disease that was diagnosable as not caused by lead. This test was of particular importance because there were no persisting signs of lead intoxication. In these lead-intoxicated patients, the mean serum urate was higher at any creatinine clearance than in patients whose renal disease was not caused by lead, and urinary uric acid excretions were particularly low.

Thus the disproportionate hyperuricemia was due to the lower urate clearance, a finding that in turn was attributed to excessive tubular reabsorption of urate. Somewhat similar findings were made in "moonshine" drinkers whose liquor was contaminated with lead, except that they usually showed persisting features of lead intoxication.

The association between industrial lead exposure and subsequent renal disease with either gout or hypertension has been examined. The EDTA test for mobilizable lead has been used to indicate excessive past lead absorption and storage. These studies were interpreted to suggest that many patients with both gout and renal disease, who might otherwise have been diagnosed as having gouty renal disease, may well be suffering from chronic lead nephropathy with secondary gout. However, no controlled epidemiologic studies have been undertaken to demonstrate the amount of industrial lead exposure needed to damage the adult kidney, and an etiologic relationship between the lead absorption and the renal disease has yet to be established unequivocally. For instance, a lead worker who was a heavy drinker and who developed chronic glomerulonephritis might show the combination of chronic renal disease, gout, and excessive lead absorption, but in his case, the disorders would not necessarily be related etiologically. Specific criteria for a lead etiology in such cases have yet to be defined. An EDTA test is usually positive in anyone with significant past industrial lead exposure and does not establish that the lead has caused any associated renal disease.

RENAL DISEASE RESULTING FROM GOUT OR URIC ACID CRYSTALS (FIG. 44.1)

In the nineteenth century and first half of the twentieth century, it was generally accepted that renal disease was a frequent sequel to gout. However, with the passage of time and the availability of effective therapies to prevent and control hyperuricemia, the association between gout and renal disease has been questioned, even to the point of doubting whether gout can induce renal disease at all, and suggesting that any associated renal disease may be due to an alternative cause such as lead intoxication or hypertension. However, there is unequivocal evidence that uric acid can induce renal disease, even though gouty renal disease is now a relatively uncommon finding in communities where gout is treated extensively by urate-lowering drugs and persistent severe hyperuricemia is avoided. This assertion can be made because of two clinical situations in which urate overproduction is the primary phenomenon and any renal disease must be secondary. First, in hypoxanthineguanine phosphoribosyl transferase deficiency, patients suffer from a primary overproduction of urate and initially have a very high urinary urate excretion. Many of these patients develop secondary renal disease. Second, patients with malignancies treated by cytotoxic agents show acute overproduction of urate and often develop acute or chronic renal disease secondary to this. Study of these types of renal disease will reveal mechanisms whereby urate and uric acid can damage the kidney.

History of Gout Nephropathy

Mention of renal involvement in gout is recorded as far back as the second century AD; and in the seventeenth century, Sydenham recorded that "gout breeds stones in the kidney." In the nineteenth century, proteinuria was noted in patients with gout, and uric acid deposits were recorded in the kidneys and joints of gouty subjects. Garrod noted deposits of urate crystals between the renal tubules and regarded urate crystal deposition as a uniform finding in gouty kidneys, being of a similar nature to that found within the joints. In 1930, a 30% incidence of nephritis was reported in gouty subjects, with an 8% death rate resulting from uremia. However, most of these patients had tophaceous gout and had suffered from gouty arthritis for more than 10 years. This was associated with degenerative vascular disease and hypertension, which appeared to contribute to the renal pathology. The most extensive study of gout nephropathy was undertaken in 1960 by Talbot and Terplan, who concluded that the only distinctive pathologic feature was the presence of urate crystals. Almost all of the 191 kidneys studied showed abnormalities, particularly microtophi, nephrosclerosis, and urinary tract infection. The authors regarded the microtophus as the distinctive pathologic feature of the gouty kidney and found renal insufficiency of "critical degree" in one-fourth of the patients.

Since then, the modern era of nephrologic investigation has occurred and effective drug control of hyperuricemia has become possible. In general, the gouty kidney has shown disproportionate impairment of tubular function, particularly concentrating power, in relation to glomerular function. Some persistent renal abnormality has been shown in most studies of gouty subjects, and these changes have usually been greater than could be attributed solely to aging, hypertensive vascular disease, or renal calculi with pyelonephritis. Persistent and significant hyperuricemia in the absence of other complications has been followed for a prolonged period without detection of deterioration of renal function. Adequate therapeutic control of hyperuricemia appears to have greatly reduced the risk of gouty renal

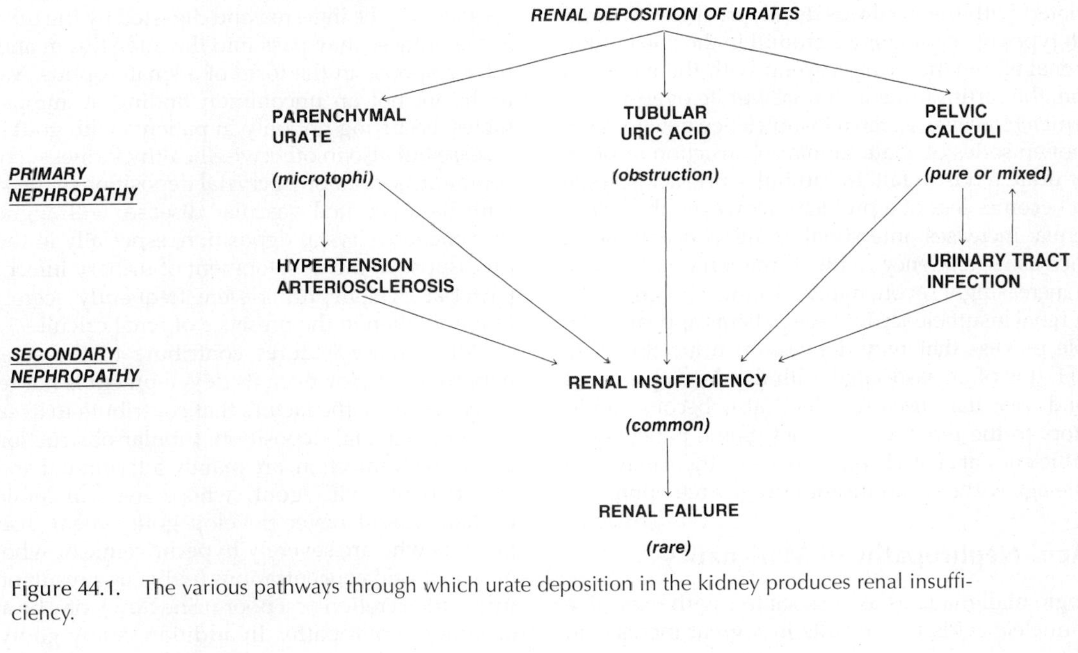

Figure 44.1. The various pathways through which urate deposition in the kidney produces renal insufficiency.

disease, and in these days, the classic gouty kidney, as seen before the development of urate-lowering agents, is uncommon.

Urate and Uric Acid Crystals

Because the pK_a of uric acid is 5.75, more than 95% of the molecules are present in the dissociated form as urate ions when the pH is 7.4. However, at the lower pH that occurs in the distal tubule, a much greater proportion of undissociated uric acid is present; if the urine is sufficiently concentrated and the pH is sufficiently low, amorphous deposits of uric acid may form within the lumina of the distal tubules or collecting ducts. The monosodium urate monohydrate or urate crystals formed at physiologic pH are acicular in shape and induce the giant cell response characteristic of the classic microtophus. Thus uric acid in the plasma, glomerular filtrate, or renal interstitium is present in the form of urate. Because there is a gradient for urate between the renal cortex and the medulla because of the countercurrent mechanism, interstitial medullary microtophi are a potential hazard in the presence of sufficient urate concentrations. X-ray diffraction studies have confirmed these two types of crystals within the kidney, namely, (a) acicular monosodium urate monohydrate crystals, occurring in the renal interstitial tissues and inducing a microtophaceous response, and (b) uric acid crystals, appearing amorphous microscopically, developing within the tubular lumen, and leading to tubular obstruction and an acute deterioration of renal function.

Renal Disease in Urate Overproduction

Patients with the inherited mutation of the purine reutilization enzyme hypoxanthineguanine phosphoribosyl transferase exhibit genetic urate overproduction. Uric acid crystals may be found in the urine shortly after birth, and renal failure may occur in infancy. Such an acute uric acid nephropathy is associated with a high ratio of uric acid to creatinine in the urine: this ratio exceeded 1.0 when calculated in mg/dl or 0.66 when calculated in mmol/L. Acute deterioration of renal function may occur at any time and be reversed by an alkaline diuresis. Follow-up of many members of these families has demonstrated a varied pattern of renal disease. Histology has demonstrated both intraluminal uric acid–containing casts, as well as typical microtophi around urate crystals situated principally in the renal interstitium and associated with the insidious development of renal insufficiency. Both types of crystal may be found in the one kidney.

As long as renal elimination can keep up with the increased urate production, the serum urate in primary urate overproduction may be normal. However, as renal insufficiency develops (either as a result of episodes of acute tubular obstruction or other causes), urinary urate tends to fall. Intratubular uric acid crystal deposition then becomes less of a problem. However, the resulting hyperuricemia increases interstitial urate concentrations, leading to an increasing tendency to the formation of interstitial microtophi and increasingly severe hyperuricemia and gout. The development of renal insufficiency in these patients appears to be an unpredictable process that may depend on urine flow rate and/or urine pH. It is often associated with the development of hypertension and vascular disease, which also become additional contributors to the renal insufficiency. Some patients develop renal insufficiency at an early age, whereas others may continue into middle age without significant nitrogen retention.

Acute Uric Acid Nephropathy of Malignancy

Many hematologic malignancies are associated with excessive degradation of nucleic acids that results in a great increase in urate production. This also occurs in an acute form when cytotoxic or cancer chemotherapeutic agents are administered. Such a urate load can cause the formation of uric acid crystals within the distal tubules and collecting ducts of the kidney, leading to an acute deterioration of renal function, unless this is prevented by alkalinizing the urine and maintaining a low urinary uric acid concentration. This can be achieved by administration of sodium bicarbonate (1 g every 6 hours) and acetazolamide at night, accompanied by high fluid intake. Urinary uric acid may also be reduced by the xanthine oxidase inhibitor allopurinol, which reduces the concentration of uric acid but increases that of its precursors xanthine and hypoxanthine. The initial dose of allopurinol during cytotoxic therapy can be large, up to 600 mg daily if renal function is normal, but because the main metabolite of allopurinol, namely, oxypurinol, is excreted principally by renal mechanisms, the dose of allopurinol should be reduced considerably in the presence of renal insufficiency. A maintenance dose of 100 mg/day of allopurinol per 30 ml/min of GFR would be a useful guide.

Urate and uric acid crystals have been observed reacting with lining tubular cells, some of which ingest the intraluminal crystals. Some experimental studies suggest that crystals may actually pass through epithelial cells into the renal interstitium. Should this occur, the crystals could form a nidus for the formation of a microtophus.

This syndrome can occur in a subacute or chronic form in which continuing overexcretion of large amounts of uric acid steadily reduces the nephron population and results in chronic renal insufficiency. Studies in animal models using the uricase inhibitor oxonic acid, together with uric acid loading, have confirmed the clinical observation that excessive excretion of uric acid by the kidneys can result in renal damage with intrarenal crystal deposition.

Chronic Gout Nephropathy

As in gouty arthritis, the essential feature of gout nephropathy appears to be the deposition of urate and/or uric acid crystals, which induces the cellular and tissue response characteristic of a tophus (Fig. 44.1). Thus interstitial microtophi may develop in the kidney as in other tissues and may affect renal function and induce hypertension. In addition to these interstitial microtophi, crystals of uric acid may form within the renal tubule and these crystals may be ingested and digested by the tubular lining cells. Some of these may pass into the interstitium and produce a cellular response in the form of a small tophus. Medullary microtophi are not an uncommon finding at autopsy in warm climates, occurring not only in patients with gout or chronic renal disease but also in otherwise healthy kidneys. Hypertension is a common association of crystal deposition in the kidney, and this, with its associated vascular disease, will aggravate any renal dysfunction. Crystal deposition, especially in the medulla, may predispose to the development of urinary infections: features of bacterial pyelonephritis were frequently seen in many gouty kidneys, often in the presence of renal calculi.

All of these features contribute to the syndrome of gout nephropathy. However, its development is not regular and consistent because the factors that contribute to it, such as uric acid and urate crystal deposition, tubular obstruction, renal calculi, and urinary infection, are mainly intermittent and variably present. Patients with gout, whose hyperuricemia is well controlled, should never develop gouty renal disease. However, patients who are severely hyperuricemic or who have high urinary uric acid concentrations (either as a result of a high urinary uric acid excretion or a poor urine flow) may be at risk of a urate or gouty nephropathy. In addition, many gouty patients have hypertension and hypertriglyceridemia, both of which may predispose to degenerative vascular disease and a vascular nephropathy.

The early features of gouty renal disease are as difficult to detect as the early stages of other renal diseases. Serial observation of the creatinine clearance is probably as satisfactory as any method before elevation of the serum creatinine concentration. Studies of more sensitive markers are few because of the infrequent occurrence of the condition at present. Prevention and treatment are by controlling the hyperuricemia and the hypertension.

It will be apparent from this consideration that there is little evidence to support the concept of a "hyperuricemic" as opposed to a gouty nephropathy unless the hyperuricemia is severe and persistent (more than 13 mg/dl or 0.8 mmol/L). Some gouty patients with serum urates of 12 mg/dl have been followed for up to 20 years without the development of renal disease, and others with serum urates of less than 10 mg/dl have been followed for prolonged periods with only mild degrees of renal insufficiency. Hyperuricosuria appears to present a greater risk to the kidney, although this is a problem only in severe overproducers or those with a concentrated urine. Patients whose hyperuricemia is due to reduced renal excretion of urate tend to have a low urinary uric acid concentration and are classified as "underexcretors" of urate. They do not exhibit a significant risk of the uric acid crystal type of nephropathy.

ASYMPTOMATIC HYPERURICEMIA AND CHRONIC RENAL DISEASE

There is no evidence that hyperuricemia of less than 10 mg/dl (0.6 mmol/L) has any deleterious effect on renal function unless there is associated hyperuricosuria. Because of the alternative extrarenal mechanism of elimination already discussed, hyperuricemia rarely exceeds this value in stable chronic renal disease. Nonetheless, a variety of nondrug options are available to reduce hyperuricemia. First, plasma volume contraction promotes a high serum urate, and this can often be corrected by adequate salt and water supplementation. Second, diuretics and other drugs that can increase the serum urate should be avoided when other therapeutic options are possible. Third, uncontrolled hypertension aggravates hyperuricemia and should be treated appropriately. Fourth, renal hyperuricemia is particularly susceptible to dietary purine restriction, so a moderate restriction of meat and alcohol intake is likely to lower the serum urate concentration. Most factors that can induce acute or chronic renal insufficiency will aggravate hyperuricemia, but such elevations are usually transient, and the serum urate will return to acceptable values when these acute factors have remitted. Allopurinol should rarely be needed in patients with renal disease without gout.

By contrast, when gout has occurred, allopurinol therapy is usually indicated, as well as a large fluid intake and control of hypertension. The main risk from the use of allopurinol is the development of an acute hypersensitivity reaction with interstitial nephritis and vasculitis, which is more frequent in patients with renal disease than in those with normal renal function. It develops particularly in patients who are given allopurinol in the dose appropriate for normal renal function. The dose of allopurinol should be reduced in proportion to the impairment of GFR, so a daily dose of 150 mg might be used at a GFR of 50 ml/min, 100 mg/day at a GFR of 30 ml/min, and 50 mg/day at a GFR of 15 ml/min. Such doses are usually effective in controlling both hyperuricemia and gout and appear not to be associated with an increased incidence of sensitivity reactions.

Selected Readings

Batuman V, Landy E, Maesaka JK, et al. Contribution of lead to hypertension with renal impairment. *N Engl J Med* 1983;309:17–21.
A report suggesting that chronic lead nephropathy may be misdiagnosed as hypertensive nephrosclerosis.

Berger L, Yu TF. Renal function in gout. IV. An analysis of 524 gouty subjects including long-term follow-up studies. *Am J Med* 1975;59:605–613.
Hyperuricemia per se is not detrimental to renal function. Gout nephropathy is largely associated with aging, vascular disease, renal calculi, or an independent primary nephropathy.

Calabrese G, Simmonds HA, Cameron HS, et al. Precocious familial gout with reduced fractional urate clearance and normal purine enzymes. *Q J Med* 1990; 75:441–450.
Emphasizes that gout, with reduced fractional excretion of urate, is often the clinical presentation of familial renal disease in young people.

Emmerson BT. Chronic lead nephropathy. *Kidney Int* 1973;4:1–5.
A detailed consideration of evidence concerning this entity, its diagnosis, and clinical associations.

Emmerson BT, Row PG. An evaluation of the pathogenesis of the gouty kidney. *Kidney Int* 1975;8:65–71.
A review of all pathogenetic mechanisms of kidney disease in gout.

Emmerson BT, Nagel SL, Duffy DL, et al. Genetic control of the renal clearance of urate. *Ann Rheum Dis* 1992;51:375–377.
Provides evidence that a reduced urate clearance is the genetic mechanism underlying the renal underexcretion of urate responsible for the common variety of primary gout.

Kelton J, Kelley WN, Holmes EW. A rapid method for the diagnosis of acute uric acid nephropathy. *Arch Intern Med* 1978;138:612–615.
The ratio of uric acid to creatinine in a random sample of urine is found to be useful in differentiation.

Talbot JH, Terplan KL. The kidney in gout. *Medicine (Baltimore)* 1960;39:405–462.
Detailed description of renal pathology in 191 cases of gouty kidneys; a major definitive study of that time. Includes reliable historical review.

Vecchio PC, Emmerson BT. Gout due to renal disease. *Br J Rheum* 1992;31:63–65.
Discusses varieties of primary renal disease that predispose to hyperuricemia and gout.

CHAPTER 45

Diabetic Nephropathy

András Mogyorósi and Fuad N. Ziyadeh

The World Health Organization estimates that there are approximately 135 million people with diabetes mellitus worldwide and that this number will increase progressively. In the United States, it is estimated that 16 million people (6% of the population) have diabetes mellitus, but a significant portion of those with type II (insulin-independent) diabetes mellitus have not yet been clinically identified. Diabetes significantly increases an individual's chance of premature death, decreasing lifespan by an average of 15 to 20 years. Diabetic nephropathy is the leading cause of end-stage renal disease in the industrialized world. Almost 30% to 40% of patients with renal failure who were admitted into renal replacement programs in the United States have diabetic kidney disease. The renal risk and the prevalence of proteinuria and renal failure are similar in type I (insulin-dependent) and type II diabetes mellitus. Because type II diabetes is a more common disease than type I, approximately 80% of all diabetic patients who develop end-stage renal failure have type II. There is also a higher prevalence of type II diabetes in the non-Caucasian population, especially in African-Americans, Native Americans, Asian-Americans, and Mexican-Americans (Fig. 45.1). In Europe, at least 20% of end-stage renal disease patients have diabetic nephropathy, but this percentage is likely to grow with the aging population, the increasing prevalence of diabetic kidney disease, and the decreasing threshold for providing renal replacement therapy to patients with multiple diabetic complications (Fig. 45.2).

The characteristic lesions of diabetic nephropathy are diffuse and nodular glomerulosclerosis. The clinical syndrome of overt diabetic nephropathy encompasses heavy proteinuria, hypertension, and renal failure. Once on renal replacement therapy, mortality among diabetic patients is 1.5 to 2.5 times higher than in nondiabetic patients, mostly due to increased cardiovascular mortality, and less than 20% of diabetic patients survive on dialysis after five years. There has been a steady improvement in the outcome of these patients over the past decade (Fig. 45.3), but the statistics remain dismal, which highlights the urgency to find more effective measures to prevent or cure diabetic nephropathy. Major progress has been made in deciphering the pathophysiology of the disease, its prevention, and treatment. Adherence to the therapeutic recommendations derived from landmark, large-scale clinical trials hold promise for significantly decreasing the morbidity and mortality associated with diabetic kidney disease. This chapter will review the following: clinical course and diagnosis, histopathology and its functional correlates, risk factors, pathogenetic mechanisms highlighting the central roles of glucose metabolism and intraglomerular hypertension, and genetic predisposition. A comprehensive survey of preventive measures, conservative management, and renal replacement therapy is provided.

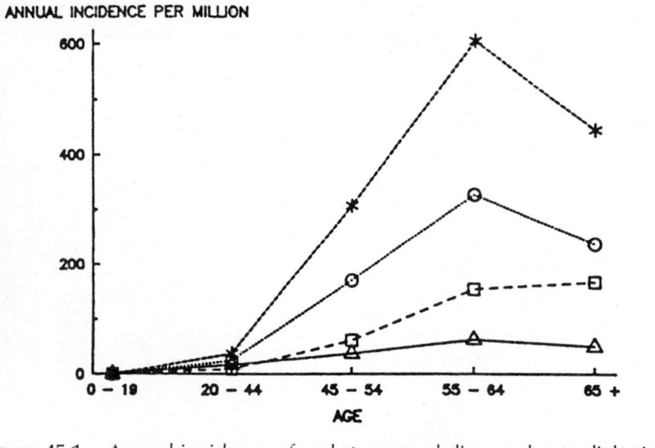

Figure 45.1. Annual incidence of end-stage renal disease due to diabetic nephropathy by age in various ethnic groups in the United States (Medicare data, 1983–1985). *Asterisk*, Native Americans; *circles*, African-Americans; *squares*, Asian-Americans; *triangles*, Caucasians. (Reproduced with permission from Teutsch S, Newman J, Eggers P. A problem of diabetic renal failure in the United States. *Am J Kidney Dis* 1989;13:11–13.)

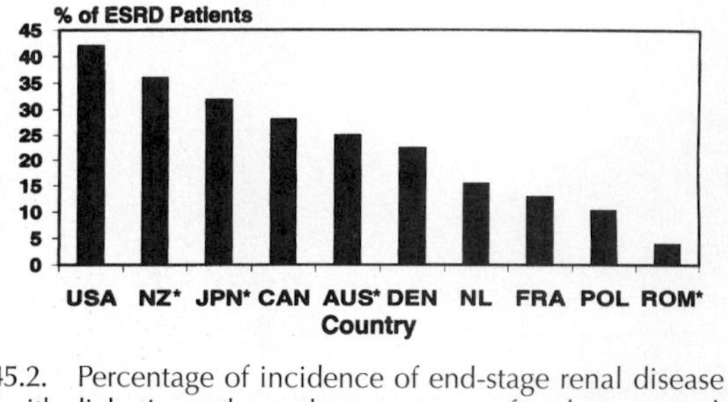

Figure 45.2. Percentage of incidence of end-stage renal disease *(ESRD)* patients with diabetic nephropathy as a cause of end-stage renal disease in 1996. United States, AU, Australia; CAN, Canada; DEN, Denmark; FRA, France; JPN, Japan; NL, the Netherlands; NZ, New Zealand; PL, Poland; ROM, Romania. *Data from New Zealand, Japan, Australia, and Romania are from 1995. [Reproduced with permission from excerpts from United States Renal Data System 1997 Annual Data Report. *Am J Kidney Dis* 1998;32(Suppl 1):S137.]

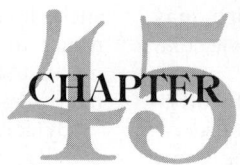

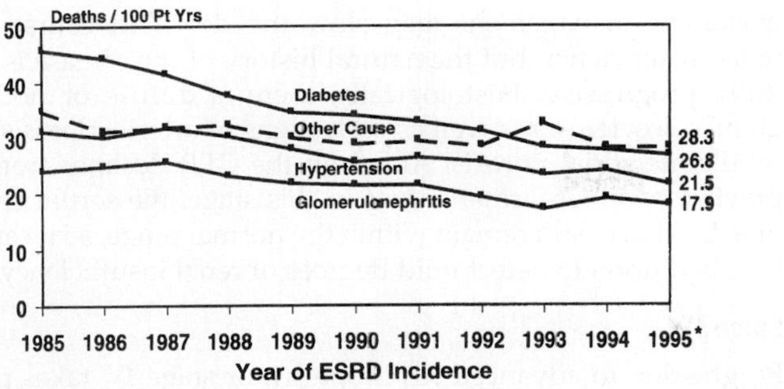

Figure 45.3. Death rates for dialysis patients (percentage of deaths per 100 patient-years) by cause and by year of incidence adjusted for age, race, and sex to the distribution of the corresponding category of the 1994 cohort. *Follow-up is preliminary. [Reproduced with permission from excerpts from United States Renal Data System 1997 Annual Data Report. *Am J Kidney Dis* 1998;32(Suppl 1):S73.]

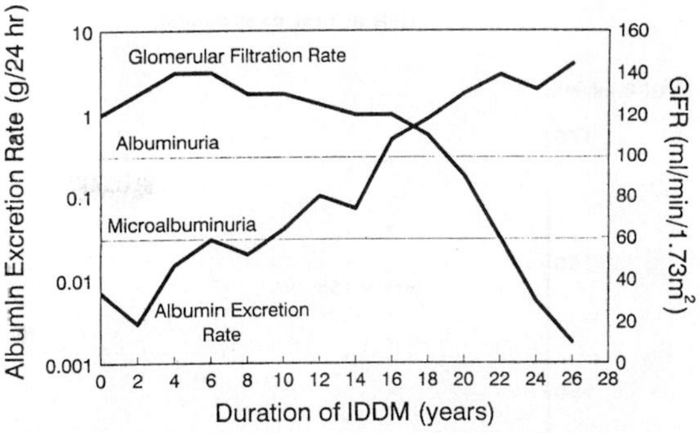

Figure 45.4. Clinical time course of urinary albumin excretion rate and glomerular filtration rate (GFR) in patients with type I diabetes mellitus (IDDM) with diabetic nephropathy. Note the development and progression of microalbuminuria to clinical or overt albuminuria many years before the fall in GFR. (Reproduced with permission from Molitch ME. Management of early diabetic nephropathy. *Am J Med* 1997;102:392–398.)

CLINICAL COURSE AND DIAGNOSIS

Clinical Course

The characteristic clinical stages of diabetic nephropathy are best understood in the setting of type I diabetes mellitus (Fig. 45.4). Most of these young patients do not have coexisting systemic illnesses that can lead to other kidney diseases, and the time of onset of diabetes is usually abrupt; therefore, the ensuing renal injury after a median period of 10 years or longer can regularly be attributed exclusively to the diabetic state without the need for a kidney biopsy. Patients with type II diabetes may have other coexisting diseases, including essential hypertension, and the renal disease in these patients can be attributed to diabetes only in approximately 75% of the cases. Premature cardiovascular mortality in many patients with type II diabetes mellitus may prevent the full manifestations of diabetic complications, including nephropathy. Furthermore, type II diabetes is usually diagnosed years after the actual onset of the disease, which is often indolent, so the characteristics of the early clinical stages of kidney involvement are more difficult to delineate. However, seminal studies in the Pima Indian community, a group with a strong genetic predisposition to developing type II diabetes in the setting of obesity around the fourth decade of life, have shown that progression of nephropathy in type II diabetes advances through similar stages as it does in type I diabetic patients.

Diabetic nephropathy in type I diabetes mellitus can be conveniently characterized into different clinical stages, which differ with respect to renal hemodynamics, systemic blood pressure, urinary albumin excretion rate (AER), and the level of glomerular filtration rate (GFR) (Table 45.1).

Stage I

Soon after the detection of diabetes mellitus in type I diabetes, the kidney manifests renal hypertrophy (nephromegaly), elevated renal blood flow, and increased GFR. Urinary AER is typically normal but transient microalbuminuria (evoked by stress, physical exercise, poor glycemic control, and intercurrent febrile illnesses) may be manifest. The blood pressure is typically within the normal range at this stage. The increase in GFR in stage I of type I diabetic patients may exceed 20% to 40% of control values. Some patients with type II diabetes mellitus have glomerular hyperfiltration at the time of discovery of hyperglycemia. Studies in Pima Indians have shown that type II diabetic patients manifest only a modest increment in GFR (about 15% above control values), a limitation imparted perhaps by the increased age of this population at the onset of the disease.

Renal hypertrophy, hyperperfusion, and the elevated GFR are potentially reversible, at least in part, with insulin therapy and tight glucose control. The relevance of renal hypertrophy and hyperfiltration, which occur in all diabetic patients, to the future development of overt renal disease in the subset of patients who are destined to have clinical nephropathy remains unclear. However, some early studies have suggested that type I diabetic patients who have extremely high GFR (above 150 to 170 ml/min) during this stage are at increased risk for future development of diabetic nephropathy (Fig. 45.5).

Stage II

Once diabetes has been present for a median of 10 years or more, a minority of patients (around 30%) can enter the stage of incipient (or latent) diabetic nephropathy, which is characterized by fixed microalbuminuria (urinary AER of at least 30 mg

TABLE 45.1. The Stages of Diabetic Nephropathy—Typical Findings

Stage	Glomerular Filtration	Albuminuria	Blood Pressure	Time Course (Years After Diagnosis)
Renal hyperfunction	Elevated	Absent	Normal	At diagnosis
Clinical latency	High normal	Absent	Rising within or above normal	5–15
Microalbuminuria (incipient nephropathy)	Normal	20–200 μg/min (30–300 mg/day)	Increased	10–15
Macroalbuminuria or persisting proteinuria (Clinically manifest nephropathy)	Decreasing	200 μg/min (300 μg/day)	—	—
Renal failure	Diminished	Massive	Increased	15–30

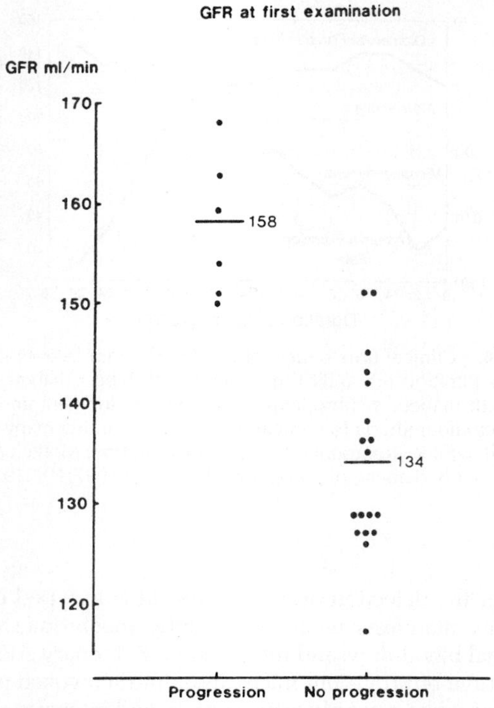

Figure 45.5. Marked glomerular hyperfiltration may predict diabetic nephropathy. The initial glomerular filtration rate (GFR) is depicted for a cohort of type I diabetic patients who were classified according to subsequent progression or nonprogression to overt diabetic nephropathy after 10 years of observation. Most patients had hyperfiltration, but the patients with very high initial GFR (at least 155 ml/min) tended to progress. (Reproduced with permission from Mogensen CE, Christensen CK. Predicting diabetic nephropathy in insulin-dependent patients. *N Engl J Med* 1984;311:89–93.)

over 24 hours). In this clinically silent stage, thickening of the glomerular and tubular basement membranes develops with some degree of mesangial matrix expansion. There is persistent hypertrophy of the glomerulus and the tubular epithelium, and the GFR may still be elevated or within the normal range. The systemic blood pressure may increase within the normal range but may not reach the level at which hypertension is established (140/90 mm Hg according to the World Health Organization). Because glomerular and tubular hypertrophy and basement membrane thickening may be present in type I and type II diabetic patients without microalbuminuria, these specific structural features of the diabetic state may not represent histologic markers for predicting the future development of clinical diabetic nephropathy. On the other hand, significant mesangial matrix expansion develops in this stage, and this is considered to be the pathologic counterpart of clinical diabetic nephropathy. A host of clinical studies have established that diabetic patients who develop fixed microalbuminuria are at a high risk of progressing in approximately five to seven years to the next phase (stage III).

Stage III

This stage typically occurs 15 years after the onset of type I diabetes mellitus and is characterized by the progression of microalbuminuria into overt proteinuria or macroalbuminuria (now detectable by a regular urinary dipstick). Macroalbuminuria refers to urinary AER of at least 300 mg/24 hr, which corresponds to overt proteinuria defined as at least 500 mg total protein in the urine per 24 hours. In this stage, the blood pressure becomes elevated. Optimal pharmacologic and nonpharmacologic management may slow the downhill course into renal insufficiency, but the natural history of the disease is typically progressive. Histologically, there is diffuse or nodular glomerulosclerosis as well as early signs of arteriosclerosis and tubulointerstitial fibrosis. Although the GFR declines from its previously supernormal values in this stage, the serum creatinine level may still remain within the normal range, so it cannot be relied upon to detect mild degrees of renal insufficiency.

Stage IV

Progression to advanced nephropathy, or stage IV, takes place in the next 4 to 6 years. End-stage renal disease requiring renal replacement therapy follows in 1 to 3 years. This stage is marked by nephrotic-range proteinuria (greater than 3.5 g of urinary protein per 24 hours), overt hypertension, and declining GFR below the normal range at an average rate of approximately 1 ml per min if the patient is not taking antihypertensive medications. The rate of loss of GFR varies considerably between individuals and can be negatively influenced by a host of factors, especially the presence and severity of hypertension. The degree of proteinuria also has a major impact on kidney survival. For instance a study in type II diabetic patients from Italy described a much worse renal prognosis when total urinary protein excretion was above a cut-off value of 2 g per 24 hours. Other complications of diabetes such as retinopathy and cardiovascular and peripheral vascular diseases greatly increase the morbidity and mortality in this stage.

Other Effects of Diabetes on the Genitourinary System

Patients may have other renal and genitourinary manifestations of the diabetic state that are not part of the clinical picture of diabetic nephropathy (Table 45.2). Renal artery stenosis due to accelerated atherosclerosis is more frequent in the diabetic patient than the general population. Such patients may experience accelerated hypertension or may develop acute renal failure when treated with angiotensin-converting enzyme (ACE) inhibitors.

The genitourinary system may be the target for recurrent bacterial or fungal infection and papillary necrosis. Autonomic neuropathy can cause impaired awareness of bladder fullness, detrusor dysfunction, and obstructive uropathy, which can contribute to the increased risk of urinary tract infections and deterioration of renal function. Management may pose particular problems in the elderly diabetic male with combined diabetic cystopathy and prostatic hypertrophy. If ureteral obstruction due to sloughing of papillary tissue is suspected, prompt relief of obstruction is necessary. Symptomatic urinary tract infec-

TABLE 45.2. Clinical Manifestations of the Diabetic Kidney of Nonglomerular Origin

Tubular proteinuria
Fluid and electrolyte disorders
Glycosuric osmotic diuresis
Hypoaldosteronism
Hyperkalemia/type IV distal renal tubular acidosis
Hypercalciuria
Obstructive nephropathy associated with neurogenic bladder dysfunction
Radiocontrast-induced nephrotoxic acute renal failure
Papillary necrosis
Pyelonephritis
Bacterial
Fungal
Emphysematous
Xanthogranulomatous

tions are more severe than in the general population. Intrarenal and perirenal abscess formation is also common among diabetic patients with urinary tract infections. Nephrectomy may be the only approach for saving the life of the patient with intrarenal and perirenal abscess. Perinephric abscess should be suspected in diabetic patients with high fever, leukocytosis, and urinary tract infection resistant to therapy. Plain film of the abdomen shows air around the kidney and the abscess could be diagnosed by CT scan.

Hyperkalemic renal tubular acidosis (type IV) develops in many diabetic patients with hypertension and preexisting renal insufficiency. The etiology of this disorder is due to hyporeninism, hypoaldosteronism, and/or impaired action of aldosterone at the distal tubular potassium-secreting sites. Patients with this tubular dysfunction may develop severe hyperkalemia when challenged by extracellular volume depletion or when certain medications are started, such as ACE inhibitors, heparin, nonsteroidal antiinflammatory agents, β-adrenergic blockers, and potassium-sparing diuretics.

For as yet unclear reasons, patients with diabetic nephropathy are particularly prone to contrast media-induced acute renal failure when they have preexisting renal impairment (a serum creatinine concentration of at least 1.5 mg/dl). Other risk factors for this complication are age older than 50 years, diabetes for more than 10 years, vasculopathy, and dehydration. The risk may be reduced but not eliminated if fluids are administered in the periprocedure period, by lowering the dosage of the radiocontrast agent, and by using nonionic rather than ionic formulations.

When patients with diabetic nephropathy develop a sharp rise in serum creatinine level, a host of causes of acute renal failure superimposed on diabetic nephropathy need to be addressed. As mentioned, this could be due to urinary tract infection with papillary necrosis, obstructive uropathy due to diabetic cystopathy, contrast media–induced nephropathy, or treatment with drugs such as ACE inhibitors and cyclooxygenase inhibitors. Other factors also need to be considered such as hypovolemia from diuretic overuse, vomiting due to gastroparesis, or diarrhea due to autonomic neuropathy, and uncontrolled hypertension and congestive hear failure.

Clinical Diagnosis

Persistent (fixed) microalbuminuria is the earliest reliable predictor and marker of diabetic nephropathy. Prospective studies have established that the risks of renal failure and cardiovascular events are clearly predicted by microalbuminuria. The normal range of total urinary protein excretion is up to 150 mg/24 hr, but the greater part is nonglomerular in origin (tubular and postrenal). Thus total urinary protein excretion is not a good indicator of the macromolecular permeability defect of the glomerulus in early stages of diabetic kidney disease. Direct measurements of urinary albumin excretion greatly improve accuracy. Microalbuminuria is measured by methods using sensitive radioimmunoassays, enzyme-linked immunoadsorbent assays, or specialized dipsticks (see Chapter 101). In healthy normal adults, urinary AER varies but averages 4 to 6 μg/min, with less than 10% of normal adults having rates exceeding 12 μg/min. A consensus group has defined microalbuminuria as urinary AER of 20 to 200 μg/min, which corresponds to AER of approximately 30 to 300 mg/24 hr. Urinary AER can vary from day to day and is temporarily increased by conditions such as intercurrent febrile illnesses, physical exercise, severe hypertension, and poor glycemic control. These conditions have to be excluded when the significance of microalbuminuria is weighed. Microalbuminuria can be diagnosed when at least two of three urine samples examined within a 6- to 12-week period show an AER of more than 20 μg/min or 30 mg/day in a 24-hour urine collection. To avoid the confounding effect of upright position on urinary AER, an albumin:creatinine ratio of at least 30 mg/g in a first-morning urine sample can also be used for diagnosis. Determination of the urinary albumin:creatinine ratio has been gaining wide acceptance as a screening method to detect microalbuminuria.

The risk for developing microalbuminuria is a function of disease duration and the presence of other microvascular complications. Proliferative retinopathy significantly increases the likelihood of diabetic nephropathy in the setting of fixed microalbuminuria. If fixed microalbuminuria is found in a diabetic patient with proven disease duration of less than 7 to 10 years, the likelihood of renal disease due to diabetes diminishes. Importantly, clinical studies have established that microalbuminuria has a much bigger specificity for diabetic kidney disease in type I than in type II diabetes. This is probably because patients with type II diabetes may have coexistent essential hypertension, and microalbuminuria may be merely a manifestation of the effect of hypertension rather than diabetes on the kidney. Up to 30% of type II diabetic patients may have diabetic nephropathy without evidence for retinopathy even by sensitive fluorescein angiography. On the other hand, type II diabetic patients may commonly have other causative factors for the proteinuria that need to be considered. Some studies have described the superimposition of other primary glomerular diseases on diabetic nephropathy in as many as 20% of patients with type II diabetes mellitus evaluated for renal replacement therapy. Therefore, if the type II diabetic patient has microalbuminuria or macroalbuminuria but no retinopathy, diabetic renal disease may or may not be the cause of the albuminuria, and a renal biopsy would be needed to determine its cause.

If diabetic nephropathy is diagnosed in later stages (stages III and IV), the patient classically demonstrates significant proteinuria (reaching the nephrotic range) and an elevated serum creatinine level. Hypertension is commonly seen, and usually there is no evidence of renal inflammation (i.e., no RBCs, WBCs, or cellular casts in the urine sediment). If the urinalysis shows evidence of inflammation in the glomerulus (RBC casts) or in the tubulointerstitium (WBCs or WBC casts), other renal disorders should be considered. Renal ultrasonography may reveal unusually large kidneys in relation to the decreased GFR. In this situation before diabetic nephropathy can be diagnosed, other diseases that can cause proteinuria, renal insufficiency, and nephromegaly, such as multiple myeloma, amyloidosis, or HIV-related nephropathy, should be ruled out. When the diagnosis is uncertain, consideration should be given to a renal biopsy. The findings on renal biopsy in the setting of diabetic nephropathy are described in the following section.

HISTOPATHOLOGY AND ITS FUNCTIONAL CORRELATES

A host of structural alterations encompass kidney involvement in diabetes. Initially, there is hypertrophy of both glomerular and tubuloepithelial elements (Table 45.3). This is followed by thickening of the glomerular and tubular basement membranes and progressive accumulation of extracellular matrix components in the glomerular mesangium. Less recognized lesions such as progressive tubulointerstitial fibrosis and renal arteriosclerosis can be present in patients with either type I or type II diabetes mellitus (Table 45.2). These extraglomerular lesions appear to be more prevalent in type II diabetic patients. The glomerular, tubulointerstitial, and arteriosclerotic lesions are all important in the

TABLE 45.3. Histopathology in Diabetic Nephropathy

Glomerular Structural Lesions
Glomerular hypertrophy
Glomerular basement membrane thickening
Mesangial matrix expansion
Diffuse glomerulosclerosis
Nodular (Kimmelstein-Wilson) glomerulosclerosis
Capsular drop
Fibrin caps
Arteriolosclerosis and hyalinosis (afferent and efferent)
Nonglomerular Structural Lesions
Tubuloepithelial cell hypertrophy
Tubular basement membrane thickening
Tubular atrophy and interstitial fibrosis
Armanni-Ebstein tubulopathy
Papillary necrosis

expression of the functional derangement that characterizes the stage of overt diabetic nephropathy, namely proteinuria, hypertension, and the progressive decline in GFR. Secondary ischemic or obliterative global glomerulosclerosis also develops, and this contributes to the marked reduction in GFR.

Glomerular Changes

Glomerular Hypertrophy and Basement Membrane Thickening

Glomerular hypertrophy is an early and persistent feature of the diabetic state. Animal studies suggest that there may be formation of new capillary segments in addition to the elongation of capillaries and the increase in the filtering surface area. The larger glomerular volume and the increase in capillary surface area maintains a higher GFR despite the development of mesangial matrix expansion.

The glomerular basement membrane (GBM) begins to increase in thickness after 2 to 3 years of diabetes. The width often exceeds 500 nm, or nearly double the control value. This thickening is potentially reversible with insulin therapy and tight glycemic control. There are specific alterations in the morphology of the GBM, such as splitting and layered thickening, as well as in its composition, such as increased abundance of type IV collagen, laminins, nidogen/entactin, and other extracellular matrix molecules. Moreover, there are qualitative changes in the composition of matrix material. Composition of type IV collagen, the most abundant matrix constituent of the GBM, may be altered so there is an increase in the subendothelial content of the novel (restricted) $\alpha3$(IV) and $\alpha4$(IV) collagen chains, whereas there is a relative decrease in the density of the classical (ubiquitous) $\alpha1$(IV) and $\alpha2$(IV) collagen chains.

The proteinuria and the permeability defects of the glomerular capillary are related to both the abnormalities in GBM composition and to alterations in the glomerular visceral epithelial cells (podocytes), which manifest as a loss in the charge-selective and size-selective permeability barriers. Polyanionic proteoglycan heparan sulfate is localized predominantly to the laminae rarae of the GBM and is believed to govern the charge-permselective properties of the filtration barrier. In diabetic nephropathy, there is a marked reduction in the number of anionic moieties such as sialic acid and heparan sulfate proteoglycan in the GBM. A decrease in the posttranslational incorporation of heparan sulfate into the core protein of the proteoglycan is a prominent mechanism for the decreased density of anionic moieties in the diabetic GBM.

The filtration barrier's loss of size permselectivity probably results from changes in podocyte structure. Longitudinal studies in Pima Indians with diabetic nephropathy have described a reduction in the number of podocytes per glomerulus and a stretching or a relative increase in the surface area covered by the remaining podocytes. Loss of podocytes and the stretching of the remaining ones causes a derangement in the filtration slit-diaphragms and shifting of the glomerular pores toward a larger size, thus explaining the filtration barrier's loss of size selectivity and enhanced trafficking of proteins into Bowman's space.

Mesangial Matrix Expansion and Glomerulosclerosis

The pathologically distinctive lesions of full-blown diabetic glomerulopathy require more time to develop than GBM thickening. The most pathognomonic lesion is nodular glomerulosclerosis, or the Kimmelstiel-Wilson lesion, which is present in up to 25% of diabetic patients at postmortem examination. A roughly similar pattern of nodular lesions may be seen in other renal diseases, notably light-chain nephropathy and amyloidosis. However, appropriate immunofluorescent staining, electron microscopy, and historical and laboratory information distinguish these conditions from the Kimmelstiel-Wilson lesion. The nodules in diabetes are centrally located in the peripheral loops of glomerular lobules, and they consist of homogeneous, well demarcated eosinophilic masses that show a laminated structure on hematoxylin-eosin and periodic acid–Schiff staining. Nodules probably form in response to injury produced by microaneurysmal dilation of glomerular capillaries and mesangial lysis.

Anecdotal reports in older literature have described the occurrence of diabetic nephropathy in nondiabetic patients based solely on the light microscopic finding of nodular sclerosis. However, these reports did not formally exclude nondiabetic causes of such lesions (e.g., light-chain nephropathy and amyloidosis) because appropriate staining techniques were not applied.

More prevalent than the Kimmelstiel-Wilson lesion, and perhaps of greater pathophysiologic significance, is the finding of diffuse glomerulosclerosis, which is a characteristic lesion of established diabetic nephropathy. Typically, the lesion is characterized by diffuse expansion of the mesangial extracellular matrix compartment, which begins to appear after at least 5 to 7 years of diabetes and accompanies the progressive thickening of the GBM. The expanded material is identified by hematoxylin-eosin and periodic acid–Schiff staining, and is distributed randomly across the glomerulus. Histomorphometric analysis on kidney specimens from patients with a wide range of disease severity has established a close correlation between the expansion of the glomerular mesangial matrix and the declining surface area available for filtration. The functional correlate of this manifestation is the reduction in GFR. Diabetic patients with hypertension and decreased GFR tend to have the highest mesangial fractional volume (Fig. 45.6). Also, diabetic patients with increasing urinary AER typically have an increase in mesangial fractional volume (Fig. 45.7).

Matrix accumulation is the result of both increased synthesis and decreased degradation of extracellular matrix molecules, especially fibronectin, laminins, and the classical collagen chains $\alpha1$ (IV) and $\alpha2$(IV). Some studies have suggested that collagen mRNA and protein content are increased in absolute amounts per glomerulus but that there may be a relative reduction in the density of certain collagen chains because of increased amounts of other matrix constituents. Fibrillary collagens that are not native to the glomerulus (e.g., collagens type I and III) may appear within the expanded mesangium. The lesions of diabetic glomerulosclerosis have traditionally been regarded as irreversible; however, reversal of these lesions has

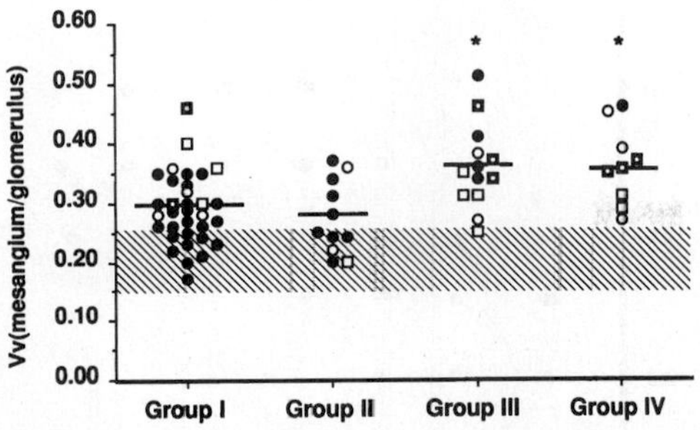

Figure 45.6. Relationship between increased mesangial fractional volume on renal biopsy in patients with type I diabetes mellitus and the clinical severity of diabetic nephropathy as assessed by the presence of hypertension and reduced GFR. The shaded area represents the means ±2 SD in a group of 52 age-matched normal control subjects. ●●, normal BP and GFR; ○○, reduced GFR (<70 ml · min^{-1} · 1.73 m^{-2}); □, hypertension ($\geq 140/85$ mm Hg); ⊡, reduced GFR and hypertension. *$P<.005$ versus groups I and II. (Reproduced with permission from Fioretto P, Steffes MW, Mauer SM. Glomerular structure in nonproteinuric IDDM patients with various levels of albuminuria. Diabetes 1994;43:1358–1364.)

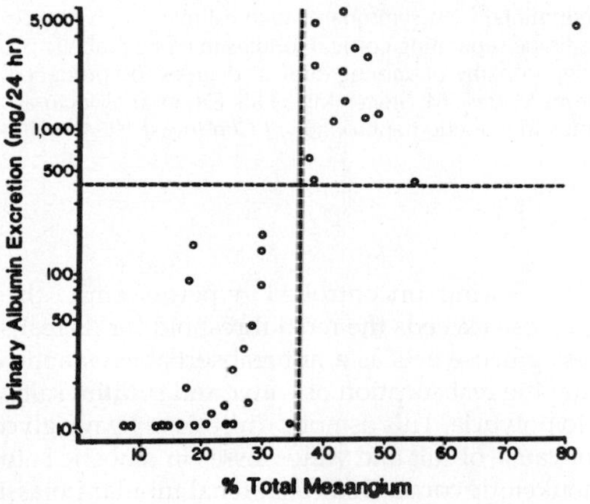

Figure 45.7. Relationship between the development of microalbuminuria and percentage total mesangium in renal biopsy specimens from type I diabetic patients with diabetic nephropathy. The interrupted lines represent the graphic limits of the chi-square, which was calculated to be 27, $P<.0005$. Note the triple log scale for the urinary albumin excretion rate; values near the abscissa (at 10 mg/24 hr) represent rates below the sensitivity range of the urinary albumin test. (Reproduced with permission from Mauer SM, Steffes MW, Ellis EN, et al. Structural-functional relationships in diabetic nephropathy. *J Clin Invest* 1984;74:1143–1155.)

proven to be possible after 10 years of successful pancreas transplants in patients with established diabetic nephropathy. Nevertheless, these lesions require several years to develop and will require several years to resolve.

Vascular hyalinosis (described in the following section) and exudative lesions in the glomerular tuft may also appear, especially when severe hypertension is longstanding. These include capsular drops, which are lens-shaped pieces of sclerosing extracellular matrix adjacent to Bowman's capsule, and fibrin caps, which are homogeneous eosinophilic masses overlying capillary loops. Globally sclerotic (obsolescent) glomeruli similar to those seen in kidneys with end-stage disease of any cause can also develop in the kidneys of patients with diabetic nephropathy. There are diverse patterns of renal lesions in patients with type II diabetes mellitus as compared with type I patients. Most type II patients have typical nodular or diffuse glomerulosclerosis, but the remaining have nonspecific chronic changes described as nephroangiosclerosis or other forms of glomerular lesions of the nondiabetic type ranging from minimal change disease to proliferative glomerulonephritis.

Tubular Changes

A host of structural and functional changes develop in the nonglomerular compartment of the kidneys of the diabetic patient (Table 45.3).

Renal Hypertrophy and Tubular Basement Membrane Thickening

Nephromegaly occurs as early as the first few months after the onset of diabetes and persists for many years even when GFR starts declining. Kidney enlargement involves both the tubules and the glomeruli, but, because of the much larger volume of tubules, it is primarily due to tubuloepithelial cellular hypertrophy (with little, if any, hyperplasia). This process also involves elongation of basement membranes. Kidney protein mass is significantly increased in diabetic renal hypertrophy due to increased synthesis and decreased breakdown.

The tubular basement membrane (TBM) thickening in the early phase of the disease increases the mass without discernible abnormalities in morphology. Conspicuous TBM thickening and occasional splitting occur after several years. Immunohistochemical techniques have revealed linear binding of albumin and IgG along the length of the thickened TBM in kidneys from diabetic subjects. These proteins are thought to have gained access to the TBM because of increased permeability of the peritubular capillaries and passive trapping. When the stage of heavy proteinuria sets in, morphologic alterations are then seen in proximal tubular cells due to enhanced protein reabsorption and lipid deposition that result in the fatty vacuolization and an increased number of protein-containing lysosomes. Renal hypertrophy and TBM thickening are seen in all patients with longstanding diabetes and are not specific signs of overt nephropathy or of the potential for progressive nephropathy to develop.

The Armanni-Ebstein Lesion

The Armanni-Ebstein lesion, the most specific morphologic tubular abnormality of diabetes mellitus, refers to glycogen accumulation in the epithelial cells of the collecting duct and Henle's loop. With hematoxylin-eosin staining, these cells appear clear and completely empty (vacuolization). Intracellular glycogen deposition can be demonstrated with periodic acid–Schiff staining. The pathophysiologic importance of glycogen accumulation in epithelial cells is unknown, but the lesion correlates with longstanding poor glycemic control and is rarely encountered.

Tubulointerstitial Fibrosis in Diabetic Nephropathy

Renal biopsies from patients with type I diabetes mellitus show subtle interstitial fibrosis at the earliest stages of diabetic nephropathy. As glomerular filtration falls, tubular atrophy and interstitial fibrosis become more prominent. These lesions may be more pronounced in type II diabetic patients. In fact, a minority of type II patients can develop more severe forms of tubulointerstitial and vascular changes with only mild degrees of the typical glomerular lesions. These nonglomerular changes, which also include prominent mononuclear cell infiltrates in the interstitium, were interpreted in the past as evidence of chronic pyelonephritis or ischemia, but they should not signify an infectious process. Tubulointerstitial fibrosis has long been recognized as the crucial histologic parameter that best correlates with chronic renal failure in a variety of renal diseases including diabetic nephropathy. The percentage of kidney volume occupied by interstitial fibrotic tissue in diabetic nephropathy correlates strongly with the rise in serum creatinine level over a wide range (Fig. 45.8). In addition, there is a direct correlation between the interstitial expansion and the severity of mesangial matrix expansion and glomerulosclerosis (Fig. 45.9). These correlations suggest a parallel, perhaps independent, process damaging the glomeruli and tubulointerstitial structures; alternatively, the changes in the interstitium could be initiating a secondary glomerular process.

Alterations in Tubular Transport Processes

Abnormalities of tubular transport are often neglected or overshadowed by the glomerular parameters that are monitored during the development of renal disease. However, the appearance of microalbuminuria in diabetic glomerulopathy and its magnitude can be modified in a major way by proximal tubular events related to the diminished capacity to reabsorb filtered albumin once the glomerular leak of albumin becomes heavy.

Abnormalities of tubular transport processes for sodium, potassium, calcium, hydrogen ion, and glucose accompany the development of diabetes mellitus. During the first few days of experimental diabetes in rodents, excess natriuresis occurs as a consequence of glycosuria; however, as early as 3 weeks after the onset of experimental diabetes, sodium balance becomes positive and blood volume increases significantly due to renal adaptive mechanisms accompanying tubular hypertrophy. In the proximal tubule, sodium reabsorption increases proportionately to the increase in GFR, thus maintaining glomerular-tubular balance. In addition, net transcellular sodium reabsorption is also stimulated as evidenced by a parallel increase in the activities of the Na^+-H^+ exchange in the luminal brush-border membrane and the Na^+-K^+-ATPase in the basolateral membrane. During uncontrolled hyperglycemia, the filtered load of glucose exceeds the renal threshold for its reabsorption. The excess glucose acts as a nonreabsorbable osmotic diuretic, preventing the reabsorption of water and sodium salts, thereby leading to polyuria. This osmotic diuresis of heavy glycosuria is the major cause of salt and water losses in diabetic ketoacidosis and in nonketotic coma. Defects in renal tubular potassium and hydrogen ion secretion related to the development of hypoaldosteronism and/or tubular unresponsiveness to the action of aldosterone are the main tubular abnormalities (type IV hyperkalemic renal tubular acidosis) associated with mild to moderate renal insufficiency due to diabetic nephropathy.

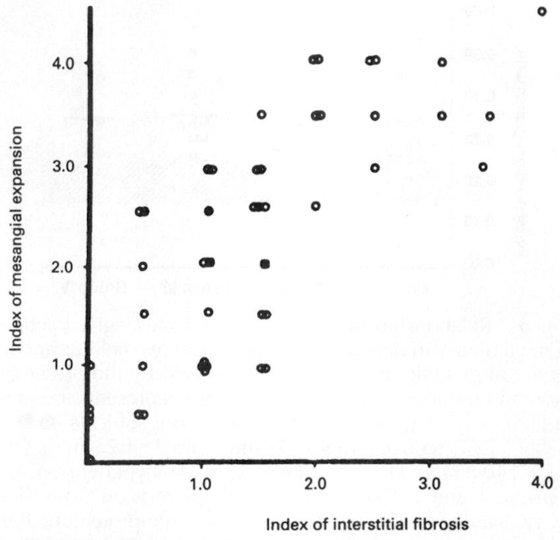

Figure 45.9. Significant positive correlation between an index of mesangial expansion, determined in renal biopsy specimens by semiquantitative estimate of mesangial zones in glomeruli, and an index of interstitial fibrosis, determined by a semiquantitative estimate of the space occupied by fibrous tissue separating cortical tubules in type I diabetic patients with diabetic nephropathy of varying clinical degrees. (Reproduced with permission from Mauer SM, Steffes MW, Ellis EN, et al. Structural-functional relationships in diabetic nephropathy. *J Clin Invest* 1984;74:1143–1155.)

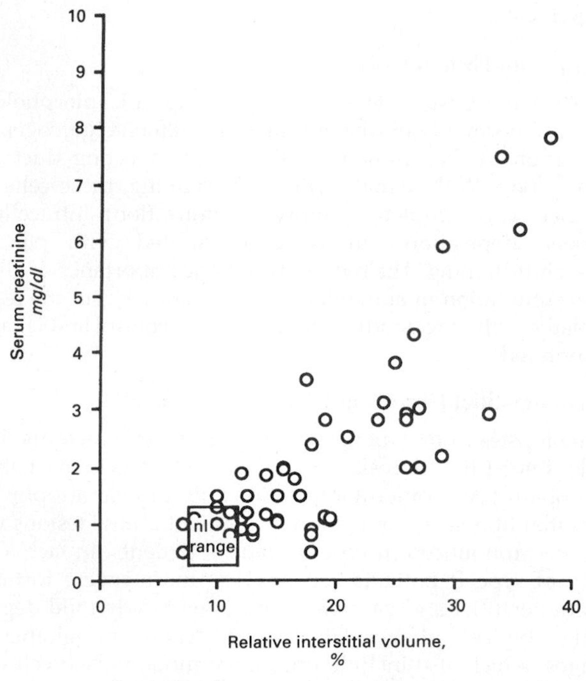

Figure 45.8. Relationship between the serum creatinine concentration (y-axis) and the percent of renal mass occupied by interstitial tissue (x-axis) in renal biopsies from patients with diabetes mellitus and various degrees of nephropathy. Normal (nl) range is indicated by the square. (Figure redrawn with permission from Bader et al. *Pathol Res Pract* 1980;167:204–2116; from Ziyadeh FN, Goldfarb S. The renal tubulointerstitium in diabetes mellitus. *Kidney Int* 1991;39:464–475.)

Arteriosclerosis and Renovascular Injury in Diabetes

In a variety of tissues in patients with diabetes, a form of ischemic injury induced by exudative hyalinosis, which progressively obliterates small- and medium-sized arterioles, may be responsible for functional organ failure. Progressive and global obliteration of glomeruli occurs in a peculiar columnarlike pattern of distribution in all levels of the renal cortex, which corresponds to the distribution of large renal interlobular vessels. Vascular lesions in the kidney are often more prevalent in type II than in type I patients, reflecting the higher incidence of hypertension in type II patients. One pathognomonic finding in established diabetic nephropathy of either type is the arteriosclerotic hyalinosis of both the afferent and efferent arterioles. In contrast, the arteriolar lesion in essential hypertension (without diabetes mellitus) is restricted to the afferent arteriole. The role of the arteriolar lesions in inducing some of the renal histopathology in diabetic nephropathy has been implied from several observations. Biopsies from patients with diabetic nephropathy show a clear correlation between the degree of diabetic glomerulosclerosis and a quantitative index of arteriolar hyalinization and occlusion. The degree of vessel obstruction and obliteration is inversely correlated with the level of renal function and directly correlates with the greater severity of both diabetic glomerular sclerosis and interstitial fibrosis. Similarly, arteriolar hyalinosis tends to be more severe in patients with overt nephropathy and increased interstitial tissue volume. However, arteriolar hyalinosis may occasionally be found in patients with milder forms of nephropathy and, therefore, cannot be used to distinguish those individuals with more severe disease.

PATHOGENESIS

The metabolic sequelae of chronic hyperglycemia comprise the central biochemical abnormalities of diabetes. Because nephropathy does not develop in all diabetic patients, genetic and hemodynamic factors in addition to hyperglycemia must be operative in those patients at risk for development of diabetic nephropathy (Table 45.4). Thus hyperglycemia is viewed as a necessary but not sufficient risk factor for the development of renal injury. Factors predicting a high risk in addition to poor glycemic control include duration of diabetes (typically more than 10 years), hemodynamic injury (systemic and intraglomerular hypertension), familial/genetic factors, and racial predisposition (see Genetic Predisposition/Markers). This section will discuss the hemodynamic factors and metabolic pathways by which elevated glucose concentration may lead to diabetic kidney disease.

Glomerular Hemodynamics in Diabetic Kidney Disease

Vascular dysfunction in diabetes is characterized by an early increase in blood flow to many organs, loss of autoregulation, and a generalized capillary hypertension, which give rise to the findings of rubeosis faciei, retinal hyperemia, and glomerular hyperperfusion. Arteriosclerotic hyalinosis and accelerated atherosclerosis cause a decrease in flow in the later stages of the disease.

In the kidney, the vascular tone of the afferent and efferent arterioles are major determinants of the glomerular capillary pressure. Classic glomerular micropuncture studies by Brenner and his coworkers demonstrated that the moderately hyperglycemic diabetic rat has increased single-nephron GFR (SNGFR) that is mediated by increased glomerular blood flow (Q_A) and an elevation of the glomerular capillary pressure (P_{GC}). The latter is mediated by a greater relaxation of the afferent arteriole than the efferent arteriole. The net result is that the enhanced glomerular blood flow is permitted to enter the glomerulus via the relaxed afferent arteriole, and because there is relatively less relaxation in the efferent arteriole, the hydrostatic pressure in the glomerular capillary increases, even when systemic arterial blood pressure is not elevated.

Patients with early diabetes (especially type I, and to a lesser degree type II) tend to have a greater GFR than nondiabetics. This hyperfiltration of early diabetes results from increases in plasma flow and, based on data obtained in diabetic animals, a concomitant increase in glomerular capillary hydraulic pressures. The mechanisms of the changes in glomerular hemodynamics are not fully understood, but a number of possible factors may be responsible including increased vasodilatory prostanoids, nitric oxide, and humoral vasodilators (glucagon and atrial natriuretic peptide). Increased sodium–glucose reabsorption in the proximal tubule leads to reduced delivery of sodium to the macula densa and alters tubuloglomerular feedback. In addition, the glomerular capillary surface area available for filtration in diabetes enlarges and contributes to the increase in the GFR.

The hemodynamic changes of diabetes may contribute to the ultimate development of end-stage renal disease. Clinical observation suggests that altered renal hemodynamics plays a permissive role in the genesis of diabetic lesions in the glomerulus. In patients who have unilateral renal artery stenosis, nodular glomerulosclerosis is noted in the contralateral kidney and not in the ipsilateral kidney, which is protected from the elevated pressure.

Micropuncture studies in diabetic rats and in subtotal nephrectomy models have formed the basis of our current understanding regarding the development of glomerular hemodynamic stress in diabetic nephropathy. They also provide a rational basis to target treatment with ACE inhibitors or low dietary protein. Direct pressure injury to the glomerular capillary wall tension leads to alterations in glomerular structure and function. The early increase in glomerular blood flow and glomerular capillary pressure enhances the shear-stress effect on the glomerular capillary wall and the mesangium. This stress may lead to endothelial dysfunction, which translates into alterations in GBM structure as well as mesangial cell dysfunction. Intraglomerular hypertension can increase the macromolecular trafficking across the mesangium that can provoke the mesangial cells to increase their production of mesangial matrix components. Besides the crowding out of the filtering surface area by the expanded mesangial matrix, the increased diameter of the glomerular capillary early in the course of diabetes may confer a mechanical disadvantage through the LaPlace relationship (tension = transmural pressure × vessel radius), in which increased capillary diameter would increase wall tension.

Mesangial expansion may be a specific example of how renal and particularly glomerular hypertrophy can be disadvantageous because disproportionate expansion of the mesangial areas appears to be an important contributor to ultimate filtration failure. A link may exist between the known intraglomerular

TABLE 45.4. Pathogenic Mediators of Diabetic Renal Involvement

Altered intrarenal hemodynamics
Activation of pathways of glucose metabolism
Increased polyol pathway (increased sorbitol)
Disordered *myo*-inositol metabolism
Increased hexosamine pathway
Increased pentose phosphate shunt (increased UDP glucose)
Increased *de novo* synthesis of diacylglycerol and stimulation of PKC
Altered cellular redox state (increased NADH:NAD$^+$)
Altered glycosphingolipid metabolism (increased glucosylceramide and ganglioside GM3)
Nonenzymatic glycation of circulating or structural proteins
Amadori glucose adducts
Advanced glycosylation end-products (AGE)
Humoral imbalance
Activation of intrarenal hormones or cytokines
Transforming growth factor-β
Angiotensin II
Endothelins
Eicosanoids (e.g., thromboxane)
Nitric oxide
Insulinlike growth factor-1
Platelet-derived growth factor
Oxidative stress
Elevation in basal level of cytosolic calcium
Genetic predisposition

hypertension of diabetic nephropathy and the stretch-induced production of the prosclerotic cytokine transforming growth factor-β (TGF-β). In fact, the production of this growth factor can be stimulated in cultured mesangial cells exposed to either high glucose concentration and/or cyclic stretch.

Superimposed on the intrarenal hemodynamic changes is the eventual development of systemic hypertension in most diabetic patients. The increase in the mean blood pressure correlates with the severity of microalbuminuria (Fig. 45.10). Arterial hypertension is one of the most important risk factors for the progression of diabetic nephropathy. The combination of arterial hypertension and afferent arteriolar vasodilation leads to especially high intrarenal and glomerular capillary pressures. In type I diabetes, blood pressure increases with the rise in urine AER. Careful 24-hour blood pressure monitoring has demonstrated that increases in both systolic and diastolic pressure, even in the top range of accepted normal values, are associated with progression from normoalbuminuria to microalbuminuria.

According to the Steno hypothesis, all diabetic microvascular complications are manifestations of increased vascular permeability and endothelial damage in various organs. This view posits that glomerular endothelial dysfunction, with the ensuing disturbance in glomerular permselectivity, is just one facet of the generalized endothelial dysfunction. Coronary artery endothelial dysfunction may explain the well known association of albuminuria with coronary artery mortality in diabetic patients.

Hyperglycemia

The most important risk factor in the development of diabetic nephropathy is hyperglycemia. One of the most convincing pieces of evidence linking glomerular lesions to hyperglycemia is the reversal of these lesions after 10 years after a successful pancreas transplant in nonuremic type I diabetic patients with established nephropathy. Experimental evidence indicates that an increase in the rate of intracellular glucose metabolism through enzymatic pathways promotes pathologic changes in genetically susceptible patients. Tissue culture studies have suggested that high ambient glucose levels increase mesangial matrix accumulation as a result of increased synthesis and possibly a decrease in degradation. A host of metabolic consequences related to hyperglycemia have been described as an explanation for the development of the renal lesions in diabetes. They include the following: increased activity of the polyol pathway, increased glucosamine metabolism, activation of protein kinase C (PKC), nonenzymatic glycation of proteins, oxidative stress, modulations in the response to hormones, cytokines or growth factors, and elevated basal levels of cytosolic calcium.

Polyol Pathway

Activation of the polyol pathway in insulin-insensitive tissues has been suspected to mediate diabetic complications such as neuropathy and retinopathy, and perhaps nephropathy. In the lens, cataract formation may be due to the osmotic swelling caused by the accumulation of intracellular sorbitol, which is converted from glucose by aldose reductase, the rate-limiting enzyme of this pathway. In tissues other than the lens, activation of the polyol pathway leads to cellular dysfunction through a mechanism that is poorly understood. Polyol pathway activation may lead to a disorder in cellular *myo*-inositol metabolism as well as provide additional reactive substrate for nonenzymatic reactions, which are important events in the vascular complications of diabetes. Increased flux of glucose through the polyol pathway leads to an increase in the redox state (high

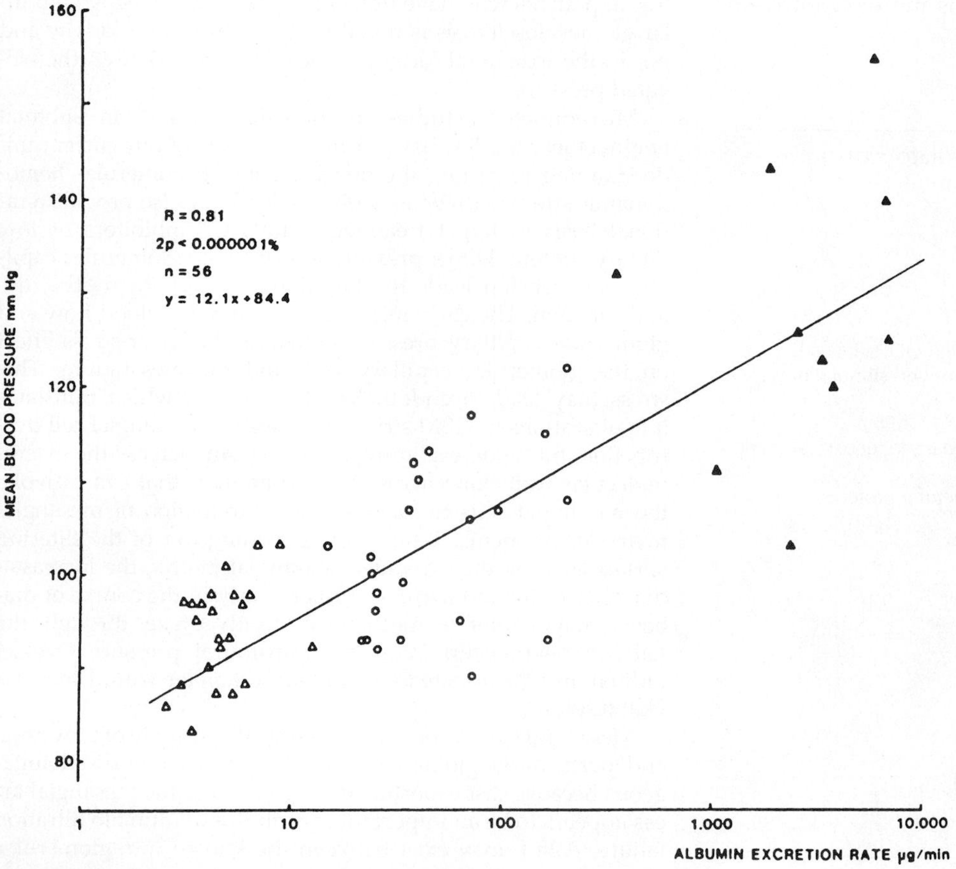

Figure 45.10. The positive correlation between the mean blood pressure and urinary albumin excretion rate in type I diabetic patients. *Open triangles,* patients with normoalbuminuria; *open circles,* patients with microalbuminuria; *closed triangles,* patients with overt proteinuria. [Reproduced with permission from Mogensen CE, Christensen CK. Blood pressure changes and renal function in incipient and overt diabetic nephropathy. *Hypertension* 1985;7(6 pt 2):1164–1173.]

NADH:NAD + ratio), which appears to be important in the stimulation of *de novo* synthesis of diacylglycerol and the subsequent activation of PKC. Treatment of experimental animals with aldose reductase inhibitors may prevent some early features of diabetic nephropathy, such as glomerular hyperfiltration and microalbuminuria. However, there is no consistent evidence that these inhibitors effectively reduce late manifestations of nephropathy in these animals.

Nonenzymatic Glycation

The early formation of Amadori products and their subsequent processing into the advanced glycosylation end-products (AGE) are considered to be major mediators of injury imposed by the hyperglycemic milieu. Nonenzymatic glycation is a condensation reaction between reducing sugars (including glucose) and reactive amino groups in target proteins (and perhaps lipids and nucleic acids). This reaction yields unstable Schiff-base intermediates that undergo Amadori rearrangement to form stable but reversible ketamine adducts (Fig. 45.11). The next step is the formation of 3-deoxyglucosone, a highly reactive Amadori-derived compound, which can glycate proteins further. Subsequent, slow, and irreversible Maillard reactions may occur resulting in the development of incompletely defined AGEs.

The concentration of Amadori products, the predominant form of circulating glycated proteins, is significantly increased in diabetes. Hemoglobin $A1_c$ ($HbA1_c$), a well-characterized Amadori product, is a widely accepted indicator of the quality of glycemic control in diabetes. Amadori-modified albumin also increases with exposure to a hyperglycemic milieu, and its level can be reduced with specific therapy directed against Amadori-modified albumin in experimental animals, resulting in the amelioration of diabetic lesions in the kidney. Such studies implicate Amadori adducts as a potential link between hyperglycemia and the pathogenesis of diabetic complications.

AGEs modify ligands on extracellular matrix components and interact with cellular receptors (e.g., RAGE; receptor for AGE) to alter intracellular function. AGEs likely upregulate a host of genes that can adversely affect protein structure and function. AGEs also cause increased cross-linking and reduced breakdown of the thickened GBM, enhanced binding of circulating plasma proteins, and activation of cells, particularly

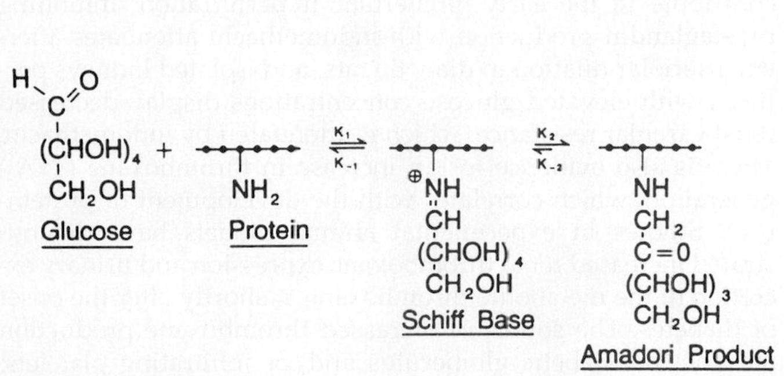

Figure 45.11. Chemical pathway for nonenzymatic formation of the early glycation products involving condensation and covalent bond formation between target proteins and glucose. The unstable aldimine Schiff base gives rise to the more stable but still reversible ketamine Amadori product. Susceptible proteins are subsequently modified by slow and irreversible Maillard browning reactions, which include rearrangement, dehydration, oxidative fragmentation, and cross-linking. This gives rise to a host of poorly defined AGE-modified proteins and cross-links. (Reproduced with permission from Brownlee M, Cerami A, Vlassara H. Advanced glycosylation end products in tissue and the biochemical bases of diabetic complications. *N Engl J Med* 1988;318:1315–1321.)

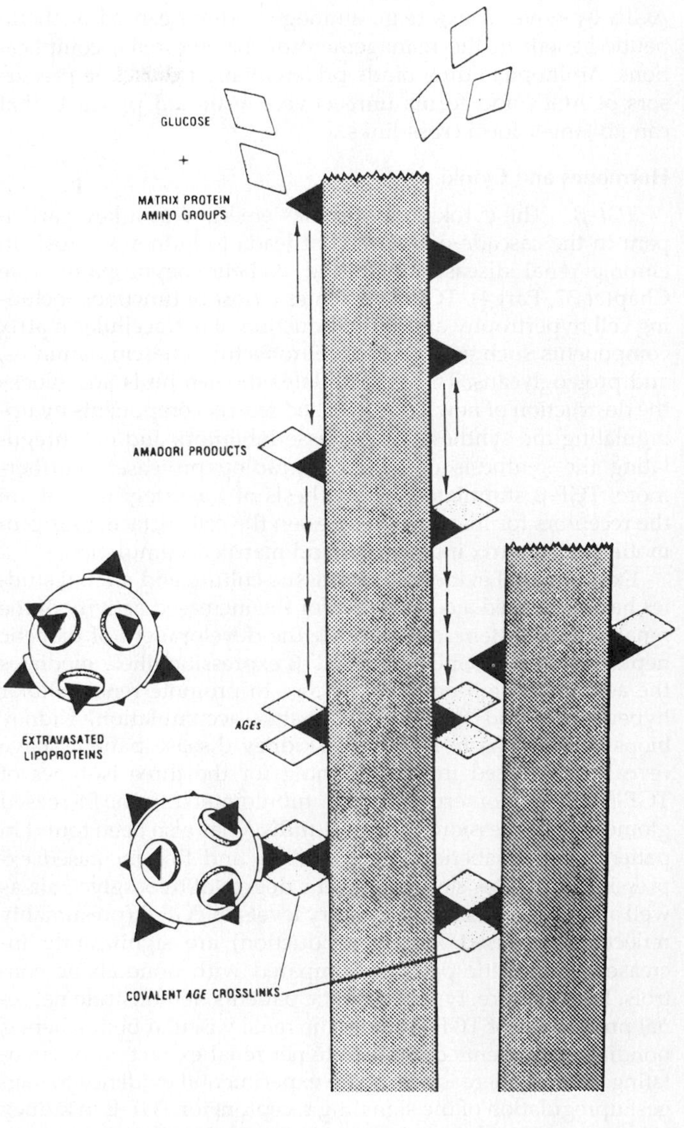

Figure 45.12. Formation of cross-links in matrix protein due to advanced glycosylation end products (AGE). The upper portion of the figure shows the formation of irreversible AGEs. The lower portion of the figure shows the accumulation of chemically reactive AGEs on long-lived matrix proteins as a function of time and glucose concentration. These accumulated end products form covalent cross-links with other matrix proteins and with extravasated plasma proteins by bonding with amino groups. (Reproduced with permission from Brownlee M, Cerami A, Vlassara H. Advanced glycosylation end-products in tissue and the biochemical bases of diabetic complications. *N Engl J Med* 1988;318:1315–1321.)

macrophages (Fig. 45.12). Type I and type II diabetic patients have increased plasma levels of AGE-modified low-density lipoprotein (LDL), which can markedly impair LDL receptor-mediated clearance. AGEs have been detected with immunohistochemical techniques in the mesangial matrix of nodular lesions and in renal vessels from diabetic patients with advanced diabetic nephropathy. Circulating AGE concentrations are dependent on normal renal function for clearance, but in diabetic patients receiving renal replacement therapy, these levels remain threefold to fourfold above normal regardless of whether high-flux dialysis, conventional hemodialysis, or chronic ambulatory peritoneal dialysis is used. Levels can be normalized by functioning renal transplants. Clinical trials are ongoing to determine whether abrogating the biologic effects of

AGEs by novel drugs (e.g., aminoguanidine) can be of therapeutic benefit in the management of diabetic renal complications. Aminoguanidine binds preferentially to reactive precursors of AGEs and forms unreactive substituted products that can no longer form cross-links.

Hormones and Cytokines

TGF-β. The cytokine TGF-β has emerged as a key participant in the cascade of events that leads to kidney sclerosis in chronic renal diseases including diabetic nephropathy (see Chapter 37, Part 4). TGF-β regulates a host of functions including cell hypertrophy and the production of extracellular matrix components such as collagens, fibronectin, tenascin, laminins, and proteoglycans. TGF-β stimulates the synthesis and blocks the destruction of newly synthesized matrix components by upregulating the synthesis of protease inhibitors and downregulating the synthesis of matrix-degrading proteases. Furthermore, TGF-β stimulates the synthesis of the integrins that are the receptors for matrix molecules on the cell surface, thus promoting cell–matrix interactions and matrix accumulation.

Experimental evidence from tissue culture and animal studies has implicated a central role for the increased activity of the renal TGF-β system in mediating the development of diabetic nephropathy. Thus increased TGF-β expression likely mediates the actions of high ambient glucose to promote renal cellular hypertrophy and to stimulate matrix accumulation. Kidney biopsy specimens from diabetic kidney disease patients have revealed increased immunostaining for the three isotypes of TGF-β in the glomeruli and the tubulointerstitium. Increased glomerular expression of TGF-β1 mRNA has also been found in patients with diabetic kidney disease, and this increased expression correlates closely with the degree of hyperglycemia as well as the sclerosis index. Urinary levels of TGF-β (presumably reflecting increased kidney production) are significantly increased in diabetic patients compared with nondiabetic controls. Furthermore, type II diabetic patients demonstrate net renal production of TGF-β across the renal vascular bed, whereas nondiabetic patients demonstrate net renal extraction of circulating TGF-β. There is also some experimental evidence to suggest upregulation of the signaling receptors for TGF-β in kidney cells exposed to a hyperglycemic milieu and in experimental diabetic kidney disease. Interventional studies in animal models have proven that the inhibition of TGF-β bioactivity by systemic treatment with a neutralizing anti–TGF-β antibody prevents the stimulation of collagen and fibronectin synthesis, ameliorates renal insufficiency, and markedly abrogates the increase in mesangial matrix fraction.

PKC. One of the earliest signal-transduction mechanisms through which high glucose stimulates matrix production is activation of PKC, presumably due to increased *de novo* synthesis of diacylglycerol. The latter reaction is driven by an increased NADH:NAD$^+$ ratio, thus shunting some glycolytic intermediates into the phosphatidic acid and diacylglycerol synthesis pathway. Increased NADH:NAD$^+$ ratio can result from increased glucose metabolism through the polyol pathway, catalyzed by the successive actions of aldose reductase and fructose dehydrogenase. The activation of PKC by diacylglycerol leads to increased production of the Jun/Fos (AP1) transcription factor complex. This complex binds and activates several gene promoters including those of growth factors and matrix molecules. A link may exist between PKC activation (induced by high glucose or other agents such as angiotensin II) and the stimulation of TGF-β action because consensus AP1-binding sites and other glucose-responsive elements have been identified in the promoter region of the TGF-β1 gene. Emerging work has implicated activation of specific PKC isozymes (e.g., α, β, delta, and zeta) in diabetic renal disease. Studies using a novel and selective PKC-β inhibitor in diabetic rats have demonstrated that chronic treatment with this oral agent is well tolerated and results in marked attenuation of proteinuria, the glomerular overexpression of TGF-β, and the increased synthesis of type IV collagen and fibronectin.

Angiotensin II. Angiotensin II is the most intensively studied factor that may underlie the altered renal hemodynamics in diabetes. The relative efferent arteriolar constriction observed in diabetes may be due to increased intraglomerular angiotensin II production. Some studies have also suggested that the receptor number for angiotensin II may be decreased in the kidney. Thus the afferent arteriole may have reduced responsiveness to angiotensin II, accounting for the observed afferent vasodilation. The fact that ACE inhibitors are renoprotective strongly suggests a role for increased systemic and intrarenal production of angiotensin II in the progression of diabetic nephropathy. Circulating angiotensin II levels are inappropriate to the prevailing blood pressure level and the amount of exchangeable sodium. Angiotensin II can also exert various nonhemodynamic effects that are relevant to the development of diabetic nephropathy. The peptide is both a renal growth factor and a profibrogenic agent that stimulates matrix synthesis, at least in part due to stimulation of TGF-β activity. Treatment with ACE inhibitors decreases the expression of TGF-β in the kidney.

Endothelin-1. Endothelins are responsible for some of the complications of diabetes. Glomerular and urinary levels of endothelin-1 are increased in diabetic rats. In animal experiments an endothelin receptor A antagonist attenuates the early increase in GFR, reduces urinary protein excretion, and decreases expression of matrix molecules and growth factors in the glomerulus. The mechanism of endothelin-1 stimulation in diabetes may involve angiotensin II, although increased TGF-β activity may also be implicated. Serum endothelin levels are higher in type II diabetic patients than the general population, especially in patients with retinopathy (but no data are available in diabetic patients with nephropathy). Interestingly, treatment with captopril reduces endothelin-1 levels in such patients.

Eicosanoids. Vasodilatory prostanoids (PGE_2, PGI_2) likely contribute to the early glomerular hyperfiltration. Inhibiting prostaglandin production with indomethacin attenuates afferent arteriolar dilation in diabetic rats, and isolated kidneys perfused with elevated glucose concentrations display decreased renal vascular resistance, which is attenuated by indomethacin. There is also evidence for an increase in thromboxane (TxA_2) generation, which correlates with the development of proteinuria. Studies in experimental animal models have demonstrated increased renal thromboxane expression and urinary excretion of the metabolite thromboxane B_2 shortly after the onset of diabetes. The source of increased thromboxane production may be the diabetic glomerulus and/or infiltrating platelets. Addition of thromboxane analogs to mesangial cells in culture results in stimulation of fibronectin production, which appears to be mediated by PKC activation. Thromboxane is also known to stimulate TGF-β production in mesangial cells. Inhibitors of thromboxane synthesis and its receptor ameliorate diabetes-induced albuminuria and mesangial matrix expansion but not GBM thickening. Short-term treatment of proteinuric type I diabetic patients with an oral thromboxane synthetase inhibitor significantly decreases proteinuria.

Other Mediators. Nitric oxide appears to be an attractive mediator of glomerular hyperfiltration because it decreases preglomerular vascular tone. There are an increased nitric oxide metabolites in the urine of diabetic rats, and inhibition of the intrarenal nitric oxide synthase system with L-arginine analogs leads to increased afferent arteriolar resistance, a decrease in hydraulic glomerular capillary ultrafiltration coefficient (K_f), and a reduction in hyperperfusion and hyperfiltration.

A role for insulinlike growth factor-1 (IGF-1) in diabetic hypertrophy has been proposed. Continuous, 12-week subcutaneous infusion of the somatostatin analog octreotide, which antagonizes release of growth hormone and therefore lowers tissue IGF-I levels, reduces renal volume and glomerular hyperfiltration in normotensive type I diabetic patients with normoalbuminuria. Growth hormone may also play a role in mediating diabetic renal pathology. Transgenic mice overexpressing growth hormone have renal and glomerular hypertrophy with associated glomerulosclerosis similar to that of diabetic nephropathy.

A renal biopsy study of diabetic patients suggests a role for interleukins in diabetic nephropathy. These patients showed a strong interleukin-6 signal intensity by *in situ* hybridization in glomeruli with moderate mesangial expansion and within areas of interstitial fibrosis. Platelet-derived growth factor-B expression has also been found to be upregulated in glomeruli from diabetic rats.

Hyperglycemia and the diabetic state may increase oxidative stress by promoting reactive oxygen species production as well as attenuating free-radical scavenging molecules. Hyperglycemia is associated with elevation in the basal levels of cytosolic calcium in almost all cells including renal proximal tubule cells. This change in cytosolic calcium has been shown to participate in the genesis of some of the diabetic complications (leukocyte and B cells dysfunction). It is possible that elevation of cytosolic calcium in renal cells contributes to the pathogenesis of diabetic nephropathy.

GENETIC PREDISPOSITION AND MARKERS OF DIABETIC NEPHROPATHY

The likely polygenic nature of diabetic renal disease in either type I or type II diabetes is unknown. However, two lines of evidence strongly suggest a genetic susceptibility to diabetic nephropathy. First, approximately only one-third of type I or type II diabetic patients will ever develop diabetic nephropathy, sometimes even if blood glucose control is excellent. Most patients will not develop renal disease even in the face of suboptimal blood glucose control and antihypertensive therapy. In fact, the incidence of diabetic nephropathy in type I patients actually declines after 25 to 30 years of diabetes, suggesting that genetic rather than metabolic factors are important in the development of nephropathy. Second, there is strong evidence for familial clustering of diabetic nephropathy. Siblings of type I diabetic patients with nephropathy have a significantly (2.5 to 5 times) higher risk for developing diabetic kidney disease. Similar findings are demonstrated among Pima Indians and African-Americans with type II diabetes. In Pima Indians there is a threefold increased risk of diabetic kidney disease if another family member has diabetic nephropathy.

Markers of Diabetic Nephropathy

Because only a minority of diabetic patients will ever develop diabetic nephropathy, identification of a predictive marker would be essential for optimal management. Several recent studies have confirmed that microalbuminuria remains the most important, albeit late, marker for diabetic nephropathy, and its detection provides a clinical index for current guidelines of disease management (Fig. 45.13). However, the clinical utility of microalbuminuria is greatly hampered because irreversible kidney damage may have already occurred by the time microalbuminuria is detected. Several recent biopsy studies attempted to relate increased AER to histopathologic lesions of diabetic nephropathy. In sequential renal biopsies performed on type I diabetic patients, changes in mesangial fraction volume correlate with increasing AER. Approximately 75% of type II diabetic patients with AER of at least 100 milligrams per day have diffuse glomerulosclerosis. Because microalbuminuria is a late marker of disease, attempts to identify earlier markers is a field of very intensive research. An ideal putative marker could be a clinical/biochemical characteristic (phenotypic marker) or it could be a DNA defect (genotypic marker) that would predict with high sensitivity and specificity the susceptibility to diabetic nephropathy before the actual development of the disease.

The Renin-Angiotensin System as a Marker

Clinical studies have mostly focused on ACE gene polymorphism as a candidate marker for the progression of diabetic nephropathy. Most authorities now agree that ACE gene insertion/deletion (I/D) polymorphism does not contribute to genetic susceptibility to diabetic nephropathy in either type I or type II diabetes but that such polymorphism may predict the severity of disease and the rate of progression once diabetic nephropathy is established. Furthermore, D/D and I/D genotypes are associated with higher risk of coronary artery disease in the setting of diabetic nephropathy. Another link to the renin-angiotensin system is the description of an association between polymorphisms of the angiotensin II–type I receptor gene and the risk of nephropathy in diabetic patients with poor glycemic control. A locus near the receptor gene appears to be involved. Other studies have concluded that it is unlikely that polymorphisms in the genes for either renin or angiotensinogen (M235T variant) confer susceptibility to diabetic nephropathy.

Membrane Transporters as Markers

The activity of the Na-H exchanger isoform-1 in skin fibroblasts and lymphoblasts from patients with diabetic nephropathy is generally higher than in patients without nephropathy. This manifestation is not due to increased expression of the transporter but rather to increased turnover number. Increased erythrocyte sodium–lithium countertransport rate has been detected in microalbuminuric children with type I diabetes. Conflicting data exist on the correlation between countertransport activity and the degree of albuminuria in type II diabetic patients. In general, there is a large overlap in transporter activities among subgroups of patients with either diabetes type, and this fact limits the utility of such tests as predictive disease markers in individual patients.

Other Phenotypic and Biochemical Markers

Congenital oligonephropathy may predispose people to the development of adult hypertension and progressive renal injury. Increased intraglomerular hydrostatic pressure is believed to be the central injurious factor. It has also been argued that low birth weight, acquired oligonephropathy, and short stature in men may pose increased risk for diabetic nephropathy, perhaps due to reduced nephron number.

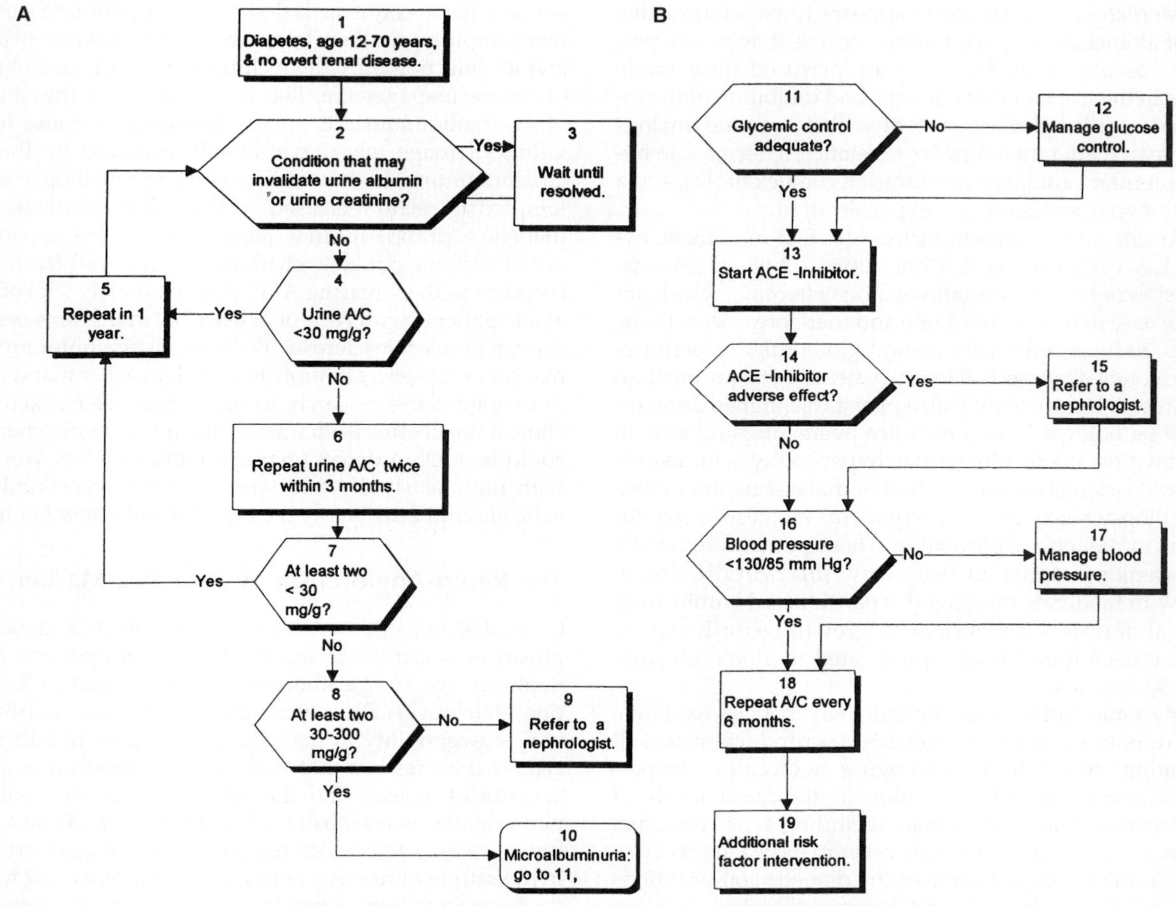

Figure 45.13. Suggested algorithm (**A** and **B**) for screening for microalbuminuria (**A/C**, albumin excretion rate per gram of urinary creatinine) in diabetic patients. (Reproduced with permission from Bennett PH, Haffner S, Kasiske BL, et al. Screening and management of microalbuminuria in patients with diabetes mellitus: recommendations to the Scientific Advisory Board of the National Kidney Foundation from the Ad Hoc Committee of the Council on Diabetes Mellitus of the National Kidney Foundation. *Am J Kidney Dis* 1995;25:101–112.)

In male type II diabetic patients, a strong univariate association was found between elevated sialic acid levels and coronary heart disease. Albuminuric type I diabetic patients have higher serum sialic acid levels than normoalbuminuric type I diabetic patients and normal controls, but there is no difference between the sialic acid levels of microalbuminuric and macroalbuminuric type I diabetic patients. Sialidase activity in mononuclear leukocytes from type I diabetic patients with retinopathy is significantly decreased.

Theoretically, blood levels of extracellular matrix proteins might serve as markers of diabetic nephropathy. However, there is only a weak correlation between plasma fibronectin level and microalbuminuria in type I diabetes. However, serum concentrations of collagen type IV and laminin, when prospectively followed in type II diabetic patients, are significantly higher in patients with worsening diabetic nephropathy. A report from Japan recently found that increased plasma levels of matrix metalloproteinase-9 predict the future development of microalbuminuria in type II diabetic patients. A Danish report has described a weak but significant association between diabetic nephropathy in type I patients and a TGF-β1 gene polymorphism (C to T transition at position 76 in exon 5 leading to a change from threonine to isoleucine in position 263).

Lipoprotein(a) levels are elevated during puberty in normoalbuminuric type I diabetic patients, and this is independent of metabolic control. In type I diabetic patients with more established nephropathy, median Lipoprotein(a) concentrations tend to be even more increased, but, when compared with normoalbuminuric control groups, the differences are small and the overlap is large.

PREVENTION OF DIABETIC NEPHROPATHY

Blood Glucose Control

The Stockholm Diabetes Intervention Study and the much larger Diabetes Control and Complications Trial (DCCT) have clearly demonstrated the beneficial effects of intensive insulin therapy on the development of the microvascular complications in type I diabetic patients, including nephropathy (Fig. 45.14). In the DCCT, the mean adjusted risk of microalbuminuria (defined in this study as AER of at least 40 mg per 24 hours) was reduced by 34% in the primary prevention cohort (patients with normoalbuminuria and without baseline retinopathy). Nevertheless, even with excellent blood glucose control approximately 16% of the primary cohort patients progressed to microalbuminuria during the study period. It is possible that the glucose control achieved in these individuals (an average blood glucose of 155 ± 30 mg per deciliter) is still not ideal and significantly surpasses the blood glucose level currently accepted for the diagnosis of diabetes mellitus (i.e., 126 mg/dl). It is also possible that genetic susceptibility to diabetic nephropathy may ultimately be responsible for diabetic complications even when the integrated blood glucose concentration is not very high. Clinically significant hypoglycemic episodes in the DCCT are three times as frequent with intensive treatment as with conventional therapy, but these events are relatively rare.

Antihypertensive Treatment

The prevalence of microalbuminuria is increased in patients with higher blood pressure levels, but whether this increase in blood pressure is a manifestation of renal disease or the microalbuminuria is a consequence of the increase in blood pressure remains unresolved. Type I diabetic patients progressing from normoalbuminuria to microalbuminuria have significantly higher mean blood pressures as documented by 24-hour ambulatory monitoring of the pressure. Overt hypertension characteristically becomes evident within three years of microalbuminuria detection in type I patients. Changes in the circadian rhythm of blood pressure may be predictive; the absence (or blunting) of the usual nighttime decrease in blood pressure that is normally found in healthy controls (10 mm Hg) is more frequent in patients developing diabetic nephropathy. Hypertension may develop at any time during the course of diabetes in type II patients and commonly is diagnosed when hyperglycemia is first detected, especially in the obese or older patient.

To achieve optimal results in the prevention of diabetic nephropathy, the daytime blood pressure has to be decreased to lower levels than what is considered to be the upper limit of normal in the general population. Because hypertension has long been established to be the most important risk factor for the progression of diabetic nephropathy, it is recommended that the blood pressure be reduced to 130/85 mm Hg or lower if possible. Obviously, the choice of antihypertensive medications has to be catered to the individual patient. Currently, there are limited data on the superiority of ACE inhibitors in the prevention of the development of microalbuminuria in normoalbuminuric diabetic patients. However, ACE inhibitors are the first choice in microalbuminuric or macroalbuminuric type I or type II diabetic patients with or without hypertension.

Modifiable Risk Factors

There is accumulating evidence that smoking, elevated cholesterol levels, and increased body mass index (at least in type II diabetes) may predispose diabetic patients to the development of nephropathy. Consequently, smoking cessation, regular physical exercise, a low–saturated fat diet, and (if necessary) cholesterol-lowering agents may, in addition to decreasing overall mortality and improving quality of life, prevent or delay the development of diabetic nephropathy.

Patient Education

For all the aforementioned preventive measures to be effective, patient cooperation is paramount. To achieve patient compliance, patients have to be educated about their disease, be treated as equal partners in the preventive and therapeutic process, and given positive reassurance and regular feedback about their condition. In fact, once patients are well educated about the potential complications of their disease and are motivated to prevent them, they predictably will take pride in monitoring their blood glucose, blood pressure, checking the urine for albumin themselves, and complying with other lifestyle-altering suggestions. The diabetic patient should be the first to detect an elevation of the blood pressure or albuminuria and bring it to the doctor's attention.

Delaying the onset of diabetes itself is the most logical maneuver to eliminate its long-term complications. This mostly pertains to type II diabetic patients where dietary prevention of

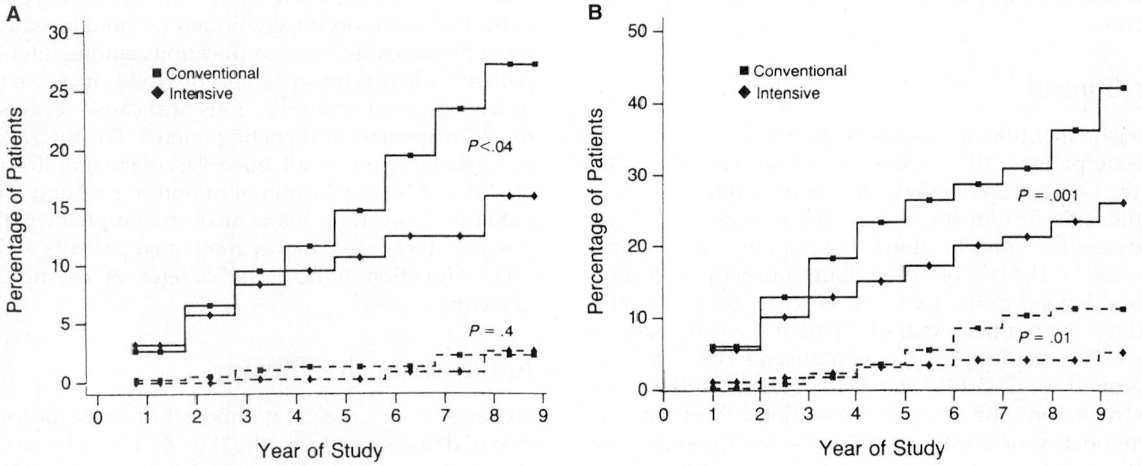

Figure 45.14. Cumulative incidence of urinary albumin excretion rate (UAE) greater than 300 mg/24 hr (*dashed line*) and greater than 40 mg/24 hr (*solid line*) in patients with type I diabetes mellitus enrolled in the DCCT and receiving intensive or conventional therapy. In the primary-prevention cohort (**A,** patients without baseline retinopathy), intensive therapy reduced the adjusted mean risk of microalbuminuria by 34% ($P > .04$). In the secondary-intervention cohort (**B,** patients with baseline retinopathy), patients with UAE greater than 40 mg/24 hr at baseline were excluded from the analysis of microalbuminuria development. Intensive therapy reduced the adjusted mean risk of overt or macroalbuminuria by 56% ($P = .01$) and the risk of microalbuminuria by 43% ($P = .001$), as compared with conventional therapy. (Reproduced with permission from The DCCT Research Group. The effect of intensive treatment of diabetes on the development and progression of long-term complications in insulin-dependent diabetes mellitus. *N Engl J Med* 1993;329:977–986.)

obesity in genetically predisposed patients will effectively delay or prevent the onset of overt hyperglycemia and insulin resistance. Unfortunately, there is an epidemic of obesity and physical inactivity in the industrialized world and prospects to decrease the incidence of type II diabetes mellitus may not be a realistic goal for the near future.

Future Perspectives

When sensitive and predictive phenotypic or genotypic markers of diabetic nephropathy (other than microalbuminuria) become available, more effective preventive measures and aggressive treatment regimens can be instituted in those patients at risk for developing nephropathy. The elucidation of the gene(s) that make type I and type II diabetic patients susceptible to nephropathy will undoubtedly raise several questions (not the least of which is the effect of screening of asymptomatic patients on their insurance coverage). The scientific and lay communities will, in time, have to find suitable answers for dealing with these issues.

THERAPY OF LATENT AND OVERT DIABETIC NEPHROPATHY

Once fixed microalbuminuria (at least 30 mg urinary albumin excretion per day) develops and other diagnoses are excluded, the patient has latent diabetic nephropathy that most likely will progress into overt disease. It became clear in the 1980s that an overwhelming majority (more than 85% of patients) of type I diabetic patients with microalbuminuria are destined to develop end-stage renal disease. Most type II diabetic patients with microalbuminuria will develop into macroalbuminuria. There is no conclusive evidence that any therapeutic modality is capable of totally preventing the progression of microalbuminuria into macroalbuminuria (overt proteinuria). However, adherence to guidelines established in landmark studies in the 1990s may significantly delay the development of overt nephropathy or decrease the rate of progression to end-stage renal disease in diabetic patients.

Glycemic Control

The previously mentioned landmark prospective studies in type I diabetic patients (the Stockholm Diabetes Intervention Study and the DCCT) convincingly demonstrated the beneficial effects of intensive insulin therapy on the progression of diabetic microvascular complications (retinopathy, neuropathy, and nephropathy). The risk of macroalbuminuria (urinary albumin excretion defined in the DCCT as at least 300 mg/day) in the secondary prevention cohort (patients with baseline retinopathy but no nephropathy) was reduced by 56% with intensive treatment (Fig. 45.14). The 44% decrease by intensive glucose control among the primary prevention cohort (patients with no retinopathy or nephropathy) was not significant because of the small number of patients who progressed to macroalbuminuria. However, subsequent subgroup analysis demonstrated that among the 73 secondary intervention cohort patients with baseline AER of more than 28 μg/min (but less than 139 μg/min), intensive therapy did not significantly reduce the progression to macroalbuminuria when compared with conventional therapy. This agrees with the findings of the Microalbuminuria Collaborative Study Group in which 70 type I diabetic patients with microalbuminuria (defined as 30 to 199 μg/min) without hypertension were followed for 3 years. Thirty-six patients received intensive insulin therapy with a target $HbA1_c$ level below 7.5% while 34 patients received conventional therapy. There was no difference in the progression to macroalbuminuria (more than 200 μg/min) between the two groups. Arterial blood pressure rather than $HbA1_c$ levels was found to be the main predictor of progression to clinical albuminuria. Taken together, these important recent studies indicate that, in terms of prevention of diabetic nephropathy, intensive glycemic control is of paramount importance in the normoalbuminuric type I diabetic patient, but it is of less clear value in patients with established microalbuminuria. However, because strict glucose control slows the development of other microvascular complications of diabetes (e.g., retinopathy and neuropathy), intensive insulin treatment can be advocated in microalbuminuric type I diabetic patients for an overall improvement in outcome.

Emerging large-scale prospective trials conducted in type II diabetic patients provide evidence that strict glucose control is likely to slow the development and progression of diabetic nephropathy. The published results in 1998 of the United Kingdom Prospective Diabetes Study (UKPDS), the largest randomized trial ever conducted in type II diabetic patients, provided the first evidence that tight metabolic control (mean $HbAl_c$ 7.0% over 9 years compared with 7.9% on conventional treatment) reduced the risk of microvascular complications in nearly 4,000 patients. Sulfonylureas and insulin produced equally good results. Metformin was more effective in obese patients but significantly doubled the mortality risk when added early on to sulfonylurea therapy as compared with conventional treatment with sulfonylureas alone.

It is still unclear what the target $HbA1_c$ should be to optimize beneficial effects of intensive therapy but minimize the risk of hypoglycemia. The risk of development of microalbuminuria in normoalbuminuric type I diabetic patients increases abruptly above a $HbA1_c$ level of 8.1%. Thus efforts to reduce the development of diabetic nephropathy should be focused on reducing $HbA1_c$ levels that are above this level. A target $HbA1_c$ level of 7% has been suggested based on the achieved glucose control in the DCCT in type I diabetic patients and the results of the UKPDS in type II patients. Even this glucose control may be insufficient based on the continued (although reduced) development of microvascular complications among intensively treated patients. Clearly, lower targets of $HbA1_c$ increase the frequency of hypoglycemic complications and cause serious problems in the management of diabetic patients. For the sake of delaying the development of all microvascular complications, a target $HbA1_c$ of 7% seems optimal in both type I and type II diabetic patients. More rigorous control in compliant patients may be possible in selected, highly motivated patients with intact autonomic function (where the danger of asymptomatic hypoglycemia is less).

Antihypertensive Therapy

Hypertension is the most important risk factor for the progression of diabetic nephropathy (Fig. 45.15). In those with type I diabetes, the incidence of hypertension rises from 5% at 10 years, to 33% at 20 years, and to 70% at 40 years. Hypertension rarely develops in type I diabetic patients who do not develop nephropathy. As documented by 24-hour ambulatory monitoring of blood pressure, type I diabetic patients with microalbuminuria or macroalbuminuria have significantly higher mean blood pressures than normoalbuminuric controls, and the increase in both systolic and diastolic pressure (even in the top range of traditionally accepted normal values) are associated with progression in albuminuria. The situation is different in type II diabetic patients. Up to 40% of newly diagnosed type II patients have overt hypertension, and in half of these patients, hypertension is detected before microalbuminuria, perhaps due to coinheritance of essential hypertension. Hypertension is strongly associated with obesity in type II patients, and it is a strong predictor of cardiovascular morbidity and mortality.

In general, the pathogenesis of hypertension in diabetes mellitus can be related to three main factors: (a) the development of renal insufficiency, (b) extracellular volume expansion, and (c) hyperinsulinemia and insulin resistance in type II diabetic patients. Obese patients with hypertension have resistance to insulin-mediated glucose uptake by skeletal muscle, which can aggravate glucose intolerance. However, it is still uncertain whether the higher peripheral insulin levels or the insulin resistance may cause hypertension. Salt retention may be due to renal insufficiency or the antinatriuretic effects of insulin therapy.

Early treatment of hypertension is particularly important in diabetic patients both to prevent cardiovascular disease and to minimize progression of renal and retinal diseases. Nonpharmacologic therapy should be encouraged, but it almost always needs to be supplemented with antihypertensive medications when renal disease appears. Nonpharmacologic therapy includes weight reduction, salt restriction, cessation of smoking, regular exercise, and no or little alcohol consumption. Based on the results of numerous studies, it is clear that antihypertensive treatment slows the progression of diabetic kidney disease in both types of diabetes irrespective of the nature of the antihypertensive regimens used. The target blood pressure for optimal results is still debated, but the Sixth Report of the Joint National Committee on Prevention, Detection, Evaluation, and Treatment of High Blood Pressure in 1997 recommended that blood pressure be reduced to a goal below 130/85 mm Hg. In principle, this should be achieved by increasing the doses of an antihypertensive agent as well as by the sequential addition of different agents in order to arrive at the target value with the least amount of undesirable side effects.

Reliance on an ACE inhibitor as the primary antihypertensive therapy in diabetic patients has been gaining wide acceptance. ACE inhibitors effectively lower the blood pressure, and they offer advantages over other classes of medications. The most widely studied agents in long-term trials are captopril, starting at 50 mg twice daily, or enalapril, starting at 5 mg daily. A host of other long-acting ACE inhibitors are now available, and they should be equally effective in terms of their antihypertensive action, their antiproteinuric effects, and theoretically, in their renoprotective action in diabetic nephropathy. Serum potassium and creatinine should be monitored after one week of initiating ACE inhibitor therapy. If the target blood pressure is not achieved by ACE inhibition alone, diuretics in low doses can be added. A higher dosage of a thiazide or loop diuretic may be necessary to counteract salt retention when there is renal or cardiac failure.

The results of the Captopril Collaborative Study Group assert that captopril is more renoprotective than other conventional antihypertensive regimens in type I diabetic patients (Fig. 45.16). In this trial, progression to renal failure was decreased by

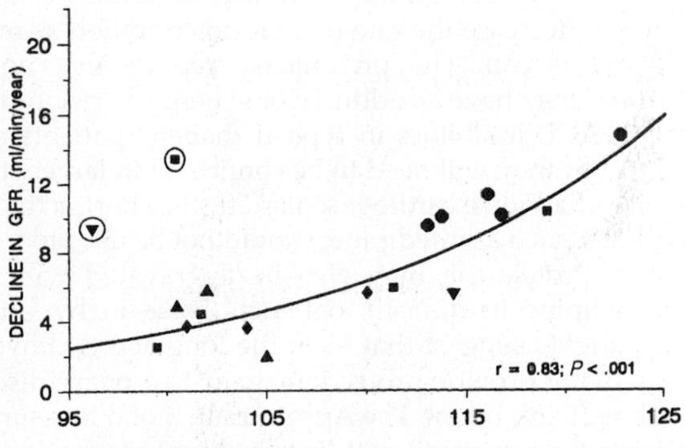

Figure 45.15. Correlation between the rate of decline in GFR and the mean arterial blood pressure (MAP) in type I diabetic patients with kidney disease untreated or treated with different antihypertensive medications. Only studies lasting at least 2 years were selected. ●, no antihypertensive treatment; ◆, β-blockers with or without diuretics; ▼, ACE inhibitors with conventional antihypertensive treatment; ▲, ACE inhibitors with or without diuretics; or □, triple or conv. tx (T). The curve is calculated without taking into account the Collaborative Study Group using captopril. The studies included are as follows: Parving HH, et al. *Br Med J* 1988;297:1086–1091; Parving HH, et al. *Am J Kidney Dis* 1993; 22:188–195; Rossing P, et al. *Kidney Int* 1994;45:S145–S149; Parving HH, et al. *Hypertension* 1985;7:114–117; Bjorck S, et al. *Br Med J* 1986;293:471–474; Mogensen CE. 285:685–688, 1982; Elving LD, et al. *Diabetologia* 1994;37:604–609. (Reproduced with permission from Deferrari G, Cheli V, Robaudo C. Treatment of diabetic nephropathy in its early stages. *Diabetes-Metabolism Rev* 1997;13:51–61.)

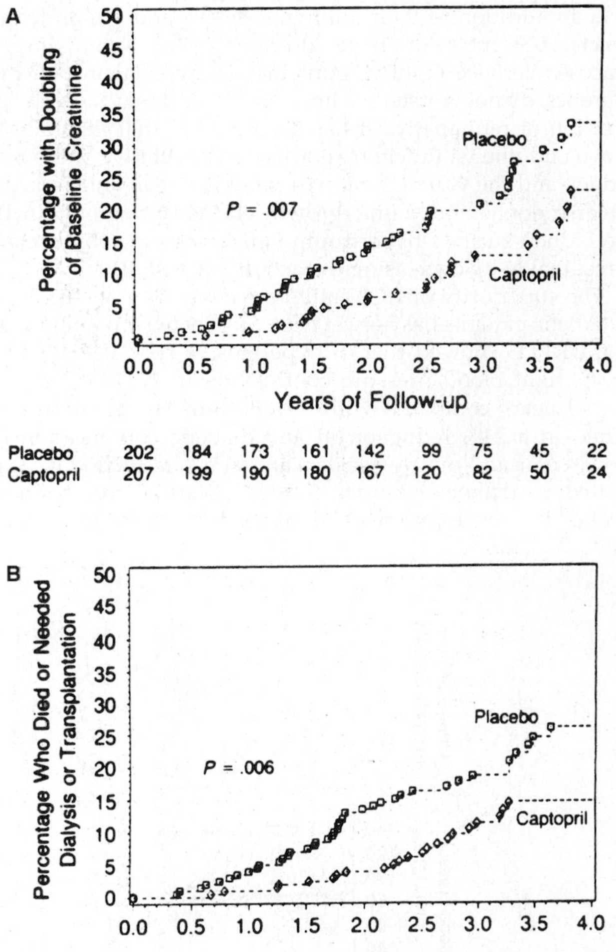

Figure 45.16. Cumulative incidence of doubling of base-line creatinine to at least 2.0 mg/dl **(panel A)** and the cumulative incidence of death or end-stage renal failure **(panel B)** in type I diabetic patients with nephropathy treated for up to 3.5 years with either captopril or placebo. Upon entry both groups had overt nephropathy as evidenced by proteinuria. All patients in the placebo group and most patients in the captopril group were hypertensive and were given traditional antihypertensive medications (but not calcium channel blockers) to achieve near-normalization of the blood pressure. The numbers of patients are given at the bottom of each panel. (Reproduced with permission from Lewis EJ, Hunsicker LG, Bain RP, et al. The effect of angiotensin-converting-enzyme inhibition on diabetic nephropathy. The Collaborative Study Group. *N Engl J Med* 1993;329:1456–1462.)

approximately 50% over a mean of 3 years of follow-up. The renoprotective response appeared to be more prominent in patients who had an elevated baseline serum creatinine (above 1.5 mg/dl). Some authorities have argued that part of the beneficial effect of captopril resulted from a slightly lower mean arterial pressure in the diabetic patients than in the control group, although this was not the initial intention of the trial. Nevertheless, captopril was clearly renoprotective. Captopril and other ACE inhibitors preserve kidney function because they are effective in lowering intraglomerular pressure due to vasodilation of the efferent arteriole. ACE inhibitors are also effective antiproteinuric agents (Fig. 45.17), and this property can further protect from progressive renal damage. As proteinuria itself is considered a progression promoter of all chronic kidney diseases including diabetic nephropathy, a decrease in proteinuria effected by ACE inhibitors is believed to contribute to their beneficial use in diabetic nephropathy. Accordingly, some authorities have suggested that ACE inhibitors be used even in normotensive patients once microalbuminuria is detected in type I diabetic patients. Studies over a 2-year period have suggested that such an approach can in fact delay the progression of renal disease. In addition to their antihypertensive and antiproteinuric effects, ACE inhibitors have additional benefits; they improve glucose tolerance slightly, counteract the hypokalemic effects of diuretics, do not worsen the lipid profile, and may slow the progression of retinopathy. It has been argued that they also improve endothelial function and decrease oxidative stress in the kidney and the vasculature. ACE inhibitors can antagonize the adverse nonhemodynamic growth effects of angiotensin II in the kidney such as hypertrophy and excess matrix formation (presumably by decreasing the activity of TGF-β).

The superiority of ACE inhibitors over other agents in type II diabetic patients has not yet been convincingly demonstrated. The UKPDS showed that in hypertensive type II diabetic patients, tight blood pressure control (mean of 144/82 mm Hg over 9 years compared with 154/87 mm Hg in controls) resulted in a 24% reduction in any diabetic complication (microvascular and macrovascular) and a 32% reduction in deaths related to diabetes (mostly from myocardial infarction and stroke). However, the effect on microalbuminuria and macroalbuminuria was not statistically significant at 9 years. Interestingly, ACE inhibitors (captopril) and β-blockers (atenolol) were equally effective. Thus lowering blood pressure in itself may be important in reducing the complications of type II diabetes regardless of the treatment used.

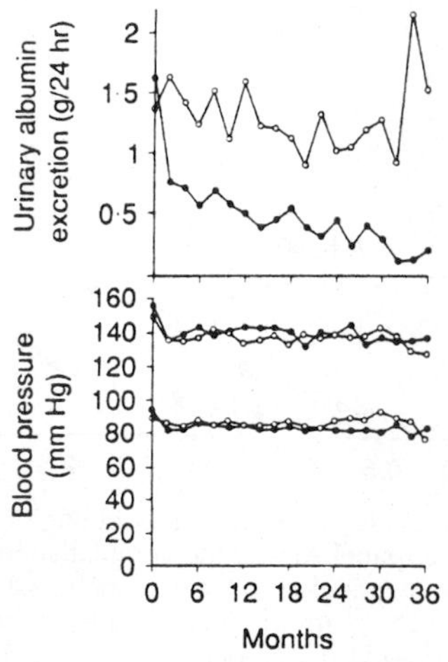

Figure 45.17. Comparison of the decline in the urinary albumin excretion rate in 40 type I diabetic patients with nephropathy and decreased GFR treated for 36 months with either enalapril (*solid squares*) or metoprolol (*open squares*). Enalapril was more antiproteinuric than metoprolol **(upper panel)** for the same degree of control of systolic and diastolic blood pressure **(lower panel).** (Reproduced with permission from Bjorck S, et al. Renal protective effect of enalapril in diabetic nephropathy. *Br Med J* 1992;304:339–343.)

The nonpeptide angiotensin II–type I (AT_1) receptor antagonists (e.g., losartan, valsartan, irbesartan, or candesartan) represent an alternative to ACE inhibitors in blocking the renin-angiotensin system, and the spectrum of their clinical indications may be similar to those of ACE inhibitors. This class of drugs provides a more complete and specific blockade of angiotensin II action at the AT_1 receptor, which mediates the pressor and growth effects of the peptide. These agents have become popular because they offer very few side effects. However, until the results of ongoing long-term prospective studies of the potential renoprotective effects of AT_1-receptor antagonists are completed in patients with diabetes, ACE inhibitors remain the drugs of choice in microalbuminuric and macroalbuminuric diabetic patients with or without hypertension. AT_1-receptor antagonists may be useful if the patient cannot tolerate the side effects of ACE inhibitors such as cough.

Therapy with calcium channel blockers for hypertension in patients with diabetes mellitus has gained popularity because this class of medications, like ACE inhibitors, offers advantages of efficacy and lack of adverse effects on lipids and glucose metabolism. Calcium channel blockers (with or without diuretics) may be particularly useful in the African-American population with hypertension who may not respond well to ACE inhibitors. Calcium channel blockers promote urinary sodium excretion even without concomitant diuretic therapy. However, unlike ACE inhibitors, calcium channel blockers have not been shown to be superior in improving cardiovascular endpoints or delaying the progression of renal insufficiency in diabetic nephropathy beyond the level achieved with conventional blood pressure–lowering regimens.

Nondihydropyridine calcium channel blockers such as verapamil and diltiazem may be used as adjunct therapy when ACE inhibitors plus diuretics do not achieve the target blood pressure. Verapamil and diltiazem can decrease the amount of urinary protein excretion, but there are no studies to indicate that they can decrease the rate of GFR deterioration as much as ACE inhibitors can. The preliminary reports that nondihydropyridines may have an additive or synergistic renoprotective effect with ACE inhibitors in type II diabetic patients are encouraging, but they will need to be confirmed in larger studies.

Because of adverse cardiovascular effects, short-acting dihydropyridines, such as nifedipine, should not be used to treat hypertension. Proteinuria may also be aggravated with short-acting nifedipine in diabetic patients. Trials in hypertensive diabetic patients suggest that even the long-acting dihydropyridines may not provide protection against coronary disease as seen with ACE inhibitors. The Appropriate Blood Pressure Control in Diabetes compared first-line therapy with enalapril and nisoldipine for 5 years. Patients treated with enalapril had fewer fatal and nonfatal myocardial infarctions. A similar conclusion was reached in the FACET study; a cardiovascular end point occurred more commonly in patients treated with amlodipine than with the ACE inhibitor fosinopril.

β-Blockers are effective therapy for hypertension in diabetes. Although β-blockers may have adverse effects on peripheral blood flow, prolong hypoglycemia, and mask hypoglycemic symptoms, patients with diabetes who are treated with diuretics and β-blockers experience a similar or greater reduction of coronary artery disease and total cardiovascular events compared with patients without diabetes. The UKPDS, mentioned earlier, showed that the long-acting, selective β_1-antagonist atenolol was as effective as enalapril in terms of both blood pressure lowering and protection against microvascular complications and cardiovascular disease. The new β-adrenergic agent carvedilol improves survival in congestive heart failure and has a favorable profile on glucose and lipid metabolism, but its role in the treatment of hypertension in diabetic nephropathy has not yet been established.

α-Blockers (prazosin, doxazosin, and terazosin) are useful adjuncts in the treatment of hypertension in diabetes mellitus because they lower blood pressure, reduce proteinuria, and improve the blood lipid profile. These drugs have the added benefit to increase urine stream in the elderly male patient with prostatic hypertrophy. The recommended dose is increased gradually to avoid symptomatic postural hypotension, which can occur especially in patients with autonomic neuropathy.

Diet

In smaller, prospective trials, reduced dietary protein intake has been shown to delay progression of diabetic nephropathy. Larger long-term trials will be required to establish efficacy and safety of restriction in dietary protein intake in diabetic patients with nephropathy. In the meantime the current recommendations of the American Diabetes Association state that nonpregnant diabetic patients should limit their protein intake to 0.8 g/kg of ideal body weight per day. When prescribing a low-protein diet in patients with renal insufficiency, a detailed assessment of nutritional requirements is mandatory to meet the specific needs of the diabetic patient who has carbohydrate intolerance and an abnormal lipid profile. It is speculative whether any beneficial effect of dietary protein restriction in diabetic nephropathy is related to inhibition of TGF-β production, although such an effect has been reported in experimental models of glomerulonephritis or tubulointerstitial injury in rats.

Antihyperlipidemic Medications

A pathogenic role for elevated LDL cholesterol, Lp(a), and triglycerides has been suggested but not yet proven in the progression of diabetic nephropathy. A trial with simvastatin to reduce hypercholesterolemia in type II patients did not affect the rate of decline of GFR. However, because cardiovascular disease is the single most common cause of mortality in the general and, in an even more pronounced way, the diabetic population, it seems reasonable to lower the risk of cardiovascular complications by antihyperlipidemic therapy. Studies in the general population with increased total and LDL cholesterol levels, with or without established cardiovascular disease, demonstrated a significant decrease by HMG-CoA reductase inhibitors in all-cause and cardiovascular mortality. Initiating antihyperlipidemic therapy in any type I or type II diabetic patient with abnormal lipid panels may eventually prove to be cost-effective in lowering cardiovascular complications. Whether this will lead to less mortalities, to decreased development of, or to slowed progression of diabetic renal disease remains to be shown. On the other hand, antihyperlipidemic therapy in diabetic patients with nephropathy but with no evidence of hyperlipidemia is not recommended at this point.

Cessation of Smoking

Although the role of smoking in the progression of diabetic nephropathy is not clearly delineated, smoking represents a modifiable lifestyle parameter that is linked to hypertension and atherosclerosis. As a result, smoking cessation likely would decrease the overall mortality rates of diabetic patients.

Summary of Treatment of Diabetic Nephropathy

The optimal approach for the management of diabetic nephropathy centers around optimal glycemic control and careful adherence to normalization of systemic blood pressure, preferably employing ACE inhibitors, with low-dose diuretics when needed. Serum potassium and creatinine should be monitored after one week of initiating ACE inhibitor therapy. Nondihydropyridines, cardioselective β-blockers, or α-blockers can be added if blood pressure control is suboptimal. Because reducing albuminuria delays progression of diabetic nephropathy, this parameter should be used as a benchmark for measuring efficacy of therapeutic interventions. Low-protein diet should be prescribed as part of a comprehensive treatment plan to address the specific nutritional needs of the diabetic state. Antihyperlipidemic therapy for patients with abnormal lipid panels and cessation of smoking are advised to reduce cardiovascular risk.

New treatment options for diabetic nephropathy will likely emerge in parallel with our expanding understanding of the mechanisms of disease progression. Ongoing clinical trials should shed light on the effectiveness of AT_1 receptor antagonists, aldose reductase inhibitors, the AGE-antagonist aminoguanidine, antioxidants (including vitamins C and E), or a novel orally active β-selective PKC inhibitor. Other approaches in the future may include selective inhibitors specifically targeting Amadori products or cytokine receptors or some form of gene therapy. Novel interventions to intercept the activity of the renal TGF-β system may prove useful in halting the progression of diabetic nephropathy.

THERAPY OF COMORBID CONDITIONS

Diabetic neuropathy, retinopathy, and nephropathy constitute the microvascular complications of type I and type II diabetes mellitus. In addition, macrovascular complications involving the cardiovascular, cerebrovascular, and peripheral vasculature are responsible for a high percentage of morbidity and mortality in diabetes.

Diabetic Neuropathy

Distal symmetric polyneuropathy is a characteristic syndrome of the diabetic patient with peripheral neuropathy. Symptoms include paresthesias and loss of temperature and pain sensation especially in a distal pattern. Cramping and aching may occur. Decreased or absent vibration, temperature, pinprick, and ankle jerk are typical findings. The severity of the disease correlates highly with diabetes duration. Nerve conduction studies disclose peripheral demyelinization. Some patients may have individual or cranial nerve involvement, especially affecting the oculomotor and median nerves. Polyradiculopathies and mononeuropathy multiplex are additional neuropathic syndromes that can affect diabetic patients.

Autonomic neuropathy is a common complication, and it may decrease or completely disrupt the sympathetic warning mechanisms of hypoglycemia. Its manifestations include postural hypotension with dizziness, gastroparesis with vomiting, and enteropathy with constipation and/or diarrhea. Excretory (urinary and fecal) incontinence may occur. The nocturnal 'non-dipping' phenomenon in patients with diabetic nephropathy may be a manifestation of autonomic neuropathy. In fact, some patients have systolic hypertension in the recumbent position and hypotension upon assuming the upright position. This poses great difficulties in the diagnosis and management of hypertension in the subset of diabetic patients with autonomic neuropathy. Cardiac denervation can occur in advanced cases of autonomic neuropathy and is associated with painless myocardial infarction and sudden death.

Diabetic genitourinary autonomic neuropathy is responsible for several syndromes including cystopathy, retrograde ejaculation, erectile dysfunction, and dyspareunia. Infrequent urination and incomplete emptying lead to dribbling, overflow incontinence, and frequent urinary tract infections. Cystometrograms confirm the diagnosis. Scheduled urination should be coupled with bethanechol. More advanced cases require intermittent catheterization, and in extreme cases resection of the internal sphincter of the bladder neck.

Once any form of diabetic neuropathy is present, its treatment is extremely difficult. One positive development was the DCCT's demonstration that tight glucose control decreases the progression of diabetic neuropathy. In addition to glucose control, multivitamin supplementation (especially vitamin B_6), promotility drugs (cisapride, metoclopramide, and erythromycin) in gastroparesis, amitriptyline or similar agents, and local anesthetics can be of value. Ongoing studies should determine if aldose reductase inhibitors would benefit diabetic neuropathy.

Diabetic Retinopathy

Diabetic retinopathy is a serious complication, often leading to blindness. It is virtually always present in type I patients with diabetic nephropathy. In fact, if retinopathy is absent, alternative diagnostic options have to be sought in the setting of proteinuria or renal insufficiency in the diabetic patient. There are two types of diabetic retinopathy: nonproliferative and proliferative retinopathy. Nonproliferative retinopathy is almost always present after more than 10 years of diabetes in patients with type I diabetes mellitus (Fig. 45.18). The nonproliferative lesion is relatively benign, but it may progress to retinal neovascularization or proliferative retinopathy. The latter lesion begins to appear after 10 to 15 years of diabetes in a fraction of the population, but the annual incident rate remains constant thereafter so that most patients become affected after 40 years of diabetes.

The DCCT found a continuous relation between the degree of glycemic control and the incidence of retinopathy (the primary end point in the trial). It should be mentioned that the DCCT confirmed that there is early exacerbation of retinopathy after intensive insulin therapy (in the first 2 to 3 years), but there is a clear overall benefit when patients are followed for the entire duration of the study. The incidence of worsening retinopathy in intensively treated patients was reduced to 25% at nine years as compared with 50% in the conventionally-treated group. Progressive retinopathy was uncommon when the $HbA1_c$ was less than 7%. Familial clustering for retinopathy was demonstrated in the DCCT; patients who had first-degree relatives with diabetes, severe retinopathy developed three times more frequently among the relatives of the retinopathy-positive patients as compared with the relatives of the retinopathy-negative patients. Adequate antihypertensive therapy, in addition to long-term tight glycemic control, can decrease the development and progression of diabetic retinopathy. However, glycemic control in advanced proliferative retinopathy, just like in overt diabetic nephropathy, offers little or no protection. Laser photocoagulation is the standard of therapy for prevention of retinal detachment, the most feared complication of proliferative retinopathy. Vitrectomy is needed when there is intravitreous body scar formation.

Macrovascular Complications

Macrovascular complications with premature atherosclerosis in diabetes involve coronary, cerebrovascular, and peripheral arteries and cause significant morbidity and mortality. Partial or complete occlusion of the renal arteries may cause worsening hypertension, 'flash pulmonary edema,' and acceleration of renal insufficiency. Cardiovascular disease is the single most frequent cause of mortality in the diabetic population with kidney disease.

There are conflicting data on the importance of glycemic control in the prevention of macrovascular disease in diabetic patients. However, certain studies suggest that there may be a benefit, especially if strict glycemic control is achieved before end-organ damage has already occurred. The DCCT found a trend toward fewer macrovascular complications with intensive insulin therapy, although these events were relatively uncommon in this young population of type I diabetic patients, and the results did not achieve statistical significance. A subanalysis of the UKPDS showed that a 1% reduction in $HbA1_c$ in type II diabetic patients was associated with an 18% reduction in myocardial infarction and a 15% reduction in stroke. Prevention and treatment of macrovascular disease generally derive from the recommendations for the general population. These include antihypertensive therapy, smoking cessation, weight loss, increased physical exercise, and antihyperlipidemic therapy. Folic acid and Vitamin B_6 in patients with homocystinemia and estrogen replacement in postmenopausal women may decrease the incidence of coronary artery syndromes.

In cardiovascular disease ACE inhibitors or angiotensin II–receptor antagonists are indicated in cases of decreased left ventricular function. β-Blockers are highly effective in decreasing mortality in coronary artery syndromes and following myocardial infarction. In non–Q-wave myocardial infarction, diltiazem is recommended. In established multivessel coronary artery disease, coronary artery bypass grafting is superior to medical therapy alone in the diabetic population. Meticulous foot care is of utmost importance in patients with peripheral neuropathy and arterial insufficiency.

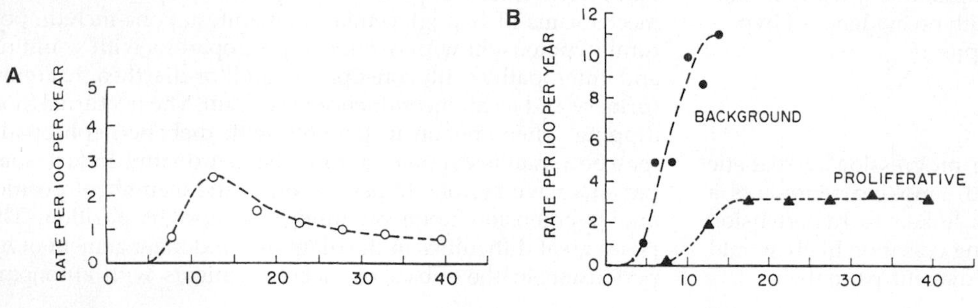

Figure 45.18. Incidence rate of nephropathy **(A)** as contrasted to the incidence rate of background and proliferative retinopathy **(B)** according to the duration of type I diabetes mellitus. Nephropathy was identified by persistent proteinuria. (Reproduced with permission from Krolewski AS, Warram JH, Rand LI, et al. Epidemiological approach to the etiology of type I diabetes mellitus and its complications. *N Engl J Med* 1987;317:1390–1398.)

RENAL REPLACEMENT THERAPY IN DIABETIC NEPHROPATHY

Dialysis

Diabetic nephropathy accounts for approximately 30% to 40% of all patients treated with dialysis or renal allografts in the United States. Nearly 82% of the total number of diabetic patients on renal replacement therapy are receiving dialysis, with a 5.7:1 ratio of diabetic patients on hemodialysis versus peritoneal dialysis in the United States. The survival of diabetic patients on either form of dialysis is lower than that of the general dialysis population. Undoubtedly, this is because of an extremely high mortality rate secondary to cardiovascular, cerebrovascular, and infectious causes. In addition, mainly because of their comorbid conditions, the quality of life (as measured by standardized surveys) is inferior in the diabetic dialysis patient as compared with the average dialysis patient. This results in a higher withdrawal rate from dialysis. Prescription of the dialysis modality should be individualized, but transplantation, because of its superior survival rate, remains the renal replacement method of choice when feasible for the diabetic patient.

Survival of diabetic patients on peritoneal dialysis is slightly worse than on hemodialysis. The difference becomes evident after 1 year of dialysis, and mainly affects patients over 55 years of age. The reason for these survival differences is not clear. High glucose in peritoneal dialysis patients' solutions may lead to inferior survival due to worse glucose control. Differences in survival may also be due to differences in levels of dialysis adequacy. Diabetic patients on hemodialysis demonstrate a decrease in mortality when the administered Kt/V is increased above 1.4. Current guidelines recommend a prescribed Kt/V of 1.3 (which will likely correspond to an actual delivered Kt/V of 1.2) in all hemodialysis patients. Peritoneal dialysis guidelines recommend a weekly Kt/V of at least 2.0 or a creatinine clearance of 60 L/wk.

Management of the diabetic patient by dialysis is generally similar to nondiabetic patients with end-stage renal disease. An important point is the timely creation of a vascular access for the patient opting for hemodialysis (serum creatinine concentration of 5 to 6 mg/dl). Arterial inflow is often poor, and venous run-off may be a problem because of venous phlebitis, occlusion, or hypoplasia. It is wise to start dialysis when the GFR is approximately 10 to 15 ml/min. Earlier treatment may be necessary (a) when volume-dependent blood pressure control becomes very difficult, (b) when the patient becomes anorectic and malnourished, or (c) when severe vomiting due to uremia and gastroparesis becomes unmanageable.

Transplantation

Eighteen percent of all diabetic patients with end-stage renal disease in the United States had functioning allografts in 1995. About 25% of new U.S. transplant recipients are diabetic (96% of whom are type I diabetic patients, reflecting the younger age of this select group). Long-term patient survival in diabetic kidney disease after transplantation is superior to that of patients on any modality of dialysis, even after correction for the selection bias that generally favors transplant patients. In addition, transplantation offers a better quality of life and higher degree of rehabilitation than other renal replacement modalities. However, long-term patient survival in the diabetic transplant population receiving a cadaver allograft is worse than in the nondiabetic transplant population, reflecting the higher prevalence of coronary artery disease and increased cardiovascular mortality of diabetic patients. For these reasons, cardiologists currently suggest preoperative clearance that includes coronary angiography and, if needed, elective coronary bypass grafting (which has been shown to be superior to percutaneous transluminal angioplasty in diabetic patients with multivessel coronary artery disease).

The Different Options for Transplantation in Diabetic Nephropathy

Living, related donors provide the best long-term results. Living unrelated donors also offer excellent results. Pancreas transplantation (partial or total) is not part of living donor transplantation procedures. However, cadaveric kidney alone, pancreas alone, or pancreas-kidney transplantation are feasible. Islet cell transplantation is still in the experimental phase. Patient and allograft survival with living donors are superior to cadaveric (kidney-alone or kidney-pancreas) transplantation. Available data regarding patient and graft survival after cadaveric kidney-alone versus pancreas-kidney transplantation are contradictory. In some centers cadaveric kidney-alone transplantations have a higher 3-year patient survival rate. Cadaveric pancreas-kidney transplantations in other centers have a higher patient and graft survival rate than cadaveric kidney transplantation alone, but selection bias may be responsible for these differences. Successful pancreas transplantation significantly improves the quality of life of the diabetic patient. It can provide improvement in the debilitating symptoms of autonomic neuropathy, the cessation of multiple daily insulin injections, and a possible improvement in diabetic retinopathy. On the other hand, 35% of patients undergoing pancreas transplantation develop major short-term surgical (especially infectious) complications; this has led some experts to restrict this form of transplantation to patients younger than 45 years old. Prospective long-term studies are needed to control for differences in criteria of patient recruitment and surgical expertise.

Posttransplant Care of the Diabetic Patient

With the advance in intraoperative and postoperative care, short-term patient survival and the rate of complications in diabetic patients after renal transplantation is gradually approaching that of other recipients. However, long-term survival still lags behind that of the general transplant population. Several medical issues have to be followed very closely in the diabetic transplant patient. The postoperative course of the diabetic patient (especially if a functioning pancreas is not transplanted) is often complicated by the difficulty of controlling blood sugar when glucocorticoids are given. Antihypertensive treatment is frequently necessary because of the blood pressure–increasing effects of both glucocorticoids and cyclosporin. Posttransplant hyperlipidemia (likely secondary to cyclosporin) is especially dangerous for type II diabetic patients with peripheral vascular, cardiovascular, and cerebrovascular disease. Urinary tract infections are more common in the diabetic transplant recipient because of a high incidence of neurogenic bladder. As a result, long-term antimicrobial prophylaxis is recommended, usually with daily oral trimethoprim-sulfamethoxazole. There is no evidence that the frequency of posttransplant lymphoproliferative disease or posttransplant erythrocytosis is different in diabetic patients.

Recurrence of Diabetic Kidney Disease and Its Prevention

It has been known that diabetic glomerulosclerosis recurs in almost all allografts from nondiabetic donors. GBM thickening and mesangial expansion are seen after 2 years, followed by hyalinization of the afferent and efferent arterioles after 4 years or transplantation. The typical nodular lesions rarely recur. Transplant patients with recurrent diabetic nephropathy typically present

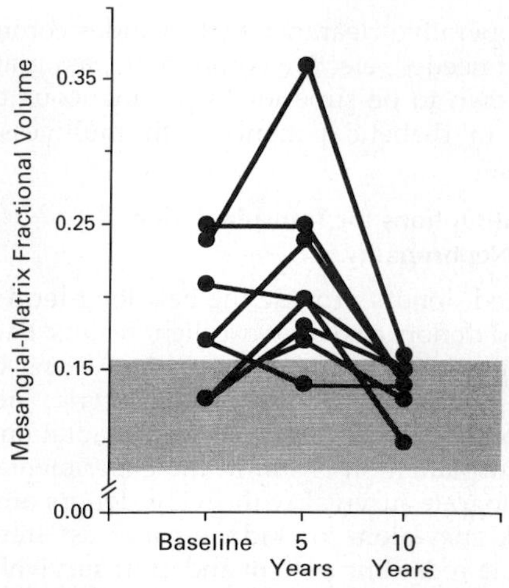

Figure 45.19. Mesangial fractional volume in sequential renal biopsies of native kidneys at baseline and after 5 and 10 years of successful pancreas transplantation in eight type I diabetic patients. Note the reversal of the increase in this volume after 10 years of euglycemia. The shaded area is the normal range in age- and sex-matched nondiabetic controls (mean ± SD). Data of individual patients are connected by lines. (Reproduced with permission from Fioretto P, Steffes MW, Sutherland DER, et al. *N Engl J Med* 1998;339:69–75.)

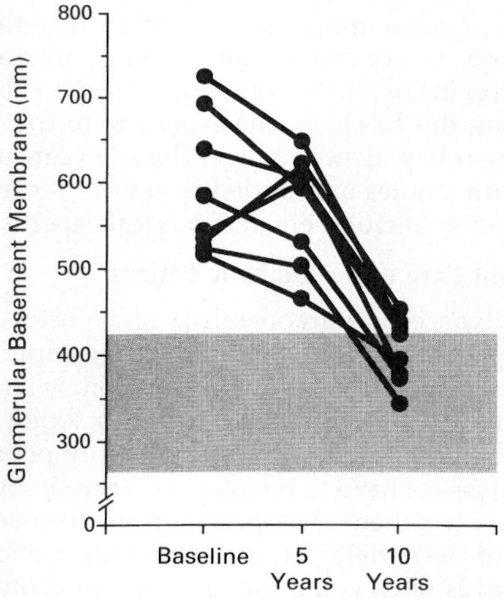

Figure 45.20. Glomerular basement membrane thickness in sequential renal biopsies of native kidneys at baseline and after 5 and 10 years of successful pancreas transplantation in eight type I diabetic patients with diabetic nephropathy but without uremia. Note the reversal of the increased thickness after 10 years of euglycemia. The shaded area is the normal range in age- and sex-matched nondiabetic controls (mean ± SD). Data of individual patients are connected by lines. (Reproduced with permission from Fioretto P, Steffes MW, Sutherland DER, et al. *N Engl J Med* 1998;339:69–75.)

with proteinuria. Graft function declines over many years, but loss of graft due to recurrent disease is unusual, occurring in fewer than 5% of cases. The redevelopment of glomerular and arteriolar lesions in the allograft can be delayed by strict glucose control either by intensive insulin therapy or by a simultaneous pancreas transplant.

A remarkable long-term study with sequential native kidney biopsies has shown that correction of hyperglycemia by pancreas-alone transplantation over a ten-year period preserves kidney function and reverses the histologic hallmarks of diabetic renal disease such as increased mesangial volume (Fig. 45.19) and basement membrane thickness (Fig. 45.20). This unexpected phenomenon highlights the important role of long-term glycemic control in the reversal and prevention of kidney disease. The long-held view that diabetic nephropathy lesions are irreversible may not be true, and this is consistent with the realization that matrix accumulation is a dynamic process encompassing a balance between synthesis and degradation. Given sufficient time and stringent metabolic control, active tissue remodeling can tip the balance toward a net decrease in the amount of extracellular matrix accumulation.

Selected Readings

Bennett PH, Haffner S, Kasiske BL, et al. Screening and management of microalbuminuria in patients with diabetes mellitus: recommendations to the Scientific Advisory Board of the National Kidney Foundation from an Ad Hoc Committee of the Council on Diabetes Mellitus of the National Kidney Foundation. *Am J Kidney Dis* 1995;25:107–112.

Useful clinical guidelines proposed by the National Kidney Foundation for the diagnosis and therapy of microalbuminuria in diabetic patients. All diabetic patients should be screened yearly with a spot urine albumin:creatinine ratio for the presence of microalbuminuria. Therapy with an ACE inhibitor is recommended for those who are diagnosed with microalbuminuria.

Brownlee M, Cerami A, Vlassara H. Advanced glycosylation end products in tissue and the biochemical basis of diabetic complications. *N Engl J Med* 1988;318:1315–1321.

This is an overview of the biochemistry of AGEs and a description of how matrix protein crosslinks are formed. AGEs interfere with normal matrix structure and alter cell function in ways that are deleterious in diabetes mellitus. Aminoguanidine's mode of action is described.

The Diabetes Control and Complications Trial Research Group. The effect of intensive treatment of diabetes on the development and progression of long-term complications in insulin-dependent diabetes mellitus. *N Engl J Med* 1993;329:977–986.

This landmark study describes the effect of intensive treatment (either with an external insulin pump or by three or more daily insulin injections) versus conventional therapy (with one or two daily insulin injections) on diabetic complications in type I diabetic patients. After a mean follow-up of 6.5 years, intensive therapy significantly reduced the development and progression of retinopathy and neuropathy as compared with conventional therapy. Similarly, intensive insulin therapy was more effective in the prevention of microalbuminuria and macroalbuminuria.

The Diabetes Control and Complications Trial Research Group. Effect of intensive therapy on the development and progression of diabetic nephropathy in the DCCT. *Kidney Int* 1995;47:1703–1720.

This subgroup analysis of the DCCT study discusses the beneficial effects of intensive therapy on development and progression of diabetic nephropathy in type I diabetic patients. Intensive therapy in patients with initial normoalbuminuria was associated with decreased incidence of microalbuminuria. However, if microalbuminuria was present at entry into the study, intensive insulin therapy did not provide a statistically different effect than conventional therapy on the subsequent progression to macroalbuminuria.

Fioretto P, Steffes MW, Brown DM, et al. An overview of renal pathology in insulin-dependent diabetes mellitus in relationship to altered glomerular hemodynamics. *Am J Kidney Dis* 1992;20:549–558.

This is a review of the pathology of diabetic nephropathy. Metabolic, systemic hemodynamic, and intraglomerular factors are mentioned as important in the pathogenesis of the disease. The argument is put forth that because renal histologic changes typical of diabetes do not develop in patients with conditions that lead to longstanding glomerular hyperfunction (e.g., unilateral nephrectomy), glomerular hemodynamic abnormalities alone cannot be the cause of diabetic nephropathy. However, the authors emphasize that there is evidence suggesting systemic hypertension increases the rate of renal functional decline in diabetes.

Hostetter TH, Troy JL, Brenner BM. Glomerular hemodynamics in experimental diabetes mellitus. *Kidney Int* 1981;19:410–415.

This animal study on streptozotocin-induced diabetic rats showed that single-nephron glomerular filtration rate (SNGFR) values were significantly lower in severely hyperglycemic rats and significantly higher in moderately hyperglycemic rats as compared to normoglycemic controls. Decreased SNGFR in severely hyperglycemic rats resulted from a decrease in glomerular plasma flow rate, while increased SNGFR in moderately hyperglycemic rats resulted from glomerular hyperfiltration. This latter hyperfiltration resulted from elevations in glomerular plasma flow and glomerular transcapillary hydraulic pressure. The authors were the first to argue that there is a deleterious role of intraglomerular hypertension in diabetic kidney disease.

Lewis EJ, Hunsicker LG, Bain RP, et al. The effect of angiotensin-converting-enzyme inhibition on diabetic nephropathy. *N Engl J Med* 1993;329:1456–1462.

Type I diabetic patients with macroalbuminuria and varying renal function (but creatinine less than 2.5 mg/dl) were randomized for treatment with captopril or placebo. The mean rate of decline in creatinine clearance was 11% per year in the captopril group and 17% per year in the placebo group. Captopril treatment was also associated with a 50% reduction in the combined risk of death, dialysis, and transplantation. This landmark study was criticized because of the high progression rate in the placebo group when compared with historic controls, as well as for the slightly better blood pressure control in the captopril treated group.

Mauer SM, Steffes MW, Ellis EN, et al. Structural-functional relationships in diabetic nephropathy. *J Clin Invest* 1984;74:1143–1155.

In renal biopsies from 45 patients with type I diabetes mellitus, a significant relationship was found between either GBM thickness or mesangial expansion and duration of diabetes. On the other hand, clinical manifestations of diabetic nephropathy related poorly to GBM thickening, while mesangial expansion related strongly to the clinical signs of progression in diabetic nephropathy. The authors concluded that mesangial expansion likely acts through crowding out glomerular filtration surface, and along with interstitial fibrosis it is a major factor in the development and progression of clinical manifestations of diabetic nephropathy.

Mogensen CE. Microalbuminuria predicts clinical proteinuria and early mortality in maturity onset diabetes. *N Engl J Med* 1984;310:356–360.

The first article that convincingly showed that the presence of microalbuminuria (30 to 140 μg of albumin/ml in this study) in type II diabetics predicts the future progression to overt proteinuria. In addition, mortality was 148% higher in the microalbuminuric group than in normal controls. Furthermore, and quite strikingly, the correlation of albuminuria and mortality was strong even among patients within the normal albumin excretion range.

Mogensen CE. Diabetic renal disease: the quest for normotension—and beyond. *Diabet Med* 1995;12:756–769.

A fascinating, thought-provoking historical overview of antihypertensive therapy in the last several decades. Putative risks of antihypertensive therapy (from a historical standpoint) are discussed. The author then discusses the recent recognition of the overriding benefits of this therapy in diabetic nephropathy. Appropriate blood pressure treatment can reduce the rate of decline in glomerular filtration rate from about 12 ml/min per year to a mean level of 2 to 5 ml/min per year, even in clinical situations where glycemic control is not perfect.

Mogyorosi A, Ziyadeh FN. Update on pathogenesis, markers, and management of diabetic nephropathy. *Curr Opin Nephrol Hypertens* 1996;5:243–253.

This recent, comprehensive article reviews new achievements in research on diabetic nephropathy. Experiments in vitro and in animal models of diabetes have provided further credence to the central role of glucose metabolism in the pathogenesis of diabetic nephropathy. Candidate phenotypic or genotypic markers for the early diagnosis of the disease are discussed, and up-to-date management recommendations summarized.

Osterby R. Early phases in the development of diabetic glomerulopathy. A quantitative electron microscopic study. *Acta Med Scand* 1974;574 (Suppl):3–82.

A landmark paper that describes in detail the different pathologic lesions in diabetic nephropathy.

Parving H, Andersen A, Smidt U, et al. Early aggressive antihypertensive treatment reduces rate of decline in kidney function in diabetic nephropathy. *Lancet*1983;ii:1175–1179.

An early report about the effect of aggressive antihypertensive therapy on kidney function in diabetic nephropathy. Ten type I diabetes patients were followed first off blood pressure medications then on strict antihypertensive therapy with metoprolol, hydralazine, and furosemide or thiazide. The rate of decline in glomerular filtration rate decreased from 0.91 ml/min per month off-treatment to 0.39 ml/min per month during treatment. An elegant study that will never be repeated for ethical reasons.

Sawicki PT, Didjurgeit U, Muhlhauser I, et al. Smoking is associated with progression of diabetic nephropathy. *Diabetes Care* 1994;17(2):126–131.

This prospective, follow-up study investigated the association between smoking and the progression of diabetic kidney disease in type I diabetics. Progression of nephropathy was less common in nonsmokers (11%) than in smokers (53%), whereas patients who quit smoking had an intermediate risk of progression (33%). The authors point out that cigarette smoking represents an important, and most of all, modifiable risk factor for the progression of diabetic nephropathy in type I diabetics.

Schmidt S, Schone N, Ritz E. Association of ACE gene polymorphism and diabetic nephropathy? *Kidney Int* 1995;47:1176–1181.

Genes of the renin-angiotensin system are obvious candidates for conferring susceptibility to diabetic nephropathy. In this large Caucasian population of type I and type II diabetic patients, ACE gene insertion/deletion polymorphism was not associated with the development of diabetic kidney disease.

Sharma K, Jin Y, Guo J, et al. Neutralization of TGF-beta by anti-TGF-beta antibody attenuates kidney hypertrophy and the enhanced extracellular matrix gene expression in streptozotocin-induced diabetic mice. *Diabetes* 1996;45: 522–530.

Streptozotocin-diabetic mice were treated with neutralizing monoclonal antibody directed against TGF-β1, β2, and β3 for 9 days. This treatment prevented glomerular hypertrophy, reduced the increment in kidney weight by about 50% and significantly attenuated the increase in mRNAs encoding TGF-β1, type II TGF-βreceptor, α1(IV) collagen, and fibronectin, without having any effect on blood glucose. This is the first demonstration that the early characteristic features of diabetic renal involvement are largely mediated by increased endogenous TGF-β activity in the kidney, and that they can be prevented by treatment with neutralizing anti–TGF-β antibodies.

Sharma K, Ziyadeh FN, Alzahabi B, et al. Increased renal production of transforming growth factor-β1 in patients with type II diabetes mellitus. *Diabetes* 1997;46:854–859.

Aortic, renal vein, and urinary levels of TGF-β and endothelin were measured in 14 type II diabetic patients and 11 control subjects who were undergoing elective cardiac catheterization. Diabetic patients demonstrated net renal production of immunoreactive TGF-β1 whereas nondiabetic patients demonstrated net renal extraction of circulating TGF-β1. Urinary levels of bioassayable TGF-β were also significantly increased in diabetic patients.

United Kingdom Prospective Diabetes Study Group. Efficacy of atenolol and captopril in reducing risk of macrovascular complications in type II diabetes: UKPDS 39. *Br Med J* 317:713–720.

In this landmark study, the largest and longest in the field of diabetes, the blood pressure lowering with captopril-based therapy was as effective as atenolol-based therapy in reducing both macrovascular and microvascular complications over a 9-year period. This study provided no evidence of any specific deleterious or beneficial effect of either drug regimen, suggesting that blood pressure reduction in itself may be more important.

Viberti GC, Hill RD, Jarrett RJ, et al. Microalbuminuria as a predictor of clinical nephropathy in insulin-dependent diabetes mellitus. *Lancet* 1982;i:1430–1432.

Another landmark article showing the importance of the presence of microalbuminuria in type I diabetic patients. Urinary protein excretion was measured twice in 63 patients with type I diabetes, 14 years apart. Clinical proteinuria developed in only 2 of 55 patients with initial normoalbuminuria and in 7 of 8 with initial microalbuminuria. Clearly, microalbuminuria is the best available marker for the development of overt diabetic nephropathy, and its screening should be a priority in the practice of all health care professionals taking care of patients with type I and type II diabetes.

Williams ME. Management of the diabetic transplant recipient. *Kidney Int* 1995;48:1660–1674.

A well written, up-to-date "Nephrology Forum" detailing the outcome and management of renal transplantation in patients with type I and type II diabetes. The author discusses the increasing percentage of diabetics among transplanted patients and their improving long-term prospects.

Zeller K, Whittaker E, Sullivan L, et al. Effect of restricting dietary protein on the progression of renal failure in patients with diabetes mellitus. *N Engl J Med* 1991;324:78–84.

The effect of reduced protein and phosphorus intake on the progression of diabetic nephropathy was studied in 35 type I diabetic patients with overt kidney disease. After 3 years, the low-protein, low-phosphorus diet containing 0.6 g of protein per kilogram of ideal body weight per day and 500 to 1,000 mg of phosphorus significantly slowed the decline of the glomerular filtration rate as compared to controls who were on daily diets of at least 1 g of protein per kilogram and 1,000 mg of phosphorus. Restriction of protein and phosphorus can alleviate the progression of kidney disease in patients with type I diabetes and clinical nephropathy.

Ziyadeh FN. Mediators of hyperglycemia and the pathogenesis of matrix accumulation in diabetic renal disease. *Miner Electrolyte Metab* 1995;21:292–302.

This review is an update on the factors that mediate diabetic kidney disease especially hyperglycemia and altered hemodynamics. The intermediary action of potent mediators include angiotensin II, thromboxane, endothelins, PDGF, and IGF-1, which all have been proposed to increase the activity of the TGF-β–TGF-β receptor system and can promote renal cell hypertrophy and extracellular matrix accumulation.

Ziyadeh FN, Han DC. Involvement of transforming growth factor-β and its receptors in the pathogenesis of diabetic nephropathy. *Kidney International* 1997;52(Suppl 60):S7–S11.

An overview of the biology of TGF-β and its receptors in the kidney, along with a detailed review of the evidence derived from cell culture and experimental animals linking the autocrine overproduction of TGF-β and diabetic renal disease.

Ziyadeh FN, Hoffman BB, Han DC, et al. Long-term prevention of renal insufficiency, excess matrix gene expression, and glomerular mesangial matrix expansion by treatment with monoclonal antitransforming growth factor-antibody in *db/db* diabetic mice. *Proc Natl Acad Sci USA* 2000;97:8015–8020.

Type II diabetic db/db *mice, which overexpress glomerular TGF-β1 and renal type II TGF-β receptor, were treated with neutralizing monoclonal antibody directed against TGF-β1, β2, and β3 for 8 weeks. This treatment prevented glomerular mesangial matrix expansion and renal insufficiency and significantly attenuated the increased mRNAs for α1(IV) collagen and fibronectin. This is the first proof-of-concept that diabetic nephropathy is mediated by increased endogenous TGF-β activity in the kidney, and that the disease can be prevented by treatment with neutralizing anti-TGF-β antibodies.*

Ziyadeh FN, Mogyorosi A, Kalluri R. Early and advanced nonenzymatic glycation products in the pathogenesis of diabetic kidney disease. *Exp Nephrol* 1997;5:2–9.

This paper reviews the evidence that accelerated nonenzymatic glycation reactions (resulting in Amadori-modified proteins and the later-developing AGEs) are linked to the pathogenesis of diabetic nephropathy. Experimental evidence is reviewed regarding the efficacy of abrogating the biologic effects of Amadori-products (e.g., using monoclonal antibodies against glycated albumin) and AGE-modified proteins (e.g., using aminoguanidine).

Ziyadeh FN, Sharma K, Ericksen M, et al. Stimulation of collagen gene expression and protein synthesis in murine mesangial cells by high glucose is mediated by activation of transforming growth factor-β. *J Clin Invest* 1995;93:536–542.

The high glucose–mediated increase in collagen synthesis in glomerular mesangial cells in culture is blocked by a neutralizing anti–TGF-β antibody. This paper provides the first evidence that the effects of high ambient glucose to stimulate matrix protein synthesis are mediated by increased production and activity of autocrine TGF-β.

CHAPTER 46

Cystic Diseases of the Kidney

PART 1
Polycystic Kidney Disease Autosomal-Dominant and Recessive Forms

Vicente E. Torres

Descriptions of cystic kidneys and livers can be traced back to antiquity. The term *polycystic kidneys* was first used by Lejars in his doctoral thesis published in 1888. The recognition of autosomal-recessive and autosomal-dominant forms as two clearly distinct entities was established in the early part of the twentieth century. Research developments in the last decade have raised hopes that elucidation of their pathogenesis and identification of effective forms of therapy may not be far away.

AUTOSOMAL-DOMINANT POLYCYSTIC KIDNEY DISEASE

Definition and Diagnostic Criteria

Autosomal-dominant polycystic kidney disease (ADPKD) is a multisystemic disorder with an autosomal-dominant pattern of inheritance characterized by (a) bilateral renal cysts; (b) frequent association with cysts in other organs, such as the liver, arachnoid membrane, and pancreas; (c) extrarenal abnormalities, such as intracranial aneurysms, mitral valve prolapse, and abdominal wall hernias; and (d) the absence of manifestations suggestive of a different renal cystic disease. In patients with a known family history of ADPKD and a compatible phenotype, the diagnosis is straight forward. Sonographic diagnostic criteria have been established for individuals known to be at 50% risk for the disease (Table 46.1.). The clinical presentation of ADPKD in the first year of life with large echogenic kidneys without distinct macroscopic cysts is an exception to these criteria. In the absence of a family history of the disease or in the presence of atypical phenotypes, other cystic diseases and benign simple cysts should be considered in the differential diagnosis. Renal cystic diseases that are occasionally confused with ADPKD include diseases associated with malformation or disruption syndromes, autosomal-recessive polycystic kidney disease, tuberous sclerosis complex (TSC), von Hippel Lindau disease, orofaciodigital syndrome type 1, localized renal cystic disease, and acquired renal cystic disease.

Epidemiology

ADPKD is the most common single-gene disorder that is potentially lethal. It has a prevalence at birth between 1:400 and 1:1,000 and affects approximately 400,000 in the United States. Of these, approximately 1,800 start renal replacement therapy every year. The annual cost of this program exceeds half a billion dollars in the United States alone. ADPKD occurs worldwide and in all races. The disease may be less common in Africa. In the United States ADPKD may be less common but more severe among African-Americans than among whites. It has been shown that the percentage of end-stage renal disease (ESRD) due to ADPKD is less among African-Americans than among whites, but this reflects a higher incidence of other causes of ESRD among African-Americans.

Genetics

ADPKD is genetically heterogeneous. There is evidence for at least three genes that result in ADPKD when mutated. Two of them (PKD1 and PKD2) have been identified by positional cloning. There is at least one more gene that is responsible for autosomal-dominant polycystic liver disease without renal involvement. This gene has been mapped but not yet identified.

TABLE 46.1. Sonographic Criteria for the Diagnosis of ADPKD in Individuals at 50% Risk

Age (yr)	At Least
<30	2 Cysts either unilateral or bilateral
30–59	2 Cysts in each kidney
>60	4 Cysts in each kidney

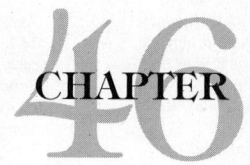

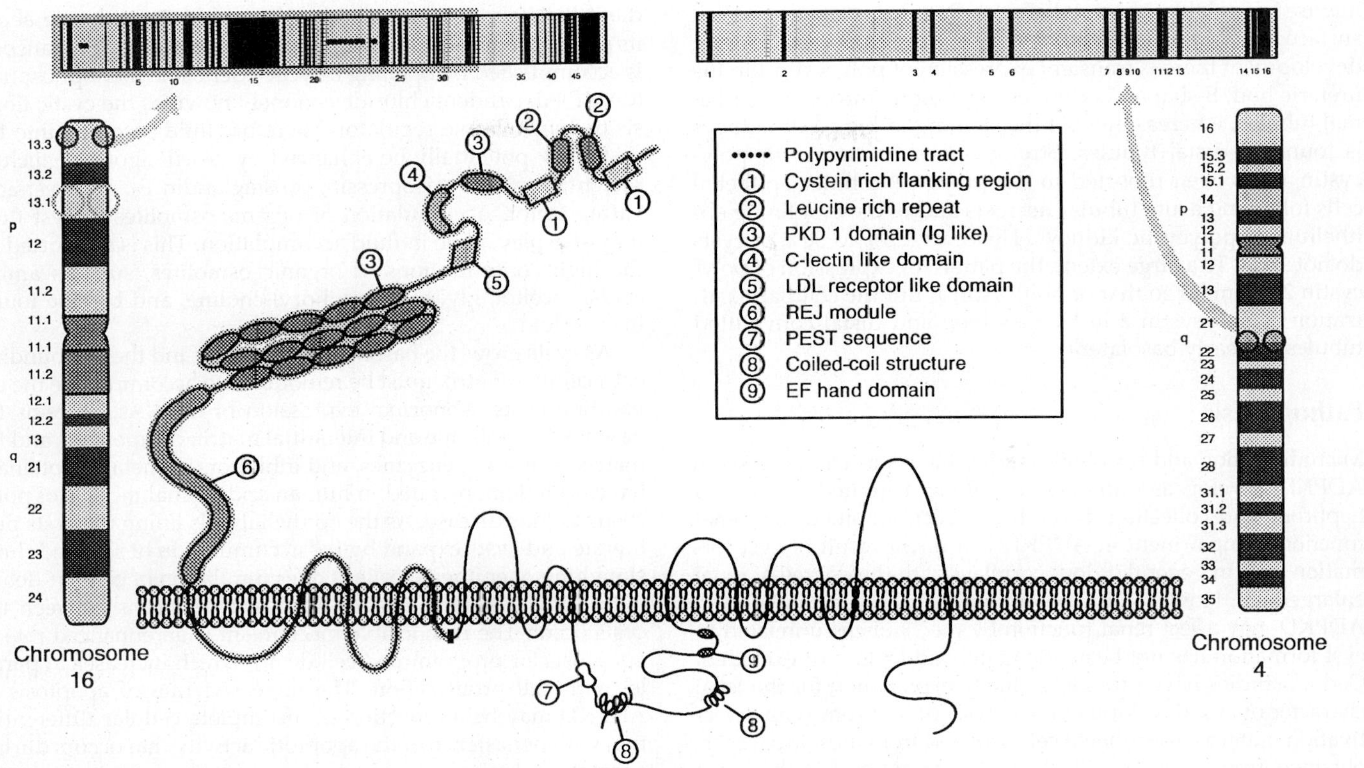

Figure 46.1. Chromosomal location and intron-exon structure of the PKD1 and PKD2 genes and sequence homologies, structural features, and possible interaction of polycystin 1 and polycystin 2. (Reproduced with permission from Torres VE. New insights into polycystic kidney disease and its treatment. *Curr Opin Nephrol Hypertens* 1998;7:159–169.)

Structure of PKD1 and PKD2 and Their Encoded Proteins, Polycystin 1 and Polycystin 2

The intron-exon structures of the PKD1 and PKD2 genes in addition to their products, sequence homologies, structural features, and possible interaction are illustrated in Fig. 46.1. Approximately 75% of the PKD1 gene (exons 1 to 34) is duplicated at least three times on the same (homologous) genes. The PKD1 gene contains three long, polypyrimidine tracts. These tracts predispose to triple helix formation, erroneous repair, and mutations during transcription.

Polycystin 1 is predicted to contain a large N-terminal extracellular region, multiple transmembrane domains, and a C-terminal cytoplasmic tail. The large N-terminal region contains many peptide motifs, which are usually associated with extracellular proteins. Based on this observation, it has been suggested that polycystin 1 may play a role in cell–cell or cell–matrix interactions. Another region of polycystin 1, which extends to the first transmembrane domain, shares significant homology with the sea urchin sperm receptor for egg jelly. Because the binding of egg-jelly glycoproteins to the receptor for egg jelly results in the acrosome reaction, an ion channel regulated event, it has been suggested that polycystin 1 may regulate an ion channel. The region containing the last four transmembrane domains of polycystin 1 has 25% identity and 50% similarity with the region containing the six transmembrane domains of polycystin 2. The C-terminal cytoplasmic tail of polycystin 1 contains a coiled-coil structure and a potential PEST. A coiled-coil structure is characterized by repeated units of seven amino acids or heptads (ABCDEFG), in which the A and D amino acids are hydrophobic and the rest are hydrophilic. A PEST sequence is an internal amino acid sequence (rich in proline, glutamic acid, serine, and threonine and flanked by positively charged amino acids) that makes a protein more susceptible to proteolysis.

Polycystin 2 is predicted to contain an N-terminal region, six transmembrane domains, and a C-terminal tail. The region of polycystin 2 that extends from the second transmembrane domain to the C-terminus has significant similarity with a voltage-activated calcium channel. The C-terminal region of polycystin 2 contains a putative EF-hand domain and a probable coiled-coil structure. An EF-hand domain has a specialized, helix-loop-helix motif that often has calcium binding activity and is important in regulating the proteins in which it occurs. Polycystin 2 is capable of forming homodimers. The coiled-coil structure in polycystin 2 appears to be essential for its homodimerization.

Using the two hybrid interaction system and coimmunoprecipitation experiments, it has been shown that polycystin 1 and polycystin 2 can physically interact. The coiled-coil structure in the C-terminal cytoplasmic tail of polycystin 1 is essential for binding to polycystin 2. This interaction suggests that polycystin 1 and polycystin 2 may function through a common signal pathway. It has also been suggested that binding of polycystin 2 is required to provide stability to polycystin 1 and prevent its rapid degradation mediated by the PEST sequence present in its C-terminal.

Polycystin 1 and polycystin 2 are expressed in many tissues in addition to the kidney and the liver, including epithelial cells of pancreatic and mammary ducts, intestinal crypts, urothelium and bronchioles, basal keratinocytes of the skin, neural crest, brain, neural plexus and adrenal medulla, myocardium, vascular smooth muscle of elastic and distributive arteries, and certain endothelial cells. In the kidney immunostaining for polycystin 1 is confined to the epithelial cells and is more intense in fetal than in adult kidneys. Both cytoplasmic and cell surface–associated localizations have been reported. During development there is transient expression of polycystin 1 in the ureteric bud, S-shaped bodies, elongating nephron, and proximal tubules, whereas most of the staining in the adult kidneys is found in distal tubules. Strong immunostaining for polycystin 1 has been reported in the proximal tubular epithelial cells following acute tubular necrosis and in the cyst lining epithelium of polycystic kidneys. However, 20% to 30% of cysts do not stain. To a large extent, the pattern of expression of polycystin 2 is similar to that of polycystin 1, but the cellular localization of polycystin 2 in Henle's loop and distal convoluted tubules is clearly basolateral.

Pathogenesis

Microdissection and histologic studies have shown that cysts in ADPKD develop as outpouchings along a limited number of nephrons and collecting ducts. It has been assumed that renal functional impairment in ADPKD is a direct result of cyst formation, and in general it does correlate with the degree of renal enlargement. However, the possibility that the genetic defect in ADPKD may affect renal function by mechanisms unrelated to cyst formation has not been adequately addressed or excluded. Certain studies have provided a likely explanation for the focal character of cyst development. Analysis of X-chromosome inactivation patterns in epithelial cells isolated from individual cysts obtained from women with ADPKD has suggested that each cyst results from clonal expansion of a single cell. In addition, analysis of PKD1 genes in the same cells has revealed loss of heterozygosity or large deletions involving the unaffected PKD1 allele in approximately 20% of renal cysts. Possibly, small deletions or point mutations could account for the inactivation of the unaffected PKD1 allele in the remaining 80%. Loss of heterozygosity has also been demonstrated in hepatic cysts. These observations are consistent with a two-hit tumor suppressor model of cystogenesis. The apparent overexpression of polycystin by immunohistochemistry can be reconciled with this hypothesis because 20% to 30% of cysts contain no detectable polycystin. Polycystin 1 immunostaining in the remaining cysts may be due to the accumulation of an abnormal protein or may reflect enhanced expression associated with cellular dedifferentiation.

Regardless of the genetic mechanism, cysts are the result of clonal expansion of partially dedifferentiated epithelial cells, characterized by dysregulation of epithelial cell proliferation, expression of a secretory phenotype, and a disarray of cell matrix interactions, which leads to interstitial inflammation and matrix accumulation. Developmental genes that are normally downregulated in mature nephron segments are persistently expressed in the epithelial cells lining the renal cysts. Many of these overexpressed proteins are involved in regulation of cell proliferation (PCNA, c-myc, c-fos, and h-ki-ras). As the cysts grow and reach a diameter of approximately 2 mm, they become disconnected from the tubular segment from which they derive. Accumulation of fluid within these cysts can only occur by a process of transepithelial fluid secretion. Certain studies indicate that active transport of chloride from the basolateral to the apical side of the epithelial cells is the driving force for secretion. The potential energy for chloride secretion is developed by the sodium pump (Na^+-K^+-ATPase) located in the basolateral membrane. A chloride entry mechanism in the basolateral membrane, most likely Na^+-K^+-$2Cl^-$ cotransporter, utilizes the gradient established by the sodium pump to bring potassium and chloride into the cells. The sodium is pumped out of the cell by the sodium pump, and the potassium exits through a selective basolateral channel, thereby establishing an electrical gradient that favors accumulation of intracellular chloride above its electrochemical equilibrium potential. Net chloride transport is accomplished by opening a cyclic adenosine monophosphate (cAMP)–dependent chloride channel known as the cystic fibrosis transmembrane regulator. Therefore fluid secretion into the cysts may potentially be enhanced by cAMP agonists, such as secretin, arginine vasopressin, prostaglandin E_2, and cyst-activating factor. Accumulation of organic osmolites in cyst fluid may also play a role in fluid accumulation. This is supported by the high concentrations of organic osmolites, such as amino acids, sorbitol, glycerolphosphoryl-choline, and betaine found in cyst fluid.

As cysts grow, the basement membrane and the surrounding extracellular matrix must be remodeled to accommodate the expanding cysts. Abnormal expression of mRNAs, proteins for basement membrane and interstitial matrix components and for matrix degrading enzymes, and inhibitors of metalloproteinase have been demonstrated in human and animal models of polycystic kidney disease. As the epithelial cells lining the cysts proliferate and cysts expand by the accumulation of secreted fluid, sloughing of epithelial cells and accumulation of cellular debris within the cysts and loss of noncystic nephrons between the cysts occur. The responsible mechanism is an enhanced rate of apoptosis, or programmed cell death, which increases in parallel with cell proliferation. The increased rate of apoptosis in ADPKD may be a reflection of incomplete cellular differentiation with persistence of the apoptotic activity that occurs during normal nephrogenesis and is downregulated during maturation. The increased apoptotic activity seen in ADPKD may explain why renal cell carcinomas do not occur more frequently in this disease.

In addition to physical compression of the surrounding parenchyma and distortion on the renal architecture, cysts produce factors capable of affecting, in a paracrine fashion, the development of neighboring cysts and other aspects of renal function. These factors include a number of cytokines (IL1, IL2, and TNF-α); cyst-activating factor, a neutral lipid with secretogogue and chemotactic activity; lactosyl ceramide, a compound with mitogenic activity that is found in increased amounts in human and experimental polycystic kidneys; and other compounds such as growth factors, renin, endothelin, proinflammatory chemokines, matrix metalloproteinase, and lysosomal enzymes.

Tubular obstruction is also a feature of some forms of polycystic kidney disease and may contribute to the growth, if not the development, of the cysts. Several investigators have drawn attention to similarities between the pathogenesis of renal cystic disease and obstructive nephropathy. These include (a) increased expression of the different components of the renin-angiotensin system; (b) increased expression of chemokines, such as monocyte chemoattractant peptide 1 and osteopontin; (c) increased expression of transforming growth factor-β and platelet-derived growth factor; (d) increased production of reactive oxygen species; and (e) reduced expression or generation of bradykinin, nitric oxide, antioxidant enzymes, and epidermal growth factor. All of these factors may contribute to the development of interstitial inflammation, matrix accumulation, and vascular lesions, which accompany the development of polycystic kidney disease.

Pathology

Polycystic kidneys are typically enlarged and diffusely cystic, but in early stages they may be of normal size and with a limited number of macroscopic cysts scattered in the cortex and medulla (Fig. 46.2). Microscopically, they are characterized by nonpolypoid and by polypoid hyperplasia of the epithelium lining the cysts. Despite the frequency of hyperplastic lesions and microscopic adenomas, the incidence of renal cell carcinoma does not appear to be increased. The tubular basement membranes surrounding the cysts are typically thickened and often laminated. The adjacent parenchyma is compressed. Interstitial fibrosis is a prominent finding, even in patients with early disease. It is associated with inflammatory infiltrates consisting of macrophages and lymphocytes. Vascular sclerosis involving both afferent arterioles and interlobular arteries is also observed.

Natural History and Clinical Manifestations of Renal Disease

Although all patients who inherit ADPKD develop cysts within the kidneys, there is substantial variability in the occurrence of renal insuffiencey and other complications of this disease. Even within the same family, significant variability in clinical presentation occurs.

Chronologically, renal manifestations of ADPKD include functional abnormalities, hypertension, pain, and renal insufficiency. Reductions in urinary-concentrating capacity and excretion of ammonia occur early and may result from the disruption of the renal architecture by the cysts, interference in the countercurrent exchange and multiplication mechanisms, and defective trapping of solutes and ammonia in the renal medulla. In the early stages of the disease, these defects are moderate, and there is significant overlap between affected and nonaffected individuals. Although the concentrating defect may not have clinical repercussions, the reduction of urinary excretion of ammonia in the presence of metabolic stresses such as dietary indiscretions may contribute to the development of uric acid and calcium oxalate stones, which, in association with low urine pH values and hypocitric aciduria, occur with increased frequency in ADPKD.

An early functional abnormality is a reduction in renal blood flow. It can be detected in young patients, when systolic and diastolic blood pressures are still normal, and precede the development of hypertension. Hypertension usually develops before any decline in glomerular filtration rate (GFR) has occurred. It is characterized by an increased renal vascular resistance and filtration fraction; normal or high peripheral plasma renin activity; resetting of the pressure–natriuresis relationship; salt sensitivity; normal or increased extracellular fluid volume, plasma volume and cardiac output; and partial correction of renal hemodynamics and sodium handling by converting-enzyme inhibition. Other vasoactive factors may also contribute to the development of hypertension. The plasma concentration of endothelin 1 has been found to be significantly increased in patients with ADPKD with or without hypertension, as compared to control subjects or to patients with essential hypertension. Immunoreactive endothelin has been detected in the cyst lining epithelial cells and in cyst fluids obtained from human ADPKD kidneys. The plasma concentration of atrial natriuretic peptide has been found to be normal or, after sodium loading or in patients with reduced renal function, elevated. Increased urinary excretion of dopamine, unaffected by changes in sodium intake, has also been reported. The early development and chronicity of hypertension in ADPKD is often responsible for significant end-organ damage. Left ventricular hypertrophy by echocardiographic criteria develops in young adults and is an independent risk factor for premature death. Hypertension increases the morbidity and mortality caused by extrarenal manifestations, such as valvular heart disease, intracranial aneurysms, and aortic dissections. Hypertensive cerebral hemorrhage is at least as, if not more, frequent as aneurysmal subarachnoid hemorrhage in these patients. Preexisting hypertension is the most important risk factor for fetal and maternal complications during pregnancy in ADPKD.

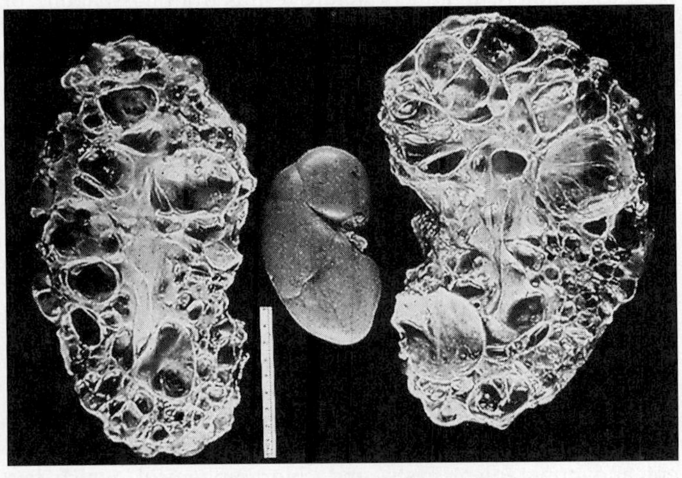

Figure 46.2. Polycystic kidney disease with marked enlargement of the kidneys without loss in their reniform appearance. The right kidney has been coronally sectioned. Note areas of preserved parenchyma between the cysts.

Pain is a common manifestation of ADPKD. Episodes of acute pain are frequent, but chronic severe pain occurs rarely. Potential etiologies for acute flank pain include cyst hemorrhage, nephrolithiasis, cyst infection, and rarely tumor.

Bleeding into a cyst can occur with or without gross hematuria. It can be accompanied by fever, raising the possibility of cyst infection. It rarely results in a retroperitoneal bleed, which may be severe and potentially require transfusion. However, most often cyst hemorrhages are self-limited, and the pain resolves within 2 to 7 days. Episodes of gross hematuria are very common and usually require no particular evaluation or treatment. Nevertheless, gross hematuria persisting more than one week or developing for the first time in a patient older than 50 should be thoroughly investigated.

Nephrolithiasis occurs in approximately 20% of patients. Most stones are uric acid and/or calcium oxalate in composition. Uric acid stones are more common in stone formers with ADPKD than without ADPKD. Small uric acid stones can be missed on nephrotomography and are best detected by computed tomographic (CT) scan. CT scan should be obtained before and after the administration of contrast material to confirm the localization within the collecting system and to differentiate calculi from parenchymal calcifications. Excretory urography can detect precalyceal tubular ectasia in 15% of ADPKD patients.

Urinary tract infections are important in ADPKD, but their prevalence may have been overestimated because of the common occurrence of sterile pyuria in these patients. Urinary tract infections occur in the form of cystitis, pyelonephritis, cyst infection, and perinephric abscesses. As in the general population, females are affected more frequently than males. Most of the infections are caused by *Escherichia coli, Klebsiella, Proteus,* and other Enterobacteriaceae. Cyst infections usually present with fever, positive blood culture, features of a complex cyst (thickened wall and content of abnormal density) on imaging studies, positive indium-111 white blood cell scan, and often an inadequate response to treatment with standard antibiotic regimens.

Renal cell carcinomas do not occur more frequently in ADPKD than in the general population. Nevertheless, when renal cell carcinomas develop in patients with ADPKD, they have

TABLE 46.2. Predictors of Disease Progression in ADPKD

PKD1 > non-PKD1
Men > women
African-American > white
Hypertension in nonaffected parent
Large renal size
Early onset of hypertension
Proteinuria
Hypercholesterolemia
ACE DD polymorphism
Sickle cell trait

a different biologic behavior with no male predominance, earlier age of presentation, frequent constitutional symptoms, and a higher percentage of sarcomatoid bilateral, multicentric, and metastatic tumors. The diagnosis of renal cell carcinoma in a polycystic kidney requires a high index of suspicion. Magnetic resonance imaging (MRI) with gadolinium enhancement is particularly helpful to detect atypical solid or cystic masses, tumor thrombi, and regional lymphadenopathy. The diagnosis of transitional cell carcinoma in a polycystic kidney is equally challenging and usually requires retrograde pyelography.

Chronic pain may be caused by stretching of the capsule and traction of the vascular pedicle by large cysts or to other poorly understood mechanisms. Massive renal enlargement can result in compression of local structures resulting in complications such as inferior vena cava compression (mainly by right renal cysts) and digestive symptoms.

Patients usually present with renal failure usually in their 30s or later. End-stage renal failure is not the inevitable outcome of ADPKD. Only 50% of ADPKD patients have reached ESRD by the ages of 57 to 73 years in large clinical series. Both genetic and environmental factors appear to play a role in the progression of renal failure. Risk factors for progressive renal insufficiency are listed in Table 46.2. Once renal insufficiency has begun, the rate of decline in renal function is linear with a loss of GFR of approximately 5.8 ml/min per year on average in patients with moderate renal insufficiency. The mechanism by which ADPKD results in renal insuffiencey is not completely understood. Histologic studies of ADPKD kidneys suggest that advanced vascular sclerosis and interstitial inflammation and fibrosis play prominent roles. Hyperfiltration may be less important because the rate of decline of renal function in ADPKD patients who underwent unilateral nephrectomy for urologic emergencies was not different from that observed in ADPKD patients with two kidneys.

Treatment of the Renal Manifestations of ADPKD

Hypertension

Early detection and control of hypertension is of the utmost importance because it may result in early end-organ damage. The antihypertensive agent of choice has not been clearly established. Because of the role of the renin-angiotensin system in the pathogenesis of hypertension in ADPKD, angiotensin-converting enzyme inhibitors or angiotensin II type 1 (AT_1) receptor antagonists are excellent agents in patients with preserved renal function. These agents and the calcium channel blockers increase renal blood flow, which is reduced in ADPKD. Other advantages include low side effect profiles and theoretical benefits such as potential reduction in vascular smooth muscle proliferation and atherogenesis. Diuretics and β-blockers, on the other hand, may cause further reduction in renal blood flow and contribute to the development of gout, increase lipid levels, and induce insulin resistance. α_1-Antagonists, central α_2-agonists, and β-blockers with intrinsic sympatheticomimetic activity have no effect on renal blood flow. The administration of converting enzyme inhibitors to patients with volume contraction, diuretic use, or advanced renal insufficiency should be done cautiously because of the risk for renal function deterioration.

Cyst Hemorrhage

Episodes of cyst hemorrhage are self-limited and respond well to conservative management with bed rest, analgesics, and adequate fluid intake to prevent clots. Rarely, the episodes of bleeding are more severe with extensive subcapsular or retroperitoneal hematoma, causing significant reductions in hematocrit and hemodynamic instability. This requires hospitalization, transfusion, and investigation by CT or angiography. In cases of unusually severe or persistent hemorrhage, segmental arterial embolization can be successful. However, surgery may be required to control bleeding.

Nephrolithiasis

Treatment of nephrolithiasis in patients with ADPKD is not different from that in patients without ADPKD. Because patients with ADPKD often have a concentrating defect and increased concentrations of circulating vasopressin could have a detrimental effect on the progression of the disease, these patients should be encouraged to drink adequate amounts of fluid. This may also reduce their risk for nephrolithiasis. Potassium citrate is the treatment of choice in the stone-forming conditions associated with ADPKD, uric acid lithiasis, hypocitraturic calcium oxalate nephrolithiasis, and distal acidification defects. When necessary, extracorporeal shock wave lithotripsy and percutaneous nephrolithotomy have proven to be approximately 80% successful without significant complication.

Urinary Tract and Cyst Infection

Prompt treatment of asymptomatic bacteriuria and symptomatic cystitis will prevent retrograde seeding of the renal parenchyma. In the case of upper tract infections, antibiotics that require glomerular filtration, such as highly polar aminoglycosides, are not effective in advanced renal insufficiency. These antibiotics should also be avoided because of their nephrotoxicity and the current availability of satisfactory alternatives. Cyst infections are often difficult to treat. High failure rates, despite prolonged therapies with antibiotics to which the organisms are susceptible, are common. Treatment failure results from the inability of certain antibiotics to successfully penetrate the cyst epithelium and achieve therapeutic concentrations within the cysts. The epithelium lining gradient type cysts have functional and ultrastructural characteristics of distal tubular epithelium. Penetration into these cysts is via tight junctions, which allow access of lipid soluble agents only. Nongradient cysts, which are more common, should allow solute access via diffusion of water-soluble agents. However, kinetic studies indicate that these agents often penetrate nongradient cysts slowly and irregularly, giving rise to unreliable drug concentrations within the cysts. Lipophilic agents have been shown to penetrate both gradient and nongradient cysts equally and reliably and have pK_a values that allow for favorable electrochemical gradients into acidic cyst fluid. Therapeutic agents of choice include trimethoprim-sulfamethoxazole and fluoroquinolones, both of which have shown favorable intracystic therapeutic concentrations in gradient and nongradient cysts, and chloramphenicol, which has shown therapeutic efficacy in otherwise resistant cases. If fever persists after 1 to 2 weeks of appropriate antimicrobial therapy, percutaneous or surgical drainage of infected cysts should be performed. If fever recurs after stopping antibiotics, complicating features such as obstruction, perinephric abscess, or stone should be considered and treated appropriately. If complicating features are not identified, the course of previously effective therapy should be extended and may require several months to eradicate the infection.

Flank Pain

After excluding causes of flank pain that may require intervention such as infection, stone, or tumor, an initial conservative approach to pain management is best. Care should be taken to avoid nephrotoxic agents such as combination analgesics and chronic use of nonsteroidal and inflammatory drugs. Tricyclic antidepressants have shown to be helpful in all chronic pain syndromes, with a generally well-tolerated side-effect profile. The mechanism is not known but is thought to involve the central descending serotonin pathway and appears to be independent of the effect on mood disorder. The use of narcotic analgesics should be reserved for the management of acute episodes of pain as chronic use can lead to physical and psychologic dependence. Splanchnic nerve blockage with local anesthetics or steroids has been shown to result in pain relief prolonged beyond the duration of local anesthetic.

When conservative measures fail, therapy can be directed toward cyst decompression by cyst aspiration and sclerosis, surgical cystic decompression, or laparoscopic cyst decompression. Cyst aspiration, under ultrasound or CT guidance, is a relatively simple procedure carried out routinely by interventional radiologists. To prevent the reaccumulation of cyst fluid, sclerosing agents such as 95% ethanol or acidic solutions of minocycline are commonly used. Excellent results have been obtained with a greater than 90% success rate in benign renal cysts. Minor complications include microhematuria, localized pain, transient fever, and systemic absorption of the alcohol. More serious complications such as pneumothorax, perirenal hematoma, arteriovenous fistula, urinoma, and infection are rare. Complications from aspiration of centrally located cysts are more common, and the morbidity of the procedure is proportional to the number of cysts treated.

In patients with many pain-causing cysts, laparoscopic or surgical cyst fenestration through lumbotomy or flank incisions may help. Surgical decompression has been shown to be effective in 80% to 90% of the patients after one year, and 62% to 77% have sustained pain relief for more than two years. Surgical intervention does not accelerate the decline in renal function as once thought, but it does not appear to prevent its decline either. Laparoscopy has been shown to be equally effective to open surgical fenestration in short-term follow-up for patients with limited disease with the advantage of a shorter, less-complicated recovery compared with open surgical intervention. Previous abdominal surgery with possible adhesion formation is a relative contraindication to the procedure.

Renal Failure

Therapeutic interventions aimed at slowing the progression of renal insufficiency in ADPKD include control of hypertension, treating hyperlipidemia, dietary protein restriction, control of acidosis, and prevention of hyperphosphatemia. There are good animal data to support careful control of hypertension and dietary protein restriction to slow down the rate of progression of renal failure in ADPKD. On the other hand, the MDRD clinical trial showed that strict blood pressure control was not better than standard blood pressure control and that a very low protein diet had only a slight beneficial effect of borderline significance. Because the interventions in this trial were introduced at a late stage in the natural history of ADPKD with (GFR 13 to 55 ml/min/1.73 m^2) the results do not exclude a beneficial effect of these interventions at an earlier stage in the disease.

Based on studies on the pathogenesis of polycystic renal disease, several interventions have been evaluated in rodents with spontaneous hereditary renal cystic disorders. In rats the disease can be aggravated by the administration of ammonium chloride, high dietary protein, or potassium depletion. These treatments cause renal epithelial cell hypertrophy in normal animals and a markedly enhanced progression to renal failure in animals with inherited renal cystic disease. The administration of buthionine sulfoximine, which causes glutathione depletion and oxidative stress, has a similar effect. Conversely the administration of sodium or potassium bicarbonate or of potassium citrate may prevent the progression to end-stage renal disease. Likewise, the administration of lovastatin and HMG-CoA reductase inhibitor and the administration of methylprednisolone have beneficial effects. Although these studies cannot be extrapolated to human ADPKD, they clearly illustrate that improved knowledge of the pathogenesis of ADPKD may lead to treatments that slow or stop disease progression.

End-Stage Renal Failure

Actual data indicate that ADPKD patients do better on dialysis than patients with renal failure from other causes. Women appear to do better than men. The reason that ADPKD patients do better may have to do with higher endogenous erythropoietin and hemoglobin concentrations. Rarely, hemodialysis can be complicated by intradialytic hypotension if there is inferior vena cava compression by a polycystic liver or a medially located right renal cyst. Despite the large renal size, peritoneal dialysis can usually be performed in ADPKD patients, although they are at increased risk for inguinal and umbilical hernias, which require surgical repair. The results of renal transplantation are as good, if not better, than in other patients with end-stage renal disease. According to the 1997 U.S. Renal Data System, the one year survival probability for cadaveric transplants in ADPKD was 87% versus 85% overall, and the 5-year graft survival probability was 68% versus 59% overall. There has been a steady increase in the relative number of living-related transplants for ADPKD from 12% in 1990 to 22% in 1995. The probability of survival for living-related transplants in ADPKD and non-ADPKD patients is also similar. Indications for bilateral nephrectomy prior to renal transplantation for ADPKD include a history of infected cysts, frequent and severe bleeding episodes, severe hypertension, and massive renal enlargement with extension into the pelvis. There is no evidence for an increased risk of renal cell carcinoma developing in native ADPKD kidneys after transplantation; therefore pre-transplant nephrectomy is not indicated as cancer prophylaxis. Living-related donors over 30 years of age can be accepted if they have a negative ultrasound or, preferably, a contrast enhanced CT of the kidneys. Genetic-linkage analysis should be considered in the evaluation of younger potential donors.

Extrarenal Manifestations

ADPKD is a systemic disorder with many extrarenal manifestations listed in Table 46.3. Thoracic aortic dissection is seven times more common at autopsy in the ADPKD population than in the general population, but actual case reports are rare. Mitral valve prolapse is the most common valvular abnormality. Pancreatic cysts occur on approximately 8% of the patients older than 30, but complications related to this (obstructive pancreatitis) are exceptional. Arachnoid cysts, which occur in 8% of the patients, are asymptomatic and require no treatment, but they may slightly increase the risk for subdural hematomas. Spinal

TABLE 46.3. Extrarenal Manifestations of ADPKD

Cysts
Liver Pancreas Arachnoid Spinal meningeal diverticula (?)
Hernias
Umbilical/ventral Inguinal Diaphragmatic (?)
Cardiac
Mitral valve prolapse Aortic insufficiency Dilated cardiomyopathy (?)
Vascular
Intracranial aneurysms Intracranial arterial dolichoectasias Aortic root dilation Dissection of ascending aorta Dissection of cervicocephalic arteries Moyamoya disease (?) Coronary artery aneurysms Other visceral aneurysms (?) Abdominal aortic aneurysms (?) Aortic coarctation (?) Arteriovenous malformations (?)
Other
Colon diverticulosis (?)

meningeal diverticula have been described and may present with intracranial hypotension presumably due to cerebrospinal fluid leak. Data on associations of ADPKD with abdominal aortic aneurysms and colon diverticula are controversial. The most important extrarenal manifestations of ADPKD are polycystic liver disease and intracranial aneurysms.

Polycystic Liver Disease

Polycystic liver disease (PLD) is often used to refer to any liver cyst in the presence of ADPKD. It has been associated with both PKD1 and PKD2 genotypes. In addition, autosomal-dominant PLD occurs as a genetically distinct disease in the absence of renal cysts. In these cases, the number of cysts helps distinguish autosomal-dominant PLD from simple hepatic cysts. Simple hepatic cysts occur in 2.5% to 4.6% of patients referred for abdominal ultrasound. They are more common among women than men and increase in frequency with age. The majority of simple hepatic cysts are solitary, and no more than three cysts are present in those with multiple cysts. Therefore autosomal-dominant PLD should be suspected when four or more cysts are present in the hepatic parenchyma.

Hepatic cysts are exceedingly rare in children with ADPKD. Their frequency increases with age with cyst formation noted in 20% of patients in the third decade and 75% in the seventh decade. Females develop more cysts at an earlier age than men, and women who have had multiple pregnancies or who have used oral contraceptives have more severe disease, suggesting a role for estrogen exposure in hepatic cyst formation. After menopause, progression of PLD slows down unless estrogen replacement therapy is used.

Typically, PLD is asymptomatic. Despite great differences in the number and size of the cysts, the volume of the noncystic parenchyma and hepatic function remain essentially normal. The development of symptoms may be due to complicated hepatic cysts or to the mass effect produced by one or several dominant cysts or by a massively enlarged polycystic liver.

Symptomatic cyst complications include hemorrhage, which occurs less frequently than renal cyst hemorrhage, cyst infection, and rarely torsion or rupture. Hepatic cyst infection typically presents with localized pain, fever, leukocytosis, elevated sedimentation rate, and often elevated serum alkaline phosphatase. Blood and cyst fluid cultures usually reveal monomicrobial infections with Enterobacteriaceae. MRI is the most sensitive technique to differentiate a complicated cyst from an uncomplicated one. ^{111}Indium-labeled leukocyte scans are more specific for cyst infection, but they may give negative results when obtained too early or too late in the course of the disease, after treatment with antibiotics, or in immunosuppressed patients. When a hepatic cyst infection is suspected, any cyst with an unusual appearance on any imaging study should be aspirated for diagnostic purposes. The management consists of drainage and antibiotic therapy. Percutaneous drainage is usually effective and safe, but surgical drainage may become necessary. Long-term antibiotic suppression or prophylaxis should be reserved for those patients with relapses or recurrences. Orally administered antibiotics that concentrate in the biliary tree and the cysts, such as trimethoprim-sulfamethoxazole or ciprofloxacin, should be used.

Symptoms typically caused by massive enlargement of the liver or by the mass effect of a single or limited number of large dominant cysts include dyspnea, early satiety, gastroesophageal reflux, mechanical back pain, uterine prolapse, and even rib fracture. Other complications may be due to hepatic venous outflow obstruction, inferior vena cava compression, portal vein compression, and bile duct compression presenting as obstructive jaundice. Hepatic venous outflow obstruction is caused by extrinsic compression of the intrahepatic inferior vena cava and hepatic veins by cysts, in rare cases with superimposed thrombosis. Recent bilateral nephrectomy or abdominal surgery may be a predisposing factor. The clinical presentation is with ascites. MRI with spin-echo and gradient-echo images is particularly useful in making the diagnosis, but when the diagnosis is in question or when superimposed thrombosis is suspected, venous catheterization for pressure measurements and venography is necessary. The outcome of hepatic venous outflow obstruction without thrombosis is usually good following hepatic resection and fenestration, whereas the outcome of patients with superimposed thrombosis is often poor.

Recurrent episodes of ascending cholangitis associated with dilation of the intrahepatic or extrahepatic bile ducts, portal hypertension with bleeding esophageal varices due to congenital hepatic fibrosis, and cholangiocarcinoma occur rarely in patients with PLD.

In general, PLD requires no treatment. Estrogens should be avoided in patients with severe PLD. H2 blockers may reduce the secretion of secretin and the secretory activity of the cystic epithelium. Cyst aspiration and sclerosis with alcohol or minocycline can be used when one or few dominant or strategically located cysts cause the symptoms. Patients with massive, severely symptomatic PLD can usually be treated with combined hepatic resection and fenestration because part of the liver is often spared. The expertise of the surgeon and the extent of the hepatic resection and fenestration are important for the

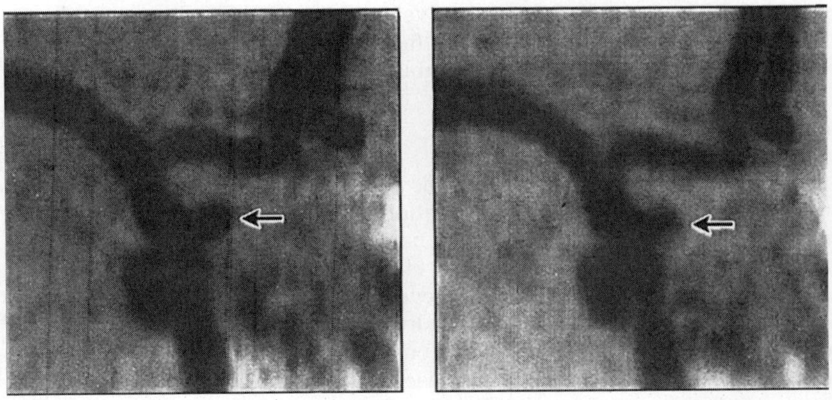

Figure 46.3. Three mm right periophthalmic aneurysm detected by MR angiography *(left panel)*. Note stability of the aneurysm on a follow-up study 2 years later *(right panel)*.

long-term outcome of this procedure. Rarely, liver transplantation may be required.

Intracranial Aneurysms

The frequency of intracranial aneurysms at autopsy and the incidence of aneurysmal subarachnoid hemorrhage are five to 10 times higher in ADPKD than in the general population. These risks may be higher in certain ADPKD families. Magnetic resonance angiography and spiral CT are sensitive, noninvasive techniques to screen for intracranial aneurysms. Asymptomatic intracranial aneurysms can be detected by magnetice resonance angiography in 22% of patients with ADPKD who have a family history of intracranial aneurysm or subarachnoid hemorrhage, but only on 5% of those without such a history. They are usually small, measuring less than 6 mm wide (Fig. 46.3). The value of detecting asymptomatic aneurysms depends on the risk of rupture, morbidity and mortality from rupture, surgical risk, and rate of formation of *de novo* aneurysms. The risk of rupture of asymptomatic aneurysms depends on their size. Rupture rates range from less than 0.5% to 4% per year. Severe morbidity and mortality from aneurysmal rupture ranges from 30% to 50% with a trend toward lower mortality in recent years. The risk of severe of morbidity and mortality from surgery depends on the number, size, and location of the aneurysms and on the presence of comorbid factors and ranges from less than 1% to 30%. Finally, the rate of development of *de novo* aneurysms is approximately 2% per year. Because most incidental, asymptomatic, intracranial aneurysms detected in patients with ADPKD are small and probably have a low risk of rupture, most investigators have concluded that generalized screening of patients with ADPKD is not cost effective or justifiable. It seems reasonable to restrict screening to patients with good life expectancy and a family history of intracranial aneurysms or subarachnoid hemorrhage and to those with a previous episode of aneurysmal rupture. Other possible indications include preparation for major elective surgery with anticipated hemodynamic instability, indeterminate symptoms that might suggest the presence of an intracranial aneurysm, high risk occupations, and patients who have been adequately informed and still want the reassurance that the screening can provide. If an aneurysm is found on presymptomatic screening, surgery is clearly indicated if the size is 10 mm or greater in diameter. Reassurance and observation are indicated for asymptomatic aneurysms measuring 5mm or less in diameter. The treatment of asymptomatic aneurysms measuring 6 to 9 mm in diameter remains controversial. Intravascular occlusion of intracranial aneurysms with detachable platinum coils may be preferable to surgery when the surgical risk is high because of the location or size of the aneurysm or because of the condition of the patient.

Presymptomatic Diagnosis and Genetic Counseling

Presymptomatic screening of patients at risk for ADPKD can be undertaken using ultrasound, genetic linkage analysis, and, when the responsible mutation has been identified in a family, direct mutation analysis. Diagnostic ultrasonographic criteria have been established to assist in the diagnosis of individuals known to be at 50% risk by positive family history (Table 46.1). Presymptomatic screening by ultrasound before age 20 may not be conclusive and is not generally recommended. Diagnosis by linkage analysis requires participation of other family members with and without the disease. It allows for prenatal diagnosis and is important in the evaluation of young, living, related kidney donors with indeterminate diagnosis by imaging studies. Prenatal diagnosis of ADPKD by chorionic sampling or amniocentesis has been performed very rarely because only a small minority of these patients would alter the course of the pregnancy if the fetus were shown to be affected. Technologic advances have also made *in vitro* fertilization with preimplantation diagnosis potentially possible, but the technical, financial, and ethical issues related to the application of this technology to ADPKD have not been adequately addressed. Direct mutation analysis is possible in most PKD2 families, but only in a few PKD1 families because of the large size of the gene and its duplication. Only individuals who have been properly informed on the advances and disadvantages of screening should be offered presymptomatic screening for ADPKD. If ADPKD is diagnosed, appropriate counseling on family planning and risk factors, such as hypertension, should be provided. If ADPKD is absent, the patient can be reassured. The disadvantages to presymptomatic screening relate to insurability and employability. As more effective therapies for ADPKD become available, these recommendations will change.

AUTOSOMAL-RECESSIVE POLYCYSTIC KIDNEY DISEASE

Definition, Genetics, and Pathology

Autosomal-recessive polycystic kidney disease (ARPKD) is characterized by various combinations of bilateral renal cystic disease and congenital hepatic fibrosis. It has a prevalence at birth of 1:10,000. The gene has been mapped to chromosome 6p21. The renal cysts result from the fusiform dilation of the collecting tubules. Congenital hepatic fibrosis, or biliary dysgenesis, a developmental abnormality that leads to portal hypertension, is characterized by enlarged and fibrotic portal areas with apparent proliferation of bile ducts, absence of central bile ducts, hypoplasia of the portal vein branches, and sometimes prominent fibrosis around the central veins. Congenital hepatic fibrosis can also occur as an isolated finding or in association with renal dysplasia and hereditary tubulointerstitial nephritis.

Clinical Manifestations

ARPKD exhibits significant phenotypic variability even within the same family. The clinical presentation of ARPKD is dominated by the manifestations of the renal disease in newborns and infants and by the manifestations of portal hypertension in older children and adolescents. However, there are cases with early childhood onset in which severe liver involvement is predominant and other cases with adult onset of ARPKD without evidence of portal hypertension. The neonatal presentation may be dominated by respiratory difficulties due to pulmonary hypoplasia (Potter's sequence) or restrictive disease caused by massive kidney enlargement. Severe hypertension is the most significant cause of morbidity and mortality among neonatal survivors and those who present in infancy. Inability to concentrate and dilute urine can cause major electrolyte abnormalities. The consequences of chronic renal insufficiency, growth failure, anemia, and osteodystrophy become a problem during childhood. Although the appearance of the kidneys on ultrasonography and other imaging studies may suggest a diagnosis of ARPKD, a definite diagnosis based on renal imaging alone is not possible. This is true particularly *in utero* and in the neonate when the appearance of the kidney may be indistinguishable from ADPKD and glomerulocystic kidney disease. The family history, the ultrasonographic or histologic evaluation of the liver, and the absence of the extrarenal malformations associated with multiple malformation syndromes and with renal dysplasia help in the diagnosis.

Prognosis and Treatment

Certain studies suggest that the prognosis of ARPKD for children who survive the first month of life is far less bleak than initially thought. Severely affected neonates may require unilateral or bilateral nephrectomy because of respiratory and nutritional compromise. Enlarged kidneys may decrease in relative size in patients who survive the neonatal phase of the disease and the renal function may remain stable for many years or slowly progress to renal failure. An aggressive nutritional program and correction of acidosis and other electrolyte disorders are required to optimize linear growth. For infants with end-stage renal failure, peritoneal dialysis is preferable, whereas either peritoneal dialysis or hemodialysis are options for children with renal failure. Renal transplantation is the treatment of choice. Pretransplant splenectomy may be indicated if there is marked leukopenia or thrombocytopenia due to hypersplenism. Surviving patients and those who present during adolescence are likely to require a portosystemic shunting procedure to prevent life-threatening hemorrhages from esophageal varices. The renal disease may progress to renal failure years after successful shunting. Patients with associated nonobstructive intrahepatic biliary dilation (Caroli's disease) may have recurrent episodes of cholangitis and may require antibiotic therapy or segmental hepatic resection.

Selected Readings

Calvet JP. Abnormal epithelial cell proliferation in renal cyst formation and growth: the maturation arrest hypothesis. *Kidney Int* 1995;47:715–716.
Review of evidence supporting the hypothesis that the tubular epithelial cells in polycystic kidney disease are trapped in a state of intermediate differentiation and share many of the phenotypic characteristics of tubular epithelial cells during development.

Germino GG. Autosomal-dominant polycystic kidney disease: a two-hit model. *Hosp Pract Off Ed* 1997;32:81–82, 85–88, 91–92.
Excellent review of recent developments in the genetics of autosomal polycystic kidney disease and underlying molecular mechanisms.

Grantham JJ. The etiology, pathogenesis, and treatment of autosomal-dominant polycystic kidney disease: recent advances. *Am J Kidney Dis* 1996;28:788–803.
Comprehensive review of recent advances in the understanding of the pathogenesis of autosomal-dominant polycystic kidney disease, including abnormal cell proliferation and apoptosis, fluid secretion, complex changes in the extracellular matrix, and renal interstitial inflammation.

Hayashi T, Mochizuki T, Reynolds DM, et al. Characterization of the exon structure of the polycystic kidney disease 2 gene (PKD2). *Genomics* 1997;44:131–136.
This study presents a description of the exon-intron structure of the PKD2 gene and of intronic oligonucleotide primers suited to amplify the entire coding sequence from genomic DNA in segments adequate for mutation analysis.

Johnson AM, Gabow PA. Identification of patients with autosomal-dominant polycystic kidney disease at highest risk for end-stage renal disease. *J Am Soc Nephrol* 1997;8:1560–1567.
PKD genotype, gender, and age of diagnosis, development of hypertension, and first episode of gross hematuria identify a subset of patients with higher risk of progression to end-stage renal failure.

Peral B, Gamble V, Strong C, et al. Identification of mutations in the duplicated region of the polycystic kidney disease 1 gene (PKD1) by a novel approach. *Am J Hum Genet* 1997;60:1399–1410.
This study presents the novel and reverse transcription-PCR approach to amplify the duplicated region of PKD1, employing one primer situated within the single copy region and one within the duplicated area.

Qian F, Watnick TJ, Onuchic LF, et al. The molecular basis of focal cyst formation in human autosomal-dominant polycystic kidney disease type I. *Cell* 1996;87:979–987.
An assay based on X-chromosome inactivation shows that individual renal cysts in ADPKD are monoclonal. In addition, loss of heterozygosity was discovered within a subset of cysts.

Sampson JR, Maheshwar MM, Aspinwall R, et al. Renal cystic disease in tuberous sclerosis: role of the polycystic kidney disease 1 gene. *Am J Hum Genet* 1997;61:843–851.
Significant renal cysts disease in tuberous sclerosis usually reflect mutational involvement of the PKD1 gene, and mosaicism for large deletions of tuberous sclerosis complex 2 and PKD1 is a frequent phenomenon.

Torres VE. New insights into polycystic kidney disease and its treatment. *Curr Opin Nephrol Hypertens* 1998;7:159–169.
Review of recent advances in the understanding of the genetics and pathogenesis of polycystic kidney disease as clues to future therapies.

Watnick TJ, Piontek KB, Cordal TM, et al. An unusual pattern of mutation in the duplicated portion of PKD1 is revealed by use of a novel strategy for mutation detection. *Hum Mol Genet* 1997;6:1473–1481.
This study presents a novel strategy that depends on long-range PCR and a specific primer from the unique region of the gene to amplify a PKD1-specific template that expands exons 23-34.

Watson ML, Torres VE, eds. *Polycystic Kidney Disease.* London: Oxford University Press, 1996.
Exhaustive review of the renal cystic diseases, from experimental animals to human disease, covering basic and clinical aspects of the disease.

Zerres K, Rudnik Schoneborn S, Mucher G. Autosomal-recessive polycystic kidney disease; clinical features and genetics. *Adv Nephrol Necker Hosp* 1996;25:147–157.
Excellent review of autosomal-recessive polycystic kidney disease.

PART 2
Medullary Cystic and Medullary Sponge Kidneys

Franz T. Winklhofer and Jared J. Grantham

MEDULLARY CYSTIC DISEASE

Medullary cystic disease and nephronophthisis are inherited diseases characterized by the development of small cysts in the renal medulla. Medullary cystic disease describes the form of the disease that develops in adults, while nephronophthisis develops in childhood. Both diseases invariably progress to chronic renal failure.

Smith and Graham first described the disease in 1945. Fanconi later used the term *familial juvenile nephronophthisis* to describe cases of chronic renal failure with tubulointerstitial nephritis and medullary cysts in children.

Etiology and Prevalence

Familial juvenile nephronophthisis is an autosomal-recessive disease. The diagnosis is typically made in childhood, with the mean age of onset at approximately 10 years of age. The gene for the disorder has been mapped to chromosome 2q13 between D2548 and D2551. Approximately 70% of patients have been shown to have deletions in this region. A gene has been isolated from this region that codes for a protein thought to be involved in interactions between other proteins, although its exact role is not understood.

Some families with the disease do not have defects at the locus 2q13 but do appear to have an inherited pattern. This suggests that there may be at least one additional chromosome abnormality in this disorder. Familial juvenile nephronophthisis can also occur sporadically. Another form of the disease occurs with retinal abnormalities, termed renal-retinal dysplasia. This also seems to have an autosomal-recessive pattern of inheritance but does not involve chromosome 2q13.

The adult-onset form of medullary cystic disease is an autosomal-dominant disorder with end-stage disease occurring between the ages of 20 and 50 and a mean age of onset of 28 to 30. An abnormality mapped to chromosome 1q21 is present in some families. The disease can also occur sporadically in 15% to 20% of cases; the gene and its product have not been identified.

The overall prevalence of medullary cystic disease is not known but is thought to be less than 1 of 1,000, yet it accounts for up to 10% of children requiring dialysis in Europe. In the United States medullary cystic disease accounts for 1% to 3% of all patients, children or adult, on dialysis.

The cause of the medullary cysts is not understood. One theory is that there may be an abnormality in the tubular basement membrane similar to what is seen in the glomeruli in hereditary nephritis, which involves an abnormality in type IV collagen. Decreased binding of antibody to tubular basement membrane has been demonstrated, which suggests that there may be an abnormality of one of the tubular basement membrane proteins. Early in the disease, the membranes appear thin and weakened, and later in the course the tubular basement membranes may become thick and laminated, which may be a response to chronic injury. Another theory suggests that tubular diverticulae and hyperplasia of the distal tubule segments lead to changes of compliance in the tubular basement membrane, as well as interstitial fibrosis. This fibrosis leads to cystic distention in the tubule segments proximal to these abnormalities.

Pathology

The gross and microscopic findings are useful for establishing the diagnosis of medullary cystic disease, however the various subtypes cannot be distinguished. On gross examination both kidneys are small, usually weighing less than 50% the normal weight. The contour is smooth, and the capsule has an irregular, granular appearance. On cross section the cortex is thinned, and there is an indistinct corticomedullary junction. Seventy-five percent of patients have numerous, grossly visible cysts at the corticomedullary junction and deeper in the medulla. The cysts range from 1 mm to 1 cm in size but are not necessary to make the diagnosis because 25% of patients have no visible cysts.

Microscopic examination shows severe tubular damage. The tubules are atrophic and may have a surrounding inflammatory infiltrate with interstitial fibrosis. On microdissection the tubules have been shown to have small diverticulae. The cysts are limited to the distal convoluted tubule and the collecting duct and are lined with cuboidal or columnar epithelium. The cysts communicate freely with the proximal and distal tubule segments. The tubular basement membrane is thickened and multilayered. The glomeruli may appear normal, but in advanced cases they usually show secondary hypertrophy and hyperplasia. Some may be obsolescent, and there is usually periglomerular fibrosis.

Clinical Manifestations

The first signs associated with medullary cystic disease are due to the chronic tubular injury. Polyuria and polydipsia are present in 80% of patients due to defects in urinary concentration (Table 46.4). These changes occur before any decline in the glomerular filtration rate is evident. If sodium intake is compromised, patients may have severe salt wasting and may become dangerously hypovolemic, hyponatremic, and azotemic. Children may develop these symptoms between the ages of 4 and 10, also associated with growth retardation and weakness. In adults the symptoms may begin in early adulthood, though they may also be delayed until the sixth and seventh decade. As patients develop progressive renal insufficiency, the clinical effects of the concentrating defect may decrease, although it is uncommon for patients to develop hypertension.

Anemia may develop and had been thought to be out of proportion for the degree of renal insufficiency. A more recent study suggests the anemia is appropriate for the level of renal function. Renal tubular acidosis may occur and has been seen in conjunction with hypokalemia or hyperkalemia. Aldosterone resistance has also been described. Flank pain, hematuria, nephrolithiasis, and urinary tract infections are all uncommon. Tubular proteinuria is common with total protein excretion usually less than 1 g/day.

Renal insufficiency is common, and most patients progress to renal failure. Children usually develop renal failure by the age of 20 or earlier. In adults, it may be delayed to the sixth and seventh decade of life. Symptoms such as nausea and anorexia occur late in the course of the disease and are due to uremia. The average time from diagnosis until dialysis is 3 to 4 years, and the rate of progression is similar in the juvenile and adult forms of the disease.

Extrarenal involvement is rare in the adult form of medullary cystic disease; however, in children many associated anomalies have been described (Table 46.5). Of cases, 15% to 20% may have retinal abnormalities including tapetoretinal degeneration, optic nerve atrophy, and retinitis pigmentosa. Senior-Loken syndrome describes patients with nephronophthisis

TABLE 46.4. Clinical Manifestations of Medullary Cystic Disease

Polyuria
Polydipsia
Renal tubular acidosis
Azotemia
Anemia
Hypokalemia
Hyperkalemia (late)

TABLE 46.5. Disorders Associated with Nephronophthisis

Retinal dysplasia
Hepatic fibrosis
Cone-shaped epiphyses
Mental retardation

and tapetoretinal degeneration. The degree of retinal dysplasia may be severe, and patients may be blind from birth. Patients may also have nystagmus, myopia, strabismus, coloboma, or amblyopia. The genetic abnormality in patients with renal-retinal involvement is distinct from the autosomal-recessive defect on chromosome 2.

Patients have also been described with hepatic fibrosis. One patient was reported with renal-retinal involvement and hepatic fibrosis. Patients may have cerebral involvement such as mental retardation, usually in conjunction with retinal degeneration. Bone abnormalities, namely cone-shaped epiphyses, have been described, almost always in association with other anomalies.

Diagnosis

Because the presentation of medullary cystic disease can be somewhat nonspecific, the diagnosis must be considered in patients with symptoms of tubulointerstitial disease and a family history of renal cysts. The urine sediment is usually bland. Urine protein excretion is usually less than 1 g/day.

Renal ultrasound usually shows normal to small-sized kidneys with increased echogenicity. The renal outline is usually smooth without localized cortical scarring. The collecting system is not dilated, but patients with polyuria may have an enlarged bladder. The cysts may be visible on sonogram although computed tomographic (CT) scanning is more sensitive. A thin section CT scan may demonstrate cysts as small as 0.5 cm. The cysts may be visualized more clearly after contrast enhancement of the CT scan. In patients without demonstrable cysts, renal biopsy may be the only reliable way to make the diagnosis. Genetic linkage analysis may allow the diagnosis to be made in approximately 70% of patients with the autosomal-recessive form of the disease.

Treatment

There is no therapy to decrease the development of cysts, interstitial fibrosis, and progression to renal failure. In the early stages of the disease, the maintenance of adequate salt and water intake is crucial. Patients who become ill and are unable to tolerate oral intake may require intravenous fluid replacement in order to prevent severe dehydration, acute renal failure, and shock.

As renal function deteriorates, patients may require treatment to manage the symptoms of chronic renal failure, including dietary alterations (including sodium restriction if salt retention develops as ongoing nephron loss occurs), antihypertensive agents, and erythropoietin to treat anemia. Acidosis and hyperkalemia may be seen later in the course of the disease and may require the use of oral alkali replacement and diuretics.

At end stage, patients may be managed by dialysis or renal transplantation. The disease does not recur in the transplanted organ. The issue of living related donors must be handled carefully. Unless the mode of inheritance can be clearly determined, it may be prudent to assume that the disease is transmitted in an autosomal-dominant manner when counseling family members. Especially with children, it is important that the family is counseled about the possibility that siblings also have the disease.

MEDULLARY SPONGE KIDNEY

Medullary sponge kidney is a disorder in which numerous small cysts develop in the terminal collecting ducts in the renal pyramids. The course of the disease is relatively benign in that patients seldom develop progressive renal failure. The renal involvement is typically diffuse and bilateral. The term *medullary sponge* was first applied in 1948 but is not a particularly accurate description of the gross appearance of the kidneys. Other terms to better describe the disorder such as *precalyceal canalicular ectasia* have not found favor.

Etiology and Prevalence

The cause of medullary sponge kidney is not known. It is believed to be a developmental abnormality. Although relatives of patients with the disorder seem to have an increased incidence of the disease, no genetic pattern has been identified. The disease has occurred in successive generations; however, only a small fraction of affected patients seem to have an autosomal-dominant pattern of inheritance. The incidence in the general population is 1 of 5,000, and the incidence is 1 of 1,000 patients studied in urology clinics. Up to 20% of women and 10% of men studied with calcium nephrolithiasis may have some degree of medullary sponge kidney. Children are rarely diagnosed, and the disorder is typically identified in the fourth or fifth decade.

There has been debate that medullary sponge kidney may be an acquired abnormality rather than a developmental one. Many of the tubules contain concretions containing calcium, and it has been suggested that the dilations form in response to hypercalcuria and deposition of intraluminal calcium with obstruction. However, hypercalcuria is frequently but not always seen with medullary sponge kidney, which weakens this explanation. Others propose that the tubular ectasia and cysts form during embryonic development perhaps from dilations in first-generation mesonephric arborizations. The frequency of concurrent developmental anomalies also supports this position.

Pathology

On gross examination, the kidneys are of normal size and appearance. When bisected there may be numerous, diffuse medullary cysts ranging in size usually from 1 to 3 mm wide. The cysts may be larger, rarely as large as 7.5 mm in diameter. The cysts are bilateral in at least 70% of cases, and involvement of a single pyramid is uncommon.

On microscopic examination the cysts are spherical or oval and involve the papillary collecting ducts. The cysts communicate proximally with the collecting duct and distally with the papillary duct or calyx. They often contain concretions of calcium oxalate or phosphate. When the cystic changes are severe, there is often surrounding interstitial fibrosis.

In addition to the small intraluminal calcifications, many patients have free renal calculi. Patients may also develop secondary obstruction and infection with subsequent pathologic changes. The kidneys are otherwise normal.

Clinical Manifestations

Most patients with medullary sponge kidney probably remain undiagnosed. The diagnosis is usually made in patients under

TABLE 46.6. Clinical Manifestations of Medullary Sponge Kidney

Nephrolithiasis
Flank pain
Hematuria
Urinary tract infection
Renal tubular acidosis

evaluation for nephrolithiasis, hematuria, or urinary tract infection (Table 46.6). Medullary sponge kidney rarely progresses to renal failure. If it does, it is typically due to complications from renal stones or infections. Most patients with medullary sponge present with nephrolithiasis. Approximately 25% of patients first present with hematuria, and 25% present with urinary tract infections.

The incidence of stones in patients with medullary sponge kidney is difficult to determine because so many patients remain undiagnosed. However, in patients with calcium nephrolithiasis, 10% to 20% may be affected. Patients most commonly have calcium stones, either calcium oxalate or calcium phosphate. Hypercalciuria occurs in up to 50% of patients, and other metabolic abnormalities such as hyperuricosuria may also be present. The hypercalciuria may be renal or absorptive in etiology, whereas other patients may have nephrolithiasis without elevated calcium excretion. Because of the variety of risk factors for stone formation, patients with medullary sponge and nephrolithiasis should undergo a formal stone evaluation.

Many patients have a partial defect in urine acidification with an inability to lower the pH to 5.5. A minority may have a frank distal tubular acidosis with hypokalemia and systemic acidosis. The combination of elevated urine pH and urinary stasis due to the cysts and tubular dilation may also predispose to stone formation.

Hematuria may be microscopic or macroscopic and may occur in the absence of nephrolithiasis. Isolated hematuria is usually painless. Urinary tract infections occur with increased frequency in medullary sponge kidney, especially women. They are often recurrent and stone formation may be a contributing factor. Females with recurrent urinary tract infections should be investigated for the possibility of medullary sponge kidney.

Many congenital diseases and disorders have been associated with medullary sponge kidney (Table 46.7). Hyperparathyroidism has been frequently described and should be tested for in patients with hypercalcemia and/or hypercalciuria. It has been suggested that the renal calcium loss may predispose patients to ionized hypocalcemia and thereby stimulate the parathyroid gland. Such chronic stimulation may lead to the development of parathyroid adenomas. Numerous cases of hemihypertrophy, Caroli syndrome, and hepatic fibrosis have been described in patients with medullary sponge kidney.

TABLE 46.7. Disorders Associated with Medullary Sponge Kidney

Beckwith-Wiedemann syndrome
Caroli syndrome
Congenital anodontia
Congenital hemihypertrophy
Congenital hepatic fibrosis
Hyperaldosteronism
Hyperparathyroidism
Renal tubular acidosis
Young's syndrome

Diagnosis

The diagnosis of medullary sponge kidney is made using intravenous urography with abdominal pressure. Contrast material fills the dilated collecting tubules causing linear streaking that gives a brushlike appearance to the renal papillae. The diagnosis can be difficult to make and may be missed if the urogram is suboptimal. Sometimes only a papillary blush may be present and in general is insufficient for the diagnosis. If the blush is reproducible, is seen before calyceal opacification, or is associated with medullary calcifications, it may be sufficient to confirm the diagnosis. Nephrocalcinosis may be present in medullary sponge kidney, especially in the presence of renal tubular acidosis or hyperparathyroidism.

CT scans and ultrasound are usually insufficient to make the diagnosis. Neither is sensitive enough to show cystic changes, although both, thin-section CT scans in particular, are capable of demonstrating medullary calcification.

Treatment

There is no particular therapy that is helpful for medullary sponge kidney because the course is generally benign in the absence of comorbid conditions. Therapy should be directed as necessary to control complications such as stone formation and urinary infection. The treatment of these disorders is no different from patients without medullary sponge kidney.

Patients with nephrolithiasis should be instructed to maintain high urine volume. Therapy to control hypercalcuria, including restriction of dietary sodium, may be helpful. Thiazide diuretics have been shown to be helpful; however, care must be taken in patients with concurrent hyperparathyroidism because hypercalcemia may develop with thiazide therapy. Additional metabolic abnormalities such as hyperuricosuria should also be treated. Renal tubular acidosis may be managed with the use of oral alkali replacement such as citrate.

Renal stones can also be managed as with other patients, including the use of extracorporeal shock wave lithotripsy. Urinary tract infections may be severe, especially when complicated by stones and obstruction. Nephrectomy may be required, especially if abscesses develop.

Selected Readings

Christodoulou K, Tsingis M, Stavrou C, et al. Chromosome 1 localization of a gene for autosomal-dominant medullary cystic kidney disease (ADMCKD). *Hum Mol Genet* 1998;7:905.

Discovery of a genetic abnormality for adult medullary cystic disease with autosomal-dominant transmission.

Cohen AH, Hoyer JR. Nephronophthisis: a primary tubular basement membrane defect. *Lab Invest* 1986;55:564.

Describes the tubular basement membrane abnormalities seen in both the juvenile and adult forms of the disease.

Elzouki AY, Al-Suhaibani H, Mirza K, et al. Thin-section computed tomography scans detect medullary cysts in patients believed to have juvenile nephronophthisis. *Am J Kidney Dis* 1996;27:216.

Report of the utility of thin section CT scanning to detect cysts in medullary cystic disease.

Holmes SA, Eardley I, Corry DA, et al. The use of extracorporeal shock wave lithotripsy for medullary sponge kidneys. *Br J Urol* 1992;70:352.

Describes the utility of extracorporeal shock wave lithotripsy in the treatment of medullary sponge kidney.

Indridason OS, Thomas L, Berkoben M. Medullary sponge kidney associated with congenital hemihypertrophy. *J Am Soc Nephrol* 1996;7:1123–1130.

A description of a patient with medullary sponge and hemihypertrophy.

Konrad M, Saunier S, Heidet L, et al. Large homozygous deletions of the 2q13 region are a major cause of juvenile nephronophthisis. *Hum Mol Genet* 1996;5:367.

A description of a 250 kb deletion seen in 70%t of patients with juvenile nephronophthisis.

O'Neill M, Breslau NA, Pak CY. Metabolic evaluation of nephrolithiasis in patients with medullary sponge kidney. *JAMA* 1981;245:1223.
Describes metabolic abnormalities in patients with medullary sponge kidney.
Parks JH, Coe FL, Strauss AL. Calcium nephrolithiasis and medullary sponge kidney in women. *N Engl J Med* 1982;306:1088.
Characterizes metabolic abnormalities in medullary sponge in women.
Senior B, Friedman AI, Braudo JL. Juvenile familial nephropathy with tapetoretinal degeneration: a new oculo-renal dystrophy. *Am J Ophthalmol* 1961;52:625.
Early report of renal-retinal dysplasia (Senior-Loken syndrome).

PART 3
Acquired Renal Cysts

Michael Schoemig, Eberhard Ritz, Irene Noronha, and Shaul G. Massry

Following the first report by Durnnill, Millard, and Oliver in 1977, acquired multicystic transformation has been widely recognized in the kidneys of dialysis patients suffering from various underlying renal diseases. Although acquired renal cysts have been considered a specific consequence of hemodialysis therapy, several lines of evidence argue against this possibility.

In 1847, the concept of renal parenchymal loss, proposed by Richard Bright to explain formation of small contracted kidneys, was challenged by Simon who claimed that in contracted kidneys "vesicles are substituted for the normal tubularity of the gland." In retrospect the vesicles described by Simon almost certainly represented dilated residual nephrons undergoing compensatory hypertrophy. However, this report prompted a careful study by Frerichs who in 1851 noted:

> In the cortex of the diseased kidneys one often finds cysts . . . their size varies from that of a millet seed to that of a hazelnut. Their content is usually watery fluid with a small amount of protein. The wall of the cyst is either denudated or covered by flat nucleated epithelia. Larger cysts have quite frequently prominent protrusions of their walls and remnants of walls separating confluent cysts. Occasionally, the content is viscous fluid of yellow, brown or black colour.

In the nineteenth century, the occurrence of cysts in contracted kidneys with Bright's disease was well known, and several authors clearly distinguished between cyst formation in "cirrhotic" kidneys and that in polycystic kidney disease. Such historical observations, which had been forgotten, are of interest because they reflect the natural evolution of cyst formation in renal failure without any therapeutic intervention.

A specific association of acquired renal cysts with hemodialysis treatment is further rendered unlikely by the observation of cyst formation in patients with early stages of renal insufficiency and in patients receiving chronic peritoneal dialysis treatment. Patients with advanced renal failure or those treated with dialysis therapy who have multiple bilateral small cysts (more than three cysts) are considered to have acquired cystic kidney disease.

PREVALENCE

The reported incidence of acquired renal cysts ranges between 10% and 95%. In a series studied in Germany (Fig. 46.4), multicystic transformation of the kidneys was found in 19% of patients with renal disease and serum creatinine of less than 2 mg/dl. The incidence rose to 28% at serum creatinine levels of less than 5 mg/dl. In parallel, the median number (but not the size) of the cysts increased with deteriorating renal function. In patients on maintenance hemodialysis therapy, the proportion with cysts increased from 35% in those treated for less than 2 years to 92% in those treated for over 8 years (Fig. 46.5). Similar observations were found in 80 dialysis patients studied in Los Angeles. Cysts occurred in 10% of those treated for less than 3 years and in 92% of those receiving hemodialysis therapy for more than 3 years. The overall incidence of renal cysts in dialysis patients is close to 45%. In men and less so in women, kidney volume increases progressively with time on hemodialysis, reaching 2.7 times the original volume over a 10-year follow-up. Cysts were also demonstrable in patients managed with chronic peritoneal dialysis treatment and persisted after transplantation. Shrinkage of the recipient's cyst-bearing kidneys occurred after transplantation, possibly because of diminished glomerular filtration and transepithelial solute movement. Despite shrinkage of the kidneys, the recipient's own kidneys with acquired cysts may be the site of renal cell carcinoma formation, as shown in Fig. 46.6. In one study renal cell carcinoma was

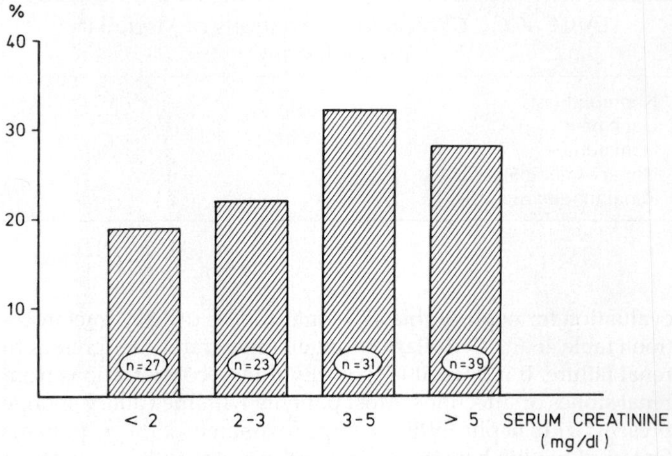

Figure 46.4. Incidence of acquired renal cysts as a function of serum creatinine in patients with renal insufficiency.

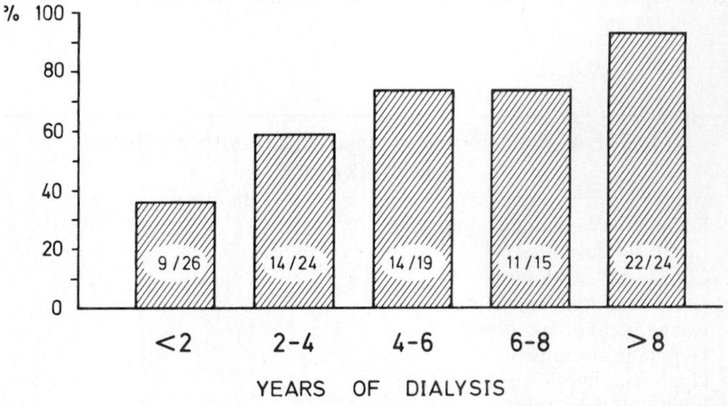

Figure 46.5. Incidence of acquired renal cysts as a function of duration of dialysis therapy.

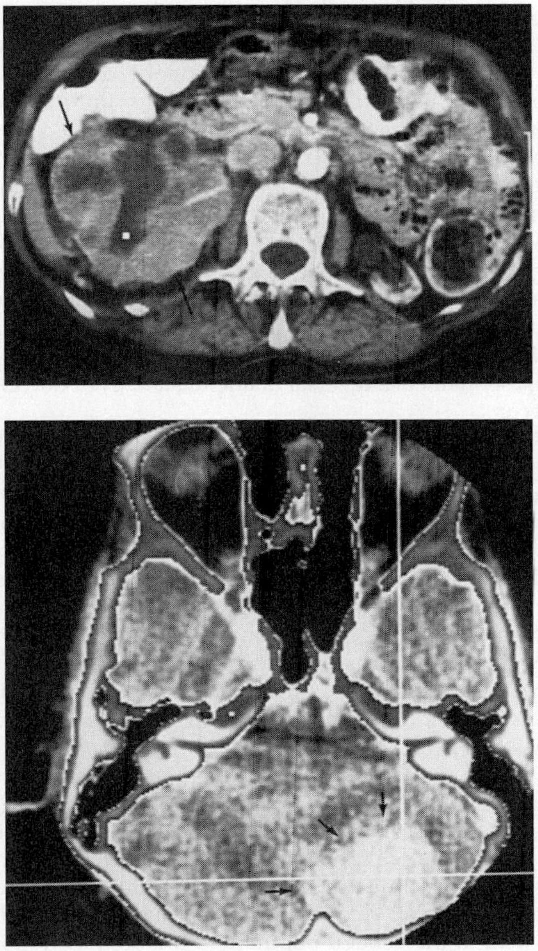

Figure 46.6. Computed tomography scans showing a right renal tumor *(top)* and cerebral metastasis in the posterior fossa *(bottom)* in a 70-year-old patient. She received a kidney graft from a homozygous twin 12 years earlier.

found in the native kidneys of 0.5% of the total transplant patient population.

Although some authors have failed to note a relation between underlying renal disease and acquired renal cyst formation, we have noted a higher prevalence in patients with analgesic nephropathy and nephrolithiasis, possibly pointing to disruption of medullary structures and tubular obstruction as one pathogenic mechanism. Furthermore, cysts were more frequent in patients with heavy proteinuria, which is reminiscent of cyst formation in partially nephrectomized proteinuric rats on high protein intake.

PATHOLOGY

Acquired cysts are present in both the cortex and the medulla and not predominantly in the outer cortex (Fig. 46.7). Occasionally, they protrude over the outer renal surface. Cyst diameters range from a few millimeters to several centimeters. Cysts are filled with clear fluid or occasionally laminated proteinaceous material with or without birefringent oxalate crystals (Fig. 46.8). Continuity between cysts and tubules has been demonstrated by microdissection analysis, suggesting that cysts begin either as fusiform tubular dilations or as saccular outpouchings, possibly arising as diverticula. Cyst fluid was shown to correspond

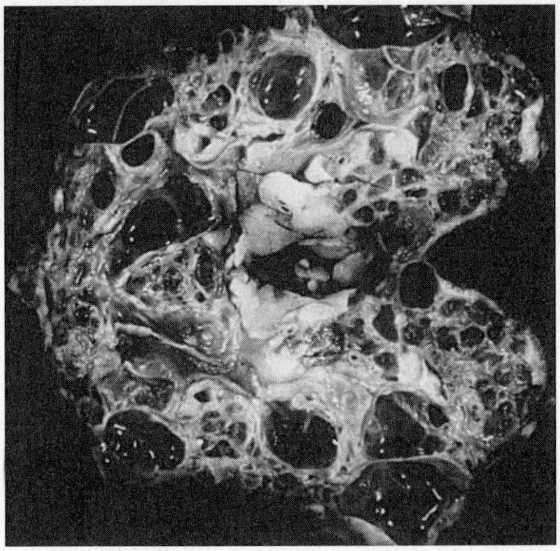

Figure 46.7. Acquired renal cysts in a 42-year-old dialysis patient as seen at autopsy. The patient had a biopsy-confirmed glomerulonephritis before beginning hemodialysis therapy.

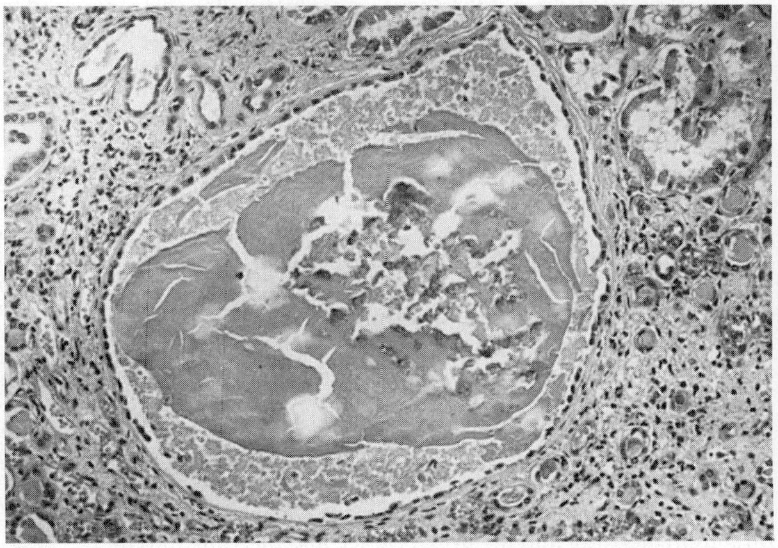

Figure 46.8. Kidney of a 55-year-old dialysis patient with glomerulonephritis who had received dialysis therapy for 7 years. Note the renal cyst lined by a single layer of epithelial cells and filled with proteinaceous material.

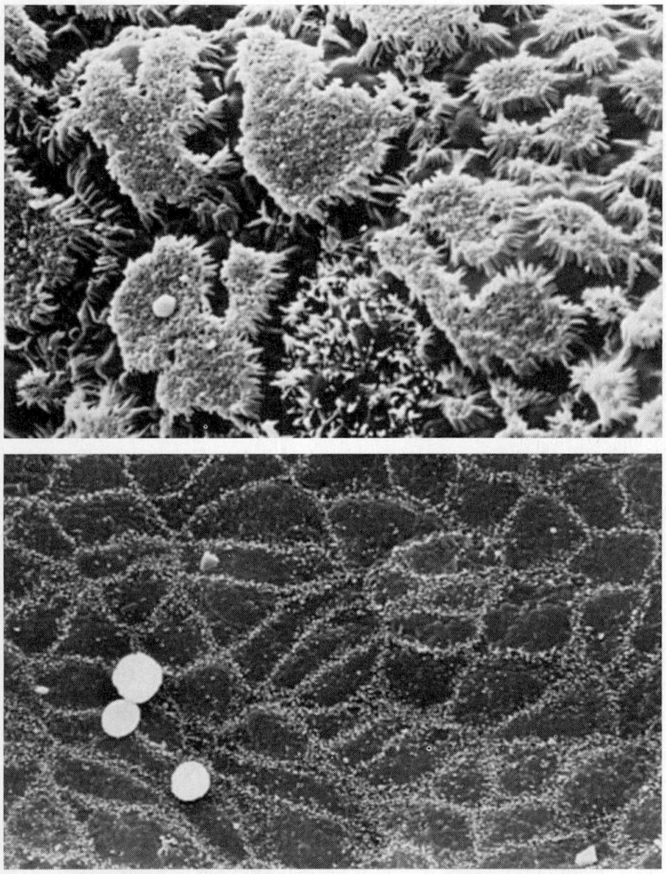

Figure 46.9. Scanning electron microscopy of a proximal tubule cyst *(top)* and a distal tubule cyst *(bottom)*. The surface of the proximal tubule cyst is studded with tightly packed microvilli. In the distal tubule cyst the microvilli delineate the luminal cell border. *Top,* × 4,750; *bottom,* × 2,500.

in composition mostly to proximal tubular equilibrium fluid. Histologically, most cysts are lined with cuboidal or columnar epithelial cells. Focal papillary hyperplasia of these lining cells frequently occurs. Severe papillary epithelial proliferations may project into the lumen of a microcyst. Such proliferations commonly bear multilayered epithelial cells with enlarged nuclei, prominent nucleoli, and frequent mitoses. We have not found that these proliferations obstruct the aboral end of the cysts, and therefore it is unlikely that they cause cysts by tubular obstruction. However, this does not exclude the possibility that tubular obstruction by proteinaceous concretions (Fig. 46.9) may contribute to cyst formation. We were able to demonstrate β_2-microglobulin–derived immunoreactivity and microfibrils in such tubular casts. An alternative or complementary mechanism of cyst formation is the progressive enlargement of preexisting diverticula, possibly favored by traction from interstitial fibrosis.

In ultrastructural studies the epithelial cells covering the walls of the cysts exhibited structural equivalents of active transepithelial transport. Cyst walls may display the characteristics of proximal or distal tubular epithelium (Fig. 46.9).

CLINICAL CONSEQUENCES

Various clinical consequences result from acquired cysts (Table 46.8). Bleeding into the cysts with flank pain, macrohematuria from bleeding into the urinary tract, and bleeding into the retroperitoneal space with exsanguination and shock have been noted. Factors contributing to the bleeding may include hemorrhagic diathesis of uremia, intermittent administration of heparin during hemodialysis treatment, and rupture of vessels that project into cysts and thus are unsupported by solid parenchyma. Nephrectomy may be required for life-threatening bleeding or uncontrollable hypertension resulting from perirenal hematoma. Suppuration of cysts with abscess formation may also occur.

In general, no relationship is found between the presence of cysts and erythropoietin levels or hematocrit in dialysis patients. However, in some patients with advanced cystic transformation of the kidneys, particularly in patients with markedly enlarged kidneys, spontaneous reversal of anemia and even polyglobulia may occur.

Potentially the most serious complication of acquired renal cysts is renal adenocarcinoma formation. Several authors have assumed that acquired renal cysts are a premalignant condition. However, most of these tumors are small (less than 3 cm in diameter) and are considered adenomas. In the first report of Dunnill, Millard, and Oliver on 14 patients with renal cysts, renal tumors were found in six, and one of these was renal cell carcinoma. Renal cell carcinoma, originating from shrunken multicystic kidneys, was described both in patients maintained with dialysis therapy and in the patient's own kidneys after renal transplantation. Bilateral renal cell carcinoma in acquired cysts has also been reported.

In patients on renal replacement therapy, the risk of renal cell carcinoma is increased 30- to 50-fold compared with the general population. In a recent series of 1,603 hemodialysis patients, the frequency of renal cell carcinoma was 2.6%. Acquired cystic kidney disease is a definite precancerous condition. Renal cell carcinoma occurs more frequently in men and is found 20 years earlier than in the general population. It is frequently bilateral (9%) and multicentric (50%).

The clinical presentation of renal cell carcinoma in dialysed patients may be bleeding, changes in hematocrit, fever, flank pain, hypoglycemia, hypercalcemia, or metastases, mostly in the lung or brain.

Based on existing data, it is difficult to give a reasonable estimate of the prevalence of renal cell carcinoma in dialysis patients and its potential association with renal cystic formation. Most authors reported that clinical evidence of renal cell carcinoma is found in approximately 1% to 2% of the dialysis population. The distinction between adenoma and carcinoma is usually based on size. Tumors less than 3 cm wide are classified as adenoma, but this distinction is arbitrary as even tumors of less than 2 cm may metastasize. We found tumors exceeding 3 cm in 3% of dialysis patients. It is also of note that incidental renal car-

TABLE 46.8. Clinical Manifestations and Complications of Acquired Renal Cysts

Asymptomatic
Palpable abdominal mass
Flank or abdominal pain
Renal colic
Macrohematuria
Retroperitoneal hemorrhage
Hypotension and shock
Acute fall in hematocrit
Infection and abscess formation in cysts
Nephrolithiasis
Polyglobulia (polycythemia)
Renal cell carcinoma with and without metastasis

cinoma is not uncommon in patients subjected to pretransplant nephrectomy. The remarkably low risk of late local recurrence or metastasis in these patients is well known. The whole spectrum of renal tumors from renal adenoma to invasive renal carcinoma is found in dialysis patients, the two often coexisting in the same patient. Upon morphologic examination, circumscribed renal tumors are found in a high proportion of contracted cyst-bearing kidneys of patients with end-stage renal failure on maintenance hemodialysis treatment (and even after successful renal transplantation). Small tumors, which are usually diagnosed as adenoma, were found in approximately 80% of our dialysed population. The point of origin of invasive carcinoma may be the noncystic portion of the kidney. This is interesting because cytologic abnormalities, proliferative lesions, and solid microadenoma are commonly noted even in noncystic tubular segments of end-stage kidneys.

In the general population, papillary renal cell carcinoma accounts for only 10% of renal cell carcinoma in contrast to uremic patients where a papillary or tubulopapillary growth pattern is noted in 50%. Deletions in the chromosome 3p region, the locus of the von Hippel Lindau gene, are common in renal cell carcinoma among nonuremic patients but infrequent among uremic patients. Based on these and other findings, it has been suggested that genetics and morphology of renal cell carcinoma in patients with end-stage renal failure differ from what is seen in renal cell carcinoma of nonuremic patients.

It has long been recommended that patients with end-stage renal disease should be subjected to renal imaging procedures at regular intervals. A decision analysis came to the conclusion that the benefit from screening is not large enough to justify this approach for all patients. Instead, it should be restricted to younger patients with low comorbidity and substantial life expectancy. However, there is no doubt that renal imaging is obligatory in the patient who has gross hematuria or *de novo* microhematuria. Ultrasonography is usually used in these cases. Computed tomography (CT) and magnetic resonance tomography are complementary procedures with higher sensitivity. In a study carried out in Los Angeles of 62 patients using both ultrasonography and CT scanning, renal cysts were detected in 19% by the former technique and in 34% by the latter. All patients who had positive findings with ultrasonography had positive CT scans. Thus CT scanning is evidently a better technique for the diagnosis of renal cysts in these patients. But the results of computed tomography and sonography do not closely correlate; therefore both procedures should be used in doubtful cases. CT scans detected enlargement of lymph nodes in several patients despite no identifiable renal tumor, presumably because the latter had escaped detection in the severely deformed kidneys. All complex cysts or solid masses must be considered as renal tumors unless proven otherwise.

Tumor nephrectomy is a worthwhile proposition if a patient is found to have renal cell carcinoma. Our own experience has been encouraging: Several patients survived up to 7 years after nephrectomy, and one patient survived for several years after surgical resection of a solitary pulmonary metastasis.

The patient who is found to have incidental renal cell carcinoma on pretransplant nephrectomy should not be disqualified from transplantation. Incidental renal cell carcinoma on pretransplant nephrectomy is found in up to 5% of patients; the remarkably low rate of local recurrence or of distant metastasis is well known. However, one should wait 2 years before transplantation is performed because most metastases occur in the first 2 years after tumor nephrectomy.

Selected Readings

Bongu S, Faubert PF, Porush JG, et al. Uncontrolled hypertension and hyperreninemia after hemorrhage in a patient with end-stage renal disease and acquired renal cysts. *J Am Soc Nephrol* 1994;5:22–26.

Report on a patient with hypertension due to persistent hematuria.

Chudek J, Herbers J, Wilhelm M, et al. The genetics of renal tumors in end-stage renal failure differs from those occurring in the general population. *J Am Soc Nephrol* 1998;9:1045–1051.

Findings using microsatellite analysis documenting differences between renal cell cancer in uremic and nonuremic patients.

Dunnill MS, Millard PR, Oliver D. Acquired cystic disease of the kidneys; a hazard of long-term intermittent maintenance haemodialysis. *J Clin Pathol* 1977;30:686–877.

The initial report on acquired renal cysts in dialysis patients that includes a report of the development of renal tumors.

Frerichs FT. *Die Bright'sche Nierenkrankheit Vieweg.* Braunschweig, 1851, p 38.

Scholarly first description of acquired renal cysts in contracted kidneys of patients with Bright's disease.

Grantham JJ. Acquired cystic kidney disease [clinical conferences]. *Kidney Int* 1991;40:143–152.

A lucid review with an in-depth discussion of potential pathogenetic mechanisms.

Hughson MD, Schmidt L, Zbar B, et al. Renal cell carcinoma of end-stage renal disease: a histopathologic and molecular genetic study. *J Am Soc Nephrol* 1996;7:2461–2468.

A study investigating the frequency with which 3p genetic changes can be found in end-stage renal disease tumors.

Ishikawa I, Saito Y, Nakamura M, et al. Fifteen-year follow-up of acquired renal cystic disease – a gender difference. *Nephron* 1997;75:315–320.

Study documenting more aggressive cyst growth in males.

Ishikawa I, Saito Y, Shikura N, et al. Ten-year prospective study on the development of renal cell carcinoma in dialysis patients. *Am J Kidney Dis* 1990;16:452–458.

Longitudinal study providing information on the risk of renal cell carcinoma in dialysis patients.

Kliem V, Kolditz M, Behrend M, et al. Risk of renal cell carcinoma after kidney transplantation. *Clin Transplant* 1997;11:255–258.

Series of 154 patients who developed a malignant tumor after kidney transplantation. The most common malignancy was renal cell carcinoma in the native kidney.

Mickisch O, Bommer S, Waldherr R, et al. Multicystic transformation of kidneys in chronic renal failure. *Nephron* 1984;38:93–99.

Study of acquired renal cysts in patients with moderate renal failure. Renal cysts were demonstrated with ultrasonography even in patients with serum creatinine levels of less than 2 mg/dl.

Noronha IL, Ritz E, Waldherr R, et al. Renal cell carcinoma in dialysis patients with acquired cystic kidney disease. *Nephrol Dial Transplant* 1989;4:763–769.

An overview on renal cell carcinoma originating in contracted kidneys with acquired renal cysts.

Sarasin FP, Wong JB, Levey AS, et al. Screening for acquired cystic kidney disease: A decision analytic perspective. *Kidney Int* 1995;48:207–219.

A study giving criteria for renal imaging as a screening procedure in dialysed patients.

Taylor AJ, Cohen EP, Erickson SJ, et al. Renal imaging in long-term dialysis patients: a comparison of CT and sonography. *Am J Roentgenol* 1989;153:765–767.

A study illustrating CT to be a better imaging modality than sonography in dialysis patients.

Terasawa Y, Suzuki Y, Morita M, et al. Ultrasonic diagnosis of renal cell carcinoma in hemodialysis patients. *J Urol* 1994;152:846–851.

A lucid discussion in the relative merits of imaging procedures in the diagnosis of renal cell carcinoma.

Truong LK, Krishnan B, Cao JT, et al. Renal neoplasm in acquired cystic kidney disease. *Am J Kidney Dis* 1995;26:1–12.

Update information on renal cell carcinoma in uremic patients.

CHAPTER 47

Nephropathies Due to Drugs, Chemicals, or Physical Agents

PART 1
Antimicrobial Nephrotoxicity

Cathryn L. Shuler and William M. Bennett

Antimicrobial agents are the most common drugs associated with nephrotoxicity in the hospitalized patient. The exact incidence of nephrotoxicity for any given agent often is difficult to determine. Antibiotics often are prescribed for critically ill patients, so concomitant factors such as volume depletion, hemodynamic instability, sepsis, and nephrotoxic drugs often are present. For this reason, the cause of acute renal failure often is multifactorial and difficult to ascribe to a single agent.

Antimicrobial agents can cause nephrotoxicity through a variety of mechanisms including direct cellular injury, immunologic or hypersensitivity reactions, and intratubular obstruction caused by precipitation of the drug. Table 47.1 summarizes antimicrobial agents that cause nephrotoxicity according to the mechanism of nephrotoxic action. The most common clinical manifestation is nonoliguric acute renal failure. Spurious elevations of the serum creatinine may result from interference with creatinine secretion or interference with the assay for creatinine. Finally, a variety of electrolyte and acid–base disturbances have been described with the use of various antimicrobials. In this chapter, acute renal insufficiency caused by antimicrobial agents is the major focus. The specific agents chosen for discussion are those that are used in everyday clinical practice and associated with a significant risk of nephrotoxicity.

TABLE 47.1. Clinical Manifestations of Antimicrobial-Induced Nephrotoxicity

Nephrotoxic Action	Antimicrobial Agent
Renal vasoconstriction	Amphotericin B
Hypersensitivity glomerular damage	Penicillin Sulfonamides
Acute interstitial nephritis	Penicillin Methicillin Ampicillin Rifampin Sulfonamides
Acute tubular necrosis	Aminoglycosides Polymyxins Cephaloridine Imipenem
Tubular syndromes	Outdated tetracycline Amphotericin B Gentamicin Demethylchlortetracycline Sulfonamides Acyclovir
Electrolyte disturbances	Carbenicillin Ticarcillin Miconazole Isoniazid
Acid–base disturbances	Amphotericin B Penicillin Nalidixic acid

SPECIFIC ANTIMICROBIAL AGENTS

Aminoglycosides

Aminoglycoside antibiotics are widely prescribed in hospitalized patients because of their superior effectiveness in combating life-threatening gram-negative infections. Unfortunately, acute renal insufficiency develops in 10% to 15% of all therapy courses and significantly affects patient morbidity and mortality, length of hospital stay, and overall treatment cost. An understanding of the renal handling of aminoglycosides and the pathogenesis and risk factors for toxicity are critical in preventing or reducing this complication.

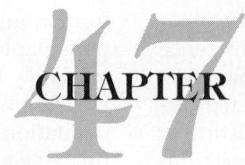

The aminoglycosides are polycations that are highly water soluble and minimally bound to plasma proteins. They are freely filtered and excreted unchanged by the kidney. A small but significant quantity of the filtered drug is reabsorbed by the proximal tubule. The aminoglycoside binds to the anionic phospholipids of the apical membrane and is taken up by pinocytosis and translocated into intracellular lysosomes. Transport into the cell also occurs at the basolateral membrane, but it appears that this is quantitatively less important. An important role of glycoprotein 330 (GP330, also known as the *Heyman nephritis*

autoantigen, or *megalin*) as a surface receptor for aminoglycosides has been identified. This anionic protein is expressed in the renal proximal tubules and the retinal and inner ear epithelium and has been shown *in vitro* to bind polybasic drugs such as the aminoglycosides.

The tissue half-life of aminoglycosides greatly exceeds the serum half-life, resulting in progressive accumulation of the drug in the renal cortex during the course of therapy. As a result, drug levels in the tissue may reach much higher concentrations than in the serum, and low-level urinary excretion may occur for weeks after a course of aminoglycoside therapy. As the aminoglycoside accumulates in the proximal renal tubular cells, alterations in membrane integrity and intracellular organelle function begin to occur. Binding to the phospholipid bilayer of the cellular membrane interferes with the signaling process associated with the phosphatidylinositol cascade. Various membrane-bound transporters such as the Na^+-Ca^{2+} exchanger (important for calcium efflux from the cell), the Na^+-K^+-ATPase, and the glucose transporter are adversely affected. Ultimately, this may lead to loss of cellular integrity, inability to repair damaged membranes, and cellular death.

Intracellular organelles also can be adversely affected by aminoglycosides. Gentamicin inhibition of endosomal fusion appears to be medicated through effects on the cytosolic tail of GP330. Lysosomal alterations in the proximal tubule cells occur early after exposure to the aminoglycoside and can affect membrane turnover and possibly result in release of damaging lysosomal contents into the cytoplasm. Divalent cations compete with aminoglycosides at transport sites in mitochondrial membranes, resulting in increased permeability. As a result, mitochondrial respiratory function is compromised, and reactive oxygen species may be generated. Finally, there is evidence that cell protein synthesis may be impaired as a very early manifestation of aminoglycoside toxicity.

There are varying degrees of toxicity, and it is probable that a subtle degree of aminoglycoside toxicity occurs in most patients exposed to the drug. However, acute renal insufficiency ultimately results in significant morbidity and mortality. Increased intratubular pressure caused by obstruction by necrotic tubular cells probably is the major mechanism through which a fall in the glomerular filtration rate (GFR) occurs. Other potential mechanisms include backleak of glomerular filtrate and enhanced tubuloglomerular feedback.

Clinically, aminoglycoside nephrotoxicity can have a variety of renal manifestations. Proximal tubular damage occurs early and initially causes an increase in the urinary excretion of brush border and lysosomal enzymes. In children, proximal tubular transport may be affected and result in glycosuria, aminoaciduria, and tubular proteinuria. Potassium and magnesium wasting sometimes occur through ill-defined effects on membrane transport or cellular permeability. A renal concentrating defect caused by interference with adenylate cyclase action on the collecting duct also is a common feature of aminoglycoside nephrotoxicity. Finally, renal dysfunction may develop, generally after 7 to 10 days of treatment.

Risk factors for aminoglycoside nephrotoxicity are summarized in Table 47.2. Higher dosages and prolonged or repeated courses of therapy result in greater accumulation of the aminoglycoside in the renal parenchyma and increase the risk of damage. Other risk factors include advanced age, preexisting renal insufficiency, hepatic failure, and volume depletion. Inaccurate renal function assessment and the use of inappropriately high aminoglycoside dosages may play a role in some cases. Decreased muscle mass in the older adult or malnourished patient with liver disease results in a lower serum creatinine for any given GFR. As a result, a "normal" serum creatinine may represent a substantial degree of renal insufficiency and thus lead to incorrect dosing if it is used as the sole parameter to assess renal function. Finally, concomitant nephrotoxin use or potassium or magnesium deficiency also increases the risk of nephrotoxicity.

Aminoglycoside nephrotoxicity usually is diagnosed clinically. As noted earlier, the patient most often presents after about a week of treatment with nonoliguric renal failure. Other reversible causes of acute renal failure such as volume depletion or obstruction should be ruled out before one concludes that a patient has aminoglycoside nephrotoxicity. Management is similar to that of other causes of acute renal failure. Close attention should be given to fluid balance and electrolytes, drug dosage adjustments, and nutritional support. Dialysis should be initiated as clinically indicated. The ongoing need for aminoglycoside therapy should be evaluated carefully and alternative agents used if possible.

Preventing aminoglycoside nephrotoxicity begins with correctly assessing renal function. The Cockroft and Gault formula should be used to estimate the creatinine clearance:

$$C_{Cr} = (140 - \text{Age}) \times \text{Lean body weight}/P_{Cr} \times 72$$

where C_{Cr} is creatinine clearance and P_{Cr} is plasma creatinine. For women this volume should be multiplied by 0.85.

In general, the loading dosage remains unchanged in patients with renal insufficiency, whereas the maintenance dosage must be adjusted. Increasing the interval between doses is the preferred method because evidence shows that large dosages given at longer intervals are less nephrotoxic than the same total daily dosage given at shorter intervals. A minimum interval of 24 hours for aminoglycoside dosing is gaining increasing acceptance. The rationale behind this regimen is that higher peak serum concentrations enhance concentration-dependent effects without increasing toxicity. The absence of detectable antibiotic levels in the serum for several hours at the end of a dosage interval does not appear to compromise antibacterial efficacy because aminoglycosides have a prolonged postantibiotic killing effect. In fact, the drug-free intervals may lower the risk of nephrotoxicity and ototoxicity. Study results are inconsistent in this regard, but once-daily dosing appears to be at least comparable to multiple-dose therapy in regard to efficacy and toxicity and certainly is more convenient and cost-effective.

Monitoring drug levels to predict nephrotoxicity is controversial. An increase in the trough level generally indicates decreased excretion of the drug because of a fall in GFR. Thus nephrotoxicity already is established by the time the trough level rises. In addition, it has been shown that peak aminoglycoside levels can be dissociated from renal failure development. Thus aminoglycoside levels are of limited usefulness in predicting nephrotoxicity. However, documented therapeutic antibacterial levels are an indication for continuing to monitor peak levels.

Patient risk factors such as volume depletion and potassium or magnesium depletion should be corrected before therapy is initiated. Once the patient is on therapy, less nephrotoxic antimicrobial agents should be prescribed as soon as the clinical circumstance and bacterial sensitivities allow. In the future, data

TABLE 47.2. Risk Factors for Aminoglycoside Nephrotoxicity
Dosage and duration of treatment
Advanced age
Preexisting renal insufficiency
Hepatic failure
Volume depletion
Potassium or magnesium depletion

TABLE 47.3. Protective Factors for Experimental Aminoglycoside Nephrotoxicity

Thyroxin
Oral calcium loading
Streptozotocin-induced diabetes mellitus
Phosphate depletion
Polyamino acid administration

from animal studies may provide some direction for preventing toxicity in humans. Table 47.3 summarizes factors that have been shown to reduce aminoglycoside nephrotoxicity. The most promising of these interventions is the use of polyamino acids. These agents have been shown to protect against aminoglycoside nephrotoxicity without sacrificing antimicrobial effectiveness. Although they inhibit aminoglycoside binding to renal brush border membranes, this does not appear to be the primary mechanism of action. In one study, protection against gentamicin nephrotoxicity was conferred despite massive drug accumulation in the renal cortex. Further studies on these agents are eagerly awaited. Other interventions, as noted in Table 47.3, have been shown to reduce aminoglycoside nephrotoxicity but are not as applicable to human use.

Amphotericin B

Amphotericin B is widely used as the most effective agent in treating life-threatening systemic fungal infections. However, nephrotoxicity remains a serious complication, affecting as many as 90% of patients who receive a full course of therapy. Amphotericin B affects a variety of tubular functions in the kidney and causes renal failure to develop. At a cellular level, amphotericin B forms complexes in the plasma membrane with cholesterol, producing aqueous pores that allow small solutes to pass through. As a result, the drug transforms the tight epithelium of the distal tubule into a leaky epithelium. Increased permeability to water produces resistance to antidiuretic hormone (ADH) (i.e., nephrogenic diabetes insipidus), and increased permeability to hydrogen ions may result in distal renal tubular acidosis. In addition, significant potassium and magnesium wasting may occur and lead to hypomagnesemia and hypokalemia.

Renal insufficiency generally is dose related and develops as a result of renal vasoconstriction and tubular injury. In animal studies, renal vasoconstriction occurs after acute and chronic amphotericin B administration and is associated with a fall in GFR and renal plasma flow. Maneuvers that prevent or reduce the fall in GFR include salt loading and calcium channel blocker or theophylline administration. On the other hand, the angiotensin II–receptor blocker Sar-Gly angiotensin II or renal denervation does not prevent the renal vasoconstriction or GFR decrease caused by amphotericin B. These observations suggest that the renin-angiotensin system or sympathetic nervous system does not play an important role in amphotericin B–induced renal vasoconstriction. Alterations in cell calcium fluxes may be an important factor. Through its effects on ion permeability, amphotericin B may affect calcium movement across the membrane and lead to vasoconstriction either directly or through mediators such as prostanoids or platelet-activating factor. The protective effect of the calcium channel blockers supports calcium fluxes as a possible factor in the renal vasoconstriction and subsequent renal failure.

Preventing amphotericin B nephrotoxicity is important because this drug often is the only possible treatment for many fungal infections. Risk factors for nephrotoxicity include volume depletion, preexisting renal insufficiency, advanced age, diuretic use, and increased cumulative dosage. Improved renal function in anecdotal cases of amphotericin nephrotoxicity has been demonstrated with repletion of sodium deficits. In addition, a double-blind trial of prophylactic salt loading with 1 L of normal saline before each dose of amphotericin B demonstrated a protective effect against a fall in GFR. Therefore, before initiating amphotericin B treatment, the patient should be well hydrated and formal salt loading should be considered if this maneuver is not contraindicated by coexisting medical conditions such as congestive heart failure. In addition, diuretic therapy should be avoided during amphotericin B therapy unless needed for volume overload. The ongoing need for amphotericin B should be reevaluated constantly and therapy discontinued as soon as the clinical circumstances dictate.

In an attempt to improve the therapeutic index of amphotericin B, newer formulations have been developed incorporating the drug into phospholipid vesicles or liposomes. Immediate side effects during infusion such as fever, rigor, or chills are ameliorated and these formulations appear to reduce nephrotoxicity while preserving antifungal efficacy. As a less expensive alternative, administering amphotericin B in a lipid emulsion, has been studied. Adding lipid emulsion reduces immediate side effects during infusion. There is evidence that nephrotoxicity also is reduced. A randomized prospective study of amphotericin B in 60 critically ill patients with *Candida* infections demonstrated a lower risk of nephrotoxicity in patients randomized to receive the drug in lipid emulsion; 20% of patients showed an increase in serum creatinine, as compared to 66.7% of those receiving the drug in dextrose. The antifungal activity of amphotericin B was preserved in the lipid diluent. The mechanism through which lipid vehicles reduce nephrotoxicity is unclear. Possibilities include altered interactions with mammalian cells, altered transfer to target cells, or a decrease in the most toxic oligomeric form of free amphotericin B. The role of these and other preventive adjuncts such as calcium channel blockers and theophyline await further study.

Vancomycin

Vancomycin is prescribed for a variety of infections caused by gram-positive organisms. Over the past few years, the use of this drug has expanded as the frequency of infections caused by methicillin-resistant *Staphylococcus aureus, Staphylococcus epidermidis,* and *Clostridium difficile* have increased. It is used often in patients on hemodialysis because the prolonged half-life in this setting allows convenient once-weekly dosing in the majority of patients. However, vancomycin-resistant enterococci have emerged.

Overall, vancomycin appears to have little nephrotoxicity potential when used alone. Animal data are conflicting depending on the dosage and route of administration, duration of treatment, and animal model. In general, only mild histologic changes are seen unless the dosage is extremely high or concomitant aminoglycosides are administered. Similarly, in humans, the potential for toxicity appears to be low. Unfortunately, it is often difficult to separate direct nephrotoxic effects from those of coexisting illness or concomitant drug therapy. An overall incidence up to 7% has been reported in various series. Increased risk of toxicity is associated with prolonged courses of therapy and high serum levels. The risk of nephrotoxicity increases if aminoglycosides are coadministered, but it is unclear whether the incidence is significantly higher than that associated with aminoglycosides alone. Rarely, vancomycin has been associated with acute interstitial nephritis (AIN). It should be noted that earlier preparations contained significant amounts of impurities. It is conceivable that at least some cases of nephrotoxicity were caused by these impurities.

Cephalosporins

The cephalosporins are an ever-expanding group of antibiotics widely used to treat a broad spectrum of infections. Most of the reported nephrotoxicity of these agents has been in association with the use of cephaloridine. Large parenteral dosages (more than 6 g/day) can cause proximal tubular necrosis and acute renal failure. As with many types of drug-induced nephrotoxicity, risk appears to be increased by volume depletion or preexisting renal dysfunction. In general, renal dysfunction is reversible upon discontinuation of the drug. The cephalosporins are secreted by the proximal tubule via the same pathway as the organic acids. Therefore it is not surprising that the experimental toxicity of cephaloridine is reduced by agents that competitively block the renal tubular uptake of the antibiotic.

Fortunately, cephaloridine has been replaced by a burgeoning list of alternative cephalosporins. Other than a few isolated cases, they do not appear to be involved in direct tubular toxicity. There is some evidence that they may act synergistically with aminoglycosides to cause acute tubular necrosis. Also, there are case reports of AIN linked to several cephalosporins. Finally, it should be noted that cefoxitin has been reported to interfere with the serum creatinine measurement, resulting in a false elevation.

Fluoroquinolones

The fluoroquinolones have a broad spectrum of activity against both gram-negative and gram-positive organisms. The incidence of nephrotoxicity with these agents appears to be low. In animal studies, high dosages have been shown to cause intratubular crystal formation and obstruction when the urine is alkaline. In humans, the risk of nephrotoxicity is low and has been limited primarily to AIN. Most cases have been reported with ciprofloxacin, but one case report was associated with norfloxacin. Most patients were nonoliguric and manifested systemic findings such as rash, fever, and eosinophilia. Drug withdrawal resulted in renal function improvement.

Sulfonamides

Early cases of nephrotoxicity caused by sulfonamides were associated with crystallization of the drug within the tubules and parenchyma. More soluble derivatives have been developed, essentially eliminating this mechanism of nephrotoxicity. AIN is a well-described complication of sulfonamide therapy. The combination of sulfamethoxazole and trimethoprim is widely used in a variety of infections, particularly urinary tract infections. The trimethoprim component competes with creatinine secretion and may result in an increase in the serum creatinine level, particularly in patients with preexisting renal failure.

Tetracyclines

Tetracycline has an antianabolic effect that may cause worsening azotemia and hyperkalemia in patients with renal failure. It interferes with protein synthesis from amino acids, and the latter are diverted for urea synthesis. Doxycycline is the preferred agent for patients with renal failure because it has minimal antianabolic effects. The use of outdated tetracycline has been reported to cause a reversible proximal tubular dysfunction. Demeclocycline inhibits the effect of ADH on the renal tubule, resulting in polyuria, and therefore has been used to treat ADH excess. A reversible decline in renal function has been observed when patients with advanced cirrhosis have been treated with this agent.

Acyclovir

Acyclovir is a nucleoside analog used to treat systemic and genital herpes or varicella infections. Acute renal failure has been observed with high-dose intravenous bolus acyclovir therapy. Intrarenal obstruction caused by crystal formation appears to be the primary mechanism of renal injury. Acute tubular necrosis also has been reported in this setting. Large intravenous boluses result in high serum drug levels and presumably high concentrations within the renal tubules that exceed the solubility product of the drug. This complication occurs quickly, often within 12 hours of the infusion, and is more likely in the setting of volume depletion, rapid high-dose infusion, preexisting renal insufficiency, or concomitant nephrotoxin exposure. In nearly all instances, renal function is recovered after the agent is discontinued. This complication may be prevented by infusing the drug slowly over 1 hour and hydrating the patient before administering the drug. Most other nucleoside analogs, including ganciclovir, do not appear to cause significant nephrotoxicity.

Foscarnet

Foscarnet is an antiviral agent that is active against cytomegalovirus and HIV and thus is prescribed commonly in patients with AIDS. The drug is poorly absorbed from the gastrointestinal tract and therefore must be administered intravenously. Because the major route of excretion is the kidneys, the dosage must be modified in patients with renal insufficiency. Nephrotoxicity is the most common adverse effect of this agent, affecting up to 65% of patients receiving the drug. Concomitant nephrotoxins, preexisting renal insufficiency, and volume depletion increase the risk of nephrotoxicity. The mode of administration also appears to be important because renal dysfunction is less common with intermittent intravenous infusion than with continuous therapy. Tubular toxicity appears to be the primary mechanism of injury, although crystal formation in glomerular capillaries also may contribute. Aggressive hydration during foscarnet therapy is crucial for preventing nephrotoxicity. In addition, careful dosing in patients with renal insufficiency and avoidance of concurrent nephrotoxin administration should be followed if possible.

Other Antiviral Agents

Indinavir is a protease inhibitor used to treat HIV infection. It is excreted by the kidney largely as the parent molecule, and its solubility decreases as the pH increases. Not surprisingly, nephrolithiasis has been reported to develop in approximately 4% of patients taking the drug. Intratubular precipitation of the drug associated with acute renal failure also has been reported. Maintaining adequate hydration while taking indinavir seems reasonable to prevent this complication. Another protease inhibitor, ritonavir, has been associated with renal insufficiency in sporadic reports. Unfortunately, the role of this drug as a causative factor has been unclear because most patients were taking other potential nephrotoxins or had concomitant clinical conditions that could cause renal failure.

Pentamidine

Pentamidine is a very effective agent for treating *Pneumocystis carinii* pneumonia in patients with AIDS. Approximately 25% of patients receiving this agent have a rise in blood urea nitrogen or creatinine. There is some evidence that the incidence is even higher in patients with AIDS and often is associated with type IV renal tubular acidosis. Coexisting illness and concurrent drug administration often make it difficult to assign an independent role for pentamidine in many cases. In general, renal failure is reversible upon drug discontinuation.

ACUTE INTERSTITIAL NEPHRITIS

A number of antibiotics have been implicated in causing AIN (Table 47.4). Methicillin is the most commonly reported, with more than 100 cases described in the literature to date. Approximately 16% of patients receiving this antibiotic develop the syndrome, whereas the risk is much lower for other penicillins. Generally, the onset of symptoms of AIN occurs approximately 2 weeks after therapy begins, although this has been reported to vary from 2 to 60 days. An earlier presentation is likely after rechallenge with a drug to which a patient has been sensitized. Systemic symptoms of AIN include fever, arthralgias, and a fleeting erythematous maculopapular rash. Acute renal failure is nonoliguric in most patients and is associated with tubular proteinuria, gross or microscopic hematuria, and usually eosinophiluria. Tubular dysfunction may be manifest, with impaired concentrating ability and renal tubular acidosis. Peripheral eosinophilia often is present. A high index of suspicion should be maintained in patients at risk because only a minority of patients present with all the classic manifestations of AIN.

On renal biopsy, light microscopy generally demonstrates diffuse interstitial infiltrates consisting of lymphocytes, plasma cells, and eosinophils. Interstitial fibrosis may be seen if a biopsy is performed late in the course of renal failure, and noncaseating granulomas with epithelioid giant cells occasionally may be present. In general, the immunofluorescence is negative and the glomeruli and vessels are normal. The exception to this is the well-described lesion associated with the use of nonsteroidal antiinflammatory agents where interstitial nephritis is seen in combination with the minimal-change lesion.

AIN should be suspected in any patient who develops acute renal failure during treatment with a potentially offending agent. The diagnosis may be difficult because patients often do not present with all the classic signs of AIN. In addition, the complex clinical picture of many patients expands the range of possible causes of acute renal failure. The presence of an active urinary sediment, eosinophilia, and eosinophiluria, in addition to extrarenal findings such as fever and rash, are highly suggestive of AIN. In many patients, however, a renal biopsy is needed for definitive diagnosis.

Overall, the prognosis for renal recovery is excellent if the offending drug is withdrawn. There is some evidence that glucocorticoids may hasten recovery. One study retrospectively reviewed the course of 14 patients with methicillin-induced AIN and found that those treated with glucocorticoids recovered renal function more rapidly than those who did not receive steroids. The use of pulse glucocorticoids, as in transplant rejection, has been shown to be effective in improving renal function in anecdotal cases. Unfortunately, a prospective randomized trial of glucocorticoid therapy to resolve this issue would be difficult because of the rarity of AIN. Nevertheless, a short course of glucocorticoids (i.e., prednisone 60 mg daily for 2 weeks) probably is reasonable and carries little risk in the patient with AIN. Obviously, the offending antibiotic should be withdrawn and future treatment with the agent avoided because the syndrome usually will recur on reexposure.

TABLE 47.4. Antibiotics Implicated in Causing Acute Interstitial Nephritis

Penicillin and derivatives
- Penicillin G
- Methicillin
- Ampicillin
- Amoxicillin
- Carbenicillin
- Oxacillin
- Nafcillin

Cephalosporins
- Cephalothin
- Cephalexin
- Cephradine
- Cefoxitin

Others
- Cotrimoxazole
- Rifampicin
- Vancomycin
- Minocycline

ANTIMICROBIAL AGENT–INDUCED DISTURBANCES OF FLUID, ELECTROLYTE, AND ACID–BASE BALANCE

Drugs may induce alterations in fluid, electrolyte, or acid–base balance. These abnormalities may or may not be associated directly with altered physiologic function of the kidney but certainly can lead to unbalanced body homeostasis.

Fluid and Electrolyte Disturbances

Increased extracellular fluid and edema may occur with high-dose parenteral use of the sodium salts of penicillin or ampicillin in patients with diminished sodium excretory capacity. The sodium contents of certain penicillins in common clinical practice are listed in Table 47.5. The problem is common in patients who need antibiotic treatment for bacterial endocarditis. When acceptable alternative antimicrobial therapy is lacking, sometimes it is necessary to combine penicillin therapy with diuretic administration. An ADH-resistant concentrating defect is a well-known effect of demeclocycline. In adults, dosages of 1,200 mg/day uniformly result in polyuria. This adverse drug effect has been used to therapeutic advantage in treating pathologic water retention such as that encountered in the syndrome of inappropriate ADH secretion. Aminoglycosides also can induce a polyuric state that can be dissociated experimentally from the acute renal failure discussed earlier. Renal potassium and magnesium wasting have been associated with amphotericin and gentamicin use. Hyperkalemia in some patients treated with trimethoprim–sulfamethoxazole has been caused by distal tubule potassium secretion inhibition by trimetho-

TABLE 47.5. Sodium Content of Penicillins

Antibiotic	Sodium Content
Penicillin G	2.0 mEq/million U
Ampicillin	3.4 mEq/g
Oxacillin	3.1 mEq/g
Carbenicillin	4.7 mEq/g
Ticarcillin	5.2 mEq/g

prim. Foscarnet is associated with a dose-dependent reduction in ionized calcium levels possibly caused by complexing of the drug with ionized calcium.

Acid–Base Disturbances

Well-characterized examples of antimicrobial agents that induce metabolic acid–base disturbances include amphotericin B, carbenicillin, and ticarcillin. The metabolic acidosis associated with amphotericin B is hyperchloremic, with the functional renal defect consisting of a failure to perform distal tubular acidification. Usually, acidosis and potassium depletion antedate the decline in glomerular filtration that often complicates antifungal therapy with amphotericin B. Supplemental potassium bicarbonate treatment is effective in correcting the hypokalemic metabolic acidosis. Conversely, ticarcillin or carbenicillin disodium administration can be complicated by hypokalemic metabolic alkalosis when large dosages are given. The apparent mechanism that leads to the alkalosis involves the semisynthetic penicillin acting as a nonresorbable anion within the distal tubular lumen. Treatment consists of reducing the dosage of the drug or substituting an equally effective antimicrobial and repleting potassium chloride. Overdosage with nalidixic acid induces a metabolic acidosis. Isoniazid overdose produces lactic acidosis. The use of outdated tetracycline causes proximal renal tubular acidosis.

Selected Readings

Becker BN, Schulman G. Nephrotoxicity of antiviral therapies. *Curr Opin Nephrol Hypertens* 1996;5:375–379.
A good overview of the nephrotoxicity of antiviral agents.

Bennet WM. Mechanisms of aminoglycoside nephrotoxicity. *Clin Exp Pharmacol Physiol* 1989;16:1–6.
A good review of the pathogenesis of renal dysfunction caused by aminoglycosides.

Choudhury D, Ahmed Z. Drug-induced nephrotoxicity. *Med Clin North Am* 1997;3:705–717.
Reviews nephrotoxicity of common drugs, including antibiotics, grouped according to pathogenetic mechanisms.

Michel DM, Kelly CJ. Acute interstitial nephritis. *J Am Soc Nephrol* 1998;9:506–515.
An excellent review of all aspects of acute interstitial nephritis.

Sorkine P, Nagar H, Weinbroum A, et al. Administration of amphotericin B in lipid emulsion decreases nephrotoxicity: results of a prospective, randomized, controlled study in critically ill patients. *Crit Care Med* 1996;24:1311–1315.
A well-designed study examining the efficacy and risk of nephrotoxicity of amphotericin B in lipid emulsion used to treat patients with Candida infections.

PART 2
Nephropathies Caused by Antineoplastic Agents

Robert L. Safirstein and Tejinder S. Ahuja

Chemotherapy, surgery, and radiation therapy are the mainstays of treatment for malignant neoplasms. One of the major limiting factors in treating these neoplasms is the toxicity of the chemotherapeutic agents. An ideal anticancer drug would eradicate cancer cells without harming normal tissue. Unfortunately, no chemotherapeutic agent meets this criterion. Bone marrow suppression and nephrotoxicity are the major dose-limiting factors in the use of these agents. As chemotherapeutic drugs are being used in high dosages in an effort to achieve a cure, nephrotoxicity of these agents has become more conspicuous. In some series of acute renal failure (ARF), cancer has been identified as the underlying disease in as many as 20% of all patients. ARF in patients with cancer results not only from antineoplastic drugs but also infections, analgesics, obstruction, products of tumor lysis (uric acid, phosphate, xanthine), and the invasion of kidney by tumor cells. In this chapter, we review the nephrotoxic chemotherapeutic agents, mechanisms of their nephrotoxicity, factors that aggravate and alleviate the nephrotoxic potential of these agents, and the prophylactic measures that should be taken. We also briefly discuss the renal manifestations of bone marrow transplantation (BMT).

FACTORS INCREASING NEPHROTOXIC POTENTIAL OF ANTINEOPLASTIC AGENTS

Many comorbid factors in patients with cancer may increase the nephrotoxic risk of antineoplastic drugs, including extracellular volume depletion, underlying hepatobiliary disease, and heart failure. Prominent among these factors is preexisting renal failure, which alters pharmacokinetics of drugs excreted primarily by the kidney. Even a small reduction in glomerular filtration rate (GFR), which could result from prior radiation therapy or chemotherapy, potentiates the nephrotoxic potential of antineoplastic agents greatly. Alterations in the extracellular fluid solute content that potentiate nephrotoxicity are prominent in patients with cancer. For example, hypercalcemia, which could result from osteolytic lesions or parathyroid hormone–related protein production, and hyperuricemia often are present in the patient with cancer. High blood concentrations of myoglobin and light chains, concomitant use of other nephrotoxic drugs, and large tumor burden (because of the risk of tumor lysis syndrome) all contribute to heightened nephrotoxicity. These risk factors should be identified and all efforts should be made to correct them before chemotherapy is administered because renal failure in these patients makes treatment much more difficult and is a predictor of bad outcome.

ANTINEOPLASTIC AGENTS THAT CAUSE ACUTE RENAL FAILURE

Antineoplastic agents can cause nephrotoxicity in a predictable dose-dependent manner, even after a single exposure. Alkylating agents such as streptozotocin and *cis*-platin, methotrexate, mithramycin, and the cytokine interleukin-2 (IL-2) belong to this category of nephrotoxic antineoplastic agents. The nephrotoxicity of other anticancer agents often occurs after chronic repeated exposures, and usually in these cases the decline in the renal failure is irreversible. Examples include the alkylating agents lomustine (CCNU) and the antitumor antibiotic mitomycin.

Alkylating Agents

Cis-Platin

Cis-platin [*cis*-diamminedichloroplatinum (II)] is an organic metal complex with two labile chloride groups. Its major antitumor activity is in genitourinary cancers, but it can also prolong survival of patients with cancer of the head, neck, and lung. Initial use of *cis*-platin not using extracellular volume expansion was limited because of unexpected and severe renal toxicity. Since its nephrotoxic potential was first recognized, much has been learned about *cis*-platin–induced renal failure, and various strategies have been used to prevent ARF.

Pharmacokinetics. Two hours after its infusion, more than 90% of the plasma platinum is protein bound and is eliminated slowly. Most of the remaining 10% is excreted by the kidney. After administration *cis*-platin accumulates in liver, spleen, and renal tubular cells, where its concentration is more than five times its extracellular concentration. The kidney accumulates *cis*-platin by peritubular uptake; there is no evidence of tubular reabsorption. The final *cis*-platin content in the kidney exceeds that in any other organ.

Pathophysiology. In animal models, the proximal tubule (specifically the S_3 segment in the outer medullary stripe) is the prominent site of *cis*-platin–induced necrosis. Focal loss of brush border, cellular swelling, and condensation of nuclear chromatin are some of the other morphologic changes seen. In humans, damage also has been noted in more distal parts of the nephron.

The exact mechanism of *cis*-platin nephrotoxicity is unclear. However, the following alterations are thought to be responsible for its toxicity. After gaining access in the cells, the labile chloride ligands of the *cis*-platin are replaced by water molecules in an aquation reaction, resulting in a highly reactive electrophilic product and possible tissue injury. *Cis*-platin inhibits DNA biosynthesis by forming crosslinks between pyrimidine nucleotides in DNA. Whether such DNA damage is responsible for nephrotoxicity is unknown. *Cis*-platin also has affinity for sulfhydryl-rich proteins and glutathione; by depleting these, it increases oxidative stress and may provoke cell damage. Another interesting mechanism, which may apply to all xenobiotics, is glutathione conjugate–mediated nephrotoxicity. Glutathione conjugates initially were thought to be detoxicants, but increasing evidence suggests that because of their physiologic function and biochemical profile, the kidneys are particularly susceptible to their toxicity. Some investigators have suggested that mitochondrial DNA might be the principal target of *cis*-platin nephrotoxicity in the kidney. However, none of these proposed mechanisms has been established definitively as the cause of *cis*-platin cytotoxicity.

Clinical Manifestations. *Cis*-platin decreases GFR in a dose-dependent manner. The onset of renal failure usually is gradual, occurring 3 to 5 days after administration, and often is nonoliguric. Urinary excretion of markers of proximal tubular injury such as B_2-microglobulin and *N*-acetyl-β-D-glucosaminidase (NAG) are increased. Mild proteinuria and glycosuria are common. *Cis*-platin also leads to magnesium wasting and hypomagnesemia in 50% of patients. Usually this is seen after repeated exposure over long periods of time, but it can occur acutely. The severity of hypomagnesemia correlates well with the cumulative *cis*-platin dosage the patient has received and often lasts for months but in a few patients can persist for years. Hypomagnesemia is much more common when *cis*-platin is given in combination with other medications that have magnesium-wasting potential such as gentamicin and amphotericin. Calcitriol therapy may aggravate magnesium wasting by an unclear mechanism in patients who have received *cis*-platin. Measurement of plasma and erythrocyte magnesium levels in patients receiving *cis*-platin showed that intracellular and serum magnesium levels are reduced. Parenteral or oral magnesium supplementation is safe and effective in treating *cis*-platin–induced hypomagnesemia, but prolonged supplementation usually is needed. The hypokalemia and hypocalcemia seen usually are related to magnesium wasting, and hypomagnesemia must be corrected. A few patients also can develop salt wasting, leading to hyponatremia and orthostatic hypotension.

Isolated cases of hemolytic uremic syndrome (HUS) have been reported in patients who have received *cis*-platin. However, the rarity of this occurrence makes it unclear whether this is a direct effect of *cis*-platin alone or is linked to other coadministered chemotherapeutic agents or factors related to the presence of the tumor.

Protective Measures. In initial studies, the frequent nephrotoxic effect of *cis*-platin was obvious. One in three patients receiving 2 mg/kg or 75 mg/m² of the drug suffered ARF. In one early series, 61% of patients receiving 100 mg/m² developed ARF. Thus it became prudent to develop strategies that diminish the severity of ARF it produces. The cornerstone of *cis*-platin nephrotoxicity prophylaxis is intravenous fluid administration. The mechanism by which intravenous hydration decreases nephrotoxicity is unclear. Although the urine concentration of the drug decreases with hydration, neither the tissue concentration nor the degree of cytotoxicity is altered. A renoprotective effect has been demonstrated when hypertonic saline solution (3%) is used as a vehicle for *cis*-platin. Although it has been suggested that raising the extracellular chloride concentration inhibits formation of aquatic forms of *cis*-platin, which is a highly reactive product, a similar protective effect is seen with mannitol, which reduces urine chloride. Administering the drug in multiple daily fractions, prolonging the infusion time, and infusing the drug directly to the target site are other maneuvers used to decrease *cis*-platin nephrotoxicity. Probenecid and other inhibitors of organic anion or cation transport may offer some degree of renal protection by decreasing the access of nephrotoxic *cis*-platin metabolites to sites of renal damage.

A variety of chelating agents have been used to reduce *cis*-platin nephrotoxicity. Sodium thiosulfate and diethyldithiocarbamate, a metabolite of disulfiram, react with and remove platinum from most binding sites. Bismuth induces metal-binding protein metallothionein. Ethyol (amifostine), an organic thiophosphate dephosphorylated by alkaline phosphatase *in vivo* into a free active thiol metabolite WR-1065, has proven to be effective in reducing *cis*-platin nephrotoxicity. However, only Ethyol is used clinically, and the recommended starting dosage is 910 mg/m² administered once daily as 15-minute intravenous infusion, starting 30 minutes before chemotherapy. Hypotension, nausea, vomiting, and hypocalcemia are its main side effects.

Carboplatin is a newer platinum compound with much less nephrotoxic potential than that of *cis*-platin. Like *cis*-platin, it produces predominantly interstrand DNA crosslinks and commonly is used in advanced ovarian cancer. The carboplatin aquation, which is thought to produce the active species, occurs at a slower rate than in the case of *cis*-platin. The development of abnormal renal function is uncommon despite the fact that carboplatin, unlike *cis*-platin, usually is administered without high-volume hydration and or diuresis. Hypomagnesemia also is less common with carboplatin use than with *cis*-platin. The main dose-limiting side effect is myelosuppression, especially thrombocytopenia. Carboplatin is as effective as *cis*-platin in several genitourinary cancers.

Cyclophosphamide

Cyclophosphamide is biotransformed principally in the liver to active alkylating metabolites by a mixed-function microsomal oxidase system. The metabolites interfere with the growth of proliferating malignant cells by cross-linking DNA and disrupting its template function. Myelosuppression is the primary dose-limiting toxicity. Hemorrhagic cystitis, sterility, and second malignancies also can occur as a result of therapy. High-dose cyclophosphamide can increase the release of and cellular response to antidiuretic hormone (ADH). Because high fluid intake is recommended to prevent hemorrhagic cystitis, the combination of increased ADH effect and hydration can lead to severe hyponatremia. Therefore isotonic saline rather than dextrose should be used to maintain high urine output.

Ifosfamide

Ifosfamide is a chemotherapeutic agent chemically related to nitrogen mustards and a synthetic analog of cyclophosphamide. Its main indication is in treating germ cell testicular cancer and certain sarcomas. Mesna often is used with ifosfamide to prevent hemorrhagic cystitis. Unlike with cyclophosphamide, tubular dysfunction after ifosfamide administration is common and can range from mild enzymuria to overt Fanconi's syndrome, especially if ifosfamide is used in conjunction with *cis*-platin or carboplatin. In children, these defects can lead to hypophosphatemic rickets. The metabolites of ifosfamide (mainly chloracetaldehyde or 4-hydroxy-ifosfamide) probably are responsible for the nephrotoxicity rather than the parent drug. By a membrane-stabilizing effect, glycine can alleviate Fanconi's syndrome induced by ifosfamide in rats. Distal renal tubular acidosis, nephrogenic diabetes insipidus (DI), and the syndrome of inappropriate ADH secretion also have been reported with ifosfamide.

Nitrosoureas

Carmustine (BCNU), CCNU, and semustine (methyl-CCNU) are highly lipid soluble and consequently have high permeability across the blood–brain barrier. For this reason they are used extensively to treat brain tumors. Nitrosoureas are rapidly and metabolized within 20 minutes of administration are cleared from the plasma. Methyl CCNU, which is not commercially available in the United States, has been associated more often with nephrotoxicity. It generates a free radical methyl group and can cause irreversible renal failure, which can occur insidiously and is not always accompanied by abnormalities on urinalysis. The risk is particularly high in patients who receive cumulative dosages greater than 1.4 to 1.5 g/m^2. Glomerular sclerosis, interstitial fibrosis, and tubular atrophy are the main histologic findings. BCNU and CCNU also can cause renal damage, but the mechanism of nephrotoxicity is unknown.

Streptozotocin is a synthetic antineoplastic agent that is chemically related to other nitrosoureas used in cancer chemotherapy. It is indicated in treating metastatic islet cell carcinoma of the pancreas. The chief limiting side effect is dose-related and cumulative nephrotoxicity, which occurs in 75% of patients receiving prolonged administration. The nephrotoxicity is characterized by mild hypophosphatemia to full-blown tubular reabsorptive abnormalities seen in Fanconi's syndrome. Mild proteinuria is one of the first signs of renal toxicity and may herald further deterioration of renal function. The drug should not be used in combination with other nephrotoxic agents, and extreme caution should be exercised in evaluating the benefit of giving the drug in the presence of preexisting renal insufficiency. Nephrogenic DI and obstructive uropathy from uric acid nephrolithiasis, caused by its uricosuric effect, also have been described.

Antimetabolites

Methotrexate

Methotrexate is a folic acid antagonist used to treat a broad spectrum of malignancies. Renal excretion by glomerular filtration and active tubular secretion is the primary route of elimination. After intravenous administration, 80% to 90% of the drug is excreted unchanged in the urine within 24 hours. Nephrotoxicity is a problem only when high dosages of the drug are used, especially in patients with underlying renal insufficiency. In these circumstances a high methotrexate concentration can lead to marked bone marrow, gastrointestinal, and renal toxicity. Although several mechanisms for nephrotoxicity have been proposed, intratubular precipitation of the methotrexate crystals in concentrated and acidic urine is the most probable mechanism. Direct tubular toxicity and hemodynamic alteration also may contribute to the nephrotoxicity. Methotrexate-induced renal failure usually is nonoliguric and resolves in a few weeks. Aggressive hydration, urine alkalinization, folinic acid (leucovorin) administration, and methotrexate level monitoring are the standard effective prophylactic measures. Removal by hemodialysis and peritoneal dialysis is poor, as is the efficacy of plasma exchange.

Cytarabine

Cytarabine, commonly known as *ara*-C, appears to act by inhibiting DNA polymerase. Its main indication is in acute nonlymphocytic leukemia, but it is also useful in acute lymphocytic leukemia and in the blast phase of chronic myelocytic leukemia. Renal failure develops in 50% of patients treated with multidrug regimens, especially in drug regimens that include *cis*-platin and hydroxyurea. The mechanism of injury is unclear but does not appear to be dose related.

5-Fluorouracil

Fluorouracil inhibits the methylation reaction of deoxyuridylic acid to thymidylic acid, thus interfering with DNA synthesis. Also, after conversion to 5-fluorouridine triphosphate it interferes with RNA processing and function. It is effective in the palliative management of gastrointestinal malignancies. Nephrotoxicity is seen only when it is used in combination with mitomycin-C, which can cause HUS. However, chronic renal failure, as a result of progressive interstitial fibrosis and glomerular sclerosis, also has been described.

5-Azacitidine

Like 5-fluorouracil, azacitidine is a pyrimidine analog that interferes with DNA, RNA, and protein synthesis. Nephrotoxicity is rare when it is used alone. In combination with other drugs, it can cause tubular reabsorptive abnormalities, leading to glycosuria and phosphaturia, but these abnormalities usually resolve on discontinuing the drug.

Antitumor Antibiotics

Mitomycin-C

Mitomycin is a naturally occurring alkylating agent that crosslinks DNA. It is used in combination protocols to treat solid tumors of genitourinary and gastrointestinal systems. Although myelosuppression is its major dose-limiting toxicity, mitomycin is the most common antineoplastic agent associated with chemotherapy-induced HUS, which occurs in 2% to 10% of treated patients. The syndrome usually occurs 1 to 2 months after the last dose, but a more delayed onset also can occur. Patients receiving a cumulative dosage of 30 to 50 mg/m^2 are at higher risk and should be monitored closely for unexplained anemia with fragmented red blood cells on peripheral smear, thrombocytopenia, and renal failure. In patients with breast cancer, concomitant use of tamoxifen with mitomycin was found to be a risk factor for HUS. Plasmapheresis has been reported to reverse the hematologic manifestations but not the renal involvement. Vincristine also can be used, but glucocorticoids and antiplatelet drugs offer no benefit. Plasma immunoadsorption with staphylococcal protein A columns can stabilize renal function and produce a beneficial hematologic response by removing immune complexes or IgG from the circulation.

Mithramycin

Mithramycin interrupts DNA-directed RNA synthesis by binding to the DNA, possibly through an antibiotic–Mg^{2+} complex. Aside for its occasional use in patients with refractory testicular cancer and malignancy-induced hypercalcemia, it currently has few other indications. A single intravenous dose of 25 μg/kg is used to treat hypercalcemia, and this rarely causes renal failure. However, repeated daily administration of the drug can cause significant nephrotoxicity in up to 40% of patients. Renal biopsy reveals necrosis of the proximal and distal tubules.

Biologic Agents

Interferons

Interferons are a group of glycoproteins with antiviral, immunomodulatory, and antitumor activities. Interferons α and β have been used increasingly to treat a wide variety of malignancies. Proteinuria is the most common abnormality, seen in 15% to 20% of patients treated with interferons. Histopathology of the kidney shows minimal-change nephropathy or focal segmental glomerulosclerosis. Interstitial nephritis, acute tubular necrosis, or HUS also can cause ARF in an occasional patient being treated with interferons.

Interleukin-2

Recombinant IL-2 is widely used in advanced cancers to enhance killer cell functions. However, frequent oliguric ARF is its main drawback. Hypotension, oliguria, decreased fractional sodium excretion, and BUN:creatinine ratio elevation all favor a prerenal cause. These findings usually resolve rapidly when the infusion is discontinued. Although capillary leak is thought to be the basis for this effect, massive infusion of the fluid does not abrogate the fall in the GFR. Also, the fall in the GFR and salt excretion precedes the fall in cardiac output, suggesting a direct effect of IL-2 on renal function. Constant infusion in repetitive weekly cycles, IL-2 administration without lymphokine-activated cells, and meticulous attention to stabilizing intravascular volume with saline and colloid, as well as low-dose dopamine, have been partially successful in decreasing the nephrotoxicity of IL-2. Nonsteroidal antiinflammatory drugs should not be used to minimize IL-2–induced nonrenal systemic effects because they can exacerbate renal failure. Isolated reports of nephrotic syndrome, nephritic syndrome from crescentic glomerulonephritis, and interstitial nephritis from use of IL-2 also have been described.

NEPHROTOXICITY RESULTING FROM INDIRECT COMPLICATIONS OF CYTOTOXIC THERAPY

Tumor Lysis Syndrome

The tumor lysis syndrome is a complication of cytoreductive therapy in rapidly growing radiochemotherapy-sensitive tumors. The blood concentrations of uric acid, xanthine, phosphate, and potassium increase out of proportion to the degree of renal failure. The subsequent filtration with intratubular precipitation of these intracellular constituents probably is responsible for ARF. A urinary uric acid:creatinine ratio of more than 1 is fairly specific for acute hyperuricemic nephropathy. The incidence and severity of acute hyperuricemic nephropathy and tumor lysis syndrome have decreased with prophylactic treatment with allopurinol, vigorous hydration, and urine alkalinization. However, prophylactic use of allopurinol can lead to an increase in xanthine concentration in the blood and xanthine crystalluria. Patients with a mild degree of hypoxanthine–guanine phosphoribosyltransferase deficiency are more predisposed to developing xanthine nephrotoxicity.

Retinoic Acid Syndrome

Tretinoin (all-*trans*-retinoic acid) has been used successfully and has become the treatment of choice for acute promyelocytic leukemia (APL). Retinoic acid syndrome is the major adverse effect of tretinoin and occurs in 25% of treated patients with APL in the absence of prophylactic measures. It is characterized by fever, respiratory distress, radiographic pulmonary infiltrates, and pleural or pericardial effusion in 25% of patients. The syndrome usually occurs 2 to 21 days after treatment begins and is associated with marked leukocytosis in two-thirds of the patients. Autopsy studies have indicated extensive infiltration of myeloid cells into various organs including kidneys. A modest elevation of serum creatinine was noticed in 20% of 51 patients in one study, but severe renal failure necessitating dialysis can occur. The pathophysiology of the syndrome is poorly understood, but a stimulatory effect of tretinoin on cytokine expression by leukemic cells is proposed because the clinical symptoms resemble adult respiratory distress and endotoxic shock syndromes. Adding intravenous dexamethasone and another antineoplastic agent (in the case of increasing leukocyte count) has decreased the incidence. Tretinoin can also induce renal failure by rapidly correcting proteolysis and fibrinolysis in APL, leading to a hypercoagulable state and occlusion of renal vessels.

RENAL FAILURE ASSOCIATED WITH BONE MARROW TRANSPLANT

BMT is an important modality for treating aplastic anemia, hematologic and nonhematologic malignancies, hereditary enzyme deficiencies, immunodeficiency states, and selected hemoglobinopathies. ARF develops in approximately 40% of the patients after transplantation, and the cause of renal failure differs depending on the time of onset of ARF.

ARF in the first 5 days after BMT probably is the result of tumor lysis syndrome, which is uncommon because of the prior cytoreductive therapy, or marrow infusion–associated toxicity. Because autologous BMT increasingly is being used after cytoreductive therapy, harvested marrow that is in a cryopreservative usually is needed. Cryopreservants such as dimethyl sulfoxide and lysis products of stored granulocytes and red blood cells usually are responsible for the marrow infusion nephrotoxicity. Hemoglobinuria occurs in 75% to 100% of these patients and is the likely cause of ARF. This complication also is rare because of the renoprotective effect of concomitant infusion of solute and alkaline diuresis.

Most cases of ARF after BMT occur 10 to 21 days after transplantation. A hepatorenallike syndrome is responsible for approximately 90% of these cases and has ominous implications. Jaundice, portal hypertension, and sodium avidity leading to weight gain invariably precede azotemia. Venoocclusive disease as a result of radiochemotherapy-induced endothelial cell injury of hepatic venules is thought to be responsible for the liver failure. The severity of hyperbilirubinemia correlates with the occurrence of renal failure; levels less than 4 mg/dl portends good renal prognosis and levels greater than 7 mg/dl predict future need for hemodialysis.

Preexisting liver and renal disease; fever with sepsis; use of estrogens, progestin, amphotericin, and methotrexate; mismatched grafts; age greater than 25 years; and protein C and anti–thrombin III deficiencies all have been identified as major risk factors for venoocclusive disease and associated ARF. Heparin and tissue plasminogen activator have shown some benefit, but therapy is limited by the high risk of hemorrhage.

HUS and cyclosporine nephrotoxicity are the major causes of late-onset renal failure after BMT. HUS occurs in 15% to 20% of patients after BMT. It can affect all age groups and can occur after either allogenic or autologous grafting. Cyclosporine treatment is not a prerequisite for the syndrome because enough cases have been identified in its absence. The severity and the time of its onset can vary widely. If the onset is with insidious development of azotemia, proteinuria, hypertension, anemia, and microscopic hematuria, the term *BMT nephropathy* has been used. However, both BMT nephropathy and HUS probably are the expression of endothelial injury from chemoradiotherapy. The main histopathologic features of BMT-associated HUS are arteriolar and glomerular capillary thrombosis and mesangiolysis, which can lead to double-contour appearance of capillary walls. Deposition of fibrin, C3 and C1q, and IgM also can be demonstrated. Total body irradiation with oxidant stress is thought to be the principal inciting agent for the syndrome.

Partial renal shielding during total body irradiation, slow radiation administration, hyperfractionation of the radiation, and administration of exogenous antioxidants all have been tried in an attempt to decrease radiation injury and the incidence of HUS. The potential problems of decreasing antitumor activity and impaired normal marrow engraftment have limited the usefulness of these measures. Although plasma exchange with or without vincristine has been used in patients with BMT-associated HUS, the results have been disappointing. Although it is not necessary to discontinue cyclosporine altogether, a dosage reduction may be considered if graft versus host disease does not appear to be life-threatening.

Selected Readings

Berns JS, Ford PA. Renal toxicities of antineoplastic drugs and bone marrow transplantation. *Semin Nephrol* 1997;17:54–66.

This is the most comprehensive review of nephropathies caused by antineoplastic agents and renal manifestations of BMT; it includes 167 references.

Cobos E, Hall RR. Effects of chemotherapy on the kidney. *Semin Nephrol* 1993;13:297–305.

A comprehensive review of nephropathies caused by antineoplastic agents; it includes 116 references.

DeFronzo RA, Calvin OM, Braine H, et al. Cyclophosphamide and the kidney. *Cancer* 1974;33:483–491.

The article reviews the effect of cyclophosphamide on fluid and electrolyte balance.

Fenaux P, Botton SD. Retinoic acid syndrome: recognition, prevention and management. *Drug Saf* 1998;18:273–279.

The review discusses the clinical features, pathophysiology, prophylaxis, and treatment of retinoic acid syndrome induced by tretinoin.

Harmon WE, Cohen HT, Schneeberger E, et al. Chronic renal failure in children treated with methyl CCNU. *N Engl J Med* 1979;300:1200–1203.

Initial report of long-term renal effects of methyl CCNU, including two patients with chronic renal failure.

Monks TJ, Lau SS. Commentary: renal transport processes and glutathione conjugate–mediated nephrotoxicity. *Drug Metab Dispos* 1987;15:437–441.

The review includes 83 references and discusses the pathways involved in the metabolism of glutathione conjugates in the kidney and the nephrotoxicity of these compounds.

Pinzani V, Bressolle F, Haug IJ, et al. Cisplatin-induced renal toxicity and toxicity-modulating strategies: a review. *Cancer Chemother Pharmacol* 1994;35:1–9.

This review includes a discussion of different renoprotective strategies that have been developed and includes the nature and mechanism of cis-platin nephrotoxicity.

Safirstein RL. Renal diseases induced by antineoplastic agents. In: Schrier RW, ed. *Diseases of the kidney.* 6th ed. Boston: Little, Brown, 1998:1153–1165.

This extensive review includes 173 references; the chapter reviews what is known about nephrotoxicity of antineoplastic agents. ARF after BMT also is discussed in brief.

Safirstein R, Winston J, Goldstein M, et al. Cisplatin nephrotoxicity. *Am J Kidney Dis* 1998;8:356–367.

The manifestations and the possible mechanism of cis-platin nephrotoxicity are discussed; the article includes 51 references.

Schacht RG, Feiner HD, Gallo GR, et al. Nephrotoxicity of nitrosoureas. *Cancer* 1981;48:1328–1334.

Insidiously progressive interstitial lesions in 17 of the 18 patients who received at least six courses of nitrosoureas for therapy of malignant brain tumors are discussed.

Suarez A, McDowell H, Niaudet P, et al. Long-term follow-up of ifosfamide renal toxicity in children treated with malignant mesenchymal tumors: an International Society of Pediatric Oncology report. *J Clin Oncol* 1991;9:2177–2182.

The renal function of 74 children with malignant mesenchymal tumors in complete remission who received an ifosfamide-containing protocol was studied; 22% of the patients had renal function abnormalities, with tubular abnormalities predominating.

Zager RA. Acute renal failure in the setting of bone marrow transplantation. *Kidney Int* 1994;46:1443–1458.

The review presents an overview of several renal syndromes that are unique to or occur with disproportionate frequency in patients receiving BMT. Tumor lysis syndrome, marrow infusion nephrotoxicity, hepatorenallike syndrome caused by venoocclusive disease of the liver, and HUS are discussed in detail. Review includes 140 references.

PART 3
Nephropathies of the Nonsteroidal Antiinflammatory Agents

Deepak K. Malhotra and William L. Henrich

The history of nonsteroidal antiinflammatory agents (NSAIAs) is fascinating. The analgesic and antipyretic properties of certain tree barks and plant derivatives have been known for centuries. In fact, it has been suggested that in the fifth century BC, Hippocrates used the bark of willow trees to treat pain and reduce fevers. Salicin was discovered by Leroux in 1827 in the bark of common white willow, *Salix alba vulgaris.* Salicylic acid was synthesized in 1899 by Piria, and Dreser subsequently synthesized acetylsalicylic acid (aspirin). One century later, this compound is widely used not only for its analgesic, antiinflammatory, and antipyretic properties but also for its ability to inhibit platelet aggregation. Because of aspirin's success, newer and more potent nonsteroidal compounds have been developed to treat rheumatologic diseases and pain associated with other conditions. Table 47.6 lists several commonly used NSAIAs, and the list is growing. It is estimated that 30 to 40 million people in the United States use an NSAIA on a daily basis. Several of these newer agents are available over the counter (e.g., ibuprofen, ketoprofen, and naproxen), enabling millions more to use these agents occasionally as needed.

The precise mechanisms by which these agents relieve pain and reduce inflammation are not known. The prostaglandin system clearly is a major pathway that leads to inflammation and is blocked by use of the NSAIAs. The prostaglandin system was described and isolated in the 1930s, and Bergstrom was able to synthesize several products of the pathway two decades later. In 1971 Vane and associates noted that aspirin inhibited the cyclooxygenation of arachidonic acid. Cyclooxygenase is an enzyme that metabolizes arachidonic acid to various prostaglandin metabolites and compounds. The pharmacologic activity of the NSAIAs involves cyclooxygenase inhibition (Fig. 47.1).

TABLE 47.6. Types of Nonsteroidal Antiinflammatory Agents

Salicylates
Aspirin
Choline magnesium trisalicylate
Diflunisal
Other Agents
Diclofenac
Etodolac
Fenoprofen
Ibuprofen[a]
Indomethacin
Ketoprofen[a]
Ketorolac
Meclofenamate
Mefenamic acid
Nabumetone
Naproxen[a]
Piroxicam
Sulindac
Tolmetin

[a] Available over the counter.

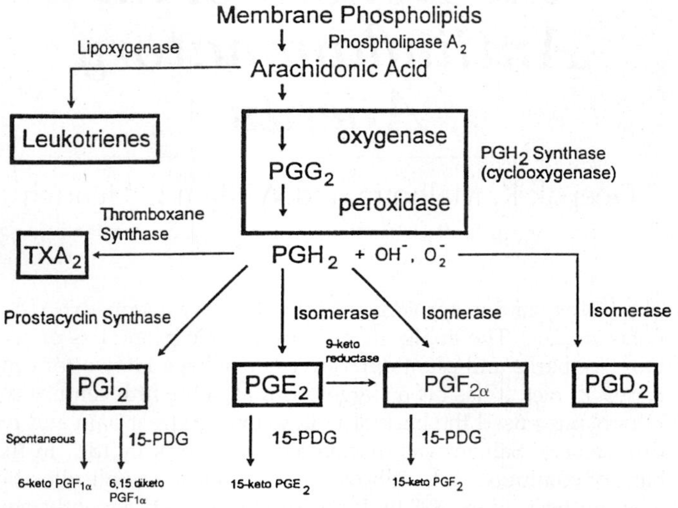

Figure 47.1. Schematic diagram illustrating the production and degradation of various prostaglandins from arachidonic acid. Cyclooxygenase catalyzes the early conversion from arachidonic acid and is blocked by the nonsteroidal antiinflammatory agents. (Reproduced with permission from Palmer BF, Henrich WL. Systemic complications of nonsteroidal antiinflammatory drug use. *Adv Intern Med* 1996;41:605–639.)

The most common toxicities associated with NSAIAs involve the gastrointestinal tract. In particular, ulcers and gastritis that result in gastrointestinal bleeding follow NSAIA ingestion in some cases. The mechanism whereby this occurs is linked to inhibition of protective prostaglandins in the stomach. Endoscopic evaluation of patients using NSAIAs at full dosages have noted that about 30% are normal, 50% have erosions or petechiae, and 5% to 30% have ulcers. The frequency with which these latter lesions result in clinically significant bleeding is unknown.

The effects of NSAIAs on other molecular systems and cellular membrane functions are unclear. With cyclooxygenase inhibition by NSAIAs, arachidonic acid metabolites may be shunted to the lipoxygenase pathway in which polyenoic acids including leukotrienes are produced. In addition, cyclooxygenase activity inhibition may result in the release of lysosomal enzymes and

TABLE 47.7. Nephrotoxicities Associated with Nonsteroidal Antiinflammatory Agents

Acute renal failure (usually reversible)
Tubulointerstitial nephritis (with or without nephrotic syndrome and renal insufficiency)
Papillary necrosis
Hypertension
Hyperkalemia
Salt and water retention

the production of oxygen free radicals. Each of these effects alone or in combination may contribute to the nephrotoxicity associated with NSAIAs. Although NSAIAs have been used for many years, the renal toxicity of these agents was not fully recognized until the late 1970s. The actual incidence of renal toxicity is not known precisely, but it is probably low. However, because of the large size of the population using these agents, nephrotoxic sequela from the drugs are not uncommon.

In both hospitalized and nonhospitalized patients, acute renal failure provoked by NSAIAs is the most common renal toxicity. The acute renal failure ranges from mild to severe in intensity, and hyperkalemia may or may not be present. The renal failure usually is reversible upon discontinuation of the NSAIAs, but a permanent decrement in renal function is possible. Patients often are asymptomatic; in some a mild decrease in urine output with a slight weight gain may occur. Therefore, mild cases of acute renal failure are easily overlooked unless a laboratory examination has been performed (i.e., serum creatinine assessment). The several different types of nephrotoxicities (Table 47.7) associated with the NSAIAs are discussed in the sections that follow.

HEMODYNAMICALLY INDUCED ACUTE RENAL FAILURE

The acute renal failure caused by NSAIAs is uncommon in the general population. In general, patients who have decreased intravascular volume or intrinsic renal disease are at increased risk for this condition. Understanding the causes of the acute renal dysfunction secondary to NSAIAs entails some understanding of prostaglandin physiology. The main categories of renal prostaglandins are prostacyclin (PGI_2), thromboxane (TXA_2), and PGE_2 (Fig. 47.2). It should be noted that prostaglandins exert a local influence (in close proximity to the region of synthesis) rather than distally (as a hormone does). Thus these molecules are designated as autocoids. PGE_2 and PGF_2 are synthesized by interstitial cells, and PGI_2 is synthesized by cortical arterioles and glomeruli. Both PGE_2 and PGI_2 are produced by the glomeruli.

Prostaglandins are central to maintaining adequate blood flow to the kidney under conditions of hypotension or volume depletion. In normal, euvolemic conditions, endogenous prostaglandin synthesis proceeds at a low rate. Prostaglandin synthesis increases under conditions in which extracellular volume declines and blood pressure is threatened (Fig. 47.2). In these situations, prostaglandins exhibit a vasodilatory, moderating influence to maintain renal blood flow and glomerular filtration rate (GFR). In these circumstances, elevated concentrations of vasoconstrictive peptides (e.g., angiotensin II and vasopressin) exist. Vasopressin and angiotensin II directly stimulate renal prostaglandin synthesis and release, thereby promoting the formation of their own antagonist. Similarly, other vasoconstrictors such as norepinephrine, endothelin, and β-adrenergic nerve stimulation also induce synthesis of the vasodilating prostaglandins. Because the effects of renal prostaglandins are to modulate the vasoconstrictor actions of peptides, inhibiting the prostaglandin system with an NSAIA sharply enhances the vasoconstrictor activity in the renal circulation, and renal blood flow and GFR decrease. A detailed discussion of the physiology of prostaglandins and their interactions with the kidney is found in Chapter 13, Part 1.

Clinical situations with increased prostaglandin activity are those associated with decreased extracellular fluid volume or effective extracellular volume and increased vasoconstrictor activity, including congestive heart failure, cirrhosis, nephrotic syndrome, some forms of hypertension, sepsis, anesthesia, and volume depletion (e.g., caused by blood loss, diuretics, or diarrhea). In addition, patients with chronic renal insufficiency may need increased prostaglandin activity to maintain renal blood flow and GFR. Therefore, administering NSAIAs in these conditions creates a condition in which unopposed vasoconstrictor activity causes decrements in renal blood flow and GFR. It has been estimated that as many as 30% of patients with chronic renal insufficiency develop an acute decrease in renal function when treated with NSAIAs. In addition, some older adults often have a decrease in renal mass as well as a tenuous intravascular volume. Thus a higher percentage of these patients may be at increased risk for acute renal failure as a result of NSAIA therapy. Another situation that may contribute to NSAIA nephrotoxicity is decreased albumin binding sites. Generally, NSAIAs are bound to albumin, and hypoalbuminemia, caused by decreased nutrition, nephrotic syndrome, or cirrhosis, results in a higher concentration of free drug in the circulation and consequently a potentially greater pharmacologic effect.

Combinations of several commonly used drugs with NSAIAs can impair kidney function. Cyclosporine and tacrolimus are immunosuppressive agents effective in preventing rejection of transplanted organs and treating autoimmune diseases. These agents induce renal vasoconstriction as part of their nephrotoxicity. NSAIAs in combination with either of these immunosuppressive agents can further compromise renal blood flow and induce further GFR reductions. In addition, angiotensin-converting enzyme inhibitors and angiotensin II–receptor blockers are used in many clinical situations including the treatment of hypertension, congestive heart failure, and nephrotic syndrome. These agents preferentially produce efferent arteriolar dilation. Concomitant use of an NSAIA (which causes afferent arteriolar vasoconstriction) may result in a loss of glomerular filtration pressure and a decline in GFR.

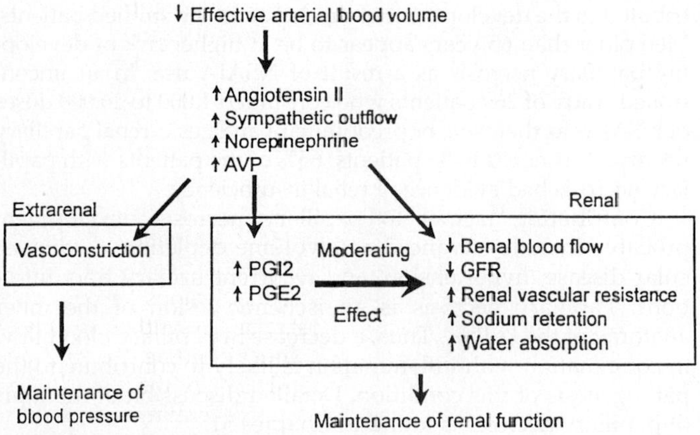

Figure 47.2. Schema depicting alterations in renal blood flow. The decrease in extracellular volume or decrease in effective extracellular volume increases angiotensin II, norepinephrine, and vasopressin *(AVP)* levels and sympathetic outflow. These factors are vasoconstrictive; however, they also induce synthesis of renal prostaglandins, which moderate the decreases in renal blood flow and glomerular filtration rate *(GFR)*. (Reproduced with permission from Palmer BF, Henrich WL. Systemic complications of nonsteroidal antiinflammatory drug use. *Adv Intern Med* 1996;41:605–639.)

TABLE 47.8. Patients at Risk for Developing Acute Hemodynamic Renal Failure with Nonsteroidal Antiinflammatory Agent Use

Patients with ineffective circulating blood volume or renal perfusion
Congestive heart failure
Cirrhosis with ascites
Hypotensive hemorrhage
Severe burns
Recent surgery or illness
Decreased blood volume (e.g., diuretics, diarrhea, gastrointestinal losses)
Patients with underlying renal disease

Intrauterine or postnatal exposure to NSAIAs (via breast milk, parentally to treat patent ductus arteriosus, or orally for various reasons) can lead to prostaglandin synthesis inhibition. This may lead to acute renal failure, salt and water retention, and hyperkalemia in the fetus or child.

In summary, prostaglandins in the kidney behave as autocoids to modulate the effects of vasoconstrictors and vasoconstrictive states. Blocking the production of prostaglandins by NSAIAs allows the vasoconstrictive state to be unopposed and thereby decreases renal blood flow and GFR. In euvolemic states, the endogenous prostaglandin synthesis is low, and prostaglandin system inhibition does not result in a decrease in renal blood flow. Patient groups at risk for the hemodynamic acute renal failure associated with NSAIAs are shown in Table 47.8.

Other Hemodynamically Induced Acute Renal Failure

Other mechanisms affecting renal hemodynamics have been postulated to occur with NSAIA therapy. One such proposed schema reasons that nonenzymatic metabolism of arachidonic acid leads to PGF_2-like products. This occurs via peroxidation of arachidonic acid by oxygen free radicals. The free radicals may be induced with acute injury such as ischemia. The PGF_2-like molecules are vasoconstrictors. If an NSAIA is present that blocks cyclooxygenase, a lower amount of the vasodilator PGI_2 is produced and a greater amount of arachidonic acid is available for peroxidation by the oxygen free radicals. Consequently, the vasoconstrictor activity is unopposed. This situation is more likely to occur in patients with renal insufficiency caused by ischemia or inflammation.

TUBULOINTERSTITIAL NEPHRITIS

Tubulointerstitial nephritis associated with NSAIAs presents in several ways. The most common is tubulointerstitial nephritis with the nephrotic syndrome and renal insufficiency. Less commonly noted are tubulointerstitial nephritis with the nephrotic syndrome without renal insufficiency and tubulointerstitial nephritis without the nephrotic syndrome with renal insufficiency (Table 47.9).

The tubulointerstitial nephritis caused by NSAIAs is different from that associated with other medications such as methicillin. In general, the interstitial nephritis associated with NSAIAs is not associated with fever, rash, eosinophilia, or eosinophiluria

TABLE 47.9. Presentation of Tubulointerstitial Nephritis

Tubulointerstitial nephritis with nephrotic syndrome with renal insufficiency (most common presentation)
Tubulointerstitial nephritis with nephrotic syndrome without renal insufficiency
Tubulointerstitial nephritis without nephrotic syndrome with renal insufficiency

TABLE 47.10. Clinical Presentation of Tubulointerstitial Nephritis

	Nonsteroidal Antiinflammatory Agent	Allergic Cause
Nephrotic syndrome	>80%	<5%
Fever	<5%	>80%
Rash	Not reported	>20%
Eosinophilia	10%	>80%
Eosinophiluria	Not reported	>50%
Hematuria	>50%	>80%
Leukocyturia	>50%	>80%
Duration of drug exposure	0.5–18 mo	2–37 days

(Table 47.10). The duration of drug exposure generally is much longer in the NSAIA type than in allergic tubulointerstitial nephritis.

Tubulointerstitial nephritis associated with the nephrotic syndrome is a unique finding associated with NSAIAs. This syndrome has been reported with nearly all NSAIAs; however, the propionic acid derivatives of NSAIAs (fenoprofen, ibuprofen, and naproxen) have been implicated most often in this complication. Patients believed to be at higher risk for developing this difficulty are those with diabetes mellitus, advanced age, hypertension, concomitant diuretic therapy, and history of episodes of tubulointerstitial nephritis with another NSAIA.

In the nephrotic syndrome associated with tubulointerstitial nephritis from NSAIAs, the kidney shows both glomerular and interstitial changes. The proximal and distal tubules show vacuolization and degeneration. The interstitium may contain a focal or diffuse predominantly lymphocytic infiltrate. In the few specimens studied, the infiltrate is composed of T cells. The glomeruli by light and fluorescence microscopy appear normal. However, electron microscopy reveals foot process fusion (i.e., the finding of minimal-change disease).

The actual pathogenesis of the tubulointerstitial nephritis occurring with NSAIAs probably is multifactorial. The process appears to be isolated to the kidney because there do not appear to be signs of a systemic hypersensitivity reaction. A primary T-cell disorder or a delayed hypersensitivity reaction may be responsible for this process. It has been proposed that noncyclooxygenase products of the arachidonic acid cascade may contribute to this phenomenon. For instance, arachidonic acid may be shunted via the lipoxygenase pathway to produce leukotrienes. Leukotrienes are proinflammatory and increase vascular permeability. They also act as chemotactic substances to attract white blood cells, thus causing the glomeruli to become leaky, allowing proteins to be filtered, and attracting inflammatory cells into the interstitium.

A diagnosis of NSAIA-induced tubulointerstitial nephritis should be entertained in a patient with a decrease in renal function taking an NSAIA in which the urine sediment contains pyuria, hematuria, and proteinuria. As noted earlier, renal function may not be reduced and the amount of proteinuria is variable. A renal biopsy may be indicated if the condition continues to worsen after the drug is discontinued and the diagnosis remains in doubt. The prognosis of NSAIA-induced tubulointerstitial nephritis, with or without the nephrotic syndrome, is good. Renal function usually recovers and the nephrotic syndrome abates once the offending agent has been stopped. However, in some patients the disease has not been reversible and dialysis therapy has been needed.

Interestingly, NSAIA agents have been used in many patients to help treat the consequences of the nephrotic syndrome resulting from other causes. Because these agents decrease renal blood flow and GFR, the amount of filtered protein is limited. Obviously, NSAIAs should be used cautiously in this setting because the number of albumin-binding sites for the NSAIAs is decreased and more of the unbound drug are pharmacologically available.

Finally, it should be acknowledged that there are several reports in the literature of nephrotic syndrome in the absence of tubulointerstitial nephritis. Most often in these cases, the renal histology is consistent with minimal-change disease, but some reports have made an association between membranous nephropathy and NSAIA use. This association between NSAIA use and isolated glomerular disease is less common than the tubulointerstitial lesion; treatment consists of discontinuing the drug and using glucocorticoids if symptoms persist or renal function deteriorates.

PAPILLARY NECROSIS

Papillary necrosis has been associated with the habitual consumption of combination analgesic medications. The term given to this disorder is *analgesic nephropathy.* Phenacetin has been seen classically as the primary culprit in generating this lesion, but this supposition has been challenged recently. Animal and human studies have supported the concept that papillary necrosis can result from NSAIAs alone or in combination with other analgesic agents.

The precise incidence of papillary necrosis in patients taking NSAIAs is not known. Autopsy studies of patients treated with NSAIAs for rheumatoid arthritis have shown this lesion to be present in 18% to 57%. However, other factors may have contributed to the development of this lesion in the studied patients. Men older than 65 years appear to be at higher risk of developing papillary necrosis as a result of NSAIA use. In an uncontrolled study of 269 patients who consumed 1,000 to 26,000 doses of NSAIAs as their sole or predominant analgesic, renal papillary necrosis was noted in 38 patients; 65% of the patients with papillary necrosis had evidence of renal insufficiency.

Contributing factors to papillary necrosis development probably include advanced age, volume depletion, cardiovascular disease, hypertension, and recurrent urinary tract infections. Papillary necrosis is an ischemic lesion of the inner anatomy of the kidney. Thus, a decrease in papillary blood flow in combination with inflammation is likely to contribute to the pathogenesis of this condition. Detailed discussion of the topic of papillary necrosis is found in Chapter 51.

SODIUM RETENTION, POTASSIUM RETENTION, AND HYPERTENSION

PGE_2 inhibits sodium chloride reabsorption in the thick ascending loop of Henle and in the collecting tubule. PGE_2 also antagonizes the antidiuretic effect of vasopressin. Therefore inhibition of prostaglandin synthesis would be expected to result in salt and water retention. A net retention of approximately 0.5 to 1.0 L ensues in up to 25% of patients using NSAIAs. Although the fluid retention is transient in most, large fluid gains have been documented in a few patients. NSAIAs also can antagonize the action of loop and thiazide diuretics. This effect could cause a compensated patient taking a diuretic to retain sodium and decompensate; patients with congestive heart failure are vulnerable to this effect.

Hyperkalemia has been noted in patients taking NSAIAs with or without antecedent renal disease. The serum potassium concentration is disproportionately high for the GFR reduction or degree of acidemia. In patients with normal renal function, hyperkalemia may result from prostaglandin inhibition. Prostaglandins have been identified as necessary for baroreceptor-mediated renal renin release. Thus NSAIA use may inhibit renin release from the juxtaglomerular cells, and a hyporeninemic state may develop. Angiotensin II formation then decreases in turn, as does aldosterone secretion. Therefore a hyporenin–hypoaldosterone state occurs and potassium excretion is diminished despite rising potassium levels. Patients who have a hyporenin–hypoaldosterone state caused by other conditions such as diabetes mellitus are at a higher risk of worsening the hyperkalemia with NSAIA therapy.

NSAIAs can also increase both diastolic and systolic blood pressure. In most large studies an increase 6 to 8 mm Hg is noted depending on the type, dosage, and duration of NSAIA therapy. The increase in blood pressure is noted in patients who are hypertensive; normotensive patients are far less likely to exhibit an increase in blood pressure. Patients taking β-receptor antagonists or diuretics for hypertension appear to be more susceptible to an increase in blood pressure with NSAIA therapy than those taking calcium channel blockers, clonidine, or direct vasodilators. NSAIAs do not appear to antagonize the hypotensive activity of angiotensin-converting enzyme inhibitors. In fact, the combination of NSAIAs and angiotensin-converting enzyme inhibitors has been used to reduce the complications of the nephrotic syndrome. However, as noted earlier, this combination of drugs has been associated with acute renal failure. Moreover, using an angiotensin-converting enzyme inhibitor and an NSAIA combines two drugs known to reduce renal potassium excretion. Therefore serum potassium and renal function should be monitored carefully in patients taking this combination, particularly if underlying renal insufficiency is present.

The cause of the increase in blood pressure is not known. Salt and water retention probably augments hypertension development. The decrease in vasodilator prostaglandins also may be a contributing factor.

Physicians and patients must remain aware of the possible loss of blood pressure control with NSAIA use. Several NSAIAs are available over the counter, and patients may not realize the potential for drug interactions.

IS THERE A SAFE NSAIA?

Sulindac initially was reported as an NSAIA with less nephrotoxicity. It was believed that this drug spared renal prostaglandin synthesis because it is converted from a prodrug to an active form by the liver. However, via mixed function oxidases the kidney also can activate the prodrug. It should be noted that vasomotor renal insufficiency and hyperkalemia have been reported with sulindac. Hence, the same precautions for all NSAIAs should be applied to sulindac.

Two isoforms of the cyclooxygenase enzyme have been identified that participate in prostaglandin synthesis: cyclooxygenase 1 and 2 (COX-1 and COX-2, respectively). COX-1 is present in nearly all tissues. Its major function involves homeostatic regulation. It is present in platelets to allow TXA_2 synthesis, and it is also present in the kidney and stomach to counteract vasoconstrictive stimuli. COX-2 is induced with inflammation and therefore is of central importance in developing pain and inflammation. Clinical trials have shown that inhibitors of the COX-2 isoform reduce inflammation in patients with arthritis. One of the COX-2 inhibitors (celacoxib) recently was approved by the U.S. Food and Drug Administration. These selective COX-2 inhibitors are appealing because they would reduce the formation of prostaglandins involved in inflammation but not perturb the prostaglandin system that provides cytoprotection in the gastrointestinal tract (the COX-1 system). Preliminary reports using COX-2 inhibitors have been encouraging in terms of preventing gastritis and ulcers. COX-2 also is present in the macula densa and interstitial cells of the medulla of the kidney. However, it remains to be determined whether these agents are associated with less nephrotoxicity because some reports of nephrotoxicity have emerged from the early trials with these drugs. More investigation is needed to determine the precise incidence and type of nephrotoxicity with COX-2 inhibitors. COX-2 also has effects on renal renin release, and it may promote renin release in response to low extracellular volume. Again, more research is needed to clarify this point.

Selected Readings

Abraham PA, Keane WF. Glomerular and interstitial disease induced by nonsteroidal anti-inflammatory drugs. *Am J Nephrol* 1984;4:1–6.

Editorial review and original report of 36 patients with glomerular and interstitial nephritis with NSAIA use.

DuBois RN, Abramson SB, Crofford L, et al. Cyclooxygenase in biology and disease. *FASEB J* 1998;12:1063–1073.

Recent review of the physiology of the cyclooxygenase (COX-1 and COX-2) enzyme system in normal and diseased states.

Harding P, Sigmon DH, Alfie ME, et al. Cyclooxygenase-2 mediates increased renal renin content induced by low-sodium diet. *Hypertension* 1997;29(2):297–302.

Study noting that the COX-2 is induced and participates in renin release with low salt intake in mice.

Kimmey MB. NSAID, ulcers, and prostaglandins. *J Rheumatol* 1992;19(Suppl 36):68–73.

Mechanisms of injury to the gastrointestinal tract mucosa by NSAIAs are reviewed.

Nadler JL, Lee FO, Hsueh W, et al. Evidence of prostacyclin deficiency in the syndrome of hyporeninemic hypoaldosteronism. *N Engl J Med* 1986;314:1015–1020.

Seven patients with hyporeninemic hypoaldosteronism were examined for urinary prostacyclin metabolite excretion and compared with normal controls and patients with chronic renal failure.

Palmer BF, Henrich WL. Systemic complications of nonsteroidal anti-inflammatory drug use. *Adv Intern Med* 1996;41:605–639.

Review of NSAIA use with emphasis on gastrointestinal and renal complications.

Perico N, Remuzzi A, Sangalli F, et al. The antiproteinuric effect of angiotensin antagonism in human IgA nephropathy is potentiated by indomethacin. *J Am Soc Nephrol* 1998;9:2308–2317.

The reduction in proteinuria with the combination of an angiotensin-converting enzyme inhibitor or an angiotensin II–blocking agent with an NSAIA is examined. The patients in this short-term study had various degrees of proteinuria caused by IgA nephropathy.

Pope JE, Anderson JJ, Felson DT. A meta-analysis of the effects nonsteroidal anti-inflammatory drugs on blood pressure. *Arch Intern Med* 1993;153:477–484.

A large meta-analysis examining the relationships of NSAIAs and blood pressure regulation.

Schlondorff D. Renal complications of nonsteroidal anti-inflammatory drugs. *Kidney Int* 1993;44:643–653.

Editorial review of the hemodynamic alterations induced in the kidney with NSAIAs.

Simon LS, Lanza FL, Lipsky PE, et al. Preliminary study of the safety and efficacy of SC-58635, a novel cyclooxygenase 2 inhibitor: efficacy and safety in two placebo-controlled trials in osteoarthritis and rheumatoid arthritis, and studies of gastrointestinal and platelet effects. *Arthritis Rheum* 1998;41:1591–1602.

Study of the efficacy of celecoxib, a COX-2 inhibitor. Primarily gastrointestinal toxicities were addressed.

PART 4
Nephropathies of Heavy Metal Intoxication

Harvey C. Gonick

Exposure to heavy metals produces various renal abnormalities. They include renal tubular dysfunction, primarily proximal, associated with chronic tubulointerstitial disease; oliguric acute renal failure; nephrotic syndrome; renal tubular dysfunction with little or no associated structural damage; chronic tubulointerstitial disease without associated tubular dysfunction; and excess metal deposition with little apparent functional or structural changes. These syndromes and the various heavy metals producing them are listed in Table 47.11. The toxic effect of the heavy metals can be modified by the organism's ability to synthesize metalloproteins in response to repeated administration of sublethal amounts of such elements. For example, cadmium administration causes the de novo synthesis of a metalloprotein named metallothionein, a low-molecular-weight (10,000 D) protein with a high sulfhydryl content, principally as cysteine. This metalloprotein is known to play an important role in the transport, organ selectivity, and detoxification of cadmium. An epidemiologic case control study has focused on occupational factors for chronic renal failure development. Increased risks of renal failure were found in workers exposed to lead, copper, chromium, tin, mercury, and silicon.

TABLE 47.11. Nephrotoxicity Syndromes Produced by Heavy Metals

Renal tubular dysfunction associated with chronic tubulointerstitial disease
Bismuth
Cadmium
Chromium
Copper
Iron
Lead
Mercury
Platinum
Uranium
Oliguric acute renal failure
Arsenic
Bismuth
Cadmium
Chromium
Copper
Gold
Iron
Lead
Mercury
Silver
Uranium
Nephrotic syndrome
Bismuth
Gold
Mercury
Lithium
Renal tubular dysfunction with little or no structural damage
Lithium
Chronic tubulointerstitial disease without tubular dysfunction
Silicon
Excess metal deposition with little functional or structural change
Silver

The characteristics of the renal lesion shared by chronic exposure to several heavy metals, including cadmium, lead, mercury, and uranium, are interstitial nephritis, selective binding by the metal to the proximal tubule, and a generalized disturbance of proximal tubular function (Fanconi's syndrome). In addition to aminoaciduria, renal tubular abnormalities include glucosuria, impaired concentrating ability, hypercalciuria, increased uric acid clearance, impaired acid excretion and hyperchloremic acidosis, and lysozymuria. Proteinuria, when present, is predominantly tubular rather than glomerular. Tubular proteinuria has been characterized by standard electrophoresis as consisting of a small albumin fraction and large α_2-, β-, and γ-globulin fractions and by ultracentrifugation, column gel filtration, or polyacrylamide gel electrophoresis as low-molecular-weight proteinuria. A radioimmunoassay developed for one of the low-molecular-weight proteins, β_2-microglobulin, has proved to be a useful screening test for detecting subtle renal damage produced by exposure to cadmium or mercury because the elevation in β_2-microglobulin excretion in these disorders is much more striking than the usually determined proteinuria.

NEPHROTOXICITY OF SPECIFIC HEAVY METALS

Cadmium

Nephrotoxicity caused by cadmium has been described in settings of industrial exposure and environmental pollution. Cadmium, a metal ordinarily obtained as a byproduct of zinc refining, is used industrially in the plating for steel, in pigments, plastics, alloys, and accumulator batteries, and in nuclear and electronic engineering. Because the biologic half-life of cadmium is long (more than 30 years), prolonged low-level exposure leads to excessive accumulation in certain tissues, with the kidney holding about one-third of the total body burden. Studies of cadmium toxicity have been performed in the accumulator battery industry, the copper–cadmium alloy industry, and cadmium pigment factories. Chronic poisoning typically was found to have occurred after several years of exposure and was characterized clinically by variable features of nasorespiratory involvement (emphysema, rhinitis, ulceration of nasal mucosa, and anosmia) and by renal tubular dysfunction. Yellow tooth discoloration, mild anemia, and disturbances in calcium metabolism (hypercalciuria, osteomalacia, and renal calculi) also were observed occasionally.

Clinically detectable proteinuria (i.e., by the sulfosalicylic or heat and acetic acid test) is not seen until at least 9 and more commonly 25 years of exposure. Initially, the proteinuria was thought to be exclusively of tubular origin (i.e., low molecular weight). Indeed, when sensitive tests for low-molecular-weight proteinuria were used (electrophoresis, immunoassays for β_2-microglobulin, α_1-microglobulin, and retinol binding protein, or enzymatic tests for lysozyme or ribonuclease), these tests were positive in workers with lesser degrees of exposure in whom clinical proteinuria was absent. Later it was found in both workers and experimental animals exposed to cadmium that the proteinuria is a mixed type, with increased excretion of both high- and low-molecular-weight proteins, indicative of both glomerular protein loss and decreased tubular reabsorption. Another low-molecular-weight protein, metallothionein, which is produced in response to the cadmium exposure, also is excreted in increased quantities when the body burden of cadmium exceeds a threshold limit. The latter is defined as a urinary cadmium level greater than 10 μg/g creatinine, although *in vivo* measurement of liver cadmium content by neutron activation analysis may yield a more precise definition. Urinary excretion of *N*-acetyl-β-D-glucosaminidase (NAG), with a molecular weight of 120,000 D, also has been reported to increase in humans exposed to cadmium. This is a lysosomal enzyme present in high concentrations in the proximal tubule. Because of its high molecular weight, its urinary origin is unlikely to occur via glomerular sieving but rather directly from damaged kidney tissue. Urinary NAG has been found to be elevated when urinary cadmium is below the threshold of 10 μg/g creatinine. Three thresholds have been noted: the first around 2 μg/g creatinine (associated with biochemical alterations), the second around 4 μg/g creatinine for high-molecular-weight proteins and some tubular antigens, and the third at 10 μg/g creatinine for low-molecular-weight proteins. Other indices of cadmium-induced renal dysfunction include increased excretion of tubular brush border antigens, thromboxane B, intestinal alkaline phosphatase, prostanoids, and glycosaminoglycans. The proteinuria induced by cadmium has been found to be irreversible, in general, even several years after cadmium exposure. However, microproteinuria may be reversible in some workers whose urinary cadmium exceeds the threshold of 10 μg/g creatinine but whose initial microproteinuria is mild (between 300 and 1,500 μg/g creatinine). The findings of generalized proximal tubular dysfunction are limited to workers with either clinically overt or subclinical tubular proteinuria.

Glomerular filtration rate (GFR) impairment was not reported in early studies of cadmium workers. However, studies from Belgium found that workers with prolonged exposure (mean 25 years) show a significant increase in serum creatinine and β_2-microglobulin with time, even when the effect of aging is factored in. The authors of the study suggest that prolonged cadmium exposure exacerbates the age-related decline in GFR. When these investigators assessed the filtration reserve capacity of the kidney (defined as the difference between baseline creatinine clearance and creatinine clearance after an acute oral load of protein), they found that cadmium workers with low-molecular-weight proteinuria had both diminished GFR and diminished filtration reserve capacity, whereas workers below age 50 without low-molecular-weight proteinuria showed neither abnormality. Although experimental evidence in rats has linked cadmium to hypertension, there is no conclusive evidence of such as an association in humans. Mortality studies from cadmium-polluted areas in Europe and Japan have demonstrated that mortality rates for nephritis and nephrosis are higher than in control areas, although no increase in the incidence of cardiovascular deaths has been reported.

The best characterized example of intoxication of a large population by environmental exposure to cadmium is *itai-itai byo*, or "ouch-ouch" disease, so named because of the crippling and painful osteomalacic component. The disease was endemic in the Jinzu River basin of the Toyama prefecture in Japan, with peak incidence shortly after World War II, and was attributable to cadmium overload. The soil and the rice fields contained large amounts of cadmium brought with the irrigation water from a polluted river. Autopsies of five patients with *itai-itai* revealed that the cadmium content of liver was 5 to 10 times higher than in age-matched controls, but the kidney values were lower than in the controls because kidney damage was present. A decrease in kidney cortex cadmium occurs with advancing age and with kidney disease of varying causes; this is consistent with a decreased metallothionein content of the kidney cortex under these conditions.

The typical patient with *itai-itai* disease was a middle-aged postmenopausal multiparous woman who had lumbar pains, leg myalgia, and ducklike gait. Pressure on bones, especially the femurs, spine, and ribs, aggravated the pain. Pseudofractures were seen on radiographic examination, and typical findings of osteomalacia were found on bone examination. Serum 1,25-dihydroxyvitamin D (1α,25(OH)$_2$D) levels were decreased and were closely related to serum concentrations of parathyroid hormone (PTH), β_2-microglobulin, and renal tubular phosphate reabsorption. Quantitative histomorphometric measurements have been consistent with the clinical impression of osteomalacia. An interesting finding was the presence of iron at mineralization fronts, detected by radiographic microanalysis, suggesting a possible synergistic adverse effect between iron and cadmium on bone mineralization. Renal findings in these patients included low-molecular-weight proteinuria, glucosuria, aminoaciduria, decreased tubular phosphorus reabsorption, low phenolsulfonphthalein excretion, and diminished concentrating ability; renal failure occurred in a few. In advanced cases, the kidneys were found to be contracted. Histologically, the kidneys showed tubular atrophy and dilation, eosinophilic casts, and interstitial fibrosis; glomeruli were normal.

Although the numbers of reported patients with full-blown *itai-itai* disease have been small and limited primarily to women, an epidemiologic survey revealed that about 45% of women and 40% of men older than 70 in the endemic area had concomitant proteinuria and glucosuria. Because the incidence of such abnormalities in younger subjects was not different from that seen in people living in a nonendemic control area, it appears that tubular dysfunctions resulted either from the protracted exposure to cadmium from an early age or from some feature of aging.

Environmental exposure to lower levels of cadmium also can pose a health risk. An epidemiologic survey of 2,327 subjects in two urban and two rural areas in Belgium with different environmental pollution by cadmium revealed a probability of tubular dysfunction of 10% when urinary cadmium levels reached 2 μg/day. There was a statistically significant dose–response relationship between the urinary cadmium excretion and five effect parameters: urinary excretion of retinol-binding protein, β_2-microglobulin, NAG, amino acids, and calcium. No statistical association was found between environmental exposure to cadmium and blood pressure elevation.

Experimental work in rabbits, rats, and mice indicates that renal functional or morphologic changes appear only after the cadmium concentration in renal cortex reaches saturation levels of about 200 to 400 ppm wet weight (approximately 100 times normal). Repeated intraperitoneal cadmium administration in small dosages to rats produces renal tubular atrophy and interstitial fibrosis, and the first pathologic alterations in cadmium-treated rabbits are seen in the proximal tubular epithelial cells. Cadmium is deposited chiefly in the renal cortex and is localized mainly in the proximal segment of the tubules. The metal deposits and renal tubular changes persist for several weeks after cessation of cadmium injections. Of particular interest is the observation that there is a long delay between initiation of cadmium injections in experimental animals and the first appearance of tubular dysfunction and increased urinary cadmium excretion. Anemia in rats appears to be related to messenger ribonucleic acid (mRNA) hypoinduction for erythropoietin in the kidneys.

The role of metallothionein, a low-molecular-weight cadmium-binding protein, is central to an understanding of cadmium nephrotoxicity. The purified protein was named metallothionein because of its high content of sulfur and metals, chiefly cadmium and zinc. Metallothionein appears to be synthesized mainly in response to exposure to cadmium and zinc. Metallothionein synthesis probably occurs through formation of a specific mRNA because both cycloheximide and actinomycin D, administered concomitantly with cadmium, block the incorporation of [^{3}H] cystine into cadmium-binding protein. Metallothionein can act as a transport protein, as well as a storage protein, for cadmium. When cadmium is injected together with metallothionein, there is selective deposition of cadmium in the kidney, and the renal tubular damage produced is greater than that seen when cadmium is given alone. The increased renal damage can be attributed to the much more profound uptake of cadmium by the kidney when cadmium is given as metallothionein rather than free cadmium. The critical concentration of cadmium–metallothionein in kidney is 10 μg/g, in contrast to that of inorganic cadmium (130 to 200 μg/g). These observations are in accord with suggestions that cadmium bound to metallothionein is preferentially filtered through the glomeruli and subsequently reabsorbed and stored in the tubules or enters the renal tubule directly from the peritubular capillaries. Zinc–metallothionein, in contrast to cadmium–metallothionein, is nontoxic when given in comparable dosage and appears to exert a protective effect against cadmium–metallothionein-induced nephrotoxicity.

In an experimental model of cadmium-induced Fanconi's syndrome achieved by repetitive intraperitoneal administration of cadmium chloride in adult rats, glucosuria and aminoaciduria were noted to appear abruptly after 3 weeks of injections, and the complete expression of the Fanconi's syndrome (i.e., diuresis, glucosuria, aminoaciduria, proteinuria, and increased sodium, potassium, calcium, magnesium, phosphate, and urate clearance) was then elicited. At the peak of Fanconi's syndrome, renal cortical adenosine 5′-triphosphate (ATP) levels were decreased and cortex homogenate Na^+-K^+-ATPase activity was significantly depressed. Ultrastructural changes at this stage paralleled the biochemical findings in that the mitochondria were dramatically altered in size and shape and there was extensive loss of the basal plasma membrane infoldings together with complex cisternal proliferation in proximal tubular cells. The structural and biochemical findings were reversed within 1 week after cessation of cadmium injections despite persistence of total renal cortical cadmium concentration at levels close to 200 ppm wet weight. Analysis of subcellular fractions of the renal cortex revealed cadmium migration from the soluble cytoplasmic fraction (where metallothionein is located) to the mitochondrial fraction and to the microsomal fraction (where Na^+-K^+-ATPase activity is maximal) at the time of appearance of Fanconi's syndrome, with reversal after cadmium injection discontinuation. Microsomal Na^+-K^+-ATPase activity decreased in tandem with the increase in microsomal cadmium concentration, and *in vivo* microsomal Na^+-K^+-ATPase inhibition was found to be precisely that predicted by *in vitro* titration of renal microsomal Na^+-K^+-ATPase with cadmium. When experimental animals were injected with cadmium-109 24 hours before death and kidney cortex soluble cytoplasm was fractionated on Sephadex G-75, the radiolabeled cadmium was found to be associated principally with high-molecular-weight proteins in control animals but with the metallothionein fraction after cadmium injections were begun. At the time of Fanconi's syndrome development, the radiolabeled cadmium was again found mainly in association with the high-molecular-weight proteins. These findings suggest that injected cadmium initially is segregated in a nontoxic complexed form as metallothionein in the cytoplasm of the proximal tubule, but when the organism's capacity to synthesize new metallothionein is exhausted, the cadmium, now less firmly bound to high-molecular-weight proteins, moves to other cell organelles, where the Na^+-K^+-ATPase transport system is affected. As indicated by other studies of experimental Fanconi's syndrome, it is likely that inhibition of this critical enzyme transport system leads to diminished proximal tubular reabsorption of sodium and of substances linked to active sodium transport.

Because of the demonstrated ability of certain heavy metals, such as gold and mercury, to produce an immune complex nephritis, and because of some evidence that cadmium-exposed workers can develop glomerular lesions, studies have been conducted in experimental animals to determine whether cadmium can also induce immune complex nephritis. In one study, oral exposure of rats to either 100 ppm or 200 ppm cadmium chloride in drinking water for 30 weeks resulted in a diffuse membranous glomerulopathy with electron-dense deposits within mesangial cells on electron microscopy and granular dense deposits of immunoglobulin G (IgG) in most glomeruli by immunofluorescence. In another study of rats given 100 ppm cadmium chloride for up to 13 months, about 25% of the rats had IgG glomerular deposits in the mesangial area. At 8 months, the rats had demonstrable circulating antilaminin antibodies, suggesting that cadmium can induce autoantibody formation.

The bone changes produced by cadmium may have a different pathogenesis than the renal lesion. Rats fed low-protein, low-calcium, cadmium-supplemented diets develop abnormal curvature of the spinal column and show diminished density of bone on radiographic examination. Analysis of ashed femurs from these animals revealed higher cadmium content and lower calcium, magnesium, and zinc than in controls. On the other hand, femurs from animals on a high-protein, calcium-sufficient diet supplemented with cadmium showed a higher cadmium content but no reduction in calcium, magnesium, or zinc. These studies suggest that dietary deficiencies could play a contributory role in *itai-itai* disease. In another experimental study in rats fed various amounts of cadmium, bones from the animals were found to show osteoporosis rather than osteomalacia, and the bone lesions preceded the onset of kidney lesions, indicating an effect of cadmium on bone not related to renal dysfunction. In a long-term (16-month) study of ovariectomized rats given low-dose (0.23 mg) cadmium intraperitoneally, decreases in bone mass and increases in fibrous tissue were noted, similar to the changes seen in *itai-itai* disease. The possibility that cadmium interference with vitamin D metabolism might contribute to the bone disease has been pursued in experimental studies. *In vitro*, small amounts of cadmium completely inhibited the renal enzymic 1-hydroxylation reaction of 25-hydroxycholecalciferol. However, the *in vivo* 1-hydroxylation proceeded without significant inhibition even in weanling animals loaded with large amounts of oral cadmium. Cadmium in kidney tissue was found to be mostly protein bound, whereas the majority of the cadmium in bone (80%) was present as free cadmium. It was concluded that the segregation of cadmium by protein binding in the kidney prevents any toxic effect on kidney enzymes but that the high level of free cadmium in bone might exert a direct toxic effect on that organ.

In contrast to the effects of prolonged chronic exposure, acute exposure to cadmium can produce acute renal failure in humans. The accidental poisoning of five construction workers by cadmium fumes while cutting cadmium-plated bolts with an oxyacetylene burner has been reported. All five developed respiratory difficulties, but four eventually recovered. Necropsy in the fatal case revealed bilateral renal cortical necrosis in addition to severe pulmonary edema and alveolar metaplasia of the lung.

Treatment for chronic or acute cadmium nephrotoxicity should be preventive. Once there is demonstrable renal disease, the worker should be removed from all further exposure to cadmium. British antilewisite (BAL) should not be administered because there is evidence that the cadmium–BAL complex is more toxic to the kidney than cadmium alone.

Of the chelating agents tested in experimental animals, after acute oral cadmium intoxication, the most effective in both enhancing survival and leaving minimal residual levels of cadmium in liver and kidney was meso-2,3-dimercaptosuccinic acid (DMSA). Esters of this agent also were effective in removing aged (more than 30 days) cadmium deposits in liver and kidney. At present there is little experience with the use of chelating agents in treating acute or chronic cadmium poisoning in humans.

Lead

Although lead, like cadmium, binds selectively to the proximal tubule and morphologic damage to this segment of the nephron is a major and early sign of lead nephropathy, there are distinctive differences between the clinical pictures produced by these two heavy metals. Fanconi's syndrome has been described in experimental animals and in children but not in adults, with the exception of aminoaciduria in some lead workers. In contrast to the hypouricemia and increased uric acid clearance found in most patients with Fanconi's syndrome, hyperuricemia and decreased uric acid clearance, in some instances associated with clinical gout, have been described in adult lead nephropathy. Another distinctive difference between the nephropathy produced by lead and that produced by cadmium is the presence in proximal tubules of a characteristic nuclear inclusion body, which has been shown to contain lead and a lead-binding protein.

There has been considerable interest in determining the factors that dictate individual susceptibility to lead. One such factor is the inducible 10-kD erythrocyte lead-binding protein found in lead workers, which appears to bind lead in a nontoxic form. A subset of workers who are incapable of responding to lead exposure by mounting a response in the 10-kD lead-binding protein demonstrate evidence of toxicity at low blood lead levels. A similar phenomenon has been described in the genotypic polymorphism of aminolevulinic acid dehydratase (ALAD). The ALAD gene contains two codominant alleles: ALAD-1 and ALAD-2. ALAD-1 is the predominant allele. Workers who are heterozygous or homozygous for ALAD-2 have blood lead values averaging 10 μg/dl higher than those of similarly exposed workers who are homozygous for ALAD-1. The difference apparently results from the greater propensity for ALAD-2 to bind lead in a nontoxic form because of less bone lead, δ-aminolevulinic acid, zinc protoporphyrin, and DMSA-chelatable lead (all markers of lead accumulation or toxicity) response in ALAD-2 patients.

In the early twentieth century, there were several reports of industrially related progressive renal failure from lead poisoning. Initial reports were scanty, suggesting the possibility that improved working conditions and medical surveillance might have aborted the development of significant renal disease. However, a 1968 study of 102 industrially exposed workers in Rumania demonstrated that 17 had evidence of renal impairment when tested by discrete renal function tests such as creatinine clearance or urea clearance. A subsequent epidemiologic survey of American lead workers revealed that after adjustment for the effect of age, there was a direct correlation of both serum creatinine and blood urea nitrogen (BUN) with the length of lead exposure. Another survey of American lead workers in 1979 found that GFR, as measured by iothalamate-125 clearances, was reduced in 21 of 57 lead workers in whom excessive body lead burdens had been shown by the urinary excretion of more than 1,000 μg lead per day during an edetate disodium calcium (calcium EDTA) lead mobilization test. A Swedish study of five lead workers with different periods of lead exposure revealed that despite an abnormal GFR in only one of five, all had abnormal renal biopsies. Proximal tubule nuclear lead inclusion bodies were found in the biopsies of two workers who had less than 1 year's exposure to lead, whereas the biopsies of the three subjects with exposures of 4 to more than 12 years did not contain these inclusions but showed varying degrees of diffuse interstitial or peritubular fibrosis.

The prevalence of lead-induced renal disease may relate to the severity of the body burden of lead. A 1992 survey of 70 active and 30 retired Swedish lead smelter workers found no evidence of renal abnormalities, as measured by plasma creatinine, creatinine clearance, β_2-microglobulin clearance, urinary albumin, or urinary excretion of the enzyme NAG, compared with a control cohort. The mean blood lead values in these workers had gradually diminished from 63 to 34 μg/dl from 1950 to 1987 as controls over lead exposure improved. Although the relationship between body burden of lead and development of chronic lead nephropathy has not been defined strictly, a World Health Organization task group concluded that prolonged lead exposure with blood lead levels greater than 70 μg/dl can result in chronic irreversible nephropathy. Several studies of low lead exposure in industry (blood lead consistently below 60 μg/dl) have failed to show convincing evidence of nephropathy. However, an epidemiologic survey of a Belgian population with known environmental exposure to both lead and cadmium (blood lead range 1.7 to 72.5 μg/dl, geometric mean 11.4 μg/dl) revealed an inverse correlation between blood lead and creatinine clearance after adjustments for age and body mass index. A 10-fold increase in blood lead was associated with a creatinine clearance reduction of 10 to 13 ml/min.

In addition to occupation-related disease, two unusual forms of lead nephropathy have been described in adults, one related to remote childhood lead exposure and the other to illicit moonshine whiskey ingestion. In both situations, there has been a high incidence of saturnine gout. Evidence indicates that a large proportion of the cases of chronic renal failure in adults in Queensland, Australia, was attributable to childhood lead poisoning. There was an unusually high incidence of acute lead poisoning in children around the beginning of the twentieth century related to ingestion of large quantities of lead-based paint, deposited as flakes in the dirt surrounding the verandas of their homes. Twenty or more years later, many of these children developed chronic renal failure, with granulated contracted kidneys. Lead was confirmed as the cause when the bone lead content of these patients with cryptogenic kidney disease was found to be significantly greater than in other patients with chronic nephropathy of recognized cause. Subsequent studies used calcium EDTA to mobilize lead from bone. Urinary lead excretion after 1 g calcium EDTA invariably exceeded 0.6 mg/day in patients with renal insufficiency attributable to childhood lead poisoning, whereas lead excretion was below this figure in normal controls and in the majority of patients with renal insufficiency resulting from causes other than lead. Although the Queensland experience seems incontrovertible, attempts to confirm that childhood plumbism leads to adult chronic renal insufficiency in other parts of the world have been unsuccessful; the difference may lie in the degree of childhood lead exposure or factors influencing the subsequent mobilization of lead from bone. Indeed, in a 50-year follow-up of childhood plumbism in the United States, studies comparing 21 lead-exposed subjects with age-, sex-, race-, and neighborhood-matched controls revealed supranormal creatinine clearance in the lead-exposed subjects, who also had a higher risk of hypertension. On the other hand, a longitudinal study of low-level lead exposure, determined by repetitive blood lead measurements in 459 men during the Normative Aging Study, found that blood lead concentration was significantly and positively associated with serum creatinine concentration; a 10-fold increase in blood lead predicted an increase of 0.08 mg/dl in serum creatinine. Furthermore, there was an acceleration of age-related changes in renal function in association with long-term low lead exposure.

The ability to confirm remote lead exposure has heretofore depended on direct measurements of lead in bone biopsies (because bone is the long-term repository for lead) or on mobilization of lead from bone with the calcium EDTA test. Today, radiographic fluorescence techniques provide a noninvasive method of measuring lead at various bone sites. Both L-line radiographic fluorescence (L-XRF) and K-line radiographic fluorescence (K-XRF) have been used to measure lead at tibial and forefinger sites, representative of cortical bone, and at patellar and calcaneus sites, representative of trabecular bone; most experience to date is with measurements at the midshaft of the tibia. The L-XRF technique uses energy of low penetrating power and measures lead primarily in the outer 0.5 mm of bone. This measurement correlates well with the results of the calcium EDTA mobilization test. On the other hand, K-XRF, which uses higher-intensity energy (derived from radioisotopes such as cobalt-57 or cadmium-109), measures the concentration of lead throughout the bone thickness. The radiographic fluorescence techniques have been used successfully for epidemiologic studies of lead exposure, as an index of cumulative exposure in occupationally exposed patients, as a measure of success of lead removal by chelation in lead-intoxicated children, and as a way to verify remote lead exposure in patients with suspected chronic lead nephropathy.

Two studies from Queensland showed that radiographic fluorescence of finger bone lead correlated well with results of the calcium EDTA test in patients with chronic renal disease secondary to childhood lead exposure, although the sensitivity of the test at this bone site was low (48%). Of interest was the finding that patients with gout and chronic renal failure (even in the absence of a known childhood exposure to lead) were more likely to have positive lead mobilization tests than those without gout.

A chronic lead nephropathy remarkably similar to the Queensland variety has been described in moonshine whiskey drinkers in the southern United States. The renal pathologic findings were similar to those seen in the Queensland cases, and intranuclear inclusion bodies were found commonly. A diagnostic infusion of calcium EDTA provided confirmatory evidence of excessive lead storage in these subjects. In addition to the high incidence of hyperuricemia and gout mentioned earlier, these patients also have unusually high rates of salt wasting, acidosis, and hyperkalemia. These findings may be attributable to hyporeninemic hypoaldosteronism, subsequent to lead intoxication, as well as to inhibition of distal tubular Na^+-K^+-ATPase.

The incidence of lead-related end-stage renal failure in the general adult population is unknown, although attempts to estimate the incidence have been made through measurements of bone lead in patients on dialysis. In one study, lead and lead:calcium ratios were measured in transiliac bone biopsies obtained from 153 patients on dialysis from units in several European countries. Elevated bone lead was found in 5% of the patients on hemodialysis, approximating levels found in active lead workers (20 μg/g in the patients on dialysis, 30 μg/g in Belgian lead workers, and 6 μg/g in normal subjects). Bone lead concentrations in patients receiving dialysis with analgesic nephropathy were comparable to control measurements in deceased subjects who had normal renal function, indicating that neither end-stage renal failure nor dialysis treatment contributes to the body burden of lead. What remains unclear is whether the 5% incidence of elevated bone lead in the patients on dialysis represents a 5% incidence of lead-induced chronic renal failure or whether 5% of patients on dialysis had increased exposure to and thus retention of lead, with the lead either playing no role or contributing to progressive renal failure initiated by other causes.

Covert lead poisoning may be responsible for sporadic cases of pre–end-stage renal failure gouty or hypertensive nephrosclerosis. In separate studies conducted in the United States, Germany, and Australia, higher urinary lead excretion after calcium EDTA mobilization was seen in patients with gout and moderate degrees of renal failure than in patients with no gout but comparable degrees of renal impairment. Elevated urinary lead was less common in patients who had gout before renal failure than in those who presented with renal failure before gout. Another study found higher mobilizable lead levels in patients with hypertension and moderate renal failure than in patients with hypertension but without renal failure and concluded that lead may have contributed to the renal impairment. However, a subsequent study compared mobilizable lead in patients with hypertensive nephropathy and in patients with other forms of mild renal failure, with a similar degree of renal dysfunction, and found no differences. Another study from Spain of 297 subjects (30 normal controls, 105 patients with essential hypertension, 132 patients with chronic renal failure and hypertension or gout, and 30 patients with chronic renal failure of known cause) revealed that groups II and III had abnormal calcium EDTA tests (15.4% in group II and 56.1% in group III). It has been suggested that the results of calcium EDTA tests in patients with renal impairment should be interpreted cautiously because the pharmacokinetics of EDTA in these patients may be different from those in patients with normal renal function. Higher chelating effectiveness may result in greater urinary lead levels in such patients than in controls. In addition, increased bone turnover secondary to hyperparathyroidism or acidosis may result in increased responsiveness to calcium EDTA.

In contrast to the adult forms of lead nephropathy, a reversible Fanconi-like syndrome with aminoaciduria, glycosuria, hypophosphatemia, and rickets has been described in children with acute lead poisoning. The pattern of aminoaciduria is generalized, as described in other causes of Fanconi's syndrome, but lead-induced Fanconi's syndrome is unique in also causing fructosuria and citruria.

The clinical characteristics of lead nephropathy are listed in Table 47.12. Unlike in most other renal diseases, proteinuria is absent or minimal and the urinary sediment is benign. The presence of renal disease is recognized primarily by abnormalities in renal function (i.e., elevated BUN or serum creatinine concentration and decreased urea or creatinine clearances). Detection improves when discrete renal function tests are used, such as inulin (or iodothalamate-125 or chromium-51 EDTA) clearance measurements of the GFR or *p*-aminohippurate (PAH) clearance measurements of renal blood flow. From a functional standpoint, lead nephropathy often is accompanied by hyperuricemia and reduced renal excretion of urate, sometimes in association with overt gouty arthritis. The pyrazinamide suppression test has demonstrated that this constella-

TABLE 47.12. Clinical and Pathologic Abnormalities of Lead Nephropathy

Reduced glomerular filtration rate
Reduced renal blood flow
Absent or minimal proteinuria
Normal urine sediment
Variable hypertension
Hyperuricemia and low urate clearance common
Acidosis and hyperkalemia sometimes seen
Fanconi's syndrome (only in acutely intoxicated children)
Interstitial nephritis and proximal tubular nuclear inclusion bodies on renal biopsy

tion of findings is caused by enhanced tubular reabsorption of urate rather than reduced secretion. As indicated earlier, lead nephropathy also can show a greater propensity toward salt wasting, acidosis, and hyperkalemia than other renal diseases with a comparable degree of renal failure. These abnormalities and the reduced uric acid clearance may be attributable to an inhibiting effect of lead on the renin-angiotensin-aldosterone system because the resultant volume depletion would be expected to increase proximal tubular urate reabsorption. Although overt manifestations of proximal tubular dysfunction are rare in adults with lead nephropathy, one study demonstrated a reduced glucose reabsorption capacity but normal bicarbonate reabsorption capacity and normal PAH reabsorption capacity in four occupationally exposed lead workers with minimally reduced GFR.

Attempts to develop early markers of renal dysfunction in patients with known lead exposure (e.g., in the industrial setting) have met with variable success. Not only is albuminuria absent in early stages of renal disease, but β_2-microglobulinuria, which has proved to be a very useful marker of cadmium nephrotoxicity, also is absent in lead-induced renal disease. The urinary excretion of certain renal tubular lysosomal enzymes, such as NAG and lysozyme, has been found to be elevated in some lead workers, with NAG but not lysozyme excretion falling after removal from exposure. A collaborative European study examined more than 20 potential indicators of renal changes in 50 workers exposed to lead (with average blood lead 48 μg/dl) and found that the most outstanding effect was a lowered urinary excretion of the eicosanoid 6-keto-$PGF_{1\alpha}$ and enhanced excretion of thromboxane (TXB_2). In another study of 81 exposed workers with a mean blood lead of 42 μg/dl, enhanced 6-keto-$PGF_{1\alpha}$ and TXB_2 excretion was found, together with enhanced intestinal alkaline phosphatase, brush border antigen (BBA), and prostaglandin $PGF_{2\alpha}$ and PGE_2 excretion and decreased fibronectin excretion. The authors claim that glomerular injury is heralded by the alterations in 6-keto-$PGF_{1\alpha}$, TXB_2, and fibronectin, proximal tubular injury by intestinal alkaline phosphatase and BBA, and collecting tubule or medullary interstitial cell injury by $PGF_{2\alpha}$ and PGE_2.

Hypertension is variably present in workers with established lead nephropathy, but the relationship between hypertension and lead exposure remains controversial. Although studies in the early twentieth century suggested an increased incidence of hypertension that appeared to correlate with lead exposure, more careful evaluations of large numbers of workers in lead-related industries have failed to establish an excessive incidence of hypertension in lead workers when these groups were carefully compared with age-matched controls. On the other hand, when blood and tap water lead levels were measured in a population of 135 hypertensive subjects and 135 sex- and age-matched normotensive subjects in west Scotland (where drinking water is soft and often is delivered and stored in lead plumbing systems), significantly higher blood lead levels were found in the hypertensive population, and there was a positive correlation between blood lead and tap water lead in this community. In addition, in two extensive epidemiologic surveys in the general population, one in the United States and the other in Great Britain, a significant positive correlation was found between blood pressure and blood lead levels within a range of blood lead generally considered to be normal. Although the increment in blood pressure produced by a doubling in blood lead was small, the relationship warrants further investigation. The observation that low but not high lead exposure levels are associated with hypertension has been confirmed in experimental animals. In rats, the discrepancy may be related to a variable effect on endothelially produced vasoactive hormones. A low lead dosage stimulates endothelin release and suppresses endothelially derived relaxing factor (EDRF), whereas a high lead dosage suppresses both endothelin and EDRF. EDRF (or nitric oxide) suppression has been shown to be related to inactivation by reactive oxygen species rather than diminished production via nitric oxide synthase. Agents that scavenge reactive oxygen species, such as DMSA or lazaroids, ameliorate the hypertension, either by restoring nitric oxide or via a direct effect of reactive oxygen species on vascular contraction.

The gross pathologic finding of chronic lead nephropathy is that of a granular, contracted kidney. Tubular atrophy and dilation with interstitial fibrosis but minimal cellular infiltration typically are seen. Glomeruli become sclerotic secondary to blood flow impairment, but there is no evidence of a primary glomerulonephritis of immune pathogenesis. Vascular lesions, with intimal proliferation and hyaline degeneration of the media, may be prominent. The eosinophilic proximal tubular nuclear inclusion body, once thought to be pathognomonic of lead nephropathy, is present only during the early years of lead exposure. Thus, the diagnosis of lead nephropathy usually is inferential, based primarily on a history of lead exposure, evidence of renal impairment by functional testing, and renal biopsy disclosure of a non–immunologically mediated interstitial nephritis.

Sporadic cases of acute lead poisoning accompanied by acute renal failure have been reported in adults. In a report of five adults poisoned by self-injection of lead and opium, hepatic failure and reversible acute tubular necrosis were prominent features.

An experimental model of lead nephropathy has helped to elucidate the effect of lead on the function and ultrastructure of renal proximal tubule lining cells. Young rats were fed a constant diet containing 1% lead as lead acetate. During the first 20 weeks, the renal changes on light microscopy were limited to proximal tubular lining cell swelling and intranuclear inclusion body development. The glomeruli are normal by light and electron microscopy at this stage, and there is no proteinuria. However, a generalized aminoaciduria reflects the functional and structural damage to the proximal tubule. By electron microscopy, the proximal tubule shows dense intranuclear inclusion bodies and swollen cytoplasmic organelles, particularly the mitochondria, which not only are altered in shape but also contain marginated cristae and a matrix of diminished granularity. Isolated mitochondrial preparations from these animals have been demonstrated to have impaired oxidative and phosphorylative abilities compared with mitochondria from control rats.

In a study in which rats were fed graded lead dosages in drinking water for 10 weeks, it was found that urinary lead excretion was nearly constant over a wide range of lead intake and despite progressively increasing amounts of lead in the renal parenchyma. Lead content analysis of organelles obtained by differential centrifugation revealed that the increment in lead concentration was highest in the nuclei and, in particular, in the nuclear inclusion bodies. It has been suggested that in lead poisoning the lead ion enters the tubule by transport across the tubule membrane in a diffusible form bound to an organic ligand. A portion of the lead becomes bound into a lead–protein complex (the inclusion body) in the nucleus, where it is no longer diffusible, and the remainder is transported into the tubular lumen, from which it is excreted in its ligand-bound form. Thus the inclusion body is seen as an important detoxification mechanism and plays a role similar to that of metallothionein for cadmium. However, the nature and subcellular location of the protein differ from those of metallothionein. Analysis of isolated bodies revealed a protein of 27,500 D that is rich in glutamic and aspartic acids, glycine, and cysteine and contains about 40 to 50 μg lead per milligram of protein. When lead-poisoned rats are treated with EDTA, the nuclear inclusion bodies are disrupted and removed from the nuclei concomitant with an increased urinary lead excretion. Thus part of the lead mobilized by EDTA treatment must come from chelation and excretion of the sequestered lead bound to nuclear protein. Renal failure in the rat model progresses via tubular atrophy and interstitial fibrosis development and, ultimately, focal and segmental glomerulosclerosis in some animals. Interestingly, GFR increases significantly in the early stages of the model, raising the question of hyperfiltration as a contributory factor in subsequent renal impairment.

Lead absorption is enhanced by concomitant dietary deficiency of zinc, iron, or calcium. In a recent study in rats of bone lesions caused by low levels of dietary lead (100 ppm), it was shown that a calcium-deficient diet both increased the absorption of lead and caused osteopenia, with elements of osteoporosis, osteomalacia, and hyperparathyroidism.

Acute lead intoxication without renal involvement or lead nephropathy ordinarily is treated with EDTA chelation. Although sodium EDTA has been shown to have toxic propensities because of its calcium chelation properties, calcium EDTA in appropriate dosages is useful and harmless. The usual recommendation is for a course of 5 to 7 consecutive days at a dosage of 50 mg/kg per day or less and an administration rate of 20 mg/min or less. A common practice is to use 1.0 g calcium EDTA in 250 ml normal saline, delivered intravenously over a 2-hour period. No adverse side effects have been reported. A small number of cases of acute tubular necrosis have been described with sodium or calcium EDTA therapy, related mainly to very large dosages, rapid administration, or severe preexisting renal or metabolic disease (e.g., hypercalcemia and multiple myeloma). Trace metal depletion, although of theoretical concern, has not yet been shown to be clinically important, although zinc excretion is known to be markedly enhanced by calcium EDTA. Advanced renal disease related to lead intoxication (GFR less than 50% of normal) must be treated cautiously because EDTA is filtered by the glomerulus, much as inulin is. In such instances, the dosage and infusion rate of EDTA should be reduced in proportion to the serum creatinine elevation. Lead nephropathy should be treated energetically, however, because treatment may stabilize or improve renal function.

Penicillamine can be used as an oral chelating agent but only when the worker has been totally removed from a lead environment because this agent can enhance gastrointestinal absorption of ingested lead. It is less effective as a chelator than calcium EDTA and, with prolonged administration, can produce renal toxicity (nephrotic syndrome), leukopenia, and anemia. Two new oral chelating agents, dimercaptopropane sulfonate (DMPS) and DMSA, water-soluble derivatives of BAL, have been shown to be effective lead chelators in experimental animals. DMSA has been approved for treating children with lead intoxication. In experimental lead-treated animals, DMSA administration has been shown to increase GFR and lower blood pressure. The renal pathologic changes produced by lead are only minimally affected by DMSA treatment, suggesting that the improvement in GFR is primarily hemodynamically mediated.

Copper

The prototype of chronic copper poisoning in humans is found in Wilson's disease (hepatolenticular degeneration), an inborn error of metabolism with an autosomal-recessive inheritance pattern. Metabolic balance and radioactive copper turnover studies in this disorder have revealed positive balance, resulting from diminished hepatobiliary excretion, and prolonged whole-body and hepatic copper retention after an intravenous radiotracer injection. Although a defect in copper-binding proteins appears to be the most likely biochemical basis of Wilson's disease, it has not been elucidated completely. The serum level of ceruloplasmin, a circulating copper-binding protein, is reduced in the vast majority of homozygotes and some heterozygotes, and the reduction appears to be caused by defective hepatic ceruloplasmin synthesis and release. However, reports of a few homozygotes with normal serum ceruloplasmin levels seem to indicate that failure to synthesize ceruloplasmin is not the primary genetically determined defect in Wilson's disease. Adult human brain, liver, and erythrocytes normally contain similar tissue copper-binding proteins in the soluble cytoplasmic fraction. Studies of brain and liver copper in Wilson's disease have disclosed markedly elevated amounts of copper in the soluble cytoplasmic fraction and smaller increases in the nuclear, mitochondrial, and microsomal fractions. However, analysis of the copper distribution in the soluble fraction of brain indicates that the amount of copper bound to the normal copper-binding protein, cerebrocuprein 1, is appropriate, whereas the pathologic copper is bound to proteins that ordinarily are copper free.

Whatever the underlying defect, the organs that appear to be most susceptible to excessive copper accumulation are the brain, liver, and kidney, and the pathologic clinical manifestations reflect damage to these organs. Clinical symptoms usually occur in the second or third decade of life but sometimes as late as the fifth decade. The characteristic metabolic abnormalities, namely hypoceruloplasminemia (less than 20 mg/100 ml), elevated urinary copper (more than 100 μg/24 hr), elevated hepatic copper (more than 100 μg/g), and elevated serum transaminase values often are seen during the latent or asymptomatic stage. Administering 1.0 g/day penicillamine increases urinary copper excretion to more than 2,000 μg/day in asymptomatic and symptomatic homozygotes but rarely more than 1,000 μg/day in normal subjects or heterozygotes. In the majority of patients with overt Wilson's disease, the predominant clinical manifestations are those related to liver and brain malfunction, including hepatosplenomegaly, spider angiomata, dysarthria, tremor, incoordination, muscle tone rigidity, gait disturbances, and mental deterioration. Kayser-Fleischer rings, copper deposits in Descemet's membrane of the cornea, are common. Early liver biopsies show periportal fibrosis, progressing to postnecrotic cirrhosis in the late stages of the disease.

Many patients with Wilson's disease, particularly those with predominant hepatic disease, also exhibit renal involvement, characterized by proximal tubular dysfunction, a decrease in GFR and effective renal blood flow, and sometimes a distal acidification defect. As in cadmium nephropathy, hypercalciuria and renal calculi sometimes are seen. Clinically overt proteinuria, when present, is minimal. Copper content of kidney tissue is markedly increased and can be shown histochemically to be localized to the cytoplasm and nuclei of the proximal tubular epithelial cells. Light microscopy reveals fatty and hydropic degeneration of the proximal tubules, whereas electron microscopy in a few cases has revealed increased numbers of electron-dense bodies in the subapical areas of proximal tubular cytoplasm (interpreted as metalloproteins) and structural alterations of mitochondria. Experimental studies of normal rats treated for prolonged periods with oral or parenteral copper have confirmed that an excess body burden of this metal can produce proximal tubule alterations manifested as lamellar lipid structures in lysosomes and loss of cristae and vacuolization of mitochondria.

Wilson's disease treatment consists of reducing the body burden of copper through a low-copper diet and cupriuresis initiated by administering 1.0 to 2.0 g/day D-penicillamine. Oral chelating agents that increase fecal copper excretion, such as diethyldithiocarbamate and carbacrylamine resin, have also been helpful. Successful Wilson's disease treatment ameliorates the renal tubular dysfunction, but treatment cessation has been shown to result in the return of kidney abnormalities.

Acute tubular necrosis from copper poisoning has been seen in fulminant Wilson's disease with active hemolysis and in cases of copper sulfate poisoning. In both instances, the increased level of copper in erythrocytes renders these cells more susceptible to hemolysis, and the resultant hemoglobinemia and hemoglobinuria contribute to the acute tubular necrosis. Copper sulfate is a chemical used most commonly as a white-washing agent and in the leather industry. It has been incriminated as a cause of accidental poisoning in children and as a means of suicide in adults. The initial clinical symptoms include a metallic taste, bluish vomitus, abdominal discomfort, diarrhea, shock, and oliguria or anuria. Both hemoglobinuria and hematuria are seen. Treatment with chelating agents alone is ineffective because of the limited urine output. Hemodialysis therapy appears to be ineffective in treating copper-induced acute renal failure because, despite a rising dialysate concentration of copper, serum levels remain constant or increase. Peritoneal dialysis therapy is the preferred treatment.

Mercury

The toxic effects of mercury depend on the compound to which the patient is exposed and the intensity and duration of exposure. Several mercury compounds, including the diuretics mercurous chloride and mersalyl and ammoniated mercury skin-lightening creams, have been reported to produce nephrotic syndrome. Renal biopsies in such cases have shown both membranous and proliferative glomerular changes on light microscopy, epimembranous electron-dense deposits on electron microscopy, and finely granular staining for IgG, IgM, and complement by immunofluorescence. These findings have been interpreted to indicate that mercury acts as a hapten, giving rise to an immune complex hypersensitivity response. However, two young children in the same family developed nephrotic syndrome attributed to mercury exposure, presumably in the form of methyl mercury, by consuming large quantities of tuna. In these patients, renal biopsies showed only increased mesangial cell ground substance and negative immunofluorescent staining.

The experimental counterpart of mercury-induced nephrotic syndrome can be produced by repeated subcutaneous administration of low-dose mercuric chloride to rats. This results in proteinuria development in association with a mesangial glomerulopathy. Kidneys from these animals show focal and segmental proliferation of the mesangial matrix, electron-dense deposits in the mesangium, and immunofluorescent staining of granular and nodular IgG, IgM, and C3 deposits in the mesangium. Although an immune complex pathogenesis appears likely in this model, the antigen has not been identified. Indeed, in a study of mercury-exposed chloralkali workers, the prevalence of abnormal autoantibodies titers or circulating immune complexes was not found to be increased. The initial hypothesis was that the renal tubular damage induced by mercuric chloride might release renal tubular antigens into the circulation, but antibodies to renal tissue antigens could not be found in sera or in glomerular eluates.

Prolonged exposure to mercurous chloride (calomel) as a cathartic may lead to chronic renal failure with elements of the Fanconi's syndrome. Patients with this disorder have watery diarrhea, tremor, and dementia in addition to nonoliguric renal failure. The renal component is characterized by moderately advanced azotemia, mild proteinuria, negative urine sediment, and renal tubular abnormalities including glucosuria, aminoaciduria, phosphaturia, and proximal and distal tubular acidification defects. At autopsy, black pigment deposits were found in the colon and renal cortex. Light microscopy of kidneys reveals the glomeruli to be normal, but moderate tubular atrophy (most severe in the proximal tubule) and diffuse deposits of lipofuscin pigment in the tubular cytoplasm are seen. Dense black deposits occur free and within macrophages in the cortical interstitium. By electron microscopy, these deposits have been resolved into the lamellated arrays of fine crystals, identified by electron diffraction as β-mercuric sulfide.

Acute exposure to large dosages of mercuric chloride leads to oliguric acute tubular necrosis. In some cases, myoglobinuria caused by rhabdomyolysis may contribute. Mercuric chloride poisoning usually occurs as an accident or suicide attempt or after its use as an abortifacient; the dosage necessary to cause acute renal failure ranges from 0.4 to 10.0 g. Acute tubular necrosis also has resulted from organic mercurial diuretic administration when given repetitively in high dosages or to patients with preexisting renal impairment. Renal oxidant injury has been demonstrated in LLC-PK-1 cells exposed to mercuric chloride, with generation of massive amounts of hydrogen peroxide. Mercuric chloride poisoning presents with a bitter metallic taste, followed by a sense of throat constriction, substernal burning, abdominal pain, nausea, vomiting, and diarrhea, often associated with ulcerative stomatitis. Oliguria or anuria develops rapidly after ingestion. Urine collected shortly after exposure shows proteinuria, red cells, glucosuria, and often aminoaciduria. The mortality rate once oliguria occurs is high. Acute poisoning is treated with BAL administration in conjunction with hemodialysis therapy. Removing the mercury–BAL complex by dialysis therapy appears to be clinically effective and sharply reduces the mortality rate if initiated within 48 hours of mercury ingestion.

Acute mercuric chloride nephrotoxicity in experimental animals has been used extensively as a model to explore the pathogenesis of acute tubular necrosis. Mercury, like cadmium, induces synthesis of the metal-binding protein metallothionein, so within 48 hours of exposure a large proportion of administered mercuric ions is bound to metallothionein within the cytoplasm of kidney tubule epithelial cells and then slowly released. Morphologic and functional evidence of renal failure occurs much earlier. At a mercuric chloride dosage of 4 mg/kg of body weight, given subcutaneously to male rats, changes by light and electron microscopy can be seen in the proximal tubules as early as 30 minutes after injection. These early changes affect the pars convoluta and pars recta of the proximal tubule; 24 hours later, the pars convoluta shows partial recovery, but there are widespread necrotic changes throughout the pars recta. Changes observed at 6 hours include focal absence of microvilli of the brush border, cytoplasmic vacuolations, appearance of small membrane-bound dense bodies, rounding and swelling of mitochondria with condensed matrices, and widened intracristal spaces. At this time, a significant GFR reduction and increased fractional sodium and potassium excretion are detectable, but these alterations in renal function are much more profound at 24 hours. Sloughing of necrotic renal tubular cell material, associated with the appearance of kidney antigens and increased enzyme activity in the urine, peaks at 48 to 96 hours, at which time flattened squamoid regenerating cells are seen in the proximal tubules. Regeneration to normal-appearing proximal tubular cells continues over the next 1 to 2 weeks.

The mechanisms of the fall in GFR have not been established clearly but have been attributed to changes in renal cortical blood blow, excessive absorption of the filtrate through an abnormally permeable tubular epithelium, obstruction of the tubular lumen by cell debris, and activation of the renin-angiotensin axis through impaired proximal sodium reabsorption and enhanced distal delivery, thereby activating the juxtaglomerular apparatus. Direct measurements have indicated that the changes in total renal blood flow, the fraction of filtrate that shows inappropriate back-diffusion, and tubular obstruction all contribute only slightly to the profound GFR decrease. On the other hand, it has been observed that blood flow is redistributed away from the renal cortex. In addition, suppressing the renin-angiotensin axis by preloading animals with saline or potassium chloride lessens the severity of renal failure after mercuric chloride. Thus the evidence is consistent with the concept that hemodynamic changes, mediated initially by the renin-angiotensin system, are predominantly responsible for the severe fall in GFR.

Some organomercurials, in which there is one covalent bond between mercury and carbon, behave similarly to inorganic mercury in that they are transformed rapidly to inorganic mercury through mercury–carbon bond cleavage by an enzyme located in the soluble fraction of the liver. These include phenyl and methoxyethyl mercury salts, which are used as fungicides, and the mercurial diuretics. Phenyl mercury has not been reported to cause acute renal toxicity in humans, but exposure to methoxyethyl mercury has resulted in a few cases of azotemia with proteinuria.

Methyl mercury, on the other hand, has been shown to produce severe toxic effects in humans, principally of the central nervous system. Poisoning has occurred through ingestion of seed grains (or meat from animals consuming such grains) treated with methyl mercury as a fungicide and through excessive consumption of fish with high levels of methyl mercury. Certain ocean fish such as tuna and swordfish, as well as some freshwater fish, have been found to have high levels of methyl mercury, the primary source of which is inorganic mercury from the natural ecosystems. It is thought that inorganic mercury is concentrated through sedimentation at the bottom of large bodies of water and then methylated by acting as a receptor for methyl groups from compounds such as cobalamin (vitamin B_{12}) secreted by various microorganisms. The methyl mercury content of canned tuna was found to average about 0.5 ppm, in contrast to the 50 ppm found in fish and up to 85 ppm in shellfish in Minamata Bay, Japan, where several cases of methyl mercury poisoning were reported. In this instance, methyl mercury was found in waste sludge of a plant that used mercuric chloride as a catalyst in producing vinyl chloride. All initial reports focused on the severe neurologic toxicity, symptoms of which included progressive paresthesias; inability to concentrate; weakness and apathy; tunnel vision; blind spots; hearing abnormalities; emotional instability with fits of anger or depression; ataxia, alexia, and agraphia; dyscoordination; spasticity; intention tremor; paralysis; coma; and death. In recent years, a renal component has been recognized. Although endogenous creatinine clearance was normal, patients with Minamata disease were found to have urinary levels of renal tubular antigen, light chains, and β_2-microglobulin higher than those in normal controls but equivalent to those in patients with tubular proteinuria. These findings indicate that methyl mercury can produce a subtle renal tubular disorder in humans. Animal experiments have revealed that methyl mercury, which accumulates rapidly and selectively in liver and kidney, is transformed slowly to inorganic mercury, perhaps accounting for the effect on renal tubular function.

Because of the long biologic half-life of methyl mercury (70 days) and irreversible nature of the damage to the central nervous system, the effect of treatment with chelating agents is doubtful. However, mercury clearance from the blood can be accelerated by D-penicillamine and *N*-acetyl-DL-penicillamine or oral administration of a nonabsorbable polythiolated resin. It has also been demonstrated *in vitro* that penicillamine, *N*-acetylpenicillamine, cysteine, and *N*-acetylcysteine can reverse the binding of methyl mercury to proteins in the red blood cells and plasma and that the thiolmethyl mercury complex is readily dialyzable. Metallic mercury exposure occurs primarily through mercury vapor inhalation, either as an industrial hazard or through accidental exposure. As with methyl mercury, the central nervous system is predominantly affected, although in some instances proteinuria, occasionally of nephrotic levels, has also been found.

In 44 workers exposed to elemental mercury for an average of 11 years, renal effects were found in those excreting more than 50 μg mercury per gram of creatinine, consisting of increased urinary excretion of tubular antigens and enzymes and decreased excretion of some eicosanoids and glycosaminoglycans. Chronic elemental mercury poisoning is an insidious disorder that characteristically results in tremor, certain personality and intellectual changes called erethism, dermatitis, gingivitis, stomatitis, and gastroenteritis. Both BAL and calcium EDTA have been used as treatment agents, with equivocal results. *N*-Acetyl-DL-penicillamine, developed as a specific chelating agent for mercury, has proved to be successful in treating elemental mercury poisoning when given in 10-day courses of 250 to 500 mg orally four times daily.

Platinum

Toxic platinum exposure occurs through the administration of the cancer chemotherapeutic agent *cis*-platin (*cis*-dichlorodiamineplatinum). Although *cis*-platin is an effective antineoplastic agent, active against several tumors, a very important dose-limiting factor has been its nephrotoxicity. In early clinical trials, it was found that single intravenous injections of *cis*-platin in a dosage of 2 mg/kg or 50 to 75 mg/m² of body surface area produced mild to moderate reversible renal impairment in one-quarter to one-third of patients treated, and at higher dosages, more frequent and severe, often irreversible nephrotoxicity was observed. Nephrotoxicity also was more likely when *cis*-platin was administered repetitively over short time intervals. It was found that the nephrotoxicity could be ameliorated significantly by hydration before and after *cis*-platin administration with intravenous saline sufficient to produce a brisk diuresis. Mannitol or furosemide often are added to the regimen to reduce the intratubular platinum concentration and, presumably, the intrarenal concentration. In addition, the interval between doses has been lengthened (e.g., to 4 weeks) to permit kidney recovery. The nephrotoxicity of high *cis*-platin dosages (100 to 120 mg/m² of body surface area) is lessened but not eliminated by such protocols. Because peak plasma platinum concentrations are seen immediately after injection and the initial decay period is rapid (half-life 25 to 49 minutes), the plasma platinum concentration at 5 minutes after injection can be a useful predictor of subsequent toxicity in such patients. In one study, 5 of 20 patients with plasma platinum concentrations greater than 6 μg/ml developed nephrotoxicity, compared with none of 26 patients with lower plasma concentrations. Further discussion on the nephrotoxicity of *cis*-platin is found in Chapter 47, Part 2.

The renal lesions produced by platinum often are compared with those produced by mercury, particularly because platinum is a heavy metal (atomic weight 195) in close proximity to mercury (atomic weight 201) in the periodic table. Characteristics common to *cis*-platin and mercuric chloride nephrotoxicity include acute tubular necrosis affecting primarily the pars recta; increased size and number of renal lysosomes, presence of membrane arrays, and focal absence of microvilli in affected tubules; early enzymuria; a low-molecular-weight metal-binding protein in kidney cytosol; and depletion of protein-bound sulfhydryl (SH) groups. In other respects, however, there are distinctive differences between *cis*-platin and mercuric chloride nephrotoxicity.

In contrast to the response to mercuric chloride (i.e., rapid-onset oliguric or anuric acute renal failure), there is in both humans and animals a time lag between *cis*-platin administration and the maximum alteration in renal function. In humans, cast formation, proteinuria, and increased urinary enzyme excretion appear early, but azotemia does not peak until day 8 to 12 and oliguria is not seen. In rats given a single injection of *cis*-platin at a dosage of 10 mg/kg intraperitoneally, serum creatinine concentration did not begin to rise until the third day and did not peak until the sixth day. Micropuncture studies have shown that whole-animal GFR decreases to a greater degree than superficial proximal single-nephron GFR. This disproportionate change was attributed to tubular fluid backleak in the S_3 or pars recta segment of the proximal tubule and possibly to some degree of intratubular obstruction.

Several discrete components of tubular dysfunction have been described in humans and experimental animals treated with *cis*-platin. Unlike the findings with mercurous chloride, these functional disturbances suggest alterations in the capacity of the distal nephron rather than the proximal nephron. Renal magnesium wasting in association with hypomagnesemia, hypocalcemia, and hypokalemia has been reported in a number of *cis*-platin–treated patients. Less frequent have been reports of severe renal salt wasting, concentrating defects, and acidifying defects consistent with incomplete distal renal tubular acidosis. In rats, the concentrating defect is associated with polyuria and a diminished corticopapillary solute gradient, related to a decrease in papilla content of both electrolyte and urea. The diminished urea content has been attributed to diminished urea recycling (secondary to the pars recta lesion) and to abnormal collecting duct function. A functional defect in the thick ascending limb of Henle's loop also has been invoked to account for the severe salt wasting and magnesium wasting and the concentrating abnormality. Polyuria in *cis*-platin–treated animals occurs in two phases: an early phase (1 day) in which the concentration defect is corrected by exogenous vasopressin and a later phase (8 days) in which the concentration defect is unresponsive to vasopressin. Animals demonstrate diminished postdehydration plasma vasopressin at day 1 but not day 8. The low plasma vasopressin levels are mediated by *cis*-platin inhibition of vasopressin release from the posterior pituitary gland rather than an effect on vasopressin synthesis. The distal tubule dysfunction is consistent with morphologic evidence in human kidneys of tubular necrosis affecting primarily the distal and collecting tubules. On the other hand, there is little agreement on this agent's morphologic effects on the distal tubule in rodents; some studies report moderate to severe damage to this segment of the nephron, and others indicate that morphologic alterations are confined to the proximal tubule.

An important aspect of treating *cis*-platin nephrotoxicity is identifying the immediate nephrotoxin. Although it seems reasonable to assume that the platinum ion, as a heavy metal, is responsible for the renal damage, certain lines of evidence indicate that this is not the complete story. First, only the *cis* isomer, not the *trans* isomer, of dichlorodiamineplatinum produces renal damage, although either agent produces similar renal platinum concentrations. In kidney slice studies, *cis*-platin uptake was found to be energy and temperature dependent and could be inhibited by drugs that inhibit base transport. Unbound platinum in blood and urine was predominantly *cis*-platin, but unbound platinum in kidney cytosol was not. The latter compound, unlike *cis*-platin, was not active as a mutagen. These studies indicate that *cis*-platin is accumulated in the kidney by a specific transport system and is biotransformed intracellularly. As discussed in earlier sections, renal Na^+-K^+-ATPase transport system inhibition may provide a biochemical basis for the toxicity of certain heavy metals. *Cis*-platin and chloroplatinic acid have been shown to inhibit human renal microsomal Na^+-K^+-ATPase by 50% at concentrations of 7×10^{-4} M and 10^{-5} M, respectively. Cysteine and glutathione (SH reagents) greatly reduced the enzyme inhibition caused by chloroplatinic acid but not *cis*-platin, again suggesting that the platinum compound configuration plays an important role in its toxicity.

At a subcellular level, platinum binding to cytosolic ligands in rat liver and kidney was found to be maximal at 24 hours. In the kidney, the cytosol contained the largest quantity of platinum (about 70%), with smaller amounts in the nuclear, microsomal, and mitochondrial fractions. In the cytosol, platinum was found as a low-molecular-weight species (less than 1,000 D), an intermediate-weight species (6,000 to 12,000 D), and a high-molecular-weight species (more than 20,000 D). The intermediate-weight species was regarded as a probable metallothionein, similar in function to cadmium–metallothionein. A further indication that metallothionein plays a protective role in *cis*-platin nephrotoxicity has been afforded by a study that compared the responses of metallothionein-null mice with those of wild-type control mice to *cis*-platin. The lethal and renal toxicities of *cis*-platin were far greater in the metallothionein-null mice.

Renal failure progression after acute or chronic *cis*-platin administration has been studied in rats. A single intraperitoneal *cis*-platin dose (6 mg/kg) induced severe focal necrosis in the proximal tubules (particularly the S_3 segment) and distal tubules, with a maximum lesion on day 7. The tubular damage was greatest in the corticomedullary region, where the platinum concentration was the highest. Repeated dosing with *cis*-platin (1 mg/kg twice weekly for 11 weeks) produced massive tubular dilation in the corticomedullary region, interstitial fibrosis, thickening of tubular basement membranes, and fibrosis of some glomeruli. In one study, proximal tubular dilation progressed (after 4 weeks) to the formation of numerous microcysts in the region of the outer stripe and later (after 6 months) to the formation of large cysts involving the entire outer stripe and extending to the subcapsular cortex. Vitamins E and C have been shown to have protective effects on *cis*-platin nephrotoxicity, with vitamin E given 12 hours before *cis*-platin diminishing the toxic effects and concomitant vitamin E and C intensifying the protection. In another study, aminoglycosides were found to produce additive nephrotoxicity when given together with a single injection of *cis*-platin. These animals showed continuous elevation of BUN and persistent tubular damage over 14 days, in contrast to animals receiving *cis*-platin only, which had diuresis onset and partial renal function recovery at this time. Other antibiotics, including penicillin derivatives and cephalothin, had no additive nephrotoxic effects. Extrapolation of these animal studies to humans emphasizes the cumulative nature of *cis*-platin nephrotoxicity and the potential hazard from simultaneous nephrotoxic antibiotic administration.

Uranium

With one exception, there have been no convincing reports of accidental or industrial uranium nephrotoxicity in humans. A survey conducted in 1956 of workers chronically exposed to certain heavy metals (cadmium, uranium, lead, and mercury) indicated that generalized aminoaciduria was a common finding suggesting subtle nephrotoxicity. The incidence and severity of the aminoaciduria were highest in the cadmium and uranium workers. The low industrial toxicity of uranium may be related in part to its limited absorption from the gastrointestinal tract (0.5% to 5%). Uranium contents of daily diets and human urine were examined from inhabitants around a uranium mine in Okayama Prefecture, Japan. In one hamlet, the mean uranium content in the diet was 4.55 μg/day per person and urinary excretion was 0.14 μg/day, as opposed to urinary excretion of 0.01 μg/day in a control area. After chronic uranium exposure, about 20% of hexavalent uranium in the blood is deposited in the kidney and a similar amount in bone; mobilization from these organs is slow. In contrast, the majority of retained uranium after acute administration is found in the kidney. The acute toxicity of hexavalent uranium (uranyl nitrate) was explored through intravenous injection in human volunteers with terminal brain tumors. Clinical findings included increased urinary catalase, proteinuria, cylindruria, impaired sodium reabsorption, and increased urine pH. At autopsy several weeks later, there were no demonstrable tubular changes, but autoradiography disclosed increased renal cortical uranium concentration.

Uranyl nitrate injections also have been used to produce animal models of acute tubular necrosis. As with mercury, the reduced GFR has been ascribed to reduced renal blood flow, increased filtrate backflow through necrotic tubular epithelium, and intratubular obstruction by necrotic debris. Although filtrate backflow has been demonstrated, recent evidence suggests that marked alterations in renal hemodynamics mediated by the renin-angiotensin system may be a more critical factor. Within 6 hours after injection, before there are significant tubular pathologic findings, decreases in total renal blood flow, renal cortical blood flow, whole-kidney GFR, and single-nephron GFR can be demonstrated. Simultaneously, plasma renin activity, renin activity in superficial and deep juxtaglomerular apparatuses, and distal tubular sodium concentration increase. Suppressing renin activity by saline loading decreases azotemia but not the later appearance of tubular necrosis, again paralleling the findings in acute tubular necrosis produced by mercury injections.

Chromium

Chromium nephrotoxicity occurs mainly as acute tubular necrosis secondary to accidental or suicidal ingestion of potassium dichromate, a compound in which chromium is present in the hexavalent form. Because intravascular hemolysis also has been reported to occur after ingestion of this agent, the acute tubular necrosis may be related to a direct toxic effect of the dichromate and to hemoglobinuria. Other toxic manifestations of acute hexavalent chromium poisoning include nausea and vomiting, diarrhea, hepatic failure, thrombocytopenia, bleeding diathesis, and central nervous system abnormalities. The lethal potassium dichromate dosage has been estimated as 0.5 to 1 g. Chromic acid, another hexavalent form of chromium, also produces acute tubular necrosis after oral ingestion or extensive chromic acid skin burns.

Chronic chromium nephrotoxicity related to industrial exposure also has been recognized. Chromium is used in chrome plating, steel welding, galvanizing, leather tanning, and dye, enamel, and paint preparation. Absorption occurs almost exclusively by respiration, and elimination occurs predominantly through the urine. Studies of workers in chromium industries reveal that diffusible chromium clearance increases in proportion to the number of years of exposure, implying a relationship between clearance and body burden. Experiments with rats given low-dose potassium dichromate repetitively over several weeks also have confirmed a direct correlation between chromium clearance and kidney chromium content. Although major renal impairment has not been documented in chromium workers, a small fraction (7%) of those tested have shown tubular proteinuria, whereas a higher percentage (17%) have shown increased urinary β-glucuronidase excretion, indicating tubular injury. By use of very sensitive immunochemical techniques to detect proximal tubular brush border antigens in urine as an index of tubular injury, a urinary chromium level of 15 μg/g creatinine has been established as an exposure threshold level for kidney disease.

Renal pathologic changes in rats or humans poisoned with potassium dichromate are confined to the proximal tubule; vacuolar changes and lysosomes with phagocytosed material are found in the cytoplasm, and the mitochondria are distorted, also with vacuolar changes. Even at late stages of cellular necrosis, the tubular basement membranes remain intact. Lesions are less prominent in sodium-loaded than sodium-depleted rats. Glutathione (GSH) is an important mediator of chromium nephrotoxicity. Chromium nephrotoxicity in mice has been shown to be accompanied by decreased renal glutathione and glutathione reductase. Pretreatment with glutathione methyl ester, a GSH-supplying agent, restored kidney GSH levels and prevented chromium-induced renal damage.

Chromium is a dialyzable substance, and acute renal failure after hexavalent chromium poisoning has been treated successfully by both hemodialysis and peritoneal dialysis. Chromium is complexed by the chelating agent BAL, but BAL has not proved to be clinically useful in treating chromium-induced acute renal failure when given alone or in conjunction with dialysis.

Arsenic

Two forms of arsenic occur in the human environment: pentavalent (arsenate) and trivalent (arsenite). The former is nontoxic, does not accumulate in human tissues, and is excreted rapidly into the urine. The latter is excreted predominantly in the bile and accumulates in tissues, with a predilection for liver, kidney, hair, nails, and skin. Toxicity is attributable to arsenic binding to dithiol groups and inhibition of thiol-containing enzymes.

As with chromium, renal toxicity can result from accidental or covert poisoning or from high levels of industrial exposure to arsenic, the former from arsenical fertilizers or pigments, the latter chiefly in the form of arsine in the chemical and petroleum industries. Both acute tubular and acute cortical necrosis have been described, with survivors often developing chronic renal insufficiency and hypertension. Intravascular hemolysis may be a complicating feature adding to the acute nephrotoxicity. Diagnosis of acute arsenic poisoning ordinarily is confirmed by the finding of elevated arsenic levels in blood, hair, or urine.

The clinical picture of acute arsenic poisoning consists of a rapid onset with nausea, vomiting, diarrhea, lethargy, anorexia, rigors, abdominal and back pain, and oliguria. The skin may develop a yellow-brown pigmentation and the hair may turn gray within 24 hours. Urine contains albumin, casts, and red and white cells. The tubular lesions pathologically resemble those of mercury nephrotoxicity. In patients who recover but are left with residual renal impairment, proteinuria persists and there may be generalized aminoaciduria.

The usefulness of BAL in treating acute arsenic poisoning is limited to patients with normal renal function because urine is the primary excretion route of arsenic and arsenic–BAL complexes. Exchange transfusions to remove the arsenic–hemoglobin complex and hemodialysis treatments have proved to be more successful as therapeutic maneuvers in the presence of acute renal failure because arsenic or arsenic complexed with BAL can be recovered from the dialysate. Arsenic dialysance as high as

87 ml/min has been reported. Meso-2,3-DMSA and 2,3-DMPS have been used successfully as alternative oral chelators.

Bismuth

Bismuth compounds have been known since the early nineteenth century to cause kidney damage, varying from asymptomatic proteinuria or nephrotic syndrome to acute or chronic renal failure. In earlier years, intoxication arose chiefly from antisyphilitic therapy, whereas currently it arises from industrial exposure or the use of soluble bismuth compounds, such as the subcarbonate and the mixed thioglycolates (Bistrimate), to treat warts, oropharyngeal infections, and infantile gastroenteritis. Anuria can result from bismuth levels as low as 1.0 mg/kg of body weight.

Like the other heavy metals, bismuth is concentrated in the kidney, and the pathologic changes are confined mainly to the proximal tubules, where swollen mitochondria and distortion of mitochondrial inner membranes are found on electron microscopy. However, a unique finding is the presence of inclusion bodies in the nuclei and the cytoplasm of proximal tubule epithelial cells. These inclusion bodies are 6 to 8 μm wide, have sharply demarcated dense margins, and are brownish yellow and refractile. They do not stain with hematoxylin and eosin but do stain with periodic acid–Schiff or Ziehl-Neelsen stain.

The clinical presentation of acute bismuth toxicity includes stomatitis, diarrhea, peripheral neuritis, obstructive jaundice, and pigmentation of the gum margins. With large dosages, oliguric renal failure is seen, but during recovery renal abnormalities may include glucosuria, aminoaciduria, and uricosuria. With lower dosages, the predominant renal manifestations may be tubular (glucosuria, aminoaciduria, phosphaturia, proximal acidification defect), with only a modest diminution in GFR. Treating bismuth intoxication with BAL has met with limited success. Recovery has followed treatment by hemodialysis therapy.

Gold

Nephrotic syndrome occurs as a complication of gold therapy for rheumatoid arthritis. The syndrome usually regresses once gold therapy is discontinued, although proteinuria resolution and renal function improvement can be accelerated by treatment with BAL and adrenocorticotropic hormone. Examination of renal biopsies from such patients by light microscopy, electron microscopy, and immunofluorescence suggests that at least in some instances, gold may induce immune complex glomerulonephritis. In a detailed study of two patients with rheumatoid arthritis who developed nephrotic syndrome with gold treatment, the first appeared to have an immunologic mechanism because light microscopy revealed membranous glomerulonephritis, electron microscopy showed slight thickening of glomerular capillary walls with the subepithelial electron-dense deposits, and immunofluorescence was positive for IgG and IgM (but not complement) in a continuous granular pattern along the peripheral glomerular capillary walls. Energy-dispersive radiographic analysis identified gold within granules in the tubular cytoplasm but not within the electron-dense deposits in the glomerular capillaries. The second patient showed prominent glomerular foot process fusion on electron microscopy but no electron-dense deposits in the glomerular capillaries. Visceral epithelial cells contained occasional vacuoles with gold particles. The authors concluded that in this second patient, a direct effect of gold on glomerular membrane permeability had occurred rather than immunologic injury. In other studies of gold nephropathy, complement, as well as IgG and IgM, has been shown to be contained within the glomerular electron-dense deposits. Gold inclusions have been identified within proximal tubular and mesangial cells but not within basement membranes or subepithelial deposits. The gold does not act directly as a hapten but apparently renders some other structure (perhaps renal tubular epithelium) antigenic and thus produces immune complex injury. Fatal anuric renal failure also has been reported after gold therapy, associated with tubular lesions and metallic inclusion bodies in tubular cells and lumen. Less severe tubular injury appears to be common; urinary markers of renal tubular damage (tubular proteinuria, tubular basement membrane antigen, renal tubular epithelial antigen, and β_2-microglobulin excretion) have been found to be significantly higher in patients with rheumatoid arthritis treated with gold therapy than in those treated with conventional therapy. Tubular proteinuria, detected by sodium dodecyl sulfate–polyacrylamide gel separation, was found in 13 of 18 gold-treated patients and only 2 of 17 patients who did not receive gold therapy.

Studies in rats injected with a single dose of gold sodium thiomalate revealed a progressive increase in BUN and serum creatinine associated with an increase in urine output, consistent with polyuric acute renal failure. Kidneys demonstrate early severe coagulative necrosis of proximal tubular epithelium, with regeneration evident by the fourth day and recovery by the eighth day.

Lithium

Interest in the renal manifestations of lithium toxicity has evolved since the introduction of lithium carbonate therapy for manic-depressive disorders and the subsequent recognition that renal toxicity limits its usefulness. Lithium is a monovalent ion belonging to the group of alkali metals, which includes sodium, potassium, rubidium, and cesium. Lithium shares some of the properties of sodium and potassium but is not handled precisely like either ion. Lithium is filtered at the glomerulus and, as with sodium, 60% to 70% of the filtered load is reabsorbed by an active transport process.

Extracellular volume contraction results in increased proximal tubular reabsorption of both sodium and lithium, but lithium reabsorption by the distal nephron is less influenced by maneuvers that normally regulate sodium reabsorption. Thus, thiazide diuretics reduce lithium excretion and result in a significant rise in serum lithium levels because of compensatory enhancement of proximal reabsorption. On the other hand, lithium excretion is unaffected by loop diuretics such as furosemide, and reabsorption is unresponsive to aldosterone.

Lithium's effect on proximal and distal tubular reabsorption of other ions has not been delineated completely, although several observations suggest that lithium may inhibit both proximal and distal sodium reabsorption. Studies in an experimental model of lithium intoxication in rats have yielded results that may account for the progressive lithium accumulation in certain patients treated with this agent for affective disorders. Lithium chloride was added to the normal rat diet in amounts corresponding to 20, 40, and 60 mmol/kg dry weight. Rats given the lowest dosage showed no adverse effects, animals given the medium dosage developed polyuria and polydipsia, and rats given the highest dosage developed potentially fatal lithium intoxication. The last group of rats was shown to have reduced GFR and evidence of salt depletion. Not only were the serum lithium levels extraordinarily high but lithium clearance was reduced disproportionately to the GFR reduction. When these animals were given additional sodium, all of these changes were reversed. Lithium-treated animals, both adrenalectomized and with intact adrenals, were shown to have a lower response to mineralocorticoid hormones. These observations suggest that the initial increase in serum lithium leads to an inhibition of distal sodium reabsorption through a lowered response to mineralocorticoids, and the resulting extracellular volume depletion leads to enhanced proximal tubular lithium reabsorption and a further increase in serum lithium levels.

The principal renal side effect of lithium treatment is diabetes insipidus, which has been observed in 10% to 30% of patients receiving this drug. Several studies have focused on the mechanisms of lithium-induced polyuria and polydipsia. Although it is clear that lithium may independently affect the hypothalamic thirst mechanism and, in some instances, the central elaboration and release of antidiuretic hormone (ADH), the predominant effect of lithium on water metabolism is through production of ADH-unresponsive nephrogenic diabetes insipidus. This effect probably is caused by diminished responsiveness of the collecting duct epithelium to ADH because lithium does not change the corticomedullary sodium gradient in dogs and does not influence diluting capacity in various species. At least part of the biochemical defect is related to lithium inhibition of adenylate cyclase, with consequent impairment of ADH-induced cyclic adenosine 3′,5′-monophosphate (cAMP) generation. An additional effect distal to cAMP generation may be operative because dibutyryl cAMP only partially reverses lithium-induced polyuria in rats. With the recent demonstration that aquaporins are water channels responsible for high water permeability in the kidney and that aquaporin-2 genetic mutations were responsible for autosomal-recessive nephrogenic diabetes insipidus, it has become evident that lithium causes marked downregulation of aquaporin-2, coincident with the development of severe polyuria.

Lithium also has been shown to affect the renal acidifying mechanism compatible with incomplete distal renal tubular acidosis. Early stop-flow studies in the dog revealed that the drop in urine pH normally seen in the distal nephron was abolished by lithium. Chronic administration of lithium to humans and rats results in urinary acidification impairment after an acid load challenge, although overt acidosis ordinarily is not seen. However, dogs given lithium chloride intraperitoneally for 3 days at a dosage of 3 mEq/kg/day developed hyperchloremic metabolic acidosis with an alkaline urine. Bicarbonate loading in these lithium-treated dogs did not produce the normal increase in urinary pCO_2, and the bicarbonate titration curve showed a small bicarbonate leak at the lower plasma concentrations of bicarbonate, a pattern identical with that described in classic distal renal tubular acidosis. A similar pattern has been described in patients receiving chronic lithium therapy, including a subgroup with short-term lithium administration in whom concentrating ability was preserved. Lithium may affect renal tubular calcium reabsorption, and hypocalciuria has been noted in patients receiving lithium therapy.

Light and electron microscopy studies of kidneys from rats given lithium-supplemented diets in a dosage sufficient to achieve therapeutic (but not toxic) serum lithium levels have revealed lesions initially in the cortical collecting tubules and adjacent portions of distal tubules and later in the medullary collecting ducts. The tubules were dilated and generally flattened but punctuated by swollen epithelial cells; these cells on electron microscopy revealed increased numbers of mitochondria (which were swollen or otherwise damaged), dilated cisternae of endoplasmic reticulum, and vacuolization of apical cytoplasm. Damage was most severe in cortical collecting tubules and less severe in distal convoluted tubules and medullary collecting tubules. No lesions were seen in glomeruli, proximal tubules, or ascending thick limbs of Henle's loop. The anatomic sites of lithium-induced pathologic findings thus corresponded to the location of lithium-induced pathophysiologic conditions.

Although the renal lesion produced by lithium initially was thought to be entirely functional, dose dependent, and completely reversible after treatment discontinuation, more recent observations indicate that this is not always true. Persistent nephrogenic diabetes insipidus has been reported in some patients years after lithium carbonate therapy was stopped and in whom serum lithium values had always remained in the therapeutic range of 0.5 to 1.5 mmol/L. In addition, renal biopsies performed in a group of 14 patients on long-term lithium therapy, referred for investigation because of acute lithium poisoning or lithium-induced nephrogenic diabetes insipidus, revealed focal nephron atrophy and interstitial fibrosis. Three of these patients showed a persistent moderate reduction in creatinine clearance after lithium was stopped.

In a later study from the same institution, it was found that 18 of 69 patients treated for more than 2 years with lithium had a marked decrease in concentrating ability, associated on renal biopsy with tubular atrophy and interstitial fibrosis in the medulla and cortex. The impairment in concentrating ability correlated with the duration of lithium therapy and the degree of tubular damage. Other investigators have questioned the specificity and frequency of lithium-related tubulointerstitial disease, pointing out that biopsies taken from patients with affective disorders before receiving lithium show a similar prevalence of tubulointerstitial disease, raising the possibility that other drugs might be responsible for the renal lesion. Nevertheless, a few patients have been reported who clearly had normal renal function at the onset of lithium therapy and who received no drugs other than lithium but progressed to chronic renal failure secondary to tubulointerstitial disease with continued lithium exposure. Renal function stabilized but did not improve substantially when lithium was discontinued. Nephrotic syndrome is another renal manifestation of lithium administration that has been reported in a few patients. The nephrotic syndrome is reversible with lithium cessation, but it reappeared in one patient when lithium was readministered. Renal biopsies disclosed minimal-change glomerular lesions without tubulointerstitial disease. Another report has described three patients with nonreversible nephrotic syndrome (two of whom were moderately azotemic), with renal pathologic findings consistent with focal segmental glomerulosclerosis.

In general it is believed that if toxic lithium levels are avoided and the serum concentration maintained in a low range (0.31 to 1.07 mmol/L), significant renal tubular dysfunction and morphologic damage rarely occur. Dehydration and concomitant use of thiazide diuretics or indomethacin can increase plasma lithium ion levels by reducing renal clearance. However, indomethacin can reduce urine flow to one-third its previous rate within hours and may be the emergency therapy of choice for diabetes insipidus.

Lithium toxicity also is associated with a variety of neurologic and cardiovascular symptoms including lethargy, muscle tremors, ataxia, hyperreflexia, muscular rigidity, visual blurring, stupor, seizures, coma, hypotension, and circulatory collapse. In a study of 55 patients with acute or chronic lithium intoxication, it was found that patients with acute intoxication may have high serum lithium levels without symptoms, whereas patients with chronic lithium intoxication may have symptoms with serum lithium levels in the therapeutic range. Dialysis is indicated when severe symptoms of toxicity are present, regardless of the lithium blood level.

Silicon

The inhalation of free silica (SiO_2) has long been recognized as a cause of lung fibrosis but has only recently been reported to cause chronic tubulointerstitial renal disease. Patients with this disorder have uniformly had prolonged heavy occupational exposure to silica dust and show high levels of silicon in renal tissue. The clinical presentation includes hypertension, glomerular proteinuria, and normal urine sediment, with no evidence of renal tubular dysfunction. GFR may be normal or low. Light microscopy of renal biopsies has disclosed a mild focal and segmental proliferative glomerulonephritis, with immunofluorescence negative (two patients) or showing focal deposits of IgM and C3 (one patient) and degenerative proximal tubular lesions. By electron microscopy, the proximal tubules were found to be filled with large vacuoles, some of which contained aggregates of dense osmiophilic particles. Similar findings have been described in experimental animals after both oral and parenteral silicon administration.

One report has described four patients with a more virulent form of *rapidly progressive silicon nephropathy* who had manifestations of a connective tissue disorder. Histologically, the kidneys showed glomerular hypercellularity and sclerosis, crescents, interstitial cellular infiltrates, and tubular necrosis, with red cell casts. Electron microscopy showed glomeruli containing electron-dense deposits and tubules containing dense lysosomes and myelinlike bodies in the cytoplasm. Two of the four patients died, one received dialysis therapy, and one responded to pulse methylprednisolone therapy.

A possible silicon-related syndrome has been described in dialysis-treated patients with excessively high levels of silicon, consisting of painful, nodular skin eruptions and aberrant hair growth, known as perforating folliculitis.

Silver

Argyria, systemic silver poisoning, occurs secondary to application or ingestion of silver-containing medicines or industrial exposure. In previous centuries, silver nitrate was advocated for treating epilepsy and central nervous system syphilis. In the early twentieth century, local silver nitrate applications were used extensively to treat nose and throat conditions. Sufficient silver was absorbed through nasal and oral mucous membranes and the gastrointestinal tract to lead in some instances to generalized argyria, a condition heralded by the bluish black discoloration of skin. The degree to which generalized argyria leads to significant organ damage is debatable. Silver is deposited as an organic silver compound in most organs of the body, with a predilection for connective tissue. The silver concentration is highest in the kidney. At autopsy examination of the kidney, silver appears primarily as granular subendothelial deposits in the connective tissue of glomerular capillaries and in the interstitial tissue around the tubules. The earlier literature indicated that the tubules were spared. However, there have been two reports of acute tubular necrosis secondary to silver exposure in photo developers; in rabbits, silver salts given intraperitoneally cause tubule degeneration, interstitial edema, and interstitial deposits of silver, with sparing of glomeruli.

A survey of 30 workers chronically exposed to silver nitrate and silver oxide found that 4 had proteinuria and 5 had creatinine clearances more than 10% lower than predicted. None of the subjects had glucosuria, aminoaciduria, phosphaturia, or acidification defects. The authors of this report agreed with earlier suggestions that argyria usually is a benign condition but thought that the question of adverse effects on the kidney is unsettled.

Iron

Renal hemosiderosis is observed in chronic intravascular hemolysis and in iron overload caused by repeated blood transfusions. This condition has been described in paroxysmal nocturnal hemoglobinuria, paroxysmal cold hemoglobinuria, autoimmune hemolytic anemia, thalassemia, hereditary spherocytosis, and chronic hemolysis secondary to prosthetic aortic valves. Hemosiderin deposits (reactive with Prussian blue stain) are found in the visceral and parietal glomerular epithelial cells, the cytoplasm of the proximal tubules and, to a lesser degree, in Henle's loop and the interstitial tissue. In most instances, the effect on renal function is negligible. However, some patients develop moderate GFR impairment, proteinuria, and concentrating defects. In such patients, renal biopsies reveal significant interstitial fibrosis and pigment deposition. In one report of three patients with renal hemosiderosis secondary to paroxysmal nocturnal hemoglobinuria, all three had concomitant glucosuria and proteinuria, and the proteinuria was shown by polyacrylamide gel electrophoresis to be low molecular weight (i.e., tubular proteinuria). Distal renal tubular acidosis also has been described in an infant with thalassemia major and an infant with thalassemia minor. In adults with thalassemia, proteinuria is common, but significant azotemia is rare except as a terminal event. In these patients, proteinuria is presumably of glomerular origin because urinary β_2-microglobulin excretion is normal.

Repeated administration of iron-dextran (Imferon) to rats produced an iron overload nephropathy characterized by lesions in the glomeruli and proximal tubules. In the glomeruli, mesangial cells and podocytes were heavily iron overloaded, whereas the endothelial cells were less affected. Proximal tubules showed greatly increased numbers of phagolysosomes (absorption droplets), which contained both periodic acid–Schiff-positive material and iron. The lumens of the proximal tubules contained extruded droplets, sloughed-off epithelial cells, and occasionally iron-loaded macrophages. Urinalysis results revealed proteinuria but no hemoglobinuria or glucosuria. It was proposed that the polycationic iron derived from the iron-dextran increased the permeability of the glomerular membrane to protein and iron, that the excess iron taken up by the cells of the glomeruli and the proximal tubule stimulated the production of the iron-binding protein ferritin, and that much of the ferritin was digested in the phagolysosomes, where the iron is incorporated into hemosiderin. Another experimental animal model of iron overload, resembling human hemochromatosis, with predominantly parenchymal cell iron overload, has been produced in rats by parenteral administration of iron complexed with nitrilotriacetate. In addition to heavy iron deposits in liver, heart, and exocrine pancreas, these animals showed moderate iron deposits in the renal cortex and histologic alterations in proximal tubules. In addition to elevated serum creatinine, indicative of impaired GFR, the animals displayed aminoaciduria and renal glucosuria, suggesting proximal tubule dysfunction. The adverse effect of iron may be ascribed to its effect on free radical generation. It is noteworthy that 21-aminosteroids (lazaroids), which act as scavengers of free radicals, appear to protect against heme protein-mediated renal injury, both *in vitro* and *in vivo,* in rats.

Oliguric acute renal failure can be seen in the chronic hemolytic anemias when there is a sudden exacerbation of hemolysis. Acute renal failure, with a high mortality rate, has also been described in children who have ingested large dosages of ferrous sulfate. Contributory factors include shock associated with hepatic damage, metabolic acidosis, and injury to the gastrointestinal mucosa.

Selected Readings

Cadmium

Gonick HC, Indraprasit S, Rosen VJ, et al. Experimental Fanconi syndrome. III. Effect of cadmium on renal tubular function, the ATP-Na-K-ATPase transport system and renal tubular ultrastructure. *Miner Electrolyte Metab* 1980;3:21–35.
A study of the effects of cadmium toxicity in rats, with evaluation of renal function, renal cortical ATP content and Na^+-K^+-ATPase activity, and ultrastructural changes in the mitochondria and basal plasma membrane infoldings of the proximal tubule. The rats developed Fanconi's syndrome when renal accumulation of cadmium was sufficient to inhibit Na^+-K^+-ATPase activity.

Klassen CD, Liu J. Role of metallothionein in cadmium-induced hepatotoxicity and nephrotoxicity. *Drug Metab Rev* 1997;29:79–102.

Examines the protective role of metallothionein in cadmium liver toxicity and the toxic role in cadmium nephrotoxicity.

Mason HJ, Davison AG, Wright AL, et al. Relations between liver cadmium, cumulative exposure, and renal function in cadmium alloy workers. *Br J Ind Med* 1988;45:793–802.

A detailed study of cadmium alloy workers that explores the relationship between liver cadmium, cumulative cadmium exposure, and glomerular and tubular renal function parameters.

Roels H, Bernard AM, Cardenas A, et al. Markers of early renal changes induced by industrial pollutants. III. Application to workers exposed to cadmium. *Br J Ind Med* 1993;50:37–48.

A detailed study of 50 workers exposed to cadmium, compared with 50 control workers. Reexamines urinary thresholds of cadmium/g creatinine in relation to urinary markers.

Lead

Gonick HC, Ding Y, Bondy SC, et al. Lead-induced hypertension. I. Interplay of nitric oxide and reactive oxygen species. *Hypertension* 1997;30(6):1487–1492.

This article examines the hypothesis that either lead-induced diminution of nitric oxide synthesis or lead-stimulated production of reactive-oxygen species may be responsible for the hypertension.

Goyer RA. Lead toxicity: a problem in environmental pathology. *Am J Pathol* 1971;64:167–181.

A discussion of environmental lead toxicity and the possible mechanism of lead nephrotoxicity. Evidence of inhibition of renal mitochondrial oxidative phosphorylation is presented.

Khalil-Manesh F, Gonick HC, Cohen AH, et al. Experimental model of lead nephropathy. I. Continuous high-dose lead administration. *Kidney Int* 1992;41:1192–1203.

Description of sequential renal functional and pathologic changes in the kidney and alterations in urinary excretion of marker enzymes, with continued exposure of rats to high-dose lead over a 12-month period.

Sharp DS, Becker CE. Chronic low-level lead exposure, its role in the pathogenesis of hypertension. *Med Toxicol Adverse Drug Exp* 1987;2:210–232.

A summary of the experimental and clinical evidence indicating that low-level lead exposure can cause hypertension.

Copper

Suzuki-Kurasaki M, Okabe M, Kurasaki M. Copper–metallothionein in the kidney of macular mice: a model for Menkes disease. *J Histochem Cytochem* 1997;45:1493–1501.

Macular mice, an experimental model of Menkes disease, an X-linked disorder of copper metabolism, have been shown by histochemistry to have deposits of copper–metallothionein in the proximal convoluted tubule.

Mercury

Cardenas A, Roels H, Bernard AM, et al. Markers of early renal changes induced by industrial pollutants. I. Application to workers exposed to mercury vapor. *Br J Ind Med* 1993;50:17–27.

A survey of several urinary markers in 50 workers exposed to elemental mercury.

Iesato K, Wakashin M, Walashin Y, et al. Renal tubular dysfunction in Minamata disease. *Ann Intern Med* 1977;86:731–737.

This article examines subtle aspects of renal tubular function in minamata disease.

Zalups RK, Knutson KL, Schnellman RG. In vitro analysis of the accumulation and toxicity of inorganic mercury in segments of the proximal tubule isolated from the rabbit kidney. *Toxicol Appl Pharmacol* 1993;119:221–227.

Describes mercury uptake by the proximal tubule and the injury produced. Glutathione, cysteine, or albumin provides protection.

Platinum

Goldstein RS, Mayor GH. Minireview. The nephrotoxicity of cisplatin. *Life Sci* 1983;32:685–690.

A concise review of the mechanism of cis-platin nephrotoxicity, its pathology, and its clinical picture, including a detailed discussion of the differences between nephrotoxicity of cis-platin and other heavy metals.

Stewart DJ, Dulberg CS, Mukhael NZ, et al. Association of cisplatin nephrotoxicity with patient characteristics and cisplatin administration methods. *Cancer Chemother Pharmacol* 1997;40:293–308.

Chromium

Franchini I, Mutti A. Selected toxicological aspects of chromium (VI) compounds. *Sci Total Environ* 1988;71:379–387.

Uses brush border antigen excretion to establish an exposure threshold for urinary chromium.

Arsenic

Shum S, Whitehead J, Vaughn L, et al. Chelation of organoarsenate with dimercaptosuccinic acid. *Vet Hum Toxicol* 1995;37:239–242.

Shows efficacy of DMSA in treating human organoarsenate poisoning.

Gold

Antonovych TT. Gold nephropathy. *Ann Clin Lab Sci* 1981;11:386–391.

A review of clinical and pathologic findings.

Lithium

Carmey SL, Ray C, Gillies AH. Mechanisms of lithium-induced polyuria in the rat. *Kidney Int* 1996;50:377–383.

Experiments demonstrate that a circulating factor inhibits arginine vasopressin action in the lithium-intoxicated rat.

Lam SS, Kjellstrand C. Emergency treatment of lithium-induced diabetes insipidus with non-steroidal anti-inflammatory drugs. *Ren Fail* 1997;19:183–188.

This paper provides details on the use of nonsteroidal antiinflammatory drugs in the treatment of diabetes insipidees due to lithium intoxication.

Marples D, Christensen S, Christensen EI, et al. Lithium-induced downregulation of aquaporin-2 water channel expression in rat renal medulla. *J Clin Invest* 1995;95:1838–1845.

Lithium downregulates aquaporin-2 in renal medulla in association with production of a urinary concentration defect.

Silicon

Bolton WK, Surratt PM, Strugill BC. Rapidly progressive silicon nephropathy. *Am J Med* 1981;71:823–828.

Describes four patients with an immunologically based rapidly progressive disease.

Gitelman HJ, Alderman FR, Perry SJ. Silicon accumulation in dialysis patients. *Am J Kidney Dis* 1992;19:140–143.

Silicon levels in normal subjects average 150 μg/L. In dialysis-treated patients, levels are up to 30 times higher, correlating with the silicon content of dialysis fluid and drinking water.

Saldanha LF, Gonick HC, Rodriguez HJ, et al. Silicon-related syndrome in dialysis patients. *Nephron* 1997;77:48–56.

Describes two patients with excessively high levels of silicon who developed painful, nodular skin eruptions associated with aberrant hair growth.

Iron

Giardina PJ, Grady RW. Chelation therapy in beta-thalassemia: the benefits and limitations of desferrioxamine. *Semin Hematol* 1995;32:304–312.

Cautions against using high-dose intravenous DFO therapy.

Landing BH, Gonick HC, Nadorra RL, et al. Renal lesions and clinical findings in thalassemia major and other chronic anemias with hemosiderosis. *Pediatr Pathol* 1989;9:479–500.

A review of the kidney pathology and renal functional alterations in several patients with iron overload secondary to the thalassemisas.

Nath KA, Balla J, Croatt AJ, et al. Heme protein-mediated renal injury: a protective role for 21-aminosteroids in vitro and in vivo. *Kidney Int* 1995;47:592–602.

Heme protein stimulates hydrogen peroxide generation, whereas 21-aminosteroids have a protective effect.

PART 5
Analgesic Nephropathy

Garabed Eknoyan

Pain is as elemental as hunger and sex. Throughout history, humankind has sought relief from pain and avidly increased consumption of painkillers as quickly as they became available. Pain-relieving plants were some of the first therapeutic agents integrated into the practice of ancient medicine. The use of henbane, opium poppy, mandragora, wintergreen, and willow bark is mentioned in medical Babylonian tablets, Egyptian papyri, and the Hippocratic corpus. Plants and their crude extracts remained part of the medical armamentarium until the nineteenth century, when the application of chemistry to medicine allowed us to isolate and synthesize their active ingredients. The shift from botanical to chemical medications heralded the dawn of a new era, nurtured by the chemical industry, in which industrial synthesis of medications, including analgesics, increased their availability. It is somewhat ironic that we are seeing a revival of the medicinal use of herbals, now marketed as dietary supplements, that rivals the use of over-the-counter synthetic drugs.

The first class of synthetic analgesics to be marketed were the salicylates. The active ingredient of willow bark, a bitter glycoside, was identified as salicin in 1830. Its acid extract, which yielded salicylic acid, was synthesized and marketed in 1860.

This paved the way for further research and synthesis of the salt of salicylic acid (sodium salicylate), introduced in 1875. The large dosages of sodium salicylate then used caused nausea, cramps, and vasoconstriction. In 1897, Felix Hoffman, a chemist working for Bayer, synthesized salicylic acid in powder form that was marketed as aspirin and ironically introduced as a painkiller that "does not affect the heart." By 1899 aspirin powder had become the number-one drug sold worldwide; in 1915 it became available over the counter.

The other principal class of analgesics, the paraaminophenol derivatives, were discovered by serendipity when acetanilid (antifibrin), inadvertently administered to a patient, was found to be antipyretic. The search for less toxic acetanilid derivatives led to the synthesis of a host of paraaminophenol acetanilid derivatives, the most satisfactory of which, phenacetin (acetophenetidin), was introduced in 1887 and dominated the market of paraaminophenols for the next 75 years. Interestingly, acetanilid also is the precursor to acetaminophen (paracetamol), which was discovered in 1878 but neglected until 1943, when it was shown to be the major deacetylated active ingredient of both phenacetin and acetanilid. In 1952, acetaminophen was approved by the U.S. Food and Drug Administration (FDA) and became available over the counter in 1960. Aggressively marketed, it soon became the best-selling analgesic, a position it has occupied since then despite the best efforts of the aspirin industry.

A third group of less potent analgesics, the pyrazolone derivatives (antipyrine, aminopyrine, and phenylbutazone) were introduced at about the same time, but because of their lower analgesic activity they were marketed primarily for their antipyretic activity. Their potential to cause agranulocytosis further limited their use. They never occupied a significant share of the analgesic market. Today, with a U.S. market for analgesics of more than $2.5 billion and gross profit margins of 60% to 80% after advertising costs, this is a competitive field in which acetaminophen occupies 41.2% of the market share, aspirin 23%, and nonsteroidal antiinflammatory drugs the balance. Aggressive marketing is used to promote analgesics to consumers who are becoming less pain tolerant than ever before.

From the outset, these two groups of analgesics were marketed as mixtures, with caffeine usually a third ingredient. Against this background of increasing use of variable and often changing analgesic mixtures, their nephrotoxic effect was recognized some 60 years after they became widely used throughout the world. In a report of autopsy findings from Switzerland published in 1953, Spühler and Zollinger suggested that the chronic use of analgesic mixtures (Kafa, Saridon) was associated with the renal lesions observed in 14 of 44 patients with chronic interstitial nephritis. A series of retrospective studies over the subsequent decade, from different countries, established this relationship. Although not mentioned in the original report, phenacetin soon was incriminated because it was the main drug common to the various analgesic mixtures then available, and this new form of kidney disease, recognized in the budding years of nephrology, was dubbed *phenacetin nephritis*. This guilt by association soon led to the voluntary or legislated withdrawal of phenacetin from analgesic mixtures and the increasing market dominance of acetaminophen in the 1960s. Since then, a host of clinical, experimental, and epidemiologic reports have provided convincing evidence that chronic and habitual use of analgesic mixtures results in progressive renal dysfunction, the characteristic lesion of which is a chronic tubulointerstitial nephritis (TIN) and renal papillary necrosis (RPN), now more appropriately called analgesic nephropathy, although the debate over the nephrotoxic potential of phenacetin continues. In addition, epidemiologic studies have led to the suggestion that analgesic exposure aggravates the progression of chronic renal insufficiency (CRI) to end-stage renal disease (ESRD), independent of the underlying cause of the CRI. These detrimental side effects can be appreciated best by reviewing these agents' handling by and action on the kidney.

ASPIRIN

In the body, aspirin is hydrolyzed rapidly to salicylate. Salicylate and its hepatic conjugated metabolites are weak organic acids. In the proximal tubule they are actively transported by the organic acid pathway, attaining a renal cortical tissue:plasma concentration ratio of 20:1. In the distal tubule, their nonionic diffusion in an acid tubular fluid that is concentrated in the medulla results in a medullary tissue:plasma concentration ratio of 60:1. This accounts for the effectiveness of a therapeutically induced high flow rate and urine alkalinization in treating aspirin overdose.

In humans, moderate dosages of aspirin result in tubular epithelial cell excretion, which reaches a maximum in 48 to 72 hours but subsides thereafter even if the drug is continued. Under normal conditions, there is no evidence of a detrimental functional effect. However, in patients with CRI, acute aspirin administration results in reversible decrements of glomerular filtration rate (GFR). This effect, which is particularly evident in sodium-retaining and high renin states (congestive heart failure, cirrhosis of the liver, and nephrotic syndrome), is related directly to the aspirin blood level. Autopsy series from the 1950s to the mid-1970s report a higher risk of RPN in aspirin-treated patients with rheumatoid arthritis. By contrast, in reports from the late 1970s of prospectively followed patients with rheumatoid arthritis and a documented history of aspirin ingestion, renal disease is said to be rare. One limitation of these latter reports is the limited duration of follow-up and the fact that a study of the living ignores the dead, hence the probable difference in results from the earlier autopsy findings. Most epidemiologic studies do not show an increased risk of ESRD caused by habitual use of aspirin as a single agent and in modest therapeutic dosages. There certainly is no known risk from regular aspirin use in the small dosages recommended for preventing cardiovascular disease.

In experimental studies, aspirin at dosages of 50 to 500 mg/kg per day failed to induce renal lesions in rats, cats, and pigs. However, its administration at higher dosages or for periods longer than 6 months resulted in TIN, RPN, and calcific deposits in 30% to 47% of rats. The importance of higher medullary aspirin concentrations in the pathogenesis of renal lesions is evidenced by the decrease in RPN from about 55% in dehydrated rats fed 200 mg/kg per day aspirin to 0% in rats undergoing water diuresis experimentally induced by free access to sugar-containing water, which rats consume avidly.

Demonstrated renal metabolic effects of aspirin that have been proposed to account for its detrimental effects are inhibition of the hexose monophosphate shunt, which diminishes tissue glutamine levels and hence the risk of covalent binding of injurious electrophilic molecules to cell proteins; blocking of fatty acid cyclooxygenase, which reduces prostaglandin generation and hence vasoconstriction and tissue glutathione levels; uncoupling of mitochondrial oxidative phosphorylation, which reduces available energy from adenosine triphosphate (ATP); and inhibition of cellular protein synthesis from amino acids.

ACETAMINOPHEN

Only a small percentage of acetaminophen is excreted as the parent compound by the kidney. Most of the ingested acetaminophen undergoes rapid first-pass metabolism to its glucuronide or sulfate conjugates in the liver. A limited portion of these metabolites is excreted in bile, and the bulk (80%) is excreted by the kidney. The glucuronide and sulfate conjugates are filtered and reabsorbed by the organic transport system of the proximal tubule, where they attain a tissue:plasma concentration of 1.5:1 to 2:1. The tissue level of acetaminophen and its conjugates increases severalfold down the corticomedullary concentration gradient. In maximally concentrating dehydrated animals, the medullary tissue:plasma concentration gradient of the conjugated metabolites is 10:1 and that of acetaminophen 16:1.

In humans, acetaminophen administration results in none of the acute untoward renal effects associated with aspirin. There is limited evidence that habitual acetaminophen use alone causes analgesic nephropathy. However, at least two case-controlled studies suggest an association between regular acetaminophen use and the progression of chronic renal failure to ESRD. Neither of these case-controlled studies distinguished between acetaminophen used alone or in combination with other analgesic agents, nor did they report on the occurrence of the classic syndrome of analgesic nephropathy. In addition, in these reports the risk of adverse effects was greater in those who used acetaminophen during the 5-year period closest to the initiation of dialysis treatment for ESRD. This is an important consideration because acetaminophen is preferentially recommended to patients with CRI because of their platelet defect and the increased risk of bleeding complications associated with aspirin in these patients. Therefore the reported association could well be an epiphenomenon as much as it may be the postulated risk factor in the reports.

In experimental studies, rats fed small dosages or large dosages of acetaminophen for short periods did not develop renal lesions. In rats fed 100 to 300 mg/kg per day, only minor tubular and interstitial changes occurred in about one-third of the rats. Larger dosages (900 to 3,000 mg/kg per day) for longer periods (5 to 12 months) resulted in papillary necrosis in 40% to 60% of dehydrated rats. Once again, the importance of attaining higher medullary tissue concentrations of the drug was evident when the lesions were shown to be completely prevented in rats allowed free access to water containing sugar.

The detrimental metabolic effects of acetaminophen have been best characterized in the liver. Oxidation of the glucuronide conjugate of acetaminophen by the hepatic cytochrome P450 system results in the production of a potentially cytotoxic metabolite, *N*-acetyl-*p*-benzoquinoneamine, which is immediately reduced by glutathione to an innocuous excretory product. Only when glutathione is deficient does covalent binding of the cytotoxic metabolite to tissue protein cause the production of reactive oxygen radicals, with consequent lipid peroxidation and hepatic cell necrosis. An analogous mechanism is postulated to operate in the kidney. Renal cytochrome P450 activity is localized to the cortex. The renal medulla, where chronic injury occurs, contains no cytochrome P450. This may account for the proximal tubular lesions that develop in rats injected with large dosages of acetaminophen (1,200 mg/kg) and the acute renal failure, in the absence of severe liver injury, encountered in clinical cases of acetaminophen overdose, particularly in those whose cytochrome P450 is stimulated (by alcohol, barbiturates, or testosterone). An analogous metabolism of acetaminophen to its cytotoxic metabolite by medullary prostaglandin endoperoxidase synthetase has been proposed as the mechanism generating a nephrotoxic radical in the medulla. Conceptually, toxic metabolites generated in the cortex may be excreted in the tubular fluid and could attain a higher toxic level down its corticomedullary concentration gradient. Under normal conditions, the medulla contains abundant glutathione, which, as in the liver, would reduce the incriminated metabolite to innocuous mercapturic acid, which is excreted in urine. On the other hand, under conditions of reduced tissue glutathione it would accumulate and cause medullary injury.

Acetaminophen also inhibits medullary synthesis of proteoglycans and glycosaminoglycans, which are necessary for maintaining the normal interstitial matrix. It has been suggested that this could contribute to the interstitial changes observed in analgesic nephropathy.

PHENACETIN

Phenacetin is a prodrug that undergoes rapid and extensive (80%) first-pass hepatic metabolism to its active form, acetaminophen (paracetamol). Only small amounts of the original drug reach the peripheral circulation. Part of the remaining phenacetin is metabolized in the liver to *p*-phenetidine, which can cause methemoglobinemia, and the rest is excreted by the kidney. Therefore most of the ingested phenacetin is presented to the kidney as acetaminophen, and its subsequent renal handling and toxicity are not different from those of acetaminophen. A major difference between the two is the significantly greater carcinogenic potential of phenacetin (relative risk 12.2 for phenacetin versus 1.3 for paracetamol), which has been linked to the increased occurrence of uroepithelial cancer in 8% to 10% of patients chronically exposed to analgesic mixtures containing phenacetin.

Phenacetin's association with nephropathy soon led to its withdrawal or banning in the 1970s. By the mid-1980s, it was evident that removing phenacetin from the market had little effect on the incidence of analgesic nephropathy. However, in a prospective study from Switzerland comparing habitual phenacetin users with controls, there was a higher risk of renal dysfunction (concentration defect, increased creatinine levels) over 10 years of follow-up.

The experimental evidence supporting phenacetin nephrotoxicity is similar to that of acetaminophen. Rats fed dosages ranging from 300 to 600 mg/kg per day develop primarily tubular epithelial degenerative changes, with only a modest increase in interstitial space. Larger dosages of 1,000 to 3,000 mg/kg per day administered for longer periods produce TIN and RPN in one-third of dehydrated rats. The lesions are preventable with forced diuresis, which abolishes the drug's corticomedullary gradient. Also, rats with congenital diabetes insipidus (Gunn rats), which cannot concentrate their urine, are protected from the renal lesions of acetaminophen and aspirin.

ANALGESIC MIXTURES

Analgesic mixtures, which allow administration of lower dosages of their constituents, have been marketed as effective pain relievers since they were first synthesized. At one time, 30 such products were introduced annually and consumed by a public seeking pain relief. The combinations vary with geography and over time. In addition to aspirin, acetaminophen, and phenacetin, a host of other derivatives (antipyrine, amidopyrine, salipyrine, salicylamide, dipyrone, and acetanilid) have been used. Most currently available formulations consist of aspirin and acetaminophen. A third compound that has been added to marketed analgesic mixtures is caffeine. In addition to its stimulatory effect, caffeine potentiates the analgesic effect of aspirin. Caffeine has no known toxic effects in the dosages (50 to 150 mg) used in analgesic mixtures. However, its stimulatory effect has been incriminated in developing dependence and the habitual use of analgesic mixtures. The habitual use of caffeine-free analgesic mixtures is just as common as that of caffeine-containing mixtures, however.

The original report of Spühler and Zollinger showed an association of chronic interstitial nephritis with analgesic mixtures. Shortly after this association became recognized, experimental evidence showed that administering aspirin with phenacetin or acetaminophen resulted in a higher incidence (80% to 100%) of RPN than when each component was administered individually and that RPN developed at lower dosages over a shorter period of time than when each agent was administered singly. Dehydration increased the severity and prevalence of the lesions, and hydration decreased their severity and incidence (20% to 30%) but did not eliminate them altogether.

In humans, two prospective cohort studies and five well-conducted case-controlled studies confirmed the association between analgesic mixtures and analgesic nephropathy. In addition, there is a positive and direct relationship between local sales of analgesic mixtures and the incidence of analgesic nephropathy. Equally convincing evidence derives from ESRD registries, which show that banning analgesic mixtures from the over-the-counter market has markedly reduced analgesic nephropathy as a cause of ESRD in Canada, Belgium, and Australia. Although clinical studies cast doubt on the role of any single agent as a cause of classic analgesic nephropathy, there is considerable support for an association between habitual analgesic mixture consumption and classic analgesic nephropathy. This is not unexpected because of the potential for a synergetic nephrotoxic effects based on the known renal metabolic action of each.

As reviewed earlier, detoxification of the potential cytotoxic metabolite of acetaminophen depends on glutathione availability. Salicylates that inhibit the hexose monophosphate shunt diminish the ability of cells to generate sufficient reducing molecules, including glutathione. When they are ingested simultaneously, acetaminophen's production of electrophilic cytotoxic molecules increases as aspirin reduces the glutathione supply. The free intermediate metabolite of acetaminophen now binds to cell protein, generates reactive oxygen radicals, and results in lipid peroxidation and cellular injury. The higher level of these agents attained down the corticomedullary concentration gradient increases papillary susceptibility to this injury and accounts for the renal protective action of water diuresis, which, by abolishing the concentration gradient, reduces the concentration of both drugs in the papillary tip. Additional effects of aspirin that would contribute to the injury are its inhibition of ATP and therefore detoxifying metabolic processes and its inhibition of prostaglandin generation, which would promote renal vasoconstriction and thus promote the added effect of ischemic injury.

THE SYNDROME OF ANALGESIC NEPHROPATHY

Pathology

The characteristic lesion of analgesic nephropathy is that of chronic TIN and RPN. Evidence indicates that focal papillary necrosis is the primary and predominant lesion, and diffuse TIN involving the cortex is a later development, secondary (at least in part) to the papillary necrosis (Fig. 47.3). Evidence of a direct cortical effect derives from experimental studies on surgically papillectomized rats, which develop cortical TIN after exposure to analgesic mixtures.

In experimental models, the earliest morphologic changes are observed at the papillary tip, which is the site of highest tissue concentration of analgesics and their metabolites. The initial lesions are patchy injury and necrosis of the medullary interstitial cells, thin loops of Henle, and vasa rectae. With time, the medullary tubular and capillary basement membranes thicken and its interstitial fibrotic space increases. At this early stage, the kidneys are normal in size and the cortex unchanged in appearance. With continued drug exposure, the papillary patchy lesions coalesce and extend to the medulla, sclerosis of the medullary vasculature and tubular atrophy and degeneration become evident, and calcium deposits develop at necrotic sites. Ultimately, the papilla becomes entirely necrotic, sequestrated, and calcified and either atrophies or sloughs into the urine. At this stage, cortical TIN becomes prominent, primarily in the cortical labyrinth overlying the necrotic papilla, while the cortical medullary rays are spared and hypertrophy. Retraction of the affected cortical tissue and compensatory hypertrophy of the unaffected medullary rays impart the characteristic cortical nodularity of the now small and shrunken kidneys (Fig. 47.4).

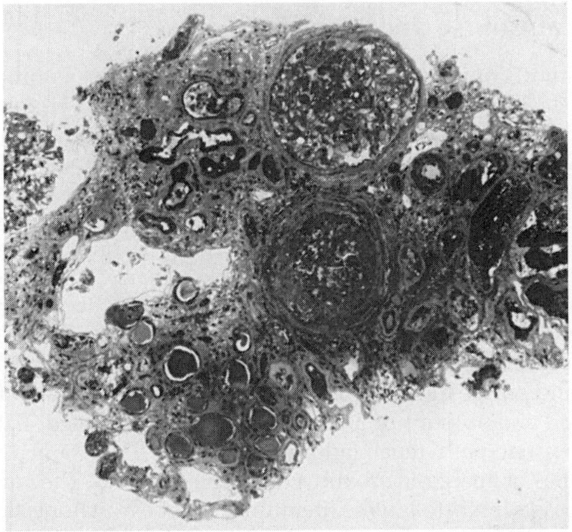

Figure 47.3. Kidney biopsy from a patient with analgesic nephropathy with changes of chronic tubulointerstitial nephritis. Note tubular degeneration, atrophy, and dilation; thickened tubular basement membrane; widened interstitial space with mononuclear inflammatory cell infiltration and fibrosis; and periglomerular fibrosis. In dilated tubules the epithelial cells are hypertrophic, and the lumen contains hyalinized casts, mimicking the appearance of thyroid follicles, hence the term *thyroidization*.

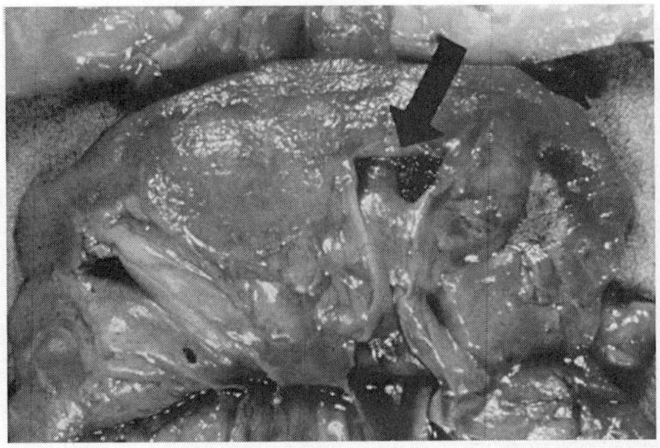

Figure 47.4. Renal papillary necrosis *(arrow)* with sloughed papilla. Note calyceal clubbing, which is considered diagnostic in intravenous pyelography; and thinned atrophic cortical tissue overlying the sloughed papilla compared with the adjacent hypertrophied cortex overlying the medullary rays. The resulting cortical bumpy contour is considered diagnostic in computed tomography.

Clinical Course and Manifestations

The clinical course and manifestations of analgesic nephropathy reflect the progressive course of the morphologic lesions found in experimental models of chronic analgesic exposure (Table 47.13). The clinicopathologic syndrome that results is insidious. Inability to concentrate and acidify the urine is an early and common manifestation of distal tubular injury. Citrate excretion is low and may promote calcification of the injured papilla and inner medulla. Proteinuria, when present, is less than 2 g/day. Severe proteinuria is an ominous finding that indicates the presence of focal glomerulosclerosis and is associated with rapid renal function deterioration. Actually, the GFR reduction is gradual. The onset and progression rate of renal insufficiency are related to the duration and amount of analgesic mixtures consumed. Patients who present with renal failure usually have consumed large quantities of analgesic mixtures over several years. The cumulative dosages reported in the literature are at best anamnestic estimates based on questionnaires. It has been estimated that the average cumulative dosage that results in clinically evident analgesic nephropathy is about 10 kg consumed over 13 years, with a range of 2 to 40 kg over 5 to 30 years. As a rule, renal injury begins after 2 to 3 kg of the index agent has been ingested over 2 to 5 years and is clinically evident after 7 kg or more has been ingested over more than 5 years. Detecting analgesic use early is extremely important because stopping analgesic use often (about 50% of cases) arrests renal dysfunction progression; in some cases (about 20%) it may result in improved renal function, but in the rest renal dysfunction progresses to ESRD.

As a rule, analgesic nephropathy is asymptomatic. Unless a high index of suspicion is maintained and an accurate history of exposure obtained, the early manifestations of sterile pyuria, urinary concentration defect, and even increases in serum creatinine may go unnoticed. In suspected cases, the urine concentration and acidification defect can be documented or gleaned from a history of polyuria and persistent urine pH higher than 6. Renal colic, caused by the passage of sloughed papilla, always should lead to a consideration of analgesic use, as should recurrent urinary tract infections caused by compromised urine flow in the scarred calyces.

Analgesic nephropathy is more common in women, with a female:male ratio of 6:1. The typical patient is older than 30 years of age. About one-third of patients have a major personality disorder, and most are dependent on other addictive substances (e.g., tobacco, alcohol, or psychotropics). They often state an organic cause of pain (headache, musculoskeletal pain, or arthralgias) for their analgesic use. But more often the drugs are used for minor complaints (sleeplessness or fatigue) and low tolerance for pain, be it organic or perceived. Because the latter is influenced by cultural factors, a family history of analgesic use is common.

Not all patients who consume analgesic mixtures regularly develop renal disease. In addition to variations in the amount consumed and variety of formulations available in a given region, personal habits may promote analgesic nephropathy. Given the importance of medullary drug concentration in the pathogenesis of renal lesions, any condition associated with higher urine concentration is expected to increase the occurrence of renal injury. Urine volume and concentration depend on the amount of fluid ingested. Those who consume less fluid have a higher urine concentration and a propensity for higher medullary drug concentration. Dehydration caused by climatic conditions has been proposed as one explanation for the geographic variability in the prevalence of analgesic nephropathy. Dehydration caused by diuretic and laxative use also has been implicated. Analgesic users with coexistent diseases that affect the medullary vasculature (e.g., diabetes, sickle hemoglobinopathy, or pyelonephritis) have been noted to have a higher propensity for analgesic nephropathy.

The two most common extrarenal manifestations of analgesic abuse are anemia and gastrointestinal symptoms. The anemia is more severe than expected for the level of renal dysfunction and usually is microcytic and secondary to the gastrointestinal blood loss associated with aspirin use. The gastrointestinal manifestations are those of dyspepsia, with documented peptic ulcer disease present in one-third of patients. Unlike other causes of TIN, hypertension is not rare in this condition. In fact, severe hypertension caused by renovascular atheromatous disease has been observed in 4% to 6% of analgesic users. Several other extrarenal manifestations recorded in the literature were caused by phenacetin and have not been encountered since its removal from the market. Historical findings attributed to phenacetin metabolites include hemolytic anemia, splenomegaly, and a yellowish discoloration of the skin, cartilage, and viscera. Patients with analgesic nephropathy have a higher risk of uroepithelial and renal cell carcinomas. These tumors may present with hematuria.

TABLE 47.13. Features of Analgesic Nephropathy

Clinical		Renal		Systemic	
Gender F:M = 6:1		Urine		Anemia	40%–60%
Age		Pyuria	50%–100%	Iron deficiency	
Mean 53 yr		Proteinuria	60%–80%	$\downarrow$ Erythropoietin	
Range 40–60 yr		Hematuria	30%–60%	Hypertension	70%
Personality disorder		$\downarrow$ Concentration	50%–100%	Severe	10%–15%
Major	35%	$\downarrow$ Acidification	20%–30%	Gastrointestinal	40%–50%
Minor	40%	Bacteria	20%–60%	Dyspepsia common	
Family history of analgesic use		$\downarrow$ Citraturia		PUD	20%–30%
Addictive tendency		$\downarrow$ GFR, RBF		Arteriosclerosis	
Smoking, alcohol, psychotropics		$\downarrow$ BUN, S_{Cr}		Renovascular	
Cause of analgesic use		RPN			
Headaches	40%–60%	ESRD			
Musculoskeletal	20%–30%	Transitional cell calcium	8%–10%		
Mood	6%–30%				

BUN, blood urea nitrogen; ESRD, end-stage renal disease; F, female; GFR, glomerular filtration rate; M, male; PUD, peptic ulcer disease; RBF, renal blood flow; RPN, renal papillary necrosis; S_{Cr}, serum creatinine.

Diagnosis

Apart from a history of analgesic abuse or recurrent detection of analgesic metabolites in the urine, the radiologic appearance of the kidney is the most reliable diagnostic tool. Traditionally, intravenous pyelography, with or without nephrotomography, has been the standard approach and remains the gold standard for early diagnosis. The classic findings are those of RPN (Chapter 51), coupled with cortical nodularity and small kidneys. Where reduced renal function limits the quality of intravenous pyelograms, retrograde pyelography is useful in visualizing the urinary tract changes. Cross-sectional imaging modalities such as ultrasound, computed tomography (CT), and, to a lesser extent, magnetic resonance imaging have been used successfully to diagnose analgesic nephropathy. Of these, the CT scan has been especially valuable in detecting the renal calcifications that characterize the early morphologic lesions of analgesic nephropathy. Careful validation in established cases of analgesic nephropathy has demonstrated that CT scans, without dye, are a convenient and accurate diagnostic tool (Fig. 47.5). CT scans have been useful in epidemiologic studies of analgesic nephropathy in Europe. However, intravenous pyelography remains a reliable method for detecting the early calyceal changes before the onset of calcification, cortical nodularity, and shrinking.

A kidney biopsy can be useful in diagnosis (Fig. 47.3). However, the typical lesions of chronic TIN are nonspecific, and the diagnosis still depends on a history of habitual analgesic mixture consumption. In addition, in performing a kidney biopsy the physician tries to obtain cortical tissue and to avoid obtaining medullary tissue, where the early changes of analgesic nephropathy occur. As a result, the chance of obtaining papillary or medullary tissue is small. Therefore a kidney biopsy is not always diagnostic in the early stages of analgesic nephropathy.

Epidemiology and Prevalence

A striking feature of analgesic nephropathy is the wide geographic variation in its incidence. Early reports clearly indicated that the disease was more common, in descending order, in Australia, New Zealand, Switzerland, Sweden, and Finland and less common in England, Canada, and the United States. It was also evident that there were regional differences within each country, with identifiable pockets of higher prevalence in a given country. A positive and direct relationship was found between local sales and estimated per capita consumption of over-the-counter analgesic mixtures and the incidence of analgesic nephropathy in a given region. The reliability of this kind of indirect association has been debated in the literature, as has the impact of phenacetin withdrawal in different countries. The composition of the marketed analgesic mixtures varies and could account for some of the differences in prevalence. Unfortunately, this is not an easy question to address because industry-initiated changes in composition confound any such studies. However, the early removal of phenacetin from analgesic

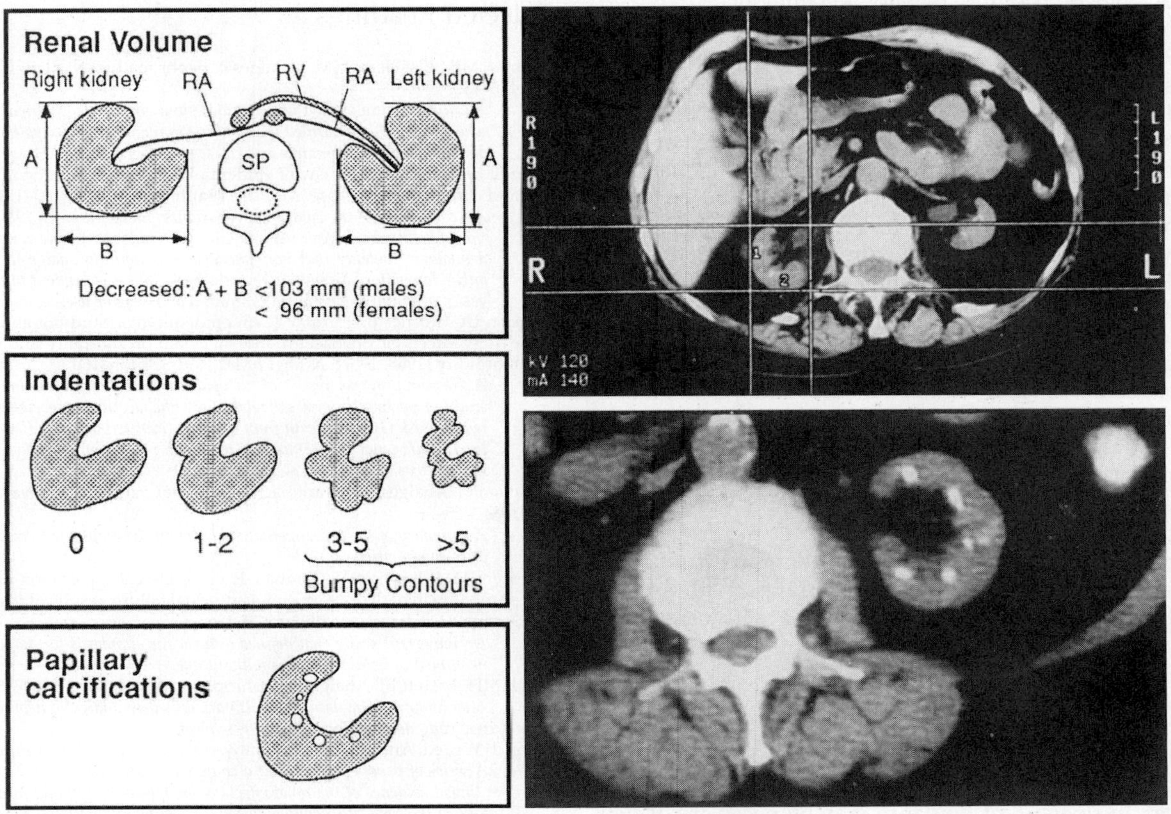

Figure 47.5. Computed tomography *(CT)* imaging criteria for diagnosing analgesic nephropathy when validated by careful history. Renal size is considered decreased if the sum of *A + B (top panel)* is less than 103 mm in men and 96 mm in women. Bumpy contours are considered significant if at least three indentations are evident *(middle panel)*. Papillary calcification *(bottom panel)* early in the course of analgesic nephropathy before the onset of atrophy or cortical indentations. RA, renal artery; RV, renal vein. (Reproduced with permission from DeBroe ME, Elseviers MM. Analgesic nephropathy. *N Engl J Med* 1998;338:446–451.)

mixtures clearly had limited impact on analgesic nephropathy as a cause of ESRD. By contrast, removing over-the-counter analgesic mixtures has been shown to reduce ESRD attributed to analgesic nephropathy. This approach, facilitated by the advent of national ESRD registries, further complicates the interpretation of epidemiologic prevalence studies. To begin with, it depends on the accuracy of the diagnosis reported to the registry. The difficulty of confirming a diagnosis of analgesic nephropathy, the general reluctance to pursue its diagnosis in patients with ESRD, and the usual tendency to rely on clinical acumen to complete registry forms all confound such data. Equally confounding are the changes in eligibility criteria for dialysis treatment that have taken place over the past decade in countries where analgesic nephropathy is more common.

Available ESRD registry data report analgesic nephropathy incidences of 0.8% in the United States, 3% in Europe, and 9% in Australia. However, limitations of registry data can be gleaned from reports using CT scan results to determine the incidence of analgesic nephropathy in patients starting dialysis, which was found to be 20% in Lisbon, 16% in Berlin, 15% in Linz, and 10.7% in the Czech and Slovak republics. For these reasons, a careful prospective multicenter study using reliable questionnaires and verifiable CT scans has been initiated by the National Institute of Diabetes, Digestive and Kidney Diseases (NIDDK).

The focus on registry data, which track only patients with ESRD, detracts from a larger issue related to habitual analgesic use: their suggested potential to aggravate preexisting renal insufficiency, independent of the underlying primary cause of renal disease. The risk reported in published cohort and case-controlled studies shows this potential to be greater for phenacetin (reported odds ratios range from 4 to 19) than for acetaminophen (reported odds ratios 2.1 to 4) and either absent or lowest for aspirin (reported odds ratios 1 to 2.5). As with classic analgesic nephropathy, all studies show a dose-dependent increased risk for ESRD and a magnified risk for analgesic mixtures (odds ratios 8 to 20).

Given widespread analgesic use, it is worthwhile to compare the risks of analgesic mixture use with those of another habitual risk factor: smoking. In a projected calculation based on available figures, it has been estimated that the risk of analgesic nephropathy in habitual analgesic mixture users (2.0:1,000) is the same as that of lung cancer in habitual smokers (2.1:1,000). The preventable risk of smoking has justifiably become a major public health concern, and that of analgesic mixtures deserves equal public health attention. Because of public health concerns about preventable causes of ESRD, the National Kidney Foundation has recommended withdrawing over-the-counter analgesic mixtures and adding warning labels to those available by prescription; using acetaminophen as the nonnarcotic analgesic of choice for episodic use in patients with underlying renal disease but discouraging its habitual use and supervising medically indicated chronic use; avoiding aspirin use in patients with impaired renal function, sodium depletion, liver cirrhosis with ascites, and acute glomerulonephritis and in children with congestive heart failure.

Treatment

The principal therapeutic goal should be to discontinue habitual analgesic consumption. This is not always easy. Psychological support and persistent guidance may be necessary. If discontinuation is not feasible, then every effort should be made to promote the use of a single agent rather than combinations. In addition, all such patients should be encouraged to increase fluid intake, even at night, to achieve a urine output of more than 2 L/day. This would be expected to reduce medullary hypertonicity and therefore the concentration of the ingested analgesics in the papillary tip. Other measures to reduce dehydration (caused by laxatives, heavy or outdoor exercise, or diuretic use) should be instituted.

Apart from these specific measures, it is important to treat urinary tract infections, particularly in patients with papillary necrosis or any evidence of compromised urine flow. As in every patient with kidney disease, controlling hypertension is an integral component of care. The anemia, usually caused by iron deficiency, should be corrected and, if necessary, treated with erythropoietin.

All patients with a history of chronic exposure to analgesics (even if their use has been discontinued), especially those exposed to phenacetin, should be monitored routinely for transitional cell carcinoma of the uroepithelium. The detection of hematuria in such patients should always lead to a thorough investigation of such an eventuality. An increased risk of adenocarcinoma of the kidney also has been noted in analgesic users. The risk ratio of renal cell carcinoma is lower than that of uroepithelial carcinoma (1.3 versus 12.2) and does not differ between patients exposed to phenacetin and those exposed to acetaminophen.

In cases that progress to ESRD, renal replacement therapy with dialysis should be initiated. Kidney transplantation is a clear alternative but is best undertaken only in patients who have discontinued analgesic use. Cases of recurrent analgesic nephropathy, manifested by RPN, in the transplanted kidney have been documented in patients who continue the habitual analgesic use after transplantation. Continuous monitoring and guidance of such patients are essential for long-term graft function.

Selected Readings

DeBroe ME, Elseviers MM. Analgesic nephropathy. *N Engl J Med* 1998;388:446–452.

A critical review of the topic that also summarizes the experience of the authors, who developed and verified the criteria for analgesic nephropathy diagnosis based on validated questionnaires and CT scans.

Deezell E, Shapiro E. A review of epidemiologic studies of nonnarcotic analgesics and chronic renal disease. *Medicine* (Baltimore) 1998;77:102–121.

An evaluation of the epidemiologic studies published since 1980 on the association of habitual analgesic use and CRI. Concludes that there is no convincing epidemiologic evidence that non–phenacetin-containing analgesics or nonsteroidal antiinflammatory drugs cause renal disease, but it is prudent to consider all analgesics nephrotoxic and avoid protracted or excessive use.

Dubach UC, Rosner B, Sturmer T. An epidemiologic study of abuse of analgesic drugs. Effects of phenacetin and salicylate on mortality and cardiovascular morbidity (1968–1987). *N Engl J Med* 1991;324:155–160.

A 20-year progress report of an epidemiologic prospective longitudinal Swiss study of phenacetin and salicylate use. Phenacetin is associated with increased relative risk (16.1) of death from urologic (cystitis) or renal disease (pyelonephritis, chronic renal failure) and an increased risk of hypertension (odds ratio 1.6). No risk was detected in salicylate users.

Eknoyan G. Analgesic nephrotoxicity and renal papillary necrosis. *Semin Nephrol* 1984;4:65–76.

A summary of the experimental evidence on the renal effects of analgesics singly or in combination.

Elseviers MM, Bosteels V, Gambier P, et al. Diagnostic criteria of analgesic nephropathy in patients with end-stage renal failure: results of the Belgian study. *Nephrol Dial Transplant* 1992;7:479–486.

An important study that defined and set the standards for diagnosing analgesic nephropathy using CT scans without dye.

Gault MH, Barrett BJ. Analgesic nephropathy. *Am J Kidney Dis* 1998;32:351–360.

A summary of the data on ESRD attributed to analgesic nephropathy based on two consensus conferences on the subject.

Henrich WL, ed. Analgesic nephropathy. *Am J Kidney Dis* 1996 (Suppl 1);28:S1–S70.

A series of papers presented at a conference that examined the experimental and clinical evidence of the renal effects of analgesics singly and in combination and formed the basis of recommendations issued by the National Kidney Foundation. An excellent resource.

Henrich WL. Analgesic nephropathy. *Am J Med Sci* 1988;295:561–568.

A review of the clinical evidence of analgesic nephropathy.

McCredie M, Stewart JH, Day NE. Different roles for phenacetin and paracetamol in cancer of the kidney and renal pelvis. *Int J Cancer* 1993;53:245–249.

An analysis of the risk of malignancy related to analgesics in a population base case-controlled study from a region (New South Wales) known for its high consumption of analgesic mixtures.

Prescott LF. Analgesic nephropathy: a reassessment of the role of phenacetin and other analgesics. *Drugs* 1982;23:75–149.

A thorough and critical review of the experimental and clinical evidence accrued in the 1970s on the subject.

PART 6
Renal Diseases Associated With Heroin Abuse

Mohammad Akmal and Shaul G. Massry

Three renal disease entities may develop in heroin users. *Glomerulonephritis* may occur secondary to bacterial endocarditis, which develops after the use of nonsterile needles and syringes for heroin injection. The clinical picture, course, and management of this glomerulonephritis are similar to those encountered in patients with other causes of endocarditis; this is discussed in detail in Chapter 39, Part 3F. *Acute renal failure* secondary to nontraumatic rhabdomyolysis is encountered after heroin abuse. Finally, proteinuria, nephrotic syndrome, and progressive deterioration of renal function may be seen in heroin users, and this entity has been called *heroin nephropathy.*

ACUTE RENAL FAILURE

The acute renal failure that occurs in heroin abusers is due to rhabdomyolysis secondary to muscle injury. It is characterized by muscle tenderness, swelling and/or necrosis, pigmenturia (red–brown urine) resulting from myoglobinuria, oliguria (occasionally the renal failure is nonoliguric), elevated blood levels of muscle enzymes [creatine phosphokinase (CPK) and aldolase], and abnormalities in serum electrolytes (including hypocalcemia, hyperphosphatemia, hyperkalemia, hypermagnesemia, acidosis, and marked hyperuricemia). Transient moderate to severe elevations in liver enzymes and bilirubinemia (several days) may also be seen in many patients with rhabdomyolysis. Leukocytosis (11,000 to 25,000 cells/mm^3) is almost always present. It must be emphasized that many heroin users who manifest rhabdomyolysis and myoglobinuria may not develop acute renal failure. The incidence of the latter among heroin abusers is not known, but it is not infrequent.

Pathogenesis

Rhabdomyolysis

The major cause of rhabdomyolysis in subjects who abuse heroin is the obtundation and/or coma that follows the injection of a large dose of heroin. The patient remains immobilized for a prolonged period, and the pressure exerted by his or her body weight against the floor damages the muscle and results in myonecrosis. The sequence of events that follow the injection of a large dose of heroin and the consequences of the rhabdomyolysis are presented schematically in Fig. 47.6. However, there is a report of a patient who developed acute renal failure after nasal sniffing of heroin and was not unconscious.

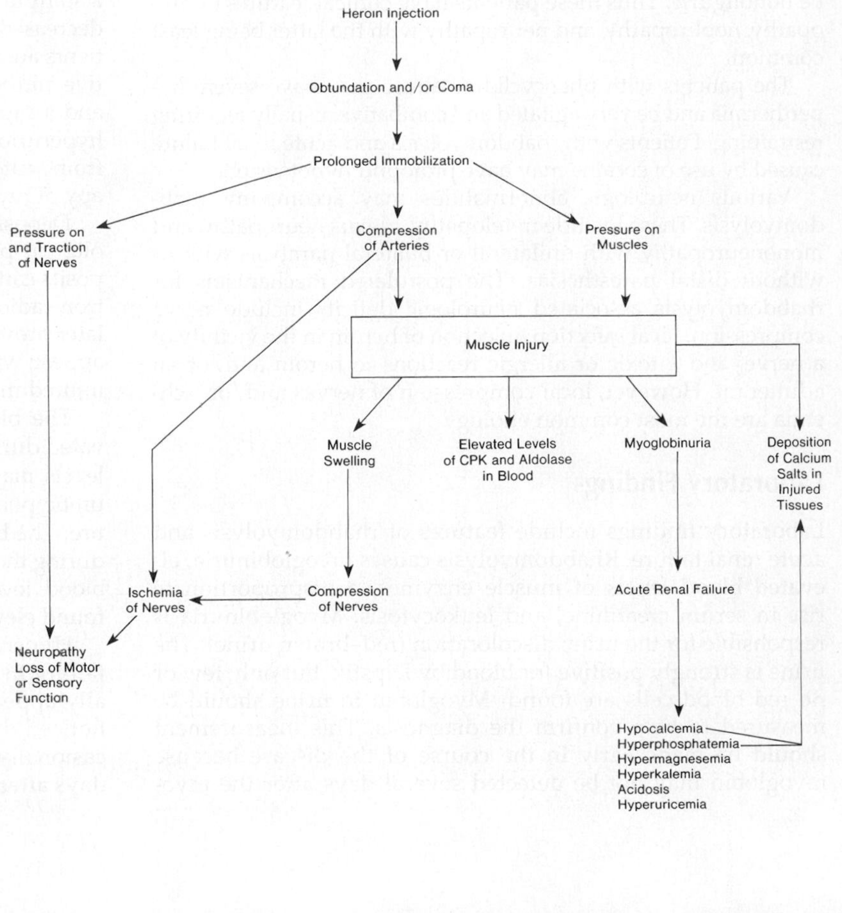

Figure 47.6. Schematic presentation of the sequence of events following an injection of a large dose of heroin. CPK, creatine phosphokinase.

Acute Renal Failure

The mechanisms of acute renal failure following rhabdomyolysis and myoglobinuria are not fully understood. The various factors that may be involved in this phenomenon are discussed in Chapter 28.

Other Causes of Rhabdomyolysis

A multitude of other conditions could also be associated with rhabdomyolysis and acute renal failure, and these are listed in Table 28.5. In the late 1970s and early 1980s, phencyclidine had been increasingly abused. This drug abuse was associated with rhabdomyolysis and acute renal failure. Among 1,000 patients with phencyclidine intoxication, 25 (2.5%) had rhabdomyolysis, and 10 of these 25 patients (40%) developed acute renal failure. Currently, cocaine is emerging as a major cause of rhabdomyolysis and acute renal failure. In a prospective study of 34 cocaine users, 8 (24%) had rhabdomyolysis as evidenced by elevated levels of CPK. In another study of 39 cocaine abusers who had rhabdomyolysis, 13 (33%) had acute renal failure.

Clinical Features

The clinical setting is that of a patient known to use heroin or cocaine and brought to the hospital obtunded or comatose. Occasionally, the patient may be awake but gives a history of recent obtundation or coma. He or she may complain of muscle tenderness or may display overt evidence of muscle injury involving one or more limbs or other parts of the body. The muscle damage may be mild or extensive and associated with marked swelling. Those with extensive muscle injury may also complain of neuropathy with motor and/or sensory deficits. Many of these patients display clinical evidence of dehydration. A decrease in urine output and the passing of red–brown urine may be reported by the patient, or oliguria and urine discoloration are detected in the hospital. The acute renal failure may be nonoliguric. Thus these patients have clinical features of myopathy, nephropathy, and neuropathy with the latter being least common.

The patients with phencyclidine abuse may have severe hyperthermia and be very agitated and combative, usually requiring restraining. Patients with rhabdomyolysis and acute renal failure caused by use of cocaine may have profound hypotension.

Various neurologic abnormalities may accompany rhabdomyolysis. These include myelopathy, plexus neuropathy, and mononeuropathy with unilateral or bilateral paralysis with or without distal paresthesias. The postulated mechanisms for rhabdomyolysis associated neurologic deficits include nerve compression, local infection, injection of heroin in the vicinity of a nerve, and a toxic or allergic reactions to heroin and/or an adulterant. However, local compression of nerves and/or ischemia are the most common etiology.

Laboratory Findings

Laboratory findings include features of rhabdomyolysis and acute renal failure. Rhabdomyolysis causes myoglobinuria, elevated blood levels of muscle enzymes, a disproportionate rise in serum creatinine, and leukocytosis. Myoglobinuria is responsible for the urine discoloration (red–brown urine). The urine is strongly positive for blood by Dipstik, but only few or no red blood cells are found. Myoglobin in urine should be measured to help confirm the diagnosis. This measurement should be made early in the course of the disease because myoglobin may not be detected several days after the myonecrosis. Red–brown urine could be produced by other disease entities such as hematuria, hemoglobinuria, and porphyria, as well as after the ingestion of exogenous pigments. The criteria for the differentiation of these conditions are provided in Table 28.4.

The blood levels of the muscle enzymes (CPK and aldolase) rise rapidly and reach high values (CPK greater than 24,000 U/L) to be followed by gradual decline. If the blood levels of these enzymes do not fall, one must suspect continued myonecrosis, which is usually encountered in the patients with extensive swelling of limbs and with marked compression of arteries and muscles. Such patients require fasciotomy of the affected limbs to relieve pressure. The levels of serum creatinine are usually disproportionately higher than those of urea nitrogen. Almost all patients with rhabdomyolysis have moderate to marked leukocytosis (11,000 to 25,000 cells/mm^3) in the absence of infection.

The features of acute renal failure are similar to those seen in patients with other causes of acute renal failure but are more marked in the patients with rhabdomyolysis. The duration of oliguria may range from 1 to 20 days, followed by diuresis and recovery of renal function. About 20% of the patients have nonoliguric renal failure. The urinary indices include high fractional excretion of sodium, isosthenuria, and low urine:plasma creatine ratio. These patients have *marked hyperphosphatemia* and *hypocalcemia,* and values of 20 and 4 mg/dl, respectively, have been encountered. In a series of 21 patients, the mean of serum phosphorus was 9.3 ± 0.9 (SE) mg/dl and that of serum calcium 6.9 ± 0.3 mg/dl. Occasionally, the concentration of serum phosphorus is not elevated, and this is seen in patients who were phosphate depleted and hypophosphatemic before the development of rhabdomyolysis. *Profound hyperuricemia* is a usual finding in these patients. We have seen a patient with a serum uric acid concentration of 49 mg/dl. The mean value in a series of 21 patients was 17.9 ± 1.3 mg/dl, compared with 10.3 ± 0.8 mg/dl in patients with other causes of acute renal failure. The mechanisms of the hyperuricemia include increased production of uric acid from its precursors released from the damaged muscles and decreased urinary excretion by the failing kidneys. These patients are usually hypercatabolic as manifested by marked negative nitrogen balance, marked hyperkalemia, severe acidosis, and a rapid rise in the blood levels of urea nitrogen. Profound hyperuricemia is also noted with acute renal failure resulting from acute pancreatitis, severe and marked dehydration, or therapy of myeloproliferative malignancies.

Deposition of calcium in the damaged muscle during the oliguric phase is common in these patients. These calcium deposits can be detected by conventional x-ray examination, electron radiography, or technetium-99m diphosphonate scan. The later provides the best diagnostic tool. The calcium deposits disappear with recovery of renal function. Calcium deposition in injured muscle occurs in the absence of renal failure as well.

The blood levels of parathyroid hormone are usually elevated during the oliguric and diuretic phase of the illness. These levels may be normal or low in many patients during the diuretic phase of the rhabdomyolysis-associated acute renal failure. The blood levels of 25-hydroxyvitamin D may be elevated during the oliguric and diuretic phase, and in many patients, the blood levels of 1,25-dihydroxyvitamin D [$1,25(OH)_2D_3$] were found elevated during the diuretic phase.

Hypercalcemia occurs in the diuretic phase of acute renal failure in about 30% of the patients. The hypercalcemia usually appears shortly after the onset of diuresis and has been noticed during the 3rd to 11th day of the diuretic phase. Occasionally, it is delayed, and in one patient, it occurred 55 days after the onset of diuresis. It is usually mild, of short duration, and relatively benign. Occasionally, it is severe, prolonged, and symptomatic. It is generally accepted that the mechanism of this hypercalcemia is the remobilization into the extracellular space of calcium previously deposited in the damaged muscle. Release of vitamin D from the damaged muscle may provide the source for the elevated blood levels of $1,25(OH)_2D_3$ seen in the diuretic phase of the acute renal failure in these patients. The available data suggest that extrarenal production of $1,25(OH)_2D_3$ may occur in these patients and/or that the renal production of this metabolite by the recovering kidney is not tightly controlled.

On rare occasions, hypercalcemia may develop during the oliguric phase of the acute renal failure and at a time when the serum phosphorus levels are also markedly elevated. This situation is very hazardous because it could cause acute widespread calcium deposition in soft tissues, including vital organs such as the lungs and heart, and could lead to severe cardiopulmonary insufficiency.

Evidence of hepatic dysfunction is commonly encountered in patients with rhabdomyolysis with acute renal failure. In a study of 119 such patients, 34 (29%) displayed evidence of severe liver dysfunction. The serum levels of lactic dehydrogenase were markedly elevated (2,500 to 40,000 U/L). The peak values occurred within 72 hours of hospitalization. There was no difference among the 22 patients with acute renal failure and the 12 patients without acute renal failure. Similarly, marked elevation in both alanine aminotransferase (ALT) and aspartate aminotransferase (AST) were observed within 72 hours after admission to the hospital. Values of up to 10,000 U/L were observed, and they were usually higher in patients with acute renal failure than in those without acute renal failure. Hyperbilirubinemia of up to 7.0 mg/dl was noted in 13 of the 22 (60%) patients with acute renal failure and in 5 of the 12 (42%) patients without acute renal failure. Prothrombin time was also significantly reduced in a large number of these patients. In another study of 33 patients with cocaine-induced rhabdomyolysis, 11 (33%) displayed evidence of hepatic dysfunction; 7 of these patients developed disseminated intravascular coagulation. The evidence of the hepatic dysfunction may last 1 to 13 days but reverses spontaneously. The pathogenesis of these abnormalities is not well defined and may be multifactorial. Hyperpyrexia, hypotension, and proteases released from injured muscle may each or all be contributory.

Clinical Course and Treatment

The clinical course of these patients is benign, and almost all of them recover from the acute renal failure. Occasionally, severe infectious complications may lead to a fatal outcome. Neurologic deficits may persist. Calcium deposition in vital organs may occur if hypercalcemia develops during the oliguric phase.

The management is the same as that for acute renal failure from other causes. Peritoneal dialysis or hemodialysis therapy may be needed during the oliguric phase. Decompression of markedly swollen limbs by fasciotomy should not be delayed to prevent loss of muscle mass and/or permanent nerve damage. The hyperuricemia does not require therapy. Hypercalcemia during the oliguric phase should be treated with dialysis therapy using calcium-free dialysate. Hypercalcemia during the diuretic phase does not require therapy unless it is marked and prolonged; the various therapeutic modalities for the treatment of hypercalcemia described in Chapter 17, Part 3 could be used.

HEROIN NEPHROPATHY

The term *heroin nephropathy* is used to describe a renal disease in heroin addicts that is manifested by proteinuria and/or nephrotic syndrome with or without renal insufficiency.

Clinical Features

The major feature of heroin nephropathy is proteinuria, which can be mild (2 g/24 hr) or severe, being in the nephrotic range; values up to 30 g/24 hr have been encountered. The proteinuria may be discovered accidentally on routine urine analysis or it may be sought in the diagnostic workup of a heroin addict who initially has peripheral edema. Microscopic hematuria and moderate leukocyturia may also be present. Many patients may have all the clinical, metabolic, and laboratory findings of nephrotic syndrome (see Chapter 39, Parts 1 and 2). Renal function may be normal, but most patients have variable degrees of renal insufficiency that may progress to end-stage renal failure. Hypertension is present, especially in those with renal failure.

Heroin nephropathy has been reported in both whites and African-Americans and in males and females. In certain series, the patients were predominantly African-Americans and especially in those with HLA-BW53. The exact duration of addiction before the appearance of the clinical manifestations of the nephropathy is not well defined, but certainly more than 1 year is required.

Amyloidosis may complicate chronic heroin use. These patients present with nephrotic syndrome, renal failure, normal urinary sediment, and frequently, tubular dysfunction such as renal tubular acidosis and/or nephrogenic diabetes insipidus.

Pathology

Almost every type of glomerular lesion has been reported in patients with heroin nephropathy. Focal or diffuse membranous, proliferative, and membranoproliferative glomerular lesions have been seen. The renal biopsy may show glomerular basement membrane thickening, hypercellularity, mesangial matrix proliferation, glomerular sclerosis, and interstitial fibrosis. The most common lesion is *focal glomerular sclerosis* and is considered by many to be the typical lesion. Immunofluorescence studies demonstrate diffuse or focal deposits of IgG, B_1C, IgA, and IgM, the latter being more common. The deposition is usually granular, but linear deposits of IgG have been reported. Electron microscopy may show focal basement membrane thickening, electron-dense deposits in the mesangial areas, and endothelial cell proliferation. Granulomatous interstitial nephritis has been reported in one patient.

Secondary renal amyloidosis is being encountered in an increasing number of patients with heroin abuse. In a study of 16 patients with heroin nephropathy, 10 had focal glomerulosclerosis, and 6 had secondary amyloidosis. It appears that the latter lesion may underlie nephrotic syndrome and renal failure in a substantial number of patients with heroin nephropathy. Patients with secondary amyloidosis have skin ulcerations and/or abscesses. It is interesting that amyloidosis has been reported predominantly in male African-American patients.

Pathogenesis

The pathogenesis of heroin nephropathy is not known. Several possibilities have been considered, including a direct effect of heroin, glomerular injury produced by a contaminant, and viral or bacterial or immune mechanisms. Mild proteinuria in heroin addicts is thought to be due to glomerular lesions secondary to viral hepatitis.

The amyloidosis is seen more commonly with skin "popping" but also follows intravenous heroin administration. It is usually seen after prolonged heroin abuse (more than 15 years) and is most likely related to chronic suppurative skin infections.

Course and Treatment

Most patients progress to end-stage renal failure and require maintenance hemodialysis therapy. Improvement or reversal of the nephrotic syndrome and of renal insufficiency may follow the discontinuation of heroin use. There is no therapeutic modality that is useful in the management of heroin nephropathy except for complete abstinence from heroin. Every effort should be made to achieve this goal. Cadaveric renal transplantation has been done in reformed heroin addicts who had heroin nephropathy and has had good outcome. Treatment of the patients who present with amyloidosis is similar to that of other causes of amyloidosis (see Chapter 42, Part 10).

Selected Readings

Akmal M, Massry SG. Reversible hepatic dysfunction associated with rhabdomyolysis. *Am J Nephrol* 1990;10:49–52.

A study of 34 patients with rhabdomyolysis with or without acute renal failure describing the presence of hepatic dysfunction in these patients.

Cunningham EE, Brentjens JR, Zielezny MA, et al. Heroin nephropathy. A clinicopathologic study. *Am J Med* 1980;68:47–53.

A clinicopathologic and epidemiologic study to determine whether heroin use and renal disease are associated. Twenty-three addicts with nephrotic syndrome and/or renal insufficiency were studied; all patients were African-American. All patients underwent renal biopsies, which uniformly showed sclerosing glomerulonephritis. End-stage renal disease developed in 15 of these patients.

Dettmeyer R, Wessling B, Madea B. Heroin associated nephropathy. A postmortem study. *Forensic Sci Int* 1998;20:109–116.

A report of postmortem findings in 179 autopsies of patients known as intravenous drug addicts from Switzerland. It is interesting that focal segmental glomerulosclerosis was not found. The latter entity was reported in the United States mainly in African-American patients.

Dubrow A, Mittman N, Ghali Y, et al. The changing spectrum of heroin associated nephropathy. *Am J Kidney Dis* 1985;5:35–41.

Biopsies were performed on 35 heroin abusers as part of the evaluation of unexplained heavy proteinuria; 80% showed focal segmental glomerulosclerosis or renal amyloidosis. The relative incidence of renal amyloidosis and focal glomerulosclerosis has changed significantly. Chronic suppurative skin infection at the site of injections seems to initiate and potentiate secondary amyloidosis.

Koffler A, Friedler RM, Massry SG. Acute renal failure due to non-traumatic rhabdomyolysis. *Ann Intern Med* 1976;85:23–28.

A study of 21 patients with acute renal failure associated with nontraumatic rhabdomyolysis. A disproportionate rise in serum creatinine concentration in relation to serum urea nitrogen was observed. Profound hyperuricemia was present in most patients; transient hypercalcemia during the diuretic phase developed in some patients. The disease has a good prognosis despite severe hypercatabolism and untreated profound hyperuricemia.

Llach F, Descoeudres C, Massry SG. Heroin associated nephropathy: clinical and histological studies in 19 patients. *Clin Nephrol* 1979;11:7–12.

A study of 19 patients with heroin addiction and renal disease. Renal biopsy revealed focal glomerulonephritis in 10 patients (5 with sclerosis); most patients demonstrated progression, and 4 patients showed marked improvement on cessation of heroin use.

Rao TKS, Nicastri AD, Friedman EA. Natural history of heroin associated nephropathy. *N Engl J Med* 1974;290:19–23.

Evidence confirming the existence of nephrotic syndrome associated with heroin abuse and description of its grim prognosis. Renal biopsies were obtained in 13 of the 14 patients; focal and segmental glomerular sclerosis were evident in 11 patients. Follow-up examinations were possible in 8 patients; in all of these, uremia developed within 6 to 48 months of detection of proteinuria.

Roth D, Alarcon FJ, Fernandez JA, et al. Acute rhabdomyolysis associated with cocaine intoxication. *N Engl J Med* 1988;319:673–677.

A study of 39 patients with acute rhabdomyolysis resulting from cocaine abuse. Thirteen developed acute renal failure. Hepatic dysfunction and disseminated intravascular coagulation were also present.

Yang C-C, Yang C-Y, Ger Jin, et al. Severe rhabdomyolysis mimicking transverse myelitis in a heroin addict. *Clin Toxicol* 1995;34:591–595.

A case report and a review of the literature regarding the neurologic abnormalities encountered in rhabdomyolysis.

PART 7
Contrast Medium–Induced Nephropathy

Oscar Fernando Pavão dos Santos, Mirian Aparecida Boim, Sandra M. Rodrigues Laranja, and Nestor Schor

Since the first report of contrast medium–induced nephropathy (CIN) in the early 1920s, many studies have been published to describe adverse effects of contrast media (CM) on kidney function. However, different experimental models, wide variability in clinical characteristics of the patients studied, different diagnostic tests used, and the type and volume of CM are all responsible for the difficult in analyzing such nephrotoxicity.

CM are freely filtered by the glomeruli, and they are not secreted or reabsorbed by the tubules. In normal people, they have a renal clearance similar to creatinine and a half-life of about 30 to 60 minutes. CM are usually safe but not free of side effects, including systemic hypersensibility reactions, cardiac adverse reactions (hypertension, tachycardia, arrhythmia), vascular effects (platelet aggregation, vasoconstriction, thrombosis), and renal effects.

The kidney is responsible for a large portion of the metabolism and excretion of many substances in the body, and it has also become a target for toxic components, including radiocontrast media. Different procedures using radiocontrast media are done with increasing frequency, and the patients submitted to them are getting older and with more comorbid conditions. Therefore the nephrotoxicity incidence of CM has increased from 5% to 30% to a very large portion of all hospital-acquired acute renal failure (ARF). Considering that 10 million procedures using CM are done yearly in the United States, an incidence of 0.1% would cause 10,000 cases of CIN per year. In this way, CM is the second most common nephrotoxic agent after aminoglicosides in clinical practice.

Multiple definitions have been used to define CIN. An absolute increase in serum creatinine from 0.5 to 1.0 mg/dl or proportional rises on creatinine from 25% to 50% are the mostly used. However, there is no consensus on the definition of CIN in the literature, making it difficult to compare the results obtained in many studies in terms of incidence, risk factors, and prognosis. Usually, the rise in serum creatinine occurs 48 to 72 hours after CM exposure, and it returns to normal values after 7 to 10 days. However, ARF may develop and last for 4 weeks as it can be seen in ARF induced by ischemia. ARF caused by CIN is nonoliguric in most patients, and the urinary sediment shows tubular epithelial cells, granular casts, and minimal proteinuria. Urinary sodium concentration is low and fractional excretion of sodium is less than 1%, particularly in oliguric patients.

The renal morphologic alterations caused by CM are not well characterized. Cytoplasm vacuolization of proximal tubular cells was found in 20% of patients submitted to biopsies. Acute tubular proximal and thick ascending limb necrosis have also been reported in animals receiving CM infusion. However, kidney tissues obtained from patients with CIN may show no significant morphologic changes.

TABLE 47.14. Main Risk Factors for Contrast Medium–Induced Nephropathy

Baseline renal insufficiency
Heart failure
Dose of contrast media
Diabetes mellitus
Volume depletion
Multiple myeloma (?)
Hypercholesterolemia (?)

RISK FACTORS (TABLE 47.14)

Many risk factors have been suggested to explain the development of CIN. Baseline renal insufficiency, heart failure, the dosage of CM, and diabetes are the most important, with preexisting renal insufficiency being the most significant of them. Indeed, the risk of developing CIN is directly correlated to the degree of renal insufficiency. Thus the lower glomerular filtration rates, the higher incidence of CIN. It was reported that a serum creatinine level greater than 1.2 mg/dl was the value at which the risk of CIN begins to increase. Actually, serum creatinine concentration higher than 2.0 mg/dl was associated with a 20% incidence of CIN.

Heart failure has also been shown to be an independent risk factor for the development of CIN. However, the intravascular volume depletion secondary to diuretic therapy and the renal vasoconstriction in patients with heart failure could play an important role in CIN in these patients.

Diabetes has also been found as an independent risk factor for CIN. However, in the absence of renal insufficiency, the risk is similar to that in nondiabetic patients. The combination of diabetes and renal insufficiency increases CIN risk compared with that observed in patients with renal insufficiency alone. Moreover, diabetic patients affected by CM develop oliguria and require dialysis more frequently. ARF after the exposure to CIN would almost certainly occur in patients with a history of diabetes of greater than 10 years, who are older than 50 years, who have incidence of vasculopathy, and who also have renal insufficiency. Dehydration will enhance the risk for CIN.

Hypercholesterolemia is another important factor that could contribute to aggravate CM nephrotoxicity.

Infusion of CM volumes larger than 125 ml appears to be a significant risk factor for CIN, especially in those volume-depleted and/or diabetic patients. Despite that multiple myeloma has been described as a potential risk factor for CIN, a recent review of myeloma patients receiving CM has failed to observe an increased risk.

Although the frequency of recovery of renal function in patients with CIN is high, it is not a benign disease. It can result in longer hospitalization, the need for dialysis in 10% to 25% of the patients, and it can affect the mortality rate. Indeed, the mortality rate in those patients who developed CIN was fivefold higher when compared with those without CIN, even after adjusting for comorbid conditions. In addition, CIN was associated with increased risk of developing many other complications, such as respiratory failure, sepsis, and bleeding.

PATHOGENESIS (TABLE 47.15)

The pathophysiology of CIN is still not well known. The pathophysiologic mechanisms involved in this disease are multiple and are related to the type, dosage, and osmolality of the CM used. The normal kidney is usually resistant to CM, and animal studies are conducted in the presence of additional risk factors, such as volume depletion, heart failure, or any other nephrotoxic agent. It seems that the main factor involved in CIN is the renal vasoconstriction, leading to a decrease in the surface available for glomerular filtration. However, it is accepted that the use of CM is associated with a biphasic hemodynamic response, an initial vasodilation followed by a period of vasoconstriction with a decrease in renal blood flow and glomerular filtration rate.

In humans, CM infusion caused an immediate elevation in renal blood flow in the absence of any change in mean arterial pressure, indicating an initial reduction in total renal vascular resistance. The administration of vasodilator substances such as dopamine or atrial natriuretic peptide (ANP) before CM exposure caused a further increase in renal blood flow. However, a multicenter, prospective, double-blind trial evaluating the efficacy of intravenous ANP (anaritide) before and during CM administration in patients with stable chronic renal failure did not reduce the incidence of ARF associated to CM. In contrast, dopamine infusion of 2.5 μg/kg (beginning 1 hour before CM administration) prevented a rise in creatinine after angiography in patients with preexisting renal insufficiency with serum creatinine greater than 2.0 mg/dl). Interestingly, it was observed that patients who developed CIN had lower baseline levels of renal blood flow and a higher increase in it after the infusion of these vasodilator substances. Because the filtration fraction was higher, these events suggest an important increase in efferent arteriolar resistance. It has also been postulated that the association of an exaggerated initial vasodilatory phase in CIN would indicate an abnormal distribution of blood flow. There may be a decrease in vascular resistance in the cortex without a similar reduction in the resistance in the medulla. This effect causes a stealing of blood flow from the medulla, leading to a decrease in medullary oxygen content compared with that of the cortex. This ischemia might cause necrosis of the medullary thick ascending limbs and a decrease in total renal filtration fraction. When the oxygen tension (Po_2) was measured in rats comparing the renal cortex and outer medulla, it was found that both low and isoosmolar CM decreases Po_2 mainly in the outer renal medulla. In addition, vasodilators could cause an elevation in glomerular filtration rate and sodium delivery to Henle's loop, leading to higher oxygen consumption. Moreover, an activation of tubuloglomerular feedback might be one of the mechanisms that affect the balance between vasodilatory and vasoconstrictive substances, including angiotensin, adenosine, endothelin,

TABLE 47.15. Main Pathophysiologic Events Related to the Contrast Medium–Induced Nephropathy

Renal vasoconstriction
Dopamine
Atrial natriuretic peptide
Endothelin
Angiotensin II
Nitric oxide
Adenosine
Insulinlike growth factor
Prostaglandins
Reactive oxygen species
Renal medullar ischemia
Activation of tubuloglomerular feedback
Direct renal toxicity of contrast media
Intracellular enzymes release
Loss of cell polarity
Apoptosis

platelet-activating factor, nitric oxide, insulinlike growth factor (IGF), ANP, and prostaglandins.

The role of endothelin in the pathophysiology of CIN is suggested by experiments using an antagonist of endothelin receptor. The antagonist was infused before CM administration, and it prevented the decrease in renal blood flow. It has also been shown that endothelin release by cultured endothelial cells treated with CM is increased, and endothelin mRNA in these cells is also increased by CM. In humans, circulating and urinary endothelin excretion increases during hours after CM exposure. Although an increase in endothelin may contribute to renal vasoconstriction following CM, simultaneous increases in endogenous ANP may offset this effect and may protect against changes in renal function. However, a further increase in ANP did not lead to significant protection against CM nephrotoxicity.

In renal circulation, adenosine is vasoconstrictive, predominantly by the A_1 receptor, although adenosine is able to induce medullary vasodilation by a different receptor, A_2. These effects can be reversed by its receptor antagonist, theophylline. In humans, CM administration is associated with an increase in urinary excretion of adenosine, and the administration of theophylline before CM ameliorates the decrease in both renal blood flow and glomerular filtration rate in patients with reduced renal function. Not only in humans but also in animals, the selective inhibition of the adenosine receptor (A_1) reduces the CIN intensity. This protective effect of A_1 inhibition is also observed during nitric oxide blocking by L-NAME.

It has also been shown that infusion of angiotensin II increases the vasoconstrictive response to CM. The use of a receptor blocker for angiotensin II partially reduced CM effects on renal microcirculation, suggesting a role for the renin-angiotensin system in the pathophysiology of CIN. It has also been shown that a complex hormonal change occurs in mesangial cells cultured from Wistar rats in the presence of CM; epinephrine and angiotensin II release are increased; vasopressin release is decreased. These events seemed to be mediated by calcium channels. Unfortunately, no controlled study has been done in humans to evaluate the role of angiotensin II on CIN.

Studies in rats suggest that IGF could be related to ARF induced by CM. Using an experimental model that combines inhibition of prostanoids and nitric oxide before CM administration, it was observed that cortical IGF-I increased, whereas medullary IGF-I mRNA decreased. The renal IGF-I–binding protein decreased. Thus it is possible that IGF-I modulates the renal medullary recovery from ARF induced by CM.

The administration of some reactive oxygen species scavenger, such as catalase or superoxide dismutase, can also attenuate the renal alterations induced by CM. Magnesium is also used to attenuate nephrotoxicity mediated by oxygen-free radicals in patients with mild renal dysfunction. Finally, the osmolar load of CM is also an important determinant of CIN. High-osmolality CM decrease renal blood flow more than low-osmolality CM do; this may be due to an effect of osmolality of CM on the release of many vasoactive substances.

Because the pathophysiology of CIN is biphasic, some vasodilator systems have also been studied to clarify these mechanisms. Inhibition of the production of vasodilator prostaglandins using indomethacin increases CM nephrotoxicity. In the same way, pretreatment with L-NAME, a nitric oxide synthase inhibitor, potentiates the medullary vasoconstrictive response to CM, affecting the oxygen tension at this region.

In addition to renal ischemia, CM could also be directly toxic to renal epithelial tubular cells. Human vascular endothelial and kidney cells exposed to CM showed an intracellular acidification. Nonionic agents caused less cellular damage than did ionic CM. The alteration in intracellular pH is involved in the immediate intracellular transduction of CM effects. It is also observed that mesangial cells are very sensitive to the cytotoxic effects of CM and hyperosmolar solutions. This direct cytotoxicity effect has been also observed in isolated tubules and on renal epithelial cells *in vitro*. It could involve a release of intracellular enzymes, disruption of epithelial cell monolayers affecting cell polarity, and modifications in the cellular energy metabolism; all of these effects may induce apoptosis. Assessing DNA fragmentation in MDCK cells by multiple techniques to evaluate apoptosis has suggested nuclear disintegration with subsequent cell death, particularly in the hypertonic/hypoxic environment of the renal medulla; these conditions could contribute to CM nephrotoxicity.

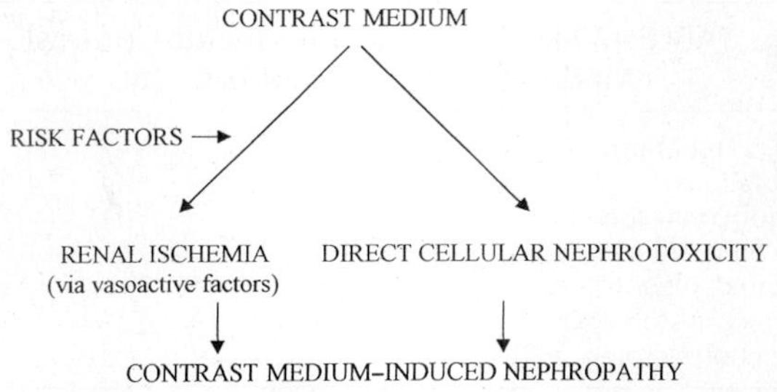

Figure 47.7. Pathophysiology of contrast medium–induced nephropathy.

It has been demonstrated that many tubular enzymes are released in the urine after CM administration. *N*-acetyl-β-D-glucosaminidase (NAG), alanine aminopeptidase (AAP), α_1-microglobulin, and β_2-microglobulin can be found in a greater amount in the urine after CM exposure. However, despite NAG, the concentration appears to correlate with structural and functional changes associated with CM; the large range of baseline values makes its measurements of dubious clinical use.

Tubular obstruction may also participate in the mechanism of CIN. It is interesting to observe that a high urine viscosity after high-osmolality contrast administration increases tubular hydraulic pressure, which causes, at least in part, decreases the single-nephron glomerular filtration rate by functional tubular obstruction as demonstrated by micropuncture technique in rats. In the presence of volume depletion, an increase in urate excretion that occurs after CM administration could also lead to a urate precipitation and elevation of hydraulic tubular pressure.

In summary, CM could induce renal ischemia by causing an imbalance of vasoactive agents, and/or it could directly affect renal function by its nephrotoxic potential at cellular and molecular levels. These two effects of CM underlie the pathogenesis of CIN (Fig. 47.7).

PREVENTION (TABLE 47.16)

Many strategies have been proposed to prevent the nephrotoxicity induced by CM. It is important is to avoid the unnecessary imaging procedures using CM in high-risk patients. Newer technologies have been developed, and the physician must look at these new imaging procedures before deciding to use CM. On the other hand, if it is necessary to expose patients to CM, it should be used in a minimum dose.

Despite some *in vitro* experiments suggesting that hyperosmolality appears to be a more important cause of cytotoxicity than the ionic strength of CM, low-osmolality agents have shown no benefit in diabetic or nondiabetic patients with normal renal function. However, these studies have used well-hydrated patients in a large prospective randomized trial. In

TABLE 47.16. Strategies to Prevent Contrast Medium–Induced Nephropathy

Use of alternative imaging technologies (no contrast media)
Low-osmolality contrast medium
Vigorous hydration before and after contrast media administration
Discontinuation of diuretics
Discontinuation of metformin
Vasodilator drugs: dopamine and theophylline
Calcium channel blockers
Magnesium (?) and atrial natriuretic peptide (?)

patients with renal insufficiency, low-osmolality contrast agents significantly reduced the incidence of CIN in both diabetic and nondiabetic patients.

The most consistent and useful approach to prevent CIN is hydration with intravenous fluid. Pretreatment with saline is effective in preventing CM nephrotoxicity as suggested by many clinical studies. It has to be initiated hours before CM exposure and must be kept for hours after the CM infusion. It has been shown that patients receiving 0.45% NaCl solution at a rate of 1 ml/kg per minute for 12 hours before and 12 hours after CM administration had a lower incidence of CIN when compared with those who received furosemide or mannitol. In another prospective trial, patients receiving furosemide had an increase in serum creatinine levels after CM infusion compared with the saline-treated group, suggesting that volume depletion occurred as a result of the furosemide treatment. Therefore diuretics should always be discontinued before the exposure to CM to prevent volume depletion. Metformin is another drug that must be discontinued in the 48 hours before or after CM administration because lactic acidosis has been seen mainly in patients with mild to severe alterations in renal function.

Several other vasodilator drugs have been widely used to prevent CM renal vasoconstriction. Both dopamine (3.0 μg/kg per minute given before and up to 24 hours after CM infusion) and theophylline (5 mg/kg given 45 minutes before CM) were effective in preventing the reduction in glomerular filtration rate. However, it must be kept in mind that vasodilator drugs could also cause a reduction of blood pressure or a preferential renal cortex vasodilation and further worsen the medullary circulation. It is worthwhile to point out that hemodialysis eliminates CM effectively; however, this procedure may not influence the incidence and/or the outcome of ARF related to CM.

Prevention of CIN may also be achieved by taking oral agents to prevent hospital admission or intravenous therapies before the procedure. Oral theophylline and calcium channel blockers were used before the administration of CM, and they attenuated the decrease in renal function according to animals and human studies.

Selected Readings

Krause W. In vivo and animal experiments in contrast media testing. *Invest Radiol* 1998;33:182–191.

Review concerning the intrinsic characteristics of CM, including physiochemical and pharmacokinetic properties and tissue tolerance.

Quader MA, Sawmiller C, Sumpio BA. Contrast-induced nephropathy: review of incidence and pathophysiology. *Ann Vasc Surg* 1998;12:612–620.

Discusses the incidence of ARF induced by CM, particularly in high-risk patients. The principal mechanisms involved in this pathology are also discussed.

Solomon R. Contrast medium-induced acute renal failure. *Kidney Int* 1998; 53(1):230–242.

This paper reviews the potential risk factors either related to CM and to the general status of the patient. The pathophysiologic mechanisms are also addressed, including the biphasic profile of the hemodynamic response to CM in humans, with an initial vasodilatory phase followed by a prolonged vasoconstrictive phase. These events contribute to the abnormal intrarenal distribution of blood flow, causing medullary ischemia. The hormonal involvement in these mechanisms is also discussed, including angiotensin II, endothelin, ANP, and nitric oxide.

Solomon R. Radiocontrast-induced nephropathy. *Semin Nephrol* 1998;18:551–557.

Discusses the ischemic injury to the medullary portion of the kidney due to the CM-induced renal vasoconstriction. Also addresses the preexisting malignancies that increase the risk of developing ARF. Finally, the author suggests the prophylaxis of high-risk patients.

Thomsen HS, Bush WH Jr. Treatment of the adverse effects of contrast media. *Acta Radiol* 1998;39:212–218.

The authors discuss the importance of the recognition and treatment of the patient who develops ARF after CM administration, and based on the literature, they suggest a treatment protocol.

Tublin ME, Murphy ME, Tessler FN. Current concepts in contrast media-induced nephropathy. *AJR Am J Roentgenol* 1998;171:933–939.

This article provides a practical overview of all aspects of CM-induced nephropathy, including epidemiology, pathophysiologic mechanisms, treatment, and prevention.

PART 8
Radiation Nephritis

Richard J. Glassock

There is little doubt that ionizing radiation can result in renal parenchymal damage. Fortunately, recognition of this fact has led to better shielding of the kidneys when radiation therapy is used to treat tumors involving tissues adjacent or near to the kidneys (e.g., Wilms' tumor, ovarian or testicular cancer, retroperitoneal lymphoma, neuroblastoma, lymphoma, or spinal or intraabdominal metastasis). As a result, radiation nephropathy, is now very rare.

The development of renal injury is related to the total dose and duration of treatment. High dosages given over short periods of time (2 to 5 weeks) are most likely to produce renal injury. Among reported cases, at least 2,000 rads (23 Gy) have been delivered to kidneys over several weeks. Lower dosages may lead to chronic injury after long latent periods. Younger patients appear to be more susceptible. Concomitant therapy with antineoplastic agents such as doxorubicin or bleomycin may enhance the likelihood of injury. It may occur after whole-body irradiation as used in bone marrow transplantation.

CLINICAL FEATURES

Acute and *chronic* forms of radiation nephropathy are recognized. The acute form usually begins within 6 to 12 months of initial radiation exposure and is characterized by the rather abrupt onset of hematuria, proteinuria, and severe or malignant hypertension. These findings are usually accompanied by a severe normochromic, normocytic anemia, often out of proportion to the degree of impairment of renal function. Nephrotic syndrome is uncommon. Microangiopathic hemolytic anemia may be present, particularly if malignant hypertension ensues. Thus acute radiation nephritis may resemble acute poststreptococcal glomerulonephritis, scleroderma renal crisis, and hemolytic uremia syndrome. During the acute injury, bone scans with technetium pyrophosphate may image the kidney. The clinical findings often slowly subside, leaving a residue of hypertension and moderate proteinuria. Most patients will later progress after intervals of 10 years or more to a chronic stage manifested by slowly worsening renal function complicated by severe hypertension.

Chronic radiation nephropathy begins more insidiously and may be manifested by stable isolated proteinuria, mild to moderate hypertension, or slowly progressive renal failure, sometimes complicated by malignant hypertension appearing years after radiation exposure. Radiation-induced fibrosis of retroperitoneal tissue, ureteric obstruction, and neurogenic bladder (from radiation myelopathy) may complicate the picture. For poorly understood reasons, uric acid excretion is severely impaired and clinical gout is occasionally seen. A microangiopathic form of hemolytic anemia may also be seen.

PATHOLOGY

In *acute* radiation nephropathy, the kidneys are often enlarged with subcapsular petechiae. The glomeruli may be enlarged and hypercellular with mesangial expansion and endothelial swelling; thus the morphologic picture may resemble acute glomerulonephritis or toxemia. Atrophy and degeneration of tubular epithelium may be present. Fibrinoid necrosis of arteries and arterioles is often found in patients with malignant hypertension. Inflammatory lesions in the interstitium are absent.

In *chronic* radiation nephropathy, the kidneys are often shrunken in size. Histologically, the hallmarks are arterial and arteriolar nephrosclerosis with marked tubular atrophy and interstitial fibrosis. The glomeruli are collapsed and appear ischemic, with mesangial sclerosis and obsolescence. Fibrinoid necrosis of arteries and arterioles is seen when malignant hypertension is present. Extrarenal arteritis may also be found. Mesangiolysis may be seen.

The pathogenesis of injury is not well understood but presumably involves the effects of ionizing radiation and toxic oxygen radicals on the integrity of endothelial smooth muscle and tubule cells.

TREATMENT

Although radiation nephropathy is a preventable disorder, excess radiation occasionally is delivered inadvertently to the renal areas. Once radiation nephropathy ensues, treatment is entirely symptomatic and supportive. Hypertension should be vigorously treated, preferably with angiotensin-converting enzyme (ACE) inhibitors. A low-protein, low-phosphorous diet accompanied by judicious salt restriction may be helpful, but this is not proven. Rarely, a salt-losing form of radiation injury may develop, requiring salt and volume repletion. Severe anemia may be treated with subcutaneous recombinant human erythropoietin. If renal arterial stenosis caused by periadventitial and retroperitoneal fibrosis develops and can be angiographically documented, reconstructive surgery rather than nephrectomy is advisable, if feasible. Despite therapy, most patients will eventually require dialysis maintenance. Because of concomitant neoplasia, patients with radiation nephropathy are generally poor candidates for renal transplantation.

Selected Readings

Crosson JT, Keane W, Anderson W. In: Tisher CC, Brenner B, eds. *Radiation nephropathy on renal pathology,* 2nd ed. Philadelphia: JB Lippincott, 1994:937–947.
A definitive account of the pathology of radiation-induced renal injury.

Luxton R. Radiation nephritis. A long-term study of 54 patients. *Lancet* 1961;2:1221–1224.
A classic description of long-term consequences of radiation nephropathy.

Madrazo A, Schwartz G, Churg J. Radiation nephritis: a review. *J Urology* 1975;114:822–827.
An excellent review with emphasis on pathology.

Tarbell N, Giunan E, Niemeyer C, et al. Late onset of renal dysfunction in survivors of bone marrow transplantation. *Int J Radiat Oncol Biol Phys* 1988;15:99–104.
Description of a rare complication of bone marrow transplantation when radiation is used to ablate marrow.

PART 9
Miscellaneous Toxic Nephropathies

Richard J. Glassock

Because of its circulatory, biochemical, and metabolic characteristics, the kidney is particularly vulnerable to the toxic effects of various chemical compounds, drugs, and physical agents. The present discussion covers miscellaneous agents that have been described as causing toxic renal lesions and that have not been discussed elsewhere in this book.

HYDROCARBONS

Ethylene glycol, an aliphatic alcohol present in antifreeze solutions, may be ingested accidentally or as a part of a suicide attempt. Overdoses cause central nervous system abnormalities (confusion, seizures, coma), high anion gap metabolic acidosis, hyperosmolality with "osmolal gap," and acute renal failure. The latter is most likely due to the metabolism of the glycol to oxalic acid with precipitation of calcium oxalate crystals in tubular cells and lumina of nephrons. Indeed, urine from patients with ethylene glycol poisoning often contains large numbers of calcium oxalate crystals. Ethyl alcohol, which competitively inhibits alcohol dehydrogenase, the major enzyme involved in the metabolism of ethylene glycol, has been used successfully in the treatment of ethylene glycol overdose. Early hemodialysis treatment is indicated to remove ethylene glycol and its toxic metabolic products, as well as to treat acidosis and renal failure.

Methoxyflurane, a volatile anesthetic compound, has been associated with acute renal failure, usually of the nonoliguric variety. Increases in plasma fluoride ion correlate best with the renal impairment, but calcium oxalate crystals have been found within the lumen and cell cytoplasm of the proximal tubule in association with necrosis. Marked impairment of urinary concentrating ability with polyuria may occur.

Carbon tetrachloride, chloroform, and *tetrachlorethylene* are well-known nephrotoxic and hepatotoxic organic solvents. Accidental inhalation of fumes by subjects, particularly while intoxicated with ethyl alcohol, is associated with acute renal failure and, to a lesser, extent hepatic failure. Because of the "first pass" effect, oral ingestion of these compounds in a suicide attempt leads to severe hepatic cell necrosis failure. Such patients may also develop acute renal failure. The renal lesion is acute tubular necrosis. In patients who inhale carbon tetrachloride, pulmonary edema may ensue because of alveolar injury. Acute renal failure is more common in inhaled intoxication with these compounds, especially in the presence of concomitant chronic ethanol consumption. Recovery can be expected in most patients unless the hepatic necrosis is very severe.

The presence of jaundice, abdominal pain, and laboratory evidence of hepatic cell necrosis in a patient with acute renal failure should give rise to a suspicion of exposure to halogenated hydrocarbons. Acute renal and hepatic failure may also be encountered in acute viral hepatitis (particularly with the delta agent), leptospirosis, mushroom poisoning, paracetamol overdose, elemental phosphorus poisoning, and hepatorenal syndrome.

Glue inhalation (glue sniffer's disease, toluene toxicity), particularly of the variety of glue used by airplane model builders (toluene, dope), may lead to a form of distal renal tubular acidosis secondary to nephron injury. Hippuric acid excretion is greatly increased as a result of the metabolism of toluene.

MISCELLANEOUS ORGANIC COMPOUNDS

Ingestion of the stems or caps of the mushroom *Amanita phalloides* containing the heptapeptide amanita toxin causes severe hepatic cell necrosis and toxic renal injury. Hepatic coma and acute renal failure may ensue. Clinically, severe watery diarrhea, vomiting, and violent abdominal pain begin 8 to 12 hours after ingestion, and within 48 hours, liver and renal damage become evident. Mannitol may be useful to prevent renal toxicity and oral charcoal may decrease absorption of the toxin. Hemoperfusion may be of benefit. Urgent liver transplantation may be lifesaving. *Toadstool poisoning* may lead to polyuria, polydipsia, and renal failure. Hepatic damage is mild.

Paraquat is an organic herbicide that is accidentally absorbed through skin exposure or ingested in a suicide attempt. Acute renal failure, often associated with multiple defects of proximal tubular function, may develop. Mortality is high because of concomitant pulmonary injury, which may be irreversible. Early hemodialysis or hemoperfusion treatment is indicated to prevent chronic pulmonary sequelae.

Paracetamol overdose is an increasingly common event because of the wide availability of the drug to the general public. Suicidal overdosage (greater than 200 mg/kg of body weight) is associated with nausea, diaphoresis, severe hepatic damage, and acute renal failure. Tissue injury is related to the accumulation of toxic metabolites through the cytochrome P450 oxygenase system. Long-term use of stimulants of this enzyme system (phenobarbital, anticonvulsants, ethanol) may enhance hepatotoxicity and nephrotoxicity. Increased availability of glutathione protects against the lesions. Oral administration of cysteine, a precursor of glutathione, as *N*-acetylcysteine (loading dose, 140 mg/kg followed by 70 mg/kg every 4 hours for 17 doses) is protective, provided it is given within 12 hours of the ingestion of paracetamol. Prompt administration of intravenous cimetidine may also prevent conversion of paracetamol to more toxic metabolites. Early dialysis or hemoperfusion therapy is indicated for severe overdosage associated with renal failure.

Infusions of *low-molecular-weight dextran* for prophylaxis of thrombosis in the postoperative period have occasionally been associated with acute renal failure. The excretion of a highly viscous urine having a high concentration of dextran suggests that the tubular lumina may be occluded with aggregated material. Alternatively, the acute increase in plasma oncotic pressure may prevent glomerular ultrafiltration by decreasing the transcapillary pressure gradient. Extracorporeal removal of the accumulated dextran may be of benefit.

Acetylsalicylic acid and methylsalicylate may provoke electrolyte and acid–base abnormalities. The diagnosis can be suspected in patients who have an elevated anion gap, respiratory alkalosis and metabolic acidosis, absence of an osmolal gap, and a positive ferric chloride test in the urine. Hypokalemia and hypophosphatemia may be encountered. Renal failure is uncommon. Confirmation of the diagnosis requires measurement of plasma salicylate levels. Mild intoxication may be managed with forced alkaline diuresis. More severe intoxication may require hemodialysis or hemoperfusion therapy (see Chapter 94).

PHYSICAL AGENTS

Two physical agents, heat and ionizing radiation, have been associated with renal injury. The renal complications of radiation are discussed in Part 8 of this chapter. Environmental heat exposure, particularly in nonacclimatized individuals, may lead to volume depletion, circulatory collapse, rhabdomyolysis, disseminated intravascular coagulation, and acute renal failure. Preexisting volume depletion, potassium depletion, poor conditioning, defects in sweating, and excessive muscular exercise predispose to the adverse consequences of excessive environmental heat exposure.

Selected Readings

Bennett WM, Plamp C, Porter GA. Drug-related syndromes in clinical nephrology. *Ann Intern Med* 1977;87:586–590.

A review of various clinical syndromes associated with renal toxic effects of drugs.

Friedman EA, Greenberg JB, Merrill JP, et al. Consequences of ethylene glycol poisoning. Report of 4 cases and review of the literature. *Am J Med* 1962;32:891–904.

An excellent study of the clinical manifestations and therapy of ethylene glycol intoxication.

Myher RK, Lee JC, Hopper J. Renal tubular necrosis caused by mushroom poisoning. *Arch Intern Med* 1964;114:196–204.

A good account of an uncommon intoxication.

Olsen S, Solez K. Acute tubular necrosis and toxic renal injury. In: Tisher CC, Brenner BM, eds. *Renal pathology,* 2nd ed. Philadelphia: JB Lippincott, 1994:769–810.

An excellent review.

CHAPTER 48

Acute Renal Failure Including Cortical Necrosis

PART 1
Pathogenesis

Karl A. Nath

The syndrome of acute renal failure arises from a rapid fall in glomerular filtration rate (GFR), occurring over hours to days, that is accompanied by derangements in solute and water transport and in acid–base homeostasis. The syndrome is detected clinically by the retention in plasma of nitrogenous waste products such as urea and creatinine, often in the setting of a declining urinary output. Mechanisms that induce acute renal failure may be prerenal, renal, or postrenal in origin. Prerenal mechanisms involve conditions that diminish true or "effective" renal perfusion, whereas postrenal mechanisms refer to obstructive lesions in the genitourinary tract that impede the egress of urine from the kidney. Renal causes of acute renal failure can arise from each of the four main anatomic structures within the kidney. Diseases of arteries and arterioles, either involving the blood vessel wall, such as vasculitides, or obstructing the vascular lumen, as seen with platelet–fibrin thrombi in hemolytic uremic syndrome/thrombotic thrombocytopenic purpura, can impair glomerular perfusion and filtration. GFR can also be profoundly depressed by diseases originating in the glomerular compartment such as rapidly progressive glomerulonephritis and other proliferative glomerulonephritides. Tubular lesions causing acute renal failure are of two main types. Those that are collectively described as acute tubular necrosis (ATN) involve, primarily, injury to the tubular epithelial cell, and are induced by ischemia or varied nephrotoxins. The other type of acute tubular lesions is occlusive lesions in the tubular lumen as seen with plasma cell dyscrasias and acute urate nephropathy. Lesions originating in the interstitium, as seen with acute interstitial nephritis, may also cause acute renal failure.

ATN is thus one of several afflictions that precipitate an acute decline in renal function. Acute renal failure is seen more commonly in hospitalized patients rather than in an ambulatory setting. In the latter instance, acute renal failure usually arises from prerenal causes and is associated with an excellent clinical outcome. In hospitalized patients, acute renal failure occurs in some 5% of admitted patients and its occurrence is even higher in certain subsets of patients, involving, for instance, some 20% to 30% of patients in intensive care settings. In hospitalized patients, prerenal mechanisms account for approximately 50% of cases of acute renal failure whereas postrenal causes account for less than 10%. The remainder of cases result from intrinsic renal causes of which the dominating contributor is ATN. The settings that predispose hospitalized patients to ATN include postoperative states (especially after cardiac surgery, repair of aortic aneurysms, or surgery involving the obstructed biliary tract), multiorgan failure, sepsis, major trauma, rhabdomyolysis, exposure to potentially nephrotoxic medications or contrast agents, burn injuries, oncologic conditions and their treatment, and the management of patients with human immunodeficiency virus infections. The mortality associated with acute renal failure in hospitalized patients is high, approximating 50% of patients, and may be substantially higher in the setting of sepsis or multiorgan failure.

This chapter reviews the pathogenesis of ATN, in particular, ischemic ATN; it also discusses the pathogenesis of acute cortical necrosis and certain forms of toxin-induced ATN such as that induced by heme pigments. The differential diagnosis and clinical features of ATN are discussed in Chapter 48, Part 2, while specific forms of ATN induced by antimicrobial agents, other therapeutic agents, and assorted toxins are discussed in relevant parts of Chapter 47.

ACUTE TUBULAR NECROSIS: CLINICAL AND EXPERIMENTAL CORRELATIONS

The Spectrum of Syndromes Arising in the Setting of Renal Hypoperfusion

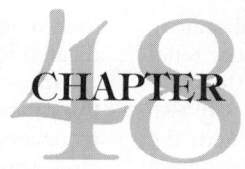

Table 48.1 lists syndromes of acute renal failure arising in the setting of renal hypoperfusion. The decline in renal function observed in prerenal forms of renal failure responds rapidly and completely to the correction of the underlying cause for the renal perfusion defect. However, renal hypoperfusion that precipitates the syndrome of ischemic ATN induces aberrant renal hemodynamic responses in conjunction with sublethal and lethal injury to renal epithelial cells, all of which have to be repaired to facilitate recovery of renal function; recovery thus necessitates reparative and regenerative mechanisms that restore the integrity of the

kidney. Of the patients with ATN who survive, recovery of renal function usually occurs. Rarely, however, renal hypoperfusion may be of such severity and type that cortical necrosis occurs, which leads, generally, to acute irreversible renal failure. In such instances the reparative and regenerative mechanisms cannot compensate for, or correct, the extensive nephron loss incurred by cortical necrosis. In a small subset of patients with cortical necrosis, hyperfunction of remnant nephrons may enable the regaining of renal function such that the need for dialysis is obviated; however, such recovery is not permanent because progressive renal dysfunction often supervenes.

Histopathology and Clinical Course

Of the terms used in the past to describe acute renal failure in humans in the setting of ischemic and nephrotoxic insults—acute tubular necrosis, lower nephron nephrosis, vasomotor nephropathy—the one that persists, and is widely used is *acute tubular necrosis*. This term, however, does not accurately reflect renal histologic changes in human ATN because necrosis of tubular epithelial cells, although emphasized in early reports, is an uncommon feature. Cellular necrosis involves few cells, in contrast to the widespread and confluent cellular necrosis observed in experimental acute renal failure; the nephron segment that most likely exhibits necrosis is the proximal tubule and, in particular, the S3 segment or the straight segment of the proximal tubule. Evidence of regenerating tubular epithelial cells may be seen in such areas. Much more characteristic of human ATN are cellular lesions reflecting sublethal rather lethal cell injury, namely, brush border loss, vacuolization of the proximal tubules, and flattening of proximal tubules. Proximal tubules are often dilated as a consequence of distally obstructing casts; the underlying tubular basement membrane may be exposed because of focal loss of cells. The interstitium is characteristically widened by edema and contains few inflammatory cells; however, congregation of leukocytes in the medulla is commonly observed. Histologic features of cell injury are also observed in the distal nephron, including the medullary thick ascending limb, and so noticeable are these changes in some studies, that the description *lower nephron nephrosis* was used. The distal tubular lumen may be occluded by casts, which are made up of cellular fragments, whole cells, and the Tamm-Horsfall protein. Swelling of tubular epithelial cells may predispose them to nephron obstruction by luminal casts. The distal nephron rather than the proximal nephron may be involved by apoptosis. Overall, these histologic changes in human ATN are generally mild compared with the marked functional impairment; nonetheless, composite scores for histologic injury correlate with renal functional impairment in ATN.

TABLE 48.1. Syndromes of Acute Renal Failure Induced Primarily by Renal Hypoperfusion

1. Prerenal renal failure
   An acute decline in kidney function that is reversed rapidly and completely by correction of the renal perfusion defect.
2. Ischemic acute tubular necrosis
   An acute decline in kidney function that is instigated by renal hypoperfusion but is sustained by aberrant hemodynamic responses, sublethal and lethal cell injury; recovery of renal function usually occurs after obligatory reparative and regenerative responses.
3. Acute cortical necrosis
   An acute decline in kidney function that is commonly irreversible because of a failure of reparative and regenerative mechanisms to correct, or compensate for, the extensive loss of functioning nephrons

From a functional standpoint, ATN progresses through three phases. The initiation phase reflects the precipitous fall in GFR, triggered by ischemia and attendant hemodynamic alterations and accompanied by sublethal and lethal tubular epithelial injury; the importance of hemodynamic abnormalities in the initiation and sustenance of ATN is emphasized by the term *vasomotor nephropathy*. The established (maintenance) phase is characterized by a persistent reduction in GFR; it is sustained by the aberrant hemodynamic responses and sublethal and lethal cell injury instigated by the original hemodynamic insult. The recovery (diuretic) phase reflects reparative and regenerative responses that restore the renal architecture and normalize GFR.

Experimental Models of Human ATN

Much of our current understanding of the pathogenesis of ATN is derived from relevant experimental models. These models lend themselves to the use of approaches in the study of the pathogenesis of ATN that are not feasible in a clinical setting, and they allow the examination of potentially beneficial and clinically relevant strategies. *In vivo* models in the rat impose occlusive clamps on the renal artery or involve the systemic administration of a vasoconstrictive substance such as norepinephrine. Simpler models include the isolated perfused kidney, isolated tubular fragments *in vitro*, and cultured renal epithelial cells *in vitro*. Because hypoxia is one of the characteristic features of ischemia, hypoxia and anoxia are regularly used in *in vitro* models; the induction of "chemical anoxia," based on the use of inhibitors of the mitochondrial electron transport, is also used in *in vitro* systems, as are methods to reduce cellular ATP levels, which are based on the reduction of ATP observed in the kidney in the ischemic or hypoxic setting.

Disparities clearly exist between settings that produce human ATN and those used experimentally. For example, the most widely applied *in vivo* model makes use of a single intervention in the rat, namely, temporary and total occlusion of the renal artery, whereas human ischemic ATN is commonly antedated by renal hypoperfusion but not by renal artery occlusion; human ATN is often multifactorial, reflecting the combined effects of nephrotoxins and sepsis; and finally, cell necrosis is uncommon in human ATN. Although simpler *in vitro* systems allow more detailed analysis of specific pathogenetic mechanisms, these *in vitro* models lack features of the *in vivo* ischemic state such as diminished delivery of substrates during the ischemic period, failure to remove metabolic products during reflow, and paracrine effects from infiltrating cells or the neighboring vasculature.

Notwithstanding these limitations, these models have provided numerous critical insights that form the basis of our current understanding of the pathogenesis of ATN. Moreover, some of the paradigms that have been derived from the use of experimental models have subsequently been validated in human disease. The continual exploration of disease models in conjunction with clinical studies that validate or refute these mechanisms represents a justified and fruitful approach in the exploration of mechanisms of ATN.

Mechanisms Accounting for the Reduction in GFR in ATN

From such a combined clinical and experimental approach, the pathogenesis of the decline in GFR in ischemic ATN can be summarized as follows. The four determinants of GFR are glomerular plasma flow rates, the glomerular transcapillary hydraulic pressure gradient, the glomerular ultrafiltration coefficient, and the plasma oncotic pressure. The latter is not appreciably altered

TABLE 48.2. Major Pathways Contributing to Functional and Structural Abnormalities in the Kidney with Acute Tubular Necrosis

1. Aberrant hemodynamic responses
2. Sublethal cell injury
3. Lethal cell injury
4. Cast formation
5. Leukocytic-dependent pathways

in ischemic ATN, whereas changes in the glomerular ultrafiltration coefficient are relatively minor; however, in nephrotoxic ATN, significant changes in the glomerular ultrafiltration coefficient may occur. The fall in GFR in ischemic ATN is determined, primarily, by reductions in the glomerular plasma flow rates and glomerular transcapillary hydraulic pressure gradient. Glomerular plasma flow rates are diminished because of increased afferent and efferent arterial resistances. The transcapillary hydraulic pressure gradient is diminished because of decreased glomerular hydrostatic pressure in conjunction with elevations in proximal tubular pressure, and proximal tubular pressures are increased because of tubular obstruction due to cast formation. These alterations in the determinants of glomerular hemodynamics impair glomerular ultrafiltration, which is further compromised by backleak of ultrafiltrate across the damaged tubular epithelium. Sublethal and lethal cell injuries profoundly impair the integrity of the tubular epithelium such that a significant portion of the glomerular ultrafiltrate is shunted across the tubular epithelium; net glomerular filtration is thereby reduced by such backleak. Thus the pathophysiologic mechanisms that contribute to the reduction in GFR in ischemic ATN represent the combined effects of alterations in glomerular hemodynamics, sublethal and lethal injuries to tubular epithelial cells, and obstructive changes due to cast formation. These mechanisms, along with leukocytic-dependent pathways, which themselves contribute to aberrant hemodynamic responses and sublethal and lethal cell injuries, are the main pathogenetic contributors to ATN (Table 48.2) and will be separately reviewed.

HEMODYNAMIC ABNORMALITIES CONTRIBUTING TO ISCHEMIC ATN

Renal hemodynamic abnormalities are recognized during the ischemic insult and in the postischemic phases of ATN. Certain characteristics of the kidney and its circulation, summarized in Table 48.3, render it prone to these hemodynamic alterations. Table 48.4 lists the major hemodynamic and vascular abnormalities in ischemic ATN.

The reductions in renal blood flow in the postischemic phase rarely exceed half of basal values and thus are outstripped by the reduction in GFR, with the latter reduced to less than 10% of basal values. The reduction in renal blood flow rates arises from increased renal vascular resistances; the functional nature of such increments in renal resistances is underscored by the capacity of certain vasodilators to relax these vascular resistances. Structural evidence of vascular injury in ischemic renal failure, such as endothelial cell swelling and damage, smooth muscle vacuolization, denudation of the vascular lining, may be present, and glomerular ultrastructural abnormalities are scant. Increased renal vascular resistances arise, mainly, from an imbalance in vasoactive species where vasoconstrictor agonists assume dominance over vasodilator species on vascular tone. An expanding number of vasoconstrictive substances are implicated in ischemic ATN, including endothelin, isoprostanes, thromboxanes, angiotensin II, leukotrienes, adenosine, and platelet-activating factor.

Considerable evidence has accrued to support a role for enhanced production of endothelin and/or enhanced effects of endothelin in renal ischemia. This vasoactive peptide, derived from the endothelium and other sites, consists of several isoforms including ET-1. Endothelin is unique because of the intensity of its vasoconstrictive action and the duration of vasoconstriction once induced. In ischemic acute renal injury, ET-1 is significantly upregulated whereas the administration of an antibody to endothelin increased single nephron GFR and decreased arteriolar resistances. Studies using blockers to endothelin receptors have also supported a role for endothelin in mediating ischemia-induced renal vasoconstriction. Endothelin receptors consist of two forms, ET_A and ET_B. The ET_A receptor mediates the vasoconstrictive effects of ET-1, in addition to other effects. Engagement of ET-1 on the ET_B receptor stimulates expression of preproendothelin mRNA. By increasing the synthesis of its preprohormone, and ultimately ET-1, such effects ultimately perpetuate the effects of endothelin itself. The ET_B receptor also has a countervailing effect in that it facilitates the release of vasodilators such as prostacyclin and nitric oxide, which oppose the vasoconstrictive effects of ET-1. Antagonists of the ET_A receptor ameliorate postischemic renal injury when administered at the time of the insult or even after the insult is

TABLE 48.3. Mechanisms Contributing to the Vulnerability of the Kidney to Hemodynamic Alterations After Ischemia

1. Renal blood flow is critically dependent upon intact endothelium-dependent vasodilation; endothelium-dependent vasodilation may be impaired by ischemia.
2. The kidney is unduly sensitive to certain vasoconstrictors such as endothelin and isoprostanes that are produced in increased amounts in the ischemic kidney.
3. Certain vasoactive species generated during ischemia such as adenosine, while vasodilatory in other organs, are vasoconstrictive in the kidney.
4. Certain regions of the kidney such as the outer stripe of the outer medulla are particularly prone to ischemia-induced hypoperfusion because of the uniqueness of the renal circulation and ischemia-induced vascular congestion in these regions.
5. Injury to nonvascular cells in the kidney may induce renal vasoconstriction:
   Impaired proximal tubular reabsorption of sodium chloride increases distal delivery of sodium chloride and water, activates tubuloglomerular feedback, and induces vasoconstriction.
   Tubular injury predisposes toward cast formation which may occlude the tubular lumen, and such nephron obstruction may induce constriction of the upstream glomerular microcirculation.

TABLE 48.4. Vascular Abnormalities in Acute Renal Failure

1. Endothelial swelling and injury, enhanced endothelial elaboration of vasoconstrictive substances, impaired endothelium-derived vascular relaxation
2. Promotion of leukocytic adherence to the injured endothelium and subsequent leukocytic infiltration
3. Increase sensitivity to vasoconstrictor species
4. Increase sensitivity to neural stimulation
5. Increased resting vascular tone
6. Impaired autoregulation

established. Simultaneous antagonism of both the ET_A and ET_B receptors is also associated with beneficial effects in renal ischemia. These latter findings indicate that the beneficial effect of blocking the ET_B receptor, partly due to the prevention of the synthesis of endothelin, prevails over the potentially adverse one of decreasing production of vasodilator species. Detailed information on endothelin and its interaction with the kidney is found in Chapter 13, Part 5.

In addition to enhanced actions of vasoconstrictors such as endothelin, impaired generation and/or actions of vasodilators also contribute to reduced renal blood flow in ischemic renal injury. Such impairment is selective because the vasculature shows a blunted response to rndothelial nitric oxide–dependent vasodilators but relative preservation of other vasodilators such as prostacyclin. In the early phase after ischemic injury, impairment in the constitutively expressed endothelial nitric oxide synthase (NOS) system may occur; this enzyme produces nitric oxide, which is critical in the maintenance of basal renal blood flow. Later on, expression and function of endothelial NOS (eNOS) are readily apparent. Thus impaired generation of nitric oxide from eNOS may initially occur; subsequently, there is recovery in the eNOS system, which mitigates the vasoconstrictive effects of increased endothelin production.

Intrinsic abnormalities in the vasculature in ischemia accompany this alteration in the vasoconstrictor/vasodilator balance. For example, *in vitro* studies of the behavior of isolated perfused arterioles harvested from kidneys subjected to norepinephrine-induced ischemia *in vivo* demonstrated augmented vasoconstriction in the basal state as well as enhanced responses to vasoconstrictors. Such arterioles demonstrate increased intracellular levels of calcium in the resting state and abnormal intracellular calcium kinetics in response to vasoconstrictors such as angiotensin II. Thus there is an inherent alteration in the vasculature induced by ischemic injury wherein intrinsic basal tone is increased in conjunction with increased responsivity to vasoconstrictors. This heightened vasoconstrictive response induced by renal ischemia may account for the particularly compromising effects of vasoconstricting agents or states, such as cyclosporine, amphotericin, contrast dye, nonsteroidal agents, and sepsis, when superimposed on a kidney already subjected to a prior ischemic insult.

Studies of afferent and efferent arterioles *in vitro* also revealed an aberrant response to changes in luminal pressure. In normal blood vessels, autoregulation serves the purpose of maintaining constancy of blood flow over a certain range of perfusion pressures: increased luminal pressure triggers a rise in the intracellular calcium concentration in smooth muscle cells, which contribute to the myogenic constrictive response; conversely, reduced renal perfusion leads to a dilation of these vessels. Such responses are reversed in the arterioles from kidneys rendered ischemic by an infusion of norepinephrine; in these arterioles, a reduction in perfusion is accompanied by a vasoconstrictive rather than a vasodilatory response. Arterioles harvested from the clamp model of ischemia demonstrate a striking unresponsivity to most vasoactive stimuli as well as an unresponsivity to alterations in renal perfusion pressure; these arterioles fail to dilate in response to reduced perfusion pressure.

This impairment in renal autoregulation is functionally significant as demonstrated by the heightened injury induced by ischemia in kidneys already subjected to ischemia several days previously. In such kidneys, a marked decline in GFR accompanied by additional histologic damage is induced by relatively mild reductions in renal perfusion that do not exert adverse effects on a healthy kidney. These experimental findings are clinically relevant. Repetitive ischemic insults, albeit mild, may extend the duration of ATN, quite possibly as a consequence of the kidney, subjected to its first ischemic insult, being unable to autoregulate to subsequent insults. Similarly, hypotensive episodes during hemodialysis of patients with acute renal failure may delay the recovery from ATN.

Reductions in renal blood after an ischemic insult may be more severe in certain areas of the kidney and may contribute to the greater histologic injury observed in these areas. Under normal conditions the countercurrent system of the kidney imposes relatively hypoxic conditions in the inner medulla (PO_2 10 mm Hg) compared with the cortex (PO_2 60 mm Hg); various segments of the nephron possess metabolic attributes and adaptations that tolerate this gradient of oxygen tension in the intact healthy state. However, ischemic insults can severely disrupt oxygenation of certain segments and thereby predispose them to ischemic injury. After ischemia, outer medullary blood flow is decreased to less than 20% of its rate before ischemia whereas cortical blood flow is decreased to 60% of preischemic basal values. This reduction of blood flow to the outer medulla arises, in part, from sludging of red blood cells as they are concentrated within the capillary due to the loss of fluid into the interstitial areas. Increased capillary leakage may be induced by activated leukocytes that are often present in this area in ischemic renal injury. Such impaired perfusion critically impairs oxygenation to tubular segments situated in the outer stripe of the outer medulla, the S3 segment of the proximal tubule and the medullary thick ascending limb. These segments, especially the S3 segment of the proximal tubule, are most likely damaged by ischemic injury. The outer stripe of the outer medulla is vascularized predominantly by the ascending vasa rectae, because the capillary supply from the efferent arteriole and the descending vasa rectae to outer stripe of the outer medulla is quite meager. Reduced perfusion of outer stripe of the outer medulla, induced by vasoconstriction and sludging of red blood cells, compromises oxygenation of nephron segments that are already tenuously oxygenated in their basal state. Regional alterations in renal hemodynamics, in addition to alterations in whole kidney hemodynamics, are thus particularly relevant to those nephron segments vulnerable to ischemic injury.

MECHANISMS OF ISCHEMIC/HYPOXIC CELL INJURY

Overview of Cell Injury: Ischemia-Dependent and Reperfusion-Dependent Processes

Table 48.5 lists mechanisms involved in ischemic/hypoxic cell injury. Although for all of these factors there is convincing experimental evidence implicating their involvement in cell injury, their relative contributions may be influenced by the experimental model under investigation. In addition, the relevance of some of these mechanisms to human ATN is under considerable debate.

TABLE 48.5. Mechanisms Contributing to Ischemic Cell Injury
1. ATP depletion
2. Alterations in the cytoskeleton
3. Increased intracellular calcium concentrations
4. Injury to plasma and cellular membranes
5. Cell swelling
6. Activation of phospholipases, proteases and endonucleases
7. Increased production of nitric oxide
8. Cast formation
9. Correction of intracellular acidosis during reperfusion
10. Increased generation of reactive oxygen species
11. Leukocytic-dependent mechanisms

The reperfusion phase after ischemic insults replenishes cells with oxygen and substrates of which they were deprived during the ischemic phase and removes metabolites generated during ischemia. Many of these mechanisms such as ATP depletion and cytoskeletal alterations arise promptly with the induction of ischemia/hypoxia and may resolve rapidly during reperfusion. However, reperfusion itself may usher in mechanisms that lead to cell injury, including processes such as the generation of reactive oxygen species, leukocytic-dependent mechanisms, and correction of intracellular acidosis; these are commonly assigned major roles in the reperfusion phase of ischemic injury. Changes in cellular pH are of interest in that during the period of ischemia, intracellular pH falls. Intracellular acidosis has been shown to protect against hypoxic injury; thus the occurrence of intracellular acidosis during ischemic/hypoxic insults is viewed as a protectant against cell injury, while the correction of cell pH during the reperfusion phase may contribute to cell injury.

Overview of Cell Injury: Sublethal and Lethal Processes

Cell injury may be sublethal or lethal in nature. Lethal cell injury damages cells irretrievably, causing the loss of these cells, and is induced by necrosis or apoptosis. Sublethal cell injury encompasses structural and functional derangements, which are potentially reversible, and represent, in the main, cytoskeletal derangements; such cytoskeletal injury results, primarily, from reductions in ATP levels. Sublethal changes include tubular epithelial brush border injury, tight junction dysfunction, disruption of the polarization of the tubular epithelial cell, and weakening in the attachment of epithelial cells to their neighbors and to the underlying basement membrane. These changes can be reversed, and these cells can resume their normal, preinjured state if the offending ischemic or nephrotoxic insult is removed, cellular stores of ATP are replenished, and ATP synthetic capability returns. However, the continued presence of the cellular insult provokes disabling reductions in ATP, progressive cytoskeletal collapse, activation of injurious enzymes, and a host of derangements in plasma membrane integrity and organellar function. Cells swell, the plasma membrane lyses, and cellular contents are released, thereby causing an inflammatory response, which removes the detritus from such necrotic cell death.

In contrast to necrosis wherein cellular viability is rapidly overwhelmed by the severity and precipitance of the given insult, apoptosis represents cellular demise in a controlled, ATP-dependent fashion, exhibiting morphologic and biochemical features that are different from necrosis (Table 48.6). Apoptosis affects individual cells rather than the confluent cell populations as is commonly seen with necrosis and is characterized by cytoplasmic shrinkage and chromatin condensation at the periphery of the nucleus. Nuclei disintegrate as DNA is lysed into fragments that are roughly 200 base pairs in size; cells are portioned off into apoptotic bodies. Unlike necrosis, which is associated with plasma membrane lysis and discharge of cellular contents, plasma membrane integrity is preserved in apoptotic cells up to the point at which apoptotic cells are phagocytosed by surrounding cells. Disposal of apoptotic cells does not cause a leukocytic inflammatory reaction.

Apoptosis is recognizable both in experimental and clinical ATN and involves principally, for reasons that are unclear, the cells of the distal nephron. Apoptotic stimuli could be categorized into three main groups. Apoptosis may be induced by many of the same stimuli that induce necrosis—for example, reactive oxygen species, various toxins, hypoxia—when these stimuli are present in much lower concentrations. In addition, apoptosis can also be induced by the loss of survival signals. The view has arisen that an apoptotic death program lurks in all cells, and this default program is overridden by any one of a variety of survival signals critical to cellular vitality. Impairment in cell–cell contact and in cell–substratum contact or the loss of specific growth factors such as insulinlike growth factor-1 (IGF-1) deprives cells of survival signals that proscribe the occurrence of the apoptotic pathway. Other growth factors, and cytokines such as tumor necrosis factor α can induce apoptosis.

In the setting of ischemic ATN, apoptosis subserves at least two critical functions. Cells that have escaped necrosis, nonetheless, may be injured to such an extent that these cells are no longer amenable to reparative mechanisms; deleting these cells by apoptotic cell death is selected in preference to efforts at cellular repair. In addition, apoptosis may be used in the repair and recovery phase of ATN when architectural demands in the refashioning of an intact nephron require the deletion of injured cells or surplus cells produced during the phase of proliferation.

TABLE 48.6. Some Contrasting Features of Necrosis and Apoptosis

Criteria	Necrosis	Apoptosis
Triggering mechanisms	Diverse insults ("high dose")	Diverse insults ("low dose") Loss of "survival" signals Certain cytokines/growth factors
Nature of the process	Precipitate, overwhelming Uncontrolled process	Sequential, protracted Controlled process
Predilection	Populations of cells Proximal nephron	Individual cells Distal nephron
ATP content	Invariably diminished	Usually preserved
Morphology	Cell swelling, nuclear karyolysis, organelles such as mitochondria are swollen and may exhibit dense calcifications, fragmentation of plasma membrane	Cytoplasmic shrinking, condensation of chromatin around the nuclear periphery, organelles such as mitochondria well preserved, plasma membrane intact
DNA fragmentation	Smear pattern usually seen; however, laddering may also be seen	Laddering of DNA commonly, but not always, seen
Effectors	Multiple—see text	Caspases, others
Modulators	Multiple—see text	Bcl-2 family of proteins
Cell fate and presence of inflammation	Lysis of plasma membrane, release of cellular contents, and instigation of inflammatory response	Formation of apoptotic bodies and phagocytosis by surrounding cells; no inflammatory response

The mechanisms that underlie apoptosis have been intensely studied, and it is now believed that key steps involve processes in the cytoplasm and mitochondrion. A critical event induced by proapoptotic stimuli is the release of cytochrome *c*, a member of the electron transport chain, from the mitochondrion into the cytoplasm. Once in the cytoplasm, cytochrome *c*, in concert with apoptosis protease-activating factor (Apaf1) activates a family of enzymes known as caspases; in addition, caspases may be activated by other pathways besides cytochrome *c*. The release of cytochrome *c* from the mitochondrion and its effects on caspases can be prevented, or enhanced, by members of the Bcl-2 family: members such as Bcl-2 and Bcl-x_L are antiapoptotic, whereas members such as Bax, Bad, and Bcl-x_S are proapoptotic. The activation of caspases has numerous injurious effects that include damage to the nuclear membrane and the cytoskeleton, degradation of antiapoptotic proteins and proteins involved in DNA repair, activation of various kinases, and factors that incur DNA fragmentation. These assorted actions of caspases, in aggregate, provide the biochemical basis for apoptosis.

Depletion of Cellular ATP Content

One of the salient features of ischemic insults is the prompt and prominent reduction of ATP. Depletion of ATP contributes, directly or indirectly, to numerous mechanisms that induce cell injury. Such ATP depletion arises, primarily, from the lack of oxygen and substrate delivery for ATP synthesis. Generation of ATP by oxidative phosphorylation provides the major cellular source of ATP and is profoundly limited by impaired oxygenation; the capacity of anaerobic sources such as glycolysis to generate ATP is limited. The reperfusion phase resupplies oxygen and metabolic substrates, which can be used to regenerate ATP, provided that mitochondrial function is sufficiently well preserved during the ischemia. If during the ischemic episode, mitochondrial function is impaired, as may occur as a consequence of the mitochondrial influx of calcium, then the recovery of cellular stores of ATP may be profoundly compromised even in the setting of renewed delivery of oxygen and substrates, and as discussed subsequently, cellular content of ATP is a critical predictor and determinant of functional and structural recovery following ischemic injury.

ATP is required for diverse and indispensable cellular processes: ATP provides energy that allows membrane pumps to work and the energy that facilitates thermodynamically unfavorable reactions required in the synthesis of proteins, nucleic acids, and carbohydrates and in aspects of lipid metabolism; and ATP is critically required in the maintenance of the cytoskeletal integrity and in cell signaling pathways. Thus the loss of ATP, as seen during ischemic and hypoxic insults, has adverse effects on myriad processes that subserve cellular vitality. For example, impaired Na^+-K^+-ATPase activity due to ATP depletion increases cellular concentrations of sodium promoting movement of water into the cell and thus cell swelling. Swelling of tubular epithelial cells predisposes them to obstruction of the nephron and compression of endothelial cells, while swelling of endothelial cells could impair perfusion of nephron segments. ATP depletion promotes the accumulation of potentially toxic lipid species, and, as will be discussed subsequently, decrements in ATP foster, in part, elevations in intracellular calcium concentration, which, in turn, could activate a number of damaging enzymes. Especially important is the fact that decreased ATP levels markedly impair the cytoskeleton. ATP metabolism by the renal cells and the role of ATP in the metabolism and function of renal cells are discussed in detail in Chapter 9.

During ischemia ATP is broken down to the nucleotides, ADP and AMP; AMP can be catabolized further to adenosine, inosine, and hypoxanthine. During reperfusion these breakdown products can be used to regenerate ATP. Generation of nucleosides and bases signifies a greater deviancy from, and compromise in, cellular energetics than that posed by the generation of nucleotides: nucleosides and bases, in contrast to the nucleotides, are membrane permeant and can be readily lost from cells, thereby depriving cells of these substrates by which to resynthesize ATP. In addition, generating ATP from these nucleosides and bases necessitates, itself, supplies of high-energy phosphate compounds.

Depletion of ATP not only instigates pathways of cell injury but also impairs reparative and regenerative responses required in the recovery from ischemic insults. The functional importance of ATP levels in the recovery from ischemic ATN is underscored by studies in which ATP–magnesium chloride or AMP–magnesium chloride is infused in the postischemic period. Nucleotides so provided are degraded to adenosine, and adenosine is subsequently converted to AMP and ATP in the kidney. By providing the precursors needed for ATP synthesis, such therapy significantly augments renal content of ATP and facilitates functional improvement. Other manipulations that foster ATP synthesis, such as the inhibition of conversion of membrane-impermeant nucleotides to permeable nucleosides and the inhibition of the degradation of adenosine, all enhance ATP synthesis and hasten the recovery, functionally and structurally, from ischemic ATN.

Alterations in the Cytoskeleton

The unidirectional transport of solutes and water by the proximal tubule from the tubular lumen to the capillaries that abut the basolateral surface is critically dependent upon its polarized structure and function. In turn such polarity, comprising as it does, an apical and basolateral domain, is dependent upon the integrity of the actin cytoskeleton. The apical domain is provided by the microvilli of the proximal tubular epithelial cells; these microvilli contain an inner core of actin microfilaments, which extend from the terminal web of the actin cytoskeleton. The basolateral domain houses the Na^+-K^+-ATPase that actively transports sodium against its electrochemical gradient across the basolateral plasma membrane. The Na^+-K^+-ATPase pump is restrained in its position in the basolateral membrane by its attachment to the neighboring cortical actin cytoskeleton via the actin-associated proteins, ankyrin and fodrin. The actin cytoskeleton also maintains the integrity of the tight junction, which separates the apical and basolateral domains, regulates reabsorption via the paracellular pathways, and provides contact between neighboring tubular epithelial cells. Finally, the actin cytoskeleton attaches the epithelial cell to its basement membrane proteins via the integrin family of transmembrane proteins.

States such as ischemia, hypoxia, and ATP depletion profoundly affect the actin cytoskeleton with far-reaching functional consequences as summarized in Table 48.7. These changes in the actin cytoskeleton underlie, in the main, cellular insults collectively described as sublethal cell injury; these cytoskeletal alterations are potentially reversible, and the cell can be restored to normalcy if the offending insult is removed.

Potential effectors for proteolytic disruption of the actin cytoskeleton and its associated proteins include calpain, a cysteine protease. The signal for the activation of calpain to its active form may reside in the increase in intracellular concentrations of calcium that occurs in these conditions. Calpain can degrade actin-binding proteins such as ankyrin and fodrin, thereby

TABLE 48.7. Adverse Functional Effects Resulting from Cytoskeletal Damage

1. Proximal tubular brush border injury impairs reabsorptive processes while sloughed fragments of the brush border promote luminal cast formation.
2. Residence of the Na^+-K^+-ATPase on the basolateral membrane is destabilized.
3. Tight junction dysfunction facilitates movement of the Na^+-K^+-ATPase to the apical domain and the loss of membrane polarization.
4. Loss of membrane polarization impairs unidirectional transport processes.
5. Impaired sodium reabsorption in the proximal tubule increases distal delivery, activates tubuloglomerular feedback, and induces vasoconstriction.
6. Tight junction dysfunction causes backleak of the glomerular ultrafiltrate, thereby decreasing glomerular filtration rate.
7. Weakening in cell–cell and cell–substratum interactions may lead to the sloughing of tubular epithelial cells into the urinary space.
8. Sloughing of tubular cells exacerbates backleak and the reduction in GFR; it also may lead to tubular obstruction, which further reduces GFR and induces vasoconstriction.

destabilizing the cytoskeleton and the residence of the Na^+-K^+-ATPase protein in the basolateral membrane. Enhanced generation of nitric oxide can also impair the cytoskeleton. Nitric oxide depletes cellular content of ATP, which is required in the maintenance of actin polymerization. Nitric oxide also stimulates the enzyme poly(ADP-ribose) synthetase, which ribosylates proteins such as actin. Thus by depleting ATP and by promoting ADP ribosylation of actin, nitric oxide could impair cytoskeleton integrity.

Increased Intracellular Concentrations of Calcium

The cytosolic concentration of calcium is in the range of 100 nM, and thus is 10^5 less than that observed in the extracellular fluid. Healthy plasma membranes are relatively impermeable to calcium and thus oppose the tendency for calcium to move down this steep concentration gradient. Other plasma membrane-residing mechanisms that safeguard the relatively low concentrations of cytosolic calcium concentrations include plasma membrane calcium ATPases and the Na^+-Ca^{2+}exchanger, both of which export calcium from the intracellular compartment. Calcium ATPases in the endoplasmic reticulum membrane take up calcium into this organelle and thereby provide an internal mechanism in the maintenance of intracellular calcium concentrations.

Ischemic and hypoxic insults increase cytosolic calcium concentrations, which can attain micromolar levels. The mechanisms contributing to the increase in intracellular calcium concentrations reside in enhanced permeability of the injured plasma membrane to calcium and to ATP depletion. The latter alteration impairs ATP-dependent extrusion of calcium from the cells, and the buffering of calcium within the endoplasmic reticulum. In addition, increments in intracellular sodium concentration due to ATP depletion stimulates activity of the Na^+-Ca^{2+}exchanger thereby further augmenting intracellular calcium concentrations. With further increments in intracellular calcium concentration, uptake by mitochondria occurs. Such mitochondrial uptake may, in the short term, mitigate further increments in cytosolic calcium, but it carries the risk of damaging mitochondria and thereby compromising generation of ATP by oxidative phosphorylation.

Plasma membrane injury per se may lead to intracellular influx of calcium; increased cytosolic calcium concentrations may represent a consequence rather than a cause of damage to plasma membranes. However, in certain models of cell injury, increments in intracellular calcium concentrations arise before appreciable lytic injury occurs, and such increments in cytosolic concentrations are implicated in attendant sublethal and lethal cell injury. Increased intracellular concentrations of calcium may contribute to hypoxic and ischemic injury by activating a number of potentially damaging enzymes, such as proteases, phospholipases, oxidases, and nucleases, and by destabilizing the actin cytoskeleton.

Injury to Plasma and Intracellular Membranes

An intact plasma membrane is a fundamental requirement for continued cellular vitality. Hypoxia-induced cell injury, culminating in cell necrosis, progressively increases membrane porosity that initiates the efflux of cellular contents into the extracellular space and the influx of substances into the intracellular space. The latter leads to increased intracellular concentrations of calcium that may be potentially injurious, as well as to cell swelling. In contrast, plasma membrane integrity is preserved for much of the course of apoptotic cell death.

Glycine is remarkably potent in suppressing the development of such porosity in the membrane in cells exposed to hypoxia and other acute insults. During the evolution of such cellular injury, the relatively high concentrations of glycine (millimolar amounts) that are normally present in the cell are lost into the extracellular space, and this loss of glycine allows the development of plasma membrane porosity. Increased membrane permeability, which occurs in models of hypoxic and other forms of acute cell injury, can be prevented by the presence of millimolar concentrations of glycine in the medium to which cells are exposed. Such addition of glycine staunches the depletion of this amino acid from the intracellular compartment that would otherwise occur and confers a protective effect on the plasma membrane. This protection against pore formation in the plasma membrane is not channeled through or obligates the maintenance of ATP levels, prevention of the increase in intracellular calcium concentrations, prevention of mitochondrial defects, or the abrogation of other pathogenetic processes involved in acute cell injury. Membrane porosity may involve the destabilization of a membrane protein that bears features of a glycine-gated chloride channel, and this destabilization is attenuated by glycine.

Activation of phospholipases is an important mechanism by which ischemia and hypoxia induce membrane injury and, ultimately, lytic cell death. While a number of phospholipases can be activated, much interest has centered on the involvement of phospholipase A_2 (PLA_2). This enzyme is present in membrane-bound and cytosolic fractions, can be activated by calcium, and degrades phospholipids to yield free fatty acids, lysophospholipids, and other lipid-derived products. Such degradation of membrane phospholipids exerts far-ranging effects on the integrity and function of plasma and intracellular membranes. The biophysical properties of the membrane lipid, the function of membrane-associated proteins, and the linkage of the membrane with the neighboring cytoskeleton can all be adversely affected as a consequence of phospholipid degradation. The detergent actions of free fatty acids and lysophospholipids may also contribute to membrane injury. Phospholipase activation locally in intracellular membranes such as those that envelope mitochondria may contribute to injury at these sites; for example, as mitochondria begin to accumulate calcium after ischemia, attendant activation of mitochondrial PLA_2 may further compromise mitochondrial membranes. Calcium-independent isoforms of PLA_2 are also activated by hypoxic injury and by degrading a type of phospholipid termed plasmalogens, such activity may contribute to hypoxic cell injury.

Activated PLA_2 also generates arachidonic acid. The kidney metabolizes arachidonic acid via enzymes such as cyclooxygenase and lipoxygenase to yield prostanoids and leukotrienes, respectively; the kidney can generate products of arachidonic acid via the cytochrome P450 system and can synthesize isoprostanes via nonenzymatic, free radical–catalyzed oxidation of arachidonic acid. These derivatives of arachidonic acid may be directly injurious or contribute to acute renal injury via their vasoactive and proinflammatory properties.

Besides these derivatives from glycerophospholipid, other phospholipids in plasma membranes may yield products that modulate ischemic injury. For example, sphingomyelin, present in the plasma membrane, may generate ceramide, which is subsequently converted into sphingosine. There is considerable interest in the involvement of ceramide and sphingosine in the response to tissue injury by virtue of the involvement of these compounds in processes such as cell death, the stress response, and cell proliferation and differentiation. Evidence has recently been presented demonstrating that during ischemic acute renal failure, there is significant depression in ceramide and sphingosine content. During reperfusion, sphingosine returns to its normal level while there is a supranormal elevation in ceramide levels that persists. Such elevation in ceramide is functionally significant because it influences the susceptibility to renal injury: for example, ceramide worsens renal injury induced by ATP depletion/calcium ionophore toxicity or PLA_2-induced renal injury. Conversely, ceramide protects against arachidonic acid cytotoxicity. These findings suggest that alterations in ceramide caused by ischemia/reperfusion injury may be a determinant of the susceptibility to injury that evolves after such insults.

Increased Production of Nitric Oxide

Depending on the sources and amounts of nitric oxide, the generation of nitric oxide in ischemic acute renal injury may be protective or deleterious. The preservation of renal blood flow is dependent upon endothelial generation of nitric oxide in low amounts by the enzyme eNOS. However, the generation of nitric oxide in large amounts by the inducible isoform of nitric oxide synthase (iNOS) worsens the course of ischemic renal injury. Studies *in vitro* involving the exposure of proximal tubule cells to hypoxia demonstrate increased amounts of nitric oxide, which contribute to tubular injury; in addition, the inhibition of the induction of iNOS in rat renal ischemic injury *in vivo* by administering antisense oligonucleotides, protects, quite convincingly, against ischemic acute renal injury.

Marked generation of nitric oxide, which occurs via iNOS, in contradistinction to the relatively low amounts produced by eNOS, induces cell injury by a number of actions. Many of these mechanisms have been seen in nonrenal cells, but they are probably applicable to acute ischemic renal injury. Nitric oxide can deplete cellular ATP content by its effects on mitochondrial respiration and glycolytic enzymes. Nitric oxide can inactivate enzymes that contain iron–sulfur clusters such as aconitase, an enzyme in the tricarboxylic acid cycle, and enzymes involved in mitochondrial electron transport. Nitrosylation of free thiols in enzymes by nitric oxide impairs enzyme activity; such a mechanism may impair glyceraldehyde-3-phosphate dehydrogenase, a critical glycolytic enzyme. Nitric oxide damages DNA, and this in turn stimulates the DNA repair enzyme poly(ADP-ribose) synthetase. Activation of this latter enzyme exacerbates ATP depletion and reduces cellular levels of NAD. By depleting ATP and by promoting ADP ribosylation, nitric oxide could impair cytoskeleton integrity. Nitric oxide may also interact with the superoxide anion, forming the peroxynitrite radical, which itself is injurious to numerous intracellular targets. Moreover, by inhibiting ribonucleotide reductase, an enzyme critical to DNA synthesis, nitric oxide can impair the regenerative processes that facilitate recovery from ATN. Thus through many actions, enhanced generation of nitric oxide could prove damaging to tissues. Additional information on the interaction between nitric oxide and the kidney is found in Chapter 13, Part 6.

Cast Formation

Cast formation contributes to the functional derangements in human and experimental ATN. A prominent component of tubular casts is the Tamm-Horsfall protein that is produced in the thick ascending limb of the loop of Henle. Several mechanisms may promote cast formation in ischemia. The Tamm-Horsfall protein provides a scaffold around which brush border fragments, tubular epithelial cells, and their fragments are congealed; such cast formation may be derived, in part, from an innate attribute of the Tamm-Horsfall protein to bind cells. Ischemia may disengage of Tamm-Horsfall protein from the apical surface of the thick ascending limb epithelial cells because of cleavage of the phospholipid moieties that tether Tamm-Horsfall protein to the apical membrane. Reduced urinary volume, which occurs in this nephron segment, promotes gel formation of the Tamm-Horsfall protein, an effect also fostered by increased luminal sodium concentrations that appear in this segment due to the failure of proximal sodium absorption. Cast formation is fostered by proteins such as Bence Jones proteins, myoglobin, and cytokines. It has also been suggested that the propensity toward ATN in sepsis, even with mild episodes of hypotension, may reflect the capacity of cytokines, which appear in the urine in septic states, to promote gel formation with Tamm-Horsfall protein.

A novel mechanism for cast formation is the involvement of cell–cell interaction in such cast formation. Tubular epithelial cells are normally anchored to the tubular basement membrane by integrins. These proteins extend from tubular epithelial cell and interact with matrix proteins in the underlying tubular basement membrane, in part, via RGD binding sequences contained in these extracellular proteins. During ischemia, integrins lose their attachment to the tubular basement membrane and are redistributed from the basolateral domain to the apical domain; these cells are sloughed off into the urinary lumen. They could bind to similarly exfoliated cells as integrins, extending from the former, and interact with matrix proteins still attached to the latter population of cells. These exfoliated cells could also interact with sublethally injured cells that are still anchored to the tubular basement membrane. In this way, progressive obstruction of the lumen could occur as exfoliated cells become attached to one another as well as to the injured epithelial cells still attached to the tubular basement membrane. Evidence in support of this mechanism is based on the demonstration that the administration of RGD-containing peptides to rats with ischemic acute renal failure diminished cast formation and prevented the functional effects, namely, the rise in tubular pressure and the fall in GFR.

Reactive Oxygen Species

A sizable literature attests to the injurious effects of reactive oxygen species on the kidney. These species include superoxide and peroxynitrite anions, hydrogen peroxide, and the hydroxyl radical. The superoxide anion is generated as oxygen accepts a single electron, while the dismutation of the superoxide ion yields hydrogen peroxide. The hydroxyl radical is generated as hydrogen peroxide interacts with the superoxide ion under the catalytic effect of the transition metal, iron. The hydroxyl ion is highly reactive, dissipating itself within the immediate environs of its site of generation. Hydrogen peroxide lacks such reactivity, freely diffusing across lipid bilayers and thus instigating oxidant effects quite distant from the site of generation. Hydrogen peroxide generates oxidants known as hypohalous acids in the presence of myeloperoxidase, an enzyme released by leukocytes. Superoxide anion reacts with nitric oxide to form the damaging species, peroxynitrite.

The reactivity of reactive oxygen species extends to lipids, carbohydrates, proteins, and nucleic acids and thus exerts injury on diverse cellular targets. Reactive oxygen species can peroxidate membrane lipid and thus perturb membrane function. Reactive oxygen species can impair transport proteins such as Na^+-K^+-ATPase activity and cytoskeletal proteins. Tethering of cells to extracellular proteins may be destabilized as integrins are redistributed in the plasma membrane under the influence of oxidative stress. Oxidants inhibit glycolytic flux and mitochondrial synthesis of ATP, increase intracellular calcium, destabilize the cytoskeleton, and damage DNA. Such attacks on multiple critical loci within cells account for the well-recognized cytotoxicity of oxidants. In addition, oxidative stress can generate vasoconstrictive substances, which can contribute to aberrant renal hemodynamics and ischemic cell injury.

A pathogenetic role for reactive oxygen species in postischemic renal injury was initially suggested by the protective effects afforded by inhibitors of xanthine oxidase, superoxide dismutase, and scavengers of the hydroxyl radical; such protection was associated with reduced oxidative stress. In addition, increased type O xanthine oxidase activity was described in the postischemic kidney, thereby providing a source for the generation of the superoxide ion in the postischemic period. In health this enzyme exists predominantly in the xanthine dehydrogenase form (type D xanthine oxidase), which uses NAD^+ as an electron acceptor in the oxidation of hypoxanthine and xanthine; however, type O xanthine oxidase enzyme used oxygen as an electron acceptor and generates superoxide ion. These two essential steps during ischemia—the conversion of xanthine dehydrogenase (type D xanthine oxidase) to xanthine oxidase (type O xanthine oxidase) and the generation of hypoxanthine from the breakdown of ATP during ischemia—may provide the basis for increased generation of superoxide ion during reperfusion.

Other sources of reactive oxygen species in ischemic injury include the electron transport chain in mitochondria and the endoplasmic reticulum, nonenzymatic processes such as the autooxidation of thiols and the plasma membrane. Arachidonic acid, liberated from membrane lipid, can generate reactive species via the cyclooxygenase or lipoxygenase pathways. Leukocytes are also involved in ischemic oxidant injury because their plasma membranes possess the enzyme NADPH oxidase, which can generate oxidants. Oxidative stress during postischemic injury may also arise from impairment of the antioxidant defense mechanisms. For example, peroxidative injury early in the postischemic period may be accompanied by impaired oxidant-scavenging enzymes, which foster the accumulation of oxidants.

The potential of iron to generate the hydroxyl anion coupled with the availability of iron presents a constant risk of iron-catalyzed oxidative stress in injured cells. Iron exists in storage and circulating plasma proteins, in a low molecular weight intracellular iron pool, and as part of the heme prosthetic group; for the most part, iron in these various forms cannot participate as a catalyst in the formation of the hydroxyl radical. However, iron, liberated from such sites, may become catalytically active and generate the hydroxyl ion with attendant cellular injury. Increased availability of iron from such sites has been described following ischemia and is implicated in postischemic renal injury.

The role of oxidative stress in the pathogenesis of ischemia-reperfusion injury has been questioned by a number of studies, which have not obtained evidence of oxidative stress in the postischemic setting or of the protective effect of various antioxidant therapies. In addition, substantial differences exist among species with regard to the involvement of oxidative stress in ischemia–reperfusion injury. Finally, the applicability of the paradigm based on the generation of superoxide anion from xanthine oxidase to clinical ATN is questioned because of the relatively low amounts of xanthine oxidase in human tissue. Oxygen species are also involved in glomerular and tubular injury and in glomerular and tubular renal disease. This issue is discussed in Chapter 37, Part 7.

Leukocytic-Dependent Processes

The activated polymorphonuclear leukocyte induces cell injury through a wide range of secreted products that include reactive oxygen species, various proteolytic and other degradative enzymes, cytokines, and numerous other proinflammatory substances. Through these potentially injurious mechanisms emanating from activated neutrophils, in conjunction with the presence, histologically, of polymorphonuclear leukocytes, most noticeably in the outer medulla, and the presence of the assorted products of these cells within the kidney, the neutrophil is implicated in the pathogenesis of ischemic ATN.

The role for neutrophils in postischemic injury has been probed by inducing neutrophil depletion. Some of these studies, but not others, support the involvement of leukocytes in postischemic injury. The occurrence of ATN in neutropenic patients has been interpreted as evidence against a critical involvement of neutrophils in such injury. However, it is possible that relatively few numbers of circulating leukocytes are needed to effect sufficient infiltration into the ischemic kidney whereby leukocyte-dependent mechanisms can contribute to renal injury.

Examination of the involvement of leukocytes in postischemic injury has also been undertaken by modulating the expression of molecules involved in leukocytic adhesion on the endothelial surface. An impressive amount of information derived from *in vivo* models of ischemic injury supports the involvement of ICAM-1 in such injury. ICAM-1 is a leukocyte adhesion molecule that is present on endothelial cells and which, because of its interaction with leukocyte integrins, can firmly immobilize leukocytes rolling across the endothelium. ICAM-1 is expressed in increased amounts in the outer medulla of rats subjected to ischemic injury, the region where polymorphonuclear leukocytes tend to congregate. The administration of an antibody to ICAM-1 before or after the induction of ischemic acute renal failure provides functional and structural protection. Other ways of manipulating ICAM-1 expression are also consistent with the involvement of this adhesion molecule in ischemic renal injury: namely, administration of ICAM-1 antisense oligonucleotides to rats significantly protects against renal injury and ICAM-1 knockout mice exhibit less postischemic renal injury. In aggregate, these data demonstrate that upregulation of ICAM-1, a molecule that immobilizes leukocytes on the endothelium, is an important mediator of ischemic injury in rodent models of postischemic injury. Interest is also directed toward upregulation in selectins—molecules that enable the rolling of leukocytes onto endothelium before immobilization—in mediating postischemic renal injury.

Added evidence in support of the involvement of neutrophils in postischemic injury is provided by studies that have administered α-melanocyte–stimulating hormone (α-MSH). This hormone is an antiinflammatory agent that inhibits the influx of neutrophils into tissues. This compound lessened functional and histologic postischemic renal injury and reduced neutrophil congregation and congestion within capillaries; α-MSH also inhibited neutrophil chemokines and the induction of iNOS and the adhesion molecule ICAM-1. Thus through a multiplicity of mechanisms including the activation and adhesion of neutrophils, α-MSH may attenuate postischemic injury.

RESISTANCE AND RESPONSE TO RENAL INJURY

The mechanistic exploration of renal injury has revealed a number of factors that confer resistance to renal injury induced by hypoxic and toxic insults (Table 48.8). Some of these factors are clinically relevant; for example, organs harvested for transplantation are preserved at low temperatures in preservation fluids that may contain adenosine (a substrate for ATP production), glutathione (a glycine-containing antioxidant), and α-ketoacids such as α-ketoglutarate.

Resistance to ischemic injury varies along the nephron. As described earlier, cellular supplies and synthesis of ATP safeguard against ischemic and hypoxic injury, and differences in ATP-generating capacity may contribute to the heterogeneity in sensitivity of nephron segments to ischemic injury. Cells that rely preponderantly on oxidative phosphorylation for generating ATP may be prone to hypoxic injury, while the presence within cells of greater glycolytic capacity provides a mechanism for generating ATP anaerobically, and one that may offer resistance to hypoxic injury. For instance, the deep medulla and papilla, regions of the kidney with enhanced glycolytic capability, are less susceptible to hypoxic injury compared with the proximal tubule, which is more dependent on oxidative phosphorylation for the supply of energy. The part of the proximal tubule that is most vulnerable to ischemic injury, however, is the S3 segment of the proximal tubule, a segment with greater capacity for glycolysis than other parts of the proximal tubule. Nonetheless, such glycolytic capacity is insufficient to compensate for the pronounced compromise in oxidative phosphorylation-dependent ATP synthesis in this segment, located as it is in the outer stripe of the outer medulla, an area that is poorly oxygenated during and after ischemic insults.

Another consideration that determines vulnerability to ischemic injury is metabolic work, as reflected by sodium transport, that the nephron segment is called upon to perform. Increased metabolic work incurs increased ATP consumption that may outstrip the capacity of a given nephron segment to generate ATP, especially under certain conditions. The medullary thick ascending limb possesses considerable glycolytic capability, but is also prone to hypoxic injury, albeit less so compared with the S3 segment of the proximal tubule. Both segments reside in areas that are poorly oxygenated following ischemic injury, and in such a circumstance, oxygenation of the medullary thick ascending limb may be burdened by demands related to metabolic work. For example, studies in isolated perfused kidney demonstrate that diminished transport in the medullary thick ascending limb and attendant less energy expenditure reduce hypoxic injury in this region, while conversely, agents that increase energy expenditure potentiate renal tubular damage. Thus increased energy expenditure necessitated by metabolic work in nephron segments with marginal tissue oxygenation may predispose these segments to ischemic injury.

Regional variation is also observed in the pattern of responses to ischemic injury. Ischemia induces sublethal and lethal cell injury, in turn accompanied by a proliferative response in the proximal tubular epithelial cells of the outer stripe of the outer medulla and in other segments of the proximal tubules. However, a complex response occurs in the cells of the distal nephron that leads to the upregulation of certain genes and the downregulation of others. The pattern of genes that are upregulated in the distal nephron in response to ischemia mimics the behavior of cells in culture exposed to such stress-inducing states as oxidants, DNA-damaging insults and increased tonicity. Cells exposed to these stressors display a rapid upregulation of a number of genes collectively called the immediate early genes; these genes can also be induced by growth factors. Stressors such as oxidants, cytokines, DNA-damaging insults and increased tonicity use the stress-activated protein kinase to induce these genes, and usually foster an antiproliferative response. Alternatively, growth factors use extracellular regulated kinases to recruit immediate early genes and foster a proliferative response. It is increasingly believed that this response in the distal nephron, one that mimics the immediate early gene response, influences the nature of recovery from acute ischemic injury.

This stress response may be adaptive or maladaptive in terms of its consequences to the kidney. For example, the cyclin-dependent kinase inhibitor, p21, which is induced by toxic and ischemic insults, is thought to prevent cells with injured DNA from progressing through the cell cycle and thus serves a protective role in renal injury. Conversely, the induction of *c-jun* following ischemia may be associated with adverse consequences for the kidney; for example, maneuvers preventing the activation of kinases that are responsible for the activation of *c-jun* protect, structurally and functionally, against ischemic renal injury.

Other genes upregulated as a stress response belong to proinflammatory genes. The upregulation of these inflammation-related genes may exert adverse or beneficial effects: genes such as *iNOS* and *ICAM-1* are implicated in the pathogenesis of ischemic injury while the recruitment of an inflammatory infiltrate, as will be discussed subsequently, provides a paracrine source of growth factors that, potentially, may contribute to the recovery from acute renal failure.

TABLE 48.8. Some Factors That Promote Resistance to Certain Types of Renal Injury

1. Availability of ATP from anaerobic sources such as glycolysis
2. Reduced temperature
3. Intracellular stores of glycine
4. Antioxidant defense mechanisms
5. Intracellular acidosis
6. Heat shock proteins
7. Sphingolipid derivatives such as ceramide
8. Heme oxygenase/ferritin
9. α-Ketoacids such as pyruvate and α-ketoglutarate
10. Prostaglandin E species
11. Certain members of the Bcl-2 family of proteins
12. Growth factors such as IGF-1 and HGF-1
13. α–MSH
14. Cyclin-dependent kinase inhibitors such as p21

REPARATIVE AND REGENERATIVE RESPONSES

Recovery from ischemic injury involves the return of normal renal hemodynamics, the resolution of vascular abnormalities, the disengagement of leukocytic-dependent mechanisms of

TABLE 48.9. Processes Involved in the Recovery from Acute Tubular Necrosis

1. Repair of renal hemodynamic and vascular abnormalities
2. Repair of sublethal cell injury
3. Replacement of cells lost by lethal injury
4. Appropriate cellular differentiation
5. Refashioning cell–cell and cell–substratum contacts
6. Disengagement of leukocytic-dependent pathways of injury
7. Removal of luminal debris

injury, and reparative responses to sublethal or lethal cell injury (Table 48.9). Sublethally injured cells require the restoration of cellular levels of ATP and ATP-generating capacity, the restoration of the cytoskeleton and recovery of polarity of the epithelial cell, the refashioning of the tight junction, and the appropriate differentiation of the surfaces into the apical and basolateral domains, the restoration of the normally low intracellular concentrations of calcium, and the deactivation of injurious enzymes such as proteases and phospholipases. What orchestrates these processes is an intriguing and largely unanswered question.

The process of recovery from tubular cell loss requires replacement of these cells and thus a mitogenic response mounted by remaining tubular epithelial cells. Three growth factors, namely, epidermal growth factor-1 (EGF-1), hepatocyte growth factor-1 (HGF-1), and IGF-1, are implicated in the proliferative responses that enable the renewal of cells lost as a consequence of the ischemic insult. Each of these growth factors, separately administered, promotes functional and structural improvement in models of ischemic acute renal failure, and based on such effects of administered growth factors, in conjunction with the presence of increased amounts of biologically active forms of these growth factors in the kidney subjected to ischemia, and in some instances, increased expression of relevant receptors, the view is evolving that regenerative responses following acute renal injury involve these, and possibly other growth factors, in the recovery process. These three growth factors may arise from autocrine sources, while paracrine sources of IGF-1 and HGF-1, as provided, in part, by inflammatory cells, may also serve as a stimulus for proliferative responses. Endocrine sources of growth factors may also exist, as is the case for HGF-1.

EGF-1 is a powerful mitogen to renal proximal tubular cells, and increased amounts of biologically active EGF appear in the postischemic kidney as it is made available from storage pools where it is largely inert; such appearance of EGF-1 is attended by increased DNA synthesis. HGF-1 is not only mitogenic to renal epithelial cells, but this growth factor, when administered to cells grown *in vitro*, can convoke renal epithelial cells into tubular structures. Ischemic injury leads to rapid and transient upregulation of HGF-1 mRNA and protein and upregulation of the mRNA for the HGF receptor. Such increased amounts of HGF-1 originate largely from paracrine sources such as endothelial cells, renal interstitial cells, and macrophages. In addition, renal injury leads to increased expression of HGF-1 in other organs such as the liver and lung, thereby providing endocrine sources of HGF-1 to aid in regenerative processes in the postischemic kidney.

IGF-1 may exert its major contributions at a somewhat later point in the regenerative and recovery process. Although not expressed in the proximal tubule of the healthy kidney, increased expression of IGF-1 mRNA and protein is observed at the site of maximal nephron injury following ischemia. These autocrine sources of IGF-1 may also be supplemented by paracrine sources provided by infiltrating mononuclear cells. The evidence that acute elevation in IGF-1 promotes a regenerative response in the kidney is supported by studies in which the administration of IGF-1 accelerates recovery from ATN. IGF-1 fosters recovery from ATN by promoting progression through the cell cycle, by upregulating expression of the EGF receptor and thereby enhancing EGF-mediated actions, and by suppressing apoptosis. Other beneficial actions of IGF-1 in the recovery from ATN include its recognized capacity to increase renal blood flow, to promote protein synthesis, to restore ATP levels, and to stimulate the expression of osteopontin, a protein involved in remodeling processes after tissue injury.

Other growth factors such as transforming growth factor (TGF), TGFβ, and fibroblast growth factor are under examination for their involvement in the reparative and regenerative responses following ischemic injury. Derivatives of ATP such as ADP and AMP may also be involved in the recovery from ATN; ADP stimulates DNA synthesis and the migration of viable epithelial cells, biologic effects that would aid in the recovery of a denuded segment of the nephron. Thus these metabolites generated from ATP during ischemia may assist in processes that restore the integrity of the nephron. Reparative and regenerative processes may also be influenced by transmembrane receptors that link epithelial cells to the extracellular matrix, namely, integrins.

In addition to regenerative processes, appropriate cell differentiation is required to restore the unique features and functions of each nephron segment damaged by ischemic injury. For example in the distal nephron, a number of genes are downregulated, including membrane transporter genes. Such downregulation may represent the relinquishing of features of differentiation not essential for cells simply attempting to survive an ischemic/hypoxic insult. Should such cells survive, restoration of these features would be necessary for the full recovery of segment-specific and cell-specific function.

ACUTE CORTICAL NECROSIS

Ischemic insults to the cortex of the kidney and attendant cortical infarction may be so severe that they outstrip the reparative and regenerative capability of the kidney; in such instances, recovery from acute renal failure does not occur. Acute cortical necrosis usually results from compromise in the perfusion of the interlobular arteries. Viability of deep nephrons often persists because of preservation of blood flow through the arcuate vessels. The majority of cases of acute cortical necrosis arise in the setting of pregnancy-related diseases such as toxemia, abruptio placentae, septic abortions, and intrauterine fetal death; other predisposing states besides pregnancy include sepsis, various gastrointestinal emergencies, dissection of aortic aneurysms, and syndromes related to hemolytic uremic syndrome/thrombotic thrombocytopenic purpura.

Mechanisms implicated in acute cortical necrosis include marked vasoconstriction and accompanying renal ischemia, the activation of the clotting cascade giving rise to endothelial injury and the formation of platelet-fibrin microthrombi. In addition, endothelial generation of nitric oxide and prostacyclin may be impaired, and these latter abnormalities are particularly implicated in those pregnancy-associated disease states that predispose to cortical necrosis. Endotoxemia is also a risk factor in those clinical and experimental conditions in which acute cortical necrosis arises. Endotoxin can induce endothelial injury and foster a procoagulant state; however, the concomitant induction of NOS by endotoxin attenuates these procoagulant effects of endotoxin because nitric oxide exerts an antiaggregatory effect on platelets, inhibits the formation of platelet-fibrin thrombi, and is vasorelaxant. Understanding the mechanisms that allow the vasoconstrictive and thrombogenic actions of endotoxin to persist relatively unopposed by commensurate generation of nitric oxide would provide important insights into the pathogenesis of cortical necrosis in this setting.

This condition presents with oliguria or anuria in the absence of urinary tract obstruction, and a urinary sediment typical for tubular necrosis or hematuria. The diagnosis may be made by ultrasonography or computed tomographic scan; it may require renal biopsy or angiography. In many cases recovery from acute renal failure does not occur. In a small subset of patients, recovery of a certain degree of kidney function is seen as surviving nephrons exhibit hyperfunction; such recovery of function, however, is often short lived.

HEME PIGMENT-INDUCED ATN

Acute renal failure can be induced by heme pigments such as myoglobin, released from injured muscle in rhabdomyolysis, and hemoglobin, released from lysed red blood cells. Heme pigment-induced ATN represents the integrated effects of three basic mechanisms—renal vasoconstriction, direct cytotoxicity, and tubular cast formation—that conspire in the evolution of renal injury.

Renal vasoconstriction in this setting involves three major pathways. Heme proteins such as myoglobin and hemoglobin possess a high affinity for nitric oxide, and thus can deprive the vasculature of its endogenous vasodilator. In addition, increased renal production of endothelin occurs in, and contributes to, renal vasoconstriction in experimental myohemoglobinuric renal injury. Another important vasoconstrictor species produced in the kidney in increased amounts as a consequence of oxidative stress involves the vasoconstrictive species, 8-isoprostanes produced via cyclooxygenase-independent oxidation of membrane lipid. Thus removal of a renal vasodilator and enhanced production of vasoconstrictors underlie vasoconstriction in this model.

Oxidative stress is implicated in the pathogenesis of tubular injury in this model. Lipid peroxidation and generation of hydrogen peroxide are both increased in the myohemoglobinuric model, and inhibitors of lipid peroxidation and scavengers of hydrogen peroxide and the hydroxyl radical are all protective. Glutathione content of the kidney is diminished, and provision of glutathione protects against renal injury. As further evidence for oxidative stress, and in particular iron-catalyzed oxidative stress in this model, chelators of iron such as deferoxamine, reduce renal injury in this model. In aggregate, these studies demonstrate that heightened generation of oxidants, impairment in antioxidant defense mechanisms as reflected by diminished content of glutathione, and increased availability of iron summate to foster iron-catalyzed oxidative stress as a pathway for heme protein-induced renal injury.

In these states, heme proteins escape across the glomerular filtration barrier into the urinary space where they are taken up by tubular epithelial cells. Once present in the tubular epithelial cells, heme proteins are broken down into heme and globin. The heme prosthetic group is lipid soluble and thus is readily transmissible to multiple cellular compartments and organelles within the kidney. In this way, heme or its contained iron could directly attack multiple compartments. Recent studies indicate that the two targets that are particularly vulnerable to such attack are the mitochondrion and the nucleus. For example, within 3 hours of the induction of the myohemoglobin model in the rat, pronounced alterations in mitochondrial function are observed in conjunction with marked increments in mitochondrial heme content. The exposure of mitochondria to comparable amounts of heme induces similar derangements in mitochondrial function. Heme itself could destabilize the cytoskeleton, the plasma membrane, and intracellular membranes.

Tubular cast formation is a prominent feature in renal failure induced by heme proteins. Such casts represent the interaction of heme pigments with the Tamm-Horsfall protein, an interaction that is enhanced by dehydration and acidosis. Cast formation can be greatly attenuated with significant improvement in renal function by the expansion of the extracellular fluid volume and the administration of bicarbonate, mannitol, and assorted antioxidants.

Several factors may contribute to the vulnerability of kidney to heme protein-induced renal injury, and these factors are summarized in Table 48.10.

TABLE 48.10. Sensitivity of the Kidney to Heme Protein-Induced Renal Injury

1. Heme proteins scavenge nitric oxide and thus deprive the kidney of its endogenous vasodilator.
2. The kidney is unduly sensitive to the vasoconstrictive effects of endothelin and isoprostanes, which are produced in increased amounts in the kidney in myohemoglobinuric renal injury.
3. The kidney concentrates heme proteins, thereby increasing renal content of a potential nephrotoxin.
4. The kidney takes up heme proteins into tubular epithelial cells and splits the protein into its heme and globulin moieties. This exposes the kidney to large concentrations of heme, which directly or via its released iron can be toxic to the kidney.
5. The kidney generates hydrogen peroxide in its basal state, a reactive oxygen species that could predispose it to heme protein toxicity and a reactive species that is produced in increased amounts in the setting of heme protein-induced renal injury.
6. The kidney reduces pH in the urinary environment, which increases the toxicity of heme proteins and promotes cast formation.

THERAPEUTIC STRATAGEMS IN ACUTE RENAL FAILURE

The current management of ATN is largely supportive care during the period within which the obligate processes of reparation and regeneration restore the functional and structural integrity of the kidney. However, the elucidation of pathogenetic mechanisms in ATN has, nonetheless, influenced our management of this disorder. For example, the recognition that the kidney with ATN is particularly vulnerable to even transient episodes of hypotension—which would be otherwise innocuous in the healthy kidney—has raised awareness with regard to myriad settings that impose additional hemodynamic insults to the kidney. Similarly, the potentially adverse effects of excessive ultrafiltration rates and other factors that predispose to hypotension during conventional hemodialysis, particularly in patients with unstable systemic hemodynamics, has influenced our dialytic prescriptions. Among the potential benefits of continuous replacement therapies compared with conventional hemodialysis is a lower risk of exposing the kidney with ATN to additional episodes of hypoperfusion. The recognition that insults besides hemodynamic ones, such as assorted nephrotoxins and septic states, may summate with ischemic insults to exacerbate renal injury has led to clinical attentiveness that minimizes such added insults. Such a consideration is also relevant to conventional dialytic management because it is now recognized that bioincompatible dialytic membranes may activate leukocytes which journey to the kidney, and thereby exacerbate renal injury in patients with ATN. The study of the pathogenesis of ATN has stimulated novel strategies in the supportive care of patients with established ATN. For example, exploration of mechanisms involved in regeneration of tubular epithelial cells led to the development of the use of the bioartificial renal tubule assist devices in which renal tubular epithelial progenitor cells are cultured onto hollow fibers impregnated with matrix substances; such an approach may provide metabolic and humoral aspects of renal function that are not replaced by current dialytic techniques.

The elucidation of pathogenetic mechanisms in ATN, however, raises the hope that our management of this disorder will advance beyond a supportive role and allow us to intervene either by lessening the severity of the renal insult and/or by hastening the recovery from these insults. Interruption of the pathways involved in the evolution of ATN—hemodynamic alterations, mechanisms contributing to sublethal and lethal cell injury, involvement of leukocytic-dependent pathways—provides strategies that may prove effective. In addition, experimental maneuvers that augment resistance to renal injury, stimulate the reparation of sublethally injured cells, promote the replacement of cells lost by lethal injury, and finally, foster the appropriate differentiation of repaired and regenerating cells, offer other possible therapeutic stratagems. Although initial attempts to improve renal function in human ATN by administering synthetic atrial natriuretic peptide or recombinant IGF-1 have not appeared to be as beneficial as was hoped, the wealth of new insights derived from the study of the pathogenesis of ATN makes it conceivable that eventually clinically effective therapies would emerge from these studies. The need for such therapies remains as pressing as ever for a disease that causes incalculable suffering and considerable cost and for which mortality has not appreciably changed since its original description.

Selected Readings

Bonventre JV. Mechanisms of ischemic acute renal failure. *Kidney Int* 1993;43: 1160–1178.

This review summarizes mechanisms contributing to ischemic renal injury, including descriptions of necrotic and apoptotic cell death, the role of increased cytosolic calcium concentrations, and phospholipase activation in ischemic cell injury.

Chiao H, Kohda Y, McLeroy P, et al. α-Melanocyte-stimulating hormone protects against renal injury after ischemia in mice and rats. *J Clin Invest* 1997;99: 1165–1172.

This experimental study provides a novel approach by which to protect against ischemic acute renal injury in rats and mice that is based on the administration of α-melanocyte-stimulating hormone.

Conger J. Hemodynamic factors in acute renal failure. *Adv Ren Replace Ther* 1997;4:25–37.

This review comprehensively discusses hemodynamic mechanisms that contribute to acute renal failure. It includes both ischemic and nephrotoxic insults and draws the pertinent clinical inferences from experimental findings.

Edelstein CL, Ling H, Schrier RW. The nature of renal cell injury. *Kidney Int* 1997;51:1341–1351.

This overview of the cell biology of renal cell injury includes discussion of calcium-dependent, calpain-dependent, and nitric oxide-dependent mechanisms of renal cell injury and other pertinent mechanisms.

Goligorsky MS, Noiri E, Kessler H, et al. Therapeutic potential of RGD peptides in acute renal injury. *Kidney Int* 1997;51:1487–1492.

This review article discusses the capacity of these peptides to interrupt cellular interactions based on the RGD sequences found in extracellular matrix proteins and the potential clinical utility of these peptides in acute renal failure.

Hammerman MR. New treatments for acute renal failure: growth factors and beyond. *Curr Opin Nephrol Hypertens* 1997;6:7–9.

This editorial review discusses the role of growth factors and other novel approaches in the treatment of acute renal failure.

Hirschberg R, Ding H. Growth factors and acute renal failure. *Semin Nephrol* 1998;18:191–207.

This comprehensive review provides a detailed analysis of the biology and pathobiology of assorted growth factors relevant to recovery from acute renal failure.

Humes HD, MacKay SM, Funke AJ, et al. Acute renal failure: growth factors, cell therapy and gene therapy. *Proc Assoc Am Physicians* 1997;109:547–557.

This review article discusses potential therapies that are being explored for acute renal failure, which are based on the administration of growth factors, cell therapy including the bioartificial tubule assist device, and gene therapy.

Hunley TE, Kon V. Endothelin in ischemic acute renal failure. *Curr Opin Nephrol Hypertens* 1997;6:395–400.

This review discusses the cell biology of endothelin and evidence supporting its role in the pathogenesis of ischemic and nephrotoxic insults.

Kumar S, Stein JH. Tubular cast formation and Tamm-Horsfall glycoprotein. In: Goligorsky MS, Stein JH, eds. *Contemporary Issues in Nephrology. Acute Renal Failure.* New York: Churchill Livingstone, 1995;30:267–286.

This review discusses the cell biology of the Tamm-Horsfall protein and the mechanisms of cast formation.

Lieberthal W. Biology of acute renal failure: therapeutic implications. *Kidney Int* 1997;52:1102–1115.

This nephrology forum provides an overview of the mechanisms of acute renal failure, focusing, in particular, on abnormalities in the cytoskeleton and on the cell biology of apoptosis.

Molitoris BA, Weinberg JM, Venkatachalam MA, et al. Experimental models of acute renal failure: imperfect but indespensable. *Am J Physiol* 2000;278:F1–F12.

This symposium provides a discussion of the applicability and the contributions of experimental models of acute renal failure to human acute renal failure.

Nolan CR, Anderson RJ. Hospital-acquired acute renal failure. *J Am Soc Nephrol* 1998;9:710–718.

This article provides a review of the predisposing conditions, clinical features and therapy for clinical ATN.

Rabb H, O'Meara YM, Maderna P, et al. Leukocytes, cell adhesion molecules and ischemic acute renal failure. *Kidney Int* 1997;51:1463–1468.

This comprehensive review discusses the cell biology of leukocyte adhesion and the evidence for, and against, the involvement of leukocytes in ischemic acute renal failure.

Racusen LC. Pathology of acute renal failure: Structure/function correlations. *Adv Ren Replace Ther* 1997;4:3–16.

This review provides a detailed description of the pathologic features of clinical and experimental ATN, correlating such structural alterations with functional ones.

Safirstein R. Renal stress response and acute renal failure. *Adv Renal Replacement Ther* 1997;4:38–42.

This review points out the nature of the renal stress response to ischemic and other insults to the kidney and provides a comprehensive description of the underlying cell biology and the implications on the recovery from acute renal failure.

Weinberg JM. The cell biology of ischemic renal injury. *Kidney Int* 1991;39:476–500.

This remarkable review summarizes quite comprehensively the body of literature that provides the basis for current understanding of ischemic renal injury.

Weinberg JM, Roeser NF, Davis JA, et al. Glycine-protected, hypoxic, proximal tubules develop severely compromised energetic function. *Kidney Int* 1997;52:140–151.

This experimental study provides continued exploration of the cytoprotective effects of glycine, demonstrating that impressive plasma membrane protection occurs in spite of profound disruption in cellular energetics.

Zager RA. Rhabdomyolysis and myohemoglobinuric acute renal failure. *Kidney Int* 1996;49:314–326.

This editorial review provides a detailed and comprehensive review of the clinical syndrome of rhabdomyolysis, mechanisms involved in such injury based on the disease models, and experimental manipulations that have proven effective in experimental models of this disease.

Zager RA, Iwata M, Conrad DS, et al. Altered ceramide and sphingosine expression during the induction phase of ischemic acute renal failure. *Kidney Int* 1997;52:60–70.

This experimental study in ischemic acute renal failure demonstrates altered levels of ceramide and sphingosine during the ischemic and postischemic phases and presents evidence that these derivatives of sphingolipid may serve as determinants of the susceptibility to injury after ischemic and nephrotoxic insults.

PART 2
Diagnosis, Clinical Presentation, and Management

Richard J. Glassock, Shaul G. Massry, and H. David Humes

Acute renal failure is a common clinical syndrome. It is defined as an abrupt decline in renal function. The clinical manifestations of this disorder are the result of a decline in glomerular filtration rate (GFR) and the inability of the kidney to excrete the toxic metabolic wastes produced by the body. It is recognized clinically by rising levels of blood urea nitrogen (BUN) and serum creatinine and may be demonstrated dramatically, with a patient who has normal metabolic parameters developing uremia within a week. Of importance, many forms of acute renal failure are reversible processes, making the correct diagnosis and management of this disorder necessary so that improvement of renal function may occur with minimal risk to the patient.

Acute renal failure arises from a vast array of causative conditions (Table 48.11) and is best understood when categorized according to the sequential process of urine formation and excretion. Acute renal failure may evolve from diminished renal blood flow (RBF), which is referred to as prerenal functional acute renal failure; from a sudden, severe renal parenchymal insult, which is referred to as intrinsic structural acute renal

TABLE 48.11. Causes of Acute Renal Failure

I. Prerenal
A. Cardiac/pulmonary
1. Severe congestive heart failure
2. Acute myocardial infarction with hypotension
3. Pericardial tamponade
4. Acute pulmonary embolism with hypotension
5. Ventricular cardiac arrhythmias with hypotension
6. Cardiac arrest
B. Volume depletion
1. Extrarenal
a. Gastrointestinal fluid losses
i. Vomiting
ii. Diarrhea
iii. Nasogastric suction
iv. Acute gastrointestinal bleeding
b. Third spacing
i. Severe necrotizing pancreatitis
ii. Peritonitis
iii. Burns
iv. Retroperitoneal hemorrhage
c. External hemorrhage
d. Excessive sweating with inadequate fluid intake (hot climate)
e. Inadequate fluid intake, especially in elderly individuals
2. Renal
a. Excessive use of diuretics
b. Marked osmotic diuresis
c. Adrenal insufficiency (excessive urinary losses of sodium)
d. Salt-wasting nephropathy
e. Central or nephrogenic diabetes insipidus
C. Reduced peripheral vascular resistance
1. Sepsis
2. Sedative overdose
3. Carcinoid syndrome
4. Interleukin-2 therapy
5. Acute and large arteriovenous fistula
6. Drugs
a. Nitrates
b. Vasodilators
7. Hepatorenal syndrome
II. Renal (intrinsic)
A. Vascular
1. Structural
a. Acute bilateral renal artery occlusion
b. Renal artery stenosis with the use of angiotensin II-converting enzyme (ACE) inhibitors
c. Aortic dissection involving the renal arteries
d. Malignant hypertension
e. Scleroderma renal crisis
f. Hemolytic uremic syndrome
g. Acute cortical necrosis (abruptio placenta)
h. Radiation nephritis
i. Atheroembolic disease
j. Acute bilateral renal vein thrombosis
2. Functional
a. Hepatorenal syndrome
b. Hypercalcemia
c. Sepsis
d. Drugs
i. Nonsteroidal antiinflammatory drugs
ii. Contrast media
iii. Cyclosporine
iv. Angiotensin-converting enzyme inhibitors
B. Glomerular
1. Acute glomerulonephritis (e.g., poststreptococcal glomerulonephritis)
2. Crescentic glomerulonephritis
3. Microscopic polyangiitis
4. Minimal change disease (adult only)
5. Lupus nephritis
6. IgA nephropathy
7. Other primary glomerular diseases associated with severe nephrotic syndrome
C. Tubulointerstitial
1. Acute hypersensitivity interstitial nephritis (drug-associated)
2. Intrarenal precipitation of insoluble substances (uric acid, myeloma light-chain proteins)
3. Acute tubular necrosis
a. Ischemic (hypotension)
b. Toxic
i. Heavy metals
ii. Halogenated hydrocarbons
iii. Solvents (e.g., ethylene glycol)
iv. Contrast media
v. Pesticides
vi. Fungicides
vii. Antibiotics
viii. Myoglobinuria or hemoglobinuria
III. Postrenal
A. Ureteropelvic junction
1. Stone (single kidney) or two stones, one each junction
2. Clots
B. Ureter
1. Trauma of both ureters
2. Intraluminal[a]
a. Stones
b. Sloughed papillae
c. Blood clots
d. Fungus ball
e. Cancer
3. Extraluminal[a]
a. Retroperitoneal fibrosis
b. Tumors (pelvic, uterine, or cervical)
c. Urinoma
d. Ureteral vasculitis
C. Bladder
1. Acute neurogenic bladder (spinal cord injury)
2. Rupture
D. Urethra
1. Prostate hypertrophy or prostate cancer causing outlet obstruction
2. Bladder cancer
3. Stone
4. Foreign body
5. Urethral valves
6. Strictures
7. Phimosis

[a] Must affect both ureters or one ureter in a patient with a single kidney.

failure; or from obstruction to urine flow, which is referred to as postrenal acute renal failure.

The initial approach in the diagnosis and management of acute renal failure is, therefore, to localize the site of dysfunction (i.e., prerenal, intrarenal, or postrenal). If the process is localized to a prerenal or postrenal site, the specific diagnosis and treatment are readily apparent, even though the causes responsible for altering renal perfusion or urine flow are numerous. If the process is localized to an intrarenal site, it is useful to further categorize the pathogenetic process into vascular, glomerular, interstitial, or tubular disease.

ETIOLOGY

Prerenal acute renal failure results from a persistent, significant decline in RBF. This decline may result from absolute or relative extracellular or intravascular fluid deficiencies, the hepatorenal syndrome, or drug-induced nephrotoxicity; the latter two are discussed in detail in Chapters 55, Part 2 and 47, respectively. Acute renal failure from obstructive disease may occur from both intrarenal and extrarenal processes and is discussed at length in Chapter 50.

Most cases of hospital-acquired intrarenal acute renal failure are the result of ischemic or nephrotoxic processes. In many clinical settings, a combination of these two processes may operate simultaneously to produce acute renal failure. An ischemic insult often potentiates renal damage produced by nephrotoxins. Rapidly progressive glomerulonephritis, acute hypersensitivity interstitial nephritis, systemic vasculitis, atheroembolic disease, and renal artery occlusion may also be seen as acute intrarenal structural renal failure and must be considered in the differential diagnosis (Table 48.11). The clinicopathologic aspects, the approach to the diagnosis, and the treatment of these entities are detailed in Chapters 39, 40, 42, Part 4, and 52.

Acute tubular necrosis is the most common name given to acute renal failure secondary to either ischemic or toxic processes. Renal failure develops from tubular cell injury that produces necrosis limited to particular nephron segments within the kidney, so that only a patchy distribution of injury is observed. Even though tubule cell injury is limited to certain nephron segments, substantial renal excretory failure may still develop, as nephrons function as segmental units in series. When widespread cortical necrosis occurs, the etiologic and pathophysiologic mechanisms involved in this process are quite different from those of nephrotoxic or ischemic acute renal failure, and the prognosis for recovery of normal renal architecture and physiologic function is poor.

Progressive renal tubular cell injury initiates alterations at the nephronal level that ultimately result in renal excretory failure. These alterations include (a) intratubular obstruction, (b) backleak of glomerular filtrate through damaged tubular epithelium, and (c) primary reductions in glomerular filtration of solutes and water. Of these factors, intratubular obstruction and backleak of filtrate appear to be the major nephronal mechanisms contributing to the decrement in GFR during acute tubular necrosis. Intratubular obstruction arises from the formation of casts composed of cellular debris from injured or necrotic renal tubular cells and Tamm-Horsfall proteins, which impede the flow of urine. The necrotic cells shed into the tubular lumen reduce renal excretory function, not only by obstructing urine flow, but also by leaving denuded regions of basement membrane along the nephron through which glomerular filtrate may reenter the circulation. The pathogenetic processes contributing to the development of these alterations are discussed in detail in Chapter 48, Part 1.

The kidney is a major excretory organ of the body for therapeutic agents. As a result, the list of drugs known to induce acute renal failure is long. As new agents are developed, additions to this list certainly will be made. The causes of nephrotoxic acute renal failure may be categorized into four major groups: antibiotics, heavy metals, radiocontrast agents, and other exogenous toxins (Table 48.11). These toxic forms of acute renal failure are discussed in Chapter 47.

Endogenous nephrotoxins include myoglobin, hemoglobin, uric acid, and calcium. When large amounts of myoglobin or hemoglobin pigments enter the circulation as the result of extensive muscle injury or hemolysis, acute renal failure may ensue. Although these substances alone do not appear to be nephrotoxic when infused into humans or animal models, they apparently interact with other toxic materials from red blood cells or muscle cells in causing renal dysfunction. Prior volume depletion seems to enhance the likelihood of development of acute renal failure with rhabdomyolysis or hemolysis. Although rhabdomyolysis was initially recognized in patients with severe crush injuries, unusually strenuous exercise, or other obvious signs of muscle injury, several instances of myoglobin-related acute renal failure have been observed in patients without obvious muscle trauma. In these cases of nontraumatic rhabdomyolysis, there frequently has been a prolonged period of immobilization while in a stuporous state such that there is subtle muscle necrosis as a result of pressure ischemia. Further discussions of acute renal failure associated with rhabdomyolysis are found in Chapters 28 and 47, Part 6.

Acute urate nephropathy is generally encountered in patients with lymphoproliferative diseases in which treatment has been recently initiated. The cytotoxic drug agents used in therapy cause massive cell lysis and an abrupt increase in the plasma urate level. Urate deposits in collecting ducts result in an intrinsic obstructive nephropathy. Hypercalcemia may be associated with acute renal failure, which is seen most frequently in patients with hypercalcemia caused by malignancies or primary hyperparathyroidism.

Renal ischemia is a common cause of acute tubular necrosis. In the clinical setting, ischemic acute renal failure has been observed after ischemic insults of variable duration and severity. In some patients, several minutes of ischemia produce acute tubular necrosis, whereas in others prolonged renal ischemia produces only transient renal dysfunction. However, regardless of the etiologic factor producing the prerenal state, if its duration is prolonged or its magnitude severe, progression to structural renal damage occurs. Most cases of ischemic acute renal failure, however, are associated with a period of frank hypotension with the highest frequency noted in patients with sepsis or patients undergoing major surgery.

Nearly half of the clinical cases of ischemic acute renal failure occur after surgery. A variety of processes, including preoperative and intraoperative fluid losses and anesthesia, result in intravascular volume depletion, with subsequent declines in RBF and GFR. If an additional hypotensive or hemolytic insult is added to these conditions, susceptible patients may develop acute tubular necrosis. Abdominal aortic aneurysmal repair, cardiac surgery, and biliary tract surgery show the highest incidence of ischemic acute renal failure. Each of these procedures is associated with a substantially greater decline in RBF than other surgical procedures. The higher frequency of acute tubular necrosis in the septic patient may relate to the major hemodynamic effects of endotoxins that have the ability to produce systemic hypotension and secondary renal vasoconstriction.

This chapter focuses predominantly on the form of acute renal failure arising from ischemic processes because other chapters have been devoted to the other forms of acute renal failure mentioned previously.

Elevated serum creatinine
Acute versus chronic renal failure?
Acute
↓
Is obstructive uropathy present?
No
↓
Are prerenal factors operative?
No
↓
Is vascular renal disease present?
Large vessel?
Small vessel?
No
Is glomerular disease present?
No
↓
Is interstital disease present?
No
↓
Is intrarenal cystal deposition present?
No
↓
Acute tubular necrosis

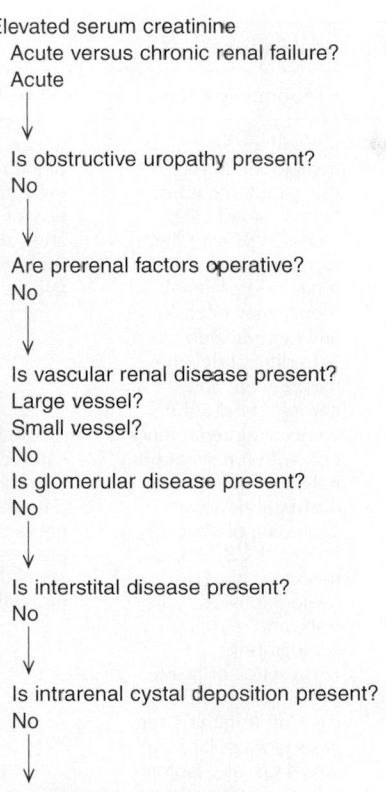

Figure 48.1. Schema for determining the cause of acute renal failure. Modified with permission from Chapter 49 of the Second Edition of the Textbook of Nephrology. Eds. Massry S.G. and Glassock R.J., Williams and Wilkins, Baltimore, 1989.

DIFFERENTIAL DIAGNOSIS

When an acute elevation of serum creatinine is encountered, a series of steps should be undertaken to evaluate possible underlying causes. These steps, which are outlined in Fig. 48.1, sequentially investigate the role of obstruction, prerenal factors, vascular, glomerular, or tubulointerstitial disease and intrarenal obstruction in the genesis of the acute renal failure. Thus a diagnosis of acute tubular necrosis of either ischemic or toxic origin is arrived at by the exclusion of other causes. The clinical and laboratory clues that are helpful in differentiating the various causes of acute renal failure are presented in Table 48.12.

CLINICAL FEATURES

In the clinical setting, a spectrum of observations has been seen, and the clinical observations seem to correlate with the severity of the decrement in renal perfusion. With systemic systolic arterial pressures as low as 90 mm Hg, adaptive intrarenal autoregulatory vasoactive mechanisms function to preserve glomerular filtration, while tubular transport mechanisms function to preserve or correct systemic intravascular volume. As systolic blood pressure decreases below 90 mm Hg, intrarenal autoregulatory vasoactive mechanisms are unable to compensate appropriately to preserve glomerular filtration. In addition, renal perfusion is compromised to the extent that reversible or irreversible renal tubular epithelial cell injury ensues. When perfusion deficits cause reversible cellular injury, synthetic repair of the reversibly injured cells restores tubular physiologic function. In situations resulting in irreversible cellular injury, proliferative repair by a resilient subpopulation of tubular cells, which have retained the capacity to undergo mitotic division and cellular differentiation, occurs, restoring both structural integrity and physiologic function. Finally, in clinical situations with severe renal perfusion deficits of extensive duration, even the viability of this resilient subpopulation of cells is compromised. The combination of the loss of these progenitor cells and the inherent inflammatory response accompanying this injurious process results in the inevitable loss of any potential replicative repair process and return of renal function. Thus the clinical spectrum resulting from the decrement in renal perfusion ranges from prerenal azotemia to acute tubular necrosis to frank cortical necrosis.

In prerenal conditions, renal function is impaired because of decreased renal perfusion, rather than intrinsic renal parenchymal alterations, whereas, with acute tubular necrosis, the intrinsic physiologic properties of the renal tubular epithelium are altered. Urinary electrolyte and solute excretion indices that are helpful in differentiating between prerenal azotemia and acute tubular necrosis are given in Table 48.13.

A decrement in the GFR secondary to intrinsic renal disease most often results in the synchronous elevation of BUN and plasma creatinine (P_{Cr}), maintaining the normal ratio between these parameters of 10:15:1. Daily creatinine production is dependent on muscle mass and ranges from 10 to 15 mg/kg per day in young healthy adult females and from 15 to 20 mg/kg per day in young adult males. With the complete cessation of effective glomerular filtration, an incremental rise in serum creatinine concentration ranges from 1 to 2 mg/dl per day, and the incremental rise in BUN ranges from 20 to 25 mg/dl per day. With less severe intrinsic renal disease, the incremental rise in plasma creatinine and BUN would also be less severe. In hypercatabolic states, situations of increased tissue breakdown or states of intracorporeal hemorrhage with reabsorption of degraded blood, the incremental rise in BUN would be expected to be more rapid. A less rapid incremental rise is expected in severe hepatic failure or states of protein malnutrition. Similarly, smaller or larger incremental rises in plasma creatinine correlate with relative muscle mass or an existing pathologic process with direct involvement of the musculature. A decrement in the GFR secondary to a prerenal state results in the compensatory increase in proximal tubular sodium and water reabsorption, promoting a disparate rise in BUN/P_{Cr} because of the passive reabsorption of BUN with water by the paracellular route. Therefore the BUN:P_{Cr} ratio increases to 20:1 or greater.

The rate of incremental rise in plasma creatinine may fluctuate in prerenal states, whereas in acute tubular necrosis the incremental rise is steadily progressive until reaching steady-state conditions. In both conditions, the decrement in glomerular filtration secondary to the alteration in intrarenal vascular resistance is a major contributing factor. However, in acute tubular necrosis additional mechanisms contribute to this incremental rise, including transtubular backleak with or without accompanying intraluminal obstruction by cellular exfoliation and aggregation.

To further assess the integrity of physiologic function, the resorptive capacity of sodium and water may be assessed by the measurement of the fractional excretion of sodium and urine osmolality. The fractional excretion of sodium (FE_{Na^+}) represents the percentage of filtered sodium ultimately excreted. During prerenal states, sodium- and water-retentive states, the FE_{Na^+} is appropriately low (less than 1.0) and the urine osmolality appropriately high (greater than 500 mOsm/kg). However, with ischemic tubular injury, the dissipation of the polar distribution of the Na^+-K^+-ATPase pump results in an elevated FE_{Na^+} (greater than 1.0 to 2.0). Renal concentrating ability may also be impaired with a decrease in urine osmolality (less than 350 mOsm/kg). A summary of urinary indices in prerenal oliguria and in oliguric and

TABLE 48.12. Differential Diagnostic Clues in Acute Renal Failure

	History	Physical Examination	Laboratory/X-Ray	Miscellaneous
? Acute versus chronic	In the absence of recent renal function tests, the differentiation of acute versus chronic renal failure is difficult. A history of ↑ BP, abnormal urinalyses, edema, recurrent UTIs, family history of renal disease, or symptoms of chronic obstruction suggest a chronic process.	There are few if any findings on physical examination that clearly differentiate acute versus chronic renal failure. The presence of peripheral neuropathy may suggest chronic renal failure.	Small kidney size,[a] low hematocrit, and urinalysis with large numbers of broad casts (>2–3 WBCs in diameter) suggest chronic renal failure. Renal biopsy may occasionally be indicated to help differentiate between acute and chronic renal failure.	The clinical course of the renal failure is the best way of differentiating acute versus chronic renal failure.
? Obstruction	Obstructive uropathy is suggested by anuria, extreme fluctuation in urine volume, known pelvic/retroperitoneal disease and/or surgery, and a history of frequency, nocturia, or urinary stream difficulties.	A distended bladder (palpation and percussion) and flank mass (distended pelvis) may suggest obstruction. Rectal and pelvic examinations are mandatory.	Deteriorating renal function with a normal urinalysis should suggest obstruction. Means of excluding obstruction include KUB film, ultrasound, infusion pyelography, isotopic tests, and retrograde pyelography.	A single bladder catheterization for residual volume should be performed in all patients with an acute decrease in renal function.
? Vascular or glomerular disease	Major vessel disease may be suggested by the presence of underlying nephrosis (renal vein thrombosis), source for arterial emboli (SBE, atrial fibrillation, recent atherosclerotic emboli provocative factor), or dissection. Small vessel disease (vasculitis/glomerulonephritis) may be suggested by underlying systemic disease symptoms. Recent onset of flank or nonspecific abdominal pain is often seen with vascular diseases of kidney.	The presence of atrial fibrillation, stigmata of SBE, and vascular disease as determined by arterial pulse palpation and auscultation suggests possible vascular disease. Physical examination for small emboli or vasculitis is needed. Neurologic evaluation and examination for jaundice, bleeding/bruising may be helpful to exclude DIC and TTP.	The presence of heavy proteinuria or RBC casts on urinalysis suggests glomerular small vessel disease. Isotopic scanning, renal venography, and arteriography may be helpful for large vessel disease. Presence of microangiopathic-hemolytic anemia, thrombocytopenia, or serologic markers may help to establish diagnosis. Renal biopsy may be helpful if small vessel disease or glomerulonephritis likely.	
? Interstitial disease	Recent drug administration, a clinical setting, or symptoms associated with hypercalcemia and symptoms of severe UTI all may suggest interstitial nephritis.	Fever and skin rash suggest possibility of allergic nephritis. Stigmata of hypercalcemia (band keratopathy) may be observed. Profound CVA pain suggests acute, diffuse pyelonephritis.	Eosinophilia and eosinophilic casts on urinalysis suggest allergic interstitial nephritis. Hypercalcemia suggests possibility of hypercalcemic nephropathy. Pyuria and bacilluria suggest possibility of acute, diffuse pyelonephritis.	
? Crystal deposits	Ethylene glycol ingestion, Penthrane anesthesia, or intestinal bypass surgery suggest potential for oxalate crystal deposition. Tumor chemotherapy suggests potential for uric acid crystal deposition. High dose methotrexate therapy suggests potential for methotrexate deposition.	Patients with ethylene glycol toxicity often have associated neurological and pulmonary diseases.	Urinalysis may demonstrate large numbers of oxalic acid or uric acid crystals. Urine-to-plasma uric acid ratio >1 suggests uric acid nephropathy. Profound metabolic acidosis accompanying acute renal failure suggests possibility of ethylene glycol. Uric acid deposition often associated with marked hyperuricemia.	

TABLE 48.12. *(continued)*

	History	Physical Examination	Laboratory/X-Ray	Miscellaneous
? Prerenal	A history of volume depletion of extrarenal (GI, skin) or renal (diuretics, ↓ adrenal function) origin, intravascular volume sequestration, or impaired cardiac output suggests prerenal factors.	Decreasing weight, orthostatic decreases in arterial pressure and increases in pulse, lack of skin turgor or moisture palpable in axilla or groin, and physical examination findings or cardiac failure suggest prerenal factors.	Deteriorating renal function with unremarkable urinalysis and the urinary chemistry indices in Table 48.13 suggest prerenal factors.	Improvement in renal function should be observed with correction of prerenal factors.

[a] Although small contracted kidney indicates chronic renal failure, the demonstration of normal size or large kidneys does not rule out chronic renal failure because this could be encountered in patients with diabetes mellitus, renal amyloid, polycystic kidneys, obstructive uropathy, and infiltrative lesions of the kidney.

BP, blood pressure; CVA, costovertebral angle; DIC, disseminated intravascular coagulation; GI, gastrointestinal; KUB, kidney, ureter, bladder; RBC, red blood cell; SBE, subacute bacterial endocarditis; TTP, thrombotic thrombocytopenia purpura; UTI, urinary tract infection; WBC, white blood cell. Reproduced by permission from Chapter 49 of the second edition of the *Textbook of Nephrology*. Eds. Massry SG and Glassock RJ. Baltimore: Williams and Wilkins, 1989

nonoliguric acute renal failure is provided in Table 48.13. In addition, Table 48.14 lists clinical conditions in which the indices of urinary sodium excretion may be misleading as a marker of prerenal azotemia or of acute tubular necrosis. Urinary output is low in prerenal states and variable with acute tubular necrosis. Thus in the latter condition one can have an oliguric or nonoliguric acute tubular necrosis. Contributing factors responsible for this variability in urine output include (a) the severity of reversible epithelial injury, (b) the extent of epithelial cell exfoliation with subsequent aggregation and intraluminal obstruction, (c) the balance of vasoregulatory mediators of the periglomerular vasculature, and (d) the adequacy of systemic arterial pressures allowing for adequate renal perfusion.

Urinalysis is generally helpful in differentiating prerenal disease from acute tubular necrosis, as well as excluding other intrinsic renal disease of glomerular origin. In prerenal conditions, qualitative glycosuria is unusual, but qualitative proteinuria occurs more frequently because of the concentrated character of the urine excreted. However, quantitative measures of proteinuria are often minimal. When appreciable quantities of protein are noted, a glomerular etiologic factor must be sought. Microscopic analysis of the urinary sediment is gener-

TABLE 48.13. Urinary Electrolytes and Solute Excretion Indices in Prerenal Azotemia and in Acute Tubular Necrosis

	Prerenal Azotemia	Acute Tubular Necrosis	
		Oliguric	Nonoliguric
Urine osmolality ($mOsm/kg\ H_2O$)	>500	<350	<350
Urine sodium (mEq/L)	<20[a]	>40	>40
Urine:plasma creatinine ratio	>40	<20	<20
Fractional excretion[b] of sodium ($FE_{Na\%}$)	<1	>>1 (usually >5)	>1 (usually >2)
Renal failure index[b]	<1	>1	>1

[a] In patients with prerenal azotemia, because of vomiting, which is associated with metabolic alkalosis, urinary sodium excretion is high due to loss of sodium bicarbonate in the urine. In such patients, urinary chloride is a better index of volume depletion. Chloride excretion is low because of the hypochloremia associated with vomiting.

[b] Fractional excretion of sodium ($FE_{Na\%}$)is calculated as follows:

$$\frac{\text{Urinary sodium in mEq/L} \times \text{Serum creatinine in mg/dl}}{\text{Serum sodium in mEq/L} \times \text{Urinary creatinine in mg/dl}} \times 100$$

Renal failure index is calculated as follows:

$$\frac{\text{Urinary sodium in mEq/L} \times \text{Serum creatinine in mg/dl}}{\text{Urinary creatinine in mg/dl}} \times 100$$

TABLE 48.14. Clinical Conditions in Which Urinary Sodium Indices May Be Misleading

1. Acute renal failure with low FE_{Na} in the absence of prerenal factors
   - Early phase of oliguric ATN in the presence of renal ischemia (e.g., sepsis)
   - Early phase of nonoliguric ATN
   - Early acute obstructive nephropathy
   - Acute glomerulonephritis
   - Radiocontrast media-associated ARF
   - Rhabdomyolysis-associated ARF
   - ARF associated with severe burns
   - Concomitant administration of nonsteroidal antiinflammatory drugs
2. Prerenal azotemia with high FE_{Na} without ATN
   - Preexisting chronic renal failure
   - Mineralocorticoid deficiency
   - Concomitant mannitol or diuretics administration
   - After contrast media due to its osmotic diuresis effect
   - Vomiting with metabolic alkalosis and hypochloremia[a]
   - Ketoacidosis with large amounts and hypochloremia[a]
   - Ketoacidosis with large amounts of ketoacids in the urine; ketoanions obligate sodium excretion[a]
   - After large doses of intravenous penicillin; urinary penicillin as an anion obligates sodium excretion[a]

[a] In these conditions urinary chloride excretion is a better index for volume depletion; FE_{Cl} is less than 1.

ARF, acute renal failure; ATN, acute tubular necrosis; FE_{Cl} fractional excretion of chloride; FE_{Na^+}, fractional excretion of sodium.

ally unremarkable in prerenal azotemia. On the contrary, numerous abnormalities of the urinalysis are seen with acute tubular necrosis. Because of the loss in renal concentrating ability the urine is isosthenuric. Glycosuria and proteinuria may be noted secondary to the alterations of phospholipid polarity and loss of the microvillus brush border. Again, significant proteinuria is not expected. Likewise, leukocyturia and hematuria are not typical features of acute tubular necrosis. Multiple dark brown granular casts, degenerating renal tubular cell casts, and exfoliated tubular cells are prominent microscopic features. A predominance of leukocytes, white blood cell casts, dysmorphic red blood cells, and/or red blood cell casts would be inconsistent with acute tubular necrosis and more representative of an intrarenal inflammatory process such as glomerulonephritis. With these findings further evaluation to determine an alternative cause for acute renal failure should strongly be considered.

The clinical problems that may occur during the developing oliguric phase of renal failure include volume overload, electrolyte and acid–base disorders (such as hyponatremia, hyperkalemia, hyperphosphatemia, hypocalcemia, and acidemia), as well as the signs and symptoms of uremia including diminished appetite with associated nausea and vomiting, generalized pruritus, alteration in mental status, pericarditis, bleeding diathesis from platelet dysfunction, and infection. In patients who have acute renal failure and a catabolic state (such as those with rhabdomyolysis, trauma, or burns or those who have undergone a major and complicated surgical procedure), the daily rise in BUN, serum creatinine, potassium, and uric acid and the decrease in serum bicarbonate are greater than in those without catabolism.

Acute renal failure is usually associated with abnormalities in the hemogram. A normocytic, normochromic anemia develops, with hematocrit values stabilizing between 20% and 30%. This anemia is due to diminished erythropoiesis and a variable degree of extracorpuscular hemolysis. Additional causes for anemia that complicate acute renal failure include hemodilution, gastrointestinal blood loss, and drug- or infection-induced marrow suppression. White blood cell counts are often elevated early in acute renal failure especially in those with rhabdomyolysis. However, persistence of leukocytosis beyond the first week of acute renal failure should suggest the possibility of infection. Thrombocytopenia resulting from diminished marrow platelet production is often observed early in acute renal failure. Associated qualitative disturbances in platelet function, combined with other poorly defined coagulation abnormalities, contribute to a tendency for enhanced bleeding in acute renal failure.

Neurologic, cardiovascular, gastrointestinal, and infectious clinical events often complicate the course of acute renal failure. Neurologic dysfunction consisting of lethargy, somnolence, confusion, agitation, asterixis, myoclonic muscle twitching, and seizures is common. These neurologic abnormalities are often observed in elderly patients, and patients generally respond well to dialysis treatment. The pathogenesis of these abnormalities has not been defined, although some investigators think they are related to high nerve tissue levels of calcium. Known causes of central nervous system (CNS) dysfunction in acute renal failure include CNS-depressant drug administration, electrolyte and arterial blood gas abnormalities, hypoglycemia, and primary neurologic disease.

The major cardiovascular complications of acute renal failure are circulatory congestion and hypertension. Salt and water overload with resultant edema and pulmonary congestion are ever-present dangers of acute renal failure, particularly the oliguric variety. This congestive state is nearly always due to excessive volume administration. Mild hypertension occurs in 15% to 25% of patients with acute tubular necrosis usually during the maintenance phase. This hypertension is also a manifestation of volume overload. Additional cardiovascular complications include supraventricular arrhythmias in 10% to 30% of patients and pericarditis. Pericarditis was formerly a major clinical problem in patients with acute renal failure. Now, perhaps because of early institution of dialytic therapy, it is rarely encountered. Because of the serious nature of the diseases predisposing to acute renal failure, myocardial infarction and pulmonary embolus occasionally complicate the course of the acute renal failure.

Gastrointestinal complications of acute renal failure are common. These complications include anorexia, nausea, vomiting, ileus, and poorly defined abdominal pains. These gastrointestinal symptoms usually respond readily to dialytic therapy. The combination of acute renal failure, stress of the underlying illness, and perhaps the poorly defined coagulopathy of acute renal failure can lead to significant gastrointestinal hemorrhage in 10% to 30% of patients. This hemorrhage is usually mild and responds to conservative therapy.

Infections are the most frequent complications of acute renal failure. Thirty percent to 70% of all patients with acute renal failure develop some clinically significant form of infection, and infections are the leading cause of mortality in patients with acute renal failure. The primary sites of infection include operative sites and the respiratory and urinary tracts. Both Gram-positive and Gram-negative organisms are encountered, and septicemia is common. The exact reason for the high frequency of infective complications remains to be determined. However, disruption of normal anatomic barriers, defective leukocyte function, impaired humoral and cellular immunity, and inappropriate use of antibiotics may all play a role.

MANAGEMENT AND CLINICAL COURSE

The goal of therapy for acute tubular necrosis is to prevent or ameliorate renal injury during the developing phase of acute renal failure and to treat established disease during the maintenance and recovery phases of the disease. Once ischemic acute tubular necrosis occurs, its treatment is similar to that of acute renal failure from other processes. The primary key steps of therapy are outlined in Table 48-15.

The use of mannitol or furosemide in the treatment of acute tubular necrosis has been controversial. Mannitol and furosemide have been shown to improve renal function in ischemic acute renal failure, if they are given before the injurious agent, but these maneuvers are usually no more beneficial than simple volume repletion. Clinical prevention of ischemic acute renal failure is difficult with these interventions, as prophylactic therapy often is not possible. Although there is no good evidence that the use of these diuretic agents can reverse acute tubular necrosis once it has developed, it is reasonable to attempt a trial of furosemide, 80 to 400 mg, or mannitol, 12.5 to 25 g, by intravenous infusion in the early phase of oliguric acute renal failure in an attempt to induce a diuresis. This enhanced urine flow may decrease the need for dialytic interventions by limiting hypervolemic and hyperkalemic complications. However, this maneuver has not been demonstrated to improve renal function, enhance renal recovery, or decrease the associated mortality risk. If no improvement in urinary flow rate occurs, the continued use of mannitol therapy is not advised given the potential side effects. Administration of large amounts of mannitol (more than 25 g) to patients with established acute renal failure who cannot excrete the mannitol may be associated with hazardous complications. The osmotic activity of mannitol (1 mOsm/180 mg) will attract water from the intracellular compartment and acutely increase blood volume, leading to pulmonary edema, and dilute the extracellular space, leading to hyponatremia in the face of hyperosmolality (hyponatremic hyperosmolar syndrome) and also dilution acidosis. The resultant intracellular dehydration increases the cellular concentration of potassium, favoring movement of potassium out of the cell and causing a rise in serum levels of potassium or worsening of an already existing hyperkalemia. Also the continued use of large amounts of furosemide may cause irreversible ototoxicity. On the other hand, in patients in whom the rise in serum creatinine and the oliguria is caused by prerenal azotemia, the use of furosemide may be hazardous. This drug will induce diuresis, worsening the volume status, a situation that would enhance the development of acute tubular necrosis. However, the use of mannitol in these patients may not be harmful because the reduction in intravascular volume secondary to the mannitol-induced diuresis would be counterbalanced by the movement of fluid from intracellular space to the vascular compartment secondary to the osmotic activity of mannitol.

Conservative therapy can control many of the complications of acute renal failure. The cornerstone of conservative therapy is careful, serial clinical and biochemical monitoring of the patient with acute renal failure to allow for early detection of potential complications (Table 48.15).

Fluid intake should equal measured output plus estimated insensible losses. Sodium and potassium administration should equal measured losses. In the well-managed patient with acute renal failure, a slight daily reduction in weight (because of mild catabolism) is often seen. Large daily weight loss (>1 kg) suggests marked catabolism or volume depletion, whereas weight gain suggests too much volume expansion.

Nutritional requirements for patients with acute renal failure should include adequate calorie intake (at least 35 kcal/kg body weight per day). The available data do not support the notion that survival of patients is improved with intravenous glucose and amino acids. Negative nitrogen balance is difficult to reverse in these patients with very large amounts of essential and nonessential amino acids. The nutritional therapy of acute renal failure is discussed in detail in Chapter 83, Part 1. Because parenteral hyperalimentation may be associated with significant mechanical, infectious, and metabolic complications, this form of therapy is best used in hospitals that have personnel experienced in hyperalimentation. Alternative methods of alimentation in patients with acute renal failure include use of gastrointestinal feeding tubes or peripheral venous alimentation with glucose and lipid solutions.

TABLE 48.15. Key Steps in the Management of Acute Tubular Necrosis

Avoid nephrotoxic antibiotics if possible, but acute tubular necrosis is not an absolute contraindication for their use.
Prevent and/or treat infectious complications (minimize indwelling catheters and vascular lines) promptly.
Provide adequate caloric intake (more than 35 kcal/kg/day).
Protein nitrogen, water, sodium, and potassium intake should match losses.
Monitor vital signs, body weight, and blood biochemistry and adjust therapy accordingly.
Institute dialytic therapy prophylactically or according to indications (Table 48.16).

Monitoring for clinical complications of acute renal failure requires serial physical examinations. The occurrence of congestive heart failure, hypertension, or edema in the patient with acute renal failure suggests volume overexpansion and should be accordingly treated. Prophylactic, non–magnesium-containing antacid therapy may help reduce "stress gastritis." In addition, selective histamine-2 receptor blockade (cimetidine or ranitidine) has been demonstrated to be of prophylactic benefit in reducing the incidence of gastrointestinal hemorrhage in some seriously ill patients with acute renal failure.

Avoidance and early detection of infection requires daily clinical and temperature-chart monitoring, minimization of interruption of normal anatomic barriers, encouragement of mouth and skin care, and early mobilization and use of aseptic techniques for intravenous line and tracheostomy care. Suspected infection should be promptly evaluated (examination, Gram stains, and cultures) and treated as specifically as possible. Careful serial neurologic evaluations with special attention to cognitive function are necessary. In patients with trauma or rhabdomyolysis, serial examinations of swollen limbs are required to detect peripheral nerve entrapment. Finally, because the metabolism and elimination of many drugs are impaired with acute renal failure, dose monitoring of drugs is needed. Chapter 85, Part 2 provides detailed information on drug regimens in patients with uremia.

In the absence of hyperglycemia or hyperlipidemia, the serum sodium concentration provides a guideline for free water administration. Hyponatremia indicates excess free water and hypernatremia denotes deficient free water. Hyperkalemia is an ever-present threat in acute renal failure. Mild elevations of serum potassium (less than 6.0 mEq/L) can best be treated by withdrawal of all sources of potassium and by continued close laboratory observation. If serum potassium increases to values of less than 6.5 mEq/L and particularly if any electrocardiogram changes appear, active therapy should be instituted (Table 48.16).

The mild metabolic acidosis associated with acute renal failure generally does not need to be treated unless serum bicarbonate falls to less than 10 mEq/L. Acute alkali administration may further decrease ionized calcium concentrations and thereby precipitate tetany. Hypocalcemia rarely requires specific therapy. Because a high calcium–phosphorus product (greater than 60) may cause soft tissue calcification, hyperphosphatemia should be controlled with gastrointestinal phosphate binders. The various forms of phosphate binders and their dosages are discussed in Chapter 77. The mild secondary hyperuricemia of acute renal failure is usually not treated with allopurinol because the low GFR limits the filtered load of uric acid and thus intratubular deposition. Also, clinical gout rarely complicates acute renal failure despite hyperuricemia because uremic serum holds more uric acid in solution than normal serum. Careful observation of the hematocrit and tests for blood in the stool are important in the early detection of gastrointestinal blood loss. Furthermore, if a decrease in hematocrit out of proportion to infection occurs, alternative causes of anemia such as hemolysis or retroperitoneal bleeding need to be evaluated.

Some patients with acute renal failure, particularly those who are nonoliguric and noncatabolic, can be successfully managed with minimal or no dialytic therapy. Indications for dialytic therapy are provided in Table 48.17. In addition, there has been an increasing tendency to use dialytic therapy early in acute renal failure in an attempt to minimize the development of complications. Early use of dialysis treatments may simplify management, allowing more liberal fluid and potassium intake and improvement in the general well-being of the patient. Thus many dialysis treatment centers attempt to keep predialysis

TABLE 48.16. Therapy of Hyperkalemia in Acute Renal Failure[a]

Modality	Dose	Onset of Effect	Duration of Effect
Calcium gluconate (10% solution)	IV, 10–30 ml given over 5 minutes	Immediate (<5 minutes)	Short (minutes)
Insulin and glucose	IV, 50% glucose solution and 5–10 units of regular insulin given over 3–5 minutes followed by 10% glucose and 20 units of regular insulin given at a rate of 50–100 ml/hr until hyperkalemia is controlled or dialysis is instituted	10 minutes	Medium (hours)
Sodium bicarbonate (44 mEq/vial)	44–132 mEq given IV over 5 minutes	10–15 minutes	Medium (hours)
Albuterol (β-receptor agonist)	10–20 mg nebulized aerosol over 15 minutes or 0.5 mg IV in 100 ml of 5% dextrose in water over 15 minutes	10–30 minutes	Short (minutes)
Sodium polystyrene sulfonate (Kayexalate)	30 g PO in 100 ml of 20% sorbitol or 60 mg in 200 of water given rectally as an enema	2 hours	Long
Dialysis	As required	30 minutes	Long (hours to days)

[a]After institution of short acting therapeutic modality, Kayexalate administration and/or dialysis should be initiated. Abrupt discontinuance of glucose and insulin therapy may be followed by a rebound hyperkalemia unless measures are undertaken to remove potassium from the body.
IV, intravenous; PO, by mouth.

TABLE 48.17 Indications for Dialytic Therapy of Acute Renal Failure

- Fluid overload (pulmonary edema)
- Hyperkalemia (serum potassium >6.5 mEq/L)
- Metabolic acidosis (pH <7.15)
- Symptomatic severe hyponatremia (serum sodium <120 mEq/L)
- Pericarditis
- Encephalopathy (confusion, myoclonic jerks, seizures, comatose)
- Symptomatic uremia
- Hypercatabolic state I[a]
- Toxin removal (ethylene glycol, salicylate, etc. intoxication)
- Severe uremic bleeding

[a] As assessed from clinical conditions, an increase in blood urea nitrogen more than 30 mg/dl/day or an increase in serum creatinine greater than 2.0 mg/dl/day; an example of this condition is acute renal failure secondary to rhabdomyolysis.

levels of BUN and serum creatinine below 80 and 8 mg/100 ml, respectively. This may require infrequent dialysis treatments in the noncatabolic, nonoliguric patient or daily dialysis treatments in the catabolic, traumatized patient. However, it is noteworthy that prospective controlled trials of prophylactic dialysis therapy have failed to consistently demonstrate a clear-cut benefit on mortality. Peritoneal dialysis therapy may be an acceptable alternative means of dialysis treatment even in the postoperative patient. It is most useful when the need for infrequent dialysis treatments is anticipated. Continuous hemofiltration could also be used. This technique is discussed in detail in Chapter 84, Part 3. It has been suggested that the use of biocompatible synthetic membranes in the dialysis therapy may enhance the recovery of renal function. However, it has not been possible to consistently demonstrate this effect.

During the maintenance phase of acute tubular necrosis, the patient most often is oliguric with a urine output of less than 500 ml/day. Nonoliguria characterized by a urine output of greater than 500 ml/day may occur in 30% to 40% of patients with acute tubular necrosis. The urine output, therefore, cannot and should not be used as an accurate reflection of GFR in developing acute tubular necrosis. It appears that nonoliguric acute tubular necrosis has a better prognosis than oliguric acute tubular necrosis, perhaps because nonoliguric infection is a reflection of a lesser degree of renal damage with less frequent progression to symptomatic infection requiring dialysis treatment.

A decrement in renal clearance and ultrafiltration function may persist for an average of 7 to 21 days, although durations of several months have been reported. At times, acute tubular necrosis may result in irreversible infection, particularly in the clinical setting of the critically ill patient where the cause of acute renal failure is often multifactorial. Because of the regenerative ability of surviving renal epithelial cells to repopulate the nephron, a return to baseline renal clearance and ultrafiltration function may occur. As renal function improves, urine output increases, and the serum creatinine levels decline. In oliguric patients, urine volume increases daily, and within a few days urine output greater than 2 L may be observed. A similar diuresis period is not observed in nonoliguric infection. Although most recovery of renal function occurs within 4 weeks of onset of improvement in the GFR, slight improvement continues to occur up to 12 months thereafter.

The prognosis for patients with acute tubular necrosis depends on the causative process. Acute tubular necrosis after a surgical procedure or traumatic injury has an overall mortality of 40% to 75%. The survival rate is much better among those patients who do not develop other medical complications, such as infection, bleeding, or respiratory failure. Patients with nephrotoxic acute tubular necrosis have an average mortality less than 10%. Because of the efficacy of dialytic interventions to correct a majority of the abnormalities associated with renal excretory failure, the dependence of patient survival on associated disease processes is not surprising.

CORTICAL NECROSIS

Acute cortical necrosis is a rare variety of acute renal failure in which diffuse necrosis of cortical structures is observed histologically. Complications of late pregnancy (abruptio placentae and septic abortion) account for the clinical setting of more than 50% of all reported cases. Cortical necrosis also occurs in the setting of sepsis, severe hypotension, and microangiopathic hemolytic anemias (e.g., hemolytic uremic syndrome). Most patients who develop cortical necrosis have undergone a severe renal ischemic insult and have biochemical evidence of intravascular coagulation. Although it was formerly thought that cortical necrosis uniformly resulted in complete, nonreversible loss of renal function, many instances of partial recovery with histologic evidence of patchy necrosis have now been observed. The diagnosis of cortical necrosis should be considered when anuria (without evidence of obstructive uropathy) occurs in the above-noted clinical settings. The diagnosis can be established by renal tissue examination or by finding diffuse cortical calcification on abdominal x-ray examination. Unfortunately, cortical calcification only occurs in 20% to 50% of patients and usually 6 weeks after the onset of illness. The finding of severely diminished interlobular and intralobar blood flow on selective renal angiography also supports a diagnosis of cortical necrosis. The therapy for this entity should be focused on controlling the inciting event. The associated renal failure should be managed as previously discussed. Additional discussion of anuria is found in Chapter 25.

Selected Readings

Abuelo JG. *Renal failure. Diagnosis and treatment.* Dordrecht, the Netherlands: Kluwer Academic Publishers, 1995.

An excellent and comprehensive volume devoted to diagnosis and management of all forms of acute renal failure.

Better OS, Stein JH. Early management of shock and prophylaxis of acute renal failure in traumatic rhabdomyolysis. *N Engl J Med* 1990:322:825–829.

A study of the effectiveness of volume replacement in the prevention of acute renal failure in crush injury.

Brosius F, Law K. Low fractional excretion of sodium in acute renal failure: role of timing of the test and ischemia. *Am J Nephrol* 1986;6:450–457.

An analysis of the factors that influence the diagnostic usefulness of urinary sodium excretion indices in acute renal failure.

Hakim RM, Lazarus JM. Hemodialysis in acute renal failure. In: Brenner BM, Lazarus BM, eds. *Acute renal failure.* Philadelphia: WB Saunders, 1993:643–688.

An excellent overview of dialysis therapy in acute renal failure.

Miller TR, Anderson RT, Linas SL, et al. Urinary diagnostic studies in acute renal failure—a prospective study. *Ann Intern Med* 1978;89:47–50.

One of the original studies of the usefulness of urinary solute excretion indices in acute renal failure.

Ronco C. Continuous renal replacement therapies for the treatment of acute renal failure in intensive care patients. *Clin Nephrol* 1993;40:187–189.

An excellent review of continuous renal replacement therapy, including hemofiltration, in acute renal failure.

Ronco C, Bellomo R, eds. *Critical care nephrology.* Dordrecht, the Netherlands: Kluwer Academic Publishers, 1998

A detailed treatise providing broad and extensive treatment of all aspects of acute renal failure, especially from the perspective of intensive care unit.

CHAPTER 49

Metabolic and Endocrine Abnormalities in Acute Renal Failure

Shaul G. Massry and Miroslaw Smogorzewski

Acute renal failure affects many metabolic and endocrine functions. It is associated with alterations in the blood levels of divalent ions, vitamin D metabolites, and hormones; derangements in carbohydrate and lipid metabolism; and dysfunction of the autonomic nervous system.

DIVALENT ION METABOLISM

Serum Levels of Phosphorus, Magnesium, and Calcium

Disturbances in divalent ion metabolism are common in patients with acute renal failure. *Hyperphosphatemia* and *hypermagnesemia* are almost always present during the oliguric phase of acute renal failure. These elevations in the serum concentrations of phosphorus and magnesium are due to retention of these ions secondary to the inability of the failing kidneys to excrete them. The magnitude of the hyperphosphatemia may vary from mild to marked (5.0 to 8.0 mg/dl), but profound hyperphosphatemia with values up to 18.0 mg/dl may be seen in patients with acute renal failure due to rhabdomyolysis. In these latter patients, the phosphorus generated by the damaged muscles enters the extracellular space and cannot be excreted by the kidneys, resulting in marked hyperphosphatemia. The hypermagnesemia is usually moderate, but levels as high as 5.0 mg/dl may be encountered, especially in patients ingesting medications containing magnesium. Because the binding of magnesium to serum proteins is not altered, the fraction of diffusible magnesium is not different from normal, but the absolute values of diffusible magnesium are increased. During the diuretic phase of acute renal failure, the serum levels of phosphorus and magnesium fall and may be normal or low in some patients, and the levels become normal in all patients after recovery of renal function.

Hypocalcemia is invariably noted during the oliguric phase of acute renal failure, and it occurs as early as 1 or 2 days after the onset of the renal failure. The lowest values of serum calcium may range between 5.0 and 7.5 mg/dl, and lower values may be noted in patients with acute renal failure due to rhabdomyolysis or acute pancreatitis. The fractions of total serum calcium identified as diffusible and ionized are the same as those observed in normal subjects, but the absolute values of these moieties are lower than normal. Hypocalcemia usually persists during the diuretic phase of the renal failure, but the values are usually higher than those observed during the oliguric phase of the disease. The concentrations of serum calcium return to normal after the recovery of renal function.

The major cause for the hypocalcemia of acute renal failure is the *skeletal resistance to the calcemic action of parathyroid hormone* (PTH). Other factors such as hyperphosphatemia, serum albumin levels, and parathyroid gland dysfunction may play a contributory role in certain patients. A relation between the concentrations of serum calcium and phosphorus during the oliguric and the diuretic phases of acute renal failure cannot be demonstrated. Hypocalcemia is observed with low, normal, or elevated serum phosphorus. Evidently the elevation in the concentration of serum phosphorus does not provide an adequate explanation for the hypocalcemia. However, the magnitude of the hyperphosphatemia may partially contribute to the degree of the hypocalcemia. For example, the marked hyperphosphatemia in patients with acute renal failure due to rhabdomyolysis enhances deposition of calcium from the extracellular space into the injured muscles, leading to more severe hypocalcemia. Indeed, calcification of the damaged muscles in these patients has been documented (Fig. 49.1). It should be noted that patients with rhabdomyolysis without acute renal failure may also display transient hypocalcemia because of deposition of calcium in injured tissues. Patients with acute pancreatitis are usually hypoalbuminemic and may have a transient state of hypoparathyroidism. These two events may contribute to the severity of the hypocalcemia in these patients when they develop acute renal failure.

Hypercalcemia may occur during both the oliguric and diuretic phases of acute renal failure. In the majority (86%) of a series of patients with elevated serum levels of calcium, the hypercalcemia occurred during the diuretic phase, whereas only a few patients (14%) had hypercalcemia during the oliguric phase of the disease. In about 75% of these hypercalcemic patients, the

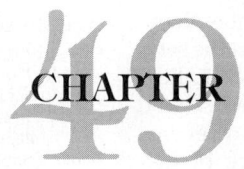

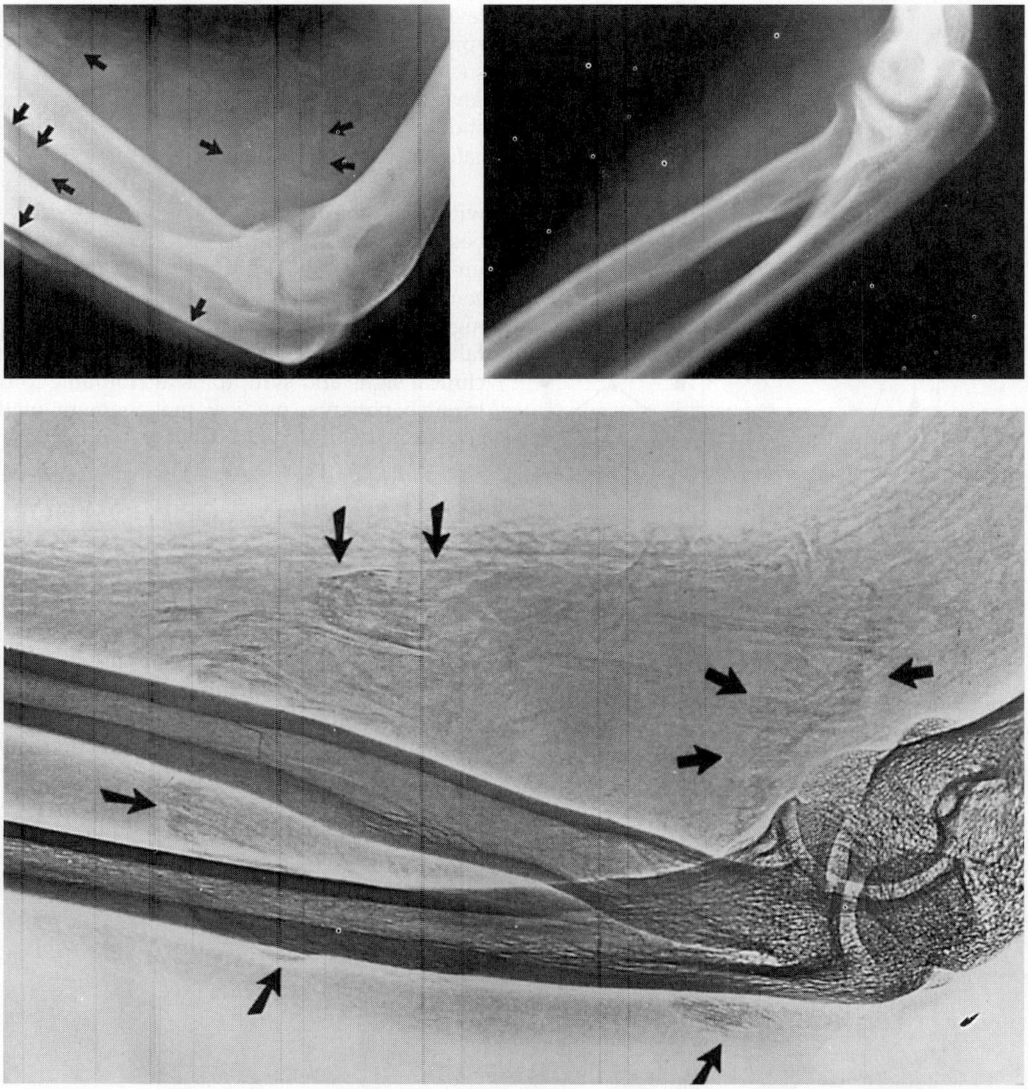

Figure 49.1. *Top left:* Calcium deposition in the soft tissues around the elbow, observed in a patient during the oliguric phase of acute renal failure resulting from rhabdomyolysis. *Top right:* Resolution of the calcifications after recovery of normal renal function. *Bottom:* An electron radiograph of the same area of the upper extremity depicted at *top left.*

acute renal failure was associated with rhabdomyolysis. In three series of patients with acute renal failure caused by rhabdomyolysis, the incidence of hypercalcemia varied between 20% and 59%. When combining all the patients from these three series, one finds that 18 of 53 patients developed hypercalcemia, giving an overall incidence of 35%. It is generally accepted that the mechanism of this hypercalcemia is the remobilization into the extracellular space of calcium previously deposited in the damaged muscles. Release of vitamin D from damaged muscles may also play a role. Indeed, elevated blood levels of 1,25-hydroxyvitamin D (1,25$(OH)_2$D) have been reported in hypercalcemic patients (Fig. 49.2). The mechanisms responsible for the elevations in the blood levels of 1,25$(OH)_2$D are not well defined. The production of 1,25$(OH)_2$D by the kidney in adults is tightly controlled; elevated levels of the metabolite occur either under conditions of stimulated production, such as hyperparathyroidism, hypophosphatemia, or hypocalcemia, or in clinical states associated with extrarenal production of 1,25$(OH)_2$D, such as sarcoidosis. Hypercalcemic patients with acute renal failure were found to have high blood 1,25$(OH)_2$D levels during the diuretic phase and at a time when their PTH levels were undetectable and when there was no hypophosphatemia. The source could be injured muscle cells and/or macrophages infiltrating the injured tissue. This possibility seems unlikely because the 1,25$(OH)_2$D levels do not increase in patients with rhabdomyolysis without acute renal failure. However, it should be mentioned that a biopsy of injured muscle with calcium deposit performed in one patient did show the presence of large multinucleated giant cells. It is equally unlikely that acute renal failure by itself is responsible because patients with acute renal failure without rhabdomyolysis do not have an increase in 1,25$(OH)_2$D levels. Thus rhabdomyolysis and acute renal failure seem to be needed. The vitamin D stored in muscles is released during muscle injury, providing more substrate for the production of 1,25$(OH)_2$D. The kidneys recovering from acute renal failure may not have regained their usual tight control of the production of 1,25$(OH)_2$D; thus this metabolite could be produced in greater quantities, and the higher the 1,25$(OH)_2$D levels, the greater the chance for the development of hypercalcemia.

Hypercalcemia developing during the oliguric phase of acute renal failure and at a time when the serum phosphorus

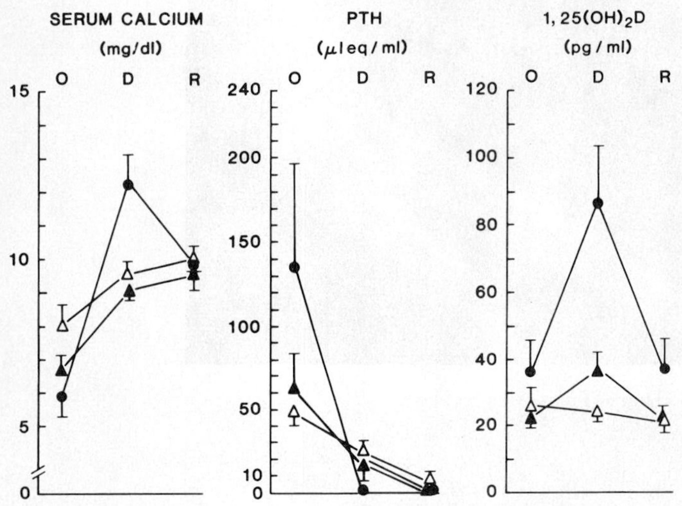

Figure 49.2. The serum levels of calcium, PTH, and 1,25$(OH)_2$D in patients with acute renal failure without rhabdomyolysis (*ARF, open triangles*) and in patients with acute renal failure and rhabdomyolysis who were normocalcemic [*RBD + ARF (NCa), solid triangles*] or hypercalcemic [*RBD + ARF (Ca), open circles*] during the diuretic phase of the disease. Data are presented as mean ± 1 SE. *O,* oliguric phase; *D,* diuretic phase; *R,* recovery phase. (Reproduced with permission from Akmal M, Bishop JE, Telfer N, et al. Hypocalcemia and hypercalcemia in patients with rhabdomyolysis with and without acute renal failure. *J Clin Endocrinol Metab* 1986;63:137–142.)

levels are also elevated could be very hazardous. Acute widespread calcium deposition in soft tissues, involving vital organs such as the lungs and heart (Fig. 49.3), may occur and can cause severe cardiopulmonary complications. Such hypercalcemia should be treated without delay with dialysis therapy using calcium-free dialysate.

The hypercalcemia of the diuretic phase usually appears within the third to the eleventh day of diuresis, but it has also been first noted as late as 35 to 55 days after the onset of the diuresis. Data from 24 such patients indicate that this hypercalcemia may last from 1 to 35 [13 ± 1.7 (SE)] days. It is usually benign because it occurs at a time when serum phosphorus is falling, but occasionally patients may have moderate-to-severe clinical signs and symptoms attributable to the hypercalcemia. In such patients, medical management of the hypercalcemia should be instituted (see Chapter 17, Part 3).

RENAL HANDLING OF PHOSPHORUS, MAGNESIUM, AND CALCIUM

During the diuretic phase of acute renal failure, there is increased fractional excretion of sodium, calcium, and magnesium. The slope for the correlation between the fraction of filtered calcium excreted and that of sodium is 0.95 (Fig. 49.4) and is similar to that seen during extracellular fluid volume expansion with saline and in patients with chronic renal failure. There is also a direct and significant correlation between the fraction of filtered magnesium excreted and that of sodium. The magnesiuria that occurs in the diuretic phase of acute renal failure leads to hypomagnesemia in many such patients. Phosphaturia is also present during the diuretic phase of acute renal failure

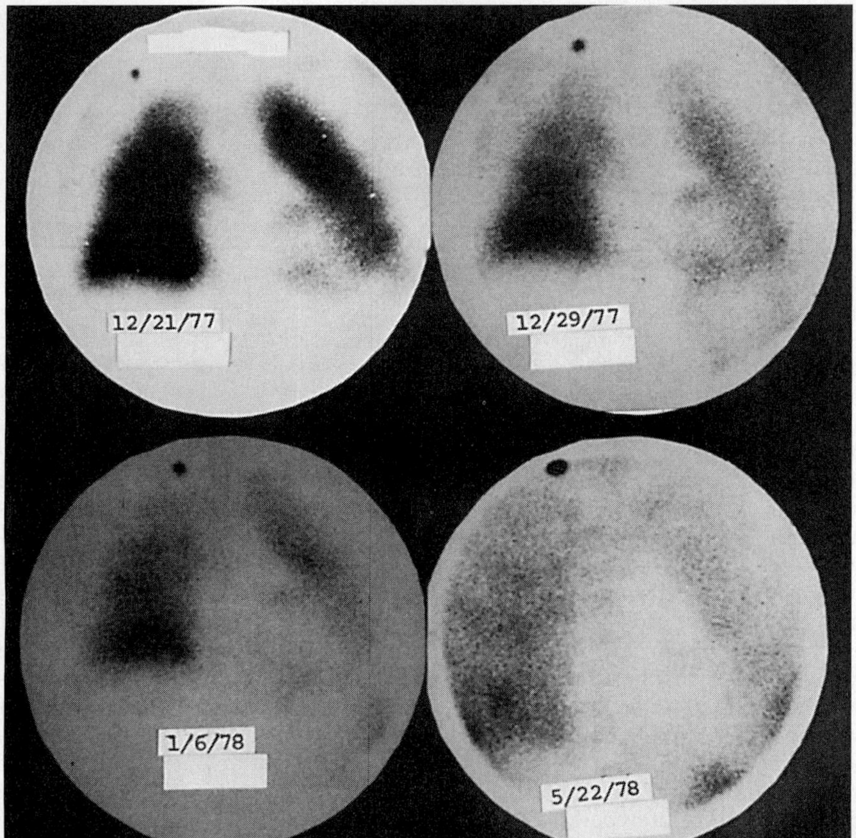

Figure 49.3. Technetium-99m diphosphate scan demonstrating marked uptake of the isotope by lungs and heart at a time of acute hypercalcemia occurring during the oliguric phase of acute renal failure caused by rhabdomyolysis (December 21, 1977). Note the improvement in subsequent scans. Uptake of the isotope by the lungs is still present 5 months later (May 22, 1978). (Reproduced with permission from Feinstein EL, Akmal M, Goldstein DA, et al. Hypercalcemia and acute widespread calcifications during the oliguric phase of acute renal failure due to rhabdomyolysis. *Miner Electrolyte Metab* 1979;2:193.)

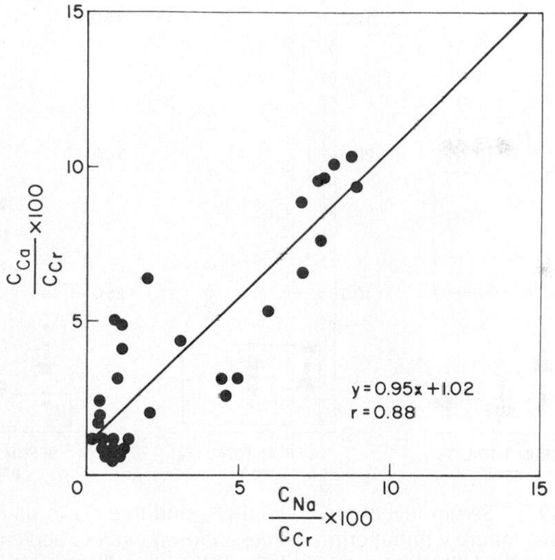

Figure 49.4. The relation between the fraction of filtered calcium excreted, ($C_{Ca/C}Cr$) × 100, and that of sodium, ($C_{Na/C}Cr$) × 100, during the diuretic phase of acute renal failure.

and is probably the cause of the hypophosphatemia that may be observed at this state of the disease.

VITAMIN D AND BONE METABOLISM

Limited data are available on the blood levels of vitamin D metabolites in patients with acute renal failure. Reduced blood levels of 25(OH)D have been observed during the oliguric and early diuretic phase of acute renal failure, most probably because of increased turnover rate. The half-life of 25(OH)D in patients with acute renal failure ranges between 1.9 and 9.2 days with a mean of 5.6 days, compared with 18 to 25 days in normal subjects. Normal or elevated blood levels of 25(OH)D have been reported during the oliguric and diuretic phases of acute renal failure resulting from rhabdomyolysis. Elevated blood levels of $1,25(OH)_2D$ were found during the diuretic phase of acute renal failure with rhabdomyolysis. The blood levels of this metabolite are usually low in the oliguric phase of acute renal failure. Evidence for a mild increase in bone resorption without an increase in osteoid was observed in bone biopsies obtained from patients with acute renal failure. In one patient with hypercalcemia during the diuretic phase of acute renal failure caused by rhabdomyolysis, a bone biopsy revealed low turnover state, no tetracycline labeling, and absent osteoclast; these findings are characteristic of adynamic bone lesion.

DISTURBANCES IN THE FUNCTION OF THE ENDOCRINE SYSTEM

Not surprisingly, acute renal failure is associated with a wide range of abnormalities in the function of the endocrine system and in the blood levels of many hormones. The reasons for this are many and include the following: (a) the kidney is an endocrine organ producing many hormones; (b) several hormones are excreted and/or metabolized by the kidney; (c) alterations in electrolyte homeostasis, such as hypocalcemia, hyperphosphatemia, and/or hyperkalemia, may affect the function of many endocrine glands; and (d) renal failure may affect the metabolism of hormones by other organs.

Parathyroid Hormone

Experimental data indicate that hyperactivity of the parathyroid glands occurs within hours after the onset of acute renal failure. In humans with acute renal failure, the blood levels of PTH are elevated during both the oliguric and diuretic phases of the disease. This change in parathyroid gland function is induced by the hypocalcemia, and indeed, an inverse and significant correlation exists between the blood levels of PTH and the concentrations of serum calcium. Also, infusion of calcium to patients with acute renal failure was associated with a fall in blood levels of PTH. Thus the parathyroid glands in patients with acute renal failure respond appropriately to the changes in serum concentrations of calcium. Decreased metabolic clearance of PTH by the failing kidneys may contribute to the magnitude of the elevation in the blood levels of the hormone. In patients with acute renal failure who develop hypercalcemia, the blood levels of PTH are elevated, normal, or low. These observations argue against an important role for PTH in the genesis of this hypercalcemia. In patients with acute pancreatitis and acute renal failure, the blood levels of PTH may be low or normal in two-thirds of the patients despite the hypocalcemia; these observations suggest that patients with acute pancreatitis may have transient failure of the parathyroid gland activity. The mRNA of the PTH-PTHrP receptor in renal tissues obtained by renal biopsies from patients with acute renal failure is reduced significantly.

Calcitonin

The serum levels of calcitonin are elevated during both the oliguric and diuretic phases of acute renal failure, but the values are usually higher during the oliguric phase of the illness. The mechanism(s) for the hypercalcitoninemia is not evident. Both increased production and decreased metabolic clearance by the failing kidneys may be operative. It is also not known whether the elevated serum levels of calcitonin represent biologically active hormone or immunologically reactive but biologically inert fragments of calcitonin. Calcium infusion in these patients produces absolute increments in calcitonin that are not different from those in normal subjects receiving similar calcium infusions.

Thyroid Hormones

Alterations in serum indices of thyroid hormones are common in patients with acute renal failure. In a detailed study performed in our laboratory the serum concentrations of total thyroxine (TT_4) and the values for the free thyroxine (T_4) index are reduced in most patients, while triiodothyronine uptake ratios (T_3UR) are normal (Fig. 49.5). The serum levels of free T_4 measured by enzyme immunoassay are normal. Others found low levels of free T_4 in 13 patients. During the oliguric phase of acute renal failure, the serum levels of TT_4 display a significant and inverse correlation with those of creatinine (Fig. 49.6). The serum levels of total triiodothyronine (TT_3) and free triiodothyronine (T_3) are markedly reduced, those of total reverse T_3 (rT_3) are normal, and those of free rT_3 are elevated (Fig. 49.7). The findings of reduced serum levels of TT_4 with normal values of free T_4 and T_3UR and normal serum levels of total rT_3 but elevated free rT_3 indicate a decrease in the binding of T_4 and T_3 to their serum carrier proteins. The low serum concentrations of TT_3 are probably due to a decreased conversion of T_4 to T_3. With the onset of diuresis, the serum levels of TT_4 and TT_3 begin to rise, and they return to normal values after the recovery of renal function.

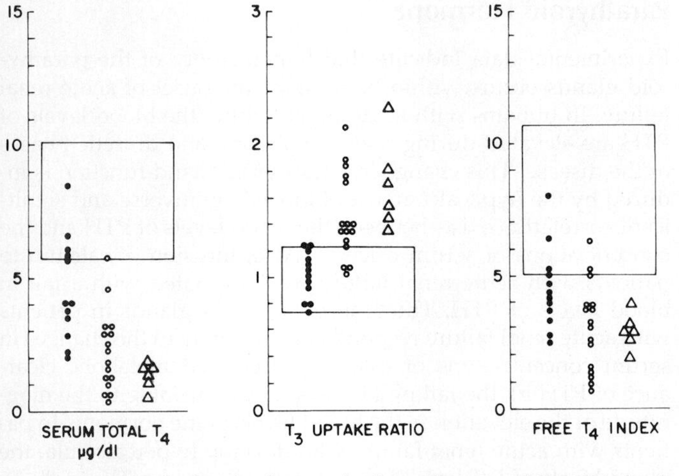

Figure 49.5. Serum levels of TT_4 and values of T_3UR and free T_4 index in patients with acute renal failure (*solid circles*), acute renal failure with critical illness (*open circles*), and critical illness without renal failure (*open triangles*). *Open rectangles* represent the normal range of values. (Reproduced with permission from Kaptein EM, Levitan D, Feinstein EL, et al. Alterations of thyroid hormone indices in acute renal failure and in acute illness with and without acute renal failure. *Am J Nephrol* 1981;1:138–143.)

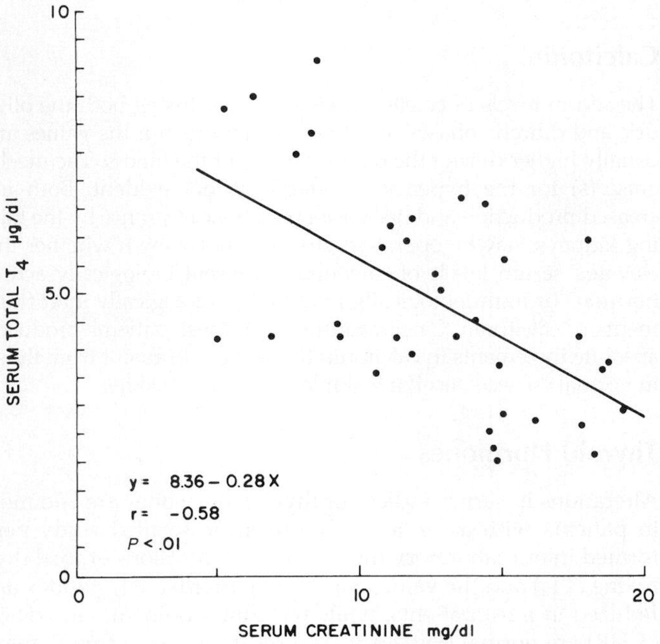

Figure 49.6. The relation between the serum concentrations of TT_4 and creatinine during the oliguric phase of acute renal failure in patients with critical illness. (Reproduced with permission from Kaptein EM, Levitan D, Feinstein EL, et al. Alterations of thyroid hormone indices in acute renal failure and in acute illness with and without acute renal failure. *Am J Nephrol* 1981;1:128–143.)

The baseline serum levels of thyroid-stimulating hormone (TSH) are within the normal range in patients with acute renal failure. The TSH response to thyroid-releasing hormone (TRH) stimulation is blunted during the oliguric phase of the illness but returns to normal after restoration of renal function (Fig. 49.8). These observations suggest mild pituitary inhibition during acute renal failure.

The changes in the serum indices of thyroid hormones in patients with acute renal failure are qualitatively similar to those

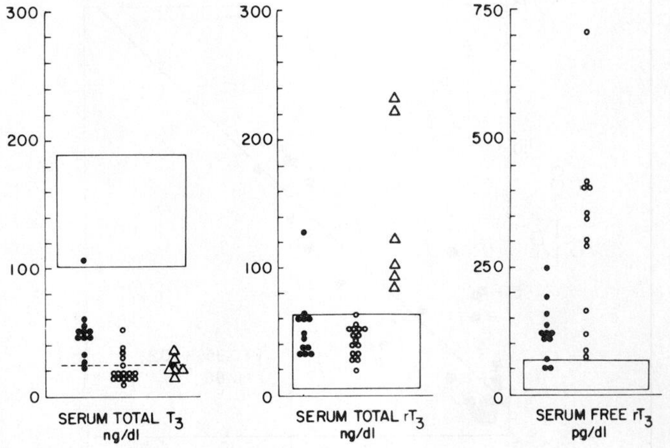

Figure 49.7. Serum levels of TT_3, total rT_3, and free rT_3 in patients with acute renal failure without critical illness (*closed circles*), acute renal failure with critical illness (*open circles*), and critical illness without renal failure (*open triangles*). *Open rectangles* represent the normal range of values. The *dashed line* represents the limit of the assay. (Reproduced with permission from Kaptein EM, Levitan D, Feinstein EL, et al. Alterations of thyroid hormone indices in acute renal failure and in acute illness with and without renal failure. *Am J Nephrol* 1981;1:138–143.)

observed in patients with acute nonthyroidal illnesses with or without renal failure, with one exception (Figs. 49.5 and 49.7). In the presence of acute renal failure, the serum concentrations of total rT_3 are normal, whereas in critically ill patients without renal failure the levels of total rT_3 are elevated.

Despite the low serum levels of TT_4 and TT_3 and sometimes of the free concentrations of these hormones, patients with acute renal failure appear to be euthyroid, which is evidenced by the normal serum levels of TSH and the blunted TSH response to TRH stimulation. This does not necessarily mean that the low T_4 and T_3 state has no clinical significance in patients with acute renal failure. It is possible that the decreased serum TT_3 levels provide a protective mechanism in the battle against the hypercatabolic state that is present during acute renal failure. Such a function has been assigned for the low serum TT_3 levels in patients with other nonthyroidal illnesses and during fasting. At present, it does not appear that the abnormalities in thyroid hormone indices in acute renal failure require therapy. Certain data, however, showed that T_4 may enhance the recovery from an acute toxic renal insult in rats. Clinical experience is needed before one can suggest the use of T_4 in humans with acute renal failure.

Growth Hormone, Glucagon, and Insulin

The basal serum levels of growth hormone are elevated in patients with acute renal failure, and the increase in growth hormone following the administration of insulin is exaggerated in these patients. The latter phenomenon occurs despite a slower decrease in plasma glucose. The abnormal growth hormone response is improved by hemodialysis therapy despite the persistence of a diminished hypoglycemic effect of insulin. Increased secretion of growth hormone and to a lesser degree decreased biodegradation are responsible for the elevated serum levels of the hormone; the latter may play a role in the carbohydrate intolerance seen with acute renal failure. The mRNA of growth hormone receptor is reduced during the initial phases of acute renal failure.

Both the serum concentrations of glucagon and the response to a test meal are normal in patients with acute renal failure. This

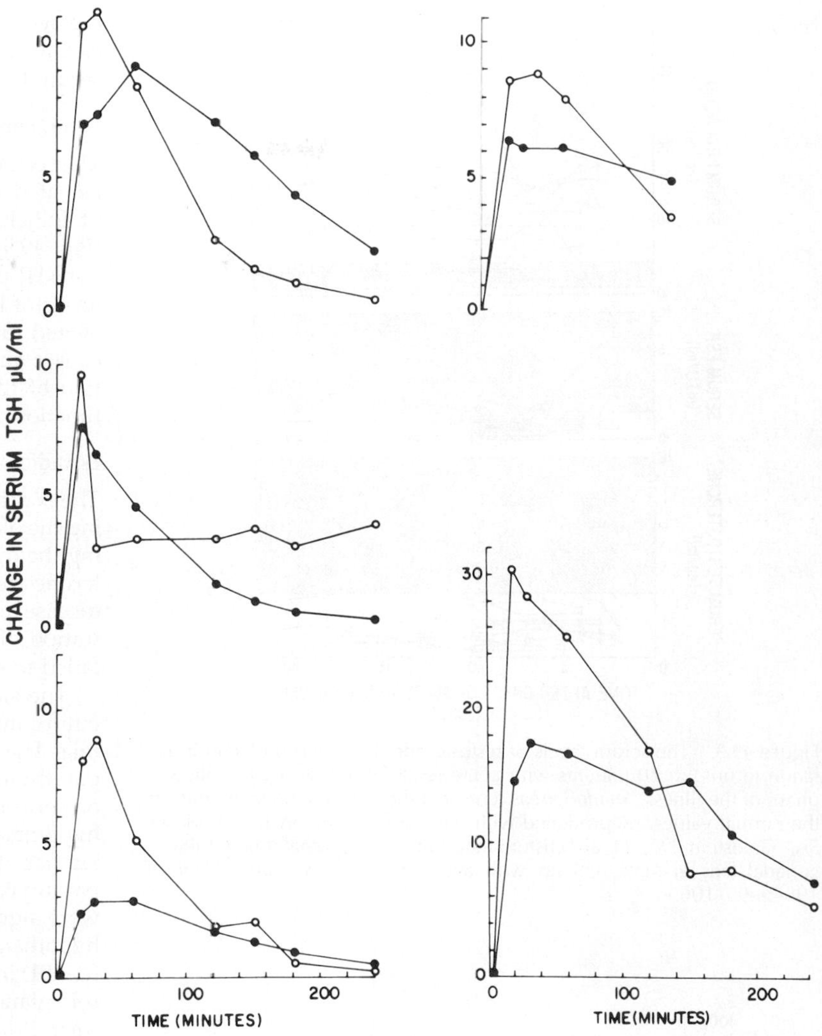

Figure 49.8. Changes in the serum concentrations of TSH in response to intravenous thyroid-releasing hormone during the oliguric phase of acute renal failure without critical illness (*solid circles*) and after recovery of normal renal function (*open circles*). (Reproduced with permission from Kaptein EM, Levitan D, Feinstein EL, et al. Alterations of thyroid hormone indices in acute renal failure and in acute illness with and without acute renal failure. *Am J Nephrol* 1981;1:138–143.)

is in contrast to reports of elevated serum levels of glucagon in experimental acute renal failure produced by ureteral ligation.

Basal serum levels of insulin are usually normal in patients with acute renal failure, but elevated levels have been reported as well. There is an exaggerated insulin response to intravenous glucose injection. Patients with acute renal failure have glucose intolerance, and hemodialysis treatment partially corrects this abnormality. Although the peak plasma glucose levels after the injection of glucose in normal subjects and in patients with acute renal failure may be similar, the fall in plasma glucose is delayed in the latter group. Thus glucose utilization is reduced in the patients with acute renal failure despite higher serum levels of insulin. It is evident, therefore, that acute renal failure is associated with resistance to the action of insulin. This resistance is responsible for the elevated plasma levels of glucose frequently observed in patients with acute renal failure. To identify the site of this insulin resistance, studies were performed to examine the effect of insulin on net glucose uptake by isolated perfused rat livers and by muscles, using a hind limb preparation. Skeletal muscles of acutely uremic animals showed a decreased insulin-mediated uptake of glucose, whereas the liver sensitivity to insulin was not affected. These studies also showed that glucose production by the liver was augmented in acutely uremic animals. Thus the glucose intolerance in renal failure is most likely due to resistance to insulin action on skeletal muscle, increased hepatic production of glucose, and elevated blood levels of growth hormone. The resistance to insulin action is most likely due to a postreceptor defect.

Because the kidneys play an important role in the metabolic clearance of insulin (see Chapters 7, Part 5, and 13, Part 12), the requirement for insulin may be markedly reduced during acute renal failure in patients with diabetes mellitus. Failure to make adjustment for this phenomenon may result in severe hypoglycemia in such patients.

Hormones of the Pituitary-Gonadal Axis

Prolactin

The serum levels of prolactin are elevated in patients with acute renal failure (Fig. 49.9), and they are much higher in patients who are critically ill than in those with uncomplicated acute renal failure. Although a relation between the serum levels of prolactin and PTH was not found in one study, others noted a direct and significant correlation between the serum levels of these hormones, suggesting that the elevated serum concentration of PTH may be partially responsible for hyperprolactinemia. Indeed, the infusion of PTH in normal subjects was associated with an increase in the serum levels of prolactin. In addition, there is a direct and significant correlation between the blood levels of prolactin and those of PTH in patients with acute renal failure (Fig. 49.10). Chlorpromazine administration to patients with acute renal failure was associated with an exaggerated increase in serum levels of prolactin, and

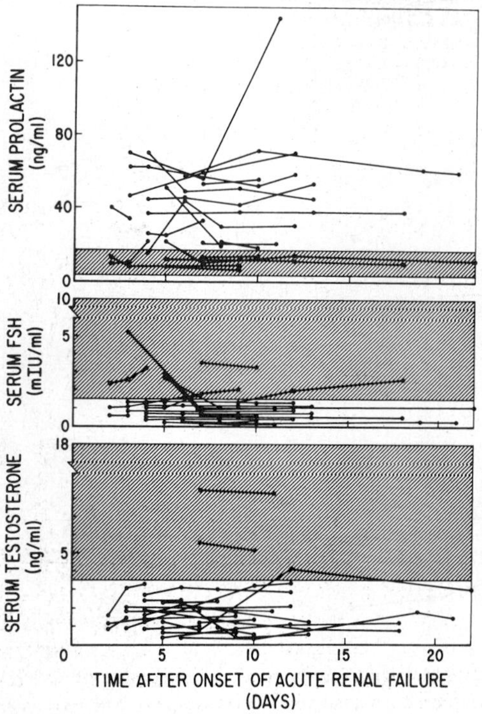

Figure 49.9. The serum levels of testosterone, FSH, and prolactin in relation to time in 20 patients with acute renal failure during the oliguric phase of the illness. *Shaded areas* represent the 95% confidence limits of the normal values. (Reproduced with permission from Levitan D, Moser SA, Goldstein DA, et al. Disturbances in the hypothalamic-pituitary-gonadal axis in male patients with acute renal failure. *Am J Nephrol* 1984;4:99–106.)

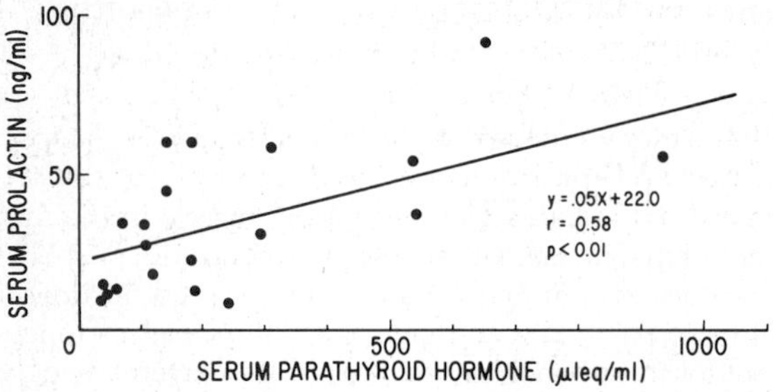

Figure 49.10. The relation between the serum levels of prolactin and parathyroid hormone in 20 patients with acute renal failure. (Reproduced with permission from Levitan D, Maser SA, Goldstein DA, et al. Disturbances in the hypothalamic-pituitary-gonadal axis in male patients with acute renal failure. *Am J Nephrol* 1984;4:99–106.)

bromocriptine produced a significant decrease in the serum concentrations of the hormone. The increment in the serum levels of prolactin during TRH stimulation in patients with acute renal failure is not exaggerated, but the levels of the hormone remain elevated for a longer period of time than in normal subjects. The response to TRH stimulation becomes normal after recovery of renal function. In a study of 26 male patients with acute renal failure, there were positive correlations between the serum levels of estradiol and prolactin and a negative correlation between the serum levels of testosterone and prolactin. Such relationships were not found in 20 patients studied by others. The hyperprolactinemia of acute renal failure is due to increased production of the hormone, but decreased metabolic clearance by the kidney may also contribute to the elevated serum levels of the hormone.

Luteinizing Hormone and Follicle-Stimulating Hormone

The serum levels of luteinizing hormone (LH) may be normal or elevated in male patients with acute renal failure, and those of follicle-stimulating hormone (FSH) are markedly reduced (Fig. 49.9). Stimulation with gonadotropin-releasing hormone (GnRH) produces normal or exaggerated increments in serum levels of LH, and the concentration of the hormone remains elevated for prolonged periods of time. Stimulation with GnRH causes a normal or blunted FSH response. The GnRH stimulation of LH and FSH becomes normal after recovery of renal function.

Estradiol and Testosterone

The serum levels of estradiol may be moderately elevated during the oliguric phase of acute renal failure and are normal during the diuretic phase of the illness. The serum levels of testosterone are markedly decreased during the oliguric phase of the disease and rise with the onset of diuresis (Fig. 49.9). Administration of human chorionic gonadotropin to oliguric patients failed to stimulate testosterone secretion.

The state of secondary hyperparathyroidism of acute renal failure may participate in the genesis of the hypotestosteronemia. The effects of 3 days of acute uremia in dogs with intact parathyroid glands and in thyroparathyroidectomized animals on serum testosterone levels and on the calcium content of the hypothalamus, pituitary gland, and the testes were examined. Similar studies were performed in normal dogs treated with parathyroid extract for 3 days. The serum levels of testosterone were significantly ($P < .01$) reduced, and the calcium levels of hypothalamus, pituitary gland, and testes were significantly ($P < .01$) increased in the acutely uremic dogs with intact parathyroid glands and in the normal dogs treated with parathyroid extract. Prior parathyroidectomy in the acutely uremic dogs prevented these abnormalities. The results of our study assign an important role for the excess blood levels of PTH in uremia in the genesis of the hypotestosteronemia. The data suggest that the effect of excess PTH on serum testosterone levels may be mediated through the accumulation of calcium in the organs that participate in synthesis and/or release of testosterone.

Renin-Angiotensin-Aldosterone System

An enlargement of the juxtaglomerular apparatus and an increase in the number of renin-containing granules were noted in patients with acute renal failure as early as 1945. Elevated plasma levels of renin activity (PRA), angiotensin immunoreactivity, and aldosterone are not infrequently noted in patients with acute renal failure and in animals with experimental acute renal failure. The rise in PRA occurs early in the course of acute renal failure, and the values may return to normal during the diuretic phase of the disease. Serial PRA determinations were made in children with acute renal failure caused by either acute poststreptococcal glomerulonephritis or the hemolytic uremic syndrome. Low PRA was found in the children with acute nephritis, all of whom were hypertensive and had evidence of fluid overload. In contrast, the hypertensive children with hemolytic uremic syndrome had elevated PRA that correlated with the extent of renal arteriolar occlusion seen on renal biopsy; such occlusions presumably reduce afferent arteriolar pressure and stimulate renin release. Other investigators also found elevated PRA in patients with noninflammatory acute renal failure and normal values in those with inflammatory acute renal failure.

Other Hormones

The plasma levels of antidiuretic hormone are frequently elevated during both the oliguric and diuretic phases of acute renal failure. Morphine administration to patients produced an early peak (30 minutes) in the levels of the hormone compared with normal subjects (60 to 90 minutes). The alterations in the plasma levels of antidiuretic hormone are not related to changes in plasma osmolality. The plasma levels of gastrin and of pancreatic polypeptides are also elevated and those of cortisol are normal.

In rats with acute renal failure resulting from renal ischemia, the blood levels of thromboxane B_2 (TXB_2) are increased and those of 6-keto-prostaglandin (PG) F1α are reduced. Others found that the urinary excretions of PGE_2, 6-keto-PGF1x, and TXB_2 are significantly increased in rats with glycerol-induced acute renal failure.

The injection of contrast media into animals is followed by an increase in the blood levels of endothelin. It is not, as yet, known whether this phenomenon participates in the genesis of contrast media–induced acute renal failure. Conclusive data on the effect of acute renal failure on blood levels of endothelin in humans are not yet available. In one preliminary report on seven patients with acute renal failure, plasma concentrations of immunoreactive endothelin were markedly elevated and decreased after recovery.

HYPERLIPIDEMIA

The serum levels of triglyceride are frequently elevated in patients with acute renal failure, whereas the serum levels of cholesterol are normal. In rats with acute renal failure, the serum levels of both triglyceride and cholesterol may be elevated; this hyperlipidemia could be prevented or ameliorated by prior parathyroidectomy and could be reproduced by the injection of PTH into parathyroidectomized acutely uremic rats. It appears that the major cause of the hyperlipidemia in acute renal failure is impaired triglyceride removal, which may be due to inhibition of lipoprotein lipase.

AUTONOMIC NERVOUS SYSTEM

Patients with acute renal failure may display dysfunctions of the autonomic nervous system similar to those seen in patients with chronic renal failure. These derangements include an abnormal Valsalva ratio, abnormal response to hand grip exercise, abnormal fall in blood pressure during orthostasis, and reduced pressor response to norepinephrine. The plasma levels of norepinephrine and epinephrine are elevated in these patients.

Selected Readings

Akmal M, Bishop JE, Telfer N, et al. Hypocalcemia and hypercalcemia in patients with rhabdomyolysis with and without acute renal failure. *J Clin Endocrinol Metab* 1986;63:137–142.

A detailed study of divalent ion metabolism, blood levels of PTH, and blood levels of 25(OH)D and 1,25(OH)$_2$D in patients with rhabdomyolysis with and without acute renal failure and in acute renal failure without rhabdomyolysis.

Akmal M, Goldstein DA, Telfer N, et al. Resolution of muscle calcification in rhabdomyolysis and acute renal failure. *Ann Intern Med* 1978;89:928–930.

The first demonstration of calcium deposition in injured tissues during the oliguric phase of acute renal failure associated with rhabdomyolysis and its resolution during the diuretic phase of the illness.

Akmal M, Goldstein DA, Kletzby OA, et al. Hyperparathyroidism and hypoaldosteronemia of acute renal failure. *Am J Nephrol* 1988;8:166–169.

Study demonstrating that the low blood levels of testosterone in dogs with acute renal failure are mediated by the state of secondary hyperparathyroidism and exploring the mechanisms through which excess PTH exerts this effect.

Chen J, Zhang J, Lin S. Down-regulation of PTH-PTHrP receptor in the kidney of patient with renal impairment. *Chinese Med J* 1998;111:24–27.

Study of renal tissues obtained by renal biopsy with relative quantitative reverse transcription/polymerase chain reaction (RT/PCR) technology showing that the mRNA of the PTH-PTHrP is downregulated in patients with acute renal failure.

Druml W. Metabolic alterations in acute renal failure. *Contrib Nephrol* 1992;98:59–66.

A good review of the subject.

Hroneck I, Hronkova B, Davenport A, et al. Thyroid hormone levels in acute renal failure. *Renal Failure* 1993;15:47–49.

A study of thyroid hormone indices in 27 patients with acute renal failure showing reduced blood levels of total T_4 and T_3 as well as free T_4 and T_3.

Kaptein EM, Levitan D, Feinstein EI, et al. Alterations of thyroid hormone indices in acute renal failure and in acute illness with and without acute renal failure. *Am J Nephrol* 1981;1:138–143.

Detailed study of thyroid hormone indices in patients with acute renal failure with and without other critical illnesses comparing the results with those from patients with critical illnesses but without acute renal failure.

Koffler A, Friedler RM, Massry SG. Acute renal failure due to nontraumatic rhabdomyolysis. *Ann Intern Med* 1978;85:23–28.

A study of a large population with acute renal failure associated with rhabdomyolysis, with emphasis on the biochemical derangements, including those in the blood levels of calcium and phosphorus.

Kokot F. The endocrine system in patients with acute renal failure. *Proc Eur Dial Transplant Assoc* 1981;18:617–629.

A short review of the disturbances in blood levels of a variety of hormones in patients with acute renal failure.

Levitan D, Moser SA, Goldstein DA, et al. Disturbances in the hypothalamic-pituitary-gonadal axis in male patients with acute renal failure. *Am J Nephrol* 1984;4:99–106.

A detailed study of the disturbances in PTH, prolactin, testosterone, LH, and FSH and in the response to GnRH and TRH in 20 patients with acute renal failure.

Llach F, Felsenfeld AJ, Haussler MR. The pathophysiology of altered calcium metabolism in rhabdomyolysis-induced acute renal failure. Interactions of parathyroid hormone, 25-hydroxycholecalciferol and 1,25-dihydroxycholecalciferol. *N Engl J Med* 1981;305:117–123.

The first demonstration that blood levels of 1,25(OH)$_2$D are elevated in the diuretic phase of acute renal failure associated with rhabdomyolysis.

Margulies KB, Hildbrand FL, Heublein DM, et al. Radiocontrast increases plasma and urinary endothelin. *J Am Soc Nephrol* 1991;2:1041–1045.

A study in dogs demonstrating that the administration of contrast media induces a rise in plasma levels and urinary excretion of endothelin.

Massry SG, Arieff AI, Coburn JW, et al. Divalent ion metabolism in patients with acute renal failure. Studies on mechanism of hypocalcemia. *Kidney Int* 1974;5:437–445.

A detailed study of the derangements in divalent ion metabolism and in blood levels of PTH in patients with acute renal failure.

Tomita K, Ujiie K, Nakanishi T, et al. Plasma endothelin in patients with acute renal failure. *N Engl J Med* 1989;321:1127.

The first report that plasma endothelin levels are elevated in acute renal failure.

CHAPTER 50

Obstructive Nephropathy

Saulo Klahr

Obstructive uropathy, obstructive nephropathy, and hydronephrosis are terms frequently used to describe the consequences of urinary tract obstruction. However, each term has a different connotation. *Obstructive uropathy* is used to describe the structural changes in the urinary tract that impair outflow of urine. Thus in the strictest sense, such changes may or may not be associated with renal parenchymal damage. Proximal to the site of obstruction, dilation occurs. The term *hydronephrosis* is used to describe this dilation. It should be stressed that a widened ureter and calyceal system do not necessarily indicate the presence of obstruction. Vesicoureteric reflux, primary megaureter, ureteral dilation associated with acute pyelonephritis, and residual ureteral dilation following surgical correction of obstruction are examples of nonobstructing causes of ureteral dilation (Table 50.1). Nevertheless, in each of these cases, renal parenchymal damage may occur. *Obstructive nephropathy* refers to the renal disease that results from impaired flow of urine. Such impedance to flow causes initially abnormal back pressure, which has a direct effect on renal parenchyma and also leads to a series of physiologic responses that contribute significantly to the pathogenesis of obstructive nephropathy.

The usual clinical features of obstructive nephropathy may be either an abrupt or a gradual and insidious decline in renal function. Such a decline may be halted and even reversed if the obstruction is relieved. Thus obstructive nephropathy, if detected promptly, is potentially curable.

INCIDENCE

Obstructive uropathy has a bimodal distribution. It is common in childhood due to congenital anomalies of the urinary tract. Obstructive uropathy is the most common cause of an abdominal mass in the neonatal period. The incidence of clinical hydronephrosis in children is highest in the first 6 years of life. It declines with age and continues to decline after age 15. In adults the incidence of obstructive uropathy at autopsy was found to be between 3.5% and 3.8%. These studies and a number of clinical observations indicate that in middle age, obstructive uropathy reaches a nadir. At age 60, the incidence begins to rise again, and males are predominantly affected because of the increase in the occurrence of prostatic hyperplasia and prostatic cancer.

TABLE 50.1. Causes of Urinary Tract Dilation

High flow states
Diabetes insipidus
Diuresis
Congenital
Congenital megacalycosis
Primary megaureter
Congenital extrarenal calyces
Extrarenal pelvis
Prune belly
Pregnancy
Postureteral anastomosis
Inflammatory (acute and/or chronic)
Postobstructive residual dilation
Vesicoureteral reflux
Bladder distension
Drugs

CLASSIFICATION

Obstructive uropathy is classified according to (a) the *degree,* (b) the *duration,* and (c) the *site* of the obstruction. The extent or degree of the obstruction is said to be *high grade* when it is complete, or *low grade* when it is partial or incomplete. When the obstruction is of *short duration* it is said to be *acute;* it is usually a reversible condition such as passage of a calculus, blood clot, or sloughed papilla. Obstruction that develops slowly and is long lasting is said to be *chronic,* as in congenital ureteropelvic or ureterovesical abnormalities and retroperitoneal fibrosis. *Upper tract* obstruction is that located above the ureterovesical junction; this type of obstruction is usually *unilateral* in nature. *Lower tract* obstruction refers to lesions located below the ureterovesical junction and by definition is *bilateral* in nature.

CAUSES OF OBSTRUCTIVE UROPATHY

The causes of obstructive uropathy can be classified as *intrinsic* or *extrinsic* (Table 50.2). The intrinsic causes in turn can be subdivided into *intraluminal,* those located in the lumen of the urinary tract, and *intramural,* those lesions that originate in the wall of the urinary tract. The *extrinsic* causes of obstructive uropathy are best divided into groups based on the organ system or anatomic location from which the obstructive lesion originates.

Intrinsic Causes of Obstructive Uropathy

Intraluminal Causes

Causes of obstructive uropathy include lesions originating in the renal parenchyma (intrarenal) or in the urinary tract (extrarenal). Probably the most common cause of intrarenal obstruction is deposition of uric acid crystals in the tubular lumen (uric acid nephropathy). This condition is seen most commonly in lymphoproliferative and myeloproliferative malignancies and bears a direct relationship to plasma uric acid levels. It is usually a complication of treating these patients with chemotherapy or ra-

TABLE 50.2. Causes of Urinary Tract Obstruction

- Intrinsic causes of urinary tract obstruction
  - Intraluminal
    - Intrarenal
      - Uric acid
      - Sulfonamides
      - Multiple myeloma?
    - Extrarenal
      - Calculi
      - Papillary tissue
      - Blood clots
      - Fungus balls
  - Intramural
    - Functional
      - Ureteral
        - Ureteropelvic dysfunction
        - Ureterovesical dysfunction
      - Bladder (neurogenic)
        - Congenital
          - Myelodysplasia
          - Spinal cord defects
        - Acquired
          - Tabes dorsalis
          - Diabetes mellitus
          - Multiple sclerosis
          - Spinal cord trauma
          - Parkinson's disease
          - Cerebrovascular disease
      - Bladder-neck dysfunction
    - Anatomic
      - Tumors
      - Infection-granuloma
      - Strictures
      - Posterior and anterior urethral valves
      - Ureteroceles
      - Urethral stones
      - Phimosis
      - Meatal stenosis
      - Periurethral abscess
- Extrinsic causes of urinary tract obstruction
  - Reproductive system
    - Males
      - Benign prostatic hyperplasia
      - Adenocarcinoma of the prostate
    - Females
      - Uterine
        - Pregnancy
        - Tumor
          - Fibroadenoma
          - Carcinoma of the cervix
        - Uterine prolapse
        - Endometriosis
      - Ovarian
        - Abscess
        - Tumor
        - Cysts
  - Gastrointestinal system
    - Crohn's disease
    - Diverticulitis
    - Pancreatitis
    - Appendiceal abscess
    - Malignancy
  - Vascular system
    - Aberrant vessels at the ureteropelvic junction
    - Aneurysmal dilation
      - Aorta
      - Iliac vessels
    - Venous
      - Ovarian (thrombophlebitis)
      - Vena cava (retrocaval ureter)
  - Retroperitoneal
    - Inflammatory
      - Idiopathic fibrosis
      - Secondary
    - Iatrogenic (surgical complications)
    - Tumor
      - Primary (lymphomas, sarcoma)
      - Secondary (e.g., cervix, bladder, colon)
    - Infection
    - Pelvic lipomatosis
    - Hemorrhage

diotherapy. The rapid lysis of malignant cells causes release of large amounts of nucleic acids, which are metabolized to uric acid. Uric acid nephropathy is discussed in detail in Chapter 44.

Intrarenal obstruction was common in patients taking long-acting sulfa drugs. This is now a rare event. Nevertheless, the presence of sulfonamide crystals in the urine of patients is an indication for increasing the degree of hydration and/or substituting antibiotics. Acyclovir administration may also cause acute intrarenal obstruction.

Deposition of Bence Jones protein in the renal tubule may play a role in causing renal insufficiency in multiple myeloma because histologic studies of end-stage renal disease in patients with multiple myeloma show laminated protein deposits in the distal tubule. Immunofluorescence techniques have shown these deposits to contain albumin, IgG, and light chains. The incidence of renal failure in multiple myeloma is higher in patients with Bence Jones proteinuria. The severity of the renal disease correlates strongly with the quantity of Bence Jones protein excreted. Evidence against this theory, however, is the observation that most patients with multiple myeloma and early renal failure have striking alterations in renal tubular morphology but no histologic evidence of protein deposition. Thus renal insufficiency in these patients may be related to toxic rather than obstructive effects of Bence Jones protein.

Renal calculi are the most common cause of ureteral obstruction in the young adult male. Calculi are three times more common in males than in females. The peak incidence of the disease occurs in the second and third decades of life. Calcium oxalate stones are the most common; these stones cause intermittent acute urinary tract obstruction and are seldom associated with any measurable decline in renal function. The less common causes of urinary lithiasis such as infection and the development of "struvite" stones, gouty nephropathy, and cystinuria are more likely to cause renal damage. Renal calculi most commonly lodge at the following locations: (a) the calyx; (b) the ureteropelvic junction, if they are larger than 1 cm in diameter; (c) near the pelvic brim, where the ureter begins to arch over the iliac vessels posteriorly into the true pelvis; (d) near the posterior pelvis, where the ureter is crossed anteriorly by the pelvic blood vessels and the broad ligament; and (e) the ureterovesical junction. Stones smaller than 0.4 to 0.5 cm in diameter seldom lodge in any of these places; they usually pass spontaneously. Although the passage of a stone must be observed carefully, it is an infrequent cause of concern to the nephrologist because the contralateral kidney is usually functioning normally and renal failure does not develop. One exception, however, is a ureteral stone in a patient with a solitary kidney. Such patients may have anuria and acute renal failure.

A less common cause of intraluminal obstruction is papillary tissue caused by papillary necrosis. Papillary necrosis occurs in sickle cell trait or disease, analgesic abuse, renal amyloidosis, and acute pyelonephritis, particularly when associated with diabetes mellitus. This latter association has the highest mortality and morbidity. Further discussion of papillary necrosis is found in Chapter 51. Such patients may have oligoanuria, fever, and septic shock. Blood clots can also cause urinary tract obstruction. An important example is the occurrence of hematuria in patients with polycystic disease of the kidney. Here, an abrupt decline in glomerular filtration rate (GFR) accompanied by a recent history of hematuria is attributable to obstruction until proven otherwise.

Intramural Causes

Intramural causes of urinary tract obstruction fall into two categories: (a) functional and (b) anatomic. The functional causes relate to dynamic abnormalities of the urinary tract. In the ureter, they usually result from inability of a peristaltic wave to be transmitted through a segment. This defect may be due to a disproportionate decrease or absence of either circular or longitudinal smooth muscle. Functional obstruction of the ureter occurs most often at the pelvic or vesical junctions. In childhood, the most common cause of urinary tract obstruction is a functional defect at the ureteropelvic junction, which is usually bilateral before the age of 1 year but unilateral thereafter. The left kidney is most commonly affected. Although the peak incidence of this lesion is seen at age 5, at least 20% of the reported cases are in adults older than 30 years. At the point of narrowing, the ureter has a preponderance of longitudinal smooth muscle fibers and a decrease or absence of circular muscle fibers. Obstruction at the ureteropelvic junction may be associated with abnormal angulation of the ureter or the presence of aberrant renal vessels. In fact, because of this close association, it is not clear whether the functional defect is a primary or secondary phenomenon.

The second most common cause of ureteral obstruction in childhood is a functional defect at the ureterovesical junction. This is a disease primarily of male children (male : female ratio, 4 : 1 to 3 : 1) and is predominantly unilateral, with the left kidney being more frequently affected. In children younger than 1 year of age, both ureters may be involved. It is an uncommon cause of obstructive uropathy in adults. As in children, it is predominantly a disease of males, although the ratio of the preponderance in adults is somewhat less (1.6 : 1). The cause of this disease is unclear. A marked predominance in circular smooth muscle with relative absence of longitudinal fibers was reported earlier; however, later studies indicated a paucity of muscular fibers, and electron microscopic studies reveal increased numbers of collagen fibers. As with ureteropelvic dysfunction, a clear histologic diagnosis is not possible because of inflammatory changes caused by dilation of the obstructed ureter. Early reports suggested that this disease was analogous to Hirschsprung's disease of the colon. However, all histologic studies indicate preservation of the nerve ganglion, and the relative prevalence of this disease in patients with Hirschsprung's megacolon is questionable. Functional defects within the calyceal system and in the midureter occur but are rare.

The urinary bladder is another site where functional obstruction can occur. Neurogenic vesical dysfunction (neurogenic bladder) can be due to upper neuron damage causing involuntary micturition (spastic bladder dysfunction) or lower spinal tract injury resulting in flaccid atonic bladder. In both settings a significant urine residual may develop, resulting in ureterovesical reflux, ureteral dilation, and a significant increase in back pressure on renal parenchymal tissue. Myelodysplasia (spina bifida cystica) is the most common cause of neurogenic bladder in childhood. If such patients survive the first year of life, renal failure is the most common cause of death. Other congenital defects of the spinal cord are less commonly associated with neurogenic bladder dysfunction in childhood. In adults, acquired bladder dysfunction is a significant cause of obstructive nephropathy. It is estimated that 90% of patients with multiple sclerosis develop bladder dysfunction. Ten percent of the population in the United States has diabetes mellitus. A significant number of these patients develop a neurogenic bladder, which compounds the adverse effects of diabetic glomerulosclerosis on renal function. Traumatic spinal cord injury, especially in postwar years, is a common cause of obstructive uropathy in young adult males. Finally, in older individuals a definite relationship exists between the incidence of cerebral vascular disease or advanced Parkinson's disease and urinary bladder dysfunction. Alterations in bladder-neck dysfunction have a peak incidence in the fourth through sixth decades of life. Anatomic lesions of the urinary tract causing obstruction are less common. Strictures of the ureter may occur after retroperitoneal surgery, although this is rare (less than 1%), or be a complication of radiation therapy in patients with cervical carcinoma (0.3% to 1.6% of treated patients). Rarely, strictures occur in association with analgesic nephropathy and/or as a consequence of the *treatment* of granulomatous disease (tuberculosis and tertiary syphilis) involving the ureter. Posterior and anterior urethral valves are an uncommon cause of lower urinary tract obstruction in childhood. Ureteroceles may also give cause obstruction. They are seen frequently in association with a reduplication of the urinary tract. Urethral strictures secondary to chronic instrumentation, surgery, or gonococcal infections are an infrequent cause of obstructive uropathy.

Malignant and benign tumors of the pelvis, ureter, and bladder can result in urinary tract obstruction. Transitional cell papillomas of the renal pelvis are by far the most common malignant lesions in this area (85%). Rarely, a metastatic lesion may cause obstruction, and sarcomas of the ureter are considered a curiosity. Benign tumors of the ureter occur in a ratio of approximately one to three carcinomatous lesions.

Extrinsic Causes of Obstructive Uropathy

The extrinsic causes of urinary tract obstruction are best classified based on the system from which the obstructive lesion originates. A pathologic change of the reproductive system is by far the most common cause of extrinsic urinary tract obstruction.

Reproductive System

In women, the most common cause of obstruction is pregnancy. The right side is more commonly affected. Renographic studies done just before delivery revealed abnormalities on the right side in nearly 70% of patients and on the left in 50% of patients. It has been suggested that ureteral stasis rather than obstruction occurs during pregnancy, and progesterone has been implicated. Large doses of progesterone can decrease ureteral peristalsis. However, blood levels of this hormone may not be high enough during pregnancy to affect the urinary tract. Furthermore, the predominance of a unilateral lesion speaks against a systemic response to elevated progesterone levels.

Pelvic malignancies, particularly carcinoma of the cervix, are the second most common cause of extrinsic urinary tract obstruction in females. Carcinoma of the cervix spreads by direct extension to contiguous tissues. The ureter may be obstructed because of its close anatomic relationship to the cervix. Metastasis from distant tumors to the pelvis, most frequently resulting from carcinoma of the breast, can cause ureteral obstruction. Hydronephrosis, urinary tract infections, and renal failure remain a common cause of death in these patients. The combination of obstructive uropathy caused by pregnancy and pelvic malignant disease accounts for the greater incidence of obstructive uropathy in young adult females than in males. Other less common disorders of the female reproductive tract that can cause urinary obstruction are listed in Table 50.2.

In males, the most common cause of extrinsic obstruction is benign hypertrophy of the prostate. About 80% of men older than 60 years have benign prostatic hyperplasia and some evidence of bladder dysfunction. Ten percent of these patients require surgery. In one large series, 24% of the patients had complete urinary retention as the initial complaint. Carcinoma of the prostate is another important cause of urinary tract obstruction. It is the combination of benign prostatic hyperplasia and adenocarcinoma of the prostate that accounts for the greater occurrence of obstructive uropathy in males older than age 60.

Gastrointestinal System

Patients with granulomatous (Crohn's) disease of the bowel may develop obstructive lesions as a result of retroperitoneal extension of the inflammatory process. The incidence of obstruction correlates with the severity of the granulomatous disease. Patients with ileocolitis are most likely to develop obstructive uropathy. It affects the right ureter exclusively and has been reported to occur in 7% to 27% of patients with this disease. Thus part of the follow-up care of patients with granulomatous disease of the bowel is a yearly intravenous pyelogram. Inflammatory disease of the appendix and large bowel diverticulitis may cause retroperitoneal scarring and extrinsic obstruction. Although both lesions are uncommon, appendicitis is more common in children and diverticulitis in patients older than 50. Similarly, chronic pancreatitis, especially when pseudocysts develop, can cause left-sided ureteral obstruction.

Vascular System

Abdominal aortic aneurysms can cause obstructive uropathy. As many as 10% of patients with aortic aneurysms may develop urologic complications. Aneurysms of external or common iliac arteries are rare causes of ureteral obstruction. Aberrant vessels may cause obstruction at the ureteropelvic junction. In one series the incidence was approximately 30%. It is not clear whether these abnormalities are merely associated with *functional* obstruction at the site or whether these vessels physically impede flow of urine at this point.

The "retrocaval" ureter is another congenital cause of urinary tract obstruction. In this instance, the right ureter passes behind the vena cava, and varying degrees of ureteral obstruction can result. Diagnosis of this disease is seldom made until the fourth decade of life. It is predominantly a disease of men (3:1), and the initial complaint is intermittent abdominal pain, which often resembles renal colic. Frequently these patients have chronic urinary tract infections. In females, dilation of the ovarian venous system, which courses close to the right ureter, is an uncommon cause of obstruction but may contribute significantly to the obstruction of pregnancy. This is particularly true in patients who have had postpartum pelvic thrombophlebitis, which resulted in incompetent valves and venous dilation of this system.

Disease of the Retroperitoneum

Diseases of the retroperitoneal space can cause obstructive uropathy. Tumor invasion from the cervix, prostate, bladder, colon, ovary, and uterus accounts for 70% of the extrinsic causes of obstruction in the retroperitoneum. Less commonly, retroperitoneal fibrosis may result in ureteral obstruction. A number of cases of unknown cause, so-called idiopathic retroperitoneal fibrosis, have been described. The entity occurs with equal frequency in both sexes with an age range from 7 to 85 years but predominantly in the fifth or sixth decades of life. The fibrosis involves the ureter in its middle third, pulling it toward the midline. Such fibrosis can also involve the aorta, vena cava, and psoas muscles and may extend from the renal pedicle to below the psoas major. The cause of this disease is unclear. A role for long-term administration of methysergide (Sansert) in the development of this disease has been suggested. Retroperitoneal fibrosis has been reported in 1% of patients taking this drug. Another ergot derivative, lysergic acid diethylamide, has also been causally implicated.

Retroperitoneal fibrosis may occur in other disease processes. Inflammatory processes of the lower extremities with ascending lymphangitis, multiple abdominal procedures, Henoch-Schönlein purpura, hemorrhage, gonorrhea, biliary tract disease, chronic urinary tract infection, tuberculosis, and sarcoidosis have all been associated with retroperitoneal fibrosis on rare occasions. In these cases the fibrosis is most commonly found at the level of the sacral promontory and within Gerota's fascia.

PATHOPHYSIOLOGIC RESPONSE TO URETERAL OBSTRUCTION

Ureteral Response to Ureteral Obstruction

The pathophysiologic events that occur after the ureter is obstructed begin with alterations in the physiologic activity of the ureter and renal pelvis. Under normal conditions, urine flows from kidney to bladder because of (a) ureteral peristalsis, (b) hydrostatic pressure (the effects of gravity), and (c) the pressure of glomerular filtration. Ureteral and pelvic peristalsis play an important role in the transport of urine down the ureter. Peristalsis generates high intraluminal pressures necessary for the propulsion of a bolus of urine without allowing transmission of these pressures to the renal parenchyma. Ureteral peristalsis consists of two dynamic forces: longitudinal and circular. The relation between these forces is illustrated in Fig. 50.1. The initial motion of the ureter in transmitting urine flow is an upward movement. Thereafter the circular fibers of the ureteral wall contract proximally and cause the formation of a bolus of urine. After these muscle fibers completely occlude the lumen, a process known as coaptation, the longitudinal forces contract and the bolus is propelled along the ureter. Thus an essential feature of normal peristalsis is bolus formation, which is only achieved by occlusion of the lumen. Baseline pressures in the ureter are

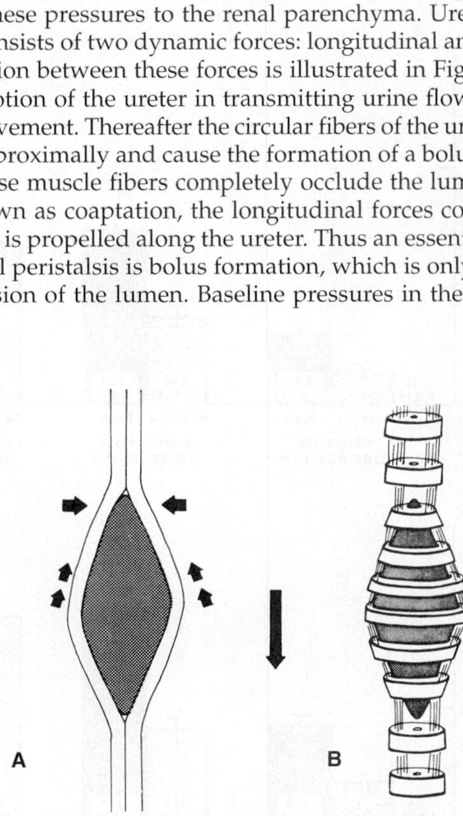

Figure 50.1. Normal ureteric peristalsis. Diagrammatic representation of the resolution of forces into **(B)** circular and **(A)** longitudinal components. (Reproduced with permission from Whittaker RH. Some observations and theories on the wide urethral hydronephrosis. *Br J Urol* 1975;47:337.)

similar to those in the renal pelvis but rise during coaptation to values between 10 and 25 mm Hg. Because of coaptation, these peak pressures are not transmitted to the renal pelvis. Thus renal pelvic pressures seldom rise above 4 mm Hg. Normal ureteral function and its neurogenic control are discussed in detail in Chapter 10. The effects of acute ureteral occlusion on the dynamics of the ureter are depicted in Fig. 50.2. Ureteral function was studied in dogs after acute occlusion. Mean ureteral pressures are shown in the lower graph of the figure. Baseline pressures averaged 7.4 mm Hg and rose during coaptation to approximately 17 mm Hg. These changes in pressure were accompanied by increases in ureteral wall tension. Three minutes after obstruction, baseline and peak measurements for both ureteral pressure and wall tension were increased nearly twofold. Five to 20 minutes after obstruction, the baseline wall tension increased and approached peak values. Thus peak ureteral wall tension and pressure changed less dramatically. One hour after obstruction, mean wall tension values at baseline and peak were threefold greater than under normal conditions but are not significantly different from each other. Similarly, baseline ureteral pressure was threefold greater than measurements obtained in control subjects but did not change during contraction. At this point, coaptation did not occur and pressures generated by ureteral wall tension were transmitted directly to the renal pelvis and parenchyma. Any further increase in pressure would result in ureteral dilation.

The effects of an increased ureteral diameter, a major consequence of obstruction, on intraluminal pressure and wall tensions are shown in Fig. 50.3. Baseline wall tensions are high and not significantly different from peak measurements. On the other hand, baseline and peak values for ureteral pressure are not significantly different from control values. This is the result of the relation between pressure and tension as expressed in Laplace's law: $P = K\ (T/R)$, where P is the transluminal pressure; K is a constant; T is the wall tension; and R is the radius of the ureter. Thus normal pressures are maintained at the expense of increasing radius. Based on these results it has been postulated that the major damage to renal tissue, which is the direct consequence of increased pressure, occurs soon after an interval narrowing of the ureteral lumen. The clinical observations that support this conclusion are as follows: (a) the highest measured ureteral pressures occur during acute obstruction as seen during the passage of stones when pressures may be as high as 40 to 50 mm Hg; (b) in patients with complete obstruction there is an inverse correlation between intrapelvic pressures and time; and (c) patients with obstructive uropathy resulting from congenital anomalies, which tend to be static, may have reasonable renal function in the fourth and fifth decades of life. Thus renal damage in the obstructed kidney will be potentiated by those conditions that acutely increase ureteral pressure, such as alterations in urine output (e.g., when fluid intake is increased or after the administration of diuretics) and/or augmentation of the degree of obstruction.

Ureteral Obstruction in Renal Transplantation

Urologic events after renal transplantation include leakage and/or obstruction of the ureter. An incidence of ureteral obstruction of 2% to 10% has been reported in renal transplant recipients. The causes of ureteral obstruction in this setting include ureteral kinking, extrinsic compression of the ureter (hematoma, abscess, lymphocele, or tumor), ureteral ischemia, previously

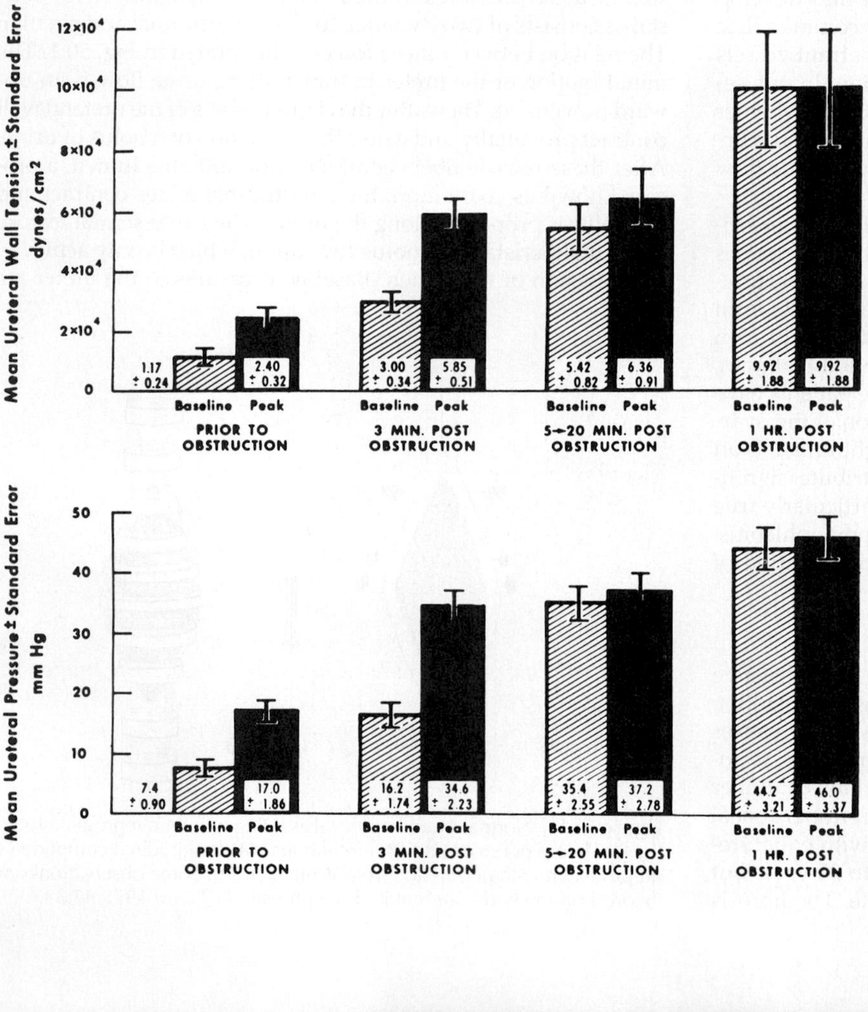

Figure 50.2. Relation of ureteral pressure and wall tension after acute obstruction. *Top:* Mean baseline and peak ureteral wall tensions at various time periods following acute ureteral obstructions in dogs. *Bottom:* Mean baseline and peak intraluminal ureteral pressures at various time periods following acute ureteral obstruction. (Reproduced with permission from Rose GR, Gillenwater JY. Pathophysiology of ureteral obstruction. *Am J Physiol* 1973;225:830.)

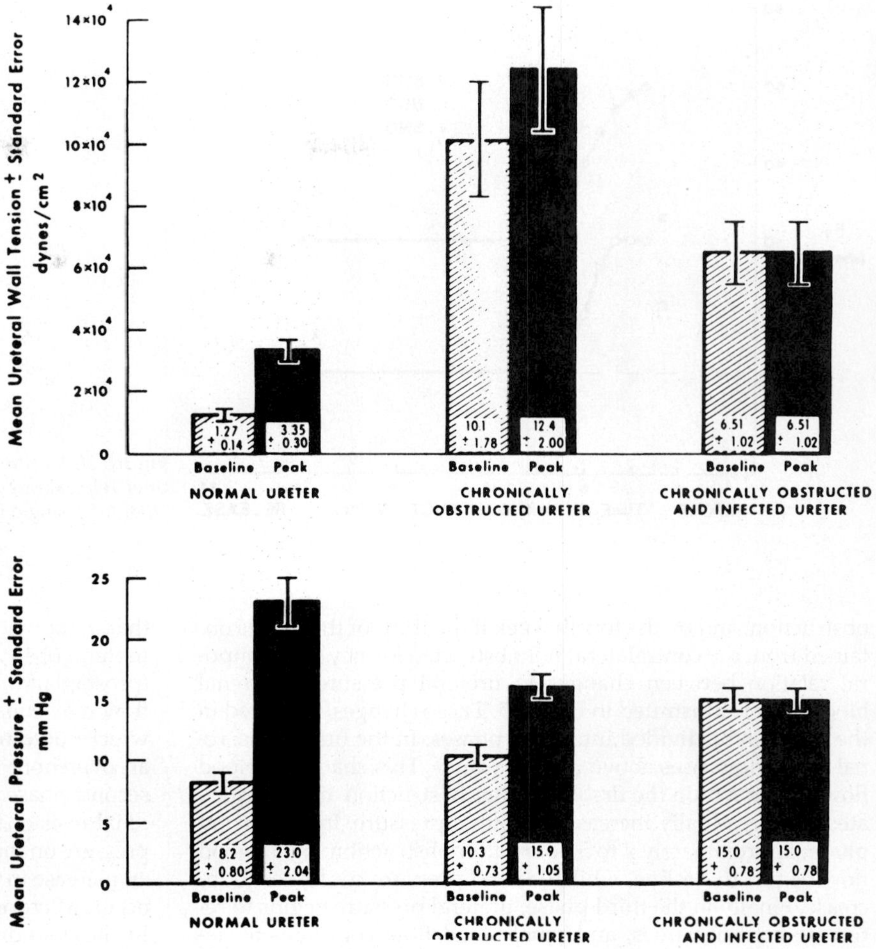

Figure 50.3. Relation of ureteral pressure and wall tension after chronic obstructions. *Top:* Mean baseline and peak ureteral wall tensions found in normal ureters, chronically obstructed ureters, and infected, obstructed ureters. *Bottom:* Mean baseline and peak intraluminal ureteral pressures obtained in the above studies. (Reproduced with permission from Rose GR, Gillenwater JY. Pathophysiology of ureteral obstruction. *Am J Physiol* 1973;225:830.)

unrecognized ureteropelvic junction obstruction, and luminal obstruction of the ureter (calculi, tumor, edema, or clots). Ureteral obstruction in the setting of renal transplantation occurs within 3 months of the surgical procedure. The urologic implications in the renal transplant recipient are discussed in detail in Chapter 89, Part 2.

Renal Response to Ureteral Obstruction

The effects of complete ureteral occlusion on ureteral and intratubular pressure, GFR, and renal blood flow are depicted in Table 50.3. The effects are related to the duration and degree of obstruction. In the rat, the immediate changes in intratubular pressure after ureteral occlusion depend on urine flow. Under hydropenic conditions pressures do not change, but when urine flow is increased, using solute diuresis or saline expansion of the intravascular space, the intratubular pressure may exceed 60 mm Hg and approximate the pressures of glomerular filtration. These initial high pressures gradually diminish over the ensuing 24 hours. Beyond 24 hours, whether intratubular pressures remain elevated is dependent on two factors: (a) alterations in the volume status of the individual and thus flow through the tubule, and (b) whether the obstruction is bilateral or unilateral (Fig. 50.4). The effects of unilateral ureteral occlusion on tubular pressure are always less profound than those of bilateral obstruction. After 24 hours of ureteral occlusion, intratubular pressures in the former group are not different from normal. On the other hand, with bilateral ureteral obstruction, intratubular pressures remain high (Fig. 50.4). It is assumed that as pressure falls within the ureter, intratubular pressures will decline accordingly.

TABLE 50.3. Renal Response to Complete Ureteral Obstruction

	P_{URET}	P_{PROX}	GFR	RBF
Bilateral				
Acute	↑↑	↑ 300%	↓	?
Chronic	↑	↑ 100%	↓	↓ 30%
Unilateral				
Acute	↑↑	NL or ↑	↓	↑ 50%
Chronic	↑	↓ 30%	↓	↓ 40%

GFR, glomerular filtration rate; NL, normal range; P_{PROX}, pressure in proximal tubule; P_{URET}, ureteral pressure; RBF, renal blood flow.

Changes in renal hemodynamics during acute or chronic ureteral obstruction contribute significantly to the pathogenesis of obstructive nephropathy. Renal blood flow falls as a function of time after ureteral occlusion. This relationship is not well appreciated clinically because the exact time of onset of ureteral obstruction in humans is seldom known. However, in experimental studies the relation between duration of obstruction and renal blood flow is clear. In most experimental models, renal blood flow falls to 50% of control values within 3 to 4 days of

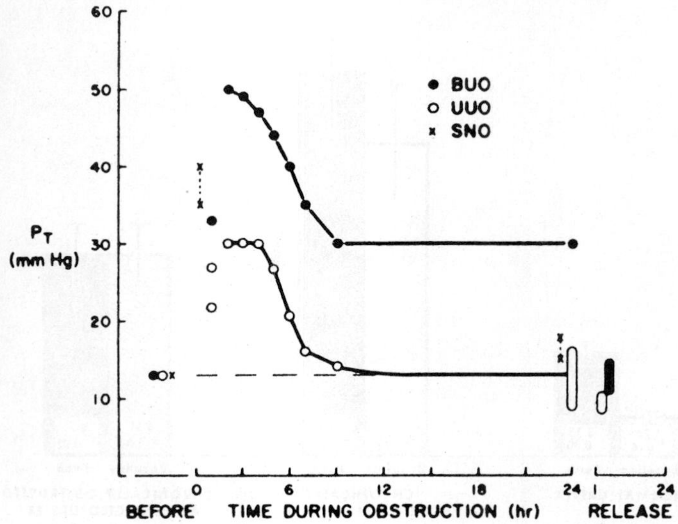

Figure 50.4. Pressure in proximal renal tubule (P_T) before, during, and after release of complete obstruction of one ureter (*UUO*), both ureters (*BUO*), or single nephrons (*SNO*).

obstruction, and by the fourth week it is a third of the values obtained from the contralateral nonobstructed kidney. The temporal relation between changes in ureteral pressure and renal blood flow is illustrated in Fig. 50.5. These changes, observed in the dog, can be divided into three phases. In the first phase, renal blood flow rises above control values. This change in blood flow occurs within the first hour after obstruction and is associated with gradually increasing ureteral pressure. In the second phase, approximately 2 to 5 hours after obstruction, renal blood flow begins to decline, while ureteral pressure continues to increase. Finally in the third phase, ureteral pressure begins to return to control values, and renal blood flow continues to decline. The physiologic explanation for this sequence of events is not clear. The first phase may be a consequence of a direct effect of ureteral pressure on inner medullary blood flow. It appears that inner medullary blood flow declines during all intervals of ureteral obstruction. Because a number of vasoactive hormones (prostaglandins) are produced in the medulla, this decline in flow may cause an alteration in intrarenal hormone regulation, which could result in abrupt changes in vascular resistance and an overshoot in renal blood flow as is seen in phase one. The second phase may be partially the consequence of augmented renal resistance, which is the direct effect of increased ureteral pressure on the interstitium. In the final phase, the chronic phase, an increase in resistance at the preglomerular level is thought to occur. Micropuncture studies in the rat support this postulate. In these studies it was found that when individual nephrons were obstructed for 24 hours in an otherwise normal kidney, stop-flow pressure decreased (Fig. 50.6). Such a decline reflects a decrease in the transcapillary pressure and implies an increase

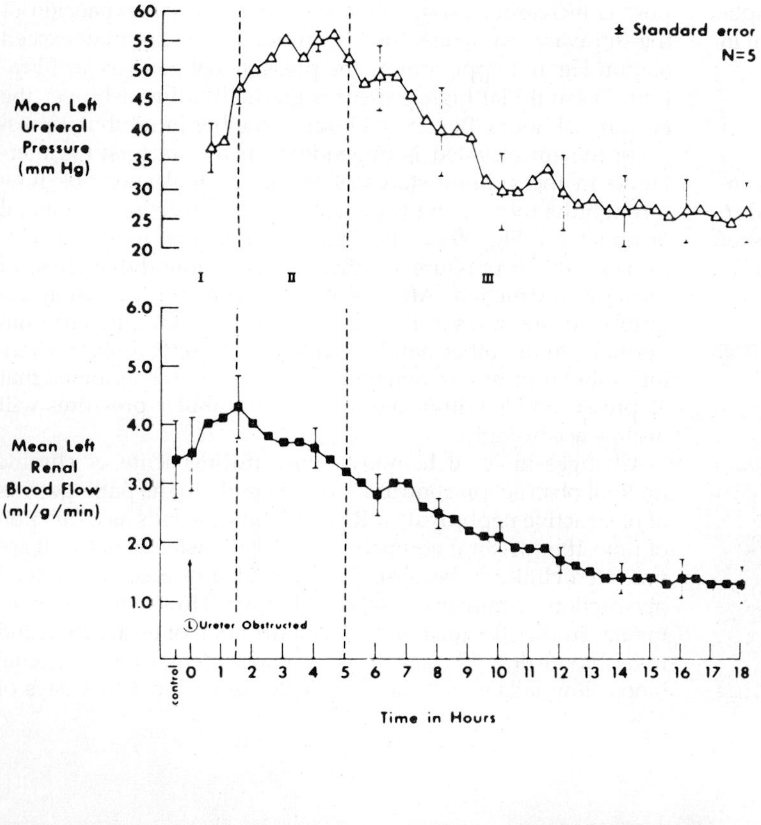

Figure 50.5. The triphasic relation between ipsilateral renal blood flow and left ureteral pressure during 18 hours of left ureteral occlusion. The three phases are designated by *roman numerals* and divided by *vertical dashed lines*. In phase I, the left renal blood flow and ureteral pressure rise together. In phase II, the left renal blood flow begins to decline, while the ureteral pressure remains elevated and, in fact, continues to rise. Phase III shows the left renal blood flow and ureteral pressure declining together. (Reproduced with permission from Moody TE, Vaughn ED Jr, Gillenwater JY. Relationship between renal blood flow and ureteral pressure during 18 hours of total unilateral ureteral occlusion. *Invest Urol* 1975;13:246. ©1975, The Williams & Wilkins Co.)

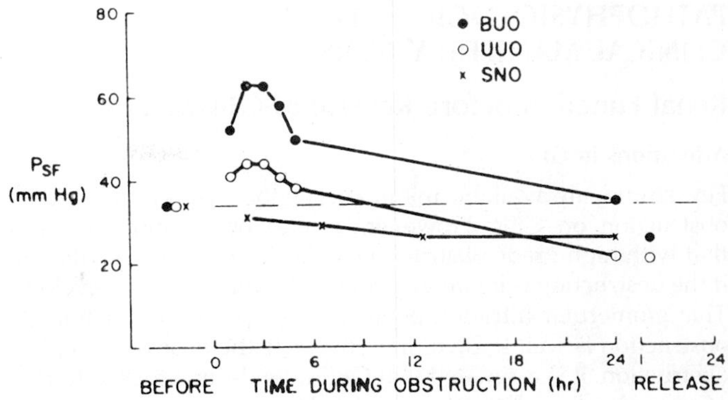

Figure 50.6. Proximal tubule stop-flow pressure (P_{SF}), a reflection of glomerular capillary pressure before, during, and after release of complete ureteral obstruction of one ureter (*UUO*), both ureters (*BUO*), or single nephrons (*SNO*).

in preglomerular resistance. Thromboxane and angiotensin, both powerful vasoconstrictors, account for most of the vasoconstriction observed after 24 hours of obstruction. Decreased production of vasodilators (nitric oxide) may also contribute to the vasoconstriction.

HISTOPATHOLOGIC CHANGES OF THE KIDNEY

The morphologic alterations in renal architecture caused by obstruction can be predicted from the major causes of parenchymal damage: (a) increased ureteral pressure, (b) decreased renal blood flow, (c) invasion by macrophages and lymphocytes, and (d) bacterial infection. Grossly hydronephrotic kidneys have a widely dilated renal pelvis with the renal papillae either flattened or hollowed out. The first structures in the kidneys to be affected are Bellini's ducts. Subsequently, other papillary structures are affected. Ultimately, there is an encroachment on renal cortical tissue, which in advanced cases may be reduced to a thin rim of renal tissue surrounding a large saccular ureteral pelvis.

Histologically, the early changes of hydronephrosis consist of dilation of the tubular system, predominantly the collecting duct and distal tubular segments. Subsequently, cellular flattening and atrophy of the cells lining the proximal tubule occur (Fig. 50.7B). In most instances there is a tendency for glomerular preservation. Acutely Bowman's space may be dilated and ultimately some periglomerular fibrosis may develop. These changes are depicted in Fig. 50.7A. Sequelae of tubular ischemia, the consequence of the combined effects of a decreased renal blood flow and obstruction, are the development of interstitial fibrosis and mononuclear infiltration (Fig. 50.7A and B). Some of mechanisms responsible for this infiltrate have been elucidated. In addition, infection (pyelonephritis) may play a role in the destruction of renal parenchyma.

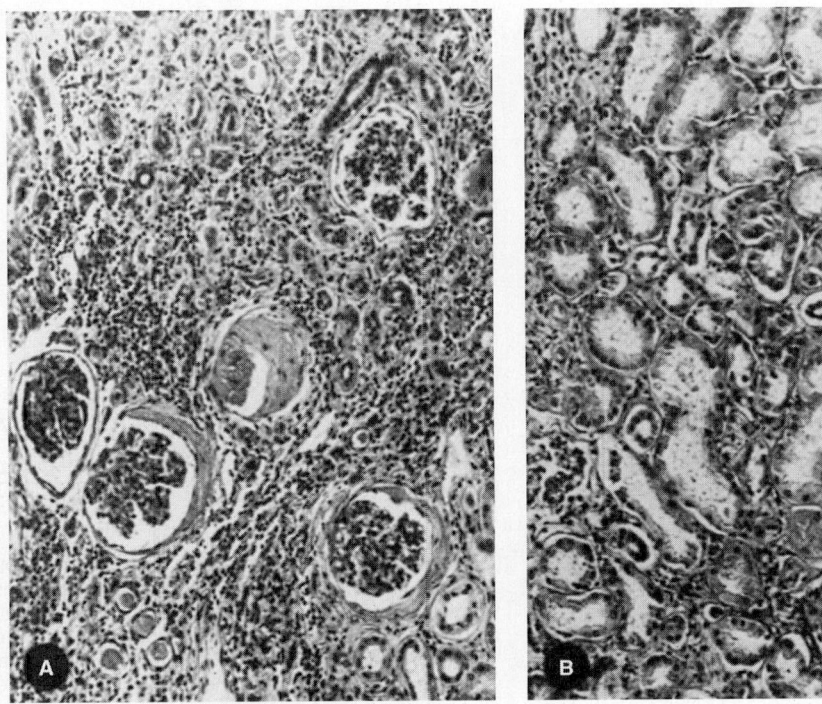

Figure 50.7. Light microscopy of kidney from a 62-year-old woman with obstructive nephropathy. Hematoxylin and eosin, ×150. Note in **A,** relatively normal glomeruli, periglomerular fibrosis, and marked mononuclear interstitial infiltration; and in **B,** the flattened epithelial cells lining the dilated lumina of proximal tubular segments.

PATHOPHYSIOLOGIC AND CLINICAL MANIFESTATIONS

Renal Function before Release of Obstruction

Alterations in GFR

Few studies are available in humans on the effects of continuing obstruction on GFR. However, several observations suggest that with high-grade obstruction, GFR decreases markedly and if the obstruction is bilateral, progressive renal failure develops. That glomerular filtration persists in the presence of complete obstruction is well known. Initially, after the onset of complete obstruction, it is estimated that GFR may decline to 30% to 50% of control values. Filtration persists because of continued renal tubular reabsorption of sodium and water, ureteral dilation, and some return of fluid through the lymphatic system.

Alterations in Renal Tubular Function

The most common sequelae of partial obstructive uropathy are abnormalities in renal tubular function. The major defects in renal tubular function are in the distal segments of the nephron. Patients with chronic obstructive uropathy have an impaired ability to concentrate their urine. Some patients have a form of nephrogenic diabetes insipidus. The magnitude of this defect is quite variable. In fact, polyuria can be an initial symptom of chronic obstructive uropathy, and children with obstructive uropathy may initially have profound dehydration and hypernatremia resulting from impaired reabsorption of free water. Observations in experimental animals suggest that decreased osmolality of the renal medulla, probably the consequence of increased medullary blood flow and decreased salt reabsorption from the thick ascending limb of Henle's loop, has a role in the concentrating defect seen immediately on release of obstruction. This concentrating defect may persist, presumably because of a permanent loss of some juxtamedullary nephrons following 24 hours of unilateral ureteral obstruction. In addition, the decreased water permeability response to vasopressin of the cortical collecting tubule is in part responsible for this abnormality. A decrease in aquaporins has been reported in obstructive uropathy. Increased solute excretion may also contribute to this polyuria and to the inability to concentrate the urine in obstructive nephropathy. An exaggerated salt-losing state may also occur in patients with hydronephrosis. However, detailed information regarding the pattern of salt excretion in obstructive nephropathy is not available.

The alterations in renal tubular function in animals with chronic obstruction are not well defined. The studies available suggest that the changes that result depend on the duration of obstruction and on whether it is bilateral or unilateral. In dogs, when acute unilateral obstruction was produced by elevating the pressure of the ureter, urine flow diminished and the absolute and fractional reabsorption of sodium and water actually increased. Similar results were obtained in the rat following acute incomplete obstruction of 30 hours' duration. In this latter case, micropuncture studies indicated increased fluid reabsorption in the proximal tubule. More chronic changes in the dog resulted in an impaired capacity to reabsorb both sodium and free water.

Another consequence of obstructive uropathy is impaired ability to secrete an acid load and to excrete potassium. These alterations may be due to decreased levels of aldosterone or unresponsiveness of distal tubular segments (cortical and medullary collecting duct) to aldosterone. Thus in most patients with obstructive nephropathy, urinary pH measurements for any given level of metabolic acidosis will be inappropriately high. This defect in urinary acidification is present with bilateral or unilateral ureteral obstruction. A hyperchloremic, hyperkalemic metabolic acidosis has been described in patients with obstruction, and at any given level of GFR, potassium excretion in the urine was decreased in these patients with obstruction when compared with other patients with renal disease and similar decrements in GFR (Fig. 50.8).

Renal Function after Release of Obstruction

Glomerular Filtration and Renal Blood Flow

In humans, the relation between duration of obstruction and degree of recovery of renal function after its release is not known. In most instances when renal function has been studied before and after correction of chronic incomplete ureteral obstruction, there is a tendency for renal blood flow to increase and GFR either to remain the same or to increase slightly. Clearly such studies do not provide information concerning the relation between the duration of obstruction and the recovery of function. Recovery of significant renal function after complete ureteral obstruction is largely anecdotal and consists of a few cases in the literature. However, in all cases there was usually some return in function as judged by the appearance of radiographic contrast medium in the renal pelvis. In one instance, GFR was actually measured following release of ureteral obstruction of 3 months' duration. In this instance the GFR of the obstructed kidney increased from 2.6 to 10.2 ml/min over a 2-week period.

In experimental animals this relationship has been more clearly defined. The long-term effects of ureteral ligation on renal function have been studied in dogs. After 1 week of complete ligation of one ureter, the ligature was removed, and serial studies were performed from 2 months to 1 year after release of obstruction. Renal function was estimated before ligation by measuring total GFR and assuming that the GFR of each kidney was one-half of the measured values. Immediately after release

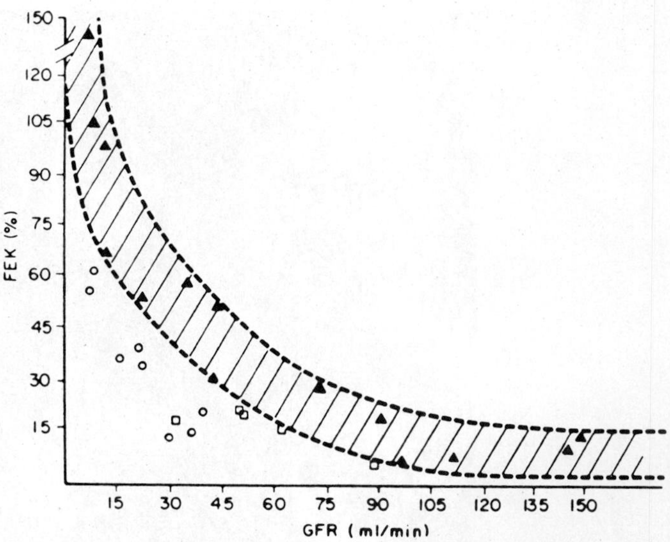

Figure 50.8. Relation of fractional excretion of potassium (*FEK*) to glomerular filtration rate (*GFR*) under baseline conditions. The area inside the broken lines depicts the normal adaptive increase in FEK observed with a chronic reduction in GFR. These data were obtained from 14 normokalemic control subjects (*solid triangles*) with different GFRs. Each patient (*open symbols*) had a baseline FEK lower than that expected for the corresponding GFR. *Open circles* denote patients with distal renal tubular acidosis (group I); *open squares* represent patients with hyperkalemic metabolic acidosis caused by selective aldosterone deficiencies (group II). (Reproduced with permission from Battle DC, Arruda JAL, Kurtzman NA. Hyperkalemic distal renal tubular acidosis associated with obstructive uropathy. *N Engl J Med* 1981;304:373–380.)

of obstruction, GFR averaged 25% of ipsilateral control values and 16% of the concurrent values for the contralateral kidney, the latter having undergone some compensatory increase in function. Follow-up studies revealed an increase in GFR of the obstructed kidney and a decrease in that of the normal kidney. However, function of both organs tended to stabilize within 2 months. In no case was there complete functional recovery of the obstructed organ. In dogs followed for a long period of time, GFR in the experimental kidney remained at approximately 50% of the simultaneous value obtained in the contralateral organ. The decrease in effective renal plasma flow estimated by *p*-aminohippuric acid clearances closely approximated the fall in GFR, and therefore the filtration fraction did not change. On the other hand, studies in rats after relief of obstruction of shorter duration (approximately 30 hours) indicated that 7 to 9 days after release, GFR in the postobstructed kidney was not significantly different from that obtained in sham-operated animals. Thus these studies suggested that the decline in GFR observed with short-term obstruction is completely reversible and that most of the early alterations are functional in nature and do not involve permanent loss of nephrons.

Studies in rats revealed that 14 days after release of unilateral ureteral obstruction of 24 hours' duration, inulin clearance values returned to levels not significantly different from those of the contralateral kidney. However, single-nephron GFR (SNGFR) was increased by about 30% to 45% in the postobstructed kidney, and the total number of filtering nephrons was decreased by about 20% to 30%, both at 8 and at 60 days after release of obstruction. These data indicate a permanent loss of nephrons with preservation of total GFR because of an increase in SNGFR in the surviving nephrons.

After release of obstruction, either bilateral or unilateral, renal blood flow is decreased. Whether this decrease is associated with an intrarenal redistribution of blood flow is controversial. Most studies in animals suggest that cortical blood flow is markedly reduced. This decline is associated with an increase or at least a return to normal of inner medullary blood flow. Micropuncture studies suggest that after release of unilateral ureteral obstruction, this redistribution of blood flow is associated with a redistribution of SNGFR. That is, GFR is significantly decreased in both nephron populations (surface and juxtamedullary), but the fall in GFR is greater in surface than in juxtamedullary nephrons. A number of studies have shown no redistribution of SNGFR after release of bilateral ureteral obstruction, although the changes in intrarenal blood flow were similar to those seen after release of unilateral ureteral obstruction. Other studies have shown that production of thromboxane A_2, a potent vasoconstrictor, can be more easily stimulated in hydronephrotic kidneys of rabbits than in control kidneys, suggesting that part of the marked decline in cortical renal blood flow seen after release of obstruction may be the consequence of intrarenal hormonal mechanisms. Dietary protein may condition the production of thromboxane A_2 after unilateral release of bilateral ureteral obstruction; following this procedure, rats fed a high-protein diet had a higher rate of thromboxane A_2 and lower renal blood flow, total GFR, and SNGFR values than rats fed a low-protein diet. Presumably increased renal synthesis of thromboxane in the high-protein–fed rats accounts for the greater decrement in renal blood flow and GFR. Inhibition of thromboxane synthesis increased glomerular plasma flow and GFR in rats fed a high-protein diet but not in rats fed a low-protein diet.

Renal Tubular Function

The functional alterations in renal tubules after release of obstruction depend in part on whether the occlusion is bilateral or unilateral. A consequence of release of complete bilateral ureteral obstruction is the development of a marked diuresis and natriuresis. The cause and incidence of this so-called "postobstructive diuresis" in humans is not clear. Several factors may be causally related to this phenomenon. One important factor is the volume status of the patients before release of obstruction. Individuals given fluid challenges in an attempt to characterize the cause of the renal failure or managed with intravenous fluids before the release of obstruction will tend to be volume expanded. Thus part of the increased water and sodium excretion that occurs after release of obstruction is a physiologic response to this expanded state. Indeed, total body sodium is increased in many of these patients. Another factor is the accumulation of relatively nonresorbable solutes such as urea, which can promote a solute diuresis and lead to losses of sodium and water.

Finally, it has been suggested that the increased diuresis seen after release of obstruction is inappropriate. It results from either an intrinsic defect in renal tubular function or a humoral agent that accumulates during the period of anuria and directly affects sodium and water reabsorption by the renal tubule.

Although the relative contribution of each of these factors cannot be clearly elucidated in humans, a variety of experimental studies in animals have been performed to characterize the pathogenesis of postobstructive diuresis. The changes in external sodium balance before, during, and after bilateral ureteral obstruction are shown in Fig. 50.9. These studies clearly demonstrate that the increase in sodium and water excretion following release of obstruction is not merely a physiologic response to volume expansion. Because this natriuresis and diuresis occur in the face of a marked decline in GFR, they must represent a decrease in reabsorption of fluid by one and most likely several segments of the renal tubule. Micropuncture studies found that after release of acute bilateral ureteral ligation, there is a decrease in the amount of water reabsorbed along the proximal and distal tubules of surface nephrons and to the bend of Henle's loop of deep nephrons. In such studies, collecting duct function appeared to be intact. That these changes are not a consequence of an increased solute load has been demonstrated by experimental studies in which urea concentrations in blood were raised to levels achieved during the period of anuria. In such studies, sodium and water excretion increased but not to the same magnitude seen after release of obstruction.

Accumulation of natriuretic factors (atrial peptide) in blood during complete ureteral obstruction may play a significant role in the ensuing postobstructive diuresis, because a natriuresis

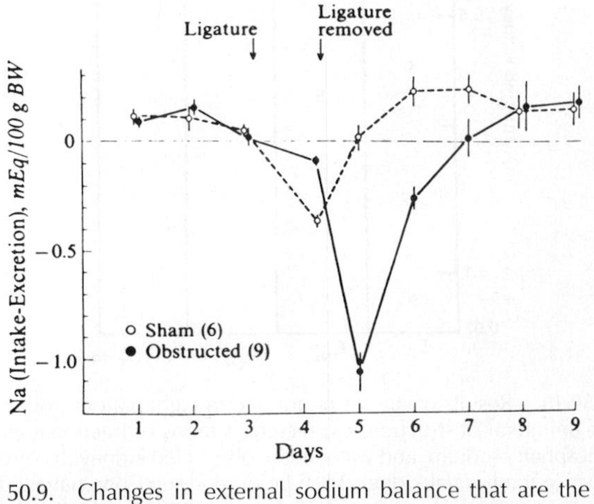

Figure 50.9. Changes in external sodium balance that are the consequence of bilateral obstruction and release or of sham operation. *BW*, body weight. (Reproduced with permission from McDougal WS, Wright FS. Defect in proximal and distal sodium transport in postobstructive diuresis. *Kidney Int* 1972;2:304.)

and diuresis comparable with those seen after release of acute bilateral ureteral obstruction can be produced in normal rats by cross-circulation with rats having complete obstruction of 24 hours' duration. Furthermore, rats subjected to unilateral ureteral obstruction and reinfusion of urine from the contralateral kidney had a marked increase in sodium and water excretion similar in magnitude to that observed after release of bilateral ureteral obstruction.

On the other hand, a postobstructive diuresis does not occur after release of unilateral ureteral obstruction. A summary of studies of renal function obtained in humans after release of unilateral ureteral obstruction is given in Fig. 50.10. These studies show that despite the marked decrease in GFR of the obstructed kidney when compared with the contralateral normally functioning kidney, in most cases there was an increase in fractional sodium and water excretion from the postobstructed kidney. The difference in the magnitude of sodium excretion seen after bilateral obstruction compared with unilateral obstruction may relate to a greater delivery of tubule fluid out of cortical nephrons after release of bilateral obstruction. A number of findings seem to support this conclusion. First, in human studies it has been shown that phosphate reabsorption is frequently greater in the postobstructed kidney than in the normally functioning contralateral kidney (Fig. 50.10). Because phosphate reabsorption occurs primarily in the proximal tubule, these studies suggest enhanced renal tubular reabsorption of sodium and water in this segment. Second, studies using micropuncture techniques demonstrated that the reabsorption of water and sodium along the proximal and distal tubular segments of surface nephrons was markedly increased after the release of unilateral ureteral obstruction compared with results obtained in normal hydropenic animals or after release of bilateral ureteral obstruction. Additional micropuncture studies suggested that increased functional sodium and water excretion after release of unilateral ureteral obstruction was due to increased delivery of sodium and water out of deep nephrons.

There is also an impaired ability to concentrate the urine after release of obstruction. This defect is unresponsive to vasopressin. An important contributing factor may be a decrease in the solute content of the papillary interstitium during obstruction. This decrease in solute content may be perpetuated by a relative increase in blood flow to papillary structures. That is, SNGFR of deep nephrons is reduced by 50% to 60%, while inner medullary plasma flow is either not different from control measurements or slightly increased. In vivo studies in normal rats and in rats subjected to bilateral ureteral obstruction for 20 hours revealed that vasopressin administration increased cyclic adenosine 3',5'- monophosphate (cAMP) excretion in control rat kidneys but not in postobstructed kidneys. These results indicate an impairment of vasopressin-dependent cAMP production in postobstructed kidneys and suggest that the concentrating defect observed after release of obstruction may relate, at least in part, to inhibition of vasopressin-dependent cAMP production within the kidney. Perfusion of dissected nephron segments from rabbits with unilateral or bilateral ureteral obstruction has revealed decreased sodium chloride reabsorption in the thick ascending limb of Henle's loop and decreased hydraulic water permeability in response to antidiuretic hormone or cAMP in the cortical collecting tubule. The concentrating defect improves markedly but is still present 60 days after release of unilateral ureteral ligation of 24 hours' duration in the rat, at a time when total GFR has returned to normal. The most likely explanation for this observation is a permanent loss of juxtamedullary or deep nephrons. A decrease in nephrons with long loops may impair the ability of the remaining nephrons to create a markedly hypertonic medulla.

In humans and experimental animals, acid excretion also is impaired following release of bilateral or unilateral ureteral obstruction. The change seen after unilateral obstruction seems to more closely reflect the intrinsic alterations in renal function, because the extrarenal manifestations of uremia seen with bilateral ureteral obstruction are not present. In this setting, urine pH from the obstructed kidney tends to be greater than 7 and is not significantly affected by an acid load (Fig. 50.11). Bicarbonate titration studies are no different after release of unilateral obstruction than after sham operation, and there is no increase in splay. Micropuncture experiments failed to demonstrate decreased reabsorption of bicarbonate in proximal or distal seg-

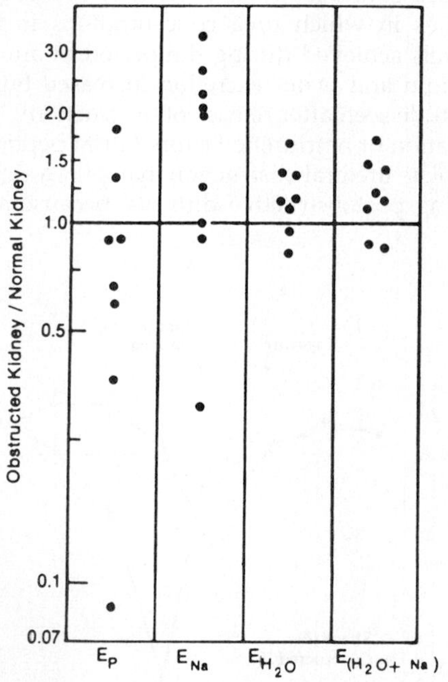

Figure 50.10. Results of studies performed in eight patients following release of unilateral obstruction, expressed as ratios of fractional excretion (*E*) of phosphate, sodium, and water in the obstructed kidney to corresponding values in the normal kidney. Each point represents one patient. (Reproduced with permission from Better OS, Tuma S, Shimeon K, et al. Enhanced tubular reabsorption of phosphate. *Arch Intern Med* 1975;135:245. ©1975, American Medical Association.)

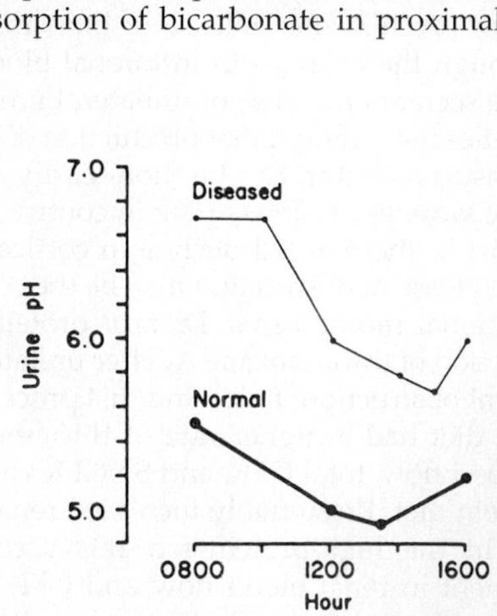

Figure 50.11. Changes in urine pH from the obstructed (*diseased*) and normally functioning kidney after the oral administration of ammonium chloride (0.1 g/kg of body weight) in a patient after release of unilateral ureteral obstruction. (Reproduced with permission from Better OS, Arieff AI, Massry SG, et al. Studies on renal function after relief of complete unilateral ureteral obstruction of three months' duration in man. *Am J Med* 1973;54:234–240.)

ments of surface nephrons. Urinary P_{CO_2} values remained low after bicarbonate loading. These data suggest that the acidifying defect observed after unilateral ureteral obstruction is due either to decreased hydrogen ion secretion in the distal tubule of surface nephrons and the collecting duct or to marked alterations in the reabsorption of bicarbonate in juxtamedullary nephrons. A hyperchloremic, hyperkalemic acidosis has been described in patients with obstruction. In some patients this defect may be due to hypoaldosteronism and in others to a decreased response to aldosterone of the medullary collecting tubule, whereby hydrogen ion secretion occurs.

Alterations in phosphate reabsorption have been reported in humans (Fig. 50.10). Phosphate and sodium excretion by the obstructed kidney differ after release of unilateral ureteral obstruction. Fractional phosphate excretion is markedly decreased, whereas fractional sodium excretion is significantly increased. These differences in the excretion of phosphate and sodium also occur in experimental animals. In rats, after relief of complete unilateral ureteral obstruction of 24 hours' duration, fractional phosphate excretion from the control kidney was greater than normal, but fractional phosphate excretion by the experimental kidney was markedly decreased. The increased excretion of phosphate by the control kidney was abolished by prior parathyroidectomy, suggesting a role for circulating parathyroid hormone (PTH) in its genesis. The study showed that the decreased urinary excretion of phosphate by the experimental kidney was apparently due to hypoperfusion and not to refractoriness of the renal tubule to the action of PTH nor to changes in the intrinsic capacity to reabsorb phosphate. Others reported a decreased responsiveness to PTH. A marked decrease in SNGFR and in the filtered load of phosphate coupled with increased proximal reabsorption of salt and water may account for the low phosphate excretion by the experimental kidney. Similar results were obtained in rats in which the filtered phosphate was decreased unilaterally by partially constricting the aorta proximal to the left renal artery. The decreased filtered load and the increased reabsorption of salt and water in the proximal tubule would markedly decrease phosphate delivery to the PTH-sensitive sites located more distally in the nephron, resulting in a marked fall in phosphate excretion. Observations in the dog suggest a loss of PTH receptors in the basolateral membrane of the proximal tubule during obstruction. Hence, a decreased response to PTH may also play a role in the decreased excretion of phosphate by the postobstructed kidney.

Hypomagnesemia has been reported in humans following relief of bilateral ureteral obstruction. In rats with unilateral ureteral ligation, relief of the obstruction resulted in a marked increase in the fractional excretion of magnesium by the experimental kidney (Fig. 50.12). This is probably due to decreased reabsorption of salt and water as well as magnesium by the thick ascending limb of Henle's loop.

Alterations in renal metabolism occur in association with urinary tract obstruction. A selective decrease of alkaline phosphatase in the proximal tubule following ureteral ligation has been described. Alkaline phosphatase activity was greatly reduced in the proximal tubule of rats after 2 days of complete ureteral obstruction. Further decreases in enzyme activity were noted after 7 days. Recovery of enzyme activity was observed 2 days following release of the obstruction, and after 6 days values were comparable to those observed preceding obstruction. Acid phosphatase activity did not change during obstruction, but its activity increased significantly early in the course of recovery from obstruction and decreased to control levels after 7 days of recovery. Glucose-6-phosphate dehydrogenase and 6-phosphogluconate dehydrogenase activities increased in the proximal tubules of obstructed kidneys. Following release of

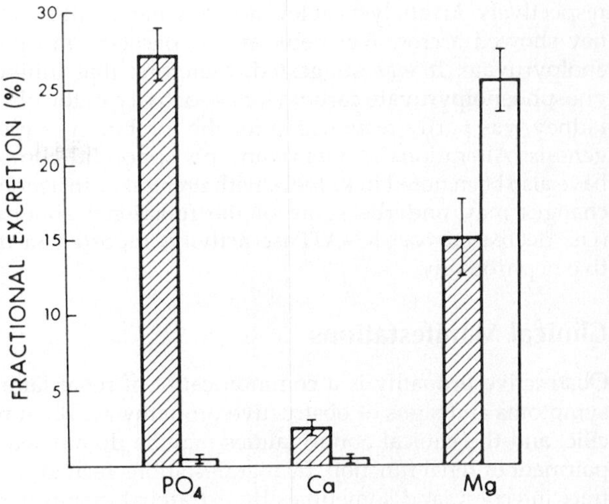

Figure 50.12. Fractional excretion of phosphate, calcium, and magnesium by the contralateral control kidney (*hatched bars*) and the postobstructed kidney (*open bars*) of rats after release of unilateral ureteral obstruction. The differences in fractional excretion between the two kidneys were significant ($P < .001$ for the three substances studied). (Reproduced with permission from Purkerson ML, Slatopolsky E, Klahr S. Urinary excretion of magnesium, calcium, and phosphate after release of unilateral ureteral obstruction in the rat. *Miner Electrolyte Metab* 1981;6:182–189.)

the obstruction, these enzyme activities remained elevated during the initial 48 hours but returned to normal after 6 days.

Unilateral ureteral ligation decreases Na^+-K^+-ATPase activity. Mg^{2+}-ATPase and Na^+-K^+-ATPase activities were assayed on microsomal fractions prepared from hydronephrotic and contralateral normal kidneys of rats at 1, 2, and 5 days following ureteral ligation. No changes in Mg^{2+}-ATPase were observed, but there was a steady decrease of Na^+-K^+-ATPase activity with longer periods of obstruction. This decrease in Na^+-K^+-ATPase activity after 24 hours of obstruction is not related to a loss of the enzyme but to alterations in the lipid composition of the basolateral membrane of proximal tubular cells.

Metabolic studies using cortical slices obtained from the control and postobstructed kidneys of rats subjected to 24 hours of complete unilateral ureteral obstruction revealed that oxygen consumption, glutamine uptake, and glutamine oxidation were considerably lower in the postobstructed kidney. No significant differences in glucose oxidation or uptake were observed in postobstructed and control kidneys. Gluconeogenesis from either glutamine or α-ketoglutarate was decreased by more than 50% in the postobstructed kidney. At the same time, ammonia production from glutamine was markedly decreased in the postobstructed kidney when compared with the contralateral control kidney. The postobstructed kidney, therefore, exhibited a marked decrease in glutamine uptake and oxidation, decreased oxygen consumption, and impaired gluconeogenesis and ammoniagenesis. A significant decrease in the steady-state levels of glutamate and adenosine 5'-triphosphate was also observed in the postobstructed kidney. No differences in the steady-state concentrations of glucose, glutamine, or lactate were noted in the two kidneys. In dogs, no significant fall in gluconeogenesis from α-ketoglutarate was observed after 6 hours of obstruction, but a marked reduction (approximately 40%) occurred after 16 to 48 hours of obstruction. The use of α-ketoglutarate, measured as $^{14}CO_2$ evolved from [1-^{14}C] α-ketoglutarate, was reduced in proportion to gluconeogenesis. The rate of aerobic glycolysis was depressed in the obstructed kidney, and glucose production from malate and pyruvate was decreased by 30% and 35%, respectively. An analysis of levels of key metabolites in the kidney showed a crossover between oxaloacetate and phosphoenolpyruvate. It was suggested, therefore, that inhibition of phosphoenolpyruvate carboxykinase activity in the obstructed kidney was partly responsible for the inhibition of gluconeogenesis. Alterations in membrane phospholipid composition have also been noted in kidneys with ureteral obstruction. These changes may underlie some of the functional abnormalities (i.e., decreased Na^+-K^+-ATPase activity) reported in obstructive nephropathy.

Clinical Manifestations

Obstructive uropathy is a common cause of renal failure. The symptoms and signs of obstructive uropathy are often nonspecific, and the clinical abnormalities may be dominated by impairment of renal function, by manifestations related to urinary tract infection, and sometimes by extrarenal manifestations of the underlying pathologic process, for example, local and distant metastases from tumors that produce obstruction in the urinary tract.

Alterations in Urine Output

If obstruction is complete and bilateral or unilateral in a patient with only one functioning kidney, *anuria* results. However, with partial obstruction, *polyuria* may occur, and when marked, it may become a prominent presenting symptom. A finding characteristic of intermittent obstruction is the sequential occurrence of oliguria or anuria and brisk polyuria. The sequence may occur in either direction and may be repetitive. When complete cessation of urine flow occurs, complete obstruction should be suspected. The clinical setting of its occurrence is important. The diagnosis should be considered in patients with previous pelvic surgery when inadvertent ligation of the ureters can occur, pelvic malignancy in which extension of the tumor with invasion of the ureters may result in obstruction, or longstanding bladder-neck obstruction, in patients who have had recent ureteric transplant, recent ileal bladder construction, or recent retrograde pyelography, and in patients with an indwelling bladder catheter that has not been irrigated.

Bladder Symptoms

Alterations in micturition are frequently associated with lower tract obstruction. Common symptoms of lower tract obstruction are hesitancy in starting urination, decreased force and size of the stream, terminal dribbling, dysuria, and acute urinary retention. These symptoms are typical of urethral stricture, benign prostatic hypertrophy, neurogenic bladder, and tumor of the bladder or prostate involving the vesical neck or its innervation.

Pain and Renal Enlargement

Pain may be the initial clinical complaint in patients with obstruction. This is usually the case in patients with acute or rapidly developing obstruction. Acute ureteral obstruction may be characterized by a steady crescendo pain radiating downward toward the groin, the testicles, or labia. It should be remembered that pain may not be present at all, especially in patients with chronic slowly progressive obstruction. Occasionally such patients may complain of dull flank pain, usually related to increased fluid intake or to the use of diuretics. Flank pain occurring during micturition is said to be pathognomonic of ureterovesical reflux. Kidney size may increase, sometimes notably, in patients with longstanding obstruction. Patients may note increased abdominal girth or a palpable flank mass. Sometimes marked hydronephrosis may be seen clinically as a flank mass on physical examination.

Deterioration of Renal Function without Apparent Cause

A number of patients who have the signs and symptoms of chronic uremia may have unrecognized longstanding urinary tract obstruction. Urinary tract obstruction may occur in patients with parenchymal renal disease of another origin and manifest itself by a change in the rate of progression of renal insufficiency. In some patients, however, obstruction is the only cause of end-stage renal failure. Occasionally, in patients with retroperitoneal fibrosis, in whom the onset of obstruction is slow and progressive, far advanced renal failure may be an initial clinical manifestation. Urinary tract obstruction should be considered in patients with uremia with no previous history of renal disease and relatively benign urine sediments. It also should be considered in patients with known renal disease who develop an abrupt decrease in renal function that is otherwise unexplained.

Symptoms of Urinary Tract Infection That Are Recurrent or Resistant to Therapy

Infection is a common complication in patients with urinary tract obstruction. Repeated infections without apparent cause should raise the suspicion of obstruction. The inability to clear urinary tract infections with adequate therapy should always raise the possibility of anatomic lesions of the urinary tract. In such patients the urinary tract should be evaluated, looking for evidence of structural abnormalities.

Polycythemia

The association of polycythemia and hydronephrosis has been reported. In a few instances the increased red blood cell count decreased following corrective surgery. The relation of hydronephrosis to increased erythropoietin levels in humans is not clear. In most instances of obstructive uropathy associated with polycythemia that have been investigated, erythropoietin levels were not determined, and in those few cases in which erythropoietin was measured, plasma levels were undetectable. However, unilateral hydronephrosis in experimental animals results in elevated plasma levels of erythropoietin that precede an increase in hemoglobin levels.

Hypertension

Acute and chronic hydronephrosis, either unilateral or bilateral, may be accompanied by a significant elevation in blood pressure. The hypertension could be coincidental or could be caused by the hydronephrosis resulting from either impaired sodium excretion or abnormal renin release.

In patients with bilateral hydronephrosis, the demonstration of increased exchangeable sodium and the usual prompt reversal of the hypertension after catheter drainage and diuresis would suggest that the hypertensive state is primarily due to excessive retention of salt and water subsequent to urinary tract obstruction. Thus these patients have a volume-dependent form of hypertension. In addition, the concentrations of renin were normal or decreased. After corrective surgery, reversal of the hypertension was associated with an osmotic diuresis and a negative sodium–water balance suggesting volume dependence.

The hypertension seen in patients with unilateral ureteral obstruction may be renin dependent. Elevated renal vein renin concentrations from unilateral hydronephrotic kidneys have been reported. After corrective surgery, the hypertension abated and the renin values returned to normal. Animal studies have demonstrated increased renin release following acute ureteral obstruction. In dogs, acute unilateral ureteral occlusion is associated with an increase in blood pressure and a rise in ipsilateral renal vein renin despite a concurrent rise in renal blood flow. A causal relation between renin release and the increase in blood pressure is suggested by the fact that pretreatment with deoxycorticosterone acetate and salt abolished the rise in renin and blood pressure. In contrast, chronic studies in animals have shown that the renin release is not sustained and that the peripheral renin value is normal with prolonged unilateral ureteral occlusion. Although it has been suggested that in unilateral obstruction, renin release is responsible for the hypertension, several studies of patients with chronic hydronephrosis revealed that the values of peripheral renin are usually normal or low. This suggests that hypertension in its established state in this setting is not due to increased renin secretion. In addition, in these studies differential measurements of renal vein renin failed to demonstrate lateralization of the renal vein renin to the hydronephrotic kidney or any contralateral suppression of renal vein secretion. Thus established hydronephrosis does not appear to be a stimulus for abnormal renin secretion. Because corrective surgery may again result in improvement of the hypertension, some other abnormalities not related to renin may occur in obstruction. Whether these abnormalities relate to subtle changes in volume or the lack of release of vasodepressor substances by the kidney has not been established.

Hyperkalemic Hyperchloremic Acidosis

Obstruction may affect the excretion of acid and potassium leading to the development of hyperkalemic hyperchloremic acidosis. Obstructive uropathy should be considered in the differential diagnosis in elderly individuals who are not diabetic and have hyperkalemic hyperchloremic acidosis.

DIAGNOSTIC APPROACH TO THE PATIENT WITH URINARY TRACT OBSTRUCTION

The diagnostic approach to a patient with urinary tract obstruction will depend on the clinical setting and initial symptoms, the spectrum of which extends from those patients who have acute onset of pain to those patients who have acute renal failure and anuria. Thus the diagnostic approach and the urgency with which the diagnosis must be made will be highly variable (Fig. 50.13). When urinary tract obstruction is suspected, certain preliminary information is essential. The past history of similar symptoms, urinary tract infection, and the kinds of drugs ingested are important. Questions focused on eliciting lower urinary tract symptoms are clearly important. If the patient is in the hospital, an attempt should be made to characterize the pattern of urine output, whether it has changed abruptly, gradually declined, or fluctuated. Such information may be obtained from input and output records, which should not only be studied for 24-hour changes but also for hourly changes. Physical examination with particular reference to the flank and abdomen is very important. Tenderness in the costovertebral angle may or may not be present. A mass in the flank area, especially in children, may be found by palpation or percussion. Muscle rigidity over the kidney may be found and rebound tenderness may be elicited, particularly if acute infection is present. Abdominal distension and diminished peristalsis usually accompany acute renal colic. In older patients, urinary outlet obstruction should be suspected when a suprapubic mass is found.

Analysis of the urine may provide important information. The presence of hematuria alone may suggest that the obstructing lesion is a calculus, sloughed papilla, or tumor. When urinary tract obstruction is suspected in conjunction with hematuria and with bacteriuria or with a urine pH greater than 7.5, it is of a more chronic nature and complicated by an infection. Bacteriuria alone may suggest stasis especially in males or in female patients who are pregnant and have not had a previous history of infection. When the bacteriuria is associated with an increased number of white blood cells and white blood cell casts, acute pyelonephritis should be suspected. It must be remembered that infection may be a complication of chronic obstruction resulting from calculi or papillary necrosis. The urine sediment should be examined carefully for the presence of crystals. Sulfonamide, cystine, or uric acid crystals may be the first indication as to the type of stone causing the ureteral obstruction or the intrarenal obstruction resulting in acute renal failure. Laboratory studies should include a measure of renal function (serum creatinine and urea nitrogen levels) in addition to the usual measurement of blood chemistries. The ratio between blood urea nitrogen and creatinine levels in blood is greater than 10.

Once this information has been collected, the course of the diagnostic evaluation of the patient will be determined by the symptom complex and by results obtained during the

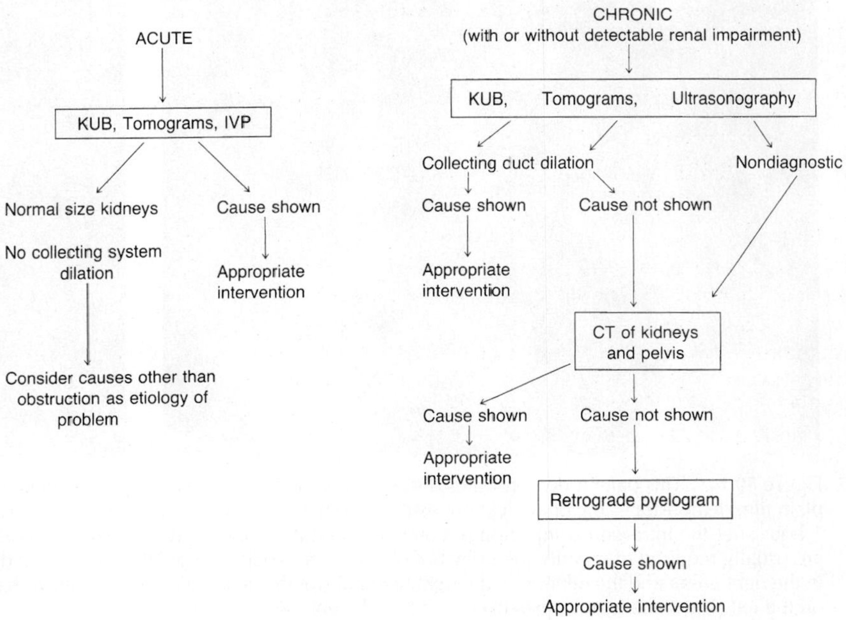

Figure 50.13. Diagnostic approach in suspected ureteral obstruction. CT, computed tomography; IVP, intravenous pyelogram; KUB, abdominal x-ray examination of kidney, ureter, and bladder.

preliminary evaluation of the patient. Two important factors are pain and whether there is evidence of diminished renal function. For patients in whom the clinical manifestation is pain without evidence of a decrease in GFR, the diagnostic emphasis should be to determine the presence or absence of a renal calculus. In these patients the next step is a radiologic evaluation of the abdomen without the injection of contrast media (Fig. 50.14A). In most cases, plain x-ray examination of the abdomen will allow the kidneys to be sufficiently outlined to comment on their size and contour. Frequently a calculus can be seen at some juncture along the urinary tract. Nearly 90% of renal stones are radiopaque. This makes them readily visible on a plain film of the abdomen unless they are very small or overlie bone. It is necessary to differentiate a renal stone from calcified mesenteric lymph nodes, calcium in the rib cage, gallstones, and solid medication (pills) in the intestinal tract. Because the plain film is two-dimensional, it has only presumptive value except in the case of a staghorn calculus, which is seldom confused with other findings. If a calculus is found or if the clinical evidence strongly suggests the passage of stone, the next step is to perform an intravenous pyelogram (Fig. 50.14B), which is needed to assess the degree of urinary obstruction and to detect radiolucent stones. The predominant radiologic findings in this setting and in the other causes of acute urinary tract obstruction reveal diminished filtration of contrast material rather than the structural effects of obstruction. Delayed parenchymal opacification compared with the nonobstructed kidney, progressive increase in the density of the nephrogram with time, and delayed opacification of the collecting system are recognized more easily than the subtle changes in calyceal or ureteric size. Uncommon but helpful findings are radiopaque and radiolucent striae in the nephrogram.

Once a diagnosis of an obstructing calculus has been made, the management is mainly supportive. Assuming a stone of less than 0.5 cm and an intact contralateral kidney, there is no immediate urgency to remove an obstructing stone. One can wait for days for it to pass spontaneously. A follow-up abdominal radiograph or intravenous pyelogram will document the movement of the stone. If an obstructing stone is stationary or if hydronephrosis is very severe, the stone must be removed by surgery or lithotripsy. Subsequent studies should include characterization of the pathogenesis of the calculus. Attempts should be made to control those factors that caused the stone. Notable exceptions to this approach are patients who have this symptom complex and are also pregnant. In these patients, radiographic evaluation may be performed when other diagnostic techniques have failed. Ultrasonography is of limited value in this situation. The utility of ultrasonography is to detect the degree of widening of the pyelocalyceal system. Widening of the collecting structures is not a major feature of acute obstruction, but does occur in 90% of pregnancies. The radiohippurate urogram is of value in studying the renal pelvis, ureter, and bladder. The renogram defines structures well enough to provide a general idea of the severity of obstruction and the level of kidney function by examining the excretory decay curves, right versus left. These studies have a low radiation exposure.

When renal function is impaired and there is no apparent reason for the decline or when renal insufficiency exists for an apparent reason but abruptly declines, the diagnosis of ureteral obstruction should be considered. The diagnostic approach to

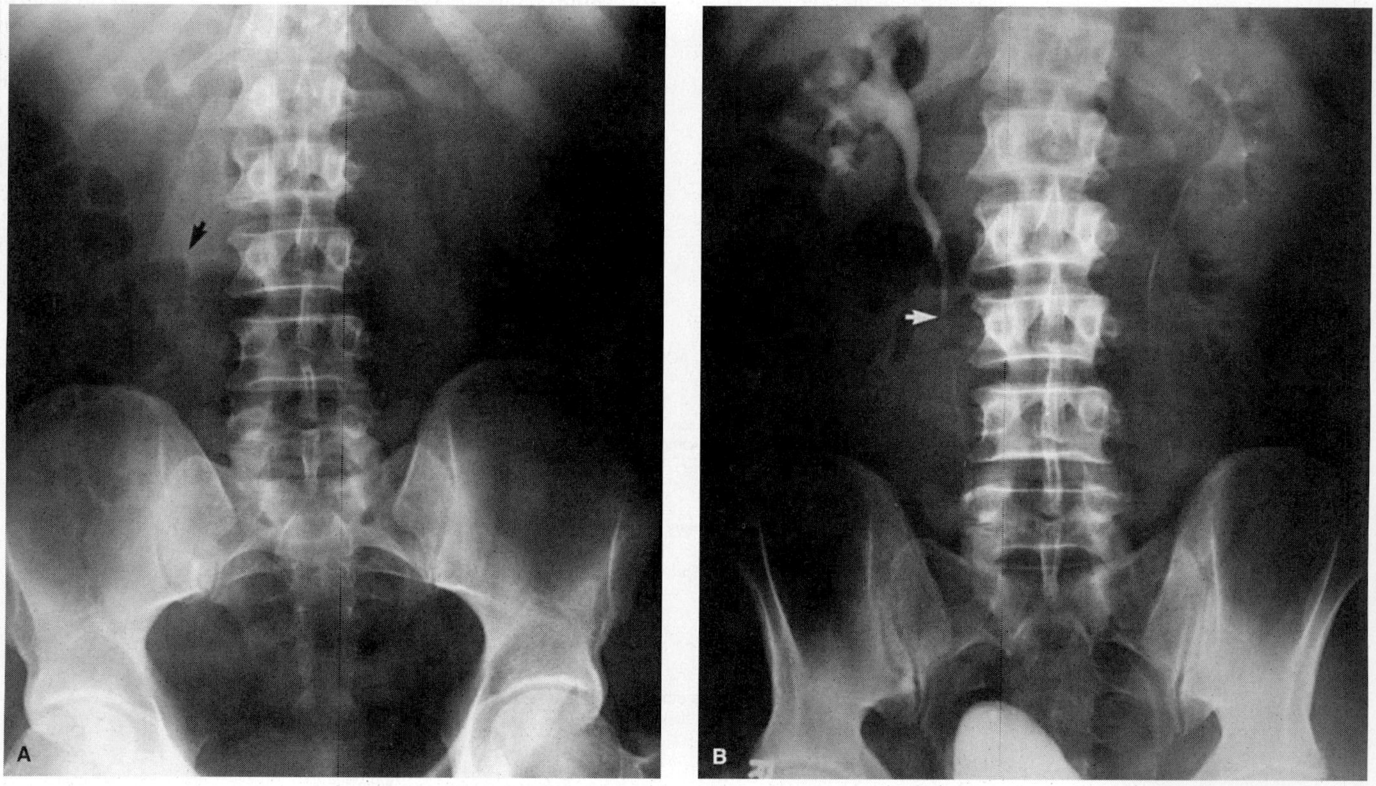

Figure 50.14. This patient demonstrates distal ureteral obstruction secondary to a renal calculus. **A:** the plain film demonstrates the opacification resulting from a stone, as indicated by the *arrow*. **B:** a film taken 1 hour after the intravenous injection of contrast material. In obstructive uropathy, delayed upright films are usually required to identify the points of obstruction. Notice the point at which the dye has stopped in the right ureter and the dilation of the right ureter above the obstruction, compared with a normal ureter on the left. The stone is now visualized as a radiolucent area (*arrow*).

these patients will depend in large part on the facilities and expertise available to the physician. We propose that the first investigation, when obstruction is suspected and renal function is impaired, should be ultrasonography to define renal size and to show collecting duct dilation. Plain films with renal tomograms should be obtained to look for calculi. Computed tomograms should be used for patients in whom the ultrasound study is not diagnostic. Using this scheme, obstruction can be diagnosed in 84% of patients, thus leaving only 16% of patients who would have to be exposed to the risk of intravenous or retrograde pyelography. If obstruction exists, it may be discerned at two points in the study using intravenous pyelography. The nephrogram phase of the study is the first point. This may be delayed, but in most cases occurs within the first hour after the injection of the contrast media. At this time, the calyces will be outlined as a negative shadow. Tomographic patterns of the fat near the renal pelvis will also be helpful; if fat is present, under normal circumstances it appears as well-defined fingerlike projections radiating from the renal hilum. When obstruction is present, this fat is displaced by the hydronephrotic calyces. The second point at which obstruction may be ascertained is in the delayed films. At this interval the radiopaque dye enters the renal pelvis. It is important to remember that using the combination of the plain films, high-dose drip or bolus intravenous injections of radiopaque dye, and tomography, renal size and calyceal dilation can be adequately assessed independent of the level of renal function.

In choosing this approach to a patient with renal insufficiency, the clinician must be aware of the possible risks involved. Acute renal failure, usually reversible, can follow intravenous pyelography or any study using radiocontrast material. The risk of this complication is greatest in patients with diabetes mellitus with or without renal insufficiency, in patients with chronic renal insufficiency of any type, and in patients with hypertension, cardiovascular disease, hematologic disorders such as sickle cell anemia or polycythemia vera. There is a strong relation between renal failure and multiple studies using any of the four contrast media procedures (intravenous and oral cholecystography, angiography, and computed tomography). Finally, there is an increased risk in elderly patients with or without azotemia. Because of this risk, less invasive approaches in the diagnosis of ureteral obstruction should be used. Detailed discussion of acute renal failure induced by contrast media is provided in Chapter 47, Part 7.

Ultrasonography is the least invasive of these procedures. Unfortunately, the success of diagnosis using this technique depends highly on the skills of the imaging technologists, on the interpretation, and on the clinical setting. Figure 50.15A and B,

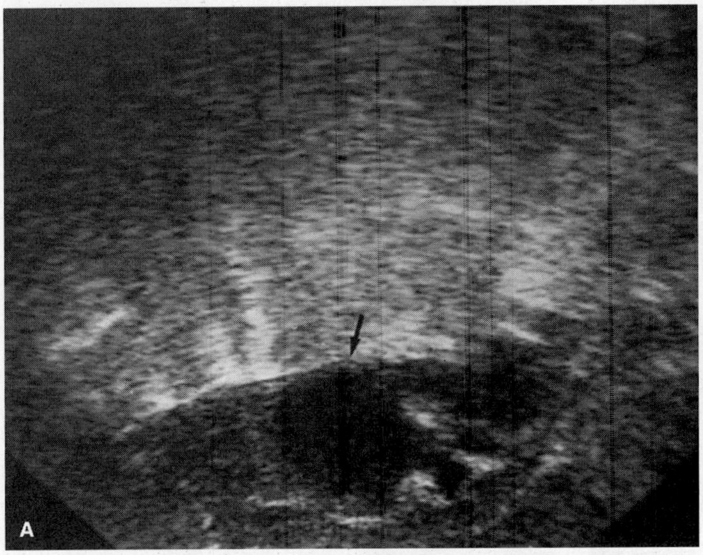

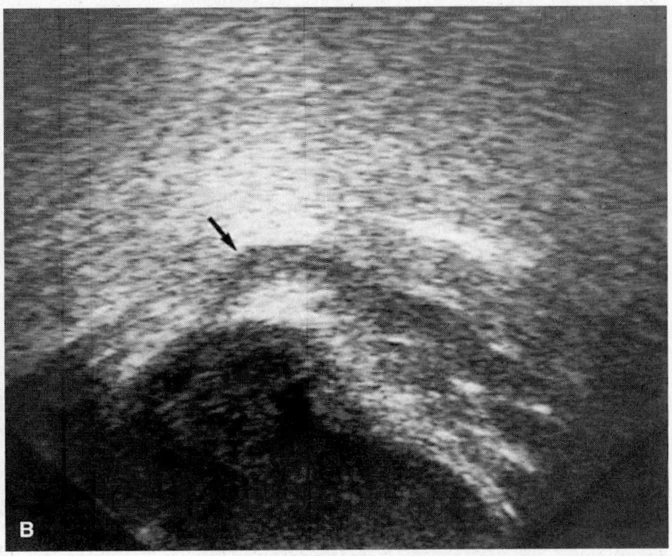

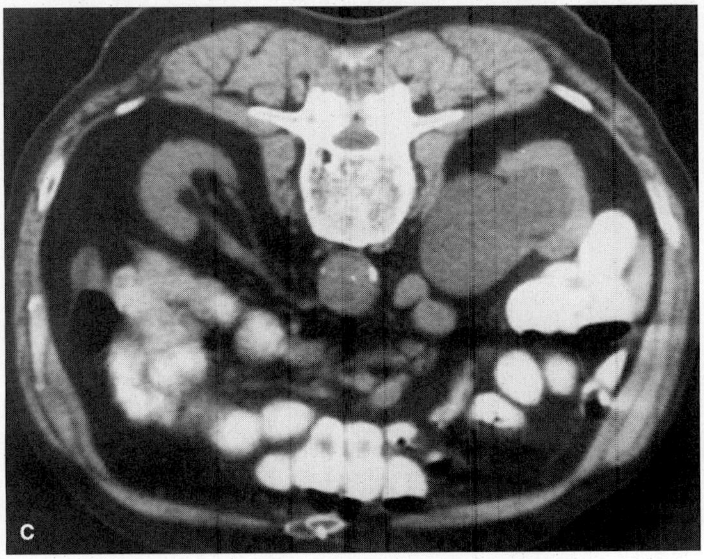

Figure 50.15. **A:** ultrasonogram, longitudinal section, of a chronically obstructed kidney caused by a large recurrent bladder neoplasm. The different echogenicity is indicated by the *arrow.* **B:** an ultrasonogram, longitudinal section, of the patient's bladder and ureter. The *arrow* denotes the widened ureter. **C:** the patient's computed tomogram, without contrast material, demonstrating chronic obstructive uropathy of the right kidney. The attenuation value of the widened pyelocalyceal system equals that of water. Note the thinning of the renal parenchyma, which is a feature of chronic obstruction.

provides an example of the sonographic findings in unilateral obstruction. In the proper hands, the diagnosis of a dilated calyceal system can be made in nearly 100% of patients. Exceptions would include patients with end-stage kidney failure or patients with high urine output states. It is important to remember that with this technique one demonstrates ureteral and calyceal dilation. Thus the diagnosis of obstruction is inferred, and further studies are indicated to determine if the dilation is a consequence of obstruction at some point along the urinary tract or is a consequence of reflux, urinary tract infection, or primary megaureter and megacalycosis.

Computed tomography scanning is also a very accurate technique for detecting widening of the collecting system. Contrast material is sometimes needed to establish that the fluid-filled structure is indeed the pyelocalyceal system rather than a parapelvic cyst. Results of such studies are shown in Figs. 50.15C and 50.16A and B. This technique may be used initially in the evaluation of the patient with suspected urinary tract obstruction from space-occupying lesions, particularly in the retroperitoneum. It provides additional information in that it can better characterize the nature and location of the obstructing lesion.

With this array of techniques it is seldom necessary to perform retrograde pyelography, which is associated with a significant morbidity, for diagnostic purposes. However, this technique remains important to characterize a lesion responsible for the calyceal widening or to relieve an obstruction by passing a ureteral catheter through a point of narrowing (Fig. 50.16C).

Although these techniques are helpful in making the diagnosis of ureteral dilation or hydronephrosis, it is frequently difficult to differentiate nonobstructing from obstructing causes of hydronephrosis. Radiologic evaluation may be helpful; a nonvisualized kidney is an extreme example of complete obstruction. Failure of the dye to pass through a point of narrowing produces additional information. Frequently, the diagnosis of obstruction may only be made in retrospect; that is, once the stenotic lesion is removed, renal function improves. The appearance and the duration of time for calyceal filling are important during intravenous pyelography. Frequently, however, such clinical approaches to the problem do not result in an answer. A test has been proposed in these situations. In this test (Whitaker test) either through a catheter placed in the renal pelvis or through a preexisting nephrostomy tube, a pressure

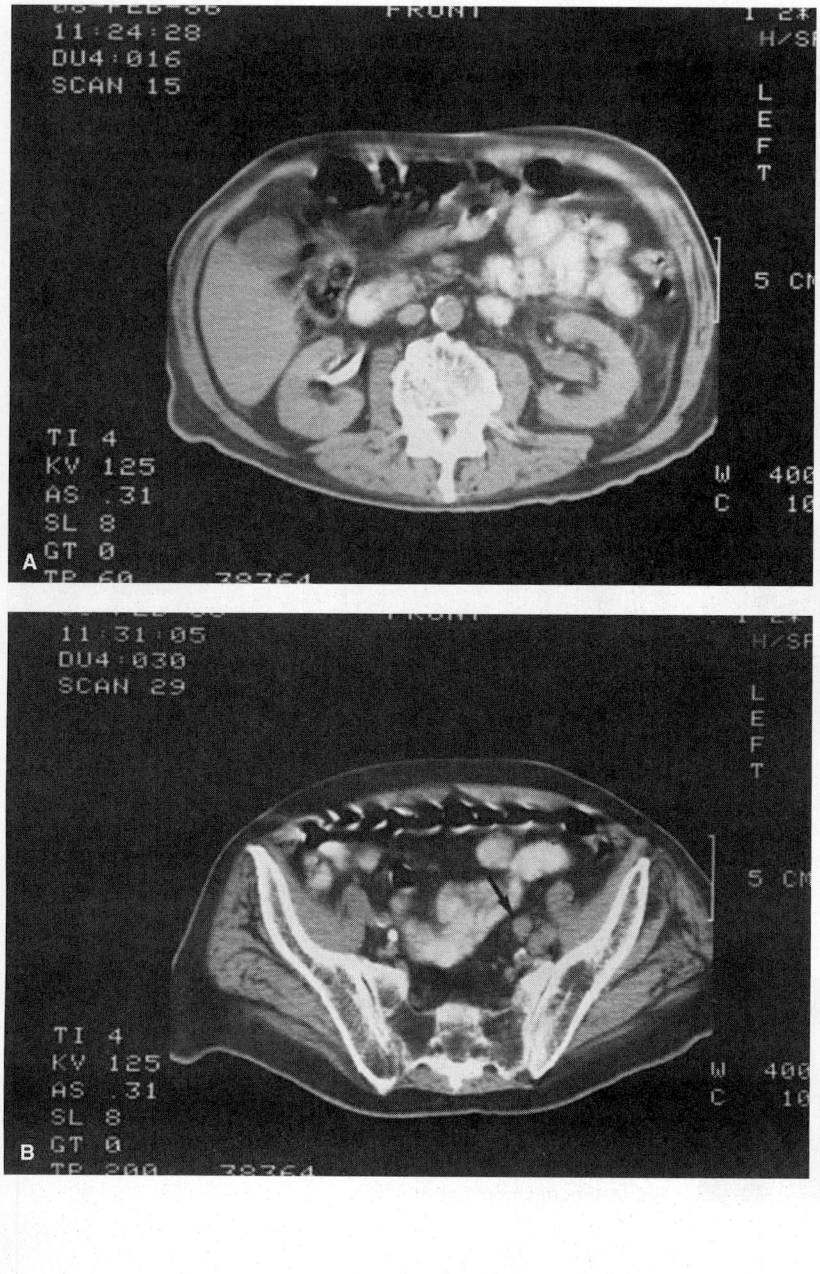

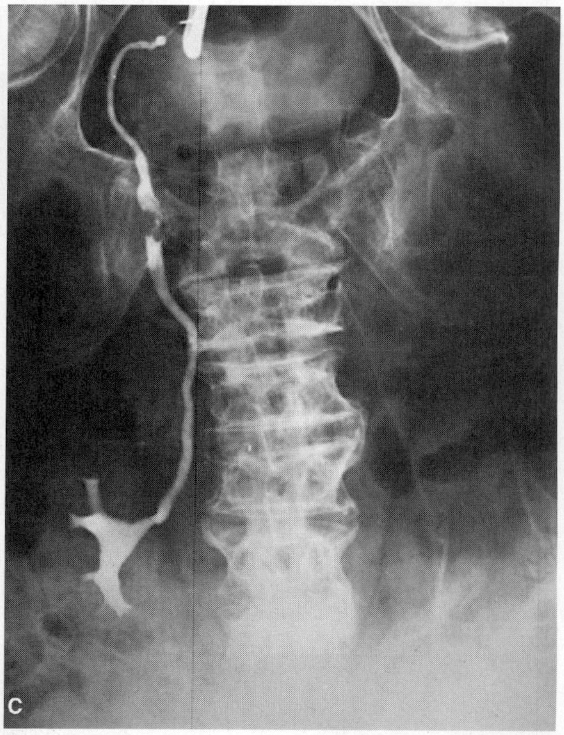

Figure 50.16. **A:** this computed tomogram demonstrates a mild hydronephrosis of the left kidney in a patient with hematuria and dull flank pain. **B:** the same computed tomogram of the level of the pelvis, showing a soft tissue density on the left (*arrow*). **C:** the retrograde pyelogram reveals an irregular mass as the cause of the symptoms, which was transitional cell carcinoma of the ureter.

gauge is placed and fluid is infused into the ureteral pelvis. Under normal circumstances the infusion rates may be increased significantly (15 ml/mm) with no real changes in or a leveling off of ureteral pressure. On the other hand, in the presence of obstruction, ureteral pressures will rise to abnormal levels and will not level off.

TREATMENT AND MANAGEMENT OF URINARY TRACT OBSTRUCTION

After establishing the diagnosis of urinary tract obstruction, a decision of when and how to decompress the obstruction needs to be made. High grade or total bilateral obstruction requires intervention as soon as possible. If clinical conditions permit, instrumentation or surgery should be carried out the same day. In some patients with bilateral obstruction and renal failure, preparatory dialysis therapy is necessary before any procedure aimed at overcoming or bypassing the obstruction is performed. In some patients with partial unilateral obstruction, especially those caused by stones, immediate intervention is not necessary. Attention should be given to pain relief, evaluation of renal function, follow-up of urine cultures to detect the presence of infection, and treatment of such infections. Repeat or serial intravenous pyelograms may allow evaluation of the progress in the location of stones. If infection is present together with obstruction, infection should be treated vigorously, and efforts to correct the obstruction should be made.

The treatment of calculi, the most common cause of ureteral obstruction, includes relief of pain, elimination of obstruction, and treatment of infection. Stones of less than 5 mm usually do not require surgical intervention or instrumentation because about 90% of these calculi will pass spontaneously. If the stones are in the range of 5 to 7 mm, however, only about half will pass, and stones larger than 7 mm usually are not passed spontaneously. High fluid intake to increase urine volume to at least 1.5 to 2 L daily may help mobilize the stone. The urine must be strained through a gauze sponge to recover the calculi for analysis.

Surgery or instrumentation for calyceal and/or ureteral calculi is indicated when there is persistent colic, urinary tract infection, complete obstruction, a calculus of more than 7 mm, or a calculus of smaller dimensions which has not moved despite a prudent period of observation and increased fluid intake.

Substantial changes in the approach to ureteral calculi have occurred in the last decade. Endourology refers to the closed controlled manipulation of the entire urinary tract. Radiologists or urologists can now place percutaneous nephrostomies and dilate the tract to as large as 12 mm. This has provided a direct conduit to the kidney for the removal of obstructing pelvic and upper ureteral calculi. Rigid or flexible endoscopes can be introduced through the nephrostomy tract to directly visualize and remove calculi of less than 1.5 cm in diameter. For larger stones, lithotriptor probes that use ultrasonic or electrohydraulic energy to disintegrate calculi have been used under direct visualization. Endourologic methods can be used to treat obstructing stones successfully in about 98% of patients. In addition, this approach shortens the hospital stay to 3 to 4 days and the convalescence period to only 4 to 7 days.

Extracorporeal shock wave lithotripsy involves the focusing of electrohydraulically or ultrasonically generated shock waves to disintegrate the stone. The method is effective for calculi of 7 to 15 mm; in 90% of patients, the stone will be disintegrated and all particulate matter will pass within a 3-month period. Morbidity is low. In selected individuals the procedure can be done on an outpatient basis. Most patients are back at their regular routine 2 to 3 days after shock wave therapy. The management of renal calculi with lithotripsy is discussed in detail in Chapter 99.

Calculi located distal to the pelvic brim can be approached from below. Calculi can be removed from the ureter using a variety of loops or baskets, and this procedure is successful in about 70% of patients. If it fails, dilation of the ureter or ultrasonic disintegration of the stone can be accomplished using the ureteroendoscope. Thus the need for open surgery for a distal ureteral calculus is rare.

Broad-spectrum antibiotics should be used when infections complicate renal calculi. The choice of antibiotic depends on the results of appropriate urine cultures and antibiotic sensitivities of the organisms. However, relief of obstruction is indispensable for antimicrobial therapy to be effective. Detailed discussion of renal stone disease is provided in Chapter 53.

Significant obstruction resulting from neoplastic, inflammatory, or neurologic disease must be treated aggressively because it is unlikely to remit spontaneously. A decision regarding urine diversion in patients with malignancy must be made on an individual basis.

In postobstructive diuresis, the management includes careful and adequate fluid replacement with frequent determinations of body weight and plasma and urine electrolyte levels. These latter measurements provide a rational basis for the amount and composition of the fluid to be administered. Urinary losses of fluid and electrolytes should be replaced only to the extent necessary to prevent hypovolemia, hypotension, hypokalemia, hypomagnesemia, and hyponatremia or hypernatremia.

Selected Readings

Berger PM, Diamond JR. Ureteral obstruction as a complication of renal transplantation: a review. *J Nephrol* 1998;11:20–23.
Causes of ureteral obstruction in renal allografts.

Butterworth PC, Horsburgh T, Veitch PS, et al. Urological complications in renal transplantation: impact of a change of technique. *Br J Urol* 1997;79(4):499–502.
The importance of surgical techniques in decreasing urologic complications in renal transplants.

Gillenwater JY. The pathophysiology of urinary tract obstruction. In: Walsh PC, Retik AB, Stamey TA, et al, eds. *Campbell's urology*, 6th ed. Philadelphia: WB Saunders, 1992:499–532.
An excellent chapter on the pathology, physiology, and experimental aspects of urinary tract obstruction with numerous references.

Klahr S. Obstructive uropathy. In: Kassirer JP, Greene HL, eds. *Current therapy in adult medicine*, 4th ed. St. Louis: Mosby 1997:1135–1140.
A detailed account of therapeutic options in patients with obstructive uropathy.

Klahr S. Obstructive nephropathy: pathophysiology and management. In: Schrier RW, ed. *Renal and electrolyte disorders*, 5th ed. Philadelphia: Lippincott-Raven, 1997:544–589.
A comprehensive and up-to date chapter on the clinical and physiologic aspects of obstructive uropathy.

Klahr S. Nephrology forum: obstructive nephropathy. *Kidney Int* 1998;54:286–300.
An up-to date discussion of the mechanisms underlying the tubulointerstitial inflammation and fibrosis of obstructive nephropathy.

Klahr S, Miller S. Acute oliguria. *N Engl J Med* 1998;228:671–675.
A review of causes of acute renal failure, its complications, and its management.

Resnick MI, Kursh ED. Extrinsic obstruction o the ureteral. In: Walsh PC, Retik AB, Stamey TA, et al., eds. *Campbell's urology*, 6th ed. Philadelphia: WB Saunders, 1992:522–569.
Very well-written description of the causes of extrinsic obstruction of the ureter.

Morrissey JJ, Ishidoya S, McCracken R, et al. Nitric oxide generation ameliorates the tubulointerstitial fibrosis of obstructive nephropathy. *J Am Soc Nephrol* 1996;7:2202–2212.
A description of the role of nitric oxide in obstructive nephropathy.

Reyes A, Martin D, Settle S, et al. EDRF role in renal function and blood pressure of normal rats and rats with obstructive uropathy. *Kidney Int* 1992;41:403–413.
A demonstration of the role of nitric oxide (endothelial-derived relaxing factor or EDRF) in the pathophysiology of obstructive nephrology.

Shoskes DA, Hanbury D, Cranston D, et al. Urological complications in 1000 consecutive renal transplant recipients. *J Urol* 1995:153:18–21.
An analyses of urologic complications in renal transplant recipients.

CHAPTER 51

Renal Papillary Necrosis

Garabed Eknoyan

Renal papillary necrosis (RPN) is a complication which develops in the course of a variety of systemic diseases (Table 51.1) that are associated with changes in the renal parenchyma in general, but in which the injury is more severe in the inner zone of the renal medulla. The basic lesion is a tubulointerstitial nephritis accompanied by compromised medullary blood flow that ultimately results in a focal or diffuse necrosis of various segments of the renal medulla. The clinicopathologic syndrome that results from this necrotic process has been recognized for well over a century and is referred to by terms such as "renal medullary necrosis," "renal necrotizing papillitis," "necrotizing pyelonephritis," and "papillary necrosis." However, the necrosis rarely involves the whole medulla. It is almost always limited to the inner zone of the medulla and often is restricted only to the papilla. Furthermore, it can develop in the absence of infection. Therefore of the different nomenclatures that have been proposed, the more appropriate term to use for this entity is *renal papillary necrosis*.

RPN has been classified into two forms, depending on the localization of the necrotic process (Fig. 51.1): a *medullary form,* in which the focal areas of the innermost medullary regions are necrotic but the fornices and papillary tip remain viable, and a *papillary form,* in which the calyceal fornices and the entire papillary tip are destroyed. An alternative nomenclature proposed is *total papillary necrosis* for the papillary form and *partial papillary necrosis* for the medullary form. Most forms of RPN start as isolated small foci of necrosis *in situ*, which with persistent injury coalesce and progress to RPN.

The exact incidence of RPN is unknown. The frequency with which the lesion is encountered at autopsy varies from one geographical region to another. In the United States, its reported incidence in large autopsy series is 0.16% to 0.26%. This is lower than that encountered in England, where its reported incidence is in the range of 0.8% to 1.3%. The highest rates are reported from Australia, where its reported incidence is about 4%.

TABLE 51.1 Clinical Conditions Associated with Renal Papillary Necrosis

Diabetes mellitus
Urinary tract obstruction
Pyelonephritis
Analgesic nephropathy
Sickle cell hemoglobinopathy
Renal transplant rejection
Infants with dehydration, hypoxia, and jaundice
Miscellaneous (see text)

Although RPN does occur in newborns and infants, the disease is principally one of older individuals, the average reported age of patients being 55 years, with nearly half of cases occurring in those older than 40 years of age. The lesion is uncommon in individuals younger than 40 years of age, except for those with sickle cell hemoglobinopathy in whom the disease occurs in a younger age group and shows the expected racial limitation to those of African-American origin.

PATHOGENESIS

The fact that the necrosis is anatomically limited to the distal segments of the renal pyramids reflects the importance of local predisposing factors unique to this region. The blood supply of the renal papilla is provided from two sources: the vasa rectae and the branches of the ureteric arteries, which supply the renal pelvis and adventitia of the minor calyces. The importance of this latter source of blood supply is reflected in the pathologic finding that the terminal portion of the affected pyramids may be viable when the rest is necrotic, presumably because of the intact blood supply from the vessels perfusing the minor calyces, which are not subject to the structural and functional changes that affect the vasa rectae.

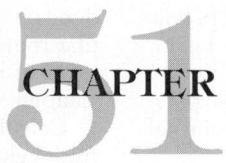

The major sources of medullary blood flow are the vasa rectae, which descend side by side, forming vascular bundles connected to each other by capillary plexuses. At the base of the pyramid, or the outer medulla, the vascular bundles are widest and the capillary plexuses richest. During the course of their descent, the vascular bundles gradually decrease in number and size such that at the tip of the papilla only single or a few communicating vessels remain. The diminution in vasculature is coupled with a 3- to 4-fold increase in interstitial space in the inner zone of the medulla relative to the cortex and outer medulla. The reduction in inner medullary blood flow is visually evident from the lighter, near whitish color, of this area compared with the beefy red hue of the cortex and outer zone of the medulla. Especially important is the fact that much of the medullary blood flow serves the countercurrent multiplier function of the vasa rectae. Nutrient blood flow is supplied by regional smaller terminal vessels that arise from the vasa rectae, whose size and frequency gradually diminish from the outer medulla to the papillary tips. The fact that the countercurrent multiplier function of the vasa rectae renders the partial pressure of oxygen lower in deeper parts of the medulla further compromises the tenuous nutrient supply to the deeper zones. The obliteration of even a few of the nutrient capillaries can result in foci of ischemic necrosis. Thus it is the relatively poor nutrient blood sup-

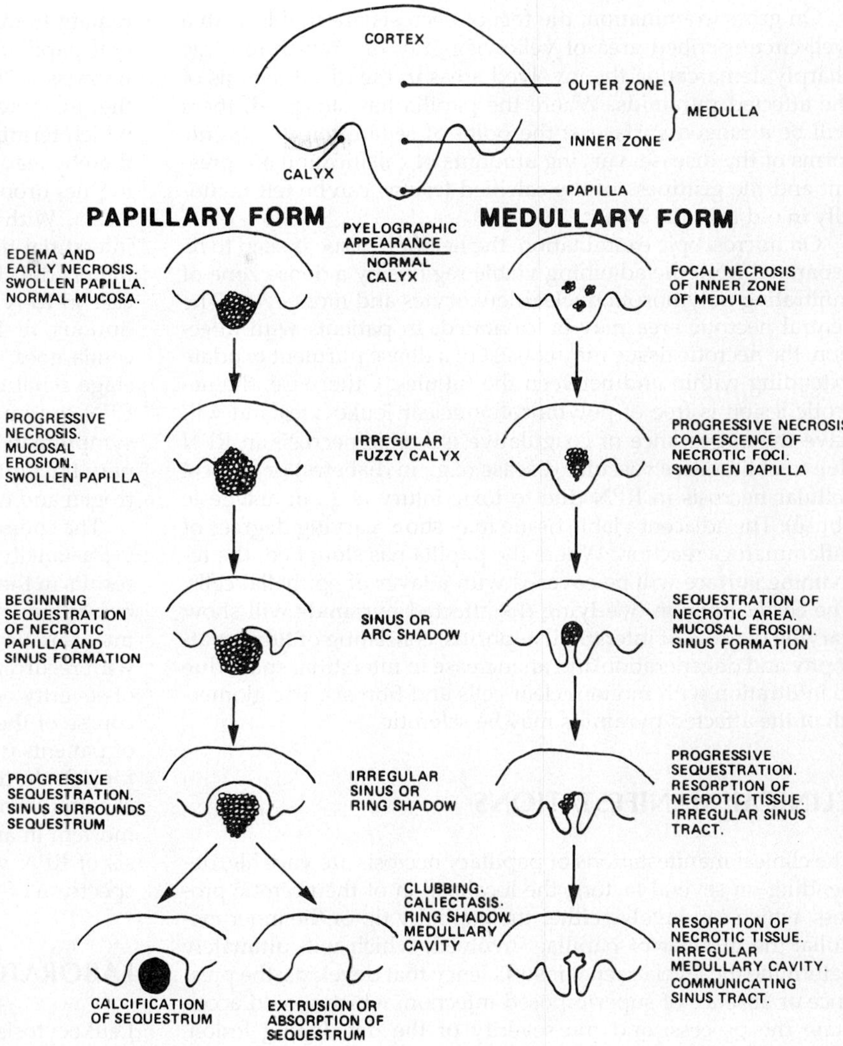

Figure 51.1. Features of the various stages of development of the papillary and medullary form of renal papillary necrosis.

ply to the papillary tip, compared with the remainder of the kidney and pyramids, which renders this anatomical segment particularly susceptible to diseases affecting the renal vasculature (arteriosclerosis, thrombosis, and inflammation) and, hence, contributes to the central role of ischemia in the development of papillary necrosis in specific clinical settings: the elderly, the diabetic, and those with sickle hemoglobinopathy and severe cases of vasculitis.

In addition, the medullary blood flow is dependent on the local generation of prostanoids (prostaglandin and thromboxane). Reduction of their synthesis by cyclooxygenase inhibitors [nonsteroidal antiinflammatory drugs (NSAIDs)] renders the papillae susceptible to ischemic necrosis when NSAIDs are consumed habitually. A condition aggravated by preexisting vascular diseases that render the papilla more dependent on prostanoids for maintaining its blood supply, such as diabetes, sickle hemoglobinopathy, and cirrhosis of the liver. It is in these clinical conditions that even a brief exposure to NSAIDs can cause RPN. This is perhaps best exemplified by the occurrence of RPN in children treated with NSAIDs, which is in sharp contrast to that due to analgesic nephropathy, which requires prolonged exposure and is not encountered in children.

Another local phenomenon that contributes to the localization of injury to the papilla is the maximal hypertonicity achieved at its tip. The function of the medullary countercurrent multiplier to achieve the medullary hypertonicity essential to normal maintenance of water balance becomes a detriment when potentially nephrotoxic agents are ingested habitually. Thus it is the higher concentration of analgesics and their metabolites at the papillary tip that accounts for analgesic nephropathy being a leading cause of RPN (Chapter 47, Part 5). Also, hypertonicity is known to compromise normal leukocyte function. Medullary hypertonicity could well account for an impairment of the ability to combat infection in necrotic foci of the papilla, rendering them all the more susceptible to bacterial loads that otherwise may be eradicated relatively easier at another site.

PATHOLOGY (SEE ATLAS OF RENAL PATHOLOGY, CHAPTER 109)

In its early phases, the necrosis appears to involve a few papillae to which RPN may remain localized, or it might become progressive and gradually involve a greater number of papillae in one or both kidneys. The lesions usually, but not invariably, involve both kidneys. RPN is bilateral in three-fourths of the cases reported in the literature. In patients in whom one kidney was involved at the time of first examination, RPN develops in the other kidney over a period of 1 to 4 years. This is not unexpected considering the systemic nature of the conditions usually associated with RPN (Table 51.1). Obviously, the lesions will be unilateral in patients in whom the principal predisposing factors, such as obstruction or infection, are localized to one kidney.

On gross examination, the foci of necrosis are friable with a well-circumscribed area of yellowish-gray or grayish-red hue sharply demarcating the involved areas in the distal regions of the affected pyramids. Where the papilla has sloughed, there will be a ragged surface at the point of separation. In chronic forms of the disease, varying amounts of calcification are present and the grittiness of the calcified lesions can be felt manually in old necrotic areas.

On microscopic examination, the necrotic tissue is seen to be separated from the adjoining viable regions by a dense zone of infiltrating polymorphonuclear leukocytes and monocytes. The central necrotic area may be cavitated. In patients with infection, the necrotic tissue may consist of a dense purulent exudate extending within and between the tubules. Otherwise, the necrotic lesion is free of polymorphonuclear leukocytes and will have the appearance of coagulative ischemic necrosis in RPN due to obliterative vascular disease (e.g., in diabetes) or of focal cellular necrosis in RPN due to toxic injury (e.g., in analgesic abuse). The adjacent viable tissue may show varying degrees of inflammatory reaction. Where the papilla has sloughed, the remaining surface will be covered with a layer of epithelial cells. The cortical region overlying the affected pyramids will show varying degrees of interstitial nephritis, consisting of tubular atrophy and degeneration and an increase in interstitial space due to infiltration with mononuclear cells and fibrosis. The glomeruli of the affected pyramids may be sclerotic.

CLINICAL MANIFESTATIONS

The clinical manifestations of papillary necrosis are variable, depending on several factors: the localization of the necrotic process, which can involve either the papillary tip or the inner medulla; the number of papillae involved, which will ultimately determine the level of renal insufficiency that develops; the presence or absence of superimposed infection, which would accelerate the process; and the severity of the developing lesion, which would determine the course of the disease as either acute or chronic.

As a rule, the necrotic lesions are well demarcated and once they develop form a sequestrum that may be sloughed and excreted into the urine, be reabsorbed leaving a sinus or cavity at their site, or remain *in situ* to become calcified and form a nidus for calculus formation (Fig. 51.1). Sinus and cavity formation is more common in the medullary form of RPN, whereas sloughing is more common in the papillary form. The passage of the sloughed papillae may be associated with lumbar pain, ureteral colic, and hematuria, which is clinically indistinguishable from that due to other causes of colic of the urinary system. Alternatively, the necrotic tissue and stagnation of urine in the cavities may become a nidus of infection. Consequently, in patients with symptomatic RPN (about 20% to 25%) the clinical manifestations are those of either nephrolithiasis or pyelonephritis. Fever and chills are the major presenting symptoms in more than two-thirds of these patients. Flank pain and dysuria are present in about half of the patients, and gross hematuria is present in less than one-fifth of them. Oliguria is an infrequent finding, being present in less than 10% of patients. The voiding of necrotic papillae, which may be recovered in the urine, is an infrequent occurrence (less than 5%), but one that can be diagnostic.

While some loss of renal function is expected to develop as a consequence of any renal parenchymal necrosis, renal failure is not common in RPN. Each human kidney contains an average of 8 pyramids, with a range of 4 to 12 pyramids per kidney. Thus even in the presence of bilateral RPN affecting one or two papillae on each side, sufficient unaffected renal lobules will remain to maintain reasonable renal function. Even when several papillae in each kidney are involved, the localization of necrosis to the inner zone of the medulla results in the loss of the juxtamedullary nephrons only; the cortical nephrons, which terminate in the outer zone of the medulla, are spared, thereby leaving in the affected lobules a multitude of functioning nephrons that are capable of maintaining normal homeostasis. With the continuous loss of several papillae, diffuse interstitial fibrosis will occur and renal insufficiency will ultimately develop and progress to renal failure. This is usually the case in RPN due to analgesic abuse, in which the insult is continuous, or RPN due to diabetes, in which chronic hyperglycemia goes uncontrolled; in both of these progression to end-stage renal disease is common. However, most patients with RPN continue to have normal renal function and patients with symptomatic RPN have acute exacerbations of renal colic or urinary tract infection, but no evidence of abnormal blood urea nitrogen and creatinine concentrations.

The course of the papillary necrosis that develops is variable. Occasionally, it may present as an acute devastating illness that results in the rapid demise of the patient due to septicemia well before the development of chronic renal insufficiency. Rarely, it may pursue a protracted clinical course of months and years, with recurrent episodes of acute symptoms of different degrees of severity occurring at intervals of varying lengths during the course of the disease. In the third and by far the largest group of patients (more than 75%), the disease may be totally asymptomatic. In these, the RPN is an incidental finding observed at excretory urography or an unexpected lesion found post mortem in an otherwise normal individual in whom a diagnosis of RPN was never suspected. Between these extremes is a spectrum of varying clinical courses that RPN may pursue.

LABORATORY FINDINGS AND DIAGNOSIS

Leukocytosis and azotemia are present in 50% to 60% of patients with symptomatic RPN. The azotemia usually is only modest, and uremia is rarely present, even when the lesions are bilateral. As documented experimentally, a finding more common than azotemia is the inability to concentrate the urine maximally, due to the damaged inner zone of the medulla where maximal urine concentration is normally attained. A history of polyuria and nocturia can be elicited in such patients.

Proteinuria, usually only modest, is the most common abnormality, being present in up to 80% of patients. Pyuria is present in 60% to 80% of patients, microscopic hematuria in 20% to 40%, and gross hematuria in some 20% of them. The hematuria may be massive, and cases of exsanguinating hemorrhage requiring nephrectomy have been reported. The urine culture is positive in about three-fourths of patients.

Because the diagnosis of RPN can be made on finding portions of the necrotic papillae in the urine, a deliberate search should be made for papillary fragments in the urine collected during or after attacks of colicky pain. This can be done best by straining the urine through a piece of gauze or filter paper and subjecting the residue to microscopic examination. In the absence of a tissue diagnosis, either of a voided necrotic papilla or of the kidneys at autopsy, the radiographic demonstration of the deformities caused by papillary necrosis is the best method available for a reliable diagnosis. Unfortunately, the radiologic changes do not become apparent until the papillae are shrunk or sequestered (Fig. 51.1). Actually, even when necrotic papillae are passed in the urine, radiograph films may remain normal. Although characteristic features of RPN have been described on ultrasound and computed tomographic imaging of the kidneys, excretory urography remains the most useful examination for the early diagnosis of RPN before the onset of renal scarring and atrophy. At earlier stages of the disease, ultrasonography is of limited value, unless obstructive uropathy is present secondary to a sloughed papilla lodged in the pelvis or urinary tract. Computed tomography is more useful because of its ability to detect early papillary calcification.

The radiologic changes of RPN are in general independent of the associated underlying primary disease and are attributable to the contrast material penetrating the regions separating necrotic areas from healthy tissue or of the spaces that develop as a result of parenchymal loss due to necrosis (Fig. 51.1). No changes will be detected early in the course of the developing lesion, but serial radiologic studies to determine relative and progressive changes can be of considerable value in establishing the diagnosis. Calyceal haziness or irregularity and failure of contrast material filling of the minor calyces are the earliest manifestations of RPN, reflecting swelling and irregularity of the involved pyramids. The subsequent sequestration of the necrotic papillae results in early cavitation and sinus formation, with the trapped contrast material providing the image of a sinus tract of varying size and shape (straight, crescentic, or arc shadow) reflecting the separation and incipient detachment of the sequestrum. The typical so-called "ring shadows," caused by the detached papilla lying in the contrast material–filled cavity, have been noted in more than 50% of patients in the presence of large papillary or medullary necrotic cavities. After the sloughing of the sequestrum, a cavity will become readily apparent. The medullary cavities are either rounded or oval while the papillary ones are triangular in appearance, with the base showing a crescentiform bulge. Obstruction of urinary drainage by the sloughed papilla will result in hydronephrotic changes. Enlargement of the medullary cavities and shrinkage of the papillary cavities will result in their merging with the adjoining calyces, giving the club-shaped appearance and caliectasis similar to those seen with pyelonephritis. Concretions will be seen in necrotic papillae that develop calcification; these will usually visualize as a radiolucent nucleus. The affected kidney is of normal size in one-quarter to one-third of patients. However, most kidneys will show a variable decrease in size, particularly in progressive disease, depending on the number of papillae destroyed. As the kidneys shrink, the cavities will also shrink in size. At these later stages computed tomography is superior to excretory urography in the diagnosis of RPN. Changes in the ureter and bladder are not common and when present are due to superimposed complicating infections or are secondary to the underlying primary infection that might have caused the RPN.

DISEASES ASSOCIATED WITH RPN

Necrosis of the renal papillae was first described as a complication of obstruction. The papillary necrosis was attributed to the increased pelvic pressure that resulted in flattening of the papillae, with the consequent angulation of the medullary blood vessels depriving the papillae of blood supply and resulting in their ischemic necrosis. Shortly thereafter, diabetes mellitus and infection were identified as the two other major causes of RPN. These three conditions—diabetes mellitus, urinary tract obstruction, and infection—to which RPN was attributed by the turn of the 20th century remained the principal causes of RPN to be considered for the next 50 years. Over the subsequent five decades, additional conditions associated with RPN have been recognized (Table 51.1), with analgesic abuse nephropathy and sickle cell hemoglobinopathy emerging as the two other leading causes of papillary necrosis. With few exceptions, patients with RPN will have a urinary tract infection. This had led to the consideration of infection as a primary cause of RPN and to the suggestion that RPN is basically a form of acute pyelonephritis whose natural course is altered by the associated diseases (diabetes mellitus or obstruction). However, while there is no doubt that urinary tract infection occurs in a majority of patients with RPN, it is not a uniform finding in all patients. In addition, in considering infection as a cause of RPN, it should be taken into account that infection itself represents a complication of papillary necrosis. Specifically, the infection develops after the primary underlying disease has initiated local injury to the renal medulla. In either case, infection, if not the cause, is a common and important finding that undoubtedly contributes to the progression and symptomatology of RPN. Unfortunately, this had led to the concept that RPN was a form of pyelonephritis, and of equating it with "necrotizing pyelonephritis." To consider RPN as an extension of severe pyelonephritis is simplistic. In patients with florid acute pyelonephritis, necrosis of the papilla does not occur. To classify RPN alongside pyelonephritis is archaic and has detracted from the recognition of RPN as a distinct entity that can develop in the absence of pyelonephritis. Perhaps the differentiation of RPN in the presence of infection from pyelonephritis is merely one of semantics. It is essential to realize, however, that RPN is a distinct syndrome that is different from acute pyelonephritis and can develop in the absence of infection.

Diabetes mellitus remains the most frequent condition associated with RPN in the United States, accounting for some 50% to 60% of cases in reported major series. This is in contrast to the 4% to 12% incidence of diabetes as the cause of RPN reported from Australia and the Scandinavian countries, where analgesic abuse is the predominant cause of papillary necrosis. The high frequency with which RPN occurs in diabetics can be appreciated from its finding in 2.7% to 7.2% of autopsies of patients with diabetes mellitus, whereas in nondiabetic patients its incidence at autopsy is less than 0.3%. Radiologic evidence of RPN has been reported in as many as 23.7% of patients with longstanding insulin-dependent diabetes mellitus. Diabetics with recurrent episodes of urinary tract infection or an acute infection of the kidney are particularly prone to development of RPN. In one series of 859 autopsied cases, RPN was found in one of every four diabetic patients with coexistent fulminant acute pyelonephritis. In diabetics, the lesion characteristically affects elderly women, with a female-to-male preponderance as high as 5:1. In diabetes, as in other causes of RPN, renal function can remain normal, and RPN can develop in the absence of other evidence of diabetic nephropathy. However, the odds of progression to end-stage renal disease due to RPN are greater in diabetics, and the 10 year survival of diabetics with RPN, independent of renal outcome, is worse than that of diabetics without RPN.

Obstructive uropathy has been reported as the cause of RPN in 15% to 40% of cases in major reviews of papillary necrosis. The general pattern of obstructive uropathy as a contributory factor to the development of RPN appears to be decreasing in frequency. This may be due to improvements in the diagnosis and therapy of obstruction, which have resulted in its earlier recognition on ultrasonography, and more effective treatment of coexistent infections with antibiotics. Obstruction as the cause of RPN is as much as three times more common in males than in females. This preponderance of males among nondiabetic patients with RPN has been a uniform finding in all series, reflecting the increased incidence of obstruction as a predisposing factor in elderly males.

Pyelonephritis, with or without coexistent obstruction or diabetes, can result in RPN. It has been noted as a cause of

RPN in 65% to 100% of cases in major reported series. In 1,023 instances of acute pyelonephritis among 32,000 consecutive necropsies, 21 were found to have bilateral or unilateral papillary necrosis. This incidence of RPN in 2.1% of patients with acute pyelonephritis is about eightfold higher than that encountered in the general population, but lower than that reported in diabetics. The development of papillary necrosis appears to be dependent on the severity of the inflammatory changes and the presence of coexistent predisposing diseases (obstruction and diabetes). It may involve only one or all the papillae and usually occurs after recurrent episodes of infection. There has been no consistency in the organisms implicated although, not unexpectedly, *Escherichia coli* is the most frequently reported organism.

Analgesic abuse accounts for about 15% to 25% of cases of RPN reported in the United States. This is in contrast to figures reported from Australia and the Scandinavian countries where analgesic abuse not only is the predominant cause of RPN, accounting for up to 70% to 90% of cases, but also is a leading cause of end-stage renal disease. Initially recognized as a cause of chronic tubulointerstitial nephritis, the principal pathologic lesion of analgesic abuse nephropathy has emerged to be that of RPN. The early changes are those of necrosis of the long loops of Henle and the vasa rectae, corresponding to the site of concentration of acetaminophen, phenacetin, and aspirin, the principal ingredients of analgesic mixtures that cause analgesic nephropathy. The development of necrosis is preceded by a decrease and disappearance of the interstitial cells and a reduction in medullary blood flow. However, unlike the coagulative necrosis seen in RPN due to ischemic lesions, those that develop in patients who abuse analgesics are those of tissue necrosis. Review of concomitant drug intake is important, because a possible contributing role in the development of nephropathy in analgesic abusers has been ascribed to a tendency for volume depletion due to the concurrent use of diuretics, cardiac glycosides, antihypertensives, and laxatives. The majority of these patients are women, with a female-to-male preponderance of 6:1. As a group, in analgesic abusers the progression to end-stage renal disease associated with RPN is second only to that of diabetes. Further discussion of analgesic abuse nephropathy is found in Chapter 47, Part 5. RPN has also been reported in individuals who are habitual users of NSAIDs (see Chapter 47, Part 3). This is due to yet another unique feature of the medullary vasculature, that is, its greater dependence on the production of vasodilator prostanoids. On a comparative mole per tissue weight basis the ratio of prostaglandin synthetase activity of the papilla to that of the medulla and cortex is 100:10:1. As such, agents that inhibit cyclooxygenase activity cause a critical compromise of the blood flow of this relatively poorly perfused region, especially in the presence of preexisting vascular lesions (e.g., in elderly patients with arteriosclerosis) and coexistent high renin states (e.g., in those with congestive heart failure, cirrhosis of the liver, or nephrotic syndrome).

The development of RPN in patients with sickle cell hemoglobinopathy was not noted until 1963. The obliterative vascular lesions that develop in the medulla of these patients result in the loss of the vasa rectae, a reduction in renal blood flow to the medulla, and ultimately an ischemic necrosis of the papilla. The incidence of radiologically demonstrable RPN in patients with sickle (S) hemoglobinopathies has been reported to be as high as 50% to 65%, independent of whether or not the patients had any symptoms. As a rule, women outnumber men in a ratio of 2:1. Urographic changes of RPN have been reported in patients with SS, SA, and S thalassemia. Typically, the RPN develops slowly in patients with S hemoglobinopathy and usually affects one papilla at a time, with the lesions being primarily those of the medullary form of RPN (Fig. 51.1). Additional discussion of the renal disease associated with sickle cell hemoglobinopathy is found in Chapter 43, Part 1.

The transplanted kidney appears to be as vulnerable to the development of RPN as is the native kidney. RPN has been diagnosed as early as the seventh day and as late as 78 months following transplantation, the average being about 28 months after transplantation. Approximately two-thirds of these cases of RPN have occurred in cadaveric transplants and the remainder in those of living-related donor kidneys. The tubulointerstitial nephritis and vascular obliteration that develops during the process of chronic rejection also affects the medulla, resulting in an ischemic necrosis of the papilla. In general, however, papillary necrosis in the renal allograft develops secondary to the usual causes of RPN (analgesic abuse, diabetes, and obstruction) and less commonly secondary to allograft rejection.

Cirrhosis of the liver has been implicated as a cause of RPN. Critical review, however, reveals only a few cases of RPN in which the underlying disease was only chronic alcoholism and cirrhosis of the liver. The possibility of another disease, particularly diabetes, must always be ruled out before implicating the liver. It is quite likely that the complicating factors associated with cirrhosis, such as sepsis, severe dehydration, jaundice, or analgesic abuse, may be critical in precipitating RPN in some patients. Evidence that chronic hyperbilirubinemia may play a contributory role is supported by the increased occurrence of RPN in the Gunn rat with a congenital defect of glucuronosyltransferase activity and consequent hyperbilirubinemia.

RPN occurs less commonly in children. The usual predisposing factors of RPN in adults are chronic conditions that are not seen in infants and children, in whom the leading causes of RPN are hypoxia, dehydration, and septicemia.

Other conditions that have been implicated as causes of RPN, primarily in isolated case reports, are systemic lupus erythematosus, renal vein thrombosis, cryoglobulinemia, arteritis, pancreatitis, hypotensive shock, rapidly progressive glomerulonephritis, renal amyloidosis, Wegener's granulomatosis, renal malacoplakia, and aplastic anemia and use of contrast media.

Actually, more than one of the individual causative factors discussed is usually present in most patients with RPN. The pathogenetic process may be viewed as an overlap phenomenon, with a combination of more than one of the conditions listed in Table 51.1 operating in concert to produce RPN. In such a scheme, whereas each condition alone may result in RPN, the coexistence of more than one predisposing condition in any one subject increases the risk for RPN. This seems to be the case for well over half of patients with RPN (Fig. 51.2) The contribution of each of the coexistent conditions to the pathogenesis of papillary necrosis would be expected to differ among individual patients and at different times during the course of the disease. Experimental evidence for an overlap phenomenon can be adduced from studies in the Gunn rat with congenital hyperbilirubinemia. RPN occurs spontaneously in these animals secondary to the deposition of unconjugated bilirubin in the tips of the renal papillae. The administration of analgesics to these animals results in acceleration of the papillary necrotic process and occurs at doses of analgesics lower than that necessary to induce RPN in other strains of rats. Similarly, in experimental animals with unilateral obstruction that are injected intravenously with *E. coli*, RPN develops only on the obstructed side, providing further evidence for the multifactorial pathogenesis of RPN. Thus whereas each of the conditions listed in Table 51.1 can cause RPN, the coexistence of more than one of them in any one individual significantly increases the risk of development

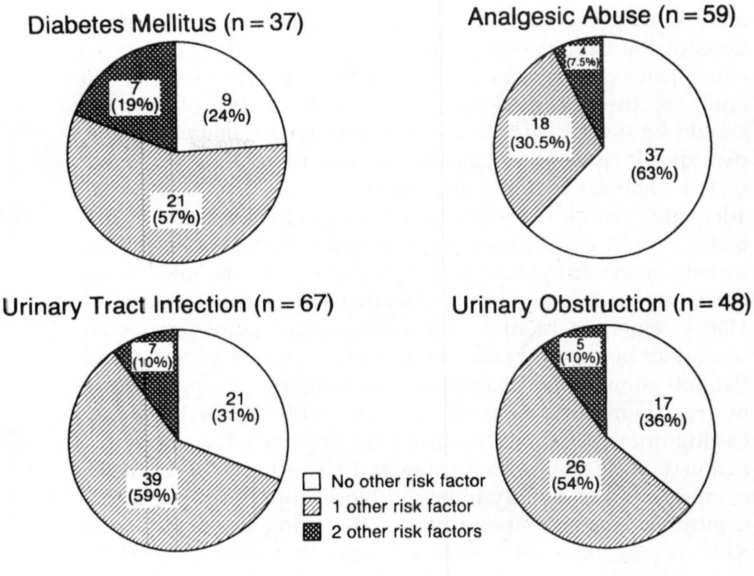

Figure 51.2. Proportion of single or combined risk factors for renal papillary necrosis of the four principal causes of this condition in a series of 165 cases. (Reproduced with permission from Griffin MD, Larson S. Renal papillary necrosis—a sixteen-year clinical experience. *J Am Soc Nephrol* 1995;6:248–256.)

of RPN. In fact, the natural course of RPN sets the stage for an overlap phenomenon, with necrosis predisposing to infection and sloughing to obstruction. In any case, whenever a diagnosis of RPN is made, a quest for more than one of the causative conditions should be made rather than attributing RPN to the first condition identified.

DIFFERENTIAL DIAGNOSIS

The differential diagnosis of RPN includes medullary cystic disease, reflux nephropathy, acute or chronic pyelonephritis, calculus with renal colic, renal tuberculosis, renal tumors, and in fulminant disease any cause of acute renal failure. Medullary cystic disease shows symmetrical involvement and usually presents with severe reduction in renal function. Reflux nephropathy will usually show extensive involvement of the ureters, which is clearly demonstrable radiologically, and a childhood history of reflux. Acute pyelonephritis without necrosis generally is less severe clinically than RPN with infection. Chronic pyelonephritis usually requires a long course of fairly characteristic recurrent history before the development of the calyceal changes that mimic RPN. The passage of a renal calculus may be confused with the passage of a sloughed necrotic papilla. Histologic examination of the excreted foreign body and radiologic examination of the urinary tract can be useful in differentiating RPN from calculus. The necrotic papillae when visualized have a radiolucent center. The differential diagnosis between renal tuberculosis and RPN can be difficult in the absence of a culture results positive for acid-fast organisms. The presence of urinary tract scarring favors a diagnosis of tuberculosis, because chronic seeding by mycobacteria almost always results in a characteristic picture of the outflow tract. By the same token, a history of symptoms or physical findings of epididymitis indicate tuberculosis. The fact that RPN is usually bilateral can be used to rule out renal tumors. Also, complaints of acute symptoms (infection or colic) favor RPN in contrast to tumors or tuberculosis.

Acute renal failure due to acute tubular necrosis must always be ruled out in those patients with RPN who are seen with oliguria and rapidly progressive deterioration of renal function. The history of predisposing factors, urine examination, and ultrasonography can be extremely useful in the diagnosis.

COURSE AND PROGNOSIS

The course and prognosis of RPN will depend on the primary underlying condition responsible for the development of the lesion. As discussed under laboratory findings, even in the presence of bilateral RPN affecting more than one papilla in each kidney, sufficient unaffected renal lobules with intact nephrons remain to maintain adequate or near normal renal function. In only some 10% of patients does RPN progress to end-stage renal disease, the majority of whom are diabetics or analgesic abusers. Symptomatic RPN can occur following institution of dialytic replacement therapy in these patients. Apart from the primary causes of RPN (diabetes and analgesic abuse), infection appears to be a major factor affecting outcome. Actually, patients with RPN who show rapid deterioration due to infected papillae will usually succumb to acute fulminant episodes of infection and septicemia well before the development of renal failure. The pessimism, perpetuated in the older literature, that surrounds the diagnosis in this latter group of patients does not appear to be entirely warranted for all patients with RPN. Early diagnosis, specific antibiotic therapy to control infection, and maintenance of adequate urine drainage will reduce mortality and improve the prognosis.

The conditions with which RPN has been associated are, in general, chronic systemic diseases, and the course of the associated RPN, therefore, can be progressive. The gradual involvement of an increasing number of papillae will ultimately result in some loss of renal function causing varying degrees of renal insufficiency. Of greater concern is the impact of RPN on life expectancy, independent of the level of renal insufficiency. The development of RPN does seem to affect adversely the survival rates of such individuals, in whom the 5- and 10-year mortality rate is twofold greater than in the absence of RPN. Hence, early detection and proper management are important even if there is no significant loss of renal function.

MANAGEMENT

In the absence of a specific etiologic factor that can be avoided (e.g., analgesics) or surgically corrected (e.g., obstruction), the therapy of RPN is focused on the associated complications. Control and eradication of any systemic or urinary tract infection are essential. Urine samples should be cultured and all infections of the urinary tract should be considered as active pyelonephritic processes and treated with a long course of specific antibiotic therapy. Evidence for adequate control of infection should be sought early in the course of antibiotic therapy and periodically thereafter once the course of treatment is completed. Diabetes mellitus, if present, should be brought under adequate control. Unnecessary bladder catheterization of diabetics should be avoided. Prompt and adequate relief of any urinary tract obstruction by surgical measures should be undertaken, keeping in mind the fact that RPN is usually bilateral. Hence, vigorous medical and conservative management are important before any radical surgical procedure is performed. Patients should be instructed to watch and report any evidence of gross hematuria to avoid uncontrollable hemorrhage with exsanguination. NSAIDs should be avoided. The inhibitory action of these agents on prostaglandin synthesis could further compromise the already impaired blood supply of the papilla. Control of hypertension, a common finding in patients with RPN, is essential as it is with any other kidney disease. Early and adequate control of hypertension will not only reduce the risk of the usual morbid events associated with hypertension, but will reduce the progression of the renal disease. Antihypertensive agents that reduce renal blood flow are best avoided.

Selected Readings

Allen RC, Petty RE, Lirenman DS, et al. Renal papillary necrosis in children with chronic arthritis. *Am J Dis Child* 1986;140:20–22.

The broader use and wider availability of NSAIDs has been associated with a more common association between these agents and RPN. Recurrent microscopic or gross hematuria was the principal manifestation in the five children reported.

Eknoyan G. Renal papillary necrosis in diabetic patients. In: Mogenson CE, ed. *The kidney and hypertension in diabetes mellitus*, 2nd ed. Boston: Kluwer Academic Press, 1997:461–468.

A discussion of the most common systemic condition associated with renal papillary necrosis.

Eknoyan G, Qunibi WY, Grissom RT, et al. Renal papillary necrosis: an update. *Medicine (Baltimore)* 1982;61:55–73.

A review of the clinical and diagnostic features of 27 patients with renal papillary necrosis, citing virtually every important reference to this subject.

Gobé GC, Axelsen RA. The role of apoptosis in the development of renal cortical atrophy associated with healed experimental renal papillary necrosis. *Pathology* 1991;23:213–223.

Description of the sequential structural changes that affect the cortex in an experimental model of RPN. The extent of initial cortical atrophy, which begins as cell deletion by apoptosis, is proportional to the extent of papillary necrosis and is accompanied by compensatory hypertrophy in adjoining areas of normal cortex.

Griffin MD, Larson TS. Renal papillary necrosis—a sixteen-year clinical experience. *J Am Soc Nephrol* 1995;6:248–256.

A summary of the clinical and laboratory findings of 165 cases of renal papillary necrosis seen at a major referral center.

Groop L, Laasonen L, Edgren J. Renal papillary necrosis in patients with IDDM. *Diabetes Care* 1989;12:198–202.

Radiologic evidence of papillary necrosis was present in 23.7% of 76 patients with longstanding diabetes. The lesion was more common in females and those with a history of urinary tract infection.

Hultengren N. Renal papillary necrosis. A clinical study of 103 cases. *Acta Chir Scand Suppl* 1961;277:1–84.

A detailed review of the clinical, pathologic, and radiologic findings in 103 patients with RPN encountered at one institution during the period of 1949 to 1959.

Kaude JV, Stone M, Fuller TJ, et al. Papillary necrosis in kidney transplant patients. *Radiology* 1976;120:69–74.

A report of RPN as a late complication of the transplanted kidney in 11 patients: In nine patients RPN was associated with diseases known to cause RPN, while in two it was due to the interstitial nephritis and vasculopathy of chronic rejection.

Kozlowski K, Brown RW. Renal medullary necrosis in infants and children. *Pediatr Radial* 1978;7:85–89.

A review of 24 cases of RPN in children.

Lauler DP, Schreiner GE, David A. Renal medullary necrosis. *Am J Med* 1960; 29:132–156.

A landmark article that provides an insightful and comprehensive examination of RPN.

Lindvall N: Radiological changes of renal papillary necrosis. *Kidney Int* 1978; 13:93–106.

A concise but thorough and well-illustrated consideration of the radiological features of RPN.

Mandel EE. Renal medullary necrosis. *Am J Med* 1952;13:322–327.

The first comprehensive review of RPN based on 160 cases reported in the literature.

Sabatini S, Eknoyan G, eds. Renal papillary necrosis. Special issue of *Semin Nephrol* 1981;4:1–106.

The seven articles comprising this issue provide a comprehensive review of RPN. The topics covered are the structure and function of the renal papilla, the pathophysiology of experimental RPN, RPN in diabetes mellitus, sickle cell hemoglobinopathies, analgesic nephropathy the radiologic manifestations of RPN, and the biochemical mechanisms by which chemicals exert their detrimental effect on the renal papillae.

Segasothy M, Sakijan AS, Zulfikar A, et al. Chronic renal disease and papillary necrosis associated with the long-term use of nonsteroidal anti-inflammatory drugs as the sole or predominant analgesic. *Am J Kidney Dis* 1994;24:17–24.

Prostaglandins are essential to maintain medullary blood flow. The chronic reduction of their synthesis by cyclooxygenase inhibitors renders the papilla susceptible to ischemic necrosis.

CHAPTER 52

Occlusive Renal Vascular Disease

Dianne Sandy and Marc A. Pohl

Renal arterial occlusion may be manifested by a variety of clinical syndromes that depend on the rate of occlusion and the caliber of the vessels involved. The spectrum of disease includes renal artery infarction, thromboembolism due to a variety of causes, and chronically progressive renal artery occlusion as a result of atherosclerosis. Arterial occlusive disease may be asymptomatic or may give rise to hypertension and/or varying degrees of renal insufficiency. This chapter will review the causes and clinical consequences of renal arterial occlusion and approaches to its diagnosis and treatment.

CLINICAL PRESENTATIONS OF RENAL ARTERY OCCLUSION

Acute Renal Artery Occlusion and Renal Infarction

Acute renal arterial occlusion may occur due to thrombosis or embolism of an artery without antecedent stenosis. In both instances, there is severe renal ischemia, which may rapidly progress to infarction unless there is a well-developed collateral circulation to the kidney. Renal artery dissection may occur spontaneously either as an extension of aortic dissection or as an isolated phenomenon. It may be secondary to traumatic injury or, more commonly, be an iatrogenic complication of catheter or balloon manipulation during angiography or angioplasty. Renal artery dissection has been reported as an isolated incident in patients who have performed strenuous physical activity. Its relationship to severe hypertension and several types of fibromuscular dysplasia has also been well-documented. Traumatic renal artery thrombosis typically occurs in the patient with multiple injuries as the result of a deceleration or twisting injury that disrupts the intima or media of the vessel. Thrombosis of previously healthy renal vessels can occur as a complication of aortic disease, in particular, aortic dissection, but renal artery thrombosis is more usually superimposed on preexisting renal artery disease. In these patients, collateral circulation may have developed, and the occlusion is often asymptomatic. Table 52.1 lists the numerous causes of renal thromboembolism that may occur at any point along the renal vasculature.

Treatment of Acute Thrombosis

In patients with traumatic renal artery thrombosis, prompt surgical thrombectomy is the procedure of choice; anticoagulation

TABLE 52.1. Classification of Arterial Thromboembolic Diseases of the Kidney

- Thrombosis
  - Spontaneous
    - Atherosclerotic diseases of the aorta and renal artery
    - Fibromuscular dysplasia of the renal artery
    - Aneurysms of the aorta or renal artery
    - Dissection of the aorta or renal artery
    - Vasculitis involving the renal artery
      - Polyarteritis nodosa
      - Takayasu's arteritis
      - Kawasaki disease
      - Thromboangiitis obliterans
      - Other necrotizing vasculitides
    - Inflammatory disease of the aorta or renal artery (syphilis, tuberculosis, mycoses)
    - Hypercoaguable states
      - Nephrotic syndrome
      - Antiphospholipid antibody syndrome
      - Antithrombin III deficiency
      - Homocystinuria
    - Thrombotic microangiopathies
      - Hemolytic uremic syndrome
      - Thrombotic thrombocytopenic purpura
      - Antiphospholipid antibody syndrome
      - Hyperacute allograft rejection
      - Postpartum nephroangiosclerosis
      - Scleroderma
      - Malignant hypertension
      - Sickle cell nephropathy
  - Induced
    - Traumatic
    - Following angiography or percutaneous transluminal angioplasty
    - Following renal arterial reconstructive surgery
    - Following renal allotransplantation
- Embolism
  - Cardiac source
    - Atrial fibrillation or other arrhythmias
    - Native and prosthetic valvular heart disease
      - Infectious endocarditis
      - Marantic endocarditis
    - Myocardial infarction with mural thrombi
    - Left atrial myxoma
  - Noncardic source
    - Atheromatous embolic disease
    - Paradoxical emboli
    - Fat emboli
    - Tumor emboli
  - Therapeutic renal embolization

and fibrinolysis are contraindicated in this situation. Iatrogenic renal artery dissection and thrombosis have been treated with either surgical thrombectomy or intraarterial fibrinolysis, but to date no comparative efficacy studies of these two approaches exist. Because fibrinolysis is less invasive and can be initiated at the time of the complication, it appears to be the preferred choice. In some patients, severe hypertension may be present. The hypertension is typically angiotensin II dependent, and antihypertensive therapy with angiotensin converting enzyme (ACE) inhibitors or β-adrenergic blockers is usually effective.

Renal Artery Embolism

Embolic renal artery occlusion can affect the main renal artery or segmental arteries depending on the size of the emboli. These embolic events may be clinically silent especially if the emboli are small and either cause partial occlusion of the vessels or lodge in very distal branches of the arterial tree. In 1940, Hoxie and Cogan studied 14,000 postmortem examinations and found a 1.4% incidence of embolic renal infarction, but only 2 of these 205 cases had been recognized clinically. More than 90% of renal emboli are cardiac in origin. Cardiac conditions favoring the development of mural thrombi include atrial fibrillation, left ventricular failure, and dilated cardiomyopathy. Other cardiac sources of emboli are vegetations on infected valves and atrial myxomas. The clinician should therefore maintain a high index of suspicion for renal emboli in the cardiac patient with flank, loin, or abdominal pain. Transthoracic echocardiography will usually demonstrate mural thrombi, but transesophageal imaging is usually required to confirm the valvular vegetations of infective endocarditis.

Clinical Features of Renal Infarction

Renal infarction characteristically presents with flank and abdominal pain, nausea, vomiting, fever recent onset, or worsening of hypertension. The presentation may mimic any of the myriad causes of an acute abdomen and therefore must be considered in the differential diagnosis of acute abdominal pain. Helpful laboratory features include leukocytosis and raised lactate dehydrogenase levels, usually more than five times the upper limit of normal. Alkaline phosphatase and transaminase levels may be mildly elevated. Mild proteinuria and microscopic hematuria are common. The serum creatinine level will be elevated if the occlusion is bilateral or involves a significant portion of a single functioning kidney. A radioisotope scan using either technetium–DTPA (diethylenetriamine pentaacetic acid) or technetium–DMSA (dimercaptosuccinic acid) will establish the diagnosis, by demonstrating a segmental or global decrease in renal perfusion. Contrast-enhanced computed tomography of the abdomen clearly delineates segmental infarction of the kidneys, the infarcted areas appearing as hypodense wedge-shaped areas. Renal angiography is the confirmatory test, but it is usually not performed unless surgical intervention or fibrinolysis is considered.

Treatment of Renal Infarction

The treatment of renal infarction depends on the cause of the occlusion and the extent of the infarcted area. With the exception of septic emboli from infective endocarditis, cardiac emboli are treated with anticoagulation unless contraindicated. The use of anticoagulation in patients with septic emboli is not recommended because of the risk of hemorrhage from cerebral emboli or mycotic aneurysms. Antimicrobial therapy is the mainstay of treatment, but the presence of emboli may hasten consideration of valve replacement. In other patients with cardiac emboli, the standard approach of intravenous heparin followed by oral warfarin (Coumadin) is used, with the goal of minimizing renal infarction and preventing further embolization. Typically the diagnosis of embolic renal infarction is delayed, and therefore when therapy is initiated, the warm ischemic time of the kidney has been exceeded. The maximal ischemic time has been estimated as between 45 and 90 minutes, and therefore optimal results require prompt diagnosis and initiation of treatment if ischemic tissue is to be preserved. This becomes clinically important if the occlusion involves a main renal artery or affects a significant proportion of the functioning renal parenchyma. In these cases, intraarterial thrombolysis with streptokinase and urokinase has been used. Up to 30 such cases have been reported in the literature, with very good technical success rates, but long-term renal function was preserved in only about half of the patients. Factors that favor the success of this procedure include prompt diagnosis and treatment, partial or segmental occlusion, and the presence of an adequate collateral circulation. The role of surgical treatment for embolic renal artery infarction is uncertain, and surgical embolectomy has not demonstrated superior functional recovery compared with anticoagulation or fibrinolysis.

ATHEROEMBOLIC RENAL DISEASE

Atheroemboli are the second most common cause of renal emboli after cardiac emboli. Atheroembolic renal disease (AERD) is characterized by the development or worsening of renal insufficiency due to showers of cholesterol from atheromatous plaques in the large arteries, to the renal microcirculation. AERD may occur spontaneously in patients with severe abdominal aortic atheroma, but at present it is more often caused by surgical or endovascular manipulation. Anticoagulation or fibrinolysis can cause hemorrhage into atherosclerotic plaques, with dislodgement of atheromatous material and subsequent embolization. AERD is an important cause of renal failure in elderly patients. It rarely causes renal infarction, but can cause acute, subacute, or chronic renal insufficiency. Elderly patients with a history of severe abdominal atherosclerosis, longstanding hypertension, hyperlipidemia, and tobacco abuse are most at risk. In many cases, there is an antecedent history of abdominal aortography, endovascular surgery or manipulation, or anticoagulation, but often no identifiable precipitating event.

Clinical Manifestations of Atheroembolism

Multiple organ systems are often involved when atheroembolic showers derive from the abdominal or thoracic aorta. Table 52.2 lists the clinical manifestations of this condition. The cutaneous findings of livedo reticularis and mottling of the toes are characteristic and should alert the physician to look for other manifestations of atheroembolism. Patients with a large embolic load may develop mesenteric and intestinal ischemia with possibly catastrophic consequences. Renal manifestations include nonoliguric renal failure and new onset or worsening of preexistent hypertension. The pattern of renal function loss is variable, depending on the severity of the embolic load. Rapidly progressive acute renal failure can occur or a slow, stepwise progression in renal failure, implying repeated small embolic showers. Other patients may have only a slight rise in serum creatinine with stabilization of renal insufficiency and no need for dialysis.

Urinalysis results in AERD are nonspecific. Many patients have a bland urine sediment, while the presence of red and white blood cells is not uncommon. Eosinophiluria (3% to 5% eosinophils) is characteristic, occurring in 70% to 80% of patients. Mild proteinuria may occur and is usually subnephrotic, but nephrotic-range proteinuria has been reported in the ab-

TABLE 52.2. The Clinical Manifestations of Atheroembolic Renal Disease

Cutaneous
Livedo reticularis Mottling of the toes—"blue toe" syndrome Focal digital ischemia
Abdominal
Secondary to emboli to the mesenteric circulation Gastric or duodenal ulceration Intestinal ischemia/infarction or perforation Pancreatitis Adrenal insufficiency
Neurological
Amaurosis fugax/transient ischemic attacks Cerebral infarction Peripheral palsies from spinal cord emboli
Coronary
Coronary ischemia (after percutaneous transluminal coronary angioplasty)
Renal
Renal insufficiency New onset/worsening hypertension Eosinophilia ± proteinuria

sence of other renal pathologic changes. Other laboratory findings include leukocytosis, eosinophilia, low serum complement levels, and a transiently elevated sedimentation rate. Because of the multisystem findings, characteristic skin rash, and the presence of renal failure, AERD may mimic systemic vasculitis.

Pathogenesis

Atheroembolism occurs when atheromatous plaques become denuded of their endothelial lining, releasing a cholesterol-rich matrix into the circulation These emboli are typically 150 to 200 μ in diameter, lodging in the lumina of arterioles and capillaries and causing partial or total occlusion. This incites an inflammatory reaction with invasion of leukocytes and complement activation within 24 to 48 hours. Over the next several days, the ischemic tissue is invaded by macrophages and multinucleated foreign body giant cells. Endothelial proliferation and intimal fibrosis follow. Over time, there may be partial dissolution of the thrombi and recanalization of the lumen.

Pathology (See Atlas of Renal Pathology, Chapter 109)

The characteristic light microscopic finding is the crystalline artifact, that is, empty elongated crystal spaces in the vessel lumen, which are due to the extraction of cholesterol and lipids during processing with organic solvents. The arteriolar lumen may be occluded by an accumulation of cells, mainly tissue macrophages, with occasional polymorphonuclear leukocytes and lymphocytes. Glomeruli show evidence of ischemia, and in chronic lesions, there may be glomerular hyalinization and global or segmental sclerosis as well as interstitial fibrosis. Focal segmental sclerotic lesions in patients with chronic disease are believed to be due to hyperfiltration injury in the remnant nephrons. Immunofluorescence examination reveals IgM and C3 in a coarsely granular or lobular pattern, while electron microscopy typically shows entrapment of electron-dense material consistent with the trapping of serum proteins in the organizing atheroemboli.

Management

Therapy of AERD focuses on controlling hypertension, preventing further embolization, and preserving remaining renal function. β-Blockers and ACE inhibitors are usually effective for hypertension control because of the high renin state caused by renal ischemia. Renal failure is managed supportively, and dialysis is initiated as needed. Anticoagulation therapy should be withdrawn or avoided. Steroid therapy to reduce the inflammatory response has been ineffective. Repeated episodes of embolic showers may prompt surgical excision or repair of the diseased aorta. In general, the prognosis for these patients is poor. A study of 52 histologically proven cases of renal atheroembolic disease revealed that 73% of patients died within 6 months of the diagnosis. The poor prognosis reflects the widespread nature of atherosclerosis in these patients, who frequently have severe comorbidities, including coronary artery disease and embolic showers to multiple organs. The mainstay of the management of this condition is prevention. Patients with known or suspected extensive atherosclerosis of the abdominal aorta should not be subjected to angiographic or other endovascular procedures unless absolutely necessary. In particular, one should avoid the correction of anatomical main renal artery stenosis unless there is firm evidence that medically uncontrollable renovascular hypertension, life-threatening "flash" pulmonary edema, or potentially reversible ischemic nephropathy is present.

CHRONIC RENAL ARTERY OCCLUSIVE DISEASE

The two main causes of chronic renal vascular occlusion are atherosclerosis and fibromuscular dysplasia of the main renal arteries. These conditions most commonly produce the syndrome of renovascular hypertension, and atherosclerotic renal artery disease in particular, is associated with ischemic renal disease. The other causes of chronic renal artery occlusion include cholesterol emboli, arterial aneurysms, arteriovenous malformations of the renal artery, neurofibromatosis, polyarteritis nodosa, and Takayasu's arteritis.

The two main causes of renal artery occlusion, however, are atherosclerosis and the fibrous dysplasias. Table 52.3 compares the clinical and anatomical features of the two main types of chronic renal occlusive disease. The natural history and clinical characteristics of these lesions are different and affect the choice of therapy.

Fibrous Renal Artery Disease

Fibrous dysplasia is the most common type of renal artery disease, causing renovascular hypertension in patients younger than 40 years of age. It is more common in women than in men and in whites as opposed to African-Americans or Asians. The etiology of the fibrous dysplasias is not understood. Its predominance in females has suggested a hormonal influence. Ischemia of the vessel wall as a result of functional defects in the vasa vasorum has also been implicated. Of the four types of fibrous dysplasias, medial fibroplasia is the most common, accounting for 75% of these lesions. Medial fibroplasia affects the distal half of the renal artery, is often bilateral, and has a typical

TABLE 52.3. Characteristics of the Two Main Types of Renal Artery Disease

Lesion Type	Frequency (%)	Sex	Age (yr)	Anatomic Location	Morphology	Natural Course
Atherosclerosis	65–70	M > F	>50	Proximal 2 cm of renal artery, ostial and adjacent aorta; branch disease uncommon; 50%–75% bilateral	Eccentric or concentric focal stenosis	Progression in 40%–50%, often to total occlusion
Fibrous dysplasias	30–35					
Medial fibroplasia	25 (65–85[a])	F	25–50	Mid and distal main renal artery and branches; 60% bilateral	Serial stenoses with intervening mural aneurysms; "string-of-beads" appearance	Progression in one-third; dissection, thrombosis, and complete occlusion rare
Perimedial fibroplasia	5 (15[a])	F	15–30	Mid and distal main renal artery or branches; 30% bilateral	Serial stenosis without mural aneurysms	Progression in most cases; dissection and/or thrombosis common
Intimal fibroplasia and medial hyperplasia	5 (5–10[a])	F > M	Children and young adults	Mid main renal artery, occasionally proximal main renal artery; rarely bilateral	Focal or tubular	Progression in most cases; dissection and/or thrombosis common

[a] Percentage of fibrous dysplasia lesions.

angiographic appearance of a "string of beads" due to multiple aneurysms. These lesions rarely progress to complete occlusion. Perimedial fibroplasia accounts for approximately 15% of the fibrous lesions, tends to progress to complete occlusion, and is frequently complicated by thrombosis and/or dissection. The other two types of fibrous dysplasia are medial hyperplasia and intimal fibroplasia, and together these account for 10% of the fibrous lesions. They are common in children and teenagers and are both characterized by linear, smooth, tight stenoses with poststenotic dilation. These lesions tend to progress to total occlusion with ipsilateral renal atrophy, and surgical renal revascularization is recommended for patients to avoid lifelong antihypertensive therapy and renal atrophy. Patients with medial fibroplasia do not develop renal insufficiency as a consequence of progression of their lesions; however, angioplasty or surgical revascularization can be performed to treat hypertension that is refractory to medical therapy.

Atherosclerotic Renal Artery Disease

Atherosclerotic renal artery disease (ASO-RAD) is the most common cause of renovascular hypertension in Western countries and accounts for 65% to 70% of renal artery lesions. Typically the patient is elderly (older than 60 years of age), often has widespread peripheral vascular disease or coronary artery disease, and has a history of tobacco use. The anatomical presence of ASO-RAD is often an incidental finding during angiography performed for other reasons. A prospective study of 395 patients who underwent abdominal and lower extremity angiography showed that more than 50% unilateral renal artery stenosis was seen in 33% to 39% of patients. Thirteen percent had severe (more than 75%) bilateral renal artery stenosis. Other observers have noted significant renal artery stenoses in 20% to 30% of patients with coronary artery disease.

The atherosclerotic lesions may occur either at the orifice of the renal artery—*ostial*—lesions, or more distally—*nonostial lesions*. The ostial lesions predominate, accounting for 75% to 80% of all atherosclerotic lesions. Several retrospective studies on the natural history of ASO-RAD have found it to be a progressive disorder. A retrospective study of 85 patients who had two or more renal angiograms in a 20-year period at the Cleveland Clinic showed that 44% of the patients had lesions which progressed over a mean follow-up period of 52 months, and 7 of 18 patients (39%) with severe stenosis showed progression to total occlusion within 24 months. Several prospective studies using serial duplex ultrasound have reported similar rates of progression but much less frequent progression to total occlusion at 2 to 3 years The clinical consequences of renal artery occlusion are renovascular hypertension or ischemic nephropathy. Detailed discussion of renovascular hypertension is found in Chapter 62.

Ischemic Nephropathy

Ischemic nephropathy is the second consequence of chronic renal arterial occlusion and is defined as a clinically significant reduction in glomerular filtration rate (GFR) caused by obstruction of renal arterial blood flow. Ischemic nephropathy is typically associated with atherosclerotic renal artery disease, but it may rarely occur as the result of the less common varieties of fibrous dysplasia. Ischemic nephropathy typically occurs in patients with severe bilateral ASO-RAD or severe atherosclerotic stenosis to a single functioning kidney. Ischemic nephropathy is currently recognized as an important cause of renal insufficiency in elderly patients and a potential contributor to the end-stage renal disease (ESRD) population. The true prevalence of ischemic nephropathy is not known. The population at risk for this condition often has other morbid conditions that may mask the presence of ischemic renal disease and which in themselves are causes of ESRD. These include hypertensive nephrosclerosis, diabetic nephropathy, and AERD.

Pathophysiology of Ischemic Nephropathy. In the presence of severe renal artery obstruction, renal perfusion pressure falls below a "critical" level, resulting in intrarenal ischemia. This critical perfusion pressure is between 70 and 80 mm Hg. Below this level, renal autoregulation fails, and the GFR falls. Repetitive episodes of renal hypoperfusion presumably produce irreversible renal parenchymal damage. The pathologic changes include glomerular collapse, basement membrane thickening, atrophic renal tubules, and a mild mononuclear interstitial infiltrate. The microvasculature may show typical atherosclerotic changes. Evidence of cholesterol embolization and hypertensive nephrosclerosis is common. In the face of total main renal artery occlusion, renal atrophy ensues. However, with slowly progressive disease, an adequate collateral circulation may develop, thereby preserving renal viability.

Clinical Features of Ischemic Nephropathy. The typical patient with ischemic nephropathy is elderly and hypertensive, with a history of peripheral or coronary artery disease and tobacco use and unexplained azotemia. Abdominal or femoral artery bruits are often observed on physical examination. Patients may be seen with deteriorating renal function after starting antihypertensive therapy, particularly with ACE inhibitors. Ischemic renal disease should be suspected in patients with uncontrolled hypertension, azotemia, and recurrent episodes of "flash" pulmonary edema. Radiographic evidence of unequal renal size or bilateral shrunken kidneys also suggests renal vascular disease.

Diagnostic Tests. Diagnostic tests for renal artery stenosis suggest either the anatomic presence of disease [e.g., duplex ultrasound, magnetic resonance angiography (MRA), and renal angiography], or the likelihood that this disease is causing renovascular hypertension (e.g., captopril renogram). In renovascular hypertension (RVHT), the peripheral plasma renin level may be elevated but is often normal. A better screening test for RVHT is the captopril provocation test, which measures the rise in plasma renin activity 1 hour after taking 25 mg of captopril. This test is, however, unreliable in patients with renal insufficiency. Determinations of renal vein renins with a ratio of at least 1.5 lateralizing to the side of the renal artery stenosis predict approximately 90% success of revascularization. Isotope renograms may be useful in selecting patients for angiography, but have low levels of sensitivity, and are even less helpful in patients with ischemic nephropathy. The sensitivity may be enhanced by the use of captopril, which accentuates the difference in function between the stenotic and the nonstenotic kidney.

The advent of duplex ultrasonography has made available a noninvasive means of detecting renal artery stenosis. It is rapidly becoming the screening test of choice. It identifies stenoses as greater or less than 60% or total occlusion. The disadvantages are that it is time-consuming and highly operator-dependent. With experienced technicians however, excellent correlations with renal angiography may be obtained. MRA is also frequently used to detect renal artery stenosis with reported sensitivity rates of 84% to 100%. However, this technique is insensitive for the detection of branch or accessory artery stenosis and tends to overestimate the degree of stenosis. The use of the nontoxic intravenous contrast agent gadolinium with three-dimensional phase contrast techniques greatly enhances the clarity of the images. With improvements in technology and expertise, MRA may become the screening test of choice for renal artery stenosis.

Definitive diagnosis of renal artery stenosis requires angiography, which can be combined, if appropriate, with therapeutic angioplasty and stenting. Conventional contrast angiography remains the gold standard for the diagnosis of renal artery stenosis but carries the risks of contrast nephrotoxicity and atheroembolism in the case of atherosclerotic disease. The technique of digital subtraction angiography (DSA) has been a major advance in renal artery imaging. It requires a smaller volume of contrast agent and is efficient because the computer-generated images can be recalled instantly. However, its spatial resolution is inferior to that of conventional angiography, and it is therefore unreliable for the detection of branch stenoses or intrarenal disease. Carbon dioxide angiography has the advantage of using a nontoxic contrast agent, but is less widely used than MRA or DSA. Before embarking on invasive diagnostic procedures in the patient with suspected ischemic nephropathy, one should first consider whether intervention is feasible, and if renal function is salvable. In general, total occlusion of the renal artery signifies irreversible ischemic damage. In some patients with gradual occlusion, collateral circulation develops that is sufficient to maintain viability of the renal parenchyma, even if the GFR is minimal. Factors that suggest a favorable result from revascularization are (a) renal size greater than 9 cm by tomography, (b) evidence of function on urogram or isotope scan, (c) adequate collateral circulation, and (d) viable glomeruli with minimal arteriosclerosis on renal biopsy. In addition, studies from the Mayo and Cleveland Clinics have shown that surgical revascularization results are much better when the renal insufficiency is not severe (serum creatinine less than 3.0 mg/dl). Patients with more severe degrees of azotemia are more likely to have irreversible parenchymal damage. Occasionally, in patients with bilateral renal artery occlusion requiring dialysis, renal function recovers with surgical revascularization, but such events are rare.

Treatment. The patient with ischemic nephropathy typically has major comorbidities and widespread atherosclerosis. The potential for benefit from surgical or endovascular revascularization must be weighed against the risks of these invasive maneuvers. The severity and extent of renal artery obstruction, the degree of renal insufficiency, the coexistence of other renal parenchymal disease, and the likelihood of progression are all factors that need consideration before exposing the patient to the risks of atheroembolism, contrast nephrotoxicity, and general anesthesia. The surgical and percutaneous approaches are the same as for renovascular hypertension. Patients with ostial atherosclerotic lesions have a high rate of restenosis with percutaneous angioplasty alone, and it is recommended that these lesions be stented at the time of angioplasty or else be repaired surgically.

ARTERIAL OCCLUSION OF THE RENAL TRANSPLANT ARTERY

Acute thrombosis is a rare complication in the renal transplant artery. It occurs within the first 2 months and is associated with a 92% graft loss rate, due to graft infarction. The process may be associated with acute or hyperacute rejection. Cyclosporine therapy is believed to increase the risk of this complication, but it is not a dose-related effect. Transplant renal artery stenosis is another vascular complication in the transplant recipient and is most common at the anastomotic site. The end-to-end anastomosis has a higher risk of stenosis compared with the end-to-side anastomosis. The condition presents with an elevated creatinine and worsening hypertension. Duplex ultrasonography is a good screening test, and angiography can be performed to confirm the diagnosis. Angioplasty is the preferred initial therapy, with surgical revascularization being performed for patients with failed angioplasties or complex stenoses.

Selected Readings

Greco BA, Breyer JA. Atherosclerotic ischemic renal disease. *Am J Kidney Dis* 1997;29:167–187.

A summary of the prevalence, etiology, pathophysiology, clinical evaluation, and treatment of atherosclerotic ischemic nephropathy.

Hallett JW Jr, Textor SC, Kos PB, et al. Advanced renovascular hypertension and renal insufficiency: trends in medical comorbidity and surgical approach from 1970–1993. *J Vasc Surg* 1995;21(5):750–759.

A review of the Mayo Clinic's experience with renovascular surgery for both renovascular hypertension and ischemic nephropathy over a period of 24 years.

Jacobson HR. Ischemic renal disease: an overlooked clinical entity? [Clinical Conference]. *Kidney Int* 1988;34:729–743.

A detailed discussion of the clinical manifestations of ischemic renal disease, and its therapy.

Llach F, Nikhatar B. Renal thromboembolism, atheroembolism, and renal vein thrombosis. In: Schrier RW, Gottschalk CW, eds. *Diseases of the kidney*, 6th ed. Boston: Little Brown, 1997:1903–1912.

A review of the causes, pathophysiology, clinical presentation, and management of renal vein thrombosis.

Novick A, Scoble J, Hamilton G, eds. *Renovascular disease.* London: WB Saunders, 1996.

A very detailed review of all aspects of renal occlusive disease including imaging techniques and all aspects of surgical and medical management.

Pohl MA. Renal artery stenosis, renal vascular hypertension, and ischemic nephropathy. In: Schrier RW, Gottschalk CW, eds. *Diseases of the kidney*, 6th ed. Boston: Little, Brown, 1997:1367–1422.

A comprehensive review of renovascular hypertension and ischemic renal disease with a focus on historical aspects of the topic as well as a detailed discussion of the pathophysiology and pathology of these conditions.

Stanley JC. Hume Memorial Lecture: Surgical treatment of renovascular hypertension. *Am J Surg* 1997;174:102–110.

A review of the contemporary surgical management of renovascular hypertension of various causes.

CHAPTER 53

Nephrolithiasis

Elaine M. Worcester and Jacob Lemann, Jr.

Descriptions of bladder stones and the surgical techniques for lithotomy have been recorded since the Hellenic epoch of Hippocrates in the fourth century BC and the comparable era of Hindu medicine. Bladder stones remained a major disorder during the Renaissance and early industrial revolution and continue to be a problem, particularly in children, in the developing nations of the modern world. By contrast, bladder stones have virtually disappeared in the populations of industrialized nations, except among patients with urethral obstruction or neurogenic bladder. At the same time, however, many studies have documented a progressive increase in the frequency of renal calculi in affluent Western nations. In the United States, the prevalence of stones reaches 10% in white males by the seventh decade and 4% in women; rates in Asians and African-Americans are lower. There is also a regional variation in stone occurrence, with the highest rates in the southeastern states. The peak age of onset is the third decade, whereas the highest incidence of stones is seen in the fifth and sixth decades. The basis for the decline in the incidence of lower urinary tract stones and the rise in frequency of renal stones has not been fully defined but may be related to increased dietary intake of animal protein and purified carbohydrates. Because of the need for hospitalization and for procedures for removal of obstructing ureteral stones, nephrolithiasis contributes significantly to morbidity but seldom results in end-stage renal failure.

GENERAL CONSIDERATIONS OF NEPHROLITHIASIS

Stone Composition

The principal crystalline constituents of urinary stones in the United States and the approximate relative frequencies of the different types of stones are listed in Table 53.1. Stones composed of calcium oxalate alone or calcium oxalate together with apatite account for about 60% to 70% of all stones, and pure apatite is found in about 7%. A small number of stones are composed of $CaHPO_4 \cdot 2H_2O$ (brushite), the solubility of which governs the solubility of calcium phosphate in aqueous biologic fluids, and which then undergoes phase transformation to apatite but also is occasionally found as the sole constituent of a stone. About 10% to20% of all stones are made of magnesium ammonium phosphate hexahydrate (struvite) together with carbonate apatite. These so-called *infection stones* or *triple phosphate* stones are the consequence of urinary infection by bacteria possessing the enzyme urease, which hydrolyzes urea to ammonium carbonate, making the urine very alkaline. Uric acid stones account for approximately 5% to 10% of all stones, whereas cystine stones are uncommon, accounting for only about 1% to 2% of calculi. There are also rare types of stones. These include xanthine stones in individuals with xanthine oxidase deficiency and 2,8-dihydroxyadenine stones in individuals with adenine phosphoribosyltransferase deficiency. Acid ammonium urate stones have been reported in patients with chronic diarrhea and hypokalemia. Oxypurinol and xanthine stones have occurred in patients treated with allopurinol and triamterene stones in patients treated with that drug. Crystalluria and stones have been reported in patients treated with indinavir, a protease inhibitor used in the treatment of human immunodeficiency virus infections and in patients who have taken large quantities of ephedrine. Stones composed solely of protein (*matrix* stones) have also been reported.

Pathogenesis of Nephrolithiasis

The formation of stones in the urinary tract occurs in several stages. The initial phase in stone formation is crystal nucleation. Crystals form by supersaturation of the urine with a potentially insoluble compound, which may occur due to either increased 24-hour urinary excretion of such solutes (calcium, oxalate, and cystine) or reduced urinary volumes secondary to accelerated extrarenal water losses or habitually low fluid intakes. Both of these processes lead to an increase in the mean urinary concentration of the sparingly soluble ions or compound and in such circumstances, the urine may become so supersaturated with the solute in question that the formation product (K_f) is exceeded and spontaneous crystal nucleation occurs. K_f is defined as the ion activity product at which crystals of the salt will spontaneously nucleate. In general, stone formers excrete urine that is more supersaturated with the constituents of their stones than is the urine of normal subjects, although normal urine is often supersaturated as well, particularly with calcium oxalate. In addition, alterations in urine pH may affect the ionization of some urinary constituents and thus their solubility. For example, at a urine pH of 6.0 to 7.0 most urinary phosphate is present as the HPO_4^- ion that readily reacts with calcium to form the sparingly soluble compound brushite ($CaHPO_4 \cdot 2H_2O$). In contrast, at a pH below 5.8, most urinary phosphate is present as $H_2PO_4^-$ and the solubility of $Ca(H_2PO_4)_2 \cdot H_2O$ is almost 4-fold greater than that of $CaHPO_4 \cdot 2H_2O$. As urine pH varies during the day, the urine of normal subjects is at least intermittently supersaturated with brushite, and the urine of stone formers may be so more often. Normal urine contains inhibitors of crystal nucleation that complex potential reactants in solution and limit their availability for crystal growth; for example, magnesium

TABLE 53.1. Composition and Frequency of Renal Calculi

Substance	Chemical Formula	Mineral Name	Frequency
Calcium oxalate			
Monohydrate	$Ca(COOH)_2 \cdot H_2O$	Whewellite	Calcium oxalate alone, 40%
Dihydrate	$Ca(COOH)_2 \cdot 2H_2O$	Weddellite	
Apatite	$Ca_{10}(PO_4)_6(OH)_2$	Hydroxyapatite	Hydroxyapatite alone, 7% Hydroxyapatite + calcium oxalate, 30%
	$Ca_{10}(PO_4)_6CO_3$	Carbonate apatite	
Calcium monohydrogen phosphate dihydrate	$CaHPO_4 \cdot 2H_2O$	Brushite	1%
Magnesium ammonium phosphate hexahydrate	$MgNH_4PO_4 \cdot 6H_20$	Struvite	Struvite + carbonate apatite 10%–20%
Uric acid	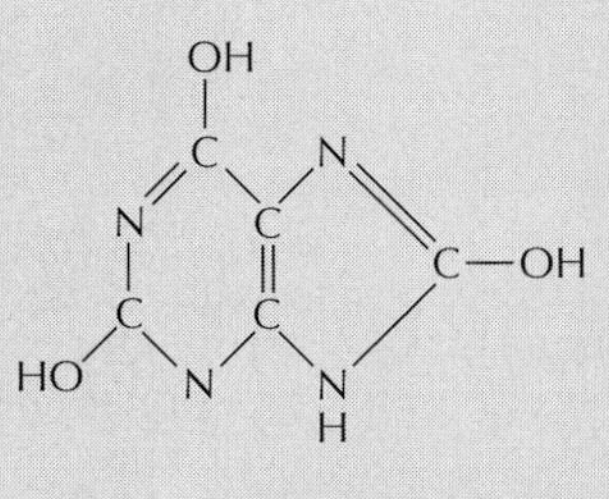		5–10%
Cystine	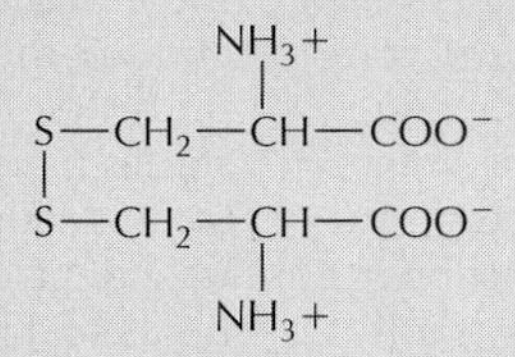		2%

complexes oxalate and citrate complexes calcium. Macromolecules may also retard nucleation. Deficiencies of these nucleation inhibitors in the urine may increase the potential for stone formation. Other data suggest that this may be true particularly for brushite in the urine of stone formers.

The formation of crystal nuclei is not in itself sufficient for stone formation. Crystals are not usually retained within the kidney but are excreted in the urine. Crystals are found more often in the urine of stone formers than of non–stone formers. The initial crystal nuclei that form in supersaturated urine can grow or aggregate with other nuclei to form larger crystals, which may be more likely to be retained. Experimental evidence also suggests that crystals may grow as a result of heterogeneous crystal nucleation or epitaxial crystal nucleation. This is the process by which one type of stone salt, such as apatite, may serve as a nucleus for the growth of another stone salt, such as calcium oxalate. Seeding of otherwise stable supersaturated solutions of calcium oxalate with apatite crystals leads to removal of calcium oxalate from solution and heterogeneous growth of calcium oxalate on the seed crystal of apatite. Because the molecular structures of calcium oxalate and apatite crystals are quite different, this effect is termed *heterogeneous nucleation* or *secondary crystal growth.* Such a mechanism probably plays a role in the pathogenesis of calcium oxalate stones because these stones frequently contain a central nucleus composed of apatite. This may derive from supersaturation of the urine with both calcium phosphate and calcium oxalate, a common occurrence. One report suggests that another source for the calcium apatite nucleus might be nanobacteria, a type of proteobacteria that form an apatetic mineral layer during growth in culture. Nanobacterial antigens were found in specimens of kidney stones, and theoretically may have provided the original seed crystal on which the stone grew. Uric acid seed crystals are also able to induce calcium oxalate crystal growth from supersaturated solutions of calcium oxalate. Because some of the crystal lattices and surfaces of uric acid and calcium oxalate are complementary on an atomic level, such an effect may be an example of epitaxial nucleation.

Urine normally contains inhibitors of the nucleation, growth, and aggregation of crystals. Such inhibitors include small molecules such as pyrophosphate and macromolecules such as ribonucleic acid, glycosaminoglycans, and acidic glycoproteins; most of the inhibitory activity appears to reside in the macromolecular fraction. One such protein inhibitor is Tamm-Horsfall protein, which inhibits the aggregation of calcium oxalate crystals *in vitro.* Tamm-Horsfall protein from some stone formers' urine reportedly has less inhibitory activity and under some circumstances may act as a promoter of aggregation. Other examples include nephrocalcin, a urinary glycoprotein that contains γ-carboxyglutamic acid, and uropontin, a phosphorylated urinary glycoprotein that is made in the kidney and inhibits calcium oxalate crystal growth and aggregation in solution. The role played by such proteins in formation of kidney stones is not yet clear; some studies suggest that impaired aggregation inhibition may be associated with increased risk of stone formation. Urinary proteins may also be incorporated in stones. Most stones contain a protein matrix, and it has been speculated that the matrix may play a role in crystal nucleation or may serve as a mechanical trap that anchors an initial crystal at the tip of a renal papilla, thereby permitting subsequent crystal growth. Both nephrocalcin and uropontin have been found in stone matrix.

Crystal attachment plays a critical role in stone formation, because without attachment to a urinary surface, crystals are not retained in the kidney long enough to form a stone. Stones are observed at the calyceal tips of renal papillae, where they have become anchored, allowing time for growth. Newer studies using cultured rat papillary collecting duct cells show that binding of calcium oxalate and apatite crystals to these cells involves attachment to specific sites and is saturable. Cell injury may be a prerequisite to attachment, exposing otherwise unavailable binding sites on the cells. Future studies will be needed to clarify the role that attachment factors play in the pathogenesis of stones.

Symptoms of Nephrolithiasis

The symptoms of nephrolithiasis are quite variable. Most often, stones totally or partially obstructing the renal pelvis or upper ureter are manifested on the affected side by flank and abdominal pain that is often of extreme severity and accompanied by nausea and vomiting. When the stone is present in the midureter to lower ureter, the pain often radiates downward toward the inguinal ligament and into the labia and urethra or testicle and penis. A stone located in the terminal intravesical segment of the ureter may be manifested by urinary frequency or dysuria and thus may be confused with symptoms of cystitis or urethritis. Passage of the stone yields immediate relief of pain. Gross or microscopic hematuria may be associated with any of these patterns of pain. Flank and back pain together with chills and fever are generally present when obstructing or partially obstructing pelvic or ureteral stones are accompanied by infection. In some patients, asymptomatic calculi are discovered when a plain abdominal radiograph, intravenous pyelogram, computerized tomogram, or ultrasonogram is obtained for other reasons.

Preliminary Evaluation of the Patient with Nephrolithiasis

The initial evaluation of patients suspected of having nephrolithiasis requires, in addition to a thorough history and physical examination, a careful urinalysis including prompt examination of the urine sediment to search for crystalluria, preferably by a physician who is acquainted with the clinical setting. The detection of crystalluria in the sediment of urine centrifuged immediately after voiding may identify the type of stone present (Table 53.2 and Figs. 53.1 through 53.6). The sediment from a urine specimen that has been refrigerated is unreliable because crystals may form in normal urine as a consequence of cooling. The initial urine specimen should be collected as a clean voided midstream specimen. A portion should be submitted for bacterial culture and the remainder used for the urinalysis. A plain abdominal radiograph, tomograms, ultrasonography, and intravenous urography may individually or in combination be required to determine whether urinary stones are radiolucent (uric acid) or radiodense (all other stone types) (Table 53.2), to determine the number of stones present, their size, and location, and to determine whether or not partial or complete ureteral obstruction is present. While these initial studies are being carried out, adequate doses of analgesics are administered to alleviate pain. Intravenous fluids may be needed to maintain adequate urine flow rates in patients who are acutely ill with nausea and vomiting. Because determination of the stone composition is crucial in guiding subsequent patient evaluation and therapy, emphasis must also be placed on attempting to recover even the smallest stones for analysis by collecting and straining all urine from the moment the patient is initially seen and suspected to have nephrolithiasis. All too often, such stones are lost in the toilet because the patient is given a container that is too small to hold the entire void volume or the stone is lost during unsupervised voiding after intravenous urography as a consequence of the osmotic diuresis induced by radiocontrast material.

TABLE 53.2. Evaluation of the Patient with Suspected Nephrolithiasis (Ureteral Colic, Hematuria, Fever)

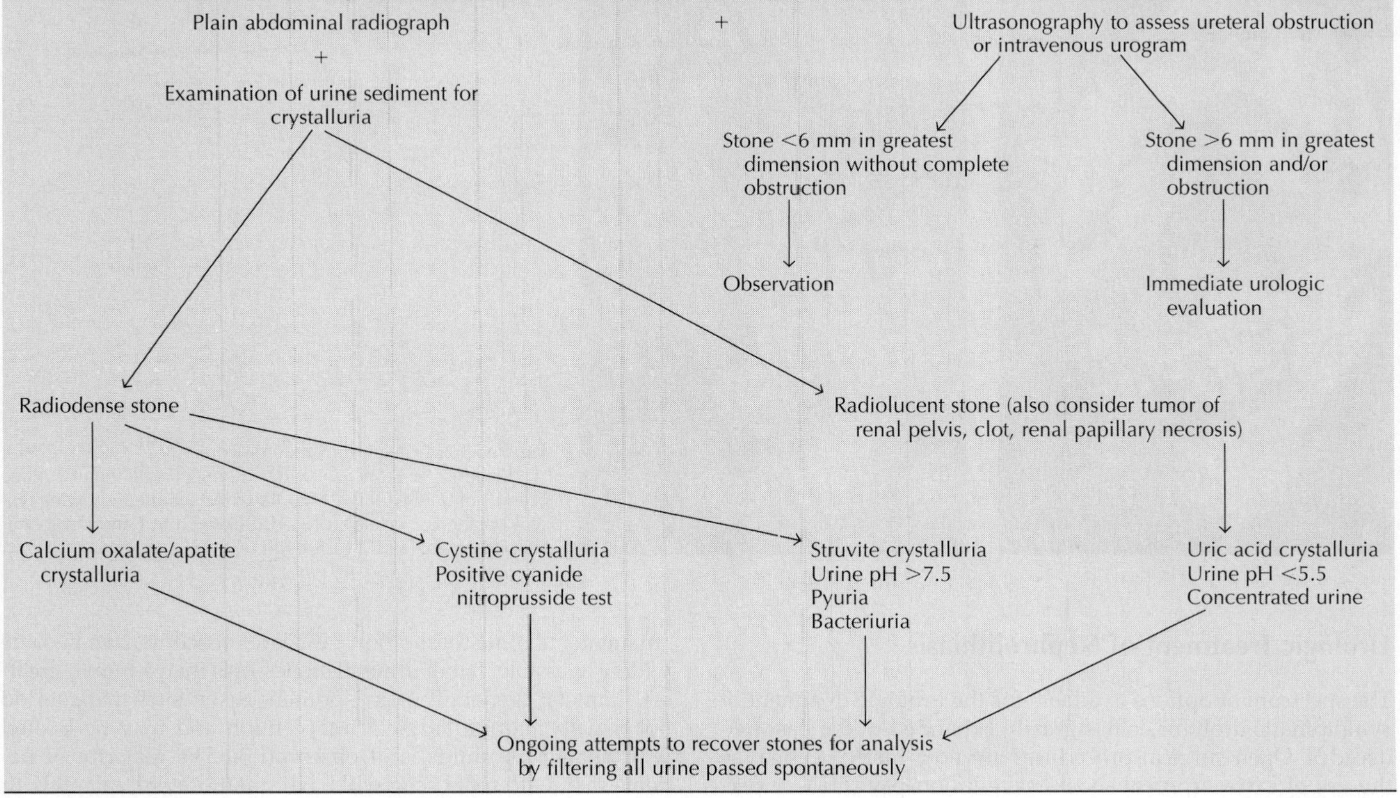

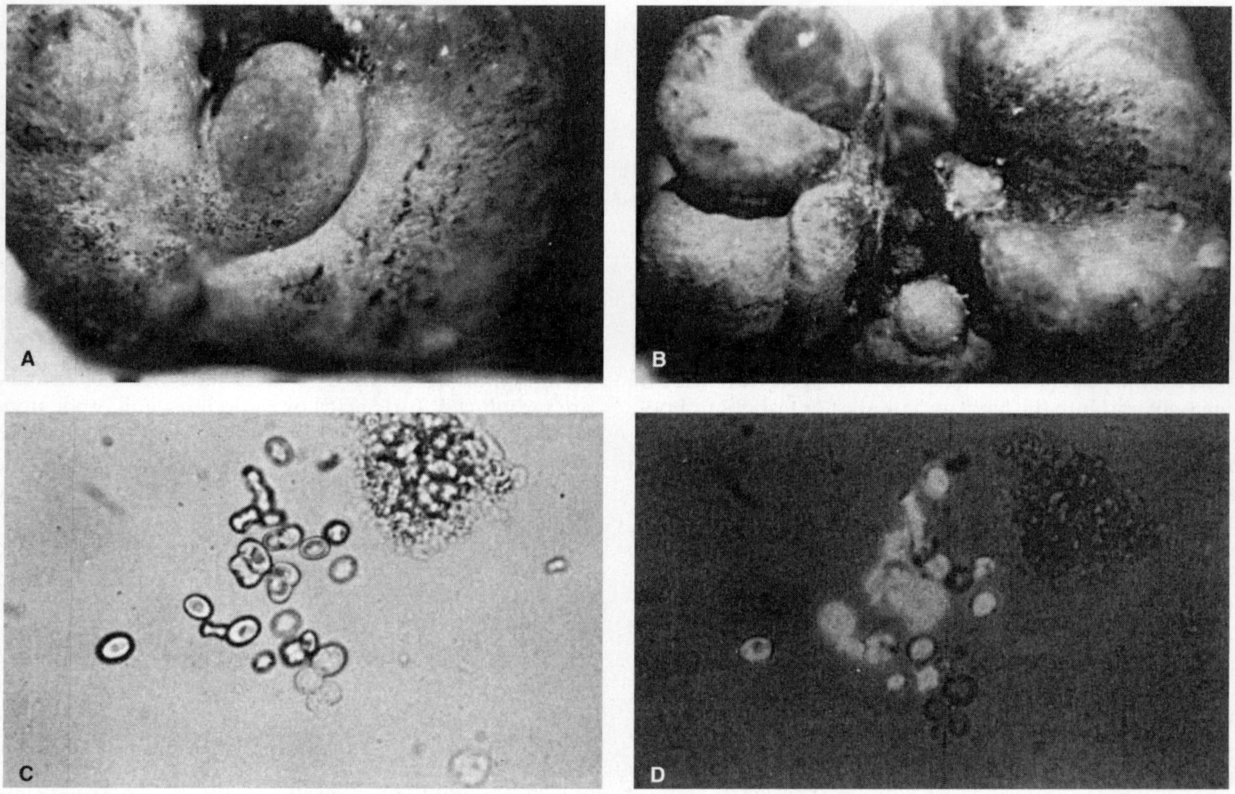

Figure 53.1. Calcium oxalate monohydrate [$Ca(COOH)_2 \cdot H_2O$; whewellite]. **A:** Typical stone of about 4 mm in diameter. **B:** Adjacent surface of the same stone showing a "papillary pit" that often, as in this instance, contains nidus of apatite. **C:** Oval and dumbbell-shaped $Ca(COOH)_2 \cdot H_2O$ crystals, about 5 mm in diameter, in urine sediment. **D:** Same field as **C** under polarized light, demonstrating high birefringence of $Ca(COOH)_2 \cdot H_2O$.

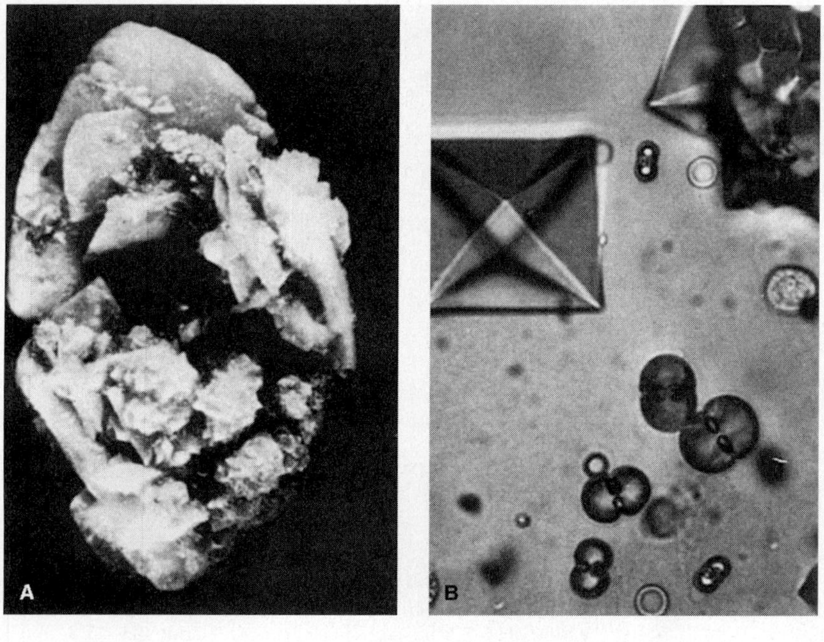

Figure 53.2. Calcium oxalate dihydrate [$Ca(COOH)_2 \cdot 2H_2O$; weddellite]. **A:** Stone showing imperfect octahedral surface crystals of $Ca(COOH)_2 \cdot 2H_2O$. **B:** Urine sediment showing typical octahedral crystals of $Ca(COOH)_2 \cdot 2H_2O$ and dumbbell-shaped crystals of $Ca(COOH)_2 \cdot H_2O$.

Urologic Treatment of Nephrolithiasis

The spectrum of options available for the urologic treatment of symptomatic urolithiasis has greatly expanded in the past two decades. Open surgical procedures are now rarely needed, as the use of extracorporeal shock-wave lithotripsy (ESWL), percutaneous nephrostolithotomy, and ureteroscopy have become widely available. Small ureteral stones, less than 5 mm in greatest diameter, generally pass spontaneously; such patients do not usually require surgical intervention and may be treated with analgesics, fluids, and observation. The majority of patients seen with renal colic will have small ureteral calculi with

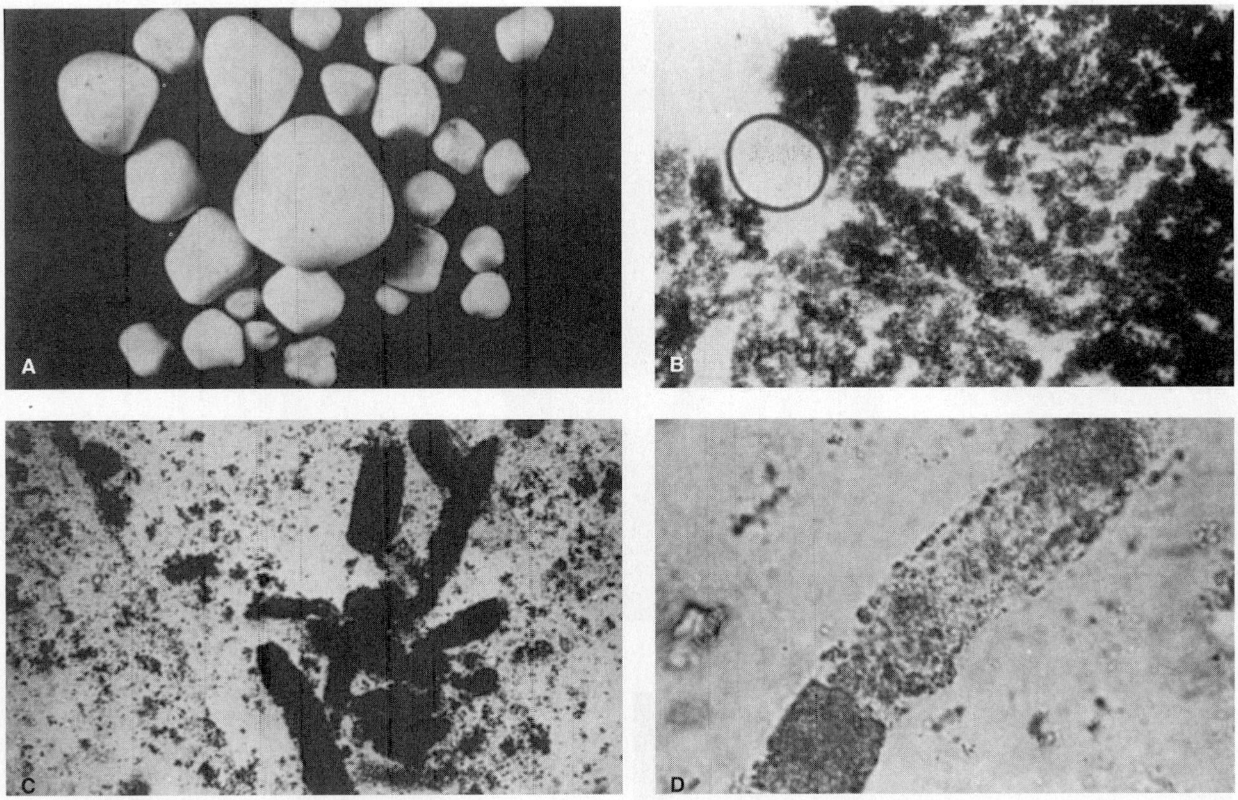

Figure 53.3. Calcium phosphate [usually apatite, $Ca_{10}(PO_4)_6(OH)_2$ or $Ca_{10}(PO_4)_6CO_3$; rarely brushite, $CaHPO_4 \cdot 2H_2O$]. **A:** Apatite stones. **B:** Calcium phosphate in urine sediment. **C:** Calcium phosphate in casts in urine sediment; original magnification ×100. **D:** Calcium phosphate in cast; original magnification ×400.

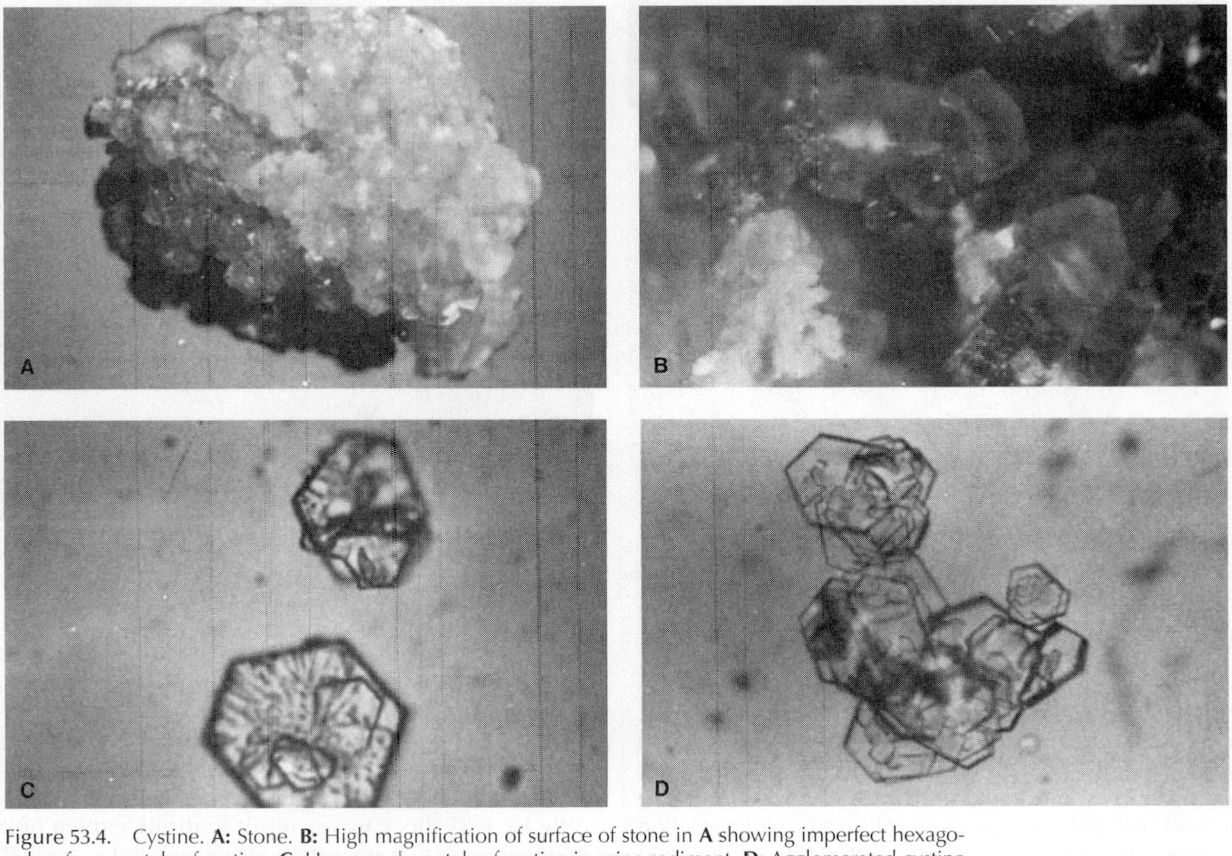

Figure 53.4. Cystine. **A:** Stone. **B:** High magnification of surface of stone in **A** showing imperfect hexagonal surface crystals of cystine. **C:** Hexagonal crystals of cystine in urine sediment. **D:** Agglomerated cystine crystals in urine sediment.

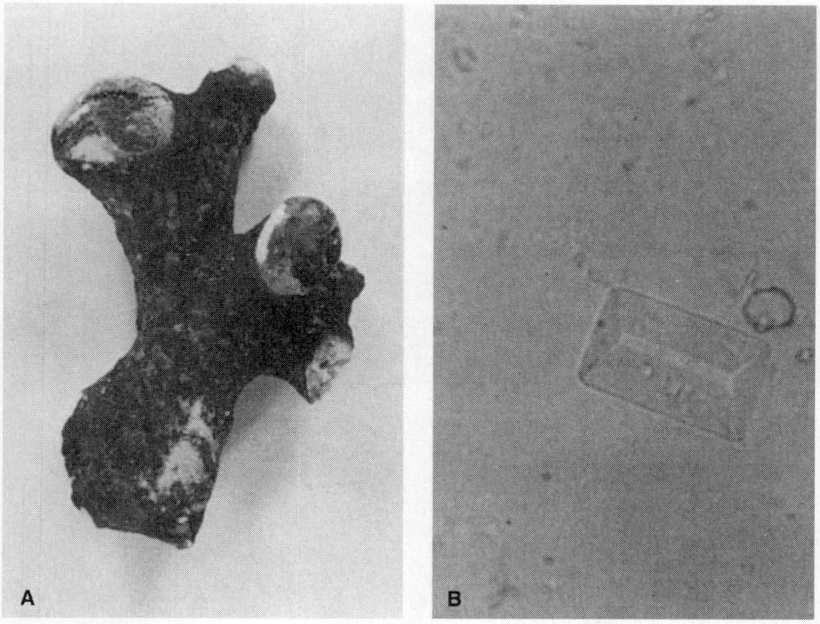

Figure 53.5. Struvite ($MgNH_4PO_4{\cdot}6H_2O$). **A:** Staghorn stone composed of struvite and carbonate apatite formed as a cast of the renal pelvis and calyces. **B:** Prismatic or "coffin-lid" crystal of struvite in urine sediment.

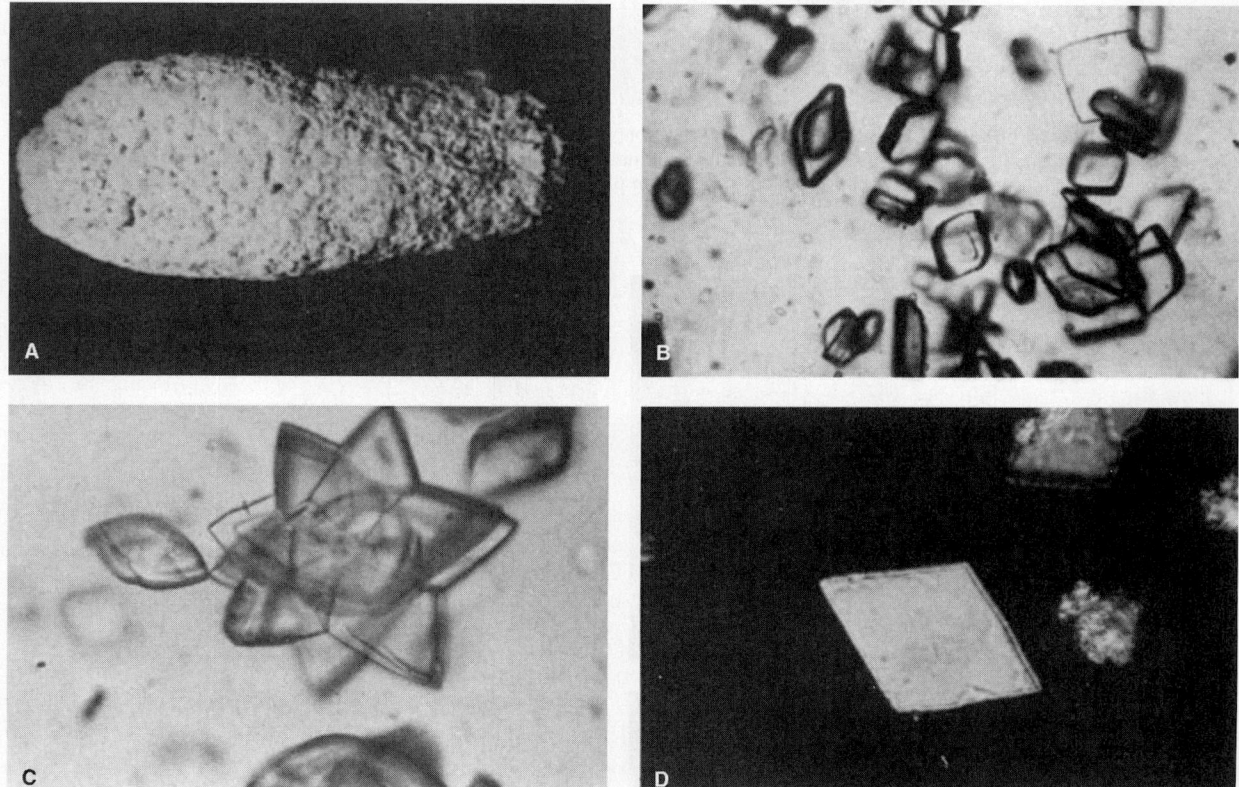

Figure 53.6. Uric acid. **A:** Stone. **B:** Rhomboidal and cuboidal uric acid crystals in urine sediment. **C:** Agglomerated uric acid crystal, rosette, in urine sediment. **D:** Rhomboidal uric acid crystal in urine sediment under polarized light demonstrating birefringence.

a high likelihood of spontaneous passage. Larger ureteral stones (greater than 7 mm), symptomatic stones in the renal pelvis, and staghorn calculi will require surgical intervention. Management of ureteral stones of intermediate size will vary depending on the presence of pain, infection, and ureteral obstruction, and such patients should be followed in collaboration with the urologist. The choice of surgical modality will depend on factors such as the location of the stone(s), their size and presumed composition, and the presence or absence of infection. Stones impacted in the lower ureter often can be extracted or fragmented using a ureteroscope. Pelvic and upper ureteral stones are most often treated by ESWL, in which fluoroscopically focused shock waves result in disintegration of the stone into fragments that are usually small enough to pass in the urine.

In the U.S. Cooperative Study of ESWL, lithotripsy rendered 78% of patients with single stones that were less than 2 cm wide free of stones within 3 months. Complications of lithotripsy include ureteral obstruction by stone fragments (*steinstrasse*), which required intervention in 7% of the US Cooperative Study patients, and pain; both are related to the size of the stone treated. Bleeding severe enough to require transfusion occurred rarely, but clinically apparent perinephric hematomas occurred in 0.66% of patients. To minimize the risk of bleeding, discontinuation of salicylates 2 weeks before ESWL is advisable. Patients with pyuria or bacteriuria may develop septic complications after lithotripsy. Prophylactic antibiotics should be instituted in such patients before ESWL and in those with a history of urinary tract infection. Percutaneous nephrostolithotomy and direct ultrasonic or laser lithotripsy may be used for stone removal or disintegration when extracorporeal lithotripsy is not feasible or successful. Large calculi, especially struvite staghorn stones, are often treated by a combination of extracorporeal and percutaneous lithotripsy. The morbidity of percutaneous techniques is higher than that of ESWL. It should be emphasized that the availability of shock-wave lithotripsy does not decrease the need for proper evaluation of stone formers to determine the cause of stone formation, followed by appropriate therapy to prevent new stone formation and, if possible, growth of retained stones, if any. Detailed discussion of lithotripsy is found in Chapter 99.

Determination of Stone Composition

Often a determination of stone type can be strongly suspected based on the initial radiographs and urinalysis, but accurate analysis of a recovered stone is required and should be performed by a laboratory with the necessary expertise and experience in the analysis of stones by optical crystallographic techniques, x-ray diffraction, and infrared spectroscopy.

Subsequent Evaluation of Nephrolithiasis

Nephrolithiasis tends to recur. Several studies have shown that, without treatment, patients with calcium oxalate stones have about a 14% chance of recurrence at 1 year, 35% at 5 years, and more than 50% by 10 years. Prevention of recurrent stones can reduce the need for hospitalization and surgery and is therefore cost-effective. A newer study estimated that adequate medical preventive therapy can result in an average saving of about $2,000/patient per year. The diagnostic evaluation of stone formers is concerned with identifying those metabolic abnormalities that raise urine supersaturation with the relevant stone salts, so that rational therapy may be selected. Therapy that is tailored to the abnormalities uncovered can lower supersaturation and decrease recurrence. Detailed evaluation of such patients is best postponed until after recovery from the acute episodes of ureteral colic and stone passage or recovery from a surgical procedure and until a time when they are generally well, free of symptoms, and eating normally.

Table 53.3 outlines a scheme for the evaluation of patients with recurrent nephrolithiasis, and subsequent sections of this chapter consider the causes of and treatment for each type of stone. Evaluation should include a history, including a complete diet history and questioning about ingestion of any nonprescription or prescription medications. The history and physical examination should focus on uncovering any underlying systemic illness that may predispose to stone formation. A urinalysis should also be performed, with attention to the urine pH. Evaluation also requires at least one and preferably two or three 24-hour urine collections, which should be analyzed for creatinine, calcium, uric acid, citrate, sodium, potassium, magnesium, pH, and volume. Oxalate excretion must also be measured, preferably in a 24-hour urine specimen preserved in acid during collection to prevent nonenzymatic conversion of ascorbate to oxalate. A qualitative screen for cystine may also be performed. At least one blood sample should be obtained for measurement of calcium, phosphate, albumin, creatinine, uric acid, potassium, sodium, chloride, and bicarbonate. Radiographs of the kidney should be reviewed to assess the size and location of any stones remaining in the kidneys.

Patients who have passed a single calcium oxalate stone may not require such an extensive workup. The history and physical examination should be reviewed to exclude factors that predispose to recurrence, such as inflammatory bowel disease, and measurement of serum calcium, phosphorus, and electrolytes should be done to exclude other systemic illnesses such as hyperparathyroidism. In the absence of such risk factors, recommendations to decrease sodium and protein intake and increase water intake may be sufficient. Patients with other types of stones, as well as children, and those with multiple stones seen on x-ray film, should have more detailed evaluation. Patients with recurrent stones need evaluation, as prolonged observation and multiple recurrences may lessen the chances for remission of stone formation.

Collection of 24-hour urine volume should be done 4 to 8 weeks after treatment has been instituted to monitor efficacy by reevaluating urine excretion rates and levels of supersaturation. Ongoing evaluation should be done at yearly intervals or more often if needed.

CALCIUM OXALATE AND APATITE STONES

Stones composed of calcium oxalate and/or apatite (Figs. 53.1, 53.2, and 53.3) may form because of (a) elevated urinary calcium or oxalate concentrations due to an increase in daily rates of calcium or oxalate excretion or a reduction in urine volume, (b) impaired urinary acidification favoring calcium phosphate precipitation, and (c) the lack of normal inhibitors, or the presence of promoters of crystal nucleation or crystal growth. Many patients have more than one abnormality. Calcium stone disease may first be manifested in childhood, especially in those with primary hyperoxaluria or distal renal tubular acidosis (RTA), but typically begins in the third and fourth decades. A family history of urolithiasis is frequent and is found in 16% to 37% of patients. The symptoms of calcium stones vary widely and include the coincidental radiographic observation of an asymptomatic stone, the passage of a single stone, the repetitive passage of gravel or small stones every few days, or the development of severe pain with partial or complete ureteral obstruction. The diagnosis of a calcium stone is suspected by the finding of a radiodense stone in a symptomatic patient. In such a patient, the presence of calcium oxalate and/or apatite crystalluria in the sediment from a fresh, warm urine specimen (Figs. 53.1, 53.2, and 53.3) provides strong support for a calcium-containing stone. Other radiodense stones (i.e., struvite and cystine) may be excluded by an acid urine pH and the absence of pyuria and bacteriuria (excludes struvite–apatite stone), together with the absence of cystine crystals and a negative cyanide nitroprusside test (excludes cystinuria). The diagnosis is confirmed by analysis of the stone. Diagnostic evaluation of patients with calcium oxalate–apatite stones is focused on detecting the possible mechanism for stone formation as outlined in Table 53.3.

TABLE 53.3. Evaluation of the Patient with Nephrolithiasis

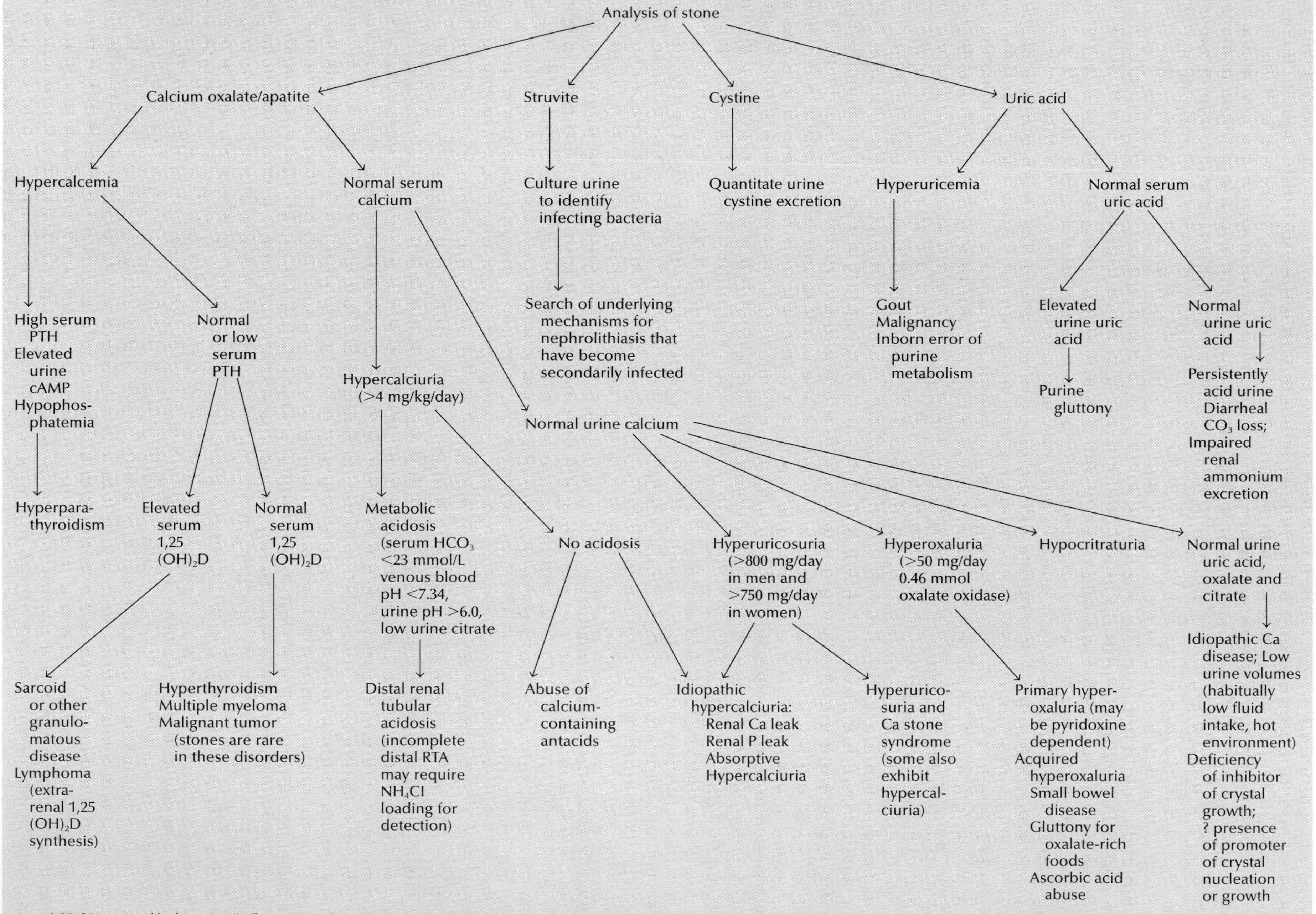

$1,25(OH)_2$, 1,25-dihydroxyvitamin D; cAMP, cyclic adenosine monophosphate; PTH, parathyroid hormone; RTA, renal tubular acidosis.

TABLE 53.4. Factors Increasing or Decreasing Urinary Calcium Excretion by Changing Either Glomerular Filtration or Tubular Reabsorption of Calcium

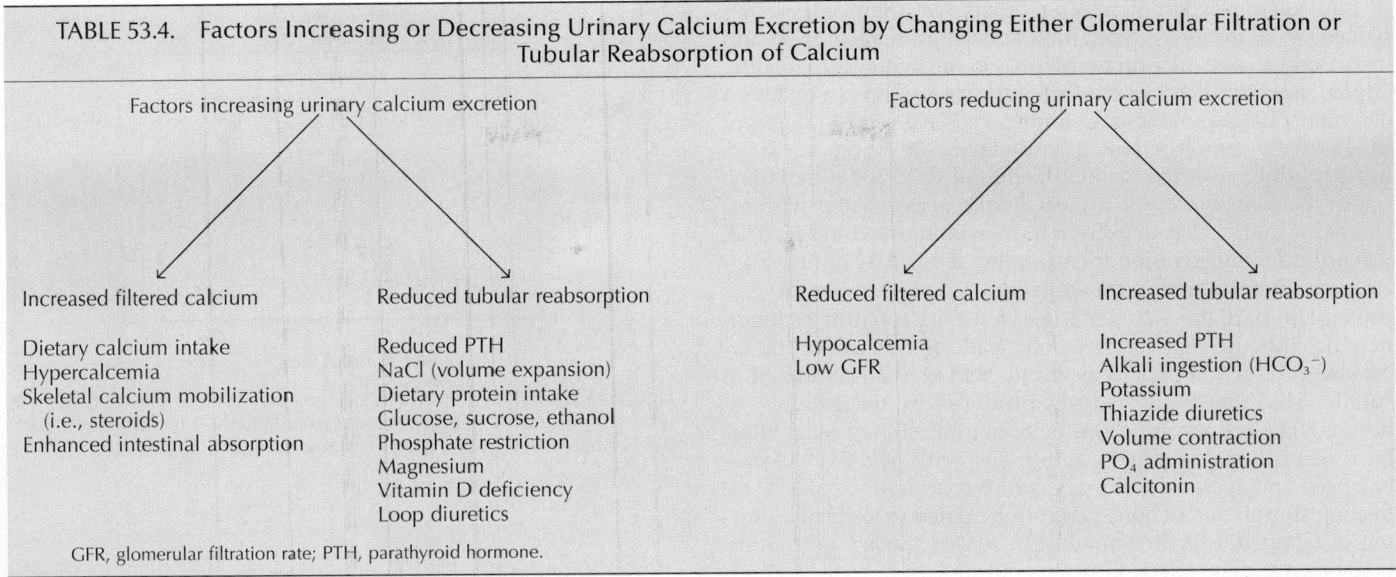

Factors increasing urinary calcium excretion		Factors reducing urinary calcium excretion	
Increased filtered calcium	Reduced tubular reabsorption	Reduced filtered calcium	Increased tubular reabsorption
Dietary calcium intake	Reduced PTH	Hypocalcemia	Increased PTH
Hypercalcemia	NaCl (volume expansion)	Low GFR	Alkali ingestion (HCO_3^-)
Skeletal calcium mobilization (i.e., steroids)	Dietary protein intake		Potassium
Enhanced intestinal absorption	Glucose, sucrose, ethanol		Thiazide diuretics
	Phosphate restriction		Volume contraction
	Magnesium		PO_4 administration
	Vitamin D deficiency		Calcitonin
	Loop diuretics		

GFR, glomerular filtration rate; PTH, parathyroid hormone.

Urinary Calcium Excretion and a Consideration of Factors Known to Influence Calcium Excretion

Ultimately urinary calcium excretion in the steady state in healthy persons must reflect the net rate of calcium entry into the extracellular fluid (ECF) from the diet via the intestine and from bone, the site of 95% or more of body stores of calcium, that is, net loss of calcium from ECF to bone during growth or skeletal repair and net gain of calcium from bone when bone formation is inhibited or bone resorption is stimulated. Intestinal absorption and renal handling of calcium is discussed in detail in Chapter 17. Increased urinary calcium excretion may be the consequence of either an increase in glomerular filtration of calcium, or inhibition of renal tubular calcium reabsorption, or both. The major factors that are known to increase or decrease urinary calcium excretion are listed in Table 53.4. The effect of dietary calcium intake on urinary calcium excretion in healthy adults is shown in Fig. 53.7 for several studies of subjects among whom dietary calcium intake was changed. On the average, urinary calcium excretion increases about 0.08 mmol/1 mmol increase in dietary calcium intake (8 mg/100 mg increase in dietary calcium). Intestinal calcium absorption rises slightly as calcium intake increases, leading to subtle increases in plasma (filterable) calcium and thus increased glomerular filtration of calcium. At the same time, an increase in plasma (ionized) calcium is accompanied by a subtle decline in parathyroid hormone (PTH) secretion and thus decreased renal tubular reabsorption of filtered calcium. Figure 53.7 also emphasizes that, on the average, urinary calcium excretion for healthy adults does not exceed 5 mmol/day (200 mg/day) even at dietary calcium intakes of 40 mmol/day (1,600 mg/day). Among healthy adults studied in metabolic wards while fed diets providing 15 to 30 mmol of calcium/day (600 to 1,200 mg/day), urinary calcium excretion averaged 3.9 ± 1.6 (SD) mmol/day (156 ± 64 mg/day). Thus the upper limit of urinary calcium excretion among healthy adults, taken as this mean ± 2 SD, is about 7.1 mmol/day (285 mg/day), similar to the generally accepted upper limit of normal of 7.5 mmol/day (300 mg/day) in men or 6.25 mmol/day (250 mg/day) in women or about 0.1 mmol/kg per day (4 mg/kg per day) regardless of sex or age.

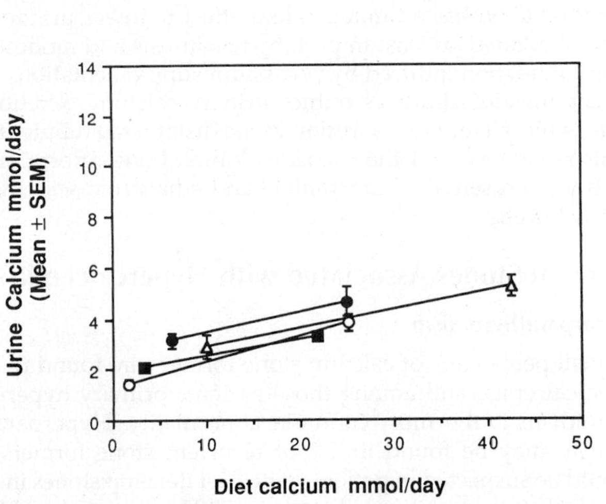

Figure 53.7. Effect of changing dietary calcium intake in healthy adults on urinary calcium excretion. (Adapted from Lemann J Jr. Idiopathic hypercalciuria. In: Coe FC, Brenner B, Stein B, eds. *Contemporary issues in nephrology*. Edinburgh: Churchill Livingstone, 1980;vol 5:86–115.)

Hypercalcemic disorders augment urinary calcium by increasing glomerular filtration of calcium. When hypercalcemia is the consequence of hyperparathyroidism, this increase is blunted by the effect of PTH to stimulate renal tubular calcium reabsorption. However, when hypercalcemia is caused by other factors, such as humoral hypercalcemia of malignancy or 1,25-dihydroxyvitamin D_3 [1,25$(OH)_2$D] excess in granulomatous diseases, PTH secretion is suppressed, and the magnitude of hypercalciuria can be expected to be exaggerated in relation to the filtered load of calcium because of the relative absence of the effect of PTH to stimulate renal tubular calcium reabsorption. 1,25$(OH)_2$D, by stimulating intestinal calcium absorption and stimulating bone resorption when dietary calcium is limited, appears to increase urinary calcium excretion by increasing plasma calcium concentrations and thus filtered calcium. Vitamin D has an independent effect on renal tubular absorption of calcium; vitamin D deficiency has been shown to reduce tubular calcium reabsorption in experimental animals, although the site of action is uncertain.

PTH is known to stimulate renal tubular calcium reabsorption in the distal renal tubule. Thus for patients with hypoparathyroidism urinary calcium excretion is higher than normal relative to serum calcium concentrations.

Infusion of NaCl or increasing dietary NaCl intake is accompanied by inhibition of renal tubular calcium reabsorption and increased urinary calcium excretion. On the average, in healthy adults, urinary calcium excretion appears to increase by about 0.6 mmol/100 mmol increase in dietary NaCl intake (25 mg of calcium/100 mmol of NaCl) as dietary salt intake varies in healthy adults over the usual extremes of 10 to 300 mmol/day.

An increase in dietary protein intake is associated with increased urinary calcium excretion. As summarized in Fig. 53.8, urinary calcium excretion increases by about 0.04 mmol/g increase in dietary protein intake (about 1.5 mg of calcium/g of protein). In part, the augmentation of urinary calcium excretion may be caused by subtle metabolic acidosis because of the increased production of acid as amino acid sulfur is oxidized to sulfate. Mild metabolic acidosis, produced by the administration of NH_4Cl, is accompanied by both inhibition of renal tubular reabsorption of filtered calcium and with negative calcium balances and increased urinary hydroxyproline excretion, reflecting stimulation of bone resorption related to skeletal buffering of retained acid. Presumably, increased dietary protein intake has a similar effect. However, administration of $NaHCO_3$ only partially corrects the effect of increased dietary protein intake to increase urinary calcium excretion. The presence in renal tubular fluid of increased concentrations of sulfate, a poorly reabsorbed anion derived from oxidation of amino acid sulfur, may also contribute to the effect of increased protein intake to augment urinary calcium excretion because of the ability of sulfate to complex calcium in solution and thereby limit renal tubular calcium reabsorption. Urinary calcium excretion is increased to a greater extent when Na_2SO_4 is infused compared with the infusion of equivalent amounts of Na as NaCl. It is noteworthy that neither NH_4Cl acidosis nor increased dietary protein intake appear to be compensated for by augmentation of intestinal calcium absorption or activation of the parathyroid–vitamin D endocrine systems. Ingestion of other rapidly metabolized nutrients such as glucose, sucrose, or ethanol augment urinary calcium excretion by inhibiting renal tubular calcium reabsorption.

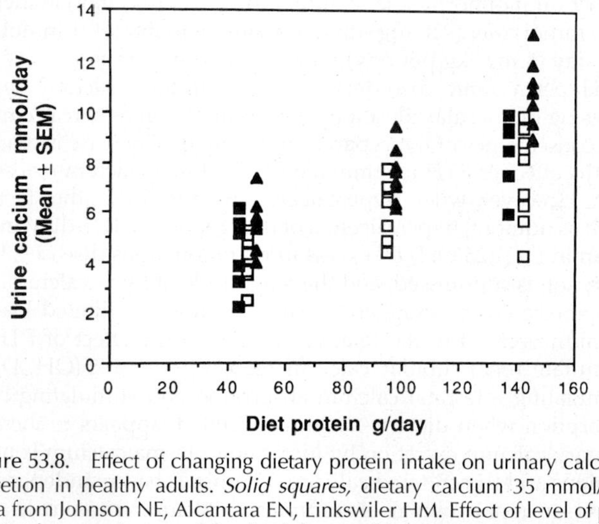

Figure 53.8. Effect of changing dietary protein intake on urinary calcium excretion in healthy adults. *Solid squares,* dietary calcium 35 mmol/day (data from Johnson NE, Alcantara EN, Linkswiler HM. Effect of level of protein intake on urinary and fecal calcium and calcium retention of young adult males. *J Nutr* 1970;100:1425–1430); *solid triangles,* dietary calcium 20 mmol/day (data from Walker RM, Linkswiler HM. Calcium retention in the adult human male as affected by protein intake. *J Nutr* 1972;102: 1297–1302); *open squares,* dietary calcium 12.5 mmol/day (data from Anand CR, Linkswiler HM. Effect of protein intake on calcium balance of young men given 500 mg calcium daily. *J Nutr* 1984;104:695–700).

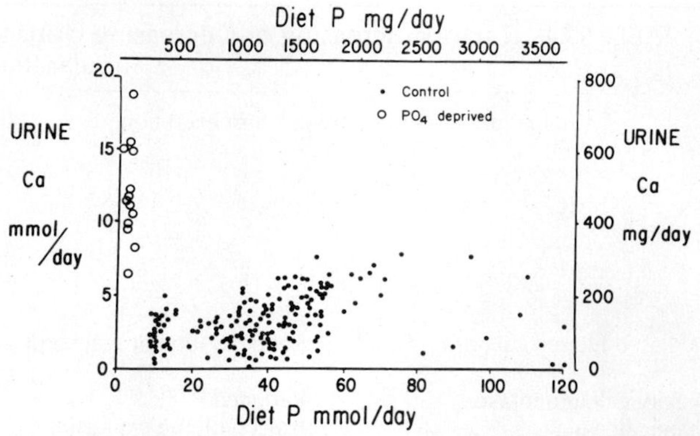

Figure 53.9. Relation of urinary calcium excretion to dietary phosphate intake. (Reproduced with permission from Lemann J Jr, Adams ND, Gray RW. Urinary calcium excretion in human beings. *N Engl J Med* 1979;301: 535–541.)

As shown in Fig. 53.9, extreme dietary phosphate restriction (less than 10 mmol or less than 300 mg of phosphorus/day) is accompanied by increased urinary calcium excretion, negative calcium balance, and a fall in serum PTH concentrations. Increased bone resorption and inhibition of renal tubular calcium reabsorption appear to contribute to the increase in urinary calcium excretion. However, it should be emphasized that variations in dietary phosphate intake over usual normal ranges of 20 to 50 mmol/day (600 to 1,500 mg/day) have little effect on urinary calcium excretion.

Urinary calcium excretion falls early in the course of established chronic kidney disease presumably in part due to the fall in glomerular filtration rate (GFR). In addition, however, renal tubular reabsorption of filtered calcium appears to be increased because the fractional excretion of filtered calcium falls early in renal failure despite a rise in the fractional excretion of filtered sodium. Secondary hyperparathyroidism that occurs in early renal failure is responsible.

As noted previously, the administration of bicarbonate reduces urinary calcium excretion and acts by directly enhancing renal tubular calcium reabsorption in the distal tubule. Alkali administered as potassium citrate or bicarbonate reduces urinary calcium excretion whereas equimolar quantities of sodium citrate or bicarbonate do not. It appears that the simultaneous sodium load blunts the anticalciuric effect of alkali. Potassium administration has an independent effect to lower urinary calcium, mediated, at least in part, by natriuresis and modest volume contraction induced by potassium supplementation.

The thiazide diuretics reduce urinary calcium excretion by increasing calcium reabsorption in the distal renal tubule. There is also evidence that the thiazides inhibit bone resorption. By contrast, furosemide, bumetanide, and ethacrynic acid are calciuric diuretics.

Calcium Stones Associated with Hypercalcemia

Hyperparathyroidism

A small percentage of calcium stone formers are found to have hypercalcemia, and among those patients primary hyperparathyroidism is the most common abnormality. Hyperparathyroidism may be found in 5% of recurrent stone formers and should be suspected in patients who first develop stones in their fifth and sixth decades and in women. The reported incidence of stones in patients with hyperparathyroidism has been falling in recent years as milder cases are recognized and varies from 4% to 40% in several recent series; over all, stones occur in about

10% to 20% of patients with clinically recognized hyperparathyroidism. Hypercalciuria and a tendency for a relatively alkaline urine (pH 6.0 or higher) appear to be the principal factors accounting for nephrolithiasis in hyperparathyroidism. The elevation of plasma calcium results in an increase in glomerular filtration of calcium that exceeds the simultaneous stimulation of renal tubular calcium reabsorption by PTH, thereby causing hypercalciuria. Furthermore, the excess PTH and associated hypophosphatemia inhibit proximal renal tubular reabsorption of bicarbonate, thus tending to make the final urine less acid. Together, these events favor brushite precipitation. Calcium oxalate stones are most often observed, perhaps because of heterogeneous nucleation of calcium oxalate crystallization by brushite. The additional calcium appearing in the urine is ultimately derived from both the skeleton and from the diet because PTH directly enhances bone resorption and stimulates renal synthesis of $1,25(OH)_2D$ thereby augmenting intestinal calcium absorption. The incidence of stones in patients with hyperparathyroidism appears to be related to the degree of hypercalciuria as determined by serum $1,25(OH)_2D$. The diagnosis of hyperparathyroidism is confirmed by the observation of persistent hypercalcemia (best assessed by ionized calcium concentration), which may be rather mild, with an elevated serum PTH concentration in the presence of a normal GFR. Other abnormalities include hypophosphatemia and a low percentage of renal tubular reabsorption of phosphorus because of the inhibition of renal tubular phosphate reabsorption by PTH. In addition, urinary cyclic adenosine monophosphate (cAMP) excretion or nephrogenous cAMP excretion (urinary cAMP minus filtered cAMP) may be elevated due to the activation of renal adenylate cyclase by PTH. Fasting hypercalciuria (urinary calcium exceeding 0.12 mg/mg of creatinine in the second morning urine specimen after overnight fasting) is also generally observed because of ongoing bone resorption and hypercalcemia. Elevation of serum alkaline phosphatase (heat-labile fraction) and radiographic evidence of subperiosteal bone resorption or other signs of bone disease secondary to excess PTH may also be observed, depending upon the duration and severity of the state of hyperparathyroidism. Treatment requires parathyroidectomy by an experienced surgeon. The majority of patients will have adenomas, usually solitary; 20% to 30% will have hyperplasia involving several glands. Patients with hyperplasia may have one of the multiple endocrine neoplasia syndromes. Postoperatively, recurrence of stone formation is unusual, especially in patients found to have adenomas at surgery.

Granulomatous Diseases

Sarcoidosis is often associated with hypercalciuria; hypercalcemia may also be present and is generally associated with mild to moderate azotemia. Urolithiasis and nephrocalcinosis occur in some patients as a result of the elevated urinary excretion of calcium. The hypercalciuria is the result of both increased bone resorption and increased intestinal calcium absorption because cystic bone lesions may be observed and increased intestinal absorption of calcium and abnormal sensitivity to administered vitamin D are well documented. Studies have provided evidence that serum levels of $1,25(OH)_2D$ are elevated due to extrarenal synthesis of $1,25(OH)_2D$ by macrophages in the granulomas, and the elevated serum $1,25(OH)_2D$ levels account for the increase in intestinal calcium absorption. Production of $1,25(OH)_2D$ in the sarcoid granulomas appears to be dependent on the availability of precursor 25(OH)D because serum $1,25(OH)_2D$ levels rise in patients with sarcoid when 25(OH)D levels are increased by the administration of vitamin D or when cutaneous vitamin D synthesis is increased by exposure to sunlight. Similar elevations of serum $1,25(OH)_2D$ resulting in hypercalciuria and hypercalcemia with or without stones have been observed in patients with other granulomatous disorders including tuberculosis, coccidioidomycosis, and extensive foreign body granulomas. In addition, some patients with lymphomas may exhibit a similar syndrome. It should be emphasized again that hypercalcemic patients with granulomatous disorders or a lymphoma are often azotemic. Thus serum $1,25(OH)_2D$ levels are high not only absolutely but also relative to the degree of renal insufficiency. Azotemia may reverse with treatment of hypercalcemia. The hypercalcemia of sarcoidosis responds very well to administration of small doses of glucocorticoids (10 to 30 mg of prednisone/day). Chloroquine and hydroxychloroquine may also reduce serum $1,25(OH)_2D$ levels and urinary calcium excretion in patients who are intolerant of glucocorticoids. Ketoconazole, an antifungal agent that interferes with synthesis of steroid hormones, has also been used successfully to treat hypercalcemia in this disorder.

Hyperthyroidism

Hyperthyroidism is often associated with bone loss and hypercalciuria and is occasionally associated with hypercalcemia caused by stimulation of bone resorption by the thyroid hormones. Serum PTH and $1,25(OH)_2D$ levels are low or low normal. Despite hypercalciuria, nephrolithiasis in association with hyperthyroidism is very rare.

Malignancies Including Multiple Myeloma

Hypercalcemia and hypercalciuria accompany a number of malignant tumors, and malignancy is the most common cause of hypercalcemia in hospitalized patients. Hypercalcemia results from osteoclast-mediated bone resorption. Bone metastases may stimulate local release of osteoclast-activating factors such as interleukin-1, lymphotoxin, and prostaglandin E. In the absence of bone metastases, tumor cells may produce humoral factors, including PTH-related peptide (PTHrP) and transforming growth factor α, that stimulate osteoclastic bone resorption. Nephrolithiasis is rare, probably because of the relatively short duration of these syndromes.

Immobilization

Hypercalciuria and, rarely, hypercalcemia occur occasionally when patients with accelerated bone turnover such as rapidly growing adolescents or individuals with Paget's disease are suddenly immobilized because of fractures or paralytic neurologic disorders. Reduced bone formation, as a consequence of the lack of normal bone stresses during weight-bearing and walking, with normal rates of bone dissolution, is thought to be the underlying cause. Early ambulation may prevent hypercalciuria and stones. Fluid intake should be increased during the period of immobilization to assure daily urine volumes of 2 L or more.

Calcium Stones Associated with Hypercalciuria without Hypercalcemia

Distal Renal Tubular Acidosis (Type 1 RTA)

RTA caused by a defect in hydrogen ion secretion in the distal tubule is a rare but important cause of recurrent stone formation. The RTA may be either hereditary or acquired and causes a hyperchloremic metabolic acidosis. Both autosomal dominant and autosomal recessive inheritance patterns have been described. The basic defect appears to involve a limitation in the capacity of the distal renal tubule to establish a normally steep hydrogen ion gradient between tubular urine and blood. As a result, the urine cannot be maximally acidified, and urine pH is relatively alkaline. Significant urinary bicarbonate wasting is not present. Hypokalemia may also be present and of sufficient severity to cause muscle weakness and paralysis. Newer work has linked the autosomal dominant form of the disorder to mutations in the basolateral chloride–bicarbonate exchanger gene AE1. Patients with proximal RTA do not form stones because they can acidify their urine maximally and do not have hypercalciuria.

Nephrolithiasis in patients with RTA is due to the presence of several risk factors, including hypercalciuria, hypocitraturia, and elevated urine pH; the combination of these abnormalities produces urine that is supersaturated with respect to calcium oxalate and calcium phosphate. Hypercalciuria is often present. In some cases it is the result of a chronically positive hydrogen ion balance and, as a consequence, loss of bone mineral because intestinal calcium absorption is apparently not increased. Since studies have demonstrated that increased bicarbonate delivery to distal tubule segments enhances net tubular calcium reabsorption, it is conceivable that the hypercalciuria is the result of reduced distal bicarbonate delivery when serum bicarbonate levels are low and proximal tubular bicarbonate resorptive capacity is normal. In other cases, the basic defect appears to be idiopathic hypercalciuria, and the RTA is believed to be secondary. Hypocitraturia is present in almost all patients with distal RTA, as a result of systemic acidosis and hypokalemia, and reabsorption of filtered citrate in the proximal tubule. Patients form both apatite and calcium oxalate stones.

Although RTA is a rare disorder, distal screening studies should be routinely carried out in patients with calcium nephrolithiasis and/or nephrocalcinosis, especially if the patient's stones contain a large amount of brushite or apatite. The diagnosis is established by the finding of (a) hyperchloremic metabolic acidosis with a plasma bicarbonate level below 24 mEq/l and a venous blood pH below 7.34, (b) urine pH persistently 5.5 or higher in the absence of urinary tract infection, and (c) hypocitraturia. The documentation of the high urinary pH should be made by the patient measuring her or his urine pH with phenaphthazine paper at each voiding throughout the day for several days. The defect in maximum acidification of the final urine can be more formally evaluated by assessing the response of urine pH to oral administration of a standard acid load in the form of ammonium chloride. Patients may be found to have an incomplete form of RTA, in which serum bicarbonate concentration is normal, but urine acidification in response to an acid load is decreased.

Alkali therapy is effective for correcting the acidosis and can decrease the stone-forming tendency. Newer studies suggest that potassium citrate is the preferred form of alkali. Alkali given as the potassium salt can decrease calcium excretion because of the effect of increased intratubular pH to increase calcium reabsorption, whereas sodium salts do not; both will increase citrate excretion. The net result is to decrease the degree of supersaturation of the urine with respect to calcium oxalate. Effective therapy is provided by the administration of sufficient alkali to maintain a normal morning serum bicarbonate concentration of 26 to 28 mEq/L. Incomplete RTA also may respond well to alkali therapy. One or 2 mEq of alkali/kg of body weight/day in divided doses may be given as potassium citrate (Polycitra-K, Urocit-K) or as a mixture of potassium citrate, acetate, and bicarbonate (K-lyte). With this therapy, recurrence of stones is decreased, nephrocalcinosis does not progress despite more alkaline urine, and bone disease, if present, often resolves. In some families, idiopathic hypercalciuria may coexist with RTA; if the urine calcium concentration does not fall with citrate therapy, additional treatment with a thiazide may be needed.

Other Renal Tubulopathies

A number of rare renal tubular disorders are known, including hypercalciuria and sometimes nephrolithiasis or nephrocalcinosis as manifestations. Newer studies have identified the molecular basis for some of these syndromes. X-linked nephrolithiasis comprises four related clinical syndromes, including X-linked recessive nephrolithiasis and Dent's disease, which share findings such as hypercalciuria, calcium stone formation, low-molecular-weight proteinuria, and eventual renal failure; rickets is also found in some kindreds. These syndromes are associated with inactivating mutations of the gene for CLC-5, a voltage-gated chloride channel. How abnormal function of this gene leads to the hypercalciuria and other tubular transport findings in these syndromes is not known.

Idiopathic Hypercalciuria

Among many series of patients with calcium oxalate–apatite kidney stones, 30% to 60% exhibit hypercalciuria in the absence of hypercalcemia, evidence of overt clinical bone disease, or distal renal tubular acidosis. Generally accepted definitions of hypercalciuria are a urinary calcium excretion of more than 7.5 mmol/day (more than 300 mg/day) in men or 6.25 mmol/day (250 mg/day) in women or more than 0.1 mmol/kg per day (more than 4 mg/kg per day) or more than 140 mg/g of creatinine in either sex. Several studies suggest that idiopathic hypercalciuria (IH) is an inherited disorder, as first-degree relatives of patients with IH have an increased incidence of hypercalciuria and kidney stones.

For a patient with a calcium stone and an elevated urinary calcium excretion rate, consideration must be given to the ultimate source of the additional calcium appearing in the urine (above the average urinary calcium excretion of 4 mmol/day in healthy adults). Clearly, the additional calcium can only be derived from the diet, from bone, or both.

Many metabolic balance studies and studies using radiocalcium have documented augmented intestinal calcium absorption among stone formers. Figure 53.10 compares net intestinal calcium absorption (dietary minus fecal calcium) during balance studies of healthy adults and of hypercalciuric calcium stone formers while both groups ate diets providing similar and normal amounts of calcium. On the average, normal subjects absorbed about 5.5 mmol of calcium/day (220 mg) while the hypercalciuric calcium stone formers absorbed about 8.5 mmol/day (340 mg) or about 50% more than the normal subjects. Furthermore, as illustrated in Fig. 53.11, urinary calcium excretion for hypercalciuric stone formers remains higher than

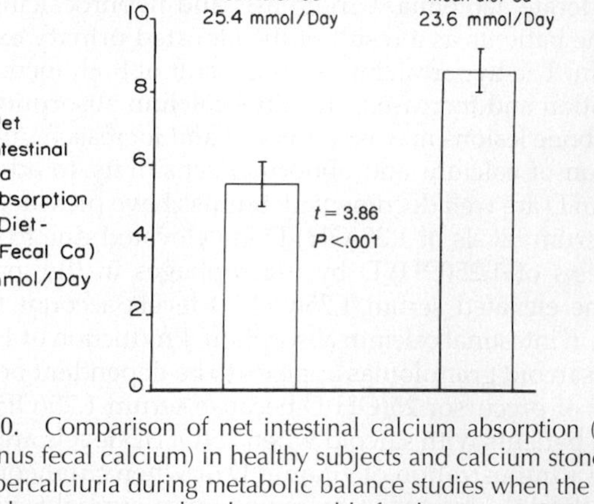

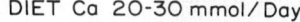

Figure 53.10. Comparison of net intestinal calcium absorption (dietary calcium minus fecal calcium) in healthy subjects and calcium stone formers with hypercalciuria during metabolic balance studies when the dietary calcium intakes were normal and comparable for the groups. (Reproduced with permission from Finlayson B, Thomas WL Jr, eds. *Colloquium on renal lithiasis*. The University Presses of Florida, 1976:280.)

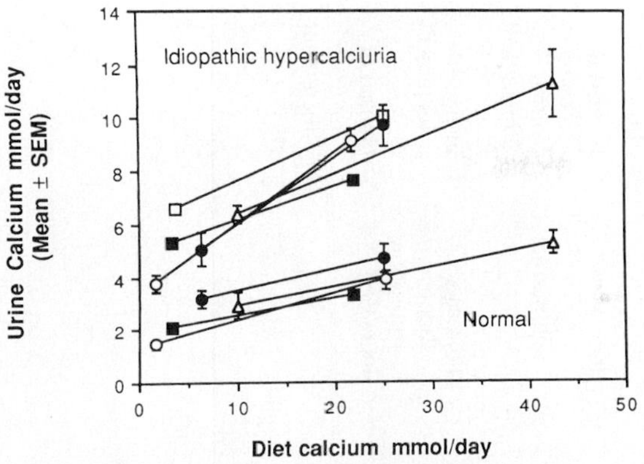

Figure 53.11. Effects of changing dietary calcium intake on urinary calcium excretion in hypercalciuric stone formers compared with healthy subjects. (Adapted from Lemann J Jr. Idiopathic hypercalciuria. In: Coe FC, Brenner B, Stein B, eds. *Contemporary issues in nephrology.* Edinburgh: Churchill Livingstone, 1980;5:86–115.)

for normal subjects when dietary calcium intake is similar. Figure 53.11 also demonstrates that urinary calcium excretion rises to a greater extent for the stone formers than for healthy adults as dietary calcium increases. For the studies depicted in Fig. 53.11, urinary calcium excretion for the stone formers increased 0.18 mmol/day for each mmol increment in dietary calcium intake (18 mg/100 mg) but only 0.08 mmol/mmol for normal subjects (8 mg/100 mg; $P < .025$). Thus for hypercalciuric stone formers intestinal calcium absorption is increased either because of augmented concentration-dependent (passive) calcium movement or an increase in active calcium transport mediated by $1,25(OH)_2D$, the only currently established stimulus for active intestinal calcium transport.

Figure 53.12 extends the evaluation of these relationships to a comparison of urinary calcium excretion as a function of net intestinal calcium absorption in hypercalciuric calcium stone formers and normal subjects while both groups ate diets providing 15 to 30 mmol of calcium/day (600 to 1,200 mg/day). For the 62 normal subjects, urinary calcium excretion averaged 3.6 ± 1.6 mmol/day, (144 ± 64 mg/day), a value less than their net intestinal calcium absorption that averaged 4.3 ± 3.1 mmol/day (172 ± 124 mg/day). Calcium balance (net intestinal calcium absorption minus urinary calcium excretion)

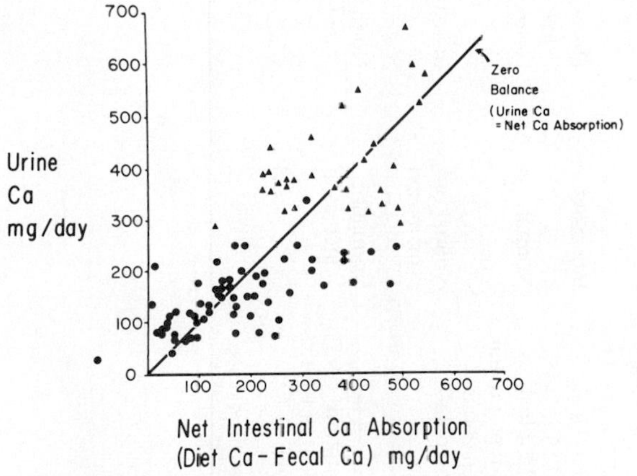

Figure 53.12. Relation between urinary calcium excretion and net intestinal calcium absorption in hypercalciuric calcium stone formers *(solid triangles)* and healthy subjects *(solid circles).* (Reproduced with permission from Lemann J Jr. Idiopathic hypercalciuria. In: Coe FC, Brenner B, Stein B, eds. *Contemporary issues in nephrology.* Edinburgh: Churchill Livingstone, 1980:5:86–115.)

for the normal subjects averaged 0.7 ± 2.4 mmol/day (28 ± 96 mg/day), a value significantly more positive than zero ($P < .05$). By contrast, for the 31 hypercalciuric calcium stone formers, urinary calcium excretion averaged 10.1 ± 2.4 mmol/day (404 ± 96 mg/day), a value greater than their average rate of net intestinal calcium absorption of 9.1 ± 2.8 mmol/day (364 ± 112 mg/day). Thus the stone formers exhibited negative calcium balances averaging −1.0 ± 2.7 mmol/day (−40 ± 108 mg/day), a value significantly more negative than zero ($P < .05$). Therefore augmentation of intestinal calcium absorption cannot be the primary or only abnormality leading to hypercalciuria among stone formers. Because of the negative calcium balances, these observations suggest that the augmentation of intestinal calcium absorption among stone formers may be part of a larger disorder that also involves a renal calcium leak and/or, speculatively, more rapid bone turnover with less efficient coupling of bone formation and bone resorption with spillage of calcium into the urine. Other studies have shown that when calcium stone formers and healthy adults were fed a very low calcium diet (0.05 mmol/kg/day or about 3.5 mmol in a 70-kg subject; 2 mg/kg per day or 140 mg), the urinary calcium excretion rates in the majority of stone formers did not decrease to levels as low as those observed for the normal subjects. These observations are also consistent with the presence of a renal calcium leak, accelerated bone turnover, or both, in addition to augmented intestinal calcium absorption. It should be said that despite the slightly negative calcium balances (Fig. 53.12) that must ultimately reflect skeletal calcium losses, bone cannot be the major source of the extra calcium appearing in the urine of hypercalciuric stone formers. If all the excess urinary calcium, approximately 5 mmol/day (200 mg/day), were derived from bone, this would result in the loss of about 7% each year of the 25,000 mmol of calcium contained in the skeleton of a normal 70-kg adult. Because hypercalciuria can be present for many years, clinically symptomatic bone loss might occur in such a circumstance, and bone disease would be expected. Clinically overt bone disease seldom occurs in hypercalciuric stone formers. On the other hand, loss of bone mineral in patients with idiopathic hypercalciuria has been found, based both on photon absorption measurements of bone density and histomorphometric evaluation of bone biopsies, as well as indirect studies demonstrating acceleration of radiocalcium kinetics and increased excretion of bone resorption markers. Several studies have shown that subjects with absorptive hypercalciuria, as well as those with fasting hypercalciuria without elevated PTH, have decreased vertebral mineral density, compared to nonhypercalciuric stone formers and normal subjects.

Table 53.5 presents a summary of proposed mechanisms accounting for hypercalciuria. Occasional patients give a history of gluttony for milk or other calcium-rich foods. As shown in the left panel of Fig. 53.13, the level of dietary calcium intake is the principle determinant of net intestinal calcium absorption when serum $1,25(OH)_2D$ levels are normal (80 pmol/L) or high (more than 130 pmol/L). Thus a large milk intake would result in augmented calcium absorption and hypercalciuria. Similarly, a patient who abused a calcium-containing antacid and used 12 tablets/day (one "roll" typically contains twelve 500-mg $CaCO_3$ tablets) would ingest 60 mmol of calcium/day (2,400 mg) and could be hypercalciuric.

Augmentation of intestinal calcium absorption due to activation of vitamin D metabolism with elevated serum levels may occur. Table 53.6 summarizes reports of serum $1,25(OH)_2D$ levels in hypercalciuric stone formers. Many researchers, although not all, have shown higher serum $1,25(OH)_2D$ levels in stone formers than in healthy subjects. Figure 53.13 shows the effect of calcitriol administration to normal subjects. When dietary calcium intake is normal, even high normal or slightly elevated

TABLE 53.5. Possible Mechanisms of Hypercalciuria

Primary Mechanism	Intestinal Calcium Absorption	Serum Calcium	Serum PTH	Urinary cAMP	Serum $1,25(OH)_2D$	Net Bone Resorption	Serum $PO_4^=$	Fasting Urine Ca/Creatinine	Urine Ca after Ca Load
Gluttony for Ca-rich food or abuse of Ca-containing antacids	Increased passive (fractional absorption of intake is low)	Normal (fasting) Increased after large Ca intake	Decreased or normal (high Ca)	Decreased	Decreased or normal	Decreased	Normal or high normal (PTH suppression)	Normal (<0.34 mmol/mmol or <0.12 mg/mg	Normal increment
Primary increased $1,25(OH)_2D$ synthesis (renal $PO_4^=$ leak and hypophosphatemia, unknown central mechanism)	Increased active (fractional absorption of intake is high)	Normal (fasting) Increased after meals	Decreased or normal (high Ca, $1,25(OH)_2D$)	Decreased	Increased	Normal (increased if diet Ca <10 mmol/day)	Normal Low if renal $PO_4^=$ leak present	Normal or increased	Increased increment
Augmented intestinal Ca absorption independent of $1,25(OH)_2D$ or enhanced sensitivity of gut to $1,25(OH)_2D$	Increased	Normal (fasting) Increased after meals	Decreased or normal	Decreased	Normal	Normal or increased	Normal or high normal	Normal or increased	Increased increment
Renal calcium "leak"—overt	Increased	Decreased or low normal	Increased	Increased	Increased	Increased	Normal	Increased	Increased increment
Subtle renal Ca leak (acidosis, high protein diet, K depletion)	Normal	Normal	Normal	Normal	Normal	? Increased	Normal	High normal	Normal increment
Primary hyperparathyroidism	Normal or increased	Increased	Increased	Increased	Increased or normal	Increased	Decreased	Increased (bone resorption)	Increased increment
Augmentation of net bone resorption independent of PTH or $1,25(OH)_2D$	Normal or increased	Normal or increased	Normal or decreased	Normal or decreased	Normal or decreased	Increased	Normal or increased	Increased	Normal or increased increment

PTH, parathyroid hormone.

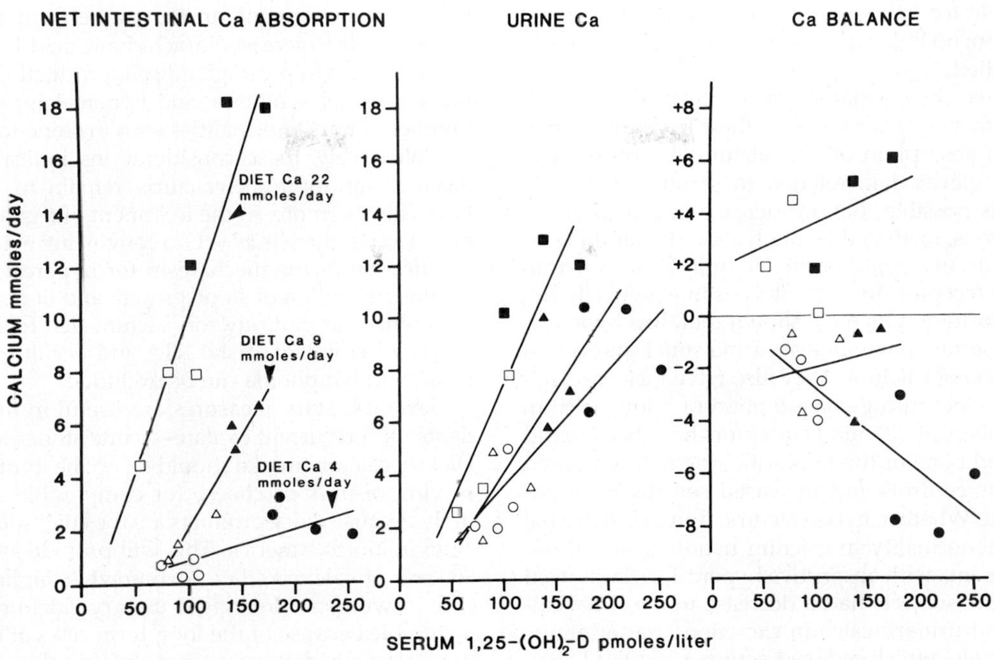

Figure 53.13. Relations of net intestinal calcium transport, urinary calcium excretion, and calcium balance to serum $1,25(OH)_2D_3$ levels in healthy men when dietary calcium intake was 22, 9, or 4 mmol/day. *Open symbols* indicate subjects who received the diet without $1,25(OH)_2D_3$; *closed symbols* indicate subjects who also received $1,25(OH)_2D$ to experimentally increase blood levels of this hormone. (Reproduced with permission from Maierhofer WJ, Lemann J Jr, Gray RW, et al. Dietary and serum $1,25(OH)_2$-vitamin D concentrations as determinants of calcium balance in healthy man. *Kidney Int* 1984;26:752–759.)

TABLE 53.6. Comparison of Serum $1,25(OH)_2$-Vitamin D Concentrations in Hypercalciuric Stone Formers and Normal Subjects

Reference	Dietary Calcium (mmol/day)	Dietary Phosphate (mmol/day)	Serum $1,25(OH)_2D$ (pmol/L) Stone Formers	Normal Subjects	*P*
Kaplan et al. (*J Clin Invest* 1977; 59:756–760)	10	26	115 ± 30 (24)	82 ± 22 (11)	<.005
Sten et al. (*J Lab Clin Med* 1977; 90:955–962)	*Ad libitum*	*Ad libitum*	130 ± 46 (15)	82 ± 17 (17)	<.001
Gray et al. (*J Clin Endocrinol Metab* 1977; 45:299–306)	*Ad libitum*	*Ad libitum*	150 ± 74 (26)	87 ± 29 (48)	<.001
Zerwekh and Pak (*Metabolism* 1980; 24:13–17)	10	26	116 ± 43 (21)	82 ± 17 (15)	<.01
Coe et al. (*Am J Med* 1982; 72:25–32)	*Ad libitum*	*Ad libitum*	99 ± 14 (27)	82 ± 17 (9)	NS
	<3.5/70 kg	22/70 kg	130 ± 14 (27)	134 ± 26 (9)	NS
Broadus et al. (*J Clin Endocrinol Metab* 1984; 58:161–169)	10	Not specified	185 ± 30 (37)	112 ± 33 (12)	<.001

serum $1,25(OH)_2D$ levels could account for increased intestinal calcium absorption and thus hypercalciuria. When the subjects given calcitriol were placed on low-calcium diets, average daily urinary calcium excretion rates exceeded dietary calcium intake, providing evidence that elevated calcitriol levels can also stimulate bone resorption. The mechanisms accounting for activation of vitamin D metabolism are not yet clear. Some patients exhibit hypophosphatemia secondary to a renal phosphate leak and studies in animals indicate that hypophosphatemia activates renal $1,25(OH)_2D$ synthesis via a growth hormone-dependent mechanism. Other patients are not hypophosphatemic, raising the possibility of other, presently unknown, mechanisms for activation of vitamin D metabolism. One study tested the hypothesis that inherited abnormalities of the 1-hydroxylase gene, which is responsible for synthesis of calcitriol, are associated with stone formation; no link was found to calciuria or stones in the 36 families studied.

Some studies have shown that serum 1,25$(OH)_2$D levels are normal in stone formers (Table 53.6) and others have shown that either radiocalcium absorption or net calcium absorption may be inappropriately elevated in relation to serum 1,25$(OH)_2$D concentrations. It is possible that an increase in sensitivity to normal calcitriol levels, mediated through altered vitamin D receptor number or affinity, could occur. Vitamin D is known to upregulate its own receptor number. Studies in genetically hypercalciuric stone-forming rats have shown that, like hypercalciuric humans, these rats have increased intestinal absorption and urinary excretion of calcium. They also have increased calcium release from bone during consumption of a low-calcium diet. Increased numbers of vitamin D receptors have been found in both intestine and bone of the hypercalciuric rats compared with normocalciuric controls and increased sensitivity to administered calcitriol. Whether hypercalciuric humans share the same generalized abnormality in calcium handling is still unclear. A study of patients with absorptive hypercalciuria showed that two-thirds of the subjects had a decrease in intestinal calcium absorption and urinary calcium excretion after administration of ketoconazole, which reduced serum 1,25$(OH)_2$D levels by 40%. The rest of the subjects had no change in calcium absorption or excretion, despite comparable reductions in calcitriol levels. Increased density of vitamin D receptors has not yet been demonstrated in hypercalciuric humans. Therefore calcitriol may play an important etiologic role in many, but not all, patients with idiopathic hypercalciuria.

As noted, many patients with hypercalciuria have accelerated bone resorption. It is conceivable that some as yet unknown signal arising in bone may stimulate intestinal calcium absorption to compensate for a primary increase in bone turnover. It has been noted that monocytes from patients with hypercalciuria elaborate increased amounts of interleukin-1, a cytokine that stimulates bone resorption by osteoclast activation, as well as other cytokines that may be involved with bone metabolism.

A small minority of hypercalciuric patients exhibit fasting hypercalciuria, a normal or low serum calcium concentration, and elevated or high-normal serum PTH levels or urinary cAMP excretion rates and high serum 1,25$(OH)_2$D concentrations. These patients have been considered to have a renal calcium leak with secondary activation of the PTH and vitamin D endocrine systems. In this circumstance, augmented intestinal calcium absorption is a physiologically appropriate compensatory mechanism. However, renal clearance studies have also demonstrated reduced tubular reabsorption of calcium compared with normal rats with the same filtered calcium load in both genetically hypercalciuric rats and in some hypercalciuric stone formers, without elevation of PTH. Several studies in humans and hypercalciuric rats have suggested that the thick ascending limb of Henle's loop may be the site of the calcium transport defect.

Finally, a more general disorder of calcium transport in patients with idiopathic hypercalciuria has been suggested by a study showing an increase in Ca^{2+}-Mg^{2+}-ATPase activity in the erythrocyte membranes of patients with hypercalciuria, regardless of whether they made stones. Other abnormalities in cellular transport of oxalate, urate, and sodium have been described in erythrocytes from patients with calcium stones. Increased erythrocyte transmembrane oxalate flux has been described in both stone formers and in their family members. These diverse transport abnormalities have been hypothesized to be due to an alteration in cell lipid content, with lower concentrations of linoleic acid and higher amounts of arachidonic acid found in the erythrocyte membranes of stone formers. The model proposes that the increased arachidonic acid level could also lead to an increase in prostaglandin E_2 production, which may stimulate calcitriol synthesis, and hypercalciuria, accounting for a number of the abnormalities seen in stone formers.

Collectively, these considerations indicate that the precise mechanisms for hypercalciuria remain to be completely defined. Furthermore, in the treatment of a given patient with hypercalciuria, there is as yet no convincing evidence that detailed clarification of the mechanism for hypercalciuria is important for the prevention of stone growth and of new stone formation, assuming that gluttony for calcium-rich foods or antacids, hyperparathyroidism, distal RTA and occult granulomatous diseases, and lymphoma can be excluded.

Several dietary measures are useful in the treatment of patients with recurrent oxalate–apatite stones and hypercalciuria. Dietary calcium intake should be not be limited to less than one serving of milk or cheese (or comparable source of calcium) daily because dairy products are the chief sources of dietary calcium in North America. This will provide an intake of roughly 800 mg of calcium/day. A somewhat higher intake is advisable in women. More rigid dietary calcium restriction is not justifiable because of the long-term risks of bone loss. In addition, very low dietary calcium intakes (less than 17.5 mmol or 700 mg/day) lead to an increase in the absorption of dietary oxalate and an increase in urinary oxalate excretion and calcium oxalate supersaturation. Two epidemiologic studies correlated a rise in urinary tract stone formation with diets that were low in calcium. The same studies found that the risk of stones increased with increasing dietary protein intake, whereas other investigators have shown that decreased bone mineral density in stone formers correlates with indices of increased protein intake. Dietary protein intake should be limited to 0.8 to 1 g of protein/kg per day to minimize the calciuric effects of protein intake. Similarly, a high NaCl intake should be avoided by eliminating salty snacks such as potato chips, pretzels, nuts, and so on, and eliminating the addition of salt to food at the table. High dietary intakes of sodium and sucrose were both associated with increased risk of stone formation in epidemiologic studies.

Patients should be advised to increase their water intake in an effort to maintain a urine volume of about 2 L/day. They should not substitute sugar-containing carbonated beverages for water because of the calciuric effects of sucrose. Grapefruit juice, but not other juices, has also been associated with increased risk of stones. A water intake of 2 to 3 L is required. After patients have increased their water intake they can be instructed to collect a 24-hour urine specimen for themselves to verify the adequacy of their daily urine volume.

In addition, specific measures to reduce urinary calcium excretion are available. These include thiazide diuretics, supplementary alkali, and supplementary inorganic phosphate. The thiazide diuretics, such as chlorthalidone, indapamide, and amiloride reduce urinary calcium excretion by 40% to 60% in hypercalciuric stone formers. Many uncontrolled studies and a few controlled trials indicated that this class of drugs is effective in reducing stone recurrence. Thiazide diuretics can be used regardless of the underlying mechanism for hypercalciuria. Hydrochlorothiazide 25 mg twice daily, chlorthalidone 25 mg once daily, and indapamide 2.5 mg daily are often used. Therapy is usually begun at a lower dose for 1 to 2 weeks to minimize the initial and transient sodium diuresis. In addition to augmenting distal renal tubular calcium reabsorption, thiazide diuretic therapy is accompanied by inhibition of bone resorption and more positive calcium balance. Chronic thiazide diuretic therapy may be accompanied by hypokalemia, hyperuricemia, hyperglycemia, and occasionally impotence. The hypokalemia is seldom symptomatic and can easily be managed by the addition of a potassium-sparing diuretic such as amiloride 5 mg/day or by potassium supplements. Potassium depletion may result in hypocitraturia. If this occurs, potassium citrate may be given, either in tablet form or as lemon juice diluted 1:16 in water. Occasionally thiazide diuretic therapy may result in hypercalcemia, which should prompt further studies for primary hyperparathyroidism. Impotence can be a significant complication of thiazide therapy, and patients should be asked about this complication as they may not complain voluntarily.

Oral administration of salts of inorganic phosphate (neutral orthophosphate) is also effective in the treatment of hypercalciuria and may reduce the incidence of stones in these patients. No controlled trial has been done, however. It is necessary to give 1 to 3 g of elemental phosphorus/day in the form of sodium or potassium salts, in three or four divided doses. Such therapy may cause troublesome diarrhea, which limits its use. Therapy with inorganic phosphate should be avoided in patients with reduced renal function because of aggravation of secondary hyperparathyroidism, accelerated loss of kidney function, and the development of soft tissue calcification.

Cellulose phosphate, which binds calcium in the intestine, has been used in the management of absorptive hypercalciuria. The dose is 10 to 15 g/day given orally in divided doses of 5 g each. These patients should also receive supplementation of 100 to 200 mg of magnesium/day because cellulose phosphate binds magnesium as well and causes a decrease in urinary magnesium excretion. Such hypomagnesuria could be hazardous because urinary magnesium, by complexing oxalate, is an inhibitor of crystallization in urine. Patients must also be placed on a low-oxalate diet to prevent hyperoxaluria. In a controlled trial, cellulose phosphate was no better than dietary calcium restriction and increased fluid intake.

Hyperuricosuria

A segment of the calcium oxalate stone-forming population exhibits hyperuricosuria, defined as a urinary excretion of greater than 4.8 mmol of uric acid/day (more than 800 mg/day) in men and more than 4.5 mmol of uric acid/day (more than 750 mg/day) in women. Many of these calcium stone formers appear to habitually ingest purine-rich diets. Some patients exhibit modest hyperuricemia, and hypercalciuria may or may not be present. The mechanisms by which hyperuricosuria leads to calcium oxalate stone formation are not yet fully defined. Both uric acid and monosodium urate seed crystals can epitaxially nucleate calcium oxalate crystal growth *in vivo* although monosodium urate crystalluria is not observed and monosodium urate has not been identified in urinary calculi. Uric acid and sodium urate crystals also may reduce urinary inhibitors (acid mucopolysaccharides) of calcium oxalate crystal growth. Despite the uncertainty regarding the ultimate causes of calcium oxalate stones in these hyperuricosuric patients, a reduction in uric acid excretion achieved by the administration of allopurinol, 200 to 300 mg/day, is effective in preventing stone recurrence. Attempts to lower dietary protein intake to normal levels (0.8 to 1.0 g/kg of body weight per day) should also be made.

Hypocitraturia

Urinary citrate excretion ranges from about 1.6 to 7 mmol/day (307 to 1,344 mg/day) in healthy adults and, by complexing calcium, citrate lowers the saturation of urine with respect to calcium oxalate and apatite. Citrate excretion has been observed to be higher for women than men, as shown in the upper panel of Fig. 53.14. This may contribute to the lower incidence of kidney stones in women. The figure also demonstrates that urinary citrate excretion increases with increased urine pH in subjects studied in the authors' laboratory who collected 24 hour volumes under mineral oil. Administration of bicarbonate as either the potassium or sodium salt will increase citrate excretion, as shown in the lower panel of Fig. 53.14. Conversely, metabolic acidosis (which may be experimentally induced by NH_4Cl administration) reduces urinary citrate excretion by stimulating proximal renal tubular reabsorption of citrate and increasing citrate metabolism. Low urinary citrate excretion (less than approximately 0.06 mmol/mmol of creatinine or 110 mg/g of creatinine) is characteristic of distal renal tubular acidosis. Reduced urinary citrate excretion also occurs in patients who form kidney stones in relation to diarrheal disease because of the acidosis that accompanies the fecal losses of bicarbonate. Hypokalemia and diets high in animal protein will also reduce urinary citrate excretion. Other studies have emphasized that on the average urinary citrate excretion is low for many patients with calcium-containing kidney stones, regardless of hypercalciuria and in the absence of systemic acidosis. Urinary citrate excretion can readily be increased by the administration of alkali, as shown previously; however the effects of sodium and potassium salts on overall urinary calcium oxalate saturation differ. $NaHCO_3$ loading raises urinary citrate excretion but does

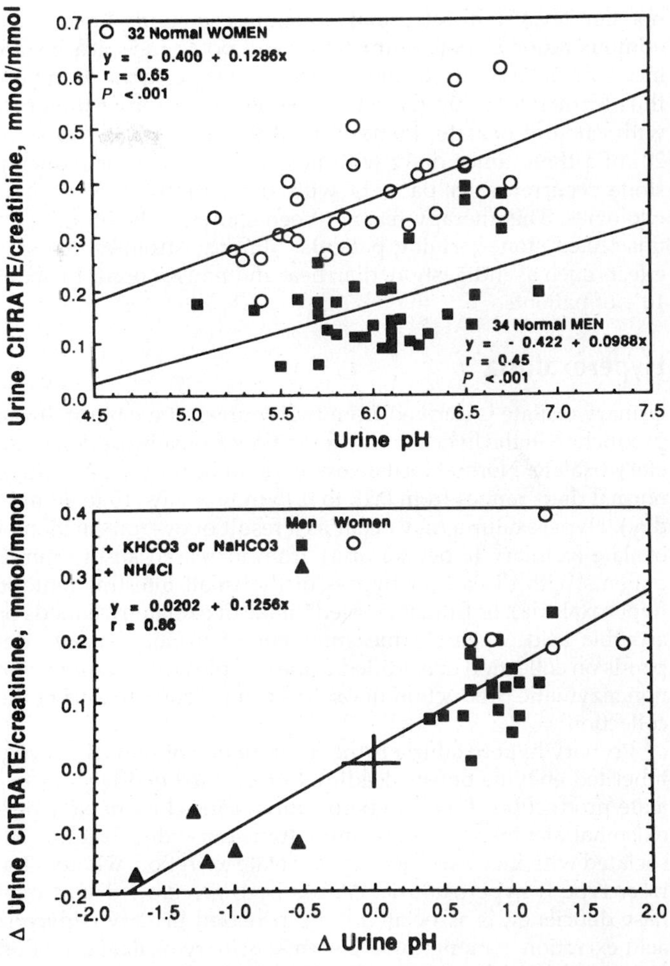

Figure 53.14. *Upper panel,* daily urinary citrate excretion/creatinine, mmol/mmol, in healthy women and men in relation to urine pH. Citrate/creatinine increases with increasing urine pH and is higher among women. *Lower panel,* the individual changes from control in urinary citrate/creatinine in relation to the changes in urine pH among men and women given $KHCO_3$ or $NaHCO_3$ and men given NH_4Cl.

not significantly lower urinary calcium excretion. By contrast, administration of potassium citrate and potassium bicarbonate increases urinary citrate and reduces urinary calcium excretion, thus further reducing the relative supersaturation of the urine with calcium oxalate. Potassium citrate therapy at a dose of 20 mEq three times daily with meals is effective for reducing stone recurrence in patients with hypocitraturia of various etiologies. This therapy has not been shown to be effective in unselected stone-forming patients. Minor gastrointestinal side effects such as indigestion, diarrhea, and nausea occur in about 10% of patients.

Hyperoxaluria

Urinary oxalate is derived from two sources: the majority from production in the liver, and the remainder from absorption of dietary oxalate. Normal oxalate excretion in healthy adults eating normal diets ranges from 0.18 to 0.45 mmol/day (16 to 40 mg/day). Hyperoxaluria may occur as a result of overproduction of oxalate (primary hyperoxaluria), from increased absorption in patients with disease or bypass of the small intestine (enteric hyperoxaluria), or from increased intake of oxalate-rich foods or ascorbic acid. Accurate measurement of urinary oxalate depends on collection of acidified urine samples to prevent *in vitro* nonenzymatic production of oxalate from ascorbate during the collection.

Primary hyperoxaluria is the result of one of two recessively inherited enzyme defects leading to increased endogenous oxalate production. Type I hyperoxaluria, caused by hepatic peroxisomal alanine:glyoxalate aminotransferase deficiency, is associated with increased urinary glycolate excretion, whereas the rarer type II hyperoxaluria, caused by D-glycerate dehydrogenase deficiency, is associated with increased urinary L-glyceric acid excretion. Among these patients, urinary oxalate excretion is generally in the range of 1.7 to 3.3 mmol/day (150 to 300 mg/day). Repetitive formation of new stones and ureteral obstruction together with soft tissue deposits of calcium oxalate, especially in the kidney, may lead to renal failure, often in childhood. In other patients with less severe hyperoxaluria, only periodic passage of stones or silent renal failure occurs. Supplementary pyridoxine, 250 to 1,000 mg/day, may lead to significant reductions of urinary oxalate excretion in some patients. These patients should also be advised to avoid oxalate-rich foods. Other therapeutic efforts, aimed at minimizing calcium oxalate supersaturation, crystal nucleation, and crystal growth, include (a) increasing water intake to reduce average urinary oxalate concentrations, (b) administration of a thiazide diuretic to reduce urinary calcium concentration, (c) administration of supplementary inorganic phosphate providing 1 to 1.5 g of elemental phosphorus/day in divided doses in the form of neutral sodium-potassium phosphate, and (d) magnesium supplements as magnesium gluconate, 1 g/day. Supplementary phosphate therapy should not be used in patients with evidence of reduced glomerular filtration because of the hazards of hyperphosphatemia that could predispose to soft tissue calcification and accelerate loss of renal function. Renal transplantation has been successful in hyperoxaluric patients with chronic renal failure, but requires careful attention to treatment of the hyperoxaluria. Definitive treatment for primary type I hyperoxaluria is liver transplantation.

Acquired hyperoxaluria may occur as a result of ingestion of oxalate-rich foods such as rhubarb, spinach, Swiss chard, beet greens, cashews, peanuts, almonds, chocolate, strawberries, and strong tea or because of the abuse of ascorbic acid (vitamin C in doses greater than 500 mg/day), which is a precursor for oxalate synthesis. Mild elevations are not rare and may be produced by a low-calcium diet, as calcium will normally complex oxalate in the gut, decreasing absorption. A low-oxalate diet should be advised for such patients.

Acquired hyperoxaluria also accompanies malabsorption in the setting of chronic inflammatory bowel disease, resection, or bypass of the distal small intestine when the colon is intact and appears to be the result of increased colonic absorption of dietary oxalate. The degree of hyperoxaluria appears to parallel the degree of fat malabsorption. Low urinary citrate excretion is often present as well because of loss of bicarbonate in the stool. Therapy in these patients is focused on reducing oxalate absorption. A low-oxalate diet and decreased intake of fat are the first steps. Administration of oral calcium carbonate or calcium citrate supplements, 0.5 to 3 g with meals, can precipitate oxalate in the gut lumen, limiting oxalate absorption. Cholestyramine, an anion exchange resin, can also bind oxalate and bile acids in the lumen of the bowel and has been used in doses of 4 g three times a day. Decreased absorption of vitamin K and some drugs may occur. Adequate water intake to maintain urine volumes of 2 L or more a day should also be advised. The efficacy of therapy should be assessed by measurement of 24-hour urine calcium and oxalate excretion.

Idiopathic Calcium Stone Formers

Approximately one-fourth of calcium stone formers do not exhibit hypercalciuria, hyperoxaluria, hyperuricosuria, hypocitraturia, or a defect in urinary acidification. For a few of these patients who are studied in their home environments, 24-hour urine volumes may persistently be only 500 to 1,000 ml, as the result of habitually low water intakes so that, even at normal excretion rates urinary concentration of calcium, oxalate, or phosphate could reach sufficiently high levels to result in crystal nucleation and crystal growth. Among this group of calcium stone formers some may have deficiencies of urinary inhibitors of crystal nucleation or crystal growth. Alternatively, the urine of stone formers could theoretically contain materials capable of evoking crystal nucleation. Therapy should include maintenance of an adequate water intake to ensure urine volumes of 2,000 ml/day or more, dietary protein intake of 0.8 to 1.0 g/kg per day and salt restriction to 2 to 3 g daily. Dietary calcium should not be restricted below 1 g daily. The administration of a thiazide diuretic as used in the management of the idiopathic hypercalciuria syndrome may be helpful in some patients. Citrate administration may also be considered.

CYSTINE STONES

The formation of renal calculi composed of the amino acid cystine is the clinical expression of a genetic abnormality of amino acid transport. Because of a defect in reabsorption from renal tubular fluid, there is increased urinary excretion of cystine and of the other dibasic amino acids lysine, arginine, and ornithine. Because cystine is only sparingly soluble, the excessive excretion rate leads to cystine crystallization within the renal pelvis and stone formation.

Cystine stone formers account for about 1% to 3% of patients with urolithiasis; the incidence of cystinuria is 1 of 15,000 births in North America. Symptoms of this inherited disorder may begin at any age but occur most commonly in the second and third decades of life. Renal colic with stone passage, flank pain with ureteral obstruction, or vague backache with large pelvic (staghorn) stones may be present. Cystine calculi are radiopaque because of the sulfur present in this amino acid although the stones are not as radiodense as calcium-containing stones. The diagnosis is confirmed directly by analysis of a stone or indirectly by either the observation of typical hexagonal cystine crystals in the urine sediment (Fig. 53.4), or by quantitation of 24-hour urinary cystine excretion. Normal subjects excrete less than 0.009 mmol cystine/mmol creatinine (20 mg/g), whereas cystinurics excrete 0.12 mmol cystine or more/mmol creatinine (more than 250 mg/g); heterozygotes fall in between. The urinary cyanide nitroprusside test is useful for screening, as it detects cystine at a concentration exceeding 0.035 mmol/mmol creatinine (75 mg/g).

Cystinuria is an autosomal recessive trait resulting in defective renal tubular and intestinal transport of cystine, lysine, arginine, and ornithine. Three subtypes of this disorder are recognized, based on the level of cystine excretion in obligate heterozygotes (the parents of affected individuals): type I, with normal cystine excretion; type II, with a marked elevation of cystine excretion; and type III, with a mild elevation. Mutations in the *SLC3A1* gene found on chromosome 2 have been associated with type I cystinuria; types II and III appear to be associated with a gene on chromosome 19. Newer work suggests that patients who are offspring of two parents with type I cystinuria have the highest levels of cystine excretion and often form stones in the first decade of life. There is a general tendency for the frequency of stone recurrence and complications to increase with higher rates of urinary cystine excretion; heterozygotes rarely form stones.

In the absence of effective and ongoing therapy, repeated stone episodes with ureteral obstruction requiring surgical procedures and accompanying urinary infection can lead to progressive renal failure as the result of hydronephrosis and pyelonephritis. Thus the first phase of treatment involves education of the patient and, in the case of a young child, his or her family about the genetic basis for cystinuria and the need for lifelong therapy.

Treatment is focused on both increasing the capacity of the urine to dissolve cystine and reducing urinary cystine excretion. The solubility of cystine over the pH range 4.5 to 7.0 is limited to about 1.25 to 1.67 mmol/L (300 to 400 mg/L). Because 24-hour cystine excretion may be in the range of 3.3 to 5.0 mmol/day (800 to 1,200 mg/day), the cystinuric patient must learn to drink sufficient water to maintain a minimum urine volume of 3 L/day. Such a program must include ingestion of sufficient water at bedtime to induce nocturia and, when the patient arises to void, an additional 300 ml of water should be drunk. Patients should collect and measure their own 24-hour urine volumes on several occasions to assure that their water intake is adequate. The solubility of cystine in urine rises sharply to about 800 mg/L as urinary pH rises from 7.0 to 8.0. Thus sustained alkalinization of the urine, in addition to ensuring large urine volumes, will assist in maintaining cystine in solution. Approximately 2 mEq/kg of body weight or 150 mEq/day of actual or potential bicarbonate in divided doses is required to maintain the urine pH in the range at 7.5 or higher. Because certain data indicate that sodium can increase cystine excretion, one half or more of the alkali should be administered as a potassium salt (potassium citrate, or potassium citrate-acetate-bicarbonate), assuming that kidney function is normal. In addition, 250 mg of acetazolamide to inhibit proximal tubular bicarbonate reabsorption may be administered at bedtime to sustain a nocturnal alkaline diuresis. An additional dose of alkali should be administered when the patient arises at night to void and drink to prevent the tendency for serum bicarbonate levels to fall and the urine to become more acid as the action of acetazolamide develops and then wanes. The patient should check the pH of each urine volume voided for several days using phenaphthazine paper to ensure that the pH is 7.5 or higher.

Urinary cystine is derived from the sulfur-containing amino acids in dietary protein, principally methionine, so that protein intake should probably be limited to 0.7 to 1.0 g/kg of body weight/day. In addition, because a high salt intake enhances urinary cystine excretion, dietary NaCl intake should be restricted.

Cystine excretion can be reduced by the administration of D-penicillamine, which undergoes a disulfide exchange reaction with cystine to form the mixed disulfide of cysteine and penicillamine, which is much more soluble than cystine. D-Penicillamine is given in doses of 250 to 500 mg four times daily. This drug can occasionally result in significant toxic side effects including fever, rash, leukopenia, thrombocytopenia, and the nephrotic syndrome. It is also expensive. Thus the use of D-penicillamine in the treatment of cystinuria is generally reserved for patients in whom stone formation cannot be adequately controlled by high fluid intake and the administration of alkali and acetazolamide. Another thiol, tiopronin, has also been shown to be effective in reducing cystine excretion and stone recurrence, and this agent appears to be better tolerated than D-penicillamine. Collectively, these measures may sometimes result in the dissolution of nonobstructing cystine stones but more often appear to be most effective in preventing further growth of existing stones and preventing new stone formation. Lithotripsy has been used in the treatment of cystine stones, but the stones are difficult to fragment.

INFECTION STONES

Stones composed of magnesium ammonium phosphate (struvite) ($MgNH_4PO_4 \cdot 6H_2O$) together with variable amounts of carbonate apatite [$Ca_{10}(PO_4)_6CO_3$], termed *infection stones* or sometimes *triple phosphate stones* (Fig. 53.5), are caused by infection of the kidney and/or bladder by bacteria that produce the enzyme urease. These stones are more common in women by a ratio of 2:1, probably because of their higher incidence of urinary tract infections. Other high-risk groups include patients who exhibit abnormal urinary drainage and/or urinary obstruction that permits establishment of urinary tract infection. Such abnormalities include congenital anomalies of the urinary tract (urethral valve or vesicoureteral reflux), bladder dysfunction (urethral obstruction due to prostatism, intrinsic motor dysfunction, or spinal cord injury or disease), chronic catheter drainage of the urinary tract (bladder, nephrostomy, or ureterostomy), or ureteral diversion to an ileal or sigmoid conduit. Infection stones may also occur as a complication in patients with other types of calculi as a consequence of infection in the setting of a foreign body. A significant number of stones contain struvite admixed with calcium oxalate or uric acid.

The symptoms of infection stones are quite variable. In many patients, stones in the renal pelvis or in the bladder apparently may be present for relatively long periods without symptoms, whereas in other patients repeated episodes of flank pain, chills, and fever may occur as a result of local urinary obstruction associated with acute exacerbation of chronic infection and bacteremia. A minority of such patients are seen with stone passage or hematuria.

The urinalysis generally demonstrates modest proteinuria (less than 1 g/day) either as caused by acute inflammation in the urinary tract or by chronic pyelonephritis. The urine is persistently very alkaline with the pH ranging from 7.5 to 8.0 or higher resulting from hydrolysis of urea by bacterial urease.

TABLE 53.7. Urease-Producing Bacteria Most Commonly Associated with Infection Stones

Proteus species
Haemophilus influenzae
Yersinia enterocolitica
Providencia species
Klebsiella pneumoniae
Pseudomonas aeruginosa
Serratia species
Bacteroides corrodens
Staphylococcus species
Corynebacterium species
Ureaplasma urealyticum

Because of infection, many white blood cells and bacilli are seen in the urine sediment, often together with struvite (Fig. 53.5) and amorphous apatite crystals (Fig. 53.3). Cultures of the urine usually demonstrate significant growth of a bacterial species that produces urease (Table 53.7), although a negative culture should suggest the presence of *Ureaplasma urealyticum*, which does not grow on standard culture media. Culture of the stone best identifies the causative agent.

Plain radiographs of the abdomen demonstrate radiopaque renal or bladder calculi that often exhibit a laminated structure. The large renal stones often have the shape of the renal pelvis and calyces; hence the term *staghorn calculi* (Fig. 53.5). Most (about 75%) of such large pelvic calyceal stones are infection stones although occasionally, large cystine, apatite, or uric acid stones have a similar shape. Intravenous or retrograde urography is required to search for sites of urinary obstruction. Depending on the duration and severity of urinary obstruction and infection, the GFR may be reduced and renal tubular function impaired as manifested by metabolic acidosis and loss of maximal renal concentrating capacity. Pathologic examination of the bladder and kidneys demonstrates variable degrees of acute and chronic inflammation, hydronephrosis, and scarring.

Bacterial urease has been found to be the fundamental cause of infection stones, leading to supersaturation of the urine with respect to $MgNH_4PO_4 \cdot 6H_2O$ and $Ca_{10}(PO_4)_6CO_3$ and thus crystallization and stone growth. Struvite–apatite stones are never formed in persistently sterile urine and do not form as a consequence of urinary infection by organisms that do not produce urease. Urinary infection by organisms that produce urease is accompanied by the hydrolysis of urea to ammonia (NH_3) and carbon dioxide (CO_2). The immediate subsequent reaction of NH_3 with water or with carbonic acid (H_2CO_3) yields ammonium (NH_4^+) and bicarbonate (HCO_3^-). Because the pK for the reaction $NH_4^+ - NH_3 + H^+$ is about 9, the urine becomes very alkaline (pH >7.5). Some carbonate ($CO_3^=$) ions also are formed because the pK for the reaction $HCO_3^- - CO_3^= + H^+$ is about 10. As the urine becomes very alkaline, most of the urinary phosphate is present as monohydrogen phosphate with small quantities of phosphate ion because the pK for the reaction $H_2PO_4^- - HPO_4^= + H^+$ is about 7 and the pK for the reaction $HPO_4^= - PO_4^{\equiv} + H^+$ is about 11. Collectively, these reactions lead to striking elevations of the urinary concentrations of NH_4^+, $PO_4^{\equiv}$, and $CO_3^=$ that together with normal concentrations of Mg^{2+} and Ca^{2+} in an alkaline solution cause precipitation of $MgNH_4PO_4 \cdot 6H_2O$ and $Ca_{10}(PO_4)_6CO_3$.

The natural history and progression of infection stones depends on whether or not the stones can be completely removed, the infection eradicated, the urinary obstruction relieved, and abnormal portals of entry in the urinary tract for new bacterial pathogens removed. The ultimate goal is to render the patient stone free, as recurrence rates are high if infected stone material remains. Although appropriate antibiotic therapy, chosen on the basis of bacterial sensitivities, may temporarily sterilize the urine, recurrence of infection is frequent due to organisms incorporated into the stones during their growth that are not reached by adequate bactericidal drug concentrations or due to new infections by urease-producing bacteria entering via urinary catheters. Thus definitive treatment requires removal of infected stone material. Clinical guidelines published by the American Urologic Association recommend a combination of shock-wave lithotripsy and percutaneous stone removal as first-line treatment. A review of the many surgical techniques that are required is beyond the scope of this chapter. At the same time, appropriate antibiotic therapy is used to eliminate tissue infections. If infection stones can be removed and the urine rendered sterile, recurrence can be prevented, although underlying structural abnormalities in the urinary tract and renal scarring often remain. When stone fragments remain, infection persists, and new stones are frequent. Nonoperative management has a poor outcome, with a high incidence of renal failure and mortality. If the urine can be sterilized, thus restoring normal urinary acidity, struvite–apatite stones can theoretically be dissolved, but antibiotic therapy alone seldom, if ever, achieves this goal. Nevertheless, long-term antibiotic therapy, has been recommended for patients in whom complete stone removal or complete correction of anatomical abnormalities in the urinary tract is not possible. The urea analog acetohydroxamic acid is an effective competitive inhibitor of urease. This agent reduces urinary ammonia and pH and when combined with appropriate antibiotics has resulted in sterilization of the urine and retarded stone growth. However, tremulousness, venous thrombosis, and anemia have necessitated stopping of treatment in 20% to 30% of patients. It probably should be reserved for use in patients who have normal kidney function but for other reasons cannot be rendered free of stones and infections.

Up to 50% of patients with struvite stones have been noted to have underlying metabolic abnormalities predisposing to stone formation, such as hypercalciuria or hyperuricosuria. This is especially true for male patients without anatomic abnormalities and for those patients with stones in which struvite is mixed with other components. For that reason, it is reasonable to search for such underlying abnormalities and treat them to reduce stone recurrence.

URIC ACID STONES

Stones composed of uric acid account for about 5% to 10% of renal stones. They are caused by disorders that lead to uric acid overproduction and hyperuricosuria, a persistently acid urine, or a persistently concentrated urine (Table 53.8). The age at which formation of uric acid stones may occur varies with the underlying causes, but they occur predominantly in middle-aged men. A family history of urolithiasis, gout, or both is common. The symptoms of uric acid crystalluria and stones likewise vary with the underlying disorder and range from the occasional passage of gravel to typical ureteral colic or to acute ureteral obstruction by stones or crystalline uric acid sludge. Uric acid stones are radiolucent and should be differentiated from tumors of the renal pelvis, blood clots, sloughed renal papillae, and xanthine stones, which are very rare. Large uric acid stones may assume a staghorn configuration.

The major determinants of uric acid crystalluria and stone formation appear to be (a) the daily urinary excretion of uric

TABLE 53.8. Causes and Mechanisms of Uric Acid Crystalluria and Uric Acid Stone Formation

Causes	Uric Acid Overproduction and Increased Urinary Uric Acid Excretion	Persistently Acid Urine (low NH_4^+ Excretion or Extrarenal HCO_3^- loss)	Persistently Concentrated Urine (Accelerated Extrarenal Water Losses or Habitually Low Water Intake)
Associated with hyperuricemia			
Primary gout (10%–20%)	+	—	—
Primary gout (80%–20%	—	0 Urinary NH_4^+	—
Lesch-Nyhan syndrome (hypoxanthine-guanine phosphoribosyltransferase deficiency) and defects in other enzymes regulating purine synthesis	+	—	—
Glycogen storage disease, type I (glucose-6-phosphatase deficiency)	+	—	—
Myeloproliferative disorders and other neoplasms	+	—	—
Without hyperuricemia			
Purine gluttony	+	±	—
Uricosuric drugs	+	—	—
Idiopathic uric acid stone disease	—	0 Urinary NH_4^+	—
Diarrheal disease	—	Intestinal HCO_3^- loss	+
Hot environments, fever	—	+	+

acid; (b) the urine volume, which determines the mean prevailing total urinary uric acid concentration; and (c) urinary pH, which in turn determines the concentration of free (undissociated) uric acid, the least soluble form of uric acid. Uric acid has two dissociable protons, the first having a pK of about 5.6 and the second having a pK of about 11. Thus at a minimum urinary pH of 4.5, approximately 95% of the total urinary uric acid will exist as undissociated uric acid whereas at a urinary pH of 7.0 approximately 95% of the total urinary uric acid will exist as urate ion. The solubility of undissociated uric acid in maximally acid urine is about 0.6 mmol/L (100 mg/L) whereas the solubility of sodium urate at pH 7.0 is about 9.5 mmol/L (1600 mg/L). Given a healthy adult who excretes a normal quantity of uric acid/24 hr (3.0 mmol or 500 mg), in a urine volume of 1 L with an average normal pH of 5.6, the estimated undissociated urinary uric acid concentration will be about 1.5 mmol/L (250 mg/L), a value clearly above the solubility of undissociated uric acid. Thus normal urine would often appear to be supersaturated with respect to undissociated uric acid, and it is perhaps surprising that uric acid crystalluria and stones are not more common. Perhaps diurnal variation in urine flow rates and the normal diurnal variation of urine pH (alkaline in late forenoon and early afternoon, acid at night and early morning) prevent uric acid crystal growth. Whether normal urine contains inhibitors of uric acid crystallization or growth is not known. Nevertheless, these considerations clearly demonstrate how increased uric acid excretion (more than 4.5 mmol or 800 mg/day), low urine volumes (less than 1 L/day), or persistently acid urine (always less than pH 5.5) can potentially lead to urine more supersaturated with respect to undissociated uric acid and, thus, crystalluria and stones.

As outlined in Table 53.8, uric acid stones are common in patients with gout, increasing in frequency as urinary uric acid excretion increases in those who overproduce uric acid. Uric acid overproduction as a consequence of rapid cell turnover in myeloproliferative and other neoplastic diseases may result in uric acid crystalluria or stones as an early symptom of the underlying malignancy, but more often crystalluria and stones occurred as a preventable consequence of cytolytic chemotherapy. Purine gluttony resulting in hyperuricosuria may occasionally be a cause for uric acid stones, and the tendency for crystal growth in this setting is probably contributed to by the concomitant high-protein intake that augments fixed acid production and acidifies the urine. Uric acid stones are also common in the majority of patients with gout who produce normal amounts of uric acid. In these individuals, persistently acid urine secondary to impaired renal synthesis and excretion of the major urinary buffer ammonium appears to be the underlying cause. A similar abnormality in renal ammonium excretion has been observed in idiopathic uric acid stone formers who do not exhibit hyperuricemia, hyperuricosuria, or gout. This defect can be suspected by the demonstration that urinary pH is 5.5 or less at each voiding throughout the day for several days. Diarrheal diseases result in accelerated fecal bicarbonate losses, a tendency toward mild hyperchloremic metabolic acidosis, and, thus persistently acid urine, which together with persistently low urine volumes caused by accelerated fecal water losses predisposes to uric acid precipitation. Similarly, accelerated cutaneous and pulmonary water losses in hot environments or during febrile illnesses that are not compensated for by increased water intake result in persistently concentrated and acid urine predisposing to uric acid crystallization and stone growth.

The diagnosis of uric acid urolithiasis can be suspected in patients with symptoms suggestive of stones who have uric acid crystals in the urine sediment under bright field illumination and polarized light (Fig. 53.6) and is confirmed by stone analysis. Factors contributing to uric acid stone formation are suggested by the clinical history and confirmed by measurements of urinary volume, pH, and 24-hour uric acid excretion. Stones may be visualized by ultrasonography.

There is general agreement regarding the prevention and treatment of uric acid stones based on the factors involved in their pathogenesis. Dietary intake of purine-rich foods should be limited or avoided (liver, kidney, brains, sweetbreads, more than 200 g/day of meat, fish, or poultry, asparagus, spinach, peas, and beans). Patients should be taught to drink sufficient quantities of water to maintain a urine volume of 2 L/day or more by having them collect and measure their own 24-hour urine volume on several occasions. If possible, the patient should drink sufficient water upon retiring to cause nocturia and be asked to drink additional water upon arising to void. Because maintenance of urine pH in the vicinity of 6.5 markedly enhances uric acid solubility as urate, alkali therapy should also be used. Generally about 1.0 mEq/kg of body weight/day or 60 mEq/day of sodium bicarbonate (1 g = 12 mEq), potassium citrate, or K-lyte (potassium bicarbonate-acetate-citrate) is sufficient when administered in divided doses three or four times a day. More may be needed if the patient is acidemic. Giving the alkali as a potassium salt may be preferred in patients with normal renal function to prevent the calciuria that may occur with sodium administration, as hyperuricosuria can predispose to formation of calcium oxalate stones. In addition, 250 mg of acetazolamide can be given at bedtime to sustain a nocturnal alkaline diuresis. The patient should be taught to monitor urine pH using phenaphthazine paper at each voiding for several days after initiation of therapy to ensure that the urine pH is maintained in the range of 6.0 to 6.5. For patients in whom these measures fail to prevent recurrence of uric acid stones, as well as for those patients whose urinary excretion of uric acid is 4.8 mmol (800 mg) or more/day or in whom such high rates of uric acid excretion can be anticipated when cytolytic drug therapy is initiated for a malignant disease, allopurinol therapy should also be used. Allopurinol, an analog of hypoxanthine, is a competitive inhibitor of xanthine oxidase and thus blocks the synthesis of uric acid. The drug also inhibits purine biosynthesis. Thus the more soluble compounds, hypoxanthine and xanthine, appear in the urine as the predominant end products of purine metabolism. Rarely, xanthine stones may complicate this therapy. Customarily, 200 to 300 mg of allopurinol is administered as a single daily dose. Allopurinol occasionally causes skin rash, leukopenia, or cholestatic jaundice, which requires stopping the drug. Increased fluid intake and alkali are generally effective in preventing new uric acid stones and together with allopurinol may result in the dissolution of nonobstructing stones that are too large to be passed spontaneously.

Selected Readings

Bataille P, Fardellone P, Ghazali A, et al. Pathophysiology and treatment of idiopathic hypercalciuria. *Curr Opin Rheumatol* 1998;10:373–388.

An excellent review of the evidence for current theories about the cause of idiopathic hypercalciuria.

Caruana RJ, Buckalew VM. The syndrome of distal (type 1) renal tubular acidosis: clinical and laboratory findings in 58 cases. *Medicine* 1988;67:84–99.

Analysis of a large number of cases from one institution and review of the literature, emphasizing the prevalence of clinical manifestations, especially stone disease, pathophysiology, and treatment.

Coe FL, Favus MJ, Pak CYC, et al., eds. *Kidney stones: medical and surgical management.* Philadelphia: Lippincott-Raven, 1996.

The most complete current reference on all aspects of the pathophysiology and management of nephrolithiasis.

Curhan GC, Willett WC, Speizer FE, et al. Comparison of dietary calcium with supplemental calcium and other nutrients as factors affecting the risk for kidney stones in women. *Ann Intern Med* 1997;126:497–504.

In more than 91,000 women without kidney stones between the ages of 30 and 55, the prospective incidence of kidney stones was inversely related to dietary intakes of calcium, fluid, and potassium; the occurrence of stones was directly related to dietary intake of sucrose. Supplemental calcium was associated with a relative risk of stones of 1.2; most supplements were not taken with meals.

Houillier P, Normand M, Froissart M, et al. Calciuric response to an acute acid load in healthy subjects and hypercalciuric calcium stone formers. *Kidney Int* 1996;50:987–997.

A study that helps elucidate the determinants of tubular calcium handling in hypercalciuric stone formers.

Lemann J Jr., Pleuss JA, Gray RW, et al. Potassium administration reduces and potassium deprivation increases urinary calcium excretion in healthy adults. *Kidney Int* 1991;39:973–983.

A short-term study showing that administration of 90 mmol/day of $KHCO_3$, but not KCl or $NaHCO_3$, decreased fasting and 24-hour calcium excretion, whereas K deprivation increased both fasting and 24-hour calcium excretion.

Lingeman JE. Mechanisms of stone disruption and dissolution. In: Coe FL, Favus MJ, eds. *Disorders of bone and mineral metabolism.* New York: Raven Press, 1992: 625–669.

An excellent survey of current methods for stone removal.

Parks JH, Coward M, Coe FL. Correspondence between stone composition and urine supersaturation in nephrolithiasis. *Kidney Int* 1997;51:894–900.

Data from a large number of stone formers demonstrating the correlation between supersaturation with various stone salts in the urine and the composition of the stones formed. The study confirms the utility (and apparent stability) of urine supersaturation measurements as a guide to treatment and points out some differences between male and female stone formers.

Thakker RV. The role of renal chloride channel mutations in kidney stone disease and nephrocalcinosis. *Curr Opin Nephrol Hypertens* 1998;7:385–388.

This paper describes the recent advances in molecular biology that have shed light on the causes of several renal tubular disorders.

CHAPTER 54

Tumors of the Kidney and Urinary Tract

PART 1
Benign and Malignant

Marc A. Lavine and Barry S. Stein

The fountainhead of renal surgery took place on August 2, 1862, at the University of Heidelberg, when Gustav Simon deliberately and successfully removed a kidney for a persistent ureteral fistula. Simon's operation was seen as huge step forward in the progress of medicine, for it was now known that one kidney could easily support human life. Only 20 years prior, the preeminent authority on the kidney at that time, Rayer, declared in his book, *Traite de Maladies des Reins*, that it would be "folly" to attempt such a procedure. In 1870, the first successful nephrectomy in the United States took place in Mobile, Alabama by Gilmore.

Although Simon died in 1876 at the age of 52 of a ruptured aortic aneurysm, his surgical boldness opened up a new world of pathology and histology for surgeons and pathologists alike. In 1855, Robin examined renal tumors and proposed renal tubular epithelium as the etiologic cell type for renal carcinoma. Grawitz, a pathologist at the Pathological Institute at Berlin and the University of Greifswald in the late 1800s, believed that renal carcinomas arose from adrenal rests within the renal parenchyma. He noted that most renal tumors were found in the upper pole of the kidney and the color of these tumors were often yellow; very similar to the adrenal gland's location and gross appearance. Even though this theory was erroneous, he made important observations regarding the hematologic spread of renal carcinoma to the skeleton and other organs. Succeeding pathologists, such as Birch-Hirschfield and Lubarch in 1894, sustained Grawitz's theory of suprarenal origin and coined the term *hypernephroma* for renal carcinomas. Albarran and Imbert opposed this explanation in 1903, and the term *Grawitz's tumor* was then used to describe renal carcinomas. In his 1926 textbook, *Young's Practice of Urology*, Young proposed the appellation of "nephroma" because, "it resembles the term in use, and commits us to no unproved theory."

RADIOLOGIC EVALUATION OF RENAL MASSES

Radiologic techniques are virtually always involved in the detection, staging, and follow-up of renal lesions. As technology has evolved, we can now identify malignant tumors that, in the not-so-distant past, may have presented only with symptoms of advanced disease. The widespread use of sonography and computed tomography (CT) has aided in the detection and earlier diagnosis of renal tumors. While improving the cure rate for malignant lesions such as renal cell carcinoma, these imaging modalities have also increased the detection rate of many benign tumors that will not need treatment. The difficulty lies in distinguishing tumors that may look similar radiologically but have different natural histories and thus different therapies.

Intravenous pyelography (IVP) and nephrotomography are often the initial diagnostic tests used in the workup of a renal mass. Despite its low sensitivity and specificity for detecting parenchymal lesions, IVP can easily detect collecting system abnormalities and is an integral part of the hematuria workup. Masses may be identified if they distort the renal outline or the collecting system. An IVP will not accurately differentiate between cystic and solid lesions.

A renal ultrasound can further characterize the mass found on IVP. Simple cysts are a common finding on IVP and are easily diagnosed by ultrasonography. A simple cyst has a smooth wall, no internal echoes, and through transmission. There are very specific diagnostic criteria set aside for simple cysts, because this condition requires no further workup. Renal ultrasound can be operator dependent, may be technically difficult due to body habitus, and may miss small intrarenal isoechoic masses. If the lesion on ultrasonography differs in any way from that of a simple benign cyst, CT is the diagnostic method of choice.

A quality CT scan includes thin renal sections (5 mm or less) and scanning with and without intravenous contrast. A CT scan has greater sensitivity in revealing the density of renal lesions and can visualize small renal masses better than ultrasound. Indeterminate cystic masses on ultrasound can be further delineated into simple or complex lesions by CT. CT scans can provide accurate tumor staging by revealing vascular thrombi, lymphadenopathy, and adjacent organ invasion. Conventional CT imaging has some disadvantages. Variations in respiration during the CT scan may distort the image. The spiral, or helical,

CT scan obtains data continuously during 20 to 40 seconds, which allows the study to be performed during one breath hold. The images can also be reconstructed into three-dimensional images, thus better defining renal masses and assisting in preoperative planning such as nephron-sparing procedures. Intravenous contrast may be contraindicated in patients with renal insufficiency. If this is the case, magnetic resonance imaging (MRI) with gadolinium administration will identify enhancing lesions. MRI is significantly more sensitive in identifying vascular invasion and local organ involvement than CT. MRI may aid in the diagnosis of angiomyolipoma because small amounts of fat are better visualized. Detailed discussion of the workup of the renal mass is found in Chapter 30.

BENIGN RENAL TUMORS

Benign renal tumors are common and usually asymptomatic. Before the development and the subsequent widespread use of sonography and CT, these masses were either found at autopsy or found when the tumors had grown large enough to be symptomatic, or even palpable. Today, our modern technology can easily uncover these renal masses but cannot reliably differentiate benign from malignant tumors. In many cases, the true diagnosis is determined at the time of pathologic examination following surgery.

Cortical Adenoma

Renal cortical adenomas are the most common renal tubular epithelial neoplasms found in 7% to 22% of autopsies or found incidentally during radiographic examination. They are rare in children and young adults but are common after age 40. The majority are less than 3 mm in size and appear gray-white or yellow on gross examination. Histologically, adenomas consist of tubular and papillary proliferations lined by single layers of basophilic or eosinophilic cells. There are no reliable cytologic criteria to distinguish papillary adenomas from small carcinomas. The presence of mitotic figures, clear cells, nuclear pleomorphism, cell stratification, or necrosis within the specimen can easily negate the diagnosis of cortical adenoma.

Although most major textbooks place these tumors in a benign category, there is significant controversy regarding the possible malignant potential of these tumors. Bell's 1950 autopsy series showed a low metastatic rate (5%) in those tumors measuring less than 3 cm in size. Thereafter, by convention, renal tumors smaller than 3 cm were considered adenomas. However, a review of Bell's original series, in addition to multiple reports of small renal tumors with proven metastases, has challenged this concept. For example, a patient with a 5 mm renal cell carcinoma with brain metastases has been reported. Thus small size alone does not guarantee a benign mass. In another autopsy review of more than 5,000 cadavers, the investigators separated two distinct groups of adenoma by size and histologic type. The researchers pointed to the larger (more than 0.5 cm), solitary adenomas that exhibited a solid or papillary pattern with clear cells as possible precancerous lesions. Smaller adenomas of the mixed tubulopapillary type did not pose a risk for malignancy. However, because the histology cannot be reliably determined preoperatively, the small, solid renal mass is best treated as a renal cell carcinoma and removed.

Oncocytoma

Renal oncocytomas account for 3% to 7% of solid renal tumors. First described in the salivary gland, these tumors can be found in multiple other organs, including the lacrimal glands, bronchial mucous glands, thyroid, parathyroid, adrenal glands, pancreas, and kidney. Oncocytomas consist of large polygonal epithelial cells with striking eosinophilic granular cytoplasm. These cells, first termed *onkocytes* by Jaffe in 1932, have abundant mitochondria rich in cristae that, under electron microscopy, are larger than those found in other renal tumors. Renal cell carcinomas may also harbor eosinophilic granular cells similar to oncocytes. Oncocytomas can be distinguished from these malignant tumors by their homogenous population of well-differentiated cells without nuclear pleomorphism.

Grossly, oncocytomas have a tan or mahogany color with a distinct fibrous capsule. On cross section a central, stellate, fibrous scar may be present. Necrosis, hemorrhage, and hypervascularity are uncommon. The tumor rarely invades the surrounding parenchyma, yet can grow to be quite large—up to 15 cm in some series. The reported median sizes range from 4 to 6 cm in diameter. Renal oncocytoma has been reported to present with bilateral synchronous tumors in 4% to 12% of cases.

The search for the histogenesis of renal oncocytoma offers an excellent example of how the rapidly evolving scientific technology, such as electron microscopy and histochemical and immunologic assays, is used to clarify medical mysteries. Originally, because of its histologic similarity to proximal renal tubular cells, it was thought that renal oncocytoma arose from this cell population. On electron microscopy, the absence of a brush border, the presence of microvilli, and the mitochondrial morphology were all consistent with a distal tubular origin for renal oncocytomas. Later, immunohistochemical staining was negative for alkaline phosphatase, also ruling out a proximal tubular origin. The increase in succinic dehydrogenase activity and the numerous mitochondria found in renal oncocytomas provided proof that the cells of origin are not the proximal tubules, but rather the collecting duct cells. Also, the majority of renal oncocytomas are positive for band 3 and carbonic anhydrase c, suggesting that the cell of origin is the intercalated cell of the collecting tubule.

Radiologic examination does not reliably differentiate these tumors from other solid renal lesions. There are no specific findings on excretory urography that will differentiate renal oncocytomas from other solid renal masses. A central scar may be demonstrated on CT or sonography, but this finding is inconsistent. Although angiography is uncommonly used today, oncocytomas can have a characteristic spoke-wheel pattern arising from the feeding interlobar arteries. Unfortunately, this finding also is unreliable and may be seen in approximately 15% of renal cell carcinomas, which are far more commonly seen. MRI has not significantly improved the preoperative radiologic diagnostic capabilities for renal oncocytomas.

A literature review showed that radionuclide imaging, such as 99m technetium glucoheptonate, ^{131}I-orthoiodohippurate, ^{123}I-iodohippinate, and others are not successful in differentiating renal oncocytomas from renal cell carcinoma. Technetium 99m sestamibi, a nuclear tracer that has an affinity for intracellular mitochondria, may have a role in aiding the preoperative diagnosis of renal oncocytomas larger than 3 cm.

The majority of oncocytomas are asymptomatic and are discovered incidentally. Occasionally patients will present with symptoms of abdominal or flank pain and gross hematuria. The median age of presentation is in the sixth to seventh decades of life, but ranges from 10 to 94 years. Oncocytoma, like renal cell carcinoma, occurs in males twice as often as in females. Renal oncocytomatosis has been reported in a postmortem case in which more than 200 small oncocytomas were found in both kidneys and has also been reported in a living patient with bilateral nephromegaly.

Though renal oncocytoma is defined as a benign epithelial tumor, a few lesions have been reported to have the potential for malignancy and metastasis. Generally, those reported malignant cases have had some degree of nuclear atypia. This led to a proposed grading system based on cellular and nuclear appearance: grade 1—regular appearing cells with smooth nuclei and eosinophilic cytoplasm, grade 2—increased cellular variation and irregular nuclei, and grade 3—nuclear atypia and mitotic figures. No patient with a grade 1 appearance had metastatic disease or died from disease. However, a review of those patients with grades 2 and 3 lesions and metastatic disease has revealed variants of renal cell carcinoma rather than malignant oncocytoma. It has been suggested that those oncocytomas that have metastasized may actually have been renal cell carcinomas exhibiting granular cell morphology, which is often difficult to separate from renal oncocytoma. Granular renal cell carcinoma, chromophobe renal cell carcinoma, papillary renal cell carcinoma, and collecting duct carcinoma are all included in the differential diagnosis of renal oncocytoma.

Atypical features such as nuclear pleomorphism, perirenal fat involvement, hemorrhage, microvascular invasion, and minimal necrosis may be present in some tumors. These are permitted in renal oncocytoma only when other characteristic cytoarchitectural features of oncocytoma are present. In one series, none of the patients, even those with "atypical" histologic features, demonstrated evidence of recurrence, metastasis, or death due to tumor at a mean follow-up of 7.6 years. In another series of 31 patients with renal oncocytomas with varying degrees of cellular pleomorphism, there were no metastases detected or deaths from oncocytoma. Therefore renal oncocytoma, if strictly defined, is a benign tumor and does not need to be graded.

Because renal oncocytoma is often histologically difficult to separate from renal cell carcinoma, and coexisting renal cell carcinoma has been reported to occur in 7% to 32% of cases, there have been many efforts to try to distinguish between the two lesions, which have markedly different prognosis, on a cellular and molecular level. Flow cytometry analysis of tumor cell deoxyribonucleic acid (DNA) ploidy can range from aneuploid to tetraploid, neither pattern accurately predicting tumor cell type. The loss of human leukocyte antigen (HLA) class I antigens has been reported to occur in most renal oncocytomas, whereas renal cell carcinomas maintain this antigen expression. Nuclear morphometric measurements can be used in differentiating between renal oncocytomas and renal cell carcinomas. Another difference between the two lesions has been found at the genetic level. The loss of chromosome Y and 1 is common in renal oncocytoma and rare in renal cell carcinoma.

Pure renal oncocytoma is difficult to diagnose preoperatively. Fine-needle aspiration has been attempted to establish the diagnosis of oncocytoma. However, it is important to remember that renal cell carcinoma can contain oncocytic cells and, conversely, large oncocytomas may harbor small foci of malignant tumor. Thus needle-core biopsy or fine-needle aspiration will probably not provide adequate tissue to subtype the renal neoplasm. Renal-sparing surgery, consisting of renal exploration and partial nephrectomy with frozen section control of margins, for young patients with tumors less than 4 cm has been advocated by several authorities. If the diagnosis of grade 1 oncocytoma is ensured in a lesion less than 3 cm, close observation rather than surgery may be allowed. However, due to the intrinsic problems in preoperatively diagnosing pure oncocytoma, radical nephrectomy remains the predominant treatment.

Angiomyolipoma

Renal angiomyolipoma is the most common mesenchymal tumor of the kidney, first described by Grawitz as "Angio-Myo-Lipoms der Niere" in 1900. Morgan coined the term *angiomyolipoma* in 1951. The tumor is composed of varying amounts of adipose tissue, smooth muscle, and thick-walled blood vessels. Originally, angiomyolipoma was thought be a hamartomatous growth, indicating a developmental rather than a neoplastic pathogenesis. Newer data suggest that renal angiomyolipoma is a clonal neoplasm that arises from the perivascular epithelial cells of the kidney.

Renal angiomyolipoma can occur either sporadically or in association with tuberous sclerosis (TS). In a large screening population from Japan, the prevalence of renal angiomyolipoma was found to be 24 tumors in 13,000 men and 5,000 women. Approximately 50% to 80% of patients with TS will develop angiomyolipomas.

The gross appearance depends on which of the three elements predominates, and varies from yellow to gray. The mass is unencapsulated and hemorrhage and necrosis are common. The lesion can extend into the collecting system as well as the perirenal fat. Approximately 12 cases have been reported of renal angiomyolipoma extending into the inferior vena cava as a tumor thrombus. Renal angiomyolipoma may also be found in the regional lymph nodes without evidence of malignant progression.

On histologic examination, the adipocytes are mature and are found in clusters, whereas the smooth muscle cells frequently grow in sheets. The vessels have thick muscular walls and are generally tortuous. Slightly pleomorphic nuclei are more common than the occasional mitotic figure. The presence of abnormal nuclei in combination with multifocality and extrarenal lymph node involvement has led to confusion regarding whether this is a malignant tumor with metastatic potential. Pure angiomyolipomas have not been reported to metastasize, and lesions seen in adjacent organs such as the spleen or liver are attributed to multicentricity.

A variant of angiomyolipoma, which contains epithelioid smooth muscle cells, can closely simulate both carcinoma and sarcoma, histologically and prognostically. The term *monotypic epithelioid malignant angiomyolipoma* has been proposed for this variant of angiomyolipoma, which has a large population of large mononuclear cells with eccentric nuclei, prominent nucleoli, and cytoplasm similar to that found in ganglion cells. Often the fat cells and the thick-walled blood vessels are absent. Immunohistochemical studies can differentiate this tumor from other malignant neoplasms if the histologic diagnosis is uncertain. This aggressive neoplasm has the capacity to locally recur, metastasize, and even cause death.

Epithelial tumors such as oncocytoma and renal cell carcinoma have been reported to coexist with angiomyolipoma. Up to 26% of patients with TS and angiomyolipomas have been reported to contain synchronous renal cell carcinoma, although other studies have reported much lower incidences. The data regarding the incidence of renal cell carcinoma in TS patients may need to be reevaluated because some of these cases may actually be the aforementioned malignant subtype of angiomyolipoma.

The tumor has a variety of presentations depending on the size of the lesion. Lesions less than 4 cm are typically asymptomatic, whereas 82% to 94% of patients with lesions greater than 4 cm are symptomatic. Abdominal or flank pain is the most common presenting symptom, followed by hematuria and hemorrhage. Hypertension and anemia may be present. Hemorrhage leading to hypovolemic shock is a rare, if not extreme, presentation. The spontaneous rupture of a renal angiomyolipoma during pregnancy is a rare, reportable phenomenon thought to be either secondary to an increase in renal vascular volume and interstitial fluid or secondary to rapid tumor growth. This event necessitates emergent nephrectomy or arterial embolization.

Before the advent of CT, angiomyolipoma was difficult to differentiate from renal cell carcinoma. The presence of fat densities (−70 to −10 Hounsfield units) on CT is classic for angiomyolipoma. However, CT is not always diagnostic for renal angiomyolipoma. There are rare reports of fat found in calcified renal cell carcinomas, atypical Wilms' tumors, and even one renal oncocytoma. Conventional CT can miss small fat deposits in tumors secondary to respiratory misregistration. A newer study found that helical CT was more sensitive than conventional CT in allowing radiologists to detect fat in masses smaller than 2 cm. Ultrasonic frequency–dependent attenuation measurement is a new, promising radiographic modality that may aid in differentiating hyperechoic renal cell carcinomas from angiomyolipomas. Extrarenal retroperitoneal angiomyolipoma or retroperitoneal liposarcoma contained within Gerota's fascia may be difficult to distinguish from a renal angiomyolipoma on CT and may only be discovered at laparotomy.

Renal angiographic findings such as hypervascularity and arteriovenous fistulas are not specific to angiomyolipomas and thus are not used diagnostically. Excretory urography cannot distinguish angiomyolipoma from other solid lesions. The tumor typically appears as an intensely echogenic mass on sonography. On T1-weighted MRI, fat will be a high signal intensity and this may aid in detecting small amounts of fat within a mass. If the radiographic findings contain calcifications, or are otherwise atypical for angiomyolipoma, the tumor should be treated as any other unknown solid mass and should be surgically removed.

The two main treatment options for renal angiomyolipoma consist of selective angiographic embolization and nephron-sparing tumor excision. The angiographic pattern, the parenchymal location of the lesion, and the patient's medical condition are some of the factors that should be considered when deciding between these treatments. Angiographic embolization is suitable for symptomatic cases, bilateral tumors, and large tumors not amenable to partial nephrectomy. A literature review found that embolization was effective in 90% of patients over a mean follow-up period of 21 months. Other reports on angiographic embolization confirm the low morbidity expected in this minimally invasive therapeutic modality. Nephron-sparing cryotherapy for a symptomatic renal angiomyolipoma in a TS patient with a single kidney has been reported. The treatment was well tolerated and there was minimal loss of parenchyma. Nevertheless, the authors note that this therapy is still experimental with a limited follow-up.

The size of the lesion often correlates with symptoms; the management varies accordingly. An isolated angiomyolipoma less than 4 cm in diameter may be observed with yearly CT or ultrasound, because these tumors are unlikely to hemorrhage or require intervention. Patients with lesions greater than 4 cm can be divided into two groups; those with symptoms and those who are asymptomatic or mildly symptomatic. The latter can be followed semiannually, but nearly 50% of these lesions will grow. Because of the high likelihood of spontaneous hemorrhage in large lesions, prophylactic treatment has been advocated. If there is significant growth or severe symptoms, as manifested by bleeding or pain, nephron-sparing surgery or embolization is warranted.

Tuberous Sclerosis

Epidemiology and Genetics

TS is one of the phakomatoses characterized by hamartomas of many organs excluding the peripheral nerves and the musculoskeletal system. The TS gene was found to be linked to the ABO locus on chromosome 9 in 1987. Other data show abnormalities in chromosome 11 and 12 as well, and a loss of heterozygosity on chromosome 16p13.3. Evidence for genetic heterogeneity exists with only 33% to 50% of cases caused by the chromosome 9 gene. There is also evidence for a gene on chromosome 16 near the ADPKD1 gene. The estimated prevalence of TS has changed from 1in 150,000 to 1 in 9,407 live births because of increasing diagnosis of individuals with a less severe phenotypic expression of the disorder. Sporadic cases are common with an estimated 60% spontaneous mutation rate. However, this too may represent failure to diagnose mild cases.

Method of Diagnosis and Clinical Characteristics

Neurocutaneous involvement and skin lesions are the most common findings followed by renal angiomyolipomas, renal cysts, and rhabdomyomas in the heart. The skin lesions occur in 95% of patients and include hypomelanotic macules (ash leaf spots), facial angiofibromas (adenoma sebaceum), ungual fibromas, and the shagreen patch.

Several brain lesions occur in TS, with subependymal nodules and cortical tubers considered pathognomonic. CT is useful for demonstrating calcified subependymal nodules, and cortical tubers are best demonstrated by MRI. Mental retardation and seizures and adenoma sebaceum were considered the classic triad of findings initially; however, mental retardation now appears in less than 25% of patients. Variable prevalence of seizures is reported in TS (48% to 84%). Renal angiomyolipomas are the most common renal finding, found in 40% to 50% of patients, followed by cysts (30%) and renal carcinoma (2%). In children, the predominant, and often the only, finding is renal involvement with cysts present. The renal lesions in TS are commonly bilateral and multifocal. Angiomyolipoma in patients with TS arises in a younger age group (25 to 35 years) and is more likely to grow, become symptomatic, and require surgery than in those patients without TS.

Isolated single renal angiomyolipomas can be found in the general population; however, bilateral or multiple angiomyolipomas are diagnostic of TS. Ultrasonography or CT should identify both renal cysts and angiomyolipomas; however, CT with thin sections (1 cm) is the most sensitive test for diagnosing small angiomyolipomas. Although renal findings are often confused with ADPKD and sometimes ARPKD, familial isolated renal cystic disease is rarely reported in TS. The presence of angiomyolipomas and careful attention to other disease manifestations should permit the diagnosis. The differentiation of angiomyolipomas from renal cell carcinoma can be difficult. Renal histology, although specific to TS, is usually not required to make the diagnosis.

Initial clinical symptoms of renal involvement include flank or back pain, hematuria, retroperitoneal hemorrhage, hypertension, and occasionally renal insufficiency. The previously reported low incidence of renal failure in patients with TS may be attributed to their early death from neurologic complications. Renal failure in TS patients is due to bilateral obstruction of the ureters by adjacent tumors or replacement of renal parenchyma by cysts and angiomyolipomas. Some authors suggest that renal failure is more likely when renal cysts predominate. Renal cell carcinoma is associated with TS occurring at a younger age than sporadic cases and may be bilateral or multiple. Indeed, in one report 14 of 53 (25%) TS patients with renal abnormalities had renal cell carcinoma.

With the advances in identifying the multiple chromosomal locations of the gene defects responsible for TS, DNA markers flanking the gene defect are now available for chromosome 9. Therefore those patients from large chromosome 9, TS families can undergo presymptomatic screening for the disease, and those unlikely to be gene carriers would be saved expensive and time-consuming screening tests for the brain and renal involvement.

Pathology and Pathogenesis

On gross inspection, kidneys are enlarged and reniform with the angiomyolipomas hamartomas composed of smooth muscle, fat, and blood vessels. Cysts are usually infrequent, although occasionally bilateral and multiple. Renal cysts are lined with characteristic hyperplastic eosinophilic epithelium that form papillary and polypoid lesions on cyst walls.

Management and Outcome

TS patients have a shortened lifespan, with 50% of affected individuals dying before the age of 20. With improved earlier diagnosis and neurosurgical techniques, renal involvement has become the leading cause of death in TS patients older than 30 years. It has been reported that of 40 patients who died from TS, 11 deaths were due to renal complications, with 2 having metastatic renal cell carcinoma, 2 severe retroperitoneal hemorrhage, and 7 renal failure. Therefore it is important to follow TS patients with renal ultrasonography and measurements of renal function. Patients with angiomyolipoma of greater than 4 cm or those who exhibit tumor growth have a high risk for hemorrhage, and therefore prophylactic renal arterial embolization or surgery should be considered.

Fibroma

Medullary interstitial fibromas are small, asymptomatic, benign tumors found in 18% to 40% of autopsies. There is no sex predilection and most are bilateral. The tumors are thought to arise from the interstitial cells of the medulla but can be found wherever there is fibrous tissue. Histologically, the tumors consist of benign sheets of fibroblasts in a loose matrix with atrophic renal tubules. The tumors are gray or white, well demarcated, and resemble uterine fibroids. There are no specific radiographic findings that distinguish fibromas from other solid tumors, and the diagnosis is frequently made at the pathologist's bench after a radical nephrectomy. If a fibroma is suspected preoperatively, nephron-sparing surgery should be considered.

Other Benign Tumors

Renin-secreting juxtaglomerular cell tumor is a rare, but significant, benign tumor of the kidney. Approximately 40 cases have been reported since this neoplasm was first characterized by Robertson in 1967. These tumors commonly present in young, predominantly female, patients with severe diastolic hypertension, usually poorly responsive to medications. Further workup reveals elevated plasma renin levels and often secondary hyperaldosteronism with hypokalemia. Radiographically, functional renin-secreting juxtaglomerular cell tumors are difficult to detect because they are usually less than 2.5 cm in diameter. CT may show masses that are isodense or hypodense with weak contrast enhancement compared with the normal renal parenchyma. Renal angiography may be used, not to identify the lesion, but to rule out renovascular hypertension and to delineate the vasculature if renal-sparing surgery is considered. Selective renal vein sampling for renin may aid in diagnosis but is not 100% diagnostic. In some cases, peripheral lesions may drain into the pericapsular veins rather than the renal veins, thus creating false-negative venous sampling.

As the name implies, these tumors arise from the smooth muscle cells of the afferent arterioles of the juxtaglomerular apparatus. Histologically, the lesion is a hemangiopericytoma with sheets of round cells with abundant pink cytoplasm. Renin granules can be detected with Bowie's stain or other immunohistochemical methods. If this benign tumor can be preoperatively distinguished from the larger, and sometimes malignant, nonfunctional renal hemangiopericytoma, partial rather than radical nephrectomy is recommended. Elevated renin levels should normalize after nephrectomy, and those patients with continued hypertension postoperatively are thought to have sustained permanent arterial damage.

Pure hemangiomas and lipomas are rare lesions that are typically asymptomatic. Hemangiomas are vascular neoplasms that can present with gross hematuria. Selective angiography will show the arteriovenous shunting in the majority of cases. These lesions can be either surgically removed or embolized. Lipomas are usually found in middle-age women and can become symptomatic as they grow. Radiographic diagnosis is most accurately accomplished with CT. Renal-sparing surgery is difficult owing to the unencapsulated nature of these tumors, and often a total nephrectomy is performed.

MALIGNANT RENAL TUMORS

Renal Cell Carcinoma

Renal cell carcinomas account for the majority (85% to 90%) of primary malignant renal tumors. This neoplasm represents approximately 3% of all adult malignancies and is more common in males by a ratio of 2:1. The American Cancer Society projected that 31,200 new cases of renal cell carcinoma would be diagnosed in 2000 and that 11,900 people would die of this disease. It is found predominantly in adults in the fifth to seventh decades of life; however, renal cell carcinoma can occur in younger age groups. There are both familial and sporadic forms of renal cell carcinoma. Patients with von Hippel-Lindau (VHL) disease, an autosomal-dominant genetic disorder, have an increased incidence of renal cell carcinoma in addition to other malignancies. Identification of the VHL gene has shown consistent deletions or mutations in both familial and sporadic cases of renal cell carcinoma.

Renal cell carcinoma is found in a greater incidence in renal transplant patients and hemodialysis patients. Acquired cystic kidney disease (ACKD), found in 40% to 90% of dialysis patients, was first associated with the development of renal cell carcinoma in 1977. Since then, many reports have attempted to conclusively show an increased incidence of malignancy in these patients. Patients with ACKD and renal cell carcinoma range from 1% to 8% of all patients on hemodialysis; one study reported a 30-fold increased risk of developing renal cell carcinoma over controls. A newer study found a 100 times greater risk of renal cell carcinoma in the native kidneys of renal transplant patients when compared with the general population. The authors did not find an increased risk of developing malignancy in patients with ACKD. This conclusion has been supported by other investigators.

Because the incidences of renal cell carcinoma are different in these two populations, the prognosis is different as well. Patients undergoing hemodialysis with renal cell carcinoma have minimal disease at presentation and their prognosis is no worse than the general population. In fact, patients receiving hemodialysis have a short life expectancy, and their morbidity and mortality may be secondary to numerous medical problems rather than renal cell carcinoma. In contrast, renal cell carcinoma in renal transplant patients is aggressive, with 53% presenting with metastatic disease. Hypotheses explaining this increased risk of malignancy in ACKD include the underlying cause of end-stage renal failure or the process of dialysis. The immunosuppressive medications taken by the transplant recipients were not a factor in developing renal cell carcinoma.

Routine renal ultrasonography has been recommended for this high-risk group of patients.

There are several reports of an increased incidence of second malignancies in renal cell carcinoma, similar to patients with other solid tumors or hematologic malignancies. Leukemias, lymphomas, and multiple myelomas have occurred either before or after the diagnosis and treatment of renal cell carcinoma. Hypotheses include a common predisposing factor such as chemical exposures or similar genetic mutations. A defect in the immune system caused by one of the malignancies that allows the other to develop is another proposed mechanism.

Etiology

The cell of origin of renal cell carcinoma is considered to be the proximal convoluted tubule. Although the etiology of renal cell carcinoma is incompletely understood, a number of factors are proposed in the development of renal cell carcinoma. Reports on smoking implicate cigarettes, whereas others find a high incidence of renal cell carcinoma in men who smoke pipes or cigars. Analytic epidemiologic studies consistently support a causal relationship between obesity and renal cell carcinoma in both males and females. Increased risk of developing renal cell carcinoma is also associated with consumption of fried/sautéed meats and low intakes of magnesium or vitamin E. Medications such as phenacetin and diuretics have been implicated in the development of renal cell carcinoma. A report suggested that medications related to the treatment of hypertension, or even the hypertension itself, may be etiologic factors. Patients with occupational exposures to chemicals such as cadmium and asbestos have also been shown to have a slightly increased incidence of renal cell carcinoma.

Molecular Genetics

As previously mentioned, renal cell carcinoma can be divided into sporadic and familial forms. The two-hit theory of carcinogenesis and the tumor suppressor gene model are the foundation upon which molecular genetics of all cancers, including renal cell carcinoma, has been built. Familial forms of cancer occurred at a younger age than the sporadic forms and the tumors were often multifocal. It was postulated that patients with the familial form inherit a mutated gene (first hit) and then later in life, the gene's other allele would become mutated through a genetic event (second hit). If these genes in question are tumor suppressor genes, then unregulated cell growth would occur and result in cancer. Sporadic tumors require two separate genetic events (mutations) for tumor formation. Therefore these patients are typically older and present with unilateral lesions.

There are three forms of inheritable renal cancer. The first is an autosomal-dominant familial clear cell renal cell carcinoma, and the second is hereditary papillary renal cell carcinoma. The third, and one of the most common inheritable types of renal cell carcinoma, is found in patients with VHL disease, an inherited cancer syndrome characterized by the development of retinal angiomas, central nervous system hemangioblastomas, pancreatic cysts and tumors, pheochromocytomas and renal cysts, and carcinomas. The familial forms of renal cell carcinoma occur at a younger age and are more commonly bilateral and multifocal than the sporadic forms.

The search for the gene for kidney cancer initiated by the National Cancer Institute has provided much of the known data on the molecular genetics of renal cell carcinoma. VHL patients with renal cell carcinomas were found to have inherited an abnormal 3p allele, and the normal or "wild-type" 3p allele from the unaffected parent was lost. The most common changes observed were deletions and translocations. The VHL tumor suppressor gene was subsequently linked to chromosome 3p and identified. The wild-type VHL gene's protein slows transcription and the mutated gene's product results in overactive transcription elongation, perhaps leading to tumorigenesis. A newer study found allelic deletions of the VHL gene in atypical and benign cysts in the VHL kidney, suggesting that these are precursors of renal cell carcinomas.

The loss of a segment of chromosome 3p is a consistent finding in cases of familial clear cell carcinomas as well as sporadic clear cell carcinomas. Loss of one copy of the VHL gene was found in 98% of sporadic renal cell carcinomas, and other VHL mutations were found in 57% of cases. Thus the association of the VHL gene in the pathogenesis of both sporadic and inherited clear cell renal carcinomas has been elucidated. In contrast, familial papillary renal carcinomas do not have chromosome 3p abnormalities. Instead, frequent trisomies of chromosomes 7,16,17 and loss of Y have been observed. In addition to the VHL mutations, there are many proto-oncogenes implicated in the development of renal cell carcinoma such as overexpression of c-*myc* and epidermal growth factor messenger ribonucleic acid (mRNA) and underexpression of HER-2 mRNA. Transforming growth factor alpha and beta are overexpressed in renal cell carcinoma and are thought to be stimulatory and inhibitory influences in tumor growth.

Pathology

Renal cell carcinomas are typically round and originate from the cortex. Compressed renal parenchyma forms a pseudocapsule around the tumor. The color of the lesion varies from gray to yellow, and hemorrhage, necrosis, and calcifications are commonly observed. Renal cell carcinoma can invade the collecting system as well as adjacent structures. The tumor frequently extends into the renal vein as a thrombus, which can enter the inferior vena cava.

Histologically, renal cell carcinomas are composed of different cell types: clear cell (nonpapillary), chromophilic (papillary or tubulopapillary), chromophobe, and collecting duct carcinoma. The clear cell type is found in 75% of renal cell carcinomas. These cells are filled with abundant lipids and glycogen, producing a transparent cytoplasm. The chromophilic type is predominantly papillary and is the second most common carcinoma of the renal tubular epithelium (10% to 15%). The third most common carcinoma type is the chromophobe variant. Chromophobe renal cell carcinoma is found in approximately 5% of renal cell carcinomas and may show better survival than clear cell renal cell carcinoma. The collecting duct carcinoma variant is the least common subtype, found in less than 1% of surgical series. It is thought to arise from the medulla and consists of often atypical, hobnail cells. Sarcomatoid histology may be found in association with other renal cell carcinoma subtypes of and is no longer considered a distinct cell type. It rather signifies a specific spindle cell growth pattern that can be found in any specimen of high-grade renal cell carcinoma. Granular cells contain eosinophilic cytoplasm due to numerous mitochondria. This term has been used to describe many of the previous subtypes as well as oncocytomas and epithelioid angiomyolipomas, thus rendering this designation vague. Therefore the American Joint Committee on Cancer (AJCC) does not recommend using the term *granular cell carcinoma.*

Clinical Presentation

Before the development and the routine use of sonography and CT, renal cell carcinoma was termed the *internist's tumor* because of its variable presentations. It could now be stated that "what was once the internist's tumor has become the radiologist's tumor." It is estimated that two-thirds of patients with locally confined tumors are now diagnosed by incidental findings on imaging studies for nonurologic problems. This is in marked contrast to earlier studies, which reported the percentage of tumors discovered incidentally as 7% from 1935 to 1965, 13% from 1961 to 1973, and 48% from 1980 to 1984. The classic triad of pain, hematuria, and a flank mass is now only found in 11% of patients with renal cell carcinoma. Hematuria, present in 60% of patients, is the most common presenting sign. Other presenting symptoms are pain, weight loss, cachexia, and fever. Approximately 25% of patients present with metastatic disease, many with the complaint of bone pain due to metastatic deposits. Paraneoplastic syndromes may accompany renal cell carcinoma but are notoriously vague and often are only appreciated after the diagnosis has been made through other means. Physical examination is usually unremarkable. A palpable flank mass or a varicocele may be present in a small number of patients.

Renal cell carcinoma is one of the few solid tumors associated with a large variety of paraneoplastic syndromes. Approximately 30% of patients with renal cell carcinoma may suffer from a paraneoplastic syndrome. Anemia is found in 20% to 40% of patients and is out of proportion to blood loss from hematuria. The normocytic, normochromic anemia may be related to an increased destruction in the circulation or possibly a decrease in erythropoietin production. Conversely, 3% to 4% of patients may present with erythrocytosis from increased erythropoietin. Renal cell carcinoma is thought to secrete an endogenous pyrogen causing fever in approximately 20% of patients. Hypertension, thought secondary to hyperreninemia, can be found in 20% to 35% of patients. Five percent to twenty percent of patients with renal cell carcinoma can be hypercalcemic. Renal cell carcinoma can produce a parathyroid hormone–related protein, which is thought to raise the serum calcium level. Increased levels of prostaglandin E, a stimulator of bone resorption, and osteolytic metastases are also associated with hypercalcemia. Stauffer's syndrome is a nonmetastatic hepatic dysfunction found in patients with renal cell carcinoma. This syndrome is characterized by abnormal liver function tests, prolonged prothrombin time, and, occasionally, hepatic necrosis. The cause is unknown. Liver function should normalize following nephrectomy; persistence of the abnormalities portends a poor prognosis. Other abnormalities associated with renal cell carcinoma include amyloidosis, polyneuromyopathy, increased levels of insulin, glucagon, and human chorionic gonadotropin.

Radiographic Diagnosis

Intravenous urography is often the first test obtained when hematuria or flank pain are the presenting signs. Renal cell carcinoma may be seen as a distortion of the calyces, or an intraluminal filling defect, or an irregularity of the renal outline. Unfortunately, an IVP may miss small tumors that do not distort the architecture of the kidney. Additionally, a benign renal cyst may cause mass effect on IVP, similar to a carcinoma. Because of the low sensitivity and specificity of IVP, all masses should be subsequently evaluated with ultrasonography or a CT scan.

Renal ultrasound can differentiate between cystic and solid lesions. A simple cyst on ultrasound requires no further studies. However, a solid or an indeterminate mass must be further delineated by CT, because the relatively low sensitivities of IVP and ultrasonography in the detection of parenchymal renal masses are 67% and 79%, respectively. Color Doppler flow ultrasound has been used to assess the extent of vascular tumor thrombus. Intraoperative ultrasound has been reported to aid in renal-sparing surgery.

Renal arteriography was used extensively in the past to evaluate renal masses. Typical angiographic findings of renal cell carcinoma are neovascularity, venous pooling, and arteriovenous fistulae. Presently, angiography is mainly used in planning nephron-sparing surgery because it delineates the arterial anatomy, providing information regarding the presence and location of upper- and lower-pole renal arteries as well as aberrant vessels. Arteriography is performed in conjunction with renal angioinfarction for similar reasons.

CT has become the most common modality used to preoperatively stage renal cell carcinoma. It is highly accurate in diagnosing renal vein involvement, inferior vena cava (IVC) extension as well as local invasion of adjacent organs or structures. Its reported accuracy rates range from 75% to 95%. Any renal mass that enhances with intravenous contrast should be considered renal cell carcinoma until proven otherwise. CT can only suggest lymph node metastases when there is extensive enlargement. Spiral CT and three-dimensional CT imaging are emerging technologies that may replace conventional CT and angiography in the delineation of renal pathology and renal vascular anatomy. Because of the rapidity of a spiral CT, scanning must be delayed until approximately 90 seconds after intravenous contrast injection to obtain a uniform nephrogram for optimal tumor visualization.

MRI is usually reserved for renal masses that are indeterminate on CT and ultrasound. This modality has been shown to be more sensitive than CT in imaging local organ extension and venous tumor involvement. MRI can be used in cases in which intravenous contrast is contraindicated. However, similar to CT, MRI cannot identify microscopic lymph node involvement or distinguish malignant from hyperplastic lymphadenopathy. The findings by various imaging techniques are provided in Chapters 105 (MRI), 106 (ultrasound), 107 (CT), and 108 (radiography).

Staging

Clinical staging of renal cell carcinoma begins with a history, physical examination, laboratory tests, and radiographic imaging. In addition to those tests discussed previously, a chest radiograph, liver function tests, and serum calcium are suitable preoperative examinations. A radionuclide bone scan may be considered in cases with elevated alkaline phosphatase, or elevated serum calcium or large, bulky tumors.

The most commonly used staging C system in the United States is that by Robson. It is simple and easy to remember. Stage I tumors are those that are confined to the renal parenchyma and contained by the capsule. Stage II tumors extend outside the renal capsule, invade the perinephric fat, and are contained by Gerota's fascia. Stage IIIa lesions involve the renal vein and/or the vena cava and stage IIIb tumors have regional lymph node metastases. Stage IIIc is the combination of IIIa and IIIb. Finally, lesions that invade adjacent organs or have distant metastases are considered stage IV tumors. Tumors that involve the ipsilateral adrenal gland are not considered stage IV, but rather are classified as stage II. However, the Robson system does not correlate well with prognosis, in part because it does not take tumor size into account, and it does not address the extent of lymphatic metastases.

The tumor, node, and metastasis (TNM) system is the most accurate and thus preferred by most modern investigators. T1 tumors are less than 7 cm and T2 tumors are greater than 7 cm, but both lesions are confined to the kidney. T3 tumors may invade the ipsilateral adrenal gland or the perinephric fat (T3a) but do not extend beyond Gerota's fascia similar to Robson's stage II tumors. In addition, T3b tumors have renal vein or vena caval involvement and T3c tumors have supradiaphragmatic vena caval extension. T4 tumors invade structures beyond Gerota's fascia. Nodal disease is stratified by size and number, and metastases are divided into two simple groups; those who have distant metastases and those who do not.

Prognostic Factorso

Prognostic factors are essential in planning therapy and predicting disease outcome. Although radiologic and pathologic studies are the gold standards in determining a patient's prognosis, recent developments in the area of biomolecular markers and molecular genetics may well advance the ability to predict the tumor's natural history to new heights. The Union Internationale Contre le Cancer (UICC) and the AJCC have divided prognostic factors into patient-related, tumor-related, and therapy-related factors. The major patient-related prognostic factors include poor performance status, symptomatic presentation, weight loss, and elevated erythrocyte sedimentation rate. Tumor-related prognostic factors include TNM classification, margin involvement, grade, histologic type, and sarcomatoid change. Gross residual disease at the time of surgery was the only major therapy-related factor of prognostic importance. Other promising, but less proven, prognostic factors include biomolecular factors such as DNA content (aneuploidy) and increased cell proliferation markers.

Pathologic stage is the sole prognostic indicator in renal cell carcinoma that is unmatched in its consistent ability to predict outcome. Reported 5-year survival rates range from 60% to 100% for tumors confined to the kidney, which then decreases to 59% for stage III tumors, and 11% to 16% for stage IV tumors. Tumors limited to Gerota's fascia but with perinephric fat invasion (T3a) have an estimated 45% to 63% 5-year survival rate. A compilation of several large studies indicated a 15% to 20% reduction in 5-year survival rates of T3a tumors when compared with T1 tumors. Lymph node involvement portends an extremely poor prognosis, with 5-year and 10-year survival rates of 5% to 30% and 0% to 5%, respectively. Metastatic renal cell carcinoma carries a dismal prognosis. The survival rates in spite of the advances in immunotherapy are still low. Metastatic renal cell carcinoma patients have 5-year and 10-year survival rates of 5% to 10% and 0% to 7%, respectively, and a median survival of less than 1 year.

Tumor size has been correlated with increased risk of metastases as early as 1938. In 1950, Bell reported that only 11% of tumors less than 5 cm metastasized, whereas 85% of tumors larger than 10 cm were associated with metastases. Since then, large retrospective studies have confirmed that larger tumors were associated with a poorer prognosis. The TNM staging system presently uses 7 cm as a primary tumor size cutoff for differentiating T1 and T2 tumors, because the previous 2.5 cm cutoff did not accurately predict survival differences. Further tinkering with the TNM system is currently being considered as nephron-sparing surgery gains a wider acceptance and a longer follow-up. No significant survival difference was found between patients undergoing radical nephrectomy or nephron-sparing surgery for lesions 4 cm or less. In light of this study and findings similar to these, the UICC and the AJCC have proposed dividing the T1 stage into T1a (tumor 4 cm or smaller) and T1b (tumor larger than 4 to 7 cm limited to the kidney).

Another proposed revision of the TNM system concerns ipsilateral adrenal involvement. The left side is predominantly affected and can be found in 1% to 10% of patients undergoing radical nephrectomy for renal cell carcinoma. Most of these patients have large, high-stage, primary tumors and have been shown to have a poorer prognosis than other T3 tumors. Based on these observations, a new stage, T3d, was proposed. It denotes those tumors with direct extension to the ipsilateral adrenal gland. Those patients with adrenal metastases separate from the primary tumor should be classified as M1.

It is unclear whether renal vein tumor thrombus in the presence of a localized tumor is a poor prognostic indicator. The propagation of a tumor thrombus into the IVC in association with renal cell carcinoma occurs in 4% to 10% of cases. Several clinical series have reported equal survival rates after radical nephrectomy and tumor thrombus extraction as compared with patients with tumors localized to the kidney. Five-year survival rates of 47% to 69% after resection of tumors confined to the kidney with vena caval thrombi have been reported, demonstrating no significant decrease in mortality for these patients. A series of 24 patients showed that renal vein involvement associated with a tumor confined to the kidney did not alter prognosis. The 5-year survival rate for patients with venous extension was 84%, and those patients with T1 and T2 tumors had a 88% survival. In contrast, other investigators state that venous extension does correlate with a poorer prognosis. The cranial extension of the thrombus into the right atrium was a significant poor prognostic indicator in patients with clinically localized renal cell carcinoma. However, the general consensus in the literature suggests that as long as the venous tumor thrombus can be safely and completely removed, and the tumor is locally confined, the survival rate should not be significantly different from T1 or T2 tumors.

Microscopic vascular invasion has been shown to be an independent prognostic factor in those patients with T2N0 and T3N0 renal cell carcinomas. The 5-year, disease-free survival was calculated as 89% with no microscopic vascular invasion and 50% with invasion. Other investigators have associated the intramural microvessel density (MMD) in renal cell carcinoma with patient survival. Decreased MMD is correlated with poor prognosis, and is thought to be secondary to the development of large vascular channels in an aggressive lesion.

Nuclear grade correlates with survival independent of pathologic stage. Several grading systems are presently in use throughout the world. Despite of this variety, all systems have shown that grading of renal cell carcinoma has prognostic value. Most pathologists in North America use the grading scheme based on nuclear size, shape, and content as proposed by Fuhrman and colleagues. In Fuhrman's study of 85 patients, the mean 5-year survival was reported to be 59% for grade 1, 30% for grades 2 and 3, and 10% for grade 4. Several studies have confirmed the utility of this grading system, although there are some discrepancies in the survival advantage cutpoints. That is to say, not all studies agreed that grade 1 tumors predicted significantly improved survival over grade 2 tumors, although overall, patients with low-grade tumors had a better prognosis than those with high-grade tumors.

Computer-aided image analysis of nuclear morphometry is a more objective method than the often subjective nuclear grading system. This technology is early in its development but has yielded promising prognostic data. The combination of mean nuclear area and mean nuclear regularity factor was found to accurately predict metastatic potential in 85% of cases studied. Other studies have found that smaller nuclear areas, shorter nuclear lengths, and less elongation are features that predict improved survival.

Histologic cell type is difficult to evaluate as a prognostic indicator because many renal cell carcinomas are composed of a mixture of cell types. However, prognosis may correlate with some specific histologic types, namely chromophobe carcinoma, collecting duct carcinoma, and tumors with sarcomatoid change. Chromophobe carcinoma, the third most common cell type, has been reported to have a better prognosis than the more common clear cell variety. The much less common collecting duct carcinoma is an aggressive lesion that rapidly develops metastases and has a poor prognosis. Sarcomatoid change in any type of renal cell carcinoma is associated with a poor prognosis. Patients with this histology will often present with bony metastatic disease. Adjuvant chemotherapy should be considered in this population, because surgery will not be curative. Whether the clinical outcome in papillary renal cell carcinoma is any different than clear cell renal carcinoma is unclear.

A number of biomolecular factors found in renal cell carcinoma are currently under investigation. These biomarkers may eventually serve to enhance the previously accepted prognostic factors or even replace them. DNA content (ploidy) of renal cell carcinomas is presently being studied in the hopes of correlating aneuploidy (different DNA content than diploid cells) with aggressive behavior and decreased survival. It has not conclusively predicted prognosis, even in locally confined tumors. Serum immunosuppressive acidic protein (IAP) has been found useful for detecting recurrence after surgery as well as predicting lymph node and distant metastasis in patients with renal cell carcinoma. The multidrug resistance (MDR-1) gene has been found to be overexpressed in a variety of tumors, and renal cell carcinoma is no exception. However, some researchers have found that the MDR-1 expression correlates directly with the differentiation of the tumor. Thus higher MDR-1 levels indicate a better prognosis. Genes promoting apoptosis, such as p53, and antiapoptotic genes, such as bcl2/bax, may correlate with renal cell carcinoma's clinical course, but these studies are still in the investigational stage.

Surgical Treatment for Localized Disease

Surgery is the only effective curative method for localized renal cell carcinoma. Radical nephrectomy, as defined by the excision of the kidney and adrenal gland *en bloc* with the perinephric fat and Gerota's fascia, is the gold standard in treating localized renal cell carcinoma.

Regional lymphadenectomy was originally described as an integral part of radical nephrectomy. Although lymph node dissection may additionally stage the patient and aid in prognosis, it is now controversial whether it confers an increased survival. Those in favor of regional lymph node dissection assert that patients with nodal involvement as their only site of metastatic disease may be cured by lymphadenectomy. A series of 328 patients that underwent radical nephrectomy with regional lymphadenectomy were retrospectively reviewed. The 5-, 10-, and 15-year survival rates for patients with nodal disease were 53%, 39%, and 16%, respectively. This survival rate was significantly lower than those patients with no nodal metastases, but the authors point to the overall high long-term survival of the N+ patients as support for the therapeutic role of lymphadenectomy. Although this concept may be initially attractive, there are several reasons why lymphadenectomy may not be beneficial. First, there are no prospective, randomized studies addressing this question at present. Furthermore, renal cell carcinoma may be microscopically present in other tissues and organs in addition to the local lymph nodes. In other words, this is an incurable situation.

Preoperative renal arterial embolization has been used in cases of bulky tumors to decrease intraoperative blood loss. Absorbable gelatin sponge, alcohol, and steel coils are the most widely used embolic agents. It was found that complete alcohol embolization within 24 hours of surgery significantly reduced the transfusion volume during nephrectomy for large, hypervascular renal cell carcinomas. Angioinfarction can also be employed in the patient with a large, symptomatic, nonresectable tumor. It may be used as a palliative treatment for spinal cord compression or tumor debulking before immunotherapy, obviating the need for open surgery. The complications associated with this procedure include pain, ileus, sepsis, and the inadvertent reflux of embolic agents into adjacent organs.

A surveillance protocol has been proposed for those patients after radical nephrectomy for renal cell carcinoma based on tumor stage and the disease's predilection for metastasizing to lungs, bone, lymph nodes, and brain. This protocol recommends an annual chest radiograph and serum liver functions and alkaline phosphatase levels for patients with T1 disease. Patients with T2 and T3 disease should have the previous studies performed at 6-month intervals, which may change to yearly intervals after a period of 3 years. CT should be performed at 2 and 5 years in patients with T2 and T3 disease or earlier as clinical symptoms or abnormal blood tests warrant. Routine yearly CT is unnecessary because no local recurrences were diagnosed via this imaging modality in the first 2 years postnephrectomy in this study.

Nephron-sparing surgery is increasingly becoming an accepted treatment option for localized renal cell carcinoma with a normal contralateral kidney. It has already become the treatment of choice for patients with bilateral renal cell carcinomas, a tumor in a solitary kidney, or a unilateral tumor with compromised renal function. In these select patients, the risks of renal-sparing surgery must be weighed against the morbidity and mortality of dialysis and renal transplantation. There are several parenchyma-preserving techniques: enucleation, partial nephrectomy, and bench surgery with autotransplantation. The technical success rate is excellent and the 5-year, cancer-specific survival rates for localized tumors after nephron-sparing surgery approach those of radical nephrectomy (87% to 100%). However, there is a 4% to 6% risk of local tumor recurrence, and the incidence of renal cell carcinoma multifocality has been reported to range from 6% to 7%. Clearly, the ability to identify which renal cell carcinomas are likely to be multifocal and/or locally recur is the key to maximizing survival benefit in patients undergoing nephron-sparing surgery.

A number of studies have attempted to find the most favorable tumor size or the most favorable tumor location for nephron-sparing surgery with a normal contralateral renal unit. It was found that a centrally located lesion is technically more difficult to excise compared with a peripherally located lesion. However, the 5-year, cancer-specific survival and the incidence of tumor recurrence have been reported as equal in nephron-sparing surgery regardless of lesion location. An increased survival rate was found in patients with unilateral, stage I tumors smaller than 4 cm compared with larger tumors; there were no postoperative recurrences and the cancer-specific survival rate was 100% for patients with tumors smaller than 4 cm. A favorable outcome for tumors less than 4 cm was confirmed in a similar patient population. An autopsy study observed a significantly increased number of multifocal malignant renal cell carcinomas associated with tumors greater than 2 cm compared with those 2 cm or less in diameter; based on these data, the investigators recommended nephron-sparing surgery for tumors less than 2 cm instead of 4 cm to lower the risk of local recurrence. Amendments in the TNM staging system were made to reflect this shift toward nephron-sparing surgery.

Two studies have compared radical nephrectomy with nephron-sparing surgery. Although they were not randomized, comparisons made between the two treatment options were favorable. The survival rates for the patients in the radical nephrectomy group and the nephron-sparing surgery group were 82% to 97% and 88% to 100%, respectively. A prospective, randomized trial is needed to definitively show that nephron-sparing surgery is equal to radical nephrectomy in terms of recurrence and survival.

The follow-up for nephron-sparing surgery has always been more aggressive based on the greater risk of local tumor recurrence when compared with radical nephrectomy. One study suggested that frequent imaging examinations are not necessary in the postoperative follow-up, and others found that the pathologic stage was a significant predictor of recurrent and metastatic disease. Tumors staged as T1 and T2 recurred locally in 0% and 2%, respectively, and 4% and 5% metastasized at 54 months postoperatively. There was a greater incidence of both local and distant tumor recurrence in T3 tumors (9% and 13%).

Based on these data, patients with T1 disease do not require any radiographic monitoring but should have yearly evaluations of serum calcium, alkaline phosphatase, liver function tests, blood urea nitrogen, serum creatinine, and electrolytes. Patients with T2 disease should have a chest radiograph annually and an abdominal CT every 2 years. Patients with T3 disease should undergo a CT every 6 months for the first 2 years postoperatively and annually thereafter.

Laparoscopic radical nephrectomy for renal cell carcinoma has been accomplished at only a few centers. The two largest series to date consist of 25 and 17 patients. Both studies noted decreased postoperative pain, shorter hospital stay, and quicker time to full convalescence in the laparoscopic group when compared with open surgery. However, the operative time was significantly longer (5 to 7 hours). There were no reports of local recurrence or port site seeding at a maximum of 4 years postoperatively.

As technology and our knowledge of this disease expands, patient survival will increase, morbidity will decrease, and normal renal parenchyma will be increasingly salvaged.

Management of Inferior Venal Caval Involvement

Renal cell carcinoma will form a thrombus in the renal vein in approximately 15% of patients and will involve the IVC in 4% to 10% of patients. The incidence of tumor thrombus is directly related to the size of the primary lesion. Preoperative delineation of the extent of the thrombus must be accomplished, either by inferior venography, CT, or MRI. Tumor thrombus with localized disease is not a poor prognostic sign. Complete hypothermic circulatory arrest with cardiopulmonary bypass can be safely performed for supradiaphragmatic extension. The 5-year survival after removal of caval extension ranges from 30% to 72%.

Treatment of Metastatic Renal Cell Carcinoma

Because surgical extirpation successfully treats localized renal cell carcinoma, there have been attempts to treat advanced renal cell carcinoma in the same fashion. The term *adjunctive nephrectomy* describes the removal of the primary tumor in patients with metastatic disease to increase survival or cause regression of the metastatic lesions. There are case reports of nephrectomies causing the regression, or even the resolution of metastatic lesions in patients with renal cell carcinoma. But the incidence of spontaneous regression is too low (less than 1%) to justify radical nephrectomy in the face of metastatic disease. In addition, increased survival after radical nephrectomy in the presence of metastases has not been definitively proven secondary to inherent selection biases. This procedure may be considered for those patients with a solitary metastasis that will be excised at the time of nephrectomy. Several investigators have shown minimally increased survival in patients with a pulmonary metastatic lesion treated with radical nephrectomy and complete surgical removal of the metastases. Palliative nephrectomy is reserved for patients with severe hemorrhage, pain, paraneoplastic syndromes, or symptomatic compression of adjacent organs. Selective renal arteriographic infarction is a reasonable alternative for nonsurgical candidates.

Despite numerous phase II trials, renal cell carcinoma remains refractory to chemotherapy either as single agents or in combination therapy. Chemotherapies have failed in part due to the intrinsic multidrug resistance of renal cells. Hormonal therapy with progestational agents was advocated in the past, but is no longer used. Radiation therapy for metastatic renal cell carcinoma is only beneficial in the palliation of bony metastases. The most promising systemic therapy for metastatic renal cell carcinoma involves immunomodulation. The various immunotherapeutic approaches to metastatic renal cell carcinoma consist of biologic response modifiers [interleukin-2 (IL-2) and interferon], adoptive immunotherapy [tumor infiltrating lymphocytes (TILs) and lymphokine-activated killer (LAK) cells], gene therapy, monoclonal antibodies, and tumor-specific vaccines.

Interferon-alpha (INF-α), a lymphokine with potent immunoregulatory properties, was the first agent to be used in clinical trials in metastatic renal cell carcinoma. Several nonrandomized trials produced an objective response in 15% to 20% of patients with metastatic disease. The responses were typically brief (6 to 10 months) and were usually found in those patients with good performance status, a long disease-free interval, lung predominant metastatic disease, and resected primary tumors. A compilation of 13 clinical trials involving more than 900 patients showed a median objective response rate of 18.4%. Interferon-gamma was investigated but it did not show a significant survival advantage when compared with placebo.

IL-2, a biologic response modifier, has no direct cytotoxic antitumor effect, rather it activates an antitumor immune response. IL-2, a T-cell growth factor, produces LAK cells and intensifies natural killer (NK) cell function *in vivo*. At present, it is the only immunotherapeutic agent approved for use in renal cell carcinoma by the United States Food and Drug Administration and is the gold standard for the treatment of metastatic disease. High-dose, bolus intravenous IL-2 produces objective response rates of approximately 20%, most of which can be durable for 3 or more years in patients with good clinical performance statuses. Low-dose IL-2 has been investigated because of significant morbidity in the high-dose preparation (hypotension, dyspnea, thrombocytopenia, malaise, and pulmonary and central nervous system effects). A 1994 randomized trial reported equal response rates in intravenous high-dose IL-2 and low-dose IL-2 at a median of 15 months follow-up, but less toxicity in the low-dose preparation. Another prospective, randomized trial comparing intravenous high-dose IL-2 with intravenous and subcutaneous low-dose IL-2 is was performed at the National Cancer Institute. At a median follow-up of 27 months, responses to high-dose IL-2 tended to be more durable. The high-dose intravenous, low-dose intravenous, and subcutaneous IL-2 protocols have produced response rates of 16%, 4%, and 11%, respectively. Perhaps as this trial is carried out further, the survival data will indicate the optimal regimen for treating metastatic renal cell carcinoma.

The toxicity of systemic IL-2 has spurred some researchers to find a different method of administration. High-dose IL-2 was used with or without coadministration of low-dose, systemic IL-2 or IFN-α in 116 patients with pulmonary or mediastinal metastatic renal cell carcinoma. The side effects were well tolerated, and the results were encouraging. The overall response rate was 16%; disease stabilized in 49% of patients for a median duration of 9.6 months.

In an effort to improve upon single-agent efficacy, many investigators have combined two or three drugs. Preclinical trials have demonstrated synergistic antitumor effects with IL-2 and IFN-α in combination. An accumulation of clinical data from 1,200 patients yielded a 20% objective response rate with IL-2 and IFN-α. A recent study comparing high dose IL-2 and IFN-α alone and in combination found a significantly higher rate of response and event-free survival in the combined therapy group, but no advantage was noted in long-term survival at 3 years. Other studies have found similar minimal effects. Low-dose, subcutaneous IL-2 in combination with INF-α showed an objective response rate of 15% to 25% with a median duration of 14 to 17 months.

Although chemotherapeutic agents have produced dismal results as single agents in advanced renal cell carcinoma, they have been combined with more efficacious immunotherapeutic agents. IFN-α combined with 5-fluorouracil (5-FU) in a small series showed a 43% objective response with a mean duration of response of 25 months. However, others have not found this combination as effective as other existing regimens. Low-dose IL-2, IFN-α, and 5-FU produced objective response rates of 39% to 47% with median durations of 11 to 15 months in some reports. Other ongoing investigations include *cis*-retinoic acid and vinblastine in addition to IL-2 and IFN-α.

Adoptive immunotherapy involves infusing lymphocytes with antitumor activity into the patient, often in combination with biologic response modifiers. TILs are isolated from the primary tumor, enhanced with IL-2 or IL-12 *in vitro* and then reinfused. High-dose IL-2 treatment with LAK cells produced a 15% to 18% objective response but also generated constitutional side effects with significant renal and cardiopulmonary toxicities. One clinical trial has demonstrated that low-dose, systemic IL-2 plus CD8+ TILs, followed by nephrectomy results in a 9% complete and a 25% partial response rate with a median duration of 14 months. Infusion of TILs, IL-2, and INF has created a high durable response rate (33%).

Gene therapy for renal cell carcinoma continues to advance rapidly due to the advances in immunotherapy and the advances in the genetic understanding of this disease. Even though the VHL gene abnormalities are only present in approximately 60% of sporadic cases of renal cell carcinoma, they have been targets for gene therapy. Some investigators replaced the defective oncogene product with normal VHL protein in malignant cells, thus inhibiting tumor cell growth *in vitro*.

Monoclonal antibodies can be used either diagnostically or therapeutically in renal cell carcinoma. The antibodies bind to tumor specific antigens and thus can deliver a cytotoxic agent directly to the lesion. A tumor-specific antigen, G250, has been identified and is approximately 90% specific to renal cells. An antibody to this antigen has been used in radionucleotide scanning in the hopes of finding tumor deposits that conventional imaging may miss. The antibody has also been labeled with I-131 to produce a local cytotoxic radiation effect with varying results.

Tumor vaccines are also a developing treatment modality for advanced renal cell carcinoma. Tumor cells are harvested from the patient and transfected with cytokine genes such as IL-2. The cells' immunogenicity is enhanced by the addition of other cytokines *in vitro* and gamma irradiation removes their ability to replicate. The cells are then reinfused into the patient in the hope that their presence will initiate an immune response against the remaining tumor. The cytokine production induces a significant inflammatory response in the tumor itself that avoids systemic toxicity. This approach has been used in patients with metastatic renal cell carcinoma using a variety of transfected genes: TNF-α, IL-2, IL-4, IL-7, granulocyte-macrophage colony–stimulating factor (GM-CSF), IFN-α, and HLA-B7. Improvements in gene therapy technology have allowed scientists to bypass the expensive and time-consuming manipulation of tumor cells in culture. Cytokine genes can now be directly injected into the primary or the metastatic tumors, producing local immune responses.

Cytoreductive surgery refers to radical nephrectomy with removal of metastatic lesions in conjunction with immunotherapy, such as IL-2. There is substantial controversy regarding the timing of the nephrectomy. Surgery before immunotherapy removes the potentially immunosuppressive tumor burden and provides fewer cells to treat. Data supporting this therapeutic sequence show that responses to IL-2 in the renal primary have been rare and immunotherapy may work better with a lower tumor burden. However, the significant morbidity secondary to cytoreductive surgery may preclude subsequent immunotherapy in 44% to 77%. Operative mortality in this patient population has been reported to range from 3% to 11%. Another disadvantage with this approach includes growth of metastatic disease during the recovery period, also eliminating immunotherapy in 11% to 23% of patients. One study evaluated 66 carefully chosen patients with excellent performance statuses and minimally advanced metastatic renal cell carcinoma who underwent cytoreductive surgery followed by systemic biologic therapy. Eighty-two percent received immunotherapy at a median of 40 days postoperatively. Although survival was not an endpoint, in a select population this therapeutic sequence may be feasible. A large trial that did record survival found that nephrectomy 6 months before IL-2 therapy and nephrectomy followed by TILs/IL-2/IFN-α was associated with a greater survival benefit than the group without surgery. Until a randomized, multicenter study is undertaken, debates will continue about which therapy is administered first.

Sarcomas

Sarcomas represent 1% to 2% of malignant renal tumors and increase in incidence with advanced age. The most common signs and symptoms are similar to those of renal cell carcinoma: flank pain, flank mass, and hematuria. CT imaging may show a soft-tissue density originating from the renal capsule or the renal sinus. The presence of fat or bone densities on CT would suggest a liposarcoma or osteosarcoma. Leiomyosarcomas are the most common sarcomas, followed by liposarcomas, malignant fibrous histiocytomas, osteogenic sarcomas, and rhabdomyosarcoma of the adult. Treatment consists of radical surgical extirpation, however prognosis is poor with surgery alone. Adjuvant therapy with chemotherapy may offer some benefit, and radiotherapy does not improve the less than 10% 5-year survival for these patients.

SECONDARY TUMORS OF THE KIDNEY

The kidney receives approximately 25% of the blood flow and is therefore a common site of metastatic tumor deposits. In fact, the incidence of secondary tumors is greater than that of primary renal tumors. Most of these lesions are not clinically evident and are often found at autopsy. Typically the metastatic lesions are small, bilateral, and multiple. Lymphomas and leukemias are the most common secondary malignancies to affect the kidney. Lung carcinoma is the most common solid tumor to metastasize to the kidney, but virtually every other solid neoplasm has been reported as well. It has been estimated that approximately 19,000 patients annually may harbor lung metastases in the kidneys. There are no specific radiologic findings that reliably differentiate secondary from primary lesions and most, if large enough, can be diagnosed by CT-guided biopsy.

Selected Readings

Belldegrun A, deKernion JB. Renal tumors. In: Walsh PC, Retik AB, Vaughan ED, et al., eds. *Campbell's urology,* 7th ed. Philadelphia: WB Saunders Co., 1998:2283–2421.

This chapter is an invaluable resource for information on both benign and malignant tumors of the kidney.

Curry NS, Bissada NK. Radiologic evaluation of small and indeterminate renal masses. *Urol Clin North Am* 1997:24(3):493–505.

A review of the frequently discovered incidental renal mass and the numerous radiologic options for further characterizing the tumor preoperatively.

Doublet J, Peraldi M, Gattegno B, et al. Renal cell carcinoma of native kidneys: prospective study of 129 renal transplant patients. *J Urol* 1997;158:42–44.

Renal transplant recipients were evaluated with renal ultrasound of the native kidneys. The risk of renal cell carcinoma was significantly greater in the transplant population, but no risk factors could be identified.

Hatcher PA, Anderson EE, Paulson DF, et al. Surgical management and prognosis of renal cell carcinoma invading the vena cava. *J Urol* 1991;145:20–25.

The authors describe a single group of patients with renal cell carcinoma and vena caval tumor thrombosis who underwent surgical resection. Prognosis was determined by the pathologic stage of the tumor and the presence or absence of vena caval invasion by the thrombus, not by the level of tumor thrombus extension.

Levy DA, Slaton JW, Swanson DA, et al. Stage specific guidelines for surveillance after radical nephrectomy for local renal cell carcinoma. *J Urol* 1998;159: 1163–1167.

A large number of patients with renal cell carcinoma treated by radical nephrectomy was evaluated for the pattern of recurrence. The risk of metastatic renal cell carcinoma was found to be stage dependent. The authors recommend tailoring the surveillance protocols to the pathologic stage of the primary tumor.

Levy DA, Swanson DA, Slaton JW, et al. Timely delivery of biological therapy after cytoreductive nephrectomy in carefully selected patients with metastatic renal cell carcinoma. *J Urol* 1998;159:1168–1173.

The majority of these carefully selected patients with metastatic renal cell carcinoma who underwent cytoreductive nephrectomy were able to receive systemic biologic therapy.

Lieber MM. Renal oncocytoma. *Urol Clin North Am* 1993;20:355.

This review describes the origin, chromosomal abnormalities, natural history, and diagnostic dilemmas associated with renal oncocytomas.

Linehan WM, Lerman MI, Zbar B. Identification of the von Hippel-Lindau (VHL) gene: its role in renal cancer. *JAMA* 1995;273(7):564–570.

The seminal work by the NCI describing the gene responsible for both sporadic and inherited renal cell carcinoma.

Mulders P, Figlin R, deKernion JB, et al. Renal cell carcinoma: recent progress and future directions. *Cancer Res* 1997;57:5189–5195.

A review describing each modern option for treating metastatic renal cell carcinoma and the attendant risks and benefits.

Naitoh J, Belldegrun A. Gene therapy—the future is here: a guide to the practicing urologist. *Urology* 1998;51(3):367–380.

A review of the most current techniques and ongoing studies involving gene therapy as they pertain to the genitourinary system.

Novick AC, Nephron-sparing surgery for renal cell carcinoma. *Br J Urol* 1998;82:321–324.

Nephron-sparing surgery in patients with localized unilateral renal cell carcinoma and a normal contralateral kidney is increasingly accepted as a therapeutic option. Radical nephrectomy and partial nephrectomy provided equally effective curative treatment for patients with a single, small renal cell carcinoma.

Pea M, Bonetti F, Martignoni G, et al. Apparent renal cell carcinomas in tuberous sclerosis are heterogeneous: the identification of malignant epithelioid angiomyolipoma. *Am J Surg Pathol* 1998;22(2):180–187.

A recently described variant of angiomyolipoma, which contains epithelioid smooth muscle cells, can closely simulate both carcinoma and sarcoma, histologically and prognostically. In the past, patients with tuberous sclerosis and angiomyolipomas have been reported to contain synchronous renal cell carcinoma. However, some of these cases may actually be the aforementioned malignant subtype of angiomyolipoma.

Srigley JR, Hutter RVP, Gelb AB, et al. Current prognostic factors—renal cell carcinoma. *Cancer* 1997;80(5):994–996.

The Union Internationale Contre le Cancer (UICC) and the American Joint Committee on Cancer (AJCC) have divided prognostic factors into patient-related, tumor-related, and therapy-related factors. The major patient-related prognostic factors include poor performance status, symptomatic presentation, weight loss, and elevated erythrocyte sedimentation rate.

Steiner MS, Goldman SM, Fishman EK, et al. The natural history of renal angiomyolipoma. *J Urol* 1993;150:1782–1786.

The authors studied a group of patients with angiomyolipoma and found that tumors greater than 4 cm were frequently symptomatic and required surgery. Patients with tuberous sclerosis presented at a younger age and had larger tumors that frequently required surgical intervention.

Zbar B, Tory K, Merino M, et al. Hereditary papillary renal cell carcinoma. *J Urol* 1994;151:561–566.

The authors describe a three-generation family affected with papillary renal carcinoma. The tumors were not linked to chromosome 3p, suggesting the presence of a renal cell carcinoma gene different than previously described.

PART 2
Neoplastic Disease of the Pelvis, Ureter, Bladder, and Urethra

Robert C. Flanigan and Fernando J. Kim

The purpose of this chapter is to review the current concepts of epidemiology, pathology, natural history, methods of diagnosis, staging, and approaches to treatment of urothelial cancer, including those tumors that arise in the upper urinary tract and the urinary bladder.

INCIDENCE AND MORTALITY RATES

In 2000, newly diagnosed bladder cancer will account for approximately 53,200 cases in the United States. Of these, 38,300 will involve males and 14,900 will involve females. Upper tract urothelial cancers are much less common, but still affect a significant number of persons. Transitional cell carcinoma (TCC) of the urinary tract is three to four times more common among men than women, and accounts for 10% of cancers among men and only 3% of cancers among women. TCC of the bladder occurs with approximately twice the incidence (cases per 100,000 person-years) among whites as compared with African-Americans (31.5 versus 16.2 when comparing white men with African-American men, and 7.8 versus 5.0 when comparing white women with African-American women). This apparent difference in incidence between white and African-American people in the United States may be explained by variables in diagnosis and reporting as suggested by studies that have shown that the increased risk in whites is limited to patients with noninvasive tumors and that among patients with muscle-invasive tumors, whites were actually at a slightly reduced risk compared with African-Americans. Mortality rates from bladder cancer (deaths per 100,000 person-years) are similar for African-Americans and whites (white men 6.0, African-American men 4.2, white women 1.7, African-American women 2.5), also suggesting that the differences in incidence may reflect variable diagnosis and reporting. Geographic distribution in the United States has been correlated with mortality rates from bladder cancer. Cigarette smokers, phenacetin usage, chronic infection or irritation, cyclophosphamide usage, living in urban areas, and other factors are associated with a higher risk of development of urothelial cancer (Table 54.1).

PATHOLOGY

Normal Urothelium

The normal bladder urothelium is composed of three to seven layers of transitional cells with large umbrella cells overlapping the cells of the intermediate cell layers that in turn rest on a basal cell layer. Below the epithelium lies the lamina propria and submucosal layer. The submucosal layer contains the muscularis mucosa and multiple vascular spaces. Below the submucosal layer lies the detrusor muscle. Tumor involvement of the muscularis mucosa must be distinguished from involvement of deep muscle (detrusor) on pathologic specimen in order to accurately stage bladder neoplasms.

A similar anatomic arrangement of layers is present in the upper urinary tract with the exception of the markedly reduced deep muscle mass. This diminished barrier to tumor extension explains the ready access of tumor to the paraureteral space.

Abnormalities of the Urothelial Layer

Abnormalities of the urothelial layer can range from hyperplasia to carcinoma. Hyperplasia may be further subdivided into epithelial hyperplasia, inverted papilloma, von Brunn's nests, and cystitis cystica.

Metaplasia

Metaplastic lesions of the urothelium include cystitis glandularis (believed to be a precursor of urothelial adenocarcinoma), nephrogenic adenoma, and squamous metaplasia.

TABLE 54.1. Other Etiologies of Urothelial Cancer

Etiologic Factor	Relative Incidence of Cancer
Cigarette smoking	30%–40% of bladder cancer may be related.
Occupational exposure	30%–35% of bladder cancer may be related to exposure to industrial chemicals.
Analgesic (phenacetin) usage	Increased risk (2.6–4.9 times normal), latency period 15–20 years.
Chronic infection/inflammation	Related to chronic catheterization or stones (typically squamous cell cancers); spinal cord patients' risk is 16–20 times normal.
Cyclophosphamide usage	Nine-fold risk; latency period short (6–13 years) due to metabolite acrolein, reduced by new protective agents, such as Mesna.
Regional differences	30%–50% higher in northern regions of the United States as compared with southern regions.
Age	Bladder cancer is uncommon in patients <50 years old and tends to be present with a more differentiated histology in younger patients.
Artificial sweeteners (saccharine, cyclamates)	These compounds have been shown in large doses to induce bladder cancers in rodents; case-controlled epidemiologic studies reveal little significant evidence of association in humans.
Pelvic irradiation	Ionizing radiation for carcinoma of the cervix has been associated with a 2- to 4-fold increase in the development of TCC of the bladder; careful epidemiologic studies have not clearly established this relationship.
Heredity	May occur in familial clusters; genetic differences in hepatic arylamine acetyltransferase may play a role (slow acetylators more susceptible to bladder tumors than fast acetylators).

TCC, transitional cell carcinoma.

Dysplasia

Dysplasia of the bladder may take the form of atypical hyperplasia, mild atypia, moderate atypia, or severe atypia. In addition, leukoplakia of the bladder may occur. Dysplastic urothelium exhibits histologic changes that are intermediate between normal urothelium and carcinoma *in situ*. It is generally felt that lesions on the severe end of this spectrum are neoplastic rather than dysplastic.

Superficial Carcinomas

Superficial carcinomas of the bladder urothelium include carcinoma *in situ* and cancers involving the epithelium and submucosal layers. Histologically, these cancers are either transitional cell, squamous, or adenocarcinomas.

Carcinoma *In Situ*

Histologically, carcinoma *in situ* is characterized by a poorly differentiated cancer involving only the urothelium. A loss of cellular cohesiveness, widening of the intracellular spaces, separation of cells from the basement membrane, and a loss of the superficial umbrella cell layer is characteristic. Carcinoma *in situ* may occur focally or diffusely within the urothelium. It is often associated with high-grade and high-stage transitional cell cancers. Although carcinoma *in situ* may occur in the absence of visible bladder tumor, its association with either a concurrent or prior bladder tumor significantly increases the risk of progression to muscle invasion of a non–muscle-invasive (superficial) TCC. In patients having a concurrent tumor, the presence of carcinoma *in situ* is associated with an approximately 80% likelihood of cancer progression to muscle invasion. Likewise, in a patient with a prior history of bladder cancer, the presence of carcinoma *in situ* is associated with an approximately 40% risk of progression.

The cystoscopic appearance of carcinoma *in situ* is often misleading in that a normal-appearing epithelium is the most common finding. A reddened or velvety patch of erythematous mucosa should, however, suggest the possibility of carcinoma *in situ*. Carcinoma *in situ*, like papillary urothelial cancer, is more common in men than in women. Because carcinoma *in situ* frequently presents with irritative voiding symptoms, the patient is often misdiagnosed as suffering from prostatism, urinary tract infection, or neuropathic bladder dysfunction. Cytopathologic studies of urine or bladder exfoliative bladder specimens are positive in 85% to 90% of patients with carcinoma *in situ*.

The natural history of carcinoma *in situ* is unpredictable. Early in its evolution, carcinoma *in situ* may produce no symptoms, and, in fact, patients with focal asymptomatic carcinoma *in situ* have been reported to generally display a protracted clinical course with a low likelihood of development of invasive bladder. In contrast, patients with diffuse or symptomatic carcinoma *in situ*, especially in association with a history of bladder cancer, often display a poor prognosis despite definitive therapy. Approximately 20% of patients, for example, who undergo cystectomy for diffuse carcinoma *in situ* are found to have microscopic evidence of muscle invasion.

Papillary Transitional Cell Carcinoma

More that 99% of bladder tumors are carcinomas. TCC represents approximately 90% of these tumors. TCC is generally graded on a scale of 1 to 3 (some systems grade from 1 to 4). Grade 1 TCCs differ from normal epithelium by having an increased number of epithelial cell layers. With increasing grade, abnormalities of nuclear morphology, loss of cellular polarity, abnormalities of the normal cellular maturation from the basal to superficial layers, nuclear crowding, and increased nuclear-to-cytoplasmic ratio are seen. In addition, prominent nucleoli with clumping of the chromatin and an increased number of mitoses may be appreciated.

Non–Transitional Cell Carcinomas (Squamous Cell Carcinoma, Adenocarcinoma)

In the United States, squamous cell carcinomas account for approximately 3% to 7% of bladder cancers. These tumors are commonly associated with a chronic inflammatory process involving the urothelium, including the presence of a chronic foreign body (e.g., an indwelling catheter, urinary tract calculi, or recurrent urinary tract infections). Generally, a greater proportion of patients with squamous cell carcinoma, as compared with TCC, present with advanced disease at the time of diagnosis. Stage for stage, however, the prognosis of patients with squamous cell carcinoma is comparable with that of patients with TCC.

Adenocarcinoma of the bladder is a rare lesion accounting for less than 2% of all bladder cancers. These highly invasive tumors do not typically present as superficial lesions. Primary adenocarcinomas can occur anywhere within the bladder and are believed to occur in response to chronic inflammation. Risk factors include bladder exstrophy, schistosomiasis, and perhaps coffee drinking. Histologically, adenocarcinomas may be varied in appearance, including signet ring and colloid carcinomas. Most are mucin producing. Adenocarcinomas are usually poorly differentiated and muscle invasive.

Adenocarcinomas arising in the urachus represent the most common type of cancer arising in this structure. Generally, these tumors arise outside the bladder and invade through the urothelium with extension into the bladder. These tumors are typically mucin producing and advanced at the time of presentation. The prognosis of urachal adenocarcinomas is worse than for primary bladder adenocarcinoma. Unexpectedly wide and deep infiltration of tumor is not uncommon on histologic examination of the surgical specimen. For this reason, partial cystectomy has been associated with local recurrence rates of 15% to 50%. Therefore the recommended treatment for all but the smallest, most well-differentiated tumors is radical cystectomy and bilateral pelvic lymphadenectomy with *en bloc* excision of the urachus. Radiation therapy is not effective in treating this lesion.

NATURAL HISTORY

TCCs are a heterogeneous group of tumors that exhibit a broad spectrum of biologic potential. Although only 10% to 15% of patients with well-differentiated superficial tumors progress to muscle invasion, invasion rates as high as 45% to 50% have been reported for high-grade lesions involving the submucosal layer.

Numerous chromosomal abnormalities have been found to be associated with the development of TCC; including chromosome 9 loss, c-*myc* amplification, Y chromosome loss, and p53, p21, and erbB-2 abnormalities. Of these, chromosome 9 loss and p53 abnormalities may be the most important. Loss of heterozygosity of chromosome 9 seems to be an early event associated with the formation of papillary tumors, whereas p53 gene deletion seems to be associated with the formation of dysplasias and carcinoma *in situ*. By the time a TCC invades the lamina propria, both of these genetic events have typically occurred. Chromosome 9 deletion is felt to result in a homozygous deletion of the MTS-1 gene (a tumor-suppressor gene), and is a frequent event in TCC but not a driving force in tumor progression. P53 is a tumor-suppressor gene located at 17p13.1, which codes for a DNA-binding protein involved in the regulation of transcription. Deletion of this gene results in an overexpression of the p53 protein (missense mutation), leading to an extension of the half-life of the protein. P53 and another transcription-mediating gene, p21, are associated with progression of TCC.

Recurrence

Approximately 70% of patients with superficial TCC will display recurrence of tumor if treated by endoscopic resection alone. Factors associated with increased risk of recurrence are shown in Table 54.2. It is believed that most recurrences are new tumors that arise in other areas of dysplastic epithelium. Some recurrences, however, undoubtedly result from inadequate treatment of preexisting tumors or from tumor cell implantation. Grade seems to be an important indicator of recurrence. Seventy-five percent of patients with grade 1 tumors are likely to be disease free at 12 months, compared with only 55% of patients with grade 3 tumors. Tumor grade is also associated with signs of urothelial abnormalities at other sites in the bladder. For example, one series showed significant distant urothelial abnormalities in association with 15% of grade 1 tumors, 59% of grade 2, and 77% of grade 3. The prevention of tumor recurrence is a major goal in the therapy of TCC.

TABLE 54.2. Factors Influencing Time to Recurrence of Superficial Transitional Cell Carcinomas

Number of visible tumors
Previous recurrence
Stage
Grade
Presence of dysplasia/hyperplasia in random biopsies
Size of largest tumor
DNA ploidy

TABLE 54.3. Risk Factors for Muscle Invasion

Stage
Grade
Carcinoma *in situ*
Chromosome analysis
DNA ploidy
p53
ABO (H) blood group

Progression to Muscle Invasion

Approximately 10% to 15% of patients presenting with superficial TCC can be expected to progress to muscle invasion. Patients with high-grade tumors invading the lamina propria, however, may display progression rates as high as 45% to 50%. Factors associated with an increased risk of muscle invasion progression are shown in Table 54.3. Reports indicate death rates at 3 years for superficial TCC of 3% for patients with grade 1 stage cancers as compared with 43% of patients with grade 3 stage lesions. Moreover, further additional studies subdivided patients with TCC by tumor stage and grade and demonstrated an increased mortality rate with increasing stage and grade of superficial TCC. In fact, once a tumor has demonstrated its aggressiveness by invasion of the lamina propria, it has already expressed its ability to metastasize. A 20% incidence of lymphatic involvement by tumors involving only the lamina propria was reported. Undifferentiated tumors are also more likely to shed cells into lymphatics and blood vessels, thereby increasing the likelihood of metastases.

Carcinoma *In Situ*

Carcinoma *in situ* of the bladder occupies a controversial area in the spectrum of bladder cancers. Patients with focal asymptomatic carcinoma *in situ* may have a relatively good prognosis, whereas patients with diffuse carcinoma *in situ*, as stated previously, often display microscopic invasion at the time of cystectomy and are at high risk for the subsequent development of muscle-invasive cancers if cystectomy is not undertaken.

Tumor Markers

Several markers are felt to be associated with an increased risk of progression to muscle invasion in patients with superficial urothelial tumors. Cellular differentiation is an important predictor of progression as described previously. In one study, for example, 19% of grade 1 superficial tumors progressed to muscle invasion as compared with 69% of grade 3 tumors.

The presence or absence of blood-group antigens on the surface epithelium has also been correlated with subsequent muscle invasion. Thus the presence of blood-group antigens in a low-grade urothelial cancer is associated with a very low likelihood of progression (3% to 5%). In contrast, the absence of blood-group antigens is associated with a 65% chance of progression.

P53 abnormalities (as described previously) are associated with progression of TCC. P53 is also closely associated with p21 in that p53 appears to mediate transcription via p21. P21 inhibits cyclin-dependent kinase (PCNA). In addition, there are p53 independent pathways that regulate p21. The University of Southern California group has demonstrated that survival of patients with muscle-invasive TCC who have p53 alterations but are wild type for p21 have a similar survival to those patients with wild-type p53.

The natural history and molecular biology of squamous cell and adenocarcinomas of the urothelium are less well understood than that of TCC. Squamous cell carcinoma is an invasive lesion with a nodular infiltrative growth pattern. It is postulated that the nitrosamines produced by bacteria in infected urine act as carcinogens and tumor promoters. Squamous cell carcinomas also occur in association with *Schistosoma haematobium* infections, presumably secondary to chronic inflammation of the bladder. Adenocarcinomas of the bladder occur in association with a retained urachal remnant or less frequently as a primary lesion of the bladder itself. Many primary adenocarcinomas are muscle invasive or metastatic at the time of presentation, whereas urachal adenocarcinomas are almost always associated with muscle invasion but are generally late to metastasize.

DIAGNOSIS

Signs and Symptoms

Hematuria is the most common presenting symptom of urothelial cancer, occurring in 85% of patients with bladder cancer. There is no correlation between the size or stage of the tumor and the degree of hematuria seen. The next most common symptom is vesical irritability including urinary frequency, urgency, and dysuria. This latter symptom complex is frequently associated with diffuse carcinoma *in situ*. Patients with hematuria and/or vesical irritability that cannot be explained on the basis of a documented urinary tract infection and does not resolve after treatment of this urinary tract infection *must* be investigated with excretory urography and cystoscopic examination. In addition, urinary cytologies including bladder wash cytologies are indicated. The mean duration of symptoms before diagnosis of tumor is typically between 3 and 8 months.

Patients presenting with ureteral obstruction and flank pain are often found on histologic evaluation to have a muscle-invasive bladder cancer. However, superficial urothelial cancers of the upper urinary tract may cause obstruction of the kidney without being associated with underlying muscle invasion.

Upper tract cancers present with hematuria in 50% to 67% of patients. Other presenting signs and symptoms are flank pain and abdominal pain (20% to 40%), and, less commonly, an abdominal mass or hydronephrosis. Frequency, dysuria, and weight loss may occur.

Excretory Urography

Excretory urography (intravenous pyelography [IVP]) is an essential facet of the evaluation of patients with presumed urothelial carcinoma whether presenting with hematuria, vesical irritability, or other symptoms. It is important to completely identify the entire upper urinary tract on the excretory urogram. Although large bladder tumors may be visualized as filling defects within the bladder or an irregularity of the bladder contour on the cystogram phase of the urogram, the excretory urogram is not an adequate test of bladder carcinoma.

Cystoscopy, Biopsy, and Transurethral Resection

Cystoscopy

Cystoscopy remains a mainstay in the diagnosis of TCC of the bladder. It is critical at the time of cystoscopic examination to identify any abnormalities involving the bladder and to map them carefully for future reference. Lesions should be identified as papillary, sessile, or nodular. Any slightly raised, velvety, or erythematous areas must be biopsied because they may portend carcinoma *in situ*. At the time of cystoscopy, bimanual examination of the bladder should be performed in patients with suspected carcinoma.

Bladder Biopsy

Biopsy of any and all abnormal areas of the bladder should be accomplished using either a cold-cup biopsy forcep (with subsequent fulguration) or a transurethral resectoscope. Small lesions are more amenable to cold-cup biopsy, so that coagulation artifact can be avoided. It is critical in any biopsy of the bladder lesion to ensure the presence of the underlying musculature within the biopsy specimen so that accurate staging of the bladder tumor is possible.

In the presence of a documented bladder tumor, selected random cold-cup mucosal biopsies from areas adjacent to the tumor, as well as the opposite bladder wall, dome, trigone, and prostatic urethra, may be indicated. The rationale for obtaining random bladder biopsies is that they provide information of significant importance regarding the likelihood of tumor recurrence, especially in patients with intermediate risk tumors. These biopsies may be shown to reveal dysplasia in approximately 25% of patients with carcinoma *in situ* and approximately 20% of patients with superficial bladder cancers. However, some investigators believe that random bladder biopsies are unnecessary, and, in fact, may be hazardous because they denude the overlying urothelium and create potential areas for tumor cell implantation. These authors generally suggest that urinary cytology is a better indicator of the presence of concurrent carcinoma *in situ* than are selected random bladder biopsies.

When superficial tumors are seen to arise in or around the area of the ureteral orifice, one must suspect the possibility of seeding of tumor from the upper urinary tract. In this case, careful excretory urography and/or retrograde urography and ureteroscopy may be necessary to identify these upper tract lesions. If the tumor occurs at the site of the ureteral orifice, resection of the tumor can be accomplished with resection of a part of the underlying ureteral submucosal tunnel. This may give rise to ureteral reflux, but if the resection is performed using a cutting current, ureteral obstruction is less likely than when extensive cauterization is performed around the ureteral orifice. If upper tract evaluation is required in a patient with a tumor at or near a ureteral orifice, it is preferable to complete the resection of the tumor before performing necessary upper tract studies in an effort to decrease the rate of implantation of tumor into the upper urinary tract. Placement of a ureteral catheter and/or guidewire before resection may, however, be helpful to allow for subsequent adequate upper tract drainage by ureteral catheterization and/or inspection of the upper urinary tract radiographically or ureteroscopically.

Because of the thin underlying muscular layer, tumors arising within a bladder diverticulum should generally be staged by cold-cup biopsy and not by transurethral resection, which is more likely to lead to perforation. In addition, these tumors are typically best treated by partial or total cystectomy rather than by transurethral resection.

Resection of tumors on the lateral bladder wall may be difficult because of stimulation of the obturator nerve. This stimulation results in contraction of the adductor muscles of the thigh. If this problem is noted, resection of the area should be performed with the patient under general anesthesia while employing intravenous muscle relaxation (pancuronium) to minimize the risk of inadvertent bladder perforation.

After resection of the bladder tumor, a urethral catheter should be left in place for some time. Although there is great controversy regarding this interval, the duration should be varied depending on the operator's impression of the depth of resection. In general, a urethral catheter is left in place for approximately 1 to 2 days if superficial muscle has been resected and for 3 to 5 days if the resection has been deep or inadvertently carried through the entire bladder thickness. If continuous bladder irrigation is felt to be necessary because of bleeding after resection of the bladder tumor, care must be taken to ensure that overdistention of the bladder does not occur secondary to occlusion of the urethral catheter because this may result in perforation of the bladder.

Evaluation of the Upper Urinary Tracts

As mentioned previously, the mainstay for the evaluation of the upper urinary tract in patients with urothelial cancer is excretory urography. If excretory urography does not evaluate the entire upper urinary tract, retrograde ureterography should be accomplished at the time of cystoscopic examination.

In cases in which retrograde urography does not supply information regarding a potential filling defect, or in cases of known urothelial cancer, ureteroscopy may be indicated. This can be accomplished using a flexible and/or rigid urethroscope. Biopsy, either cytologic or histologic cold cup, should be obtained of any abnormal lesions seen during ureteroscopy.

Brush biopsies for cytologic evaluation of potential upper tract lesions should be accomplished under fluoroscopic control whenever possible. This minimizes the risk of perforation of the upper urinary tract that may occur during blind manipulation of the brush biopsy catheter.

Urinary Cytology

Urinary cytology is a useful technique for identifying malignant cells that are exfoliated into the urine or that are obtained by washing with normal saline from the upper or lower urinary tract. Malignant transitional cells have enlarged nuclei with irregular, coarsely textured chromatin. Cytologic identification of these tumors is easier in patients with poorly differentiated cancers than well-differentiated tumors that are cytologically normal in appearance, more cohesive, and not readily shed into the urine. Thus low-grade papillary tumors most often display a negative cytology, whereas 50% of grade 2 and the majority of grade 3 tumors are associated with a positive cytology. On the other hand, urinary cytology, even in the face of high-grade tumors, may be falsely negative in 20% of cases.

Flow Cytometry

Flow cytometry and imaging analysis are techniques that allow for the identification of the DNA content of the urothelial cells. Most superficial low-grade tumors are diploid, thus leading to false-negative results. This problem is further complicated by the presence of inflammatory cells and other cellular debris within the urinary specimen that may make the identification of small populations of aneuploid tumor cells difficult. In contrast, aneuploidy is common in high-grade lesions. Flow cytometry is capable of detecting carcinoma *in situ* with an accuracy of more than 90%.

TABLE 54.4. Tumor Markers

Marker	Characteristics
Cytology	30%–60% sensitive
Flow cytometry	70% sensitive (89% if either positive cytology or positive flow cytometry used together)
Bladder tumor Ag	65% sensitive; high false-positive rate with inflammation
Nuclear matrix protein	70% positive in post-TURBT patients who recur, near 100% positive in T2 disease
Fibrin-degradation products	70% sensitive; nearly 100% positive in muscle-invasive disease

Other Tumor Markers

A great deal of investigation has occurred in the last decade with the goal of enhancing tumor detection using exfoliated urinary specimens. Although a thorough discussion of this area is beyond the scope of this chapter, the reader should be aware of these markers and their potential use in clinical practice (Table 54.4). In a recent head-on-head trial of four of the markers (NMP-22, BTA, telomerase TRAP assay, and cytology), the NMP-22 and TRAP assays appeared to perform better in both clinical stage Ta and T1 or greater tumors (approximately 80% overall sensitivity compared with approximately 40% for BTA and cytology).

STAGING

An accurate staging of urothelial cancers is critical to the development of a carefully planned therapeutic approach to these tumors. The mainstay of staging is a thorough biopsy of the identified lesions, including resection of underlying bladder muscle. Computed tomography (CT) scanning, ultrasound, and magnetic resonance imaging (MRI) may also be used to evaluate the local extent of bladder tumors, although all of these studies provide limited accuracy in determining the presence or absence of microscopic muscle invasion or minimal extravesical tumor spread. Furthermore, postoperative changes induced by transurethral resection and/or other therapies, including radiation and chemotherapy, may make interpretation of these studies extremely difficult.

In general, if adequate histologic biopsies identify a superficial urothelial cancer, CT scanning will probably provide limited useful clinical information. The major usefulness of CT scanning would be to detect regional lymph nodes. It is important to recognize that enlarged lymph nodes do not always indicate the presence of metastases and that CT scans have failed to detect lymph node metastasis in 40% to 75% of node-positive patients in some studies.

The American Joint Committee on Cancer (AJCC)–Union Internationale Contre le Cancer (UICC) classification is subdivided into clinical and pathologic stages (Table 54.5). Clinical staging is referred to as the *T stage* and pathologic staging as the *P stage.* Clinical carcinoma *in situ* is stage Tis, noninvasive papillary tumors involving only the urothelium is stage Ta, and tumor with lamina propria invasion is stage T1. The pathologic counterparts in this system are identical.

TABLE 54.5. Staging Systems of Urothelial Cancer

Stage Description	AJCC-UICC Clinical	AJCC-UICC Pathologic
Carcinoma *in situ*	Tis	Pis
Papillary tumor—no invasion	Ta	Pa
Papillary tumor—lamina propria invasion	T1	P1
Superficial	T2	P2
Deep muscle invasion		
Invasion of perivesical fat	T3	T3
Invasion of contiguous viscera	T4	P4
Involvement of pelvic nodes		N1–3
Involvement of juxtaregional nodes		N4
Distant metastases		M1

AJCC, American Joint Committee on Cancer; UICC, Union Internationale Contre le Cancer.

MANAGEMENT OF SUPERFICIAL UPPER URINARY TRACT CANCERS (TIS, TA, AND T1)

Urothelial lesions of the upper urinary tract may or may not occur in association with synchronous or metachronous urothelial carcinoma of the bladder. Upper urinary tract cancers are most frequently TCCs. Upper tract urothelial lesions occur in association with prior bladder cancer in only 2% to 5% of patients, whereas patients with an initial upper tract lesion develop tumors in the bladder in 50% to 75% of cases. These data imply that urothelial cancer is a field disease. Approximately 80% of renal pelvic transitional cell tumors are papillary and grade 1 or 2. High-grade lesions are therefore infrequent but are associated with rapid invasion and a poor prognosis. Because of the relatively thin ureteral muscle layer (as compared with bladder), tumor penetration results in a higher stage of disease more quickly.

The diagnosis of upper urinary tract cancers relies on the evaluation of the upper urinary tract as previously discussed. Although microscopic or gross hematuria occurs in 50% to 67% of patients with upper urinary tract cancers, up to 15% of the patients are asymptomatic and the diagnosis is established serendipitously as a result of studies initiated for other reasons. Flank pain occurs in 30% to 40% of patients and is usually a dull ache, although acute renal colic and the passage of long, thin clots indicative of upper tract bleeding may occur. A palpable flank mass is present in less than 15% of patients and usually indicates and extensive lesion.

Excretory urography reveals an abnormal filling defect suspicious for intrinsic lesion in 50% to 75% of patients with upper urinary tract cancers. A large variety of other lesions can produce similar filling defects including nonopaque calculi, blood clots, sloughed renal papillae, fungus balls, fibroepithelial polyps, hemangiomas, and extrinsic compression by renal vessels. Ultrasonography or CT scanning can be used to reliably distinguish a radiolucent stone from other causes of a filling defect. Indications for upper urinary tract endoscopy have been discussed previously. Percutaneous nephrostomy has also been advocated by some authors. However, as with other antegrade studies, the risk of tumor spillage contraindicates this approach except in highly selected patients.

TREATMENT OF UPPER TRACT CANCERS

To date, there have been no controlled, randomized series that have evaluated the optimum therapy for upper tract urothelial cancer. In particular, the treatment of cancers that do not invade the muscle or renal parenchyma can be approached in several different fashions, including ureteroscopic or nephroscopic biopsy and fulguration, segmental ureterectomy or pyelectomy, simple nephrectomy, and radical nephroureterectomy. Patients with low-grade, low-stage lesions may be appropriately treated by local therapies including endoscopic biopsy and fulguration and/or segmental resection of the lesion. If local therapy is employed, care must be taken to analyze the surrounding tissues and to assess the entire upper urinary tract carefully using all available modalities. Carcinoma *in situ* of the upper tract may occur in conjunction with a papillary urothelial cancer. If carcinoma *in situ* of the upper urinary tract is found in a patient with a low-grade, low-stage lesion, nephroureterectomy is generally preferable in a patient with a normal contralateral kidney.

In patients with high-grade lesions of the upper urinary tract, simple nephrectomy and subtotal ureterectomy results in a substantial local recurrence in the renal bed (30% to 40%) and distal ureteral stump (30% to 60%). These patients are therefore probably best treated by nephroureterectomy with removal of the associated bladder cuff in most patients. The role of formal retroperitoneal lymphadenectomy in this setting in undetermined. It would appear to be unnecessary in patients with low-stage, low-grade disease, and may be only of prognostic value in high-grade, high-stage lesions. With improvement in adjunctive therapy [i.e., methotrexate–vinblastine adriamycin–cisplatinum (MVAC) chemotherapy], the presence or absence of regional lymphatic metastases may direct the use of these therapies.

The standard surgical approaches to nephroureterectomy are a retroperitoneal flank incision plus a second low midline or Gibson incision, a single extended flank incision, or a single transperitoneal abdominal incision. The kidney, ureter, and bladder cuff should be delivered as a single unit whenever possible. The entire ureter, including the intramural portion, should be removed to prevent recurrence. The retention of a ureteral stump has been associated with an overall 20% likelihood of recurrence in the stump (30% to 60% for high-grade cancers).

Intravesical therapeutic agents will be discussed in detail later. These agents may play a role in the treatment of upper urinary tract urothelial cancers. Bacille Calmette-Guérin (BCG), mitomycin-C, and thiotepa may be given safely by a percutaneous route to patients with upper urinary tract cancers. In addition, reflux of an intravesical agent into the ureter may be possible in some patients where vesicoureteral reflux has occurred or when a ureteral stent is placed.

Prognosis of Upper Tract Cancers

The 5-year survival rate for all patients with transitional cell upper tract tumors approaches 50% to 60%. High-grade and high-stage tumors are associated with a poorer prognosis. In one series, grade 1 and 2 tumors had a 63% 5-year survival compared with a 13% survival for grade 3 and 4 lesions. Squamous cell cancers are associated with a dismal prognosis with few 5-year survivals.

MANAGEMENT OF SUPERFICIAL BLADDER CANCER (STAGES TIS, TA, AND T1)

Approximately 70% to 80% of bladder cancer patients have low-grade superficial tumors at the time of their initial presentation. The great majority of these patients can be treated adequately by simple transurethral resection or biopsy and fulguration. The overall 5-year survival rate of patients with superficial cancers treated with transurethral resection alone approaches 70%. Nonetheless, because of the high likelihood of recurrence of superficial bladder cancers (approximately 50% to 75%), many trials have been undertaken to define the efficacy of intravesical therapy, not only to destroy existing bladder cancer (definitive therapy) but also to reduce the recurrence rate (suppressive therapy).

It is important to recognize that this group of superficial cancers is a very heterogeneous group in terms of the likelihood that the patient will progress to muscle invasion, and in fact, succumb to their bladder cancer. For example, the patient with grade 1 Ta lesion (low-risk tumor), although prone to recurrence, has only approximately a 2% chance of progressing to muscle invasion. Similarly, patients with a grade 2 Ta lesion have only approximately a 6% chance of proceeding to muscle invasion. It is therefore possible to withhold intravesical therapy in this group of patients unless they present initially with four or more tumors or develop multiple, rapid recurrences of their cancer. On the other hand, high-risk tumors, including the unusual patient with a high-grade, low-stage cancer (grade 3, stage Ta) are very prone to progress to muscle invasion and should be treated with intravesical therapy at the time of initial presentation. Similarly, patients with invasion of the lamina propria are generally treated with intravesical therapy at initial presentation.

External beam irradiation therapy has not been proven effective in controlling superficial bladder cancer and does not prevent the recurrence of new lesions.

Most studies favor the use of intravesical therapy in patients with focal carcinoma *in situ,* especially if cytologies are not cleared after tumor resection.

Patients with diffuse or symptomatic carcinoma *in situ* should be treated with intravesical therapy at the time of initial presentation. Careful reassessment using endoscopically controlled biopsies and urinary cytologies is critical in this group of patients.

It would appear that BCG immunotherapy is superior to other intravesical therapies in the treatment of carcinoma *in situ*. Failures of intravesical therapy are common in this group and one must always remember the extremely high reported incidence of ureteral and prostatic urethral recurrence during intravesical therapy for carcinoma *in situ*. Therefore these areas of the urothelium must be carefully evaluated, including sequential prostatic urethral biopsies.

Studies have shown that the presence of a recurrent stage T1 TCC occurring at the 3-month cystoscopy after a single 6-week course of BCG therapy is an extremely poor prognostic sign that is associated with a high incidence of progression to muscle invasion and a high mortality rate. In this situation, early cystectomy may be beneficial. Other authors favor the use of a second 6-week course of BCG therapy.

One group analyzed the result of cystectomy for patients with high-grade, superficial bladder cancer. They reviewed 160 patients who underwent cystectomy and were found to have pathologic stage P_2 or less, including 11 patients with positive nodes. The survival rates at 95% confidence limits were 100% for stage $P_{0/a}$, 80% for stage P_1, and 76% for stage P_2. This study suggested that cystectomy is highly effective in curing patients with high-grade, superficial disease, including those with lymph node metastases. Others also reviewed a large experience with cystectomy in high-risk, non–muscle-invasive TCC patients. In 182 patients, pathologic upstaging occurred in 34% with metastases in 8% overall. The disease-specific survival in their study was: 94.2 (93.2%) at 2 years, 85.3 (83.6%) at 5 years, and 69.8 (74%) at 10 years.

Follow-Up of Non–Muscle-Invasive Tumors

An International Consensus Conference has offered the following guidelines for the follow-up of non–muscle-invasive tumors:

Low-risk tumors (unifocal Ta): Regular cystoscopy at 3 months and then at 6- to 12-month intervals for 3 years. If free of recurrence, follow-up cystoscopy, cytology, and/or ultrasonography is suggested yearly for 10 years.

High-risk tumors (Grade 3 Ta, any T1 multifocal or recurrent CIS, or tumor size more than 5 cm): After intravesical therapy, cystoscopy at 3-month intervals for 1 year, at 6-month intervals to year 5, and annually for the patient's lifetime. Upper tracts should be evaluated periodically (usually yearly).

Intermediate-risk tumors (all others): Cystoscopy at 3-month intervals for 1 year, every 6 months until year 3, and then annually for 10 years. Upper tract evaluation should be done in the case of recurrence in the bladder. Excretory urography is probably warranted every 1 to 2 years after initial treatment. Patients with reflux are at higher risk of upper tract recurrence and may be evaluated more frequently using voiding cystourethrography.

Despite the aforementioned recommendations, the frequency of upper tract surveillance after diagnosis of superficial bladder cancer remains debatable. A review revealed the development of upper tract disease in 4.8% of cases with a mean time to upper tract disease of 5.4 years.

Intravesical Therapy for Non–Muscle-Invasive Tumors

The use of intravesical therapy employing either chemotherapeutic agents or immunotherapeutic agents has arisen in response to the extremely common problem of recurrence in patients with superficial bladder cancer and the definite (10% to 15%) risk of progression to muscle invasion. Intravesical agents have been used as definitive therapy for the treatment of tumor left in the bladder after transurethral resection of non–muscle-invasive tumors (Table 54.6) as well as in an attempt to decrease the rate of subsequent recurrence in patients who have had complete resection of all cystoscopically visible tumor (prophylactic or suppressive therapy).

Bacille Calmette-Guérin. Intravesical BCG therapy was introduced by Morales in 1976 using the Pasteur strain of BCG given both intravesically and intradermally. BCG is an attenuated tuberculin bacillus that is known to be effective in treating superficial cancers left *in situ* as well as in reducing the recurrence rate in patients whose tumor has been completely resected. Several different strains of BCG have been used including Pasteur, Tice, Dutch, Connaught, and Moreau. The viability and density of the tubercule bacilli per milliliter of vaccine may vary with the strain used and may vary from lot to lot within the same strain. Various routes of administration of BCG have been employed including intravesical, intradermal, and oral. All routes have been reported to be successful, but the intravesical route is routinely used.

TABLE 54.6. Agents for Intravesical Chemotherapy–Definitive Treatment

Agent	CR (%)	PR (%)	CR + PR (%)
Thiotepa	30–41	35–53	72–85
Mitomycin C	47–49	30–35	79–82
Adriamycin			45–71
BCG	17–83	10–27	58–83

BCG, bacille Calmette-Guérin; CR, complete response; PR, partial response.

The mechanism of action of BCG is believed to be immunologic. Several authors have reported increased urinary interleukin-2 levels after BCG therapy. BCG appears to induce an immune response in the bladder after being attached to the bladder via fibronectin. It creates the features of a T-cell–dominated cystitis [predominantly CD4+ helper cells activated by major histocompatibility complex (MHC)-II antigens]. Intravesical BCG has also been shown to induce a chronic granulomatous response in the bladder in many patients. Although there may be an increased trend for favorable response to BCG in patients who have either developed granulomas within the urinary tract or converted their purified protein derivative (PPD) test, this correlation is not reliably predictive for the individual patient.

The principal toxicity of intravesical BCG therapy is vesical irritability. Patients commonly complain of dysuria, urinary frequency, hematuria, fever, malaise, nausea, chills, and arthralgia. Granulomatous prostatitis is a common occurrence following BCG therapy and approximately 6% of these patients have severe enough symptoms to require treatment with isoniazid (INH). A small number of deaths have been reported in patients treated with BCG therapy due to apparent disseminated BCG infection. Lamm has cataloged the toxicity associated with BCG, and has reported that BCG sepsis is a rare event, occurring in only 0.4% of treatments. Nonetheless, the clinician must be aware of the risk factors for BCG sepsis and withhold treatment in the face of high fever (more than 103° F), concomitant cystitis, and especially any evidence of urethral or bladder trauma. The current treatment algorithm for the management of presumed BCG sepsis includes isoniazid (300 mg/day), rifampin (600 mg/day), and prednisone (40 mg/day). It is also important to cover the patient with broad-spectrum antibiotics to treat a potential urosepsis.

Several prospective, randomized trials have evaluated BCG for prophylaxis of recurrent tumors. It has been reported that BCG reduced the tumor recurrence rate to 17% as compared with 42% in control patients treated with transurethral resection alone. Other trials are summarized in Table 54.7. High-risk patients display a delay in disease progression, prolonged bladder preservation, and improved survival when treated with BCG. Responses to BCG treatment appear to be durable rather than simply delaying eventual tumor recurrence.

TABLE 54.7. Bacille Calmette-Guérin (BCG) Trials

Trials of BCG for Prophylaxis

Rx	Number	Recurrence Rate (%)	Time to Recurrence
BCG	(67)	33[a]	13.4 ± 6
Control	(33)	58	9.9 ± 5

Prospective Trials of Prophylactic BCG versus Other Agents

Rx	Recurrence Rate (%)	Recurrence/ 100 Patients/Month
BCG	13.4[a]	0.53
Thiotepa	35.7	1.55
Adriamycin	44.2	1.7
BCG	0.33	
Mitomycin C	0.29	
BCG	19[a]	
Adriamycin	54	

[a] Statistically significant difference.

Intravesical BCG has also been extensively evaluated for the therapy of carcinoma *in situ*. A complete response rate can be expected to occur in approximately 70% of treated patients. Complete responses are usually associated with the resolution of irritative voiding symptoms.

The dilemma of how much BCG therapy to provide still remains. Some evidence points to the usefulness of a second induction course of BCG, particularly in patients who have responded to the initial treatment.

A randomized, controlled trial by the Southwest Oncology Group (SWOG) has demonstrated the enhanced efficacy of maintenance BCG given as 3 weekly treatments at 3, 6, 12, 18, 24, 30, and 36 months after completion of the induction course (6 weekly treatments). This trial demonstrated an enhanced recurrence and progression-free survival for the maintenance arm.

Other agents have been employed in the management of TCC, both in the bladder and the upper urinary tracts. A complete discussion of the agents and their efficacy is beyond the scope of this chapter. The most useful drugs clinically at this time include mitomycin-C, adriamycin, interferon-α, and thiotepa.

TREATMENT OF MUSCLE-INVASIVE DISEASE

The tumors discussed previously have a marked tendency to progress to muscle invasion. When they do so, they are commonly no longer effectively managed by simple transurethral resection and the use of topical immunotherapy or chemotherapy. Typically, more extensive surgery, radiation, or systemic chemotherapies are required, either alone or in combination. Muscle-invasive lesions of the bladder are typically treated by radical cystectomy including the removal of the prostate and seminal vesicles in men, and the uterus, ovaries, and the tubes with part of the vagina in women. Most experts also favor the removal of the regional lymph nodes. Muscle-invasive cancers of the upper urinary tract are treated primarily by radical nephrourectomy including the removal of a cuff of bladder around the ureteral orifice (in selected cases, partial ureterectomy may be performed). Urethral cancers, when invasive, also frequently require cystectomy in addition to urethrectomy. Other modalities of treatment for bladder cancers are possible, including partial cystectomy, radiation alone, radiation with concomitant chemotherapy, and chemotherapy followed by transurethral resection. To date, most would agree that an aggressive surgical approach with cystectomy is the gold standard of treatment. Nonetheless, advances using combined chemotherapy, radiation, and transurethral resection have demonstrated results that appear similar to those seen historically with radical surgery in selected patients, while preserving the bladder in the majority of patients. Long-term follow-up is still needed to demonstrate the value of these approaches. Ultimately, further studies including randomized trials would be useful in demonstrating the relative efficacy of these multimodality approaches as compared with cystectomy (with or without neoadjuvant or adjuvant chemotherapy). In a first attempt to use a molecular marker in bladder cancer to determine therapeutic options, a multiinstitutional trial is currently underway, which stratifies the use of adjuvant chemotherapy after cystectomy based on the patient's p53 status within the tumor.

TREATMENT OF METASTATIC DISEASE

The management of metastatic TCC has primarily centered around the use of chemotherapies given in combination regimens. The National Comprehensive Cancer Network currently recommends the use of MVAC as standard treatment for good risk patients. This combination has resulted in overall response rates of 50% to 70% and complete response rates of 10% to 20%. Median survival, however, continues to be approximately 1 year despite significant toxicity following treatment with these agents.

Combinations of paclitaxel (Taxol) and platinum-based doublets or triplets (especially carboplatin) have seemed to indicate similar efficacy with markedly reduced toxicity. These agents have resulted in expanded use of chemotherapy for patients with poorer performance status initially and improved tolerance of the regimen for all. An on-going phase III trial comparing paclitaxel–carboplatin and MVAC should clarify the roles of these treatments.

Selected Readings

Anderstrom C, Johansson S, Nilsson S. The significance of lamina propria invasion on the prognosis of patients with bladder tumors. *J Urol* 1980;124(1):23–26.

This study indicates that patients with grades 1 to 3 bladder tumors, which are confined to the mucosa or do not infiltrate deeper than into the lamina propria, should be managed by transurethral resection. However, if lymphatic invasion is present, combined treatment of supervoltage irradiation and an extensive operation may be considered in these patients.

Blot WJ, Fraumeni JF Jr. Geographic patterns of bladder cancer in the United States. *J Natl Cancer Inst* 1978;61(4):1017–1023.

Age-adjusted rates of mortality during 1950 to 1969 from bladder cancer were correlated with demographic and industrial indexes for the 3,056 counties of the contiguous United States. Rates among whites and nonwhites of both sexes rose sharply with urbanization. Industrial factors may explain at least part of the geographic clustering, inasmuch as rates among males were significantly higher in U.S. counties where the chemical industry is heavily concentrated.

Goffinet DR, Schneider MJ, Glatstein EJ, et al. Bladder cancer: results of radiation therapy in 384 patients. *Radiology* 1975;117(1):149–153.

Approximately 30% to 40% of deeply invasive tumors confined to the bladder can be controlled with radiation therapy alone, directed solely to the bladder itself.

Heney NM, Ahmed S, Flanagan MJ, et al. Superficial bladder cancer: progression and recurrence. *J Urol* 1983;130(6):1083–1086.

In this study, 249 patients presenting initially with stages Ta and T1 bladder cancer were only treated with transurethral resection and/or fulguration. Progression according to stages Ta and T1, and grades 1, 2, and 3 was 4%, 30%, 2%, 11%, and 45%, respectively, and also correlated with nontumor dysplasia and size. High tumor grade, lamina propria invasion, atypia elsewhere in the bladder, positive urinary cytology, tumor multiplicity, and large tumors were associated with shorter intervals free of disease.

Johansson S, Wahlqvist L. A prognostic study of urothelial renal pelvic tumors: comparison between the prognosis of patients treated with intrafascial nephrectomy and perifascial nephroureterectomy. *Cancer* 1979;43(6):2525–2531.

The study shows that the 5-year survival for patients operated with intrafascial nephrectomy was 51%, and 84% in the patients operated with perifascial nephrectomy. The main difference in prognosis between the two series was in patients with high-stage tumors. Therefore aggressive attitude against urothelial renal pelvic tumors is recommended.

Johnson DE, Schoenwald MB, Ayala AG, et al. Squamous cell carcinoma of the bladder. *J Urol* 1976;115(5):542–544.

Clinical and morphologic features of 90 cases of squamous cell carcinoma of the bladder was reviewed demonstrating an overall 5-year survival rate of only 10.6%. Seventeen patients with no therapy expired before 2 years. Supervoltage radiation therapy for patients with stages B2 and C lesions yielded a 5-year survival rate of only 17.7% and preoperative radiotherapy followed by simple total cystectomy and urinary diversion in a small number of patients with stages B2 and C lesions resulted in a 5-year survival rate in excess of 34%.

Kantor AF, Hartge P, Hoover RN, et al. Epidemiological characteristics of squamous cell carcinoma and adenocarcinoma of the bladder. *Cancer Res* 1988;48(13):3853–3855.

This study indicates that in the United States transitional cell carcinoma accounts for the vast majority (95%) of bladder tumors, with squamous cell carcinoma (less than 3%) and adenocarcinoma (less than 2%) comprising nearly all the remaining cases. Rates of squamous cell carcinoma and adenocarcinoma were higher in African-Americans compared with whites, whereas the reverse was true for transitional cell carcinoma.

Koss JC, Arger PH, Coleman BG, et al. CT staging of bladder carcinoma. *AJR Am J Roentgenol* 1981;137(2):359–362.

This study revealed that the overall accuracy of computed tomography (CT) in predicting lymph node metastasis was 92%, the sensitivity 60%, and the specificity 100%. Most diagnostic errors in this series were related to the determination of perivesical fat involvement by tumor.

Lantz EJ, Hattery RR. Diagnostic imaging of urothelial cancer. *Urol Clin North Am* 1984;11(4):567–583.

Technologic advances in diagnostic imaging, such as, CT, ultrasound, and magnetic resonance imaging (MRI) offer new ways to evaluate urothelial tumors.

Lutzeyer W, Rubben H, Dahm H. Prognostic parameters in superficial bladder cancer: an analysis of 315 cases. *J Urol* 1982;127(2):250–252.

A retrospective study of 315 patients with superficial transitional cell carcinoma (stages Ta to T2) with follow-up of 3 years or longer revealed that stage Ta tumors can be treated sufficiently by transurethral resection even in the case of several recurrences; however, more aggressive therapy should be considered when multifocal or recurrent stage T1 or T2 tumors recur as invasive carcinomas.

Malkowicz SB, Nichols P, Lieskovsky G, et al. The role of radical cystectomy in the management of high grade superficial bladder cancer. *J Urol* 1990;144(3):641–645.

This study demonstrates that radical cystectomy has been highly effective in curing patients with high-grade, superficial disease, including those with superficially invasive disease associated with nodal metastases.

Strong DW, Pearse HD. Recurrent urothelial tumors following surgery for transitional cell carcinoma of the upper urinary tract. *Cancer* 1976;38(5):2173–2183.

When nephroureterectomy is performed for carcinoma of the renal pelvis and ureter, a cuff of bladder that includes the ureteral orifice should be removed to obviate recurrent disease in the ureteral stump. Because single-incision nephroureterectomy did not include the intramural ureter in 50% of the cases in which it was performed, a second incision may be required for adequate exposure.

PART 3
Prostate Cancer

Bernard H. Bochner and Gary Lieskovsky

Prostate cancer is the most commonly diagnosed cancer in men in the United States and the second leading cause of male cancer deaths. Prostate cancer is a disease whose prevalence increases with age. More than 90% of prostate cancers are diagnosed in men between the ages of 45 and 90. As the general population ages, an increase in the number of newly diagnosed cases is anticipated. Increased awareness of the importance of prostate cancer and advances in diagnostic strategies has been largely responsible for the increased incidence observed as well as a stage migration wherein fewer men are presenting with advanced disease.

EPIDEMIOLOGY

Autopsy studies have demonstrated that 15% to 30% of men 50 years of age will have histologic evidence of prostate cancer; however, by age 80 the incidence of latent prostate cancer increases to 60% to 70%. Age-adjusted incidence rates and death rates vary significantly among countries and racial ethnic groups. African-American men demonstrate incidence rates among the highest in the world with age-standardized rates 50% to 60% greater than Caucasian-Americans. Caucasians demonstrate an intermediate incidence, whereas Asian men demonstrate very low incidence rates, approximately 5% of that in African-Americans. Causative factors responsible for these regional and ethnic variations include genetic, environmental, and endogenous factors.

Genetic Studies

One of the most consistent risk factors associated with prostate cancer is a positive family history in which first-degree relatives are effected. Men with a single, effected first-degree relative (father, brother, or son) demonstrate a 2 to 2.5 times increased risk of developing clinically detected disease. If two or more first degree relatives are involved, a 4-fold increased risk is observed in Caucasians and Asians, whereas as much as a 10-fold increased risk is found in African-Americans. Familial clustering of prostate cancer is well documented clinically. Familial cases of prostate cancer, although presenting at an earlier age compared with sporadic cases, do not demonstrate a more aggressive histologic phenotype or pathologic stage. Furthermore, familial cases do not appear to exhibit an increased risk of recurrence following definitive local therapy (i.e., surgery).

A hereditary form of prostate cancer has been identified and is thought to encompass 9% of prostate cancer patients. Hereditary prostate cancer is thought to be the result of inheritance of susceptibility genes, which predispose to the development of prostate cancer. Linkage analysis has identified one such candidate susceptibility gene on chromosome 1q, designated the *human prostate cancer gene-1 (HPC-1)*. Chromosomal analyses have demonstrated regions of deletions by loss of heterozygosity studies to 8p, 10q, 13q, 16q, 17p, and 18q, suggesting the location of putative genes with tumor-suppressor activity, such as the cellular-adherence protein, e-cadherin. Although p53 tumor-suppressor gene alterations, located on 17p, are the most common genetic changes found in most types of cancer, they are not commonly identified in low-grade, low-stage prostate tumors. In contrast, 50% of metastatic prostate cancer lesions do demonstrate p53 gene alterations.

CLINICAL PRESENTATION

The natural history of prostate cancer varies greatly. Some tumors demonstrate a slow-growing, indolent course, whereas others invade locally and rapidly metastasize. Clinical symptoms are typically not present in most men with localized prostate cancer. The peripheral location of the majority of prostate cancers, unlike the central, periurethral position of benign prostatic hypertrophy (BPH), does not lead to obstructive voiding symptoms until the tumor has progressed locally. Once the lesion is large enough to impinge on the urethra or bladder neck, hesitancy, decreased force of stream, and urinary retention may occur. As the tumor further progresses locally, hematospermia from ejaculatory duct or seminal vesicle involvement may be found. Tumor extension onto the bladder trigone and periureteral tissues can lead to ureteral obstruction and progressive azotemia. Lower extremity edema can be a manifestation of pelvic lymph node involvement or venous thrombosis secondary to iliac vein compression by locally advanced tumor. The neurovascular structures responsible for erectile function lie immediately adjacent to the prostatic capsule and may be involved by locally extensive disease leading to impotency. Metastatic disease will commonly involve the axial skeleton and typically manifest as bone pain and/or as a pathologic fracture. Acute paralysis or other neurologic symptoms of spinal cord compression can result from a fractured vertebral body infiltrated by tumor and represents a tragic presentation of advanced disease.

DIAGNOSTIC MODALITIES

Currently, three tests are the mainstay diagnostic modalities used to detect cancer of the prostate: digital rectal examination (DRE), serum prostate-specific antigen (PSA), and transrectal ultrasound (TRUS) with biopsy. Large studies have confirmed that the combination of DRE and serum PSA serve as the best clinical predictor of the presence of prostate cancer. The risk of cancer found by TRUS and biopsy is related to the degree of elevation of the serum PSA and the presence of an abnormal DRE. The use of PSA and DRE in combination in the screening for prostate cancer has lead to a significant stage migration in which many more men are initially diagnosed with organ-confined disease, which is amenable to definitive local therapy.

Digital Rectal Examination

DRE has been established as a useful tool in the diagnosis of prostate cancers. Variations in examiner experience and the ability of benign prostatic conditions to mimic the feel of malignancy limits its overall sensitivity and specificity. DRE allows for palpation of the posterior aspect of the prostate, the location of 75% of prostate cancers. DRE is, however, ineffective at identifying tumors originating in the anterior lobe of the prostate gland, thought to be involved in up to 25% of prostate cancers. Lesions detected by DRE often have extended beyond the confines of the prostate, suggesting they have already progressed beyond curability by local therapy alone (surgery or radiation).

Serum Prostate-Specific Antigen Testing

PSA, a 30Kd serine protease responsible for the liquefaction of the seminal coagulum, was discovered in the 1960s and has since become one of the most valuable tumor markers ever discovered. Although initially thought to be prostate-tissue specific, immunohistochemical and immunoassay techniques have detected PSA in male and female periurethral glands, sweat glands, breast milk, benign and malignant breast tissues, and salivary gland neoplasms. PSA is secreted by normal and hyperplastic prostate as well as primary and metastatic prostate cancer. Any condition that is capable of disrupting the normal prostate architecture will cause PSA to leak into the surrounding tissues and facilitate its entry into the systemic circulation. Benign prostatic conditions such as BPH and prostatitis, as well as carcinoma of the prostate all lead to detectable elevations in serum PSA, which limits the specificity of serum PSA determinations in screening men at risk. Manipulation of the lower urinary tract (catheterization, cystoscopy, or prostatic biopsy) or urinary retention also elevates serum PSA concentrations. Studies demonstrate that DRE does not produce a clinically significant rise in serum PSA, whereas ejaculation may transiently elevate levels within the first 24 hours. Treatments that decrease the volume of prostatic epithelium will lower serum PSA levels. This includes treatments for BPH and cancer with androgen withdrawal strategies that decrease the production or activity of the potent androgens, testosterone and dihydrotestosterone (DHT). Use of 5 α-reductase inhibitors, which prevent the conversion of testosterone to DHT (i.e., finasteride), will decrease serum PSA levels by 50% following 12 months of treatment.

Serum PSA concentration is determined by immunologic (polyclonal or monoclonal) assays that detect several forms of the protein. Most PSA within the circulation is complexed to serine protease inhibitors (α_1-antichymotrypsin, α_2-acroglobulin). Monoclonal assays are the most commonly used tests and detect both free and complexed (specifically bound to α1-antichymotrypsin) forms of PSA. Significant variation between PSA assays exists with respect to the forms and extent of PSA detected. A total serum PSA value of less than 4.0 ng/ml, when measured by the monoclonal assays, is considered normal. To improve the detection of prostate cancers in younger men (sensitivity) while increasing the specificity in older men, age-specific PSA ranges have been proposed. Although PSA determination is currently the single best test for the detection of prostate cancer, 25% of prostate cancers will present with a normal PSA (less than 4.0 ng/ml), highlighting the importance of the combination of PSA and DRE in accurately assessing prostate cancer risk. Newer concepts have been developed that combine serum PSA with ultrasound-obtained prostate volumes (PSA density), the rate of PSA elevation with time (PSA velocity). The amount of free versus complexed PSA (percent free PSA) is demonstrating great promise to increase specificity of PSA as a screening tool to limit the number of negative biopsies performed in men with PSA elevations. Serum PSA level also serves as a useful marker to evaluate response to therapy for either local or distant disease. Elevations in serum PSA following definitive local therapy correlates with the identification of subsequent clinical recurrences.

Transrectal Ultrasound of the Prostate

Detection of an abnormality of the DRE and/or serum PSA level suggests the presence of cancer that must be confirmed histologically. The use of transrectal ultrasound of the prostate (TRUSP) to guide needle-directed biopsy has become the standard method of obtaining tissue for pathologic diagnosis. Although TRUSP may aid in the identification of suspicious regions (hypoechoic lesions) within the gland that can be targeted for biopsy, the main benefit of TRUSP rests in its ability to direct accurate, bilateral systematic sampling of the gland from its apex to base.

Radiographic Staging Modalities

A variety of imaging studies have been evaluated to stage prostate cancer including TRUS, computed tomography (CT), magnetic resonance imaging (MRI), and bone scintigraphy. TRUS, CT, and MRI have demonstrated a low sensitivity in assessing the extent of disease beyond the capsule of the prostate as well as involvement of the surrounding pelvic lymph nodes. Radionucleotide scintigraphy is useful for clinical staging by identifying metastatic bone involvement. Low-risk patients for bone metastases (serum PSA values less than 10 ng/ml and well to moderately differentiated disease) need not undergo a routine bone scan as part of their staging evaluation.

CLASSIFICATION

Histologic Characteristics

Adenocarcinoma comprises the vast majority of cancers of the prostate gland. Squamous cell carcinoma, neuroendocrine, and primary prostatic sarcomas are described but rare histologic variants. Adenocarcinoma of the prostate typically involves the peripheral lobes of the gland, making these lesions amenable to identification by DRE. Multifocality is typical of prostate cancers, identified in 85% of tumors. Although no definite preinvasive lesion such as carcinoma *in situ* has been identified, prostatic intraepithelial neoplasia (PIN) is a premalignant lesion of the prostatic epithelium that may be a precursor lesion to some invasive tumors. High-grade PIN in the absence of cancer on a needle biopsy signifies a high likelihood that cancer is present in the gland and warrants repeat biopsy.

The Gleason's system is the most widely used histologic criteria for grading prostate cancer. It is based on the glandular pattern of the tumor rather than cytologic and nuclear features. The Gleason's system grades tumor patterns from 1 (most differentiated) to 5 (poorly differentiated). The primary (predominant) and secondary pattern grades are added to give a Gleason's score that will range from 2 to 10. Gleason's score has proven to be a useful and independent predictor of outcome in patients with prostate cancer. Tumors are also commonly grouped into a three grade system: well (Gleason's score 2 to 4), moderate (Gleason's score 5 to 7), and poorly (Gleason's score 8 to 10) differentiated lesions. One disadvantage of the three grade system is the grouping of Gleason's 7 tumors, which demonstrate a biologic aggressiveness between moderate and poorly differentiated lesions.

Clinical Staging

The initial staging system by Whitmore and Jewett consisted of an A, B, C, D system and incorporated information on the status of the primary lesion and regional lymph nodes. Stage A tumors were detected following transurethral resection of the prostate for BPH. Stage B lesions were palpable on DRE, felt confined to the prostate, and were designated as B1 or B2 if tumor involved one or both sides of the gland, respectively. Stage C tumors were locally advanced lesions that extended beyond the prostatic capsule. Stage D disease designated metastatic involvement of the regional lymph nodes. Currently, the tumor, node, and metastasis (TNM) system is the most commonly used clinical staging system in which the extent of the primary tumor is designated by a T stage. T1 lesions are described as T1a (less than 5% of specimen involved) and T1b (more than 5% involvement) if the tumor was discovered following transurethral resection of prostate. T1c lesions are clinically inapparent lesions that are nonpalpable and detected solely on the basis of an elevated serum PSA value. T1c lesions make up the majority of patients in contemporary prostate cancer patient series. T2 lesions are palpable on DRE and designated T2a and T2b corresponding to the B1 and B2 lesions of the Whitmore-Jewett system. T3 lesions demonstrate focal (T3a) or extensive (T3b) extracapsular extension or invasion of the seminal vesicles (T3c). T4 disease involves adjacent organs (T4a) (bladder neck, rectum) or the pelvic side wall (T4b). Nodal status is N0 if uninvolved or N1 to N3 depending on the dimensions of the involved regional nodes.

TREATMENT

Localized Disease

Management options for patients with localized disease include conservative and curative interventions. Given that many men with histologic evidence of prostate cancer will remain asymptomatic from their tumor and die as a result of other medical causes, careful clinical judgement is needed to select appropriate candidates for treatment. Important selection criteria in determining a particular patient's treatment recommendations include patient age and anticipated life expectancy, comorbidity, and clinical tumor characteristics (grade and stage). The natural history of prostate cancer patients can be surmised from mortality data in countries that practice a watchful waiting policy. These data demonstrate that most men followed conservatively for 15 years will die of prostate cancer. The metastasis-free survival at 10 years for men followed conservatively depends on the grade of the tumor. Metastatic disease will be observed in 19%, 42%, and 74% of men with well, moderate, and poorly differentiated tumors, respectively, if followed conservatively for 10 years. The indolent nature of some small, well-differentiated tumors make many older men with less than 10 years life expectancy reasonable candidates for a watchful waiting approach. Patients are monitored for symptoms of progressive disease with palliative treatment provided at the time of progression or the development of symptoms. Patients with more than 10 years life expectancy and clinically localized disease are candidates for curative intervention, including surgery or radiation therapy.

The surgical removal of the prostate for cancer is referred to as a *radical prostatectomy* and involves the removal of the prostate and surrounding seminal vesicles. The pelvic lymph nodes (obturator, hypogastric, iliac) that serve as the primary landing area for lymph node metastases are also sampled at the time of surgery, which provides important staging and prognostic information. Radical prostatectomy may be performed through a lower midline, extraperitoneal incision (retropubic approach) or via the perineum (perineal approach). Improved understanding of the anatomic structures responsible for urinary continence and erectile function has led to surgical advances that have decreased the morbidity and mortality associated with surgery compared with historic series. Nerve-sparing surgical procedures were introduced in 1982 in which the parasympathetic innervation responsible for erectile function is preserved. Potency rates following nerve-sparing radical prostatectomy are dependent on presurgical erectile function, age, and whether bilateral or unilateral nerve sparing was performed. Functional erections can be obtained by 50% to 70% of younger patients with normal preoperative erectile function after bilateral nerve-sparing surgery. Oral and injectable vasoactive medications and prosthetic devices are available to return erectile function in those men with postoperative impotency. Urinary incontinence following surgery is usually transient and related to physical exertion (stress incontinence); however, severe incontinence effects approximately 5% of postsurgical patients. Other complications of radical prostatectomy include urethral anastomotic stricture, rectal injury, lymphocele formation, and lymphedema. Tumor progression rarely occurs following surgery without a PSA elevation. The progression-free survival (undetectable PSA and no clinical evidence of recurrence) following radical prostatectomy for clinically organ-confined prostate cancer is 70% to 85% at 5 years and 50% to 75% at 10 years.

Radiation

Radiation delivered to the prostate via external beam or interstitial implants can be effective at treating a subset of prostate tumors. Currently, early-stage prostate cancer is treated for cure with various radiation techniques including three-dimensional conformal external beam therapy; radioactive iodine, palladium, or iridium implantation with or without external beam radiation therapy; and proton beam radiation. Controversy exists regarding the definition of a favorable outcome following radiotherapy. Criteria includes a stable serum PSA following treatment, a nadir total PSA value of less than 0.5 to 1.5 ng/ml, and a negative postradiation biopsy more than 1 year following the completion of treatment. External beam doses of less than 75 Gy are used to decrease serious local complications and late sequelae including radiation cystitis, incontinence, impotency, urethral stricture, and proctitis. Up to 50% of patients will demonstrate residual tumor on biopsy following external beam therapy. The finding of a rising postradiation PSA and the presence of a positive biopsy are directly correlated. To improve the outcomes in patients undergoing radiotherapy, newer strategies including conformal field therapy with dose escalation, brachytherapy followed by external beam boosting, and combination of neoadjuvant and adjuvant hormone-deprivation therapy have been proposed.

Brachytherapy using radioactive implants such as iodine-125 (I-125), palladium-103 (Pd-103), gold-198 (Au-198) and iridium-192 (Ir-192) have been used to increase the local dose of radiation received by the tumor by placing the radioactive source in intimate proximity to the malignancy. Theoretic advantages of brachytherapy over external sources include the delivery of high local doses to the prostate while limiting exposure to surrounding structures. Methods for implantation vary and can be divided into temporary and permanent implants. Early series using retropubically implanted permanent I-125, demonstrated suboptimal local control rates. With the advent of transperineal CT or ultrasound-guided permanent implants, the accuracy of isotope placement has improved to provide more homogenous dosimetry to the gland. The recent introduction of these technical improvements has led to a renewed interest in this modality for patients with early-stage localized disease; however, although short-term data are encouraging, longer follow-up is necessary to assess its therapeutic efficacy. The absence of large, randomized clinical trials make direct comparisons between outcomes following radiation therapy and surgical series difficult. Although the risk of biochemical recurrence is greater in patients that received radiation therapy compared with surgically treated patients, the overall survival data at 10 years do not demonstrate a clear advantage for either treatment modality. An additional important use for localized external beam radiation therapy in the management of prostate cancer patients is to provide palliation of pain from bone involvement by metastatic disease.

Locally Advanced Prostate Cancer

The optimal treatment of locally advanced prostate cancer (stage T3) remains uncertain. Lesion that are palpated to extend beyond the confines of the gland or involve seminal vesicles or periprostatic tissues demonstrate poor results following definitive radiotherapy or surgery. Up to 50% of locally advanced lesions will demonstrate pathologic evidence of regional lymph node metastases. Treatment strategies involving a combination of surgery, radiation, and hormonal deprivation have been proposed. Pretreatment cytoreduction using hormone deprivation allows for a reduction in the treatment field when followed by radiation therapy and improves pathologic outcomes (surgical margin status) following surgery. Significant improvements in long-term survival have yet to be demonstrated with these combination strategies.

Metastatic Disease

The prostate is dependent on androgens for its embryonic development, growth, and normal function. Testosterone, the major androgen produced by the testis, is responsible for 90% of the DHT within the prostate. Adrenal-produced androgens, which consist of the less potent androgens, androstenedione and dehydroepiandrosterone, are the precursors for the remaining 10% of prostatic DHT. Dihydrotestosterone is produced from testosterone within the prostate cell by the enzyme 5α-reductase. Once produced, DHT binds to androgen receptors that then activate the expression of specific genes responsible for cell differentiation and growth. Androgen withdrawal therapy, introduced in 1941 by Huggins and Hodges, remains the most effective means of decreasing prostate tumor growth. The majority of prostate cancer cells are dependent on androgens for survival and will undergo apoptosis, or programmed cell death, following androgen withdrawal. Objective responses and symptomatic relief are observed in up to 80% of patients following androgen withdrawal. The duration of these responses are variable with a mean time to progression between 18 and 36 months. Inevitably, the emergence of androgen independence occurs through an incompletely understood mechanism that involves the selective growth of androgen-independent clones, increased genetic instability, mutations of the androgen receptor, and the reliance on alternative growth factors (fibroblast growth factor, insulinlike growth factors, and transforming growth factor-β). Androgen withdrawal therapy centers on the ability to induce castrate levels of androgens within the circulation. Surgical castration involves the removal of the testicles and has the advantages of immediate effectiveness, low cost compared with prolonged medical therapy, and alleviates the concerns over compliance with long-term medical therapy.

Medical castration can be obtained through a variety of mechanisms including oral estrogens, luteinizing hormone-releasing hormone (LH-RH agonists), and antiandrogens (hormone receptor antagonists, steroid synthesis inhibitors). Combination therapy to eliminate the effects of testicular- and adrenal-derived androgens results in maximal androgen blockade. Evidence suggests that maximal androgen blockage will provide improved progression-free survival when LH-RH agonists are combined with pure antiandrogens.

Effective therapeutic options for patients with hormone refractory disease are limited. Following confirmation that castrate levels of testosterone are present, elevations in serum PSA levels confirm the onset of androgen independence in patients receiving hormone withdrawal therapy. Patients that progress while receiving maximal androgen blockade should initially undergo discontinuation of the antiandrogen. Up to 40% of patients will experience a biochemical, symptomatic, and/or objective response following antiandrogen withdrawal (antiandrogen withdrawal syndrome), which is proposed to be mediated by tumor clones expressing a mutated androgen receptor. Maintenance of gonadal-androgen suppression is recommended despite evidence of androgen independence. Several chemotherapeutic substances have demonstrated modest single-agent antitumor effects on hormone-resistant disease. Among these are cyclophosphamide, *cis*-platin, 5-flurouracil, and doxorubicin. Growth factor stimulation of prostate cancer growth has been proposed as a mechanism of hormone resistance. Suramin, a polysulfonated napthylurea, is a multifunctional agent with growth factor binding activity. Suramin has demonstrated effectiveness at inhibition of hormone-resistant tumor growth; however, its toxicity pattern and complex pharmacology has limited its widespread use.

Selected Readings

Chodak GW, Thisted RA, Gerber GS, et al. Results of conservative management of clinically localized prostate cancer. *New Engl J Med* 1994;330:242–248.

The authors provide a pooled analysis of 828 patients with prostate cancer followed conservatively. Risk for experiencing metastatic disease at 10 and 15 years are provided. This demonstrates the natural history of prostate cancer and the outcomes of untreated patients followed long term.

Gleason DR, Mellinger GT. Prediction of prognosis for prostatic adenocarcinoma by combined histological grading and clinical staging. *J Urol* 1974;111:58–64.

Histologic grading of prostate cancer remains one of the strongest prognostic variables available. In this early study, the authors provided data demonstrating the close correlation between histologic classification and mortality.

Pound CR, Partin AW, Epstein JI, et al. Prostate-specific antigen after anatomic radical retropubic prostatectomy. Patterns of recurrence and cancer control. *Urol Clin North Am* 1997;24:395–406.

The authors provide a single institution experience with nearly 1,700 prostate cancer patients that have undergone radical prostatectomy for clinically organ-confined disease. This large series provides clear evidence of the efficacy of radical prostatectomy, including anatomic nerve-sparing procedures, in the long-term control of this disease.

Smith DS, Catalona WJ, Herchman JD. Longitudinal screening for prostate cancer with prostate-specific antigen. *JAMA* 1996;276:1309–1315.

The authors relate their experience with a community-based PSA screening program for prostate cancer. More than 10,000 men were followed serially to determine, among other variables, cancer detection rates and pathologic characteristics of PSA-detected cancers. This study demonstrates the important stage migration in PSA-detected lesions in which most lesions are organ confined and potentially curable tumors.

CHAPTER 55

Effects of Heart and Liver Disease and Neoplasia on Kidney and Electrolyte Metabolism

PART 1
Heart Disease

Richard J. Glassock

Disease of the heart may affect fluid and electrolyte metabolism through perturbations of kidney function mediated by diverse mechanisms. The principal cardiac disturbance influencing kidney function is the failure of the heart to deliver blood flow required for the maintenance of oxygen and nutrients supplies to tissues. Thus defined, cardiac failure can arise from many disorders including congenital anomalies, ischemia, hypertension, acquired valvular disease, inflammatory, degenerative or infiltrative cardiomyopathies, pericardial constriction or tamponade, arteriovenous fistula, beriberi, hyperthyroidism, severe anemia, or Paget's disease. Both high and low output varieties exist, and the pumping function of the left or right side of the heart may be independently affected. Heart failure may also be due to the inability of the ventricles to maintain the systolic ejection phase (systolic heart failure) or to the inability of the ventricles to fully relax and fill during diastole (diastolic heart failure). Regardless of the cause or the underlying pathophysiology of the heart failure, a complex series of interacting endocrine, paracrine, autocrine, and neural responses are elicited which, in turn, have effects on the heart, peripheral vasculature, and kidney as well as many on other organs (Table 55.1). Many of these responses to cardiac failure can be viewed as *compensatory* in that they are designed to restore the capacity of the heart to deliver blood flow to vital tissues. These compensatory processes augment myocardial contractility and enhance venous return and thereby promote a restoration of cardiac output. Because cardiac failure and reduced perfusion pressure and flow (e.g., reduced cardiac output) are sensed by the body as a defect or deficit in "effective arterial blood volume (EABV)," many of these compensatory responses result in a retention of fluids by the kidney and in vasoconstriction. However, as with most short-term compensatory responses, there may be long-term maladaptive features in which the response has undesirable effects, which can then evoke new complications or even aggravate the underlying disorder. Examples of the latter include increased impedance to blood flow depressing systolic ventricular function. These positive feedback mechanisms may complete a vicious cycle (Fig. 55.1). These compensatory mechanisms and their beneficial and deleterious effects will be the subject of this chapter. Particular

TABLE 55.1. Neurohormonal Changes in Heart Failure

Activation of the sympathetic nervous system
Increased renin-angiotensin system activity
Increased aldosterone secretion
Increased antidiuretic hormone release
Increased endothelins release
Increased prostaglandin (PGI_2 and PGE_2) production
Increased inducible nitric oxide synthase activity

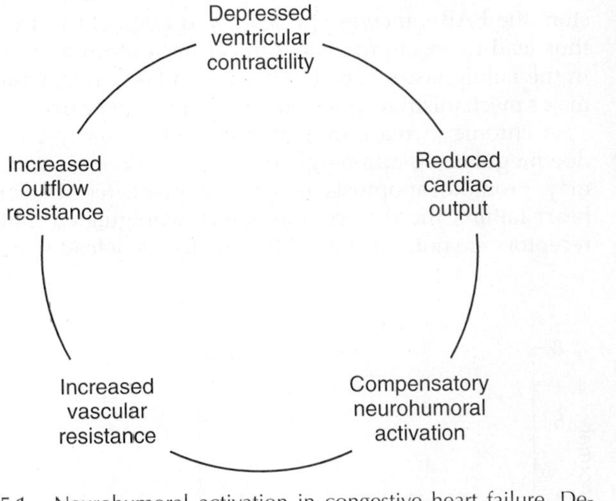

Figure 55.1. Neurohumoral activation in congestive heart failure. Depressed ventricular contractility, induced by the underlying cardiac disease, leads to neurohumoral activation (moving clockwise) that is initially adaptive in that it maintains blood pressure and tissue perfusion. Over the long term, however, the increase in outflow resistance (afterload) hastens the rate of myocardial deterioration and worsens ventricular performance. This leads to a vicious cycle of increasing release of norepinephrine, angiotensin II, and ADH that further increases afterload. (Reproduced with permission from *Up to Date*, Boston, MA, version 7.0, CD-ROM.)

emphasis will be placed on alteration of kidney function and fluid and electrolyte disorders. The pathophysiology of edema in heart failure is discussed further in Chapter 31.

NEURAL ACTIVATION AND ITS CONSEQUENCES

It is well established that the sympathetic nervous system is activated in cardiac failure. This seems to be due to an activation of the carotid sinus and aortic baroreceptors, which sense reduced cardiac output and perfusion pressure and thereby tonically modulate the outflow of sympathetic nerve traffic from vasomotor centers in the central nervous system. Additional sensors in the renal circulation send afferent signals to the central nervous system, which also promote sympathetic nervous system activity. These renal sensors are similar to those involved in the renal response to extracellular volume depletion. They also activate hormonal responses, which include activation of the renin-angiotensin system, promotion of excretion of aldosterone, and enhancement of antidiuretic hormone release. The activation of stretch receptors located in the left atrium act in a counterregulatory fashion to reduce sympathetic nervous system outflow and to inhibit the renin-angiotensin system and antidiuretic hormone release. However, the response initiated in the left atrium is either overridden by the aortic– and carotid sinus–mediated mechanisms or is attenuated by downregulation of the sensitivity of the atrial receptors. There may also be a cardiac-specific increase in efferent sympathetic activity.

The activation of the sympathetic nervous system in cardiac failure leads to increased plasma levels of norepinephrine (Fig. 55.2). Measurements of norepinephrine levels can be used as a crude indicator of the severity of cardiac failure. Increased sympathetic nervous system activity leads to arterial and venous vasoconstriction, an increase in myocardial contractility (inotropy), and a rise in heart rate (chronotropy). Renal vasoconstriction, mediated by increased neural sympathetic traffic, increased plasma norepinephrine levels, and activation of the renin-angiotensin system cause an increase in the resistance of the efferent glomerular arteriolar bed. This change leads to an increase in filtration fraction [glomerular filtration rate (GFR)/renal blood flow (RBF)]. Proximal tubular reabsorption of sodium chloride is also enhanced. These changes tend to restore the EABV, increase preload, and augment heart rate and thus lead to an improvement in cardiac output and perfusion. In the failing heart, it is the increase in heart rate, which is the major mechanism responsible for maintaining cardiac output.

A chronic increase in sympathetic nervous system activity downregulates β-adrenergic receptors in the myocardium and may promote apoptosis of cardiac myocytes. In congestive heart failure, the β_1 receptors are downregulated, but the β_2-receptors are not. The loss of β_1 function may lead to depressed cardiac function. β_2-Receptors lead to greater intracellular calcium accumulation and may predispose to ventricular arrhythmias. β-Receptor blockade (with nonselective β-receptor antagonists such as carvedilol, bucindolol, and propranolol) reduce the proarrhythmic state and also improve cardiac function. Arterial vasoconstriction leads to an increase in aortic impedance (afterload), which depresses myocardial performance. The peripheral vascular system in congestive heart failure is associated with a chronically vasoconstricted state, leading to decreased perfusion of the kidney, splanchnic bed, skin, and skeletal muscle.

RENIN-ANGIOTENSIN-ALDOSTERONE SYSTEM

The renin-angiotensin-aldosterone system (RAAS) is activated in cardiac failure partly as the consequence of heightened sympathetic nerve traffic but also by local effects in the kidney. The intrarenal renin-angiotensin system may be activated to a greater extent than the systemic RAAS. Measurement of plasma renin activity in cardiac failure may underrepresent the degree of activation of the renin-angiotensin system within the kidney. Plasma renin activity is frequently, but not universally, increased in cardiac failure (Fig. 55.1). The intracardiac renin-angiotensin system is also activated in congestive heart failure.

Angiotensin II thus produced causes increased sodium reabsorption by the kidney in part by a direct effect on proximal tubular reabsorption and in part by an effect on distal sodium reabsorption mediated by enhanced release of aldosterone from the adrenal gland. Angiotensin II also directly causes myocardial hypertrophy, which, although beneficial in the short term, has long-term deleterious consequences on cardiac function. Individuals possessing the deletion or DD angiotensin-converting enzyme (ACE) genotype have higher ACElevels and may be at higher risk for cardiac complications including acute myocardial infarction, left ventricular hypertrophy, and mortality from congestive heart failure. Increased conversion of angiotensin I to cleavage peptides (angiotensin II, III, and IV) may promote thrombosis by elevating levels of plasminogen activator inhibitor-1 and tissue thromboplastin. It may also promote cardiac fibrosis by increasing transforming growth factor β_1 synthesis. Long-term angiotensin II antagonism (by administration of ACE inhibitors or angiotensin II–receptor antagonist) and the use of inhibitors of aldosterone action (spironolactone) have favorable effects on mortality in congestive heart failure.

ANTIDIURETIC HORMONE

Activation of the carotid sinus baroreceptors by decreased cardiac output results in enhanced release of antidiuretic hormone

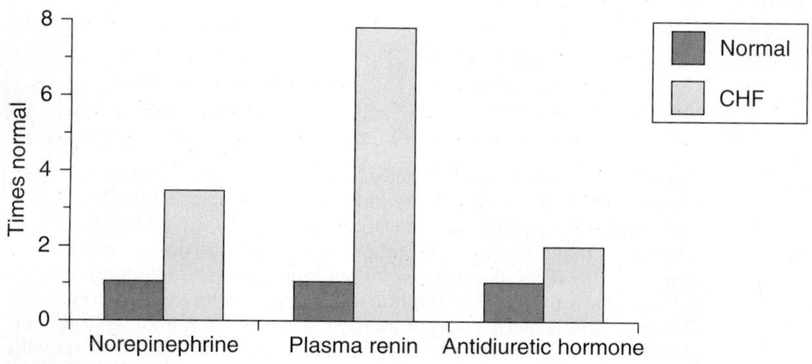

Figure 55.2. Hormone levels in congestive heart failure. Plasma levels of norepinephrine, renin activity, and antidiuretic hormone are increased twofold to eightfold (when compared with those in normal subjects) in patients with stable congestive heart failure treated with digitalis, but not diuretics or vasodilators. (Data reproduced with permission from Francis GS, Goldsmith SR, Levine TB, et al. *Ann Intern Med* 1984;101:370.)

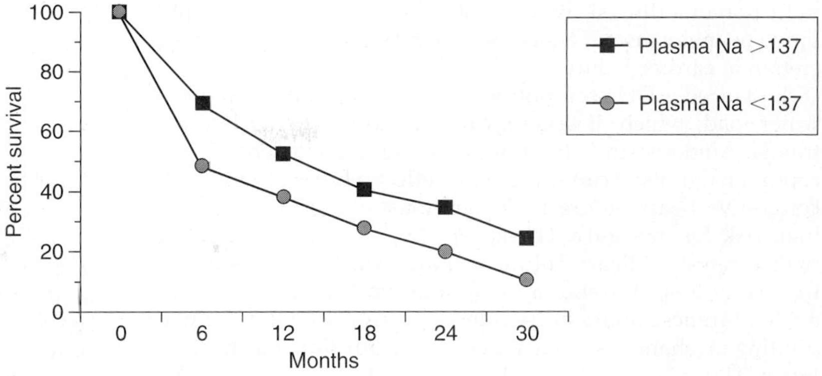

Figure 55.3. Hyponatremia associated with reduced survival in congestive heart failure. Survival over time in patients with severe heart failure and a normal plasma sodium concentration (*squares*) or hyponatremia (*circles*). Survival was significantly reduced in patients with hyponatremia. (Reproduced by permission from Lee WH, Packer M. *Circulation* 1986;73:257.)

(ADH). Thirst is also augmented, in part by a direct effect of angiotensin II on the central nervous system and in part by increased neural traffic impinging on central thirst centers. The increased levels of ADH may participate in the increase in renal vascular resistance, via V_1 receptors (Fig. 55.1). Through the hydroosmotic effects of activation of V_2 receptors, the principal action of elevated ADH levels is to reduce renal water excretion, an effect that parallels the severity of the cardiac failure. The combined effects of increased thirst and a heightened antidiuretic state promote the development of dilutional hyponatremia. Indeed, the degree of hyponatremia parallels the severity of congestive heart failure and can be used to predict the risk of mortality (Fig. 55.3).

NATRIURETIC PEPTIDES

The secretion of both atrial natriuretic peptide (ANP) and brain natriuretic peptide (BNP) are increased in cardiac failure. Left atrial stretch receptors promote ANP release. The physiology and the action of natriuretic peptides are discussed in detail in Chapter 13, Part 8. Plasma levels increase in proportion to the severity of cardiac failure but due to acquired resistance to physiologic actions, the effectiveness of these natriuretic peptides in promoting sodium excretion and relaxing the vasculature is blunted. Both ANP and BNP tend to counteract the actions of norepinephrine and angiotensin II on systemic vasoconstriction and renal sodium retention. Ureodilatin, also known as renal natriuretic peptide, is a locally acting natriuretic peptide synthesized in distal tubular epithelial cells. It may have actions governing sodium excretion in cardiac failure.

ENDOTHELINS

The physiology and actions of endothelins are discussed in Chapter 13, Part 5. The plasma level of endothelins is increased in cardiac failure in rough proportion to the degree of left ventricular dysfunction. Interaction with endothelin A receptors promotes vasoconstriction while interaction with endothelin B receptors mediates vasodilatation via prostanoids and nitric oxide. Elevated plasma levels of endothelins downregulate endothelin receptors. *In vivo* the vasoconstrictive effect of endothelins is dominant. Endothelins also cause sodium retention and reduced water excretion and lead to the activation of ANP and aldosterone secretion. Endothelins also have a positive inotropic effect on myocardium and over long periods may induce ventricular hypertrophy and exhibit myocardial cell toxicity. Inhibitors of endothelins improve outcome in congestive heart failure.

PROSTAGLANDINS

Plasma levels of vasodilatory prostaglandins, PGI_2 and PGE_2, are greatly elevated in congestive heart failure in proportion to its severity. Synthetic rates of these prostanoids are increased largely in response to increased sympathetic nervous system traffic, increased norepinephrine levels, and increased activity of the renin-angiotensin system and elevated ADH. They serve to blunt the usual vasoconstrictor effects of congestive heart failure and blunt the hydroosmotic affect of ADH. Inhibition of cyclooxygenase I by nonselective, nonsteroidal antiinflammatory agents therefore results in increased renal vascular resistance, decreased renal blood flow and glomerular filtration rate, and augmented sodium and fluid retention. Hyponatremic patients, representing the most severe forms of congestive heart failure, are at particular risk of manifesting the deleterious effects of nonsteroidal antiinflammatory agents.

FLUID AND ELECTROLYTE DISTURBANCES

Congestive heart failure, from its very early to advanced stages, is characterized by an impaired ability to excrete sodium chloride and water and by reduced RBF relative to GFR (Table 55.2). The augmentation of renal sodium chloride reabsorption is mediated by increased proximal and distal tubular reabsorption. The increase in filtration fraction leads to a change in physical forces governing the uptake of proximal tubular fluid. Increased angiotensin II and sympathetic nervous system activity also augment proximal tubular fluid reabsorption. Distal tubular reabsorption is increased by enhanced aldosterone action and perhaps by other factors. Inhibition of angiotensin II action promotes renal sodium excretion as do inhibitors of aldosterone action. Marked proximal tubular fluid reabsorption accompanied by depression of GFR may limit the capacity of distally acting diuretics to cause a natriuresis. Agents that inhibit the augmented proximal tubular fluid reabsorption can facilitate the

TABLE 55.2. Renal Function and Fluid and Electrolyte Disorders in Cardiac Failure

Change	Clinical Consequence
Reduced glomerular filtration rate and renal blood flow	Azotemia
Increased sodium chloride reabsorption	Edema
Decreased water excretion	Hyponatremia

induction of a diuresis with a distally acting agent. Thus, inhibition of angiotensin II action has salutary effects on sodium excretion in cardiac failure.

Enhanced ADH secretion leads to impaired excretion of a water load, which, if severe, can lead to dilutional hyponatremia. Angiotensin II inhibitors and aquaretic agents (V_2 receptor antagonists) can reverse this effect. Hyponatremia with congestive heart failure is an ominous sign and indicates a high risk for mortality. Therapy of hyponatremia in patients with congestive heart failure includes water restriction and the use of loop diuretics and angiotensin II antagonists. Thiazide diuretics should be avoided because they interfere with diluting mechanisms while leaving concentrating mechanisms intact. Thirst is also blunted by the use of A2 antagonists. Vasodilators (e.g., Apresoline), angiotensin II antagonists (e.g., ACE inhibitors or angiotensin II–receptor blockers), and nonselective β-antagonists can lead to improved cardiac function by reducing afterload and improving myocardial performance. These changes in myocardial function may be translated into an improvement in the kidney to handle sodium and water loads and by improved renal function. On the other hand, in patients with severe congestive heart failure, the use of potent diuretics to promote renal fluid loss, may result in temporary reductions in preload sufficient to cause a reduction in cardiac output. This reduction in cardiac output, consequent to overaggressive diuresis, may further impair renal function, manifested by declining GFR and rising serum creatinine levels.

Selected Readings

Andersson, B, Sylven, C. The DD genotype of the angiotensin-converting enzyme gene is associated with increased mortality in idiopathic heart failure. *J Am Coll Cardiol* 1996;28:162.

A study showing that polymorphisms of the gene for angiotensin II–converting enzyme may be associated with increased mortality in cardiac failure.

Dzau VJ. Vascular and renal prostaglandins as counter-regulatory systems in heart failure. *Eur Heart J* 1988;9(suppl H):15–19.

A brief review of the role of vasodilatory prostaglandins in modulating renal circulatory and functional alterations in heart failure.

Ichikawa I, Yoshioka T, Fogo A, et al. Role of angiotensin II in altered glomerular hemodynamics in congestive heart failure. *Kidney Int* 30(Suppl 30):S123–S126, 1990.

A review of experimental studies on the role of the renin-angiotensin system in the renal microcirculatory alterations observed in heart failure.

Mulder P, Richard V, Derumeaux G, et al. Role of endogenous endothelin in chronic heart failure. Effect of long-term treatment with an endothelin antagonist on survival, hemodynamics, and cardiac remodeling. *Circulation* 1997;96:1976.

A study demonstrating increased blood levels of endothelins in cardiac failure and the beneficial effects of endothelin antagonists.

Packer M. The neurohormonal hypothesis: a theory to explain the mechanism of disease progression in heart failure. *J Am Coll Cardiol* 1992;20:248–254.

An insightful discussion of the role of neurohumoral activation in the maladaptive compensatory mechanisms in heart failure.

Perrella MA, Margulies KB, Burnett JC Jr. Pathophysiology of congestive heart failure: role of atrial natriuretic factor and therapeutic implications. *Can J Physiol Pharmacol* 1991;69:1576–1581.

A review of human and experimental studies concerning the role of atrial natriuretic factor in the circulatory and renal adaptations to heart failure.

Oster JR, Materson BJ. Renal and electrolyte complications of congestive heart failure and effects of therapy with angiotensin-converting enzyme inhibitors. *Arch Intern Med* 1992;152:704–710.

An excellent review of complications observed in patients with congestive heart failure treated with ACE inhibitors.

Schrier RW. Pathogenesis of sodium and water retention in high-output and low-output cardiac failure, nephrotic syndrome, cirrhosis and pregnancy. *N Engl J Med* 1988;319:1065–1072, 1126–1134.

An excellent review of the various factors that mediate sodium and water retention in edema forming disorders.

Schrier RW, Fasset RG, O'Hara M, et al. Vasopressin release, water diuresis, and vasopressin antagonism in cardiac failure, cirrhosis and pregnancy. *Proc Assoc Am Physicians* 1998;110:407–411.

A scholarly review of the role of altered vasopressin release and its antagonism in cardiac failure.

PART 2
Liver Disease

Murray Epstein

Liver disease is frequently accompanied by a variety of alterations in renal function and electrolyte metabolism (Table 55.3). These complications of liver disease are diverse and vary from those that have little clinical significance to others that constitute serious derangements requiring therapeutic intervention. In this discussion, emphasis is placed on abnormalities of renal sodium and water handling, on the syndrome of acute vasomotor nephropathy and the hepatorenal syndrome, and on the immune complex glomerulonephritides that complicate liver disease.

RENAL SODIUM HANDLING

Clinical Features

The majority of data regarding renal sodium handling come from studies of patients with Laënnec's cirrhosis. Patients with Laënnec's cirrhosis manifest a *remarkable* capacity for sodium chloride retention; indeed, they frequently excrete urine that is virtually free from sodium. Extracellular fluid accumulates excessively and eventually becomes evident as clinically detectable ascites and edema. It should be emphasized that cirrhotic patients who are unable to excrete sodium will continue to gain weight and accumulate ascites and edema as long as dietary sodium content exceeds maximal urinary sodium excretion. If access to sodium is not curtailed, the relentless retention of this ion may lead to the accumulation of vast amounts of ascites (on occasion up to 30 L). Weight gain and ascites formation promptly cease when sodium intake is limited.

The abnormality of renal sodium handling in cirrhosis should not be regarded as a static and unalterable condition. Rather, patients with cirrhosis may undergo a spontaneous diuresis followed by a return to avid salt retention. Although a significant number of patients who are maintained on a sodium-restricted dietary program may demonstrate a spontaneous diuresis, there is inadequate information concerning the incidence of this phenomenon and the predictability of its occurrence in any particular patient. Sometimes, spontaneous diuresis occurs within a few days, but more often within a few weeks, after hospital admission.

Although ascites is often viewed as an indicator of decompensated hepatic disease, this caveat does not always obtain. Sometimes the onset of ascites can be related directly to increased dietary sodium intake and is more a reflection of salt loading than of progressive alterations in hepatic function. Oc-

TABLE 55.3. Renal Abnormalities in Liver Disease
Deranged renal sodium handling
Deranged renal water handling
Impaired renal acidification
Hepatorenal syndrome
Acute renal failure
Glomerulopathies

casionally, a history of increased intake of salted foods in the period before entry into the hospital can be elicited, whereas in other patients the use of sodium-containing remedies may be the culprit. Even when such precipitating events are ruled out, there is evidently a poor relationship between abnormalities in renal sodium handling and the presence or absence of decompensated liver disease. The presence or magnitude of the impairment of renal sodium handling in the cirrhotic patient cannot be predicted merely on the basis of the absence of ascites and/or edema. It should be emphasized that the primary renal excretory abnormality causing fluid retention is a disturbance of sodium, rather than water excretion. Many sodium-retaining patients with ascites and edema can excrete large volumes of dilute urine when given excessive amounts of water without sodium. Finally, it should be underscored that the bulk of available data on renal sodium handling in liver disease in humans have been derived from studies in patients with Laënnec's cirrhosis. The prominent sodium-retaining state commonly observed in Laënnec's cirrhosis may not be manifested in patients with primary biliary cirrhosis.

Pathogenesis

The pathogenetic events leading to the deranged sodium homeostasis of cirrhosis are exceedingly complex and remain the subject of continuing controversy. At least two hypotheses have been advanced. Traditionally, it has been proposed that ascites formation in cirrhotic patients begins when a critical imbalance of Starling forces in the hepatic sinusoids and splanchnic capillaries causes an excessive amount of lymph formation, exceeding the capacity of the thoracic duct to return this excessive lymph to the circulation. Consequently, excess lymph accumulates in the peritoneal space as ascites. Simultaneously, vasodilation and opening of arteriovenous shunts expand the space in which the plasma volume is contained; renal sodium retention is activated, and the relative disparity between plasma volume and the circulatory space is perceived as "effective" plasma volume contraction. The renal retention of sodium may be successful in restoring absolute total plasma volume to a normal or even supranormal value; however, because of the enlargement of the circulatory space in which this volume is contained, a state of relative or "effective" plasma volume contraction persists. This may explain the apparent paradox of unremitting renal sodium retention even with an apparently expanded absolute plasma volume. The term *effective* plasma volume refers to the part of the total circulating volume that is effective in stimulating volume receptors. The concept is somewhat elusive because the actual volume receptors remain incompletely defined. A diminished effective volume may reflect subtle alterations in systemic hemodynamic factors such as decreased filling of the arterial tree, diminished central blood volume, or both. Because the stimulus is unknown and the afferent receptors are incompletely elucidated, alterations in effective volume must be defined in a functional manner such as the kinetic response to volume manipulation. The diminished effective volume is thought to constitute an afferent signal that triggers events leading to augmentation of salt and water reabsorption by the renal tubule. Thus the traditional formulation implies that the renal retention of sodium is a secondary rather than a primary event.

In contrast, the *overflow* hypothesis for ascites formation suggests that the primary event is the inappropriate retention of excessive sodium by the kidneys with a resultant expansion of plasma volume. In the setting of abnormal Starling forces (both portal venous hypertension and a reduction in plasma colloid osmotic pressure) in the portal venous bed and hepatic sinusoids, the expanded plasma volume is sequestered preferentially in the peritoneal space with ascites formation. Thus according to this formulation, renal sodium retention and plasma volume expansion precede rather than follow the formation of ascites.

A third hypothesis to account for renal sodium and water retention in cirrhosis has been proposed. This theory, termed the *peripheral arterial vasodilation hypothesis*, postulates that peripheral vasodilation is the initial determinant of intravascular underfilling (i.e., that an imbalance between an expanded capacitance and the available volume constitutes a diminished effective volume).

Although I believe that the presently available evidence favors a prominent role for a diminished effective plasma volume in mediating the avid sodium retention and ascites formation in many cirrhotic patients, it is important to underscore that the two hypotheses (i.e., diminished effective volume and overflow) may not be mutually exclusive. Virtually all the available clinical studies of deranged sodium homeostasis in cirrhosis were carried out at a time when decompensation of liver disease and ascites were well established, with little information available during the incipient stage of sodium retention. The two ostensibly differing explanations may be reconciled by viewing the pathogenesis of abnormal sodium retention in cirrhosis as a complex clinical constellation in which differing forces participate in varying degrees as the derangements in sodium homeostasis evolve. Thus a primary defect in renal sodium handling may assume a more prominent role in the early stages of cirrhosis, and a diminished effective volume may constitute the major determinant of sodium retention in many patients once hepatic decompensation and ascites are established.

Efferent Factors

The initial attempts to explain the renal abnormalities responsible for sodium retention focused on the decrement in glomerular filtration rate (GFR) that occurs frequently in patients with advanced liver disease. A number of observations indicated, however, that a decrease in GFR cannot constitute the major determinant of the abnormalities in renal sodium handling, because sodium retention occurred despite normal or supranormal GFR. Thus renal sodium retention accompanying cirrhosis is due primarily to enhanced tubular reabsorption rather than to alterations in the filtered load of sodium. Avid reabsorption of filtrate along the proximal tubule is probably responsible in large part for the sodium retention of cirrhosis, but sodium reabsorption at more distal sites is also important.

The mediators for the enhanced tubular reabsorption of sodium in cirrhosis and their relative role in this process have not been elucidated completely. Several mechanism(s) have been suggested, including (a) hyperaldosteronism, (b) alterations in intrarenal blood flow distribution, (c) an increase in sympathetic nervous system activity, (d) alterations in the endogenous release of renal prostaglandins, (e) changes in the kallikrein-kinin system, (f) alterations in atrial natriuretic peptide (factor), and (g) modulation of a possible humoral natriuretic factor. These mechanism(s) and their interrelationships are summarized schematically in Figure 55.4.

Aldosterone. Cirrhosis is frequently associated with increased levels of aldosterone in the urine and plasma. The elevation of plasma aldosterone is attributable to both an increase in the adrenal secretion secondary to stimulation of the renin-angiotensin system and to a decrease in the metabolic degradation of the hormone. The rate of hepatic degradation is related directly to hepatic blood flow, which is markedly decreased in

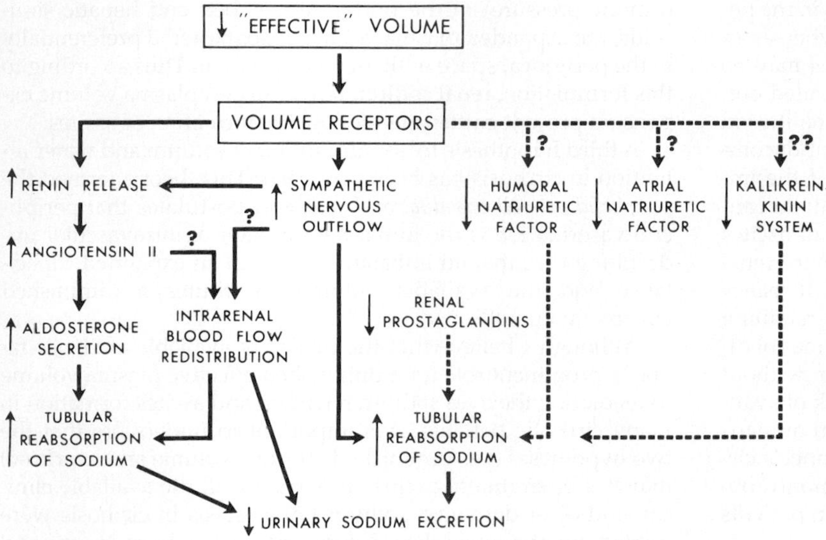

Figure 55.4. Schematic drawing of possible mechanisms whereby a diminished "effective" plasma volume results in sodium retention. The *heavy arrows* indicate pathways for which evidence is available. The *dashed lines* represent proposed pathways, the existence of which remains to be established. (Reproduced with permission from Epstein M. Renal sodium handling in liver disease. In: Epstein M, ed. *The kidney in liver disease,* 4th ed. Philadelphia: Hanley & Belfus, 1996:3–30.)

patients with decompensated cirrhosis. The etiologic relation between the hyperaldosteronism and the sodium retention encountered remains a subject of continuing debate. The traditional viewpoint holds that aldosterone is a major determinant of the sodium retention. However, many lines of evidence have demonstrated a dissociation between sodium excretion and plasma aldosterone under a number of experimental conditions, thereby challenging the predominance of elevated plasma aldosterone levels in mediating the sodium retention of cirrhosis. The model of head-out water immersion has been particularly illuminating in this regard. Water immersion results in a prompt and sustained increase in central blood volume comparable to the infusion of 2 L of isotonic saline without changes in plasma composition. When patients with cirrhosis who were receiving chronic spironolactone treatment were subjected to water immersion, marked natriuresis ensued. However, chronic spironolactone treatment alone produced only a modest increase in sodium excretion. The observations and the further demonstration of a dissociation between the suppression of circulating aldosterone and the absence of the natriuresis during water immersion favor the notion that hyperaldosteronism plays a permissive role in the sodium retention of cirrhosis, and the major factor underlying this abnormality is reduced distal delivery of filtrate.

Renal Prostaglandins

The possibility that prostaglandins participate in mediating the sodium retention of cirrhosis must be considered. Because both natriuretic and antinatriuretic effects of prostaglandins have been described, it is conceivable that alterations in renal prostaglandin synthesis may contribute to the derangements in renal handling of sodium in cirrhosis. The administration of agents that impair the synthesis of prostaglandins (e.g., indomethacin or ibuprofen) is associated with pronounced decrements in renal blood flow, GFR, and sodium excretion. Thus alterations in vasodilatory prostaglandins might best be viewed as playing an adaptive role, blunting the vasoconstrictive and antinatriuretic effects of activation of the renin-angiotensin axis and the sympathetic nervous system by the diminished effective volume that characterizes the decompensated cirrhotic state. There is little evidence to suggest that an alteration in renal prostaglandin synthesis plays a primary role in the sodium retention of cirrhosis.

Role of Atrial Natriuretic Peptide

Mammalian atria have been shown to contain potent natriuretic and vasoactive peptide(s), which have been referred to as *atrial natriuretic peptides* (ANPs) (see Chapter 13, Part 8).

In the light of several lines of evidence suggesting that stretch receptors residing in the atria may participate in regulating volume homeostasis, it is tempting to attribute a role to this peptide in modulating renal sodium handling in both normal subjects and those with edematous disorders. Specifically, the sodium retention and activation of the renin-angiotensin-aldosterone system in patients with cirrhosis may result from a failure to elaborate ANP. The blood level of ANP is normal or elevated in cirrhosis with ascites. The observations during studies with water immersion, in concert with the results of studies using ANP infusions in patients with cirrhosis, indicate that the sodium retention of cirrhosis may be related in part to a reduced renal responsiveness to ANP. It is conceivable that renal vasoconstriction mediated by diverse mechanisms, including activation of the renin-angiotensin axis and the sympathetic nervous system, impedes the ability of ANP to promote a natriuresis. The resistance to ANP action is most likely due to events beyond the coupling of the hormone to its renal receptor.

Other Humoral Natriuretic Factors

Several lines of evidence have suggested the possibility that a circulating natriuretic factor other than ANP constitutes a component part of the biologic control system regulating sodium excretion in humans. These natriuretic factors has been demonstrated in normal subjects during acute or chronic expansion of extracellular fluid volume, such as water immersion, saline infusion, or chronic mineralocorticoid administration. Thus deficiencies of these factors in cirrhosis might participate in the complex process leading to sodium retention (Fig. 55.4). Indeed, it was shown that plasma from cirrhotic patients neither altered sodium transport in epithelial membranes *in vitro* nor enhanced urine flow rate or sodium excretion in the rat. Taken together, these preliminary observations warrant additional studies to assess the possibility that a deficiency of a natriuretic factor plays a role in the pathogenesis of the sodium retention of cirrhosis.

Sympathetic Nervous System

The sympathetic nervous system is stimulated in decompensated cirrhosis and may play a role in enhancing the activity of the renin-angiotensin axis (Chapter 13, Part 3), as well as directly influencing renal tubular sodium handling (Chapter 5).

Studies with tracer kinetic techniques using radiolabeled norepinephrine have demonstrated that the elevated plasma norepinephrine concentrations in patients with cirrhosis are attributable to higher overall rates of spillover of the neurotransmitter to plasma and not to reduced plasma clearance caused by liver disease. The administration of clonidine reduced previously elevated norepinephrine overflow rates for the whole body, kidneys, and hepatomesenteric circulation. This sympathetic inhibition was accompanied by two potentially clinically beneficial effects: the lowering of renal vascular resistance and an augmentation of GFR.

Management of Ascites and Edema

Ascites is associated with many unwanted side effects in the patient with liver disease. Ascites enhances the two prime precipitants of variceal bleeding: high portal pressure, which predisposes to rupture of the varices, and gastroesophageal reflux, which may lead to the erosion of the varices. Furthermore, ascites is suggested to be the *sine qua non* of spontaneous bacterial peritonitis. Finally, the frequent association of ascites with the development of the hepatorenal syndrome raises the possibility that ascites may play an essential role in its pathogenesis. However, it should be emphasized that removal of ascites has not been demonstrated to increase life expectancy.

The approach to the cirrhotic patient with ascites should be grounded on the realization that ascites, unless massive, may not require treatment per se. The initial goal of any treatment program should be an attempt to obtain spontaneous diuresis by consistent and scrupulous adherence to rigid dietary sodium restriction (500 mg/day). Although the frequency with which such dietary management successfully relieves ascites is unsettled, such a diet should be prescribed for all patients because it is impossible to predict which patients will respond. When the response to dietary management is inadequate or when the imposition of rigid dietary sodium restriction is not feasible because of cost or unpalatability of the diet, the use of diuretic agents may be considered.

The rational basis for diuretic therapy lies in an understanding of the mechanism(s) and sites of action of the diuretic agent, coupled with an understanding of the pathophysiology of sodium retention in cirrhosis. Because the attributes and efficacy of varying diuretic agents are reviewed elsewhere in this book, I will focus solely on therapeutic considerations that are unique to the cirrhotic patient. When diuretics are used, the therapeutic aim is a slow and gradual diuresis not exceeding the capacity for mobilization of ascitic fluid. The decrease in the volume of ascites during spontaneous diuresis usually averages 300 to 500 ml/day with the maximum of 700 to 900 ml/day. Any diuresis that exceeds 900 ml/day in the patient with ascites but *without* edema occurs at the expense of the plasma compartment with resultant volume contraction. Therefore an appropriate goal of diuretic therapy is to achieve a negative fluid balance of about 700 ml/day in patients with ascites and no edema. In the presence of edema, greater losses, up to 1000 ml/day, can be well tolerated. The objectives may be achieved with the use of spironolactone, 100 to 400 mg/day. More potent diuretics, such as furosemide, should be used with caution because of enhanced risk of complications.

The hazards of diuretic use in patients with cirrhosis include hypokalemia, hyponatremia, impaired GFR, and encephalopathy. The danger of diuretic-associated hypokalemia should be emphasized. Because total body potassium depletion is frequently associated with cirrhosis, the use of any diuretic that acts proximal to the distal potassium secretory site may result in profound hypokalemia. Because of the frequently observed temporal relationship between diuretic therapy and the induction of hepatic encephalopathy and the probability that the enhanced renal ammonia production during hypokalemia may be related to the encephalopathy, great care should be exercised in monitoring potassium derangements in the cirrhotic patient who is receiving diuretics. The risk of hypokalemia is lessened but not eliminated by the sole or adjunctive use of potassium-sparing diuretics such as spironolactone or amiloride. The overriding consideration in diuretic therapy, however, is that its use for the sole indication of cosmetic improvement is contraindicated.

Paracentesis for diagnostic purposes (e.g., culture, cytology, or enzyme levels) is not contraindicated; however, controversy surrounds the question whether repeated removal of large volumes of ascitic fluid could be hazardous and may precipitate encephalopathy, volume depletion, and/or hepatorenal syndrome. Loss of protein with such repeated paracenteses may worsen the hypoalbuminemia often present in patients with decompensated cirrhosis. Because of the putative risk of hypovolemia, hyponatremia, renal failure, and encephalopathy, therapeutic paracentesis has not enjoyed much popularity in the treatment of refractory ascites. However, several groups of investigators have evaluated the effects of large-volume (4 to 15 L) paracentesis. The results of these studies suggest that therapeutic paracentesis can be used in the treatment of refractory ascites. In patients without peripheral edema, albumin infusions may be necessary to avoid concomitant decreases in renal function. The use of peritoneal–jugular shunts (LeVeen shunt) or other surgical procedures should be reserved for the relief of chronic intractable ascites. The morbidity and mortality associated with these procedures are high, and their long-term beneficial effects have not as yet been fully established in carefully controlled randomized trials.

RENAL WATER HANDLING IN CIRRHOSIS

Clinical Features

Impairment in renal excretion of free water occurs frequently in cirrhosis. Hyponatremia, the expression of this impaired capacity to excrete water, is a commonly encountered clinical problem in cirrhotic patients. Although it has been suggested that this abnormality may reflect the severity of the hepatic disease, the available data raise some difficulty in correlating the impairment of maximal water diuresis with a specified clinical feature, such as the degree of ascites or the level of jaundice.

Most patients with compensated liver disease excrete water normally, whereas those with decompensated hepatic illness manifest widely varying responses to oral water loading. Furthermore, prospective studies have indicated that the transition from compensation to decompensation, or vice versa, is not necessarily accompanied by concomitant changes in renal water handling.

Pathogenesis

The mechanism(s) responsible for the impairment of water diuresis in cirrhosis have not been fully established. Four factors have been implicated: (a) enhanced antidiuretic hormone (ADH) activity, (b) a decreased delivery of filtrate to the diluting segments of the nephron, (c) alterations in renal prostaglandins, and (d) an increase in sympathetic nervous system activity.

Increased ADH Activity

Several lines of evidence have suggested that the impairment in water excretion is attributable to increased levels of ADH, with a resultant increased back diffusion of free water in the collecting tubule. In 1956, Maurice Strauss demonstrated that the ingestion of alcohol increased urine flow and decreased urine osmolality in severely decompensated cirrhotic patients with normal GFR, raising the possibility that the alcohol inhibited the release of ADH. Further support for this contention is found in the demonstration that drugs interfering with the action of ADH on the kidney (e.g., demeclocycline) also augment the capacity to excrete water in patients with cirrhosis. Measurement of plasma levels of ADH with sensitive and specific radioimmunoassays has shown that patients with decompensated cirrhosis display a wide spectrum of ADH levels, varying from normal to elevated values. The factors underlying elevated plasma levels of ADH in cirrhosis include enhanced release secondary to a reduction in effective plasma volume, impaired degradation secondary to hepatocellular damage, or both. The frequency of elevations in plasma levels of ADH and their contribution to the impaired water handling in liver disease have not as yet been fully delineated.

Decreased Delivery of Filtrate to the Diluting Segments of the Nephron

The avid reabsorption of filtrate along the proximal tubule is responsible in great part for the impaired water diuresis of cirrhosis. The demonstration that free water generation is improved in some cirrhotic patients following extracellular fluid volume expansion with infusions of hypotonic saline, isotonic mannitol, or saline and albumin or by water immersion supports a role for increasing distal delivery of filtrate in the enhancement of water excretion. The concomitant suppression of endogenous ADH release during these maneuvers may also be a contributing factor.

Decreased Renal Prostaglandins

Evidence has pointed to an additional role of renal prostaglandins in mediating the water retention of cirrhosis. The overall action of prostaglandins appears to promote free water excretion. To the extent that there is a "relative" diminution of renal prostaglandins in cirrhosis, this may contribute to the renal water retention.

In summary, it is apparent that renal water retention in patients with advanced liver disease has a complex pathophysiology with numerous causes. The dissociation between elevated arginine vasopressin levels and the attendant changes in renal water handling under diverse experimental conditions and the demonstration of an impairment in renal water excretion in response to prostaglandin synthetase inhibition underscore the multifactorial nature of the derangement.

Treatment of Hyponatremia

An impaired diluting ability has important management implications for many patients with advanced liver disease. Because hyponatremia connotes a dilutional state secondary to an impaired capacity to excrete water, fluid restriction constitutes the basis for treatment. Appropriate fluid restriction will eventually repair this abnormality, regardless of the degree of dilutional impairment.

Unfortunately, this seemingly simple goal is often elusive. In many hospitals the physician's orders for fluid restriction are not always properly adhered to. Because paramedical and nursing personnel may not consider the fluids administered with medication as part of fluid intake, patients who are supposedly on rigid fluid restriction regimens may be receiving as much as 1,500 and even 2,000 ml of fluid/day. Because of this problem, it is sometimes necessary to resort to absolute fluid restriction (0 to 200 ml/day) for the first few days to initiate normalization of serum sodium.

A development that holds promise in the management of dilutional hyponatremia is the potential future availability of vasopressin receptor antagonists that act as specific water diuretic (aquaretic) agents.

SYNDROMES OF ACUTE AZOTEMIA

Acute renal failure occurs with increased frequency in patients with hepatic and biliary disease. Although acute azotemia may often represent classic acute renal failure, cirrhotic patients may also develop a unique form of renal failure called the hepatorenal syndrome, for which a specific cause cannot be elucidated.

Hepatorenal Syndrome

Progressive oliguric renal failure commonly complicates the course of advanced hepatic disease. Although this condition has been designated by any names including *functional renal failure* and *the renal failure of cirrhosis,* the more appealing, albeit less specific, term *hepatorenal syndrome* (HRS) has been used. HRS may be defined as unexplained renal failure occurring in patients with liver disease in the absence of clinical, laboratory, or anatomic evidence of other known causes of renal failure.

Clinical Features

The clinical manifestation and course of HRS are characterized by marked variability. HRS develops usually in patients who have advanced chronic hepatic failure and portal hypertension. Although this form of renal failure can complicate the course of virtually all forms of severe liver disease, most studies performed in the United States have identified alcoholic cirrhosis as the underlying disorder. In contrast, European reports describe postnecrotic, primary biliary, and idiopathic cirrhosis with greater frequency. These differences probably reflect the overall incidence patterns of those diseases in the specific populations studied rather than a specific predilection for the development of HRS. This syndrome may also develop in patients with acute hepatitis and hepatic malignancy.

Renal failure may develop with great rapidity, occasionally occurring in patients in whom normal GFR and concentrating ability were documented a few days before the onset of HRS. Although HRS may follow events that reduce effective blood volume, including abdominal paracentesis, vigorous diuretic therapy, and gastrointestinal bleeding, it can occur in the absence of an apparent precipitating factor. Patients with cirrhosis often develop HRS after admission to the hospital, raising the question whether events in the hospital might precipitate HRS. However, prehospital development of HRS also occurs. Generally, HRS develops in patients who have ascites (often tense) and other clinical stigmata of portal hypertension and chronic liver disease. Rarely, HRS can occur with little evidence of severe hepatic dysfunction.

Laboratory studies confirm the severity of hepatic disease. Prothrombin time is prolonged, serum albumin concentration is reduced, and bilirubin concentration is increased although the degree of jaundice is extremely variable. Most patients have a modest decrease in systemic blood pressure. Urine volume is reduced (less than 800 ml/day), oliguria is common (less than 400 ml/day), but anuria is rare. The serum creatinine and blood urea nitrogen (BUN) levels are elevated but seldom approach the high values seen in patients with end-stage renal failure re-

TABLE 55.4. Differential Diagnosis of Acute Azotemia in the Patient with Liver Disease: Important Differential Urinary Findings

	Prerenal Azotemia	Hepatorenal Syndrome	Acute Renal Failure
Urine sodium concentration (mEq/L)	<20	<10	>40
Urine:plasma creatinine ratio	>40.1	>40.1	<20:1
Urine:plasma osmolality ratio	>1.2	>1.2	1.0 ± 0.1
Urine sediment	Normal	Unremarkable	Casts, cellular debris

Adapted with permission from Epstein M. Hepatorenal Syndrome. In: Epstein M, ed. *The kidney in liver disease,* 4th Ed. Philadelphia: Hanley & Belfus, 1996:75–108.

sulting from primary renal disease. The degree of renal impairment is underestimated by our reliance on the BUN and serum creatinine concentrations as indices of renal function. These parameters are misleading because BUN levels tend to be depressed in cirrhotic patients owing to reduced protein intake from anorexia and limited hepatic synthesis of urea. Similarly, endogenous creatinine production declines as muscle wasting develops in protein-malnourished cirrhotic patients, thereby lowering serum creatinine concentration at any level of creatinine clearance. The urine is usually acid; mild proteinuria, granular casts, and microscopic hematuria are not infrequent. The urine is virtually free of sodium chloride (less than 10 mEq/L) and modestly concentrated (500 to 700 mOsm/kg H_2O). Occasionally, urine sodium concentrations of 20 to 30 mEq/L may be seen. This may be due to superimposed acute tubular necrosis (ATN) or acute metabolic alkalosis caused by vomiting; in the former, urinary chloride would be commensurate with that of sodium, while in the latter, urinary chloride would be low. Toward the end of the clinical course, urinary sodium excretion may increase and urine osmolality decrease toward isotonicity, probably as a result of superimposed ATN. Urinary lysozyme, a marker of tubule cell injury, is also low in contrast to the levels in typical ATN. Data regarding fractional sodium excretion are not generally available, although in the author's experience, these indices are typical of prerenal azotemia (Table 55.4).

The prognosis of HRS is grave. The majority of patients die within a few weeks of onset of azotemia, although 5% to 10% of the patients may survive several months of mild azotemia. Complete recovery in those with advanced renal failure is rare.

Pathogenesis

Several lines of evidence have lent strong support to the concept that the renal failure in HRS is functional in nature. Despite the severe derangement of renal function, pathologic abnormalities are minimal and inconsistent. Furthermore, tubular functional integrity is maintained during the renal failure as manifested by a relatively unimpaired sodium reabsorptive capacity and concentrating ability. Finally, more direct evidence is derived from the demonstration that kidneys transplanted from patients with HRS are capable of resuming normal function in the recipient.

Despite extensive study, the precise pathogenesis of HRS remains obscure. Many studies using diverse hemodynamic techniques have all documented a significant reduction in renal perfusion. Because a similar reduction of renal perfusion is compatible with urine volumes exceeding 1 L/day in many patients with chronic renal failure, it is unlikely that a reduction in mean blood flow per se is responsible for the oliguria encountered.

In our laboratory, the ^{133}Xe washout technique and selective renal arteriography have been applied to the study of HRS, and we have demonstrated a significant reduction in both calculated mean blood flow and preferential reduction in cortical perfusion. In addition, cirrhotic patients manifested marked vasomotor instability that was characterized not only by variability between serial xenon washout studies but also by instability within a single curve. This phenomenon has not been encountered in renal failure of other origins. Selective renal arteriograms disclosed marked beading and tortuosity of the interlobar and proximal arcuate arteries and an absence of both distinct cortical nephrograms and of vascular filling of the cortical vessels (Fig. 55.5A). Postmortem angiography carried out on the kidneys of five patients studied previously during life disclosed a striking normalization of the vascular abnormalities (Fig. 55.5B). These findings provide additional strong evidence for the functional basis of the renal failure, operating through active renal vasoconstriction.

Although renal hypoperfusion with preferential renal cortical ischemia has been shown to underlie the renal failure of HRS, the factors responsible for sustaining the reductions in cortical perfusion and the suppression of glomerular filtration in HRS have not been elucidated. Several major factors have been implicated, including (a) activation of the renin-angiotensin system, (b) an increase in renal sympathetic nervous system activity, (c) alterations in the endogenous release of renal prostaglandins, (d) changes in the kallikrein-kinin system, and (e) endotoxemia. These proposed mechanisms and their interrelationships are summarized schematically in (Fig. 55.6).

Renin-Angiotensin System. Patients with decompensated cirrhosis with or without HRS frequently manifest marked elevations of plasma renin activity attributable to both decreased hepatic inactivation of renin and to increased renin secretion by the kidney (Fig. 55.7). Often, the elevation of plasma renin activity occurs despite the presumed failure of hepatic synthesis of the α_2-globulin renin substrate. There are at least two alternative explanations for the persistence of high plasma renin activity in cirrhosis. First, the renal hypoperfusion may be the primary event with a resultant activation of the renin-angiotensin system. Alternatively, the activation of the renin-angiotensin system, perhaps in response to diminished effective blood volume, may constitute the main pathogenetic factor. In the light of compelling experimental evidence that angiotensin II plays an important role in the control of the renal circulation, it is tempting to speculate that elevated plasma angiotensin II levels contribute to the renal vasoconstriction and reduction in GFR of renal failure in cirrhosis (Fig. 55.7).

Renal Prostaglandins. The role of prostaglandins in the genesis of HRS is not established. Inhibition of the synthesis of vasodilatory prostaglandins with indomethacin or ibuprofen is followed by a marked decline in GFR in many patients with cirrhosis and ascites. This raises the possibility that a relative diminution in the levels of renal prostaglandins may be involved in the development of HRS. The renal synthesis of vasoconstricting prostaglandins (thromboxanes) is increased in cirrhosis with ascites, and it may play a role in HRS.

Endotoxins. Systemic endotoxemia in patients with cirrhosis might result from incomplete hepatic inactivation and/or portal-systemic shunting of material originating in the gastrointestinal tract of the patients. A high frequency of positive *Limulus* assays for circulating endotoxins has been observed in patients with cirrhosis and renal failure, but not in those without renal failure. Thus endotoxins might contribute to the

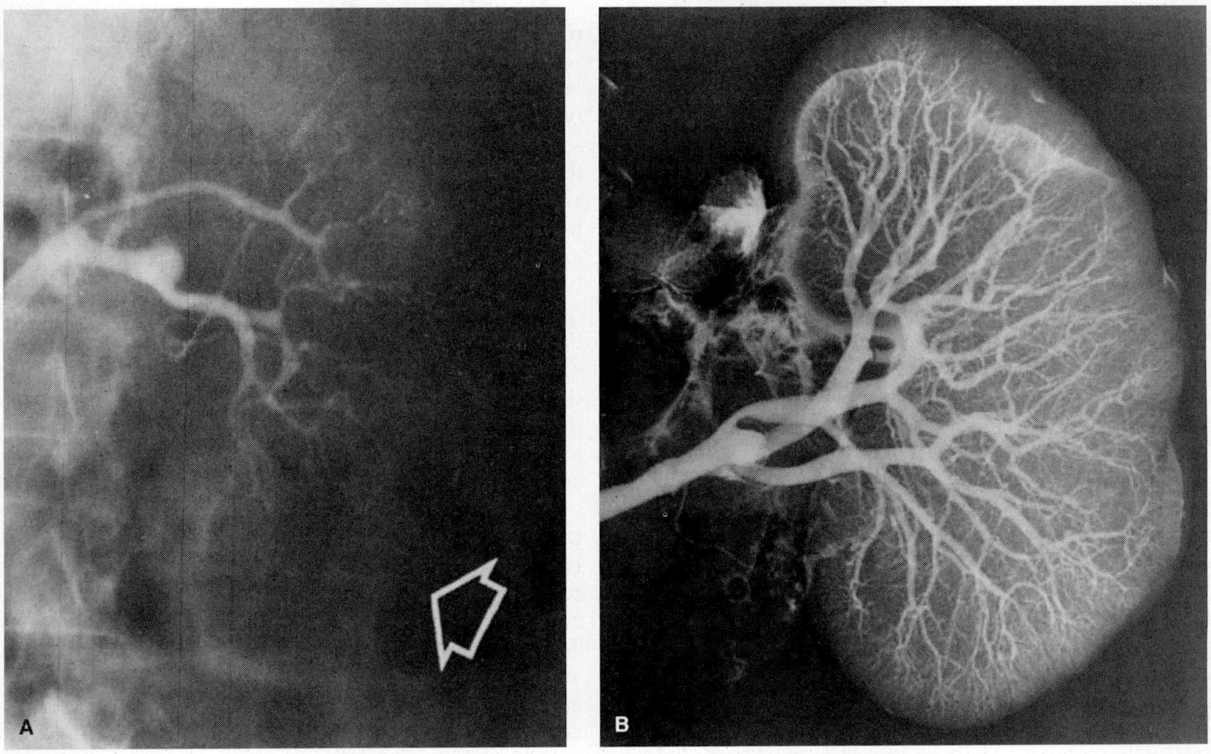

Figure 55.5. **A:** Selective renal arteriogram carried out in a patient with oliguric renal failure and cirrhosis. Note the extreme abnormality of the intrarenal vessels including the primary branches off the main renal artery and the interlobar arteries. The arcuate and cortical arterial system is not recognizable, nor is a distinct cortical nephrogram present. The *arrow* indicates the edge of the kidney. **B:** Angiogram carried out at postmortem examination on the same kidney, with the intraarterial injection of Micropaque in gelatin as the contrast agent. Note the filling of the renal arterial system throughout the vascular bed to the periphery of the cortex. The vascular attenuation and tortuosity are no longer present. The vessels were also histologically normal. (**A** and **B** reproduced with permission from Epstein M, Berk DP, Hollenberg NK, et al. Renal failure in the patient with cirrhosis. The role of active vasoconstriction. *Am J Med* 1970;49:175–185.)

pathogenesis of HRS. In light of the florid systemic hemodynamic disturbances that accompany the HRS, including a hyperdynamic circulation, increased heart rate and cardiac output, and decreased blood pressure and systemic vascular resistance, attention has focused on the role of nitric oxide (NO) as a mediator of these changes. An inducible NO synthase that occurs in response to bacterial lipopolysaccharide endotoxin releases NO for many hours. It has been postulated that the induction of this synthase may cause the vasodilation of endotoxemia and that inhibition of NO synthesis should restore

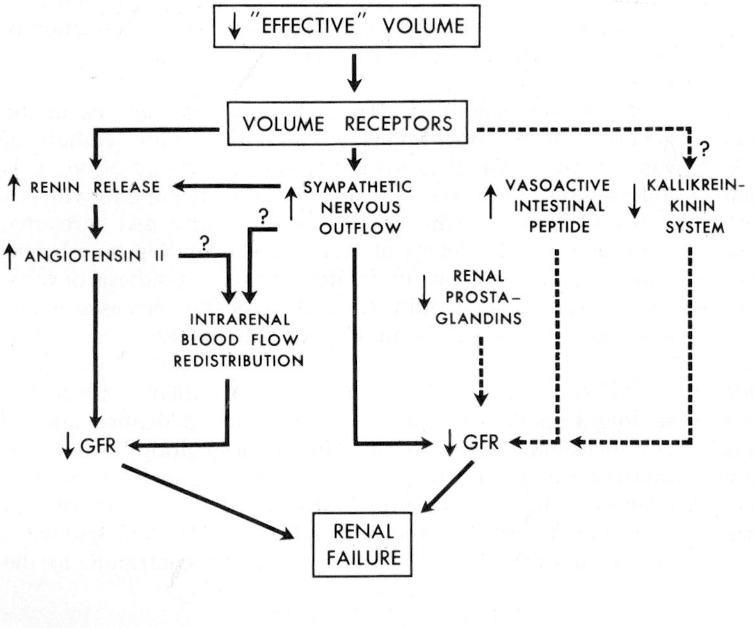

Figure 55.6. Schematic representation of possible mechanisms whereby a diminished "effective" plasma volume might modulate a number of hormonal effectors, resulting in renal failure. The *heavy arrows* indicate pathways for which evidence is available. The *dashed lines* represent proposed pathways, the existence of which remains to be established. GFR, glomerular filtration rate. Adapted with permission from Epstein M. Hepatorenal Syndrome. In: Epstein M, ed. *The kidney in liver disease,* 4th Ed. Philadelphia: Hanley & Belfus, 1996:75–108.

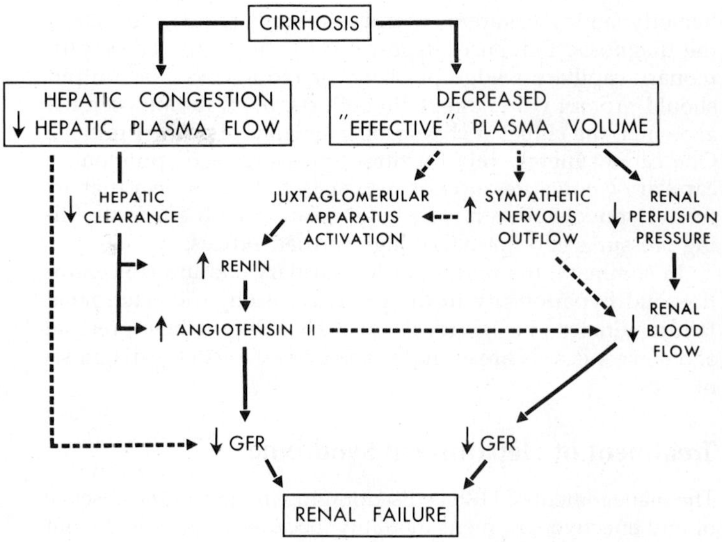

Figure 55.7. Schematic drawing of probable mechanisms whereby the renin-angiotensin system and the sympathetic nervous system interact to produce renal failure. Both a diminished "effective" plasma volume and impaired hepatic clearance of renin-angiotensin result in a marked enhancement of circulating plasma renin activity with a resultant decrease in glomerular filtration rate *(GFR)*. An increase in sympathetic nervous system activity (attributable primarily to decreased effective plasma volume) decreases GFR both by diminishing renal perfusion and by activating the renin-angiotensin system. (Reproduced with permission from Epstein M, ed. *The kidney in liver disease,* ed 3. Baltimore: Williams & Wilkins, 1988:100.)

sensitivity to vasoconstrictors and reverse these hemodynamic abnormalities. Proof of this hypothesis is, as yet, not available.

Endothelin. In the past one and one-half decades endothelins (ETs) have emerged as an important new peptide family in the hormonal regulation of body fluid and cardiovascular homeostasis (see Chapter 13, Part 5). During the past few years increasing attention has been focused on the possibility that alterations in ETs may play a pathogenetic role in the renal failure of the HRS. Several investigators have reported that patients with HRS had markedly elevated plasma ET-1 and ET-3 concentrations compared with normal subjects, patients having acute or chronic renal failure, and patients with liver disease without renal dysfunction. Although such findings are consistent with the pathogenetic role of ET, it is equally possible if not probable that the results merely represent *pari passu* events. The recent availability of several chemically diverse ET antagonists, including agents that block the generation of ET and agents that antagonize its binding to cellular receptors, provides an opportunity for using such pharmacologic probes in delineating the pathogenetic role of ET.

Acute Renal Failure (Synonym: Acute Tubular Necrosis)

Although much attention has been directed to HRS, it should be borne in mind that cirrhotic patients are no less vulnerable than noncirrhotic patients to the development of ATN. Renal failure occurring in patients with cirrhosis is more commonly due to ATN than to HRS. The increased frequency of ATN may relate to the hypotension, bleeding dyscrasias, infection, and multiple metabolic disorders that complicate the course of cirrhosis. In addition, jaundice may predispose to ATN. The incidence of ATN in patients undergoing surgery for relief of obstructive jaundice is many times greater than that in a comparable group of nonjaundiced patients undergoing abdominal surgery. It also appears that the more severe the jaundice, the greater the risk of ATN. Experimental data suggest that an increase in the level of circulating conjugated bilirubin is responsible for the predisposition to ATN. In addition, studies of the metabolic and renal tubular effects of bile fractions (using both *in vivo* and *in vitro* techniques) indicate that a nephrotoxin may also be retained in obstructive jaundice. The clinical and biochemical features of ATN accompanying cirrhosis are not different from those of ATN in patients without cirrhosis.

Differential Diagnosis of Acute Azotemia in Cirrhosis

The abrupt onset of oliguria and azotemia in a cirrhotic patient does not necessarily imply the presence of HRS. Prerenal causes of oliguria and azotemia should be excluded, particularly because they constitute reversible conditions if recognized and treated in the incipient phase of renal failure. Volume contraction or cardiac failure may manifest as a "pseudohepatorenal" syndrome. It is important to search for clinical clues such as decreased tissue turgor, orthostatic hypotension, jugular venous distention, gallop rhythm, cardiomegaly, and pulmonary rales. It should also be emphasized that patients with alcoholic cirrhosis commonly develop oliguria and azotemia as a result of classic ATN of either ischemic or nephrotoxic origin. In many instances the differentiation from HRS can readily be made by recognition of the precipitating event and by characteristic laboratory findings. Laboratory features helpful in differentiating the three principal causes of acute azotemia in the patient with liver disease are listed in Table 55.4. The most uniform finding in the urine of HRS patients is a strikingly low sodium concentration, usually less than 10 mEq/L, and occasionally as low as 2 to 5 mEq/L. Similarly, prerenal azotemia is associated with low urinary sodium concentrations. In contrast, patients with oliguric ATN frequently have urinary sodium concentrations exceeding 30 mEq/L and usually even higher. Both HRS and prerenal azotemia manifest well-maintained urinary concentrating ability characterized by a urine-to-plasma osmolality ratio exceeding 1.0, whereas ATN patients excrete an isoosmotic urine. The urine-to-plasma creatinine ratio is more than 30:1 in both prerenal failure and HRS, whereas it is less than 20:1 in ATN. Proteinuria is absent or minimal in HRS.

Differentiation of HRS from prerenal azotemia may be extremely difficult. As previously noted, the presence of advanced liver disease frequently blurs the distinction between HRS and prerenal azotemia. Under these circumstances, hemodynamic measurements are commonly required to clarify the diagnosis. Evidence of postural hypotension, a low pulmonary capillary wedge pressure, or reduced cardiac output should prompt volume repletion efforts. In excluding prerenal azotemia, the clinician should be cognizant of several pitfalls. One cannot merely rely on filling pressures (i.e., pulmonary capillary wedge pressure) or cardiac indices. It is clear that arterial hypovolemia can exist in association with adequate filling pressures and normal or high cardiac indices.

In summary, the finding of low urinary sodium concentration and hypertonicity in the presence of oliguric acute renal failure vitiates the diagnosis of ATN. Only when prerenal azotemia and ATN are excluded can one establish the diagnosis of HRS.

Treatment of Hepatorenal Syndrome

The management of HRS is discouraging in view of the absence of any effective treatment modality. Because knowledge about the pathogenesis of HRS is inferential and incomplete, therapy is empirical and supportive. The initial step is not to equate decreased renal function with HRS, but rather to search diligently for and treat correctable causes of azotemia such as volume contraction, cardiac decompensation, and urinary tract obstruction. Because HRS and prerenal azotemia have similar urinary diagnostic indices, one must often use a functional maneuver (i.e., administration of volume expanders) to differentiate between these two entities. In this regard, it should be underscored that our frame of reference for the cirrhotic patient may be quite different from that of other disease states. The degree of volume expansion necessary for repletion of the cirrhotic patient may at times be marked, occasionally requiring the infusion of massive amounts of colloids. The diagnosis of ATN should be considered because the cirrhotic patient with ATN may recover if supported with dialytic therapy.

Once the correctable causes of renal functional impairment are excluded, the mainstay of therapy is careful restriction of sodium and fluid intake. Although a number of specific therapeutic measures have been attempted, none has proved to be of practical value. Attempts to expand volume with different colloid or crystalloid solutions have resulted in only transient improvement in renal hemodynamics and function without significant improvement in the outcome. Similarly, attempts for reinfusion of ascites using peritoneal fluid that has been concentrated have not provided any lasting improvement.

Dialysis has been reported to be ineffective in the management of HRS. Increasing experience, however, suggests that such a sweeping condemnation should be qualified. Although most of the early published literature indeed suggested a dismal prognosis for patients who undergo dialysis, such reports dealt with patients who had chronic end-stage liver disease. In a few instances, dialysis was performed in patients with HRS who had *acute* hepatic disease with an ultimately favorable outcome. These observations indicate that in patients with acute hepatic dysfunction in whom there is reason to believe that renal failure may reverse with resolution of the acute hepatic insult, dialytic therapy is indicated. The role of dialysis has been expanding dramatically as a supportive measure for patients awaiting hepatic transplantation.

More than 20 years ago, there was a flurry of enthusiasm for the use of the peritoneal–jugular shunt (LeVeen shunt) in the management of HRS. Because the underlying abnormality is thought to be maldistribution of extracellular fluid with a resultant diminished effective blood volume, attention has focused on developing procedures that can redistribute body fluids between compartments, so that the central compartment is replenished at a time when ascites is decreasing. Unfortunately, based on the available data, the peritoneal–venous (PV) shunt does not favorably alter survival in patients with HRS.

Transjugular Intrahepatic Portosystemic Shunt

Few anecdotal reports have appeared describing improvement in renal function in patients with HRS following insertion of a transjugular intrahepatic portosystemic shunt (TIPS). The rationale for this procedure is similar to that for the establishment of a side-to-side portacaval shunt: to create a portal to the systemic vascular pathway that decompresses the portacaval system. Although a TIPS obviates the need for performing major vascular surgery, insertion of a TIPS is not a simple and innocuous procedure as some of its adherents suggest. A skilled and experienced interventional radiologist is needed for successful insertion of a TIPS. It should also be noted that the available data consist in great part of a few preliminary and anecdotal reports.

Orthotopic Liver Transplantation

Orthotopic liver transplantation (OLTX) has become the accepted treatment for end-stage liver disease. Of interest, many of these patients have varying degrees of concomitant renal dysfunction, including HRS. OLTX has been reported to reverse HRS acutely. A review of the extensive experience of the Baylor University transplant group reported good, long-term survival with return of acceptable renal function for prolonged periods. Of more than 800 patients undergoing transplantation in Dallas, 59 had HRS. Of the patients surviving liver transplant, 4 required subsequent renal transplant for nonreturn of function. Of the remaining patients without HRS (more than 650), 2 required subsequent kidney transplant. The results from Dallas and other centers clearly indicate that patients with HRS have good survival rates following liver transplant but that the rates are statistically inferior compared with patients without HRS. These investigators concluded that with aggressive pre- and posttransplant management, one could anticipate good survival rates following OLTX in patients with HRS.

There has been renewed interest in the florid hemodynamic derangements and attempts to improve renal function by countervailing this hyperdynamic state. The effects of infusion of ornipressin on renal and circulatory function and preliminary data showed that ornipressin reversed the hyperdynamic state. Concomitantly there was improvement in renal function as assessed by more than 70% increase in creatinine clearance and doubling in urine flow. These preliminary observations lend support to the concept that the peripheral vasodilation of liver disease has an important contribution to the renal dysfunction. Consequently, maneuvers that counter the vasodilation may possibly prove to be beneficial in improving renal function.

Figure 55.8 summarizes my recommended approach to the management of acute renal failure in cirrhosis. As discussed above, the three important diagnostic considerations are prerenal azotemia, ATN, and HRS. Thus FE_{Na^+} or the urinary sodium concentration in a spot urine specimen and the pulmonary capillary wedge pressure (PCWP) or the central venous pressure (CVP) may help to distinguish among these diagnostic possibilities. There is, however, considerable overlap between the three categories, and more than one diagnosis may be applicable to a given patient. For example, patients with HRS often exhibit ATN, and HRS and prerenal failure often coexist. In fact, the response to colloid infusion is the only feature that helps differentiate the latter two conditions. Of note, because of the low pe-

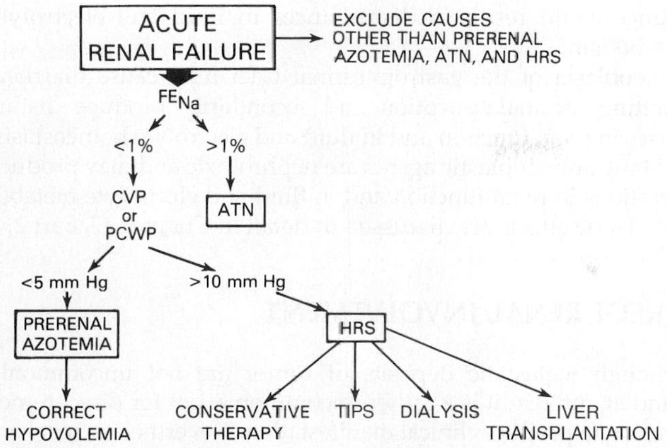

Figure 55.8. Algorithm for the evaluation and the management of a cirrhotic patient with acute renal failure. Abbreviations are explained in text. (Reproduced with permission from Epstein M, ed. *The kidney in liver disease,* ed 3. Baltimore: Williams & Wilkins, 1988:89–117.)

ripheral resistance associated with cirrhosis, volume expansion frequently does not result in a marked increase in CVP or PCWP. Intensive hemodialysis and/or hemoperfusion therapy is indicated for the management of HRS complicating acute (reversible) liver injury. In patients with chronic cirrhosis, dialysis therapy may maintain the patient's condition until a suitable liver donor is found. Otherwise, good-risk patients may be treated by TIPS insertion.

GLOMERULAR CHANGES IN LIVER DISEASE

Glomerular changes occur primarily in patients with cirrhosis and acute and chronic viral hepatitis.

Cirrhosis

The first report of glomerular changes in patients with cirrhosis of the liver appeared more than 30 years ago. Subsequent studies have demonstrated that glomerular changes are quite common in these patients, and both proliferative and nonproliferative abnormalities occur.

The changes *without proliferation* are characterized by sclerosis and an increase in mesangial matrix. Electron microscopy reveals electron-dense deposits that are mainly mesangial but frequently extend into the subendothelial space. IgA is the main immunoglobulin in the glomerular deposits, often accompanied by IgG and/or IgM. These glomerular changes are usually not associated with urinary abnormalities. However, some of these patients may have proteinuria, microscopic hematuria, or both.

Glomerular changes *with proliferation* are characterized by slight mesangial hypercellularity, endocapillary and extracapillary proliferation, and mesangial interposition, giving a pattern similar to that of membranoproliferative glomerulonephritis. IgA is the major immunoglobulin in the deposits. Patients with endocapillary proliferation have a clinical picture similar to that of acute glomerulonephritis, whereas those with membranoproliferative alterations may have no urinary abnormalities or may have proteinuria and microscopic hematuria. Although it is possible for a patient with cirrhosis to develop *de novo* glomerulonephritis, the available evidence suggests that the glomerular changes in these patients are usually related to the liver dysfunction.

VIRAL HEPATITIS

In most patients with acute viral hepatitis, renal function is only mildly impaired. The most common findings include a modest degree of proteinuria, hematuria, and a mild reduction in GFR. The concentrating ability is usually unimpaired in these patients. Renal biopsy specimens from patients with acute viral hepatitis reveal mild proliferative glomerulonephritis. Immunofluorescence studies disclose the presence of IgG, IgM, and complement as discrete nodular deposits. Electron microscopy demonstrates the presence of dense deposits, primarily near the mesangial areas. In most of these patients, GFR will return to normal and proteinuria will disappear after recovery from hepatitis.

In contrast, more severe impairment of renal function has been reported in patients with persistent HB_sAg antigenemia associated with chronic active hepatitis. The characteristic glomerular lesion in such patients with progressive deterioration of renal function has been a membranoproliferative glomerulonephritis or membranous glomerulopathy. Clinically, these patients demonstrate proteinuria, nephrotic syndrome, or renal failure. The renal lesions associated with HB_sAg hepatitis are due to an immune complex-mediated glomerulonephritis. The severity of the renal lesion and its accompanying clinical disease may depend on the duration of HB_sAg antigenemia. The prognosis of the glomerulonephritis in patients with persistent HB_sAg has not as yet been defined, but the disease tends to be progressive. The glomerular changes in viral hepatitis are discussed in detail in Chapter 39, Part 3B.

ABNORMALITIES OF RENAL ACIDIFICATION

Defects in renal acidification are seen in many patients with chronic liver disease. Distal renal tubular acidosis of the complete or incomplete type is encountered, particularly in autoimmune liver disease (e.g., primary biliary cirrhosis), but the complete form with systemic hyperchloremic acidosis is not common in patients with Laënnec's cirrhosis. This is attributable in part to low rates of excretion of both creatinine and phosphate, which in turn may be the result of the diminished protein intake and reduced muscular mass in these patients. The sequelae of renal tubular acidosis in chronic liver disease may include nephrolithiasis, nephrocalcinosis, osteomalacia, and potassium wasting. It has been suggested that the acidification impairment enhances the susceptibility of patients with liver disease to hepatic encephalopathy by diverting ammonia from the inappropriately alkaline urine to the blood.

Selected Readings

Epstein M. Derangements of renal water handling in liver disease. *Gastroenterology* 1985;89:1415–1425.
A comprehensive review of deranged water homeostasis in liver disease.

Epstein M. Renal prostaglandins and the control of renal function in liver disease. *Am J Med* 1986;80(Suppl 1A):46–55.
A review of the pathogenetic role of derangements in renal prostaglandins in mediating the renal complications of liver disease.

Epstein M. Hepatorenal syndrome: emerging perspective of pathophysiology and therapy. *J Am Soc Nephrol* 1994;4:1735–1753.
A comprehensive recent review of emerging perspectives of pathophysiology and therapy of patients with HRS.

Epstein M. Renal sodium handling in liver disease. In: Epstein M, ed. *The kidney in liver disease,* 4th ed. Philadelphia: Hanley & Belfus, 1996:1–31.
A comprehensive review of the clinical features and pathogenesis of deranged sodium homeostasis in liver disease.

Epstein M. Hepatorenal syndrome. In: Epstein M, ed. *The kidney in liver disease,* 4th ed. Philadelphia: Hanley & Belfus, 1996:75–108.
A comprehensive recent review of emerging perspectives of pathophysiology, and therapy of patients with HRS.

Epstein M. Atrial natriuretic factor and liver disease. In: Epstein M, ed. *The kidney in liver disease,* 4th ed. Philadelphia: Hanley & Belfus, 1996:339–358.
A definitive review of the topic.
Epstein M. Role of peritoneovenous shunt in the management of ascites and the hepatorenal syndrome. In: Epstein M, ed. *The kidney in liver disease,* 4th ed. Philadelphia: Hanley & Belfus, 1996:491–506.
A definitive review of the topic.
Epstein M, Berk DP, Hollenberg NK, et al. Renal failure in the patient with cirrhosis. The role of active vasoconstriction. *Am J Med* 1970;49:175–185.
A classic paper delineating the florid renal hemodynamic derangements in HRS.
Epstein M, Goligorsky MS. Endothelin and nitric oxide in hepatorenal syndrome: a balance reset. *J Nephrol* 1997;10:120–135.
An in-depth and critical review of the possible pathogenic role of endothelin and nitric oxide in mediating the renal dysfunction of liver disease.
Epstein M, Levinson R, Sancho J, et al. Characterization of the renin-aldosterone system in decompensated cirrhosis. *Circ Res* 1977;41:818–829.
An in-depth study of renin-aldosterone responsiveness in decompensated cirrhosis, providing important insights into the role of this hormonal system in mediating sodium retention.
Esler M, Dudley F, Jennings G, et al. Increased sympathetic nervous activity and the effects of its inhibition with clonidine in alcoholic cirrhosis. *Ann Intern Med* 1992;116:446–455.
An in-depth study of sympathetic nervous system activation in cirrhosis applying tracer kinetic techniques.
Perez GO, Golper TA, Epstein M, et al. Dialysis, hemofiltration and other extracorporeal techniques in the treatment of the renal complications of liver disease. In: Epstein M, ed. *The kidney in liver disease,* 4th ed. Philadelphia: Hanley & Belfus, 1996:517–528.
A contemporary review of the spectrum of extracorporeal techniques that may be needed to successfully manage patients with liver disease who have sodium retention and renal failure.
Shear L, Ching S, Gabuzda GJ. Compartmentalization of ascites and edema in patients with hepatic cirrhosis. *N Engl J Med* 1970;282:1391–1396.
A classic study of the compartmentalization of ascites and its relevance to rational diuretic therapy.
Warner L, Skorecki K, Blendis LM, et al. Atrial natriuretic factor in liver disease. *Hepatology* 1993;17:500–513.
A recent comprehensive review of atrial natriuretic factor in decompensated cirrhosis, providing important insights into the role of this hormonal system in mediating sodium retention.

PART 3
Neoplasia

Shaul G. Massry, Richard J. Glassock, and Miroslaw Smogorzewski

Neoplastic disorders may affect the kidney, urinary tract, and fluid and electrolyte homeostasis in a variety of ways. These neoplasia-associated disorders can be broadly categorized as parenchymal renal disease, urinary tract obstruction, fluid and electrolyte disturbances resulting from excess or deficiency of hormones, disturbances in gastrointestinal tract function, and nephrotoxicity from antineoplastic therapy.

The renal parenchymal disease could arise from (a) invasion of the renal parenchyma by distant malignancy or extension of primary renal neoplasia into the renal venous supply; (b) deposition within glomeruli of tumor-associated antigen–antibody complexes or amyloid, leading to nephrotic syndrome; or (c) nephrotic syndrome and minimal change disease possibly caused by elaboration of a permeability factor from deranged neoplastic cells, most commonly lymphoid cells.

Obstructive nephropathy may arise from (a) extrinsic compression of the urinary tract by pelvic or retroperitoneal tumors or metastasis of distant tumors, (b) intrinsic urinary tract tumor, or (c) intranephronal obstruction from deposition of crystals or protein aggregates.

Many tumors produce excessive amounts of various hormones, and neoplasia may destroy endocrine glands (e.g., pituitary and adrenal). The consequent changes in the hormonal balance could result in disturbances in fluid and electrolyte metabolism.

Neoplasia of the gastrointestinal tract may cause diarrhea, vomiting, or malabsorption and secondarily produce disturbances in renal function and in fluid and electrolyte homeostasis.

Many antineoplastic agents are nephrotoxic and may produce alterations in renal function and in fluid and electrolyte metabolism. These effects are discussed in detail in Chapter 47, Part 2.

DIRECT RENAL INVOLVEMENT

Although metastatic deposits of tumor are not uncommonly found at autopsy, it is a rather uncommon event for direct tumor invasion to produce clinical manifestation. Nevertheless, renal enlargement, pain, urinary abnormalities, and even renal failure may be observed, particularly with leukemia, lymphoma, and Hodgkin's disease and in aggressive B-cell lymphomas found in patients with acquired immunodeficiency syndrome. Such renal involvement may be unilateral or bilateral and is often accompanied by hepatomegaly. Treatment of the neoplastic condition (e.g., x-ray therapy or chemotherapy) may cause some improvement, but secondary fibrosis may ultimately lead to irreversible impairment of renal function. Renal cell carcinoma may produce acute renal failure as a result of invasion of both renal veins. Metastatic disease of the kidney of nonrenal origin is usually not associated with clinical renal manifestations, but at times a palpable mass may be found and hematuria may be present. Carcinoma of the breast metastasizes to the kidney and around the ureters.

INDIRECT RENAL INVOLVEMENT

Impairment of renal venous drainage by extrinsic compression from retroperitoneal tumors may occur. As noted above renal cell carcinoma may also invade one or both renal veins and lead to acute renal failure. Ureteric, bladder, or urethral involvement leading to obstruction in urinary flow is dealt with elsewhere. The etiology, diagnosis, consequences, and management of urinary tract obstruction are discussed in detail in Chapter 50.

GLOMERULAR DISEASES

The association between various malignant and benign neoplasms and glomerular diseases was first suggested by Gallaway in 1922 and since then several hundred case reports and collected series have confirmed this relationship. Although a cause and effect relationship has been established for some of the instances of malignancy in glomerular disease, many of the data simply point to an association without defining the mechanism. The strongest evidence for a cause and effect relationship is the contemporaneous appearance of glomerular lesions concomitantly with malignancy and the resolution of glomerular disease with eradication or substantial control of the tumor. Relapse of glomerular disease with recurrence of the neoplastic process provides further proof of the intimate relationship between tumor growth and glomerular disease. The presumed mechanisms underlying this association are varied. In some instances relapse is clearly associated to glomerular deposition of tumor-associated antigen-containing immune complexes. Indeed, in several patients with malignancy and membranous glomerulonephritis, immune complexes composed of antigens such as carcinoembryonic antigen and antibodies have been reported in the basement membrane of the glomeruli. Also vascular permeability factors elaborated by the tumor itself or

TABLE 55.5. Types of Glomerular Diseases Associated with Malignancy

Type of Tumor	Type of Glomerular Disease
Lymphomas and leukemias	
Hodgkin's lymphoma	Majority with minimal change disease; few cases of membranoproliferative or crescentic glomerulonephritis, IgA nephropathy, or glomerulosclerosis
Non-Hodgkin's lymphoma	Same as Hodgkin's lymphoma but membranous glomerulonephritis is more common
Leukemias	Same as Hodgkin's lymphoma
Solid tumors	
Bronchogenic, gastrointestinal, breast, thyroid, head, and neck, genitourinary, kidney, pheochromocytoma, neuroblastoma, mesothelioma, malignant melanoma, and Wilms tumor	Almost always membranous glomerulonephritis but occasionally minimal change disease, IgA nephropathy, or membranoproliferative glomerulonephritis
Multiple myeloma[a]	Amyloid type AL, membranoproliferative and mesangioproliferative glomerulopathy, crescentic glomerulonephritis, and occasionally minimal change disease

[a] The renal involvement in multiple myeloma is discussed in detail in Chapter 42, Part 12.

infiltrating cells have been proposed. The nature of the latter factors is largely unknown. Amyloidosis is another mechanism through which malignancy may cause glomerular disease. The various types of glomerular diseases associated with malignancy are listed in Table 55.5.

Clinical Presentation

The clinical presentation of the glomerular diseases associated with malignant tumors is usually the nephrotic syndrome. The latter may precede the clinical presentation of the malignant tumor. It should be mentioned, however, that proteinuria and nephrotic syndrome are rare in patients with malignant tumors (about 1%). In contrast, the prevalence of malignancy in patients with nephrotic syndrome could be as high as 20%. Therefore there is no benefit to screening all patients with malignancy for proteinuria, but it may be prudent to investigate certain patients with nephrotic syndrome for the potential presence of a malignant disease. We stated in 1991 that "Patients over the age of 50 years with nephrotic syndrome in whom membranous glomerulonephritis is demonstrated by renal biopsy should be scrutinized carefully for underlying carcinoma, especially that of the lung, stomach, colon, or breast." It is our opinion that such patients should have a thorough medical history, careful physical examination, blood chemistry evaluation, chest radiograph, and cancer screening procedures such cancer markers, occult blood, flexible sigmoidoscopy if occult blood test is positive, abdominal ultrasound, and mammography. Even if these results of these tests are negative, the patient should be followed carefully. Occasionally, renal insufficiency, acute renal failure, and rapidly progressive glomerulonephritis may be the presentation of the renal disease associated with malignancy.

Glomerular Diseases in Lymphomas and Leukemias

By far the most common lymphoma associated with glomerular disease in the past has been Hodgkin's disease. The most common clinical manifestation is nephrotic syndrome, and the most common underlying glomerular lesion is minimal change disease. Numerous case reports describing this association can be found in the literature; however, the incidence of glomerular lesions in Hodgkin's disease has been decreasing for several decades, and at the present time it is an exceedingly rare event. It is likely that the decreasing incidence of glomerular lesions in Hodgkin's disease is a reflection of earlier recognition of neoplasia and better therapeutic regimens. The presence of glomerular lesions appears to relate to tumor mass, although cases of minimal change disease have been reported in patients with stage IA and widespread stage IVB Hodgkin's disease. Treatment that is successful in reducing tumor burden is generally successful in ameliorating the nephrotic syndrome. Recurrences of the nephrotic syndrome may herald recurrence of Hodgkin's disease. Morphologically, the minimal change lesions seen in Hodgkin's disease cannot be distinguished from the idiopathic disorder. Other less common glomerular lesions also occur in Hodgkin's disease. These include membranous, focal sclerosing, proliferative, crescentic, and membranoproliferative glomerulonephritis. Amyloidosis may appear in some patients, but this is uncommon. A number of patients have been described in which crescentic glomerulonephritis was associated with circulating antiglomerular basement membrane antibody. Non-Hodgkin's lymphoma may be also associated with minimal change disease and a variety of other glomerular lesions. However, in comparison with Hodgkin's disease, patients with non-Hodgkin's lymphoma and glomerular lesions have a higher prevalence (approximately 20%) of membranous glomerulonephritis. Angioimmunoblastic lymphadenopathy may be associated with cryoglobulinemia, and membranoproliferative glomerulonephritis and glomerular lesions have been observed in patients with Burkitt's lymphoma.

Chronic lymphocytic leukemia is the most common leukemia associated with glomerular lesions that are similar to those found in lymphomas. Renal amyloidosis may occur in association with a monoclonal gammopathy.

Glomerular Diseases Associated with Carcinomas and Sarcomas

When studied at autopsy by sensitive techniques (e.g., immunofluorescence or electron microscopy), glomerular involvement in patients with carcinoma (or sarcoma) is common. Nevertheless, light microscopic alterations and clinical manifestations are relatively rare. With the exception of localized intracranial neoplasms and tumors arising in bone, the spectrum of carcinomas and sarcomas associated with glomerular lesions is extremely broad. Not surprisingly, the most common neoplasias are carcinoma of the lung, breast, and colon. Squamous and basal cells carcinoma of the skin have occasionally been reported to be associated with glomerular lesions, although, of course, they also may arise as a consequence of immunosuppressive therapy designed to eradicate the glomerular lesion. Other tumors reported to be associated with glomerular lesions include carcinoma of the oral pharynx, thyroid carcinoma, mesothelioma, hepatoma, carcinoma of the pancreas, carcinoma of the stomach, carcinoma of the bladder, carcinoma of the ovary, cervical cancer, prostatic carcinoma, malignant melanoma, carcinoma of the stomach, renal cell carcinoma, Wilms tumor, and mesothelioma. In approximately two-thirds of the reported cases, the malignant neoplasia has been diagnosed before the onset of or simultaneously with the renal disease. In about one-third of patients, the underlying neoplasia was not evident or was overlooked at the time of presentation with clinical manifestations of glomerular involvement, principally nephrotic syndrome. As expected, the association between malignancy and renal disease rises with increasing age, and the great majority of cases are found in patients older than age 55. However, young children with Wilms tumor or gonadoblastoma in association with membranoproliferative glomerulonephritis (Drash syndrome) have been reported.

The glomerular lesions observed in patients with carcinoma or sarcoma are diverse but most commonly fall into one of five categories, namely, membranous glomerulonephritis, membranoproliferative glomerulonephritis, crescentic glomerulonephritis, minimal change disease, or amyloidosis.

The most common glomerular lesion is membranous glomerulonephritis accounting for almost two-thirds of the total glomerular lesions in patients with carcinoma. Carcinomas of the lung, stomach, breast, ovary, cervix, and thyroid and undifferentiated carcinoma are the most common underlying neoplasias. Overall, approximately 6% (range 4% to 19%) of patients with membranous glomerulonephritis may be found to harbor an underlying malignancy. However, the prevalence rises to about 19% in patients older than age 60. The histologic appearance by light, immunofluorescence, and electron microscopy is very similar to, if not identical with, the idiopathic lesion. However, in unusual circumstances a tumor-associated antigen may be detected in the glomerular deposits (carcinoma of the lung, colon, breast, and melanoma). Membranoproliferative glomerulonephritis may be observed with the Drash syndrome of nephroblastoma (Wilms' tumor) and pseudohermaphroditism. Amyloidosis is a rather uncommon lesion associated with underlying carcinoma or sarcoma. Nevertheless, renal cell carcinoma is strongly associated with the development of amyloidosis. Concomitant hepatomegaly and proteinuria are common clinical manifestations. About 25% of all tumors associated with amyloidosis are renal cell carcinoma. Crescentic glomerulonephritis may rarely arise in the context of an underlying malignancy. Occasionally, instances of IgA nephropathy associated with malignancy (mycosis fungoides and carcinoma of the lung) have been reported. Minimal change disease has been observed in patients with mesothelioma, colon carcinoma, lung carcinoma, prostatic carcinoma, pancreatic carcinoma, and renal cell carcinoma. Surgical removal of the tumor in one patient has lead to a remission of nephrotic syndrome.

VASCULAR DISEASES ASSOCIATED WITH MALIGNANT TUMORS

Vascular involvement in association with neoplasia takes two forms: (a) thrombotic microangiopathy and (b) vasculitis. Thrombotic microangiopathy (e.g., hemolytic uremic syndrome) is very likely a complication of chemotherapeutic agents used in the treatment of the malignancy. On the other hand, a true renal vasculitis may be a direct consequence of the malignant process. In some of these, a common etiologic agent has been implicated; hepatocellular carcinoma caused by chronic hepatitis C–related liver disease with concomitant cryoglobulinemic vasculitis is an example. Rarely, Henoch-Schönlein purpura, a form of microscopic vasculitis, may appear in patients with underlying carcinoma of the lung.

GLOMERULAR DISEASE IN PATIENTS WITH BLOOD DYSCRASIAS

As discussed in greater detail in Chapter 42, Part 12, plasma cell dyscrasias including multiple myeloma, Waldenström's macroglobulinemia, and benign monoclonal gammopathies may be associated with a wide variety of glomerular lesions including amyloidosis and proliferative glomerulonephritis. The renal involvement in cryoglobulinemia is discussed in detail in Chapter 42, Part 11.

RENAL INVOLVEMENT IN PATIENTS WITH BENIGN TUMORS

A wide variety of benign tumors have been associated with the occurrence of glomerular disease and nephrotic syndrome. The tumors include uterine leiomyoma, dermoid cyst, pheochromocytoma, and carotid body tumors. The exact cause and effect relationship between benign neoplasia and glomerular lesions is difficult to prove.

FLUID AND ELECTROLYTE DISTURBANCES

Many tumors produce hormones or humoral factors that can affect fluid and electrolyte homeostasis resulting in hypercalcemia, hyponatremia, hyperkalemia, hypokalemia, hypophosphatemia, hyperchloremic acidosis, metabolic alkalosis, or hyperglycemia (Table 55.6).

Hypercalcemia and Hypocalcemia

Hypercalcemia is common in patients with malignant disease (10% to 20%), and 50% of women with disseminated breast carcinomas have hypercalcemia. The mechanisms responsible for such hypercalcemia are many. They include increased bone destruction by metastases or enhanced bone resorption secondary to the production by the tumor of bone-resorbing agents such as transforming growth factors, parathyroid hormone (PTH)-related peptide, a family of osteoclastic activating factors [interleukin-1 (α and β), lymphotoxin, and tumor necrosis factor], colony transforming factor(s), 1,25-dihydroxyvitamin D_3, and prostaglandins of the E series (Table 55.6). These factors are discussed in more detail in Chapter 17, Part 3.

The PTH-related peptide responsible for the humorally mediated hypercalcemia of malignancy has been identified. A full-length complementary DNA responsible for its synthesis has been cloned, and cell lines have been transfected with an expression vector. The synthesized peptide has a molecular weight of 16,000 and consists of a single chain of 141 amino acids. The N-terminal portion of this protein shows significant sequence homology with PTH. This may explain the ability of the PTH-related peptide to react with the PTH receptor and stimulate adenylate cyclase activity in bone and/or kidney. The full-length peptide represents a prepro form of this PTH-related factor, and cleavage of the full-length molecule is required for full expression of its activity. The lack of amino acid sequence homology between PTH and the PTH-related peptide at the C-terminal end of the molecule may explain the lack of or poor reactivity with antibody directed to intact or C-terminal fragments of PTH. Further discussion of PTH-related protein is found in Chapter 17, Part 3. The PTH-related peptide receptor has been cloned. The hypophosphatemia not infrequently encountered in patients with malignant tumors (especially breast cancer) is, at least in part, due to the phosphaturic action of the PTH-related protein produced by the tumor.

Excess PTH could be produced by adenoma or carcinoma of the parathyroid glands. The biochemical disturbances in such patients are related to the actions of PTH. These patients will have hypercalcemia, hypophosphatemia, phosphaturia, and hypercalciuria. However, the fraction of filtered calcium excreted for any given level of serum calcium is less than in patients without excess PTH. An increased association between carcinoma of the breast and parathyroid adenoma exists; thus the biochemical manifestations of excess PTH could be seen in patients with carcinoma of the breast despite the fact that the tumor is not producing PTH. Patients with parathyroid adenoma may have hyperchloremic acidosis (20% to 40%), nephrolithiasis (20% to 60%), and hypertension (30% to 55%). The renal stones may cause urinary tract obstruction, leading to renal failure and uremia with the attendant abnormalities in fluid and electrolyte metabolism. In patients with tumors and non–PTH-induced hypercalcemia, the latter suppresses the activity of the parathyroid gland, resulting in reduced urinary excretion of phosphate with mild to moderate hyperphosphatemia and metabolic alkalosis.

TABLE 55.6. Humoral Factors Associated with Hypercalcemia of Malignancy[a]

- Parathyroid hormone
  - Parathyroid adenoma
  - Parathyroid carcinoma
  - Small cell carcinoma of lung
  - Ovarian adenocarcinoma and primitive ectodermal cancer
- Parathyroid hormone–related peptide
  - Carcinoma of breast
  - Carcinoma of the lung (squamous)
  - Renal cell carcinoma
  - Hepatoma
  - Squamous cell carcinoma
  - Carcinoma of colon, ovary, and pancreas
  - Reticulum cell sarcoma
- Transforming growth factor-α (TGF-α)
  - Most solid tumors associated with hypercalcemia
  - TGF-β stimulates release of TGF-α by breast cancer
- Osteoclastic activating factors
  - Multiple myeloma
  - Malignant lymphoid cell lines
    - Lymphosarcoma
    - T-cell lymphoma
- Prostaglandins (E series)
  - Epidermoid carcinoma of tonsils, lung, and penis
  - Carcinoma of pancreas and kidney
  - Hepatoma
  - Melanoma
- 1,25-dihydroxyvitamin D_3
  - Hodgkin's disease
  - T-cell lymphoma
  - Leiomyoblastoma
  - Carcinoma of the breast

[a] This table provides examples and is not intended to be all inclusive.

Hypercalcemia per se may cause disturbances in renal function; these include a fall in renal blood flow and glomerular filtration rate (GFR); a decrease in the concentrating ability and hence polyuria; a reduction in tubular reabsorption of sodium and magnesium, and therefore natriuresis and magnesiuria; and on occasion nephrocalcinosis. Hypercalcemia causes nausea and vomiting, resulting in hypochloremic alkalosis, volume depletion, and renal potassium wasting. Finally, acute renal failure may occur in patients with marked hypercalcemia.

Hypocalcemia resulting from malignancy is extremely rare. It is not seen even seen in patients with medullary carcinoma of the thyroid, which produces calcitonin, because secondary hyperparathyroidism develops in these patients.

Hyponatremia and Hypernatremia

Increased blood levels of antidiuretic hormone (ADH) occur in association with many tumors (Table 55.7). These patients are unable to excrete free water adequately and therefore develop the biochemical abnormalities of the syndrome of inappropriate ADH release, which includes hyponatremia, hyposmolality of blood, urine osmolality that is usually higher than that of blood, and high urinary excretion of sodium. Complete removal of the tumor is associated with the correction of the hyponatremia, but this is not always possible, especially if there are metastases. Demeclocycline in doses of 800 to 1,200 mg/day produces a resistance to the action of ADH on the kidney and results in an acquired nephrogenic diabetes insipidus state. The drug may provide a promising approach for the management of patients with excess ADH resulting from neoplasia. Salts of lithium can induce the same effect, but the toxicity of lithium may preclude its use for treatment of such patients. An oral nonpeptide selective V2 receptor antagonist (OPC-31260) is now available and has been used successfully to interfere with the action of ADH on the kidney. It has reversed the hyponatremia of the syndrome of inappropriate ADH secretion. Hyponatremia may develop during the course of treatment of tumors with drugs that may enhance ADH release (vincristine) or impair free water excretion (cyclophosphamide).

Hypernatremia occurs in patients with malignant diseases when their water losses exceed their intake. Such an imbalance in water homeostasis my occur in patients with neoplasia of the diencephalopituitary region, which may destroy the site of production and storage of ADH and possibly damage the thirst center. The most common lesions are craniopharyngioma and metastases from carcinoma of the breast. The clinical picture is that of diabetes insipidus. Hypernatremia was noted in patients with hypothalamic tumors or pinealoma; these patients do not have diabetes insipidus and their kidneys can concentrate urine normally, but they display total absence of thirst.

Tumors may also cause disturbances in fluid and electrolyte metabolism and in renal function and structure that by themselves may render the kidney resistant to the action of ADH, resulting in a state of acquired nephrogenic diabetes insipidus.

TABLE 55.7. Tumors Associated with Increased Blood Levels of Antidiuretic Hormone

Oat cell carcinoma of lung	Carcinoma of colon
Carcinoma of esophagus	Carcinoma of ovary
Carcinoma of duodenum	Carcinoma of nasopharynx
Carcinoma of pancreas	Hodgkin's disease
Thymoma	Cholangiocarcinoma
Primary central nervous system tumors	Cancer of breast

Examples include hypercalcemia and hypokalemia associated with malignancy, the diuresis following the relief of obstructive uropathy secondary to tumors, and deposition of amyloid in renal tubules in patients with multiple myeloma. In some of these patients, polyuria, dehydration, and hypernatremia may develop. Patients with obstruction of the esophagus caused by primary tumor or to extraesophageal neoplasia are unable to ingest water and develop severe dehydration and hypernatremia.

Hypokalemia and Hyperkalemia

Excessive losses of potassium in urine and/or stool may occur in patients with various neoplastic diseases. The tumors producing adrenocorticotropic hormone, renin, or aldosterone are listed in Table 55.8. In patients with these tumors, there are excessive losses of potassium in the urine, leading to hypokalemia. Ectopic adrenocorticotropic hormone production stimulates the release of various adrenal corticoids, with deoxycorticosterone and corticosterone (compound B) responsible for the urinary losses of potassium. Hypokalemia occurs in 50% of these patients. Excessive renin production stimulates aldosterone release, which in turn induces kaliuresis and hypokalemia. Prolonged potassium deficiency may result in a defect in the renal concentrating ability and polyuria. The patients develop a state of acquired nephrogenic diabetes insipidus. Hypokalemia may also enhance thirst and cause polydipsia and, secondarily, polyuria.

Abnormalities in water and electrolyte metabolism that occur in primary aldosteronism or other states of excess mineralocorticoids include hypokalemia, mild elevation in serum sodium, metabolic alkalosis, and inappropriate excretion of potassium in relation to its level in blood. There is usually a mild degree of extracellular fluid volume expansion, and urinary sodium excretion is equal to intake. Many of these patients may not display a persistent and consistent hypokalemia, but if the level of serum potassium is followed for an adequate period of time while the patient is consuming a normal salt intake, hypokalemia can usually be demonstrated.

Augmented urinary losses of potassium and hypokalemia have also been noted in patients with Hodgkin's disease, multiple myeloma, and myelomonocytic leukemia. Renal tubular acidosis may occur in patients with Hodgkin's disease (distal type) and in those with multiple myeloma (proximal type). Both types of renal tubular acidosis are associated with renal potassium wasting and hypokalemia. Patients with myelomonocytic leukemia may have multiple defects in proximal tubular reabsorption, kaliuresis, and lysozymuria.

Increased losses of potassium in stool and hypokalemia occur in patients with villous adenoma of the rectum and in those with non–β-cell adenoma of the pancreas. The latter tumor may produce gastrin resulting in Zollinger-Ellison syndrome or vasoactive intestinal polypeptide (VIP), causing pancreatic cholera. Both of these clinical entities are associated with diarrhea with excessive losses of potassium. The VIP may also be produced by extrapancreatic tumors such as bronchogenic carcinoma, pheochromocytoma, and ganglioneuroblastoma. Patients with tumors producing VIP may also have hypercalcemia, hyperglycemia, and episodes of flushing. Tumors of the stomach may cause vomiting and, consequently, hypochloremic alkalosis and hypokalemia. In all these conditions, the patients may also have contraction of extracellular fluid volume, which in turn stimulates aldosterone release causing further urinary losses of potassium and contributing to the magnitude of the hypokalemia.

Hyperkalemia may be seen in patients with malignant diseases under the following circumstances: (a) adrenal insufficiency secondary to metastasis or deposition of amyloid associated with other neoplasms, (b) renal failure resulting from obstruction of ureters or secondary to sludging of the renal tubules with uric acid during the use of chemotherapy, and (c) *tumor lysis syndrome* arising from rapid necrosis of the tumor during chemotherapy or radiation treatment; these patients also display acute renal failure, hyperphosphatemia, hypocalcemia, and hyperuricemia. False elevations in the levels of *serum* potassium (pseudohyperkalemia) may be noted in patients with myeloproliferative disorders such as polycythemia vera, myelogenous leukemia, and myelomonocytic leukemia. This is due to release of an excessive amount of potassium from the increased number of platelets or white blood cells during the clotting of the blood samples. *Plasma* potassium is normal in these patients.

TABLE 55.8. Tumors Producing Adrenocorticotropic Hormone, Renin, or Aldosterone

Adrenocorticotropic hormone
Carcinoma of lung, esophagus, prostate, parotid, thymus, thyroid, breast, ovary, pancreas
Bronchial adenoma, pheochromocytoma, ganglioma, paraganglioma, carcinoid, melanosarcoma
Renin
Wilms' tumor, hemangiopericytoma (juxtaglomerular cell tumor), carcinoma of lung, pancreas
Aldosterone
Adrenal adenoma, adrenal carcinoma

Hypophosphatemia and Hyperphosphatemia

Hypophosphatemia may occur in adults with benign sclerosing hemangiomas. These patients have phosphaturia, hypophosphatemia, normal blood levels of PTH, severe bone pain, and osteomalacia. Resection of the tumor is followed by the disappearance of the syndrome, suggesting that the tumor produces a humoral factor responsible for the observed derangements. A similar syndrome has been reported in patients with giant cell granuloma, osteoid tumor, cavernous hemangioma, prostatic carcinoma, and giant cell carcinoma. In some patients, the administration of 1,25-dihydroxyvitamin D_3 reversed the renal losses of phosphate. This observation suggests that the tumor may produce a factor that inhibits the renal synthesis of 1,25-dihydroxyvitamin D_3. Hyperphosphatemia occurs in patients with tumors associated with non–PTH-induced hypercalcemia or in patients in whom the tumor or its therapy caused acute renal failure.

OBSTRUCTIVE UROPATHY

External

Neoplasms of the pelvic organs and genitourinary tract, malignancies of retroperitoneal structure, and metastases from distant tumors (especially carcinoma of the breast) may produce obstruction of the upper or lower urinary tract. Retroperitoneal tumors may provoke marked retroperitoneal fibrosis, which by itself can cause ureteral obstruction. All these lesions may result in unilateral or bilateral obstructive uropathy. Nocturia, polyuria, and a history of periods of oliguria followed by polyuria suggest an obstructive lesion. Anuria occurs with total bilateral obstruction. Occasionally, hypertension may develop. Hyperchloremic, hyperkalemic (type IV) renal tubular acidosis may occur. Progressive azotemia leading to uremia is common and may progress rapidly. After relief of bilateral obstruction, the patient may have massive diuresis and the kidney may display functional abnormalities such as decreased reabsorption of sodium, impaired response to ADH, inability to acidify the urine, and hypophosphaturia.

The decision to undertake palliative diversion of the urinary tract in patients with advanced malignancy causing bilateral urinary tract obstruction must be made on an individual basis, taking into account the responsiveness of the tumor to therapy and the overall prognosis.

Internal

Uric acid is the most common cause of intrarenal obstruction that may occur in patients with neoplasia. Uric acid production and urinary excretion are increased in most patients with myeloproliferative and lymphoproliferative disease. Uric acid excretion may be increased to five times normal in acute lymphotic leukemia and twice normal in acute and chronic myelogenous leukemia, Hodgkin's disease, and reticulum cell sarcoma, and is usually normal or only slightly elevated in chronic lymphocytic leukemia and multiple myeloma. During treatment with radiation or with chemotherapy, uric acid excretion may increase dramatically, particularly in patients with very responsive tumors. Under these circumstances, uric acid may precipitate in the lumen of the nephrons, leading to intrarenal obstruction and to a clinical syndrome called *acute hyperuricemic nephropathy*. The incidence and severity of this syndrome are determined by the rates of uric acid excretion, the pH of the urine, and the presence of other endogenous solutes and pharmacologic agents that affect the transport processes for urate in the nephron. The patient develops oliguria or anuria; hematuria is common, and uric acid crystals are frequently detected in the urinary sediment. Although ureteric obstruction occurs in few patients, the obstruction is intrarenal in most patients, and therefore cystoscopy and retrograde pyelography are of limited value in the diagnosis and therapy.

Appropriate measures should be taken to prevent acute hyperuricemic nephropathy in patients at risk. These measures include hydration and increased urinary flow, avoidance of uricosuric agents, alkalinization of urine, and inhibition of uric acid biosynthesis. Urine volume could be increased by water or osmotic diuresis; it should be remembered that antitumor agents such as cyclophosphamide and vincristine impair water excretion and may precipitate severe hyponatremia in a patient ingesting large volumes of fluid. Alkalinization of the urine to obtain a urinary pH of 7.0 could be achieved by prescribing sodium bicarbonate, 20 to 30 mEq every 6 hours during the day (three times), and 500 mg of acetazolamide every evening. Allopurinol (300 mg/day) is an effective inhibitor of uric acid production. If any of the purine analogues (mercaptopurine or azathioprine) are given to the patient with allopurinol, the amount of these former drugs must be reduced to one-third of the usual dose.

Once oliguric renal failure has developed in the course of acute hyperuricemic nephropathy, the goals of therapy are to reduce urate production with allopurinol and to diminish urate pool size by dialysis therapy. These two therapeutic approaches have reduced markedly the mortality resulting from this syndrome. Hemodialysis therapy is more effective than peritoneal dialysis therapy in removing uric acid.

Other compounds can produce intrarenal obstruction in patients with malignant disease. Precipitation of Bence Jones protein in the lumen of the nephrons has been associated with oliguria or anuria in patients with multiple myeloma. Acute renal failure secondary to intranephronal obstruction by precipitates of mucoproteins has been noted in a patient with carcinoma of the pancreas; apparently, the pancreatic tumor secreted the mucoproteins.

MISCELLANEOUS

Increased renal clearance of uric acid (greater than 15% of GFR) and hypouricemia (less than 2.0 mg/dl) have been noted in patients with Hodgkin's disease; glioblastoma; carcinoma of the cervix, tongue, and lungs; and anaplastic carcinoma. Some patients may also display evidence for impairment of other proximal tubule transport processes resulting in Fanconi syndrome. This has been observed in patients with carcinoma of the bronchus and pancreas, multiple myeloma, and monocytic or myelomonocytic leukemia associated with lysozymuria. Lactic acidosis of malignancy has been described in Hodgkin's lymphoma; acute leukemia, oat cell carcinoma and osteogenic sarcoma with hepatic metastasis. Abnormalities in renal function, in structure, and in fluid and electrolyte metabolism secondary to medications used in the treatment of cancer are discussed in detail in Chapter 47, Part 2.

Selected Readings

Beaufils H, Jauanneau C, Chomette G. Kidney and cancer: results of immunofluorescence microscopy. *Nephron* 1985;40:303–308.
An autopsy study of immune deposits in the kidney in 129 subjects with solid tumors and 55 control subjects, emphasizing the frequent occurrence of IgA deposits.

Dabbs D, Morel-Maroger Striker L, Mignon F, et al. Glomerular lesions in lymphomas and leukemias. *Am J Med* 1986;80:63–70.
An in-depth review article on glomerular lesions encountered in lymphoid malignancies and leukemias.

Dafnis EK, Laski ME. Fluid and electrolyte abnormalities in the oncology patient. *Semin Nephrol* 1993;13:281–296.
An excellent review of the topic.

Davison A, Thomson D. Malignancy associated glomerular disease. In: Cameran S, Davison A, Grunfeld, JP, et al., eds. *Oxford textbook of clinical nephrology.* Oxford: Oxford Medical Publishing, 1993:475–486.
An excellent summary and source of references.

Eagen JW, Lewis EJ. Glomerulopathies of neoplasia. *Kidney Int* 1977;11:297–306.
A classic review article on glomerular lesions in malignancy.

Glassock RJ. Secondary membranous nephropathy. *Nephrol Dial Transplant* 1992;7:64–71.
An excellent overview of cancer in membranous nephropathy.

Glassock RJ, Friedler RM, Massry SG. Kidney and electrolyte disturbances in neoplastic diseases. *Contrib Nephrol* 1977;7:2–41.
A thorough discussion of changes in fluid and electrolyte metabolism in patients with cancer.

Habib R, Loirat C, Gubler MC, et al. The nephropathy associated with male pseudohermaphroditism and Wilms' tumor (Drash syndrome): a distinctive glomerular lesion. Report of 10 cases. *Clin Nephrol* 1985;24:269–278.
A clinical and pathologic study of 10 children with Drash syndrome, emphasizing the distinctive glomerular lesion: diffuse mesangial sclerosis.

Lee JC, Yamauchi H, Hopper J. The association of cancer and the nephrotic syndrome. *Ann Intern Med* 1966;64:41–51.
The original article calling attention to the association of cancer with the nephrotic syndrome, particularly that caused by membranous glomerulonephritis.

Norris SH. Paraneoplastic glomerulopathy. *Semin Nephrol* 1993;13:258–272.
An excellent review of the topic.

Rieselbach RE, Garnick MB, eds. *Cancer and the kidney.* Philadelphia: Lea & Febiger, 1982.
An excellent book dealing with aspects of neoplasia and the kidney.

Schrier RW, Fasset RG, Ohara M, et al. Vasopressin release, water diuresis, and vasopressin antagonism in cardiac failure, cirrhosis and pregnancy. *Proc Assoc Am Physicians* 1998;110:407–11.
An excellent overview of pathophysiology.

Suva LJ, Winslow GA, Weltenhall REH, et al. A parathyroid hormone-related protein implicated in malignant hypercalcemia: cloning and expression. *Science* 1987;237:893–896.
The first demonstration that a preprohormone resembling parathyroid hormone can be expressed from the cloned DNA to protein in mammalian cell.

CHAPTER 56

Kidney in Nutritional Disorders

PART 1
Malnutrition

Saulo Klahr

Primary malnutrition is dietary in origin, with intake deficient in specific or overall nutrients. Secondary malnutrition is due to disease processes that interfere with the utilization or disposition of nutrients, for example, gastrointestinal diseases that decrease food absorption or malignancies that increase energy utilization. Sometimes anorexia caused by illness may lead to primary malnutrition through decreased food intake. In developing countries, primary malnutrition predominates. In industrialized nations, secondary malnutrition is more common, particularly among hospitalized patients. Hypoalbuminemia, a common manifestation of chronic protein-calorie malnutrition, may occur in as many as 40% of hospitalized patients. No clearly defined criteria exist to determine the degree or severity of malnutrition. The terms *mild, moderate,* and *severe* are frequently used, especially regarding protein-energy malnutrition. Protein-calorie malnutrition comprises a spectrum of diseases with severe forms manifesting themselves clinically as marasmus or kwashiorkor. Several million new clinical cases are estimated to occur annually. Marasmus is characterized by a deficiency of calories and all nutrients, whereas kwashiorkor results from a deficiency of protein and, to a lesser extent, other nutrients, in the presence of adequate or even excessive caloric intake. The clinical consequences of protein-energy malnutrition depend on several factors: (a) the severity and duration of the nutritional deficiencies of protein and calories, (b) the proportion of protein intake to caloric intake, (c) the nature and severity of other associated nutritional deficiencies, (d) the age of the person affected, and (e) the frequency of occurrence of infections or other morbid events that increase energy requirements. Mild and moderate forms of protein-energy malnutrition frequently go unrecognized and are primarily characterized by inadequate growth and development.

EFFECTS OF PROTEIN INTAKE ON RENAL FUNCTION

Short- or long-term administration of amino acids or a protein-rich diet increases glomerular filtration rate (GFR) between 22% and 100% in animals and humans; the magnitude of the rise depends in part on the amount ingested, the timing of the study in relation to when the food was eaten, and the basal dietary conditions. Most studies reveal a significant but less pronounced rise in renal blood flow, although two groups found no change in renal blood flow 1 to 2 hours after the ingestion of a protein-rich meal. Experimental animals fed a high-protein diet have higher basal GFR values than animals fed a low-protein diet. However, kidney weight is greater in rats fed a high-protein diet than in rats fed a low-protein diet. When expressed per gram of kidney, GFR did not differ between animals fed a high- or a low-protein diet. This result suggests that decreased protein intake reduces kidney mass and that this reduction is the main factor responsible for the lower GFR in growing rats. In normal adult humans, it has been found that increased protein intake raises GFR, effective renal plasma flow, and the maximum transport of *p*-aminohippurate. Table 56.1 summarizes the effects of ingesting one of three different protein diets for 1 week on GFR and effective renal plasma flow (RPF) in humans. Normal subjects fed a calorie-deficient diet in which the distribution of calories among protein, fat, and carbohydrate was not controlled had a fall in GFR when measured by creatinine clearance. The renal hemodynamic response to a meat meal has been studied in humans. Ten volunteers were studied after eating an average of 3.5 g/kg of body weight of lean cooked beefsteak and on a separate day after ingestion of an amount of sodium and water equivalent to that in the meat meal. The GFR increased 28% at 3 hours after the meat meal compared with the same time period after the control salt solution. Compared to basal values, the GFR increased by 15% at 3 hours after the meat meal, but this difference did not achieve statistical significance. Not all subjects demonstrated an increase in GFR, and in those in whom the increase was seen, it ranged from 5% to 46%. The increase in renal plasma flow was nearly proportional to the rise in GFR. The increase in renal blood flow could be explained en-

TABLE 56.1. Influence of Dietary Protein Intake on Renal Function in Normal Humans[a]

Diet (g protein/kg BW/day)	GFR (ml/min)	ERPF (ml/min)	T_mPAH (mg/min)
0.1–0.4	95.2 ± 3.1	538.2 ± 21.2	69.5 ± 3.2
1.0–1.4	104.2 ± 2.9	570.8 ± 17.6	75.9 ± 4.5
2.3–3.0	117.3 ± 4.3	640.2 ± 18.5	86.3 ± 3.1

[a] Data are means and standard errors of the mean.

Adapted from Pullman et al. The influence of dietary protein on specific renal functions in normal man. *J Lab Clin Med* 1954;44:320–332.

BW, body weight; ERPF, effective renal plasma flow; GFR, glomerular filtration rate; T_mPAH, maximum transport of *p*-aminohippurate.

TABLE 56.2. Effects of Chronic Protein-Calorie Malnutrition on Renal Function

1. Decreased renal plasma flow and glomerular filtration rate
2. Impaired concentrating ability (polyuria) with normal diluting capacity
3. Impaired ability to excrete acid loads
4. Normal ability to lower urine pH
5. Markedly decreased titratable acid excretion due to a substantial reduction in phosphate excretion in urine

Adapted with permission from Klahr S, Davis T. Changes in renal function with chronic protein-calorie malnutrition. In: Mitch W, Klahr S, eds. *Nutrition and the kidney.* Boston: Little, Brown, 1988: 59–79.

tirely on the basis of decreased renal vascular resistance. Sodium excretion was significantly greater after the meat meal, indicating a natriuretic effect of the meal beyond that expected from its sodium and water content.

EFFECTS OF CHRONIC PROTEIN-ENERGY MALNUTRITION ON KIDNEY FUNCTION

The effects of nutritional disturbances on renal function are summarized in Table 56.2 but remain poorly understood. The urine of most patients with malnutrition usually does not contain protein, glucose, or formed elements such as casts and red or white blood cells. The plasma of malnourished individuals does not exhibit the chemical changes that characterize renal insufficiency [i.e., the levels of blood urea nitrogen (BUN), creatinine, and other substances that accumulate in renal disease are not elevated]. Such negative evidence, however, neither proves the full normality of the kidney nor provides an accurate picture of renal function in chronic protein-energy malnutrition. The renal consequences of malnutrition are more evident in children than in adults. Disturbances of water and electrolyte metabolism frequently occur in children with malnutrition, and it seems likely that altered renal function plays a major role in initiating and prolonging these abnormalities.

EFFECTS ON GFR AND RPF

In both adults and children with malnutrition, GFR and RPF as assessed by the clearances of inulin and PAH, respectively, are markedly decreased. Both values increase with protein repletion. There are, however, a few reports in which malnourished subjects had no substantial decrements in GFR. Although the data in children with protein-energy malnutrition indicate a universal decrease in both GFR and RPF, in adults with protein malnutrition conflicting results have been reported for GFR and RPF values. These different results may reflect differences in the severity and duration of the malnutrition.

The mechanisms underlying the decrease in GFR and RPF in chronic protein-calorie malnutrition have not been completely elucidated. Several factors may be involved, including a decrease in cardiac output and systemic blood pressure. In this respect, a reduced total blood volume and stroke volume may contribute to the reduced cardiac output and blood pressure. Those changes may lead to decreases in intraglomerular pressure and in the net filtration pressure necessary for filtration. In addition, studies in experimental animals have revealed a decrease in the ultrafiltration coefficient (K_f) and in plasma flow per nephron. Single-nephron GFR is decreased in animals fed a low-protein diet compared with those fed a normal-protein diet. These changes occurred despite modest changes in serum albumin, and they also were seen before any major changes in total blood volume or arterial pressure. Morphologic studies revealed a decrease in the surface area of glomerular capillaries, suggesting that the decrease in K_f may be related to a decrease in surface area available for filtration. It has been reported that inhibition of angiotensin II in animals with protein malnutrition may increase GFR and RPF. Also, low-protein diets decrease the excretion of prostaglandins in the urine and prostaglandin synthesis in isolated glomeruli. However, no effect of inhibiting the synthesis of angiotensin II on the production of prostaglandins was observed in animals fed a low-protein diet compared with those fed a high-protein diet. Whether a decrease in renal prostaglandin synthesis contributes to the decrease in RPF and GFR observed in malnutrition has not been established. The potential decrement in arginine concentrations as a consequence of a markedly decreased amount of protein in the diet may result in impaired production of nitric oxide and consequently to vasoconstriction of the renal circulation. Again, no information in humans is available to support a potential role of arginine deficiency and alterations in the endothelial production of nitric oxide.

PLASMA LEVELS OF CREATININE AND BUN

A decrease in GFR results in increased plasma levels of creatinine and urea nitrogen. When production of urea or creatinine is decreased, however, moderate to severe impairment of renal function may not result in increased plasma levels of either of these two compounds. Patients with moderate to severe protein-energy malnutrition usually have low or normal plasma levels of creatinine and urea nitrogen, despite marked reductions in GFR. As the urine excretion of both creatinine and urea is markedly reduced in patients with protein-calorie malnutrition, it may be concluded that production of both of these substances is diminished in subjects with malnutrition. The decrease in creatinine production is probably the result of a marked decrease in muscle mass. The low levels of urea presumably result from decreased protein intake, slower tissue breakdown, and/or urea reutilization.

During protein repletion both BUN and plasma creatinine levels increase despite a rise in GFR. This increase in the levels of BUN and creatinine presumably reflects increased entry of both end products of the metabolism of protein and creatine into body fluids. Hence, during the period of repletion, urea and creatinine production exceeds their excretion.

CONCENTRATION AND DILUTION OF URINE

Polyuria and nocturia are common complaints of patients with malnutrition. The polyuria is due, at least in part, to the inability of the kidneys of patients with protein-calorie malnutrition to adequately concentrate urine. In a group of adult patients with malnutrition, urine osmolality never exceeded 600 mOsm/kg of water after 14 hours of fluid deprivation. (Values in normal subjects usually exceed 800 mOsm/kg water.) Protein repletion increased urine osmolality progressively after overnight fluid deprivation in each patient. Values for solute-free water reabsorption (TC_{H_2O}) were also decreased in malnourished patients given mannitol and vasopressin. Values for TC_{H_2O} rose after protein repletion in all patients studied. A renal concentrating defect that improves after protein repletion has also been described in malnourished children. On the other hand, patients with malnutrition can dilute the urine adequately. During water loading, urine osmolality in malnourished adults averaged

57 mOsm/kg body water, a figure comparable to that observed in normal subjects. Mean values for free water clearance corrected for GFR averaged 15.8 ml, a figure also similar to that reported in healthy subjects.

The decreased ability of the kidneys of malnourished subjects to concentrate urine is most likely due to decreased osmolality of the renal medulla. This is probably the result of a lower urea concentration in this area of the kidney. The concentrating defect is corrected slowly with protein repletion. This slow correction is most likely due to a markedly positive nitrogen balance in the initial weeks of protein repletion; consequently, urea excretion in the urine does not rise greatly for several weeks after the increase in dietary protein intake is effected. Thus rapid restoration of an osmolar gradient in the renal medulla would not be expected. On the other hand, the oral administration of urea led to a rapid increase in the ability to concentrate the urine after fluid deprivation. This increase in concentrating ability was accompanied by an increase in BUN and in the excretion of urea in the urine. Discontinuation of urea administration resulted in a fall in the values for maximal urine osmolality after overnight fluid deprivation. The response to antidiuretic hormone appears to be intact because in malnourished subjects undergoing a water diuresis, administration of vasopressin markedly decreased free water clearance. In addition, the central release of vasopressin is intact in such subjects, as determined by changes in urine osmolality occurring during water diuresis as a consequence of the administration of hyperosmolar loads or nicotine, both known stimulators of the release of vasopressin.

The correction of the concentrating defect observed in malnourished subjects during protein repletion and the dramatic change observed with the oral administration of urea suggest that an anatomic alteration is not responsible for the concentrating defect. Rather, a functional disorder seems to account for the inability of kidneys of malnourished subjects to concentrate urine. Impaired reabsorption of sodium in the ascending loop of Henle may explain the concentrating defect; however, the finding of a normal capacity to dilute the urine in such subjects argues against such a postulate. Most likely, a decrease in urea as an effective osmolal particle that promotes the reabsorption of water from the cortical and medullary collecting ducts is responsible for the concentrating defect seen in patients with protein-energy malnutrition. A good correlation was found between values for urine osmolality and the concomitant 24-hour nitrogen excretion in the urine in malnourished subjects undergoing protein repletion. These data support the notion that decreased urea concentration in the renal medulla accounts for the renal concentrating defect seen in patients with chronic protein malnutrition.

REGULATION OF ACID–BASE BALANCE

Subjects with chronic protein-calorie malnutrition have normal values for blood pH and serum bicarbonate. However, the total net acid excretion, as measured by the sum of urine ammonium plus titratable acid minus urine bicarbonate is markedly decreased in such patients. The finding of reduced acid excretion in the presence of normal blood pH and bicarbonate values supports the postulate that endogenous acid production is reduced in malnutrition. On a diet containing 1.5 to 2 g of protein/kg of body weight, the metabolic production of hydrogen ions (H^+) usually equals 50 to 100 mEq/day. Three major sources of H^+ from metabolism have been identified. First, metabolism of dietary sulfoproteins produces sulfuric acid. Second, phosphoproteins from the diet are broken down to yield phosphoric acid. Third, H^+ are produced in association with certain organic acid ions, notably urate, which are not further degraded by the body and therefore are excreted in the urine. The generation of H^+ from metabolism and the relative contribution of each of the sources enumerated previously to H^+ production will vary with the type and quantity of protein in the diet and with the rate of nonmetabolizable organic acid production. In a normal person who consumes a diet with a constant daily composition, the rate of metabolic H^+ production will be constant and the quantity of H^+ excreted in the urine will equal the rate of H^+ production. As mentioned above, patients with severe malnutrition have a decreased production of H^+. When subjects with malnutrition are given protein repletion, they retain nitrogen, and in severely malnourished children there is a marked positive balance after protein administration. Thus fewer amino acids will be catabolized. An adaptive change in protein metabolism also occurs in malnutrition. There is reduced protein turnover in muscle, while protein turnover in liver is reduced to a small extent. However, there is a rise in the activity of amino acid–activated enzymes of liver and a decrease in urea cycle enzymes; thus amino acids from muscle are preferentially incorporated into protein and there is less wasteful degradation. The net effect of all these adaptations is a reduction in the metabolic production of acids. Renal excretion of acid as measured by the sum of ammonium plus titratable acid minus bicarbonate increases in malnourished subjects during protein repletion without a detectable change in the serum levels of bicarbonate or in blood pH. Ammonium chloride administration produces a greater degree of metabolic acidosis in patients with protein malnutrition than in the same subjects after protein repletion. After NH_4Cl loading the increase in ammonia excretion in the urine is similar before and after protein repletion. However, the excretion of titratable acid is markedly increased, by about fourfold, after protein repletion compared with the malnourished state. This increment in titratable acid is related to the greater excretion of phosphate in the urine after protein repletion. A similar pattern of acid excretion has been reported in children. Total H^+ excretion in the urine was greater in children who had recovered from protein malnutrition than in the same children during their malnourished state. The percentage of H^+ excretion contributed by ammonia was approximately 75% in the malnourished state and 58% in children after recovery from malnutrition. In adults with malnutrition the urine can be acidified to a pH as low as 4.5 during ammonium chloride administration, suggesting no defect in the kidney's ability to produce an acid urine. However, it has been found that infants with malnutrition and gastroenteritis have a lower urine pH when they are well nourished than when they are malnourished. Therefore, malnourished children have a defect in urine acidification. Despite a normal bicarbonate level and blood pH, malnourished patients have an impaired ability to handle acid loads and develop marked metabolic acidosis after trauma. This greater acidosis may be due to a decrease in the total buffer capacity of the body in the malnourished state.

EFFECTS ON SODIUM HOMEOSTASIS

Edema is not always present in patients with chronic protein-energy malnutrition. Dietary intake of salt seems to determine the presence or absence of edema in malnourished subjects. All children with kwashiorkor have some degree of edema; it is usually present in the lower extremities, hands, and face. Edema-forming states are characterized by the renal retention of salt and water. Thus, in the edema-forming syndromes, the rate of excretion of sodium and water from the body is less than the concurrent rate of acquisition. Common to all edema-forming states is the apparent need for expansion of effective extracellular fluid volume. Sodium conservation is adequate in malnourished subjects fed diets containing 10 mEq of sodium/day. By contrast, when fed a diet containing 170 mEq of sodium/day, patients with malnutrition demonstrated a mean positive balance of 420 mEq and a weight gain of 2.8 kg after 5 days of such a diet. After protein repletion the same subjects fed an identical diet demonstrated a mean positive balance of only 150 mEq of sodium and a weight gain of 1.2 kg. The results of these balance studies indicate that subjects with protein malnutrition demonstrate impaired excretion of sodium loads. The capacity to excrete an equivalent sodium load improves after protein repletion. The acute, intravenous administration of sodium chloride results in greater retention of sodium in malnourished subjects than in the same subjects after protein repletion. In the malnourished state fractional sodium excretion rose from 0.5% to 0.8% with acute saline administration. When the same individuals were studied after protein repletion sodium excretion rose from 1.1% to 11% after saline expansion. These data demonstrate that during the malnourished state, the rapid intravenous administration of saline results in an almost negligible increase of fractional sodium excretion. When the same studies were repeated after protein repletion a pronounced increase in fractional sodium excretion was observed. Similar observations have been obtained in malnourished children.

The mechanisms underlying sodium retention and edema formation in patients with chronic protein malnutrition have not been completely elucidated (Fig. 56.1). Decreased protein intake usually leads to hypoalbuminemia. However, it is controversial whether plasma volume is decreased in malnourished subjects. Available evidence indicates that cardiac output is decreased. A fall in cardiac output in turn would decrease arterial blood pressure, leading to a fall in peritubular hydrostatic pressure and increased tubular reabsorption of salt and water. In addition, renal blood flow and GFR are greatly diminished in malnourished subjects, leading to a decrease in the filtered load of salt and water. At the same time, there is increased renin-

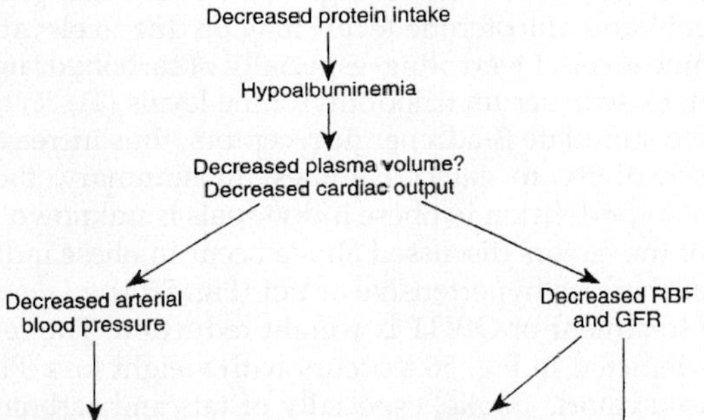

Figure 56.1. Possible mechanisms for the development of edema in patients with chronic protein-calorie malnutrition. GFR, glomerular filtration rate; RBF, renal blood flow. (Reproduced with permission from Klahr S, Alleyne GAO. Effects of chronic protein-calorie malnutrition on the kidney. *Kidney Int* 1973;3:129–141.)

angiotensin production and presumably elevated levels of circulating aldosterone which in turn will increase the tubular reabsorption of salt and water. The combination of a decreased filtered load of salt and water plus increased tubular reabsorption leads to net sodium retention and edema formation. Studies performed in adults with malnutrition before and after protein repletion have revealed a decrease in free water clearance values after correction of the protein deficit. These results suggest that proximal sodium reabsorption may actually be decreased in the malnourished state. If so, most of the increased retention of sodium observed in malnourished subjects could be the consequence of forces acting beyond the proximal tubule, presumably at the level of the ascending limb of Henle's loop and the distal tubule. The decrease in GFR and the increase in reabsorption of solutes observed in malnourished individuals would minimize the loss of nutrients in the urine. In addition, the decrease in the filtered load of sodium would reduce the metabolic requirements for sodium reabsorption in the kidney and consequently lower the basal energy expenditure of patients with chronic protein-energy malnutrition.

Selected Readings

Benabe JE, Martinez-Maldonado M. Renal effects of dietary protein excess and deprivation. *Semin Nephrol* 1991;11:76–85.

A review of the effects of diets with a high or a low protein content on renal function.

Klahr S. Effect of malnutrition and of changes in protein intake on renal function. In: Kopple JD, Massry SG, eds. *Nutritional management of renal disease.* Baltimore: Williams & Wilkins, 1997:229–244.

A description of protein as an important modulator of renal hemodynamics and the potential role of circulation and local factors.

Klahr S, Alleyne GAO. Effect of chronic protein-calorie malnutrition on the kidney. Editorial. *Kidney Int* 1973;3:129.

A classic and comprehensive review of the effects of chronic protein-calorie malnutrition on renal function and structure.

Klahr S, Davis T. Changes in renal function with chronic protein-calorie malnutrition. In: Mitch W, Klahr S, eds. *Nutrition and the kidney.* Boston: Little, Brown, 1988:59–79.

A detailed description of the changes in renal blood flow, GFR, and tubular function in chronic protein-calorie malnutrition.

PART 2
Obesity

Leslie P. Dornfeld

Every decade the weight of the population in the United States is increasing and more and more of these individuals are obese. This could potentially represent as many as one-third of all Americans. With such a large number of potential patients having this metabolic derangement, deciding whether a coexistent renal abnormality is causally related or merely coincidental is difficult. Obesity per se has only rarely been associated with overt renal disease. However, because of the variety of dietary, surgical, and self-administered treatments for obesity, a significant number of renal, electrolyte, and acid–base problems have arisen (Tables 56.3 and 56.4).

RENAL FUNCTION

The absolute glomerular filtration rate (GFR) has been reported to be elevated in obese subjects, but corrected for the increase in

TABLE 56.3. Renal and Electrolyte Disturbances Associated with Obesity Hypertension

Asymptomatic proteinuria
Nephrotic syndrome
Renal vein thrombosis
Diabetic nephropathy
Contralateral renal and urethral displacement associated with incisional hernia
Respiratory acidosis (Pickwickian syndrome)
Carcinoma of the kidney

TABLE 56.4. Renal and Electrolyte Consequences of Obesity Therapy and Bulimia

Jejunoileal bypass surgery
Nephrocalcinosis
Nephrolithiasis
Interstitial nephritis
Hyperchloremic acidosis
Hypokalemia
Hypocalcemia
Hypomagnesemia
Dehydration
Bulimia complications
Hypokalemia
Hypomagnesemia
Metabolic alkalosis
Hypochloremia
Fasting
Natriuresis
Ketonemia
Hypokalemia
Hypomagnesemia
Hyperuricemia

body surface area, GFR appears to be normal. There may be a correlation between GFR, plasma cortisol, and urinary excretion of free cortisol. No functional changes have been described in humans despite the fact that genetically obese Zucker rats develop glomerular enlargement and glomerular sclerosis.

Autopsy studies in obese patients reveal glomerular enlargement, mild hypercellularity, and variable widening of mesangial regions. It is postulated that the glomerular enlargement is due to a combination of tissue hypoxia secondary to hypoventilation or hypoxemia, increased blood volume, and the effect of right ventricular hypertrophy causing arteriolar and capillary dilatation. Despite these findings, most patients have no proteinuria or functional changes.

HYPERTENSION AND OBESITY

The relationship between hypertension and obesity has been clearly established. The mechanisms by which an obese person becomes hypertensive are multifactorial and still have not been fully elucidated. (Table 56.5). An increased food intake, whether it be total calories, fat, sugar, or protein, leads to numerous hormonal and sympathetic nervous system changes, which in turn may lead to the development of hypertension. Absolute weight does not always correlate with blood pressure. Weight distribution does appear to be a significant factor in the incidence of hypertension as well as type II diabetes mellitus. So-called android obesity (upper body fat distribution: abdomen, neck, and shoulder) has a higher association with hypertension than gynecoid obesity (lower body fat: hips and thigh).

TABLE 56.5. Possible Factors in the Etiology of Obesity-Related Hypertension[a]

Absolute weight
Weight distribution
Error in sphygmomanometer cuff size
Sodium
Sympathetic nervous system
Catecholamines
Renin-aldosterone
Insulin
Thyroid hormones
Hemodynamic changes
Others

[a] Many factors may contribute to the development of hypertension in obese individuals; no single factor can be implicated as being more important than any other.

Frequently, blood pressure is measured in obese people using a normal size sphygmomanometer cuff. There is a significant diastolic error, which increases with increasing arm circumference (Fig. 56.2). Care must be taken to establish that hypertension truly exists.

The role of sodium intake on the pathogenesis of obesity-related hypertension (OBHT) is still an open question. If one restricts salt and not calories, blood pressure falls. Similarly, if one significantly reduces caloric intake and not salt, blood pressure falls. If calories are only moderately restricted, the change in blood pressure may not be as great regardless of sodium intake. Most people now accept weight and sodium as independent factors in the etiology and treatment of OBHT.

Obese individuals usually have elevated insulin levels and therefore a stimulus to retain sodium, because insulin enhances tubular sodium reabsorption. With a fall in serum insulin levels due to weight loss or exercise, there is a natriuresis that may contribute to the fall in blood pressure seen with both exercise and dieting. Insulin also stimulates plasma catecholamine levels, which could further elevate blood pressure.

Available evidence has shown inappropriately high levels of renin and aldosterone in obese individuals, which falls in response to weight reduction (Fig. 56.3). These inappropriately high renin and aldosterone levels may be due to elevated catecholamine levels. Overeating, especially of carbohydrates, leads to an increase in serum triiodothyronine levels (T_3). T_3 has been shown to stimulate β-adrenergic receptors, thus increasing vascular sensitivity to catecholamines. In summary, the actual cause of hypertension in obese individuals is unknown because many of the factors discussed above occur in obese individuals whether they are hypertensive or not (Fig. 56.4).

The treatment of OBHT is weight reduction. The reverse of events depicted in Fig. 56.4 occurs with weight loss (Fig. 56.5). Decreased caloric intake, especially of fats and carbohydrates, leads to a decrease in insulin secretion, circulating catecholamine levels, and sympathetic activity. These in turn lead to a natriuresis, a decrease in the activity of the renin-aldosterone system, decreased cardiac output, and thus lowering of arterial blood pressure. If weight loss is not possible, or the hypertension does not respond to weight reduction, pharmacologic agents should be used.

In deciding which pharmacologic agent to use, one should consider the mechanisms of action of each class of antihypertensive agent to avoid exacerbation of the changes discussed above and to block these known abnormalities.

Long-term follow-up of obese patients shows that if weight loss is maintained, patients remain normotensive even though they are consuming a higher calorie, higher sodium diet. If patients begin to regain weight, blood pressure rises modestly by

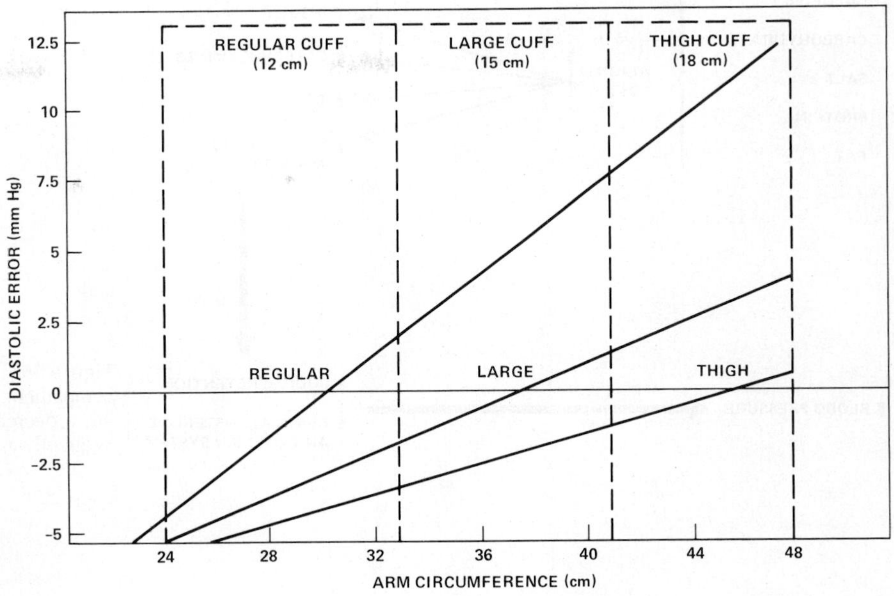

Figure 56.2. Measuring blood pressure in obese individuals can lead to significant technical error if arm size is not taken into account. Which arm cuff to use can be determined with the above graph.

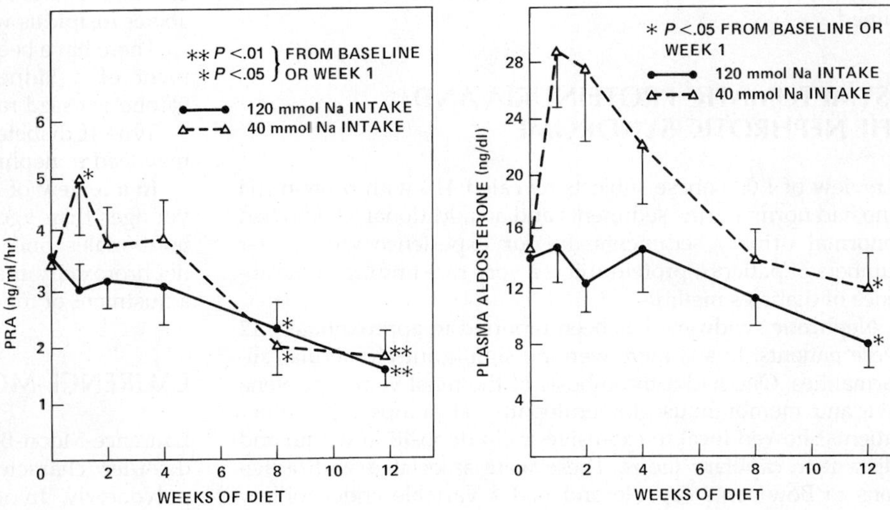

Figure 56.3. Changes in plasma renin activity (*PRA, left panel*) and plasma aldosterone (*right panel*) during fasting. Renin and aldosterone levels are inappropriately high in obese individuals, considering that their sodium intake is 200 mEq/24 hr. There is a paradoxical fall in both substances with a concomitant weight loss while patients are consuming lower sodium diets.

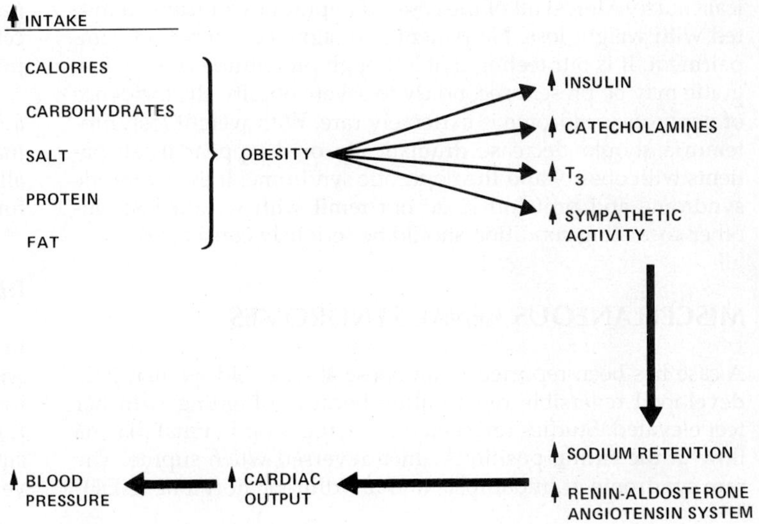

Figure 56.4. Pathogenetic mechanisms of obesity-related hypertension. Increased ingestion of food substances or sodium leads to an increase in body weight and secondary metabolic changes, which in turn lead to an increase in renin-aldosterone activity and salt retention. T_3, triiodothyronine.

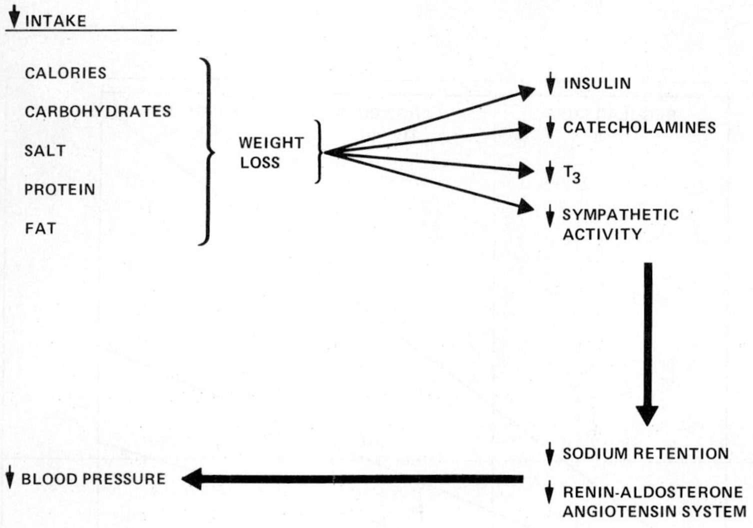

Figure 56.5. With weight loss, obesity-associated endocrine and sympathetic nervous system changes reverse, leading to a natriuresis, a decrease in renin-aldosterone-angiotensin activity, and consequently a fall in blood pressure. T_3, triiodothyronine.

an amount equal to approximately 30% of the original decrease in blood pressure. It is not until a significant amount of weight is regained that blood pressure rises proportional to the weight gained.

ASYMPTOMATIC PROTEINURIA AND THE NEPHROTIC SYNDROME

A review of 1,000 obese subjects revealed 410 with proteinuria who had normal urine sediments and an additional 53 who had abnormal urinary sediments. In our experience with larger numbers of patients, proteinuria is a very rare finding in the absence of diabetes mellitus.

Nephrotic syndrome has been reported in approximately 12 obese patients. In six, there were no significant glomerular abnormalities. One had a thrombosis of the renal veins and vena cava and membranous glomerulopathy at autopsy. The other patients showed focal to extensive fibrin deposition within and adjacent to capillary loops. These were associated with adhesions to Bowman's capsule and had a variable endocapillary proliferative response. Although these changes had some similarities to focal sclerosing glomerulonephritis, there were many features that were not typical of this condition including the clinical course. Almost all of the cases of nephrotic syndrome remitted with weight loss. No patient had significant functional impairment. It is our feeling that although proteinuria of very low grade may be present secondary to severe obesity, the incidence of nephrotic syndrome is extremely rare. With weight loss, proteinuria should decrease dramatically or disappear in all patients with obesity and the nephrotic syndrome. If the nephrotic syndrome and proteinuria do not remit with weight loss, another coexisting condition should be seriously considered.

MISCELLANEOUS RENAL SYNDROMES

A case has been reported of an obese 48-year-old woman who developed reversible renal failure because of sitting with her feet elevated. Studies revealed a dramatic drop in renal plasma flow in the sitting position, which reversed when supine. The rare syndrome of hypodipsia and antidiuretic hormone (ADH) resistance resulting in hypernatremia with subsequent muscle weakness and paralysis has been reported in an obese 24-year-old man. This is thought to be due to a hypothalamic lesion. Diabetes insipidus was not present in this patient.

There have been a number of cases of contralateral displacement of a kidney and ureter due to an incisional hernia (pseudocrossed renal ectopy).

Type II diabetes mellitus occurs in obese patients, and this may lead to nephrotic syndrome and renal failure.

In a review of risk factors for renal cell carcinoma in people younger than age 55, obesity was a significant risk factor for both males and females. The incidence of aminoglycoside nephrotoxicity may be increased in obese patients despite the adjustment of the drug dosage.

LAURENCE-MOON-BIEDL SYNDROME

Laurence-Moon-Biedl syndrome is a rare autosomal recessive disorder characterized by obesity, pigmentary retinopathy, polydactyly, hypogonadism, and mental retardation. Renal structural or functional abnormalities are found in almost every patient with this syndrome and many go on to develop end-stage renal disease, requiring hemodialysis. Fifty percent of the patients have hypertension. In most patients urine is not concentrated above 750 mOsm/kg of body weight after vasopressin and urinary pH is not lowered after an acid load.

Structural changes include calyceal clubbing and blunting in almost all patients. Many had calyceal cysts or diverticula, and many had lobulated renal outlines of the fetal type. Therefore, all patients with this syndrome should be evaluated carefully for the presence of structural abnormalities.

RENAL TRANSPLANTATION COMPLICATIONS

In comparing obese cadaveric transplant recipients with normal-weight control subjects, it was found that overall mortality was increased from 2% to 11% in obese recipients, immediate graft function decreased to 38% compared with 64% in nonobese subjects, and 1-year graft survival was 66% in obese recipients versus 84% in nonobese recipients.

PICKWICKIAN SYNDROME

The Pickwickian syndrome (named after Joe, the fat boy in Dickens' *Pickwick Papers*) is frequently associated with respiratory insufficiency. Eighteen of 22 patients in one series had an arterial P_{CO_2} greater than 50 mm Hg; 14 of 22 had a decreased arterial P_{O_2}.

END-STAGE RENAL DISEASE

Chronic ambulatory peritoneal dialysis is equally effective in obese and normal weight patients with end-stage renal disease (ESRD); however, the death rate is higher in patients who lose weight irrespective of their initial weight.

Leptin, which is produced by fat cells and thought to be the "satiety" hormone, has been implicated in the obesity of humans and genetically obese mice. Leptin is primarily degraded in the kidney (80%). This may account for the anorexia associated with chronic renal failure, because with the greater percentage of body fat the leptin levels become higher. Detailed discussion on leptin is found in Chapter 74, Part 5.

CONSEQUENCES OF JEJUNOILEAL INTESTINAL BYPASS SURGERY

Renal Complications

Although the use of gastrointestinal bypass has diminished considerably in the past 5 years, there are still many patients who had undergone gastrointestinal bypass surgery for the treatment of morbid obesity. As many as 30% of these patients develop calcium oxalate renal calculi.

Gastrointestinal bypass leads to steatorrhea and subsequent hyperoxaluria. The hyperoxaluria is a result of increased oxalate absorption from the large bowel. Normally, 20 to 40 mg of oxalate is excreted in the urine each day as a result of oxalate absorption from the large bowel. Most ingested oxalate is eliminated in the stool as insoluble calcium oxalate. In the post-bypass state, or for that matter in steatorrhea from any cause, large quantities of unabsorbed fatty acids are present in the lower bowel. These fatty acids combine with available calcium ions to form insoluble calcium soaps. Because the oxalate is no longer bound to calcium, it is free to be absorbed into the circulation and therefore excreted by the kidney. With this increased load of oxalate, crystals form in both the urine and the kidney. The deposition of oxalate crystals in the renal parenchyma leads to a tubulointerstitial nephritis and potential renal failure. Dismantling of the bypass reverses the hyperoxaluria, but the renal failure is often irreversible.

The treatment of post-bypass hyperoxaluria consists of a diet low in oxalate, an increase in fluid intake, and in many cases a low-fat diet. Substitution of medium-chain triglycerides for dietary fat may reduce oxaluria by as much as 30% because of the reduced complexing effects with calcium. Paradoxically, the oral administration of calcium in large quantities permits the formation of calcium soaps and yet provides surplus calcium in the bowel to be bound to oxalate. The precipitating insoluble calcium oxalate complex in the bowel or in the stool leads to a decrease in the oxalate available for absorption. Cholestyramine is also a viable alternative because it absorbs soluble oxalate salts.

In a significant number of patients, no oxalate crystals are found after bypass surgery; however, a focal interstitial nephritis with tubular atrophy, fibrosis, and glomerular hyalinization may be present. IgM and C3 granular deposits have been found in the glomerular capillaries and the mesangium of several patients, suggesting that immune complex injury may be playing a role. The antigen for the immune complexes probably arises from the overgrowth of colonic bacteria. Antibody against *Klebsiella pneumoniae* was found in the glomeruli of a patient with renal and skin vasculitis accompanied by cryoglobulinemia, polyarthritis, and acute renal failure. Cryoglobulins with IgG antibodies to *Escherichia coli* and *Bacillus fragilis* have been found in similar patients with a multisystem disease characterized by mixed cryoglobulinemia, polyarthritis, dermatitis, and renal insufficiency. A clinically similar syndrome has been described, consisting of fevers, myalgia, polyarthralgias, and aseptic joint swellings but with granulomas in the kidney and liver. No immunoglobulins were found in the kidneys.

One case of granulomatous interstitial nephritis and renal failure has been reported following intestinal bypass surgery. In this case. oxalate crystals and interstitial nephritis with giant cells relating to the crystalline material was found. Renal function improved following the reversal of the intestinal bypass.

Electrolyte Disturbances

Following bypass surgery, many fluid and electrolyte changes may be anticipated. During this initial period, most patients develop diarrhea, and if adequate water intake is not maintained, dehydration will occur. Over time, however, total body water frequently increases, leading to overhydration. This may be the result of protein malnutrition. As many as 40% of patients develop signs of electrolyte depletion during the first year following bypass surgery. With time, the incidence of electrolyte depletion decreases to a low of approximately 5%.

The most frequently reported electrolyte derangement seen after bypass surgery is potassium depletion. Somewhere between 20% and 30% of patients will develop hypokalemia (defined as a potassium level of less than 3.5 mEq/L) despite potassium supplementation. Potassium levels of less than 3.0 mEq/L occurred in approximately 18% of patients in one series. The potassium depletion is due to fecal loss. If there is accompanying volume depletion, elevations in aldosterone levels occur, and urinary potassium losses ensue. Symptoms such as muscle weakness, cramping, tingling, and other paresthesias are common as in other hypokalemic states. Although sodium is frequently lost in the stool of patients with diarrhea, sodium absorption in the colon and ileum is relatively more efficient. With elevated aldosterone levels, sodium retention in exchange for potassium occurs and losses of sodium are not as great as those of potassium. Hyponatremia and hypernatremia have been reported in patients after bypass surgery, but these abnormalities are usually very rare. More commonly, hyperchloremia is found and in some patients, a severe hyperchloremic acidosis may be present. This may also be a clue to the existence of the interstitial nephritis seen after bypass surgery as discussed previously.

Calcium losses following bypass surgery may be marked. Fecal calcium loss increases in steatorrheic conditions in which there is rapid transit, short bowel syndrome, or reduced vitamin D levels. Gastrointestinal absorption of calcium in some patients has been as low as 8% of ingested calcium after bypass surgery, compared with normal obese patients whose calcium absorption is around 20%. Because magnesium is absorbed throughout the small bowel and absorption decreases in proportion to reduction in bowel length, losses of magnesium in stool after bypass surgery are substantial and increase when diarrhea is severe. As much as 30 mEq of magnesium/24 hr may be lost in the stool. Desspite these large losses of magnesium and calcium, clinical manifestations of depletions are rare.

Hypocalcemia (defined as less than 8.5 mEq/L) has been observed in 20% to 25% of patients after bypass surgery.

Dehydration after bypass surgery must obviously be handled initially with intravenous solutions. Once a patient is eating, oral supplementation of calcium, magnesium, potassium, or vitamin D is recommended as maintenance therapy. Often, bulk-forming agents and/or cholestyramine may be used to slow down the diarrhea. If there is significant enteropathy, systemic antibiotics against bowel flora may be used.

BULIMIA AND ANOREXIA NERVOSA

The incidence of eating disorders is said to be reaching epidemic proportions in some populations. Bulimia is a syndrome characterized by a pattern of episodic binge eating frequently followed by self-induced vomiting or laxative abuse. Patients with anorexia nervosa differ in that they do not ingest the large amount of food that bulimic patients do; however, they do induce vomiting, abuse laxatives, and, in addition, often abuse diuretics. Frequently, the two syndromes overlap. As a result, patients are frequently seen with dehydration, metabolic alkalosis, hypochloremia, hypocalcemia, or hypokalemia. Many are also likely to show magnesium depletion. The mechanisms for the fluid and electrolyte problems are the same as in any patient with vomiting, diuretic use, or laxative abuse. Plasma renin concentration and aldosterone levels are often elevated. Frequently in these patients, urinary electrolyte measurements are extremely helpful in establishing the diagnosis.

FLUID AND ELECTROLYTE COMPLICATIONS OF FASTING

Fasting has been practiced throughout history. People have fasted for political as well as religious reasons. Fasting has also been used as a therapeutic modality for various medical conditions. During wartime, many people have been forced to fast, and many survivors of catastrophes at sea or in the air have also fasted. For a period of time, total fasting was used in the hospital setting for morbidly obese patients. A modified fast, that is, a supply of 400 to 800 kcal/24 hr, has also been used as a therapeutic modality in the morbidly obese patient. As a result of these experiments, many physiologic alterations have been studied. A thorough knowledge of the pathophysiology of fasting is necessary before considering this treatment for any patient. Without adequate supervision, total fasting or even modified fasting can lead to severe fluid and electrolyte disturbances.

Water Balance

During the initial 5 to 7 days of a total fast, patients undergo a spontaneous and marked diuresis. Obese patients lose as much as 12 L of fluid in the course of a 1 month's total fast. This diuresis is partially blunted with the introduction of calories. The major part of the water loss occurs in the first 5 days, diminishing rapidly over the next 5 to 7 days. Approximately two-thirds of the early water loss originates in the extracellular compartment. There is also a contraction of the intravascular volume, estimated to be between 12% and 20%.

Sodium

Sodium losses in the urine are marked in the first week of fasting, after which a balance is gradually achieved. If a patient was consuming a low-sodium diet before fasting, the natriuresis will be much less. The etiology of this natriuresis involves decreasing serum insulin levels, increasing plasma glucagon levels, acidemia, and changes in renin and aldosterone.

Potassium

During the initial phases of fasting, urinary potassium loss occurs as long as the sodium and water diuresis is maintained. Significant amounts of potassium are lost; during a total fast the amount of potassium lost for a 1-month period is between 500 and 800 mEq.

Magnesium and Calcium

With total fasting, significant amounts of magnesium are lost in the urine. Magnesium losses in the first 1 to 2 months of fasting can be as much as 450 mEq, with the average loss being approximately 400 mEq. Urinary calcium losses also occur in the initial phases of fasting but to a much lesser degree. Total losses of calcium during a 50-day period of fasting have ranged from 500 to 900 mEq.

Acid–Base Balance

Initially, there is a dramatic rise in serum ketone levels, primarily β-hydroxybutyric acid. Blood pH frequently falls to between 7.30 and 7.36 at the end of the first week of fasting and then slowly rises. Serum bicarbonate falls to as low as 16 mEq/L and then gradually rises to normal over the next 2 to 3 weeks. Respiratory compensation does occur, with the P_{CO_2} falling to between 30 and 35 mm Hg. This respiratory compensation usually subsides within 3 weeks, after which complete acid–base equilibrium is maintained.

Uric Acid

Primarily because of the competition for excretion between keto acids and uric acid at renal tubular transport sites, serum uric acid rises in the first 2 weeks of fasting. Thereafter, serum uric acid levels fall. Rarely, uric acid renal calculi may form during this period. Patients with a history of uric acid calculi or acute gouty arthritis probably should be treated with allopurinol during fasting.

Modified Fasting and Refeeding

Modified fasting, that is, the provision of 400 to 800 kcal/24 hr, is still associated with diuresis. However, because lean tissue is spared in modified fasting relative to total fasting, the losses of magnesium, potassium, and calcium are of a lesser magnitude.

During refeeding, there is a dramatic change in many of the hormonal and hemodynamic changes that have occurred during fasting. Insulin levels rise, volume expansion occurs, catecholamine levels rise, and there is a retention of salt and water, causing many individuals to actually become edematous. After the ingestion of food for a number of days, the patient usually undergoes spontaneous diuresis of the retained fluid.

Management of Electrolyte Problems Incurred by Fasting

Obviously, in the first 1 to 2 weeks of fasting adequate fluid intake must be maintained. Although there is a dramatic water diuresis, a considerable amount of sodium chloride is also lost. For this reason, patients may need to be given salt, especially if they are not edematous. Often, this is not necessary because the patient already shows volume expansion and has hypertension and/or edema. In any circumstance, potassium, usually as sugarless 10% potassium chloride, should be given in divided doses to equal at least 40 to 60 mEq/day. If there is no source of magnesium or calcium in the diet, supplementation of these cations along with vitamins and other minerals must be provided. Total fasting is not acceptable as a therapeutic modality. Modified fasting however, with appropriate vitamin and mineral supplementation has been found to be an acceptable therapy for morbidly obese patients.

Selected Readings

Bendezu R, Wieland RD, Green SG, et al. Certain metabolic consequences of jejunoileal bypass. *Am J Clin Nutr* 1976;29:366–370.

Discussion of metabolic changes, including calcium and magnesium, in patients after jejunoileal bypass.

Cohen AH. Massive obesity and the kidney. *Am J Pathol* 1975;81:117–127.

Review of pathology of the kidney in obese patients.

Drenick EJ, Stanley TM, Border WA, et al. Renal damage with intestinal bypass. *Ann Intern Med* 1978;89:594–599.

Renal pathology and pathophysiology in patients after intestinal bypass.

Hall J. The Kidney, Obesity, and Essential Hypertension Symposium. *Hypertension* 1992;(Suppl 1):I1.

Excellent update on problems relating to blood pressure, obesity, and the kidney.

Maxwell MH, Schroth PC, Waks AU, et al. Error in blood-pressure measurement due to incorrect cuff size in obese patients. *Lancet* 1982;2:33–36.

Discussion of the problem of blood pressure measured in obese subjects, with an excellent chart of arm size versus blood pressure.

Mitchell JE, Pyle RL, Eckert ED, et al. Electrolyte and other physiological abnormalities in patients with bulimia. *Psychol Med* 1983;13:273–278.

Review of acid–base, fluid, and electrolyte changes in bulimic patients.

Sowers JR, Whitefield LA, Catania RA, et al. Role of the sympathetic nervous system in blood pressure maintenance in obesity. *J Clin Endocrinol Metab* 1982;54:1181–1186.

Discussion of problems involving the sympathetic nervous system in obese patients.

Tuck ML, Sowers JR, Dornfeld LP, et al. The effect of weight reduction on blood pressure, plasma renin activity, and plasma aldosterone levels in obese patients. *N Engl J Med* 1981;304:930–933.

Analysis of renin-aldosterone response to weight reduction.

Weinsier RL, James LD, Darnell BE, et al. Clinical studies: Obesity-related hypertension: evaluation of the separate effects of energy restriction and weight reduction on hemodynamic and neuroendocrine status. *Am J Med* 1991;90:460–468.

Summary of obesity, insulin, and kidney relationship.

PART 3
Lipoprotein Disorders

Hiroaki Oda and William F. Keane

LIPOPROTEIN ABNORMALITIES IN PATIENTS WITH RENAL DISEASE

A number of investigations have characterized the abnormalities in circulating lipoproteins that are associated with renal disease (Table 56.6). Increased serum concentrations of total cholesterol and low-density lipoprotein (LDL) cholesterol have been the most frequently reported abnormalities in patients with nephrotic syndrome. Alterations in the composition, including increased phospholipids and cholesterol esters, as well as increased apolipoprotein B, have been described. The level of high-density lipoprotein (HDL) may be low, normal, or high. However, the HDL subtypes are abnormally distributed. Specifically, the level of HDL_2 is reduced while the level of HDL_3 is frequently increased. Clinically, reduced HDL_2 levels have been associated with increased risk of atherosclerosis. Triglyceride levels are also commonly elevated, particularly when the degree of proteinuria is severe or when renal insufficiency is present. Patients with proteinuria were also shown to have an increase in the putative atherogenic lipoprotein a [Lp(a)]. Lp(a) is under genetic control separate from LDL, and its presence in the circulation of nephrotic patients may further increase the risk of atherosclerosis. The mechanisms for these abnormalities in proteinuric patients are incompletely understood, but increased synthesis and altered receptor-dependent and receptor-independent catabolism have been demonstrated. Further discussion of the hyperlipidemia in nephrotic syndrome is found in Chapter 39, Part 2C.

The cardiovascular implications of these lipid abnormalities in patients with nephrotic syndrome have been considered controversial. However, given the magnitude and frequency of these changes, it is difficult to ignore their potential for vascular injury, particularly when they persist over many years. In a preliminary report of adults with chronic proteinuria, the relative risk for death related to coronary artery disease and the risk for an acute myocardial infarction was more than fivefold greater than that for age-matched and sex-matched nondiabetic control patients. In addition, in children with proteinuric renal diseases who died at a mean age of 14.9 + 7.7 years, more than 75% had evidence of coronary artery disease, and 13% had greater than 50% narrowing of coronary arteries. Unfortunately, lipid analysis were not routinely performed in these young patients.

Patients with both type I and type II diabetes have abnormalities in circulating lipoproteins that are evident with the onset of microalbuminuria (Table 56.6). In this setting both an increase in LDL cholesterol and a reduction in HDL cholesterol have been reported. Other data suggest that diabetic patients with microalbuminuria also have an increased Lp(a) level. These observations are of particular note because it has been established that the presence of microalbuminuria in type I and type II diabetes has been associated with a dramatic increase in mortality from cardiovascular diseases. Perhaps more important than the levels of lipoproteins, are the potentially injurious alterations in lipoprotein composition that are associated with diabetes. Decreased density, increased size, triglyceride enrichment, decreased apolipoprotein content, and glycosylated as well as oxidized lipoproteins have all been reported in diabetic patients.

Decreased renal function also appears to be associated with abnormal lipoprotein metabolism. In patients with glomerular filtration rates (GFRs) less than 60 ml/min, triglyceride levels are usually elevated and HDL concentrations are lower. These lipoprotein abnormalities may be the result of decreased lipoprotein lipase activity and could possibly be injurious to vascular and renal tissues. In patients with renal failure an increase in Lp(a) has been reported, and this might also contribute to the high incidence of cardiovascular disease in patients with

TABLE 56.6. Lipoprotein Abnormalities in Patients with Renal Disease[a]

	Very-Low-Density Lipoproteins	Low-Density Lipoproteins	High-Density Lipoproteins
Nephrotic syndrome	↑	↑↑	N/↓
Diabetes with nephropathy	↑	↑/↑↑	↓
Renal insufficiency	↑	N	↓

[a] Arrows indicate direction and magnitude of lipoprotein alteration. *N*, not different from normal.

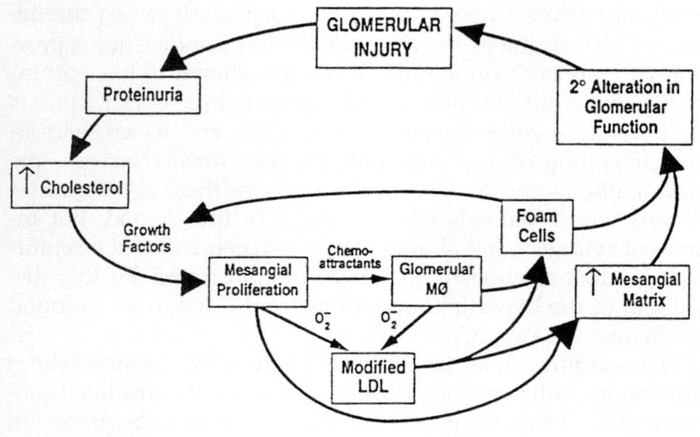

Figure 56.6. Experimental evidence suggests that increased lipids *(cholesterol)* as a result of proteinuria leads to a number of changes in the glomerulus that result in an increased influx of macrophages, formation of modified (oxidized) LDL, foam cell development, and progressive expansion of the mesangial matrix, ultimately leading to glomerulosclerosis. LDL, low-density lipoprotein; MÆ, macrophage; O_2^-, superoxide.

end-stage renal failure. Detailed discussion of lipid abnormalities in patients with chronic renal failure is provided in Chapter 74, Part 2.

The mechanisms whereby lipids contribute to glomerular injury are incompletely understood (Fig. 56.6). Experimental evidence for a role of glomerular macrophages, modified (oxidized) LDL, and glomerular cell growth has been found. Foam cells, which are believed to result from nonreceptor-regulated uptake of modified lipoproteins by macrophages, are frequently found in sclerotic segments of glomeruli of patients with focal glomerulosclerosis. The finding of lipoproteins in glomeruli of patients with nephrotic syndrome suggests that these lipoproteins may indeed be modified. In addition, experimental data have indicated that modified LDL may alter vasoactive substances. Specifically, a reduction in vasodilator substances such as nitric oxide and an increase in vasoconstrictor substances such as endothelin and thromboxane A_2 have been demonstrated.

LIPIDS AND THE PROGRESSION OF HUMAN RENAL DISEASE

The incidence of overt renal disease in patients with the most common forms of hyperlipidemia, although unknown, is presumably low. One study suggested that there is no increased incidence of microalbuminuria in patients with primary lipid abnormalities. On the other hand, an autopsy study showed that there is a significant relationship between global glomerulosclerosis and atherosclerosis, suggesting that potentially important relationships exist between factors leading to atherosclerosis and those leading to glomerulosclerosis. This evidence suggests, in part, that lipid abnormalities are more important modulators of progressive renal injury than primary initiators of kidney disease.

Genetically, apolipoprotein E polymorphism may play a role in the progression of renal dysfunction in lipoprotein glomerulopathy. Histologically this form of glomerular injury is characterized by the presence of laminated thrombi consisting of lipid droplets with mesangial expansion, endothelial cell swelling, and segmental sclerosis. Immunofluorescence studies showed apolipoprotein B and E staining in the dilated lumina of glomeruli, and granular deposits have been observed in the capillary lumina by electron microscopy. The clinical features of lipoprotein glomerulopathy are the presence of nephrotic syndrome with relatively rapid progression of renal impairment and development of glomerulosclerosis and tubulointerstitial fibrosis. Reported patients with lipoprotein glomerulopathy have been mostly Japanese and have apolipoprotein ϵ2 as shown by isoelectric focusing. Interestingly, some of these patients carry a specific phenotype of apolipoprotein E Sendai, which shows apolipoprotein ϵ2 by isoelectric focusing, but apolipoprotein ϵ3 by DNA sequence analysis. These data indicated that a point mutation had occurred which altered the electrophoretic mobility, resulting in a misclassification of the phenotype, but this relatively minor change also resulted in altered apolipoprotein E receptor binding. Recurrence of lipoprotein glomerulopathy has occurred in transplanted kidneys, suggesting that this disease is caused by extrarenal factors. The prevalence of the apolipoprotein ϵ2 phenotype in nondiabetic Japanese patients with end stage renal disease was higher than that found in normal Japanese subjects, and a higher prevalence of the apolipoprotein ϵ2 phenotype in Japanese patients with type II diabetes and renal failure was similarly reported. Whether a similar preponderance of apolipoprotein phenotypes occurs in the non-Japanese population remains controversial.

There are other uncommon lipoprotein abnormalities that appear to lead to glomerular lipid deposition, the accumulation of glomerular foam cells, and the development of glomerulosclerosis. In patients with a deficiency of lecithin–cholesterol acyltransferase (LCAT) activity cholesterol is not normally esterified and develop abnormally large, lipid-laden HDLs develop. Patients with an inherited deficiency of the LCAT enzyme have abnormal lipoproteins, and in the majority of these patients progressive glomerulosclerosis develops. Electron micrographs of renal tissue obtained from these patients show dense deposits in the glomerular capillary basement membrane and the mesangium that resemble the abnormal circulating LDL. In addition, apolipoprotein B has been detected in the mesangium and along the glomerular capillary loop in a patient with LCAT deficiency. It has been suggested that the physiochemical alterations of LDL resulting from diminished LCAT activity may lead to the deposition of LDL in the glomerulus. Interestingly, reductions in LCAT activity also have been reported to cause formation of abnormal lipoproteins and glomerular disease in some patients with congenital or acquired liver disease.

In nondiabetic patients with proteinuria, hypercholesterolemia, and hypertriglyceridemia, the rate of loss of renal function was nearly twofold greater than in control patients. This effect was independent of blood pressure control. Other studies have also shown that apolipoprotein B–containing lipoproteins contribute to the progression of renal disease. Triglyceride-rich apolipoprotein B–containing lipoproteins had a positive association with the rate of a yearly decline of GFR in nondiabetic patients with renal insufficiency. In addition, in black and Hispanic children with focal glomerulosclerosis, the rate of loss of renal function was related to the level of cholesterol. Whether other lipid fractions, such as Lp(a), which is also elevated in patients with nephrotic syndrome, play a role in progressive nephron injury remains to be established. The study of the modification of diet in renal disease has also demonstrated that lipids were an independent predictor of progression of renal disease. In this study patients with higher HDL levels had slower rates of progressive loss of renal function.

In some studies of patients with type I and type II diabetic nephropathy, a significant independent correlation between total serum cholesterol and the rate of decline of renal function was observed in retrospective analyses.

Other studies have suggested that the dyslipidemia present in patients after renal transplantation also predicts loss of renal allograft function. Transplant recipients with hypercholesterolemia have a higher plasma creatinine level, lower creatinine clearance, greater histologic changes including interstitial fibrosis, and more severe vascular intimal changes, consistent with chronic graft damage. Hypertriglyceridemia has been reported also to be a significant and independent risk factor for chronic renal allograft loss.

LIPID-LOWERING STRATEGIES

A variety of lipid-lowering agents have been shown to reduce cholesterol levels in patients with hypercholesterolemia and proteinuria. All of these studies have been short term and designed to show the safety and efficacy of the agent. Preliminary, uncontrolled studies have suggested that lipid-lowering therapy may be of clinical benefit to patients. In large part, these studies have used the newer 3-hydroxy-3-methylglutaryl coenzyme A (HMG-CoA) reductase inhibitors. In one uncontrolled study, therapy for nearly 1 year with this class of agents was associated with a reduction in proteinuria, whereas in another study no change in proteinuria was observed although patients with only a modest reduction in renal function had a significant improvement in glomerular filtration rate. A preliminary trial in patients with hypercholesterolemia and proteinuria treated for 1 year with an angiotensin-converting enzyme inhibitor to which an HMG-CoA reductase inhibitor was then added showed a further reduction in the rate of loss of renal function. Uniquely, angiotensin-converting enzyme inhibitors decrease proteinuria which secondarily will also decrease the degree of hyperlipidemia seen in proteinuric patients. In conclusion, although these studies suggest that, in human renal diseases, treatment of hyperlipidemia may be of benefit to patients, it is imperative that prospective and controlled studies with clinically appropriate functional and morphologic end points be developed. The impact of these agents on cardiovascular disease is unknown.

Extracorporeal LDL cholesterol removal or LDL apheresis has been reported to lower serum cholesterol, reduce proteinuria, and improve renal function in a small group of patients with nephrotic syndrome. Of note is the fact that repeat renal biopsy specimens from these patients demonstrated a decrease in lipoprotein deposits in glomeruli and a reduction in the number of glomerular foam cells.

In addition to their lipid-lowering effects, the HMG-CoA reductase inhibitors suppress the inflammatory response caused by certain cytokines and growth factors by inhibiting *Ras* isoprenylation. Experimental evidence suggests that HMG-CoA reductase inhibitors affect at least two important processes involved in the development of glomerulosclerosis, that is, proliferation and glomerular monocyte infiltration. Thus the lipid-lowering strategies may influence progression of renal disease by both direct (lipid-lowering) and indirect mechanisms (decreasing inflammatory response).

Selected Readings

Attman P-O, Samuelsson O. Lipid abnormality in progressive renal insufficiency. *Contrib Nephrol* 1997;120:1–10.

In this study a significant independent correlation between rate of loss of renal function and plasma levels of apolipoprotein B–containing lipoproteins was demonstrated.

Chan PCK, Robinson JD, Yeung WC, et al. Lovastatin in glomerulonephritis patients with hyperlipidemia and heavy proteinuria. *Nephrol Dial Transplant* 1992;7:93–99.

This is a recent study demonstrating a longer term benefit of lipid-lowering therapy in patients with nephrotic syndrome. Specifically, improvement in renal function was observed in a subset of these patients.

Jenkins AJ, Steele JS, Janus ED, et al. Increased plasma apolipoprotein (a) levels in IDDM patients with microalbuminuria. *Diabetes* 1991;40:787–790.

In this study diabetic patients with microalbuminuria had significantly elevated apolipoprotein (a) levels compared with control diabetic patients without microalbuminuria. The clinical implications of this association need to be established in prospective studies.

Jensen T, Borch-Johsen K, Kofoed-Enevoldsen A, et al. Coronary heart disease in young type I (insulin-dependent) diabetic patients with and without diabetic nephropathy: incidence and risk factors. *Diabetologia* 1987;30:144–148.

This study demonstrates the development of potentially atherogenic lipid profiles in diabetic patients with nephropathy as indicated by the presence of albuminuria.

Joven J, Villabona C, Vilella E, et al. Abnormalities of lipoprotein metabolism in patients with the nephrotic syndrome. *N Engl J Med* 1990;323:579–584.

This is a comprehensive study of lipoprotein abnormalities in patients with nephrotic syndrome. In addition, this study addresses the mechanism of the abnormalities in lipid metabolism present in patients with nephrotic syndrome.

Keane WF. Lipids and the kidney. *Kidney Int* 1994;46:910–920.

This recent review details experimental and clinical insights as to how lipids contribute to renal injury. The mechanisms of lipid-lowering agents such as HMG-CoA reductase inhibitors in modulation of cell proliferative response to mitogenic cytokines are also well described.

CHAPTER 57

The Kidney and Aging

David A. Maddox, Fred K. Alavi, and Edward T. Zawada, Jr.

The geriatric population (65 years of age or older) in the United States is rapidly increasing. As a consequence of age-related infirmities, more than 40% of hospital admissions are associated with this segment of society, which currently comprises only about 15% of the total population. Among the pathologic consequences associated with normal aging are a number of structural and functional changes in the kidney. These changes complicate common illnesses of elderly patients, add to the length of hospital stays in older individuals, add morbidity and mortality in this population, and influence the cost of care of those older than age 65. It is therefore of great importance to consider potential ways of slowing the development of these age-related changes.

The subject matter of the aging kidney is the foundation for the geriatric subspecialty area, geriatric nephrology. As in previous editions we will cover the new findings that explain renal senescence. In addition, we will review the most common acquired renal diseases of older adults, such as hypertension, reviewing their management not only from the perspective of the nephrologist but also from the perspective of the geriatrician. From this latter point of view, treatment that does not improve the patient's quality of life or that worsens functional status because of side effects is considered futile and may not be continued. Although end-stage renal disease (ESRD) is covered in other chapters, we will specifically examine the newest developments in management of the elderly patient with this disease as it relates to the subspecialty of geriatric nephrology.

FUNCTIONAL CHANGES IN THE AGING KIDNEY

Glomerular Hemodynamics

Progressive age-dependent declines in glomerular filtration rate (GFR) and renal blood flow (RBF) are observed in nearly everyone as they age past 30 to 40 years. As shown in Fig. 57.1, the decline in GFR between 35 and 55 years of age is approximately 1 ml/min × year, accelerating to about 1.4 ml/min × year beyond 55 years of age. Nevertheless, the loss of filtration capacity is slow enough that even in very elderly patients GFR is more than adequate to sustain life. Moreover, GFR may not decline with age in as many as one-third of all individuals. This suggests that factors other than aging, such as immunologic injury, drug or toxic chemical exposure, environmental factors, diet, infections, ureteral obstruction, or other pathologic insults may contribute, in part, to the age-related decline in GFR seen in the rest of the population. More than likely a decline in GFR with age in most people is linked to normal exposure of the glomerulus to a variety of factors. These include lifelong repeated high-protein meals (yielding routine episodes of hyperfiltration and glomerular capillary hypertension) and the presence of glucose in the blood [yielding, with time, advanced glycosylated end products (AGEs) even at normal glucose concentrations and accelerated in the face of high concentrations]. Chronic exposure to oxygen free radicals and oxidized low-density lipoproteins and periodic exposure to a variety of diseases and drugs may also contribute.

The determinants of GFR are discussed in Chapter 4, but a brief summary is presented as a prelude to the discussion of age-related changes in GFR. GFR is determined by the product of the surface area available for filtration (S), the hydraulic conductivity of the filtering area (k), and the mean net pressure for ultrafiltration (P_{UF}). P_{UF} is the difference between the mean transcapillary hydraulic and colloid osmotic pressure differences (ΔP and $\Delta\pi$, respectively) averaged along the length of the glomerular capillary. ΔP equals the mean glomerular hydraulic pressure (P_{GC}) minus the pressure in Bowman's space and $\Delta\pi$ equals the mean glomerular capillary oncotic pressure minus Bowman's space oncotic pressure (which is essentially zero). The four primary determinants of GFR are glomerular capillary plasma flow rate (Q_A), ΔP, K_f, and plasma oncotic pressure. In humans, the decline in GFR with age is accompanied by a marked reduction in RBF and hence Q_A because of a marked increase in renal vascular resistance. The degree of reduction in Q_A is greater than the reduction in GFR, thereby resulting in an increase in filtration fraction. The decrease in blood flow is confined primarily to the cortex, with juxtamedullary blood flow

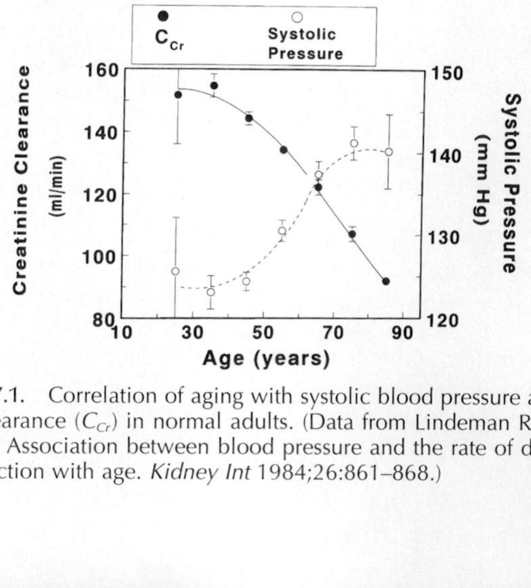

Figure 57.1. Correlation of aging with systolic blood pressure and creatinine clearance (C_{Cr}) in normal adults. (Data from Lindeman R, Tobin J, Shock N. Association between blood pressure and the rate of decline in renal function with age. *Kidney Int* 1984;26:861–868.)

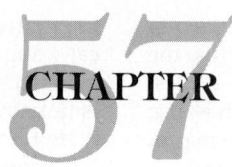

being better preserved. Micropuncture measurements in the rat indicate that P_{GC} and ΔP are relatively unchanged as a consequence of aging until the animals are very old at which point both P_{GC} and ΔP are markedly elevated. Similarly, K_f is relatively unchanged until rats reach a very advanced age at which point there is a marked decline in K_f and an increase in proteinuria and glomerular sclerosis. Thus, in humans, it might be predicted that the age-related decline in GFR is caused by a combination of a marked reduction in renal plasma flow and possibly K_f with GFR being sustained as well as it is because of concomitant increases in P_{GC} and ΔP. A chronic increase in P_{GC} is thought to play an important initiating role in the development of glomerular injury in many disease states. If P_{GC} is increased with aging in the human, the net result might then be a progressive loss of more and more glomeruli and a further reduction in GFR.

RBF and GFR are under the direct control of a variety of vasoconstrictor and vasodilator substances, and alterations in the production of these vasoactive agents occur with aging. There is increased renal sympathetic nerve activity due to a blunting of the arterial baroreceptor reflex that could increase renal vascular tone. Although systemic renin levels appear to decline with age, intrarenal angiotensin II production may actually increase, again resulting in increased renal vascular resistance. Furthermore, endothelin (ET-1) production by vascular endothelial cells is increased with aging, although vascular smooth muscle sensitivity to the peptide may decline. Both angiotensin and ET-1 initiate a cascade of events leading to mesangial expansion. Vascular endothelial cell production of the potent vasodilator prostaglandin prostacyclin (PGI_2) is decreased with aging, leading to an increase in the ratio of thromboxane production, a vasoconstrictor, relative to PGI_2 and prostaglandin E_2. This may also contribute to the reduction in RBF observed. Nitric oxide (NO), a powerful vasodilator released from vascular endothelial cells, is reduced in peripheral blood vessels in aging animals. In the kidney, however, basal NO production appears to be high and may be working overtime to protect the kidney against the other vasoconstrictor influences working to reduce blood flow.

The reduced GFR and RBF due to aging may become problematic in the event of additive loss caused by concomitant diseases such as diabetes, hypertension, and obstructive uropathy. At the least, the reduced GFR will contribute to altered pharmacokinetics, thus complicating medical therapy of elderly patients. Greater attention must be paid to dosages when elderly patients are given drugs excreted by the kidney, and elderly patients are at increased risk for ischemic and toxin-induced renal injury. It should be noted that serum creatinine concentrations do not increase with age due to a concomitant reduction in muscle mass, so this parameter becomes an unreliable indicator of the extent of the decline in GFR in elderly patients. Formulas have been developed for estimating creatinine clearance in elderly individuals based upon serum creatinine, body weight, and age that are reasonably reliable. One commonly used estimate for creatinine clearance in elderly individuals is given by the Cockroft and Gault formula:

$$\text{GFR (ml/min)} = \frac{[(140 - \text{age in yr}) \times \text{body weight (kg)}]^*}{(72 \times \text{Serum creatinine, mg/dl})}$$

Although this equation may be useful in everyday clinical practice to obtain a quick estimate of renal function, the values obtained are unacceptable predictors for true GFR in the aging population. When a precise estimate of GFR is required, only a timed measurement of creatinine or inulin clearance will provide accurate information.

*Multiply by 0.85 for females.

Fluid and Electrolyte Balance

Fluid Balance

Older individuals are more susceptible to dehydration than younger people and they recover more slowly from dehydration than young people. Some studies have shown that a similar degree of dehydration results in a greater rise in plasma osmolality and sodium in healthy older individuals than in young subjects. When allowed water *ad libitum* to rehydrate, young subjects have a greater sense of thirst and consume an amount of water necessary for complete rehydration more rapidly than the elderly subjects. Elderly individuals thus appear to have a greater thirst threshold and a lower thirst sensitivity to hypertonicity than young persons. In addition to alterations in the thirst response, elderly subjects have decreased renal concentrating ability in response to dehydration (Fig. 57.2). This could be due in part to the decline in GFR, but studies indicate that it is also related to a defect in response to antidiuretic hormone by the collecting duct and a defect in solute transport in the thick ascending limb of Henle's loop. The constancy of medullary blood flow combined with age-related declines in cortical blood flow and GFR may result in a greater medullary blood flow relative to medullary solute delivery, thereby tending to wash out the medullary hypertonicity. Some studies have shown that elderly patients experience a greater increase in plasma arginine vasopressin (AVP) levels in response to hypertonic sodium chloride infusion or dehydration. This suggests that the decrease in renal concentrating ability is due to an intrarenal defect rather than to a failure to release AVP in response to an osmotic stimulus. This enhanced AVP secretion may compensate for the reduced ability of the kidney to form concentrated urine with age. In association with decreased ability to conserve water and a diminished thirst response, plasma volume tends to be lower and plasma osmolality higher in older than in young subjects (Fig. 57.3). Renal diluting ability is also impaired in aging subjects and solute-free water clearance is decreased. The decrease in free water clearance is due in part to the reduction in GFR. Inadequate suppression of AVP release in response to lowering of plasma osmolality combined with an impairment of solute transport in the thick ascending limb may also play a role in the blunting of renal diluting capacity.

Sodium Balance

As shown in Fig. 57.4, when faced with sodium restriction normal young subjects are able to conserve sodium much more rapidly than elderly subjects. This may be related, in part, to

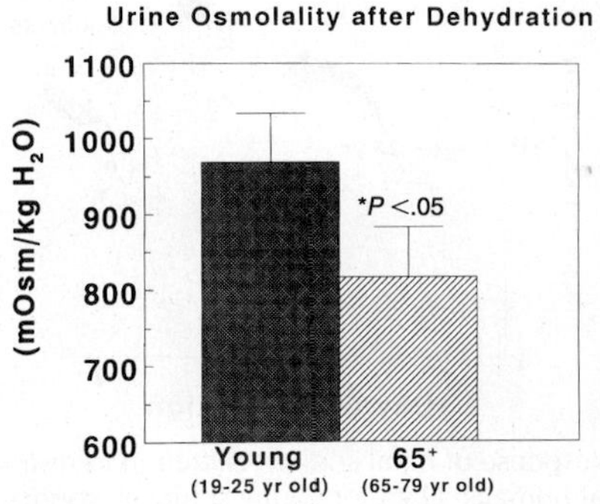

Figure 57.2. Dehydration (2.2% to 2.5% body weight induced by simultaneous exposure to heat and exercise for 105 minutes) results in the production of a more concentrated urine in young subjects compared to those older than 65 years of age. (Data from Mack GW, Weseman CA, Langhans GW, et al. Body fluid balance in dehydrated healthy older men: thirst and renal osmoregulation. *J Appl Physiol* 1994;76:1615–1623.)

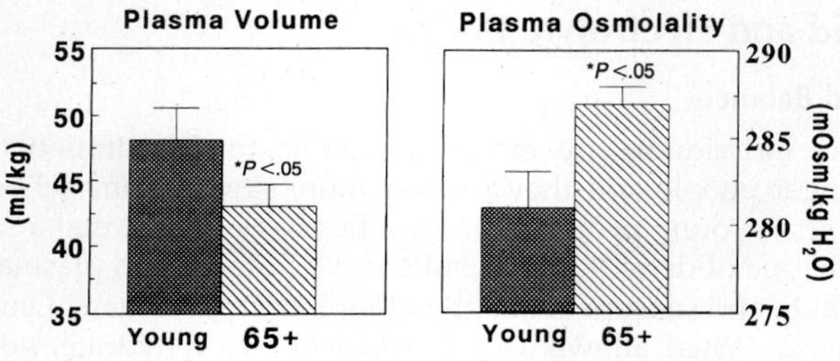

Figure 57.3. Plasma volume (*left panel*) and plasma osmolality in young subjects compared with those older than 65 years of age. (Data from Mack GW, Weseman CA, Langhans GW, et al. Body fluid balance in dehydrated healthy older men: thirst and renal osmoregulation. *J Appl Physiol* 1994;76:1615–1623.)

age-related changes in the renin-aldosterone system. Plasma renin activity declines with age in both sexes, and plasma renin and aldosterone activities increase less in elderly versus young subjects in response to sodium restriction. Thus during sodium restriction, the impaired ability to conserve sodium may be related both to decreased angiotensin II– and aldosterone-induced sodium transport.

The ability to excrete a sodium load is also impaired in elderly subjects. In part this is related to the reduction in GFR. Filtration fraction is higher in elderly subjects, thereby increasing efferent arteriolar oncotic pressure and hence increasing the physical forces favoring reabsorption in the proximal tubule. This may partially counterbalance the diminution of renin/angiotensin II levels, a factor that would tend to decrease proximal Na^+-H^+ exchange. In addition, there appears to be an age-related diminution in the responsiveness to atrial natriuretic peptide (ANP). Indeed, healthy elderly individuals have basal circulating levels of ANP that are three to five times that of young individuals, and these already high levels are stimulated to a greater extent in elderly than in young subjects in response to saline loading or head-out water immersion. Despite high circulating levels of ANP, which should enhance the ability to excrete a sodium load, there is a blunted renal response to the peptide, probably due to an age-related postreceptor defect.

Potassium Balance

Total body potassium stores and exchangeable potassium decrease with age in humans, possibly related in part to decreasing muscle mass. The risk of hyperkalemia in response to a potassium challenge, however, is theoretically increased in the elderly population because the decrease in GFR and the decreases in renin and aldosterone impede the ability of the kidney to eliminate potassium. In addition, elderly individuals may have impaired α-adrenergic–related potassium influx into skeletal muscle, resulting in a more rapid increase in plasma potassium in response to exercise. In aged rats maintained on a high-potassium diet, the ability to excrete an additional acute potassium load is diminished, resulting in a more marked elevation in plasma potassium. There is also extrarenal (gastrointestinal tract) impairment in potassium adaptation. In both the intrarenal and extrarenal components, it is thought that a reduction in Na^+-K^+-ATPase activity may be involved in the age-associated impairment of potassium adaptation. This may be related, in part, to the reduction in aldosterone seen with aging. Studies to examine whether age-dependent declines in the ability to adapt to potassium loads or potassium deprivation occur in humans have not been performed, but presumably that is the case. Indeed, elderly individuals are at increased risk for hyperkalemia when subjected to potassium-sparing diuretics, converting enzyme inhibitors, nonsteroidal antiinflammatory drugs (NSAIDs), or potassium supplements.

Acid–Base Balance

Elderly individuals have an impaired ability to increase acid excretion in response to an acute acid load as well as impaired excretion of an alkali load. The age-related impaired ability to excrete an acid load is related to a defect in NH_4^+ excretion. As a consequence, elderly individuals are at risk for longer persistence of acid–base disorders and may have a greater disturbance in acid–base homeostasis in response to a variety of medications taken for other diseases. Medications frequently prescribed for elderly patients that may cause acid–base disturbances are shown in Table 57.1.

Calcium and Phosphorous Balance

Elderly individuals may display a wide variety of disturbances in divalent ion metabolism including hypocalcemia, mild hypophosphatemia, high blood levels of parathyroid hormone (PTH), low blood levels of 25-hydroxyvitamin D_3 and 1,25-dihydroxyvitamin D_3, hypocalciuria, and hyperphosphaturia. Aging does not significantly alter renal tubule reabsorption of filtered calcium, but intestinal absorption of calcium is significantly

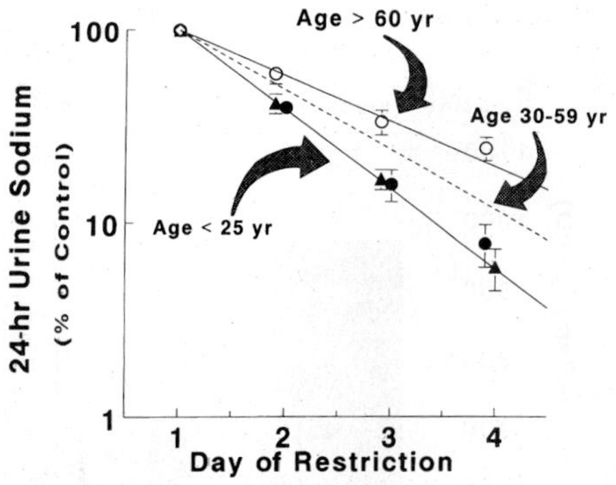

Figure 57.4. Response of renal sodium excretion to restriction of sodium intake in normal humans. Data for young subjects (younger than 25 years old) were obtained from New England (*filled circles*) and Texas (*filled triangles*) while those for the elderly subjects (older than 60 years of age, *open circles*) were obtained from New England residents. *Dashed line* denotes rate of response in people 30 to 59 years old. (Modified from Epstein M, Hollenberg NK. Age as a determinant of renal sodium conservation in normal man. *J Lab Clin Med* 1976;87:411–417.)

TABLE 57.1. Medicines That Predispose Elderly Individuals to Acid–Base Disorders

Acid–Base Disorder	Medication	Mechanism
Metabolic acidosis	Acetazolamide	Carbonic anhydrase inhibition
	Aspirin	Metabolic disruption
	Laxatives	Diarrhea
	NSAIDs	Aldosterone inhibition
Metabolic alkalosis	Digoxin	Vomiting
	Diuretics	Bicarbonate production and retention; volume contraction
	Antacids	Exogenous alkali
	Chemotherapy	Vomiting
	Estrogen	Increased renin/aldosterone
Respiratory alkalosis	Sedatives	Respiratory center depression
	Opiates	Respiratory center depression
Respiratory alkalosis	Aspirin	Respiratory stimulation

depressed as a consequence of age-related reductions in 1,25-dihydroxyvitamin D_3. The disturbed vitamin D metabolism is caused by an age-related reduction in renal 1α-hydroxylase activity (decreasing α-hydroxylation of vitamin D), a lack of exposure to sunlight, and dietary deficiency of vitamin D. Because of this disturbed vitamin D metabolism and diminished intestinal absorption of calcium, serum calcium levels are lower in elderly patients. The lower serum calcium levels stimulate PTH secretion, resulting in secondary hyperparathyroidism. Also, the decline in GFR in elderly individuals contributes to the elevation in blood levels of PTH. The mechanisms through which renal insufficiency causes an increase in PTH are discussed in Chapter 77.

Renal tubule reabsorption of phosphate is reduced with aging, an effect mediated by a decrease in the *V*max for Na^+ gradient–dependent phosphate transport associated with a decrease in the abundance of the Na^+-PO_4^{3-} transporter in the brush border membrane. The relative abundance of the Na^+-PO_4^{3-} transporter mRNA in the renal cortex is also lower in aged rats fed a normal phosphate diet than in young rats. When young and old rats were exposed to a low-phosphate diet for 7 days the Na^+-PO43– transporter mRNA increased markedly in the young rats and to a much lesser degree in the old animals. The inhibition of sodium-dependent phosphate transport may be mediated, in part, by age-dependent alterations in membrane cholesterol and fatty acid composition, resulting in a decrease in membrane fluidity, modulation of protein trafficking to and from the plasma membrane, and modulation of transcriptional regulation. Intestinal absorption of phosphate is also impaired. Transport of both renal and intestinal phosphate is improved in vitamin D–deficient animals by the administration of 1,25-dihydroxyvitamin D_3, suggesting that the deficiencies in vitamin D and 1,25-dihydroxyvitamin D_3 in elderly individuals may contribute to the declines in intestinal and renal phosphate transport in this population. In addition, 1,25-dihydroxyvitamin D_3 has been shown to increase membrane fluidity as well as phosphate transport, suggesting that even in the absence of changes in membrane lipid composition the decline in 1,25-dihydroxyvitamin D_3 may trigger a reduction in phosphate transport by this mechanism. Also, the elevation in blood levels of PTH may contribute to the decrease in tubular reabsorption of phosphate.

Several bone diseases are commonly seen in elderly individuals including osteoporosis, Paget's disease, and osteomalacia. Disturbances in renal and gastrointestinal calcium and phosphate handling, elevated PTH levels, and deficiencies in vitamin D and 1,25-dihydroxyvitamin D_3 in elderly persons, make bone disease worse in elderly individuals. In addition, the prevalence of diseases that cause hypercalcemia such as malignancy is greater in the older population. Thus the nephrologist is frequently called upon to assist in the management of bone disease in elderly patients because of familiarity with bone-mineral balance in patients with renal disease in general.

ANATOMICAL CHANGES IN THE AGING KIDNEY

Glomerular Morphology

The gradual decline in GFR and RBF seen with aging is associated with a reduction in both renal mass and the number of functional glomeruli. The loss of renal mass appears to be primarily cortical, with a decrease in size of both the glomerulus and the proximal convoluted tubule in nephrons with glomerulosclerosis (the remaining functioning nephrons probably have an increase in glomerular size). Even in the absence of clinical evidence of hypertension or renal disease, there is an age-related increase in the incidence of glomerulosclerosis and proteinuria accompanied by significant basement membrane thickening. Glomerular size in the human increases between the ages of infancy to middle age (approximately 40 years) but decreases during senescence. The number of sclerotic glomeruli increases from approximately 5% of the total at age 40 to two to six times that amount by age 80 to 90 years. In experimental animals such as the rat, age-induced glomerular damage includes thickening of the glomerular basement membrane (GBM), an increase in mesangial matrix, and an increase in mesangial cell number. Also seen is obliteration of the capillary spaces, fusion of the foot processes, progressively more interstitial infiltration with mononuclear cells, progressive thickening of Bowman's capsule, and adhesions of the glomerular tufts to the capsule. Proteinuria, thickening of the GBM, accumulation of extracellular matrix, and epithelial foot process fusion precedes the development of sclerotic glomeruli. In addition, data in experimental animals indicate that males may be more susceptible to glomerular injury than females. This sex-related difference appears to be the consequence of androgens rather than the absence of estrogens because both the ovariectomized female and the castrated male as well as the intact female are protected from age-related glomerular injury.

The accumulation of mesangial matrix with age is dictated both by the rate of matrix production and the rate of matrix degradation; the latter is controlled by glomerular metalloproteases. As shown in Fig. 57.5, in the young rat glomerular metalloprotease concentrations are equivalent in male and female animals. With aging glomerular metalloprotease levels increase in female but not in male rats, and the latter develop glomerular injury. In castrated old males and in ovariectomized old females glomerular metalloprotease activities increase as they do in the aging intact female and these animals are also protected from glomerular injury. Thus alterations in the ability to degrade mesangial matrix components may play a key role in the development of glomerular senescence, at least in the rat. Also important in age-related declines in renal function is atherosclerotic disease of the renal vasculature.

Tubular Morphology

Beyond the fourth decade of life renal mass declines, with the loss of cortical mass greater than that of medullary mass. By the ninth decade the loss of renal mass may exceed 25% and is accompanied by total sclerosis of more than 10% of all glomeruli. With age there is a steady loss of tubular length and volume and

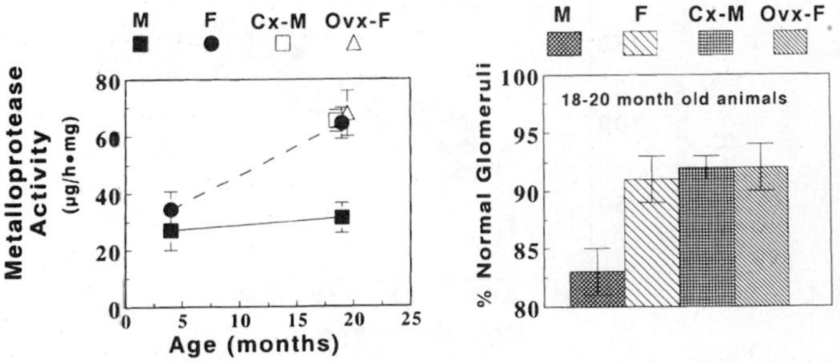

Figure 57.5. Glomerular metalloprotease activity and glomerular injury in the aging kidney. *Left panel:* Metalloprotease activity in intact aging male (*M*) and female (*F*) Munich-Wistar rats and in old castrated males (*Cx-M*) or old ovariectomized females (*Ox-F*). *Right panel:* Percentage of normal glomeruli remaining at 18 to 20 months of age in these animals. (Data from Reckelhoff JF, Baylis C. Glomerular metalloprotease activity is suppressed by androgens in the aging kidney. *J Am Soc Nephrol* 1993;3:1835–1838.)

an increase in tubulointerstitial fibrous tissue. As in the case of GBM, tubule basement membrane thickens and undergoes biochemical alterations. These include a decrease in lysine and hydroxylysine content, an increase in 3-hydroxyproline and 4-hydroxyproline content, and an increase in glycosylation of basement membrane proteins resulting in the formation of AGEs. Proteinaceous casts and hydronephrosis have also been reported.

MODULATION OF GLOMERULAR SENESCENCE: IMPACT OF DIET

Effect of Dietary Protein

Increased protein ingestion results in renal vasodilation, particularly of the afferent arteriole, thereby increasing RBF and glomerular capillary pressure. The result is an increase in GFR. Such an outcome would enhance the ability to eliminate nitrogenous wastes as well as excess minerals and water that may be consumed with the protein meal. Fig. 57.6 shows the effects of a range of spontaneous chronic dietary protein intakes on creatinine clearance in young (20 to 50 years of age, mean = 32) and old (55 to 88 years old, mean = 70) healthy humans (most of the elderly subjects studied were female). The young subjects ingesting a low-protein diet (less than 0.85 g/kg per day) were primarily vegetarians, while the old subjects presumably were ingesting a low-protein diet due to a generalized decreased intake. No information was given regarding chronicity of the diet or total caloric intake. High protein intake resulted in an increase in GFR in both young and old male and female humans. As can be seen, at any given dietary protein intake, older subjects had lower GFR values than younger subjects, but in both groups, the greater the protein intake, the higher the GFR, just as has been observed in experimental animal models.

The magnitude of the renal vasodilatory and hyperfiltration response to an acute protein load is termed the *renal functional reserve* (RFR), and RFR in rats is blunted in old versus young animals. In human studies RFR appears to be preserved in elderly subjects (as might be predicted from the results shown in Fig. 57.6), but the elderly subjects in the human studies of RFR have generally included a broad range of ages (61 to 80). Perhaps if studies in humans were limited to the oldest of the old (ages greater than 75 to80) one would see a reduction in RFR as is observed in the old rat.

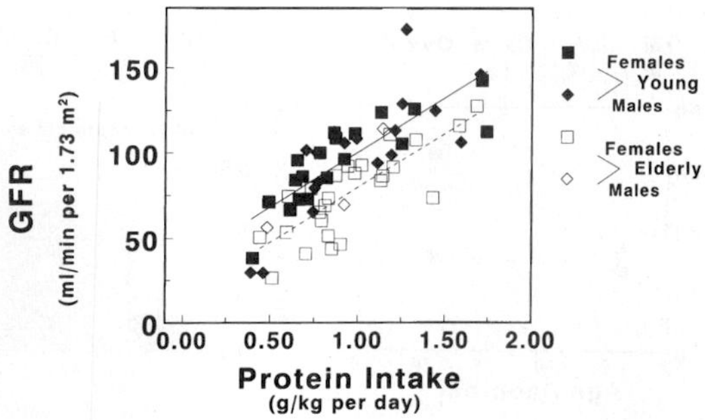

Figure 57.6. Relationship between protein intake and glomerular filtration rate (*GFR*) in young (mean age 31.4 years; range 20 to 50 years) and elderly (mean age 70 years; range 55 to 88 years) healthy humans. *Closed symbols* indicate young subjects; *open symbols* indicate elderly subjects; *squares* indicate females; and *diamonds* indicate males. (Data from Lew SQ, Bosch JP. Effect of diet on creatinine clearance and excretion in young and elderly healthy subjects and in patients with renal disease. *J Am Soc Nephrol* 1991;2:856–865.)

Thus studies in humans and animals have shown that GFR increases in direct relation to dietary protein intake. The tradeoff, glomerular capillary hypertension and hyperperfusion, appears to be damaging when a high-protein diet is consumed over a lifetime. Studies in a variety of animal models have shown that chronic feeding of a high-protein diet accelerates the progression of renal disease in young and middle-aged animals while chronic dietary protein restriction prevents progression. Dietary protein restriction is also thought to slow the progression of chronic renal failure in humans, although the effects are less dramatic than in animal models. The largest, best controlled trial, the Modification of Diet in Renal Disease study, analyzed the effect of moderate dietary protein restriction (0.7 versus 1.1 g/kg per day) in 585 patients with nondiabetic chronic renal disease. The projected mean decline in GFR over a 3-year period did not differ significantly between diet groups, but it could be argued that 3 years is not sufficient to draw firm conclusions. Other meta-analyses of the role of dietary protein restriction in progression of chronic renal disease concluded that dietary protein restriction is beneficial in slowing diabetic and nondiabetic chronic renal disease. Whether dietary protein restriction can be prescribed safely and influence the outcome of progressive renal disease in elderly individuals remains to be tested. A more effective way to prevent age-related renal disease in the first place might be moderation of protein intake over an entire lifetime rather than waiting until age-related renal disease is already underway. Additional discussion on the factors that affect progression of renal failure in general is found in Chapter 67, Part 2.

Effect of Dietary Lipids

The typical human diet in the United States today is approximately 12% to 15% protein, and 46% carbohydrates and has 4 to 10 times as much sodium as the late Paleolithic diet. An important fact is that major changes in dietary fat consumption have occurred in the past 100 years, and today we derive approximately 40% of our calories from fat sources rather than the approximately 20% our ancestors ate. Moreover, the ratio of polyunsaturated to saturated fats was about 1.5 in the late Paleolithic diet but only about 0.5 in the modern diet. In addition, the polyunsaturated fatty acid composition of our diet has shifted from an ω-6:ω-3 ratio of about 1 to a ω-6:ω-3 ratio of 20 to 40:1. Our total fat consumption has therefore increased dramatically, and it is important to note that we have significantly altered the types of fat that we eat.

Role of Hypercholesterolemia in Glomerular Senescence

Obesity in humans and experimental animals is associated with hyperlipidemia and hypercholesterolemia. Progressive hypercholesterolemia tends to develop with age even in the absence of frank obesity and is associated with proteinuria and glomerular disease. Elevated plasma cholesterol levels presented to the glomerular mesangium, separated from the plasma only by the highly fenestrated endothelium without an intervening basement membrane, sets off a cascade of events. An increase in low-density lipoprotein (LDL), particularly oxidized LDL, brought about by high plasma cholesterol levels stimulates the infiltration and differentiation of monocytes into macrophages within the mesangium. This leads to increased production of cytokines and growth factors and subsequent mesangial proliferation and increased production of mesangial matrix including fibronectin, collagen, and proteoglycans. The result is mesangial expansion, thickening of the basement membrane, increased glomerular capillary pressures, deposition of lipid material in the mesangium, proteinuria, and glomerulosclerosis.

Lowering of serum cholesterol in obese animals by long-term treatment with lipid-lowering agents (e.g., clofibric acid and mevinolin, a 3-hydroxy-3-methylglutaryl coenzyme A reductase inhibitor), largely prevents the usual age-related development of proteinuria, mesangial expansion, and glomerular sclerosis. Thus it has generally been observed that an elevation in serum cholesterol and lipoprotein levels, resulting from age-related hypercholesterolemia, excess food consumption, hereditary hypercholesterolemia, or disease, has a detrimental effect on glomerular function and morphology that exacerbates other stimuli for injury.

Role of Dietary Fatty Acids in Age-Related Glomerular Injury

Polyunsaturated fatty acids (PUFAs) derived from either plant sources (principally ω-6 fatty acids) or fish oils (high in ω-3 fatty acids) lower plasma cholesterol and triglycerides. Studies of the Greenland Eskimos in the 1970s indicated that they had a low risk of atherosclerosis and coronary heart disease (CHD) despite a high dietary fat intake. This was postulated to be related to their high consumption of fish containing large amounts of the ω-3 fatty acid eicosapentaenoic acid, which has antithrombotic effects and decreases serum cholesterol. There are many similarities between atherosclerosis and glomerulosclerosis, and as a consequence, in addition to studies devoted to dietary fatty acid influences on atherosclerosis and CHD, many studies have now examined the influence of dietary fatty acids on kidney disease and, to a lesser extent, on age-related glomerular injury.

Diets high in ω-3 PUFAs such as fish oil have indeed been found to be protective in preventing proteinuria and glomerulosclerosis in a variety of renal diseases. Data regarding the influence of ω-3 PUFAs in preventing age-related glomerular senescence in humans are limited. Epidemiologic studies strongly suggest that consumption of a diet low in saturated fatty acids combined with increased ω-3 PUFA intake is beneficial in preventing CHD. Based on the beneficial effects of this class of fatty acids on a variety of glomerular disease processes, it seems likely that increased consumption of ω-3 PUFAs would provide significant protective effects and would markedly reduce the loss of renal function seen with aging. Further long-term studies are required to examine whether age-related glomerular senescence can be prevented with high PUFA diets. The beneficial effects of high PUFA diets may be related to the relative production of vasodilator versus vasoconstrictor prostaglandins, endothelial derived relaxing factor, and membrane fluidity. In that regard, membrane fluidity decreases with age, possibly related to elevated cholesterol levels, and a diet high in PUFAs might reverse that effect. A great deal of work remains to elucidate the mechanisms for the beneficial effects of PUFAs in the progression of renal disease and age-related glomerular senescence. Additional discussion on the interaction between lipids and the kidney is found in Chapter 56, Part 3.

Effect of Dietary Carbohydrates

Chronic administration of a high-sucrose diet (60% to 80%) to rats accelerates age-related glomerulosclerosis relative to that seen in animals ingesting a normal-carbohydrate diet. High-sucrose diets fed to obese Zucker rats are associated with elevated blood pressure (perhaps related to elevated catecholamine release), higher total lipids, triglycerides and total cholesterol levels, and a shorter life span than for animals ingesting a normal-carbohydrate diet. High-sucrose diets given chronically have also been shown to produce insulin resistance in normal rats, and high-sucrose diets over a lifetime result in a slight chronic increase in blood glucose levels. Diabetes is increasingly prevalent in our society and is associated with an elevation of blood glucose levels. Diabetic nephropathy is one of the leading causes of renal disease, occurring in 30% to 40% of patients with type I (insulin-dependent) diabetes mellitus and 40% to 50% of patients with type II diabetes mellitus. Type II diabetes mellitus occurs in the aging population. The classical pathologic hallmarks of diabetic nephropathy include thickening of the GBM and mesangial cell expansion (leading to obliteration of the vascular spaces), an increase in kidney size, glomerular hypertrophy, and proteinuria, findings reminiscent of those observed in age-related glomerular injury. High-fructose diets result in significantly impaired insulin action, elevations in blood pressure, and increased serum triglyceride levels, suggesting that it too will adversely affect glomerular function.

A key biochemical event that occurs when proteins are exposed to glucose or fructose over a prolonged period of time is the chemical association of the sugars and proteins by a process of nonenzymatic glycosylation. These final products are called *advanced glycosylation end-products* (AGEs). The accumulation of AGEs depends upon two factors: the absolute concentration of glucose and time. In diabetes the process is accelerated due to an increase in glucose concentration. In aging, although the concentration of glucose may not be elevated, the factor of time may become important, and the formation of AGEs might play a role in the deleterious consequences of aging on glomerular senescence.

Glycosylation of collagen causes cross-linking that might result in alterations and architectural distortion of the filtration barrier. In addition, glycosylated collagen has a greater affinity for LDL than normal collagen, suggesting that the accumulation of AGEs in glomeruli of elderly individuals may cause the mesangial extracellular matrix to trap more LDL, accelerating the development of glomerulosclerosis. In addition, mesangial cell membranes have receptors for AGE proteins, and exposure of the mesangium to AGE-modified albumin yields enhanced production of matrix proteins, an increase in glomerular volume, basement membrane thickening, proteinuria, and glomerulosclerosis. These effects may be mediated by the interactions of AGE-modified proteins with AGE-specific receptors that induce the infiltration of monocytes into the mesangium, leading to the synthesis and release of cytokines and growth factors. These effects are remarkably similar to those seen with normal aging. Even in the absence of elevated blood glucose, AGEs increase with advancing age in long-lived proteins such as collagen. Thus an important mechanism by which a diet restricted in monosaccharides and disaccharides might slow age-related glomerular senescence is through decreased production of AGEs.

Effect of Dietary Food Restriction

As of 1991, 33% of U.S. adults 20 years and older were overweight, a direct result of increased availability and consumption of food products. Obesity is associated with type II diabetes, hypertension, and hyperlipidemia, all potential risk factors for glomerular injury. In the early stages of chronic obesity, GFR and RBF are increased. Ultimately, the hyperfiltration, hyperlipidemia, and hypertension associated with obesity lead to a progressive decrease in GFR, proteinuria, and glomerulosclerosis. Limiting total caloric intake by decreasing the quantity of food consumed over a lifetime (without limiting any one particular food group) is one method to restrict body size. A number of animal studies have demonstrated a beneficial effect of food limitation on longevity (provided the limitation is not too severe), blood pressure control, and age-related glomerular senescence. The obese (hyperphagic) Zucker rat is insulin resistant, hypertensive, and hyperlipidemic, and dies of kidney disease. We have examined the effects of limiting dietary food

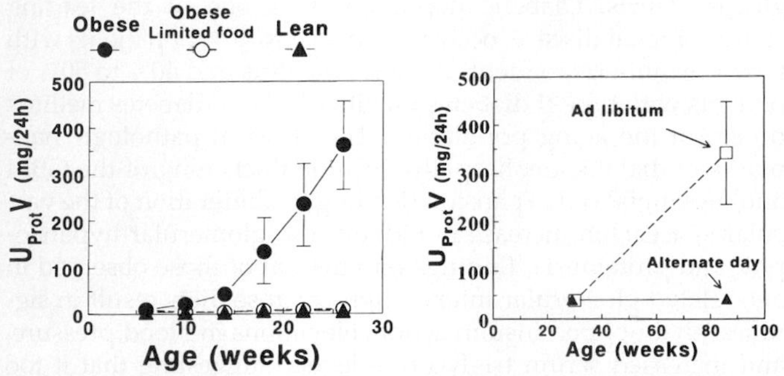

Figure 57.7. *Left panel*: Proteinuria in the aging obese female Zucker rat fed *ad libitum* versus lean and obese Zucker rats limited in food intake to 14 g/day from 6 weeks of age (14 g/day is the normal food intake for lean rats). (Preliminary data from a recent study by Maddox DA, Alavi FK, Leyse JW, et al. At what point will limiting food intake no longer be effective in preventing age-related hypertension and kidney disease in the obese Zucker rat? *Am J Hypertension* 1997;10:196A.) *Right panel*: Proteinuria in the aging male Sprague-Dawley rat fed *ad libitum* or maintained on alternate day feeding from the age of 4 to 6 weeks. (Data from Gehrig JJ, Ross J, Jamison RL. Effect of long-term, alternate day feeding on renal function in aging conscious rats. *Kidney Int* 1988;34:620–630.)

intake in these animals from their *ad libitum* intakes (approximately 28 g/day) to 14 g/day (that normally consumed by their lean littermates). As shown in Fig. 57.7, obese rats fed *ad libitum* developed progressive glomerular injury (as evidenced by an increase in proteinuria) compared with their lean counterparts. When food was limited in obese rats to that consumed by their lean littermates, proteinuria and glomerular injury were almost completely prevented. The prevention of glomerular injury in the obese rats limited in food intake appeared to be most closely associated with a marked reduction in GFR from the hyperfiltration state observed in the obese *ad libitum* group to values equal to those seen in the lean animals. In the normal Sprague-Dawley rat alternate day feeding for 80 weeks almost completely prevented the age-associated proteinuria and glomerular sclerosis that develops in these animals when fed *ad libitum* (Fig. 57.7). This long-term protective effect of reduced food (and hence protein) intake was associated with significantly lower values of GFR and renal plasma flow early in life in these animals (as measured at 30 weeks of age). These data indicate that reduced food intake for a lifetime in normal animals protects the kidneys from glomerular senescence just as it does in the genetically obese animal. By analogy, a lifetime of overeating is very likely responsible for part of the glomerular senescence observed with aging (Fig. 57.1).

ALTERED PHARMACOKINETICS

Elderly individuals experience adverse reactions to drugs more frequently than all other age groups, a problem compounded by the fact that it is relatively commonplace for elderly patients to take three or more medications every day. Up to 24% of patients older than age 80 have complications with drug treatments compared with half that number for patients 40 to 50 years of age. Double dosing, occurring when two or more medications used to treat more than one disease contain the same active ingredient, can also contribute to increased drug side effects elderly patients. In 1994 an estimated 33 million Americans (13% of the population) were aged 65 and older. With better medical care and the aging baby boomer population, it has been estimated that by year 2030 this number will reach 70 million (21% of the population). With age, there is a decrease in the functional capacity of many vital organs (e.g., kidney, liver, heart). When this age-associated decrease in organ function is superimposed with disease processes, complications from medications are more likely. With the unprecedented increase in the elderly population, particular emphasis must be placed on adverse drug reactions in elderly individuals. The great majority of clinical studies for new therapeutic agents are done in young, healthy individuals. Elderly patients, however, become the direct recipients of a great majority of new medications. This population needs to be included, when possible, in the clinical trials to expand our understanding of drug sensitivity, interaction, and dosage requirements of elderly patients.

A number of factors contribute to the increased toxicity and adverse drug effects in elderly patients. These include (a) age-dependent declines in glomerular filtration, (b) increased renal disease, (c) decreased tubular function manifested by reduced tubular transport capacity, (d) decreased capacity to acidify the urine, (e) greater use of medication, (f) drug interactions, (g) changes in central nervous system function, and (h) double dosing. Age-dependent decreases in RBF and glomerular filtration reduce the amount of drug filtered by the kidney, thus extending the half-time for elimination of the drug, leading to sustained high steady-state plasma levels. When renal dysfunction due to renal disease is superimposed on normal age-dependent declines in renal function, even more significant alterations in drug pharmacokinetics and drug toxicity occur. The most frequently reported alterations in pharmacokinetic parameters in elderly individuals are changes observed in half-life ($t_{½}$), volume of distribution (V_d), drug clearance (Cl), and plasma protein binding. Drug $t_{½}$ is given by the following formula:

$$t_{½} = \frac{0.693 \times V_d}{Cl}$$

Because GFR is reduced in elderly individuals, the clearance of many drugs by this route is also reduced leading to an increased $t_{½}$ and a prolonged elevation in plasma levels of many drugs. An increase in V_d in elderly patients is also observed, especially for lipophilic (fat-soluble) drugs because of the increase in body fat as a percentage of body weight that occurs with age. Thus drugs such as benzodiazepines, taken at night, will have a higher V_d and therefore a prolonged $t_{½}$, resulting in hangover-like effects the next day. In addition to filtration, the renal capacity to eliminate drugs by tubular secretory mechanisms may diminish with age, both as a consequence of some glomeruli becoming sclerotic and nonfunctional as well as through decreased transport capacity of the remaining functional nephrons. Again, the result is an altered $t_{½}$ and consequently an increase in the potential for adverse drug reactions.

Many drugs undergo biotransformation and metabolism in the liver and, to a lesser extent, in the kidney by the microsomal mixed-function oxidase system (MFOS). Evidence indicates that with aging there is a decline in both renal and hepatic MFOS function. This would suggest that in addition to a decline in renal filtration, the renal capacity to metabolize drugs may be compromised with aging, thus delaying elimination. Animal studies also show that age plays a significant role in susceptibility to metabolic insults in renal ischemia. Thus the decline in renal metabolic capacity, when superimposed on a decline in renal filtration and transport capacity, leads to a prolonged half-life and much higher plasma drug concentrations than would obtain in the young individuals.

Body composition changes with aging; there is less lean mass and increased body fat. In an average 25-year-old individual compared with an average 70-year-old, fat increases from approximately 15% to 30% of body weight, muscle mass decreases from approximately 19% to 12% of body weight, and total body water decreases from approximately 61% to 53% of body weight. The initial concentration of an administered drug (C_i) is a function of the dose given and the volume of distribution (V_d) and is given in the following equation:

$$C_i = \frac{\text{Dose}}{V_d}$$

As a result of the altered body composition in elderly individuals, plasma concentrations of lipophilic drugs may be at subtherapeutic levels because of the increased volume of distribution due to increased body fat. In contrast, concentrations of hydrophilic (water-soluble) drugs that distribute primarily into the extracellular compartment (primarily plasma) may reach toxic levels. In addition to changes in body composition, dehydration and a reduction in plasma volume are frequently observed in elderly individuals. Thus for drugs that distribute to the extracellular fluid space, a given dose will result in a higher than desired plasma concentration, exacerbating drug toxicity in elderly patients. Diuretics, commonly used in elderly hypertensive patients, pose a similar problem, by further reducing extracellular volume and V_d. Other physiologic changes in elderly patients that exacerbate the alterations in extracellular volume and V_d are the declines in the renin-angiotensin system and aldosterone secretion, the relative renal resistance to vasopressin, and the inability of the kidneys to produce maximally concentrated urine as discussed earlier.

Protein binding of an ingested drug is primarily dependent on the physicochemical properties of that drug. Because plasma protein binding of a drug reduces the availability of unbound free drug, plasma concentrations of proteins (e.g., albumin) can play an important role in the buffering of a drug dosage. Serum albumin, an abundant plasma protein, can bind to a variety of drugs and metabolites. An evaluation of the Elderly Nutrition Program of the Older American Act indicates that 67% to 88% of elderly Americans have a moderate to high risk for nutritional deficiencies. With a diminished quality of nutrition (due to loss of appetite or a low-protein diet) plasma protein levels may decline enough to alter the ratio of unbound (free drug) to bound drug. As a result, a normal therapeutic dose of a drug may lead to an unexpected increase in the unbound (free) drug levels and increased undesirable effects.

In elderly individuals, reduced renal clearance, reduced renal transport capacity, dehydration, poor nutritional status, and increased number of medications consumed by this patient population can lead to potentially harmful plasma levels of drugs. By adjusting the initial dose, reducing the frequency of administration, or reducing the dosage levels, most of the adverse reaction can be easily prevented. With an increasing number of elderly patients and frequent use of medication, it is critical to monitor renal function, overall nutritional status, plasma drug levels, and the concomitant use of other drugs in the elderly population.

GERIATRIC HYPERTENSION

Hypertension is a risk factor for renal disease, and hypertension is more prevalent in the elderly population, averaging 1 of 3 for individuals older than 65 years of age compared with 1 of 4 for society as a whole. In some subgroups of our population, for example, elderly black females, the prevalence can reach 80%. As shown in Fig. 57.1, systolic blood pressure tends to increase with age while diastolic pressure tends to remain constant or decline somewhat (data not shown). Not surprisingly, isolated systolic hypertension is common in the latter decades of life. Many large studies including the Systolic Hypertension of the Elderly Prevention Trial have shown that control of hypertension of all types reduces the risk of stroke, coronary events, and congestive heart failure, and total mortality by 12% to 30%. It is paramount to treat hypertension in elderly patients based on these findings.

Several etiologic factors may contribute to the greater prevalence of hypertension in the elderly age group than in younger age groups. Obesity, dietary disturbances, and concomitant medications should be investigated first. Weight loss has not been shown to lower blood pressure in elderly individuals per se, although such studies are ongoing. In younger age groups weight reduction can lower blood pressure significantly. Weight reduction where possible may lead to the need for fewer medications, lower dosing of medications, or even discontinuation of drug therapy in some elderly individuals with hypertension. Weight loss may require both caloric restriction and increased exercise, both of which should be explored in obese elderly hypertensive patients.

Many meta-analyses concerning dietary factors and the amelioration of hypertension are now available. Sodium, potassium, and calcium are the most well-known dietary factors that may influence hypertension. These analyses conclude that sodium restriction, potassium supplementation, and calcium supplementation each may influence blood pressure from 1 to 7 mm Hg, affecting systolic more than diastolic blood pressure.

Finally, the most common medical problem reported by elderly patients in surveys is arthritis. Consequently, it is not surprising that many individuals older than age 65 consume prescription or over-the-counter analgesics, including NSAIDs. Our studies have suggested that renal prostanoid production may be impaired in elderly individuals compared with younger people. Studies have also shown frankly low urinary prostanoid excretion in elderly male hypertensive patients compared with younger hypertensive persons and older persons without hypertension. Because prostanoids influence sodium excretion, renal perfusion, renin release by the juxtaglomerular apparatus, and subsequent aldosterone levels, it is not surprising that discontinuation of NSAIDs has by itself been associated with a reduction in blood pressure of up to 5 mm Hg in some hypertensive individuals. Elimination of these agents must be sought in elderly hypertensive patients. Finally, other concomitant medications that may contribute to blood pressure elevation include α-adrenergic agonists used for stress incontinence in elderly women and β-agonists used for patients with chronic obstructive lung disease.

After such nonpharmacologic measures have been exhausted in the management of hypertension in elderly patients, pharmacologic therapy should proceed using the geriatric principle of "start low and go low." Methods of of choice include diuretics, renin-angiotensin blockade agents, and calcium channel blockers. All of the large worldwide multicenter trials have shown excellent efficacy and safety for low-dose diuretics. They remain the drugs most commonly used in initial therapy. Efficacy does not generally increase with increased dosing, but side effects such as hypokalemia do. Therefore only low-dose therapy should be used. Thiazides may also have a beneficial effect on calcium homeostasis; the reduced urinary calcium excretion contributes to positive cumulative calcium balance and has been shown to decrease the incidence of hip fractures due to improvement of osteoporosis. Thiazide therapy for elderly patients has the potential for aggravation of incontinence and an increased likelihood of falling due to a higher incidence of orthostatic hypotension. Greater urinary urgency, especially in the middle of the night with concomitant impaired vision, increases the potential for tripping and falling and thus increases the risk for hip fracture or other traumatic injury.

Calcium channel blockers have been shown to have an age-related increase in efficacy per dose. Clearly they will be efficacious, but low dosages should be prescribed. Converting enzyme inhibitors and angiotensin receptor blockers are efficacious, have few side effects, and are well tolerated by patients, thereby improving compliance. Beneficial effects on the heart are also common. With advanced renal arteriosclerosis, however, reduction of glomerular filtration by these agents may create azotemia and hyperkalemia.

Common diuretic doses for elderly patients might be 12.5 mg of hydrochlorothiazide three times weekly. Enalapril should be started at a dose of 2.5 mg daily. Amlodipine should be started at 5 mg daily. At every visit a reevaluation of all medications should be undertaken with a goal to reduce doses and limit them so that patients take no more than three or four medications in total, consistent with the geriatric principle called *med/red* or *medication reduction*. With greater numbers of medications, side effects become inevitable and drug–drug interactions will occur. Attempts must always be made to see which new agents may have been added by other subspecialists and which over-the-counter medication or supplements the patient may have added because of hearsay or popular magazine articles. Finally, patients may often experiment with their spouse's medication, searching for an improvement in well-being. All these sources of drug–drug interactions must be sought. It is often key for the patients to bring their medications to each visit. The "brown bag" or "shoebox" syndrome is often uncovered in patients who have been experimenting with a variety of medications that were long ago discontinued and are often outdated. Only with a careful med/red strategy can there be good long-term safety and efficacy in the management of hypertension in elderly patients. Geriatric hypertension is discussed in detail in Chapter 65.

RENAL DISEASE IN ELDERLY PATIENTS

Ischemic Renal Disease

Ischemic nephropathy has now emerged as a clinical syndrome in elderly individuals. There are several acute and chronic conditions in this category. They most often include small vessel injury due to chronic hypertension, renal artery atherosclerosis, thromboemboli to the kidneys, atheroemboli to the kidneys, renal vasculitis, aortic dissection, and coagulopathies causing microangiopathy.

There are several common clinical presentations of patients with this important cause of acute and chronic renal failure. Most often these patients develop rising blood urea nitrogen (BUN) and creatinine levels after the initiation of antihypertensive therapy, particularly with angiotensin-converting enzyme inhibitors and to a lesser extent with angiotensin II–receptor inhibitors. The reduction of blood pressure leads to reduced renal perfusion pressure, reduced RBF, and reduced glomerular filtration. Other presentations include progressive azotemia in a patient with documented or suspected renovascular disease due to ongoing worsening renal atherosclerosis in the major renal arteries or the renal microcirculation. Main renal artery atherosclerosis may also cause frequent paroxysms of hypertension with recurrent episodes of pulmonary edema (flash pulmonary edema).

Often patients have chronic stable renal insufficiency with concomitant atherosclerotic disease elsewhere with either long-standing hypertension or recent onset of hypertension. Diagnosis is confirmed, usually by imaging studies of the kidneys. These studies include Doppler studies showing reduced RBF and renal artery lesions and renal scans showing reduced perfusion and reduced blood flow. Magnetic resonance angiography or spiral computed tomography (CT) may show the renal atherosclerosis and finally angiography with contrast medium or with carbon dioxide may reveal the definitive diagnosis.

The renal pathologic changes associated with this condition include not only the vascular lesions themselves and cholesterol clefts in small vessels, but also several glomerular and tubular changes as well. The glomerular changes include wrinkling of the basement membrane, implosion or collapse of open capillary loops, thickening and duplication of Bowman's capsule, and atubular glomeruli. The tubular changes include atrophy, patchy inflammation and fibrosis.

Atheroembolic disease has been better diagnosed as a common clinical problem of elderly individuals in the past few years and deserves special emphasis in a review of the topic of ischemic nephropathy. Although worsening renal function due to this problem can occur spontaneously, it mostly follows instrumentation of the vascular system in which an atherosclerotic plaque is mechanically disturbed and embolizes to the renal microcirculation. Accompanying the worsening azotemia are volatile, often malignant, levels of hypertension in most but not all patients, probably due in part to the renin-angiotensin system response to the renal microcirculatory ischemia. Also accompanying the azotemia is evidence of embolization to other tissues, most notably the lower extremities. The skin is often mottled, and the toes are cyanotic due to sluggish circulation and may develop frank gangrene. The "blue toe" sign in the setting of azotemia may be the only clinical clue to the syndrome of atheroembolic ischemic nephropathy when blood pressure is not a problem. Laboratory testing reveals eosinophilia and eosinophiluria and reductions of complement levels, that is, C_3 and C_4. The latter represents the result of an inflammatory response to the intrarenal cholesterol deposition histologically demonstrated as cholesterol clefts in the vascular wall. Original reports suggested a very poor outcome with rapid deterioration progressing to death in a very short time, a matter of weeks. Patient survival is possible but digits may be lost due to autoamputation or surgical debridement and amputation. Renal failure is most often relentlessly progressive and permanent. After the wave of ischemia has passed over several weeks, many patients do survive for many years with dialysis treatment. In the authors' experience, one patient who survived the renal failure and loss of multiple toes after atheroemboli due to coronary angioplasty went on to receive a cadaveric renal transplant 3 years later. He is alive and enjoys a fully functional and independent life in his late 70s 10 years after the transplant, although he required coronary artery bypass surgery in his early 70s and has developed insulin-dependent diabetes mellitus. Detailed discussion of occlusive renal vascular disease is provided in Chapter 52.

Glomerulonephritis

Glomerulonephritis is not common in elderly individuals. However, when elderly individuals have this problem, there are often delays in recognizing it. The prognosis is usually less favorable than in younger patients. In large reviews of patients older than age 60 with glomerulonephropathies, crescentic glomerulonephritis, focal proliferative/mesangial glomerulonephritis, and membranous glomerulonephritis have been the common entities diagnosed in those elderly patients who have the nephritic syndrome. Of these, idiopathic rapidly progressive glomerulonephritis (RPGN) has been the most common in large series in the literature. In our experience, the crescentic RPGNs have been the most common but are fairly equally distributed between Wegener's granulomatosis, Goodpasture's disease, crescentic nephritis associated with systemic vasculitis, and idiopathic RPGN. In our experience, NT-neutrophil cytoplasmic auto-antibodies [ANCA]–positive Wegener's granulomatosis is the most common form of crescentic glomerular nephritis. In a report of crescentic nephritis in an elderly patient who died from disseminated prostatic adenocarcinoma, there were positive immunoperoxidase stains for both prostatic specific acid phosphatase and prostatic specific antigen in addition to immune deposits in the glomeruli observed at autopsy. This patient had renal failure without obstructive uropathy. Another unusual association has been the occurrence of crescentic anti-GBM glomerulonephritis in a patient who had undergone extracorporeal shock-wave lithotripsy (ESWL) 7 months earlier. The authors speculated whether the ESWL induced an injury to GBM that rendered it antigenic, leading to an immune response and linear deposition of anti-GBM antibodies.

The high incidence of crescentic glomerulonephritis in elderly patients with rapid progression to renal failure is not widely appreciated by nonnephrologists. It is important to be wary of this possibility in patients with acute renal failure because the primary care physician may confuse it with acute tubular necrosis. Without a high degree of suspicion, the opportunity for renal biopsy, accurate diagnosis, and appropriate treatment may be missed. In a large series, membranous nephropathy has been the most common entity found in aged individuals who have nephrotic syndrome. The largest numbers of these patients have an underlying malignancy, and in many cases there has been evidence for tumor antigen in the immune complexes deposited in the glomeruli. The membranous nephropathy is then similar to a paraneoplastic syndrome and its course can be used as a marker for remission of the malignancy with therapy.

A somewhat newer entity manifesting as nephrotic syndrome in patients including elderly patients is that associated with intraglomerular immunoglobulin fibrils that are not amyloid and are Congo red–negative; fibrillary glomerulonephritis is described in detail in Chapter 39, Part 10. These deposits are reactive for polyclonal immunoglobulins and are thought to result from local production and deposition of abnormal paraproteins, often associated with hematuria and hypertension. The condition progresses to end-stage renal failure in 5 years or less in many cases and may recur after renal transplantation.

Newer techniques make renal biopsy somewhat easier and safer in elderly individuals. Use of the fluoroscope, ultrasound, CT scans, and the new biopsy gun leads to better localization to the lower pole away from the collecting system. Renal tissue is now rarely missed and fewer entries into the kidneys are required. The new biopsy guns cut a smaller core with speed and precision such that renal trauma is minimized. Most large series reports of biopsies in elderly individuals indicate very low incidences of serious complications with these new techniques.

Tubular Diseases in Elderly Individuals

Acute and chronic tubulointerstitial nephritis produce the syndromes of acute and chronic renal failure, and they are seen in every age group including the elderly. This disease entity is discussed in detail in Chapter 40. One important cause of acute inflammatory renal failure in elderly individuals is drug-induced acute interstitial nephritis (AIN). Drugs known to produce AIN include antibiotics (especially the penicillins), antituberculosis drugs, NSAIDs, diuretics, and anticonvulsants. Antibiotic-induced AIN has been found to occur with the newest category of widely used antibiotics, the fluoroquinolones, with documentation in patients treated with ciprofloxacin. Because elderly individuals have a higher likelihood of drug exposure because of concomitant diseases, they are at greater risk for drug-induced AIN than other age groups. AIN associated with NSAIDs differs from other forms of AIN in that fever, rash, and eosinophilia are uncommon, the duration of exposure is usually much longer, and it is often associated with a glomerulopathy and nephrotic-range proteinuria. Ketorolac is a NSAID developed primarily as an alternate to opiates for pain management, especially perioperatively. An increasing number of reports now document AIN resulting from use of this agent as well. In elderly patients, the antineoplastic agents, myeloma kidney, and hypercalcemia associated with malignancy are particularly noteworthy causes of AIN. Chronic tubulointerstitial nephritis is more often due to chronic intermittent obstructive uropathy, which is most often caused by prostatic hypertrophy or malignancy in men, pelvic malignancies in women, or recurrent urolithiasis in both sexes. Next in order of frequency of causes of chronic tubulointerstitial nephritis is recurrent infections in patients with neurogenic bladder dysfunction caused by diabetes mellitus, degenerative neurologic diseases, or spinal cord trauma. Finally, chronic tubulointerstitial injury is still seen with recurrent crystal-induced injuries such as severe cases of gout and severe recurrent episodes of hypercalcemia (usually associated with malignancies) or excessive calcium and vitamin D intake. Oxalate-induced injury due to longstanding inflammatory bowel diseases or surgical bypass of the small intestine, especially the terminal ileum, can also induce chronic tubulointerstitial injury.

Acute Renal Failure in Elderly Individuals

Acute renal failure is a common problem in elderly hospitalized patients in part because they have less renal reserve as a result of reductions in RBF and GFR due to aging and also to concomitant diseases such as hypertension, diabetes, ischemic renal disease, and obstructive uropathy. With elderly patients being considered for more aggressive therapy including surgical treatment of coronary artery disease, peripheral vascular diseases, and aneurysm repair, there is frequent exposure to contrast media in the diagnosis. Frequent atheroembolic disease as a consequence of instrumentation, including angioplasty and stent placement, and occasional hypotension due to hemorrhage and perioperative cardiac decompensation also occur. This commonly results in acute tubular necrosis (ATN) and the requirement for dialysis therapy. Gastrointestinal disease and nephrotoxic antibiotics are other common risks for ATN. Cholelithiasis, cholecystitis, ulcerative disease, diverticular disease, and gastrointestinal cancers also frequently require contrast diagnostic studies such as CT scanning, increasing the risk for ATN. Hypotension caused by sepsis or severe volume contraction due to fluid and electrolyte disorders or hemorrhage may complicate these diseases and further increase the risk for ATN. Finally, aggressive medicosurgical or radiation therapies for malignancies create renal ischemia and nephrotoxicity that often results in ATN.

Besides the reduced renal reserve, other factors that increase the risk of acute renal failure in elderly individuals are the tendency for volume contraction due to impaired renal salt and water conservation during a time of increased fluid losses and reduced oral intake during acute illness. In an elderly patient receiving therapy with NSAIDs and diuretics or antihypertensive therapy, there is an increased risk of renal ischemia (and additive nephrotoxicity) during any acute illness, which may lead to dehydration or hemorrhage. Similarly such therapy increases the risk of nephrotoxicity if such a patient were exposed to a second nephrotoxic agent such as an antibiotic, a chemotherapy agent, or intravenous contrast medium. We have hypothesized that renal tubular mitochondrial DNA mutations can develop in elderly individuals that may lead to an inability to respond to oxidative stress as well as younger individuals, resulting in a predisposition to worse tubular ischemia associated with hypotension or toxins that produce free radicals.

Dialysis issues in elderly patients with acute renal failure are beyond the scope of this chapter. Nephrologists are faced daily with ethical decisions concerning the initiation of dialysis strategies for elderly individuals with acute renal failure. These decisions may become quite logistically difficult, requiring face-to-face visits or teleconferencing with family who have durable power of attorney for medical care for elderly patients unable to give consent. Situations such as acute renal replacement therapy for delirium, dementia, stupor, or coma all occur and are more common in elderly patients with acute illnesses. One principle that must be kept in mind is that a patient may have a physiologic age that suggests the need to proceed with heroic life support measures even if chronologic age would tend to deter proceeding with renal replacement therapy.

Conventional dialysis is still most often performed to sustain patients during the acute renal failure episode. Continuous renal replacement in the form of chronic venovenous hemofiltration (CVVH) is becoming quite common, even since the last edition of this book. Manufacturers have now developed complete modular units for CVVH, which have simplified the setup time and effort by staff. The amount of maintenance by staff is often quite minimal once a successful initiation has passed the therapeutic trial stage and has been in progress for several hours. Patients who have low blood pressure, reduced cardiac output, and severe hypotension due to sepsis can often be sustained well for weeks with interventions to change the filter once a week under the best case scenarios. Addition of dialysis to create CVVHD is also possible. The metabolic and hemodynamic benefits of this therapy in general are described elsewhere in this text, but clearly apply to the group of elderly patients in a fragile condition with acute renal failure, often accompanied by multiple system chronic disease.

Dialysis in Elderly Individuals for Chronic Renal Failure

There are differences in the causes of ESRD in elderly patients, compared with younger patients. In young patients, the most common cause is diabetes mellitus, followed by hypertension, then glomerular disease. Hereditary or familial causes of renal diseases such as polycystic kidney disease are the fourth most common with tubulointerstitial disease completing the top five causes. In elderly individuals, hypertension is followed by obstructive uropathy with or without recurrent pyelonephritis as the most common causes of renal failure. Diabetes and ischemic nephropathy described above are next in importance. Finally, failure to recover from acute renal failure caused by the common circumstances described above, polycystic kidney disease with a late onset of renal failure, glomerular disease, and multiple myeloma are all frequent causes of ESRD.

Elderly individuals, especially the old-old (older than age 80), are the age group with the greatest increase in numbers presenting for ESRD management. Nephrologists are gaining increasing experience with patients older than 85 to 90 who are undergoing dialysis. More reports are appearing in the literature about dialysis of patients older than 95 and even 100. All age groups including those older than 65 are living longer with dialysis treatment. Most geriatric patients with ESRD receive in-center hemodialysis. They often do not have the visual skills or manual dexterity to perform home dialysis, that is, peritoneal dialysis, and probably do not have a capable helper for home dialysis. Although life span is increasing for elderly patients receiving dialysis, life expectancy is still reduced compared with individuals of similar age who are not receiving dialysis. In old-old patients, life expectancy is often greater than 3 years, with nearly 80% of patients older than 80 who are receiving dialysis living more than 3 years. When home dialysis is possible, selection factors may create a bias for healthier individuals choosing this modality, and so comparison of their survival to that of patients who are less independent and receiving in-center hemodialysis may not be accurate.

Access for dialysis is often a problem in elderly patients. Advanced concomitant vascular disease often makes natural fistulas, even synthetic graft fistulas, impossible. As a result the access of last resort is often a cuffed central vein dual lumen catheter. Although muscle mass is often decreased in these individuals, there is often a problem in getting an adequate dialysis prescription with this form of dialysis access. Flow may be limited, and recirculation limits efficiency, so increased time may be the only solution. Fortunately, such individuals are almost always retired and willing to put in the necessary time, that is, comply well with all aspects of ESRD management including diet and blood pressure control. Logistical problems may arise with long dialysis times if patients require family members to transport them to and from the dialysis center. Many assisted living centers provide such transportation as part of their patient assistance services for all their residents to get them to and from doctors and hospitals for all medical diagnostic, and therapeutic needs. For discussion on chronic hemodialysis in elderly patients, the reader is referred to Chapter 84, Part 1H.

Renal Transplantation in Elderly Individuals

A brief case report will be used to illustrate several issues associated with renal transplant in elderly individuals. A 68-year-old white male had developed ESRD as his creatinine clearance level was steadily declining as seen at periodic clinic visits over many years. When a colonic resection was performed for a villous adenoma, a renal biopsy revealed focal sclerosis of the glomeruli. In the subsequent year, access for dialysis was placed and in-center hemodialysis was initiated without difficulty. The patient did extremely well for the next 1½ years without any major medical or surgical problems. A decision was made to consider a renal transplant as he had been free of any recurrent colon malignancy for 3 years and his advancing age would soon disqualify him from being a transplant candidate. A living donor transplant was not possible. After repeat gastrointestinal and cardiovascular evaluations, he was listed on the active cadaver transplant list. Aortic stenosis was noted but not believed to preclude transplantation. Rather it was likely to be corrected later. Cardiac clearance was given because the stress test was normal. At age 72, he received a cadaveric transplant from an elderly donor with 15% sclerosis of glomeruli. With prednisone, azathioprine, and cyclosporine immunosuppression, he was discharged with his serum creatinine level stabilized at 2.3 mg/dl while doses of the medications were being tapered. His main problem was lower extremity edema, which required high doses of diuretics, primarily furosemide. One month later he developed malaise and lethargy that lasted for 1 day and was admitted to the hospital with a glucose level of 1,300 mg/dl. His edema continued as well. After discharge from this admission tapering of the immunosuppressives was continued. Insulin was required for the next 3 months but glucose levels remained controlled. Edema began to improve. Diuretic therapy was markedly decreased but not discontinued. Ultimately, insulin was discontinued and has not been needed again. One and one-half years later, his serum creatinine level slowly increased to the 2.5 to 2.7 mg/dl range, and exercise tolerance began to diminish. When his serum creatinine level rose to more than 3.5 mg/dl, he was hospitalized. The aortic stenosis was felt to have reached critical gradient and reduced valve area to necessitate aortic valve replacement. Transplant function improved to 2.5 to 2.7 mg/dl after a surgical procedure that was surprisingly uneventful. Three months later he was hospitalized with fever to 103°F, which was ultimately diagnosed as urosepsis and required urinary bladder catheterization to overcome some urinary retention. Mild to moderate prostate hypertrophy was treated with long-acting α-blocker therapy. Several years later the patient at age 78 is alive and well, independent in usual activities of daily living and instrumental activities of daily living and has a serum creatinine level of 2.8 mg/dl.

The preceding case illustrates several key points about performing transplants in elderly patients. No matter how stable the patient's condition appears before transplantation, there are an increased number of perioperative and postoperative complications. In the case above, it is likely that cyclosporine and corticosteroids were the cause of the self-limited period of insulin requirement. Pretransplant evaluation requires careful attention to the risk of malignancy and risk of cardiovascular disease, both of which may be accelerated posttransplant. The patient above received a kidney from an aged donor that might otherwise not have been used. Posttransplant function was not as good as that from a younger donor but the patient's reduced muscle mass still allowed an acceptable posttransplant result in terms of serum creatinine and BUN levels. He has felt better and been able to function better than when receiving dialysis. He clearly has more time for independent activities and recreation. Infection risk remains high because of immunosuppression. His prostate hypertrophy was an unexpected problem posttransplant as well in light of the lack of symptoms with his low urine flow while receiving dialysis.

There has been a tremendous growth in transplantation in the elderly, not only in patients older than 55, a one-time limit, but also groups older than 60, 65, 70, 75, and now even older than 80 years of age. The upper limit of age at this time would appear to be in the low 80s at any center in this country. Transplantation has included not only cadaveric donors, but there has also been an increase in living-related donation, including that from children to parent. This increase in demand for transplantation has led to an increase in time on the waiting list for patients of all ages, because the donor pool has not kept pace. Larger waiting lists and longer times for all potential recipients have led to exploration of expanded donor criteria, older aged donor kidneys, and dual kidney donation. One recent advance has been the use of two cadaver kidneys harvested from older individuals to be transplanted into older recipients. Results to date suggest better renal function when assessed initially, that is, serum creatinine level was 1.7 versus 2.4 mg/dl in recipients of single kidneys at 1 month and 1.4 versus 1.8 mg/dl at 1 year. One-year graft survival seems comparable to that of age-matched recipients of single kidneys. This appears to be an excellent way to achieve improved renal function while accelerating the opportunity for transplant of the willing older recipient.

Finally, new immunosuppression regimens are being designed to markedly reduce cumulative corticosteroid doses that will minimize subsequent risks of metabolic derangements, infection, congestive heart failure, cataracts, and osteoporosis. Newer strategies are attempting to avoid calcineurin antagonists that would also minimize risks of renal toxicity and posttransplant diabetes. These new prospects for immunosuppression that rely heavily on mycophenolate and rapamycin will allow easier perioperative management of elderly patients receiving transplants in the future. Further discussion on renal transplantation in elderly individuals is found in Chapter 90.

Selected Readings

Baylis C, Corman B. The aging kidney: insights from experimental studies. *J Am Soc Nephrol* 1998;9:699–709.

Summary of current knowledge of glomerular structural and functional changes that occur with age with a focus on experimental findings in the rat, including a discussion of the hormonal adaptations with age, particularly those that influence renal vascular resistance and GFR (151 references).

Epstein M. Aging and the kidney. *J Am Soc Nephrol* 1996;7:1106–1122.

Review of glomerular and tubular structural and functional changes with age, including a discussion of hormonal changes, age-dependent alterations in fluid and electrolyte homeostasis, and renal disease in elderly individuals (135 references).

Greco B, Beyer JA. Atherosclerotic ischemic renal disease. *Am J Kidney Dis* 1997; 29:167–187.

Excellent review of new syndrome with emphasis on definition, differential diagnosis, pathology, pathophysiology, and treatment (144 references).

Palmer BF, Levi M. Effect of aging on renal function and disease. In: Brenner BM, ed. *The kidney*, 5th ed. Philadelphia: WB, 1996:2274–2296.

Comprehensive review of renal anatomical and functional changes that occur with aging, including renal hemodynamics, fluid and electrolyte balance, and clinical renal diseases in the aged (280 references).

Salmone J, Piccoli GB, Quarello F, et al. Dialysis in the elderly: improvement in survival results in the eighties. *Nephrol Dial Transplant* 1995;10(Suppl 6): 60–64.

European experience with demographics and treatment of elderly patients receiving dialysis (19 references).

Scandling JD. Emerging options for renal transplantation in the older patient. *Nephrol Rounds* 1998;2:1–6.

Excellent review of the demographics and outcomes in transplantation as a function of age, which presents new options for organ procurement in elderly patients (15 references).

Schmucker DL. Aging and drug disposition: an update. *Pharmacol Rev* 1985; 37:133–148.

Comprehensive review of age-dependent alterations in drug absorption, distribution, metabolism, and excretion (224 references).

Singh PJ, Santella RN, Zawada ET. Mitochondrial genome mutations and kidney disease. *Am J Kidney Dis* 1996;28:140–146.

Presents anatomy and function of mitochondrial genome and review of diseases with mutations of these genes (47 references).

Tumer N, Scarpace PJ, Lowenthal DT. Geriatric pharmacology: basic and clinical consideration. *Annu Rev Pharmacol Toxicol* 1992;32:271–302.

Excellent comprehensive review of geriatric pharmacology including clinical examples (189 references).

Whelton PK, Appel LJ, Espeland MA, et al. Sodium reduction and weight loss in the treatment of hypertension in older persons. *JAMA* 1998;279:839–846.

Report of a randomized trial of nonpharmacologic interventions in the control of hypertension in elderly patients (39 references).

Zawada ET Jr, Alavi FK, Santella RN, et al. Influence of dietary macronutrients on glomerular senescence. In: Gonick HC, ed. *Current nephrology.* St Louis: Mosby, 1997;20:1–47.

Comprehensive review of the factors leading to glomerular senescence and the role of dietary macronutrients in this process, including discussion of the effects of dietary protein, carbohydrates and AGEs, dietary lipids, and food restriction on the aging glomerulus (272 references).

CHAPTER 58

Kidney Diseases and Hypertension in Pregnancy

Mark S. Paller

Pregnancy holds many fascinations and hazards for the nephrologist. Remarkable hemodynamic and renal functional adaptations continue to fascinate physiologists. An increasing number of women with renal diseases are becoming pregnant and present additional challenges for clinicians. It is becoming increasingly common for renal transplant recipients and even chronic dialysis patients to become pregnant. An understanding of the normal physiology in pregnancy is useful in understanding how diseases of the kidneys are affected by pregnancy.

HEMODYNAMIC CHANGES

A fundamental pregnancy alteration is a decrease in peripheral or vascular resistance that results in a decrease in blood pressure, an increase in cardiac output, and an increase in renal blood flow (Table 58.1). As discussed later in this chapter, renal sodium retention may also be a consequence of peripheral vasodilation. Alterations in endothelial cell function contribute to systemic and uterine vascular changes. Increased synthesis of vasodilator prostaglandins and other vasodilator substances such as nitric oxide produce resistance to the vasoconstricting effects of circulating vasoconstrictors such as angiotensin II and norepinephrine. By the end of the first trimester of pregnancy blood pressure falls to an average of 103 ± 11 mm Hg systolic and 56 ± 10 mm Hg diastolic. After the 28th week of pregnancy, there is a small rise in systolic and diastolic blood pressure such that average values at term are 109 ± 12 mm Hg systolic and 69 ± 9 mm Hg diastolic. Systemic vasodilation and an increase in blood volume cause cardiac output to increase. Compared with nonpregnant values, cardiac output in midpregnancy is 30% to 40% greater. Even when hypertension complicates pregnancy, cardiac output usually remains higher than the nonpregnant level, although it falls from the very high values observed in normal pregnancy. Blood volume increases approximately 50% in pregnancy. Although both plasma volume and red blood cell volume increase, there is a proportionately greater increase in plasma volume resulting in a "physiologic anemia" of pregnancy. Cumulative sodium retention throughout pregnancy ranges between 500 and 900 mEq. The sodium retention results in a mean weight gain of 12.5 kg. It is believed that the major stimulus for renal sodium retention is the decrease in peripheral vascular resistance resulting in baroreceptor stimulation. Pregnant baboons studied with serial Swan-Ganz catheter determinations from the onset of pregnancy demonstrated early decreases in right atrial pressure and systemic and pulmonary vascular resistance well before expansion of the plasma volume occurred. Women monitored closely during a planned pregnancy demonstrated significant decreases in arterial pressure within 6 weeks of gestation. Cardiac output began to rise by the sixth week of gestation and was maximum in the second trimester. Plasma volume began to increase at 6 weeks gestation and reached a maximum value at 36 weeks.

TABLE 58.1. Hemodynamic Changes in Pregnancy

Peripheral vascular resistance	Decreased
Cardiac output	Increased
Blood pressure	Decreased
Renal vascular resistance	Decreased
Renal blood flow	Increased
Cerebral or hepatic blood flow	No change

Parallel Changes Occur in Renal Hemodynamics

Renal blood flow measured by clearance of *para*-aminohippurate increases by 40% to 75% beginning at 6 weeks of gestation. The increase in renal blood flow is not nearly a passive consequence of the increase in cardiac output because not all organs show a similar increase in blood flow. Therefore renal vasodilation allows the increase in cardiac output to translate into an increase in renal blood flow. A consequence of increased renal blood flow is an increase in glomerular filtration rate (GFR) (Fig. 58.1).

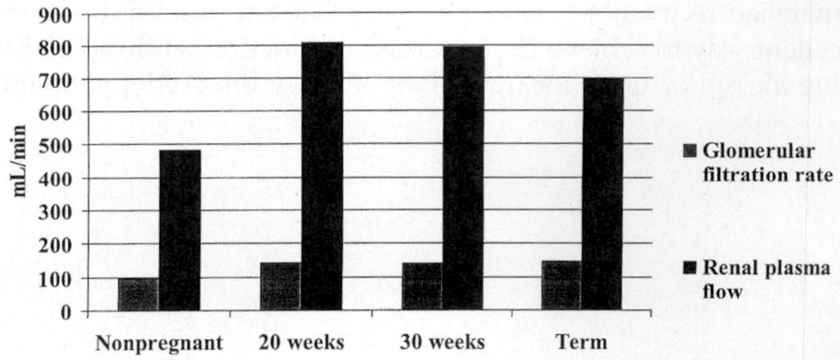

Figure 58.1. Effects of pregnancy on glomerular filtration rate and renal plasma flow. (Data from Davison JM, Dunlop W. Renal hemodynamics and tubular function in normal human pregnancy. *Kidney Int* 1980;18: 152–161.)

GFR also begins to rise as early as 6 weeks of gestation and reaches a plateau in the second trimester. Micropuncture studies of pregnant rats suggest that both afferent and efferent arteriolar resistances decrease.

The specific causes of pregnancy-mediated systemic and renal vasodilation are undefined. Similar changes in hemodynamics occur in pseudopregnant rats and in women during the luteal phase of the menstrual cycle. Prostaglandins and cyclic adenosine monophosphate (cAMP) are candidate mediators of these vascular changes.

Glomerulotubular Balance Is Maintained During Pregnancy

The renal adaptation to a 50% increase in GFR during pregnancy is remarkable (Table 58.2). Although the daily filtered load of sodium in midpregnancy may increase by 10,000 mEq, renal sodium retention increases by only 3 to 5 mEq/day to contribute to plasma volume expansion and fetal development. Despite these remarkable requirements for an alteration in sodium handling, pregnant women adapt reasonably well to alterations in dietary sodium intake. Thus when dietary sodium intake was decreased experimentally to 10 mEq per day, pregnant women reduced urinary sodium excretion as well as did nonpregnant women and did not experience excessive weight loss. Conversely, when the diet of pregnant women was experimentally increased to 300 mEq/day, they came into sodium balance within 4 days. Pregnant women also secrete an intravenous sodium load as rapidly as do nonpregnant women. Thus despite changes in the baseline values in renal function and renal and systemic hemodynamics, pregnant women maintain sodium balance in a normal manner.

Water Balance Is Also Maintained "Normally" During Pregnancy

The ability to concentrate and to dilute the urine is not affected by pregnancy. This may be surprising because increased renal prostaglandin production and increased renal blood flow would otherwise tend to impair urinary concentrating ability. Renal diluting ability is not affected by pregnancy and excretion of a water load is similar in pregnant and nonpregnant women. In midpregnancy, 24-hour urine volumes in pregnant women have been observed to be increased by as much as 25%. This would suggest that water intake mediated by increase thirst is responsible for increased urine volumes.

Although renal concentrating and diluting ability is not changed in pregnancy, plasma osmolality decreases by approximately 10 mOsm/kg H_2O. This decrease in plasma osmolality (and of serum sodium concentration) is the consequence of an alteration in the osmotic threshold for vasopressin secretion by the pituitary. Whereas nonpregnant women secrete vasopressin when plasma osmolality exceeds 285 mOsm/kg H_2O, pregnant women secrete vasopressin when plasma osmolality rises higher than 276 to 278 mOsm/kg H_2O. In addition to a change in the osmotic threshold for vasopressin release, there also appears to be a parallel alteration in the osmotic thirst threshold. Therefore pregnant women sense thirst and begin to drink water at a plasma osmolality 10 mOsm/kg H_2O lower than that for nonpregnant women. The mediator for the resetting of thirst and vasopressin osmoreceptors has not been identified. Unlike the mediators of changes in systemic and renal hemodynamics, a fetal–placental unit does appear necessary to produce these changes in osmoregulation.

TABLE 58.2. Pregnancy-Induced Changes in Renal Function

Parameter	Change	Normal Value
Renal blood flow	Increased	
Glomerular filtration rate	Increased	Creatinine (serum) 0.5 mg/dl
Renal prostaglandin synthesis	Increased	
Renin-angiotensin system activity	Increased	
Filtered load of sodium	Increased	
Renal sodium excretion	No change (slight decrease)	
Renal concentrating ability	No change	
Renal diluting ability	No change	
Urine volume	Increased	
Plasma osmolality	Decreased	Osmolality (plasma) 276 mOsm/kg H_2O; Sodium (plasma) 135 mEq/L
Potassium excretion	No change	
Urate clearance	Increased	Uric acid (serum) 2.5 to 4 mg/dl
Albumin excretion	Increased	Less than 250 mg/24 hr

Other Changes in Solute Metabolism and Renal Function

Pregnancy requires the cumulative retention of approximately 350 mEq of potassium for fetal–placental development and expansion of the maternal red cell mass. Plasma aldosterone levels are increased during pregnancy, but renal potassium wasting does not ensue. Progesterone may inhibit the kaliuretic effect of mineralocorticoids. This effect may even result in reversal of potassium wasting in women with primary hyperaldosteronism who become pregnant. However, this is not a universal finding. Some women with primary hyperaldosteronism develop severe sodium retention and hypertension during pregnancy. On the other hand, pregnancy-induced antagonism of mineralocorticoid action occasionally unmasks otherwise inapparent defects in potassium excretion resulting in hyperkalemia. This has been observed in patients with sickle cell anemia, diabetes, and renal insufficiency, and in women using β-adrenergic antagonists.

Progesterone also seems to be a major factor by stimulating the respiratory center of the brain. Arterial P_{CO_2} decreases by approximately 10 mm Hg and arterial pH rises slightly to 7.44. Plasma bicarbonate usually decreases to 18 to 20 mEq/L. The increase in renal blood flow results in an increase in urate clearance so that serum uric acid falls to 2.5 to 4 mg/dl early in pregnancy. When renal blood flow falls late in pregnancy, urate clearance also falls and the serum uric acid level rises.

A combination of an increase in the filtered load of glucose plus a mild decrease in renal tubule reabsorption of glucose may cause glucosuria. Fractional reabsorption of some amino acids such as glycine, histidine, threonine, serine, and alanine results in specific amino aciduria. Although the increase in GFR causes an increase in the urinary excretion of albumin, 24-hour urinary excretion usually remains less than 200 to 250 mg. These physiologic alterations in renal function are accompanied by anatomic changes. Renal size increases because of increased vascular volume and collecting system volume, as well as hypertrophy of the kidney. During pregnancy this results in an increase in length of approximately 1 cm and an increase in volume by up to 30%. These changes rapidly reverse within 1 week of delivery. Increased estrogen and progesterone results in dilation of the renal collecting system, a process know as *physiologic hydronephrosis* of pregnancy. This is more pronounced in the right side. This phenomenon becomes evident by the end of the first trimester and becomes more marked at term when it is discovered in up to 90% of pregnant women. Muscle relaxation within the ureter may result in vesicoureteral reflux. Unlike the changes in renal volume, these changes in the renal pelvis and ureter may persist for as long as 3 months postpartum.

HYPERTENSION IN PREGNANCY

Hypertension should be classified as either chronic or pregnancy induced. When hypertension is recognized before 20 weeks of gestation it is chronic. Pregnancy-induced hypertension occurs only in the second half of pregnancy. This separation has clinical utility because hypertension presenting early in pregnancy is the result of an underlying condition, either essential of secondary hypertension or renal in origin. Essential hypertension or secondary hypertension due to hyperaldosteronism or pheochromocytoma can be generally classified as chronic hypertension. When hypertension becomes apparent in the second half of pregnancy it may either be a specific consequence of a pregnancy-induced process or a resulting interaction of pregnancy with renal disease or chronic hypertension causing a clinically apparent exacerbation of hypertension. Many obstetricians would further characterize hypertension in pregnancy as being related to one of four conditions: preeclampsia, preeclampsia superimposed on chronic hypertension or renal disease, chronic hypertension, or gestational hypertension (Table 58.3). Gestational hypertension is hypertension that is manifest only during pregnancy, but without features of systemic illness characteristic of preeclampsia.

Normal pregnancy values for blood pressure have been given previously. Although a blood pressure of 140/90 mm Hg is a useful epidemiologic criterion for hypertension, perinatal mortality increases for every increment in blood pressure above a diastolic blood pressure of 85 mm Hg. In the past, it was stated that a pregnancy-related increase in systolic blood pressure of 30 mm Hg or a diastolic blood pressure increase of 15 mm Hg also represented hypertension complicating pregnancy. Many authors now believe that these criteria are invalid because there is considerable variability of blood pressure when measured under usual clinical conditions in healthy normotensive women.

Maternal death still complicates child birth in approximately 9 in 100,000 deliveries. Pregnancy-induced hypertension is the leading cause of maternal death. Perhaps 15% of maternal deaths are the result of hypertension. Pregnancy is also often the first sustained contact between a young woman and the health care system. It is not unusual for asymptomatic hypertension or renal disease to be first recognized during a prenatal visit.

Preeclampsia

Preeclampsia is a pregnancy-specific disease. It is a poorly understood illness whose major manifestations may be those of diffuse endothelial cell injury. Clinically, these manifestations are hypertension, edema, proteinuria, and seizures. Hypertension is the defining, but not invariable, manifestation of preeclampsia. Women who have higher blood pressures in the first trimester of pregnancy have a greater risk of developing overt preeclampsia at the end of pregnancy. Thirty-three percent of women with a mean arterial pressure greater than 90 mm Hg in the second trimester will develop preeclampsia compared with only 2% of those with a mean arterial pressure less than 90 mm Hg. Ambulatory blood pressure monitoring has also revealed increased blood pressure variability in women destined to develop preeclampsia, although ambulatory blood pressure monitoring does not have clinical utility in diagnosing preeclampsia.

TABLE 58.3. Classification of Hypertension in Pregnancy

Preeclampsia
Preeclampsia superimposed on chronic hypertension (essential hypertension, secondary hypertension, or renal disease)
Chronic hypertension (essential hypertension, secondary hypertension, or renal disease)
Gestational hypertension

Etiology

Preeclampsia is characterized by two pathophysiologic abnormalities that are presumed to mediate its development: impaired placentation and diffuse endothelial cell dysfunction. Indeed, impaired placentation may be a consequence of localized endothelial cell abnormalities. When the placenta develops, trophoblast cells from the embryo invade the uterine vessels. Columns of cytotrophoblasts invade the decidual layer of the endometrium aided by the secretion of proteolytic enzymes from these migrating and proliferating cells. The fetal–maternal circulation is established when cytotrophoblasts invade the spiral arteries of the myometrium. If trophoblast invasion is not adequate, development of the spiral arteries fails and uteroplacental hypoperfusion results. Such findings are characteristic of preeclampsia and may be pathogenetic. Abnormal placentation is also a feature of intrauterine growth retardation in the absence of hypertension. The possible link between abnormal placentation and endothelial cell function has been proposed. Invading cytotrophoblasts usually transform from an epithelial to an endothelial phenotype. Cytotrophoblasts obtained from placentas of women with preeclampsia do not express the cell adhesion molecules characteristic of endothelial cells and do not behave normally when placed in cell culture.

Generalized endothelial dysfunction also characterizes preeclampsia. Hypertension, a consequence of systemic vasoconstriction, and coagulopathy are the most prominent manifestations of endothelial dysfunction. Endothelial cells produce both vasodilators, such as prostacyclin and nitric oxide, and vasoconstrictors, such as thromboxane and endothelin. In normal pregnancy the synthesis and/or the effects of the vasodilators predominate. As noted previously, this increased vasodilator tone induces a resistance to the vasoconstrictive effects of angiotensin II and norepinephrine. Women who ultimately develop preeclampsia show an increased vascular sensitivity to infused angiotensin II well before they develop overt hypertension.

Another manifestation of endothelial cell injury is activation of the coagulation system. Patients with preeclampsia develop thrombocytopenia, microangiopathic hemolytic anemia, fibrin deposition in the kidney and liver, and consumptive coagulopathy. Fulminant consumptive coagulopathy is rare, but evidence of a lesser degree of intravascular coagulation is common. Not only is this reflected by changes in the serum level of coagulation factors, but also in flow cytometric analysis of platelets, which demonstrate increased expression of activation markers. These changes in the coagulation system are mediated in part by a decrease in prostacyclin synthesis in endothelial cells without an accompanying reduction in platelet thromboxane synthesis.

Preeclampsia may be part of a spectrum of diseases occurring in pregnancy caused by endothelial cell injury and dysfunction. The HELLP (Hemolysis, Elevated Liver enzymes, Low Platelet) syndrome, a more severe variant of preeclampsia, and acute fatty liver of pregnancy have features shared with preeclampsia consistent with endothelial cell injury. Pregnant women are also susceptible to postpartum acute renal failure (or postpartum hemolytic uremia syndrome), another disease

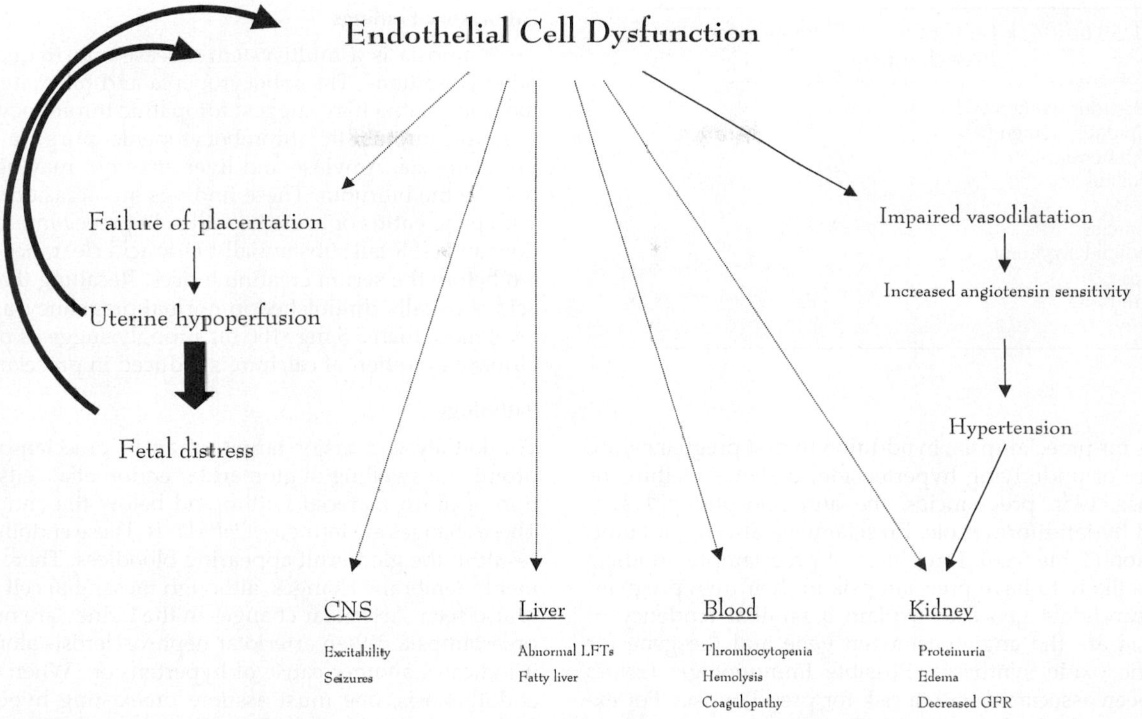

Figure 58.2. Hypothetic scheme for the pathogenesis of preeclampsia. The two central processes are diffuse endothelial cell dysfunction and failure of placentation.

characterized by hypertension and coagulation abnormalities consistent with endothelial cell injury.

Although both changes in coagulation and in vascular reactivity and tone can be explained by diffuse endothelial injury, the relationship between impaired uteroplacental blood flow and the health and function of the systemic endothelium is not understood. Figure 58.2 demonstrates an hypothesized scheme to explain the multiple features of preeclampsia.

Clinical Features

Preeclampsia sometimes develops abruptly, but more often develops insidiously. Common symptoms are headache, visual disturbances, epigastric pain, and apprehension (Table 58.4). Weight gain and edema usually accompany rising blood pressure and proteinuria. However, because as many as 83% of healthy pregnant women develop localized edema and up to 10% develop generalized edema, these findings are not diagnostic for preeclampsia. Proteinuria may be minimal (500 mg/24 hr) or in the nephrotic range. Hypertension occurs in preeclampsia. The clinical characteristics of diseases associated with hypertension in pregnancy are provided in Table 58.5. Preeclampsia usually develops after the thirty-second week of pregnancy. Sometimes it begins earlier, particularly in women with chronic hypertension or renal disease. In some cases preeclampsia develops postpartum. Preeclampsia usually resolves within 10 days of delivery.

An interesting feature of preeclampsia is its epidemiology. Preeclampsia has a bimodal frequency affecting younger primiparous and older (more than 40 years) multiparous women.

TABLE 58.4. Clinical Features of Preeclampsia

Symptoms
Headache
Visual disturbances
Epigastric pain
Apprehension
Signs
Hypertension
Hyperactive deep tendon reflexes
Edema
Pulmonary edema
Laboratory Findings
Thrombocytopenia
Microangiopathic hemolytic anemia
Increased serum uric acid
Proteinuria
Increased serum creatinine
Abnormal liver function tests

TABLE 58.5. Clinical Features of Diseases Causing Hypertension in Pregnancy

	Preeclampsia	Chronic Hypertension	Renal Disease
Hypertension	?/+	?/+	?/+
Proteinuria	−/+	−/−	+/+
Microscopic hematuria	−/−	−/−	?/?
Increased serum creatinine	−/?	−/−	?/?
Increased serum uric acid	−/+	−/−	?/?
Coagulopathy	−/?	−/−	−/−
Neurologic abnormalities	−/?	−/−	−/−
1st 20 weeks/ 2nd 20 weeks			

+, usually present; ?, may be present; −, usually absent.

TABLE 58.6. Risk Factors for the Development of Preeclampsia
Young primiparous women (<18 yr)
Older multiparous women (>40 yr)
Essential hypertension
Diabetes mellitus
Renal disease
Twin pregnancies
Antiphospholipid syndrome
Fetal hydrops
Hydatidiform mole
Family history

Risk factors for preeclampsia, in addition to first pregnancy, are the presence of underlying hypertension, diabetes mellitus or renal disease, twin pregnancies, the anti–phospholipid syndrome, and hydatidiform mole. Preeclampsia also has a familial association (Table 58.6). Daughters of preeclamptic mothers are twice as likely to have preeclampsia in their own pregnancies. Two candidate genes to explain a familial tendency of preeclampsia are the angiotensinogen gene and the gene for eNOS (nitric oxide synthase). Possible immunologic factors have also been associated with a risk for preeclampsia. For example, women who had previously received blood transfusions or had a long period of cohabitation before conception were found to be less likely to develop preeclampsia.

Laboratory Findings

Preeclampsia is a multisystem disease and frequently mimics other conditions. Thrombocytopenia and microangiopathic hemolytic anemia may suggest idiopathic thrombocytopenic purpura or thrombotic thrombocytopenic purpura rather than preeclampsia. Amylase and liver enzymes may be elevated as may be the bilirubin. These findings are occasionally confused with pancreatitis or acute hepatitis. In preeclampsia renal blood flow and GFR fall substantially. Uric acid clearance also falls, often before the serum creatinine rises. Recalling that serum uric acid is usually diminished in normal pregnancy, a serum urate level more than 5.5 mg/100 ml strongly suggests preeclampsia. Urinary excretion of calcium is reduced in preeclampsia.

Pathology

The kidney is a major target organ in preeclampsia. There is prominent swelling of glomerular endothelial cells and deposition of fibrin material within and below the endothelial cells. These changes are termed *endotheliosis*. These endothelial changes result in the glomeruli appearing bloodless. There are no basement membrane changes, although mesangial cell proliferation is also seen. Arteriolar changes in the kidney are not part of the preeclampsia. When arteriolar nephrosclerosis alone is present, it indicates another cause of hypertension. When present with endotheliosis, one must assume preexisting hypertension before pregnancy. Immunofluorescent examination of kidneys in preeclampsia reveals fibrinogen in glomeruli (Fig. 58.3). Glomerular endotheliosis tends to disappear soon after delivery,

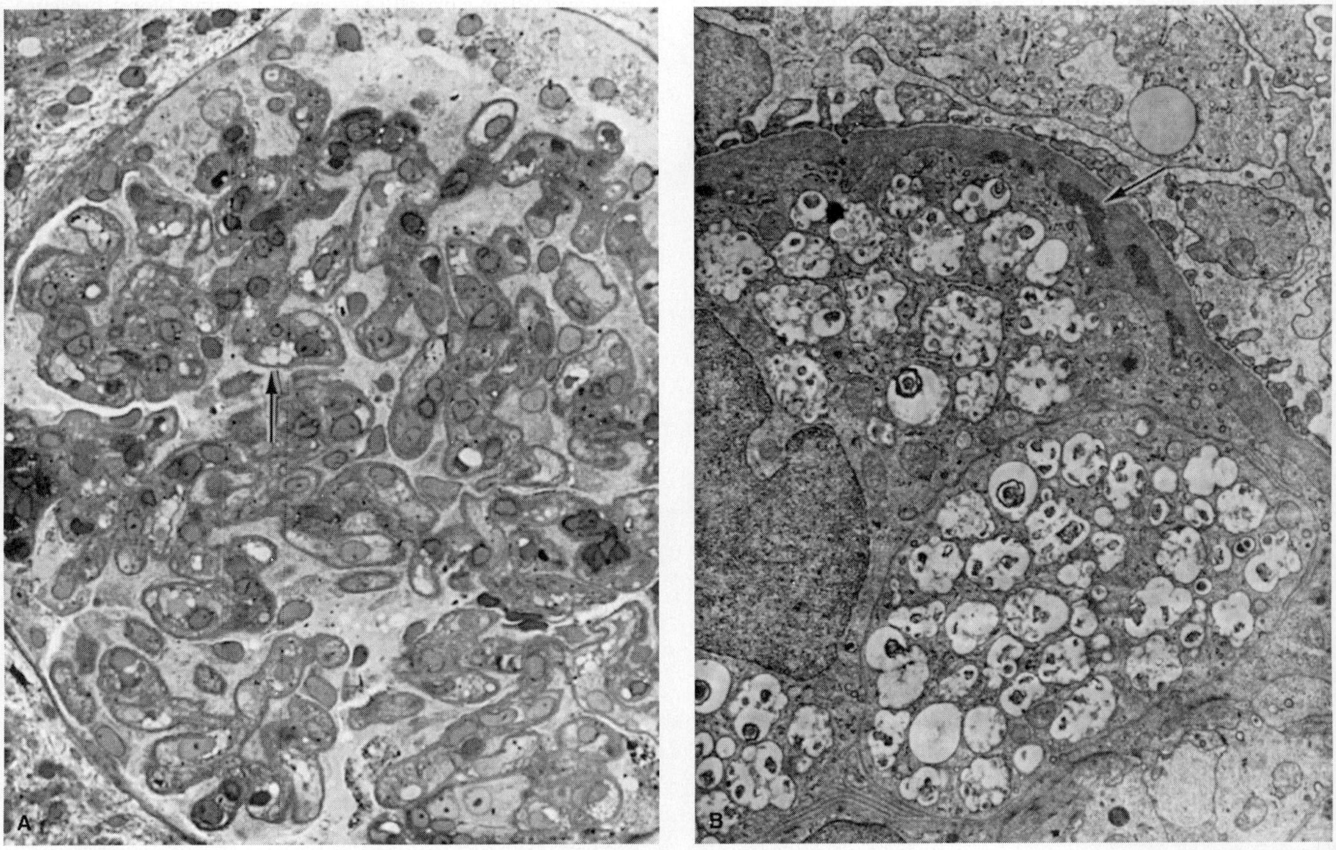

Figure 58.3. The renal lesion in preeclampsia. **A:** Capillary lumina are encroached upon by swollen endothelial cells, which show prominent vacuolization (*arrow*). **B:** Electron micrograph demonstrating complete obliteration of capillary lumen by swollen endothelium filled with lipid-containing vacuoles, some of which contain myelinlike figures. Small subendothelial accumulations of fibrin are evident (*arrow*). (Courtesy of Dr. BH Spargo, The University of Chicago, Chicago, IL.)

and the glomerulus is usually normal by the end of 2 to 4 weeks.

Liver biopsies demonstrate patchy areas of necrosis with fibrin deposit; some liver biopsies in patients with preeclampsia show microvascular fat, necrosis, and cholestasis, which are the typical findings of acute fatty liver in pregnancy. Many hepatologists believe that acute fatty liver of pregnancy is a hepatic manifestation of preeclampsia. The brain in women who die after preeclampsia usually shows cerebral edema and may show petechial or larger hemorrhages.

Treatment of Preeclampsia

Prevention. Several early studies of low-dose aspirin suggested a beneficial effect to prevent preeclampsia. Unfortunately, larger multicenter studies have not uniformly demonstrated such a benefit. Some studies suggested that the greater the risk of developing preeclampsia, the greater the benefit of low-dose aspirin. However, a recent National Institutes of Health study focusing on 2,539 high-risk women failed to demonstrate a reduction in the incidence of preeclampsia by treatment with low-dose aspirin. That study did not evaluate a large number of women with preexisting renal disease. In addition, it remains possible that the negative results of that study can be explained by a failure to control the timing of aspirin administration. One other study suggested that low-dose aspirin lowered blood pressure in pregnant women when given at midday or at bedtime, but not when given in the morning. Therefore there is still an opportunity to further evaluate low-dose aspirin to prevent preeclampsia in high-risk women. For now, the use of low-dose aspirin to prevent preeclampsia can not be recommended. It is important to note, however, that a number of very large studies have demonstrated the safety of using low-dose aspirin in pregnant women. Calcium supplementation has also been suggested to prevent the development of preeclampsia. Again, large, multicenter, prospective studies have failed to confirm this benefit.

Treatment. There is no evidence that salt restriction alters the odds for developing preeclampsia or its severity when it occurs; on the contrary, current nutritional recommendations emphasize the importance of adequate salt intake during pregnancy. The definitive treatment for preeclampsia is delivery. When preeclampsia occurs at term this does not represent a significant problem. When preeclampsia occurs between the 32nd and 34th weeks of gestation there is some flexibility in management because long-term fetal outcome is likely to be good. If preeclampsia is not severe, conservative therapy with antihypertensive medication and bed rest can be tried. Because fetal survival is less predictable at 28 to 34 weeks of gestation, medical management is usually first attempted. Management of preeclampsia occurring between 18 and 28 weeks is an unsettled issue. Claims can be made for both terminating the pregnancy or for attempting conservative management, which occasionally results in prolongation of pregnancy with an acceptable outcome. Almost all obstetricians would recommend terminating pregnancy if preeclampsia develops before the eighteenth week of gestation.

Hypertension is a risk factor for both the fetus and the mother. There are concerns about the effects of antihypertensive therapy on the fetus. However, hypertension needs to be treated to prevent cerebral hemorrhage in the mother. There are fears that aggressive antihypertensive therapy will result in compromise of uteroplacental blood flow if maternal blood pressure falls quickly because of the limited ability of the placenta to autoregulate blood flow. There is no unanimity of opinion as to the diastolic blood pressure goal. Published values have ranged as low as 90 to as high as 110 mm Hg. Unfortunately, there are only a small number of prospective trials of antihypertensive therapy in women who developed hypertension in the last trimester. The majority of these studies suggest that fetal morbidity and mortality is reduced by antihypertensive therapy when the pretreatment diastolic blood pressure is more than 90 mm Hg. Under these circumstances, antihypertensive therapy reduces the incidences of prematurity, intrauterine growth retardation, and perinatal death. In one carefully performed study, the investigators treated pregnancy-induced hypertension in women whose blood pressure increased to only 126/82 mm Hg. Relative to placebo, clonidine therapy reduced third-trimester complications and prematurity by 80%. Most of studies that have demonstrated improvement in fetal outcome have instituted antihypertensive therapy in the second or third trimester of pregnancy. The benefits of antihypertensive therapy when begun in the first trimester of pregnancy are less clear.

Mild hypertension is usually treated with bed rest. Part of the evaluation of such a patient is to evaluate for the presence of serious disease. Such an evaluation includes determining urinary protein excretion, renal function (serum creatinine), serum uric acid, liver function tests, and coagulation parameters. When pregnancy is at 32 weeks of gestation or greater, development of any of these complication is an indication for delivery. In the absence of additional complications, moderate hypertension (diastolic blood pressure of 95 to 100 mm Hg) should be treated with an antihypertensive agent if it is desirable to delay delivery because of prematurity.

The antihypertensive agents used in pregnancy are many of the same employed for the general treatment of hypertension (Table 58.7). One major difference is that older agents that have a longer track record of successful use in pregnancy are favored despite undesirable side effect profiles. Methyldopa, not often used in essential hypertension because of side effects of dry mouth, fatigue, depression, and orthostatic hypertension, is the agent of first choice in pregnancy hypertension because of its extensive experience in pregnancy. The dosage is 0.5 to 3.0 g/day. Many years ago, it was demonstrated that relative to placebo, methyldopa effectively controlled blood pressure and yielded better fetal outcomes. Methyldopa therapy resulted in fewer midpregnancy abortions, but did not prevent preeclampsia. Infants born to mothers who have received methyldopa had small head circumference for gestational age, which presented a serious initial concern. However, when these infants were reevaluated at 1 year, growth and head circumference were normal. More importantly, the infants of women who had received methyldopa scored higher on the Denver Developmental Screening Test than did infants whose mothers received placebo. Reevaluated at 4 years of age, this trend persisted. This long-term study raises the interesting possibility that maternal hypertension may lead to mild developmental delays in children and that methyldopa, by effectively treating hypertension, prevented this unfavorable outcome. No other study of antihypertensive therapy has evaluated long-term outcomes in children so well. Nevertheless, many studies have demonstrated that antihypertensive therapy does improve short-term maternal and fetal outcome.

An acceptable alternative to methyldopa is a β-adrenergic blocker. Atenolol (50 to 100 mg/day), metoprolol (50 to 225 mg/day), and propranolol (40 to 240 mg/day) have been most thoroughly studied. Labetalol, a combined α- and β-adrenergic blocker is also commonly used. Previous concerns about β-adrenergic blockade–inducing fetal bradycardia have not been sustained. One concern about the use of β-blockers when given early in pregnancy is the possibility of a decrease in birth weight. It was found that although atenolol reduced perinatal

TABLE 58.7. Use of Antihypertensive Agents in Pregnancy

Category	Specific Agent	Potential Complications
β-Adrenergic blockers	Atenolol	Fetal bradycardia
	Metoprolol	Low birth weight when used in first trimester
α,β-Adrenergic blockers	Labetalol	
Calcium channel blockers	Nifedipine, isradipine, verapamil	Avoid near term; prolongation of labor
	Diltiazem	Avoid near term; prolongation of labor
Centrally acting adrenergic agents	Methyldopa	Side effects (dry mouth, fatigue, orthostatic hypotension)
	Clonidine	
Vasodilators	Hydralazine	Maternal tachycardia
	prazosin	
Thiazides	HCTZ	Volume depletion (use in combination therapy)
Angiotensin-converting enzyme inhibitors		Do not use in pregnancy; switch to other agents if pregnancy occurs during therapy with these agents; they are associated with fetal loss, fetal renal dysplasia, other congenital abnormalities, and perinatal acute renal failure in the infant

mortality when used to treat pregnancy-induced hypertension developing in the third trimester, atenolol administered beginning in the first trimester to women with chronic essential hypertension resulted in intrauterine growth retardation. A major difficulty in evaluating these findings is the different underlying nature of the hypertension. It is just as likely that chronic hypertension that is present throughout pregnancy is more detrimental to fetal development than is hypertension that only develops late in pregnancy. Nevertheless, a concern about the effects of antihypertensive therapy, per se, suggests caution in the use of antihypertensive medications for mild hypertension.

Other hypertensive agents can also be used for treating hypertension in pregnancy. Hydralazine (50 to 200 mg/day) is used as adjunctive therapy with methyldopa. This combination therapy has been shown to be a safety practice in pregnancy. Clonidine, α-adrenergic antagonists, and dihydropyridine calcium channel blockers (such as nifedipine) all have published experience in pregnancy. The phenyl alkylamine and benzothiazepine calcium channel blockers (verapamil and diltiazem) have not been as widely utilized in pregnancy, particularly in the prepartum period because of the possibility of retarding labor. Combination therapy is effective for severe hypertension. Angiotensin-converting enzyme (ACE) inhibitors are contraindicated in pregnancy.

Diuretics are not first-line agents for treating hypertension caused by preeclampsia. The preeclampsia-induced decrease in GFR does result in sodium retention. However, compared with normotensive pregnancy, plasma volume is sometimes diminished in preeclampsia. This is likely a consequence of a shift in extracellular volume from the vascular to the interstitial space, a phenomenon that also occurs in pheochromocytoma, malignant hypertension, and renal artery stenosis. Therefore, because preeclampsia is predominately a disease of vasoconstriction, vasodilators are much more appropriate than are diuretics. On the other hand, thiazides have been extensively studied in preeclampsia because they were once given prophylactically to prevent preeclampsia. Although they have a limited ability to prevent preeclampsia, diuretics certainly do not have adverse effects on fetal outcome. For women who have increased intravascular volume, thiazides can and should be used as one component of combination antihypertensive therapy. This is certainly true of women who have pulmonary edema in whom Swan-Ganz catheter determinations of pulmonary capillary wedge pressure has often confirmed increased intravascular volumes.

Severe hypertension (diastolic blood pressure of more than 100 mm Hg) requires delivery, as discussed previously, and the use of parenteral agents to prevent maternal complications (Table 58.8). Intravenous labetalol may be the best choice for parenteral treatment of severe hypertension in pregnancy. Hydralazine has been used more frequently but has a major side effect of reflex tachycardia, and headache and neonatal thrombocytopenia have been reported. This reflex tachycardia of hydralazine can be eliminated by the concomitant use of a β-adrenergic blocker. The therapy with hydralazine begins with 5 mg followed with 5 to 10 mg every 20 to 30 minutes until the goal blood pressure is achieved. Oral nifedipine is a useful alternative whose use should be restricted to those situations in which severe hypertension needs to be treated but use of parenteral agents is problematic, such as in primary care clinics or during emergency transfer of patients to a tertiary care center. Very severe or resistant hypertension can be treated by infusion of sodium nitroprusside. The use of sodium nitroprusside must be limited in duration because of the risks of fetal cyanide toxicity.

Women with severe preeclampsia should also be given magnesium sulfate to prevent the development of seizures. Magnesium sulfate has mild antihypertensive effects, perhaps through the induction of prostacyclin synthesis. More importantly, magnesium sulfate is superior to phenytoin in preventing seizures in women with preeclampsia. Magnesium sulfate must be ad-

TABLE 58.8. Agents for Severe Hypertension in Pregnancy

Agent	Benefits	Risks
Hydralazine	Safety record	Maternal tachycardia
Labetalol	Effective	Newer agent (less experience)
Nifedipine	Effective orally	Erratic blood pressure lowering (use only when patient cannot receive parenteral agents)
Magnesium sulfate	Prevents seizures	Respiratory paralysis; weak antihypertensive
Sodium nitroprusside	Very effective	Fetal cyanide toxicity (use for short duration)
Diazoxide		Rarely used; erratic blood pressure lowering

ministered carefully because of the frequent impairment in ventilatory function that occasionally leads to respiratory arrest. Use of continuous infusions of magnesium sulfate in women with impaired renal function is particularly risky. If muscular or respiratory paralysis develops, intravenous calcium should be administered.

Outcomes

Because of its association with abnormal placentation, preeclampsia causes perinatal morbidity and mortality, including intrauterine growth retardation and prematurity. As noted previously, the major maternal risks are pulmonary edema and cerebral hemorrhage. Women who develop preeclampsia in a first pregnancy but experience normotensive subsequent pregnancies have no long-term morbidity or mortality related to the initial episode of preeclampsia. In such women, life expectancy is normal and there is no increase in the long-term risk of developing hypertension. In marked contrast, if preeclampsia develops in second or multiple pregnancies, there is an adverse effect on morbidity and mortality. Women who have experienced multiple episodes of preeclampsia have a twofold increase in the prevalence of hypertension when evaluated more than 20 years after their initial pregnancy. These women also have an excess incidence of vascular disease and premature death believed to be related to hypertension. In such women, preeclampsia was probably not idiopathic but rather a manifestation of underlying chronic hypertension, renal disease, or diabetes. Therefore in women who develop preeclampsia in the first half of pregnancy a strong association with other diseases such as chronic hypertension and renal disease requires long-term follow-up.

Chronic Hypertension

Essential Hypertension

Essential hypertension is a common disease and may not have been previously diagnosed in women without regular medical contacts. Pregnancy may represent the first opportunity for an adult to seek medical care. In the absence of blood pressure determinations before pregnancy, it is possible to overlook the failure of blood pressure to decrease in the first half of pregnancy. Thus it is possible to initially overlook chronic hypertension, a diagnosis that might not be obvious until postpartum. Because chronic hypertension is a risk factor for the development of preeclampsia, it is not uncommon for such women to have an exacerbation of hypertension late in pregnancy that is difficult to differentiate from idiopathic or primary preeclampsia. Hypertension due to preeclampsia should resolve within 10 days of delivery. Blood pressure may decrease somewhat in women with chronic hypertension only to again increase years later or during a subsequent pregnancy. Table 58.4 suggests differentiating features of chronic hypertension and preeclampsia.

Antihypertensive medications should be continued throughout pregnancy in women who were previously treated. This recommendation includes the use of a diuretic if one was part of the antepartum antihypertensive regimen. The only exception to this rule is that ACE inhibitors should be discontinued as soon as pregnancy is recognized. ACE inhibitors have been associated with fetal loss, fetal renal dysplasia, other congenital abnormalities, and perinatal acute renal failure in the infant. These findings have not been seen in infants whose exposure to ACE inhibitors were limited to the first trimester of pregnancy, if ACE inhibitors were subsequently not administered during the second and third trimester. Therefore if a woman using an ACE inhibitor becomes pregnant, the drug should be discontinued. It does not appear necessary to terminate the pregnancy intentionally.

The proper management of mild chronic hypertension during pregnancy is more controversial. There do not appear to be major short-term risks of mild blood pressure elevations to either the mother or fetus. Maternal risks of cerebral hemorrhage and fetal risks of intrauterine growth retardation and death are related to the absolute blood pressure. When diastolic blood pressure exceeds 100 mm Hg, there is little argument about the institution of antihypertensive therapy. However, because fetal mortality increases even when blood pressure exceeds 85 to 90 mm Hg, some practitioners would begin the use of medication at these blood pressure levels. Prospective, randomized, controlled trials for the treatment of mild chronic hypertension in pregnancy have demonstrated both beneficial effects and lack of effect. These studies have suffered because of small sample sizes and may have missed both beneficial and harmful effects of therapy. Beneficial effects of antihypertensive therapy in moderate to severe hypertension are less controversial.

Secondary Hypertension

Secondary causes of hypertension (renal artery stenosis, hyperaldosteronism, or pheochromocytoma) often present difficult management scenarios or interesting presentations. For example, progesterone has the ability to antagonize the kaliuretic effect of mineralocorticoids and sometimes reverses potassium wasting in hyperaldosteronism.

Pheochromocytoma has been documented on several occasions to present suddenly and dramatically during pregnancy. Maternal and fetal mortality may be as high as 25% if pheochromocytoma is not recognized. When diagnosed, pheochromocytoma should be managed with the use of α- and β-adrenergic blockers, and maternal mortality can be prevented.

KIDNEY DISEASES AND PREGNANCY

Bacteriuria

Although urinary tract infection is no more frequent in pregnant women compared with nonpregnant women, the consequences are far more serious during pregnancy. When untreated, bacteriuria evolves into urinary tract infection and becomes symptomatic in approximately 30% of pregnant women. Women with diabetes or sickle cell trait or sickle cell disease have a greater risk of developing urinary tract infection during pregnancy. In all pregnant women, the increased capacity of the urinary collecting system, slower emptying, and usual development of vesicoureteral reflux also predispose to urinary tract infection.

Bacteremia, septic shock, and impaired renal function are the maternal risks of urinary tract infection. Fetal risks are even more serious. Midtrimester abortions have been linked to bacteriuria. Bacteriuria occurring near term has been associated with perinatal mortality. Because only half of pregnant women with bacteriuria are symptomatic, all pregnant women should have a screening urine culture at an initial prenatal visit. Not all women with symptoms suggestive of bacteriuria have infection. Nocturia, polyuria, and stress incontinence are common complaints in uncomplicated pregnancy.

Women with a history of asymptomatic bacteriuria during childhood have an increased frequency of complications during pregnancy. These women more frequently develop bacteriuria and pyelonephritis in pregnancy. Asymptomatic bacteriuria during childhood may also result in subtle renal damage that is unmasked during pregnancy. Women with known renal scars because of renal injury occurring during childhood have an increased risk of preeclampsia. These women are more likely to require induction of labor or operative delivery compared with those having no such history.

Bacteriuria should be treated even if asymptomatic. The organism and its sensitivity to antibiotics should be determined with urine culture. Long-term cure rates after short courses of therapy for 5 to 10 days are approximately 65%. Some single-dose regimens have been recommended, although 3 days of therapy may be superior to single-dose regimens. Women with symptomatic urinary tract infection usually require more prolonged (usually 10 to 14 days) therapy to eradicate infection. If the infection recurs, 3 to 5 weeks of therapy is needed. All women who develop urinary tract infection during pregnancy require close follow-up during the remainder of pregnancy. Because urinary tract infection usually develops in pregnancy in the absence of underlying structural abnormalities, only when infection is difficult to eradicate or when there is history suggestive of underlying disease should the presence of structural abnormalities be sought. Therapy with amoxicillin may be initiated awaiting the results of the urine culture. Most patients respond promptly, and defervescence occurs within 1 to 3 days.

Asymptomatic Urinary Abnormalities

Proteinuria developing during pregnancy may indicate worsening of preexistent renal disease, the *de novo* development of renal disease, or preeclampsia, which includes renal involvement as part of a systemic disorder. The increase in GFR occurring during normal pregnancy results in an increase in urinary excretion of albumin. Nevertheless, in otherwise healthy pregnancy women, the 24-hour urinary excretion of protein does not usually exceed 250 mg. Trace positive results for protein by dipstick testing (false positive) will occasionally be seen in concentrated urine specimens, but a random urine protein:creatinine ratio can be used to detect significant proteinuria in pregnancy. Urinary protein excretion greater than 2 g/24 hr suggest a glomerular process. Although pregnancy does not predispose to the development of renal disease, renal diseases such as membranous nephropathy, focal glomerulosclerosis, minimal-change nephropathy, diabetic nephropathy, and systemic lupus erythematosus (SLE) will occasionally occur during pregnancy.

Hematuria usually indicates an organic process. Despite the development of glomerular lesions and proteinuria in preeclampsia, hematuria is not characteristic of preeclampsia. Therefore the finding of red cells or, in particular, red cell casts in a patient with preeclampsia suggests the coexistence of underlying renal disease.

When glomerulonephritis or other renal disease develops during pregnancy, renal biopsy is often considered. Although many authors would argue for an empiric trial of corticosteroids in a patient with uncomplicated nephrotic syndrome, in some cases, such as rapidly progressive glomerulonephritis, renal biopsy is desirable. If clinical opinion is such that renal biopsy should not be delayed until after delivery, the procedure can be safely performed during pregnancy. Complications are no more frequent than those in nonpregnant women when the usual guidelines are followed.

Acute Renal Failure

Acute renal failure is an impairment in renal function and reduction in urine output that develops over a period of hours to days. In pregnancy, acute renal failure usually takes the form of one of three renal diseases: acute tubular necrosis (ATN), renal cortical necrosis, or postpartum acute renal failure. On occasion, obstructive uropathy or acute fatty liver of pregnancy also cause acute renal failure. The approach to acute renal failure occurring during pregnancy is the same as that for nonpregnant women. There are often clues as to what renal disease is responsible for the acute renal failure. However, a systematic approach should always be taken. This requires evaluating the patient for the possibility of prerenal azotemia by performing a careful physical examination evaluating volume status, careful physical and laboratory evaluation, and evaluation of the urinary tract collecting system to rule out obstructive uropathy.

Acute Tubular Necrosis

ATN complicates many conditions, but most commonly sepsis or hypotension. This disease is now rare because of the low incidence of septic abortion in the industrialized world. In late pregnancy, ATN may complicate preeclampsia or abruptio placenta. ATN is a rare complication of preeclampsia occurring in only 1% to 2% of cases. In the HELLP syndrome, a clinical variant of preeclampsia, acute renal failure occurs more frequently (5% to 10%).

Abruptio placenta causes both ATN and renal cortical necrosis. The volume depletion because of hemorrhage is presumed to be the cause of acute renal failure in abruptio placenta. The urine sediment will contain renal tubular epithelial cells, dark or muddy granular casts, and other cellular debris characteristic of ATN.

Renal Cortical Necrosis

Risk factors for the development of renal cortical necrosis are similar to those for ATN. Abruptio placenta, septic abortion, severe preeclampsia, amniotic fluid embolism, and retained fetus have been associated with renal cortical necrosis. Anuria is far more common in renal cortical necrosis than in ATN. Renal cortical necrosis should also be suspected when severe oliguria or anuria persists for more than 1 week. Hematuria is more suggestive of renal cortical necrosis than of ATN. Renal arteriogram or radionuclide renal scan show patchy blood flow or the absence of a nephrogram. Renal cortical necrosis has also been diagnosed by computed tomography (CT) scan, which demonstrates a lucent area below the renal capsule representing an ischemic zone.

Postpartum Acute Renal Failure

Postpartum acute renal failure or postpartum hemolytic uremic syndrome is a disease characterized by coagulation abnormalities, hypertension, and acute renal failure. It occurs in otherwise uncomplicated pregnancies between 1 to 2 days and several months after delivery. Microangiopathic hemolytic anemia is recognized by the finding of schistocytes and burr cells on peripheral blood smear. Thrombocytopenia is usually present, but bleeding times are not usually prolonged. Neurologic symptoms may be present and suggest thrombotic thrombocytopenic purpura. Some believe that hemolytic uremic syndrome and thrombotic thrombocytopenic purpura are different syndromes along a continuum of disease caused by diffuse endothelial cell injury. As noted previously, several pregnancy-related diseases, including preeclampsia, the HELLP syndrome, postpartum acute renal failure, and acute fatty liver of pregnancy, are characterized by acute endothelial cell injury. Hemolytic uremic syndrome also has developed in women taking oral contraceptives, suggesting a causal link with the hormonal alterations of pregnancy. Postpartum acute renal failure usually requires supportive therapy with dialysis. Uncontrolled studies suggest a benefit of plasma exchange or infusion of fresh-frozen plasma, but these therapies are unproven.

TABLE 58.9. Pregnancy Complications in Women with Renal Disease

Increased frequency of fetal loss
Intrauterine growth retardation
Prematurity
Superimposed preeclampsia
Progression of renal disease

Pregnancy in Women with Renal Disease

Renal disease in pregnant women presents potentially serious consequences for both maternal health and fetal outcome regardless of whether the renal disease is preexistent or has developed during pregnancy (Table 58.9). In addition, pregnancy may have adverse effects on renal function that persist after pregnancy has been completed. Both of these aspects must be considered when counseling a patient as to the advisability and risks of pregnancy. No simple recommendations are possible. However, any pregnant women with underlying renal disease should be managed by an obstetrician experienced in high-risk pregnancies and by a nephrologist.

Effects of Renal Disease on Fetal Outcome

Although fertility is impaired by renal dysfunction, pregnancy occasionally occurs in women with severe renal insufficiency and even in patients on chronic dialysis. A survey of dialysis units in the United States found that approximately 2% of women of childbearing age became pregnant during a 4-year observation. Maternal renal disease results in an increased frequency of fetal loss, intrauterine growth retardation, and prematurity. Hypertension is the major risk factor for these adverse outcomes. Additional risk factors are renal insufficiency and the presence of nephrotic syndrome. The more chronic and stable the course of renal disease, the better the fetal outcome. When preeclampsia is superimposed on preexistent renal disease, fetal loss is increased. Women with impaired renal function and superimposed preeclampsia may have fetal loss rates approaching 40% to 60%. Even in women with preserved renal function and mild or no hypertension, renal disease results in an increase in fetal wastage. Compared with women who have no renal disease, women with renal disease have perinatal mortality rates that are increased three to four times, and comparable increases in preterm deliveries and infants that are small for gestational age. It is important to note that it is the manifestations of renal disease and not the specific diagnosis that has the greatest influence on fetal outcome (Table 58.10). To demonstrate the importance of impairment in renal function and the presence of severe hypertension or nephrotic syndrome, one may review a published retrospective report. This review of 25 years of experience comprising 398 pregnancies revealed a perinatal mortality rate of 30% when one of the three aforementioned risk factors was present compared with perinatal mortality of only 5% if renal function was preserved and hypertension and nephrotic syndrome were absent. In general, even for high-risk pregnancies fetal outcomes have improved over time.

TABLE 58.10. Risk Factors for Poor Fetal Outcome in Women with Renal Disease

Hypertension
Renal insufficiency
Nephrotic syndrome

Underlying renal disease predisposes to the development of superimposed preeclampsia. The risk varies between 20% and 40%. When renal disease causes preeclampsia, it may affect multiparous women as well as nulliparous women. Importantly, preeclampsia may also appear earlier than 32 weeks. In one study, one-fourth of all cases of preeclampsia had an onset earlier than 37 weeks of gestation. Of these, 90% were women who had chronic renal disease or essential hypertension. As discussed previously, women with renal disease are a very high-risk group for the development of preeclampsia and would be most appropriate for intervention. Unfortunately, prophylactic agents such as aspirin or calcium have not been demonstrated to be useful in preventing preeclampsia, although their evaluation in women with renal disease has been quite limited to date.

The Risk of Progression of Renal Disease in Pregnancy

It is now well recognized that once a certain threshold of renal injury has been reached, renal disease may progress inexorably. One of the major factors contributing to progressive renal insufficiency is hypertension with transmission to the glomerular capillaries leading to intraglomerular hypertension. This suggests the possibility that hypertension complicating pregnancy might cause further deterioration in preexistent renal disease. This might be especially true in pregnancy because pregnancy is associated with afferent arteriolar dilation. Thus systemic blood pressure would be more likely to be transmitted into the glomerulus resulting in intraglomerular injury. This has been difficult to prove because not all laboratory rats with renal disease develop afferent arteriolar dilation, although this change is characteristic of pregnancy in control laboratory rats.

It is clear that women with mild renal insufficiency respond to pregnancy with changes in renal hemodynamics similar to those in normal women. Thus women with mild renal insufficiency develop an increase in GFR and renal blood flow during pregnancy. As renal function becomes more severely impaired, the magnitude of these changes is diminished.

A general statement can be made that women who have renal disease with preserved renal function (usually defined as a serum creatinine less than 1.4 mg/dl in most studies) experience no permanent deterioration in renal function due to pregnancy. On the other hand, up to one-third of women who have renal impairment seem to suffer a more rapid decline in renal function after pregnancy than would have been predicted by their prior course (Table 58.11). It should be pointed out that there has been no systematic investigation of the effects of rigorously controlling hypertension in women with moderate renal insufficiency who become pregnant to determine whether this reduces the chances of a permanent deterioration in renal function. Many women who suffer permanent deterioration in renal function during pregnancy experience severe hypertension. In

TABLE 58.11. Risk Factors for Progression of Renal Disease During Pregnancy

Renal insufficiency (serum creatinine >1.4 mg/dl)
Proteinuria
Hypertension
Specific renal diseases (possibly):
Membranoproliferative glomerulonephritis
IgA nephropathy
Focal sclerosis
Reflux nephropathy

addition to the baseline level of renal function at the time of pregnancy, proteinuria may represent an additional risk factor for pregnancy-related declines in renal function. In one study of 30 pregnancies in women with renal disease, proteinuria greater than 2 grams per day better predicted which 10 pregnancies would be complicated by worsening of renal function than did the level of blood pressure or the absolute level of renal function.

Some claims have been made that specific renal diseases are more likely to result in accelerated progression of renal disease during pregnancy. Such claims have been made for membranoproliferative glomerular nephritis, IgA nephropathy, focal sclerosis, and reflux nephropathy. For the most part, the number of such women observed has been small. The already defined risk factors of level of renal function, hypertension, and amount of proteinuria are probably more robust predictors of the effects of pregnancy on long-term renal outcomes than the specific renal diagnosis.

Periarteritis nodosa and scleroderma with renal involvement imparts high risks for the mother and the fetus largely because of the hypertension that worsens markedly. Maternal mortality from rapidly progressive renal failure is high and fetal prognosis is dismal. It is better to terminate the pregnancy in such patients.

SLE commonly affects women of childbearing age. Historically, there were concerns that pregnancy induced exacerbations of SLE. Modern studies have not generally borne out historic fears of extremely high fetal wastage. Clinical exacerbations or relapses occur in between 9% and 60% of pregnancies. However, the rate of disease exacerbations is not different in concurrent nonpregnant control groups. The major factor determining whether pregnancy results in an exacerbation of lupus is the stability of the disease before the pregnancy. Thus when SLE is in remission or well controlled for a period of more than 6 months, the chance of a clinical flare during pregnancy is low. On the other hand, when pregnancy occurs in close temporal association with an exacerbation of SLE, exacerbations are also frequently seen during or shortly after pregnancy.

Fetal survival is also closely related to the clinical status of SLE before conception. In a prospective study of planned pregnancy in women with inactive SLE, the live birth rate was 96%. Nevertheless, prematurity was common. In another report, fetal survival rate was only 64% when SLE was active at the beginning of pregnancy. The presence of anti–cardiolipin antibodies is certainly related to an increased likelihood of spontaneous abortion and may be associated with certain types of congenital heart disease such as heart block and endocardial fibroelastosis. However, it is controversial whether fetal outcome beyond the first trimester is adversely affected by the presence of antiphospholipid antibody.

As is true for all women with renal disease, hypertension may worsen during pregnancy. Similarly, proteinuria increases in half of pregnancies complicated by SLE, but this increase is rarely irreversible. An irreversible deterioration in renal function was observed in fewer than 10% of pregnancies occurring in women whose SLE was not active at conception. Exacerbation of SLE may occur after delivery and some authors advocate the administration of glucocorticoids a few days before delivery. The consensus is that pregnancy should not be prohibited in patients with SLE but the patient should be monitored carefully for the clinical course, renal function, and blood pressure during gestation and puerperium; if exacerbation occurs, the patient should be managed appropriately.

Treatment of Renal Failure in Pregnancy

Dialysis. As previously noted, although some women on chronic dialysis do become pregnant, it is more common for women to develop end-stage renal disease during pregnancy and to then require dialytic therapy. No firm recommendations regarding dialysis regimens can be made but some general guidelines are possible (Table 58.12). A study from Belgium suggested a positive correlation between hemodialysis dose and birth weight. Outcomes do not appear to be remarkably different between hemodialysis and peritoneal dialysis. In general, outcomes have improved since the institution of erythropoietin to treat anemia. Prematurity and low birth weight always occur. A successful outcome to pregnancy occurs in approximately 40% to 50% of pregnancies occurring in chronic dialysis patients and in 74% to 80% of women who develop end-stage renal disease during pregnancy. The timing of initiation of dialysis in women with severe renal insufficiency during pregnancy is unknown. Although some clinicians begin dialysis therapy before the GFR falls below 10 ml/min, there have also been successful case reports of pregnancy in women with advanced renal failure treated conservatively.

TABLE 58.12. Management of Pregnancy in End-Stage Renal Disease Patients

Avoid pregnancy in dialysis patients, if possible.
Continue antihypertensive agents and erythropoietin as needed.
Maximize dialysis adequacy.
Refer all patients to obstetrician with expertise in high-risk pregnancies.
When possible, plan pregnancies to occur after renal transplantation (with stable function for 1 to 2 years).

Transplantation. The experience of pregnancy in transplant recipients is dramatically different from that in hemodialysis patients (Table 58.13). Pregnancies are successful in more than 90% of kidney transplant recipients. Renal function increases in transplanted kidneys in a manner similar to that in native kidneys. Acute rejection is no more frequent in pregnant than in nonpregnant women. Hypertension or preeclampsia is more common in transplant recipients complicating approximately 30% of pregnancies. Preterm delivery is also frequent in transplant recipients, occurring in 45% to 60% of cases. Results with the use of cyclosporine are similar to those experienced in the precyclosporine era. One exception is that women treated with cyclosporine tend to have slightly smaller infants than those treated without cyclosporine. In addition, cyclosporine levels often decline during pregnancy and require closer monitoring.

Pregnancy does not appear to adversely affect the long-term survival of renal allografts. Because the outcomes of pregnancy in transplantation are so different than those in chronic dialysis, unless maternal age is an overwhelming factor, it is advisable to treat end-stage renal disease patients with transplantation and wait until renal function has been stable for 1 to 2 years before undertaking a planned pregnancy. Such planning affords the mother and fetus the best chance of favorable outcomes.

TABLE 58.13. Consequences of Pregnancy in Renal Transplant Recipients

Prematurity (45%–60%)
Small for gestational age infants (20%–30%)
Superimposed preeclampsia (30%)
No increased risk of acute rejection
No increased risk of loss of graft function

Selected Readings

ACOG Technical Bulletin. Hypertension in pregnancy. *Int J Gynecol Obstet* 1996;53:175.

A succinct, easy-to-read review of pregnancy-induced hypertension detailing epidemiology, findings, and therapy.

Armenti VT, Ahlswede KM, Ahlswede AB, et al. National transplantation pregnancy registry—outcomes of 154 pregnancies in cyclosporine-treated female kidney transplant recipients. *Transplantation* 1994;57:502.

A report of current experience of pregnancy in cyclosporine-treated renal transplant recipients. This is a registry report and, unfortunately, not the result of a prospective study. The overall findings are that cyclosporine appears to be reasonably safe for use in this setting.

Bagon JA, Vernaeve H, deMuylder X, et al. Pregnancy and dialysis. *Am J Kidney Dis* 1998;31:756.

A very recent review of pregnancy (15 cases) in 1,472 women of childbearing age receiving chronic hemodialysis from Europe. This article discusses the authors' practice to use erythropoietin and increase dialysis dose when pregnancy occurs in dialysis patients.

Butters L, Kennedy S, Rubin PC. Atenolol in essential hypertension during pregnancy. *Br Med J* 1990;301:587.

An important report suggesting an adverse effect of β-blockers when used to treat chronic hypertension in the first trimester, as opposed to beneficial effects when employed to treat pregnancy-induced hypertension in the second or third trimester.

Davison JM. Dialysis, transplantation, and pregnancy. *Am J Kidney Dis* 1991;17:127.

A discussion of the consequences of pregnancy on renal transplant function and survival in women becoming pregnant after transplantation.

Hou SH, Grossman SD, Madias NE. Pregnancy in women with renal disease and moderate renal insufficiency. *Am J Med* 1985;78:185.

One of the first careful studies to evaluate the effects of pregnancy on the course of renal disease in women with moderate renal insufficiency. When prepartum creatinine was greater than 1.4 mg/dl, there was an almost 30% chance of permanent deterioration in renal function greater than expected from the natural history of the disease.

Jones DC, Hayslett JP. Outcome of pregnancy in women with moderate or several renal insufficiency. *N Engl J Med* 1996;335:226.

A recent version of the same population studied by Hou et al. Findings were also similar. Forty-three percent of women with a creatinine greater than 1.4 mg/dl suffered a decline in renal function related to pregnancy. In 10% of pregnancies, the decline in renal function was rapid.

Morbidity and Mortality Weekly Report. Post-marketing surveillance for angiotensin-converting enzyme inhibitor use during the first trimester of pregnancy—United States, Canada, and Israel, 1987-1995. *MMWR Morb Mortal Wkly Rep* 1997;46:240–242.

A review of several databases suggesting a lack of obvious long-term fetal toxicity in women exposed to ACE inhibitors in the first trimester (and subsequently stopping the medication before the second half of pregnancy). This experience contrasts with the known fetal toxicity when the drug is administered later in pregnancy.

National High Blood Pressure Education Program Working Group report on high blood pressure in pregnancy. *Am J Obstet Gynecol* 1990;163:1691–1712.

A consensus report produced by obstetricians and internists defining hypertensive disorders of pregnancy, reviewing pathophysiology, and setting guidelines for therapy. A complete and very helpful document.

Okundaye I, Abrinko P, Hou S. Registry of pregnancy in dialysis patients. *Am J Kidney Dis* 1998;31:766.

The recent U.S. experience of pregnancy occurring in chronic dialysis patients based on self-reporting by dialysis units. Over a 2-year period, pregnancy occurred in 2% of women of childbearing age. Maternal and fetal complications are summarized.

Packham DK, North RA, Fairley KF, et al. Primary glomerulonephritis and pregnancy. *Q J Med* 1989;71:537.

A thorough review of the consequences of pregnancy in women with glomerulonephritis. Hypertension complicated 52% of 395 pregnancies, with 7% worsening despite continuation of antihypertensive therapy throughout pregnancy. Different outcomes depending on specific type of glomerulonephritis is also discussed.

Phippard AF, Fischer WE, Horvath JS, et al. Early blood pressure control improves pregnancy outcome in primigravida women with mild hypertension. *Med J Aust* 1991;154:378.

A carefully performed placebo-controlled trial of antihypertensive therapy in the early third trimester in women with mild hypertension. Fetal morbidity was significantly reduced by antihypertensive therapy.

Redman CWG, Beilin LJ, Bonnar J, et al. Fetal outcome in trial of antihypertensive treatment in pregnancy. *Lancet* 1976;ii:753–756.

One of the first prospective, placebo-controlled trials to demonstrate a benefit of early treatment of hypertension complicating pregnancy. Methyldopa was begun in women before 28 weeks gestation when blood pressure exceeded 140/90 mm Hg. Fetal loss was reduced by antihypertensive therapy.

Remuzzi G, Ruggenenti P. Prevention and treatment of pregnancy-associated hypertension: what have we learned in the last 10 years? *Am J Kidney Dis* 1991;18:285–305.

A nephrologic viewpoint of hypertension in pregnancy. These authors, who have a strong interest in systemic disorders of endothelial dysfunction such as thrombotic thrombocytopenic purpura and hemolytic uremic syndrome, focus on that aspect of pathophysiology in preeclampsia. Therapy is also carefully reviewed.

Sibai BM. Treatment of hypertension in pregnant women. *N Engl J Med* 1996;335:257.

A single author review of the most important published papers testing the effects of treatment of hypertension in pregnancy. Chronic hypertension and pregnancy-induced hypertension are appropriately treated separately, as are mild and severe hypertension, a more arbitrary distinction.

Zhou Y, Damsky CH, Fisher SJ. Preeclampsia is associated with failure of human cytotrophoblasts to mimic a vascular adhesion phenotype. One cause of defective endovascular invasion in this syndrome? *J Clin Invest* 1997;99:2152.

Recent highly compelling studies to determine the pathophysiology of preeclampsia. This paper and several related ones by the same scientists provide support for the hypothesis that endothelial cell dysfunction is the fundamental cause of preeclampsia.

SECTION VII

Hypertension

CHAPTER 59

Pathophysiology of Essential Hypertension

Vito M. Campese

Blood pressure is regulated by neurogenic, hormonal, nutritional, biochemical, and structural mechanisms. Alterations of any of these mechanisms may result in elevation of blood pressure.

The development of essential hypertension is thought to depend on the interrelation between multiple genes (polygenic trait) and environmental factors. The genetic factors responsible for essential hypertension are largely unknown. Relatively few linkage studies examining the potential role of "candidate genes" in hypertensive patients have been reported. This issue is discussed in Chapter 60. In addition, in its initial phase, hypertension may be sustained by mechanisms other than those responsible for its long-term maintenance. Functional or structural abnormalities may occur during the life of an individual patient that may alter the course of the disease. Obesity, hypokalemia, and hypomagnesemia represent examples of functional factors that may alter the pathogenetic profile of hypertension. Development of an atherosclerotic plaque in one renal artery and development of renal insufficiency are examples of structural abnormalities that can complicate the pathogenetic profile of hypertension.

Because of the complexity of these interrelations, the mechanism(s) responsible for the development and maintenance of essential hypertension remains elusive despite intensive and relentless efforts. This chapter reviews the mechanisms involved in normal blood pressure regulations and the known aberrations of these regulatory mechanisms that have been implicated in the pathophysiology of essential hypertension.

REGULATION OF BLOOD PRESSURE

Blood pressure depends on the blood volume and peripheral vascular resistance. The regulation of peripheral vascular resistance depends on neurogenic, hormonal, nutritional, structural, and biochemical factors. The regulation of circulating volume depends on kidney function. However, kidney function and sodium retention can be affected by the same neurogenic, hormonal, nutritional, biochemical, and structural factors responsible for the regulation of peripheral vascular resistance.

The Kidney and Sodium–Blood Volume State

One of the most important function of the kidneys is to maintain relatively constant extracellular fluid volume and composition, even in the face of wide variations in daily fluid and electrolyte intake and excretion. The composition of body sodium and blood volume are important regulators of blood pressure homeostasis. Sodium and volume depletion tend to decrease blood pressure. On the contrary, sodium retention and volume expansion tend to increase blood pressure. A rise in blood pressure, in turn, tends to increase sodium excretion (pressure natriuresis). This ultimately results in volume depletion and normalization of blood pressure, unless adaptive renal mechanisms ensue. Thus any long-term rise in blood pressure, whether sodium-volume dependent or caused by a rise in systemic vascular resistance, must be accompanied by a rightward shift (toward higher levels of blood pressure) of the pressure natriuresis relationship.

Guyton was the first to suggest a primacy of the kidney in the genesis or in the maintenance of hypertension and that hypertension may be necessary to maintain a normal sodium balance in the presence of a reduced ability of the kidney to excrete a salt load. One postulate to explain the genesis of hypertension is that humans ingest sodium in excess of the amount that their kidneys are capable of excreting. Hypertension becomes a necessary adjustment to maintain a relatively normal sodium and blood volume balance and to prevent volume expansion. To validate this concept, one must be able to demonstrate that abnormalities in renal function precede the development of hypertension and that a relationship is present between dietary salt (NaCl) intake and blood pressure in the hypertensive population. Despite extensive epidemiologic and interventional studies, controversy still remains regarding the pathophysiologic role of dietary NaCl intake in essential hypertension.

The Concept of Salt Sensitivity

It is now apparent that NaCl raises blood pressure only in some patients with essential hypertension. Based on their blood pressure response to an NaCl load, patients with essential hypertension are classified as salt sensitive or as salt resistant. We have classified as salt sensitive those patients who manifest a rise in blood pressure of at least 10 mm Hg during a 200 mEq/day sodium (Na^+) diet for 1 week, compared with a diet of 10 to 20 mEq of Na^+ per day, and have found approximately 50% of patients with essential hypertension to be salt sensitive.

The prevalence of salt sensitivity appears to be greater in African-Americans and in older patients than in whites or in younger hypertensive patients, and it appears also to be more frequent among obese patients or those with concomitant diabetes mellitus.

The mechanisms for salt sensitivity are complex. One hypothesis proposed to explain salt sensitivity postulates the existence of an inherited reduced ability of the kidneys to excrete a sodium load. This notion is supported by the frequent finding that salt-sensitive patients retain more sodium when exposed to a high dietary NaCl intake. Most studies, however, have failed to show a significant relationship between the amount of sodium lost during depletion or retained during NaCl loading and changes in arterial pressure.

Sequential hemodynamic characterization of patients with essential hypertension has shown that sodium retention results in volume expansion and increased cardiac output without any concomitant change in peripheral resistance, and this results in hypertension. Subsequently, peripheral vascular resistance progressively rises, so that the chronic elevation of NaCl-induced hypertension is dependent on an increase in peripheral vascular resistance rather than in cardiac output (Fig. 59.1). This notion is supported by studies showing that cross-transplantation of a kidney from a young prehypertensive rat into a normotensive rat results in chronic elevation of blood pressure in the latter animal, whereas transplantation of a kidney from a young normotensive rat into a hypertensive animal results in normalization of blood pressure. Transplantation of a kidney from normotensive donors into patients with severe hypertension and end-stage renal disease (ESRD) caused by nephrosclerosis also can result in complete normalization of blood pressure. In addition, there is evidence both in hypertensive strains of rats and in human subjects that a resetting of kidney function occurs very early or may even precede the development of hypertension because renal hemodynamic abnormalities can be observed in normotensive offspring of hypertensive patients. Subjects with positive family history of hypertension exhibit a blunted natriuretic response and an exaggerated blood pressure response to an acute saline load when compared with subjects with negative family history of hypertension. Renal vascular resistance was shown to be greater during both a low and a high NaCl intake and during an acute intravenous saline load in sons of two hypertensive parents compared with sons of two normotensive parents, suggesting that alterations of renal hemodynamics may represent an inherited abnormality that may be involved in the development of hypertension. Studies in identical twins have shown that the trait of salt sensitivity has a strong inheritance. To investigate the influence of heredity on blood pressure and the renal excretion of sodium following volume expansion and contraction in humans, Grim studied 37 pairs of homozygotic and 18 pairs of dizygotic twins under conditions of acute volume expansion or contraction; he observed that urinary sodium excretion, fractional excretion of sodium, and blood pressure response revealed evidence of significant genetic influence. In another study, salt-sensitive patients showed a 2.5-fold higher incidence of a positive family history of hypertension than salt-resistant patients.

To explain the greater prevalence of salt sensitivity and hypertension among African-Americans, some have proposed that African-Americans evolved in a tropical or subtropical environment where dietary NaCl intake was low and salt and water depletion caused by sweating, vomiting, and diarrhea was very common. In this environment, selective pressures favored survival of those who carried the sodium-retaining genotype. During the slave trade, African-Americans were suddenly exposed to an environment rich in sodium. In addition, the adverse conditions of slavery may have favored survival and selection of those with an enhanced ability to conserve sodium, and descendants of these individuals are at greater risk for salt-sensitive hypertension.

The slope of the renal function (pressure natriuresis) curve is significantly flatter in salt-sensitive than in salt-resistant patients (Fig. 59.2), suggesting a disturbance in renal-tubular sodium reabsorption. There are other substantial differences in renal hemodynamic adaptation to a high dietary sodium intake between salt-sensitive and salt-resistant patients. Glomerular filtration rate (GFR), does not change and renal vascular resistance decrease during high compared with low dietary NaCl intake in salt-resistant patients. In salt-sensitive patients, on the other hand, there are significant renal hemodynamic changes during high compared with low dietary sodium intake. GFR does not change, renal vascular resistance increases, RBF decreases, and filtration fraction increases, suggesting a parallel rise in intraglomerular pressure. Calculations of glomerular capillary pressure by the Gomez formulae revealed a decrease in response to high NaCl intake in salt-resistant patients but an increase in salt-sensitive patients (Fig. 59.3). Although results obtained with these formulae must be regarded as approximations and interpreted with caution, it is of interest that they substantiate the differences in filtration fraction that we have observed in salt-sensitive and salt-resistant patients in response to a high dietary sodium intake.

Measurements of renal hemodynamics in a group of patients with essential hypertension and normal plasma renin activity (PRA) showed that with changes in dietary NaCl intake some of those patients failed to modulate their RBF and aldosterone response to angiotensin II. In these patients, called *nonmodulators,* RBF failed to increase in response to high NaCl intake, whereas in normal subjects and in hypertensive

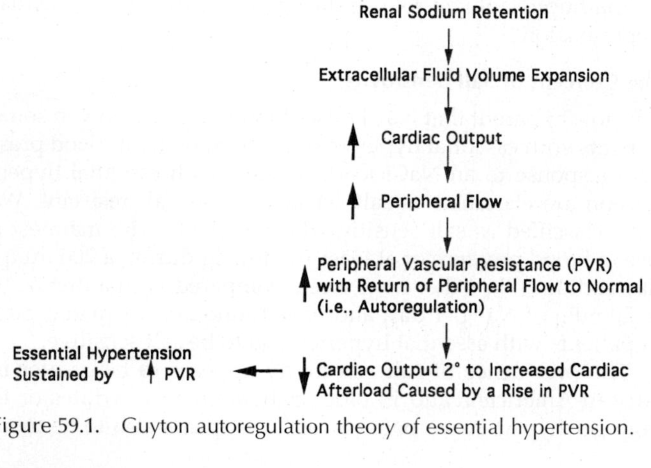

Figure 59.1. Guyton autoregulation theory of essential hypertension.

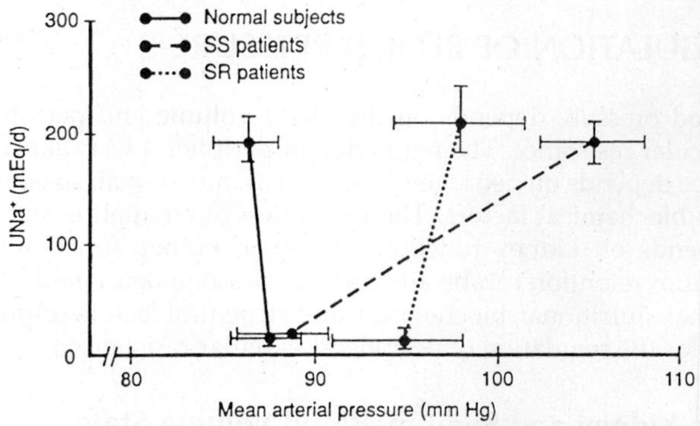

Figure 59.2. Plot showing the renal function (pressure natriuresis) relationship in normal subjects and in salt-sensitive *(SS)* and salt-resistant *(SR)* patients with essential hypertension.

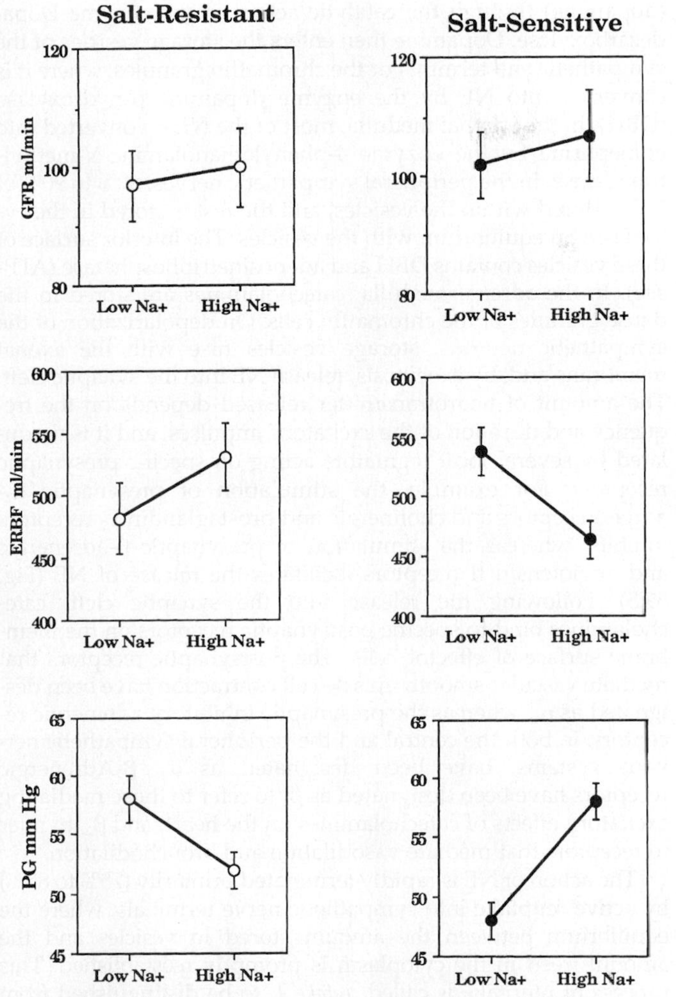

Figure 59.3. Glomerular filtration rate *(GFR)* in ml/min/1.73 m², effective renal blood flow *(ERBF)* in ml/min/1.73 m², and calculated glomerular capillary pressure *(PG)* in mm Hg in salt-resistant and in salt-sensitive patients with essential hypertension during a low (20 mEq/day) and a high (200 mEq/day) dietary sodium (Na^+) intake.

patients with normal renal vascular and adrenal modulation, RBF increased by at least 120 ml/min/1.73 m². Nonmodulators also manifested a derangement in the capacity to handle sodium, along with an increase in blood pressure, during high NaCl intake.

Studies in African-American patients, who are more commonly salt sensitive, have shown a difference in blood volume or cardiac output compared with whites, but African-Americans had significantly lower RBF and higher renal vascular resistance than whites.

Evidence from very young, spontaneously hypertensive rats (SHR) indicates that alteration of the pressure natriuretic relationship is associated with inhibition of tubular reabsorption of sodium in deep nephrons and with changes in renal medullary vascular resistance, blood flow, and renal interstitial pressure. The changes in renal medullary hemodynamics may participate in resetting the pressure natriuretis relationship in this genetic model of hypertension. On the other hand, the relationship between papillary blood flow and renal perfusion pressure appears to be similar in prehypertensive Dahl S and Dahl R rats of the Rapp strain, suggesting that the abnormal pressure natriuretis relationship in this strain of rats occurs independently of alterations in renal medullary hemodynamics and perhaps are caused by a primary alteration of renal-tubular sodium reabsorption. Because nitric oxide (NO)–induced formation of cyclic guanosine monophosphate (cGMP) appears to be a major factor linking changes in renal medullary blood flow with sodium excretion, some have proposed that salt-sensitive essential hypertension may be the result of deficient production of NO by endothelial cells.

The Tubuloglomerular Feedback Mechanism

The delivery of Cl^- to the macula densa regulates the tone of renal afferent arterioles, renal perfusion, and GFR. Volume expansion following a saline load will increase Cl^- delivery to the juxtaglomerular apparatus resulting in inhibition of the tubuloglomerular feedback (TGF). This results in increased GFR and sodium excretion. Some have proposed that a reduced sensitivity of the TGF could be responsible for sodium retention and for salt-related hypertension.

The Sympathoadrenal System

Physiology

The sympathoadrenal system comprises a central (brain) and a peripheral component. The role of the brain in the control of the cardiovascular system has been recognized since the seventeenth century. However, many questions still remain regarding the structure, function, and neurotransmitters involved in integrative areas of the central nervous system (CNS) that regulate blood pressure. Not until the early 1980s was the nucleus tractus solitaries (NTS) in the brainstem identified as a major integrating center. The NTS receives afferent input from sensory receptors in the cardiovascular system, skeletal muscle, skin, kidney, various cranial nerves, hypothalamic nuclei, the A2 group of neurons, the locus coeruleus, and, most importantly, the afferent baroreceptor neurons. The NTS projects efferent neurons to higher centers in the forebrain and to the intermediolateral cell column in the spinal cord, which is considered the origin of the sympathetic efferent neurons. The connecting center between these two structures was called the *vasomotor center* but was not clearly identified nor localized to any specific area of the brainstem. It was established that the rostral part of the ventral medulla (RVM) is the pressor region from which bulbospinal sympathetic neurons descend to the intermediolateral cell column. The caudal ventrolateral medulla (CVLM), on the other hand, is a depressor region that modulates the activity of the RVM.

It is now believed that baroreceptor afferent neurons synapse into second-order neurons in the NTS. The second order of neurons projects to the CVLM, where they synapse with inhibitory neurons that, in turn, project to the RVM, where they synapse with bulbospinal excitatory neurons (Fig. 59.4). The area postrema, which lies immediately dorsal to the NTS, also receives baroreceptor information, and its ablation causes a sustained decrease in blood pressure in all mammals except the rat. Several other hypothalamic nuclei may play an important role in regulation of the cardiovascular system. In the rat, the area postrema is substituted by a region in the anterior hypothalamus, labeled the *anteroventral third ventricle (AV3V)*. Lesions in this region prevent or attenuate hypertension in several experimental models. The lateral and posterior hypothalamic nuclei have been identified as pressor regions, whereas the anterior hypothalamic area has been identified as a depressor region. The paraventricular and supraoptic nuclei of the hypothalamus release vasopressin and oxytocin into the portal blood and the cardiovascular nuclei of the brainstem and may participate in the pathogenesis of hypertension in the SHR.

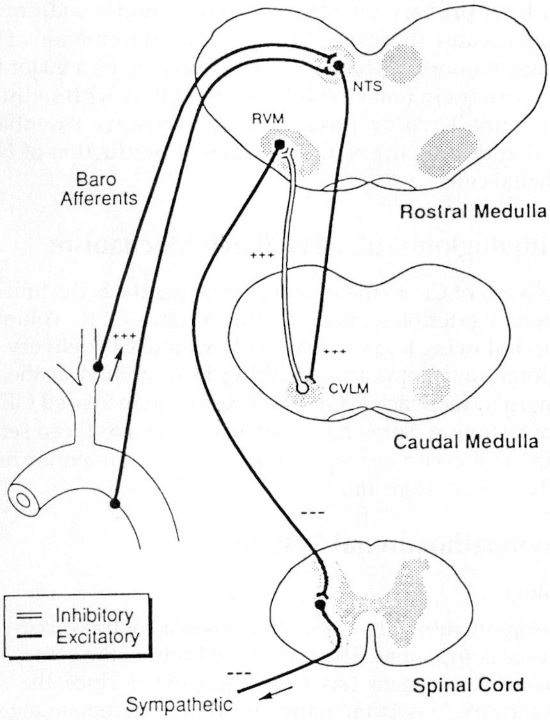

Figure 59.4. Schematic representation of neurons involved in the baroreceptor sympathetic reflex. Baroreceptor afferent neurons establish synapses with neurons in the nucleus tractus solitarius *(NTS)*. Neurons from the NTS project to the caudal ventrolateral medulla *(CVLM)*, where they synapse with inhibitory neurons that, in turn, project to the rostral ventrolateral medulla and synapse with bulbospinal sympathetic excitatory neurons located in the rostral ventral medulla *(RVM)*. The + and − signs indicate changes in the activity of the neurons following an acute increase in arterial blood pressure. Black neurons are excitatory, and white neurons are inhibitory. (Reproduced with permission from Chalmers J, Pilowsky P. Brainstem and bulbospinal neurotransmitter systems in the control of blood pressure. *J Hypertens* 1991;9:675–694.)

The peripheral component of the sympathetic nervous system is composed of the thoracolumbar system, with cell bodies of the preganglionic myelinated fibers arising in the intermediolateral gray portion of the spinal cord and being distributed to the sympathetic ganglia and to the adrenal medulla via the anterior roots of the spinal nerves.

The major known neurotransmitters of the sympathetic nervous system are norepinephrine (NE), epinephrine, and dopamine. NE is the main neurotransmitter of the sympathetic nerves and acts locally on effector cells in almost every organ in the body where it activates specific receptors. Epinephrine is synthesized mainly in the adrenal medulla and is released in the circulation to act as a hormone on distant target organs. Dopamine is a precursor of NE and an important neurotransmitter in the CNS, particularly in the corpus striatum, basal ganglia, and substantia nigra, areas of the brain involved in the coordination of motor activity.

The biosynthesis of these amines occurs in the CNS in the postganglionic sympathetic fibers, and in the chromaffin cells of the adrenal medulla. The amino acid precursor of these amines is L-tyrosine, which is taken up by the axonal membranes or by the chromaffin cells and converted to L-dihydroxyphenylalanine (L-Dopa) by the enzyme thyroxin hydroxylase. The activity of the enzyme is believed to be the rate-limiting step in the biosynthesis of catecholamines and is directly influenced by the concentration of catecholamines in the axoplasm. L-Dopa is subsequently converted to 3,4-dihydroxyphenylethylamine (dopamine) through the catalytic action of the enzyme Dopa-decarboxylase. Dopamine then enters the storage vesicles of the sympathetic end terminal or the chromaffin granules, where it is converted into NE by the enzyme dopamine β-hydroxylase (DBH). In the adrenal medulla, most of the NE is converted into epinephrine by the enzyme 4-phenylethanolamine-*N*-methyltransferase. In the peripheral sympathetic nerves, 80% to 90% of NE is stored within the vesicles, and the rest is stored in the cytoplasm, in equilibrium with the vesicles. The interior surface of these vesicles contains DBH and adenosinetriphosphatase (ATPase). In the adrenal medulla, catecholamines are stored in the dense granules of the chromaffin cells. On depolarization of the sympathetic neurons, storage vesicles fuse with the axonal membrane and, by exocytosis, release NE into the synaptic cleft. The amount of neurotransmitter released depends on the frequency and duration of the excitatory impulses, and it is modulated by several local regulators acting on specific presynaptic receptors. For example, the stimulation of presynaptic α_2-adrenoreceptors and cholinergic and prostaglandin E_2 receptors inhibits, whereas the stimulation of presynaptic β-adrenergic and angiotensin II receptors facilitates the release of NE (Fig. 59.5). Following the release into the synaptic cleft, catecholamines bind to specific postsynaptic receptors on the membrane surface of effector cells. The postsynaptic receptors that mediate vascular smooth muscle cell contraction have been designated as α_1, whereas the presynaptic inhibitory adrenergic receptors, in both the central and the peripheral sympathetic nervous systems, have been designated as α_2. β-Adrenergic receptors have been designated as β_1 to refer to those mediating excitatory effects of catecholamines on the heart, and β_2, to refer to receptors that mediate vasodilation and bronchodilation.

The action of NE is rapidly terminated primarily (75% to 80%) by active reuptake into sympathetic nerve terminals, where the equilibrium between the amount stored in vesicles and the amount freed in the cytoplasm is promptly reestablished. This process of reuptake is called *uptake 1*, to be distinguished from *uptake 2*, which occurs in extraneural peripheral tissues, such as cardiac muscle cells, vascular smooth muscle cells, collagen, elastin, and certain glandular tissues. Uptake 1 has higher affinity for NE, whereas uptake 2 has higher affinity for epinephrine. The uptake of catecholamines in extraneuronal sites is rapidly

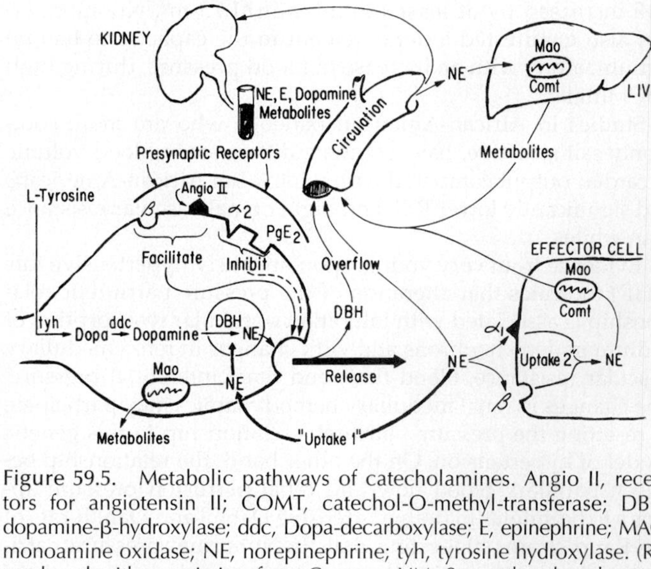

Figure 59.5. Metabolic pathways of catecholamines. Angio II, receptors for angiotensin II; COMT, catechol-O-methyl-transferase; DBH, dopamine-β-hydroxylase; ddc, Dopa-decarboxylase; E, epinephrine; MAO, monoamine oxidase; NE, norepinephrine; tyh, tyrosine hydroxylase. (Reproduced with permission from Campese VM. Sympathoadrenal system and the kidney in hypertension. *Am J Nephrol* 1983;3:128–138.)

followed by intracellular catabolism by the enzymes monamine oxidase and catechol-O-methyltransferase and not by storage.

A small fraction of the catecholamines released from the sympathetic nerve terminals overflows into the circulation. This, in conjunction with the catecholamines released from the adrenal medulla, constitutes the measurable pool in the plasma. The amount of NE that overflows into the circulation depends not only on the rate of release from the sympathetic nerve terminals but also on the density, distribution, and width of the neuroeffector junctions. Circulating catecholamines are metabolized mainly in the liver by the enzymes monoamine oxidase and catechol-O-methyltransferase. The half-life of intravenously infused NE is about 2 minutes. In the normal human, approximately 29% of total plasma NE and epinephrine and less than 1% of total dopamine are free in the blood, the rest being predominantly sulfoconjugated by the enzyme phenolsulfotransferase.

The main metabolites of NE and epinephrine detectable in the urine are vanillylmandelic acid (VMA) and 4-hydroxy-3-methoxyphenylglycol (MHPG). Normetanephrine and metanephrine are excreted in the urine in smaller amounts, but they reflect more closely the amount of NE and epinephrine released by the peripheral sympathetic nerves. The main metabolites of dopamine found in the urine are homovanillic acid (HVA) and methoxytyramine. Only small quantities of catecholamines appear intact in the urine: 1% to 5% of NE and approximately 1% of epinephrine.

Environmental, emotional, nutritional, or pathologic factors can alter the activity of the sympathetic nervous system and the plasma concentrations of these amines. The plasma concentration of NE increases with age in normal subjects but not in patients with essential hypertension. Upright posture also increases the activity of the sympathetic nervous system and plasma levels of NE. Plasma NE levels undergo significant diurnal variations. They reach the lowest levels between 4 and 6 a.m., increase abruptly before awakening, and reach peak concentrations at approximately 9 a.m. These diurnal variations of plasma NE levels correlate with diurnal variations of blood pressure. Caloric intake and obesity are associated with increased levels of NE in the plasma that are reversible with fasting or loss of body weight. Caffeine consumption, smoking, cold, pain, anxiety, anger, ovulation, hypoglycemia, hypercapnia, burns, immobilization, social isolation, hemorrhage, hypotension, diabetic ketoacidosis, surgical and traumatic stress, anesthesia, myocardial infarction, iron deficiency, neural crest tumors, and quadriplegia are some of the conditions that can increase plasma NE levels. Finally, a large number of drugs such as diuretics, vasodilators, and β-blockers, can increase plasma NE levels. All the factors that can affect plasma NE levels need to be taken into account when evaluating plasma NE levels in physiologic and pathologic conditions.

The Sympathetic Nervous System Activity and the Kidney

The kidneys have an extensive adrenergic, dopaminergic, and cholinergic innervation. Sympathetic nerve fibers have been shown in direct contact with the juxtaglomerular apparatus and the basement membranes of proximal and distal renal tubules in various mammalian species. α-Receptors, β-receptors, and dopaminergic receptors have been described in the renal vasculature. Infusion of NE into the renal artery increases renal vascular resistance and decreases RBF, whereas infusion of isoproterenol increases RBF. There is considerable evidence that dopamine has potent natriuretic and vasoactive properties. In normal subjects, low dosages of dopamine increase RBF and the urinary excretion of prostacyclin and sodium. An acute volume expansion stimulates dopamine release, and the natriuresis associated with acute volume expansion can be attenuated by dopamine receptor antagonists. These studies have led to the commonly held notion that renal dopamine participates in the homeostatic regulation of sodium balance. Thus a decrease in renal dopamine production could decrease both RBF and urinary sodium excretion. Locally produced dopamine causes a reversible and dose-dependent inhibition of Na^+ -K^+-ATPase activity in rat proximal tubule segments, and this inhibitory effect is enhanced by high NaCl diet.

An increase in renal sympathetic nerve activity inhibits renal sodium excretion, and this action can result from a decrease in RBF, redistribution of blood from the superficial cortex to the juxtaglomerular cortex and outer medulla, activation of the renin-angiotensin system, or a direct action on the renal tubules. Low-level activation of renal sympathetic outflow may alter renal function and significantly alter the normal relationship between arterial pressure and natriuresis and diuresis without significant alterations of RBF or GFR.

The renal sympathetic nerves appear to be under the control of integrative areas in the CNS. Stimulation of the hypothalamus or midbrain produces an increase in renal sympathetic nerve activity and renal vasoconstriction. Stimulation of the parabrachial region of the dorsal rostral pons or of certain areas of the hypothalamus selectively activates the renal sympathetic nerves without any effect on sympathetic efferent inputs to other organs. Efferent stimuli from the CNS to the kidney may be important in the maintenance of blood pressure because they may inhibit sodium excretion. Detailed discussion of renal nerves and their role in modulating renal function is found in Chapter 5.

Afferent Renal Sympathetic Activity and Blood Pressure Regulation

The kidney is richly innervated with baroreceptors and with chemoreceptors and renal afferent nerves that project directly or indirectly to a number of areas in the CNS that contribute to blood pressure regulation. Stimulation of renal receptors by adenosine, urea, or electrical impulses evokes reflex increases in sympathetic nerve activity and blood pressure. Renal afferent impulses play an important role in the genesis of hypertension in one kidney–one clip and two kidney–one clip Goldblatt hypertension in rats, but not in the deoxycorticosterone acetate-salt (DOCA-salt) hypertension in rats; in the one kidney–one wrap Grollman hypertension in the rat; or in the SHR.

Renal afferent impulses may also play a role in the pathogenesis of hypertension in rats with experimentally induced chronic renal failure. In these animals, bilateral dorsal rhizotomy, at the level T-10 to L-3, completely prevented the increase in blood pressure. This suggests that increased renal sensory inputs from the injured kidney to the CNS may contribute to the development of hypertension and to the progression of renal disease in CRF rats. The decrease in arterial pressure in patients with bilateral nephrectomy is associated with lower sympathetic nerve firing and regional vascular resistance. These findings support the notion that increased afferent nervous inputs from kidneys with renal diseases may send signals to integrative sympathetic nuclei in the CNS and contribute to the pathogenesis of hypertension. The normalization of blood pressure that follows bilateral nephrectomy may be largely due to elimination of these afferent impulses.

A renal injury caused by the injection of phenol in the kidney raises blood pressure and the secretion of NE from the posterior hypothalamic nuclei. Renal denervation prevents the increase in blood pressure and in NE secretion from the hypothalamus caused by the intrarenal injection of phenol (Fig. 59.6). The effects of the phenol-induced renal injury on blood pressure are long lasting and can be reverted by ablation of the injured

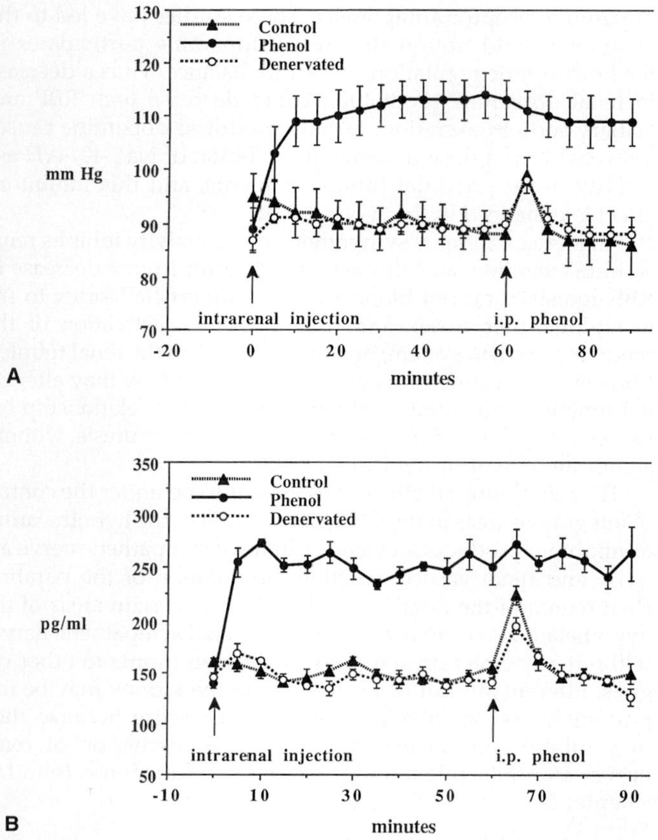

Figure 59.6. **A:** The line graphs show levels of mean arterial pressure in Sprague-Dawley rats who received 50 μL of 10% phenol in the lower pole of the right kidney *(closed circles),* those who received only the vehicle *(closed triangles),* and those with renal denervation. After 60 minutes of observation, all rats received an intraperitoneal injection of 50 μL of 10% phenol. Each group comprised 6 rats. Values are expressed as means ± SEM. **B:** The line graphs show levels of norepinephrine in Sprague-Dawley rats who received 50 μL of 10% phenol in the lower pole of the right kidney *(closed circles),* those who received only the vehicle *(closed triangles)* and those with renal denervation. After 60 minutes of observation, all rats received an intraperitoneal injection of 50 μL of 10% phenol. Values are expressed as means ± SEM. (Reproduced with permission from Ye S, Ozgur B, Campese VM. Renal afferent impulses, the posterior hypothalamus, and hypertension in rats with chronic renal failure. *Kidney Int* 1997;51:722–727.)

kidney. These studies have demonstrated that a limited injury to one kidney may activate renal afferent pathways and cause a permanent elevation of blood pressure mediated by increased sympathetic nervous system activity.

Mechanisms Through Which Abnormalities in Sympathetic Nervous System Activity Cause Hypertension

Disturbances of the neurogenic control of the circulation may be responsible for the development of hypertension. Alterations of the sympathetic nervous system leading to hypertension may involve the arterial baroreceptors or other afferent pathways to the CNS, central integrative structures in the CNS, efferent sympathetic pathways, or effector cells.

Arterial Baroreceptors. Higher threshold and reduced sensitivity of arterial baroreceptors have been observed in experimental animals as well as in human subjects with hypertension. The decreased sensitivity of arterial baroreceptors could increase peripheral sympathetic nerve activity and cause hypertension. A significant resetting of baroreceptors has been demonstrated in the early stages of hypertension, suggesting that it might be causative. However, the resetting of the baroreceptors may be a consequence of hypertension, because it occurs within hours after the rise in blood pressure.

High NaCl diet sensitizes cardiopulmonary baroreceptor reflexes in salt-resistant but not in salt-sensitive hypertensive patients, suggesting that the lack of compensatory augmentation in cardiopulmonary baroreceptor reflex function may contribute to salt sensitivity. Similarly, high NaCl diet sensitized the cardiopulmonary baroreceptor reflex modulation of sympathetic nerve activity in Dahl R but not in Dahl S rats.

The Central Nervous System. Central noradrenergic neurons are involved in the pathogenesis of hypertension. Intracerebroventricular administration of a neurotoxin, 6-hydroxydopamine, prevents the development of hypertension in young SHR. The concentration of NE was increased in the brainstem and hypothalamus, and DBH activity was greater in the locus caeruleus, A2 area, and thoracointermediolateral cells of SHR when compared with Wistar Kyoto (WKY) rats. NE turnover was increased in the hypothalamus and brainstem of neonatal SHR. Lesions of the AV3V area may prevent or retard the development of deoxycorticosterone acetate (DOCA)-salt hypertension and the development of hypertension in Dahl salt-sensitive rats but not in spontaneously hypertensive rats. Destruction of inhibitory inputs to the CVLM, a depressor area, results in disinhibition of descending bulbospinal sympathoexcitatory neurons and causes a sustained rise in blood pressure. Dietary NaCl supplementations elevate blood pressure and increase peripheral sympathetic nervous system activity in salt-sensitive SHR. Evidence indicates that the increase in blood pressure in this animal model may be caused by decreased noradrenergic activity of sympathoinhibitory neurons in the anterior hypothalamic area.

An increase in neurogenic tone has been observed in a subset of young patients with borderline hypertension. Hemodynamically, the increase in blood pressure in these patients is sustained primarily by a rise in cardiac output, whereas peripheral vascular resistance remains normal but inappropriately high in relationship to the level of cardiac output. Complete autonomic blockade with a β-blocker and atropine caused a greater reduction in cardiac output in patients with borderline hypertension than in normotensive subjects. With prolonged duration of hypertension, cardiac output tends to normalize, whereas peripheral vascular resistance progressively rises, so that in most patients, the chronic maintenance of blood pressure is dependent on a rise in peripheral vascular resistance. In these patients, the sympathetic nervous system activity is usually normal. To explain the transition from a neurogenic to a nonneurogenic form of hypertension, some have proposed the concept of *total body autoregulation.* According to this concept, an increase in cardiac output and the ensuing tissue overperfusion trigger a rise in peripheral vascular resistance that, in turn, reduces blood flow. This notion has been refuted by other investigators on the basis of patients with high cardiac output manifesting an increase in oxygen consumption. An alternative explanation is that the normalization of cardiac output may result from downregulation of cardiac adrenergic receptors caused by enhanced sympathetic nervous system activity.

To explain the progressive reduction in sympathetic activity in patients with hypertension, it has been postulated that the CNS may tightly regulate blood pressure. Accordingly, when structural changes occur in the peripheral circulation as a result of hypertension, vascular responsiveness to agonists increases, and lesser neurogenic influence on the peripheral circulation may be required to sustain the same degree of blood pressure elevation.

Efferent Pathways. Increased renal sympathetic nerve activity may contribute to the development and maintenance of hypertension through inhibition of sodium excretion. Renal denervation of young SHR leads to an increase of urinary sodium excretion and retards the development of hypertension. In rats with established hypertension, however, renal denervation does not alter urinary sodium excretion or blood pressure.

The evidence available in humans for a role of the sympathetic nervous system in the pathogenesis of essential hypertension is in large part indirect. Plasma NE levels have been shown to be increased in approximately 30% of patients with essential hypertension, mostly younger patients. The increase in plasma NE in response to orthostasis or isotonic or isometric exercise also is greater in hypertensive than in normotensive subjects. Administration of antiadrenergic agents decreases blood pressure and increases urinary sodium excretion in patients with essential hypertension, suggesting that increased renal sympathetic nerve activity and the attendant sodium retention may contribute to the maintenance of hypertension in these patients. Other studies have shown an increase in sympathetic discharge in the peroneal nerve of patients with essential hypertension when compared with normotensives.

Extensive evidence also suggests that in salt-sensitive subjects, sodium retention and hypertension may be related to increased activity of the sympathetic nervous system or to an increase in the NE:dopamine secretion ratio. Several years ago, we observed that salt-sensitive patients with essential hypertension displayed an abnormal relationship between urinary sodium excretion and plasma NE levels. A high NaCl diet was accompanied by a decrease in plasma concentrations of NE in normal subjects and in salt-resistant patients, but by a rise, no change, or a decrease in salt-sensitive patients (Fig. 59.7).

An increase in renal sympathetic nerve activity could shift the pressure natriuretic relationship toward higher pressure and could be responsible for the sodium retention observed in patients with essential hypertension. Dopamine and fenoldopam, a dopamine-1 (DA-l) receptor agonist, do not increase RBF or PGI_2 production in patients with essential hypertension, suggesting an alteration in dopaminergic tone, characterized by a defect in dopamine-receptor sensitivity. Exogenous administration of dopamine to anesthetized Sprague-Dawley rats may affect the pressure natriuresis response by altering the magnitude of arterial pressure–induced changes in tubular sodium reabsorption via an action of DA-1 receptors. The natriuretic effect of DA-1 agonists and the antinatriuretic effects of DA-1 antagonists are reduced in SHR compared with normotensive controls. DA-1 agonists stimulate adenylate cyclase activity to a lesser extent in the proximal convoluted tubule of SHR than WKY rats, suggesting a defect in the DA-1 receptor second-messenger coupling mechanism. No difference in urinary dopamine excretion or in natriuretic response to infused dopamine was observed in Dahl S compared with Dahl R rats.

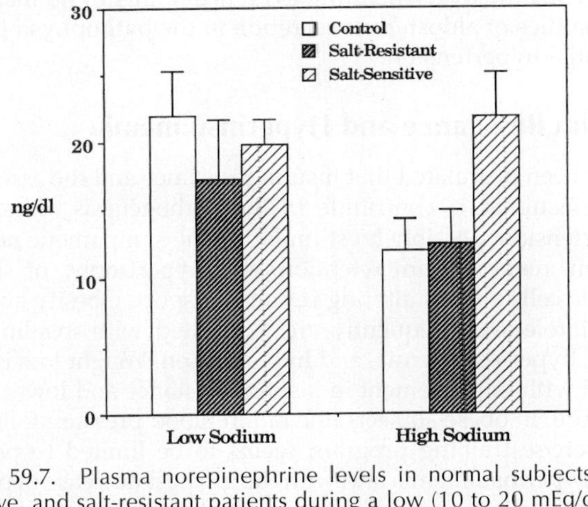

Figure 59.7. Plasma norepinephrine levels in normal subjects, salt-sensitive, and salt-resistant patients during a low (10 to 20 mEq/day) or a high (200 mEq/day) sodium intake. (Reproduced with permission from Campese VM, Romoff MS, Levitan D, et al. Abnormal relationship between sodium intake and sympathetic nervous activity in salt-sensitive patients with essential hypertension. *Kidney Int* 1982;21:371–378.)

Dopamine and NE exert opposite effects on renal sodium handling, so an increase in NE:dopamine ratio may result in sodium retention. Dahl S rats, compared with Dahl R rats, have a higher adrenal synthesis of NE following injection of tyrosine, a higher adrenal NE and epinephrine content, but a lower content of dopamine in the kidney and heart and lower urinary excretion of dopamine. This suggests that during high NaCl intake, Dahl S rats may be unable to turn off the increase in adrenal NE synthesis from dopamine. A decrease in urinary dopamine and an increase in NE excretion has been described in salt-sensitive patients, suggesting that a reduction in dopamine secretion may contribute to salt sensitivity and hypertension in these patients.

Because a rise in intracellular calcium ($[Ca^{2+}]i$) in the sympathetic nerves may stimulate NE release, it is possible that an Na^+-linked rise in$[Ca^{2+}]i$ in the renal sympathetic nerves may alter the normal ratio between NE and dopamine release and contribute to the derangements of renal hemodynamic and Na^+ excretion in salt-sensitive hypertensive patients.

Effector Cells Response to Norepinephrine. The effect of sympathetic stimulation on the cardiovascular system depends on the vascular reactivity to adrenergic stimuli. The increase in sympathetic nervous system activity in response to a decrease in peripheral vascular response may be a physiologic attempt to maintain normal blood pressure. On the other hand, an increased vascular response in the face of normal or increased sympathetic nervous system activity may result in hypertension. Several investigators have observed an exaggerated blood pressure responses to NE in patients with essential hypertension and have postulated that this mechanism may contribute to the maintenance of hypertension.

Salt-sensitive patients exhibit an even greater blood pressure response to NE than do salt-resistant patients, irrespective of the dietary NaCl intake (Fig. 59.8). These studies indicate that increased reactivity to the pressor action of NE may contribute to the maintenance of hypertension in salt-sensitive patients. Some investigators have shown a relationship between changes in blood pressure response to a high dietary NaCl intake and changes in the ratio between α_2- and β_2-receptors in platelets of hypertensive subjects and have suggested that the rise in blood pressure in response to high NaCl intake in predisposed patients may be the result of enhanced vasoconstriction caused by an increased ratio of α_2- and β_2-receptors in blood vessels and by enhanced sympathetically mediated renal sodium reabsorption.

The Renin-Angiotensin-Aldosterone System

Physiology

Renin is a proteolytic enzyme that cleaves angiotensinogen, a glycoprotein produced by the liver, to produce angiotensin I, an inactive decapeptide. Angiotensin I is converted into the active octapeptide, angiotensin II, by the converting enzyme, a dipeptidylcarboxypeptidase localized in the membrane of vascular endothelial cells, lungs, placenta, testicles, kidneys, and brain. The angiotensin-converting enzyme (ACE) is structurally identical to kininase II, an enzyme that metabolizes bradykinin. Thus inhibition of this enzyme will result in increased tissue accumulation of

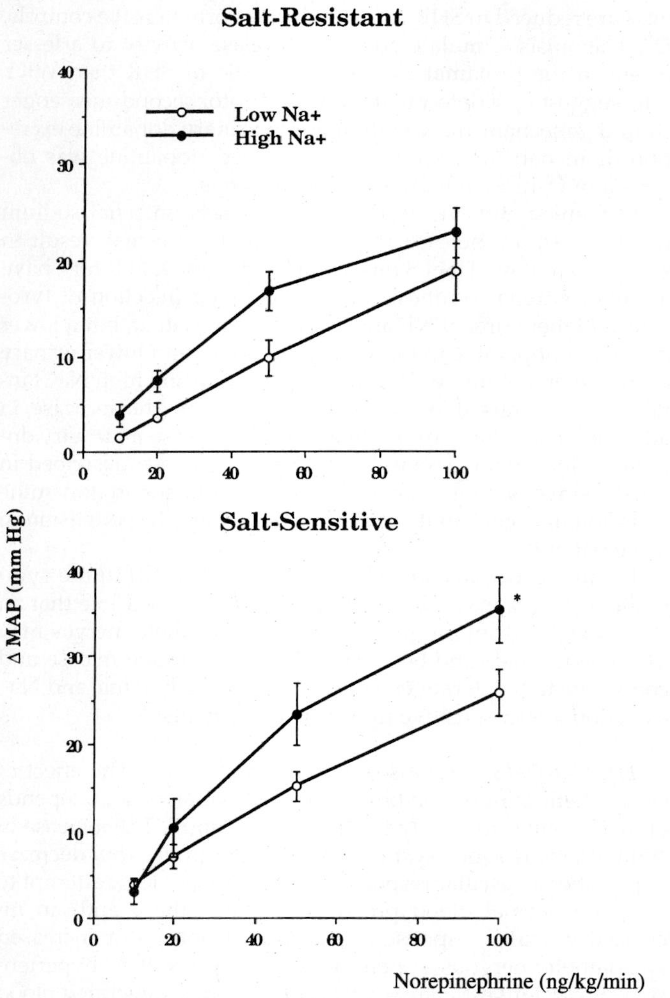

Figure 59.8. Effect of norepinephrine infused in increasing doses of 20, 50, and 100 ng/kg/min on mean arterial pressure (MAP) in salt-resistant and in salt-sensitive patients with essential hypertension. Values are means ± SEM. *$P < .05$ compared with salt-resistant patients. (Reproduced with permission from Campese VM, Karubion F, Chervu I, et al. Pressor reactivity to norepinephrine and angiotensin in salt-sensitive hypertensive patients. *Hypertension* 1993;21:301–307.)

bradykinin. Angiotensin II has several important functions. It is a powerful vasoconstrictor; stimulates aldosterone secretion; can stimulate the sympathetic nervous system both centrally (the area postrema) or peripherally (by facilitating NE release from the sympathetic nerve terminals and the adrenal glands); stimulates the release of antidiuretic hormone and oxytocin from the pituitary gland; increases thirst; exerts a negative feedback on renin release; and exerts trophic actions on myocardial cells, smooth muscle cells, and glomerular mesangial cells. Detailed discussion of the physiology of this system is provided in Chapter 13, Part 3.

Pathophysiology in Hypertension

The role of the renin-angiotensin system in essential hypertension remains controversial partially because PRA can be normal, high, or low. PRA is high only in approximately 10% to 15% of patients, mostly young and with evidence of increased sympathetic nervous system activity. In most patients, PRA is either normal or low. Those with low PRA represent approximately 25% of patients, mostly older, and African-Americans. Several hypotheses have been proposed to explain the low renin status in these patients, but none has been proven. Sodium retention and volume expansion are the most obvious candidates, but no evidence exists that blood volume is expanded in older or African-American patients with hypertension. Decreased sympathetic nervous system activity, decreased sensitivity of β-adrenergic receptors, structural abnormalities of the juxtaglomerular apparatus, increased plasma levels of atrial natriuretic peptide, and increased $[Ca^{2+}]i$ in the juxtaglomerular cells are some of the many hypotheses proposed by different investigators. The vascular response to angiotensin II appears also to be normal in most patients with essential hypertension, and it is modified by dietary sodium intake but to the same degree as in normal subjects.

These findings do not support a primary role for the renin-angiotensin system in the pathogenesis of most cases of essential hypertension. There are, however, several counter-arguments to this conclusion. The first is that in experimental models of hypertension, such as the one kidney–one clip model, the chronic maintenance of blood pressure can be, at least in part, renin mediated even though PRA may be decreased. The second derives from observations in dogs that constant infusion of minute amounts of renin may increase blood pressure even without any significant change in PRA. Low-level infusions of angiotensin II that do not alter the levels of blood pressure can cause a shift of the pressure natriuresis relationship to the right. The antinatriuretic action of angiotensin II may result from stimulation of aldosterone secretion or from direct action on proximal tubular cells. Thus even low elevations of the levels of angiotensin II in relation to sodium intake may alter the pressure natriuresis relationship and result in a sustained elevation of blood pressure. Local production of renin within the kidneys may contribute to shifting the relationship between pressure and natriuresis in patients with hypertension.

A role for angiotensin II in the pathophysiology of malignant hypertension is well established. Evidence also points to a role for the renin-angiotensin system in myocardial and vascular remodeling that occurs with the development of hypertension.

In patients with essential hypertension, plasma aldosterone levels may range from low to high. In those with slightly increased levels, it is not clear whether this results from increased secretion or decreased liver clearance. Reduced suppressibility of aldosterone during volume expansion also has been observed in some patients. In normotensive offspring of patients with hypertension, plasma aldosterone levels are normal. Thus the overwhelming evidence points to no major abnormalities of aldosterone secretion in the pathophysiology of essential hypertension.

Insulin Resistance and Hyperinsulinemia

It has been postulated that insulin resistance and the associated hyperinsulinemia contribute to the pathogenesis of essential hypertension, possibly by stimulating the sympathetic nervous system, renal sodium retention, and hypertrophy of smooth muscle cells and by altering cation transport. Obesity and glucose intolerance frequently are associated with insulin resistance, hyperinsulinemia, and hypertension. Weight loss is associated with improvement in insulin resistance and lower blood pressure. In obese subjects, the fall in blood pressure following an exercise training program seems to be limited to patients with hyperinsulinemia and with the greatest decrease in plasma insulin levels.

More controversial are the data in patients with essential hypertension. Certain studies have demonstrated that nonobese adult subjects of either sex with moderate to severe essential hypertension have reduced sensitivity to insulin and that a direct correlation between insulin resistance or plasma insulin concentration with severity of hypertension exists. However, several other studies among whites in Rancho Bernardo, California, as well as Pima Indians, New Caledonians, and Polynesians have failed to demonstrate an association between insulin levels and hypertension. The prevalence of hypertension among populations with a high incidence of obesity, insulin resistance, and hyperinsulinemia, such as Pima Indians, and Mexican-Americans, is lower than among whites who are, on the average, leaner and more insulin sensitive. Conversely, African-Americans who are known to have a higher prevalence of hypertension, display a lower prevalence of insulin resistance than whites, and no association between blood insulin levels and blood pressure can be found in this group. Even among white hypertensives, hyperinsulinemia is present in only approximately 40% of patients. Finally, patients with insulinoma who are exposed to severe elevations in blood insulin levels do not manifest an increase in blood pressure, and removal of the tumor does not lower blood pressure. All these studies clearly suggest that the presence of hyperinsulinemia is not a prerequisite for the development of hypertension.

Conflicting findings have been described in experimental models of hypertension. Some have shown that the integrated blood insulin response to an oral glucose challenge was significantly greater in SHR, whereas the ability of a similar blood concentration of exogenous insulin to stimulate glucose disposal was reduced in these rats compared with WKY rats. Fasting and postglucose load hyperinsulinemia suggestive of insulin resistance have been described in Dahl S rats. However, other investigators, using the intravenous glucose tolerance test or the euglycemic clamp technique, found enhanced glucose disposal when SHR were evaluated while conscious and unrestrained to avoid the possible hyperglycemic effects of stress. No abnormalities in insulin sensitivity were found in rats with the one clip–one kidney or the one clip–two kidney models of renovascular hypertension.

Several mechanisms have been postulated to mediate the hypertensive effect of insulin. Acute and chronic infusion of insulin in the absence of changes in serum glucose may cause sodium retention, may stimulate the activity of the sympathetic nervous system, may alter cation transport, and may stimulate hypertrophy of smooth muscle cells. Acute infusions of low doses of insulin usually cause vasodilation in both humans and experimental animals. Infusion of supraphysiologic doses of insulin can raise blood pressure in humans. Chronic infusions of insulin increased blood pressure in the rat but not in the dog. The rise in blood pressure in the rat was not associated with a positive sodium balance. Insulin may exert antinatriuretic effects. This was first observed while instituting insulin therapy in diabetic patients with poorly controlled diabetes. Subsequent studies with a euglycemic clamp technique in humans and rats have shown that insulin may promote sodium retention through a direct effect on the kidney, independent of changes in renal hemodynamics. On the basis of this observation, some have postulated that if insulin resistance to glucose disposal in the muscle and the concomitant hyperinsulinemia were to be associated with a normal response to insulin in the kidneys, this could result in sodium retention, volume expansion, and hypertension. This appealing concept is not fully substantiated by the available evidence. Following a glucose load, salt-sensitive young normotensive subjects with a genetic predisposition to develop hypertension manifested greater blood levels of both glucose and insulin compared with salt-resistant subjects during a high, but not during a low, NaCl intake. An association of hyperinsulinemia and blood pressure sensitivity to NaCl has been shown in young normotensive and borderline hypertensive African-Americans by some but not by others. Obese adolescents when compared with nonobese adolescents tended to be salt sensitive, as attested by a shallow slope of the renal function relation, and fasting blood insulin levels predicted salt sensitivity. Loss of body weight in these subjects was accompanied by decreased plasma insulin levels and by an increase in the slope of the pressure natriuresis relationship. Other investigators, however, have shown that hyperinsulinemia and decreased sensitivity to insulin were seen most commonly in hypertensive patients with low salt sensitivity. Chronic administration of insulin in the dog does not cause sodium retention or hypertension. Chronic hyperinsulinemia in Sprague-Dawley rats produced a shift of the pressure natriuresis relation, but hypertension in these rats was not salt sensitive and not dependent on sodium retention or increased renin secretion. Moreover, an association between insulin resistance and hyperinsulinemia has been observed in whites but not in African-Americans, whereas salt sensitivity is more frequent in the latter than in the former.

Insulin infusion in humans causes an increase in sympathetic nervous system activity, as reflected by an increase in plasma NE levels and in sympathetic discharge measured by microneurography in the peroneal nerves. On the basis of these observations, some have suggested that chronic hyperinsulinemia may increase blood pressure through activation of the sympathetic nervous system. Other studies, however, have shown that the increase in sympathetic activity during insulin infusion is not accompanied by an increase in blood pressure, and it may actually be a consequence of peripheral vasodilation.

Insulin stimulates the activity of the Na^+-H^+ antiport, a cell membrane system involved in maintaining a normal intracellular concentration of sodium and pH. An increase in the activity of this system may lead to an increase in intracellular Na^+ and Ca^{2+}, resulting in increased vascular tone and pressor response to NE and angiotensin II. In addition, intracellular pH may increase, resulting in smooth muscle cell growth and increased peripheral vascular resistance. There is also evidence that insulin may stimulate proliferation of smooth muscle cells directly or through stimulation of an insulin growth factor.

An alternative hypothesis for the relationship between hyperinsulinemia and hypertension is that insulin and blood pressure are not causally related but both are either inherited or caused by a common factor. For example, insulin resistance and hypertension could both be caused by an increase in sympathetic nervous system activity. An alternative explanation is that a decrease in intracellular magnesium could cause both abnormalities.

Hyperinsulinemia is a major risk factor for the development of cardiovascular diseases, and its effects seem to be independent of blood pressure and plasma lipid levels. The structure of an atherosclerotic plaque is characterized by excessive amounts of lipids and collagen, foam macrophages, and proliferation of smooth muscle cells. Insulin could cause all these abnormalities. Insulin infusion into one femoral artery in animals induced intimal and medial proliferation and accumulation of cholesterol and fatty acids, whereas the contralateral femoral artery was unaffected. Insulin, by itself or through the mediation of growth-promoting factors, can stimulate the proliferation of smooth muscle cells and collagen deposition *in vitro*. Insulin can increase cholesterol and triglyceride synthesis and enhance low-density lipoprotein receptor activity in arterial smooth muscle cells, fibroblasts, and mononuclear cells.

Membrane Transport and Intracellular Ions in Hypertension

The Sodium Pump

Increased intracellular concentrations of sodium have been shown in erythrocytes, leukocytes, and lymphocytes of hypertensive patients. The sodium pump maintains sodium and potassium gradients across the cell membranes by an electrogenic and active transport, and this pump is inhibited by cardiac glycosides, such as ouabain. It has been proposed that in hypertensive salt-sensitive subjects, sodium retention and volume expansion may lead to increased secretion of a circulating substance with ouabainlike properties, capable of inhibiting Na^+-K^+-ATPase activity. On one hand, this factor would increase natriuresis and reestablish sodium balance; on the other hand, this factor would cause increased contractility of vascular smooth muscle cells due to increased intracellular sodium and calcium, and increased NE release from sympathetic nerve terminals. The end result would be hypertension. This notion has led many investigators to study the Na^+-K^+-ATPase activity and the sodium pump density in cells isolated from hypertensive patients. In addition, an exhausting search has been undertaken to detect circulating inhibitors of the sodium pump. This search has led to conflicting results. Some studies have shown reduced activity of the sodium pump (determined by the rate constant of ouabain-sensitive ^{22}Na efflux) in patients with hypertension. Other studies, however, have failed to show any abnormalities. In one large study of 247 subjects, a negative correlation was found between levels of blood pressure and erythrocyte Na^+-K^+-ATPase activity, and a positive correlation was found between blood pressure and intracellular sodium. African-Americans appear to have lower levels of ouabain-sensitive cation transport in red blood cells than whites, and it is possible that pump suppression may predispose African-Americans to salt sensitivity and hypertension. The V_{max} of Na^+-K^+-ATPase activity was found to be decreased in erythrocyte membranes of Nigerians with newly identified essential hypertension.

Several investigators have described increased serum and urine levels of Na^+-K^+-ATPase inhibitors in essential hypertension. The plasma from salt-sensitive patients showed significantly higher levels of Na^+-K^+-ATPase inhibitors and plasma NE levels. Other studies have shown that salt-sensitive patients display higher serum levels of digoxinlike factor than salt-resistant patients, and a significant correlation of those levels with blood pressure. However, high NaCl diet failed to increase the serum levels of the digoxinlike factor in both groups of patients. African-American girls with hypertensive parents had very low binding affinity for ouabain in erythrocytes. A cause and effect relationship between inhibitors of Na^+-K^+-ATPase activity and salt sensitivity in hypertension has not been conclusively established.

Na^+-K^+-$2Cl^-$ Cotransport

This system cotransports Na^+ and K^+. It is electrically neutral, because it also transports Cl^-, and it is inhibited by furosemide. In several mammalian cells, such as vascular smooth muscle cells and renal tubular epithelial cells, the transport is in an inward direction. Erythrocytes, on the other hand, have this transport in an outward direction. The data on this transport system in hypertension are conflicting. Different strains of hypertensive rats display rates of erythrocyte Na^+-K^+ cotransport different from their controls. Erythrocyte Na^+-K^+ cotransport is low in SHR, high in the Milan strain, and normal in Dahl salt-sensitive rats. The data in patients with essential hypertension are equally conflicting. Some have shown a decrease and some an increase in the V_{max} of the Na^+-K^+ cotransport system. Some have shown a direct relationship among severity of hypertension, decrease in venous compliance, and V_{max} of the Na^+-K^+ cotransport. The reason for these conflicting data is not readily apparent. It has been shown that a bimodal distribution of the Na^+-K^+ cotransport exists in hypertensive patients, with 75% manifesting a distribution similar to that of normal subjects and 25% manifesting a distribution into higher levels. Patients with high Na^+-K^+ cotransport had lower plasma renin activity and fractional uric acid excretion, whereas GFR and urinary sodium and potassium excretion were the same as in normotensive individuals. These patients also have greater blood pressure response to furosemide than normotensive subjects or hypertensives with normal Na^+-K^+ cotransport. Similarly conflicting are the data on the effect of different dietary NaCl intakes on this transport system. Some have found no significant effects, others observed a lower V_{max}, and K_m in hypertensive patients on a low compared with a high NaCl diet. The K_m for Na^+ at the inner face was significantly lower in salt-sensitive than in salt-resistant African-American adolescents. The studies suggest that dysregulation of the Na^+-K^+ cotransport in vascular smooth muscle and endothelial cells may predispose to hypertension in response to high NaCl intake.

The Na^+-H^+ Antiport

The Na^+-H^+ antiport is a ubiquitous cell-membrane transport system that promotes an electroneutral 1:1 exchange of intracellular H^+ for extracellular Na^+ and is activated by an increase in cytosolic proton concentration. This transport system is inhibited by amiloride and its N-substituted analogs. The Na^+-H^+ exchanger accepts Na^+ as the physiologic substrate, but it can also accept Li^+ and $NH4^+$. The system is involved in the regulation of intracellular pH, cell volume, stimulus-response coupling, and cell proliferation. Red blood cell Na^+-H^+ exchanger exhibits, in most hypertensive patients, abnormal kinetics of activation. Increased activity of the Na^+-H^+ antiport has been described in leukocytes and platelets from hypertensive compared with normotensive individuals and in cultured fibroblasts from normotensive African-Americans compared with whites. The increase in Na^+-H^+ antiport activity does not correlate with the increase in blood pressure and does not regress when blood pressure normalizes. Na^+-H^+ antiport activity during an acid load *in vitro* was found to be increased, and skeletal muscle acidification was found to be decreased in hypertensive patients. If an increase in Na^+-H^+ antiport activity were to be expressed in renal tubular cells, it could provide an explanation for the propensity of African-American subjects to retain sodium and to develop hypertension in response to an NaCl load. This hypothesis, however, is not supported by recent findings because all changes in Na^+-H^+ antiport activity reported thus far refer to the isoform, which is not involved in epithelial Na^+ transport.

Enhancement of the Na^+-H^+ antiport activity should result in alkalinization of cells. However, studies in red blood cells have shown a decrease in pH, those in leukocytes have shown an increase in pH, and most studies in platelets have shown no difference in pH between normotensive and hypertensive subjects. Studies in resting skeletal muscle *in vivo* also have failed to show any difference in pH between normotensive and hypertensive subjects, although the recovery of pH after maximal exercise was faster in hypertensive than it was in normotensive individuals. No difference in pH was observed in resistance vessels from normotensive and hypertensive individuals.

The increased activity of the Na^+-H^+ antiport has been linked to increased cell proliferation. Smooth muscle cells from SHR display a faster replication compared with cells from the WKY rats, and this is associated with increased activity of the Na^+-H^+ exchanger. A significant correlation between increased Na^+-H^+ antiport activity in lymphocytes and left ventricular hypertrophy has been described in patients with essential hypertension.

The mechanisms for the potential increase in the activity of the Na^+-H^+ exchanger are unclear. This could represent a primary defect, or it could be secondary to alterations of intracellular pH, to vasoconstrictors, or to changes in $[Ca^{2+}]$i. A rise in $[Ca^{2+}]$i caused by ionophores activates the Na^+-H^+ antiport. However, well-known stimuli of the Na^+-H^+ exchanger, such as phorbol myristate acetate and ammonium chloride, had no effect or actually decreased $[Ca^{2+}]$i in vascular smooth muscle cells. The activation of the Na^+-H^+ antiport could, however, be secondary to an agonist-mediated rise in Ca^{2+} inside of vascular smooth muscle cells. Insulin and NE, which increase $[Ca^{2+}]$i, also activate the Na^+-H^+ exchanger. This raises the possibility that an increase in NE or in insulin secretion may be responsible for the sodium-dependent rise in $[Ca^{2+}]$i and blood pressure in salt-sensitive patients with hypertension. One study has shown that erythrocyte Na^+-H^+ exchanger activity did not correlate with blood pressure or with blood insulin levels but did correlate with body-mass index. Because differences in plasma lipids may affect membrane fluidity and the activity of the Na^+-H^+ antiport, some have speculated that hyperlipidemia may increase Na^+-H^+ antiport activity in hypertensive patients. A direct correlation has been observed between serum levels of triglycerides and cholesterol and Na^+-H^+ antiport activity in hypertensive patients. Administration of lovastatin, an HMG-CoA reductase inhibitor, decreased Na^+-H^+ antiport activity in hypertensive patients.

Red Blood Cell Na^+-Li^+ Countertransport

This cell transport system is measured by the rate of exchange of external Li^+ for internal Na^+, and it has been suggested that this transport system is the same as the Na^+-H^+ antiport, even though some believe that they represent different entities. Both systems mediate an influx of Na^+, Li^+, and H^+, and both systems are inhibited by acidic extracellular pH. However, the Na^+-Li^+ countertransport is not amiloride sensitive. There is a considerable amount of variability in the activity of erythrocyte Na^+-Li^+ countertransport in normotensive and hypertensive subjects. However, the weight of evidence indicates increased activity of this transport system in patients with essential hypertension. It has been shown that patients who demonstrate the greatest degree of elevation of blood pressure in response to changes from a low salt to a high salt diet have a significant elevation in the V_{max} of erythrocyte Na^+-Li^+ countertransport. These investigators have also shown a positive correlation between Na^+-Li^+ countertransport and peripheral vascular resistance and a negative correlation with renal clearance of lithium, which may represent increased Na^+ reabsorption by the renal proximal tubule. A direct correlation has been observed between Na^+-Li^+ countertransport and body-mass index, plasma uric acid, and triglyceride concentrations.

The Sodium Channel

Liddle's syndrome has been attributed to a mutation of the Na^+ channel in the distal tubule leading to sodium retention and hypertension. Attempts to implicate an abnormality of this channel in the genesis of essential hypertension have thus far failed to provide convincing evidence.

Abnormalities in Intracellular Calcium Regulation in Hypertension

The concentration of $[Ca^{2+}]$i in platelets of hypertensive patients is greater than in normotensive subjects. In addition,

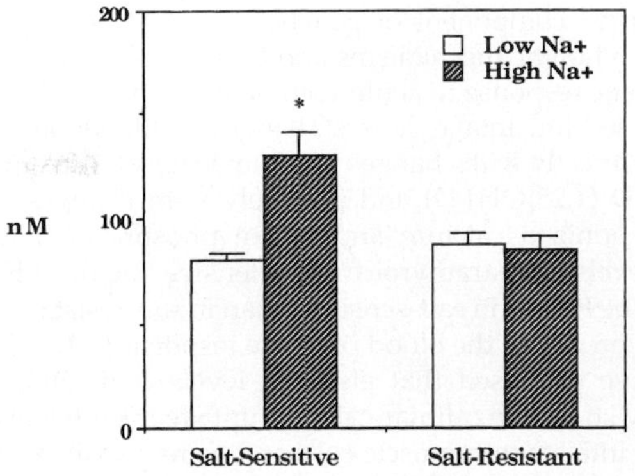

Figure 59.9. The concentration of $[Ca^{2+}]$i in lymphocytes of salt-sensitive and salt-resistant patients during a low Na^+ intake (20 mEq/day) and during a high Na^+ intake (200 mEq/day). *$P < .01$. (Reproduced with permission from Alexiewics JM, Gaciong Z, Parise M, et al. Effect of dietary sodium intake on intracellular calcium in lymphocytes of salt-sensitive hypertensive patients. *Am J Hypertens* 1992;5:536–541.)

some agonists cause a greater increase in the entry and mobilization of Ca^{2+} in platelets of hypertensive patients compared with normotensive subjects. In salt-sensitive patients, the rise in blood pressure during high NaCl diet was associated with an increase in $[Ca^{2+}]$i in lymphocytes (Fig. 59.9). In salt-resistant patients, on the other hand, there were no changes in mean arterial pressure or in $[Ca^{2+}]$i during NaCl loading. In addition, a direct and significant correlation was present between the changes in $[Ca^{2+}]$i and the changes in mean arterial pressure. These studies suggest the existence of a linkage between dietary NaCl intake, $[Ca^{2+}]$i, and blood pressure in salt-sensitive patients with essential hypertension.

The mechanisms for the rise in $[Ca^{2+}]$i are not clear. Increased entry into cells because of greater serum levels of agonists, such as NE or angiotensin II, could be responsible for this rise. The mechanisms whereby a high NaCl intake increases $[Ca^{2+}]$i also are unclear. Several investigators have proposed that the Na^+-linked rise in $[Ca^{2+}]$i may be caused by increased secretion of a circulating inhibitor of the Na^+-K^+-ATPase pump. This would increase intracellular sodium and, in turn, alter the Na^+-Ca^{2+} exchange system, resulting in increased $[Ca^{2+}]$i in vascular smooth muscle cells. Red blood cell lysates of hypertensive subjects have decreased activity of the Ca^{2+}-ATPase pump, whereas platelets of hypertensive patients have increased activity of this calcium pump. This increase may be an adaptive response to agonist-mediated rise in Ca^{2+} entry into platelets. The reason for the different activity of the Ca^{2+}-ATPase pump between erythrocytes and platelets of hypertensive patients and normotensive subjects is unknown, but it could be because of the absence of calcium organelles and of receptors to most agonists regulating calcium entry in erythrocytes.

Calcium Metabolism in Hypertension

Evidence has accumulated suggesting a relationship between low calcium intake, abnormalities in calcium metabolism, and hypertension in animal models, as well as in patients with essential hypertension. Salt-sensitive individuals are more likely to manifest disturbances of calcium metabolism, such as low serum ionized calcium and serum magnesium, increased urinary excretion of calcium and magnesium, and elevation of serum parathyroid hormone and vitamin D, and they are more likely to display a reduction in arterial pressure in response to increased dietary calcium intake. High calcium intake prevents the salt-sensitive hypertensive component of genetically mediated hypertension via sympatholytic mechanisms and by increasing the natriuretic and diuretic response to acute volume loading.

High sodium intake causes changes in blood pressure that correlate directly with changes in serum levels of 1,25-dihydroxyvitamin D (1,25[OH]$_2$D) and inversely with changes in serum levels of ionized calcium and serum phosphate. In addition, serum levels of parathyroid hypertensive factor (PHF) were found to be higher in salt-sensitive than in salt-resistant patients, and they predicted the blood pressure response to NaCl loading. Some have proposed that elevated levels of 1,25(OH)$_2$D and PHF may stimulate cellular calcium uptake from the extracellular space into smooth muscle cells and be responsible, at least in part, for salt-sensitive hypertension. Consistent with this hypothesis is the demonstration of 1,25(OH)$_2$D receptors in vascular smooth muscle cells and of 1,25(OH)$_2$D-induced increase in the uptake of calcium in cultured rat aortic myocytes. Finally, acute and chronic hypercalcemia are associated with hypertension, and acute hypocalcemia may cause hypotension. The relationship between blood pressure and plasma calcium is discussed in Chapter 17, Part 3.

PROSTAGLANDINS AND THE KALLIKREIN-KININ SYSTEM

The physiology of the prostaglandins and the renal kallikrein-kinin system is discussed in detail in Chapter 13, Part 1, and Chapter 13, Part 4, respectively.

Pathophysiology in Hypertension

The production of thromboxane β_2 by renal cortical microsomes is increased in SHR, and administration of thromboxane synthase inhibitors may increase papillary blood flow and retard the development of hypertension. On the other hand, urinary excretion and renal papillary content of prostaglandin E_2 (PGE_2) are reduced in SHR. Dahl salt-sensitive rats also manifest lower urinary excretion of pseudocholinesterase (PCE_2) than do salt-resistant rats. Reduced urinary excretion of PCE_2 and 6-keto-$PGF_{1\alpha}$ have been described in essential hypertension. However, the role of prostaglandins in essential hypertension remains elusive.

A reduction in urinary kallikrein excretion has been demonstrated in both clinical and experimental hypertension, and this reduction correlates with the severity of hypertension. In addition, urinary kallikrein excretion is lower in African-American than in white patients with essential hypertension. This has lead to the suggestion that a blunted activity of the vasodilating renal kallikrein-kinin system may be partially responsible for sodium retention and participate in the pathophysiology of hypertension.

ATRIAL NATRIURETIC PEPTIDE

The physiology of atrial natriuretic peptide (ANP) is reviewed in Chapter 13, Part 8.

Pathophysiology in Hypertension

ANP has diuretic, natriuretic, vasodilator, sympatholytic, and renin- and aldosterone-suppressing activities. Because of these properties, ANP is considered an important regulator of the sodium-volume status and blood pressure. The possibility has been raised that hypertension and, particularly, salt sensitivity, might be a consequence of reduced secretion or action of ANP. However, the role of ANP in the pathophysiology of experimental and human hypertension and salt sensitivity remains elusive.

A disruption of the pro-ANP gene in mice caused salt-sensitive hypertension. Homozygous mutants had no circulating ANP, and manifested high blood pressure whether mice were fed a standard or an intermediate salt diet. In contrast, the heterozygotes were normotensive and had normal blood ANP levels, but became hypertensive only when fed a high salt diet. By contrast, in NPRa knockout mice, blood pressure also increased, but this model of hypertension was not salt sensitive. Transgenic mice overexpressing the genes for ANP or brain natriuretic peptide had lower blood pressure than normal littermates.

Studies in rats showed increased ANP levels in response to NaCl loading in WKY but not in NaCl-sensitive rats. ANP infusion in a dose that achieves plasma ANP levels well within the physiologic range abolished the NaCl-induced exacerbation of hypertension in salt-sensitive, spontaneously hypertensive rats. ANP secretion in response to increased atrial pressure was impaired in prehypertensive Dahl salt-sensitive rats but it was exaggerated in more advanced phases when hypertension was complicated by left ventricular hypertrophy. In hypertension caused by excess mineralocorticoid, the concentration of ANP increases in coincidence with the phenomenon of "escape." Blockade of endogenous atrial natriuretic factor (ANF) with specific monoclonal antibodies increases the severity of hypertension in stroke-prone SHR and DOCA-salt–sensitive rats.

Previous measurements of plasma ANP levels in patients with essential hypertension have provided conflicting results. Some studies have shown low to normal plasma ANP levels, whereas others have shown increased levels. Some have shown an increase in plasma ANP levels during high Na^+ intake in patients with essential hypertension, but others have shown a blunted increase in plasma ANP in response to high dietary NaCl intake in salt-sensitive compared with salt-resistant patients. Some have observed markedly reduced plasma ANP during high sodium intake in the offspring of hypertensive parents compared with the offspring of normotensive parents, and have suggested that a relative ANP deficiency may potentially predispose individuals to the development of essential hypertension.

We have demonstrated that salt-sensitive, hypertensive African-Americans manifest abnormal ANP secretion in response to increased dietary Na intake. Salt-resistant patients failed to manifest the expected rise in ANP, whereas salt-sensitive patients manifested a paradoxic decrease in ANP. In these patients, reduced atrial secretion of ANP could be responsible, at least in part, for the reduced ability to excrete Na and for the Na-induced rise in blood pressure. In whites, we noticed a similar tendency for ANP to decrease during high salt intake, but the decrease did not reach statistical significance.

All of these studies suggest that a deficiency in circulating endogenous ANP may play a role in the NaCl-sensitive component of hypertension in SHR and in patients with essential hypertension. Further studies, however, are needed to ascertain the role, if any, of ANP in the pathophysiology of salt-sensitive hypertension. The use of inhibitors of ANP, such as the endopeptidase 24-11, may help to clarify the pathogenetic role of these peptides in hypertension.

The discrepancy in ANP findings in the literature could be partly due to methodologic discrepancies in ANP measurements, to differences in age and dietary NaCl intake, to the presence of left ventricular dysfunction, or to genetic differences of the populations studied.

The Vascular Endothelium and Hypertension

As the interface between the circulating blood and the vascular smooth muscle cells, the endothelial cells have several key functions: (a) they serve as a first barrier to circulating antigens and actively participate in the defense reactions; (b) they play a cardinal role in both preventing and promoting clot formation through their interaction with platelets, the fibrinolytic system, and the clotting cascade; (c) they clear from the blood such substances as NE and serotonin; (d) they activate peptides, such as angiotensin, and inactivate others, such as bradykinin; and (e) they may play a key role in promoting thickening and fibrosis of blood vessels through mitogenic effects. In addition, the endothelium plays a crucial role in regulating regional blood flow and vascular resistance. The endothelium is the major source of prostacyclin, and acetylcholine-induced arterial relaxation is endothelium dependent and is caused by generation of a diffusible and transferable substance that relaxes smooth muscle cells. This substance was initially called *endothelium-derived relaxing factor (EDRF)* and later characterized to be *NO*.

Prostacyclin is activated by bradykinin, and it increases cyclic adenosine monophosphate (cAMP) levels in the vascular smooth muscle cells leading to vasodilation. It also inhibits platelet adhesion and has thrombolytic and cytoprotective actions. Prostacyclin and NO potentiate each other's vascular and platelet antiaggregating effects even at subthreshold concentrations.

An endothelium-dependent hyperpolarization factor (EDHF) was discovered in the canine femoral artery in 1988. This factor decreases the responsiveness of vascular walls to vasoconstrictor hormones and is released by the endothelium in response to acetylcholine. The activity of EDHF is attenuated by ouabain, an Na^{+}-K^{+}-ATPase inhibitor.

Endothelin is the most potent vasoconstrictor isolated thus far. Other endothelium-derived contracting factors (EDCF) being studied include prostaglandin H, and epidermal growth factor (EGF), which is a mitogen for smooth muscle cells *in vitro* and causes arterial strips to contract.

A number of investigators have speculated that these vasoactive peptides may play a role in disease states, such as hypertension. The possibilities include (a) altered balance between EDRF and EDCF, resulting in a rise in renal and systemic vascular resistance and hypertension; (b) hypertensive vascular endothelial damage, leading to abnormal production of endothelium-derived vasoactive factors; and (c) endothelium effects on systemic hemodynamics by secreting substances that have effects on other key regulators.

Endothelium-Derived Vasoconstrictor Factors

Of the various vasoconstrictor factors mentioned, endothelin (ET) has attracted the most attention in the genesis of hypertension. The physiology of ET is discussed in detail in Chapter 13, Part 5.

Compelling evidence that ET-1 might play a role in the pathophysiology of hypertension derives from the observation that patients with hemangioendothelioma, a rare malignant vascular neoplasm, have hypertension and plasma levels of ET 10-fold to 15-fold greater than in normal and hypertensive subjects; surgical removal of the tumor led to resolution of hypertension. In one patient, the tumor recurred, along with a rise in plasma ET level and hypertension. ET may play a role in cyclosporine-induced hypertension. Cyclosporine increases ET release from endothelial cells in culture and increases blood levels of ET in patients. Some have speculated that ET may be responsible for the decrease in RBF observed during administration of cyclosporine and possibly, for its nephrotoxicity.

Intravenous administration of ET-1 into animals initially leads to peripheral vasodilation and decrease in blood pressure, probably because of release of prostanoids and NO. The depressor response is followed by a sustained and prolonged vasoconstriction and rise in blood pressure. Controversy exists in the literature about the vascular response to ET in experimental models of hypertension. In isolated blood vessels, such as the aorta or mesenteric arteries from rats with spontaneous hypertension or DOCA-salt hypertension, a reduction in sensitivity to ET has been observed. This has been attributed to downregulation of ET receptors. In the perfused, intact mesenteric arteries of SHR, however, the pressor response to ET is increased. In addition, ET enhances the pressor response to angiotensin II and NE. Thus the pressor response to this substance may also depend on the circulating levels of other vasopressor hormones. Infusion of ET causes profound reductions in RBF and GFR. Because the kidneys play a critical role in the long-term maintenance of hypertension through the pressure natriuresis and the tubulo-feedback mechanisms, these effects of ET may be extremely important in the pathophysiology of hypertension.

The circulating levels of ET are not increased in several forms of experimental hypertension unless malignant hypertension develops. The studies performed thus far in human subjects with stage 1 or 2 hypertension are inconclusive. Increased plasma ET-1 levels have been shown by some investigators but not by others. Normal circulating levels of ET, however, do not rule out a role of this peptide in the maintenance of hypertension because circulating levels do not necessarily reflect the local vascular production. Hypertensive patients with chronic renal failure have higher plasma ET-1 levels than normotensive subjects, which could be because of either the uremic state or exposure of the cells to an extracorporeal circuit during hemodialysis.

Evidence also exists indicating that circulating ET levels are elevated in patients with myocardial infarction and with atherosclerotic vascular disease. This has led some to suggest that ET may play a role in the complications of the hypertensive process. Further studies using ET-1 receptor blockade may be necessary to prove whether ET-1 plays an etiologic role in the hypertension of uremic patients.

Endothelium-Derived Vasodilator Factors

The endothelium-derived relaxing factor (EDRF) was discovered in 1980. This followed the observation that preconstricted arterial ring preparations relaxed in response to acetylcholine when the endothelium was kept intact but not when the endothelium had been removed. This EDRF is now known as NO. The physiology of NO is discussed in detail in Chapter 13, Part 6.

In the kidney, NO contributes to the regulation of renal hemodynamics and sodium excretion. Impaired NO synthesis may lead to sodium retention, to salt-sensitive hypertension, and to cardiovascular morbidity and mortality. Impaired NO production in the endothelium and the kidneys could be responsible, at least in part, for the reduced ability to excrete sodium and the greater propensity to cardiovascular damage in African-Americans. Certain evidence supports this hypothesis.

First, there is substantial evidence that NO participates in the control of renal medullary blood flow, water and sodium excretion, tubuloglomerular feedback, and blood pressure. Chronic inhibition of endogenous NO increases renal vascular resistances and decreases RBF and sodium excretion, resulting in a salt-sensitive form of hypertension. Some have suggested that a deficient NO production in the macula densa cells may lead to an increase in TGF-β sensitivity, increased sodium and water retention, and elevated blood pressure. Salt-sensitive hypertensive patients exhibit increased renal vascular resistance and impaired ability to produce NO in the renal vasculature compared with salt-resistant patients. In all, these studies are in keeping with the notion that a defect in NO production may participate to the genesis of blood pressure sensitivity to salt.

Second, studies in hypertensive human subjects have shown great variability in endothelial function. Some researchers have observed a normal vasodilator response to acetylcholine, whereas others have reported an abnormal response. Accordingly, it is unclear whether endothelial dysfunction uniformly occurs in individuals with essential hypertension and whether NO deficiency plays a role in the development and/or maintenance of hypertension, or whether it is a consequence of high blood pressure. It appears that a decrease in NO is more prevalent among salt-sensitive than among salt-resistant subjects. We have shown that infusion of L-arginine decreases blood pressure more in salt-sensitive than in salt-resistant hypertensive subjects and normotensive controls; on the other hand, L-arginine caused a smaller increase in RBF in salt-sensitive than in salt-resistant hypertensive subjects and normotensive controls. Others observed that the dose-dependent vasodilation induced by acetylcholine was significantly reduced in salt-sensitive compared with salt-resistant patients regardless of sodium loading. In salt-sensitive hypertensives, an increase in plasma levels of the endothelium-derived substances E-selectin, von Willebrand factor, and ET-1 compared with salt-resistant subjects was observed, and these levels were affected by dietary salt intake. In all, these studies support the hypothesis that salt sensitivity is correlated with evidence of increased endothelial damage and decreased NO production.

Several studies have also demonstrated that the incidence of cardiovascular events varies in different populations; it is more prevalent among African-Americans than it is among Caucasians, and this difference cannot be explained solely on the basis of differences in blood pressure levels. Certainly, an impairment of endothelial NO production could cause greater vascular damage. This possibility is supported by experimental evidence. Abnormal endothelial function has been described in many experimental models of hypertension, and it appears to be more common in salt-sensitive than in salt-resistant models. Dietary salt supplementation does not increase NO production in Dahl/Rapp S rats, although it does so in salt-resistant rats. Some investigators have observed lower cNOS activity in the aorta and left ventricle of Dahl S rats than in SHR and normotensive WKY rats. Dahl S rats also manifested greater left ventricular hypertrophy, proteinuria, and renal injury than SHR despite similar levels of blood pressure. Exogenous L-arginine, the substrate for NO synthase, decreased blood pressure to normotensive levels in Dahl/Rapp S rats, but it did not alter blood pressure in SHR. Taken together, these observations lend strong support to the hypothesis that a genetic defect in endothelial (e) NO production may predispose to salt sensitivity, and to greater cardiovascular and renal injury.

It is still open for discussion whether cellular impairments in NO production are primary, that is, dependent on genetic mutations of the three NO synthase genes, or are secondary to other genetically determined cellular abnormalities or to hypertension. It is possible that a genetically conditioned heterogeneity in vascular endothelial nitric oxide synthase (eNOS) activity may be responsible, at least in part, for the heterogeneity in endothelial-dependent vasorelaxation and in end-organ injury in human subjects with hypertension. Existing evidence supports this possibility. The offspring of hypertensive patients exhibit a reduced response to acetylcholine suggesting that a defect in NO production may precede the development of hypertension. Also, some investigators identified a missense variant of eNOS (Glu298Asp) in exon 7 of the eNOS gene in a Japanese population, and demonstrated a strong association of this variant with essential hypertension and coronary heart disease. This study suggests that variants of the eNOS gene may impart genetic susceptibility for essential hypertension, for salt sensitivity, and for cardiovascular disease. Unfortunately, all attempts thus far to detect a possible association or linkage between NOS gene polymorphisms and hypertension, both in rats and in humans, have failed to demonstrate any positive results. These negative findings, however, are not conclusive and do not rule out the possibility that other, as yet undetected, polymorphisms within or in close vicinity with the NOS genes might be responsible for reduced NO production in hypertension, particularly if selected groups of patients, such as salt-sensitive African-Americans, are studied. Further studies are necessary to confirm these relationships and to support our hypothesis. It should be mentioned that a highly significant cosegregation of alleles at the inducible, but not the constitutive, NOS locus with systolic blood pressure has been observed in Dahl S rats, but no linkage between eNOS and blood pressure was demonstrated in the same rats.

Chronic inhibition of NO synthesis by NwL-nitro-L-arginine-methylester (L-NAME) has been used as a new approach to induce arterial hypertension in animals. Administration of nitro-L-arginine to rats caused systemic hypertension, marked renal vasoconstriction, and hypoperfusion, as well as a 30% fall in GFR and a 39% increase in filtration fraction and a rise in PRA, which could be responsible in part for the severe vasoconstrictor activity. Renal histologic examination revealed widespread arteriolar narrowing, focal arteriolar obliteration, and segmental fibrinoid necrosis of the glomeruli. Administration of a NOS inhibitor to WKY rats increases renal sympathetic nerve activity and causes systemic hypertension. It has been shown that the increase in renal sympathetic nerve activity and in blood pressure induced by this compound could be reduced by spinal C1-C2 transection, implying that NO may also play a role in central regulation of sympathetic tone.

NO synthesis, both *in vitro* and *in vivo*, can be inhibited by an endogenous compound, NGNG-dimethylarginine [asymmetrical dimethylarginine (ADMA)]. Significantly higher plasma levels of ADMA and significantly lower plasma arginine/dimethylarginine ratios have been found by some investigators in uremic patients on chronic hemodialysis, raising the intriguing possibility that hypertension in these patients might result, at least in part, from inhibition of NO synthesis caused by increased levels of this circulating endogenous inhibitor. Other investigators, however, have observed increased content of NO in platelets and increased blood arginine levels in uremic patients.

Dietary salt intake may also affect NO production at the level of the endothelium. In normotensive rats, dietary salt loading enhanced NO production, measured by the excretion of NO_2 and NO_3 (NO_x), as well as cGMP, but did not affect NO production in the hindquarter circulation. In Dahl/Rapp salt-resistant rats, ingestion of a high NaCl diet impaired the myogenic response of renal afferent arterioles, and the dilation of large cerebral collateral arterioles in response to cerebral occlusion, two hemodynamic responses thought to be endothelium dependent. In addition, high dietary NaCl intake attenuated the flow-dependent arteriolar dilation in rat spinotrapezius muscle, an action partly mediated by endogenous NO. In hypertensive African-Americans, we have shown that under condition of high NaCl intake, plasma NOx decrease compared with a low NaCl intake. High dietary salt intake reduced serum NOx both in normotensive and hypertensive individuals, independently of their blood pressure response to changes in dietary NaCl intakes. One could speculate that the reduction in NOx levels during high dietary NaCl intake is a physiologic response to decreased secretion of pressor hormones, such as NE and angiotensin II. Alternatively, high NaCl intake may have some as yet unknown effects on vascular endothelial cells leading to suppression of NO production.

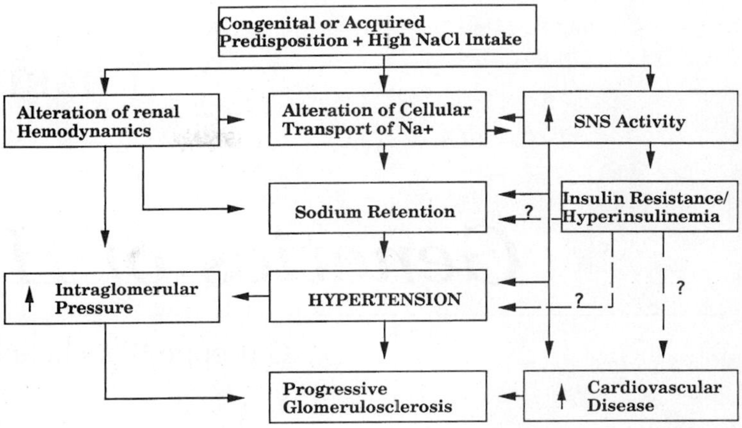

Figure 59.10. Salt-sensitivity and cardiovascular and renal complications: a hypothesis. (Reproduced with permission from Campese VM. Salt sensitivity in hypertension: renal and cardiovascular implications. *Hypertension* 1994;23:531–550.)

CONCLUSION

Several mechanisms have been implicated in the pathophysiology of essential hypertension. Because these mechanisms are strictly interrelated, it remains difficult, when evaluating established hypertension, to determine which factor is primary and which is secondary. In addition, different mechanisms may be involved in different patients, and mechanisms that are responsible for the onset of hypertension may be different from those that sustain blood pressure. Defining pathophysiologic mechanisms may be easier in subsets of patients with well-defined phenotypic characteristics. For example, in salt-sensitive patients with essential hypertension, we have proposed a hypothesis that interrelates alterations of cellular ion transport with hemodynamic and hormonal abnormalities (Fig. 59.10). In these patients, an increased activity of the sympathetic nervous system may play an important role in the alterations of renal hemodynamics, insulin resistance, and NaCl-dependent rise in blood pressure. All these factors combined may lead to the greater propensity of salt-sensitive patients to develop renal and cardiovascular complications.

Selected Readings

Campese VM, Parise M, Karubion F, et al. Abnormal renal hemodynamics in black salt-sensitive patients with hypertension. *Hypertension* 1991;18:805–812.

This study demonstrates that in salt-sensitive hypertensive patients, high NaCl intake reduces renal blood flow and increases intraglomerular pressure. It is suggested that this abnormal renal hemodynamic adaptation to changes in dietary sodium intake may underlie the greater propensity of salt-sensitive hypertensive patients to develop renal failure.

Campese VM, Romoff MS, Levitan D, et al. Abnormal relationship between Na^+ intake and sympathetic nervous system activity in salt-sensitive patients with essential hypertension. *Kidney Int* 1982;21:371–378.

This study demonstrates the existence of an abnormal relationship between plasma norepinephrine levels and urinary sodium excretion in salt-sensitive patients with essential hypertension. This study demonstrated for the first time that high NaCl intake may raise blood pressure by activating the sympathetic nervous system.

Chalmers J, Pilowsky P. Brainstem and bulbospinal neurotransmitter systems in the control of blood pressure. *J Hypertens* 1991;9:675–694.

This is an editorial review of the brainstem and bulbospinal neurotransmitter systems that regulate blood pressure.

Furchgott RF, Zowadski JV. The obligatory role of endothelial cells in the relaxation of arterial smooth muscle by acetylcholine. *Nature* 1980;299:373–376.

This is the first demonstration that relaxation induced by acetylcholine is endothelium dependent.

Grim CE, Robinson M. Blood pressure variation in blacks: genetic factors. *Semin Nephrol* 1996;16:83–93.

In this article, Dr. Grim formulates his hypothesis of a relationship between the slave trade, salt-sensitivity, and hypertension in African-Americans.

Guyton AC. Dominant role of kidney and accessory role of whole-body autoregulation in the pathogenesis of hypertension. *Am J Hypertens* 1989;2:575–585.

This article reviews the theory of Guyton supporting a key role of the kidney in the pathogenesis of hypertension.

Kurokawa K. Tubuloglomerular feedback: its physiological and pathophysiological significance. *Kidney Int* 1998;54(Suppl 67):S71–S74.

This article reviews the experimental evidence supporting a derangement of the tubuloglomerular feedback mechanism in the pathogenesis of hypertension.

Ye S, Gamburd M, Mozayeni P, et al. A limited renal injury may cause a permanent form of neurogenic hypertension. *Am J Hypertens* 1998;11:723–728.

These studies have shown that a limited renal injury to one kidney caused by intrarenal injection of phenol may raise blood pressure permanently and this is associated with increased sympathetic nervous system activity.

CHAPTER 60

Genetics of Hypertension

Giuseppe Bianchi and Daniele Cusi

A long series of genetic epidemiologic studies have demonstrated the importance of genetic factors in causing primary or essential hypertension. However, many problems have to be addressed when trying to establish a cause-and-effect relationship between a given genetic polymorphism and essential hypertension. These problems may be grouped into three categories:

(a) *Hypertension is caused by many genes with locus heterogeneity or inheritance that is polygenic or oligogenic.* Although there is general agreement that essential hypertension is caused by many genes, two alternatives are possible. Different forms of essential hypertension share only the same final phenotype but have different pathogenetic genetic-molecular mechanisms. In this case, only one of the many possible mutated genes is needed to express the disease, as in the case of monogenic forms of hypertension. Alternatively, more than one gene with at least one deleterious allele must be simultaneously present in an individual to cause essential hypertension. In the first case, we are dealing with locus heterogeneity, whereas in the second case, we are dealing with polygenic or oligogenic inheritance. Both alternatives may be true for essential hypertension, although it is highly likely that it is polygenic and heterogeneous. In other words, the phenotype is determined by allelic variation at more than one gene at a time. Moreover, different sets of allelic variation of different genes may cause a similar final phenotype. To further complicate the picture, multigenic inheritance may be additive or epistatic. For example, the effect of a given mutation may be added to or subtracted from that of another mutation (additive), or when the mutation of interest is inherited with a mutation in another gene, a synergistic effect either positive or negative may occur—that is, the effect of the two mutations is larger than the sum of the individual mutations (epistatic).

(b) *Environmental factors.* The environment can alter the sequence of events that lead from the primary DNA mutation to the final blood pressure level acting at all the different levels of biologic organization. Therefore when assessing the role of a given genetic polymorphism, the environment must be defined in order to obtain biologically meaningful and comparable data.

(c) *Compensatory factors.* No biologic function operates in a closed system so that any malfunctioning protein may influence (induce or inhibit) transcription of other proteins, which, in turn, may have an effect on blood pressure, so the pathogenic mutation of any gene may be obscured by the redundancy of compensatory mechanisms and the disease phenotype may be determined only by compensatory overexpression or inhibition of another gene whose DNA sequence is indeed normal. Therefore the effect of a given genetic polymorphism must be assessed within the framework of the other genes whose products interact with the protein coded by the gene of interest. In genetic terms, this means that one needs to evaluate all the possible epistatic interactions, as suggested previously.

Although the complexity of the picture may appear discouraging because of the large number of potential candidate genes and possible confounding interactions among the many physiologic and/or biochemical mechanisms that affect blood pressure, only relatively few are involved in its long-term control. Whatever the initiating event, some alteration in kidney function must occur to produce a permanent blood pressure increase. Guyton called this phenomenon the *overriding role of the kidney on blood pressure control.* Other findings on the genetics of monogenic forms of hypertension seem to support this notion. Indeed, the few genes thus far found to be associated with blood pressure regulation in humans are all directly or indirectly involved in the renal control of sodium balance (Fig. 60.1). This does not, of course, exclude the possibility that other genetic defects operating through nonrenal mechanisms may be discovered in the future, but it underlines the importance of the renal genetic-molecular mechanisms of essential hypertension. This importance is also supported by the overwhelming amount of data, collected over a period of more than 30 years, that deal with the crucial interaction between body sodium and the renin-angiotensin-aldosterone system in determining the final level of blood pressure and kidney function. Careful studies of sodium handling by the kidney, the renin-angiotensin-aldosterone system, the pressor response to sodium load or depletion, or other aspects of renal function under different experimental conditions may help to cluster hypertensive patients into discrete subgroups whose members should all have the same more clearly identifiable renal genetic-molecular mechanisms. This consideration underlines the crucial role that the clinical and experimental nephrologist may play in clarifying the pathogenetic mechanisms of essential hypertension.

MONOGENIC FORMS OF HUMAN HYPERTENSION

Monogenic forms of human hypertension are very rare syndromes in which mutations in single genes are sufficient to produce large blood pressure changes. Although the majority of patients have essential forms of hypertension, a brief description of monogenic forms of hypertension is included in this section because knowledge of these forms may provide new insights into blood pressure regulation.

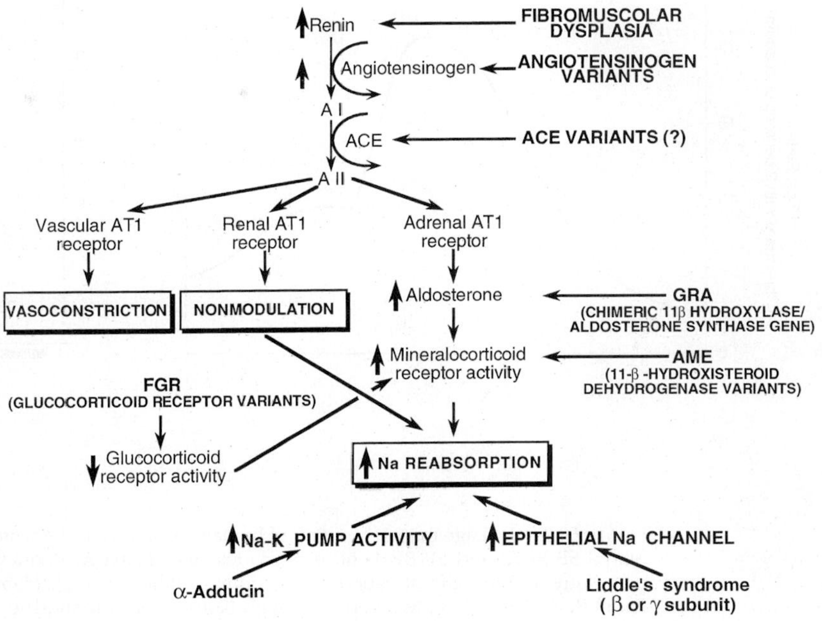

Figure 60.1. Most of the known genetic polymorphisms involved in both monogenic forms of hypertension or primary hypertension affect a sequence of events leading to an increase of renal tubular reabsorption or renal vascular resistances. In other words, the concept of the pressure natriuresis mechanism as the crucial component of the "overriding role of the kidney in blood pressure control" is strengthened by the recent findings on genetics of hypertension. AME, apparent mineralocorticoid excess; FGR, familial glucocorticoid resistance; GRA, glucocorticoid remediable aldosteronism. For details see text. (Modified from Lifton RP. Molecular genetics of human blood pressure variation. *Science* 1996; 272:676–680.)

Liddle's Syndrome

Liddle's syndrome is an autosomal-dominant form of salt-sensitive hypertension characterized by early onset, hypokalemia, and low renin and aldosterone levels. It can be treated by salt restriction and amiloride, the selective inhibitor of the epithelial Na channel. A linkage study in Liddle's original pedigree demonstrated linkage to a segment of chromosome 16 containing two genes, the β and γ subunits of the epithelial Na channel, which were considered plausible candidates because sodium reabsorption through this channel is one of the major determinants of tubular sodium reabsorption. Different mutations causing truncation of the cytoplasmic C-terminus of the β or γ subunit have subsequently been described as responsible for Liddle's syndrome in different pedigrees. In all cases, premature truncation of the cytoplasmic C-terminus of either the β or γ subunit results in constitutive activation of the channel (i.e., loss of normal negative regulation of the channel, and hence increased net renal sodium reabsorption). The critical role of the epithelial Na channel in maintaining salt and extracellular fluid balance and controlling blood pressure is confirmed by the finding of different mutations in both the α and β subunits, either of which cause pseudohypoaldosteronism type I, a rare autosomal-recessive disease characterized by neonatal salt wasting, low blood pressure, hyperkalemia, and metabolic acidosis. Sodium is lost as the mutations cause a striking decrease of the opening time of the Na channel (and hence of the sodium reabsorption).

Pseudohypoaldosteronism Type II, or Gordon's Syndrome

Pseudohypoaldosteronism type II is another rare form of dominant familial hypertension with low renin, high serum K, normal glomerular filtration rate, and good response to salt restriction and/or thiazide diuretic treatment. Linkage analysis demonstrated locus heterogeneity, with significant linkage to chromosome 17q21 in some families, which is syntenic with a segment of rat chromosome 10 that contains at least one or two blood pressure QTLs. Interestingly, the locus is also in linkage with essential hypertension (Fig. 60.2).

Apparent Mineralocorticoid Excess

Apparent mineralocorticoid excess (AME) is an autosomal-recessive form of hypertension, phenotypically similar to Liddle's syndrome (low renin and low aldosterone levels) but responsive to mineralocorticoid (type 1) receptor inhibition by spironolactone. Different mutations in the gene of the 11β-hydroxysteroid dehydrogenase kidney isozyme cause different degrees of loss of function of the enzyme. The kidney isozyme of 11β-hydroxysteroid dehydrogenase is expressed in distal and cortical collecting tubules, where the mineralocorticoid receptor is also present. It converts cortisol to cortisone, which has no mineralocorticoid activity, at the prereceptor level. When the enzymatic activity is defective, normal circulating cortisol can thus produce a large mineralocorticoid effect by direct stimulation of the mineralocorticoid receptor. Due to the enzyme defect, affected patients have an elevated urinary tetrahydrocortisol plus allo-tetrahydrocortisol to tetrahydrocortisone ratio. A case of a heterozygous hypertensive father of an affected homozygous proband has been described in a Brazilian kindred. The interest of this case is that the father, who also has an altered urinary steroid ratio, had previously been defined as having essential hypertension although with low renin and aldosterone levels and suboptimal response to conventional antihypertensive treatment (diuretics and β-blockers). The urinary steroid ratio has also been reported as abnormal in some essential hypertensive individuals, therefore it is possible that subtle defects in 11β-hydroxysteroid dehydrogenase activity play some role also in essential hypertension.

Glucocorticoid Remediable Aldosteronism

Glucocorticoid remediable aldosteronism (GRA) is an autosomal-dominant form of hypertension with low renin but high aldosterone levels, whose secretion is controlled by adrenocorticotropic

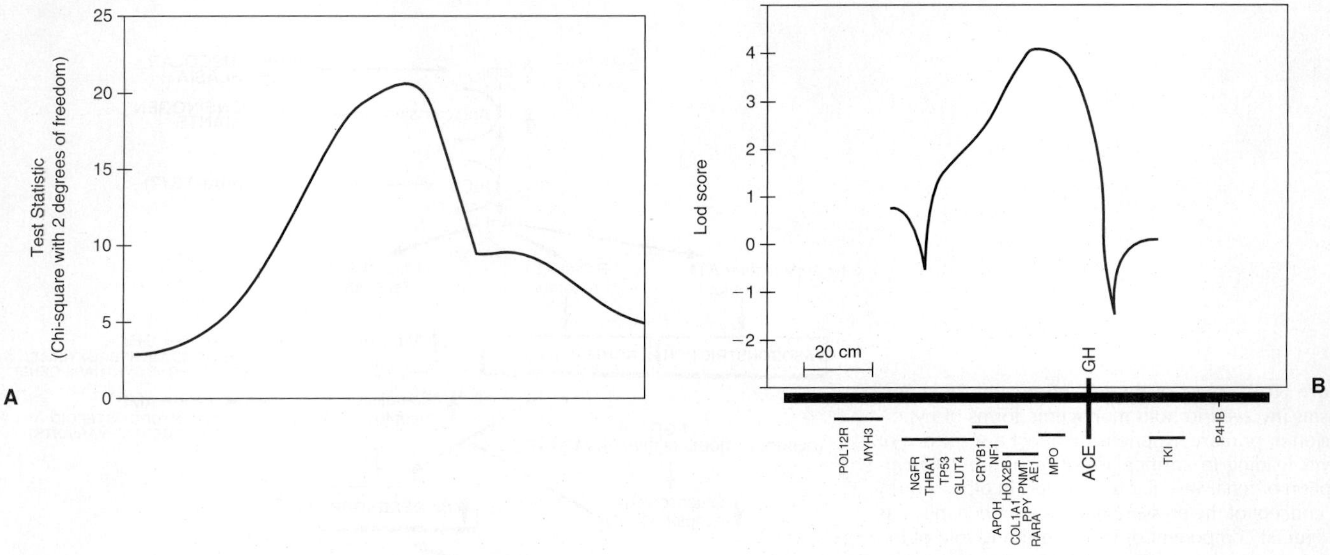

Figure 60.2. Linkage map of a region of human chromosome 17 syntenic to that of rat chromosome 10, where SP-BP1a and SP-BP1b have been detected. **Panel A:** Redrawn and simplified from a sibling-pair study in 518 pairs of hypertensive siblings. (Julier C. et al. *Hum Mol Genet* 1997;6:2077–2085). **Panel B:** Redrawn from two pedigrees with Gordon's syndrome. The symbols on the X axis refer to the genes identified in the region (Mansfield TA, et al. *Nature Genet* 1997;16:202–205).

hormone (ACTH) and not by angiotensin II. The disease is caused by unequal crossing-over of chromosome 8 between the aldosterone synthase and 11β-hydroxylase genes, which are tightly linked. The crossing-over produces a novel "chimeric" gene, which contains the proximal (regulatory) sequence of 11β-hydroxylase and the distal (coding) sequence of aldosterone synthase. In this way the chimeric gene is under the control of ACTH but its gene product has aldosterone synthase activity.

GENETICS AND PATHOGENESIS OF PRIMARY HYPERTENSION

For a long time, research for the pathogenetic mechanisms of primary hypertension focused only on the search for biochemical and physiologic differences between hypertensive and normotensive humans or between spontaneously hypertensive rats and their respective normotensive control strains. Many differences were found and many biochemical and physiologic mechanisms for hypertension have been proposed. Probably much of that work did not yield meaningful conclusions. In the case of humans, the population of hypertensives is too heterogeneous and, in the case of rats, many of the observed differences between hypertensive and control strains were simply due to chance selection and fixation of specific biochemical and physiologic traits, rather than real causal differences relevant to the pathogenesis of hypertension. Genetic approaches are indispensable for detecting primary pathogenetic mechanisms both in animals or humans with primary, or essential, forms of hypertension. With the various approaches many, relatively short (containing from 50 to 200 genes) DNA segments have been shown to be involved in animal primary hypertension. Almost all chromosomes contain at least one of this DNA segment. In humans a long list of candidate genes has been studied with variable results, particularly with the case-control method in association studies. An allele B at a given locus is said to be associated to hypertension if it occurs at a significantly higher frequency among hypertensives compared with normotensives. This method has many drawbacks. Differences in population stratification between cases and controls may be an important cause of variability because the frequency of a given allele at a given locus may vary in the different populations independently from hypertension.

As mentioned previously, differences between cases and controls in the allelic distribution of other genes with additive or epistatic interaction with the gene of interest may either enhance or blunt the differences we are looking for in the allele of the gene of interest. For instance, as compared with the other alleles, if an allele B of a gene involved in renal Na handling favors hypertension by increasing renal sodium retention for any given level of the other genetic or environmental factors affecting this renal function, this effect must be evaluated by taking into account all of these factors including the epistatic interactions with the other genes affecting renal Na handling. In fact, in large pedigrees of GRA monogenic hypertension it is possible to find individuals with the mutated allele but without hypertension. The results of more than 8-year studies have weakened the hope of finding a candidate gene with such an overwhelming influence on blood pressure control that could be detected in all the population studies independently from the difference in the other genes or environmental factors affecting its function. With current knowledge of these limitations, variants (or alleles) of the angiotensinogen, angiotensin-converting enzyme (ACE), and adducin genes seem to contribute to the genetic component of hypertension in humans. For these last two genes, at least one positive linkage study and two association studies in independent populations gave positive results, even though the published data describing an association between ACE or adducin genotype and hypertension are as numerous as those that have not found such an association. As discussed previously, many problems weaken the biologic significance of association studies. The role of a given polymorphism in causing a polygenic disease such as hypertension must be assessed through a complex strategy involving five independent groups of approaches:

1. Genetic animal models, appropriate to evaluate the relationship between the polymorphism of interest and blood pressure
2. Pathophysiologic link between the altered gene product and the sequence of events leading to hypertension
3. The effect of the pharmacologic blockade on this sequence
4. All the methods of statistical genetics aimed at the genetic dissection of the complex traits and the association studies is only the most weak type of these methods
5. Epistatic interaction with the gene polymorphisms whose products modulate the gene product of interest.

At present, only for angiotensinogen and α-adducin, positive results in all five approaches have been provided even though some of them have been presented only at scientific meetings and not yet published in full papers, therefore caution is mandatory.

Relation Between Genetics and Pathophysiologic Mechanism of Hypertension

The mechanism linking the variants of the aforementioned genes (angiotensinogen, ACE, and adducin) to primary hypertension or its organ complication are still open for discussion. Discussion of the proposed mechanisms thus far follows. The mutated allele of angiotensinogen is in linkage disequilibrium with a mutation within the promoter region that produces an increased level of plasma angiotensinogen, which, in turn, may raise blood pressure by increasing the levels of angiotensin II. For the mutated (D for deletion) allele of ACE, the pathophysiologic link is even more controversial because the suggestion that the D allele is associated to higher plasma and tissue levels of ACE, which in turn favors higher tissue levels of angiotensin II, has been disputed. For the cytoskeleton protein adducin, the pressor mechanism is related to renal handling of Na, in line with a growing body of experimental evidences showing an involvement of cytoskeleton proteins in the regulation of cellular Na transport.

In the Milan strain of rats, which develop a primary form of hypertension, the mutated allele of α-adducin seems to increase tubular Na reabsorption for any given level of all of the other factors affecting this function by enhancing the overall Na^+-K^+ pump activity in the basolateral plasma membrane. In humans, a missense mutation on α-adducin is associated with and linked to hypertension, at least in some cohorts. When compared with patients with the wild allele, hypertensive patients carrying the mutated allele display a less steep pressure natriuresis curve (i.e., a higher blood pressure is needed to excrete the same amount of sodium) together with greater fall in blood pressure after acute sodium depletion or chronic diuretic treatment. The findings in rats and in humans point to the same genetic renal mechanism in two species that diverged almost 40 million years ago.

Clinical Implications of Genetic Studies

The main characteristic of primary or essential hypertension is heterogeneity in terms of organ complications, response to therapy, and underlying genetic mechanisms. Due to such heterogeneity, it is not possible to say whether a given patient, with recent onset of hypertension, will develop organ complication later in life or will respond to a given drug or to a given dietary change such as a reduction of dietary sodium intake. The understanding of the genetic mechanisms of hypertension, including the appropriate epistatic interaction, is the only approach that will give us a clear solution to this problem. In this regard, studies with adducin polymorphism, including its interaction with ACE genotype, furnish interesting results. The fall in blood pressure on diuretics is greater in patients with the "mutated" variants of α-adducin than in patients with the "normal" variant. Also the rise in blood pressure after Na load is greater in patients with mutated adducin, and the inclusion of ACE genotype in the analysis allows better separation of responders and nonresponders to this treatment. Further explorations are needed before the results of these studies can be applied to day-to-day practice; however, they constitute a promising approach. The influence of ACE genotype on organ complication is also an important area with promising results. Even though conclusive data on the genetics of cardiac complication in hypertension are not available, the demonstration on an association between ACE D/D genotype and myocardial infarction or greater increase in cardiac mass after exercise may be taken as a clear suggestion that the variability in cardiac response to pressure overload may be caused, at least in part, by a genetic component, and ACE genotype may be a part of it.

Acknowledgments

This work was supported in part by Ministero Universitê Ricerca Scientifica of Italy (ex MPI 60% years 1993–1996 to Daniele Cusi and Giuseppe Bianchi; ex MPI 40% years 1993–1996 to Daniele Cusi) and by Telethon grant E.C516.

Selected Readings

Barlassina C, et al. Synergistic effect of α-adducin and ACE genes causes blood pressure changes with body sodium and volume expansion. *Kidney Int* 2000; 57:1083–1090.

Cusi D, et al. α-Adducin polymorphism in primary hypertension: linkage and association study; relationship to salt sensitivity. *Lancet* 1997;349:1353–1357.

The results of both linkage and association studies are consistent with a role of adducin in human primary hypertension; moreover in patients with "mutated" adducin the blood pressure fall after acute or chronic reduction of body sodium is greater than in patients with "wild" adducin.

Guyton AC, et al. The dominant role of the kidneys in the long-term regulation of arterial pressure in normal and hypertensive states. In: Laragh JH, Brenner BM, eds. *Hypertension: pathophysiology, diagnosis and management*. New York: Raven Press, 1990:1029–1052.

An analysis of the most significant experimental data on the relationship between the factors involved in renal Na and H_2O excretion, blood pressure, and body fluids regulation, with the aim of enlightening the most significant mechanism controlling the set point of blood pressure and renal Na excretion.

Jeunemaitre X, et al. Molecular basis of human hypertension: role of angiotensinogen. *Cell* 1992;71:169–180.

The first clear demonstration of the role of the mutation within the angiotensinogen gene as a possible cause of "primary" form of hypertension.

Julier C, et al. Genetic susceptibility for human familial essential hypertension in a region of homology with blood pressure linkage on rat chromosome 10. *Hum Mol Genet* 1997;6:2077–2085.

This study shows the involvement in human blood pressure regulation of some genes mapping within a short segment of human chromosome 17, which is syntenic to the rat chromosome 10 region previously shown to be involved in genetic rat hypertension.

Lander ES, Schorl NJ. Genetic dissection of complex traits. *Science* 1994;265: 2037–2045.

A comprehensive review that discusses all of the possible approaches to the genetic dissection of a complex trait, such as hypertension, from the view point of statistical genetics.

Lifton RP. Molecular genetics of human blood pressure variation. *Science* 1996;272: 676–680.

A concise review of the most significant findings in monogenic forms of hypertension that points to the genetic alteration of tubular sodium reabsorption or of renal circulation as possible causes of both rare forms of hypertension with some abnormalities of plasma electrolytes or the renin-angiotensin-aldosterone system or other not yet well-defined forms of "primary" hypertension in which no electrolytes or hormonal abnormalities are present.

Lifton RP, et al. A chimaeric 11 beta-hydroxylase/aldosterone synthase gene causes glucocorticoid-remediable aldosteronism and human hypertension. *Nature* 1992;1355:262–265.

A brilliant genetic explanation of hypertension accompanied by a form of glucocorticoid-remediable aldosteronism.

Mansfield TA, et al. Multilocus linkage of familial hyperkalaemia and hypertension, pseudohypoaldosteronism type II, to chromosomes 1q31-42 and 17p11-q21. *Nature Genet* 1997;16:202–205.

The first description of the genetic cause of familial hyperkalemia and hypertension.

Manunta P, et al. α-Adducin polymorphism and renal sodium handling in essential hypertensive patients. *Kidney Int* 1998;53:1471–1478.

Demonstration that patients with "mutated" adducin need a higher renal perfusion pressure to excrete the same amount of Na than patients with "wild" adducin.

Mune T, et al. Human hypertension caused by mutations in the kidney isozyme of 11B-hydroxysteroid dehydrogenase. *Nat Genet* 1995;10:394–399.

The first description of a genetic defect in the 11β-hydroxysteroid dehydrogenase responsible for a type of hypertension associated with hypokalemia.

Shimkets RA, et al. Liddle's syndrome: heritable human hypertension caused by mutations in the β subunit of the epithelial sodium channel. *Cell* 1994;79: 407–414.

The first description of the genetic cause of Liddle's syndrome.

Soubrier F. Blood pressure gene at the angiotensin I-converting enzyme locus. Chronicle of a gene foretold. *Circulation* 1998;97:1763–1765.

The controversy about the role of angiotensin-converting enzyme polymorphism in hypertension is summarized in this editorial.

CHAPTER 61

Essential Hypertension

PART 1
Clinical Aspects of Essential Hypertension and its Management

George L. Bakris

DEFINITION AND MEASUREMENT OF BLOOD PRESSURE

Although the distribution of blood pressure in the general population adheres to a Bell curve, the association with fatal and nonfatal cardiovascular diseases, including stroke, renal disease, and ischemic heart disease, follows a linear distribution by blood pressure level. Significant increases in cardiovascular events start to occur at blood pressure levels greater than or equal to 140/90 mm Hg. Thus hypertension is defined by the Joint National Committee Report VI (JNC VI) as a systolic blood pressure of 140 mm Hg or greater or a diastolic blood pressure of 90 mm Hg or greater in anyone on or off antihypertensive medication.

The classification of blood pressure in adults ages 18 and older is summarized in Table 61.1. These definitions are obtained from the most recent JNC VI report on the prevention, detection, evaluation, and treatment of high blood pressure. It is clear from this report that blood pressure levels of even 130/85 mm Hg suggests that a person has the potential for developing hypertension and may, if elevated pressure is sustained, develop some degree of end-organ injury.

Hypertension detection begins with proper blood pressure measurements that should be obtained at each physician or nurse encounter. Repeated blood pressure measurements will determine whether initial elevations in blood pressure persist and require prompt attention.

Blood pressure should be measured using equipment that meets certification criteria and with proper technique. The following techniques for measuring blood pressure are recommended.

(a) Patients should be seated, with bare arms and both their backs and arms supported at heart level.
(b) Measurements should begin after a 5-minute rest period. The practice of having patients come in and rest for 30 minutes in a darkened room or other such procedures should be *avoided*. This procedure will not yield a blood pressure reflective of a patient's everyday activities.
(c) In diabetic patients and those with neurologic disorders, both supine and standing pressures should be obtained. This is also important in patients in whom you suspect volume depletion.
(d) The most important factor is to ensure that cuff size is appropriate. The bladder within the cuff should encircle at least 80% of the arm. Many adults will require a large cuff.
(e) Using a cuff that is too small will give you a *falsely elevated* blood pressure. Blood pressure measurements should be taken preferentially with a mercury sphygmomanometer. Home blood pressures using a calibrated aneroid or validated electronic device may be used to compare blood pressure readings with those in the office.
(f) The first appearance of a sound (phase 1) should be used to define systolic blood pressure. Total disappearance of the sound (phase 5) should be used to define diastolic blood pressure.
(g) To ensure accuracy of blood pressure measurements, two or more readings separated by at least 2 minutes should be averaged. If the first two readings differ by more than 5 mm Hg, additional readings should be obtained and averaged.

TABLE 61.1. Classification of Blood Pressure for Adults Age 18 and Older[a]

Category	Systolic (mm Hg)		Diastolic (mm Hg)
Optimal[b]	<120	and	<80
Normal	<130	and	<85
High-normal	130–139	or	85–89
Hypertension[c]			
Stage 1	140–159	or	90–99
Stage 2	160–179	or	100–109
Stage 3	>180	or	>110

[a] Not taking antihypertensive drugs and not acutely ill. In addition to classifying stages of hypertension on the basis of average blood pressure levels, clinicians should specify presence or absence of target organ disease and additional risk factors.

[b] Optimal blood pressure with respect to cardiovascular risk is below 120/80 mm Hg. However, unusually low readings should be evaluated for clinical significance.

[c] Based on the average of two or more readings taken at each of two or more visits after an initial screening.

Adapted from the Joint National Committee Report on the Diagnosis and Treatment of Hypertension (JNC VI). *Arch Intern Med* 1997;157:2413–2446.

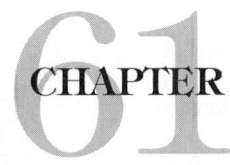

There are certain conditions in which blood pressure values may be incongruous with the clinical milieu of the patient. The three most prominent conditions are bilateral subclavian artery stenosis, pseudohypertension, and "white-coat" hypertension.

Bilateral subclavian artery stenosis is an extremely rare condition, but should be suspected in anyone with normal blood pressure values bilaterally who has clear evidence of ischemic heart disease with other physical findings of systemic hypertension such as retinopathy or peripheral vascular disease. An additional aid to help distinguish this diagnosis from unilateral stenosis is to measure the circumference of the arms. If one arm has a normal blood pressure and the other is markedly elevated, the diagnosis of unilateral subclavian artery stenosis should be suspected.

Pseudohypertension is a diagnosis that should be suspected in elderly patients. The definition of pseudohypertension is the measurement, by blood pressure cuff, of a substantially elevated arterial pressure with intraarterial measurements that are relatively normal. A way to distinguish this problem is by use of the Osler maneuver. This maneuver consists of inflating the blood pressure cuff well above the measured systolic blood pressure. When this is done, the brachial and radial arteries remain palpable. Obviously, this should not occur under normal circumstances. Thus if this occurs, the maneuver is considered positive and it indicates that the cuff method is overestimating the true intraarterial pressure.

The third and last confounder for blood pressure measurement is the "white-coat syndrome" or white-coat hypertension. White-coat hypertension was initially thought to be a benign condition not associated with a higher cardiovascular risk. Long-term studies, however, demonstrate that this group manifests an intermediate degree of target-organ injury between normotensive and hypertensive patients. Specifically, this group of individuals has a greater degree of left ventricular hypertrophy, microalbuminuria, and retinopathy in comparison with normotensive individuals, but less than individuals with established hypertension. This diagnosis should be suspected in patients who have no obvious evidence, on either physical examination or history, of cardiovascular disease but who have high arterial pressures in an office setting with normal arterial pressures at home.

Two methods of ruling out white-coat hypertension should be employed. These include: (a) 24-hour blood pressure monitoring or (b) a comparison between home and office blood pressure readings. If a discrepancy of more than 10 mm Hg diastolic or 20 mm Hg systolic is noted, a clear diagnosis of white-coat hypertension should be made. In this circumstance, if patients have an average blood pressure of more than 130/85 mm Hg in an outpatient setting, they should be strongly encouraged to modify their lifestyle, especially if they are under very high stress conditions. If this is not possible, biofeedback or psychologic stress management should be strongly encouraged to help these individuals reduce their arterial pressure. Evidence from small, uncontrolled studies has suggested that these techniques reduce blood pressure levels and reduce the large fluctuations in pressures seen on an outpatient basis. It should be noted, however, that at least two large studies demonstrated that patients with white-coat hypertension do not necessarily have blood pressure elevations in other "real life" stress situations.

EPIDEMIOLOGY

The National Health and Nutrition Examination Survey started in 1976 to assess the percentage of Americans who are aware that they have high blood pressure. Moreover, they assessed who was receiving treatment and, further, who actually achieved adequate blood pressure control, defined as a blood pressure of less than 140/90 mm Hg. The results have been resoundingly disappointing. Despite 25 years of Joint National Committee recommendations for the assessment, treatment, and diagnosis of hypertension, only 27% of individuals being treated for hypertension have actually achieved blood pressure control. This is a relatively small percentage of patients considering that hypertension is present in more than 50 million Americans.

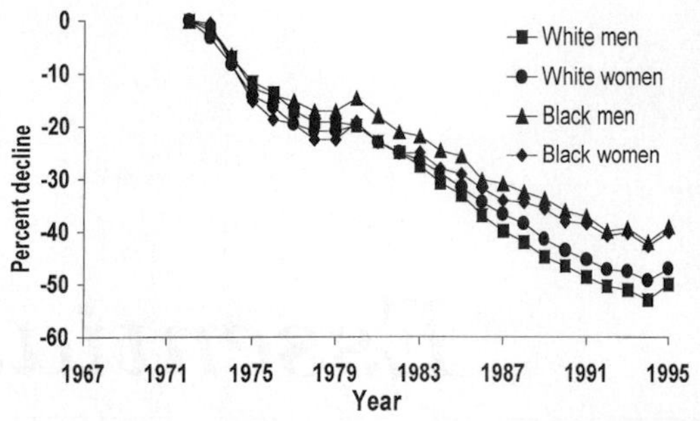

Figure 61.1. The age-adjusted rates of coronary heart disease in the United States over the past 25 years.

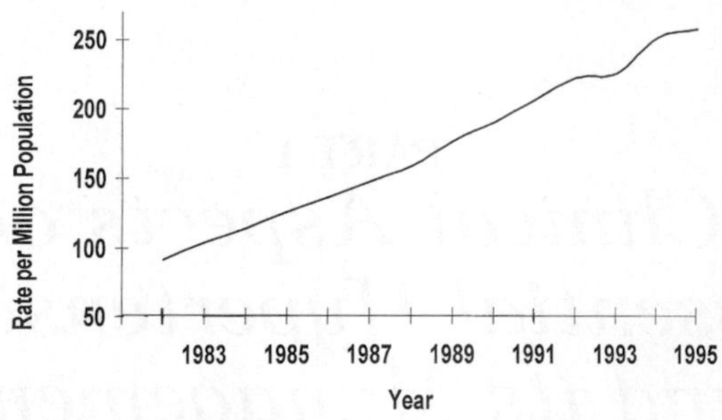

Figure 61.2. The age-adjusted rates of new end-stage renal disease cases over the past 25 years.

The good news, however, is that the number of patients controlled to levels below 140/90 mm Hg has increased from 10% to 27% over the last 2 decades. These changes have contributed to dramatic reductions in cardiovascular morbidity and mortality attributed to hypertension (Fig. 61.1). This benefit, however, has not been as dramatic as it may appear. Since 1992, the age-adjusted stroke rates have been rising slightly and the slope of age-adjusted decline in coronary heart disease events has also reached a plateau (Fig. 61.1). Furthermore, incidence rates for end-stage renal disease have not been significantly affected by any of these recommendations (Fig. 61.2). Further concern comes from a study in Iowa in which the average blood pressure in a cohort that has been serially evaluated and age adjusted has demonstrated an increase in the average blood pressure over time. Therefore these results indicate that although patients and physicians are putting some effort into reducing blood pressure, all this decrement is doing is reducing mortality enough to substantially increase morbidity and thus increase health-care costs.

CLINICAL EVALUATION AND FOLLOW-UP

The recommendations by the Joint National Committee for follow-up based on initial blood pressure measurements are summarized in Table 61.2. Once a diagnosis of hypertension has been established three main objectives should be clear:

TABLE 61.2. Recommendations for Follow-Up Based on Initial Blood Pressure Measurements for Adults

Systolic	Diastolic	Follow-up Recommended[b]
Initial Blood Pressure (mm Hg)[a]		
<130	<85	Recheck in 2 years
130–139	85–89	Recheck in 1 year[c]
140–159	90–99	Confirm within 2 months[c]
160–179	100–109	Evaluate or refer to source of care within 1 month
≥180	≥110	Evaluate or refer to source of care immediately or within 1 week depending on clinical situation

[a] If systolic and diastolic categories are different, follow recommendations for shorter time follow-up (e.g., 160/86 mm Hg should be evaluated or referred to source of care within 1 month).

[b] Modify the scheduling of follow-up according to reliable information about past blood pressure measurements, other cardiovascular risk factors, or target-organ disease.

[c] Provide advice about lifestyle modifications.

Adapted from the Joint National Committee Report on the Diagnosis and Treatment of Hypertension (JNC VI). *Arch Intern Med* 1997;157:2413–2446.

(a) Identify known causes of high blood pressure. (b) Assess the presence or absence of target-organ damage in the renal and cardiovascular systems to determine the response to therapy, if any. (c) Identify other cardiovascular risk factors or concomitant disorders that may define prognosis and guide treatment. The data for evaluation of these objectives are acquired through the medical history, physical examination, laboratory tests, and other diagnostic procedures.

Medical History

Factors that should be included in the medical history are summarized in Table 61.3. It is vitally important in taking a medical history from such patients that symptoms suggesting the causes of hypertension, including secondary causes, should be sought. This should include a good history for over-the-counter medications such as herbal remedies and decongestant medications, as well as nonsteroidal antiinflammatory drugs. These agents along with illicit drugs clearly increase blood pressure and, in those with high normal values, actually generate hypertension.

TABLE 61.3. Information That Must Be Sought from the Medical History

- Family history of high blood pressure, premature coronary heart disease, stroke, diabetes, dyslipidemia, or renal disease
- Known duration and levels of elevated blood pressure
- Patient history or symptoms of coronary heart disease, heart failure, cerebrovascular disease, peripheral vascular disease, renal disease, diabetes mellitus, dyslipidemia, other comorbid conditions, gout, or sexual dysfunction
- Symptoms suggesting causes of hypertension
- History of recent changes in weight, leisure-time physical activity, and smoking or other tobacco use
- Dietary assessment including intake of sodium, alcohol, saturated fat, and caffeine
- History of all prescribed and over-the-counter medications, herbal remedies, and illicit drugs, some of which may raise blood pressure or interfere with the effectiveness of antihypertensive drugs
- Psychosocial and environmental factors (e.g., family situation, employment status and working conditions, educational level) that may influence hypertension control
- Results and adverse effects of previous antihypertensive therapy

TABLE 61.4. Information That Must Be Obtained by the Physical Examination

- Two or more blood pressure measurements separated by 2 minutes with the patient either supine or seated, and after standing for at least 2 minutes in accordance with the recommended techniques mentioned previously
- Verification in the contralateral arm (if values are different, the higher value should be used)
- Measurement of height, weight, and waist circumference
- Funduscopic examination to determine hypertensive retinopathy
- Examination of the neck for carotid bruits, distended veins, or an enlarged thyroid gland
- Examination of the heart for abnormalities in rate and rhythm, increased size, precordial heave, clicks, murmurs, and third and fourth heart sounds
- Examination of the lungs for rales and evidence for bronchospasm
- Examination of the abdomen for bruits, palpable kidneys, masses, and abnormal aortic pulsation
- Examination of the extremities for diminished or absent peripheral arterial pulsations, bruits, and edema
- Neurologic assessment

Physical Examination

The most important physical findings that should be sought in a patient with hypertension are summarized in Table 61.4. The physician or health-care provider should ensure that blood pressure is the same in both arms, that the appropriate size cuff is used, and that there is no evidence of either end-organ or vascular disease.

Laboratory Tests and Diagnostic Workup

A summary of the routine and optional laboratory tests for evaluation of hypertension in a patient is summarized in Table 61.5. It should be noted that if proteinuria is present at baseline, it is vitally important to reduce proteinuria because it has been shown to not only be predictive of renal disease progression but also of mortality from cardiovascular disease. In addition, proteinuria may be a causative agent in the genesis of renal disease, especially diabetic nephropathy.

It is also well known that certain antihypertensive agents affect proteinuria to a greater degree than do others. Moreover, this antiproteinuric effect may be dependent on sodium intake.

TABLE 61.5. Laboratory Tests Required for the Evaluation of Hypertension

Basic (Essential)
Urinalysis (including microalbuminuria)[a]
Complete blood count
Blood chemistries (electrolytes, BUN, creatinine, fasting glucose, total and HDL cholesterol)
12-lead electrocardiogram
Optional
Creatinine clearance
24-hour urinary sodium and protein
Serum [Ca^{2+}], uric acid, fasting triglycerides, LDL cholesterol, HbA1c[b], thyroid-stimulating hormone, limited echocardiography (for left ventricular hypertrophy assessment), plasma renin

[a] Spot urine for microalbuminuria or protein/creatinine value.

[b] Should be performed in everyone who is obese and suspected of diabetes

BUN, blood urea nitrogen; HDL, high-density lipoprotein; LDL, low-density lipoprotein.

Therefore urinary sodium should be included in a spot urinalysis for microalbuminuria in the basic workup of these patients.

IDENTIFIABLE CAUSES OF HYPERTENSION

Medically treatable causes of hypertension are listed in Table 61.6. In addition to these, a number of secondary causes of hypertension are also listed in this table, most of which require surgical intervention. These include primary hyperparathyroidism, pheochromocytoma, either adrenal adenomas or bilateral adrenal hyperplasia leading to primary aldosteronism, Cushing syndrome, congenital adrenal hyperplasia, and enzyme defect such as 11-β-hydroxylase. Finally, the most common surgically treatable causes of secondary hypertension are renal vascular disorders. These include renal arterial disease and atherosclerotic disease. These secondary causes are covered in other chapters in this book and will not be discussed in this chapter.

TABLE 61.6. Treatable Causes of Hypertension

I. Primary (essential)
II. Renal
  A. Parenchymal diseases
    1. Diabetic nephropathy
    2. Glomerulonephritis
    3. Pyelonephritis
    4. Tubulointerstitial nephritis, lead nephropathy
    5. Acute tubular necrosis?
    6. Cystic diseases
    7. Nephrocalcinosis
    8. Neoplasms
    9. Radiation nephritis
    10. Renal trauma
  B. Obstructive uropathies[a]
  C. Renin-secreting tumors[a] (Hemangiopericytoma, Wilms', renal cell, pancreatic, or ovarian tumors)
  D. Renovascular diseases
III. Aortic diseases
  A. Coarctation[a]
  B. Takayasu's arteritis[a]
  C. Atherosclerosis (systolic hypertension of the elderly)
IV. Adrenal
  A. Pheochromocytoma[a]
  B. Primary aldosteronism (bilateral adrenal hyperplasia)
  C. Cushing's syndrome[a]
  D. Congenital adrenal hyperplasia[a] (defects of 11β-hydroxylase or 17α-hydroxylase
V. Other endocrine disorders
  A. Obesity
  B. Insulin resistance/hyperinsulinemia
  C. Thyrotoxicosis
  D. Hypothyroidism
  E. Hypercalcemia
  F. Primary hyperparathyroidism[a]
  G. Acromegaly
  H. Carcinoid syndrome
VI. Neurogenic
  A. Excessive stress, psychogenic
  B. Increased intracranial pressure
  C. Cerebrovascular accidents
  D. Encephalitis, Guillain-Barré syndrome
  E. Autonomic hyperreflexia associated with cord injury, polio
VII. Toxemia of pregnancy
VIII. Drugs
  A. Oral contraceptives
  B. Alcohol abuse
  C. Glucocorticoid therapies
  D. Cocaine, nonsteroidal antiinflammatory agents (NSAIDs)
  E. Black licorice (glycyrrhizic acid), Florinef
  F. Sympathomimetics used as decongestants, amphetamines
  G. MAO inhibitors in combination with tyramine-containing foods
  H. Tricyclic antidepressants
IX. Other causes
  A. Sleep apnea
  B. Acute intermittant porphyria

[a] Indicates surgical intervention is usually required.

GENETICS OF HYPERTENSION

Blood pressure levels are correlated among family members, a fact attributable to common genetic background, shared environment, or lifestyle habits. The transmission of high blood pressure appears to be polygenic and does not follow classic Mendelian rules. A few rare forms of hypertension are exceptions to this rule, including a chimeric 11-β-hydroxylase/aldosterone synthase gene.

A number of potential candidate genes have been implicated in the genesis of hypertension, including the angiotensin-converting enzyme (ACE) gene and genes involving the kallikrein-kinin and the sympathetic nervous systems.

CARDIOVASCULAR RISK STRATIFICATION

A number of risk factors are associated with the presence of hypertension that confer an increase in cardiovascular risk. These are summarized in Table 61.7. These factors independently modify the risk of subsequent cardiovascular events and development of renal disease in persons with hypertension. Based on this assessment in concert with laboratory findings at a given blood pressure level, risk stratification and treatment as recommended by the JNC VI should be employed. These recommendations are summarized in Table 61.8. The reader will note in this table that anyone with evidence of target-organ disease or clinical cardiovascular disease, defined as angina or heart failure, should automatically be treated with antihypertensive medications.

TABLE 61.7. Components of Cardiovascular Risk Stratification in Patients with Hypertension

Major Risk Factors
Smoking
Dyslipidemia
Diabetes mellitus
Age older than 60 years
Sex (men and postmenopausal women)
Family history of cardiovascular disease: women under age 65 or men under age 55
Target-Organ Damage/Clinical Cardiovascular Disease
Left ventricular hypertrophy
Angina/prior myocardial infarction
Prior coronary revascularization
Heart failure
Stroke or transient ischemic attack
Nephropathy
Peripheral arterial disease
Retinopathy

TABLE 61.8. Risk Stratification and Treatment in Patients with Hypertension[a]

Blood Pressure Stages (mm Hg)	Risk Group A (No Risk Factors; No TOD/CCD)	Risk Group B (At Least One Risk Factor Not Including Diabetes; No TOD/CCD)	Risk Group C (TOD/CCD and/or Diabetes, With or Without Other Risk Factors)
High-normal (130–139/85–89)	Lifestyle modification	Lifestyle modification	Drug therapy[c]
Stage 1 (140–159/90–99)	Lifestyle modification (up to 12 months)	Lifestyle modification[b] (up to 6 months)	Drug therapy
Stages 2 and 3 (≥160/≥100)	Drug therapy	Drug therapy	Drug therapy

[a] Lifestyle modification should be adjunctive therapy for all patients recommended for pharmacologic therapy.
[b] For patients with multiple risk factors, clinicians should consider drugs as initial therapy plus lifestyle modifications.
[c] For those with heart failure, renal insufficiency, or diabetes.
CCD, clinical cardiovascular disease; TOD, target-organ disease.

TARGET-ORGAN INJURY (TABLE 61.9)

It is clear that most markers of target-organ injury are, in fact, surrogate markers and their management may potentiate the benefit obtained from the control of hypertension in the reduction in either cardiac or renal mortality. Specifically, reductions in arterial pressure and proteinuria are associated with a reduction in cardiovascular mortality and, in the case of proteinuria, slowed renal disease progression. However, it has been widely assumed that blood pressure reduction alone confers the major benefit on mortality reduction and it was further assumed that reductions in these surrogate markers of cardiovascular risk are not necessarily required to reduce risk for mortality. However, evidence suggests that although blood pressure control certainly does confer a major benefit with regard to cardiovascular mortality reduction, the benefit obtained through additional reduction in proteinuria or left ventricular hypertrophy potentiate the reduction seen in mortality. This section presents a brief overview of the data supporting these observations.

There is no question that reduction in arterial pressure, regardless of the antihypertensive agents used, generates a clear and absolute benefit, in that it reduces the incidence of strokes. This is not as obvious when one looks at the outcome of ischemic heart disease. There have been many secondary prevention trials in patients, following myocardial infarction, documenting a clear reduction in mortality with most antihypertensive agents. No randomized, double-blind, placebo-controlled trial, however, has documented a reduction in mortality from ischemic heart disease with a dihydropyridine calcium antagonist. Interestingly, this subclass of antihypertensive agents does not reduce proteinuria. Therefore simply reducing blood pressure does not necessarily translate into a maximum benefit in the reduction of cardiovascular events.

TABLE 61.9. Manifestations of Target-Organ Disease in Patients with Hypertension

Organ System	Manifestations
Cerebrovascular	Transient ischemic attack or stroke
Cardiovascular	Clinical, electrocardiographic, or radiologic or coronary heart disease; myocardial infarction
Peripheral vascular	Absence of one or more major pulses in the extremities (except for dorsalis pedis) with or without intermittent claudication; abdominal
Renal	Serum creatinine ≥130 μmol/L (1.4 mg/dl); microalbuminuria (>30mg/day) or proteinuria (≥300 mg/day)
Retinopathy	Grade 1: vascular spasm (vein/artery ratio >3.2) Grade 2: arteriolar narrowing and arteriovenous nicking Grade 3: hemorrhage and cotton-wool exudates Grade 4: papilledema

Left Ventricular Hypertrophy

Development of left ventricular hypertrophy (LVH) permits cardiac adaptation to the increased afterload imposed by elevated arterial pressure. However, LVH is a major independent risk factor for sudden cardiac death, myocardial infarction, stroke, and other cardiovascular morbid and mortal events. Here again, evidence demonstrates that antihypertensive agents other than vasodilators such as hydralazine and minoxidil, weight reduction, and a decrease in excessive salt intake are capable of reducing left ventricular mass and wall thickness. No controlled studies, however, demonstrate that reversal of LVH offers additional benefits beyond that offered by reduction in blood pressure.

The electrocardiogram remains the most cost-effective tool for detecting both left atrial and left ventricular hypertrophy, as well as for identifying myocardial ischemia and arrhythmias. However, echocardiography is much more sensitive for identifying LVH, but is too expensive for routine use.

One of the major problems with LVH is that it markedly reduces coronary reserve even in the absence of stenosis of larger coronary arteries. This may predispose patients with LVH to development of congestive heart failure and sudden death. There are many factors that play a role in development of LVH, which are beyond the scope of this chapter. However, use of antihypertensive agents in an appropriate "cocktail" to lower pressure will improve cardiac function and regress LVH through eliminating or attenuating the effects of various neurohumoral forces.

Proteinuria

Proteinuria results from an increase in intraglomerular pressure as well as an increase in membrane permeability of the glomerulus and leakage through the proximal tubule of the kidney. Results of large clinical trials have implicated proteinuria itself as predictor of renal disease progression (Fig. 61.3). Data from randomized, blinded trials and open-labeled trials suggest that if blood pressure is lowered and proteinuria is not reduced, renal failure progression is not maximally slowed.

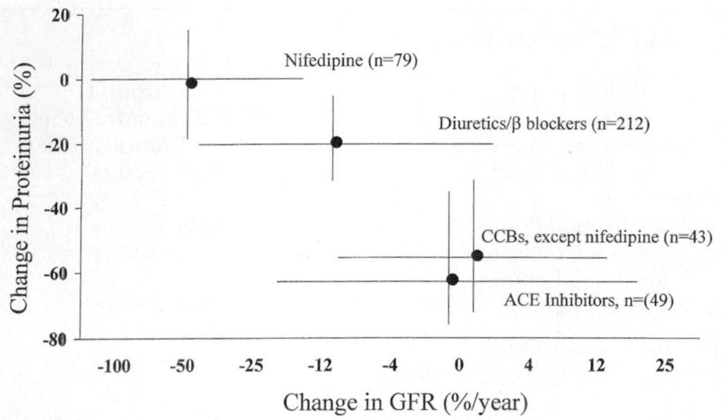

Figure 61.3. A meta-analysis of clinical trials and studies that demonstrates the relationship between reductions in proteinuria and progression in renal disease, assessed by change in glomerular filtration rate (GFR). (Adapted from Remuzzi G, Benigni A. Understanding of the nature of renal disease progression. *Kidney Int* 1997;51:2–15.)

There are many reasons for this association including direct evidence from *in vitro* studies that proteinuria, especially in its glycated state, stimulates matrix protein production such as collagen IV, laminin, and fibronectin. In addition, it increases macromolecular trafficking not only in the glomerulus, but also through leakage from the proximal tubule into the interstitial space, leading to interstitial inflammation and fibrosis. This is important because interstitial disease is a harbinger of a poor renal prognosis. Therefore reducing the protein load through reducing membrane permeability and intraglomerular pressure clearly would have adjunctive benefits in preserving renal function.

Development of proteinuria may relate more to the patient's lipid profile than to his or her renal function or blood pressure. In a recent analysis of more than 1,500 patients with nondiabetic renal disease, it was noted that those who had higher levels of low-density lipoprotein (LDL) cholesterol and who were obese had a higher level of proteinuria when compared with patients without these attributes. Interestingly, duration of hypertension and level of blood pressure did not correlate with the severity of proteinuria. This provides indirect evidence that abnormal lipid profiles may contribute to the genesis of proteinuria.

Moreover, in a meta-analysis of clinical trials, it was noted that antihypertensive agents that had the most dramatic effect on reducing proteinuria [i.e., ACE inhibitors and nondihydropyridine calcium antagonists (verapamil and diltiazem)] yielded the greatest impact on slowing renal disease progression. Conversely, agents that did not have significant effects on proteinuria such as dihydropyridine calcium antagonist, in spite of blood pressure reduction, offered the least benefit in terms of renal disease progression (Fig. 61.3). Thus the goal of proteinuria reduction should be an integral part of antihypertensive therapy. This will be discussed in greater detail later in this chapter.

Retinopathy

Physicians should clearly take time to fully examine the retina and vessels of patients with hypertension. This relates to the fact that funduscopic examination is the only true view of the vasculature without an invasive procedure. Vascular changes are graded according to the criteria of Keith and Wagner. Grade I retinopathy consists of arteriolar constriction. A vein/arteriole ratio of 3:2 is considered normal. A ratio more than 4:1, however, suggests significant hypertension and, unless treated, a poor outcome. Grade II consist of narrowing and tortuosity of the arterioles leading to stiffening of the adventitial layers, which results in compression of the column of blood in the accompanying venules and genesis of so-called arterial venous nicking. Grade III is characterized by cotton-wool exudates resulting from anoxia and retinal tissue and in hemorrhage in the deeper retinal layers given the appearance of a flicker of a candle (flame hemorrhages). Grade IV is simply the presence of grade III with papilledema.

TREATMENT

Lifestyle Modification

Lifestyle modifications such as weight reduction, dietary sodium restriction, moderation of alcohol intake, and increase in physical activity must accompany all recommendations for treatment of blood pressure. Moreover, the biggest problem facing treatment of hypertension in the United States is the geometric increase in obesity. Obesity is associated with an increase in insulin resistance, salt sensitivity, and a more volume-dependent hypertension.

From among this group of factors, weight reduction is probably the most important single factor that will contribute to reductions in blood pressure. This, along with sodium restriction and other factors, should absolutely be entertained as initial therapy before initiation of drugs. This is especially true in patients with stage 1 hypertension (Table 61.1) and no other risk factors. In addition, dietary potassium supplementation is critical in people who are on diuretics or who have poor potassium intake. Low potassium is known to generate increases in diastolic blood pressure of as much as 6 mm Hg. Moreover, high potassium intake has been demonstrated to have an antihypertensive effect in a number of animal models as well as in humans. In one study, addition of 60 mmol/day of potassium caused an average of a 4% decrease in blood pressure. In a separate study, 40 mmol/day of potassium supplementation resulted in a 14/10.5-mm Hg decrease in blood pressure. Perhaps the best evidence to support the notion that serum potassium levels should be maintained above 3.8 mEq/L comes from a double-blind, crossover trial. This trial showed an average decrease in mean arterial pressure of 5.5 mm Hg after potassium supplements were given to a group of hypertensive patients who developed hypokalemia as a result of diuretic therapy. Taken together with results of previous studies, these data strongly suggest that serum potassium levels should remain in the normal range to ensure adequate blood pressure control.

Excessive alcohol intake is an important risk factor that elevates blood pressure and can cause resistance to antihypertensive therapy. Alcohol intake should be limited to a maximum of 1 oz (30 ml) of ethanol, for example, 24 oz of beer, 10 oz of wine, or 2 oz of 100-proof whiskey, per day.

Sodium, in the form of sodium chloride or table salt, clearly elevates pressure or hinders its reduction in people with frank hypertension. This is especially true in people that are "salt sensitive." Salt-sensitive individuals have a rise in systolic blood pressure of more than 10 mm Hg for a given amount of salt, compared with individuals who have less than that rise in blood pressure, who are called salt resistant. African-Americans, older people, and patients with diabetes mellitus are more salt sensitive than other individuals. Epidemiologic data demonstrate a positive association between sodium intake and the level of blood pressure. Meta-analyses of clinical trials reveal that a reduction of sodium intake to 75 to 100 mmol/day lowers blood pressure over a period of several weeks. These effects are greater for older people and those with elevated blood pressure.

Moreover, in an analysis of 17 published, randomized, controlled trials involving patients ages 45 or older with hypertension found an average decrease of 6.3/2.2 mm Hg with urinary sodium reduction of 95 mmol/day.

Available data suggest that dietary calcium supplements may cause a modest decrease in blood pressure, especially in salt-sensitive hypertensives and in those with low plasma renin activity. However, there is no rationale to increase calcium intake above the daily recommended allowance, but low calcium intake should be avoided.

Pharmacologic Therapy

There is no question that treatment of hypertension reduces cardiovascular morbidity and mortality. It is also clear that most clinical trials that have examined the incidence of cardiovascular events have used diuretics and β-blockers as primary modes of therapy to reduce blood pressure.

There is a wide range of antihypertensive medications commonly used for control of hypertension. The more commonly used agents are summarized in Table 61.10. Treatment

TABLE 61.10. Pharmacologic Properties of Commonly Used Antihypertensive Agents

Drug	Dosage (mg/day)	Doses/Day	Mechanisms of Action	Special Consideration
		Diuretics		
Thiazides and related drugs				
Hydrochlorothiazide	12.5–25	1	Decrease body sodium and extracellular fluid volume	Effective antihypertensive unless serum creatinine is ≥2 ml/min or creatinine clearance ≤50 ml/min
Loop diuretics			Inhibit 2Cl/Na pump ascending Henle's loop	Effective even in patients with advanced renal or congestive heart failure
Furosemide	20–320	2		
Bumetanide	0.5–5	2		
Ethacrynic acid	25–100	2		
Torsemide	5–20	1		
Fixed-dose diuretics (Potassium sparing)			Increase K reabsorption	Weak diuretics
Hydrochlorothiazide/Amiloride (Moduretic)				
Hydrochlorothiazide/Triamterene (Maxzide, Dyazide)				
Spironolactone	25–100	2–3	Aldosterone antagonist	May cause hyperkalemia in patients with serum creatinine >2.5 mg/dl, particularly when combined with ACE inhibitors, K^+ supplements, or NSAIDs; Spironolactone may cause menstrual irregularities, gynecomastia, mastodynia, and decreased libido in males
Triamterene	50–100	2		
		Adrenergic Inhibitors		
β-Blockers				
Cardioselective			Inhibit β_1-receptors; decrease CO; increase SVR; decrease plasma renin activity (PRA)	In higher doses, will also inhibit β_2-receptors
Atenolol	25–100	1		
Metoprolol	50–200	1–2		
Noncardioselective			Inhibit β_1- and β_2-receptors	More likely to cause metabolic side effects
Nadolol	20–240	1		
Propranolol	40–240	1–2		
Timolol	20–40	2		
With intrinsic sympathomimetic activity (ISA)				
Acebutolol	200–1200	2	Partial agonist activity on β-adrenergic receptors	No clear advantage except for less bradycardia and metabolic side effects than other β-blockers
Pindolol	10–60	2		
		Antiadrenergic Agents		
Centrally acting				
α-Methyldopa	250–1500	2	Stimulate α_2-adrenergic receptors in the brainstem resulting in inhibition of efferent sympathetic activity; decrease SVR	Sudden withdrawal may result in hypertensive crisis
Clonidine	0.1–0.6	2		
Clonidine TTS	0.1–0.3	Once/week		
Guanfacine	1–3	1		
Peripherally acting				
Guanethidine	10–100	1	Inhibit norepinephrine release from sympathetic nerve terminals; decrease SVR	Frequently cause orthostatic hypotension and sexual dysfunction
Reserpine	0.05–0.25	1	Depletion of norepinephrine	Causes frequent neurologic symptoms

(continued)

TABLE 61.10. *(continued)*

Drug	Dosage (mg/day)	Doses/Day	Mechanisms of Action	Special Consideration
α_1-Receptor blockers				
Doxazosin	2–16	1	Inhibit α_1-adrenergic receptors; decrease SVR; CO same or increases	First-dose effect; postural hypotension; useful for prostatic hypertrophy
Prazosin	2–20	1–2		
Terazosin	1–20	1		
ACE inhibitors				
Benazepril	10–40	1–2	Block convertion of angiotensin I to angiotensin II; decrease aldosterone; may increase bradykinin and vasodilatory prostaglandins; decrease SVR; no change in CO	When added to diuretics may cause hypotension; may cause hyperkalemia in patients with renal failure, in those with hypoaldosteronism, and in those receiving K-sparing diuretics or NSAIDs; may increase serum creatinine
Captopril	12.5–100	2–3		
Cilazapril	2.5–5	1–2		
Enalapril	2.5–40	1–2		
Fosinopril	10–40	1		
Lisinopril	5–40	1		
Perindopril	1–16	1–2		Can cause acute renal failure in patients with bilateral renal artery stenosis, renal artery stenosis of a solitary kidney, creatinine >3 mg/dl, or severe CHF
Quinapril	5–80	1–2		
Ramipril	1.25–20	1		
Spirapril	12.5–50	1–2		
Trandolapril	1–4	1		
Calcium antagonists				
Diltiazem	90–360	3–4	Blocks entry of calcium into smooth muscle cells resulting in vasodilation; decrease SVR; blunt increases in exercise heart rate	
Diltiazem CD	180–360	1		
Verapamil	80–480	2–3		May cause heart block, particularly when combined with β-blocker
Verapamil SR	120–480	1–2		
Verapamil-Covera HS	180–240	1 (at bedtime)		
Dihydropyridines				
Amlodipine	2.5–10	1	Same as diltiazem and verapamil	More potent vasodilators than diltiazem and verapamil; may cause dizziness, headache, tachycardia, flushing, edema
Felodipine	5–20	1	Do not blunt increase in exercise heart rate	
Isradipine	2.5–10	2		
Nicardipine	60–120	3		
Nifedipine	30–120	3		
Nifedipine (GITS)	30–120	1		
Nisoldipine	10–10	1–2		
Direct vasodilators				
Hydralazine	50–200	2–4	Direct relaxation of smooth muscle cells, causing arteriolar vasodilation secondary to opening [K^+] channels	Limited efficacy if given alone due to fluid retention and reflex vasodilation; should be combined with a diuretic and a β-blocker to prevent edema and tachycardia; Minoxidil causes hirsutism and occasionally pericarditis
Minoxidil	2.5–80	1		

ACE, angiotensin-converting enzyme; CHF, congestive heart failure; CO, cardiac output, NSAIDs, nonsteroidal antiinflammatory drugs; SVR, systemic vascular resistance; TTS, transdermal therapeutic system.

of hypertension should also incorporate factors dealing with patient compliance. Based on large surveys, it is clear that monotherapy will only adequately treat approximately 45% to 50% of the patients with hypertension. This means that more than half the patients require at least two medications. There are a whole host of antihypertensive medications that are available at various fixed-dose combinations (Table 61.11). These agents are ideal for treating poorly compliant patients because they can be given once daily and reduce the number of pills required to lower pressure by 50%.

Based on criteria outlined in Table 61.1, patients with an established diagnosis of hypertension should be managed in a manner recommended by the JNC VI report (Fig. 61.4). However, in the presence of renal disease and/or diabetes, an ACE inhibitor should be part of their antihypertensive cocktail.

A number of trials in type 1 diabetes clearly provide evidence that ACE inhibitors slow progression of renal disease. Moreover, many studies in type 2 diabetes have shown that ACE inhibitors reduce proteinuria, and although they may not be superior to other classes of antihypertensive medications, they certainly have a positive impact on slowing progression of renal disease. However, the data with ACE inhibitors in nondiabetic renal disease are not as clear cut. A meta-analysis of available data showed that there was no clear benefit or superiority of ACE inhibitors over other forms of antihypertensive agents for slowing progression of nondiabetic renal disease. In contrast to this meta-analysis, however, the Ramipril Efficacy in Nephrology (REIN) trial shows evidence that, in fact, ACE inhibitors have a benefit in slowing progression of nondiabetic renal disease. These observations are further corroborated by the Angiotensin Converting Enzyme Inhibition in Progressive Renal Insufficiency

TABLE 61.11. Combination Drugs for Hypertension

Drug	Trade Name
β-Adrenergic Blockers and Diuretics	
Atenolol, 50 or 100 mg/chlorthalidone, 25 mg	Tenoretic
Bisoprolol fumarate, 2.5, 5, or 10 mg/hydrochlorothiazide, 6.25 mg	Ziac*
Metoprolol tartrate, 50 or 100 mg/hydrochlorothiazide, 25 or 50 mg	Lopressor HCT
Nadolol, 40 or 80 mg/bendroflumethiazide, 5 mg	Corzide
Propranolol hydrochloride, 40 or 80 mg/hydrochlorothiazide, 25 mg	Inderide
Propranolol hydrochloride (extended release), 80, 120, or 160 mg/hydrochlorothiazide, 50 mg	Inderide LA
Timolol maleate, 10 mg/hydrochlorothiazide, 25 mg	Timolide
ACE Inhibitors and Diuretics	
Benazepril hydrochloride, 5, 10, or 20 mg/hydrochlorothiazide, 6.25, 12.5, or 25 mg	Lotensin HCT
Captopril, 25 or 50 mg/hydrochlorothiazide, 15 or 25 mg	Capozide*
Enalapril maleate, 5 or 10 mg/hydrochlorothiazide, 12.5 or 25 mg	Vaseretic
Lisinopril, 10 or 20 mg/hydrochlorothiazide, 12.5 or 25 mg	Prinzide, Zestoretic
Angiotensin II–Receptor Antagonists and Diuretics	
Losartan potassium, 50 mg/hydrochlorothiazide, 12.5 mg	Hyzaar
Calcium Antagonists and ACE Inhibitors	
Amlodipine besylate, 2.5 or 5 mg/benazepril hydrochloride, 10 or 20 mg	Lotrel
Diltiazem hydrochloride, 180 mg/enalapril maleate, 5 mg	Teczem
Verapamil hydrochloride (extended release), 180 or 240 mg/trandolapril 1, 2, or 4 mg	Tarka
Felodipine, 5 mg/enalapril maleate, 5 mg	Lexxel
Other Combinations	
Triamterene, 37.5, 50, or 75 mg/hydrochlorothiazide, 25 or 50 mg	Dyazide, Maxzide
Spironolactone, 25 or 50 mg/hydrochlorothiazide, 25 or 50 mg	Aldactazide
Amiloride hydrochloride, 5 mg/hydrochlorothiazide, 50 mg	Moduretic
Guanethidine monosulfate, 10 mg/hydrochlorothiazide, 25 mg	Esimil
Hydralazine hydrochloride, 25, 50, or 100 mg/hydrochlorothiazide, 25 or 50 mg	Apresazide
Methyldopa, 250 or 500 mg/hydrochlorothiazide, 15, 25, 30, or 50 mg	Aldoril
Reserpine, 0.125 mg/hydrochlorothiazide, 25, or 50 mg	Hydropres
Reserpine, 0.10 mg/hydralazine hydrochloride, 25 mg/hydrochlorothiazide, 15 mg	Ser-Ap-Es
Clonidine hydrochloride, 0.1, 0.2, or 0.3 mg/chlorthalidone, 15 mg	Combipres
Methyldopa, 250 mg/chlorothiazide, 150 or 250 mg	Aldoclor
Reserpine, 0.125 or 0.25 mg/chlorthalidone, 25 or 50 mg	Demi-Regroton
Reserpine, 0.125 or 0.25 mg/chlorothiazide, 250 or 500 mg	Diupres
Prazosin hydrochloride, 1, 2, or 5 mg/polythiazide, 0.5 mg	Minizide

ACE, angiotensin-converting enzyme.
*Approved as first-line antihypertensive therapy by FDA.

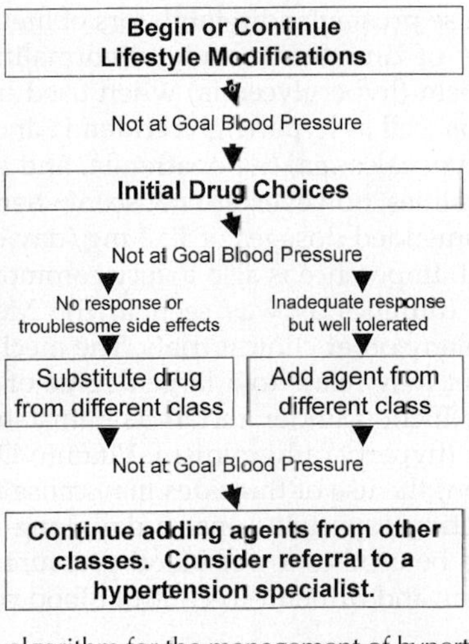

Figure 61.4. An algorithm for the management of hypertension. [Adapted from the Joint National Committee Report on the Diagnosis and Treatment of Hypertension (JNC VI). *Arch Intern Med* 1997;157:2413–2446.]

(AIPRI) trial of patients with nondiabetic renal disease. Therefore ACE inhibitors absolutely should be included in the antihypertensive cocktail for controlling blood pressure in patients with renal disease.

In addition, the recommendations of the JNC VI suggest that three groups of patients must have blood pressure controlled or reduced to levels of less than 130/85 mm Hg, and in the case of nondiabetic renal disease perhaps as low as 125/75 mm Hg. These patients include African-Americans with renal disease, those with diabetes mellitus, and anyone who has renal insufficiency with proteinuria of more than 1g. An analysis of long-term clinical trials in diabetes suggests that a minimum of four different, antihypertensive agents with complementary mechanisms of action are required to achieve these lower levels of blood pressure control. Additionally, a similar number of different antihypertensive medications are required in those with nondiabetic renal disease. Therefore an optimal antihypertensive cocktail for anyone with renal disease should include a diuretic, either loop or thiazide, depending on level of renal function; an ACE inhibitor in moderate doses; a calcium antagonist, preferably a nondihydropyridine agent; and some type of vasodilator, either an α-blocker, hydralazine, or minoxidil, along with possibly a sympatholytic agent such as clonidine. Given the advent of fixed-dose combination medications, the number of pills that any given patient takes can be limited to as few as three and at the same time receive five different medications.

It is vitally important that clinicians understand that ACE inhibitors will slow progression of renal disease regardless of the preexisting level of renal function. Moreover, data from clinical trials support the notion that those with the highest levels of serum creatinine are the ones that will garner the greatest benefit. Thus individuals with a serum creatinine of 2.5 mg/dl may get a greater benefit than those with a value of 1.2 mg/dl.

Although it is not common for serum creatinine to increase by 20% to 25 % after ACE inhibitors are given, this rise will lead many clinicians to withdraw ACE inhibitors. This unfortunately is not based on clinical fact of poor outcome. Moreover, withdrawal may be doing more harm than good. Evidence from three separate, long-term follow-up studies, one as long as 7 years, demonstrates that this rise in serum creatinine results in a benefit, not a detriment, in renal outcome.

The concept is simple—what β-blockers do to the heart in terms of reducing cardiac work load and myocardial oxygen demand is similar to what the ACE inhibitors do to the kidney by reducing nephron pressure and work load. If this is done in a setting of preexisting renal insufficiency without altering dietary intake of protein, clearly serum creatinine and blood urea nitrogen (BUN) will increase. A patient who is not volume depleted (the most common cause of a rise in serum creatinine with ACE inhibitors) should not have more than a 20% to 25% increase in serum creatinine within a span of 3 to 4 weeks. Thus ACE inhibitors should not be discontinued as long as *hyperkalemia* or *acidosis* does not develop. If increases of more than 25% occur or these increases continue after a 3- to 4-week period, patients should be evaluated for bilateral renal artery stenosis. This diagnosis, however, is uncommon and seen most prominently in older patients (60 years or older) who have a smoking history, or continue to smoke, and a history of hypercholesterolemia.

As previously mentioned, it is clear that pharmacologic therapy is necessary to reduce arterial pressure in anyone with hypertension and target-organ damage. Moreover, based on the particular type of target-organ injury and concomitant disease states present in an individual, therapy should be tailored using specific types of antihypertensive medications. Based on clinical trials, particular types of antihypertensive therapies have compelling indications for their use in certain diseases; these are listed in Tables 61.12 and 61.13. These agents should be included in the "antihypertensive cocktail" of any patient with that particular problem. For example, not only should ACE inhibitors be part of the "antihypertensive cocktail" for treatment of hypertension in diabetes, but diuretics and nondihydropyridine calcium antagonists also should be included as part of the "cocktail" to achieve the desired lower level of blood pressure reduction. Thus antihypertensive therapies can be broken into specific classes and studied in regard to their complementary effects on reducing blood pressure.

TABLE 61.12. Initial Drug Choices for Specific Preexisting Conditions[a]

Compelling Indications
Heart failure
ACE inhibitors ↓
Diuretics
Myocardial infarction
β-Blockers (non-ISA)
ACE inhibitors (with systolic dysfunction)
Diabetes mellitus (type 1) with proteinuria
ACE inhibitors
Isolated systolic hypertension (older persons)
Diuretics preferred
Long-acting dihydropyridine calcium antagonists

[a] Based on randomized controlled trials.
ACE, angiotensin-converting enzyme; ISA, intrinsic sympathomimetic activity.

TABLE 61.13. Specific Indications for Certain Medications

Angina
β-Blockers
Calcium antagonists
Diabetes mellitus (types 1 and 2) with proteinuria
ACE inhibitors (preferred)
Calcium antagonists
Diabetes mellitus (type 2)
Low-dose diuretics
Dyslipidemia
α-Blockers
Renal insufficiency (caution in renovascular hypertension and creatinine > 3 mg/dl [> 265.2 μmol/L])
ACE inhibitors
Myocardial infarction
Diltiazem
Verapamil

ACE, angiotensin-converting enzyme.

Diuretics

Diuretics very clearly have natriuretic effects. However, the exact mechanism by which they reduce arterial pressure is not precisely understood. Thiazide diuretics inhibit sodium chloride reabsorption in the cortical diluting segment of the early distal tubule. The initial effect of these agents is a mild degree of sodium loss leading to a decrease in plasma and extracellular fluid volume. The kidney reequilibrates and establishes a new level of homeostasis (i.e., a new steady state with modest volume contraction).

Other potential mechanisms by which diuretics may lower arterial pressure include (a) increased production of prostacyclin and (b) indirect activation of the kinin system as indicated by an increase in urinary kallikrein excretion. Animal data does exist indicating that thiazide diuretics cause a vasodilatory effect in hypertensive animal models. This may be secondary to prostaglandins because prostaglandin inhibitors obliterate this effect.

Side effects of diuretics include abnormalities in carbohydrate metabolism (hyperglycemia) when used in dosages of 25 mg or higher as well as hypertriglyceridemia and electrolyte abnormalities (hypocalcemia, hyponatremia, and hyperuricemia). These abnormalities, however, are not seen when the commonly used or recommended dosages of 12.5 mg/day of a thiazide diuretic are used. Impotence is also a very common side effect associated with diuretics as was seen in the Medical Research Council and many other clinical trials. The mechanisms for this are unclear, but may relate to a large degree of blood pressure control and reduction under certain circumstances of increase bone turnover (hyperparathyroidism, Vitamin D therapy, phosphate depletion) the use of thiazides may cause hypercalcemia.

Loop diuretics, especially once-a-day, long-acting loop diuretics, should be used to lower blood pressure in people with renal sufficiency and difficult-to-control blood pressure.

β-Blockers

β-Blockers have been shown in many clinical trails to reduce mortality and morbidity in people with myocardial infarctions.

However, their efficacy in the elderly, especially among smokers, is at best questionable. Clearly, however, they do have an important role in mitigating against increases in the sympathetic nervous system.

The mechanisms through which β-blockers lower blood pressure are not clear. β-Blockers reduce heart rate, myocardial contractility, atrioventricular conduction time, and automaticity. Thus the antihypertensive action may be, in part, a result of decreased cardiac output. Peripheral vascular resistance initially rises, presumably because of inhibition of β-receptors that mediate vasodilation and unopposed stimulation of α-receptors or to stimulation of the sympathetic nervous system as a secondary adaptive response to a fall in cardiac output. After prolonged therapy, some found a persistent increase of peripheral vascular resistance, whereas others found a decrease in peripheral vascular resistance in those patients in whom blood pressure fell.

β-Blockers reduce plasma renin activity, and some studies have shown a relationship between their hypotensive action and pretreatment renin levels or degree of renin suppression. Other studies, however, suggest that renin suppression is not a necessary condition for the antihypertensive action of these drugs because even patients with low renin may respond to β-blockers. Moreover, agents such as pindolol may effectively lower blood pressure without decreasing renin levels. Additionally, the hypotensive action of β-blockers reaches its peak after several days of treatment, whereas the decrease in plasma renin occurs more rapidly.

Other mechanisms postulated to lower blood pressure include penetration of β-blockers into the central nervous system. β-Blockers may lower blood pressure by stimulating α-adrenergic receptors in the locus caeruleus of the brain that result in inhibition of sympathetic discharge from the central nervous system. Infusion of propranolol directly into the cerebral ventricle of dogs caused a fall in blood pressure in direct proportion to the increase in norepinephrine in the cerebrospinal fluid. This mechanism, however, does not appear to be essential for the antihypertensive action of β-blockers because predominantly water soluble agents, such as atenolol with little penetrance into the brain, exert equal antihypertensive action. In addition, β-blockers usually increase plasma levels of catecholamines rather than causing a decrease, as one would expect from a reduction of sympathetic outflow from the brain. The mechanism for the increase in circulating levels of plasma catecholamines is also unclear and can be explained only partially by a decrease in clearance from the circulation.

Special Indications for β-Blockers. β-Blockers are particularly useful in the treatment of hypertension in patients with hyperdynamic circulation, characterized by increased cardiac output, or those with associated tachycardia, tremor, anxiety, and increased sweating. These agents are also beneficial in patients with angina pectoris or arrhythmias. They are the drugs of choice in patients with previous myocardial infarction. Secondary prevention trials have shown as much as a 25% decrease in recurrence of myocardial infarction in patients treated with β-blockers.

The most frequent side effects of β-blockers are bradycardia, muscular fatigue, tiredness, atrioventricular blocks, sick sinus syndrome, heart failure, cold extremities and Raynaud's phenomenon, and bronchospasms. They should be avoided in patients with asthma. Bradycardia and heart failure are less likely to occur with β-blockers with intrinsic sympathomimetic activity (ISA). β-Blockers increase serum triglycerides and decrease serum levels of high-density lipoprotein (HDL) cholesterol, whereas they do not significantly affect serum levels of LDL cholesterol. β-Blockers with ISA, however, cause little or no increase in triglycerides. β-Blockers can cause several central nervous system symptoms, including insomnia, nightmares, hallucinations, and depression. Because β-blockers increase the number of receptor sites on vascular smooth muscle cells, caution must be exercised when these drugs are acutely withdrawn because coronary artery spasm or arrhythmias may complicate such withdrawal. *Simultaneous administration of β-blockers with nondihydropyridine calcium antagonists must be avoided in patients with preexisting atrioventricular (AV) conduction abnormalities because of increased incidence of AV block.*

Labetalol. Labetalol is a nonselective β-blocker with little ISA but with α_1-blocking properties. The ratio of α- to β-blocking activity is about 1:7. This drug lowers blood pressure by decreasing both peripheral vascular resistance and cardiac output. After prolonged therapy, the decrease in blood pressure is sustained primarily by a fall in peripheral vascular resistance, whereas cardiac output returns to pretreatment levels. Acutely, the drug may cause slight reflex tachycardia, but chronic use decreases heart rate. This agent can be used both orally and intravenously. The intravenous form has been used with some success in hypertensive emergencies, even though its efficacy is not as predictable and immediate as that of sodium nitroprusside. The oral form can be used in the management of mild to moderate form of hypertension, and it appears to be more effective than propranolol in African-Americans.

The most common side effect is orthostatic hypotension, which is related to the α-blocking properties. As with all β-blockers this drug can cause sodium retention and is more suitable for use in combination with diuretic. Labetalol is less likely to cause bronchospasm and has no deleterious effects on serum lipids. Occasionally, it can increase the titer of antinuclear and antimitochondrial antibodies. Last, liver function abnormalities (increased transaminases) have been noted with the drug. In four separate cases in which the drug was terminated and then reintroduced, liver failure occurred in all cases. Therefore increased transaminases should result in permanent discontinuance of the drug.

Centrally Acting Antiadrenergic Agents

α-Methyldopa. α-Methyldopa is the α-methylated derivative of dopa, the precursor of dopamine and norepinephrine. This drug lowers blood pressure by activating α_2-adrenergic receptors in inhibitory centers of the sympathetic nervous system localized in the brainstem and, partially, by biotransformation into a false neurotransmitter. It also lowers plasma renin activity, but this is not considered to be of primary importance for the antihypertensive action of this drug. It lowers blood pressure primarily by decreasing peripheral vascular resistance and has little effect on cardiac output. The efficacy of α-methyldopa has been well tested, but its use has decreased substantially, primarily because of the relatively high incidence of side effects. However, it remains the most commonly prescribed agent to treat pregnant hypertensive women, particularly in the United States. Among the most common side effects are somnolence, dry mouth, orthostatic hypotension, and impotence. Occasionally, the drug can cause Coombs-positive hemolytic anemia or hepatitis. Fever has also been reported with the use of methyldopa.

Clonidine. Clonidine is an imidazoline derivative that lowers blood pressure primarily by activation of presynaptic α_2-adrenergic receptors in the medulla oblongata, resulting in decreased sympathetic nervous system activity. The inhibition of renin secretion contributes to the hypotensive action of the drug to a lesser extent. The drug is readily absorbed from the intestine and reaches peak plasma levels within 1 hour. The antihypertensive action appears within 30 minutes, and it peaks within 2 to 4 hours. In addition to the oral form, clonidine is available as a transdermal therapeutic system (TTS), which allows steady and continuous transdermal delivery of the drug for 1 week. This limits fluctuation in blood pressure commonly observed with oral dosing, improves compliance, and reduces the incidence of side effects.

The use of this drug had substantially decreased because of the high incidence of untoward side effects related to the central nervous system, including drowsiness, lethargy, dry mouth, impotence, and orthostatic hypotension. In addition, hypertensive crisis may occur if the drug is discontinued abruptly, particularly in patients on a combination of clonidine and β-blockers or in those receiving doses greater than 0.8 mg/day. In this instance, the surge of catecholamines occurring after withdrawal of the drug will bind preferentially to unoccupied α-receptors and have little binding capacity for the occupied β-receptors, resulting in greater vasoconstriction and in more severe hypertension. The transdermal form of delivery can cause skin rash at the site of adherence of the patch. Alternatively, guanfacine is a longer-acting agent that works like clonidine to decrease pressure. Thus it can be given once daily. However, all other aspects associated with clonidine are associated with this agent.

The use of this drug for hypertensive urgencies secondary to profound reductions in blood pressure has increased with the substantial decreased use of sublingual nifedipine. The decrease of this latter agent was related to an increase in cardiovascular events following its use.

Peripherally Acting Antiadrenergic Agents

α_1-Adrenergic Receptor Blocking Agents. Selective α_1-adrenergic receptor blocking agents such as prazosin, terazosin and doxazosin bind reversibly with α_1-receptor sites, thus decreasing peripheral vascular resistance and lowering blood pressure. Unlike nonselective α-blockers, such as phentolamine, selective α_1-blockers do not inhibit the α_2-mediated inhibition of norepinephrine release. Maintenance of this negative feedback loop prevents the undesired side effects of increased norepinephrine release observed with nonselective α-blockers. Unlike β-blockers, α-blockers do not lower cardiac output, and they cause minimal change of plasma renin activity, heart rate, plasma catecholamines, and renal blood flow.

Terazosin has a longer half-life and can be given twice daily, and doxazosin with the longest half-life (10 to 12 hours), may be given once daily. The prototype of this group of agents is prazosin. It has a short half-life (2 to 3 hours) and needs to be administered twice daily. These drugs are metabolized extensively by the liver and require little dose adjustment with worsening of renal function.

Urapidil is a peripheral α_1-adrenergic receptor blocking agent with an additional central component, which is different from that of clonidine because it does not involve stimulation of central α_2-adrenoreceptors. This compound stimulates serotoninergic receptors in the 5-hydroxytryptamine (5HT)-1A subtype, located in the ventral region of the medulla oblongata. Stimulation of these receptors lowers blood pressure without causing sedation.

The most troublesome side effect of prazosin is the first-dose phenomenon, consisting of significant orthostatic hypotension, which occurs after administration of the first dose. This phenomenon is particularly common in patients who are volume depleted because of previous diuretic therapy and in elderly patients. The incidence of orthostatic hypotension can be minimized by administering a small test dose, by slowly increasing the dose during titration, and by administering the drug at bedtime.

Common side effects include dizziness, headache, diarrhea, nausea, and asthenia. α_1-Blocking agents decrease LDL and increase HDL cholesterol. In addition, they have no untoward effects on glucose metabolism.

α_2-Adrenoreceptor Antagonists. Traditionally, α_2-adrenoreceptor antagonists have not been considered as good potential candidates for antihypertensive therapy because of the commonly held belief that presynaptic and postsynaptic α_2-adrenoreceptors were structurally very similar. Thus any antihypertensive effect would be counterbalanced by increased release of norepinephrine from presynaptic sites. However, some functional dissimilarities have been identified between presynaptic and postsynaptic α_2-adrenoreceptor activation in vascular smooth muscle, but not prejunctional α_2-adrenoreceptor activation on sympathetic nerve endings, which is now known to use a pertussis toxin-sensitive guanine nucleotide-binding regulatory (Gi) protein. This discovery has led to the identification of some selective postsynaptic α_2-adrenoreceptor antagonists, such as SK&F 104078 [6-chloro-9-[(3-methyl-2-butenyl) oxy]-3-methyl-1H-2, 3,4,5-tetrahydro-3-benzazepine]. This compound has manifested potent vasodilator and hypotensive action in rat without causing an increased release of norepinephrine from presynaptic sites. This and other similar compounds have not been tested in humans.

Angiotensin-Converting Enzyme Inhibitors

Angiotensin-converting enzyme (ACE) inhibitors, a class of antihypertensive agents, inhibit kininase I (ACE) and, thereby, the conversion of angiotensin I to angiotensin II. The prototype of this group of substances was isolated from the venom of the Brazilian arrowhead viper, Bothrops iaracaca. Since then, several molecules belonging to the same class have been isolated, and several have already reached the American market. ACE inhibitors can be classified into three main chemical categories: sulfhydryl-, carboxyl-, and phosphoryl-containing compounds.

The sulfhydryl agents are prodrugs that are converted *in vivo* into active compounds—captopril is an example. Newer sulfhydryl-containing compounds have a slower onset and longer duration of action than captopril. Zofenopril has greater potency and is partially eliminated by the liver.

The carboxyl-containing ACE inhibitors (of which enalapril is an example) are also prodrugs converted *in vivo* to the active metabolite. The kidney principally excretes this subgroup of ACE inhibitors. Compared with enalapril, benazepril has an earlier peak time and a slightly shorter terminal half-life, whereas perindopril has a peak time and half-life similar to those of enalapril. Lisinopril is not a prodrug but has the poorest oral bioavailability (37%) of all ACE inhibitors.

The last class of ACE inhibitors, the phosphoryl-containing group, includes fosinopril, a drug that is partially eliminated by the liver and does not require dose adjustment in the presence of renal failure. Newer agents such as trandolapril and ramipril also do not need dosage adjustment in the presence of renal insufficiency.

All ACE inhibitors reduce plasma levels of angiotensin II and aldosterone and increase renin secretion. Thus to the extent that blood pressure is dependent on the renin-angiotensin system, these agents are effective in reducing blood pressure. This explains the greater efficacy of these agents in patients with increased plasma renin activity (PRA), albeit they can also effectively decrease blood pressure in patients with low PRA. Because kininase II also blocks the degradation of kinin, some have postulated that the antihypertensive action of these drugs may depend in part on increased levels of bradykinin at the tissue level. A summary of all ACE inhibitors defined by both pharmacology and clinical trial data is shown in Table 61.14.

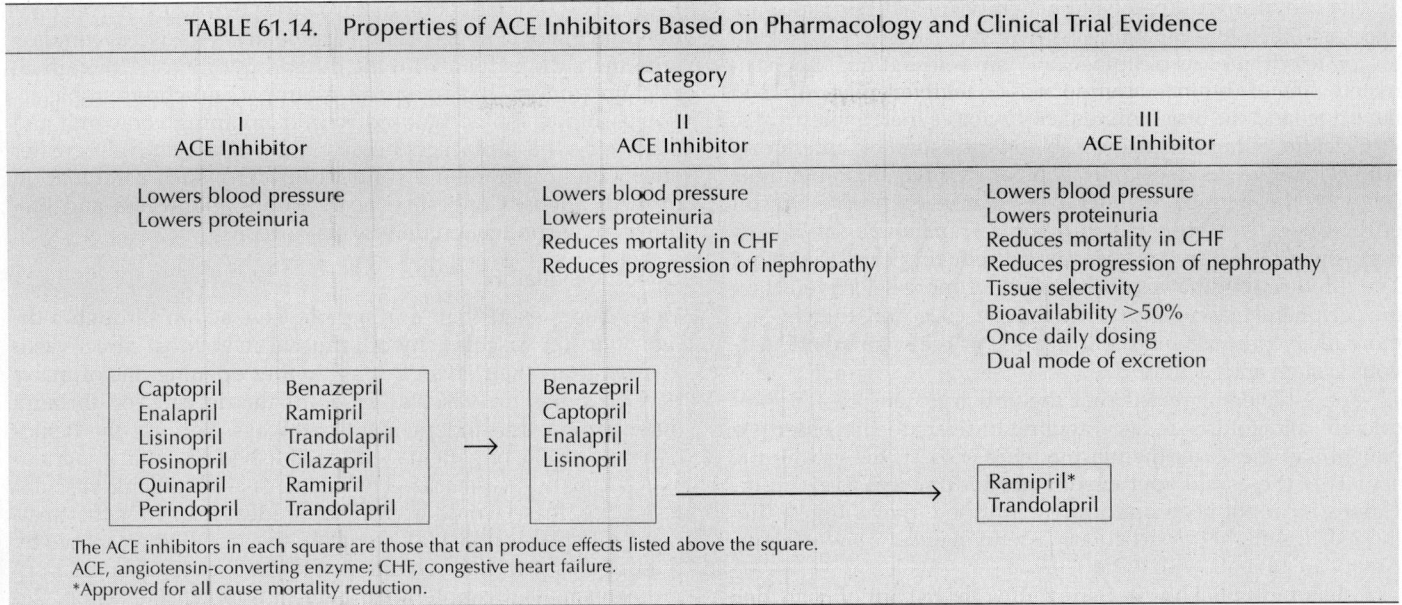

TABLE 61.14. Properties of ACE Inhibitors Based on Pharmacology and Clinical Trial Evidence

Category		
I ACE Inhibitor	II ACE Inhibitor	III ACE Inhibitor
Lowers blood pressure Lowers proteinuria	Lowers blood pressure Lowers proteinuria Reduces mortality in CHF Reduces progression of nephropathy	Lowers blood pressure Lowers proteinuria Reduces mortality in CHF Reduces progression of nephropathy Tissue selectivity Bioavailability >50% Once daily dosing Dual mode of excretion
Captopril, Enalapril, Lisinopril, Fosinopril, Quinapril, Perindopril, Benazepril, Ramipril, Trandolapril, Cilazapril, Ramipril, Trandolapril →	Benazepril Captopril Enalapril Lisinopril →	Ramipril* Trandolapril

The ACE inhibitors in each square are those that can produce effects listed above the square.
ACE, angiotensin-converting enzyme; CHF, congestive heart failure.
*Approved for all cause mortality reduction.

ACE inhibitors decrease peripheral vascular resistance without increasing heart rate, cardiac output, or pulmonary wedge pressure and without reflex activation of the sympathetic nervous system. Cerebral blood flow usually remains unchanged. These drugs reduce proteinuria and microalbuminuria more effectively than any other class of antihypertensive agents. This has been shown in patients with diabetes mellitus, essential hypertension, and a variety of glomerulonephritis. The mechanism of their effect on proteinuria relates to both their ability to reduce glomerular membrane permeability as well as their effect on reducing intraglomerular pressure.

The most common side effects include cough, skin rash, angioedema, and leukopenia. Neutropenia is more likely to occur after 3 to 12 months of therapy in patients with collagen vascular disease. In patients with chronic renal failure, ACE inhibitors may cause an acute deterioration of renal function and hyperkalemia. In addition, they may aggravate anemia. This is not associated with decreased levels of erythropoietin or increased hemolysis. However, it appears to be related to interference by angiotensin II with the erythropoietin signal transduction at the cellular level. Evidence suggests that this is due to tremendous increases in IGF-3 binding protein associated with ACE inhibitors.

Angiotensin II–Receptor Antagonists

Saralasin was the first competitive antagonist of angiotensin II to be discovered and introduced in the market. This agent, however, has had limited clinical use in the management of hypertension because it could be administered only intravenously because of its peptide structure. In addition, this drug has 10% of the agonist activity of angiotensin II and is therefore considered a partial agonist, and it has a very short half-life.

Losartan (DuP 753), a derivative of imidazole, has been discovered to be an orally active and highly specific angiotensin II–receptor antagonist with vasodilator and antihypertensive activity. Because losartan does not affect the activity of kininase II, it is possible that cough, a well-known adverse reaction to ACE inhibitors considered to be secondary to accumulation of bradykinin, may be less frequent with this compound. In human pharmacokinetic studies, losartan has been shown to have a half-life of 1.5 hours. The active metabolite has a longer half-life of 9 hours. Preliminary studies in healthy volunteers using doses of 20 to 40 mg have shown that losartan blocks angiotensin II–induced responses. Antihypertensive activity was seen with doses of 50 to 150 mg given once daily for 5 days to hypertensive patients. To date, the drug appears to be well tolerated.

Since the discovery of losartan, five other AT_1-receptor antagonists—valsartan, irbesartan, candesartan, eprosartan and telmesartan—have been approved. All of these agents appear to reach an asymptote in their dose-response curve for blood pressure reduction early in their dosing. The exceptions to this may be candesartan and telmesartan.

Molecular techniques, AT_1 and AT_2, have identified at least two angiotensin II–receptor subtypes. Losartan is a selective AT_1-receptor antagonist, and AT_1 receptors mediate the vasoconstriction of resistance vessels. Several types of nonpeptide AT-receptor antagonists have now been developed, including selective AT_2-receptor antagonists (e.g., PD 123177). Losartan has an approximately 10,000-fold selectivity for the AT_1 receptor, whereas PD 123177 is approximately 3,500 times more specific for the AT_2 receptor. AT_2 receptors appear to be important in the regulation of vascular homeostasis and are altered by sodium intake. Thus they may contribute to a variety of factors in which sodium has been found to be important.

Calcium Channel Antagonists

Intracellular calcium exerts critical functions in all organ systems and, in the cardiovascular system, it regulates the excitation-contraction coupling, the activity of cardiac pacemaker, and atrioventricular conduction. In addition, intracellular calcium regulates the secretion of several pressor or depressor hormones, such as catecholamines, renin, aldosterone, and prostaglandins. Several membrane channels regulate the movement of calcium from the extracellular to the intracellular compartment. Calcium channel antagonists inhibit the cellular entry of calcium primarily through voltage-dependent calcium channels and to a lesser extent through receptor-operated channels.

It is now well established that there are multitudes of calcium channels, structurally different and with different affinity for different calcium channel antagonists. Several classifications of these agents have been proposed. However, the divisions into two types, type I and type II agents, is used most often. Type I refers to the dihydropyridines, such as nifedipine, amlodipine, and felodipine-type agents. Type II agents include diltiazem, which is structurally related to the benzodiazepines, and verapamil, which is structurally similar to papaverine.

The dihydropyridines have a significant hepatic first-pass effect, and their bioavailability is between 6% and 30%. Less than 1% of felodipine, nisoldipine, and nimodipine and approximately 10% of the other compounds is excreted unchanged in the urine, and the rest is excreted as inactive metabolites.

Calcium antagonists lower blood pressure by interfering with calcium-dependent contraction of vascular smooth muscle cells, and they reduce peripheral vascular resistance. As a result of their negative chronotropic action, verapamil and diltiazem may lower blood pressure in part by reducing cardiac output. The dihydropyridine derivatives have a more selective action on peripheral vascular smooth muscle cells and thereby are more likely to cause reflex stimulation of the sympathetic nervous system and tachycardia.

Some have suggested that the antihypertensive action of calcium antagonists is age- and renin-related—the older the patient and the lower the plasma renin activity, the greater the activity of these antihypertensive agents. Although these observations have not been uniformly confirmed, they suggest that these drugs might be particularly useful in elderly and African-American patients with hypertension.

Calcium channel blockers are more effective in salt-sensitive than in salt-resistant patients with hypertension. As discussed previously, categories of patients more likely to display salt sensitivity are African-American, elderly, and obese patients as well as those with diabetes mellitus. The greater efficacy in these subgroups of patients may be related to interference with the sodium-linked rise of cytosolic calcium in vascular smooth muscle cells during high salt intake. In addition, salt-sensitive patients are more likely than salt-resistant patients to manifest increased natriuresis during administration of calcium channel antagonists. The mechanisms for the natriuretic action of these compounds have not been totally ascertained, but the possibility of a direct interference with proximal tubular reabsorption of sodium has been suggested.

Some calcium channel antagonists may provide the advantage of treating comorbid conditions in addition to their primary antihypertensive efficacy. For example, verapamil and, to a lesser extent, diltiazem may prolong atrioventricular conduction and are thereby useful in the treatment of supraventricular tachycardia. Verapamil is also useful in the treatment of supra-ventricular tachycardia. Verapamil is useful for the prophylaxis of migraine.

Nimodipine, on the other had, appears to have more selective action on the cerebral circulation and seems to be useful in the setting of cerebrovascular accidents. Some studies have shown that these drugs may prevent ischemia-induced mitochondrial overload of calcium during reperfusion. As a result of peripheral vasodilation, dihydropyridines may reduce the incidence of Raynaud's phenomenon. Experimental evidence indicates that calcium channel antagonist may inhibit the progression of atherosclerosis. However, the clinical significance of these observations remains to be established.

These agents, however, do not all demonstrate the same efficacy for reducing cardiovascular events in clinical trials. Two separate trials have documented the efficacy of verapamil to reduce mortality in the post–myocardial infarction setting. A separate study has documented this for diltiazem in the same setting. The reasons for this may have to do with a reduction in sympathetic activity by verapamil and diltiazem and not by dihydropyridines. However, this has not been shown for any dihydropyridine agent. Moreover, only the Systolic Hypertension in Europe (SYS-EUR) trial, with nitrendipine, suggests that dihydropyridine calcium blockers reduce mortality associated with ischemic cardiovascular events among elderly hypertensives.

These drugs usually are well tolerated. The dihydropyridines are more likely to cause flushing, headache, tachycardia, ankle edema, and nausea. Verapamil on the other hand, is more likely to cause conduction disturbances, bradycardia, constipation, and gingival hyperplasia. Peripheral edema is less common with these drugs than with the dihydropyridines. Although all calcium blockers have negative inotropic and chronotropic actions, caution should be used when combining verapamil and diltiazem with β-blockers because they have relatively greater effects on heart rate and contractility with such combination of medications. Congestive heart failure and severe and life-threatening conduction defects may occur.

Direct Vasodilators

Vasodilators exert their antihypertensive action through a direct effect on vascular smooth muscle cells. Most direct vasodilators exert their effect through either opening one of many [K^+] channels on vascular smooth muscle cells or through other nitric oxide–independent pathways. Because the hemodynamic profile of patients with established essential hypertension is usually characterized by an increase in systemic vascular resistance, these would appear to be ideal drugs for the treatment of hypertension. Unfortunately, the vasodilation caused by these agents results in activation of normal reflex compensatory mechanisms that counteract the direct hypotensive action. Reduction in arterial pressure through vasodilation activates baroreceptor mechanisms and results in increased activity of the sympathetic nervous system, tachycardia, increased myocardial contractility, and cardiac output; all effects can interfere with as much as 75% of the hypotensive action of these agents. The attendant reflex increase in heart rate and cardiac output may also precipitate feelings of alarm and anxiety and attacks of angina pectoris in patients with coronary artery disease. In addition, vasodilators cause sodium retention and volume expansion, in part, because of stimulation of renin secretion and because of direct action on renal proximal tubular cells.

The concomitant use of β-blockers may prevent the effects of reflex stimulation of the sympathetic nervous system on the heart and may decrease renin secretion. Diuretic therapy is needed to prevent sodium and water retention and to overcome the tolerance to vasodilators that otherwise would develop. Alternatively, ACE inhibitors may be used in combination with vasodilators to counteract the increased activation of angiotensin II.

Some vasodilators, such as sodium nitroprusside, hydralazine, and diazoxide, are available for intravenous use and are more suitable for the treatment of hypertensive emergencies. On the other hand, oral vasodilators, such as hydralazine and minoxidil, are more suitable for chronic therapy of hypertension.

Hydralazine was the most widely used oral vasodilator before the advent of calcium antagonists. The drug is predominantly an arteriolar vasodilator, with little effect on capacitance vessels. Thus this drug decreased almost exclusively the afterload, with little or no impact on preload of the heart. Daily dosages of 200 mg should not be exceeded because of the possibility of lupuslike syndrome. The most frequent side effects are headache, nausea, vomiting, tachycardia, palpitations, dizziness, fatigue, angina pectoris, sleep disturbances, nasal congestion, and lupuslike syndrome.

Minoxidil, an oral vasodilator, is more potent than hydralazine. It dilates arterioles with no capacitance vessels. This results in reflex activation of the sympathetic nervous system and of the renin-angiotensin system, resulting in tachycardia, increased cardiac output, and sodium retention. Some patients, particularly those with advanced renal failure or those with cardiomyopathy, may develop severe sodium retention, volume expansion, and congestive heart failure that, at times, are unresponsive even to high doses of loop diuretics. In such patients, discontinuation of the drug may be necessary.

Even anuric patients on maintenance hemodialysis treated with minoxidil display an increase in body weight during the interdialytic periods and in the long term. This is thought to be secondary to increased thirst and salt appetite caused by stimulation of the renin-angiotensin system. The liver primarily metabolizes the drug, and dose adjustment is not required with advanced renal failure. The most common side effects are edema, hypertrichosis, tachycardia, angina pectoris, and pericardial effusion. The increased hair growth (hirsutism) makes it unacceptable to female patients.

Sodium nitroprusside is the most effective intravenous vasodilator, with action on both arterioles and veins, resulting in decreased afterload and preload of the heart without any significant change in cardiac output. The antihypertensive action ensues immediately, and it also terminates rapidly because the drug is promptly biotransformed into inactive metabolites, such as thiocyanate and cyanogen. In patients with renal failure, these toxic metabolites can accumulate in the blood and cause delirium, seizures, coma, and hypothyroidism. To prevent these toxic effects in patients with renal failure, the drug should not be administered for more than 2 or 3 days unless patients are undergoing hemodialysis. Hydroxocobalamin appears to prevent transfer of cyanide from red cells to tissues and may reduce cyanide toxicity.

Endothelin-Receptor Antagonists

Endothelin is a newly discovered potent endothelium-derived vasoconstrictor agent. Three different isoforms of endothelin have been identified. All three isoforms have the 21–amino acid structure in common. ET-1 acts predominantly on the endothelin A (ET_A) receptor, the major subtype on vascular smooth muscle cells. Activation of these receptors leads to sustained and profound vasoconstriction. The role of endothelin in the physiologic maintenance of vascular tone and in some pathologic disorders, such as hypertension, acute myocardial infarction, and Raynaud's disease, remains to be established.

Specific antagonists of both the ET_A and ET_B receptors, as well as a selective antagonist for the ET_A receptor, have provided new insights in understanding the role of endothelin in various diseases such as hypertension associated with cyclosporine and heart failure. BQ 123, BQ 162, and BQ 153 have a greater affinity for ET_A and cause a dose-dependent decrease in ET-1–induced pressor response. A multicenter, international, clinical trial noted that the nonspecific endothelin receptor antagonist, bosentan, reduced blood pressure in patients with essential hypertension without concomitant increases in sympathetic tone. In addition, other small studies demonstrate that these agents are useful for reducing blood pressure in transplant patients who are receiving cyclosporine. Clearly, these agents will have a special place in the methodology of blood pressure reduction in specific subgroups of hypertensive patients.

Initiating Drug Therapy

The major factors that should be considered for initiating drug therapy are ethnic origin of the patient, concomitant disease states, presence of target-organ injury, and, obviously, cost of medications. Elderly patients with hypertension and cardiovascular disease should be started with diuretic therapy. This includes those who have either isolated systolic or diastolic hypertension. Additional therapy such as calcium antagonists should be given for better control of blood pressure if goal blood pressures are not achieved with the diuretic only.

Diabetic patients with hypertension should always be given an ACE inhibitor or, if contraindicated, possibly an AT_1-receptor antagonist as part of their antihypertensive cocktail. In this circumstance, diuretics and nondihydropyridine calcium antagonists should always be offered as second- and third-line agents to maximally protect against progression of renal disease. African-American patients should not be denied ACE inhibitors if they are diabetic because ACE inhibitors have clearly been shown to lower blood pressure in such patients when given in higher-than-usual doses.

Treatment of blood pressure and heart failure should obviously include a diuretic, ACE inhibitor, and β-blocker. It is clear in this era of antihypertensive management that the level of blood pressure control is probably as, if not more, important than the agents used to control it. No matter what class of antihypertensive agents is used, however, if blood pressure control is not achieved the ultimate benefit in cardiovascular and renal risk reduction will not be garnered.

In short, physicians should try to adhere to the JNC VI guidelines that state: Blood pressure goals should be achieved by the least intrusive means possible in order to reduce morbidity and mortality. In high-risk patients such as African-Americans, diabetics, and those with renal insufficiency with proteinuria, the goal blood pressure should be less than 130/85 mm Hg.

Last, inadequate response to antihypertensive therapy may be due to many factors. These are summarized in Table 61.15. Patient noncompliance and a relative lack of aggressiveness on the part of the physician to increase medication dose account for the most common causes of poor blood pressure control. It

TABLE 61.15. Causes of Inadequate Responsiveness to Therapy

Pseudoresistance
"White-coat hypertension" or office elevations
Pseudohypertension in older patients
Use of regular cuff on very obese arm
Nonadherence to Therapy
Volume overload
Excess salt intake
Progressive renal damage (nephrosclerosis)
Fluid retention from reduction of blood pressure
Inadequate diuretic therapy
Drug-Related Causes
Doses too low
Wrong type of diuretic
Inappropriate combinations
Rapid inactivation (e.g., hydralazine)
Drug actions and interactions
Sympathomimetics
Adrenal steroids
Nasal decongestants
Licorice (may be found in chewing tobacco)
Appetite suppressants
Cyclosporine, tacrolimus
Cocaine and other illicit drugs
Erythropoietin
Caffeine
Antidepressants
Oral contraceptives
Nonsteroidal antiinflammatory drugs (NSAIDs)
Associated Conditions
Smoking
Increasing obesity
Sleep apnea
Insulin resistance/hyperinsulinemia
Ethanol intake of more than 1 oz (30 ml) per day
Anxiety-induced hyperventilation or panic attacks
Chronic pain
Intense vasoconstriction (arteritis)
Organic brain syndrome (e.g., memory deficit)

is the physician's responsibility to use his or her knowledge and put together the best available combinations of antihypertensive agents so as to reduce blood pressure into the range that the patient can tolerate and that will reduce cardiovascular and renal disease progression. Additional discussion on the management of hypertension in children is found in Chapter 64, on hypertension in the elderly in Chapter 65, and on hypertension in African-Americans in Chapter 66.

Selected Readings

Bakris GL. Microalbuminuria: prognostic implications. *Curr Opin Nephrol Hypertens* 1996;5(3):219–223.

An overview of data from long-term clinical and epidemiologic studies that evaluate the role of microalbuminuria as a risk factor for renal disease progression as well as cardiovascular risk. Data are reviewed from both diabetic and nondiabetic studies.

Bakris GL, Weir MR. Salt intake and reductions in arterial pressure and proteinuria: is there a direct link? *Am J Hypertens* 1996;9:200s–206s.

This article reviews the impact of high sodium intake on the antiproteinuric effect of ACE inhibitors and nondihydropyridine calcium agonists.

Curb JD, Pressel SL, Cutler JA, et al. Effect of diuretic-based antihypertensive treatment on cardiovascular disease risk in older diabetic patients with isolated systolic hypertension. *JAMA* 1996;276:1886–1892.

This paper presents data from the Systolic Hypertension in the Elderly Program (SHEP) trial. It clearly indicates that diuretics reduce mortality when blood pressure is controlled among elderly persons.

Epstein M, Bakris GL. Newer approaches to antihypertensive therapy: use fixed-dose combination therapy. *Arch Intern Med* 1996;156:1969–1978.

A historic review and perspective of fixed-dose antihypertensive therapy in the armamentarium of blood pressure control.

Joint National Committee Report on the Diagnosis and Treatment of Hypertension (JNC VI). *Arch Intern Med* 1997;157:2413–2446.

The most recent consensus report on the diagnosis and treatment of hypertension in all commonly encountered clinical settings.

Kasiske BL, Ma JZ, Kalil RSN, et al. Effects of antihypertensive therapy on serum lipids. *Ann Intern Med* 1995;122:133–141.

This is a meta-analysis of studies that evaluate the effects of lipids and their subfractions on renal disease progression.

Lazarus JM, Bourgoignie JJ, Buckalew VM, et al. Achievement and safety of a low blood pressure goal in chronic renal disease, The Modification of Diet in Renal Disease Study Group. *Hypertension* 1997;29:641–650.

Post-hoc analysis of the Modification of Diet in Renal Disease (MDRD) trial with a focus on the level of blood pressure reduction on renal disease progression among African-American subjects with hypertension and renal insufficiency.

Makrilakis K, Bakris GL. New therapeutic approaches to achieve the desired blood pressure goal. *Cardiovasc Rev & Reports* 1997;18:10–16.

This article reviews the newer modalities of fixed-dose combination therapy and presents a newer approach to lower pressure in patients with difficult-to-control hypertension.

Muntzel M, Drueke T. A comprehensive review of the salt and blood pressure relationship. *Am J Hypertens* 1992;5:1s–42s.

This article reviews concepts of salt sensitivity and other related issues in the context of race and sex as they relate to blood pressure reduction and impact on the efficacy of antihypertensive medication.

Perry HM, Miller JP, Fornoff JR. Early predictors of 15-year end-stage renal disease in hypertensive patients. *Hypertension* 1995;25:587–594.

Results of a retrospective analysis of more than 11,000 patients from Veteran's Administration Medical Centers that clearly demonstrate that systolic hypertension is one of the strongest predictors of renal disease progression and development, stronger than diastolic pressure.

Remuzzi G, Ruggenenti P, Benigni A. Understanding the nature of renal disease progression. *Kidney Int* 1997;51:2–15.

A meta-analysis of clinical studies that evaluates the impact of different classes of antihypertensive medications on renal disease progression in the context of proteinuria reduction.

Silverman M, Bakris GL. Treatment of renal failure and blood pressure. *Curr Opin Nephrol Hypertens* 1997;6:237–242.

This paper presents an overview of the pathophysiologic changes that occur in chronic renal failure and an approach to optimize antihypertensive and related therapies.

Tarif N, Bakris GL. Preservation of renal function: the spectrum of effects by calcium channel blockers. *Nephrol Dial Transpl* 1997;12:2244–2250.

This article presents a comprehensive review of all aspects of calcium antagonists as they relate to the prevention of renal disease progression. The focus is on why differences exist between the calcium channel blockers and how this translates into different renal outcomes given similar blood pressure control.

Villarosa I, Bakris GL. Antihypertensive treatment in type 2 diabetes with nephropathy. In: Ritz E, Fliser D, eds. *Nephropathy in type II diabetes.* London: Oxford University Press, 1999:111–136.

This paper reviews the importance of lower levels of blood pressure reduction as well as how to achieve this in diabetic patients without compromising glucose control.

Weir MR, Bakris GL, Toto RD, et al. Hypertension. In: Gonick H, ed. *Current nephrology.* St. Louis: Mosby-Year Book, 1997;20:209–241.

This paper reviews the major risk factors associated with renal disease development and progression among patients with hypertension.

PART 2
White Coat Hypertension

Yahya Sagliker

DEFINITION AND PREVALENCE

The prevalence of hypertension around the world varies among different ethnic group and countries, ranging between 20% and 23%. Hypertension occupies the third place as a cause of morbidity and mortality among the general population.

Blood pressure variability in response to environmental influences may be considered in five categories defined as follows:

1. *Normal blood pressure:* These subjects have blood pressure measurements of less than 140/90 mm Hg at home as well as when measured in medical environment or during stress.
2. *Sustained hypertension:* These are patients who have a blood pressure readings of greater than 140/90 mmHg on repeated measurements.
3. *"White-coat" phenomenon:* These are subjects whose blood pressure reading is less than 140/90 mm Hg in their regular daily life, but equal or higher while they are in any medical environment and particularly when the measurement of blood pressure is done by a doctor or a nurse wearing a white coat. However, this definition does not always reflect the total reality because the blood pressure levels of these subjects always increase when they face doctors or nurses, whether or not they are wearing a white coat, and these patients also display a rise in blood pressure when they visit medical facilities. In contrast, these subjects do not have an elevation in their blood pressure when they visit their butcher shops, attend movie theaters, or meet religious personnel. Thus this phenomenon is quite far from that of "white-coat" hypertension. It is more related to medical environment and/or devices. Some of these patients are aware of this phenomenon and refuse to attend medical facilities or subject themselves to medical devices. Their fear is more related to the device used for measuring blood pressure than the color of the coat of the person measuring the blood pressure.
4. *"White-coat" hypertension:* These patients are already hypertensive in their routine daily life but develop higher levels of blood pressure when they are exposed to a medical environment and/or devices.
5. *Stress hypertension:* These subjects have blood pressure levels below 140/90 mm Hg during their daily routine but display significant elevation in their blood pressure when exposed to psychologic or emotional stresses during days or nights; these stresses include hearing door bells; hearing phones ring; receiving bad news; going to courts, financial districts, or funerals; and facing monetary crises.

The concept of white-coat phenomenon was first described in 1940. The prevalence of white-coat hypertension in large studies varies between 16% and 60%, and it increases with age irrespective of gender; indeed it is more pronounced in the elderly, particularly in those with isolated systolic hypertension.

Some studies have shown that blood pressure levels measured by doctors are higher than those measured by nurses in the same patient (Fig. 61.5). Similarly, blood pressure may increase in male adolescents when measured by a woman compared with that measured by a man (Fig. 61.6).

The mechanisms responsible for white-coat hypertension are not well defined. However, a strong relationship between white-coat hypertension and psychologic and emotional factors has been demonstrated. A study from Japan showed that in patients with white-coat hypertension, blood pressure increases when the patients are presented with a mental arithmetic challenge.

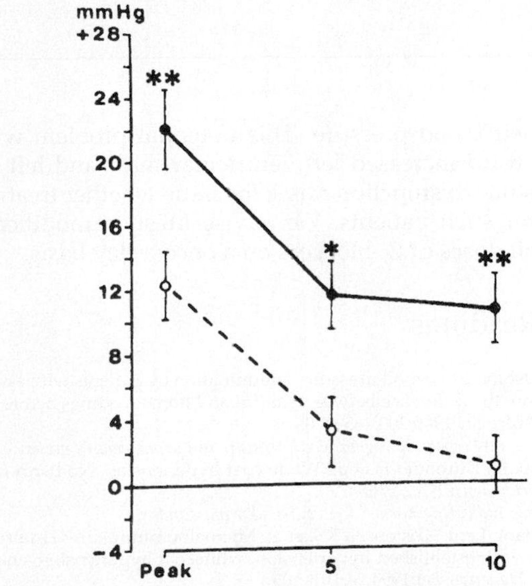

Figure 61.5. Differences between blood pressure levels taken by doctor and nurses. *Solid line:* Taken by doctors. *Dashed line:* Taken by nurses. (Adapted with permission from Mancia G, Parati G, Pomidossi G, et al. Alerting reaction and rise in blood pressure during measurement by physician and nurse. *Hypertension* 1987;9:209–215.)

TARGET ORGAN DAMAGE

Observations on the effect of white-coat hypertension on microalbuminuria have been inconsistent and conflicting. Thus there is no clear relationship between white-coat hypertension and microalbuminuria.

There are no consistent data on abnormalities in glucose and lipid metabolism in patients with white-coat hypertension. However, we found that blood levels of cholesterol, low-density lipoprotein cholesterol, and triglycerides increase gradually in such patients as they progress from a normotensive state to that of white-coat hypertension and then to sustained hypertension.

It was reported that blood vessels elasticity, compliance, and stiffness in patients with white-coat hypertension are different from normal subjects. Some studies, including our own, have shown an abnormality in left ventricular muscle mass in patients with white-coat hypertension compared with subjects with normal blood pressure (Table 61.16). Indeed, it was reported that a correlation between white-coat blood pressure levels and left ventricular hypertrophy exists (Fig. 61.7). There is also a trend toward impairment in left ventricular diastolic function in patients with white-coat hypertension compared with normal subjects (Table 61.16).

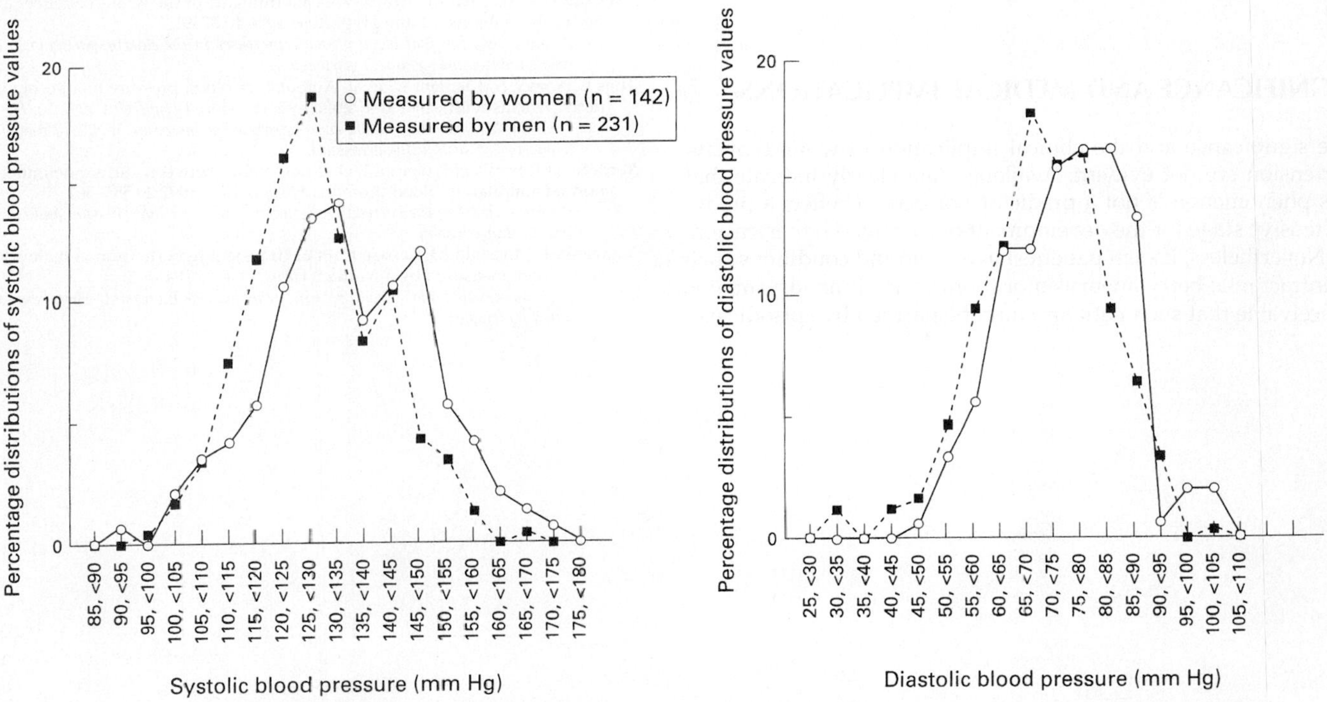

Figure 61.6. A reverse relation for the blood pressure levels taken by women and men. (Adapted with permission from Yamazaki T, Miyazaki M, Kanase H, et al. Transient hypertension in male adolescents when measured by a woman. *Heart* 1998;79:104–105.)

TABLE 61.16. Systolic and Diastolic Functions in Normal Subjects, Patients with White-Coat Hypertension, or Those with Sustained Hypertension

	IVS (mm)	PWD (mm)	LVMI (g/m²)	E/A
PHP	11.7±1	11.4±1.0	137.5±8.3	0.86±0.01
WCHP	11.0±1.2	11.0±0.8	131.3±14.4	1.12±0.4
CS	10.0±1.0	9.5±1.2	107.0±2.0	1.60±0.2
P value (PHP vs. WCHP)	>.05	>.05	>.05	<.02
P value (PHP vs. CS)	>.05	<.04[a]	<.03[a]	<.002α
P value (WCHP vs. CS)	>.05	<.01[a]	<.05[a]	<.001α

A, atrial contribution peak to diastole; CS, control subjects; E, early atrial filling peak; IVS, interventricular septum; LVMI, left ventricular mass index; PHP, sustained hypertension; PWD, posterior wall dimension; WCHP, white-coat hypertension.
[a] Significant difference ($p < 0.05$) compared with controls.

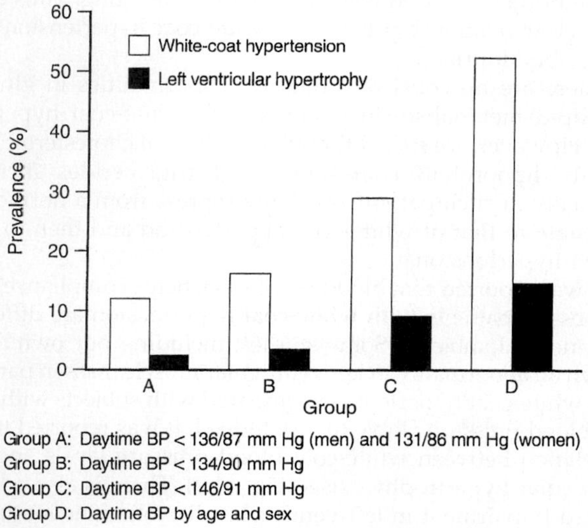

Figure 61.7. Correlations between blood pressure and left ventricular hypertrophy levels. (Adapted with permission from Verdecchia P, Schillaci F, Zampi I, et al. Variability between current definitions of normal ambulatory blood pressure. *Hypertension* 1992;20:555–562.)

SIGNIFICANCE AND MEDICAL IMPLICATIONS

The significance and the clinical implication of white-coat hypertension are not evident. Available data clearly indicate that this phenomenon is not a predictor nor does it reflect a prehypertensive stage for the development of sustained hypertension.

Nevertheless, if such patients have comorbid conditions such as intracranial berry aneurysm or thoracic aortic aneurysm, it is conceivable that such patients could be harmed by episodic elevation in their blood pressure. This potential problem with a tendency toward increased left ventricular mass and left ventricular diastolic dysfunction raises the issue whether treatment is needed for such patients. We advise lifestyle modification and/or small doses of β_1-blockers on a once-a-day basis.

Selected Readings

Ayman D, Goldshine AD. Blood pressure determination by patients with essential hypertension: the difference between clinical and home readings before treatment. *Am J Med Sci* 1940;200:465–470.
The first study reporting higher blood pressure in the physician's presence.

Gosse P, Promax H, Durondet P, et al. White coat hypertension. No harm for the heart. *Hypertension* 1993;22:766–770.
A research indicating normal left ventricular mass index.

Hoegholm A, Bang Lem, Kristensen KS, et al. Microalbuminuria in 411 untreated individuals with established hypertension, whitecoat hypertension, and normotension. *Hypertension* 1994;24:101–105.
A study showing no increased levels of microalbuminuria.

Kuwajima I, Suzuki Y, Fujisawa A, et al. Is whitecoat hypertension innocent? *Hypertension* 1993;22:826–831.
A study showing impaired left ventricular diastolic function.

Mancia G, Parati G, Pomidossi G, et al. Alerting reaction and rise in blood pressure during measurements by physician and nurse. *Hypertension* 1987;9:209–215.
Research showing an alerting reaction and rise in blood pressure during measurements by physician and nurse.

Mansoor GA, McCabe EJ, White WB. Determinants of the whitecoat effect in hypertensive subjects. J Hum Hypertens 1996;10:87–92.
A study showing that blood pressure increases in the elderly, particularly those who have isolated systolic hypertension.

Thijs L, Amery A, Clement D, et al. Ambulatory blood pressure monitoring in elderly patients with isolated systolic hypertension. *J Hypertens* 1992;10:693–699.
A study demonstrating white-coat hypertension increases in elderly people who have isolated systolic hypertension.

Verdecchia P, Schillaci F, Zampi I, et al. Variability between current definitions of normal ambulatory blood pressure. *Hypertension* 1992;20:555–562.
Research showing the correlation between white-coat hypertension and left ventricular hypertrophy.

Yamazaki T, Miyazaki M, Kanase H, et al. Transient hypertension in male adolescents when measured by a woman. *Heart* 1998;79:104–105.
A study showing that blood pressure in males was increasing when being measured by females.

CHAPTER 62

Renovascular Hypertension

Christopher S. Wilcox

DEFINITION

Renovascular hypertension defines a functional subset of hypertension that is caused by reduced renal perfusion pressure. Its operational definition is hypertension that is improved or cured by reversal of a renal artery stenosis. *Renal artery stenosis* is an anatomic diagnosis: a narrowing of one or both renal arteries or their branches. The great majority of patients with renovascular hypertension have renal artery stenosis. *Renovascular disease* is a generic term encompassing renovascular hypertension, renal artery stenosis, and a poorly defined condition referred to as vascular or ischemic nephropathy or azotemic renovascular hypertension. Some related conditions that do not fall strictly within this definition and are not considered in this chapter include hypertension caused by small vessel disease within the kidney and renin-secreting tumors.

The definition of renovascular hypertension is unsatisfactory, both for the practicing nephrologist and for the clinical investigator. Several points require emphasis. First, the finding of a renal artery stenosis, even of high grade, in a hypertensive patient does not necessarily imply causality. Thus the stenosis may represent coexistence of a functionally unimportant renal artery stenosis and essential hypertension. Alternatively, the stenosis may have been the original cause of the hypertension, but the condition has progressed to a very late stage in its natural history when hypertension has become autonomous and persists despite correction of the renal artery stenosis. Second, the apparent degree of stenosis may be exaggerated by catheter tip spasm during arteriography or by turbulent blood flow during magnetic resonance angiography. Third, failure of hypertension to improve or reverse following an intervention to correct renal artery stenosis does not negate the possibility that the stenosis was the cause of the hypertension. The intervention may not have been successful in reversing the stenosis, or the stenosis may have recurred or another stenosis may have developed in the intervening time. Failure of blood pressure to decrease after an intervention to correct renal artery stenosis can only be taken as evidence that the stenosis was unimportant if the angiography is performed again and the renal artery stenosis is seen to have been corrected. Moreover, renal artery stenosis is often superimposed on underlying essential hypertension. Because this is a progressive condition, a remission of hypertension that is only temporary may reflect the progression of the underlying essential hypertension, especially when this is complicated by impairment of renal function and progressive azotemia. This uncertainty in the diagnosis of renovascular hypertension contributes to the lack of precision apparent in the results of clinical trials of tests or interventions for this condition. Even a test with perfect accuracy would be evaluated as flawed if the patient's diagnosis was wrong.

Renovascular hypertension is defined by the response of hypertension to correction of renal artery stenosis. Yet nephrologists increasingly have as their primary goal the stabilization or improvement of renal function rather than a decrease in hypertension. For these patients, a term such as *vascular nephropathy* may be preferred. *Ischemic nephropathy* is a less satisfactory term because it implies that the renal tissue has a low oxygen tension, yet this cannot be assessed adequately with current methods.

PATHOPHYSIOLOGY

Animal Models

Immediately after a constricting clip or clamp is placed around one renal artery, there is an autoregulatory vasodilation of the afferent arterioles that maintains the renal blood flow and the glomerular filtration rate (GFR), providing that the mean renal perfusion pressure is not reduced below approximately 70 mm Hg. The fall in renal perfusion pressure is accompanied by a brisk release of renin within the kidney, leading to increased secretion of renin into the renal vein and increased generation of angiotensin I (Ang I) and angiotensin II (Ang II) within the renal parenchyma, as reflected in measurements in renal lymph. Both the renal arteriolar vasodilation and the renin secretion increase in proportion to the reduction in renal perfusion pressure. Release of renin into renal venous plasma and renal lymph of the clipped kidney increases the circulating plasma renin activity (PRA). Renin acts on its substrate, angiotensinogen, which is formed predominantly in the liver, to increase the circulating levels of Ang I. Further metabolism by angiotensin-converting enzymes (ACEs) located on vascular endothelium and in most tissues leads to the formation of the octapeptide, Ang II. Further metabolism by peptidases leads to other active peptides, such as angiotensin III, but ultimately to inactive fragments.

Activation of the renin-angiotensin system (RAS) is critical for determining the early pathophysiologic events. First, the generation of Ang II within the clipped kidney counteracts the effects of autoregulation and maintains the renal vascular resistance. This effect of Ang II in the clipped kidney is expressed predominantly on the efferent arterioles. The ensuing increase in the postglomerular vascular resistance is critical for the maintenance of adequate glomerular capillary hydraulic pressure (P_{GC}) and GFR when the perfusion pressure is falling. The combination of reduced renal perfusion pressure and high local Ang II levels ensure a high rate of renal tubular sodium chloride reabsorption in the poststenotic kidney, despite systemic hypertension. The level of sodium reabsorption by the contralateral kidney is also inappropriately high for the degree of hypertension. This can be seen as a blunted pressure natriuresis or a shift to the right in the relationship between sodium excretion and perfusion pressure. The enhanced tubular sodium reabsorption at the contralateral kidney also can be ascribed in large part to Ang II because this is reduced after blockade of Ang II generation with an ACE inhibitor. However, unlike the clipped kidney, the renin secretion and local Ang II production by the contralateral kidney are strongly suppressed. The effects of Ang II on this kidney are due to Ang II generated in the circulation in response to renin secreted from the clipped kidney.

Within hours or days of placement of a unilateral renal artery clip or clamp, the blood pressure begins to rise progressively. During this early phase, the hypertension is strictly dependent on the circulating RAS because blockade of Ang II generation with an ACE inhibitor or of Ang II receptors with a nonselective Ang II antagonist (e.g., saralasin) or with a selective Ang II type I (AT_1) receptor antagonist (e.g., losartan) entirely prevents the development of hypertension or, when hypertension has developed, reverses it abruptly.

Subsequent events depend on several factors, including the species of the experimental animal, the presence of a normal contralateral kidney, the level of dietary salt intake, and the time after clipping. In the dog, it is hard to induce consistent and sustained hypertension with a unilateral renal artery clamp unless the contralateral kidney is removed or the clamp is tightened progressively to further restrict renal perfusion pressure. In the rat, placement of a unilateral renal artery clip, with the contralateral kidney intact, leads to progressive hypertension. This is termed *two-kidney, one-clip Goldblatt hypertension*, which is a model for hypertension caused by a unilateral renal artery stenosis in humans. In this model, the level of dietary NaCl intake influences the PRA but not the development of hypertension. After 10 to 12 weeks, the hypertension enters an intermediate phase characterized by a further rise in arterial pressure but a return of PRA and plasma Ang II concentrations to, or toward, the preclip values. However, during this phase, the clipped kidney is still secreting renin, as evidenced by a high renal venoarterial gradient for PRA across this kidney. Renin secretion by the contralateral kidney is fully suppressed. Tissue levels of renin, renin mRNA, and Ang II follow the pattern of renin secretion. They are increased in the clipped kidney but severely reduced in the contralateral kidney. During this intermediate phase, the RAS exerts a complicated effect on blood pressure control mechanisms reflected in the variable effects of an ACE inhibitor or Ang II receptor antagonist on blood pressure. Thus, in some studies the PRA remains elevated, and in these rats, interruption of the RAS reduces the blood pressure abruptly and in proportion to the level of PRA. When the PRA is not elevated, interruption of the RAS has little immediate effect on blood pressure. More prolonged administration of an ACE inhibitor over many hours or days can completely reverse hypertension during this phase even in rats that did not have an abrupt fall in blood pressure with the first dose of the ACE inhibitor. Importantly, the administration of an ACE inhibitor can reduce the GFR of the clipped kidney, despite little or no short-term antihypertensive effect. This indicates that Ang II may have important actions on blood pressure and renal function that outlive the effects of elevated circulating Ang II levels. This may reflect the effects of Ang II generation in the tissues of the kidney, blood vessel walls, and brain. Removal of the clip or of the clipped kidney leads to prompt reversal of hypertension in the early and intermediate phases of two-kidney, one-clip hypertension.

Some 4 to 9 months after clipping, the hypertension enters a chronic phase characterized by sustained hypertension despite normal or even suppressed levels of PRA and circulating Ang II. The administration of a renin-angiotensin antagonist during this phase causes a slow reduction in blood pressure to near-normal values over 3 to 4 days. However, unclipping of the kidney does not normalize blood pressure. Thus blood pressure remains Ang II dependent, but has become somewhat autonomous. This may be due to the development of structural lesions of glomerulosclerosis in the contralateral kidney and of hypertrophy, proliferation, and fibrosis in the blood vessels.

When a clip is placed around both renal arteries (two-kidney, two-clip hypertension) or the contralateral kidney is removed after clipping (one-kidney, one-clip hypertension), the intermediate phase of the hypertension has a different pathophysiology. This has been used as a model for hypertension caused by stenosis of both renal arteries or of stenosis to a single or dominant kidney (e.g., renal transplant stenosis). If dietary salt levels are high, the PRA is barely elevated in these models. Administration of an ACE inhibitor or AT_1 antagonist has only a transient antihypertensive action, even in the early phase. However, Ang II dependence can be uncovered in animals ingesting a salt-restricted diet. In the earlier phases of hypertension in the two-kidney, one-clip model there is less salt sensitivity than with the two-kidney, two-clip or one-kidney, one-clip models because the presence of a normal unclipped contralateral kidney provides a route, albeit blunted, for NaCl excretion in response to the rise in blood pressure (pressure natriuresis).

The critical ingredients in the various models of Goldblatt hypertension include reduced renal perfusion pressure in the clipped kidney and enhanced action of Ang II in both kidneys. These together limit NaCl elimination and promote sustained hypertension. ACE inhibitors are natriuretic in rats with two-kidney, one-clip renovascular hypertension, despite causing a sharp fall in the blood pressure. The antihypertensive response to unclipping in the early or intermediate phases of two-kidney, one-clip hypertension is paralleled by a reduction in circulating Ang II and a marked natriuresis by the previously clipped kidney.

Actions of Angiotensin II on Blood Pressure Regulatory Mechanisms

Ang II coordinates many prohypertensive actions. First, it has important actions on the nervous system. Its actions within the brain release arginine vasopressin, stimulate thirst and salt appetite, enhance the tone of the sympathetic nervous system, and blunt the baroreflex. These effects are quantitatively important because an ACE inhibitor or AT_1 antagonist given in low dose into the brain is almost as effective in lowering blood pressure in rats with early or intermediate two-kidney, one-clip hypertension as an intravenous infusion of these drugs. Brain Ang II is derived in part from circulating Ang II, which can penetrate the blood–brain barrier at certain sites. However, the brain has a complete RAS and can generate Ang II locally, independent of the circulating system. Ang II also promotes the peripheral sympathetic nervous system by enhancing ganglionic transmission, peripheral sympathetic neurotransmission, norepinephrine release, and the contractile response of norepinephrine on vascular smooth muscle cells.

Second, Ang II promotes renal salt retention. It has a direct effect on the early proximal tubule to enhance the activity of the Na^+-H^+ antiporter, thereby facilitating $NaHCO_3$ and fluid reabsorption. Its effects on renal hemodynamics, which include an increase in the filtration fraction, may increase the interstitial protein concentration and further enhance the reabsorption of

NaCl and fluid by the proximal nephron. It stimulates the secretion of aldosterone and inhibits the secretion of atrial natriuretic peptide, which facilitates NaCl reabsorption by the collecting ducts.

Third, Ang II interacts with various tissue autocoid systems, including prostaglandin (PG). Ang II activates phospholipases, which stimulate the release of arachidonate, whose metabolism by cyclooxygenase yields PG endoperoxides such as PGH_2. Subsequent metabolism to PGE_2 or prostacyclin produces agents that buffer the actions of Ang II on renal and systemic vasoconstriction, enhancement of the sympathetic nervous system, and renal NaCl retention. In contrast, metabolism to thromboxane A_2 (TxA_2) provides a powerful contractile agent, which also stimulates NaCl reabsorption in the kidney and activates the sympathetic nervous system. TxA_2 and PGH_2 promote several of the hypertensive actions of Ang II. The net effect of activation of this PG system is variable. Thus blockade of cyclooxygenase with aspirin or indomethacin can enhance the pressor and renal vasoconstrictor actions of Ang II, thereby demonstrating the overriding importance of the vasodilator PGs (PGE_2 and PGE_1) in this setting. In contrast, indomethacin and aspirin can be antihypertensive agents in rats with two-kidney, one-clip hypertension or humans with renovascular hypertension. These actions probably reflect the importance of prohypertensive PGs (TxA_2 and PGH_2) and a reduction in renin secretion.

Some rats with two-kidney, one-clip hypertension develop a hyponatremic malignant hypertensive syndrome characterized by reduced urine output, severe hypertension, azotemia, and vascular damage. During this phase, the PRA is markedly elevated, and the blood pressure can be reduced abruptly by an ACE inhibitor. However, ACE inhibitors can worsen azotemia. Administration of saline can reduce the blood pressure, at least temporarily.

Thus hypertension in the Goldblatt model is a complex interaction between the direct effects of the clip to increase vascular resistance in the kidney and reduce the perfusion pressure downstream and the effects of local and systemic Ang II. The hemodynamic actions of Ang II within the kidney further increase the renal vascular resistance, yet maintain the GFR. The systemic effects of Ang II on blood vessels raise the blood pressure directly, and its actions on the clipped and contralateral kidneys sustain the elevated blood pressure by retaining NaCl and fluid. The actions of Ang II in the brain interrupt the homeostatic reflex mechanisms that normally buffer changes in blood pressure and enhance sympathetic tone and arginine vasopressin release. A complex set of actions of Ang II in the tissues, blood vessels, and kidneys, involving generation of PGs and other autocoids, can promote or blunt the ultimate degree of hypertension achieved. With time, maladaptive and irreversible processes become predominant in sustaining hypertension through vascular proliferation of resistance vessels and, ultimately, sclerosis in the contralateral kidney.

Human Renovascular Hypertension

In the rare instance in which the onset of renovascular hypertension can be clearly dated, subjects typically have an elevated PRA and hypertension that is strongly Ang II dependent. More often, a renal artery stenosis develops insidiously over months or years before diagnosis. In these patients, the PRA and plasma Ang II concentrations often are elevated. However, about one-third of patients have a normal PRA value, although low renin values are quite exceptional. The immediate antihypertensive response to an ACE inhibitor is proportional to the log of the PRA. However, ACE inhibitors have an additional and delayed antihypertensive action in patients with essential or renovascular hypertension that is not so clearly related to PRA values. There is a significant correlation between the blood pressure during ACE inhibitor monotherapy and that achieved after a technically successful reversal of renal artery stenosis by percutaneous transluminal renal angioplasty (PTRA) or reconstructive surgery.

As with the animal model, PRA is often elevated in the renal vein draining the stenotic kidney, despite a less impressive elevation of systemic PRA. This is explained by a suppression of renin secretion by the contralateral kidney. A more reliable index of renovascular hypertension than PRA is a reduction in GFR or a prolongation in nephron tubular fluid transit time of the poststenotic kidney after administration of an ACE inhibitor. These findings indicated that Ang II action in the poststenotic kidney is closely related to the development of hypertension. As in the chronic rat model of two-kidney, one-clip hypertension, hypertension in patients with very advanced, prolonged renal artery stenosis with marked atrophy of the poststenotic kidney may no longer respond to successful reversal of the stenosis. There is evidence of enhanced sympathetic nervous system activity in human renovascular hypertension because plasma norepinephrine levels may be elevated and there is an exaggerated antihypertensive response to interruption of sympathetic tone with clonidine.

As in the two-kidney, two-clip rat model, patients with bilateral renal artery stenosis may have severe hypertension without elevated PRA levels. However, these subjects often retain the characteristic reduction in GFR after administration of an ACE inhibitor, which can be sufficiently severe to lead to acute renal insufficiency during ACE inhibitor therapy. Patients with stenosis of a single functioning kidney (e.g., renal transplant recipients) may have marked blood pressure dependency on circulating Ang II, especially if diuretics and salt restriction are used to control the hypertension. Thus the rat models of Goldblatt hypertension are helpful in understanding the pathophysiology of the human condition, but it is harder to place human subjects on a continuum between early, intermediate, and late phases. Moreover, renal artery stenosis is often progressive in human subjects. Some patients develop a rapid elevation of blood pressure with vascular damage, oliguria, thirst, and hyponatremia. These patients with accelerated or malignant hypertension frequently have very high values for PRA, analogous to the hyponatremic hypertensive syndrome in the two-kidney, one-clip rat model.

PREVALENCE

The prevalence of renal artery stenosis among unselected patients with mild hypertension in the community is less than 1%. Its prevalence becomes much higher among certain categories of patients seen by nephrologists or referred to a hospital setting. The prevalence rises some 10-fold among patients with moderate hypertension seen in a referral clinic. Prevalence rates of 10% to 35% are reported in patients with severe, accelerated, or malignant hypertension and in those who remain hypertensive despite therapy with three or more antihypertensive agents. The prevalence of renal artery stenosis in hypertensive patients investigated for aortoiliac occlusive vascular disease or coronary artery disease is 15% to 35%. It is greater than 50% in hypertensive patients with a paraumbilical bruit. Renovascular hypertension is seen quite frequently among patients with hypertension and impaired renal function, but the true prevalence in this patient population is uncertain. Other studies have reported a 30% prevalence of unsuspected renal artery stenosis among elderly patients in whom renal disease is progressing to end-stage and a 34% prevalence in elderly patients with congestive heart failure.

ETIOLOGY AND PATHOLOGY

The main causes of renovascular hypertension are shown in Table 62.1. The cause of renovascular hypertension is atherosclerosis or fibromuscular disease in more than 95% of patients. Atherosclerotic lesions of the renal artery typically occur at the ostium or the proximal segment of the renal artery and complicate generalized atherosclerosis. In contrast, fibromuscular disease can affect any part of the renal artery or its intrarenal branches. Fibromuscular disease often is confined to the renal arteries but may involve other vessels. The lesions of fibromuscular disease are frequently multiple. Areas of local stenosis are succeeded by aneurysmal dilation, leading to a string-of-beads appearance on arteriography. The renal artery may be elongated, and the kidney may show nephroptosis. Not infrequently, prolonged hypertension resulting from neglected fibromuscular disease is complicated by superimposed atherosclerosis. Both conditions are frequently bilateral.

Fibromuscular disease usually affects the media of the blood vessel wall. Medial or paramedial fibroplasia accounts for 85% and medial hyperplasia for 10%. Occasional patients display medial dissection, intimal fibroplasia, or periarterial fibroplasia. In many patients medial fibroplasia shows no progression over many years, and complete occlusion or thrombosis of the renal artery is unusual.

Fibromuscular disease is the most common cause of renovascular hypertension among young subjects. It occurs eight times as frequently in females as in males. In contrast, atherosclerosis accounts for an overwhelming number of cases in the elderly population. Black subjects have a lower prevalence of renovascular hypertension. In Asians, Takayasu's arteritis can cause renovascular hypertension. Other forms of arteritis, including polyarteritis nodosa or progressive systemic sclerosis, are occasional causes of renovascular hypertension. They are important to diagnose because they require specific therapy.

Renovascular hypertension may be caused by ureteral obstruction, for example, secondary to malignant involvement of the ureter. A simple renal artery cyst may lead to hypertension by compromising renal perfusion pressure. Hypertension can be reduced after cyst drainage. However, simple renal cysts and hypertension are both very common diseases. It is only rarely that the cyst is the cause of the hypertension. Patients with polycystic kidney disease often have hypertension. The etiology of their hypertension is complex, but ACE inhibitors can reduce the blood pressure and the GFR abruptly, which suggests that some may have a form of renovascular hypertension. Abdominal aortic aneurysms may cause renovascular hypertension by compromising the renal perfusion pressure because of involvement of the origin of one or both renal arteries. Coarctation of the aorta is a form of hypertension caused in part by a persistent reduction in renal perfusion pressure. Indeed, any condition that limits transmission of arterial pressure to the afferent arterioles and glomeruli may be a cause of renovascular hypertension.

The sudden development of hypertension after renal trauma or after car accidents should prompt consideration of renovascular hypertension. This may be secondary to a renal artery dissection or thrombosis or to an intrarenal arteriovenous fistula. Hypertension may also develop more insidiously following a perirenal hematoma that compresses the kidney as it heals by fibrosis and scarring (Page kidney).

The kidney downstream from a renal artery stenosis has a relatively well-preserved vasculature. Glomeruli may appear normal or show ischemic atrophy. With advanced disease, there is tubular atrophy and interstitial fibrosis that ultimately becomes extensive. The contralateral kidney shows the typical features of sustained, severe hypertension. The vessels show medial hypertrophy and endothelial hyperplasia, with an increased vessel wall/lumen ratio. Glomeruli show sclerosis and ischemic atrophy. Ultimately, this kidney may develop the features of generalized nephrosclerosis.

TABLE 62.1. Etiology of Renovascular Hypertension

	Frequency (%)
Atherosclerosis of the renal artery	75
Fibromuscular disease	20
Abdominal aortic aneurysm	2
Rarer causes	3
Vasculitis (including Takayasu's disease, polyarteritis nodosa, and progressive systemic sclerosis)	
Renal embolism or infarction	
Intrarenal arteriovenous fistula	
Renal or perirenal neoplasm	
Simple renal cyst	
Polycystic kidney disease	
Subcapsular hematoma (Page kidney)	
Renal arterial trauma	
Renal outflow obstruction	
Coarctation of the aorta	

NATURAL HISTORY

Renovascular hypertension frequently is more severe and rapidly progressive than essential hypertension, although exceptions are seen. Indeed, some patients with advanced congestive heart failure can have severe renal artery stenosis and normal or low levels of blood pressure. Severe renovascular hypertension is frequently associated with impaired renal function. Renovascular hypertension appearing in adolescence or early adulthood, especially in a female subject, should always raise the possibility of fibromuscular disease. Conversely, hypertension appearing for the first time in an elderly subject suggests atherosclerosis of the renal arteries. Fibromuscular disease is usually stable over long periods, although certain uncommon subcategories presenting in childhood can progress more rapidly to renal artery occlusion. In contrast, atherosclerosis of the renal artery, like that elsewhere, typically progresses relentlessly. Over a 2-year period, in approximately half of such patients a higher grade lesion will develop, and in one-tenth will progress to complete occlusion of the renal artery. Thus the risk with a decision to delay intervention in a patient with known atherosclerotic renal artery stenosis is that renal function may become irreparably impaired. Detailed discussion of occlusive renal vascular disease is provided in Chapter 52.

CLINICAL FEATURES

Clinical features are reviewed in Table 62.2. Some features are highly discriminatory. For example, an abdominal bruit, especially when prolonged and heard in the flank, is 5- to 20-fold more frequently seen in renovascular hypertension than in essential hypertension. Fifty percent of hypertensive patients with a bruit are found to have renal artery stenosis. The presence of severe, accelerated, or malignant hypertension or evidence of

TABLE 62.2. Clinical Features of Renovascular Hypertension

Features not typical of essential hypertension
Age of onset before 25 years, especially in females (suggests fibromuscular disease)
Age of onset after 55 years (suggests atherosclerotic disease)
Severe two or more drug-resistant hypertension
Accelerated or malignant hypertension
High grades of retinopathy
Absence of a family history of hypertension
Unexplained features of renal involvement
Azotemia
Heavy proteinuria
Renal size disparity of >1.5 cm in the long axis
Reversible azotemia during ACE inhibitor or AT_1 receptor antagonist therapy
Recurrent flash pulmonary edema, especially if the EF is preserved
Features of hyperaldosteronism
Hypokalemia
Alkalosis
Features of atherosclerosis elsewhere
History of coronary, carotid, cardiovascular, aortoiliac, or peripheral vascular disease
Severe CHF
Decreased or absent peripheral pulses
Peripheral vascular bruits
Heavy use of tobacco products
Features of turbulent renal artery blood flow
Abdominal bruit (especially when prolonged into diastole)
Flank bruit

ACE, angiotensin-converting enzyme; EF, ejection fraction; CHF, congestive heart failure.

unexplained renal functional impairment or hypokalemia, severe atherosclerosis elsewhere, or heavy use of tobacco should alert the physician to the possibility of renovascular hypertension. Other studies have shown a 30% prevalence of renal artery stenosis in patients whose hypertension is not controlled even with more than two antihypertensive agents. Unfortunately, no clinical algorithm has been developed that has sufficient accuracy to provide a reliable diagnosis of renovascular hypertension from the clinical features alone. Nevertheless, these clinical features remain critical in selecting patients for screening for renovascular hypertension.

DIAGNOSIS

Selection of Patients for Screening

Ideally, the detection and evaluation of patients with renovascular hypertension should start with an evaluation of clinical criteria and proceed to a screening test, to an anatomic diagnosis of renal artery stenosis and, if necessary, to a final functional test before intervention. Screening tests should be safe, inexpensive, and convenient for the patient because they must be applied to large numbers of patients. They must detect virtually all those with the condition (i.e., they must have a very high sensitivity) without including too many false-positive test results in those with essential hypertension (i.e., they must have quite a high specificity). Unfortunately, all tests are fallible and lack accuracy. Therefore a policy of blanket application of a screening test to an unselected population of patients with mild hypertension with a prevalence of renovascular hypertension of about 1% would yield many more false-positive than true positive results. If arteriograms were performed on these patients, the great majority of these expensive, invasive, and potentially harmful tests would be undertaken in patients with essential hypertension who had false-positive results from their screening tests. Therefore the clinician must first select a population of patients by reference to clinical features of renovascular hypertension (Table 62.2), before proceeding to screening.

Screening and Functional Tests

PRA, Intravenous Pyelogram, and Hippuran Renogram

The unstimulated peripheral PRA, intravenous pyelogram (IVP), and basal hippuran renogram have been extensively evaluated for use as screening tests. The PRA is a more discriminating test when it is related to the patient's dietary salt intake by comparison with a concurrent 24-hour sodium excretion measurement (renin/sodium profile). The patient should be studied after withdrawal of antihypertensive agents and diuretics for 2 weeks and after 30 minutes of sitting. Unfortunately, even in these ideal circumstances, the PRA value has limited accuracy because some 15% of patients with essential hypertension have high PRA values (high-renin hypertension). More seriously, up to 30% of patients with renovascular hypertension, especially those with bilateral renal artery stenosis or stenosis of a solitary kidney, have normal PRA values. Therefore the peripheral PRA value is a rather poor guide to the presence of renovascular hypertension.

Features of the IVP that suggest renal artery stenosis include a size disparity of greater than 1.5 cm in the long axis, a delay in the appearance and disappearance of the nephrogram phase, a delay in the excretion of contrast material into the renal pelvis and ureter, an enhancement of cortical contrast and evidence of collateral vessels supplying the kidney. These features are the consequences of reduced renal perfusion pressure at the affected kidney. A rapid sequence IVP should be used to screen for renovascular hypertension, but has limited accuracy.

Features of the hippuran renogram that suggest renovascular hypertension include a delay in the time to peak of greater than 40 seconds between the two kidneys, a delay in the elimination of hippuran from the renal cortex, and an unexplained difference in the size or in plasma flow between the two kidneys.

Extensive evaluation of the accuracy of the rapid sequence IVP and the hippuran renogram has shown that they have limited sensitivity and specificity of approximately 75% and 85%, respectively. This is inadequate for screening for renovascular hypertension.

Post-ACE Inhibitor PRA Test

Administration of an ACE inhibitor increases the PRA to a greater extent in patients with renovascular hypertension than in those with essential hypertension. This is caused by a sharp increase in secretion of active renin from the poststenotic kidney because of blockade of the negative feedback restraint on renin secretion by high levels of interstitial Ang II and a selective reduction in the GFR in the poststenotic kidney. A fall in GFR, leading to a fall in macula densa NaCl delivery and reabsorption, stimulates renin secretion. ACE inhibitors maintain or increase the GFR (and presumably also the macula densa NaCl delivery and reabsorption) in contralateral and normal kidneys. This may explain the selective stimulus to renin secretion after administration of ACE inhibitors in poststenotic kidneys. Regardless of the mechanism, the PRA after ACE inhibitor administration is a more discriminating test for renovascular hypertension than is a basal PRA.

Currently, the captopril PRA test is undergoing evaluation. The details of a simplified captopril test, suitable for conducting in the clinic setting, are given in Table 62.3. The test is very safe

TABLE 62.3. Simplified Captopril Test for Renovascular Hypertension

Exclusion criteria
Heart failure or edema
Cardiovascular instability
Severe hypertension not amenable to manipulation of drug therapy
Allergy to ACE inhibitors
Moderate or severe renal functional impairment (S_{cr} >2.5 mg/dl)
Absolute requirement for ACE inhibitor therapy
Preparation
No restriction of dietary salt
Diuretics and ACE inhibitors withdrawn for 2 weeks
Antihypertensive regimen switched to calcium antagonist and/or labetalol
Check renal function
Conduct of test
No antihypertensive drugs on day of the study
Patient seated throughout
Check BP three times: proceed only if hypertensive and BP stable
Administer captopril (50 mg crushed and suspended in water)
Draw blood for PRA before and 60 min after captopril
Check lying and standing BP
Discharge if stable
Interpretation
Test is positive if the post-captopril PRA >5.4 ng/ml/h (PRA assay by Smith-Kline or Mayo Medical Laboratory methods)

ACE, angiotensin-converting enzyme; PRA, plasma renin activity.

in patients selected as in Table 62.3. Unfortunately, renal functional impairment limits the test characteristics. Dietary salt restriction should not be undertaken. Diuretics and ACE inhibitors should be withdrawn 2 weeks previously. Where necessary, hypertension should be controlled with a calcium antagonist and/or an α- and β-blocking drug, such as labetalol. These drugs should not be administered on the day of testing. The patient should be seated throughout the test. Captopril should be administered only if the patient is hypertensive and the blood pressure is stable. Evaluation of the captopril test in 100 consecutive patients with hypertension in the author's hospital indicated that the PRA measured 1 hour after captopril was the single most discriminating function for renovascular hypertension. Others have developed a more complicated interpretation depending on the baseline PRA, the increase in PRA with captopril, and the fractional change with captopril. The use of multiple requirements for a positive test increases its specificity, yet limits its sensitivity and thereby its ability to detect renovascular disease in the patients who have it. Therefore we routinely undertake the simplified test in which only the postcaptopril PRA is evaluated. There is significant variability in PRA values between different laboratories. The cutoff value for PRA for a positive test is 5.4 ng of Ang I/ml per hour or more in the assay using the Smith-Kline or Mayo Medical Laboratory methods.

There is considerable variation between studies in the evaluation of the captopril test. However, among the largest studies of 100 or more patients, most have found a high sensitivity for diagnosis of renovascular disease (greater than 90%) but a limited specificity (85% to 90%). Application of a test with these characteristics to an unselected group of hypertensive patients with a prevalence of renovascular hypertension of less than 2% would yield a very low positive predictive value of less than 5%. This implies that only 5% of the patients with positive test results will have renovascular hypertension. The remaining 95% will have false-positive results. Therefore neither this test, nor any other noninvasive test currently evaluated, has a sufficiently high accuracy in different studies for diagnosis of renovascular hypertension when applied to an unselected population of hypertensive patients. In contrast, when applied to a group of subjects selected on clinical criteria (Table 62.2) with a prevalence of renovascular hypertension of 10% to 35%, the positive predictive value increases to 30% to 70%. Note that at all reasonable levels of prevalence of renovascular hypertension, the negative predictive value of a test with these characteristics is extremely high (about 99%). This implies that only about 1% of patients with a negative test result will have renovascular hypertension. It follows that a positive test result is not generally helpful in decision making, because even in a selected group of patients, it may identify incorrectly a patient with essential hypertension. In contrast, a negative test result is helpful because it implies that the patient has an extremely low probability of having renovascular hypertension. Unless there are compelling reasons to the contrary, the workup may be terminated after a negative test result, providing that the patient can be followed carefully thereafter.

Renal Vein Renin Test

Renal vein renin determinations have been evaluated as tests of functional significance of renal artery stenosis, but they have limited diagnostic accuracy. A positive test is indicated by an increase in the renal vein PRA of the affected side, compared with the vena cava, of 45% or more, accompanied by a renal vein PRA of the contralateral kidney that is not more than 10% above that of the vena cava. These differences are exaggerated after ACE inhibitor administration. The disadvantages of this test are its limited accuracy, its expense, the need to administer radiologic contrast agents, and the inconvenience to the patient. ACE inhibitor renography is now preferred by most physicians.

ACE Inhibitor Renogram

Administration of ACE inhibitors to rats with two-kidney, one-clip Goldblatt hypertension causes a selective reduction in the GFR, urine flow rate, and sodium excretion in the clipped kidney. The contralateral kidney shows the opposite changes.

[^{99m}Tc]-Diethylenetriaminepentaacetic acid (DTPA) is a GFR marker. Its plasma disappearance is proportional to the global GFR, and its initial renal uptake is proportional to the single kidney fraction of global GFR. Therefore DTPA can be used to estimate the single-kidney GFR. Functionally important unilateral renal artery stenosis is detected as a reduction in the single-kidney GFR after ACE inhibitor administration relative to that at the contralateral kidney. The functional importance of bilateral renal artery stenosis is indicated by a reduction in the global GFR. ACE inhibitor administration delays the cortical elimination of DTPA in the poststenotic kidney.

o-[^{131}I]-Iodohippurate (hippuran) is a marker of renal plasma flow. After administration of an ACE inhibitor to a two-kidney, one-clip Goldblatt hypertensive rat, the renal plasma flow of the clipped and contralateral kidneys is increased. Therefore the delivery of hippuran to the proximal tubule cells and its secretion into the tubular lumen are increased. However, if the renal artery stenosis is functionally important, ACE inhibitors cause a sharp reduction in the GFR and therefore of the tubular fluid flow rate. Thus hippuran secretion is maintained, but its elimination from the nephron is impaired. Therefore ACE inhibitors delay the time to peak of the hippuran renogram or, in extreme cases, cause a progressive accumulation of hippuran throughout the period of the renogram. Either a reduction in single-kidney DTPA uptake or a delay in hippuran or DTPA elimination from the renal cortex after ACE inhibitor can detect functionally important renal artery stenosis.

Most nuclear medicine units now use [^{99m}Tc]-mercaptoacetyltriglycine (MAG_3), which combines excellent imaging quality and the short half-life of ^{99m}Tc. This limits radiation exposure to patients with renal failure. It yields a renographic picture that is quite similar to that with hippuran. However, the radiopharmaceutical is more expensive, and its renal uptake and extraction are not as high as those of hippuran. Therefore [^{99m}Tc]-MAG$_3$ cannot be used to calculate renal plasma flow.

A post–ACE inhibitor renogram can be used to screen. A second renogram, undertaken without an ACE inhibitor, is obtained only if the initial study is abnormal. This reduces costs and inconvenience to the patient. However, the most accurate data from these tests are the ACE inhibitor–induced changes in a renogram parameter (e.g., single-kidney GFR with [^{99m}Tc]-DPTA, time to peak, or delay in washout with [^{131}I]-hippuran or [^{99}mTc]-MAG$_3$). This requires two separate scans.

There are widely varying reports of the sensitivity and specificity of these tests. They can have an excellent sensitivity and specificity under protocol conditions. This has encouraged investigators to recommend that these tests be performed in screening before any arteriogram or intervention for renal artery stenosis. They have the advantage over post–ACE inhibitor PRA values of locating which kidney is functionally involved. However, they have the disadvantage of greater cost, inconvenience, and the use of a radiochemical. Both types of tests can have similar sensitivities that exceed 90% under ideal protocol conditions.

OVERVIEW OF FUNCTIONAL TESTS FOR RENOVASCULAR HYPERTENSION

The appropriate use of tests for renovascular hypertension depends on the clinical circumstances. For example, it is particularly important to detect fibromuscular dysplasia, which has a high rate of cure following PTRA. Paraumbilical bruits and/or severe or drug-resistant hypertension in female patients (Table 62.2) should be investigated.

Planning functional screening tests for renovascular hypertension before radiologic tests for renal artery stenosis is appealing. However, reevaluations of ACE inhibitor renography in large series have shown a disappointing sensitivity of only approximately 80%. Moreover, functional tests have never been evaluated for their ability to predict which patients are at risk for developing progressive ischemic nephropathy. It is probable that anatomical criteria will be of most value in this assessment. Ischemic nephropathy is being found to be a far more common cause of renal failure than was previously believed, especially among elderly patients, those with congestive cardiac failure, or those with coronary or peripheral artery disease. Finally, some studies have documented a significant increase in the GFR of patients with fibromuscular dysplasia or atheromatous renal artery stenosis 1 year after PTRA. Although not blinded and controlled, these results are encouraging and suggest that improvement in renal function in addition to blood pressure may be a realistic goal of intervention for renal artery stenosis. These new data have led the author to use an algorithm outlined in Fig. 62.1. This bypasses functional testing in certain categories of patients who are judged to have a very high probability of benefiting from PTRA to preserve renal function, even if its principal effects are not for hypertension, and in patients who are judged to have a high probability of renovascular hypertension. In patients with a moderate probability of renovascular hypertension and in those with a high probability but who have a high risk for complications from arteriography,

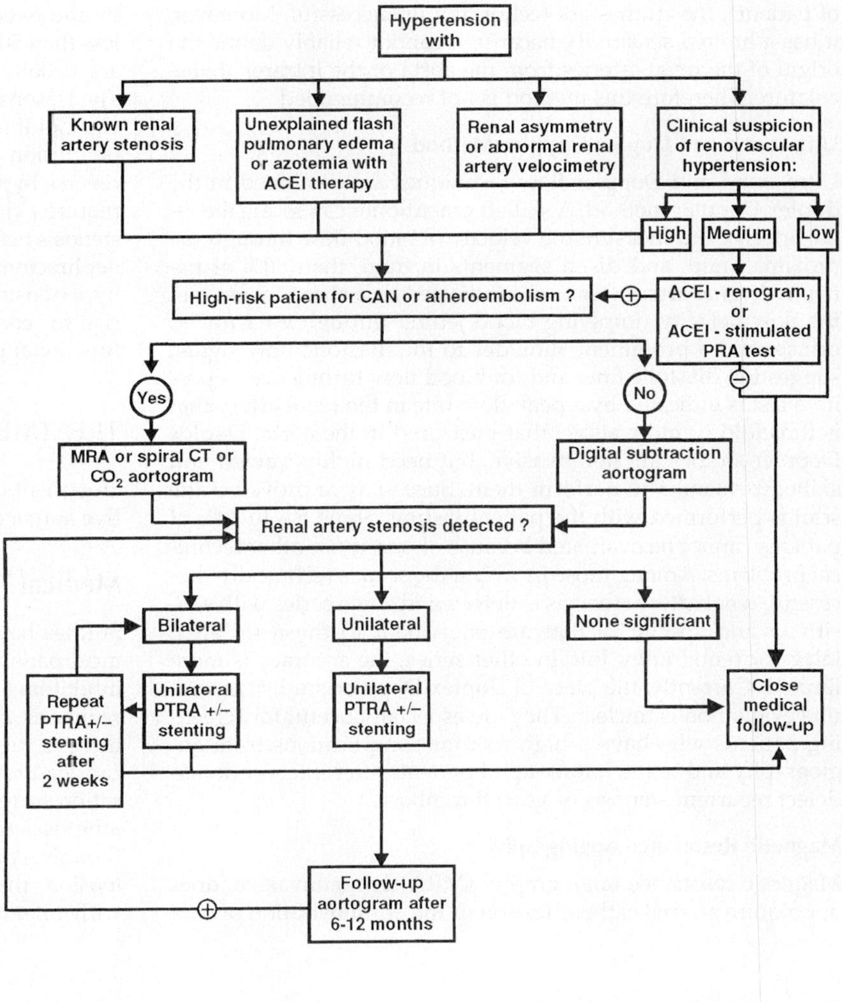

Figure 62.1. An algorithm for detection and management of renovascular hypertension or renal artery stenosis.

functional testing with ACE inhibitor–induced changes in PRA or the renogram is undertaken. Patients with negative functional tests and those with a low probability of renovascular hypertension are referred for close medical follow-up.

Radiologic Tests

Arteriography

A positive result from a screening test and/or strong clinical suspicion of renovascular hypertension should prompt radiologic evaluation for renal artery stenosis. The gold standard is an aortogram with selective renal arteriograms studied with posteroanterior and oblique films. The dye load is minimized by digital subtraction methods. Aortography can be undertaken using small diameter catheters. Only high-risk patients need to be admitted to the hospital, providing that patients can be followed after the procedure and have close clinical follow-up, including a measurement of blood urea nitrogen (BUN) and serum creatinine levels within 3 to 5 days. Patients with significant renal functional impairment or diabetes mellitus, or those taking nephrotoxic drugs, such as aminoglycosides, or those with uncompensated heart failure, are at increased risk for radiologic contrast material–induced nephropathy (Chapter 47, Part 7). It is prudent to admit such patients to the hospital and to give them hydration with saline at 2 ml/min for 2 to 4 hours before, during, and for 6 hours after the aortogram under close clinical surveillance. The risks of nephropathy are reduced further in high-risk patients by use of a nonionic contrast agent.

Digital Subtraction Intravenous Angiography

Unfortunately, digital subtraction intravenous angiography has two limitations: it requires a larger quantity of radiologic contrast agent than is required for angiography and in 10% to 25% of patients, the studies are technically unsuccessful. Moreover, it has a limited sensitivity because it cannot reliably define the origin of the renal arteries from the aorta or the intrarenal vasculature. Therefore this method is not recommended.

Ultrasound and Duplex Doppler Method

Ultrasound and Doppler flow techniques are combined in the duplex Doppler method. A skilled practitioner can locate the renal arteries and measure the velocity of blood flow through the proximal, mid, and distal segments in more than 80% of patients. A renal artery stenosis is indicated by a sharp increase in the flow velocity (implying blood jetting through a narrowed orifice) and a prominent shoulder to the diastolic flow signal, suggesting diastolic flow and/or blood flow turbulence. A positive test is indicated by a peak flow rate in the renal artery that is threefold or more above that measured in the aorta. Duplex Doppler studies are noninvasive, but need highly trained and skilled personnel to perform them. Success is improved if the scan is performed with the patient fasting. Some 5% to 20% of patients cannot be evaluated because of obesity or other technical problems. Among those in whom the scan is technically successful, renal artery stenosis is detected in some series with sensitivity and specificity that are equivalent to those for ACE inhibitor renography, but, in other series, the accuracy is more limited. Currently, the place of duplex Doppler studies in routine evaluation is unclear. They are especially useful for screening patients who have a high risk for complications from angiography and in the follow-up of patients after intervention to detect recurrent stenosis or graft thrombosis.

Magnetic Resonance Angiography

Magnetic resonance angiography (MRA) is noninvasive, does not require arterial catheterization or the administration of contrast agents or radioactive tracers, and does not use x-rays. Providing that there are no contraindications to magnetic resonance imaging (e.g., implanted pacemaker), most patients can be evaluated successfully. MRA has high sensitivity and specificity of >95% for detection of renal artery stenosis, compared with arteriography. The main limitations are a failure to detect stenosis of intrarenal vessels, overreporting of the degree of renal artery stenosis because turbulence distorts the flow signal and exaggerates the apparent degree of luminal narrowing, and high costs.

Carbon Dioxide Angiography

CO_2 angiography appears to be safer than using radiologic contrast material and may not cause nephrotoxicity. It is helpful for detecting renal artery stenosis in patients at high risk for contrast material–associated nephropathy. The best results are obtained when the CO_2 is delivered from a controlled injector.

OVERVIEW OF RADIOLOGIC TESTS FOR RENAL ARTERY STENOSIS OR RENOVASCULAR HYPERTENSION

Even a high-quality renal arteriogram cannot by itself be used to diagnose renovascular hypertension. The degree of renal artery stenosis is hard to quantitate from an arteriogram. This is especially so if there are multiple stenoses, as in most patients with fibromuscular dysplasia or long and irregularly stenosed segments. Moreover, the resistance offered by a stenosis varies with the flow characteristics and with the downstream vascular resistance. Therefore the hemodynamic consequences even of a well-defined stenosis cannot be predicted accurately. Ostial lesions originating within the wall of the aorta may be obscured by the overlying shadow of the aorta. Although a stenosis of less than 50% is rarely significant and those of greater than 75% are usually significant, many fall in an intermediate category. The lessons learned from the chronic phase of two-kidney, one-clip Goldblatt hypertension in the rat suggest that the correction of a lesion that was originally causative may ultimately fail to reverse hypertension. For all these reasons, many nephrologists require evidence of the functional importance of a renal artery stenosis before recommending PTRA, reconstructive surgery, or nephrectomy when the indication is improvement or cure of hypertension. This is especially true in patients who are at high risk for complications from intervention and those with renal functional impairment.

TREATMENT

Treatment options include medical therapy, PTRA, reconstructive surgery, nephrectomy, and renal ablation.

Medical Therapy

Studies have indicated that hypertension can be controlled in most patients with renovascular disease, especially where ACE inhibitors are used, providing that high doses or multiple drug regimens are used. However, with antihypertensive therapy there is the risk of progressive renal arterial occlusion, which can lead to renal artery thrombosis or to progressive deterioration in renal function. The risk of progression is greater in atherosclerotic than in fibromuscular renal artery disease. Although ACE inhibitors often are effective in controlling hypertension, there is the real risk of causing azotemia in patients with bilateral renal artery stenosis or stenosis of a single or dominant kidney. Even in those with unilateral renal artery stenosis, ACE inhibitors may reduce the GFR of the poststenotic kidney. The long-term consequences of ACE inhibitor–induced reduction in GFR have not been established in humans. Therefore these drugs are not recommended except in patients whose hypertension cannot be controlled with other antihypertensive medications. Calcium antagonists block the actions of Ang II on systemic arterioles, the renal afferent arteriole and mesangium, and the zona glomerulosa of the adrenal cortex. However, they do not fully block the actions of Ang II on the efferent arteriole. Therefore in contrast to ACE inhibitors, calcium antagonists maintain the GFR of poststenotic kidneys yet are also effective antihypertensive agents. Studies in limited numbers of patients have confirmed these predictions. Antihypertensive regimens based on β-blockers are logical because these drugs inhibit renin secretion yet do not appear to have the specific risks of ACE inhibitors for decreasing the GFR of the poststenotic kidney. Diuretics are sometimes required, especially in patients with resistant hypertension or those with bilateral renal artery stenosis and fluid retention. They are generally not very effective as single-agent antihypertensive agents in patients with unilateral renal artery stenosis. A trial of medical therapy may be appropriate for patients with fibromuscular dysplasia who are reluctant to undergo intervention. However, in those with atherosclerosis, the stenosis often worsens with time. Therefore it is wise not to delay intervention unnecessarily.

Percutaneous Transrenal Angioplasty

PTRA has been evaluated extensively. The technical success rate is greater than 95% for patients with fibromuscular disease and is about 80% for those with atherosclerosis. Osteal lesions more frequently require either the placement of a stent or repeated PTRA because of recurrent stenosis. Approximately 20% of patients with atherosclerosis and 35% of those with fibromuscular dysplasia are cured of hypertension after PTRA. About half the patients with renal artery stenosis have improved blood pressure control. The rest (25% to 35% of patients with atherosclerosis and 15% to 25% of those with fibromuscular dysplasia) derive no significant antihypertensive benefit. Some of those who failed to respond probably had a functionally insignificant renal artery stenosis and coexisting essential hypertension. Others had entered the chronic phase, when hypertension is no longer dependent on the continued presence of a renal artery stenosis. Others had developed a recurrent stenosis or a stenosis of the artery to the contralateral kidney or had a decrement in renal function.

The complications of PTRA include some degree of acute renal insufficiency in up to 25% of patients. Fortunately, this is often mild and reversible. Complications caused by atheroemboli include progressive azotemia and proteinuria, small vessel vasculitis, and digital gangrene accompanied by eosinophilia and complement consumption. This syndrome may be difficult to differentiate from a vasculitis. Biopsy of affected tissues shows small vessel vasculitis and the characteristic cholesterol crystals in the small vessels or glomeruli. Local complications produced by the catheter or guidewire within the renal artery and aorta include trauma leading to intimal tears, flaplike occlusion of the artery, arterial thrombosis, arterial puncture, and perirenal or exit site hematomas. The mortality is less than 2% in most series, but major complications requiring surgical intervention occur in 2% to 5% of patients and minor complications in up to 40%. Patients should be observed in the hospital overnight. Blood for BUN and serum creatinine concentrations should be sampled the next day and if any increase has occurred after 3 to 5 days to ensure that the patient has not developed acute renal insufficiency.

Surgery

A variety of surgical revascularization techniques are available. Overall, the success rate for cure of hypertension is usually rather better than that with PTRA. Recurrent renal artery stenosis is less common than with PTRA, but graft thrombosis can occur and necessitate nephrectomy. As with PTRA, success rates are better for fibromuscular disease because patients generally are younger, have a better cardiovascular status, and have disease limited to the renal arteries. However, vascular surgery is very expensive and is accompanied by higher morbidity and mortality than PTRA. The mortality is increased further when more extensive surgery is undertaken for simultaneous correction of disease in the aorta and renal arteries. After PTRA or reconstructive surgery, patients should be given a low maintenance dose of aspirin, unless there is a specific contraindication because this may reduce the rate of graft thrombosis.

Renal Ablation

Renal ablation by intraarterial injection of alcohol or nephrectomy is occasionally indicated in high-risk patients who are not candidates for PTRA or reconstructive surgery. However, elimination of a small kidney (less than 7.5 cm in the long axis) can help to improve hypertension.

OVERVIEW OF CHOICES OF TREATMENT FOR RENAL ARTERY STENOSIS

Medical therapy is preferred for very high-risk patients or those with advanced renal insufficiency in whom arteriography or intervention is judged to have an unacceptable risk of renal insufficiency. Nevertheless, reliance on medical therapy will deny some patients the opportunity for an improvement in renal function following a successful reversal of renal artery stenosis. Therefore an intervention should be seriously considered in all patients with known or suspected renal artery stenosis. PTRA is the preferred modality for most patients, especially those with fibromuscular disease. If hypertension recurs and arteriography indicates a recurrent renal artery stenosis, PTRA with stenting is still effective in improving or curing hypertension in approximately 50% of patients. In all patients, the risks of renal insufficiency, local complications, contrast material–induced nephropathy, or atheroembolism must be weighed against the benefits of reduced blood pressure.

Renal revascularization performed by an experienced surgeon is indicated in selected patients with complete occlusion of the renal artery, providing that they have evidence on arteriography of distal filling of the artery from collateral vessels, or those who have had technically unsuccessful PTRAs.

All patients should be closely followed-up, with regular measurements of blood pressure and renal function. Deterioration in blood pressure control, especially when accompanied by a reduction in renal function, should prompt a fresh search for recurrent or *de novo* renal artery stenosis. Periodic analysis of PRA and duplex Doppler studies of the kidneys and renal arteries are helpful noninvasive tests to screen for restenosis. Because restenosis often can be treated successfully by another PTRA or the placement of a stent, another arteriogram should be considered in all patients who have not responded satisfactorily at 6 to 12 months after PTRA.

An important, although unresolved, issue is how best to detect and treat patients with renal insufficiency caused by a renal artery stenosis. Most studies indicated that PTRA or reconstructive surgery does not improve overall renal function.

However, within this group are some patients who show a striking reversal of renal insufficiency. The prevalence of such patients in the population with chronic renal failure and hypertension remains to be established. The advent of functional tests that are appropriate for use in patients with impaired renal function (before and after ACE inhibitor renography) and of visualizing techniques that do not require administration of contrast dye (e.g., CO_2 angiography, MRA, or duplex Doppler scanning) has provided the potential means for approaching this unresolved clinical problem.

Selected Readings

Datseris IE, Bomanji JB, Brown EA, et al. Captopril renal scintigraphy in patients with hypertension and chronic renal failure. *J Nucl Med* 1994;35:251–254.

An evaluation of ACE inhibitor renography in patients with impaired renal function.

Davidson RA, Wilcox CS. Newer tests for the diagnosis of renovascular disease. *JAMA* 1992;268:3353–3358.

A review of tests that can be used to diagnose renal artery stenosis or renovascular hypertension.

Derkx FHM, van Jaarsveld BC, Krijnen P, et al. Renal artery stenosis towards the year 2000. *J Hypertens* 1996;14:S-167–S-172.

Overview of the field of renal artery stenosis.

Erbsloh-Moller B, Dumas A, Roth D, et al. Furosemide-^{131}I-hippuran renography after angiotensin-converting enzyme inhibition for the diagnosis of renovascular hypertension. *Am J Med* 1991;90:23–29.

Description of how to undertake a hippuran renogram study to detect renovascular hypertension, containing the criteria for a positive test and methods to distinguish renovascular hypertension from renal parenchymal disease.

Frederickson ED, Wilcox CS, Bucci CM, et al. A prospective evaluation of a simplified captopril test for the detection of renovascular hypertension. *Arch Intern Med* 1990;150:569–572.

Description of how to undertake a simplified captopril challenge test to detect renovascular hypertension and the results obtained in one large referral center where 100 patients with hypertension were studied prospectively.

Krijnen P, van Jaarsveld BC, Steyerberg EW, et al. A clinical prediction rule for renal artery stenosis in drug-resistant hypertension. *Ann Intern Med* 1998;129:705–711.

Paper concluding that a weighted clinical prediction rule is as successful as ACE inhibitor renography in screening for renal artery stenosis.

MacDowall P, Kaira PA, O'Donoghue DJ, et al. Risk of morbidity from renovascular disease in elderly patients with congestive cardiac failure. *Lancet* 1998;352:13–16.

Demonstration of a prevalence of 34% of renal artery stenosis in elderly patients with severe congestive heart failure.

Mailloux LU, Napolitano B, Bellucci AG, et al. Renal vascular disease causing end-stage renal disease, incidence, clinical correlates, and outcomes: a 20-year clinical experience. *Am J Kidney Dis* 1994;24:622–629.

The experience of one center showing a high prevalence of renal artery stenosis in patients developing end-stage renal disease.

Mann SJ, Pickering TG. Detection of renovascular hypertension. State-of-the-art: 1992. *Ann Intern Med* 1992;117:845–853.

A current review of tests that may be used to detect renovascular hypertension.

Mann SJ, Pickering TG, Sos TA, et al. Captopril renography in the diagnosis of renal artery stenosis: accuracy and limitations. *Am J Med* 1991;90:30–40.

Description of the methods used to diagnose renovascular hypertension with ACE inhibitor–induced changes in the DTPA renogram.

Martinez-Maldonado M. Pathophysiology of renovascular hypertension. *Hypertension* 1991;17:707–719.

Overview of the pathophysiology of renovascular hypertension with insights from animal models.

Pickering TG, Mann SJ. Is there a role for non-invasive screening tests in diagnosing renal artery stenosis? *J Hypertens* 1996;14:1265–1266.

Provocative analysis of the role of functional testing.

Pickering TG, Sos TA, Vaughan ED Jr. Predictive value and changes of renin secretion in hypertensive patients with unilateral renovascular disease undergoing successful renal angioplasty. *Am J Med* 1984;76:398–404.

Description of the use of renal vein renin estimations to diagnose renovascular hypertension and their reversibility following correction of the stenosis.

Ploth DW. Angiotensin-dependent renal mechanisms in two-kidney, one-clip renal vascular hypertension. *Am J Physiol* 1983;14:F131–F141.

Useful review of the pathophysiology of renovascular hypertension in the animal model.

Rudnick MR, Berns JS, Cohen RM, et al. Nephrotoxic risks of renal angiography: contrast media-associated nephrotoxicity and atheroembolism—a critical review. *Am J Kidney Dis* 1994;24:713–727.

Reviews the risks of contrast nephropathy and strategies for its prevention.

Taylor A, Nally J, Aurell M, et al. Consensus report on ACE inhibitor renography for detecting renovascular hypertension. *J Nucl Med* 1996;37:1876–1882.

An overview by a select panel of nuclear medicine specialists.

Taylor ATJ, Fletcher JW, Nally JVJ. Procedure guideline for diagnosis of renovascular disease. *J Nucl Med* 1998;39:1297–1302.

A review of the current recommendations of renal nuclear medicine physicians for the evaluation of suspected renovascular hypertension.

van Jaarsveld BC, Krijnen P, Derkx FHM, et al. The place of renal scintigraphy in the diagnosis of renal artery stenosis: fifteen years of clinical experience. *Arch Intern Med* 1997;157:1226–1234.

An important review of the practical experience of nuclear medicine tests from the pioneer group.

Wilcox CS. Use of angiotensin-converting-enzyme inhibitors for diagnosing renovascular hypertension. *Kidney Int* 1993;44:1379–1390.

Summary of the physiologic basis for the use of ACE inhibitors in the diagnosis of renovascular hypertension and evaluation of the different tests based on ACE inhibitor–induced changes in blood pressure, PRA, renal vein renins, and nuclear medicine studies.

Zierler RE, Bergelin RO, Isaacson JA, et al. Natural history of renal artery stenosis: a prospective study with ultrasound. *J Vasc Surg* 1994;19:250–257.

The value of renal ultrasound and duplex Doppler to follow outcomes in patients with renal artery stenosis.

CHAPTER 63

Endocrine Hypertension

Steven A. Atlas

Endocrine disorders, particularly those of the adrenal gland, are the major cause of secondary hypertension arising outside the kidney. Although relatively uncommon (accounting for only 1% to 2% of all cases of hypertension), recognition of these conditions is clinically important because they respond best to specific therapies and because they are often surgically correctable, particularly early in their course. Moreover, elucidation of the mechanisms underlying certain rare genetic disorders has provided important insight into basic physiologic processes as well as the pathophysiology of hypertensive syndromes. This chapter will focus on the pathophysiology, diagnosis, and management of adrenal disorders and will also briefly consider other endocrine abnormalities associated with an increased prevalence of hypertension.

ADRENOCORTICAL DISORDERS

Mineralocorticoid Hypertension

Physiologic Regulation of Mineralocorticoids

Aldosterone is the major mineralocorticoid hormone released from the adrenal cortex. Its synthesis is normally restricted to cells of the outermost zone (zona glomerulosa) of the cortex, owing to the unique expression of the gene for aldosterone synthase (CYP11B2), a cytochrome P450–linked mixed function oxidase that is responsible for the conversion of deoxycorticosterone (DOC) to aldosterone by sequential oxygenation steps at the 11- and 18-carbon positions of the steroid nucleus (Fig. 63.1). Steroidogenesis in this zone is regulated mainly by the renin-angiotensin system and by potassium. Stimuli to renin secretion (e.g., upright posture, low sodium intake, or other causes of volume contraction) lead to increased plasma angiotensin II, which stimulates aldosterone biosynthesis. Physiologic increases in plasma potassium (e.g., due to intake or metabolic status) are also sufficient to stimulate aldosterone production (and vice versa).

Aldosterone and other mineralocorticoids bind to mineralocorticoid (type 1 corticosteroid) receptors in their target cells. Genomic effects in transport epithelia include activation of sodium channels in the luminal membrane and of Na^+-K^+-ATPase in the serosal (basolateral) membranes, which lead in the distal nephron (cortical collecting duct) to increased reabsorption of sodium and increased excretion of potassium and hydrogen ion. Aldosterone thus promotes volume retention, which in turn suppresses renin secretion, and also tends to decrease extracellular potassium, thereby exerting negative-feedback effects on its own synthesis. In this manner the renin-angiotensin-aldosterone system functions as a closed-loop system involved in both volume and potassium homeostasis. Changes in adrenocorticotrophic hormone (ACTH) normally play a secondary role in aldosterone regulation. A diurnal rhythm for aldosterone is not nearly as apparent as it is for cortisol; furthermore, there is no known major feedback effect of aldosterone on the hypothalamic-pituitary axis. A variety of additional factors have the potential to modulate aldosterone production, although the physiologic importance of these pathways is still uncertain. Several pituitary peptides derived from pro-opiomelanocortin, as well as vasopressin and serotonin, are known to stimulate aldosterone release *in vitro*. Other substances, including dopamine, somatostatin, and atrial natriuretic peptide (ANP), have been shown to inhibit aldosterone synthesis. Of these, ANP has been shown clearly to inhibit aldosterone at physiologic levels, and its own regulation by intravascular volume would fit well with a role in the aldosterone-volume homeostatic loop.

The aldosterone precursors DOC and corticosterone (Fig. 63.1) have weaker mineralocorticoid effects. These biosynthetic intermediates are not appreciably released by the zona glomerulosa because of nearly complete conversion to 18-hydroxycorticosterone and aldosterone; however, substantial amounts of DOC, corticosterone, and other 17-deoxysteroids such as 18-hydroxy-DOC are also synthesized and released by the zona fasciculata-reticularis under ACTH control. The P450-linked 11β-hydroxylase in these zones (which also has 18-hydroxylating activity) is derived from a distinct gene (CYP11B1), which is nonetheless highly (approximately 95%) homologous with aldosterone synthase (CYP11B2); these two genes are located close together (approximately 40 kbases apart) on the same chromosome (8q21-q22). Of the fasciculata steroids, DOC has the greatest mineralocorticoid activity. Its circulating levels are similar to those of aldosterone, but it is more highly protein bound (more than 95% versus approximately 40% to 60%) and thus contributes minimally to normal volume regulation. Under normal circumstances, cortisol and corticosterone have little or no mineralocorticoid action *in vivo*, mainly because they are largely inactivated by mineralocorticoid target cells (see "Syndrome of Apparent Mineralocorticoid Excess" later in this chapter).

Pathophysiology of Mineralocorticoid Excess

Primary mineralocorticoid excess is typically characterized by hypertension associated with potassium wasting and alkalosis.

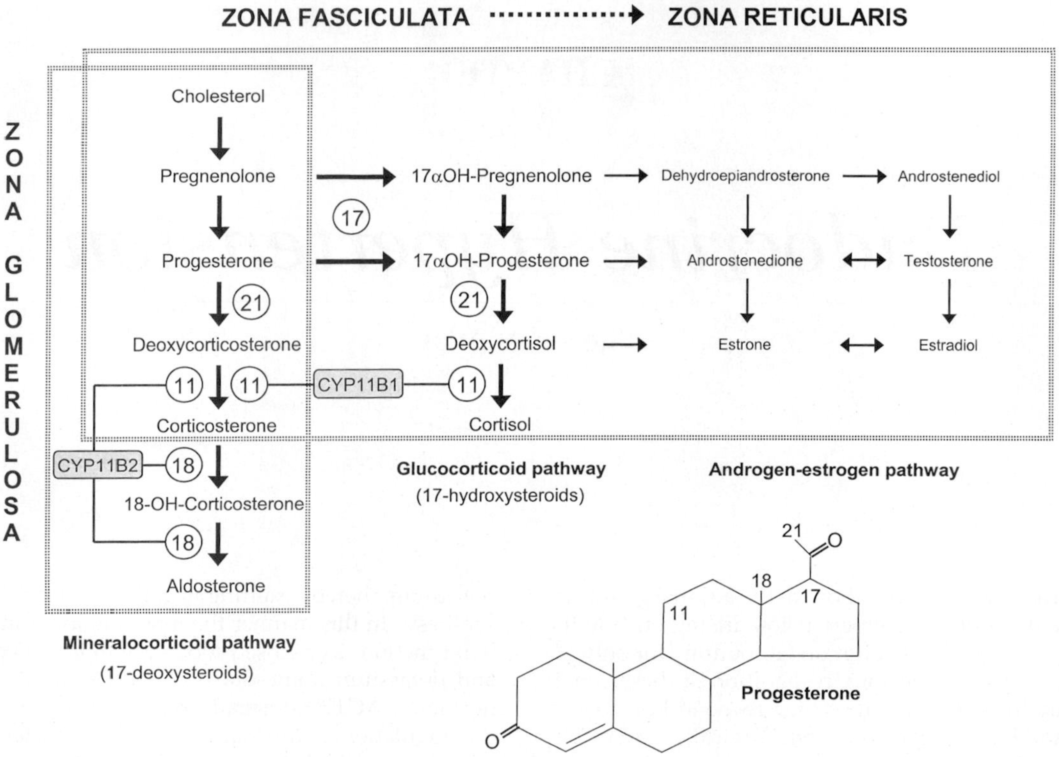

Figure 63.1. Steroid biosynthetic pathways in the normal adrenal cortex. *Vertical box,* Mineralocorticoid pathway of the zona glomerulosa. *Overlapping horizontal box,* Pathways operant in the remaining inner zones of the cortex (zona fasciculata-zona reticularis), including a truncated mineralocorticoid pathway (stopping at corticosterone). *Circled numbers,* Enzymatic hydroxylation steps at the respective carbon atoms of the steroid nucleus (illustrated for progesterone at bottom). In the mineralocorticoid pathway of the zona glomerulosa, both the 11- and 18-hydroxylation steps are catalyzed by the aldosterone synthase complex (previously termed *corticosterone methyl oxidase*) derived from the CYP11B2 gene. In the fasciculata-reticularis, 11-hydroxylase activity is derived from the distinct, but related CYP11B1 gene; this enzyme is also capable of some 18-hydroxylating activity, leading to the production of 18-OH-DOC (not shown) and possibly small amounts of 18-OH-corticosterone, but not of aldosterone.

Of the numerous causes listed in Table 63.1, primary aldosteronism resulting from either an aldosterone-producing adenoma (Conn's syndrome) or bilateral adrenocortical hyperplasia (idiopathic hyperaldosteronism) is by far the most common. The pathogenesis of hypertension is similar in all the syndromes listed.

A primary increase in mineralocorticoid levels enhances distal sodium reabsorption in exchange for potassium and hydrogen ions. Sodium retention leads to generalized volume expansion and increased blood pressure, both of which suppress renin secretion. Most adenomas are autonomous with respect to the renin-angiotensin system, thus the fall in angiotensin II concentration fails to reduce aldosterone production. Excess mineralocorticoid production is thus sustained, but volume expansion is limited because the kidney eventually "escapes" from the sodium-retaining effect. Therefore edema is absent in patients with primary mineralocorticoid excess. The mechanisms of mineralocorticoid escape are incompletely understood, but important components serving to increase natriuresis include: (a) the inhibitory effect of increased renal perfusion pressure (leading to increased peritubular capillary hydrostatic pressure) on sodium reabsorption and (b) the homeostatic increase in ANP secretion by the cardiac atria. In contrast, wasting of potassium and hydrogen ions continues, and the maintained increment in extracellular volume is sufficient to induce progressive hypertension. Plasma and extracellular volumes as well as cardiac output are increased, but these may tend to return toward normal over the long term, at which point the hypertension is maintained by increased peripheral vascular resistance. The mechanisms by which this transition occurs are controversial, but the established hypertensive state remains "volume dependent" because it is specifically reversed by volume contraction (or prevented from the outset by sodium restriction). In addition, however, aldosterone may have other direct actions (e.g., on the central nervous system) that contribute to blood pressure elevation.

In contrast to this limited volume retention (and lack of edema), aldosterone induces progressive sodium retention in the edematous disorders (heart failure, cirrhosis, and nephrotic syndrome), in which conditions aldosterone production is increased secondary to an increase in renin secretion resulting from reduced renal perfusion. Other causes of reduced renal perfusion (e.g., renovascular disease or diuretic therapy) may similarly cause "secondary aldosteronism" (Table 63.1) and may coexist with hypertension. For this reason measurement of plasma renin activity (PRA) is a key diagnostic step in identifying patients with primary mineralocorticoid excess, in whom PRA is suppressed.

Clinical Features

Patients with these disorders are commonly asymptomatic and present for evaluation because of hypertension found on routine examination. The signs and symptoms are related to the electrolyte disturbance and hypertension. Aside from hypokalemia, which may not always be present, mild hypernatremia, alkalosis and evidence of renal magnesium wasting are com-

TABLE 63.1. Causes of Adrenocortical Hypertension

	Serum K^+	Renin	Aldosterone
Primary Aldosteronism	Low	Low	High
Aldosterone-producing adenoma (Conn's syndrome)			
Autonomous (majority)			
Renin-responsive			
Aldosterone-producing carcinoma			
Adrenocortical hyperplasia (usually bilateral)			
Idiopathic hyperaldosteronism			
Primary adrenal hyperplasia			
Glucocorticoid-remediable hyperaldosteronism			
Other Mineralocorticoid Excess	Low	Low	Low
Deoxycorticosterone (DOC) excess syndromes			
Congenital adrenal hyperplasia			
11β-hydrolase deficiency			
17α-hydroxylase deficiency			
DOC-producing adenoma or carcinoma			
Androgen- or estrogen-producing tumors			
Apparent mineralocorticoid excess syndrome			
Licorice intoxication			
Exogenous mineralocorticoids			
Other endogenous mineralocorticoids?			
Pseudomineralocorticoid excess (Liddle's syndrome)			
Cushing's Syndrome	Normal or Low	Normal or Low	Varies
Pituitary microadenoma or macroadenoma (Cushing's disease)			
Ectopic ACTH syndrome			
Adrenocortical adenoma, carcinoma or nodular hyperplasia			
Exogenous glucocorticoids			
Secondary Aldosteronism	Normal or Low	High	High
Renovascular hypertension			
Accelerated or malignant hypertension			
Renin-secreting tumors			
Pheochromocytoma			
[a][Diuretic use]			
[a][Laxative abuse, other gastrointestinal losses]			
[a][Edematous disorders]			

[a] These conditions may coexist with hypertension of other etiology. In other causes of secondary aldosteronism (e.g., Bartter's syndrome, Gitelman's syndrome, renal tubular disorders), blood pressure is normal or low.
ACTH, adrenocorticotropic hormone.

mon. Symptoms include nonspecific complaints such as muscle weakness, fatigue, or lassitude. Nocturia is common and, if hypokalemia is severe or prolonged, patients may report polyuria and polydipsia, which results from renal insensitivity to vasopressin (nephrogenic diabetes insipidus). Severe hypokalemia may also induce or potentiate glucose intolerance and cardiac arrhythmias, and may lead to autonomic dysfunction manifested by orthostatic hypotension without reflex tachycardia. Muscle paralysis has been reported rarely, and signs of tetany (e.g., positive Chvostek or Trousseau signs) may be present in patients with severe alkalosis and/or hypomagnesemia. Hypertension ranges from mild to severe, but advanced (grade III or IV) retinopathy or malignant hypertension is rare.

Initial Diagnosis

The diagnostic hallmark is unprovoked hypokalemia as a manifestation of renal potassium wasting. This is associated with mild to moderate elevations of serum bicarbonate, thus excluding metabolic acidosis or renal disorders as a cause of hypokalemia. Because hypokalemia may be intermittent or subtle, particularly early in the disease, the diagnosis should also be considered in hypertensive patients with serum K^+ in the low-normal range (i.e., 3.6 to 4.0 mmol/L) or with a history of significant diuretic-induced hypokalemia. In hypokalemic patients who have recently discontinued diuretic therapy, measurements should be repeated after 3 to 6 weeks with an adequate sodium intake (5 to 6 g NaCl per day). Low sodium intake may mask the hypokalemic alkalosis because mineralocorticoid-induced K^+ and hydrogen losses depend on adequate distal sodium delivery. To confirm renal K^+ wasting (i.e., excretion greater than intake), serum K^+ measurement should be repeated in conjunction with a 24-hour urine for sodium, potassium, and creatinine. With ordinary dietary K^+ intake, urinary K^+ excretion greater than 40 mmol/24 hours is inappropriate in the setting of hypokalemia. Low urine K^+ excretion suggests renal K^+ conservation, consistent with extrarenal losses (e.g., gastrointestinal, due to vomiting or diarrhea), recent discontinuation of diuretic use, or, rarely, prolonged dietary deprivation.

The next diagnostic step should be measurement of PRA, because a normal or low aldosterone level does not necessarily rule out a diagnosis of mineralocorticoid hypertension. A low or suppressed PRA confirms the suspicion of primary mineralocorticoid excess. On the other hand, an elevated PRA is diagnostic of secondary hyperaldosteronism and obviates the need for steroid measurements. A normal PRA is highly unusual in untreated patients with pure mineralocorticoid hypertension (unless explained by antecedent therapy with spironolactone); however, if documented renal K^+ wasting persists and remains otherwise unexplained, further workup for adrenal steroid abnormalities (including Cushing's syndrome) should nonetheless be undertaken.

Measurements of urine or plasma aldosterone concentrations are performed to confirm the diagnosis of primary aldosteronism. Many experts recommend simultaneous measurement of plasma aldosterone and PRA, using the ratio of aldosterone to renin as a diagnostic criterion. This is not an unreasonable approach to screening of populations, but there are pitfalls in applying it too rigidly because too low a cutoff (e.g., a ratio of more than 25) would include many patients with low-renin essential hypertension who have normal levels of aldosterone and no evidence of renal potassium wasting, and because too high a cutoff (e.g., more than 50) will miss patients who have aldosterone levels in the high normal range (see following). In addition, plasma aldosterone levels may fluctuate widely with time of day, posture, or food intake. Measurements of 24-hour urine aldosterone excretion are more reliable because they reflect the integrated daily secretion rate. Many authorities favor measurement of the minor metabolite aldosterone 18-glucuronide in urine because of the relative simplicity and extreme specificity of available methods. Particularly in patients ingesting a high-salt diet (more than 200 mmol/day), a urine aldosterone greater than 14 μg/day is considered diagnostic of primary aldosteronism. Methods for measurement of other metabolites (e.g., tetrahydroaldosterone) or urinary free aldosterone are also available and preferred by some investigators. Simultaneous measurement of urinary sodium is advisable because normal levels of aldosterone and PRA vary reciprocally with sodium intake. It is important to remember that an aldosterone level within the normal range does not rule out the diagnosis, particularly if the patient is severely hypokalemic. This is because aldosterone production by most adenomatous or hyperplastic glands remains under the influence of extracellular potassium. Therefore repeat measurements should be obtained after attempts at potassium repletion.

Primary Aldosteronism

The triad of renal potassium wasting, suppressed PRA, and elevated aldosterone levels in a hypertensive patient establishes the diagnosis of primary aldosteronism. The causes of this syndrome are listed in Table 63.1. In a majority (60% to 70%) of cases this is attributable to an ***aldosterone-producing adenoma*** (APA) or Conn's syndrome, which generally becomes manifest between 30 and 50 years of age and is somewhat more common in women. APA is nearly always unilateral, although cases of bilateral tumors have been reported. ***Aldosterone-producing carcinomas*** are exceedingly rare. The remainder of cases are largely attributable to adrenal hyperplasia, typically bilateral; included in adrenal hyperplasia are a heterogeneous disorder termed ***idiopathic hyperaldosteronism*** (IHA), which frequently presents later in life, and a rare autosomal-dominant disorder termed ***glucocorticoid-remediable hyperaldosteronism*** (GRH), which is more common in males and usually presents before adulthood.

Further diagnostic workup should aim to identify patients with APA, which is often surgically remediable, especially early in its course. In general, patients with APA have a greater degree of hyperaldosteronism than patients with IHA, which leads to greater suppression of PRA and more pronounced hypokalemia. A variety of ancillary biochemical and physiologic tests, to be described later, have been used to further distinguish these disorders. Since the advent of high-resolution imaging techniques, however, these ancillary procedures are often reserved for confirmation of "autonomous" hyperaldosteronism or for those patients in whom anatomic evidence of an adenoma is equivocal or absent.

Of available imaging techniques, computed tomography (CT) with thin (3 to 5 mm) sections is the most sensitive procedure for adrenal cortical tumors, which are often less than 1 cm in diameter. With present technology it still offers somewhat better spatial resolution and less motion artifact than does magnetic resonance imaging (MRI), although advances in this area are occurring at a rapid pace. Adrenal scintigraphy using a radioiodinated cholesterol metabolite is also used in some centers; the study is done after dexamethasone pretreatment in order to decrease uptake by the normal fasciculata-reticularis. This technique is less sensitive because of its poorer resolving power, and it involves greater radiation exposure; it should be avoided in women of childbearing potential because of the risks of ovarian irradiation. Because this is a functional test, however, it may be useful as a confirmatory procedure in some instances.

Nonfunctioning adrenocortical adenomas are relatively common in the adult population and increase in frequency with age. Therefore the finding of a small tumor by CT or MRI is insufficient reason to recommend adrenalectomy without evidence of functional significance, particularly if the ancillary tests discussed later in this chapter are equivocal. Adrenal scintigraphy is used for this purpose but provides less sensitivity and specificity than does adrenal venous sampling, where aldosterone and cortisol levels are compared in adrenal and peripheral venous blood samples. Lateralization of aldosterone to one side, with levels often more than 50-fold higher than in peripheral blood, provides highly specific evidence for adenomatous aldosterone production. Proper interpretation requires that there be evidence of bilateral adrenal venous increments of cortisol, because cannulation of the right adrenal vein is often difficult; erroneous sampling of the inferior vena cava or hepatic vein will result in steroid levels that are, respectively, similar to or lower than peripheral levels. When performed properly, this technique can localize small functioning tumors that are undetectable by CT or MRI. This approach should be considered when results of the ancillary tests are suggestive of an adenoma.

The ancillary procedures that have been used are listed in Table 63.2. Of the tests that evaluate the relative autonomy of aldosterone production, the postural response is most widely used at present. The normal pattern of an increase in plasma aldosterone levels, in parallel with PRA, during upright posture is nearly always preserved in patients with IHA but is lost in those with APAs because of the insensitivity of most adenomas to angiotensin II or the pronounced suppression of PRA. When this maneuver is performed with supine and upright sampling at 8 AM and noon, respectively, patients with APAs may even have a paradoxic fall in aldosterone levels because of diurnal variation in ACTH, to which adenomas usually retain sensitivity. Other typical responses of patients with APAs such as nonsuppressibility of aldosterone by captopril, saline infusion, or exogenous mineralocorticoid administration or lack of stimulation by spironolactone (Table 63.2) similarly reflect relative autonomy from the renin-angiotensin system. Although responses indicating autonomy are highly suggestive of APAs (or, as discussed later, certain rare forms of hyperplasia), normal or equivocal responses to these maneuvers occur in at least 10% to 20%

TABLE 63.2. Ancillary Tests in the Diagnosis of Primary Aldosteronism

	Autonomy of Aldosterone Production	
	APA GRH PAH	RR-APA IHA
	Posture Test	
Measurement of plasma aldosterone, cortisol, and PRA at 8 AM (after overnight recumbency) and at noon (after 2-hour ambulation)	Plasma aldosterone fails to increase (or falls) despite upright posture	Plasma aldosterone increases by >30% with upright posture
	Captopril Test	
Steroid responses to a single oral dose of captopril (25–50 mg) over a 60- to 90-minute period	Plasma aldosterone/cortisol ratio is unaffected	Plasma aldosterone/cortisol ratio falls
	Suppressive Maneuvers	
Steroid responses to acute saline infusion (2 L over 2–4 hours) or to dietary salt loading or exogenous mineralocorticoid (DOC acetate or fludrocortisone) over 3 days	Failure to suppress plasma aldosterone (to <10 ng/dl) or urine aldosterone excretion (to <14 μg/day)	Variable suppression of aldosterone
	Spironolactone Response	
Response of aldosterone levels during long-term (4 weeks or more) treatment with spironolactone	Aldosterone levels generally unaffected	Aldosterone levels increase markedly
	Other Steroid Measurements	
	Aldosterone Precursors	
Plasma 18-hydroxycorticosterone Other precursors (DOC, corticosterone)	Frequently >100 ng/dl May be increased	Nearly always <100 ng/dl Generally normal
	C-18 Oxygenated Cortisol Metabolites	
Urine levels of 18-hydroxycortisol and of 18-oxo(tetrahydro)cortisol	>60 μg/day[a] >17 μg/day[a]	<60 μg/day <12 μg/day

[a] Median values approximately 200 μg/day and 45 μg/day, respectively, in APA. Median values are approximately fivefold higher in patients with GRH, but there is overlap with the upper end of the range found in patients with APA.

APA, aldosterone-producing adenoma; DOC, deoxycorticosterone; GRH, glucocorticoid-remediable hyperaldosteronism; IHA, idiopathic hyperaldosteronism; PAH, primary adrenal hyperplasia; PRA, plasma renin activity; RR-APA, renin-responsive APA.

of patients with surgically remediable adenomas. Therefore when the diagnosis of APA is strongly suspected (e.g., in a patient with a probable adenoma by CT), additional confirmatory tests such as adrenal venous sampling may still be required.

Several biochemical features also help to distinguish APA from IHA. In patients with APA, the 8 AM plasma aldosterone level is nearly always greater than 20 ng/100 ml, and plasma levels of precursor steroids, particularly 18-hydroxycorticosterone, are usually elevated. In addition, APAs typically synthesize unusual "hybrid" steroids—18-hydroxycortisol and 18-oxocortisol—because these tumors, which are often histologically "fasciculatalike," possess some 17α-hydroxylase activity and therefore synthesize small amounts of cortisol, which acts as a substrate for the aldosterone synthase complex that normally converts corticosterone to aldosterone (Fig. 63.1). Elevated urinary levels of such oxygenated cortisol metabolites are typical of patients with APA or GRH but are rare in patients with IHA and may offer one of the best tests to discriminate these conditions. An exception may be the uncommon examples of angiotensin II–responsive APAs, which are composed predominantly of glomerulosalike cells and respond to angiotensin infusion and upright posture.

IHA is a heterogeneous disorder. Adrenocortical hyperplasia may be either anatomically diffuse (micronodular) or macronodular. In a majority of patients the hypertension is not fully explained by mineralocorticoid excess. This was recognized in early clinical series in which bilateral or subtotal adrenalectomy corrected the hypokalemia but often failed to ameliorate hypertension. It is now recognized that rare patients with macronodular hyperplasia exhibit a response pattern typical of APA-like autonomous hyperaldosteronism, a subset that has been termed *primary adrenal hyperplasia.* This disorder is generally bilateral but may also account for rare reports of unilateral adrenal hyperplasia, where reduction of adrenal mass (or spironolactone therapy) has substantial antihypertensive benefit.

The rare syndrome of GRH, which is inherited in an autosomal-dominant pattern and frequently presents in childhood or adolescence, should be considered in patients with a family history of hypertension and hypokalemia as well as in those with an autonomous pattern in whom an adenoma cannot be identified.

The name of this syndrome derives from the unique ability of exogenous glucocorticoid therapy to normalize aldosterone production, which is fully under the control of ACTH and hence not subject to feedback control by changes in sodium balance. A diagnostic hallmark is extreme elevation in levels of the hybrid 18-oxygenated cortisol metabolites mentioned earlier. These features would suggest that GRH is caused by acquisition of aldosterone synthase activity by otherwise normal fasciculata cells. This has now been demonstrated in several kindreds in which fasciculata cells express a chimeric gene formed by unequal crossover of the highly homologous CYP11B1 and CYP11B2 genes, in which the hybrid contains the 5′ regulatory end of the normal fasciculata 11β-hydroxylase or CYP11B1 gene (which confers ACTH responsiveness) and the coding sequence of CYP11B2 (which confers aldosterone synthase activity). The adrenal glands may be either mildly hyperplastic or anatomically normal. The clinical features are similar to those of APA or IHA, except that hypokalemia is more variable. In fact, in GRH, the plasma potassium concentration is normal in more than half of the patients. Hypertension may be severe and associated with a strong familial history of cerebral hemorrhage or other vascular insult. Patients with GRH have a high frequency of hemorrhagic stroke due to rupture of intracranial aneurysms. The diagnosis of GRH is confirmed by a therapeutic trial of dexamethasone or other glucocorticoid, which promptly suppresses urine aldosterone and normalizes blood pressure over a period of several days to weeks. Genetic diagnosis is possible by molecular biological techniques that detect the chimeric gene. Glucocorticoid replacement may also be used for chronic treatment. It has been suggested that carriers of the GRH gene be periodically screened for intracranial aneurysms by magnetic resonance angiography.

A practical approach to the differential diagnosis is summarized schematically in Fig. 63.2. The finding of a discrete adrenal nodule by CT leads to a presumed diagnosis of APA that should generally be confirmed by selected ancillary tests (e.g., abnormal postural response, elevated 18-oxocortisol levels), adrenal vein sampling, or a therapeutic trial of spironolactone (see the following section, "Management") before recommending surgery. Radiologic evidence of hyperplastic or apparently normal adrenal glands leads to a tentative diagnosis of IHA, but if subsequent evaluation indicates autonomy, further workup for the possibility of surgically remediable disease or GRH is recommended. Finally, in a hypokalemic patient with suppressed PRA, the unexpected finding of a low aldosterone level should prompt further evaluation for the even rarer syndromes of DOC excess or other forms of mineralocorticoid hypertension.

Other Forms of Mineralocorticoid Hypertension

Deoxycorticosterone Excess Syndromes. Excess production of DOC (probably together with other fasciculata steroids with mineralocorticoid activity) leads to a syndrome clinically indistinguishable from primary aldosteronism except that aldosterone production is typically suppressed. Classic examples are provided by two of the rarest forms of ***congenital adrenal hyperplasia,*** autosomal-recessive disorders in which inherited defects in cortisol production result in stimulation of ACTH and lead to hyperplasia of the zona fasciculata-reticularis and excessive production of all steroids proximal to the defect (Fig. 63.1). These conditions nearly always present in childhood or adolescence. *11β-Hydroxylase deficiency* leads to accumulation of DOC, 11-deoxycortisol, and adrenal androgens and causes mineralocorticoid hypertension associated with virilization (females) or with precocious puberty (males). In contrast, *17α-hydroxylase deficiency* leads to accumulation of all fasciculata 17-deoxysteroids and deficiency of glucocorticoids and adrenal (and gonadal) androgens and estrogens and causes hypertension associated with primary amenorrhea and lack of secondary sex characteristics (females) or with pseudohermaphroditism (males). In each case, aldosterone synthesis is depressed because DOC-induced volume retention suppresses the renin-angiotensin system and leads to zona glomerulosa atrophy. Plasma DOC is elevated in both

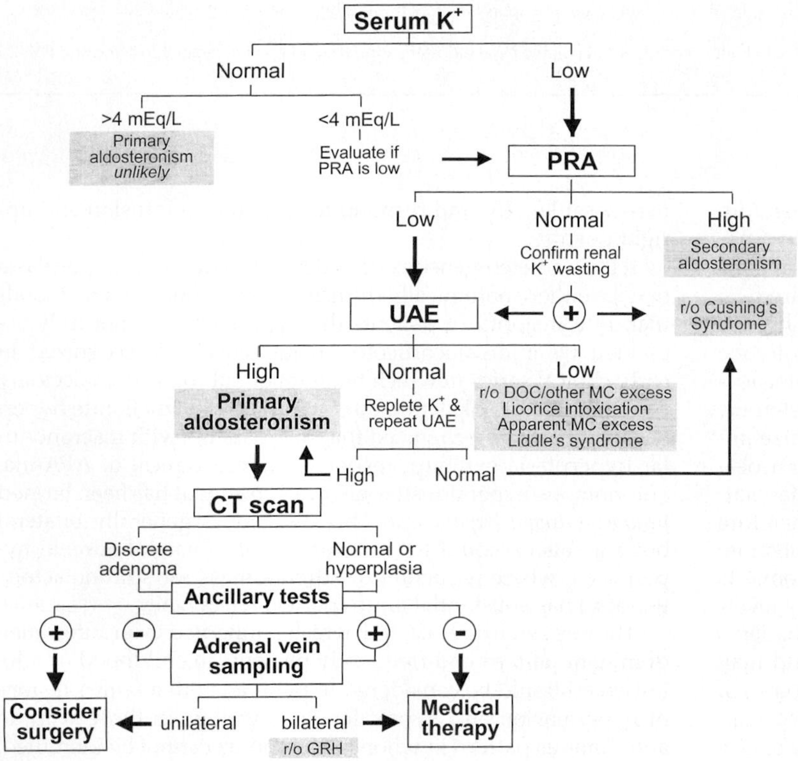

Figure 63.2. Approach to the evaluation of suspected mineralocorticoid hypertension. The ancillary tests (see Table 63.2 for description) are considered positive (+) if the results indicate autonomy or abnormal levels of other steroids. According to this scheme, surgery should be considered if the CT scan demonstrates an adenoma and either the ancillary tests are positive or adrenal vein sampling provides evidence of unilateral secretion; if the CT scan fails to demonstrate an adenoma, the possibility of surgically remediable disease should still be considered if ancillary tests are positive and sampling is unilateral (see text for further discussion). CT, computed tomography; DOC, desoxycorticosterone; GRH, glucocorticoid remediable hyperaldosteronism; K+, potassium; MC, mineralocorticoid; PRA, plasma renin activity; R/O, rule out; UAE, urinary aldosterone excretion.

defects. 11β-Hydroxylase deficiency is further distinguished by elevated plasma 11-deoxycortisol and urine 17-ketosteroids, whereas in 17α-hydroxylase deficiency, corticosterone is increased in parallel with DOC. Glucocorticoid replacement suppresses ACTH release in each condition and thereby reverses the biochemical abnormalities.

There have also been rare reports of predominantly DOC-producing tumors of the adrenal gland, both adenomas and carcinomas. Although aldosterone is usually suppressed by the same mechanism described previously for congenital adrenal hyperplasia, normal levels have also been observed in some cases, possibly because of the multifunctional nature of such tumors. Cortisol levels are usually normal but may be suppressed if excess production of weaker glucocorticoids (e.g., corticosterone) is sufficient to inhibit ACTH release. Finally, virilizing or feminizing adrenal tumors may also be associated with DOC excess; the mechanism appears to be androgen- or estrogen-induced inhibition of 11β-hydroxylase activity leading to some accumulation of DOC (and 11-deoxycortisol).

Syndrome of Apparent Mineralocorticoid Excess. This rare autosomal-recessive disorder is characterized by mineralocorticoidlike hypertension with suppressed aldosterone levels but no detectable abnormality in steroidogenesis other than a decrease in cortisol turnover. Nearly all cases have presented in childhood with severe hypokalemia and hypertension, with some reports of cerebrovascular accident at a young age. The syndrome responds well to the specific mineralocorticoid antagonist, spironolactone, and early studies pointed to cortisol itself, at normal circulating levels, as the offending mineralocorticoid. Deficiency of cortisol-inactivating enzymes, responsible for either conversion of cortisol to cortisone or reduction of the A-ring, appears to account for two forms of this disorder. Insights gained from this disorder, together with the discovery that licorice also impairs conversion of cortisol to cortisone by inhibiting 11β-hydroxysteroid dehydrogenase, led to the revolutionary concept that metabolic inactivation of cortisol (which has a similar binding affinity to the mineralocorticoid receptor *in vitro* as does aldosterone) plays a major role in mineralocorticoid hormone specificity *in vivo*. The well-known form of 11β-hydroxysteroid dehydrogenase, a low-affinity, bidirectional oxidoreductase present in liver, kidney, and elsewhere, is not localized to mineralocorticoid target cells, a finding that led to the discovery of a distinct renal (type 2) isoform that binds cortisol with very high affinity and causes unidirectional conversion to the inactive steroid cortisone. The prominence of this enzyme in the endoplasmic reticulum of mineralocorticoid target cells is believed to prevent cortisol from reaching the type 1 (mineralocorticoid) receptor. Several mutations of the gene for this enzyme have been identified among patients with apparent mineralocorticoid excess, each of which leads to enzymatic deficiency. Studies to date indicate that unrelated kindreds each carry a unique mutation, and the frequency of heterozygotes (who are unaffected) in the general population is extremely low.

Pseudomineralocorticoid Excess (Liddle's Syndrome). Several kindreds have been identified with features similar to the original description by Liddle and colleagues of members of a family with hypertension, hypokalemic alkalosis, and suppression of aldosterone or other mineralocorticoids. The disorder is transmitted in autosomal-dominant fashion. Affected patients have a renal abnormality causing distal sodium conservation even in the absence of mineralocorticoids. The mineralocorticoid antagonist, spironolactone, is without effect, and the abnormality is specifically reversed by the potassium-sparing diuretics, triamterene and amiloride, which are now known to work by blocking the epithelial sodium channel. It has been shown that the disorder is explained by mutations in either the β or γ subunits of the sodium channel, which renders it constitutively in the active conformation, leading to unregulated distal sodium reabsorption.

Other Conditions. Exogenous mineralocorticoid ingestion is another cause of hypertension and hypokalemia in which aldosterone is typically suppressed (Table 63.1). Fluorinated steroid nasal sprays and topical ointments have been reported to cause this syndrome. Licorice intoxication was initially thought to produce hypertension by this means, because licorice contains glycyrrhizinic acid and closely related compounds that are known to have weak direct mineralocorticoid action. Studies suggest that their mineralocorticoidlike effect *in vivo* is mainly accounted for by inhibition of the renal (type 2) isoform of 11β-hydroxysteroid dehydrogenase, providing an acquired counterpart to the syndrome of apparent mineralocorticoid excess discussed previously.

Overproduction of a number of unusual mineralocorticoids have been postulated in hypertensive disorders, including even low-renin "essential" hypertension without hypokalemia. Such additional steroids may contribute to the hypertension of primary aldosteronism or Cushing's syndrome, but no unique clinical syndromes have been clearly described.

The genetic basis of GRH, apparent mineralocorticoid excess, Gordon's syndrome, and Liddle's syndrome are also discussed in Chapter 60.

Management of Mineralocorticoid Hypertension

The specific mineralocorticoid antagonist, spironolactone, is useful in the preoperative management of patients with surgically remediable forms and can also be used for long-term medical therapy of all conditions caused by true mineralocorticoid excess. Doses of 25 to 50 mg/day are usually well tolerated, but higher doses (100 to 400 mg) are often necessary and may induce side effects (gynecomastia, impotence, gastrointestinal upset). Preoperative treatment is important to correct the metabolic abnormalities and hypertension (and thereby reduce perioperative complications) and also to minimize postoperative hypoaldosteronism, which is caused by atrophy of the normal glomerulosa due to the suppressed renin-angiotensin system. These effects may be reversed during prolonged spironolactone administration (2 to 6 months, or less at high doses). A therapeutic trial may also help to predict surgical outcome, because a poor blood pressure response may reflect the existence of other factors (e.g., renal or vascular damage, coexisting essential hypertension) that could sustain hypertension, thereby diminishing enthusiasm for recommending surgery. A therapeutic failure must not be overinterpreted, however, if adverse reactions limit the dose of spironolactone.

Unilateral adrenalectomy is commonly recommended for patients with APA or other mineralocorticoid-producing tumors unless surgery is contraindicated. This has conventionally been performed via a flank incision, but a laparoscopic approach is increasingly being adopted at some centers. Postoperative hypoaldosteronism, manifest by fatigue, lassitude, hyperkalemia, and variable hyponatremia, may occur despite prior treatment with spironolactone; this can usually be managed with a high-salt diet alone, but occasionally may require treatment for several months with the mineralocorticoid agonist, fludrocortisone. Adrenalectomy may also be beneficial in cases in which evidence of "autonomy" is equivocal, provided that unilateral (or markedly asymmetric) aldosterone secretion is documented by adrenal venous sampling and that hypertension is improved with spironolactone. The same criteria may also be used to justify subtotal adrenalectomy in the small subset of patients with presumed IHA who show an autonomous pattern. In all cases, evidence of advanced renal damage or hypertensive vascular disease poses relative contraindications to surgery because the chances for a cure are diminished.

Spironolactone is the mainstay of medical therapy in nonsurgical candidates or in patients with IHA. Other potassium-sparing diuretics (amiloride, triamterene), which work by blocking the apical sodium channel, may be used in patients intolerant of spironolactone. Although these agents can ameliorate hypokalemia, they are rarely sufficient to normalize blood pressure, except in patients with Liddle's syndrome, where they specifically correct consequences of the underlying genetic abnormality. In some patients with IHA, converting enzyme inhibitors may lower aldosterone secretion (because of a presumed increased adrenal sensitivity to angiotensin II) and thereby improve potassium balance and blood pressure to some extent. Hypertension is often not controlled in this disorder by correction of hyperaldosteronism alone. Other agents that are frequently effective include calcium channel blockers (particularly dihydropyridines) and α_1-adrenergic blockers. The rarer forms of mineralocorticoid hypertension usually respond to spironolactone, but glucocorticoid replacement therapy (e.g., with dexamethasone or prednisone) is more specific treatment for GRH and is mandatory in congenital adrenal hyperplasia.

Cushing's Syndrome

Clinical Presentation and Nosology

The diverse manifestations of Cushing's syndrome result from excessive production of glucocorticoids and, occasionally, other steroids from the zona fasciculata-reticularis of the adrenal cortex. Cortisol is the major glucocorticoid in humans, whereas corticosterone is more important in some species; the terminal biosynthetic step for each is catalyzed by the fasciculata form of 11β-hydroxylase, or CYP11B1 (Fig. 63.1). In contrast to the zona glomerulosa, synthesis of fasciculata steroids is governed almost exclusively by ACTH, whose elaboration by the anterior pituitary is regulated in turn by the hypothalamic release of corticotropin-releasing hormone (CRH). Synthesis and/or secretion of both CRH and ACTH are subject to feedback inhibition by blood-borne cortisol, leading to the so-called hypothalamic-pituitary-adrenal neuroendocrine axis. The dominant circadian rhythm of cortisol synthesis is determined by central nervous system influences on CRH release. This spontaneous rhythm can be interrupted, both acutely and chronically, by a variety of emotional and physical stresses, including many illnesses, and is characteristically lost in all forms of chronic hypercortisolism.

Mild to moderate hypertension occurs in the majority of patients with Cushing's syndrome, and is occasionally quite severe, but it is rarely the sole presenting complaint. Clinical suspicion is usually aroused by the more typical features of glucocorticoid excess present on examination (centripetal obesity, moon facies, buffalo hump, hirsutism, purplish striae, proximal muscle weakness) or identified by history or laboratory evaluation (easy bruisability, menstrual irregularity, loss of libido, mood alterations, impaired glucose tolerance or frank diabetes, and spontaneous fractures due to osteoporosis). The mortality rate is increased significantly in all forms of the disorder, and appears to be substantially worsened by hypertension.

The principal causes of this syndrome are listed in Table 63.1. Secondary hypercortisolism resulting from ACTH excess (which leads to bilateral adrenal hyperplasia) accounts for approximately 80% of all cases of noniatrogenic Cushing's syndrome. This is usually due to a *pituitary microadenoma* or *macroadenoma* (Cushing's disease), which is more common in women and typically occurs before the age of 50. The syndrome is occasionally caused by *ectopic ACTH production* by small-cell bronchogenic carcinomas of the lung, or less commonly by pancreatic or carcinoid tumors, thymomas, medullary carcinoma of the thyroid, bronchial adenomas, chromaffin tumors, or, rarely, other carcinomas (breast, ovary, prostate); very rarely, *ectopic CRH production* by such tumors has been reported. Primary cortisol excess accounts for approximately 20% of cases and is usually due to an *adrenal adenoma* or less commonly to an *adrenal carcinoma* or to *macronodular adrenal hyperplasia*. These forms are characterized by feedback suppression of ACTH release and resultant atrophy of the contralateral adrenal cortex. Carcinomas frequently produce a variety of steroids in addition to cortisol.

Pathogenesis of Hypertension

Hypertension occurs in all forms of the disorder but is less common in iatrogenic Cushing's syndrome (i.e., resulting from chronic administration of exogenous steroids) than in patients with pituitary or adrenal disease. The reasons for this are not fully defined but probably reflect the more complex nature of endogenous adrenal dysfunction and the complete lack of mineralocorticoid activity of commonly used synthetic steroids (e.g. prednisone, dexamethasone). Some component of functional mineralocorticoid excess probably occurs in all forms of endogenous hypercortisolism but usually does not fully explain the hypertension. Cortisol, when markedly elevated, may directly activate mineralocorticoid receptors, particularly if inactivation or clearance pathways are overwhelmed as discussed previously. This mechanism appears to contribute to the dominant mineralocorticoid pattern (i.e., hypertension associated with hypokalemia and suppressed PRA) that occurs in some patients with the ectopic ACTH syndrome and very high cortisol levels; DOC excess may also be present in such patients, due to the intense stimulation of fasciculata pathways by markedly elevated ACTH levels. A dominant mineralocorticoid pattern is also seen on occasion with adrenal carcinomas that, in addition to cortisol, may produce substantial amounts of DOC, corticosterone, or rarely, aldosterone or other mineralocorticoids.

Several glucocorticoid actions can also contribute to blood pressure elevations. Even in the absence of positive sodium balance, glucocorticoids can increase plasma and extracellular fluid volumes by causing a shift in fluid from the intracellular to the extracellular compartments. This may contribute to the increase in cardiac output observed in some patients with Cushing's syndrome. Glucocorticoids also stimulate hepatic synthesis of angiotensinogen (renin substrate), which tends to counter the suppression of plasma angiotensin–forming activity caused by mineralocorticoid-induced inhibition of renin secretion. As a result, PRA and angiotensin II are typically normal (or even slightly elevated) and are clearly inappropriate for the volume status. Glucocorticoids may also exert permissive effects on catecholamine action by enhancing vascular reactivity, in part because of inhibition of reuptake or of extraneuronal metabolism. They also appear to have a generalized sensitizing effect to a variety of vasoconstrictor substances. Finally, they are reported to have inhibitory effects on potential vasodilatory (kallikrein-kinin and prostaglandin) systems.

Diagnosis

The screening tests generally used for glucocorticoid excess are either measurement of 24-hour urinary free cortisol or the overnight dexamethasone suppression test; in the latter, the synthetic glucocorticoid dexamethasone, which normally suppresses ACTH, fails to reduce plasma cortisol to subnormal levels. Both tests are extremely sensitive, but false-positive results are common (e.g., due to stress, depression or other psychiatric disturbance, strenuous exercise, pregnancy). Confirmation is obtained with the standard low-dose (2 mg/day for 2 days) dexamethasone suppression test; if this is positive, a high-dose test (8 mg/day) can distinguish pituitary Cushing's disease (in which significant but incomplete suppression occurs) from other forms (Table 63.3). A variety of other indirect tests (e.g., metyrapone test, CRH infusion) have been used for further diagnosis, but with the advent of more specific and sensitive assays, measurement of plasma ACTH is often able to discriminate adrenal adenomas or carcinoma (ACTH suppressed) from ectopic ACTH or CRH production (ACTH elevated). Levels are usually normal in patients with pituitary Cushing's disease. Pituitary tumors can sometimes be localized by brain MRI (or CT), but petrosal sinus sampling to determine lateralization of ACTH production is often needed for smaller microadenomas (i.e., less than 1 cm). Adrenal tumors are usually detected by abdominal CT or iodocholesterol scintigraphy, as described previously.

Therapeutic Approaches

Surgical intervention is the treatment of choice for operable conditions. Resection of an isolated adrenal tumor is usually curative. Transsphenoidal resection of a pituitary adenoma is the favored approach for patients with Cushing's disease, most of whom have a microadenoma. Glucocorticoid replacement therapy is commonly given perioperatively and for up to 6 months afterward to prevent hypoadrenalism due to the sudden reduction in ACTH. Among patients whose hypercortisolism remits, approximately 10% to 20% will have recurrence within 5 years,

TABLE 63.3. Diagnosis of Cushing's Syndrome

Screening Tests
Urine Free Cortisol Excretion
Urine free cortisol excretion >100 μg/day is highly suggestive of Cushing's syndrome and nearly 100% sensitive.
Overnight Dexamethasone Suppression Test
Failure to suppress 8 AM plasma cortisol to <5 μg/dl following a bedtime 1-mg dose of dexamethasone is also highly sensitive, but has a higher false-positive rate (e.g., due to stress, depression, or obesity, or due to more rapid hepatic metabolism of dexamethasone induced by alcohol or certain drugs).
Confirmation
Low-Dose Dexamethasone Suppression Test
Failure to suppress plasma or urine cortisol (or metabolites) following low-dose dexamethasone (0.5 μg every 6 hours) for 2 days. Normal suppression of urine free cortisol (to <10 μg/day) or of urine 17-hydroxycorticoids (to <2.5 μg/day) excludes a diagnosis of Cushing's syndrome.
Differential Diagnosis
High-Dose Dexamethasone Suppression Test
Normal suppression of urine cortisol and 17-hydroxycorticoids (as above) following high-dose dexamethasone (2 mg every 6 hours) for 2 days occurs in most patients with pituitary Cushing's disease (because ACTH hypersecretion is generally mild and not truly autonomous). Failure to suppress occurs in the ectopic ACTH syndrome or in adrenal tumors. This classic test is now commonly being replaced by measurement of plasma ACTH, but may still be useful if those results (or imaging studies) are ambiguous.
Plasma ACTH
Normal to modestly elevated levels, which are suppressible by high-dose dexamethasone (see above), are characteristic of pituitary Cushing's disease. Levels are grossly elevated in the ectopic ACTH syndrome and are suppressed in adrenal tumors.
CRH Stimulation Test
If plasma ACTH levels are equivocal, the ACTH response to CRH administration may distinguish patients with pituitary Cushing's disease (normal ACTH stimulation) from those with ectopic ACTH secretion or adrenal tumors.
Petrosal Sinus Sampling
Sampling of the inferior petrosal venous sinus blood for ACTH may be helpful in confirming pituitary Cushing's and in helping to localize a pituitary microadenoma.
Imaging Studies
When hormonal studies suggest Cushing's disease, brain MRI (especially gadolinium enhanced), or alternatively, CT is performed to localize a pituitary tumor. The sensitivity is low (<50%) for microadenomas, so if results are negative, petrosal sinus sampling should be done. When plasma ACTH is suppressed, abdominal CT or MRI should be done to localize an adrenal tumor; bilateral adrenal hyperplasia can also sometimes be identified, but it may be difficult to distinguish primary adrenal disease from ACTH-dependent disease. Adrenal scintigraphy with [^{131}I]-iodomethyl-19-norcholesterol may occasionally detect tumors that are too small to be identified by CT or MRI. When plasma ACTH is greatly elevated, a source of ectopic ACTH secretion may be identified by CT of the chest and abdomen. Because many such tumors contain somatostatin receptors, octreotide scintigraphy may also be helpful.

ACTH, adrenocorticotropic hormone; CRH, corticotropin-releasing hormone; CT, computed tomography; MRI, magnetic resonance imaging.

particularly in those with macroadenomas. Total hypophysectomy is occasionally required for larger tumors. External proton-beam irradiation of the pituitary or implantation of yttrium or gold seeds are alternative approaches for patients with either adenomas or diffuse corticotrope hyperplasia. Bilateral adrenalectomy used to be a common approach for pituitary Cushing's and is extremely effective; however, as many as 25% of patients develop Nelson's syndrome (a more aggressive, locally invasive pituitary tumor associated with hyperpigmentation and visual field defects) unless the pituitary is also irradiated, thus this option should be reserved for patients who fail to respond to other therapies, or for those with metastatic ACTH-producing neoplasms.

Although there are several agents that may modify pituitary ACTH release or inhibit adrenal steroidogenesis, there are at present no satisfactory medical approaches for long-term management of glucocorticoid excess. Agents that interfere with ACTH release include the serotonin antagonist, cyproheptadine; the dopaminergic agonist, bromocriptine; and the long-acting somatostatin analog, octreotide; cyproheptadine in particular has had some limited success in patients with Cushing's disease. Inhibitors of steroidogenesis include the 11β-hydroxylase inhibitor, metyrapone, as well as agents that block at several biosynthetic steps (ketoconazole, aminoglutethimide, and trilostane). Such agents may be useful for temporary, rapid reduction in cortisol in preparation for definitive treatment, but careful titration is required to avoid adrenal insufficiency. Mitotane or *o,p'*-DDD [2,2-bis(2-*o*-chlorophenyl-4-*p*-chlorophenyl)-1,1-dichloroethane] is an adrenolytic agent that destroys the zona fasciculata-reticularis while sparing the zona glomerulosa. Although slow in onset, and often poorly tolerated (nausea, depression, ataxia), its prolonged action (due to accumulation in adipose tissue) makes it quite effective in suppressing steroid production in patients with metastatic adrenal carcinoma, which it may also destroy. Lastly, glucocorticoid-receptor antagonists (e.g., RU 38486) may have some utility in modifying tissue responses to cortisol excess, but experience has been limited.

For medical management of the associated hypertension, logical choices include spironolactone or a calcium channel blocker (particularly if a major mineralocorticoid component is suspected), α_1-adrenergic blockers or sympatholytic agents, and angiotensin-converting enzyme inhibitors.

PHEOCHROMOCYTOMA AND RELATED DISORDERS

Catecholamine-secreting tumors are extremely rare, accounting for less than 0.1% of all cases of hypertension, but represent an important category of secondary hypertension because of the serious and often fatal consequences if they are left unrecognized. In addition, they are nearly always curable. Although the diagnosis may still at times be difficult and elude even the most diligent physician, advances in biochemical screening and radiographic procedures over the past 2 decades have greatly simplified the approach to this problem.

Origin

Pheochromocytomas account for most catecholamine-producing tumors. These arise from chromaffin cells of the adrenal medulla (85% to 90% of cases) or from extraadrenal chromaffin cells (10% to 15% of cases) found in the organ of Zuckerkandl or associated with the sympathetic chain in the abdomen, chest, and neck (Table 63.4). Bilateral adrenal tumors or multiple extra-adrenal tumors each occur in approximately 10% of cases, the frequency being higher (up to 40%) in children. In familial forms [i.e., those associated with multiple endocrine neoplasia (MEN) and other syndromes listed in Table 63.4], bilateral tumors occur in more than 60% of cases; these are inherited as autosomal-dominant traits and have been associated with a variety of reported chromosomal abnormalities.

TABLE 63.4. Catecholamine-Producing Neural Crest Tumors

Pheochromocytoma
Location
~90% Adrenal ~8% Extraadrenal abdominal sites (sympathetic chain, organ of Zuckerkandl, urinary bladder) ~2% Chest (posterior mediastinum) or neck
Characteristics ("Rule of Tens")
~10% Familial (MEN type 2 or type 3) ~10% Bilateral adrenal (higher in children or familial cases, uncommon in sporadic cases) ~10% Extraadrenal or multifocal, or both (higher in children) ~10% Malignant (higher in extraadrenal sites)
Inherited Syndromes
MEN type 2, or Sipple's syndrome (pheochromocytoma [often bilateral], medullary thyroid carcinoma, parathyroid adenoma or hyperplasia) MEN type 3 (pheochromocytoma [often bilateral], medullary thyroid carcinoma, mucosal neuromas, thickened corneal nerves, alimentary ganglioneuromas, marfanoid habitus) von Hippel-Lindau disease (retinal angiomas, cerebral hemangioblastoma, renal and pancreatic cysts; pheochromocytoma in ~15%) von Recklinghausen's disease (neurofibromatosis ± café-au-lait spots, pheochromocytoma in ~1%)
Other Neural Crest Tumors (occasionally catecholamine producing)
Neuroblastoma (80% abdominal, 100% malignant) Ganglioneuroma (80% abdominal, 10% malignant) Chemodectoma (90% in neck, rarely malignant)

MEN, multiple endocrine neoplasia.

Approximately 10% of pheochromocytomas are malignant (i.e., locally invasive and occasionally metastatic to lymph nodes, liver, bone, and lung), but these are histologically similar to benign tumors. The frequency of malignancy is increased with extraadrenal tumors (30% to 40%) and is particularly high in those secreting dopamine. Rarely, other tumors of neural crest origin may be responsible for excessive catecholamine production (Table 63.4). These produce a clinical syndrome indistinguishable from pheochromocytoma.

Pathophysiology

Hypertension and other manifestations are mainly attributable to excessive catecholamine production, but a great variety of peptide hormones may be elaborated by some tumors (e.g., ACTH, α-melanocyte–stimulating hormone, opioid peptides, vasoactive intestinal polypeptide, and neuropeptide Y, to name a few), and these may cause additional symptoms. The complete catecholamine biosynthetic pathway (Fig. 63.3) is present in most adrenal tumors, but unlike the normal adrenal medulla,

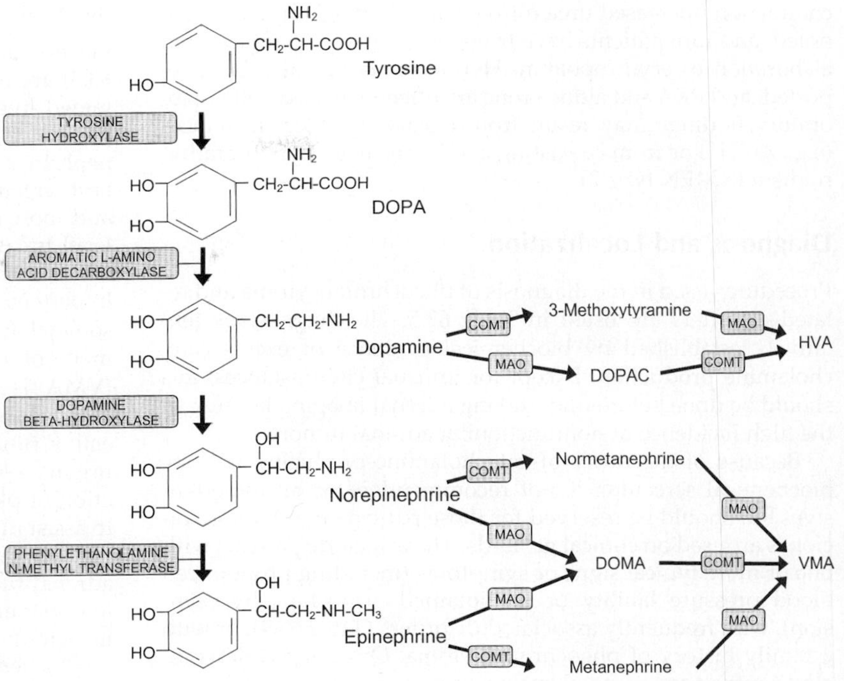

Figure 63.3. Pathways of catecholamine biosynthesis and metabolism. The vertical pathway *on the left* shows the structures of tyrosine and the catechol metabolites derived from it; the enzymes catalyzing each step are named in the shaded boxes to the left of each arrow. The horizontal pathways *on the right* indicate the major metabolites of each catecholamine produced by two enzymes, catechol O-methyltransferase (COMT) and monoamine oxidase (MAO). DOMA, dihydroxymandelic acid; DOPA, dihydroxyphenylalanine; DOPAC, dihydroxyphenylacetic acid; HVA, homovanillic acid; VMA, vanillylmandelic acid.

norepinephrine is the predominant secretory product, as it is in most extraadrenal tumors. Tumors that secrete mainly epinephrine are occasionally found, and these are almost always of adrenal origin. Dopamine-producing tumors are rare, but are associated with increased prevalence of malignancy.

Norepinephrine induces hypertension through the hemodynamic responses to α- and β-adrenergic receptor activation (i.e., systemic vasoconstriction, venoconstriction, and increased cardiac output). Although α-adrenergic effects on the kidney tend to promote sodium conservation, patients with sustained hypertension often have reduced extracellular volume because of the phenomenon of pressure natriuresis. PRA and angiotensin II are often increased as a result of β-adrenergic stimulation of the kidney. Hyperreninemia is even more pronounced in patients who develop malignant hypertension, and may be associated with hypokalemia due to secondary aldosteronism. β-Adrenergic effects (e.g., tachycardia, increased cardiac output, increased PRA) are typical of all pheochromocytomas but predominate in epinephrine-secreting tumors. These patients may rarely exhibit episodic hypotension because of β-mediated vasodilation.

Depending on the pattern of catecholamine secretion and other modifying influences, hypertension (and other symptoms) may be either episodic or sustained, with the latter pattern often accompanied by superimposed paroxysms of hypertension. No morphologic features are known to predict either pattern, which occur with roughly equal frequency. There is considerable variability in both tumor size (from less than 1 to several thousand grams) and catecholamine content, but neither parameter correlates with plasma catecholamine levels or clinical manifestations. Thus small tumors may release large amounts because of rapid catecholamine turnover, whereas very large tumors may release only small amounts due to sluggish turnover and increased intratumoral catabolism.

Clinical Presentation

The signs and symptoms are attributable to catecholamine excess, to the complications of hypertension, and, occasionally, to the elaboration of specific peptide hormones. In the episodic form, attacks may occur several times a day or as infrequently as every few months; these may be spontaneous or provoked by a variety of factors, including abdominal pressure, exercise, posture, bladder distension or decompression, certain foods (e.g., tyramine-containing cheeses or wines) and drugs (e.g., phenothiazines, metoclopramide, histamine, glucagon, and tyramine), or general anesthesia. The most common symptoms are headache, generalized sweating, and palpitations or tachycardia; reflex bradycardia sometimes accompanies paroxysms of hypertension in patients with mainly norepinephrine-secreting tumors. Anxiety, tremulousness, lightheadedness, nausea and vomiting, and chest or epigastric pain are also frequent complaints, especially in patients with paroxysms. Weight loss caused by a hypermetabolic state may be notable in some patients. Untreated patients suffer typical hypertensive complications such as stroke, renal insufficiency, heart failure, dissecting aneurysm, and encephalopathy. In addition, a unique form of potentially reversible cardiomyopathy that is attributable to catecholamine-induced cardiac toxicity occurs in patients with severely elevated levels. Occasional patients have an explosive or fulminant course, sometimes precipitated by a sudden increase in catecholamine release because of spontaneous hemorrhagic necrosis of the tumor. Such patients may present with malignant hypertension; acute pulmonary edema; encephalopathy; or, occasionally, unexplained shock, lactic acidosis, and multisystem failure.

The incidence of cholelithiasis is increased in patients with pheochromocytoma for reasons that are unknown. Several other conditions or lesions are associated with familial forms, as noted in Table 63.4, some of which may be detected on physical examination. Typical signs of catecholamine excess (tachycardia, hyperhidrosis, pallor, tremor, and pupillary dilation) are often present on examination, and the blood pressure and heart rate are often very labile. Orthostatic hypotension may also be notable; this is due to a blunting of sympathetic reflexes induced by adrenergic receptor downregulation and may be accentuated by coexisting volume contraction.

Laboratory evaluation frequently provides evidence of impaired glucose tolerance or even frank diabetes. Signs of volume contraction (increased urea nitrogen and hemoglobin) are often noted, and rare patients have true polycythemia resulting from elaboration of erythropoietin. Hypokalemia has also been reported, and PRA and aldosterone are often increased. Other laboratory findings may result from release of other substances (e.g., ACTH) or from coexisting conditions (e.g., hyperparathyroidism in MEN type 2).

Diagnosis and Localization

Procedures used in the diagnosis of pheochromocytoma and related disorders are listed in Table 63.5. The diagnosis is tentatively established by biochemical evidence of excess catecholamine production. Except for unusual circumstances, this should be done before undertaking adrenal imaging because of the high incidence of nonfunctioning adrenal tumors.

Because of the rarity of catecholamine-producing tumors, biochemical screening is not recommended for all hypertensives but should be reserved for those patients in whom suspicion is aroused on clinical grounds. These include patients with one or more typical signs or symptoms (including pronounced blood pressure lability or unexplained orthostatic hypotension), with frequently associated disorders (Table 63.4), or with a family history of pheochromocytoma. Other indications include refractory or accelerating hypertension, particularly if associated with glucose intolerance; evidence of a hypermetabolic state (including weight loss); infrequent or unusual complications (e.g., dissecting aneurysm, unexplained cardiomyopathy) or a history of hypertensive crises (e.g., induced by anesthesia, surgery, angiography); paradoxic response to antihypertensive therapy (e.g., β-blockers); or unexplained circulatory collapse.

TABLE 63.5. Diagnosis of Pheochromocytoma

Biochemical Identification
Plasma catecholamines[a]
Urinary metanephrines,[a] catecholamines, VMA, homovanillic acid
Pharmacologic Testing
Clonidine suppression test
Useful for confirming autonomous catecholamine production
Regitine (phentolamine) test
Not specific and rarely needed but may be useful in patients with hypertensive crises
Provocative testing (glucagon, histamine, tyramine)
Unnecessary (and contraindicated) in patients who are hypertensive
Localization Techniques
Computed tomography (CT)
Most sensitive imaging procedure for adrenal and extraadrenal tumors
Magnetic resonance imaging (MRI)
Resolution somewhat less than CT, but unique signal intensity on T_2-weighted images (due to hemorrhage or necrotic foci) may be useful (e.g., to distinguish from adrenocortical tumors)
Scintigraphy
Meta-[^{131}I]iodobenzylguanidine scanning is highly specific for chromaffin tissue but has less sensitivity than CT or MRI
Central venous blood sampling
Helpful in localization or confirmation of extraadrenal tumors when imaging results are negative or equivocal

[a] Recommended screening tests.
VMA, vanillylmandelic acid.

Biochemical Identification

Plasma and urinary catecholamines or their metabolites (Fig. 63.3) are nearly always clearly increased in patients with sustained hypertension induced by catecholamine-producing tumors. Of the tests listed in Table 63.5, urinary total metanephrines or plasma catecholamines are widely considered the best screening tests. Plasma measurements are more convenient and more sensitive, but less specific; a plasma norepinephrine level greater than 2,000 pg/ml is virtually diagnostic, but at lesser elevations there is considerable overlap with essential hypertension. Urinary measurements are less expensive and somewhat more specific. If clinical suspicion is high, measurement of urinary catecholamines and vanillylmandelic acid (VMA) is also advisable because metanephrines are not invariably increased; for instance, in patients with large, relatively inactive tumors with much intratumoral catabolism, increased urinary VMA may rarely be the only positive finding. Fractionation of plasma or urinary catecholamines is often performed to assist in localization because a major increase in epinephrine (or its metabolite metanephrine) is highly suggestive of an adrenal tumor. Urinary homovanillic acid (HVA) is increased in dopamine-producing tumors and may be associated with an increased incidence of malignancy.

Biochemical diagnosis may be more difficult in patients with purely episodic hypertension because measurements can be entirely normal between attacks. Measurement of plasma catecholamines during a paroxysm is ideal but often unfeasible. A useful alternative procedure is to instruct the patient to begin a timed (2 to 4 hour) urine collection at the onset of symptoms after emptying the bladder; an increase in the urinary catecholamine-to-creatinine ratio is nearly always diagnostic, and provocative testing rarely is needed.

Pharmacologic Testing

The *clonidine suppression test* is a useful procedure for confirming autonomous catecholamine production in patients with mild increases in catecholamines because values of plasma norepinephrine up to twice the upper limit of normal are not uncommon in patients with essential hypertension. The basis for this test is that clonidine acts centrally to decrease sympathetic outflow, thereby lowering plasma norepinephrine to normal limits (or by more than 50%) when attributable to increased neurogenic drive but has no effect when due to autonomous production by a tumor.

The *Regitine (phentolamine) test,* which assesses the blood pressure response to acute α-adrenergic blockade, is not specific and is rarely used now. *Provocative testing* with agents known to stimulate tumoral release of catecholamines used to be performed commonly in patients suspected of having episodically secreting tumors, but this is rarely necessary and potentially dangerous; it is absolutely contraindicated in patients with sustained hypertension. It should be considered only if the diagnosis eludes repeated attempts at biochemical diagnosis or in normotensive individuals at increased risk because of family history (e.g., MEN syndromes). Of the agents listed in Table 63.5, glucagon is probably the safest; the test entails far less risk if performed during α-blockade (e.g., with phentolamine infusion) to blunt the pressor response, with a rise in plasma catecholamine levels (rather than in blood pressure) being the end point.

Localization Techniques

Although tiny tumors occur, the average size of adrenal pheochromocytomas is quite large (approximately 5 cm) at the time of diagnosis. As with adrenocortical tumors, *CT* is the most sensitive imaging technique, and this may identify extraadrenal as well as adrenomedullary pheochromocytomas. *MRI scans,* although perhaps having somewhat poorer resolution, are widely used because pheochromocytomas often produce a unique signal intensity as a result of their vascularity and propensity for intratumoral hemorrhage and necrosis. Although not specific for pheochromocytoma, this feature may be helpful in localizing extraadrenal tumors, and its absence may help to distinguish cortical adenomas. *[^{123}I]Meta-iodobenzylguanidine (MIBG) scintigraphy* has lesser sensitivity (approximately 85%) but is highly specific for chromaffin tissue and is sometimes used for functional confirmation or for localization of extraadrenal tumors. The latter may, however, elude all imaging techniques, particularly if small, in which case *venous sampling* of vena cava blood at various levels for plasma catecholamine measurements may successfully identify the tumor site.

Medical and Surgical Management

Surgical resection is the treatment of choice for all patients with nonmetastatic disease unless surgery is contraindicated. With rare exception, however, a period of preoperative medical management is mandatory in order to establish adrenergic blockade and to restore euvolemia, because this significantly reduces intraoperative and postoperative morbidity.

The mainstay of medical management is the establishment of α-adrenergic blockade. β-Adrenergic blocking agents are also sometimes indicated as adjunctive therapy, but β-blockers should *never* be administered until α-blockade is achieved because of the high risk of potentiating α-mediated vasoconstriction and inducing a pronounced blood pressure rise.

When rapid α-blockade is indicated, intravenous phentolamine (a nonselective α-antagonist) may be administered as intermittent boluses (1 to 5 mg) or by continuous infusion; however, in patients with hypertensive crisis caused by pheochromocytoma, sodium nitroprusside is also usually effective and is easier to titrate. The most commonly used oral agent is phenoxybenzamine, a long-acting, noncompetitive antagonist that acts by alkylating α-receptors; the usual initial dose is 10 mg once or twice daily, and this can be increased by 10-mg increments every 3 to 5 days according to the response. A therapeutic dose (to reduce seated blood pressure to near-normal levels) should generally be maintained for several weeks before surgery. Side effects include dizziness (orthostatic hypotension), nasal congestion, lassitude, and drowsiness. Competitive α_1-blocking agents (e.g., prazosin, terazosin, doxazosin) have also been used and may be better tolerated; however, these agents are less effective in blocking the effects of a pronounced catecholamine surge (e.g., during anesthesia induction or intraoperative tumor manipulation) and should not be used alone. Combined α- and β-blocking agents (e.g., labetalol) have also been used; however, pressor responses to labetalol have been reported, thus this approach to initial therapy is not recommended. Some combination of phenoxybenzamine and an α_1-antagonist may be logical when side effects limit the dose of the former agent. Overzealous treatment (i.e., to the point of subnormal seated pressures or obvious orthostatic hypotension) should be avoided because incomplete blockade allows blood pressure fluctuations during surgery to be used as a guide to tumor localization or to the existence of multiple tumors.

Addition of β-adrenergic blocking agents may be helpful in patients who have severe tachycardia, hazardous arrhythmias (unless the latter are escape rhythms that occur after reflex bradycardia), or coexisting angina. They may also be indicated in patients with catecholamine-induced cardiomyopathy. The use of cardioselective agents (e.g., atenolol, metoprolol) is probably more logical because nonselective β-blockers are more likely to offset β_2-mediated vasodilation.

α-Methyl-L-tyrosine, known commercially as metyrosine (Demser), is a competitive inhibitor of tyrosine hydroxylase that has been used to inhibit catecholamine biosynthesis, mainly in chronic medical management of inoperable cases. It may also be useful in patients who are unable to tolerate α- and β-blockers, and is probably of value in preoperative management of patients with cardiomyopathy, particularly when catecholamine elevations are extreme. Although its usefulness may be limited by serious side effects (sedation, extrapyramidal signs, psychic disturbances, and diarrhea), some experts have also incorporated this agent into a more routine preoperative regimen. The drug must be given with adequate hydration to minimize the risk of crystalluria.

Another important aspect of preoperative management is restoration or frank expansion of extracellular volume, mainly to minimize the profound hypotension that often follows tumor removal. A high-salt diet over a several-week period as blood pressure is lowered by adrenergic blockade usually produces adequate positive sodium balance. However, some also recommend additional volume expansion with colloid or whole blood in the immediate preoperative period.

The classic surgical approach for an adrenal pheochromocytoma is through a midline abdominal incision, even if a unilateral tumor has been identified, thus allowing the surgeon to explore the contralateral gland and extraadrenal sites for possible additional tumors. This is thus the preferred approach for children or for patients with familial pheochromocytoma. With the advent of better imaging techniques, however, some surgeons now consider laparoscopic adrenalectomy or even a unilateral (thoracolumbar) approach, particularly if the probability of multiple tumors is low (e.g., in patients with sporadic pheochromocytoma). Special precautions and expertise are required during induction and maintenance of anesthesia and in the immediate postoperative period, particularly with regard to cardiovascular instability and volume and metabolic status.

Long-term treatment with adrenergic blocking agents or metyrosine can be effective in controlling hypertension and other symptoms in inoperable cases. Tumor debulking or embolization is also sometimes recommended in patients with malignant pheochromocytomas to reduce catecholamine output. Conventional radiotherapy (e.g., to painful bony metastases), ^{131}I-MIBG administration, and combination chemotherapy have been used with various success to treat metastatic disease.

RENIN-SECRETING TUMORS

Renin-secreting tumors are an extremely rare cause of curable hypertension with fewer than 100 cases having been reported in the English-speaking literature. Most of these have been small, benign, juxtaglomerular cell tumors (hemangiopericytomas) of the kidney. Nearly all such cases have presented before 30 years of age with often severe or accelerating hypertension and hypokalemia caused by secondary aldosteronism (Table 63.1). PRA is usually greatly elevated, and renin secretion is unilateral by renal venous sampling, similar to unilateral renovascular disease. Suspicion should be aroused when a vascular cause (e.g., main or branch renal artery stenosis, segmental renal infarct, subcapsular hematoma) cannot be identified, and the tumors can be usually localized by CT scan. Other renal tumors can occasionally cause hypertension by hypersecretion of renin, including Wilms' tumor in children and rare cases of renal cell carcinoma in adults. Hypertension is usually cured by resection of the tumor, but also responds very well to drugs that block the renin-angiotensin system (i.e., angiotensin-converting enzyme inhibitors, angiotensin-receptor blockers).

Ectopic renin production by extrarenal hemangiopericytomas, other sarcomas, or certain malignancies (adenocarcinoma of pancreas, ovary, and lung) has also been reported. A diagnostic hallmark that may be helpful in distinguishing this syndrome from renovascular and other high-renin forms of hypertension is pronounced elevations in plasma prorenin levels. Prorenin normally accounts for 70% to 90% of the total renin in blood, with levels generally being 3 to 5 times higher than active renin levels in high-renin states. But in renin-secreting tumors, prorenin levels may sometimes be as much as 50- to several hundred–fold higher than active renin. This is particularly so in extrarenal malignancies and in Wilms' tumor, but higher than expected prorenin levels have also been reported in some juxtaglomerular cell tumors as well.

OTHER ENDOCRINE DISORDERS ASSOCIATED WITH HYPERTENSION

The prevalence of hypertension is increased twofold to threefold in a variety of other endocrine disorders. Particularly with hypothyroidism and acromegaly, treatment of the primary condition often corrects the hypertension, thus implying a causal relationship. As with other secondary forms, cure of hypertension is more likely if the underlying disorder is recognized and treated early in its course.

Thyroid Disorders

Thyroid hormone has profound actions on the cardiovascular system, causing an increase in heart rate, stroke volume, and cardiac output, effects that are associated with a fall in peripheral vascular resistance and increased intravascular volume. The cardiac effects are due to a direct effect of thyroid hormone and to an increase in β-adrenergic sensitivity (mediated in part by increased receptor density). As a consequence, in *hyperthyroidism* of any cause (e.g., Grave's disease, autonomous thyroid nodule, toxic goiter) the pulse pressure is widened, and approximately one-third of patients develop mild to moderate systolic hypertension. These signs generally resolve with restoration of the euthyroid state, particularly in younger patients. Exactly the opposite hemodynamic profile occurs in *hypothyroidism,* with the increase in peripheral vascular resistance leading to true diastolic hypertension in approximately 50% of cases. Vascular resistance is increased because of structural changes induced by thyroid-hormone deficiency and perhaps also because of an imbalance of sympathetic innervation, with a relative increase in α-adrenergic tone resulting from a decrease in β-adrenergic–receptor density. Thyroid hormone replacement is often sufficient to normalize blood pressure.

Acromegaly

Excess production of growth hormone by pituitary adenomas is the most common cause of acromegaly in adults (and gigantism in prepubertal children). Rarer causes include ectopic production by hypothalamic, carcinoid, or pancreatic islet cell tumors. Approximately 40% to 50% of patients have hypertension, which is probably explained by a combination of sodium retention and vascular hypertrophy induced by growth hormone or other mediators [e.g., insulinlike growth factor-1 (IGF-1)]. In addition to hypertension, chronic acromegaly is associated with a specific cardiomyopathy, and cardiovascular mortality is high in untreated cases.

Parathyroid Disorders and Hypercalcemia

The prevalence of hypertension is more than doubled among patients with primary hyperparathyroidism due either to parathyroid adenoma or hyperplasia. It is uncertain whether the association with hypertension is direct, because the response of blood pressure to parathyroidectomy is highly variable, with some series reporting amelioration of hypertension in the majority of patients and others in only a small fraction. The pathogenesis of hypertension is likely to be multifactorial, but the underlying mechanisms are poorly understood. Some investigators report that plasma renin and aldosterone levels are frequently increased and tend to normalize following parathyroidectomy. Hypercalcemia is also likely to play a role. Calcium infusion has been shown to raise blood pressure acutely, perhaps because of enhanced sensitivity to noradrenergic and other vasoconstrictive mechanisms that depend on an increase in cytosolic calcium. Indeed, certain other causes of hypercalcemia (e.g., *milk-alkali syndrome, hypervitaminosis D, sarcoidosis*) are commonly associated with hypertension even though parathyroid hormone (PTH) levels are suppressed. On the other hand, increased PTH levels are also thought to contribute to hypertension by some investigators. Although PTH has a vasorelaxant effect in some isolated vessel preparations, infusion into intact humans has been shown to raise blood pressure. In support of a role for PTH itself, mention is often made of disorders associated with hypertension in which increased PTH levels occur in the setting of hypocalcemia, for example, *secondary hyperparathyroidism* (most often in the setting of chronic renal insufficiency), and the type I variant of *pseudohypoparathyroidism,* a rare inherited disorder due to target organ resistance to PTH (in which abnormal G-protein coupling to adenylate cyclase may affect receptor transduction for other hormonal systems as well). As should be obvious, however, each of these conditions is too complex to permit the conclusion that the hypertension is caused by PTH excess *per se.* Further discussion on the relation between PTH, serum calcium, and hypertension is provided in Chapter 17, Part 3.

Selected Readings

Atlas SA, Hesson TE, Sealey JE, et al. Characterization of inactive renin ("prorenin") from renin-secreting tumors of non-renal origin: similarity to inactive renin from kidney and normal plasma *J Clin Invest* 1984;73:437–447.

Description and characterization of markedly elevated levels of prorenin in patients with ectopic renin production. Disproportionate increases in plasma prorenin levels serve to distinguish patients with renin-secreting tumors from those with other high-renin forms of hypertension.

Biglieri EG, Melby JC. *Endocrine hypertension.* New York: Raven Press, 1990.

A comprehensive monograph providing many excellent chapters by experts in the field on all aspects of adrenocortical and adrenomedullary hypertension. Particularly noteworthy are several chapters by Biglieri and colleagues detailing their extensive experience in patients with various subforms of primary aldosteronism and other forms of mineralocorticoid hypertension, and chapters on Cushing's syndrome, apparent mineralocorticoid excess, and the role of other steroids in hypertensive disorders.

Bravo EL. Evolving concepts in the pathophysiology, diagnosis, and treatment of pheochromocytoma. *Endocr Rev* 1994;15:356–368.

An outstanding, up-to-date review of the pathophysiology, clinical features, diagnostic approach, and management of patients with pheochromocytoma.

Bravo EL, Tarazi RC, Fouad FM, et al. Clonidine-suppression test: a useful aid in the diagnosis of pheochromocytoma *N Engl J Med* 1981;305:623–626.

A classical description of the effects of oral clonidine on plasma catecholamine levels in patients with pheochromocytoma and with essential hypertension. These data form the basis for a useful clinical test that can distinguish patients with pheochromocytoma (i.e., relatively autonomous production of catecholamines by a tumor) from those with modest elevations of catecholamines due to increased neurogenic drive, which are suppressed by clonidine.

Corvol P, Pinet F, Plouin P-F, et al. Renin-secreting tumors. *Endocrinol Metab Clin North Am* 1994;23:255–270.

A careful literature review of renin-secreting tumors, providing a thorough description of clinical and pathologic features, laboratory abnormalities, diagnostic procedures, and therapeutic responses.

Edwards CRW, Stewart PM, Burt D, et al. Localisation of 11β-hydroxysteroid dehydrogenase, tissue specific protector of the mineralocorticoid receptor. *Lancet* 1988;2:986–989.

Elegant description of the fundamental concepts regarding specificity of mineralocorticoid action that derived from prior studies on the syndrome of apparent mineralocorticoid excess and on the mechanism of licorice-induced hypertension. Although it has been subsequently shown that a different isoform of 11β-hydroxysteroid dehydrogenase is actually responsible for these observations, the important insights derived from the work of these investigators remain unchallenged.

Gennari C, Nami R, Gonnelli S. Hypertension and primary hyperparathyroidism: the role of adrenergic and renin-angiotensin-aldosterone systems. *Miner Electrolyte Metab* 1995;21:77–81.

Analysis of the incidence of hypertension in 34 consecutive patients with primary hyperparathyroidism. Provides evidence for abnormalities in the renin-angiotensin-aldosterone system in affected patients, which may play a role in the pathogenesis of hypertension.

Lifton RP, Dluhy RG, Powers M, et al. A chimeric 11β-hydroxylase-aldosterone synthase gene causes glucocorticoid remediable aldosteronism and human hypertension. *Nature* 1992;16:262–265.

Identification of the genetic abnormality in glucocorticoid-remediable hyperaldosteronism (GRH), in which a gene duplication arising from unequal crossing over two highly homologous genes leads to a chimeric gene that fuses the 5′ regulatory end of the steroid 11β-hydroxylase gene to the coding sequences of the aldosterone synthase genes. The abnormal gene is thus expressed by fasciculata cells where it confers aldosterone synthesizing ability under the control of ACTH. This discovery provides an excellent example of genetic research inspired by insightful clinical observation and physiologic and biochemical studies.

Manger WM, Gifford RW Jr. *Clinical and Experimental Pheochromocytoma,* 2nd ed. Cambridge, MA: Blackwell Science, 1996.

An outstanding, highly readable, and comprehensive monograph providing detailed discussion of all aspects of pheochromocytoma and related disorders.

Orth DN. Cushing's syndrome. *N Engl J Med* 1995;332:791–803.

An up-to-date review that provides a particularly clear and thorough consideration of the approaches to diagnosis and management of these disorders.

Saito I, Saruta T. Hypertension in thyroid disorders. *Endocrinol Metab Clin North Am* 1994;23:379–386.

Concise review article that considers the pathophysiology of hemodynamic disturbances in states of thyroid-hormone deficiency and excess. The responses of blood pressure to treatment of the primary disorders are also reviewed.

Tunny TJ, Gordon RD, Klemm SA, et al. Histological and biochemical distinctiveness of atypical aldosterone producing adenoma responsive to upright posture and angiotensin. *Clin Endocrinol* 1991;34:363–369.

Characterization of so-called renin-responsive APAs, providing evidence of a link between the ability of these tumors to respond to angiotensin II or upright posture with a relative paucity of the fasciculatalike cells that are characteristically predominant in classical ("autonomous") APAs. The presence of such cells probably also accounts for the overproduction of oxygenated cortisol metabolites seen in classical APAs (see following reference).

Ulick S, Blumenfeld JD, Atlas SA, et al. The unique steroidogenesis of the aldosteronoma in the differential diagnosis of primary aldosteronism. *J Clin Endocrinol Metab* 1993;76:873–878.

In a large series of patients with primary aldosteronism, elevated levels of 18-oxocortisol and 18-hydroxycortisol provide a diagnostic hallmark for patients with the classic form of APA, as well as for rare patients with unilateral hyperplasia (i.e., PAH). On the other hand, levels are uniformly normal in patients with IHA or with atypical, "renin-responsive" APA. Although the analytic methods involved are difficult, these analyses offer a promising approach to identifying patients who are likely to benefit from adrenalectomy (or who have the rare familial syndrome of GRH).

Ulick S, Levine LS, Gunczler P, et al. A syndrome of apparent mineralocorticoid excess associated with defects in the peripheral metabolism of cortisol. *J Clin Endcrinol Metab* 1979;49:757–764.

A classic description of a rare disorder and its underlying biochemical abnormalities. These observations have had profound impact in leading not only to identification of the genetic abnormality in the disorder but also to revolutionary new concepts concerning the specificity of mineralocorticoid hormone action.

Ulick S, Wang JZ, Blumenfeld JD, et al. Cortisol inactivation overload: a mechanism of mineralocorticoid hypertension in the ectopic adrenocorticotropin syndrome. *J Clin Endcrinol Metab* 1992;74:963–967.

Studies in two patients with the ectopic ACTH syndrome reveal that, in addition to hypersecretion of DOC, cortisol can contribute to mineralocorticoid hypertension by a mechanism similar to that of the apparent mineralocorticoid excess syndrome. In this case, overwhelming of inactivating pathways by other steroids secreted in response to ACTH is postulated to permit cortisol access to the mineralocorticoid receptor.

Wenting GJ, Man in't Veld AJ, Schalekamp MADH. Recurrence of hypertension in primary aldosteronism after discontinuation of spironolactone. Time course of changes in cardiac output and body fluid volumes. *Clin Exp Hypertens* 1982; 4:1727–1748.

Demonstration of the sequential volume and hemodynamic changes during the development of mineralocorticoid hypertension in humans by careful study of 10 patients with primary aldosteronism following discontinuation of spironolactone therapy. Cardiac output, blood volume, and sodium space increased initially in all patients, and these changes were sustained in half of them (all under 50 years old). In the remaining older patients, although sodium space remained expanded, cardiac output and blood volume returned toward baseline by 6 weeks, at which point a rise in peripheral resistance accounted for sustained hypertension.

White PC. Inherited forms of mineralocorticoid hypertension. *Hypertension* 1996; 28:927–936.

A lucid and comprehensive review of the hypertensive syndromes associated with congenital adrenal hyperplasia, GRH, and apparent mineralocorticoid excess. Provides an excellent discussion of the pathophysiology and genetic bases for these disorders and of the current concepts of mineralocorticoid hormone regulation and specificity.

CHAPTER 64

Pediatric Hypertension

Ellin Lieberman

Childhood hypertension is a distinct pediatric problem. The requirements for blood pressure measurements and their interpretation in young people have been delineated. Numbers have arbitrarily been chosen to define normal, high normal, and abnormal levels integrating age, sex, and height. The impact of body mass on blood pressure levels during childhood is known. The special problems of neonatal hypertension are beyond the scope of this chapter. Selected issues relevant to hypertension in pediatric patients are addressed.

Abnormal blood pressure patterns, that is, those levels that consistently track in the upper percentiles are present during childhood and adolescence and presage adult hypertension. Consensus has not been reached concerning the utility of investigations that separate primary from secondary hypertension. Moreover, considerations of cost versus yield now influence clinical decision making. Treatment regimens for young individuals with primary hypertension use nonpharmacologic measures; pharmacotherapy is reserved for failure to achieve therapeutic objectives. Controversy persists as to the pros and cons of pharmacologic intervention for children with blood pressure in the upper percentiles. Therapy of secondary, nonsurgically remediable hypertension is more difficult. Controlled trials of adequate cohorts of pediatric patients with long follow-up do not exist. Providers caring for children therefore have extrapolated from adult experience and revised regimens as needed.

NORMAL AND ABNORMAL BLOOD PRESSURE LEVELS

Guidelines regarding normal and abnormal blood pressure levels in infants, children, and adolescents are available, based on data that include adequate sample size, sex distribution, maturational stage, height, and information regarding selected minorities. Consensus exists that blood pressure increases with age and that, as with adults, blood pressure levels track although the correlation coefficient is greater for systolic than for diastolic levels. The IV Korotkoff or muffling sound has been chosen, as of 1996, as the best indirect reflection of diastolic blood pressure. Blood pressure measure on the right arm with the patient seated is the norm for all measurements. Height, weight, and stage of puberty have now been integrated into the interpretation of levels. For example, if an adolescent male has a diastolic or systolic blood pressure level just above the 90th percentile and his height also falls into the 90th percentile, his blood pressure is not considered abnormal. The 1996 Update on Blood Pressure Control in Children did not revise the guidelines on significant and severe hypertension throughout the childhood years, which were provided in 1987 (Table 64.1). Recommendations from the 1996 Task Force and those from the Subcommittee on Atherosclerosis and Hypertension in Childhood provide a foundation for health care providers on measures for the maintenance of cardiovascular health beginning in childhood. The Subcommittee emphasized the prevention of childhood obesity, the limitation of fat calories to less than 30% of caloric intake, the reduction of excessive salt intake, and the encouragement of an active physical exercise program. In the pediatrics age range, the major predictors for future hypertension are obesity, an elevated blood pressure level, and a positive family history for hypertension. The major factor amenable to modification is prevention or reduction of obesity.

TABLE 64.1. Classification of Hypertension by Age Groups

	Age (yr)	Systolic/Diastolic (mm Hg) Significant	Severe
Newborn		104	110
Infant	<2	112/74	118/82
Children	3–5	116/76	124/84
	6–9	122/78	130/86
	10–12	126/82	134/90
Adolescents	13–15	136/86	144/92
	16–18	142/92	150/98

BLOOD PRESSURE MEASUREMENTS

Blood pressure measurements in children require use of cuffs appropriate for the size of the child's extremity (Table 64.2). Accurate blood pressure measurements in infants, children, and adolescents require the bladder of the blood pressure cuff to encircle 80% to 100% of the girth of the upper arm and to cover 40% of the length from the olecranon to the acromion. The right upper arm is used for repetitive measurements. Documentation of blood pressure levels in this manner permits comparisons over time. Care should be taken to avoid blood pressure cuffs that are too small and result in spuriously high blood pressure measurements.

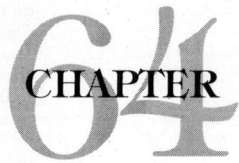

TABLE 64.2. Blood Pressure Measurements in Children and Adolescents

Environment
- Quiet and comfortable.

Cuff size
- Cuffs differ in width and in length. The rubber bladder should encircle 80% to 100% of girth of upper arm and cover 40% of length of upper arm. If the cuff is too small, use of the next larger size will avoid falsely elevated readings.

Procedure
- The technique is similar to that for adults. The IV Korotkoff sound is used as the best indirect reflection of diastolic pressure. Blood pressure should be measured in both arms, standing, sitting and supine, and in the leg.

Sources of error
- These include arm not at heart level, malfunctioning manometers, and observer bias and/or hearing deficit.

IDENTIFICATION AND INTERPRETATION OF ELEVATED BLOOD PRESSURE LEVELS

When the blood pressure has been carefully measured three times and on three separate occasions, the measurements should be compared with the guidelines provided in Table 64.1. Levels can be categorized as normal, high normal, or elevated. Children with borderline levels require repeat measurements every 6 months or more frequently if warranted by higher levels or a change in clinical condition. Borderline levels should be recorded and follow-up monitoring should be planned, but interpretation of these levels as abnormal or the need for investigation should be avoided in otherwise healthy youngsters. Mild hypertension is defined as levels that persistently exceed these guidelines by up to 10% for systolic and/or diastolic pressures, assuming that the child's height is less than the 90th percentile and that the child is not obese. Such patients require careful assessment, as outlined in Table 64.3. Children whose measurements exceed the guidelines by 10% or more are categorized as having moderate hypertension unless they are very

TABLE 64.3. Evaluation of Asymptomatic Hypertensive Children and Adolescents

Blood pressure
- Systolic and or diastolic levels that exceed guidelines at least three times on three separate occasions

History
- Excessive calorie or salt intake
- Exposure to pressor agents, birth control pills (adolescents)
- Menstrual history
- Family history of primary hypertension and its complications
- Past history of renal disease or other disorders associated with hypertension

Physical examination
- Clues to primary hypertension: obesity, increased pulse rate
- Clues to secondary causes: external physical findings associated with known underlying secondary causes (e.g., Cushing's syndrome)
- Clues to target-organ changes: evidence of hypertensive retinopathy and/or left ventricular hypertrophy

Laboratory evaluation
- Urinalysis and culture
- Serum electrolytes
- Hemoglobin and hematocrit
- Serum creatinine (must be interpreted for sex, age, height, weight)
- Triglycerides and cholesterol (fasting)

Diagnostic evaluation
- Echocardiogram

TABLE 64.4. Evaluation of Moderate Persistent Hypertension in Children and Adolescents

History
- Headaches: frequency, severity ± vomiting
- Dizziness; localizing neurologic signs
- Blurred or double vision
- Sweating, palpitations, tremor
- Renal trauma: recent or past
- Urinary tract infection with or without symptoms of obstruction
- Umbilical artery catheterization
- Growth retardation
- Presence of polydipsia and polyuria
- Diet: excess energy intake, excess salt intake
- Medication or drug use
  - α-Adrenergic agonists: phenylephrine, ephedrine
  - Amphetamines
  - Corticosteroids
  - Oral contraceptives (adolescent)
  - Cyclosporine
  - Methamphetamines, street drugs
  - Withdrawal of specific antihypertensive agents
- Family history: primary hypertension and its complications; pheochromocytoma, familial nephritis, polycystic kidney disease

Physical examination (focused on hypertension)
- Blood pressure
  - Correct cuff size and blood pressure measurement technique are essential for accurate recordings.
- Height and weight
  - Overweight (weight in excess for height by 20% or more) has been correlated with high blood pressure or primary hypertension; growth retardation is most often associated with structural renal and/or renovascular abnormalities.
- Pulse
  - A tendency toward higher pulse rates in primary or borderline primary hypertensive chidren and adolescents is documented; hyperthyroidism is an exceedingly rare cause of hypertension in pediatric age groups.
- Skin
  - Café au lait spots, adenoma sebaceum, or striae are important clues to secondary etiologies.
- Funduscopy
  - The most common changes that reflect longstanding hypertension of moderate severity include arteriolar narrowing, tortuosity, and arteriovenous nicking.
- Cardiovascular examination
  - Physical evidence of left ventricular hypertrophy or a hyperdynamic heart is rare. If both are present, diagnosis of pheochromocytoma must be sought. Careful attention should be paid to femoral pulses, which may be present but reduced and/or delayed in coarctation of the thoracic or abdominal aorta.
- Abdominal examination
  - Presence of midline or lateral bruits suggests renal artery stenosis; abdominal bruits do not occur in children with primary hypertension.
  - Palpably enlarged kidney(s) is unusual but if present indicates obstruction or cystic renal disease.
  - Costovertebral tenderness may be seen in renal infection.
  - Palpable bladder may be present in bladder outlet obstruction.
- Peripheral edema
  - This may indicate extracellular volume expansion, which occurs in chronic and acute renal failure.

Laboratory evaluation
- Urinalysis and culture
- Serum creatinine (interpreted for age, sex, height, weight)
- Complete blood count
- Serum electrolytes (adrenal cause more likely in patients older than 13 years)
- Fasting cholesterol and triglycerides
- Renal ultrasound (unless nonrenal diagnosis established)
- Echocardiogram
- Chest x-ray study
- Radionuclide scans
- Renal vein renin studies
- Arteriography with selective angiograms (see text for indications)

TABLE 64.5. Secondary Causes of Hypertension in Children and Adolescents

- Renal
  - Acute acquired renal disorders
    - Acute renal failure with hypervolemia
    - Acute glomerulonephritis
    - Acute obstruction
    - Anaphylactoid purpura (Henoch-Schönlein) nephritis
    - Hemolytic uremic syndrome
    - Interstitial nephritis
    - Renal calculi
    - Renal trauma
  - Chronic acquired renal disorders
    - Chronic glomerulonephritis
    - Chronic pyelonephritis
    - Chronic renal disease
    - End-stage renal disease
    - Hemolytic uremic syndrome
    - Interstitial nephritis (analgesic abuse)
    - Radiation nephritis
    - Reflux nephropathy
    - Renal trauma
  - Tumors
    - Renin-secreting tumors
    - Wilms' tumor
  - Congenital or genetic renal disorders
    - Alport's syndrome (familial nephritis)
    - Asymmetrical renal disease
    - Cystic dysplasia
    - Obstructive uropathy
    - Polycystic kidney disease (dominant or recessive types)
    - Tuberous sclerosis
  - Renal vascular abnormalities
    - Neurofibromatosis (von Recklinghausen's disease)
    - Renal arterial disease
    - Renal vein thrombosis
    - Thrombosis, embolism, and renal infarction
- Cardiovascular
  - Aortic insufficiency
  - Arteriovenous fistula
  - Coarctation of the thoracic or abdominal aorta
  - Hypoplasia of the abdominal aorta
  - Patent ductus arteriosus
  - Takayasu's arteritis
- Endocrine
  - Adrenal
    - Adrenal cortical defects (of unclear origin)
    - Cushing's disease
    - 11- and 17-hydroxylase deficiencies
    - Neuroblastoma
    - Pheochromocytoma
    - Primary aldosteronism
  - Other
    - Diabetes mellitus
    - Gonadal dysgenesis (Turner's syndrome)
    - Hyperparathyroidism and other hypercalcemic states
    - Hyperthyroidism
- Connective tissue disorders
  - Dermatomyositis
  - Ehlers-Danlos syndrome
  - Juvenile rheumatoid arthritis
  - Mixed connective tissue disease
  - Scleroderma
  - Systemic lupus erythematosus
- Central nervous system disorders
  - Dysautonomia (Riley-Day syndrome)
  - Guillain-Barré syndrome
  - Meningitis
  - Poliomyelitis
  - Space-occupying lesions
- Drug-related
  - Drug withdrawal hypertension (clonidine, atenolol, minoxidil, propranolol)
  - Oral contraceptives
  - Methamphetamines and street drugs
  - Poisonings (lead, mercury)
  - Steroids (corticosteroids, mineralocorticoids)
  - Sympathomimetics (amphetamines, Dexedrine, ephedrine, phenylephrine eye drops in neonates)
- Orthopedic injuries and procedures
  - Harrington rod placement for scoliosis
  - Leg lengthening
  - Trauma
- Miscellaneous
  - Burns
  - Porphyria
  - Stevens-Johnson syndrome

tall. Such children require more extensive evaluation (Table 64.4). The differential diagnosis of major causes of hypertension forms the basis for test ordering with an awareness of cost and of yield. Beyond these considerations, physicians must be sensitive to the needs of youngsters undergoing normal maturation. Accordingly, discussion of abnormal levels of blood pressure, of the need for diagnostic testing, and of the possible underlying etiologies requires time, patience, and insight into the milestones of childhood and of adolescence (Table 64.5).

ASYMPTOMATIC HYPERTENSIVE CHILDREN AND ADOLESCENTS

Evaluation

Hypertension is estimated to affect approximately 1% of prepubertal children and approximately 12% of postadolescents less than 20 years of age. Such frequency in young individuals mandates careful assessment and management because a significant proportion will have lifelong primary hypertension and others will have remediable secondary causes. Once criteria for abnormal blood pressure levels have been met, a stepwise approach can be adopted (Table 64.3). Children and adolescents with primary hypertension often have a lifelong history of obesity. In addition, their parents are also likely to be significantly overweight. A positive family history for primary hypertension or one of its complications (i.e., stroke, myocardial infarction, or renal failure) is found in 50% of children with primary hypertension. Physical examination is focused on findings correlated with primary hypertension or, conversely, those that support the possibility of a secondary cause. Obesity and high pulse rates have been found in children with primary hypertension.

Management

Because these patients are young and are asymptomatic, therapeutic options for the child and for the family require careful consideration. For those children who are overweight or who ingest an excessive amount of sodium, dietary intervention may result in gradual weight reduction and in a gradual change in appetite for salt. Reduction in salt intake with resulting blood pressure lowering is only effective in a subset of patients with salt-sensitive hypertension. However, this regimen requires enthusiastic endorsement by the medical team and a change in lifestyle of the child and his or her family. A motivated family may require 1 year to reach these goals, but the lifelong benefit for the child's and family's health is inestimable.

The major recommendations for prevention of cardiovascular disease should be integrated during this period of dietary intervention. These include (a) avoidance of foods high in cholesterol or in saturated fatty acids to provide a total diet with less than 30% of calories from fat, (b) participation in an active sports program, (c) avoidance of agents known to exacerbate hypertension or to contribute to cardiovascular disease, with special emphasis on cigarette smoking, over-the-counter remedies such as adrenergic agonists (e.g., phenylephrine and ephedrine), steroids, and street drugs [amphetamines, phencyclidine (PCP)], and (d) provision of information for pubertal girls about the use of oral contraceptives and encouragement to seek consultation.

If the child (and/or family) cannot alter eating habits, if the child's blood pressure levels remain in the abnormal range throughout an observation period, or if the child shows symptoms of hypertension, pharmacotherapy is warranted. Long-term studies of pediatric patients treated with antihypertensive agents do not exist. Because these youngsters will undoubtedly require lifelong treatment, their experience with drug-taking beginning in childhood should be structured to favor long-term compliance. Accordingly, the agent selected should have the fewest side effects and should be given the least number of times per day. Our experience with low-dose thiazides or low-dose atenolol has been favorable. Clonidine patches have been used for selected patients.

Occasionally, thiazides prove inadequate for blood pressure control, and a long-acting β-blocker is substituted in those without asthma or other contraindications. Long-term studies of adverse biochemical effects in children and adolescents, especially attributable to hyperlipidemia, are not available. It is prudent to monitor all children receiving these agents for lipid elevations or a decrease in high-density lipoprotein cholesterol. If these abnormalities are encountered, the importance of fat intake and the types of fat ingested should be reemphasized. Future needs include an assessment of the prevalence of secondary hyperlipidemia and whether it is amenable to dietary alterations or whether pharmacologic intervention is indicated. Because these individuals face decades of medications, the significance of secondary adverse effects should be taken into account. Usually, one agent given once a day provides adequate blood pressure control, allows the patient to remain symptom-free, and most important, does not introduce unpleasant or intolerable side effects.

When possible, the child's caregivers are taught to measure blood pressure and to keep a record of home blood pressure measurements. Whenever the measurements deviate from the established pattern, a telephone consultation can establish whether (a) the child has received his or her medication, (b) intervening illnesses or stresses exist, (c) the dose is adequate, or (d) the patient needs to be reevaluated. Ambulatory blood pressure monitoring is not yet available for pediatric patients but has promise for providing objective data so that regimens can be revised and include diurnal changes in blood pressure.

MODERATE PERSISTENT HYPERTENSION IN CHILDREN AND ADOLESCENTS

Evaluation

Children and adolescents whose blood pressure is moderately elevated typically are symptomatic. These patients require the studies outlined in Table 64.4 because of the likelihood of a secondary cause (Table 64.5). The younger the child and the higher the blood pressure the greater the odds of a secondary cause. The most frequent cause is renal and the investigation is straightforward. Recognition of a renal etiology is usually evident after minimal, noninvasive studies. In prepubertal children, urinalysis, measurement of serum creatinine, and renal ultrasound are the primary methods of screening for a renal etiology. If one or more of these studies is abnormal, further investigation is easily organized to identify a specific underlying disorder.

The differential diagnosis does, however, include diverse etiologies (Table 64.5), which can be systematically considered once a thorough history, physical examination, and routine laboratory studies (urinalysis with culture; blood urea nitrogen, serum creatinine and serum electrolyte levels; and hemoglobin and hematocrit) have been completed. Subsequently, a focused and a selective strategy for the investigation of a specific child can be employed. This approach minimizes the number of extensive and invasive studies for hypertension of unknown etiology. A stepwise approach also yields significant cost savings because only selected patients will be subjected to all-inclusive studies.

If, on the basis of screening studies, a renal etiology cannot be excluded, renal ultrasound (US) examination is required. In experienced hands, with currently available equipment, US can delineate kidney size, differences in size between two kidneys, hydronephrosis, large focal scars, and ureteral dilatation if it is severe and proximal. Limitations of US include lack of detection of mild parenchymal scarring, lack of discrimination between congenital anomalies such as duplicated systems and hydronephrosis, and lack of sensitivity for the detection of vascular abnormalities. Doppler renal US is not a reliable test for renal artery stenosis in the pediatric age group. If renal arterial disease is suspected, additional useful tests include plasma renin activity (PRA) and radionuclide scans (with or without captopril and/or furosemide (Lasix) before arteriography.

PRA has been used to develop renin profiles in patients with primary hypertension or as a discriminator for renal artery stenosis. Several problems beset the interpretation of PRA values in children: PRA is age-related, samples must be obtained under controlled conditions, and PRA values may be normal when significant renal scarring or renal ischemia exists. For these reasons, PRA measurements should be reserved for those hypertensive pediatric patients whose diagnosis is elusive, who have coexistent hypokalemia, or who are suspected of having renal artery stenosis. Normal PRA values however do not exclude the diagnosis of renal artery stenosis.

Radionuclide scans of the kidney have a limited role in the investigation of hypertension because of either a lack of sensitivity and or of specificity. The results with [^{99m}Tc]-diethylenetriamine pentaacetic acid (DTPA) or with ^{131}I-orthoiodohippurate have been disappointing. The use of ^{99m}Tc succimer (DMSA) scans may provide information concerning pyelonephritic scars or segmental areas of ischemia suggestive of renal artery stenosis. If the DMSA scan suggests renal arterial disease or if this diagnosis cannot be excluded, renal arteriography is warranted.

Renin ratios comparing levels from individual renal veins in relation to peripheral and vena caval levels have proven valuable. Traditionally the affected:nonaffected ratio is 1.5:1 or greater, although important exceptions exist with achievable surgical cures despite ratios less than 1.5. Renal vein renin levels are useful in several clinical circumstances including when one kidney appears atrophic and is regarded as ischemic, when segmental disease is present, and when a renin-secreting tumor is suspected. In our experience, if the index of suspicion is high that renal artery stenosis exists, arteriography with selective angiography remains the study of choice and is mandatory. Small children require the expertise of a radiologist with experience in the catheterization of small vessels, so that complications are avoided and high-quality studies are obtained. Adequate blood

TABLE 64.6. Treatment of Chronic Hypertension in Children and Adolescents

Drug	Drug Dose[a]	Comment
Hydrochlorothiazide	1 mg/kg q12hr	Ordinarily not effective in patients with renal insufficiency; usually need furosemide
Furosemide	1 mg/kg q6hr	Especially valuable in patients with reduced renal function; reduced dosage for neonates
Hydralazine	0.5–1 mg/kg q8hr	Frequently causes reflex tachycardia, abdominal discomfort, and headache; lupuslike syndrome rare
Prazosin	20-25 μg/kg q8hr	No studies of drug in pediatric patients; clinical experience indicates that drug is well tolerated; first-dose effect dictates that patient receives initial dose supine; some children have hair loss with chronic use
Minoxidil	0.025–0.05 mg/kg q12hr	Salt and water retention modulated or prevented by concomitant diuretics, hypertrichosis important problem in pediatric patients; resolves with discontinuation of drug; rebound hypertension with abrupt discontinuation
Captopril	0.25–0.5 mg/kg q8hr	Modification of dose needed in patients with azotemia; may cause decreased platelets, plus neutropenia; close blood pressure monitoring needed because of potency
Methyldopa	10 mg/kg q6hr	Dose adjustment required with reduced renal function, interferes with mental concentration and induces sleepiness when started, rebound hypertension with drug interruption
Propranolol	0.5–1 mg/kg q12hr	May have problem with bradycardia, bronchospasm; hypoglycemia reported, especially in patients with inadequate oral intake; rebound hypertension with drug interruption
Atenolol	1-2 mg/kg q24hr	No published experience in pediatric patients; may be associated with bronchospasm or bradycardia; advantage over other adrenergic agents is a lack of central nervous system effects and a once-only daily dosage
Clonidine	0.1–0.2 mg q24hr	May be effective once daily; initial drowsiness; rebound hypertension with abrupt discontinuation
Nifedipine, XL	0.25–0.5 mg/kg/24 hr	Chronic usage not studied in chidlren, but drug is effective; tachycardia may occur

[a] Lowest starting dosage is given.

pressure control is a prerequisite to avoid hypertensive spikes during and after the procedure. Blood pressure levels must be monitored throughout the procedure and prompt intervention for elevations must occur with a rapidly acting agent. All children should be monitored carefully for 24 hours either as an inpatient or outpatient depending on individual circumstances.

Management

Patients with chronic essential hypertension or hypertension secondary to renal parenchymal diseases are the most difficult to manage. Most drugs are marketed without controlled studies in children because of the problems in conducting therapeutic trials in the pediatric age group. Furthermore, the pharmaceutical industry customarily includes caveats in package inserts that exclude the use of such agents in individuals younger than 12 years of age. The physician who treats affected children must use data available from published pediatric studies and, as needed, extrapolate from adult experience (see Chapter 61). Selection of agents should be based on the underlying pathophysiology and knowledge of effects and of adverse effects of the medications and with an emphasis on those agents that are best tolerated. The lowest oral starting dosages of various antihypertensive agents are presented in Table 64.6. Dosages for all agents are presented on a per kilogram per dose basis. Increases in dosages should be made judiciously; modifications as needed should be integrated in regimens for all children with abnormal glomerular filtration rates.

HYPERTENSIVE EMERGENCIES IN CHILDREN AND ADOLESCENTS

The number of conditions associated with abrupt elevations of blood pressure in pediatric patients is limited (Table 64.7). The most prevalent underlying cause is renal disease. *Acute* renal disorders with rapid onset of blood pressure elevation include acute glomerulonephritis, hemolytic uremic syndrome, urinary tract acute obstruction, and trauma. *Chronic* renal disorders in which blood pressure elevation may abruptly occur include chronic renal disease, end-stage renal failure, posttransplant hypertension, reflux nephropathy, segmental hypoplasia, and renal artery stenosis. Pheochromocytoma is rare in pediatric patients; in a 30-year period at a tertiary pediatric center, 30 tumors were diagnosed. Presenting symptoms are similar to those in adults with orthostatic hypotension and weight loss as major markers.

Signs and symptoms associated with hypertensive emergencies include seizures, severe headaches (often frontal), blurred vision, peripheral facial palsy (unlike adults), hypertensive retinopathy, congestive heart failure, and peripheral edema. Epistaxis, syncope, and physical findings attributable to intracranial bleeding are uncommon in children. Pharmacologic management of hypertensive emergencies in children is exhibited in

TABLE 64.7. Etiology of Hypertensive Emergencies in Children and Adolescents

- Renal
  - Acute glomerulonephritis
  - Acute hydronephrosis
  - Chronic renal failure
  - End-stage renal disease
  - Hemolytic uremic syndrome
  - Posttransplant hypertension
  - Reflux nephropathy (previously termed chronic atrophic pyelonephritis)
  - Renal artery disease
  - Trauma
  - Unilateral dysplasia (unilateral asymmetrical renal disease)
  - Volume overload (iatrogenic)
- Nonrenal
  - Exogenous agents
    - Phencyclidine (PCP)
    - Amphetamines
    - Drug withdrawal from antihypertensive agents
  - Pheochromocytoma

TABLE 64.8. Treatment of Hypertensive Emergencies in Pediatric Patients

Drug	Onset of Action	Dose and Route[a]	Comments
Captopril	Minutes	0.1–0.2 mg/kg PO q6hr	Do not use in hyperkalemic patients; lower dose needed in azotemic patients; may produce acute increases in creatinine with solitary kidney and renal artery stenosis
Diazoxide	Minutes	1–5 mg/kg (rapid bolus IV) or by continuous infusion	Lower dose for acute disorders; salt and water retention; do not use more than 4 times per 24 hr.; do not repeat dose in less than 1 hr.
Hydralazine	Minutes	0.15–0.25 mg/kg (IV)	Reflex tachycardia, flushing, headache
Sodium nitroprusside	Seconds	0.5–1 μg/kg/min (IV)	Must be given by constant infusion with solution wrapped in foil in an ICU; thiocyanate levels must be monitored after 24 hr
Labetalol	Minutes	1–3 mg/kg (IV)	May be given by constant infusion for maintenance

[a] Once adequate or initial blood pressure lowering has occurred with parenteral therapy, oral therapy as shown in Table 62.6 may be introduced.

Table 64.8. General guidelines are to reduce the elevation by one-third of the difference between the abnormal pressure and normal pressure within the first 6 to 8 hours and to treat significant signs/symptoms (i.e., seizures), the second one-third within the next 16 hours, and then to construct a nonemergency management plan with long-term goals for blood pressure control. The last objective is the most difficult because many patients have underlying chronic renal failure not amenable to medical therapy.

Selected Readings

Goonasekera CDA, Shah V, Wade AM, et al. *Lancet* 1996;347:640–643.

This publication represents a 15-year follow-up of 55 patients seen with reflux nephropathy at Great Ormond Street, London, England. Of the 55, 5 had systolic and 2 had diastolic hypertension. PRA showed an increasing dissociation from the emergence of blood pressure elevation and could not be used as a predictor for which patient was at risk for the development of hypertension.

Kaplan NM. *Clinical hypertension*, 7th ed. Baltimore: Williams & Wilkins, 1997:1–444.

This latest edition covers all aspects of clinical hypertension in adults with one chapter on pediatrics.

O'Neill JA Jr. Long-term outcome with surgical treatment of renovascular hypertension. *J Pediatr Surg* 1998;33:106–111.

Of 136 patients evaluated for severe hypertension, 53 had renovascular lesions. Of these 45 had fibromuscular hyperplasia of whom 17 had midaortic involvement. Treatment included surgery for 50 of 53; as of a 16-year follow-up, 70% were cured, 26% improved, and in 4% treatment failed.

Rocchini AP, ed. Childhood hypertension. *Pediatr Clin North Am* 1993;40:1–219.

This volume has been written primarily by cardiologists and updates information concerning genetics, epidemiology, prevention, and obesity. Special emphasis is given to cardiovascular risk factors identifiable during childhood, notably obesity, hyperlipidemia, and hypertension. In addition, separate chapters focus on neonatal hypertension, endocrine causes of hypertension, renovascular hypertension, imaging, and pharmacologic management.

Rosen PR, Treves S, Ingelfinger J. Hypertension in children. *Am J Dis Child* 1985; 139:173–177.

Renal scintigraphy with DMSA was superior to that with DTPA in detecting renal abnormalities in 80 hypertensive pediatric and adolescent patients. DMSA scintigraphy had a sensitivity of 92% and a specificity of 97%.

Stringer DA, deBruyn R, Dillon MJ, et al. Comparison of aortography, renal vein renin sampling, radionuclide scans, ultrasound and the IVU in the investigation of childhood renovascular hypertension. *Br J Radiol* 1984;57:111–121.

In a review of all 17 patients with primary renovascular hypertension who underwent renal angiography at the Hospital for Sick Children, London, over a 3-year period before January 1981, the studies that proved most useful were DMSA scans, segmental renal vein renin estimations, and anteroposterior and oblique selective renal arteriograms with macroradiography.

Subcommittee on Atherosclerosis and Hypertension in Childhood of the Council on Cardiovascular Disease in the Young, American Heart Association. Integrated cardiovascular health promotion in childhood. *Circulation* 1992;85: 1638–1650.

This article provides strategies for promotion of cardiovascular health that can be integrated into routine pediatric care, emphasizing cigarette smoking, physical activity, obesity, hypertension, and levels of cholesterol.

Update on the 1987 Task Force Report on High Blood Pressure in Children and Adolescents: A Working Group Report from the National High Blood Pressure Education Program. *Pediatrics* 1998;98:649–658.

This further revision of the original 1977 Task Force report includes normative blood pressure data integrating age, gender, and height, revision of guidelines for blood pressure measurements, guidelines for detecting children with elevated levels, and strategies for appropriate diagnostic evaluation along with nonpharmacologic and pharmacologic treatment.

CHAPTER 65

Geriatric Hypertension

William C. Cushman

Until 1991 there was uncertainty whether hypertension, especially from elevated systolic blood pressure (SBP), should be treated in older persons. The decade of the 1990s has clarified our perspective on treating hypertension in geriatric patients, and many studies have provided a wealth of information to assist in the management of elevated blood pressure (BP) in older persons.

EPIDEMIOLOGY

Cardiovascular events and mortality are more common, and hypertension is the most important cardiovascular risk factor in elderly patients. SBP and diastolic BP (DBP) have continuous, graded, strong, and independent significant relationships to a variety of outcomes, including coronary heart disease, stroke, cardiac abnormalities, end-stage renal disease (ESRD), and mortality, but for middle-aged and older persons SBP relates even more strongly to risk than DBP. Persons with stage 2 or higher (Table 65.1) isolated systolic hypertension (ISH) (SBP ≥ 160 mm Hg and DBP less than 90 mm Hg) are at particularly high risk of experiencing cardiovascular events or death, but even persons with stage 1 ISH (SBP 140 to 159 mm Hg and DBP less than 90 mm Hg) have a 47% increase in risk of cardiovascular events and 57% increase in cardiovascular death. Stage 2+ SBP is also a potent risk factor for ESRD, although ESRD is much less common than cardiovascular complications of hypertension.

High pulse pressure, a result of increases in large artery stiffness, is associated with even higher cardiovascular risk, especially for coronary heart disease. Hypertensive patients in the upper tertile of pretreatment pulse pressure (63 mm Hg or greater) had a greater incidence of myocardial infarction than those in the lower tertiles in one study, and this relationship was stronger than for SBP or DBP. SBP and pulse pressure are highly correlated and both are usually better predictors of risk than DBP. Because pulse pressure has not been used as a specific entry criteria in prospective clinical trials, pulse pressure should not replace elevated SBP as an indication to initiate antihypertensive treatment. In the presence of elevated SBP, however, low DBP should only further encourage treatment of the SBP elevation.

The Sixth Joint National Committee on Prevention, Detection, Evaluation, and Treatment of High Blood Pressure (JNC VI) has classified and stratified risk for hypertension based on levels of SBP and DBP (Table 65.1), the presence or absence of other risk factors, and the presence or absence of target organ damage or clinical cardiovascular disease (Tables 65.2 and 65.3). Hypertension, defined in JNC VI as SBP 140 mm Hg or greater or DBP 90 mm Hg or greater or both is present in more than 50% of the American population older than 60 years of age. SBP increases on average with advancing age, while DBP increases until the sixth decade and declines thereafter because

TABLE 65.1. Classification of Blood Pressure and Hypertension for Adults

	Systolic Blood Pressure (mm Hg)	Diastolic Blood Pressure (mm Hg)
Optimal blood pressure	<120	<80
Normal blood pressure	<130	<85
High-normal blood pressure	130–139	85–89
Hypertension		
Stage 1	140–159	90–99
Stage 2	160–179	100–109
Stage 3	≥ 180	≥ 110

Reprinted with permission from Joint National Committee on Prevention, Detection, Evaluation, and Treatment of High Blood Pressure. The Sixth Report of the Joint National Committee on Prevention, Detection, Evaluation, and Treatment of High Blood Pressure (JNC VI). *Arch Intern Med* 1997;157:2413–2446.

TABLE 65.2. Components of Cardiovascular Risk Stratification in Patients with Hypertension

Major Risk Factors	Clinical Cardiovascular Disease/ Target Organ Damage
Smoking	Heart diseases
Dyslipidemia	Stroke or transient ischemic attack
Diabetes mellitus	Nephropathy
Age older than 60 years	Peripheral arterial disease
Sex (men or postmenopausal women)	Retinopathy
Family history of cardiovascular disease	

Reprinted with permission from Joint National Committee on Prevention, Detection, Evaluation, and Treatment of High Blood Pressure. The Sixth Report of the Joint National Committee on Prevention, Detection, Evaluation, and Treatment of High Blood Pressure (JNC VI). *Arch Intern Med* 1997;157:2413–2446.

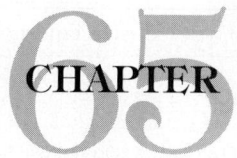

TABLE 65.3. Risk Group Classification

Risk Group A	Risk Group B	Risk Group C
No risk factors	At least one risk factor, not including diabetes	Target organ disease, clinical cardiovascular disease and/or diabetes
No target organ disease or clinical cardiovascular disease	No target organ disease or clinical cardiovascular disease	

Reprinted with permission from Joint National Committee on Prevention, Detection, Evaluation, and Treatment of High Blood Pressure. The Sixth Report of the Joint National Committee on Prevention, Detection, Evaluation, and Treatment of High Blood Pressure (JNC VI). *Arch Intern Med* 1997;157:2413–2446.

of arterial stiffening. In Americans older than 60 years of age, stage 1 ISH (SBP 140 to 159 mm Hg with DBP less than 90 mm Hg) is present in 25% and stage 2 to 3 ISH (SBP 160 mm Hg or greater with DBP less than 90 mm Hg) in 10% of this population. ISH is the predominant form of hypertension in elderly patients, followed by systolic-diastolic hypertension or very uncommonly diastolic-only hypertension. Thus treatment of hypertension in older individuals almost always involves treatment of SBP elevation.

LIFESTYLE INTERVENTION

Several lifestyle interventions have been shown to lower BP or prevent hypertension in elderly persons. The JNC VI lifestyle modifications recommended are (a) lose weight if overweight, (b) limit alcohol to no more than 1 oz (30 ml) of ethanol/day (28 g or 2 drinks/day), or 0.5 oz of ethanol/day for women and lighter weight people, (c) increase physical activity (30 to 45 minutes most days of the week), which for older individuals most often can be with brisk walking, (d) reduce sodium intake to no more than 100 mmol/day (2.4 g of sodium or 6 g of salt), (e) maintain adequate levels of potassium, calcium, and magnesium for general health, and (f) stop smoking and reduce intake of saturated fat and cholesterol for overall cardiovascular health.

MORBIDITY AND MORTALITY TRIALS IN ELDERLY PERSONS

The hypertension morbidity and mortality trials completed before 1990 were all based on DBP inclusion criteria, but consistently demonstrated reductions in cardiovascular events in the subgroups of older hypertensive patients included. SBP was often elevated in these older individuals and treatment lowered SBP as well as or better than DBP. These trials proved that treatment of hypertension in elderly individuals based on diastolic entry criteria (above 90 to 95 mm Hg) reduces cardiovascular morbidity and mortality.

Trials in the 1990s have proven that treating entry SBP levels of 160 mm Hg or above, regardless of DBP levels, reduces cardiovascular morbidity and mortality (Table 65.4). In the Systolic Hypertension in the Elderly Program (SHEP) trial, 4,736 older (60 years or older) persons with SBP 160 to 219 mm Hg and DBP less than 90 mm Hg (stage 2+ ISH) were randomly assigned to receive active treatment or placebo. Active therapy was begun with the diuretic chlorthalidone 12.5 to 25 mg/day and atenolol or reserpine could be added in low doses if needed. Strokes were reduced by 36% (P = .0003), coronary events by 27% (P <.05), and heart failure by 49% (P <.001) over 4 to 5 years of follow-up. Heart failure was reduced by 81% (P = .002) in participants with a history or electrocardiogram (ECG) evidence of myocardial infarction. The reduction in events were seen in many subgroups: (a) all levels of entry SBP; (b) patients aged ≥ 80 years (P <.01), as well as those aged 60 to 79 years; (c) all race and sex subgroups, including white women; (d) all three baseline cholesterol strata; (e) patients receiving or not receiving antihypertensive drug therapy at screening; (f) patients with or without baseline ECG abnormalities; (g) those receiving a diuretic alone or a diuretic plus atenolol; (h) those with the highest serum creatinine levels (1.4 to 2.4 mg/dl); and (i) the 583 patients with type II diabetes. In diabetic patients, major cardiovascular disease events were reduced by 34%, the same risk reduction as in nondiabetic patients, but with twice the absolute risk reduction.

TABLE 65.4. Reduction in Major Cardiovascular Events in Placebo-Controlled Trials of Systolic Hypertension in Elderly Patients

Event	Event Reduced (%)				
	SHEP (n = 4,736)	STOP (n = 1,627)	MRC Elderly (n = 4.396)		Syst-Eur (n = 4,695)
Initial active drug	Chlorthalidone	HCTZ/amiloride or β-blocker	HCTZ/amiloride	Atenolol	Nitrendipine
Stroke	36[a]	47[a]	31[a]	17	42[a]
Coronary heart disease	27[a]	13	44[a]	+1	30
Heart failure	49[a]	51 (NR)	NR	NR	29
Cardiovascular disease	32[a]	40[a]	35[a]	2	31
Mortality	13	43[a]	19	+7	14

[a] Significant reduction.

HCTZ, hydrochlorothiazide; MRC Elderly, Medical Research Council trial of treatment of hypertension in older adults; NR, not reported; SHEP, Systolic Hypertension in the Elderly Program; STOP, Swedish Trial in Older Persons with Hypertension; Syst-Eur, Systolic Hypertension in Europe Trial.

In the Medical Research Council (MRC) trial of Great Britain (Table 65.4), 4,396 men and women aged 65 to 74 years with entry SBP of 160 to 209 mm Hg and DBP less than 115 mm Hg (43% had ISH) were randomly assigned to receive a diuretic (hydrochlorothiazide 25 mg plus amiloride 2.5 mg once daily), a β-blocker (atenolol 50 mg once daily), or placebo. The diuretic group had 31% fewer strokes (*P* <.05), 44% fewer coronary events (*P* <.001), and a 35% reduction in all cardiovascular events (*P* <.001) compared with the placebo group, but the atenolol group experienced no benefits.

The Swedish Trial in Older Persons with Hypertension (STOP-Hypertension) was conducted in 1,627 men and women aged 70 to 84 years with SBP of 180 to 230 mm Hg and DBP 90 mm Hg or higher (or DBP 105 to 120 mm Hg, regardless of SBP) (Table 65.4). Therefore this did not include any patients with ISH. Therapy with a diuretic (same as the MRC study) or one of three β-blockers (investigator's choice) significantly reduced stroke (47%), all cardiovascular events, and deaths (43%), but not coronary events alone; heart failure was also reduced by 51%.

The Systolic Hypertension in Europe (Syst-Eur) Trial was a randomized, placebo-controlled trial of 4,695 Europeans aged 60 years or older with SBP 160 to 219 mm Hg and DBP less than 95 mm Hg (Table 65.4), who were randomly assigned to receive the moderately long-acting dihydropyridine calcium antagonist, nitrendipine 10 to 40 mg/day, with the addition of enalapril 5 to 20 mg/day and hydrochlorothiazide 12.5 to 25 mg/day if necessary, or matching placebos. Active treatment reduced stroke by 42% (*P* = .003) and all cardiovascular events by 31% (*P* <.001), but reductions in heart failure (29%) and myocardial infarction (30%) were not statistically significant. The importance of treating hypertension in older persons has been well established by the evidence from these trials of persons with systolic or diastolic hypertension or both. There are few areas of medicine where treatment is as evidence-based as pharmacologic treatment of hypertension in elderly patients.

BLOOD PRESSURE LEVELS FOR INITIATION OF DRUG THERAPY

Because several of the diastolic hypertension trials demonstrated reduction in events for older individuals with DBP 90 mm Hg or higher, it is reasonable to initiate antihypertensive drug therapy in an older person with persistent DBP 90 mm Hg or greater. For patients with stage 2 to 3 diastolic hypertension, drug therapy should be initiated after confirmation within days to weeks. If the individual patient with stage 1 diastolic hypertension does not meet his or her goal within 6 months by making lifestyle changes, then drug therapy should be started.

SBP levels persistently above 160 mm Hg (stages 2 to 3) should be treated with antihypertensive drugs. Although stage 1 ISH is associated with increased risk of cardiovascular events, no prospective randomized controlled trials have been completed to test whether treating SBP of 140 to 159 mm Hg reduces events. Indirect evidence comes from diastolic hypertension trials or the in-study BP levels in systolic hypertension trials. In SHEP, for example, the 5-year average SBP was 155 mm Hg for the placebo group and 143 mm Hg for the active treatment group. Because cardiovascular morbidity was substantially reduced in the treated group compared with the control group, this suggests that lowering SBP below approximately 150 mm Hg would be beneficial. The prevalence of stage 1 ISH increases with age and because it is present in 25% of the population older than 60 years, initiating a randomized, controlled trial of drug treatment of stage 1 ISH should be a high public health priority. Aggressive lifestyle modifications and treatment of other cardiovascular risk factors are clearly appropriate for patients with stage 1 ISH. Because of the indirect evidence, however, JNC VI recommends drug therapy for patients with stage 1 systolic hypertension in Risk Group B or C if SBP is greater than 140 mm Hg after a maximum of 6 months of lifestyle modification (Tables 65.1, 65.2, and 65.3).

BLOOD PRESSURE GOALS OF THERAPY

The morbidity trials of treatment of hypertension in elderly patients have used DBP goals of less than 90 mm Hg and SBP goals of less than 150 to 160 mm Hg and at least a 20 mm Hg reduction from a baseline SBP of 160 mm Hg or higher. Therefore less than 150 mm Hg should be the (highest) goal for treatment of systolic hypertension. Lower SBP goals may be reasonable, but have not yet been tested in completed prospective studies.

There has been concern, especially in hypertensive patients with preexisting ischemic heart disease, that coronary events might be increased if DBP was lowered too far. In SHEP, however, the average on-treatment DBP was 68 mm Hg for the active treatment group, who had fewer events than those less aggressively treated in the placebo group, including the subgroup with prior myocardial infarction. The Hypertension Optimal Treatment (HOT) study was specifically designed to address whether there is benefit or harm in lowering DBP to lower than usual DBP goals: 18,790 hypertensive patients, aged 50 to 80 years with DBP 100 to 115 mm Hg were randomly assigned to target DBP goals of less than or equal to (a) 90, (b) 85, or (c) 80 mm Hg. The on-treatment BP averaged 144/85, 141/83, and 140/81 mm Hg, respectively. There were no significant differences in major cardiovascular, coronary, or cerebrovascular events among the three groups. The in-trial BP for this somewhat elderly population suggested increased risk with a DBP above 90 mm Hg and an SBP greater than 160 mm Hg. HOT suggests that there is neither benefit nor harm with these lower DBP goals.

In the 1,501 diabetic participants in HOT, however, major cardiovascular events were significantly lower in the those randomly assigned to a DBP goal of 80 mm Hg or lower compared with 90 mm Hg or lower (*P* = .005). Subsequently, the United Kingdom Prospective Diabetes Study Group (UKPDS) trial (1,148 hypertensive type II diabetics) compared tight control of BP (less than 150/85 mm Hg) with less tight control (less than 180/105 mm Hg) over a median of 8.4 years: diabetes-related endpoints were reduced 24% (*P* = .005), deaths related to diabetes 32% (*P* = .019), strokes 44% (*P* = .013), and microvascular endpoints 37% (*P* = .009). Average BPs over 9 years were 144/82 mm Hg and 154/87 mm Hg in the tight and less tight BP control groups, respectively. In the Appropriate Blood Pressure Control in Diabetes (ABCD) trial, the effects of moderate control of BP (DBP 80 to 89 mm Hg) were compared with intensive control of BP (DBP 75 mm Hg) on the incidence and progression of complications of diabetes in a hypertensive diabetic population. There were no differences in cardiovascular or microvascular events in the two groups. Therefore, these three trials support a BP goal in older diabetic hypertensive patients of 140/180 mm Hg, somewhat higher for SBP and lower for DBP, than the recommendation from JNC VI (130/85 mm Hg).

SELECTION OF ANTIHYPERTENSIVE DRUGS

Many drugs are available that lower BP effectively either as a single drug or in combination therapy. Factors that may be considered when selecting a drug for treatment of hypertension in el-

TABLE 65.5. Considerations in the Selection of Antihypertensive Drug Therapy in Elderly Patients

Hypertension morbidity trial experience
Diuretic-based regimen strongly preferred
Second choice in ISH: long-acting dihydropyridine calcium antagonist
Compelling indication for comorbid condition
Heart failure: ACE inhibitors, diuretics
Myocardial infarction: beta-blockers (non-ISA), ACE inhibitors
Other indications and contraindications
Predicted antihypertensive efficacy
Economic considerations
Quality of life and symptomatic adverse effects

ACE, angiotensin-converting enzyme; ISA, intrinsic sympathomimetic activity; ISH, isolated systolic hypertension.

derly patients (Table 65.5) include (a) Has the drug reduced major events in trials of antihypertensive therapy in elderly patients? (b) Is there an important comorbid condition for which there is a compelling indication for an antihypertensive agent based on randomized, controlled trials? (c) Are there other important indications or contraindications for drugs or drug classes? (d) Do patient characteristics, such as age, sex, or race, predict the antihypertensive response to a drug? (e) Can the patient afford the drug? and (f) Will it affect his or her quality of life?

Other considerations, such as effects on left ventricular mass or on a patient's renin profile, have not been proven to be important differentiating factors in making a drug selection. For example, the Veterans Affairs (VA) Cooperative Study Group on Antihypertensive Agents has reported that the combination of age and race of a hypertensive patient was a better predictor of BP control with antihypertensive drugs than renin profiling, and several groups have shown that diuretic therapy is as good or better at reducing left ventricular mass than other drug classes. But it is the benefit of diuretics in reducing major cardiovascular events that makes them the drug class of choice for most older persons with hypertension. In most situations, the first factor, morbidity and mortality trial experience, should be the only consideration, but there are other situations when one or several of the others will take precedence.

Morbidity/Mortality Trial Experience

The older subgroups in the hypertension trials with diastolic entry criteria all showed reductions in cardiovascular events with diuretic-based therapy. Cardiovascular events were also reduced with the diuretic-based therapy in SHEP and the diuretic arm of the MRC elderly trial (Table 65.4). In the MRC elderly trial, the β-blocker atenolol did not reduce events (Table 65.4). On the basis of this, the National High Blood Pressure Education Program Working Group on Hypertension in the Elderly and JNC VI recommended that β-blocker monotherapy not be used in elderly patients unless a comorbid condition requiring a β-blocker was present, even though β-blockers are recommended in middle-aged and younger individuals because of morbidity trial results in these age groups. Because most of the patients in STOP were receiving a β-blocker and a diuretic, the mortality and cardiovascular benefits in STOP do not confirm or contradict the lack of benefit observed with the β-blocker in the MRC trial in elderly patients (Table 65.4).

Nitrendipine, a dihydropyridine calcium antagonist, reduced strokes by 42% and cardiovascular events by 31% in older patients with ISH in the Syst-Eur study (Table 65.4). Although moderately long-acting or long-acting dihydropyridine calcium antagonists are an acceptable alternative to diuretics in patients with ISH, the number of studies and patients studied, the confirmed benefit in reducing coronary events and heart failure in addition to stroke, the lower cost, and the proven benefit in combination regimens argue that a diuretic-based regimen should be preferred for elderly patients with ISH and other forms of hypertension until further evidence is available to the contrary.

There are a number of current ongoing morbidity trials that compare two or more antihypertensive agents, especially in elderly patients. The largest of these is the Antihypertensive and Lipid Lowering to Prevent Heart Attack Trial (ALLHAT), sponsored by the National Heart, Lung and Blood Institute. Begun in 1994 and projected to be completed by 2001, it is a randomized, controlled trial comparing a diuretic (chlorthalidone), a calcium antagonist (amlodipine), an angiotensin-converting enzyme (ACE) inhibitor (lisinopril), or an α_1-blocker (doxazosin) in 42,000 high-risk hypertensive patients at least 55 years of age. In early 2000, the doxazosin arm was stopped because cardiovascular events were significantly higher than in the chlorthalidone arm. Until ALLHAT or other trials are completed, we will not know whether other classes of drugs will reduce cardiovascular events in older individuals with systolic or diastolic hypertension as well as or better than diuretics.

In type II diabetics with hypertension several relatively small trials have reported lower rates of cardiovascular events with an ACE inhibitor than a calcium antagonist. However, in the 758 patients in the tight control group of the UKPDS the ACE inhibitor captopril and the β-blocker atenolol were similarly effective in reducing the incidence of diabetic macrovascular and microvascular complications. ALLHAT, with more than 15,000 hypertensive diabetics, should be able to address with clarity whether major cardiovascular events are different in older patients with diabetes treated with a diuretic, ACE inhibitor or calcium antagonist. Until data from ALLHAT or other data are available, it is reasonable to include a diuretic and an ACE inhibitor or possibly a β-blocker (because of UKPDS results) in antihypertensive regimens for older diabetics. In clinical practice it is likely that the overwhelming majority of hypertensive diabetics will require more than one drug to meet the BP goals recommended by various consensus committees.

Other Indications or Contraindications

Some conditions have *compelling* indications (based on randomized, controlled trials) for drugs that are also used for the treatment of hypertension (Table 65.5). A patient with hypertension who also has systolic dysfunction (low ejection fraction) heart failure should almost always be treated with ACE inhibitors and diuretics. For a patient with myocardial infarction, β-blockers without intrinsic sympathomimetic activity or ACE inhibitors or both are indicated for at least several years. Type I diabetes mellitus with proteinuria is considered a compelling indication for ACE inhibitors, but this form of diabetes is uncommon in the elderly. There are other situations in which an antihypertensive agent is indicated or contraindicated. Examples of indications include β-blockers for migraine headache and α_1-blockers for benign prostatic hyperplasia, but an α_1-blocker should not be used by itself in hypertension because of the ALLHAT results. There are some situations where indications or contraindications are less relevant; for example, the uric acid–raising effect of a diuretic may be of little importance if a patient's gout is well controlled with allopurinol. If there is a compelling reason to use one agent and a specific indication for a different agent, then both drugs should be used if tolerated.

Predicted Antihypertensive Efficacy

Not all elderly patients with hypertension can be treated with the "preferred" agent or agents. Another class of drug may be

TABLE 65.6. One-Year Treatment Success and Short-Term Systolic Blood Pressure Reduction in Older (Age ≥ 60 years) African-Americans and Whites and Drug Intolerance Rates with Different Classes of Antihypertensive Agents in the VA Single-Drug Therapy of Hypertension Study

	HCTZ	Atenolol	Captopril	Clonidine	Diltiazem	Prazosin	Placebo
Success[a] in African-Americans (%)	64	45	33	58	85	49	27
Success[a] in whites (%)	68	72	62	73	72	69	38
SBP reduction (mm Hg) in African-Americans	16	9	7	17	15	13	3
SBP reduction (mm Hg) in whites	13	12	11	17	12	17	3
Drug intolerance (%)	3	5	7	14	4	12	6

[a] Success = diastolic blood pressure <90 mm Hg during titration, <95 mm Hg for 1 year, and tolerating medication in each randomized group.

Reprinted with permission from Madhaven S, Ooi WL, Cohen H, et al. The relationship of pulse pressure and blood pressure reduction to the incidence of myocardial infarction. *Hypertension* 1994;23:395–401.

HCTZ, hydrochlorothiazide; SBP, systolic blood pressure.

necessary to control BP if the preferred one is contraindicated, ineffective, or not tolerated. If a compelling indication exists for a drug that is not controlling BP, then one or more other drugs should be added without stopping the first. For others, the choice of drug for a given patient often will be based on a prediction of how well it is likely to lower BP. Age and race seem to be the most helpful factors in predicting the response to some classes of antihypertensive medications. In the VA Single-Drug Therapy for Hypertension Study, 1,292 men with diastolic hypertension were randomly assigned to receive a placebo or one of six classes of agents (Table 65.6). The 1-year DBP control rate in older African-Americans was best for diltiazem and hydrochlorothiazide and worst for atenolol and captopril. In older whites, all the active drugs were very effective, and there were no differences in efficacy among them. However, clonidine and prazosin had to be discontinued in substantially more patients than the other agents (Table 65.6). Combining antihypertensive drugs with at least additive effects will control BP in almost all stage 1 and 2 hypertensive patients and, especially if a diuretic is included, eradicate any age–race differences in response rates.

Economic and Quality of Life Considerations

The cost of antihypertensive medications is often a cause of nonadherence and apparent resistance to therapy because hypertension is usually an asymptomatic condition. Fortunately, most of the medications that have been used in outcome trials, such as diuretics, β-blockers, and reserpine, are now inexpensive, and most classes of antihypertensive agents have relatively inexpensive members. There is little evidence that other costs of management should differ significantly between drugs, based on the experience in blinded trials.

There are some reports of differences in quality of life among antihypertensive drugs, but the clinical or long-term effects of these differences have not been documented, other than adverse effects leading to drug discontinuation, as is more frequent with central α_2-agonists, such as clonidine or methyldopa. Other commonly used antihypertensive drugs are well tolerated in older men and women. When symptoms may be caused by a preferred medication, a trial of a lower dose or a drug-free period may allow continuation of the medication. A serious or life-threatening adverse effect believed to be caused by a medication should certainly lead to its permanent discontinuation.

CONCLUSION

Elevated SBP or pulse pressure is associated with considerable risk in older persons. Drug treatment of SBP or DBP has been demonstrated to substantially lower the occurrence of cardiovascular events in many randomized, controlled trials. Lifestyle modifications are reasonably effective in reducing BP in elderly patients, but drug therapy, usually diuretic-based, is necessary for most older patients with hypertension. Because many hypertensive elderly patients are not treated or do not have adequate BP control, prevention and control of hypertension will remain a major challenge for the twenty-first century as the numbers and proportion of elderly individuals in the U.S. population and the world markedly increase.

Selected Readings

Applegate WB, Miller ST, Elam JT, et al. Nonpharmacologic intervention to reduce blood pressure in older patients with mild hypertension. *Arch Intern Med* 1992;152:1162–1166.

This randomized, controlled trial demonstrated that lifestyle changes significantly reduced SBP and DBP in older men and women with hypertension who were not taking antihypertensive medications. The intervention was primarily weight and sodium reduction, but included limitation of excess alcohol intake and increased physical activity as part of the weight reduction intervention.

Curb JD, Pressel SL, Cutler JA, et al. Effect of diuretic-based antihypertensive treatment on cardiovascular disease risk in older diabetic patients with isolated systolic hypertension. *JAMA* 1996;276:1886–1892.

This article describes the 583 patients in SHEP with type II diabetes at baseline. In diabetic patients major cardiovascular disease events were reduced by 34%, the same risk reduction as in nondiabetics. The absolute risk reduction, however, was twice that of the nondiabetics.

Dahlof B, Lindholm LH, Hansson L, et al. Morbidity and mortality in the Swedish Trial in Old Patients with Hypertension (STOP-Hypertension). *Lancet* 1991; 338:1281–1285.

The STOP-Hypertension trial was conducted in 1,627 men and women aged 70 to 84 years with SBP 180 to 230 mm Hg and DBP ≥ 90 mm Hg (or 105 to 120 mm Hg, regardless of SBP). A diuretic or one of three β-blockers (clinic choice, but most patients assigned β-blockers also required a diuretic) significantly reduced stroke, heart failure, all cardiovascular disease events, and deaths, but not coronary heart disease as a separate endpoint.

Davis BR, Cutler JA, Gordon DJ, et al. Rationale and design for the Antihypertensive and Lipid Lowering Treatment to Prevent Heart Attack Trial (ALLHAT). *Am J Hypertens* 1996;9:342–360.

ALLHAT, the largest hypertension morbidity trial ever conducted, begun in 1994 and projected to be completed by 2001, is a randomized, controlled trial comparing a calcium antagonist (amlodipine), an ACE inhibitor (lisinopril), or an α_1-blocker (doxazosin) with a diuretic (chlorthalidone) in 42,000 high-risk hypertensive patients at least 55 years of age. The primary endpoint is nonfatal myocardial infarction plus fatal coronary heart disease. Part of this study population is also participating in a randomized, controlled trial of lipid lowering with pravastatin—total mortality is the primary endpoint of the lipid portion.

Franklin SS, Gustin WG, Wong ND, et al. Hemodynamic patterns of age-related changes in blood pressure. The Framingham Heart Study. *Circulation* 1997; 96:308–315.

This is a report from the Framingham Heart Study that characterizes age-related changes in blood pressure to infer underlying hemodynamic mechanisms. The early rise and later fall in DBP with age and the continual rise in SBP were greatest for the subjects with the highest baseline SBP and was consistent with increased large artery stiffness.

Hansson L, Zanchetti A, Carruthers SG, et al. Effects of intensive blood-pressure lowering and low-dose aspirin in patients with hypertension: principal results of the Hypertension Optimal Treatment (HOT) randomised trial. HOT Study Group. *Lancet* 1998;351:1755–1762.

In the HOT study, 18,790 hypertensive patients with DBP 100 to 115 mm Hg were randomly assigned to target DBP goals of ≤ 90, ≤ 85, or ≤ 80 mm Hg.

Major cardiovascular, coronary, or cerebrovascular events were not significantly different among the three groups. The results suggest neither benefit nor harm with these lower DBP goals. In the 1,501 diabetic participants, however, major cardiovascular events were significantly lower in the those randomly assigned to the DBP goal of ≤ 80 mm Hg.

Joint National Committee on Prevention, Detection, Evaluation, and Treatment of High Blood Pressure. The Sixth Report of the Joint National Committee on Prevention, Detection, Evaluation, and Treatment of High Blood Pressure (JNC VI). *Arch Intern Med* 1997;157:2413–2446.

The most recent U.S. consensus hypertension recommendations are based in large part on evidence from clinical trials, but also include consensus opinions of experts in some areas not adequately addressed by major outcome trials. Drug treatment is recommended for elderly patients with SBP ≥ 160 mm Hg based on randomized, controlled trials and 140 to 159 mm Hg based on epidemiologic and other indirect evidence. Diuretics are recommended as the preferred initial therapy, especially for ISH, for which a long-acting calcium channel blocker is recommended as an alternative.

Madhavan S, Ooi WL, Cohen H, et al. The relationship of pulse pressure and blood pressure reduction to the incidence of myocardial infarction. *Hypertension* 1994;23:395–401.

High pulse pressure is a result of increases in large artery stiffness. This was an observational study of the relationship between pulse pressure, SBP, and DBP and cardiovascular risk in treated hypertensive patients from a work-site program. Hypertensive patients in the upper tertile of pretreatment pulse pressure (≥ 63 mm Hg) had a greater incidence of myocardial infarction than those in the lower tertiles in this study. The relationship with pulse pressure was stronger than for SBP or DBP.

Materson BJ, Reda DJ, Cushman WC, et al. Single-drug therapy for hypertension in men: a comparison of six antihypertensive agents with placebo. *N Engl J Med* 1993;328:914–921.

This randomized, controlled trial compared the antihypertensive efficacy of six different classes of antihypertensive agents and placebo in 1,292 men. Single-drug therapy was successful in a majority of patients. In older African-Americans the proportion with DBP control and who tolerated the medication after 1 year was best for diltiazem (85%) and hydrochlorothiazide (64%) and worst for atenolol (45%) and captopril (33%); results for clonidine and prazosin were intermediate. In older whites all the drugs were very effective (62% to 73% success rates), and there were no differences in efficacy among them. However, clonidine and prazosin caused substantially more adverse effects and drug intolerance than the other agents.

MRC Working Party. Medical Research Council trial of treatment of hypertension in older adults: principal results. *BMJ* 1992;304:405–412.

In this trial, 4,396 men and women in the United Kingdom aged 65 to 74 years with entry SBP of 160 to 209 mm Hg and DBP less than 115 mm Hg were randomly assigned to receive a diuretic (hydrochlorothiazide/amiloride), a β-blocker (atenolol), or placebo. The diuretic group had significantly fewer strokes (31%), coronary events (44%), and all cardiovascular events (35%) compared with the placebo group, but the atenolol group experienced no benefits. These results show that a diuretic is preferred over a β-blocker as the initial therapy for the treatment of hypertension in elderly patients.

National High Blood Pressure Education Program Working Group. National High Blood Pressure Education Program Working Group report on hypertension in the elderly. *Hypertension* 1994;23:275–285.

This consensus report reviews the observational and clinical trial basis for identification and treatment of hypertension in elderly patients and provides recommendations for prevention and management of hypertension in geriatric patients based on this evidence.

Pahor M, Shorr RI, Somes GW, et al. Diuretic-based treatment and cardiovascular events in patients with mild renal dysfunction enrolled in the Systolic Hypertension in the Elderly Program (SHEP). *Arch Intern Med* 1998;158:1340–1345.

This was a subgroup analysis of the effect of antihypertensive treatment on cardiovascular events in patients with ISH according to baseline serum creatinine levels, as an estimate of renal function, in SHEP. Cardiovascular events were reduced by diuretic-based treatment in the subgroup with the highest serum creatinine levels (1.4 to 2.4 mg/dl), even more than in those with more normal renal function. Hypokalemia was also less common in this subgroup.

Preston RA, Materson BJ, Reda DJ, et al. Age-race subgroup compared with renin profile as predictors of blood pressure response to antihypertensive therapy. *JAMA* 1998;280:1168–1172.

This analysis of the VA Cooperative Study Group on Antihypertensive Agents Single-Drug Therapy Study found that the combination of age and race of a hypertensive patient, was a better predictor of blood pressure control with antihypertensive drugs than renin profile determination. Renin profiling tended to predict response, but not as well as demographics. Thus plasma renin assay, while useful for evaluating some patients suspected of having secondary hypertension is unnecessary in most workups for hypertension.

Sagie A, Larson MG, Levy D. The natural history of borderline isolated systolic hypertension. *N Engl J Med* 1993;329:1912–1917.

This report from the Framingham Heart Study showed that stage 1 ISH (SBP 140 to 159 mm Hg and DBP less than 90 mm Hg) was the most common form of untreated hypertension in elderly patients, predicted progression to more severe forms of hypertension (80% in 20 years), and was associated with a significantly increased risk of cardiovascular disease (47%) and death from cardiovascular disease (57%) compared with normotensive participants.

SHEP Cooperative Research Group. Prevention of stroke by antihypertensive drug treatment in older persons with isolated systolic hypertension: final results of the Systolic Hypertension in the Elderly Program (SHEP). *JAMA* 1991; 265:3255–3264.

This article gives the primary results of SHEP, the first trial to demonstrate the marked benefit of treating ISH in elderly patients. A total of 4,736 older persons with SBP 160 to 219 mm Hg and DBP less than 90 mm Hg were randomly assigned to receive diuretic-based treatment or placebo. With an average follow-up of 4.5 years, the percentages of strokes (36%), coronary events (27%), and heart failure (49%) were all significantly reduced. The reduction in events were seen in numerous subgroups (some reported in subsequent articles), including patients aged ≥ 80 years, patients with or without baseline ECG abnormalities, and patients with type II diabetes.

Staessen JA, Fagard R, Thijs L, et al. Randomised double-blind comparison of placebo and active treatment for older patients with isolated systolic hypertension. *Lancet* 1997;350:757–764.

In the Syst-Eur Trial 4,695 older Europeans with ISH, SBP 160 to 219 mm Hg, and DBP less than 95 mm Hg were randomly assigned to receive the calcium antagonist nitrendipine or a matching placebo. Active treatment significantly reduced stroke (42%) and all cardiovascular events (31%), but reductions in heart failure (29%) and myocardial infarction (30%) were not statistically significant. This confirms the benefit of treating ISH in elderly patients and is the first trial to show reductions in major morbid events with a calcium antagonist.

United Kingdom Prospective Diabetes Group. Tight blood pressure control and risk of macrovascular and microvascular complications in type 2 diabetes. *BMJ* 1998;317:703–713.

The UKPDS trial compared tight control of blood pressure (less than 150/85 mm Hg) with less tight control (less than 180/105 mm Hg) over a median of 8.4 years in 1,148 hypertensive type II diabetics. Significant reductions were seen with diabetes-related endpoints (24%), deaths related to diabetes (32%), strokes (44%), and microvascular endpoints (37%). There were no differences in endpoints between patients within the tight blood pressure control group randomly assigned to receive captopril or atenolol. This demonstrates the value of treating diabetic hypertensive patients to a blood pressure goal of less than 150/90 mm Hg and suggests that there is no difference between ACE inhibitor and β-blocker therapy.

CHAPTER 66

Hypertension in African-Americans

Donald E. Wesson

Hypertension is one of the most common chronic health conditions in industrialized societies and is the single most important contributor to the high rate of cardiovascular disease in these societies compared with nonindustrialized societies. The prevalence of hypertension among U.S. residents is one of the highest of industrialized nations, and Americans of African descent have a higher incidence and prevalence of hypertension compared with other U.S. population groups. Recognizing that there are some regional differences, African-Americans have about 1.7 times the incidence of hypertension compared with age- and sex-matched Americans of European descent. The reasons for this high rate of hypertension in industrialized societies are not entirely clear and the reasons for the excess incidence among African-Americans compared with other U.S. population groups are even less understood. More disturbing, end-organ damage from hypertension is more frequent in African-Americans compared with other U.S. population groups with the same level of hypertension. This disparity is most evident with regard to the risk for hypertension-associated end-stage renal disease (ESRD), which hypertensive African-Americans are at least four times more likely to develop than other U.S. population groups. Thus greater prevalence combined with higher rates of end-organ disease means that hypertension exacts a disproportionately greater toll on African-Americans. These data lend urgency to the goal of eradicating this syndrome and its devastating complications.

HISTORICAL ISSUES

The higher prevalence of hypertension in African-Americans compared with Americans of European descent was first reported in 1932. Blood pressure was higher in African-Americans of all age groups, and there was a tendency toward higher pressure in female than in male African-Americans. Since this landmark observation, subsequent studies showed that compared with European-Americans, African-Americans have higher blood pressure earlier in life, have a higher incidence of hypertension that is manifest earlier in life, have hypertension that is more severe, and have hypertension that is associated with a greater risk for cardiovascular complications. Mortality rates from 1950 census data showed higher hypertension-related mortality in African-Americans compared with European-Americans with similar blood pressures. These important findings have been confirmed by numerous subsequent studies. Newer studies show that cardiovascular disease predominantly accounts for the excess hypertension-associated mortality in African-Americans compared with European-Americans. Within the spectrum of cardiovascular disease, the two major contributors to this excess mortality are cerebrovascular accident (stroke) and ischemic heart disease. Improved control of hypertension has reduced hypertension-associated mortality in all U.S. population groups, but the reduction has been less for African-Americans. The first systematic study of possible physiologic differences in hypertension between North Americans of African and European descent showed that hypertensive persons of African descent more commonly had low plasma renin activity, a finding confirmed by many subsequent studies. Many investigators reported that hypertension in African-Americans is more likely to be salt-sensitive (i.e., to be improved with restricted dietary sodium and/or exacerbated with an increase in sodium intake) than for other U.S. population groups. Another consistent finding that characterizes the hypertension of African-Americans compared with other U.S. population groups is increased sympathetic nervous activity, particularly that mediated by α-receptors. Despite these physiologic insights, successful pharmacologic treatment of hypertension in African-Americans differs little from that in other U.S. population groups. As indicated earlier, African-Americans with hypertension are much more likely than other U.S. population groups to develop ESRD associated with this syndrome. This recognition has led to a lower threshold for treatment of hypertension in African-Americans and encourages the clinician to be more aggressive in attaining the target blood pressure in this population group. Despite significant research efforts, the reasons for the increased hypertension incidence and prevalence and for the increase in hypertension-associated complications in African-Americans remain unknown.

PATHOGENESIS

When considering the pathogenesis of hypertension, it is important to recognize that it is clearly not a single "disease" but is more accurately described as a syndrome. The elevation in blood pressure that characterizes this syndrome is probably due to the combination of multiple factors interacting against a background of susceptibility determined in part by genetics and environmental factors. Furthermore, when considering the etiology of hypertension in African-Americans as a group, it is important to remember that the excess incidence of hypertension in African-Americans occurs within the context of an overall higher incidence of hypertension in industrialized societies compared with nonindustrialized ones. Hence, despite some genetic influences, hypertension is probably induced by factors related to life in industrialized societies that remain poorly understood. It follows that factors that contribute to the excess incidence of hypertension in African-Americans compared with European-Americans probably do not affect African-Americans exclusively or in an entirely unique fashion, but do so disproportionately compared with whites. This analysis suggests that there is probably no "black" mechanism for hypertension that is limited to this population group. Instead, it is more likely that hypertension mechanisms in African-Americans have application to the syndrome and its complications in other population groups. Nevertheless, the higher prevalence and complication rates for hypertension in African-Americans make this population group an important one in which to study this syndrome. The following section discusses mechanisms that were suggested by many published studies to contribute to hypertension in African-Americans. The list of topics is by no means an exhaustive one.

Social, Cultural, and Psychologic Contributors

Hypertension is virtually nonexistent in nonindustrialized societies. Such societies with a very low incidence of hypertension include those of Western Africa, the ancestral home of most African-Americans. The latter point suggests that genetics alone do not explain the excess incidence of hypertension in African-Americans but might instead provide the necessary background upon which important environmental factors interact to induce hypertension. Levels of blood pressure vary dramatically among individual members of all North American population groups including African-Americans. Blood pressure correlates inversely with socioeconomic status within all these population groups although socioeconomically disadvantaged African-Americans have higher blood pressure than do age-matched European-Americans. Examining social and psychologic factors within the context of low socioeconomic status shows that blood pressure directly correlates with the degree to which an individual struggles to achieve and maintain valued social and personal goals in a setting of limited means by which these goals can be attained. In other words, many African-Americans chronically struggle against a persistently discriminatory and occasionally hostile environment in an effort to achieve a measure of perceived self-worth. Those African-Americans who are actively engaged in this struggle are more likely to be hypertensive than are African-Americans who are not. By contrast, those African-Americans who are engaged with supportive community institutions like church and extended family are less likely to be hypertensive. Although studies in this area show strong associations, direct causal links have yet to be established. In addition, the relative contribution of these conditions as etiologic factors for hypertension in African-Americans and other population groups is not established. Nevertheless, this continues to be a fruitful area of study.

Cardiovascular Reactivity

Investigations show that the cardiovascular system reacts to stressful stimuli in well-defined and measurable ways, some of which increase blood pressure acutely. In most individuals, this blood pressure increase is not sustained, and blood pressure returns to its baseline within minutes to hours. These studies show that the components of this vascular reactivity are characteristic for an individual and are reproducible over time. Because of the chronic environmental stresses discussed earlier that are faced by many African-Americans, investigators have begun testing the hypothesis that aberrant physiologic responses to stressful stimuli might play a role in the development of human hypertension, including that in African-Americans. These investigators show ethnic differences in cardiovascular reactivity to stress, including greater vascular reactivity (vasoconstriction) in African-Americans and greater cardiac (predominately tachycardia) reactivity in European-Americans. Nevertheless, neither stress nor the cardiovascular reactivity to it has been shown to have a causal role in human hypertension, but this remains an active investigative area.

Genetic Factors

African-Americans as a group have higher blood pressure than both the indigenous Africans from which they are descended and their fellow inhabitants of the Western Hemisphere. Although debate continues as to the relative importance of genetics compared with environment in yielding this higher pressure, available data leave little doubt for a genetic contribution to the generally higher blood pressures in African-Americans compared with other population groups. Physiologic studies show that hypertension in many African-American is "salt sensitive" as discussed earlier. Because most individuals, including most African-Americans, can ingest a high NaCl diet without increased systemic blood pressure, salt-sensitive hypertension can be viewed as a failure to avoid an increase in blood pressure in response to high NaCl intake. Two physiologic mechanisms that contribute to this normal response to increased dietary NaCl are increased renal NaCl excretory ability and dilation of resistance blood vessels. Many investigations have focused on possible genetic differences in factors that might affect these physiologic phenomena. Some studies support genetic differences in components of the renin–angiotensin–aldosterone system in a minority of hypertensive African-Americans. These differences include the renin and angiotensinogen genes on human chromosome 1 and the angiotensin-converting enzyme on human chromosome 17. In general, studies show a higher frequency of hypertension-associated gene alleles for these substances in some but clearly not in all hypertensive African-Americans. It is apparent that abnormalities in some or all of these gene products might limit renal NaCl excretory ability. Similar data have been reported with regard to human genes for kallikrein (chromosome 19) and the α_2-adrenergic receptor (chromosome 10) that might affect the vasoactive state of resistance vessels.

Mitochondrial DNA is exclusively maternally inherited and studies in this area allow for accurate tracking of maternal ancestry. Twin studies show that the African mitochondrial DNA phenotype is associated with the faster age-related blood pressure increase that occurs in African-Americans as described earlier compared with other U.S. population groups. The physiologic mechanisms that mediate the faster blood pressure increase are not known.

Dietary Factors

Epidemiologic and experimental data suggest that dietary constituents are among the environmental factors that contribute to the higher prevalence and severity of hypertension in African-Americans compared with those of other population groups. Epidemiologic studies in populations ingesting their usual diets have highlighted aggregate dietary constituents that are associated with a given range of blood pressures in a particular population. These studies show that hypertension is virtually nonexistent in societies whose dietary sodium (Na^+) content is very low. By contrast, populations ingesting diets very high in Na^+ have some of the world's highest hypertension rates. Such studies must be interpreted with caution, however, when attempting to link a particular dietary constituent and/or level thereof with the observed population blood pressure. Diets among human population groups are rarely distinguished by differences in the presence and/or level of a single constituent. More commonly, these diets differ in many constituents in addition to the one or ones being examined as a possible mediator of or contributor to hypertension. Therefore the question as to the role of a particular dietary constituent on blood is best answered with prospective studies done on patients ingesting well-defined diets in which the constituent being studied is altered in its presence or amount while all others remain unchanged. Studies done in this way show that normal blood pressure is maintained in response to a high Na^+ diet in most individuals including African-Americans. Nevertheless, a higher proportion of African-Americans compared with European-Americans show significant increases in their blood pressure in response to a high Na^+ diet, thereby characterizing their blood pressure as salt-sensitive. Conversely, a reduction in dietary Na^+ reduces blood pressure in these individuals. Yet, large population studies show that dietary Na^+ intake is comparable in African-Americans and other U.S. population groups. Together, available data support the fact that dietary Na^+ in excess of the amount needed to maintain normal extracellular volume is not sufficient to induce hypertension in most if not all individuals with this syndrome. Even so, other factors must combine with dietary Na^+ to lead to this abnormal increase in blood pressure. These other factors include genetic makeup and most probably other environmental, including other dietary, factors.

Other dietary factors that have been implicated as mediators of hypertension in general and of that in African-Americans in particular include potassium (K^+), calcium (Ca^{2+}), and caloric intake. Potassium depletion is associated with increased blood pressure and a number of studies show lower dietary K^+ intake in African-Americans compared with other U.S. population groups. In addition, K^+ repletion in depleted individuals lowers blood pressure. The quantitative contribution of K^+ depletion to the high prevalence of hypertension in African-Americans, however, is not known. Similar epidemiologic studies show an inverse relationship between dietary intake of Ca^{2+} and risk for hypertension. To date, it has not been clearly demonstrated that this relationship between intake of Ca^{2+} and hypertension risk is a causal one, but this continues to be an active area of research. High caloric intake increases the risk for obesity, a state that is associated with hypertension. Conversely, weight reduction in obese individuals reduces blood pressure. Obesity is more prevalent in African-Americans compared with other U.S. population groups, thereby making it a likely contributor to the high prevalence of hypertension in African-Americans. Recognizing that obesity increases the risk for cardiovascular disease for all individuals, it is imperative that clinicians encourage weight reduction for their hypertensive patients.

Substance Use and Abuse

Excessive alcohol consumption and tobacco use of any amount are associated with increased blood pressure. Moderate alcohol intake (one or two drinks per day) lowers blood pressure and is associated with reduced mortality from coronary artery disease. By contrast, excessive alcohol intake increases blood pressure and its cessation reduces it. Similarly, tobacco smoking increases blood pressure acutely and chronically, providing yet another reason not to ingest tobacco products. African-Americans are disproportionately represented among the American poor who consume proportionately more alcohol and tobacco products than the nonpoor. This association possibly contributes to higher hypertension prevalence in individuals of lower socioeconomic status.

Renal Factors

Extensive autopsy studies show that the age-related increase in blood pressure is preceded by and associated with progressive fibroplasia of renal interlobular arteries. This process occurs, on average, faster in African-Americans than in European-Americans. Supporting these anatomic studies are physiologic studies showing that hypertensive African-Americans have lower renal blood flow and higher renal vascular resistance than hypertensive European-Americans. African-Americans with salt-sensitive hypertension who ingest a high-salt diet rather than a low-salt diet exhibit decreased renal blood flow, increased glomerular pressure, and increased urine albumin excretion, the latter being a possible indicator of renal injury. Hypertensive African-Americans also have delayed excretion of administered Na^+ compared with hypertensive European-Americans. These data are consistent with the many studies showing a vasoactive hormonal profile in hypertensive African-American consistent with an expanded extracellular fluid volume. Furthermore, it has been reported that six African-Americans with hypertension-associated ESRD became normotensive after transplantation of kidneys from normotensive donors. Additionally, there is a strong familial association of hypertension-associated renal disease among African-Americans with ESRD. These data are consistent with the hypothesis that underlying but clinically inapparent renal disease contributes to hypertension in African-Americans. Nevertheless, only classical hypertensive nephrosclerosis was found in a renal biopsy study of hypertensive African-Americans who entered into the National Institutes of Health-sponsored African American Study of Kidney Disease. Thus it appears unlikely that primary renal disease other than that associated with hypertension contributes to the hypertension of African-Americans. Identification of the molecular abnormalities of the amiloride-sensitive Na^+ channel in patients with Liddle's syndrome and the salt-sensitive nature of this disorder raise the possibility that abnormalities in this renal membrane channel contribute to hypertension in African-Americans. Although it has been shown that sodium channel mutations occur more frequently in hypertensive than in normotensive African-Americans, this mutation accounts for only a small minority of those with apparently essential hypertension.

Summary of Pathogenesis

Investigations to date confirm that hypertension in African-Americans, like that in other populations, is multifactorial and probably not mediated by the same mechanism(s) in every patient. Nevertheless, the data to date support the idea that hypertension in many if not most African-Americans is mediated by an inherited or acquired increased Na^+ avidity combined with a shift of the dose-response curve of vascular reactivity. This shifted dose-response curve for vascular responsivity yields relative vasoconstriction in the setting of a prevailing expanded extracellular fluid volume.

CLINICAL PRESENTATION

Hypertension in African-Americans is detected, as it is in all individuals with hypertension, through its measurement, preferably confirmed with at least one follow-up measurement. Hypertension is not commonly symptomatic except when it is severe and causes acute end-organ damage. Because hypertensive African-Americans have a higher rate of end-organ damage, it is important for the clinician to look for evidence of this damage. African-Americans, for example, have a higher risk for left ventricular hypertrophy (LVH) and its associated higher risk for cardiovascular complications. An electrocardiogram, by which LVH might be detected, should be a part of the initial workup of all hypertensive patients although echocardiography does so with greater sensitivity. The greater risk for renal disease in hypertensive African-Americans supports measuring of plasma creatinine and blood urea nitrogen levels and performing a urinalysis to look for evidence of associated renal injury. The latter can be indicated by the presence of cells and/or casts but more commonly by proteinuria. The presence of proteinuria detectable with the conventional dipstick is consistent with a daily albumin excretion of at least 300 mg. This level of urine albumin excretion is now termed *macroalbuminuria* and greatly exceeds that excreted by normal individuals. The finding of macroalbuminuria is consistent with significant renal injury and/or inflammation. If urine albumin excretion is in the nephrotic range (greater than 3 g/day), the clinician should consider a renal biopsy to explore the possibility of primary renal disease because nephrotic-range proteinuria is not a common presentation for hypertensive nephrosclerosis. Ongoing studies are evaluating the meaning of urine albumin excretion that is greater than normal but less than macroalbuminuria (urine albumin excretion of 30 to 300 mg/day, called *microalbuminuria*) with respect to risk for hypertension-associated ESRD and/or cardiovascular complications. All hypertensive patients should also have a serum lipid profile done as a gauge to their risk for cardiovascular disease. Patients with elevated low-density lipoprotein and/or low high-density lipoprotein levels have a higher risk for cardiovascular complications when these biochemical abnormalities occur in conjunction with hypertension. Thus the clinician should not only intervene to lower blood pressure but also to correct the abnormal lipid profile. This is particularly true for hypertensive African-Americans who, as stressed earlier, have a higher rate of cardiovascular complications.

MANAGEMENT

Because hypertension in African-Americans is salt sensitive, restriction of sodium intake and the use of diuretics, such as hydrochlorothiazide, when renal function is normal represent a reasonable therapeutic approach. In association with this regimen, the patient should be encouraged to refrain from smoking and excessive alcohol ingestion. If the patient is obese, weight reduction should be attempted.

In patients for whom diuretics are not adequate to control the hypertension, a β-blocker is a reasonable choice. β-Blockers are effective in lowering blood pressure in hypertensive African-Americans. Calcium channel antagonists are also effective in this group of patients. Angiotensin-converting enzyme inhibitors are less effective hypertensives but remain good reno- and cardioprotective agents in this population. Loop diuretics (furosemide) should be substituted for hydrochlorothiazide in patients with renal failure (serum creatinine level greater than 2.5 mg/dL).

Hypertension in African-Americans is a greater risk factor for progression of renal failure than in whites. Therefore the goal for blood pressure control in African-Americans is 130/85 mm Hg or less. The goal for those with macroproteinuria should be 125/75 or less.

Selected Readings

Adrogue HJ, Wesson DE. Role of dietary factors in the hypertension of African Americans. *Semin Nephrol* 1996;16:94–101.

Data linking dietary constituents as etiologic factors in hypertension of African-Americans.

Bergman SM, Curtis JJ. Possible mediators in hypertension: renal factors. *Semin Nephrol* 1996;16:134–139.

Discussion of studies that investigated possible renal contributions to hypertension in African-Americans.

Dressler WW. Hypertension in the African American community: social, cultural, and psychological factors. *Semin Nephrol* 1996;16:63–70.

Description of studies linking social, cultural, and psychologic factors to hypertension and provides support for these factors as contributing causes.

Falkner B. The role of cardiovascular reactivity as a mediator of hypertension in African Americans. *Semin Nephrol* 1996;16:117–125.

Discussion of data supporting a contributing role of aberrant and/or sustained cardiovascular reactivity to environmental stress to hypertension in African-Americans.

Grim CE, Robinson M. Blood pressure variation in blacks: genetic factors. *Semin Nephrol* 1996;16:83–93.

Discussion of studies that explore the genetic contributions to hypertension in African-Americans.

SECTION VIII

Uremia and the Effects of Dialysis

CHAPTER 67

Progression of Renal Insufficiency

PART 1
Methods of Assessment

Mark J. Sarnak and Andrew S. Levey

Over many years, it is relatively straightforward to document the decline in renal function in chronic renal disease. However, precise measurement of the rate of change in renal function over shorter intervals has proved more difficult. This is mainly because of the slow rate of progression of most renal diseases and the limited accuracy, sensitivity, and specificity of the renal function measurements used to document progression.

Accurate measurement of the rate of decline in renal function is necessary in clinical research. Appreciation of the methods for serial measurement of renal function, as well as the statistical methods to interpret them, are essential to evaluate the efficacy of therapeutic interventions. In clinical practice, accurate measurement of the rate of decline in renal function would be useful to assess the response to therapy in individuals with chronic renal disease. In addition, knowing the rate of decline in renal function would help predict future rates of decline and thereby the interval until the onset of end-stage renal disease (ESRD).

In this chapter, we focus our discussion on the estimation of glomerular filtration rate (GFR) from the clearance of radionuclide-labeled filtration markers as well as from creatinine clearance and serum creatinine. These concepts are more thoroughly discussed in Chapter 103. We briefly review the attributes of these measurements to highlight concepts necessary for discussion of serial measurements to estimate progression. We then consider various statistical issues common to assessment of longitudinal data. Definitions of some of the statistical terms used throughout the chapter are included in the chapter appendix. Finally, we conclude with recommendations for both clinical practice and clinical research.

GFR AS AN INDEX OF RENAL FUNCTION

In principle, the level of GFR is the sum of the filtration rates of all the nephrons, as expressed in the following formulas.

(1) $$GFR = n \times SNGFR$$

where *SNGFR* is single-nephron GFR and *n* is the total number of nephrons in both kidneys and:

(2) $$SNGFR = K_f \times \Delta P \text{ and } SNGFR = A \times P\,(\Delta P_H - \Delta P_O)$$

where K_f is the ultrafiltration coefficient, defined as the product of glomerular surface area *(A)* available for filtration and its hydraulic permeability *(P)*; and ΔP is the net filtration pressure, defined as the difference between the transglomerular hydrostatic (ΔP_H) and oncotic (ΔP_O) pressure gradients.

Progression of renal disease is usually defined as the loss of functioning nephrons, which is ultimately reflected by a decrease in GFR. However, it is well recognized that SNGFR in experimental renal diseases can increase secondary to an increase in ΔP_H (glomerular capillary hypertension) or in surface area (glomerular hypertrophy). These increases in SNGFR blunt the decline in GFR following a reduction in nephron number, thereby decreasing the sensitivity of changes in GFR to detect the onset and progression of renal disease.

Conversely, changes in GFR can occur due to hemodynamic effects on SNGFR, rather than effects on nephron number (Table 67.1). Therefore changes in GFR may not be specific for the progression and remission of renal disease. It is especially important to point out some of the interventions used to slow the progression of renal disease, such as intensive glycemic control in patients with diabetes, dietary protein restriction, strict blood pressure control, and angiotensin-converting-enzyme inhibition, induce changes in SNGFR. As discussed later, interpretation of changes in GFR after introduction of these therapies can be especially difficult.

Despite these limitations, the level of GFR remains the gold standard in evaluating the level of renal function in patients with chronic renal disease. In some renal diseases, measures other than the rate of decline in renal function may be preferable in

TABLE 67.1. Conditions Other Than Renal Disease That Affect Glomerular Filtration Rate

Pregnancy
Reduced renal perfusion
Marked surfeit or deficit of extracellular fluid volume
Nonsteroidal antiinflammatory drugs
Acute protein load and habitual protein intake
Blood glucose control (in diabetic patients)
Level of arterial blood pressure and class of antihypertensive agent used for therapy

Reprinted from *Primer on kidney diseases,* 2nd ed. Academic Press, 1997:21.

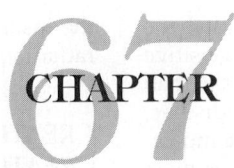

assessing the rate of progression. For example, in early diabetic nephropathy, the rise in albumin excretion is a more sensitive and specific indication of the progression of renal disease than changes in GFR. Similarly, in early polycystic kidney disease, renal enlargement may be a more sensitive and specific indication of progression than changes in GFR. However, for most other renal diseases, specific markers of disease progression are not available; therefore changes in the level of GFR are the gold standard in evaluating the rate of progression.

EXOGENOUS FILTRATION MARKERS FOR MEASUREMENT OF GFR

As described in Chapter 103, GFR is estimated from renal clearance of an ideal filtration marker, as defined by the following equation:

(3) $$C_x = U_x \times V/P_x$$

where C_x is the clearance of substance x (measured in ml/min), V is the urine flow rate (measured in ml/min), U_x is the urinary concentration of x (measured in mg/dl), and P_x is the average plasma concentration of x during the interval of urine collection (measured in mg/dl). If substance x is freely filtered across the capillary wall and excreted only by glomerular filtration, its rate of filtration is equal to its rate of urinary excretion:

(4) $$GFR \times P_x = U_x \times V$$

where the term $GFR \times P_x$ is the filtered load of x. Therefore, by substitution:

(5) $$C_x = GFR$$

Hence, substance x would be defined as an "ideal filtration marker" whose renal clearance could be used to assess the level of GFR. Inulin fulfills all the criteria for an ideal filtration marker, and its renal clearance has long been considered the gold standard in measuring GFR. However, the protocol for measuring inulin clearance is inconvenient, thus it is usually performed only in research settings. Techniques using radionuclide-labeled filtration markers are simpler and have been used in clinical trials and clinical research.

Renal ^{125}I-iothalamate clearance slightly exceeds renal inulin clearance, probably because of secretion of iothalamate to a minor degree. The renal clearance of iothalamate after subcutaneous injection and spontaneous bladder emptying has been extensively studied. In the Modification of Diet in Renal Disease (MDRD) Study, accuracy was excellent: the mean and standard deviation of the difference between inulin and ^{125}I-iothalamate clearances were only 0.65 and 2.77ml/min/1.73m^2, respectively. In addition, the precision of ^{125}I-iothalamate clearances was acceptable. The median coefficient of variation (CV) among four successive urine collection periods was 9.4%, and the median CV between repetitive measurements in a single patient was only 6.3%. ^{125}I-iothalamate has a long half-life, which is ideal in clinical trials using a central laboratory. The main drawbacks of ^{125}I-iothalamate include radiation exposure, its short shelf-life, and expense. In addition, multiple blood and urine measurements are required.

^{99m}Tc-DPTA has also been widely studied in research studies. It is usually administered as an intravenous bolus, and either plasma or renal clearance can be measured. The renal clearance of ^{99m}Tc-DTPA approximates that of renal inulin clearance. The principal drawbacks of using ^{99m}Tc-DPTA are its instability and short shelf-life. Consequently, it must be used immediately after preparation, and plasma and urine samples must be counted soon after completion of the clearance measurement. This makes its use difficult when there is a central laboratory. Conversely, the instability and short half-life are advantageous in limiting radiation exposure and hazardous waste.

CREATININE CLEARANCE AND SERUM CREATININE AS INDICES OF RENAL FUNCTION

In clinical practice, it is more convenient to estimate the level of GFR from the renal clearance or plasma levels of the endogenous filtration marker, creatinine. Assumptions underlying use of creatinine clearance (C_{cr}) and serum or plasma creatinine (P_{cr}) as indices of GFR are given in Table 67.2. If these assumptions are valid, then:

(6) $$C_{cr} = GFR$$

(7) $$P_{cr} = k/GFR$$

where k is a constant that is proportional to urine creatinine excretion. Unfortunately, in patients with chronic renal disease, these assumptions are often not valid; therefore the true relationships of creatinine clearance and serum creatinine with GFR are considerably more complex. In the following sections, we briefly review the renal handling and metabolism of creatinine and derive the more appropriate relationships of creatinine clearance and serum creatinine to GFR.

Renal Creatinine Handling

Creatinine (molecular weight of 113 D) is freely filtered by the glomerulus. However, it is also secreted by the proximal tubule. Therefore urine creatinine excretion is the sum of the filtered and secreted creatinine, as shown in the following equation:

(8) $$U_{cr} \times V = GFR \times P_{cr} + Ts_{cr}$$

where TS_{cr} is the rate of secretion of creatinine (measured in mg/min or mg/day). Dividing by P_{cr}:

(9) $$C_{cr} = GFR + C_{TScr}$$

where C_{TScr} is the clearance of creatinine due to tubular secretion (measured in ml/min). Thus it is clear that creatinine clearance exceeds GFR at all levels of renal function.

The overestimation of GFR by creatinine clearance is approximately 5% to 10% in individuals with normal GFR, but it is greater and more unpredictable in patients with chronic renal disease. The greatest difference occurs in patients with GFRs of 40 to 80 ml/min/1.73 m^2. Creatinine secretion is also affected by factors other than the level of GFR. It is higher in patients with glomerular diseases and lower in patients with polycystic kidney disease or diabetes. Interventions used in clinical trials are also known to affect the secretion of creatinine. For example, in the MDRD Study, the low-protein diet and usual blood pressure goal reduced creatinine secretion. Treatment with calcium channel blockers was associated with lower creatinine secre-

TABLE 67.2. Assumptions Underlying Use of Creatinine Clearance (C_{cr}) and Plasma Creatinine (P_{cr}) as Indices of Glomerular Filtration Rate

	Assumption for C_{cr}
1	Creatinine is an ideal filtration marker.
	Assumptions for P_{cr}
1	Creatinine is an ideal filtration marker.
2	Urine creatinine excretion is similar among patients.
3	GFR and $U_{cr}V$ are constant during the interval in which P_{cr} is measured.

TABLE 67.3. Clinical Conditions That Affect Tubular Secretion of Creatinine (TS_{cr}), Generation of Creatinine (G_{cr}) and Extrarenal Elimination of Creatinine (E_{cr})

Condition/Intervention	TS_{cr}	G_{cr}	E_{cr}
Chronic renal disease	↑	↓	↑
Glomerular disease	↑		
Polycystic kidney disease	↓		
Diabetes	↓	↓	
Increased muscle mass		↑	
Muscle wasting		↓	
Low-protein diet	↓	↓	
Conventional versus strict blood pressure control	↓		
Calcium channel blocker	↓		
Broad-spectrum antibiotics			↓
Trimethoprim	↓		
Cimetidine	↓		

tion, whereas other classes of antihypertensives had no significant effect on creatinine secretion. Finally, creatinine secretion is known to be inhibited by various medications, for example, cimetidine and trimethoprim. Thus the assumption that creatinine is an ideal filtration marker (Table 67.2, assumption 1) is not valid in chronic renal disease, and many factors can affect creatinine secretion, thereby altering the relationship between creatinine clearance and GFR (Table 67.3).

Creatinine Metabolism

Urine creatinine excretion reflects the difference between creatinine generation (G_{cr}) and extrarenal creatinine elimination (E_{cr}), both measured in mg/min or mg/day.

$$U_{cr} \times V = G_{cr} - E_{cr} \tag{10}$$

Substituting into equation 8 and rearranging to solve for P_{cr} or its reciprocal ($1/P_{cr}$) yields the following expressions:

$$P_{cr} = (G_{cr} - TS_{cr} - E_{cr})/GFR \tag{11}$$

$$1/P_{cr} = GFR/(G_{cr} - TS_{cr} - E_{cr}) \tag{12}$$

Thus the relationship between serum creatinine and GFR is affected by the generation, secretion, and extrarenal elimination of creatinine.

Creatinine is largely derived from the metabolism of creatine in muscle. Therefore creatinine generation parallels total muscle mass. Consequently, mean creatinine generation is higher in younger than in older individuals, in men than in women, and in African-Americans than in whites. These differences lead to differences in serum creatinine concentration according to age, gender, and race, even after controlling for the level of GFR (Fig. 67.1). Muscle wasting is associated with reduced creatinine generation, and individuals with malnutrition have lower serum creatinine concentration than would be expected for the level of GFR. To a lesser extent, creatinine generation is also affected by meat intake because the process of cooking meat converts a variable fraction of creatine to creatinine. Meat intake is often restricted in conjunction with a low-protein diet in patients with chronic renal disease. In addition, anorexia, weight loss, and muscle wasting are common findings in patients with chronic renal disease. Patients with diabetic renal disease also have a lower urine creatinine excretion, most likely due to a greater reduction in creatinine generation (Table 67.3).

Extrarenal creatinine elimination is negligible in individuals with normal renal function, but it is increased in patients with chronic renal disease due to degradation of creatinine by bac-

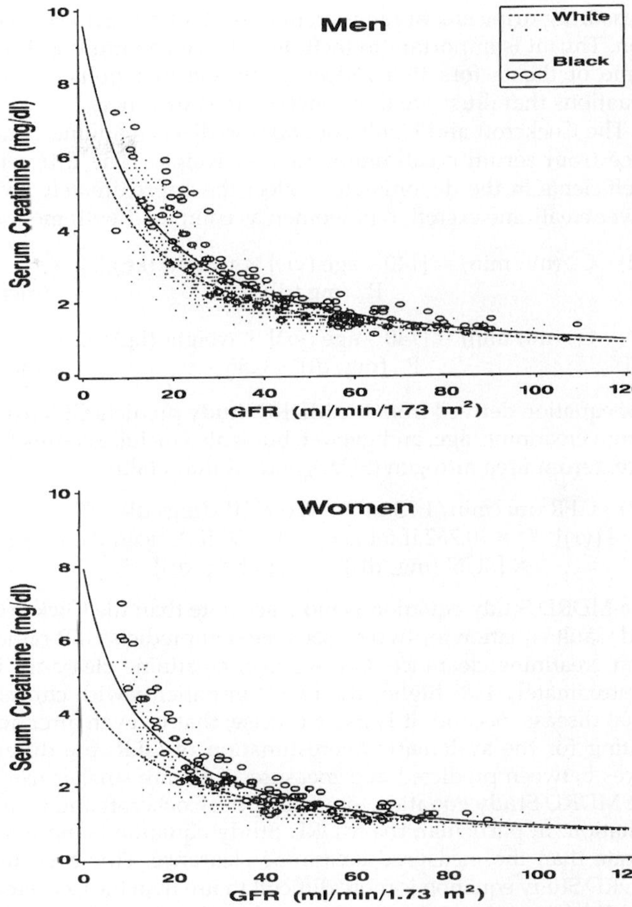

Figure 67.1. Relationship of serum creatinine concentration to measured GFR. Each point represents the baseline measurement for one patient during the MDRD Study. GFR was measured as the renal clearance of ^{125}I-iothalamate. Serum creatinine (P_{cr}) concentration was measured using a kinetic alkaline picrate assay. Values are shown separately by race for men (*upper panel, n* = 915) and women (*lower panel, n* = 586). Regression lines were computed from the relationship $1/P_{cr}$ versus GFR. At any given level of GFR, men have higher serum creatinine values than women (*P* <.001). Among men, African-Americans (*n* = 113) have higher serum creatinine values than whites (*n* = 802, *P* <.001). Similarly, among women, African-Americans (*n* = 84) have higher serum creatinine values than whites (*n* = 502, *P* <.001). (Reproduced with permission from Levey AS, Bosch JP, Breyer-Lewis J, et al. A more accurate method to estimate glomerular filtration rate from serum creatinine: a new prediction equation. Modification of Diet in Renal Disease Study Group. *Ann Intern Med* 1999;130(6):461–470.)

terial overgrowth in the small bowel. Clearance of creatinine due to extrarenal elimination (E_{cr}/P_{cr}) varies from approximately 1 to 7 ml/min. Depending on the level of renal creatinine clearance, up to two-thirds of total daily creatinine excretion can occur by extrarenal elimination. Possibly, treatment with broad-spectrum antibiotics may increase serum creatinine due to decreased extrarenal elimination of creatinine in chronic renal disease (Table 67.3).

These two factors, reduced generation and increased extrarenal elimination of creatinine, lead to reduced urine creatinine excretion. Clearly, the assumption of a constant urine creatinine excretion (Table 67.2, assumption 2) is not valid in patients with chronic renal disease. A corollary of this finding is that it can be difficult to determine the completeness of 24-hour urine collections by quantitating urine creatinine excretion.

Equations to Estimate GFR from Serum Creatinine

It remains of considerable interest to estimate GFR from equations using serum creatinine, without the inconvenience of measuring urine creatinine excretion in a 24-hour urine collection. Thus it is important to include in these equations at least some of the factors that reflect creatinine metabolism. Two equations that illustrate this concept are shown here.

The Cockcroft and Gault equation predicts creatinine clearance from serum creatinine, age, and weight. The different coefficients in the denominator reflect the approximately 15% lower creatinine excretion in women as compared with men.

(12) C_{cr} (ml/min) = [140 – age (yr)] × weight (kg)/72 × P_{cr} (mg/dl) (men)

C_{cr} (ml/min) = [140 – age (yr)] × weight (kg)/72 × P_{cr} (mg/dl) × 0.85 (women)

The equation derived from the MDRD Study predicts GFR from serum creatinine, age, and gender, but it also includes terms for race, serum urea nitrogen (SUN), and albumin (alb).

(13) $GFR\ (ml/min/1.73\ m^2) = 170 \times [P_{cr}\ (mg/dl)]^{-.999} \times [age\ (yr)]^{-.176} \times [0.762 \text{ if female}] \times [1.180 \text{ if African-American}] \times [SUN\ (mg/dl)]^{-.170} \times [alb\ (g/dl)]^{+.318}$

The MDRD Study equation is more accurate than the Cockcroft and Gault equation for two reasons. First, it predicts GFR rather than creatinine clearance. On average, creatinine clearance is approximately 15% higher than GFR in patients with chronic renal disease. Second, it is more precise; that is, even after adjusting for the systematic overestimation of GFR, the differences between predicted and measured GFR are smaller using the MDRD Study equation than using the Cockcroft and Gault equation. In particular, the MDRD Study equation is more accurate than the measured creatinine clearance. However, the MDRD Study equation is more difficult to use than the Cockcroft and Gault equation. It is easiest to apply if the clinical laboratory performs the computations as well as the measurements and reports "predicted GFR," in addition to serum creatinine. The Cockcroft and Gault equation remains a useful bedside tool for estimating GFR from serum creatinine concentration.

Steady-State Assumption

Of course, renal function (GFR and creatinine secretion) and creatinine metabolism (creatinine generation and extrarenal elimination) must be constant during the interval in which serum creatinine is measured (Table 67.2, assumption 3). Otherwise, none of the equations relating serum creatinine to GFR are valid. For example, in acute renal failure, GFR is declining rapidly and serum creatinine is rising. Estimating GFR from these equations will underestimate the decrement in GFR. The converse result occurs during the resolution of acute renal failure, when GFR is rising and serum creatinine is falling. Similarly, abrupt changes in creatinine metabolism can also lead to errors in estimation of GFR from serum creatinine. For example, after the ingestion of cooked meat, serum creatinine can rise by 0.5 to 1.0 mg/dl, without a corresponding decline in GFR. During acute tubular necrosis induced by rhabdomyolysis, it has been speculated that the abrupt rise in serum creatinine reflects its release from injured muscle, in addition to its retention because of decreased GFR.

Estimating Changes in GFR Over Time from Serial Measurements of Creatinine Clearance or Serum Creatinine

Inspection of equations 9 and 12 reveals that the rate of decline in creatinine clearance or reciprocal serum creatinine will equal the rate of decline in GFR only if the generation, secretion, and extrarenal elimination of creatinine are constant over time. However, based on the previous discussion, all three terms vary over time during the course of chronic renal disease, as well as among individuals (Table 67.3). Thus changes in creatinine clearance or serum creatinine may not accurately reflect changes in GFR. This is especially important in studies using dietary protein restriction, which can affect both creatinine generation and secretion. In the MDRD Study, the correlation between rates of decline in GFR with both rates of decline in creatinine clearance (r = 0.64) and rates of decline in reciprocal serum creatinine (r = 0.79) were significant, although relatively weak. More important, the use of different measures of renal function as the outcome variable in the clinical trial would have led to opposite conclusions regarding the efficacy of the low-protein diet (Fig. 67.2). Two recent clinical trials on the efficacy of angiotensin-converting enzyme (ACE) inhibitors used the doubling of serum creatinine as the outcome variable. Although ACE inhibitors are not known to affect the generation, secretion, or extrarenal metabolism of creatinine, the level of blood pressure and other classes of antihypertensive agents have been shown to affect creatinine secretion. For this reason, it is necessary to consider the effects of

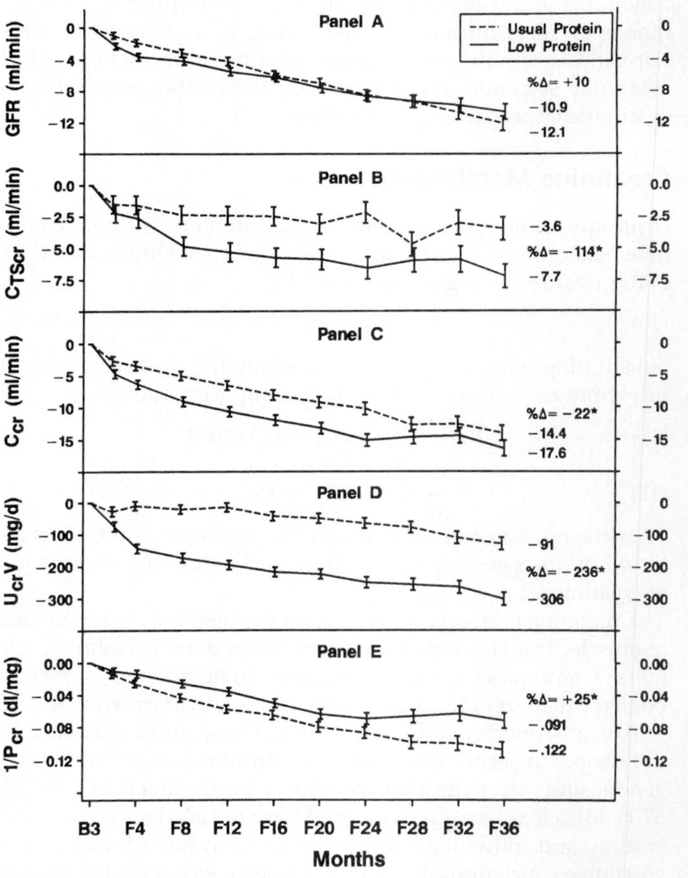

Figure 67.2. Comparison of diet groups in study A of the MDRD Study. Usual protein diet *(dashed lines)*, low-protein diet *(solid lines)*. **A:** Effects on GFR. **B:** Effects on creatinine secretion (C_{TScr}). **C:** Effects on creatinine clearance (C_{cr}). **D:** Effects on creatinine excretion rate ($U_{cr}V$). **E:** Effects on reciprocal serum creatinine concentration ($1/P_{cr}$). Also shown are the estimated mean (± SE) changes at 3 years for each diet group. %Δ indicates the percentage difference in estimated mean change between the low- and usual-protein diet groups. A positive value indicates a lesser decline in the low-protein diet. A negative value indicates a greater decline in the lower-protein diet. *$P<0.05$. (Reproduced from Levey AS, Bosch JP, Coggins CH, et al. Effects of diet and antihypertensive therapy on creatinine clearance and sodium creatinine in Modification of Diet in Renal Disease Study. *J Am Soc Nephrol* 1996;7:556–565.)

therapeutic interventions on creatinine secretion and excretion if serum creatinine is to be used as an outcome measure in clinical trials.

ESTIMATING THE RATE OF PROGRESSION FROM SERIAL MEASUREMENTS OF RENAL FUNCTION

In this section, we review statistical issues related to assessment of longitudinal data. We consider five different issues and how they relate to assessment of the rate of decline in renal function.

Assumption of a Constant Rate of Decline (Slope) and Observed Changes in the Rate of Decline (Breakpoints)

The use of linear regression to estimate the rate of change in renal function over time rests on the assumption of a nearly constant rate of decline. In a series of observational studies, the proportion of variability in reciprocal serum creatinine that could be attributed to variability in time (r^2) was greater than 0.7 in 90% of patients. Approximately linear declines in GFR and C_{cr} have also been documented in observational studies. Nonetheless, many studies have shown that changes in the rate of decline commonly occur.

We examined whether two or more slopes would fit the data better than a single slope in three retrospective studies in which the rate of decline in reciprocal serum creatinine was apparently constant. Results demonstrated spontaneous changes in the slope (breakpoints) in one-third to one-half of patients (Fig. 67.3). The magnitude of the changes in slope was large enough to cause errors in predicting the interval to ESRD as well in assessing the effectiveness of therapy.

There are several possible causes for breakpoints. Possibly, the rate of decline in renal function is not truly constant. Based on the previous discussion of alterations in SNGFR in the initial stages of renal disease and changes in creatinine secretion, generation, and extrarenal elimination in the later stages of renal disease, it is likely that neither GFR, creatinine clearance, nor reciprocal serum creatinine declines at a constant rate throughout the entire course of chronic renal disease. Therefore two or more slopes would fit the data better than a single slope.

Intervention studies often demonstrate short-term effects of the interventions on renal function, which are opposite in direction of their long-term hypothesized beneficial effects. For example, the MDRD Study found a two-slope model with a breakpoint at approximately 4 months after randomization fit the data better than a single-slope model. Similar changes have been observed in studies of intensive glycemic control in diabetes, strict blood pressure control, and ACE inhibition. Possibly, changes in therapy during these observational studies were the cause of breakpoints. Another possible cause of breakpoints is the development of a new or superimposed renal disease.

In prospective studies, regression to the mean can cause apparent breakpoints when comparing the rate of decline before and after the study begins. This concept was analyzed in the MDRD Pilot Study to assess the cause of the slowing in the mean rate of decline in reciprocal serum creatinine after enrollment in the study. In patients with moderate renal disease, 35% of the change in mean decline could be explained by regression to the mean, whereas in the group with advanced renal disease, 100% of the change in mean decline could be explained by regression to the mean.

The occurrence of nonlinear declines in renal function and breakpoints suggests that patients should not be used as their

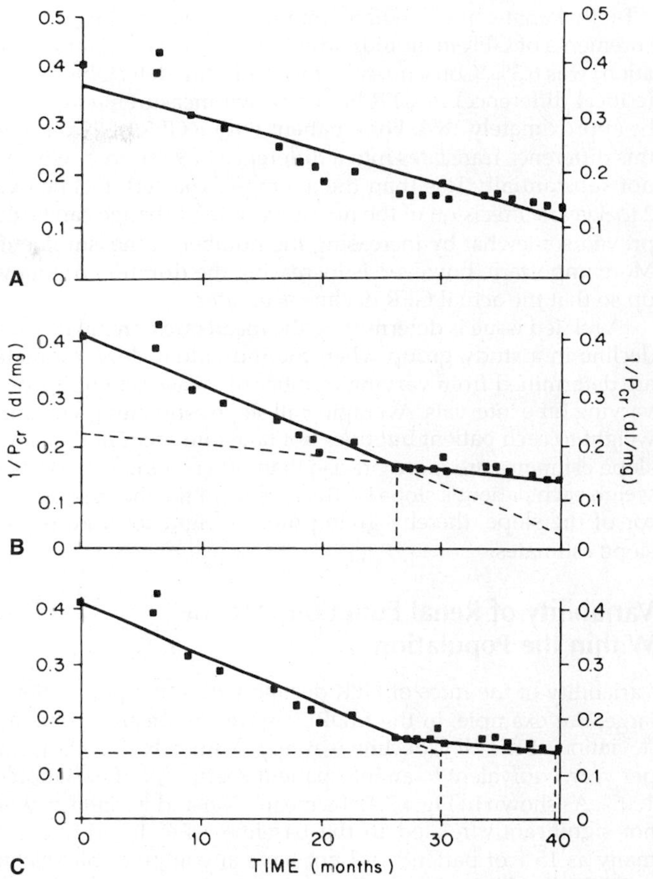

Figure 67.3. Plot of $1/P_{cr}$ versus time in a representative patient. **A:** *Solid line* is the single best fit regression line. **B:** *Solid lines* are the two best-fit regression lines with an intersection (breakpoint) at 26 months *(vertical dashed line)*. *Diagonal dashed lines* are extrapolations of the regression lines to earlier and later times. **C:** Calculation of prediction error. *Solid lines* are the two best-fit regression lines. The *diagonal dashed line* is an extrapolation of the first regression line to the time when the final value for $1/P_{cr}$ (0.132 dl/mg) was obtained. The interval predicted from the first regression line was 30 months *(left vertical dashed line)*. The actual interval was 40 months *(right vertical dashed line)*. The prediction error (difference between the actual and predicted intervals) was 10 months (25% of the actual interval). (Reproduced with permission from Shah BV, Levey AS. Spontaneous changes in the rate of decline in reciprocal creatinine: Errors in predicting the progression of renal disease from extrapolation of the slope. *J Am Soc Nephrol* 1992;2:1186–1191.)

own controls in cross-over studies of the effect of interventions to slow the progression of renal disease. Even if treatment and control periods were assigned randomly, the possibility of carry-over effects would limit the interpretation of cross-over studies.

Imprecision of Slope Estimates

If changes in renal function over time are large, then almost any measure of renal function will be sufficient to document the change. The problem arises when the decline in GFR is slow and only a limited duration of follow-up is practical. In this situation, small errors in measurement of GFR can lead to large errors in the estimation of the change in GFR.

Using currently accepted therapies, the mean rate of decline in renal function in most studies of chronic progressive renal diseases is slow, approximately 4 ml/min per year. Thus, over a 2- to 3-year follow-up interval that is typical of most clinical trials, the decline in mean GFR will be only approximately 8 to 12 ml/min. As discussed earlier, using the renal clearance of

^{125}I-iothalamate, the median time-to-time variability in measurements of GFR in an individual (intertest coefficient of variation) was 6.3%. Consequently, the minimum detectable change (critical difference) in GFR between two measurements would be approximately 18%. For a patient with a GFR of 50 ml/min, this difference translates into a difference of 9 ml/min, which is not substantially less than the average expected decline over 2 to 3 years. Precision of the measured rate of change can be improved somewhat by increasing the number of measurements. More important, however, is increasing the duration of follow-up so that the actual GFR decline is greater.

A related issue is determining the mean rate of renal function decline in a study group when the individual slope estimates are determined from varying number of measurements or over varying time intervals. Averaging all slope estimates gives equal weight to each patient but does not take into account that some slope estimates are more precise than others. One method is to weigh each patient's slope by the inverse of the mean square error of the slope, thereby giving more weight to more precise slope estimates.

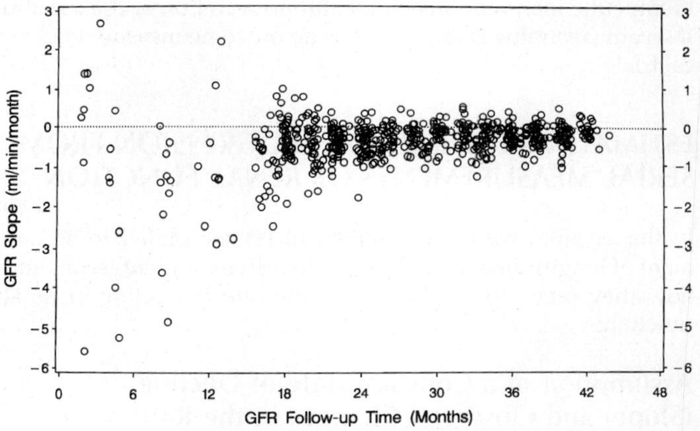

Figure 67.5. Relationship between GFR slope variability and duration of follow-up in MDRD Study A. (Reproduced with permission from Levey A, Greene T, Lau. In: Neilson EG, Couser WG, eds. *Immunologic renal diseases.* Philadelphia: Lippincott-Raven, 1997:899.)

Variability of Renal Function Decline Within the Population

Variability of the rates of GFR decline within the population is large. For example, in the MDRD Study, the mean ± standard deviation of the GFR decline was approximately 4 ± 4 ml/min per year, equivalent to an interpatient coefficient of variation of 100%. As shown in Fig. 67.4, the mean level and variability were not significantly related to the baseline GFR. In addition, as many as 15% of patients did not have any appreciable decline in GFR over the 2- to 4-year interval of follow-up.

There are several reasons for this large variability in GFR decline among patients. First, at least some of the variability appears to be due to "outlier values," that is, single measurements that are very different from other measurements in the same individual. This results in extreme values for slope estimates that are based on few measurements. Figure 67.5 shows the relationship between the duration of follow-up in the MDRD Study and observed variability in GFR declines. With longer follow-up and more GFR measurements, fewer patients had extreme values (i.e., either rapidly declining or rising GFR).

Second, some of the variability in GFR declines can be attributed to patient characteristics. Stepwise regression analysis of baseline factors related to subsequent GFR decline in the MDRD Study revealed six factors that were independent predictors of the rate of progression (Table 67.4). The most important predictors of a faster GFR decline were greater urine protein excretion and the diagnosis of polycystic kidney disease. African-American race, higher mean arterial pressure, lower serum transferrin, and lower high-density lipoprotein (HDL) cholesterol level were also significant, but weaker. After taking these variables into account, neither age, gender, baseline level of GFR, nor the cause of renal disease (other than polycystic kidney disease) were significant. Altogether, these baseline factors accounted for only about one-third of the variability in subsequent GFR decline in the MDRD Study. Thus it is difficult to

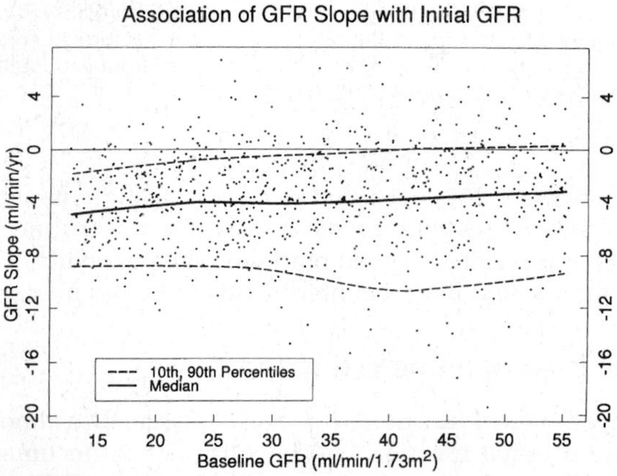

Figure 67.4. Follow-up GFR slopes as a function of baseline GFR. The best linear unbiased predictors of mean GFR slope over 3 years in Study A or overall GFR slope in Study B are shown as a function of GFR. The *lower, middle, and upper lines* indicate the 10th, 50th, and 90th percentiles of the estimated GFR slopes, respectively. The slope estimates were computed using a two-slope mixed-effects model in Study A and an informative censoring model in Study B. The higher variability of the GFR slopes is higher at higher levels of GFR. (Reproduced with permission from Hunsicker LG, Adler S, Caggiula A, et al. Predictors of progression of renal disease in the Modification of Diet in Renal Disease Study. *Kidney Int* 1997;51:1908–1919.)

TABLE 67.4. Cumulative Variance of Glomerular Filtration Rate Slopes in Study A and Study B Explained by Successive Entry of Covariates into the Predictive Model[a]

Baseline Covariate Added	Study A Cumulative Variance Explained %	Study B Cumulative Variance Explained %
Baseline urine protein (g/day)	14	13.2
Polycystic kidney disease	32	27.1
Baseline transferrin (mg/dl)	32.9	30
African-American race	32.7	31.2
Baseline mean arterial pressure (mm Hg)	33.3	31.9
Baseline high-density lipoprotein (mg/dl)	34.2	32.1

[a] Cumulative variance explained is defined as the percent reduction in the between-patient variance component for the estimated slope over 3 years in Study A and for the overall glomerular filtration rate slope in Study B due to the indicated baseline covariates. Unlike the R^2 in standard multiple regression analysis, the cumulative variance explained as defined here can decrease slightly when a new variable is added to the model.

Modified from Hunsicker LG, Adler S, Caggiula A, et al. Predictors of progression of renal disease in the Modification of Diet in Renal Disease Study. *Kidney Int* 1997;51:1915.

TABLE 67.5. Relationship of Effect Size, Variability, and Sample Size for Comparison of Mean Glomerular Filtration Rate Slopes Between Two Groups[a]

SD	Minimum Detectable Effect Size[b]		
(ml/min/yr)	20%	30%	50%
3.0	592	264	96
4.5	1,330	592[c]	214
6.0	2,362	1,050	378

[a] Total sample size required in both groups, based on a two-sided test with 5% type I error and 90% power. For purposes of illustration, equal follow-up times assumed for all patients with no loss of follow-up.
[b] Effect sizes expressed as a percentage of assumed mean slope of −4 ml/min/yr in the control group.
[c] Approximately equivalent to the parameters for MDRD Study A.

predict the rate of progression of renal disease based on patients' clinical characteristics.

Determinants of Sample Size in Clinical Trials

This large variability among patients has important implications for determining the sample size in clinical trials comparing the mean slopes between randomized groups. In these studies, the difference in mean slope between randomized groups is the "effect size." In general, for any given effect size, the greater the variability among patients, the larger the number of patients required in clinical trials to test the effect of interventions (Table 67.5). Obviously, large numbers of patients and a long duration of follow-up are required in clinical trials of interventions to slow the rate of decline in renal function.

Time-to-Event Analysis Versus Comparison of Mean Slopes

Time-to-event analysis is also known as *survival analysis* and refers to the method of measuring the rate of occurrence of discrete outcomes. In studies of progressive renal disease, examples of time-to-event analyses are determining the rate of ESRD or doubling of serum creatinine. Clinical trials using this method of analysis typically compare curves showing "event-free survival" or cumulative incidence of events between randomized groups. The relative risk (or relative hazard) of the event in any given time interval is the estimate of effect size. Time-to-event analysis has been used successfully in several important clinical trials of interventions to slow the progression of renal disease.

If the benefit of the intervention is proportional to the underlying rate of progression, it can be shown that the time-to-event analysis has greater statistical power than the comparison of mean slopes and therefore requires a smaller sample size. For example, in the comparison of mean slopes, if 10% to 15% of patients have no detectable change in GFR during 2 to 4 years of follow-up, the beneficial effect of the intervention in patients with declining GFR is diluted by the lack of effect in patients with stable or rising GFR. Thus a larger sample size is often needed to detect the beneficial effect of the intervention.

However, there are limitations of time-to event analyses in clinical trials. First, the relative risk of doubling of serum creatinine or ESRD does not lead to a straightforward computation of the rate of decline in renal function, which may lead to difficulty in interpreting the effect size. Second, the relative risk of reaching the end-point principally reflects differences in proportion of patients with more rapidly declining renal function. Thus the relative risk may overestimate the effect size in patients with more slowly declining renal function. Third, time-to-event analysis is not applicable in cross-over studies.

APPLICATIONS AND CONCLUSIONS

Clinical Practice

Serum creatinine is easy to measure and is widely used as an index of renal function in clinical practice. In most circumstances, serum creatinine provides a rough estimate of the level of GFR and is adequate for clinical assessment of renal function. Because of the limitations of serum creatinine in the elderly and in patients with chronic renal disease, formulas based on serum creatinine and factors related to creatinine excretion, such as the Cockcroft and Gault equation or the MDRD Study equation, should be used to estimate the level of renal function. In malnourished or debilitated patients, these formulas may overestimate the level of renal function. In these individuals, as in patients not in the steady state, measurements of creatinine clearance or clearance of an exogenous filtration marker may be necessary if accurate assessment of renal function is necessary. Changes in serum creatinine, especially if they are large, provide adequate information to assess whether renal function is worsening or improving. However, the rate of change in serum creatinine does not accurately reflect the rate of change in GFR. In particular, substantial disease progression can occur despite a minimal increase or no increase in the serum creatinine. If an accurate estimate of disease progression is required, serial measurement of GFR using a radionuclide-labeled filtration marker is recommended. It is extremely difficult to predict the future rate of decline in GFR or the interval until the onset of ESRD. The level of renal function is not related to the subsequent rate of GFR decline. On average, patients with greater urine protein excretion have faster rates of disease progression, but neither the level of proteinuria nor other patient characteristics provide sufficient information to permit accurate predictions in individual patients with chronic renal disease. Over a long period, the rate of decline in renal function follows a roughly linear decline, but extrapolation of the slope to predict the interval until the onset of ESRD has not proven successful. In our view, knowledge of the previous rate of decline, in combination with clinical characteristics, can provide a rough idea of the prognosis but do not substitute for repetitive measurement and careful interpretation of serum creatinine.

Clinical Research

Determining the effect of therapeutic interventions requires randomized trials. Cross-over studies are not appropriate because of the possibility of nonlinear declines in renal function, breakpoints, and carry-over effects. Parallel studies require a large sample size and long duration of follow-up because of the slow mean rate and wide variability in progression rates in most chronic renal diseases. If the hypothesized beneficial effect is proportional to the underlying rate of renal function decline, a time-to-event analysis would have greater statistical power than a comparison of mean slopes. Doubling of serum creatinine has been a useful end-point in clinical trials of antihypertensive agents but has been misleading in clinical trials of dietary protein restriction. Studies using doubling of serum creatinine as the end-point should assess the effects of the proposed interventions on creatinine secretion and excretion. Irrespective of the type of statistical analysis, large, multicenter collaborative studies will be required for the conduct of clinical trials, in most cases, requiring prioritization of use of national resources.

APPENDIX: EVALUATION OF A DIAGNOSTIC TEST

Precision is defined by the degree of spread of a series of observations or the degree to which a variable has nearly the same value when measured multiple times. The relative spread of distributions can be compared using the coefficient of variation (CV), which is defined as the standard deviation divided by the mean.

Bias in a study is a systematic (nonrandom) deviation that leads to an incorrect conclusion. Therefore a study can be unbiased but have low precision and vice versa.

Accuracy reflects the degree to which a variable represents what it is supposed to represent. Accuracy encompasses both precision and unbiasedness. It is often defined as how the measure compares to a gold standard.

Sensitivity is the proportion of patients with the disease in whom the test is positive. It indicates how good the test is at identifying the diseased.

Specificity is the proportion of patients without the disease in whom the test is negative. It indicates how good the test is at identifying nondiseased.

Convenience is defined by technical difficulty, as well as the expense and risk of performing the measurement.

Regression to the mean is the tendency of an extreme value when it is remeasured to be closer to the mean, because the original value was likely to have been unduly influenced by random variation. As an example, consider patients selected for enrollment into a clinical trial because of more rapid decline in renal function. After enrollment, repeat measurement of the decline in renal function would reveal a less rapid mean decline because of random variation.

Acknowledgment

The authors are grateful to Tom Greene, Ph.D., whose contributions have influenced the development of the ideas expressed in this chapter.

Selected Readings

Hunsicker LG, Adler S, Caggiula A, et al. Predictors of progression of renal disease in the Modification of Diet in Renal Disease Study. *Kidney Int* 1997;51:1908–1919.

This article describes the univariate and multivariate analysis of factors that are predictive of renal function decline in the MDRD Study.

Levey AS. Measurement of renal function in chronic renal disease. *Kidney Int* 1990; 38:167–184.

This is a detailed review of the measurement of renal function in chronic renal disease. It describes GFR as an index of renal function, the relationship between GFR and the reciprocal of the serum creatinine, applications of the rate in decline in renal function in studies of the progression of renal disease, and the outlook for the future.

Levey AS, Gassman JJ, Hall P, et al. Assessing the progression of renal disease in clinical studies: effects of duration of follow-up and regression to the mean. *J Am Soc Nephrol* 1991;1:1087–1094.

This article emphasizes that the mean rate of decline of renal function is slow and that rates are highly variable amongst individuals. Precision of individual rates of decline in renal function are low but improve with follow-up. Regression to the mean explains a significant proportion of the observed change of rate of decline in renal function over time.

Levey AS, Greene T, Schluchter MD, et al. Glomerular filtration rate measurements in clinical trials. *J Am Soc Nephrol* 1993;4:1159–1171.

This study describes the utility and precision of using ^{125}I-iothalamate in the MDRD Study and the Diabetes Control and Complications Trial (DCCT). Intratest and intertest coefficients of variation and convenience of the technique are discussed.

Levey AS, Bosch JP, Coggins CH, et al. Effects of diet and antihypertensive therapy on creatinine clearance and serum creatinine concentration in the Modification of Diet in Renal Disease Study. *J Am Soc Nephrol* 1996;7:556–565.

This manuscript describes the variable effects of diet and different antihypertensives on tubular secretion of creatinine and creatinine excretion. Through the latter effects, diet and antihypertensives have different effects on plasma creatinine, creatinine clearance, and reciprocal plasma creatinine. The article explains how incorrect conclusions would have been obtained if creatinine clearance or reciprocal plasma creatinine, rather than GFR, were used as the measures of renal function.

Levey AS, Bosch JP, Breyer Lewis J, et al. A more accurate method to estimate glomerular filtration rate from serum creatinine: a new prediction equation. Modification of Diet in Renal Disease Study Group. *Ann Intern Med* 1999; 130(6):461–470.

This article describes an equation derived from the MDRD Study that can accurately predict GFR using plasma creatinine, age, gender, race, blood urea nitrogen, and serum albumin.

Meyer TW, Baboolal K, Brenner BM. Nephron adaptation to renal injury. In: *Brenner and Rector's the kidney*, 5th ed. Philadelphia: WB Saunders, 1996:2011–2048.

This chapter reviews the adaptive mechanisms of a nephron during chronic renal disease. This includes mechanisms to maintain total GFR (i.e., by increasing SNGFR) despite a decrease in the number of nephrons.

Mitch WE, Walser M, Buffington GA, et al. A simple method of estimating progression of chronic renal failure. *Lancet* 1976;2(7999):1326–1328.

This paper was the first to point out that in most patients reciprocal serum creatinine declines linearly as renal disease progresses.

Shah BV, Levey AS. Spontaneous changes in the rate of decline in reciprocal creatinine: errors in predicting the progression of renal disease from extrapolation of the slope. *J Am Soc Nephrol* 1992;2:1186–1191.

This paper emphasizes the frequency of breakpoints in the slope of reciprocal serum creatinine versus time. These breakpoints can cause both errors in assessing the effectiveness of therapy and in extrapolating the slope to predict the interval until the onset of end-stage renal disease.

Walser M. Progression of chronic renal failure in man. *Kidney Int* 1990;37: 1195–1210.

This article reviews quantitation of renal function and determinants of progression of renal disease. It also discusses the issue of whether all patients with chronic renal disease progress, the acute effects of protein restriction on GFR, and whether GFR decline progresses linearly. Finally, it discusses the design of clinical trials used to assess the effects of treatment on progression of chronic renal disease.

PART 2
Mechanisms

Mauro Abbate and Giuseppe Remuzzi

Patients with almost any form of renal disease are at risk of progressively declining renal function over variable periods of time. Risk factors and disease modifiers have been recognized and they are listed in Table 67.6. The rate of disease progression is relatively independent of the type of initial insult to the kidney and, to some extent, of the severity of renal damage actually seen by the pathologist at the time of the diagnosis. At one end of the spectrum, the kidney in renal syndromes, such as some forms of proliferative glomerulonephritis or acute tubular necrosis, recovers even spontaneously despite the presence of severe lesions, by effective processes of repair in the relatively short term. In other conditions, however, repair of a critical amount of nephrons may fail. Responsible for the consequent progressive destruction of nephron units that culminates in uremia are processes of inflammation and remodeling that occur in the renal parenchyma while replacing the function of the lost nephrons. These processes are shared by experimental and human progressive nephropathies and are accelerated if functioning units are low due to congenital or acquired nephron loss. That functional responses in the surviving nephrons are instrumental to perpetuate renal injury forms the basis of the "common pathway" theory of chronic renal disease progression elaborated in the early 1970s. Newer animal and human studies have indicated that central in this process can be an enhanced passage of proteins through the glomerular barrier as a consequence of persistent injury to the glomerular filtration compartment. Other coexisting factors have importance and include

TABLE 67.6. Factors Leading to Increased Risk of Progressive Renal Insufficiency

Renal lesion progression as a consequence of persistent immune insult to the glomerulus or disease gene abnormality
Coexisting modifiers of risk (infection, obstruction, drugs toxic to the kidney)
Systemic hypertension promoting glomerular capillary hypertension and hyperperfusion, in turn responsible for enhanced intrarenal traffic of protein and structural injury
Proteinuria
Low number of nephrons (congenital or resulting from extensive reduction of renal mass or nephropathy) and other factors (high-protein diet, diabetes) leading to glomerular hemodynamic changes and proteinuria
Hyperlipidemia
Metabolic factors facilitating tubulointerstitial injury (phosphate, calcium and urate deposition)
Others (cigarette smoking, male sex, African-American race)

systemic arterial hypertension, hyperlipidemia, and interstitial deposition of crystal and salts. This chapter approaches the topic of the mechanisms of renal progressive injury from the point of view that the common pathway determinants emerging from basic and experimental research, specifically glomerular capillary hypertension and hyperperfusion, abnormal intrarenal protein traffic, and consequent inflammatory and fibrogenic signalling, must be the primary targets of a strategy to arrest disease progression, together with targeting secondary amplifiers of risk commonly sought in clinical practice.

SYSTEMIC HYPERTENSION

A role for hypertension in the induction of renal damage was suggested 40 years ago in a long-term study on 500 patients diagnosed with arterial hypertension. Proteinuria was present in 42% of the patients, and chronic renal failure developed in 18%. Increased urinary excretion of albumin in arterial hypertension correlates with blood pressure levels and is decreased with antihypertensive therapy. There is a vicious circle relationship between systemic hypertension and deteriorating renal function. Secondary hypertension occurs early in many progressive renal diseases and is present in virtually all patients by the time renal replacement therapy is initiated. Findings from the Multiple Risk Factors Intervention Trial revealed that the risk of developing or dying of progressive renal failure was 22-fold higher in patients whose systolic blood pressure at screening averaged 210 mm Hg compared with those with values less than 120 mm Hg. It also showed that the risk correlated at intermediate levels of blood pressure. The high prevalence of proteinuria points to a role of hypertension in facilitating chronic renal injury. Tight control of blood pressure in accelerated hypertension preserves and may improve renal function. Reducing blood pressure to normal or near normal levels slows the rate of progression of renal failure in diabetic nephropathy and in many renal diseases.

The mechanisms by which increased blood pressure may play a contributory role in the progression of renal disease include injury to preglomerular arteries, leading to glomerular ischemia with progressive luminal narrowing and hence fall in glomerular blood flow. Glomerular sclerosis, however, is not prominent in rats with hypertension alone. In experimental models of essential hypertension, the increase in afferent arteriolar resistance attenuates the transmission of systemic hypertension to the glomerulus and may limit hypertension-induced renal injury. Studies of linkage analysis to localize genes responsible for blood pressure regulation and early onset renal failure in the fawn-hooded hypertensive rat model suggest that the "renal failure" genes (Rf-1 and Rf-2) responsible for renal damage are different from those influencing blood pressure or they act through an independent mechanism. Renal vessels and glomeruli appear susceptible to the adverse effects of systemic hypertension when there is proteinuria or when there is glomerular inflammation and vascular damage. In nephroangiosclerosis and diabetic nephropathy, the onset of *de novo* proteinuria, after a number of years of stable renal function, is an indicator of subsequent renal function decline.

Cellular mechanisms of hypertensive renal injury may partly overlap with those of vascular damage in severe arteriosclerosis and include endothelial dysfunction and increased permeability to plasma constituents mediated by angiotensin II, nitric oxide, endothelin, and growth factors. Concentrations of angiotensin II are often elevated in patients with hypertension. Hypertension has also proinflammatory actions, increasing the formation of hydrogen peroxide and free radicals. These include superoxide anion and hydroxyl radicals in plasma that reduce the formation of nitric oxide by the endothelium and increase leukocyte adhesion. In the glomerulus, the transmission of high levels of hydraulic blood pressure is thought to exacerbate preexisting increments of glomerular capillary pressure owing to compensation from nephron loss, reduced glomerular filtering area, or diabetic hyperfiltration.

GLOMERULAR CAPILLARY HYPERTENSION, HYPERPERFUSION, AND INJURY TO THE GLOMERULAR CAPILLARY

Role of Angiotensin II

The pathogenetic mechanisms of renal scarring after the loss of a critical amount of nephrons are thought to be unique to the kidney and probably account in large part for injury processes in the early stages of experimental renal disease progression. The common histologic lesions are glomerulosclerosis, atrophy of the renal tubules (which are surrounded by inflammatory cells and fibroblasts), and accumulation of extracellular matrix in the renal interstitium. In chronic proteinuric nephropathies, such lesions are indistinguishable from those resulting from a diversity of insults that primarily affect the glomerulus. Our knowledge of the underlying mechanisms of injury is derived primarily from experimental studies in the rat. One of the main models is the remnant kidney after reduction of renal mass performed by unilateral nephrectomy and removal or infarction of approximately two-thirds of the remaining kidney. Other disease models, including streptozotocin-induced diabetes, Heymann nephritis, and spontaneous glomerular sclerosis, have been widely investigated and share with the remnant kidney most of the functional and structural consequences of reducing the functional kidney mass, with differences inherent to specific features in each model. Such consequences are not unique to rodents. In humans, they are usually less obvious because of the slow time course, but in patients undergoing extensive surgical resection of renal mass for neoplasm, both the functional and structural changes are identical to those found in the rat model consistent with progression by nephron dropout. In all conditions, in addition to foci of diseased nephrons with contracted glomeruli and atrophic tubules foci of healthier but hypertrophied nephrons are also present and presumably carry a greater functional load.

When the number of nephrons is reduced to a critical extent, there is a compensatory increase in renal plasma flow and an increase in the amount of filtrate in each of the remaining nephrons. Increased flow rates result from a dilation of the afferent arteriole to a greater extent than the efferent arteriole, which is under the vasoconstrictive influence of angiotensin II. These changes in arteriolar tone produce an increase in the hydraulic pressure in the glomerular capillaries, with the subsequent increase in single-nephron glomerular filtration rate (GFR). The adaptive response while serving to maintain GFR in the failing kidney may be a maladaptive response in the long term and cause renal functional and structural damage.

Strong evidence in support of the pathogenetic role of changes in renal hemodynamics in progressive renal injury has been provided by seminal studies in rat models documenting that interventions that control glomerular hypertension effectively limit the decline of GFR and minimize structural damage. They include low-protein diets and angiotensin-converting enzyme (ACE) inhibitors. Low-protein diets, in addition to reducing the load of nitrogenous metabolic end-products, limit the adaptive changes in remnant nephrons and slow the tendency to renal disease progression. In addition to reducing intraglomerular capillary pressure more effectively than other antihypertensive drugs, ACE inhibitors protected rats with reduced renal mass or streptozotocin-induced diabetes from progressive renal injury.

Why should glomerular hypertension lead to progressive renal injury? One possible explanation is that the high glomerular capillary pressure impairs the permselective function of the glomerular filtration barrier, mimicking those diseases in which the initiating insults to the intact kidney lead to both proteinuria and chronic parenchymal injury. Other mechanisms and coexisting factors include enhanced angiotensin II generation, glomerular hypertrophy, mesangial stretching, and macrophage infiltration.

The presence of proteinuria or microalbuminuria serves as a marker of glomerular capillary hypertension even more than does systemic arterial hypertension. Several studies have documented that elevations in glomerular capillary pressure do enlarge the radius of the pores in the glomerular membrane, leading to impaired permselectivity for albumin. Acute increases in glomerular capillary pressure were accompanied by a sudden impairment of barrier-size selectivity in a model of renal vein obstruction. In a study aimed at mathematically dissociating hemodynamics from the intrinsic permeability properties of the membrane, structural modifications were required to explain findings of increased dextran clearances obtained upon increasing the glomerular pressure in passive Heymann nephritis.

In addition to mediating preferential constriction of the efferent arteriole and consequent glomerular capillary hypertension, angiotensin II increases the permeability of the glomerular barrier both in intact rat kidney and in isolated perfused kidney preparation. By implication, the mechanism underlying proteinuria in response to enhanced glomerular capillary pressure can be mediated at least in part by angiotensin II. Interestingly, angiotensin II also increases vascular permeability in other vascular beds. In the kidney, it appears that local generation of angiotensin II, possibly formed in excessive amounts during hemodynamic injury to the endothelium and physical stretching of the tuft, shifts glomerular unselective pores toward larger dimensions.

Angiotensin II influences other physiologic and cellular processes in the glomerulus whereby excessive angiotensin II formation or action may promote functional and structural injury. In conjunction with its effect to increase the permeability of the glomerular barrier, excess angiotensin II may promote injury by increasing macromolecular flux into the mesangium, thereby inciting cytokine release, glomerular cell proliferation and macrophage influx, and mesangial matrix formation. Under some conditions, angiotensin II may directly induce expression of transforming growth factor-β (TGF-β), which is thought to play a ubiquitous role in mediating extracellular matrix overproduction, raising the possibility that TGF-β is an alternative target of ACE inhibitors in addition to their beneficial hemodynamic and antiproteinuric actions.

Glomerular hypertension in the remnant kidney is associated with perturbation of endothelial cell function and structure following the early hypertrophic response of the glomerulus. The glomerular endothelium is a potential cellular source of TGF-β along with other cytokines and growth factors [platelet-derived growth factor (PDGF) and basic fibroblast growth factor (bFGF)] inducible by angiotensin II. Endothelial cells, particularly in the dilated capillaries, expressed angiotensinogen and TGF-β1 mRNAs, as well as fibronectin and laminin β1 mRNA transcripts. Such expression became prominent and more diffuse over time, particularly for matrix protein mRNAs in the regions of evolving sclerosis, and it was blocked by treatment of animals with angiotensin II–receptor antagonists.

Finally, enhanced renal angiotensin II possibly by activation of nuclear factor κB (NF-κB)-dependent intracellular signalling may activate the transcription of chemoattractant cytokines, thus facilitating leukocyte infiltration at the glomerular site of excess angiotensin II production. Angiotensin II stimulates endothelial cells to upregulate the synthesis of RANTES, a mononuclear cell chemoattractant. In the glomerulus, such effect may favor mononuclear cell recruitment and activation, leading to synthesis of additional permeabilizing factors and of prosclerosing cytokines. One study found that angiotensin II also increases MCP-1 mRNA expression through NF-κB activation in mesangial cells. NF-κB–dependent gene transcription is part of a putative common pathway mechanism for the induction of cellular responses in the glomerulus as well as the tubulointerstitium.

Hypertrophy and Mesangial Stretching

Glomerular enlargement, which almost invariably accompanies augmented glomerular hemodynamics during the adaptive response of the kidney to nephron loss, precedes and may predispose to glomerular scarring. However, hypertrophy was dissociated from both altered glomerular hemodynamics and glomerulosclerosis by experimental maneuvers or in certain strains of rats. Thus a substantial body of data supports the notion that the hemodynamic determinant is central in disease progression and that glomerular hypertrophy is a coexisting factor that may exacerbate injury. Hypertrophy may damage the glomerulus by increasing wall tension proportional to the increase in the glomerular capillary radius. The precise cellular mechanisms by which glomerular enlargement may concur to glomerular injury have not been clarified yet. Interestingly, glomerular hypertrophy per se may have a role in the induction of injury in some disease models even independent of altered glomerular hemodynamics. Capillary distension may lead to deposition of hyaline material. This is associated with damage of the visceral glomerular epithelial cells consisting of vacuolization, hyalin droplet formation, and cell detachment from the basement membrane, thus predisposing to local formation of capsular adhesions, mesangial expansion, and sclerotic lesions.

In the condition of altered glomerular hemodynamics, it has been postulated that expansion of the glomerular capillaries and stretching of the mesangium in response to glomerular hypertension might be a force that translates high glomerular capillary pressure into increased mesangial matrix formation. Various cell culture systems have been developed to address the question of whether mechanical stimuli due to glomerular capillary hypertension may lead to glomerular structural injury. Part of these studies point to the hypothesis that increased glomerular capillary pressure and plasma flow rates alter the growth and activity of glomerular cells, inducing the elaboration or expression of cytokines and other mediators, which then stimulate mesangial matrix production and promote structural injury. Hemodynamic physical forces, such as pulsatile pressure, changes in blood flow, and shear stress, may increase the activity or expression of a number of prosclerosing mediators, possibly still mediated by angiotensin II. Thus controlling glomerular hypertension ameliorates the production of mediators, which would include TGF-β1, PDGF, and endothelin. It is unknown whether a "common pathway" type of signalling can be responsible for such putative response and to what extent this might be dissociated from enhanced protein traffic as an additional target to the action of antihypertensive and antiproteinuric therapy with ACE inhibitors. An intriguing possibility is that TGF-β is an effector of injury promoted by glomerular capillary hypertension. In support of this, cyclic mechanical stretching of cultured mesangial cells upregulates the expression of TGF-β, linking glomerular hypertension to the generation of a common putative factor of mesangial matrix overproduction. In contrast to other consequences of glomerular hypertension, fluid shear stress seems to be essential to adaptation of nephron loss at least in the early time, as suggested by the finding that in mice lacking vimentin, in which shear stress was impaired, subtotal nephrectomy was lethal.

Increased Glomerular Permeability to Macromolecules

The breach of the glomerular barrier to protein is perhaps the most threatening consequence of increased glomerular capillary pressure. Importantly, a sustained passage of excessive amounts of protein through the altered glomerular membrane is the common feature of experimental models characterized by glomerular hemodynamic changes as well as almost any form of chronic progressive nephropathy following a primary insult to the glomerular filtration barrier (Fig. 67.6). There is a ubiquitous association between injury to the glomerular capillary filter, proteinuria, and progressive renal failure. Remarkable exceptions are minimal-change disease and certain experimental diseases, all of which share self-limited proteinuria and no progression to renal failure.

Certain studies suggested that abnormally filtered proteins have intrinsic renal toxicity, which perhaps is a key factor of disease progression when the primary immune or nonimmune insult to the kidney has ceased. Aging is associated with progressive proteinuria and glomerulosclerosis, which lead to renal insufficiency in certain strains of rats. Interestingly, the degree of proteinuria predicts the development of renal damage. Rats with urinary protein excretion values of less than 60 mg/day had no glomerular sclerotic lesions in the kidney, whereas rats with urinary protein excretion values of more than 100 mg/day during the same period had glomerulosclerosis and tubulointerstitial changes proportional to the severity of proteinuria. Several studies in other rat models, including the remnant kidney, revealed a close link between abnormal permeability of the glomerular capillary barrier to proteins and the subsequent renal structural injury. Examples are streptozotocin-induced diabetes, the BioBreeding/Worchester (BB/W) rat, and the spontaneous nephropathy of Zucker rats. Of interest, the extent of tubulointerstitial injury correlated with the proportion of glomeruli showing reabsorption droplets in podocytes, taken as a marker of enhanced protein traffic across the altered glomerular capillary wall.

Finally, support to the pathogenic potential of enhanced protein filtration has been derived from the evidence in a diversity of models that the renoprotective effect of low-protein diets or pharmacologic manipulation with ACE inhibitors cannot be dissociated from their ability to limit proteinuria as well as the underlying defect of the glomerular permselective barrier. Besides the remnant kidney or streptozotocin-induced diabetes typically characterized by altered glomerular hemodynamics, this was also observed in aging rats, male MWF/Ztm rats, and passive Heymann nephritis. In all models, proteinuria is the earliest sign of injury to the glomerular capillary barrier, preceding the onset of structural lesions.

The mechanisms underlying the permselective defect that are interrupted by ACE inhibitor therapy are not clear. Data in the male MWF/Ztm rat model indicate that ACE inhibitors may prevent abnormalities in the cellular distribution or expression of ZO-1 and presumably other functional proteins normally associated with the slit diaphragm, a key component of the glomerular filtration barrier provided by the podocyte. Possibly relevant to the permselective function of the glomerular barrier, ACE inhibitors also reduce the expression of extracellular matrix components, both in experimental diabetes and in immunologic models of massive proteinuria of immune origin.

More steps are being taken in understanding the cellular mechanisms that may mediate detrimental effects of filtered proteins on the kidney. We mainly summarize experimental data supporting the possibility that the abnormal transit of plasma proteins into the tubule induces functional abnormalities of proximal tubular cells, including the overexpression of proinflammatory and vasoactive mediators.

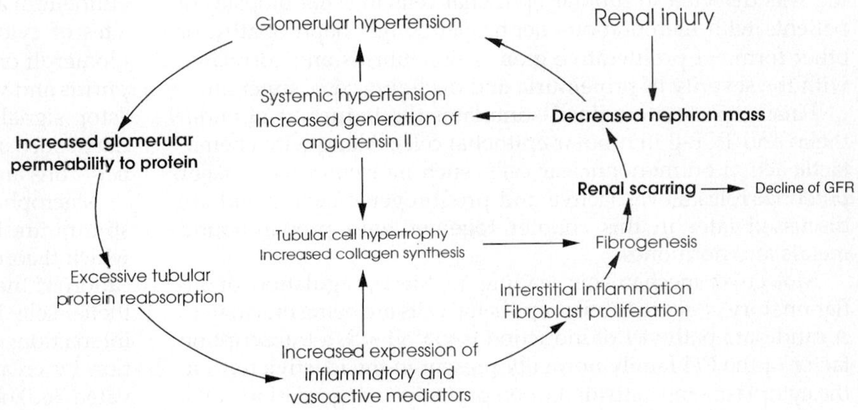

Figure 67.6. Schematic representation of mechanisms that may perpetuate renal damage in progressive renal disease initiated by injury to the glomerular barrier to protein or after renal mass ablation.

Insights were derived from findings that in the kidneys of proteinuric rats with adriamycin nephrosis the accumulation of filtered proteins in the cytoplasm of proximal tubular cells and in luminal casts was associated with focal breaking of the tubular basement membrane and extravasation of the tubular content into the renal interstitium. Such alterations were taken to reflect events of protein overload of tubular epithelial cells, which may have a role in the induction of interstitial injury. A cause-and-effect relationship between protein traffic and interstitial inflammation was also suggested by studies in models of protein overload proteinuria. Repeated injections of albumin, which is then filtered in large amounts, did cause tubulointerstitial lesions and renal scarring. Excessive proteinuria can also be induced in rats by transplanting a pituitary tumor that causes liver hyperplasia with overproduction of albumin and consequent hyperalbuminuria, followed by tubular damage and interstitial inflammation.

High concentrations of albumin and other less abundant plasma proteins in proximal tubular lumen effectively transmit to the tubular epithelial cells information of an increased passage of protein across the perturbed glomerular filter, which can elicit an inflammatory response independently of the nature of the primary insult to the glomerulus. Highlights have been provided by *in vitro* studies with proximal tubular cells maintaining a polarized phenotype such that the cellular effects of apical exposure to ultrafiltered protein can be assessed. Thus albumin, transferrin, or immunoglobulin G (IgG) stimulates proximal tubular epithelial cells in culture to upregulate monocyte chemoattractant protein 1 (MCP-1), one of the most powerful mononuclear cell attractants characterized so far. The RANTES gene displayed the same type of gene upregulation and chemokine secretion mainly polarized toward the basal compartment of the cultured cells.

Effects on chemokines were not confined to *in vitro* studies. Indeed, other reports indicate that the same pathways of chemokine induction by ultrafiltered protein are activated in the renal tubule and predictably induce the relevant cellular responses in the interstitium in experimental nephropathies. Enhanced MCP-1 mRNA expression was localized to proximal tubules in rats with protein overload proteinuria or immune nephrosis. In puromycin nephrosis, an anti–MCP-1 antibody attenuated macrophage infiltration.

Other genes are upregulated in kidneys upon protein challenge, including the proinflammatory glycoprotein osteopontin, which may play important roles in tubulointerstitial injury in various models. The osteopontin gene was upregulated in the kidneys of rats with protein overload proteinuria. Cells showing positive intracellular staining for both IgG and osteopontin were surrounded by inflammatory infiltrates of macrophages, suggesting that protein overreabsorption may cause osteopontin-dependent macrophage recruitment. Increased osteopontin staining was detected in tubular epithelial cells in renal biopsies of patients with membranous nephropathy, IgA nephropathy, or other forms of proliferative glomerulonephritis and correlated with the severity of proteinuria and declining renal function.

Finally, protein overload stimulates the induction of endothelin and TGF-β in tubular epithelial cells. Along with chemotactic action on mononuclear cells, such molecules have major potential roles as vasoactive and profibrogenic factors and are discussed later in this chapter together with protein-bound metals and hormones.

Molecular mechanisms leading to the upregulation of inflammatory genes in tubular epithelial cells are being elucidated. A candidate pathway of induction is via NF-κB, a transcription factor of the Rel family normally present in the inactive form in the cytoplasm and activated upon proteolytic degradation of the inhibitory molecule I-*k*B. In proximal tubular cells, increasing concentrations of albumin caused a dose-dependent increase in NF-*k*B that was abolished by blocking I-*k*B degradation.

Complement factors can be filtered across the altered glomerular barrier and form deposits (C3, C5b-9) along the luminal side of proximal tubular cells in rats with protein overload nephropathy, aminonucleoside nephrosis, and remnant kidneys, a pattern that is observed in the kidneys of patients with nonselective proteinuria and that correlates with urinary complement excretion. Components of the complement cascade from C3 to C9 after ultrafiltration can be activated and generate C5b-9 membrane attack complex. Proximal tubular cells possess alternative pathway activity that *in vitro* mediates the assembly of the components of C5b-9 complex on the plasma membrane, followed by synthesis of inflammatory cytokines such as interleukin (IL)-6 and tumor necrosis factor-α (TNF-α).

C3 may have additional and independent proinflammatory actions in proteinuric settings. The renal tubulointerstitium is likely to be susceptible to C3-dependent injury due to a relative lack of complement regulatory proteins. In addition to activating exogenous complement, proximal tubular cells can synthesize C3. Other studies suggest that both functional properties of C3 activation and local C3 synthesis in proximal tubular cells are in a unique pathway to mediate interstitial injury in response to protein load. The possibility that the activation of C3 may occur at tubular sites, in which protein traffic and reabsorption are enhanced, is suggested by findings of colocalization of C3 and other ultrafiltered proteins in proximal tubular cells in rats after 5/6 renal mass ablation. A soluble form of recombinant human complement receptor type 1 (sCR1) that inhibits complement activation by decay acceleration of C3 convertase reduced tubulointerstitial cell infiltration and injury in rats with aminonucleoside of nephrosis or anti-Thy1.1 nephritis.

INTERSTITIAL INFLAMMATION

The accumulation of mononuclear cells into the renal interstitium is a common feature of diseases evolving to progressive renal scarring and loss of function. In humans with diabetic or nondiabetic renal diseases, the degree of tubulointerstitial infiltration of monocytes and lymphocytes have predictive value along with proteinuria in determining the rate of progression. Studies in animal models have found that an influx of mononuclear cells into the interstitium occurs in the relative early stage of progressive disease in primarily nonimmune or immune glomerulopathies as well as in rats with remnant kidneys. Responsible for the initial accumulation of mononuclear cells into the interstitium are chemoattractant molecules and cytokines released by resident parenchymal cells. Current evidence, as discussed previously, indicates that a major source is the tubular epithelium after a primary insult to the glomerulus. Additional sites of cytokine synthesis may include persistently inflamed glomeruli or vessel walls usually seen in chronic glomerulonephritis and vascular disease. Much less is known about whether "stop signals" of repair exist and whether inflammatory reactions, once initiated, inevitably causes destruction of individual nephrons and adjacent parenchyma.

Macrophages and lymphocytes once recruited into the interstitium are in turn a source of cytokines and growth factors, which theoretically participate in the maintenance and amplification of the inflammatory reaction. Studies with tubular epithelial cells in culture have suggested that leukocyte–epithelial interactions would play a contributory role in renal inflammation by creating amplification loops. IL-1α, a product of activated leukocytes, which is predictably released by recruited cells into the interstitium, can stimulate tubular epithelial cells in culture to produce the cytokine TNF-α. Another cytokine of lymphocyte origin, interferon-γ (IFN-γ), stimulated human tubular epithelial cells to produce inflammatory molecules such as IL-6, granulocyte-macrophage colony-stimulating factor (GM-CSF), and PDGF.

Specific functions of T lymphocytes are antigen recognition by T-cell surface-antigen receptors and induction of inflammation at the recognition sites. In immune nephritis, this can occur as a consequence of intrarenal processing of self epitopes. It is unclear whether T cells may interact specifically with other immune or renal cell types in the environment of those nephrons carrying a greater functional load or exposed to the signalling of persistent glomerular injury. The trigger for local lymphocyte activation is the interaction of peptide epitope–MHC-II complexes at the surface of dendritic cells or other antigen-presenting cells with the T-cell receptors at the surface of lymphocytes. Interestingly, infiltrating inflammatory and immune cells at tubular sites of protein reabsorption express high levels of MHC class II antigen in rats with passive Heymann nephritis, as well as in the remnant kidney in which a primary immune mechanism can be excluded. Both in experimental and in human nephropathies, interstitial infiltrates contain cells with dendritic phenotype, which may imply roles for these highly immunogenic cells in capturing and processing antigens and initiate responses in the kidney. In rats with a remnant kidney, the increase in urinary protein excretion over time was associated with interstitial infiltration of cells positive for a rat dendritic cell marker, macrophages, CD4+ cells, and CD8+ cells, and MHC II upregulation in the kidney. Cells positive for p55, a dendritic cell-associated antigen, were detected in the cellular infiltrates in renal biopsies in patients with severe interstitial disease associated with focal segmental glomerulosclerosis or diabetic nephropathy, similar to the pattern found in patients with acute renal allograft rejection or chronic pyelonephritis.

Other studies addressed the possibility that immune-dependent mechanisms contribute to severe renal injury in proteinuric rats. Given in combination with ACE inhibitors, the immunosuppressive drug mycophenolate mofetil suppresses interstitial inflammation and immune injury after extensive renal mass reduction, despite the nonimmune nature of the primary insult. Source of self epitopes may include endogenous cellular proteins normally cryptic to the immune system or endocytosed ultrafiltered proteins that are processed and presented in association with MHC II molecules to T cells either directly by the tubular cells or after release into the interstitium. Key interactions between antigen-presenting cells and the lymphocyte are mediated by costimulatory molecules such as CD40L or ICAM1. Proximal tubular cells express these molecules, and ICAM1 was consistently upregulated in kidneys in experimental and human progressive nephropathies.

Inflammatory cells can profoundly perturb the interaction of tubular cells, fibroblasts, and interstitial matrix, facilitating fibrogenesis and nephron loss back to glomerular sites of altered hemodynamics and protein filtration. In the remnant kidney, the initial wave of inflammation is associated with the initial change in fibroblast phenotype, interstitial cell proliferation, and early progressive interstitial accumulation of collagen I and IV, laminin, and fibronectin. In less rapidly progressive models of renal disease, an influx of macrophages and lymphocytes commonly precedes fibrosis and tubular atrophy in the long term. T lymphocytes and macrophages driven into the interstitium by chemoattractant proteins of tubular cell origin or other sources at different stages may synthesize and secrete fibrogenic cytokines such as TGF–β, IL-4, and TNF-α, which act as stimuli for interstitial fibroblast mitogenesis, migration, and phenotypic change to myofibroblast, a characteristic phenotype associated with exuberant scar formation. T lymphocytes, by releasing IL-2, can also stimulate macrophages to secrete growth factors (TGF-β, PDGF). In turn, interstitial cells can produce regulatory molecules such as SPARC (secreted protein acidic and rich in cysteine), which might have a role in resolution of injury. Macrophage overproduction of tissue inhibitors of metalloproteinases (TIMPs) eventually leads to decreased matrix degradation. Such events can spread to the periglomerular regions, and the intact parenchyma, particularly in the presence of abnormal extracellular matrix, and this may thereafter promote lesion progression independently of continuing inflammation.

Epithelial-Fibroblast Interactions and Phenotypic Alterations Leading to End-Stage Accumulation of Extracellular Matrix and Remodeling

Proteins of the extracellular matrix by accumulating within the interstitial space substantially contribute to alter the normal tubulointerstitial architecture. Collagen types I and III, fibronectin, laminin, and various proteoglycans are the main components of the expanding interstitial matrix. Both the increased synthesis and decreased degradation play important roles in this process. The renal interstitial fibroblast is thought to be the main cellular effector of matrix synthesis and overproduction. However, several other studies have documented that the recruited inflammatory cells and the tubular epithelium can play crucial roles in the early steps of interstitial fibrogenesis. An important concept is that the early inflammation and matrix overproduction are potentially reversible, and if the common signalling pathways were interrupted by effective therapy, actual regression of lesions can be anticipated.

Studies with cultured cells and in experimental models found evidence that the proximal tubular cells synthesize profibrogenic cytokines, which in turn activate a collagen-producing phenotype of interstitial fibroblasts. In the remnant kidney, signals for such synthesis can be delivered by mediators of the adaptive response to nephron loss. The increase in the synthesis of angiotensin II by the kidney as a result of injury may lead to an increase in the expression of the gene for TGF-β in tubular cells, eventually inducing hypertrophy of these cells and increasing the synthesis of type IV collagen. Importantly, both after extensive reduction of the renal mass and in chronic proteinuric glomerulopathies, other fibrogenic stimuli, such as endothelin, insulinlike growth factor-I (IGF-I) or complement factors, are generated in proximal tubular epithelial cells. These mediators can substantially contribute to renal scarring along with other growth-promoting factors and profibrogenic stimuli of inflammatory cell origin. Proximal tubular epithelial cells generate effective signals to neighbouring cortical fibroblasts in coculture and conditioned media experiments. In response to TGF-β and PDGF released from the tubular cells, fibroblasts proliferate, synthesize collagen, and release matrix degrading enzymes (metalloproteinases). Such early kind of activation in some experimental models is followed by overexpression of protease inhibitors, such as tissue inhibitor of metalloproteinases (TIMP1) and plasminogen activator inhibitors (PAI1), resulting in enzyme suppression and additional accumulation of excess matrix proteins.

Endothelin (ET-1) was initially studied both as a candidate stimulus for fibroblast proliferation and matrix production and because of its chemotactic properties. ET can bind specifically to receptors at the cell surface of renal interstitial fibroblasts. Human fibroblasts respond to ET-1 by proliferation and new synthesis of matrix. Interestingly, ET can also stimulate the transcription of the α-smooth muscle actin gene via activation of *cis*-acting elements in the promoter in smooth muscle cells, a pattern of induction that in fibroblasts and other cell types is associated with myofibroblast phenotype and collagen overproduction. Finally, ET by virtue of its vasoactive properties can promote ischemic injury, in turn leading to imbalance of matrix degrading enzymes and their inhibitors and consequently less degradation of matrix.

One potent stimulus to endothelin gene activation and secretion toward the basolateral compartment of tubular cells is luminal protein exposure. Such response contributes to progressive renal injury. In passive Heymann nephritis, proximal tubular epithelial cells were a major site of ET-1 synthesis. After renal mass ablation, renal ET-1 gene expression and urinary excretion of the peptide increased over time, along with increasing proteinuria and tubulointerstitial damage. ET-1 mRNA expression was detectable in tubular epithelial cells during the early proteinuric stage. Subsequent severe proteinuria was associated with an additional increase in tubular ET-1 mRNA expression and severe tubulointerstitial damage. In the kidneys of rats made diabetic by streptozotocin, ET-1 mRNA levels were also increased in parallel with the progression of nephropathy. Importantly, blocking the ET-1 receptor with a specific antagonist prevented renal structural damage. The ETA–ETB receptor antagonist bosentan exerted similar beneficial effects. Another gene relevant to fibrogenic stimulation is TGF-β, now ubiquitously recognized as putative central mediator of wound healing and tissue scarring. The exposure of proximal tubular epithelial cells to albumin caused upregulation of TGF-β mRNA expression. However, the role of TGF-β, either of tubular cell or inflammatory cell origin, has been studied in a rat model of glomerulonephritis in which injury is usually nonprogressive. In proximal tubular cells, TGF-β may simultaneously inhibit chemokine and complement synthesis. Thus TGF-β, while upregulating IL-8 production in proximal tubular cells *in vitro,* downregulated MCP-1 and the complement components C3 and C4.

Complement components and protein-bound hormones can promote fibrogenesis. In human tubular epithelial cells in culture, C5b-9 MAC stimulated the synthesis of fibronectin driven by the cyclic adenosine monophosphate (cAMP)–responsive element of the gene. After filtration, IGF-I dissociates from binding proteins and stimulates mitogenesis and synthesis of collagen type I and IV in proximal tubular cells. Such effects were retained by the tubular fluid collected from nephrotic rats and were partially prevented by neutralizing IGF-I receptor antibodies.

An emerging concept in organ fibrosis is the conversion of epithelial cells to a fibroblast phenotype at sites of injury. In models of progressive nephropathy and human glomerulonephritis, tubular epithelial cells express α-smooth muscle actin, a form of actin expressed in the myofibroblast. Mouse tubular epithelial cells, after transfection with the gene for the fibroblast specific protein (FSP-1), showed signs of differentiation to a fibroblastlike phenotype with loss of an epithelial specific protein and gain of vimentin expression. *De novo* expression of FSP-1 became detectable in the tubular epithelium of mice with persistent renal inflammation elicited by anti–basement membrane antibodies. The conversion of tubular cells to fibroblast phenotype is a presumptive step of tubular atrophy in areas of inflammation and fibrogenesis. TGF-β and possibly PDGF, IGF-I, and ET may act as inducers. However, changes in phenotype with *de novo* expression of FSP-1 occurred in the absence of stimulating factors in three-dimensional gels, enforcing the notion that in some stages the altered matrix directly transduces fibrogenic signals through the cell membrane.

The extracellular matrix influences functional properties of many cell types, including the renal tubular epithelial cell and the fibroblast. For example, fibronectin acts as a chemotactic stimulus for fibroblasts, is an adhesive protein, and provides a scaffold for collagen deposition. Different matrix components on which the renal tubular cells and fibroblasts were cocultured (collagen IV, laminin) influenced differentially matrix turnover. One major question for future studies is whether the altered extracellular matrix surrounding individual nephrons after sustained glomerular damage or inflammation becomes itself a source of signals for changes in epithelial cell and fibroblast phenotype, perpetuating tubular atrophy and nephron destruction.

Finally, tubular atrophy and interstitial fibrogenesis can proceed in parallel with phenotypic changes within the glomerulus, including myofibroblast formation from resident glomerular cells, and they converge at the sites of evolving sclerosis. In the remnant kidney model, the glomerular overexpression of PDGF-B chain and upregulation of the PDGF receptor b-subunit may have importance in mesangial cell proliferation concomitant to downstream tubulointerstitial events. Inflammatory cells and interstitial fibroblasts can theoretically migrate from sites of recruitment or proliferation and propagate cytokine signalling and consequent parenchymal injury. Phenotypic changes and architectural remodeling eventually lead to expansion of interstitial space and obliteration of postglomerular capillaries, ischemic injury, and tubular destruction typical of irreversible nephron loss and declining GFR.

HOW THERAPEUTIC TRIALS HAVE SUPPORTED THE HYPOTHESIS OF PROGRESSION

The evidence that ACE inhibitors effectively slowed the GFR decline in experimental nephropathies opened the way to clinical trials and to studies specifically designed to clarify the possible underlying mechanisms of renoprotective action in humans. A landmark trial on more than 400 proteinuric patients concluded that the ACE inhibitor therapy can slow the rate of decline of the GFR in insulin-dependent diabetes. Hypertension was not an entry requirement. The ACE inhibitor exerted a marked antiproteinuric action and caused a minimal difference in the reduction in blood pressure (2 or 3 mm Hg) compared with placebo. Other studies and metaregression analysis in type II diabetes suggested that part of the renoprotective effect could reflect favorable changes in glomerular hemodynamics equivalent to those produced by ACE inhibitors in animal studies.

A meta-analysis of studies of nondiabetic renal disease found that ACE inhibitors reduced the risk of progressing to end-stage renal failure by about 30%. However, it was not clear whether the risk reduction was an effect of better blood pressure control than in conventional therapy groups. The same question was left unanswered in a study on 583 patients with renal insufficiency due to various nephropathies, in which a better control of blood pressure by ACE inhibitors reduced the number of patients at risk of doubling of the baseline serum creatinine.

Insights into the mechanisms underlying renoprotection with tight control of blood pressure have emerged from secondary analysis of data in the Modification of Diet in Renal Disease (MDRD) trial, designed to assess the effects of dietary protein intake or blood pressure control on the rates of GFR decline in 840 nondiabetics with chronic renal failure. Over the entire study period, the decline in the GFR that occurs immediately after the institution of blood pressure control was reversible and therefore consistent with hemodynamically mediated effects. Importantly, however, the correlation between higher mean blood pressures during follow-up and steeper decline in the GFR depended on the level of baseline proteinuria, becoming apparent at about 98 mm Hg in patients with baseline proteinuria of 0.25 to 3 g/24 hr, and 92 mm Hg in patients with baseline proteinuria of more than 3 g/24 hr. The results of the MDRD study together with a body of evidence from other clinical studies have generated consensus that proteinuria is the most potent independent risk factor for renal disease progression in humans.

Unlike previous trials, the Ramipril Efficacy in Nephropathy (REIN) study was designed to formally address whether glomerular protein traffic influenced renal disease progression and whether an ACE inhibitor was superior to conventional therapy, at comparable blood pressure control, in reducing proteinuria, limiting GFR decline, and preventing end-stage renal failure. The decline of the GFR was found to correlate with the degree of proteinuria, and this phenomenon was independent of the nature of the underlying disease or blood pressure. Remarkably, in patients with proteinuria of 3 g/24 hr or more, the ACE inhibitor ramipril reduced the risk of doubling serum creatinine or end-stage renal failure as compared with other antihypertensive drugs at the same level of blood pressure control. The results of the REIN follow-up trial indicate that if the treatment period is long enough (36 months or longer) in patients with heavy proteinuria, the ACE inhibitor can reverse the tendency of the GFR to decline and halt the disease progression to terminal renal failure. Consistent with evidence from animal models, in patients with diabetes or IgA nephropathy, ACE inhibitors lowered the mean dimensions of unselective pores, thus reinforcing the possibility that the superior effect of the ACE inhibitor is due to amelioration of the glomerular barrier size-selective function.

Selected Readings

Anderson S, Rennke HG, Brenner BM. Therapeutic advantage of converting enzyme inhibitors in arresting progressive renal disease associated with systemic hypertension in the rat. *J Clin Invest* 1986;77:1993–2000.

The original report of the protective effect of ACE inhibitors against progressive renal disease.

Brenner BM, Meyer TW, Hostetter TH. Dietary protein intake and the progressive nature of kidney disease: the role of hemodynamically mediated glomerular injury in the pathogenesis of progressive glomerular sclerosis in aging, renal ablation, and intrinsic renal disease. *N Engl J Med* 1982;307:652–659.

The first unifying hypothesis suggesting that renal diseases can progress via "common pathway" mechanisms of injury linked to glomerular hemodynamic changes which prove maladaptive.

Eddy AA. Expression of genes that promote renal interstitial fibrosis in rats with proteinuria. *Kidney Int* 1996;49(Suppl 54):S49–S54.

A detailed review of the cellular and molecular mechanisms of inflammation and fibrosis in models of proteinuric nephropathies.

Ketteler M, Noble NA, Border WA. Transforming growth factor-beta and angiotensin II: the missing link from glomerular hyperfiltration to glomerulosclerosis? *Annu Rev Physiol* 1995;57:279–295.

The authors provide a commentary on the putative role of TGF-β as a common pathway mediator of renal scarring.

Nomura A, Morita Y, Maruyama S, et al. Role of complement in acute tubulointerstitial injury of rats with aminonucleoside nephrosis. *Am J Pathol* 1997;151: 539–547.

Demonstration that the treatment with soluble recombinant complement receptor (sCR1) attenuates the severity of tubulointerstitial injury associated with proteinuria at least partially by inhibiting complement activation in proximal tubular cells.

Remuzzi G, Bertani T. Pathophysiology of progressive nephropathies. *N Engl J Med* 1998;339:1448–1456.

A comprehensive review of the effect of increased glomerular permeability to proteins on progressive renal injury and of relevant clinical studies in diabetic and nondiabetic nephropathies.

Riser BL, Cortes P, Heilig C, et al. Cyclic stretching force selectively up-regulates transforming growth factor-beta isoforms in cultured rat mesangial cells. *Am J Pathol* 1996;148:1915–1923.

An interesting study demonstrating that mechanical stretching can be a force that stimulates mesangial cells in culture to selectively release and activate TGF-β1, possibly leading to enhanced extracellular matrix synthesis in the setting of loss of glomerular pressure autoregulation.

Ruggenenti P, Perna A, Gherardi G, et al, on behalf of GISEN. Renal function and requirement for dialysis in chronic nephropathy patients on long-term ramipril: REIN follow-up trial. *Lancet* 1998;352:1252–1256.

Evidence that in patients with heavy proteinuria that ACE inhibitors can reverse the tendency of GFR to decline and halt the disease progress to renal failure.

Wang Y, Chen J, Chen L, et al. Induction of monocyte chemoattractant protein-1 in proximal tubule cells by urinary protein. *J Am Soc Nephrol* 1997;8:1537–1545.

An important study in support of the notion that ultrafiltered protein is a "common pathway" stimulus for chemokine signalling in proximal tubular cells that may promote interstitial inflammation in chronic proteinuric nephropathies.

Zoja C, Liu X-H, Abbate M, et al. Angiotensin II blockade limits tubular protein overreabsorption and the consequent upregulation of endothelin 1 gene in experimental membranous nephropathy. *Exp Nephrol* 1998;6:121–131.

Evidence that limiting protein traffic with an angiotensin II–receptor antagonist given to proteinuric rats while reducing proteinuria prevents the upregulation of the endothelin gene and preserves the structural integrity of the kidney in the long term.

Zoja C, Morigi M, Figliuzzi M, et al. Proximal tubular cell synthesis and secretion of endothelin-1 on challenge with albumin and other proteins. *Am J Kidney Dis* 1995;26:934–941.

The first demonstration that a protein challenge can stimulate proximal tubular epithelial cells to release vasoactive and profibrogenic substances into the medium at the basal aspect of the cell.

PART 3
Therapeutic Interventions

Francis J. Kelly and Sharon Anderson

Progressive renal injury is associated with high rates of morbidity and mortality as a consequence of end-stage renal disease (ESRD). Recognizing the pathogenesis of progressive renal injury is key to rational intervention. Since the early 1980s, the development of first micropuncture techniques, and later sophisticated cell biologic and molecular techniques, has enabled investigators to more clearly define the mechanisms of progressive renal injury, which are discussed in Part 2 of this chapter. Understanding of the basic mechanisms of disease has led to the development and study of rational therapeutic interventions. As experimental studies and clinical trials reveal effective interventions to slow the progression of renal disease, nephrologists and particularly primary care providers need to understand and use these strategies at the earliest possible stages, before irrevocable renal injury is present. To provide patients with the best chance for prolonged renal survival, some useful interventions have been identified, interventions that are effective and well-tolerated by the patients. Until the late 1980s, many attempted clinical trials were fraught with the hazards of incomplete patient compliance and participation and inadequate or controversial methods for assessing changes in glomerular filtration rate (GFR) and rates of progression. However, newer, well-designed clinical trials, as well as meta-analyses, are providing guidance as to effective therapeutic strategies. This chapter defines progress in three general categories: antihypertensive therapy, dietary interventions, and other pharmacologic approaches.

ANTIHYPERTENSIVE THERAPY

An important risk factor contributing to the acceleration of renal disease is systemic hypertension, which may be both a cause and a consequence of chronic renal disease. Patients with chronic renal failure exhibit not only higher blood pressures but also loss of the usual nocturnal blood pressure decline, so the mechanisms of hypertensive injury are more continuously operable. Clinically, faster rates of decline in renal function were noted in the most hypertensive patients in several large, prospective studies, including the MRFIT study and the Hypertension Detection and Follow-Up Program trial. Hypertension may also initiate renal disease; the incidence of ESRD presumably secondary to essential hypertension is considerable, particularly in African-Americans.

Level of Blood Pressure Reduction

The first important question relates to the blood pressure goal; that is, how far should blood pressure be lowered to afford maximal renal protection? Current evidence clearly indicates that traditional blood pressure targets (140/90 mm Hg) are too conservative in patients at risk. The Joint National Committee ("JNC-6") placed patients with renal disease in the highest risk category, recommending institution of pharmacologic therapy once the blood pressure reaches a value of 130/85 mm Hg. Similar recommendations were given for all patients with diabetes; this recommendation was similar to that reached by the American Diabetes Association.

The basis for these aggressive recommendations comes from numerous epidemiologic studies but also from randomized clinical trials (RCTs). In the Modification of Diet in Renal Disease (MDRD) Study, 840 patients with various nondiabetic renal diseases were followed for a mean of 2.2 years. Patients were randomly assigned to a "usual" blood pressure goal [target mean arterial pressure (MAP) of 107 to 113 mm Hg] or a low blood pressure goal (target MAP of less than 92 mm Hg for younger patients, less than 98 mm Hg for older patients). At the end of the study, there were no significant differences in rates of decline of GFR overall, although specific subgroup analyses were more positive. There was a trend toward a slower rate of decline in African-American patients assigned to the lower blood pressure target and particularly a significant slowing of functional decline in patients with proteinuria of more than 1 g/24 hr. The greater beneficial effect of aggressive blood pressure reduction in proteinuric patients was also noted by the Northern Italian Cooperative Study Group.

The Choice of Antihypertensive Agent

Angiotensin-Converting Enzyme Inhibitors

The renin-angiotensin system (RAS) contributes to renal injury by a number of mechanisms, and animal studies have shown that drugs that block the RAS protect the kidney in a wide variety of animal models. Although clinical studies are not so uniform in showing a preferential benefit of angiotensin-converting enzyme (ACE) inhibitors, many studies do find such a benefit, and no class of drugs has been shown to be superior to ACE inhibitors in ability to protect the kidney. For this reason, ACE inhibitors are the drugs of choice in patients with diabetic nephropathy and in some forms of progressive nondiabetic renal disease. The JNC-6 also generally recommends ACE inhibitor therapy for patients with progressive nondiabetic renal disease, in the absence of contraindications to their use.

The basis for this recommendation comes from numerous short-term clinical studies showing a beneficial effect of ACE inhibitors on the surrogate marker, proteinuria, as well as from RCTs and meta-analyses. The Ramipril Efficacy in Nephropathy (REIN) trial examined the effects of the ACE inhibitor ramipril on rate of decline in GFR in 352 patients with proteinuria and chronic renal disease. The ACE inhibitor slowed the decline of GFR and reduced the risk of ESRD, particularly in those with the highest levels of proteinuria. Similarly, the Angiotensin Converting Enzyme Inhibition in Progressive Renal Insufficiency (ACEPRI) trial studied some 583 patients with chronic renal failure and randomized patients to the ACE inhibitor benazepril or placebo. Renal survival at 3 years was greater in the group receiving ACE inhibitors, and again, the greatest benefit accrued to those patients with the highest levels of proteinuria. One meta-analysis examined 10 clinical RCTs evaluating the effects of ACE inhibitor therapy in nondiabetic renal disease and found that overall, the relative risk of progression was reduced by 30% in patients receiving ACE inhibitors. However, the pooled analysis showed a slight but significant difference in achieved blood pressures, with values in the ACE inhibitor–treated group being about 5 mm Hg lower than those in other groups; therefore a contributing effect of blood pressure level per se (in addition to choice of specific agent) cannot be readily excluded.

The specific beneficial effect of ACE inhibitors in the setting of diabetic nephropathy is discussed elsewhere in this book (see Chapter 45), but it is worth noting that both RCTs and a meta-analysis have shown a specific benefit of these agents in slowing the progression of diabetic nephropathy. Both the JNC-6 and the American Diabetes Association practice guidelines strongly urge the use of these drugs in patients with diabetic nephropathy, as well as the importance of aggressive blood pressure control.

Other Antihypertensive Regimens

Relatively little information is available regarding the specific renoprotective potential of other antihypertensive agents, although as stated earlier, none has been shown to be superior to ACE inhibitors. The angiotensin II (AT_1) receptor antagonists have been shown to reproduce the beneficial effects of ACE inhibitors in animal models, and short-term clinical studies have shown that these agents lower proteinuria in patients with renal disease. Long-term RCTs are in progress to determine whether these drugs slow the progression of renal disease when evaluated by more stringent criteria. In the meantime, it seems reasonable to consider use of these agents in patients who cannot tolerate ACE inhibitors due to cough because the mechanism of ACE inhibitor–induced cough does not involve the RAS and such patients can successfully tolerate the receptor antagonists.

Calcium channel blockers have proven particularly controversial in the setting of diabetes, where there is growing evidence that the dihydropyridines are less effective than ACE inhibitors in reducing proteinuria and in protecting against cardiovascular events, whereas the nondihydropyridines have been shown in very small studies to replicate the renoprotective effects of ACE inhibitors. Using proteinuria as a short-term endpoint, some initial studies have shown that addition of a dihydropyridine calcium channel blocker does not attenuate the antiproteinuric efficacy of ACE inhibitors, whereas addition of the nondihydropyridine verapamil has an additive effect with the ACE inhibitor in further reducing proteinuria. In nondiabetic renal disease, the dihydropyridines have been less convincingly disadvantageous, but the available RCTs are flawed, and meta-analyses have not shown a convincing benefit.

There is almost no information available regarding other classes of antihypertensive agents, although a small prospective trial found no particular benefit of a β-blocker in slowing progression of diabetic nephropathy.

DIETARY INTERVENTIONS

Protein Restriction

There is a surfeit of protein in the typical Western diet, and the excess beyond that which is needed biochemically is excreted as urea and other nitrogenous wastes. For decades, researchers have recognized the potential benefit of protein restriction in the setting of advanced renal disease as a way to delay or minimize the clinical syndrome of uremia. Attention has turned to the potential renoprotective effect of protein restriction but also to the potential dangers of excessive limitation of this essential nutrient. Key to safe dietary protein restriction is recognition of the importance of maintaining positive nitrogen balance.

After a number of smaller trials, the MDRD was designed to prospectively study the benefits of dietary protein restriction in terms of preservation of GFR. Patients were randomized to a usual protein diet (1.3 g/kg per day), a low-protein diet (0.58 g/kg per day), or a very-low-protein diet (0.28 g/kg per day, with supplemental ketoacid–amino acids). On the lower protein intakes, patients exhibited a decline in GFR during the first 4 months of therapy, after which GFR stabilized, but there were no statistical differences seen at the end of the study. The findings and main conclusions of the MDRD have been hotly debated, with some advocates noting that the slope of loss of GFR were indeed improved, after that initial decline (which may have reflected hemodynamic adjustments). A meta-analysis of 13 randomized controlled trials (n = 1,919) found that dietary protein restriction reduced the decline of GFR significantly, but only by 0.53 ml/min per year. At this point, there is no clear benefit to protein restriction per se as a strategy to ameliorate the decline in GFR. Of note, however, is the fact that the recommended daily allowance for the U.S. population as a whole is just 0.8 g/kg per day, and the general U.S. diet contains far more protein than is needed for good health. Given the strong animal evidence of an adverse effect of a high-protein diet and the fact that such a diet usually contains more fat and phosphate than is advisable, it seems prudent to consider some degree of protein restriction in patients whose protein intake is excessive. However, caution must be taken to avoid malnutrition, particularly in the more advanced stages, because malnutrition at the onset of dialysis has been shown to be a potent risk factor for cardiovascular mortality in ESRD patients. In patients with massive urinary protein losses due to nephrotic syndrome, there is some value in restricting protein, but care should be taken to replace urinary losses as well. The role of dietary protein intake in patients with diabetes has been less well studied, but the five available RCTs and a recent meta-analysis all indicate that protein restriction does offer a specific benefit in preserving renal function in this population.

Lipid Intake

High-fat diets and hyperlipidemia have received significant experimental support as mediators of glomerular injury (see Chapter 56, Part 3). In experimental animals and humans, glomerular deposits of lipids have been described in the course of nephropathy. In numerous animal models of progressive renal disease, consuming a high-cholesterol diet accelerates injury, whereas lipid control therapy retards progression. As in atherosclerosis, hyperlipidemia appears to act synergistically with other risk factors, such as hypertension.

There are as yet no strong RCT studies addressing the potential renoprotective effect of cholesterol lowering in patients with renal disease. However, epidemiologic evidence strongly points to hyperlipidemia as a risk factor for development or progression of diabetic nephropathy. Furthermore, the hugely increased cardiovascular risk in patients with renal disease should prompt aggressive treatment of hypercholesterolemia.

Other Dietary Therapies

Experimentally, nutritional interventions, including phosphate restriction, total caloric restriction, and water supplementation, have all been shown to slow the progression of renal disease. Most of these have not been seriously tested in clinical trials, so their potential clinical importance remains to be determined. Small clinical trials of dietary protein restriction with or without concomitant phosphate restriction (6.5 mg/kg per day) have suggested a beneficial effect of phosphate restriction but have been criticized on methodologic grounds. Clinically, however, dietary phosphate restriction is generally advocated as a means to maintain normal mineral homeostasis.

OTHER INTERVENTIONS

Glycemic Control

In patients with diabetes, tight glycemic control slows the progression of virtually all microvascular complications, including nephropathy. Such benefit has been shown in type 1 diabetic patients in the Diabetes Control and Complications Trial (DCCT) and in type 2 patients in the United Kingdom Prospective Diabetes Study (UKPDS). In most of these studies, patients were followed for a few years in the earliest stages of diabetic nephropathy. Although effects on microalbuminuria were quite positive, long-term effects (e.g., delaying the onset of ESRD) remain to be determined. Nevertheless, small studies have shown that institution of good glycemic control can slow the onset of even advanced nephropathy.

Nonsteroidal Antiinflammatory Drugs

Experimentally, drugs that limit the production of vasodilatory prostaglandins have shown some benefit in slowing the progression of renal disease. Clinically, they have been demonstrated to reduce proteinuria in patients with nephrotic syndrome. However, in general, the potent deleterious effects on renal blood flow and GFR make these drugs difficult to use safely in patients with renal insufficiency.

Antiplatelet Agents and Anticoagulants

These drugs have also shown some promise in experimental models of renal disease. However, most clinical trials (usually in various forms of glomerulonephritis) have provided disappointing results, together with a high incidence of hemorrhagic complications. Accordingly, these drugs are not currently useful in slowing the progression of renal disease, although the cardioprotective effects of low-dose aspirin warrant their use in these patients at high cardiovascular risk.

Immunosuppressive Therapy

Various immunosuppressive agents have been successfully used in slowing the progression of experimental renal disease, even in models considered nonimmunologic in nature. Mycofenamate mofetil and tacrolimus appear to be promising in this regard. However, although immunosuppressive agents are routinely used for specific glomerulonephritides, their roles in more generic forms of progressive renal disease have not been clearly evaluated.

Other Therapies

A number of cytokines and vasoactive mediators have been implicated in the pathogenesis of progressive renal disease in experimental models. A number of new pharmacologic agents have been used to great benefit in these models, including anti–transforming growth factor-β (TGF-β) agents, endothelin-receptor antagonists, platelet-activating factor (PAF) antagonists, and protein kinase C (PKC) inhibitors. None of these have been tested clinically. However, as described in the preceding part of this chapter, major advances in our understanding of the pathogenesis of progressive renal disease are generating great excitement that specific new combinations of therapies may slow the progression of clinical renal disease in the future.

CURRENT STRATEGIES

Based on the available clinical information, a number of guidelines are available for slowing the progression of renal disease. First, early detection of patients at risk is key; prompt recognition of proteinuria or a slight increase in serum creatinine should trigger an aggressive approach. Second, strict blood pressure control is of paramount importance. All patients with renal disease or with diabetes, even in the absence of clinically detectable renal disease, should receive institution of pharmacologic antihypertensive therapy as soon as the blood pressure rises above 130/85 mm Hg. For patients with proteinuria of more than 1 g/24 hr, the target blood pressure level is 125/75 mm Hg. For patients with evidence of diabetic nephropathy or nondiabetic proteinuria (even if normotensive), ACE inhibitors should be used as first-line therapy. Maximal doses should be used, and then diuretic therapy and/or sodium restriction added, as this latter intervention may increase both the antihypertensive and antiproteinuric efficacy of ACE inhibitors. Furthermore, continued volume overload will impair the efficacy of most antihypertensive drugs and make hypertension more difficult to control. If blood pressure is not adequately controlled with ACE inhibitors and a diuretic, other agents should be added to achieve the blood pressure goal. Dietary protein restriction may be considered, at least to the level recommended for the U.S. population as a whole (0.8 g/kg per day). In diabetic patients, glycemic control should be optimized. Because of enhanced cardiovascular risk, and perhaps to protect the kidney, aggressive lipid-lowering therapy should be used. Use of low-dose aspirin should also be considered to reduce cardiovascular risk. Smoking cessation will also reduce cardiovascular risk. Smoking is a strong epidemiologic risk factor for progression of renal disease; therefore smoking cessation may someday be shown to reduce renal risk as well. Finally, there is increasing evidence documenting the value of early referral to a nephrologist. Available data clearly shows that pre-ESRD referral reduces the use of temporary hemodialysis access, as well as initial hospital length of stay.

Selected Readings

Bakris GL, Copley JB, Vicknair N, et al. Calcium channel blockers versus other antihypertensive therapies on progression of NIDDM associated nephropathy. *Kidney Int* 1996;50:1641–1650.

Randomized, controlled trial of atenolol versus ACE inhibitors versus nondihyropyridine calcium channel blockers on rate of loss of GFR in 52 hypertensive patients with type 2 diabetes and renal insufficiency.

Gansevoort RT, de Zeeuw D, de Jong PE. Is the antiproteinuric effect of ACE inhibition mediated by interference in the renin-angiotensin system? *Kidney Int* 1994;45:861–867.

Short-term clinical trial in patients with nondiabetic renal disease showing equivalent antiproteinuric efficacy of the AT_1 receptor losartan as compared with the ACE inhibitor lisinopril.

Giatras I, Lau J, Levey AS. Effect of angiotensin-converting enzyme inhibitors on the progression of nondiabetic renal disease: a meta-analysis of randomized trials. *Ann Intern Med* 1997;127:337–345.

Meta-analysis of 10 prospective trials, involving 1,594 patients, of the relative benefit of ACE inhibition in slowing the progression of nondiabetic renal disease.

GISEN Group. Randomized placebo-controlled trial of effect of ramipril on decline in glomerular filtration rate and risk of terminal renal failure in proteinuric, non-diabetic nephropathy. *Lancet* 1998;349:1857–1863.

Prospective, randomized controlled trial of the benefits of ramipril versus placebo in 352 patients with chronic renal disease and proteinuria of more than 1 g/24 hr.

Kasiske BL, Kalil RSN, Ma JZ, et al. Effect of antihypertensive therapy on the kidney in patients with diabetes: a meta-regression analysis. *Ann Intern Med* 1993;118:129–138.

Meta-analysis of 100 controlled and uncontrolled prospective trials, involving 2,494 patients, of the relative benefit of ACE inhibition in slowing the progression of diabetic renal disease.

Kasiske BL, Lakutua JDA, Ma JZ, et al. A meta-analysis of the effects of dietary protein restriction on the rate of decline in renal function. *Am J Kidney Dis* 1998;31:954–961.

Meta-analysis of 13 prospective trials, involving 1,919 patients, of the benefits of dietary protein restriction on the progression of renal disease.

Klahr S, Levey AS, Beck GJ, et al. The effects of dietary protein restriction and blood pressure control on the progression of chronic renal disease. Modification of Diet in Renal Disease Study Group. *N Engl J Med* 1994;330:877–884.

Prospective, randomized controlled trial of the benefits of aggressive blood pressure lowering and of dietary protein restriction in 840 patients with nondiabetic renal disease.

Lewis EJ, Hunsicker LG, Bain RP, et al, for the Collaborative Study Group. The effect of angiotensin-converting enzyme inhibition on diabetic nephropathy. *N Engl J Med* 1993;329:1456–1462.

Prospective, randomized controlled trial of the benefits of captopril versus placebo in 407 patients with type 1 diabetes and proteinuria exceeding 0.5 g/24 hr.

Maschio G, Alberti D, Janin G, et al. Effect of the angiotensin-converting-enzyme inhibitors on the progression of renal insufficiency. *N Engl J Med* 1996;334:939–945.

Prospective, randomized controlled trial of the benefits of benazepril versus placebo in 583 patients with chronic renal disease and proteinuria greater than 1 g/24 hr.

The Sixth Report of the Joint National Committee on Prevention, Detection, Evaluation and Treatment of High Blood Pressure. *Arch Intern Med* 1997;157:2413–2446.

A comprehensive analysis of the available evidence base for hypertension risk and therapy, with specific attention to other cardiac risk factors and individualized therapy in specific population groups.

CHAPTER 68

Uremic Toxicity

PART 1
Parathyroid Hormone as a Uremic Toxin

Shaul G. Massry

A variety of signs and symptoms listed in Table 68.1 constitute the uremic syndrome. The mechanisms for such a widespread organ dysfunction in patients with advanced chronic renal failure (CRF) are not well delineated. However, a multitude of factors have been implicated. These include anemia, acidosis, fluid overload, electrolyte disturbances, accumulation of end products of protein metabolism, malnutrition, increased aluminum burden, as yet unidentified uremic toxin, and hormonal imbalances.

One of the major hormonal disturbances in uremia is the state of secondary hyperparathyroidism and the elevation in blood levels of parathyroid hormone (PTH). In an editorial published in 1977, Massry suggested that the state of chronic excess of PTH in patients with CRF may exert a widespread adverse effect on many organs. Thus this *Massry hypothesis* implicated PTH as a major uremic toxin participating in the genesis of many of the manifestations of the uremic syndrome. Since then, a large body of evidence has accumulated demonstrating the multiple effects of PTH and its role in the overall pathogenesis of uremia. Indeed, the available data show that PTH satisfies the strict criteria of a uremic toxin, in that its nature and structure is known, its blood levels are elevated, a relationship between it and the uremic manifestation(s) exists, an improvement in many signs and symptoms of uremia follows a reduction in its blood levels, and administration of PTH to experimental animals with normal renal function produces derangements similar to those seen in uremic patients.

TABLE 68.1. The Manifestations of Uremic Syndrome

Encephalopathy	Carbohydrate intolerance
Neuropathy	Impaired insulin secretion
Dialysis dementia	Anemia
Bone disease	Bleeding tendencies
Soft tissue calcification	Immunologic disturbances
Soft tissue necrosis	Myocardiopathy
Pruritus	Myopathy
Hyperlipidemia	Sexual dysfunction

ACUTE EFFECTS OF PARATHYROID HORMONE ON CYTOSOLIC CALCIUM

Earlier studies showed that PTH enhances the entry of calcium into cells, and newer data demonstrated that PTH causes an acute rise in cytosolic calcium ($[Ca^{2+}]i$) in pancreatic islets, thymocytes, cardiac myocytes, hepatic cells, adipocytes, kidney cells, and osteoblasts. This effect of PTH is receptor mediated and uses several cellular pathways. However, the pathways that are involved in this action of the hormone are not uniform among these cells (Table 68.2). These potential pathways are depicted in Fig. 68.1. In all these cells, PTH activates voltage-dependent and other calcium channels, and hence the hormone-mediated calcium influx into cells is blunted or prevented by calcium channel blockers such as verapamil or nifedipine.

It is of interest that some of these cells respond only to the intact molecule of PTH [PTH-(1–84)], whereas in other cells the response to PTH-(1–84) is significantly greater than equimolar amounts of its aminoterminal fragment [PTH-(1–34)]. These observations suggest that the biologic activity of PTH assessed by the calcium movement into cells resides not only in its aminoterminal fragment but in a bigger moiety containing the 1–34 amino acid sequence or in both the 1–34 fragment and another part of the carboxyterminal sequence of the hormone. Figure 68.2 shows a dose-response relationship between the rise in $[Ca^{2+}]i$ of rat renal proximal tubule cells and equimolar concentrations of PTH-(1–34) or PTH-(1–84). Note the greater effect of the latter at higher concentrations.

The aforementioned data indicate that the traditional (kidney and bone) and the nontraditional cells for PTH action must have the molecular machinery for the production of PTH receptors. Available data have demonstrated that the messenger ribonucleic acid (mRNA) for the PTH-PTH related protein (PTH-PTHrP) receptor is present in the kidney, bone, heart, brain, spleen, aorta, ileum, skeletal muscle, lung, and testis (Fig. 68.3). Thus both physiologic and molecular evidence exists supporting the notion that almost all body organs are targets for PTH action; and, therefore it is not surprising that chronic excess of PTH in CRF may exert a widespread deleterious effect on body function in uremia.

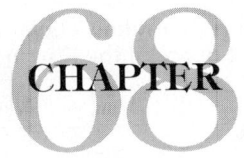

TABLE 68.2. The Effects of PTH on $[Ca^{2+}]i$ of Various Cells, the Cellular Pathways that Are Involved in This Action of PTH, and the Source of the Rise in $[Ca^{2+}]i$

				Cellular Pathways						
Cell Type	PTH 1–84	PTH 1–34	Generation of cAMP	Inhibition by PTH Antagonist	Voltage-Dependent Calcium Channels	cAMP	G Protein(s)	Protein Kinase C	Source of Calcium: Extracellular	Source of Calcium: Intracellular
Cardiac myocytes	++	+	+	+	++	–	+	–	+	+
Pancreatic islets	++	+	+	+	+	+	+	+	+	–[b]
Thymocytes	++	–	+	+	+	+		+	+	–[b]
Hepatocytes	++	+	+	+	+	++	+	+	+	–[b]
Adipocytes	++	–	–	+	+	–	+	+	+	+
Renal cells	++	+	+	+	+	–[a]	+	+	+	+
Osteoblasts[c]		+	+	+	+	+	+	+	+	+

[a] cAMP pathway participates in the PTH-induced rise in $[Ca^{2+}]i$ of rabbit connecting tubular cells.

[b] PTH failed to increase $[Ca^{2+}]i$ in these cells when they were incubated in a free calcium media. It should be mentioned that cells incubated in free calcium media are calcium depleted (low basal levels of $[Ca^{2+}]i$) and therefore mobilization of calcium from intracellular stores may be limited. However, other agonists were able to cause a rise in $[Ca^{2+}]i$ in cells incubated in calcium free media when PTH failed to do so; examples include arginine vasopressin and angiotensin II in hepatic cells, and AVP in adipocytes. It appears therefore that if PTH raises $[Ca^{2+}]i$ by mobilizing intracellular calcium in these cells, such an action would depend on PTH-induced calcium influx, which is important in intracellular calcium mobilization (calcium–calcium release phenomenon); absence of such influx, when cells are incubated in a free calcium media, may impede intracellular calcium mobilization.

[c] The data on osteoblasts are derived from studies on rat osteosarcoma cell line UMR-106 and rat osteoblastlike cells ROS 17/2.8.

AVP, arginine vasopressin; cAMP, cyclic adenosine 3′,5′-monophosphate; PTH, parathyroid hormone.

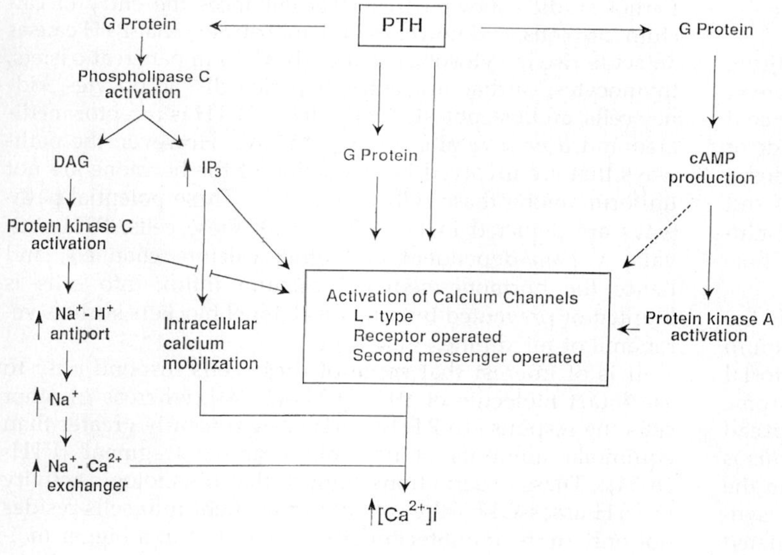

Figure 68.1. The potential cellular pathways through which parathyroid hormone (PTH) may mediate its action on $[Ca^{2+}]i$ of cells. DAG, diacylglycerol. (Reproduced with permission from Massry SG, Smogorzewski M. The mechanisms responsible for the PTH-induced rise in cytosolic calcium in various cells are not uniform. *Miner Elect Metab* 1995;21:13–28).

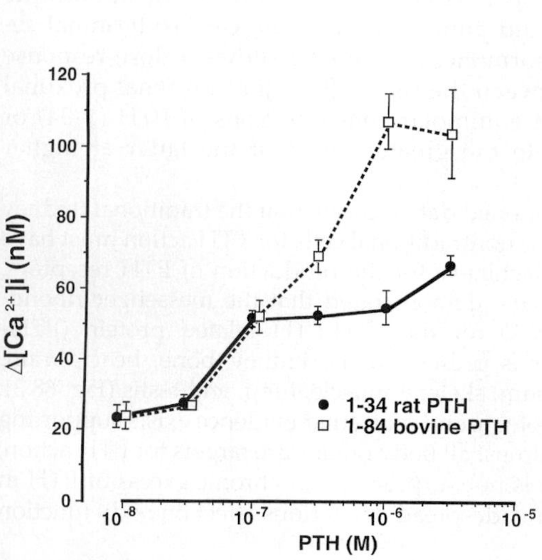

Figure 68.2. Dose-response relationship between rise in $[Ca^{2+}]i$ of renal proximal tubule cells and concentration of parathyroid hormone (PTH). Each datum is the mean of 8 to 18 studies; brackets denote ± 1 SE. Changes in $[Ca^{2+}]i$ with PTH 1–34 represent the peak value (20 seconds), and those with PTH 1–84 represent the time when the initial rapid rise reached its maximum (90 seconds). (Reproduced with permission from Tanaka H, Smogorzewski M, Koss M, et al. Pathways involved in PTH-induced rise in cytosolic Ca^{2+} concentration of rat renal proximal tubule. *Am J Physiol* 1995;268:F330–F337.)

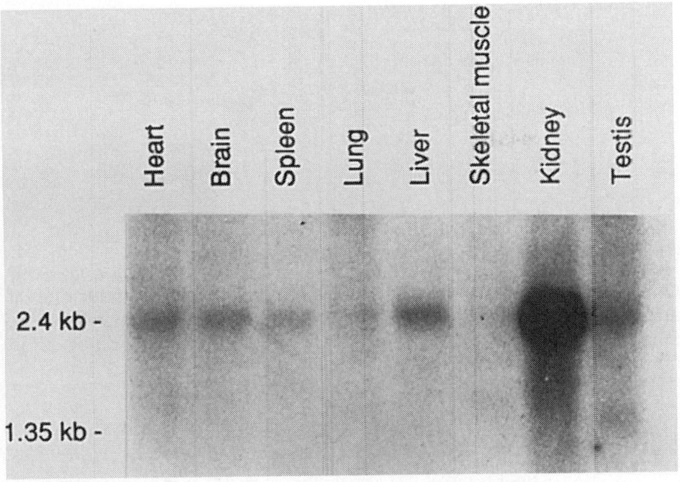

Figure 68.3. Northern blot analysis of poly A$^+$ RNA prepared from various tissue of rat. Transcripts of approximately 2.4 Kb of PTH-PTHrP were found in all these tissues with the strongest expression in the kidney tissue. In addition, a smaller band was detected in the kidney (approximately 1.8 Kb) and testis (approximately 1.5 Kb). (Reproduced with permission from Tian J, Smogorzewski M, Kedes L, et al. Parathyroid hormone related protein receptor messenger RNA is present in many tissues besides the kidney. *Am J Nephrol* 1993;13:210–213.)

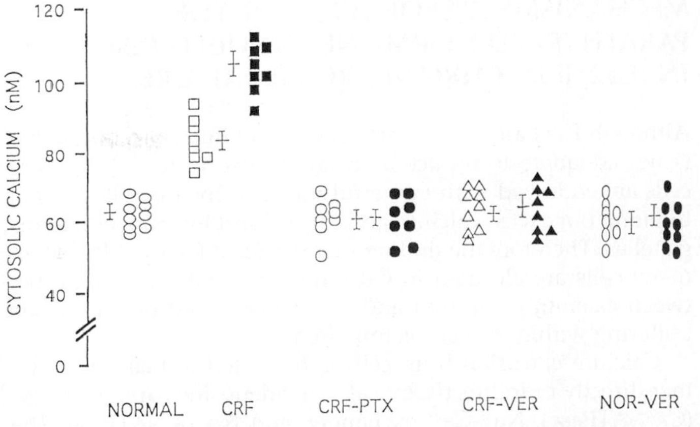

Figure 68.4. Cytosolic calcium in cardiac myocytes of rats. Each *datum point* represents one animal. *Brackets* denote mean ± 1 SE. *Open symbols* are data after 3 weeks of study and *closed symbols* after 6 weeks of study. CRF, chronic renal failure; PTX, parathyroidectomized; VER, verapamil; NOR, normal. (Reproduced with permission from Zhang Y-B, Smogorzewski M, Ni Z, et al. Altered cytosolic calcium homeostasis in rat cardiac myocytes in CRF. *Kidney Int* 1994;45:1113–1119.)

CHRONIC EFFECT OF PARATHYROID HORMONE ON TISSUE CALCIUM CONTENT AND BASAL LEVELS OF [Ca^{2+}]i

Soft tissue calcification is a common finding in uremic patients, and increased calcium content was found in the cornea, skin, blood vessels, brain, peripheral nerves, heart, lungs, pancreas, liver, epididymal fat, and testis of patients and animals with renal failure. These abnormalities have been attributed to the state of secondary hyperparathyroidism of CRF, because parathyroidectomy prevented the calcium accumulation in these tissues. These observations are consistent with the ability of PTH to augment entry of calcium into cells.

Newer data have further documented that the increased calcium burden of the tissues in CRF is also associated with significant elevation of the basal levels of [Ca^{2+}]i of various cells including brain synaptosomes, pancreatic islets, cardiac myocytes hepatocytes, adipocytes, thymocytes, B cells, T cells, leukocytes, and platelets. An example of the changes in the basal levels of [Ca^{2+}]i of the cardiac myocytes of uremic rats is shown in Fig. 68.4. This chronic and sustained elevation in [Ca^{2+}]i of these cells is prevented or reversed by parathyroidectomy and/or by treatment with the calcium channel blocker, verapamil. Again these observations are in agreement with the property of PTH to augment entry of calcium into cells and with the finding that this action of the hormone uses voltage-dependent calcium channels that are blocked by verapamil.

EFFECT OF PARATHYROID HORMONE ON PHOSPHOLIPIDS OF CELL MEMBRANE

In addition to the effect of PTH on [Ca2$^+$]i of cells, chronic excess of the hormone may affect the phospholipid contents of cell membrane, and alterations in these compounds may affect membrane fluidity, permeability to ions, and agonist–receptor interaction. Indeed, PTH enhances phospholipid turnover in the kidney. We found that PTH also affects phospholipid content of human red blood cells. Also, chronic exposure of brain synaptosomes to excess PTH in the presence or absence of CRF in rats was associated with significant reduction in their total content of phospholipids as well as in the content of phosphatidylserine, phosphatidylethanolamine, and phosphatidylinositol (Fig. 68.5). This effect is prevented by parathyroidectomy of the CRF rats (Fig. 68.5) or by their treatment with verapamil.

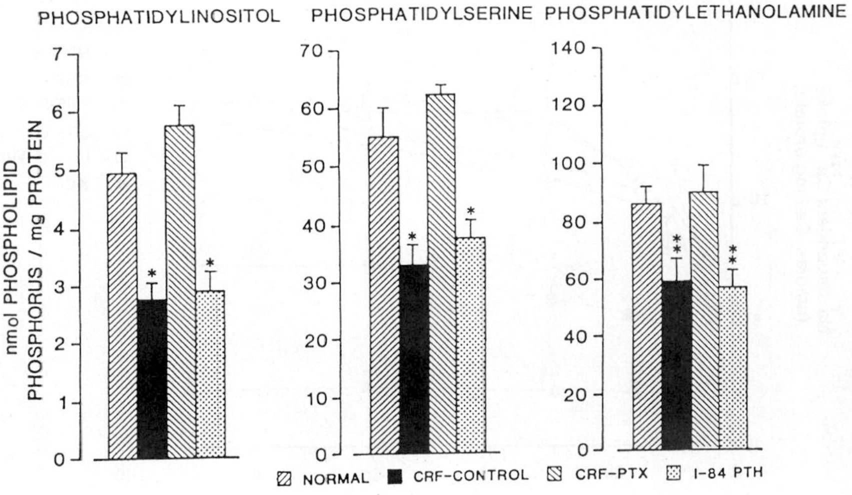

Figure 68.5. Content of various phospholipids in brain synaptosomes. Assays of synaptosomes obtained from one animal of each group were performed on the same day. Each *column* represents mean value of data obtained from four animals in each group, and *bracket* denotes SE. *, $P < .01$; **, $P < .02$ from normal and parathyroidectomized *(CRF-PTX)* rats. CRF, control rats with chronic renal failure; PTH 1–84, rats treated with PTH 1–84. (Reproduced with permission from Islam A, Smogorzewski M, Massry SG. Effect of chronic renal failure and parathyroid hormone on phospholipid content of brain synaptosomes. *Am J Physiol* 1989;206:F705–F710.)

MECHANISMS RESPONSIBLE FOR THE PARATHYROID HORMONE–INDUCED RISE IN [$Ca2^+$]i IN CHRONIC RENAL FAILURE

Although PTH augments entry of calcium into cells, this action is not adequate to induce a sustained rise in [Ca^{2+}]i because cells are endowed with powerful mechanisms that allow them to pump out excess calcium and/or buffer it by intracellular organelles. Therefore the finding that the basal levels of [Ca^{2+}]i of many cells are elevated in CRF indicates that the balance between calcium entry into and its extrusion out of cells or its buffering within the cells is impaired.

Calcium extrusion from cells is regulated in major part, either directly or indirectly, by calcium adenosine triphosphatase (Ca^{2+}-ATPase), Na^+-Ca^{2+} exchanger, and Na^+-K^+-ATPase. The activities of Ca^{2+}-ATPase and of Na^+-K^+-ATPase of many cells are impaired in CRF; this has been demonstrated in pancreatic islets, brain synaptosomes, cardiac myocytes, hepatocytes, adipocytes, red blood cells, and lymphocytes. Figures 68.6 and 68.7 show these changes in adipocytes in CRF. Additional studies demonstrated that the activity of Na^+-Ca^{2+} exchanger is also impaired in CRF in many cells such as cardiac myocytes, hepatocytes (Fig. 68.8), and adipocytes. The changes in Ca^{2+}-ATPase, Na^+-K^+-ATPase, and Na^+-Ca^{2+} exchanger are prevented by parathyroidectomy of the CRF animals or by their treatment with a calcium channel blocker (Figs. 68.6 to 68.8).

The mechanisms responsible for the impaired activities of Ca^{2+}-ATPase and Na^+-K^+-ATPase are not fully understood. Several possibilities should be considered. *First,* it is well documented that the functional integrity of both enzymes requires adenosine triphosphate (ATP), and the ATP content of cells in CRF is significantly reduced because of inhibition of mitochondrial oxidation. Therefore this significant reduction in ATP content of cells (Fig. 68.9) could be responsible, at least in part, for the reduced activity of these enzymes. It could be argued that this decrease in ATP is not adequate to affect the activity of these enzymes because the decrease in ATP content is in the millimolar range, whereas the affinity of the enzymes to ATP is in the micromolar range. However, there may be compartmentalization of ATP with the submembrane pool being considerably lower than that in other cytosolic pools of ATP, and therefore a decrease in this submembrane pool could affect the enzymes' activity.

Second, we found that the increase in V_{max} of Ca^{2+}-ATPase in response to calmodulin is impaired in CRF animals (Fig. 68.10). This phenomenon may also contribute to the reduced V_{max} of this enzyme. *Third,* CRF is associated with reduced phospholipid contents of cells; it was found that the V_{max} of Ca^{2+}-ATPase is directly related to the concentration of phosphatidylinositol and phosphatidylserine. Thus a decrease in the contents of these phospholipids in CRF could also play a role in the reduction of the activity of this enzyme. A similar effect may be present in regard to Na^+-K^+-ATPase as well.

The changes in ATP content and in the activity of Ca^{2+}-ATPase, Na^+-K^+-ATPase, and Na^+-Ca^{2+} exchanger are also most likely mediated by the state of secondary hyperparathyroidism and the PTH-induced entry of calcium into cells. This proposition is supported by two observations. *First,* excess PTH in the absence

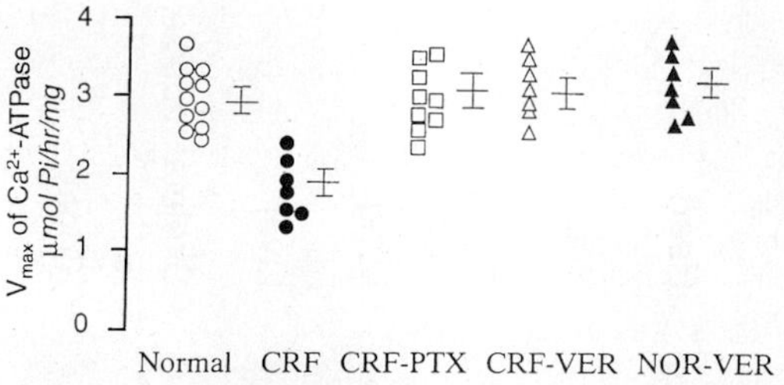

Figure 68.6. The V_{max} of Ca^{2+}-ATPase of adipocytes from normal, CRF, CRF-PTX, CRF-V, and normal-V rats. Each *datum point* represents one rat and *brackets* denote ± 1 SE. (Reproduced with permission from Ni Z, Smogorzewski M, Massry SG. Elevated cytosolic calcium of adipocytes in chronic renal failure. *Kidney Int* 1995;47:1624–1629.)

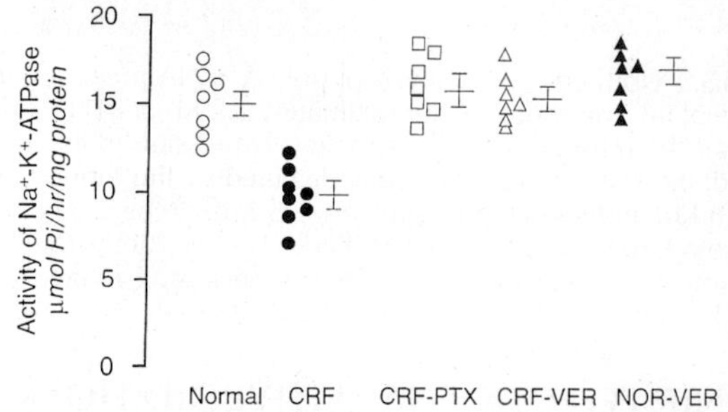

Figure 68.7. The activity of Na^+-K^+-ATPase of adipocytes from normal, CRF, CRF-PTX, CRF-V, and normal-V rats. Each *datum point* represents one rat and *brackets* denote ± 1 SE. (Reproduced with permission from Ni Z, Smogorzewski M, Massry SG. Elevated cytosolic calcium of adipocytes in chronic renal failure. *Kidney Int* 1995;47:1624–1629.)

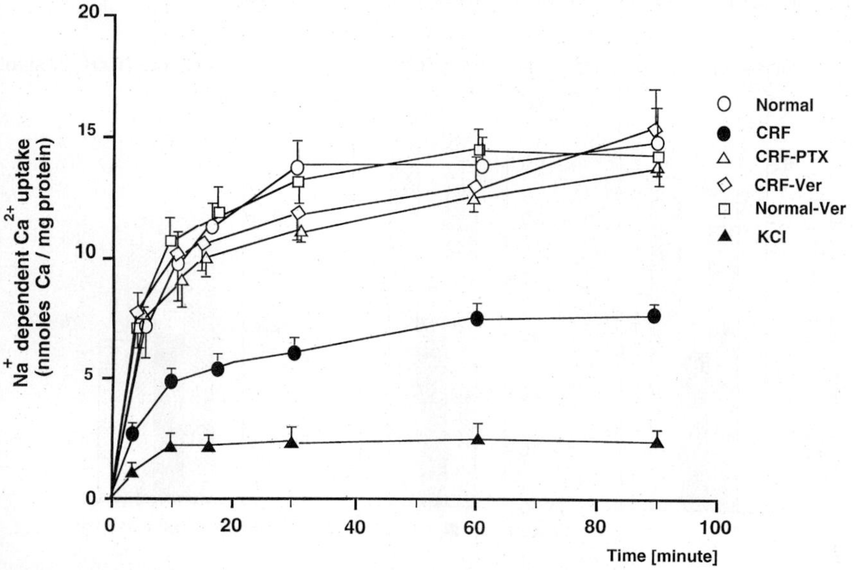

Figure 68.8. Time course of Na^+-dependent ^{45}Ca uptake by membrane vesicles of hepatocytes of normal CRF, CRF-PTX, CRF-VER, and NOR-VER rats. Each *datum point* represents mean of 7 to 10 rats and *brackets* denote ± 1 SE. Values in the CRF animals at all times are significantly ($P < .01$) lower than in the other four groups. (Reproduced with permission from Klin M, Smogorzewski M, Massry SG. Chronic renal failure increases cytosolic Ca^{2+} of hepatocytes. *Am J Physiol* 1995;269:G103–G109.)

of CRF also causes a reduction in ATP content of cells and impairs the activity of their Na^+-K^+-ATPase. *Second,* parathyroidectomy of CRF rats or their treatment with verapamil prevented these derangements. It should also be mentioned that some investigators found that a circulating inhibitor of Ca^{2+}-ATPase of red blood cells is present in the blood of CRF patients; the nature of this compound is not yet well defined.

The data presented previously permit the formulation depicted in Fig. 68.11, which provides a scheme for the events that occur in the cells in CRF and lead to the increase in their basal levels of $[Ca^{2+}]i$. It appears that the initial event is a PTH-induced augmentation of calcium entry into the cells, which would impair mitochondrial production of ATP. The subsequent decrease in ATP content of cells would impair the activities of Ca^{2+}-ATPase and Na^+-K^+-ATPase. The decrease in the phospholipid contents of cell membrane would contribute to the inhibition of the activity of Ca^{2+}-ATPase and Na^+-K^+-ATPase. The reductions in the activity of Ca^{2+}-ATPase, Na^+-K^+-ATPase, and Na^+-Ca^{2+} exchanger lead to a decrease in calcium extrusion out of the cells. Such an effect in the face of a continued PTH-induced increase in calcium entry would result in calcium accumulation in the cells and to an increase in their $[Ca^{2+}]i$ levels.

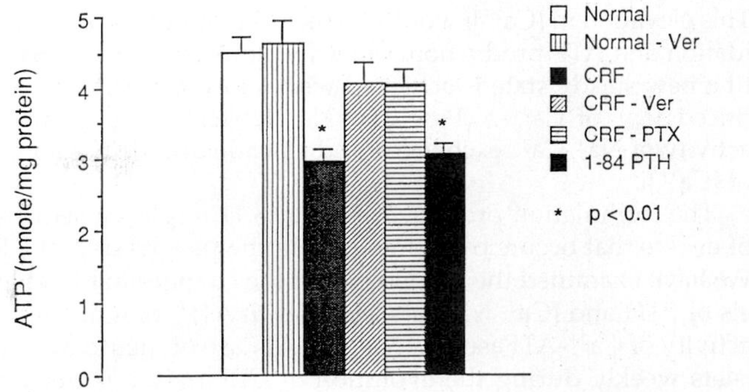

Figure 68.9. The ATP content of brain synaptosomes obtained from rats of various groups of animals studied. Each *column* represents the mean value, and *brackets* denote 1 SE. (Reproduced with permission from Smogorzewski M, Koureta P, Fadda GZ, et al. Chronic parathyroid hormone excess *in vivo* increases resting levels of cytosolic calcium in brain synaptosomes: studies in the presence and absence of chronic renal failure. *J Am Soc Nephrol* 1991;1:1162–1168.)

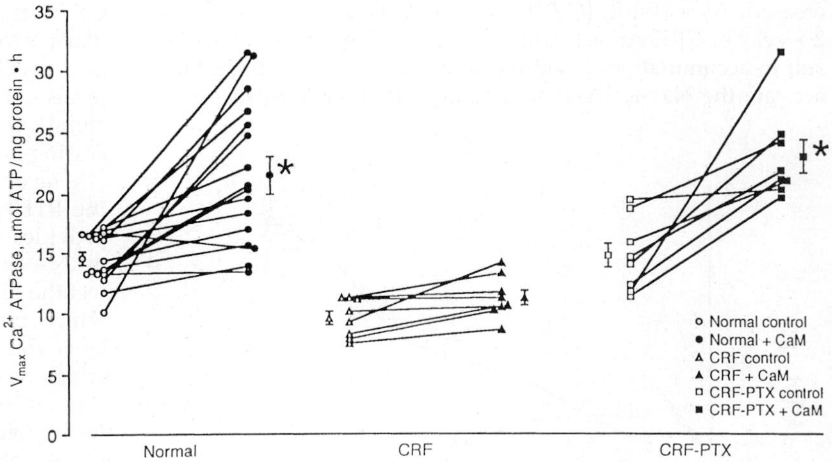

Figure 68.10. The basal levels of the V_{max} of Ca^{2+}-ATPase of pancreatic islets and the response of the enzyme to calmodulin (CaM). Each *line* represents a study in one rat; *open symbols* denote basal values; *closed symbols* represent values after calmodulin; *brackets* denote mean ± 1 SE; and * indicates a $P < .01$ versus basal levels. (Reproduced from Ozbasli CF, Fadda GZ, Massry SG. Effects of chronic renal failure with and without excess parathyroid hormone on calmodulin content of pancreatic islets and on the response of their Ca^{2+}-ATPase to calmodulin. *Contrib Nephrol* 1993;102:135–143.)

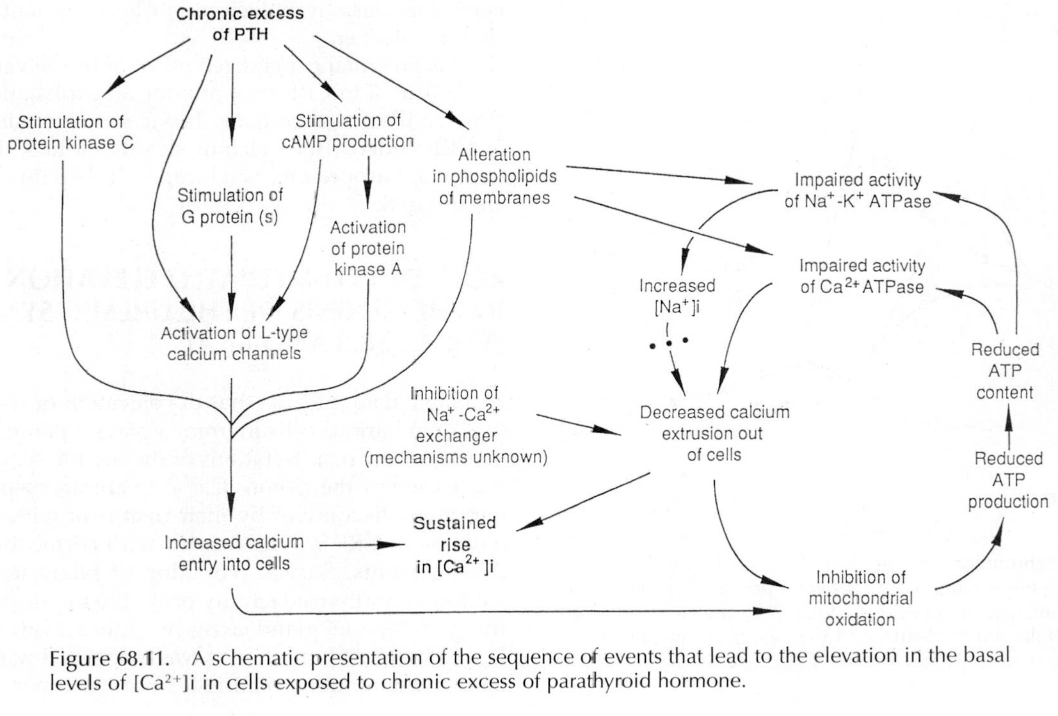

Figure 68.11. A schematic presentation of the sequence of events that lead to the elevation in the basal levels of $[Ca^{2+}]i$ in cells exposed to chronic excess of parathyroid hormone.

This elevation in $[Ca^{2+}]i$ would further inhibit mitochondrial oxidation and ATP production. Thus a vicious circle develops until a new steady state is achieved with a low ATP content, a reduced V_{max} of Ca^{2+}-ATPase and Na^+-K^+-ATPase, a decreased activity of Na^+-Ca^{2+} exchanger, and elevation in the basal levels of $[Ca^{2+}]i$.

The formulation presented in Fig. 68.11 implies a sequence of events that occurs over time during the progression of CRF. We have examined the chronology of the changes in blood levels of PTH and $[Ca^{2+}]i$ in rats, changes in ATP content, and the activity of Ca^{2+}-ATPase and Na^+-K^+-ATPase of their pancreatic islets weekly during the evolution of CRF over a 6-week period. The results of this study are shown in Fig. 68.12. The serum levels of PTH begin to rise during the first week of CRF. The V_{max} of Ca^{2+}-ATPase was higher during weeks one to two, and of Na^+-K^+-ATPase during weeks one to three of CRF, but both activities fell to low levels thereafter. At week 3 of CRF, the ATP content started to fall, and the basal level of $[Ca^{2+}]i$ began to rise. Thus these data support the formulation shown in Fig. 68.11 and indicate that as serum levels of PTH begin to rise, calcium entry into islets is augmented; this in turn will stimulate the activity of Ca^{2+}-ATPase and the Na^+-Ca^{2+} exchanger, and hence, calcium extrusion out of the islets is increased. As a result, $[Ca^{2+}]i$ remains normal during the first 2 weeks of CRF. An activation of Na^+-Ca^{2+} exchanger may result in accumulation of sodium into islet, an event that would activate the Na^+-K^+-ATPase. As calcium entry is further augmented by the progressive rise in serum PTH levels, mitochondrial oxidation and ATP production would be reduced, resulting in lower ATP content. This fall in ATP causes a reduction in the V_{max} of Ca^{2+}-ATPase and Na^+-K^+-ATPase, and therefore calcium extrusion out of the islets is reduced; consequently, $[Ca^{2+}]i$ rises.

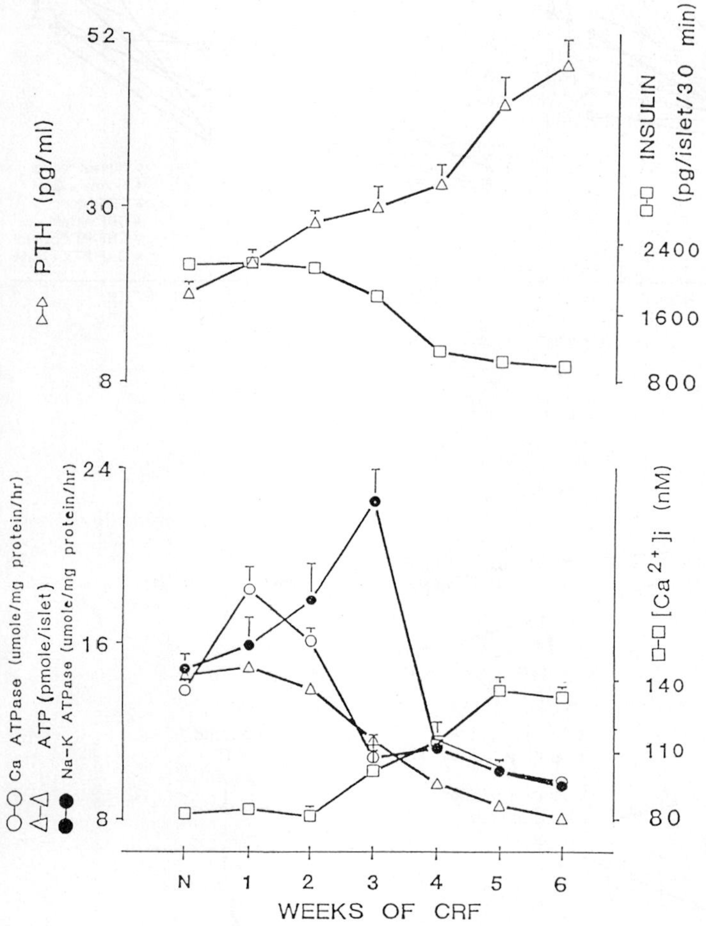

Figure 68.12. The chronologic relationship between the various parameters studied during the evolution of CRF over a period of 6 weeks. (Reproduced with permission from Levi E, Fadda GZ, Thanakitcharu P, et al. Chronology of cellular events leading to derangements in function of pancreatic islets in chronic renal failure. *J Am Soc Nephrol* 1992;3: 1139–1146.)

It is of interest that the sequence of events described in Fig. 68.11 does not continue, but stabilizes at a new steady state. This may be due to downregulation of the PTH receptors in CRF, an adaptive process that would protect the cells from further actions of the high blood levels of PTH and consequent continued accumulation of calcium, which may eventually lead to cell death. Indeed, studies have demonstrated that the PTH-PTHrP receptor mRNA is downregulated in CRF, an event that would lead to reduced receptor synthesis and hence a decrease in the number of receptors. The reduction in the amount of mRNA of the PTH-PTHrP receptors was found in both the traditional (kidney) and the nontraditional organs (liver and heart) for PTH action.

The downregulation of the mRNA of the PTH-PTHrP receptor in various organs in uremia is prevented by parathyroidectomy or by treatment with a calcium channel blocker. Because these latter procedures normalize the basal levels of $[Ca^{2+}]i$ in CRF, one may suggest that the elevation of $[Ca^{2+}]i$ in CRF plays a major role in the downregulation of the PTH-PTHrP receptor. Such an effect may be mediated by the interference of the high levels of $[Ca^{2+}]i$ with the molecular machinery of the cells. The chronic increase in $[Ca^{2+}]i$ may impair the transcription or processing or turnover of the mRNA of the receptor.

The available data are consistent with the proposition that the PTH-mediated rise in the basal levels of $[Ca^{2+}]i$ in CRF provides a negative feedback mechanism through which the mRNA of the PTH-PTHrP receptor is downregulated to protect the cells against continued increase in blood levels of PTH, which further augments the elevation in $[Ca^{2+}]i$ to reach a level that would result in cell death. However, this useful adaptive process is not without an adverse effect. The trade-off may be a downregulation of other hormone receptors, if their molecular machinery is affected in a similar manner by the elevated $[Ca^{2+}]i$ of CRF. Indeed, the mRNA of angiotensin II (AT_1) and of vasopressin (AV1a) are downregulated in CRF. Again, this downregulation of these two receptors is prevented by parathyroidectomy or by treatment with a calcium channel blocker.

This potential generalized effect of the elevation in the basal levels $[Ca^{2+}]i$ in CRF may provide an explanation for the resistance to the action of many hormones commonly encountered in CRF. Indeed, the calcium signals induced by PTH, angiotensin II, vasopressin, or glucagon in hepatocytes of CRF rats are reduced.

ROLE OF PTH-MEDIATED ELEVATION IN [Ca2+]i IN THE GENESIS OF THE UREMIC SYNDROME (TABLES 68.3 AND 68.4)

Available data indicate that the elevation of the basal levels of $[Ca^{2+}]i$ in various cells in uremia plays a paramount role in the genesis of the manifestations of the uremic syndrome. *First,* the prevention of the rise in $[Ca^{2+}]i$ in animals with CRF by prior parathyroidectomy or by their treatment with verapamil from day one of CRF was associated with correction of the uremic derangements. *Second,* reduction of blood levels of PTH by subtotal parathyroidectomy or by the medical suppression of the parathyroid gland activity with 1,25-dihydroxyvitamin D_3 [$1,25(OH)_2D_3$] in humans was associated with improvement of the uremic abnormalities. *Third,* treatment of humans or

TABLE 68.3. Uremic Manifestations Attributed to PTH-Mediated Rise in $[Ca^{2+}]i$ in Animals With CRF

Organ	Derangement	Prevented or Reversed by: Total Parathyroidectomy	Prevented or Reversed by: Calcium Channel Blocker	Induced by PTH Administration in Normal Animals
Brain	Abnormal EEG	+		+
Brain synaptosomes	Decreased NE content	+	+	+
	Decreased NE release	+	+	+
	Decreased NE uptake	+	+	+
	Reduced V_{max} of tyrosine hydroxylase	+		
	Increased K_m of monoamine oxidase	+		
	Reduced total phospholipid content, phosphoinositol phosphatidylserine, and phosphatidylethanolamine	+	+	+
	Increased Ach content and release	+	+	
	Reduced choline kinase activity	+	+	
	Decreased choline content	+	+	
	Increased choline uptake	−	−	
	Increased choline release	−	−	
Peripheral nerves	Prolonged motor nerve conduction velocity	+		+
Heart	Impaired mitochondrial oxidation	+	+	+
	Impaired energy shuttle[a]	−		+
	Impaired energy utilization[a]	−		+
	Impaired fatty-acid oxidation	+	+	+
	Decreased cardiac output[a]	−		+
	Right ventricular hypertrophy	+		
Lungs	Impaired diffusion capacity	+		
	Increased mean pulmonary wedge pressure	+		
Pancreas	Impaired glucose-induced insulin secretion	+	+	+
	Reduced leucine-induced insulin secretion	+	+	
	Decreased potassium-induced insulin secretion	+	+	
Lipid metabolism	Triglyceridemia	+	+	
	Impaired fat tolerance	+	+	
	Reduced postheparin lipolytic activity	+	+	
	Decreased hepatic lipase (HL) activity	+	+	
	Downregulation of mRNA of HL	+	+	
	Decreased production of HL	+	+	+
	Decreased release of HL	+	+	+
	Decreased LPL activity	+	+	
	Downregulation of mRNA of LPL	+	+	
	Reduced production of LPL	+	+	
	Decreased release of LPL	+	+	+
Nitric oxide metabolism	Reduced NOS activity in kidney and aorta	+	+	
	Reduced eNOS and iNOS protein mass in kidney and aorta	+	+	
Polymorphonuclear leukocytes	Impaired phagocytosis	+	+	
	Reduced oxygen consumption	+	+	
Erythrocytes	Shortened survival	+		
Testes	Reduced blood levels of testosterone	+		+
B cells	Impaired immunoglobulin production	+		
Blood testosterone reduced		+		+

[a]Total parathyroidectomy did not correct these abnormalities because normal amounts of PTH are required for the synthesis of creatinine phosphokinase.
Ach, acetylcholine; EEG, electroencephalogram; eNOS, endothelial NOS; iNOS, inducible NOS; LP, lipoprotein; LPL, lipoprotein lipase; mRNA, messenger ribonucleic acid; NE, norepinephrine; NOS, nitric oxide synthase.

animals with preexisting CRF with calcium channel blockers (verapamil or nifedipine) reversed the uremic manifestations.

Additional support for the proposition that elevated basal levels of $[Ca^{2+}]i$ is the culprit in the genesis of organ dysfunction in uremia is provided by other observations. Phosphate depletion, which is a state with elevated basal levels of $[Ca^{2+}]i$, hypoparathyroidism, and normal renal function, is also associated with a wide range of organ dysfunction similar to those seen in CRF; and the normalization of $[Ca^{2+}]i$ in phosphate-depleted animals by therapy with a calcium channel blocker that normalizes $[Ca^{2+}]i$ is also followed by correction of the organ dysfunction (Chapter 19, Part 3). Also, diabetes mellitus with even normal renal function is a state in which $[Ca^{2+}]i$ is elevated in many cells, and this abnormality is associated with cell dysfunction similar to those seen in uremia. Calcium channel blockers can prevent the elevation in $[Ca^{2+}]i$ and this correction is followed by normalization of the diabetic complication that was studied (i.e., polymorphonuclear dysfunction). In addition, chronic treatment of normal animals with PTH was also associated with a rise in $[Ca^{2+}]i$ and organ dysfunction despite the absence of CRF.

It appears therefore that a large body of evidence indicates that the secondary hyperparathyroidism of CRF generates a state of cell calcium toxicity that is responsible, in major part, for many of the uremic manifestations. The clinical implication of this formulation is that the signs and symptoms of uremic syndrome could be ameliorated, prevented, or reversed either by reduction of blood levels of PTH or by blocking the action of the hormone on $[Ca^{2+}]i$ by therapy with a calcium channel blocker.

TABLE 68.4. Uremic Manifestations Attributed to Excess PTH in Patients with Chronic Renal Failure

		Improved or Normalized by		
Organ	Derangements	Parathyroidectomy	Suppression of Parathyroid Glands' Activity by $1,25(OH)_2D_3$ or Vitamin D_3	Calcium Channel Blocker
Brain	Abnormal EEG	+	+	
Peripheral nerve	Prolonged motor nerve conduction velocity[a]			
Heart	Decreased cardiac index	+	+	
	Reduced left ventricular ejection fraction	+		
	Decreased percent fiber shortening	+	+	
Pancreas	Impaired insulin secretion	+	+	
Polymorphonuclear	Impaired phagocytosis			+
	Impaired glycogen metabolism		+	+
Itching		+		
Tissue necrosis		+		
Soft tissue calcification		+	+	
Bone resorption		+	+	
Sexual function (impotence)		+	+	

[a] A relationship between the derangement in motor never conduction velocity and blood levels of PTH was documented.
EEG, electroencephalogram; PTH, parathyroid hormone.

OTHER PATHWAYS THROUGH WHICH PTH MAY EXERT TOXIC ACTIONS IN UREMIA

As mentioned previously, PTH affects phospholipids of cell membrane, and alterations in these phospholipids may affect agonist–receptor interactions and cell membrane fluidity. These latter alterations may be associated with adverse effects on cell function.

PTH could be a catabolic agent and, as such, play a role in the wasting syndrome of uremia and contribute in a modest manner to the accumulation of nitrogenous compounds in blood. Indeed, administration of PTH to humans is associated with a negative nitrogen balance, and nitrogen balance is usually negative in patients with primary hyperparathyroidism; the nitrogen balance becomes significantly more positive after removal of the adenoma. Thus it is possible that the elevated blood levels of PTH not only are directly toxic by affecting cell function but may contribute to uremic toxicity by enhancing catabolism and by augmenting the accumulation of nitrogenous compounds in the blood.

SPECIFIC ORGAN DYSFUNCTION IN UREMIA AND THE ROLE OF PTH IN THEIR GENESIS

Neurotoxicity of PTH in Uremia

Neurobehavioral abnormalities, disturbances in electroencephalogram (EEG), and peripheral neuropathy are frequently seen in uremia (see Chapter 69). A multitude of experimental and clinical data point toward the neurotoxicity of PTH in uremia.

Studies in dogs have shown that (a) acute uremia increases the calcium content of both brain and peripheral nerves, (b) acute uremia is associated with slowing of the EEG and prolongation in motor nerve conduction velocity (MNCV), (c) parathyroidectomy before the induction of uremia prevents the rise in calcium content of both brain and peripheral nerves and averts the disturbances in EEG and MNCV, and (d) administration of PTH to dogs with normal renal function increases the calcium content of brain and peripheral nerves and induces changes in EEG and MNCV similar to those seen with acute uremia; these changes are reversed after the discontinuation of PTH administration.

We have also examined the effect of a comparable degree of chronic uremia of 8 to 16 months' duration on brain and peripheral nerve calcium content and on the EEG and MNCV in dogs with intact parathyroid glands and in parathyroidectomized animals maintained normocalcemic. Calcium contents of these organs were markedly increased in the dogs with intact parathyroid glands. The percentage of slow waves (less than 7 Hz) in the EEG was significantly increased and MNCV was significantly prolonged in uremic dogs with intact parathyroid glands, but both functions were not different from normal in the parathyroidectomized uremic dogs.

Further support for the neurotoxic effects of PTH is provided by a number of clinical observations. (a) Patients with chronic renal failure, who usually have elevated blood levels of PTH, have increased calcium content of the brain. (b) The EEG abnormalities in patients with chronic renal failure were found to be reversed 3 months after parathyroidectomy (Fig. 68.13). (c) A

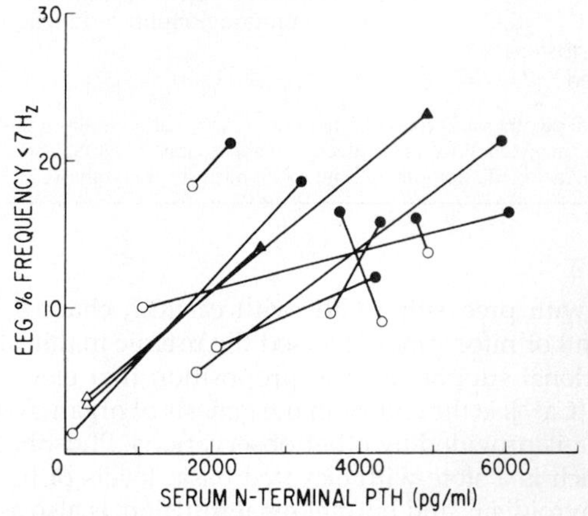

Figure 68.13. The effect of the fall in blood levels of the N-terminal fragment of parathyroid hormone induced by $1,25(OH)_2D_3$ treatment *(circles)* or parathyroidectomy *(triangles)* on the percentage of EEG frequencies below 7 Hz. *Solid symbols,* data before treatment; *open symbols,* data after treatment. (Reproduced with permission from Goldstein DA, Feinstein EI, Chui IA, et al. The relationship between the abnormalities in electroencephalogram and blood levels of PTH in dialysis patients. *J Clin Endocrinol Metab* 1980;51:130–134.)

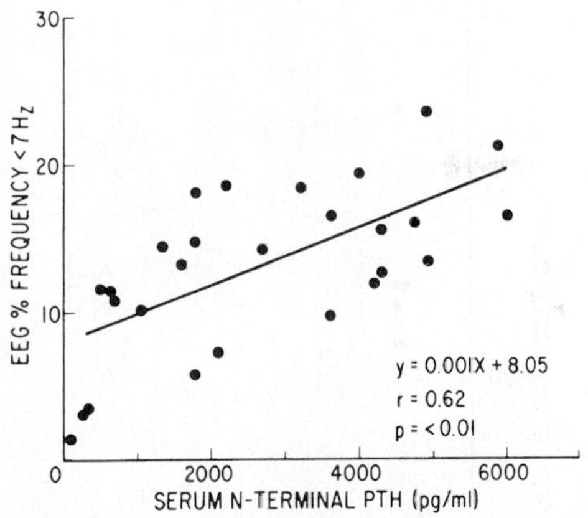

Figure 68.14. The relationship between blood levels of the N-terminal fragment of parathyroid hormone and the percentage of EEG frequencies below 7 Hz in dialysis patients. (Reproduced with permission from Goldstein DA, Feinstein EI, Chui IA, et al. The relationship between the abnormalities in electroencephalogram and blood levels of PTH in dialysis patients. *J Clin Endocrinol Metab* 1980;51:130–134.)

direct and significant relationship exists between the EEG abnormalities and the blood levels of the N-terminal fragment of PTH (Fig. 68.14), and amelioration of secondary hyperparathyroidism by treatment with $1,25(OH)_2D_3$ is associated with improvement of the EEG (Fig. 68.13). (d) Patients with primary hyperparathyroidism and normal renal function display EEG abnormalities similar to those observed in uremia, and these derangements progressively improve following parathyroidectomy, with the EEG recordings being normal within 2 to 3 weeks after surgery. (e) MNCV is reduced in dialysis patients with elevated blood levels of PTH, but it is within the normal range in age-matched dialysis patients who have markedly lower blood levels of PTH. (f) A careful review of the literature reveals that several investigators have reported slowing of MNCV and segmental demyelination of peripheral nerve in humans during the early course of acute renal failure, a condition associated with elevated blood levels of PTH. It is of interest that some investigators failed to demonstrate abnormalities in MNCV in 10 patients with acute renal failure; this does not necessarily vitiate the notion that excess PTH is toxic to peripheral nerve function. Patients with acute renal failure are hypocalcemic, and hypocalcemia accelerates MNCV. Thus a hypocalcemic acute renal failure patient with normal MNCV could have a slow conduction velocity if blood levels of calcium were normal. Indeed in dogs with acute renal failure and prolonged MNCV, the blood calcium was maintained at normal levels. Finally, certain data also point toward a possible role of PTH in the pathogenesis of dialysis encephalopathy. Aluminum toxicity resulting in increased aluminum content of the brain has been implicated in the cause of dialysis encephalopathy. It has been reported that the accumulation of aluminum in the brain is increased by PTH, suggesting that the hormone may play a role in the overall process underlying the development of this syndrome. Interestingly, a patient with dialysis encephalopathy improved markedly after parathyroidectomy.

Other studies have demonstrated that acute or chronic renal failure in rats is associated with accumulation of calcium in brain synaptosomes. Indeed, the basal levels of $[Ca^{2+}]i$ of brain synaptosomes in rats with CRF is significantly elevated. This derangement is mediated by the state of secondary hyperparathyroidism of CRF; it is prevented by prior parathyroidectomy of CRF animals or by their treatment with verapamil, which blocks the PTH-induced rise in $[Ca^{2+}]i$, and chronic administration of PTH to rats with normal renal function is associated with a rise in $[Ca^{2+}]i$ of synaptosomes. The elevation in $[Ca^{2+}]i$ of brain synaptosomes causes significant derangements in their metabolism and function.

The brain synaptosomes of CRF rats display the following: (a) decreased total phospholipids, phosphatidylinositol, phosphatidylserine, phosphatidylethanolamine (Fig. 68.5), and ATP; (b) impaired activity of Na^+-K^+-ATPase and Ca^{2+}-ATPase; (c) decreased norepinephrine content, uptake, and release; (d) reduced V_{max} of tyrosine hydroxylase and increased K_m of monoamine oxidase; (e) increased acetylcholine content and release; (f) reduced choline kinase activity; and (g) decreased choline content and increased choline uptake. These derangements are prevented by prior parathyroidectomy of the CRF rats or by their treatment with verapamil (Table 68.3). The abnormalities in brain synaptosomes of CRF rats may be produced in rats with normal renal function after chronic treatment with PTH.

Thus the available data provide support for a cause-and-effect relationship between excess PTH and certain metabolic and functional disturbances of the nervous system in uremia. The various pieces of evidence satisfy all the criteria for a uremic toxin: excess PTH is present in the blood of the patients; the hormone can be assayed; administration of PTH to experimental animals with normal renal function induces changes similar to those seen in uremia; and prevention of secondary hyperparathyroidism of CRF, reduction in the blood levels of the hormone, or blocking of the action of PTH by a calcium channel blocker is associated with amelioration of the abnormalities.

Role of PTH in the Genesis of the Anemia of Uremia

The factors responsible for the anemia of uremia are multiple and are discussed in detail in Chapter 72, Part 1. Clinical data suggest that PTH may play a role in the genesis of the anemia in patients with CRF. It has been reported that the hematocrit and reticulocyte count increased and the blood transfusion requirements decreased after subtotal parathyroidectomy in dialysis patients with secondary hyperparathyroidism. Also, a significant rise in hemoglobin may follow suppression of parathyroid gland activity by treatment with $1,25(OH)_2D_3$.

Effect on Erythropoiesis

Several observations provide evidence that PTH inhibits erythropoiesis. First, intact PTH (1–84 PTH), in concentrations (7.5 to 30 U/ml) comparable with those found in the blood of uremic patients, produced marked inhibition of human peripheral blood and mouse bone marrow erythroid burst-forming units (BFU-E) but had no effect on mouse bone marrow erythroid colony-forming units. Inactivation of 1–84 PTH abolished its action on erythropoiesis. Increasing the concentration of erythropoietin in the media from 0.67 to 1.7 U/ml overcame the inhibitory effect of 1–84 PTH on BFU-E. The N-terminal fragment of PTH (1–34 PTH) and the C-terminal fragment of PTH (53–84 human PTH) had no effect on BFU-E. These data demonstrate that (a) either the intact PTH molecule or a C-terminal fragment(s) bigger than the 53–84 moiety exerts the inhibitory effect on erythropoiesis and (b) adequate amounts of erythropoietin can overcome this action of PTH. Second, 8 U/ml of parathyroid extract inhibited RNA synthesis and 2 U/ml inhibited heme synthesis by mouse embryonic liver erythroid precursors. Third, red blood cell production as measured by ^{59}Fe incorporation was reduced in rats with excess PTH compared with control rats. Other investigators were unable to demonstrate an inhibition of erythropoiesis by PTH.

If PTH interferes with erythropoiesis, one would expect patients with primary hyperparathyroidism and normal renal function to have anemia. Indeed, 5% to 21% of patients with primary hyperparathyroidism have a moderate degree of chronic normocytic anemia, which improves or normalizes after removal of the adenoma. The lower incidence and the milder degree of anemia in patients with primary hyperparathyroidism than in patients with uremia should not be construed as evidence against a role for PTH in the pathogenesis of anemia. The presence of normal kidneys and hence normal production of erythropoietin in patients with parathyroid adenoma counterbalances the action of PTH on erythropoiesis. In contrast, patients with CRF are in double jeopardy: the excess blood levels of PTH inhibit erythropoiesis, and the inability to generate adequate erythropoietin permits the inhibitory action of PTH to proceed unchecked.

Effect on Osmotic Fragility of Human Red Blood Cells

Both the N-terminal (1–34) PTH and the intact (1–84) PTH but not the C-terminal (53–84) PTH have been shown to produce significant increases in osmotic fragility of human red blood cells (RBCs). This effect was abolished by prior inactivation of the hormone. There was a dose-response relationship between both moieties of PTH and the increase in osmotic fragility. This action of PTH required calcium, was mimicked by calcium ionophore, and was partially blocked by verapamil, and PTH caused significant influx of ^{45}Ca into RBCs. Scanning electron microscopy revealed that the incubation of RBCs with PTH was associated with the appearance of membrane filamentous extensions that anchor RBCs together. PTH did not affect water content of RBCs. Inhibition of glycolytic activity of RBCs with NaF or inhibition of Na^+-K^+-ATPase with ouabain did not abolish the effect of PTH on osmotic fragility. PTH did not stimulate RBC Na^+-K^+-ATPase or Mg-dependent ATPase but caused marked and significant stimulation of Ca-activated ATPase. This acute effect of PTH on Ca^{2+}-ATPase activity is different from the chronic effects of the hormone; Ca^{2+}-ATPase activity of RBCs in CRF is reduced. The basal activity of RBC adenylate cyclase was low, and PTH produced only a modest stimulation of this enzyme. Both cyclic adenosine 3′,5′-monophosphate (cAMP) and dibutyryl cAMP had no effect on osmotic fragility. These observations indicate that (a) the human RBC is a target organ for PTH, (b) the hormone increases osmotic fragility of RBCs, and (c) this effect of PTH is due to enhanced calcium entry into RBCs. It is possible that the increased calcium influx may affect the spectrin-actin of the cytoskeletal network of the RBCs and alter the stability and integrity of the cell membrane.

The implications of the effects of PTH on RBCs were examined in the *in vivo* setting in experimental animals and humans. ^{51}Cr RBC survival was evaluated in six normal dogs, in six animals with CRF and secondary hyperparathyroidism, and in six parathyroidectomized dogs with comparable degrees and duration of CRF (Fig. 68.15). In the normal dogs, the ^{51}Cr RBC survival ranged between 22 and 35 (25.6 ± 1.9) days. In the animals with renal failure and intact parathyroid glands, the ^{51}Cr survival was shortened, with values ranging between 16 and 20 (18.4 ± 0.6) days, which were significantly (P <.01) lower than that in normal dogs. In the parathyroidectomized, normocalcemic dogs with CRF, the ^{51}Cr RBC survival ranged between 20 and 33 (25.2 ± 1.8) days, a value not different from that in normal dogs but significantly higher (P <.01) than that in dogs with renal failure and intact parathyroid glands. These data demonstrate that excess blood levels of PTH and not other consequences of the uremic state are responsible for the shortened RBC survival in CRF. Further support for this notion is found in humans: a significant inverse relationship (r = −0.67, P <.01) between RBC survival, as measured by ^{51}Cr, and blood levels of PTH was demonstrated in 27 hemodialysis patients.

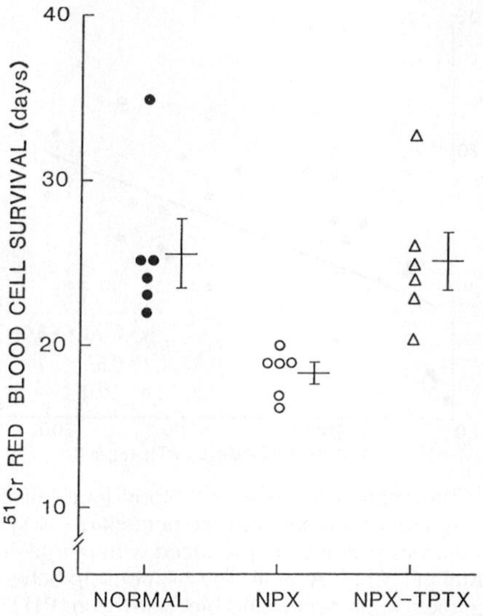

Figure 68.15. Red blood cell survival in normal dogs *(solid circles)*, dogs with chronic renal failure *(NPX) (open circles)*, and normocalcemic, thyroparathyroidectomized dogs with chronic renal failure *(NPX-TPTX) (open triangles)*. Each *data point* represents one animal and *brackets* denote mean ± 1 SE. (Reproduced with permission from Akmal M, Telfer N, Ansari AN, et al. Red blood cell survival in chronic renal failure. Role of secondary hyperparathyroidism. *J Clin Invest* 1985;76:1695–1698.)

Role of PTH-Induced Marrow Fibrosis

Excess PTH induces moderate to marked degrees of bone marrow fibrosis and therefore limits the availability of red marrow, hence reducing the number of red cell-forming units. Myelofibrosis in dialysis patients has been noted, and its relation to anemia has been documented.

Summary of the Role of PTH in the Genesis of Anemia of Renal Failure

PTH may participate in the genesis of the anemia of uremia through at least four pathways: inhibition of erythropoiesis, reduction of survival of RBCs, inhibition of platelet aggregation, and fibrosis of bone marrow cavity (Fig. 68.16).

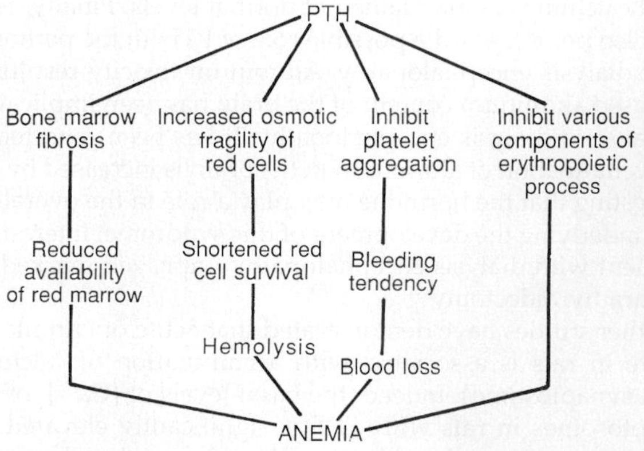

Figure 68.16. A schematic presentation of the pathways through which parathyroid hormone may participate in the genesis of the anemia of chronic renal failure.

Effect of PTH on Polymorphonuclear Leukocyte Function

Uremic patients have an increased susceptibility to infection. This may be partly due to defective leukocyte function. Indeed, polymorphonuclear leukocytes (PMNLs) from uremic patients display impaired migration and defective phagocytic and bactericidal activities. The pathogenesis of these derangements is not evident. Certain clinical observations suggest that PTH affects leukocyte function. It has been reported that random migration and chemotaxis of PMNLs were impaired in patients with primary hyperparathyroidism and normal renal function, and these defects disappeared after removal of the adenoma. Others found that sera from uremic patients with high blood PTH levels stimulated chemiluminescence of PMNLs, and the decrease in blood levels of PTH after parathyroidectomy was associated with a reduction in this stimulatory effect.

Studies from our laboratory have demonstrated that PMNLs are targets for PTH action. Indeed, acute exposure of leukocytes to 1–84 PTH increased elastase release from these cells and impaired their random migration. The aminoterminal fragment of the hormone was inert in regard to PMNLs function, and the 19–84 aminosequence fragment of PTH increased elastase release from PMNLs as did the 1–84 PTH.

A large body of evidence exists implicating the state of secondary hyperparathyroidism in the genesis of PMNLs dysfunction in uremic patients. Random migration of PMNLs is impaired in CRF patients, and an inverse relationship exists between random migration of PMNLs and blood levels of PTH in these patients. PMNLs of CRF patients and those treated with hemodialysis have elevated basal levels of $[Ca^{2+}]i$, reduced ATP content, and impaired phagocytosis (Fig. 68.17). These derangements are due to the state of secondary hyperparathyroidism of CRF. Studies in CRF rats support this conclusion and further demonstrate that these derangements are prevented by prior parathyroidectomy of CRF animals or by their treatment with

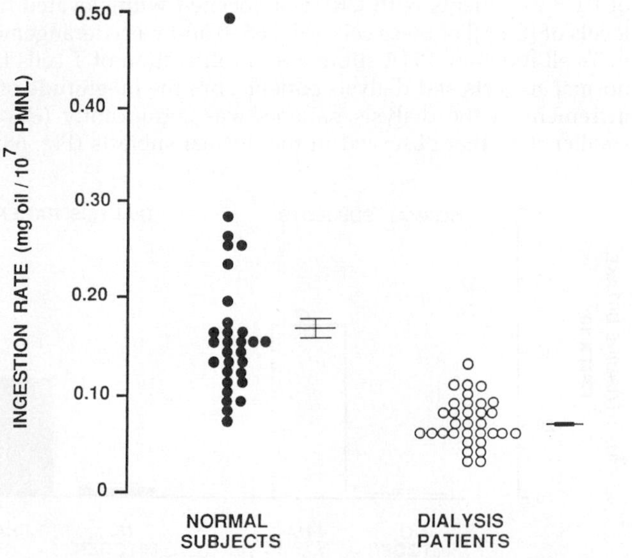

Figure 68.17. Ingestion of lipopolysaccharide-coated oil droplet by PMNL from normal subjects and dialysis patients. Each *datum point* denotes one individual and *brackets* represent mean ± 1 SE. (Reproduced with permission from Alexiewicz JM, Smogorzewski M, Fadda GZ, et al. Impaired phagocytosis in dialysis patients: studies on mechanisms. *Am J Nephrol* 1991;11:102–111.)

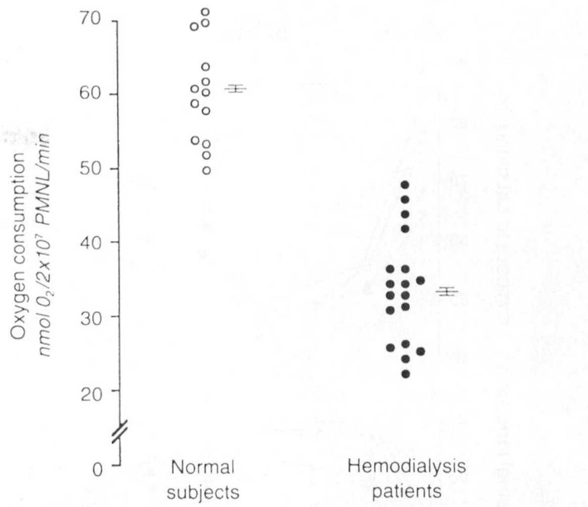

Figure 68.18. Oxygen consumption in response to FMLP by polymorphonuclear leukocytes *(PMNL)* from normal subjects and hemodialysis patients. Each *datum point* represents one subject and *brackets* denote mean ± 1 SE. (Reproduced with permission from Kierszteјn M, Thanakitcharu P, Fadda GZ, et al. Decreased O_2 consumption by PMNL from humans and rats with CRF: role of secondary hyperparathyroidism. *Kidney Int* 1992;42:602–609.)

verapamil. Also, glucose uptake by and glycogen content of PMNLs are reduced and the activity of their glycogen synthetase is impaired in patients with CRF. The treatment of these patients with verapamil or $1,25(OH)_2D_3$ (which suppresses the activity of the parathyroid glands) reversed these abnormalities. Finally, oxygen consumption by PMNLs from humans (Fig. 68.18) and rats with CRF is decreased; this abnormality is due to the state of secondary hyperparathyroidism of CRF, and is prevented by prior parathyroidectomy of the CRF animals or by their treatment with verapamil. The treatment of rats with preexisting CRF with verapamil reversed the derangement in the oxygen consumption by these cells.

The demonstration in animals with CRF that their treatment with verapamil normalizes the ATP content, the basal levels of $[Ca^{2+}]i$, and phagocytosis of PMNLs was confirmed in a study of two groups of hemodialysis patients. Indeed, the PMNLs of hemodialysis patients without therapy with a calcium channel blocker displayed elevated basal levels of $[Ca^{2+}]i$, reduced ATP content, and impaired phagocytosis. In contrast, the PMNLs of hemodialysis patients who were receiving nifedipine had normal levels of $[Ca^{2+}]i$, ATP content, and phagocytosis.

In a prospective study of hemodialysis patients, the basal levels of $[Ca^{2+}]i$ and phagocytosis of PMNLs were examined before, monthly for 2 months during treatment with nifedipine (30 mg/day), and monthly for an additional 2 months after discontinuation of the drug. Therapy with amlodipine reversed the derangements in the PMNLs, $[Ca^{2+}]i$ and phagocytosis, with the values being normal during the treatment period. However, the abnormalities in $[Ca^{2+}]i$ and phagocytosis of the PMNLs reemerged after discontinuation of the treatment with the calcium channel blocker (Fig. 68.19).

These observations and others cited earlier demonstrate that calcium channel blockers are effective in reversing the effects of uremia on the metabolism ($[Ca^{2+}]i$, ATP content, glucose uptake, glycogen content, glycogen synthetase) and function (phagocytosis) of PMNLs in humans. The therapy with the calcium channel blocker should be continued in order to maintain their beneficial effects.

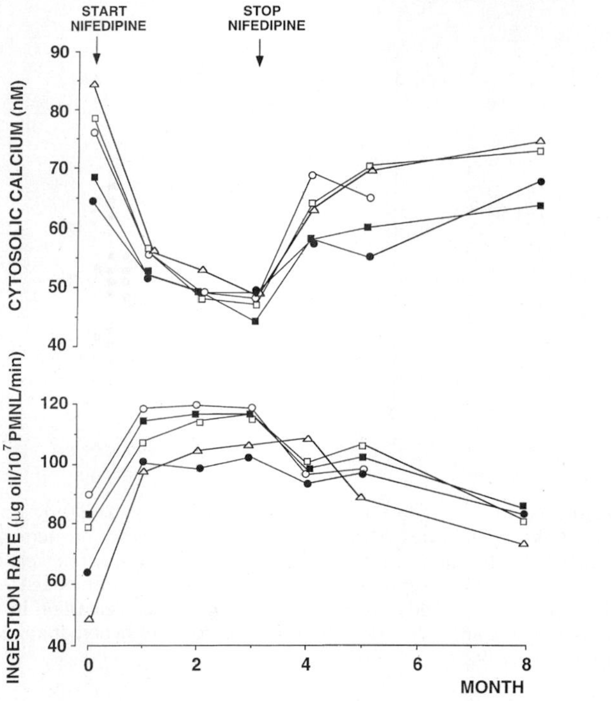

Figure 68.19. The changes in $[Ca^{2+}]i$ of PMNLs *(upper panel)* and phagocytosis *(lower panel)* observed in the five hemodialysis patients before, during, and after cessation of nifedipine therapy. Each *line* represents one patient. (Reproduced with permission from Alexiewicz JM, Smogorzewski M, Gill S, et al. Time course of the effect of nifedipine therapy and its discontinuation on $[Ca^{2+}]i$ and phagocytosis of polymorphonuclear leukocytes from hemodialysis patients. *Am J Nephrol* 1997; 17:12–16.)

ROLE OF PTH IN THE GENESIS OF THE ABNORMALITIES OF THE IMMUNE SYSTEM IN UREMIA

Abnormalities in the immune system are encountered in clinical and experimental CRF, and both cellular and humoral immunity are impaired. These derangements are discussed in Chapter 80. The mechanisms responsible for these derangements are not fully delineated. Metabolic and toxic consequences of CRF and/or the compounding effects of malnutrition, vitamin deficiency, drug therapy, and dialysis treatment may each alone, or in any combination, contribute to the genesis of the deranged immune system in CRF.

Available data indicate that lymphocytes have receptors for PTH. It is therefore reasonable to suggest that the function and/or metabolism of lymphocytes (both T and B cells) could be affected by PTH. It has been shown that 1–34 PTH activated mononuclear leukocytes, most likely T cells, and caused them to produce a substance(s) that enhances bone resorption. In addition, it was reported that PTH stimulates proliferation of thymic lymphocytes. It is plausible that the state of excess PTH in patients with CRF adversely affects the function of T and B cells and as such contributes to the impaired cellular and humoral immunity in these patients. We have examined the function of T and B cells from dialysis patients and the effects of the intact molecule of PTH (1–84 PTH) and its aminoterminal fragment (1–34 PTH) on T- and B-cell function in an effort to delineate the interactions between PTH and T and B cells and to investigate the role of excess PTH in the genesis of the deranged immune system in CRF.

PTH and T-Cell Function

1–84 PTH produced a small and significant ($P < .01$) increase in the proliferation of unstimulated lymphocytes. In addition, 1–84 PTH caused significant ($P < .01$) increments in phytohemagglutinin (PHA)-induced lymphocyte proliferation in a dose-dependent manner, and the inactivation of the hormone abolished this effect. Higher doses of 1–34 PTH were required to enhance PHA-induced proliferation of lymphocytes, and the magnitude of the increment (+28% ± 5%) by 1–34 PTH was significantly ($P < .01$) less than that noted with equimolar concentration (4×10^{-7} M) of 1–84 PTH (+51% ± 9%). It is of interest that PTH did not stimulate pokeweed mitogen (PWM)–induced lymphocyte proliferation. The hormone did not alter CD4:CD8 ratio.

PTH augmented interleukin-2 (IL-2) production by PHA-activated T cells but did not increase expression of IL-2 receptors. The phorbol ester TPA increased PHA-induced T-cell proliferation, but the addition of PTH to the culture stimulated by PHA or TPA did not augment further the proliferation of T cells. Staurosporine reversed the stimulation by PTH of the PHA-induced T-cell proliferation. Both 1–34 and 1–84 PTH stimulated cAMP production by lymphocytes. Forskolin did not affect PHA-induced T-cell proliferation although it did stimulate cAMP generation.

These observations show that lymphocytes are targets for both 1–84 PTH and 1–34 PTH and that both moieties of the hormone augment PHA-induced lymphocyte proliferation. This effect of the hormone is related to its biologic activity because inactivation of the hormone abolished its stimulatory effect. This action of PTH is most likely due to the ability of the hormone to enhance entry of calcium into cells and/or stimulation of protein kinase C, but is independent of cAMP production.

We must emphasize that the studies detailed previously dealt with the effect of the acute exposure of the T cells to PTH. However, in patients with advanced CRF, there is chronic exposure to markedly elevated blood levels of PTH. Such sustained exposure may result in a calcium overload of the lymphocytes, downregulation of their PTH receptors, and altered phospholipid metabolism of their cell membrane. Either or any combination of such events may have adverse effects on lymphocyte function. Indeed, the chronic exposure of T cells to high levels of PTH in patients with CRF is associated with elevated basal levels of $[Ca^{2+}]i$ of these cells (Fig. 68.9) and with derangements in T-cell function. PHA stimulated proliferation of T cells from normal subjects and dialysis patients, but the magnitude of the increment in the dialysis patients was significantly ($P < .01$) smaller than that observed in the normal subjects (Fig. 68.20).

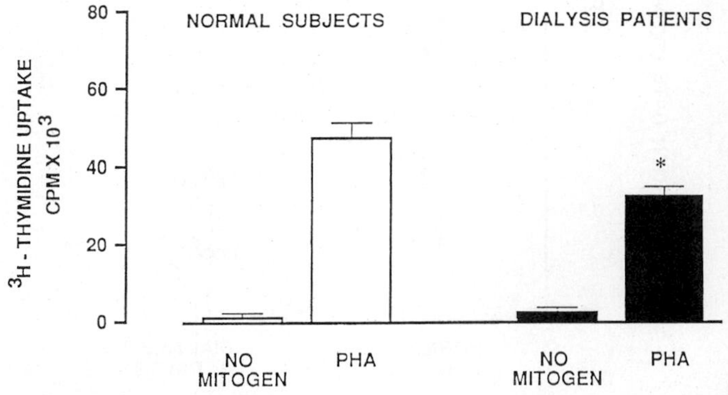

Figure 68.20. Basal levels of $[Ca^{2+}]i$ of B cells from normal subjects and hemodialysis patients without treatment with nifedipine *(HD)* and those treated with nifedipine *(HD + NIF)*. Each *datum point* represents one individual and *brackets* denote mean ± 1 SE. (Reproduced with permission from Alexiewicz JM, Smogorzewski M, Akmal M, et al. Nifedipine reverses the abnormalities in $[Ca^{2+}]i$ and proliferation of B cells from dialysis patients. *Kidney Int* 1996;50:1246–1254.)

Although both 1–84 PTH and 1–34 PTH in a dose of 4×10^{-7} M stimulated PHA-induced proliferation of T cells from normal subjects, they failed to stimulate PHA-induced proliferation of T cells from dialysis patients.

T cells from dialysis patients failed to produce a significant increment in IL-2 after 48 hours of culture with PHA. In contrast, T cells from normal subjects produced a significantly ($P < .05$) greater amount of IL-2 than T cells from dialysis patients. Also, 1–84 PTH produced further augmentation ($P < .02$) in PHA-induced IL-2 production by T cells from normal subjects, but failed to increase PHA-induced IL-2 production by T cells from dialysis patients.

The effects of PHA; exogenous IL-2; PHA and exogenous IL-2; PHA and PTH; and PHA, PTH, and exogenous IL-2 on the proliferation of T cells from normal subjects and dialysis patients are given in Fig. 68.21. In both groups of subjects, exogenous IL-2 alone stimulated T-cell proliferation, and the magnitude of the stimulation was similar to that of PHA alone. Although IL-2 significantly ($P < .05$) increased the PHA-induced proliferation of T cells from normal subjects, it failed to enhance PHA-induced proliferation of T cells from dialysis patients. In addition, exogenous IL-2 did not reverse the failure of PTH to augment the PHA-induced proliferation of T cells from dialysis patients and did not succeed to further enhance the PTH-induced augmentation of the stimulation of T-cell proliferation by PHA in normal subjects.

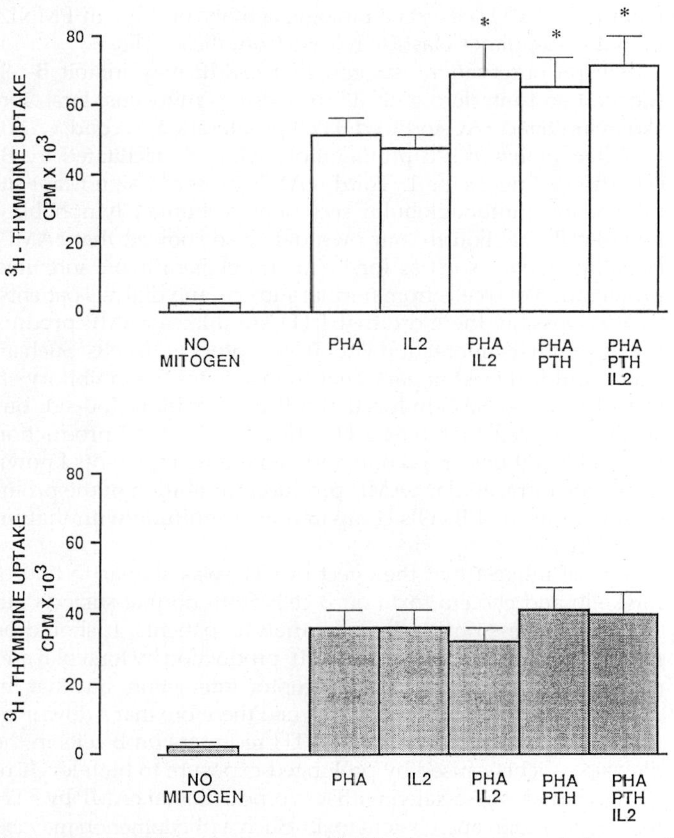

Figure 68.21. Effect of exogenous IL-2 in the presence and absence of PHA or 4×10^{-7} M 1–84 PTH on T-cell proliferation from six normal subjects *(upper panel)* and from eight hemodialysis patients *(lower panel)*. Each *column* represents mean value, and *vertical bars* denote 1 SE. *, $P < .01$ versus PHA or IL-2. (Reproduced with permission from Alexiewicz JM, Klinger M, Linker-Israeli M, et al. Evidence of impaired T cell function in hemodialysis patients. Potential role for secondary hyperparathyroidism. *Am J Nephrol* 1990;10:495–501.)

These observations show that PHA-induced T-cell proliferation is impaired in the dialysis patients. These data are in agreement with reports of others. The mechanisms responsible for this defective response of T cells are not well understood. The proliferation of T cells requires the presence of monocytes and their production of IL-1, the production of IL-2 by the T cells, and the action of IL-2 on its surface receptors in the T cells. Also, normal antigen-receptor interaction and intact cellular signals that follow such an interaction are required for normal proliferation. A defect in one or more of these steps could be present in hemodialysis patients and could be responsible for the impairment in PHA-induced T-cell proliferation.

Available data regarding production of IL-1 by stimulated monocytes from hemodialysis patients are controversial. A normal or increased production of IL-1 has been reported by some authors, whereas others found defective production of IL-1 by monocytes of hemodialysis patients. Our observations and those of others demonstrate that the impaired IL-2 production could be, at least in part, responsible for the defective T-cell proliferation in these patients. It has been shown that IL-2 production by T cells is stimulated by a rise in $[Ca^{2+}]i$. It is, theoretically, possible that the chronic elevation in $[Ca^{2+}]i$ of T cells could interfere with the magnitude of the rise in $[Ca^{2+}]i$ and/or with the ratio between the calcium signal and the resting levels of $[Ca^{2+}]i$ in response to stimulation of T cells, and hence the production of IL-2 would be impaired. Indeed, we found that both the magnitude of the rise in $[Ca^{2+}]i$ and the ratio between this rise and basal levels of $[Ca^{2+}]i$ in response to exposure of 500 ng/ml of anti-CD3 antibody are significantly lower in hemodialysis patients than in normal subjects (Fig. 68.22). It should be mentioned that this latter observation could also suggest that either the interaction between the antibody and its receptors is impaired, the number of the receptors are reduced, and/or the postreceptor events leading to the generation of the calcium signal are defective.

If the impairment in the production of IL-2 by T cells of hemodialysis patients is the only defect responsible for the impaired T-cell proliferation in these patients, one would expect that exogenous IL-2 corrects this defect. Indeed, certain studies showed that exogenous IL-2 reversed the defect in PHA-induced proliferation of peripheral blood mononuclear cells

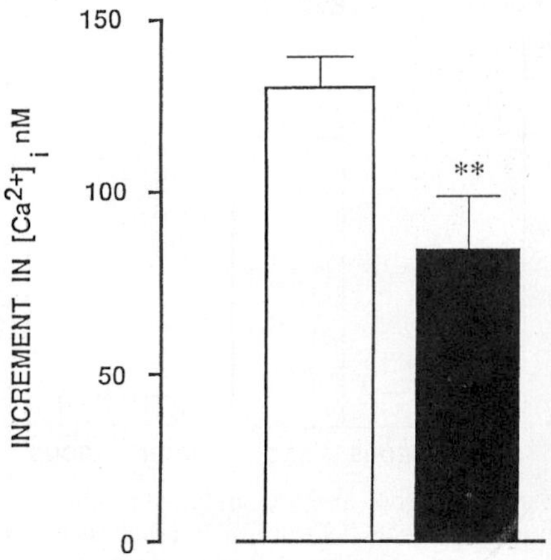

Figure 68.22. The increment in $[Ca^{2+}]i$ of T cells from normal subjects *(open columns)* and dialysis patients *(black columns)* after the exposure of the cells to anti-CD3 antibody. Each *column* represents mean value and *brackets* denote 1 SE. **, $P < .02$. (Reproduced with permission from Alexiewicz JM, Klinger M, Linker-Israeli M, et al. Evidence of impaired T cell function in hemodialysis patients. Potential role for secondary hyperparathyroidism. *Am J Nephrol* 1990;10:495–501.)

(PBMC) from hemodialysis patients. In addition, others reported that the addition of IL-2 to spontaneous culture of PBMC from hemodialysis patients produced a greater proliferative response than in PBMC from normal subjects; these investigators also found that T cells from hemodialysis patients have increased spontaneous expression of IL-2 receptors and that these cells displayed greater response to the exogenous IL-2. In contrast, one group of investigators could not find a difference in the expression of IL-2 receptors in T cells from normal subjects and hemodialysis patients. Our observations are also different from those of others in that exogenous IL-2 did not correct the defect in PHA-induced proliferation of PBMC from dialysis patients, nor did it cause greater proliferation of spontaneous culture of these cells. The reasons for these differences are not evident, and the question of whether T cells from hemodialysis patients respond to IL-2 like those from normal subjects awaits further clarification.

PTH and B-Cell Function

Studies were also conducted to examine the potential effects of PTH on B cells because patients with CRF display variable degrees of impaired humoral immunity. Indeed, the antibody response to viral, but not bacterial, antigens may be reduced, and the number of total B cells has been reported to be normal or decreased. Furthermore, it was found that in dialysis patients, both the T-cell–dependent and T-cell–independent B-cell proliferation are reduced.

B-Cell Proliferation. Available data indicate that *Staphylococcus aureus Cowan* I (SAC)–induced lymphocyte proliferation represents T-cell–independent B-cell proliferation. SAC induced a significant ($P < .01$) increase in proliferation of B cells from both normal subjects and dialysis patients, but the increment in the dialysis patients was significantly ($P < .01$) lower than in normal subjects (Fig. 68.23).

Both 1–34 PTH and 1–84 PTH produced a dose-dependent inhibition of SAC-induced B-cell proliferation, but the effect of 1–84 PTH was significantly greater ($P < .01$) than that produced by an equimolar dose of 1–34 PTH. At a dose of 4×10^{-7} M, the

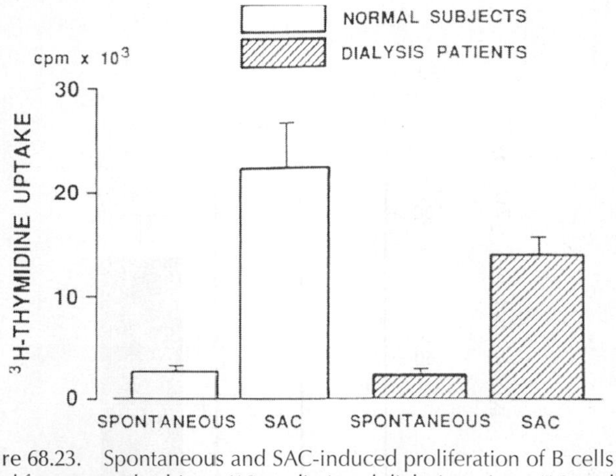

Figure 68.23. Spontaneous and SAC-induced proliferation of B cells obtained form normal subjects (19 studies) and dialysis patients (16 studies). Each *column* represents the mean value, and *bars* denote 1 SE. The values with SAC are significantly higher ($P < .01$) than the spontaneous values in both normal subjects and dialysis patients, but the value with SAC in dialysis patients is significantly lower ($P < .01$) than that in normal subjects. (Reproduced with permission from Alexiewicz JM, Klinger M, Pitts TO, et al. Parathyroid hormone inhibits B cell proliferation: implications in chronic renal failure. *J Am Soc Nephrol* 1990;1:236–244.)

decrement in B-cell proliferation was $-9.7\% \pm 3.8\%$ with 1–34 PTH and $-55.2\% \pm 6.9\%$ with 1–84 PTH ($P < .01$).

1–84 PTH also inhibited SAC-induced proliferation of B cells from dialysis patients, but the decrement ($-47.3\% \pm 3.9\%$) in the dialysis patients was significantly smaller ($P < .05$) than that in normal subjects ($-58.4\% \pm 2.5\%$). In 12 dialysis patients, the percentage inhibition of SAC-induced B-cell proliferation with 1–84 PTH was inversely and significantly correlated with the blood levels of PTH ($r = -0.78$, $P < .01$).

1–84 PTH also produced a significant ($P < .01$) increase in the production of cAMP by B cells from normal subjects. It is of interest that agents that increased cAMP without receptor interaction (forskolin and cholera toxin) also inhibited SAC-induced proliferation of B cells from normal subjects and dialysis patients, and this effect was not different between the two groups.

These observations indicate that B cells are targets for PTH. It is worthwhile to mention again that the effect of the intact hormone is greater than that of its aminoterminal fragment. This phenomenon is similar to the effects of these two moieties of PTH on T-cell function. As we suggested earlier, this difference between the magnitude of the effects of 1-84 PTH and 1-34 PTH is consistent with the notion that the intact hormone may attach more tightly to its receptor or that other parts of PTH, in addition to its aminoterminal fragment, may possess biologic activity. Certain data exist supporting such possibilities. For example, binding sites with specificity for the middle region or the carboxy-terminal fragment of PTH have been described in canine and chicken renal membranes and in cloned rat osteosarcoma. Also, we have found that the carboxy-terminal fragment (19–84 PTH) exerts a biologic activity on human PMNLs in that it stimulates elastase release from these cells.

Several observations suggest that cAMP may inhibit B-cell function and interfere with its response to mitogens. First, forskolin inhibited SAC-induced B-cell proliferation. Second, cAMP inhibited mouse B-cell proliferation, which is facilitated by B-cell–stimulating factor 1. Third, cAMP caused a significant inhibition of immunoglobulin secretion by human lymphoblastoid–B-cell line. Fourth, our own data also showed that cAMP-elevating agents, such as forskolin and cholera toxin, inhibited proliferation of B cells from normal subjects and dialysis patients.

It is possible therefore that PTH stimulates cAMP production through its interaction with its receptors on B cells. Such an event could, at least in part, be responsible for the inhibitory effect of PTH on SAC-induced B-cell proliferation. Indeed, our studies showed that 1–84 PTH stimulated cAMP production by B cells and both forskolin and cholera toxin, agents known to elevate intracellular cAMP, produced inhibition of the proliferation of normal B cells compared in magnitude with that induced by PTH.

It is of interest that the effect of PTH was similar to that of forskolin and cholera toxin on B cells from normal subjects but significantly less on B cells from dialysis patients. It should be mentioned that the increase in cAMP production by forskolin and cholera toxin does not require receptor interaction, but that induced by PTH does. It could be argued therefore that a downregulation or desensitization of the PTH receptors on B cells in the dialysis patients caused by prolonged exposure to high levels of PTH in blood is associated with less production of cAMP by PTH than by forskolin and cholera toxin. Such a phenomenon may explain the differences in the action of PTH and forskolin or cholera toxin on the proliferation of B cells of the dialysis patients.

Antibody Production by B Cells. The inhibition of B-cell proliferation by PTH may also lead to impaired antibody production by these cells. We examined the production of IgG,

IgM, and IgA by B cells stimulated with SAC or with PWM after 8 days of culture and evaluated the effect of PTH on this process in 34 hemodialysis patients and 44 normal subjects. IgG, IgM, and IgA production by B cells from patients was lower ($P <.01$) than by B cells from normal subjects (Fig. 68.24). Both 1–34 and 1–84 PTH inhibited ($P <.01$) immunoglobulin production by B cells from normal subjects and dialysis patients. However, this inhibitory effect was evident in dialysis patients only with the higher dosage of PTH. The inhibition of immunoglobulin production by PTH occurred only when the hormone was added in the initiation of the B-cell culture. Inactivation of PTH abolished its inhibitory effect on immunoglobulin production. Agents that stimulate cAMP production (forskolin, cholera toxin) and the cAMP analog, 8-bromoadenosine 3′,5′ cyclic monophosphate inhibited immunoglobulin production by B cells from both normal subjects and dialysis patients, and the degree of inhibition was not different between the two groups. The calcium ionophore A23187 also inhibited IgG, IgA, and IgM production by B cells from normal subjects and dialysis patients; there was no difference in the degree between the two groups. As mentioned previously, the resting levels of $[Ca^{2+}]i$ of B cells from dialysis patients is significantly higher than in normal subjects. These observations show that: (a) immunoglobulin production by B cells from dialysis patients is impaired; (b) PTH inhibits IgG, IgA, and IgM production and this effect is, at least, partly mediated by PTH-induced cAMP generation and by alterations in $[Ca^{2+}]i$ of B cells; (c) this inhibitory effect is mediated by events that affect the initial stages of B-cell proliferation and maturation; and (d) the requirement for high doses of PTH for its inhibitory effect on B cells from dialysis patients is probably due to desensitization and/or downregulation of PTH receptors on B cells. The results are consistent with the proposition that impaired immunoglobulin production by B cells from dialysis patients is, at least partly, due to the state of secondary hyperparathyroidism in these patients.

The observations that PTH inhibits immunoglobulin production *in vitro* do not provide definite proof for a role of excess PTH in the genesis of the abnormality in the *in vivo* immunoglobulin production. It is possible that other consequences of the uremic state and/or another, as yet unidentified, factor accumulates in the blood of uremic patients and underlies the impaired humoral immunity. To definitely incriminate excess PTH in the genesis of impaired humoral immunity in CRF, one must document that reduced antibody production in response to antigens is normal in a CRF state without excess PTH.

We examined *in vivo* antibody production in response to sheep red blood cells (SRBCs), bovine serum albumin (BSA) and influenza vaccine in normal rats, CRF rats, and parathyroidectomized (PTX)-CRF rats maintained normocalcemic. The antibody response to all three antigens in CRF rats were significantly and markedly lower than in normal or CRF-PTX rats (Figs. 68.25 to 68.27). The response to SRBC, the IgG anti-BSA

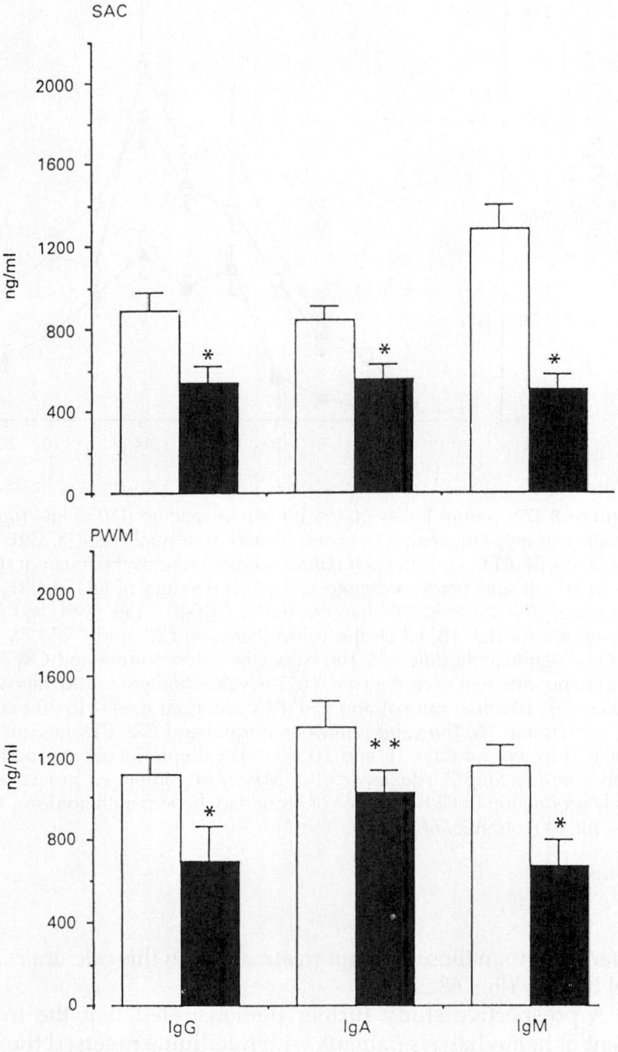

Figure 68.24. SAC (*upper panel*) and PWM-induced (*lower panel*) immunoglobulin production by B cells from normal subjects (□) and dialysis patients (■). Each *column* represents mean value and *brackets* denote 1 SE. *, $P<.01$; **, $P<.05$ versus normal subjects. (Reproduced with permission from Gaciong Z, Alexiewicz JM, Linker-Israeli M, et al. Inhibition of immunoglobulin production by parathyroid hormone. Implications in chronic renal failure. *Kidney Int* 1991;40:96–106.)

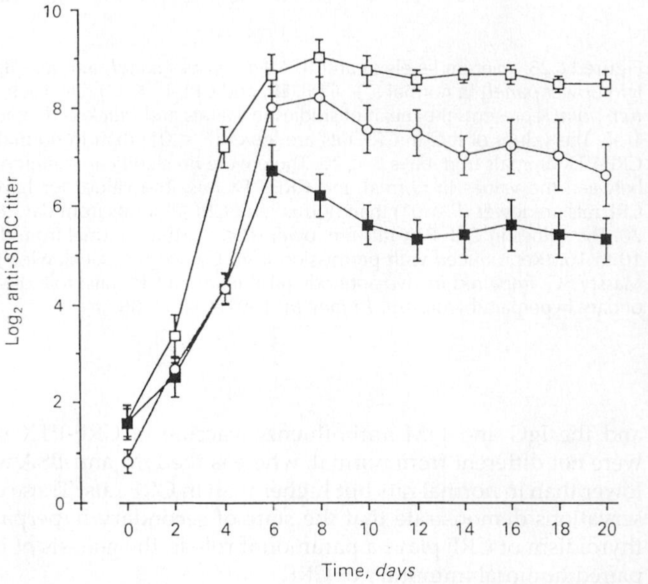

Figure 68.25. Serum levels of anti-SRBC titer in normal (□), CRF (■) and CRF-PTX (○) rats. Each *datum point* represents the mean value of studies in 10 rats and *brackets* denote ± 1 SE. The values in CRF rats are lower ($P <.05$ to $<.01$) than in normal and CRF-PTX animals from days 8 to 18. On day 20, the values in CRF and CRF-PTX rats are not different and the values in CRF-PTX rats are lower than normal rats ($P <.05$) (Reproduced with permission from Gaciong Z, Alexiewicz JM, Massry SG. Impaired *in vivo* antibody production in CRF rats: role of secondary hyperparathyroidism. *Kidney Int* 1991;40:862–867.)

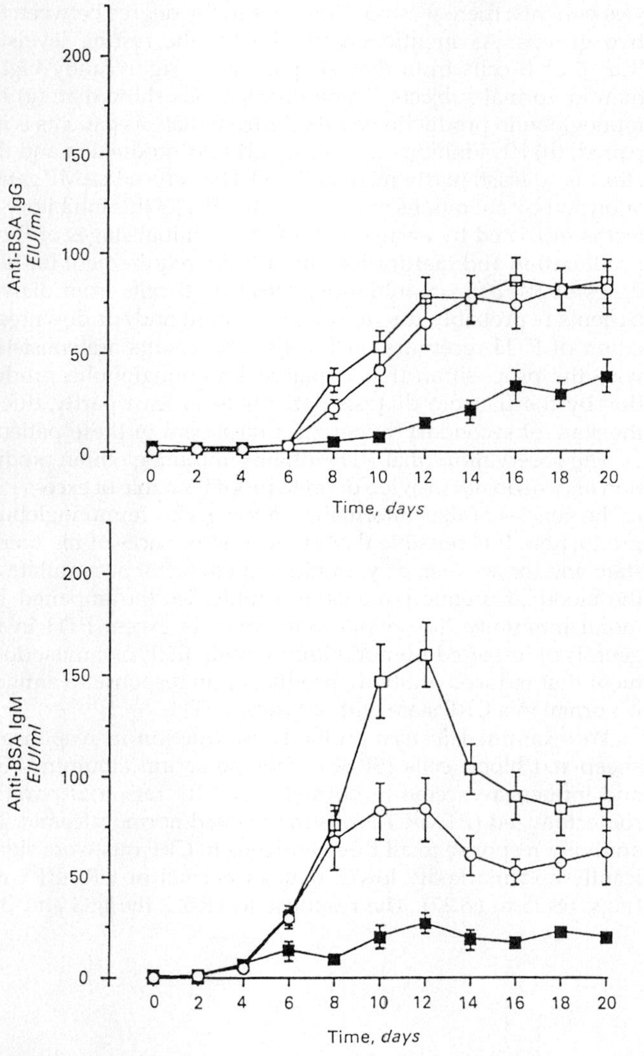

Figure 68.26. Serum levels of anti BSA-IgG (*upper panel*) and anti BSA-IgM (*lower panel*) in normal (□), CRF (■), and CRF-PTX (○) rats. Each *datum point* represents the mean of studies in 10 rats and *brackets* denote ± 1 SE. The values of IgG in CRF rats are lower ($P < .01$) than in normal or CRF-PTX animals from days 8 to 20. There were no significant differences between the values in normal and CRF-PTX rats. The values for IgM in CRF rats are lower ($P < .01$) than normal and CRF-PTX rats from days 6 to 20. The values in CRF-PTX rats are lower ($P < .01$) than normal from days 10 to 16. (Reproduced with permission from Gaciong Z, Alexiewicz JM, Massry SG. Impaired *in vivo* antibody production in CRF rats: role of secondary hyperparathyroidism. *Kidney Int* 1991;40:862–867.)

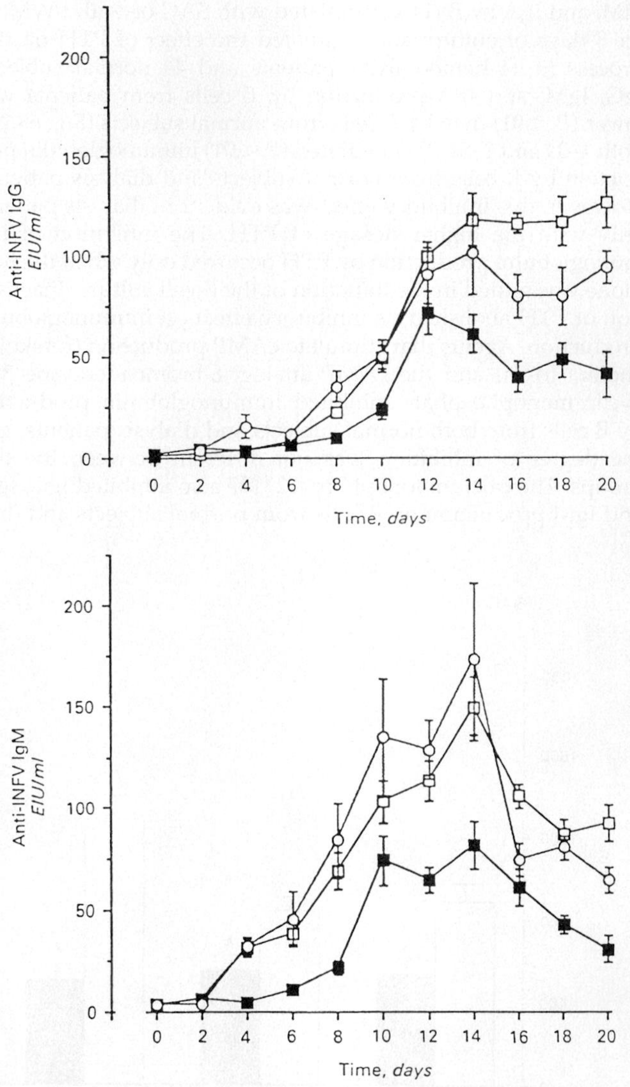

Figure 68.27. Serum levels of anti-influenza vaccine *(INFV)* IgG (*upper panel*) and anti-influenza IgM (*lower panel*) in normal rats (□), CRF rats (■), and CRF-PTX rats (○). Each *datum point* represents the mean of studies in 10 rats and *brackets* denote ± 1 SE. The values of IgG in CRF rats are lower ($P < .05$ to $< .01$) than normal or CRF-PTX rats from days 8 to 20, except for day 18, when the values between CRF and CRF-PTX rats are not significantly different. The values between normal and CRF-PTX rats are not different except on day 16. The values for IgM in CRF rats were lower ($P < .01$) than normal and CRF-PTX rats from days 4 to 20 except for day 10 and 16. The values between normal and CRF-PTX rats are not different except for days 16 and 20 ($P < .01$). (Reproduced with permission from Gaciong Z, Alexiewicz JM, Massry SG. Impaired *in vivo* antibody production in CRF rats: role of secondary hyperparathyroidism. *Kidney Int* 1991;40:862–867.)

and the IgG and IgM antiinfluenza vaccine in CRF-PTX rats were not different from normal, whereas the IgM anti-BSA was lower than in normal rats but higher than in CRF rats. These observations demonstrate that the state of secondary hyperparathyroidism of CRF plays a paramount role in the genesis of impaired humoral immunity of CRF.

Treatment of hemodialysis patients with the calcium channel blocker nifedipine produced marked and significant improvement in the basal levels of $[Ca^{2+}]i$ and ATP content of B cells and in their proliferation in response to SAC as compared with hemodialysis patients who were not receiving treatment with nifedipine. The values of all these parameters of B-cell metabolism and function in the group of patients treated with nifedipine approached the normal values. Furthermore, the blood levels of IgG were significantly higher in patients receiving nifedipine than those without treatment with this calcium channel blocker (Fig. 68.28).

A prospective study further demonstrated that the treatment of hemodialysis patients with nifedipine reversed the abnormalities in B cells cited previously within 2 months and that these derangements reemerged after discontinuation of therapy with the drug (Figs. 68.29 and 68.30). It appears therefore that the treatment of hemodialysis patients with a calcium channel blocker is beneficial in combating the adverse effects of uremia on the function of B cells. The treatment must be maintained in order to maintain the benefit of the treatment.

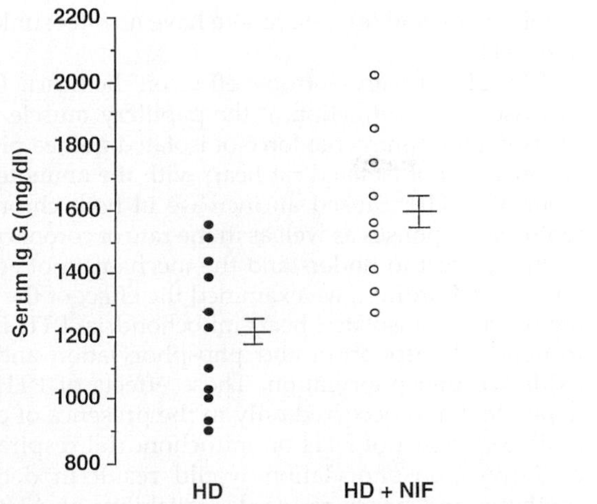

Figure 68.28. The serum levels of IgG in hemodialysis patients with and without therapy. Each datum point represents one patient and the brackets denote mean ± SE. The values between the two groups are significantly different ($P < 0.01$). (Reproduced with permission from Alexiewicz JM, Smogorzewski M, Akmal M, et al. Nifedipine reverses the abnormalities in $[Ca^{2+}]$i and proliferation of B cells from dialysis patients. *Kidney Int* 1996;50:1249–1254.)

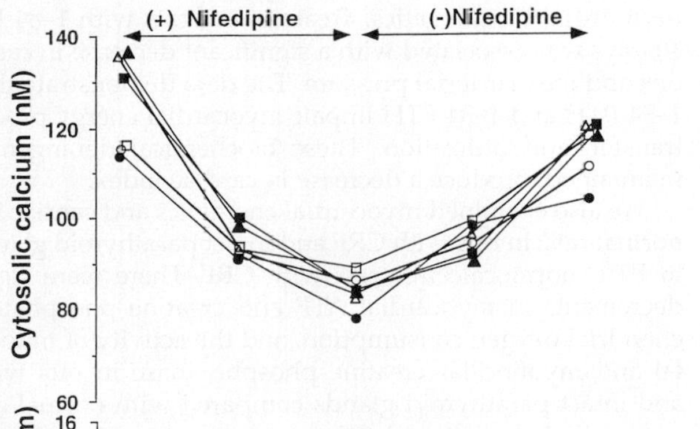

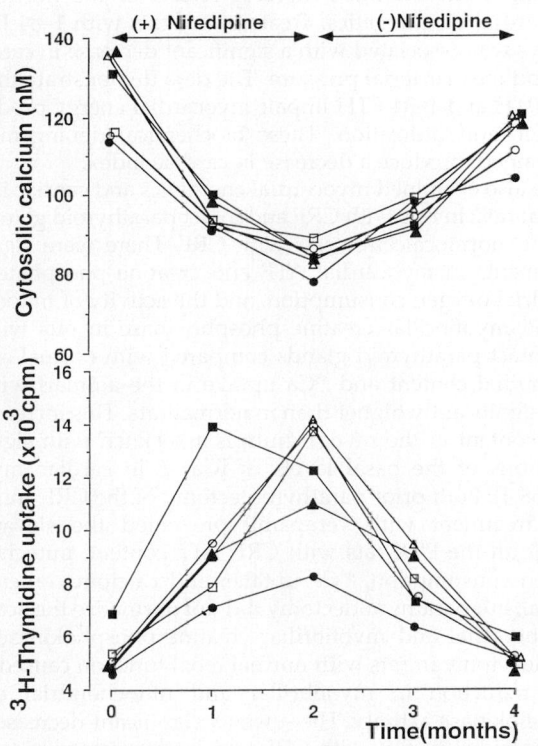

Figure 68.29. The changes in $[Ca^{2+}]$ of B cells *(upper panel)* and of B-cell proliferation in response to mitogen *(lower panel)* of six hemodialysis patients before, during, and after cessation of nifedipine therapy. Each *line* represents one patients. (Reproduced with permission from Alexiewicz JM, Smogorzewski M, Akmal M, et al. A longitudinal study on the effect of nifedipine therapy and its discontinuation on $[Ca^{2+}]$i and proliferation of B lymphocytes of dialysis patients. *Am J Kidney Dis* 1997;29:233–238.)

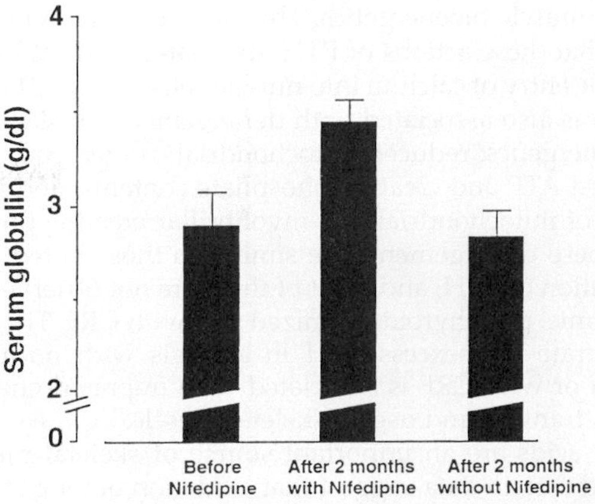

Figure 68.30. The changes in the serum globulin in six dialysis patients before, during, and after cessation of nifedipine therapy. Each *column* represents the mean of data from six hemodialysis patients and *brackets* denote 1 SE. (Reproduced with permission from Alexiewicz JM, Smogorzewski M, Akmal M, et al. A longitudinal study on the effect of nifedipine therapy and its discontinuation on $[Ca^{2+}]$i and proliferation of B lymphocytes of dialysis patients. *Am J Kidney Dis* 1997;29:233–238.)

EFFECT OF PTH ON PLATELET FUNCTION

Bleeding tendencies are not infrequent in uremic patients, and this abnormality is thought to be due to many factors among which is impaired platelet aggregation (see Chapter 72, Part 2). We have found that 1–84 PTH, and not 1–34 PTH, inhibits platelet aggregation induced by adenosine 5′-diphosphate (ADP), fibrin, and collagen. Similar observations were reported by others. The state of secondary hyperparathyroidism of uremia may contribute to the pathogenesis of the bleeding tendencies and blood loss in these patients. This phenomenon may provide an additional pathway through which PTH participates in the etiology of the anemia of uremia (Fig. 68.16).

PTH AND UREMIC MYOPATHY

Uremic patients may experience muscle dysfunction (see Chapter 78), and patients with primary hyperparathyroidism may display diffuse neuromuscular defects and prominent myopathy. These clinical observations suggest that the state of secondary hyperparathyroidism of renal failure could play an important role in the etiology of uremic myopathy. Indeed, available data indicate that the skeletal muscle is a target organ for PTH action, and the hormone may affect its protein metabolism, bioenergetics, and fatty-acid oxidation.

Both intact PTH and its aminoterminal fragment exert marked effects on the metabolism of skeletal muscle protein, amino acids, and cyclic nucleotides. PTH stimulates the production of both cAMP and cyclic guanosine 3′,5′-monophosphate (cGMP), enhances the release of alanine and glutamine from muscle without altering their intracellular levels, and decreases the incorporation of $[^3H]$ leucine into muscle protein.

Studies in our laboratory showed that the administration of PTH for 4 days to normal rats caused a significant increase in ^{45}Ca uptake by the skeletal muscle and was associated with a significant decrease in the muscle content of inorganic phosphorus, creatine phosphate, and ATP. The hormone also significantly reduced mitochondrial oxygen consumption and impaired the activity of mitochondrial and myofibrillar creatine phosphokinase. Verapamil abolished all these adverse effects of

PTH on muscle bioenergetics. The data are consistent with the notion that these actions of PTH are related to its ability to enhance the entry of calcium into muscle cells. CRF of 21 days' duration was also associated with derangements in skeletal muscle bioenergetics: reduced mitochondrial oxygen consumption, decreased ATP and creatine phosphate contents, and impaired activity of mitochondrial and myofibrillar creatine phosphokinase. These derangements are similar to those noted with administration of PTH, and most of them are not observed in normocalcemic, parathyroidectomized rats with CRF. The findings demonstrate that excess PTH in animals with normal renal function or with CRF is associated with impaired energy production, transfer, and use by skeletal muscle.

Fatty acids are an important source of skeletal muscle energy, and certain data suggest that oxidation of long chain fatty acids (LCFA) may be impaired in uremia. Such an abnormality may contribute to uremic myopathy. Studies in our laboratory showed that the administration to rats of either 1–84 or 1–34 PTH for 4 days was associated with impaired oxidation of LCFA and with reduced activity of carnitine-palmitoyl transferase; inactivation of PTH abolished these effects. CRF of 21 days' duration in rats was also associated with impaired oxidation of LCFA and impaired carnitine-palmitoyl transferase activity; parathyroidectomy in rats with CRF normalized these disturbances. Carnitine content of the muscle was not altered. These data show that PTH excess in normal rats or in rats with CRF is associated with impaired oxidation of LCFA; this effect is due to a reduction in the activity of carnitine-palmitoyl transferase, a key enzyme for the transport of LCFA, but not of short chain fatty acids (SCFA), to the mitochondrial matrix for β-oxidation.

EFFECT OF PTH ON MYOCARDIUM

Patients with advanced renal failure may have myocardiopathy of unexplained origin. A large body of evidence obtained from experimental data suggests that the excess blood levels of PTH in uremia adversely affect the heart. Uremia is associated with cardiac lesions and accumulation of calcium in the heart. Administration of PTH enhanced the progression of these lesions, and parathyroidectomy prevented their evolution as well as the accumulation of calcium.

Detailed information on the interaction between PTH and the myocardium has been obtained by studying the effect of the hormone on rat heart cells grown in culture. Both N-terminal (1–34) PTH and intact (1–84) PTH produced an immediate and sustained significant rise in beats per minute, and the cells died earlier than control cells. The effect was reversed if PTH was removed from medium, and the effect was abolished by inactivation of the hormone. There was a dose-response relationship between both moieties of PTH and the rise in heartbeats, but the effect of 1–84 PTH was significantly greater than that of the 1–34 moiety. PTH stimulated cAMP production within 1 minute and cAMP remained elevated thereafter. The effect of PTH required calcium, was mimicked by calcium ionophore, was prevented by verapamil, and was not abolished by α- or β-adrenergic blockers. PTH action was additive to an α-adrenergic agonist and synergistic with a β-adrenergic agent. Sera from uremic PTX rats did not affect heartbeats, but sera from uremic rats with intact parathyroid glands or from uremic PTX rats treated with PTH had effects similar to PTH. These observations indicate that (a) the heart cell is a target organ for PTH and may have receptors for PTH, (b) PTH increases the beating rate of heart cells and causes early death of the cells, (c) the PTH effect appears to be due to calcium entry into heart cells, (d) the locus of action through which PTH induces calcium entry is different from that for catecholamines, and (e) uremic sera have no effect unless they contain PTH.

PTH also has an inotropic effect on the heart. The hormone increased the contraction of the papillary muscle and affected the isometric contractile force of isolated guinea pig auricles.

Perfusion of isolated rat heart with the aminoterminal fragment of PTHrP caused an increase in both chronotropic and inotropic responses as well as in the rate of coronary blood flow.

In an effort to understand the mechanism of action of PTH on the myocardium, we examined the effect of the hormone on the function of isolated heart mitochondria. PTH inhibited mitochondrial respiration and phosphorylation and uncoupled oxidative phosphorylation. These effects of PTH were dose dependent and occurred only in the presence of calcium. The inhibitory effect of PTH on mitochondrial respiration and on oxidative phosphorylation would result in decreased ATP synthesis and hence reduced availability of ATP. Such a sequence of events may provide an explanation for potential long-term adverse effects of the hormone on the myocardium. Support for such a notion came from additional studies carried out in our laboratory evaluating the *in vivo* effect of PTH on myocardial metabolism.

Administration of 1–84 and 1–34 PTH to rats for 4 days significantly reduced mitochondrial oxygen consumption without altering the ADP:oxygen ratio, indicating reduced phosphorylation. Myocardial contents of inorganic phosphorus, ATP, and creatine phosphate were significantly lower in 1–84 PTH–treated animals. Both moieties of the hormone significantly reduced mitochondrial and myofibrillar creatine phosphokinase. There were also significant increments in myocardial ^{45}Ca uptake and total calcium content. Inactivation of PTH and administration of verapamil, a calcium channel blocker, abolished these adverse effects of the hormone on myocardial bioenergetics. Treatment of rats with 1–84 PTH for 10 days was associated with a significant decrease in cardiac index and mean arterial pressure. The data demonstrate that both 1–84 PTH and 1–34 PTH impair myocardial energy production, transfer, and utilization. These biochemical derangements, if maintained, produce a decrease in cardiac index.

We also examined myocardial energetics and cardiac index in normal rats; in rats with CRF and intact parathyroid glands; and in PTX, normocalcemic rats with CRF. There were significant decrements in myocardial ATP and creatine phosphate, mitochondrial oxygen consumption, and the activity of mitochondrial and myofibrillar creatine phosphokinase in rats with CRF and intact parathyroid glands compared with normal animals. Myocardial content and ^{45}Ca uptake in the animals with CRF were significantly higher than in normal rats. This increased calcium content in the myocardium is associated with significant elevations of the basal levels of $[Ca^{2+}]i$ in cardiac myocytes (Fig. 68.4). Both prior parathyroidectomy of the CRF animals or their treatment with verapamil prevented the elevation in $[Ca^{2+}]i$. In the PTX rats with CRF, ATP content, mitochondrial oxygen consumption, ^{45}Ca uptake, and calcium content were normal, but parathyroidectomy did not normalize the activity of mitochondrial and myofibrillar creatine phosphokinase. Parathyroidectomy in rats with normal renal function caused significant reduction in myofibrillar and mitochondrial creatine phosphokinase activity. There was a significant decrease in the cardiac index in rats with CRF and intact parathyroid glands, and the cardiac index did not normalize in PTX rats with CRF.

These data allow the following conclusions: (a) In the state of CRF with excess PTH, there is impaired myocardial energy production, transfer, and utilization, and a fall in cardiac index. (b) The decrease in energy production is due to excess PTH and not CRF. (c) The impaired energy transfer and utilization is most likely due to excess PTH, but absence of the hormone did not correct these abnormalities, because parathyroidectomy even in rats with normal renal function was followed by reduced activity of mitochondrial and myofibrillar creatine phosphokinase. (d) The effect of PTH on myocardium is partially mediated by enhanced entry of calcium into the heart. (e) The optimal activity of creatine phosphokinase of heart mitochondria and myofibrils requires PTH, and either excess or lack of the hormone is deleterious. (f) Total parathyroidectomy is not the procedure of choice for the prevention of uremic myocardiopathy.

Fatty acids constitute an important substrate used by the myocardium as a major fuel for energy production; impaired oxidation of fatty acids may result in myocardial dysfunction. As in the case of skeletal muscle, excess PTH in normal rats or in rats with CRF is associated with impaired oxidation of LCFA and SCFA, and this effect is due to reduction in the activity of carnitine-palmitoyl transferase and inhibition in the β-oxidation sequence, respectively. No changes in carnitine content of the myocardium were observed, and parathyroidectomy in rats with CRF normalized these derangements in fatty-acid oxidation.

Several clinical studies examined the relationship between primary hyperparathyroidism or secondary hyperparathyroidism of CRF on myocardial function. It was found that reductions in blood levels of PTH in dialysis patients by parathyroidectomy was followed by significant improvement in cardiac function. Indeed, cardiac index, left ventricular ejection fraction, and percent fiber shortening increased 6 to 14 days after parathyroidectomy. Others examined the effects of reduction of blood PTH levels on left ventricular function in dialysis patients, either after 6 weeks of treatment with $1,\alpha(OH)_2D_3$ or after total parathyroidectomy. They found that these medical or surgical procedures were followed by improvements in fractional fiber shortening and mean velocity of fiber shortening; there was also a significant inverse relationship between the ratio of preejection period/left ventricular ejection time (an index of left ventricular function) and blood levels of PTH. We have previously provided experimental data indicating that total parathyroidectomy in CRF may not be beneficial for cardiac function. These experimental data appear to contradict the results of the aforementioned study; however, it seems that the total parathyroidectomy performed in the patients was not complete, because the blood levels of PTH after the surgical procedure were normal. Other investigators studied 37 hemodialysis patients and found that 62% of them had abnormal left ventricular function, including enlargement of left ventricular cavity, a reduction of myocardial contractility, and thickening of left ventricular posterior wall. In 7 of these 37 patients, congestive myocardiopathy was present, and these patients had severe secondary hyperparathyroidism. These authors concluded that secondary hyperparathyroidism plays an important role in the genesis of congestive myocardiopathy.

In 1985, an interesting finding was presented by British investigators. They reported that 15 of 16 patients with primary hyperparathyroidism and without renal insufficiency or hypertension had hypertrophic cardiomyopathy (5 patients), asymmetric septal hypertrophy (6 patients), and symmetric left ventricular hypertrophy (4 patients). This was not due to the hypercalcemia of the primary hyperparathyroidism because 6 patients with hypercalcemia related to other causes did not have cardiac hypertrophy. These authors also found that in 5 of 18 (28%) patients who had hypertrophic myocardiopathy not caused by CRF, the blood levels of PTH were elevated. These data clearly demonstrate an effect of excess PTH on the myocardium even in the absence of CRF.

Canadian investigators studied 217 nondiabetic dialysis patients and renal transplant recipients with echocardiography and gated cardiac scan. They then compared dialysis patients with and without low-output left ventricular failure and found that the most important of the three factors associated with left ventricular failure was high serum levels of alkaline phosphatase. These authors considered this parameter to be an index of the hyperparathyroidism in their patients. They therefore concluded that the severity of hyperparathyroidism is a risk factor for low-output left ventricular failure in CRF.

Others concluded that the major derangement in cardiac function in uremia is an inappropriate change in the left ventricular wall in response to alterations in chamber size resulting in higher ventricular radius:wall thickness ratio. They found a direct and significant correlation between this ratio and the blood levels of PTH, and an inverse relationship between left ventricular posterior wall thickness and blood levels of PTH. These observations incriminate secondary hyperparathyroidism of CRF patients in the genesis of myocardial dysfunction. It should be mentioned that these observations are at variance with those of others, demonstrating that dialysis patients frequently display left ventricular thickening. The reasons for these differences are not clear. Also, these observations differ from those demonstrating left ventricular hypertrophy in primary hyperparathyroidism. It is possible that the response of the myocardium to excess PTH in the presence or absence of CRF is different.

In contrast to the aforementioned data, others reported that parathyroidectomy in 10 dialysis patients did not modify the various aspects of left ventricular function. However, it should be indicated that all the parameters of left ventricular function were normal before parathyroidectomy, and therefore improvement should not be expected.

Taken together, the available experimental and clinical data clearly demonstrate that the heart is a target for PTH and that chronic excess of the hormone in the presence or absence of CRF exerts adverse effects on the metabolism, structure, and function of the myocardium. PTH satisfies all the criteria described earlier in this chapter for a cardiotoxin in CRF. Its structure is identified, its blood levels are elevated in CRF, a relationship between its blood level and various parameters of cardiac dysfunction is documented, the reduction of its blood levels is followed by improvement in cardiac function, and its administration to experimental animals with normal renal function produces cardiac alterations similar to those seen in CRF. Also, excess PTH in humans with normal renal function causes myocardial disease. In addition, it was found that left ventricular hypertrophy among patients with essential hypertension and normal renal function is independently affected by blood PTH levels, and there is a strong positive correlation between left ventricular mass index and blood level of PTH. *We would like to emphasize, however, that this conclusion in no way means that PTH is the only cardiac toxin or the only factor underlying the myocardiopathy of uremia.*

Finally, it should be mentioned that it may not always be possible to demonstrate a direct relationship between the various components of left ventricular function and the blood levels of PTH, for several reasons. First, in CRF, there are a multitude of factors besides PTH that could be harmful to the myocardium. Second, the derangements in cardiac metabolism, structure, and function in CRF are due to chronic and progressive processes, and it may not always be possible to correlate the outcome of such chronic processes with a single measurement of blood PTH. Third, it is also possible that chronic excess of PTH may cause in certain CRF patients irreversible myocardial damage; therefore a reduction in blood levels of PTH may not be followed by improvement in cardiac function.

PTH AND VASCULAR REACTIVITY IN UREMIA

PTH is known to be a vasodilator and to exert a hypotensive action. We evaluated the possible mechanisms involved in this action, with special emphasis on the role of vasodilatory prostaglandins. The effects of intact 1–84 PTH and of its N-terminal (1–34 PTH) fragment on mean arterial pressure and on the vascular response to norepinephrine or angiotensin II were examined in rats before and after pretreatment with indomethacin. Bolus injections of 1–84 and 1–34 PTH produced a significant decrease in mean arterial pressure; however, the hypotensive response to 1–34 PTH was more marked than the response to 1–84 PTH. Both 1–84 and 1–34 PTH antagonized the pressor effects produced by bolus injection of norepinephrine or angiotensin II. Pretreatment with indomethacin abolished the inhibitory effect of 1–84 and 1–34 PTH on the response of mean arterial pressure to norepinephrine or angiotensin II. The infusion of 1–84 and 1–34 PTH produced a significant rise in urinary excretion of 6-keto-$PGF_{1\alpha}$. These data are consistent with the hypothesis that the effect of PTH on blood vessels is mediated by increased prostaglandin production. Others have found that PTH may block the calcium channels in vascular smooth muscle cells and suggested that this action underlies the vasodilatory effect of the hormone.

Patients with acute or chronic renal failure manifest reduced pressor response to norepinephrine. This abnormality is at least partly responsible for some of the manifestations of autonomic nervous system dysfunction in these patients (see Chapter 69, Part 3). Because uremia is associated with increased blood levels of PTH, and because PTH blunts the pressor effect of norepinephrine, most likely by the activation of prostaglandins, we studied the relationships between blood levels of PTH and the magnitude of the reduction in the pressor response to norepinephrine in uremic patients. We also examined the effect of treatment with indomethacin on the response to norepinephrine in these patients. There was a significant negative correlation between the changes in blood pressure and the blood levels of PTH in the uremic patients (Fig. 68.31). Treatment with indomethacin was followed by significant improvement or normalization of the pressor response to norepinephrine. These data are consistent with the notion that the decreased pressor response to norepinephrine in uremia is due to increased production of prostaglandins induced by excess PTH and provide a therapeutic tool for the treatment of some of the manifestations of autonomic nervous system dysfunction in uremia.

To evaluate further the role of PTH in the genesis of this abnormality in uremia, we examined the pressor responses to norepinephrine in rats with experimental CRF with and without (CRF-PTX) parathyroid glands. The pressor response to norepinephrine was significantly reduced in CRF rats compared with normal rats was significantly less than in CRF-PTX rats, in which the pressor responses were the same as those in control rats (Fig. 68.32). Treatment of CRF rats with indomethacin normalized the pressor responses to norepinephrine. We also examined the dose-response curves between norepinephrine and perfusion pressure of the hind-limb preparation. There was a significant shift to the right in the dose-response curve in CRF rats compared with controls and CRF-PTX rats, indicating a decreased sensitivity to norepinephrine in CRF rats. No significant difference was observed between the dose-response curves in control and CRF-PTX rats. Thus excess PTH and not other consequences of CRF plays a paramount pathogenetic role in the reduced pressor response to norepinephrine, and this effect of PTH is due to direct action on the blood vessels. Furthermore, this action of the hormone is most likely to be mediated by increased production of vasodilating prostaglandins. It is also possible that downregulation of norepinephrine and/or angiotensin II receptors in CRF, as discussed earlier, play an important role in the reduced pressor response to those vasoconstrictor agonists.

All the data detailed previously provide evidence for the role of PTH in the genesis of the reduced pressor response to norepinephrine in uremia. Thus these observations are consistent with the idea that excess blood levels of PTH contribute to the pathogenesis of some of the manifestations of autonomic nervous system dysfunction in CRF.

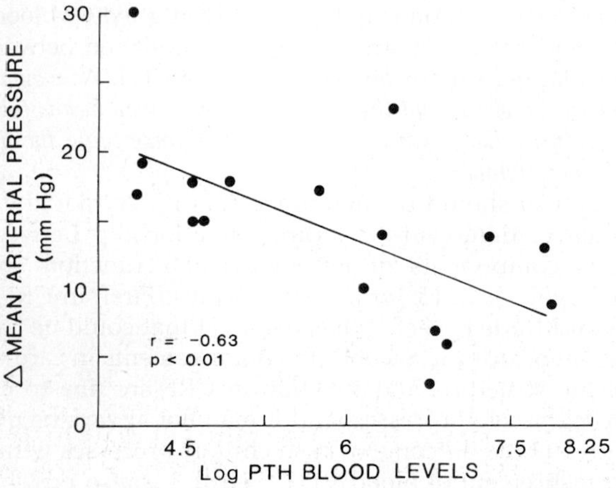

Figure 68.31. The relationship between the changes in mean arterial pressure produced by infusion of norepinephrine and the log of blood levels of PTH in 17 patients with chronic renal failure. (Reproduced with permission from Collins J, Massry SG, Campese VM. Parathyroid hormone and the altered vascular response to norepinephrine in uremia. *Am J Nephrol* 1985;5:110–113.)

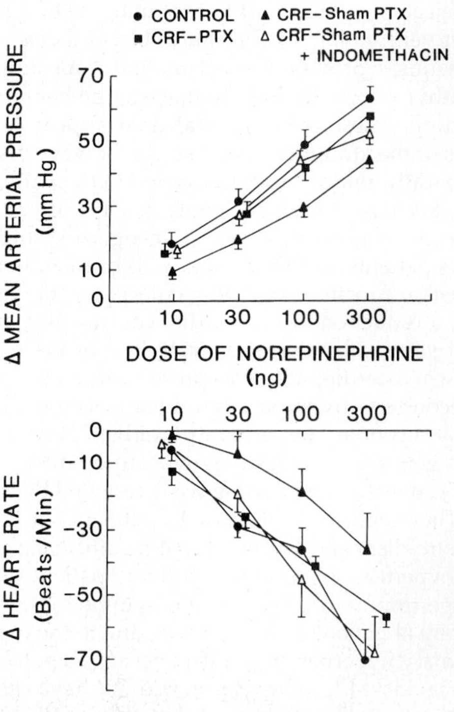

Figure 68.32. The relationship between the changes in mean arterial pressure (*upper panel*) and heart rate (*lower panel*) and the injected dose of norepinephrine in control rats; in rats with chronic renal failure and intact parathyroid glands (*CRF*-sham *PTX*), with and without indomethacin; and in normocalcemic, parathyroidectomized rats with chronic renal failure *(CRF-PTX)*. Each *datum point* represents mean value, and *brackets* denote ± 1 SE. (Reproduced with permission from Iseki K, Massry SG, Campese VM. Evidence for a role of PTH in the reduced pressor response to norepinephrine in chronic renal failure. *Kidney Int* 1985;28:11–15.)

ROLE OF PTH IN THE CARBOHYDRATE INTOLERANCE OF UREMIA

Abnormal glucose metabolism is present in uremia. This is due to impaired insulin secretion by pancreatic islets and to resistance to the peripheral resistance to the action of insulin. Convincing evidence has been mounted indicating that the state of secondary hyperparathyroidism of CRF inhibits insulin secretion by pancreatic islets. Furthermore, chronic exposure to excess PTH in the presence or absence of CRF inhibits insulin secretion. Excess PTH, however, is not responsible to the peripheral resistance to insulin action.

The cellular and metabolic derangements in pancreatic islets that are induced by excess PTH and that are responsible for impaired insulin secretion are discussed in detail in Chapter 74, Part 1.

PTH AND THE HYPERLIPIDEMIA OF UREMIA

Hyperlipidemia is usually present in patients with chronic uremia, and it has been reported in the oliguric phase of an acute renal failure. A rise in blood lipids also occurs in animals rendered uremic by either bilateral nephrectomy or bilateral ureteral ligation. An increase in production of triglyceride-rich lipoproteins by the liver, reduction in their removal by peripheral tissues, or a combination of both may be operative. In 1965 Cantin provided experimental evidence suggesting that PTH is involved in the genesis of the lipidemia of uremia. He found that removal of the parathyroid glands partially inhibited the rise in blood lipids observed after bilateral nephrectomy, and the administration of parathyroid extract to PTX rats restored the hyperlipidemia.

Both clinical and experimental data indicate that PTH can affect lipid metabolism. (a) PTH stimulates adipose tissue lipase in animals and in humans. (b) The N-terminal fragment of PTH stimulates basal and GMP (PNP)-liganded adenylate cyclase of human fat cells. (c) A state of endogenous hyperparathyroidism, induced in rats by feeding them a calcium-poor diet, caused a significant increase in serum cholesterol and triglyceride concentrations, a significant decrease in the rate of serum clearance of intravenously infused lipids, and a significant increase in hepatic tissue triglyceride content, compared with the values obtained in control animals. The administration of parathyroid extract to normal rats was also associated with a modest increase in serum cholesterol and triglyceride concentrations. In the aparathyroid state, a significant decrease in serum levels of cholesterol and triglycerides and a significant increase in plasma postheparin lipolytic activity were observed. These studies show that *(1)* hyperparathyroidism induces an increase in serum cholesterol and triglyceride levels, the latter being due to decreased peripheral removal; and *(2)* the aparathyroid state induces opposite changes. The authors concluded that normal parathyroid function is required for normal lipid metabolism in the rat. (d) Type IV hyperlipoproteinemia was found in a large number of patients with primary hyperparathyroidism. (e) Other studies showed that parathyroidectomy ameliorated the hyperlipidemia of chronic uremia, and the presence of excess PTH enhanced the magnitude of the hyperlipidemia of CRF. The authors of these studies suggested that PTH plays a permissive role in the genesis of the hyperlipidemia of uremia. Indirect evidence from these studies also suggested that PTH may affect serum lipids in experimental uremia by modulating hepatic synthesis of lipoproteins.

Despite the impressive information implicating PTH in the genesis of abnormal lipid metabolism, certain clinical data argue against such a notion. Patients with primary hyperparathyroidism may have low serum levels of cholesterol and triglycerides. In some patients, blood levels of both cholesterol and triglycerides rose after surgical removal of the parathyroid adenoma, despite the lack of change in body weight or serum thyroxine.

We examined the interaction between PTH and adipocytes and investigated the role of excess PTH in CRF on lipid metabolism. Acute exposure of adipocytes to 1–84 but not 1–34 PTH causes a rise in their $[Ca^{2+}]i$ (Table 68.2), and *in vivo* exposure to chronic excess of PTH was followed by a significant elevation in the basal levels of $[Ca^{2+}]i$ of adipocytes. This latter effect is prevented by prior parathyroidectomy of the CRF rats or by their treatment with verapamil. Both dogs and rats with CRF have fasting triglyceridemia, impaired fat tolerance test, and reduced postheparin lipolytic activity (Figs. 68.33 to 68.35).

The available data indicate that the hyperlipidemia of CRF is due to impaired removal of lipids from the circulation. This derangement is secondary to abnormalities in the metabolism of both hepatic lipase (HL) and lipoprotein lipase (LPL).

We have found that CRF is associated with (a) reduced V_{max} (Fig. 68.36) and increased K_m (Fig. 68.37) of HL in liver homogenate, (b) lower-than-normal activity of HL after 8 hours of

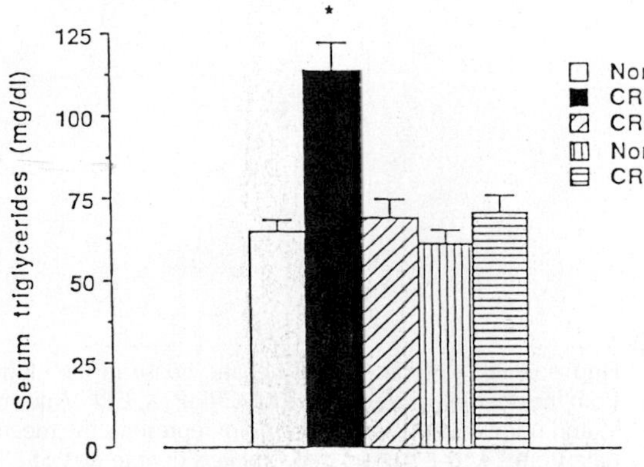

Figure 68.33. Serum levels of triglycerides in five groups of rats. Each *column* represents mean value and *brackets* denote 1 SE. Ver, verapamil, *, $P < .01$ versus other groups. (Reproduced with permission from Akmal M, Perkins S, Kasim S et al. Verapamil prevents renal failure-induced abnormalities in lipid metabolism. *Am J Kidney Dis* 1993;22:158–163.)

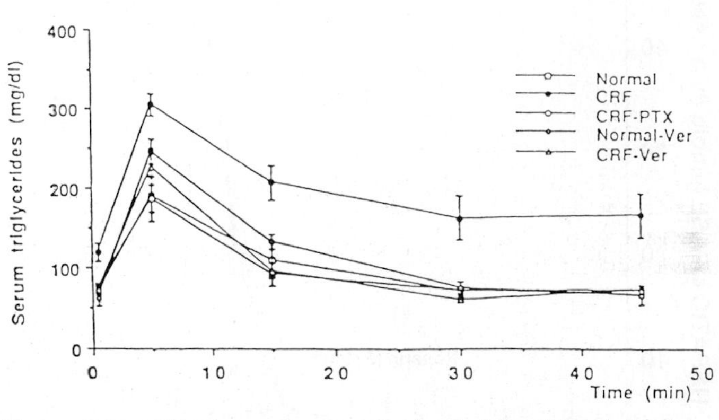

Figure 68.34. The change in serum levels of triglycerides during intravenous fat tolerance test in five groups of rats. Each *datum point* represents mean value and *brackets* denote ± 1 SE. Ver, verapamil. (Reproduced with permission from Akmal M, Perkins S, Oh H-Y et al. Verapamil prevents chronic renal failure-induced abnormalities in lipid metabolism. *Am J Kidney Dis* 1993;22:158–163.)

culture of hepatic cells, (c) downregulation of the expression of mRNA of HL, (d) marked reduction of the heparin-induced release of HL in *in vitro* hepatic perfusion system (Fig. 68.38). All these derangement in HL were prevented by parathyroidectomy of the CRF animals or by their treatment with verapamil. Furthermore, perfusion of the liver with PTH 1–84 or PTH 1–34 inhibited the heparin-induced release of HL. These observations show that the molecular machinery of HL, its production, its activity, and its release are impaired in CRF. These abnormalities are most likely caused by the PTH-mediated elevation in the basal levels of $[Ca^{2+}]$i of hepatic cells.

We and others also found that CRF is associated with alterations in the molecular machinery of LPL in both adipose tissue and myocardium; both the expression of the mRNA and the protein mass of LPL are reduced. In addition, the activity of LPL and its release by heparin are impaired. Again these abnormalities are prevented by parathyroidectomy of the CRF animals or by their treatment with verapamil, indicating that the im-

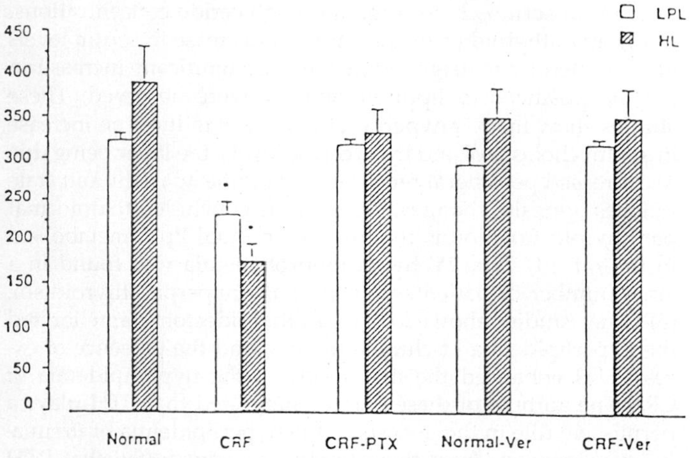

Figure 68.35. The postheparin plasma lipoprotein lipase (*open bars*) and hepatic lipase (*shaded bars*) in five groups of rats. Each *column* represents mean value and *brackets* denote 1 SE. *, $P < .01$ versus all groups. (Reproduced with permission from Akmal M, Perkins S, Oh H-Y, et al. Verapamil prevents chronic renal failure-induced abnormalities in lipid metabolism. *Am J Kidney Dis* 1993;22:158–163.)

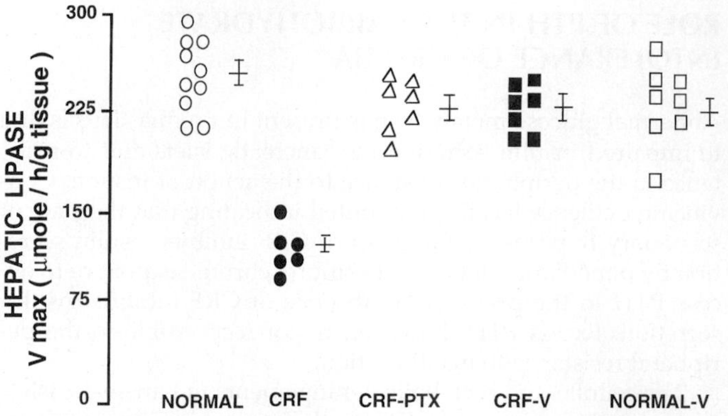

Figure 68.36. The V_{max} of hepatic lipase of liver homogenate from normal, CRF, CRF-PTX, CRF-V, and normal-V rats. Each *datum point* represents one rat and *brackets* denote mean ± 1 SE. Values in CRF animals are significantly ($P < .01$) lower than those of the other groups of animals. (Reproduced with permission from Klin M, Smogorzewski M, Ni Z, et al. Abnormalities in hepatic lipase in chronic renal failure: Role of excess parathyroid hormone. *J Clin Invest* 1996;97:2167–2173.)

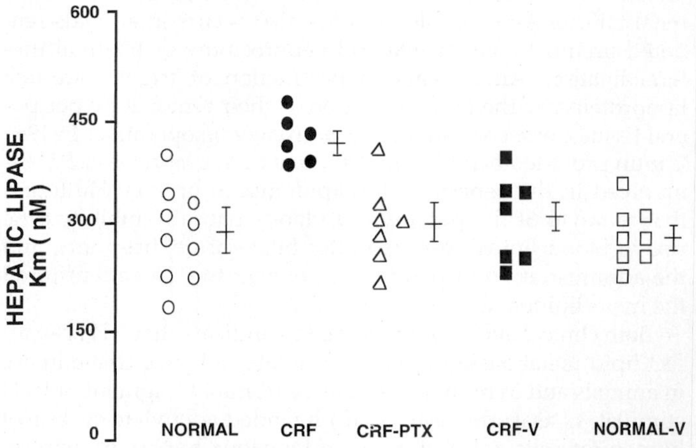

Figure 68.37. The K_m of hepatic lipase of liver homogenate from normal, CRF, CRF-PTX, CRF-V, and normal-V rats. Each *datum point* represents one rat and *brackets* denote mean ± 1 SE. Values in CRF animals are significantly ($P < .01$) higher than those of the other groups of animals. (Reproduced with permission from Klin M, Smogorzewski M, Ni Z et al. Abnormalities in hepatic lipase in chronic renal failure: Role of excess parathyroid hormone. *J Clin Invest* 1996;97:2167–2173.)

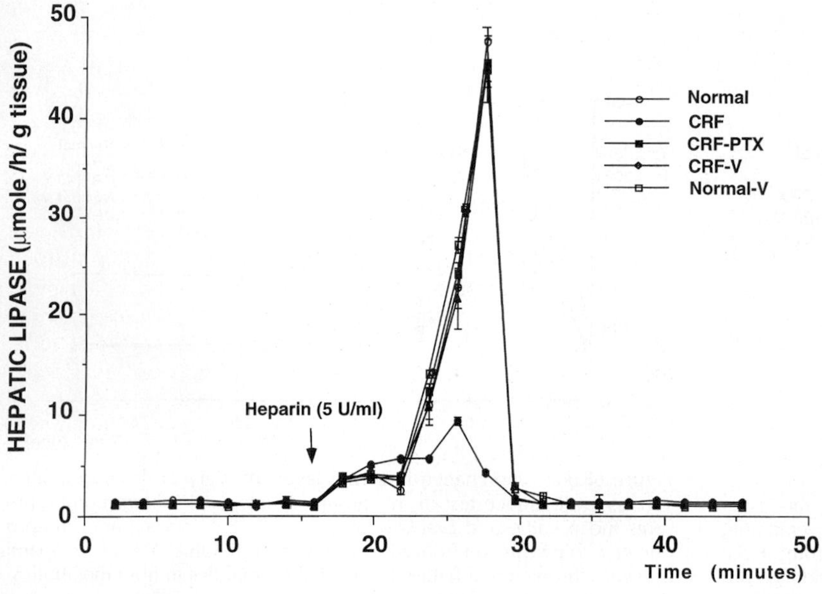

Figure 68.38. The activity of hepatic lipase in the effluent from liver perfusion studies in CRF, CRF-PTX, CRF-V, normal-V, and normal rats. Each *datum point* represents the mean of data from 11 to 7 studies and *brackets* denote ± 1 SE. (Reproduced with permission from Klin M, Smogorzewski M, Ni Z, et al. Abnormalities in hepatic lipase in chronic renal failure: Role of excess parathyroid hormone. *J Clin Invest* 1996:2167–2173.)

pairment in the metabolism and function of LPL are mediated by the PTH-induced rise in $[Ca^{2+}]i$ of adipocytes and cardiac myocytes.

It is of interest that an *in vitro* study demonstrated that $1,25(OH)_2D_3$ antagonizes the effect of PTH on LPL activity of adipocytes. Because CRF is associated with both reduced blood levels of $1,25(OH)_2D$ and elevated blood levels of PTH, animals or human with CRF are in double jeopardy for developing derangements in LPL metabolism and activity.

EFFECT OF PTH ON EXTRARENAL DISPOSITION OF POTASSIUM IN CRF

The translocation of potassium loads from extracellular fluid (ECF) space into cells is an important mechanism involved in potassium homeostasis. This process assumes greater importance in clinical conditions associated with reduced renal function or with inability of the kidney to excrete potassium. The movement of potassium from ECF space into the intracellular compartment is regulated by a variety of hormones such as aldosterone, catecholamine, and insulin (Chapter 16, Part 2). Several studies showed that the permeability of the cellular membrane to potassium is affected by $[Ca^{2+}]i$. Therefore it is reasonable to assume that factors that may affect $[Ca^{2+}]i$ may alter extrarenal disposal of potassium loads. We and others have examined the effect of excess PTH in CRF on the disposition of a potassium load. The results of these studies demonstrated that the state of secondary hyperparathyroidism of CRF interferes with extrarenal disposal of potassium. This derangement could be prevented by parathyroidectomy or by treatment with verapamil.

Patients with CRF have varying degrees of secondary hyperparathyroidism. Therefore those with higher blood levels of PTH may be at a greater risk of hyperkalemia when exposed to a potassium load than those with lower levels of PTH. Thus it appears prudent that in developing dietary regimens for potassium intake to patients with CRF, their blood levels of PTH should be considered in such dietary planning.

EFFECT OF PTH ON NITRIC OXIDE SYNTHASE IN CRF

CRF in rats is associated with reduced activity of nitric oxide synthase (NOS). This abnormality was accompanied by a significant reduction in both endothelial NOS (eNOS) and inducible NOS (iNOS) proteins. These derangements were prevented by parathyroidectomy of the CRF animals or by their treatment with the calcium channel blocker felodipine. These observations again assign to a PTH-mediated rise in $[Ca^{2+}]i$ a critical role in the genesis of the abnormalities of NOS.

Role of Parathyroid Hormone in the Pathogenesis of Other Uremic Manifestations

PTH may play a role in the genesis of the impotence of male uremic patients; the evidence for this role of PTH is discussed in Chapter 74, Part 6.

Necrosis of soft tissue is a serious and life-threatening complication of uremia. It was first seen in renal transplant recipients with secondary hyperparathyroidism and later reported in patients with chronic uremia. These lesions are progressive, and in most cases, healing occurs only after parathyroidectomy. It has been suggested that this lesion is a manifestation of calciphylaxis induced by PTH.

Pruritus is a common manifestation among patients with advanced renal failure and has been attributed to the toxic effect of uremia on the skin. The amelioration of uremia by dialysis is not always associated with alleviation of pruritus, and the latter may even worsen despite dialysis therapy. It has been demonstrated that in patients with persistent pruritus, the itching may rapidly disappear after subtotal parathyroidectomy, assigning a possible role for PTH in the etiology of uremic pruritus.

PTH has been shown to promote the deposition of calcium in the myocardium or in and around the conduction system. Such an event may cause cardiac block and arrhythmias. Pulmonary calcification may reduce the vital capacity and diffusion functions of the lung and may even lead to pulmonary fibrosis. This may cause an increase in pulmonary artery pressure and right ventricular hypertrophy. Thus by promoting soft-tissue calcification, PTH participates in the genesis of the cardiac and pulmonary dysfunction of uremic patients.

Osteitis fibrosa caused by excess PTH is an important component of renal osteodystrophy. Enhanced bone resorption and variable degrees of fibrosis of the bone marrow cavity are almost always observed in bone biopsy specimens from uremic patients. Removal of the parathyroid glands or medical suppression of their activity is usually associated with healing of the osteitis fibrosa. Another bone disorder that may be related to excess PTH in the blood is aseptic necrosis. In a study of 60 renal transplant recipients, 7 of 16 patients who had persistent secondary hyperparathyroidism and elevated blood levels of PTH developed aseptic necrosis of the head of the femur, whereas only 2 of the remaining 46 patients had this complication, despite no significant differences in glucocorticoid regimen between the two groups. Furthermore, aseptic necrosis of the femoral head has been reported in 22 dialysis patients who had secondary hyperparathyroidism and who had not been treated with glucocorticoid.

CLINICAL IMPLICATIONS

The interactions of PTH with the function of so many organ systems assign to the hormone a deleterious role when it accumulates in pharmacologic quantities in the blood of uremic patients. The documentation of the uremic toxicity of PTH has tremendous clinical implications because we have means to prevent the development of secondary hyperparathyroidism and the accumulation of PTH in blood as renal failure progresses. This could be done by appropriate dietary-phosphate restriction or by supplementation of small dosages of $1,25(OH)_2D_3$. Thus it is theoretically possible to have patients with renal disease reach end-stage renal failure without secondary hyperparathyroidism. Such patients may not display or may have an ameliorated version of the uremic syndrome, would feel better, and could easily be rehabilitated, with the quality of their lives as well as their contribution to society greatly improved. In addition, medical and surgical therapeutic modalities are available to manage an already existing state of severe secondary hyperparathyroidism in patients with advanced renal failure and those treated with hemodialysis. Furthermore, the use of calcium channel blockers can prevent or reverse the action of PTH on cells. Thus it is also possible to ameliorate the uremic manifestations in those who already have the uremic syndrome. *The concept that PTH is a uremic toxin is unique because it is the first time in the history of the search for uremic toxins that we can identify a toxin whose source could be controlled, allowing us to prevent its accumulation and to reduce its level or its action if it is already elevated.*

Selected Readings

Akmal M, Brandt RR, Ansari AN, et al. Excess PTH in CRF induces pulmonary calcification, pulmonary hypertension and right ventricular hypertrophy. *Kidney Int* 1995;47:158–163.

Excess PTH in CRF dogs causes pulmonary calcification, pulmonary hypertension, impairment in diffusing capacity of lung, and right ventricular hypertrophy. Parathyroidectomy of CRF dogs prevented these abnormalities.

Akmal M, Perkins S, Kasim SE, et al. Verapamil prevents chronic renal failure-induced abnormalities in lipid metabolism. *Am J Kidney Dis* 1993;22:158–163.

A study in rats with CRF demonstrating the role of excess PTH in the pathogenesis of lipid abnormalities and the usefulness of the treatment with verapamil in preventing the hyperlipidemia of CRF.

Alexiewicz JM, Gaciong Z, Klinger M, et al. Evidence of impaired T cell function in hemodialysis patients: potential role for secondary hyperparathyroidism. *Am J Nephrol* 1990;10:495–501.

A study in dialysis patients and normal subjects examining the role of PTH in the genesis of the abnormality of T-cell function in CRF.

Alexiewicz JM, Smogorzewski M, Akmal M, et al. Nifedipine reverses the abnormalities in $[Ca^{2+}]i$ and proliferation of B cells from dialysis patients. *Kidney Int* 1996;50:1249–1254.

Treatment of hemodialysis patients with nifedipine produced significant improvements in the derangements in $[Ca^{2+}]i$ of B cells and in their proliferation in response to Staphylococcus aureus Cowan I (SAC). The blood levels of IgG were higher in patients treated with nifedipine than in those not receiving such therapy.

Alexiewicz JM, Smogorzewski M, Akmal M, et al. Longitudinal study on the effect of nifedipine therapy and its discontinuation on $[Ca^{2+}]i$ and proliferation of B lymphocytes of dialysis patients. *Am J Kidney Dis* 1997;29:233–239.

A prospective study demonstrating that treatment of hemodialysis patients with nifedipine corrects the abnormalities in $[Ca^{2+}]i$ of B cells, their proliferation in response to SAC, and blood levels in IgG and that those derangements reemerge after discontinuation of the drug.

Alexiewicz JM, Smogorzewski M, Fadda GZ, et al. Impaired phagocytosis in dialysis patients. Studies on mechanisms. *Am J Nephrol* 1992;11:102–111.

The first study pointing toward the role of secondary hyperparathyroidism of CRF in the genesis of impaired phagocytosis in CRF patients.

Alexiewicz JM, Smogorzewski M, Gill S, et al. Time course of the effect of nifedipine therapy and its discontinuation on $[Ca^{2+}]i$ and phagocytosis of polymorphonuclear leukocytes from hemodialysis patients. *Am J Nephrol* 1997;17:12–16.

A prospective study demonstrating that treatment of hemodialysis patients with nifedipine corrects the abnormalities in $[Ca^{2+}]i$ and phagocytosis of polymorphonuclear leukocytes, and discontinuation of therapy is followed by reemergence of the abnormalities.

Alexiewicz JM, Smogorzewski M, Klin M, et al. Effect of treatment of hemodialysis patients with nifedipine on the metabolism and function of polymorphonuclear leukocytes. *Am J Kidney Dis* 1995;25:440–444.

A study showing that the polymorphonuclear leukocytes of hemodialysis on nifedipine therapy have normal $[Ca^{2+}]i$, ATP content, and phagocytosis compared with patients not receiving nifedipine and who display abnormalities in these parameters.

Chervu I, Kiersztejn M, Alexiewicz JM, et al. Impaired phagocytosis in chronic renal failure is mediated by secondary hyperparathyroidism. *Kidney Int* 1992; 41:1501–1505.

A study in rats with CRF examining the PTH-induced cellular derangements in polymorphonuclear leukocytes leading to impaired phagocytosis.

Fadda GZ, Hajjar SM, Perna AF, et al. On the mechanisms of impaired insulin secretion in chronic renal failure. *J Clin Invest* 1991;87:255–261.

A detailed study examining the cellular derangements in pancreatic islets that underlie the impairment in insulin secretion in CRF.

Fadda GZ, Thanakitcharu P, Smogorzewski M, et al. Parathyroid hormone raises cytosolic calcium in pancreatic islets: study on mechanisms. *Kidney Int* 1993; 43:559–560.

A study examining the cellular pathways through which PTH augments calcium entry in pancreatic islets.

Gaciong Z, Alexiewicz JM, Linker-Israeli M, et al. Inhibition of immunoglobulin production by parathyroid hormone: implications in chronic renal failure. *Kidney Int* 1991;40:96–106.

The first study demonstrating the inhibitory effect of PTH on the immunoglobulin production by B cells.

Kiersztejn M, Smogorzewski M, Thanakitcharu P, et al. Decreased O_2 consumption by polymorphonuclear leukocytes from humans and rats with CRF. Role of secondary hyperparathyroidism. *Kidney Int* 1992;42:602–609.

A study in CRF rats demonstrating impaired O_2 consumption by polymorphonuclear leukocytes and the role of excess PTH of CRF in the genesis of this abnormality.

Klin M, Smogorzewski M, Massry SG. Chronic renal failure increases cytosolic $[Ca^{2+}]i$ of hepatocytes. *Am J Physiol* 1995;269:G103–G109.

This paper details the mechanisms responsible for the rise in basal levels of $[Ca^{2+}]i$ of hepatocytes in CRF. It demonstrates that both increased entry of calcium into and decreased exit of calcium out of hepatocytes are responsible for the elevation in the basal levels of $[Ca^{2+}]i$.

Klin M, Smogorzewski M, Ni Z, et al. Abnormalities in hepatic lipase in chronic renal failure. *J Clin Invest* 1996;97:2167–2173.

This study demonstrates that CRF is associated with downregulation of hepatic lipase, and with a decrease in the production activity and the heparin-induced release of the enzyme. These derangements are prevented by parathyroidectomy of the CRF animals or by their treatment with verapamil.

Massry SG. Is parathyroid hormone a uremic toxin? *Nephron* 1977;19:125–130.

The original editorial report putting forward the hypothesis that PTH could be a major uremic toxin.

Massry SG. The toxic effects of parathyroid hormone in uremia. *Semin Nephrol* 1983;3:306–328.

A detailed review of the data pertaining to the toxic effects of PTH in uremia; contains 214 references.

Massry SG, Fadda GZ. Chronic renal failure is a state of cellular calcium toxicity. *Am J Kidney Dis* 1993;21:81–86.

A review of evidence supporting the concept that the uremic syndrome is a state mediated by the PTH-induced elevation in $[Ca^{2+}]i$ of cells.

Massry SG, Klin M, Ni Z, et al. Impaired agonist-induced calcium signaling in hepatocytes from chronic renal failure rats. *Kidney Int* 1995;48:1324–1331.

This study demonstrates that CRF with excess PTH is associated with downregulation of the mRNA of the receptors for PTH-PTHrP, angiotensin II (AT_1) and vasopressin (V1a) in the liver. These changes are associated with reduction in the calcium signal induced by these hormones. The data provide an explanation for the resistance to the action of many hormones in CRF.

Massry SG, Smogorzewski M. Mechanisms through which parathyroid hormone mediates its deleterious effect on organ function in uremia. *Seminars in Nephrol* 1994;14:219–231.

A review of the mechanisms underlying the toxic effects of PTH in CRF. It contains 105 references.

Ni Z, Smogorzewski M, Massry SG. Derangements in acetylcholine metabolism in brain synaptosomes in chronic renal failure. *Kidney Int* 1993;44:630–637.

A detailed study evaluating the derangements in acetylcholine metabolism in brain synaptosomes of CRF rats. The report also demonstrates that these abnormalities are due, in large part, to a state of secondary hyperparathyroidism of CRF.

Smogorzewski M, Zayed M, Zhang Y-B, et al. Parathyroid hormone increases cytosolic calcium concentration in adult rat cardiac myocytes. *Am J Physiol* 1993;264:H1998–H2006.

A study evaluating the cellular pathways involved in mediating the PTH-induced rise in $[Ca^{2+}]i$.

Tian J, Smogorzewski M, Kedes L, et al. Parathyroid hormone related protein receptor messenger RNA is present in many tissues besides the kidney. *Am J Nephrol* 1993;13:210–213.

The first demonstration that the mRNA of the PTH-PTHrP is present in large number of tissues.

Tian J, Smogorzewski M, Kedes L, et al. PTH-PTHrP receptor is down-regulated in chronic renal failure. *Am J Nephrol* 1994;14:41–46.

A study demonstrating that the mRNA of the PTH-PTHrP receptor in traditional (kidney) and nontraditional (liver) organs is downregulated in CRF. This phenomenon is, in major part, due to the PTH-induced elevation in $[Ca^{2+}]i$ because verapamil, which normalizes $[Ca^{2+}]i$, also prevents the downregulation of the mRNA of the receptor despite the presence of CRF and excess PTH.

Urena P, Kubrusky M, Mannstadt M, et al. The renal PTH/PTHrP receptor is down-regulated in rats with chronic renal failure. *Kidney Int* 1994;45:605–611.

Another study demonstrating downregulation of PTH-PTHrP receptor mRNA in the kidney in CRF.

Vaziri ND, Ni Z, Wang XQ, et al. Downregulation of nitric oxide synthases in chronic renal insufficiency: role of excess PTH. *Am J Physiol* 1998;274: F642–F649.

This study shows that CRF in rats is associated with reduction in the protein of both endothelial and inducible nitric oxide synthases in aorta and in kidney and that these derangements are due to the state of secondary hyperparathyroidism of CRF because parathyroidectomy reversed these abnormality.

Vaziri ND, Wang XQ, Liang K. Secondary hyperparathyroidism downregulates lipoprotein lipase expression in chronic renal failure. *Am J Physiol* 1997;273: F925–F930.

The authors demonstrated that CRF in rats is associated with downregulation of the mRNA of lipoprotein lipase and causes a reduction in the protein of the enzyme. Parathyroidectomy of the CRF rats prevented these abnormalities.

PART 2
Aluminum

João M. Frazão and Jack W. Coburn

The major syndromes that arise as a consequence of aluminum loading in patients with renal failure include (a) dialysis encephalopathy (dialysis dementia); (b) acute aluminum neurotoxicity; (c) aluminum-related bone disease; and (d) aluminum-induced microcytic anemia. Myocardial dysfunction may arise from aluminum loading, but this is poorly delineated. This chapter reviews these clinical syndromes, their clinical and laboratory features, and pathogenesis. As will be apparent, the syndrome that develops depends on the intensity and rapidity of aluminum loading. Thus the manifestations of aluminum toxicity that are encountered vary substantially, with major differences arising due to different sources and varying intensity of the aluminum burden. The biology of aluminum will be considered briefly before reviewing the various syndromes of aluminum toxicity.

BIOLOGY OF ALUMINUM

Aluminum is ubiquitous in nature and is the third most prevalent cation in the earth's crust; however, it is a "trace substance" in biologic systems. In nature, almost all aluminum exists as part of complex compounds with oxygen, sulfur, fluorine, and silicon. Most aluminum compounds are highly insoluble, and the concentrations of aluminum are very low in most biologic systems. The skin is quite impervious to aluminum, and only tiny fractions of the ingested aluminum are absorbed from the intestinal tract. Indeed, nature may protect both cells and the organism from exposure to excess aluminum. The solubility of many aluminum compounds varies with pH and increases markedly as the pH either rises or falls from neutral.

In man, the total body burden of aluminum is 30 to 35 mg, and the intake of aluminum in foods is 2 to 3 mg/day, with only 10 to 30 μg/day absorbed. In humans with normal renal function, the aluminum levels of tissues other than lung are 1 to 4 mg/kg dry weight. The lungs contain the largest amount; this arises from dust that is trapped in pulmonary macrophages and the amount increases slowly with age. After the lungs, the highest concentrations of aluminum are found in the liver, bone, spleen, myocardium, and parathyroid glands. Tissue levels are above normal in most patients with renal failure and in those treated with dialysis.

For many years, there has been some controversy about the quantitation of intestinal absorption of aluminum. Until it was shown that urinary aluminum increases following loading with oral aluminum hydroxide, it had been believed that there was little or no absorption of aluminum. From results of net intestinal absorption from a metabolic balance study (i.e., the measurement of the amount of aluminum in the diet less the amount recovered in the feces), it had been concluded that the body absorbs a substantial amount after oral aluminum loading. However, the methodology for measuring aluminum is not accurate enough to detect absorption of less than 1% to 2% of ingested aluminum. Thus indirect methods provided the best information on absorption. After parenteral aluminum loading, most aluminum excretion occurs in the urine, with a minute fraction in the bile. In normal subjects, there is little or no increase of tissue aluminum content (except in the lungs) with aging; this suggests that the body is in neutral balance. If this is the case, urinary aluminum excretion may approximate the amount absorbed. On the basis of this hypothesis, it has been estimated that the amount of aluminum normally absorbed is 10 to 30 μg/day, the quantity normally excreted in the urine. After oral loading with aluminum hydroxide (3.8 g/day), urinary aluminum increases to as high as 100 to 400 μg/day in normal subjects. These studies suggest that aluminum absorption is only 0.01% to 0.5% of the ingested load.

Until recently the only aluminum isotope available was ^{29}Al with a half-life of 6.5 minutes, which is far too short for use as a tracer in biologic systems. The advent of accelerator mass spectrometry has permitted the ultrasensitive detection of the extremely long-lived isotope, ^{26}Al, thereby permitting the study of aluminum absorption and kinetics with adequate accuracy. Studies in rats with normal renal function have shown that the fractional absorption of ^{26}Al is 0.1% after an oral load of aluminum hydroxide and 0.7% after aluminum citrate, but the latter increases markedly to 5% when it is given with additional sodium citrate. Other studies used this isotope to measure the intestinal absorption of aluminum and its compartmentalization in uremic rats compared with rats with normal renal function; uremia augmented the fractional absorption of aluminum to 0.175%, compared with 0.133% in controls. Uremia also increased the deposition of aluminum into bone but not in the liver and spleen. As yet, aluminum absorption has not been studied using ^{26}Al in patients with renal failure, but such experiments are feasible. Thus this technique represents an important breakthrough in the study of aluminum metabolism and it may provide important insights into the pathophysiology of aluminum intoxication.

The factors that affect the absorption of aluminum include citrate, a low gastric pH, fasting, and to a lesser degree, lactate; parathyroid hormone (PTH) and vitamin D may have a small effect. Of these factors, citrate is by far the most important; it can enhance absorption as much as 10- to 30-fold. Thus citrate-containing compounds are dangerous in uremic patients who are ingesting any aluminum compound. Also, fluoride may impair the absorption of aluminum, and aluminum absorption may be high in premature infants. The presence of dissolved silica in water leads to reduced aluminum absorption, presumably by reducing even further the solubility of aluminum in the solution. Finally, certain factors associated with uremia, per se, may enhance the absorption of ingested aluminum, but the mechanism for this effect is not understood.

The quantity of aluminum leaving the body via the enteral route is unknown; the increment in biliary aluminum in dogs after parenteral aluminum loading is very small and biologically insignificant. In patients ingesting no food but receiving inadvertent aluminum loading via intravenous solutions used in total parenteral nutrition, the fecal excretion of aluminum was only 5 to 71 μg/day despite a daily aluminum load of 2,000 to 3,000 μg from the parenteral solution. Such observations suggest that the enteral excretion of aluminum is very small. In contrast, others concluded that a considerable fraction of aluminum was absorbed and later excreted via the enteric route after the long-term ingestion of aluminum hydroxide.

The kidney is the major organ responsible for the elimination of aluminum that enters the body, and reported renal clearances of aluminum vary from 2% to 50% of glomerular filtration rate; newer observations indicate that the correct value is less than 10%. The binding of a large fraction of plasma aluminum to plasma proteins, particularly transferrin and albumin, likely accounts for the low renal clearance of aluminum. However one study suggests there is tubular reabsorption of aluminum. When renal function is normal, months to years may be required before a large aluminum load can be excreted; this slow exit of aluminum from the body is related not only to its low renal clearance but also to the slow egress of aluminum from various tissue stores, including bone.

SOURCES OF ALUMINUM IN PATIENTS WITH RENAL INSUFFICIENCY

Parenteral Sources

Initial outbreaks of *dialysis osteomalacia* were first reported in locations with very high aluminum concentrations in the water used to prepare dialysate. In certain areas, large amounts of alum (aluminum sulfate) are added to precipitate particulate matter and to "clarify" the appearance of the water in a storage reservoir, and this process can produce aluminum concentrations as high as 100 to 600 μg/L (3.7 to 20 μMol/L). When such high aluminum concentrations exist, the lack of an adequate water treatment system or the failure of an existing purification system will produce serious aluminum toxicity in the dialysis patients. At least 85% to 95% of the aluminum in plasma is tightly bound to plasma proteins (particularly transferrin); also most plasma transferrin is free and not bound to iron, hence it is available to bind aluminum. This leads to a concentration gradient producing significant aluminum transfer from dialysate into the blood when the dialysate aluminum exceeds the ultrafiltrable concentration in the blood. Before the introduction of adequate water purification systems, aluminum toxicity and aluminum-related bone disease were common when the dialysate aluminum levels reached 30 to 75 μg/L, and such values were not uncommon in areas of the northeastern United States, where acid rain increases the solubility of aluminum in water. Under such conditions, the plasma aluminum levels can rise by 50% to 70% during a single hemodialysis procedure. Such observations underscore the importance of using adequate water purification before the preparation of dialysate solutions.

Other sources for aluminum exist: In one outbreak of encephalopathy, aluminum was derived from an aluminum-containing anode used to protect the boiler in a hospital water supply from corrosion; after the dialysis unit was moved to another building, no new cases of encephalopathy occurred. An earlier form of the Redy cartridges employed to regenerate dialysis fluid added aluminum to dialysate and produced aluminum loading and bone disease; this problem was rectified in Redy cartridges manufactured after 1982. Peritoneal dialysate solutions have been contaminated with aluminum in the past, but this has been corrected. Indeed, all peritoneal dialysate solutions we have tested have had aluminum concentrations below 5 μg/L. The use of an aluminum-contaminated replacement solution for hemofiltration can also be a source.

Commercially prepared albumin solutions for intravenous use can have substantial concentrations of aluminum, as can several other constituents of intravenous solutions. If a patient with reduced renal function were to receive such products repeatedly (e.g., as a replacement solution during repeated plasma-exchange procedures), significant aluminum loading can develop.

Enteral Sources

The slow but toxic accumulation of aluminum can occur via intestinal absorption in patients with renal insufficiency. The potential danger from oral aluminum-containing compounds was initially raised in 1961, but this warning was overlooked. Adequate means for water purification have been in use in many dialysis units in the United States since the mid-1970s; despite this, aluminum-related bone disease was observed sporadically—this was almost certainly due to the intestinal absorption of aluminum. The dietary intake of phosphate is higher in North America than in many European and Asian countries, and the amount of aluminum hydroxide prescribed as a phosphate binder for dialysis patients in North America often exceeds that used in Europe, Japan, and other countries with large dialysis populations. This factor probably accounts for the significant incidence of bone disease even when the water used to prepare dialysate is adequately purified.

A small but significant amount of aluminum is absorbed by normal humans, and giving standard dosages of aluminum hydroxide leads to a 4- to 10-fold increment of urinary aluminum and a small but variable rise in plasma aluminum in normal subjects. Although aluminum is excreted in the urine by normal persons, it will accumulate in patients with renal failure. Close correlations have been observed between serum aluminum levels and the amount of aluminum-containing gels ingested in both children and adults undergoing dialysis. In children with renal failure, the ingestion of doses of aluminum hydroxide containing more aluminum than 75 mg/kg per day was associated with plasma levels of aluminum above 100 μg/L, and features of aluminum toxicity were common. Based on these retrospective observations, it was recommended that the aluminum dose in children should be below 50 to 75 mg/kg per day. However, a prospective study in pediatric patients assigned to this dose of aluminum hydroxide or to calcium carbonate for 1 year showed evidence of significant aluminum loading in the children ingesting the aluminum gels; indeed, aluminum-related bone disease developed in one patient. Moreover, when all aluminum gels are withdrawn from patients who previously ingested aluminum gels and dialysis is performed with dialysate containing "no" aluminum (less than 5 to 10 μg/L), serum aluminum levels fall strikingly and the histologic features of aluminum loading and low bone turnover disappear or return toward normal. Such observations prove that the intestinal absorption of aluminum causes aluminum toxicity in certain renal failure patients with an impaired ability to excrete aluminum.

Features of aluminum toxicity, either encephalopathy or aluminum-related bone disease, have also occurred in patients with advanced renal failure but not undergoing dialysis. Almost all of these patients were also ingesting substantial quantities of citrate (Shohl's solution, Bicitra, or Alka-Seltzer), which markedly augments the intestinal absorption of aluminum. For this reason, citrate or citrate-containing compounds must be avoided in renal patients who are taking any amount of aluminum gels. The ingestion of large amounts of orange juice, as can occur in a continuous ambulatory peritoneal dialysis (CAPD) patient, can augment aluminum absorption markedly and cause aluminum accumulation.

CLINICAL SYNDROMES OF ALUMINUM TOXICITY

Dialysis Encephalopathy

Dialysis encephalopathy was the first syndrome linked to aluminum accumulation in patients maintained on long-term hemodialysis. It first appeared in epidemic proportions in certain geographic areas and was rarely, if ever, observed in others. The "classical syndrome" developed insidiously after at least 1 to 2 years of dialysis. The clinical features included subtle personality changes and a progressive speech disturbance characterized by a stuttering, stammering, hesitant speech or even the total inability to speak. There were motor disturbances with twitching, myoclonic jerks, and motor apraxia. Distinct auditory and visual hallucinations were sometimes present and were commonly associated with paranoid behavior. Symptoms tended to fluctuate widely and were typically much worse in the immediate postdialysis period. As time passed, the symptoms became more persistent and convulsive seizures were common. With further time of exposure, most patients became mute, immobile, and obtunded; almost all died within 6 to 12 months after the appearance of symptoms.

No distinct laboratory features were noted, although the serum aluminum levels were elevated to ranges from 100 to 350 μg/L. A useful test to aid in the diagnosis of dialysis encephalopathy is the electroencephalogram (EEG); this shows a normal background rhythm, but superimposed are multifo-

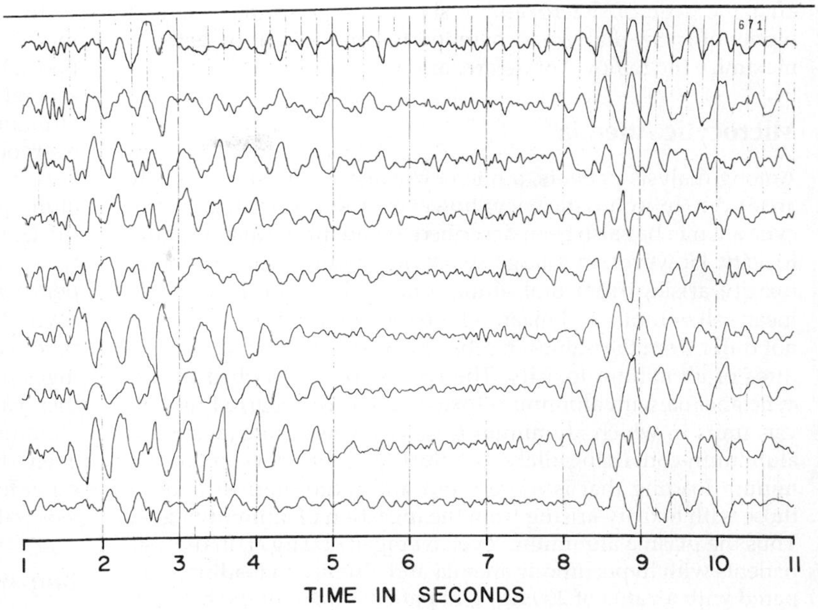

Figure 68.39. Classic EEG changes observed with dialysis encephalopathy, demonstrating bursts of spike and slow wave activity with relatively normal background between the bursts.

cal bursts of slow or delta waves that are accompanied by spike activity. This finding contrasts with the generalized slowing of the EEG noted in most other metabolic encephalopathies (Fig. 68.39). Computed tomography reveals nonspecific cortical atrophy. Evidence of aluminum-related bone disease is often present, as is a hypochromic, microcytic anemia with the presence of normal iron stores; moreover, this anemia was refractory to erythropoietin or required large doses.

The proof that aluminum is the cause was derived from several epidemiologic observations: (a) substantially elevated aluminum content of the gray matter of the brain, (b) elevated dialysate aluminum levels in all units noting outbreaks of encephalopathy, and (c) the disappearance of new cases after the introduction of water purification methods that removed aluminum. Also, the usual fatal course was ameliorated by therapy with deferoxamine, a chelating agent that augments aluminum removal during dialysis. Subsequently it was found that dialysis encephalopathy can occasionally develop as a result of the absorption of aluminum from aluminum gels. The latter usually required a substantially longer time to develop (e.g., often more than 5 to 10 years), and clinically overt bone disease was usually present as well.

Because of its progressive and often fatal course, it is imperative to recognize the disorder, identify and remove the source of aluminum loading, and initiate proper treatment. The diagnosis is made based on the clinical and EEG findings supported by evidence of increased aluminum burden from serum aluminum levels, the increment of serum aluminum after a deferoxamine infusion, and aluminum loading on bone biopsy. The methods to identify loading of bone with aluminum and the treatment of aluminum toxicity are detailed in the following section.

Acute Aluminum Neurotoxicity

The syndrome of acute aluminum toxicity or acute aluminum neurotoxicity is a nearly uniformly fatal disorder brought about by marked aluminum loading or an acute change in the distribution of a large burden of aluminum within the body. It is characterized by the relatively abrupt onset of agitation, confusion, myoclonic jerks, and major motor seizures. These symptoms are commonly followed by coma and death. This syndrome has appeared under several circumstances: (a) hemodialysis with markedly elevated aluminum levels in dialysate (150 to as great as 1,000 μg/L), (b) after the initiation of deferoxamine in patients with markedly elevated plasma aluminum levels and with very high levels of deferoxamine-aluminum complexes, and (c) in uremic patients ingesting aluminum gels in combination with citrate of various types (Shohl's solution, Bicitra, calcium citrate, or Alka-Seltzer). Most cases of acute aluminum toxicity that developed in renal failure patients not yet treated with dialysis involved the concomitant ingestion of aluminum hydroxide and a form of citrate. The cases of acute aluminum neurotoxicity that arose from contaminated dialysate or the ingestion of citrate plus aluminum have uniformly been fatal, and the course was not modified by deferoxamine therapy. This clinical syndrome that appears soon after initiating treatment for aluminum toxicity with deferoxamine is probably due to redistribution of aluminum within the body. Although most cases are fatal, some patients improved and survived when the drug was temporarily discontinued and later restarted at a much lower dose. In cases arising from oral aluminum plus citrate, the patient often died before the results of serum aluminum levels were known. In these cases, the serum aluminum levels were often markedly elevated, with values of 300 to 1,000 μg/L reported, and the characteristic EEG findings described previously were often present.

The treatment of this disorder is largely unsatisfactory except in patients developing the syndrome during deferoxamine therapy. Thus the prevention of acute aluminum toxicity is essential. Attention to water treatment is important to prevent the marked contamination that sometimes occurs. Also, renal failure patients who are prescribed aluminum-containing compounds must be cautioned to avoid completely any citrate-containing compound, including calcium citrate, Bicitra, Shohl's solution, Alka-Seltzer, and perhaps citrus juices, as well. When deferoxamine therapy is deemed necessary for aluminum toxicity, it is desirable to avoid marked elevations of the aluminum-deferoxamine complex. To avoid this problem with deferoxamine treatment, the dosage should be kept to a minimum, that is, 250 to 500 mg per dose, and 7 to 10 days should elapse between doses. Therapy can also be given intramuscularly, 6 to 8 hours before dialysis, rather than infusing the deferoxamine 48 hours before dialysis, as was generally done. The first dialysis after the dose of deferoxamine should be performed using a highly efficient dialyzer, a hemoperfusion system, or both, to maximize the removal of deferoxamine.

Microcytic Anemia

Among dialysis patients, a microcytic anemia most commonly arises due to iron deficiency; however, a hypochromic, microcytic anemia has also been described in patients with aluminum toxicity. However, in a large series of patients with aluminum toxicity arising from oral aluminum loading, the hematocrit, mean cell volume, and mean cell hemoglobin concentration did not differ from the values in other dialysis patients with no features of aluminum toxicity. The reports that described microcytic anemia with aluminum toxicity have all occurred in dialysis units in which aluminum toxicity arose from exposure to aluminum-containing dialysate. Such patients developed aluminum loading that is more rapid and more marked than in those with toxicity arising from the ingestion of aluminum gels. Thus the plasma aluminum level averaged 450 μg/L in dialysis patients with hypochromic anemia and aluminum loading compared with a value of 200 μg/L in patients without the hematologic abnormality but with aluminum-related bone disease that arose from oral aluminum gels. The aluminum-induced anemia is resistant to erythropoietin therapy.

Aluminum-Related Bone Disease

Osteomalacia due to aluminum accumulation is well recognized as a complication in dialysis patients. The bone biopsies from these patients often show increased trabecular surface covered with osteoid and increased osteoid width. Such features of osteomalacia can also arise from vitamin D deficiency, but the bone disease occurring in aluminum-loaded dialysis patients fails to respond to treatment with active vitamin D sterols. Aluminum-related bone disease has been recognized under three conditions: (a) clusters of cases or "epidemics" in certain dialysis units or in geographic areas where untreated tap water or "softened" water is used to prepare dialysate or where there is malfunction of a water-treatment system leading to excessive aluminum in the water used for dialysate preparation; (b) sporadic cases in end-stage renal disease (ESRD) patients using properly purified water for dialysis but ingesting large amounts of aluminum-containing phosphate binders for long periods of time; and (c) ingestion of a combination of aluminum gels and some form of citrate, which ***markedly enhances*** aluminum absorption by either uremic patients not yet on dialysis or by dialysis patients.

Aluminum accumulation has accounted for most cases of vitamin D–resistant osteomalacia observed in dialysis patients. Evidence for the role of aluminum includes epidemiologic observations, the quantity and localization of aluminum on bone biopsy, the production of osteomalacia in animal models by aluminum loading, and the favorable response to the removal of aluminum, either by chelation therapy or by the total withdrawal of aluminum gels combined with water purification.

The syndrome *fracturing osteomalacia* was first described in patients undergoing hemodialysis in the United Kingdom. The syndrome *dialysis encephalopathy* was common in these locations, and it had been shown earlier that dialysis encephalopathy was associated with the accumulation of aluminum in the brain. This led to the suspicion that aluminum might cause fracturing osteomalacia, as well; epidemiologic surveys showed a strong association between the occurrence of dialysis osteomalacia and concentrations of aluminum above 100 μg/L in the water used to prepare dialysate. Similar outbreaks related to water contamination were identified elsewhere.

In California and Washington state, sporadic cases of vitamin D–refractory osteomalacia were noted among dialysis patients, but there were only one or two cases observed in each of several large dialysis centers that used water free of elevated aluminum levels; also, dialysis encephalopathy was rarely, if ever, observed. Because of this, an etiologic role of aluminum was not readily accepted. Subsequently, the incidence of aluminum-related bone disease was found to be much higher in the United States than the 3% to 4% initially proposed, and surveys with bone biopsies of dialysis patients disclosed the incidence of aluminum-related bone disease to be as high as 30% in asymptomatic patients and up to 75% in patients who had hypercalcemia and skeletal symptoms. When the etiologic role of ingesting large quantities of aluminum gels was recognized and then calcium carbonate or calcium acetate was substituted for aluminum gels as phosphate binders, a dramatic reduction or even disappearance of aluminum-related bone disease and other features of aluminum toxicity was observed among dialysis patients.

Biopsy Features of Aluminum Bone Disease

The aluminum content of both trabecular and cortical bone is above normal in most dialysis patients, whether measured by neutron activation, atomic absorption spectroscopy, electron probe analysis, laser microprobe mass analysis, or histochemical staining. In dialysis patients with osteomalacia, the bone aluminum content directly correlated with the extent of unmineralized osteoid. In *symptomatic* dialysis patients with either osteomalacia or the low turnover "aplastic" or "adynamic" bone, histochemical staining revealed that aluminum was located along the mineralizing surface of trabecular bone. Moreover, the clinical manifestations of pain, weakness, and fractures have occurred only in those with adynamic bone who have more than 25% to 30% of the bone surface stained with aluminon stain. The bone surfaces with aluminum staining often fail to show normal bone formation as indicated by the absence of tetracycline uptake at the same site. Bone apposition rate has been correlated inversely with both the trabecular surface showing aluminum staining and the bone aluminum content, although it correlates much more closely with the former.

In most dialysis patients, the total content of aluminum in bone is above normal, although there is wide variation. The content is much higher in those with osteomalacia and many of those with adynamic bone in comparison with that in patients with osteitis fibrosa or the mixed disorder. In patients with osteitis fibrosa and normal or high bone turnover, aluminum staining may be either negative or occur only along the cement lines; however, ultrastructural methods reveal inclusion bodies containing aluminum within osteoblasts. These findings contrast to the trabecular surface localization of aluminum and the virtual absence of both osteoblasts and osteoclasts along bone surfaces in patients with aluminum-induced osteomalacia. Such observations have led to the view that the localization of aluminum along bone surface is the major factor that inhibits mineralization; however, it is also likely that the surface deposition of aluminum is increased substantially as a result of the markedly reduced or absent bone formation.

Aluminum Toxicity and Adynamic or Aplastic Bone Disease

Some dialysis patients with bone pain, fractures, and muscle weakness have lacked the widened osteoid and other features of osteomalacia on bone biopsy. A few showed "patchy" areas of widened osteoid but the total osteoid volume was not above normal. Bone formation, as assessed by double tetracycline labelling, was subnormal or absent, the numbers of osteoclasts and osteoblasts were reduced or absent, and there was substantial surface staining for aluminum. This condition has been called *aplastic* or *adynamic bone*. It is now known that such a low bone-turnover state occurs in renal failure patients whose biopsies show little or no surface staining with aluminum. This has been termed *aplastic bone without aluminum* or *idiopathic adynamic bone*. In contrast to the features in patients with significant aluminum staining, these patients exhibit no bone pain, no muscle weakness, nor a higher incidence of fractures; however, they do have an increased tendency to hypercalcemia and they are prone to develop aluminum accumulation if they ingest aluminum gels. Oversuppression of the PTH levels, that arises from an high calcium level in dialysate and the ingestion of calcium-containing phosphate binders, is a major factor in the pathogenesis of this condition, which is a common finding on bone biopsy among patients with advanced renal insufficiency and in those on dialysis.

The histologic criteria for aluminum toxicity in bone are arbitrary. The most consistent features on bone biopsies are significant surface accumulation of aluminum and reduced bone formation. A few symptomatic patients have exhibited a mixed lesion on bone biopsy, with features of both osteomalacia and osteitis fibrosa; they may have significant peritrabecular fibrosis, and even a normal rate of bone formation, but with substantial surface staining for aluminum. These observations indicate that aluminum can exert a pathogenic effect without bone formation being subnormal. Among dialysis patients whose bone biopsies showed osteitis fibrosa, a high rate of bone formation, and negative surface staining for aluminum, the bone formation rate was inversely related to the total aluminum content of bone (Fig. 68.40). The effect of aluminum on bone formation probably depends on the previous state of bone turnover, and aluminum toxicity may pass through a transition period and show a normal bone formation rate in a patient who previously had osteitis fibrosa and an elevated bone formation rate. The accumulation of aluminum thus represents a spectrum in patients with renal failure, and the pathologic effects of aluminum also may show a continuum.

A newly introduced method for staining aluminum, which uses acid solochrome azurine, is much more sensitive than the standard aluminon method. Almost all dialysis patients exhibit significant positive staining with this method whether or not

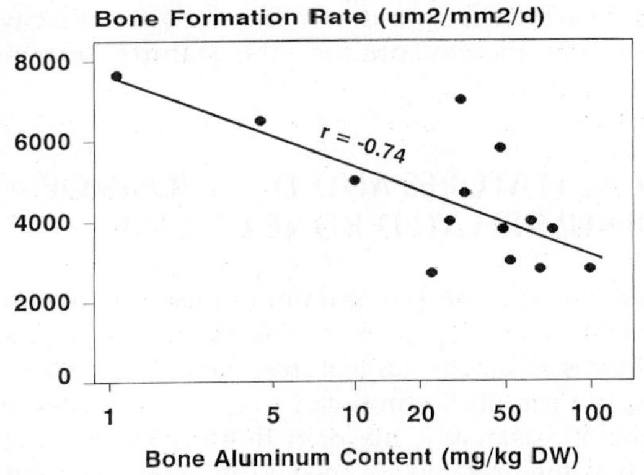

Figure 68.40. Bone formation rate was inversely related to the total aluminum content of bone in these dialysis patients whose bone biopsies showed osteitis fibrosa, a high rate of bone formation, and negative surface staining for aluminum. (Reproduced from Salusky IB, Coburn JW, Brill J, et al. Bone disease in pediatric patients undergoing dialysis with CAPD or CCPD. *Kidney Int* 1988;33:975–982.)

there is evidence of aluminum toxicity. It would seem more appropriate to employ the staining method that has a predictive value for clinical disease.

It is possible that other metals can also cause osteomalacia. An increase in the strontium content of bone has been reported in hemodialysis patients with osteomalacia. Furthermore, in an animal model, strontium administration led to the accumulation of strontium at the border between osteoid and calcified bone and the development of osteomalacia. The extrapolation of such animal data to the earlier observations of aluminum in the dialysis population raises the possibility that strontium may also be an etiologic factor in the development of osteomalacia. Iron has been found along the mineralizing surface, either alone or in conjunction with aluminum, in patients with symptomatic osteomalacia; however, this finding is quite uncommon. It has been suggested that silicon and sulfur may exhibit bone surface localization, but proof of their pathogenicity is lacking. There has been no relationship between the accumulation of lead in the bone of dialysis patients and any type of bone disorder.

Parathyroid Hormone and Aluminum-Related Bone Disease

There are several interactions between parathyroid gland activity and aluminum toxicity. Serum PTH levels are lower in patients with aluminum-related bone disease than is expected for dialysis patients. When hypocalcemia is induced in patients with aluminum toxicity, the PTH levels fail to show the expected increment in response to hypocalcemia. The parathyroid glands accumulate aluminum preferentially compared with many other tissues, and adding aluminum to parathyroid cells directly inhibits PTH secretion. Serum calcium levels are commonly elevated in patients with aluminum-related bone disease. Thus low serum PTH levels in aluminum-loaded patients may arise from a direct effect of aluminum to inhibit PTH secretion, may occur due to the high serum calcium levels, or may arise from a combination of both effects. It should be remembered that serum PTH levels are not low in all patients with aluminum toxicity, and serious aluminum loading and even symptomatic aluminum-related bone disease can occur in patients with markedly elevated intact PTH levels.

The manifestations of aluminum overload are modified by the existing state of the parathyroid glands. Thus symptomatic aluminum-related bone disease has appeared in dialysis patients shortly after total or subtotal parathyroidectomy or after serum PTH levels were reduced by treatment with an active vitamin D sterol, including 25-hydroxyvitamin D_3 or calcitriol [1,25(OH)$_2$D$_3$]. In dialysis units that employed aluminum-containing dialysate, patients with severe osteitis fibrosa rarely developed osteomalacia despite being exposed to the same toxic aluminum levels as those with symptomatic osteomalacia. Thus hyperparathyroidism seems to protect the bone from the toxic effect of aluminum. Moreover, the bone biopsy from an aluminum-loaded patient who has a parathyroidectomy often shows an increase in surface stainable aluminum, a further reduction of bone formation, and more symptomatic bone disease. Thus some factor associated with high serum PTH levels and/or an increased bone turnover retards or inhibits the appearance of aluminum toxicity. The same quantity of aluminum can be toxic when serum PTH and/or bone turnover are reduced. How parathyroid hormone protects from this syndrome and how a reduction in serum PTH levels precipitate the appearance of aluminum toxicity is uncertain.

PTH affects the distribution of aluminum in experimental animals. Injection of PTH increases the retention of parenterally administered aluminum, it may augment the intestinal absorption of aluminum to a small degree, and it enhances the deposition of aluminum in bone following its parenteral administration. The last may occur because the bone turnover is high. After serum PTH levels are reduced by medical therapy or after parathyroid surgery, bone turnover slows; this allows aluminum to localize on the mineralization front, which is associated with greater inhibition of matrix synthesis and bone mineralization.

Aluminum and Bone Disease in Patients on Total Parenteral Nutrition

The development of symptomatic low-turnover bone disease in patients with gastrointestinal diseases who received parenteral nutrition solutions that were contaminated with aluminum provides further evidence that aluminum causes skeletal toxicity. Despite normal renal function and substantial improvement of these patients' nutritional status, periarticular bone pain and fractures appeared within 1 to 3 years after initiation of treatment with long-term total parenteral nutrition (TPN). Serum calcium and phosphorus levels were normal or slightly increased; serum PTH and calcitriol levels were low or undetectable; and hypercalciuria was prominent. Bone biopsies disclosed reduced numbers of osteoblasts and osteoclasts and little or no tetracycline uptake, indicating markedly reduced bone formation. Bone biopsies sometimes showed *patchy osteomalacia*, characterized by focal areas of widened osteoid on the trabecular surface but with the total osteoid surface being normal. These patients were receiving aluminum, 2,000 to 3,000 μg/day, in the casein hydrolysate used as a protein source in the TPN solution. Bone biopsies showed prominent aluminum staining along trabecular surfaces. Plasma aluminum levels were markedly elevated (100 to 150 μg/L, versus normal, less than 8 μg/L), and aluminum also accumulated in bone and liver despite normal renal function. After substitution of amino acids, with much lower aluminum content than casein, in the TPN solution, serum aluminum decreased after a few weeks; however, 2 to 3 years were required before the bone aluminum content fell and bone formation improved. These observations indicate that parenteral aluminum loading can produce bone disease in humans with normal renal function and that the process is reversed only very slowly after aluminum loading is stopped.

Bone Disease in Aluminum-Loaded Animals

Parenteral aluminum loading in experimental animals has produced histologic alterations in bone similar to that of dialysis patents with aluminum-related bone disease. Aluminum-loaded rats and dogs developed osteomalacia involving both cancellous and trabecular bone, and the skeletal lesions were more severe when renal function was impaired. Short-term aluminum loading of rats impaired the mineralization of cortical bone, measured by tetracycline labelling, but caused no widening of osteoid seams; this lesion may be analogous to the "dynamic" lesion observed in dialysis patients. In aluminum-loaded dogs, the severity of osteomalacia correlated with the extent of aluminum staining on bone, and aluminum loading of pigs led to osteomalacia with reduced numbers of active osteoblasts that was independent of the inhibition of osteoid calcification. In dogs, PTH levels were stable or slightly increased, but the plasma levels of $1,25(OH)_2D$ fell. The aluminum content of the renal cortex was markedly increased, which could account for the mild decrease in renal function and the reduced synthesis of $1,25(OH)_2D_3$.

In summary, the administration of parenteral aluminum to experimental animals induces a bone disease that is remarkably similar to that found in aluminum-loaded uremic patients; the aluminum content of bone and its localization are similar to the findings in uremic patients with aluminum toxicity, and removal of aluminum leads healing of bone.

MECHANISMS OF ALUMINUM TOXICITY

The mechanisms of aluminum toxicity on bone and other tissues are largely unknown. Metals, such as aluminum, may become biochemically active as a result of being attached to a protein or cofactor, and aluminum could exert its toxicity because it substitutes for magnesium in certain biologic systems. Several magnesium–adenosine triphosphate (Mg-ATP)–dependent kinases are inhibited by aluminum, perhaps as aluminum-ATP. Enzymes that have been reported to be affected by aluminum include hexokinase, adenylate cyclase, feroxidase (Ceruloplasmin), magnesium–adenosine triphosphatase (Mg-ATPase), and many others. Aluminum can also affect the calcium-binding effect of calmodulin by causing its denaturation; this could reduce the capacity of calmodulin to activate the phosphodiesterase that inactivates cyclic adenosine 3′,5′-monophosphate (cAMP). Aluminum has a high affinity for the nucleus of the cell, perhaps accounting for its effects in certain organs, particularly the brain. Thus several biochemical processes may be deranged by aluminum when it bypasses the normal barriers that prevent or retard its entry into the body or into the cell.

Aluminum may affect bone via two mechanisms: it may "poison" osteoblasts directly and/or it may retard or even block the process of mineralization. Very low aluminum concentrations increase the alkaline phosphatase activity of fetal bone, whereas higher concentrations inhibit its activity. Ultrastructural studies of bone show that aluminum is localized within vesicles of the osteoblast; such intracellular localization may be responsible for altered cell metabolism. Aluminum may directly block the mineralization of bone as well: In cell free solutions, aluminum directly inhibits both the formation of hydroxyapatite crystals from calcium phosphate and the growth of existing apatite crystals. Also, aluminum citrate directly inhibits the precipitation of calcium phosphate. In tissue cultures, the addition of aluminum inhibits mineralization without inhibiting matrix formation or protein synthesis. The wide osteoid seams of typical dialysis osteomalacia may be an example of inhibition of both mineralization and matrix synthesis, with the former impaired more than the latter. The aluminum-induced, adynamic bone lesion may arise because matrix synthesis and mineralization are equally impaired. It is not certain which factors determine the effect that will predominate and thereby produce the features seen on bone biopsy.

CLINICAL FEATURES AND DIAGNOSIS OF ALUMINUM-RELATED BONE DISEASE

Typically, the symptoms of aluminum-related bone disease include axial bone pain, proximal muscular weakness, and recurrent fractures. Such clinical features, themselves, are rarely diagnostic, but certain findings can suggest the existence of this syndrome. Occasionally, the pain first occurs at a peripheral site, such as the heel, leg, or knee. More often, the pain is generalized or localized to the back, hips, shoulders, and/or ribs. Proximal weakness, particularly of the lower extremities, is common, making it difficult for the patient to rise from a low chair or to climb stairs. Occasionally, proximal muscular weakness is pronounced and pain is absent; this has led to the search for a neurologic cause of weakness before a metabolic bone disease was suspected.

Fractures of the ribs, femoral necks, vertebral bodies, and shafts of the femur, humerus, or metatarsal are not unusual in patients with aluminum-related bone disease. Severe pain on any motion against gravity may restrict the patient to a wheelchair or bed. Physical findings are often absent, although skeletal deformities, such as a funnel chest deformity, sternal bowing due to rib fractures, or kyphosis, can occur. The musculoskeletal symptoms of patients with aluminum-related bone disease are often more severe than those of patients with secondary hyperparathyroidism, except for the rare patient with fractures or spontaneous tendon rupture due to severe secondary hyperparathyroidism. Fractures are more common in patients with aluminum-related bone disease than in those with severe osteitis fibrosa. Periarticular pain around a major joint, such as the knee or ankle, and spontaneous variation in the location and intensity of the pain are more common in patients with symptomatic osteitis fibrosa, whereas it is unusual for aluminum-related bone disease to show spontaneous improvement.

Certain background or risk factors are more prevalent in patients with aluminum-related bone disease than in dialysis patients with other types of bone disease. These include previous parathyroidectomy, an earlier kidney transplant that was rejected, and earlier bilateral nephrectomy. Also, patients with diabetes mellitus as the cause of ESRD are at great risk to develop aluminum toxicity. Each of these factors (e.g., parathyroidectomy, diabetes mellitus, glucocorticoid therapy for a renal transplant, and bilateral nephrectomy) can lower the rate of bone turnover, contrasting to the usual high bone turnover of osteitis fibrosa.

Certain biochemical findings are common in patients with aluminum-related bone disease, but most are neither sensitive nor specific. Serum calcium levels are in the upper range of normal or above; such hypercalcemia can appear spontaneously or during treatment with an active vitamin D sterol or oral calcium salts, or with use of dialysate calcium level above 3.0 mEq/L. The findings of fractures, bone pain, hypercalcemia, and PTH levels that are above the "normal range" have led to parathyroid surgery for presumed secondary hyperparathyroidism in patients later shown to have aluminum-related bone disease; this syndrome has been termed *pseudohyperparathyroidism*. In a comparison of (a) patients with aluminum-related bone disease, (b) patients with severe hyperparathyroidism, and (c) those with "mild" bone disease, serum calcium levels did not differ between those with aluminum-related bone disease and those with osteitis fibrosa; however, the mean serum calcium levels of both groups exceeded that of asymptomatic patients with mild hyperparathyroidism. Serum calcium levels exceeded 10.4 mg/dl in 45% of patients with symptomatic aluminum-related bone disease and were above 10.9 mg/dl in 20%. Serum phosphorus levels do not distinguish between these groups of dialysis patients, although the values tend to be lower in patients with aluminum-related bone disease, perhaps because of greater adherence to the large dosages of aluminum gels that were prescribed.

Alkaline phosphatase levels have varied in different reports of patients with aluminum-related bone disease: they were normal or only slightly elevated in patients whose disease was due to aluminum-contaminated dialysate, but they were higher than normal in most symptomatic patients with aluminum toxicity arising from intestinal absorption through the aluminum gels. In the latter patients, the plasma alkaline phosphatase levels were not different from the group with osteitis fibrosa.

In patients with aluminum toxicity, the PTH levels are usually lower than expected for patients on dialysis; however, 10% to 20% of those with aluminum toxicity have PTH levels as high as those with significant osteitis fibrosa. The mean serum-midregion PTH levels were higher in hemodialysis patients with osteitis fibrosa than in those with aluminum-related bone disease, and the PTH in the latter was lower than that observed in patients with mild hyperparathyroidism. The midregion PTH levels did not differ according to the type of bone disease in a population study of pediatric patients undergoing CAPD. This latter finding may be related to an effect of CAPD to modify the midregion PTH levels because of high removal of these PTH fragments by peritoneal dialysis.

The plasma levels of 1,25(OH)D are normal, an observation that helps to exclude nutritional vitamin D deficiency in a renal patient. The serum levels of $1,25(OH)_2D$ are low or undetectable, an expected finding with ESRD; however, the levels may be even lower than those from dialysis patients without aluminum loading.

As stated previously, a hypochromic, microcytic anemia has been described in patients with aluminum toxicity due to aluminum-containing dialysate. It was even suggested that the hemogram might be useful to identify patients with aluminum toxicity. However, the hematocrit, mean cell volume, and mean cell hemoglobin concentration of patients with aluminum toxicity from oral aluminum gels were not different from values of hemodialysis patients with no evidence of aluminum toxicity.

The various clinical features observed in patients with aluminum toxicity are, in large part, due to differences in the rate and magnitude of aluminum loading: Thus serum aluminum levels rise rapidly to values above 100 to 200 μg/L in patients who acquire aluminum from dialysate or those who ingest aluminum gels with citrate; in contrast, patients who accumulate aluminum gradually from intestinal absorption develop clinical manifestations more gradually and have serum aluminum levels that are less elevated. Anemia, encephalopathy, and even acute aluminum neurotoxicity occur with the former, and the bone disease is often overshadowed by the symptoms of encephalopathy; on the other hand, patients who absorb aluminum slowly most often exhibit aluminum-related bone disease, have anemia that is consistent with renal failure and a low risk of encephalopathy, and may have alkaline phosphatase levels that are above normal.

In patients with aluminum-related bone disease, the skeletal radiographs show highly variable findings. Demineralization or fractures of various sites, including the ribs, hips, and vertebral bodies, are common. Typical pseudofractures are uncommon, although a scintiscan can show nondisplaced pseudofractures that are undetectable on initial radiographs and only apparent from the subsequent callus formation. Subperiosteal erosions can be observed: they represent erosions of earlier osteitis fibrosa that failed to mineralize as aluminum toxicity appeared and serum PTH levels fell. The overall uptake of radiolabeled bisphosphonate by bone is often lower than that of patients with osteitis fibrosa, but the lack of adequate quantitation does not allow clear separation between aluminum-related bone disease and osteitis fibrosa.

Serum Aluminum Levels. Improved methodology using endothermic atomic absorption spectroscopy permits the accurate measurement of aluminum in biologic fluids, and serum aluminum levels have been evaluated in renal patients suspected of aluminum toxicity. Compared with normal values of less than 8 μg/L, the serum aluminum levels are increased in nearly all dialysis patients. Initial reports noted a lack of correlation between serum aluminum levels and the aluminum content of bone; however, low-order but significant correlations were observed in subsequent series. Plasma aluminum levels are useful in the clinical evaluation of uremic patients suspected of aluminum toxicity. The laboratory should be carefully chosen; a laboratory reporting normal values above 8 to 10 μg/L or a normal range for dialysis patients should be used with caution.

Serum aluminum levels reflect the load of aluminum over the previous few weeks to months; the finding of serum aluminum levels that are persistently higher than 75 to 100 μg/L indicate that a patient has had recent, significant exposure to aluminum. Such a value may exist in a patient with aluminum toxicity or indicate substantial risk of future toxicity unless the exposure to aluminum is stopped. When aluminum exposure is stopped under such circumstances, serum aluminum levels can fall by 50% to 70% after 6 to 12 months. In contrast, aluminum toxicity is quite unlikely in dialysis patients with serum aluminum levels below 30 to 40 μg/L unless several months have elapsed without any exposure to aluminum or the function of the parathyroid glands is depressed.

For an accurate interpretation of the baseline serum aluminum level, the iron status of the patient should be taken into consideration. Patients with iron deficiency may exhibit high serum aluminum levels in the presence of only a modest increase in the body burden of aluminum, as evaluated by a deferoxamine infusion test. On the other hand, patients with severe iron overload, as manifested by a serum ferritin level above 1,000 μg/L, may have a positive deferoxamine test and significant bone accumulation of aluminum and yet exhibit serum aluminum levels below 30 μg/L. Such findings are probably due to the interference of iron with the protein binding of aluminum, which can modify the distribution of aluminum. Aluminum and iron both are transported by transferrin, which has a greater affinity for iron than aluminum. These two facts may explain the negative relationship observed between the serum iron levels and/or transferrin saturation and the serum aluminum levels that are reported. When serum iron levels are elevated in iron-loaded patients with increased iron binding to transferrin, there is a limited capacity for the transferrin to bind aluminum. There may be increased binding of aluminum to citrate, which has a larger space of distribution than transferrin; the result may be lower serum aluminum levels.

Some animal data suggest that iron loading may interfere with the intestinal absorption of aluminum. Iron and aluminum share a common pathway for their intestinal absorption, and they compete for binding to the same protein, transferrin, which may promote their cellular uptake and absorption. Also, preliminary data suggest that iron deficiency may augment the intestinal absorption of aluminum.

The benefits of periodic measurement of serum aluminum in all patients in a dialysis unit include: (a) the identification of defective water purification, which causes aluminum levels to rise in all patients and (b) the detection of either excess aluminum intake or unusually high aluminum absorption in individual patients. In geographic locations where the aluminum levels in the water supply commonly exceed 20 to 50 μg/L (e.g., areas that use surface water or have acid rain), serum aluminum levels should be measured more frequently than in areas where water aluminum levels are rarely if ever increased (e.g., the Pacific Northwest and other parts of the far western United States). Serum aluminum levels should be measured at 3- to 4-month intervals in dialysis patients who ingest aluminum gels.

Deferoxamine Infusion Test. The increment of urinary iron following an infusion of the chelating agent, deferoxamine, correlates with tissue stores of iron, and it was postulated that the increment in serum aluminum following a standard infusion of deferoxamine would predict the presence of aluminum loading. The maximum increment in serum aluminum occurs by 8 to 24 hours after a deferoxamine infusion, and initial reports, with aluminum toxicity in a high fraction of patients, reported the reasonable identification of the afflicted patients; however, the sensitivity of the test was not high, and others did not recommend this test.

A large series of nearly 300 unselected dialysis patients with bone biopsies, studied in Toronto, provides useful information on the value of this test, particularly when evaluated in conjunction with the level of intact PTH, measured with an immunoradiometric assay. An increment of serum aluminum of more than 100 μg/L after a deferoxamine infusion, 40 mg/kg body weight, had a positive predictive value for aluminum bone disease of 75% to 88%, but the sensitivities were low (10% and 37% for peritoneal dialysis and hemodialysis patients, respectively). The combination of an intact PTH (iPTH) level less than 200 pg/ml (normal, less than 65 pg/ml) and an increment in serum aluminum of more than 150 μg/L provided excellent positive predictive value that exceeded 95%, but the sensitivity was only 35% to 45%. They evaluated other cut-off values for the increment in plasma aluminum after deferoxamine of 100 μg/L or more, and in excess of 50 μg/L combined with the same iPTH limit. There was a modest reduction of positive predictive value, but the sensitivity rose substantially (Fig. 68.41). The sensitivity of the procedure was substantially lower in patients who had withdrawn from all aluminum gels for longer than 6 months (Fig. 68.42). These authors suggest that this evaluation is of most value in ESRD patients who continue to ingest aluminum gels. Under such circumstances, performing a deferoxamine infusion test combined with intact PTH levels at intervals would be useful to identify those with increasing aluminum loading and thus a higher risk of toxicity.

The iron status of the patient may also be important for the correct interpretation of a deferoxamine infusion test. Available data suggest that the peak aluminum level after a deferoxamine infusion test is higher in patients with iron deficiency (ferritin less than 300 μg/L) than in those with normal to high iron stores (ferritin levels more than 300 and less than 1,000 μg/L) and in those with iron overload (ferritin levels more than 1,000 μg/L).

A lower deferoxamine dose, 5 mg/kg body weight, compared with the 40 mg/kg body weight previously employed,

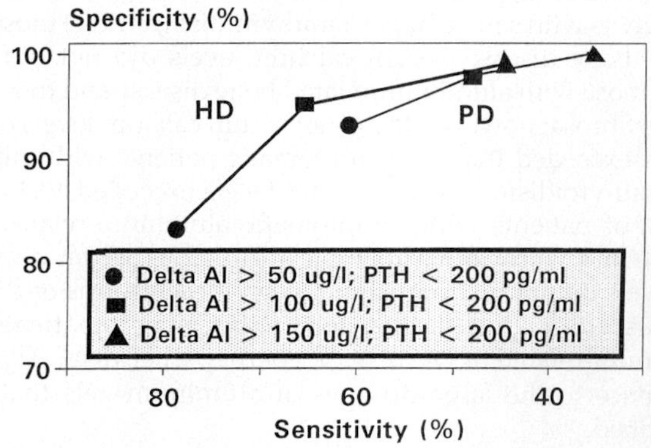

Figure 68.41. Predicting aluminum bone disease based on Delta aluminum and intact PTH. Specificity and sensitivity of the deferoxamine infusion test combined with an intact PTH level less than 200 pg/ml for the diagnosis of aluminum-related bone disease, as determined by bone biopsy, in patients treated with hemodialysis (HD) and peritoneal dialysis (PD). Several different "cut-off" limits are shown for the Delta aluminum, indicating the maximum increment in plasma aluminum following the infusion of deferoxamine, 40 mg/kg body weight. (Reproduced from Pei Y, Hercz G, Greenwood C, et al. Non-invasive prediction of aluminum bone disease in hemo-and peritoneal dialysis patients. *Kidney Int* 1992;41:1374–1382.)

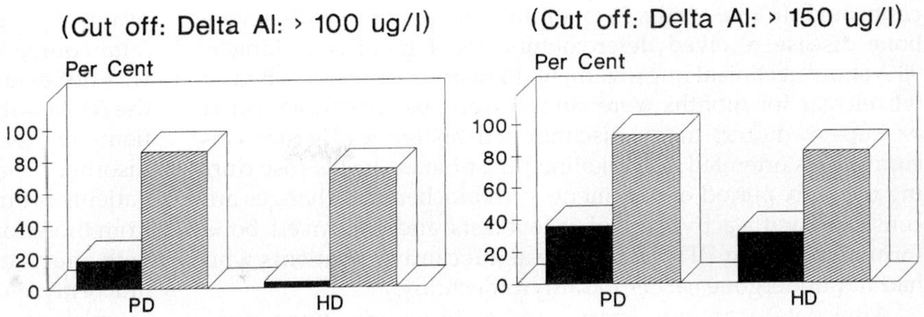

Figure 68.42. Influence of the recent ingestion of aluminum gels on the false-negative rate for the deferoxamine infusion test combined with intact PTH level for the diagnosis of aluminum-related bone disease in dialysis patients. The *solid bars* represent patients who had received aluminum gels during a period of 6 months before the deferoxamine infusion test, whereas the *cross-hatched bars* represent those who had discontinued the ingestion of aluminum 6 or more months before the test. Two different "cut-off" limits are given for Delta serum aluminum, Delta aluminum more than 100 μg/L *(left panel)* and Delta aluminum more than 150 μg/L *(right panel)*, which represents the maximum increment in plasma aluminum after the infusion of deferoxamine, 40 mg/kg. (Adapted from Pei Y, Hercz G, Greenwood C et al. Non-invasive prediction of aluminum bone disease in hemo-and peritoneal dialysis patients. *Kidney Int* 1992;41:1374–1382.)

was reported to be effective for the detection of aluminum overload; one benefit of this lower dosage is less potential risk of side effects. The combination of this low deferoxamine dose and certain iPTH levels separated patients with (a) aluminum-related bone disease, (b) aluminum loading with a high risk of toxicity, and (c) aluminum overload combined with either hyperparathyroid or mixed bone disease. The first group had an increment of serum aluminum above 50 μg/L and an iPTH below 150 pg/ml; the second and third categories had similar increments of serum aluminum level (more than 50 μg/L increment) plus an iPTH level of 150 to 650 pg/ml or above 650 pg/ml, respectively.

Certain clinical risk factors and biochemical findings should alert a nephrologist to a greater probability that an ESRD patient may have aluminum toxicity. The measurement of serum iPTH, plasma aluminum, and the results of the deferoxamine infusion test can provide important clues to whether aluminum toxicity exists. In patients with substantially elevated plasma aluminum levels (more than 70 μg/L) and serum intact PTH levels greater than 5-fold normal, a bone biopsy may be necessary to distinguish between aluminum toxicity and osteitis fibrosa as the primary skeletal disease. Thus a bone biopsy, carried out with double tetracycline labelling and aluminum staining, is often needed to provide a specific diagnosis and a guide to the proper therapy.

TREATMENT OF ALUMINUM TOXICITY

The outcome of the dialysis patients initially identified as dialysis osteomalacia, which was later identified as aluminum-related bone disease, was poor. These patients often exhibited progressive deterioration and many died; treatment with vitamin D or its active analogs was largely ineffective. An initial report described symptomatic improvement following combined treatment with calcitriol and 24,25$(OH)_2D_3$; however, trials in additional patients failed to show substantial improvement except in isolated cases. With identification of the etiologic role of aluminum, further trials were abandoned.

During the early 1980s, severe aluminum loading was recognized in increasing numbers of dialysis patients, and the value of various therapeutic modalities arose from retrospective analysis. With the introduction of effective water purification, new cases of symptomatic aluminum toxicity no longer appeared; however, patients with symptomatic disease rarely improved. It was believed at that time that dialysate was the only source of aluminum, and most clinicians continued to give aluminum gels as phosphate binders. From the observation that relatively small amounts of aluminum were removed by standard dialysis procedures, it was concluded that such removal by standard dialysis was inadequate to manage aluminum toxicity effectively. This conclusion was compounded by the fact that most patients continued to receive substantial doses of aluminum gels; thus an alternative therapy for aluminum toxicity was desperately needed.

In patients undergoing CAPD, aluminum toxicity has been less common than during long-term hemodialysis. Because of aluminum binding to plasma proteins, particularly transferrin, and because of the losses of such plasma proteins into the peritoneal dialysate, the removal of aluminum bound to these proteins can be substantial. The aluminum levels in peritoneal dialysate correlate with serum aluminum levels, with the dialysate level being 20% to 25% of the corresponding serum level. The total amount of aluminum removed by CAPD in patients regularly ingesting aluminum gels as phosphate binders was found to be 100 to 400 μg/day, an amount considerably greater than the 10 to 30 μg/day lost in the urine of normal individuals; these data also provide insight into the amount of aluminum absorbed by these patients.

Treatment with Deferoxamine

Following the initial report of successful treatment of dialysis encephalopathy with deferoxamine, other reports documented the substantial increase of aluminum removal by dialysis after a deferoxamine infusion. Patients with encephalopathy often improved, and refractory bone disease was reversed. During the early and mid-1980s, deferoxamine was used widely to treat aluminum toxicity, although this indication was never approved by the Food and Drug Administration in the United States.

Deferoxamine enhances aluminum removal in dialysis patients by two mechanisms: first, it mobilizes aluminum from tissue stores and thereby raises the total serum aluminum level, and second, deferoxamine forms the ultrafiltrable deferoxamine–aluminum complex, aluminoxamine, that permits increased removal across the dialysis membrane. The amount of aluminum removed during a 4 hour dialysis increased from a basal value of 50 to 300 μg before deferoxamine to as great as 4 to 8 mg during a dialysis treatment 48 hours after infusing deferoxamine. Because of aluminoxamine's relatively large size (molecular weight, approximately 620 D), its removal is relatively slow across a standard dialysis membrane, and three to four dialysis treatments are needed to remove the aluminoxamine arising from a single infusion of deferoxamine.

The initial favorable results with deferoxamine treatment for aluminum toxicity, particularly the bone disease, were confirmed. In one study, 27 symptomatic patients with severe bone disease received deferoxamine for 4 months or longer; 93% showed clinical improvement. Patients confined to a bed or wheelchair for months were able to walk, bone pain vanished or improved, and many discontinued analgesics. Serum calcium levels often fell and alkaline phosphatase levels rose during the early period of treatment; such biochemical changes are consistent with activation of osteoblasts and improved bone formation. Serum PTH levels rose significantly in patients who had not undergone earlier parathyroidectomy.

After deferoxamine therapy for 4 to 14 months, bone biopsies showed reduced surface staining with aluminum and increased bone formation. The degree of histologic improvement was less in patients who previously underwent parathyroidectomy. However, the clinical reversal of pain and weakness was independent of the changes noted on bone biopsy. Among CAPD patients, the intravenous infusion or the intramuscular injection of deferoxamine or its intraperitoneal instillation caused similar and large increments in aluminum removal via CAPD. Long-term deferoxamine therapy for CAPD patients with aluminum-related bone disease led to both clinical and biochemical improvement, independent of whether the deferoxamine was given by the intravenous or intraperitoneal route.

Side Effects of Deferoxamine. Despite these substantial benefits of such treatment, deferoxamine therapy is associated with certain adverse effects, some very serious. Hypotension, usually managed by slowing the infusion rate, occurs in a small but significant fraction. Rarely, the hypotension is marked and necessitates a dose reduction and/or extending the infusion over a longer period of time. Certain ophthalmic complications, including cataracts and retinal abnormalities, have been reported in nonrenal patients receiving large doses of deferoxamine for hematologic disorders and in hemodialysis patients treated with deferoxamine. Acute visual loss that was irreversible has been reported after a single dose of 40 mg/kg of deferoxamine. Rarely, skin rashes or thrombocytopenia can occur.

One serious complication is the precipitation of acute aluminum neurotoxicity that develops within the first few weeks of deferoxamine therapy for the management of aluminum-related bone disease. In some cases, this syndrome has been fatal; in other patients, cessation of treatment followed by use of a substantially lower doses of deferoxamine was followed by improvement of both neurologic features and bone disease.

A very serious problem encountered in deferoxamine-treated dialysis patients is the increased prevalence of fatal mucormycosis (Fig. 68.43). The disseminated or rhinocerebral type

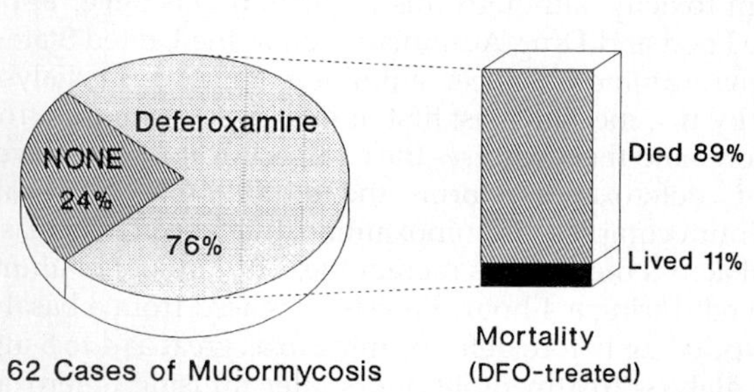

Figure 68.43. Prevalence of deferoxamine therapy among 62 dialysis patients who developed mucormycosis and the very high mortality among the patients receiving deferoxamine. [Reproduced with permission from Coburn JW. Treatment and prevention of aluminum toxicity. *Nephrologia* 1993;13(Suppl. 3):123–128; as adapted from Boelaert JR, Fenves AZ, Coburn JW. Deferoxamine therapy and mucormycosis in dialysis patients: report of an international registry. *Am J Kidney Dis* 1991;18:660–667.]

of mucormycosis is most common, with a fulminant, rapidly fatal course. In many cases, the cause or nature of the illness was not even suspected until autopsy. It is also probable that the 60 identified cases among deferoxamine-treated dialysis patients represent a small fraction of the true prevalence of this disorder. The infection encountered in deferoxamine-treated patients is limited to certain specific *Rhizopus* species that differ from those found in diabetics or immune-compromised patients with mucormycosis. In animals with experimentally induced mucormycosis, deferoxamine treatment causes a rapidly fatal course compared with infected animals not given deferoxamine. The pathogenic mechanism responsible for this susceptibility to mucormycosis has been delineated: Deferoxamine is a microbial siderophore that promotes assimilation of iron from the environment by the microbe. The parenteral administration of deferoxamine produces chelates of both iron, forming feroxamine, and aluminum, generating aluminoxamine. With normal renal function, these chelates are rapidly excreted in the urine; however, their circulating half-life is greatly prolonged with renal failure or during dialysis. Moreover, feroxamine can promote both the growth and pathogenicity of specific *Rhizopus* species with receptors for feroxamine. The prolonged plasma half-life of feroxamine in dialysis patients undoubtedly accounts for these patients' enhanced susceptibility to mucormycosis; this contrasts to its rarity among hematologic patients with normal renal function, who received deferoxamine for treatment of iron overload.

Hypersensitivity to deferoxamine has been reported; when this occurs and therapy is absolutely essential, the patient can be desensitized and then given the drug. Serum ferritin levels do not fall significantly in most dialysis patients treated with deferoxamine; however, in a rare patient who develops iron deficiency, it may be necessary to discontinue deferoxamine and administer parenteral iron.

Deferoxamine Use: Minimizing Treatment Complications and Side Effects. To minimize the risk of deferoxamine treatment, the dose should be kept to a minimum (i.e., 0.25 to 0.5 g/dose), and 7 to 10 days should elapse between doses. Therapy can also be given intravenously or intramuscularly, 6 to 8 hours before the dialysis procedure, rather than infusing the deferoxamine 48 hours before dialysis, as is generally done. To maximize the removal of feroxamine, the first dialysis after the deferoxamine dose should be performed using a highly efficient dialyzer, a hemoperfusion system, or a combination to maximize the removal of feroxamine.

A favorable outcome was reported on the use of low-dose deferoxamine to treat 41 hemodialysis patients with severe acute aluminum toxicity arising from contaminated water. Initially, the patients were treated for 6 weeks with intensive 6 day per week hemodialysis and hemoperfusion and withdrawal of all aluminum-containing phosphate binders, but no deferoxamine was given. During these 6 weeks, the mean serum aluminum level (±SD) decreased from 506 ± 255 μg/L to 121 ± 46 μg/L. Then, a deferoxamine test was performed using 5 mg/kg given during the last hour of hemodialysis with the serum aluminum measured before the next dialysis. The patients were then grouped according to the serum aluminum levels after deferoxamine. Among the 11 patients with serum aluminum of more than 300 μg/L, acute neurologic and/or ophthalmologic side effects were observed in 9 patients, whereas such side effects occurred in only 2 of the 30 patients with a postdeferoxamine serum aluminum level below 300 μg/L. Two different treatment approaches were devised: The most severely intoxicated patients included the patients with postdeferoxamine serum aluminum levels above 300 μg/L plus the two patients with serum aluminum levels below 300 μg/L but with neurologic or ophthalmologic symptoms after the deferoxamine test. The second group included those with postdeferoxamine serum aluminum levels below 300 μg/L and no symptoms after the test. The most severely intoxicated patients received deferoxamine, 5 mg/kg, given intravenously 5 hours before a dialysis procedure that used both charcoal hemoperfusion and hemodialysis. The patients in the less intoxicated group received deferoxamine, 5 mg/kg, infused during the last hour of hemodialysis and then hemoperfusion and hemodialysis were performed 44 hours later. There were no side effects with the use of this protocol. Over the next 6 months, both a significant decrease in the basal serum aluminum levels and a reduction in the serum aluminum level after the deferoxamine infusion were seen in both groups of patients. The serum iPTH levels and the mean corpuscular volume of erythrocytes rose in both groups.

These various maneuvers designed to minimize the risks of deferoxamine therapy have not been proven to prevent the occurrence of mucormycosis, although new cases have not been identified or reported using the low dosages and the highly efficient dialysis. For this reason, we recommended that deferoxamine therapy be restricted to patients with the serious and potentially fatal forms of aluminum toxicity (e.g., dialysis encephalopathy or acute aluminum neurotoxicity). For patients with symptomatic bone disease there should be a trial period with the total withdrawal of exposure to aluminum before this potentially dangerous treatment is started. Patients who pose a significant management problem are those with severely symptomatic bone disease; hypercalcemia; significant secondary hyperparathyroidism, as indicated by iPTH levels more than 10- to 15-fold normal; and evidence of significant recent aluminum loading from results of serum aluminum level and/or a large increment in serum aluminum after the infusion of deferoxamine. Parathyroidectomy should definitely be postponed until there is substantial reduction of the aluminum burden. If the skeletal symptoms are severe in such patients, it is justified to use low doses of deferoxamine, a maximum of 250 mg given a few hours before dialysis, but only before every third or fourth dialysis. Alternative recommendations have been made, and the interested reader is referred to the Consensus Conference of the European Dialysis and Transplant Association–European Renal Association; they suggest a more liberal use of deferoxamine therapy.

The major disadvantages of deferoxamine are its life-threatening side effects and the necessity of its parenteral administration; therefore there is interest in finding an alternative chelating agent. One such compound, deferiprone, has been shown to be effective in the management of iron overload, both clinical and experimental. *In vitro* observations and *in vivo* data in experimental animals suggest that this drug is an effective chelator of aluminum; further studies with this agent will be followed with interest.

Management of Aluminum-Toxicity with Total Aluminum Withdrawal

Most trials of deferoxamine therapy of aluminum toxicity were performed after dialysate aluminum levels were properly reduced, but most patients continued to ingest aluminum gels. With the introduction and extensive use of calcium salts as phosphate binders, it was possible for the first time to evaluate the effect on aluminum toxicity of the total withdrawal of all exposure to aluminum. When dialysis patients with bone biopsy features of aluminum toxicity were changed from aluminum gels to calcium carbonate and underwent hemodialysis using dialysate aluminum less than 5 μg/L, there was a substantial fall in serum aluminum levels and a reduced increment of plasma aluminum after a deferoxamine infusion (Fig. 68.44). Moreover, the histologic features of aluminum toxicity on bone biopsy either improved substantially or disappeared (Fig. 68.45). Therefore it is recommended that this procedure should be the first approach to aluminum bone disease, particularly in patients with adequate parathyroid function (e.g., intact PTH above 2- to 3-fold normal). If improvement fails to occur after this approach, a brief trial with deferoxamine therapy would be justified. It is essential that a period of "aluminum-free" therapy precedes parathyroid surgery in any patient with features of both aluminum loading and secondary hyperparathyroidism.

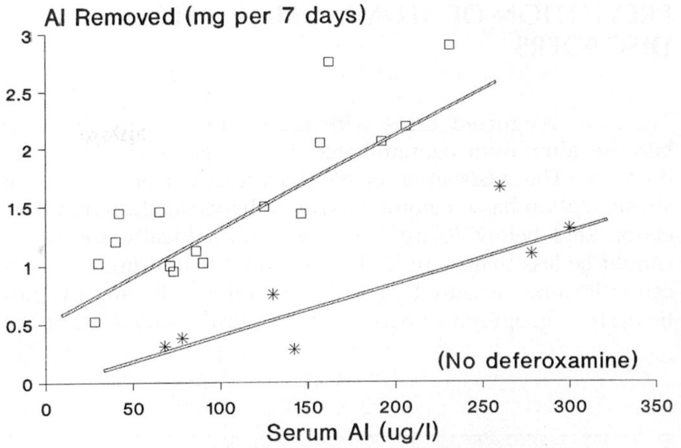

Figure 68.44. Comparison of aluminum removal by hemodialysis (*) versus CAPD (®) in patients with end-stage renal disease not receiving deferoxamine. Data are shown according to the level of plasma aluminum and each point represents a different patient who was regularly ingesting aluminum-containing gels. [Reproduced with permission from Coburn JW. Mineral metabolism and renal bone disease: effects of CAPD versus hemodialysis. *Kidney Int* 1993;43(Suppl 40):S92–S100.]

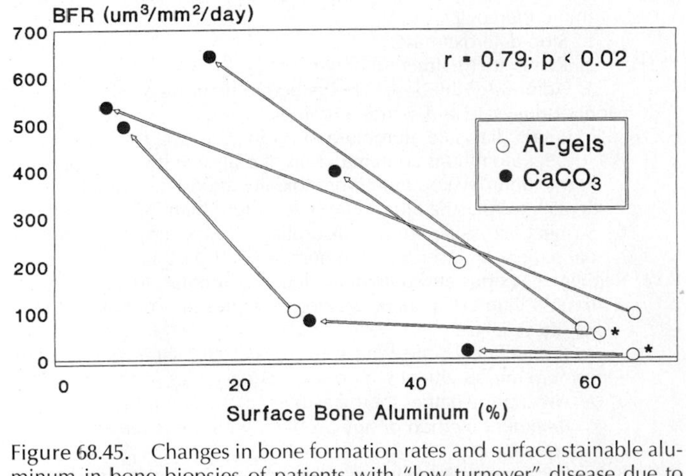

Figure 68.45. Changes in bone formation rates and surface stainable aluminum in bone biopsies of patients with "low turnover" disease due to aluminum accumulation in six dialysis patients who had calcium carbonate substituted for aluminum-containing phosphate binding agents. The two patients who had previously undergone subtotal parathyroidectomy are indicated by the asterisk (*). (Adapted from Hercz G, Andress DA, Norris K et al. Improved bone formation after replacing aluminum gels with calcium carbonate in dialysis patients with aplastic bone disease. *Trans Assoc Am Physicians* 1988;100:139–146.)

PREVENTION OF ALUMINUM-RELATED DISORDERS

The first recognized cases with aluminum toxicity occurred because aluminum contaminated the water used to prepare dialysate. The Association of the Advancement of Medical Instrumentation has recommended that dialysate aluminum levels be kept below 10 μg/L (0.4 μMol/L). Ideally, the levels should be less than 5 μg/L. It is essential that aluminum concentrations be measured periodically in the water supply, particularly in geographic areas in which alum is added to surface water to remove particulate matter or where the water aluminum concentrations exceed 30 to 40 μg/L, including areas where acid rain lowers the pH and increases the solubility of aluminum. Thus appropriate water purification methods must be installed and employed before dialysate is prepared. The choice of a specific method to purify water must take into consideration the specific local problems and requirements; only general principles are included here. Of the water purification methods available, water softeners (ion exchanger) remove moderate amounts of aluminum. Mixed-bed deionization is effective under some circumstances; however, reverse osmosis is the most effective, widely available method to reduce the alumi-

TABLE 68.5. Treatment and Prevention of Aluminum Toxicity

Treatment of Aluminum Toxicity	Prevention of Aluminum Loading and Toxicity
I. Eliminate/minimize intake of all aluminum-containing agents. A. Discontinue intake of the following: 1. Aluminum hydroxide 2. Aluminum carbonate 3. Sucralfate II. Avoid excessive aluminum absorption. A. Avoid all types of citrate salts with aluminum: 1. Shohl's solution 2. Bicitra 3. Calcium citrate 4. Alka-Seltzer 5. Excess citrus juice III. Enhance removal of tissue aluminum. A. Dialysis with aluminum-free dialysate (<5 μg/L) B. Net aluminum removal might be greater with peritoneal dialysis than with standard hemodialysis C. Deferoxamine therapy (0.250–0.5 g every 7–10 days) 1. This should be limited to symptomatic encephalopathy and bone disease not responsive to aluminum-free dialysis. D. With concomitant severe secondary hyperparathyroidism, treat aluminum toxicity first before parathyroidectomy or vigorous vitamin D therapy IV. Manage associated complications. A. Hypercalcemia: Discontinue calcitriol. 1. Reduce dialysate calcium to 2.5 or even 2.0 mEq/L. B. Encephalopathy or seizures (may appear or worsen with deferoxamine therapy). 1. Stop deferoxamine. 2. Reinitiate treatment at lower dose, 5 mg/kg. 3. Administer the dose 5 hours before hemodialysis. V. Monitor dialysate and serum aluminum. A. Maintain dialysate aluminum <5 μg/L. B. Suspect aluminum contamination of dialysate if several patients in one unit develop aluminum toxicity and/or almost all patients have plasma aluminum levels more than 75–100 μg/L. C. Suspect excess aluminum absorption or exposure in an individual patient with serum aluminum >70–100 μg/L. VI. Recognize serious and potentially lethal aluminum toxicity. A. If more than one patient develops seizures or abnormal behavior after dialysis: 1. **Immediately** send both serum and water samples for aluminum measurement with results requested as soon as possible. 2. Ascertain whether there has been a change in the water-treatment method or any problem with the reverse osmosis equipment. B. If effectiveness of the water treatment is questionable or if serum aluminum levels exceed 150–200 μg/L or dialysate aluminum level exceeds 75–100 μg/L: 1. Find alternative dialysis facilities for patients. 2. Use dialysate regeneration cartridges (Redy) and small volumes of pure aluminum-free water.	I. Control serum phosphorus levels without use of aluminum gels. A. Almost all patients (95%–98% of dialysis patients) 1. Use $CaCO_3$ calcium acetate sevelamer HCl alone or in combination. 2. Use adequate doses of these compounds to control serum phosphorus. 3. Maintain dietary phosphorus intake below 800 mg/day. 4. Use dialysate calcium of 2.5 mEq/L to minimize hypercalcemia. B. If aluminum gels are absolutely necessary: 1. Keep dose <1.5–3 g/day. 2. Combine with calcium salts and/or $MgCO_3$ with low magnesium dialysate. 3. Avoid iron deficiency that may enhance aluminum absorption (keep transferrin saturation at 30%–40%). II. Eliminate all sources of aluminum. A. Proper water treatment for preparation of dialysate: 1. Ideal: water aluminum concentration <5 μg/L 2. Permitted: 5–10 μg/L B. Eliminate unnecessary intake of all aluminum-containing drugs. C. Avoid citrate ingestion. III. Monitor serum aluminum in dialysis patients (three to four times per year). A. With serum aluminum >75–100 μg/L but no symptoms: 1. Stop *all* aluminum exposure. 2. Follow serum aluminum at monthly intervals to observe the expected decrease. B. Goal: serum aluminum <20–30 μg/L in all dialysis patients

Adapted from Frazao JM, Coburn JW. Aluminum toxicity in patients with end-stage renal disease: diagnosis, treatment and prevention. *Rev Port Nefrol Hipert* 1996;10(Suppl 1):S85–S112.

num concentration in water. Distillation methods can also be highly effective, but these are rarely available. It should be noted that reverse osmosis "rejects" only 85% to 95% of the aluminum in a solution; thus the aluminum concentration entering the reverse osmosis system must be below 100 to 125 μg/L (3.7 to 5.0 μMol/L) before reverse osmosis is effective. When the aluminum levels in the fluid exceed this level, a deionizer must be used to pretreat the water before it enters the reverse osmosis system.

When the concentrations of aluminum in the water supply are checked frequently, they can show variability from day to day, and it is impossible to monitor the water aluminum levels frequently enough to detect periodic but dangerous increments in aluminum levels. The measurement of plasma aluminum levels in all patients in a dialysis unit at 3- to 4-month intervals will permit monitoring of a water purification system, and it will identify individual patients who ingest excessive amounts of aluminum or absorb a high fraction of ingested aluminum. The finding of elevated or rising serum aluminum levels in all patients points to a problem with water purification, whereas an elevation of serum aluminum in only a few patients can focus attention to the source of aluminum loading in these specific patients (e.g., excessive oral intake or enhanced absorption). In either situation, the source of the aluminum loading should be found and corrected.

Aluminum absorption from aluminum-containing gels is the major source of aluminum accumulation in the United States and other advanced countries. Plasma aluminum levels correlate roughly with the amount of aluminum being ingested; if serum aluminum levels rise to 75 to 100 μg/L, aluminum gels should be discontinued or the dosage should be markedly reduced. Dietary phosphate should be restricted below 800 to 900 mg/day to lower the required doses of phosphate-binding agents. The total quantity of aluminum hydroxide ingested should not exceed six capsules per day (i.e., 3 g/day), and one should question such patients regarding their intake of any citrate-containing food or medication. Ideally, any patient with serum aluminum higher than 40 to 50 μg/L should discontinue aluminum gels and substitute a calcium salt, either calcium acetate or calcium carbonate. A small fraction of patients cannot tolerate either calcium carbonate or calcium acetate, either because of hypercalcemia or other side effects, particularly nausea, diarrhea, or constipation. To reduce absorption of calcium from calcium carbonate or calcium acetate, these compounds should be taken with meals and the dose with each meal should be adjusted in proportion to the amount of phosphate in the specific meal. For patients who are unable to restrict the phosphate in the diet or to take adequate quantities of calcium carbonate or calcium acetate, a combination of aluminum gels (in low dosages) and calcium carbonate may be employed. Hypercalcemia can be managed by employing dialysate containing calcium in a concentration no higher than 2.5 mEq/L. Some patients tolerate dialysate calcium levels as low as 2 mEq/L; the use of such dialysate permits the more aggressive use of calcium-containing phosphate binders.

The use of phosphate binders other than calcium carbonate and calcium acetate are limited to relatively small trials. Some recommend the use of magaldrate (Riopan), which contains less aluminum than aluminum hydroxide, a moderate amount of magnesium, and yet provides phosphate binding. Magnesium carbonate, given in conjunction with a magnesium-free dialysate solution, has also been used as an alternative phosphate-binding agent; when this is done, the dialysate magnesium concentration should not exceed 0.5 mEq/L. Its use can reduce the need for calcium-based phosphate binders. In general, most attempts to control serum phosphate levels with magnesium carbonate or magnesium hydroxide have not been successful, or was associated with the development of significant hypermagnesemia. Results of trials using sevelamer HCl, a polymer, poly[allylamine hydrochloride] (Renagel), a noncalcemic phosphate binder, show promise and this agent may be a useful alternative to the calcium-based compounds.

In summary, aluminum toxicity can be avoided when appropriate methods for water purification are used and when aluminum gels are replaced by alternative phosphate binders. Calcium carbonate and/or calcium acetate can be safe, effective phosphate binders when there is a reduction of dialysate calcium to 2.5 mEq/L or in rare instances even lower; aluminum gels can be avoided in more than 90% to 95% of patients. In the 5% to 10% of patients who require aluminum gels, their dose should be restricted substantially and plasma aluminum levels should be monitored frequently.

Continued awareness and surveillance is necessary to avoid the tragic but accidental outbreaks of fatal acute aluminum toxicity that still occur, usually in association with adverse climatic conditions that lead to markedly elevated aluminum levels in the water supply and the unrecognized failure of a water treatment system. A summary of methods to prevent aluminum toxicity is provided in Table 68.5.

Selected Readings

Andress DL, Nebeker HG, Ott SM, et al. Bone histologic response to deferoxamine in aluminum-related bone disease. *Kidney Int* 1987;31:1344–1350.

This paper reports bone biopsy features of 28 patients with symptomatic aluminum-related bone disease who were treated with deferoxamine.

Bakir AA, Hryhorczuk DO, Berman E, et al. Acute fatal hyperaluminemic encephalopathy in undialyzed and recently dialyzed uremic patients. *Trans Am Soc Artif Intern Organs* 1986;32:171–176.

This sentinel paper describes four patients with stable chronic renal failure who received a combination of aluminum–hydroxide to treat hyperphosphatemia and Shohl's solution to treat acidosis; they developed the frightening syndrome of acute aluminum neurotoxicity that proved fatal despite deferoxamine therapy.

Barata JD, D'Haese PC, Pires C, et al. Low dose (5 mg/kg) desferrioxamine treatment in acutely aluminum-intoxicated haemodialysis patients using two drug administration schedules. *Nephrol Dial Transplant* 1996;11:125–132.

This prospective study shows the safety of low-dose deferoxamine (5 mg/kg) in a group of dialysis patients with severe acute aluminum toxicity. The deferoxamine treatment had been preceded by 6 weeks of intensive hemoperfusion and hemodialysis with aluminum-free dialysate, which reduced serum aluminum by half. Two separate deferoxamine treatment schedules were then used according to the severity of the aluminum loading.

Boelaert JR, Fenves AZ, Coburn JW. Deferoxamine therapy and mucormycosis in dialysis patients: report of an international registry. *Am J Kidney Dis* 1991; 18:660–667.

This records known cases of mucormycosis, both published and collected through an international registry, among dialysis patients. The important pathogenic role of deferoxamine therapy is documented with a rapidly fatal course in the deferoxamine-treated cases.

Cannata JB, Diaz Lopez JB. Insights into the complex aluminum and iron relationship. *Nephrol Dial Transplant* 1991;6:605–607.

Editorial review on the interactions between aluminum and iron and the importance of this interaction in the pathogenesis, diagnosis, and management of aluminum toxicity.

De Broe ME, Drueke TB, Ritz E. Consensus conference—diagnosis and treatment of aluminum overload in end-stage renal failure patients. *Nephrol Dial Transplant* 1993;8:1–4.

Summarizes the recommendations reached during a Consensus Conference on the diagnosis and treatment of aluminum overload organized under the auspices of the European Dialysis and Transplant Association–European Renal Association.

D'Haese PC, Couttenye M-M, Goodman WG, et al. Use of the low-dose desferrioxamine test to diagnose and differentiate between patients with aluminum-related bone disease, increased risk for aluminum toxicity, or aluminum overload. *Nephrol Dial Transplant* 1995;10:1874–1884.

This paper shows the usefulness of a combination of low-dose deferoxamine (5 mg/kg) and various iPTH levels to separate patients with aluminum-related bone disease, aluminum loading with a high risk of toxicity, and aluminum overload combined with either hyperparathyroid or mixed bone disease. This approach may avoid the necessity of a bone biopsy in many patients.

Frazao JM, Coburn JW. Aluminum toxicity in patients with end-stage renal disease: diagnosis, treatment and prevention. *Rev Port Nefrol Hipertens* 1996; 10(Suppl 1):S85–S112.

This thorough review of the diagnosis, treatment, and prevention of aluminum toxicity. Includes many original and recent references.

Ittel TH, Steinhausen C, Kislinger G, et al. Ultrasensitive analysis of the intestinal absorption and compartmentalization of aluminum in uremic rats: a ^{26}Al tracer study employing accelerator mass spectrometry. *Nephrol Dial Transplant* 1997;12:1369–1375.

This study reports the ultrasensitive measurements of the isotope ^{26}Al using accelerator mass spectrometry to evaluate the intestinal absorption and compartmentalization of aluminum in rats. They showed that uremia enhances both the fractional absorption of aluminum and its subsequent deposition in bone.

Molitoris BA, Froment DH, Mackenzie TA, et al. Citrate: a major factor in the toxicity of orally administered aluminum compounds. *Kidney Int* 1989;36:949–953.

An editorial review summarizing the important role of citrate to enhance aluminum absorption and produce aluminum toxicity in uremic patients ingesting aluminum-containing compounds.

Pei Y, Hercz G, Greenwood C, et al. Non-invasive prediction of aluminum bone disease in hemo-and peritoneal dialysis patients. *Kidney Int* 1992;41:1374–1382.

A study of 279 dialysis patients, with similar numbers treated with hemodialysis versus peritoneal dialysis, provides data on the ability to predict aluminum bone disease from intact PTH levels and results of the deferoxamine infusion test.

Salusky IB, Foley J, Nelson P, et al. Aluminum accumulation from recommended doses of aluminum hydroxide in dialyzed children. *N Engl J Med* 1991;324: 527–531.

A prospective, controlled study of pediatric patients demonstrated that a presumed "safe" dose of aluminum gels leads to aluminum accumulation and is less effective than calcium carbonate in controlling secondary hyperparathyroidism.

Simoes J, Barata JD, D'Haese PC, et al. Cela n'arrive qu'aux autres (Aluminum intoxication only happens in the other nephrologist's dialysis centre). *Nephrol Dial Transplant* 1994;9:67–68.

This paper is a must read for every nephrologist. It reports a recent outbreak of severe acute aluminum toxicity that occurred in a dialysis unit under adverse climatic conditions and unrecognized failure of the water treatment system.

PART 3
Homocysteine

Alessandra F. Perna

Evidence is accumulating on the deleterious effects of hyperhomocysteinemia in both renal and nonrenal patients. These effects are related to a substantial increase in cardiovascular risk, even with modest elevations of homocysteine in plasma. The (putative) underlying biochemical mechanisms include three broad categories: (a) homocysteine (Hcy) oxidation, with H_2O_2 generation; (b) hypomethylation through S-adenosylhomocysteine (AdoHcy) accumulation; and (c) acylation of free amino groups in proteins, particularly those of lysine residues, by Hcy thiolactone. All of these mechanisms potentially interfere with the activity of several enzymes, structural proteins, and other biologic molecules.

HOMOCYSTEINE METABOLISM

Hcy is a sulfur amino acid that cannot be used as a building block by the protein biosynthesis machinery within the cell. Nevertheless, Hcy enters the metabolism of the essential amino acid methionine, in the methionine-Hcy cycle (Fig. 68.46). Methionine, unlike Hcy, becomes part of newly synthesized proteins, or alternatively is converted into the nucleoside S-adenosylmethionine (AdoMet). This reaction is catalyzed by the enzyme methionine adenosyl transferase, with adenosine triphosphate (ATP) consumption. AdoMet possesses a highly reactive methyl group, which is enzymatically transferred to many potential acceptors. AdoMet thus represents the universal methyl donor in *transmethylation* reactions. The aminopropyl moiety of decarboxylated AdoMet is instead necessary for polyamine biosynthesis.

The demethylated derivative of AdoMet is the thioether AdoHcy, which is a powerful inhibitor of the numerous AdoMet-dependent methyl transfer reactions, acting with a competitive mechanism toward the relevant enzymes. In spite of the numerous AdoMet-dependent reactions taking place intracellularly, which therefore produce stoichiometric amounts of AdoHcy, product inhibition is effectively counteracted under physiologic conditions. In fact, AdoHcy is readily metabolized to Hcy through a reversible enzymatic hydrolysis reaction, which splits this compound into Hcy and adenosine.

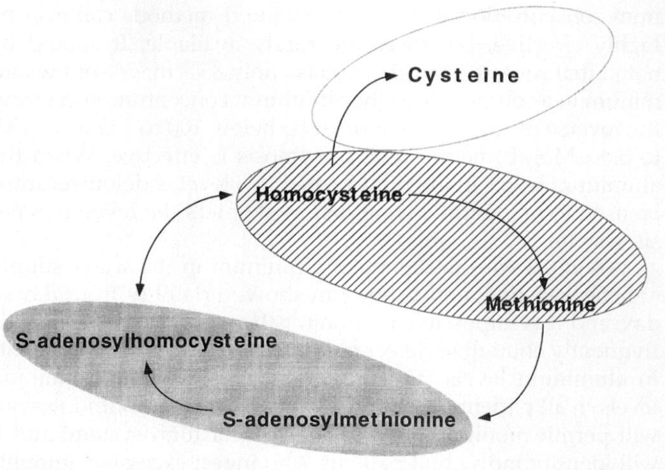

Figure 68.46. This scheme shows the remethylation pathway *(shaded area)*, the transmethylation pathway *(gray area)*, and the transsulfuration pathway *(white area)* of methionine-Hcy metabolism.

Hcy, in turn, is metabolized through two major pathways. The first is named *transsulfuration*, and represents a vitamin B_6–dependent pathway that yields cysteine as the final product. The enzyme cystathionine β-synthase binds serine and Hcy to produce cystathionine, and then a cystathioninase, which also requires vitamin B_6, cleaves cystathionine to 2-ketobutyrate and cysteine. Cysteine is eventually converted to glutathione, taurine, and other sulfur-containing metabolites.

The second pathway requires the enzyme methyltetrahydrofolate (MTHF)-Hcy methyltransferase (methionine synthase), leading to methionine synthesis *(remethylation)*. Cofactors in this reaction are folate in its active form and vitamin B_{12}. The active form of folate is MTHF, which donates the methyl group in the reaction catalyzed by methionine synthase, thus representing a true substrate. MTHF is formed from methylenetetrahydrofolate by enzymatic reduction catalyzed by methylenetetrahydrofolate reductase (MTHFR). The liver and kidney can also use betaine as a methyl donor, in an alternative pathway, for methionine biosynthesis.

As for the relative importance of the transsulfuration pathway and the remethylation pathway, the first metabolizes Hcy prevalently in the fed state, as represented by a methionine loading test for example, whereas the second assumes higher significance during fasting conditions. AdoMet crucially regulates the partitioning of Hcy between transsulfuration and remethylation through allosteric inhibition of MTHFR, and activation of cystathionine β-synthase.

A 2- to 4-hour methionine loading test can identify a substantial portion of hyperhomocysteinemic patients, who display methionine intolerance despite their normal fasting plasma Hcy levels.

CAUSES OF HYPERHOMOCYSTEINEMIA

Although not all cases of hyperhomocysteinemia can be explained by them, basically three causes of hyperhomocysteinemia are known. These causes include (a) genetic deficiencies of the relevant enzymes, (b) dietary related, and (c) chronic renal failure.

In the rare syndrome of homocystinuria, most cases are due to cystathionine β-synthase deficiency and are treated with high amounts of vitamin B_6, which probably acts by straining the metabolic pathway, and the little available enzyme. This was in fact the first model ever studied of hyperhomocysteinemia, where Hcy can reach, in the fasting state, a 400 μM concentration ("normal" value 10 μM). Most untreated patients affected by each genetic defect of the methionine-Hcy cycle succumb at an early age to cardiovascular accidents, and it was soon recognized that Hcy could be the culprit in the genesis of the disease. In fact, if in the classic form of homocystinuria (i.e., cystathionine β-synthase deficiency), hypermethioninemia accompanies hyperhomocysteinemia, whereas in other genetic diseases such as MTHFR deficiency and methionine synthase deficiency, where high plasma Hcy is detected as well, hypermethioninemia usually is absent. Among all of these rare genetic disorders, a much more common one has been described, which can give rise to hyperhomocysteinemia when associated with a reduction in folate intake. The thermolabile mutated enzyme (223Alafi→Val), in the case of this MTHFR variant, due to a C to T transition at gene position 677, is less active compared with the product of the normal allele. The allelic frequency is approximately 35%, whereas homozygous subjects represent approximately 12% of the general population. Mutants were probably selected during evolution because of their natural advantage in times of dietary-folate deficiency (thus saving folates necessary for purine biosynthesis) but are at risk of developing high Hcy levels. There is some evidence in fact that this mutation increases the individual's folate requirement, in order to keep plasma Hcy at low levels.

A relative or an absolute deficiency of folates and vitamins B_6 and B_{12} in the diet can also induce Hcy increases, through inadequate ingestion (diet poor in meats and green vegetables, food overcooking), inadequate absorption (chronic alcoholism, gastric atrophy), increased requirement (infancy), or therapy with methotrexate. As of January 1, 1998, folate fortification of foods such as cereals, breads, and the like is mandatory in the United State as a preventive measure for neural tube defects.

Among the acquired causes of hyperhomocysteinemia, renal failure is almost constantly associated with high levels of Hcy, with an 85 % prevalence. These patients have also an increased risk of vascular disease, with event rates for stroke or myocardial infarction 5 to 10 times higher than in the general population. The classic cardiovascular risk factors (e.g., hypertension, smoking, diabetes mellitus, hyperlipidemia), although in some instances more prevalent in these patients, and the presence of risk factors typical of the uremic state (e.g., hyperparathyroidism, anemia, atrioventricular fistula, hypoalbuminemia), cannot entirely explain by themselves such an increase in cardiovascular accidents (Fig. 68.47).

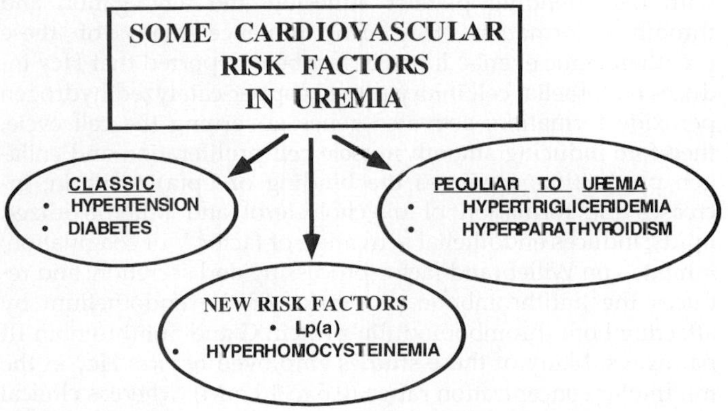

Figure 68.47. Some of the cardiovascular risk factors present in uremia: among the classic ones, diabetes and hypertension; among the ones peculiar to uremia, hyperparathyroidism and hypertriglyceridemia; among the new risk factors, Lp(a) and Hcy.

HYPERHOMOCYSTEINEMIA AS A RISK FACTOR FOR CARDIOVASCULAR DISEASE

In 1991, the first study in which it was concluded that even moderately increased homocysteinemia is an independent risk factor for vascular disease appeared. It would therefore not be necessary to have very high levels of Hcy in blood to elevate the cardiovascular disease risk; in fact several investigations, including large prospective population studies (such as the 5-year U.S. Physician's Health Study, with a few notable exceptions, such as the 10-year Multiple Risk Factor Intervention Trial), demonstrate that even a moderate Hcy increase is an independent risk factor for coronary artery disease, cerebrovascular disease, peripheral artery disease, venous thromboembolism, neural tube defects, and placental infarcts. Even if the normal range for plasma Hcy has been fixed to 8 to 10 μM for women and 10 to 12 μM for men, the epidemiologic evidence is in favor of a graded effect for Hcy. It has been calculated that any increment in 5 μM units (μmol/L of plasma) of Hcy is equivalent to a 20 mg/dl cholesterol elevation in terms of risk increase, and that hyperhomocysteinemia is the most likely explanation in at least one of five cardiac infarction cases. The April 1998 Second International Conference on Homocysteine Metabolism resulted in a consensus statement that more large prospective studies, done with the most appropriate sample collection (blood should be immediately centrifuged and plasma separated, because of Hcy release from red cells, up to 5 μM/hr), storage, and assay validation, are necessary.

Associations built on epidemiologic evidence must be strongly supported by basic research in adequately controlled models. A causative link between Hcy and vascular disease is supported by the observation that (a) the association is always present, regardless of the nature of the metabolic defect that caused hyperhomocysteinemia, and (b) *in vivo* studies show that baboons infused with Hcy develop vascular lesions; and mild dietary-induced hyperhomocysteinemia in mini-pigs or cynomolgus monkeys induces vascular damage and dysfunction.

The mechanism of the pathophysiologic link between Hcy and atherosclerosis is still actively investigated. Hypotheses concerning Hcy metabolic interferences and molecular targets, and the relevant biochemical evidence fall into the three categories mentioned previously. Hcy can *directly* react with different compounds ranging from small molecules such as nitric oxide, to several macromolecules including proteins. For example, the formation of adducts with proteins, through oxidation of key-free thiol groups, could explain their inactivation. Criticism to this model has been raised concerning Hcy specificity. In fact, other thiols are detectable at even higher concentrations than Hcy, nevertheless they do not appear to be related to the development of atherothrombosis. The second and third categories of proposed mechanisms sustain the role of Hcy precursors and/or derivatives as the true mediators of the effects of this amino acid. Hcy thiolactone, a highly reactive Hcy species, is produced as the result of proof-reading activity of methionyl transfer ribonucleic acid (tRNA) synthetase in order to prevent Hcy misincorporation within proteins in place of methionine during protein biosynthesis. Another key compound in this respect is AdoHcy, the *in vivo* Hcy precursor, whose respective concentrations are tightly regulated through the enzymatic equilibrium reaction described previously. It has been shown that in end-stage renal disease (ESRD), hyperhomocysteinemia is accompanied by a significant elevation of AdoHcy concentration in erythrocytes, a typical cell model for these studies, with a severely decreased AdoMet/AdoHcy ratio (Fig. 68.48). This, in turn, causes a significant impairment of an AdoMet-dependent membrane protein methylation reaction (Fig. 68.48), which is catalyzed by L-isoaspartate protein *O*-methyltransferase (or

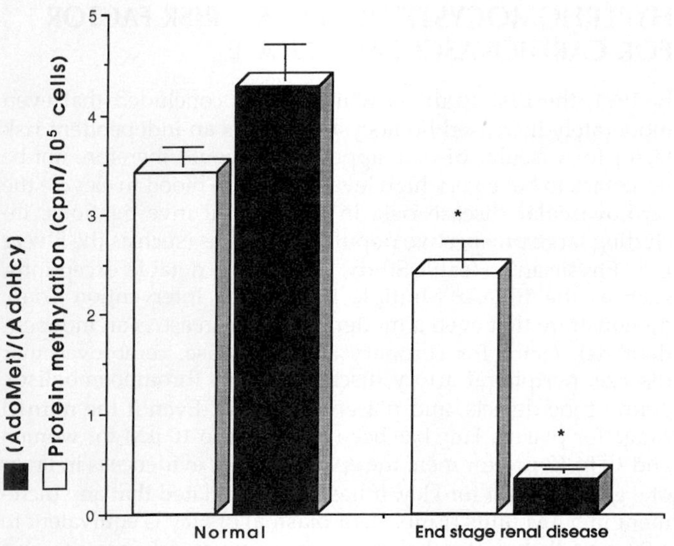

Figure 68.48. Enzymatic methyl esterification of erythrocyte membrane proteins was measured in end-stage renal disease (ESRD) patients and in normal controls. The results show that, in ESRD, methylation levels were significantly decreased compared with normal. In addition, a dramatic increase in the intracellular concentration of methylation inhibitor AdoHcy could also be detected in ESRD patients. This latter result is expressed as [AdoMet]/[AdoHcy] ± SE.

PCMT, EC 2.1.1.77), an enzyme involved in the repair of molecular damages spontaneously occurring in proteins through deamidation of asparagine residues. As a final result, the inadequate repair of such structural alterations can be evidenced and monitored by a significant reduction of D-isoaspartyl residues, a side-product of the repair enzyme activity, in membrane proteins.

It should be pointed out that (a) this protein repair mechanism is ubiquitous, as well as the type of structural damages recognized by PCMT in protein substrates, and (b) AdoMet-dependent methyltransferases are widespread enzymes, regulating the activities of several hundreds of methyl acceptors, which can all be inhibited by the increased AdoHcy concentration. Functional consequences of hyperhomocysteinemia may therefore involve, in different cells, not only proteins, but also other classes of biomolecular targets, ranging from DNA to phospholipids. For example, DNA methylation represents a strong modulator of cell growth and oncogene expression. Therefore a reduction of the AdoMet/AdoHcy ratio can potentially interfere with a number of different processes in which AdoMet acts as the methyl donor. In this regard, Hcy, at a concentration comparable with that present in uremic patients, inhibits through AdoHcy accumulation, cell growth, and methylation of protein p21^{ras} in cultured vascular endothelial cells. P21^{ras} hypomethylation leads to reduced membrane association of this important regulator of cell cycle, thus it may have an important effect on arteriosclerotic lesion formation through reduced endothelial cell proliferation. These effects appear to be cell specific because they are not reproduced in vascular smooth muscle cells and fibroblasts, thus reflecting cell differences in Hcy metabolism.

These models show how Hcy (and its parent compounds) has multiple sites of interference in various target organs and tissues, hence fully supporting the denomination of multisystemic toxin.

Atherosclerosis is the ultimate result of various events. From the time when Virchow conceived the triad composed of vascular injury, blood flow slackening, and coagulopathy, we now

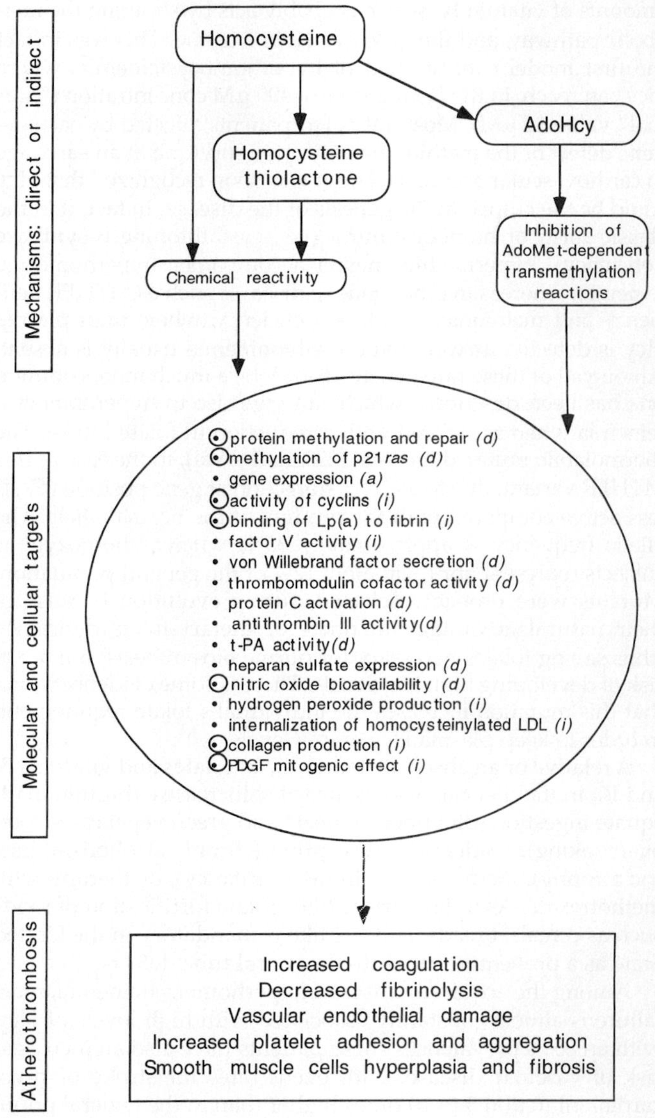

Figure 68.49. Synopsis of molecular mechanisms underlying Hcy proatherosclerotic actions. The *circles* surrounding the black points indicates effects tested under micromolar Hcy concentrations (i.e., in the range clinically detected in renal failure patients). a, altered; d, decreased; i, increased.

understand the role played by smooth muscle cell proliferation, high levels of oxidized cholesterol, and plaque generation, with the attending platelet adhesion and aggregation and thrombus formation. Hcy can influence many of these proatherogenic events. It has in fact been reported that Hcy induces endothelial cell injury due to copper-catalyzed hydrogen peroxide formation; activates genes governing the cell cycle, therefore inducing smooth muscle cell proliferation and collagen production; increases the binding of Lp(a) to fibrin; increases the formation of oxycholesterol and other oxidized lipids; induces endothelial activation of factor V of coagulation; inhibits von Willebrand factor processing and secretion; and reduces the antithrombotic properties of the endothelium by affecting both thrombomodulin-protein C and antithrombin III pathways. Many of these studies employed *in vitro* Hcy in the millimolar concentration range (0.5 to 10 mM), whereas clinical observation can attribute meaningful relevance only to situations in which Hcy is present in the micromolar range. Keeping these constraints in mind, it is likely that Hcy exerts its toxic effects in more than one way, not mutually exclusive (Fig. 68.49).

HYPERHOMOCYSTEINEMIA IN RENAL FAILURE

ESRD subjects have Hcy plasma levels between 25 and 40 μM or more, a high range indeed, considering that Hcy plasma levels of more than 15 μM puts patients at very high risk for cardiovascular disease.

Prospective studies established that hyperhomocysteinemia is also an independent risk factor for cardiovascular morbidity and mortality in ESRD [hemodialysis and continuous ambulatory peritoneal dialysis (CAPD)] patients; as well as in predialysis chronic renal failure patients, confirming its relation with the uremic state per se. In addition, it could play a role in recurrent vascular access thrombosis in hemodialysis patients.

Several studies show excess prevalence of both fasting and postmethionine loading hyperhomocysteinemia in stable renal transplant recipients. Hcy levels depend on residual renal function and on cyclosporine treatment, as demonstrated by the observation that heart transplant recipients treated with cyclosporine show moderate hyperhomocysteinemia. Whether Hcy levels influence renal graft outcome is still under investigation.

As for the cause of high Hcy levels, it has become clear that renal excretion is negligible (less than 2% of an oral Hcy load is eliminated by the kidneys), whereas total body metabolic clearance of this amino acid is reduced in chronic renal failure patients. Nevertheless, the role played by the kidneys in the metabolism of Hcy is highly debated. Kidneys possess the major enzymes for Hcy remethylation and transsulfuration, and the concentration of this amino acid is lower in the renal vein than in the renal artery in a rat model. In rats, however, Hcy is mostly represented by its free form, although in humans the opposite is true. In fact, studies in humans suggest that there is no net renal extraction of Hcy.

Among the determinants of Hcy plasma levels, we find vitamins B_{12} and B_6, and folic acid in its active form, that is, MTHF. The concentration of folic acid in plasma and in erythrocytes (which represents a more stable folate pool disjointed from daily fluctuations) in uremic patients is higher than normal control values in uremic patients. We must remember that these patients often receive vitamin supplementation in order to manage the losses of water-soluble vitamins during dialysis. However, it has been shown that the negative correlation between Hcy and folic acid levels is maintained. B vitamin levels, in particular folic acid, are lower in renal failure patients with vascular complications than those without. Of note, Hcy in its non–protein-bound form can be dialyzed; in fact, after a hemodialysis session it decreases by approximately 30%, but the levels return to the predialysis level before the next dialysis session.

Regarding the management of hyperhomocysteinemia in uremia, folic acid has been used as a means to reinforce the remethylation reaction of Hcy to methionine. Other compounds, such as betaine, *N*-acetylcysteine, or vitamin B_6, have also been used in the attempt to lower Hcy, with discouraging results. Apparently, uremic patients are resistant to folic acid at low dosages, that is, 1 to 2 mg (which is instead sufficient in the general population), thus leading to the concept of a "relative" folate deficiency in the face of an increased plasma and/or erythrocyte concentration. The mechanism of such resistance to folate needs to be clarified, but alterations of folate-dependent metabolism have been described in uremia, which may contribute to alter the bioavailability of the active form MTHF for Hcy metabolism.

Independent investigators used folates at a 15 mg/day dose by mouth for 2 months in hemodialysis patients. In one study, vitamins B_6 and B_{12} were also employed at low dosages, and in another study, MTHF, the direct precursor of the methyl moiety for methionine resynthesis from Hcy, was used. This choice of MTHF was done also in order to circumvent spurious effects due to the presence of the thermolabile variant of MTHFR, which is present in uremic patient with a frequency not different from the normal population. In the first study, therapy was effective and lowered Hcy (in the 12 patients who had Hcy above 20 μM) below the level of 15 μM in 3 patients. In the second study, this result was attained in 5 of 12 patients with Hcy levels above 20 μM, with the response correlated to pretreatment Hcy levels (Fig. 68.50). In addition, MTHF ameliorates the erythrocyte AdoMet/AdoHcy ratio, thus inducing a beneficial effect on AdoMet-dependent transmethylation reactions. Clearly, this dose is not effective in order to lower Hcy to normative levels in all patients.

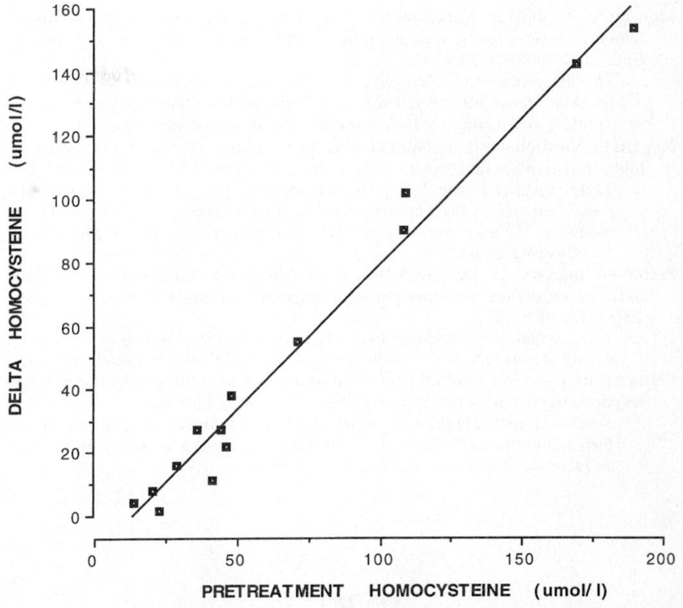

Figure 68.50. The higher the pretreatment Hcy levels, the greater the response in terms of Hcy reduction (Delta Hcy) after 2 months of MTHF therapy.

A placebo-controlled trial on renal transplant patients showed that the combination of vitamins B_6 and B_{12} and folic acid is the most effective in order to lower both postmethionine loading and fasting Hcy.

Regarding the inherent risks of folate therapy (excluding uncontrolled claims of neurotoxicity and zinc deficiency with high-dose folates), a definite "masking" effect of folates on the hematologic abnormalities develops early in the clinical picture of vitamin B_{12} deficiency (as in pernicious anemia), leaving the diagnosis to the detection of the much more damaging later neurologic complications (as many as 1% of elderly people may be affected). Therefore vitamins relevant to hematopoiesis, that is, folic acid and vitamin B_{12}, should be measured, along with Hcy determination, before being supplemented in conjunction.

Hcy levels can be reliably assessed by high-performance liquid chromatography (HPLC) separation and fluorescence detection, or by various recently marketed enzymatic immunoassays, whereas vitamins are easily measured by radioimmunoassay with commercially available kits.

Selected Readings

Bostom AG, Lathrop L. Hyperhomocysteinemia in end-stage renal disease: prevalence, etiology, and potential relationship to arteriosclerotic outcomes. *Kidney Int* 1997;52:10–20.

A thorough review of hyperhomocysteinemia, especially with respect to clinical implications.

Moustapha A, Naso A, Nahalawi M, et al. Prospective study of hyperhomocysteinemia as an adverse cardiovascular risk factor in end-stage renal disease. *Circulation* 1998;97(2):138–141.

This prospective study shows that high Hcy is an independent cardiovascular risk factor in uremic patients followed for 17 months. The follow-up is of reasonable duration, considering the high mortality rates in this patient group.

Nygård O, Nordrehaug JE, Refsum H, et al. Plasma homocysteine levels and mortality in patients with coronary artery disease. *N Engl J Med* 1997;337:230–236.

This prospective 5-year study on 587 angiographically confirmed coronary artery disease patients shows a strong graded relation between plasma Hcy levels and mortality. The mortality ratio was 2.8 for Hcy between 15 and 20 μM, and 4.5 for Hcy above 20 μM.

Perna AF, Ingrosso D, De Santo NG, et al. Metabolic consequences of folate-induced reduction of hyperhomocysteinemia in uremia. *J Am Soc Nephrol* 1997;8(12):1899–1905.

Therapy with pharmacologic doses of folate in its active form is effective in reducing plasma Hcy and in ameliorating the normal flow of transmethylations.

Perna AF, Ingrosso D, Galletti P, et al. Membrane protein damage and methylation reactions in chronic renal failure. *Kidney Int* 1996;50:358–366.

A thorough review of the basic science findings on protein fatigue and repair, and their relation with chronic renal failure, the first described in vivo model in which an impairment of protein methylation and repair is present.

PART 4
Products of Nitrogen Metabolism

Joel D. Kopple

Compared with normal sera, uremic sera are toxic to a wide variety of biologic systems and enzymes. The list of reported toxic effects of uremic sera in *in vitro* studies is long and continues to grow. A partial list of these toxic effects of uremic sera includes its ability to impair glucose uptake by rat diaphragm, reduce oxidation of glucose by white cells, decrease glucose use by red cells, inhibit adenosine diphosphate (ADP)-induced platelet factor 3 activation, decrease calcification of rachitic rat cartilage, reduce activity of serum lactate dehydrogenase, inhibit ouabain-sensitive adenosinetriphosphatase (ATPase) activity in red cells, impair activity of brain sodium-potassium activated ATPase, and reduce protein synthesis in Krebs II ascites tumor cells.

On the other hand, the clinical effects of uremic sera on biologic systems *in vivo* are not well defined. However, they may be responsible for many of the alterations in carbohydrate, fat, and amino acid and protein metabolism; impaired ion transport; decreased muscle membrane potential; hypothermia; and other manifestations of the uremic syndrome. The mechanisms by which compounds in uremic sera exert their toxic effects are not known. It is possible that some compounds may act after they enter the cell, whereas others may stimulate receptors or alter membrane transport.

Only some of the specific compounds responsible for uremic toxicity have been identified. Altered plasma and tissue hormone and electrolyte concentrations, edema, and acidemia contribute to the uremic syndrome. However, metabolic products of protein and amino acid metabolism are probably also toxic. Fats and carbohydrates are almost completely oxidized to carbon dioxide and water, which may be excreted through the lungs and skin as well as the kidneys. In contrast, many products of protein and amino acid metabolism are not completely oxidized in the body to carbon dioxide and water. These compounds are less volatile or diffusible, and, hence, the kidney plays a greater role in the excretion of these metabolites. Thus the number of compounds derived from proteins and amino acids that are increased in uremic plasma far exceed those derived from fats and carbohydrates. Table 68.6 lists major classes of products of nitrogen metabolism that are increased in uremic plasma or tissues.

The challenges of identifying the compounds that are toxic in uremia are difficult for the following reasons: (a) the lack of sensitive and reproducible techniques for assaying toxic effects of specific compounds, (b) the difficulties in accurately measuring many of these compounds at the intracellular and extracellular concentrations found in uremia, and (c) uremic toxins may exert their effects slowly, over days, weeks, or months, and possibly only in concert with other toxic compounds or in the absence of normal tissue levels of protective compounds. Potential uremic toxins, including homocysteine-advanced glycosylation

TABLE 68.6. Partial List of Nitrogenous Compounds and Products of Nitrogen Metabolism That Are Increased in Uremic Plasma or Tissues

Certain amino acids	Guanidines	Catecholamines
Ammonia[a]	Indoles	Peptide hormones
Aromatic acids	Inorganic anions	Cholecystokinin
Benzoic acids	Nucleic acid derivatives	Follicle-stimulating hormone
Cinnamic acids	Oxalate	Gastrin
Hippuric acids	Phenols	Glucagon
Mandelic acids	Polyamines	Growth hormone
Phenylacetic acid	Carbonyl compounds	Luteinizing hormone
Phenyllactic acid	Advanced glycosylation end products	Leptin
Phenylpyruvic acid	Peptides, bound amino acids, middle molecules	Parathyroid hormone
Aliphatic amines	Urea	Prolactin
Aromatic amines	Proteins	Cytokines, inflammatory mediators
Cyanate	Bence Jones proteins	Tumor necrosis factor-α
	β_2-Glycoprotein	Soluble tumor necrosis factor receptors
	β_2-Microglobulin	Interleukin-1
	Lysozyme	Interleukin-6
	Retinol-binding protein	Interleukin-1β
	Ribonuclease	Interleukin-1RA
	Insulinlike growth factor binding proteins—2, 4	C-reactive protein
		Serum amyloid A

[a] Although blood ammonia is generally not elevated in uremia, ammonia may be increased in the gastrointestinal tract and at mucosal sites.
RA, receptor antagonist.

end-products and "carbonyl stress" compounds are also discussed in Chapter 68, Parts 3 and 7.

UREA

Urea is the most abundant nitrogenous end-product of protein metabolism. Urea accounts for approximately 80% of the urinary nitrogen excreted in clinically stable renal failure patients who ingest 40 g protein/day, and at least 90% of urinary nitrogen when such patients ingest at least 60 g protein/day. In normal individuals, approximately 10% to 15% of the urea synthesized each day is degraded in the gastrointestinal (GI) tract to ammonia and carbon dioxide. Urea is hydrolyzed in the GI tract by bacterial ureases; in renal failure, bacterial urease activity in the gut is increased.

Although it was formerly believed that degradation of urea in the gut was increased in renal failure, a number of studies have provided evidence to the contrary. Most of the ammonia released in the GI tract from the hydrolysis of urea is reabsorbed where it is reincorporated into urea in the liver; a small proportion of this ammonia may combine, often by transamination, with precursor compounds to form amino acids. It appears that a relatively small amount of the ammonia derived from urea hydrolysis in the gut is used for *de novo* synthesis of amino acids in either normal or uremic subjects. Urea therefore does not seem to be an important nutritional source of nitrogen for amino acid and protein synthesis in renal failure. Because the ammonia released from urea degradation in the gut is largely reconverted to urea in the liver, the enterohepatic recycling of urea seems to have little influence on the body economy of urea. In the nonedematous uremic patient, the volume of distribution of urea, which approximates 60% of the body mass, is similar to that of normal individuals.

Animal and human studies provide evidence for and against the toxicity of urea. Many of these studies were of short duration, and methods for assessing adverse effects were often crude. Also, the oral administration of urea to normal subjects or animals may have caused an osmotic diuresis (polyuria) or local irritation of the GI tract with some of the resulting symptoms interpreted as being caused by uremic toxicity. These factors may have led to the varying conclusions drawn concerning the toxicity of urea.

Some investigators added urea to dialysate in order to prevent changes in the serum urea levels of patients undergoing hemodialysis. Despite the addition of urea to dialysate, the researcher noted an excellent clinical response to hemodialysis. Elasmobranchii fish, which include sharks, may have blood urea concentrations of 2,000 mg/dl, and these fish do not appear to be anorectic.

On the other hand, most studies seem to indicate that urea is a uremic toxin. The most impressive studies perhaps were those carried out in uremic patients in whom urea was added to dialysate for periods of 7 to 90 days. With high levels of serum urea, malaise, lethargy, pruritus, headache, vomiting, and bleeding tendencies were noted. The lowest levels of serum urea nitrogen (SUN) at which symptoms began to appear were 100 to 150 mg/dl. Urea has also been implicated as a cause of altered carbohydrate metabolism in uremia. Elevating the serum urea in normal or azotemic humans or dogs by administering urea orally, subcutaneously, or through dialysate causes glucose intolerance. *In vitro* studies indicate that urea nitrogen concentrations in excess of 370 mg/dl impair glucose uptake by rat diaphragm or human red cells. Creatinine seems to potentiate the inhibitory effects of urea on glucose uptake. However, not all investigators confirmed these observations.

Urea, in concentrations often higher than present in uremic patients, has been shown to inhibit *in vitro* a number of metabolic processes or enzyme activities. Urea may suppress protein synthesis in lymphocytes; increase cell membrane permeability to various compounds, some of which may be toxic; inhibit platelet aggregation; and decrease acetylcholine-stimulated relaxation of rabbit thoracic aorta rings *in vitro*. Elevated urea levels may increase the synthesis rate of guanidinosuccinic acid.

Studies in nondiabetic patients with far-advanced chronic renal failure (CRF) and glomerular filtration rates of 1 to 3 ml/minute who are fed very-low nitrogen diets suggest that when the SUN is maintained below 70 to 80 mg/dl, individuals usually maintain a good appetite with no nausea, vomiting, or diarrhea. However, they may have profound malaise, weakness, tremulousness, fasciculations, and twitching. These observations suggest that urea may be a cause of the GI symptoms of renal failure but may play a smaller role in the neurologic or other clinical manifestations of uremia.

Despite its rather mild toxicity, the urea concentration in serum is often considered to be a good marker for uremic toxicity. The net rate of urea generation (urea appearance) is considered to roughly reflect the rate of generation of toxic products of protein metabolism and, in clinically stable patients, may also be used to estimate the dietary protein intake (see Chapter 83, Part 2). In comparison with nondiabetic patients, individuals with diabetes mellitus often seem to develop frank uremic toxicity (i.e., nausea, vomiting, profound malaise) with somewhat lower SUN levels (e.g., 65 to 75 mg/dl). At present, one of the most common techniques for quantitating the dose of hemodialysis and peritoneal dialysis treatments is by calculating the daily or weekly clearance of urea adjusted for its volume of distribution in the patient (K_t/V) or, for hemodialysis, calculating the urea reduction ratio (URR), which is the product of 100 and the difference between the initial and final SUN during a hemodialysis treatment divided by the initial SUN. The rationale for the use of urea for these quantification procedures is based on the perception that the rate of urea generation and the body urea pool correlate with the generation rate and pool sizes of other organic uremic toxins.

In summary, although the role of urea in the pathogenesis of the uremic syndrome is not precisely known, the preponderance of evidence suggests that urea does have pathophysiologic effects. At the concentrations of urea that occur in patients with renal failure, urea does not appear to be a major toxin. Serum urea may roughly indicate the degree of uremic toxicity, and the urea nitrogen appearance may reflect the rate of generation of toxic products of protein metabolism.

CYANATE AND CARBAMYLATED COMPOUNDS

Urea spontaneously undergoes partial degradation in aqueous solutions to form ammonium, carbonate, and cyanate. Cyanate (CNO) has been considered another potential uremic toxin. CNO can react irreversibly with the end-aminoterminal groups of many proteins and amino acids. This reaction is called *carbamylation.* In individuals with advanced renal failure and high SUN levels, carbamylation of proteins and amino acids increases markedly. High concentrations of carbamylated proteins can inhibit activities of certain enzymes. Carbamylation of albumin may decrease its ability to form ligands as a carrier protein. Carbamylated low-density lipoprotein (LDL) may have a reduced plasma clearance and hence lead to increased serum LDL levels. Carbamylation may inhibit polymerization of actin and lead to alterations in the filament structure and shape of fiber cells in the lens of the eye. It has been proposed that carbamylation of leukocyte proteins may cause abnormal leukocyte function. A large proportion of the free amino acids in plasma of maintenance dialysis patients are carbamylated. Indeed, the techniques for measuring plasma amino acids normally do not measure the carbamylated ones. In individuals who have advanced renal failure with high SUN levels, the plasma free carbamylated–amino acid concentrations may be greater than the free noncarbamylated amino acids. Whether carbamylated amino acids have adverse effects is not yet certain.

The effects of urea and cyanate were examined in nephrectomized dogs undergoing peritoneal dialysis with solutions of normal composition, 1% urea, and 0.015% potassium isocyanate. The dogs undergoing dialysis with normal dialysate survived for an average of 14 days; those dialyzed against 1% urea survived an average of 7 days, and those who received dialysate containing isocyanate survived an average of 6 days. Dogs dialyzed with urea and isocyanate developed hypothermia, lethargy, anorexia, diarrhea, and seizures. There is little information concerning the potential toxicity of isocyanate in patients with renal failure.

GUANIDINES

Next to urea, guanidino compounds are the most abundant group of nitrogenous products of protein metabolism. Guanidino compounds include guanidine, methylguanidine, dimethylguanidine, creatinine, creatine, guanidinoacetic acid, guanidinosuccinic acid, guanidino-proprionic acid, and 1,3-diphenylguanidine. There is a striking similarity between the structure of urea and the guanidino nucleus, which is indicated in Fig. 68.51. Like urea, at least some of the guanidines are derived from the urea cycle.

Guanidines are among the more likely candidates for uremic toxins. Many guanidino compounds inhibit a large variety of enzymes and interfere with a number of biochemical and physiologic processes. However, with few exceptions, these effects of guanidino compounds have only been shown to occur at concentrations greater than have been observed in sera of uremic patients.

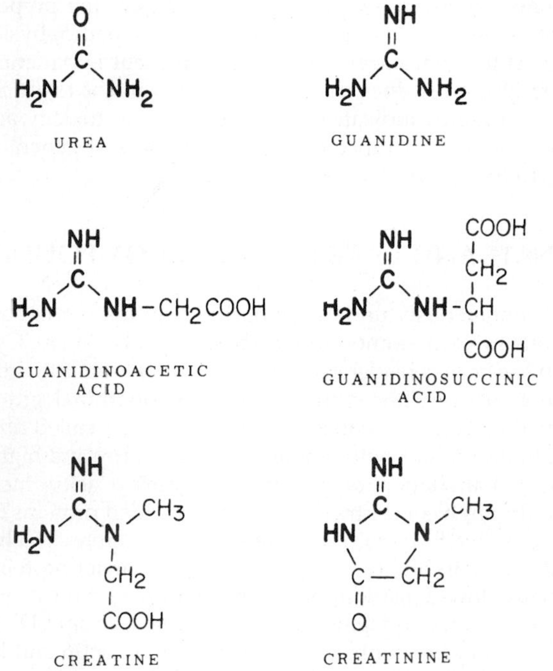

Figure 68.51. The chemical structure of urea and some guanidine compounds. The guanidino nucleus in the guanidine compound is indicated by heavier type.

Guanidine

Guanidine can inhibit mitochondrial respiration by uncoupling oxidative phosphorylation; can decrease oxygen consumption in rat brain, liver, and kidney; and can increase glucose uptake by rat diaphragm, glucose use by human red cells, and autohemolysis of normal blood *in vitro*. Experimental guanidine intoxication in animals may cause elevated blood pressure and a number of neuromuscular and GI effects. Administration of guanidine to animals can produce salivation, vomiting, diarrhea, incoordination, muscle tremors, twitching, spasms, convulsions, apathy, coma, and death.

Creatinine and Creatine

Urinary creatinine excretion is reduced in individuals with CRF when their serum creatinine level is increased to approximately 6 to 7 mg/dl or greater. This may be due to several factors: The degradation of creatinine is increased in patients with renal failure. Such patients may degrade up to 72% of the creatinine produced each day, presumably in the gut. Creatinine is degraded in uremic patients to methylamine, sarcosine, methylhydantoin, and CO_2. Also, in uremia, creatinine can be reconverted to creatine. A substantial amount of urinary creatinine is derived from the creatine and creatinine present in ingested skeletal muscle. Also, reduced dietary intake of meat (skeletal muscle) and a reduction in skeletal muscle mass may each decrease urinary creatinine excretion in individuals with CRF.

Creatinine is considered to be rather nontoxic, and administration of large quantities of creatinine to animals or healthy human subjects is well tolerated. However, some studies indicate that large quantities of creatinine may enhance hemolysis, decrease platelet adherence, inhibit oxygen uptake by brain slices, or impair glucose tolerance. Creatinine at concentrations similar to those found in uremic plasma were reported to suppress erythrocyte proliferation and maturation. This was not confirmed in another study.

Creatine is the metabolic precursor of creatinine and is primarily located intracellularly. In uremia, creatine is increased in plasma and cerebrospinal fluid. Although serum creatine is increased in renal failure, it is unclear whether creatine is elevated intracellularly in uremia. Creatine is formed in the liver from guanidinoacetic acid, which is also elevated in uremic sera. In acutely uremic rats, creatine production appears to be reduced or creatine metabolism increased. However, in patients with renal insufficiency, urinary creatine is normal, which suggests that creatine production may not be reduced in uremic patients. Creatine may increase autohemolysis *in vitro* and inhibit glucose oxidation in brain slices, but this occurs at concentrations higher than are found in uremia. Normal individuals have eaten up to 20 g of creatine/day for about 5 days without ill effects. Blood phosphocreatine is also reported to be increased in renal failure.

Guanidinoacetic Acid

Guanidinoacetic acid is elevated in sera and reduced in urine in renal failure. Thus either its production is reduced or its degradation is increased in uremia. Guanidinoacetic acid is formed from arginine and glycine. This reaction is catalyzed by the enzyme, transaminidase. Activity of this enzyme is inhibited by creatine, which is elevated in uremic sera, and possibly by guanidinoacetic acid itself. The kidney is a major site for transaminidase activity. Hence, it is possible that production of guanidinoacetic acid in uremia is decreased by two mechanisms: enzyme repression secondary to product inhibition and impairment of enzyme activity in the kidney due to parenchymal damage. Guanidinoacetic acid is reported to increase autohemolysis of red cells *in vitro* at concentrations greater than occur in uremia and may also have minor inhibitory effects on glucose uptake by diaphragm and glucose use by red cells.

Guanidinosuccinic Acid

This compound is increased in serum, cerebrospinal fluid, and urine of patients with renal failure. This suggests that production of guanidinosuccinic acid is increased in uremia. Guanidinosuccinic acid is poorly degradable, and it appears to be primarily removed by urinary excretion. Urine guanidinosuccinic acid excretion is directly correlated with dietary protein intake. Several theories have been proposed for the biosynthetic pathway of guanidinosuccinic acid. It has been suggested that canavaninosuccinic acid, which is synthesized from ingested canavanine by intestinal flora, may be converted to guanidinosuccinic acid in the liver. It appears more likely that guanidinosuccinic acid is a metabolic product of the urea cycle enzymes in the liver. A strong relationship between urea and guanidinosuccinic acid concentrations has led to the theory that urea is involved in the synthesis of the latter compound. Hence, elevated urea concentrations in CRF would enhance the rate of guanidinosuccinic acid synthesis. Newer studies suggest that guanidinosuccinic acid is formed by the transfer of the amidino group of arginine to aspartic acid. In renal failure, the decreased synthesis of guanidinoacetic acid from arginine and glycine may increase the availability of arginine for transamidation to aspartic acid.

Guanidinosuccinic acid is reported to inhibit ADP activation of platelet factor 3, ADP-induced transformation of platelet structure, and secondary irreversible platelet aggregation induced by ADP, L-epinephrine, and collagen, and to cause minor changes in platelet fine structure. These effects were observed at concentrations similar to those found in plasma of uremic patients. Thus guanidinosuccinic acid may be a cause of the bleeding defect in uremia. However, one investigator has been unable to confirm that elevated guanidinosuccinic acid alters platelet aggregation. Guanidinosuccinic acid is reported to suppress 1-alphahydroxylase activity in monocytes that were stimulated by inflammatory cytokines and to inhibit growth of cultured promyelocytic and erythroleukemia cell lines; creatinine and guanidinoproprionic acid (see following discussion) also suppressed growth of these latter cell lines. Guanidinosuccinic acid, at concentrations similar to those found in uremic sera, may inhibit the transformation of lymphocytes to lymphoblasts.

Methylguanidine

This compound is elevated in serum, in cerebrospinal fluid, intracellularly, and in urine of patients with CRF. Methylguanidine may accumulate in renal cells against a concentration gradient. Methylguanidine clearance may exceed that of creatinine, suggesting that there may be renal tubular secretion of methylguanidine. The finding that both serum and urinary methylguanidine are elevated in renal failure suggests that methylguanidine production may be increased in uremia. Methylguanidine is formed from creatinine, which undergoes oxidation when it is boiled. Hence, methylguanidine can be ingested in diets containing cooked foods that are high in creatinine, such as beef. Studies in germ-free rats and in rats treated with antibiotics suggest that gut bacteria probably do not participate in this reaction. Methylguanidine synthesis may also occur nonenzymatically.

Methylguanidine is synthesized from creatinine and arginine in hepatic microsomes and several other organs. The increased plasma concentration and urinary excretion of methylguanidine in renal failure may be due to increased synthesis caused by the elevated serum creatinine levels. Methylguanidine synthesis also appears to be related to protein intake; low protein or essential amino acid diets lower serum and urinary methylguanidine levels, possibly by reducing the degradation rate of arginine. The intermediary metabolite, 5-hydroxycreatinine, is produced during the synthesis of creatinine to methylguanidine. 5-hydroxycreatinine has been identified in urine of uremic patients and has been proposed to be a uremic toxin.

Although injection of methylguanidine into dogs caused a syndrome resembling uremic toxicity, this occurred at concentrations that far exceeded the plasma levels in uremic patients, which usually are less than 3 μmol/L. *In vitro* studies indicate that methylguanidine may enhance glucose use by rat diaphragm and human red cells; increase autohemolysis of human red cells (this has not been confirmed by others); inhibit red cell globin formation; impair pancreatic (Na^+-K^+)-ATPase, Mg^{2+}-ATPase, and Ca^{2+}-ATPase; inhibit DNA synthesis in lymphocytes and norepinephrine transport in synaptic vesicles of sympathetic nerves; impair serum activity of diamine oxidase; inhibit ^{59}Fe uptake in bone marrow cultures; impair glucose-6-phosphate dehydrogenase activity in normal red cells; suppress nitric oxide production in macrophages; and stimulate relaxation of contracted aortic rings. In most of these assay systems, higher concentrations of methylguanidine were used than are found in uremic sera. It has been suggested that methylguanidine may play a causal role in neuropathy of the sympathetic nervous system in renal failure.

Guanidinoproprionic Acid

This guanidino compound is also elevated in uremic serum and has been implicated as a cause of autohemolysis and depression of red cell glucose-6-phosphate dehydrogenase. In rats given guanidinoproprionic acid, atrophy of type II muscle fibers has been observed. In uremic patients, plasma guanidinoproprionic acid is reported to correlate inversely with the reduced red cell glutathione concentrations.

AROMATIC COMPOUNDS

Compounds containing a benzene, phenol, or indole ring have also been considered potential uremic toxins. These compounds are often metabolic products of the aromatic amino acids, phenylalanine, tyrosine, and tryptophan. Phenylalanine and tyrosine may be deaminated and oxidized to form phenolic or hydroxyphenolic acids or may be conjugated with glycine, glucuronic acid, or sulfate to form potentially less toxic phenol compounds. The aromatic amino acids may also be decarboxylated to form aromatic amines. Tryptophan is degraded primarily by two pathways in mammals. It is hydroxylated and decarboxylated to form serotonin, which may be metabolized to indolic compounds. Also, the ring structure of tryptophan may be oxidized to form kynurenine, which may be degraded further to form a number of other products that are normally excreted in the urine.

Phenolic and Hydroxyphenolic Acids

Normally, most phenolic and hydroxyphenolic acids, aromatic amines, and indoles are excreted in the urine and are present in plasma at very low levels. However, many of these compounds accumulate in plasma in uremia. At least 45 aromatic compounds have been identified in hemodialysate of uremic patients; in contrast, only 6 of these have been identified in dialysate collected from a woman with no evidence of renal disease. Evidence concerning the toxicity for the large number of free and conjugated phenolic and hydroxyphenolic acids in renal failure is less definite. Toxicity of phenolic compounds has been particularly related to symptoms of neurologic depression in uremia. Several investigators have reported a close association between the onset or severity of uremic symptoms, particularly those of neurologic depression, and the blood or cerebrospinal fluid phenol levels. Others, however, found no close correlation. The conjugated phenols are believed to be relatively nontoxic.

Many aromatic compounds identified in dialysate from uremic subjects inhibit oxygen consumption in guinea pig brain slices, anaerobic glycolysis in rat brain, and a variety of enzymes present in brain and kidney. Hydroxyphenylacetic acid and phenyllactic acid competitively inhibit rat red cell Na^+-K^+-ATPase. Reduced activity of this enzyme and elevated ATP levels in red cells also have been observed in uremic patients. Thus it is possible that toxic phenolic compounds could cause elevated red cell–sodium concentrations and altered red cell–sodium transport in uremia. However, as with many other studies concerning uremic toxins, the concentrations of these compounds that cause physiologic alterations or enzyme inhibition were often far greater than those found in uremic plasma.

Hydroxyphenylacetic acid may prolong platelet factor 3-A time and inhibit secondary platelet aggregation. The concentrations of the phenolic acids that inhibit platelet factor 3-A time are similar to the levels that have been observed in uremic plasma.

Aromatic Amines

Total, free, and conjugated aromatic amines are increased in uremic plasma and decrease with dialysis. Among these is tyramine, which is elevated in plasma and cerebrospinal fluid of uremic patients. High concentrations of a number of aromatic amines inhibit oxidative reactions in brain and certain enzyme systems. However, these effects were only noted at concentrations much greater than are found in uremic plasma.

Indoles

A side chain of tryptophan may be oxidized by bacteria in the colon to form a number of products including tryptamine, indoleacetic acid, skatole, skatoxyl, indole, and indoxyl. Mammalian tissues also may convert tryptophan to tryptamine and indoleacetic acid. When formed in the colon, some of these compounds may be absorbed, conjugated with sulfate or glucuronic acid in the liver, and excreted in the urine. Indoxyl, formed in the colon, may be absorbed and esterified in the liver with sulfate to form indoxylsulfate and then excreted in the urine as the potassium salt, indican. Achlorhydria, liver disease, intestinal obstruction, and paralytic ileus may increase serum or urinary indican. Urinary indican excretion is increased with higher protein intakes and decreased with fasting; this may have relevance for the treatment of kidney failure. Broad-spectrum antibiotics may decrease indoleacetic acid excretion, probably by decreasing activity of GI bacteria.

Serum indican correlates with serum creatinine and urea levels, and serum indoleacetic acid correlates with serum urea. Other indolic compounds increased in plasma of uremic patients include indoxyl phosphate, indoxyl sulfate (see Chapter 68, Part 5), 5-hydroxyindoleacetic acid, 5-hydroxytryptophan, and 6-hydroxyskatole; these compounds decrease during dialysis. A number of other indolic compounds have also been described in dialysate from patients with acute or chronic renal failure. 5-Hydroxyindoleacetic acid is reported to be increased and serotonin is reported to be normal in the brain of chronically azotemic rats. Platelet serotonin is decreased in chronically uremic patients. Increased levels of indoles inhibit insulinase and also oxidation in brain slices. Indoxyl may inhibit transport of thyroxin by hepatocytes. Rats with CRF given indoxyl sulfate manifested increased gene expression of transforming growth factor-β1 (TGF-β1), tissue inhibitor of metalloproteinases (TIMP-1), and pro-α1 (I) collagen in their kidneys; increased glomerulosclerosis; and more rapid loss of renal function (see Chapter 68, Part 5). Kynurenate and 3-carboxyanthralinic acid inhibit phosphoenolpyruvate carboxykinase, thereby suppressing the Embden-Meyerhof pathway.

ALIPHATIC AMINES

Chemical measurements for the general class of aliphatic amines have demonstrated increased concentrations in sera, spinal fluid, and GI fluid of patients with acute and chronic renal failure. Serum concentrations of methylamine, dimethylamine, trimethylamine, ethanolamine, pyrrolidine, piperidine, and choline are elevated in renal failure. Methylamine, dimethylamine, ethanolamine, propylamine, isobutylamine, and butylamine are increased in gastric juice of patients with acute renal failure. Dimethylamine and trimethylamine are probably present intracellularly as well. Aliphatic amines are synthesized by bacteria in the gut. Monomethylamine is formed from sarcosine, creatinine, and homomethylguanidine. Trimethylamine is synthesized from lecithin and choline. Dimethylamine may be formed from trimethylamine and also monomethylamine. Protein intake increases production of piperidine, but appears to have little effect on dimethylamine or methylamine. Suppression of bacterial growth in the gut decreases serum concentrations of dimethylamine and trimethylamine and may decrease asterixis and myoclonus and increase alertness. Elevated serum choline levels in uremia may reflect decreased degradation of choline by the diseased kidney.

Certain aliphatic amines may reduce oxygen consumption by brain slices or red cells, increase hemolysis, or inhibit succinate oxidation and glutamic acid decarboxylase. As with many other putative toxins, these effects occur at amine concentrations far higher than are found in uremia. However, serum dimethylamine and trimethylamine concentrations are reported to correlate with choice reaction time, and the latter compound also correlates with the electroencephalographic changes. Dimethylamine has been found in the breath of uremic patients and causes a fishy odor. We have found increased activity of the enzyme, monoamine oxidase, in platelets, and of diamine oxidase in the platelet-free fraction of plasma of uremic patients.

POLYAMINES

The polyamines, putrescine, spermidine, and spermine, are compounds that appear to have many biologic actions. Polyamines appear to play a role in ribonucleic acid (RNA) and DNA synthesis and tissue growth. Putrescine is formed from the decarboxylation of the urea cycle amino acid, ornithine. Putrescine is converted to spermidine and then spermine; both of these biochemical reactions involve S-adenosylmethionine. Urinary excretion of putrescine, spermidine, and spermine are reduced in patients with renal failure. Plasma putrescine, spermidine, spermine, and cadaverine concentrations are increased in uremic patients and tend to fall with a hemodialysis treatment. Red cell spermidine concentrations are also increased.

Spermine, in concentrations similar to those observed in uremic plasma, has been shown to decrease red cell colony formation (CFU-E) *in vitro*. Uremic sera has the same effect, but when antispermine antibodies are added to uremic sera to remove spermine concentrations, the inhibitory effect of uremic sera on CFU-E disappears. These findings suggest that spermine may, by suppressing erythropoiesis, be a cause of the anemia of uremia and of resistance to erythropoietin. It has been hypothesized that due to their growth-stimulating actions, increased polyamine concentrations may stimulate proliferation of arterial smooth muscle cells and thereby promote cardiovascular and cerebrovascular disease.

AMMONIA

There is net synthesis of ammonia by the kidney that forms ammonium from amino groups derived from glutamine and other amino acids. Although ammonia is excreted in the urine, the kidney serves as a source of blood ammonia. In renal failure, the generation of ammonia by the kidney decreases. Hence, blood ammonia levels are generally not increased in uremic patients.

On the other hand, the ammonia concentrations in the GI tract are proportional to the SUN levels and are increased in renal failure. Urea, which undergoes hydrolysis by GI bacteria, is the major source of gut ammonia. Because urea turnover in the uremic patient appears to be normal or at most only slightly increased, it is unclear why GI ammonia concentrations are increased in renal failure. Ammonia excretion in the feces is also elevated in renal failure. Ammonia is cleared efficiently by hemodialysis.

Increased gastric ammonia concentrations may cause gastric hypoacidity. It has been suggested that markedly increased GI ammonia concentrations, such as occurs in severe uremia, can cause stomatitis, gastritis, and ulcerative enteritis and colitis.

NUCLEIC ACID DERIVATIVES

Uric Acid

The kidney normally excretes into the urine about two-thirds of the uric acid produced daily in the body. The major nonrenal route for elimination of uric acid is the GI tract, where bacteria metabolizes uric acid to allantoin, allantoic acid, carbon dioxide, and ammonia. Individuals with CRF have increased plasma concentrations of uric acid and also of inosine, xanthine, and hypoxanthine. In patients with hyperuricemia and CRF, the fractional renal excretion of uric acid may increase. In addition, the extrarenal elimination of uric acid, presumably in the GI tract, rises. Formation of uric acid is usually normal in renal failure but may decrease when severe uremia is present. This may be due to reduced purine intake by the sick patient or altered nucleic acid or purine metabolism.

Toxicity studies have generally failed to demonstrate a toxic effect of uric acid in uremia. Hyperuricemia is very common in patients with advanced renal failure and in those undergoing maintenance dialysis, but episodes of gouty arthritis or formation of uric acid tophi are uncommon. Renal failure patients with uremic pericarditis have higher serum uric acid levels than those without pericarditis. It has been suggested that hyperuricemia may accelerate the progression of renal failure in patients with chronic kidney disease. Uric acid and theophylline decrease calcitriol synthesis in rats and inhibit receptor binding affinity for DNA. Allopurinol treatment, which decreases plasma uric acid levels, is associated with increased calcitriol concentrations. Thus elevated plasma urate may play a role in uremic osteodystrophy. Hyperuricemia has been associated with hypertension, hypertriglyceridemia, and atherosclerotic vascular disease. Whether hyperuricemia contributes to these disorders in renal failure is not established.

Cyclic Adenosine Monophosphate

Cyclic adenosine monophosphate (cAMP) is a mediator through which a number of hormones exert their actions. Plasma cAMP is elevated in uremia and correlates with plasma creatinine levels. Elevated plasma cAMP in renal failure may reflect both impaired urinary excretion and increased production secondary to elevated hormone levels. cAMP is a relatively small molecule, and plasma concentrations fall during hemodialysis. cAMP inhibits platelet aggregation *in vitro*.

Other Compounds

Pseudouridine, 4-amino-5-imidazole carboxamide, 1-methylhypoxanthine, and a number of pyridine derivatives have been identified in increased quantities in hemodialysate or blood from patients with acute or chronic renal failure. Plasma concentrations of at least some of these compounds decrease during hemodialysis. *N*-methyl-2-pyridone-5-carboxylic acid and *N*-methyl-2-pyridine-5-formamidoacetic acid are reported to inhibit protein synthesis in liver homogenates.

OXALIC ACID

Plasma oxalic acid concentrations are elevated in uremia and correlate with plasma urea nitrogen. Hemodialysis decreases plasma oxalate. Whole blood oxalate levels exceed those in plasma, which suggests that red cell oxalate concentrations exceed those in plasma. Oxalic acid is normally absorbed to a small degree from the intestinal tract and may also be formed *in vitro*. The two main pathways for oxalate synthesis are from ascorbic acid and from glyoxylate, which is a metabolic product of glycine or glycolate. Normally, oxalate is excreted in the urine, and it is possible that impaired urinary clearance may be the cause of increased plasma and tissue levels. Plasma oxalate appears to correlate directly with plasma ascorbic acid levels and ascorbic acid intake. Patients with renal failure who ingest moderate or large quantities of ascorbic acid (e.g., 500 mg/day or greater) also may increase their plasma oxalate concentrations. Hence, only the Recommended Dietary Allowance for vitamin C, 60 mg/day, is recommended as an ascorbic acid supplement for renal failure patients. Treatment with large doses of pyridoxine HCl is reported to lower plasma oxalate levels in some maintenance hemodialysis patients.

Because oxalate is very insoluble, there is concern that high concentrations of plasma oxalate may cause calcium oxalate precipitation in soft tissues and urinary calcium oxalate calculi. Calcium oxalate crystals have been found in kidneys and myocardium of patients dying with kidney failure; congestive heart failure caused by calcium oxalate deposition in the myocardium has been reported in maintenance dialysis patients. Oxalic acid inhibits activity of lactic acid dehydrogenase *in vitro*, but it is not known whether it does this *in vivo* in uremia.

CARNITINE

Carnitine, a quaternary amine, plays an essential role for the transfer of long- and some medium-chain fatty acids into the mitochondria for β-oxidation. Carnitine is synthesized in humans in the liver, kidney, and brain from two essential amino acids, lysine and methionine. Four micronutrients are required for its enzymatic synthesis: vitamin C, niacin, vitamin B_6, and iron. In patients undergoing maintenance hemodialysis or peritoneal dialysis, plasma free carnitine is reduced, whereas both short-chain and long-chain acylcarnitine (fatty acid–carnitine compounds) are increased. In patients with mild-to-moderate renal insufficiency, (i.e., glomerular filtration rate approximately 35 ml/min/1.73 m^2), plasma-free carnitine is usually normal or modestly increased. Red blood cell carnitine is normal, and skeletal muscle carnitine is normal or low and acylcarnitine increased in hemodialysis patients. Although reduced free carnitine was considered to be due to losses from dialysis, the weekly removal of free carnitine by hemodialysis is similar to the amount of carnitine excreted in normal urine. The low concentrations of plasma free carnitine in hemodialysis patients are considered to be largely due to impaired renal synthesis and reduced intake of carnitine, its amino acid precursors, or the cofactors necessary for enzymatic synthesis. It is speculated that the elevated plasma acylcarnitines may reflect impaired excretion or catabolism by the kidney. The possible clinical benefits of treating CRF patients with L-carnitine are discussed in Chapter 83, Part 2.

MIDDLE MOLECULES, PEPTIDES, AND BOUND AMINO ACIDS

It has been known for many years that a number of oligopeptides and polypeptides are excreted in the urine of normal individuals. These compounds can be observed as chromatographic peaks after column separation. Similar chromatographic peaks can be obtained in plasma of patients with renal failure and in dialysate from patients undergoing hemodialysis or peritoneal dialysis. Glycine and glutamic and aspartic acid residues are particularly abundant in many of these bound amino acids and peptides in the urine of healthy subjects and in plasma and dialysate of uremic patients. These observations suggest that some of these compounds are retained in renal failure at least partly because of impaired urinary excretion.

In the early 1970s, it was noted that patients undergoing long-term intermittent peritoneal dialysis appeared to do well clinically and did not develop neuropathy even though they had a relatively low clearance of small-sized molecules. On the other hand, with peritoneal dialysis the weekly clearance of peptides and small proteins is similar to or greater than that with hemodialysis. Moreover, it has long been recognized that there is a poor correlation between uremic toxicity and serum concentrations of urea, creatinine, and other smaller molecules (i.e., compounds with a molecular weight less than 200 D). Finally, animal and *in vitro* studies with these small compounds do not provide clear evidence that these compounds are highly toxic. These observations gave rise to the concept of toxicity of "middle molecules," which are considered to be compounds of molecular weight varying between 200 and 3,000 D, probably most commonly between 500 and 2,000 D. Middle molecules are reported to increase measurably in plasma when the creatinine clearance falls to less than 11 ml/minute.

This theory engendered a large number of research studies designed to identify those molecules and to demonstrate their role in uremic toxicity. Studies were conducted in which dialysis regimens were varied so that hemodialyzers with large pore sizes, which would clear greater quantities of middle molecules, were compared with dialyzers with small pore sizes, which were highly efficient at removing smaller molecules. Patients underwent dialysis with one or the other of these dialyzers and with dialysis treatments of different durations. The patients' clinical response was used to judge the potential toxicity of these middle-sized molecules. In some studies, patients underwent longer dialysis treatments that were designed to remove greater quantities of middle molecules without changing the predialysis values of urea and creatinine. Although some studies were interpreted to confirm a toxic effect of middle molecules, others did not demonstrate this.

Despite the large number of studies carried out, there is still relatively little known about the clinical significance of middle molecules. A number of studies indicate toxic effects of middle molecules. However, no uremic symptom or adverse event has been unequivocally related to the accumulation of a specific middle molecule. Plasma concentrations of certain chromatographic peaks in the middle-molecule range were reported to be greater in "sick" uremic patients as compared with those patients who are less symptomatic, although there is considerable overlap. Reversal of neuropathy has been attributed to removal of a greater quantity of middle molecules either by treatment with longer dialysis or with dialyzers that were more permeable to compounds of middle-molecular size. Toxic effects of middle-molecule fractions obtained from plasma, urine, or dialysate have also been described. Injecting mice with middle-molecule fractions that are estimated to give blood levels comparable with those of uremic patients are reported to decrease hemoglobin concentrations and lower the incorporation of ^{59}Fe into red cells. Middle molecules may also increase osmotic fragility of red cells. Hence, middle molecules may be among the uremic toxins responsible for anemia.

Middle molecules have been reported to inhibit lymphoblastic transformation and erythrocyte rosette formation. Middle-molecule fractions injected into rats delayed rejection of skin allografts and inhibited the graft-versus-host rejection. Middle molecules may inhibit migration of leukocytes. These observations suggest that middle molecules might play a role in inhibiting cell-mediated immunity and other aspects of the immune system.

Middle molecules are also reported to inhibit *in vitro* glucose utilization, proliferation of fibroblasts, phagocytic activity of leukocytes, proliferation of stem cells, formation of granulocyte colonies, and aggregation of platelets. These compounds are alleged to cause uncoupling of oxidative phosphorylation in mitochondria and may inhibit activity of a number of enzymes including lactic acid dehydrogenase, adenylate cyclase, (Na^+-K^+)-ATPase, and lipoprotein lipase. In summary, despite the extensive number of studies with middle molecules, the role of these compounds in the genesis of uremic toxicity is still not well defined.

PEPTIDE HORMONES

Plasma concentrations of many hormones are elevated in patients with advanced CRF, as indicated in Table 68.6. The elevated hormones are usually peptides. The increased plasma concentrations of these hormones are due in part to impaired degradation by the diseased kidney. In addition, for some hormones, such as parathyroid hormone and probably insulin, secretion is increased. The metabolic and clinical effects of the elevated parathyroid hormone concentrations on the renal failure patient have been extensively studied (see Chapter 68, Part 1).

CYTOKINES AND INFLAMMATORY MEDIATORS

Plasma concentrations of a number of cytokines and mediators of inflammation are elevated in maintenance hemodialysis or chronic peritoneal dialysis patients and in individuals with chronic renal insufficiency. Elevated plasma concentrations have been observed for tumor necrosis factor-α (TNF-α), soluble TNF receptors, interleukin-1 (IL-1), IL-1β, IL-6, IL-1 receptor antagonist (RA), and soluble markers of the activation of T cells, B cells, and monocytes (sCD25, sCD23, and neopterin). It has been suggested that these increased plasma levels may be due to enhanced production stimulated by intercurrent illnesses, bioincompatible membranes, endotoxin-contaminated dialysate, dialysis tubing, or arteriovenous grafts. Indeed some of these proteins increase further during the course of a hemodialysis treatment. Blood monocytes obtained from maintenance dialysis patients and stimulated *in vitro* by phytohemagglutinin, lipopolysaccharide, or tuberculin purified protein derivative (PPD) secrete increased quantities of TNF-α, IL-1β, IL-8, and IL-10 as compared with blood monocytes from normal controls. The cause for the increased levels of these cytokines has not yet been clearly defined.

There is epidemiologic evidence that increased levels of these cytokines may exert antianabolic effects. In a report in chronic peritoneal dialysis patients, high plasma TNF-α has been associated with anorexia and lower serum concentrations of retinol-binding protein, transferrin, cholesterol, urea, and cholecystokinin. TNF-α increases protein catabolism. In this regard, the dietary protein requirement of maintenance hemodialysis and chronic peritoneal dialysis patients is greater than that of normal adults, and the increment in the dietary protein requirement cannot be entirely accounted for by the increased protein, peptide, and amino acid losses in hemo- or peritoneal dialysate.

In another study of maintenance hemodialysis patients, elevated predialysis serum IL-6 levels were associated with lower serum albumin, serum cholinesterase, and midarm muscle area, and decreases in body weight. These epidemiologic studies are consistent with a causal role for inflammation in the protein-energy malnutrition, morbidity, and mortality of maintenance dialysis patients. However, the data are also consistent with other possibilities. For example, some of the effects of inflammation on morbidity and mortality may be mediated through the malnutrition engendered by inflammatory cytokines. Alternatively, malnutrition may predispose to an inflammatory state. Also, it is possible that elevated plasma cytokines, malnutrition, and clinical outcome may be independently caused by one or more other common factors. Serum TNF-α and IL-6 do not decrease during the course of a hemodialysis treatment. On the other hand, serum concentrations of soluble TNF receptors seem to increase and IL-1RA seems to decrease with the hemodialysis procedure.

ACUTE-PHASE REACTANTS

The increase in inflammation-related cytokines (e.g., interleukin) causes increased production of acute-phase reactants, including C-reactive protein and serum amyloid A protein but also fibrinogen, ceruloplasmin, plasminogen activator inhibitor-I, and ferritin. Increased serum levels of C-reactive protein in uremic and dialysis patients are associated with low serum albumin concentrations and increased mortality and greater risk of cardiovascular disease.

Selected Readings

Brunner H, Mann H. What remains of the "middle molecule" hypothesis today? *Contrib Nephrol* 1985;44:14–39.

An excellent overview of the development of the middle molecule concept.

Descamps-Latscha B, Herbelin A, Nguyen AT, et al. Balance between IL-1β, TNF-α, and their specific inhibitors in chronic renal failure and maintenance dialysis. *J Immunol* 1995;154:882–892.

This paper describes the plasma levels of certain inflammatory cytokines and soluble cytokine receptors in patients with chronic renal failure and individuals undergoing maintenance hemodialysis or chronic peritoneal dialysis.

Kaizu Y, Kimura M, Yoneyama T, et al. Interleukin-6 may mediate malnutrition in chronic hemodialysis patients. *Am J Kidney Dis* 1998;31:93–100.

This paper shows a relationship between serum interleukin-6 concentrations and measures of nutritional status in patients undergoing maintenance hemodialysis.

Kaysen GA. Inflammation, nutritional state and outcome in end stage renal disease. *Miner Electrolyte Metab* 1999;25:242–250.

This paper describes epidemiologic interactions between markers of inflammation and measures of nutritional status in patients with chronic renal failure.

Miyata T, Oda O, Inagi R, et al. β_2-Microglobulin modified with advanced glycation end-products is a major component of hemodialysis-associated amyloidosis. *J Clin Invest* 1993;92:1243–1252.

A study indicating that advanced glycation end-products of β_2-microglobulin are a cause of hemodialysis-associated amyloidosis.

Miyazaki T, Ise M, Seo H, et al. Indoxyl sulfate increases the gene expressions of TGF-β1, TIMP-1 and pro-α1(I) collagen in uremic rat kidneys. *Kidney Int* 1997;62:S15–S22.

This paper provides evidence that indoxyl sulfate may promote progressive renal injury by stimulating gene expression of certain growth factors in the kidney.

PART 5
Indoxyl Sulfate

Toshimitsu Niwa

METABOLISM

Indoxyl sulfate (indican, 213 D) is synthesized in the liver from indole absorbed from the intestines (Fig. 68.52). Indole is produced in the large intestines from dietary protein–derived tryptophan by intestinal bacteria such as *Escherichia coli*. Indoxyl sulfate is normally excreted into the urine at an amount of approximately 60 mg/day primarily by proximal tubular secretion through the organic anion secretory pathway, and partly by glomerular filtration. However, indoxyl sulfate markedly accumulates in uremic serum due to its reduced renal clearance. The serum levels of indoxyl sulfate are markedly increased in undialyzed patients with chronic renal failure (CRF) (1.8 ± 1.5 mg/dl, mean ± SE), and in uremic patients on hemodialysis (prehemodialysis 5.3 ± 2.1 mg/dl, posthemodialysis 3.5 ± 1.1 mg/dl) as compared with normal subjects (0.064 ± 0.086 mg/dl). Indoxyl sulfate cannot be efficiently removed from blood by hemodialysis as compared with creatinine and urea, because approximately 90% of indoxyl sulfate is bound to serum albumin.

An oral sorbent (AST-120; Kremezin, Kureha-Chemical Co., Tokyo) absorbs indole, and the other indolic and phenolic metabolites in the intestines, and stimulates their excretion into feces, thus suppressing indole absorption from the intestines (Fig. 68.52). Consequently, the oral sorbent reduces the production of indoxyl sulfate in the liver accompanied by a reduction in the serum and urine levels of indoxyl sulfate. Oral administration of antibiotic-resistant lactic acid bacteria to uremic patients also reduces the serum levels of indoxyl sulfate by decreasing bacterial production of indole through balancing the disturbed composition of intestinal microflora.

The derivative of indoxyl sulfate, indoxyl-β-D-glucuronide, an emitter of chemiluminescence, is also accumulated in uremic serum due to its reduced renal clearance and increased production. High serum level of indoxyl sulfate may stimulate the glucuronide conjugation pathway of indole for the synthesis of indoxyl-β-D-glucuronide. The ratio of serum indoxyl-β-D-glucuronide to serum indoxyl sulfate gradually increases as the

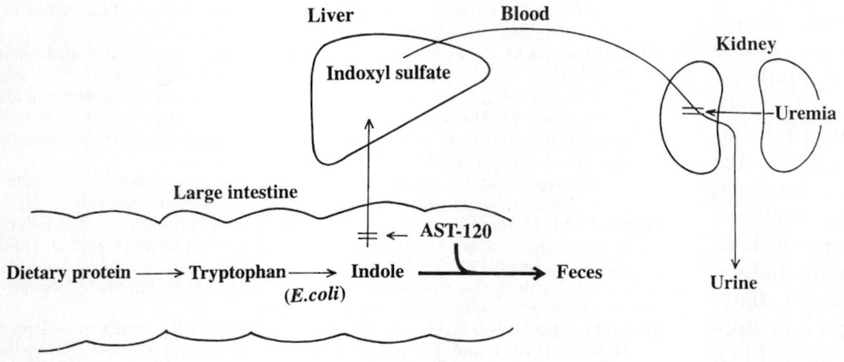

Figure 68.52. Metabolic pathway for the production of indoxyl sulfate and the suppressive effect of an oral sorbent (AST-120) on its production.

duration of hemodialysis treatment increases. AST-120 administration decreases the serum and urine levels of indoxyl-β-D-glucuronide as well as indoxyl sulfate. Although the protein binding of indoxyl-β-D-glucuronide is as high as approximately 50%, it can be efficiently removed by hemodialysis in contrast to markedly less dialyzable indoxyl sulfate, suggesting that the binding affinity of indoxyl-β-D-glucuronide to serum albumin is weak. Thus the glucuronide conjugation of indole is favorable for uremic patients to eliminate the indole metabolites from blood by hemodialysis.

The other indolic metabolites such as indole acetic acid, 5-hydroxyindoleacetic acid, 5-hydroxytryptophol, and *N*-acetyltryptophan are also accumulated in uremic serum not only in free but also protein-bound form. However, because the serum levels of these indolic metabolites including indoxyl-β-D-glucuronide in uremic patients are less than one-tenth of that of indoxyl sulfate, indoxyl sulfate is the most important uremic toxin among the indole metabolites.

UREMIC TOXICITY

The uremic toxicity of indoxyl sulfate includes (a) stimulation of CRF progression, (b) inhibition of drug binding to serum albumin, and (c) inhibition of thyroxine–hepatocyte transport.

Uremia is associated with defective protein binding of tryptophan and weakly acidic drugs (e.g., phenytoin, salicylate, penicillins, cephalosporins, sulfonamides, barbiturates, furosemide, clofibrate, and warfarin), whereas the protein binding of basic drugs, except certain basic drugs (diazepam and triamterene), is normal. The defective protein binding of drugs is due to the accumulation of drug-binding inhibitors that compete for binding sites on serum albumin; the blood levels of these inhibitors rise as a result of their reduced renal excretion. Thus far, the major inhibitors of drug binding are identified as 3-carboxy-4-methyl-5-propyl-2-furanpropionic acid, indoxyl sulfate, and hippuric acid. Indoxyl sulfate is demonstrated to inhibit the albumin binding of drugs such as diazepam, warfarin, methylred, methylorange, 2-(4′-hydroxybenzeneazo)benzoic acid, L-tryptophan, furosemide, salicylic acid, and ketoprofen. Indoxyl sulfate and hippuric acid bind to site 2 of serum albumin, whereas 3-carboxy-4-methyl-5-propyl-2-furanpropionic acid binds to site 1. The compound 3-carboxy-4-methyl-5-propyl-2-furanpropionic acid shows the strongest binding affinity for serum albumin, followed by indoxyl sulfate, and then by hippuric acid.

Uremic patients sometimes show thyroid abnormalities most commonly characterized by a reduction in the serum levels of total and free triiodothyronine (T_3). The low T_3 is a result of impaired peripheral conversion of T_4 to T_3, whereas the degradation rate of T_3 is normal. Indoxyl sulfate and 3-carboxy-4-methyl-5-propyl-2-furanpropionic acid at concentrations present in uremic patients inhibit cellular transport and subsequent deiodination of T_4 in rat hepatocytes. Thus these substances may account for the low T_3 levels in uremic patients.

Indoxyl Sulfate Stimulates the Progression of Chronic Renal Failure

Indoxyl sulfate is a stimulating factor for the progression of CRF because oral administration of indoxyl sulfate or its precursor, indole, stimulated the progression of CRF in 5/6-nephrectomized uremic rats. Oral administration of indoxyl sulfate for 6 weeks increased the serum levels of creatinine and urea nitrogen and glomerular sclerosis index, and decreased renal clearances of creatinine, inulin, and *p*-aminohippurate in 5/6-nephrectomized uremic rats. In the indoxyl sulfate–administered uremic rat, a global collapse of the glomerular capillaries, a hyaline material, and mesangial expansion were found, and the renal tubules were dilated with casts.

Tubulointerstitial injury is of equal or greater importance than glomerular sclerosis in determining whether progressive renal dysfunction will ensue in various renal diseases. Thus the expressions of genes related to tubulointerstitial fibrosis such as transforming growth factor-β1 (TGF-β1), tissue inhibitor of metalloproteinase-1 (TIMP-1), and pro-α1 (I) collagen were examined in the renal cortex of 5/6-nephrectomized uremic rats given indoxyl sulfate. The administration of indoxyl sulfate for 5 weeks significantly upregulated the mRNA levels of TGF-β1, TIMP-1, and pro-α1 (I) collagen in the uremic rats given indoxyl sulfate compared with the control uremic rats; these changes were accompanied by a significant decline in renal function, and worsening of glomerular sclerosis. Furthermore, the administration of indoxyl sulfate for 2.5 weeks also upregulated the expression of these mRNA levels even when no significant decline in the renal function was observed (Fig. 68.53). Thus the overload of the protein metabolite indoxyl sulfate on remnant nephrons increased bioactivity of TGF-β1 in uremic kidneys, which enhanced the renal expression of TIMP-1, and type 1 collagen, and consequently stimulated the progression of CRF. The mechanisms through which indoxyl sulphate stimulates TGF-β1 is not known. One possible mechanism is the direct effect of indoxyl sulfate on proximal tubular cells, because the addition of indoxyl sulfate in cultured proximal tubular cells increased the synthesis of TGF-β1 by the cells. Either way, the overload of indoxyl sulfate on the uremic kidneys increases the synthesis of TGF-β1 in the renal cortex.

A Low-Protein Diet Suppresses Indoxyl Sulfate Levels and the Progression of Chronic Renal Failure

A low-protein diet reduces the serum and urine levels of indoxyl sulfate in both uremic rats and undialyzed uremic patients. These findings suggest that a smaller portion of proteins or peptides reaches the large intestines under these circum-

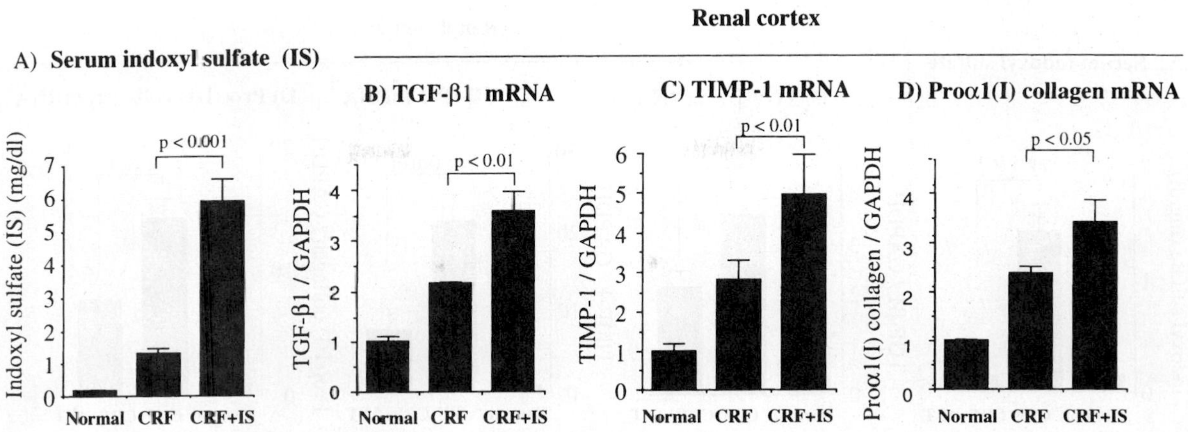

Figure 68.53. Effects of indoxyl sulfate administration for 2.5 weeks on the serum level of indoxyl sulfate **(A)**, and the mRNA levels of TGF-β1 **(B)**, TIMP-1 **(C)**, and pro-α1 (I) collagen **(D)** in the renal cortex. CRF: 5/6-nephrectomized uremic rats, CRF + IS: 5/6-nephrectomized uremic rats administered indoxyl sulfate. The administration of indoxyl sulfate significantly increased the serum level of indoxyl sulfate, and upregulated the gene expression of TGF-β1, TIMP-1, and pro-α1 (I) collagen in the renal cortex of the uremic rats.

stances, and a smaller amount of tryptophan is released *in situ* by their further digestion; it is then metabolized into indole by tryptophanase in intestinal bacteria. However, orally administered tryptophan was not metabolized to indole by intestinal bacteria because it was rapidly absorbed in the small intestines, and consequently did not reach the large intestines. On the other hand, the serum and urine levels of indoxyl sulfate increased by administering tryptophan directly into the large intestines of uremic rats, and thus indole can be produced from tryptophan by the intestinal bacteria in the large intestines. In contrast to tryptophan, oral administration of indole increased urinary excretion of indoxyl sulfate. The administered indole was absorbed from the intestines, and was then metabolized to indoxyl sulfate in the liver.

In our studies, the serum and urine levels of indoxyl sulfate were measured, and protein intake was calculated from urinary amounts of urea nitrogen using Maroni's equation in undialyzed uremic patients with creatinine clearance less than 30 ml/min. The uremic patients were classified into the following four groups according to dietary protein intake: (a) 0.25 to 0.50 g/kg per day, (b) 0.50 to 0.75 g/kg per day, (c) 0.75 to 1.00 g/kg per day, and (d) 1.00 to 1.25 g/kg per day, and the effects of low-protein diet on the urine and serum levels of indoxyl sulfate were studied. There were no significant differences in renal function (serum creatinine and creatinine clearance) among the four patient groups. Both serum levels and urinary excretion of indoxyl sulfate were significantly reduced as the protein intake decreased to less than 0.75 g/kg per day. Serum urea nitrogen and urine protein were also significantly reduced in the low-protein diet groups. Thus a low-protein diet reduced the serum and urine levels of indoxyl sulfate, which is a stimulating factor for the progression of CRF in undialyzed uremic patients.

A low-protein diet delays the progression of renal disease in laboratory animals and humans. High-protein intake accelerates the development of glomerular sclerosis in uremic rats, leading to a more rapid loss of renal function. A high-protein diet induces renal vasodilation, leading to glomerular hyperfiltration and glomerular hypertension, which are considered to play an important role in the development of glomerular sclerosis. A low-protein diet reduces the serum and urine levels of indoxyl sulfate in both undialyzed uremic patients and experimental uremic rats. Indoxyl sulfate stimulates the progression of CRF in uremic rats by upregulating the gene expression of TGF-β1. A low-protein diet attenuates the gene expression of TGF-β1 and reduces the prevalence of glomerular sclerosis in the rat kidneys and of focal glomerulosclerosis induced by puromycin aminonucleoside. Thus the decreased production of indoxyl sulfate by a low-protein diet may, at least partly, explain the suppression of CRF progression by a low-protein diet.

An Oral Sorbent Suppresses Indoxyl Sulfate Levels and the Progression of CRF. Clinically, the oral administration of AST-120 to undialyzed uremic patients prolongs the period until the induction of dialysis therapy, and thus markedly delays the progression of CRF (Fig. 68.54). AST-120 has already been approved in Japan for slowing the progression of CRF in undialyzed uremic patients. AST-120 also prevents the progression of CRF in experimental uremic rats. Oral administration of AST-120 reduces the serum levels of indoxyl sulfate in uremic rats, and undialyzed and hemodialyzed uremic patients (1,5).

The gene expression of TGF-β1, TIMP-1, and pro-α1 (I) collagen in the renal cortex was markedly increased in 5/6-

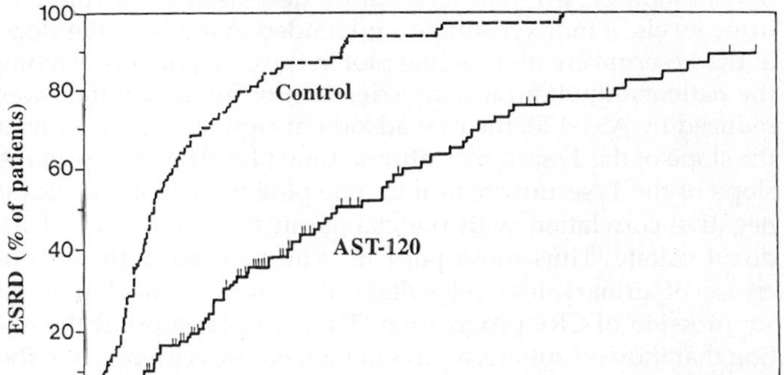

Figure 68.54. Clinical effects of AST-120 on the occurrence of end-stage renal disease (ESRD), which requires dialysis therapy, in uremic patients with the serum creatinine levels of 6 mg/dl (ranging from 5.5 to 6.4 mg/dl): a retrospective study. Oral administration of AST at a dose of 6 g/day to undialyzed uremic patients (n = 129) markedly prolonged the period until the induction of dialysis therapy, and thus delayed the progression of CRF as compared with control uremic patients (n = 71). Time-to-event analysis was conducted with the use of the Kaplan-Meier method to estimate cumulative-incidence curves and with log-rank tests.

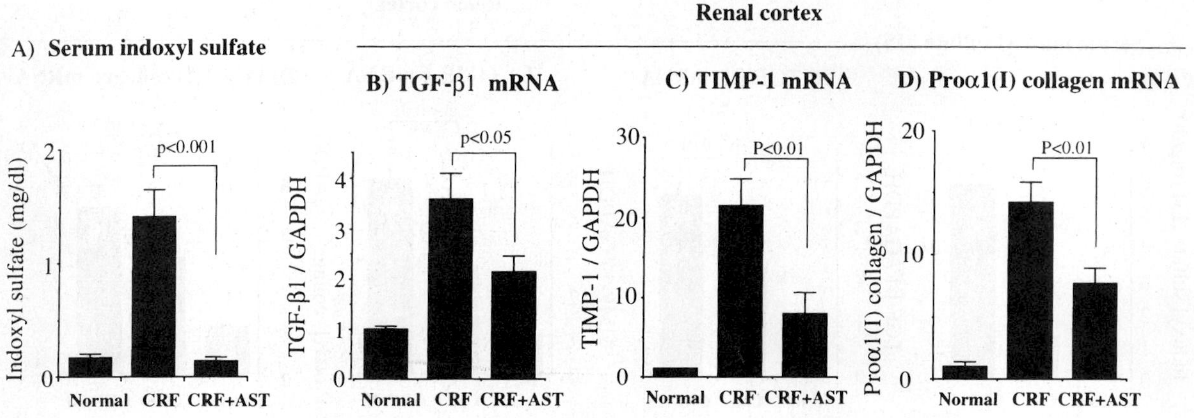

Figure 68.55. Effects of the administration of AST-120 for 11 weeks on the serum levels of indoxyl sulfate **(A),** and the mRNA levels of TGF-β1 **(B),** TIMP-1 **(C),** and pro-α1 (I) collagen **(D)** in the renal cortex. CRF: 5/6-nephrectomized uremic rats, CRF + AST: 5/6-nephrectomized uremic rats fed with the diet containing 5% AST-120. The administration of AST-120 to the uremic rats significantly decreased the serum level of indoxyl sulfate, and downregulated the gene expression of TGF-β1, TIMP-1, and pro-α1 (I) collagen in the renal cortex.

nephrectomized uremic rats as compared with normal rats. Oral administration of AST-120 for 11 weeks suppressed the gene expression of TGF-β1, TIMP-1, and pro-α1 (I) collagen in the renal cortex of the uremic rats (Fig. 68.55). The uremic rats given AST-120 showed significantly lower levels of serum and urine indoxyl sulfate, serum creatinine, serum urea nitrogen, and urinary protein, and higher levels of creatinine clearance than control uremic rats. Further, the administration of AST-120 suppressed glomerular sclerosis index, interstitial fibrosis area, and the incidence of atrophic tubules. Thus AST-120 suppressed glomerular sclerosis and interstitial fibrosis by reducing the serum and urine levels of indoxyl sulfate, and consequently reducing the gene expression of TGF-β1, TIMP-1, and pro-α1 (I) collagen in the kidneys.

Furthermore, to determine whether AST-120 could reduce the serum and urine levels of indoxyl sulfate, and suppress the progression of CRF in undialyzed uremic patients, 25 undialyzed uremic patients were given AST-120 at a dose of 6 g/day for 6 months, and 10 undialyzed uremic patients were not given AST-120 and served as controls. The effects of the oral adsorbent on the slope of the 1/serum creatinine-time plot and the serum and urine levels of indoxyl sulfate were evaluated. Administration of AST-120 significantly decreased the serum and urine levels of indoxyl sulfate, and tended to improve the slope of the 1/serum creatinine-time plot in the CRF patients. Among the patients in whom urinary excretion of indoxyl sulfate was reduced by AST-120, the oral adsorbent significantly improved the slope of the 1/serum creatinine-time plot. The change in the slope of the 1/serum creatinine-time plot showed a significant negative correlation with the change in the urine level of indoxyl sulfate. Thus those patients who showed a greater decrease of urinary indoxyl sulfate also showed more marked suppression of CRF progression. These results support the notion that indoxyl sulfate, a protein metabolite, is involved in the progression of CRF, and that the oral adsorbent can delay progression at least partly by reducing the serum and urine levels of indoxyl sulfate.

Selected Readings

Miyazaki T, Ise M, Seo H, et al. Indoxyl sulfate increases the gene expressions of TGF-β1, TIMP-1 and pro-α1 (I) collagen in kidneys of uremic rats. *Kidney Int* 1997;52(Suppl 62): S15–S22.

The administration of indoxyl sulfate to 5/6-nephrectomized uremic rats increased the mRNA levels of TGF-β1, TIMP-1 and pro-α1 (I) collagen in the kidneys. Thus the overload of indoxyl sulfate on remnant nephrons is involved in the increased bioactivity of TGF-β1 in uremic kidneys, which enhances the renal expression of TIMP-1 and type 1 collagen, leading to the progression of CRF.

Niwa T, Ise M. Indoxyl sulfate, a circulating uremic toxin, stimulates the progression of glomerular sclerosis. *J Lab Clin Med* 1994;124:96–104.

The oral administration of indoxyl sulfate to 5/6-nephrectomized uremic rats increased serum creatinine, blood urea nitrogen, and glomerular sclerosis index, and decreased creatinine clearance, inulin clearance and p-aminohippuric acid clearance.

Niwa T, Ise M, Miyazaki T. Progression of glomerular sclerosis in experimental uremic rats by administration of indole, a precursor of indoxyl sulfate. *Am J Nephrol* 1994;14:207–212.

The oral administration of indole to 5/6-nephrectomized uremic rats increased serum creatinine, blood urea nitrogen, and glomerular sclerosis index, and decreased creatinine clearance, inulin clearance and para-aminohippuric acid clearance.

Niwa T, Nomura T, Sugiyama S, et al. The protein metabolite hypothesis, a model for the progression of renal failure: an oral sorbent lowers indoxyl sulfate levels in undialyzed uremic patients. *Kidney Int* 1997;52(Suppl 62):S23–S28.

Administration of AST-120 decreased the serum and urine levels of indoxyl sulfate and improved the slope of the 1/serum-creatinine versus time plot in CRF patients. Those patients who showed a greater decrease of urinary indoxyl sulfate also showed more marked suppression of the progression of CRF.

Niwa T, Tsukushi S, Ise M, et al. Indoxyl sulfate and progression of renal failure: effects of a low-protein diet and oral sorbent on indoxyl sulfate production in uremic rats and undialyzed uremic patients. *Miner Electrol Metab* 1997;23: 179–184.

Fasting or AST-120 administration decreased the serum and urine levels of indoxyl sulfate in 5/6-nephrectomized uremic rats. A low-protein diet or AST-120 also decreased the serum and urine levels of indoxyl sulfate in CRF patients.

PART 6
Metabolic Acidosis

Harold A. Franch and William E. Mitch

Until the blood pH falls below 7.2, adults tolerate metabolic acidosis with minimal acute complications. Indeed, the acid-induced increase in tissue oxygen delivery (because of the Bohr effect and respiratory compensation) may be beneficial in some acutely or critically ill patients. At blood pH levels below 7.2, cardiovascular function can be affected, including increased susceptibility to arrhythmias, decreased cardiac output, and resistance to the effects of catecholamines. Other complications occur at even lower blood pH levels, including obtundation

TABLE 68.7. Endocrine Effects of Chronic Metabolic Acidosis

1. Increased plasma cortisol concentration
2. Increased plasma aldosterone concentration
3. Insulin resistance in nonhepatic organs
4. Decreased plasma insulinlike growth factor 1 concentration
5. Increased serum parathyroid hormone concentration (clinically apparent in uremia only)
6. Increased serum 1,25 vitamin D concentration (nonuremic only)

and coma. These complications largely arise because hydrogen ions disrupt the structure and function of cellular protein.

In contrast, even small degrees of chronic metabolic acidosis have been linked with major, long-term complications. The best described complications, abnormalities of calcium and protein metabolism, (Table 68.8), arise from changes in endocrine function and the homeostatic responses that compensate for the acidosis. Hormones, including cortisol, insulin, insulinlike growth factor-1 (IGF-1), and parathyroid hormone (PTH), play a prominent role in mediating some important chronic complications of acidosis as do the homeostatic responses responsible for acid buffering in bone and for increasing net acid excretion. In many cases, uremia interacts with acidosis to exacerbate these problems. This makes acidosis an excellent target for therapies to relieve complications of uremia.

ENDOCRINE ABNORMALITIES (TABLE 68.7)

The best described hormonal alteration in acidosis is an increase in adrenal cortical hormones, ascribed to a hypothalamic mechanism. There are high circulating adrenocorticotropin (ACTH) levels in chronic acidosis; whether this is related to increased ACTH production or a prolonged half-life is unknown. The high ACTH level drives the overproduction of both glucocorticoids and aldosterone. This rise in ACTH occurs in response to an acute infusion of organic or inorganic acids but in uremia, the increase is not solely due to acidosis; glucocorticoid excretion returns to normal in nonuremic acidotic subjects who are infused with bicarbonate, but in those with uremic acidosis given bicarbonate, glucocorticoid excretion does not normalize. Glucocorticoid excess plays an important role in inducing abnormalities of calcium and protein metabolism. The clinical significance of the elevated circulating mineralocorticoids is unclear, but this may raise potassium excretion by the kidneys and intestines.

Insulin and IGF-1 signaling are affected in different ways by acidosis. Insulin secretion is not changed by acidosis, but there is resistance to insulin action in peripheral tissues; reversal of acidosis by bicarbonate infusion improves insulin sensitivity in normal or uremic animals or humans. In skeletal muscle, it appears that insulin resistance occurs at a postreceptor level. IGF-1 resistance is not induced by acidosis because the IGF-1 resistance that occurs in uremia does not improve with correction of acidosis, but acidosis does cause decreased circulating IGF-1. The fall in IGF-1 is probably partly due to decreased hypothalamic growth hormone releasing factor (GRF) production, because there is decreased IGF-1 production and other parts of the growth hormone (GH)/IGF-1 axis are intact. IGF-1 formation in response to GH is unchanged by acidosis, and the rise in serum GH in response to an exogenous dose of GRF is increased. In addition to this hypothalamic defect, the half-life of IGF-1 is shortened due to increased renal metabolism. Thus decreased GRF production and increased renal metabolism account for the decreased IGF-1 levels in acidosis. Abnormalities in insulin and IGF-1 may play a role in the decreased growth, abnormal bone metabolism, and increased muscle proteolysis.

Acidosis directly stimulates the release of PTH by increasing the sensitivity of the gland to changes in ionized calcium. In patients with normal renal function, chronic acidosis decreases tubular phosphate reabsorption resulting in hypophosphatemia and a secondary elevation of 1,25 vitamin D levels. The rise in 1,25 vitamin D and calcium absorption can suppress or even reverse the effect of acidosis on PTH. Because rats with parathyroidectomy have impaired renal acid excretion, it appears that the increase in PTH secretion in response to acidosis is part of a homeostatic response. In patients with end-stage renal disease, acidosis will have little or no effect on phosphate or 1,25 vitamin D levels because of the loss of kidney mass, and it would be expected that chronic acidosis would stimulate PTH release. Although this hypothesis has not been directly proven, correction of acidosis in hemodialysis patients with secondary hyperparathyroidism improves the response of the parathyroid glands to calcium.

Other hormones are affected by acidosis: in normal adults, acidosis lowers serum levels of free T_3 and T_4, whereas the concentration of reverse T_3 is unchanged. Thyroid-stimulating hormone (TSH) levels are mildly increased and there is an increased TSH response to nasal thyroid-releasing hormone. The clinical significance of this mild hypothyroidlike response has not been demonstrated, but theoretically, it could affect both calcium and protein metabolism.

TABLE 68.8. Complications of Chronic Metabolic Acidosis and Possible Mechanisms

I. Dissolution of Bone
   A. Direct effect of acid on bone mineral content
   B. Increased osteoclast and decreased osteoblast activity
   C. Glucocorticoids, PTH, and other hormones
II. Hypercalciuria and Hyperphosphaturia Leading to Hypophosphatemia
   A. Increased filtered load of calcium and phosphorous
   B. Decreased tubular reabsorption of calcium and phosphorous
III. Nephrolithiasis
   A. Hypercalciuria
   B. Hypocitraturia (decreases calcium solubility)
   C. Decreased urine pH (decreases urate solubility)
IV. Protein Malnutrition and Muscle Wasting
   A. Activation of the ubiquitin-proteasome system
      1. pH
      2. Glucocorticoids
      3. Other hormones
   B. Activation of Branched-Chain Keto Acid Dehydrogenase
      1. pH
      2. Glucocorticoids
   C. Increased Hepatic Glutamine Synthesis and Renal Glutamine Metabolism

PTH, parathyroid hormone.

CALCIUM METABOLISM

The direct effect of acidosis on calcium metabolism occurs in the bone. An acid load is immediately buffered by the bicarbonate system, proteins, and bone. Bone buffering involves the direct release of alkali by two mechanisms. First, bone is dissolved when acid reacts with carbonates in bone mineral and when there is ion exchange of hydrogen ions for sodium and potassium. For example, acidifying the media by bathing isolated mouse calvariae with acid increases the release of calcium even if the osteocytes have been killed. In contrast, acidifying the media with CO_2 only barely increases calcium release, suggesting that with respiratory acidosis, the high carbonic-acid concentration in the blood inhibits the release of carbonate from bone. Second, metabolic acidosis causes higher osteoclast and lower osteoblast activity in isolated calvariae, whereas respiratory acidosis has little effect on osteocyte activity. *In vivo,* cell-mediated calcium release may be more significant in chronic compared with acute acidosis.

Metabolic acidosis also raises PTH and glucocorticoid levels but suppresses thyroxine, and each of these could contribute to loss of bone mineral. Moreover, the increase in bone resorption is independent of and additive with the response to hyperparathyroidism, because parathyroidectomy does not block acid's direct effect on calcium release from bone. Acidosis increased the influence of PTH to release calcium, to raise osteoclast β-glucuronidase activity, and to decrease collagen synthesis in isolated mouse calvariae. As discussed previously, phosphaturia and elevated 1,25 vitamin D levels may also play a role in the bone demineralization and osteomalacia that occur in patients with intact renal function.

Mobilizing calcium from bone increases serum calcium and hence, renal filtered load of calcium. This leads to hypercalcuria because acidosis directly inhibits tubular calcium reabsorption independently of the increase in filtered load or of PTH. This decrease in reabsorption has both a proximal and a distal component under slightly different regulatory mechanisms. Both a lower plasma and luminal pH decrease calcium reabsorption by the proximal tubule. In contrast, luminal, not plasma, pH appears to regulate absorption in the distal segment, because even in the presence of metabolic acidosis, increased distal delivery of bicarbonate stimulates calcium absorption. Thus acidosis contributes directly to negative calcium balance by causing dissolution of bone and renal calcium loss.

Given these mechanisms, it is not surprising that correction of acidosis has been shown to improve both bone mineralization and histology in patients with acidosis. Administration of alkali to hemodialysis dialysis patients improves both biochemical and histologic markers of renal osteodystrophy. Still, a correlation with fracture rates or other outcome measurements and acid–base status has not been documented in dialysis patients.

NEPHROLITHIASIS

Because acidosis can cause hypercalciuria, it is not surprising that it plays a major role in kidney stone formation. However, hypocitraturia and a low urinary pH probably contribute as much or more than hypercalciuria to the increased incidence of nephrolithiasis. Citrate is a major inhibitor of calcium oxalate and calcium phosphate crystallization. Freely filtered, citrate in the urine is largely regulated by proximal tubular reabsorption. Because citrate is metabolized to bicarbonate, the loss of citrate in the urine is a loss of potential base. To avoid the loss of this potential bicarbonate, the activity of the proximal tubule brush boarder Na/citrate cotransporter rises to decrease citrate excretion. Mild degrees of acidosis cause profound hypocitraturia, and even when plasma pH is normal, a diet yielding acid (e.g., a diet rich in protein and low in organic base) can reduce citrate excretion.

Uric acid is much less soluble at a low pH and can precipitate; uric acid crystals not only form stones themselves, but also can act as a nidus to form calcium stones. Clinically, the importance of acidosis on stone formation is clear. Patients with chronic metabolic acidosis either from distal renal tubular acidosis or intestinal bicarbonate loss have a much greater incidence of calcium stones and may have nephrocalcinosis and progressive renal damage.

PROTEIN MALNUTRITION

Although anorexia complicates the assessment of protein malnutrition in patients with metabolic acidosis, several lines of evidence suggest that excessive protein catabolism is the dominant mechanism. First, infants with metabolic acidosis grow poorly and have increased nitrogen excretion that occurs independently of protein intake. Normal adults fed NH_4Cl to induce metabolic acidosis exhibit both increased oxidation of the essential, branched-chain amino acids (BCAA) plus increased protein degradation. In fact, metabolic acidosis has been identified as a principal catabolic factor suppressing growth and stimulating loss of lean-body mass associated with chronic uremia. In both hemodialysis and continuous ambulatory peritoneal dialysis (CAPD) patients, correction of acidosis improves indices of nutrition even though protein intake does not increase. This suggests that correction of acidosis suppresses protein catabolism. Studies of amino acid metabolism have directly demonstrated a catabolic response to acid in patients with uremia. In predialysis patients fed a low-protein diet (0.6 to 0.8 g/kg body weight), correction of metabolic acidosis improved nitrogen balance and raised the plasma concentrations of the BCAA. Similarly, in hemodialysis patients there was a strong linear correlation between the plasma bicarbonate measured just before a dialysis treatment and the free-valine concentration in a muscle biopsy; there also was a direct correlation between the plasma bicarbonate concentration and the plasma level of α-ketoisocaproate, the keto acid of leucine.

Experimental studies have begun to reveal how acid causes protein catabolism. One response to metabolic acidosis is to stimulate renal ammonia excretion. The kidney extracts glutamine from plasma and forms ammonia in order to excrete acid. Because the plasma concentration of glutamine does not fall dramatically, glutamine production must increase. Increased glutamine production results from increased muscle-protein degradation leading to a supply of amino acid precursors for glutamine synthesis by the liver. BCAA are oxidized to provide much of the nitrogen for hepatic glutamine synthesis. Plasma levels of BCAA in uremic rats are low and are linked to increased oxidation of the BCAA. The influence of acidosis in these processes was proven by adding $NaHCO_3$ to the diet to correct the metabolic acidosis: both normal plasma levels of BCAA and normal rates of muscle leucine oxidation were restored. These relationships suggest that metabolic acidosis activates the rate-limiting enzyme for the irreversible decarboxylation of BCAA, branched-chain keto acid dehydrogenase (BCKAD), and in acidotic rats, metabolic acidosis lowered plasma and muscle BCAA levels and increased the rates of valine and leucine transamination and oxidative decarboxylation by stimulating the activity of BCKAD in muscle. Human studies confirm these results. When normal subjects were fed an acid diet, there was a 25% stimulation of BCAA decarboxylation.

Muscle, the largest store of protein in the body, appears to be the source for the BCAA used by the liver for glutamine synthesis, because acidosis stimulates breakdown of protein in muscle. In chronically uremic rats, protein degradation was increased in isolated muscle, but correction of acidosis reduced protein degradation to normal levels; there was no correction of impaired protein synthesis. A recent study of protein turnover in predialysis patients confirmed that correction of the metabolic acidosis reduces both whole body protein degradation and BCAA oxidation. In fact, switching patients with chronic renal failure and metabolic acidosis to an isocaloric, low-protein diet (0.6 g protein/kg body weight per day) also decreased skeletal muscle and whole body protein degradation, presumably because the low-protein diet reduced the accumulation of acid. This is important because metabolic acidosis will override the body's normal adaptive responses to low protein intake. These adaptations include suppression of the oxidation of essential amino acids and degradation of protein. Thus there is abundant evidence from rat models and patient studies demonstrating that metabolic acidosis accelerates irreversible oxidation of BCAA and skeletal muscle protein degradation.

When the pH of the media of cultured myocytes is lowered, there is a slight decrease in protein synthesis plus an increase in protein degradation compatible with a direct effect of acidosis. However, the high levels of glucocorticoids stimulated by metabolic acidosis also play a role. In rats, adrenalectomy blocked the effect of acidosis on catabolism, whereas replacing glucocorticoids restored the effect of acid and indeed, both elevated glucocorticoids and acidosis are needed *in vivo* to accelerate skeletal muscle proteolysis. In support of this conclusion, both acidosis and glucocorticoids are required to increase the activity of protein and BCKAD. Correction of the acidosis associated with chronic renal failure blocked the accelerated protein degradation occurring in muscle without reducing urinary glucocorticoid excretion.

Metabolic Acidosis Stimulates the Ubiquitin–Proteasome Proteolytic Pathway

In all tissues and cell types, including skeletal muscle, there are multiple proteolytic pathways. These pathways include the acidic proteases found in lysosomes, the calcium Ca^{2+}-activated proteases in the cytoplasm, plus adenosine triphosphate (ATP)-independent and ATP-dependent cytosolic pathways. The best described ATP-dependent cytosolic pathway is the ubiquitin/proteasome system. Acidosis accelerates the ATP-dependent pathway in muscle, whereas lysosomal protein degradation and Ca^{2+}-activated proteolysis do not play a major role. In the ATP-ubiquitin–dependent pathway, proteins are targeted for degradation by conjugation to ubiquitin, a small protein found in all cells. This conjugation occurs in an ATP-dependent reaction involving one of several ubiquitin-conjugating enzyme complexes. Protein-ubiquitin conjugates are then degraded, in an ATP-dependent process, to small peptides and constituent amino acids by the 26S proteasome, a large, multicatalytic, multiple subunit proteolytic complex. The proteasome is found in the nucleus and cytoplasm of virtually all cells.

Activation of the ATP-dependent ubiquitin–proteasome pathway in acidosis also requires glucocorticoids; the rise in ATP-dependent proteolysis occurring in skeletal muscle of acidotic rats was abolished by adrenalectomy, and restored by administration of dexamethasone. Interestingly, the response to acidosis includes activation of gene transcription. The abundance of ubiquitin mRNA increased in skeletal muscles from acidotic rats and this change was accompanied by increased levels of mRNA encoding for subunits of the proteasome. These changes in mRNA require glucocorticoids, and studies with the promoter region of the proteasome C3 gene show that acid and glucocorticoids synergistically increase transcription of the mRNA for this subunit. Thus metabolic acidosis appears to upregulate skeletal muscle protein degradation through a coordinate increase in the expression of the genes for proteins responsible for ATP-ubiquitin–dependent protein degradation.

The role of other hormonal abnormalities in stimulating protein degradation are more controversial. Insulin and IGF-1 are anabolic hormones that improve body protein metabolism; insulin can regulate cellular proteolysis *in vitro* and insulin resistance occurs with acidosis. Rats with streptozotocin-induced diabetes have increased muscle proteolysis that occurs via the ubiquitin-proteasome system, suggesting that reduced insulin activity could contribute to activation of this important pathway causing muscle protein wasting. The relative contribution of acidosis to insulin resistance in uremia and of insulin resistance to protein wasting in acidosis still remain to be determined. It also is uncertain whether acidosis contributes to lack of IGF-1 action in uremia, but at pharmacologic doses, growth hormone is effective therapy for growth retardation in both uremic and nonuremic acidosis. The roles of thyroid hormone and PTH on protein metabolism in acidosis have not been fully identified.

Selected Readings

Alpern RJ, Sakhaee K. The clinical spectrum of chronic metabolic acidosis: homeostatic mechanisms produce significant morbidity. *Am J Kidney Dis* 1997;29:291–302.

A review of complications arising from the bone and renal response to acidosis with a focus on nonuremic effects on bone, nephrolithiasis, and eubicarbonatemic acidosis.

Bushinsky DA. Bone disease in moderate renal failure: cause, nature, and prevention. Annu Rev Med 1997;48:167–176.

A review of renal osteodystrophy highlighting the role of acidosis.

Mitch WE, Goldberg AL. Mechanisms of muscle wasting: the role of the ubiquitin proteasome system. *N Eng J Med* 1996;335:1897–1905.

A general review of the ubiquitin-proteasome system in muscle wasting and protein malnutrition in chronic disease. The effects of pH and glucocorticoids in acidosis and uremia are placed in the larger context of factors that regulate proteolysis.

Price SR, Mitch WE. Metabolic acidosis and uremic toxicity: protein and amino acid metabolism. *Semin Nephrol* 1994;14:232–237.

A comprehensive review of the effect of acidosis on protein and amino acid metabolism in uremic and nonuremic subjects.

PART 7
Carbonyl Stress in Uremia: Alterations in Nonenzymatic Biochemistry of Carbohydrates and Lipids

Toshio Miyata and Kiyoshi Kurokawa

The long-term survival and quality of life of uremic patients undergoing renal replacement therapy is determined largely by complications, such as cardiovascular diseases and bone disease. Factors responsible for these complications have been intensively investigated. The recognition that uremic complications are related to the accumulation of toxic metabolites in blood and tissues has led to efforts to identify the causal substances and to enhance their detoxification or accelerate their removal by dialysis procedures.

The discovery that proteins are progressively and irreversibly modified with advanced glycation end-products (AGEs), by nonenzymatic Maillard reaction during the normal process of aging, and in diabetes mellitus has opened new avenues for research on uremic toxicity, because it has been known that this nonenzymatic process is markedly accelerated in renal failure.

In this part, we will summarize the evidence that nonenzymatic modification of carbohydrates and lipids is profoundly altered in renal failure and discuss its role in uremic joint and vascular complications. We will advance our thesis that the accumulation of AGEs in renal failure is only one facet of a much broader derangement in reactive carbonyl chemistry. We describe the accumulation in uremia of reactive carbonyl compounds derived not only from carbohydrates but also from lipids, and propose that these alterations, best described as *carbonyl stress,* underlie the development of many uremic complications.

ADVANCED GLYCATION END-PRODUCT

The nonenzymatic reaction of carbohydrates with proteins has been a topic of great interest in food and nutrition biochemistry. The Maillard reaction is initiated by the attachment of carbohydrates to protein amino groups and proceeds from reversible Schiff base adducts to reversible Amadori products. The AGEs eventually form irreversibly, leading to covalent cross-linking of amino groups of proteins.

Research on the role of AGEs in human pathology focused initially on diabetes with sustained hyperglycemia. The causal role of hyperglycemia is confirmed by the relationship between the tissue content of AGEs and the serum levels of fructose-lysine and hemoglobin A1c, well-known and widely used clinical and molecular markers of prevailing plasma glucose concentration. In diabetic patients, high plasma glucose is thought to accelerate the Maillard reaction and to increase generation of AGEs. The demonstration that tissue and plasma AGE levels are correlated with the severity of diabetic complications suggests the clinical relevance of AGEs.

INCREASED AGE IN UREMIA

Recently, it was discovered that AGEs accumulate markedly in normoglycemic uremic patients. Several AGE products have been chemically identified, including pentosidine and N^{ϵ}-carboxymethyllysine (CML), and specific chemical methods have been developed to quantify these products, using high-performance liquid chromatography or gas chromatography/mass spectrometry instruments. Pentosidine and CML accumulate in plasma and tissue proteins of uremic patients. Levels of pentosidine and CML in plasma proteins, however, do not differ between diabetic and nondiabetic hemodialysis patients. Furthermore, in uremic patients, there is no correlation between serum fructose-lysine and pentosidine or CML in plasma or tissue proteins, in contrast to diabetic patients. The plasma pentosidine and CML levels in uremia thus appear unrelated to plasma glucose levels. The markedly elevated levels of AGEs in proteins of nondiabetic uremic patients indicates that factors other than hyperglycemia determine the rate of formation of AGEs.

Pentosidine and CML are markedly increased in uremic plasma and are more than 90% bound to serum albumin. The remaining fraction is in free rather than peptide-bound form. Pentosidine and CML accumulation in plasma proteins thus cannot be attributed to decreased renal clearance of protein-linked CML and pentosidine. Both hemodialysis and peritoneal dialysis could clear only the free form and do not significantly modify protein-bound form of these AGE products.

INCREASED OXIDATIVE STRESS IN UREMIA

Obviously, uremic sera contain either unknown precursor(s) and/or catalyst(s) of the Maillard reaction. Newer studies emphasized that pentosidine and CML are products of the combined processes of glycation and oxidation (glycoxidation). They require oxygen for their formation. The formation of pentosidine and CML on proteins is considered to result from a second-order chemical reaction with a rate dependent on the concentrations of precursors and of reactive oxygen species (oxidative stress). Pentosidine is derived exclusively from carbohydrates. CML, by contrast, originates not only from carbohydrates but also from metal-catalyzed oxidation of polyunsaturated fatty acids in lipoproteins and from hypochlorous acid–mediated oxidation of the hydroxy amino acid, L-serine. CML may thus be formed by autoxidation of lipids and amino acids as well as carbohydrates.

In diabetic patients, age-adjusted increases in pentosidine and CML in skin collagen can be explained by the duration of disease and the long-term severity of hyperglycemia. Thus there is no need to implicate an increase in oxidative stress in diabetes. Indeed, age-adjusted levels of *ortho*-tyrosine (*o*-Tyr) and methionine sulfoxide (MetSO), markers of oxidative protein damage, are not increased in the skin collagen of diabetic patients.

In nondiabetic uremic patients, by contrast, the increase in pentosidine and CML in skin collagen and plasma proteins, in the absence of hyperglycemia, suggests that oxidative stress may be increased in uremia. Evidence for an uremia-associated oxidative stress may include increased serum ratios of oxidized to total ascorbate, of oxidized to reduced glutathione, and of oxidized to reduced serum albumin; increased serum levels of advanced oxidation protein products (AOPP) and of protein carbonyls; and decreased serum activity of glutathione-dependent enzymes. Furthermore, serum levels of the lipid peroxidation marker, malondialdehyde (MDA)-lysine, are elevated. There are significant correlations between serum levels of pentosidine and oxidative markers such as AOPP and dehydroascorbate, and between the levels of CML and MDA-lysine in plasma proteins. Altogether, these findings are consistent with a generalized increase in oxidative stress in chronic uremia.

INCREASED CARBONYL MODIFICATION OF PROTEINS (CARBONYL STRESS) IN UREMIA

Proteins may be modified either directly by reactive oxygen species with the eventual formation of oxidized amino acids, or indirectly by reactive carbonyl compounds generated by the autoxidation of carbohydrates, lipids, or amino acids. Autoxidation of carbohydrates yields reactive carbonyl compounds, precursors of glycoxidation products, such as glyoxal, and glycolaldehyde, as well as dehydroascorbate formed on oxidation of ascorbate. Lipid peroxidation yields other reactive carbonyl compounds, some of which are identical to those formed from carbohydrates, such as glyoxal, whereas others are characteristic to lipids, such as MDA and 4-hydroxynonenal (HNE). The latter reactive carbonyl compounds produce MDA- and HNE-protein adducts, also termed *lipoxidation products* or *advanced lipoxidation end-products (ALEs).* Oxidation of hydroxy amino acids, L-serine and L-threonine, yields glycolaldehyde and acrolein, two carbonyl compounds highly reactive with proteins, leading to formation of CML and acrolein-protein adducts, respectively. Polyunsaturated fatty acids are also sources of acrolein that cause the production of acrolein-protein adduct.

In addition to oxidative chemistry, nonoxidative pathways also contribute to formation of reactive carbonyl compounds, such as 3-deoxyglucosone and methylglyoxal. Both 3-deoxyglucosone and methylglyoxal react with protein amino groups and form AGEs on proteins. The increase in 3-deoxyglucosone and methylglyoxal, and their protein adducts in uremic serum is evidence of the contribution of nonoxidative chemical reaction to the formation of reactive carbonyl compounds and AGEs in uremia.

In vitro studies indicate that there are elevated levels of low–molecular-weight AGE precursors in uremic plasma. Plasma samples, obtained from normal and nondiabetic hemodialysis patients, have been incubated under air for several weeks. Generation of pentosidine is monitored during the incubation. Protein-linked pentosidine rises much more in uremic than in control plasma. This difference is still observed for plasma ultrafiltrates (5,000 Dalton cut off) incubated with normal human albumin. The pentosidine yield in the ultrafiltrate is also significantly higher in plasma samples of predialysis than those of postdialysis. The known inhibitors of AGE formation, aminoguanidine and OPB-9195, could inhibit the *in vitro* production of pentosidine in uremic plasma. Because aminoguanidine and OPB-9195 act by capturing carbonyl compounds, these results point to an increase in reactive carbonyl compounds in plasma as precursors of AGEs on plasma proteins. Direct evidence for an elevated plasma level of carbonyl compounds was obtained by exposure of ultrafiltered plasma to 2,4-dinitrophenylhydrazine. Hydrazones formed by interaction with carbonyl groups are detected by a spectrophotometric assay. The hydrazone yield is several times higher in uremic, compared with control subjects.

The levels of glyoxal and methylglyoxal and their of the imidazolium cross-links, glyoxal-lysine dimer and methylglyoxal-lysine dimer, are all increased in plasma proteins of uremic patients. Altogether, these findings indicate that uremic plasma contains elevated levels of low–molecular-weight carbonyl compounds. The increased levels of these carbonyl compounds together with those of pentosidine, CML, and MDA-lysine suggest a generalized increase in circulating carbonyl compounds formed by both oxidative and nonoxidative chemical processes in uremic plasma. Thus the metabolic and chemical imbalances characteristic of uremia may be described more appropriately as carbonyl stress, rather than singly advanced glycation or oxidative stress.

The increased carbonyl stress observed in uremia is the consequence either of an increased production (oxidative stress) or of a decreased renal detoxification or clearance of reactive carbonyl compounds. The latter hypothesis may be more likely, because carbonyl compounds, derived from both oxidative and nonoxidative chemical modification of both carbohydrates and lipids, have a rather low molecular weight and rise simultaneously in uremic plasma without concomitant changes in glycemia or lipemia.

PATHOLOGY OF CARBONYL STRESS

The relevance of carbonyl stress in uremia has been suggested in the pathogenesis of bone and joint destruction associated with chronic renal failure, known as β_2-microglobulin amyloidosis or dialysis-related amyloidosis, and in accelerated atherosclerosis.

Dialysis-Related Amyloidosis

Dialysis-related amyloidosis is a serious complication occurring most commonly in patients undergoing long-term hemodialysis, but also in patients undergoing continuous ambulatory peritoneal dialysis. This complication occurs even in those patients with renal failure before the initiation of dialysis therapy. Amyloid fibrils consisting of β_2-microglobulin deposit preferentially in the osteoarticular tissues and then, over the years, lead to bone and joint destruction. Two stages may be considered in the development of dialysis-related amyloidosis. The preclinical stage is characterized by histologic evidence of β_2-microglobulin deposits in the joints several years before the onset of clinical or radiologic signs. Amyloid deposits, already present in 20% of patients within 2 years after the start of dialysis, are not surrounded by macrophages or evidence of bone destruction. The clinical stage emerges subsequently and is characterized by arthralgias, carpal tunnel syndrome, and radiologically visible bone cysts. At this stage, the amyloid deposits are surrounded by macrophages and bone resorption is observed in adjacent regions.

The cause of β_2-microglobulin–amyloid fibril deposition is not fully elucidated. The role of elevated plasma β_2-microglobulin levels is controversial, because there is no significant difference in the plasma β_2-microglobulin levels between dialysis patients with and those without clinical evidence of amyloidosis. Efforts have therefore been directed toward the identification of chemical modifications of β_2-microglobulin. Although these studies are not complete, immunohistochemical and chemical analyses indicate that β_2-microglobulin–amyloid deposits are modified by a range of carbonyl stress–modified protein products. β_2-Microglobulin–amyloid plaques react not only with anti-AGE and antireceptor for AGE (anti-RAGE) antibodies, but also with antibodies specific for the glycoxidation products, pentosidine and CML, and for the lipoxidation products, MDA-lysine and HNE-protein adduct. β_2-Microglobulin isolated from plasma and urine of uremic patients also reacts with these antibodies. The issue of β_2-microglobulinemia in uremic patients is further discussed in Chapter 84, Part 1E.

Thus at present, it is fair to state that it remains unknown whether carbonyl stress actively plays a role in the pathogenesis, or is merely long-term transformation of, long-lived amyloid fibrils of chronic dialysis patients. Still, as described in the following section, recent studies have demonstrated the biologic activities of carbonyl stress, which can at least in part account for the bone and joint destruction associated with amyloidosis. Uremic arthropathies might be thus the combined result of carbonyl stress accumulation in long-lived amyloids linked to activation cellular responses. The progressive accumulation of carbonyl stress in amyloid deposits might be responsible in transforming the silent early deposits into clinically manifest osteoarticulitis at the advanced stage.

Atherosclerosis

Levels of AGEs in arterial tissues are higher in dialysis patients than in normal subjects. Immunohistochemical examination reveals the presence of CML, pentosidine, MDA-lysine, and HNE-protein adducts in the thickened neointima of arterial walls. The staining pattern for these compounds corresponded with that for protein carbonyls, a biomarker of oxidative protein damage. Colocalization of carbonyl stress–modified protein products and protein carbonyls in the vascular tissue of uremic patients indicates a wide range of chemical modifications in vascular matrix proteins.

Biologic Activities of Carbonyl Stress

The presence of carbonyl stress–modified protein products on β_2-microglobulin in amyloid plaques and on lipoproteins in vascular lesions may play a role in the pathogenesis of joint and vascular complications in uremia. Carbonyl stress–modified protein products (AGE and/or ALE) initiate a range of inflammatory responses, including stimulation of monocyte chemotaxis, secretion of inflammatory cytokines from macrophages, stimulation of collagenase secretion from synovial cells, stimulation of osteoclast-induced bone resorption, proliferation of vascular smooth muscle cells, and acceleration of platelet aggregation.

Carbonyl stress not only induces local inflammatory responses, but also initiates biologic responses effects in parenchymal cells. AGE-RAGE interaction produces intracellular oxidative stress and enhances the expression of cytokines. Carbonyl compounds *per se* react covalently with matrix or cell-surface proteins and alter their structures and functions or stimulate cellular responses perhaps by cross-linking to cell-surface proteins. Exposure of cells to carbonyl compounds (e.g., MDA, glyoxal, or HNE) results in phosphorylation of the tyrosine residues of a number of intracellular proteins.

Selected Readings

Miyata T, Jadoul M, Kurokawa K, et al. β_2-Microglobulin in renal disease. *J Am Soc Nephrol* 1998;9:1723—1735.

This article reviews the clinical manifestation, diagnosis, treatment, and especially recent advances in the understanding of the pathogenesis of dialysis-related amyloidosis. A newly identified modification of β_2-microglobulin, AGEs and carbonyl stress, is discussed.

Miyata T, van Ypersele de Strihou C, Kurokawa K, et al. Alterations in nonenzymatic biochemistry in uremia: origin and significance of "carbonyl stress" in long-term uremic complications. *Kidney Int* 1999;55:389—399.

A review article that describes that nonenzymatic biochemistry of carbohydrates and lipids is profoundly disturbed in renal failure. The clinical relevance of "carbonyl stress" in uremia is discussed in the pathogenesis of dialysis-related amyloidosis and atherosclerosis.

CHAPTER 69

Central and Peripheral Nervous System in Uremia

PART 1
Psychiatric and Psychosocial Considerations

Norman B. Levy and Lewis M. Cohen

Progressive uremia and its treatment modalities are associated with major stressors and psychologic sequelae. The dialysis patient is the paradigm for this chapter, but much of what is said is also applicable to the transplant patient. Differences between the two modalities are pointed out. It is important to understand that dialysis only partially corrects the uremic state equivalent to less than 10 ml/min glomerular filtration rate, and in hemodialysis, this clearance is provided only intermittently. This limited amount of clearance of uremic toxins is enough to prevent death; however, many uremic symptoms may remain. Furthermore, dialysis therapy can unfortunately produce a multiplicity of additional symptoms.

The federal government is appreciative of the psychosocial considerations of end-stage renal disease (ESRD) and has mandated clinical social work involvement in all dialysis programs. However, it is still the unusual unit that forges a close working relationship with a psychiatric consultant.

MAJOR PSYCHOLOGIC AND PSYCHIATRIC STRESSORS

Dependency/Interdependency Conflicts

Dialysis requires lifelong dependency on a procedure and, in the case of hemodialysis and continuous cycle peritoneal dialysis, dependency on a machine. At dialysis centers, patients find themselves dependent on a group of individuals, whereas the dependency in home dialysis is focused usually on a single person. For many individuals, independence is severely compromised, and this may pose a formidable obstacle for the enjoyment of life. Dialysis may reinforce dependency and the sick role, making rehabilitation for some patients difficult or impossible.

Medical Regimen

Some people never adjust to the restricted fluid intake or the high-protein, low-potassium, low-phosphate, and sodium-restricted dietary requirements of dialysis. Patients need to juggle complex and expensive medication regimens, while balancing the many complications, time constraints, and impositions of illness and procedure. For example, as many as 15 to 20 calcium tablets taken with meals as phosphate binders may be necessary to maintain normal blood levels of phosphorus.

Procedure

Dialysis staff members accept the procedure of dialysis as being an everyday matter. However, for the patient, this is the method by which life is renewed and extended. Although complications are not common during dialysis treatments, patients are aware that they do occur. It is the rare patient receiving dialysis therapy for any reasonable period of time who has not witnessed someone suffer severe hemorrhage, loss of graft function, cardiopulmonary resuscitation, syncope, or vomiting, or has not experienced the death of a fellow patient. Although these are not common occurrences, they threaten people's psychologic stability. For some individuals, the 4 hours of confinement in a dialysis chair is sheer torture; no one could reasonably be expected to look forward to the compromised mobility, muscle cramps or dizziness, and diminished time for family, pleasure, and work. Patients often will cope by means of deniallike processes, avoidance, and repression. Visitors to dialysis centers discover large rooms filled with people who are trying to lose themselves in television, crocheting, and sleep.

PSYCHIATRIC COMPLICATIONS

Organic Mental Disorders

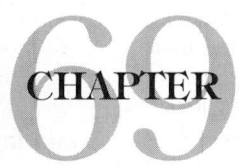

The term *organic mental disorders* refers to the group of mental illnesses directly resulting from destruction of brain tissue or interference with brain function by other causes, such as metabolic disorders, anemia, infection, circulatory compromise, or toxic states such as uremia. Other causes of these disorders include hyperparathyroidism, cardiac decompensation, and toxic states from intercurrent infections and surgical procedures.

As in the case of all organic mental disorders, the major effect is on the individual's intellectual (cognitive) functions. This is characterized by diminished ability to recall recent events, inability to perform simple arithmetic, difficulties in abstraction, irritability, difficulty concentrating, reduced level of consciousness, and confabulation.

Organic mental disorders may present as delirium or dementia. In severe cases of dementia, there may be other disturbances of higher cortical functions such as aphasia, apraxia, and agnosia. There may also be personality changes, which tend to accentuate the premorbid traits of individuals. On occasion, patients suffering from organic mental disorders may present with signs and symptoms of overt psychosis.

The basic treatment of organic mental disorders involves recognition and correction of the underlying pathologic condition. Intensified dialysis, suppression of parathyroid gland activity, parathyroidectomy, or improved control of diabetes mellitus can all prove to be helpful. Neuroleptics or benzodiazepines may provide symptomatic treatment of agitation and delusions. However, even well-dialyzed patients have subtle abnormalities of cognitive function.

Depression

Depression may be precipitated by loss, be it real, fantasized, or threatened. Patients with ESRD face many such losses, including loss of good health; loss of productivity in work, school, or household; loss of energy; loss of sexual abilities; loss of income; loss of freedom; loss of life expectancy; and lost opportunities.

Depression is the most common psychologic problem seen in the medically ill. Here we refer not only to a depressed mood or transient state of depression, but also to additional symptoms that constitute a major depressive disorder. This disorder often includes feelings of low self-esteem, worthlessness, hopelessness, and/or helplessness; sleep and/or eating disturbances; and sometimes suicidal ideation or acts.

The evaluation of depression in people with renal failure is complicated by the fact that the symptoms of ESRD and its treatment may produce the identical somatic signs and symptoms that are components of the criteria for depression. Although many patients have vegetative signs and diminished sexual interest, they still maintain that they are not necessarily depressed. The sensitivity of the Beck Depression Inventory and other assessment measures is only modest for this population.

A worthwhile measure of depression in these patients is the obvious presence of depressive affects, such as poor self-esteem, worthlessness, hopelessness, helplessness, and suicidality. Our own approach entails describing the criteria for a major depressive disorder, eliciting the patient's opinion as to whether he or she believes himself or herself to be depressed, and then documenting the existence of associated factors, such as episodes of depression before the onset of renal failure, a family history of affective disorders, and past suicide attempts.

Anxiety

Anxiety is a natural protective mechanism in which the body responds to perceived threats. Patients undergoing dialysis and transplantation recipients may experience anxiety in a number of settings. The procedure of dialysis, with its potential for mishap, may itself present the patient with the threat of impending disaster. Many other situations connected with renal failure and its treatment, such as the experience of repeated bouts of peritonitis from peritoneal dialysis, may be similarly viewed. The renal transplant patient may experience a "Sword of Damocles" syndrome, awaiting a major rejection of the graft with considerable anxiety.

Maladaptive and Uncooperative Behavior

The availability and democratization of dialysis has permitted people from all walks of life to receive treatment. This is a vast improvement over the early days of the field, when selection criteria excluded the aged, the very ill, and the disenfranchised. Even today, some authorities ask whether women or minority patients receive proportionate opportunities for transplantation. Nevertheless, whether it is the substance abuser, the demented, the sociopath/criminal, or the average American who has become mistrustful of organized medicine, staff members now work with a large percentage of individuals who have problems cooperating with authority.

Noncompliance, or the preferable term, *nonadherence*, is presently commonplace. It is not unusual for some patients to miss treatments; require emergency, middle-of-the-night dialysis due to excessive fluid gains; or demand control over the length of dialysis treatments, amount of fluid removal, or heparin administration. Staff learn on a daily basis the limits of their control over patients; maybe this is the patients' way of communicating the lack of control that they experience with their disease. Aggressive behavior has also become an issue in some dialysis programs, reinforcing the axiom that the primary responsibility of a dialysis or transplant center is not only to treat the afflicted but also to protect them and their caretakers from harm.

Like beauty, maladaption or uncooperativeness is often in the eyes of the beholder. Like beauty, there will be general agreement as to both extremes. What a physician may consider uncooperative, a fellow patient may consider an act of good consumerism or of healthy assertiveness. It is important therefore to be wary about labeling patients as being uncooperative because this itself may be seen as a provocation. We live in a very consumer-oriented medical environment. Although most health professionals prefer to think of themselves as being open-minded, the patient who questions the validity of recommendations or who asks for a second opinion may be viewed by some medical staff as being particularly difficult or nonadherent.

When patient–staff relationships deteriorate, it is worthwhile to consider the depths of misery and unhappiness that accompany ESRD. People take good health not only for granted, but virtually as a right. Many individuals see the deprivation of good health as something unfair, and they would like to personify their difficulties in terms of individuals. A small error on the part of a staff member may evoke an exaggerated response on the part of the patient. Therefore finding a medical professional who has made a mistake in some way or who has not acted in a manner that the patient may consider as being optimal may cause patients to displace their anger on to that person. Medical professionals cannot expect to be complimented for their efforts, and their sense of accomplishment must come primarily from within. Gratitude is a rarity and a blessing when it does occur. Most staff will fortunately never know the terror, deprivation, and hardship that patients experience, but compassion and empathy can go a long way toward improving strained treatment relationships.

Psychosis

There is no evidence that the stresses and strains of kidney disease and its treatment are likely to produce psychosis. Liberalization of the criteria for initiating dialysis has led to substantial numbers of patients who premorbidly suffered from schizophrenia, dementia, major affective disorders, and substance abuse. Some of these psychiatric disorders or their treatments, such as intravenous drug abuse or lithium maintenance of bipolar affective disorder, may cause renal failure. Initiation of high dosages of glucocorticoids, acyclovir, clarithromycin, and cyclosporine can also lead to exacerbation of underlying psychiatric disorders or the precipitation of delirium, manic, hypomanic, paranoid, or depressive episodes.

Additional Symptoms and Disorders

There are several problems that trouble the lives of patients receiving dialysis but that may remain undetected unless they are the subject of active inquiry by the nephrologist. Sleep disorders are common, and in one hemodialysis unit, they were found to be present in 83% of the patients. Daytime drowsiness, restless leg syndrome, insomnia associated with a painful neuropathy, and symptoms of sleep apnea are common problems. Because of the similarity of uremic symptoms to those of the sleep apnea syndrome, differential diagnosis can be difficult. Polysomnography is cumbersome and expensive; however, it may also be beneficial and invaluable.

Patients receiving dialysis therapy and, to a lesser extent, recipients of a renal transplant, have greater sexual difficulties than patients with comparable medical and surgical disorders. Men and women experience diminished sexual interest. Although impotence is common in men, women can experience diminished orgasm during sexual intercourse and are commonly infertile.

The cause of these problems is not completely understood. Research points in the direction of organic factors, with endocrinopathies including hyperparathyroidism playing a significant role. Much of our knowledge is based on studies of nocturnal penile tumescence, which show that in a large percentage of men receiving dialysis treatment, there is total or partial inability to get an erection during phase 1 REM sleep. While ESRD is associated with a decrease in testosterone and increase in other hormones such as prolactin, this is not sufficient to explain the extent of patients' sexual difficulties; testosterone replacement usually does not help. Medications for the treatment of hypertension may be an iatrogenic cause of sexual dysfunction, producing diminished libido in both men and women and causing impotence in men.

Psychologic factors may also play an important role, and depression is often associated with decreased sexual interest. The cessation of urination may affect the sense of masculinity of men, and the cessation of menses and reduced fertility may compromise the feminine identity of women. All patients, but especially those who receive peritoneal dialysis, experience changes in their appearance. This may markedly affect their self-esteem.

Numerous psychosocial problems are also associated with dialysis; these are subsumed under the generic term *quality of life*. The impact of fatigue on one's capacity to work or to enjoy daily activities, financial distress, and family discord can each present critical challenges to patient management. It is important to keep in mind that although the patient is the person who receives the treatment, the entire family is impacted by the illness.

TREATMENT

Preventive Measures

The evaluations of patients before starting treatment should include a careful social and psychologic assessment. Individuals who have had psychologic problems before dialysis treatment or who had difficulty coping with life before renal failure should be given close attention by a social worker and/or psychiatric consultant. Selection of individual treatment modalities, such as continuous peritoneal dialysis or a transplant, should follow identification of the patient's basic personality type (are they independent?) and the availability of social supports.

Patients need to be adequately informed concerning the medical and psychologic problems that are associated with ESRD. Patients should be told that sleep disorders and diminished sexual interest, pleasure, and/or sexual ability are problematic and commonly associated with maintenance dialysis therapy. Although transplant patients experience improvement in sexual interest and function, many do not resume prerenal failure status. Staff are interested in hearing about patient concerns, whether these are physical, psychologic, spiritual, or existential. A patient who is informed previously that a sexual disorder may be a complication of treatment is more likely to seek the advice of staff members. Patients who understand that concentration or memory may be impacted by renal failure will be more able to seek help. Finally, family members who are educated about ESRD will also be less hesitant to seek assistance.

Use of Psychologically Active Medications

With the exception of lithium and barbiturates, virtually all psychotropic medications are fat soluble, pass the blood–brain barrier, and are broken down by the liver and removed in the bile. They may be used in patients with renal failure if attention is paid to dosage. A major factor connected with dosage is the diminished capacity of blood protein to bind drugs and the fact that psychotropic medications are largely protein bound. Pharmacologists recommend that the maximum dosage of a psychotropic agent be no greater than two-thirds of the maximum dose that one would give a patient with normal kidney function.

Many excellent medications can address problems of anxiety and/or depression. The chances of amelioration or cure of major depressive disorders by the use of antidepressants is about 75%. Although the greatest body of experience is with the tricyclics, the selective serotonin reuptake inhibitors (SSRIs) appear to be highly effective in this patient population. There is an unfortunate dearth of systematic research involving psychotropic medications and patients with impaired or absent renal function. Of the new generation of drugs, fluoxetine is the best studied. Neither its pharmacokinetics nor that of its major metabolite norfluoxetine are materially altered by the process of hemodialysis. Despite the cautionary warnings of the manufacturer, we have clinically observed that ordinary maintenance dosages are tolerated and necessary. This has also been our experience with the other SSRIs.

Benzodiazepines are a mainstay in the treatment of anxiety and have a very high therapeutic/toxic ratio. They are quite safe in this group of patients. On the other hand, nefazodone hydrochloride should be used with caution in patients who have chronically impaired renal function, and administration of bupropion hydrochloride and buspirone hydrochloride cannot be recommended.

Psychotherapy

Motivated individuals with psychologic problems should be considered for formal psychotherapy. This involves relating to a therapist, talking about problems, and working out practical solutions based on understanding the underpinnings of these problems. Depending on the circumstances, individual, family, couples, or group therapy may each offer benefits.

Talking therapies may have value for patients whose problems are connected with self-esteem and gender identity. Although anecdotal reports suggest a role for sildenafil (Viagra), many dialysis and transplant patients receive nitrates for coronary insufficiency and are not candidates for this medication. All patients experiencing sexual dysfunction should be considered for behavioral therapy. The best known form of this treatment was developed by Masters and Johnson and modified by Helen Singer Kaplan and others. These techniques encourage intimacy and do not necessarily aim at sexual intercourse as a goal. This is especially important because individuals experiencing sexual difficulties often withdraw from their partners and do not engage in the physical intimacies that can still be enjoyed.

Treatment of Maladaptive Behavior

Dangerous behavior should not be tolerated in dialysis programs. In all cases of aggressive behavior, an energetic attempt should be made to find the source or precipitant. In addition to limit setting and empathic responses, environmental maneuvers may at times be helpful or even curative. These include a change of dialysis hours, rearrangement of seating patterns to minimize interpatient conflict and patient–staff problems, and the setting of lesser expectations for those individuals who cannot adhere to particular medical regimens. Noncompliance or substance abuse can be addressed with greater leverage in patients who are seeking transplantation as preconditions for acceptance to the transplantation list. It is reasonable to set clearly defined expectations concerning attendance at dialysis, follow-through with counseling, and maintenance of sobriety.

End-of-Life Issues and Palliative Medicine

Considerable attention in nephrology is now focusing on end-of-life issues. There is renewed interest in this area throughout all of medicine, but it is especially pertinent to the dialysis population, which is aging and has multiple associated and progressive disorders, such as hypertension and diabetes. Despite all of the treatment advances, the adjusted annual mortality rate is greater than 20% for people who require dialysis. Nephrologists are being increasingly confronted with issues related to decisions to discontinue dialysis. Not surprisingly for such life-and-death decisions, it is essential that patient competency be assessed and, in the case of the demented, that trust be established between staff, family members, and designees or health care proxies. It is important to differentiate these decisions from ordinary suicide and to recognize that cessation of life support is sanctioned by most organized religions and a growing majority of the population.

Preliminary psychiatric studies suggest that most patients who decide to stop dialysis and die do not have active major depressions or past histories that are significant for psychiatric disorders, psychologic treatment, or suicide attempts. Interestingly, prospective studies have shown that some of these patients will change their minds and resume dialysis; they may also decide to finally terminate the treatment in the future. Psychiatric consultants can assume a beneficial role in these complex and difficult evaluations; in rare cases, their involvement is necessary for the direct treatment of individuals who have active psychiatric conditions.

There is also growing recognition that advances in palliative medicine, based on clinical experience with cancer or AIDS, should be applied to ESRD. Both the psychiatric and the pharmacologic aspects of symptom management, such as pain or nausea, need to be mastered. Future management protocols will likely incorporate symptom and quality of assessment tools to identify problems and focus attention on their treatment. Likewise, advanced and repeated discussions of end-of-life treatment preferences between patients, family members, and staff will likely become incorporated into clinic guidelines. Achievement of good deaths as well as good lives are worthy goals for nephrology; this will require a heightened appreciation of patient autonomy, sensitivity, flexibility, and psychologic sophistication.

Selected Readings

Blumenfield M, Levy NB, Spinowitz B, et al. Fluoxetine in depressed patients on dialysis. *Int J Psychiatry* 1997;27:71–80.

This is one of the few empirical drug studies of an antidepressant medication in this population.

Cohen LM. Renal disease. In: Rundell JR, Wise M, eds. *American Psychiatric Press textbook of consultation liaison psychiatry*. Washington, DC: American Psychiatric Press, 1996:573–578.

This is a recent review of the psychiatric aspects and complications of renal dialysis and transplantation.

Cohen LM, Fischel S, Germain M, et al. Ambivalence and dialysis discontinuation. *Gen Hosp Psychiatry* 1996;18:431–435.

Case reports and literature review suggesting that patients will often vacillate about this decision.

Cohen LM, McCue J, Germain M, et al. Dialysis discontinuation: a "good" death? *Arch Intern Med* 1995;155:42–47.

The first prospective study of this phenomenon. This pilot project has been replicated at seven sites in Canada and the United States, with the conclusion that the availability of palliative medicine interventions could improve the quality of dying of the ESRD population.

Devins GM, Binik YM, Hutchinson TA, et al. The emotional impact of end-stage renal disease: Importance of patient's perceptions of intrusiveness and control. *Int J Psychiatry Med* 1983–1984;13:327–343.

An examination of the patient's perspective of the different forms of dialytic treatment. Intrusiveness did not significantly differ with dialysis modality.

Gutman RA, Stead WW, Robinson RR. Physical activity and employment status of patients on maintenance dialysis. *N Engl J Med* 1981;304:309–313.

An excellent, large-scale study that pointed out the high frequency of the poor rehabilitative outcome in maintenance hemodialysis patients. Diabetic patients were noted to have especially marked problems. More recent statistics have not shown an improvement in this area.

Kjellstrand CM, Dossetor JB. *Ethical problems in dialysis and transplantation*. Boston: Kluwer Academic Publishers, 1992.

An erudite monograph on this subject.

Kramer L, Madl C, Stockenhuber F, et al. Beneficial effect of renal transplantation on cognitive brain function. *Kidney Int* 1996;49:833–838.

This study shows that in comparison to dialysis, renal transplantation patients have a marked improvement in cognitive functions.

Levy NB. Psychopharmacology in patients with renal failure. *Int J Psychiatry Med* 1990–1991;20:303–312.

A comprehensive review of pharmacokinetics, indications, and dosages of psychiatrically active medicines.

Levy NB, Cohen LM. End stage renal disease and its treatment: dialysis and transplantation. In: Stoudemire A, Fogel BS, Greenberg D, eds. *Psychiatric care of the medical patient*, 2nd ed. New York: Oxford University Press, 2000:791–799.

This is an overview of the field of psychonephrology.

Neu S, Kjellstrand CM. Stopping long-term dialysis: an empirical study of withdrawal of life supporting treatment. *N Engl J Med* 1986;314:14–20.

An important retrospective study that investigated the factors that entered into the decision to stop maintenance dialysis.

PART 2
Brain Abnormalities and Peripheral Neuropathy

Cosmo L. Fraser and Allen I. Arieff

One of the most common complications in patients with renal failure is nervous system dysfunctions. It is one of the most debilitating complications that contributes to the overall morbidity and mortality of patients with renal failure. Patients with renal failure often manifest a variety of neurologic disorders that can occur before, during, and after the initiation of adequate dialysis. Patients with chronic renal failure who are yet to begin dialysis may develop symptoms that could be as mild as sensorial clouding or as severe as coma and even death. Because of the use of routine blood work these days, patients are often picked up with renal disease before gross symptoms are evident. However, even after the initiation of adequate maintenance dialysis, patients may continue to manifest subtle nervous system dysfunction such as impaired mentation, generalized weakness, sexual dysfunction, and peripheral neuropathy. Hemodialysis itself has also been associated with distinct disorders of the central nervous system (CNS). These include dialysis disequilibrium syndrome, dialysis dementia, and progressive intellectual dysfunction. Dialysis disequilibrium syndrome occurs in a small number of patients and is a consequence of the initiation of dialysis. Dialysis dementia is a progressive and generally fatal encephalopathy that can affect patients receiving chronic hemodialysis as well as children with chronic renal failure who have not yet started dialysis. The incidence of dialysis dementia has decreased dramatically over the years because of improvements in the delivery of chronic hemodialysis. Progressive intellectual dysfunction and peripheral neuropathy may also occur in patients who are being treated with maintenance dialysis therapy.

UREMIC ENCEPHALOPATHY

The term *uremic encephalopathy* describes the central neurologic signs and symptoms that are manifested by patients with rapidly developing end-stage renal failure. Symptoms are usually seen when glomerular filtration rate falls below 10% of normal. These patients usually display variable disorders of consciousness that can affect psychomotor behavior, thinking, memory, speech, perception, and emotion (Table 69.1). The severity and rate of progression of symptoms varies directly with the rapidity with which renal failure develops. In patients with acute renal failure (ARF), neurologic symptoms are generally more severe and progress more rapidly than in patients with chronic renal failure. In progressive chronic renal failure, the number and severity of symptoms are quite variable, and symptoms may occur in a cyclic manner in that there are intervals of well-being in an otherwise inexorable downhill course.

Diagnosis

Uremic encephalopathy should be suspected in any patient with renal failure if there are clinical signs and symptoms consistent with CNS dysfunction. However, the presenting symptoms of uremic encephalopathy may be similar to those of many other types of metabolic encephalopathies, so there is always a risk of misdiagnosis. Uremic encephalopathy may also be difficult to diagnosis because patients with renal failure may also have other illnesses that can cause encephalopathy. In addition, if a patient with renal insufficiency is taking a drug with potential CNS toxicity that is excreted or metabolized by the kidney, the CNS symptoms could be caused either by the drug, which has reached toxic levels at ordinary dose rates, or by uremia, or a combination of both factors. It may also be difficult to differentiate whether the encephalopathy is due to hepatic or renal causes or both in patients with both advanced liver and renal diseases. In such patients, the blood urea nitrogen (BUN) and serum creatinine do not always adequately reflect the degree of renal function impairment.

TABLE 69.1. Clinical Manifestations of Uremia

Subtle
Anorexia Nausea Insomnia Restlessness Decreased attention span Inability to manage ideas Decreased sexual interest
Moderate
Vomiting Sluggishness Easy fatigue Drowsiness Sleep inversion Volatile emotions Paranoia Decreased cognitive function Inability to decipher abstractions Decreased sexual performance
Severe
Itching Disorientation Confusion Bizarre behavior Slurring of speech Hypothermia Myoclonus Asterixis Convulsions Stupor Coma

Clinical Manifestations

Mental status abnormalities are early signs and symptoms to indicate that a patient with renal failure may need to be started on dialysis (Table 69.1). Patients with ARF may present with signs of toxic psychosis, abnormal mental status, lassitude, lethargy, disorientation, and confusion. Physical findings may include cranial nerve signs, nystagmus, dysarthria, abnormal gait, and abnormalities of skeletal muscles manifested by weakness, fasciculations, and asymmetric variation in deep tendon reflexes. Later findings may include asterixis, hyperreflexia, and unsustained ankle clonus. If uremia is left untreated and allowed to progress, seizures, coma, and death will be certain.

Despite the fact that there are fairly characteristic electroencephalographic (EEG) patterns in patients with end-stage renal disease, the EEG is not used to make the diagnosis of renal failure. Patients who present with elevated BUN and creatinine and mental status changes do not require an EEG to make the diagnosis of uremic encephalopathy. EEGs in patients with ARF are generally grossly abnormal when the diagnosis of ARF is first made. In most instances, the percentage of EEG frequency less than either 5 Hz or 7 Hz and is 20 times greater than normal value. The abnormal percentages of EEG frequencies both above 9 Hz and below 5 Hz are not usually improved by dialysis within the first few weeks of treatment, although they may return to normal with recovery of renal function. If renal failure continues, the EEG may transiently worsen during and after hemodialysis, and this pattern may continue for up to 6 months after the initiation of dialytic therapy.

The neurologic manifestations of chronic renal failure are also numerous, and impairment of cognitive function is believed to be a major abnormality. These abnormalities include decreased attention span, speed of decision making, short-term memory, and mental manipulation of symbols. The EEG findings are usually not as severe as those reported in patients with ARF. In general, there is good correlation between the percentage of EEG frequencies and power below 7 Hz and the decline of renal function. After the initiation of dialysis, there may be an initial period of clinical stabilization of the patient, during which time the EEG continues to deteriorate. However, after approximately 6 months of adequate dialysis treatment, the EEG tends to normalize. Normal values may not be reached, however, unless the patient receives a transplanted kidney.

Pathogenesis

Parathyroid Hormone

Although many factors may contribute to uremic encephalopathy, there is no known precise correlation between the degree of encephalopathy and any of the commonly measured blood chemistries that are associated with renal dysfunction (e.g., BUN, creatinine, bicarbonate, pH). However, there is a substantial amount of evidence to suggest that parathyroid hormone (PTH) is a uremic neurotoxin.

In uremic animals, both the EEG and brain calcium abnormalities observed can be prevented by parathyroidectomy. Conversely, many of the CNS abnormalities observed in uremia can be reproduced by administration of PTH to normal animals. Similarly, in humans, PTH has been shown to produce CNS effects even in the absence of impaired renal function. Patients with either primary or secondary hyperparathyroidism have EEG changes that are similar to those observed in patients with ARF. In uremic patients, both the EEG changes and abnormalities of psychologic testing are improved by parathyroidectomy or medical suppression of PTH. Thus, based on current evidence, it appears that PTH is indeed a bonified uremic toxin.

Membrane Transporters in Uremia

Studies carried out in metabolically active brain synaptosomes have shown that both the Na^+-K^+-ATPase pump and the plasma membrane–bound calcium pumps are affected by uremia. The alterations of the function of the calcium pumps are believed to be due in part to the action of PTH acting through cyclic adenosine monophosphate (cAMP)-independent pathways, as well as to the uremic milieu. Because the calcium pumps at the nerve terminals (synaptosomes) mediate neurotransmitter release, their abnormal function in uremia may result in impairment of the processing of information in the uremic state. The basal levels of cytosolic calcium of brain synaptosomes is elevated significantly. This effect is also mediated by PTH.

COMPLICATIONS OF DIALYSIS THERAPY

Dialysis Dementia

Dialysis dementia is a progressive, often fatal neurologic disease that is seen almost exclusively in patients who are being treated for chronic hemodialysis. Although early studies focused on the distinctive neurologic findings of this disorder, later reports have suggested that some forms of dialysis dementia may be part of a multisystem disease that includes dementia, osteomalacic bone disease, proximal myopathy, and anemia.

The etiology of dialysis dementia remains controversial, but it most likely represents a symptom complex that is the final common pathway for a variety of abnormal metabolic processes resulting from long-term hemodialysis. Dialysis dementia can be subdivided into three groups (Table 69.2). These include an epidemic form, an endemic form, and dementia associated with childhood renal disease. Initial reports of dialysis dementia were all of the endemic form, which occurred in patients who had been receiving chronic hemodialysis for more than 2 years. The most common initial symptoms are dysarthria, apraxia, slurring of speech, stuttering, and hesitancy. As the disease progresses, symptoms also progress to include personality changes, psychosis, myoclonus, seizures, and eventually dementia and death within 6 months of the onset of symptoms.

TABLE 69.2. Neurologic Manifestations of Uremia

Uremic encephalopathy	Acute central nervous system signs and symptoms of uremia Asterixis usually present Indication to initiate dialysis
Dialysis disequilibrium syndrome	Idiogenic osmoles result in brain to plasma osmolar gradient Caused by aggressive initial hemodialysis treatments
Dialysis dementia	Epidemic, endemic, and childhood forms Aluminum associated with epidemic form Frequently fatal Prevented by deionization of dialysis water and restriction of oral aluminum
Intellectual function	Generally impaired
Peripheral neuropathy	Motor and sensory impairment
Autonomic dysfunction	Postural hypotension, impaired sweating, gastrointestinal disturbances, impotence

Early in dialysis dementia, the EEG shows multifocal bursts of high-amplitude delta activity with spikes and sharp waves, intermixed with runs of more normal-appearing background activity. These EEG changes may precede overt clinical symptoms by up to 6 months. However, as the disease progresses, the normal background activity of the EEG will deteriorate to a predominance of slow frequencies. With the appropriate clinical symptoms, this EEG pattern is pathognomonic of dialysis dementia; however, these EEG patterns by themselves may be seen in other metabolic encephalopathies. Because there are no specific markers for dialysis dementia, the diagnosis depends on the presence of the typical clinical picture, the characteristic EEG findings, and most importantly, exclusion of other causes of dementia.

Role of Aluminum in Dialysis Dementia

Aluminum intoxication was implicated in this disorder when it was observed to be markedly elevated in brain gray matter in patients with dialysis dementia. Aluminum content in brain is also more than threefold greater in patients with dialysis dementia than in those receiving chronic hemodialysis who do not have dementia. The reasons for the increased brain aluminum remain controversial, although the actual source of the aluminum is quite evident. Aluminum is the second most common element in the earth's crust, and in the United States, the typical dietary intake of aluminum is 10 to 100 mg/day. This aluminum intake is substantially greater in individuals who are taking aluminum-containing antacids. Normally, only a small amount of orally administered aluminum is absorbed, but for unknown reasons, absorption appears to be increased in patients with renal failure. Before the routine deionization of the water used in dialysis, most of the aluminum in dialysis patients came from the water. Because aluminum is normally excreted by the kidney, renal failure leads to aluminum retention in such patients. Thus the problem is not where the aluminum comes from, but rather how it gets into the brain and how it causes dementia. In dialysis dementia, abnormalities of the blood–brain barrier may play some role in the entry of aluminum into brain.

Elevated brain aluminum levels are also present in several other groups of patients who are not demented, including patients with ARF, hepatic encephalopathy, and metastatic cancer, as well as individuals who are older than 60 years of age. However, the levels of aluminum are generally lower than that observed in dialysis dementia patients. In patients with dialysis dementia, aluminum appears to be important in the development of the epidemic form; however, whether aluminum plays an important role in the other types of dialysis dementia (endemic, childhood) is still unresolved. The water used to prepare dialysate is now deionized as a preventive measure to reduce aluminum concentration in dialysate fluid. However, deionization removes not only aluminum from the water but also other ions as well (cadmium, mercury, lead, manganese, copper, nickel, thallium, boron, and tin).

Despite these unresolved questions, most outbreaks of the epidemic form of dialysis dementia have been associated with high levels of aluminum in the dialysate. Thus therapy has been directed toward removing aluminum not only from the dialysate but orally as well. Lowering the dialysate aluminum levels to less than 20 μg/L by deionization and reverse osmosis appears to be beneficial for patients who are starting dialysis. In patients with overt disease, eliminating the source of aluminum has only rarely resulted in improvement. Diazepam or clonazepam appear to be useful in controlling initial seizure activity associated with the disease; however, they usually become ineffective later in the course of the disease and do not appear to alter the usually fatal outcome. Improvement in symptoms has recently been reported in several patients treated with deferoxamine, which chelates serum aluminum and reduces tissue burden of aluminum. However, it has been suggested that deferoxamine without diazepam may worsen symptoms of dementia because it promotes aluminum removal from other tissues, which may in turn facilitate brain deposition.

Deferoxamine is also associated with a number of side effects, including fatal fungal mucormycosis in approximately 10% of treated dialysis patients, cataracts, retinal changes, and thrombocytopenia. In general, it appears that the removal of aluminum from dialysate water largely prevents the occurrence of dialysis dementia (epidemic form); however, removal of aluminum from dialysate in patients with established dialysis dementia has not been as helpful. Treatment of sporadic cases, in which the etiology of the encephalopathy is unclear, is more difficult. In this instance, it is most important to differentiate dialysis dementia from other metabolic encephalopathies and from structural lesions such as strokes and intracerebral hemorrhages.

Finally, dialysis dementia has also been reported in several children with renal failure, many of who were not yet receiving dialysis while some were exposed to aluminum-containing compounds. Therefore the cause of encephalopathy in such children cannot be ascribed to aluminum alone and may represent developmental neurologic defects resulting from exposure of the growing brain to a uremic environment. However, dementia did develop in many predialysis patients who were taking aluminum hydroxide phosphate binders. Additional discussion on the toxicity of aluminum in uremia and dialysis patients is found in Chapter 67, Part 5.

Dialysis Disequilibrium Syndrome

Dialysis disequilibrium syndrome is a clinical disorder that occurs exclusively in patients who are being treated with hemodialysis. The syndrome was first characterized in the early 1960s, and symptoms may include headache, nausea, emesis, blurring of vision, muscular twitching, disorientation, hypertension, tremors, seizures, muscle cramps, anorexia, restlessness, and dizziness. Although dialysis disequilibrium syndrome has been reported among all age groups, it is more common among younger patients, particularly the pediatric age group. Dialysis disequilibrium syndrome is one of several CNS abnormalities that may occur in patients with chronic renal failure. It is most often associated with rapid hemodialysis of patients who have recently started hemodialysis. Symptoms may also occur but are far less common after maintenance hemodialysis for up to 6 months. The incidence of dialysis disequilibrium syndrome is very high among patients with preexisting neurologic disease, such as head trauma, recent stroke, or malignant hypertension.

Symptoms of Dialysis Disequilibrium Syndrome

Mild forms of dialysis disequilibrium may be manifested by no more than restlessness and severe headache, which may occur during or soon after hemodialysis. This is commonly followed by nausea, vomiting, and blood pressure elevation. These symptoms may be accompanied by disorientation and tremors. Seizures and cardiac arrhythmias have been reported in the older literature but are uncommon today. The symptoms are usually self-limited, but recovery may take several days. In severe cases, patients may develop seizures and coma. The symptoms of dialysis disequilibrium syndrome reported since about 1970 have generally been milder than previous reports. These usually consists of nausea, weakness, headache, fatigue, and muscle cramps. These milder symptoms are probably due to the greatly improved management of patients with renal failure undergoing hemodialysis. It is unclear whether any patient actually died from dialysis disequilibrium syndrome or rather from associated neurologic complications such as acute stroke, subdural hematoma, subarachnoid hemorrhage, head trauma, or malignant hypertension. Recently, the diagnosis of dialysis disequilibrium syndrome has become a "wastebasket" for a number of disorders that can occur in patients with renal failure and may affect the CNS. It should be stressed that the diagnosis of dialysis disequilibrium syndrome should be one of exclusion.

Pathogenesis of Dialysis Disequilibrium Syndrome

Early clinical investigation in patients with dialysis disequilibrium syndrome included evaluation of pressure and composition of the cerebrospinal fluid (CSF). In patients with dialysis disequilibrium syndrome, findings included a persistent elevation of CSF pressure and levels of urea that were higher in CSF than in blood. These findings led to the early speculation that cerebral edema was responsible for most of the manifestations of dialysis disequilibrium syndrome. Based on subsequent evidence, it is now clear that many of the clinical manifestations of dialysis disequilibrium syndrome are in fact due largely to brain swelling, which occurs as a consequence of the dialysis procedure. Brain edema has been confirmed both at autopsy and by computed tomographic (CT) scanning in humans with renal failure who have undergone dialysis.

Reverse Urea Effect. The presence of brain edema in some patients with dialysis disequilibrium syndrome, along with the observation that in patients undergoing rapid hemodialysis, urea levels are higher in CSF than in blood led to formulation of the "reverse urea" hypothesis. In general, the reverse urea effect assumes that concentrations of urea are similar in plasma, CSF, and brain tissue water. With rapid hemodialysis, it was assumed that clearance of urea would be more rapid from plasma than from brain tissue. This assumption was based on the observation that urea was cleared more slowly from the CSF than from plasma in patients who were undergoing rapid hemodialysis. This decrement of plasma urea leads to a fall in plasma osmolality relative to the CSF. It was postulated that, with a slower clearance of urea from brain, the osmolality of brain tissue remained elevated above that of plasma, and this led to a net movement of water from plasma into brain, the result of which is cerebral edema. However, the reverse urea hypothesis has not been supported experimentally. In both uremic patients and animals subjected to rapid hemodialysis, urea levels in CSF are consistently higher than those of plasma. However, there appears to be no significant difference between urea concentrations in the plasma and brain. As originally described, urea levels after hemodialysis are higher in CSF than in plasma. However, the elevated urea levels in CSF do not reflect brain tissue levels and are probably a function both of the small surface area available for exchange of CSF with blood and the "sink" action of the CSF.

Role of Brain Intracellular pH in the Pathogenesis of Dialysis Disequilibrium Syndrome. To understand how changes of brain intracellular pH (pHi) could play a role in the pathogenesis of dialysis disequilibrium syndrome, it is first necessary to briefly review certain aspects of brain acid–base regulation. Intracellular acid–base status has been extensively evaluated in both uremic humans and animal models of acute and chronic renal failure. Currently, the gold standard for measurement of brain pHi is by magnetic resonance spectroscopy (MRS), a noninvasive technique suitable for repeated measurements in the same animal. Although there were certain theoretical problems with the older DMO method, the values for brain pHi are very similar to those obtained using the newer MRS technique. In animals with ARF and metabolic acidosis, the pHi in brain and skeletal muscle is normal. In patients with chronic renal failure, pHi has been reported to be normal in skeletal muscle, leukocytes, and the "whole body." In dogs with chronic renal failure, despite a metabolic acidosis, the pHi is normal in several different parts of the brain, as well as in the liver and skeletal muscle. The pH of CSF has also been shown to be normal in both patients and laboratory animals with renal failure. Thus, in uremic animals and humans, the intracellular buffering capacity of brain, muscle, and other tissues is capable of maintaining pHi in the normal range despite the presence of extracellular metabolic acidosis.

In dogs with ARF, pHi is normal in brain and skeletal muscle. However, after rapid hemodialysis, there is no change in the pHi of muscle, but a significant decrement is observed in the pHi of both CSF and cerebral cortical gray matter. The increased H + ion activity in the brain is accompanied by an increase of brain osmole content, which secondarily results in an increase of brain water. The cerebral edema that occurs is probably an important cause of the clinical manifestations of dialysis disequilibrium syndrome. The source of the increased brain H^+ ion is not known. Cerebral hypoxia is an unlikely source for the CSF H^+ ion, as the Po_2 in CSF and brain is normal in both CSF and brain. Furthermore, cerebral hypoxia would lead to increased brain lactate, and such a phenomenon does not occur. In uremia, brain and CSF lactate levels are normal. It is theoretically possible that hemodialysis could lead to increased oxygen–hemoglobin binding as a result of increased blood pH and decreased red blood cell 2,3-diphosphoglycerate. The red cell levels of 2,3-diphosphoglycerate are lower than normal in chronic hemodialysis patients. Following hemodialysis, there is a decrease in the *in vivo* P_{50}, which impairs tissue oxygen delivery. However, most chronic dialysis patients are able to increase their cardiac output, which would serve to increase oxygen delivery back to normal. Thus dialysis-induced alterations of red cell 2,3-diphosphoglycerate with subsequent hypoxia are unlikely to contribute to CSF acidosis.

Dialysis Disequilibrium Syndrome

The management of dialysis disequilibrium syndrome can be divided into preventative modalities and therapeutic maneuvers. In general, symptoms of dialysis disequilibrium syndrome are treated by adding an osmotically active solute (glycerol, albumin, NaCl, mannitol) to the dialysate or by substituting sodium bicarbonate for sodium lactate (or acetate) in the dialysate. The technique of hemofiltration is now in common use. When this technique is used, the patient is subjected to ultrafiltration without dialysis, with the net result a loss of fluid without the patient undergoing dialysis. This procedure can then be followed by conventional dialysis without ultrafiltration. With the use of hemofiltration followed by dialysis, the incidence of dialysis disequilibrium syndrome is substantially reduced. The reason for the reduction in symptoms by this procedure is presently unknown but may be due to the reduced dialysis time because fluid is removed before the initiation of hemodialysis. Chronic ambulatory peritoneal dialysis (CAPD) is currently in use worldwide. When this technique is used, patients undergo continuous low-volume peritoneal dialysis with incremental removal of solutes per unit time. To date, there have been no reports of dialysis disequilibrium syndrome occurring in patients receiving CAPD. Thus, in both humans and experimental animals, the occurrence of dialysis disequilibrium syndrome can best be prevented either by use of "slow" dialysis (i.e., low blood flow rates at frequent intervals), by a combination of hemofiltration followed by conventional slow hemodialysis, or by peritoneal dialysis. Patients with certain preexisting neurologic conditions, particularly intracranial lesions (head trauma, recent stroke, brain tumor, subdural hematoma) or conditions characterized by cerebral edema (hyponatremia, hepatic encephalopathy, malignant hypertension) are at particular risk for the development of dialysis disequilibrium syndrome.

INTELLECTUAL FUNCTION

The impairment of intellectual function is another commonly recognized complication in many patients with chronic renal failure who are being treated with dialysis. However, the syndrome is not well defined, and there is no anatomic lesion that can be correlated with intellectual deterioration, nor are there any associated neurologic abnormalities. The methods of assessing intellectual function include the full Wescher Adult Intelligence Scale, the Walton-Black Modified Word Learning Test, and the Block Design Learning Test. Although some studies suggest that the overall intellectual level in chronic renal failure patients does not differ significantly from normal, others have suggested that the Wescher Adult Intelligence Scale full-scale IQ in dialysis patients is below that of the general population. Based on psychologic testing, the consensus is that chronic renal failure is often associated with organiclike loss of intellectual function.

PERIPHERAL NEUROPATHY IN UREMIA

There are two broad categories of peripheral neuropathy associated with uremia, and these are described in terms of their pattern of neuronal involvement. The first is bilaterally symmetric disturbance of nerve function, often designated as *polyneuropathies*. Polyneuropathy is said to be associated with toxic substances; metabolic disorders such as uremia, diabetes, and deficiency states; and certain immune reactions that diffusely affect the peripheral nervous system. The second pattern consists of isolated or multiple isolated lesions of the peripheral nerves and is termed *mononeuropathy*. In severe symmetric polyneuropathies, a generalized loss of peripheral nerve function may occur, and the impairment is usually worse distally. It is characterized as a mixed motor and sensory polyneuropathy with a distal distribution. It often results in weakness and muscle wasting of the arms and legs. There may also be distal sensory changes of a "glove and stocking" distribution associated with this type of neuropathy. Motor nerve conduction velocity was once frequently used to assess peripheral neuropathy; however, the test is somewhat unreliable in uremia because the procedure itself has a normal daily variation of up to 20%. Thus motor nerve conduction velocity has very limited utility in detecting moderately impaired peripheral nerve function. Although sensory nerve conduction velocity is more sensitive than motor nerve conduction velocity, the procedure is not routinely performed because it is so painful.

Neuropathy of some degree is present in about 65% of patients with end-stage renal disease who are receiving dialysis. When the glomerular filtration rate is greater than approximately 10% of normal, peripheral neuropathy is fairly uncommon. Many asymptomatic patients with chronic renal failure have autonomic neuropathy on physical examination, which can be manifested as impotence and postural hypotension. Moreover, abnormal nerve conduction may be present in the absence of symptoms or physical findings.

In summary, uremic neuropathy is a distal, symmetric, mixed polyneuropathy that belongs to a group known as *dying-back polyneuropathies* or *central-peripheral axonopathies,* the etiology of which includes toxic insults due to diabetes, amyloidosis, multiple myeloma, and hereditary polyneuropathies, in addition to uremia. Uremic neuropathy is also associated with a secondary demyelinating process in the posterior columns of the spinal cord and CNS. Motor and sensory modalities are both generally affected, and lower extremities are more severely involved than are the upper extremities. Clinically, uremic neuropathy cannot easily be distinguished from the neuropathies associated with diabetes mellitus, chronic alcoholism, and other deficiency states. The occurrence of uremic neuropathy bears no relationship to the type of the underlying kidney disease. However, certain diseases that can lead to renal failure may simultaneously affect peripheral nerve function separately from the manifestations of uremia. Such diseases include amyloidosis, multiple myeloma, systemic lupus erythematosus, polyarteritis nodosa, diabetes mellitus, and hepatic failure.

Clinical Manifestations

The restless leg syndrome is a common early manifestation of chronic renal failure. Clinically, patients experience crawling sensations, prickling, and pruritus in their lower extremities. The sensations are generally worse distally and are usually more prominent in the evening. The burning foot syndrome, which is present in fewer than 10% of patients with chronic renal failure, actually represents swelling and tenderness of the distal lower extremities. The physical signs of peripheral nerve dysfunction often begin with loss of deep tendon reflexes, particularly in the knee and ankle. There is also impaired vibratory sensation and loss of sensation in the lower leg in the from of "stocking glove" anesthesia. Affected patients usually experience diminished sensations of pain, light touch, vibration, and pressure.

Uremic Toxins as Causes of Neuropathy

A number of potential uremic toxins might lead to symptoms. Although any or all of these agents may play a role in the development of uremic neuropathy, the evidence that any one of them are true "neurotoxins" is scant. "Middle molecules" (molecular weights of 500 to 2,500 D), once believed to be uremic toxins, have not stood the test of time. Of the several other potential "uremic toxins" that have been suggested, PTH has received much of the attention. Suggestions that PTH may be a uremic neurotoxin are based on studies that showed a correlation between plasma PTH levels and motor nerve conduction velocity in patients and animals with chronic renal failure. However, in patients with hyperparathyroidism without uremia, there is no consistent effect of PTH on peripheral nerve function. At present, no single uremic toxin has been shown to affect peripheral nerve function in a consistent manner. Most of the present evidence suggests that uremic neuropathy may be related to anatomic nerve damage or to cumulative effects of multiple toxic agents, which usually takes months to years to develop.

Selected Readings

Andreoli SP, Bergstein JM, Sherrard DJ. Aluminum Intoxication from aluminum containing phosphate binders in children with azotemia not undergoing dialysis. *N Engl J Med* 1984;310:1079–1084.

An excellent article showing that young children with renal failure who are taking aluminum containing phosphate binders can develop dementia. Evidence to implicate aluminum as an etiologic factor in dialysis dementia and that dialysis may not be a requirement in this disorder.

Arieff AI, Massry SG. Calcium metabolism of brain in acute renal failure: effects of uremia, hemodialysis and parathyroid hormone. *J Clin Invest* 1974;53:387–392.

This paper shows the effect that PTH has on brain intracellular calcium. The increased brain calcium seen in acute uremia was reversed by prior parathyroidectomy of uremic animals and reproduced by administering PTH to normal animals.

Fraser CL, Arieff AI. Nervous system complications in uremia. *Ann Intern Med* 1988;109:143–153.

An excellent review of the neurologic manifestations of renal failure and uremia. It contains descriptions of dialysis disequilibrium syndrome, dialysis dementia, and intellectual function impairment associated with renal failure. Extensive discussions of the roles of PTH and aluminum in the pathogenesis of uremic encephalopathy.

Fraser CL, Arieff AI. Nervous system manifestations of renal failure. In: Schrier RW, Gottschalk CW, eds. *Diseases of the kidney,* 5th ed. Boston: Little, Brown, 1993;2789–2816.

In-depth and most current review of the neurologic manifestations of uremia. Exhaustive bibliography on the subject matter. Extensive discussions of complications of dialysis therapy and of the roles of PTH and aluminum in the pathogenesis of uremic encephalopathy.

Olivieri NF, Bungig RJ, Chew E, et al. Visual and auditory neurotoxicity in patients receiving subcutaneous deferoxamine infusions. *N Engl J Med* 1986;314:869–873.

This paper describes complications that can develop in dialysis patients who are receiving deferoxamine infusion for iron overload. Because of the possibility of the development of visual and auditory neurotoxicity, deferoxamine should be administered only when absolutely indicated and while the patient's clinical condition is being carefully monitored.

Prior JC, Cameron EC, Knickerbocker WJ, et al. Dialysis encephalopathy and osteomalacic bone disease. *Am J Med* 1982;72:33–42.

This paper shows that patients with dialysis encephalopathy had more rib fractures than dialysis patients without encephalopathy, suggesting a common etiology for the two disorders.

Rotundo A, Nevins TE, Lipton M, et al. Progressive encephalopathy in children with chronic renal insufficiency in infancy. *Kidney Int* 1982;21:486–491.

This paper shows that 20 of 23 infants with renal failure during the first year of life developed profound neurologic abnormalities. No patients were dialyzed and four had not received aluminum salts prior to the development of symptoms. This suggests that the developing brain may be more susceptible to the development of encephalopathy than are the brains of adults. These data also put into question the role of aluminum and dialysis as etiologic causes of chronic uremic encephalopathy.

PART 3
Autonomic Nervous System

Vito M. Campese, Adina Tanasescu, and Shaul G. Massry

Patients with chronic renal failure often display a variety of disturbances in the function of the autonomic nervous system (ANS) (Table 69.3). Some patients display a decrease in the number of functioning eccrine sweat glands and a reduction in the volume of sweat and its chloride concentration. Other patients manifest reduced baroreceptor sensitivity, which may result in paroxysmal hypertension, postural hypotension, persistent hypotension, and hypotensive episodes during hemodialysis unresponsive to volume repletion. Autonomic dysfunction may also be responsible for dysfunction of gastrointestinal motility, impotence, and abnormal circadian variations of blood pressure with

TABLE 69.3. Clinical Manifestations of Autonomic Nervous System Dysfunction in Uremia

Defective sweat gland function
Reduced baroreceptor sensitivity
Orthostatic hypotension
Persistent hypotension
Nonvolume-responsive hypotension during dialysis
Abnormal circadian patterns of blood pressure
Reduced pressure response to vasoconstrictor agonists
Impotence
Arrhythmias
Dysfunction of gastrointestinal motility

a reduced fall of blood pressure during the night. Certain evidence also indicates that ANS dysfunction may increase the risk for significant arrhythmias and sudden death. In all, abnormalities of the ANS may play an important role in the morbidity and mortality of patients with end-stage renal disease.

PATHOGENESIS

The pathogenesis of ANS dysfunction in uremia is complex and most likely multifactorial. Careful studies have ruled out a role for the state of chronic illness in the genesis of these abnormalities. Studies in our laboratory have also excluded an important role of anemia in the genesis of these abnormalities, as no difference in the degree of anemia was observed between uremic patients with normal and those with reduced Valsalva ratio. In addition, patients with anemia from other chronic illnesses usually do not manifest abnormalities of the ANS. However, newer evidence indicates that improvement of anemia after treatment with erythropoietin may result in partial or total regression of several clinical manifestations of autonomic dysfunction. The "uremic state" has been implicated to be toxic for the central and peripheral nervous systems. Among the uremic "toxins," parathyroid hormone (PTH) may play a role in the genesis of ANS dysfunction in patients with end-stage renal disease.

Lesions of several segments of the baroreceptor reflex arc have been described in uremic patients. These include reduced baroreceptor sensitivity, alterations of central integrative structures of the ANS, alterations of both the efferent sympathetic and parasympathetic pathways, and reduced end-organ response to vasopressor agonists.

BARORECEPTOR DYSFUNCTION

Functional derangement of both the low- and high-pressure baroreceptors have been described in uremic patients. First, uremic patients display a blunted heart rate response to changes in blood pressure induced by phenylephrine, norepinephrine, or angiotensin II. The slope of the line relating R-R intervals to systolic blood pressure during infusion of angiotensin II is lower in dialysis patients than in normal subjects. Second, the heart rate does not change in uremic patients in response to occlusion of the arteriovenous fistula, a maneuver that acutely lowers cardiac output. Third, the heart rate response to inhalation of amyl nitrate, a peripheral vasodilator with direct action on vascular smooth muscle cells, is blunted in many uremic patients. Finally, the blood pressure overshoot and bradycardia that normally occur during the release phase of the Valsalva maneuver are blunted or absent in many uremic patients.

The heart rate response to the Valsalva maneuver has been used by many investigators to evaluate the overall function of

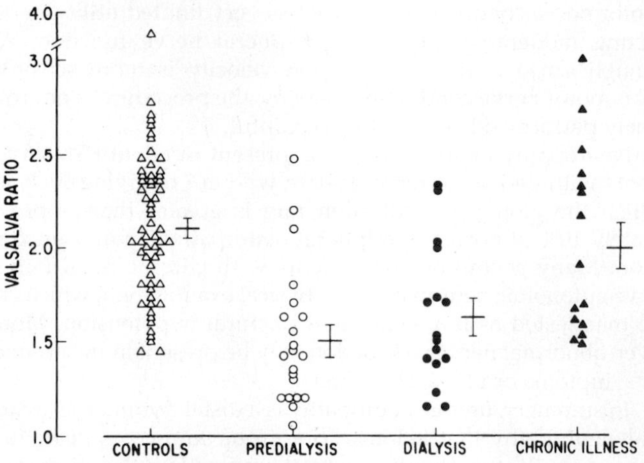

Figure 69.1. The Valsalva ratio (i.e., the ratio between the longest R-R interval during the release phase and the shortest R-R interval during the strain phase of the Valsalva maneuver) in 60 normal subjects, 21 uremic nondialysis patients (predialysis), 16 patients receiving maintenance hemodialysis therapy, and 15 patients with chronic illnesses but with normal renal function. The *bars* denote mean ± SE. (Reproduced with permission from Campese VM, Romoff MS, Levitan D, et al. Mechanisms of autonomic nervous system dysfunction in uremia. *Kidney Int* 1981;20:246–253.)

the baroreceptor reflex arc. The Valsalva ratio is defined as the ratio between the longest R-R interval during the release phase and the shortest R-R interval during the strain phase of the Valsalva maneuver. We have observed a reduced ratio in approximately 50% of patients with end-stage renal disease, whether receiving maintenance hemodialysis or not (Fig. 69.1). The abnormality in the Valsalva ratio is mainly due to smaller decrements in heart rate during the release phase of the Valsalva maneuver (Fig. 69.2) and is more pronounced in uremic

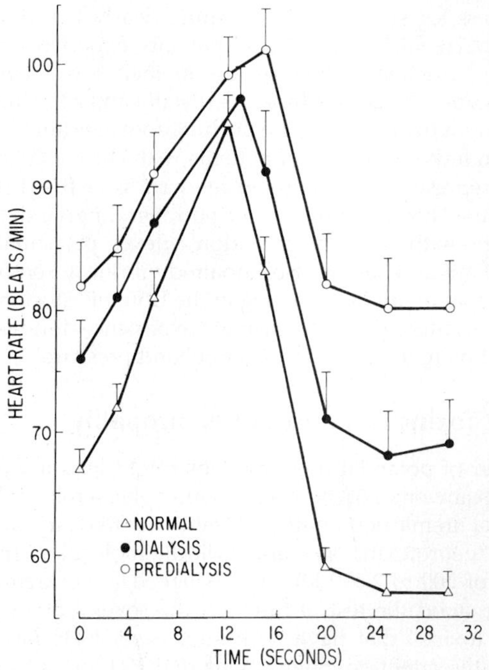

Figure 69.2. Heart rate before and during the Valsalva maneuver in normal subjects and predialysis and dialysis patients. During the release phase, heart rate was significantly lower in normal subjects than in the two groups of uremic patients ($P < .01$) and lower in dialysis than in uremic predialysis patients ($P < .05$). Data are presented as mean ± SE. (Reproduced with permission from Campese VM, Romoff MS, Levitan D, et al. Mechanisms of autonomic nervous system dysfunction in uremia. *Kidney Int* 1981;20: 246–253.)

patients not treated with dialysis than in those receiving maintenance hemodialysis. It must be pointed out, however, that the Valsalva maneuver is a complex test that involves the function of several integrative structures of the baroreceptor reflex arc. Thus a reduction in the heart rate response during this maneuver could be the result of reduced baroreceptor sensitivity, failure of blood pressure to rise during the release phase due to inappropriate changes in peripheral vascular resistance, or a derangement of the parasympathetic efferent pathway.

EFFERENT PARASYMPATHETIC FUNCTION

Several studies point to functional abnormalities of the parasympathetic nervous system in uremia. All the abnormalities in heart rate response to baroreceptor stimulations described previously could be the result either of reduced baroreceptor sensitivity or of impaired efferent parasympathetic discharge.

The beat-to-beat variation of heart rate during inspiration is impaired in uremic patients. The R-R interval variability contains two components: a high-frequency component (greater than 0.15 Hz) that reflects parasympathetic control and can be inhibited by atropine and a low-frequency component (0.04 to 0.15 Hz) that reflects sympathetic and parasympathetic function and can be inhibited by atropine and propranolol. The ratio of the low- and high-frequency components has been proposed as an index of sympathetic nervous system function. In uremic patients, a reduction in the heart rate power spectrum was observed in all frequency ranges, including those mediated by the sympathetic nervous system and those mediated by the parasympathetic nervous system. Another test used to measure parasympathetic activity is the diving test. During immersion of the face in water, trigeminal nerve receptors of the face are stimulated, resulting in apnea and sinus bradycardia. The bradycardia occurring during this test is reduced in many uremic patients.

EFFERENT SYMPATHETIC PATHWAY

Controversy exists regarding the activity of the efferent sympathetic pathways in uremic patients. Evidence for increased or decreased activity is available. Part of the confusion derives from the limitations of the methods used to determine the activity of the sympathetic nervous system and/or from the belief that these derangements are uniform in all uremic patients and in all districts. Most studies have relied on indirect indices of sympathetic nervous system activity, such as blood pressure response to cold pressor test and hand-grip exercise, or biochemical markers, such as plasma concentrations of catecholamines or of dopamine-β-hydroxylase (DBH).

The blood pressure response to the cold-pressor test is usually normal, whereas the heart rate and blood pressure response to hand-grip exercise are often impaired in uremic patients. The changes in heart rate occurring during hand-grip exercise appear to be due to parasympathetic inhibition (vagus release), whereas the rise in blood pressure appears to be mediated by an increase in systemic vascular resistance secondary to sympathetic nervous system activation. Thus the abnormal heart rate response during hand-grip exercise described in uremic patients points to a disturbance of the parasympathetic pathway, whereas the abnormal pressor response suggests a disturbance in the efferent sympathetic pathways. The reasons for the discrepancy between the findings with the cold-pressor test and those with the hand-grip exercise are not clear. It is possible that the disturbance in blood pressure response during the hand-grip exercise is due to derangements of the afferent rather than the efferent pathways of this reflex.

Measurements of plasma norepinephrine (NE) levels have been extensively used to determine sympathetic nervous system activity in patients with renal failure. Plasma NE levels are usually normal in patients with mild renal insufficiency but are commonly increased in patients with advanced renal failure. In predialysis patients with renal failure, baseline levels of NE measured in the supine position are almost universally raised. When these patients assume the upright posture, there is an almost threefold increase in plasma NE levels, a change significantly greater than that observed in normal subjects. By contrast, plasma NE levels are usually normal both during supine and upright posture in patients receiving maintenance hemodialysis.

However, when plasma NE levels are corrected for methylation index, they are usually elevated even in patients receiving maintenance hemodialysis. During regular hemodialysis, plasma levels of NE usually do not increase in response to volume depletion with ultrafiltration. During hemofiltration, however, plasma levels of NE increase in response to volume depletion. This difference may partly explain the lower incidence of hypotensive episodes during hemofiltration compared with hemodialysis.

The significance of increased plasma concentrations of NE in uremic patients is uncertain, and it does not necessarily indicate increased sympathetic nervous system activity. In fact, the amount of NE reaching the blood is only a fraction (perhaps 10% to 20%) of the total amount released into the synaptic clefts and the concentration in the blood is not only a reflection of the amount released, but also of NE turnover, reuptake, spillover to plasma, and metabolism.

Experimental evidence suggests that profound abnormalities in the synthesis and metabolism of NE may be present in uremia, pointing to decreased activity of the system. The activity of thyrosine hydroxylase, the rate-limiting enzyme of NE synthesis, was found to be significantly reduced in myocardial homogenates and brain synaptosomes of uremic rats. DBH, the enzyme that catalyses the conversion of dopamine to NE, was significantly lower in dialysis patients than in normal subjects. This enzyme is stored along with NE in the secretory granules of the terminal varicosities of the sympathetic nerves. During depolarization, both NE and DBH are released into the synaptic space, but there is no reuptake for DBH. For this reason, the plasma levels of DBH have been considered a marker of the tonic activity of the sympathetic nervous system.

A depletion of catecholamine stores has been shown in the parotid glands of uremic patients and in the brain of uremic rats. In our laboratory, we have shown a decrease in the content, release, and reuptake of NE in brain synaptosomes isolated from the cerebral cortex of rats with 5/6 nephrectomy. These derangements are due to the secondary hyperparathyroidism of uremia. Evidence from our laboratory, however, also suggests that the turnover rate of NE in the posterior hypothalamic nuclei and locus ceruleus of uremic rats was significantly faster than in control rats. Inhibition of NE synthesis in the posterior hypothalamus by 6-hydroxy dopamine, caused a significant decrease in blood pressure, whereas injection of the vehicle caused no changes. The turnover rate of NE in the anterior and lateral hypothalamus and in the nucleus tractus solitarius did not differ between uremic and control rats.

These studies demonstrate the presence of increased efferent sympathetic nerve discharge from these brain nuclei to the cardiovascular system, and such an event may play a role in the pathogenesis of hypertension in uremia.

The studies on degradation and clearance of NE in uremia are conflicting and inconclusive. On one hand, some investigators have shown diminished degradation of NE secondary to reduced catechol-*O*-methyl transferase activity or to diminished reuptake from the sympathetic neuron end terminals, suggesting that decreased degradation and/or disposition of NE may contribute to the increase in plasma levels. On the other hand, metabolic turnover studies performed by two-step steady-state cold NE infusion have shown an increase in the appearance rate and clearance rate in patients on maintenance hemodialysis when compared with normal subjects, suggesting an increase in sympathetic nervous system activity. However, kinetic studies with cold NE are not reliable because they require the administration of doses of NE large enough to cause hemodynamic changes and to interfere with NE release and disposition. The increased clearance of NE in uremic patients has been attributed to increased transhepatic extraction and metabolism secondary to high cardiac output.

Direct microelectrode recordings of postganglionic sympathetic action potentials in peroneal nerves of chronic hemodialysis patients with and without bilateral nephrectomy have shown that the rate of sympathetic nerve discharge was much higher in dialysis patients with their native kidneys than in those who had undergone bilateral nephrectomy or in control subjects. In both groups of uremic patients, plasma NE levels varied widely and no correlation was found between plasma NE levels and sympathetic nerve discharge in the peroneal nerves. In patients with bilateral nephrectomy, the decrease in mean arterial pressure was associated with lower sympathetic nerve firing and regional vascular resistance. These findings support the notion that increased afferent nervous input from the kidney to the central nervous system may play a role in the pathogenesis of hypertension in uremic patients. This notion is supported by experiments performed in our laboratory showing that bilateral dorsal rhizotomy from T-10 to L-3 at the time of partial nephrectomy prevents blood pressure elevation in rats with 5/6 nephrectomy. These studies have demonstrated that increased renal sensory feedback to the central nervous system may contribute to the development of hypertension in rats with chronic renal failure. To further evaluate the role of renal afferent nerves in the regulation of blood pressure and whether renal afferent pathways integrate with the posterior hypothalamus, we studied the effects of an intrarenal injection of 50 μL of 10% phenol on blood pressure and NE secretion from the posterior hypothalamus of Sprague Dawley rats. We showed that the injection of phenol in the kidney raises blood pressure and the secretion of NE from the posterior hypothalamic nuclei, whereas renal denervation prevented the increase in blood pressure and in NE secretion from the hypothalamus caused by the intrarenal injection of phenol. The effects on blood pressure of phenol-induced renal injury are long-lasting, suggesting that a limited injury to one kidney may cause a permanent elevation of blood pressure, which is associated with increased sympathetic nervous system activity.

VASCULAR RESPONSE TO AGONISTS

A major role in the genesis of ANS dysfunction in uremia can be attributed to reduced end-organ response to *vasoconstrictor agents*. Several observations support this notion. First, before initiation of dialysis therapy, uremic patients experience a marked and greater fall in blood pressure during upright posture than normal subjects, and this occurs despite greater increments in plasma NE concentrations. Second, the pressor response during infusion of NE is blunted in uremic patients. Similarly, a reduced vascular response to NE both *in vivo* and in the isolated perfused hindlimbs and in isolated aortic strips has been observed in rats with experimental chronic renal failure. This abnormality is due, at least in part, to downregulation of α-adrenergic receptors.

A substantial body of evidence suggests that postreceptor aberrations, related to excessive levels of PTH may be partially responsible for the decreased pressor response to NE in uremia. First, PTH is a vasodilator, and it blunts the pressor action of NE and angiotensin II both *in vivo* and *in vitro* in the rat. Second, parathyroidectomy normalizes the pressor response to NE in uremic rats. Third, a correlation was present between PTH levels and degree of hyporesponsiveness to NE in uremic subjects. Because PTH increases the urinary excretion of $PGF_{1\alpha}$ (a stable metabolite of prostacyclin) in rats and the administration of indomethacin restores a normal pressor response to NE in uremic subjects and rats, it stands to reason that the excessive levels of PTH in uremia may stimulate the production of prostacyclin, resulting in reduced pressor response to agonists.

The heart rate and blood pressure response to stimulation of β-adrenergic receptors induced by isoproterenol is normal in uremic patients, indicating an intact β-receptor function.

AUTONOMIC DYSFUNCTION AND CARDIOVASCULAR INSTABILITY DURING HEMODIALYSIS

Symptomatic hypotension is a common complication of hemodialysis treatment, particularly in patients who have normal or low blood pressure before initiation of dialysis and in patients who have large interdialytic weight gains. Some investigators have advanced the hypothesis that dialysis hypotension is a consequence of involvement of the sympathetic nervous system in the generalized uremic neuropathy. Most studies, however, have shown that in uremic patients, although the reflex control of heart rate may be abnormal, the reflex control of blood pressure was not affected. Moreover, most studies have shown no difference in autonomic function between patients with and without dialysis hypotension. Uremic diabetic patients are an exception because the involvement of autonomic dysfunction in these patients is more severe and often involves the sympathetic nervous system, compromising the control of peripheral vascular resistance in response to volume depletion.

Several investigators have drawn attention to the fact that in concomitance with dialysis-induced hypotension, some patients develop bradycardia, rather than tachycardia, suggesting that hypotension during dialysis may be induced by the activation of a vagal-sympathoinhibitory reflex originating in the heart (Bezold-Jarish reflex) that causes bradycardia, vasodilation, and hypotension. This has been clearly demonstrated by Converse and colleagues, who documented a precipitous fall in sympathetic nervous activity, registered by direct measurement of sympathetic activity in the peroneal nerve, and in heart rate in concomitance with the episode of dialysis-induced hypotension. This suggests that vigorous contraction of the heart around an almost empty chamber may trigger the vagal-sympathoinhibitory reflex that leads to hypotension and bradycardia. Whether uremic patients are more predisposed to this reflex than normal individuals remains a subject of speculation.

It is important to emphasize that most of the episodes of dialysis-induced hypotension are characterized by tachycardia and not by bradycardia. What determines one type of response versus the other and whether bradycardia occurs only in the most severe forms of dialysis-induced hypotension remains to be investigated. The management in all cases is administration of normal saline because blood pressure in both cases increases with volume expansion. In patients with dialysis-induced bradycardia, atropine increases heart rate but does not increase blood pressure, suggesting that volume depletion is the principal factor responsible for bradycardia and hypotension.

Selected Readings

Converse RL, Jacobsen TN, Jost CMT, et al. Paradoxical withdrawal of reflex vasoconstriction as a cause of hemodialysis-induced hypotension. *J Clin Invest* 1992;90:1657–1665.

These investigators measured blood pressure, vascular resistance, and sympathetic nerve activity (by intraneural microelectrodes) during sessions of hemodialysis in 7 patients with and 16 patients without a history of hemodialysis-induced hypotension. With continued hemodialysis, in hypotensive-prone subjects the precipitous decrease in blood pressure was accompanied by decreases in sympathetic nerve activity, vascular resistance, and heart rate. They suggest that dialysis-induced hypotension is caused by an acute, paradoxical withdrawal of sympathetic vasoconstriction producing vasodepressor syncope.

Converse RL, Jacobsen TN, Toto RD, et al. Sympathetic overactivity in patients with chronic renal failure. *N Engl J Med* 1992;327:1912–1918.

Using direct recording of sympathetic nervous system activity in the peroneal nerve, this study demonstrates an increase in sympathetic nervous system activity in human subjects with chronic renal failure. In patients with bilateral nephrectomy, peripheral sympathetic activity was normal, suggesting a possible role for renal afferent pathways in the genesis of increased sympathetic activity in these patients.

Iseki K, Massry SG, Campese VM. Evidence for a role of PTH in the reduced pressor response to norepinephrine in chronic renal failure. *Kidney Int* 1985; 28:11–15.

This study demonstrates that the pressor response to NE is reduced in rats with 5/6 nephrectomy and that this abnormality may be corrected by prior parathyroidectomy.

Ye S, Ozgur B, Campese VM. Renal afferent impulses, the posterior hypothalamus, and hypertension in rats with chronic renal failure. *Kidney Int* 1997; 51:722–727.

These studies show that a renal injury caused by an intrarenal injection of phenol raises blood pressure and increases the secretion of NE from the posterior hypothalamic nuclei. These nuclei are important in the noradrenergic control of blood pressure. Renal denervation prevents the rise in blood pressure and NE secretion from the posterior hypothalamus.

CHAPTER 70

Cardiovascular System in Uremia

PART 1
Uremic Pericarditis

A. Peter Lundin

Pericarditis is due to an inflammation of the pericardium, the serous membrane enclosing the heart and the roots of the great blood vessels. The association of pericarditis with renal failure was first described by Richard Bright in his landmark observation of 100 cases of patients with "albuminous urine," which appeared in the Guys Hospital Report of 1836. Autopsy studies demonstrated pericarditis or pericardial effusion in 37 of these patients. Although more commonly seen in patients with chronic renal failure, pericarditis can also be found in patients with acute nephropathies.

In azotemic patients pericarditis is due to a number of causes including bacterial, viral, or tubercular infections; diseases involving serous membranes, such as systemic lupus erythematosus; or to some condition of azotemia itself. In the azotemic patient, uremic pericarditis usually appears late in the course of renal failure when the glomerular filtration rate has dropped below 5 ml/min. Pericarditis can also be a consequence of a failing or poorly functioning kidney transplant. In the first 2 months after renal transplantation, one group reported 2.4% of patients to have pericarditis. Causes were identified as uremia (14 patients), cytomegalovirus (4) or bacterial infection (3), and tuberculosis (1).

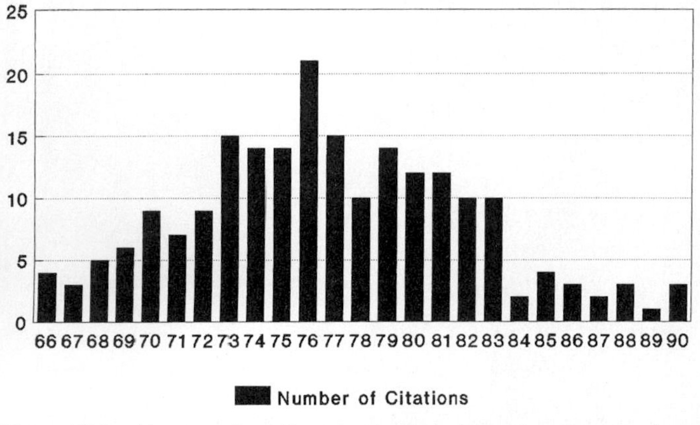

Figure 70.1. Number of publications dealing with pericarditis in patients with chronic renal failure and in those treated with dialysis (1966–1990).

Pericarditis due to uremia clears quickly when dialysis is started, but has been noted to recur at varying periods of time after patients begin dialysis. Over the past 40 years with the advent of dialysis therapy for the treatment of acute, and later for chronic, renal failure, the occurrence of uremic pericarditis has declined dramatically.

The impression that uremic pericarditis is decreasing in incidence is supported by personal experience and a virtual disappearance of the topic from the medical literature (Fig. 70.1). Most of the reports since 1966 pertain to dialysis-associated pericarditis. The greatest number of papers occurred between 1970 and 1983, the peak years of frequency being between 1973 and 1979. The dramatic decrease since 1983 would suggest that either there was nothing new to report or the incidence of disease was decreasing. During 1995 and 1998, less than 1% of the 702 papers discussing pericarditis were specifically related to uremic pericarditis. It has become enough of a medical curiosity to be treated as a case report in a French journal titled *Clinical Case of the Month, Uremic Pericarditis in a Dialysis Patient.*

Circumstantial evidence implicates inadequate dialysis as a permissive factor for uremic pericarditis. This evidence includes a number of clinical observations of pericarditis often occurring in patients who have not received their full dialysis prescription for various reasons, and the frequent beneficial response to more dialysis. Also it is interesting to note that in the early 1980s, hollow-fiber dialyzers, more efficient than the flat-plate and coil dialyzers that were employed at the time, came into wider utilization, probably leading to better dialysis delivery. In general, details of the dialysis prescription including type of dialyzer used, frequency, time, and blood flow have been ignored in literature reports, indicating a widespread lack of realization that these parameters of the prescription require careful attention for dialysis efficiency (Table 70.1). Considering that the maximum dosage of dialysis available today achieves only a

TABLE 70.1. Dialysis Problems Associated with Uremic Pericarditis

Dialyzer clearance of uremic too low for metabolic needs of patient
Time and/or frequency of dialysis inadequate by prescription or patient noncompliance
Blood and/or dialysate flow insufficient by prescription or intradialytic complications
Inadequate blood access

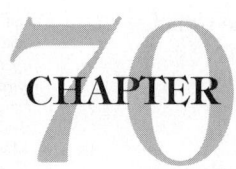

TABLE 70.2. Factors Contributing to or Complicating Pericarditis in Patients with Renal Failure

Late start of or inadequate hemodialysis
Retained uremic toxins
Loss of residual renal function
Parathyroid hormone
Underlying systemic disease
Infection: viral, tubercular
Platelet dysfunction with intrapericardial bleeding
Anticoagulation causing tamponade

small proportion of normal kidney function, it does not require much of a decrease in any of these parameters for a patient to become subadequately dialyzed and thus at risk for recurrent pericarditis. Early detection and correction of problems with blood access and maximization of the dialysis prescription according to increasingly well-defined standards should prevent episodes of pericarditis in the dialysis patient.

PATHOLOGY AND PATHOGENESIS (TABLE 70.2)

Fibrinous, aseptic inflammation is the hallmark of uremic pericarditis. Distribution of the inflammation can be diffuse or localized with areas of adhesion between the parietal and visceral layers of the pericardium. An increase in vascularity occurs as the pericardial membranes thicken. With movement between the layers, blood vessels are broken causing formation of a serosanguinous effusion loculated between adherent fibrous bands. The volume of effusion may grow if the time of inflammation is prolonged; as the patient becomes edematous with extravascular movement of fluid into the pleural, peritoneal, and pericardial spaces; or heparin is given for dialysis treatments. Serious, life-threatening consequences result from acute or chronic compression of the heart, which causes a decrease in cardiac output. This can happen rapidly due to accumulation of fluid in a limited space (tamponade) or slowly from chronic thickening and scarring of the membrane (constriction).

Because pericarditis appears late in the course of renal failure and is reversed by dialysis, it can be assumed that both the presence of dialyzable toxins and the time of exposure to these toxins have etiologic roles. As with other signs or symptoms of uremia, no single toxin has been implicated. Small molecules that clear rapidly with conventional hemodialysis are likely responsible but there is some indirect evidence that larger molecules might also be involved. When pericarditis appears in dialysis patients it is usually after a period of time on treatment and under conditions of catabolic stress, such as infection or as a result of inadequate dialysis. In the first situation the patient is probably receiving dialysis of borderline adequacy, and in the latter, loss of native residual kidney function may expose an inadequate prescription.

SYMPTOMS AND SIGNS (TABLE 70.3)

The first presentation of pericarditis is usually chest pain. The patient will report a substernal discomfort that is typically worse when lying down, and is alleviated by sitting up and leaning forward. This may be due to the frequent posterior location of the pathologic changes, explaining an associated atrial arrhythmia (fibrillation or flutter) that is noted by the patient as a new, irregular heartbeat with or without chest pain. If the inflammation affects the inferior wall, the pain may be located in areas reflecting involvement of the diaphragm, which is supplied by the phrenic nerve, such as superior border of the trapezius muscle in the neck.

TABLE 70.3. Clinical Features of or Associated Findings with Uremic Pericarditis

Symptoms
Chest pain with or without radiation
Dyspnea, irregular heart beat
Loss of pulse in fistula
Orthostatic dizziness and decrease in urine output
Rapid weight gain
Signs
Pericardial friction rub
Fever
Mental confusion
Edema, anasarca, ascites
Hypotension and intolerance of ultrafiltration
Pulsus paradoxus, distension of neck veins
Lab Results
Enlarged cardiac profile on chest radiograph
Leukocytosis
Pericardial effusion, thickened pericardial membrane
Atrial arrhythmias

In the dialysis patient it is not unusual to have other manifestations of uremia that are expected in the undialyzed patient when pericarditis appears, such as marked urochrome pigmentation, poor appetite, and weight loss. However, the most severe symptoms or signs of uremia, such as nausea and vomiting and uremic encephalopathy with obtundation, are usually prevented by even minimal dialysis.

When the patient is examined a pericardial friction rub is usually noted. The rub is of two or three components timed with the heart cycle. The sound is scratchy or grating, like rubbing two pieces of sandpaper together, and can be accentuated by having the patient sit to bring the heart closer to the chest wall. A pleural rub indicating pleuritis, particularly in the predialysis, uremic patient, may be more notable. The pericardial rub may appear or disappear depending on patient position when listened for, or because an effusion separating the inflamed pericardial membranes goes or comes. Disappearance of the pericardial rub is not always an indication that the pericarditis is improving because the appearance of pericardial effusion may abolish the rub. Low-grade fever and leukocytosis may also be noted, but high temperatures and marked elevation of white blood cells with a leftward shift should prompt a search for a bacterial infection elsewhere in the body either precipitating uremic pericarditis or as a cause itself.

COMPLICATIONS

Cardiac tamponade is the most serious, life-threatening acute complication. Fluid accumulating rapidly in a poorly compliant compartment with thickened membranes leads to a decrease in cardiac output and hypotension. The neck veins are engorged but the lungs are usually clear. The heart is enlarged on percussion, the point of maximal impulse (PMI), if palpable, is diffuse, and the cardiac sounds muffled; a rub, if previously noted, has probably disappeared. A paradoxic pulse is often present, identified as a drop of the pulse pressure of more than 10 mm Hg during inspiration. This fall can sometimes be palpated as an exaggerated waxing and waning of the pulse volume, but is more reliably measured by a sphygmomanometer. With the inflated cuff held at a point 10 mm Hg below the maximum systolic pressure, the pulse is felt or heard during normal expiration and disappears with normal inspiration in the presence of a regular cardiac rhythm.

In dialysis patients, clotting of a previously well-functioning fistula or graft or unexpected hypotension may mark the onset of tamponade. The event may be precipitated by rapid bleeding into the pericardial space induced by heparin or by removal of fluid. Hemodialysis is contraindicated if there is evidence of or concern for tamponade. Treatment is by surgical drainage by the subxiphoid approach, if there is time, or by needle pericardiocentesis with electrocardiogram (ECG) monitoring if not.

Long-standing, asymptomatic, subclinical pericarditis can lead to constriction of the heart as the pericardial membrane tightens. The symptoms are the same as those with tamponade but less acute and therefore often missed until the late stages. Treatment is surgical stripping of the pericardium. Similar treatment is indicated in patients with pericardial effusion unresponsive to therapy.

When patients who receive a dialysis dose of more than 1.2 of Kt/v or who experience a 65% reduction of urea develop symptoms of pericarditis, infectious causes should be strongly suspected. Viral infections due to coxsackieviruses A and B, influenza A and B, and echovirus usually appear in epidemic form. High, spiking fevers with a neutrophil-predominant leukocytosis suggest a bacterial cause. Delay of specific therapy by pursuing a course of intensive dialysis alone may prove fatal. Uremia can reactivate tuberculosis, which can cause an indolent pericarditis, later presenting with signs and symptoms of constriction.

DIAGNOSIS

As the most specific diagnostic evidence for predialysis, uremic pericarditis is the symptom and sign with which most patients present. These findings may be muted in the underdialyzed patient who may present with other complications discussed previously. In the catabolic uremic patient who is losing weight and presenting with obvious symptoms, or the dialysis patient who is missing or shortening dialysis treatments or having access problems, uremic pericarditis should be suspected. In other patients, infectious causes of pericarditis should be looked for.

Pericardial effusion is frequently present with but is not diagnostic of uremic pericarditis. Therefore tests that demonstrate pericardial effusion will support the diagnosis only if other symptoms or signs are present. The pericardial sac is a potential site for storage of extra fluid in patients with impaired or no kidney function. Transudative fluid may be found there as well as in the pleural and peritoneal spaces even in the absence of peripheral signs of fluid retention. A sterile, serosanguinous fluid obtained by pericardiocentesis is typically the result of uremia. One prospective study of a large number of patients showed that pericardial effusion of small, moderate, or even large amount is present when the patients present themselves for the first time.

A triangular shaped, "water bottle," heart may be noted by chest radiograph, signaling the possible presence of intrapericardial fluid. Subsequent radiographs showing an enlargement of the cardiac silhouette with clear lung fields are strongly indicative. ECG is the definitive diagnostic procedure for detecting fluid in the pericardial space. Computed tomography and magnetic resonance imaging can more specifically indicate the presence of chronic pericarditis, most frequently seen today in the underdialyzed patient, by identifying a thickened pericardial membrane and presence of fibrous adhesions, or calcium deposits in the constricting membrane.

Changes in the ECG with low voltage across the precordium are also typical for effusion or membrane thickening. Elevated ST segments present in most leads may indicate injury due to inflammation. New onset atrial fibrillation or other atrial arrhythmias may be the presenting finding.

TREATMENT

The best treatment is prevention. Starting dialysis treatments before the onset of catabolism in uremic patients, and prescribing and ensuring delivery of a dialysis prescription reducing blood urea nitrogen by greater than 65% will prevent uremic pericarditis. Uremic pericarditis should be a problem limited to the noncompliant patient.

On the occasion when noninfectious pericarditis is diagnosed in the uremic or dialysis patient, initiation or intensification of dialysis is usually efficacious, suggesting that dialysis was started late or given insufficiently. Some patients, particularly those on hemodialysis for a period of time, may not respond to more dialysis. This persistence of pericarditis is likely due to a more prolonged subclinical course in which other symptoms and signs of uremia have been minimal or overlooked, leading to a greater extent of intrapericardial adhesion formation. When fluid is present, surgical drainage has been recommended, with or without the placement of a pericardial window, to diminish the risk of progression to tamponade. Because of the apparent inflammatory nature of uremic pericarditis, some have advised oral treatment with or injection of nonsteroidal antiinflammatory agents directly into the pericardial effusion to reduce the extent of the adhesions. Others have recommended a combination of intensified dialysis with drainage and instillation of antiinflammatory agents. Any intrusion into the pericardial sac is not without risk, however, and includes secondary infection and cardiac laceration, particularly when the transcutaneous route is used. Treatment of tamponade and constriction has been described previously. Persistent chronic pericarditis and/or recurrent pericardial effusion despite adequate dialysis require pericardial stripping.

Selected Readings

Bailey GL, Hampers CL, Hager EB, et al. Uremic pericarditis: clinical features and management. *Circulation* 1968;38:582–591.

A look at pericarditis in the early years of dialysis. Instances of pericarditis that developed during regular dialysis were attributed to metabolic stresses such as surgery, infection, or inadequate dialysis.

Comty CM, Cohen SL, Shapiro FL. Pericarditis in chronic uremia and its sequels. *Ann Intern Med* 1971;75:173–183.

In this article, it is noted that episodes of pericarditis were associated with infection and inadequate dialysis; it is also seen more frequently in younger female patients and those with hyperparathyroidism.

Minuth ANW, Nottebohm GA, Eknoyan G, et al. Indomethacin treatment of pericarditis in chronic hemodialysis patients. *Arch Intern Med* 1975;135:807–810.

Although the efficacy of nonsteroidals in treating uremic pericarditis is disputed and risks underestimated, this paper shows successful treatment of symptoms without requiring invasive procedures. Whether dialysis efficiency was coincidentally improved is not stated.

Rutsky EA, Rostand SG. Pericarditis in end-stage renal disease: clinical characteristics and management. *Semin Dial* 1989;2:25–30.

This paper reviews a clinical experience in 148 of 1257 patients who experienced 173 episodes of pericarditis.

Sever MS, Steinmuller DR, Hayes JM, et al. Pericarditis following renal transplantation. *Transplantation* 1991;51:1229–1232.

An analysis of 27 years of investigating the frequency, etiology, and outcome of pericarditis developing during the first 2 months following renal transplantation.
Ventura SC, Garella S. The management of pericardial disease in renal failure. *Semin Dial* 1990;3:21–26.
This paper is a recent review of the management of pericarditis comparing treatment of pericarditis occurring in the predialysis period with that appearing after onset of dialysis. Recommendation for dialysis in pericarditis is intensification of dialysis followed by surgical procedures in cases in which dialysis is unsuccessful.

PART 2
Cardiomyopathy

Patrick S. Parfrey and Robert N. Foley

In chronic uremia, cardiomyopathy may manifest as concentric left ventricular hypertrophy (LVH) or left ventricle (LV) dilation, and may result in diastolic or systolic dysfunction. These disorders are associated with the subsequent development of cardiac failure and with death. Ischemic heart disease, which may be atherosclerotic or nonatherosclerotic in origin, may present with myocardial infarction or angina, but it is also intimately associated with the development of cardiac failure. It is likely that LVH predisposes to the development of ischemic symptoms and that ischemia also predisposes to the development of cardiac failure (Fig. 70.2).

PATHOPHYSIOLOGY

Left Ventricular Hypertrophy

LVH is an adaptive process occurring in response to long-term increase in myocardial work caused by pressure or volume overload, and results from the interaction between mechanical stimuli and locally generated growth factors and vasoactive substances. LVH usually develops in a pattern specific to the inciting mechanical stress. Pressure overload results in parallel addition of new sarcomeres and is characterized by an unchanged or smaller internal diameter of the LV and an increased wall thickness (concentric hypertrophy). Volume overload results in addition of new sarcomeres in series, increasing LV diameter with a proportional increase in LV wall thickness (eccentric hypertrophy).

LVH is both beneficial and detrimental. The benefit is linked to increased numbers of sarcomeres and ventricular wall thickness, which maintain stable parietal tensile stress, and thus has an energy-sparing effect. This permits the generation of high intraventricular pressures without a large increase in wall stress. According to Laplace's law, the relationship between the parietal stress (S), the ventricular pressure (P), and the LV internal diameter (D) is: $S = PD/Th$, where Th is LV wall thickness.

Detrimental effects of LVH are related to decreased capillary density, decreased coronary reserve and subendocardial perfusion, and development of myocardial fibrosis. The principal consequences of these alterations are electrophysiologic abnormalities and abnormal ventricular relaxation. Arrhythmias are caused in part by conduction in homogeneity and prolongation of the action potentials because of increased slow, inward calcium current. Abnormal diastolic function is linked to fibrosis and increased stiffness of the LV wall, and to slow relaxation and uptake of calcium by sarcoplasmic reticulum. Finally, in conditions of chronic and sustained overload, the deleterious effects of hypertrophy and fibrosis become prominent, leading to development of cardiomyopathy of overload and LV failure.

Initially LVH is an adaptive response to pressure or volume overload. Eventually LVH becomes maladaptive, and cell death occurs, which predisposes to cardiac failure. Overstretching of papillary muscles is coupled with oxidant stress, programmed cell death, architectural rearrangement of myocytes, and impairment in force development of the myocardium. The chronic uremic state in hemodialysis patients is a model for the development of overload cardiomyopathy because LV pressure and/or volume overload is maintained for prolonged periods. The death of myocytes in chronic uremia may be exacerbated by diminished perfusion, malnutrition, hyperparathyroidism, and perhaps inadequate dialysis (Fig. 70.3). Such cell death in the presence of LVH and continuing pressure and volume overload may be catastrophic, leading to further LV dilation and eventually systolic dysfunction.

When the increase in LV mass is appropriate to the LV volume for a given ventricular or aortic systolic pressure, a direct correlation is seen between pressure and the LV mass/volume ratio. This correlation is found in the normal population, as well as in physiologic situations of volume and pressure overload. In conditions in which the relative parietal thickness is insufficient for a given systolic pressure (decreased LV mass/volume ratio) the hypertrophy is termed *inadequate hypertrophy.* This occurs in hemodialysis patients and may be associated with an adverse outcome. In dialysis patients with LV dilation, adverse survival is associated with a low LV mass/volume ratio, whereas in

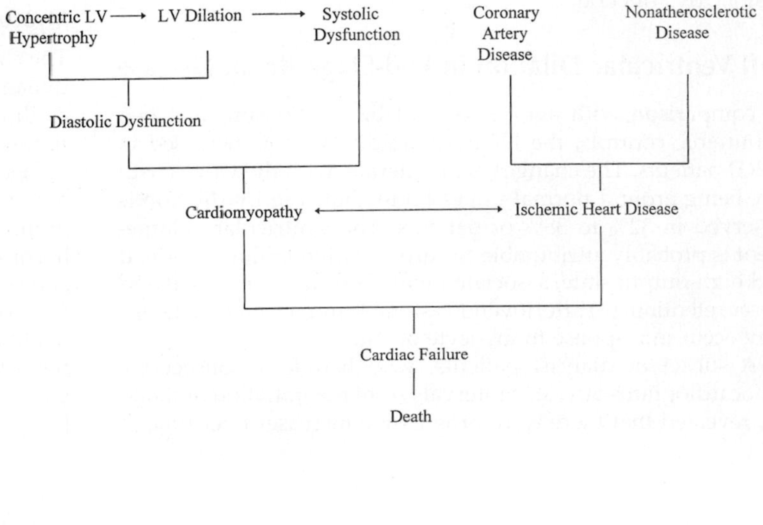

Figure 70.2. The cause of heart failure in chronic uremia.

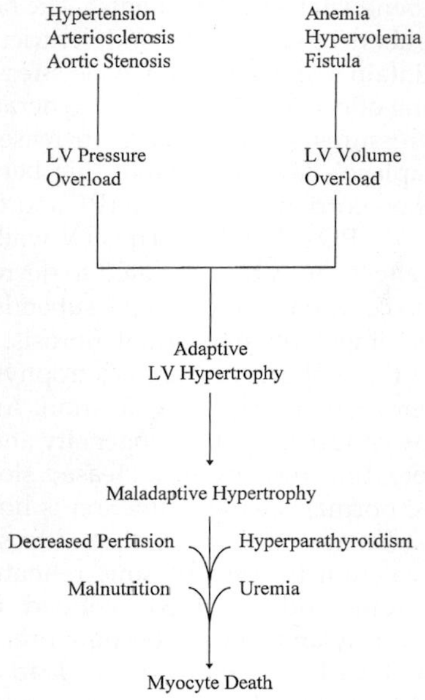

Figure 70.3. Myocyte death in chronic uremia.

patients with concentric LVH, the opposite occurs: adverse survival is associated with high LV mass/volume ratio.

Left Ventricular Geometry in End-Stage Renal Disease Patients

The study of LV morphology and function in end-stage renal disease (ESRD) patients on dialysis is difficult because of the absence of steady-state conditions, associated with cyclic variations in blood volume and humoral balance. The internal dimensions of the LV are influenced by volume status. Body fluid volume contraction during a dialysis session decreases the LV diameter, and dialysis-induced changes in loading conditions or inotropic state could modify the functional indices of ventricular function. Although hemodynamic factors cannot account entirely for increased LV mass, the cardiac hypertrophy in ESRD patients results principally from an association of volume and pressure overload and combines features of eccentric and concentric hypertrophy, that is, a moderate increase in LV diameter, and a more marked increase in LV wall thickness. The relative importance of pressure overload, volume overload, cell death, and ischemic heart disease in the development of cardiomyopathy will vary from patient to patient. Furthermore, during follow-up of an individual patient, cardiomyopathy may be manifest as concentric LVH, LV dilation, or eventually systolic dysfunction.

Left Ventricular Dilation in End-Stage Renal Disease

In comparison with age-, sex-, and blood pressure–matched nonuremic controls, the LV diastolic diameter is increased in ESRD patients. The changes are moderate, with the values usually being around normal upper limits, but true LV dilation is observed in 32% to 38% of patients. The ventricular enlargement is probably attributable to chronic volume/flow overload and high-output state, associated with three factors: (a) salt and water retention, (b) arteriovenous shunts, and (c) anemia. It also may occur in response to myocyte death.

A subset of dialysis patients, who had four consecutive echocardiograms at yearly intervals from the initiation of dialysis, revealed that there were progressive increases over time in posterior wall thickness, LV end-diastolic diameter, LV mass index, and LV cavity volume. LV mass-to-volume ratios did not change. The biggest changes in LV mass index and LV volume index occurred between baseline and year 1, although increases in both were seen after 1 year. Hemodialysis versus peritoneal dialysis and anemia were associated with progressive LV enlargement. Partial correction of anemia with erythropoietin induces a regression of the hemodynamic state and of the size of the LV.

When chronic uremia patients with LV dilation were compared with those with normal echocardiograms, independent associations of higher LV volumes included ischemic heart disease, anemia, hypertension, and hypoalbuminemia. Furthermore, low serum albumin levels were significantly associated with progressive LV dilation between baseline and follow-up echocardiograms 1 year later. This is consistent with the hypothesis that diminished perfusion, as defined by the presence of ischemic symptoms, and malnutrition, as suggested by low serum albumin levels, predisposes to LV dilation, which may result from myocyte death.

Concentric Left Ventricular Hypertrophy

LV pressure overload results from hypertension, aortic stenosis, and/or arteriosclerosis. Several determinants of systolic and pulse pressure are altered in ESRD patients, including decreased arterial compliance and an early return of arterial wave reflections, which are independent factors associated with the extent of LVH. Decreased arterial compliance and functional alterations observed in ESRD are associated with remodeling of conduit arteries, characterized by arterial dilation and intima-media hypertrophy. These arterial changes resemble those that occur with aging, such as arteriosclerosis, which is primarily medial, characterized by diffuse dilation and stiffening of major arteries. These changes must be distinguished from atherosclerosis, which is focal, nonuniformly distributed, primarily intimal, inducing occlusive lesions and compensatory focal enlargement of arterial diameters.

In ESRD, the increased arterial diameters and intima-media hypertrophy are associated with flow overload and increased blood flow velocity. Arterial walls are exposed to the influence of mechanical factors, such as flow and pressure stresses, which act as mechanical stimuli for remodeling. Experimental and clinical studies have shown that chronically increased arterial flow leads to increased internal arterial dimensions and arterial wall remodeling, with a compensatory increase in arterial wall thickness. The consequence of structural and functional changes of the arterial system in uremic patients is increased pulsatile work of the heart, which accounts in part for the development of parallel LV, and vascular adaptation in chronic uremia.

Myocardial Fibrosis in End-Stage Renal Disease

The clinical spectrum of the LV hypertrophic response to hemodynamic overload is wide and influenced by many factors, including gender, race, age, and the development of myocardial fibrosis. Myocardial fibrosis is not an obligatory consequence of hemodynamic stress and is more marked in pressure overload than in volume overload. The causes of myocardial fibrosis are multifactorial and include senescence, ischemia, and effects of hormones such as catecholamines, angiotensin II, aldosterone, and so forth. Other studies have demonstrated that parathyroid hormone is a permissive factor in the genesis of cardiac interstitial fibrosis. The extensive intramyocardial fibrosis in ESRD patients with elevated parathyroid hormone could be responsible for attenuation of the hypertrophic response to pressure overload and the development of high-stress cardiomyopathy and cardiac failure. Interstitial myocardial fibrosis is a prominent finding in uremia. Clinical studies have shown that the extent of myocardial fibrosis in ESRD patients is more marked than in patients with diabetes mellitus or essential hypertension with similar LV mass.

Systolic Dysfunction

The influence of loading conditions on systolic and diastolic function complicates the assessment of LV function. This is particularly true in hemodialysis patients because of changing volume status and variations in humoral parameters during a dialysis session. Decreased systolic function is observed frequently in patients with cardiac diseases preexisting before ESRD therapy or in patients with sustained and marked hemodynamic overload. Diminished myocardial contractility may be a result of overload cardiomyopathy. This manifestation of cardiomyopathy has a substantially worse prognosis than either concentric LVH or LV dilation with normal systolic function. In dialysis patients, systolic dysfunction is associated with the presence of ischemic heart disease and with anemia. However, systolic dysfunction may also be a manifestation of uremia per se and thus reversible when the uremic environment is removed. Uremic serum reduces inotropy of cultured heart cells in a concentration-dependent manner. Renal transplantation normalizes systolic function in dialysis patients with systolic dysfunction.

Diastolic Dysfunction

In ESRD patients without cardiac antecedents, the indices of systolic function are normal and may be increased in a subset of patients (hypertrophic hyperkinetic disease). However, diastolic filling is frequently altered in dialysis patients. Hemodialysis patients with LVH have some impairment in LV diastolic function, but the degree of the disturbance is similar to that observed in those with hypertensive heart disease, but milder than that observed in those with hypertrophic cardiomyopathy. The abnormal ventricular filling in ESRD results from increased LV stiffness caused by intramyocardial fibrosis and delayed relaxation. It is highly likely that patients with concentric LVH or LV dilation have diastolic dysfunction, which predisposes to the development of heart failure.

Atherosclerotic Disease

Because of the high prevalence of hypertension, LVH, diabetes, and lipid abnormalities in dialysis patients, it has been suggested that these patients have an accelerated rate of coronary atherogenesis. However there was no difference in the rate of appearance of ischemic heart symptoms in dialysis patients compared with nondialysis subjects with similar risk factors who were part of the Framingham study. In addition, a cohort study of 432 patients followed for an average of 41 months identified 336 dialysis patients who did not have ischemic heart disease on starting dialysis. Only 41 patients subsequently developed *de novo* ischemic heart disease. Thus the incidence of *de novo* symptomatic ischemic heart disease was 2.8% per year in this cohort. The suggestion that atherogenesis may not be accelerated in ESRD populations is strengthened by the observation that rates of death from myocardial infarction in these populations are not different from those described in the general population.

Multiple factors contribute to the vascular pathology of chronic uremia, including injury to the vessel wall, prothrombotic factors, lipoprotein interactions, proliferation of smooth muscle, hyperhomocysteinemia, increased oxidant stress, and diminished antioxidant levels (Fig. 70.4). There is evidence of chronic *in vivo* endothelial activation and injury in uremia.

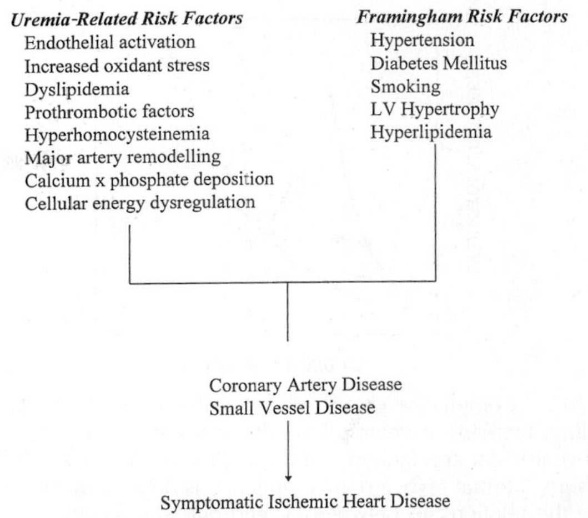

Figure 70.4. The cause of ischemic heart disease in chronic uremia.

More information on prothrombotic factors may be obtained in Chapter 72, Part 2, on lipid abnormalities in Chapter 74, Part 2, and on hyperhomocysteinemia in Chapter 68, Part 3.

Oxidant Stress

The oxidative modification of low-density lipoprotein (LDL) in the vascular wall may be an important step in atherogenesis. Reactive oxygen species may initiate LDL oxidation. Ingestion of oxidized LDL by monocytes leads to foam cell development. In addition, oxidized LDL may be cytotoxic for endothelial cells and may stimulate vascular smooth cell proliferation. In uremia, oxidant activity can be identified, and endogenous oxidant activity may occur as a byproduct of acidosis and abnormal metabolism. This suggests that increased oxidant stress may occur, particularly if there are reduced concentrations of endogenous antioxidants and if there are ongoing low-grade inflammatory processes. Dysregulation in the balance between proinflammatory cytokines and their inhibitors has been shown, which may contribute to the uremia-related chronic immunoinflammatory disorder. The evidence to support the presence of oxidized LDL in dialysis patients is contradictory, although increased titers of autoantibodies against oxidized LDL, compared with normal controls, have been reported.

Congestive Heart Failure

Congestive heart failure (CHF) may result from systolic failure, usually caused by dilated cardiomyopathy, or from diastolic dysfunction, usually caused by LVH. In fact, diastolic dysfunction is almost as frequent a cause of recurrent or persistent CHF in dialysis patients as is dilated cardiomyopathy.

Among patients with diastolic dysfunction, CHF results from impaired ventricular relaxation, which leads to an exaggerated increase in LV end-diastolic pressure for a given increase in LV end-diastolic volume (Fig. 70.5). As a result, a relatively small excess of salt and water intake leads rapidly to a large increase in LV end-diastolic pressure, culminating in pulmonary edema.

In dilated cardiomyopathy, cardiac output is maintained at the expense of an increase in both the end-diastolic fiber length and end-diastolic volume (i.e., through the Frank-Starling mechanism). As ventricular volume increases, however, a constant wall stress requires (by Laplace's law) a proportionate increase in LV end-diastolic pressure. This increase in LV end-diastolic pressure leads to increased pulmonary capillary pressure and dyspnea.

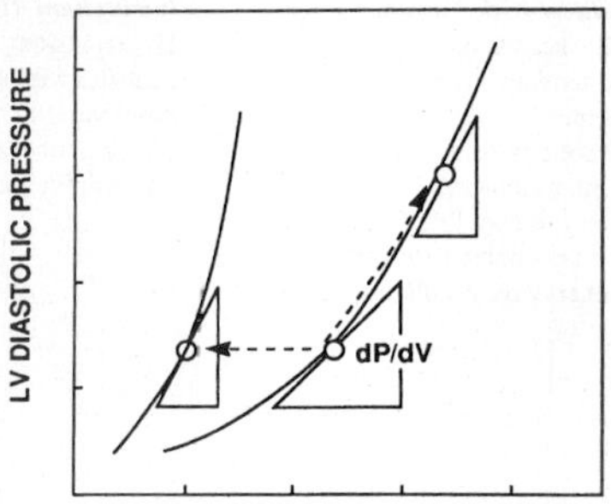

Figure 70.5. Compliance characteristics of the left ventricle during diastolic filling. Increase in ventricular volume results in an increase in the force of ventricular contraction and consequently an increase in ventricular pressure. Normal myocardial compliance is defined by the right curve showing the relationship between LV end-diastolic volume and LV end-diastolic pressure. In chronic uremia, myocardial compliance is decreased, and the pressure-volume relationship is shifted to the left and operates within a narrow range. Consequently, changes in plasma volume lead to congestive heart failure, and a decrease leads to hypotension. (Reproduced with permission from Palmer BF, Henrich WL. The effect of dialysis on left ventricular contractility. In: Parfrey PS, Harnett JD, eds. *Cardiac dysfunction in chronic uremia.* Boston: Kluwer Academic, 1992.)

Ischemic Heart Disease

Myocardial infarction and angina result from decreased perfusion of the myocardium. Although symptoms of ischemic heart disease are most often due to the presence of coronary artery disease, they may also result from nonatherosclerotic disease, in which a reduction in coronary vasodilator reserve and altered myocardial oxygen delivery and use predispose to ischemic symptoms. In dialysis patients the presence of LVH predisposes to nonatherosclerotic ischemia. As the demand for oxygen increases, the coronary vasculature dilates above baseline, and a further increase in myocardial oxygen requirement may not be met with adequate increase in coronary flow, especially if there are pathologic changes in the large coronary arteries or in the small coronary vessels. Small vessel smooth muscle hypertrophy and endothelial abnormalities have been described in LVH, which further predisposes to ischemia.

Dialysis Hypotension

The pathophysiology of dialysis hypotension is multifactorial and not fully understood. It may occur in the presence of systolic failure, diastolic dysfunction, or ischemic disease. In the latter condition, whether it be atherosclerotic or nonatherosclerotic in origin, hypotension is usually associated with chest pain.

In dilated cardiomyopathy, hypotension during dialysis will only occur in patients who are unable to augment intrinsic myocardial contractibility in response to plasma volume depletion. Such patients usually have severe systolic failure because the dialysis procedure actually improves myocardial performance in most patients with depressed LV function.

LVH may also be a contributing factor to dialysis hypotension. Because of diminished LV compliance, the relationship between LV end-diastolic pressure and volume is exaggerated (Fig. 70.5). As a result, during dialysis, relative hypovolemia may lead to a disproportionately large decrease in LV end-diastolic pressure, which in turn leads to a decreased stroke volume and hypotension, if a compensatory increase in peripheral resistance does not occur. A number of investigators have documented an excess prevalence of LVH among dialysis patients prone to dialysis hypotension. Further discussion of dialysis hypotension is found in Chapter 70, Part 3.

Arrhythmias

Twelve percent of patients starting dialysis treatment are on therapy for either atrial or ventricular arrhythmias. These patients have a significantly higher mortality than those without such a predictor. In three studies of 100 or more maintenance dialysis patients, the prevalence of atrial arrhythmias ranged from 68% to 88%, ventricular arrhythmias ranged from 59% to 76%, and complex premature ventricular contractions ranged from 14% to 21%. This high occurrence of arrhythmias is probably associated with the high incidence of sudden death. In an analysis of more than 50,000 cases of death in European dialysis patients, cardiac arrest of unknown cause accounted for 9.5% of deaths in women and 9.0% in men.

Coronary artery disease, dilated cardiomyopathy, and LVH all predispose to arrhythmias. In one study of 105 ESRD patients, 75% with coronary artery disease had complex ventricular arrhythmias, as had 63% with severe LVH, compared with approximately 20% in the total population. In nonrenal patients, increasing LV mass has been associated with more frequent and more malignant arrhythmias on 24-hour Holter monitoring.

Epidemiology

The survival rate of dialysis patients is worse than that of patients with colon or prostate cancer, and the cause of death is cardiac in approximately 40% of cases. Table 70.4 shows the annual percentage of cardiovascular mortality by gender, race, and diastolic status in hemodialysis, peritoneal dialysis, and renal transplant patients, compared with the general population. In hemodialysis patients the mortality rate is 35 times higher than in the general population.

TABLE 70.4. Cardiovascular Mortality by Gender, Race, and Target Population (Annual Mortality, %)

	All	Men	Women	White	African-American	Diabetic	Nondiabetic
GP[a]	0.27	0.27	0.27	0.29	0.23	NA	NA
HD[b]	9.47	9.66	9.28	11.50	7.03	11.74	8.20
PD[b]	9.70	10.76	8.52	11.15	6.36	13.85	7.54
RTR[b]	0.59	0.66	0.49	0.57	0.77	1.22	0.45

[a] Data from NCHS 1993 Multiple Causes of Death File.
[b] Data from United States Renal Data System. *1997 Annual Data Report, Bethesda, MD, US Department of Health and Human Services.* National Institutes of Health, 1997.
GP, general population; HD, hemodialysis; NA, not available; PD, peritoneal dialysis; RTR, renal transplant recipients.
Reproduced with permission from Levey AS, Beto JA, Coronado BE. Controlling the epidemic of cardiovascular disease in chronic renal disease. What to do? What do we need to learn? Where do we go from here? *Am J Kid Dis* 1998;32:853–906.

TABLE 70.5. Approximate Prevalence (%) of Cardiovascular Disease by Target Population

	CAD (clinical)	LVH (echo)	CHF (clinical)
General population	5–12[a]	20[b]	5[c]
Chronic renal insufficiency	NA	20–25 (varies with renal function)[d]	NA
Hemodialysis	40[e]	75[f]	40[e]
Peritoneal dialysis	40[e]	75[f]	40[e]
Renal transplant recipient	15[g]	50[h]	NA

[a] Lower value, ages 45 to 64; higher values, ages 65 or older. Data from *NHLBI Morbidity and Mortality Chartbook* 1996.
[b] Data from Levy. *N Engl J Med* 1990;322:1561.
[c] Age 60. Data from *NHLBI Morbidity and Mortality Chartbook* 1996.
[d] Data from Levin. *Am J Kidney Dis* 1996;27:347-351.
[e] Data from USRDS Case-Mix Adequacy Study. *Am J Kidney Dis* 1992; 20:32–38.
[f] Data from Foley. *Kidney Int* 1995;47:186–192.
[g] Data from Kasiske. *Am J Med* 1988;84:985–952.
[h] Data from Weinrauch. *Am J Med* 1992;93:19–28.
CAD, coronary artery disease; CHF, congestive heart failure; LVH, left ventricular hypertrophy; NA, not available.
Reproduced with permission from Levey AS, Beto JA, Coronado BE. Controlling the epidemic of cardiovascular disease in chronic renal disease. What to do? What do we need to learn? Where do we go from here? *Am J Kidney Dis* 1998;32:853–906.

Table 70.5 shows the approximate prevalence of ischemic heart disease, LVH, and clinical heart failure in chronic renal insufficiency, dialysis, and renal transplant patients compared with the general population. The prevalence of LVH in chronic renal insufficiency with glomerular filtration rate greater than 50 ml/min is approximately 27%; it is 45% in those with glomerular filtration rate less than 24 ml/min, and 75% in patients starting dialysis. Clinical manifestations of cardiac disease, such as ischemic heart disease and heart failure, in patients starting dialysis are frequently present.

Figure 70.6A shows the survival of patients starting dialysis by echocardiographic diagnosis. Those with systolic dysfunction had significantly worse survival than those with normal echocardiogram through all time frames, whereas those with concentric LVH and LV dilation had significantly worse late survival, after 2 years on dialysis. CHF has been consistently shown to be a strong independent risk factor for death (Fig. 70.6B), whereas the adverse impact of ischemic heart disease is not a significant risk factor for death independent of age, diabetes, and presence of heart failure. This suggests that the adverse impact of ischemic heart disease exerts its effect through compromising LV pump function.

Diagnosis

Echocardiography provides useful information concerning cardiac cavity, wall dimensions, wall movement, valvular function, and pericardial fluid. It should be performed in all dialysis patients with clinical manifestations of cardiac disease because it will accurately diagnose LVH, systolic failure, aortic and mitral disease, and pericardial effusion. It should also be undertaken as a baseline in all ESRD patients starting dialysis therapy, especially because the prevalence of echocardiographic disease is so high.

Systolic failure is measured more accurately using radionuclide angiography, as is the detection of regional wall abnormalities. The diagnosis of coronary artery disease is more problematic because of the relatively high prevalence of nonatherosclerotic ischemic heart disease and because the sensitivities and specificities of most noninvasive tests for coronary artery disease in dialysis patients are not optimal. Some have found that a negative dipyridamole or dobutamine thallium scan is helpful in ruling out coronary artery disease. However, the gold standard remains coronary angiography.

Fewer than one-fifth of patients have normal left ventricular and left atrial dimensions on starting ESRD therapy. Substantial proportions have dilated cardiomyopathy and severe LVH. Systolic failure (ejection fraction 40% or less) is most often due to dilated cardiomyopathy, which on echocardiograph is diagnosed by the presence of an increased LV end-diastolic diameter (5.7 cm or more) and a decreased fractional shortening (less than 25%). Diastolic dysfunction is often associated with LVH, in which the LV wall is thickened in diastole (1.2 cm or more), and systolic function is maintained. In epidemiologic studies of nonrenal patients, LV mass has been calculated, the upper limits of normal being 130 g/m² for adult men and 102 g/m²

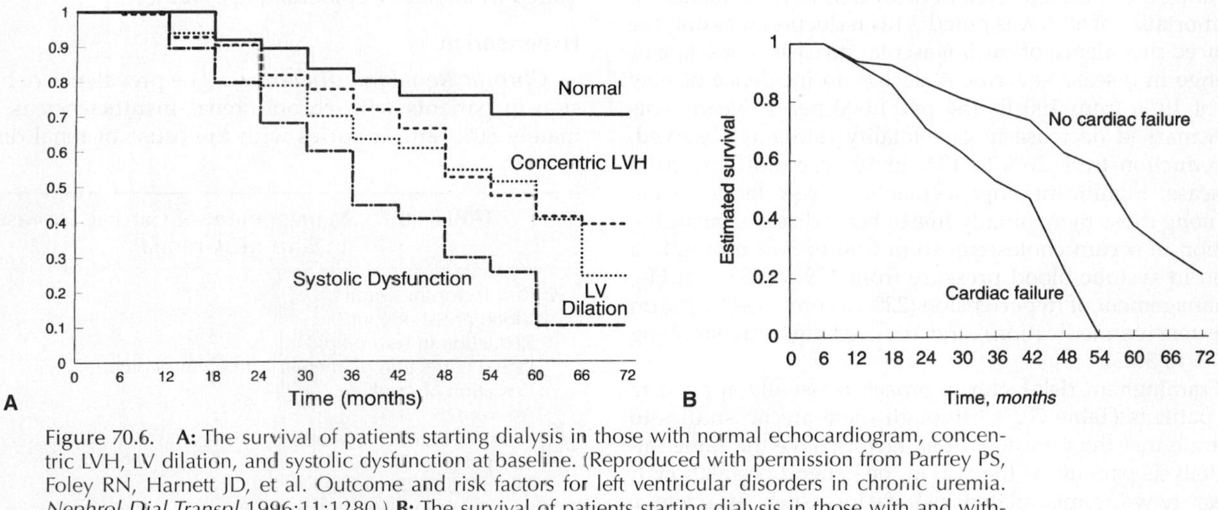

Figure 70.6. **A:** The survival of patients starting dialysis in those with normal echocardiogram, concentric LVH, LV dilation, and systolic dysfunction at baseline. (Reproduced with permission from Parfrey PS, Foley RN, Harnett JD, et al. Outcome and risk factors for left ventricular disorders in chronic uremia. *Nephrol Dial Transpl* 1996;11:1280.) **B:** The survival of patients starting dialysis in those with and without cardiac failure at baseline. (Reproduced with permission from Foley RN, Parfrey PS, Harnett JD, et al. Clinical echocardiographic cardiovascular disease in patients starting end-stage renal disease therapy: prevalence, associations and prognosis. *Kidney Int* 1995;47:189.)

for adult women. LV mass index is calculated by the following formula:

$$\text{LV mass index} = \frac{1.04\,[(\text{LVIDD} + \text{IVST} + \text{PWT})^3 - (\text{LVIDD}^3)] - 13.6}{\text{Body surface area}}$$

where *LVIDD* is diastolic LV internal diameter, *IVST* is diastolic LV septal wall thickness, and *PWT* is diastolic posterior wall thickness.

Diastolic LV function can be assessed noninvasively using pulsed Doppler analysis of flow across the mitral valve during diastole. Normally, as the mitral valve opens, ventricular relaxation occurs, with a rapid increase in flow leading to an E (or "early") peak, followed by a later increase, the A (or "atrial") peak, which reflects atrial contraction. Assuming normal atrial function, the increased stiffness of the hypertrophic LV leads to a smaller E peak, and a larger A peak, expressed conveniently as a decreased E/A ratio.

Echocardiography should be performed when the patient is considered to be euvolemic, because the increase in LV end-diastolic diameter, which occurs as plasma volume increases between hemodialyses, will increase the LV mass index calculation by approximately 25 g/m². The LV wall thickness in diastole does not change between dialyses and is a more stable assessment of LVH.

Differentiating between CHF caused by underlying heart disease and that caused by salt and water overload is not straightforward in dialysis patients. Therefore it is vital to know the "dry" weight (i.e., the patient's weight at which he or she is considered to be euvolemic). The examination of the dyspneic dialysis patient, outlined in Table 70.6, will help decide whether symptoms result from myocardial dysfunction.

TABLE 70.6. Investigation of Congestive Heart Failure in Chronic Uremia

A. Physical examination
  Number of kg above dry weight
  ? Volume overload
  Pulse rate and rhythm
  ? New arrhythmia
  Hypotension
  ? Severe systolic failure
  ? Silent infarction
  ? Pericardial effusion
  Hypertension
  ? Volume overload
  ? LV hypertrophy

B. Blood chemistry:
  Acidosis
  Hyperkalemia — Reversible causes of myocardial depression
  Hypocalcemia
  Hypophosphatemia
  Hypermagnesemia
  Hypoalbuminemia

C. Chest x-ray examination
  Heart size, pulmonary hypertension, interstitial edema

D. Electrocardiogram
  Infarction, ischemia, arrhythmia, LV hypertrophy, LA enlargement

E. Echocardiogram:
  LV hypertrophy
  LV systolic failure
  Segmental dyskinesia
  Valvular disease
  Pericardial effusion

Question: What is the cardiac diagnosis?

1. Systolic failure → Radionuclide angiography
2. Ischemic heart disease → Dipyridamole or dobutamine thallium scan
   If positive
   ↓
   Coronary arteriography
3. ? Diastolic dysfunction → Doppler echocardiography

LA, left atrial; LV, left ventricular.

Risk Factors

Risk-factor intervention has probably reduced cardiovascular mortality in the general population during the past 3 decades. Between 1950 and 1980, there has been a 30% decrease in cardiovascular deaths in the United States, two-thirds of which have occurred since 1970.

In an attempt to clarify the causes of this decline, a report from the Framingham study compared males who were 50 to 59 years of age on January 1, 1950, with a similar cohort from 1970. Among those initially free of heart disease, a reduction in 10-year mortality of 60% was noted. This reduction was not due to a reduced prevalence of cardiovascular disease at baseline or to a change in disease severity. A decline in incidence of new disease of 19%, from 190 to 154 per 1,000 per 10 years, was noted. A marked decrease in case-fatality rate was observed, with a reduction from 26% to 13% in 10-year mortality from new disease. Significant improvements in risk factors were noted among those men initially free of heart disease, including a reduction in serum cholesterol from 5.90 to 5.72 mmol/L, a reduction in systolic blood pressure from 139 to 135 mm Hg, better management of hypertension (22%, as opposed to 0%, on antihypertensive medication), and reduced cigarette smoking (from 56% to 34%).

The Framingham risk-factor approach is usually applied to dialysis patients (Table 70.7), although there are no studies to demonstrate that the traditional risk factors have the same impact in dialysis patients as they do in the general population. It is unclear how uremia-related risk factors such as anemia, weight gains between dialyses, volume removal during dialysis, fistula, hyperparathyroidism, divalent ion abnormalities, aluminum, iron, and acidosis impact on cardiac prognosis, hypertension, LVH, diabetes mellitus, hyperlipidemia, obesity, and smoking. Furthermore, the dialysis population is substantially different from the general population, having a high prevalence of cardiac disease at the start of dialysis, and a higher proportion with multiple cardiac risk factors. Accurate data on the most important, reversible, cardiac risk factors on dialysis patients is required from quality epidemiologic studies.

Hypertension

Chronic Renal Insufficiency. The prevalence of hypertension in patients with chronic renal insufficiency is approximately 80%, and it varies with the cause of renal disease. In

TABLE 70.7. Management of Cardiac Disease in Chronic Uremia

A. Risk-factor interventions
  Blood pressure control
  Reduction in serum lipids
  Partial correction of anemia with erythropoietin
  Cessation of smoking
  Aspirin

B. Uremia-related interventions
  Adequate dialysis
  Choice of ESRD modality
  Prevention of malnutrition
  Prevention and treatment of divalent ion abnormalities
  Prevention of hemodynamic overload

ESRD, end-stage renal disease.

the Modification of Diet in Renal Disease (MDRD) study, although 91% of patients were treated with antihypertensive agents, only 54% had blood pressure less than or equal to 140/90. Hypertension was associated with increased risk of progression of renal disease and onset of dialysis. A lower-than-usual target blood pressure (less than 125/75 mm Hg) was more effective than the usual goal (less than 140/90 mm Hg) in patients with proteinuria (more than 1 g/day), but not in patients without proteinuria. In both diabetic and nondiabetic patients, angiotensin-converting enzyme (ACE) inhibitors in combination with other drugs appear to be more effective in improving chronic renal disease outcomes than antihypertensive regimens not including ACE inhibitors. Further discussion on hypertension in chronic renal failure is found in Chapter 70, Part 3.

Dialysis Patients. The prevalence of hypertension is approximately 80% in hemodialysis patients, but the prevalence is lower in peritoneal dialysis patients (approximately 50%). The 1996 Core Indicators project reported that 53% of prevalent adult hemodialysis patients had predialysis systolic blood pressures in excess of 150 mm Hg, and 17% had predialysis diastolic blood pressures of 90 mm Hg or more. The comparable rates in peritoneal dialysis patients were 29% and 18%, respectively. In dialysis patients, hypertension is associated with increased risk of developing LVH, *de novo* ischemic heart disease, and *de novo* cardiac failure. Although these cardiac outcomes have an adverse impact on mortality, low blood pressure has been shown repeatedly to be associated with increased mortality. It is likely that low blood pressure is a marker for the presence of cardiac failure (and other disorders with an adverse outcome), which confounds the analyses assessing the relationships between blood pressure and death. A reasonable target blood pressure for antihypertensive treatment is predialysis blood pressure less than 140/90, unless the patient develops symptomatic hypotension or low blood pressure during or after dialysis. The mainstay of therapy is maintenance of normal extracellular fluid volume. Patients whose blood pressure is higher than 140/90 mm Hg following achievement of dry weight should have antihypertensive drugs prescribed. For further discussion of the topic, the reader is referred to Chapter 70, Part 3.

Hyperlipidemia

Virtually 100% of patients with nephrotic syndrome have hyperlipidemia, including approximately 30% of patients with chronic renal insufficiency without nephrotic syndrome, approximately 50% of hemodialysis patients, and 70% of peritoneal dialysis and renal transplant patients. Few longitudinal studies examine the relationship between lipid abnormalities and cardiac outcomes, although hyperlipidemia has been linked to progression of renal disease. The National Kidney Foundation Task Force on Cardiovascular Disease has recommended that the National Cholesterol Education Program (NCEP) Adult Treatment Panel General Population guidelines for initial classification, treatment initiation, and target cholesterol levels for diet and drug therapy should be used in patients with chronic renal disease, particularly because these patients are in the highest risk group for cardiac disease. Patients with serum cholesterol of more than 200 mg/dl or HDL cholesterol of 35 mg/dl or less should have a fasting lipid profile. LDL-cholesterol levels in excess of 100 mg and 130 mg/dl or more indicate treatment initiation values for diet and drug therapy, respectively. Target LDL-cholesterol levels are less than or equal to 100 mg/dl for both types of therapies. The HMG-CoA reductase inhibitors are the most effective drugs to lower LDL cholesterol in chronic renal disease and should be agents of first choice. Fibric acid analogs are also effective, but dosage reduction is required due to reduced renal function. Elevated serum triglyceride or low HDL cholesterol, in the absence of increased LDL cholesterol, should be treated by diet and increased physical activity, but drug therapy to reduce cardiac risk is not recommended. Further discussion on hyperlipidemia in nephrotic syndrome is found in Chapter 39, Part 2C, on the effects of lipid abnormalities on the kidney in Chapter 56, Part 3, and on the type, pathogenesis, and management of lipid abnormalities in chronic renal failure in Chapter 74, Part 2.

Diabetes Mellitus

Glycation of collagen may induce cross-linking of collagen fibers and cause not only large vessel and small vessel disease, but also myocardial dysfunction. However, the diabetic patient with chronic uremia has multiple other risk factors for cardiomyopathy including hyperlipidemia, hypertension, LVH, and chronic uremia.

Diabetes mellitus is an independent risk factor for the development of heart failure and coronary artery disease. Diabetic patients have more widespread coronary artery disease than do age- and sex-matched controls. Some diabetic patients with ESRD have impairment of LV function despite normal coronary arteries, perhaps because of a diabetic cardiomyopathy. In addition to coronary artery disease and systolic dysfunction, echocardiographic LVH is probably a more frequent finding in hypertensive diabetic patients than in hypertensive nondiabetic patients. In diabetic patients, this increased LV mass seems closely related to the level of blood pressure. A comparison of the pathologic spectrum of hypertensive, diabetic, and hypertensive-diabetic heart disease shows that the latter group had a significantly higher heart weight and a higher total fibrosis score than either of the other two groups.

In a cohort of dialysis patients who survived at least 6 months following the initiation of dialysis, 15% had insulin-dependent diabetes and 12% had non–insulin-dependent diabetes. On starting dialysis therapy, the prevalence of clinical manifestations of cardiac disease was significantly higher in diabetic patients compared with nondiabetic patients. Only 11% of diabetic patients had normal echocardiographic dimensions compared with 25% of nondiabetic patients, predominantly because of the prevalence of severe LVH (34% versus 18%). Echocardiographic determination of LV size and function was a good predictor of survival. Diabetic patients receiving dialysis therapy with abnormal LV wall motion and abnormal LV internal diameter had the lowest mean survival (8 months), a mortality rate not matched by any subgroup defined by coronary anatomy, ventricular function, or clinical manifestation.

In patients with chronic renal insufficiency due to diabetic renal disease, strict glycemic control may slow the progression of renal disease, and in transplant recipients it may slow the recurrence of diabetic renal disease. Therefore intensive glucose control may be beneficial in these two groups. However in dialysis patients, strict glycemic control is more difficult, the risk of hypoglycemia is greater, and the consequences of hypoglycemia are greater.

Tobacco Use

The prevalence of tobacco use in chronic renal disease is similar to that observed in the general population. Tobacco use is associated with a higher risk of cardiovascular outcomes. Therefore the general population guideline for counseling and nicotine replacement should be applied in patients with chronic renal disease.

Anemia

Anemia is associated with LV dilation and LVH in chronic renal insufficiency and in dialysis patients. It is a risk factor for the development of *de novo* cardiac failure and death in dialysis patients. It is not a risk factor for *de novo* ischemic heart disease.

The number of dialysis patients entered in studies of the effect of erythropoietin on cardiac structure and function have been few. It is likely that correction of anemia will induce regression of hypertrophy, but whether it will normalize mass is not clear. Furthermore, irreversible myocardial fibrosis is probably responsible for some increase in LV mass and is likely to persist despite amelioration of anemia. If so, correction of anemia may not prevent all of the clinical consequences of LVH. Furthermore, the impact of erythropoietin on various subsets of dialysis patients with other cardiac disease is unknown.

A large, randomized, controlled, clinical trial was undertaken in the United States in hemodialysis patients with preexisting ischemic heart disease or cardiac failure, in which normalization of hemoglobin with erythropoietin was compared with partial correction of anemia. The primary outcome was death or myocardial infarction. The trial was stopped early because of increased mortality and increased vascular access loss in the group randomized to normalization of hemoglobin level. Therefore the target hemoglobin for patients with preexisting symptomatic cardiac disease should be approximately 10 to 11 g/L.

Another multicenter, randomized, controlled trial was undertaken in Canada in which hemodialysis patients without symptomatic cardiac disease were allocated to normalization of hemoglobin with erythropoietin or to partial correction of anemia. Two groups were studied, patients with preexisting LV dilation and patients with concentric hypertrophy. In the former group, mean LV volume was high at baseline (approximately 120 mg/m^2) and a substantial minority had systolic dysfunction. Normalization of hemoglobin failed to induce regression of LV dilation. In the latter group, normalization of hemoglobin failed to induce regression of LVH but it did prevent progressive LV dilation. These two studies suggest that normalization of hemoglobin will not be effective when cardiac disease progresses to severe LV dilation or to symptomatic presentation. Further studies are necessary to demonstrate whether normalization of hemoglobin in patients with less-severe cardiac disorders may be efficacious in the prevention of adverse cardiac outcomes.

Hypoalbuminemia and Therapy of Uremia

There is no evidence to suggest that continuous ambulatory peritoneal dialysis (CAPD) is better than hemodialysis in prolonging life in those with cardiac disease, or in predisposing to the development of cardiac diseases. It is unclear whether further improvements in dialysis technology are necessary to diminish the uremic component of cardiac disease. The effect of inadequate dialysis and malnutrition on the development or progression of cardiac disease is unknown, and awaits the performance of good prospective cohort studies. Nonetheless, it is imperative that we prescribe optimal dialysis prescription to our patients. Frequent determination of dialysis adequacy should be performed and acted upon.

Uremia

The hemodialysis state constitutes a condition of hemodynamic overload and metabolic perturbation lethal in its impact on the heart. Renal transplantation is the best model of what happens to the heart when uremia is treated properly. Although hypertension usually persists, as does the fistula and perhaps hypervolemia, anemia is corrected, as is the metabolic perturbation. Following renal transplantation, concentric LVH and LV dilation improve, but the most striking observation is the improvement in systolic dysfunction. It is not known which adverse risk factors characteristic of the uremic state have been corrected to produce the improvement in LV contractility. Dialysis provides inadequate treatment of the uremic state, but the target quantity of dialysis, which may limit the contribution of "uremic toxins" to cardiac dysfunction, is unknown. The current trial ongoing in the United States comparing two quantities of hemodialysis may be helpful in this regard.

Hypoalbuminemia

Hypoalbuminemia has been shown repeatedly to be a most potent predictor of outcome in ESRD patients. Hypoalbuminemia is associated with LV dilation, which may reflect the impact of malnutrition in predisposing to myocyte death. Hypoalbuminemia predisposes to *de novo* cardiac failure and to *de novo* ischemic heart disease. Is hypoalbuminemia a marker for malnutrition, or inadequate treatment of uremic cardiotoxins, or a prothrombotic state, or a dyslipidemic state, or a chronic inflammatory state, or vitamin deficiencies? How hypoalbuminemia predisposes to cardiac disease is clearly an area for research because interventions may then be developed to reverse the culprit risk factors.

Hypoalbuminemia is more characteristic of peritoneal dialysis than of hemodialysis, and may result from different mechanisms in patients treated by these different modalities of dialysis therapy. It is likely that the path to death is different in hemodialysis patients because a higher proportion of this group developed cardiac failure (presumably due to the more adverse hemodynamic environment), which predisposed to earlier death.

Abnormal Divalent Ion Metabolism

In our study, hypocalcemia was strongly associated with ischemic heart disease, even after adjusting for age, diabetes, blood pressure, hemoglobin, and several other covariates. The effect was as marked in peritoneal dialysis patients as in hemodialysis patients, and was only partly explained by the relationship between mean serum calcium and time spent on dialysis therapy. Another group has shown that low calcium levels are independently associated with mortality in a large cross section of dialysis patients.

Death of myocytes may be caused by hyperparathyroidism, as may interstitial myocardial fibrosis. Extensive fibrosis may be responsible for attenuation of the hypertrophic response to pressure overload, and may contribute to the development of dilated cardiomyopathy and heart failure in subjects with secondary hyperparathyroidism. Although the circumstantial evidence supports a role for abnormalities of divalent ion metabolism in the development of cardiac disease in dialysis patients, the implications of these observations for patient care are less obvious. The absence of detailed longitudinal data in large numbers of patients precludes the identification of precise risk factors, which would permit studies of relevant interventions. The effect of secondary hyperthyroidism and of excess parathyroid hormone on the myocardium is discussed in Chapter 68, Part 1.

Our current armamentarium of vitamin D analogs, phosphate binders, and high-flux dialyzers should diminish the incidence of hyperparathyroidism. The increased acceptance of early parathyroidectomy in those with nonresponsive hyperparathyroidism should reduce the duration of time that the heart is exposed to high levels of this cardiotoxic hormone. Thus it is likely that the impact of hyperparathyroidism as a potentially important cardiac toxin will diminish. Our current decreased use of aluminum–phosphate binders should have a similar result on the potentially toxic effect of aluminum on the heart.

Hyperhomocysteinemia

Homocysteine levels in blood are elevated in patients with chronic renal disease in inverse proportion to the reduction in renal function. Elevated levels are a risk factor for cardiovascular disease in the general population and appear to be associated with increased risk in patients with chronic renal disease. A combination of high-dose folic acid, vitamin B_{12}, and vitamin B_6 lower homocysteine levels by 25%, which may restore normal levels in patients with chronic renal insufficiency or in renal transplant recipients, but not in dialysis patients. Whether this intervention will provide clinical benefit is unknown. Further discussion on the metabolism of homocysteine in chronic renal failure and on the adverse effects of hyperhomocysteinemia in these patients is found in Chapter 68, Part 3.

Prothrombotic Factors

Decreased platelet aggregation and increased bleeding time occur in patients with chronic renal disease, especially chronic renal insufficiency and hemodialysis patients. Elevated levels of fibrinogen and other procoagulant factors are also observed in chronic renal disease. There is no evidence concerning the relationship of these abnormalities in platelet function and procoagulant activity to cardiac outcomes in chronic renal disease. In the general population the percentage reduction of cardiac disease by aspirin in patients with prior myocardial infarct, stroke, transient ischemic attacks, unstable angina, coronary bypass graft surgery, coronary angioplasty, atrial fibrillation, valvular heart disease, and peripheral vascular disease is approximately 25%. Aspirin therapy probably worsens the platelet defect in chronic renal disease and increases the risk of bleeding. Despite these risks in chronic renal disease, patients with overt cardiovascular disease should probably be prescribed aspirin (81 mg/day) to reduce the risk of subsequent cardiovascular events. However in renal patients without clinical cardiac disease, although they are at high risk of developing cardiac disease, it is not possible to recommend universal use. Individual treatment decisions must be based on considerations of patients' individual risks, likely benefits, and preferences.

Management

Drug Therapy for Heart Failure (Fig. 70.7)

Angiotensin-Converting Enzyme Inhibitors. ACE inhibitors have been clearly shown to improve symptoms, morbidity, and survival in nonuremic individuals with heart failure. It seems reasonable to extrapolate these results to the dialysis population and to recommend their use. The benefit of ACE inhibition is applicable to those with diastolic and systolic dysfunction. ACE inhibitors should also be used to prevent CHF in asymptomatic patients whose LV ejection fraction is less than 35% and in post–myocardial infarction patients with an ejection fraction of 40% or less.

Digoxin. Digoxin improves symptoms in nonrenal subjects with heart failure, and clinical deterioration may occur when it is discontinued. Based on these results, it is recommended for use in dialysis patients with heart failure who have systolic dysfunction, with or without atrial fibrillation. It should be avoided in those dialysis subjects with diastolic dysfunction because increased contractility induced by digoxin could worsen diastolic function. It should be used cautiously in this group if atrial fibrillation with a rapid ventricular response is present. Care should be taken to avoid low dialysate potassium levels, because the resultant hypokalemia may predispose to arrhythmias in the presence of digoxin. Other inotropic agents, with the possible exception of dobutamine in intractable cases, are not recommended.

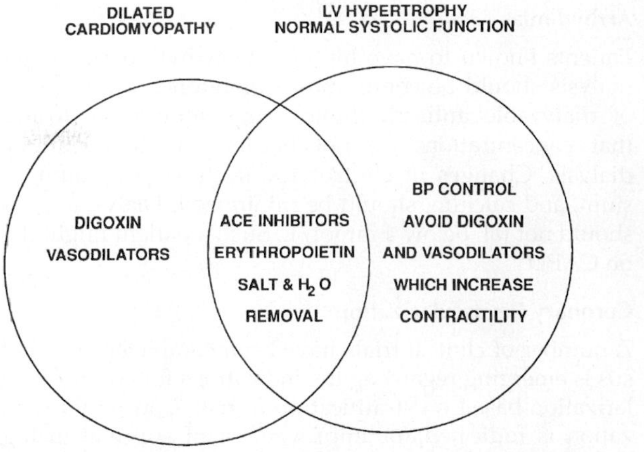

Figure 70.7. Treatment of congestive heart failure in chronic uremia for patients with dilated LV and systolic failure and for patients with LV hypertrophy and normal systolic function. BP, blood pressure.

Other Drugs. Nitrates and hydralazine can be used as adjunctive therapy or in subjects intolerant of ACE inhibitors. They have been shown to improve symptoms and survival in the nonuremic population with heart failure. They are not of proven benefit in subjects with diastolic dysfunction and should probably be avoided because they increase contractility. When nitrates are prescribed, the patient should avoid the use of the antiimpotence drug sildenafil (Viagra).

The Canadian Cardiovascular Society Consensus Conference on the diagnosis and management of heart failure recommends that the results of larger trials with clinically important end points be awaited before recommending routine use of β-blockers. This would appear to be wise advice to apply to the dialysis population. In individual patients who remain refractory to usual treatment, careful use of a β-blocker may be reasonable. At this time, there is inadequate evidence to support the use of calcium channel blockers in heart failure.

Drug Therapy for Angina

Nitrates are the mainstay of treatment for acute anginal episodes. The response to long-acting nitrates is comparable to that seen in nonuremic patients, and nitrate tolerance is usually not a major problem. When angina occurs during dialysis, however, administration of sublingual nitrate may predispose to hypotension. Therefore whenever possible, this should be avoided. Other measures such as nasal oxygen administration, decreasing ultrafiltration rate, and fluid replacement may alleviate the symptoms of angina. β-Blockers and calcium channel blockers are useful adjuncts to the medical therapy of angina. Short-acting calcium channel blockers should be used with caution, because they may cause unpredictable changes in blood pressure.

Arrhythmias

Patients known to have high-grade arrhythmia during hemodialysis should be continuously monitored. Dosing schedules of dialyzable antiarrhythmic drugs should be arranged so that concentrations do not become subtherapeutic during dialysis. Changes in electrolytes, such as potassium, magnesium, and calcium, should be minimized. Dialysate potassium should not fall below 4 mmol/L. Such a patient might do better on CAPD.

Coronary Revascularization

A number of clinical trials have been completed and a consensus is emerging regarding the indications for coronary revascularization based on stratification of risk. Coronary revascularization is indicated for improvement of survival in high-risk patients or relief of symptoms as an alternative to medical therapy in low-risk patients. High-risk patients include patients with left main coronary artery disease; three-vessel disease, moderate symptoms and reduced LV function; and two-vessel disease and involvement of proximal left anterior descending coronary artery. In high-risk patients, coronary artery bypass graft (CABG) surgery reduces the rate of subsequent myocardial infarct and improves survival, compared with medical therapy. CABG is generally preferred to percutaneous transluminal coronary angioplasty (PTCA) in high-risk patients. Low-risk patients include those with single-vessel disease and normal LV function. In these patients, a strategy of initial medical therapy is reasonable for relief of symptoms. PTCA provides greater alleviation of symptoms, but does not improve rates of mortality or acute myocardial infarct. Moderate-risk patients include those with multivessel coronary artery disease and normal LV function. Coronary revascularization is often necessary for relief of symptoms. In these patients, PTCA and CABG produce roughly equivalent rates of mortality and acute myocardial infarct, but PTCA-treated patients require more revascularization procedures.

The benefits and risks of coronary arteriography and revascularization have not been carefully studied in chronic renal disease. Some differences from the general population are apparent. First, impairment in renal function is a risk factor for contrast-induced acute renal insufficiency; thus patients with chronic renal insufficiency or renal transplant recipients are at higher risk for this complication. In patients with severe impairment in renal function, infusion of radiocontrast during cardiac catheterization may precipitate ESRD, and in dialysis patients, it may cause a reduction in residual renal function. The risk of contrast-induced acute renal insufficiency may be lessened by nonionic contrast media and by saline infusion. Further discussion on contrast media nephropathy is found in Chapter 47, Part 7.

Second, in hemodialysis patients, the perioperative mortality of CABG surgery is approximately three times higher than in the general population, even when adjustment for other comorbid factors is not performed. Third, PTCA is successful in dilating stenotic vessels, but is associated with frequent recurrence of symptoms, usually resulting from restenosis. Early results from stenting of dilated vessels suggest a lower restenosis rate with this procedure. However, the initial technical success and relief of symptoms obtained by revascularization is similar to the general population. In one randomized trial of a small number of diabetic transplant candidates, an approach using screening coronary arteriography and CABG surgery reduced acute myocardial infarct and cardiac mortality. Whether revascularization improves survival in other high-risk subgroups or target populations is not known.

Overall, the indications for coronary revascularization in chronic renal disease are generally similar to those in the general population. In high-risk patients, and in patients with persistent symptoms of myocardial ischemia despite maximal medical therapy, whose life expectancy is greater than 6 months, revascularization appears to be beneficial. CABG is probably the revascularization procedure of choice, although angioplasty with stenting may prove to be a reasonable alternative in single-vessel disease or multi-vessel disease with culprit lesions. In the latter, antiplatelet therapy used with stenting could possibly exacerbate the bleeding diathesis of uremia. As in the general population, coronary arteriography should be reserved for patients in whom revascularization would be undertaken if critical coronary artery disease were identified.

Conclusions

The burden of cardiac disease in dialysis patients is high. Multiple Framingham-derived risk factors and potential uremia-related risk factors for cardiac disease exist. The impact of the latter on the development and progression of cardiac diseases and their interrelationships are virtually unknown. Severe LVH, dilated cardiomyopathy, and coronary artery disease occur frequently and predispose to CHF, myocardial infarction and angina, arrhythmias, dialysis hypotension, and death. Echocardiography is a useful diagnostic tool in chronic uremia. Interventions that should be considered in dialysis patients with cardiac disease include drugs that lower blood pressure and induce regression of hypertrophy, correction of anemia with erythropoietin, prevention and treatment of hyperparathyroidism, lipid-lowering agents, and drugs that improve systolic function.

Selected Readings

Foley RN, Parfrey PS. Cardiac disease in chronic uremia: clinical outcome and risk factors. *Adv Renal Replac Ther* 1997;4:234–248.

This paper reviews the multiple publications arising from a cohort study of 433 end-stage renal disease (ESRD) patients who survived at least 6 months on ESRD therapy and were followed for a mean of 41 months.

Levey AS, Beto JA, Coronado BE, et al. Controlling the epidemic of cardiovascular disease in chronic renal disease. What do we know? What do we need to learn? Where do we go from here? *Am J Kidney Dis* 1998;32:853–906.

This is the final report of the National Kidney Foundation Task Force on Cardiovascular disease in chronic uremia, which provided recommendations for risk-factor intervention and clinical management of cardiac disease in the various groups of patients with chronic renal disease.

London GM, Parfrey PS. Cardiac disease in chronic uremia: pathogenesis. *Adv Renal Replac Ther* 1997;4:194–211.

This paper is a distillation of patient-related research performed in France and Canada on cardiac disease in dialysis patients. References for the pathogenesis section of this chapter can be obtained from this paper.

Murphy SW, Foley RN, Parfrey PS. Recommendations for the screening and treatment of cardiovascular disease in patients with chronic renal disease. *Am J Kidney Dis* 1998;32:S184–S199.

This review was performed for the National Kidney Foundation Task Force on Cardiovascular Disease in chronic renal disease. It contains an up-to-date reference list.

Sytkowski PA, Kannel WB, D'Agostino RB. Changes in risk factors and the decline in mortality from cardiovascular disease: the Framingham study. *N Engl J Med* 1990;322:1634–1641.

The Framingham study is one of the most important clinical studies undertaken since the Second World War. It has had a major impact on the management of cardiac disease in nonrenal patients, and its conclusions have been extrapolated to ESRD patients. Every nephrologist should have intimate knowledge of this magnificent project.

United States Renal Data System. *1997 Annual Data Report, Bethesda, MD, US Department of Health and Human Services.* National Institutes of Health, 1997.

This huge registry of ESRD patients in the United States is a mine of information concerning prognosis and cause of death analyzed by year of starting ESRD therapy, modality of ESRD therapy, and primary renal diagnosis.

PART 3
Hypertension

Robert G. Luke and Max C. Reif

Our goal is to address hypertension as both a cause of renal failure and a result of parenchymal renal disease. Essential (Chapter 61), renovascular (Chapter 62), endocrine (Chapter 63), pediatric (Chapter 64), and geriatric (Chapter 65) hypertension, as well as the genetics of hypertension (Chapter 60) and hypertension in African-Americans, are discussed elsewhere in this text. Hypertension frequently complicates acute and chronic renal failure, and malignant or accelerated hypertension virtually always affects the kidney. Hypertension is the most important risk factor for increasing rate of loss of renal function in patients with chronic renal failure; in turn, absent specific treatment for the primary cause of chronic renal failure, treatment of hypertension is the most important therapeutic intervention to slow progression of renal disease. Treatment of hypertension is especially beneficial if it is associated with a persistent reduction in proteinuria. In patients with end-stage renal disease (ESRD) who are receiving renal replacement therapy, hypertension remains an important risk factor for cardiovascular morbidity and mortality, which continues to account for half of the deaths in dialysis and transplant patients. Early and intensive treatment of hypertension in the pre-ESRD stage is also necessary if we are to reduce cardiovascular mortality in ESRD patients.

HYPERTENSION AS A CAUSE OF RENAL FAILURE: HYPERTENSIVE NEPHROSCLEROSIS

Primary malignant or accelerated hypertension with grade 4 or grade 3 hypertensive retinopathy can cause acute and chronic renal failure. The pathognomonic feature of this syndrome in the kidney is arteriolar fibrinoid necrosis. The syndrome is seen much less commonly today than previously because of earlier detection and treatment of essential hypertension by effective drugs. Even before the development of such therapy, only 1% to 3% of patients with so-called benign essential hypertension entered the malignant phase. In Caucasians, primary malignant hypertension is more likely to be due to hypertension secondary to, for example, renovascular causes, primary renal disease, or systemic vasculitis.

Hypertensive nephrosclerosis is the renal lesion associated with long-standing nonmalignant essential hypertension, formerly—and wrongly—called *benign hypertension.* Clinical studies before the availability of efficacious antihypertensive drugs in the 1950s revealed an approximately 60% mortality over a 20-year follow-up in such patients, mainly attributable to heart failure and stroke, but also to chronic renal failure in as many as 25% of patients dying from hypertension. The classic histologic lesions are myointimal hyperplasia and hyaline arteriosclerosis in small arteries and arterioles, predominantly in the preglomerular arterioles. The vascular lesions are associated with ischemic glomerular "wrinkling collapse." The renal lesions can be seen after 5 years of hypertension and occur in other arteries and arterioles in the body, but are most severe in the kidneys. These vascular lesions can also occur in the absence of, or before the onset of, hypertension in patients with chronic primary renal disease such as glomerulonephritis, especially focal glomerulosclerosis. They are also seen with aging, diabetes mellitus, and states of prolonged vasoconstriction.

Hypertension now accounts for approximately 26% of the annual incidences of ESRD, according to the data from the U.S. Registry. In Caucasians, such ESRD usually occurs after the age of 60 years with a peak incidence at 70 to 75 years. The annual incidence of ESRD due to hypertension continues to increase, especially in the elderly. Because few of these patients have other primary renal diseases excluded by renal biopsy, some experts question the accuracy of the diagnosis of primary hypertensive nephrosclerosis. It is admittedly likely that a minority of patients also have related contributory factors to renal functional deterioration such as renovascular renal failure (potentially treatable by angioplasty or surgery), atheroembolic renal disease, and segmental renal infarction. A strong association between increasing severity of essential hypertension in males initially examined between 1973 and 1975 and the incidence of ESRD over an average period of 16 years has also been shown. Increasing evidence also supports both a genetic basis for essential hypertension via various renal mechanisms and for, by separate genetic mechanisms, a susceptibility for progressive renal disease in response to hypertensive damage. Both hypertension and hypertensive nephrosclerosis are more common in African-Americans.

It has been much easier to show a reduction (now amounting to 60%) in mortality resulting from stroke and heart failure due to hypertension over the past 2 decades than it has been to show a reduction in ESRD secondary to hypertension. As noted, the latter has, at least currently, increased. Even if ESRD is not yet being prevented, it is essential to obtain the protective effects of antihypertensive therapy on the systemic cardiovascular system. Hypertensive patients with evidence of any impairment in renal function or of proteinuria should be regarded as being at enhanced cardiovascular risk ("vasculopaths") and they require meticulous blood pressure control. Available data support the recommendations that call for a target blood pressure of 125/75 mm Hg (mean blood pressure of 92 mm Hg) in patients with proteinuria more than 1 g/day.

A diagnosis of hypertensive nephrosclerosis depends on a history of hypertension for some time, at least 5 years and probably longer, along with initially normal renal function and urinalysis. In contrast, the majority of patients with primary parenchymal renal disease, the most common cause of secondary hypertension, have an abnormal urinalysis with proteinuria or microscopic hematuria, pyuria, or casts before the onset of hypertension. Hypertension secondary to underlying renal disease is a certain risk factor for renal failure and must be treated, whereas watchful waiting might be employed in many patients with essential hypertension, with borderline elevation of blood pressure, and with no evidence of hypertensive target-organ diseases or other cardiovascular risk factors.

In cases in which the patient is seen initially with hypertension and chronic renal failure, the differential diagnosis can be difficult (Table 70.8). Renal ultrasound reveals polycystic kidney disease, reflux nephropathy (chronic pyelonephritis), or obstructive uropathy. A history of nephrotic syndrome, gross hematuria, or previous acute nephritic syndrome suggests primary renal disease. Symptoms of chronic renal failure are, of course, nonspecific for primary or secondary hypertension. Findings of left ventricular hypertrophy and hypertensive retinopathy lend some support to the diagnosis of primary hypertension because it is unusual for mild to moderate hypertension to cause substantial renal impairment without evidence of target-organ damage elsewhere.

Renal biopsy confirmation of the accuracy of a diagnosis of hypertensive nephrosclerosis based on these clinical features

TABLE 70.8. Clinical Features Favoring a Diagnosis of Primary Hypertensive Nephrosclerosis over Primary Parenchymal Renal Disease in Hypertensive Patients[a]

- African-American race
- Onset of hypertension before proteinuria
- Hypertension documented for at least 10 years or previous accelerated hypertension
- Family history of hypertension or ESRD due to hypertensive nephrosclerosis
- Left ventricular hypertrophy
- 24-hour urinary protein excretion less than 2 g
- Except for accelerated hypertension, an "active" urinary sediment

[a] After ruling out obvious primary renal diseases such as glomerulonephritis with nephrotic syndrome, polycystic kidney disease, Alport's syndrome, reflux nephropathy, and so on.
ESRD, end-stage renal disease.

has been provided in preliminary studies for the African American Study of Kidney Disease (AASK) Trial, at least in African-Americans with nonnephrotic proteinuria. In older Caucasians, the clinical diagnosis is also likely feasible but, as noted, other vascular causes must be considered.

There are likely two mechanisms of glomerular damage in primary nonmalignant hypertension. The first is due to ischemia, characterized by afferent arteriolar hyalinization and luminal narrowing and wrinkling collapse of the basement membranes of the glomerular capillaries. There is progressive glomerular dropout because of global sclerosis, and the less severely involved nephrons undergo hypertrophy. These "adapted" nephrons are then subject to glomerular hypertrophy, hyperperfusion, and the ultimate development of focal glomerulosclerosis. Based on animal studies, one could make a case for preferring calcium channel blockers to dilate the afferent arteriole for the ischemic lesion and for angiotensin-converting enzyme (ACE) inhibitors to reduce glomerular capillary pressure via efferent dilation in hyperperfused nephrons. Such acquired focal glomerular sclerosis likely accounts for the heavier proteinuria and worse prognosis seen in some patients with hypertensive nephrosclerosis and renal failure; these patients merit ACE inhibitors as primary therapy for their hypertension.

We urgently need identifiable risk factors for hypertensive nephrosclerosis in patients with mild to moderate hypertension. Perhaps the best indicators of the risk for hypertensive renal disease in patients with less-severe hypertension are African-American race, a family history of hypertensive ESRD, left ventricular hypertrophy, and the presence of even slight fixed proteinuria (i.e., more than 150 mg/24 hr). Confirmed microalbuminuria (more than 30 mg/24 hr), unlike diabetic nephropathy, is a likely but not yet a proven harbinger of progressive hypertensive nephrosclerosis, but certainly indicates a much increased cardiovascular risk and justifies more intense antihypertensive treatment.

ACUTE RENAL FAILURE

Acute intrinsic renal failure is commonly accompanied by new onset of hypertension in acute nephritic syndrome, rapidly progressive glomerulonephritis, hemolytic-uremic syndrome, and atheroembolic renal failure. Likewise, many connective tissue disorders leading to acute renal impairment such as scleroderma, systemic lupus erythematosus, or polyarteritis nodosa often also cause new hypertension. The most common causes of intrinsic acute renal failure, acute tubular necrosis, and acute interstitial nephritis do not lead to hypertension unless the renal failure results in marked retention of sodium chloride and water. Such hypertension remits with diuresis or dialysis.

Very severe primary hypertension with arteriolar fibrinoid necrosis can cause acute renal failure. Even when less-severe hypertension than this is treated with antihypertensive drugs, an acute fall in glomerular filtration rate (GFR) can occur. This relates to an impaired autoregulatory response for GFR during reduced renal perfusion as blood pressure is brought down into the normal range. This is likely, in turn, secondary to impaired vasodilation of the nephrosclerotic or necrotic afferent arteriole. Severe hypertension should be reduced gradually over a few days or weeks into the normal range, but the physician should persist with antihypertensive therapy despite an immediate deterioration of renal function, because the latter may return to the level of GFR before the development of accelerated hypertension. This rule also holds even in cases in which dialysis is needed; patients with accelerated hypertension compose one of the groups most likely to recover some renal function, presumably because of resolution of arteriolar fibrinoid necrosis with maintained blood pressure control. Physicians should attempt to prevent accelerated hypertension; however, one series showed that 50% of patients developed a further elevation of serum creatinine over the 5 years following an accelerated phase of hypertension, even with good antihypertensive treatment, presumably as a result of the long-term effects of acute vascular injury.

There are two exceptions to this policy of persisting with antihypertensive therapy despite an initial drop in GFR. First, if the blood pressure is reduced below the normal autoregulatory range, therapy should be reduced or temporarily discontinued. Second, when the renal perfusion pressure in a hypertensive patient is reduced in a clinical setting in which the afferent arteriole cannot relax or dilate to maintain glomerular capillary pressure, the latter, and hence GFR, becomes dependent on the ability of the efferent arteriole to constrict. Afferent dilation is often already complete (in an attempt to maintain GFR) distal to a functionally significant severe renal artery stenosis (RAS); the afferent arteriole may not be able to relax if the patient is taking nonsteroidal antiinflammatory drugs (failure to produce vasodilatory prostaglandins) or cyclosporine (which induces constriction of vascular smooth muscle in the afferent arteriole); and in very severe arteriolar vascular disease (resulting from scleroderma or diabetes, for example), preglomerular arteriolar vasodilation may be inadequate. Under these circumstances, efferent arteriole constriction becomes important in the maintenance of intraglomerular pressure. Because efferent arteriolar vasoconstriction is highly dependent on the effect of angiotensin II, the use of ACE inhibitors in these clinical situations may precipitate acute renal failure. Thus this acute renal failure is a form of hemodynamic prerenal failure with no change in urinary sediment and a low excretion of sodium, and it usually responds quickly to withdrawal of the drug. The phenomenon is due to an *intrarenal* hemodynamic event and can occur at normal or even high blood pressure levels. Concomitant use of any two, or all three, of the nonsteroidal antiinflammatory drugs, cyclosporine, and ACE inhibitors should be approached with great caution. Acute renal failure during treatment of hypertension with an ACE inhibitor in an elderly hypertensive patient with diffuse atherosclerotic disease should lead the clinician to consider a diagnosis of renovascular renal failure (ischemic nephropathy) in which all remaining functional nephrons are distal to a significant renal artery stenosis.

PARENCHYMAL RENAL DISEASE AND HYPERTENSION

Prevalence

The prevalence and severity of hypertension increases steadily as renal function deteriorates, until 95% of patients are hypertensive as they approach ESRD. If one looks at all presenting hypertensive patients, approximately 5% relate to underlying renal parenchymal disease. Thus renovascular hypertension is the most common remediable cause of hypertension, and parenchymal renal disease is the most common secondary cause of hypertension. Patients with tubulointerstitial disease, such as medullary cystic kidney disease, leading to salt wasting even at normal levels of dietary salt intake, are usually "protected" from hypertension up to or close to the need for renal replacement therapy. Renal diseases associated with proliferative glomerular processes (e.g., membranoproliferative glomerulonephritis) or with severe involvement of the renal vasculature (e.g., polyarteritis nodosa or scleroderma) may be associated with early onset of hypertension even before a measured increase in blood urea nitrogen or serum creatinine levels become evident. In glomerulonephritis caused by a nonproliferative process such as membranous glomerulopathy, hypertension may develop much later, when the GFR has fallen significantly. In "malignant" focal glomerulosclerosis, which progresses to ESRD within a few years, early onset of hypertension may relate to the commonly accompanying hyaline arterial sclerosis of the preglomerular vessels. In autosomal-dominant, adult polycystic kidney disease, hypertension also may be the first manifestation of the disease at a time when GFR is still in the normal range.

Pathogenesis (Table 70.9 and Fig. 70.8)

As compared with essential hypertension, elevated blood pressure secondary to parenchymal renal disease is much more likely to progress to a malignant phase, to be associated with left ventricular hypertrophy, and to cause more cardiovascular disease. In contrast to the "normal" circadian rhythm in essential hypertensive patients with a fall in blood pressure and pulse rate at night, in hypertensive chronic renal failure patients there is an actual *increase* in nighttime blood pressure and pulse rate. The association of hypertension, chronic renal disease, and increased cardiovascular risk may reflect extracellular fluid and plasma volume expansion, enhanced renin-angiotensin activity (both systemic and organ based), hyperlipidemia, insulin resistance, secondary hyperparathyroidism, and a resetting of

TABLE 70.9. Mechanisms of Hypertension Secondary to Primary Renal Disease

Retention of NaCl and H_2O[a] (see Fig. 70.11)[a]
High renin-angiotensin activity relative to ECF volume[a]
Stimulation of SNS by kidney[a]
Increased vascular sensitivity to vasopressors[b]
Defective NO formation[b]
Enhanced endothelin release[b]
High parathyroid hormone levels[b]
Renoprival mechanisms—low VMDL[b]
Insulin resistance[b]

[a] Most important mechanisms
[b] Less important or putative mechanisms
ECF, extracellular fluid; NO, nitric oxide; SNS, sympathetic nervous system; VMDL, vasodepressor medullary lipid.

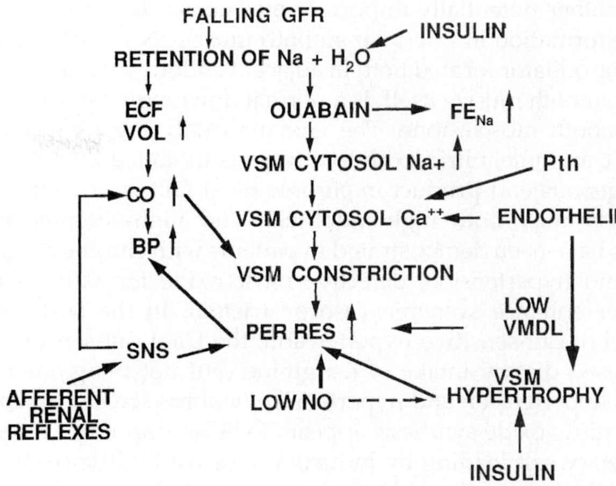

Figure 70.8. Mechanisms of hypertension in renal parenchymal disease. Heightened sensitivity to vasoconstrictors may also be important. CO, cardiac output; ECF vol, extracellular fluid volume; NO, nitric oxide; PER RES, peripheral resistance; PTH, parathyroid hormone; SNS, sympathetic nervous system; VSM, vasodepressor medullary lipid.

endothelial-derived factors influencing vascular smooth muscle endothelins to favor vasoconstriction and hypertrophy. There is experimental evidence that elevated intrarenal and systemic angiotensin II levels may be associated with increased renal endothelin, reduced nitric oxide, and elevated systemic and renal transforming growth factor (TGF)-β levels. The latter is a cytokine that can lead to glomerular and tubulointerstitial fibrosis. Some genetic polymorphisms of the ACE gene appear to be associated with a tendency to progression of renal disease.

Studies in humans from the stage of mild renal insufficiency to ESRD patients on dialysis, and in various experimental animal models of chronic renal failure, show an overall pattern of extracellular fluid volume expansion with a level of activity of the renin-angiotensin system elevated above that seen in normal subjects with an equivalent degree of retention of sodium chloride. The normal inhibitory effects of plasma volume expansion and hypertension on renin synthesis and release are clearly impaired.

Most patients with chronic renal failure and hypertension have salt-sensitive hypertension. As nephrons are lost in progressive renal disease, the remaining nephrons must excrete progressively greater fractions of the filtered load of sodium chloride to maintain sodium balance. The mechanisms by which this occurs are likely multiple, but include release from the central nervous system of a natriuretic ouabainlike substance that inhibits Na^+-K^+-ATPase. This helps natriuresis but increases vascular smooth muscle cytosol sodium and calcium concentrations with enhanced sensitivity to vasoconstrictors. In a minority of patients, induction of a negative balance of sodium and chloride by diuretics or dialysis leads to a marked elevation of renin levels and hypertension, at least in the supine position. Such patients have been considered to have renin-dependent hypertension. The concept of either volume-dependent or renin-dependent hypertension is an oversimplification; however, and it now appears that there is a spectrum of causation in both of these situations.

Plasma norepinephrine levels are elevated in chronic renal failure. Enhanced activity of the peripheral sympathetic nervous system in dialysis patients, terminated by bilateral nephrectomy, has now been clearly demonstrated. Both chemoreceptor and baroreceptor afferent signals from the damaged kidneys appear to be involved.

Another potentially important mechanism is defective nitric oxide formation in arteriolar smooth muscle. Nitric oxide, a potent vasodilator formed both in adjacent endothelium and in vascular smooth muscle itself, is a normal downregulator of arteriolar smooth muscle tone. The enzyme catalyzing its formation from L-arginine, nitric oxide synthase, is inhibited by a retained nitrogenous end product in chronic renal failure, dimethylarginine. Because both high-endothelin and high-norepinephrine levels have been demonstrated in patients with chronic renal failure and hypertension, defective nitric oxide formation would further enhance systemic vasoconstriction. In the best animal model of salt-sensitive hypertension, the Dahl salt-sensitive rat, increased dietary intake of L-arginine (but not D-arginine) prevents hypertension and hypertensive nephrosclerosis. Enhanced renal nitric oxide synthesis appears to be an important response to dietary salt loading by induction of a renal nitric oxide synthase. Activity of this enzyme in response to salt loading in the Dahl salt-sensitive rat is defective, and the defect can be overcome by dietary loading of the substrate L-arginine. Renal nitric oxide formation is important for both vasodilation and natriuresis and for modulation of GFR by tubuloglomerular feedback. Thus defective nitric oxide formation in the kidney would inhibit natriuresis, and defective nitric oxide formation in the peripheral vasculature would increase peripheral vasoconstriction. High levels of endothelin in the systemic and renal circulation may also contribute to renal and systemic vasoconstriction.

Most studies in experimental animal models of chronic renal failure have shown an initial increase of cardiac output as a cause of the hypertension with subsequent normalization of cardiac output and an increase in peripheral vascular resistance. In humans, although this pattern has also been seen, it appears that high cardiac output–high peripheral resistance, normal cardiac output–high peripheral resistance, and high cardiac output–normal peripheral resistance mechanisms of hypertension can all be seen in different patients and even at different stages in the same patients both before dialysis and during renal replacement therapy. Indeed, expansion of extracellular fluid volume caused by sodium chloride retention does not result in hypertension in a few patients receiving dialysis therapy.

Role of Hypertension in Progression of Renal Failure

The onset of hypertension often accompanies an increase in the rate of deterioration of GFR, probably as both a consequence and a cause of that deterioration. The concept of vicious circle hypertension is an important one. In addition to the mechanism of damage described under primary hypertension, vicious circle hypertension may act in a synergistic manner to increase glomerular damage caused by other primary processes such as diabetic glomerulopathy and immune complex glomerulonephritis. Support for this is based on animal studies and on the clinical documentation of protection of a kidney distal to a significant renal artery stenosis with expression of the primary disease process in the contralateral kidney exposed to systemic hypertension.

Both retrospective and prospective studies in patients with chronic renal failure and hypertension and studies in experimental animal models suggest that effective treatment of hypertension offers the best opportunity to slow the rate of progression of chronic renal disease. Reduction in systemic blood pressure at least stops vicious circle hypertension. As discussed for primary hypertensive renal damage, it is likely that secondary hypertension also damages the kidney in patients with primary renal disease by at least two mechanisms: primary ischemic global glomerulosclerosis and hemodynamic stress in adapted nephrons (Fig. 70.9). Adaptation in surviving nephrons is associated with preglomerular dilation and glomerular hypertrophy. In that setting, systemic hypertension would be transmitted to the glomerular capillary bed and would further contribute to the development of focal glomerular sclerosis (segmental hyalinosis). In such circumstances, antihypertensive drugs that increase preglomerular dilation might not adequately protect the glomerulus. Hypertension plays a pivotal role in the development and progression of diabetic glomerulosclerosis and in adult onset autosomal-dominant polycystic kidney disease.

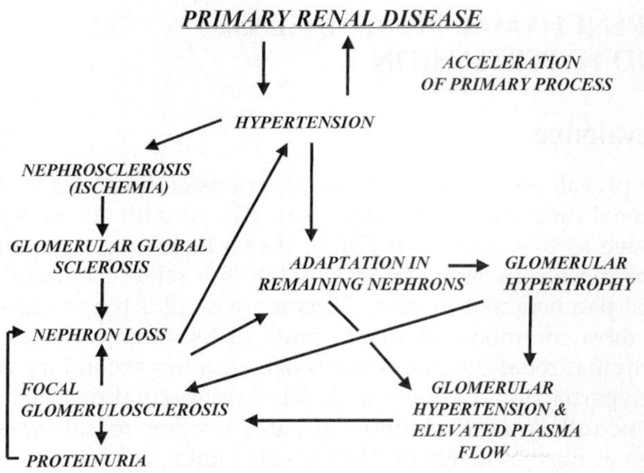

Figure 70.9. Mechanisms by which secondary hypertension contributes to progression of renal parenchymal disease.

TREATMENT

Essential hypertensive patients are sometimes classified as salt sensitive or salt resistant. Regardless of the initial mechanisms of hypertension, once renal failure develops the renal pathogenetic mechanisms responsible for hypertension predominate.

Even modest increases in blood pressure within the normal range should be treated at least by dietary restriction of sodium chloride to a 2-g sodium (5-g sodium chloride) intake per day. More severe restriction may be associated with failure to conserve sodium appropriately and continuing negative sodium balance with a deleterious effect on renal function. Initially, thiazide diuretics are appropriate, but when the serum creatinine approaches 2 mg/dl, loop diuretics must be employed. It is difficult to obtain blood pressure control in patients with chronic renal failure without the use of diuretic therapy. In patients with nephrotic syndrome or proteinuria, ACE inhibitor therapy may have additional benefits by reducing urinary protein excretion by approximately 50%. Possible deleterious effects on GFR can occur in certain clinical circumstances in which GFR is reduced may be dependent on efferent arteriolar constriction. Chronic antihypertensive therapy with ACE inhibitors is best avoided in the presence of renovascular renal failure, renovascular hypertension, or hyporeninemic hypoaldosteronism. In the presence of renal impairment, the serum potassium should be monitored. With early renal insufficiency, only approximately 10% of patients will develop ACE inhibitor–related hyperkalemia; great care is necessary with concomitant use of nonsteroidal antiinflammatory drugs, K-sparing diuretics, and β-blockers, especially in the elderly.

All hypertensive diabetics who develop microalbuminuria should receive ACE inhibitors or, if the latter are not well tolerated due to a side effect such as cough, angiotensin-II receptor blockers such as Losartan should be considered. Progression to diabetic glomerulosclerosis is likely to be at least delayed, and possibly prevented. Once fixed proteinuria (more than 0.5 g/24 hr) develops, ACE inhibitors are also obligatory. It should be emphasized that the effects of ACE inhibitors are only partly due to the antihypertensive actions and likely relate to blocking other intrarenal effects of angiotensin II such as elevated intraglomerular pressure, increased endothelin levels, increased TGF-β levels, and increased glomerular permeability.

In nondiabetic renal disease, hypertension should also be treated initially with ACE inhibitors especially if proteinuria is more than 1 g/24 hr. The slowing of progression of renal disease correlates directly with the degree of reduction in proteinuria and the degree of initial hemodynamic fall in GFR. Indeed, even after years of ACE inhibitors the GFR may show a small hemodynamic rise after withdrawal of these agents. ACE inhibitors are also the drugs of choice for initial treatment of hypertension in polycystic kidney disease.

Calcium channel blockers may also be renal protective by mechanisms independent of reduction of blood pressure. Such mechanisms may include a more effective inhibition of the effects of endothelin, inhibition of glomerular hypertrophy in the adapted nephron, and other cytoprotective effects due to reduction of cytosol calcium.

The actual level of blood pressure control achieved remains important. Studies suggest that if proteinuria is more than 1 g/24 hr, target blood pressure should be 125/75 mm Hg, and if proteinuria is less, target blood pressure should be 130/85 mm Hg. These levels are achievable and safe in the absence of severe ischemic cerebral or cardiac vascular disease.

As renal disease progresses, hypertension usually requires the use of several antihypertensive agents. We favor a loop diuretic, then an ACE inhibitor followed by a calcium channel blocker for the aforementioned reasons. If these are inadequate, either a central acting α2-blocker (e.g., Clonidine) and/or a small dose of the potent vasodilator Minoxidil can be added. It must be remembered that the goal of therapy is not only to slow the rate of progression of renal disease but also to protect from subsequent cardiovascular disease.

END-STAGE RENAL DISEASE

Up to 95% of patients reaching ESRD are hypertensive and many have advanced cardiovascular disease. Twenty-four hour ambulatory blood pressure monitoring has shown that hemodialysis patients lose the normal circadian blood pressure pattern, no longer displaying a drop in nighttime blood pressure. Both systolic and diastolic blood pressures rise to pretreatment values within 12 to 24 hours after dialysis. Postdialysis blood pressure appears to correlate better with average interdialytic blood pressure than does predialysis blood pressure, but neither provides a truly accurate assessment of blood pressure status in hemodialysis patients. Lacking a nighttime blood pressure drop ("nondipping pattern"), the true blood pressure load is often greater than might be estimated from casual readings in the dialysis unit.

At the initiation of chronic dialysis, more than 20% of patients have clinically manifest ischemic heart disease, and an additional 10% will develop coronary artery disease during their life on dialysis. More than 40% of new dialysis patients have left ventricular hypertrophy and many have signs or symptoms of congestive heart failure. Other signs of vascular damage include reduced aortic and large artery compliance and a past history of stroke that is significantly more prevalent than in a control population of the same age.

Surprisingly, in dialysis patients a clear statistical association of hypertension with cardiovascular mortality could not be demonstrated, possibly due to the fact that patients with low blood pressures also have increased mortality. However, given the overwhelming evidence that hypertension contributes to cardiovascular disease in the general population, hypertension in ESRD must be treated aggressively. Patients with ESRD represent a group at particularly high cardiovascular risk. Acute myocardial infarction, cardiac arrest, and other forms of heart disease together with cerebrovascular disease cause half of all deaths in the dialysis population. As the dialysis population ages, the prevalence of cardiovascular disease is expected to increase, and the importance of aggressive management of hypertension can only increase.

Consequences of Hypertension in End-Stage Renal Disease

Hypertension accelerates atherosclerosis, leading to coronary artery disease and myocardial infarction, and is the main cause of left ventricular hypertrophy. Both mechanisms can cause progression to congestive heart failure, placing hypertension upstream of a dangerous pathogenic synergy (Fig. 70.10). The heart of dialysis patients is not only exposed to pressure overload, but also to chronic volume expansion predisposing to cardiac decompensation. Left ventricular hypertrophy is an independent predictor of coronary ischemia, congestive heart failure, and stroke. Hypertension leads to vascular remodeling causing increased peripheral vascular resistance and impaired endothelial function. The resulting decrease in arterial compliance predisposes the patient to predominantly systolic hypertension, with a decreased ability to respond to rapid volume changes such as may occur during hemodialysis. The decrease in arterial compliance results in an increased pulse wave pressure that, in a vicious cycle, leads to further arterial damage. Other causes of increased arterial stiffness in dialysis patients are calcification and fibroelastic intimal thickening.

In the general population, systolic hypertension with a wide pulse pressure carries a worse prognosis than do other forms of hypertension with smaller pulse pressures. Isolated systolic

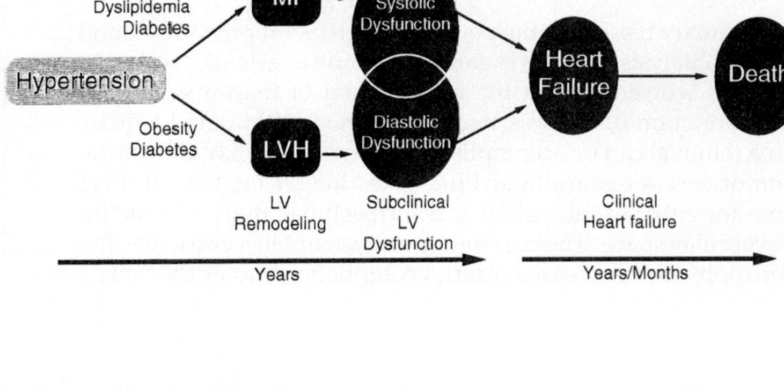

Figure 70.10. The pivotal role of hypertension in the development of congestive heart failure. MI, myocardial infarction; LV, left ventricle; LVH, left ventricular hypertrophy. (Adapted with permission from Vasan RS, Levy D. The role of hypertension in the pathogenesis of heart failure: a clinical mechanistic overview. *Arch Int Med* 1990;156:1789–1796.)

hypertension is notoriously difficult to control, often requiring several antihypertensive medications, which further complicates management. Hemodialysis patients are subject to chronic volume and pressure overload and to rapid swings in extracellular volume and left ventricular filling. Hypertensive vascular disease reduces the patient's ability to respond to these acute changes. High blood pressure with its consequences is one of the great threats to the dialysis patient. Unfortunately, many nephrologists continue to accept elevated blood pressures in their dialysis patients. This trend may have worsened because of economic considerations, patient preference for short dialysis times, and/or the physician's lack of appreciation of the seriousness of hypertension in patients with ESRD.

Other Cardiovascular Risk Factors

Most dialysis patients are elderly and the majority already have several cardiovascular risk factors at onset of dialysis. More than one-third of all new ESRD patients in the United States are diabetic. In the general population, the presence of diabetes mellitus doubles cardiovascular morbidity and mortality. Dyslipidemia, such as high triglyceride levels, low high-density lipoprotein (HDL) levels, and high low-density lipoprotein (LDL) levels, as well as high lipoprotein(a) levels are common in ESRD. Uremia can cause myocardial interstitial fibrosis, but the question whether uremia per se, in the absence of other risk factors, accelerates atherosclerosis has not been definitively answered.

Anemia can aggravate myocardial ischemia and hasten the development of congestive heart failure. Hyperparathyroidism leads to myocardial fibrosis, increased myocardial and vascular calcification, and impaired myocardial function. Hypercalcemia, more common in renal failure since the introduction of high calcium dialysate and intravenous $1,25(OH)_2D_3$ (calcitriol), has been found to be independently associated with ischemic heart disease. Homocysteine has been identified as an independent risk factor for atherosclerosis in both the general population and in dialysis patients. Patients with ESRD have elevated homocysteine levels. Most multivitamin preparations prescribed for dialysis patients contain between 0.8 and 1 mg of folic acid, but greater amounts are needed to reduce homocysteine levels effectively. Whether lowering homocysteine levels in dialysis patients reduces morbidity and mortality remains to be determined.

The high prevalence of cardiovascular risk factors in the dialysis population is a major challenge for the nephrologist. The patient with new ESRD requires not only dialysis therapy but also reversal or at least arrest of ongoing cardiovascular disease. Despite progress in dialysis technique, morbidity and mortality from cardiovascular disease remains high.

Cardiovascular risk can be reduced by successful renal transplantation but both the prevalence of hypertension and cardiovascular mortality remain elevated when compared with normal subjects. Mechanisms of posttransplant hypertension and its therapy are discussed in Chapter 89, Part 7.

Pathogenesis of Hypertension in End-Stage Renal Disease

The primary reason for the persistent high blood pressures found in hemodialysis patients is chronic volume overload. This problem has worsened with the introduction of high-flux dialysis and reduction of dialysis treatment times. Although adequate urea removal can be accomplished relatively quickly, ultrafiltration of excess extracellular fluid takes longer because of a lag time for entry of interstitial and intracellular fluid into the intravascular space. The common presence of left ventricular hypertrophy and decreased arterial compliance impair the body's ability to maintain adequate circulating volume during dialysis, leading to hypotension. The loss of blood pressure in turn makes it difficult to achieve true dry weight. Support for this view comes from two observations: (a) patients receiving more than 12 hours of hemodialysis per week are less hypertensive and have a lower mortality rate than patients who receive fewer hours of treatment, and (b) patients on continuous ambulatory peritoneal dialysis with more consistent volume removal have better blood pressure control.

Up to 80% of hemodialysis patients with elevated predialysis blood pressure can be made normotensive with ultrafiltration performed at optimal rates, but the remaining 20% cannot. When the "refractory" (volume-independent) patient's weight is lowered by ultrafiltration, hypotension develops and hypertension immediately reappears with a return to dry weight. The pathogenesis of refractory hypertension probably relates not only to the renin-angiotensin system, but also to uremic toxins, parathyroid hormone, altered sympathetic responses, defects in nitric oxide formation, and erythropoietin therapy. Other causes may include arterial stiffness and left ventricular diastolic dysfunction, both of which can lead to hypotension as soon as a critically low threshold level of circulating volume is reached, thereby preventing optimal volume control.

The introduction of recombinant human erythropoietin has improved quality of life for dialysis patients. On the other hand, treatment with erythropoietin can elevate blood pressure. One-third of patients receiving erythropoietin therapy will show worsening or *de novo* appearance of hypertension. Increased blood viscosity, increased blood volume, changes in peripheral tissue autoregulation, and a direct effect of erythropoietin on vascular reactivity have been implicated. The vasoconstriction in peripheral tissues that follows the increased oxygen-carrying capacity is greater than the corresponding drop in cardiac output, causing a rise in blood pressure. In some patients, a reduction in dosage is sufficient to control blood pressure, whereas others will require antihypertensive therapy. Table 70.10 summarizes the major causes of hypertension in dialysis patients.

Dialysis Hypotension (Table 70.11)

Hypotension is the most common acute complication of hemodialysis. The presence of diabetes and atherosclerotic diseases increase the risk for hypotensive episodes.

The principal cause of hypotension during hemodialysis is excessive volume loss by ultrafiltration. If volume removal is more rapid than reequilibration from the extravascular space, hypovolemia with decreased cardiac filling and, ultimately, hypotension will result. Short dialysis times, even if adequate for urea removal, require more rapid fluid equilibration from intracellular and interstitial spaces. A drop in serum osmolality caused by rapid solute removal or the use of low sodium dialysate interferes with refilling of the vascular space from the interstitium. In addition, the normal response to acute volume loss during dialysis may be impaired due to a noncompliant left ventricle, inadequate sympathetic vasoconstriction, anemia, or

TABLE 70.10. Causes of Hypertension in Dialysis Patients

Expanded intravascular volume
Elevated angiotensin II levels
Decreased vascular compliance (especially systolic hypertension)
Erythropoietin therapy
Increased sympathetic activity
Hyperparathyroidism
Deficient nitric oxide production

TABLE 70.11. Factors Responsible for Dialysis Hypotension

Intravascular volume loss
Ultrafiltration
Solute loss
Low dialysate sodium
Acute blood loss
Venous pooling
Food ingestion
Low muscle tone
Elevated body temperature
Drop in cardiac output
Left ventricular hypertrophy
Pericardial tamponade
Acute myocardial infarction
Arrhythmia
Uremia
Acute loss of calcium
Acetate dialysate
Loss of catecholamines
Loss of peripheral vascular resistance
Antihypertensive drugs
Increase in nitric oxide production
Hyperparathyroidism

poor lower-extremity muscle tone with venous pooling. The presence of hyperparathyroidism can reduce the vascular response to epinephrine and angiotensin II.

Additional mechanisms predisposing patients to dialysis hypotension include the release of cytokines caused by the interaction of the dialysis membrane with blood. Interleukin-1 can induce the synthesis of endothelium- and vascular smooth muscle–derived nitric oxide, a potent vasodilator. Ingestion of food during the treatment may cause vasodilation. Acetate used in dialysate can cause vasodilation and has a negative inotropic effect, a problem not seen with the use of bicarbonate dialysate. Higher dialysate temperatures can dilate cutaneous arterioles, and the removal of catecholamines by hemodialysis may further impair the sympathetic response to volume decreases. Rapid drops in serum calcium levels caused by low calcium dialysate can impair myocardial contractility.

The perceived risk of hypotension during dialysis makes drug therapy of hypertension more difficult. Agents that reduce the heart rate and contractility, such as β-blockers and diltiazem, can contribute to hypotensive episodes, but the chronotropic and inotropic responses of the heart probably play a minor role in dialysis hypotension. Many nephrologists withhold antihypertensive agents on the day of dialysis, but the efficacy of this strategy has not been established. Most newer antihypertensive agents have long half-lives, which are further prolonged by absent renal function, and holding the drug on the day of dialysis may do little to prevent hypotension.

The most serious consequence of dialysis hypotension is the inability to achieve true dry weight. Chronic volume overload in turn worsens hypertension and left ventricular hypertrophy. The vicious cycle of dialysis hypotension and chronic volume overload is shown in Fig. 70.11. It is clear that some patients are more prone to hypotensive episodes than others. The episodes are usually treated easily by placing the patient in the supine position, discontinuing ultrafiltration, and administering normal saline. Even if usually reversible, the symptoms of dialysis hypotension are unpleasant and should be prevented if possible. Patients with frequent episodes of dialysis hypotension have an increased risk of cardiovascular death. Furthermore, acute hypotension can precipitate seizures, myocardial ischemia, or stroke. It should be kept in mind that early, severe, or refractory hypotension on dialysis can be the result of a serious medical problem, such as acute myocardial infarction, pericardial tamponade, or gastrointestinal bleeding.

Treatment

Persistent hypertension leads to reduced survival in dialysis patients. The optimal blood pressure level in dialysis patients has not been established. The Sixth Report of the Joint National Committee on Prevention, Detection, Evaluation and Treatment of High Blood Pressure (JNC-VI) proposes a goal blood pressure of 130/85 mm Hg for patients in high-risk groups (i.e., with diabetes and/or heart failure) and advocates immediate drug therapy without waiting for the effect of lifestyle modifications. In our view, ESRD is a major cardiovascular risk factor, comparable to diabetes, and we advocate a goal blood pressure of 130/85 mm Hg or lower. The only exceptions are patients with symptomatic coronary or cerebral artery disease in which a higher blood pressure may have to be accepted to avoid underperfusion of poststenotic tissue (J curve phenomenon).

Volume Control

The importance of appropriate volume removal and establishing the correct dry weight has been understood since the early days of chronic hemodialysis. The *dry weight* of a patient has been defined as the weight at which a patient is normotensive and free of edema, but develops hypotension by further acute

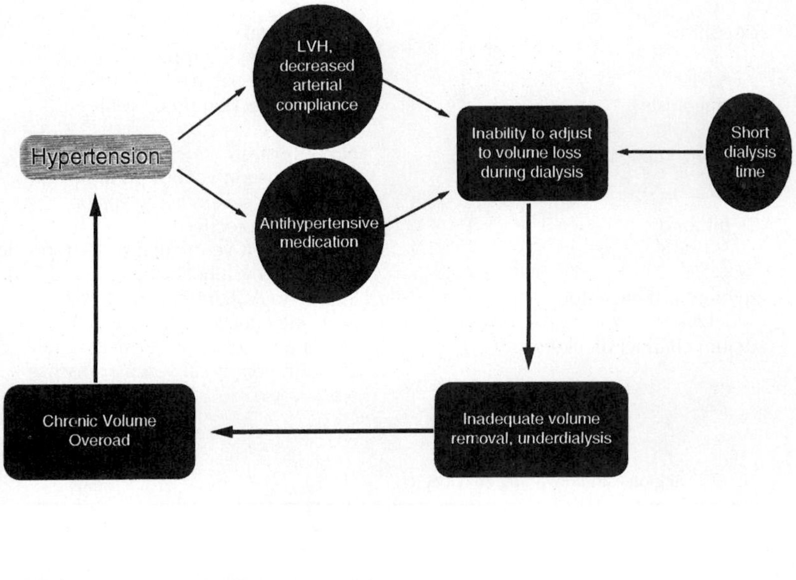

Figure 70.11. The vicious circle of hypertension and chronic volume overload in hemodialysis.

weight reduction. During the past few years it has become clear that the speed with which extracellular fluid volume is being removed during dialysis has to be taken into account. A report from the Centre de Rein Artificiel in Tassin, France, where patients are dialyzed 8 hours three times weekly, has shown that of 445 dialysis patients, only 7 required long-term antihypertensive medication. These and other data indicate that longer dialysis times may indeed permit more complete fluid removal with better control of extracellular fluid volume and blood pressure. As mentioned previously, more than 90% of new dialysis patients are hypertensive. Upon starting dialysis, careful assessment of the hemodynamic status and stepwise lowering of the target weight should be accompanied by gradual withdrawal of antihypertensive drugs.

The majority of ESRD patients should be able to come off antihypertensive medication with consistent and meticulous fluid management. It is also important to keep interdialytic fluid gain in the range of 0.5 kg/day, especially when shorter dialysis times are used. Moderate restriction of dietary salt intake is sufficient for most patients.

Antihypertensive Medications (Table 70.12)

Many dialysis patients are unwilling to increase the time spent receiving hemodialysis, and there will always be patients whose blood pressure cannot be controlled, even with optimal fluid management. Patients with systolic hypertension and a wide pulse pressure often need aggressive volume removal in combination with carefully chosen antihypertensive medications. The potential of promoting dialysis hypotension and other side effects has to be kept in mind, however.

Most antihypertensive agents, with the exception of diuretics, are effective in dialysis patients. Some patients have residual renal function, and loop diuretics can be given to maintain urine output. Even modest amounts of daily urine output permit a commensurate liberalization of fluid intake.

β-Blockers, although effective, must be used with caution in dialysis patients because they have the potential to promote dialysis hypotension and to increase peripheral vascular constriction and Raynaud's phenomenon. β-Blockers have been shown to reduce mortality and reinfarction rates following a myocardial infarction. Therefore β-blockers represent an excellent choice in patients with a history of angina or myocardial infarction. β-Blockers are less well suited for dialysis patients with diabetes mellitus, severe peripheral vascular disease, or a propensity to dialysis hypotension. Agents with intrinsic sympathomimetic activity (ISA), such as pindolol or acebutolol, are preferable in patients with low–resting heart rates or cold extremities. Some β-blockers are dialyzable (nadolol, acebutolol, and its active metabolite, diacebutolol) and should be given after dialysis. Nadolol and acebutolol require a 75% reduction in dosage in dialysis patients, whereas propranolol, metoprolol, and atenolol can be given at a moderately decreased dose. Labetalol has nonselective β-adrenergic blocking activity (without ISA) and is also a peripheral α_1-blocker. Labetalol is useful in cases of severe hypertension and in hypertensive emergencies. Labetalol may be given once daily in patients with ESRD.

α_2-Adrenergic agonists decrease both cardiac output and total peripheral vascular resistance and should be used with caution in patients prone to dialysis hypotension. Members of this drug class share several side effects. Drowsiness, dry mouth, and constipation can be particularly bothersome to hemodialysis patients. Abrupt withdrawal can cause severe rebound hypertension. Clonidine is available as a transdermal patch, an advantage for patients taking a large number of pills. The patch appears to be better tolerated than the oral form. The dosages of clonidine and methyldopa have to be reduced in renal failure, whereas guanabenz and guanfacine can be given at the low end of their usual dose range. With the possible exception of methyldopa, α_2-adrenergic agonists do not cause orthostatic hypotension.

Peripheral α_1-adrenergic blockers do not cause reflex tachycardia. These drugs improve the lipid profile, albeit on a small scale. Possible side effects important to dialysis patients include fatigue, dizziness, and orthostatic hypotension. The dosage of doxazosin can be kept unchanged in renal failure.

Direct vasodilators, which include hydralazine and minoxidil, are potent antihypertensive agents. The normal sympathetic

TABLE 70.12. Antihypertensive Agents in Dialysis Patients

Agent	Pros	Cons
β-Blockers	Cardioprotective after myocardial infarction	Negative inotrope Worsen peripheral vascular disease Central nervous system depression Not recommended in diabetes mellitus
α_2-Agonists	No orthostasis Not negative inotrope Available in patch	Constipation Drowsiness, dry mouth Rebound hypertension
α_1-Antagonists	Positive effect on lipid profile	Fatigue, drowsiness Orthostasis
Direct vasodilators	No orthostasis No increase in venous pooling Effective in severe hypertension	Tachycardia Hypertrichosis (minoxidil) Pericardial effusion (minoxidil)
ACE inhibitors	Vascular protective Useful in left ventricular hypertrophy and systolic dysfunction	Chronic cough ? Hyperkalemia
Angiotensin II–receptor blockers	Similar to ACE inhibitors Few side effects	New drug class, no long-term data
Calcium channel blockers	Potent antihypertensive effect Good in peripheral vascular disease No adverse metabolic effects	Negative inotrope (L channel blockers) Tachycardia (dihydropyridines) Bradycardia (verapamil, diltiazem, and mibefradil)

ACE, angiotensin-converting enzyme.

response is not altered by theses agents, and the tachycardia induced via the baroreceptor reflex usually requires the concomitant administration of a β-blocker. However, because of the intact baroreceptor reflex, orthostatic hypotension is unusual. The half-life of hydralazine is short and not substantially prolonged in renal failure. Minoxidil can be given once a day but is dialyzable and should be taken following dialysis. Minoxidil is highly effective in cases of severe hypertension, but may cause hypertrichosis, an annoying side effect, especially to women. It is not clear if the risk of pericardial effusion in the hemodialysis patient is truly potentiated by minoxidil, but all patients on this drug require close observation for this potential complication.

ACE inhibitors are clearly effective in most nonnephrectomized dialysis patients, both as monotherapy and in combination with other antihypertensive agents. Their vasodilatory and cardioprotective actions provide additional benefits to patients with congestive heart failure and left ventricular hypertrophy. ACE inhibitors reduce morbidity and mortality, independent of their antihypertensive action, in symptomatic and asymptomatic heart failure and following myocardial infarction. ACE inhibitors may be superior to other agents in promoting regression of left ventricular hypertrophy. ACE inhibitors have a general "vascular protective" effect that goes beyond blood pressure control. In our estimate, ACE inhibitors are often underdosed in dialysis patients. ACE inhibitors that contain a sulfhydryl group (e.g., captopril) should be avoided in dialysis patients. The doses of enalapril, lisinopril, benazepril, quinapril, or ramipril have to be adjusted downward in dialysis patients, and it is prudent to start therapy at the lowest end of their recommended dosing ranges. The half-life of fosinopril is not affected by renal failure.

At present, use of angiotensin-II receptor blockers should be reserved for patients who are intolerant of or do not respond adequately to ACE inhibitors. The possibility of combining an angiotensin II–receptor blocker with an ACE inhibitor is currently under study. No data are available regarding their long-term usefulness in dialysis patients.

Calcium channel blockers are excellent agents in cases of ischemic heart disease, severe or systolic hypertension, and peripheral vascular disease. Short-acting calcium channel blockers should be avoided. There have been reports of myocardial infarction and stroke following their use, and a retrospective drug utilization study has linked short-acting calcium channel blockers to increased risk of myocardial infarction. No such links have been documented with long-acting preparations. All calcium channel blockers must be used with caution in patients with congestive heart failure. Verapamil and diltiazem are useful in cases of left ventricular hypertrophy with diastolic dysfunction. A drawback to their use is the common side effect of constipation. The dose of nicardipine must be reduced in renal failure, but the doses of nifedipine, felodipine, verapamil, and diltiazem require no adjustment. However, their half-life can be prolonged in the presence of liver disease, and serious toxicity has been described in such patients. Calcium channel blockers are not removed by hemodialysis.

The most important factors to be considered when choosing an antihypertensive drug in a dialysis patient is the property of the drug and its side effects (Table 70.12). Dialysis patients often take large numbers of pills and once-a-day regimens are an important convenience. Many combination preparations have become available. The use of combination drugs has several advantages, such as a reduction in number of pills, synergistic action (e.g., combination of an ACE inhibitor and a calcium channel blocker), improved side-effect profile (because submaximal doses can be used), and sometimes lower cost. It is important to reevaluate the drug regimen of dialysis patients frequently, in concert with assessment of true body weight, cardiac function, comorbidity, and compliance.

For dialysis patients in need of antihypertensive medication, we propose the following approach:

1. ACE inhibitor (increase dose stepwise, avoid underdosing)
2. Calcium channel blocker (choose agent according to heart rate, presence of systolic and/or diastolic dysfunction, presence of peripheral vascular disease)
3. β-Blocker for patients with ischemic heart disease and/or history of myocardial infarction
4. Add α_1-blocker, α_2-agonist, or labetalol if blood pressure is still not controlled
5. For severe hypertension, add minoxidil, preferably in combination with a β-blocker or heart rate lowering calcium channel blocker; minoxidil can be given once or twice daily.

Patients whose blood pressures cannot be controlled even with a combination of agents at maximum dosages as outlined previously need reassessment of their dialysis prescription and modality. In our view, with the availability of ACE inhibitors and angiotensin II–receptor blockers, nephrectomy is no longer necessary for blood pressure control.

Selected Readings

Abuelo JG. Diagnosing vascular causes of renal failure. *Ann Intern Med* 1995; 123:601–614.

A good clinical description of renovascular renal failure, atheroembolic renal disease, hemolytic-uremic syndrome, and other vascular causes of hypertension and both acute and chronic renal failure.

Fogo A, Breyer JA, Smith MC, et al. Accuracy of the diagnosis of hypertensive nephrosclerosis in African-Americans: a report from the African-American Study of Kidney Disease (AASK) Trial. *Kidney Int* 1997;51:244–252.

Careful selection of African-American patients on clinical criteria for a diagnosis of hypertensive nephrosclerosis is supported by renal biopsy in 90% of patients selected for a clinical trial.

Foley RN, Parfrey PS. Risk factors for cardiac morbidity and mortality in dialysis patients. *Curr Opin Nephrol Hypertens* 1994;3:608–614.

A comprehensive review of prevalence and significance of cardiovascular risk factors in end-stage renal disease, with 64 references.

Giatras I, Lau J, Levey AS. Effect of angiotensin-converting enzyme inhibitors on the progression of nondiabetic renal disease: a meta-analysis of randomized trials. *Ann Intern Med* 1997;127:337–345.

A summary of all randomized studies of ACE-inhibitor treatment in this population. The beneficial effects are likely due to both nonspecific antihypertensive effects and specific antiproteinuria mechanisms.

Klag MJ, Whelton PK, Randall BL, et al. Blood pressure and end-stage renal disease in men. *N Engl J Med* 1996;334:13–18.

In a follow-up of 330,000 men screened for the Multiple Risk Factor Intervention Trial (MRFIT), hypertension was a strong, independent risk factor for ESRD. Approximately 0.25% of this population developed ESRD over a mean period of 16 years.

Peterson JC, Adler S, Burkart JM, et al. Blood pressure control, proteinuria, and the progression of renal disease. *Ann Intern Med* 1995;123:754–762.

Data from the MDRD study suggests that proteinuria is a risk factor for progression of renal disease, both of which can be ameliorated by lowering of blood pressure to normal levels.

Remuzzi G, Ruggenenti P, Benighi A. Understanding the nature of renal disease progression. *Kidney Int* 1997;51:2–15.

Discusses the evidence that nonselective proteinuria contributes to progression of renal disease likely through cytotoxic effects on the proximal tubule, perhaps via increased renal endothelin and TGF-β production.

Ritz E, Weidmann PU. Hypertension and the kidney. *Nephrol Dial Transplant* 1995; 10 (Suppl 9)1–65.

This supplement provides experimental animal and human data on the differing effects of ACE inhibitors and calcium channel blockers in the progression of hypertension and proteinuric renal disease. A good case can be made, although not yet proven, for their synergistic use in such patients.

Sixth Report of the Joint National Committee on prevention, detection, evaluation and treatment of high blood pressure. *Arch Intern Med* 1997;157:2413–2446.

A complete account of expert views on the management of hypertension. This is the most important review of this therapeutic area available today.

Wolfe RA, Port FK, Web RL, et al. Incidence and prevalence of ESRD. *Am J Kidney Dis* 1999;34:S1–S176.

The latest available summary of the report of the U.S. Renal Data system, which includes virtually all U.S. dialysis and renal transplant patients. It provides a wealth of data regarding incidence, prevalence, morbidity, and mortality in end-stage renal disease.

CHAPTER 71

Pulmonary Complications of Uremia

R. Scott Morehead and Peter E. Morris

The lungs are in intimate contact with the external environment (air) and the internal environment (blood) at all times. It is therefore to be expected that the lungs can become diseased by derangements in either of these environments. The internal environment can be drastically modified by the failure of any organ, not the least of which is the kidney. With the altered immune status of uremia or renal transplantation, the external environment then becomes much more threatening, particularly with regard to infectious agents. The surprise is not that the lung is frequently affected by renal failure but that the lung is so frequently spared.

UREMIC LUNG

The butterfly or batwing distribution of pulmonary infiltrates seen in uremic lungs is a radiologic diagnosis and is thought to represent edema. Most investigators conceive of fluid and solute filtration across the walls of capillaries in the lungs as occurring through holes or "pores" between endothelial cells, with some transport occurring by way of intracytoplasmic vesicles. The forces that control transvascular fluid flux are governed by principles outlined in the Starling equation:

$$Qv = K_f\,(Pmv - Ppmv) - Jpd\,(\pi mv - \pi pmv)$$

where Qv is the net fluid volume filtered per unit time; K_f is the filtration coefficient; Pmv is the hydrostatic pressure within the pulmonary microvessels; $Ppmv$ is the hydrostatic pressure surrounding the microvessels; Jpd is the osmotic reflection coefficient for plasma proteins, which is an index of the permeability of the microvascular membrane to these proteins; πmv is the oncotic pressure exerted by the plasma; and πpmv is the oncotic pressure exerted by the interstitial fluid.

The forces at play in the pulmonary capillary are illustrated in Fig. 71.1. As the equation shows, net fluid flux (Qv) is determined by the interplay of transmural hydrostatic pressure differences (ΔP), transmural oncotic pressure differences $(\Delta\pi)$ and the filtration coefficient, which describes both the porosity of the filtering membrane and its surface area (K_f).

Normally, the relationship between transmural hydrostatic and oncotic pressures is such that any net filtration into the interstitium is handled easily by the lymphatics. Primary pulmonary edema occurs when the membrane coefficient changes to increase membrane "leakiness" to the point where lymphatic drainage is overwhelmed. Secondary pulmonary edema occurs when either net transmural oncotic $(\Delta\pi)$ or hydrostatic pressures (ΔP) change to cause efflux of large amounts of fluid from the lung capillaries and venules into the interstitium. Frequently, there is a combined primary and secondary edema. In patients with uremia, serum proteins are often reduced, and this possibly alters transmural oncotic pressures. Volume retention is also common in uremia, potentially altering transmural hydrostatic pressures.

The question of whether lung capillary permeability is increased in uremia is an interesting one. In support of the view that permeability is increased are the data that demonstrate that alveolar edema fluid in uremia is often rich in protein. However, well-designed, controlled animal studies do not appear to support the hypothesis of an increase in pulmonary capillary permeability due to uremia alone. A few, small, nonrandomized studies have examined lung epithelial permeability by using a technetium-99 DTPA inhalation technique that is very sensitive to epithelial permeability/damage. These studies looked at asymptomatic chronic renal failure patients with normal chest radiographs and demonstrated abnormal permeability immediately after hemodialysis but normal values more than 24 hours afterward. The patients that were predialysis were similar except for a reversal of the apex-base gradient of the lung seen in normal individuals, possibly indicating subclinical epithelial damage in the lower lungs. Although these data raise questions regarding pulmonary epithelial function in chronic renal failure patients, further work is necessary to resolve whether increased epithelial permeability plays a role in

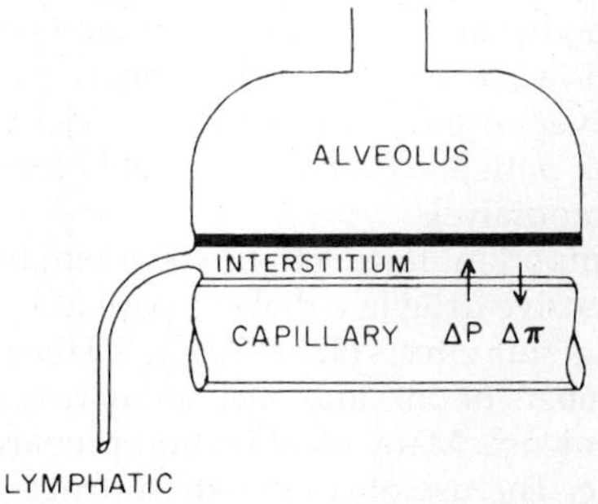

Figure 71.1. Schematic representation of the fluid exchanging unit in the lung. ΔP denotes transmural hydrostatic pressure difference and $\Delta\pi$ represents the transmural oncotic pressure difference.

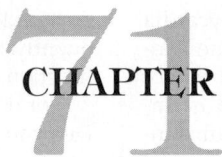

the entity "uremic lung." The combination of altered hydrostatic and oncotic pressures probably accounts for much of these infiltrates, and the favorable effects of dialysis may result from decreased intravascular volume with the consequent decrease in hydrostatic pressure.

EFFECTS OF CHRONIC RENAL FAILURE ON PULMONARY FUNCTION

Patients with chronic renal failure often develop metabolic acidosis, which may have a profound effect on oxygen transport. Metabolic acidosis shifts the oxygen–hemoglobin dissociation curve to the right, which promotes release of oxygen at the tissues. With chronic acidosis, erythrocyte 2,3-diphosphoglycerate decreases, which tends to shift the dissociation curve back to the left, negating the beneficial rightward shift. Vigorous treatment of chronic metabolic acidosis can cause a further shift of the curve to the left, possibly adversely affecting oxygen delivery.

Acidosis in patients with renal failure is believed to affect ventilatory drive. The effect depends on whether acidosis is respiratory or metabolic. Carbon dioxide stimulates ventilation, and because its diffusion into the central nervous system (CNS) occurs rapidly, there is a rapid equilibration of CNS pH with circulatory pH when the acidosis is caused by carbon dioxide retention. When bicarbonate is infused into the bloodstream to correct the acidemia, the response of ventilatory drive lags behind blood pH changes because bicarbonate crosses the blood–brain barrier slowly.

Changes in lung mechanics and lung hemodynamics may occur without overt pulmonary signs or symptoms in patients with chronic renal failure. A study of patients with chronic renal failure but without primary lung disease showed (a) decrease in vital capacity (VC) indicative of mild restriction, and no evidence of obstructive disease, and (b) significant negative correlations between diffusing capacity (DL_{CO}) and blood urea nitrogen and a positive correlation with creatinine clearance after correction of anemia.

The effects of hemodialysis on pulmonary function in chronic renal failure appear mainly attributable to changes in fluid volumes. One report postulated that the effect of dialysis was an increase of ventilation to basilar areas of the lung, a decrease in closing capacity, and in patients with edema, an increase in vital capacity. These changes were explained by a decrease in lung water content because interstitial edema around small airways causes airway closure at relatively high lung volumes, and interstitium and alveolar edema can account for the other pulmonary function abnormalities. Because increased lung water is often present in patients with chronic renal failure even without detectable abnormalities of radiographs or pulmonary function, this most likely accounts for the modest abnormalities occasionally reported.

Diffusion capacity, unlike other pulmonary function tests, measures the ability to transfer gas from air to blood. This measure depends on the nature of the alveolar–capillary barrier as well as the amount of hemoglobin in the alveolar capillary. As anemia is commonly associated with renal failure, DL_{CO} is often reduced. However, after correction for anemia, the DL_{CO} remains subnormal in many, often those on longstanding hemodialysis, raising the question of whether this therapy or prolonged uremia somehow injures the alveolar–capillary membrane. It has been shown that there is an initial decrease in DL_{co} during dialysis, followed several hours later by an increase above predialysis values. The notion of a progressive hemodialysis-related lung disease was supported by workers specifically examining the membrane component of diffusion using a nitric oxide–carbon monoxide technique and finding a correlation between membrane diffusion abnormality and time on dialysis.

Respiratory muscle strength was assessed in a small group of nonsmoking, hemodialysis patients, who on routine spirometry achieved normal values. Maximal static inspiratory (PI_{max}) and expiratory pressures (PE_{max}) and maximal voluntary ventilation (MVV) were significantly lower than the age-, sex-, weight-, and height-matched controls. This decrease was found to correlate with an elevation of inorganic phosphorus in 9 of the 10 patients with chronic renal failure. This correlation may reflect the presence of calcium deposition in the lungs.

Recombinant human erythropoietin (rHuEPO) and renal transplantation are commonly used therapies in chronic renal failure patients. Use of rHuEPO has been associated with increased exercise capacity, improved MVV and forced vital capacity (FVC), and DL_{CO}. It is important to note that the studies reporting these findings were nonblinded, and inasmuch as exercise capacity, MVV, and FVC are dependent both on diaphragmatic strength and motivation, they need further validation. Because rHuEPO increases blood hemoglobin by design, it is to be expected that the DL_{CO} increases during therapy, approximately 9% per gram rise in hemoglobin in one study. One small study of renal transplantation patients showed no significant change in pulmonary function other than a slight decrease in DL_{CO} from a supranormal pretransplant value.

Earlier studies suggested that patients with limited respiratory reserve should not be placed on peritoneal dialysis therapy because some reports showed significant decreases in VC during the placement of 2 L of dialysate in the peritoneal cavity of patients with chronic lung disease. Newer studies have shown no decrease in VC, expired residual volume, forced expiratory volume in one second, maximal midflow, maximal expiratory flow at 50%, or closing volume per vital capacity, and no changes in arterial blood gas values. There was a decrease in functional residual capacity during dialysis that returned to baseline after peritoneal dialysis. It is hypothesized that the decrease in VC in earlier studies was secondary to pain. Based on available data, it would seem all but the most decompensated patient with chronic obstructive lung disease can safely undergo peritoneal dialysis.

PULMONARY INFECTION IN UREMIA

Concern for infection is paramount in patients with uremia. It is a major cause of death in acute renal failure and also increases the morbidity and mortality of chronic renal failure. Several factors may account for the increased propensity of uremic patients for infection. There is a decrease in cell-mediated immunity, possible suppression of antibody production, and peripheral blood lymphocytopenia.

Uremic Pleuritis

Pleural effusions are a common problem in patients with uremia. In a recent retrospective study of adult hospitalized patients on long-term hemodialysis, radiographic evidence of pleural effusion was found in 21%. Congestive heart failure accounted for almost half the effusions in this series, with uremic pleurisy, parapneumonic effusion, and atelectasis comprising most of the others.

The clinical diagnosis of uremic effusion remains one of exclusion. One must rule out other causes, especially infection, before the diagnosis can be made. The clinical diagnosis of uremic pleuritis rests on several findings. On physical examination, dullness to percussion and decreased breath sounds indicate

TABLE 71.1. Findings in Pleural Effusion Due to Uremia Per Se or Secondary to Infection

	Empyema	Uremia
Gram's stain, culture	+	−
White blood cells	↑↑↑	↑
Red blood cells	↑	↑ or ↑↑
Protein	↑ or ↑↑	↑
Glucose	↓	Normal
Lactate dehydrogenase	↑	↑
pH	<7.3	>7.3

From Wilson WR, Cockerill FR, Rosenow EC. Pulmonary disease in the immunocompromised host: second of two parts. *Mayo Clin Proc* 1985;60:610–631.

fluid in the chest. These findings may be absent if the effusion is small. Frequently, a pleural and/or pericardial friction rub is heard and occasionally may be bilateral. Most patients will complain of pleuritic-type pain. Fever may be present in a few but is usually low grade. As with many other manifestations of uremia, uremic pleural effusions do not correlate directly with the degree of blood urea nitrogen and the elevation in serum creatinine concentration.

The laboratory diagnosis of uremic effusions rests on thoracentesis and pleural biopsy findings. Although there are many potential causes of pleural effusion in uremia, infection must always be considered, especially in light of the immunocompromised state of patients with renal failure and their blunted febrile response to systemic infection. The differentiation between infectious and uremic causes of pleural effusions is shown in Table 71.1. In uremia, the pleural biopsy will show only nonspecific inflammatory changes. Uremic pleural effusions are usually clear but occasionally are bloody, especially in dialysis patients. Such bloody effusions may organize and on occasion have been reported to require surgical decortication.

PULMONARY CALCIFICATION IN CHRONIC RENAL FAILURE

Virchow first described metastatic calcification in 1855. Of the visceral organs, the lungs, kidneys, stomach, and heart are the most common sites of calcification. There has been an increase in the number of case reports of metastatic pulmonary calcification, probably because of the increased survival of patients with chronic renal failure treated with hemodialysis. Pulmonary calcification, which is rarely visible on chest radiograph, occurs primarily in alveolar septae and is often associated with fibrosis. Pulmonary calcification is present in about 50% of patients with chronic renal failure who have other evidence of soft tissue calcification. Patients may even have severe abnormalities of pulmonary function without clear-cut evidence of calcification on chest radiograph. Because the calcifications are only occasionally visible on plain films, tomography or radionuclide scanning are more helpful in the detection of pulmonary calcification; increased uptake of technetium-99 is seen when pulmonary calcifications are present.

It has been generally accepted that the incidence of calcification does not correlate with severity or duration of chronic renal failure, and calcification is seen in both dialysis-treated and untreated patients. The mechanisms responsible for pulmonary calcification in uremic patients are not fully understood but may be related to factors underlying the propensity for soft tissue calcification in uremia. The state of secondary hyperparathyroidism of uremia may be important. Indeed, pulmonary calcification in dogs with chronic renal failure is prevented or ameliorated by prior parathyroidectomy.

Pulmonary calcification may be associated with respiratory distress, and restrictive abnormalities in pulmonary function even affect the function of the right side of the heart secondary to elevated pulmonary artery pressure.

Diseases such as sarcoidosis, miliary tuberculosis, pulmonary microlithiasis, occupational lung disease, *Pneumocystis* infection, pulmonary edema, and many others could be interpreted as metastatic calcification on chest x-ray examination. Many of these entities are much more common in uremia than metastatic calcification, which presents a relatively unchanging pattern on chest x-ray film that can be a clue to the diagnosis, especially for distinguishing calcification from infection and other acute processes.

Pulmonary calcification in rare cases can be fulminant and rapidly fatal, permitting little time for diagnosis, and the calcium–phosphorus product may be below the recognized threshold for tissue calcification (60 mg^2/dl^2) in biopsy-proven cases. Nevertheless, discontinuation of *calcium-containing* phosphorus-binding agents and vitamin D to avoid significant elevations in serum calcium is advisable, and minimizing alkalosis during dialysis may be of benefit.

HEMODIALYSIS-ASSOCIATED HYPOXEMIA

Hypoxemia during dialysis is a well-documented phenomenon. Not so clear is the etiology of this transient fall in arterial Po_2 that occurs almost immediately with the start of hemodialysis. Initially, it was thought that the cellophane dialyzer membranes activated complement, which in turn caused granulocyte activation and pulmonary leukostasis. This leukostasis was presumed to cause ventilation-perfusion mismatch, resulting in hypoxemia. Although the data indicating complement activation are convincing enough, the cause-and-effect relationship between it and hemodialysis-associated hypoxemia has not been established. Carbon dioxide loss across the dialyzer membrane has also been implicated. This loss would cause alveolar hypoventilation and alteration of the respiratory quotient (RQ) with resultant arterial hypoxemia.

A proposal that combines these hypotheses suggests that the hypoxemia seen during dialysis has membrane-independent as well as membrane-dependent mechanisms. Membrane-independent factors include those etiologic agents that decrease the RQ, such as carbon dioxide loss across the dialyzer. Membrane-dependent factors are related to blood interaction with the cellophane membrane, causing more complement activation and a larger decline in arterial Po_2 than when other types of membranes are used, such as the polyacrylonitrile membrane. Regardless of the cause, the hypoxemia is rarely clinically significant. However, during dialysis of a patient with an already low Po_2, the effect could become significant. The hypoxemia is usually readily corrected by administration of oxygen.

CHRONIC PULMONARY CHANGES

Little is known about the effects of chronic renal failure and/or hemodialysis on the lung parenchyma. A retrospective autopsy study noted that there was an increased incidence of interstitial fibrosis, pleural fibrosis and/or pleuritis, pulmonary arteriosclerosis, thromboembolism, and calcification in chronic hemodialysis patients. Electron microscopy studies on the lungs of chronic renal failure patients have shown the irregular thickening of the alveolar–capillary basement membrane, with occasional laminations and fragmentation. Alterations in the basement membrane have been suggested as the cause of increased capillary membrane permeability. Other lesions include alveolar epithelial degenerative changes and detachment from the basement membrane with capillary endothelium swelling, vacuolization, and occasionally loosening of intercellular junctions. Whether these changes are related to the underlying disease or to transient but repetitive injury that may occur during dialysis is unclear.

Selected Readings

Akmal M, Barndt RR, Ansari AN, et al. Excess PTH in CRF induces pulmonary calcification, pulmonary hypertension, and right ventricular hypertrophy. *Kidney Int* 1995;47:158–163.

A study demonstrating the role of secondary hyperparathyroidism in the genesis of pulmonary calcifications in uremia.

Bark H, Heimer D, Chaimovitz C, et al. Effect of chronic renal failure on respiratory muscle strength. *Respiration* 1988;54:153–161.

Respiratory muscle strength and endurance is described in 10 patients with chronic renal failure undergoing dialysis.

Bush A, Gabriel R. Pulmonary function in chronic renal failure: effects of dialysis and transplantation. *Thorax* 1991;46:424–428.

Describes the results of pulmonary function tests in 80 patients. These patients were categorized as predialysis, dialysis, or postcadaveric renal transplantation.

Conger JD, Hammond WS, Alfrey AC, et al. Pulmonary calcifications in chronic dialysis patients: clinical and pathological studies. *Ann Intern Med* 1975;83:330–336.

Study of 31 patients who developed pulmonary calcification in the course of chronic hemodialysis. It includes complete descriptions of the pathologic and radiologic findings in these patients.

Jarrat MJ, Sahn SA. Pleural effusions in hospitalized patients receiving long-term hemodialysis. *Chest* 1995;108:470–474.

Retrospective study of 100 hospitalized adult patients with chronic renal failure undergoing long-term hemodialysis with pleural effusion. The most common etiologies and percentages of each are as follows: heart failure 46%, uremic pleurisy 16%, parapneumonic effusion 15%, and atelectasis 11%.

Lee YS. Ultrastructural observations of chronic uremic lungs with special reference to histochemical and x-ray microanalytic studies on altered alveocapillary basement membranes. *Am J Nephrol* 1985;5:255–266.

Presentation of data that may be used to relate ultrastructural changes in the lung to pulmonary physiologic alterations.

Moinard J, Guenard H. Membrane diffusion of the lungs in patients with chronic renal failure. *Eur Resp J* 1993;6:225–230.

Study of 15 patients hemodialyzed for 1 to 10 years without symptoms, history, or chest x-ray evidence of lung disease. Using a nitric oxide–carbon monoxide technique, the membrane component of the diffusion capacity (DL_{CO}) was found to be reduced proportionate to time on dialysis. This finding is consistent with the notion of hemodialysis-induced lung disease, possibly due to a bioincompatible dialysis membrane (Cuprophane) used in all study patients.

Slutsky RA, Day R, Murray M. Effect of prolonged renal dysfunction on intravascular and extravascular pulmonary fluid volumes during left atrial hypertension. *Proc Soc Exp Biol Med* 1985;179:25–31.

Study of development of pulmonary edema during experimental renal dysfunction. Left atrial pressure was elevated in 14 study animals, 7 of which had surgically induced renal failure. Greater accumulations of extravascular lung water occurred at lower levels of left atrial pressure in the renal failure group; presumed causes included lower protein oncotic pressure in the renal failure group and possibly altered pulmonary microvascular permeability.

Tarasuik A, Heimer D, Bark H. Effect of chronic renal failure on skeletal and diaphragmatic muscle contraction. *Am Rev Resp Dis* 1992;146:1383–1388.

Study of rat diaphragm and skeletal muscle to examine the effect of chronic uremia on the force of contraction, twitch characteristics, and fatigability. Fatigability was increased in diaphragms of the most severely uremic rats.

Ücok K, Gökbel H, Yeksan M, et al. The effect of rHUEPO administration on pulmonary functions in haemodialysis patients. *J Artif Organs* 1996;19:336–338.

A study of 13 hemodialysis patients demonstrating that the treatment with erythropoietin and the amelioration of the anemia was associated with significant improvement in pulmonary tests as evidenced by an increase in the diffusing capacity, maximal voluntary ventilation, forced vital capacity, and peak expiratory flow rate values.

CHAPTER 72

Hematopoietic System in Uremia

PART 1
Anemia

David B. Van Wyck

Anemia in the patient with chronic renal failure poses a diagnostic and management challenge rich in ambiguity. Among patients with chronic renal failure, not all suffer anemia, nor do all show erythropoietin deficiency. Among those who suffer anemia, erythropoietin deficiency is not the only cause. Erythropoietin replacement therapy in sufficient doses corrects most anemia regardless of cause, but iron deficiency, which responds to simple iron supplementation, and inflammation, which otherwise resists treatment, each commonly contribute to anemia in chronic renal failure. Regrettably, the presence of renal failure renders laboratory evaluation of both iron deficiency and inflammation unreliable. Other factors that contribute to the anemia of chronic renal failure include shortened red cell survival (hemolysis) inhibition of erythropoiesis by uremic toxins (PTA, spermine, and others), aluminum toxicity, and blood loss due to increased bleeding tendency.

The appearance of erythropoietin deficiency, iron deficiency, and inflammation in the natural history of anemia in chronic renal failure is, moreover, variable. In general, a progressive decline in GFR involves a commensurate fall in renal erythropoietin secretion. When erythropoietin secretion is insufficient to maintain circulating red cell mass, erythropoietin deficiency anemia results. In the absence of erythropoietin replacement (Epoetin) therapy, average hemoglobin concentrations in end-stage renal disease range from 6 to 8 g/dl, corresponding to a hematocrit of 18% to 24%. As many as 40% of patients require red cell transfusions annually. Only 5% to 10% of untreated hemodialysis patients show hemoglobin levels within normal range. The two additional pathogenic factors are introduced by hemodialysis: iron depletion from dialysis-related blood loss and inflammation from recurrent infection or surgery. Iron depletion, in the absence of iron replacement therapy, progresses to iron deficiency erythropoiesis, which contributes to worsening anemia. Finally, despite appropriate Epoetin and iron therapy, a substantial fraction of patients fail to achieve target hemoglobin range (11 to 12 g/dl). These patients often show evidence of inflammation: low hemoglobin despite high-dose Epoetin, low transferrin saturation despite normal or elevated ferritin levels, hypoalbuminemia, and elevated levels of C-reactive protein.

The Anemia Work Group of the National Kidney Foundation Dialysis Outcomes Quality Initiative (NKF-DOQI) has provided comprehensive, evidence-based clinical practice guidelines for anemia management in patients with chronic renal failure. Their recommendations, which are exhaustively referenced and widely available electronically and in print, cover diagnostic evaluation, erythropoietin (EPO) therapy, iron management, and causes of Epoetin resistance. The causes of resistance to EPO therapy in patients with chronic renal failure are provided in Table 72.1. The clinical practice of anemia management borrows heavily from our understanding of the normal regulation of erythropoiesis and iron metabolism, as well as from the pathogenesis of anemia in patients with kidney disease. This information, much of which has only recently come to light, has particularly important implications for guiding the administration and monitoring of Epoetin and iron therapy.

TABLE 72.1. Causes of Resistance to Erythropoietin Replacement Therapy in Patients with Anemia of Chronic Renal Failure

Bleeding
Iron deficiency
Inflammatory syndromes
Infection
Trauma
Surgery
Autoimmune disorders
Solid tumors
Pregnancy
Drugs
Myelosuppressive agents
ACE inhibitors
Angiotensin II–receptor blockers
Aluminum intoxication
Nutritional disorder
B_{12} deficiency
Folate deficiency
Hyperparathyroidism
Hemolysis
Hemoglobinopathy
Thalassemia
Sickle cell disease
Hemoglobin S
Myelodysplastic syndrome
Multiple myeloma
Leukemia
Inadequate dialysis

ACE, angiotensin-converting enzyme.

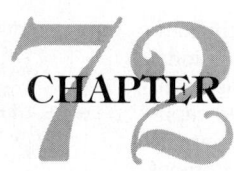

REGULATION OF ERYTHROPOIESIS

Regulation of Erythropoietin Secretion

The kidney produces EPO to maintain effective circulating red cell mass much the way it produces renin to maintain effective circulating volume: specialized cells anatomically positioned to sense subtle rheologic changes trigger a sequence of events that begins with a molecular signal to promote gene transcription and proceeds, in steps, from elaboration of hormonal mRNA to secretion of circulating hormone, activation of distant cells, and finally restoration of homeostasis. EPO-producing cells are strategically located in the interstitium of the renal cortex, closely juxtaposed with the convoluted tubules. Despite high renal arterial blood flow, the high oxygen demand of proximal tubular epithelium coupled with preglomerular arteriovenous shunting render tissue oxygen delivery to the cortex marginally adequate. Tissue oxygen tension falls progressively with increasing depth from the renal capsule. Thus, under optimal conditions, inner cortical cells specialize to produce EPO balance at the threshold of tissue oxygen levels sufficient to provoke a hypoxic signal. Small decrements in effective oxygen delivery recruit these cells to hypoxia-induced EPO secretion. Further decrements in oxygen delivery expand the area subject to low-tissue oxygen tension, advancing the recruitment of EPO-producing cells progressively from inner toward outer cortex.

The hypoxia-sensing molecule within EPO-producing cells is a hemelike factor that undergoes conformational change in the absence of oxygen to cause it to bind regulatory elements on the EPO gene, thereby initiating transcription of EPO mRNA. Secretion of circulating EPO quickly follows. In humans and animals, increases in EPO concentration in serum are detectable within 2 hours after exposure to hypoxia. The rate of renal EPO production and the level of EPO in circulating blood reflect the total number of cells recruited to produce EPO, rather than the rate of production per cell.

An important distinction is that EPO secretion is regulated not by absolute hematocrit but by effective oxygen delivery, as determined by the molecular hypoxia sensor in renal peritubular interstitial cells. Secondary polycythemia, a set of disorders characterized by persistent EPO production and hypoxia-sensor activation despite a pathologically increased hematocrit, best illustrates this concept. Polycythemia due to increased EPO secretion may be associated with continuous hypoxemia in patients with lung disease, intermittent hypoxemia in patients with sleep apnea, renal ischemia in patients with renal artery stenosis, and impaired oxygen dissociation in patients with chronic carbon monoxide poisoning or inherited hemoglobinopathy.

Mechanism of Erythropoietin Action

Erythropoietin increases red cell production by salvaging red cell precursors from preprogrammed cell death (apoptosis), by sparing immature erythroblasts from destruction mediated by mature erythroblasts and macrophages (Fas/Fas ligand dependent cytolysis), and by priming erythroblasts to increase iron supply for erythropoiesis.

Erythropoiesis takes place in functionally autonomous islands of cells that include both erythroid precursors and one to two macrophages. These erythroblastic islands feature the full lineage of cells that participate in forming the mature circulating reticulocyte, including, in expanding sequence, pluripotent stem cells, blast-forming cells (BFU-E), colony-forming cells (CFU-E), immature erythroblasts, mature erythroblasts, and early, noncirculating reticulocytes (Fig. 72.1). Expansion of the erythropoietic cascade through proliferation, differentiation, and maturation takes place concentrically, with the earliest precursors forming the center of the island and the most mature at the periphery. EPO receptors are found in highest concentration on CFU-E and in higher concentration on immature than mature erythroblasts. Thus EPO exerts its role strategically at the early stages of erythropoiesis, where small changes in proliferation rates among relatively few cells can be amplified throughout subsequent generations of lineage-committed erythroid precursors. Proliferation is regulated by the binding of EPO to EPO receptors on precursor cell surfaces. In the presence of EPO, precursors survive to proliferate, differentiate, and populate successive generations, and thereby preserve or expand precursor mass. In the absence of EPO, cells succumb to apoptosis within hours after formation, and total precursor mass contracts or fails to expand. The effect of EPO on proliferation, precursor mass, red cell mass and their clinically useful measures, reticulocyte index, hemoglobin and hematocrit are directly related to serum EPO concentration.

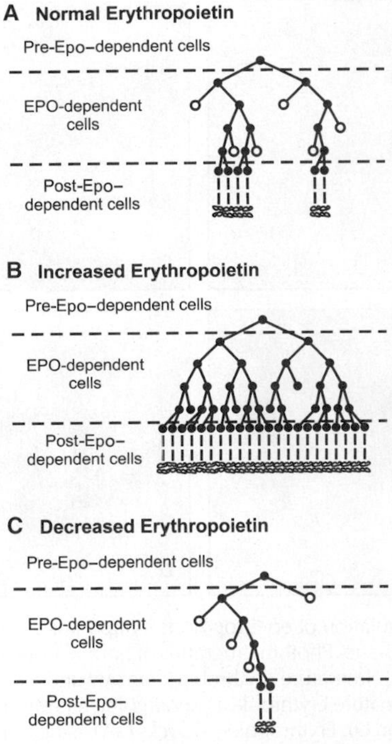

Figure 72.1. Role of erythropoietin and apoptosis in regulating expansion of red cell precursors. Erythropoietin promotes expansion of erythroid precursor mass in part by salvaging cells bearing erythropoietin receptors from apoptosis. The higher the level of circulating erythropoietin, the greater the activation of erythropoietin receptors and the greater the proportion of cells surviving to proliferate, differentiate, and mature. (Reproduced with permission from Koury MJ, Bondurant MC. The molecular mechanism of erythropoietin action. *Eur J Biochem* 1992;210:649–663.)

Immature erythroblasts require EPO to prevent not only self-destruction by apoptosis but also cytolysis by neighboring macrophages. Mature erythroblasts, which are Fas insensitive, express Fas ligands, which, when bound to Fas receptors on the surface of immature erythroblasts, target the Fas/Fas ligand-bearing cell for ingestion and killing by nearby macrophages (Fig. 72.2). The interaction of the Fas "death receptor," Fas ligand, erythroid precursors, and macrophages constitute a negative feedback loop, internal to the erythroblastic island, which acts to curtail further precursor expansion once a sizeable generation of mature erythroblasts is established. Binding of EPO to EPO receptors blocks the cytotoxic effect of Fas/Fas

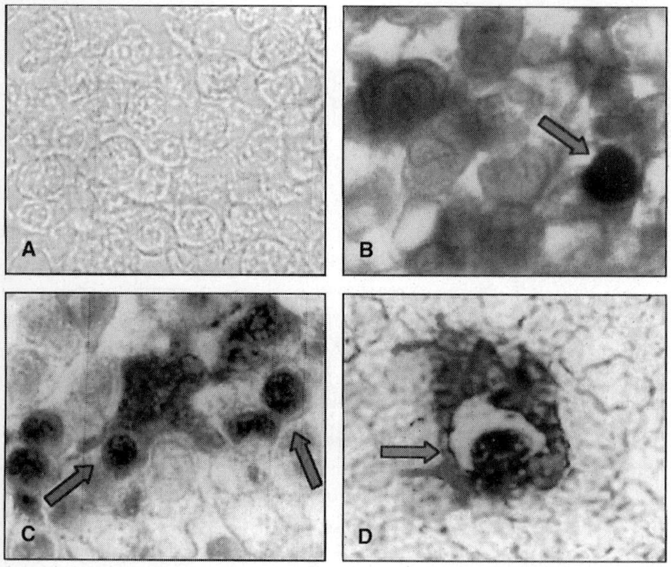

Figure 72.2. Regulation of erythropoiesis by apoptosis and phagocytosis of apoptotic erythroblasts. Photomicrographs of normal bone marrow show unstained control **(A)**, immature erythroblast *(arrow)* undergoing apoptosis **(B)**, and apoptotic immature erythroblasts undergoing ingestion by a neighboring macrophage **(C** and **D)**. Erythropoietin blocks Fas/Fas-ligand mediated phagocytosis. (Reproduced with permission from De Maria R, Testa U, Luchetti L, et al. Apoptotic role of Fas/Fas ligand in the regulation of erythropoiesis. *Blood* 1999;93:796–803; Copyright American Association of Hematology.) (See Color Figure 72.2.)

ligand, thereby interrupting the negative feedback and ensuring survival of immature erythroblasts.

EPO exerts a third effect on erythropoiesis by acting to enhance iron uptake in erythroid precursors. EPO directly activates cytosolic iron-regulatory protein (see Intracellular Iron Disposition) and thereby increases expression of the transferrin receptor on erythroid cell surfaces. This finding is in keeping with the clinical observation that intravenous iron administration boosts hemoglobin content of reticulocytes but does not affect total reticulocyte production in iron-replete patients undergoing acute Epoetin administration. In short, EPO enhances avidity of erythroid cells for available iron, and intravenous iron administration ensures optimal iron availability. Additional discussion on the physiology and metabolism of EPO is found in Chapter 13.

Implications for Erythropoietin Replacement Therapy

The physiology of erythropoietin secretion and action suggests practical guidelines for designing EPO replacement therapy in patients with chronic renal failure (Tables 72.2 and 72.3). The short plasma half-life of recombinant EPO (e.g., Epoetin alfa, 6 to 8 hours) after intravenous injection and the rapid destruction of red cell precursors after EPO deprivation support measures that prolong effective half-lives and minimize the likelihood of EPO withdrawal. The prolonged half-life of Epoetin after subcutaneous compared with intravenous administration probably explains why subcutaneous adminis-

TABLE 72.2. Physiologic Approach to Clinical Problem Solving: The Patient with Widely Fluctuating Hgb/Hct Values

Governing Physiologic Principle	Possible Cause of the Clinical Problem	Recommended Approach
1. Erythropoiesis is normally regulated by small, incremental changes in EPO secretion.	a. Epoetin dosage adjustments are disproportionately large. b. Epoetin vial sizes are being used to determine Epoetin dosage adjustments. c. Sliding scale is being used to determine Epoetin dosage adjustments.	a. Confine Epoetin dosage adjustments to 75% or 125% of previous dose. Initiate Epoetin at 120–180 u/kg/wk (IV) or 80–120 u/kg/wk (SC), then adjust upward or downward. b. Calculate initial Epoetin dosage as above, then adjust. Using vial size to determine dose requires disproportionate dosage adjustments. c. Avoid sliding scale. Adjusting Epoetin dosage to hematocrit level leads to disproportionately large dose adjustments.
2. EPO secretion responds to changes in effective tissue oxygen delivery to maintain Hgb within normal range.	a. Epoetin dosages are being adjusted on the basis of a single Hgb/Hct value, usually the latest available. b. Epoetin dosage determinations are being made on the basis of Hct rather than Hgb.	a. Evaluate at least 3–4 previous Hgb values to discern trend. If values suggest a trend toward out-of-range, adjust Epoetin dosage to prevent progression to out-of-range values. b. Use Hgb to monitor anemia management. Target range is 11–12 g/dl. Hgb more stable than Hct because results are less affected by patient volume status, blood sample transportation, and instrumentation.
3. The delay between changes in EPO secretion and changes in Hct/Hgb is long: 2–4 wk.	a. Epoetin dosages are being adjusted too frequently to adequately gauge response to each dosage change.	a. Adjust Epoetin no more frequently than twice monthly when initiating therapy, once monthly when patient has achieved target range.
4. EPO deprivation results in rapid loss of immature erythroblasts by apoptosis and cytolysis.	a. Epoetin dosages have been withheld, commonly in response to above-target Hgb/Hct values.	a. Adjust Epoetin downward for above-target hemoglobin values, avoid holding doses.
5. Adequacy of iron supply for erythropoiesis and efficacy of EPO are inextricably linked at the cellular and molecular level.	a. Iron deficiency has been permitted to develop, leading to below-target Hgb/Hct, elevated Epoetin dosage, or both. If EPO dosage has also been increased, simultaneous intravenous iron therapy may lead to overshoot of Hgb/Hct. b. Iron and Epoetin orders are being determined separately. Failure to recognize iron deficiency may lead to increased Epoetin dosage, then Hgb/Hct overshoot after intravenous iron administration.	a. Maintain iron indices in target range (transferrin saturation 20%–50%, ferritin <800 ng/ml) using regular iv iron administration. b. Consider Epoetin and iron therapy together. If iron deficiency develops, give loading dose of intravenous iron; avoid simultaneous Epoetin dosage adjustment.

TABLE 72.3. Physiologic Approach to Clinical Problem Solving: The Patient with High Epoetin Dosage, Low Hgb/Hct, or Both

Governing Physiologic Principle	Possible Cause of the Clinical Problem	Recommended Approach
Adequacy of iron supply for erythropoiesis and efficacy of EPO are inextricably linked at the cellular and molecular level.	Iron deficiency is unrecognized and untreated.	Maintain iron sufficiency by giving regular intravenous iron to maintain iron indices within target range (transferrin saturation 20%–50%, ferritin <800 ng/ml). Treat iron deficiency (saturation <20%) by intravenous iron 1 g in divided doses.
Intestinal iron transport is downregulated at levels of transferrin saturation associated with optimal Epoetin therapy.	Oral iron agents are inappropriately being relied on for iron therapy.	Avoid oral iron as a source of iron supplement in all but predialysis and peritoneal dialysis patients.
Inflammatory mediators impair erythropoiesis, shift intracellular iron from heme synthesis to storage ferritin.	Patient harbors unrecognized inflammatory disease or infection or has other causes for high levels of inflammatory mediators.	Determine C-reactive protein (CRP). If elevated, exclude obvious causes (infection, inflammatory disease, cancer, recent trauma or surgery), correct if possible. Do not hold Epoetin.
Nonhematologic disorders that adversely affect bone and bone marrow often adversely affect erythropoiesis.	Hyperparathyroidism with or without radiographic bone disease is present.	Calcitriol, oral or intravenous, may be effective in lowering parathyroid hormone levels and increasing sensitivity to Epoetin.

tration is associated with lower Epoetin dosages to maintain target-range hematocrits. New erythropoiesis-stimulating proteins and gene-activated EPO delivery systems, currently under investigation, take advantage of the mode of action of native EPO by prolonging effective half-life. These strategies promise the erythropoietic and practical benefits of subcutaneous injection without the attendant patient discomfort.

The long delay between the onset of Epoetin action and the apparent clinical response as a change in hemoglobin/hematocrit requires that dosages of Epoetin be adjusted infrequently, cautiously, and by iteration: the new dosage should be either 75% or 125% of the previous dosage and should be reviewed for effectiveness once a month (Table 72.4). Dosages should certainly not be adjusted more frequently than once every 2 weeks. For the same reasons, Epoetin dosages should be adjusted according to trends to anticipate projected values rather than respond to current results alone. In this way, Epoetin doses need never be held, a practice that leads to a rapid collapse of early red cell progenitors, followed by a delayed but sudden fall in hemoglobin/hematocrit. This in turn is followed by higher-than-needed Epoetin dosages, and finally by a delayed but sudden rise in hemoglobin/hematocrit, which threatens to overshoot the target range. When anemia management is characterized by pronounced oscillations of hemoglobin and hematocrit above and below target range, failure to observe and anticipate trends, to make Epoetin dosage adjustments in small increments, or to refrain from withholding Epoetin doses should be suspected (Table 72.2).

REGULATION OF IRON METABOLISM

External Iron Balance

Regulation of intestinal iron absorption maintains iron sufficiency while avoiding either deficiency or overload, despite constantly changing dietary iron supply. In the absence of substantial bleeding, body iron status varies little throughout adult life. Although iron deficiency remains common among females of reproductive age, a measure of the success of intestinal iron

TABLE 72.4. Epoetin Dosage Recommendations for Patients with Anemia of Chronic Renal Failure

Situation	Hgb[a] (g/dl)	Anemia Status	Recommended Epoetin Therapy: Predialysis and Peritoneal Dialysis	Recommended Epoetin Therapy: Hemodialysis
Initial therapy	<10.0	Presumed erythropoietin deficiency	100 u/kg SC weekly; adjust downward 25% if Hgb rise >1.3 g/dl/mo	100 u/kg IV three times weekly; adjust downward 25% if Hgb rise >1.3 g/dl/mo
	11.0–12.5	Target range achieved	Adjust dosage downward at Hgb 12–12.5	Adjust dosage downward 25% at Hgb 12–12.5
Maintenance therapy	>12.5	Above target range	Adjust dosage downward 25%	Adjust dosage downward 25%
	<11.0	Below target range	Adjust dosage upward 25%	Adjust dosage upward 25%
	<7.0–8.0	Meets transfusion criteria	Consider transfusion 25%	Consider transfusion 25%

[a] Monitored twice monthly.

regulation is the observation that iron deficiency among North American adult males is less common than even homozygous hereditary hemochromatosis. A useful clinical conclusion is that iron deficiency occurs only when iron losses outstrip iron absorption, due to bleeding, and that iron overload occurs spontaneously only when iron absorption fails to decrease appropriately as iron stores increase, due to a genetic disorder.

When tissue iron stores are adequate, intestinal iron absorption ensures neutral iron balance by matching the approximately 1 mg lost daily by unregulated intestinal iron excretion. Iron absorption increases dramatically in the presence of either iron deficiency, hypoxia, or accelerated erythropoiesis. Neither serum iron, transferrin, transferrin saturation, nor ferritin act directly to regulate iron absorption. Nevertheless, markers of body iron status yield indirect information about intestinal iron avidity. Indices consistent with iron deficiency (Tf-saturation less than 20% and ferritin less than 30 ng/ml in normal individuals or less than 50% in patients with chronic renal failure) are associated with increased iron absorption, whereas indices optimal for Epoetin efficacy (Tf-saturation 20% or greater) are associated with minimal iron absorption.

The primary transporter responsible for bringing iron into enterocytes has been identified as Nramp2, a molecule that functions in the brush border of the intestinal epithelium (Fig. 72.3). In keeping with the known physiology of iron absorption, expression of Nramp2 mRNA dramatically increases in the presence of iron deficiency, mutations of the Nramp2 gene in mice produce iron deficiency anemia, transfection of Nramp2 cDNA promotes increased iron uptake in cells, and the gene product transports other heavy metals in addition to iron. Interestingly, Nramp2 also plays a key role in facilitating uptake of iron in erythroid cells.

Another protein, Hfe, which is structurally related to class I MHC molecules, also participates in the regulation of iron absorption. Although the precise role of Hfe has not been elucidated, mutation of the Hfe gene appears to be responsible for the failure to appropriately downregulate iron absorption in the face of tissue iron excess in most patients with hereditary hemochromatosis. Presumably, intact Hfe attenuates iron absorption by regulating the function or expression of Nramp2 in intestinal epithelium.

Finally, effective intestinal iron absorption requires iron to be presented to the apical transporter in the ferrous (Fe^{2+}) state. High luminal acidity is also required, both to maintain iron in the ferrous state and to prevent formation of unabsorbable polynuclear iron hydroxide complexes. Some reduction of ferric (Fe^{3+}) to ferrous iron takes place within the duodenal brush border.

Thus iron supplements containing ferrous salts are more readily absorbed than ferric forms. Failure to adequately acidify gastric secretions, whether by pharmacologic antagonism or by primary achlorhydria, impairs iron absorption. Food and phosphate binders also block iron absorption, presumably by forming nonabsorbable polymolecular complexes.

Internal Iron Balance

The bulk of body iron, approximately 2,500 mg, resides in circulating hemoglobin. Intracellular iron stores, in the form of iron–ferritin complex, amount to only 200 to 1,200 mg. The total amount of iron in the extracellular fluid space averages only 5 mg and is found exclusively on the extracellular transport protein transferrin. Approximately 20 mg of iron is used daily for new hemoglobin formation, matching the amount returned daily to stores as aging red cells are removed from circulation. The process of iron cycling, from storage cells to erythroid precursors to red cells and back to stores (Fig. 72.4) is remarkable for the safety with which a large quantity of a highly reactive element is moved safely. Storage cells rely on rapid-acting post-transcriptional synthesis of ferritin to enfold intracellular iron in a protein coat, thereby preventing intracellular free iron to exceed 10^{-15} M, a threshold above which lipid peroxidation occurs. In the extracellular space, iron sequestration is even more potent: the stability constant for Fe^{3+} binding to transferrin is on the order of 10^{22}, which is sufficient to ensure that spontaneous dissociation of iron from a molecule of transferrin takes place no more often than once every 20 years.

Because transferrin (Tf) is the exclusive iron-binding protein in plasma under usual conditions, plasma iron-binding capacity is determined entirely by the concentration of transferrin, and all plasma iron is transferrin bound. The proportion of total iron-binding capacity (TIBC) that is occupied by plasma iron (P_{Fe}) is therefore expressed as the percentage of transferrin saturation ($[P_{Fe} \div TIBC] \times 100\%$). Each Tf molecule has two potential binding sites for iron and therefore exists in one of three forms: apoTf, monoferric Tf, and differic Tf. Compared with apoTf or monoferric Tf, differic Tf displays a pronounced conformational advantage in binding affinity to Tf receptors (TfR) on cell surfaces. Because internalization of Tf-bound iron first requires Tf-TfR binding, the rate of donation of iron to cells,

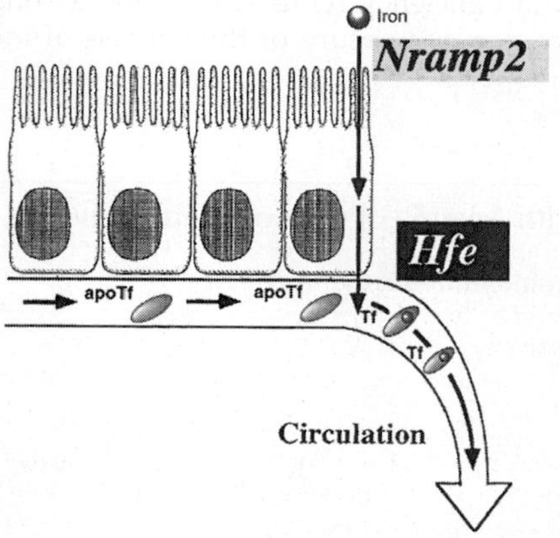

Figure 72.3. Physiology of intestinal iron transport. Iron transport by intestinal epithelium involves uptake of divalent (ferrous) iron by a transporter, Nramp2, on the luminal surface. Hfe acts to regulate basolateral iron transfer to plasma transferrin (Tf). Nramp2 also acts to transport iron from transferrin cycle endosomes (see Fig. 72.5). (Adapted with permission from Andrews NC, Levy JE. Iron is hot: an update on the pathophysiology of hemochromatosis. *Blood* 1998;92:1845–1851. Copyright American Society of Hematology.)

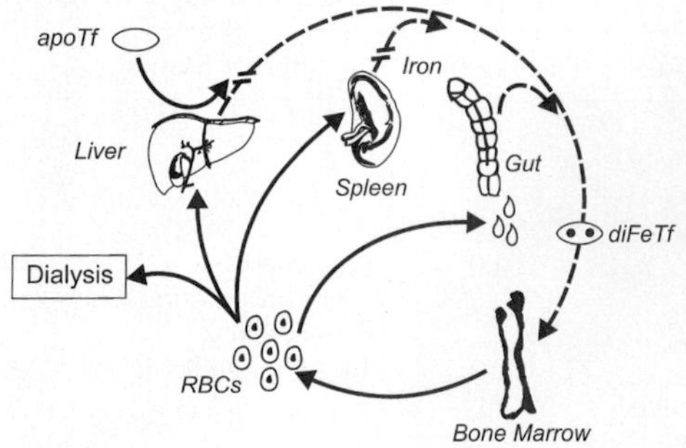

Figure 72.4. Internal and external iron balance. Internal iron balance is maintained by cycling approximately 20 mg of iron daily between red cells, reticuloendothelial macrophages and RES iron stores, and erythroid precursors. External iron balance is maintained by adjusting iron absorption to match intestinal iron excretion, normally 1 mg/day, or other iron losses.

and therefore the supply of iron for erythropoiesis, depends crucially on the concentration of differic Tf. The proportion of Tf present in the differic form increases directly with the percentage of transferrin saturation. At saturation levels below 20%, insufficient differic transferrin exists to support rates of erythropoiesis normally found during Epoetin treatment for dialysis-associated anemia. At saturation levels above 60%, on the other hand, iron donation to cells exceeds iron needs and, if allowed to persist, may eventually produce tissue iron overload and iron-mediated heart, liver, and endocrine failure.

Intracellular Iron Disposition

Binding of Tf to cell-surface Tf-receptor triggers surface invagination, endosome formation, and internalization of the complete iron–Tf-TfR complex (Fig. 72.5). Acidification of the endosome subsequently results in the release of iron from the tight Tf bond, making the iron available for use in mitochondrial heme synthesis and eventual hemoglobin formation. Iron not needed for heme synthesis is stored in cytosolic ferritin. The cell iron cycle is completed when the endosome returns the Tf-TfR complex to the cell surface and apoTf is released back to the circulation to acquire iron from storage cells.

Intracellular iron regulation maintains the balance between iron availability, iron needs for erythropoiesis, and iron storage. When iron requirements for erythropoiesis exceed iron availability, TfR expression increases to promote acquisition of iron, synthesis of erythroid-5-aminolevulinic acid synthase (eALAS) decreases to limit heme synthesis, and synthesis of ferritin declines to shift iron away from stores. When more iron is available than is needed, the process reverses: TfR expression declines, and eALAS and ferritin expression rises. The reciprocal relationship between TfR on the one hand and eALAS and ferritin on the other is due to differing effects of iron, iron-regulatory proteins (IRPs), and iron-responsive elements (IREs) on expression of the three products' respective mRNAs (Fig. 72.6). An IRE is an RNA stem-loop structure that activates when bound by IRP. IRP-1, a form found in erythroid precursors, cannot bind IRE in the presence of iron. Under conditions of iron deprivation, however, IRP-1 loses a crucial conformational feature: a central iron–sulfur cluster. Loss of the iron–sulfur cluster precipitates a conformational change that increases affinity of IRP-1 for IRE, facilitates binding, and thereby activates IRE. The effect of activated IRE on mRNA expression depends on whether the IRE resides in the 5′ or 3′ region. IREs residing in the 3′ untranslated region, as found in TfR mRNA, enhance mRNA stability when activated: thus the effect of activation is to increase effective TfR expression. IRE residing in the untranslated 5′ region, as found in ferritin and eALAS mRNA, slow mRNA translation when activated: the effect of activation is to decrease effective expression. In short, the iron–sulfur complex in IRP-1 provides an exquisitely sensitive sensor of intracellular iron. Erythroid precursor cells use IRP-1, binding of IRP-1 to IRE, or release of IRP-1 from IRE to maintain intracellular iron homeostasis by controlling, at the posttranscriptional level, how cells take up, use, and store iron.

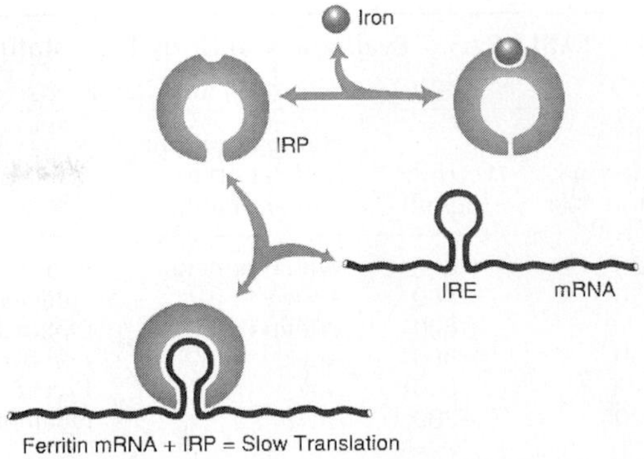

Figure 72.6. Translational control of cellular iron acquisition and utilization. Intracellular iron deprivation produces a conformational change in IRP (iron-regulatory protein), which permits it to bind to IRE (iron-responsive element), an mRNA stem-loop structure, which, when activated by IRP, affects mRNA translation. The effect on protein expression depends on the position of the IRE on mRNA. IREs residing in the 3′ untranslated region, as found in TfR mRNA, enhance mRNA stability when activated: thus the effect of activation is to increase effective TfR expression. IRE residing in the untranslated 5′ region, as found in ferritin and eALAS mRNA, slow mRNA translation when activated: the effect of activation is to decrease effective expression. (Adapted with permission from original artwork by R&D Systems, Inc.)

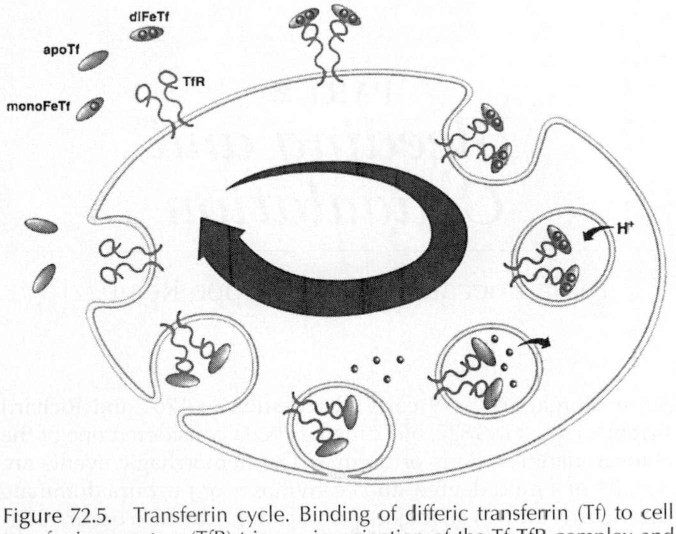

Figure 72.5. Transferrin cycle. Binding of differic transferrin (Tf) to cell transferrin receptors (TfR) triggers invagination of the Tf-TfR complex and subsequent endosome formation. Acidification of the endosome releases iron from Tf for use by mitochondria in heme synthesis or cytosolic ferritin for storage. To complete the cycle, the Tf-TfR complex is then returned intact to the cell surface, where apo-Tf is released to the circulation, and TfR again becomes for binding differic Tf. (Adapted with permission from original artwork by R&D Systems, Inc.)

EPO, oxidative stress, and nitric oxide (NO) all affect intracellular iron disposition through the IRP–IRE pathway. The effect of erythropoietin-mediated activation of IRP binding to IRE in erythroid precursors is to increase TfR expression and thereby enhance iron availability for erythropoiesis.

Oxidative stress and NO both modestly activate IRP-1, the main form of IRP found in erythroid cells. However, these factors exert their most prominent effect on iron metabolism by downregulating activity of IRP-2, a form of IRP that lacks an iron–sulfur cluster and is found in abundance in macrophages. Because IRP-2 acts to suppress ferritin synthesis and increase TfR expression, the negative effect of NO and oxidative stress on IRP-2 activity presumably explains the elevated intracellular ferritin and reticuloendothelial iron sequestration characteristic of inflammatory disease states.

Implications for Monitoring Iron Status and Managing Iron Replacement

The principles that govern normal intestinal iron absorption, internal iron disposition, and intracellular iron homeostasis have direct implications for monitoring iron status and managing iron

TABLE 72.5. Evaluation of Body Iron Status and Recommended Iron Therapy in Patients with Anemia of Chronic Renal Failure

Transferrin Saturation[a] (%)	Ferritin[a] (ng/ml)	Hemoglobin[b] in Relation to Target Range	Body Iron Status	Recommended Iron Therapy (intravenous iron dextran, gluconate, or sucrose)
<20	≤800	Within or below	Iron deficiency	1,000 mg in divided doses
≤50	≤800	Above	Sufficient iron present in excess Hgb	Withhold iron; adjust Epoetin dosage downward
20–50	≤800	Within or below	Optimal iron target range	100–200 mg intravenous iron per month
>50	>800	Any	Iron overload	Withhold iron
20–50	>800	Any	Excess iron stores	Withhold iron
<20	>800	Any	Inflammatory syndrome	Withhold iron

[a] Monitored monthly.
[b] Monitored twice monthly.

replacement in patients with the anemia of chronic renal failure (Tables 72.1 and 72.2). The need for intensive iron replacement in patients undergoing chronic hemodialysis is well established. Without iron supplementation, these patients are subject to iron depletion secondary to ongoing dialysis-associated blood loss. Estimates of cumulative iron losses in hemodialysis patients range from 1 to 5 g/yr.

Intestinal iron absorption, even under optimal conditions, is insufficient to manage iron losses of such magnitude. Oral iron supplements do not help. Oral iron agents fail to prevent negative iron balance in hemodialysis patients, are substantially inferior to intravenous iron therapy in minimizing Epoetin doses, and provide no benefit compared with no iron therapy at all. Reasons for the failure of oral iron agents are numerous: a flat dose–response curve and prominent adverse gastrointestinal effects limit effective doses to 60 to 150 mg of ferrous iron daily; gastritis and constipation contribute to a high rate of noncompliance with ferrous iron salts; simultaneous ingestion of food or phosphate binders impairs iron absorption; administration of antacids, H_2-blockers, or proton pump inhibitors hinder acidification needed for iron absorption; and nonferrous iron preparations commonly substituted for ferrous salts show better patient compliance but poor bioavailability. Finally, the inverse relationship between iron absorption and iron stores ensures minimal iron absorption at levels of body iron status associated with optimal Epoetin efficacy.

Because EPO acts at the cellular level to promote erythroid precursor survival, stimulate expansion of red cell mass, and enhance cell surface TfR, the central objective of iron monitoring and iron replacement must be to maintain adequate iron supply for Epoetin-stimulated erythropoiesis. Because erythroid iron uptake depends on binding of differic Tf to TfR and differic Tf is not present in appreciable concentrations below a transferrin saturation of 20%, the serum transferrin saturation should be maintained above that threshold (Table 72.5).

Selected Readings

Andrews N, Levy J. Iron is hot: an update on the pathophysiology of hemochromatosis. *Blood* 1998;92:1845–1851.

An extensive review of the physiology of normal iron metabolism, the molecular and cellular biology of iron transport, and the pathophysiology of iron loading diseases.

Barany P, Divino Filho JC, Bergstrom J. High C-reactive protein is a strong predictor of resistance to erythropoietin in hemodialysis patients. *Am J Kidney Dis* 1997;29:565–568.

The observation that high C-reactive protein levels are associated with impaired responsiveness to Epoetin therapy firmly establishes the importance of inflammatory mediators in managing dialysis associated anemia.

Cazzola M, Ponchio L, Benedetti FD, et al. Defective iron supply for erythropoiesis and adequate endogenous erythropoietin production in the anemia associated with systemic-onset juvenile chronic arthritis. *Blood* 1996;87:4824–4830.

Convincing evidence that inflammation impairs iron supply for erythropoiesis, even when ferritin levels are normal or elevated. This work, together with those by Barany et al. (above) and Gabay and Kushner (below), sheds light on a disorder that commonly contributes to anemia in patients with chronic renal failure. In anemic children with chronic inflammatory arthritis, as in anemic patients with chronic renal failure, intravenous iron therapy frequently unmasks iron deficiency erythropoiesis.

De Maria R, Testa U, Luchetti L, et al. Apoptotic role of Fas/Fas ligand system in the regulation of erythropoiesis. *Blood* 1999;93:796–803.

Expands the known actions of erythropoietin to include protecting immature erythroblasts from the cytotoxic effects of mature erythroblasts and macrophages, and describes a negative feedback loop that regulates erythropoiesis at the level of the erythroblastic island.

Eschbach JW, et al. NKF-DOQI Clinical Practice Guidelines for the Treatment of Anemia of Chronic Renal Failure. *Am J Kidney Dis* 1997;30(Suppl 3):S192–S240.

This document, also available online at http://www.kidney.org/doqi/doqi/doqianemia.html, provides comprehensive, evidence-based clinical practice guidelines for the management of the anemia of chronic renal failure.

Gabay C, Kushner I. Mechanisms of disease: Acute-phase proteins and other systemic responses to inflammation. *N Engl J Med* 1999;340:448–454.

A comprehensive review of the pathophysiology of inflammation and the clinical evaluation of inflammatory disease.

Weiss G, Houston T, Kastner S, et al. Regulation of cellular iron metabolism by erythropoietin: activation of iron-regulatory protein and upregulation of transferrin receptor expression in erythroid cells. *Blood* 1997;89:680–687.

This original work makes the important observation that the cellular and molecular effects of erythropoietin include actions that enhance iron availability for erythropoiesis. The introduction features a lucid explanation of intracellular iron metabolism, and the conclusion supports clinical practice guidelines recommending regular parenteral iron administration to optimize Epoetin efficacy.

PART 2
Bleeding and Coagulation

Paola Boccardo and Giuseppe Remuzzi

Since Morgagni's very early observation in 1764 and Richard Bright's report in 1827, bleeding has been considered one of the clinical manifestations of uremia. The hemorrhagic events are usually of a mild degree, and ecchymoses or purpura dominate the picture. However, major complications can also occur, ranging from epistaxis or bleeding from the gums to hemorrhagic pericarditis and retroperitoneal, gastrointestinal, and intracranial bleeding. The modern management of renal failure has definitely reduced the incidence of severe hemorrhages, but bleeding complications still represent a problem for uremic patients, particularly during surgery or invasive procedures.

The pathogenesis of uremic bleeding has still not been completely elucidated. The available data indicate that, in uremia, the main defect is in primary hemostasis, whereas no major alterations of plasma coagulation factors have been reported, except for notations of increased plasma fibrinogen and factor VIII/von Willebrand factor–related properties. There are data, however, showing that major natural inhibitors of coagulation are modified in uremia. Conflicting results have been reported on antithrombin III levels; although previous reports demonstrated increased levels of this natural anticoagulant, subsequent studies showed reduced levels of antithrombin III in uremic patients. Protein C anticoagulant activity, like protein S is decreased; this may contribute to thrombotic tendency observed in uremic patients. Thrombin is also continuously generated as demonstrated by increased levels of thrombin–antithrombin III complex, D-dimer, and fibrinopeptide A, further suggesting a hypercoagulable state.

Reports on fibrinolysis in uremia are also controversial: findings of decreased fibrinolytic activity at least relative to the extent of activation of coagulation are available, but others found an activation of fibrinolysis, with an increase of plasmin–antiplasmin complexes, fibrinogen, and fibrin degradation products, as well as decreased activity of plasminogen activator inhibitor. This may reflect a fibrinolytic response secondary to fibrin deposition, even if the overall fibrinolytic activity is depressed. These abnormalities paradoxically predispose uremic patients to thrombosis.

A complex cascade of events operating in concert is essential for normal hemostasis: (a) vessel wall contraction, (b) platelet adherence to the injured vessel wall, (c) platelet aggregation, and (d) formation and stabilization of fibrin clots. Thus primary hemostasis results from a combination of vasoconstriction, platelet adherence, and aggregation. The earliest event following vessel wall injury is the adhesion of platelets to exposed collagen fibers. In the next few minutes, platelets degranulate and become more closely packed in a plug mainly consisting of interdigitated platelets. These processes are impaired in uremic patients, and early studies referred to increased "capillary fragility" and prolonged bleeding time (BT), two constant abnormalities typical of uremia. Because both tests are influenced by the platelet number, the question of whether uremic bleeding depends on a decreased platelet number was soon addressed. Platelet count is in fact generally lower in uremic patients than in the control population, but thrombocytopenia rarely develops to such an extent as to impair primary hemostasis. As the problem of uremic bleeding was addressed with modern techniques, it soon became apparent that platelet function rather than number is abnormal. Virtually all the laboratory tests exploring platelet function gave abnormal results in patients with severe renal insufficiency. Defects in platelet factor 3 availability, clot retraction, and platelet retention on foreign surfaces in native whole blood were all reported in early studies. Reductions in platelet serotonin and adenosine diphosphate (ADP), elevation of cyclic adenosine monophosphate (cAMP), and reduced platelet ability to generate thromboxane $A_2(TXA_2)$, as well as an abnormal mobilization of platelet Ca^{2+} content have all been reported. Furthermore, additional studies have documented that nitric oxide (NO), a labile humoral agent formed by vascular endothelial cells from L-arginine, is produced in excessive amounts in uremia.

Studies focusing on the platelet–vessel wall interaction found several abnormalities. Vascular prostacyclin (PGI_2) is formed in excessive amounts in human and experimental uremia and structural and functional changes in von Willebrand factor (vWF), which normally mediates platelet adhesion to subendothelium and is mainly generated by endothelial cells, have been reported.

TABLE 72.6. Possible Factors Involved in the Pathogenesis of Uremic Bleeding

Platelet Dysfunction
Decreased platelet factor 3 availability
Reduction in intracellular serotonin and adenosine diphosphate (ADP)
Elevation in intracellular cyclic adenosine monophosphate (cAMP)
Reduced thromboxane A_2 generation
Defective cyclooxygenase activity
Abnormal mobilization of platelet Ca^{2+}
Uremic toxins, especially parathyroid hormone
Abnormal Platelet-Vessel Wall Interactions
Enhanced vascular PGI_2 production
Altered PGI_2 degradation
Altered factor VIII/von Willebrand factor
Anemia
Altered platelet adhesion
Altered blood rheology
Abnormal Production of Nitric Oxide

It has also been found that the hemorrhagic tendency in uremia is influenced by the low hematocrit. Red blood cells are certainly pivotal in primary hemostasis, and the anemia of renal failure may adversely influence the rheologic component of the platelet–vessel wall interaction.

Thus the pathogenesis of bleeding in uremia is multifactorial, with the complex platelet biochemical changes and multiple abnormalities of platelet–vessel wall interaction probably being the most important determinants. The various factors that may contribute to the pathogenesis of bleeding in uremia are listed in Table 72.6. Several studies have been aimed at finding a global measure of primary hemostasis that could predict the patient risk of bleeding. Among the various tests, the most valuable is skin BT, which has been demonstrated to correlate with clinical bleeding. Besides the various abnormalities in the hemostatic system that are related to the uremic condition itself, the hemorrhagic risk in today's patients is exacerbated by the technology currently used for the treatment of chronic renal failure. The interaction between blood and artificial surfaces contributes to platelet dysfunction and thrombocytopenia through platelet adhesion to and activation by the dialysis membranes. Heparin, commonly used to prevent coagulation in the extracorporeal circuit, can occasionally induce platelet activation and thrombocytopenia. In this chapter, we attempt to define the pathogenic mechanisms involved in the abnormal bleeding of uremia and discuss the approaches for the management of bleeding abnormalities.

PATHOGENESIS OF UREMIC BLEEDING

Platelet Functional Abnormalities and the Role of Dialyzable Factors

Among the platelet biochemical abnormalities reported, those likely to have clinical relevance are the reduction in platelet serotonin and ADP, elevation of cAMP levels, and altered platelet arachidonate metabolism leading to a reduced capability of uremic platelets to generate TXA_2.

Serotonin and ADP, which are extruded with other substances from endogenous stores during the platelet release reaction, play a pivotal role in platelet aggregation and plug formation. A defect in platelet serotonin and adenine nucleotide metabolism, storage, or release can alter platelet function. In view of the prime importance of platelet aggregation in platelet–platelet interaction, it is conceivable that the low platelet serotonin and ADP observed in uremia may contribute to the hemorrhagic diathesis of patients with chronic renal failure. Moreover, the observation that many inhibitors of platelet aggregation and adhesion to injured vessels exert their effects by altering the level of intraplatelet cAMP suggests that the high cAMP content in uremia might play a role in the platelet refractoriness to aggregation and adhesion and may thus be important in uremic platelet dysfunction. Another clue to the pathogenesis of the altered platelet function in chronic renal failure derives from the detection of an abnormal platelet arachidonic acid metabolism; platelet malondialdehyde production in response to arachidonic acid or thrombin was reduced *in vitro*. Because normal plasma partially corrects the defective production, uremic plasma would appear to be responsible for the derangement.

Defective platelet TXA_2 production in response to endogenous as well as exogenous stimuli has been described. The defect was not corrected by adding thrombin to the system *in vitro*, thus suggesting an intrinsic platelet defect. Because aspirin given to healthy volunteers reduces platelet thromboxane production to the same level as in uremic patients, a functional cyclooxygenase defect has been hypothesized. A similar threshold concentration of a TXA_2 agonist (U-46619) induced aggregation of normal and uremic platelets, indicating a normal TXA_2 receptor site in uremic platelets. It has been suggested that the abnormal platelet TXA_2 formation in uremia might be attributed to a defect proximal to cyclooxygenase (i.e., in the steps involved in the release of arachidonic acid by membrane phospholipids). This cannot be excluded on the basis of the available evidence. In a subpopulation of uremic patients, irreversible platelet activation does not occur in response to platelet-activating factor (PAF). This abnormality is independent of factor(s) of plasma origin but likely due to a reduced capability of platelets to form TXA_2 in response to PAF.

Experimental and clinical data have suggested that bleeding tendency in uremia is associated with an excessive formation of NO, a potent vasoactive molecule. Plasma concentrations of the stable NO metabolites, nitrites, and nitrates are higher than normal in rats with prolonged bleeding time. High systemic NO likely derives from vessels as documented by the increased nitric oxide synthase (NOS) activity and higher expression of both inducible NOS (iNOS) and constitutive NOS (cNOS) in the aorta of uremic animals. Besides its vasoactive properties, NO inhibits platelet aggregation *in vitro* and platelet adhesion to cultured endothelial cells. *In vivo*, a prolongation of skin bleeding time was observed in healthy volunteers given NO by inhalation. The possibility that high systemic NO may play a role in the abnormal primary hemostasis in uremia is supported by the observation that the *N*-monomethyl-L-arginine, a competitive inhibitor of NO synthesis, normalized the prolonged bleeding time in uremic rats. In the same model, the shortening effects of either conjugated estrogens mixture or its active component 17-β estradiol, was abolished by L-arginine administration and was associated with a complete normalization of plasma concentrations of NO metabolites and vascular expression of NO synthase isoenzymes. Experimental data were confirmed in humans. Patients with chronic renal failure (CRF) have a defective platelet aggregation associated with higher-than-normal platelet NO synthesis. In addition, plasma from uremic patients induces NO synthesis in human umbilical vein endothelial cells much more than plasma from healthy subjects. The same results have been recently obtained in cultured human microvascular endothelial cells exposed to uremic plasma. The aforementioned findings suggest that substances accumulate in plasma of uremic patients capable of upregulating vascular NO synthesis. The stimulatory activity was attributed to cytokines, such as tumor necrosis factor-α (TNF-α) and interleukin (IL)-1β, which are potent inducers of the inducible isoform of NO synthase and circulate in increased amounts in the plasma of patients with chronic renal failure or those treated with maintenance hemodialysis.

Two adhesive proteins, fibrinogen and vWF, and two adhesion receptors, the glycoprotein (GP) Ib and the GP IIb–IIIa complex, are thought to play a crucial role in hemostasis by initiating and mediating the formation of platelet thrombi at sites of vascular injury. GP Ib binding to vWF is normal in uremic patients, as well as the surface expression of the receptor. In CRF patients, a decrease in total content of platelet GP Ib has been documented, accompanied by an increase of soluble glycocalicin, a soluble proteolytic fragment of GP Ib, probably due to proteolytic damage to membrane GP Ib. The normal surface expression of this receptor and the total content decrease account for a redistribution from the intraplatelet pool to the surface pool. The activation-dependent receptor function of the GP IIb–IIIa complex is defective in uremia, as shown by decreased binding of both vWF and fibrinogen to stimulated platelets. The number of GP IIb–IIIa receptors expressed on the platelet membrane is normal. Removal of components present in uremic plasma markedly improved the GP IIb–IIIa defect. Altogether these findings suggest that a reversible abnormality of the activation-dependent binding activity of GP IIb–IIIa, likely due to dialyzable toxic substance(s) or due to receptor occupancy by fibrinogen fragments present in uremic plasma, is likely to be a major component of the altered platelet function in uremia.

It is relevant in this context that several dialyzable "toxins," including urea, creatinine, phenol, phenolic acids, and guanidinosuccinic acid, have been considered as possibly being involved in the genesis of uremic platelet dysfunction. Urea infused into healthy volunteers caused headache but did not influence BT. Very high concentration of urea may impair platelet aggregation to a very mild extent. Guanidinosuccinic acid, which accumulates in uremic plasma, inhibits the second wave of platelet aggregation to ADP when added to normal platelet-rich plasma. Platelet aggregation in response to collagen and ADP-induced platelet factor 3 release is also inhibited. These effects can be overcome by raising the ADP and collagen concentrations. Phenolic acid, at the concentrations found in uremic plasma, also impairs kaolin-activated platelet factor 3 release and primary aggregation to ADP. All these observations would suggest that reducing the blood levels of these compounds may correct the abnormal hemostasis of patients with renal failure. However, no correlation has been found between BT or platelet retention on artificial surfaces and the serum level of the dialyzable compounds accumulating in uremia, namely urea, creatinine, uric acid, and phosphorus. Thus the uremic "milieu" probably contributes to bleeding tendency, but some other nondialyzable factors seem to play an equally important role in determining uremic bleeding. Consistent with the preceding interpretation are data that an adequate dialysis program often is not enough to normalize BT and platelet retention nor is uniformly effective in preventing or treating hemorrhages.

Altered Platelet–Vessel Wall Interaction and the Role of Nondialyzable Factors

Increased formation of vascular PGI_2, a potent vasodilator and inhibitor of platelet function, was demonstrated in uremic patients as well as in rats with experimental uremia. Plasma of uremic patients have high vascular PGI_2 stimulant activity. The responsible factor in plasma could be parathyroid hormone (PTH) in view of findings that PTH increases urinary excretion of the PGI_2 metabolite 6-keto $PGF_{1\alpha}$.

Plasma levels of factor VIII/vWF are high in uremia. vWF is required to fully bind platelets to subendothelial collagen and is present in the circulation as multimers of different molecular weight. Multimers are thought to interact with specific thrombocyte receptors and to promote both platelet adhesion and aggregation. It has been suggested that a quantitative and/or qualitative abnormality of the vWF molecule causes an altered platelet–vessel wall interaction that may, in turn, contribute to the hemorrhagic tendency of uremia.

Functional and structural studies of the vWF in uremia have given conflicting results. Some investigators found elevated vWF antigen levels in patients with CRF, but a lower-than-normal ristocetin cofactor activity and suggested that a functional abnormality of vWF was the reason for bleeding in uremia. Additional studies found higher-than-normal levels of vWF functional activity. In only one study was the vWF activity, although above normal, lower than the antigen level. The multimeric structure of vWF has been closely studied too, and no abnormalities have been reported. All these *in vitro* findings apparently do not support the concept that vWF is structurally or functionally abnormal in uremia. Nevertheless, the observation that both cryoprecipitate (a plasma derivative enriched in factor VIII and vWF components) and desmopressin (a synthetic derivative of the antidiuretic hormone that induces autologous vWF release from the storage sites) increase vWF plasma concentration and significantly shorten BT in uremic patients is strongly suggestive of an abnormality in vWF structure or function as the cause of bleeding in these patients. In summary, the present knowledge as a whole suggests that abnormalities in vWF metabolism, structure, and/or function may indeed be important in the bleeding tendency of CRF patients, but the exact nature of the defect has not been fully clarified.

Red blood cells have long been suspected to play a crucial role in platelet–vessel wall interactions. In an *in vitro* system, a rise in the red cell concentration in the flowing blood is accompanied by enhanced platelet adhesion to subendothelium. The red cell per se plays an important role in platelet adhesion and thrombus formation in that its deformability influences the rheology of blood and modifies the transport mechanisms in flowing blood. The possible role of anemia in the bleeding tendency of uremia has been investigated. A significant negative correlation was found between BT and packed cell volume (PCV) in 52 patients receiving chronic hemodialysis. A BT of more than 270 seconds was found in 90% of patients with a PCV of less than 30% but in only 45% of patients with a PCV of more than 30%. In 15 patients with anemia without uremia, a statistically significant negative correlation between the two parameters has also been found, but BT was significantly shorter than in uremic patients. Increasing the PCV over 30% by red cell transfusion in uremic patients is associated with a significant shortening of BT. Also, correction of the anemia with erythropoietin treatment was associated with improvement and/or normalization of BT and platelet aggregation.

THERAPEUTIC STRATEGIES FOR UREMIC BLEEDING

The approach to uremic bleeding must be considered in two contexts: the prevention of bleeding in patients at high risk because of invasive procedures or surgery and the treatment of patients with active bleeding. The strategy depends on the urgency of the situation, the severity of uremia, and the previous therapy used (Table 72.7).

Dialysis

Although some investigators have found that both hemodialysis and peritoneal dialysis partially improve the hemostatic abnormality of uremia, both can potentially produce adverse effects on hemostasis. Peritoneal dialysis has been reported to cause platelet hyperreactivity, which may be related in some cases to the development of hypoalbuminemia. Hemodialysis is often accompanied by transient platelet activation due to interaction of platelets with both dialyzer membranes and the vascular access itself. Dialysis patients have an accelerated platelet turnover, supporting the concept that platelets are chronically activated by dialytic treatment. Repeated platelet activation on dialysis membranes may induce refractoriness to further platelet stimulation, thereby contributing to the clinical bleeding sometimes observed temporally related to the dialysis procedure.

It has been documented that plasma levels of the potent NO inducers TNF-α and IL-1β rise during dialysis; they are generated *in vivo* by circulating monocytes during hemodialysis with complement-activating membranes. Increased cytokines production may also be triggered by intact endotoxin, endotoxin fragments, and other bacterial toxins that may cross the dialysis membranes, and also by acetate-containing dialysate. Apart from the triggering factor, the result of the massive release of cytokines during dialysis is an increase of NO synthesis. Thus it has been found that in a subgroup of uremic patients, NO production

TABLE 72.7. Possible Therapeutic Strategies for Patients with Uremic Bleeding

	Red Blood Cell Transfusions	Recombinant Human Erythropoietin	Cryoprecipitate	Desmopressin	Conjugated Estrogens
Dosage	Depending on the severity of anemia	50 U/kg IV	10 bags	0.3 μg/kg IV or SC 3.0 μg/kg intranasal	3 mg/kg IV in 5 daily infusions
Effect					
Start	Ht = 30%	Ht = 27%–32%	1 hr	1 hr	6 hr
Maximum			4–12 hr	2–4 hr	5–7 days
End	According to RBC life span		24–36 hr	6–8 hr	21–30 days
Indication	Prophylaxis of bleeding in high-risk patients with anemia	Prophylaxis of bleeding in high-risk patients with anemia	Acute, severe bleeding episodes	Acute, severe bleeding episodes	Major surgery or when a long-lasting effect is required

markedly increased during hemodialysis. In addition, it was found that plasma collected after hemodialysis appears to stimulate NO synthesis by cultured endothelial cells more than plasma from the same patients before dialysis. Thus the capability of dialysis procedure to remove uremic toxins is negatively counterbalanced by its effects on platelet activation and NO synthesis.

In addition, heparin may also present a problem. "Regional" heparinization has been used to minimize the effects of systemic anticoagulation, but it is not always practical, and rebound phenomena can cause delayed bleeding. As an alternative, heparin can be administered as to keep constant levels by frequent injections of low-dose heparin during dialysis. Usually, a dose ranging from 40 to 50 IU/kg of heparin at the beginning of hemodialysis is followed after 1 hour by 60% of the initial dose, after 2 hours again by 60% of the initial dose and after 3 hours by 30% of the initial dose. The level of anticoagulation can be monitored by the whole blood activated partial thromboplastin time, which is measured at hourly intervals during dialysis. It is generally believed that the desired level of anticoagulation should prolong whole blood activated partial thromboplastin time to 1.5 to 2 times the basal value.

An interesting approach to the hemodialysis of patients at high risk of bleeding is the use of an ethylene-vinyl alcohol copolymer hollow-fiber dialysis membrane. This membrane does not require systemic anticoagulation with heparin provided that blood flow is greater than 200 ml/min. Double access must be available, with separate needles for arterial and venous return, and blood products must be administered into a different intravenous line. Dialysis with such a membrane has been successfully carried out in patients at high risk for clinical bleeding.

A possibility to prevent systemic anticoagulation is to use hollow-fiber dialyzers and blood tubings coated with covalently bound heparin. The efficacy of this approach is being investigated, and so far, the results have been encouraging. Low-molecular-weight heparin has a more favorable effect than the unfractionated heparin in patients receiving chronic hemodialysis or hemofiltration who are at high risk for bleeding. These data need careful evaluation in controlled clinical trials before low-molecular-weight heparin can be used in routine hemodialysis. As an alternative to heparin, the infusion of dermatan sulfate has been proposed in view of its property to cause less bleeding than heparin in animal models. This may be due to its reduced effect on platelet function. A comparative short-term clinical study has been performed on 10 hemodialysis patients, demonstrating that dermatan sulfate doses can be individually titrated to suppress clot formation during hemodialysis as efficiently as does individualized heparin. However, clinical experience with this agent is limited.

In the search for real alternatives to heparin, antiplatelet drugs such as sulfinpyrazone, adenosine, and PGE_1 have been used for regional infusion during extracorporeal circulation, but they appear to have no advantage over heparin. Aspirin and dipyridamole analogs reduce fibrin and cellular deposition on the filter membrane, but with aspirin, the risk of gastrointestinal bleeding is greatly enhanced. PGI_2 seems to be a very promising alternative to heparin. In animals, PGI_2 has been successfully used to prevent clotting in cardiopulmonary bypass and during hemodialysis. In humans, given as a continuous infusion during the dialysis session at a mean dose of 5 ng/kg per minute, PGI_2 completely inhibited platelet aggregation without causing bleeding. Unfortunately, the use of PGI_2 is associated with serious adverse reactions, such as headache, flushing, tachycardia, and chest and abdominal pain, which require careful hemodynamic monitoring and a physician's supervision. Thus it is advisable to limit the use of PGI_2 to patients at particular risk of hemorrhagic complications.

Red Blood Cell Transfusions and Recombinant Human Erythropoietin

Because there is a close correlation between low PVC and prolonged BT, red cell transfusions have been used in the management of uremic bleeding. Available data indicate that CRF patients with prolonged BT consistently benefited from red cell transfusions. The effect was independent of changes in platelet function tests or in the level of factor VIII-vWF–related properties. A threshold of PVC between 26% and 30% had to be reached for red cell transfusion to be effective in shortening BT.

Similar findings have been reported from several studies in which partial correction of the anemia associated with CRF was accomplished using recombinant human erythropoietin (starting dose of 50 U/kg three times per week). A randomized study established the minimum level of hematocrit necessary to achieve the correction of the prolonged BT of uremic patients with erythropoietin. A threshold of hematocrit between 27% and 32% has to be obtained for BT to become normal. In some studies, it was documented as an increase in platelet adhesion to subendothelium, whereas no consistent changes in platelet number, platelet aggregability, and platelet TXA_2 formation were observed. Other studies showed that the correction of anemia with erythropoietin improved or normalized platelet aggregation. No thromboembolic complications were reported in any of the published studies, but several anecdotal reports have raised the possibility of an increased risk for thromboembolic complications in uremic patients receiving erythropoietin treatment.

Cryoprecipitate and Desmopressin

Cryoprecipitate is a plasma derivative rich in factor VIII and vWF, fibrinogen, and fibronectin that has traditionally been used in the treatment of hemophilia A, von Willebrand's disease, hypofibrinogenemia, and dysfibrinogenemia. The observation that cryoprecipitate shortened the BT of patients with platelet storage pool disease prompted the use of cryoprecipitate in uremic patients with BT of more than 15 minutes. The effect of cryoprecipitate was detectable as early as 1 hour after the infusion, with the maximum effect being obtained between 4 and 12 hours. The BT returned to pretreatment levels by 24 to 36 hours after infusion in all patients. The mechanism of action of cryoprecipitate is unknown. It seems to be unrelated to the protein infusion itself or to changes in platelet aggregation. A small rise in platelet levels of fibrinogen and factor VIII-vWF–related properties was the only change noted after cryoprecipitate infusion. This favorable effect of cryoprecipitate on BT has not been uniformly observed, probably because different preparations of cryoprecipitate were used. On the basis of the available data, it seems that the most effective commercial preparation is that obtainable from the American Red Cross.

The disappointing results with cryoprecipitate and the risk of inducing hepatitis associated with blood product administration prompted a search for therapeutic alternatives. Desmopressin (1-deamino-8-D-arginine vasopressin) is a synthetic derivative of the antidiuretic hormone, which induces the release of autologous vWF from the storage sites. A randomized, double-blind, cross-over trial showed that desmopressin can temporarily correct the prolonged BT in patients with CRF. Desmopressin was given intravenously at a dosage of 0.3 μg/kg body weight in 50 ml of physiologic saline over 30 minutes. The shortening of BT was significant 1 hour after the end of the infusion, and the effect lasted 6 to 8 hours. Subsequently, BT returned to basal values. No appreciable side effects were noted. Desmopressin loses its efficacy when repeatedly administered. This has been ascribed to depletion of vWF storage sites or negative feedback exerted by high circulating vWF levels on further release. An alternative route of desmopressin administration to uremic patients could be the intranasal route, as used in patients with hemophilia or von Willebrand's disease. Intranasal administration is well tolerated and quite safe; 10 to 20 times the intravenous dose is required. Intranasal desmopressin (3 μg/kg) given to uremic patients shortens the prolonged BT and decreases clinical bleeding. No adverse effects on serum sodium or systemic blood pressure are observed. Desmopressin can also be given subcutaneously at the dosages used for the intravenous route. Peak responses are achieved 30 to 90 minutes later than after intravenous injection.

Conjugated Estrogens

One oral dose of 25 mg of conjugated estrogen preparation (Premarin, Ayerst) normalizes BT for 3 to 10 days without apparent clinical side effects. Conjugated estrogens, given intravenously at the cumulative dose of 3 mg/kg divided over 5 consecutive days, shorten BT in uremics, and the hemostatic effect was long-lasting. The administration of estrogens was safe and well tolerated. Moreover, it was found that the estrogen therapeutic activity could not apparently be ascribed to an effect on vWF multimeric structure, platelet aggregation in citrated plasma in response to different stimuli (ADP, arachidonic acid, calcium ionophore A23187), or platelet TXA_2 generation. The minimum dose of estrogen (0.6 mg/kg) able to reduce BT was determined by a subsequent dose–response study. Four or five infusions spaced 24 hours apart were needed to decrease BT by at least 50%. The effect of estrogens on BT in experimental uremia was completely reversed by giving to uremic animals the NO precursor L-arginine, suggesting that the effect of estrogens on primary hemostasis in uremia might be mediated by changes in the NO synthetic pathway. These results suggest that estrogens could offer a good alternative to cryoprecipitate or desmopressin infusions in the treatment of uremic bleeding, especially when a long duration of action is required.

Selected Readings

Aiello S, Noris M, Todeschini M, et al. Renal and systemic nitric oxide synthesis in rats with renal mass reduction. *Kidney Int* 1997;52:171–181.

An excellent study aimed to clarify the pathophysiology of NO synthesis in uremia.

Castaldi PA. Homeostasis and kidney disease. In: Ratnoff OK, Fobes CD, eds. *Disorders of hemostasis*. Orlando, FL: Grune & Stratton, 1984:473–483.

A comprehensive general review of uremic bleeding.

Himmelfarb J, Holbrook D, McMonagle E, et al. Increased reticulated platelets in dialysis patients. *Kidney Int* 1997;51:834–839.

A study demonstrating a marked increase in circulating reticulated platelets in dialysis patients, indicating accelerated platelet turnover, which may contribute to the qualitative platelet dysfunction observed in patients receiving dialysis.

Janson PA, Jubelier SJ, Weinstein MS, et al. Treatment of bleeding tendency in uremia with cryoprecipitate. *N Engl J Med* 1980;303:1318–1322.

A study of the use of cryoprecipitate in the treatment of uremic bleeding, showing a beneficial effect.

Liu KY, Kosfeld RE, Marcum SG. Treatment of uraemic bleeding with conjugated oestrogen. *Lancet* 1984;2:887–890.

The original report of the beneficial effects of estrogen on uremic bleeding diathesis.

Livio M, Benigni A, Remuzzi G. Coagulation abnormalities in uremia. *Semin Nephrol* 1985;5:82–90.

An excellent comprehensive review of the subject of uremic bleeding.

Livio M, Gotti E, Marchesi D, et al. Uraemic bleeding: role of anaemia and beneficial effect of red cell transfusion. *Lancet* 1982;2:1013–1015.

A study of the beneficial effect of blood transfusion on uremic bleeding.

Mannucci PM, Remuzzi G, Pusinieri F, et al. Deamino-8-D-Arginine vasopressin shortens the bleeding time in uremia. *N Engl J Med* 1983;308:8–12.

Demonstration of the beneficial effect of desmopressin on bleeding abnormalities in uremia.

Mezzano D, Tagle R, Panes O, et al. Hemostatic disorder of uremia: the platelet defect, main determinant of the prolonged bleeding time, is correlated with indices of activation of coagulation and fibrinolysis. *Thromb Haemost* 1996;76(3): 312–321.

An excellent and comprehensive study about hemostatic disorder of uremia.

Viganò G, Benigni A, Mendogni D, et al. Recombinant human erythropoietin to correct uremic bleeding. *Am J Kidney Dis* 1991;18:44–49.

A randomized study in 20 patients with anemia and CRF showing that a partial correction of renal anemia (PCV between 27% and 32% to be reached) achieved with erythropoietin treatment is enough to normalize the prolonged bleeding time.

Zusman RM, Rubin RH, Cato AE, et al. Hemodialysis using prostacyclin instead of heparin as the sole antithrombotic agent. *N Engl J Med* 1981;1:934–939.

A study of the usefulness of prostacyclin as an alternative to heparin in hemodialysis.

CHAPTER 73

Gastrointestinal Tract in Uremia

PART 1
Gastrointestinal Abnormalities

Nicholas J. Nickl

The nephrologist and gastroenterologist often collaborate in the treatment of patients who experience concurrent illness involving both organ systems. From an etiologic perspective, gastrointestinal (GI) symptoms or pathology may be associated with renal disease in several ways. The GI tract and the kidney both may be targets of a common independent disease process, as is the case in concomitant diabetic nephropathy and diabetic gastroparesis. The GI tract may be secondarily affected by primary renal disease or its treatment; examples include hepatitis B acquired during dialysis and renal medication side effects such as constipation associated with aluminum-containing antacids. As these examples show, the GI illness in such cases is often not specific to the type of kidney disease but is related to renal dysfunction and its treatment per se. Sometimes, the kidney is a target of primary GI disease or its treatment; the hepatorenal syndrome in chronic liver failure is a good example. Finally, the GI and kidney diseases may represent coexistent but independent illnesses. Regardless of the pattern of causation, concurrent renal and GI disease poses special challenges in patient management because of interdependent factors in these two important organ systems.

From the dialysis patient's perspective, digestive complaints are among the most common symptoms. Nausea or vomiting may occur in three-fourths of patients, abdominal pain or heartburn in half, and diarrhea or constipation in two-thirds. The nephrologist must become adept at dealing with digestive complaints, with or without the assistance of a gastroenterologist, to maintain both excellent patient care and personal sanity.

This overview will travel "downstream" through the GI tract, making a side trip at the pancreas. The liver requires its own discussion, which follows in Part 2 of this chapter. For the most part, the discussion concentrates on pathologic processes; treatment is usually well described elsewhere in the gastroenterology and nephrology literature.

THE UPPER GASTROINTESTINAL TRACT

The Esophagus

Dysgeusia

Dysgeusia (disordered taste, including both diminished taste and taste perversion) has long been reported in renal failure; the symptom does not respond to dialysis, and in some cases, associated food avoidance may lead to protein and calorie malnutrition. Recent studies have linked this symptom with zinc deficiency, a condition often seen in other situations, including aging. Supplementation with oral zinc results in both return of serum zinc levels to normal and improvement in dysgeusia. Nutritional status has also improved in some studies after amelioration of dysgeusia.

Gastroesophageal Reflux Disease

Heartburn and dyspepsia are common complaints among patients with renal disease, and gastroesophageal reflux disease (GERD), along with complications such as hemorrhagic esophagitis, is often reported in uremic patients. This raises the question of whether renal disease is a predisposing factor for GERD. The issue is not as well investigated as is GERD in the general population; older studies in selected populations, such as autopsy series, have suggested a substantially higher prevalence of GERD. However, although some newer endoscopic series have reported esophagitis prevalence rates of approximately 25%, other studies in less highly selected populations have suggested little or no increase in endoscopic GERD among patients with renal failure. Possible pathophysiologic mechanisms for uremia-associated GERD (assuming it exists) include an observed higher prevalence of hiatus hernia among dialysis patients, alterations of GI hormones that influence lower esophageal sphincter tone or control, and abdominal distension among peritoneal dialysis patients. Studies correlating symptoms with endoscopic reflux, or involving ambulatory esophageal pH monitoring, have not been reported. When GERD is present, the bleeding complication rate may be higher if a significant degree of coagulopathy is present as a result of concomitant renal failure or dialysis, but this question has also not been well studied.

Infectious Esophagitis

Infectious esophagitis appears to have a higher incidence among renal failure patients if there is a concurrent immunocompromised state. *Candida* esophagitis, sometimes but not always associated with oral thrush, is often observed and has been reported with catastrophic upper GI hemorrhage. Viral esophagitis, associated with herpes simplex virus (HSV) or cytomegalovirus (CMV), is more common in renal transplant patients but is also sometimes seen in dialysis patients. Herpetic esophagitis is more common than CMV, and the presence or absence of herpetic stomatitis is not a reliable marker of HSV esophagitis.

Esophageal Motility

Subtle disorders of esophageal motility have been reported in a few small series of dialysis patients, primarily contraction abnormalities. Importantly, such studies have documented preservation of the reflux barrier of lower esophageal sphincter function. Although early reports suggested a higher incidence of major motility disorders such as achalasia in this population, current thinking is that subtle variations in motility, if present, are unlikely to produce symptoms.

The Stomach

Gastritis

Upper digestive symptoms, such as nausea, vomiting, anorexia, and dyspepsia, are common among patients with end-stage kidney disease, particularly those with clinical uremia. Such complaints often lead to endoscopy, at which time, gastritis is a common finding, including acute gastritis, chronic gastritis, atrophic gastritis, and intestinal metaplasia. Interestingly, the endoscopic appearance of gastritis correlates poorly with histologic findings; this has led some to advocate that endoscopy in this setting should always include biopsies regardless of the mucosal appearance. Balancing this perspective, however, is the observation that histologic abnormalities and symptoms correlate poorly. Often, digestive symptoms improve in uremic patients after correction of fluid and electrolyte imbalances or initiation of symptomatic treatment, but no change is seen in the gastritis. Confusing the picture still further is the known association of both atrophic and chronic gastritis with *Helicobacter pylori* colonization, an association that holds true in uremic patients: most of those with gastritis show evidence of *H. pylori* infection. However, several studies have shown that there is no increased incidence of *H. pylori* infection among chronic dialysis patients when compared either with patients with other chronic illness or with controls who do not have chronic illness. Nevertheless, eradication of *H. pylori* is effective in reversing gastritis, an observation that remains true among patients with chronic renal disease.

All this may lead to uncertainty about whether "uremic gastritis" exists. Reports from the predialysis era of severe gastric pathology among patients with untreated uremia are of uncertain relevance in understanding contemporary gastritis. In many renal disease patients with gastritis, recognized causes can be found, such as *H. pylori* infection or ulcerogenic drug use. However, there remains a group of renal disease patients with otherwise unexplained gastritis. One suggestion is that alterations in mucosal perfusion during dialysis may lead to ischemia, causing a kind of gastritis. Others have invoked coagulopathy as an important factor. Much work remains to be done to understand the epidemiology and pathophysiology of this condition.

Serum Gastrin

Elevated serum gastrin levels are observed in about half of renal failure patients; although decreased renal catabolism of gastrin has a role to play in this process, newer investigations have also linked this finding with chronic *H. pylori* infection and its associated gastric hypochlorhydria. This line of reasoning is supported by the epidemiologic association of hypergastrinemia with *H. pylori* infection, as well as the observation of an inverse correlation between serum gastrin level and gastric acid output. More importantly, eradication of *H. pylori* by appropriate antibiotic regimens has been reported to result in improvement of serum gastrin levels to normal in many cases; gastric acid production likewise often returns to normal. Some studies have also reported that *H. pylori* eradication causes improvement of nonspecific symptoms such as nausea or dyspepsia, even in the absence of a proven peptic ulcer. However, this finding is much less well documented, and controversy continues to surround this issue.

Peptic Ulcer Disease

Some earlier reports had suggested that dialysis patients have a greater prevalence of peptic ulcer disease. Such reports used radiographic methods; newer endoscopic studies have failed to demonstrate a higher incidence of peptic ulcer disease among dialysis patients. The exception may be patients with acute renal failure associated with acute tubular necrosis; gastric ulcers are common in such patients and may be linked in many to the underlying pathologic condition that caused the acute tubular necrosis (e.g., hypotension). When peptic ulceration is found in renal patients, the usual causes should be sought, including ulcerogenic drugs, tobacco use, and *H. pylori* infection.

Although the prevalence of peptic ulcers is not higher among dialysis patients, the rate of bleeding complications is higher; this may be related in part to coagulopathy, which is often present among patients with renal disease. Upper GI hemorrhage from all causes is a common source of morbidity and mortality among this group. When bleeding occurs, the mortality is twofold to threefold higher among patients with renal disease. The worst outcomes are seen among patients with GI hemorrhage and acute renal failure; in this group, mortality may exceed 60%.

Arteriovenous Malformations

Arteriovenous malformations (AVMs) are also a common cause of upper GI hemorrhage among renal failure patients, accounting for more than 10% of bleeding cases and in some reports more than 30%. These are particularly troublesome lesions: GI AVMs may be as much as 10-fold more common among dialysis patients and, when present, appear to bleed more commonly in such patients. They are difficult to find, may be distributed throughout the GI tract (including areas not accessible by endoscope), and often respond poorly to endoscopic treatment. Both acute high volume bleeding and slow chronic GI blood loss may be seen with this condition. Again, the greater risk of bleeding may relate in part to concomitant coagulopathy.

Gastroparesis

Gastroparesis is a common source of symptoms in dialysis patients. Undoubtedly, the most common cause of gastric dysmotility associated with renal failure is diabetes. Studies of gastric emptying in renal disease that exclude diabetic patients have shown mixed results, with delayed, normal, and accelerated emptying all being reported. Moreover, as is the case with other causes of gastric dysmotility, symptoms correlate poorly with the results of motility testing. The complex effects of sympathetic and parasympathetic neuropathy and changing balances in renal failure of GI hormones affecting motility such as gastrin, CCK, and secretin may all combine to create alterations in gastric emptying; all authorities agree that much work remains to be done in this area.

The Pancreas

Pancreatic Enzymes

Alterations of serum pancreatic enzyme levels in patients with renal failure raises considerable confusion when pancreatic disease is being considered. Serum amylase levels are above the upper limit of normal in up to three-fourths of hemodialysis patients without overt pancreatic disease, and both pancreatic isoamylase and lipase levels are elevated in one-fourth to half of such patients. Amylase elevation correlates in some studies with glomerular filtration rate (GFR), while it has been speculated that the elevated serum lipase levels are partially related to heparin-induced lipoprotein lipase stimulation associated with hemodialysis. Elevated lipase levels have also been observed in patients receiving continuous ambulatory peritoneal dialysis. Serum amylase and lipase levels more than three times the upper limit of normal are uncommon in hemodialysis patients without pancreatic disease, and this has been suggested as a threshold value for the diagnosis of pancreatic disease; pancreatic isoamylase and prehemodialysis lipase levels may be more sensitive than total amylase or random lipase in this respect. Other serum pancreatic enzyme levels as well as urinary clearance levels (in nonanuric renal failure patients) have also been examined, but none offer consistently superior performance in identifying the presence of pancreatic disease in this group.

Pancreatic Histology

Autopsy studies of patients receiving chronic dialysis show changes in pancreatic histology, including interstitial and periductal fibrosis, acinar dilation, and ductectasia. These findings exist in more than half of patients and have been observed in both hemodialysis and peritoneal dialysis patients. The mechanism is not understood; it has been thought to be related to chronic or intermittent uremia, but newer work has suggested that chronic hyperstimulation by elevated GI hormone levels such as cholecystokinin may be an important factor. This theory is supported by observed changes in alterations of trypsin and lipase in pancreatic juice, which are consistent with a chronically stimulated state. Whether these histologic changes have a clinical correlate is unclear. Studies examining pancreatic imaging (e.g., by transabdominal ultrasound) do not demonstrate consistent changes compared with controls. Similarly, there is not a clear increase in the prevalence or incidence of either acute or chronic clinical pancreatitis among renal failure patients, although this observation may be obscured by chronic elevations of serum pancreatic enzyme levels seen in renal failure. On the other hand, pancreatic exocrine insufficiency has been found in some otherwise asymptomatic renal failure patients and has been linked with adverse nutritional status.

THE LOWER GASTROINTESTINAL TRACT

The Small Intestine

Intestinal Absorption

Considerable attention has been paid to intestinal absorption of minerals in renal failure, particularly calcium and phosphate, but less is known about other aspects of small bowel absorptive function in renal disease. Detailed discussions of intestinal absorption of calcium and phosphate in uremia are provided in Chapters 18, Part 1, and 19, Part 1, respectively. Bacterial overgrowth, with levels comparable to those seen in blind loop syndromes, has been reported and may cause nutritional malabsorption. As noted earlier, absorptive function may also be impaired in renal failure by pancreatic exocrine insufficiency. Alterations of small bowel disaccharidase activity has been investigated in chronic renal failure and appears not to be more common than in the general population. Iron absorption appears to be normal.

Small Bowel Anatomy

Small bowel anatomy and histology do not appear to be altered by chronic renal disease. An exception is the unusual condition of duodenal pseudomelanosis, which consists of a blackened endoscopic appearance of the duodenum caused by pigment-laden macrophages. It has been reported in patients with renal failure and also among patients with conditions associated with renal failure, such as hypertension and diabetes mellitus. The condition is of unknown clinical significance but presents a striking endoscopic appearance. Also, there is reduction in the villus height, increased crypt depth, and increased number of inflammatory cells. Deficiency in $1,25(OH)_2D_3$ may be at least partly responsible. Indeed, administration of $1,25(OH)_2D_3$ caused reversal of these abnormalities.

The Colon

Constipation

Undoubtedly, the most common colonic symptom among patients with renal failure is constipation, usually related to phosphate-binding antacids containing aluminum. A sustained medication regimen is important among such patients to maintain regular bowel habits; usually, a combination regimen includes a bulk agent such as psyllium along with a nonabsorbable sugar such as sorbitol or lactulose. Regular use of anthraquinone or phenolphthalein laxatives must be avoided because habituation and tolerance rapidly develop.

Bleeding

As is the case in the upper GI tract, lower GI bleeding is more often associated with AVMs in patients with renal disease and may cause either overt or occult bleeding. Some have speculated that hemodynamic alterations accompanying dialysis are responsible for the formation of these minute vascular lesions; however, because they also occur in patients receiving peritoneal dialysis, other factors are likely to be operative. Diverticulosis may also be a source of rapid painless lower GI hemorrhage as well as diverticulitis; colonic diverticula are associated with polycystic kidney disease. Positive occult blood in uremic patients was thought to be due to the bleeding abnormalities of uremia. Newer studies showed positive occult blood in well-dialyzed patients is most likely associated with an organic lesion. In contrast, in uremic patients who are not treated with dialysis, such a likelihood is significantly less. Therefore a positive occult blood in dialysis patients requires a GI workup.

Intestinal Infarction

The catastrophic complication of intestinal infarction has been observed in both hemodialysis and peritoneal dialysis patients. Concomitant atherosclerotic disease is often present, but nonocclusive intestinal ischemia is identified in up to half of such patients. In nonocclusive ischemia, antecedent hypotension or low flow states are often present, and pathology in such cases demonstrates submucosal small vessel congestion with nonoccluded mesenteric vessels. Watershed circulation zones such as the descending colon are often the site of ischemia. Although early diagnosis is critical to a favorable outcome, several authors have emphasized that the presentation may be confusing, particularly among peritoneal dialysis patients in whom peritoneal signs may be attributed to dialysate contamination.

Obstructive Uropathy

Obstructive uropathy has been reported in conjunction with Crohn's disease, usually associated with inflammatory masses. Other inflammatory masses of GI origin reported to cause obstructive uropathy include diverticulitis and pancreatitis.

Selected Readings

Chalasani N, Cotsonis G, Wilcox CM. Upper gastrointestinal bleeding in patients with chronic renal failure: role of vascular ectasia. *Am J Gastroenterol* 1996;91: 2329–2332.

This study highlights the prominent role of AVMs in upper GI hemorrhage among renal failure patients and comments on current controversies in this condition.

Etemad B. Gastrointestinal complications of renal failure. *Gastroenterol Clin North Am* 1998;27:875–892.

This is an excellent general review of the topic, including both basic and clinical discussions. There is a particular focus on the upper GI tract.

Gladziwa U, Koltz U. Pharmacokinetic optimisation of the treatment of peptic ulcer in patients with renal failure. *Clin Pharmacokinet* 1994;27:393–408.

The authors review the pharmacologic treatment of acid peptic disease in patients with renal failure, including adjustment of dosage requirements for H_2-receptor antagonists, proton pump inhibitors, and other commonly used agents.

Pardi DS, Tremaine WJ, Sandborn WJ, et al. Renal and urologic complications of inflammatory bowel disease. *Am J Gastroenterol* 1998;93:504–514.

This article provides a thorough review of nephrologic complications of inflammatory bowel diseases, including a discussion of appropriate preventive measures.

PART 2
Hepatitis and the Renal Patient

Laurence Chan, Stephen K.L. Mo, and Wei Wang

Patients with end-stage renal disease (ESRD) may have acute or chronic hepatitis, and the types of hepatitis that are caused by several of the hepatitis viruses could be transmitted to other patients, as well as to the staff of the dialysis unit. Furthermore, hepatic enzymes abnormalities and hepatitis are commonly seen in the ESRD population during pretransplant evaluation. Serologic evaluation for multiple etiologic viruses is obtained in all patients with persistent increased in serum transaminase, and screening for hepatitis B and C is routine.

Classic acute viral hepatitis is caused by one of six etiologic agents: hepatitis A virus (HAV), hepatitis B virus (HBV), hepatitis C virus (HCV), hepatitis D virus (HDV), hepatitis E virus (HEV), or hepatitis G virus (HGV). The history of the various types of the hepatitis viruses is given in Table 73.1. All six viruses can cause acute hepatitis, but only four—HBV, HCV, HDV, and HGV—can lead to chronic infection. A number of viruses that cause systemic illnesses may also affect the liver. These viruses include cytomegalovirus and Epstein-Barr virus. In addition, hepatitis syndromes can be caused by certain drugs and toxins. In the United States, approximately 50% of reported cases of acute viral hepatitis in adults are classified as HBV infection, 30% as HAV infection, and 20% as HCV infection. HDV infection (delta hepatitis) occurs either as a superinfection in chronic HBV carriers or as a coinfection during acute HBV infection. The purpose of this chapter is to give an overview of hepatitis in the context of patients with ESRD. In addition to brief descriptions of etiology and differential diagnoses, strategies are described for the prevention and control of viral hepatitis.

TABLE 73.1. History of the Various Types of Hepatitis Virus

1973	Identification of hepatitis A virus, antigen, and antibody
1978	Enzyme-linked immunosorbent assay for anti-HAV
1983	Molecular cloning of HAV cDNA
1992	Description of inactivated hepatitis A vaccine
1965	Discovery of HBsAg, anti-HBs
1970	Radioimmunoassay for HBsAg
1971	Development of hepatitis B immunoglobulin
1972	Identification of HBeAg, anti-HBe
1979	Cloning of HBV DNA
1980	Establishment of efficacy of HBV vaccine in humans
1984	Recombinant HBV vaccine
1989	Identification of HCV genome
1989	First assay for anti-HCV
1990	Detection of HCV genome by polymerase chain reaction
1977	Identification of delta antigen and antibody
1980	Radioimmunoassay for detection of delta antigen and antibody
1982	Effect of acute HDV infection on severity of acute hepatitis B
1986	Cloning of cDNA fragment of delta RNA genome
1989	Agent named hepatitis E virus
1990	HEV cloned by recombinant DNA techniques
1991	Diagnostic tests for HEV
1995	Hepatitis GB virus C cloned
1996	Hepatitis G virus cloned

HAV, hepatitis A virus; HBV, hepatitis B virus; HCV, hepatitis C virus; HDV, hepatitis D virus; HEV, hepatitis E virus.

DIFFERENTIAL DIAGNOSIS

Patients with ESRD who initially have symptoms of hepatitis that include anorexia, fatigue, arthralgias with or without jaundice, and elevated blood levels of transaminases need to clearly have the cause of the disease determined. In the case of viral hepatitis, there may be a necessity for certain infection control strategies to prevent transmission of infection to other patients and to dialysis staff members. It is important to note that some renal patients who are infected with hepatitis viruses have no signs or symptoms of hepatitis. Although hepatitis is generally characterized by biochemical evidence of elevated aminotransferase levels or histologic evidence of liver inflammation, these two features may not necessarily occur together. For example, chronic hepatitis patients sometimes have normal or fluctuating liver enzymes.

Among the many different causes of hepatitis, viral etiology remains the most important in long-term dialysis patients. Nevertheless, other nonviral and potentially treatable causes such as drug-induced hepatitis and autoimmune hepatitis should be borne in mind. The clinical course of hepatitis in dialysis patients may be different from that in the normal population. Aminotransferase levels also tend to be lower in patients with renal failure, which may pose diagnostic problems.

Viral Hepatitis

The agents of viral hepatitis A to E account for 90% of posttransfusion and community-acquired hepatitis cases. The existence of other infectious etiologic factors is presumed.

Hepatitis A

The hepatitis A virus is a picornavirus with a single molecule of RNA surrounded by a small 27-nm diameter protein capsid.

About 100,000 to 200,000 Americans contract hepatitis A each year. There is only one serotype but at least seven genotypes. It is highly contagious, with worldwide distribution. Transmission is by the fecal–oral route. Parenteral transmission is very rare, probably because of the very short viremic phase. Hepatitis A infections occur in both epidemic and sporadic fashions. The incubation period is from 2 to 6 weeks, with a mean of 30 days. This depends on the number of infectious particles consumed. The period of infectivity extends from early incubation period to about 1 week after the development of jaundice. Highest infectivity is in the middle of incubation period well before the onset of symptoms. Clinical features include fever, malaise, anorexia, nausea, abdominal discomfort, and jaundice. Fulminant hepatitis can occur. Many infections do not result in clinical disease, particularly in children. Fewer than 0.4% of reported cases in the United States are fatal, usually in the elderly. Acute infection always resolves with no carrier state. Anti-HAV induced by infection or vaccination protects against infection or reinfection.

Diagnosis is by finding IgM anti-HAV during acute or early convalescent phase. This antibody arises early and is almost invariably present when the patient first presents. It disappears within 6 to 12 months. Serologic studies in 15 dialysis centers in the United States showed similar prevalence in patients and staff compared with the general population. Hepatitis A is not a recognized problem in dialysis units.

Renal patients who travel to endemic areas may ask about prevention. Hepatitis A vaccine or immune globulin is recommended for susceptible travelers. Two types of hepatitis A vaccines are licensed in the United States: HAVRIX and VAQTA. Both are inactivated vaccines adsorbed to aluminum hydroxide as adjuvants. The efficacy rate is near 90% in the normal population. Patients at risk who travel less than 4 weeks after initial dose of vaccine should be given immune globulin.

Immunity increases with age. In the United States, it is 10% in those aged 18 to 19 and 65% if older than 50. As standard of hygiene and sanitation improves the age at exposure increases. Adults are increasingly susceptible to clinical attacks.

Hepatitis B

The hepatitis B virus is a double-stranded DNA virus in the Hepadnaviridae family. In the United States, about 100,000 to 300,000 new cases of HBV infection occur yearly, and there are 1 to 1.25 million chronic infected patients. From 5% to 10% become chronic carriers, and 25% of carriers develop chronic active hepatitis. Cirrhosis and liver failure develop in 3,000 to 4,000, while 1,000 to 1,500 deaths due to HBV-related liver cancer occur annually. Transmission of HBV is by parenteral, mucosal, sexual, and vertical routes. The virus is found in all body fluids except stool. HBeAg positivity increases infectivity and is associated with the presence of other markers of replication such as HBV DNA. In about 30% of patients, no risk factors can be identified.

HBsAg is detectable several weeks after acute infection (Fig. 73.1.). The antigen has several subtypes—a, d/y, w/r of epidemiologic interest. HBcAg, a part of the nucleoprotein center, is not detectable in blood. HBeAg also develops early following HBsAg. It disappears soon in self-limited disease but persists for years in chronic carriers before eventual disappearance in the majority of patients. IgM anti-HBc is positive in the early and window phase but negative in late convalescence. Its level may also increase during exacerbation of chronic hepatitis B infection. IgG anti-HBc lasts for years whether or not HBV infection clears. Anti-HBs is a convalescent phenomenon and confers protective immunity. HBsAg becomes undetectable as

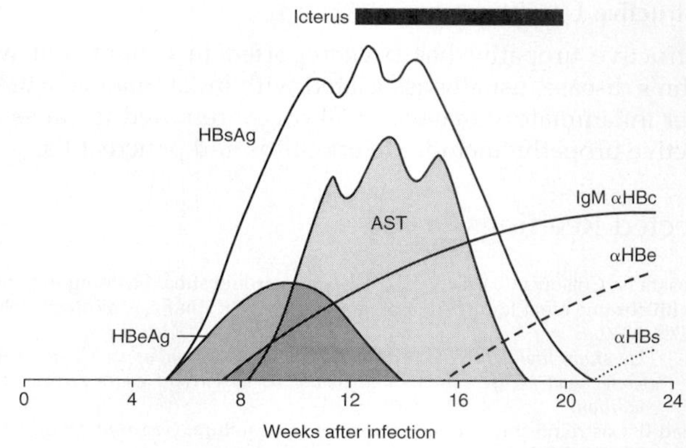

Figure 73.1. The course of acute type B hepatitis. AST, aspartate transaminase; αHbe, antibody against hepatitis e antigen; αHBs, antibody against hepatitis B surface antigen; HbeAg, hepatitis Be antigen; HbsAg, hepatitis B surface antigen; IgM αHbc, IgM antibody against hepatitis B core antigen.

acute infection resolves. Immunoassay for detecting HBsAg has sensitivity and specificity of more than 98%.

Chronic infection can be either replicative or nonreplicative. In the replicative state, HBeAg is positive and the HBV DNA level is high. Progression to cirrhosis and hepatocellular carcinoma is more likely. Most chronic cases will become nonreplicative with time and lose serum HBeAg and develop anti-HBe. The HBV DNA level will become low. However, the two states can switch in an individual. In rare strains with mutation of precore gene, replicative state can be HBeAg negative. HBV replication and viral gene expression are not directly cytopathic. Pathogenesis is predominantly immune mediated. Factors determining individual clinical course of HBV infection are not clearly defined.

Hepatitis B is a major problem in dialysis centers. In dialysis units, HBsAg carrier rates and overall exposure to HBV are substantially higher than those in the general population. Hemodialysis patients follow a different course than normal individuals after HBV infection. They have a greater tendency to develop initially asymptomatic but chronic HBV infection. This is likely due to depressed cell-mediated immunity. From 60% to 80% fail to clear the acute infection, compared with 5% to 10% in the general population and dialysis staff. Chronicity occurs more often after a mild anicteric attack than an icteric or fulminant course. More than one-third of HBV carrier hemodialysis patients have chronic elevations in aminotransferases. However, the overall survival of HBsAg-positive dialysis patients does not differ from their noncarrier counterparts. This may be due to death from other causes that precede the progression of liver disease. End-stage liver disease is not common, and fewer than 10% of liver biopsies in HBsAg-positive hemodialysis patients show cirrhosis. Most chronic carriers have no inflammation on liver biopsy.

Dialysis staff are at high risk of HBV infection because of exposure to patients and their body fluids. Conversely, transmission of hepatitis B from carrier health care workers to patients has been reported, but only infrequently. Prospective studies, however, failed to demonstrate HBV transmission from staff to patients. HBsAg carrier state is not a contraindication to employment in dialysis units. Prevention and education about potential mechanisms of transmission are of utmost importance.

CDC Recommendations. In 1977, the Center for Disease Control and Prevention (CDC) issued recommendations for controlling the spread of HBV in dialysis units. In essence, HBsAg-positive hemodialysis patients are dialyzed in isolated areas with dedicated machines. Regular serologic screening of staff and patients are performed. Routine cleaning and disinfection procedures are emphasized. There has been a significant decline in HBsAg seropositivity among dialysis patients and staff since then. In patients, HBsAg seropositivity was 3% in 1976, 0.5% in 1982, and 0.1% in 1989. In staff, corresponding figures were 2.6%, 0.5%, and 0.1%. The major decline in HBV transmission rate preceded the widespread availability of HBV vaccines.

Prophylaxis. The plasma-derived HBV vaccine was introduced in 1982. It is no longer distributed in the United States. Currently, two types of recombinant HBV vaccines are licensed in the United States: Engerix-B and Recombivax HB. The usual recommended dose in dialysis patients is twice the normal amount. Three doses are given at 0, 1, and 6 months. Four-dose series at 0, 1, 2, and 12 months was approved for Engerix-B vaccine. In hemodialysis patients, however, the fourth dose can be given at 6 months after the first dose instead of 12 months. Both three- and four-dose regimens confer the same level of immunity. For hemodialysis patients, 1 ml of special formulation of Recombivax HB containing 40 μg or two 1-ml doses of Engerix B is injected intramuscularly into the deltoid muscle. HBV vaccines can be given at the same time, but at a different site, with HBIG and other vaccines. Side effects are mild and include local pain and low-grade fever in 1% to 6% of patients. Guillain-Barré syndrome was reported at 0.5 per 100,000 for plasma-derived vaccine but was not associated with recombinant vaccines. For optimal potency, HBV vaccine should be stored at 2° to 8°C (36° to 46°F) but not frozen. Seroconversion occurs in 90% of healthy individuals and in 99% of those 2 to 19 years old. The seroconversion rate is lower in dialysis patients, and rates around 30% to 80% have been reported. The level of anti-HBs is 20-fold higher in staff than in patient responders. Younger patients and females show better response. Inclusion in the vaccine of a more extended portion of HBV genome containing pre-S2 may increase response rate. Revaccination with one or more additional doses can be given for inadequate initial responses. Vaccination before advanced chronic renal failure has also been recommended to improve effectiveness. Routine testing for anti-HBs and booster vaccination if the antibody level falls below 10 mIU/ml, the level considered as protective, are recommended for hemodialysis patients. Cases of acute HBV developing in hemodialysis patients who previously had protective anti-HBs levels have been reported. In the normal population, protection appears to be of long duration even if antibody levels decline or become undetectable, which occurs in up to 50% of patients. All susceptible dialysis patients and staff should be vaccinated. Following percutaneous or mucosal exposure, HBIG should be administered as soon as possible and within 14 days, but effectiveness is uncertain after 7 days or more. A dose of 0.06 ml/kg is given intramuscularly, preferably in deltoid muscle. It is 75% effective. HBIG should be followed by the usual HBV vaccination in HBsAg-negative individuals. The risk of acquiring HBV in hemodialysis units has practically disappeared after implementation of various preventive measures, including screening of blood products for HBV, isolation of HBsAg-positive patients, and vaccination policies.

Treatment. At present, interferon alpha is the only drug approved in the United States for treatment of chronic hepatitis B. Interferon is recommended for replicative disease with HBeAg and HBV DNA positivity, elevated aminotransferases, and chronic hepatitis on liver biopsy. It is usually given for 3 to 6 months. Responders will lose serum HBeAg, followed by HBsAg in some. Patients who lose HBsAg may have undetectable HBV DNA in serum. Sustained response is associated with a decrease in inflammatory activity in liver biopsies and normalization in aminotransferase levels. It is effective in fewer than 40% patients, must be given by injection, and has dose-limiting side effects. To increase response rate, various methods have been attempted, such as prednisone priming. Results are not yet conclusive.

Nucleoside analogs provide a promising alternative approach. Lamivudine is an oral 2′3′-dideoxynucleoside. It interferes with reverse-transcriptase activity of HBV and inhibits viral DNA synthesis. At concentrations that block HBV DNA synthesis, lamivudine does not inhibit mitochondrial DNA or marrow progenitor cells. This accounts for the low toxicity. Side effects are mild, and the drug is well tolerated. Suppression of HBV DNA is dose dependent. Sustained suppression is associated with sustained normalization of plasma alanine aminotransferase (ALT) levels. It is also effective in patients unresponsive to interferon, including those with high HBV DNA levels and normal ALT levels. Doses above 100 mg result in almost complete suppression of HBV DNA. However, rebound occurs in most patients after treatment is stopped and HBV DNA returns to pretreatment levels. The aim of treatment in HBsAg carriers is permanent viral suppression. This may reduce immunologic damage to the liver and retards progression to cirrhosis and hepatocellular carcinoma. To achieve this, lamivudine may have to be administered on a long-term basis. This is feasible in view of its oral administration and low side effect profile. However, possibility of escape mutations emergence with prolonged treatment exists and is being studied in trials of longer duration. Whether permanent HBV DNA suppression can be achieved by long-term treatment awaits further trials. Although interferon use in renal transplant patients is associated with increased rejection, lamivudine use in HBV DNA–positive transplant patients has no significant adverse effects, including renal function deterioration.

Penciclovir is a deoxyguanosine analog. Famciclovir is the oral form of penciclovir and is well absorbed orally. Bioavailability is 77%, with a prolonged intracellular half-life of 9 to 10 hours. Intracellular formation of penciclovir triphosphate inhibits HBV replication by interfering with viral DNA polymerase activity. A much higher concentration is required to inhibit host DNA polymerase. The affinity for viral polymerase is 4,000-fold higher. It suppresses HBV DNA and is well tolerated with long-term treatment. In liver transplant HBV reinfections, famciclovir 500 mg three times per day suppresses HBV DNA, with a concomitant decrease in aminotransferase levels. Results of an integrated safety analysis of 13 completed clinical studies showed no differences in hematology parameters, renal and liver functions, muscle and bone metabolism, glucose levels, and urinalysis compared with placebo group.

Hepatitis C

HCV is a linear, single-stranded, positive polarity, 9,400 nucleotide RNA virus encoding a polyprotein of approximately 3,000 amino acids (Fig. 73.2). The 5′ end of the genome consists of an untranslated region adjacent to the genes for structural proteins, the nucleocapsid core, and the viral envelope. The 5′ untranslated and core genes are highly conserved among genotypes. The envelope proteins, coded for by the hypervariable region, varies among isolates and even within the same agent isolated over time from the same patient. This allows the virus to evade host immunologic mechanisms directed at virus-envelope

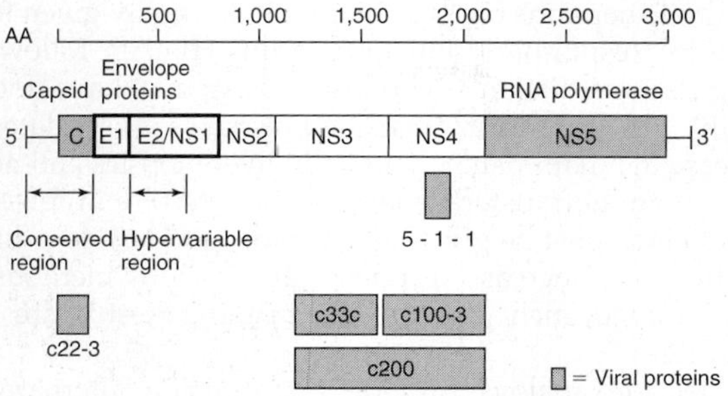

Figure 73.2. Structural genes at the 5′ end include the nucleocapsid region, C, and the envelope regions, E1 and E2. The 5′ untranslated region and the C region are highly conserved among isolates, while the envelope domain E2/NS1 contains the hypervariable region. At the 3′ end are five nonstructural (NS) regions. Viral proteins included in the first-generation (c100-3) and second-generation (c200, a fusion protein of c100-3 and c33c, and c22-3) immunoassays and in the recombinant immunoblot assay (5-1-1, c100-3, c33c, c22-3) are presented below their corresponding genes. AA, amino acid.

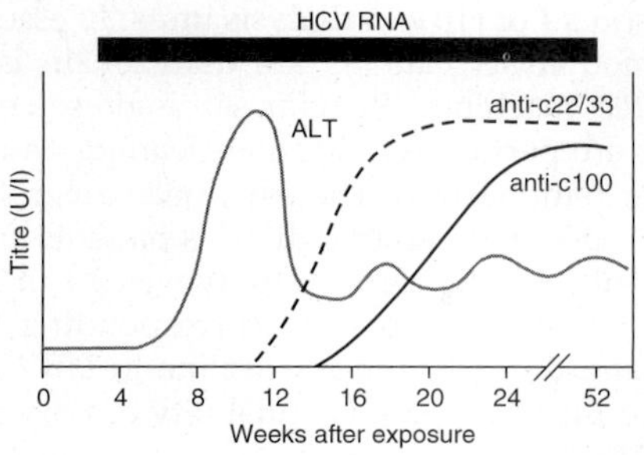

Figure 73.3. The serologic course of chronic hepatitis C infection. Note that HCV RNA appears early, before the rise in alanine transferase (ALT), and persists. Anti-c22/33 appears at 12 weeks and anti–HCV-100 only appears about 20 weeks after exposure.

proteins. The 3′ end of the genome contains the genes for nonstructural (NS) proteins 1 through 5. The original clone, 5-1-1, and the nucleotide sequence coding for C100-3 reside within the NS4 gene.

Hepatitis C was found to be responsible for 80% to 90% of cases of non-A non-B hepatitis. About 4 million people in the United States are infected. Currently, around 30,000 acute new infections occur yearly. It is primarily transmitted by blood and blood products or via intravenous drug use. Perinatal transmission is relatively low (below 6% to 10%) but possible. Many of those infected have no obvious risk factors. The incubation period is 5 to 12 weeks. Only 25% to 35% have symptoms such as anorexia, malaise, or jaundice. Most acute infections are clinically silent, but rarely, it can cause liver failure. Of infected patients, 85% fail to clear the virus in 6 months and become chronic. Recovery is characterized by disappearance of HCV RNA from the blood and normalization of liver function. Approximately 25% of chronic cases will progress to cirrhosis, and 1% to 4% of cirrhotic patients develop hepatocellular carcinoma annually. HCV infection is the leading cause of liver transplant in the United States. The hepatitic C antibody–positive patient is at risk for progression to end-stage liver disease, but interpretation of the antibody test must be considered in light of the sensitivity and specificity of the test.

Diagnostic Testing of HCV. The screening tests marketed by Ortho Diagnostic System and Abbot Laboratory use material derived from the original Chiron Corporation isolate. Other manufacturers in Europe and North America have independently cloned HCV genomes and marketed screening and supplementary tests. The various available tests for the screening of HCV antibodies include ELISA-I, ELISA II, recombinant immunoblot assay (RIBA), and HCV RNA, which detects the presence of the virus.

In some cases, anti-HCV antibodies can be present immediately after transfusion due to passive transfer from the donor. This antibody disappears over the next few weeks in keeping with the half-life of IgG. Anti-HCV antibodies will then reappear if the patient becomes infected. ELISA-I is the first-generation assay introduced, which detected antibodies to C100-3, which is a recombinant polypeptide derived from the NS4 region of the genome. This assay detects anti-HCV antibodies between 4 to 6 months and even 1 year after HCV infection. ELISA-II is the second-generation assay and incorporates C22-3, 5-1-1, C33c (expressed in combination with C100-3 as C200). It is more sensitive (by approximately 20%) and detects anti-HCV 30 to 90 days earlier, during the period of acute hepatitis. From 70% to 95% of ELISA-II–positive patients have detectable HCV RNA. RIBAs serve as more specific supplementary tests. RIBA-2 contains the same antigens as in ELISA-II in immunoblot format and detects individual antibodies to nonstructural and structural viral proteins. Third-generation assays for anti-HCV are now available. Both ELISA-III and RIBA-3 assays incorporate more immunogenic epitopes and additional antigens encoded by the NS5 region. It remains to be proven whether third-generation assays for anti-HCV are more sensitive and specific than second-generation assays. Still, detection of anti-HCV is insufficient to identify all persons infected with HCV.

The most sensitive indicator is the presence of HCV RNA, which requires molecular amplification by polymerase chain reaction or the newer branched chain DNA (bDNA) signal amplification assay, which provides a direct measure of viral load. HCV RNA can be detected 1 to 3 weeks after exposure to HCV, well before the appearance of anti-HCV antibodies, and tends to persist for the duration of HCV infection. The serologic course of chronic hepatitis C infection is shown in Fig. 73.3.

Variability in the HCV Genome. HCV genome is substantially more variable than other hepatitis viruses. The nucleotide sequences of HCV variants worldwide show considerable diversity. Six major genotypes and more than 40 different subtypes have been identified. Individual genotypes may be limited to a particular geographic area or more widespread. Coinfection with different HCV genotypes has been demonstrated. Antigenic variation of HCV can also occur within a genotype. *Quasispecies* refers to the genetic heterogeneity of the population of HCV genomes coexisting in a single infected individual. High replicative activity (10^{10} to 10^{11} viral particles are produced daily) and lack of proofreading function of viral RNA-dependent RNA polymerase explains in part the rapid emergence of viral variants. These genotypic variations may lead to false-negative test results for host antibody to HCV or viral RNA by means of polymerase chain reaction (PCR) assays, in which the primers and probes used may fail to recognize the nucleotide sequences of the particular isolate. This genomic variability may also account for the lack of immunity against reinfection in naturally acquired HCV infection, high rate of chronicity, and multiple infection with different HCV strains. These characteristics may impede HCV vaccine development and influence responsiveness of HCV infection to preventive measures and to therapy. For example, HCV genotype 1b shows more severe liver disease and significantly less therapeutic response to interferon alpha treatment. However, other confounding factors such as duration of infection need to be considered.

Prevalence in ESRD Patients. Dialyzed patients are at high risk of acquiring HCV infection, with higher prevalence of anti-HCV positivity than in the general population. Using a first-generation ELISA, the prevalence of anti-HCV in dialysis units ranges from 8% to 36% in North America, 10% to 50% in South America, 1% to 31% in Europe, 17% to 51% in Asia, and 1% to 10% in Australia and New Zealand. ELISA-II tests reveal even higher prevalence. Documentation of active HCV infection may be difficult in dialysis patients because there is an inconsistent correlation between anti-HCV antibodies and either HCV RNA or plasma ALT levels in this setting. HCV RNA in plasma has been found in only 52% to 93% of anti-HCV antibody–positive patients but also in 2.5% to 12% of anti-HCV antibody–negative patients receiving maintenance dialysis. Furthermore, only 83% of all HCV RNA–positive patients have circulating anti-HCV antibodies. In general, 85% to 95% of patients infected with HCV by blood transfusion will test positive for anti-HCV within 6 months. Also, anti-HCV can disappear spontaneously despite the presence of HCV RNA.

Plasma ALT levels are a poor predictor of HCV infection or active liver disease. Studies in blood donors found elevated ALT levels in only 20% of anti-HCV antibody–positive blood products and 33% of the anti-HCV antibody–positive blood donors. Similarly, ALT levels are elevated in only 4% to 67% of anti-HCV antibody–positive dialysis patients and only 30% of those who had biopsy-proven hepatitis. Chronic HCV hepatitis characteristically has fluctuating ALT levels. Elevated ALT levels have also been observed in 4% to 23% of anti-HCV antibody–negative dialysis patients. Some of these patients could be carriers of HCV infection without antibody production in addition to non-HCV causes. Hence, liver biopsy is the only reliable method of confirming the presence of liver disease. However, ALT levels may be of diagnostic utility in two settings. First, higher ALT and other liver enzyme levels increase the probability of histologic liver disease. Second, seroconversion in initially anti-HCV antibody–negative hemodialysis patients is almost always preceded by a sustained elevation in ALT levels.

Anti-HCV antibody prevalence among dialysis personnel ranges from 0% to 3.6%, comparable to or higher than that in blood donors. The infective risk after accidental needlestick exposure to an anti-HCV antibody positive patient is only about 2.7% to 10 % versus a 67% risk in HBeAg-positive individuals.

Anti-HCV antibody prevalence correlates directly with the number units of blood transfused. The advent of erythropoietin therapy for anemia of chronic renal failure and the implementation of screening of blood products for anti-HCV antibody should markedly reduce HCV infection from blood transfusion. The duration the patient receives hemodialysis has a stronger correlation with HCV prevalence than total unit of blood transfusion and itself is an independent risk factor for HCV infection. Anti-HCV antibody positivity increases considerably after the tenth year of dialysis, about 10% per year on dialysis. This suggests that factors other than transfusion alone are involved.

In patients receiving continuous ambulatory peritoneal dialysis, anti-HCV antibody prevalence is significantly lower than that in patients receiving hemodialysis. Respective values from pooled data were 1.8% to 5% with peritoneal dialysis compared with 16.4% to 44% with hemodialysis. Peritoneal dialysis is primarily a home procedure in a more isolated environment. Furthermore, there is less blood transfusion compared with hemodialysis. The absence of vascular access site and extracorporal blood circuit also reduces the risk of parenteral exposure to the virus. Similarly, anti-HCV antibody prevalence is lower in home hemodialysis patients compared with those treated at a hemodialysis center.

Preventive Measures. The implementation of standard (universal) precautions as well as measures to reduce the spread of HCV in dialysis units has led to a parallel decline in the incidence of non-A, non-B hepatitis. Outbreaks of HCV infection in individual dialysis units have been linked to breaks in infection control procedures. Cross-infection appears to be an important mode of transmission in dialysis units. A high incidence of seroconversion after the start of dialysis has been reported. Several studies performed before the availability of anti-HCV antibody testing documented outbreaks of non-A, non-B hepatitis in hemodialysis patients and implicated blood transfusions, person-to-person, and contaminated environmental surfaces. Clustering of seroconversion appears to occur only in dialysis units in which anti-HCV antibody–positive patients were being treated. The risk of seroconversion is highest in patients dialyzed at a station adjacent to that of an antibody-positive patient. However, the absence of seroconversion in most dialysis units dialyzing anti-HCV–positive patients suggests that isolation of such patients is not yet warranted.

CDC Guidelines. Strict adhesion to CDC guidelines is recommended. CDC recommendations emphasized that universal (standard) precautions should be followed. Routine screening of dialysis staff and patients is not required except for epidemiologic purposes. Patient isolation is not recommended. Dedicated machines are not recommended. Reuse of dialyzers is not prohibited. Policies will have to be reevaluated as more sensitive and specific tests become available. Nevertheless, some physicians have suggested isolation of anti-HCV antibody–positive patients. Some dialysis centers have noted a decrease in the incidence of HCV seroconversion following the use of dedicated areas for antibody-positive patients in association with other infection control measures. However, the lack of cross-immunity between the different strains limits the usefulness of this strategy. Furthermore, grouping of antibody-positive patients might lead to superinfection with multiple HCV strains. Thus most hemodialysis units apply conventional infection control strategies to prevent environmental contamination and do not isolate anti-HCV antibody–positive patients. Sharing of dialysis machines may be another risk factor for HCV transmission. The use of dedicated machines and areas for anti-HCV–positive patients has in some studies led to a marked reduction in the incidence of seroconversion from 20% to 25% to almost zero. However, the efficacy of dedicated machines remains controversial because other investigators have found that conventional cleansing and sterilization are sufficient to prevent the spread of HCV infection within the unit as long as other infection control measures are also followed. Intact dialysis membranes are safe barriers against HCV passage. Nevertheless, an increase in pore size due to disruption of membrane integrity during filter assembly, the dialysis session itself, or dialyzer reuse could theoretically permit the passage of HCV into the blood compartment. At present, however, the prevalence of anti-HCV–positive patients among hemodialysis patients has not been found to be linked to reuse of dialyzers or to any particular dialysis membranes. In units with low prevalence, standard precautions probably suffice. However, in units with high prevalence and incidence, additional measures may be required.

Treatment. If antiviral therapy is being considered, a firm diagnosis of active HCV infection should be made by PCR testing for HCV RNA, ELISA-II, or RIBA positivity with histologic evidence of chronic hepatitis. A 6-month course of interferon alpha is approved by the Food and Drug Administration. It results in 40% to 50% complete response with ALT normalization and clearance of serum HCV RNA. However, about 50%

responders will relapse when treatment is stopped resulting in long-term response of 15% to 25% only. Interferon therapy should be stopped if no response is seen after 3 months. Higher response rates have been reported with ribavirin in combination with interferon than with interferon monotherapy. Liver histology improves in 80% to 100% of responders. However, the long-term outcome is still not adequately defined. No effective vaccine is available at present. Interferon therapy is associated with increased graft rejection, often steroid resistant, in renal transplant patients even after years of stable graft function. Therefore it is considered safer to start interferon treatment in dialysis patients before renal transplantation.

Hepatitis D

HDV, also called *hepatitis delta virus*, is a small, circular RNA virus. It is replication defective, and infection occurs only in the presence of HBV infection. The viral particle is composed of an outer lipoprotein envelope made of HBsAg and inner HDV genome. Transmission is parenteral, and risk factors for infection are similar to those for HBV. HDV most often affects intravenous drug users. HDV acquired simultaneously with HBV infection is called *coinfection*. HDV infection in an HBsAg carrier is called *superinfection*. Coinfection is usually self-limited. Superinfection tends to enhance the severity of preexisting HBV liver disease and causes rapid progression to cirrhosis.

Clinical features vary from benign acute hepatitis to fulminant hepatitis, and from asymptomatic carrier state to progressive chronic liver disease. Approximately 5% of coinfections become chronic; more than 70% and up to 100% of superinfections become chronic. HBsAg positivity is necessary for diagnosis of HDV infection. IgM anti-HBc is necessary for diagnosis of acute HBV/HDV coinfection. Serum HDAg appears early in acute HDV infection but is very short lived. HDV RNA is an early and sensitive marker in acute infection. IgM anti-HDV is transient and delayed in self-limited disease, and it may not be detectable. In chronic HDV infection, anti-HDV is present in high titer. Chronic HDV patients usually have absent markers of HBV replication. They are typically HBeAg negative and anti-HBe positive.

HDV infection is not a significant problem in dialysis units, but cases had been reported. HDV-infected hemodialysis patients should be isolated, especially from HBsAg-positive ones.

Interferon alpha is the only approved drug for treatment of chronic hepatitis D and hepatitis B infection. Overall response is poor. Some studies suggested that a dosage higher than that usually used for hepatitis B may be beneficial. Prevention of HDV infection relies on that of HBV infection and reduced exposure to blood.

Hepatitis E

HEV is a nonenveloped, calicilike RNA virus. It is the main agent of enterically transmitted non-A, non-B hepatitis. The viral genome has been cloned in 1990. Serologic assays for detection of antibody to recombinant expressed HEV antigen have been developed. Only one type of HEV exists, but several strains are recognized. In one study, one-third of acute non-ABC hepatitis were positive for IgM anti-HEV. Six percent of acute hepatitis A patients were also IgM anti-HEV positive. Coinfection of both HEV and HAV is possible. Prevalence of IgG anti-HEV increases with age, but the antibody may disappear with time, within a year of the onset of hepatitis. On the contrary, IgG anti-HAV usually persists for life. Variable persistence of IgG anti-HEV makes it difficult to determine accurately the frequency of previous exposure in any population and raises the possibility of reinfection after disappearance of the antibody. It is also unclear whether the IgG anti-HEV detected is a neutralizing antibody.

Geographic and epidemiologic features are close to those of hepatitis A. Both are transmitted by the fecal–oral route. Vertical transmission had also been observed. Theoretical possibility of transmission in endemic areas via a parenteral route was suggested. For example, one study found anti-HEV antibody to be more common in transfusion recipients. However, hemophiliacs showed low prevalence. Water-borne outbreaks and sporadic cases can occur. No outbreaks in the United States have been reported. HEV usually causes acute, icteric self-limiting hepatitis clinically indistinguishable from hepatitis A with no chronic sequelae. It generally occurs in young to middle-age adults. The incubation period is 2 to 9 weeks. The fatality rate is 0.1% to 1%. However, there is a very high mortality rate up to 20% in pregnant women infected during the last trimester of pregnancy.

Data concerning anti-HEV prevalence among chronic dialysis patients are few, and results are conflicting. It was found in 11% of one and 2.8% of another French dialysis center, 3% among 204 Italian chronic hemodialysis patients, and 6.3% in a Spanish hemodialysis center. Anti-HEV prevalence in European blood donors is 1% to 3% but as high as 7% in blood donors in Mexico and Thailand. More studies are necessary to investigate whether HEV infection has a nosocomial origin or is transmitted by parenteral routes in dialysis patients. HEV seems to play no role in the development of liver disease in hemodialysis patients.

No specific treatment is available. Immune globulin is not useful for prophylaxis. There is no evidence of immunity against HEV in the American population. Potential for spread in the United States is great. Good sanitation and personal hygiene are the best preventive measures.

Hepatitis G

From 10% to 15% non-A, non-B hepatitis patients have no evidence of HCV after extensive evaluation. The search for other viral hepatitis agents continues. In 1995, a putative HGV and its strain hepatitis GB virus C were cloned. They belong to a new genus of the family Flaviviridae. The viral genome consists of a single-stranded RNA molecule of positive polarity and is about 9,400 nucleotide in length, encoding a polyprotein precursor of around 2,900 amino acids. The geographic distribution of HGV/GBV-C is not yet clear. Approximately 1% to 2% of voluntary blood donors in the United States are infected. The corresponding prevalence figure is 0.9% in Japan and 3% in Spain. HGV/GBV-C is parenterally transmitted. Higher prevalence was found in hemophiliacs and intravenous drug users (18%) and multiple transfused patients. Comparison of nucleotide sequence of helicaselike region of HGV clones suggested patient-to-patient transmission. Vertical transmission from mother to child was reported.

Prevalence of HGV RNA in blood donors with normal or abnormal ALT levels is not different. The association of HGV/GBV-C with liver disease may be based on its epidemiologic relationship with parenteral risk factors and concurrent infection with HCV or other agents. In fact, HGV was cloned from a patient infected with HCV. However, there is still lack of evidence that this agent causes biochemical or clinical liver injury. To call HGV/GBV-C a hepatitis virus may be premature. The relevance of HGV in some reported cases of fulminant hepatitis, especially in Japan, is still under investigation. Clinical and pathologic significance of HGV/GBV-C infection needs better evaluation, especially in patients coinfected with other hepatitis viruses such as HBV or HCV.

Diagnosis is by HGV RNA analysis through PCR. More recently, antibody to the envelope region E2 of HGV/GBV-C was developed. This E2 antibody appears when HGV RNA levels have diminished or become absent as the virus is cleared. It was demonstrated that a humoral response to HGV envelope may be associated with loss of viremia and occurs in a substantial proportion of intravenous drug users or posttransfusional cases. Persistence of HGV RNA observed in longitudinal studies of hemodialysis patients may be related to the immunodeficiency associated with ESRD. HGV/GBV-C seems to be able to establish chronic infection in humans.

There is a high risk of HGV/GBV-C in dialysis patients. Reports of HGV/GBV-C prevalence in hemodialysis patients showed figures of 3% in Japan, 16% in Belgium, 26% in Spain, and 19% in Italy. In another Italian study, HGV RNA was found to be 6% in hemodialysis, 17% in continuous ambulatory peritoneal dialysis, and 36% in renal transplant patients. Recognition of a new frequent infection makes it increasingly unfeasible to isolate in terms of organizational and material resources. Improving standards and rigorous application of infection control measures remain the most important strategy.

Nonhepatotropic Viruses

Other nonhepatotropic viruses that do not primarily affect the liver can be associated with hepatitis as part of a systemic infection. Epstein-Barr virus can cause a hepatitis that mimics acute HAV or HBV in adolescents to adults. Cytomegalovirus infection has a diverse clinical picture, including acute hepatitis, and is a rare cause of posttransfusion hepatitis. Herpes simplex virus types I and II and varicella-zoster virus infections may be complicated by hepatitis in both normal and immunocompromised patients. These viruses are prominent pathogens in renal transplant recipients but are not of great epidemiologic importance in dialysis units. Nevertheless, they should be considered in the differential diagnosis if no apparent cause can be identified. Liver disease in renal transplant recipients is discussed in detail in Chapter 89, Part 5.

Drug-Induced Hepatitis

Chronic renal failure and dialysis patients can also be affected by other nonviral causes of hepatitis encountered in the general population. About 2% of all cases of jaundice in hospitalized patients are drug induced. Early suspicion and diagnosis of a drug-induced hepatic reaction is essential, even in patients with viral hepatitis markers. Liver damage is greatly increased if the offending drug is continued after symptoms develop. Many drugs are related to hepatitis. Examples of drugs causing acute hepatitis are isoniazid, rifampicin, methyldopa, and halothane. Chronic hepatitis can develop with methyldopa, isoniazid, nitrofurantoin, and ketoconazole, to name but a few. Drug-induced chronic hepatitis is almost invariably associated with prolonged drug use rather than due to a self-perpetuating process after cessation of the drug. The clinical picture can resemble that of viral hepatitis, and a high index of suspicion is essential. Clinical and biochemical improvement usually follows drug withdrawal.

Chronic Hepatitis

Renal failure patients may also suffer from chronic hepatitis of various causes. *Chronic hepatitis* is a chronic inflammatory reaction in the liver continuing without improvement for at least 6 months. The new classification of chronic hepatitis is based on etiology, clinical grade, and histologic severity (necroinflammatory activity) and the stage (extent of fibrosis). Causes include hepatitis B, C, and D; autoimmune hepatitis; and drugs. Type 1 autoimmune hepatitis (lupoid hepatitis) is the most common form of nonviral chronic hepatitis in the United States, constituting at least 80% of adult cases. Type 2 autoimmune hepatitis is characterized by the presence of autoantibodies against liver/kidney microsome type 1. It can be anti-HCV negative (type 2a) or associated with HCV infection (type 2b).

SUMMARY OF INFECTION CONTROL STRATEGIES

Strategies for the control of blood-borne viral agents basically have evolved from those developed for the control of HBV in the dialysis setting. In 1977, the CDC published a set of guidelines for the recommended basic barrier precautions to prevent the spread of HBV from patient to patient and from patient to staff members. These strategies included the avoidance of needlesticks, wearing of protective clothing, eye and face protection, and gloves to minimize exposure to blood and body fluids. Additional recommendations included serologic screening of patients for HBsAg/Anti-HBs, separate machines and area of dialysis for HBsAg-positive patients. Over the years, studies have shown that these infection control strategies are effective and do indeed help minimize transmission of HBV among patients in the dialysis center.

In 1987, CDC recommended an infection control strategy referred to as "Universal Precautions" for the control of blood-borne infections in health care settings. Basically, these strategies are the same ones that had been used for years in dialysis centers. The prevalence of anti-HCV antibody–positive patients on dialysis is consistently higher than in general population (8% to 30% in North America, 10% to 50% in South America, 1% to 31% in Europe, 17% to 51% in Asia, and 1% to 10% in Australia and New Zealand). Because of this increase in incidence, various strategies have been recommended to reduced the incidence of HCV infection in dialysis unit.

The recommendations include the following:

1. *Standard infection-control practices:* The implementation of universal precautions as well as measures to reduce the spread of HBV in dialysis units has led to a parallel decline in the incidence of non-A and non-B hepatitis. On the other hand, outbreaks of HCV infection in individual dialysis units have been linked to sharing of a multidose heparin or erythropoietin vial by patients on the same shift and to other breaks in infection control procedures.
2. *Nosocomial transmission:* Cross-infection appears to be an important mode of transmission of HCV infection in dialysis units. A number of studies have reported high incidences of seroconversion after the start of dialysis. Several studies performed before the availability of anti-HCV antibody testing documented outbreaks of non-A, non-B hepatitis in hemodialysis patients and implicated blood transfusions, person-to-person, and contaminated environmental surfaces. One outbreak of non-A, non-B hepatitis in dialysis unit correlated with anti-HCV antibody testing. Of 56 potentially susceptible patients being dialyzed in a single unit, 11 (20%) seroconverted to anti-HCV antibody positive between 1987 and 1989. No associations were found with dialysis on a particular schedule, incidence of dialysis complication, or exposure to a bleeding event from anti-HCV antibody–positive patient, contact with a nurse who also cared for an anti-HCV–positive patients, or use of multidose medications. Routine equipment maintenance record documented a problem with sporadic overload of transducer protectors resulting in reflux of patient blood across the transducers between 1985 and 1989. Furthermore, inadequate infection control measures, such as lack of glove use and poor handwashing, occurred during the exposure period. Overall, neither a common source nor direct person-to-person transmission could be documented. It was concluded that strict adherence to standard infection control strategies was sufficient to control the spread of HCV in the dialysis setting. A multicenter trial in Belgium reported that the yearly incidence of seroconversion for HCV averages

1.7%. They found that 38% of hemodialysis patients who seroconverted had never been transfused and had no other risk factor for HCV infection. Furthermore, clustering of seroconversion appears to occur only in dialysis units in which anti-HCV antibody–positive patients were being treated. The risk of seroconversion is highest in patients dialyzed at a station adjacent to that of an antibody-positive patient. The absence of seroconversion in most units dialyzing ELISA-tested anti-HCV antibody–positive patients suggest that isolation of such patients is not yet warranted. Strict adhesion to the CDC guidelines is recommended. Thus most hemodialysis units apply conventional infection control strategies to prevent environmental contamination and do not isolate anti-HCV antibody–positive patients.

3. *Dialysis machines:* It has been proposed that sharing of dialysis machines may be another factor that contributes to the transmission of HCV infection. In some studies, for example, the use of dedicated dialysis machines and areas for anti-HCV antibody–positive patients has led to a marked reduction in the incidence of seroconversion. However, the efficacy of dedicated machines remains controversial because other investigators have found that conventional cleansing and sterilization are sufficient to prevent the spread of HCV infection.
4. *Dialyzer membranes:* The possibility of HCV passage through an intact dialysis membrane appears to be negligible. The particle diameter of HCV has been estimated at 35 nm, which is much larger than the pore size of the most porous dialysis membranes, which range from 1.7 to 7 nm. Thus intact hemodialysis membranes are safe barriers against the passage of the virus. Nevertheless, an increase in pore size due to disruption of membrane integrity could theoretically permit the passage of HCV into the blood compartment. Microfractures of the membrane are often associated with the process of filter assembly, the dialysis session itself, or dialyzer reuse. At present, however, the prevalence of anti-HCV antibodies among hemodialysis patients has not been found to be linked to reuse of dialyzers or to any particular dialysis membranes. Thus the CDC recommendation for HCV patients in the dialysis unit are as follows:
   - "Universal Precautions" should be followed.
   - Routine screening of dialysis staff and patients is not required except for epidemiologic purposes.
   - Patient isolation is not recommended.
   - Dedicated machines are not recommended.
   - Reuse of dialyzers is not prohibited.
   - Policies will have to be reevaluated as more sensitive and specific tests become available.

The CDC recommendations for patients in dialysis units are as follows:

1. Universal precautions and appropriate labeling of all specimens and equipment
2. Surveillance for hepatitis B surface antigen (HBsAg) and antibody every 3 to 6 months for susceptible individuals (those not antibody positive)
3. Surveillance of anti-HBs–positive patients every year
4. Use of separate rooms and dedicated machines for hemodialysis of HBsAg-positive patients and avoidance of dialyzer or blood line reuse
5. Vaccination of susceptible patients and staff. To increase the chances of successful vaccination, the dosage of hepatitis B vaccine in dialysis patients should be twice the normal amount. Table 73.2 describes these measures in more detail.)

TABLE 73.2. CDC: Hepatitis-Control Measures for Hepatitis B in Dialysis Centers

A. Surveillance-Serologic Testing
   1. Routine surveillance of patients and staff for HBV infection
   2. Candidates for dialysis and potential employees are screened for HBsAg and anti-HBs
   3. To know the HBsAg status of visiting and home patients on admission
   4. Sensitive tests for HBsAg and anti-HBs used
   5. Seronegative patients tested regularly for aminotransferases, HBsAg, and anti-HBs
   6. HBsAg-negative, anti-HBs–positive patients and staff receive annual test for anti-HBs

B. Record Keeping
   1. Dialysis records should have the following clearly noted:
      - Lot number of blood and blood products used
      - Blood leaks and spills, dialysis machine malfunction
      - Number and location of each dialysis machine
      - Name of staff who connect and disconnect patient and machine
   2. A log of all aminotransferase hepatitis serologic results of all patients and staff
   3. A log of all accidental needle punctures and prophylactic measures

C. Education

   Continuing educational program for hepatitis infection control

D. Control and Prevention
   1. HbsAg-positive patients isolated and dialyzed on dedicated machines
   2. Staff not attending to both HBsAg-positive and HBsAg-negative patients during the same shift
   3. Dialysis equipment not used for both HBsAg-positive and HBsAg-negative patients
   4. Patients assigned to specific dialysis chairs or beds and machines
   5. Items such as tourniquets, antiseptics, pencils, and blood pressure cuffs not shared
   6. Nondisposable items such as clamps and scissors used only in a single patient unless disinfected
   7. Disposable gloves worn by staff when handling patients and equipment; fresh pair of gloves with each patient
   8. Gloves worn when handling blood specimens
   9. Protective eye glasses and masks used if splattering of blood is possible (e.g., cleaning dialyzers)
   10. Gowns or scrub units worn in the unit
   11. Disinfection/sterilization of nondisposable equipment, cleaning of control knobs after each dialysis
   12. Rinsing and disinfection of dialysis machines according to procedure
   13. Venous pressure isolators or in-line filters not reused
   14. Staff should not eat, drink, or smoke in dialysis area
   15. Patients should not share food, drink, or smoke items
   16. Immediate thorough cleaning and disinfection after a blood spill, cleaning equipment used in dialysis units not be used in other areas
   17. Avoidance of overcrowding of patients and machines
   18. Blood specimens and charts from HBsAg-positive patients labeled

E. Housekeeping
   1. Proper bagging of disposable items for incineration or disposal
   2. Puncture-proof containers for used needles
   3. Contaminated linen be handled with glove and bagged properly

F. Sterilization and Disinfection
   1. Thorough and mechanical cleaning before sterilization and disinfection
   2. Sterilization treatment to inactivate HBV; always use sterilization except for noncritical items

Selected Readings

Centers for Disease Control and Prevention. Control measures for hepatitis B in dialysis centers. In: *Viral Hepatitis Investigation and Control Series*, November 1977.

This classic article is the earliest published comprehensive guidelines for controlling hepatitis B in dialysis centers.

Fabrizi F, Lunghi G, Bacchini G, et al. Hepatitis E virus infection in hemodialysis patients: a seroepidemiological survey. *Nephrol Dial Transplant* 1997;12: 133–136.*A study of the prevalence of hepatitis E virus in a large cohort of chronic hemodialysis patients in a single dialysis unit. Conflicting results in other studies were also discussed.*

Garner JS, the Hospital Infection Control Practices Advisory Committee. Guideline for isolation precautions in hospitals. *Infect Control Hosp Epidemiol* 1996;17:53-80.

Revised guideline by the CDC and the Hospital Infection Control Practices Advisory Committee to assist hospitals in maintaining up-to-date isolation practices based on the latest epidemiologic information on transmission of infection in hospitals.

Martin P, Friedman LS. Chronic viral hepatitis and the management of chronic renal failure. *Kidney Int* 1995;47:1231–1241.

A balanced review of hepatitis B and C in dialysis and renal transplant patients.

Pereira BJG, Levey AS. Hepatitis C virus infection in dialysis and renal transplantation. *Kidney Int* 1997;51:981–999.

A concise review of hepatitis C in renal patients. Virology, interpretation of different HCV tests, epidemiology in dialysis units, and control measures are well addressed.

Seeff LB. Diagnosis, therapy and prognosis of viral hepatitis. In: Zakim D, Boyer TD, eds. *Hepatology a textbook of liver disease*, 3rd ed. Philadelphia: WB Saunders, 1996:1067–1145.

A comprehensive description of all aspects of viral hepatitis, including highlights on histories of various agents.

Sheng L, Widyastuti A, Kosala H, et al. High prevalence of hepatitis G virus infection compared with hepatitis C virus infection in patients undergoing chronic hemodialysis. *Am J Kidney Dis* 1998;31:218–223.

This article investigated the prevalence of HGV-RNA and anti-E2 antibodies in chronic hemodialysis patients and healthy blood donors.

Sherlock S, Dooley J. Virus hepatitis. In: *Diseases of the liver and biliary system*, 10th ed. Oxford: Blackwell Scientific, 1997:265–302.

An updated and detailed account of all types of viral hepatitis, including hepatitis A to G and nonhepatotropic viruses.

CHAPTER 74

Metabolic and Endocrine Disturbances in Uremia

PART 1

Glucose and Insulin Metabolism

Shaul G. Massry and Miroslaw Smogorzewski

Chronic renal failure (CRF) is associated with many disturbances in carbohydrate metabolism. The characteristic of glucose and insulin metabolism in uremia is presented in Table 74.1. Studies in humans have demonstrated that both insulin resistance and impaired insulin secretion contribute to the pathogenesis of carbohydrate intolerance. The insulin resistance is almost always present in patients with uremia, whereas insulin secretion, as evaluated by the blood levels of insulin in response to hyperglycemia, may be normal, increased, or decreased. These variations appear difficult to reconcile but may reflect different responses of β-cells to hyperglycemia and/or different degrees of impairment in insulin degradation.

The normal response of β-cells to the presence of insulin resistance is to enhance their secretion of insulin. If for any reason the β-cells are unable to augment their secretion of insulin appropriately, an impaired glucose tolerance would ensue. Indeed, glucose intolerance is usually encountered in uremic patients in whom both impaired tissue sensitivity to insulin and impaired β-cell secretion of insulin coexist.

PERIPHERAL RESISTANCE TO THE ACTION OF INSULIN

The first indirect and convincing evidence for the presence of impaired peripheral action of insulin was provided in 1962 by studies showing that glucose uptake by the forearm of uremic patients is reduced. This phenomenon was confirmed by studies using an euglycemic clamp technique, which demonstrated that the amount of glucose metabolized per unit of insulin in dialysis patients is reduced.

TABLE 74.1. Characteristics of Glucose and Insulin Metabolism in Uremia

Clinical presentation
Impaired glucose tolerance[a]
Decreased requirement for insulin by diabetic patients with diabetic nephropathy and uremia
In blood
Normal fasting blood glucose
Spontaneous hypoglycemia
Fasting hyperinsulinemia[b]
Normal, elevated, or decreased blood insulin levels in response to hyperglycemia induced by oral or intravenous glucose administration
Elevated blood levels of proinsulin or C-peptide
Elevated blood levels of immnunoreactive glucagon
In pancreatic islets
Elevated basal levels of cytosolic calcium
Reduced calcium signal and response to glucose and potassium
Impaired glycolytic pathways
Reduced basal and glucose-stimulated ATP content
Decreased V_{max} of Ca^{2+} ATPase and Na^{+}-K^{+}-ATPase
Impaired insulin secretion in response to glucose, potassium or amino acids[c]
In liver
Normal hepatic glucose metabolism
Normal suppression of hepatic glucose production by insulin
In peripheral tissues
Resistance to the peripheral action of insulin
Number and affinity of insulin receptor and insulin receptor tyrosine kinase activity unchanged
Abundance of glucose transports protein (GLUT4) in muscle not reduced
Postreceptor defect, which may be due to derangement in the downstream signaling that leads to impaired insulin mediated glucose transport

[a] This is present only when glucose-induced insulin secretion is impaired in the presence of resistance to the peripheral action of insulin.
[b] Normal blood levels may be encountered.
[c] This occurs in the presence of established secondary hyperparathyroidism.

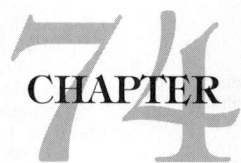

The two tissues that are involved in most of the peripheral uptake of glucose are the liver and the skeletal muscle. Therefore resistance to insulin action may result from (a) impaired uptake of glucose by these tissues and/or (b) increased production of glucose by the liver. However, glucose uptake by the liver is small compared with that of skeletal muscle, and it is not impaired in uremia. Also, glucose production by the liver and its suppression by insulin is not affected by uremia. Therefore it is evident that the major site for the decreased sensitivity to insulin action is the skeletal muscle.

The insulin action on glucose transport by muscle is mediated through a complex process. First, insulin must bind to its receptor, which is made of two dimmers (α and β) connected by a disulfide bond. The α subunit is located extracellularly and represents the ligand-binding site. The β subunit is a transmembrane protein and contains an extracellular transmembrane and cytoplasmic domains; this β subunit has a tyrosine kinase activity. After insulin binding to the subunit, a signal is transmitted to the β subunit, resulting in autophosphorylation of the tyrosine residues, which causes a marked increase in tyrosine kinase activity. This is followed by tyrosine phosphorylation of insulin receptor substrate 1 (IRS1). The IRS1 is thought to operate as a multisite docking protein linked with insulin receptor, and it subsequently serves an important signaling role in the pathways for the various actions of insulin. One of these is the phosphatidylinositol 3-kinase pathway, which is involved in the modulation of glucose transport.

Available data indicate that the number and the affinity of the insulin receptors in uremia are unchanged and may even be increased. Furthermore, the insulin receptor kinase activity in the skeletal muscle of patients with CRF or in the skeletal muscle of uremic rats is unchanged. It is evident, therefore, that a postreceptor defect due to derangement in the downstream signaling most likely leads to impaired insulin-mediated glucose transport. Such a defect is responsible for the resistance to the peripheral action of insulin in uremia. This notion would imply that even very high levels of insulin may not correct the defect in glucose uptake by skeletal muscle, and available data show that this indeed may be the case.

Skeletal muscles and adipose tissue posses a glucose transporter (GLUT-4), which is regulated by insulin. A defect in this system, including a reduction in the abundance of the GLUT-4, its translocation to cell surface, and/or its intrinsic activity, may contribute to the reduced glucose uptake by skeletal muscle in response to insulin. However, the abundance of GLUT-4 in the muscle of uremic patients is not different from that of normal individuals.

The peripheral resistance to insulin action occurs early in the course of renal failure and before the onset of signs and symptoms of the uremic syndrome become apparent. It is observed in the majority of patients with advanced renal failure and those treated with hemodialysis. This defect is markedly improved after 10 weeks of hemodialysis therapy and following treatment with continuous ambulatory peritoneal dialysis (CAPD). Furthermore, treatment of uremic patients with dietary protein restriction and supplementation with keto and amino acids for 6 months was followed by marked amelioration of the peripheral resistance to insulin action. These observations are consistent with the notion that the defect in peripheral action of insulin is at least partly due to a dialyzable compound(s) produced by protein breakdown. It has been reported that the sera of uremic patients contain a compound with a molecular weight of 1,000 to 2,000 D, which inhibits glucose metabolism by normal rat adipocytes. This compound appears to be specific for uremia because it is absent in the blood of patients with insulin resistance but without uremia. Others proposed that hippurate, which accumulates in the blood of patients with renal failure, contributes to the insulin resistance in these patients; indeed, hippurate inhibits glucose utilization by the diaphragm, brain, kidney cortex, and erythrocytes in rats.

Uremic patients are weak, lead a sedentary lifestyle, and engage in little exercise if any. The sedentary lifestyle could contribute to the resistance of insulin action, and certain studies have demonstrated that uremic patients displayed improvement in insulin sensitivity after exercise training.

INSULIN SECRETION AND PANCREATIC ISLET METABOLISM

Insulin secretion by β-cells of the pancreatic islets is a complex process. The β-cells are stimulated by nutrients (glucose, amino acids, or fatty acids) or nonnutrient agents such as hormones and neurotransmitters. The scope of this chapter does not permit a detailed presentation of this process. Although, the mechanisms of recognition by the β-cells of nutrient and nonnutrient stimuli may be different, the secretory process of insulin utilizes the same intracellular processes when the β-cells are activated by nutrient or nonnutrient secretagogues.

In the case of glucose-induced insulin secretion, the process begins by the uptake of glucose by the β cells. Glucose is then metabolized to produce adenosine triphosphate (ATP). The latter facilitates the closure of ATP-dependent potassium channels, which is followed by cell depolarization and subsequent activation of voltage-sensitive calcium channels. As a consequence, calcium enters the islets, causing a rise in cytosolic calcium concentration that triggers cellular events that lead to insulin secretion. Others proposed that the ATP:adenosine diphosphate (ADP) ratio is important factor in the sequence of events just described, and a rise in the ATP:ADP ratio initiates the closure of the ATP-sensitive potassium channel and the depolarization of islets. Thus a lower ATP content and/or a lower ATP:ADP ratio in islets in CRF, both in the resting state or after the stimulation with glucose, may contribute to the reduced insulin secretion.

As indicated, reduced insulin sensitivity is common in uremic patients. Hence glucose intolerance is found only in those who display reduced insulin secretion, and one must conclude that insulin secretion is impaired in a substantial segment of patients with renal failure.

In Table 74.1, it is stated that the blood levels of insulin in patients with renal failure may be normal, elevated, or decreased in response to hyperglycemia. These observations may suggest that insulin secretion in these patients may not be reduced. However, it must be remembered that the blood levels of insulin are determined by insulin secretion and its metabolic clearance rate. Because the latter is impaired in patients with CRF, changes in the blood levels of insulin in response to hyperglycemia are not a reliable indicator of insulin secretion. Evaluation of insulin secretion is better estimated by the hyperglycemic clamp technique. Studies in humans or animals with CRF using this technique reported a normal initial and exaggerated late response, an exaggerated early and late response, or decreased initial and late responses. In all these studies, glucose utilization was lower than normal, indicating that insulin secretion is inappropriate relative to the insulin resistant state.

Direct evidence for impaired insulin secretion in CRF was provided by *in vitro* dynamic perfusion studies of pancreatic islets obtained from rats with CRF. Both the initial and the late phases of glucose-induced insulin secretion were markedly reduced (Fig. 74.1).

MECHANISMS OF IMPAIRED INSULIN SECRETION

Available data indicate that in renal failure, there is a generalized failure of the pancreatic islets to respond to glucose, amino acids, or potassium. The mechanisms for this phenomenon are not totally understood. However, a substantial body of evidence has accumulated, incriminating the chronic excess of parathyroid hormone (PTH) and/or the reduced blood levels of $1,25(OH)_2D$ in the genesis of the impaired insulin secretion in chronic renal failure.

Role of Secondary Hyperparathyroidism

Hyperglycemic clamp studies in dogs with CRF with elevated blood levels of PTH showed that both the initial and late plasma insulin levels were reduced; however, insulin responses were normal in normocalcemic-parathyroidectomized CRF animals. These observations were confirmed in uremic children treated with hemodialysis. These studies showed marked improvement in insulin secretion after normalization of the blood levels of PTH by the medical suppression of the parathyroid glands by treatment with $1,25(OH)_2D_3$ or after the surgical removal of the glands. Furthermore, others showed that glucose-induced insulin secretion by islets from CRF rats is impaired but is normal by islets obtained form normocalcemic parathyroidectomized rats with similar degree and duration of renal failure (Fig. 74.1). It has also been reported that the daily administration of PTH for 6 weeks to rats with normal renal function caused a marked impairment in insulin secretion by their pancreatic islets (Fig. 74.2). Also, the impairment in L-leucine and potassium-induced insulin secretion in CRF is due to chronic excess of PTH. All these observations clearly demonstrate that states with chronic excess of PTH inhibit insulin secretion whether renal failure is present or not.

Patients with CRF display variability in regard to glucose intolerance. This may be due in part to the variations in the severity of secondary hyperparathyroidism among these patients. It is reasonable to propose that patients with moderate elevations in blood levels of PTH may secrete adequate insulin in response to hyperglycemia and hence have normal glucose tolerance. On the other hand, in patients with marked secondary hyperparathyroidism, insulin secretion is significantly reduced and glucose intolerance is present.

Chronic excess of PTH in renal failure is associated with a rise in basal levels of cytosolic calcium $[Ca^{2+}]i$ in many cells, including the pancreatic islets; furthermore, chronic excess of PTH without renal failure also causes a rise in the basal levels of $[Ca^{2+}]i$ of pancreatic islets (Fig 74.3). The mechanisms responsible for this phenomenon are complex and are discussed in detail in Chapter 68, Part 1. In short, there are both a PTH-mediated increase in calcium entry into the islets and decreased calcium exit out of the islets because of impaired activity of both Ca^{2+}-ATPase, $Na^{-+}K^{+}$-ATPase and Na^{+}-Ca^{2+} exchange.

The elevation in the basal levels of $[Ca^{2+}]i$ of pancreatic islets in CRF appears to be responsible, in major part, for the

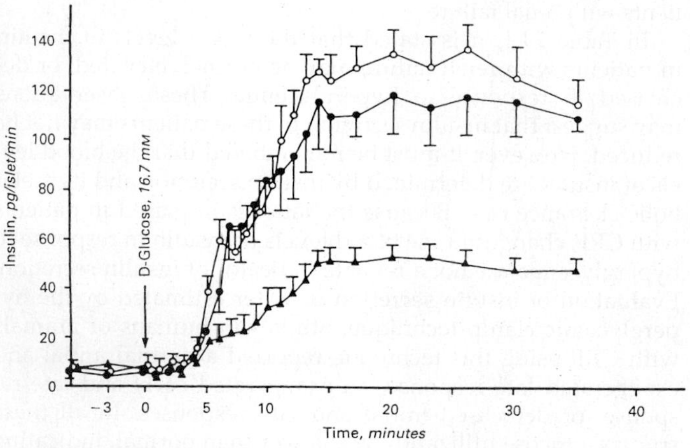

Figure 74.1. Dynamic insulin release from perfused pancreatic islets in normal rats *(O)*, CRF animals *(△)*, and CRF normocalcemic parathyroidectomized rats *(●)*. Each datum point represents the mean value and brackets denote 1 SE. Note that both initial and late phases of glucose-induced insulin secretion are impaired. (Reproduced with permission from Fadda GZ, Akmal M, Permdas FH, et al. Insulin release from pancreatic islets: effects of CRF and excess PTH. *Kidney Int* 1988;33:1066–1072.)

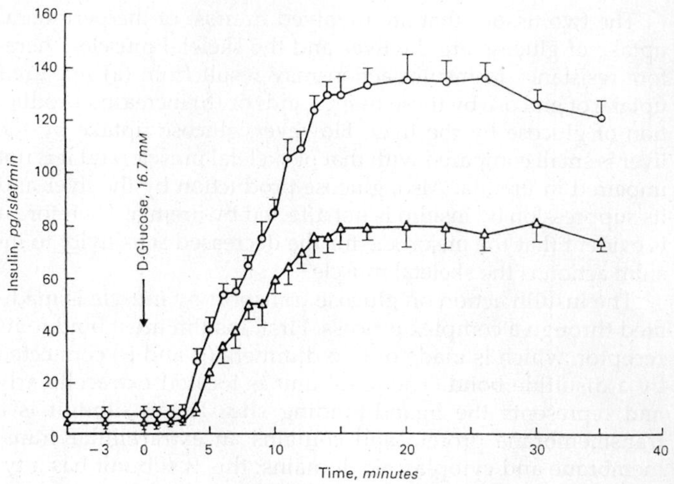

Figure 74.2. Dynamic insulin release from perfused pancreatic islets in normal rats *(O)* and PTH-treated rats with normal renal function *(△)*. Each datum point represents mean value and brackets denote 1 SE. Note the impaired insulin secretion in the PTH-treated animals. (Reproduced with permission from Fadda GZ, Akmal M, Premdas FH, et al. Insulin release from pancreatic islets: effects of CRF and excess PTH. *Kidney Int* 1988;33:1066–1072.)

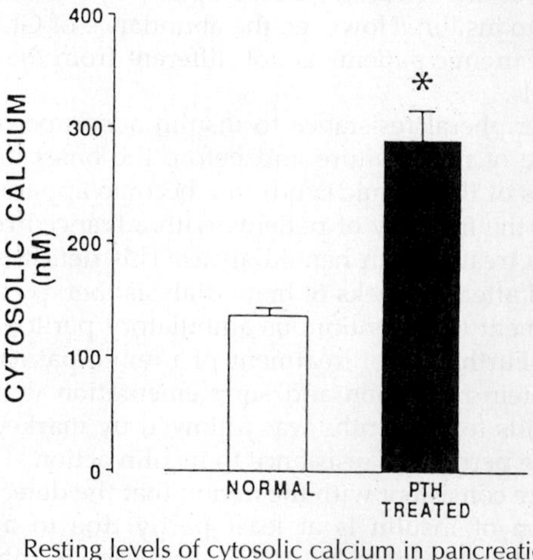

Figure 74.3. Resting levels of cytosolic calcium in pancreatic islets from normal rats and PTH-treated animals with normal renal function. Each column represents mean value and brackets denote 1 SE. $*P < .01$. (Reproduced with permission from Perna AF, Fadda GZ, Zhou X-J, et al. Mechanisms of impaired insulin secretion after chronic excess of parathyroid hormone. *Am J Physiol* 1990;259:F210–F216.)

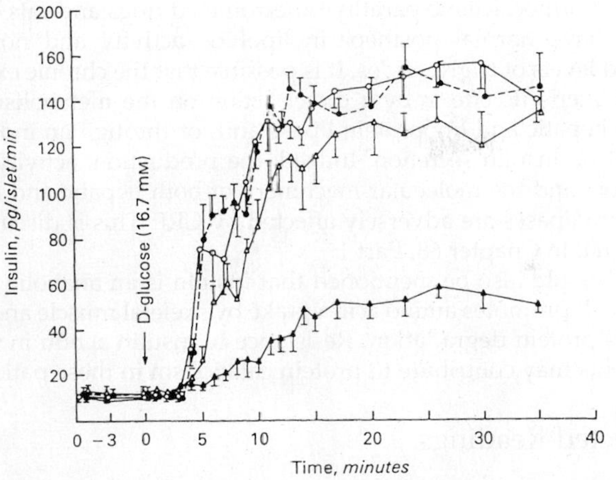

Figure 74.4. Dynamic insulin release from perfused pancreatic islets. Each datum point depicts mean value and brackets denote 1 SE. Symbols are *(O)* normal rats; *(●)* normal animals treated with verapamil; *(▲)* CRF rats; *(△)* CRF rats treated with verapamil. (Reproduced with permission from Fadda GZ, Akmal M, Soliman AR, et al. Correction of glucose intolerance and the impaired insulin release of chronic renal failure by verapamil. *Kidney Int* 1989;36:773–779.)

impairment in their insulin secretion by glucose, potassium, or L-leucine. Indeed, normalization of $[Ca^{2+}]$i of pancreatic islets of CRF rats by prior parathyroidectomy or by their treatment with verapamil, an agent that blocks the PTH-mediated entry of calcium into the islets, prevented the impairment in insulin secretion (Fig. 74.4). Also, treatment of rats with established CRF with verapamil reversed the elevation in the basal levels of $[Ca^{2+}]$i of their pancreatic islets and normalized the glucose-induced insulin secretion by these islets. Finally, in rats with phosphate depletion that have normal renal function and low blood levels of PTH, the basal levels of $[Ca^{2+}]$i of the islets are elevated, and both glucose or L-leucine–induced insulin secretion are impaired (see Chapter 19, Part 3). Thus an elevation in basal levels of $[Ca^{2+}]$i of pancreatic islets is associated with impaired insulin secretion in the presence or absence of renal failure and whether blood levels of PTH are elevate or not.

Pancreatic Islet Metabolism

Several aspects of the metabolism of pancreatic islets are altered in CRF (Table 74.1). These changes provide for the understanding of the cellular pathways that lead to impairment in the glucose-induced insulin secretion.

The basal and glucose-induced rise in ATP contents of pancreatic islets of CRF rats are significantly reduced. This is mediated by the rise in $[Ca^{2+}]$i of islets because normalization of the latter by prior parathyroidectomy of these animals or by their treatment with verapamil prevents the fall in ATP content of the islets. The role of ATP in permitting calcium influx in pancreatic islets has already been discussed. The low ATP content of pancreatic islets in CRF would be associated with reduced acute rise in $[Ca^{2+}]$i after exposure of the islets to secretagogues. Indeed, the calcium signal rise in $[Ca^{2+}]$i after the exposure of the pancreatic islets to glucose or potassium is reduced in CRF.

To generate ATP after the exposure of the pancreatic islets to glucose, the latter must enter the islets and be metabolized normally. Available data indicate that glucose entry into the islets is normal in CRF but its metabolism within the islet is impaired.

After its entry into the islets, glucose is phosphorylated to glucose-6-phosphate, converted by an isomerase to fructose-6-phosphate and further phosphorylated by phosphofructokinase-1 (PFK-1) to fructose-1,6-bisphosphate. Both an adequate amount of ATP and intact function of PFK-1 are essential for this phosphorylation process to proceed normally. However, ATP content of pancreatic islets from patients with CRF is low and the V_{max} of their PFK-1 is reduced. Therefore it appears that glucose metabolism by pancreatic islets from chronic renal failure rats is impaired at steps of the glycolytic pathways before the production of glyceraldehyde-3-phosphate. This notion is supported by two findings. First, glucose-induced ATP and lactic acid production by pancreatic islets are impaired in CRF; second, glyceraldehyde, which enters the glycolytic pathways after the PFK-1 step, induces normal insulin secretion by islets from CRF rats. All these metabolic derangements of the islets appear also to be due to the elevation in basal levels of $[Ca^{2+}]$i of the islets. Indeed, glucose metabolism of islets is normal in normocalcemic parathyroidectomized CRF rats (no elevation in blood levels of PTH and normal $[Ca^{2+}]$i of the islets) and in CRF rats treated with verapamil (elevated blood levels of PTH but normal $[Ca^{2+}]$i of the islets).

Derangements in the metabolic pathways, involved in leucine-induced insulin secretion, are also present in islets from CRF rats. Both leucine uptake and α-ketoisocaproic acid–induced insulin secretion by islets from CRF rats are normal; however, both the activation of glutamate dehydrogenase by leucine or by 2-amino-bicyclo-[2-1-1]-haptene and the utilization of α-ketoglutarate are impaired, and the maximal reaction velocity (V_{max}) of glutaminase is reduced.

Role of $1,25(OH)_2D_3$

Certain data indicate that $1,25(OH)_2D_3$ interacts with the pancreatic islets and modulates their insulin secretion. In the chick, the pancreatic islets possess receptor proteins for $1,25(OH)_2D_3$ and for vitamin D–dependent calcium-binding protein. Both of these proteins are localized in the β-cells of the islets. Also, vitamin D–deficient rats with normal renal function display impaired insulin secretion, and this defect is corrected with administration of vitamin D.

Therefore it is theoretically possible that the deficiency of $1,25(OH)_2D_3$, commonly present in patients with CRF plays a role in the impaired insulin secretion observed in these patients. Studies are available showing that the acute intravenous administration of $1,25(OH)_2D_3$ to dialysis patients caused a significant increment in early and late phases of insulin secretion and corrected the glucose intolerance as well; this effect of $1,25(OH)_2D_3$ occurred without changes in blood levels of PTH.

INSULIN CLEARANCE

Insulin is metabolized and cleared by the kidney. The hormone is filtered by the glomeruli and is reabsorbed by the proximal tubule. The renal clearance of insulin in normal subjects (200 ml/min) is greater than the glomerular filtration rate. This observation indicates peritubular uptake of insulin. The daily renal clearance of insulin (6 to 8 units) is about 25% to 40% of that secreted by the pancreatic islets.

It is not surprising, therefore, that impaired metabolic clearance of insulin is encountered in patients with CRF. This defect in insulin clearance becomes apparent when the glomerular filtration rate falls below 40 ml/min. In patients with more advanced renal failure (glomerular filtration rate below 20 ml/min), the half-life of insulin is markedly prolonged. In addition, insulin is also cleared by the muscles and liver; these latter processes may be affected by as yet unidentified uremic toxin(s) because treatment of uremic patients with dialysis is followed by marked improvement in insulin clearance, presumably due to increased removal of the hormone by liver and muscles. Further discussion on insulin metabolism and clearance is found in Chapter 12.

The impairment in the clearances of insulin in patients with CRF is responsible for the fasting hyperinsulinemia, for the higher blood levels of insulin after glucose administration, for the decreased requirement of insulin in patients with diabetic nephropathy and uremia, and at least in part, for the hypoglycemia that is occasionally encountered in nondiabetic patients with CRF.

HYPOGLYCEMIA

Hypoglycemia is encountered in diabetic and nondiabetic patients with CRF. The reduced degradation of the administered insulin to diabetic patients with CRF results in higher blood levels of insulin than those expected; consequently, hypoglycemia may develop. Careful adjustment of the dosage of insulin therapy is needed in these patients.

The mechanisms of spontaneous hypoglycemia in nondiabetic uremic patients are not clear. In one such patient, a reduction in hepatic glucose output caused by diminished alanine availability for gluconeogenesis was found. In another patient, spontaneous hypoglycemia occurred after parathyroidectomy, which was followed by a significant increase in insulin secretion.

Also, uremic diabetic patients treated with oral hyperglycemic agents, which are cleared by the kidney, may require appropriate adjustment of the dosage of these drugs to avoid hypoglycemia. It is also advisable to use short-acting oral hypoglycemic agents.

Clinical Consequences

The state of secondary hyperparathyroidism and the elevated blood levels of PTH in patients with CRF impair the extrarenal disposal of potassium. This derangement may reduce entry of potassium into pancreatic islets and may therefore interfere with insulin secretion because potassium stimulates insulin secretion. Indeed, potassium-induced insulin secretion is markedly impaired in CRF. Because insulin is an important regulator of extrarenal disposal of potassium, it is plausible to propose that the interactions between PTH, impaired insulin secretion, as well as extrarenal potassium disposal may contribute to the development of hyperkalemia in patients with CRF.

The disturbances in glucose metabolism, insulin secretion, and secondary hyperparathyroidism may all contribute to the increased risk for atherogenesis in patients with CRF. Postprandial hyperglycemia in the glucose-intolerant uremic patient may, by itself, be a risk factor for the atherosclerotic cardiovascular disease. Hyperinsulinemia and insulin-resistant state may be associated with hypertension, which is an important risk factor for cardiac disease in uremia.

Lipoprotein lipase activity is regulated by insulin, and a deficiency of the hormone or a resistance to its action is associated with reduced availability of the enzyme, which plays a major role in triglyceride removal from the blood. Indeed, in CRF, the postheparin lipolytic activity is reduced, and this defect is the primary cause of hypertriglyceridemia in these patients. Support for the role of insulin in this regard comes from studies that showed that the administration of insulin to rats with CRF corrected the defect in postheparin lipolytic activity as well as the hypertriglyceridemia.

Data from our laboratory have demonstrated that chronic excess of PTH plays a significant role in the genesis of the reduced postheparin lipolytic activity and in the hypertriglyceridemia of CRF. Normocalcemic parathyroidectomized dogs and rats with CRF have normal postheparin lipolytic activity and normal blood levels of triglycerides. It is possible that the chronic excess PTH exerts its effects by a direct action on the metabolism of both hepatic and lipoprotein lipase and/or through an indirect effect on insulin secretion. Indeed, the production, activity, secretion, and the molecular machinery of both hepatic and lipoprotein lipases are adversely affected by CRF. This is discussed in detail in Chapter 68, Part 1.

It should also be mentioned that insulin is an anabolic hormone. It promotes amino acid uptake by skeletal muscle and inhibits protein degradation. Resistance to insulin action in CRF patients may contribute to protein catabolism in these patients.

Selected Readings

Akmal M, Massry SG, Goldstein DA, et al. Role of parathyroid hormone in the glucose intolerance of chronic renal failure. *J Clin Invest* 1985;75:1037–1044.

The first demonstration that excess blood levels of PTH in CRF impair insulin secretion and contribute to the carbohydrate intolerance of uremia.

Akmal M, Perkins S, Kasim SE, et al. Verapamil prevents CRF induced abnormalities in lipid metabolism. *Am J Kidney Dis* 1993;22:1158–1163.

A detailed study in rats with CRF demonstrating that excess PTH is a major factor in the genesis of the defect in postheparin lipoprotein lipase activity and in the hypertriglyceridemia of CRF.

Cheatham B, Khan CR. Insulin action and the insulin signaling network. *Endocr Rev* 1995;16:117–142.

An excellent review of the cellular pathways that are involved in insulin action.

DeFronzo RA, Alvestrand A, Smith D, et al. Insulin resistance in uremia. *J Clin Invest* 1981;67:563–568.

Studies in normal volunteers, patients with CRF, and dialysis patients demonstrating insulin resistance.

DeFronzo RA, Andres R, Eager P, et al. Carbohydrate metabolism in uremia: a review. *Medicine* 1973;52:469–481.

An excellent review of the various aspects of carbohydrate intolerance in CRF.

Fadda GZ, Akmal M, Premdas FH, et al. Insulin release from pancreatic islets: effects of CRF and excess PTH. *Kidney Int* 1988;33:1066–1072.

The first direct evidence that insulin secretion is impaired in CRF as documented by in vitro perfusion of pancreatic islet. It also provides information on the role of excess PTH in this process.

Fadda GZ, Hajjar SM, Perna AF, et al. On the mechanism of impaired insulin secretion in chronic renal failure. *J Clin Invest* 1991;87:255–261.

Detailed study on the derangement in the cellular metabolism of pancreatic islet leading to impaired insulin secretion in CRF.

Fadda GZ, Thanakitcharu P, Smogorzewski M, et al. Parathyroid hormone raises cytosolic calcium in pancreatic islets: study on mechanisms. *Kidney Int* 1993; 43:554–560.

A detailed study examining the cellular pathways through PTH augments entry of calcium into the pancreatic islets.

Jones M, Persaud SJ. Protein kinase, protein phosphorylation, and the regulation of insulin secretion from pancreatic islets. *Endocr Rev* 1998;19:429–461.

An excellent review of the cellular pathways responsible for insulin secretion.

Mak RHK. Renal disease, insulin resistance and glucose intolerance. *Diabetes Rev* 1994;2:19–28.

A crisp review on carbohydrate metabolism in CRF.

Perna AF, Fadda GZ, Zhou X-J, et al. Mechanisms of impaired insulin secretion following chronic excess of parathyroid hormone. *Am J Physiol* 1990;259:F210–F216.

A study in normal rats demonstrating that chronic excess of PTH impairs insulin secretion and causes derangements in the cellular metabolism of islets similar to those noted in CRF.

PART 2
Lipid Metabolism

Bernard Lacour, Ziad Massy, and Tilman B. Drüeke

Dyslipidemia is a common complication of patients with chronic renal failure (CRF). Because a variety of changes in the level and the composition of lipoproteins have been recognized as cardiovascular risk factors, a detailed analysis of the lipid anomalies associated with the uremic state is in order. Moreover, the precise knowledge of their pathogenesis and the definition of their relative contribution to the atherosclerosis of patients with CRF are prerequisites for therapeutic interventions and prophylactic measures. Because the predominant quantitative lipoprotein anomaly is an accumulation of very-low-density lipoproteins (VLDL) together with hypertriglyceridemia, in the absence of an increase of serum total cholesterol, the question has long been asked to which extent this type of anomaly is atherogenic. The answer to this question, the hypothesis of a deleterious role of triglyceride (TG)-rich lipoproteins per se, has received considerable support. It is of note that this role appears to be linked to discrete atherogenic species within the TG-rich lipoproteins. The latter should be defined precisely for the evaluation of cardiovascular risk.

Another important problem is that the understanding of the link between lipid disturbances and atherosclerosis in uremia is confounded by the presence of numerous other interacting risk factors, such as age, gender, ethnic origin, underlying nephropathy, diabetes, hypertension, endocrine anomalies, modality of dialysis treatment, drug therapy, diet, smoking, and alcohol habits.

Newer findings of an association of CRF with lipoprotein modifications resulting from lipid peroxidation and the formation of advanced oxidation protein products (AOPP) and advanced glycation end-products (AGEs) allow one to envisage a role of modified lipoproteins in the often severe atheromatous complications of uremic patients. This area represents a new, promising avenue of research in the attempt to identify the relative place of each factor potentially involved in the dramatically high cardiovascular morbidity and mortality of uremic patients.

LIPOPROTEIN ANOMALIES IN CHRONIC RENAL FAILURE

CRF is generally associated with disturbances of lipoprotein metabolism. Many of these disturbances are already present in patients with a moderate degree of renal failure, and most of them are not corrected by hemodialysis. The dyslipoproteinemia of renal disease has characteristic abnormalities of apolipoprotein (apo) profile and lipoprotein composition.

Lipid and Lipoprotein Anomalies

Hypertriglyceridemia is the most common lipid abnormality in CRF patients. Its degree is moderate because serum TG concentration is roughly twice that of healthy subjects. It may affect up to 70% of the uremic population. It is present in children as well as in adults. Its prevalence, however, varies greatly according to geography, probably in relation to dietary habits. In most instances, serum TG start to increase during moderate to advanced renal failure, that is, the prevalence of hypertriglyceridemia increases when the glomerular filtration rate is reduced to below 50 ml/min or less. There is, however, no tight correlation between serum TG and renal function in terms of serum creatinine, nor between serum TG and the nature of nephropathy. The hypertriglyceridemia of uremic patients is due to an accumulation of VLDL, of the metabolically derived intermediate-density lipoproteins (IDL), and also of residual particles of intestinal origin.

In contrast, total serum cholesterol is either normal or only slightly increased in CRF. The mean serum concentration of low-density lipoproteins (LDL) is generally normal, whereas that of high-density lipoproteins (HDL) is diminished in correspondence with the increase of serum TG concentration, with a more marked decrease in HDL2 than in HDL3 (46% versus 24%). Thus cholesterol is redistributed from HDL to VLDL and LDL.

Qualitative analysis of lipoproteins, which can be isolated by density gradient, has shown that the VLDL of uremic patients have a relative enrichment in protein and cholesterol ester (CE), together with a decrease in TG. This CE enrichment may result in prolonged action of transfer proteins on VLDL, the metabolism of which is slowed. According to the literature, the uremic IDL are enriched either in proteins or in TG. The uremic LDL are characterized by a reduced size, by a relative decrease in CE, and a relative increase in TG content compared with normal LDL. This anomaly is predominant within mature LDL of a density of 1.043 g/ml, in which the CE:TG ratio is three times lower in uremic than in normal subjects. Another newly described change of LDL structure is their modification by AGE, oxidation, or carbamylation. Finally, both HDL2 and HDL3 of uremic patients are enriched in TG, whereas HDL3 are more specifically deficient in CE. The frequent reduction in HDL particle size has been found to be linked with insulin resistance.

Separation of lipoproteins by electrophoresis established that the hyperlipoproteinemia of CRF is most often of type IV according to Fredrickson's classification, and more rarely of type III. Isolated lipoproteins often have abnormal electrophoretic mobility. Thus in uremic patients the VLDL isolated by ultracentrifugation migrate in the beta position, whereas normal VLDL migrate in the pre-beta position.

Abnormalities of Apolipoproteins and of Lipoparticles

The serum apo pattern has been found to be in general accordance with the lipid findings. A significant reduction of apoAI and apoAII levels may be detected in early renal insufficiency and in normolipidemic uremic patients. This decrease is in direct relation with the decrease of HDL because only the latter lipoproteins contain these apo species. The decrease of apoAI is due to a reduction of lipoparticles (Lp) AI-AII rather than of LpAI alone. However, in continuous ambulatory peritoneal dialysis (CAPD) patients, a greater reduction in the levels of LpAI was reported compared with that of LpAI-AII. Finally, in uremic patients there is an increase of free apoAI levels in the serum fraction of a density greater than 1.21 g/ml, corresponding presumably to a weaker link of apoAI to uremic HDL particles than to normal HDL.

The serum concentration of apoB is normal or moderately increased, together with either normal or moderately increased total cholesterol. However, there is an increase of oxidized apoB100 in CRF patients. ApoB is distributed within VLDL, IDL, and mainly LDL. Therefore a moderate increase of apoB in the uremic patient may be associated with an accumulation of VLDL and IDL. The significance of apoB-containing Lp is different depending on the other apos associated with them. LpB, which contain only apoB as protein constituent and which are rich in CE, are normally predominant within LDL and remain in the normal concentration range in CRF. In contrast, LpB-CIII, which constitute part of residual particles formed during VLDL and chylomicron catabolism, may accumulate to a considerable extent (up to 5-fold) in uremic patients. LpB-E however, which also correspond to residual particles originating from the catabolism of TG-rich lipoproteins, do not increase during CRF. Unlike CRF patients not yet on dialysis, hemodialysis patients have a preferential accumulation of LpB-C-E (up to three times normal) and of LpB-E. The reason for such differences in Lp profiles between uremic patients not yet receiving dialysis and patients receiving hemodialysis treatment is still unknown.

Median Lp(a) concentration is increased in uremic patients. This increase is only observed in uremic patients with a high-molecular-weight isotype of apo(a), whereas patients with low-molecular-weight phenotypes show unchanged Lp(a) values in relation to apo(a) phenotype-matched controls. The increase in Lp(a) concentration already occurs in moderate renal failure and is always present in hemodialysis patients. Lp(a) concentrations increase with the progression of renal failure, as documented by the correlation existing between Lp(a) and serum creatinine or glomerular filtration rate. In hemodialysis patients Lp(a) is characterized by an elevated content in TG and apoCIII in comparison with that of controls. Lp(a) levels are higher in patients treated by CAPD than those treated by hemodialysis. A stimulation of hepatic synthesis consecutive to the loss of protein through dialysis or to an increased cytokine production has been postulated as a possible explanation for the higher levels found in CAPD patients.

Concerning exchange apo, the characteristic element of the uremic profile is a considerable increase of apoCIII, reminiscent of the augmentation observed in type IV hypertriglyceridemia in which apoCIII and TG are tightly associated. In the uremic patient, the increase of apoCIII is, however, disproportionate compared with that of serum TG and has even been observed in patients with normal serum TG values. In contrast, plasma apoCI concentration is subnormal and that of apoCII more moderately increased than that of apoCIII. This leads to a decrease of CII:CIII ratio corresponding to the ratio of activator/inhibitor of lipoprotein lipase (LPL). Moreover, the apoCIII molecules are abnormally rich in sialic acid in uremic patients. This leads to a disequilibrium of the ratio between the isoforms $CIII_2$, $CIII_1$, and $CIII_0$.

Plasma apoAIV concentrations are markedly increased in CRF, with an abnormal distribution within VLDL, IDL, and LDL.

The mean plasma concentration of apoE is normal or only slightly diminished in uremia. The absence of an increase in apoE in the face of hypertriglyceridemia suggests a preferential formation from VLDL of LpB-C rather than B-E. This could be due to the reduction of apoE synthesis in association with a reduced functional nephron mass. Concentrations of total apoE are only moderately, even though significantly, elevated in hemodialysis patients, perhaps by stimulation of apoE synthesis by interleukins due to activation of lymphocytes and monocyte/macrophages. The distribution of apoE phenotypes and apoE allelic frequency among the CAPD patients corresponds to that of the healthy population, as reported in a Swedish study.

Analysis of apo distribution within lipoprotein classes allows identification of anomalies that may be involved in the disturbances of lipoprotein metabolism in uremic patients. The TG-rich lipoproteins, namely VLDL and IDL, are characterized by the presence of apoB48, with a decrease of the CII:CIII ratio and an increase of the CIII:E ratio within the lipoproteins. Uremic LDL contain an excessive amount of apoE, whereas normal LDL are nearly devoid of apoE. Uremic HDL are characterized by a relative diminution of their apoAI and apoAII content, an enrichment in apoCIII content, and a relative deficit of apoCII leading to a decrease in CII:CIII ratio. The apoCIII of HDL could have taken the place of apoAI within these lipoproteins and correspond to the nonexchangeable pool of apoCIII. In normolipidemic subjects, more than 60% of apoCIII and apoE are present in HDL, whereas the remaining apos occur in VLDL and LDL. In CRF patients, approximately 60% to 80% of the apoCIII and apoE are present in VLDL and LDL, characterizing an inefficacy of processes responsible for the degradation of TG-rich lipoproteins.

The importance of apo as markers of uremic dyslipoproteinemia is illustrated by the fact that certain abnormalities of the apo profile already exist during the initial stage of CRF. Thus a decrease in apoAI and apoAII and an increase in apoC-III are observed even before hypertriglyceridemia occurs. The apoAI:apoCIII ratio is the most discriminating parameter between control subjects and uremic patients.

Taken together, uremic patients have a special type of dyslipoproteinemia that is characterized by hypertriglyceridemia with an accumulation of VLDL and particularly of IDL, and TG enrichment of LDL and HDL, together with a decrease of HDL cholesterol. There is a different relative distribution of the principal apos, compared with healthy subjects. The wide distribution of TG within the various lipoprotein classes is highly suggestive of a prolonged stagnation in plasma of particles originating from VLDL catabolism, with a preferential accumulation of LpB-C and LpB-C-E within VLDL, IDL, and even LDL. The most characteristic feature of dyslipoproteinemia in CRF is the accumulation of partially delipidized, TG-rich, apoB-containing lipoproteins enriched in apoC peptides and distributed characteristically in the IDL density range, irrespective of fasting TG concentrations.

DISTURBED LIPOPROTEIN METABOLISM IN CHRONIC RENAL FAILURE

Lipoproteins are useful for the transport of hydrophobic lipids TG and CE in the circulation, which are hidden in a core under a layer of hydrophilic surface components containing free cholesterol, phospholipids, and apos. The latter play an important role in the orientation of the metabolism of the different lipoproteins, either by allowing their recognition by receptors, or by controlling the activity of enzymes that are involved in lipoprotein metabolism. The normal endogenous lipoprotein metabolism can be considered as the sum of two pathways. The first is that of VLDL and LDL metabolism, which allows at its terminal step the influx of cholesterol into peripheral tissues. The second is that of HDL metabolism, which corresponds to the efflux of cholesterol from peripheral tissues and also to the delivery of cholesterol to at least some tissues, particularly the liver and endocrine tissues. Both pathways are disturbed in uremia. Figure 74.5 schematically represents the metabolism of TG (VLDL, IDL, and LDL) and that of cholesterol (HDL2 and HDL3), as well as the interactions that exist between the two metabolic pathways.

VLDL and LDL Metabolism

There is a decrease in the clearance of lipid emulsions in CRF and a decrease in VLDL turnover rate, in close inverse correlation with serum TG concentrations. These findings clearly indicate that the catabolism of TG-rich particles is diminished in the uremic patient.

Lipoprotein Lipase Activity in Uremia

Numerous studies have established a marked decrease of LPL activity in uremia. This decrease has been found in several tissues, including the vascular endothelium. The LPL associated with the glycosaminoglycans of the vascular endothelium can be explored by the standardized heparin test, LPL having a higher affinity for heparin than heparan sulfate of the capillary wall. Postheparin lipolytic activity (PHLA) is markedly dimin-

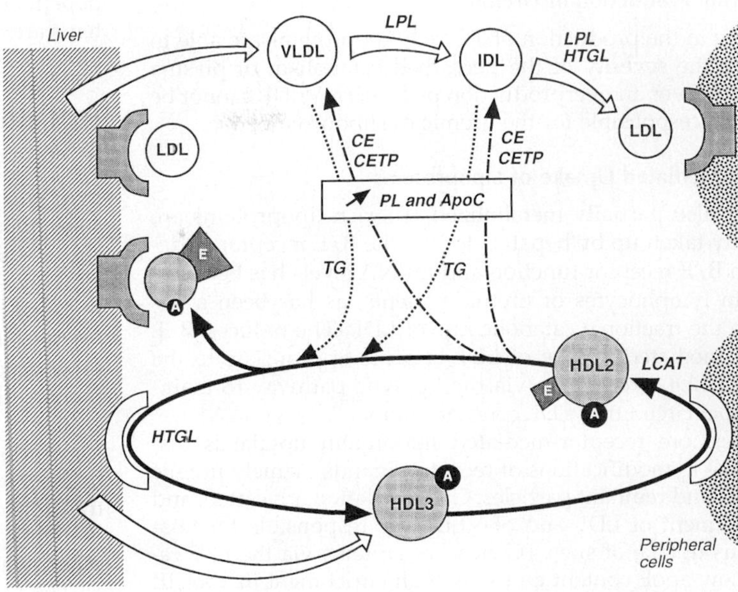

Figure 74.5. Schematic representation of the metabolism of TG (VLDL, IDL, and LDL) and cholesterol (HDL2 and HDL3), as well as of the interactions between these two metabolic pathways.

ished in uremic plasma. This decrease is already observed at a glomerular filtration rate of 50 ml/min, even in the absence of any increase in TG serum concentrations. It is always present in uremic patients treated by hemodialysis. Several mechanisms explain this decrease.

First, the decrease in LPL activity may be due to a defect in the synthesis of the enzyme itself. LPL is synthesized by the parenchymal cell under the influence of insulin and then transported in its active dimer form by an unknown mechanism to the luminal side of the capillary endothelium. Reduced LPL synthesis in uremic patients can be attributed to the well-known state of insulin resistance or a relative cellular deficit of insulin. LPL activity is already reduced at early stages of renal failure, in coincidence with the appearance of abnormal insulin metabolism and insulin resistance. The reduction of LPL activity precedes the increased plasma TG levels. In dialysis patients, an inverse correlation between postheparin fractional clearance rates of ultralipid and plasma concentrations of insulin has been established. Thus uremia results in a marked downregulation of LPL expression, with the decline in LPL activity being directly related to LPL mRNA in all tissues tested. Furthermore, in the uremic rat, the administration of insulin leads to an increase in LPL activity of adipose tissue and normalizes the hypertriglyceridemia.

It appears that the state of secondary hyperparathyroidism of CRF plays a major role in low LPL activity, and parathyroidectomy may improve hyperlipidemia. Similarly, in CRF animals, parathyroidectomy can completely normalize LPL mRNA, protein mass, and catalytic activity, and partially ameliorate hypertriglyceridemia. Parathyroid hormone (PTH) could exert its effect via a direct action on LPL secretion, as reported in mature 3T3-L1 adipocytes *in vitro.* Additional discussion on the interaction between excess PTH and LDL metabolism is found in Chapter 68, Part 1. Furthermore, calcitriol induces LPL expression in these cells, probably by improving insulin sensitivity of peripheral tissues. The decrease of calcitriol synthesis already present in early CRF could contribute to low LPL activity.

Second, the low LPL activity of uremia is also due to the existence of circulating inhibitors of the enzyme. Thus sera from uremic patients inhibit LPL activity in various *in vitro* models. They also activate LPL from human PHLA less efficiently than sera from healthy controls. An improvement in lipoprotein profile has been associated with high-flux dialysis, which is assumed to increase the removal of LPL inhibitor(s). ApoCIII and pre-β-HDL, described as apoAI associated with phospholipids in the nonlipoprotein fraction of plasma, have been suggested to be inhibitors of LPL activity. No free CIII accumulation has been documented, but pre-β-HDL was markedly increased in uremic patients.

Third, VLDL that accumulate in uremia are bad substrates for LPL. Moreover, the extent of lipolysis is reduced with uremic VLDL as compared with normal VLDL, in agreement with the accumulation of remnant particles. This can be attributed to the disturbed apo composition of uremic VLDL, namely an increase of apoCIII as well as a decrease of the apoCII : apoCIII ratio within VLDL leading to decreased LPL activity. Moreover, the excess of sialylation of apoCIII makes TG-rich particles particularly poor substrates for LPL. Other modifications such as carbamylation, oxidation, and terminal glycation are probably involved as well, decreasing VLDL affinity for LPL. Finally, in hemodialysis patients an intermittent depletion of tissue LPL stores occurs due to the thrice weekly administration of heparin (see following discussion).

Hepatic Lipase and Lecithin-Cholesterol Acyltransferase Activity in Uremia

Considering various studies about the role of hepatic lipase (HL) in VLDL and LDL metabolism, it is possible that this enzyme participates only at the last step of their conversion to LDL. Its role in the impairment of TG-rich catabolism probably is of minor importance, perhaps via the level of surface-material exchange with HDL3. The decreased catabolism of TG-rich lipoproteins could be aggravated by a reduced lecithin-cholesterol acyltransferase (LCAT) activity responsible for the diminution of apoC and apoE transfer from HDL to VLDL and IDL. HL metabolism and activity are impaired in uremia due, in major part, to the state of secondary hyperparathyroidism. This issue is discussed in Chapter 68, Part 1.

Triglyceride Production in Uremia

Variations in the production of TG-rich lipoproteins are able to modulate the severity of the perturbed catabolism of plasma lipids. However an overproduction of TG-rich VLDL cannot be held solely responsible for the uremic dyslipoproteinemia.

Receptor-Mediated Uptake of Lipoproteins

LDL and also partially metabolized, TG-rich lipoproteins are essentially taken up by hepatocytes via the B/E receptor. A decrease in B/E receptor function and mRNA levels has been observed in lymphocytes of uremic patients, as has been a decrease in the fractional catabolic rate of LDL. The reduced B/E receptor–mediated uptake of LDL appears appropriate to the decreased LDL production via the lipolytic pathway to maintain normal circulating LDL concentrations.

Furthermore receptor-mediated lipoprotein uptake is disturbed due to modifications of receptor ligands, namely uremic LDL, IDL, and remnant particles. Carbamylation, glycation, and TG enrichment of LDL and of VLDL are responsible for less-efficacious uptake of such TG-rich lipoproteins via the B/E receptor. Low apoE content and very high enrichment in apoCIII of TG-rich lipoproteins constitute two other reasons for retarded removal of such particles via the B/E receptor, leading to the accumulation of TG-rich lipoproteins in the circulation and hypertriglyceridemia.

In addition to disturbed endogenous lipoprotein metabolism, postprandial lipoprotein metabolism is also delayed, as evidenced by a vitamin A loading test revealing a long-term retention of chylomicron remnants in the circulation of uremic subjects. These particles are taken up by an apoE-specific receptor, and uremic particles with a low apoE content constitute ligands with low affinity for this receptor. A receptor with high affinity for VLDL, named *VLDL receptor,* was identified. It binds apoE-containing lipoproteins, but not LDL, and is mainly expressed in skeletal muscle, heart, adipose tissue, and brain tissue, which use fatty acids for energy metabolism. The distribution of the VLDL receptor is remarkably similar to that of LPL. A marked decrease of VLDL-receptor mRNA and protein expression has been shown in the heart and skeletal muscle of chronically uremic rats. This downregulation probably participates in the disturbed lipid metabolism of uremia.

Finally, uremic serum also contains a factor(s) that enhance(s) macrophage scavenger receptor activity by increasing the amount of receptor protein, at least in U 937 cells. This receptor mediates uptake of modified LDL, such as oxidized LDL, by macrophages. The enhancement could be due to elevated plasma macrophage colony-stimulating factor. Enhanced uptake of modified LDL obviously would favor uremia-associated atherosclerosis.

Lp(a) Metabolism in Uremia

Lp(a) is taken up by B-E receptors less effectively than LDL. The longer sojourn in the plasma increases the risk of infiltration of the arterial intima and hence the risk of oxidation and/or uptake by smooth muscle cells and macrophages. Moreover, it has a high affinity for gangliosides and proteoglycans in the arterial wall. The high thrombogenic and atherogenic action of Lp(a) could also be explained by competition between Lp(a) and plasminogen for the plasminogen receptors located at the endothelial cell surface and by inhibition of the activation of plasminogen by tissue-type plasminogen activator.

It would appear important to define precisely whether the augmentation of serum Lp(a) concentration is related to the decrease of uremic LDL uptake via altered affinity or activity of the B-E receptors during CRF. However Lp(a) metabolism is independent of that of LDL. Thus the fate of these two lipoproteins after renal transplantation is opposite, possibly due to the effect of immunosuppressive drugs.

HDL Metabolism and the Reverse Cholesterol Transport

In uremia, the generally observed decrease in HDL is merely the consequence of hypertriglyceridemia. Even in normolipemic subjects there is a correlation between LPL activity and HDL cholesterol or between lipolytic activity and the magnitude of the intravascular HDL2 pool. Given these interdependencies, uremic HDL2 are diminished because lipolysis is decreased due to reduced LPL activity and because HDL3 levels, which are the precursors of HDL2, are diminished.

The cholesterol esterification rate in uremic plasma is significantly decreased, probably not only due to weak LCAT activity in these patients, but also to the inhibition of cholesterol ester transfer toward VLDL and LDL. The decreased LCAT activity of uremia, in contrast to other hypertriglyceridemic states, is explained, at least in part, by the decrease of apoAI concentration.

The rate of esterified cholesterol transfer between lipoproteins is diminished in hemodialysis patients. The lipoprotein-devoid fraction is responsible for the decrease of CE transfer protein (CETP) activity, because it contains a high concentration of inhibitor. The transfer of cholesterol from HDL toward VLDL and LDL plays an essential role in reverse cholesterol transport, allowing depletion of cells of cholesterol and transport to the liver. The defect of such a mechanism leads necessarily to cholesterol accumulation in peripheral tissues, favoring the development of atherosclerosis. In CAPD patients, CETP activity has been reported to be increased, possibly due to increased synthesis in response to protein loss into the dialysate.

HDL3 binding to cellular receptors is a high affinity, saturable process, mediated by apoAI. If spatial configuration is an important factor in HDL3 recognition by the receptor, replacement of apoAI by apoCIII in uremia may lead to inhibition of HDL binding and thereby disturb HDL metabolism as well as reverse cholesterol transport. Furthermore, the decrease in LpAI is important to consider because only LpAI is responsible for cholesterol efflux and reverse cholesterol transport from peripheral tissues to the liver.

Thus reduced LCAT activity in connection with reduced HL activity and decreased apoAI and apoAII concentrations contribute to retarded conversion of HDL3 to HDL2 by decreasing the rate of cholesterol esterification.

HORMONAL, NUTRITIONAL, AND TREATMENT-RELATED FACTORS INVOLVED IN THE DYSLIPOPROTEINEMIA OF CRF PATIENTS

Several of the endocrine disturbances of CRF contribute to the uremic hyperlipidemia. Moreover, decreased nutrient intakes and malnutrition, either due to recommended dietary changes or to the uremic state, may also play a role. Finally, a number of drugs prescribed to uremic patients on a regular, long-term basis may alter lipoprotein metabolism.

Hormonal and Metabolic Dysregulation (Table 74.2)

Several hormones play an important role in lipoprotein metabolism, including insulin, glucagon, the thyroid hormones, PTH, and adrenal steroids.

TABLE 74.2. Hormonal and Metabolic Factors Involved in the Dyslipoproteinemia of Uremic Patients

Factor	Principal Effect(s)
Insulin resistance	↓ LPL synthesis and activity
Glucagon (↑)	ND
Parathyroid hormone (↑)	↓ LPL and HL synthesis
Thyroid hormones (↓)	≠ TG; ≠ total cholesterol; ≠ Lp(a) (?)
Testosterone (↓)	↓ HDL cholesterol; ≠ TG
Leptin (↑)	ND
Growth hormone resistance	≠ Lp(a)
Carnitine (↓)	≠ TG (?)

HDL, high-density lipoprotein; HL, hepatic lipase; Lp, lipoparticles; LPL, lipoprotein lipase; ND, not determined; TG, triglyceride.

Insulin and Glucagon

LPL synthesis is mainly regulated by insulin. Disturbances of insulin secretion or its action on target tissues lead therefore to changes in the activity of this enzyme. The downregulation of LPL synthesis in uremia is probably largely due to peripheral-tissue resistance to the action of insulin, even in the presence of hyperinsulinemia. To what extent the increase in plasma glucagon levels in CRF also contributes directly to the disturbances of lipoprotein metabolism or only indirectly via its contribution to an abnormal carbohydrate metabolism remains to be seen.

The abnormal carbohydrate metabolism has been shown to favor the excessive formation of AGE not only in diabetic, but also in nondiabetic uremic patients. AGE transformation of LDL slows their catabolism and probably also enhances their uptake by macrophages via the AGE receptor (RAGE), thereby favoring the formation of foam cells and atheromatous lesions. Whether excessive serum levels of AGE-transformed apoB, the main apo component of LDL, can be more effectively removed by high-flux than by low-flux dialysis membranes, as has been reported in recent studies, and if so whether this will result in a decreased incidence of atheromatous lesions in uremic patients remains to be demonstrated.

Parathyroid Hormone

The secondary hyperparathyroidism of uremia also adversely influences lipoprotein metabolism. Thus dialysis patients with severe hyperparathyroidism often have a more-marked degree of hypertriglyceridemia than euparathyroid patients, and parathyroidectomy can correct this anomaly at least partially. High plasma PTH levels delay TG metabolism by interfering with LPL and HL action. This effect is attributed to reduced synthesis and/or secretion of LPL and HL enzyme protein. In the uremic animal, the downregulation of the expression of these two enzymes can be reversed by parathyroidectomy. Because severe parathyroid overfunction is associated with insulin deficiency, at least in experimental uremia, this pathway is one of the possible mechanisms of insufficient LPL activity. A direct, PTH/PTH-related protein (PTHrP) receptor–mediated effect of PTH via an elevation of intracellular free-calcium concentration is also possible. Thus decreased LPL activity in uremic rats could be corrected by administration of the calcium channel blocker, verapamil, *in vivo*, and treatment of adipose cells by PTH led to a reduction of LPL secretion *in vitro*. Further discussion on this topic is found in Chapter 68, Part 1.

Thyroid Hormones

The role of disturbed thyroid function is generally considered as being of only minor importance because the prevalence of hypothyroidism in dialysis patients has been estimated to be between 0% and 10%, depending on centers and regions of each study. Hypothyroid dialysis patients have serum TG levels that are generally higher than those of euthyroid dialysis patients. This is due to a defect in TG catabolism and a change in lipoprotein composition. Because in the general population hypothyroid patients have high serum total cholesterol and Lp(a) levels and clinical observations indicate that treatment with thyroid hormones reduces both serum total cholesterol and Lp(a) concentrations in such patients, a study has been carried out in hemodialysis patients to see whether the non–hormonally active isomer of L-thyroxine, namely dextro-thyroxine (D-thyroxine) might have similar effects on serum Lp(a) as the endogenous hormone. This was indeed the case because the administration of D-thyroxine reduced elevated Lp(a) levels by nearly 30%.

Testosterone

The decrease of plasma testosterone levels in uremia could also contribute to lipoprotein anomalies because a positive correlation has been observed between serum testosterone and HDL cholesterol, and a negative correlation has been seen between serum testosterone and TG. The prolonged administration of the nor-17α-alkylated androgen, nandrolone decanoate, has been shown to decrease median serum Lp(a) concentration in hemodialysis patients by more than 60%, although concomitantly serum apoB and TG increased and serum HDL cholesterol and apoAI decreased.

Leptin

Leptin functions as a lipostat mechanism through modulation of satiety signals. Obese individuals have markedly elevated leptin levels. Leptin is partly cleared by the kidney and is not removed by hemodialysis using modified cellulose membrane. Serum leptin concentrations (mostly free leptin) have been found to be approximately three to four times higher in dialysis patients than in healthy volunteers matched for age, gender, and body mass index. The highest leptin levels were observed in uremic patients with signs of inflammation. Of interest, serum leptin correlates with serum insulin in dialysis patients independently of body fat. On the other hand, however, serum leptin is also associated in them with body mass index. Thus even in CRF serum, leptin appears to be a good marker for body fat content. Detailed discussion on leptin in uremia is found in Chapter 74, Part 5.

Growth Hormone

It must be outlined that, in uremic patients, the treatment with growth hormone is able to increase markedly Lp(a) serum levels.

Carnitine

A deficit in carnitine may develop in patients with longstanding, severe CRF not yet on dialysis, and in dialysis patients suffering from malnutrition. It is observed only exceptionally in well-nourished patients. Because carnitine is involved in the transport of long-chain fatty acids across the mitochondrial membrane for subsequent oxidation, a deficit in carnitine leads to an increase in TG synthesis through the elevation of free fatty acids in serum. Another potential mechanism, involving carnitine indirectly, is the reported decrease in CRF of muscular carnitine palmitoyl transferase activity, which also leads to free fatty acid accumulation and hypertriglyceridemia. The activity of this enzyme has been shown to be inhibited by parathyroid overfunction. Several uncontrolled trials suggested a beneficial effect of exogenous carnitine administration with respect to hypertriglyceridemia correction in selected dialysis patients. In contrast, a large, prospective, controlled trial has not been able to confirm this in the standard dialysis patient population.

However, a metaanalysis of 25 studies in hemodialysis patients showed a beneficial effect of carnitine on serum TG levels.

Nutritional Factors

A low-protein diet is generally recommended to arrest or slow down the progression of CRF. Long-term follow-up with this type of diet showed no change in plasma lipid or apo levels. However, because such a diet implies the ingestion of large amounts of complex sugars and low amounts of saturated fat, it may lead to a decrease in serum TG concentration. Similarly, the supplementation of such regimens with essential amino acids results in a reduction of serum TG and cholesterol levels, as well as the correction of decreased HDL cholesterol and apoAI levels in patients with CRF.

On the other hand, simple dietary restriction of carbohydrates and cholesterol, without changing protein intake, also leads to a reduction of hypertriglyceridemia via a significant decrease of TG production, especially in case the intake of polyunsaturated fatty acids is increased concomitantly. An increase in the polyunsaturated, nonesterified fatty acids:saturated fatty acids ratio may improve the lipid anomalies of hemodialysis patients by increasing the catabolism of TG-rich particles.

Treatment-Related Factors

Dialysis Treatment

The hemodialysis procedure itself appears to play only a minor role in the various disturbances of lipoprotein metabolism in chronic uremia, although it may improve some of them. Compared with the patient in terminal renal failure who is not yet treated by dialysis, the hemodialysis patient has lower LDL cholesterol and apoB, and higher apoAI, apoAII, and apoE levels. Moreover, there are differences with respect to Lp accumulating within VLDL and IDL.

The composition of the dialysis fluid, including type of buffer and presence or absence of glucose, is of importance and may contribute to the degree of hyperlipidemia. Thus proatherogenic serum lipoprotein levels are higher in hemodialysis patients treated with an acetate buffer than in those dialyzed against a bicarbonate buffer.

The use of highly permeable, synthetic dialysis membranes has been shown to induce an increase in serum LPL activity, a decrease in serum TG, and an increase in serum HDL, compared with use of cellulosic membranes.

CAPD is responsible for the aggravation of several lipoprotein anomalies, that is, an increase in serum total cholesterol, LDL cholesterol, TG and VLDL levels, and a decrease in HDL cholesterol. This type of lipoprotein disturbance is correlated with the amount of glucose instilled into and absorbed from the peritoneal cavity during dialytic exchanges. The continuous absorption of glucose leads to hyperinsulinemia with an increase in VLDL synthesis and hence in serum TG levels. However, CAPD may improve other lipid disturbances of uremia, such as cholesterol ester transfer from peripheral tissues to the liver, which becomes close to normal, in contrast to what is observed in patients treated by hemodialysis. Finally, more or less marked amounts of LDL and HDL are lost into the peritoneal space on a day-to-day basis, resulting in a continuous depletion of apoAI, apoAII, apoCII, apoCIII, and even apoB. This loss may vary from negligible to important, depending on the overall protein loss across the peritoneal membrane. The regular loss of albumin by the same route could play an additional role in the frequently more severe hyperlipoproteinemia of CAPD patients than that of hemodialysis patients.

The use of heparin is an integral part of each hemodialysis session. Its intravenous injection leads to a reduced cellular pool of the two lipolytic enzymes, LPL and HL, by stimulating their release from the vascular endothelium into the circulation. This action aggravates the LPL deficit associated with the uremic state. Moreover, heparin inhibits LCAT activity via an increase in circulating nonesterified fatty acids. Several studies in chronic hemodialysis patients have shown an advantage of low-molecular-weight (LMW) heparin over standard heparin. Thus the long-term use of LMW heparin led to a decrease in serum total cholesterol and TG levels compared with conventional heparin, probably via a less marked induction of LPL release from the vessel wall.

Drug Therapy

It is well known that thiazide diuretics used for the treatment of arterial hypertension may cause several anomalies of lipid metabolism, including an increase in serum TG and LDL cholesterol. Similarly, β-adrenergic blockers may worsen hypertriglyceridemia because they reduce lipolytic activity and thereby retard the catabolism of TG-rich particles. However, the negative effects of the β-adrenergic blockers have not been found consistently in all studies.

LIPOPROTEIN OXIDATION ABNORMALITIES IN CRF PATIENTS

Oxidative stress, which occurs when there is excessive free-radical production and/or low antioxidant defense, may lead to the oxidation of lipoproteins, including LDL. The generation of lipid peroxides is followed by their breakdown and release of aldehydes and ketones, such as malondialdehyde (MDA) and 4-hydroxynonenal, which can modify lysine residues on apoB. The oxidation of the protein moiety of LDL also occurs, directly modifying apoB. The clinical relevance of each oxidized moiety remains to be determined. Oxidized lipoproteins may contribute to atherogenesis by several mechanisms. The balance between the production of free-oxygen radicals and antioxidant defense mechanisms determines the formation of the biologically active, oxidized lipoproteins.

Several lines of evidence indicate that excessive oxidation of lipoproteins occurs in CRF patients. The evidence includes (a) the demonstration that lipid peroxidation markers such as MDA or conjugated diene concentrations are increased in plasma (although not in all reports), and particularly in lipoproteins, peripheral blood cells, and adipose tissue and (b) the observation of increased levels of circulating oxidized LDL, as well as reactive circulating antibodies directed against them. Yet, there is no demonstration by immunohistochemistry methods to date that atherosclerotic lesions in CRF patients contain materials reactive with antibodies generated against oxidized LDL, as shown in the general population. Moreover, the precise role of oxidized lipoproteins as cardiovascular risk factors and the potential benefit of antioxidant therapies in CRF patients, as well as in the population at large, need to be evaluated. It should be noted that several studies in CRF patients have assessed the susceptibility of LDL to oxidation *in vitro*, with conflicting results. However, the factors influencing the duration of the lag-phase, which was used in these studies to measure the resistance of LDL to oxidation, may differ between *in vitro* and *in vivo* conditions. Thus it remains to be seen whether determinations of the susceptibility of LDL to oxidation *in vitro* are a good means to assess the increase of LDL oxidation present in CRF patients *in vivo*.

Free Radical Production in CRF Patients

Free radicals, which are continuously formed *in vivo* from a number of sources, are likely to be increased in CRF. The presence of oxidizing species in the plasma of CRF patients has been detected using electron spin resonance spectroscopy. Moreover, the presence of numerous oxidative products in the plasma of CRF patients other than lipid peroxidation materials (e.g., methylguanidine, a peroxidative product of creatinine, and AOPP) has been well documented.

The origin(s) of this increased free-radical production in CRF patients remains unsettled at present. Nicotinamide adenine dinucleotide (NADH)/nicotinamide adenine dinucleotide phosphate (NADPH) oxidase is the major source of superoxide anion ($O_2^{\cdot -}$) in polymorphonuclear (PMN) cells, endothelial cells, and smooth muscle cells (Fig. 74.6). When evaluating $O_2^{\cdot -}$ production by PMN cells from CRF patients with chemiluminescent methods, many authors found a decrease in their capacity to produce $O_2^{\cdot -}$, except during the dialysis session. This defect can probably be attributed to impaired hexose monophosphate shunt pathway activity, delivering energy to NADPH oxidase in PNM cells. However, the role of vascular NADH/NADPH oxidase in $O_2^{\cdot -}$ production, which differs from that of neutrophils in many respects, remains to be evaluated in CRF patients.

Iron ions are themselves free radicals, and ferrous iron takes part in electron transfer reactions with molecular oxygen to generate $O_2^{\cdot -}$. Generation of $O_2^{\cdot -}$, in the presence of iron ions of any source, can lead to the formation of hydroxyl radical (OH^-) by Fenton chemistry and could initiate lipid peroxidation (Fig. 74.6). In the absence of iron supplementation, CRF patients often develop a state of iron deficiency. Iron supplementation has been shown to increase lipid peroxidation in them, except in the case of a concomitant treatment with recombinant human erythropoietin. Copper ions also catalyze formation of OH^{Σ} from hydrogen peroxide (H_2O_2). Conflicting results have been reported concerning the copper status of CRF patients.

The myeloperoxidase (MPO), which is present in azurophil granules of neutrophils and monocytes, can generate a variety of reactive oxygen species, including hypochlorus acid (HOCl) (Fig. 74.6). The latter is a potent oxidizing agent. These highly reactive species lead to the generation of several protein adducts, including *p*-hydroxyphenyl-acetaldehyde, glycolaldehyde, 2-hydroxy-propanol, and 3-chloro-tyrosine, which act on

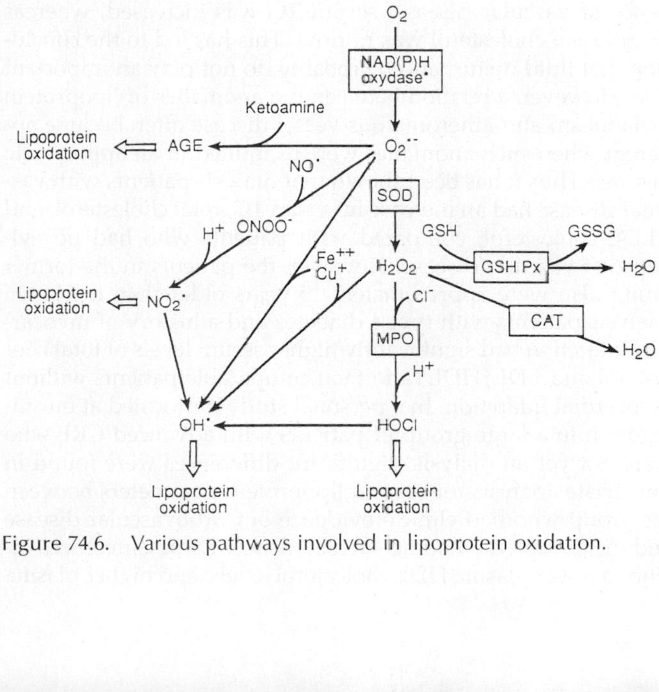

Figure 74.6. Various pathways involved in lipoprotein oxidation.

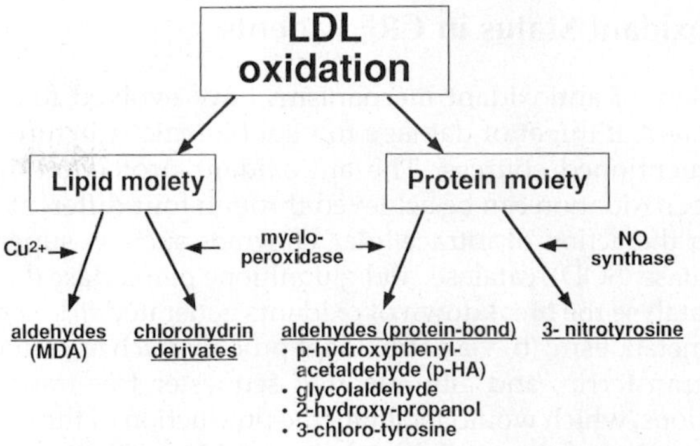

Figure 74.7. Generation of modified lipid and protein products by various oxidation mechanisms, including copper ion, myeloperoxidase, and NO synthase.

a variety of target tissues, which in turn are powerful oxidizing agents (Fig. 74.7). Tyrosyl radicals also may undergo lipid peroxidation. Enzymatically active MPO, and oxidatively modified lipoproteins and proteins by the action of MPO have been detected in human atherosclerotic vascular lesions. Moreover, LDL isolated from atherosclerotic tissue in such patients are not enriched in protein-oxidation products characteristically induced by the action of free-metal ions, pointing to the importance of amino acid–derived aldehydes generated by MPO in the formation of atherosclerosis. Few data are available concerning MPO activity and oxidation products in the plasma and the arterial vessels of CRF patients. Increased plasma MPO activity in hemodialysis patients has been shown in one study. In another study, AOPP, which are probably chlorinated products, have been found to be present at high levels in the plasma of CRF patients. The presence of HOCl-modified lipoproteins and other proteins has been demonstrated in diseased kidney tissues as well, including vascular structure.

Increased AGE levels may be another source of free-radical production in CRF patients. AGE formation involves oxidative modification of fructolysine (a compound containing a ketoamine link) and the formation of the AGEs, carboxymethyllysine, and pentosidine (Fig. 74.7). However, AGEs may be formed also nonoxidatively by interactions between proteins and dissociation products of fructolysine. Elevated AGE levels lead in turn to the generation of reactive oxygen intermediates. In CRF patients, there is an increased rate of LDL modification by AGE, independent of glucose level. AGE moieties are present on both the apo and the lipid components of LDL in such patients. Experimental data suggest that circulating AGE peptides can impair plasma clearance kinetics of native LDL, and may increase LDL susceptibility to oxidative changes. However, there is yet no data concerning the role of AGE-modified LDL on free-radical production in CRF patients.

Nitric oxide (NO) is a relatively stable free radical that plays a central role in the regulation of vasomotor tone and a wide variety of other biologic events. However, NO also reacts with $O_2^{\cdot -}$ to yield peroxynitrite ($ONOO^-$), a reactive nitrogen species that promotes LDL oxidation via the formation of nitrogen dioxide gas (HNO_2^-) and OH^- (Fig. 74.6). This latter reaction leads to inactivation of NO. In CRF patients, there is evidence in favor of NO deficiency, which presumably results both from reduced arginine availability (because the kidney is a major site of endogenous arginine synthesis) and accumulation of endogenous NO inhibitors secondary to decreased renal clearance. Thus it is unlikely that NO metabolism plays an important role in free-radical production in CRF.

Antioxidant Status in CRF Patients

A variety of antioxidant mechanisms have evolved to combat the potential threat of damage to vital biologic structures from aforementioned sources. The antioxidant protection against lipid peroxidation can be achieved through four different ways: (a) via the action of intracellular enzymes such as superoxide dismutase (SOD), catalase, and glutathione peroxidase (GSHPx) that catalyse the breakdown of oxidants generated *in situ* by cellular metabolism; (b) via antioxidant proteins such as ceruloplasmin, transferrin, and albumin that sequester free-transitional metal ions, which would facilitate the production of the OH^-; (c) via the action of water-soluble, chain-breaking antioxidants such as ascorbate (that however may also function as an oxidant), and lipid-soluble, chain-breaking antioxidants such as tocopherol, ubiquinone, vitamin A (retinol), and carotenoids that prevent the propagation phase of lipid peroxidation; and (d) via the action of HDL enzymes such as paraoxonase and platelet-activating factor acetyl hydrolase that cause the destruction of the oxidized lipids.

Conflicting data have been reported in the literature regarding the levels and/or the activities of SOD, glutathione, glutathione-related enzymes, trace elements (selenium, zinc, copper), ceruloplasmin, and transferrin in CRF patients. Consequently, it is difficult to assess their role in antioxidant defense of CRF patients. Of note, the deficit of hexose monophosphate shunt pathway activity may cause a reduction in antioxidant reserve in CRF patients because NADPH is a cofactor required to recycle the oxidized glutathione back to the effective reduced form. Moreover, serum albumin, which can bind copper and scavenge HOCl, is frequently decreased in some CRF patients, especially in those who suffer from malnutrition.

Vitamin C deficiency has been observed in CRF patients due to dietary restriction of fresh fruit and vegetables to avoid hyperkalemia, and due to vitamin C loss during dialysis. However, others reported plasma vitamin C concentrations within the normal range, in the absence of any supplementation. Because vitamin C plays a key role in recycling tocopherol at the aqueous lipid interface, a depletion of vitamin C is therefore likely to lead to rapid loss of LDL tocopherol in an oxidizing environment.

Vitamin E (alpha-tocopherol) appears to be the most important molecule, providing protection against free-radical–induced oxidative damage of LDL and biologic membranes. Plasma and LDL vitamin E concentrations in CRF patients have been shown to be usually normal, whereas erythrocyte and mononuclear cell concentrations appear to be decreased. The reported inefficiency of vitamin E in CRF patients to protect LDL particles against oxidation, despite a normal level, may be due to an alteration of its function resulting from vitamin C deficiency.

High plasma, liver, and skin concentrations of retinol occur in CRF patients, and probably result from the elevated concentrations of retinol-binding protein that accumulates in CRF, and from reduced urinary excretion of polar vitamin A metabolites. A normal plasma α- and β-carotene status has been reported for CRF patients. However, in one study a significant deficiency of plasma lycopene, which is the most reactive antioxidant carotenoid found in physiologic amounts in humans, was observed in such patients.

Preliminary reports have shown decreased plasma ubiquinone (CoQ_{10}) levels in CRF patients. Extracellular CoQ_{10} is incorporated and transported within lipoprotein particles, particularly within LDL. It has been found to inhibit the initiation and propagation of lipid peroxidation. It is possible that the decreased plasma CoQ_{10} levels in CRF patients are due to an elevated consumption of CoQ_{10} to scavenge free radicals.

Paraoxonase is an HDL-associated enzyme capable of hydrolyzing lipid peroxides. Its activity has been found to be decreased in CRF patients. The activity of platelet-activating factor acetyl hydrolase in CRF patients remains to be evaluated.

LIPID DISTURBANCES AS RISK FACTORS FOR ATHEROGENESIS IN CRF

The numerous quantitative and qualitative derangements of lipoprotein metabolism should, at least theoretically, contribute to the pathogenesis of the atherosclerosis of CRF. Abnormal concentrations of apoCIII probably play an important role because uremic patients with vascular disease have a significant increase in the apoCIII concentration of their LpB, compared with uremic patients free of vascular lesions. Partially degraded TG-rich LpB-C also have been shown to be strongly associated with the development of small coronary artery atherosclerotic disease, whereas the level of cholesterol-rich LpB was associated with large coronary artery lesions.

The role of the TG-rich lipoproteins as cardiovascular risk factor remains controversial. However, hemodialysis patients with coronary heart disease (CHD) generally have increased serum TG levels together with a diminished serum HDL cholesterol concentration. The results of the CLAS-study showed that the progression of myocardial ischemia was associated with increased circulating levels of TG-rich lipoproteins. However, the relatively low degree of hypertriglyceridemia that is seen in the majority of uremic patients corresponds only to a small increase in cardiovascular risk in the general population without renal insufficiency. On the other hand, there is an association between IDL, cholesterol-rich VLDL, and the degree of severity of CHD. In addition, the cholesterol-rich uremic VLDL have a greater atherogenic potential than normal VLDL. Furthermore, clinical conditions with an accumulation of residual Lp and IDL, such as are seen in chronic uremia, represent an increased risk for the development of ischemic cardiomyopathy.

Only a small number of systematic studies have been performed with the most powerful exploration techniques to test the hypothesis of an association between disturbances of lipoprotein metabolism and atherosclerosis in a large population of chronically uremic patients. In the majority of studies with a sufficient sample size that are available, only serum levels of total cholesterol and TG have been measured for this purpose; it was found that in most of the patients who had clinical evidence of vascular disease, serum TG was increased, whereas serum total cholesterol was normal. This has led to the conclusion that lipid disturbances probably do not play an important role. However, a relation between the anomalies of lipoprotein metabolism and atheromatous vessel disease often became apparent when such anomalies were examined in an appropriate manner. Thus it has been shown that dialysis patients with vascular disease had an increase in serum TG, total cholesterol, and VLDL cholesterol, compared with patients who had no evidence of vascular disease. However, the patients in the former group also were approximately 15 years older than the latter. Dialysis patients with type I diabetes and a history of myocardial infarction had significantly higher serum levels of total cholesterol and LDL:HDL ratio than comparable patients without myocardial infarction. In a personal study performed at our institution in a large group of patients with advanced CRF who were not yet on dialysis, significant differences were found in univariate analysis for several lipoprotein parameters between the group who had clinical evidence of cardiovascular disease and the group who had no such evidence. These differences included lower plasma HDL cholesterol levels, and higher plasma

TABLE 74.3. Independent Risk Factors for Cardiovascular Accidents in Predialysis Chronic Renal Failure Patients[a]

Independent Risk Factors	Relative Risk (95% CI)	*P* value
Cigarette smoking (5 pack-years)	1.11 (1.06–1.14)	.008
Systolic blood pressure (10 mm Hg)	1.25 (1.13–1.37)	.026
HDL cholesterol (0.2 mmol/L)	0.79 (0.71–0.88)	.032
Fibrinogen (0.5 g/L)	1.23 (1.18–1.30)	.000

[a] Variables not predictive of cardiovascular accidents in chronic renal failure patients by multivariate analysis were age, gender, diabetes, diastolic blood pressure, total cholesterol, triglycerides, apolipoproteins A and B, lipoprotein(a), and rate of decline in creatinine clearance.

Reproduced with permission from Jungers P, Massy ZA, Nguyen-Khoa T, et al. Incidence and risk factors of atherosclerotic cardiovascular disease in predialysis chronic renal failure patients: a prospective study. *Nephrol Dial Transplant* 1997;12:2597–2602.

CI, cancer incidence; HDL, high-density lipoprotein.

LDL cholesterol, TG, apoB, and Lp(a) levels in patients with cardiovascular disease. However, in multivariate analysis only HDL cholesterol remained as a significant risk factor among the lipid anomalies (Table 74.3).

In a study from Italy in which chronic hemodialysis patients were examined using carotid ultrasonography, a significant association was observed between the intima/media thickness of the vessel wall and the serum concentration of LDL cholesterol. In contrast, in two other ultrasonographic studies performed in dialysis patients no association was found, based on multivariate regression analysis, between the degree of severity of atheromatous lesions of the carotid and the femoral artery and the serum levels of a variety of lipid parameters, including apoAI, apoB, total or HDL cholesterol, LDL cholesterol, and TG. Similarly, in another study, no difference in commonly measured serum lipid levels was observed between hemodialysis patients with or without ultrasonographically proven atheromatous plaques of the carotid artery. However, in none of these studies was a comparison made between lipid parameters and clinically evident cardiovascular or cerebrovascular events. Moreover, the plaques could be the result of longstanding lipid abnormalities that have been changed with the advent of uremia or dialysis. Thus, for instance, the serum level of total cholesterol decreases in case of malnutrition. Consequently, this parameter then probably loses its predictive value for vascular risk.

Another independent, genetically determined, vascular risk factor is the serum level of Lp(a). However, its predictive value remains controversial. In accord with the findings in the population at large, higher serum Lp(a) concentrations were also found in uremic patients with a history of cardiac ischemia. Surprisingly, a correlation existed on the one hand between the serum level of Lp(a) and the number of ultrasonographically demonstrated lesions of the carotid artery, and on the other hand between the apo(a) phenotype and the presence of atheromatous vessel changes. The complex relationship between serum Lp(a) and atherogenesis in CRF requires further scrutiny.

Increased lipoprotein oxidation, carbamylation, and AGE-transformation theoretically favor atherogenesis as well. The presence in human atherosclerotic lesions of various hypochlorite-modified and NO-modified protein adducts, including oxidized LDL, has been demonstrated. The findings of these studies suggest that the oxidative mechanisms that participate at the atherogenic process probably involve, to a larger extent than previously thought, the protein moieties of lipoproteins as well as lipid moieties.

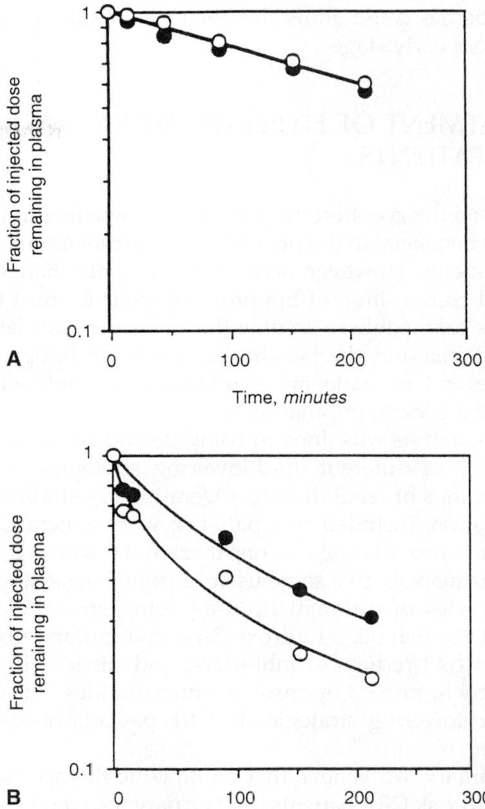

Figure 74.8. Plasma clearance of native and AGE-transformed human LDL in normal control mice **(A)** and in transgenic mice for the human LDL receptor **(B).** The animals were injected either native LDL (o) or AGE-LDL (l). The control mice without the human LDL receptor exhibit a slow decrease of native as well as of AGE-LDL **(A).** In contrast, the transgenic mice were able to eliminate relatively rapidly native LDL, but not AGE-transformed LDL. The latter therefore accumulate in serum. (Reproduced from Bucala R, Makita Z, Vega G, et al. Modification of low density lipoprotein by advanced glycation end products contributes to the dyslipidemia of diabetes and renal insufficiency. *Proc Natl Acad Sci* 1994;91: 9441–9445.)

Oxidized LDL may be taken up more readily in dialysis patients than in healthy subjects because of an increased expression of type I scavenger receptor. An enhanced formation of atheromatous lesions ensues. Similarly, AGE-LDL may be available for uptake into the vessel wall to a larger extent than normal LDL because such transformed particles have a prolonged stay in the circulation. Figure 74.8 shows the pathologically slowed clearance of AGE-transformed LDL particles in the experimental animal, compared with that of native LDL particles. AGE-transformed lipoproteins might participate in the genesis of vascular lesions, especially in diabetic patients, via binding to their endothelial receptor, RAGE; the induction of the vascular adhesion molecule, VCAM-1; and the attraction of circulating monocytes to the vessel wall. It could be shown that RAGE was expressed in arterial and capillary endothelial cells of uremic patients, whereas it was not constitutively expressed in endothelial cells sampled from nonuremic control individuals. However, the role of oxidized or AGE-modified lipoproteins as cardiovascular risk factors is not yet evaluated in CRF patients.

A profound immunologic response against various epitopes of oxidized LDL generally occurs in patients with atherosclerotic lesions. The identification of the specific epitopes inducing this response probably will be assessable in the near future with the help of natural monoclonal autoantibodies, and the use of such antibodies could allow the diagnosis of atheromatous lesions at very early stages.

MANAGEMENT OF HYPERLIPIDEMIA IN CRF PATIENTS

There are no intervention trials examining whether antilipemic therapy is beneficial in the prevention of cardiovascular disease in CRF patients. However, because atherogenic changes in the levels and composition of lipoproteins occur in most CRF patients, it is reasonable to assume that the risks associated with hyperlipidemia and the benefits of correcting lipoprotein abnormalities in CRF patients are at least comparable with those found in the general population.

A metaanalysis was done to compare and contrast the relative efficacy of different lipid-lowering strategies in various clinical settings of renal disease. Overall, these studies were of short duration, included few patients, were generally uncontrolled, and most investigated one therapy. However, the results of the metaanalysis give some useful insights regarding the relative efficacies of different lipid-lowering strategies in CRF patients. Diet, fish oil, 3-hydroxy-3-methyl-glutaryl-coenzyme A (HMG-CoA) reductase inhibitors, and fibric acid analogs consistently improved lipoprotein abnormalities. The safety of other lipid-lowering strategies in CRF patients needs further evaluation.

In summary, we believe that antilipemic therapy is reasonable in high-risk CRF patients, that is, patients who have multiple risk factors for cardiovascular disease, and particularly in CRF patients who have preexistent cardiovascular disease. In patients with predominant hypertriglyceridemia (in excess of 1.75 mM or 150 mg/dl), low calorie intake, low-fat diet, and, in some cases, fish oil may help to reduce TG levels. A fibric acid analog (e.g., gemfibrozil) may also effectively reduce TG, but the dose must be reduced in patients with decreased renal function. A low dose of an HMG-CoA reductase inhibitor appears to be the best choice for therapy to reduce LDL. It is reasonable to target LDL cholesterol of less than 3.30 mM or 130 mg/dl for primary prevention and of 2.55 mM or 100 mg/dl or less for secondary prevention. Whether combination therapy is safe and effective in reducing lipids in CRF patients requires further studies.

Selected Readings

Attman PO, Alaupovic P, Tavella M, et al. Abnormal lipid and apolipoprotein composition of major lipoprotein density classes in patients with chronic renal failure. *Nephrol Dial Transplant* 1996;11:63–69.

This is a recent description of the characteristic features of dyslipoproteinemia in uremic patients, with particular emphasis on partially delipidized TG-rich apoB-containing lipoproteins, which are characteristically distributed in the IDL density range.

Heinecke JW. Mechanisms of oxidative damage of low density lipoprotein in human atherosclerosis. *Curr Opin Lipid* 1997;8:268–274.

Excellent outline of the mechanisms through which oxidatively damaged LDL contribute to the pathogenesis of vascular lesions, with particular emphasis on various protein oxidation products isolated from atherosclerotic lesions and analyzed by mass spectrometry including tyrosyl radicals and reactive nitrogen intermediates and the role of hydrochlorous acid in their generation.

Kronenberg F, Konig P, Neyer U, et al. Multicenter study of lipoprotein(a) and apolipoprotein(a) phenotypes in patients with end-stage renal disease treated by hemodialysis or continuous ambulatory peritoneal dialysis. *J Am Soc Nephrol* 1995;6:110–120.

This is a large, multicenter study investigating serum lipoprotein(a) levels and apolipoprotein(a) isoforms in a group of 702 end-stage renal disease patients. It shows for the first time that the higher lipoprotein(a) levels observed in such patients is not explained by differences in isoform frequencies, but that the increase in lipoprotein(a) is apolipoprotein(a)-type specific.

London GM, Drüeke TB. Atherosclerosis and arteriosclerosis in chronic renal failure (Editorial Review). *Kidney Int* 1997;51:1678–1695.

The authors proceed to schematic, mechanistic distinction between two different types of arterial wall changes in uremic patients: early focal changes of conduit function (atheromatous plaques) leading eventually to vessel wall occlusion versus early diffuse changes of cushion function (arterial stiffening) responsible for increased pulse-wave velocity, systolic hypertension, and end-organ damage. Exhaustive description of underlying mechanisms.

Massy ZA, Kasiske BL. Hyperlipidemia and its management in renal disease. *Curr Opin Nephrol Hypertens* 1996;5:141–146.

This is a critical overview of hyperlipidemia and renal disease that also considers correlations of hyperlipidemia with cardiovascular disease and the progression of renal disease observed in various renal pathologies. Moreover, it includes practical guidelines for the management of hyperlipidemia in such patients.

Massy ZA, Ma JZ, Louis TA, et al. Lipid-lowering therapy in patients with renal disease. *Kidney Int* 1995;48:188–198.

In this metaanalysis the authors compared and contrasted the relative efficacy of different lipid-lowering strategies in various clinical settings of renal disease. The study included 3,065 patients and control subjects in 198 study groups. The results of the analysis provide a useful framework for choosing antilipemic therapy in patients with renal disease.

Ni Z, Smogorzewski M, Massry SG. Elevated cytosolic calcium of adipocytes in chronic renal failure. *Kidney Int* 1995;47:1624–1629.

This study demonstrates that adipocytes in uremic rats exhibit an overload in systolic calcium, which is probably responsible for the observed reduction of LPL secretion. The calcium increase is mainly mediated by secondary hyperparathyroidism. It is reversible on parathyroidectomy or by treatment with calcium channel blocking agents. This observation adds to previously obtained evidence that parathyroid overfunction greatly contributes to lipoprotein disturbances in chronic renal failure.

Witko-Sarsat V, Friedlander M, Capeillére-Blandin C, et al. Advanced oxidation protein products as a novel marker of oxidative stress in uremia. *Kidney Int* 1996;49:1304–1313.

The occurrence of advanced oxidation protein products (AOPP) is described in patients with chronic renal failure. These compounds probably are more reliable markers of oxidative stress than presently available markers. The hypothesis is also made that AOPP may constitute a novel family of modified proteins, which are capable of exerting noxious effects on various target tissues including the vessel wall.

PART 3
Amino Acid and Protein Metabolism in Chronic Renal Failure

Joel D. Kopple

In renal failure, there are a number of abnormalities in amino acid and protein metabolism. This chapter reviews the status of these disorders in chronic uremia.

AMINO ACID METABOLISM IN CHRONIC RENAL FAILURE

The plasma amino acid pattern in chronic renal failure (CRF) is pathognomonic of this condition (Table 74.4). Typically, there is decreased plasma tryptophan, valine, and tyrosine and reduced ratios of essential to nonessential amino acids, tyrosine to phenylalanine, and serine to glycine. Plasma cystine, citrulline, N^{π}-methylhistidine (1-methylhistidine), and N^{τ}-methylhistidine (3-methylhistidine) levels are increased. Tryptophan is the one essential amino acid that is substantially protein bound in plasma. In CRF, total and bound plasma tryptophan is reduced, whereas free tryptophan is increased. Concentrations of most other amino acids are usually normal both in clinically stable chronically uremic patients who are not dialyzed and in patients undergoing maintenance hemodialysis or chronic peritoneal dialysis (PD).

TABLE 74.4. Typical Amino Acid Patterns in Nondialyzed Patients with Chronic Renal Failure and in Patients Undergoing Maintenance Dialysis

	Plasma	Red Cells	Granulocytes[a]	Muscle
Essential				
Histidine	N-L	H	N	N-H
Isoleucine	N-L	N	N	N-L
Leucine	N-L	N-L	N	N-L
Lysine	N	N	N-H	N-H
Methionine	N-L	N-H	N	N
Phenylalanine	N-H	N-H	N	H
Threonine	N	N	N	L
Tryptophan	L	—[b]	N	—
Valine	L	L	N-L	L
Cystine[c]	H	H	—	—
Tyrosine[c]	L	L	N	L
Nonessential				
Alanine	N-L	N	N-H	H
Arginine	N	N-H	N-H	H
Asparagine	N	N-H	—	N-H
Aspartic acid	N	L	N	N-H
Citrulline	H	H	H	H
Glutamic acid	N	H	H	N
Glutamine	N	N	—	N-H
Glycine	N-H	H	H	N-H
Ornithine	N	H	N	H
Proline	N	N	—	—
Serine	N-L	N	—	N
Taurine	H-N-L	H	N	L
Homocysteine	H	—	—	—
N^{π}-methylhistidine	H	H	—	—
N^{τ}-methylhistidine	H	H	—	H
Ratios				
Essential/nonessential	L	N	—	—
Tyrosine/phenylanine	L	L	N	L
Serine/glycine	L	L	—	—

[a] Data obtained from patients undergoing continuous ambulatory peritoneal dialysis; amino acid concentrations for other cell types refer primarily to nondialyzed patients with advanced chronic renal failure and maintenance hemodialysis patients.
[b] Indicates data are not available.
[c] Semiessential amino acids.
H, high; L, low; N, normal.

There are many abnormalities in sulfur amino acid concentrations in renal failure. Plasma free cystine, free homocystine, cysteine-homocysteine mixed disulfide, protein-bound cysteine, protein-bound homocysteine, and cysteinesulfinic acid are elevated in hemodialysis patients. Methionine is reported to be normal or reduced. Plasma taurine is variously reported as elevated, normal, or reduced, possibly reflecting the degree of contamination or leakage from platelets or other cellular elements in blood. In patients with chronic renal insufficiency who do not have end-stage renal disease, the number and severity of altered plasma amino acid concentrations increase as the glomerular filtration rate (GFR), measured by the clearances of ^{125}I-iothalamate or similar markers, is reduced. Some plasma amino acid concentrations begin to become abnormal when the GFR is as high as 30 to 40 ml/min/1.73m^2. This was particularly observed for the inverse relation between GFR and plasma $N^{\tau\tau}$-methylhistidine, cystine, citrulline, and the glycine:serine ratio.

The intracellular amino acid patterns in red cells, leukocytes, and muscle are also abnormal (Table 74.4). With regard to the sulfur amino acids, taurine is reported to be elevated in erythrocytes, normal in granulocytes and lymphocytes, and reduced in platelets. In muscle, valine, threonine, tyrosine, and taurine frequently are low, whereas phenylalanine, alanine, arginine, citrulline, and ornithine often are increased.

There are several causes for altered amino acid pools in renal failure (Table 74.5). In nonuremic individuals as well as patients with CRF, low-protein diets or poor nutritional intake will lead to decreased concentrations of such amino acids as histidine, isoleucine, leucine, valine, and tyrosine; the ratio of essential to nonessential amino acids often falls. Because protein calorie malnutrition occurs commonly in renal failure, the plasma amino acid pattern of the typical patient with advanced renal failure has many similarities to that of patients with malnutrition. Plasma levels of some amino acids display a direct or inverse correlation with protein intake, and for several amino acids this relationship is different in chronically uremic or hemodialysis patients as compared with normal subjects. Thus the response of plasma concentrations of certain amino acids to protein restriction also is abnormal in uremia.

Serum albumin is a transport protein, and in renal failure, competitive binding by compounds that accumulate in this

TABLE 74.5. Causes of Altered Amino Acid Pools in Chronic Renal Failure

Causes of Alteration	Example of Altered Amino Acid Concentrations or Ratios
Low protein diets or inadequate nutrition intake	Low plasma valine, tyrosine, and total essential amino acid levels; essential/nonessential ratio
Reduced binding to serum albumin	Low plasma-bound and total-tryptophan concentrations; increased plasma free tryptophan level
Decreased urinary excretion of amino acids	Increased plasma and red cell N^{π}-methylhistidine and plasma, red cell, and muscle N^{T}-methylhistidine concentrations
Impaired renal amino acid metabolism due to damaged renal parenchyma	High plasma, red cell, granulocyte, and muscle citrulline levels; low plasma and red cell serine/glycine ratio and tendency to low-serine and high-glycine concentrations in plasma
Enhanced bone reabsorption	Increased plasma-free and -bound hydroxyproline levels
Impaired cellular amino acid transport or decreased capacity to maintain cellular concentration gradients	Possibly altered taurine concentration
Acidemia	Low intracellular muscle isoleucine, leucine, and valine concentrations
Abnormal metabolism of amino acids	Theoretical in organs due to (a) accumulated toxins and/or (b) altered hormone levels or activities

condition can alter albumin binding. The reduction in normal albumin binding probably accounts for the low plasma total tryptophan and increased plasma free (unbound) tryptophan concentrations in renal failure. Decreased urinary excretion of certain amino acids also contributes to altered amino acid levels. Reduced excretion probably accounts for increased plasma and red cell N^{π}-methylhistidine and plasma, red cell, and muscle N^{T}-methylhistidine concentrations. The urinary clearance of some amino acids in patients with advanced renal failure may be markedly increased relative to the GFR, but the absolute rate of urinary excretion of amino acids is reduced, normal, or, at most, only slightly increased.

Decreased metabolic activity of the kidney may contribute to altered amino acid pools in renal failure. The kidney normally metabolizes glycine and several other amino acids to serine. In renal failure, the reduced ability to convert glycine to serine may account for the low plasma serine:glycine ratio. Altered renal amino acid metabolism may also lead to reduced conversion in the kidney of citrulline to arginine and may account for the high plasma, red cell, granulocyte, and muscle citrulline concentrations. Moreover, although most of the phenylalanine hydroxylase activity in the body appears to reside in the liver, a small amount of the activity of this enzyme is present in the kidney and the pancreas. Impaired activity of this enzyme in the kidney may contribute to the low plasma, red cell and muscle tyrosine concentrations and tyrosine:phenylalanine ratios and to the high plasma, red cell or muscle phenylalanine levels.

Cysteinesulfinic acid is the metabolic precursor of taurine. The finding that, in CRF, plasma cysteinesulfinic acid is increased and, in some reports, plasma taurine is low has led some researchers to hypothesize that activity of cysteinesulfinic acid decarboxylase may be decreased. This enzyme is rate limiting for the conversion of cysteinesulfinic acid to taurine.

Plasma total, free, and peptide-bound hydroxyproline may be elevated in renal failure. Impaired urinary excretion of these compounds may contribute to the elevated plasma levels. Collagen is a major reservoir for hydroxyproline, and in conditions of enhanced bone reabsorption, such as renal hyperparathyroid bone disease, there may be increased release of hydroxyproline from bone. Hence, urine free and peptide-bound hydroxyproline may be elevated in renal failure. There is a correlation between the severity of renal hyperparathyroid bone disease and the degree of elevation of plasma free and peptide-bound hydroxyproline concentrations. It has been suggested that impaired activity of hepatic hydroxyproline oxidase may contribute to increased plasma free hydroxyproline levels.

Other possible causes of altered amino acid pools in renal failure include uremic toxins and abnormal concentrations or activities of hormones. These factors may alter enzyme activities and cause abnormal metabolism of amino acids in various organs. One such toxin appears to be hydrogen ion. Acidemia increases activity of branched-chain amino acid dehydrogenase, the enzyme that causes irreversible degradation of isoleucine, leucine, and valine. In maintenance hemodialysis patients, isoleucine, leucine, and valine concentrations are often decreased in skeletal muscle cells and in plasma (Table 74.5). Muscle valine levels correlate directly with the serum bicarbonate. It has been reported that treatment of nine maintenance hemodialysis patients with dialysis providing a high-bicarbonate dialysate was associated with a significant increase in intracellular concentrations of isoleucine, leucine, and valine in the quadriceps femoralis muscle. These observations suggest that acidemia may affect both amino acid metabolism and tissue amino acid concentrations.

The finding that in CRF, the altered pattern of amino acids in plasma differs from that in muscle, suggests that the transcellular movement of amino acids or the capacity to maintain intracellular amino acid gradients may be abnormal in renal failure. Indeed, abnormal system A amino acid transport has been described in rats with CRF. Others reported that in nondialyzed patients with CRF and maintenance hemodialysis patients who were infused with the nine essential amino acids plus arginine and glucose, the whole body clearances of several amino acids were abnormally increased or decreased.

Decreased gastrointestinal absorption has been suggested as a cause of altered plasma amino acid levels in uremia. In our experience, fecal nitrogen excretion is not increased in renal failure. Metabolic studies in 11 chronically uremic men and 7 healthy male subjects who ingested 40-g protein diets showed that fecal nitrogen excretion was 1.32 ± 0.29 (SD) and 1.37 ± 0.39 g/day, respectively. This observation suggests that gastrointestinal absorption of amino acids or peptides is not markedly altered in uremia. Losses of amino acids into hemodialysate and peritoneal dialysate may also contribute to altered amino acid pools in maintenance dialysis patients if the patient's protein intake is low.

PROTEIN METABOLISM IN CHRONIC RENAL FAILURE

Mild to moderate protein or energy malnutrition occurs in approximately 33% of maintenance hemodialysis or chronic peritoneal dialysis patients, and severe malnutrition occurs in an additional 6% to 8% of these individuals. Growth is impaired in chronically azotemic rats as well as in children with renal insufficiency. Although reduced-calorie and/or protein intake is a cause of the growth retardation, growth also is impaired in chronically azotemic rats as compared with sham-operated, pair-fed controls. Growth hormone can stimulate both normal growth and catch-up growth in most children with CRF; pharmacologic doses of growth hormone are often required for a sustained effect. These observations, as well as the aforementioned evidence that adults with CRF often have protein-energy malnutrition, have stimulated a number of studies of protein metabolism in CRF.

The metabolism and pool sizes of body proteins, particularly albumin, is of great concern in maintenance hemodialysis and peritoneal dialysis patients, because serum albumin is one of the most powerful predictors of mortality in these individuals. Patients with CRF usually have a normal or increased intravascular pool of albumin. However, in those patients who have serum albumin concentrations less than 3.5 g/dl, the intravascular albumin pool tends to be decreased. Extracellular albumin pools often are reported to be decreased and total body albumin to be normal or low in CRF patients. The absolute rates of synthesis and degradation of albumin are reduced. The serum albumin concentrations are more likely to be normal in CRF patients if they are given more aggressive nutritional management and if they are inaugurated on maintenance dialysis therapy earlier, before frank uremia supervenes. It has not been ascertained whether the size of the albumin pools also is normal in these latter individuals.

In clinically stable patients undergoing maintenance hemodialysis, the intravascular pool and absolute catabolic rate of intravascular albumin are somewhat increased and the fractional catabolic rate is normal. Serum albumin concentrations are often normal (i.e., 4 to 5 g/dl), but commonly fall during periods of poor nutritional intake, catabolic stress, and increased urinary albumin losses. Serum albumin and albumin pools in patients undergoing chronic peritoneal dialysis are frequently normal. Serum albumin is particularly likely to fall rapidly during acute catabolic illness or reduced nutrient intake in these latter patients because of their superimposed chronic protein losses into peritoneal dialysate of about 9 g/day. If such individuals develop peritonitis, peritoneal protein losses can increase dramatically; protein losses often rise to approximately 15 g/day. We observed peritoneal protein losses of more than 100 g/day in one patient with well-established severe peritonitis. Peritoneal protein losses may not return to normal for as long as several weeks after the peritoneal infection has been eradicated. In normal adult humans, acidemia appears to suppress albumin synthesis. Hence, it is possible that acidemia contributes to the reduced albumin pools in patients with CRF.

The data regarding serum transferrin levels are conflicting. Some studies indicate that serum transferrin is low in many chronically uremic and maintenance dialysis patients, even when they appear to be rather well nourished. Serum transferrin is even lower when such individuals are wasted or malnourished. Other studies indicate that serum transferrin usually is normal. The reason for this discrepancy is not clear. Iron stores may affect transfer in concentrations. In some of these latter studies, serum transferrin was estimated from the serum total iron-binding capacity; in other studies, transferrin was measured directly, which may give more accurate results. As with serum albumin, serum transferrin is a negative acute-phase protein and will decrease in response to catabolic or inflammatory illnesses. Several centers have reported a close correlation between serum total iron-binding capacity and serum transferrin measured by radial immunodiffusion. However, the slopes or intercepts defining this relationship vary substantially from center to center.

Because there is a strong epidemiologic association between markers of protein-energy malnutrition and the risk of death in maintenance dialysis patients, a number of researchers have examined whether the malnutrition is the cause of death or is the result of underlying illnesses that independently cause both malnutrition and fatality. Interest in this question is due, in part, to the recognition that the most common causes of death in maintenance dialysis patients are cardiovascular and cerebrovascular diseases, and it is unclear why protein-energy malnutrition *per se* should increase the death rate from cardiovascular and cerebrovascular disorders.

Most research on this matter has examined the relationship between indicators of inflammation, such as C-reactive protein (CRP) or serum amyloid A (SAA), and serum albumin levels. Catabolic cytokines, such as tumor necrosis factor-alpha and interleukin I, are elevated in serum of both nondialyzed CRF patients and in individuals undergoing maintenance dialysis. Several studies indicate that CRP, SAA, or other inflammatory markers correlate inversely with the serum albumin levels in maintenance dialysis patients. Serum albumin is a negative acute-phase protein and, in some studies, is also directly correlated with the dietary protein intake, as indicated by the normalized protein total nitrogen appearance (nPNA or PCRn). These considerations are consistent with the possibility that underlying diseases that promote chronic inflammation and poor nutrient intake both engender protein-energy malnutrition and also mortality.

Although this latter hypothesis is attractive and is gaining wide acceptance, it is far from proven. The following are among the unresolved questions relating to this matter: (a) the correlation of inflammatory markers with serum albumin concentrations is of a low order; usually correlation coefficients are between about 0.35 and 0.55. (b) Protein-energy malnutrition is associated with increased levels of acute-phase proteins; this may reflect the fact that malnourished patients are at increased risk for infection and other catabolic diseases. (c) Some of the nutritional parameters that predict mortality are indicators of body composition or body mass, such as the body mass index or weight-for-height percentiles, or are indicators of skeletal muscle mass or protein intake, such as the predialysis–serum creatinine concentration or the nPNA. Although chronic inflammation could lead to inadequate nutrient intake and tissue wasting, it is less obvious that inflammation, as opposed to poor nutrient intake, will decrease total body or muscle mass. (d) The fact that the correlation between nPNA and serum albumin is of a low order does not, in itself, contradict the possibility that low-nutrient intake decreases serum albumin. Moreover, no epidemiologic study in maintenance dialysis patients has attempted to correlate the dietary energy intake with serum albumin levels. In studies of the baseline phase of the Modification of Diet in Renal Disease (MDRD) study in which 1,785 clinically stable patients with mild to moderate renal insufficiency were evaluated, dietary energy and protein intake were each correlated with the serum albumin levels and also with a number of other parameters of nutritional status. (e) In all of these foregoing studies, the data analyzed were epidemiologic or associative in nature. In order to prove that there is a causal relationship between either nutritional intake or inflammation and outcome, interventional protocols will be necessary. Such studies, for example, could test whether in maintenance dialysis patients with protein-energy malnutrition, an increased nutrient intake or an antiinflammatory treatment will decrease morbidity or mortality.

Although acute-phase proteins or catabolic cytokines may be elevated in the nondialyzed patient with advanced CRF, there is little evidence that advanced CRF *per se* is a state of hypercatabolism. Indeed, when such individuals are fed diets very low in protein, with or without essential amino acids or ketoacid supplements, or diets providing very low quantities of the nine essential amino acids, they are able to conserve protein very efficiently. Such conservation is indicated by their low total-nitrogen output, neutral or positive nitrogen balance, or reduced rates of amino acid oxidation; whole-body protein degradation also may decrease with these low-nitrogen diets, but this is not as well documented in patients with advanced CRF.

In contrast to the nondialyzed CRF patient, nitrogen balance studies clearly indicate that maintenance hemodialysis patients and chronic peritoneal dialysis patients are unable to conserve nitrogen normally and have an increased dietary protein requirement. The increased dietary protein needs in these individuals are greater than can be accounted for by the amino acid, protein, and peptide losses in dialysate. These findings are consistent with the existence of a chronic, low-grade catabolic state in maintenance dialysis patients. Such a catabolic state could be due to the accumulation of catabolic uremic toxins, altered hormonal pattern, inhibition of anabolic hormonal activity (e.g., resistance to insulin and insulinlike growth factor-I [IGF-I]), or the presence of a chronic state of inflammation with increased levels of inflammatory, catabolic cytokines. It is possible that this condition is engendered by the dialysis process itself because, as indicated previously, it is not observed in patients with advanced CRF.

Serum concentrations of many small proteins and peptides are increased in renal failure. These include α_1-microglobulin; β_2-microglobulin; β_2-glycoprotein; lysozymes; retinol-binding protein; IGF binding proteins 1, 2, 3, and 6; fragments of some of these binding proteins; α_1-acid glycoprotein; prealbumin; ribonuclease; fibrinogen-degradation products; gamma-globulin light chains; and Bence Jones proteins. Many small proteins and peptides are normally degraded or excreted by the kidney, and loss of these latter activities in CRF probably contributes to the increased serum concentrations. The urinary excretion of some proteins may be increased in renal failure, possibly because of impaired ability of renal tubular cells to degrade the filtered protein.

Some small proteins, when present in increased concentrations, may be toxic. Ribonuclease may inhibit lymphocyte proliferation, impair growth of red and white cells in bone marrow cultures, and inhibit cultured fat cells. Elevated serum β_2-microglobulin may cause deposits of this protein in soft tissue and bone of uremic patients, particularly in those individuals undergoing maintenance dialysis therapy. These protein deposits may cause an amyloidlike syndrome, which is discussed in greater detail in Chapter 84, Part 1G.

Protein Metabolism in Specific Organs

The kidney normally degrades many peptide hormones. These include parathyroid hormone, insulin, proinsulin, glucagon, growth hormone, somatostatin, calcitonin, C-peptide, thyrotropin, prolactin, luteinizing hormone, leptin, and gastrin. Increased secretion is a cause of elevated serum levels of some of these hormones; however, decreased degradation by the diseased kidney probably contributes more to the increased serum levels of most hormone levels. Elevated serum concentrations of some hormones cause adverse effects in uremia. This may be particularly true for parathyroid hormone, glucagon, and possibly leptin. The toxicity of excess parathyroid hormone in uremia is discussed in detail in Chapter 68, Part 1.

Studies in animal models of CRF indicate that hepatic albumin synthesis is reduced. This effect may be due, at least in part, to acidemia. It has been shown that when chronically azotemic and sham-operated, ad lib–fed, control rats were fasted for up to 36 hours, there was a greater reduction in skeletal muscle–protein synthesis in the azotemic animals. Indirect evidence indicates that the rate of leucine metabolism during fasting is increased in chronically azotemic rats versus control animals. Also, others reported increased N^T-methylhistidine appearance (the sum of urinary excretion plus body accrual) in rats with CRF that were fasted in comparison with fasting controls.

Other investigators have described increased net-protein degradation (i.e., an increase in the difference between the absolute rates of protein degradation and protein synthesis) in rats with chronic renal insufficiency. It has been suggested that alterations in net-protein degradation in uremic muscle may be caused at least partly by impaired activation of adenylate cyclase and release of cyclic adenosine monophosphate (cAMP) in the muscle. In the epitrochlearis muscle of azotemic rats, there was resistance to the (a) generation of cAMP and (b) suppression of alanine and glutamine release by serotonin and epinephrine. In rats with renal insufficiency, there was normal suppression of muscle alanine release (net-protein degradation) by insulin when the animals were fed a 10% or 20% casein diet. However, insulin did not suppress muscle alanine release normally in azotemic rats fed a 40% casein diet as compared with controls given the same intake. This suggests that high-protein diets may be less able to promote protein balance in skeletal muscle in CRF than in the normal state. Possibly, the less anabolic effect of high-protein diets might be due to the generation of acid metabolites.

Studies of polysomal profiles were performed in isolated polysomes from liver and muscle of rats with renal insufficiency of 2 weeks' duration. The results showed that in muscle of the azotemic as compared with control rats that were starved for 18 hours, there was extensive disaggregation of polysomes. This may help to explain the previously described inability of azotemic rats to conserve muscle protein normally during starvation. The azotemic rats that were not starved showed evidence for impaired hepatic-protein synthesis. Interpretation of these results must be qualified because animals were not pair fed, and the azotemic rats may have eaten less food. Hence, reduced food intake in addition to or instead of azotemia may have influenced the findings.

Other investigators showed that chronically azotemic rats have increased skeletal muscle–protein degradation and reduced muscle–protein synthesis. At least part of the enhanced skeletal muscle degradation in rats with CRF appears to be due to acidemia. Acidemia increases skeletal muscle–protein degradation by activating the ATP-dependent ubiquitine-proteosome system, which is responsible for much of the protein catabolism that occurs intracellularly. Acidemia increases the gene expression of segments of both ubiquitin and the proteosome. The enhanced muscle–protein degradation could be prevented by treatment with sodium bicarbonate. On the other hand, Ding and coworkers found increased protein degradation and suppressed protein synthesis in epitrochlearis muscle of chronically azotemic rats given bicarbonate in comparison with sham-operated, pair-fed, control rats. The arterial blood pH of these two groups of rats were similar, indicating that acidemia is not the only cause of the enhanced degradation and suppressed synthesis of skeletal muscle protein in these animals. The toxic effect of acidosis on muscle metabolism in uremia is discussed in detail in Chapter 68, Part 6.

There is resistance to the actions of insulin in CRF that can only partly be attributed to acidemia. We have described resistance *in vitro* to the IGF-1–induced stimulation of protein synthesis and suppression of protein degradation in epitrochlearis muscle of chronically azotemic rats as compared with sham-operated, pair-fed controls. These effects were not considered to be due to acidemia because the azotemic rats were given sodium bicarbonate and their arterial blood pH was not different from control rats. We also observed that injection of recombinant human IGF-1 into maintenance dialysis patients suppressed plasma amino acid levels and insulin to a lesser degree than in normal adults. There are probably several causes of resistance to IGF-1 in CRF. These include accumulation of small, dialyzable compounds and larger-sized proteins in plasma that suppress the actions of IGF-1; these inhibitory proteins may be IGF-1 binding proteins or fragments of these proteins. Other probable causes include disorders of the signal transduction system such as impaired phosphorylation of the beta subunit of the IGF receptor, decreased phosphorylation of insulin-related substrate I by the beta subunit, and elevated basal cytosolic calcium. Inhibition of insulin and IGF-1 may contribute to protein wasting in patients with CRF.

It has been reported that regular exercise in chronically azotemic rats causes a reduction in basal muscle–protein catabolism. The muscles of these exercised azotemic rats showed improved sensitivity to the anticatabolic effects of pharmacologic doses of insulin.

Selected Readings

Nutrition and Metabolism in Renal Disease. Proceedings of the 7th International Conference on Renal Nutrition and Metabolism. Stockholm, Sweden, May 29–June 1, 1994. *Mineral Electrolyte Metabolism* 1996;22:1–202.

These are the proceedings of a symposium and contain a number of articles on amino acid, protein, and nitrogen metabolism in renal failure.

Nutrition and Metabolism in Renal Disease. Proceedings of the 8th International Conference on Renal Nutrition and Metabolism. Naples, Italy, October 9–12, 1996. *Mineral Electrolyte Metabolism* 1997;23:125–318.

This is a series of papers concerning metabolic and nutritional disorders in renal disease and renal failure.

Ding H, Gao X-L, Hirschberg R, et al. Impaired actions of insulin-like growth factor 1 on protein synthesis and degradation in skeletal muscle of rats with chronic renal failure: evidence for a postreceptor defect. *J Clin Invest* 1996;97:1064–1075.

This paper describes mechanisms for the resistance to the anabolic effects of IGF-1 in chronic renal failure.

Franch HA, Mitch WE. Catabolism in uremia: the impact of metabolic acidosis. *J Am Soc Nephrol* 1998;9(Suppl):S78–S81.

This paper gives a brief and concise review of the effects of acidemia on protein and calcium metabolism and endocrine disorders.

Kaysen GA, Rathore V, Shearer GC, et al. Mechanisms of hypoalbuminemia in hemodialysis patients. *Kidney Int* 1995;48:510–516.

This paper describes mechanisms responsible for hypoalbuminemia in maintenance hemodialysis patients.

Kaysen GA, Stevenson FT, Depner TA. Determinants of albumin concentration in hemodialysis patients. *Am J Kidney Dis* 1997;29:658–668.

This paper evaluates, in a prospective fashion, statistical relationships between serum albumin, serum acute-phase proteins, dose of dialysis, and the normalized protein–nitrogen appearance and assesses whether these factors influence serum albumin levels in maintenance hemodialysis patients.

Kuhlmann MV, Kopple JD. Amino acid metabolism in the kidney. *Semin Nephrol* 1990;5:445–447.

This article reviews the metabolism of amino acids in the kidney under normal conditions and in renal failure.

Laidlaw SA, Berg RL, Kopple JD, et al. Prepared for the Modification of Diet in Renal Disease (MDRD) Study. Patterns of fasting plasma amino acid levels in chronic renal insufficiency: results from the feasibility phase of the MDRD study. *Am J Kidney Dis* 1994;23:504–513.

This manuscript describes the relationships between the glomerular filtration rate and plasma amino acid concentrations in 78 patients with chronic renal insufficiency.

Masud T, Young VR, Chapman T, et al. Adaptive responses to very low protein diets: the first comparison of ketoacids to essential amino acids. *Kidney Int* 1994;45:1182–1192.

Tom K, Young VR, Chapman T, et al. Long-term adaptive responses to dietary protein restriction in chronic renal failure. *Am J Physiol* 1995;268:E668–E677.

These two papers examined turnover of [1-^{13}C]leucine and [5-5-5-$^{2}H_3$]leucine in patients with chronic renal failure who were fed low-protein diets. The studies describe mechanisms by which patients with chronic renal failure adapt to low-protein diets.

PART 4
Thyroid Hormone Metabolism

Victoria S. Lim

Chronic renal failure (CRF) affects thyroid function in multiple ways, including low-circulating thyroid hormone concentration, altered peripheral hormone metabolism, disturbed binding to carrier proteins, reduction in tissue hormone content, increased iodine store in the thyroid gland, and others. These derangements, although they do not have serious physiologic consequences, make interpretation of thyroid function tests difficult.

SERUM THYROID HORMONE PROFILE AND THYROID HORMONE KINETICS IN END-STAGE RENAL DISEASE PATIENTS

Table 74.6 summarizes thyroid hormone profile in end-stage renal disease (ESRD) patients before and after initiation of maintenance hemodialysis and following successful renal transplantation. The most obvious abnormality is a reduction in serum

TABLE 74.6. Serum Thyroid Hormone Profile in Normal Subjects as Compared with ESRD Patients Before and After Initiation of Maintenance Dialysis and Renal Transplant Patients

Group	TT_4 µg/dl	FTI	TBG capacity µgT_4/dl	TT_3 ng/dl	TT_4/TT_3	TSH µU/ml
Normal	6.6 ± 1.4	7.1 ± 1.0	18.3 ± 5.4	128 ± 25	55 ± 17	2.8 ± 1.2
pre-HD	6.2 ± 2.5	7.0 ± 2.4	16.4 ± 3.0	63 ± 17[a]	102 ± 43[a]	3.2 ± 1.5
HD	5.6 ± 1.2[a]	6.6 ± 1.5	16.5 ± 4.0	83 ± 22[a]	72 ± 28[a]	2.7 ± 2.5
RT	7.9 ± 1.6	7.8 ± 1.1	22.0 ± 6.4	134 ± 20	58 ± 13	3.3 ± 2.1
Anova:*P*	<.01	ns	ns	<.001	<.001	ns

Values (mean ± SD) from all groups were tested by analysis of variance, and the *P* values are listed in the bottom line.

[a] Significant differences between the means of each patient group and the normal controls, tested using mean square within value. (Reproduced with permission from Lim VS, Fang VS, Katz AI, et al. Thyroid dysfunction in chronic renal failure: a study of the pituitary-thyroid axis and peripheral turnover kinetics of thyroxine and triiodothyronine. *J Clin Invest* 1977;60:522–534.)

ESRD, end-stage renal disease; FTI, free T_4 index; HD, hemodialysis; RT, renal transplant; TBG, thyroxine-binding globulin; TSH, thyroid-stimulating hormone; TT_3, total triiodothyronine; TT_4, total thyroxine.

TABLE 74.7. T_4 and T_3 Kinetics in ESRD Patients Before and After Initiation of Maintenance Hemodialysis Treatment and After Successful Renal Transplantation as Compared with Normal Subjects

				T_4 Kinetics					T_3 Kinetics			
Group	Serum Creatinine mg/dl	Body Weight kg	Plasma Volume L	TT_4 µg/dl	k %/day	DS L	MCR L/day	D µg/day	TT_3 ng/dl	MCR L/day	D µg/day	T_4–T_3 conversion %
Normal	1.0 ± 0.2	65 ± 13	3.8 ± 0.5	9.1 ± 1.2	10.2 ± 0.9	11.7 ± 1.1	1.2 ± 0.2	109 ± 12	184 ± 25	18.6 ± 3.6	33.8 ± 6.1	37.2 ± 5.8
pre-HD	10.0 ± 2.3[a]	65 ± 16	4.0 ± 0.9	9.5 ± 0.8	7.0 ± 1.1[a]	15.8 ± 2.4	1.1 ± 0.1	103 ± 2	94 ± 17[a]	14.6 ± 3.0	13.5 ± 2.6[a]	15.7 ± 3.1[a]
HD	12.2 ± 3.5[a]	75 ± 7	4.1 ± 1.6	9.1 ± 2.9	9.6 ± 1.9	15.0 ± 5.2	1.4 ± 0.4	122 ± 31	105 ± 24[a]	12.5 ± 3.1[a]	12.9 ± 3.1[a]	12.8 ± 1.7[a]
RT	1.6 ± 0.6	75 ± 16	4.0 ± 1.0	10.2 ± 1.5	9.9 ± 2.3	11.5 ± 1.4	1.2 ± 0.3	117 ± 34	168 ± 24	17.9 ± 2.4	30.0 ± 7.1	34.0 ± 14.7
Anova:*P*	<.001	ns	ns	ns	<0.05	ns	ns	ns	<.0001	<.01	<.0001	<.0001

[a] Significant difference between each patient group and the normal controls, tested using the mean square within values.

Values (mean ± SD) from all four groups were tested by analysis of variance and the *P* values are listed in the bottom line.

TT_4 is elevated because the experiment was done during LT[4] replacement. (Data derived from Lim VS, Fang VS, Katz AI, et al. Thyroid dysfunction in chronic renal failure: a study of the pituitary-thyroid axis and peripheral turnover kinetics of thyroxine and triiodothyronine. *J Clin Invest* 1977;60:522–534.)

D, daily degradation rate; DS, distribution space; ESRD, end-stage renal disease; HD, hemodialysis; k, daily fractional degradation; MCR, metabolic clearance rate; RT, renal transplant; TT_3, total triiodothyronine; TT_4, total thyroxine.

total triiodothyronine (TT_3). Serum free T_3, not listed in the table but reported by several groups of investigators, is also significantly reduced. Serum total thyroxine (TT_4) is frequently reduced, especially in hemodialysis patients, though to a lesser extent. Free T_4 index (FTI), an indirect estimate of serum free T_4, is reduced proportionally as TT_4. T_4 binding capacity or thyroxine-binding globulin (TBG) is normal. Serum thyroid-stimulating hormone (TSH) is not elevated. The high TT_4:TT_3 ratio in the renal failure patients suggests a selective T_3 deficiency. Rarely TT_4 and free T_4 are elevated in the absence of hyperthyroidism.

The low serum TT_3 and free T_3 is not due to increased T_3 degradation or decreased thyroidal T_3 secretion, but is a result of impaired extrathyroidal conversion of T_4 to T_3. Table 74.7 summarizes the T_4 and T_3 kinetics following ^{125}I-T_4 and ^{131}I-T_3 injections in groups of ESRD patients before and after initiation of maintenance hemodialysis and after successful renal transplantation as compared with the normal controls. To suppress endogenous thyroid hormone secretion and to prevent uptake and recirculation of the labeled iodide, the study was performed with 0.2 mg/day of LT_4 (Synthroid) replacement and saturated iodide solution administration. With LT_4 replacement, serum TT_4 rose equally in all study groups, indicating that thyroxine absorption in the ESRD and renal transplant patients is similar to that of the normal subjects. By contrast, serum TT_3 increased significantly only in the normal subjects and in the renal transplant patients, and remained subnormal in the two groups of renal failure patients. T_4 metabolism, including daily fractional degradation, metabolic clearance rate (MCR), and degradation rate (D) are comparable in the normal controls, ESRD patients, and kidney transplant recipients. T_3 kinetics, on the other hand, are distinctly abnormal in both the predialysis and hemodialysis patients, and are characterized by a decrease in LT_3 metabolic clearance and degradation rates, and more importantly, a drastic reduction in T_4 to T_3 conversion. Figure 74.9 illustrates the difference between serum TT_4 and TT_3 before and after LT_4 replacement showing that although serum TT_4 increased to similar extent in all study subjects, the increment in serum TT_3, is more marked in the normals and the posttransplant subjects and much less in the two groups of renal failure patients. In other words, the rise in serum TT_3 during LT_4 replacement is proportional to the pre-LT_4 replacement levels. This further confirms that there is a selective defect in T_4 to T_3 conversion.

The reduced TT_4 is generally attributed to the presence of serum inhibitors that impair binding of T_4 to TBG. Yet free T_4, calculated indirectly as the free T_4 index, and free T_4 measurements provided by commercial kits, also frequently yielded low values. It is the current belief that the putative serum-binding inhibitors, which inhibit binding of T_4 to TBG *in vivo*, also inhibit the binding of T_4 to the solid-phase matrices, such as resin or activated charcoal used in *in vitro* assays. This phenomenon could be further aggravated by ingestion of medication such as salicylate and phenytoin. Uremia decreases the binding of these medicines to serum proteins, leaving higher free fractions of these drugs, which then secondarily displaced T_4 from TBG and prealbumin. Tracer equilibrium dialysis has been touted to offer the most accurate free T_4 quantitation. Unfortunately, even this technique is influenced by TBG content and T_4 binding capacity, and 5% to 10% of ESRD patients may still have reduced serum free T_4 measured by tracer equilibrium dialysis technique. The ultimate method of measuring serum free T_4 is by nontracer or direct dialysis equilibrium technique. This latter technique should not be affected by binding inhibitor and should be most specific, but data using this technique of measurement are not yet available.

In peritoneal dialysis patients, serum total T_3 is reduced and serum total T_4 is in the normal range. TBG, T_4, and T_3 are lost in the peritoneal fluid effluent. The documented losses, however, are quite small; less than 10 μg of T_4 and less than 0.1 μg of T_3 each day, representing less than 10% and less than 1%, respectively, of T_4 and T_3 production rates. The daily production rates of T_4 and T_3 in ESRD patients are, respectively, approximately 120 and 13 μg. Thus no replacement is necessary for the peritoneal dialysis patients.

THYROID-PITUITARY AXIS

Despite a marked decrease in serum T_3 and a modest reduction in serum T_4, serum TSH is not elevated in renal failure patients. This absence of TSH elevation is not due to dysfunction of the hypothalamopituitary axis because truly hypothyroid ESRD patients can mount a very high TSH response. Conversely, hyperthyroid ESRD patients showed appropriate TSH suppression. Furthermore, subtle and minute changes in serum T_3 by

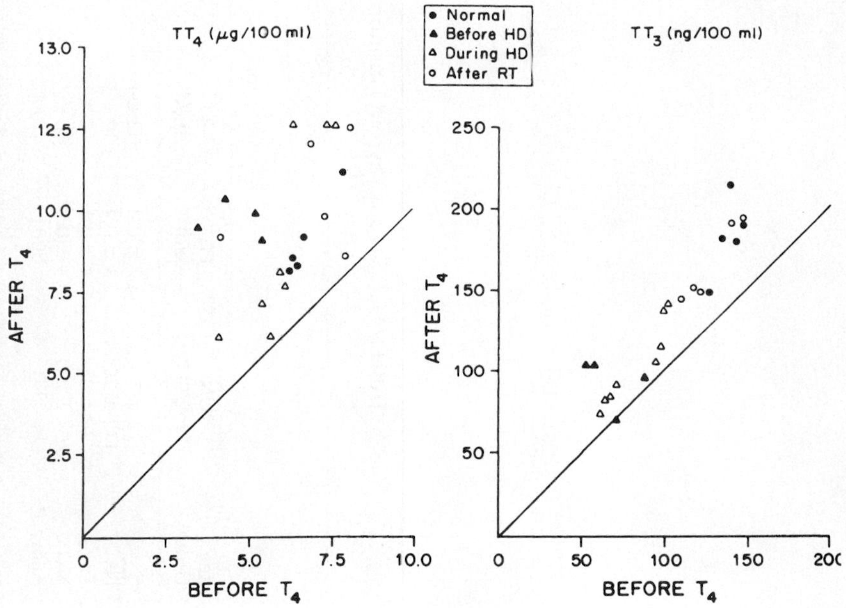

Figure 74.9. Serum TT_4 *(left panel)* and TT_3 *(right panel)* before *(X axis)* and after *(Y axis)* LT_4 replacement in the normal subjects, ESRD patients before and after maintenance hemodialysis, and patients after successful renal transplantation. All subjects received 0.2 mg of LT_4 orally every day for 7 days before and during the entire kinetic study period. While serum TT_4 concentration before and after LT_4 replacement did not show any correlation, that of TT_3 showed a significant correlation between the pre- and post-LT_4 treatment values ($r = 0.943$, $P < .001$). The incremental rise in serum TT_3 concentration was proportional to the pre-LT_4 replacement values, being higher in the normal and transplant subjects and lower in the two ESRD patient groups. (Reproduced with permission from Lim VS, Fang VS, Katz AI, et al. Thyroid dysfunction in chronic renal failure: a study of the pituitary-thyroid axis and peripheral turnover kinetics of thyroxine and triiodothyronine. *J Clin Invest* 1977;60:522–534.)

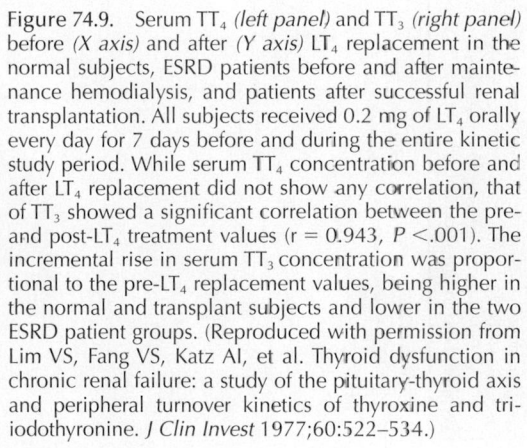

TABLE 74.8. Serum Thyroid Hormone Profile: Liver and Pituitary Thyroid Status in Control, Nephrectomized, Thyroidectomized, and Nephrectomized-Thyroidectomized Rats

		Serum			Liver						Pituitary
					T_3						
Rat/ Group	BUN mg/dl	TT_4 μg/dl	TT_3 ng/dl	TSH ng/ml	ng/g liver	pg/mg protein	αGPD ΔOD/min/ mg protein	MDH units/mg protein	Nuclear T_3 pg/g liver	C_{max} pg/g liver	T_3 pg/mg pituitary
C	22 ± 1	4.7 ± 0.3	52 ± 6	703 ± 61	2.5 ± 0.2	19 ± 1	1.7 ± 0.1	0.037 ± 0.003	308 ± 45	355 ± 29	7.0 ± 1.5
Nx	112 ± 20[a]	3.3 ± 0.4[a]	30 ± 7[a]	441 ± 87[a]	1.5 ± 0.1[a]	12 ± 1[a]	1.1 ± 0.1[a]	0.024 ± 0.003[a]	163 ± 19[a]	233 ± 18[a]	13.0 ± 3.6
Tx	28 ± 2[a]	0.4 ± 0.1[a]	18 ± 2[a]	2249 ± 136[a]	0.5 ± 0.05[a]	4 ± 0.4[a]	0.6 ± 0.05[a]	0.019 ± 0.002[a]	43 ± 11[a]	244 ± 28[a]	3.1 ± 0.9[a]
NxTx	203 ± 24[a]	0.4 ± 0.2[a]	10 ± 0[a]	2525 ± 292[a]	0.4 ± 0.04[a]	5 ± 0.4[a]	0.6 ± 0.12[a]	0.020 ± 0.001[a]	33 ± 10[a]	187 ± 26[a]	—
Anova:*P*	<.0001	<.0001	<.0001	<.0001	<.0001	<.0001	<.0001	<.0005	<.0001	<.0005	<.05

[a] Significant differences between the means of each experimental rat group and the controls were assessed by the Student's t test.

Values (mean ± SEM) of the four groups of rats were tested by analysis of variance and the *P* values are listed in the last line of the table. (Data derived from Lim VS, Henriquez C, Seo H, et al. Thyroid function in a uremic rat model: evidence suggesting tissue hypothyroidism. *J Clin Invest* 1980;66:946–954, and Lim VS, Passo Y, Murata E, et al. Reduced triiodothyronine content in liver but not pituitary of the uremic rat model. *Endocrinology* 1984;114:280–286.)

αGPD, α-glycerophosphate dehydrogenase; BUN, blood urea nitrogen; C, control; C_{max}, T_3-binding capacity derived from Scatchard plot analysis; MDH, cytosoic malate dehydrogenase; Nx, nephrectomized; NxTx, nephrectomized-thyroidectomized; OD, optical density; TT_3, total triiodothyronine; TT_4, total thyroxine; Tx, thyroidectomized.

pharmacologic manipulation can induce appropriate TSH responses. After administration of thyrotropin-releasing hormone (TRH) to normal subjects, serum TSH rises rapidly in the normal subjects, reaching a peak in 30 minutes, and returned to baseline in 3 hours. In the renal failure patients, the response is delayed and blunted. In the posttransplant subjects, TSH response is markedly suppressed; the latter attributable to glucocorticoid administration. Serum T_3 increment following TRH, nevertheless, is positive and comparable between the different study groups indicating that the thyroid gland responds appropriately to its trophic hormone in ESRD patients.

IODINE METABOLISM AND THYROID DISEASES

Because of decreased urinary iodide excretion, both serum inorganic iodide level and thyroidal iodine content, the latter estimated by fluorescent thyroid scanning, are unequivocally increased in ESRD patients. As a result, thyroid gland enlargement is frequently encountered. The incidence of goiter has been reported to be higher in ESRD patients as compared with normals, and goiter frequency is not related to age, race, or the presence of thyroid disease, but to the duration of hemodialysis; the latter is thought to be related to increased cutaneous absorption of povidone-iodine. Autoimmune thyroid disease is not more frequent in ESRD patients because the incidence of positive thyroglobulin and thyroid microsomal antibodies is low. The incidence of hypothyroidism is higher in ESRD patients. It is usually seen in female diabetic patients with ESRD. The frequency of hyperthyroidism is similar to that of the general population. Treatment for hypothyroidism is similar to that of normal subjects; that is, LT_4 replacement. For hyperthyroidism, the antithyroid drugs do not required dose adjustment because they are not dependent on the kidneys for excretion or metabolism. Treatment with ^{131}Iodide could be done, but the dose and the procedure need to be carefully planned ahead with nuclear medicine colleagues. The dose of radioactive iodide should be determined on an individual basis because the blood clearance half-time is markedly prolonged in renal failure patients. Removal of ^{131}Iodide by dialysis varied with the clearance of the dialysis procedure. In the past, we first used a test dose of 10-30 μCi of isotope to assess its kinetics during at least three hemodialysis sessions, and from that we then determined the actual treatment dose, which is likely to be in the 4 to 8 millicurie range. The dialysate for the next two to three sessions needs to be disposed in the same manner as any other radioactive material and requires assistance from the Radiation Protection Service.

THYROID HORMONE METABOLISM IN THE PARTIALLY NEPHRECTOMIZED UREMIC RAT MODEL

In the partially nephrectomized rat model (Table 74.8), serum thyroid hormone profile mimics that of the ESRD patients showing elevated blood urea nitrogen, decreased serum TT_4, and TT_3. Serum TSH is likewise not elevated, and, in fact, is reduced. Analysis of the liver in these uremic rats showed a reduction in T_3 content as well as a decrease in the activity of two thyroid hormone–dependent enzymes, mitochondrial α-glycerophosphate dehydrogenase (αGPD) and cytosolic malate dehydrogenase (MDH), compared with the liver of age-matched normal rats. The reduction in the activity of these enzymes correlates with the decrease in T_3 content. Figure 74.10 depicts such a relationship between liver T_3 content and mitochondrial αGPD in

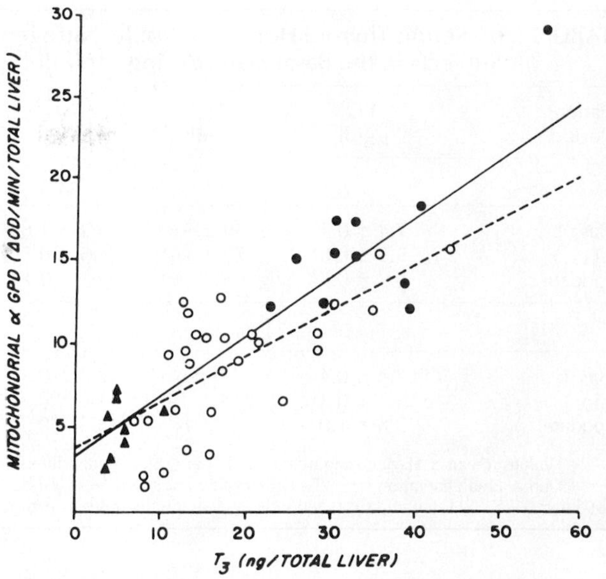

Figure 74.10. Correlation between liver T_3 content and liver mitochondrial α-glycerophosphate dehydrogenase (αGPD) activity. Two regression lines are presented, the *solid line* was derived from control (●) and thyroidectomized (▲) rats (n = 19, r = 0.896, $P < .01$), and the *dotted line* from nephrectomized (○) rats (n = 29, r = 0.666, $P < .01$). There is no statistical difference between these two lines. (Reproduced with permission from Lim VS, Henriquez C, Seo H, et al. Thyroid function in a uremic rat model: evidence suggesting tissue hypothyroidism. *J Clin Invest* 1980;66:946–954.)

control, nephrectomized, and thyroidectomized rats. Moreover, in the liver of the same rat model, nuclear T_3 content was reduced. Scatchard plots showed a reduction in T_3-receptor binding capacity, but the binding affinity is unaltered. Thus it appears that in this uremic rat model, biochemical evidence of hypothyroidism is unequivocally present at the tissue level.

In thyroidectomized, nonuremic rats, the reduction in liver T_3 content and enzyme activity are more pronounced than that found in nephrectomized rats. Moreover, serum thyroid hormones are profoundly low and TSH is elevated to an astounding degree. The nephrectomized-thyroidectomized rats showed data akin to that of the thyroidectomized rats, including an enormous TSH elevation.

The pituitary behaves differently from the liver, its T_3 content is similar between the normal and the nephrectomized rats, and is reduced only in the thyroidectomized rats. This normal pituitary T_3 content in the nephrectomized rats suggests that the ability of the pituitary to convert T_4 to T_3 may not be impaired as in the case of the liver, and thus could explain the absence of TSH elevation in uremia. Others have demonstrated that a greater fraction of nuclear T_3 in the pituitary is produced locally as compared with the liver. The dissociation between liver and pituitary T_3 generation is also seen after propylthiouracil administration, when liver T_4 5′deiodination is markedly inhibited, whereas intrapituitary T_3 generation is not affected.

BIOLOGIC SIGNIFICANCE OF THE CHANGES IN THYROID HORMONE METABOLISM IN END-STAGE RENAL DISEASE PATIENTS

Although we have no data on tissue T_3 content in humans, extrapolation of data from the uremic rat model showing reduced liver T_3 content and decreased thyroid hormone–dependent enzyme activity, would support the concept of peripheral tissue

TABLE 74.9. Serum Thyroid Hormone Profile, Nitrogen Metabolism, and Leucine Flux in Hemodialysis Patients and Normal Subjects in the Basal State, during L-triiodothyronine Replacement, and Sodium Ipodate Administration

Patient/ Period	TT_4 μg/dl	TT_3 ng/dl	TSH μU/dl	Nin g/24 hr	Nb g/24 hr	G urea mg/min	Q^2H_3 leu μmol/kg/min	$Q^{15}N$ leu μmol/kg/min
Hemodialysis								
Basal	7.4 ± 0.4	79 ± 5	5.2 ± 1.6	9.2 ± 0.8	0.58 ± 0.3	4.6 ± 0.6	1.4 ± 0.1	2.5 ± 0.2
LT_3	5.5 ± 0.8[a]	172 ± 16[a]	1.5 ± 0.5	9.2 ± 0.8	−0.80 ± 0.4[a]	6.0 ± 0.5[a]	1.7 ± 0.1[a]	3.4 ± 0.2[a]
Ipodate	8.9 ± 0.7[a]	66 ± 9[a]	9.1 ± 2.4[a]	8.7 ± 0.8	0.87 ± 0.4	4.7 ± 0.6	—	—
Normal								
Basal	7.4 ± 0.4	111 ± 6	2.2 ± 0.3	14.7 ± 1.1	0.02 ± 0.5	—	1.2 ± 0.1	2.1 ± 0.2
LT_3	5.3 ± 0.3[a]	214 ± 12[a]	1.0 ± 0.3	14.8 ± 1.1	0.22 ± 0.7	—	1.4 ± 0.1	2.5 ± 0.1
Ipodate	9.6 ± 1.0	74 ± 8	2.4 ± 0.5	14.6 ± 0.9	0.05 ± 0.6	—	—	—

[a] Values (mean ± SEM) during treatment that are significantly different from those of the basal period as assessed by paired t test.

Gurea, urea generation rate; LT_3, L-triiodothyronine; Nb, nitrogen balance; Nin, nitrogen intake; TSH, thyroid-stimulating hormone; TT_3, total triiodothyronine; TT_4, total thyroxine. Q^2H_3 leu and $Q^{15}N$ leu indicate leucine flux rates as measured using two stable isotopes.

"hypothyroid" state in CRF patients. We speculate that this functionally hypothyroid state serves to defend against protein wasting in a precarious situation in which protein/caloric intake is limited and protein amino acid loss is significant via dialysis procedures.

To test the validity of this hypothesis, we treated CRF patients having low serum TT_3 with a slightly higher than physiologic dose, 50 μg/day, of L-triiodothyronine (LT_3), Cytomel. Table 74.9 compares the serum thyroid hormone profile of hemodialysis patients and normal controls in their basal state, during LT_3 replacement and sodium ipodate administration; the latter is an oral cholecystographic agent that inhibits liver T_4 to T_3 conversion. LT_3 replacement raises serum TT_3 uniformly. Serum TSH and TT_4 are reduced in both CRF and control subjects; the former due to elevated serum TT_3, and the latter, to suppression of TSH secretion. Although LT_3 replacement in the normal controls did not affect nitrogen balance or leucine flux, it resulted in a lesser (more negative or less positive) nitrogen balance, a greater urea generation rate, and an increase in leucine flux in the renal failure patients. Leucine flux is linearly proportional to protein turnover, and when the experiment is performed in the postabsorptive state, as in the study cited here, it represents protein degradation. Ipodate administration changes thyroid hormone profile in directions opposite than during LT_3 replacement; serum TT_3 decreases and TSH and TT_4 are increased, but the effects on protein/nitrogen metabolism are negligible.

Thus in CRF patients with low serum thyroid hormone, misguided attempts to replete thyroid hormone stores may worsen the situation of protein malnutrition because of their greater sensitivity to the catabolic effects of thyroid hormones. A similar phenomenon has been observed in normal human subjects undergoing starvation. When patients with starvation are supplemented with 40 μg/day of LT_3, urinary urea nitrogen excretion rose significantly compared with starvation without LT_3 supplement. We believe that this decrease in serum thyroid hormones represents a metabolic adaptation for protein/nitrogen conservation.

The absence of TSH elevation in the face of low circulating levels of T_3 and T_4 has been an enigma and raised issue regarding whether there might be concomitant hypothalamo-pituitary disturbance. Yet in the experiments in which we gave CRF patients and normal controls LT_3 and sodium ipodate, we found that the pituitary gland is exquisitely sensitive to minute changes in serum T_3 concentration. As shown in Table 74.9, serum T_3 rose during LT_3 administration, and resulted in suppression of TSH; ipodate treatment, on the other hand, reduces serum T_3 slightly, and serum TSH rises. Most interestingly, we found that, in contrast to the liver, the pituitary in the uremic rats have normal T_3 content. As discussed previously, it appears that there is a dissociation in the *in situ* T_3 generation of the pituitary and the liver in the uremic rats. Such dissociation between liver and pituitary T_3 production is also seen after propylthiouracil administration, when liver T_4 5′-monodeiodination is markedly inhibited, but intrapituitary T_3 generation is not affected. These findings provide a logical explanation for the failure to observe an increase in serum TSH in patients with renal failure, starvation, and other chronic illnesses. If one accepts the theoretic construct that a state of protein conservation is achieved in uremia through reduction of thyroid hormone in the peripheral tissue, this can be accomplished only if thyroid gland stimulation by the pituitary is prevented. Had the pituitary shared with the liver in the reduction in T_3 production, the resulting increase in TSH secretion would have led to an increase in thyroid hormone production and secretion, and restoration of peripheral tissue T_3 content.

ALTERED THYROID FUNCTION IN OTHER NONTHYROIDAL ILLNESSES

Thyroid hormone changes similar to those found in uremic patients are also found in a number of medical conditions including starvation, liver cirrhosis, chronic obstructive pulmonary diseases, and others. The major difference between uremia and other nonthyroidal illnesses is serum reverse T_3 (rT_3), which is normal in the former and elevated in the latter. Hypothyroid patients have unequivocally reduced serum rT_3. In renal failure patients and patients with other nonthyroidal illnesses, there is a preferential inner ring monodeiodination of thyroxine producing rT_3 instead of T_3. The absence of rT_3 elevation in renal failure patients is due to an increased exit of rT_3 from plasma to the extravascular compartment. Metabolically, T_3 is many times more active than its parent hormone, T_4, whereas rT_3 has minimal calorigenic activity. Table 74.10 summarizes the directional changes in serum thyroid hormone profile in patients with CRF; nonrenal, nonthyroidal illnesses; and hypothyroidism as compared with euthyroid normal subjects.

TABLE 74.10. Directional Changes in Serum Thyroid Hormone Profile in Patients with Chronic Renal Failure, Nonthyroidal Illness, and Hypothyroidism as Compared with Normal Controls

	ESRD	Nonrenal Nonthyroidal Illnesses	Hypothyroidism
TT_4	↓N	↓N	↓
FT_4I	↓N	↓N	↓
FT_4-RIA	↓N	↓N	↓
FT_4-ED	↓N	↓N	↓
TT_3	↓	↓	↓
FT_3	↓	↓	↓
rT_3	N	↑	↓
TSH	N	N	↑
TRH test	↓N	↓N	↑

ESRD, end-stage renal disease; FT_3, free serum T_3; FT_4-ED, free serum T_4 measured by equilibrium dialysis assay; FT_4I, free thyroxine index; FT_4-RIA, free serum T_4 measured by radioimmunoassay; N, normal; rT_3, reverse T_3; TRH, thyrotopin-releasing hormone; TSH, thyroid-stimulating hormone; TT_3, total triiodothyronine; TT_4, total thyroxine; ↓, decreased; ↑, increased.

ACKNOWLEDGMENT

The author is grateful to the patients at the University of Chicago and University of Iowa Hospitals for their trust and confidence, to Dr. Samuel Refetoff and Dr. Fredric Coe at the University of Chicago for their guidance and support, and to Dr. Michael Flanigan at the University of Iowa for his friendship.

Selected Readings

Kaptein EM, Feinstein EI, Nicoloff JT, et al. Serum reverse triiodothyronine and thyroxine kinetics in patients with chronic renal failure. *J Clin Endocrinol Metab* 1983;57:181–189.

In most nonthyroidal illnesses, serum reverse T_3 is elevated in proportion to the reduction in serum T_3. In the ESRD patients, serum rT_3 is not elevated despite reduced serum T_3. Kinetic studies showed that the normal rT_3 level is explained by an increase in rT_3 exit from the vascular to the extracellular compartment.

Lim VS, Fang VS, Katz AI, et al. Thyroid dysfunction in chronic renal failure: a study of the pituitary-thyroid axis and peripheral turnover kinetics of thyroxine and triiodothyronine. *J Clin Invest* 1977;60:522–534.

This is a comprehensive study on thyroid function in the ESRD patients before and after maintenance hemodialysis and after successful renal transplantation showing low circulating T^4 and T_3 and normal TSH. The low T_3 is due to impaired peripheral T_4 to T_3 conversion. TSH is not elevated despite low T_4 and T_3.

Lim VS, Flanigan MJ, Zavala DC, et al. Protective adaptation of low serum triiodothyronine in patients with chronic renal failure. *Kidney Int* 1985;28:541–549.

During LT_3 (Cytomel) treatment, ESRD patients with low serum T_3 normalized their serum levels, but nitrogen balance became less positive or more negative. Parallel studies in control subjects showed no significant changes in nitrogen balance.

Lim VS, Henriquez C, Seo H, et al. Thyroid function in a uremic rat model: evidence suggesting tissue hypothyroidism. *J Clin Invest* 1980;66:946–954.

Thyroid function was studied in a partially nephrectomized, chronic uremic rat model showing a serum thyroid hormone profile that mimics that of the ESRD patients. Additionally, T_3 content and two T_3-dependent enzyme activities are reduced in the liver, suggesting tissue hypothyroidism in this rat model.

Lim VS, Passo C, Murata Y, et al. Reduced triiodothyronine content in liver but not pituitary of the uremic rat model: demonstration of changes compatible with thyroid hormone deficiency in liver only. *Endocrinology* 1984;114:280–286.

In the partially nephrectomized uremic rat model, liver T_3 content and nuclear T_3 binding capacity are reduced. By contrast, pituitary T_3 content is normal, thus providing an explanation for the absence of TSH elevation in renal failure setting despite low-circulating thyroid hormone.

Lim VS, Tsalikian E, Flanigan MJ. Augmentation of protein degradation by L-triiodothyronine in uremia. *Metabolism* 1989;38:1210–1215.

Nitrogen balance and leucine flux were measured in ESRD patients and control subjects before and during LT_3 treatment. The treatment resulted in greater increments in nitrogen output and leucine flux in the ESRD patients as compared with the controls.

Nelson JC, Wilcox RB, Pandian MR. Dependence of free thyroxine estimates obtained with equilibrium tracer dialysis on the concentration of thyroxine-binding globulin. *Clin Chem* 1992;38:1294–1300.

Serum free T_4 were measured by two methods, equilibrium tracer dialysis and direct equilibrium dialysis. The former method yielded higher free T_4 values, which is in direct proportion to thyroxine globulin or thyroxine-binding capacity.

Robey C, Shreedhar K, Bautman V. Effect of chronic peritoneal dialysis on thyroid function tests. *Am J Kidney Dis* 1989;13:99–103.

In peritoneal dialysis patients, serum total T_3 is reduced and total T_4 is in the low-normal range. Peritoneal effluent T_4 and T_3 losses are modest and remained far below their respective production rate.

Silva JE, Dick TE, Larsen PR. The contribution of local tissue thyroxine monodeiodination to the nuclear 3,5,3′-triiodothyronine in pituitary, liver and kidney of euthyroid rats. *Endocrinology* 1978;103:1196–1207.

In the rats, the fraction of intracellular T_3 generated from T_4 in the pituitary is proportionally much greater than that found in the liver and the kidney. As a result of this property, the amount of nuclear T_3 and the fraction of nuclear T_3-receptor saturation are higher in the pituitary.

PART 5
Leptin

Peter Stenvinkel

The notion that the brain regulates food intake and body weight dates back to the beginning of this century when it first was observed that in some cases damage to the human hypothalamus resulted in extreme obesity. A genetic trait that results in profound obesity and type 2 diabetes mellitus was identified in a particular type of mice (*ob/ob* mice) in the early 1950s. Subsequent parabiosis experiments in which obese, mutant homozygote *ob/ob* mice and normal mice were cross-connected circulatorily resulted in decreased food intake and weight loss in the obese mice, suggesting that these mice were deficient of a blood-borne factor regulating nutrient intake and metabolism. A major breakthrough was achieved in November 1994, when Friedman and collaborators used positional cloning to identify and sequence this blood-borne factor, the obesity (*ob*) gene protein named *leptin* from the Greek word *leptos* ("thin").

Leptin (16 kD) is almost exclusively produced by adipocytes, and a strong positive correlation exists between the body fat mass and serum leptin levels. In lean subjects, the majority of leptin circulates in the bound form, whereas in obese subjects, the majority of leptin is present in the free form. Leptin reaches the brain by a saturable transport mechanism via the blood–brain barrier and, via direct effects on the hypothalamus, decreases appetite and increases metabolism (Fig. 74.11). The leptin receptor (OB-R) belongs to a class 1 cytokine–receptor family and up until now at least six alternatively spliced forms of leptin receptor–mRNA have been discovered. The short-length OB-Ra receptor is present in virtually all tissues examined but it is unknown if this receptor has any functional signalling activity. The full-length variant of the leptin receptor (OB-Rb), contains characteristic second messengers for receptor signalling and is expressed at a high level in the hypothalamus.

Administration of recombinant leptin elicits impressive biologic effects in the *ob/ob* mice. It has been demonstrated that after 4 days on daily injections with recombinant leptin, the obese *ob/ob* mice consumed 60% less food and their physical activity increased compared with untreated *ob/ob* mice. No obvious side effects of leptin were observed and the metabolic control improved considerably during the treatment period. Available data suggest that weight-reducing effects of leptin may be mediated by signal transduction through leptin receptors in the hypothalamus that modulate the activity of neuromodulators known to affect feeding behavior such as neuropeptide Y (NPY)

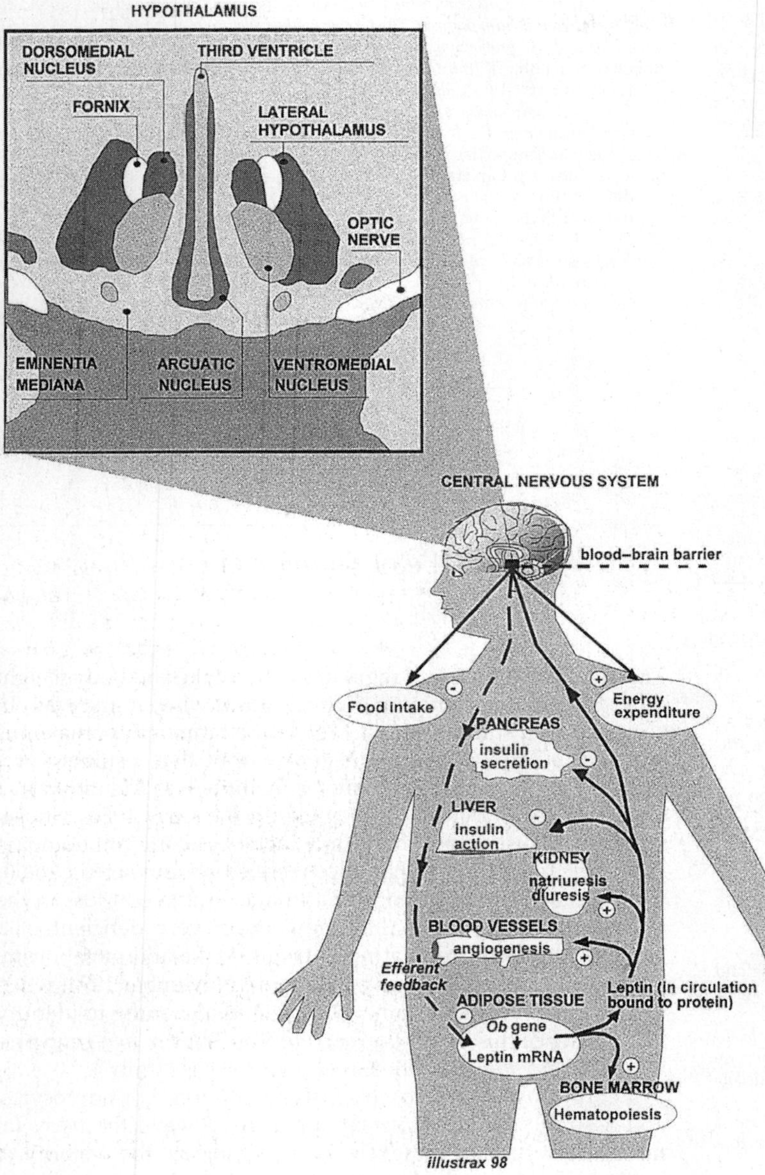

Figure 74.11. Hypothetic role of leptin in humans. Adipose tissue secretes the *ob* gene protein, leptin, which travels in the circulation bound to protein. Leptin is actively transported over the blood–brain barrier and reaches the hypothalamus, where it binds to specific leptin receptors at various hypothalamic nuclei. Such binding decreases the release of neuropeptide Y (NPY) and possibly also affects other neuromodulators, thereby affecting appetite and energy expenditure. Available evidence suggests that leptin also influences the function of various peripheral target organs such as the liver, pancreas, kidney, bone marrow, and blood vessels. (Modified with permission from Meister B, Arvidsson U. The hormone leptin reduces body weight. A mutant gene makes the mouse obese. *Läkartidningen*. 1996;93:247–251.)

and melanocortin. It is of interest that certain evidence suggests that besides an effect on body weight homeostasis, leptin also modulates other physiologic actions such as hematopoiesis, pancreatic β-cell function, angiogenesis, ovarian function, and thermogenesis.

STUDIES ON LEPTIN IN HUMANS

Compared with rodents, much less is known about the role of leptin in humans. The human *ob* gene homolog is 84% identical to the mouse gene. Markedly elevated leptin mRNA expression has been demonstrated in subcutaneous tissue in obese subjects. It is of interest that although leptin is predominantly secreted by widely dispersed adipocytes, it has been demonstrated that serum leptin levels are highly organized and pulsatile with diurnal variation. Meal ingestion does not acutely regulate serum leptin levels. However, a nocturnal rise of leptin has been observed, probably due to cumulative hyperinsulinemia of the entire day, indicating that leptin may have a role in suppressing appetite at night. Serum leptin concentrations are correlated with the percentage of body fat, suggesting that most obese persons are insensitive to endogenous leptin production. However, in spite of a strong correlation between body fat and leptin levels, there is great heterogeneity in leptin levels at any given index of body fat. It has been proposed that in obese patients there is a defective transport of leptin across the blood–brain barrier indicating a resistance to the central actions of leptin. Accordingly, if only small amounts of leptin reach the brain, satiety is not obtained and the obese patient continues to eat. Leptin has been thought to have dual regulation in human physiology. During the periods of weight maintenance, when energy intake and energy output are equal, leptin levels reflect total body fat mass. However, in conditions of negative (weight loss) or positive (weight gain) energy balances, the changes in leptin levels are thought to function as a sensor of energy imbalance.

A number of factors have been shown to affect *ob* gene expression and leptin levels in humans (Table 74.11). One of the most important hormonal modulators of leptin is insulin, which has a direct stimulatory effect on leptin mRNA. Consequently, in humans long-term hyperinsulinemia increases leptin levels by approximately 40%, probably through a trophic effect on

TABLE 74.11. Physiologic Factors Associated with Changes in Leptin Secretion

Increased Leptin Secretion	Decreased Leptin Secretion
Obesity	Fasting
Female gender	Exercise
Insulin	Menopause
Cytokines (IL-1α, TNF-α)	Senescence
Corticosteroids	
Puberty	

IL-1α, interleukin-1α; TNF-α, tumor necrosis factor-α.

adipocytes. Leptin receptors are present in the pancreas and, in *ob/ob* mice, leptin inhibits pancreatic insulin secretion in a dose-dependent manner. Leptin has also been shown to inhibit insulin mRNA expression in cultured cells and rat islets. This may imply that markedly elevated serum leptin levels impair the pancreatic insulin secretion and that hyperleptinemia could be a factor contributing to impaired glucose tolerance. Another important modulator of leptin mRNA is glucocorticoids, and within 48 hours of dexamethasone treatment, leptin levels rise approximately 100%. Moreover, available data suggest that there are important gender-based differences in the regulation and action of leptin in humans, and for any given measure of obesity, leptin levels are higher in women than in men. Because postmenopausal women have lower leptin levels than do premenopausal women, and ovariectomy decreases leptin mRNA in rats, it is probable that also ovarian steroid hormones are important modulators of leptin mRNA.

LEPTIN IN END-STAGE RENAL DISEASE

Soon after leptin became measurable in humans, several studies demonstrated that uremic patients, with and without ongoing dialysis treatment, have elevated serum leptin levels clearly out of proportion with the body fat mass. Possible mechanisms for hyperleptinemia in end-stage renal disease (ESRD) patients (Table 74.12) include impaired clearance and/or increased synthesis. Because the kidneys are important in clearing several other polypeptide hormones such as insulin, parathyroid hormone, and glucagon, it seems reasonable to surmise that leptin also accumulates in the case of renal failure due to reduced renal clearance. Indeed, the kidney appears to be responsible for approximately 80% of elimination of circulating leptin in healthy subjects and urinary leptin levels are usually below the detection of the assay. It has also been demonstrated that renal transplantation normalizes leptin levels in uremic humans. Other *in vivo* studies in rats have demonstrated that uptake of leptin by renal tissue rather than glomerular filtration is the predominant elimination mechanism. However, one must bear in mind that some patients with ESRD [especially males with low body mass index (BMI) and low plasma insulin levels] maintain normal or even low leptin levels. One can therefore assume that counterregulatory mechanism(s) may become operative in ESRD and it is possible that nonrenal (i.e., splanchnic) organs contribute to some of the leptin removal. Another possible reason for elevated leptin levels in ESRD is increased leptin synthesis in adipocytes. However, leptin mRNA expression has been demonstrated to be lower in patients with ESRD than in controls, which suggests that a decreased renal catabolism, by a feedback mechanism, downregulates leptin mRNA expression in ESRD.

TABLE 74.12. Factors That May Affect Leptin Levels in End-Stage Renal Disease

Impaired glomerular filtration rate
Hyperinsulinemia
Obesity
Chronic inflammation
Corticosteroid treatment

Other factors shown to stimulate leptin mRNA expression in nonuremic subjects, such as markedly increased body fat mass and hyperinsulinemia, are probably also important factors that determine serum leptin levels in patients with ESRD. Leptin, insulin concentrations, and body weight are interrelated and there is a direct correlation between insulin and leptin levels in nonuremic as well as uremic patients. Accordingly, results of certain studies demonstrate that ESRD patients with high leptin levels could be separated from those with normal leptin levels based on their fasting plasma insulin levels. Moreover, results suggest that also other hormones, such as rh insulinlike growth factor-1 (IGF-1) and rhGH, regulate serum leptin levels in dialysis patients. Also gender could possibly have some impact on leptin levels in ESRD because sex hormones have been demonstrated to affect leptin production. Another possible reason for elevated leptin levels in ESRD is chronic inflammation, which is a common feature in uremic patients. It has been demonstrated that ESRD patients with elevated C-reactive protein (CRP) levels have an increased expression of leptin mRNA compared with patients with no or minor elevation in CRP. Studies in animals have demonstrated that administration of endotoxins or cytokines, such as tumor necrosis factor-α (TNF-α) and interleukin (IL)-1, induce an increase in leptin mRNA levels along with a decreased food intake. Taken together, this suggests that elevated leptin levels may be one of the mechanisms by which anorexia is induced during inflammatory conditions.

LEPTIN AND BODY COMPOSITION IN ESRD

Protein-calorie malnutrition can be found in up to 40% to 50% of patients with advanced ESRD and is associated with increased morbidity and mortality. Numerous factors contribute to malnutrition in ESRD, but reduced food intake due to anorexia is probably the most important one. The documented spontaneous reduction in food intake seems to appear before the onset of ESRD, and studies have reported a linear energy and protein intake decrease with the decline of renal function over time. The mechanism(s) causing decreased appetite in uremia are not well known. However, because leptin is thought to be an inhibitor of appetite it has been speculated that elevated serum leptin levels could act as a "lipostat" mechanism through modulation of satiety signals and cause anorexia. In ESRD patients an excellent correlation between leptin and body fat mass, but not with lean body mass, has been documented. This suggests that leptin may be used as a nutritional marker to assess the body fat content in patients with ESRD. Moreover, the increase in the body fat content during peritoneal dialysis is closely related to changes in serum leptin concentrations, suggesting that longitudinal changes in leptin may be used to determine whether a change in body weight is caused by changes in the body fat mass. A detailed discussion of the changes in appetite in renal failure is found in Chapter 82.

Effects of Dialysis Treatment on Serum Leptin Levels

Anorexia, one of the major symptoms of uremia, is only partly corrected by dialysis. Even if the majority of leptin circulates in the unbound form, the size of leptin (16 kD) suggests that it will not be cleared by ordinary synthetic dialysis membranes. Certain studies have also demonstrated that leptin levels are not reduced by low-flux dialysis membranes, whereas high-flux dialysis membranes decrease leptin levels by 30% to 40%. In general, patients treated by peritoneal dialysis have higher leptin levels compared with patients treated by hemodialysis. In a 12-month prospective study, serum leptin levels were unchanged following hemodialysis, whereas leptin levels increased markedly in patients treated by peritoneal dialysis. Whether peritoneal dialysis may be less efficient in clearing leptin, or may be associated with a greater stimulation of leptin synthesis, than in hemodialysis is not known. However, the peritoneal clearance of leptin is higher than expected from the molecular weight (16 kD), which suggests the existence of local intraperitoneal leptin production. A markedly enhanced peritoneal leptin clearance has been observed in diabetic peritoneal dialysis patients treated with intraperitoneal insulin, which suggests that insulin stimulates the intraperitoneal leptin production. It remains to be proven whether elevated leptin concentrations contribute to the low eating drive in peritoneal dialysis patients despite their great need for protein and calories.

Possible Clinical Consequences of Hyperleptinemia in ESRD

The pathophysiologic significance of elevated circulating leptin levels in ESRD is not clear. However, it could be postulated that hyperleptinemia could affect several metabolic processes if leptin receptors are not downregulated. Because leptin-receptor antagonists are likely to be developed for future clinical use, it would be of obvious clinical importance if hyperleptinemia could be proven to contribute to uremic anorexia. However, for leptin to suppress the appetites of ESRD patients, we have to assume that leptin is present mostly in its unbound, bioactive form and that there is a normal transport of leptin across the uremic blood–brain barrier. At present, available data suggest that increased leptin levels in ESRD are not due to the accumulation of leptin-degradation products but further studies are needed to confirm this finding. Although there is not yet any direct evidence that increased levels of leptin may cause anorexia, some indirect evidence suggests that leptin may mediate anorexia in uremic patients. First, a significant negative relation between the serum leptin:body fat ratio and the dietary protein intake in dialysis patients has been demonstrated, which is consistent with the concept that leptin contributes to malnutrition. Moreover, an inverse linear correlation between standardized leptin levels and the spontaneous energy intake has been demonstrated in uremic children, and a significant correlation between leptin levels and serum albumin and the protein catabolic rate has been described in dialysis patients. Finally, it has been suggested that elevated serum leptin levels may induce anorexia in uremic patients with an ongoing inflammatory process. However, others have found that leptin is a marker of good nutritional status rather than a cause of malnutrition. Thus, at present, there is some evidence indicating that elevated leptin levels may mediate anorexia in ESRD, but it is obvious that further studies are necessary to substantiate this suggestion. In addition to its effects on appetite, leptin also increases energy expenditure by a stimulatory effect on the sympathetic nervous system. It also has been suggested that leptin, by acting on the vascular endothelium as an angiogenic factor, may facilitate energy expenditure. Because an elevated energy expenditure has been demonstrated in hemodialysis patients, it could be speculated that elevated leptin levels is one factor that contributes to a negative energy balance in uremia.

The kidney has been shown to express leptin receptors, and it has been demonstrated that leptin in high doses increases diuresis and natriuresis without significant effects on renal blood flow and glomerular filtration rate in rats, which suggests a direct tubular effect. It has been suggested that some of the peripheral actions of leptin may act as a signalling mechanism to activate compensatory mechanisms for the potentially deleterious effects of an increased body fat mass. Chronic increases in leptin levels in the central nervous system increase heart rate and blood pressure in rats, which could suggest a possible role of leptin in obesity hypertension. One might therefore speculate that if obese and uremic patients with hyperleptinemia are resistant to the facilitative effects of leptin on insulin sensitivity and sodium excretion, but not resistant to the stimulatory effects of leptin on the sympathetic activity, then this explains why sodium-sensitive hypertension and insulin resistance are such frequent accompaniments of both obesity and uremia. Thus leptin has multiple actions that are potentially relevant not only to the control of eating behavior but also to cardiovascular regulation.

In addition to its role in fat regulation, other research suggests that leptin also may be able to regulate aspects of hematopoiesis and macrophage function. It has been reported that the leptin receptor (OB-R/B219) is associated with a variety of hematopoietic lineages. *In vitro* studies have suggested that leptin can induce proliferation and differentiation of hematopoietic stem cells and there might be a synergy between leptin and erythropoietin (rHuEPO). Furthermore, leptin has also been shown to activate the function of mature macrophages. Adipocytes participate in the bone marrow microenvironment but their exact role has not yet been determined. It is therefore of interest that a high expression of leptin was demonstrated in human bone marrow adipocytes and it has been suggested that bone marrow adipocytes could contribute to hematopoiesis via the secretion of leptin in the vicinity of hematopoietic stem cells. It has been demonstrated that the levels of the stem cell factor increases with deterioration of renal function, therefore further studies are needed to determine whether hematopoietic factors, such as leptin, will be increasingly important in stimulating erythropoiesis in ESRD, characterized by anemia and insufficient production of rHuEPO.

SUMMARY AND PERSPECTIVES

The discovery of the *ob* gene product leptin has markedly increased our understanding of the complex physiologic system that regulates satiety and eating behaviors. Moreover, because leptin-receptor isoforms have now been reported in several peripheral organs, it may be conjectured that leptin, besides having central effects, also has a pleiotropic action. This suggests that the functional role of leptin appears to extend beyond the regulation of feeding and metabolism to include other organs and biologic functions. Indeed, certain findings indicate that besides regulating appetite, leptin may play a role in sympathicoactivation, insulin secretion and sensitivity, renal sodium handling, and hematopoiesis. Because patients with ESRD in general have an inappropriate elevation of leptin levels, further research is necessary to determine the potential biologic effects of hyperleptinemia in this condition.

Selected Readings

Haalas JL, Gajiwala KS, Maffei M, et al. Weight-reduction effects of the plasma protein encoded by the obese gene. *Science* 1995;269:543–546.

In this important work it was demonstrated that daily intraperitoneal injections of leptin for 2 weeks reduced body weight of ob/ob mice by 30% with no apparent toxicity.

Haynes WG, Sivitz WI, Morgan DA, et al. Sympathetic and cardiorenal actions of leptin. *Hypertension* 1997;30(part 2):619–623.

This is an excellent review in which the sympathetic and cardiorenal actions of leptin are discussed.

Heimbürger O, Lönnqvist F, Danielsson A, et al. Serum immunoreactive leptin concentrations and its relation to the body fat content in chronic renal failure. *J Am Soc Nephrol* 1997;8:1423–1430.

This is one of several studies from 1997 that reported elevated serum leptin levels in most patients with ESRD. Prospective data in this study demonstrate that leptin levels increase markedly in patients that start peritoneal dialysis, whereas no change in serum leptin levels are observed following 12 months of hemodialysis.

Sinha MK, Caro JF. Clinical aspects of leptin. *Vitam Horm* 1998;54:1–30.

This is an excellent review of current basic and clinical aspects of leptin and its metabolism.

Zhang Y, Proenca R, Maffei M, et al. Positional cloning of the mouse gene and its human homologue. *Nature* 1994;372:425–432.

This is the original work from 1994 in which Friedman and colleagues isolated mouse ob gene by positional cloning.

PART 6
Sexual Dysfunction

Shaul G. Massry, Guido Bellinghieri, Vincenzo Savica, and Miroslaw Smogorzewski

Patients with chronic renal failure and those treated with hemodialysis manifest a multitude of abnormalities in their sexual function (Table 74.13). Most attention has been directed toward the evaluation of impotence and the disturbances in the hypothalamic-pituitary-gonadal axis in male uremic patients.

TABLE 74.13. The Various Manifestations of Sexual Dysfunction in Uremic Patients and Patients Treated with Hemodialysis

Female patients
Delayed sexual maturation
Amenorrhea
Menorrhagia
Conception rare
Spontaneous abortion usual if conception occurs[a]
Decreased libido
Frigidity
Male patients
Delayed sexual maturation
Decreased libido
Reduced frequency of intercourse
Partial or total impotence
Reduced nocturnal penile tumescence
Gynecomastia
Atrophic testes
Oligospermia or azoospermia
Unconcealed masturbation among dialysis patients
Priapism
Disturbance in function of hypothalamic-pituitary-gonadal axis

[a] Among 142 patients with chronic renal failure and pregnancy, there was no fetal survival in those with blood urea nitrogen above 28 mg/dl. Pregnancy carried out successfully to term has been reported in a 26-year-old dialysis patient who became pregnant 4 years after initiation of dialysis therapy.

PHYSIOLOGY OF ERECTION

Several events must occur before erection develops. There must be (a) a direct genital stimulation leading to reflexogenic erection or supraspinal psychogenic impulses, (b) a relaxation of the corporal smooth muscles of the penis, (c) an increase of 5- to 10-fold in penile arterial flow, and (d) occlusion of venous outflow from the penis.

These processes are controlled and coordinated by complex neurohormonal mechanisms that involve both the sympathetic and the parasympathetic nervous systems, the pituitary-gonadal axis, and arterial vasodilators such as prostaglandins, nitric oxide, or others.

Thus impotence can result from abnormalities in the neurohormonal control system, dysfunction of the corporal smooth muscles or in their response to relaxing stimuli, and/or from derangements in the arterial supply or the venous drainage of the penis.

IMPOTENCE

Incidence

Impotence is defined as the inability to obtain or maintain erection satisfactorily for completing intercourse in 50% or more of sexual attempts. Such total or partial impotence is common among patients with advanced chronic renal failure, and it may first appear or worsen after initiation of maintenance dialysis. Most attempts to evaluate the incidence of impotence among these patients were made either by psychiatric interviews with patients and/or their spouses or by sending questionnaires to the patients. These observations revealed that (a) reduced or partial impotence was present in 38% to 80% of the dialysis patients studied, and total impotence was observed in 20% to 55% of the patients and (b) the frequency of intercourse was decreased as uremia supervened and further decrements occurred during treatment with hemodialysis. A more objective evaluation of impotence was performed in 25 patients with advanced renal failure and in 23 dialysis patients, using a combined approach of psychiatric interviews and the examination of erectile activity by monitoring nocturnal penile tumescence (NPT). About half of the patients complained of erectile dysfunction and reported a significant and marked decline in the frequency of intercourse. Also, 50% of the patients had values for NPT lower than the lowest value observed in normal subjects (Fig. 74.12). NPT appears to provide a good indication of erectile function because it significantly correlated with the frequency of intercourse in 23 patients who did not have evidence of depression and who had available and active sexual partners (Fig. 74.13). The age of the patient should also be considered in the interpretation of the value of NPT because NPT declines significantly after the age of 40 years in normal subjects and in patients with renal failure (Fig. 74.14).

Mechanism of Impotence

The mechanisms responsible for the pathogenesis of impotence are not fully elucidated and several potential factors have been implicated (Table 74.14).

State of Chronic Illness

Patients with chronic and protracted illnesses but with normal renal function do not complain of significant erectile difficulties or a decline in frequency of intercourse, and they have normal

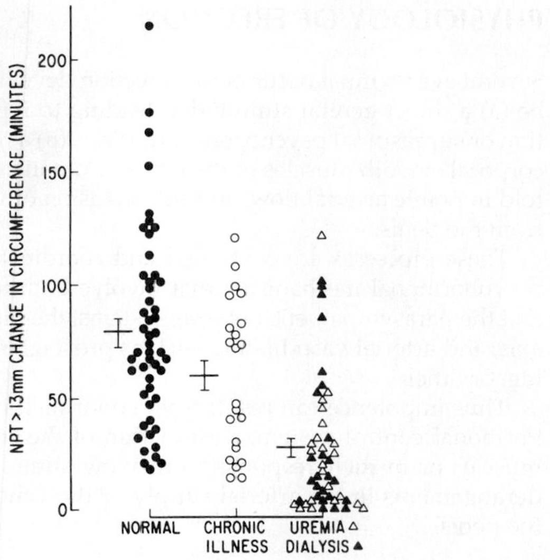

Figure 74.12. Nocturnal penile tumescence *(NPT)* in normal subjects, patients with chronic illness and normal renal function, patients with advanced renal failure (uremia), and dialysis patients. The *bars* represent mean ± SE. (Reproduced with permission from Procci WR, Goldstein DA, Adelstein J, et al. Sexual dysfunction in the male patient with uremia. A reappraisal. *Kidney Int* 1981;19:317–323.)

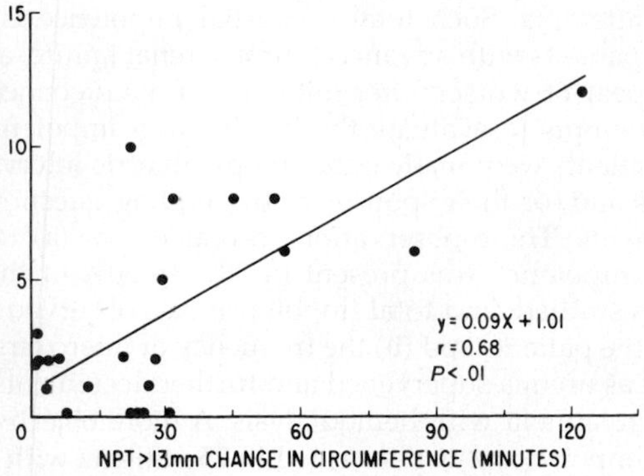

Figure 74.13. Relationship between frequency of intercourse per month and nocturnal penile tumescence *(NPT)* in 23 patients with chronic renal failure who had no evidence of depression and had permanent and active sexual partners. Each *point* represents one patient. (Reproduced with permission from Procci WR, Goldstein DA, Adelstein J, et al. Sexual dysfunction in the male patient with uremia. A reappraisal. *Kidney Int* 1987;19:317–323.)

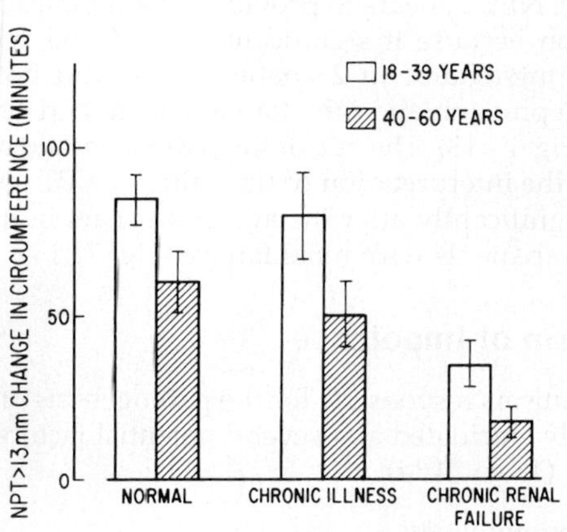

Figure 74.14. Effect of age on nocturnal penile tumescence *(NPT)* in normal subjects, patients with chronic illness and normal renal function, and patients with chronic renal failure. (Reproduced with permission from Procci WR, Goldstein DA, Adelstein J, et al. Sexual dysfunction in the male patient with uremia. A reappraisal. *Kidney Int* 1987;19:317–323.)

TABLE 74.14. Potential Factors Involved in the Pathogenesis of Impotence in Uremic Male Patients[a]

State of chronic illness
Psychologic Factors
Zinc deficiency
Autonomic neuropathy
Abnormalities in arterial blood supply or venous drainage of the penis
Dysfunction of corporal smooth muscles
Hormonal disturbances
Abnormalities in hormones of the hypothalamic-pituitary-gonadal axis
Follicle-stimulating hormone
Luteinizing hormone
Prolactin
Testosterone
Secondary hyperparathyroidism
Anemia
Medications for hypertension

[a] The relative role of these various factors and the evidence supporting or refuting their role in the pathogenesis of impotence are discussed in the text.

NPT (Fig. 74.12). Thus it appears that the state of chronic illness of patients with renal failure is not responsible for their impotence.

Depression

Primary depression may affect sexual function, and depressed individuals may have reduced libido and decreased frequency of intercourse. Patients with uremia and those undergoing hemodialysis could be depressed, and it had therefore been suggested that depression may play an important role in the genesis of sexual dysfunction in these patients. Indeed, we have found an overall incidence of mild to severe depression in 43% of 50 patients evaluated by three different tests. However, we could not find a significant difference in the complaints of erectile difficulties, frequency of intercourse, or NPT between the depressed and the nondepressed patients. These observations support the notion that depression is not a major factor in the pathogenetic processes underlying the impotence in uremic patients. Similarly, the presence or absence of depression is not associated with differences in the frequency of sexual intercourse or NPT in patients with chronic illness. Thus the effects on sexual potency of the depression associated with chronic illnesses with and without renal failure may be different from the effects of primary depression.

Zinc Deficiency

A state of zinc deficiency has been incriminated in the pathogenesis of impotence. This claim is based on two observations. First, the treatment of four impotent uremic patients for several months with dialysate containing zinc was associated with hyperzincemia and improvement in their sexual function. This may not necessarily mean that zinc deficiency is responsible for impotence but rather that hyperzincemia improves sexual performance. Second, oral zinc administration to uremic patients was associated with normalization of serum levels of testosterone and a fall toward normal of the serum levels of follicle-stimulating hormone (FSH) and luteinizing hormone (LH). It should be mentioned that neither of these observations has been confirmed by others. Also, the serum levels of zinc are not always reduced in patients with renal failure, and the majority of these patients have normal blood zinc levels. Thus the potential role of a possible zinc-deficient state in uremia in the causation of impotence awaits further studies.

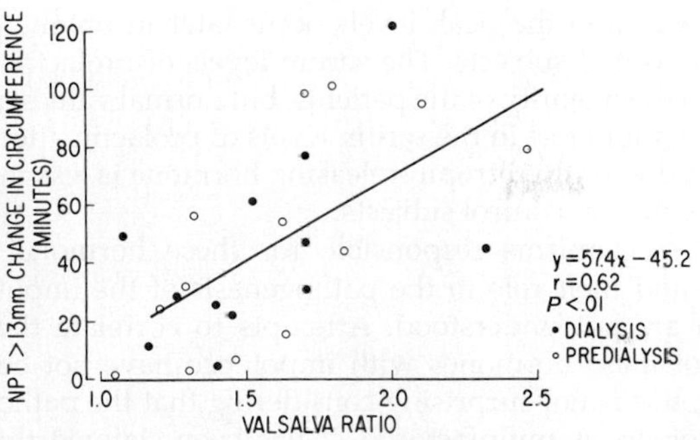

Figure 74.15. The relationship between nocturnal penile tumescence *(NPT)* and Valsalva ratio in male uremic patients. Each *point* represents one patient. (Reproduced with permission from Campese VM, Procci WR, Levitan D, et al. Autonomic nervous system dysfunction and impotence in uremia. *Am J Nephrol* 1682;2:140–143.)

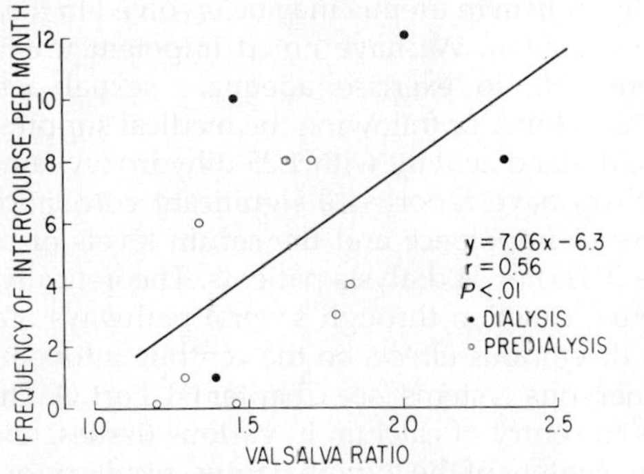

Figure 74.16. The relationship between frequency of sexual intercourse and Valsalva ratio in male uremic patients who are not depressed and have steady and active sexual partners. Each *point* represents one patient. (Reproduced with permission from Campese VM, Procci WR, Levitan D, et al. Autonomic nervous system dysfunction and impotence in uremia. *Am J Nephrol* 1982;2:140–143.)

Autonomic Nervous System Dysfunction

A significant portion of uremic patients and those treated with hemodialysis display abnormalities in the function of the autonomic nervous system (see Chapter 69, Part 3). Such derangements may participate in the genesis of the impotence in uremia. Indeed, a significant correlation exists between both NPT and frequency of intercourse and autonomic nerve function as evaluated by the Valsalva ratio (Figs. 74.15 and 74.16).

Arterial and Venous Abnormalities

Arterial penile insufficiency is associated with impotence. Indeed, obstructive vascular disease of the internal iliac arteries and/or pudendal arteries and pelvic arterial steal syndrome are associated with erectile dysfunction. Patients with end-stage renal disease have vascular calcifications, and such a derangement has been reported in the vessels of the penis. Also, these patients have hyperlipidemia and increased incidence of atherogenesis that could affect the penile arterial system. In addition, many of them have hypertension and are treated with medications that affect the vascular tone. All of these factors may interfere with the arterial blood flow to the penis and therefore adversely affect the erectile process. Venous occlusion or disturbances in venous vascular tone may also impair erection.

The hypogastric cavernous arterial bed and/or venoocclusive dysfunction of the corpora cavernosa was evaluated in 20 patients with end-stage renal failure and impotence. The study used pharmacocavernosometry, pharmacocavernosography, and pharmacoarteriography. Almost all of the patients had vascular disease of the penis as evidenced by abnormal intracavernous pressure response to repeated intracavernous injections of vasoactive agents. Other findings included cavernous artery occlusive disease; atherosclerotic disease of the distal penile arteries; corporal venoocclusive dysfunction; diffuse pan-cavernous leakage involving the dorsal, cavernous, and crural veins, glans penis; and corpus spongiosum.

Dysfunction of Corporal Smooth Muscles

The function of the corporal musculature is controlled by adrenergic and cholinergic neurotransmitters. As mentioned previously, dysfunction of the autonomic nervous system is common in uremia, and it is not surprising that the relaxation of the corporal muscles that is essential for erection may be defective. Also the response of these smooth muscles to local relaxant agonists may be impaired. Finally, the production of these relaxants may be reduced.

Also structural alterations in the corporal smooth muscle cells may occur in uremia. Fine-needle biopsy of the cavernous bodies demonstrated deposits of membrane debris, vacuoles, and granular material in the perinuclear region (Fig. 74.17) as compared with normal (Fig. 74.18). More extensive changes

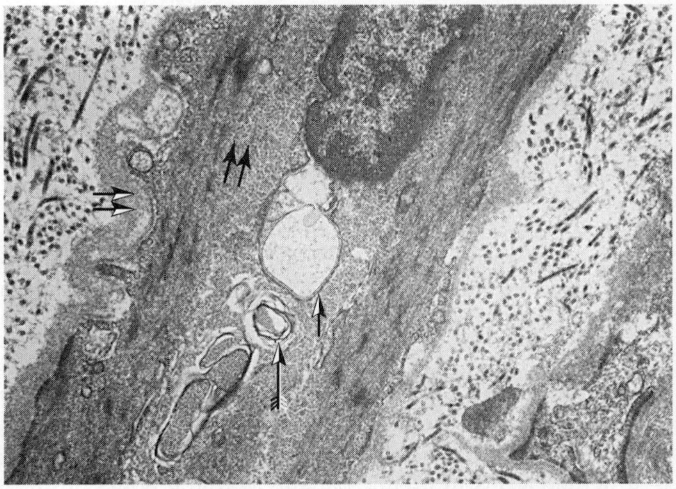

Figure 74.17. Early changes in smooth muscle cell in a uremic patient. Deposits of membrane debris (⤜), vacuoles (→), and glycogen (⇉) are seen in the perinuclear region. The basal lamina is irregularly thickened. (⇉)

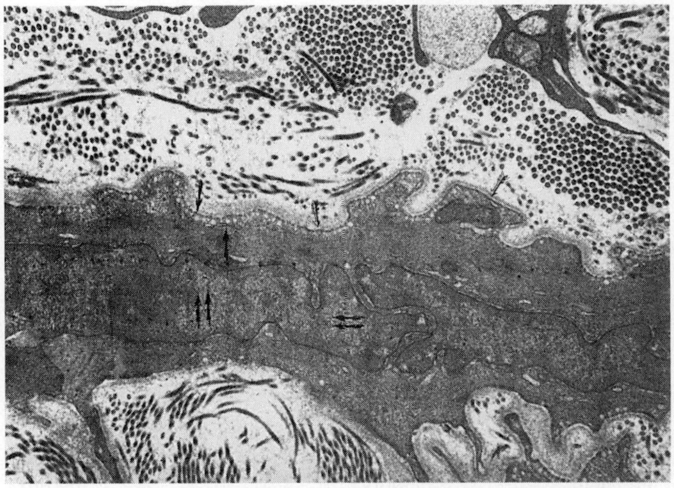

Figure 74.18. Normal smooth muscle cell (SMC). A thin, regular basal lamina surrounds the cell profile (⤜). The elongated nucleus is deeply indented (⇉). Note the abundant pinocytotic vesicles (→). Uranyl acetate and lead citrate, original magnification × 18,000.

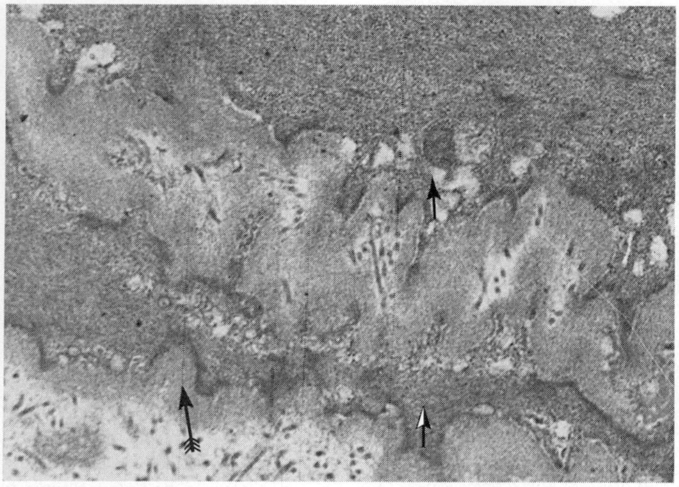

Figure 74.19. More extensive changes in a diabetic uremic patient. Some smooth muscle cell (SMC) profiles are thin (→), exhibiting subplasmalemmal vesicles (→). The basal lamina is regularly and significantly thickened (→).

included significant thickening of basal lamina and subplasmalemmal vesicles (Fig. 74.19).

Hormonal Abnormalities

Derangements in the serum levels of testosterone, FSH, LH, and prolactin have been observed in patients with uremia and those treated with hemodialysis (Table 74.15). Most of these patients have low serum levels of testosterone, but normal values are encountered. Testosterone production is reduced, but its metabolic clearance rate is normal except in dialysis patients with significant arteriovenous shunt; the latter patients may have an accelerated metabolic clearance rate. The conversion of testosterone to dihydrotestosterone is normal, but the serum levels of dihydrotestosterone are reduced. The serum levels of estradiol are normal. The free testosterone:estradiol ratio is reduced. Administration of human gonadotropin for 4 days did not increase testosterone levels in uremic patients within 8 hours but produced a twofold to threefold rise after 4 days. This observation suggests a sluggish Leydig cell function in uremic patients. The serum levels of FSH are usually normal, but some patients may have elevated values. The serum levels of LH are high in the majority of patients, but normal values are encountered. The maximum increments in the serum levels of FSH and LH following the administration of gonadotropin-releasing hormone are greater, and the peak levels occur later in uremic patients than in normal subjects. The serum levels of prolactin are elevated in the majority of the patients, but normal values are seen. The maximum rise in the serum levels of prolactin after the administration of thyrotropin-releasing hormone is less in uremic patients than in control subjects.

The mechanisms responsible for these hormonal disturbances and their role in the pathogenesis of the impotence of uremia are not understood. Attempts to correlate the serum levels of these hormones with impotence have not been successful; this is not surprising considering that the pathogenesis of impotence is multifactorial. It has been claimed that treatment of a few impotent uremic patients with bromocriptine, a drug that suppresses prolactin release, was associated with a fall in the serum levels of prolactin and an improvement in sexual function, assigning a role for the elevated serum levels of prolactin in the pathogenesis of the impotence.

Several observations suggest that the state of secondary hyperparathyroidism in uremia may be involved in the etiology of sexual dysfunction. We have noted impotent uremic patients who were able to exercise adequate sexual activity after parathyroidectomy or following the medical suppression of the parathyroid gland activity with 1,25-dihydroxyvitamin D_3 treatment. Others have reported a significant correlation between the degree of impotence and the serum levels of parathyroid hormone (PTH) in 24 dialysis patients. Theoretically, PTH may affect sexual function through several pathways (Table 74.16). PTH has deleterious effects on the central, autonomic, and peripheral nervous systems (see Chapter 68, Part 1). The hormone enhances the entry of calcium in various tissues, and a change in calcium content of the hypothalamus, pituitary, or testes may affect their secretory function. Indeed, calcium deposits in the testes of dialysis patients have been reported. Also, acute uremia of 3 days' duration in dogs produced a significant increment in the calcium content of the hypothalamus, anterior pituitary, and testes, and a significant fall in the serum levels of testosterone. These abnormalities in the uremic dogs could be prevented by prior parathyroidectomy and could be produced in dogs with normal renal function by the administration of PTH. The hormone may directly affect prolactin release. Indeed, the administration of PTH or the stimulation of endogenous PTH release in normal subjects produced an immediate rise in the serum levels of prolactin. Also, a significant and direct correlation exists between the serum levels of prolactin and those of PTH in patients with acute renal failure. These interactions between PTH, the function of the hypothalamic-pituitary-gonadal axis, and impotence require further exploration before a definite role for PTH in the pathogenesis of the impotence in uremia is accepted.

Medications

Uremic patients receive many medications. Some of these drugs interfere with the erectile process and may cause impotence. Table 74.17 provides a list of such medications.

TABLE 74.15. Abnormalities in the Hormones of the Hypothalamic-Pituitary-Gonadal Axis in Uremic Patients and Patients Treated with Hemodialysis

	Serum Levels	Response to GnRH	Response to TRH
Testosterone	Majority ↓		
Follicle-stimulating hormone	Majority normal, some ↑	↑ and delayed	
Luteinizing hormone	Majority ↑	↑ and delayed	
Prolactin	Majority ↑		↓ and prolonged

GnRH, gonadotropin-releasing hormone; TRH, thyrotropin-releasing hormone.

TABLE 74.16. Possible Mechanisms by Which Parathyroid Hormone May Affect Sexual Potency

Disturbances in central nervous system
Disturbances in autonomic nervous system
Disturbances in peripheral nervous system
Alterations in cellular content of calcium in hypothalamus, pituitary, or testes, affecting hormonal synthesis and/or release
Direct stimulation of prolactin release

TABLE 74.17. Drugs that May be Responsible for Impotence in Patients with Chronic Renal Failure[a]

β-Blockers
Atenolol
Propanolol
Lebatalol
Pindolol
Metoprolol
Diuretics
Thiazides
Aldactone
Antihypertensive agents
Clonidine
Guanethidine
Reserpine
Methyldopa
Hydralazine

[a] This list is not all inclusive but provides for medications commonly used with chronic renal failure.

Diagnosis and Management

Figure 74.20 provides an algorithm for the diagnostic and therapeutic approaches in the uremic patients with impotence. Of course some patients may have more than one factor responsible for the erectile dysfunction.

Testosterone injections (100 to 200 mg/day) have provided inconsistent results. Bromocriptine (1.25 to 5.0 mg/day) or clomiphene (100 mg/day) have been reported to improve potency and sexual performance. Certain data suggest that the correction of the anemia of chronic renal failure with erythropoietin has been associated with improvement in potency. Others found that dialysis patients with similar hematocrits with or without treatment with erythropoietin did not differ in their sexual performance, although some patients claimed an increase in their libido. However, those with erythropoietin therapy had elevated blood levels of testosterone and sex hormone–binding globulin but normal free testosterone.

A major advance in the treatment of impotence in general, and in patients with renal failure as well, is the introduction of intracavernosal pharmacotherapy. This requires the injection of relaxant agents into the corpora cavernosa of the penis. The best approach uses polytherapy, which includes the injections of several relaxants. In most patients two agents are adequate. The most widely used are prostaglandin E_1 (20 mg/ml) and phentolamine (1.25 mg/ml). This therapy is usually followed by a successful erection permitting a successful intercourse culminating into an orgasm. In some patients, pharmacotherapy is needed before every intercourse, whereas in others several therapies may be followed by restoration of the erectile function and no further therapy is needed; this is especially true in those with psychogenic impotence. Failure of pharmacotherapy may then necessitate surgical treatment of impotence; this requires the implantation of penile prostheses.

The discovery of sildenafil (Viagra) constitutes a breakthrough in the medical treatment of impotence. This drug is a selective inhibitor of cyclic guanosine monophosphate (cGMP)–specific phosphodiesterase type 5, which is the predominant isoform in the corpus cavernosum. cGMP stimulates relaxation of the smooth muscles of the cavernous body. Therefore Viagra allows relaxation of corporal smooth muscle and facilitates erection after sexual stimulation. Its effect occurs within 1 to 2 hours after its administration. Doses of 25, 50, or 100 mg may be effective. The use of Viagra is contraindicated in patients taking nitrates. Medications that inhibit cytochrome P450 reduce the

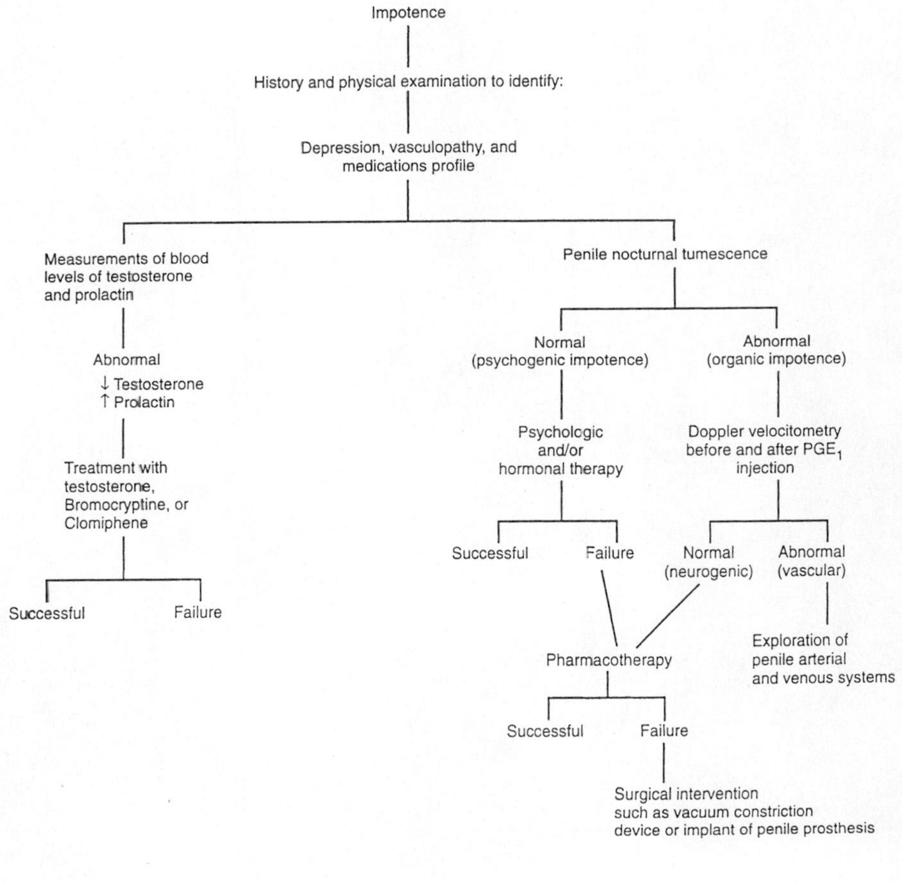

Figure 74.20. Algorithm for the diagnosis and management of impotence in patients with uremia.

clearance of Viagra and result in higher blood levels of the drug for any given dose. These medications include cimetidine, erythromycin, ketoconazole, and itraconazole. Cardiac arrhythmias, myocardial infarction, and death have been reported in elderly patients with the use of Viagra.

As of the end of 1998, there were no reported studies on the use of Viagra in patients with end-stage renal failure. If Viagra is effective in this patient population, it may cut short the need for the diagnostic algorithm described in Fig. 74.20. Such a diagnostic approach may be necessary only in those in whom Viagra is not effective.

GYNECOMASTIA

Variable degrees of gynecomastia are frequently encountered in the male uremic patient treated with maintenance hemodialysis. The gynecomastia is less common in uremic patients who are not receiving dialysis therapy. It may be transient or may last for periods of several months. The mechanism of the gynecomastia is not known. The etiology may be related to the improvement in the nutritional status of the uremic patients with dialysis therapy and, as such, is similar to the mechanism of refeeding gynecomastia. It must be emphasized that in almost all cases of gynecomastia, there is an alteration either in the ratio between the serum levels of androgen and estrogen, in favor of the latter, or in the ratio between the action of androgen and estrogen at the tissue level. Indeed in patients with advanced chronic renal failure and those treated with hemodialysis, the ratio between the serum levels of free testosterone and estradiol is reduced because of a decrease in testosterone levels.

Selected Readings

Bennett AH. *Impotence: diagnosis and management of erectile dysfunction.* Philadelphia: WB Saunders, 1994.

An excellent book dealing with all aspects of impotence. Highly recommended for informative reading.

Campese VM, Procci WR, Levitan D, et al. Autonomic nervous system dysfunction and impotence in uremia. *Am J Nephrol* 1982;2:140–143.

A study of the relationship between autonomic nervous system dysfunction and impotence and NPT in patients with advanced chronic uremia.

Goldstein I, Lue TF, Padma-Nathan H, et al., for the Sildenafil group. Oral sildenafil in the treatment of erectile dysfunction. *N Engl J Med* 1998;338:1397–1404.

The original report that demonstrated the efficacy of sildenafil (Viagra) in the management of impotence. The study did not include patients with end-stage renal failure.

Kaufman JM, Hatzichristou DG, Mulhall JP, et al. Impotence of chronic renal failure: a study of the hemodynamic pathophysiology. *J Urol* 1994;151:612–618.

A study that examined the arterial and venous circulation of the penis with pharmacocavernosometry, pharmacocavernosography, or pharmacocavernosometry. A variety of organic lesions were found.

Lawrence IG, Price DE, Howlett TA, et al. Erythropoietin and sexual dysfunction. *Nephrol Dial Transplant* 1997;12:741–747.

The study examined the hormones of the pituitary-gonadal excess and sexual function in two groups of dialysis patients with similar hematocrits with and without treatment with erythropoietin. They found no difference in sexual performance among the two groups.

Massry SG, Goldstein DA, Procci WR, et al. Impotence in patients with uremia. A possible role for parathyroid hormone. *Nephron* 1977;19:305–319.

An editorial review on the potential role of the state of secondary hyperparathyroidism in the genesis of the impotence of uremia.

Padma-Nathan H. Intracavernosal pharmacotherapy. *Curr Opin Urol* 1993;3:492–495.

A short review of the current status of intracavernosal pharmacotherapy for the treatment of impotence.

Procci WR, Goldstein DA, Adelstein J, et al. Sexual dysfunction in the male patient with uremia. A reappraisal. *Kidney Int* 1981;19:317–323.

A study of NPT in a large number of normal subjects, patients with chronic renal failure, dialysis patients, and patients with chronic illnesses but without renal failure.

CHAPTER 75

The Skin in Uremia

G. Reza Babapour and Arnold W. Gurevitch

Cutaneous signs of uremia are usually present in fairly advanced stages of chronic renal failure. In this chapter, a review of cutaneous changes related to uremia and in patients treated with hemodialysis is presented. These are listed in Table 75.1.

PRURITUS

Among the various cutaneous symptoms associated with uremia and in patients receiving hemodialysis, pruritus is certainly the most disturbing. Pruritus is an unpleasant, vexing sensation that leads to an intense desire to scratch. Although patients commonly present with generalized itching, uremic pruritus can be localized, affecting only parts of the body. In some patients, it is persistent and extensive, whereas in others it is transient. Symptoms can vary from mild to severe. The effect of hemodialysis on pruritus is variable. Although hemodialysis can initiate pruritus, it can also improve the symptoms. In general, pruritus in patients receiving long-term hemodialysis appears to be more severe. Pruritus may be caused by the metabolic derangements and/or the marked alterations in the central and peripheral nervous systems in uremia.

Despite numerous studies, the cause of uremic pruritus remains unknown, although several hypotheses have been suggested. Histologically, the skin of these patients may have an increase in the density of cutaneous mast cells, which may release mediators that produce pruritus. Although blood levels of serotonin and histamine are elevated in uremic and dialysis patients, there is no compelling evidence for a role of these compounds in the genesis of uremic pruritus. In addition, there may be decreased function of sweat and sebaceous glands and hence increased dryness, which may contribute to extreme itching. Other possible factors include allergic sensitization, erythropoietin deficiency (anemia), hypervitaminosis A, neuropathy and neurogenic changes, and secondary hyperparathyroidism. Uremic patients with severe secondary hyperparathyroidism appear to be more often affected by pruritus. Subtotal parathyroidectomy has been associated with almost immediate relief of pruritus in these patients. The direct role of parathyroid hormone (PTH) as a pruritogenic agent, however, has been questioned because patients with primary hyperparathyroidism do not develop pruritus. However, in primary hyperparathyroidism without uremia, the blood levels of PTH are only mildly elevated, whereas in uremia the PTH levels are markedly elevated. Other studies have also pointed to the possibility that patients receiving hemodialysis may have abnormal patterns of cutaneous innervation, thus accounting for their pruritus. In summary, despite numerous studies, the pathophysiology of pruritus still remains unclear. It is possible that more than one mechanism may be involved.

TABLE 75.1. Abnormalities in Skin and Skin Appendages in Uremia

Skin Abnormalities
Pruritus
Xerosis
Pallor
Gray–yellow discoloration
Brown hyperpigmentation
Cutaneous calcification
Acquired perforating disease
Bullous lesions of porphyria cutaneous tarda
Bullous dermatosis of hemodialysis
Drug-induced bullous dermatosis
Furosemide
Nalidixic acid
Tetracycline
Pseudo-Kaposi's sarcoma
Squamous cell carcinoma
Basal cell carcinoma
Skin necrosis
Abnormalities of Skin Appendages
Atrophy of sweat and sebaceous glands
Alopecia of skull
Patchy hair loss on extremities
Dry, fine, and brittle hair
Nail pigmentation, which manifests as Muehrcke's lines
Mee's lines, half-and-half nails

The treatment of uremic pruritus is a challenge because conventional antipruritic therapies do not appear to ameliorate the symptom. Antihistamines, cholestyramine, activated charcoal, lidocaine, topical corticosteroids, and other conventional antipruritic agents are not effective. Ultraviolet B, however, has now become the standard therapeutic regimen for uremic pruritus. Topical antipruritic agents, including emollients and pramoxine, may provide adjunctive benefit. In one study, erythropoietin appeared to improve pruritus by decreasing plasma histamine concentration. In hemodialysis patients with marked elevation in blood levels of PTH and severe pruritus unresponsive to therapy, subtotal parathyroidectomy may be the treatment of choice and should be considered.

XEROSIS

Xerosis, or generalized dry skin, is a common feature in patients with uremia and those receiving dialysis. As noted, xerosis may contribute to the development of pruritus. The most severely affected areas of the body are commonly the extensor surfaces of the extremities as well as the trunk (Fig. 75.1). Patients may develop scales of variable size and thickness with subsequent desquamation. Histologically, atrophy of sweat glands and sebaceous glands are noted in the skin of these patients. Although the functional abnormalities of eccrine sweat glands may account for xerosis, some studies have questioned whether any epidermal dehydration actually exists in uremic patients. It is possible that xerosis in patients with uremia may develop in response to a keratinization disorder.

Patients with chronic renal failure are known to have higher serum levels of vitamin A. Alterations in vitamin A metabolism may produce abnormal keratinization and thus play a role in the causation of xerosis in uremic patients.

The treatment of xerosis in uremic patients is palliative and includes the use of conventional moisturizing and keratolytic agents following short, lukewarm baths or showers. A moisturizing skin cleanser is also helpful.

SKIN COLOR CHANGES

Alterations in skin color are among the most widely reported cutaneous changes in uremic patients. Pallor is a common feature because of the anemia associated with chronic renal failure. A sallow, yellowish discoloration of the skin has been attributed to the deposition of urochrome pigment. Diffuse hyperpigmentation is also commonly seen in patients with uremia, thought to be associated with an accumulation of β-MSH. This causes an increase in melanin production, especially in sun-exposed areas.

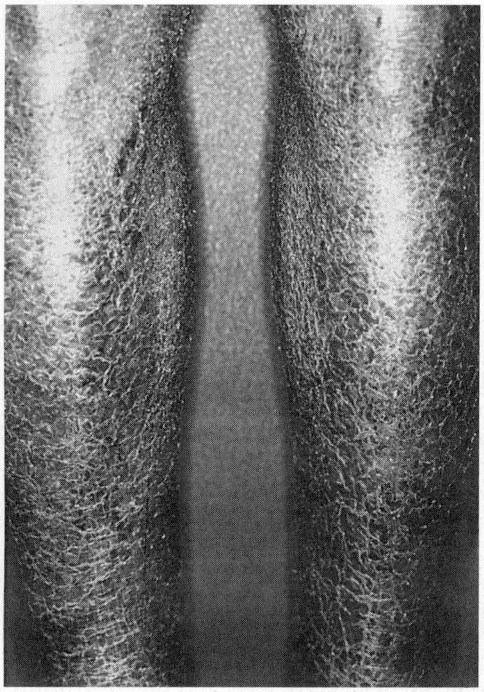

Figure 75.1. Dry, scaling skin on legs.

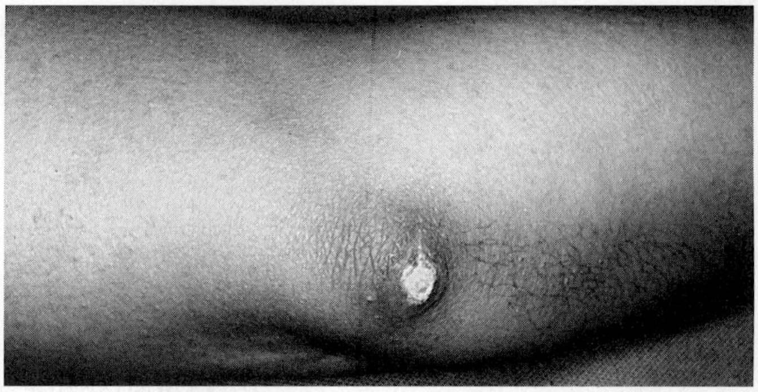

Figure 75.2. Calcinosis cutis exhibiting white, chalky material extruding from the skin (elbow).

CALCIFICATION

Metastatic cutaneous calcification (calcinosis cutis), a rare phenomenon occurring in uremia, is a result of high calcium-phosphorus product (more than 60) and secondary hyperparathyroidism (Fig. 75.2). Clinically, firm papules, nodules, or plaques, often with typical chalky discharge, may be seen chiefly around periarticular and flexural sites. If metastatic calcification involves blood vessel walls, it may lead to cutaneous ulceration and gangrene.

Calciphylaxis is a rare condition involving calcification of small- and medium-sized blood vessels of the skin and subcutaneous tissue. This results in painful erythematous subcutaneous nodules and plaques, most commonly located on the extremities, buttocks, thighs, or abdomen. These lesions subsequently develop purpura on a livedolike background, followed by progressive necrotic ulcerations (Fig. 75.3). It is potentially life-threatening and is seen most commonly in patients with secondary hyperparathyroidism and end-stage renal disease. Septicemia and organ failure are common causes of death. A large incisional skin biopsy is a very helpful diagnostic tool.

Early treatment of calciphylaxis is important. Parathyroidectomy is the treatment of choice, although some studies do not support a beneficial result. Wound debridement to prevent sepsis is also important. Hyperbaric oxygen has also been occasionally effective in healing the ulcers. Detailed discussion of cutaneous calcification and calciphylaxis is provided in Chapters 68, Part 1 and 77.

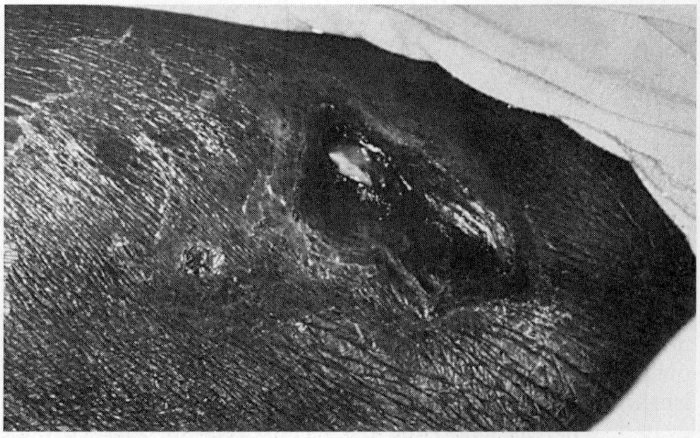

Figure 75.3. Cutaneous ulceration secondary to metastatic calcification in a blood vessel.

VESICULOBULLOUS DISEASES

Bullous eruptions in patients with uremia who are receiving hemodialysis may be due to porphyria cutanea tarda (PCT) or to a relatively unique bullous dermatosis of hemodialysis (BDH).

True porphyria cutanea tarda (Fig. 75.4) is a disorder in porphyrin heme metabolism, in which a decrease in the activity of uroporphyrinogen decarboxylase results in an overproduction of oxidized heme precursors. Clinically, patients present with vesicles and bullae on sun-exposed skin, especially the dorsum of the hands. Lesions heal with scarring and milia. Hirsutism and hyperpigmentation are also common. Many cases of PCT in uremic patients receiving dialysis have been reported. Normally, the diagnosis is made by quantification assays of urinary uroporphyrins. In dialysis patients, who are essentially anuric, the standard diagnostic approach involves measurement of plasma porphyrins.

Bullous dermatosis of hemodialysis resembles the cutaneous features of PCT except that milia and hirsutism usually are absent. Histologically, the bullae are indistinguishable from lesions of PCT. Patients with BDH have normal uroporphyrinogen decarboxylase activity as well as normal fecal and plasma porphyrin levels. The cause of this condition is unknown. Sun exposure appears to be either a contributory or aggravating factor in these patients. A similar process occurring in patients with renal failure has occasionally been associated with certain medications, including furosemide, nalidixic acid, and tetracycline. The bullous eruptions heal after discontinuation of these drugs.

There is no optimal treatment for these bullous disorders. Patients with PCT usually have excessive total body iron stores. In addition, porphyrins are poorly dialyzable because of their high-affinity plasma protein binding. Therefore phlebotomy is the treatment of choice for patients with PCT. Most patients with uremia, however, suffer from severe anemia, making phlebotomy an impractical treatment modality. Antimalarial drugs also appear to be ineffective because the porphyrins removed from the liver by these drugs are not sufficiently cleared by hemodialysis.

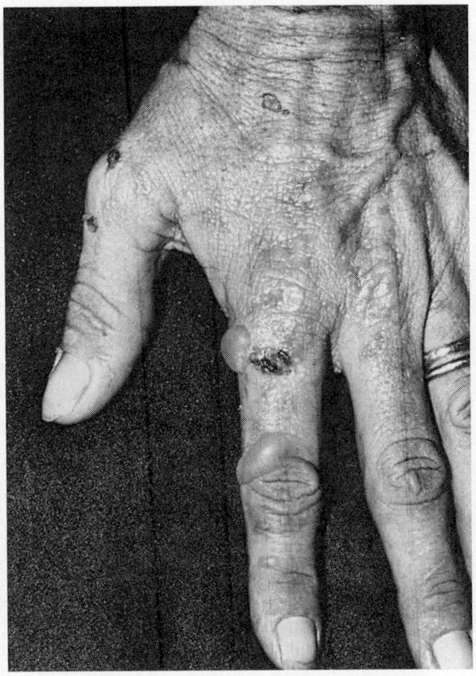

Figure 75.4. Typical lesions of porphyria cutanea tarda.

Avoidance and protection from sun exposure are the mainstays of therapy in these patients. In addition, avoidance of PCT-precipitating agents such as alcohol, iron, and estrogen should be considered. The use of erythropoietin has produced clinical and laboratory improvement in some patients with PCT. Erythropoietin stimulates red blood cell production, which leads to a decrease in total body iron stores. Also, by correcting the anemia, erythropoietin can make therapeutic phlebotomies possible in these patients.

ACQUIRED PERFORATING DISEASE OF CHRONIC RENAL FAILURE

Acquired perforating disease (APD) is reported with increasing frequency in uremic patients, both those who are and are not receiving hemodialysis (Fig. 75.5). Most of these patients have diabetes mellitus. Clinically, patients present with pruritic dome-shaped papules and nodules with central keratin-filled craters. These lesions can aggregate to form hyperkeratotic plaques. The eruption tends to be chronic, and the lesions typically are distributed over the extensor surfaces of the extremities, the trunk, and rarely, the forehead and scalp. The cause of APD remains unknown. Because patients with uremia as well as diabetes mellitus suffer from extreme pruritus, it is believed that trauma from scratching may be a predisposing factor.

Treatment of this condition is difficult. Various therapeutic approaches have been described and include topical corticosteroids, topical retinoic acid, keratolytic agents, and ultraviolet B phototherapy for control of uremic pruritus.

NAIL AND HAIR CHANGES

A distinctive nail pigmentation abnormality associated with uremia is referred to as *half-and-half nails* (Fig. 75.6). This condition is characterized by red, pink, or brown discoloration of the distal half of the nail combined with a white appearance of the proximal half. Fingernails and toenails may be involved. When pressure is applied to the distal area of the nail, the discoloration does not completely fade. This abnormality is seen in uremic patients before dialysis therapy in 10% to 35% of dialysis patients.

Another nail change may be associated with chronic severe hypoalbuminemia, often secondary to nephrotic syndrome. Referred to as *Muehrcke's lines,* this condition is characterized by

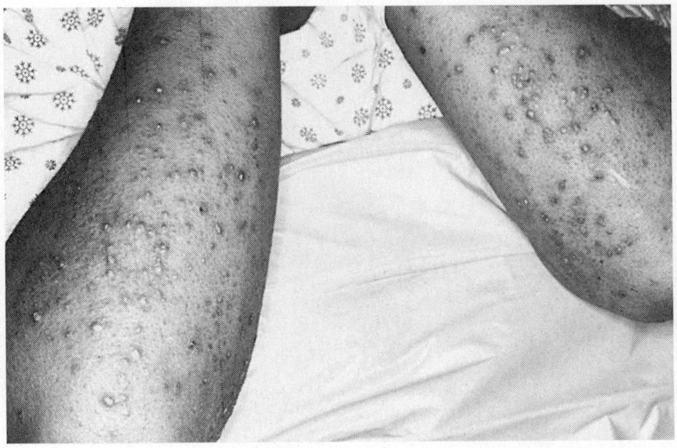

Figure 75.5. Acquired perforating disease with keratotic follicular papules on extensor surfaces.

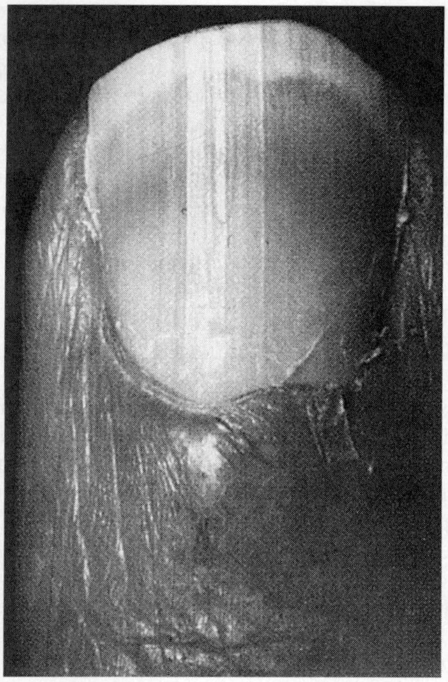

Figure 75.6. Half-and-half nail.

paired narrow white transverse bands in the nail bed, running parallel to a lunula, separated from the lunula and from each other by normal appearing pink nail. Compression of the affected fingernails will cause the lines to temporarily disappear. Although the exact pathogenesis of the Muehrcke's line is still unknown, edematous changes in the nail bed may explain the nail discoloration.

Other nail changes such as occurrence of splinter hemorrhage in patients receiving hemodialysis, as well as onycholysis, nail thickening, and yellow or gray discoloration of the fingernails and toenails, have also been described but are not specific to uremic patients.

Multiple hair abnormalities have also been associated with uremia and include alopecia of the scalp, patchy hair loss on the extremities, and dry, fine, brittle hair. These hair changes are not specific to uremic patients and are more indicative of severe chronic illness.

PSEUDO-KAPOSI'S SARCOMA

These are purplish nodules or papules, slowly evolving into scaly, crusted, violaceous patches, which rarely develop in the vicinity of arteriovenous fistulas or shunts. Histologic features include vascular and fibroblast proliferation in the superficial dermis, vascular slits, mitotic figures, and extravasated red blood cells.

Selected Readings

Faver IR, Daoud MS, Su WPD. Acquired reactive perforating collagenosis. *J Am Acad Dermatol* 1994;30:575–580.

This article reviews clinical features of reactive perforating collagenosis, including diagnostic criteria, histopathologic findings, and treatment modalities.

Ivker RA, Woosley J, Briggaman RA. Calciphylaxis in three patients with end-stage renal disease. *Arch Dermatol* 1995;131:63–68.

This article discusses the pathogenesis of calciphylaxis in the setting of end-stage renal disease. The relationship between calciphylaxis and the serum parathormone levels is discussed, and the article stresses the need for prompt early diagnosis and treatment.

Pico MR, Lugo-Somolinos A, Sanchez JL, et al. Cutaneous alterations in patients with chronic renal failure. *Int J Dermatol* 1992;31:860–863.

This article deals with the prevalence of various dermatologic problems in patients with chronic renal failure who are undergoing dialysis. The most common cutaneous disorders and underlying pathogenesis are discussed.

Stahle-Backdahl M. Uremic pruritus. *Semin Dermatol* 1995;14:297–301.

This article discusses various clinical aspects of uremic pruritus as manifested in the setting of chronic and end-stage renal disease. Pathophysiologic considerations as well as treatment modalities are reviewed.

Stevens BR, Fleischer Jr AB, Piering F, et al. Porphyria cutanea tarda in the setting of renal failure. *Arch Dermatol* 1993;129:337–339.

This article deals with a report of cases and description of clinical features of bullous dermatosis in the setting of renal failure. The authors recommend, in refractory cases, renal transplantation may be indicated.

CHAPTER 76

Disturbances in Fluid, Electrolyte, and Acid-Base Balance

PART 1
Patients with Chronic Renal Failure

Arthur Greenberg and Paul M. Palevsky

Adaptation to the progressive loss of renal function is highly effective, and there is considerable renal reserve. Nearly 90% of renal function may be lost before patients develop uremic symptoms. Abnormalities of hydrogen ion, calcium, and phosphorus concentrations are usually not manifest until the glomerular filtration rate (GFR) falls below 30 ml/min. In the absence of mineralocorticoid deficiency, specific tubular defects, or dietary discretion, hyperkalemia may not have developed even at the time dialysis is required for uremic symptoms. Sodium and water balance are also generally preserved until late in the course of renal failure. Water balance depends not only on renal water excretion but also on intake, as determined by thirst. The latter is generally unaffected by the development of renal failure, except when hyperreninemia is present. In humans, intake of solutes, however, is neither stimulated nor suppressed by deficiency or surfeit. For these solutes, the kidney and the signaling systems that affect renal excretion are solely responsible for the remarkable and persistent preservation of the internal milieu that continues despite advanced renal failure. The ability of these adaptive responses to keep up with sudden or extreme changes in solute intake is limited, however. As a result, patients with advanced chronic renal failure are at increased risk for volume depletion or overload, hyponatremia, and hyperkalemia whenever abrupt or extreme changes in sodium, water, or potassium load occur.

PROGRESSIVE LOSS OF RENAL FUNCTION

Ablation of five-sixths or more of renal mass is a frequently used animal model of chronic renal insufficiency. Immediately after ablation, the fall in GFR is proportionate to the tissue loss, but within a few days, renal plasma flow and GFR rise. Completion of compensation for uninephrectomy occurs over several weeks, by which time GFR in the remaining kidney rises approximately 50%, and the GFR will be roughly 70% of the original value. The increase in function is due to an increase in blood flow as well as hypertrophy of glomeruli and tubular cells. Renal afferent and efferent arteriolar vasodilation are responsible for the increase in renal plasma flow. Because the number of nephrons does not increase, the GFR change must represent an increase in GFR per nephron, or single-nephron GFR (SNGFR). In animal studies, the increase in SNGFR may be due to a rise in glomerular perfusion pressure, particularly if systemic hypertension is present, or due to an increase in glomerular membrane permeability.

Studies of animals and humans undergoing uninephrectomy indicate that a loss of 50% of renal mass is well tolerated over the long term. With greater loss, however, the hemodynamic changes that restore GFR are maladaptive and result in damage to and loss of the remaining nephrons. In human disease, either because of this effect or because of ongoing loss of nephrons due to the primary process, compensatory increases in SNGFR will not sustain an adequate GFR indefinitely and GFR falls progressively.

The loss of functioning renal tissue is "pan-nephronal" even though a disease process may be primarily glomerular or tubular. Detailed anatomic studies confirm that those glomeruli that continue to function drain into intact tubules. Conversely, atrophic tubules incapable of reabsorption are matched with severely diseased glomeruli that filter little. Progressive renal insufficiency does not result in chaotic and unpredictable loss of function or regulation. Rather, remaining nephrons function in a fashion appropriate to the need for excretion or retention of a particular solute. This behavior is termed the *intact nephron hypothesis*.

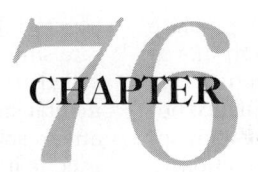

The normal kidney adapts proximal tubular function to changes in SNGFR over a wide range in a process termed *glomerulotubular balance*. The purpose of glomerulotubular balance is to minimize the effect of GFR changes on absolute solute excretion. For instance, if a transient rise in blood pressure raises GFR, fluid delivery to the proximal tubule increases. If absolute reabsorption remained constant, distal delivery of fluid would rise as well. However, because of glomerulotubular balance, reabsorption increases in parallel and the change in distal delivery is minimized. Glomerulotubular balance is preserved in renal insufficiency as well. Because SNGFR is increased, proximal tubular reabsorption increases, largely as a result of Starling forces. The rise in filtration fraction is associated with a drop in peritubular capillary pressure, thus promoting solute and fluid reabsorption. Tubule cell hypertrophy also results in augmented reabsorption. Together, these influences return distal delivery to near normal. Were glomerulotubular balance not preserved, the distal nephron might be overwhelmed with solute, potentially impeding precise control of solute excretion.

If diet remains constant as renal failure progresses, the amount of a solute such as sodium or phosphate that must be excreted per day remains constant. Consequently, and separate from the increased reabsorption, the absolute amount of solute excreted per nephron must rise. For the body as a whole, this is expressed quantitatively as the clearance of the solute divided by the GFR, or the fractional excretion (FE) of that solute. Studies in animals show that the required increase in FE occurs under the influence of the same hormones and other control mechanisms that adjust excretion to dietary load under usual circumstances. However, the changes required are much greater. Consider how a normal individual maintains balance for an ingested solute such as sodium. Because GFR remains constant, a doubling of sodium intake will be matched by a doubling of sodium excretion. Filtered load is unchanged because neither GFR nor serum sodium concentration change, so tubular reabsorption falls enough to permit the necessary doubling of fractional sodium excretion. Halving the intake would have to be matched with a halving of the FE. Sodium excretion and FE vary over a fourfold range in this example.

In an individual with a GFR only 20% of normal, a fivefold increase in FE over baseline would be required simply to maintain balance. To accommodate the same doubling of intake would require that the FE increase to a level 10 times that of the normal individual under basal conditions. It is clear that at some point, the ability of FE to increase will be exceeded and positive salt balance will commence. At a GFR of 5 ml/min with a serum sodium concentration of 140 mEq/L, the daily filtered load of sodium is 1,000 mmol, limiting the maximal sodium excretion to 400 to 500 mmol, because FE_{Na} cannot rise above 40% to 50%. Similar constraints apply to other solutes. The relationship between dietary intake and FE_{Na} required to excrete that load is shown for two GFR values in Fig. 76.1. An additional

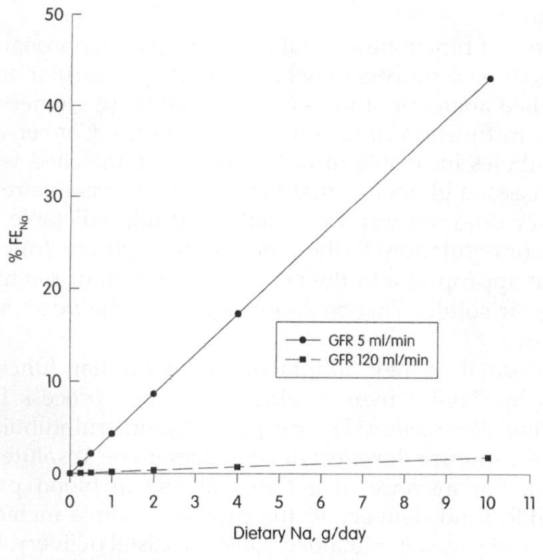

Figure 76.1. Fractional excretion of sodium *(FE_{Na})* shown as a function of dietary sodium intake for normal subjects (GFR of 120 ml/min) and subjects with advanced renal failure (GFR of 5 ml/min). Note that the FE_{Na} required to excrete a sodium load varies directly with the size of the load and that the slope of the curve for the patients with renal failure is 24-fold higher (120:5) than the curve for the normal subjects. This need for a greater change in fractional excretion with renal failure for any given change in intake is termed the magnification phenomenon.

constraint follows from operating at a near maximum excretory rate simply to maintain ordinary balance. Little reserve can be called upon when an augmented response is needed. Experimental studies in animals with renal insufficiency confirm that after a solute load is ingested with a meal, the time required to excrete it increases as GFR falls.

The changes required to promote sodium excretion are not harmful. However, some adaptive mechanisms are potentially deleterious, and for them, the "trade-off hypothesis" applies. This is illustrated by phosphate excretion. To excrete the daily intake of phosphate, FE must increase. According to this scheme, phosphorus accumulates and the serum phosphate level rises as GFR falls. This leads to a drop in serum calcium concentration with a secondary rise in parathyroid hormone (PTH). Because PTH inhibits renal phosphate reabsorption, the rise in PTH level causes phosphate excretion to increase with a drop in serum phosphate. The "trade-off" is a significant rise in bone dissolution owing to the increase in PTH. The progression can be mitigated by phosphate restriction. Subsequent studies have shown that in early renal failure, before phosphate rises, a fall in 1,25-dihydroxyvitamin D levels and numerous other factors also contribute to the observed rise in PTH. Isolated tubule studies show diminished phosphate reabsorption independent of changes in PTH levels. Thus phosphate handling cannot be explained simplistically on the sole basis of a trade off with PTH, but clearly the latter is an important element. The interaction between phosphate retention, $1,25(OH)_2D_3$, and PTH is discussed in detail in Chapter 77.

HOMEOSTASIS OF SPECIFIC SOLUTES AND WATER

Sodium

As noted, a wide range in FE_{Na} is required to match salt excretion to salt intake and maintain balance. The principal hormonal regulators of sodium balance are the renin-angiotensin-aldosterone system and atrial natriuretic peptide (ANP) as well as other factors (see Chapter 15, Part 2). ANP is released from the cardiac atria when intravascular volume is increased. Its principal action is to decrease distal convoluted tubule sodium reabsorption. ANP levels are elevated in renal failure when sodium overload is present, rise after a sodium meal, and fall with sodium restriction. Aldosterone levels are elevated in renal insufficiency and increase further when dietary salt is restricted. Although spironolactone administration to patients with chronic renal insufficiency may cause natriuresis, studies of sodium loading of humans with graded degrees of chronic renal failure show that supplemental mineralocorticoid administration does not interfere with handling of a sodium load. All patients increased FE_{Na} to the degree required and expected to excrete the added salt. This is fortunate and probably not fortuitous as aldosterone release is independently stimulated by hyperkalemia. Its level may not fall in chronic renal failure despite volume expansion if the potassium level is elevated. Resistance to its sodium retentive effect makes good sense teleologically.

In contrast to normal individuals, in whom GFR and renal plasma flow remain constant, the response to salt restriction in patients with mild chronic renal insufficiency also involves changes in these hemodynamic parameters. GFR falls and the filtration fraction increases following institution of a sodium-restricted diet in individuals with impaired renal function due to glomerulonephritis, but not in normal individuals or patients with glomerulonephritis and normal renal function. The reduction in GFR reduces filtered load of sodium. The increase in the filtration fraction reduces hydrostatic pressure in peritubular capillaries and favors proximal tubular fluid reabsorption. Thus

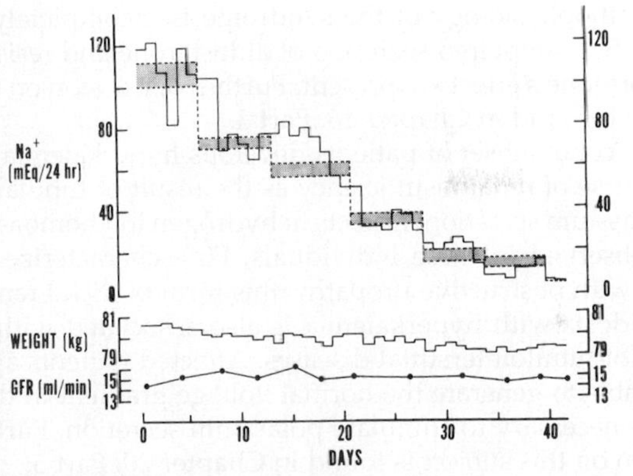

Figure 76.2. Na^+ refers to daily urinary sodium excretion *(solid lines)* and daily dietary sodium intake *(dashed lines)*. The *shaded areas* represent the range of dietary sodium intake. As daily sodium intake was slowly and incrementally reduced on a metabolic ward, sodium excretion fell to as low as 5.6 mEq/day. The subjects remained free of evidence of volume depletion. (Reproduced with permission from Danovitch GM, Bourgoignie J, Bricker NS. Reversibility of the "salt-losing" tendency of chronic renal failure. *N Engl J Med* 1977;296:14–19.)

the effect of these hemodynamic changes is to promote sodium retention. This effect may only be a matter of degree, as a drop in GFR and increase in filtration fraction do occur when normal individuals have frank volume depletion.

Clinicians have long recognized that patients with chronic renal insufficiency are at risk for developing volume depletion with consequent prerenal azotemia if sodium intake drops abruptly or if intercurrent vomiting or diarrhea develop. Rarely, a patient with tubulointerstitial disease or polycystic kidney disease wastes salt and develops spontaneous hypovolemia unless the dietary sodium is supplemented. Such patients were believed to have an intrinsic inability to drop sodium excretion to low levels. Careful studies (Fig. 76.2) have shown that most patients with chronic renal insufficiency can reduce sodium excretion to levels as low as 5 mEq/day, as can normal individuals, but only when the intake is reduced gradually over an extended period of up to 3 months with careful monitoring of blood pressure and renal function. The mechanism for this slow "readaptation" to low salt intake has not been elucidated. It could be that time is required to fully inhibit ANP production. Distal tubule hypertrophy with augmented sodium reabsorption occurs in animals subjected to protracted treatment with furosemide. It may be that similar hypertrophy is required in patients with chronic renal insufficiency who must conserve sodium and that it requires time to develop. In practical terms, caution should be exercised before reducing sodium intake in individuals with chronic renal failure. In the absence of hypertension or evidence for fluid overload such as congestive heart failure or edema, salt restriction is not necessary. When required, patients can be placed on a no-added-salt diet (4 g sodium per day) or a tighter restriction (2 g sodium per day), and they will usually be able to maintain balance. Lower intakes, an abrupt cessation of all intake due to nausea and vomiting, development of salt losses from diarrhea, and continued diuretic therapy are risk factors for the development of negative sodium balance. Prerenal azotemia may result and should be suspected in any patient with stable chronic renal failure who presents with a sudden drop in function to a level below that expected from progression alone.

Potassium

Potassium homeostasis is well preserved until late in the course of chronic renal disease. In the absence of tubular defects in potassium secretion or aldosterone deficiency, the failing kidney is able to excrete the usual daily potassium load and maintain a normal serum potassium concentration until the GFR falls to approximately 10% to 15% of normal. The adaptation to renal failure that permits the preservation of potassium homeostasis occurs at the expense of increased potassium secretion by the remaining functional nephrons. However, the ability to further augment potassium secretion in response to an increased exogenous load is severely limited, and hyperkalemia may result from even modest increases in potassium intake.

In the normal kidney, renal potassium excretion is more dependent on distal tubular potassium secretion than on glomerular filtration. Approximately 90% of the filtered potassium load is reabsorbed in the proximal tubule and Henle's loop. Potassium secretion in the distal nephron, primarily the connecting tubule and cortical collecting duct, is responsible for the final regulation of renal potassium excretion. In response to an increased dietary potassium load, distal tubular potassium secretion can be markedly augmented. In experimental animals subjected to chronic potassium loading, the excretion of potassium may exceed the filtered load.

In chronic renal insufficiency, the adaptive processes that facilitate preservation of potassium excretion are believed to be similar to the adaptive processes that occur in response to increased dietary potassium intake in normal individuals. Fractional excretion of potassium increases as the result of increased potassium secretion in the late distal tubule and the collecting duct. This functional adaptation is accompanied by tubular hypertrophy with proliferation of principal cell basolateral membranes and increased activity of the basolateral Na^+-K^+-ATPase.

The mechanisms responsible for this adaptation have not been completely elucidated but are believed to involve transient increases in extracellular potassium following dietary ingestion as well as increased mineralocorticoid activity. After ingestion of a potassium load, serum potassium increases by approximately the same increment in patients with moderate renal insufficiency as in subjects with normal renal function. This is accompanied by an increase in distal tubular potassium secretion and excretion of the potassium load. In dogs with experimental renal insufficiency induced by partial nephrectomy, the absolute rate of excretion of a potassium load was markedly attenuated as compared with normal controls, although the fractional excretion of potassium in both groups was similar (Fig. 76.3). As a result, the time required to excrete the potassium load was prolonged in renal insufficiency and was accompanied by prolongation of the transient increase in the plasma potassium concentration and elevation of plasma aldosterone levels.

Significant variability in the plasma aldosterone concentration is characteristic of patients with chronic renal disease, primarily as the result of associated hyporeninemia and variations in sodium intake. However, an inverse correlation of aldosterone levels and renal function has been observed. When normalized for the plasma renin activity, aldosterone levels remain within the normal range when the GFR is greater than 50 to 60 ml/min. However, a progressive increase in plasma aldosterone levels is observed when the GFR falls below 50 ml/min (Fig. 76.4).

In a subset of patients, hyperkalemia develops early in the course of renal insufficiency as the result of suppressed plasma aldosterone levels. In most of these patients, the low aldosterone levels are associated with reduced plasma renin activity. Multiple mechanisms appear to mediate this syndrome of hyporeninemic hypoaldosteronism, including direct damage to the juxtaglomerular apparatus, chronic extracellular volume expansion, and treatment with certain medications. Incipient diabetic nephropathy is present in approximately 60% to 65% of

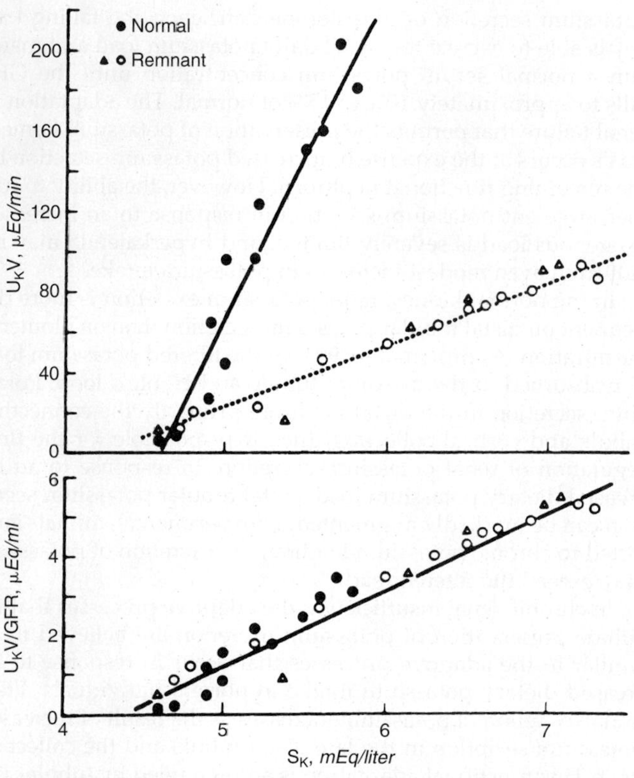

Figure 76.3. Urine potassium excretion *(U_KV) (upper panel)* and fractional potassium excretion *(U_KV/GFR) (lower panel)* as a function of serum potassium concentration *(S_K)* in normal dogs *(solid circles)* and uremic dogs *(open circles)* receiving 50 or 100 mEq of potassium per day and uremic dogs receiving 15 mEq of potassium per day *(open triangles)*. Fractional excretion of potassium as a function of the serum potassium concentration is similar in all groups. (Reproduced with permission from Bourgoignie JJ, Kaplan M, Pincus J, et al. Renal handling of potassium in dogs with chronic renal insufficiency. *Kidney Int* 1981;20:482–490.)

these patients, but patients with obstructive uropathy or systemic lupus erythematosus are also at risk. The syndrome may be reversibly induced by treatment with nonsteroidal antiinflammatory drugs. β-Adrenergic blockers have a similar effect.

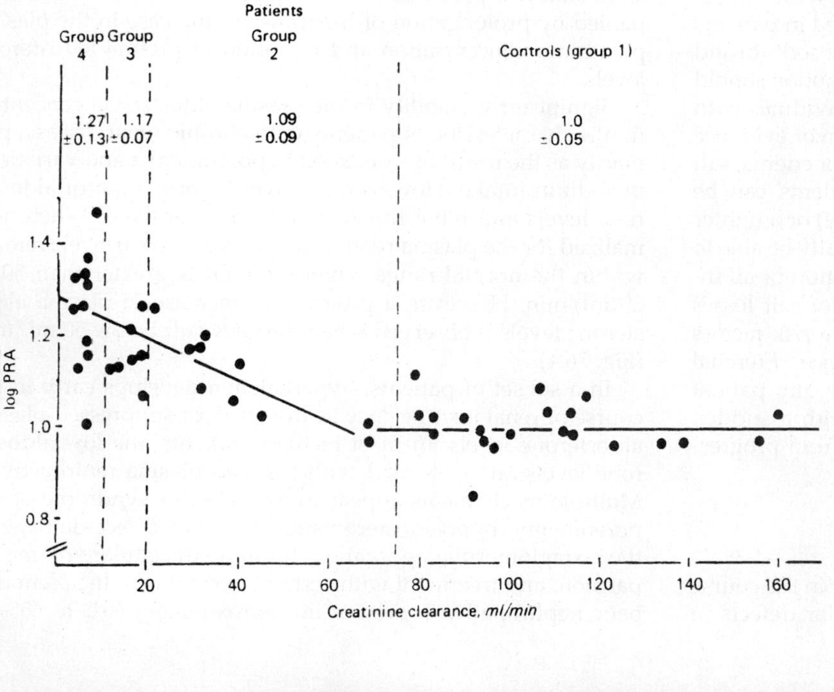

Figure 76.4. Relationship between the plasma aldosterone concentration *(P_{ALDO})* and the creatinine clearance in patients with varying degrees of chronic renal insufficiency. On the vertical axis, the plasma aldosterone concentration has been plotted as a function of the plasma renin activity *(PRA)* as log P_{ALDO}/log PRA. Group 1 patients have a creatinine clearance of 78 to 160 ml/min; group 2, 21 to 70 ml/min; group 3, 11 to 20 ml/min; and group 4, 3 to 10 ml/min. Below a creatinine clearance of 50 to 60 ml/min, a progressive increase in plasma aldosterone concentration is observed. (Reproduced with permission from Hene RJ, Boer P, Koomans HS, et al. Plasma aldosterone concentrations in chronic renal disease. *Kidney Int* 1982;21:98–101.)

The pathophysiology of the syndrome is incompletely understood. Both impaired secretion of aldosterone and resistance to the hormone's effect are present. Further discussion on this syndrome is found in Chapter 16, Part 3.

A second subset of patients develops hyperkalemia early in the course of renal insufficiency as the result of tubular defects in potassium secretion. Defects in hydrogen ion homeostasis are also observed in these individuals. First characterized in patients with obstructive uropathy, this form of distal renal tubular acidosis with hyperkalemia is also associated with a wide range of tubulointerstitial diseases. Affected patients appear to be unable to generate the normal voltage gradient in the distal tubule necessary to stimulate potassium secretion. Further discussion on this subject is found in Chapter 20, Part 5.

Several approaches may be used to manage potassium balance and treat hyperkalemia in patients with advancing renal insufficiency. In the absence of hypoaldosteronism or tubular defects in potassium secretion, overt hyperkalemia will develop with excessive potassium intake during a drop in urine output (oliguria), severe constipation, and digitalis toxicity, as well as with the ingestion of certain medications, such as angiotensin-converting enzyme inhibitors or nonsteroidal antiinflammatory agents. For most patients with moderate renal insufficiency, dietary potassium restriction to approximately 60 mEq/day is sufficient. In patients with defects in potassium excretion, loop diuretics in combination with liberalization of dietary sodium intake may be beneficial. Mineralocorticoid replacement with fludrocortisone acetate, a synthetic mineralocorticoid, may normalize the serum potassium in resistant cases, but at the expense of sodium retention and increased hypertension. In patients in whom renal excretion cannot be adequately augmented, sodium polystyrene sulfonate (Kayexalate) may be used as an exchange resin in the gastrointestinal tract. In addition, careful attention must be paid to the avoidance of medications, such as angiotensin-converting enzyme inhibitors or nonsteroidal antiinflammatory drugs, which can interfere with potassium homeostasis and exacerbate hyperkalemia.

Acid–Base Homeostasis

In the absence of a marked change in diet, the daily acid load in chronic renal failure is unchanged from normal and approximates 1 mEq/kg hydrogen ion per day. Acid is excreted after binding to a buffer, either titratable acid, which is largely phosphate and to a lesser degree creatinine, or ammonia. Three conditions must be satisfied to maintain normal acid excretion: Filtered bicarbonate must be reabsorbed completely in the proximal nephron, adequate buffer must be available, and secretion of hydrogen ion in the collecting duct must be normal. The major lesion in chronic renal failure is deficiency of buffer, although selected subsets of patients may have an impairment of distal proton secretion.

The buffer lacking in chronic renal insufficiency is ammonia. Although proximal tubule production of ammonia per nephron increases in response to acidosis, total ammonia production falls because of the marked drop in renal mass. This results in a decrease in buffer availability and a reduction in net acid excretion. Absolute excretion of titratable acid and ammonia fall with GFR despite the rise in excretion factored for GFR. In patients with hyporeninemic hypoaldosteronism, ammonia excretion decreases to a degree disproportionate to the severity of renal failure. This disorder, which is also termed *type IV renal tubular acidosis,* is characterized by hyperkalemic, hyperchloremic metabolic acidosis in association with diminished renin and aldosterone levels. In these patients, acidosis occurs at a much higher level of renal function than would be expected solely from renal insufficiency. Hyperkalemia induced by aldosterone deficiency suppresses proximal tubular ammonia production. The lack of buffer leads to proton accumulation and hyperchloremic acidosis.

As defined in the classic studies of Wrong and Davies, ammoniagenesis is reduced, but proton secretion and the ability to lower urine pH is normal in progressive chronic renal failure. Patients with mild renal failure and acidosis due to distal renal tubular acidosis with hyperkalemia are an exception. This disorder has been best characterized in obstructive uropathy. In these patients, a voltage-dependent impairment in collecting duct proton and potassium secretion due to diminished sodium reabsorption is suspected. Maneuvers such as sodium sulfate infusion or furosemide administration stimulate delivery of solute to the collecting duct and thereby augment distal sodium reabsorption. As a result, the magnitude of the lumen negative electrical charge increases. This more favorable electrochemical gradient increases potassium and proton secretion, leading to a resolution of the hyperkalemia and correction of the inappropriately high urine pH in some affected individuals.

Except for rare patients whose underlying disease is complicated by proximal renal tubular acidosis, proximal bicarbonate handling is normal in progressive renal failure and bicarbonaturia does not occur. In normal individuals, a transient increase in bicarbonate excretion after an oral protein load may result from the increase in GFR and filtered load. In patients with chronic renal insufficiency, fractional bicarbonate reabsorption is increased, and this "alkaline tide" does not occur.

Studies on patients with graded degrees of chronic renal failure show an inverse correlation between serum creatinine and bicarbonate. The change is apparent with mild degrees of renal impairment, as it has been documented in careful studies of individuals whose only renal insufficiency is the modest decrement in renal function seen with aging. Similarly, the anion gap increases as serum creatinine rises. Patients with less severe renal functional impairment tend to have hyperchloremic metabolic acidosis due to impaired excretion of protons. As renal function progresses, accumulation of fixed acid anions such as phosphate and sulfate results in an anion gap acidosis. However, such an orderly progression of hyperchloremic acidosis followed by anion gap acidosis is not invariable. One study of the serum electrolyte patterns of patients at the time they began dialysis showed hyperchloremic acidosis in 30%, high anion gap acidosis in 20%, hyperchloremia together with an elevated anion gap in 16%, acidosis with normal chloride and anion gap in 14%, and normal electrolytes in 20%. Patients in the latter group were mainly diabetics and had the lowest serum creatinine values. Early studies suggested that hyperchloremic acidosis was more common in tubulointerstitial disease, such as chronic pyelonephritis, than in glomerular disease and that hyperchloremia could be taken as a marker for tubulointerstitial disease. Some of these patients probably had hyporeninemic hypoaldosteronism. Later reports have not borne out this view.

To what extent patients with chronic renal insufficiency are in positive hydrogen ion balance is an unresolved question. It was long thought that the decrease in daily acid excretion required that patients be in considerable positive balance. The drop in serum bicarbonate concentration that should result was mitigated by release of alkali from bone. Careful calculations suggest that the amount of potential buffer in bone is insufficient to the task. Furthermore, buffering by bone would release calcium. In chronic renal failure, however, the urine calcium excretion is reduced. One analysis of the available data reports that a significant portion of the acid excreted in normals is present to balance excreted organic anions rather than to effect an increase in net acid excretion. In chronic renal failure, excretion of these anions (largely citrate) is decreased due to augmented reabsorption, with a consequent drop in the need to excrete protons. Thus a good deal of the drop in acid excretion observed in chronic renal insufficiency

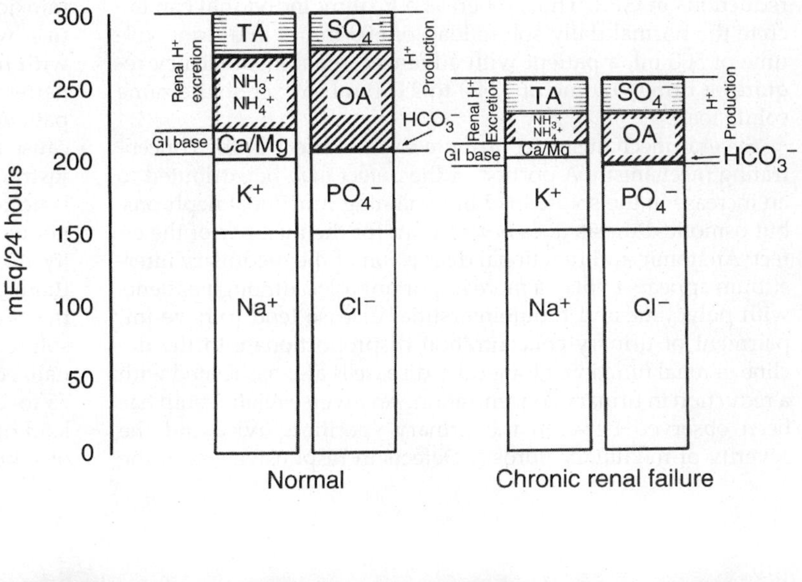

Figure 76.5. Gamblegram showing urinary electrolytes with normal renal function and chronic renal failure. Electrolytes directly relevant to acid–base excretion are shaded. The reduced excretion of divalent cations in renal failure is a result of diminished intestinal calcium absorption. In normal individuals, daily acid production exceeds the renal proton output by an amount equal to base absorption from the gut. In renal failure, acid–base balance is maintained despite the decrease in renal proton output because there is an equimolar decrease in the net production of organic acids. The latter results in a decrease in excretion of organic anions (bicarbonate equivalents). OA, organic anions; TA, titratable acid. (Reproduced with permission from Cohen RM, Feldman GM, Fernandez PC. The balance of acid, base and charge in health and disease. *Kidney Int* 1997;52:287–293.)

does not represent proton accumulation and does not require bone buffering.

Nonetheless, the serum bicarbonate concentration in individuals with renal failure does vary directly with net acid generation, and bicarbonate concentration falls as renal failure progresses. Sustained metabolic acidosis can lead to anorexia and nausea with diminished intake and malnutrition. Thus it is appropriate to treat acidosis with sodium bicarbonate. To prevent a high sodium load, it is customary to give sufficient bicarbonate to maintain blood bicarbonate at 20 to 23 mEq/L rather than to attempt to bring it fully into the normal range. Only modest doses are required (0.5 to 1 mEq/kg) because there is no bicarbonaturia.

Water

Renal water homeostasis in chronic renal insufficiency is characterized by a reduced capacity both to conserve and to excrete solute-free water. Renal concentrating ability is lost early in the course of chronic renal disease, limiting renal water conservation. Systemic hypertonicity, however, is uncommon because the regulation of water ingestion by thirst is not impaired. The primary clinical manifestation of the concentrating defect is nocturia, resulting from the loss of the normal nocturnal rise in urine osmolality and a corresponding decrease in nocturnal urine volume.

In contrast, the ability to excrete a dilute urine remains intact until late in the course of renal disease. Maximal solute-free water excretion, however, decreases in proportion to the decline in GFR. Because maximal solute-free water excretion in normal individuals is many-fold greater than that required to maintain water balance, overt hyponatremia is not common until the GFR is less than 10 ml/min.

RENAL CONCENTRATING MECHANISM

Urinary concentration requires generation and maintenance of a hypertonic gradient in the medullary interstitium and utilization of this gradient for water reabsorption from the medullary collecting duct in response to arginine vasopressin (AVP). Chronic renal disease is generally associated with structural and functional disruption of the medullary countercurrent multiplier. It is therefore not surprising that limitation of urinary concentration is an early manifestation of chronic renal disease. Maximal urine osmolality declines from approximately 1,200 mmol/kg H_2O in individuals with normal renal function to 600 mmol/kg H_2O when the GFR is reduced by approximately one-third, and it approaches isosthenuria with further reductions in GFR. Thus, whereas a healthy individual can excrete the normal daily solute load of 600 mmol in a urine volume of 500 ml, a patient with advanced renal insufficiency requires a urine volume of 1,500 to 2,000 ml to excrete the same solute load.

Several mechanisms contribute to this defect in the concentrating mechanism. A portion of the defect may be attributed to an increase in the solute load in remaining functional nephrons, but osmotic diuresis does not account for the majority of the effect. Anatomic and functional disruption of the medullary interstitium appears to play a more important role. Although patients with polycystic and tubulointerstitial disease tend to have impairment of urinary concentration disproportionate to the decline in renal function, glomerular disease is also associated with a reduction in urinary concentration. An inverse relationship has been observed between the urinary specific gravity and the severity of medullary fibrosis. Defects in responsiveness of the collecting duct to AVP also contribute to impaired urinary concentration. Microperfusion of collecting duct segments from rabbits subjected to renal ablation suggest that uremia may impair vasopressin-mediated water permeability through inhibition of adenylate cyclase activity. In addition, the increased tubular flow rate in the remaining functional nephrons limits the fractional reabsorption of water in response to vasopressin.

RENAL DILUTING MECHANISM

The elaboration of a dilute urine depends on the generation of solute-free water in the thick ascending limb of Henle's loop and the distal convoluted tubule and on the maintenance of low water permeability in the collecting duct. In contrast to the defects in the concentrating mechanism, the functional integrity of the diluting mechanism remains intact in most patients with chronic renal insufficiency. The generation of solute-free water, expressed as a fraction of GFR, is maintained at a normal rate of approximately 12 ml/100 ml of glomerular filtrate, even in the setting of advanced renal insufficiency. However, this constancy of fractional solute-free water generation means that overall solute-free water clearance declines in proportion to the fall in GFR. Thus, with a GFR of 150 L/day (100 ml/min), maximal free-water generation is approximately 18 L/day. In contrast, when the GFR falls to 15 L/day (10 ml/min), maximal free-water excretion is only 1.8 L/day.

A second implication of the constancy of fractional solute-free water generation is a reduction in maximal urinary dilution. Under conditions of maximal water diuresis, the urine volume may be considered to consist of two components: a volume of solute-free water and a volume of isotonic urine containing the obligate solute load (approximately 600 mmol/day corresponding to a volume of 2 L at a concentration of 300 mmol/kg H_2O). With normal renal function, the daily urine volume during maximal water diuresis would be approximately 20 L with an osmolality of 30 mmol/kg H_2O. With a reduction in GFR to 10 ml/min, this urine volume is reduced to 3.8 L with a corresponding minimal urine osmolality of approximately 160 mmol/kg H_2O. Mechanistically, the diminution in urinary dilution is primarily attributable to the increase in solute load per residual functional nephron.

Specific involvement of the diluting segments by an underlying disease process, resulting in more severe defects in urinary dilution, has been described in a small number of patients. More commonly, diluting capacity is iatrogenically impaired by the administration of loop diuretics such as furosemide.

The reduction in the ability to excrete solute-free water places the patient with renal insufficiency at increased risk for water intoxication. Excessive water intake, which would result in polyuria without associated electrolyte disturbances in a patient with normal renal function, may result in symptomatic hyponatremia in the setting of advanced renal disease. In general, patients do not require imposition of a fixed water intake because the thirst mechanism remains intact, and they should be instructed to drink in response to thirst. Specific fluid restriction is necessary only when habitual water intake (i.e., water intake not mediated by thirst) exceeds water excretion and hypotonicity develops. For hospitalized patients requiring intravenous fluids, the fluid prescription should provide sufficient solute-free water to replace obligate insensible and urinary water and solute losses. Although the fluid prescription must be individualized for each patient, the administration of 0.45% saline at 75 to 100 ml/hr is usually sufficient, providing a daily sodium load of approximately 3 to 4 g while providing 900 to 1,200 ml of solute-free water.

Selected Readings

Bourgoignie JJ, Kaplan M, Pincus J, et al. Renal handling of potassium in dogs with chronic renal insufficiency. *Kidney Int* 1981;20:482–490.

This study examines the dynamics of renal potassium excretion in dogs with experimental chronic renal insufficiency. Although fractional excretion of potassium at any given level of serum potassium remains normal in chronic renal failure, the ability to excrete a potassium load is impaired, resulting in transient elevations in plasma potassium.

Cohen RM, Feldman GM, Fernandez PC. The balance of acid, base and charge in health and disease. *Kidney Int* 1997;52:287–293.

A provocative new analysis of hydrogen ion balance in renal insufficiency. Reexamination of the original papers on acid excretion in normal individuals suggests that the methods used overestimated endogenous acid production and underestimated organic anion (bicarbonate equivalent) excretion. The authors suggest that the drop in total acid excretion observed in renal failure is largely due to the drop in organic acid excretion and the degree of hydrogen ion accumulation is negligible.

Danovitch MB, Bourgoignie J, Bricker NS. Reversibility of the "salt-losing" tendency of chronic renal failure. *N Engl J Med* 1977;296:14–19.

This classic and carefully conducted study refuted the notion that patients with chronic renal insufficiency are obligate salt wasters. Slow and stepwise reduction in dietary sodium was accompanied by a matching drop in excretion to very low levels. Patients developed no ill effects and did not become volume depleted even as sodium intake fell from 350 to 5 mEq/day.

Frassetto LA, Morris RCJ, Sebastian A. Effect of age on blood acid-base composition in adult humans: role of age-related renal functional decline. *Am J Physiol* 1996;271:F1114–F1122.

In detailed balance studies on patients with varying ages, these investigators found that plasma bicarbonate concentration fell as net acid excretion rose or GFR fell. Low grade acidosis may accompany the low-grade renal insufficiency seen with aging.

Hene RJ, Boer P, Koomans HS, et al. Plasma aldosterone concentrations in chronic renal disease. *Kidney Int* 1982;21:98–101.

This study demonstrates the relationships between plasma aldosterone levels, plasma renin activity, and GFR in patients with chronic renal insufficiency. When adjusted for plasma renin activity, aldosterone levels increase once the creatinine clearance falls below 50% of normal.

Kleeman CR, Adams DA, Maxwell MH. An evaluation of maximal water diuresis in chronic renal disease: 1. Normal solute intake. *J Lab Clin Med* 1961;58:169–184.

A detailed study of the concentrating and diluting capacity of subjects with chronic renal disease demonstrating that there is no specific defect in urinary dilution and that the loss of maximal urine diluting capacity is consistent with the increase in solute load in the remaining nephrons. In contrast, the authors demonstrate that the defect in concentrating ability could not be attributed to the increased osmotic diuresis per nephron.

Martinez-Maldonado M, Yium JJ, Eknoyan G, et al. Adult polycystic kidney disease: studies of the defect in urine concentration. *Kidney Int* 1972;2:107–113.

A detailed study of the defects in urinary concentration in patients with polycystic kidney disease, with and without renal insufficiency, relating the defects in urinary concentration to the presence of corticomedullary disease.

Wallia R, Greenberg A, Piraino B, et al. Serum electrolyte patterns in end-stage renal disease. *Am J Kidney Dis* 1986;8:98–104.

We studied the electrolyte patterns of patients with renal failure at the time they began dialysis. In contrast to the prevailing view at the time, a high anion gap acidosis was not the most common abnormality. Hyperchloremia with or without a high anion gap was seen in 46% of individuals and 20% had normal electrolytes.

PART 2
The Dialysis Patient

F. John Gennari and Jeffrey M. Rimmer

In end-stage renal disease, control of fluid, electrolyte, and acid–base balance passes from regulation by the kidneys to a unique new relationship between the patient and dialytic therapy, whether in the form of hemodialysis or peritoneal dialysis. With the initiation of chronic dialysis, interactions between the patient and treatment develop, establishing new equilibria that are dependent on patient intake and on the particular dialysis prescription the patient is receiving. Because dialysis therapy is less versatile than our native kidneys in responding to variations in intake, patients receiving dialysis treatments must consciously regulate their diet to prevent major disruptions in balance. Despite this limitation, the new equilibria are readily achieved in most patients and are remarkably stable, resulting in maintenance of body fluid volume and blood electrolytes at reasonable, if not normal, levels. In this chapter, we review how these equilibria develop and are maintained, and how one can recognize and manage superimposed disorders in fluid, electrolyte, and acid–base balance.

FLUID BALANCE AND SODIUM CONCENTRATION

Dynamics of Fluid Balance and Maintenance of Blood Pressure

Without renal function, all fluid and Na^+ ingested is retained, except for minor insensible losses and the small amount lost in stool. Thus maintenance of normal extracellular fluid (ECF) volume and tonicity devolves to control of intake and to regulation of output during dialysis. Because dialysis therapy is limited in its ability to dissociate Na^+ and water removal, ECF volume and osmolality are more tightly linked in the end-stage renal disease patient than in individuals with normal renal function. Fluid removal is a critical part of any dialytic therapy. Movement of water across the dialysis membrane is driven by a hydrostatic pressure gradient in hemodialysis and by an osmotic gradient (generated by the addition of dextrose to the dialysate) in peritoneal dialysis. With either process, Na^+ is removed with water in an amount approximately equivalent to that in a comparable volume of ECF fluid. Although the goals are the same in peritoneal and hemodialysis, differences between the two techniques (e.g., continuous versus intermittent) are significant and issues surrounding salt and water balance are discussed separately in the following sections.

Hemodialysis

The intermittent nature of hemodialysis requires that fluid and Na^+ be removed rapidly over the short period of treatment. The ability to achieve this goal during hemodialysis is limited by vascular volume depletion and hypotension. Fluid is removed rapidly from the vascular compartment and must be replenished continuously with fluid from the interstitial and intracellular compartments. In addition to these fluid shifts, rapid adjustments in vascular tone and cardiac output must occur to maintain arterial pressure. The normal hormonal and neurologic mediators of these adjustments are probably disordered in the uremic state. Many vasoactive substances, such as eicosanoids, catecholamines, and peptides, are present in abnormal concentrations or respond inappropriately to stress in end-stage renal disease. The anemia of end-stage renal disease may also contribute to the impaired vascular response to fluid removal. Elements of the dialysate, such as acetate, appear to alter the vascular response to fluid removal. Finally, blood interaction with the dialysis membrane may lead to the release of cytokines that cause vasodilation and hypotension. Given the complexity of the response to the rapid efflux of fluid from the vascular space, it is remarkable that in most patients 1 to 3 L of fluid can be removed routinely during a 3- to 4-hour hemodialysis session with few symptoms. When larger volumes must be removed, symptomatic hypotension and cramps are the rule rather than the exception.

Many approaches have been developed to minimize hemodialysis-induced hypotension. Acetate with its capacity to cause vasodilation and depress myocardial function has virtually disappeared as a major constituent of the dialysis bath. In the early years of hemodialysis, bath [Na^+] was deliberately kept low (130 mmol/L) to promote some additional Na^+ removal by diffusion. However, this practice was associated with a high frequency of dialysis-induced hypotension, presumably because the low bath [Na^+] facilitated movement of water from the extracellular to intracellular compartment. Transcellular water shifts are particularly a problem early in the dialysis procedure because as urea is rapidly removed from the ECF, a transient disequilibrium develops in which urea concentration, and therefore osmolality, is higher in cells, promoting water entry. Increasing dialysate [Na^+] reduces the likelihood of hypotension, most likely by increasing the osmolality of the ECF compartment and retarding the shift of water into cells. In some centers, bath [Na^+] has been increased to as high as 155 mmol/L at the beginning of the treatment to achieve this goal. During the treatment, bath [Na^+] is gradually reduced to a final value of 140 mmol/L, avoiding postdialysis hypernatremia and excessive thirst. A high dialysate [Na^+] may also enhance the osmotic driving force for vascular refilling during the later stages of the dialysis treatment.

In addition to varying bath [Na^+], attempts have been made to vary the rate of ultrafiltration during the procedure to minimize hypotension. High rates of ultrafiltration are used early in the procedure, on the assumption that entry of fluid from the interstitial space to the vascular compartment will occur more rapidly when fluid volume excess is the greatest. A linkage between rapid fluid removal and high bath [Na^+] may also enhance vascular refilling. Another technique that has been tried is to alternate periods of high and low ultrafiltration, in theory, to allow for vascular refilling during the low fluid removal phase. Despite all these maneuvers, dialysis-induced hypotension remains a problem. In problem cases, cooling the dialysate bath sufficiently to cause vasoconstriction of the blood vessels to the skin has been used in some patients with success.

New methods are currently being tested to provide a better evaluation of extracellular and vascular volume during hemodialysis. These methods include continuous measurements of electrical impedance and hematocrit. The former measurement allows estimation of intracellular volume, total body water, and intrathoracic volume. From these values, one can estimate cardiac output and peripheral vascular resistance. Continuous hematocrit measurements allow one to estimate the rate of change in vascular volume during hemodialysis. As these techniques improve, algorithms can be developed that drive preemptive changes in ultrafiltration rate, bath [Na^+], and dialysate temperature to maximize hemodynamic stability.

Most patients receiving hemodialysis pass through the period between dialysis treatments with only modest increases in ECF volume and small changes in sodium concentration [Na^+], indicating that fluid and Na^+ intake can be regulated. This regulation is probably achieved in part by unconscious control mechanisms (e.g., renin-angiotensin system, neural reflexes sensing ECF volume), as well as by conscious choice.

Peritoneal Dialysis

During treatment with peritoneal dialysis, fluid and Na^+ removal are relatively continuous and gradual processes. Because the sieving coefficient for Na^+ across the peritoneal membrane is low and would result in hypernatremia if convection were the only means of Na^+ removal, peritoneal bath [Na^+] is reduced to 132 mmol/L, allowing for additional Na^+ loss by diffusion. The result of this adjustment in bath [Na^+] is that fluid loss is isotonic during dialysis. Regulation of isotonic fluid loss is achieved by adjusting bath dextrose concentration, and thereby the osmotic driving force for fluid removal. Two forms of therapy are currently in use: chronic ambulatory peritoneal dialysis (CAPD) and chronic cycling peritoneal dialysis (CCPD). In the CAPD, 2 to 3 L are exchanged at evenly timed intervals four to five times a day. In CCPD, most of the exchanges are accomplished overnight, with shorter dwell times (see Chapter 84, Parts 2C and 2D). Serum [Na^+] is maintained in the normal range during CAPD and appears to be unaltered by the newer CCPD technique despite differences in dwell time and in the total volume of exchanges each day. With either technique, fluid removal is a more gradual process than in hemodialysis; therefore hypotension is usually not a problem unless ECF volume is depleted excessively.

Abnormalities in Fluid Balance and Sodium Concentration

Assessment of ECF Volume

Determining the ECF volume status in patients receiving dialysis therapy is a continual challenge. In current practice, patients are assigned a "dry weight," which is an estimate of the weight at which ECF volume is at or near normal. Typically, the weight chosen is one that is associated with minimal signs of ECF volume overload or depletion. With hemodialysis therapy, fluid removal is adjusted to achieve this weight at the end of each treatment. With peritoneal dialysis, the osmotic concentration of each day's exchanges is adjusted to maintain this weight. Signs of an increase in ECF volume are similar to those in individuals with functioning kidneys and include hypertension, edema, basilar rales, and eventually orthopnea and an S_3 gallop. ECF volume depletion is associated with orthostatic hypotension and tachycardia. Unfortunately, comorbid conditions such as heart failure, neuropathy, and advanced age often make physical findings unreliable. The blood pressure response to the removal of fluid during dialysis and chest x-ray examination offer some additional clues to volume status. In the acutely ill dialysis patient, direct measurements of pulmonary artery and capillary wedge pressures are often required for ECF volume assessment.

New techniques are currently being tested to help in the clinical assessment of ECF volume. Elevated levels of atrial natriuretic peptide (ANP) and cyclic guanosine 3′,5′-monophosphate (cGMP) have been shown to correlate with excess ECF volume. The diameter of the inferior vena cava, assessed by ultrasound, also appears to correlate with ECF volume. As discussed earlier, electrical impedance measurements allow estimation of body fluid volume. In the future, one or more of these techniques may become a routine part of the management of patients with end-stage renal disease.

ECF Volume Excess with Normal or Near Normal [Na^+]

The most common abnormality in the dialysis patient is isotonic volume expansion due to excess Na^+ and fluid intake. In most individuals, thirst responds appropriately to Na^+ intake and little change in serum [Na^+] occurs. ECF volume expansion is often associated with an increase in blood pressure, but typically, there are few other signs of volume overload. The diagnosis is made primarily on the basis of an excessive increase in weight, and dialysis therapy is then adjusted to increase fluid removal. If volume expansion is such that it results in symptomatic dialysis or worsening hypertension, the best approach is to reinforce the importance of Na^+ and fluid restriction. A more insidious form of ECF volume overload occurs in the patient who has an unrecognized loss of lean body mass. If the "dry weight" is not adjusted downward in this situation, ECF volume will obviously increase over time. In such cases, as much as 5 to 7 kg of fluid may be retained before symptoms become evident.

ECF Volume Excess with Hyponatremia

If water intake is excessive but Na^+ intake is not, serum [Na^+] will fall in association with the increase in fluid volume. Excess water intake most often occurs in two groups of patients: those with diabetes mellitus and those with congestive heart failure. In both groups, excessive thirst probably occurs as a result of systemic disease. In the diabetic patient, hyperglycemia and the attendant increase in serum osmolality stimulate thirst; in the patient with congestive heart failure, high levels of angiotensin II, catecholamines, and antidiuretic hormone all contribute to stimulate thirst. As with isotonic volume expansion, the extent of associated hypertension, edema, and pulmonary congestion depends on a complex set of variables, including cardiac function, serum albumin, and the degree of volume expansion.

Hemodialysis is a very effective means for returning serum [Na^+] to normal levels if hyponatremia is mild to moderate ([Na^+] 125 to 135 mmol/L, Table 76.1). Correction of hyponatremia occurs regardless of the requirement for fluid removal. As a result, severe hyponatremia is unlikely to occur from excess water intake in the interdialytic period unless water ingestion is massive and salt intake is virtually nil. If hyponatremia and excess weight gain recur, reinforcement of the importance of fluid restriction may be helpful in management along with concrete methods of monitoring fluid intake. Improved blood sugar control may reduce thirst in the diabetic patient, and maneuvers that improve cardiac performance can blunt thirst in those with heart failure. Because fluid removal occurs continually in patients receiving peritoneal dialysis, hyponatremia from excess water ingestion is less likely to occur. Once established, however, hyponatremia is more difficult to correct because the low bath [Na^+] limits the diffusive transfer of Na^+ from the bath to the patient.

Even when hyponatremia is more severe ([Na^+] less than 125 mmol/L), further reductions during the intervals between hemodialysis treatments do not appear to produce neurologic symptoms or damage. However, initiation of hemodialysis therapy in a patient with severe hyponatremia can induce central pontine myelinolysis, and caution must be exercised during the first treatment. One can slow the rise in serum [Na^+] by reducing bath [Na^+], although present dialysate delivery systems prevent a reduction below 132 mmol/L. The rate of change can also be slowed by reducing blood and dialysate flow rates. Frequent monitoring of serum [Na^+] should be carried out during the treatment and water administered to slow the rise if necessary.

Hyponatremia can also occur without a concomitant reduction in serum osmolality, in association with ECF volume expansion. Hyperglycemia is the most common cause for this clinical picture. The high ECF glucose concentration provides an osmotic force for fluid to shift out of cells, increasing ECF volume and decreasing ECF [Na^+]. Because patients with renal failure are unable to excrete excess ECF glucose, its concentration can rise rapidly to very high levels when insulin levels are low or absent. An increase of 1,000 mg/dl will reduce serum [Na^+] by approximately 15 mmol/L. This problem is easily corrected with the administration of insulin, which facilitates glucose removal from the ECF and allows water to reenter cells, restoring ECF volume and [Na^+] to normal. With solutes such a mannitol where there is no route of metabolism, dialysis is required to reverse the abnormality.

TABLE 76.1. Effect of a 3.5-hr Hemodialysis Treatment on Serum [Na^+][a]

Serum [Na^+] mmol/L		
Predialysis	Postdialysis	Change
160	144	−16
150	141	−9
140	137	−3
130	134	+4
120	130	+10
110	127	+17
100	123	+23

[a] Assumes the following: (a) blood flow rate = 300 ml/min, (b) bath [Na^+] = 140 mmol/L, (c) dialysance$_{Na^+}$ = 219 ml/min, (d) Na^+ distributed in a single compartment, and (e) equivalent to 0.6 × body weight (kg).

ECF Volume Excess with Hypernatremia

Hypernatremia coupled with an increase in ECF volume can occur only through the inadvertent administration of hypertonic fluids to patients with end-stage renal disease. This extremely rare problem requires dialysis treatment for correction (Table 76.1).

ECF Volume Depletion with Normal or Near Normal [Na^+]

Volume depletion without a major change in ECF [Na^+] is usually the result of overly aggressive fluid removal during dialysis, most commonly due to an incorrect estimate of the dry weight. In a patient whose nutrition has improved with dialysis treatment, lean body mass increases. If the dry weight is not appropriately increased, ECF volume depletion will occur. This problem is easily corrected by adjusting the dry weight. Gastrointestinal hemorrhage, vomiting, or diarrhea can also cause ECF volume depletion without major changes in [Na^+]. In these settings, blood products or isotonic fluid replacement are required to replenish ECF volume.

ECF Volume Depletion with Hyponatremia

If water and electrolyte losses from the gut or by ultrafiltration are replaced with only water, hyponatremia and hypoosmolality with a normal or reduced ECF volume can result. Because serum [Na^+] can be increased rapidly by hemodialysis (Table 76.1), sustained severe hyponatremia is unlikely to occur in patients receiving this form of renal replacement therapy. Nonetheless, care should be taken in treating hyponatremia if the condition is severe ([Na^+] less than 125 mmol) because rapid correction can cause neurologic damage if the disorder is sustained for more than 2 to 3 days.

ECF Volume Depletion with Hypernatremia

Because thirst is such a strong driving force when serum tonicity is increased, this clinical picture develops only when the patient is confused, comatose, or unable to gain access to water. In addition, because renal water loss is minimal in the dialysis patient, development of hypernatremia requires the loss of water in excess of [Na^+] from the gut or skin, a rare event. In patients receiving acute peritoneal dialysis with rapid fluid exchanges, hypernatremia can occur because of the low sieving coefficient for Na^+ across the peritoneal membrane. Inadvertent failure to reduce dialysate [Na^+] during a planned "variable [Na^+]" hemodialysis treatment can also result in postdialysis hypernatremia. Treatment in all instances is repletion with water or hypotonic fluids as needed.

POTASSIUM BALANCE

Serum potassium concentration ([K^+]) is determined by (a) control of K^+ partition between cells and the ECF compartment and

TABLE 76.2. K^+ Balance in Dialysis Patients Adhering to a 2-g K^+ Diet

Intake: 50 mmol/day
Excretion:
A. Peritoneal dialysis (CAPD)
  1. By dialysis: daily efflux (L) × serum [K^+]
     10 L × 4 mmol/L = 40 mmol/day
  2. Stool = 10 mmol/day (20% of intake)
B. Peritoneal dialysis (using cycler, CCPD)
  1. By dialysis: daily efflux (L) × 0.8 × serum [K^+][a]
     15 L × 3.2 mmol/L = 48 mmol/day
  2. Stool = 2 mmol/day (4% of intake)
C. Hemodialysis
  1. By dialysis: using standard glucose containing 2 mmol/L [K^+] bath
     60 mmol/treatment = 180 mmol/wk or 26 mmol/day
  2. Stool = 24 mmol/day (48% of intake)

[a]Assuming only 80% equilibration with serum [K^+] due to shorter dwell time.
CAPD, continuous ambulatory peritoneal dialysis; CCPD, chronic cycling peritoneal dialysis.

(b) regulation of external K^+ balance through modulation of renal excretion. Both processes are disrupted by renal failure. The uremic state impairs K^+ entry into cells by reducing the activity of cell membrane Na^+-K^+-ATPase. Renal regulation of external K^+ balance is reasonably preserved until very late in the course of most renal diseases. Thus external K^+ balance is well maintained, but hyperkalemia is seen in patients with renal insufficiency. When renal failure reaches end stage, the ability to excrete K^+ is also lost, and maintenance of external K^+ balance depends on matching dietary intake with the limited excretion of K^+ into the stool and its removal by dialysis therapy (Table 76.2). Gastrointestinal K^+ secretion is increased adaptively in renal failure and may account for as much as 70% of K^+ excretion in some patients.

Dialysis therapy may correct the impairment of cell membrane Na^+-K^+-ATPase, but it is unlikely that transcellular K^+ balance is restored to normal. Transfer of extracellular K^+ into cells depends on a variety of factors, including insulin, β-adrenergic activity, acid–base status, and parathyroid hormone. Aldosterone also plays a role in regulating serum [K^+], but its influence is probably confined to stimulation of K^+ secretion into the colon. Virtually all of these factors may be disordered in end-stage renal disease. In the absence of the ability to excrete K^+ readily, any defect in K^+ uptake by cells will result in sustained hyperkalemia. Perhaps the best evidence that such defects are present is the virtually ubiquitous presence of some degree of hyperkalemia in hemodialysis patients, despite measurements of total body K^+ that are normal or below normal.

Potassium removal by dialysis therapy is determined primarily by the transmembrane [K^+] gradient and is relatively inflexible (Table 76.2). Estimation of K^+ removal during chronic peritoneal dialysis is straightforward because the bath contains no K^+. When exchanges are carried out every 5 to 6 hours (CAPD), the concentration of K^+ in the dialysate approaches equilibrium with the concentration of K^+ in plasma water. If serum [K^+] is stable at 4 mmol/L and 9 to 12 L of dialysate effluent are drained from the peritoneal space in a typical 24-hour period, a maximum of 36 to 48 mmol of K^+ can be removed each day. With the larger daily volume exchanges achieved in CCPD (12 to 18 L/day), more K^+ is probably lost, although dwell times are shorter and bath [K^+] is probably not in equilibrium with plasma [K^+]. Even if bath [K^+] is only 80% of plasma [K^+], however, more than 50 mmol of K^+ will be removed in 18 L of dialysis effluent. Because of the gradual rate of K^+ removal during peritoneal dialysis, ECF K^+ is readily replenished by K^+ from cells, and large changes in serum [K^+] do not occur. In addition, other factors influencing transcellular K^+ movement, such as insulin and acid–base status, remain relatively stable. Therefore the major factor influencing K^+ removal is the prevailing serum [K^+].

With intermittent hemodialysis, the factors influencing K^+ removal are more complex. The driving force for K^+ removal is the same, that is, the transmembrane [K^+] gradient. However, because of the rapid diffusive movement from serum to bath, K^+ exit from cells cannot replenish ECF stores during dialysis, and serum [K^+] falls precipitously, limiting its removal. In addition, countervailing forces actually promote K^+ entry into cells during dialysis. Bicarbonate and glucose diffuse from the bath to the patient, alkalinizing the plasma and stimulating insulin release, changes that enhance cellular K^+ uptake. Failure to achieve normal equilibrium between cells and ECF during hemodialysis is reflected by a rebound rise in serum [K^+] of 0.5 to 1 mmol/L in the immediate postdialysis period.

Potassium removal during hemodialysis varies widely from patient to patient but averages 60 mmol per treatment when bath [K^+] is 2 mmol/L. Removing glucose from the bath can increase K^+ removal by 20% to 25% by preventing the insulin surge during dialysis. Elimination of K^+ from the bath can also increase K^+ removal, but it reduces serum K^+ rapidly to very low levels during treatment and may precipitate cardiac arrhythmias in susceptible patients.

Hyperkalemia

Diet

The most common cause of hyperkalemia in dialysis patients is dietary indiscretion. This is easily understood given the limitation on K^+ removal by dialysis and the care required to maintain dietary K^+ intake at 50 mmol/day (2-g K^+ diet). The limitation is most severe with hemodialysis. Approximately 60 mmol are removed with each hemodialysis treatment, or only 180 mmol/wk, the equivalent of 26 mmol/day or 52% of a 2-g K^+ diet (Table 76.2). Thus patients receiving hemodialysis are dependent on significant K^+ excretion in the stool to maintain balance even when K^+ intake is successfully restricted. Because this excretory route has limitations as well, these patients are almost always poised at the edge of positive K^+ balance, and even a small positive balance of K^+ will increase serum [K^+] to more than 6 mmol/L.

Drugs

Table 76.3 lists a variety of drugs that can increase serum [K^+] in dialysis patients. Drugs that inhibit insulin release, β-adrenergic activity, or directly inhibit Na^+-K^+ ATPase activity impair entry of K^+ into cells. Even partial inhibition of K^+ entry can cause significant hyperkalemia in patients with end-stage renal disease because the excess extracellular K^+ has no ready route for excretion. A second group of drugs promote K^+ exit from cells by depolarizing cell membranes, by causing outward fluid and K^+ movement (hypertonic solutions), or by less clearly defined mechanisms (arginine, fluoride). A third group of drugs inhibit aldosterone secretion. Whether these drugs impair K^+ entry into cells or act by decreasing K^+ excretion in the stool is unknown, but all have been shown to increase serum [K^+].

Transcellular Shifts

Catabolic states or tissue disruption of any sort will add K^+ to the ECF compartment and can rapidly increase serum [K^+]. In diabetic patients, hyperglycemia causes water and K^+ move-

TABLE 76.3. Drugs That Can Increase Serum [K^+] in Dialysis Patients

By Impairing K^+ Entry into Cells
β-Adrenergic blockers Digoxin Somatostatin analogs
By Promoting K^+ Exit from Cells
Depolarizing neuromuscular blockers Arginine Fluoride intoxication Hypertonic glucose or mannitol
By Inhibiting Aldosterone Secretion
Angiotensin-converting enzyme inhibitors Heparin Nonsteroidal antiinflammatory drugs Cyclosporine

ment from cells to the ECF. Severe hyperkalemia is a notable feature of uncontrolled diabetes mellitus in dialysis patients. Even in dialysis patients without diabetes, suppression of insulin release by prolonged fasting can increase serum [K^+] by as much as 1 mmol/L. Extreme exertion can also increase serum [K^+] by stimulating α-adrenergic activity.

Dialysis

A reduction in the efficiency of dialysis or noncompliance with the dialysis prescription will reduce the removal of K^+. The former can occur with a poorly functioning fistula in hemodialysis or a change in peritoneal permeability or surface area in peritoneal dialysis. When hyperkalemia is due to inadequate dialysis, it should be associated with an increase in urea concentration or other signs, such as worsening acidosis.

Therapy

The cornerstone of therapy for chronic hyperkalemia is dietary assessment, instruction, and reinforcement with frequent reminders. In the new dialysis patient, medicinal or dietary sources of K^+, such as "salt substitutes," should be sought for and eliminated. Drugs that inhibit cellular K^+ uptake or aldosterone secretion (Table 76.3) should be discontinued. Potassium removal during dialysis can be augmented by increasing blood and dialysate flow rates, by increasing the time of treatment, or by instituting maneuvers that reduce extracorporeal recirculation. Eliminating K^+ from the dialysate solution will also increase K^+ removal but with the risk of more severe intradialytic hypokalemia. In dialysis patients with persistent severe hyperkalemia ([K^+] = 6 to 7 mmol/L) in whom the aforementioned maneuvers have been ineffective, sodium polystyrene sulfonate can be given by mouth on a regular basis to increase K^+ excretion by the gut.

If hyperkalemia is severe (serum [K^+] greater than 6.5 mmol/L or rising rapidly), urgent attention is indicated. There is no evidence that dialysis patients are less susceptible to the depolarizing and arrhythmic effects of severe hyperkalemia. Administration of calcium gluconate or chloride provides immediate cardiac protection and is the treatment of choice if conduction abnormalities are present on electrocardiogram. ECF [K^+] can be lowered within 15 to 30 minutes by the administration of insulin or albuterol. In patients with end-stage renal disease, sodium bicarbonate administration has only a minimal effect on serum [K^+] and is not recommended for acute treatment. Sodium polystyrene sulfonate should be given by mouth or by enema to begin to remove excess K^+. In most instances, emergency dialysis is required to control the hyperkalemia.

Hypokalemia

Sustained hypokalemia is rare in patients receiving hemodialysis for all the reasons outlined previously, although transient hypokalemia occurs during the course of each treatment. In patients with underlying heart disease, the rapid fall in K^+ that occurs in the first 2 hours of dialysis is associated with an increased incidence of cardiac arrhythmias. Arrhythmias may be more likely to occur in patients taking digoxin. Intradialytic hypokalemia can be avoided by increasing dialysate [K^+], but this maneuver obviously limits K^+ removal and increases the risk of subsequent positive K^+ balance and hyperkalemia. Hypokalemia can occur when K^+ losses from the gut (e.g., diarrhea) are increased or with extremely poor dietary intake. Correction of the causes in such instances should lead to repair of the deficit. Potassium administration is rarely indicated in patients receiving hemodialysis and is potentially dangerous.

In contrast, sustained hypokalemia is occurring with increasing frequency in patients receiving peritoneal dialysis treatments, particularly when large volumes are exchanged each day.

The hypokalemia is due in most instances to poor dietary intake as well as increased losses into the dialysate each day (Table 76.2). For example, in a patient ingesting only 40 mmol of K^+ each day and having an effluent of 15 L/day, serum [K^+] would have to drop to approximately 3.0 mmol/L to maintain external K^+ balance. In such patients, oral potassium supplements are occasionally required on a sustained basis to maintain serum [K^+] in the normal range.

ACID–BASE HOMEOSTASIS

Strong acids produced by metabolic processes in the body are buffered transiently by alkali stores (primarily HCO_3^-), and the buffers are then regenerated by renal acid excretion. In patients with end-stage renal disease, the buffer response is unaffected but acid excretion is lost. As a result, acids are retained and body buffer stores are depleted, with consequent metabolic acidosis an invariable feature. Dialysis therapy restores the capacity for buffer replenishment, not by acid excretion, but by the direct addition of alkali (or alkali precursors) during treatment. With the institution of dialysis, a new equilibrium is achieved, allowing for maintenance of a stable serum [HCO_3^-]. In patients receiving peritoneal dialysis, the steady-state serum [HCO_3^-] values are at or near the normal range for patients with functioning kidneys. With hemodialysis, however, predialysis serum [HCO_3^-] is significantly lower than normal, averaging only 20 mmol/L (Table 76.4). Dialysis therapy is much less flexible than our kidneys in responding to variations in acid production, and therefore serum [HCO_3^-] varies more in patients with end-stage renal disease than in individuals with normally functioning kidneys. In addition, no adaptive adjustments are made by the dialysis therapy when superimposed acid–base disorders arise, resulting in unique issues relating to diagnosis and management. The dynamics of alkali addition during renal replacement therapy and the special issues relating to the management of superimposed acid–base disorders are discussed in the following sections.

TABLE 76.4. Acid–Base Values in Stable Dialysis Patients

	Hemodialysis[a]	N	Peritoneal Dialysis[b]	N
Venous [Total CO_2]	—		26 mmol/L	109
Fistula [Total CO_2]	20 mmol/L (15–25)	104	—	
Fistula [HCO_3^-]	20 mmol/L	36	—	
Arterial/fistula pH	7.38 (7.28–7.48)	36	7.42 (7.39–7.44)	20
P_{CO_2}	34 mm Hg (30–38)	36	42 mm Hg (40–44)	20
Anion gap	19 mmol/L (13–25)	66	15 mmol/L (9–21)	56

[a] Bath [HCO_3^-] = 35 mmol/L, predialysis values.
[b] Bath [lactate$^-$] = 40 mmol/L, steady-state values in patients receiving four exchanges per day (continuous ambulatory peritoneal dialysis).
Numbers in parenthesis = ± 2 SD, N = number of patients.

Dynamics of Alkali Addition During Dialysis

With either hemodialysis or peritoneal dialysis, the amount of alkali delivered is determined by the transmembrane concentration gradient and by the dialysance of the substance used (HCO_3^-, lactate, or acetate). Because the bath concentration of these substances is fixed and the factors determining dialysance (membrane permeability, surface area, and blood flow rate) are also fixed to maximize urea clearance, serum [HCO_3^-] sets the transmembrane concentration gradient and is therefore the variable that regulates net alkali addition. When the dialysis bath solution contains HCO_3^-, serum [HCO_3^-] determines the amount of HCO_3^- added. When the bath contains no HCO_3^-, serum [HCO_3^-] determines the amount lost into the bath solution. Serum [HCO_3^-] in turn is determined by the rate of endogenous acid production. In patients receiving dialysis therapy, a new balance is struck between acid production and alkali addition. In this new steady state, serum [HCO_3^-] is determined by the interplay between endogenous acid production and the specific characteristics of the dialysis therapy used. Table 76.5 illustrates this relationship in a patient receiving hemodialysis with a bicarbonate-containing bath solution (final concentration of 35 mmol/L). In this example, hemodialysis treatments are given 3 times weekly with a polysulfone membrane and 400 ml/min blood flow rate, and the patient retains 2 L of fluid between each treatment. The relationship shown in Table 76.5 is a theoretical one, based on the assumption of a stable rate of acid production and a stable buffer response in the period between treatments. Acid production in patients with end-stage renal disease cannot be measured directly, but the buffer response to added acid or alkali appears to be unchanged from normal. As shown in the table, variations in net acid production over a reasonable range can result in variations in steady-state predialysis serum [HCO_3^-] of up to 6 mmol/L. These variations in acid production could be due to variations in dietary intake of acid precursors or to the catabolic state of the patient. In addition to the rate of acid production, the amount of fluid retained (without alkali) in the period between treatments influences the predialysis serum [HCO_3^-] (Table 76.5) by changing the space of distribution of the body alkali stores. If a similar analysis is made for peritoneal dialysis, the predicted serum [HCO_3^-] will be higher for any given rate of acid production because of differences in the dynamics of net alkali addition. In patients receiving CAPD (four 2-L exchanges per day), in fact, acid production has been measured and the type of theoretical analysis presented in Table 76.5 has been validated.

TABLE 76.5. Predicted Effect of Variations in Acid Production and Fluid Retention on Predialysis Serum [HCO_3^-][a,b]

Net Acid Production (mmol/day)	Fluid Retention[c] (L)	Predialysis [HCO_3^-] (mmol/L)
40	2	23.4
80	2	20.4
120	2	17.3
60	0	23.1
60	3	21.3
60	6	19.8

[a] Assumes weight of 70 kg, postdialysis serum [HCO_3^-] of 28 mmol/L, and HCO_3^- buffer space of 0.5 × body weight.
[b] Predialysis serum [HCO_3^-] after long interval between hemodialysis treatments (68 hr).
[c] Liters of alkali-free fluid retained during the interval between treatments.

Normal Values

A summary of published values for [HCO_3^-] or [Total CO_2] obtained from artereo-venous fistulas or grafts in patients receiving hemodialysis and venous [Total CO_2] in patients receiving peritoneal dialysis is shown in Table 76.4. These values are useful guides for assessing whether patients have a "normal" or expected serum [HCO_3^-], but it should be emphasized that the levels vary widely from patient to patient. Such variability is not surprising because endogenous acid production, the type of membrane used, the amount of fluid removed, and blood flow rate vary from patient to patient. The values in the table for peritoneal dialysis are for patients carrying out four exchanges a day (CAPD). No published information is available concerning the effect on serum [HCO_3^-] of using larger bath volumes and shorter dwell times (CCPD), but informal observations suggest that this technique does not alter the values notably. If serum [Total CO_2] is measured at regular intervals in individual dialysis patients, changes can quickly be detected and can be used to identify new metabolic acid–base disorders. In the absence of such measurements, one should use the values in Table 76.4 as a basis for defining superimposed acid–base disturbances.

Diagnosis and Management of Acid–Base Disorders

In the dialysis patient, as in the patient with normal renal function, one must first identify a primary acid–base disturbance (metabolic acidosis, metabolic alkalosis, respiratory acidosis, respiratory alkalosis) and then determine whether the adaptive response is appropriate. To identify the primary disturbance, the following guidelines can be used in dialysis patients.

1. Metabolic acidosis—serum [Total CO_2] or [HCO_3^-] lower than the usual value by 4 mmol/L or more.
2. Metabolic alkalosis—serum [Total CO_2] or [HCO_3^-] higher than the usual value by 4 mmol/L or more.
3. Respiratory acidosis—P_{CO_2} 5 mm Hg or higher than predicted for the prevailing [Total CO_2] or [HCO_3^-]. (See the following for evaluation equation.)
4. Respiratory alkalosis—P_{CO_2} 5 mm Hg or lower than predicted for the prevailing [Total CO_2] or [HCO_3^-]. (See the following for evaluation equation.)

The compensatory ventilatory response to metabolic acid–base disorders is unaffected by renal failure. The rules of thumb for evaluating whether P_{CO_2} is appropriate for a given serum $[HCO_3^-]$ are as follows:

1. For $[HCO_3^-]$ less than 24 mmol/L:

$$P_{CO_2}\ (\text{mm Hg}) = 40 - 1.3 \times (24 - [HCO_3^-])$$

2. For $[HCO_3^-]$ greater than 24 mmol/L:

$$P_{CO_2}\ (\text{mm Hg}) = 40 + 0.7 \times ([HCO_3^-] - 24)$$

If the primary disorder is respiratory acidosis or alkalosis, the normal adaptive response (which is mediated by the kidney) does not occur. Thus serum $[HCO_3^-]$ does not change, and diagnosis depends on clinical suspicion and measurement of P_{CO_2}.

Metabolic Acidosis

As indicated earlier, virtually all patients receiving hemodialysis have a mild to moderate metabolic acidosis when compared with individuals who have normal renal function. Whether this chronic disorder contributes to dialysis morbidity remains a subject of continued debate and is not addressed here. The important management issue is to identify patients with very low values for serum [Total CO_2] (less than 17 mmol/L) and to identify the presence of a new superimposed metabolic acidosis, defined by a fall in [Total CO_2] or $[HCO_3^-]$ by 4 mmol/L or more. In the patient with a persistently low serum [Total CO_2], one should evaluate dietary intake, explore potential causes for increased catabolism, and assess whether organic acid production during dialysis is excessive. Almost all new acidoses in dialysis patients are associated with a further increase in anion gap. The most common cause is diabetic ketoacidosis, which is readily corrected by appropriate insulin treatment. Other causes include lactic acidosis and certain toxin ingestions. For any severe metabolic acidosis, dialysis therapy can replenish alkali stores rapidly because alkali addition is greatest when serum $[HCO_3^-]$ is the lowest.

Metabolic acidosis without a further increase in anion gap can occur as a result of gastrointestinal HCO_3^- losses or from expansion of the ECF volume with saline. For gastrointestinal HCO_3^- losses, management involves fluid and alkali replacement. Expansion acidosis is usually a milder problem, and management involves long-term adjustments in fluid and salt intake.

Metabolic Alkalosis

Metabolic alkalosis has only two causes in dialysis patients: (a) gastrointestinal HCl loss and (b) exogenous alkali administration. The most common cause is vomiting or nasogastric suction. Exogenous alkali can come in a variety of forms, from HCO_3^- (baking soda, Alka-Seltzer) to organic anions. Citrate, lactate, acetate, and other organic anions are contained in various parenteral solutions and can all increase $[HCO_3^-]$. The increase in serum $[HCO_3^-]$ engendered by either HCl loss (vomiting) or alkali intake limits HCO_3^- addition during dialysis, but metabolic alkalosis is nonetheless sustained because dialysis therapy is designed to ensure alkali delivery, with high levels of HCO_3^- or HCO_3^- precursors in the dialysate. At the same time, dialysis limits the increase in $[HCO_3^-]$ to approximately 35 mEq/L in most instances (unless HCl losses are very large) and tends to blunt the development of severe alkalosis. Unless the alkalosis is unusually severe (serum $[HCO_3^-]$ greater than 35 mEq/L), it does not usually require correction by adjustments in dialysis. Removal of the cause will lead to eventual correction of the disorder. In the rare instance in which rapid correction is required, one can adjust bath $[HCO_3^-]$ to facilitate HCO_3^- removal, carry out isolated ultrafiltration and replace the fluid lost with saline, or titrate excess HCO_3^- with parenteral HCl.

Respiratory Acidosis

Hypercapnia produces a sustained and severe fall in pH in dialysis patients because the adaptive increase in $[HCO_3^-]$, normally brought about by renal mechanisms, does not occur. Serum $[HCO_3^-]$ is determined by the nature of the dialysis prescription, and this dynamic is unaffected by changes in pH or P_{CO_2} in the patient. Respiratory acidosis is always due to impaired CO_2 excretion with one rare exception. In patients maintained on a ventilator kept at a fixed rate, increased CO_2 production can cause hypercapnia because excretion of CO_2 is fixed. The first approach to management of respiratory acidosis is to improve ventilation and reduce P_{CO_2} if possible. If hypercapnia cannot be ameliorated, increasing $[HCO_3^-]$ by adjustments in dialysis therapy or oral supplementation may mitigate the degree of acidemia, although the ability to increase serum $[HCO_3^-]$ is limited.

Respiratory Alkalosis

Hypocapnia induces severe and sustained alkalemia in dialysis patients because, as in respiratory acidosis, alkali addition during dialysis is not influenced by pH or P_{CO_2}. In this instance, the added alkali maintains serum $[HCO_3^-]$ at an inappropriately high level. Respiratory alkalosis has multiple causes, including hypoxemia, anxiety, central nervous system disease, pulmonary disease, and hepatic failure. Because serum $[HCO_3^-]$ is not changed, diagnosis requires clinical suspicion and measurement of P_{CO_2} and pH. Management is directed at correction of the underlying disorder. If the alkalemia is severe (pH greater than 7.65), hypocapnia can be corrected acutely using a rebreathing device. Management of sustained hypocapnia is difficult but can be ameliorated by reducing bath $[HCO_3^-]$ in patients receiving hemodialysis or by carrying out isolated ultrafiltration and replacing losses with NaCl.

Selected Readings

Daugirdas JT. Dialysis hypotension: a hemodynamic analysis. *Kidney Int* 1991;39:233–246.

Comprehensive review of the factors contributing to hypotension during hemodialysis.

Franz M, Pohanka E, Tribl B, et al. Living on chronic hemodialysis between dryness and fluid overload. *Kidney Int* 1997;51(Suppl 59):S39–S42.

Review of new techniques being developed to assess ECF volume in dialysis patients.

Gennari FJ. Acid–base homeostasis in end-stage renal disease. *Semin Dial* 1997;9:404–411.

Review of the factors influencing acid–base homeostasis in patients receiving peritoneal dialysis or hemodialysis.

Gennari FJ, Rimmer JM. Acid–base disorders in end-stage renal disease, parts I and II. *Semin Dial* 1990;3:81–85, 161–165.

Complete review of acid–base balance and acid–base disorders in patients receiving hemodialysis or peritoneal dialysis.

Hou S, McElroy PA, Nootens J, et al. Safety and efficacy of low-potassium dialysate. *Am J Kidney Dis* 1989;13:137–143.

Original study examining the kinetics of K^+ removal during hemodialysis and the effects of altering bath $[K^+]$.

Ketchersid T, Van Stone J. Dialysate potassium. *Semin Dial* 1991;4:46–51.

Review of the special issues of potassium removal by hemodialysis.

Sargent JA, Gotch FA. Principles and biophysics of dialysis. In: Maher JF, ed. *Replacement of renal function by dialysis.* Boston: Kluwer Academic Publishers, 1989:87–144.

Complete description of the dynamics of fluid and electrolyte transfer during dialysis therapy.

van Ypersele de Strihou C. Potassium homeostasis in renal failure. *Kidney Int* 1977;11:491–504.

Excellent review of the changes in internal and external potassium balance that occur in renal failure.

Ward RA, Wathen RL, William TE, et al. Hemodialysate composition and intradialytic metabolic, acid–base and potassium changes. *Kidney Int* 1987;32:129–135.

Original study examining the effects of glucose addition to the bath and using acetate or bicarbonate as alkali precursors, on metabolic events, acid–base status, and K^+ removal during hemodialysis.

CHAPTER 77

Divalent Ion Metabolism and Renal Osteodystrophy

Shaul G. Massry and Miroslaw Smogorzewski

Disturbances in divalent ion metabolism are common in patients with renal failure. The major features of these abnormalities are listed in Table 77.1. The processes causing disordered divalent ion metabolism and osteodystrophy have their onset in the early stages of renal insufficiency, continue throughout the life of the patient, and may be influenced beneficially or adversely by various therapeutic approaches used.

TABLE 77.1. Major Features of Disordered Divalent Ion Metabolism in Renal Failure

Hyperphosphatemia
Hypocalcemia
Secondary hyperparathyroidism
Defective intestinal absorption of calcium
Altered vitamin D metabolism
Bone disease
Soft tissue calcification
Alterations in renal handling of phosphate, calcium, and magnesium
Pruritus
Proximal myopathy
Skin ulceration and soft tissue necrosis

PATHOGENESIS

Hypocalcemia and Secondary Hyperparathyroidism

Patients with renal failure almost always have secondary hyperplasia of the parathyroid glands, resulting in elevated blood levels of parathyroid hormone (PTH). This abnormality is due to the *hypocalcemia* that develops during the course of renal insufficiency and/or to a *deficiency of 1,25-dihydroxycholecalciferol* [1,25(OH)$_2$D] that may directly affect the function of the parathyroid glands. As renal failure progresses, there is a decrease in the number of vitamin D receptors (VDR) and calcium sensing receptors (CaR) in the parathyroid glands, rendering them more resistant to the action of vitamin D and calcium. These events will allow secondary hyperparathyroidism to worsen. At least three hypotheses have been proposed to explain the pathogenesis of the hypocalcemia. These include (a) phosphate retention, (b) skeletal resistance to the calcemic action of PTH, and (c) altered vitamin D metabolism. The zeal and vigor with which the proponents of these hypotheses have defended their concepts have created the impression that a major controversy exists. We believe that these possibilities are not mutually exclusive but rather interrelated, and together form a unified and integrated explanation for the hypocalcemia of renal failure.

Role of Phosphate Retention

Several lines of evidence suggest that phosphate retention may provoke secondary hyperparathyroidism. First, a disorder called *sneezing disease* was described in piglets; this disease is characterized by labored respiration and sneezing and is due to deformities of turbinate nasal bones caused by generalized osteitis fibrosa. This disease was reproduced in horses fed high-phosphate, low-calcium diets. The animals developed lameness and "big head" secondary to swelling of facial bones; both abnormalities were due to osteoclastic bone resorption. Initially, the animals developed hyperphosphatemia and hypocalcemia followed by hypophosphatemia and hypercalcemia. The parathyroid glands were diffusely hyperplastic. These observations demonstrate that the ingestion of an excessive amount of phosphate is associated with secondary hyperparathyroidism, even in the absence of renal failure.

Second, the acute ingestion of inorganic phosphate by normal subjects causes a transient rise in the levels of serum phosphorus, a fall in the concentration of ionized calcium, and a significant elevation in the blood levels of PTH.

Third, the development of secondary hyperparathyroidism in dogs with experimental renal failure is influenced by the magnitude of dietary phosphate intake; secondary hyperparathyroidism was prevented when dietary intake of phosphate was reduced in proportion to the fall in the glomerular filtration rate (GFR).

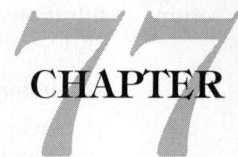

It appears, therefore, that phosphate retention and hyperphosphatemia can provoke secondary hyperparathyroidism in the absence or presence of impaired renal function. Because secondary hyperparathyroidism occurs early in the course of renal failure, hyperphosphatemia should develop at an early stage of renal insufficiency. However, the available data indicate that patients with moderate renal insufficiency are not hyperphosphatemic but are either normophosphatemic or mildly hypophosphatemic. To overcome this discrepancy, Bricker and Slatopolsky postulated that a transient and possibly undetectable increase in serum phosphorus occurs early in renal failure with each decrement in renal function. Such a transient hyperphosphatemia would directly decrease the blood levels of ionized calcium, which then stimulates the parathyroid glands to release more hormone. PTH would decrease the renal tubular reabsorption of phosphate, with a return of serum phosphorus and calcium levels to normal at the expense of a new steady state characterized by elevated blood levels of PTH.

This postulate implies that these adaptive changes occurring in patients with incipient renal failure and leading to secondary hyperparathyroidism are geared to maintain normal phosphate homeostasis. However, ample evidence exists that phosphate homeostasis in renal failure can be maintained without secondary hyperparathyroidism. First, in thyroparathyroidectomized dogs with renal failure in which the serum calcium was maintained at a normal level by vitamin D supplementation, the fraction of filtered phosphate excreted increased and the serum concentration of phosphorus remained normal despite the renal failure. Second, rats immunized against tubular basement membrane developed interstitial nephritis and renal failure and lost the response of renal adenylate cyclase to PTH. Despite these changes, the fraction of filtered phosphate excreted increased markedly. Third, studies in rats with renal failure have clearly demonstrated that PTH is not the main regulator of the renal handling of phosphate in renal failure. Fourth, a very high fractional excretion of phosphate is present in patients with chronic renal failure (CRF) even after total parathyroidectomy.

If the sequence of events described by the Bricker-Slatopolsky hypothesis does occur, the basal serum levels of phosphorus and calcium should display one of the following combinations: hyperphosphatemia and hypocalcemia, normophosphatemia and normocalcemia, or hypophosphatemia and hypercalcemia; the latter may occur if the adaptive response of the parathyroid glands is exaggerated, as in the case of nutritional secondary hyperparathyroidism in horses. However, the available data show that the mean levels of both serum phosphorus and calcium in most patients with early and moderate renal failure are significantly lower than the values in normal subjects. These observations cannot be explained by the Bricker-Slatopolsky postulate. Thus other factors must also be operative and contribute to the genesis of the hypocalcemia in early renal failure.

These considerations do not necessarily mean that phosphate retention is not an important factor in the pathogenesis of the hypocalcemia and secondary hyperparathyroidism in early renal failure. They suggest rather that phosphate retention in early renal failure may contribute to the hypocalcemia by mechanisms other than a direct effect of hyperphosphatemia on serum calcium.

It should be mentioned that with more advanced renal failure when hyperphosphatemia develops, the elevated blood levels of phosphorus may suppress blood levels of calcium and contribute to the hypocalcemia of advanced renal failure. In addition, experimental evidence indicates that the very high levels of phosphorus may directly affect the function of the parathyroid glands; such high phosphorus may induce hyperplasia of the parathyroid glands independent of calcium or $1{,}25OH_2D_3$, and by posttranscriptional mechanism increases PTH synthesis and secretion.

Role of Skeletal Resistance to the Calcemic Action of PTH

Hypocalcemia is frequently encountered in patients with renal failure despite the elevated blood levels of PTH, suggesting a skeletal resistance to the calcemic action of the hormone. The calcemic response to the infusion of PTH or to an acute rise in the blood levels of endogenous PTH is markedly blunted in patients with mild to moderate renal failure, indicating that this skeletal resistance occurs early in the course of renal insufficiency. This abnormality has also been documented in patients with advanced renal failure, in those treated with hemodialysis, and in many renal transplant recipients.

Skeletal resistance to the calcemic action of PTH occurs in patients with acute renal failure. Hypocalcemia is almost always observed in these patients (see Chapter 49). The degree of the hypocalcemia is moderate to marked, occurs early in the course of the oliguric phase of the disease, and persists through the diuretic period. The hypocalcemia is observed in patients with low, normal, or elevated serum concentrations of phosphorus, indicating that the hyperphosphatemia of acute renal failure is not a major determinant of the hypocalcemia. Also, the hypocalcemia cannot be attributed to a failure in the function of the parathyroid glands because the blood levels of PTH are elevated and display an inverse correlation with the concentrations of serum calcium. The infusion of PTH fails to elicit a normal rise in serum calcium. All these derangements are reversed after the return of renal function to normal.

All the observations cited thus far indicate that there is skeletal resistance to the calcium-mobilizing action of PTH, an abnormality that occurs early in the course of both acute and CRF and is not reversed by hemodialysis. This derangement is an important factor contributing to the hypocalcemia in renal failure, and hence it plays a role in the pathogenesis of secondary hyperparathyroidism in these patients.

A series of studies in thyroparathyroidectomized dogs with acute renal failure produced by bilateral ureteral ligation, bilateral nephrectomy, or diversion of both ureters into the jugular veins has demonstrated that the skeletal resistance to the calcemic action of PTH is partially due to a deficiency of $1{,}25(OH)_2D$, and its complete correction requires adequate amounts of both $1{,}25(OH)_2D$ and $24{,}25(OH)_2D$. Other studies suggest that the skeletal resistance to the calcemic action of PTH is, at least in part, due to downregulation of PTH receptors. Indeed, several studies have shown that the PTH–PTHrP receptors are downregulated in many organs in uremia; these include the kidney, liver, and heart. This downregulation of the PTH–PTHrP receptors is not due to the high levels of PTH but rather to the PTH-induced elevation in the basal levels of cytosolic calcium.

Role of Altered Vitamin D Metabolism

The experimental data cited previously suggest that alterations in vitamin D and/or a deficiency of one or more of the vitamin D metabolites are present in patients with early renal failure because these patients display skeletal resistance to the calcemic action of PTH. Indeed, disturbances in the functional integrity of the target organs for vitamin D (impaired intestinal absorption of calcium and/or defective mineralization of osteoid) have been found in patients with mild to moderate renal insufficiency, indicating that a state of relative or absolute vitamin D deficiency exists in these patients.

The blood levels of $1{,}25(OH)_2D$ are usually normal or modestly elevated in patients with moderate renal failure, although low levels have also been noted in both adults and children with early renal insufficiency. Therefore it appears that absolute deficiency of and/or resistance to vitamin D [normal blood levels of $1{,}25(OH)_2D$] develop early in the course of renal failure. As mentioned, as renal failure progresses, the number of VDRs decreases, resulting in resistance to vitamin D action.

It is intriguing that despite the presence of adequate functioning renal mass in patients with moderate renal insufficiency, the production of $1{,}25(OH)_2D$ is not increased adequately to meet the needs of the target organs for vitamin D. Because the regulation of the renal 1α-hydroxylase, the enzyme responsible for $1,25(OH)_2D$ production, is influenced by alterations in phosphate homeostasis, it is possible that phosphate retention, which may develop with declining renal function, plays a major role in the disturbances in $1,25(OH)_2D$ production. Indeed, dietary phosphate restriction in proportion to the reduction in GFR in adults with moderate renal failure has been associated with a significant increase in the blood levels of $1,25(OH)_2D$ and with biologic evidence for the normalization of the target organ response to vitamin D. Similar observations were also reported in children with moderate renal insufficiency.

The mechanisms through which dietary phosphate restriction in patients with early renal insufficiency is associated with increased production of $1,25(OH)_2D$ are not evident. This effect does not seem to be mediated by changes in the serum concentration of phosphorus because no significant changes in this parameter were found in the studies of adults and children. The effect of dietary phosphate on renal production of $1,25(OH)_2D$ could be mediated through changes in transcellular flux of phosphate and/or in the concentration of inorganic phosphorus in renal cortical cells. Indeed, studies in rats have shown that the level of inorganic phosphorus in the renal cell is reduced during feeding with phosphate-restricted diet.

Interaction Between $1,25(OH)_2D$ and Parathyroid Glands

Available data indicate that $1,25(OH)_2D$ may have a direct effect on the parathyroid glands. First, prolonged exposure to $1,25(OH)_2D$ both *in vivo* and *in vitro* may directly suppress the activity of the parathyroid glands. Second, $1,25(OH)_2D$ renders the parathyroid glands more susceptible to the suppressive action of calcium. Such an effect of $1,25(OH)_2D$ may correct the abnormal shift in set point for calcium of the parathyroid glands in patients with renal failure. Third, $1,25(OH)_2D$ decreases prepro-PTH messenger RNA in a dose-dependent manner. Thus it is possible that deficiency of $1,25(OH)_2D$ may initiate secondary hyperparathyroidism even in the absence of overt hypocalcemia; this has been demonstrated in dogs with a 70% decrease in GFR.

Regulation of the Parathyroid Hormone Gene by Vitamin D, Calcium, and Phosphorus

The secondary hyperparathyroidism in uremia is due to increased synthesis and secretion of PTH secondary to an increase in PTH gene expression and parathyroid cell proliferation. $1,25(OH)_2D_3$ acts directly on the PTH gene, causing a decrease in its transcription and hence in the synthesis of PTH. Hypocalcemia increases and hypophosphatemia decreases PTH gene expression by an effect on the stability of the mRNA of PTH. Thus there is an increase in the stability mRNA of PTH with hypocalcemia, resulting in increased synthesis of the PTH protein. In contrast, the stability of mRNA of PTH is decreased during hypophosphatemia, leading to increased degradation of the mRNA of PTH and hence decreased production of PTH. Thus the effects of hypercalcemia and hypophosphatemia on PTH synthesis is posttranscriptional.

Integration of the Various Pathogenetic Factors

The clinical and experimental evidence discussed thus far allow a new formulation for the mechanisms of secondary hyperparathyroidism in renal insufficiency. It appears that phosphate retention, which may develop as renal insufficiency ensues, may interfere with the ability of the patients to augment the renal production of $1,25(OH)_2D$ to meet their increased need. A state of absolute or relative vitamin D deficiency develops, leading to defective intestinal absorption of calcium and impaired calcemic response to PTH. These two abnormalities produce hypocalcemia and, subsequently, secondary hyperparathyroidism. Although this formulation still assigns an important role to phosphate retention in the genesis of secondary hyperparathyroidism of renal failure, the pathway through which such phosphate retention mediates its effect is different from that originally proposed; the original theory maintained that phosphate retention in early renal failure is associated with a rise in serum phosphorus and a consequent fall in serum calcium, which in turn stimulates the parathyroid gland activity. However, it must be emphasized that if marked hyperphosphatemia does develop in a patient with renal failure, it could directly lower the level of serum calcium and contribute to the severity of the hypocalcemia and the secondary hyperparathyroidism. Hyperphosphatemia per se may stimulate parathyroid hormone synthesis by a posttranscriptional effect of PTH gene expression. An Na-P cotransporter is present in the parathyroid gland, and this transporter may play a role in the processes that allows the parathyroid gland to sense the level of extracellular phosphorus.

An additional pathway through which an absolute or relative deficiency of $1,25(OH)_2D$, independent of hypocalcemia, may mediate secondary hyperparathyroidism is related to the interaction between this vitamin D metabolite and the parathyroid glands, as discussed earlier.

This integrated formulation for the pathogenesis of secondary hyperparathyroidism has important clinical implications. It is evident that dietary phosphate restriction in proportion to the fall in GFR in patients with early renal failure is adequate to reverse and correct secondary hyperparathyroidism and other abnormalities in divalent ion metabolism. However, achieving the proper and adequate dietary phosphate restriction and successful patient compliance with the dietary regimen may prove difficult. Because the available data indicate that dietary phosphate restriction exerts its effect through the increased production of $1,25(OH)_2D$ and because this vitamin D metabolite also exerts a direct effect on the parathyroid glands, an alternative therapeutic approach would be supplementation of $1,25(OH)_2D_3$. Indeed, treatment of patients with moderate renal failure with $1,25(OH)_2D_3$ for 6 to 12 months was associated with improvement or normalization of the disturbances in divalent ion metabolism, including secondary hyperparathyroidism and bone disease.

Hyperphosphatemia

Hyperphosphatemia is a common finding in patients with advanced renal failure, and it usually becomes evident when the GFR falls to 20% to 30% of normal. Several factors may affect the level of serum phosphorus in patients with renal failure (Table 77.2).

The dietary intake of phosphate and the fraction of the ingested phosphate absorbed by the intestine have an important

TABLE 77.2. Factors Affecting the Level of Serum Phosphorus in Uremia

Magnitude of residual renal function
Dietary intake of phosphate
Degree of secondary hyperparathyroidism and the responsiveness of the skeleton to parathyroid hormone
Ingestion of phosphate-binding antacids
Magnitude of vitamin D deficiency and treatment with vitamin D or its metabolites
Balance between degradation and synthesis of body proteins
Frequency, duration, and adequacy of dialysis
Parenteral alimentation
Intake of large supplements of calcium

effect on the serum levels of phosphorus in uremic patients. These patients have only mild impairment in intestinal absorption of phosphate, and their kidneys are unable to adequately handle phosphate loads. Thus an increase in phosphate intake can cause a marked rise in serum phosphorus levels in such patients.

Intestinal absorption of phosphate is enhanced by $1,25(OH)_2D_3$, and administration of this metabolite to patients with advanced renal failure may produce or worsen hyperphosphatemia. In patients who have substantial osteomalacia, the levels of serum phosphorus may remain unchanged or even fall during therapy with $1,25(OH)_2D_3$. This is due to the deposition of calcium and phosphorus into bone because $1,25(OH)_2D_3$ improves mineralization of osteoid and heals osteomalacia.

Phosphate-binding antacids render dietary phosphate and phosphate contained in swallowed saliva and intestinal secretions unabsorbable. Thus patients receiving these antacids may have normal levels of serum phosphorus or modest hyperphosphatemia. It should be emphasized that these compounds are most effective when dietary intake of phosphate is below 1.0 g/day. With higher phosphate intake (more than 2.0 g/day), their effectiveness is reduced and hyperphosphatemia may persist despite their use.

An important factor determining the level of serum phosphorus in advanced uremia is the degree of hypersecretion of PTH and the response of the skeleton to the high levels of this hormone. Normally, PTH decreases the renal tubular reabsorption of phosphate, increases urinary phosphate excretion, and consequently reduces serum phosphorus. This effect becomes progressively limited as renal failure advances. For example, with GFR of 5 ml/min and serum phosphorus of 8.0 mg/dl, the maximal urinary excretion of phosphate that can be achieved is less than 600 mg/day, even when no phosphate is reabsorbed. Under such conditions, the severely damaged kidneys cannot respond to a further increase in PTH with additional augmentation in phosphate excretion. The enhanced bone resorption, which is induced by the high levels of PTH, liberates calcium and phosphorus from the skeleton into the extracellular fluid. This phosphorus cannot be excreted by the kidney, and hence serum phosphorus concentration rises. Several clinical observations support this view. First, the levels of serum calcium and phosphorus are higher in patients with advanced uremia and severe secondary hyperparathyroidism than in other patients with comparable renal failure but without severe hyperparathyroidism. Second, following total or subtotal parathyroidectomy in patients with renal failure and severe secondary hyperparathyroidism, the serum concentrations of calcium and phosphorus fall (Fig. 77.1). Third, when patients with CRF and overt secondary hyperparathyroidism are treated with hemodialysis, the serum phosphorus levels not only may remain above normal but may rebound rapidly after dialysis to predialysis levels.

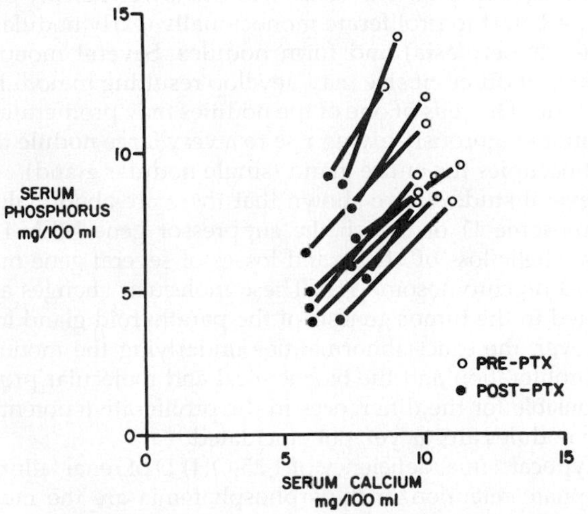

Figure 77.1. Changes in total serum calcium and inorganic phosphorus observed in 11 uremic patients before and after subtotal parathyroidectomy *(PTX).* (Reproduced with permission from Massry SG, Caburn JW, Popovtzer MM, et al. Secondary hyperparathyroidism in chronic renal failure. *Arch Intern Med* 1969;124:431.)

A shift in the balance between protein synthesis and breakdown toward catabolism, as occurs with infection, trauma, starvation, and the administration of glucocorticoids or tetracycline, can cause an increase in serum phosphorus concentration. The parenteral administration of solutions containing large quantities of glucose and amino acids can cause an abrupt reduction in serum phosphorus levels. Also, the concentration of serum phosphorus may fall during refeeding after a period of calorie or protein malnutrition.

ALTERED VITAMIN D METABOLISM

The normal metabolism of vitamin D, the mechanisms controlling and regulating the renal production of $1,25(OH)_2D$ and $24,25(OH)_2D$, their biologic actions, and their altered metabolism in patients with renal failure are discussed in Chapter 13, Part 11. Patients with mild renal failure may have a vitamin D–resistant state and/or a relative vitamin D–deficient state. As renal failure progresses, an absolute vitamin D–deficient state develops, with the blood levels of $1,25(OH)_2D$ being reduced when GFR falls below 50 ml/min in children and below 30 ml/min in adults. In anephric patients and in those treated with dialysis, the blood levels of $1,25(OH)_2D$ are usually undetectable. Patients with renal failure and granulomatous diseases such as sarcoidosis or tuberculosis may have elevated blood levels of $1,25(OH)_2D$ caused by extrarenal production of this metabolite by the granulomatous tissue. In advanced renal failure, the number of VDRs is reduced, leading to vitamin D resistance. Thus, in patients with CRF, there is vitamin D deficiency and vitamin D resistance as well. The blood levels of 25-hydroxyvitamin D [25(OH)D] in patients with advanced renal failure and those treated with hemodialysis are usually normal. Low levels of 25(OH)D may be encountered in patients with advanced renal failure who have nephrotic-range proteinuria [loss of 25(OH)D in urine, Chapter 39, Part 2A], those who are treated with peritoneal dialysis [loss of 25(OH)D in peritoneal fluid], or those who have nutritional vitamin D deficiency. The biologic consequences of vitamin D deficiency are multiple and are manifested by disturbances in the function of its target organs: parathyroid glands, skeleton, intestine, and skeletal muscle (Table 77.3). Because other organs such as testes, myocardium, and pancreas have receptors for $1,25(OH)_2D$, it is

TABLE 77.3. Biologic Consequences of Vitamin D Deficiency

Shift in set-point of calcium for the parathyroid gland
Secondary hyperparathyroidism
Skeletal resistance to the calcemic action of parathyroid hormone
Impaired mineralization of osteoid
Abnormalities in formation and maturation of collagen
Retarded growth in uremic children
Defective intestinal absorption of calcium and phosphorus
Abnormalities in the structural integrity of the intestinal mucosa
Proximal myopathy

possible that a deficiency of this vitamin D metabolite plays a role in the dysfunction of these organs in uremia.

The factors responsible for the decrease in the number of VDRs in uremia are not fully elucidated but may include (a) reduced levels of $1,25(OH)_2D_3$ because this metabolite affects the production of VDRs (low levels of $1,25(OH)_2D_3$, downregulate the mRNA of VDR); (b) hyperparathyroidism of renal failure may also play a role because high levels of PTH interfere with the $1,25(OH)_2D_3$-induced upregulation of VDR; and (c) uremic toxins, which may decrease the stability of the mRNA of VDRs, resulting in transcriptional reduction of VDR protein.

The action of vitamin D is mediated by its binding with its cytosolic receptor, VDR. The DNA binding site for VDR is a nuclear receptor that contains two "zinc fingers" that mediate the binding of VDR to a regulatory promotor regions of DNA 5'-flanking sequence of vitamin D–responsive genes. This domain is the VDR element (VDRE). Thus the binding of the vitamin D–VDR complex to the VDRE results in the transcription of specific mRNAs. In renal failure, there are impairments in the binding of vitamin D to VDR as well as in the binding of the vitamin D–VDR complex to the VDRE. Both of these events in addition to the reduced number of VDR are responsible for the vitamin D–resistant state of renal failure.

INTESTINAL ABSORPTION OF CALCIUM

The processes involved in the regulation of intestinal absorption of calcium and the various factors that affect the absorption of this ion are discussed in Chapter 17, Part 1. Metabolic balance studies carried out in patients with renal failure indicate that fecal calcium equals or even exceeds the amount ingested, suggesting diminished intestinal absorption of calcium. With the introduction and the use of radioisotopic methods, intestinal absorption of calcium has been found to be reduced in most patients with advanced renal failure, but normal values are also encountered. Indeed, a great deal of overlap with normal values is noted. This may be due to variations in habitual dietary intake, known to affect intestinal absorption of calcium, and to variations in the degree of renal failure. In a study of a large population of patients with CRF and patients treated with hemodialysis, in whom intestinal absorption of calcium was evaluated in relation to their habitual calcium intake, 54 (57%) of the 96 uremic patients and 21 (36%) of 58 dialysis patients had impaired absorption. A defect in intestinal absorption of calcium may become evident in patients with mild renal failure; however, in most patients with serum creatinine of less than 2.5 mg/dl, the fractional calcium absorption is not different from normal.

Evaluation of intestinal calcium absorption in uremic patients with ^{47}Ca showed that absorption was markedly reduced below normal only during the first 2 hours after ingestion of the isotope, whereas absorption equalled or surpassed that of normal subjects after 4 hours. These observations are consistent with those showing that intestinal absorption of calcium is impaired in the duodenum and jejunum of uremic patients. This defect is largely due to (a) reduced availability of $1,25(OH)_2D$, which is involved in the various steps of the active intestinal transport of calcium, and (b) structural abnormalities of the intestinal mucosa, which are usually encountered in uremic patients. These structural changes are most likely also due to a deficiency of $1,25(OH)_2D$ because vitamin D has a trophic effect on intestinal mucosa. Indeed, therapy of uremic patients with $1,25(OH)_2D_3$ restores the structural integrity of the intestinal mucosa and augments intestinal absorption of calcium.

The defect in intestinal calcium absorption in uremic patients is most evident when they ingest normal or small quantities of calcium. These patients can absorb amounts of calcium similar to those absorbed by normal subjects when their calcium intake is markedly increased to 4 to 10 g/day. Under such circumstances, most calcium absorption probably occurs through simple ionic diffusion, a process that may be unaffected by uremia, and a defect in active or carrier-mediated transport may be obscured.

Intestinal absorption of calcium is either unchanged or only slightly improved following therapy of uremic patients with regular hemodialysis. This failure to restore calcium absorption to normal with improvement of uremia by hemodialysis is consistent with the view that impairment of a metabolic rather than excretory function of the kidney accounts for the abnormalities in calcium absorption. On the other hand, the slight improvement of calcium absorption following treatment with hemodialysis suggests that uremia per se also contributes to reduced intestinal absorption of calcium. After renal transplantation, calcium absorption returns to normal following the restoration of normal or near normal renal function. Calcium absorption may remain reduced in renal transplant recipients with serum creatinine levels of more than 2.0 mg/dl.

STRUCTURE AND FUNCTION OF THE PARATHYROID GLANDS

Hyperplasia of the parathyroid glands is almost always present in patients with renal failure, but the increase in volume and mass of the glands varies among patients and among the four glands in the same patient. The size of the glands may reach 10 to 50 times normal. The parathyroid glands may occasionally be of normal size in patients with CRF. Histologically, the glands show chief cell hyperplasia with or without oxyphil cell hyperplasia. The usual cell is the vacuolated or chronically stimulated chief cell, 6 to 8 μm wide, with a sharply defined plasma membrane. Nodular or adenomatouslike masses may be found within the hyperplastic glands. These nodules are well circumscribed and surrounded by a fibrous capsule. The cells in the nodular hyperplasia have less VDR density and calcium-sensing receptors (CaR) and higher proliferative potential then the cells of diffuse hyperplasia. The change in the structure of the parathyroid glands begins as polyclonal diffuse hyperplasia. The cells with the lower density of VDR and CaR start to proliferate monoclonally (early nodularity in diffuse hyperplasia) and form nodules. Several monoclonal nodules of different size may develop resulting in nodular hyperplasia. The cells of one of the nodules may proliferate faster and more vigorously giving rise to a very large nodule that almost occupies the entire gland (single nodular gland).

Several studies have shown that there are abnormalities in chromosome 11 on which the suppressor gene MEN-1 is located, allelic loss of 11q13, and losses of several gene markers located on chromosome 11p. These molecular changes are implicated in the tumor genesis of the parathyroid gland in CRF. However, the exact abnormalities underlying the monoclonal cell proliferation and the biochemical and molecular processes responsible for the differences in the proliferative potentials of these nodules are, as yet, not elucidated.

Hypocalcemia, deficiency of $1,25(OH)_2D$ of renal failure, and phosphate retention or hyperphosphatemia are the most important factors responsible for the hyperplasia of the parathyroid glands. Because hypocalcemia and relative or absolute deficiency of $1,25(OH)_2D$ (vitamin D resistance) may develop early in the course of renal failure, hyperactivity of the parathyroid glands is also encountered in the early stages of renal insufficiency. Indeed, elevated blood levels of PTH may be noted when the GFR falls below 70 ml/min.

The appearance of spontaneous and persistent hypercalcemia in uremic patients has led to the suggestion that the parathyroid glands in these patients may become autonomous. However, after calcium infusion, the blood levels of PTH in patients with advanced renal failure and in those treated with hemodialysis invariably fall, although not to normal levels. Thus the parathyroid glands in these patients are suppressible by hypercalcemia. The appearance of spontaneous hypercalcemia and the failure of the blood levels of PTH to fall to normal values after calcium infusion in uremic patients are most likely due to the large mass of the gland. Malregulation of PTH release at the cellular level may also be present. Indeed, studies of dispersed cells of parathyroid glands from patients with renal failure showed that a higher concentration of calcium was required to achieve a suppression of PTH secretion similar to that of cells from normal parathyroid glands. This has been interpreted to indicate a shift in the set point for calcium; this abnormality is at least in part due to deficiency in $1,25(OH)_2D$. True adenomas may develop and function autonomously in certain cases of secondary hyperparathyroidism, but such cases are probably not common. The use of the term *tertiary hyperparathyroidism* should be limited to those cases in which it is documented that a true adenoma has developed in a previously hyperplastic gland.

Pro-PTH (90 amino acids) is synthesized in the rough endoplasmic reticulum of the chief cells of the parathyroid glands. PTH, which is a single-chain polypeptide containing 84 amino acids, is produced by proteolytic cleavage of the pro-PTH in the Golgi apparatus. The PTH is then stored in secretory granules from which it is secreted into the circulation. Pro-PTH is usually not secreted into the circulation. A precursor to pro-PTH known as *prepro-PTH* (115 amino acids) has also been found. The prepro-PTH mRNA is inhibited by $1,25(OH)_2D$ in a dose-dependent manner.

Multiple factors control the release of PTH from the glands, and they do so by inducing changes in the intracellular content of cyclic adenosine monophosphate (cAMP). Any factor that increases cAMP content (hypocalcemia, β-adrenergic agonists, dopaminergic agents, secretin, prostaglandin E, and cholera toxin) enhances PTH secretion. On the other hand, factors that reduce intracellular cAMP (hypercalcemia, hypermagnesemia, α-adrenergic agonists, prostaglandins of the F series, and nitroprusside) inhibit PTH release. Calcium is the most important regulator of PTH secretion, and the effect is mediated by changes in intracellular concentration of calcium. An increase in the concentration of intracellular calcium influences PTH secretion through several mechanisms: (a) inhibition of cAMP accumulation, (b) inhibition of cAMP action, and (c) stimulation of intracellular degradation of preformed PTH.

The cells of the parathyroid glands possess CaR. This receptor protein is located in the membrane of these cells. The levels of serum calcium and $1,25(OH)_2D_3$ as well as dietary phosphate do not appear to regulate the synthesis of CaR. In renal failure, there is reduced density of CaR in the parathyroid gland cells.

The CaR interacts with calcium as well as with other divalent, trivalent, and plications. This receptor protein plays an important role in the ability of parathyroid glands to recognize changes in the concentration of calcium ion in the blood; and as such, CaR mediates the effect of calcium on the secretion of PTH from the parathyroid glands. A decrease in the concentration of calcium ion in blood is recognized by a G-protein–coupled CaR and subsequently leads to PTH release. An increase in the concentration of calcium in the blood activates the CaR, an event that leads to an increase in the concentration of cytosolic calcium secondary to mobilization of calcium from intracellular calcium stores. This rise in cytosolic calcium results in inhibition of PTH release from the parathyroid glands.

The relationship between calcium concentration and the parathyroid gland in the modulation of PTH secretion is altered in patients with renal failure. In normal subjects, this relationship is sigmoidal over a narrow range of calcium concentration, but in patients with renal failure, higher calcium concentration is needed to suppress the secretion of PTH than in normal subjects. Also, in the renal failure patients, the susceptibility of adenyl cyclase of the parathyroid gland to the inhibitory effect calcium is reduced; such an effect would impair the ability of calcium to inhibit PTH secretion. These abnormalities between calcium and PTH secretion could be evaluating the changes in set-point for calcium. The latter is defined as the calcium concentration that produces half the maximal inhibition of PTH and that is the midpoint between the maximal and minimal PTH secretions. Indeed, alterations in set-point for calcium with a shift to right (i.e., 50% inhibition of PTH secretion occurs at higher calcium concentration) were observed in parathyroid glands of patients with primary or secondary hyperparathyroidism. Administration of $1,25(OH)_2D_3$ to dialysis patients was associated with suppression of PTH secretion and with a shift of the set-point to the left, supporting the notion that deficiency of this vitamin D metabolite plays an important role in the genesis of secondary hyperparathyroidism in CRF.

It appears that in patients with renal failure, the structural change in the parathyroid glands (increase in their mass due to diffuse and nodular hyperplasia) and the functional abnormality (shift in set point of calcium to the right) are responsible to increase production and release of PTH. Because the changes in the structure and function of the parathyroid glands occur early in the course of renal failure, the blood levels of PTH are elevated when the GFR falls below 10 ml/min.

The peripheral metabolism of PTH after its secretion from the glands is discussed in Chapter 13. The intact hormone is cleaved by the liver into an N- and a C-terminal fragment. The half-life of both the intact hormone and its N-terminal fragment is short (about 5 minutes), whereas that of the C-terminal fragment is much longer. Renal failure is associated with alterations in PTH metabolism. Both the hepatic removal of the intact hormone and the renal clearance of the C-terminal fragment are impaired. Thus the elevated blood levels of PTH in patients with renal failure are due to both increased secretion and impaired degradation. The major component of the elevated blood levels of the immunoreactive PTH in these patients is the C-terminal fragment(s) and particularly the midmolecule or midregion of C-terminal fragments.

Hyperplasia of the parathyroid glands in patients with CRF are not easily reversed even after the correction of its causes. Indeed, after renal transplantation, the regression of the size of the glands and the reversal of secondary hyperparathyroidism is very slow. We found that 16 of 60 renal transplant recipients have persistent secondary hyperparathyroidism for up to 1 to 7 years after renal transplantation. This slow regression process may accelerate by the use of intravenous $1,25(OH)_2D_3$ pulse therapy. Some investigators found that parathyroid gland hyperplasia regresses in all patients in whom PTH secretion was successfully suppressed. The mechanisms underlying this regression process are not well understood. Apoptosis has been proposed, and certain *in vitro* studies indicate that high concentrations of $1,25(OH)_2D_3$ induce apoptosis of parathyroid gland cells. Such a phenomenon may occur *in vivo* as well. Spontaneous hemorrhage in the hyperplastic glands do occur and may be responsible for the regression of the hyperplastic glands in some patients.

TABLE 77.4. Possible Reasons for Variations in Bone Disease Among Patients with Chronic Renal Failure

Age of the patient
Type of underlying renal disease
Duration of renal failure
Relative severity of the pathogenetic processes underlying the derangement in bone metabolism
Differences in dietary habits
Type of therapy used
Treatment with dialysis and its duration
Aluminum burden

Bone Disease

The nature and type of bone disease that develops in uremic patients may vary from one patient to another. Multiple reasons may account for these variations (Table 77.4). The two major types of bone disease that are commonly encountered in patients with renal failure are *enhanced bone resorption* and *defective mineralization*. Some patients may have one of these types predominantly, whereas others may have a mixed type of bone disease. Mild forms of these derangements in bone metabolism may be observed in the early stages of renal insufficiency, and they become more severe as renal failure progresses. Osteosclerosis may also occur, whereas *osteoporosis* is not common. Another form of bone disease seen in renal failure patients and those treated with dialysis is adynamic bone disease.

Bone Lesion of Excess PTH (High Turnover Bone Disease)

The elevated blood levels of PTH with contribution of locally derived cytokines, such as interleukin (IL)-1, IL-4, IL-6, IL-11, endothelin, tumor necrosis factor-α, and nitric oxide, are responsible for the enhanced number and activity of osteoclasts leading to increased bone resorption. As this process increases in severity, marked fibrosis involving the marrow space develops, with the histologic picture of *osteitis fibrosa* becoming evident. The marrow fibrosis is caused by activation of marrow mesenchymal cells, which differentiate into fibroblastlike cells, which forms fibrous tissue. In this condition, there is also increased bone formation as evidenced by increased amounts of osteoid. This ostitis fibrosa is a high turnover bone disease. Osteoclastic bone resorption occurs along subperiosteal and endosteal surfaces, within the haversian canals of cortical bone, and also on the surfaces of trabecular bone. These alterations are more readily identified in cortical (compact) bone and are less commonly seen in trabecular bone. Resorption of cortical bone may also occur because of increased activity of osteocytes, that is, osteocytic osteolysis, a process that is also stimulated by PTH. The degree of enlargement of osteocytic lacunae correlates with the blood levels of PTH. The hormone also stimulates the activation of osteoblasts, which are increased, but the individual rate of activity of these cells may be suppressed in the uremic patient. Hyperparathyroidism also elicits the appearance of woven osteoid and woven bone. In woven osteoid, collagen fibers of varying dimensions are randomly arranged. This osteoid does not display normal mineralization and shows speckled mineralization and diffuse fluorescence after administration of tetracycline. It is possible that the amorphous calcium phosphate deposited in woven osteoid does not mature to hydroxyapatite. *Thus the manifestations of excess PTH in the bone of uremic patients include increased numbers of osteoclasts and osteoblasts, osteoclastic bone resorption, enlarged haversian lacunae, endosteal fibrosis, and accumulation of woven osteoid and woven bone.*

Bone Lesion of Defective Mineralization

Defective mineralization of osteoid leads to rickets in children and osteomalacia in adults. Histologically, osteomalacia can be accurately diagnosed only by the evaluation of undecalcified bone specimens. Osteomalacia is due to a delay in the rate of skeletal mineralization, resulting in accumulation of excess unmineralized osteoid. However, it must be emphasized that the presence of excess osteoid does not necessarily mean osteomalacia. Hyperosteoidosis may be (a) secondary to abnormalities in normal mineralization (osteomalacia) or (b) caused by an increased rate of synthesis of bone collagen, which is normally mineralized. The use of double tetracycline labeling can differentiate between these two possibilities and is thus critical for the diagnosis of osteomalacia. Two doses of tetracycline are administered, separated by a known period of time (10 to 14 days). Diffuse uptake of the antibiotic denotes impaired mineralization, whereas double linear uptake reflects a normal mineralization process. The mean distance between the two linear labels divided by the time interval separating the two doses of tetracycline provides the rate at which the average osteoblast is synthesizing bone. The total rate of bone formation can also be calculated by multiplying the cellular rate by the linear extent of bone formation. Uremic patients may have a decreased cellular rate and an increased linear extent of bone formation.

Several mechanisms may underlie the defective mineralization of osteoid and hence the development of osteomalacia in patients with renal failure. First, relative or absolute deficiency of vitamin D or its active metabolites and/or resistance to their action are major factors responsible for the osteomalacia of uremia. Vitamin D may affect mineralization through several pathways; it may affect collagen synthesis and maturation, directly stimulate bone mineralization, and/or increase the levels of calcium and phosphorus in the extracellular fluid surrounding the bone. This latter effect is the result of the action of vitamin D on intestinal absorption of these minerals. It is not evident whether a deficiency in one or more of the vitamin D metabolites is critical. For example, few anephric patients with undetectable blood levels of $1,25(OH)_2D$ did not show histologic evidence of osteomalacia. On the other hand, long-term therapy with $1,25(OH)_2D_3$ improved or healed osteomalacia in many patients with advanced renal failure. Osteomalacia may be more frequently encountered in uremic patients with low blood levels of 25(OH)D. A role for alteration in $24,25(OH)_2D$ metabolism in the genesis of the osteomalacia of uremia has not yet been established.

Second, abnormalities in the formation and maturation of collagen have been found in rats with experimental uremia and in patients with CRF. These derangements result in a defect in collagen cross-linking and may affect bone mineralization. These abnormalities in collagen metabolism are most likely due to vitamin D deficiency. Indeed, treatment of uremic patients with $25(OH)D_3$ reversed these defects.

Third, inhibition of maturation of amorphous calcium phosphate to its crystalline phase is another defect participating in the genesis of the osteomalacia of uremia. The magnesium content of the bones of uremic patients is increased, and this may interfere with the process of normal mineralization. Magnesium stabilizes the amorphous calcium phosphate and inhibits its transformation into hydroxyapatite. The bone content of pyrophosphate is also increased in uremia, and pyrophosphate may inhibit mineralization.

Fourth, aluminum toxicity may be responsible for a certain type of mineralization defect that is resistant to vitamin D therapy. This type of bone disease has been called *low turnover bone disease* or *low turnover osteomalacia*. This is mainly seen in dialysis patients who have a large content of aluminum in bone and in whom the aluminum is localized in the mineralization front (i.e., the limit between osteoid and calcified tissue). The effect of aluminum excess on bone in patients with renal failure is discussed in detail in Chapter 68, Part 2. With a decrease in the use of aluminum-containing compounds for the control of hyperphosphatemia, the incidence and prevalence of osteomalacia have been decreasing. Increased burden of iron alone or in combination with aluminum cause osteomalacia in renal failure patients.

The skeleton in osteomalacias is weakened, and patients with this bone disease have skeletal deformities, bone pain, fractures, and musculoskeletal disability.

Adynamic Bone Disease

The exact mechanisms underlying adynamic bone disease (ADB) are not fully elucidated. It is seen in renal failure patient before and after treatment with peritoneal dialysis or hemodialysis. The prevalence of ADB varies between 15% and 60% among the dialysis patient, whereas 30% of bone biopsies from predialysis patients displayed finding consistent with ADB. This entity is characterized by a defect in bone matrix formation and mineralization, increased osteoid thickness, and a decrease in the number of both osteoblast and osteoclast on bone surfaces. There is no excessive amounts of aluminum in the mineralization front. Patients with ABD have lower blood levels of PTH than those with other forms of bone disease. Thus suppression of the parathyroid gland activity with high calcium intake and/or administration of $1,25(OH)_2D_3$ with decrement of blood levels of PTH to normal value may be a factor in the genesis of ADB. This entity of bone disease is also encountered after parathyroidectomy, in renal failure patients with diabetes, and in those with increased aluminum burden; in all those clinical settings, the blood levels of PTH are low. This relationship between the PTH level and ADB is understandable because hypersecretion of PTH in renal failure patients is needed to maintain normal rates of bone formation. It is generally accepted that the blood levels of PTH in the range of two to three times normal are necessary to maintain normal rates of bone formation and prevent the emergence of ADB.

Patients with ADB have increased rates of overt fractures and microfractures. The latter causes bone pain. Calcium uptake by the adynamic bone is reduced, and therefore patients with ABD may develop hypercalcemia if calcium intake is increase or if dialysate calcium is high.

Osteosclerosis and Osteoporosis

A peculiar feature of renal osteodystrophy is osteosclerosis, which appears as increased bone density in roentgenographic studies. Histologically, osteosclerosis is most likely due to accumulation of unmineralized trabecular bone with an increase in total bone mass. Because osteosclerosis affects trabecular bone, it is most evident in the vertebrae, pelvis, ribs, clavicles, and metaphyses of long bones, which are made predominantly of cancellous (trabecular) bone. In patients with osteosclerosis, no correlation is found between the bone lesion and any specific pattern of change in serum levels of calcium, phosphorus, or alkaline phosphatase. Certain experimental and clinical evidence suggests that osteosclerosis could be induced by excess PTH. Indeed, patients with primary hyperparathyroidism may display radiographic evidence of osteosclerosis.

Osteoporosis is defined as a decrease in the mass of normally mineralized bone. Because bone mass may increase in patients with advanced renal failure and osteopenia in these patients is usually associated with increased quantities of osteoid, osteoporosis is uncommon. Immobilization, calcium deficiency per se, and chronic protein depletion may be causes of the osteoporotic component of renal osteodystrophy. In patients older than 50 years, factors that cause postmenopausal, idiopathic, or senile osteoporosis may contribute to the skeletal abnormalities of uremia.

Role of Acidosis in Bone Disease

Acute acidosis produces a significant loss of the acid-soluble calcium carbonate from the skeleton and is usually associated with negative calcium balance. Rats fed a diet rendering them permanently acidotic were found to have less calcified bone than control animals despite adequate intake of calcium. Patients with stable CRF show a persistent positive retention of hydrogen ion, with the skeleton providing the buffer. Indeed, evaluation of the composition of bone in CRF reveals a loss of calcium carbonate. These observations imply that uremic acidosis may contribute to negative balance and the development of skeletal demineralization. However, there is no evidence that the chronic acidosis observed in renal failure can produce continued loss of bone minerals once the labile calcium carbonate component of bone is lost. Although there may be a slight improvement in negative calcium balance following treatment of the chronic acidosis of uremia with alkali, a positive balance for calcium usually does not occur, and hypocalcemia, bone pain, and radiographic abnormalities are not corrected. Moreover, no data are available suggesting that chronic acidosis can cause defective mineralization. It appears that the chronic acidosis of uremia does not play a major role in the pathogenesis of renal osteodystrophy.

Soft Tissue Calcification

Various factors present in uremia may predispose to soft tissue calcification (Table 77.5). An increase in the calcium–phosphorus product in the extracellular fluid is probably the most important pathogenetic factor. The incidence of soft tissue calcification is high when the calcium–phosphorus product (each in mg/dl) exceeds 75, and soft tissue calcification is infrequently noted when the calcium–phosphorus product is below 70. It is recommended, however, that the product be maintained below 55. Alkalemia, which often occurs after hemodialysis, may persist during the interdialytic period and may predispose to precipitation of calcium salts in soft tissues. An increase in local pH due to loss of CO_2 from the exposed part of the eye may bring about the observed conjunctival and corneal calcifications. PTH enhances movement of calcium into cells, and the state of secondary hyperparathyroidism plays an important part in the *genesis* of soft tissue calcification in uremia. Certain factor(s) that may act locally to inhibit calcification and are present in the blood of uremic patients may possibly be removed during hemodialysis. Local tissue injury may also predispose to calcification when the calcium–phosphorus product is normal or only slightly elevated. Expression of genes coding for certain

TABLE 77.5. Factors That May Predispose to Soft Tissue Calcification in Uremia

An increase in calcium–phosphorus product in serum
Secondary hyperparathyroidism
Local tissue injury
A rise in local pH of tissue
Removal of calcification inhibitors by dialysis

proteins involved in prevention of calcification has been demonstrated in macrophages and smooth muscle cells of blood vessels wall. One of these proteins is matrix gla protein (MGP). Its deficiency permits medial calcification of blood vessels. Indeed, MGP knockout homozygous mice displayed extensive and severe vascular calcification. It is possible that downregulation of the production of this protein occurs in uremia and participates in the genesis of the vascular calcification seen in patients with end-stage renal failure.

The chemical nature of soft tissue calcification may vary in different tissues. Thus the calcification found in nonvisceral tissue (periarticular and vascular calcification) consists of hydroxyapatite, with a molar Ca:Mg:P ratio similar to that of uremic bone. In contrast, the calcification found in visceral organs (skeletal and myocardial muscle) is made of amorphous $(CaMg)_3(PO_4)_2$, which has a much higher magnesium content. These observations suggest that the mechanisms responsible for the calcification of various tissues in uremic patients may be different.

Magnesium Homeostasis

Disturbances in magnesium metabolism may occur in patients with renal failure. These include changes in serum levels of magnesium and in its renal handling, intestinal absorption, and tissue content. The alterations in the serum concentrations of magnesium and the renal handling of this ion are discussed in later sections of this chapter.

Intestinal Absorption of Magnesium

Data from balance studies indicate that net magnesium absorption in relation to dietary intake in normal subjects is not different from that in uremic patients. Thus it appears that CRF does not reduce intestinal magnesium absorption, and this ion is readily absorbed by these patients independently of the presence of hypermagnesemia and the body need for magnesium. As in normal subjects, the amount of ingested magnesium absorbed by uremic patients increases as dietary magnesium is augmented. This provides an explanation for the development of hypermagnesemia in such patients as their magnesium intake is increased. $1.25(OH)_2D_3$ has no or little effect on intestinal absorption of magnesium in uremic patients.

In contrast to data from balance studies, evaluation of intestinal absorption of magnesium with *in vivo* intestinal perfusion techniques showed that patients with end-stage renal disease have impaired magnesium absorption in the jejunum and ileum. The reason for this discrepancy is not evident. It is possible that the defect in magnesium absorption is limited to certain segments of the intestine, while the absorption in other parts is normal or increased, resulting in an overall normal absorption as evaluated by balance studies.

Tissue Content of Magnesium

The content of magnesium in red blood cells of uremic patients undergoing treatment with hemodialysis is usually higher than in normal subjects and correlates well with the serum concentration of magnesium.

The magnesium content of skin in patients treated with hemodialysis is affected by the concentration of magnesium in dialysate. We have evaluated magnesium content of skin in two populations of patients treated with hemodialysis for periods of 2 months to 5 years with dialysate containing magnesium in concentrations of either 1.8 or 0.6 mg/dl. Although there was an overlap between the individual values, the magnesium content of skin was significantly higher in the group treated with dialysate containing 1.8 mg/dl. The magnesium content of muscle in patients with advanced renal failure can be low, normal, or elevated.

Magnesium content of both cortical and trabecular bone is increased in uremia. The excess magnesium is found in both the exchangeable and nonexchangeable pools of bone magnesium. The most probable cause for the increase in bone magnesium in these patients is the hypermagnesemia usually present. Indeed, a direct relationship exists between the magnesium content of bone and the serum levels of magnesium.

Renal Handling of Divalent Ions

Calcium

Hypocalciuria is almost always present in patients with CRF, and it is observed in the early stage of renal insufficiency. Occasionally, patients with CRF caused by polycystic kidney diseases or chronic pyelonephritis may lose sizeable amounts of calcium in their urine.

In patients with early renal failure, the fraction of filtered calcium excreted is low, but it increases as renal failure progresses. It thus appears that the factors regulating the renal handling of calcium may differ at various stages of renal failure. Possibly, the hypocalciuria and the decreased fractional excretion of calcium are produced by the high circulating levels of PTH, which increase the tubular reabsorption of calcium and reduce its urinary excretion. In patients with advanced renal failure, the increase in the fractional excretion of calcium correlates very closely with that of sodium. This relationship is almost identical with that observed in normal dogs undergoing extracellular fluid volume expansion with saline infusion. A factor that depresses the tubular reabsorption of sodium has been isolated from the plasma of uremic patients. It is possible that such a factor is responsible for the decrease in the fractional reabsorption of both sodium and calcium. Under such circumstances, the effect of PTH in reducing fractional excretion of calcium is overcome. The interdependence between the clearances of sodium and calcium persists in patients undergoing maintenance hemodialysis who have only vestigial renal function and form small amounts of urine.

Phosphorus

The fraction of filtered phosphorus excreted increases as renal failure progresses. This phenomenon has been attributed to the elevated blood levels of PTH. In patients with advanced renal failure, the number of functioning nephrons is small, and the effect of PTH on the tubular reabsorption of phosphorus by the nephron is maximal. Therefore further elevation in the blood levels of PTH is no longer effective in maintaining body phosphorus homeostasis. Indeed, administration of PTH to patients with advanced renal failure does not augment phosphorus excretion.

Clinical and experimental evidence discussed earlier in this chapter indicate that an increase in fractional excretion of phosphorus occurs, and phosphorus homeostasis can be maintained even in the absence of PTH. These observations indicate that factors other than the elevated blood levels of PTH may affect the renal handling of phosphorus in uremia.

The use of T_mP/GFR, where T_mP is the maximum capacity to transport phosphorus, instead of percentage of tubular reabsorption of phosphorus (%TRP) provides a better understanding of the renal handling of phosphorus in renal failure. Calculation of the predicted levels of serum phosphorus and %TRP in patients with impaired renal function, assuming that T_mP/GFR remains constant (i.e., without factors that decrease T_mP/GFR, such as PTH), showed that a fall in GFR to 50 ml/min would cause little change in serum phosphorus levels or in %TRP; a further decrease in GFR would produce a large increase in serum phosphorus levels and a decrease in %TRP. These predictions are similar to actual data observed in patients with CRF. Thus it appears that the change in the serum levels of phosphorus and %TRP can be explained by a fall in GFR per se, without the need to implicate factors that decrease T_mP/GFR. However, PTH may affect T_mP/GFR in patients with renal failure and contribute to the changes in the renal handling of phosphorus in these patients. Indeed, the available data from patients with renal failure show that a small reduction in T_mP/GFR is present in early renal insufficiency, but a considerable decrease in T_mP/GFR occurs in advanced renal failure.

Magnesium

The daily urinary excretion of magnesium is usually reduced in patients with advanced renal failure. In patients with uremia and salt wasting, such as those with polycystic kidney disease or chronic pyelonephritis, the 24-hour urinary excretion of magnesium may be normal or high, and renal magnesium wasting has been encountered in few such patients.

The fraction of filtered magnesium excreted increases as renal failure progresses, and the increment is more marked when the GFR is less than 10 ml/min. There is a positive and significant correlation between the fraction of filtered magnesium excreted and that of sodium in patients with a GFR of less than 40 ml/min.

BIOCHEMICAL FEATURES

Serum Calcium

Hypocalcemia is common but not invariably present in patients with advanced renal failure, and modest reductions in the concentration of serum calcium may be noted in patients with mild renal insufficiency. The hypocalcemia may be more pronounced in uremic patients with marked and widespread osteomalacia. In contrast, the serum levels of calcium may be normal or elevated in the patients with marked secondary hyperparathyroidism and generalized osteitis fibrosa.

In a study of 100 patients with advanced renal failure, about 40% had serum calcium concentrations below the 95% confidence limit (less than 9.4 mg/dl) of values observed in normal subjects. Levels of serum calcium below 6.5 mg/dl are less commonly encountered. Very low levels of serum calcium (less than 5.0 mg/dl) have been seen in patients whose renal failure is due to amyloidosis. In such patients, amyloid deposits in the parathyroid glands cause hypoparathyroidism, leading to profound hypocalcemia.

Usually, the levels of total, diffusible, and ionized calcium are reduced, whereas those of complexed calcium are elevated. The percentages of diffusible and ionized fractions are not different from normal. There is a tendency for a direct relationship between the serum levels of ionized calcium and the degree of reduction in GFR; the patients with marked decreases in the serum concentrations of ionized calcium are those who have the lowest levels of GFR. Acidosis may increase the serum levels of ionized calcium, but the relative contribution of uremic acidosis to the values of ionized calcium in patients with renal failure is unknown. Occasionally, a sudden rise in blood pH produced by alkali therapy of a uremic acidotic patient may precipitate a seizure, presumably caused by a fall in the serum level of ionized calcium.

TABLE 77.6. Causes of Hypercalcemia in Patients with Chronic Renal Failure

Severe secondary hyperparathyroidism
Pure low turnover osteomalacia
High dietary calcium intake and/or supplementation
Use of high-calcium dialysate (<8.0 mg/dl)
Use of calcium-cycle ion exchange resin
Treatment with vitamin D or one of its metabolites
Administration of thiazide diuretics
Marked lowering of serum levels of phosphorus to <2.0 mg/dl
Immobilization
Coexistent disease causing hypercalcemia

Within 3 to 5 months after initiation of regular hemodialysis, predialysis concentration of serum calcium generally reaches levels between 9.0 and 10.0 mg/dl. Thus a rise in serum calcium occurs in patients with hypocalcemia, whereas little or no change is seen in those having initial levels within the normal range. This phenomenon occurs independently of the changes in serum phosphorus concentrations and despite the use of dialysate containing low calcium concentration.

To obtain a reliable measure of blood calcium in uremic patients undergoing hemodialysis, it is important that serum rather than plasma be obtained, and measurement should be made shortly after the samples are taken. Calcium levels in samples of stored serum and especially stored heparinized plasma may be spuriously low because of adsorption of calcium onto the tube or its loss in precipitates within the sample.

Hypercalcemia may be encountered in patients with CRF and in those treated with hemodialysis (Table 77.6). Spontaneous and persistent hypercalcemia is occasionally observed in patients with severe secondary hyperparathyroidism or after the initiation of hemodialysis. In the latter situation, transient hypercalcemia, which regresses spontaneously, may be noted more frequently. Persistent hypercalcemia has also been seen in dialysis patients who have pure low turnover osteomalacia without osteitis fibrosa and who have normal or undetectable serum levels of PTH; in these patients, the hypercalcemia may appear or worsen when they are given calcium supplement or vitamin D or are treated with dialysate containing a high calcium concentration. Patients with CRF may also develop hypercalcemia after the reduction of serum phosphorus with the use of phosphate-binding antacids, during the ingestion of large quantities of calcium carbonate, after the administration of calcium-cycle exchange resin or thiazide diuretics, and following treatment with vitamin D or one of its active metabolites [$25(OH)D_3$ or $1,25(OH)_2D_3$].

Serum Phosphorus

The concentrations of serum phosphorus during the fasting state are usually normal or lower than normal in the early stages of renal failure. Hyperphosphatemia becomes apparent when the GFR falls below 20 ml/min. Even at this degree of renal failure, many patients may have a normal or low serum phosphorus level. Many factors (Table 77.2) affect the serum concentration of phosphorus in patients with advanced renal failure and are responsible for the wide variations noted.

The levels of serum phosphorus decrease during dialysis secondary to its removal by the dialytic procedure. The dialysance of phosphorus is 25% to 35% of that of urea. Serum phosphorus concentration increases during the interdialytic period, the rapidity of the rise depending on the dietary intake of phosphorus, the adherence to therapy with phosphate-binding antacids, and the severity of secondary hyperparathyroidism.

Serum Magnesium

The concentration of serum magnesium is usually normal in patients with early renal failure, but hypermagnesemia is common in patients with advanced renal failure. The hypermagnesemia becomes apparent when the GFR falls below 30 ml/min. Abrupt increases in serum magnesium may occur when these patients consume magnesium-containing antacids or laxatives. It should be mentioned that hypomagnesemia has also been encountered in patients with advanced renal failure. The percentage of diffusible magnesium in the serum of the uremic patient is not different from that in normal subjects.

The concentration of serum magnesium in dialysis patients is determined by the concentration of dialysate magnesium and by the dietary intake of this ion. Magnesium readily crosses the dialysis membrane, and its movement depends on the gradient between the concentrations of diffusible magnesium in serum and that in dialysate. Patients treated with dialysate containing a low concentration of magnesium have lower predialysis serum magnesium levels than those treated with dialysate containing a higher concentration of magnesium.

Alkaline Phosphatase

Patients with advanced renal failure and those treated with hemodialysis may have normal, moderately elevated, or markedly increased serum levels of alkaline phosphatase. This enzyme is increased in skeletal conditions associated with enhanced osteoblastic activity. Patients with renal failure have osteomalacia and/or secondary hyperparathyroidism, both of which are associated with increased bone turnover rate; therefore it is not surprising that the serum levels of alkaline phosphatase are elevated in these patients. Indeed, the serum levels of alkaline phosphatase in a large number of dialysis patients correlate with osteoid surface covered with osteoblasts, osteoclastic resorption surface, number of osteoclasts, and percentage of osteoid seams labeled with tetracycline.

Although the serum levels of alkaline phosphatase are usually elevated in renal failure patients with osteitis fibrosa, osteomalacia, or mixed lesions, marked elevations are commonly seen in those with severe osteitis fibrosa. Measurements of the serum levels of alkaline phosphatase every 1 or 2 months can provide a useful guide to the progression of bone disease or to its healing during therapy with vitamin D.

It must be emphasized that because renal failure patients with significant bone disease may have normal serum levels of alkaline phosphatase, normal serum values of this enzyme should not be considered evidence for the absence of bone disease. Finally, alkaline phosphatase is also produced in the liver, intestine, kidney, and placenta, and disorders of these organs may also be associated with a rise in the serum levels of this enzyme. The skeletal origin of alkaline phosphatase can be determined only by the evaluation of its isoenzymes.

A monoclonal antibody specific for bone alkaline phosphatase (bAP) has been developed and is used in radioimmunologic and immunoenzymatic assays of bAP. Available data indicate that bAP is more sensitive that total alkaline phosphatase, osteocalcin, and osteonectin in the assessment of bone remodeling in patients with CRF. Indeed, in adult hemodialysis patients, values of bAP higher than 20 ng/ml are associated with histologic or biologic evidence of high bone turnover and bone disease due to secondary hyperparathyroidism, and these values exclude the presence of low or normal bone turnover.

Serum Osteocalcin

Serum osteocalcin (OC) is a noncollagenous (GLA) protein that contains γ-carboxy amino acids. The γ-carboxylation of the glutamic acid residues depends on vitamin K, which acts as a cofactor. The human form of OC contains 49 amino acids, and its production is under the control of $1,25(OH)_2D_3$.

OC is secreted by osteoblasts, incorporated into the matrix, and released from the matrix into the blood during bone resorption. Therefore its blood levels may reflect both bone formation and bone resorption (i.e., bone turnover).

In the blood, OC is present as intact molecule and as aminoterminal, carboxyterminal, and midregion fragments. In patients with renal failure, intact OC comprises about 30% of total OC in blood. OC is measured by immunoradiometric (IRMA) assay, which recognizes both the aminoterminal moities (i.e., intact and aminoterminal fragments) as well as the midregion fragments.

The blood levels of OC are higher in hemodialysis patients than in those treated with continuous ambulatory peritoneal dialysis. It is useful in differentiating patients with high turnover bone disease (osteitis fibrosa) from those with low turnover bone disease such as ABD; indeed, the blood levels of OC are many times higher in the former than in the latter groups of patients. In studies of hemodialysis patients in whom bone biopsies were obtained, a correlation between the blood levels of OC and parameters of bone turnover and peritrabecular fibrosis was found. The blood levels of the intact molecule or of the large aminoterminal fragment of OC provided greater reliability as a bone turnover marker.

Serum Hydroxyproline

Bone resorption is associated with degradation of bone collagen, which in turn results in the liberation of free hydroxyproline and peptides containing hydroxyproline. Both free and peptide-bound hydroxyprolines are excreted in the urine. The plasma and urinary concentrations of free hydroxyproline reflect the ingestion of foods containing hydroxyproline and the rate of collagen degradation.

In patients with advanced renal failure, the serum levels of both free and peptide-bound hydroxyproline are elevated because of increased bone resorption and decreased renal excretion. The normal plasma levels of free hydroxyproline range between 0.12 and 0.26 mg/dl, whereas the values in uremic patients range from 0.25 to 4.0 mg/dl. It has been suggested that the serum levels of hydroxyproline can provide an index for assessing the extent of bone resorption and for evaluating the effectiveness of therapy. The serum levels of hydroxyproline usually fall in association with healing of osteitis fibrosa after subtotal parathyroidectomy or after therapy with $1,25(OH)_2D_3$. Because some of the free and peptide-bound hydroxyprolines may be lost in dialysate, blood samples for their measurement should be obtained before dialysis.

Other collagen breakdown products (pyridinolines and deoxypyridinolines) are detected in the blood of CRF patients and those treated with dialysis. The blood levels of these compounds, like hydroxyproline, reflect bone resorption.

Other compounds that are released into the circulation during bone resorption are tartarate-resistant acid phosphatase and type I collagen cross-linked telopeptide.

Serum Parathyroid Hormone

As indicated earlier in this chapter, the serum levels of PTH in patients with renal insufficiency are elevated. The rise in the serum concentration of PTH occurs early in the course of renal failure and becomes more marked as renal failure progresses. There is marked variation in the serum concentrations of PTH in patients with advanced renal failure and in those treated with hemodialysis; the levels may be 2 to 200 times normal. Low or undetectable levels of PTH may be encountered in patients with advanced renal failure who are hypomagnesemic and magnesium deficient, those who have low turnover osteomalacia, and those who have primary hypoparathyroidism and aluminum. Patients with diabetes mellitus and renal failure may have lower levels of PTH than those with renal failure resulting from other causes. The serum levels of PTH in the dialysis patient may be affected by the concentration of calcium in dialysate; patients treated with high-dialysate calcium may have lower serum levels of PTH than those treated with lower-dialysate calcium.

Most of the PTH in the serum of the renal failure patient is made up of the C-terminal fragments and midregion of the C-terminal fragment. Therefore assays using an antibody directed toward this moiety of PTH yield high values; in contrast, the use of an antibody to the N-terminal fragment may reveal a modest elevation in the serum levels of PTH. Two other sensitive assays for intact PTH have been developed. These are the IRMA and the chemiluminescence assay. These assays use saturation kinetics and two region-specific antibodies. A very good correlation ($r = 0.93$) was obtained between the results of these two assays in a population of 104 patients treated with hemodialysis. These assays provide the best correlation with secondary hyperparathyroidism, enhanced bone resorption, and high turnover bone disease. Indeed, serum levels of PTH greater than 450 pg/ml (IRMA assay) have a 100% predictive value for enhanced bone resorption and high turnover bone disease. In contrast, serum levels of less than 65 pg/ml in the absence of conditions that are associated with low serum levels of PTH are seen in patients with ABD.

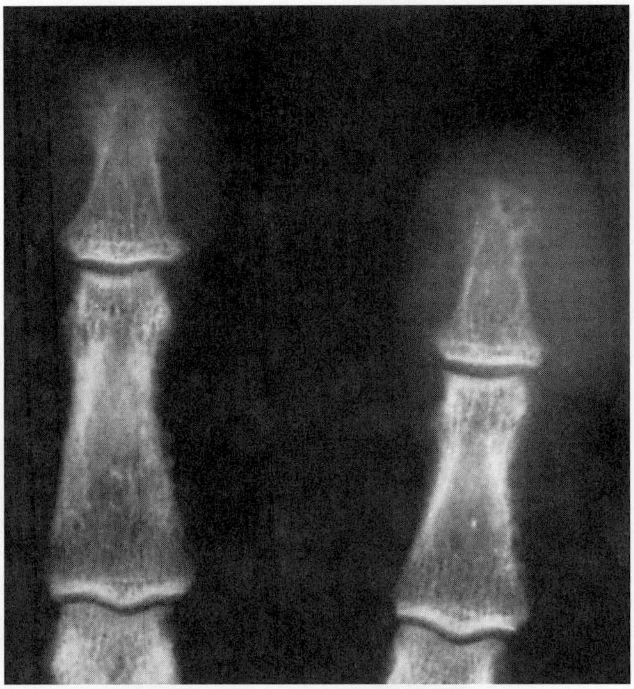

Figure 77.2. Subperiosteal resorption predominantly affecting radial borders of the second and third digits of the left hand in a uremic patient about to start treatment with hemodialysis. (Reproduced with permission from Massry SG, Coburn JW. Divalent ion metabolism and renal osteodystrophy. In: Massry SG, Sellers AL, eds: *Clinical aspects of uremia and dialysis.* Springfield, IL: Charles C. Thomas, 1976:304–387.)

LABORATORY FINDINGS OF BONE DISEASE

Radiographic Findings in Bone

There is a wide variation in the reported incidence of radiographic abnormalities in the skeleton of patients with advanced renal failure. Several factors may contribute to this variability: the method of evaluation, the level of interest of the radiologist reviewing the x-ray films, the type of x-ray film used, the nature of the patient population studied, and the type of therapy used. The use of fine-grain industrial x-ray film, prolonged exposure, and magnification techniques increase greatly the yield of detection of skeletal abnormalities. The major radiographic findings in the bone of renal failure patients are those produced by secondary hyperparathyroidism. Evidence for osteomalacia may also be encountered.

Secondary Hyperparathyroidism

The radiographic features of secondary hyperparathyroidism in renal failure include endosteal, intracortical, and subperiosteal resorption; erosion of tufts of terminal phalanx; cyst formation; periosteal neoostosis; and osteosclerosis. The radiographic abnormalities of secondary hyperparathyroidism are seen in about 50% of the patients with renal failure who almost always have increased bone resorption by bone biopsy.

Subperiosteal bone resorption is probably the most readily recognizable radiographic feature of secondary hyperparathyroidism. Such erosions are most commonly seen in the phalanges of the hand (Figs. 77.2 and 77.3) and are

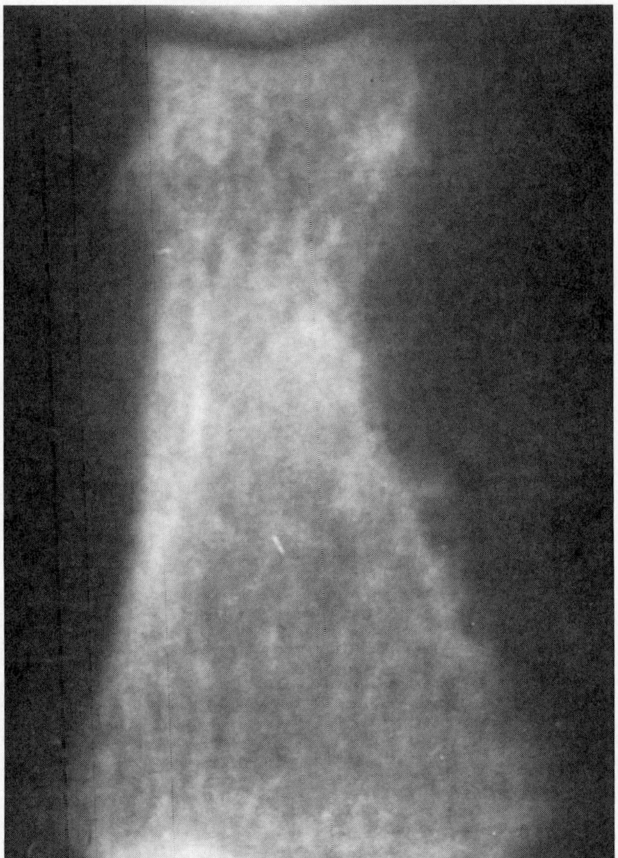

Figure 77.3. Magnification of the radiograph of the middle phalanx of the second digit of the same patient shown in Fig. 77.2.

observed in the pelvis (Fig. 77.4), the distal end of the clavicles (Figs. 77.5 and 77.6), and the inferior surface of ribs, femur, ulna, tibia (Fig. 77.7), and mandible (Fig. 77.8). The earliest change in the phalanges is haziness and irregularity of the borders, followed by disruption of the contour lines of the periosteum and subsequently by the appearance of scalloped erosions. These changes are initially noticed near the proximal and distal ends of the phalanges and on the medial surface of the middle phalanx of the second or third digit of the dominant hand. The lesions then progress to other phalanges and may appear on their ulnar borders as well. Resorption of the phalanges is less common in children. Erosion of the tuft of the terminal phalanx of the second or third finger is commonly noted, but lesions may occur in the tufts of the other fingers as well (Fig. 77.9). Severe erosion of the tuft may result in collapse of soft tissues, giving the appearance of clubbing of the finger. In the long bones, such as the tibia and femur, subperiosteal resorption usually appears at the outer

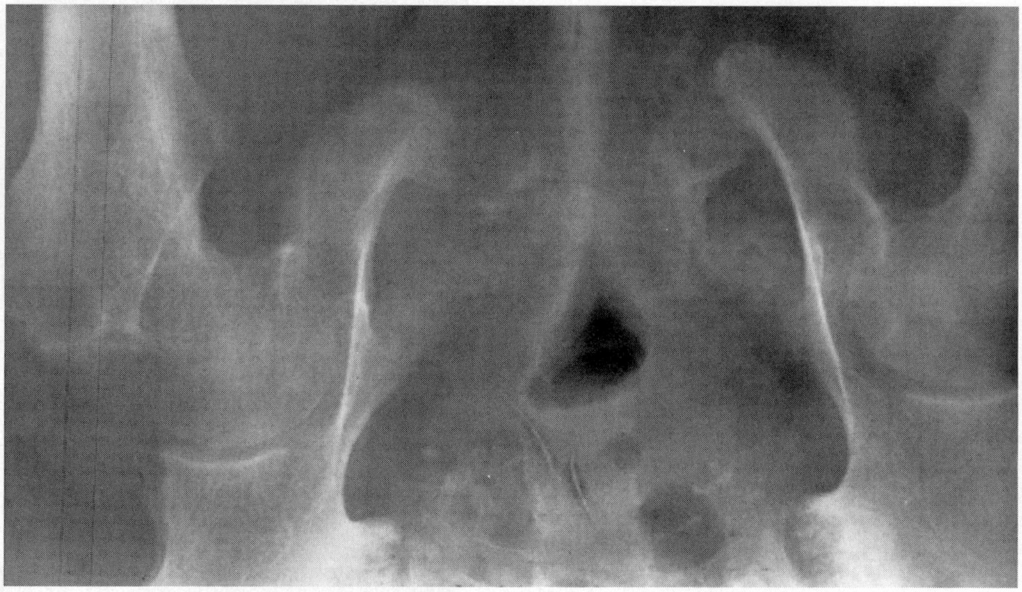

Figure 77.4. Resorption of the pubic rami in a patient with advanced renal failure before initiation of hemodialysis therapy.

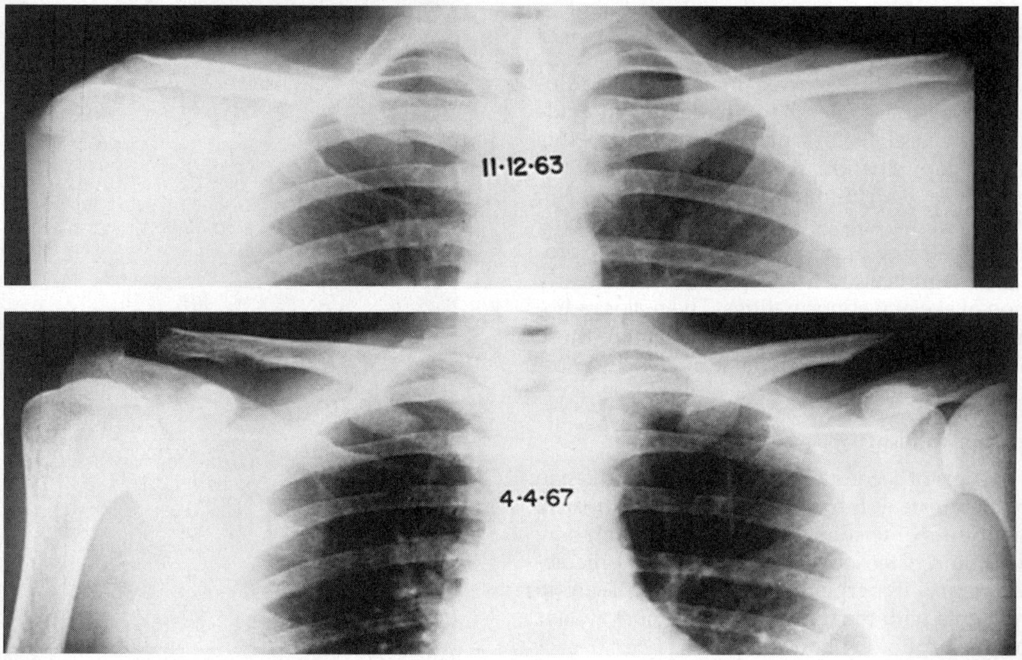

Figure 77.5. The development of severe resorption of the distal ends of the clavicles over a period of 3½ years in a patient with advanced renal failure. (Reproduced with permission from Massry SG, Coburn JW, Popovtzer MM, et al. Secondary hyperparathyroidism in chronic renal failure. *Arch Intern Med* 1969;124:431.)

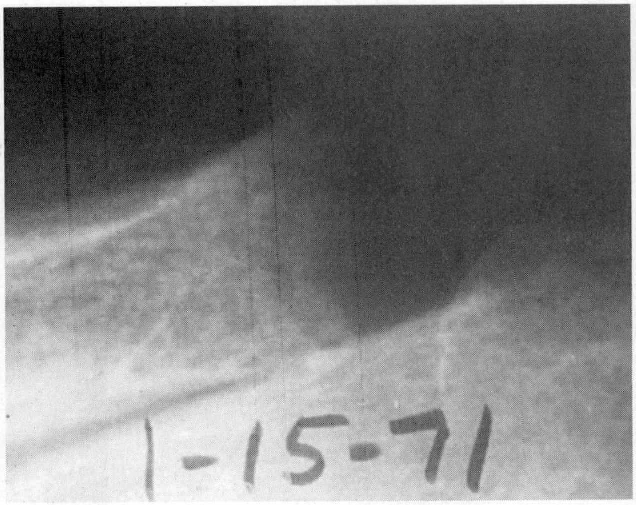

Figure 77.6. Magnification of a radiograph of the latter end of the clavicle, depicting bone resorption in a patient with advanced renal failure.

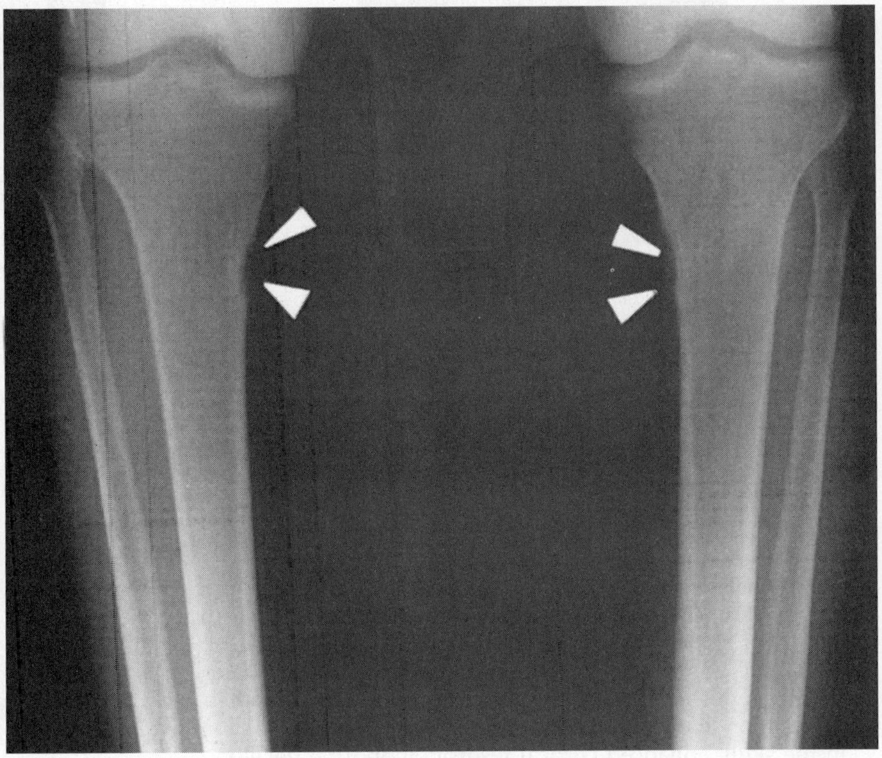

Figure 77.7. Subperiosteal bone resorption of the upper ends of both tibias in a patient with advanced renal failure.

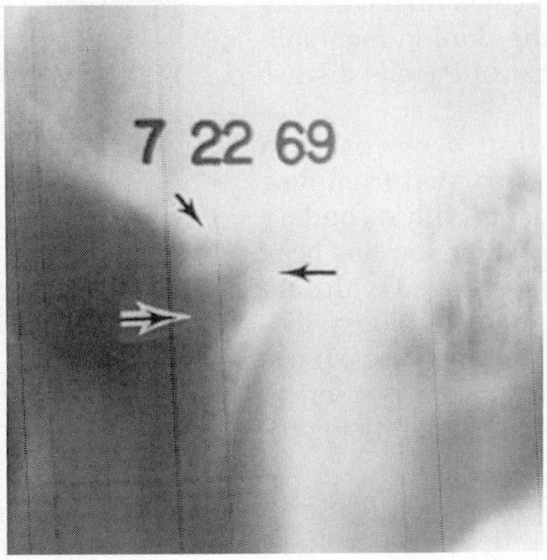

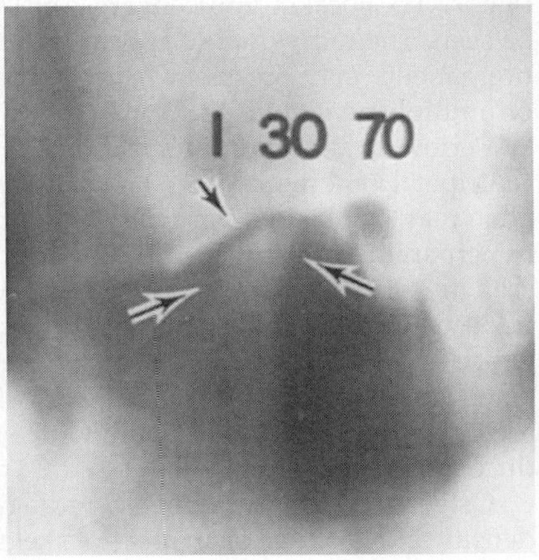

Figure 77.8. *Left:* Total dissolution of the head of the left mandible in a dialysis patient. *Right:* Three months after subtotal parathyroidectomy, extensive reformation of the head of the left mandible occurred. *Arrows* point to the lesion. (Reproduced with permission from Sellers AL, Winfield AC, Massry SG. Resorption of condyloid process of the mandible. *Arch Intern Med* 1973;131:727.)

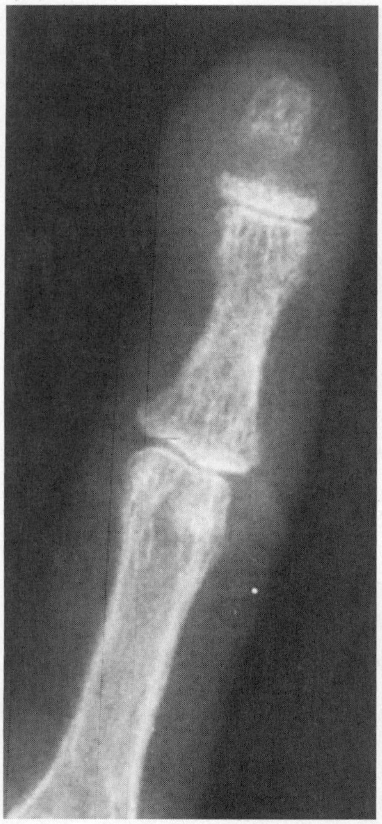

Figure 77.9. Resorption of the luft of the terminal phalanx in a patient with advanced renal failure.

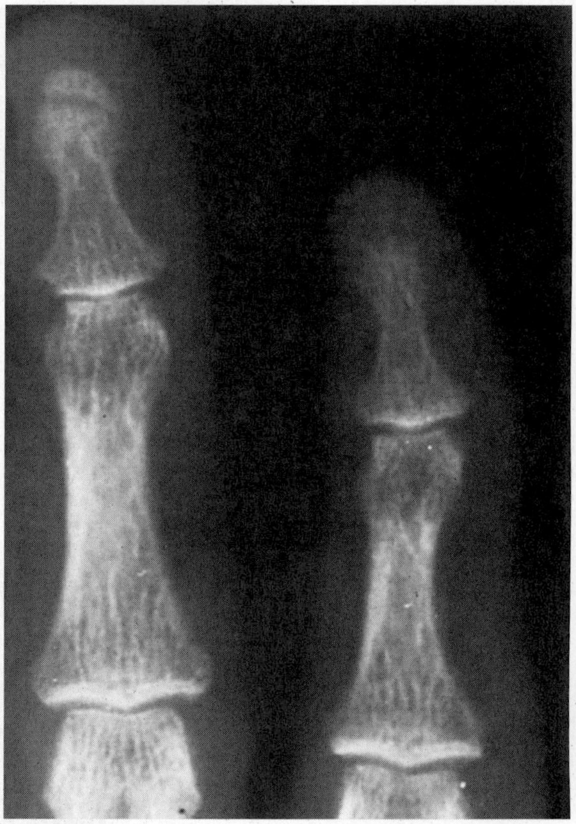

Figure 77.10. Coarse striation, endosteal resorption, subperiosteal resorption, and resorption of the tuft of the terminal phalanx in a patient with advanced renal failure.

circumference of the metaphysis (Fig. 77.7). This occurs because there is normally an active collar of osteoclasts that act to reduce the diameter of the epiphyseal growth plate to that of the shaft of the bone. The radiographic areas of subperiosteal bone resorption may represent active osteoclastic process or may reflect radiolucent osteoid filling previously resorbed areas of bone.

In the phalanges and in the long bones, enhanced bone resorption within the haversian canals and along the endosteal surface gives rise to exaggerated striation and to scalloping of the endosteal border on x-ray examination (Fig. 77.10). In our experience, endosteal bone resorption is noted earlier and is more common than subperiosteal bone resorption.

In the skull, enhanced cortical resorption and the development of areas of increased trabecular density give rise to granularity and a mottled appearance (the "salt and pepper" skull) (Fig. 77.11). Focal radiolucent areas of 1 to 3 cm in diameter may be seen. The radiographic appearance of the skull in renal failure patients may occasionally resemble that of Paget's disease or multiple myeloma.

Periosteal new bone formation (periosteal neostosis) of a centripetal type with periosteum initially separated from new bone may be observed in renal failure patients with secondary hyperparathyroidism (Fig. 77.12). This phenomenon has been seen in 8 of 117 patients surveyed and was associated with subperiosteal resorption of the phalanges and bone biopsy evidence of osteitis fibrosa and osteoid excess in most cases. It has been proposed that periosteal neostosis is a manifestation of secondary hyperparathyroidism with a sustained ability to produce mineralized bone.

Osteosclerosis is recognized radiographically by increased density and is observed in areas of skeleton where cancellous or trabecular bone predominates over cortical bone. These areas

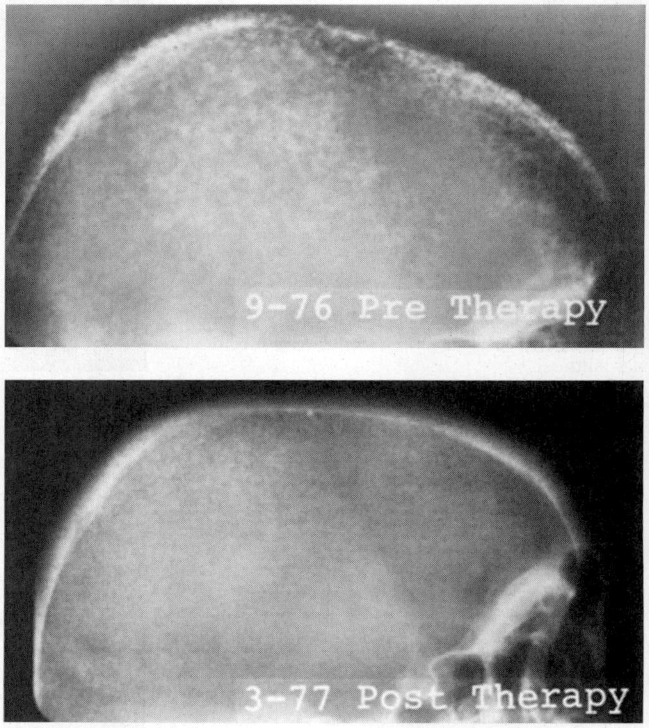

Figure 77.11. *Top:* Radiograph of the skull of a patient treated with hemodialysis for 8 years. Note the bone resorption, the mottling, and the salt and pepper appearance of the skull. *Bottom:* Radiograph of the skull of the same patient following therapy with $1,25(OH)_2D_3$ for 6 months. Note the marked improvement. (Reproduced with permission from Goldstein DA, Malluche HH, Massry SG. Management of renal osteodystrophy with $1,25(OH)_2D_3$. *Miner Electrolyte Metab* 1979;2:35.)

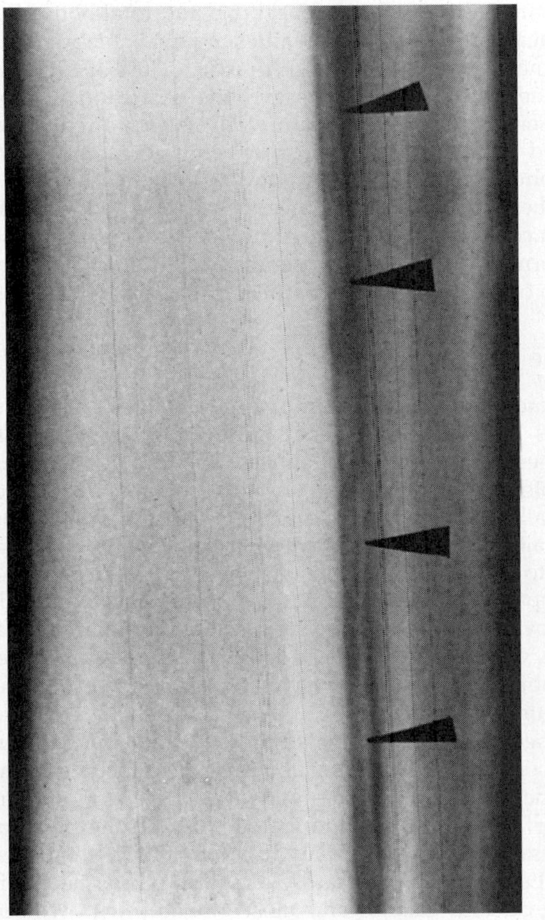

Figure 77.12. Periosteal new bone formation (periosteal neostasis) in the tibia of a patient treated with hemodialysis. (Reproduced with permission from Massry SG, Coburn JW. Divalent ion metabolism and renal osteodystrophy. In: Massry SG, Sellers AL, eds. *Clinical aspects of uremia and dialysis* Springfield, IL: Charles C. Thomas, 1976:304–387.)

include vertebral bodies, pelvis, ribs, clavicles, and the metaphyses of various long bones. In the vertebral bodies, where osteosclerosis is most often evident on x-ray examination, dense sclerotic bands are evident along the upper and lower borders of the body, with radiolucency of the central portion ("rugger jersey" appearance). Cystic lesions of the skeleton (Figs. 77.13 and 77.14) and brown tumors are seen in patients with renal failure. Erosion of lamina dura is less common in secondary than in primary hyperparathyroidism.

Osteomalacia

The diagnosis of osteomalacia should be made by bone biopsy. The only pathognomonic radiographic finding of osteomalacia is Looser's zones or pseudofracture. These are linear radiolucent bands, usually observed at right angles to the surface of the bone and seen in pubic rami, the inferior angle of the scapula, the lower ribs, and the metatarsal shafts. They represent areas of unmineralized woven bone and may occur in areas of mechanical stress or at sites of entry of nutrient vessels. Looser's zones are usually not a common finding in patients with renal failure, although they have been reported in high frequency in Australia. The most consistent but nondiagnostic x-ray feature of osteomalacia is decreased density of bone. Defective mineralization in children with renal failure leads to radiographic abnormalities that are typical of rickets; widening of the epiphyseal growth plate and bone deformities occur.

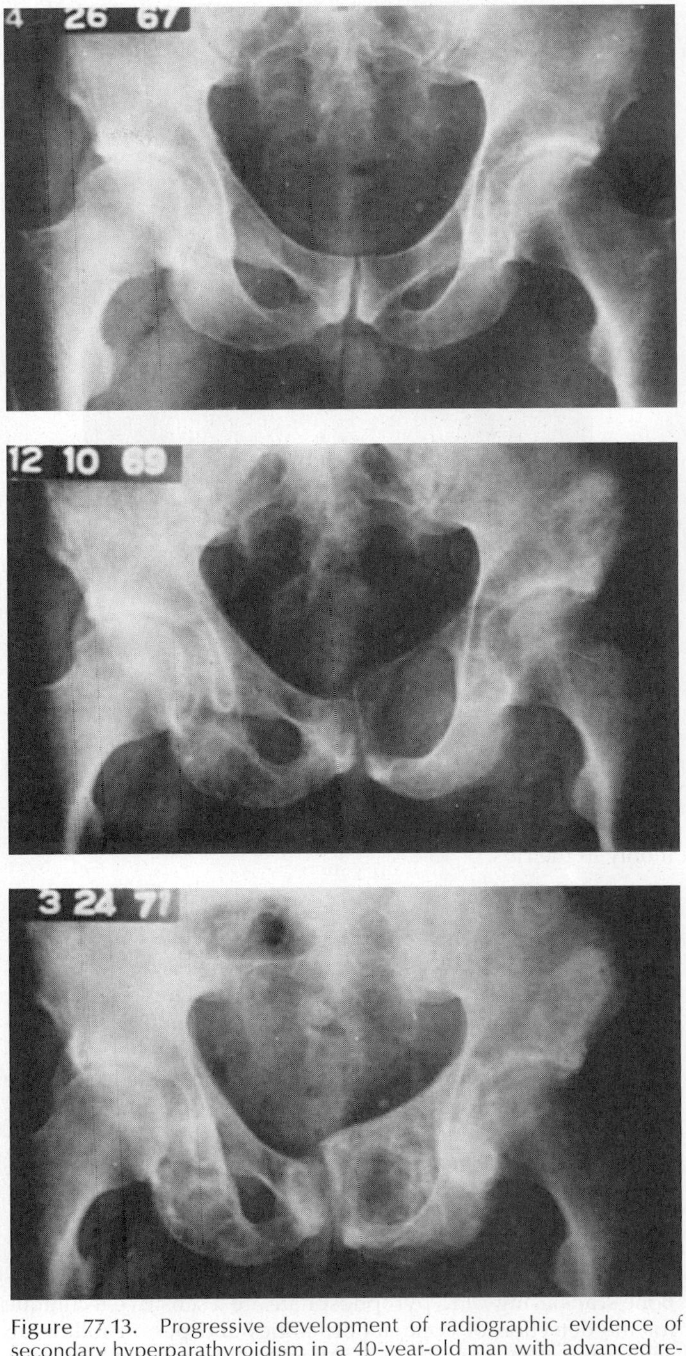

Figure 77.13. Progressive development of radiographic evidence of secondary hyperparathyroidism in a 40-year-old man with advanced renal failure. Note the disappearance of the left ischium and cystic areas of the right pubic ramus (12/10/69). Treatment with hemodialysis was begun in November 1970, and subtotal parathyroidectomy was performed in December 1970. This was followed by remineralization of the left ischium, but the cystic changes of the pubic ramus persisted (3/24/71). (Reproduced with permission from Massry SG, Caburn JW. Divalent ion metabolism and renal osteodystrophy. In: Massry SG, Sellers AL, eds: *Clinical aspects of uremia and dialysis*. Springfield, IL: Charles C. Thomas, 1976:304–387.)

Osteopenia

The term *osteopenia* denotes decreased density of bone seen by x-ray examination. Osteopenia is a common finding in patients with longstanding renal failure and those treated with hemodialysis. Osteomalacia, secondary hyperparathyroidism, and osteoporosis can each lead to decreased density of bone on radiographs, and it is difficult to determine the cause of osteopenia by x-ray characteristics alone. Fractures occur occasionally

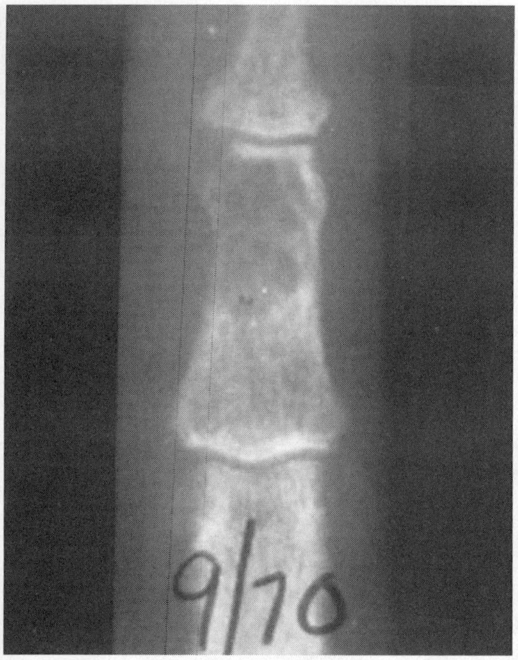

Figure 77.14. Cystic formations in the second phalanx of a digit of a patient with advanced renal failure. This is a manifestation of secondary hyperparathyroidism.

in patients with renal osteodystrophy and are seen most commonly in the ribs.

Effect of Hemodialysis

The reported incidence of radiographic evidence of bone disease in 524 hemodialysis patients treated for 3 to 108 months with dialysate containing 4.6 to 8.0 mg of calcium per deciliter of dialysate was 6% to 66%. Available data from the 1970s indicate that prolonged treatment with maintenance hemodialysis is associated with worsening of radiographic evidence of bone disease in most patients, irrespective of the calcium concentration in dialysate. Adequate control of the serum levels of phosphorus within the normal range and the use of $1,25(OH)_2D_3$ may possibly ameliorate or reverse this trend.

Skeletal Scintigraphy

Bone scans using ^{99m}Tc-pyrophosphate are a sensitive technique for the detection of bone abnormalities and permit follow-up evaluation of therapy. The pyrophosphate accumulates in areas of increased bone turnover; thus this technique could be useful in the diagnosis and follow-up of bone resorption. In contrast, diffuse reduction of pyrophosphate uptake is seen in renal failure patients with aluminum bone disease. Others, however, were unable to differentiate between aluminum bone disease and osteitis fibrosa with bone scintigraphy. Pseudofractures of ribs and other bones due to osteomalacia could also be detected by this technique. Positive bone scans may be obtained before the appearance of radiographic evidence of bone disease. It should be emphasized that bone scintigraphy does not provide adequate information on the type and severity of bone disease in renal failure patients. Therefore bone biopsy remains the gold standard for the evaluation of bone disease in these patients.

Bone Mineral Content

Several techniques are available for the measurement of bone mineral content. They include (a) metacarpal index, which is the ratio between the cortical bone and total bone width of a metacarpal bone (normal values are available for the second left metacarpal; it is reduced in 20% to 40% of CRF and those treated with hemodialysis and the reduction in this index worsens with the duration of dialysis); (b) quantitative computed tomography; (c) positron emission tomography; and (d) photon absorptiometry.

These techniques may assess changes in bone mass or calcium content but do not determine the underlying cause of the abnormality. They can be useful as guides for follow-up evaluation of the response to a particular therapy.

Bone Histology

Histologic evidence of abnormalities in bone is apparent in patients with moderate renal failure, and bone disease progresses as renal failure advances. The finding of normal bone histology in patients with chronic uremia is uncommon. The overall incidence of bone disease in patients with advanced renal failure and those treated with maintenance hemodialysis is 90% to 100%. These patients display evidence of enhanced bone resorption, bone marrow fibrosis, osteomalacia (including low turnover osteomalacia induced by aluminum accumulation in bone, Chapter 68, Part 2), and osteosclerosis. A high degree of variability exists, and any given type of lesion may be more severe or more prevalent.

Specific conditions related to hemodialysis therapy may affect bone structure and metabolism. These include calcium and magnesium content of dialysate, use of heparin, impurities of water and the use of fluoridated water in the preparation of dialysate, and adequacy and duration of the hemodialysis therapy. Low-calcium dialysate (5.0 mg/dl) is associated with negative calcium balance and most probably with worsening of secondary hyperparathyroidism. However, the use of a higher calcium concentration (6.0 to 7.0 mg/dl) does not prevent secondary hyperparathyroidism or bone disease. High-magnesium dialysate may result in increased bone magnesium, and such an event may not be desirable.

Both clinical and experimental studies indicate that heparin given repeatedly may cause decreased mineralization of bone and predispose to fractures. In patients receiving 15,000 to 30,000 U of heparin daily for long periods, osteoporosis, multiple fractures, and pseudoarthrosis have been observed. Because dialysis cannot be performed without the use of heparin, it is impossible to know whether heparin administration plays a role in the pathogenesis of dialysis-related bone disease. With the use of more efficient dialyzers and shorter periods of dialysis, the quantity of heparin needed is less, and hence any potential deleterious effects on the skeleton are reduced.

The use of fluoridated water in the preparation of dialysate has been reported by some to cause worsening of bone disease, but others failed to confirm such a deleterious effect. It is our opinion that fluoridated water should not be used; in communities in which water is fluoridated, purification of the water with a method capable of removing fluoride (reverse osmosis) should be used. Impurities in water used for the preparation of dialysate may produce severe bone disease. Indeed, in Newcastle upon Tyne, England, and Charlottesville, Virginia, a remarkably high incidence of bone disease in dialysis patients was present, and bone disease decreased significantly after the introduction of water purification. It was later found that aluminum was the culprit in the water in Newcastle upon Tyne.

Aluminum accumulation in bone may be associated with a specific type of bone lesion called *pure low turnover osteomalacia.* It is characterized by accumulation of osteoid exclusively of the lamellar type, minimal osteoid–osteoclast interface, reduced tetracycline uptake, no evidence of current enhanced bone resorption, and no endosteal fibrosis. The serum levels of PTH are low or undetectable. This lesion is seen almost exclusively in dialysis patients but has also been noted in a patient before dialysis therapy. Its exact incidence is not known. This is discussed in detail in Chapter 68, Part 2.

Certain data in the literature and our own experience permit evaluation of the effect of duration of hemodialysis on various indices of bone. *Bone mass* is not affected by hemodialysis, and it seems that loss of bone is not a common consequence of hemodialysis. *Osteoid volume* and fraction of mineralizing osteoid seams are not affected by duration of dialysis; this observation would suggest that defective mineralization of bone does not necessarily worsen with dialysis, and the severity of the abnormality after years of hemodialysis in any particular patient may not be different from the degree of the derangement at the time therapy was initiated. The *osteoid–osteoblast* interface increases significantly with the duration of dialysis; this is consistent with the interpretation that the amount of bone matrix produced by each osteoblast is reduced, dictating the need for an increased number of osteoblasts if bone mass is to be maintained. Alternatively, the increase in the number of osteoblasts may represent a response to the increase in the number of osteoclasts.

Parameters of hyperparathyroid bone disease, including surface density of osteoclasts (bone resorption), accumulation of woven osteoid, and endosteal fibrosis, display a significant increment with the duration of dialysis. However, it is difficult to attribute these changes to duration of dialysis per se because these parameters correlated well with the serum levels of PTH. Thus the worsening of the state of secondary hyperparathyroidism after long-term therapy with hemodialysis appears to be responsible for the worsening of the histopathologic changes. These observations are consistent with the radiographic evidence of worsening of bone resorption with hemodialysis. It is possible that the introduction of $1,25(OH)_2D_3$ in the management of these patients would reverse this worsening trend in osteitis fibrosa.

The indications and techniques for bone biopsy and its value in the evaluation of bone disease in patients with renal failure are discussed in detail in Chapter 98.

CLINICAL FEATURES

Patients with advanced renal failure display a variety of signs and symptoms related to the disturbances in divalent ion metabolism (Table 77.7).

Pruritus

Itching is common in patients with advanced renal failure, but it generally improves or disappears with adequate treatment with hemodialysis. However, pruritus may persist despite dialysis, and itching may be of such intensity that it prevents sleep and interferes with normal activities. This type of pruritus is common in patients with marked secondary hyperparathyroidism and usually disappears within 48 hours to 7 days after subtotal parathyroidectomy. This procedure is now recommended for the management of severe pruritus that does not respond to adequate maintenance dialysis and is associated with markedly high serum levels of PTH. In some uremic patients, itching may be relieved by treatment with lidocaine or ultraviolet light.

The mechanisms responsible for such pruritus remain unknown. Elevated levels of calcium in the skin were observed in these patients, but it is unlikely that the increase in skin calcium is primarily responsible. Itching improves within a few days after subtotal parathyroidectomy, but skin calcium requires a much longer time to decrease. Excess serum levels of PTH also affect the function of both the central and peripheral nervous systems and as such may alter the threshold for sensation, causing itching in some patients in response to stimuli that do not elicit pruritic sensation in others. Most uremic patients with pruritus were found to have levels of serum calcium above 9.5 mg/dl, and the levels of calcium in blood or extracellular fluid probably predispose to itching. This postulate is supported by the observation that pruritus may reappear after subtotal parathyroidectomy when hypercalcemia develops following vitamin D therapy or during calcium infusion.

Some investigators found that the plasma levels of histamine are markedly elevated in patients with renal failure who suffer from pruritus. Because histamine is a potent inducer of pruritus, it was suggested that elevated levels of plasma histamine may play a role in the genesis of uremic pruritus. Support for this proposal was provided by the observation that treatment with human recombinant erythropoietin was associated with a reduction in plasma histamine and improvement in pruritus in patients with CRF. This effect was independent of the changes in the level of hematocrit.

TABLE 77.7. Clinical Signs and Symptoms Related to Disturbances in Divalent Ion Metabolism

Uremic symptoms caused by excess parathyroid hormone (Chapter 68, Part 1)
Myopathy and proximal muscle weakness (Chapter 78)
Pruritus
Arthritis and periarthritis (Chapter 79)
Bone pain and fractures
Spontaneous tendon rupture
Growth retardation
Skeletal deformities
Soft tissue necrosis (calciphylaxis)
Soft tissue calcification

SPONTANEOUS TENDON RUPTURE

The state of secondary hyperparathyroidism in uremia is most likely responsible for spontaneous tendon rupture because this complication has also been noted in patients with other causes of secondary hyperparathyroidism and in those with primary hyperparathyroidism. Other possible causes include abnormal collagen synthesis secondary to vitamin D deficiency or chronic metabolic acidosis, which may cause elastosis of the tendons. Microfractures in the bone at the site of tendon insertion may be a contributor to the pathogenesis of tendon rupture.

The spontaneous tendon rupture may develop in the quadriceps, triceps, or Achilles tendons or in the extensor tendons of the fingers. The rupture of the quadriceps tendons may occur during walking, stumbling, or descending the stairs. The patient experiences pain and is unable to extend the leg, and a palpable gap and ecchymosis is encountered above the tendon. This complication can be satisfactorily corrected by surgery, but recovery is slow.

Bone Pain and Fractures

Bone pain is not uncommon. Patients with osteitis fibrosa or osteomalacia may develop skeletal pain, which may progress, making the patient totally disabled. The pain is often described as a vague, deep ache aggravated by pressure, sudden movement, or weight bearing. The pain may be located in the low back, hips, legs, or knees. Occasionally, the pain is sudden and is localized around the knees or ankles, suggesting acute arthritis, tendonitis, or synovitis. Physical findings are often absent. Pain in the chest area may be the initial symptom of a rib fracture, and low back pain may be due to a compression fracture of a vertebral body. Fractures are more common in patients with marked osteopenia and in those with low turnover osteomalacia.

Bone Deformities

Skeletal deformities can occur in uremic children and adults. Children may develop bone deformities as a result of vitamin D deficiency (rickets) or secondary hyperparathyroidism (slipped epiphysis). The deformities of rickets result in bowing of the long bones, which occurs early in childhood and becomes more severe at adolescence. Slipped epiphysis is seen more commonly in children with longstanding renal failure. This complication most commonly affects the hip and usually appears during preadolescence. Pain may be present or absent, and a limp is almost always present. Slipped epiphysis may also affect the radius, ulna, lower humerus, lower femur, and lower tibia. Local swelling and ulnar deviation develop when the radius and ulna are involved.

Skeletal deformity in adults is seen most commonly in those who have severe osteomalacia. The patient may develop lumbar scoliosis, thoracic kyphosis, and deformities of the thoracic cage. Compression fractures of several vertebral bodies result in loss of height.

Growth Retardation

Most children with advanced renal failure have reduced heights, and hemodialysis does not produce marked improvement in growth velocity. Malnutrition, vitamin D deficiency, anemia, chronic metabolic acidosis, defective intestinal absorption of calcium, bone disease, low blood levels of somatomedin, and resistance to the action of growth hormone may all contribute to growth retardation in children. Initial reports showed that treatment with $1,25(OH)_2D_3$ has produced improvement and even "catch-up" growth in many children; however, subsequent studies did not confirm these observations. The use of recombinant growth hormone in prepubertal children with CRF increased growth velocity.

Skin Ulcerations and Tissue Necrosis

An unusual syndrome, characterized by the development of progressive ischemic skin ulcerations involving the fingers, toes, thighs, legs, and ankles has been observed in a small number of patients with advanced renal failure (Figs. 77.15 and 77.16). This syndrome occurs in patients after successful renal transplantation, in those treated with hemodialysis, and less frequently, in patients with advanced renal failure. It appears that this entity is less common among patients treated with continuous ambulatory peritoneal dialysis.

The patients almost always have vascular calcification involving the media of the arteries, and they usually exhibit x-ray evidence of subperiosteal bone resorption. Serum calcium is usually normal and occasionally elevated. A period of hyperphosphatemia has been present for some time before the appearance of the syndrome. The lesions may be preceded or accompanied by severe pain. Before the appearance of the ulcer or the tissue necrosis, tender, slightly erythematous, subcutaneous nodules may develop, or there may be blotchy, bluish discoloration. Raynaud's phenomenon may also precede the lesions of the fingers or toes. The ulcers may develop slowly over several months, or skin and muscle necrosis may appear and progress rapidly over a few weeks. Infection may supervene, leading to sepsis and death. In one renal transplant recipient, the gangrenous skin lesions of the trunk and thighs were associated with painful proximal myopathy and ischemic perforation of the small bowel. Histologic examination of the lesions of the skin and soft tissues revealed calcification of the media of arteries and arterioles (Fig. 77.17), thrombosis of both arteries and veins, and varying degrees of ischemic necrosis. The original reports of this entity assigned the name of *calciphylaxis* because of an apparent similarity to the calciphylaxis described by Seyle in 1962. Other investigators have argued that the name should be changed to *calcific uremic arteriolopathy.*

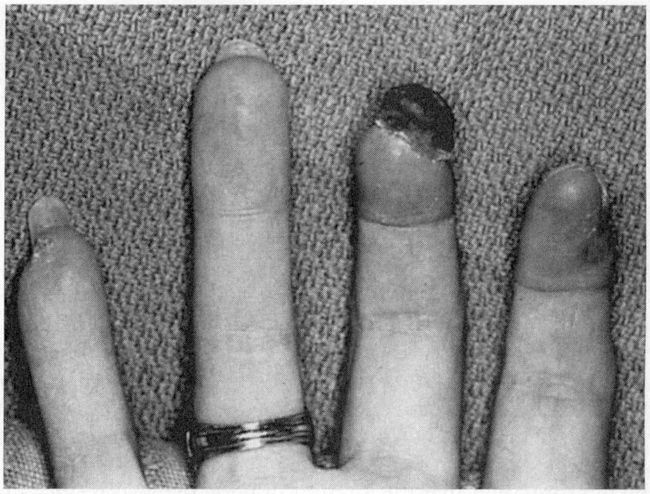

Figure 77.15. Ischemic lesions of the second, third, and fifth digits of the right hand of a uremic patient. The second and fifth digits show mottling and bluish discoloration, while the third digit has marked ischemic necrosis. Following subtotal parathyroidectomy, there was complete healing of the lesions. (Reproduced with permission from Massry SG, Coburn JW. Divalent ion metabolism and renal osteodystrophy. In: Massry SG, Sellers AL, eds: *Clinical aspects of uremia and dialysis.* Springfield, IL: Charles C. Thomas, 1976:304–387.)

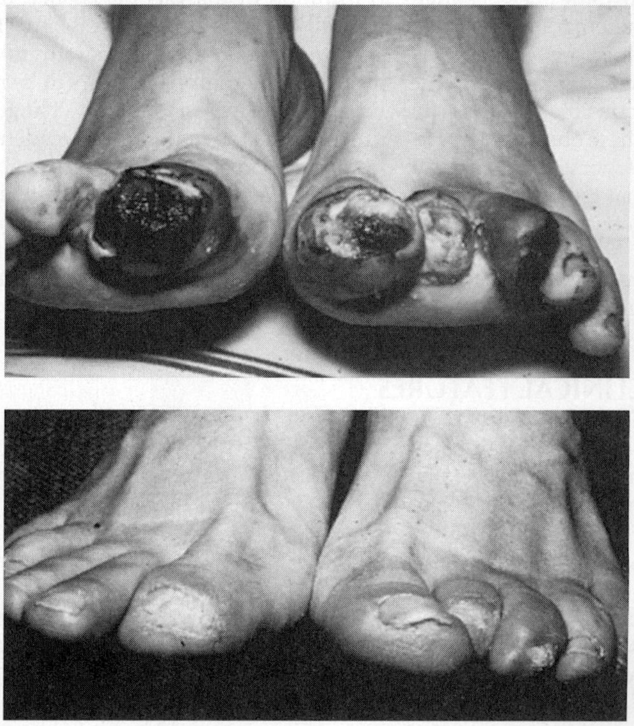

Figure 77.16. *Top:* Necrosis of the toes in a patient with severe hyperparathyroidism that developed after successful renal transplant. *Bottom:* Healing of all the necrotic lesions 3 to 4 months after subtotal parathyroidectomy. (Reproduced with permission from Massry SG, Coburn JW, Popovtzer MM, et al. Secondary hyperparathyroidism in chronic renal failure. *Arch Intern Med* 1969;124:431.)

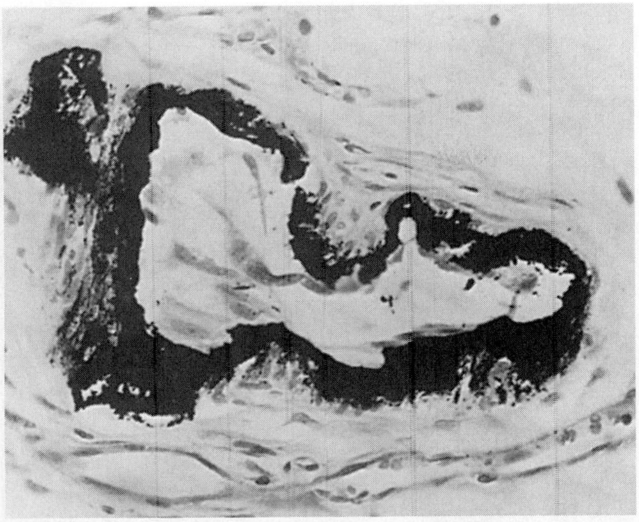

Figure 77.17. Dense medial calcification of a subcutaneous artery seen in a skin biopsy specimen obtained from the toe lesions of the patient in Fig. 77.16. von Kossa stain, ×400. (Reproduced with permission from Massry SG, Gordon A, Caburn JW, et al. Vascular calcification and peripheral necrosis in a renal transplant recipient. *Am J Med* 1970;49:416.)

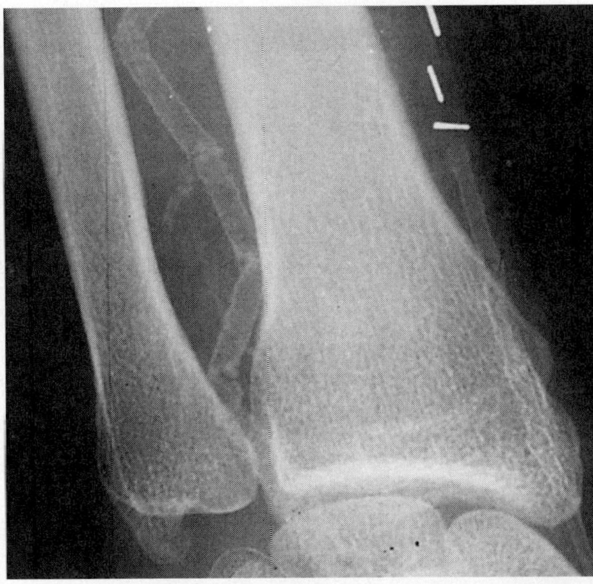

Figure 77.18. Calcification of the media of the radial and ulnar arteries of a 46-year-old woman treated with hemodialysis for 2 years. The metal clips mark the site of earlier surgery for vascular access. (Reproduced with permission from Massry SG, Caburn JW. Divalent ion metabolism and renal osteodystrophy. In: Massry SG, Sellers AL, eds: *Clinical aspects of uremia and dialysis.* Springfield, IL: Charles C. Thomas, 1976:304–387.)

This complication of advanced renal failure could be life-threatening and requires aggressive therapeutic attention. The lesions do not respond to treatment with local measures but have healed following subtotal parathyroidectomy in most patients. In some patients, the lesions did not heal after parathyroidectomy, and in others, the lesions were aggravated. However, we recommend this procedure for any patients who develop these lesions if other therapies do not heal the lesions, if the patients have severe secondary hyperparathyroidism, and if no other cause for this entity is found.

Although disturbances in divalent ion metabolism, secondary hyperparathyroidism, and vascular calcification appear to play an important role in the genesis of this entity, other factors may also contribute to its emergence and progression. Acquired protein C deficiency has been reported in patients with CRF, and such a derangement may lead to a hypercoagulability state and consequently to vascular occlusion and tissue necrosis. Therefore it is important that the blood levels and the activity of protein C be measured in patients with calciphylaxis. It is interesting that obesity, especially in white women, predisposes to calciphylaxis, and the relative risk for calciphylaxis rises with weight increase. Local trauma may be a contributory factor as to site where the lesion may appear; indeed, in some patients, the necrotic lesions began in areas where insulin, heparin, or iron dextran were injected.

Soft Tissue Calcification

Soft tissue calcification, which may be detected clinically or radiographically, constitutes a serious problem in uremic patients. These extraskeletal calcifications may be localized in the arteries (vascular calcification), in the eyes (ocular calcification), in the visceral organs (visceral calcification), around the joints (periarticular calcification), and in the skin (cutaneous calcification).

Vascular Calcification

Vascular calcification is detected radiographically. The calcification appears as a fine, granular density outlining a portion of the entire artery, giving it a pipestem appearance (Figs. 77.18 and 77.19). This x-ray appearance is due to deposition of calcium within the media and the internal elastic membrane of the

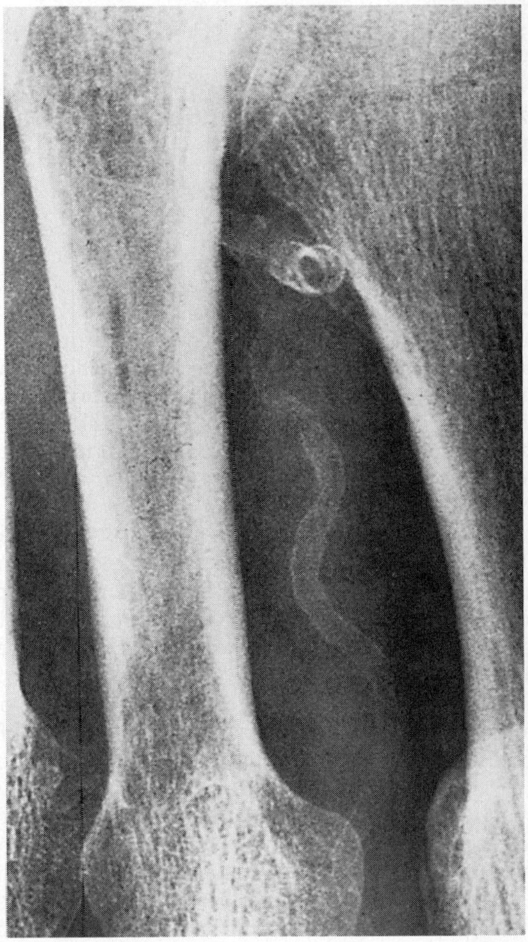

Figure 77.19. Calcification of the dorsalis pedis. Note the ring sign. (Reproduced with permission from Tatler GLV, Baillod RA, Varghese Z, et al. Evolution of bone disease over 10 years in 135 patients with terminal renal disease. *Br J Med* 1973;4:315.)

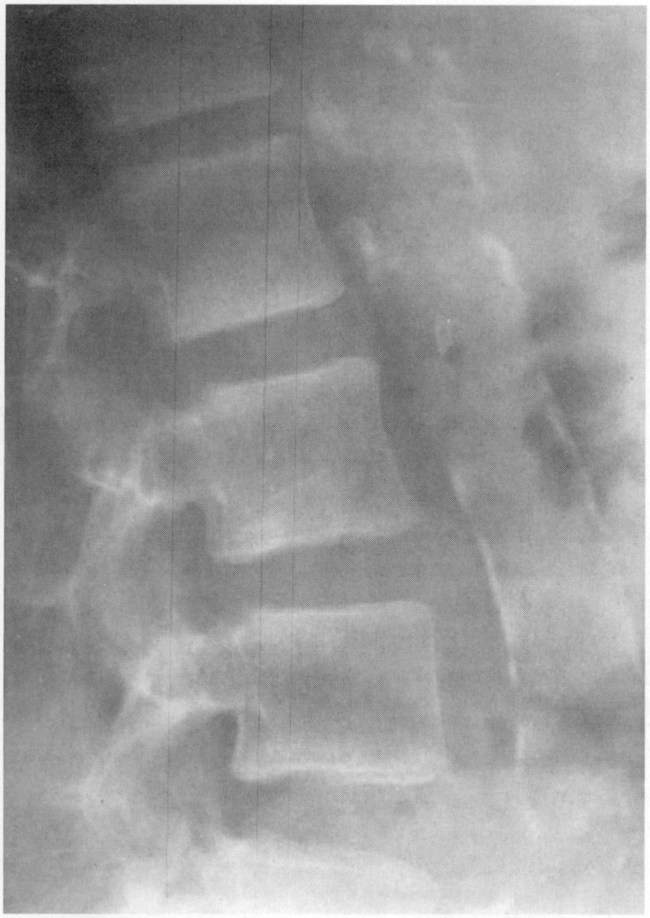

Figure 77.20. Radiographic appearance of calcified atherosclerotic plaques involving the abdominal aorta in a patient treated with hemodialysis.

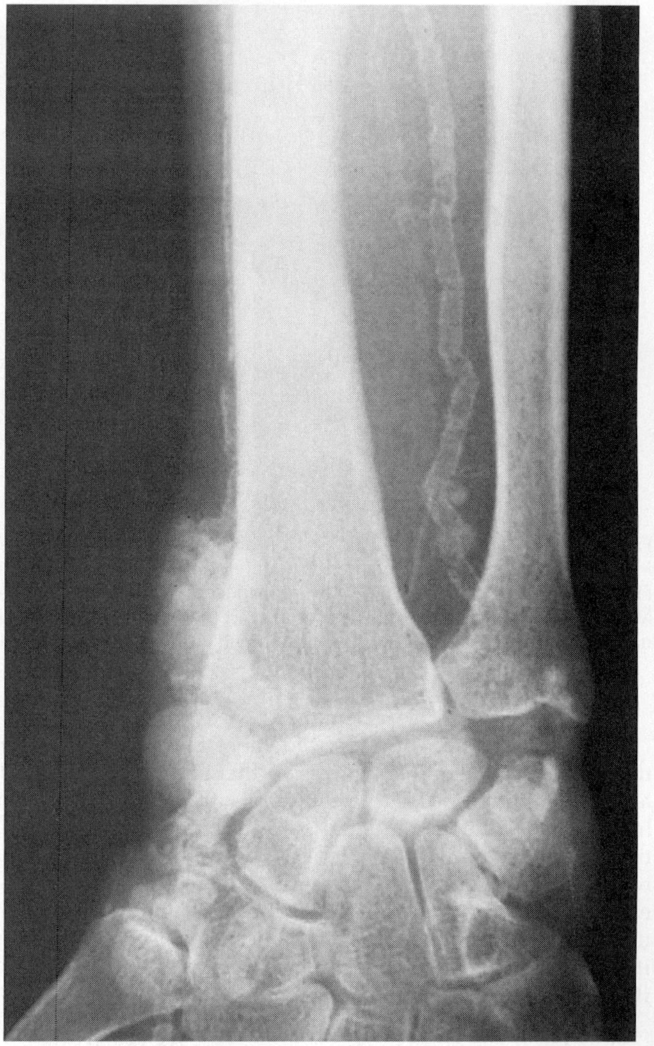

Figure 77.21. A roentgenogram from a patient with advanced uremia and severe clinical hyperparathyroidism. Vascular and periarticular calcifications were present before dialysis. (Reproduced with permission from Massry SG, Coburn JW, Popovtzer MM, et al. Secondary hyperparathyroidism in chronic renal failure. *Arch Intern Med* 1969;124:431.)

artery. The lumen of the vessel is usually not involved. This medial calcification may first be seen in the dorsalis pedis as a ring or a tube as it descends between the first and second metatarsals (Fig. 77.19). As mentioned earlier, the medial calcification may be due, in part, to a deficiency of gla protein (MPG). Calcification can also occur in atherosclerotic plaques in the intima of large vessels. The radiographic appearance is that of discrete, irregular densities (Fig. 77.20). It is possible that uremic patients are more prone to this type of calcification because of the presence of hypertension and a propensity to accelerated atherosclerosis.

Arterial calcification is rare in children, uncommon in patients between 15 and 30 years of age, and common in those older than 40. Vascular calcifications are seen in uremic patients and in those treated with hemodialysis, and they persist after renal transplantation. The incidence of arterial calcification in dialysis patients has varied from 3% to 83%. In general, the incidence of arterial calcification increases with duration of dialysis treatment. In a series of 135 patients, the incidence of vascular calcification increased from 27% in those treated for less than 1 year to 83% in patients treated for more than 8 years.

Vascular calcification may involve almost every artery and has been seen in arteries of the forearm, wrist, hands, eyes, feet, abdominal cavity, breasts, pelvis, and brain (Figs. 77.21 through 77.24). The calcification may be very extensive, rendering the artery so rigid that the pulse is not palpable and the Korotkoff sounds may be difficult to hear during the measurement of the blood pressure. Such calcification may also present difficulties during surgery for the creation of arteriovenous shunts or fistulas for maintenance hemodialysis or during renal transplantation. The arterial calcification shows little tendency to regress; in some patients, improvement or disappearance of arterial calcification occurs within months to years after subtotal parathyroidectomy or renal transplantation.

Ocular Calcification

Ocular calcifications are the most common types of soft tissue calcification seen in uremic patients and in those treated with hemodialysis. Calcium deposition in the eye may produce visible inflammation and local irritation, resulting in the *red eye* of uremia (Fig. 77.25). This is a transient phenomenon and may last only a few days. Recurrence of the red eye phenomenon is not infrequent, and it becomes apparent each time a new calcium deposition occurs in the conjunctiva. More commonly, conjunctival calcium deposits are asymptomatic and are seen as white plaques or as small punctate deposits on the lateral or medial segment of the bulbar conjunctiva. Also, calcium deposits may occur within the cornea at the lateral or medial segments of the limbus, the so-called band keratopathy. Slitlamp examination permits easier recognition of these lesions, which are common and may occur in the absence of soft tissue calcification elsewhere. The loss of CO_2 through the conjunctival sur-

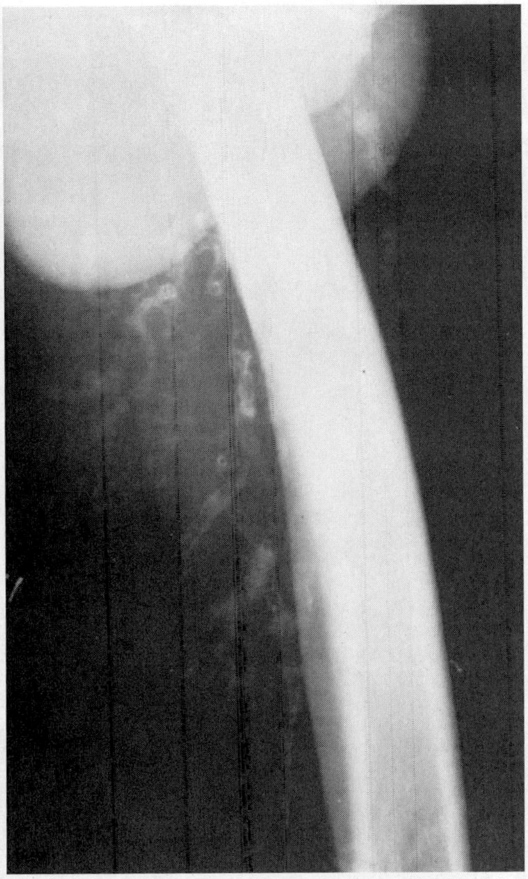

Figure 77.22. Extensive calcification involving the arteries of the thigh of a patient with longstanding advanced renal failure. (Reproduced with permission from Massry SG, Coburn JW. Divalent ion metabolism and renal osteodystrophy. In: Massry SG, Sellers AL, eds: *Clinical aspects of uremia and dialysis.* Springfield, IL: Charles C. Thomas, 1976:304–387.)

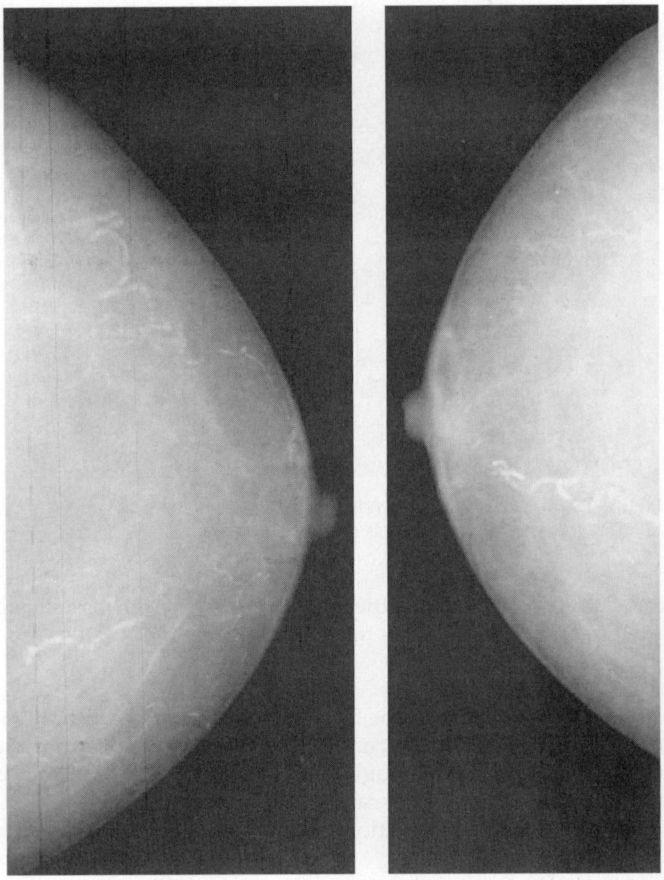

Figure 77.23. Vascular calcification in the breasts of a uremic patient with hyperparathyroidism. Calcifications of the vessels of the forearms, hands, and feet were also present in this patient. (Reproduced with permission from Massry SG, Coburn JW, Popovtzer MM, et al. Secondary hyperparathyroidism in chronic renal failure. *Arch Intern Med* 1969;124:431.)

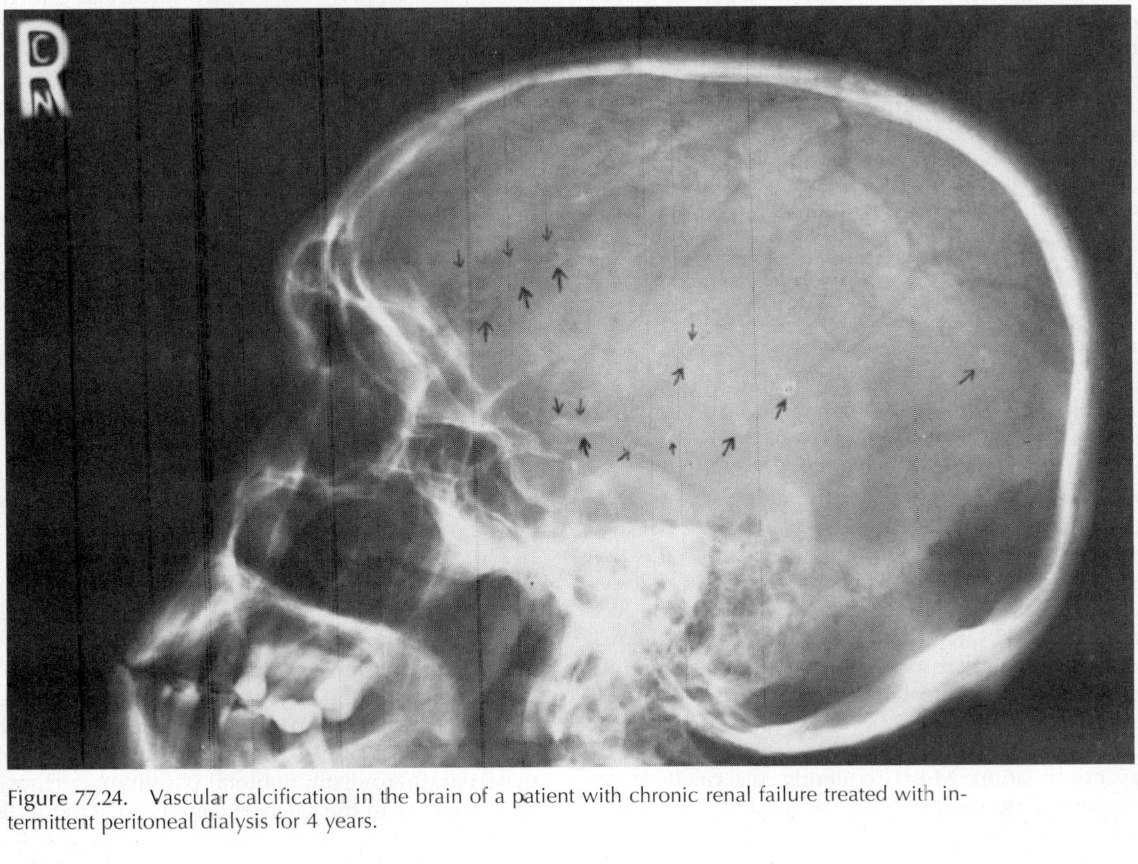

Figure 77.24. Vascular calcification in the brain of a patient with chronic renal failure treated with intermittent peritoneal dialysis for 4 years.

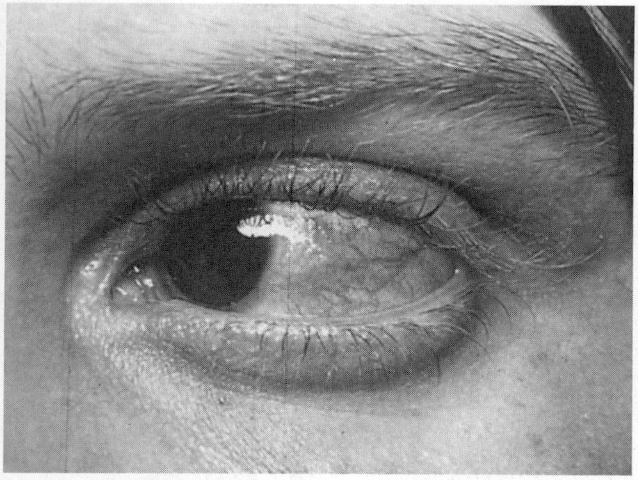

Figure 77.25. The red eye syndrome in a patient with advanced renal failure. Note the injected vessels of the conjunctiva.

face into the air increases the local pH of the ocular tissue, and this rise in pH predisposes to calcium deposition.

Visceral Calcification

Deposits of calcium may be found in the lungs, stomach, myocardium, skeletal muscles, and kidney. These calcifications are usually not evident radiographically but could be detected by ^{99m}Tc-pyrophosphate scan. They are recognized at postmortem by gross examination, microscopically, or by chemical analysis.

Visceral calcification may cause serious clinical complications. Congestive heart failure, cardiac arrhythmias, and heart block may occur in patients with calcium deposition in the myocardium or in and around the conduction system of the heart or the mitral anulus. Abnormal pulmonary function may be noted in patients with pulmonary calcification. Such patients may have reduced vital capacity and reduced carbon monoxide diffusion. Improvement in pulmonary function has been noted after subtotal parathyroidectomy in these patients. Extensive pulmonary calcification may lead to severe pulmonary fibrosis, pulmonary hypertension, and right ventricular hypertrophy.

Increased oxalate burden may occur in uremic or dialysis patients, especially if they receive large amounts of ascorbic acid. This may be associated with marked deposition of calcium oxalate in soft tissues. Such deposition in the myocardium, or mitral and aortic valves (Figs. 77.26 and 77.27), would cause myocardiopathy and congestive heart failure, eventually leading to the demise of the patient.

Periarticular Calcification

Periarticular calcification, with or without symptoms, may develop in patients with advanced renal failure and in those treated with hemodialysis (Figs. 77.21 and 77.28). The incidence of periarticular calcifications varies widely among dialysis patients. These calcifications were absent in one report but were encountered in up to 52% of the patients in other series of dialysis patients. The incidence of the periarticular calcification may increase with the duration of dialysis. In a study of 135 patients published in 1973, the incidence of these calcifications increased from 9% to 42% from the first to the eighth year of dialysis. In recent years, their incidence has decreased significantly as a result of better control of hyperphosphatemia.

Periarticular calcification may be detected because of the pain induced by the deposition of calcium or may be noted by routine x-ray examination. Most frequently, the calcifications appear as small discrete radiodensities around the shoulders,

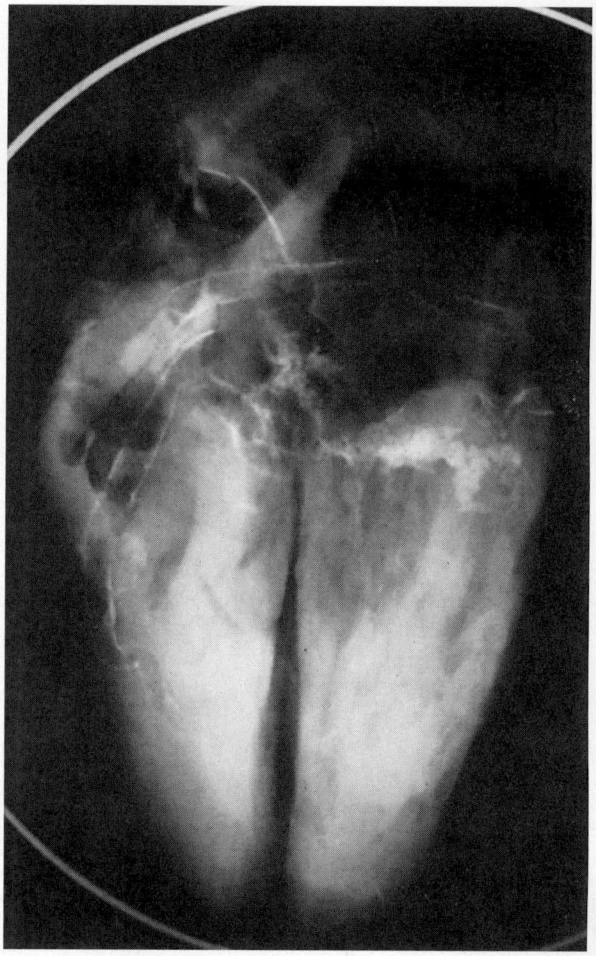

Figure 77.26. Postmortem radiograph of the heart showing calcification of the mitral and aortic valves and coronary arteries and diffuse calcinosis of the myocardium. (Reproduced with permission from Zazgornik J, Blacke P, Rokitansky A, et al. Excessive myocardial calcinosis in a chronic hemodialyzed patient. *Klin Wochenschr* 1987;5:97–100.)

wrists, phalangeal joints, hips, or ankles (Fig. 77.29). Tendosynovitis or tendonitis with abrupt pain may develop, presumably caused by deposition of microcrystals of hydroxyapatite. The synovial fluid of the involved joints is clear with normal viscosity and number of cells. This acute periarticular illness is called *calcific periarthritis.*

Occasionally, large tumoral masses develop adjacent to joints of patients with advanced renal failure (Figs. 77.30 and 77.31). The lesions are usually painless, but they may restrict movement of the joint by virtue of their size. These tumoral masses are encapsulated and filled with chalky fluid or pastelike material. The intake of food with high phosphorus content such as milk may enhance the development of tumoral calcification. These lesions often regress with the control of serum phosphorus levels by phosphate-binding antacids or following subtotal parathyroidectomy.

Cutaneous Calcification

These lesions may appear as small macules or papules composed of firm calcium deposits. However, calcium deposition in the skin of uremic patients is better detected by the chemical analysis of small skin biopsy specimen. Calcium content of skin is increased in most uremic patients and such increments are more commonly seen in patients with severe secondary hyperparathyroidism. Subtotal parathyroidectomy is followed by a decrease in the calcium content of skin, underscoring the

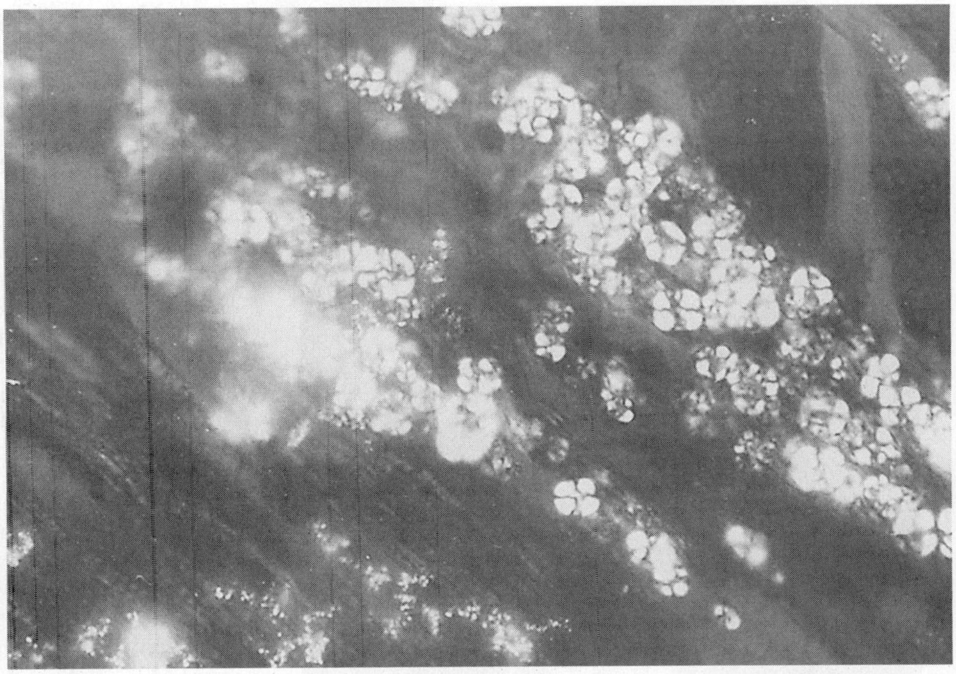

Figure 77.27. Section of myocardium of the patient shown in Fig. 77.26, depicting diffuse calcification under polarized light. ×100. (Courtesy of Professor J. Zazgornik.)

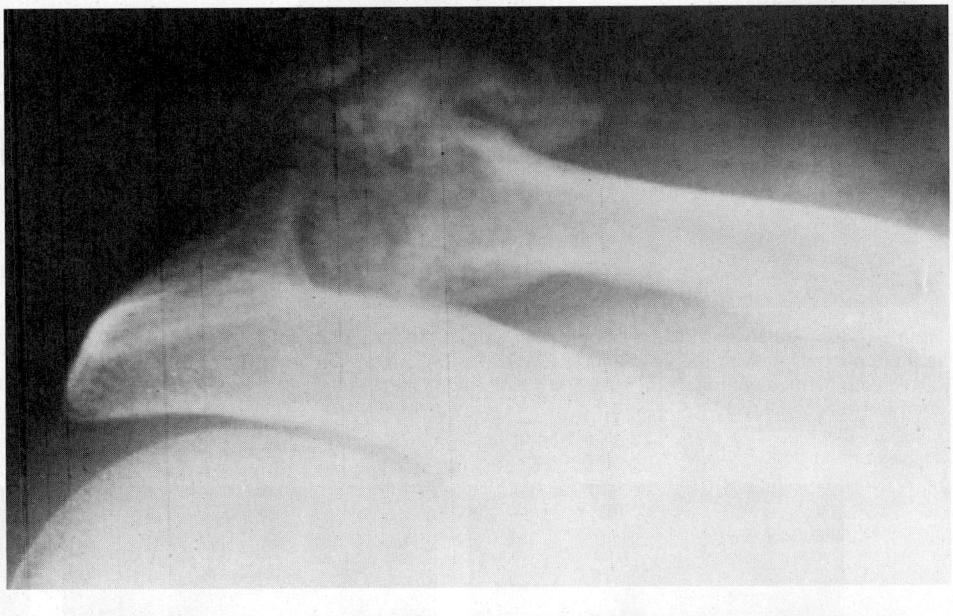

Figure 77.28. Calcium deposition around the shoulder and bone resorption of the distal end of the clavicle in a patient with advanced renal failure.

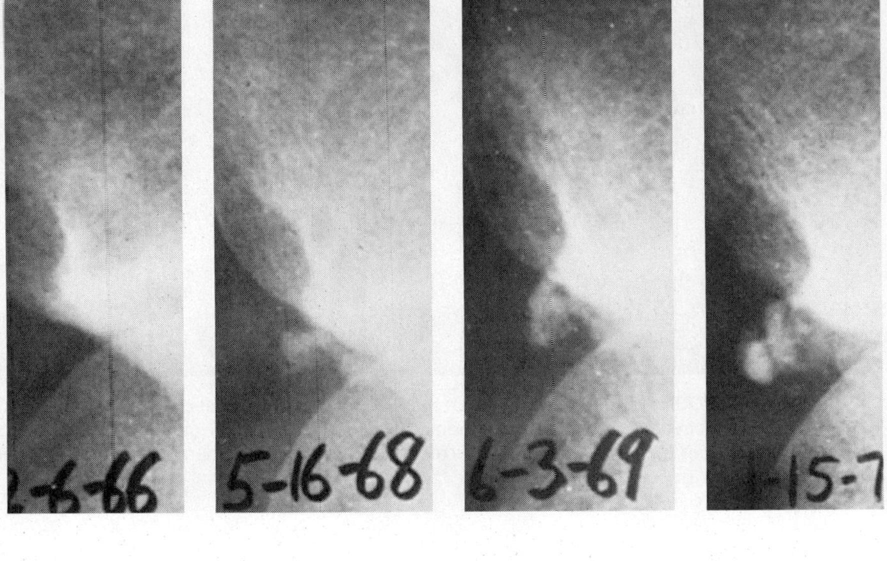

Figure 77.29. The development of asymptomatic areas of soft tissue calcification around the right hip of a 44-year-old man who was treated with regular hemodialysis but rarely consumed the prescribed quantities of aluminum hydroxide gel. (Reproduced with permission from Massry SG, Coburn JW. Divalent ion metabolism and renal osteodystrophy. In: Massry SG, Sellers AL, eds: *Clinical aspects of uremia and dialysis*. Springfield, IL: Charles C. Thomas, 1976:304–387.)

role of secondary hyperparathyroidism in the genesis of the cutaneous calcification. In uremic children, who exhibit evidence of soft tissue calcification far less frequently than adults, the calcium content of skin is significantly lower than that observed in adults being treated with hemodialysis.

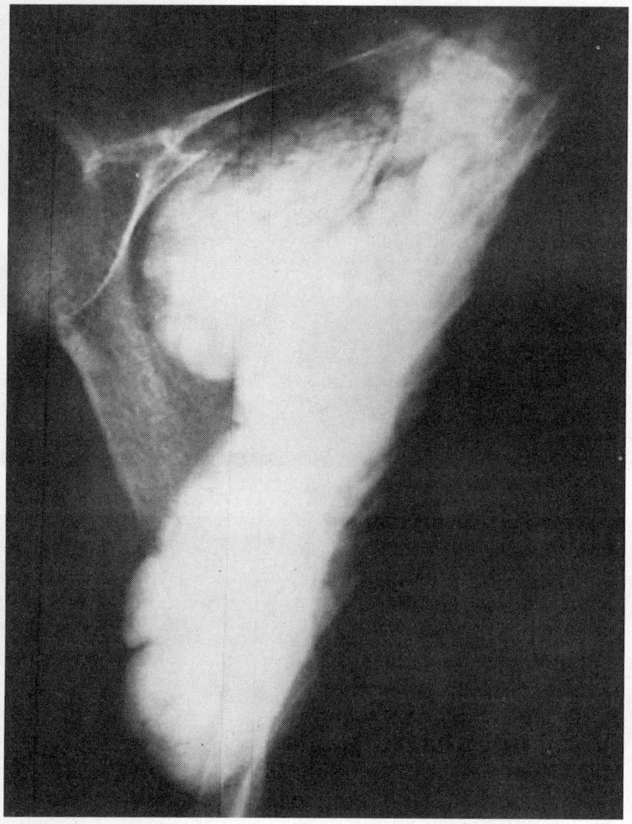

Figure 77.30. Massive soft tissue calcification around the shoulder joint in a uremic patient with severe secondary hyperparathyroidism. (Reproduced with permission from Parfitt AM. Soft-tissue calcification in uremia. *Arch Intern Med* 1969;124:544–546.)

PREVENTION AND TREATMENT

The goals of the therapy of disorders in divalent ion metabolism and osteodystrophy in patients with renal failure are (a) to maintain the blood concentrations of calcium and phosphorus as near normal as possible; (b) to prevent the development of secondary hyperparathyroidism and, if the latter already exists, to suppress the activity of the parathyroid glands; (c) to heal bone disease; (d) to prevent and reverse soft tissue calcification; and (e) to ameliorate or reverse the proximal myopathy, bone pain, pruritus, and soft tissue necrosis.

Despite the increase in our knowledge on the pathogenesis of the deranged divalent ion metabolism in patients with renal failure, there is still no unified approach to optimal therapy. The various therapeutic modalities currently in use are neither perfect nor without hazards. The overall management includes the use of one or more of the following therapeutic approaches: (a) control of phosphate retention and hyperphosphatemia, (b) supplementation of calcium, (c) treatment with vitamin D or one or more of its metabolites, (d) parathyroidectomy, and (e) appropriate dialysate composition in the dialysis patients.

Control of Phosphate Retention and Hyperphosphatemia

As indicated earlier, phosphate retention and hyperphosphatemia play an important role in the pathogenesis of the disorders of divalent ion metabolism of renal failure. The prevention of phosphate retention in patients with mild or moderate renal insufficiency and the control of hyperphosphatemia in those with advanced renal failure represent important parts of the management of these patients.

The hyperphosphatemia of uremia may be reduced by dietary restriction of phosphate, the use of phosphate-binding antacids, increased frequency of hemodialysis, and the inhibition of PTH-mediated bone resorption.

The dietary intake of phosphate is a function of the meat and dairy products ingested by the patient. The usual phosphate intake by a normal adult in the United States ranges between 1.0 and 1.8 g/day. One can reduce dietary intake of phosphate by

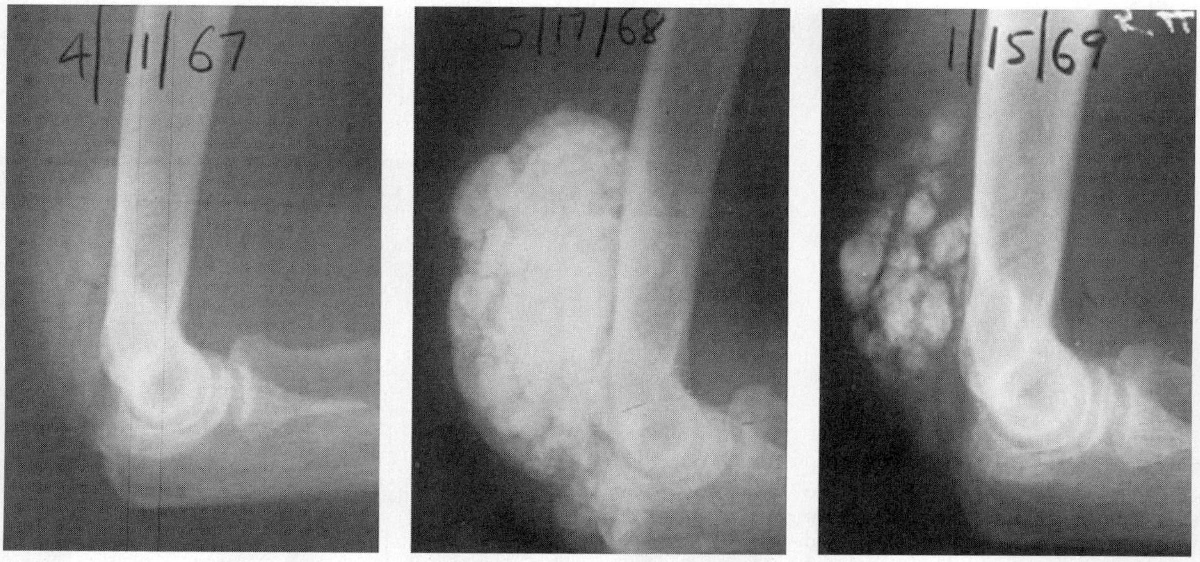

Figure 77.31. The development of massive tumoral calcifications around the right elbow of a 49-year-old man treated with regular hemodialysis. In May 1968, he began to follow the prescribed treatment with aluminum hydroxide gel. After this regimen, there was considerable regression of the calcification.

40% (600 to 900 mg/day) by eliminating dairy products and restricting protein intake. Further reduction may be difficult to achieve without jeopardizing adequate protein intake or compromising the palatability of the food. Thus restriction of dietary phosphate intake in proportion to the decrease in GFR as the sole measure for the prevention of phosphate retention is feasible only in patients with moderate renal failure (GFR of 60 to 30 ml/min). Indeed, this approach has been successful in reversing many of the abnormalities in divalent ion metabolism in such patients.

In patients with advanced renal failure, dietary phosphate restriction alone is not adequate to control the hyperphosphatemia. In a group of patients with creatinine clearances of 2 to 10 ml/min who were treated with rigid protein restriction of 20 or 40 g/day for 30 to 60 days, serum phosphorus levels remained elevated, with mean levels of 7.2 ± 0.86 and 7.3 ± 0.72 mg/dl, respectively, despite continued negative phosphorus balance in some of the patients. It is evident that in patients with advanced renal failure, other measures are needed to maintain serum phosphorus within the normal range. This could be achieved with the use of phosphate-binding antacids, which would render the ingested phosphate and the phosphate contained in the saliva (12 mmol/L), bile (5 mmol/L), and intestinal juices (1 mmol/L) unabsorbable.

Several compounds that bind phosphate in the intestinal tract are available in liquid, tablet, and capsule forms. The capsules are less effective than liquid gels in binding phosphate, but patient compliance is easier to achieve with capsules than with either the liquid or the tablets. The most commonly used compounds were Alu-Cap, Amphojel, and Basaljel concentrate. The latter is tasteless and only a small volume is necessary per dose, hence the patients more readily follow the prescribed regimen. The goal of the treatment is to reduce the level of serum phosphorus to near normal. Care should be exercised to prevent a fall in serum phosphorus to very low levels and the production of phosphate depletion with these agents. Phosphate depletion per se may aggravate bone disease and even cause osteomalacia. Therapy may be started with two to three tablets of Amphojel or capsules of Alu-Cap, or 5 to 10 ml of Basaljel, with each meal. The levels of serum phosphorus should be monitored at least twice per month, and the dose of the phosphate binders should be adjusted accordingly. Continued coaxing and emphasis on the importance of this treatment are essential to obtain adherence to this therapy by the patients. These compounds are ineffective in controlling the concentration of serum phosphorus if phosphate intake exceeds 2.0 g/day.

The fall in serum phosphorus concentration during therapy with dietary phosphate restriction and phosphate-binding antacids is usually associated with a rise in the level of serum calcium; if the magnitude of the latter is adequate, a fall in the blood levels of PTH may occur, and this in turn will contribute to the maintenance of lower levels of serum phosphorus.

The aluminum in the phosphate-binding antacids is absorbed by the intestine and may accumulate in various tissues of the body such as brain and bone. Increased aluminum burden of brain has been incriminated in the pathogenesis of dialysis encephalopathy (see Chapter 69, Part 2) and accumulation of aluminum in bone may be responsible for the low turnover osteomalacia that is refractory to therapy (see Chapter 68, Part 2). Anemia could also be a consequence of increased aluminum burden. These toxic effects resulted in a significant reduction in the use of aluminum compounds in the treatment of hyperphosphatemia in patients with advanced renal failure and in those treated with dialysis. One approach that may minimize the hazards of aluminum toxicity is to begin therapy with aluminum compounds and then replace these with calcium carbonate once serum phosphorus is reduced toward normal. The use of magnesium-containing compounds should be avoided because of the risks of hypermagnesemia. If these compounds are used, the patient should undergo dialysis with a magnesium-free dialysate.

Calcium salts are effective phosphate binders. They should be ingested with meals. The doses of the various calcium salts necessary for effective control of the hyperphosphatemia depend on the phosphate intake per day and on the efficacy of the various calcium salts to bind phosphorus. The most commonly used calcium salts as phosphate binders are calcium carbonate and calcium acetate. Calcium carbonate contains 40% elemental calcium, whereas calcium acetate contains 25% elemental calcium. Each gram of calcium in calcium carbonate binds 43 mg of phosphorus, whereas each gram of calcium in calcium acetate binds 106 mg of phosphorus. The dosage of calcium carbonate ranges from 1 to 12 g/day and for calcium acetate, 2 to 6 g/day. These dosages could be adjusted upward or downward depending on the degree of the control of the hyperphosphatemia. Calcium acetate is poorly tolerated, and therefore compliance is worse than with calcium carbonate. Hypercalcemia is more common with calcium carbonate than with acetate. The aggressive use of calcium salts in the management of hyperphosphatemia has been associated with ABD most likely due to oversuppression of PTH production leading to blood levels of PTH below 65 pg/ml. Calcium citrate is also an effective phosphate binder but is not used frequently because it enhances intestinal absorption of aluminum, and combination of calcium citrate and aluminum compounds has been associated with acute aluminum intoxication manifested by acute encephalopathy. Caution should be exercised with calcium salts administration in patients with blood levels of phosphorus greater than 7.0 mg/dl.

A newer phosphate binder is sevelamer hydrochloride (RenaGel, marketed by Genzyme). It is a polymeric phosphate binder (cross-linked poly [allylamine hydrochloride]). It also lowers the levels of low-density lipoprotein (LDL) and total cholesterol in blood. Clinical trial demonstrated that sevelamer is a very effective phosphate binder without the side effects of calcium salts or aluminum compounds. The dose of sevelamer necessary to control the hyperphosphatemia depends on blood levels of phosphorus. The starting dose for patients with blood of phosphorus between 6 and 7.5 mg/dl is two capsules of RenaGel three times a day; this dose is increased to three capsules three times per day in patients with blood levels of phosphorus between 7.5 and 9 mg/day and to five capsules three times per day in those with blood phosphorus greater than 9 mg/day. These doses could be adjusted upward or downward depending on the changes in the blood levels of phosphorus. RenaGel may also bind certain medication and as such may decrease their bioavailability. Because such interactions have not been studied in detail, it is recommended that drugs be administered at least 1 hour before or 3 hours after the ingestion of renagel; special caution should be exercised in patients taking antiarrhythmic or antiseizure medications. RenaGel is contraindicated in patients with intestinal obstruction, and it is not recommended for pregnant women or nursing mothers.

Calcium Supplementation

The low dietary intake of calcium and the defect in intestinal calcium absorption that is more evident at low calcium intake put renal failure patients in double jeopardy regarding their calcium balance. Evidence exists that normal amounts of calcium could be absorbed by the gut of these patients when their calcium intake is high. Indeed, long-term calcium supplementation has been associated with beneficial effects such as a rise in the concentration of serum calcium, a fall in the serum levels of alkaline phosphatase and PTH, and a reduction in bone resorption and the number and incidence of fractures; such therapy, however, did not achieve normal mineralization of osteoid. Thus there is a good rationale for calcium supplementation, but the time in the course of renal insufficiency at which such therapy should be initiated is not evident. It is reasonable to suggest that patients with a GFR between 40 and 10 ml/min should receive 1.2 to 1.5 g of calcium per day. Calcium supplements may be given to these patients to bring their total daily intake to this level. Patients with advanced renal failure (GFR of less than 10 ml/min) may need a calcium supplement of 1.0 to 2.0 g/day.

Treatment with calcium salts is not without hazards. It is dangerous to administer large quantities of oral calcium compounds in the face of marked hyperphosphatemia because of the danger of an elevation in calcium–phosphorus product, predisposing to soft tissue calcification. Thus it is imperative that hyperphosphatemia be controlled and the level of serum phosphorus be less than 5.5 mg/dl before treatment with calcium salts. As discussed earlier, this could be achieved by a short duration therapy with aluminum compound or sevelamer. Also, hypercalcemia may appear during therapy with large doses of oral calcium, especially in patients with advanced renal failure; this is particularly true when there has been a concomitant reduction in the levels of serum phosphorus to 2.0 mg/dl or in those receiving vitamins or being dialyzed with high-calcium dialysate. Various symptoms may accompany even mild hypercalcemia in uremic patients. Nausea, vomiting, mental confusion, lethargy, pruritus, dysesthesias, and severe hypertension have been encountered. Therefore weekly or bimonthly monitoring of the concentration of serum calcium and phosphorus is advisable. If the serum concentration of calcium exceeds 10.5 mg/dl, calcium supplements may be cut in half or may even be discontinued temporarily.

Elemental calcium constitutes 40% of calcium carbonate, 25% of calcium acetate, 12% of calcium lactate, and 8% of calcium gluconate. Calcium chloride should be avoided in uremic patients because of its acidifying properties. Calcium citrate should not be given to patients receiving aluminum salts because citrate augments aluminum absorption, increases the body burden of aluminum, and enhances the risk of aluminum toxicity. Alka Seltzer contains citric acid and should also be avoided by renal failure patients ingesting aluminum salts. Calcium carbonate is inexpensive, tasteless, and relatively well tolerated. Calcium carbonate is available in several proprietary preparations such as Titralac, Tums, or Os-Cal. Titralac provides 0.42 g of calcium carbonate and 0.18 g of glycine per tablet (160 mg of elemental calcium per tablet). Neo-Calglucon syrup is another preparation well accepted by patients, but it is costly; each 4 ml contains 92 mg of calcium ion. To maximize calcium absorption, the amount prescribed should be ingested in several small doses divided throughout the day rather than in one or two large doses. Calcium acetate is also an effective phosphate binder with lower calcium (25%) content than calcium carbonate. The risk of hypercalcemia is therefore less with the use of calcium acetate.

Use of Vitamin D Compounds

Because many of the features of abnormal calcium metabolism in uremia resemble those of vitamin D deficiency, this compound and its related steroids have been used in the management of renal osteodystrophy. The currently available forms of vitamin D metabolites for clinical use in the United States are vitamin D_2 (ergocalciferol); vitamin D_3 (cholecalciferol), which is the naturally occurring form of the steroid in mammals; dihydrotachysterol; $25(OH)D_3$ (calcifediol), $1,25(OH)_2D_3$; (calcitriol, the intravenous form called Calcijex), 19-nor-$1,25(OH)_2D_2$ [Zemplar]). Another vitamin D analog, $1a(OH)D_3$, is available for clinical use outside the United States. In Japan, 22-oxa-$1,25(OH)_2D_3$ is being evaluated for clinical use.

Because of its low cost, vitamin D_2, a steroid obtained from plant sources, has been most widely used in medicine. Vitamin D_3 can now be prepared inexpensively, but it does not enjoy widespread use. Moreover, there is little evidence to indicate that vitamin D_2 differs in activity from vitamin D_3 in humans.

Vitamins D_2 and D_3

There is a great variability in the required amount of vitamin D by patients with advanced renal failure. Dosages as high as 50,000 to 200,000 IU/day (1.25 to 5.0 mg) may be needed to achieve beneficial effects. The long-term therapy with large doses of vitamin D causes a rise in the serum calcium levels and may be followed by a fall in serum levels of alkaline phosphatase and PTH, reduced bone resorption, and amelioration or healing of rickets in uremic children or of osteomalacia in uremic adults. Because of the need for large doses of vitamin D, hypercalcemia is a real and frequent hazard. Such *hypercalcemia may persist for weeks* after the discontinuation of therapy. In addition to the clinical side effects of hypercalcemia, the elevation in the serum levels of calcium in a hyperphosphatemic patient would cause a marked rise in calcium–phosphorus product, predisposing to soft tissue calcification. Therapy with vitamin D should not be started before the normalization of the serum levels of phosphorus. Frequent monitoring of the levels of serum calcium and phosphorus during such therapy is advisable.

25-Hydroxyvitamin D_3 (Calcifediol)

Despite the block in the conversion of 25(OH)D to $1,25(OH)_2D$, therapy with 50 to 100 μg of $25(OH)D_3$ per day has been shown to be beneficial. Treatment with this metabolite was associated with amelioration of bone pain and proximal myopathy, a rise in serum calcium concentration, and a fall in serum levels of alkaline phosphatase and PTH. A decrease in the degree of osteitis fibrosa and even improvement in bone mineralization have been noted.

1,25-Dihydroxyvitamin D_3

A relative deficiency of $1,25(OH)_2D_3$ is present in patients with mild and moderate renal failure, and absolute deficiency exists in those with advanced renal failure. Furthermore, the kidney is required to convert the parent vitamin D to this active metabolite; therefore it is rational to treat renal failure patients with this metabolite to correct the vitamin D–deficient state. Indeed, such therapy has proven beneficial. It is important to emphasize that some or most of the beneficial effects of $1,25(OH)_2D_3$ in the management of renal osteodystrophy could be produced by other vitamin D compounds. However, the smaller dose of $1,25(OH)_2D_3$ that is needed to achieve beneficial effects and its shorter half-life make it a better and safer agent than other vitamin D compounds. On the other hand, the high biologic potency of $1,25(OH)_2D_3$ causes the early appearance of hazardous side effects (hypercalcemia and elevation in calcium–phosphorus product) with even very small doses. Thus close monitoring of patients receiving $1,25(OH)_2D_3$ is mandatory.

The suggested initial dosage for oral therapy is 0.5 μg/day, although it may be safer to begin therapy with 0.25 μg/day.

The changes in the concentrations of serum calcium provide the best clinical guide for modification of the dosage. Failure of the level of serum calcium to rise by at least 0.5 mg/dl with any particular dosage given for 4 to 6 weeks justifies increasing the dosage by 0.25 μg/day. Such an approach may be used until serum calcium reaches the upper normal range (10.0 to 10.5 mg/dl). When this is achieved, frequent monitoring of serum calcium is needed, and if the latter approaches hypercalcemic range, a reduction of the dosage or temporary discontinuation of therapy should be considered. In our and others' experience, the requirement of and the tolerance for $1,25(OH)_2D_3$ may decrease progressively during treatment in many patients; therefore reduction of the maintenance dosage after a prolonged period of therapy may be needed.

Among the most disturbing clinical symptoms of renal osteodystrophy are muscle weakness and bone pain. The muscle weakness is a clinical manifestation of uremic myopathy, which is at least partly due to vitamin D deficiency. The myopathy of renal failure is discussed in detail in Chapter 78. The exact cause of bone pain is not known, but it may be related to the presence of osteomalacia and/or osteitis fibrosa or to a potential *algesic effect* of excess blood levels of PTH. These disturbances may interfere seriously with the daily activity of patients and may even render them totally disabled. Improvement in these symptoms appears rapidly after initiation of therapy with $1,25(OH)_2D_3$. The improvement in muscle strength may become noticeable within 2 to 5 weeks of treatment. A significant amelioration or complete disappearance of bone pain may also occur in some patients within 1 to 3 weeks. This clinical improvement produces a remarkable change in the physical disability of patients; many become symptom free and are able to perform their daily activity without limitation.

The most consistent effect of $1,25(OH)_2D_3$ in uremic and dialysis patients is the elevation in the serum concentration of calcium. Although it is reasonable to assume that the higher the dose of the metabolite, the greater the rise in serum calcium concentration, many variables in addition to the dose may modify the calcemic response to therapy with $1,25(OH)_2D_3$. These variables may include duration of treatment, dietary calcium intake, changes in intestinal absorption of calcium, type of bone disease and its response to treatment, and the severity of the state of secondary hyperparathyroidism. Occasionally, serum calcium concentration may fall during the first 1 to 2 weeks of therapy, probably because of rapid remineralization of the skeleton.

Hypercalcemia is a common complication of treatment with $1,25(OH)_2D_3$. It has been reported that 30% to 67% of the patients treated with this metabolite developed one or more hypercalcemic episodes during the course of their therapy. The overall incidence of one episode was 42%. Hypercalcemia occurred with a dosage of 0.5 to 3.0 μg/day. Certain patients are more prone to develop hypercalcemia: (a) patients with osteitis fibrosa and pretreatment serum calcium concentration of greater than 10.5 mg/day; (b) patients with low turnover osteomalacia, low serum concentration of PTH, and absent bone marrow fibrosis; (c) patients receiving large amounts of calcium supplementation; and (d) patients dialyzed with high-calcium (more than 6.0 to 7.0 mg/dl) dialysate. Hypercalcemia may appear at any time during therapy with $1,25(OH)_2D_3$. It usually occurs after 2 to 3 months of therapy but has been encountered as early as 5 days and as late as 6 to 18 months after treatment. A high starting dose may be the cause for the early appearance of hypercalcemia. Early hypercalcemia within 1 to 4 weeks of therapy may also occur in patients with severe osteitis fibrosa and pretreatment serum calcium concentration of 10.5 mg/dl. Extreme caution should be exercised in the management of such patients with $1,25(OH)_2D_3$. *The incidence of hypercalcemia increases as serum alkaline phosphatase activity returns to normal, and a reduction in the dosage of $1,25(OH)_2D_3$ is recommended when serum levels of alkaline phosphatase normalize.* The hypercalcemia is usually mild and asymptomatic, but serum calcium concentrations of more than 13.0 mg/dl and occasionally even more than 15.0 mg/dl have been encountered during therapy with $1,25(OH)_2D_3$. The elevated levels of serum calcium usually return to normal shortly after reduction of the dose or discontinuation of therapy. Occasionally, the hypercalcemia may persist for several weeks. It is advisable to stop treatment completely rather than to reduce the dose when hypercalcemia appears and to reinstitute therapy with a small dose as serum calcium concentrations return to normal.

The effect of $1,25(OH)_2D_3$ treatment on the concentration of serum phosphorus in uremic or dialysis patients is not consistent. An increase, a decrease, and no change have been reported. This variability in the various patient populations may be related to differences in dietary intake of phosphate and/or the ingestion of phosphate-binding antacids, the dosage of $1,25(OH)_2D_3$, the effect of the metabolite on intestinal absorption of phosphate, the degree of suppression of parathyroid gland activity, and the status of the remineralization of bone. Monitoring of serum phosphorus concentrations during therapy with $1,25(OH)_2D_3$ is mandatory because the development of hyperphosphatemia, especially in the face of rising serum calcium concentration, would result in elevation of calcium–phosphorus product and augment the hazards of soft tissue calcification. If hyperphosphatemia occurs and calcium–phosphorus product approaches 55, every effort should be made to control the levels of serum phosphorus with phosphate-binding antacids. If this procedure is not successful, the dose of $1,25(OH)_2D_3$ should be reduced or temporary cessation of therapy should be considered. The calcium–phosphorus product should be maintained below 55.

Serum alkaline phosphatase activity usually decreases during therapy with $1,25(OH)_2D_3$, but several months may elapse before its level returns to normal. Occasionally, serum alkaline phosphatase may rise during the initial phase of therapy. *Monitoring the serum alkaline phosphatase can provide an additional guide for the adjustment of the dosage of $1,25(OH)_2D_3$ for two reasons. First, normalization of serum levels of alkaline phosphatase reflects improvement in bone disease, and second, the occurrence of hypercalcemia increases as serum alkaline phosphatase returns to normal.*

Long-term therapy with $1,25(OH)_2D_3$ may be associated with a marked fall in or even normalization of the serum levels of PTH. No change, or even an increase, in serum levels of the hormone has also been encountered during therapy with this metabolite. On the average, the blood levels of PTH fall by 50% to 60% with 1 to 2 years of oral therapy with $1,25(OH)_2D_3$. The reduction in the serum levels of PTH during oral therapy with $1,25(OH)_2D_3$ is probably due to the rise in the concentration of serum calcium, but a direct effect of $1,25(OH)_2D_3$ on the activity of the parathyroid glands also play a role. We have found an inverse correlation between the percentage change in serum calcium concentrations and PTH levels (Fig. 77.32). Caution should be exercised in not lowering serum levels of PTH below 65 pg/ml (IRMA assay) in order to prevent the emergence of ABD.

Intestinal absorption of calcium is usually increased in most uremic patients during therapy with $1,25(OH)_2D_3$. The increment in calcium absorption is most evident during the first 2 hours after the ingestion of the ^{47}Ca, suggesting that the metabolite exerts its effect in the duodenum and proximal part of the small intestine. The metabolite may also affect calcium absorption in the jejunum because this segment of the

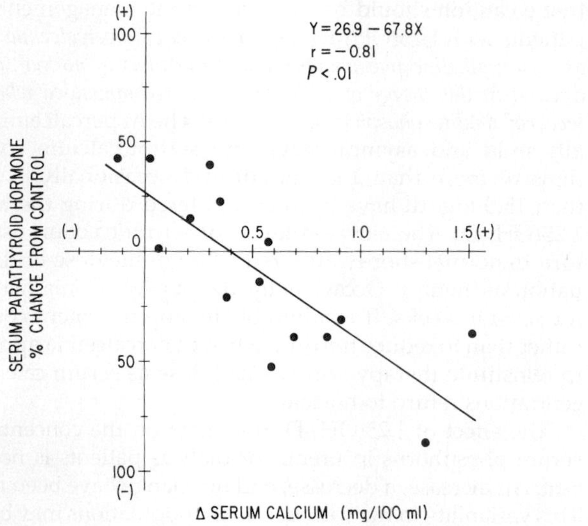

Figure 77.32. Relationship between the changes in the concentration of serum calcium and the percentage change in serum parathyroid hormone (PTH) levels during therapy with $1,25(OH)_2D_3$. Each data point represents one patient. (Reproduced with permission from Goldstein DA, Malluche HH, Massry SG. Management of renal osteodystrophy with $1,25(OH)_2D_3$. *Miner Electrolyte Metab* 1979;2:35.)

intestine has receptors for $1,25(OH)_2D_3$. There is a dose–response relationship between $1,25(OH)_2D_3$ and intestinal absorption of calcium. Finally, the quantity of the sterol required to elicit an increase in intestinal calcium absorption in the uremic patient is greater than in normal subjects, suggesting that uremia per se may interfere with the action of the sterol on the gut. $1,25(OH)_2D_3$ also augments intestinal absorption of phosphate. The metabolite may produce a modest rise in urinary calcium in uremic patients.

Therapy with oral $1,25(OH)_2D_3$ for several months may be associated with a decrease in bone resorption, and treatment for 2 to 3 years may result in complete healing. The effect on bone resorption reflects the degree of success in suppressing the activity of the parathyroid glands. Endosteal fibrosis is either markedly reduced or completely reversed after several months of treatment, irrespective of whether serum levels of PTH are decreased or not. This observation raises the possibility that endosteal fibrosis is not entirely the result of excess PTH but could also be related to vitamin D deficiency as well. The osteomalacia in patients with mixed bone disease (osteomalacia and osteitis fibrosa) responds well to therapy with $1,25(OH)_2D_3$. Long-term treatment usually results in marked improvement or healing of the osteomalacia. In patients with pure low turnover osteomalacia, the response to $1,25(OH)_2D_3$ is poor; these patients may respond better to a long-term therapy (4 to 6 months) of both $1,25(OH)_2D_3$ and $24,25(OH)_2D_3$ (2.5 to 10 μg/day). The healing of the bone lesions during treatment with $1,25(OH)_2D_3$ may also be evidenced by improvement in the radiographic findings of the skeleton (Fig. 77.11).

Failure of therapy with $1,25(OH)_2D_3$ to improve clinical signs and symptoms has been reported. The treatment failure group appeared to be heterogeneous and did not display a specific biochemical pattern of bone disease. Although patients had higher serum calcium concentrations than those who responded to treatment, the serum levels of PTH were normal, moderately elevated, or very high, and the bone lesions varied from pure osteomalacia in some to marked osteitis fibrosa in others. Further analysis of the data, however, indicates two distinct subgroups among these patients. The first group consists of patients with severe osteitis fibrosa and marked elevation of serum PTH; the second group consists of patients with normal serum levels of PTH and pure osteomalacia without evidence of hyperparathyroid bone disease. Both types of patients rapidly develop hypercalcemia. Because this complication requires cessation of treatment, it would preclude long-term therapy; hence the failure to improve the clinical and histologic abnormalities of renal osteodystrophy.

An intravenous preparation of $1,25(OH)_2D_3$ (Calcijex; Abbott Laboratories Inc.) is available for use in dialysis patients. This metabolite, given in doses of 1.0 to 2.5 μg three times per week, almost normalized blood levels of PTH within 2 to 3 months. It appears that intravenous administration of $1,25(OH)_2D_3$ is more effective than oral therapy. This is most likely due to a greater delivery of $1,25(OH)_2D_3$ to the parathyroid glands and a direct inhibitory effect on their activity. Indeed, the blood levels of PTH begin to fall before a significant rise in the concentrations of serum calcium becomes evident. *Others have used oral pulse therapy of $1,25(OH)_2D_3$ (i.e., large doses 2.0 to 4.0 μg given three times a week) and found that this approach is as effective as intravenous therapy.* $1,25(OH)_2D_3$ could be given to children in the peritoneal dialysis fluid; the metabolite should be delivered into the peritoneal cavity in a small volume of peritoneal dialysis (20 ml) and 20 minutes later the total volume of the dialysate fluid could be delivered.

$1,25(OH)_2D_3$ could also be used for the prevention of the secondary hyperparathyroidism and other derangements of divalent ion metabolism in patients with early to moderate renal failure. In a double-blind control study, it was found that 0.5 to 2.0 μg of $1,25(OH)_2D_3$ per day given for 1 year to patients with a GFR ranging between 15 and 55 ml/min was associated with a rise in blood concentrations of calcium, a fall in alkaline phosphatase, a marked reduction in blood levels of PTH (50% to 60%), and healing of hyperparathyroid bone disease and osteomalacia. Blood levels of serum calcium should be monitored carefully during this therapy, and hypercalcemia should be avoided.

It has been claimed that the administration of $1,25(OH)_2D_3$ to patients with moderate renal failure produced a significant reduction in GFR by a direct adverse effect. Analysis of all available and pertinent data does not support the contention that $1,25(OH)_2D_3$ has a direct deleterious effect on renal function. The metabolite could produce a reversible or permanent fall in GFR, however, if sustained hypercalcemia developed during its administration. The use of the proper dosage, the frequent monitoring of serum calcium and creatinine concentrations, and the discontinuation of therapy as hypercalcemia develops are the precautionary measures to reduce the likelihood of a harmful effect on renal function.

19-nor-$1,25(OH)_2D_2$ (Paricalcitol)

This is a new vitamin D analog marketed by Abbott laboratories Inc. under the name of Zemplar. Three double-blind, placebo-controlled trial evaluating the efficacy of paricalcitol in suppressing the blood levels of PTH in 78 dialysis patients (40 received the drug and 38 took a placebo) were conducted. Paricalcitol was effective in reducing blood levels of PTH with fewer hypercalcemia or hyperphosphatemia. No studies are available on the effect of paricalcitol on bone disease of patients with renal failure, as yet, are available. The recommended initial dose is 0.04 to 0.1 μg/kg (2.8 to 7 μg for a 70-kg patient) given as a bolus intravenous injection no more than every other day. The dose may be increased by 2 to 4 μg at 2- to 4-week intervals if a satisfactory response is not achieved. Blood levels of calcium, phosphorus, and calcium–phosphate product should be monitored. Overdosage of paricalcitol may cause hypercalcemia.

Studies in animals have shown that 22 oxa $1,25(OH)_2D$ is effective in suppressing secondary hyperparathyroidism of renal failure with little hypercalcemia. In early clinical trials, 22 oxa $1,25(OH)_2D$ therapy was not devoid of hypercalcemia. This metabolite of vitamin D, however, suppressed blood levels of PTH effectively and in a dose-dependent manner, but substantial number of patients had hypercalcemic episodes. This compound is not approved for use in the United States, and it is not evident that it has therapeutic advantages over the use of $1,25(OH)_2D_3$.

Dialysate and Its Composition

There is evidence for considerable geographic variations in the incidence of bone disease in patients undergoing hemodialysis. Various impurities and trace elements such as fluoride or aluminum may be responsible for these geographic variations. It is now accepted that water treatment and purification should be used before the preparation of dialysate.

Variations in the concentration of calcium in dialysate may affect the course of renal osteodystrophy. All calcium present in dialysate is ionized and diffuses freely across the membrane of the dialyzer. This contrasts with calcium in blood: only 60% of the total amount is not bound to protein and is able to move across the membrane. Depending on the gradient, the dialysate calcium level, and the concentration of diffusible calcium in blood, there will be either a loss or a gain of this ion by the patient. The use of dialysate containing calcium concentrations of 5.0 to 5.5 mg/dl was associated with a high incidence of radiographic evidence of bone disease, progressively rising serum levels of alkaline phosphatase, loss of calcium from bones, and persistently elevated serum levels of PTH. For these reasons, use of dialysate containing such low concentrations of calcium has been abandoned. The use of dialysate containing 8.0 mg/dl may be hazardous in that it may cause hypercalcemia and enhance soft tissue calcification. Most authorities recommend a calcium concentration of 6.0 to 7.0 mg/dl. Occasionally, the use of this level of calcium in the dialysate in patients treated with $1,25(OH)_2D_3$ may be associated with hypercalcemia. If this occurs, either the dose of $1,25(OH)_2D_3$ is reduced or the dialysate calcium is decreased.

Most centers have used dialysate containing magnesium in a concentration varying between 0.5 and 1.8 mg/dl (0.5 to 1.5 mEq/L). With the lower-magnesium dialysate, predialysis levels of magnesium are usually normal and are slightly below normal immediately after dialysis. Patients treated with dialysate containing the higher concentration of magnesium have moderate hypermagnesemia all the time. There is no evidence that variations in dialysate magnesium within this range have an effect on the incidence, course, or severity of skeletal disease, soft tissue calcification, or symptoms related to altered divalent ion metabolism.

Parathyroidectomy

The various medical therapeutic modalities detailed earlier can result in suppression of the hyperplastic parathyroid glands in uremic patients. However, these measures may not be successful, and parathyroidectomy may be the only way to treat the clinical, biochemical, and skeletal manifestations of secondary hyperparathyroidism. Subtotal parathyroidectomy should be considered (a) when persistent hypercalcemia develops in the absence of other causes of hypercalcemia such as excessive intake of calcium and/or vitamin D, malignancy, or sarcoidosis; (b) when severe intractable pruritus that is unresponsive to dialysis is present, especially when the blood levels of PTH are markedly elevated; (c) when marked soft tissue calcification (especially vascular) and radiographic evidence of marked osteitis fibrosa are present and cannot be adequately controlled with conservative therapy; and (d) when ischemic lesions of soft tissues with ulcerations and necrosis develop in the presence of vascular calcification and no other cause for the tissue necrosis (normal blood levels and activity of protein C) is present. It should be mentioned that parathyroidectomy does not always cure this lesion.

The amount of parathyroid tissue to be removed at surgery depends on the size of the parathyroid glands in any particular patient. We recommend that all four glands be first identified; three glands are then removed and weighed. By comparing the size of the fourth gland with those removed, one can roughly estimate the weight of the fourth gland. The surgeon should leave only 150 to 200 mg of this remaining gland. Because the residual parathyroid tissue may undergo further hyperplasia and a second operation may be required, it is recommended that the residual tissue be marked by a metal clip and long black silk suture. An alternative approach is to remove all four glands and transplant part of a gland in the forearm. Occasionally, this has been associated with recurrent hyperparathyroidism caused by development of sheets of parathyroid tissue along the entire arm, a situation that is not amenable to surgical correction. The use of this procedure is decreasing. If fewer than four glands are identified in the neck, they should all be removed. Rarely, removal of three identified glands will result in a state of permanent hypoparathyroidism. Total parathyroidectomy may be considered in patients who will be maintained with hemodialysis and are not suitable for renal transplantation. However, one must be cautioned that total parathyroidectomy may be followed by a fall of PTH levels to less than 65 pg/ml, a situation that may lead to the development of ABD. Also, it must be stressed that patients with aluminum toxicity may develop and/or have worsening of ADB after parathyroidectomy.

The technical problems during the surgical procedure are few. The glands are grossly enlarged and easily identifiable. In the hands of an experienced surgeon, the operation is not hazardous, and the patient leaves the hospital within a week. The patients should be treated with dialysis 1 day before surgery.

A major problem during the postoperative period is the control of serum calcium concentration. Its level invariably falls after the removal of three or more parathyroid glands. The magnitude and the duration of the hypocalcemia vary from one patient to another. Those with marked periarticular calcification usually maintain serum levels of calcium between 8.0 and 9.0 mg/dl until the ectopic calcifications disappear. Also, the use of dialysate containing calcium levels of 7.0 mg/dl causes a rise in serum calcium concentration during dialysis and may alleviate the hypocalcemia during the interdialytic intervals. Profound hypocalcemia may develop in certain patients, especially those with radiographic evidence of bone resorption; treatment of such patients with $1,25(OH)_2D_3$ may reduce the severity of the postoperative hypocalcemia. Tetany may occur in those who develop severe hypocalcemia. When the level of serum calcium falls below 7.5 mg/dl, oral calcium supplementation may prevent a further decrease. The amount of oral calcium needed is usually quite large. The initial treatment should provide at least 2.0 g of calcium, and the dose can be increased at intervals of 3 to 7 days until an adequate rise in serum calcium concentration is achieved. If the concentration of serum calcium falls to lower levels and if tetany appears, intravenous calcium should be given in addition to the oral supplements of calcium. In patients with profound and sustained hypocalcemia, $1,25(OH)_2D_3$ may be needed; careful monitoring of serum calcium and phosphorus should be undertaken with this therapy. Serum levels of phosphorus almost always fall after parathyroidectomy. Therefore phosphate-binding antacids should be withheld if serum levels of phosphorus decrease to less than 3.0 mg/dl. Also, serum levels of phosphorus should not be allowed to rise above 4.0 mg/dl because the hyperphosphatemia may aggravate the hypocalcemia in the parathyroidectomized patient.

Selective Percutaneous Ethanol Injection (PEIT) or $1,25(OH)_2D_3$ into the Parathyroid Glands

PEIT was introduced by Italian workers in 1980, and the technique was perfected by Japanese scientists. This procedure has been used in Japan to treat secondary hyperparathyroid in more than 600 patients with CRF by the end of 1996.

PEIT is usually reserved for the treatment of nodular hyperplasia of the parathyroid glands because patients with this abnormality are resistant to medical therapy. The indications for PEIT are the same as for parathyroidectomy. However, additional criteria should be satisfied: (a) blood levels of PTH greater than 400 pg/ml (IRMA assay) in the presence of normal blood levels of calcium, (b) ultrasonographic evidence of the presence of at least one significantly enlarged parathyroid gland which could be reached by the PEIT needle, and (c) consent of the patient for the procedure.

Certain conditions must be satisfied before embarking on the use of such therapy. First, a high-resolution electrosonographic machine is available to define the location and size of the glands; second, the physician must be highly experienced in the performance of the procedure; third, the availability of color Doppler imaging equipment is required to confirm the destruction of the parathyroid tissue; and fourth, a special needle with side holes that would permit homogenous distribution of the ethanol must be available.

All glands larger than 1 cm in diameter or 0.5 cm^3 in volume should be injected slowly with 90% ethanol with 1% lidocaine under ultrasound observation after confirming that the tip of the needle is inside the center of the gland. The volume of the initial injection should not exceed 80% of the calculated volume of the gland.

The success of the procedure is ascertained by following of the blood levels of PTH. If the reduction of the blood levels of PTH is not adequate, reinjection of ethanol may be considered. A major side effect of this procedure is a leak of ethanol to the surrounding tissues, which may lead to tissue necrosis and may be associated with recurrent laryngeal nerve palsy. The Japanese Working Group on PEIT recommends that patients with three large glands with nodular hyperplasia should not be treated with PEIT but should be managed with parathyroidectomy.

The advantages of PEIT over parathyroidectomy are avoidance of the risks of the surgical procedure, lack of hypoparathyroidism after PEIT, and the destruction of the parathyroid glands with nodular hyperplasia, which renders the patient with the remaining glands with diffuse hyperplasia more amenable to medical therapy.

Also injection of 1 μg of $1,25(OH)_2D_3$ into the nodular hyperplastic gland, using the same technique described for ethanol injection, has been successful in reducing the blood levels of PTH. Several injections, may be needed. Leakage of $1,25(OH)_2D_3$ to the surrounding tissues during its injection does not cause necrosis or recurrent laryngeal nerve palsy.

Other Therapeutic Modalities

The use of β-adrenergic blocking agents (propranolol) may cause a decrease in the serum levels of PTH, but this action is variable and is not successful in complete reversal of secondary hyperparathyroidism. Claims that cimetidine may be effective in controlling secondary hyperparathyroidism in uremic patients have not been convincingly substantiated. Occasionally, treatment with diphosphonate (disodium ethane-1-hydroxy-1,1-diphosphonate) may cause regression of ectopic calcification resistant to the usual therapy (control of the hyperphosphatemia, suppression of parathyroid gland activity, or parathyroidectomy). Treatment with disodium ethane-1-hydroxy-1,1-diphosphonate, by itself, may produce osteomalacia. A calcimimetic agent (R-568) that activates the CaR of the parathyroid glands has the potential of suppressing the activity of the parathyroid glands and reducing the blood levels of PTH in patients with CRF. Preliminary data indicate that this is indeed the case. This agent has not been, as yet, for clinical use.

Selected Readings

Arnoud CD. Hyperparathyroidism and renal failure. *Kidney Int* 1973;4:89–95.
A study demonstrating that blood levels of PTH begin to rise in early renal failure.

Bricker NS, Slatapalsky E, Reiss E, et al. Calcium phosphorus and bone in renal disease and transplantation. *Arch Intern Med* 1969;123:543–553.
The original publication implicating phosphate retention in the genesis of secondary hyperparathyroidism in early renal failure.

Coburn JW, Elangovan L, Goodman WG, et al. Calcium-sensing receptor and calcimimetic agents. *Kidney Int* 1999;73:S52–S58.
A detailed review of the potential uses of calcimemtic agents in the management of primary and secondary hyperparathyroidism.

Coburn JW, Mischel MG, Goodman WG, et al. Citrate markedly enhances aluminum adsorption from aluminum hydroxide. *Am J Kidney Dis* 1991;6:708–711.
A study demonstrating aluminum absorption by the intestine is augmented in the presence of citrate.

De Marchi S, Cecchin E, Villata D, et al. Relief of pruritus and decrease in plasma histamine concentrations during erythropoietin therapy in patients with uremia. *N Engl J Med* 1992;326:969–974.
A study examining the role of histamine in the genesis of uremic pruritus.

Fukagawa M. Cell biology of parathyroid hyperplasia in uremia. *Am J Med Sci* 1999;317:377–382.
A discussion of the pathways that lead to diffuse and modular hyperplasia of the parathyroid glands in patients with CRF.

Fukagawa M, Kitaoka M, Tominaga Y, et al. Selective percutaneous ethanol injection ther (PEIT) of the parathyroid in chronic dialysis patients—the Japanese strategy. *Nephrol Dial Transpl* 1999;14:2574–2577.
A detailed review of the indication, technique, and results of PEIT in patients with CRF treated by hemodialysis.

Llach F. Calcific uremic arteriopathy (calciphylaxis): an evolving entity? *Am J Kidney Dis* 1998;32:514–518.
An editorial revisiting the issue of calciphylaxis.

Llach F, Massry SG. On the mechanism of secondary hyperparathyroidism in moderate renal insufficiency. *J Clin Endocrinol Metab* 1985;61:601–606.
A study in patients with early renal failure delineating the interaction between phosphate retention, skeletal resistance to the calcemic action of PTH, and vitamin D metabolism in the genesis of secondary hyperparathyroidism.

Martin KJ, Gonzalez EA, Gellens M, et al. 19-nor-1-a-25 dihydroxyvitamin D_3 (Paricalcitol) safely and effectively reduces the levels of intact parathyroid hormone in patients on hemodialysis. *J Am Soc Nephrol* 1998;9:1427–1432.
A detailed description of the results of three double-blind, placebo-controlled trials on the effect of Paricalcitol in hemodialysis patients with secondary hyperparathyroidism. Paricalcitol effectively reduced the blood levels of PTH with fewer hypercalcemia.

Massry SG, Coburn JW, Lee DBN, et al. Skeletal resistance to parathyroid hormone in renal failure: study in 105 human subjects. *Ann Intern Med* 1973;78: 357–367.
The first detailed study demonstrating skeletal resistance to the calcemic action of PTH in patients with early and advanced renal failure, in patients treated with hemodialysis, and in transplant recipients.

Massry SG, Goldstein DA, Malluche HH. Current status of the use of $1,25(OH)_2D_3$ in the management of renal osteodystrophy. *Kidney Int* 1980;18:409–418.
An editorial review analyzing the data on the use of $1,25(OH)_2D_3$ in the treatment of derangements of divalent ion metabolism in patients with renal failure and in patients treated with dialysis.

Massry SG, Kopple JD. Requirements for calcium, phosphorus, and vitamin D. In: Mitch WE, Klahr S, eds: *Nutrition and the kidney,* 2nd ed. Boston: Little, Brown, 1993:96–113.

A detailed discussion of the metabolism of calcium, phosphorus, and vitamin D in normal subjects and in patients with renal failure. Has with 85 references.

Parfitt AM. Soft-tissue calcification in uremia. *Arch Intern Med* 1969;124:544–556.

An excellent description of the pathogenesis and clinical manifestations of soft tissue calcification in patients with advanced renal failure and patients treated with hemodialysis.

Proudfoot D, Shanahan CM, Weissberg PL. Vascular calcification: New insights into an old problem. *J Pathol* 1998;185:1–3.

An editorial discussing the molecular bases for intimal and medical vascular calcifications.

Sherrard DJ, Hercz G, Peiy M, et al. The spectrum of bone disease in end stage renal failure—on evolving disorder. *Kidney Int* 1993;43:436–442.

An excellent study on bone disease in patients with renal failure.

Statopolsky E, Weerts C, Thielan J, et al. Marked suppression of secondary hyperparathyroidism by intravenous administration of 1,25-dihydroxycholecalciferol in uremic patients. *J Clin Invest* 1984;74:2136–2143.

The first report on the use of intravenous $1,25(OH)_2D_3$ in dialysis patients. This made of therapy proved more effective than the oral use of this vitamin D metabolite in suppressing the activity of the parathyroid glands.

Slatopolsky EA, Burke SK, Dillon MA, The RenaGel Study Group. RenaGel, a nonabsorbed calcium- and aluminum-free phosphate binder, lowers serum phosphorus and parathyroid hormone. *Kidney Int* 1999;55:299–307.

It describes the results of a study on the effect of RenaGel on serum levels of phosphorus and PTH in 172 patients treated with hemodialysis. This phosphate binder is effective in controlling the hyperphosphatemia of renal failure patients.

Urena, P, de Vernejoul M-C. Circulating biochemical markers of bone remolding in uremic patients. *Kidney Int* 1999;55:2141–2156.

A review on the usefulness of the various blood markers for the detection of the state of bone turn over in patients with CRF.

CHAPTER 78

Uremic Myopathy

Eberhard Ritz, Michael Schoemig, and Shaul G. Massry

Patients with chronic renal failure may experience muscle dysfunction for a variety of reasons (Table 78.1). However, some uremic patients manifest a specific myopathy, presumably caused by abnormal vitamin D metabolism, and it usually improves or reverses after therapy with active metabolites of the vitamin. It is this muscle disease that we refer to as *uremic myopathy.*

PATHOGENESIS

Vitamin D deficiency is the main cause of uremic myopathy. Other factors such as secondary hyperparathyroidism, disturbances in the concentrations of calcium and phosphorous in the extracellular and/or intracellular compartments, and vascular calcification are contributory.

Clinical and experimental evidence indicate that vitamin D is important for the normal function and structural integrity of the skeletal muscle, and its deficiency may be associated with myopathy even in the presence of normal renal function. Indeed, in rachitic children and in adult patients with nutritional vitamin D deficiency or those treated with anticonvulsant medications, myopathy is not uncommonly encountered. It is characterized by asthenia and muscle wasting without fascination of fibrillation and by low serum concentrations of muscle enzymes. The changes are most prominent in the proximal muscles of the lower extremity.

Studies of muscle from experimental animals with uremia demonstrated abnormalities of force generation, disturbed calcium transport in subcellular membranes (sarcoplasmic reticulum), abnormal polypeptide chains of the troponin molecules, disturbed function of actinomycin ATPase, and abnormal adenosine nucleotides and creatinine phosphate content. Many of these abnormalities disappeared after administration of vitamin D or its metabolites, notably 1,25-dihydroxyvitamin D_3 [1,25$(OH)_2D_3$], despite persisting uremia. Available data suggest that both 25(OH)D and 1,25$(OH)_2$D are important for muscle function, and these metabolites may affect different aspects of muscle metabolism. *In vitro* studies showed that 25(OH)D, but not 1,25$(OH)_2$D, stimulated protein synthesis in muscle. However, in other experimental models, including experimental uremia, 1,25$(OH)_2$D acted on muscle in the absence of added 25(OH)D. The effects of vitamin D metabolites on muscle are not surprising in view of the demonstration that skeletal muscle phenotypically expresses receptors for 1,25$(OH)_2$ vitamin D_3. 1,25(OH)2D3 has been shown to influence subcellular calcium fluxes and total calcium content of myocytes.

There is also evidence for direct actions of parathyroid hormone (PTH) on muscle cells, mediated by adenylate cyclase–independent, protein kinase C–dependent pathways. PTH raises intracellular calcium uptake via voltage-dependent transmembrane Ca channels and causes metabolic abnormalities, for example, diminished oxidation of long-chain fatty acids, by reducing the activity of carnitine palmitoyl transferase and by diminishing fatty acid transport into the mitochondrial matrix. PTH also impairs energy production, shuttle, and utilization by skeletal muscle in rats, and it enhances muscle proteolysis and increases the release of alanine and glutamine from skeletal muscle. Also, muscle dysfunction is encountered in patients with primary hyperparathyroidism. It is therefore possible that the state of secondary hyperparathyroidism in uremia participates in the genesis of uremic myopathy. Further discussion of the interaction between PTH and skeletal muscle is provided in Chapter 68, Part 1.

Histochemical studies of muscle of uremic patients invariably show atrophy of individual muscle fibers, which preferentially affects type II rather than type I fibers. Type II fibers (white) are large, fast-contracting fibers that contain little myoglobin and have predominantly glycolytic metabolism. These fibers are involved in phasic contractions of muscle. They un-

TABLE 78.1. Causes of Muscle Dysfunction in Chronic Uremia

Peripheral neuropathy
Muscle cramps
Restless leg syndrome
Myopathy as a manifestation of disease underlying uremia
Lupus erythematosus
Polyarteritis nodosa
Systemic sclerosis
Diabetes mellitus
Amyloidosis
Carcinomatosis
Drug toxicity
Glucocorticoids
Clofibrate
Phosphate binders causing severe hypophosphatemia
Aluminum toxicity
Iron overload
Colchicine
Myopathy related to disturbances of uremic states
Catabolism
Inactivity
Hyperparathyroidism
Ischemia (vascular calcification)
Uremic toxins?
Myopathy related to disturbed vitamin D metabolism

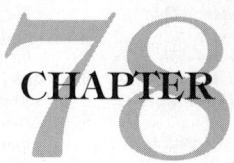

dergo preferential atrophy after various forms of neuronal damage. In contrast, type I fibers (red) are small, myoglobin-rich fibers that contain numerous mitochondria and have predominantly oxidative metabolism. Such fibers contract slowly and are involved in tonic contractions of muscle. These fibers can be classified on the basis of Ca-activated myosin ATPase (pH 9.4) and NADH-diaphorase activities. Preferential atrophy of type II fibers in uremic patients is presumably the consequence of neuronal damage secondary to neuropathy. Obvious myopathic features (e.g., necrosis and phagocytosis of fibers or pronounced increase of endomysial tissue) are usually lacking. However, several discrete additional findings point to the coexistence of some nonneuronal damage. These include abnormal cytoarchitecture (i.e., localized areas of severe disorganization of the myofibrillar pattern with the moth-eaten appearance of type I fibers, decay of mitochondria or lysosomes at the cell periphery, appearance of fragments of myofilaments, and dispersion of Z-line material). The aforementioned abnormalities of muscle fiber cytoarchitecture in uremic patients normalize after the administration of vitamin D metabolites.

In some uremic patients, the electromyogram (EMG) reveals abnormal polyphasic motor unit potentials of brief duration and small amplitude. Such findings are analogous to the observations in myopathy of vitamin D deficiency or hyperparathyroidism. These findings in themselves are not diagnostic of myopathy and merely indicate functional or structural fractionation and decreased size of the motor unit (i.e., a diminished number of fibers). They may either result from loss of function of some, but not all, axonal endings of many motor units (neurogenic) or else from random loss of muscle fibers (myopathic). Consequently, the EMG in itself is not helpful in establishing the presence of a primary (i.e., nonneurogenic) form of muscle disease.

METABOLIC ABNORMALITIES

Studies on muscle protein turnover and amino acid exchange across skeletal muscle of uremic patients showed increased release and reuptake of phenylalanine reflecting a concomitant increase of both proteolysis and protein synthesis. Both processes were related to acidosis and plasma cortisol concentration. For more details, the reader is referred to Chapter 68, Part 6. The net amino acid balance across the muscle was not changed. Low intracellular concentrations of several amino acids (e.g., threonine, valine, tyrosine, and a high glycine : valine phenylalanin : tyrosine ratio) were noted. Resistance to insulinlike growth factor 1, secondary to a postreceptor defect, has also been documented.

Using ^{31}P magnetic resonance spectroscopy, it was noted that the calculated maximal oxidative capacity was significantly reduced in subjects with terminal renal failure, and it remained abnormal despite partial correction of anemia.

During exercise, increased phosphocreatine breakdown was accompanied by rapid intracellular acidification and increased lactic acid accumulation, suggesting that glycolysis predominated over oxidative phosphorylation.

Studies measuring contractile properties of the quadriceps muscle found muscle weakness, which was present even when weakness was subtle or absent on clinical examination. This abnormality was correlated to low serum albumin concentration, suggesting that muscle function depends on nutritional state. Exercise training partially reverses muscle atrophy in renal patients and causes an increase in the proportion of type II fibers and muscle fiber area. Because of the availability of rhEPO treatment, the potential relation of abnormal muscle function to anemia commands great interest. Despite partial correction of anemia, peak V_{O_2} (oxygen uptake) increased only moderately by erythropoietin, which is largely explained by reduced peak blood flow to exercising muscle limiting the gain in oxygen transport. Flow limitation is due to exhypoxic vasoconstriction.

Several other abnormalities of muscle metabolism have been demonstrated in experimental uremia. Increased proteolysis was observed in muscle of uremic animals during the fasting state. Also, *in vitro* studies showed increased release of alanine and some other amino acids from muscle of uremic animals. The amino acid release varied with protein intake and administration of insulin and could be modified by administration of vitamin D metabolites. Finally, loss of muscle glycogen was observed in acute experimental renal failure, and impaired lactate production after ischemic forearm exercise was found in uremic patients.

CLINICAL MANIFESTATIONS

In addition to easy fatigability and asthenia, patients with uremic myopathy experience difficulty in performing acts involving tonic contractions of shoulder or pelvic girdles such as climbing or descending stairs, arising from a squatting or kneeling position, negotiating curbstones, getting out of a bathtub, combing hair, putting an object on a high shelf, or cleaning windows. An aching sensation in fatigued muscles may be noted. Of particular importance is the propensity of patients with uremic myopathy to fatigue of respiratory muscles. The latter has repeatedly been shown to respond to parathyroidectomy.

On physical examination, patients exhibit muscle weakness, particularly of the proximal muscles of the lower extremities. Weakness of the thighs commonly begins before and is more severe than weakness of the arms. Muscles that are weak appear flaccid to palpation. The tendon reflexes, in contrast, may occasionally be hyperactive, unless neuropathy is present. Objective evidence of impaired muscle strength may be obtained by dynamometry.

DIAGNOSIS

Complaints of asthenia and loss of muscular force are nonspecific and common in uremic patients. The presence of the uremic myopathy can be established by the characteristic history, by the coexistence of severe uremic osteodystrophy (particularly osteomalacia), and by maneuvers that elicit dysfunction of tonic contraction of the muscles of the shoulder and pelvic girdles.

The serum levels of muscle enzymes (creatine phosphokinase and aldolase) are normal both in the basal state and after exercise. The changes in EMG are characteristic but nonspecific. There are no other clinical procedures to diagnose uremic myopathy. Muscle histology, histochemistry, electron microscopy, and biochemical measurements of muscle energetics such as inorganic phosphorus, adenine nucleotides, and creatine phosphate levels may be useful. These compounds usually occur in lowered concentrations in uremic myopathy.

DIFFERENTIAL DIAGNOSIS

The most important differential diagnosis is between vitamin D–responsive uremic myopathy and muscle dysfunction caused by neuropathy because both abnormalities may coexist in the same patient. Some helpful differentiating features are listed in Table 78.2.

TABLE 78.2. Features Differentiating Uremic Myopathy from Muscle Dysfunction Caused by Neuropathy

Feature	Uremic Myopathy	Muscle Dysfunction Caused by Neuropathy
Preferential localization	Proximal muscle of lower extremity and upper extremity	Distal muscle of lower extremity
Sensory disturbances	None	++
Decreased nerve conduction velocity	None	++
Electromyogram	Polyphasic, brief duration, small amplitude potentials	Defective recruitment during maximal voluntary effort
Muscle wasting	±	++
Tendon reflexes	Present	Absent
Therapy	Vitamin D metabolites	Adequate dialysis

Disturbances in muscle function secondary to metabolic myopathy or neuropathy must also be distinguished from several other muscle dysfunctions that may be encountered in uremic patients (Table 78.1). *Diminished muscular strength,* as evaluated by standard dynamometric tests, is occasionally encountered even in asymptomatic, well-rehabilitated patients being treated with hemodialysis. This may be the result of redistribution of fiber composition, structural damage, loss of training, subclinical neuropathy, anemia, and abnormal muscle metabolism.

Muscle cramps unrelated to myopathy are a common complication of hemodialysis and are less commonly observed in uremic patients not receiving hemodialysis. Cramps may be extremely painful. They usually involve the lower limbs. The patients commonly lack evidence of neuropathy or tetany. Although cramps are unimportant with respect to the patient's survival, they may be of paramount importance for the patient's rehabilitation. The pathogenesis of these cramps has not been completely elucidated, but clinical observations suggest that hyponatremia and hypovolemia play a major role in their development. These problems may respond to administration of magnesium salts and quinine.

Restless leg is an ill-defined sensation of discomfort in the feet and lower legs, which is partially relieved by frequent movement of the lower extremities. Its appearance is not necessarily followed by other evidence of neuropathy such as paresthesia of the soles of the feet, loss of distal reflexes, or loss of position and vibratory sense. The relationship, if any, of the restless leg syndrome to neuropathy is still controversial. Promising therapeutic results have been described after administration of pergolide and pramipexole.

Myopathic changes secondary to *steroid* therapy are common in patients with renal failure. Steroid myopathy causes wasting and diminution of muscle strength, which primarily affect the proximal muscles of the lower extremities without muscle pain. The electromyogram shows small but abundant action potentials. Muscle biopsy results reveal evidence of atrophy that preferentially affects type II fibers, an increase of muscle glycogen content, and few degenerating and regenerating muscle fibers without infiltrates. Serum levels of muscle enzymes are normal or slightly elevated. There is no clear-cut relation to steroid dose, but the myopathy appears to be more common after therapy with fluorinated steroid derivatives.

Clofibrate has been used in the therapy of uremic hyperlipoproteinemia. Because the metabolite of clofibrate, clofibrinic acid, is excreted by the kidneys, it accumulates in the blood of patients with chronic renal failure. In uremic patients treated with clofibrate, severe myalgia may be observed when the levels of the drug are in the toxic range. Muscle histologic examination shows muscle fiber necrosis. The serum levels of muscle enzymes and heart enzymes are elevated. These changes are reversed when clofibrate is withheld.

Postoperative rhabdomyolysis has also been observed in patients with end-stage renal failure. It has been ascribed to precipitating factors (e.g. opiates, anaesthetic agents, and surgical position).

THERAPY

The administration of 0.5 to 1.5 μg/day of $1,25(OH)_2D_3$ is beneficial in the treatment of uremic myopathy. The initial dose is 0.5 μg/day and could be increased gradually to achieve the beneficial effect. Improvement in muscle weakness usually occurs within 2 to 5 weeks, and complete disappearance of the clinical manifestations of uremic myopathy occurs in most patients within a few months of therapy. Occasionally, prolonged therapy for periods of 1 to 2 years and large doses of $1,25(OH)_2D_3$ up to 2.5 to 3.0 μg/day are required before improvement or cure of the myopathy ensues. Finally, a small group of patients may fail to respond to treatment with $1,25(OH)_2D_3$. A hazardous complication of treatment with $1,25(OH)_2D_3$ is the development of hypercalcemia. Therapy should be discontinued when hypercalcemia appears and reinstituted at a smaller dose upon the return of serum calcium to a normal level. In the patient whose muscle performance is reduced in the absence of overt abnormalities of calcium metabolism, one should consider physical exercise, correction of anemia, optimal nutrition, and intensified dialysis treatment (if polyneuropathy is present). The administration of L-carnitine is still controversial.

Selected Readings

Baczynski R, Massry SG, Magott M, et al. Effect of parathyroid hormone on energy metabolism of skeletal muscle. *Kidney Int* 1985;28:722–727.

Original publication on effects of PTH on energy production, mitochondrial creatine phosphokinase, and Mg-ATPase, and myofibrillar creatine phosphokinase in skeletal muscle.

Birge S. Vitamin D, muscle and phosphate homeostasis. *Miner Electrolyte Metab* 1978;1:57–64.

State-of-the-art review of the field.

Ding H, Gao XL, Hirschberg R, et al. Impaired actions of insulin-like growth factor 1 on protein synthesis and degradation in skeletal muscle of rats with chronic renal failure. Evidence for a postreceptor defect. *J Clin Invest* 1996; 15:1064–1075.

An experimental study documenting a hormonally mediated defect in protein metabolism in skeletal muscle of uremic rats.

Durozard D, Pimmel P, Baretto S, et al. ^{31}P NMR spectroscopy investigation of muscle metabolism in hemodialysis patients. *Kidney Int* 1993;43:885–892.

A human study providing information on energy metabolism in exercising and resting muscle.

Garibotto G, Russo R, Sofia A, et al. Skeletal muscle protein synthesis and degradation in patients with chronic renal failure. *Kidney Int* 1994;45:1432–1439.

Study on 9 hemodialysis patients showing changes in muscle protein turnover and amino acid exchange by using the arterio-venous difference technique.

Goodhue WW, Davis JN, Porro RS. Ischemic myopathy in uremic hyperparathyroidism. *JAMA* 1972;221:911–912.

Description of ischemic myopathy in uremic patients with advanced secondary hyperparathyroidism.

Marrades RM, Roca J, Campistol JM, et al. Effects of erythropoietin on muscle O2 transport during exercise in patients with chronic renal failure. *J Clin Invest* 1996;97:2092–2100.

An excellent study providing information on limitations of oxygen supply when hematocrit is raised.

Moore GE, Bertocci LA, Painter PL. ^{31}P-magnetic resonance spectroscopy assessment of subnormal oxidative metabolism in skeletal muscle of renal failure patients. *J Clin Invest* 1993;91:420–424.

Another study on skeletal muscle metabolism in uremic patients.

Ori Y, Korzets A, Gruzman C, et al. Postoperative rhabdomyolysis in patients with end-stage renal failure. *Am J Kidney Dis* 1998;31:539–544.

Description of muscular complications in hemodialyzed patients after major surgery.

Perma AF, Smogorzewski M, Massry SG. Verapamil reverses PTH- or CRF-induced abnormal fatty acids oxidation in muscle. *Kidney Int* 1988;34:774–778.

An excellent study confirming a role for PTH in abnormal muscle metabolism in uremia.

Ritz E, Boland R, Kreusser W. Effects of vitamin D and PTH on muscle-potential role in uremic myopathy. *Am J Clin Nutr* 1980;33:1522–1529.

State-of-the-art review of the interactions of PTH and vitamin D metabolites with skeletal muscle; includes description of clinical syndromes and molecular mechanisms.

Smogorzewski M, Piskorska G, Borum PR, et al. Chronic renal failure, parathyroid hormone, and fatty acids oxidation in skeletal muscle. *Kidney Int* 1988;33:556–560.

One of the original studies showing an effect of PTH on oxidation of long-chain fatty acids via an effect of mitochondrial enzymes.

Thompson CH, Kemp GJ, Barnes PR, et al. Uraemic muscle metabolism at rest and during exercise. *Nephrol Dial Transplant* 1994;9:1600–1605.

NMR spectroscopy study on muscle metabolism in uremic patients.

CHAPTER 79

Articular Complications in Uremia

Shaul G. Massry, Miroslaw Smogorzewski, and Glenn R. Ehresmann

Articular and rheumatic disorders are major complications of uremia and are more frequently seen in dialysis patients. The most common causes of arthropathy in patients with end-stage renal failure are listed in Table 79.1.

Uremic patients with articular complaints may have true arthritis manifested with swelling, pain, limitation of range of motion, and warmth of the involved joints, or they may have periarticular involvement with periarteritis or tendonitis. In patients with periarteritis, the swelling of the joints is less pronounced and active motion is difficult, while passive motion is usually preserved.

Arthritis in the uremic patient could manifest itself as a monoarthritis or polyarthritis. When true arthritis is present, the differential diagnosis should take into account the underlying diseases that may cause arthritis and lead to renal failure, as well as the metabolic and/or immunologic disturbances in the uremic patient that may be associated with arthritis. Another form of arthropathy, which is encountered mainly in the dialysis patients, is due to dialysis-associated amyloidosis, and this type of arthropathy is called *dialysis-associated arthropathy* (DAA).

TABLE 79.1 Causes of Arthritis in Uremia

Crystal-Induced Arthritis: Monoarticular or Polyarticular
Gout—monosodium urate crystals
Pseudogout—calcium pyrophosphate dihydrate crystals
Hydroxyapatite crystal deposition disease
Calcium oxalate crystal synovitis
Septic Arthritis
Polyarthritis
Rheumatoid arthritis
Systemic lupus erythematosus
Scleroderma
Spondyloarthropathy
Ankylosing spondylitis
Reiter's syndrome
Inflammatory bowel disease
Psoriasis
β_2M amyloid arthropathy

CRYSTAL-ASSOCIATED ARTHRITIS

Crystal deposition in joints is a common cause for arthritis in uremic patients. These crystals may be monosodium urate causing gout, calcium pyrophosphate dihydrate causing pseudogout, basic calcium phosphate such as hydroxyapatite or osteocalcium phosphate (these crystals may also cause periarthritis), and calcium oxalate.

Gout

Gout may antedate the uremia or develop as a consequence of prolonged hyperuricemia in patients with renal failure. It is more common in patients with renal insufficiency than in those with advanced renal failure, and it is rare in patient treated with dialysis. Typically, gouty episodes begin at nighttime with acute and severe pain in one or more joints. About 50% of patients initially have metatarsal-phalangeal swelling and pain, but patients with uremia initially have atypical features. Attacks tend to occur and resolve without specific treatment, generally within 5 to 15 days. Often, the patient will have a history of smaller episodes before a severe episode precipitates physician consultation. Confirmation of suspected gout is made by diagnostic joint aspiration; this procedure also excludes the possibility of infection and assesses whether the clinical symptoms are caused by other crystal arthropathies.

The synovial fluid of a patient with gouty arthropathy demonstrates mild inflammatory changes with white blood cell (WBC) counts ranging from 2,000 to 40,000 WBCs, principally polymorphonuclear cells. The polarizing microscope will be necessary to demonstrate the negatively birefringent crystals.

Attacks of gouty arthritis occur after renal transplantation and result from the use of cyclosporine. Indeed, cyclosporine impairs renal urate clearance, so hyperuricemia occurs in up to 90% and gouty arthritis in up to 24% of cyclosporine recipients.

Pseudogout

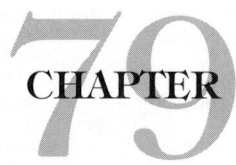

Pseudogout is also a common acute crystalline arthritis seen in patients with uremia. It results from the deposition of calcium pyrophosphate crystal, and it less common than arthropathy caused by urate or basic calcium crystal deposition and is rare in dialysis patients. Symptoms may occur acutely after trauma to individual joints or after metabolic changes associated with surgery or acute medical illnesses. Pseudogout has been reported after parathyroidectomy. The symptoms may be as severe as an acute gouty episode, but they typically involve the knee or the wrist more often than the first metatarsal-phalangeal joint. The radiographic features of this disease with the chondrocalcinosis in the meniscal cartilage of the knees or the triangular cartilage of the wrists is particularly helpful in evaluating for the possibility of pseudogout. The calcium pyrophosphate crystals appear as punctate and linear calcification and may involve joint capsules, ligaments, and tendons in addition to the joint cartilage. However, the appearance of chondrocalcinosis on the radiograph is not diagnostic of pseudogout. The joint must be aspirated to demonstrate the presence of weakly positively birefringent crystals by polarizing microscopy to confirm the diagnosis and exclude the possibility of infection.

Calcium Oxalate Crystals

This form of arthropathy is rare in dialysis patients and results from the formation calcium oxalate crystals within the joints or from deposition of these crystals in the joints. It has been observed especially in patients ingesting large amounts of ascorbic acid, which subsequently metabolized to oxalate. Thus excessive intake of vitamin C should be avoided. There is a report of a patient who developed widespread deposition of calcium oxalate in the skin and joints even though the patient did not ingest vitamin supplementation.

Typically, patients with calcium oxalate arthropathy have an acute monoarticular arthritis, although subacute and more chronic polyarticular symptoms may also be present. The crystals can be seen by examination of the synovial fluid with polarizing light microscopy. These patients may have diffuse swelling of an involved finger, or occasionally, a large joint will have effusion and inflammatory fluid.

Basic Calcium Phosphate

Occasionally, a uremic patient will manifest an acute arthritis, typically monoarticular, with inflammatory joint fluid, but evidence of crystals will not be found on polarizing microscopy. In the absence of evidence for infection, the possibility of basic calcium phosphate crystals should be considered. These crystals are ill defined and nonbirefringent. Because of their small size, they are not seen on usual polarizing microscopy of synovial fluid. It is necessary to stain the joint fluid with Alizarin red to detect calcium-containing particles. A more sensitive and specific assay for these crystals is done by incubating the joint fluid with [^{14}C]ethane-1-hydroxy-1,1,diphosphonate (EHDP). This binds to the crystal surface and makes it possible to sediment the crystals in the fluid for direct visualization.

Hydroxyapatite Crystals

Another crystal that results in musculoskeletal symptoms is hydroxyapatite. This results in a calcific periarthritis in uremic patients rather than an actual acute arthritis. The distinction between these two can be difficult clinically at times. The usual patient with calcific periarthritis has marked redness and swelling of the overlying skin, but in a periarticular distribution, or alone in a known anatomic tendonous distribution. Typically, one area is involved, but at times, there may be several areas. These calcific hydroxyapatite deposition episodes are seen in patients who have an elevated plasma calcium-phosphorous product, especially when the latter exceeds 70. Patients who are at risk for metastatic soft tissue calcium deposition are particularly prone to such attacks. X-ray examination of the involved area may demonstrate signs of soft tissue swelling and some speckling with fluffy radiopaque deposits.

Treatment of Crystal-Induced Arthropathy

Treatment of the uremic patient with crystalline arthropathy must be individualized. Aspiration of the joint is important for diagnosis, but it also may relieve considerable symptoms by reducing the crystal burden. The patients may have some additional response by splinting to rest an involved joint such as a wrist for several days. It is important to be sure that the patient does not develop a contracture, and daily range of motion of the involved joint should be encouraged.

Specific therapies for crystalline arthritis include nonsteroidal antiinflammatory agents or occasionally intravenous colchicine with the dosage reduced to one-third to half normal because of potential severe multisystem toxicity. Colchicine, which has been most useful for episodes of gout or pseudogout, is less effective for calcium hydroxyapatite or calcium oxalate arthritis. Oral colchicine at reduced dosage can be used briefly as well, but diarrhea and occasionally cytopenia are problematic. Long-term use of colchicine should be discouraged because of the potential development of myopathy.

The nonsteroidal medications are used with caution in patients with uremia, and their dosage should be reduced because most of these drugs are excreted by the kidney. Indomethacin, which has principal hepatic excretion, may be a consideration. The physician and the patient must be aware of potential gastrointestinal complications of these drugs. All of the magnesium-containing salicylate preparations are to be avoided in patients with renal failure because they induce hypermagnesemia. The nonsteroidal medications should be given for a brief course titrated to the patient's acute symptoms and then discontinued.

In joints where crystals have been demonstrated and there is no evidence of infection, local installation of corticosteroid is very effective for acute crystal arthritis and may be safer than systemic use of nonsteroidal medications.

POLYARTHRITIS

Uremic patients with common causes of inflammatory arthritis such as rheumatoid arthritis, systemic lupus erythematosus, and various spondyloarthropathies may have substantial decrease in their symptoms as their uremia progresses. Often, such patients can be maintained with much less medication, generally nonsteroidal antiinflammatory agents, than they required before the onset of uremia and/or dialysis. Medications commonly used to treat rheumatoid arthritis, such as gold compounds and D-penicillamine, should be avoided in the uremic patient because of the renal excretion of these agents and the potential of bone marrow and other toxicities. Patients with calcium pyrophosphate dihydrate crystal deposition disease may have associated hyperparathyroidism; 5% of these patients will have a chronic polyarthritis resembling rheumatoid arthritis. Symptoms may fluctuate with metabolic and medical illnesses associated with their uremia.

ARTHROPATHY DUE TO SECONDARY HYPERPARATHYROIDISM

Patients with uremia and secondary hyperparathyroidism develop erosive changes of large and small joints, and they are subject to episodes of recurring arthritis, which are typically associated with noninflammatory joint fluids. It is suspected that basic calcium phosphate crystals are involved in the pathogenesis of this process, which results in proteolytic enzymes being released to damaged cartilage, bone, and tendons. Lesions are typically seen in the shoulders of such patients, but other areas are also frequently involved. Severe hyperparathyroidism in dialysis patients is associated with aseptic necrosis of the head of the femur and cause pain in the hip joints.

UNEXPLAINED JOINT INFLAMMATORY EFFUSIONS

Occasionally, unexplained joint inflammatory effusions are encountered in dialysis patients. This condition may mimic other inflammatory joint disease, but no cause could be identified. Joint fluid may revel the presence of aluminum, iron, and/or liquid lipid crystals. All these compounds may induce joint inflammation

AMYLOID-ASSOCIATED ARTHROPATHY

Amyloid-associated arthropathy is seen in patients treated with hemodialysis or continuous ambulatory peritoneal dialysis for a long period. Indeed, its prevalence increases with the duration of the dialysis therapy. Its prevalences also rises with increased age of the patients. It results from deposition of β_2-microglobulin (β_2M) amyloid fibrils in osteoarticular locations. β_2M blood levels in dialysis patients are high, and the mechanisms for this phenomenon are not fully understood; they are discussed in detail in Chapter 84, Part 1E. Apparently, the β_2M fibrils are modified by a nonenzymatic combination of protein amino groups with sugar aldehyde groups to form advanced glycated end-products (AGEs). The AGEs may be generated in the blood or in the sites of β_2M deposition, and the generation of these AGEs may be enhanced by the oxidative stress associated with chronic uremia (see Chapter 68, Part 7). These AGEs would bind to AGE receptors on monocytes and macrophages, resulting in the release of tumor necrosis factor-α and interleukin-1β; these compounds may be the mediators of β_2M-related bone disease. This arthropathy is commonly called *DAA.* It presents clinically with pain and stiffness of various joints such as the shoulder, knee, wrist, and small joints of the hand. The patient may experience restriction of movement of these joints. Another feature of DAA is chronic joint swelling, recurrent hemarthrosis, and chronic tenosynovitis of the finger flexors.

β_2M amyloid deposition may involve the cervical vertebrae, causing destructive spondyloarthritis. This event may be asymptomatic or associated with mild cervical pain. Rarely, this may cause compression of nerve root.

Another clinical presentation of DAA is carpal tunnel syndrome, which presents with pain and numbness of the hand. This syndrome could be unilateral or bilateral.

The roentgenographic findings of DAA are multiple subchondral bone cysts and articular erosions as a result of the replacement of subchondral bone by β_2M amyloid (see Chapter 84, Part 1E, Fig. 84.22).

Several tools have been used for the diagnosis of DAA. These tools include regular x-ray examinations, ultrasound, computed axial tomography (CAT) scan, or magnetic resonance imaging (MRI). Plain radiography and MRI provide the most useful information. Bone scan using radiolabeled diphosphonate may be useful in detecting increased uptake of involved areas, but this test is not specific. Scintigraphy using ^{123}I-radiolabeled P component (SAP) or ^{131}I-radiolabeled β_2M is a better technique for localization of the β_2M amyloid. These radiolabeled compounds are no longer in use and have been replaced by ^{111}In-radiolabeled β_2M. Aspiration of synovial fluid may not provide definite diagnosis of β_2M amyloid arthropathy but may help to rule out crystal-associated arthropathy.

Patients with carpal tunnel syndrome may have positive Phalen's and Tinel's signs. The Phalen's sign is elicited by holding the patient's wrist in acute passive flexion for a minute. If positive, tingling and paresthesia in the median nerve region would be felt by the patient. Positive Tinel's sign is the production of tingling and paresthesia over the volar radial aspect of the hand by percussing the volar wrist over the carpal tunnel. Electromyography and nerve conduction test will confirm the diagnosis.

There is no specific treatment of DAA. Therefore therapy is aimed at relieving pain. This could be achieved by use of nonsteroidal antiinflammatory drugs. Acute monoarthritis may be treated with local or systemic glucocorticoids. Carpal tunnel syndrome may be treated with local splinting; and in refractory patients, the treatment is surgical to achieve decompression.

Once β_2M amyloid has been deposited, it cannot be removed. Therefore successful renal transplantation cannot reverse the disease, but it certainly can arrest its progression. However, symptomatic improvement occurs after transplantation. The mechanism(s) for this improvement are not evident but may be related to the routine use of glucocorticoids in transplant recipients.

Selected Readings

Bardin T, Lebail-Darne JL, Zingraph J, et al. Dialysis arthropathy: outcome after renal transplantation. *Am J Med* 1995;99:243–248.

Discusses the effect of renal transplantation on β_2M amyloid arthropathy. Renal transplantation may arrest progression of the disease and is associated with symptomatic improvement.

Caner J, Decker J. Recurrent acute arthritis in chronic renal failure treated with periodic hemodialysis. *Am J Med* 1964;36:571–582.

This original article describes the acute periarticular calcifications associated with hydroxyapatite crystals.

Drüeke T. Extraskeletal problems and amyloid. *Kidney Int* 1999;56:S89–S93.

An excellent review of β_2M arthropathy in dialysis patients. He sites β_2 relevant references.

Goldstein S, Winston E, Chung T, et al. Chronic arthropathy in long-term hemodialysis. *Am J Med* 1985;78:82–86.

This is a review article recognizing the high frequency of joint symptoms in patients receiving chronic hemodialysis treatment, with 9 of 11 patients completing more than 10 years of dialysis demonstrating either acute or chronic joint involvement with radiographic correlation.

Nakazawa R, Hamaguchi K, Hosaka E, et al. Cutaneous oxalate deposition in a hemodialysis patient. *Am J Kidney Dis* 1995;25:492–497.

A case report and a review of the literature of calcium oxalate deposition arthropathy in a dialysis patient and a review of the literature.

Reginato A, Ferreiro Seoane J, et al. Arthropathy and cutaneous calcinosis in hemodialysis oxalosis. *Arthritis Rheum* 1986;29:1387–1396.

This is a report of the dactylitis associated with calcium hydroxylate deposition.

CHAPTER 80

Immunological Disturbances in Uremia

Lucienne Chatenoud and Béatrice Descamps-Latscha

The Increased Frequency of Infections in Patients with End-Stage Renal Disease

Patients undergoing a progressive deterioration of renal function invariably exhibit a complex immunodeficiency syndrome that is secondary to uremia and that represents a major cause of morbidity and mortality. Thus it is this immunodeficiency state that explains the high frequency of bacterial, mycobacterial, and viral infections observed in patients with end-stage renal disease (ESRD). In some reported series, infections accounted for 36% of mortality both in old and young ESRD patients (40 years of age or younger). These infectious processes were mostly due to commonly occurring microorganisms and not to opportunistic agents; their elective target sites and causal pathogens were frequently dictated by repetitive exposure to certain obvious risk factors (e.g., urinary tract infections mediated by *Escherichia coli*). The immunodeficiency syndrome also accounts for the increased incidence of infections due to intracellular pathogens (tuberculosis, listeriosis) observed in ESRD. Other reports have confirmed that ESRD patients are at increased risk for developing active tuberculosis after primary infection and have pointed out the need for a more regular tuberculin skin test assessment and isoniazid prophylaxis. The abnormal response of ESRD patients to viral infections is also well established, one of the best examples being the hepatitis B virus (HBV) infection. Until 1982, when the vaccination became available, hepatitis B was a source of considerable morbidity and mortality among ESRD patients. In the absence of active immunization, ESRD patients were unable to eradicate HBV and easily become chronic carriers (30% as compared with 5% in the normal population). We shall also allude later to the well-known poorer response to HBV vaccination that ESRD patients exhibit as compared with normal subjects; this requires the use of reinforced vaccination protocols to induce and maintain protective antibody levels, especially in aged patients. Needless to say, the other hepatitis viruses, including the C virus (HCV), are now posing almost the same problem HBV represented in before a vaccination was available.

It is important to stress at this point that the improvements in renal replacement therapies, and particularly hemodialysis, did not reverse uremia-induced immunodeficiency syndrome and the various clinical problems linked to it. Thus patients treated with hemodialysis show severely impaired humoral and cellular immune responses as illustrated by their cutaneous anergy and the completely inadapted response to bacterial, mycobacterial, and viral infections. Albeit indirectly, these epidemiologic facts indicate that the initiating pathogenetic event responsible for the immunodeficiency is directly linked to uremia.

The aim of this chapter is to discuss the various immunologic disturbances found in ESRD patients, before and after the institution of renal replacement therapy. We shall first introduce some general principles that govern immune responses, and then we will address, in the context of ESRD, the abnormalities of both specific and nonspecific immunity pathways, with particular attention being focused on T lymphocytes mediating cellular immunity; B lymphocytes mediating humoral immunity; monocyte and macrophages, which are major antigen-presenting cells (APC) but also play an important role in inflammatory responses; and polymorphonuclear neutrophils. Throughout this discussion, it will become clear that one converging although puzzling feature is that the ESRD immunodeficiency syndrome is associated with clear-cut signs of immune cell activation. Finally, based on the available data, some etiologic hypotheses will be discussed.

MECHANISMS OF B- AND T-CELL–MEDIATED IMMUNITY

Effective immune responses ensue from an effective cooperation between functionally distinct cell types that are APCs: B and T lymphocytes, which communicate through an intricate network of cell receptors and soluble mediators, namely, cytokines. Cell-to-cell cooperation links involve a number of surface receptors interacting with their specific ligands as well as a variety of soluble mediators (Figs. 80.1 and 80.2). The stimuli elicited trigger the transduction of intracellular signals, which, depending on the context, lead to immune cell activation, differentiation, functional inactivation (anergy), or programmed death (apoptosis). The characterization of murine monoclonal antibodies specifically directed to human T-lymphocyte surface antigens and/or receptors represented a fundamental advance. They provided the tools to probe simply and reliably for the distinct human T-cell subsets.

Among the major receptors that may be characterized at the surface of human lymphocytes one must distinguish the following:

1. Receptors and coreceptors involved in antigen recognition: Surface immunoglobulins are the antigen receptor for B

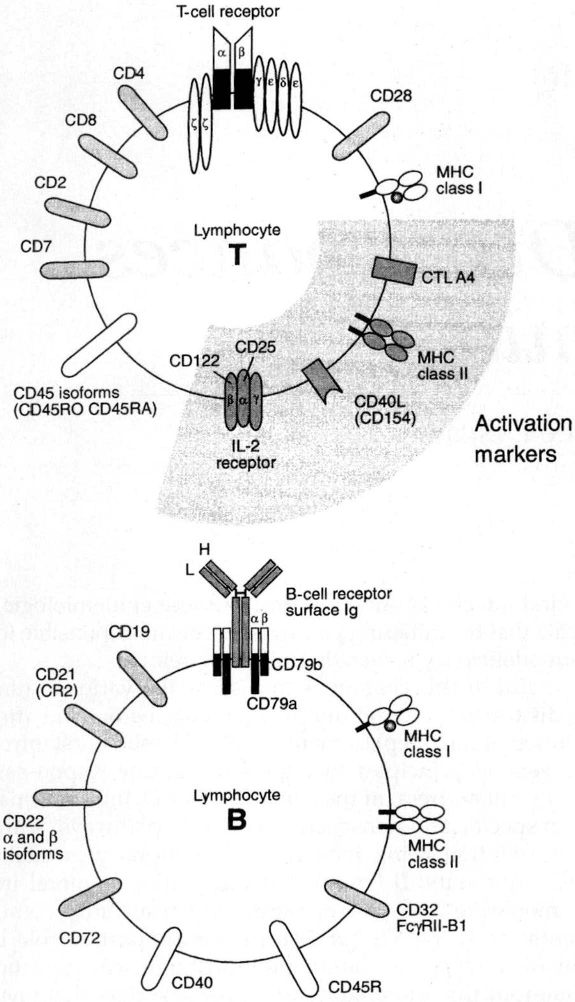

Figure 80.1. Schematic representation of the principal membrane receptors that have been identified at the surface of B and T lymphocytes. Receptors exclusively expressed at the surface of activated T lymphocytes are highlighted.

lymphocytes; the CD19, CD20, and CD21 act as coreceptors. T cells bind peptides presented in the context of major histocompatibility (MHC) molecules via specialized dimeric receptors: the T-cell receptor (TCR) α and β chains. The CD3 molecular complex composed of five invariant membrane proteins designated γ, δ, ϵ, ζ, and η regulates the assembly and expression of TCR and is responsible for transducing TCR αβ signals. The CD4 and CD8 receptors that bind MHC class II and I products, respectively, represent important "coreceptors" of CD3-TRC that actively participate to the delivery of activation signals.

2. Receptors delivering "costimulatory" signals: Although lymphocyte activation is initiated through the antigen receptor, this signal is not sufficient to sustain full activation of naive cells, and in contrast, upon rechallenge, it can result in a state of unresponsiveness or anergy. To allow sustained lymphocyte activation, costimulatory signals derived from specialized receptors must be delivered. In the case of naive T cells, CD28 is one important receptor mediating costimulation upon interaction with the B7 family (B7.1, B7.2) of ligands expressed on APCs. Some receptors delivering costimulatory signals are also essential for the cooperation between activated T lymphocytes and immunoglobulin-producing B cells. This is in particular the case for the CD40 receptor, which is expressed at the surface of B cells that specifically bind to the CD40 ligand (CD40L), which is expressed by activated T cells.
3. Receptors selectively expressed by activated cells: Cytokine receptors probably best illustrate the case of membrane molecules present at the membrane of activated immune cells. Of particular interest in the field of uremia was the analysis of the expression of the interleukin (IL)-2 receptor, especially on T lymphocytes, and of the CD23 molecule, which is the low-affinity receptor for the Fc potion of IgE on B lymphocytes.

Cytokines are essential mediators of immunity and inflammation (Fig. 80.2). A major concept emerged in the mid 1980s, which proposed that CD4+ T lymphocytes providing help for humoral (i.e., B-cell dependent) or cellular (i.e., T-cell depen-

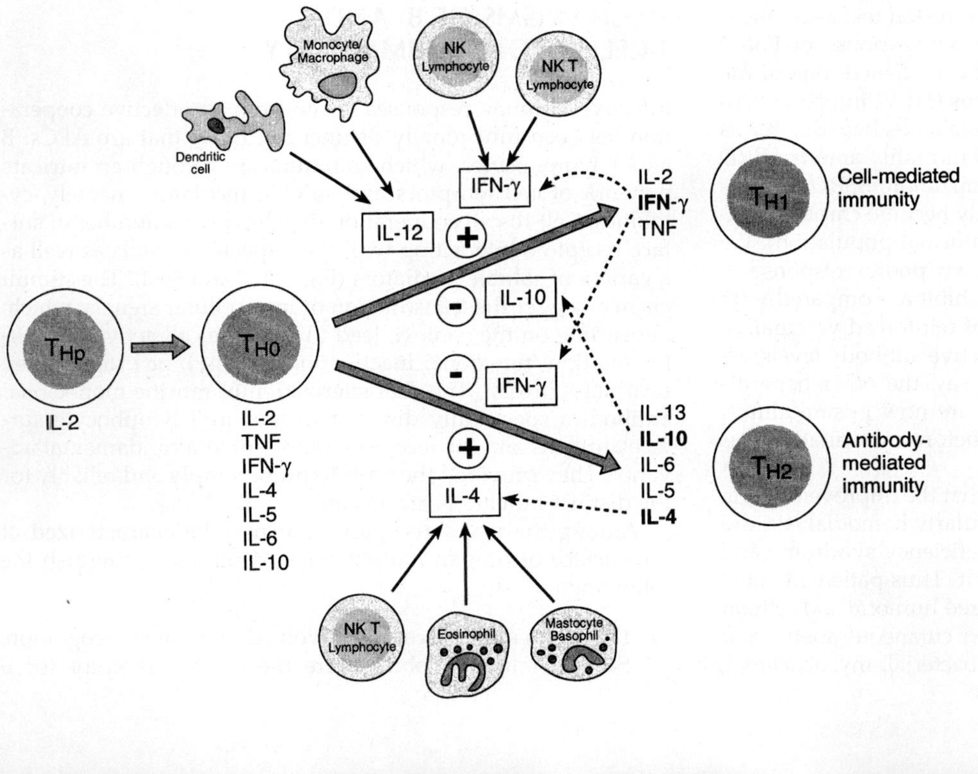

Figure 80.2. The differentiation pathways of the two main subsets of CD4+ cytokine producing helper T lymphocytes.

dent) responses were in fact distinct and could be differentiated on the basis of the cytokines they produced. Thus two lymphokine patterns, termed Th_1 (type 1 helper T cell) and Th_2 (type 2 helper T cell) were identified. Activation of the Th_1 cells [IL-2 and interferon-γ (IFN-γ) producers] supports macrophage activation and cell-mediated delayed-type hypersensitivity responses. Activation of Th_2 cells (IL-4, IL-5, IL-6, and IL-10 and IL-13 producers) provides efficient B cell help, thus favoring humoral responses. Fully differentiated Th_1 and Th_2 subsets do not preexist in the naive immunologically unprimed host. Among the various factors that direct naive T-helper precursors to differentiate upon antigen encounter into a Th_1 or a Th_2 cell are the type of antigen and its dose, the nature of the APC, the genetic background [both major histocompatibility (MHC) and non-MHC genes] and, interestingly enough, the environmental cytokines by themselves. IFN-γ, produced by Th_1 cells, inhibits the proliferation of Th_2 cells; conversely, IL-10, produced by Th_2 cells, inhibits the synthesis of cytokines by Th_1 cells by acting at least in part on APCs. IL-12, an APC-derived cytokine (dendritic cells, monocyte/macrophages), is a key factor driving the differentiation of Th_1 cells, at least in part through its capacity to induce IFN-γ. Conversely, IL-4 strongly directs the development of Th_2 cells and together with IL-10 show a strong inhibitory capacity on Th_1-type response development. Finally, in addition to IL-12, several other monocyte-/macrophage-derived cytokines potentiate immune function. Among those are IL-1, IL-6, and tumor necrosis factor (TNF) (Fig. 80.3).

Abnormalities in T Cell-Mediated Responses Associated with ESRD

Various clinical observations point to the crucial role of a T-cell defect in the ESRD immunodeficiency syndrome, including the very well-described cutaneous anergy to different antigens, the defective capacity of uremic patients to reject skin allografts, and as we previously discussed, the incapacity of ESRD patients to mount adequate humoral responses upon vaccination with T-dependent antigens such as HBV. A moderate decline in peripheral T cell numbers is generally observed in ESRD patients, and it has been reported that this lymphopenia may improve during maintenance dialysis. At variance with the situation observed in other secondary immunodeficiency syndromes, no imbalances between major T-lymphocyte subsets (CD4+, CD8+) has been observed. *In vitro* studies have shown decreased proliferative capacities of T lymphocytes from ESRD patients to both mitogens and alloantigens. These alterations were more marked when cultures were performed in the presence of autologous serum, an observation that led some authors to look for circulating "immunosuppressive" molecules in uremic sera, which, at least until now, could not be identified as such.

Contrasting with this evident decrease of T-cell responsiveness, data initially published by our laboratory, and subsequently largely confirmed by others, demonstrated that peripheral T cells from uremia without and with dialysis treatment showed clear-cut biologic signs of activation. In particular, they expressed increased levels of high-affinity receptors for IL-2 at their surface. In addition, significantly increased levels of circulating soluble receptors for IL-2, probably released from these activated T cells, were also found.

A hypothesis to reconcile these two paradoxical facts proposed that a decreased bioavailability of IL-2 was generated through its increased adsorption to the specific cell-associated and/or soluble receptors.

As previously described, it is now possible to distinguish various subsets of CD4+ helper T lymphocytes based on their cytokine production pattern. A more detailed analysis of the circulating T cells recovered from uremic patients using this tool may allow to get further interesting insights.

ABNORMALITIES IN B CELL-MEDIATED RESPONSES ASSOCIATED WITH ESRD

Plasma levels of immunoglobulins (IgG, IgM, IgA, and IgE) are usually normal in ESRD patients. As we previously discussed, the abnormal response to various T-cell–dependent vaccines is

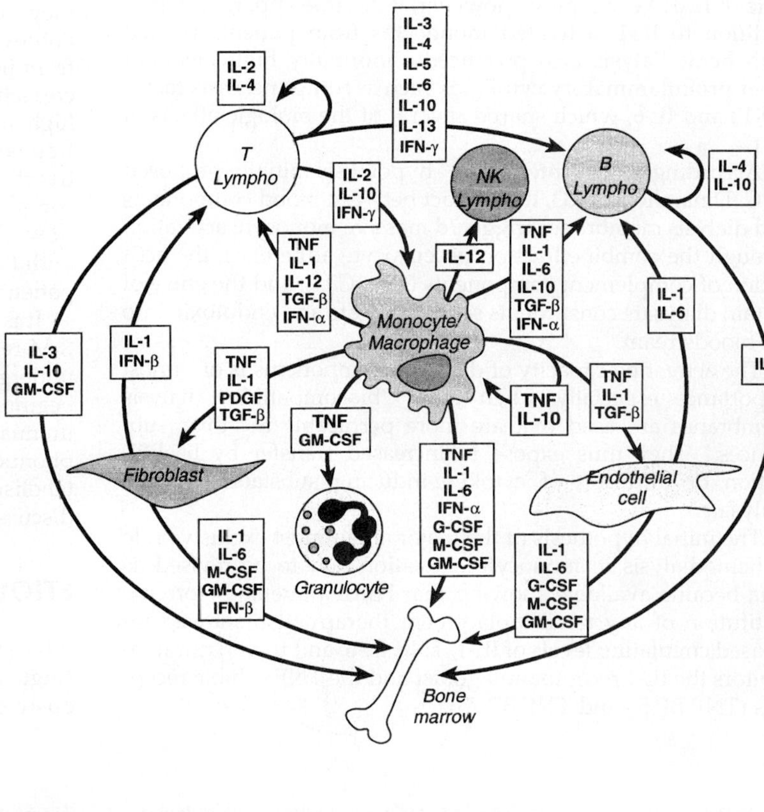

Figure 80.3. Schematic representation of the various cytokines produced by monocytes/macrophages and of their principal targets.

probably more related to the defective T-cell response than to an intrinsic B-cell abnormality. This is further supported by the normal humoral responses that had been reported in ESRD patients upon vaccination with T-independent antigens (pneumococcal). Some interesting clinical studies have demonstrated that the *in vivo* administration of recombinant erythropoietin was efficient in improving the immune response to vaccination with T-cell–dependent antigen such as tetanus toxoid.

Just as we discussed for T lymphocytes, there is compelling evidence to show that B cells from ESRD patients also show clear-cut biologic signs of activation. Thus uremic patients and those treated with hemodialysis exhibit increased levels of the soluble form of the low-affinity Fc receptor for IgE (FcϵRII/CD23), which is predominantly expressed on activated B cells. Moreover, recent data also demonstrated that ESRD B lymphocytes show significantly higher levels of cytosolic Ca^{2+} as compared with normal lymphocytes. This was correlated to an abnormally decreased sensitivity of ESRD B cells to the inhibitory activity of parathyroid hormone (PTH) on their proliferative capacity. Interestingly, these "biologic" defects were totally corrected upon treatment with the calcium channel blocker nifedipine. The capacity of such treatment to improve *in vivo* immune responses in ESRD patients is presently under study. Further discussion of B-cell function and metabolism in uremia is found in Chapter 68, Part 1.

THE ACTIVATION OF MONOCYTES/MACROPHAGES ASSOCIATED WITH ESRD: SOMETHING MORE THAN A MARKER OF "BIOCOMPATIBILITY"

It was mainly through the study of IL-1 that the potential pathophysiologic role of monocyte activation in the acute and chronic inflammatory manifestations associated with hemodialysis was first highlighted. These manifestations, which include an increase in body temperature 3 to 4 hours from initiation of hemodialysis, a characteristic sleepiness that follows the sessions, a negative nitrogen balance, and high circulating levels of acute reactive proteins, totally fit with the biologic effects of IL-1. Very rapidly, however, it became apparent that in addition to IL-1, activated monocytes from patients treated with hemodialysis also produced abnormally high levels of other proinflammatory cytokines such as tumor necrosis factor (TNF) and IL-6, which shared several of the biologic effects of IL-1.

According to the "interleukin" hypothesis initially proposed by C. Dinarello in 1983, the contact between blood components and dialysis membranes triggered massive monocyte activation through the combined action of leucocyte adherence, the activation of complement components (C5a, C3a), and the entry of certain dialysate constituents such as acetate and endotoxin into the bloodstream.

The activating capacity of dialysate components is of utmost importance especially when more "biocompatible" dialysis membranes are used that are more permeable to "toxic substances." They thus expose to increased transfer by backfiltration or diffusion of cytokine-inducing substances in the dialysate.

The initial hypothesis of the major and almost exclusive role of hemodialysis in monocyte activation had to be revised as data became available showing that ESRD patients before the institution of any renal replacement therapy also showed increased circulating levels of IL-1, TNF, IL-6, and their natural inhibitors the IL-1 receptor antagonist and the TNF soluble receptors (TNF BP 55 and TNF BP 75).

ABNORMALITIES OF POLYMORPHONUCLEAR NEUTROPHILS ASSOCIATED WITH ESRD

Polymorphonuclear neutrophils, which are central mediators of nonspecific immunity, play a central role in host resistance to bacterial pathogens and also represent a very good example of the biologic paradox of uremia we just alluded to.

On one hand, it has been extensively demonstrated that neutrophils from uremic patients exhibit impaired chemotaxis, adherence, phagocytosis and oxidative metabolism, and metabolic glycolysis in response to phagocytosis. The oxidative metabolism of phagocytes induced by opsonized zymosan, which mimics neutrophil–cell–membrane/bacteria interaction through IgG and C3b receptors, assessed by means of luminol-dependent chemiluminescence, is significantly decreased in uremic hemodialyzed patients. A prospective cross-sectional study showed that both uremia and the type of dialysis membrane affect the ability of neutrophils to mount oxidative responses to phagocytic challenge and that the risk of infections is increased in advanced uremia and is worsened by the use of less biocompatible cellulose membranes. This deficiency is in keeping with the impaired capacity of macrophages from hemodialyzed patients to clear sensitized IgG-coated autologous red cells, pointing to a defect of the Fcγ receptor functional capacity.

Dialysis sessions trigger neutrophil activation, which leads to the liberation of their cytosomal enzymes, an increased expression of adhesion molecules (CD11/CD18) favoring the trapping of neutrophils in the lung, and the generation of reactive-oxygen species (ROS). The physiopathologic relevance of this increased ROS generation is well established. In fact, it has been demonstrated that both the oxidative stress induced by ROS and the proinflammatory effect of monocyte-derived cytokines such as IL-1 and TNF largely contribute to β_2-microglobulin (β_2M) amyloidosis arthropathy and accelerated atherosclerosis, which are causes of morbidity and mortality in ESRD. β_2M is the 11-kDa constant chain of HLA class I molecules, expressed at the surface of all nucleated cells. It is released in the serum and essentially circulates as a monomeric form not bound to any transporter serum protein; it is filtered and metabolized by the kidney. Normal levels range from 1 to 3 mg/L, and they very significantly increase with the progression of renal failure. *In vitro* data suggest that peripheral blood cells collected from hemodialyzed patients at the end of a session exhibit increased levels of β_2M-specific transcripts and cultures release high amounts of β_2M in the supernatant. ROS contribute to the fragmentation and polymerization of β_2M, which favors its intraarticular deposit to constitute one serious osteoarticular complication. Based on clinical and radiologic criteria, the prevalence of osteoarticular lesions attributed to β_2M increases with the duration of dialysis and beyond 15 years virtually all patients exhibit clear-cut lesions.

It is of interest to mention that, as one could expect, cases of β_2M-related amyloidosis have also been reported in patients undergoing peritoneal dialysis or even in ESRD patients before beginning any renal replacement therapy, showing again that uremia per se favors the activation of monocytes and polymorphonuclear neutrophils. Further discussion on leukocyte metabolism and function can be found in Chapter 68, Part 1, and discussion on β_2M can be found in Chapter 84, Part 1E.

ETIOLOGIC FACTORS

It is difficult to propose a unicist theory that can reconcile in one single and simple scheme all the abnormalities we have previously discussed. There are probably several nonmututally exclusive processes that differentially affect, alone or in combination, the various components of the immune system. However, any good hypothesis should consider the "apparent" paradox that the ESRD immunodeficiency syndrome does not translate at the single immune cell level as a hyporesponsiveness but rather as a major hyperresponsiveness. It may be relevant to quote at this point other pathologic situations, quite diverse from ESRD, in which a superimposable pattern is observed such as advanced type II diabetes and some non–organ-specific autoimmune diseases such as systemic lupus erythematosus. Interestingly, in both these conditions, just as in ESRD, immune cells show a clear-cut hyperactivation (e.g., expression of activation markers, an increase of intracytosolic Ca^{2+} concentrations, basal hyperproduction of immunoglobulins by B cells *in vitro*), although when adaptive immune responses to particular foreign antigens have to be mounted they are totally inadapted.

Is it really so paradoxical that a state of cellular hyperactivation does translate at the level of the whole organism into a global hyporesponsiveness? Probably not. It is a well-known phenomenon in cellular biology that when a given cell is in a state of chronic hyperactivation, it becomes, due to complex feedback mechanisms, unresponsive to otherwise normal stimulations. The molecular basis for this includes, among other features, the down-modulation of some key cell-surface receptors and the inactivation of intracellular enzymes involved in the transduction of signaling pathways. Coming back to ESRD, there is evidence to show that the hyperactivation of B cells correlates with a down-modulation of PTH receptors, which probably explains their *in vitro* insensitivity to the antiproliferative effect of the hormone. Concerning T cells, it has been reported that some uremic T-lymphocyte subsets exhibit a lower density of TCRs at their surface, which could be secondary to their intrinsic activation state and could account for inadequate antigen-driven responses. The interesting feature is that this concept applies not only at the single cell level but also for global immune responses. The best example that is worth recalling at this point is that of "antigenic competition." According to this concept, described in the early 1960s, an immune stimulation, usually driven by an antigen, but also possibly by nonantigenic (polyclonal) stimuli, would automatically depress any concomitant immune response elicited in the host. This well-confirmed observation did not yet find a satisfactory mechanistic explanation. Several hypotheses were proposed, among which are the production of suppressor cytokines, or perhaps, more relevant to uremia, the exhaustion through increased consumption of "nutrient" cell factors, namely, cytokines; a good example for T cells being IL-2, as previously discussed. Evidence has also established that cytokine deprivation not only may lead to the unresponsiveness of the immune cell but also constitutes, especially in the case of activated T cells, one major element triggering apoptosis or activation-induced cell death (AICD). Although it is purely speculative, it is tempting to propose that the lymphocytopenia seen in uremia could be due, at least in part, to this sort of mechanism.

Thus one could conclude that when a physiologic immune response develops in some part of the body, the natural fate of the involved immune cells is to undergo activation upon the delivered stimuli, a period in which they are refractory to any concomitant stimulation, and then, as the stimulus is eliminated, the response progressively vanishes, leaving behind committed memory cells. The problem with the situation in ESRD is that the activation is generalized to the vast majority of immune cells and that, probably because of the nature of the stimulant(s), it is chronic.

The key question is then which is (are) the factor(s) triggering this deleterious immune cell activation, which, as we previously discussed, are already present in uremic non hemodialyzed patients because most of the activation markers are readily identified in patients presenting with mild or moderated renal failure? Of course, hemodialysis provides a further important stimulus to amplify and entertain this immune cell activation but in no case, and in clear contrast to the hypothesis initially proposed, does it constitutes the first and unique immunopathologic causal event.

Important efforts were devoted to the molecular characterization of "uremic toxins," initially considered as products issued from physiologic metabolic pathways that were not cleared in patients with chronic renal failure even upon hemodialysis. This concept has evolved over the years to also embrace "modified" soluble products. Data from our group demonstrated the presence of abnormally high concentrations of both advanced oxidation products (AOPPs) and advanced glycation end-products (AGEs) in ESRD patients before the institution of renal replacement therapy. Concentrations of AOPPs increased with progression of chronic renal failure, they were related to those of AGEs, and tightly correlated with conventional markers of monocyte activation (neopterin, IL-1–receptor antagonist, TNF, and TNF-soluble receptors). Importantly, *in vitro*–produced AOPP-human serum albumin and AGE-human serum albumin were capable of stimulating the oxidative burst of cultured human monocytes, thus pointing to the active role of this novel class of proinflammatory mediators in the vicious circle that self-perpetuates immune cell activation in ESRD.

Aside from "uremic toxins," one must also mention several other well-known factors that, in a nonmutually exclusive way, may have an impact on the immune function of ESRD patients. Among those are the various hormonal or metabolic deficiencies, the anemia (which is still a problem only in patients not receiving EPO), the malnutrition, and iron overload. Iatrogenic factors such as vitamin D (which, as extensively reported in the literature, is an immunosuppressant) can also be added to this list.

Selected Readings

Alexiewicz JM, Smogorzewski M, Akmal M, et al. Nifedipine reverses the abnormalities in [Ca2+]i and proliferation of B cells from dialysis patients. *Kidney Int* 1996;50:1249–1254.

An interesting study that illustrates, at the molecular level, the activation state of circulating B lymphocytes in uremic patients as assessed by abnormally increased levels of intracytoplasmic Ca^{2+}. Importantly, the authors also demonstrate that the calcium channel blocker nifedipine fully reverses the defect.

Birmingham DJ, Shen XP, Hartman JA, et al. Effect of chronic human recombinant erythropoietin therapy on antibody responses to immunization in chronic hemodialysis patients. *Kidney Int* 1996;50:543–549.

This paper describes the data from a well-conducted clinical study showing that recombinant erythropoietin administration significantly improves the in vivo response of uremic patients to vaccination with T-cell–dependent antigens such as tetanus toxoid.

Beaurain G, Naret C, Marcon L, et al. In vivo T cell activation in chronic uremic hemodialyzed and non-hemodialyzed patients. *Kidney Int* 1989;36:636–644.

Evidence for T-cell preactivation, as assessed by the presence of high-affinity IL-2 receptors, in both uremic hemodialyzed and nonhemodialyzed patients.

Chatenoud L, Dugas B, Beaurain G, et al. Presence of preactivated T cells in hemodialyzed patients: their possible role in altered immunity. *Proc Natl Acad Sci USA* 1986;83:7457–7461.

The first description of the presence of circulating preactivated T cells in hemodialyzed patients.

Dammin GJ, Couch NP, Murray JE. Prolonged survival of skin homografts in uremic patients. *Ann NY Acad Sci* 1957;64:967–976.

This historical paper was the first description of the impact of the in vivo immunodeficiency characteristic of uremia: a significant prolongation of the survival of skin allografts was evidenced in uremic recipients.

Descamps-Latscha B, Herbelin A, Nguyen AT, et al. Balance between IL-1 beta, TNF-alpha, and their specific inhibitors in chronic renal failure and maintenance dialysis. Relationships with activation markers of T cells, B cells, and monocytes. *J Immunol* 1995;154:882–892.

Study of a large cohort of uremic patients showing first, an imbalance between monocyte-derived cytokines and their inhibitors and second, that the cellular activation state is present at an early stage of uremia, regularly worsens with the progression of renal failure and is exacerbated by dialysis therapy.

Dinarello CA. Interleukin-1—its multiple biological effects and its association with hemodialysis. *Blood Purif* 1988;6:164–172.

In this review, the author presents in a clear and comprehensive way his hypothesis on the role of proinflammatory cytokines, and IL-1 in particular, in the pathophysiology of hemodialysis acute and chronic complications.

Mailloux LU, Bellucci AG, Wilkes BM, et al. Mortality in dialysis patients: analysis of the causes of death. *Am J Kidney Dis* 1991;3:326–335.

A study that points to one of the major clinical consequences of the immunodeficiency syndrome observed in uremic patients, namely, the high incidence of infections.

Witko-Sarsat V, Friedlander M, Capeillere-Blandin C, et al. Advanced oxidation protein products as a novel marker of oxidative stress in uremia. Kidney In 1996;49:1304–1313.

First description of circulating oxidized proteins in human plasma: based on their biochemical characteristics, this novel class of molecules were designated "advanced oxidation protein products."

Witko-Sarsat V, Friedlander M, Nguyen Khoa T, et al. Advanced oxidation protein products as novel mediators of inflammation and monocyte activation in chronic renal failure. *J Immunol* 1998;161:2524–2532.

The first study showing that I) in vivo AOPP are present in the plasma uremic patients prior to dialysis therapy and are closely related to the levels of advanced glycation end products (AGE) and monocyte but not T or B cell activation markers and II) in vitro produced AOPP do promote activation of human monocytes.

Woeltje KF, Mathew A, Rothstein M, et al. Tuberculosis infection and anergy in hemodialysis patients. *Am J Kidney Dis* 1998;31:848–852.

A recent and interesting epidemiologic study showing that mycobacterial infection still represents a major clinical problem in uremic patients.

CHAPTER 81

Cancer in Uremia

Spiros Vamvakas and August Heidland

In 1975, it was reported that over a short period of observation of 6 to 36 months, nine tumors were detected in 646 patients with chronic renal insufficiency (serum creatinine greater than 2.5 mg/100 ml), resulting in a cancer incidence (CI) seven times higher than in an age-matched control population. This first report on increased incidence of malignancies in patients with moderate to advanced renal disease has been confirmed in most of the subsequent studies; however, some studies failed to reveal this association.

A meta-analysis examined the cancer risk in a total of 15 studies with more than 100,000 patients with end-stage renal disease (ESRD): in 10 studies (72,484 ESRD patients), the relative risk expressed as observed over expected cancer cases averaged 7.6 (values between 1.4 and 22.8). In contrast, in the remaining five studies (35,407 ESRD patients), the average risk was 0.98 (0.45 to 1.3). It has to be stressed, however, that in various studies without an enhanced overall cancer risk, certain malignant diseases, such as non-Hodgkin's lymphomas and carcinomas of the kidney, prostate, and uterus, showed an enhanced prevalence compared with the general population.

In particular, excess incidence of renal cell carcinomas was observed in ESRD patients. One study reported a fourfold to fivefold increase of renal cancers in the 4,161 ESRD patients of the Michigan Kidney Registry. In a study conducted in 1990 and covering 65% of the 88,534 Japanese patients treated with maintenance hemodialysis (MHD), the renal cancer incidence was even increased 41-fold. Considering all available data, one finds a threefold to sixfold increase of renal cell tumors in patients receiving MHD compared with the general population.

The increased incidence of renal cancer and of the other malignancies frequently observed in uremic patients was also confirmed in a report on the cancer incidence in MHD patients in the Lombardy region in Italy during the 4-year period of 1983 to 1987. Of a total of 21 examined cancer sites, increased odds-ratios (ORs) were found for kidney cancer (2.82), primary liver cancer (2.41), multiple myeloma (2.39), thyroid tumors (2.22), and lymphoma (2.19). Significantly decreased risks of cancer were found in the MHD patients for cancer of the oral cavity and larynx (0.40), and a nonsignificant decrease was obtained for esophagus cancer. The incidences of the other sites did not differ from those in control patients.

RENAL DISEASES AS PREDISPOSING FACTORS OF CANCERS OF THE KIDNEY AND URINARY TRACT

Acquired cystic kidney disease (ACKD) is observed in patients with advanced renal failure and in those treated with hemodialysis or peritoneal dialysis. Increased cell proliferation to replace nephron loss together with the uremic milieu and renal ischemia favor cyst formation, which finally may lead to malignant transformation. In autosomal-dominant polycystic kidney disease (ADPKD), however, the renal cancer incidence is much lower, which correlates with the comparatively low cell proliferation rates. In contrast, in von Hippel-Lindau syndrome, multiple, bilateral cysts of the kidney are usually found together with renal cell tumors (see also Chapter 54, Parts 1 and 2).

Depending on the region, long-term analgesic abuse comprises the cause of renal failure in about 5% to 20% of MHD patients; analgesic nephropathy is associated with urothelial carcinomas and also, albeit less so, with renal cell carcinomas in particular after renal transplantation. In a study carried out in 65 patients after renal transplantation whose renal failure was due to analgesic nephropathy, the following cancers were observed: urothelial carcinoma in 15.4%, bladder cancer in 10.8%, and pelvic cancer in 9.1%.

Furthermore, Balkan endemic nephropathy is associated with increased formation of urinary tract tumors. Of 923 patients with chronic renal failure, 45 (4.9%) developed malignancies over a period of 10 years in certain regions in Serbia. The tumors in the patients with Balkan endemic nephropathy were usually cancer of the urinary tract (see also Chapter 47, Part 5).

POTENTIAL MECHANISMS

The pathogenetic mechanisms responsible for the increased cancer incidence in uremia have not been fully elucidated as yet. The available data indicate that several factors directly or indirectly associated with advanced renal disease and the MHD treatment may favor malignant transformation and tumor development (Table 81.1).

Impaired Function of the Immune System

The strong association of an impaired immune function with increased cancer risk has been repeatedly demonstrated, and this

TABLE 81.1. Potential Mechanisms Involved in Tumor Formation in End-Stage Renal Disease

Impaired function of the immune system
Impaired antioxidant defense in association with increased formation of reactive-oxygen species
Chronic infections and inflammations
Medication: prior immunosuppressive therapy, analgesic abuse, diuretics, calcium channel blockers (?)
Disturbed DNA repair
Parathyroid hormone excess and deficiency of 1,25-dihydroxycholecalciferol
Accumulation of carcinogenic heterocyclic amines and nitrosodimethylamine
Hypomethylation
Factors associated with the dialysis treatment

is specially evident in patients with acquired immunodeficiency syndrome (AIDS). In ESRD, both cellular and humoral immune responses are impaired despite major improvement in renal replacement therapy in the last decades. Uremic patients show reduced circulating B and T lymphocytes, reduced ratio of helper to suppressor T cells, delayed cutaneous hypersensitivity, decreased response to immunization (e.g., incomplete protection and response variability upon vaccination against hepatitis B), and prolonged graft survival. In addition to the underlying renal disease, the type of renal replacement therapy may also modulate the function of the immune system. In MHD patients, inducibility of the interleukin (IL)-2 gene is lost and that of the interferon (IFN) gene is decreased; in contrast, in peritoneal dialysis (PD) patients, IL-2 mRNA expression is normal, and IFN mRNA expression is enhanced.

Circulating levels of IL-1β and IL-1Ra, tumor necrosis factor-α (TNF-α), and its soluble receptors (TNF-sR55 and TNF-sR75), as well as activation markers of T cells (soluble CD25), B cells (soluble CD23), and monocytes (neopterin) increase with progression of chronic renal failure. Compared with undialyzed patients, levels of IL-1β, TNF-sR55, and TNF-sR75 were even higher than those treated with MHD; only IL-1Ra levels were decreased by MHD. This is in line with a subsequent investigation showing increased levels of macrophage colony-stimulating factors (M-CSF) in patients with ESRD as well as in MHD patients. Furthermore, marked elevation of advanced glycation end-products (AGEs) due to loss of renal function and oxidative stress may contribute to activation of macrophages.

MHD patients show a diminished proliferative response to phytohemagglutinin. Compared with healthy controls, stimulated peripheral blood mononuclear cells from MHD patients produced similar amounts of T-cell–derived cytokines such as IL-2 and IFN-γ, but greater amounts of monocyte-derived inflammatory cytokines (IL-1β, IL-8, and TNF-α) and of a regulatory cytokine (IL-10). IL-10 production was positively correlated with IL-1β and TNF-α in healthy controls, whereas no correlation was observed in MHD patients.

The abnormalities of the immune system in uremia are not reversed by dialysis therapy. Detailed discussion of the derangements of the immune system in uremia can be found in Chapter 80. It is possible that these abnormalities in the immune system contribute to the increased incidence of cancer in uremia.

REDUCED ANTIOXIDANT DEFENSE AND INCREASED FORMATION OF REACTIVE-OXYGEN SPECIES

Oxidative DNA lesions from endogenous and exogenous sources are one of the major causes of aging and malignant transformation. A complex defense machinery aims to detoxify the daily formed reactive-oxygen species, including the enzymes superoxide dismutase, glutathione peroxidase, glutathione *S*-transferase, and catalase, as well as the dietary antioxidants ascorbate, carotenoids, tocopherol, and coenzyme Q 10. In ESRD, plasma glutathione peroxidase activity is reduced mainly due to its deficient synthesis in the damaged proximal tubule cells, which are the main source of plasma glutathione peroxidase. Selenium is part of the enzyme's active center, and thus the frequently reduced serum selenium level in ESRD may contribute to the decreased glutathione peroxidase activity. A survey in 146 MHD patients in Wuerzburg revealed a lower serum selenium by 34% and a decline of serum glutathione peroxidase activity by 56%. A direct correlation was evident between the decrease in serum selenium levels and the reduced serum albumin and prealbumin concentrations. This suggests that malnutrition might be an important causal factor in the reduction of the serum levels of selenium. Low serum selenium levels have been incriminated as a risk factor for developing cancer in several epidemiologic studies. The protective effect of selenium supplementation against tumor development may rely on its action as a radical scavenger and also as an inhibitor of the activation of procarcinogens to carcinogens. In line with these mechanistic considerations, selenium supplementation exerted preventive effects against tumor development in animal models certain. It should be mentioned that a low serum selenium level is not always found in uremic or dialysis patients. MHD patients often also display a decline of superoxide dismutase activity.

The dietary intake of the antioxidants ascorbate, tocopherol, and coenzyme Q10 may be reduced in MHD patients compared with the general population because of the prescribed lower consumption of fruits and vegetables to prevent the risk of hyperkalemia. Because the cancer-preventing effect of the natural "cocktail" in fruits and vegetables has been clearly demonstrated by many epidemiologic studies, decreased consumption of these dietary components in MHD patients may also be a factor for their increased cancer risk.

Furthermore, accumulation of stable oxidizing components has been demonstrated in the plasma of MHD patients, whereas these components were not present in the plasma from subjects with normal renal function. Physiologic plasma concentrations of vitamin C or a water-soluble congener of vitamin E or reduced glutathione could not eliminate these oxidizing components of the uremic plasma.

After adding serum from prehemodialysis and posthemodialysis patients and from healthy controls to a system producing hydroxyl radicals, the signal intensities for reactive-oxygen species of the reaction mixture containing prehemodialysis sera were significantly stronger than those of the reaction mixture containing posthemodialysis or healthy sera. These observations suggest that the uremic state promote the generation of oxygen species.

Chronic Infections and Inflammations

In ESRD patients, chronic immunosuppression and impaired antioxidant defense favor infections by viruses and bacteria. Enhanced phagocytic activity in the course of chronic inflammations with increased release of nitric oxides (NO), superoxide ($\cdot\, O_{2-}$), hydrogen peroxide (H_2O_2), and hydroxyl radicals ($\cdot$ OH) contributes to DNA damage, induction of mutations, and cancer. Chronic inflammations are also associated with forced cell proliferation, an additional factor favoring the cascade DNA-adducts → mutations → malignant transformation, because DNA replication is not an error-free process and time for repair of DNA damage is shortened in the course of rapid DNA replication, thus facilitating the manifestation of mutations.

MHD patients have an increased incidence of hepatitis B and C infections, which can give rise to chronic hepatitis and, in certain cases, to liver cirrhosis and hepatocellular carcinoma. In Japan, increased adult T-cell leukemias were described in MHD patients due to an activation of oncogenic human T-cell leukemia virus type I.

Reactivation of Epstein-Barr virus (EBV) infection is a common finding in immunocompromised patients. Serologic evidence of reactivated or chronic persistent EBV infection was found in 18% of patients with chronic renal failure not yet receiving renal replacement therapy, in 11% of peritoneal dialysis patients, in 25% MHD patients, in 24% of renal transplant recipients, but in only 6% of healthy controls.

Medications

Some MHD patients were treated with immunosuppressive drugs in the past for the management of glomerulonephritis or due to a prior unsuccessful renal transplantation. Immunosuppressive therapy with azathioprine, methotrexate, cyclophosphamide, and particularly cyclosporine may give rise to enhanced prevalence of carcinomas of the skin, lips, uterus, bladder, and liver, as well as lymphomas and sarcomas.

The association between analgesic abuse and transitional cell tumors of the urinary tract was already mentioned. In addition, analgesic nephropathy may also be associated with renal cell tumors.

In several studies, chronic intake of diuretics was revealed as a risk factor for renal cell cancer, especially in women. The risk was proportional to the number of prescriptions and remained elevated even if the intake of diuretics was started more than 10 years before the cancer diagnosis. However, in another study, increased risk for renal cancer was attributed to the use of antihypertensive medications in general and not only to diuretics and was associated with the severity of hypertension. Also, in this study, the results were significant only in women. Risk was not significantly increased for either men or women who had not been receiving antihypertensive medication or who used only diuretics with or without hypertension.

Furthermore, elderly patients (average age of 79 years) with chronic intake of calcium channel blockers (verapamil, nifedipine, or diltiazem) for any indication had increased relative risk for most of the common cancers except skin and lung cancer. In another study in women age 65 years or older, an association was found between the use of calcium channel blockers and the incidence of invasive breast carcinoma. However, in a systematic review of all published randomized controlled trials to assess the risk of cancer or death in 11,201 patients receiving verapamil, no statistically significant increase in risk for cancer was found. Furthermore, a small increase in the relative cancer risk for calcium channel blockers (1.27; 95%) was not considered a proof of a causal relationship because there was no increase in risk with increasing duration of calcium channel blocker use.

Impaired DNA Repair After Long-Term Hemodialysis Treatment

Because cellular ability to repair DNA damage is a major defence mechanism against cancer, we investigated DNA repair in freshly isolated lymphocytes from short-term and long-term MHD patients with and without cancer, as well as from healthy subjects and patients with carcinomas and normal renal function. Ultraviolet (UV) light radiation of freshly isolated peripheral blood lymphocytes was used as a model of DNA damage. Suppressed DNA repair was observed in the long-term (more than 120 months) MHD group and in the MHD patients who had developed carcinomas during dialysis treatment Surprisingly, the short-term hemodialysis groups of our study (up to 12 months renal replacement therapy) showed a tendency to an even increased DNA repair compared with control subjects, while DNA repair of patients with an intermediate duration in hemodialysis (60 months) was comparable to that of controls. This data is similar to results observed by Israeli investigators in MHD patients treated for an average of 45 months. It additionally showed that pre-ESRD patients also display a decreased DNA repair. The impaired DNA repair may be the result of various factors, including DNA hypomethylation as well as increased intracellular calcium concentration. Indeed, acute elevation of lymphocyte calcium content by a calcium-ionophore inhibited the DNA repair *in vitro.* In uremic patients, the cellular calcium concentration is elevated due to the state of chronic excess of parathyroid hormone (see Chapter 68, Part 1), and this derangement may contribute to impaired DNA repair. Furthermore, advanced glycation end-products, which are extremely elevated in ESRD, have been shown to induce DNA damage and this may be an additional burden for the cellular DNA repair system (see Chapter 68, Part 7).

Taking into consideration the results of the aforementioned studies, the following hypothesis on the impact of renal disease on DNA repair can be postulated: DNA repair seems to be depressed in pre-ESRD patients. This abnormality is reversed (occasionally even to supranormal levels) within the first year of hemodialysis treatment, probably due to elimination of as yet unidentified uremic toxins. However, after long-term (more than 10 years) hemodialysis treatment, impairment in DNA repair recurs; the reason for this phenomenon is not defined as yet.

Parathyroid Hormone Excess and Deficiency of 1,25-Dihydroxy-Cholecalciferol

Primary hyperparathyroidism has been repeatedly shown to be associated with an increased frequency of malignancies. In four surgical series, the incidence ranged between 16% and 34%, whereas carcinomas were found in 42% of the cases in an autopsy series. In particular, thyroid, breast, and gastrointestinal tract tumors were linked with primary hyperparathyroidism. Because secondary hyperparathyroidism is often found in patients with ESRD, involvement of parathyroid hormone (PTH) excess in the enhanced cancer incidence in these patients is possible.

At the cellular level, excess PTH increases proliferation of various cells including T lymphocytes *in vitro.* However, in the physiologic situation, PTH stimulates the secretion of 1,25-dihydroxycholecalciferol, the active form of vitamin D, which appears to suppress cell proliferation and promote differentiation of immature or neoplastic cells. Hence, because of the deficiency of the counterregulatory 1,25-dihydroxycholecalciferol in chronic renal failure, the protumor action of excess PTH may act unopposed contributing to increased tumor formation.

Accumulation of Carcinogenic Compounds

Accumulation of carcinogenic heterocyclic amines such as dietary pyrolysis products of tryptophane and glutamic acid (Trp-P1/Trp-P2; Glu-P1, Glu-P2) and imidazoquinoline compounds (IQ, MelQ, MelQx) has been observed in ESRD patients. The highest levels were found in patients immediately before starting dialysis treatment.

Furthermore, elevated blood levels of the potent carcinogen nitrosodimethylamine are found in serum after consumption of ethanol. In uremia, there is an enhanced formation of nitrosodimethylamine in the small intestine due to bacterial overgrowth. Consumption of ethanol in chronic uremia unmasks the increased gastrointestinal formation of nitrosodimethylamine by inhibiting its first-pass metabolism. Pretreatment of the patients with oral ascorbic acid or freeze-dried *Lactobacillus acidophilum* counteracts the enhanced formation of nitrosodimethylamine.

Hypomethylation

Another potential factor involved in the increased tumor formation in ESRD patients is hypomethylation. An intracellular accumulation of the natural methyl transferase inhibitor *S*-adenosylhomocysteine (*S*-AdoHcy) was found in hemodialysis patients. *S*-AdoHcy impairs methylation-dependent repair of protein and peptide damage induced by spontaneous deamidation in erythrocytes. The formation of the highly toxic *S*-AdoHcy is directly related to the blood concentration of homocysteine, which is increased in ESRD. Fortunately, homocysteine levels can be reduced with treatment with folic acid, which decreases the toxic *S*-Ado-Hcy concentrations as well. Hypomethylation of DNA favors cellular dedifferentiation and malignant transformation (see Chapter 68, Part 3).

Factors Associated with the Dialysis Treatment

Factors directly associated with the dialysis procedure itself may also contribute to an increased risk of malignancy. In particular, bioincompatibility reactions due to complement activating dialysis membranes may induce granulocyte and platelet activation, increased formation of oxygen-free radicals, as well as release of proteases and cytokines. In follow-up studies, no significant difference in cancer incidence among complement activating and nonactivating membrane types was observed. However, tumor mortality was greater in MHD patients than in PD patients, which fits to the better immune state of PD patients and supports a potential role of bioincompatibility reactions in MHD patients.

Selected Readings

Ames BN, Shigenaga MK, Hagen T. Oxidants, antioxidants, and the degenerative diseases of aging. *Proc Nat Acad Sci USA* 1993;90:1915–1922.

An excellent editorial review on the role of endogenous oxidant byproducts of normal metabolism in the damage to DNA, proteins, and lipids. This damage (the same as that produced by radiation) is a major contributor to aging and to degenerative diseases such as cancer, cardiovascular disease, and immune-system decline.

Cohen SM. Role of cell proliferation in regenerative and neoplastic disease. *Toxicol Lett* 1995;82/83:15–21.

DNA replication occurs with a high, albeit not 100% fidelity (i.e., cell replication is a potential source of mutations). Consequently, a chemical can increase the risk of cancer not only by directly damaging DNA, but also by increasing the number of cell replications.

Finkle WD, McLaughlin JK, Rasgon SA, et al. Increased risk of renal cell cancer among women using diuretics in the United States. *Cancer, Causes, Control* 1994;4(6):555–558.

Strong and significant association between renal cell cancer and prescription diuretics (odds ratio adjusted for hypertension, smoking, and obesity = 2.9) in a group of 400 women. Risk tended to increase with dose, measured by number of prescriptions.

Grantham JJ. Polycystic kidney disease: neoplasia in disguise. *Am J Kidney Dis* 1990;15:110–116.

In both the autosomal-dominant polycystic and the acquired cystic kidney disease the central process in the initiation and progressive enlargement of renal cysts is proliferation of renal cells. Hence, these conditions resemble neoplastic disorders, except that in these conditions the "tumors" are filled with fluid instead of cells.

Heidland A, Hörl WH, Heller N, et al. Proteolytic enzymes and catabolism: enhanced release of granulocyte proteinases in uremic intoxication and during hemodialysis. *Kidney Int* 1983;24:S27–S36.

Granulocytes of pre-ESRD and ESRD patients have reduced proteolytic activities as compared with normal controls. On the contrary, increased serum levels of plasma elastase α_1-proteinase inhibitor complex were found, indicating granulocyte activation.

Iseki K, Osawa A, Fukiyama K. Evidence for increased cancer deaths in chronic dialysis patients. *Am J Kidney Dis* 1993;22:308–313.

Increased mortality from cancer in a group of about 2,000 renal hemodialysis patients compared with the general population in Japan. The risk ratio was increased to approximately 2.5 in males and 4 in females. Colon cancer (both sexes) as well as cancer of the uterus and breast (females) showed particularly increased incidences.

Ishikawa I. Renal cell carcinoma in chronic hemodialysis patients—a 1990 questionnaire study in Japan. *Kidney Int* 1993;41:S167–S169.

A very extensive study (more than 80,000 patients) on renal cancer in hemodialysis patients showing a 40 times higher incidence compared with the general population.

Kallistratos G, Evangelou A, Seferiadi K, et al. Selenium and hemodialysis: serum selenium levels in healthy persons, non-cancer and cancer patients with chronic renal failure. *Nephron* 1985;41:217–222.

Data on the possible role of low selenium levels as one of the factors responsible for the increased incidence of malignancy in hemodialysis patients are presented.

Kopple JD, Massry SG. Is there an association between neoplasia and primary or secondary hyperparathyroidism? *Am J Nephrol* 1988;8:437–448.

With regard to the association of hyperparathyroidism with neoplasias of other endocrine glands (multiple endocrine neoplasia) as well as with the increased CI in primary hyperparathyroidism, a hypothesis is presented that also secondary hyperparathyroidism may be involved in carcinogenesis in patients with ESRD, particularly due to the concomitant low levels of 1,25-cholecalciferol, as a counterregulatory hormone.

Malachi T, Zevin D, Gafter U, et al. DNA repair and recovery of RNA synthesis in uremic patients. *Kidney Int* 1993;44:385–389.

UV light–induced and γ-irradiation–induced DNA repair in freshly isolated lymphocytes was markedly suppressed in patients with chronic renal failure not yet receiving hemodialysis. In contrast, patients receiving hemodialysis (mean duration of 47 months) displayed DNA repair values similar to control levels.

Manabe S, Suzuki M, Kusano E, et al. Elevation of levels of carcinogenic tryptophan pyrolysis products in plasma and red blood cells of patients with uremia. *Clin Nephrol* 1992;37:28–33.

Certain tryptophan pyrolysis products (heterocyclic amines) are mutagenic and carcinogenic in experimental animals. In a group of hemodialysis patients, the concentrations of tryptophan pyrolysis products were several-fold higher compared with healthy controls. Hence, they may contribute to the increased cancer incidence in uremic patients.

Marple JT, MacDougall M. Development of malignancy in the end-stage renal disease patient. *Semin Nephrol* 1993;13:306–314.

Increased prevalence of malignancy in ESRD patients. Certain tumors such as renal carcinoma, prostate carcinoma, cutaneous melanoma, uterine carcinoma, and non-Hodgkin's lymphoma are particularly increased.

Marple JT, MacDougall M, Chonko AM. Renal cancer complicating acquired cystic kidney disease. *J Am Soc Nephrol* 1994;4:1951–1956.

The incidence of renal cancer is markedly increased in end-stage renal failure patients with acquired cystic disease of the kidney.

Massry SG, Alexiewicz JM, Gaciong Z, et al. Secondary hyperparathyroidism and the immune system in chronic renal failure. *Semin Nephrol* 1991;11(2):186–201.

A detailed study of the mechanisms involved in the alterations of the immune system induced by PTH excess in chronic renal failure.

Matas AJ, Simmons RL, Kjellstrand CM, et al. Increased incidence of malignancy during chronic renal failure. *Lancet* 1975;1:883–886.

First report on a sevenfold higher incidence of cancer in patients with ESRD.

Neumann HPH, Zbar B. Renal cysts, renal cancer and von Hippel-Lindau disease. *Kidney Int* 1997;51:16–26.

Excellent review on the increased incidence of renal cancer in patients with von Hippel-Lindau disease. Patients develop renal tumors at a very early age (35 to 40 years) and renal cancer is the cause of death in 50% of patients with this syndrome.

Pahor M, Guralnik JM, Ferrucci L, et al. Calcium-channel blockade and incidence of cancer in aged populations. *Lancet* 1996;348:493–497.

First observation about an association of chronic intake of calcium channel blockers (nifedipine, verapamil, or diltiazem) with a weakly increased risk for cancer.

Perna AF, Ingrosso D, De-Santo NG, et al. Mechanism of erythrocyte accumulation of methylation inhibitor S-adenosylhomocysteine in uremia. *Kidney Int* 1995;47(1):247–253

A very careful study about an intracellular accumulation of a methyltransferase inhibitor S-adenosylhomocysteine in hemodialysis patients that may impair methylation-dependent repair of protein and DNA damage.

Port FK, Ragheb NE, Schwartz AG, et al. Neoplasms in dialysis patients: a population-based study. *Am J Kidney Dis* 1989;14:119–123.

High incidence of renal, endometrial, and prostate cancer was observed in dialysis patients in a population-based study.

Roselaar SE, Nazhat NB, Winyard PG, et al. Detection of oxidants in uremic plasma by electron spin resonance spectroscopy. *Kidney Int* 1995;48:199–206.

Increased oxidizing activity was detected in the plasma of uremic patients compared with healthy controls with a very sensitive method. Reactive-oxygen species have been demonstrated to contribute to aging, atherosclerosis, and tumor formation.

Vamvakas S, Bahner U, Becker P, et al. Impairment of DNA repair in the course of long-term hemodialysis and under cyclosporine immunosuppression after renal transplantation. *Transplant Proc* 1996;28:3468–3473.

First demonstration that in long-term hemodialysis patients (more than 120 months therapy) and in hemodialysis patients with cancer UV light–induced DNA repair in freshly isolated lymphocytes is markedly suppressed.

CHAPTER 82

Appetite in Chronic Renal Failure

Jonas Bergström

BACKGROUND

Protein-energy malnutrition is common in patients with chronic renal failure (CRF). Among patients treated with hemodialysis (HD) or continuous ambulatory peritoneal dialysis (CAPD), the prevalence of malnutrition is as high as 30% to 70%. Several reports suggest that anthropometric and biochemical signs of malnutrition are risk factors for infection, morbidity, and mortality in HD and CAPD patients. Malnutrition in patients with renal failure may have many causes, including disturbances in protein and energy metabolism, hormonal disturbances, various forms of comorbidity, and psychosocial factors. Suboptimal food intake has a major role in the development of malnutrition in patients with CRF. Dialysis patients are recommended a protein intake of 1.2 g/kg per day and an energy intake of 35 kcal/kg, but a large proportion of these patients ingest considerably lower amounts. This chapter summarizes mechanisms by which appetite is regulated in general, discusses various factors that may potentially be involved in appetite suppression in CRF, and various measures to be taken to increase nutritional intakes.

GENERAL REGULATION OF APPETITE

The Depletion–Repletion Model

In principle, two types of model have dominated the study of food intake. The first type of model, the so-called depletion–repletion model, proposes that some parameters of immediately available nutritional substrates (e.g., glucose, lipids, amino acids) are constantly monitored, with declining amounts triggering meal onset, and that the meal is terminated when substrates are sufficiently replenished. Both the liver and the brain have been proposed to be involved in this process. Several factors, such as habits, learned associations, opportunity, and time of the day, may induce meal onset. Meal size, once eating has begun, is regulated by various satiety factors. Gastric distension and meal volume may have a direct effect. Moreover, there are endogenous satiety factors secreted in response to a meal. Best known of these is the gut peptide cholecystokinin (CCK), but several other peptides from the gut, such as glucagon and members of the bombesin family, may also be involved. They may inhibit gastric motility and signal the central nervous system (CNS) via peripheral nerves (vagal afferent fibers), as well as through receptors within the nucleus of the solitary tract within the brainstem area, where the satiety signals are integrated with afferent signals from the tongue and the gastrointestinal system.

Although it was suggested long ago that protein intake is physiologically regulated by amino acids accumulating after a meal, comparatively little work has been done to elucidate its mechanisms. It has been suggested that the inhibitory effect of amino acids is mediated in the liver and by neurotransmitters and receptors in the CNS.

The Lipostatic Model

The depletion–repletion models can account for both meal onset and meal termination, but they do not explain the matching of intakes with expenditures that results in the long-term stability of body composition. The so-called lipostatic model links food intake to the amount of stored energy (fat mass) in the body. According to this model, signals proportional to the size of fat stores become integrated with other regulators of food intake. Critical elements of this control system are hormones secreted in proportion to body fat mass, including leptin and insulin, the circulating concentration of both being proportional to adiposity, although leptin is mainly generated by adipocytes and insulin is secreted from pancreatic β-cells. In addition to its effect on appetite, leptin induces a relative elevation of energy expenditure, associated with increased sympathetic nervous system outflow. No long-term integrating system similar to the lipostatic system has been identified that regulates protein balance. Further discussion on leptin is found in Chapter 74, Part 5.

Role of the Central Nervous System

Long-term regulation of energy balance is accomplished by integration of signals secreted in proportion to body adiposity (leptin and insulin) and the short-term signals regulating meal size. The major integration site is the paraventricular nucleus in the hypothalamus. Neuropeptide Y (NPY) is a neurotransmitter, which is so far the most potent appetite stimulant described and it also reduces energy expenditure. Its generation is inhibited by insulin and leptin. Glucocorticoids appear to be antagonists of leptin and insulin in the control of energy homeostasis by effects on NPY. Several other hypothalamic neuropeptides are also involved in the regulation of energy homeostasis.

The amino acid profile in the CNS in uremia may be of major importance for ingestive behavior because amino acids may act as neurotransmitters (e.g., glycine and glutamate), whereas others (e.g., tryptophan and tyrosine) are precursors of monoamine neurotransmitters such as serotonin and catecholamines. The monoamines serotonin, dopamine, and under certain conditions, norepinephrine and epinephrine are involved in appetite suppression, apparently operating through hypothalamic receptor mechanisms.

Nitric Oxide

Nitric oxide (NO) has been demonstrated to stimulate appetite. Food deprivation increases NO synthase and depresses brain serotonin levels in rats and inhibition of the enzyme results in anorexia, but there is conflicting opinion whether NO exerts its stimulating effect on appetite by interfering with the serotonin system or by other mechanisms.

Proinflammatory Cytokines

Interleukin (IL)-1, IL-6, tumor necrosis factor (TNF), and other proinflammatory cytokines, generally produced and secreted in a cascade pattern, also exert a negative effect on appetite, in addition to other negative effects on protein homeostasis. They inhibit feeding by causing a decrease in gastric motility and emptying and intestinal motility, by modifying gastric secretion, and by eliciting taste aversion, either resulting from direct effects or mediated by the CNS. Cytokines stimulate glucagon and CCK release as well as the release of leptin and insulin. They may act in the CNS by interacting with the secretion of NPY, while increasing the secretion of serotonin, catecholamines, and their metabolites.

LOSS OF APPETITE IN CHRONIC RENAL FAILURE

Appetite suppression in CRF patients is multifactorial. Some factors that may contribute to a low intake of protein and energy are listed in Table 82.1. Low nutritional intakes may be due to unpalatable or inadequate diets, medications, gastropathy, and reduced intestinal motility [e.g., in diabetic patients with autonomic neuropathy], congestive heart failure, infections (peritonitis in peritoneal dialysis patients), and other forms of comorbidity. Psychosocial and socioeconomic factors, such as loneliness, depression, ignorance, and poverty, especially in elderly patients and those with alcohol and drug problems, may also be causes of low nutritional intakes. Nausea and vomiting during and immediately after HD, which are often associated with cardiovascular instability and postdialysis fatigue, may lead to a reduction in food intake during the days on dialysis. In CAPD, the presence of dialysate in the peritoneal cavity may interfere with gastric emptying and intestinal motility, resulting in discomfort or pain, as may the peritoneal catheter. It is also possible that glucose or amino acids absorbed from the dialysis fluid may exert an inhibiting effect on food consumption, as has been shown in experimental studies in rats.

TABLE 82.1. Causes of Low Nutritional Intake in Chronic Renal Failure

Uremic toxicity (underdialysis)
Unpalatable or inadequate diets
Complicating illness
Gastrointestinal illness
Cardiovascular disease
Inflammation, infection, sepsis
Medications
Psychosocial and socioeconomic factors
Loneliness
Depression
Ignorance
Poverty
Poor dental status
Alcohol and drug abuse
Effects of hemodialysis
Cardiovascular instability
Nausea, vomiting
Postdialysis fatigue
Effects of peritoneal dialysis
Abdominal distension and pain
Dialytic uptake of glucose or amino acids

Uremic Toxicity and Appetite

Anorexia, nausea, and vomiting are hallmarks of uremic intoxication, which typically develop when the glomerular filtration rate is less than 10% to 15% of normal and increase in severity with progression toward end-stage renal failure. However, patients with CRF may reduce their protein and energy intake already at a glomerular filtration rate of 25 to 30 ml/min as has been demonstrated in prospective, randomized studies. A plausible explanation of this is that inhibition of appetite is caused by retention in body fluids of one or more toxic substances as a consequence of reduced renal function. Conservative treatment of renal failure with a low-protein diet may alleviate temporarily or forestall uremic symptoms in the form of anorexia, nausea, and vomiting, suggesting that one or more of these toxins are generated by breakdown of dietary protein. After dialysis therapy is started, these symptoms are partly relieved or disappear within a few days. Underdialyzed patients, on the other hand, tend to have a low intake of protein as evaluated from studies of urea appearance rate. Such observations indicate that one or more uremic factors causing these symptoms have a molecular size that permits their transport through conventional hemodialysis membranes (i.e., less than 10,000 D). Experimental data in support of this conclusion demonstrate that ingestion of carbohydrate or protein is suppressed in rats by plasma ultrafiltrate from uremic hemodialysis patients and normal urine ultrafiltrate injected intraperitoneally, but not by ultrafiltrate from normal controls.

The pivotal role of residual renal function for elimination of anorexigenic uremic compounds is supported by longitudinal studies showing that protein intake (estimated from urea appearance rate) decreases along with the loss of residual renal function. It is conceivable that the natural kidneys are superior to any form of dialytic treatment regarding blood purification. However, it is still an open question to what extent an increase in dialysis dose (by more frequent exchanges and/or larger filling volumes) may compensate for the gradual loss of renal function with ensuing anorexia in long-term CAPD patients.

The mechanisms by which uremic toxins exert their effects on appetite are not known. In addition to less specific effects, there may be more specific ones such as food aversion, altered taste acuity, gastric distension, impaired gastric emptying, bowel obstruction, and constipation.

Factors Regulating Appetite in Renal Failure

Malnutrition in patients with CRF is generally of mixed type with low body weight, loss of somatic protein (low muscle mass), low plasma levels of serum albumin, and other visceral proteins as well as depletion of energy (adipose tissue) stores. Hence, insofar that appetite suppressors contribute to uremic malnutrition, they should inhibit both protein and energy intake.

Elevated concentration in plasma or CNS of several potentially anorexigenic compounds have been reported in patients

TABLE 82.2. Putative Appetite-Suppressing Compounds in Uremia

Leptin
Insulin
Cholecystokinin
Glucagon
Serotonin
Catecholamines
Amino acid imbalances
Nitric oxide–synthase inhibitors
Proinflammatory cytokines (tumor necrosis factor, IL-1, IL-6)
Middle molecules

with end-stage renal disease (Table 82.2). However, their exact role in uremic appetite suppression is not well defined.

Leptin and Insulin

Several studies demonstrated that plasma leptin concentrations are elevated in patients with CRF. Reduced renal elimination seems to play a major role, but other factors seems to be in operation as well, such as infection/inflammation (cytokines), which triggers release of leptin from the fat cells. However, there is only indirect evidence that hyperleptinemia is involved in appetite suppression in uremia. For more details about the role of leptin in uremia, see Chapter 74, Part 5.

Circulating insulin levels are elevated in CRF patients and might potentially suppress appetite in synergism with leptin. However, the role of hyperinsulinemia as an appetite-suppressing factor in uremia is unsettled. Peripheral insulin resistance is a feature of uremia, but it is currently unknown whether the resistance also involves effects of insulin in the CNS.

Gastrointestinal Hormones

The plasma levels of several peptide hormones are elevated in renal failure, which is at least partly due to reduced renal catabolism. Among the satiety factors, the plasma concentrations of immunoreactive glucagon and CCK have been reported to be elevated in CRF patients, but there is no direct evidence that they are involved in uremic appetite suppression.

Amino Acids, Neurotransmitters, and Their Metabolites

Several amino acid abnormalities have been observed in CRF patients, with imbalances between individual amino acids, which may contribute to appetite suppression. Total plasma tryptophan levels are low in end-stage renal disease patients, whereas free tryptophan in plasma and total tryptophan in red blood cells and muscle are elevated. In rats with chronic uremia, elevated levels of tryptophan and serotonin have been observed in the hypothalamus and medulla. Humans with CRF have been reported to have elevated levels of tryptophan, serotonin, and 5-HIA in cerebrospinal fluid. The role of these findings for appetite suppression in renal failure patients remains to be defined.

Nitric Oxide

NO has been implicated as a potentially adverse factor in renal failure that may cause cardiovascular instability and hypotension, especially in HD patients, because of its vasodilatory action. There is evidence that the dialysis procedure stimulates generation of NO, which might enhance appetite. On the other hand, uremic plasma inhibits NO synthase activity *in vitro*, but the mechanism for this has not been elucidated. In view of these conflicting results, the role of NO in appetite regulation of uremic patients is unsettled.

Proinflammatory Cytokines

Several reports point out that there is an association between malnutrition and inflammation, evaluated as elevated plasma levels of C-reactive protein in nondialyzed CRF patients and HD patients. Assuming that acute-phase proteins reflect the activity of proinflammatory cytokines, such findings suggest a role of these cytokines in malnutrition. Elevated plasma concentrations of TNF, IL-1, and IL-6 are observed in nondialyzed CRF patients and in HD and CAPD patients. High circulating IL-6 levels are associated with loss of body weight and reduced arm-muscle circumference, and TNF-α levels are more elevated in anorectic peritoneal dialysis patients than in patients without anorexia.

The origin of elevated plasma cytokine levels remains unclear. Reduction in renal function seems to play a role. Chronic bacterial or viral infections and congestive heart failure, which are common complications among patients with CRF, may trigger the generation of proinflammatory cytokines. In summary, several studies suggests that cytokines may have a major role in the development of malnutrition in renal failure patients, but it is not clear to what extent this is due to their role as appetite suppressors.

Middle Molecules

Several studies in HD and CAPD patients report a correlation between the dose of dialysis for small molecule removal (Kt/V_{urea}) and protein intake, especially in the lowest dose interval. However, in CAPD patients, an adequate protein intake, estimated from urea appearance rate, is achieved with much lower weekly Kt/V_{urea} than with HD. One explanation might be that molecules of larger molecular weight than urea (so-called middle molecules) might cause anorexia. Such hypothetical molecules should be dialyzed more efficiently by the peritoneal membrane than by dialysis with conventional hemodialysis membranes.

There is some evidence from experimental studies that compounds within the molecular weight range of 1 to 10 kD are involved in uremic appetite suppression. Among fractions of various molecular sizes prepared by molecular filtration of uremic and normal ultrafiltrate and urine from healthy subjects, injected intraperitoneally in rats, a 1- to 5-kD fraction from uremic ultrafiltrate and the corresponding fraction from normal urine inhibited both carbohydrate and protein ingestion in a dose-dependent manner, whereas fractions with lower molecular weight as well as all fractions from normal ultrafiltrate were without effect. These results lend strong support for the hypothesis that appetite-suppressing middle molecular compounds that are normally excreted by the kidneys accumulate in plasma of patients with renal failure. Other data suggest that the uremic middle molecules may exert their effects on appetite by splanchnic signaling as well as directly on the feeding center in the brain. Further investigations are needed to elucidate their chemical structure, transport through the blood–brain barrier, and molecular basis for their action.

MEASURES TO INCREASE FOOD INTAKE AND STIMULATE APPETITE

Because uremia per se may cause anorexia, nausea, and vomiting, a prerequisite for successful intervention is that uremic intoxication is alleviated or eliminated. In nondialyzed patients, this may be achieved by ordering a low-protein diet. Such a diet should have a high energy content and may need to be supplemented with essential amino acids or their ketoanalogs to prevent protein malnutrition. In addition, the nutritional status has to be monitored regularly to detect signs of malnutrition. Low-protein diets are not recommended for patients with advanced renal failure without back up by dedicated dietitians and doctors; instead, early start of dialysis is then recommended. In maintenance dialysis patients who are underdialyzed, the dose of dialysis should be increased so that it becomes adequate because this may restore appetite and improve general well-being. If this is ignored, all other measures aimed at improving appetite may be futile.

Because low nutritional intake in renal failure patients may be related to comorbidity apart from underdialysis (Table 82.2), comorbidity factors such as infection, cardiac failure, and gastrointestinal dysfunction need to be identified and if possible remedied to ensure an adequate nutritional intake. Psychosocial and economic support should be provided when needed. Dietary advice with the aim of increasing the quantity, quality, and palatability of the food consumed may be helpful. Attention should be paid not only to the protein intake but also to the energy intake, which needs to be adequate for the optimal utilization of protein. Correction of anemia by treatment with recombinant human erythropoietin is also reported to improve appetite in dialysis patients.

More specific measures to intervene with mechanisms that may inhibit appetite are theoretically possible, for example, by attenuating the generation of anorexigenic factors, stimulating the generation of orexigenic factors, supplying exogenous orexigenic agents, and interfering with receptor mechanisms involved. However, until now, a lack of basic knowledge of which specific mechanisms are involved the uremic appetite suppression has precluded the development of efficient therapies along these lines. Insofar that proinflammatory cytokines are involved in appetite suppression, various forms of anti-inflammatory and anticytokine therapies might be potentially beneficial, especially because cytokines also enhance muscle protein catabolism and reduce albumin generation. Among potentially applicable agents along these lines are active synthetic derivatives of progesterone, such as megestrol acetate, which have been used successfully for treatment of the cancer-related anorexia/cachexia syndrome, characterized by high serum levels of proinflammatory cytokines, proposed as mediators of the cachectic process. These agents downregulate the synthesis and release of IL-1, IL-6, and TNF, and they increase hypothalamic release of neuropeptide Y. Administration of cytokine-receptor antagonists, soluble receptors to cytokines, or cytokine antibodies are other therapeutic options that may deserve to be studied.

Selected Readings

Aguilera A, Codoceo R, Selgas R, et al. Anorexigen (TNF-a, cholecystokinin) and orexigen (neuropeptide Y) plasma levels in peritoneal dialysis (PD) patients: their relationship with nutritional parameters. *Nephrol Dial Transplant* 1998;13: 1476–1483.

The results of this study show that plasma cholecystokinin and TNF levels are elevated in renal failure patients and that high TNF levels are associated with appetite suppression, nausea, and vomiting.

Anderstam B, Mamoun A-H, Södersten P, et al. Middle-sized molecule fractions isolated from uremic ultrafiltrate and normal urine inhibit ingestive behavior in the rat. *J Am Soc Nephrol* 1966;7:2453–2460.

Experimental evidence that middle molecules isolated from uremic ultrafiltrate inhibit ingestion of carbohydrate and protein in the rat.

Kaizu Y, Yoenama T, Miyaji M, et al. Interleukin-6 may mediate malnutrition in chronic dialysis patients. *Am J Kidney Dis* 1998;31:93–100.

A longitudinal study demonstrating that elevated plasma levels of proinflammatory cytokines are associated with development of malnutrition.

Plata-Salamán CR. Cytokines and anorexia: a brief overview. *Semin Oncol* 1998; 25(Suppl 1):64–72.

This paper summarizes the various mechanisms by which proinflammatory cytokines may cause anorexia and presents a brief outline of potential therapeutic approaches.

Woods SC, Seeley RJ, Porte D Jr, et al. Signals that regulate food intake and energy homeostasis. *Science* 1998;280:1378–1383.

General overview of the current models of regulation of food intake, the generation and action of various satiety factors and neuropeptides, and the integration of the various signals in the CNS.

SECTION IX

Management of the Uremic State

CHAPTER 83

Nutritional Management

PART 1
Acute Renal Failure

Joel D. Kopple

THE NUTRITIONAL AND METABOLIC STATE OF PATIENTS WITH ACUTE RENAL FAILURE

The metabolic and nutritional status of the patient with acute renal failure (ARF) varies markedly. Some patients are hypercatabolic, are acidemic, and have markedly increased serum urea, potassium, phosphorus, urate, and total body water. Net protein degradation can be massive, up to 200 to 250 g/day or more, and basal energy expenditure may be increased. ARF in these patients is often associated with shock, sepsis, surgery, or severe polytrauma, and oliguria or anuria is often present. They are not uncommon among the most ill patients in an intensive care unit. On the other hand, some ARF patients maintain nitrogen balance and have normal body water, serum electrolytes, and acid–base status. These latter patients often are not oliguric. The causes of their ARF usually do not induce hypercatabolism, and such causes include toxic effects of aminoglycoside antibiotics or radiocontrast media.

Animal studies indicate that ARF per se causes many abnormalities in amino acid and protein metabolism, and it also induces resistance to insulin. The activities of many amino acid catabolizing enzymes are increased. In addition, there is increased activity of serine dehydratase, which catalyzes the degradation of the gluconeogenic amino acid serine and of phosphorylase a, which catalyzes glycogenolysis. Glycogen synthase 1, which catalyzes glycogen synthesis, displays reduced activity in muscle of acutely uremic rats. These alterations may explain the reduced muscle glycogen content observed in acutely uremic patients.

There are many causes for hypercatabolism in ARF. First, underlying catabolic conditions such as sepsis, hypotension, surgery, polytrauma, or rhabdomyolysis may cause increased plasma concentrations of counterregulatory hormones, including epinephrine, norepinephrine, cortisone, and glucagon. Indeed, these hormones are often elevated in patients with ARF. Underlying catabolic illnesses may also stimulate the release of endotoxin and such cytokines as tumor necrosis factor and interleukin-1; these compounds may induce catabolism. Second, ARF itself can increase serum levels of certain catabolic hormones, including glucagon and parathyroid hormone. Third, acidemia promotes catabolism of proteins and amino acids. Fourth, there are increased plasma concentrations of many metabolic products; some of these compounds may be toxic. Fifth, increased basal energy expenditure may promote amino acid and protein catabolism if energy intake is inadequate.

Protein-energy malnutrition may be accentuated by the following factors in patients with ARF: (a) Many ARF patients ingest little or no nutrients. This may occur because they have anorexia or vomiting. Underlying medical or surgical illnesses may impair the patient's food intake or gastrointestinal function. Altered consciousness or frequent diagnostic studies also may reduce the patient's ability to eat or to receive nutrients by tube feeding or parenterally. (b) Loss of nutrients in dialysate (amino acids, peptides, proteins, water-soluble vitamins, and with glucose-free dialysate, glucose) may promote protein malnutrition. (c) Bioincompatible membranes in the hemodialyzer may stimulate the release of cytokines that promote protein catabolism. (d) Blood drawing, gastrointestinal bleeding (which may be occult), blood lost into the dialyzer, and draining fistulae or wounds are other sources of protein loss.

PAST EXPERIENCE WITH NUTRITIONAL THERAPY IN ACUTE RENAL FAILURE

Because many patients with ARF are hypercatabolic and malnourished and nutritional therapy may affect the rate of generation of metabolites of protein and amino acids, a number of researchers have evaluated the effects of nutritional support in this condition. Only about six prospective randomized clinical trials of nutritional support have been carried out in patients with ARF. These trials all involve rather small numbers of patients; the largest trial randomized 53 patients to two treatment groups. In some studies, patients were not very ill and almost all individuals survived, whereas in other studies, most patients died. Different nutritional formulations were also used in these studies, including essential amino acids, mixtures of essential and nonessential amino acids, or no amino acids; thus it is difficult to compare the results from different studies.

In one study, patients receiving total parenteral nutrition (TPN) that provided about 16 g of eight essential amino acids (not including histidine), as compared with parenteral nutrition without amino acids, showed increased survival until recovery of renal function, but hospital survival was not significantly greater. Other studies have not confirmed that nutritional support increases survival in patients with ARF. In the former study, there was a suggestion that renal function may have recovered earlier when TPN with essential amino acids was given; however, this observation was not clearly proven, nor has it been confirmed in other studies in ARF patients. Some studies in animals with experimental ARF also suggest that nutritional support can enhance the rate of recovery of renal function; other animal research has not confirmed this. Several studies conducted in small numbers of ARF patients suggest that TPN with small amounts of essential amino acids may reduce the urea nitrogen appearance (UNA, net urea generation) without worsening protein balance. TPN with small amounts of essential amino acids also may decrease the rate of rise of serum potassium and phosphorus in these patients.

The lack of a clear-cut benefit of nutritional therapy on outcome in patients with ARF may be due to the following factors: First, the numbers of patients studied in each clinical trial were small. Given the great heterogeneity in the clinical status of patients with ARF and their usual high mortality rate, it could be anticipated that the numbers studied would be insufficient to demonstrate a difference in the treatment outcome if one existed. Second, no research has compared nutritional support with no nutritional support in randomized, prospective studies. In each study, patients receiving TPN were compared with a control group that received parenteral nutrition without amino acids or TPN with a different amino acid formulation. It is possible that the nutritional therapy given to the control patients also increased their survival, thereby reducing the difference in outcome between the control and treatment groups. Third, in some studies, patients probably were not very ill. It would be difficult in these studies to show an effect of nutritional support on mortality, particularly when only small numbers of patients were studied. Fourth, the optimal formulations for nutritional support may not have been developed. Finally, it is possible that nutritional support is not sufficiently effective to reduce mortality by itself, and other measures (e.g., compounds that suppress or inhibit inflammatory or catabolic cytokines, growth factors, immune-enhancing agents) may need to be applied in association with nutritional therapy.

AIDS IN THE DELIVERY OF NUTRITIONAL THERAPY

Use of Continuous Renal Replacement Therapy

Continuous renal replacement therapy is a commonly used alternative to hemodialysis or hemofiltration. It is usually performed as continuous venovenous hemofiltration (CVVH) or CVVH with continuous hemodialysis (CVVHD). CVVH and CVVHD are primarily used for the treatment of sick patients with ARF or other disorders causing water, electrolyte, or nitrogen intolerance, such as severe liver or congestive heart failure. CVVH or CVVHD offers the following advantages to the patient with ARF: (a) large amounts of water, electrolytes, and metabolites may be removed each day; (b) because the rate of removal of water and electrolytes is slow, CVVH or CVVHD is less likely to cause or worsen hypotension; (c) because large quantities of water and small molecules, including metabolic waste products, can be removed over a 24-hour period with CVVH or CVVHD, one may safely administer greater amounts of amino acids and other nutrients to the patient; (d) patients with ARF who are receiving CVVH or CVVHD usually have high daily clearances of molecules and therefore may require hemodialysis therapy less frequently and usually may avoid it altogether; and (e) CVVH or CVVHD may be administered by nurses who are not specifically trained in hemodialysis (although special training of nursing personnel is required). Thus CVVH or CVVHD may be more convenient to use, and the cost for this therapy may be no more or possibly even less expensive than for intermittent hemodialysis. It is unclear whether CAVH or CAVHD or CVVH or CVVHD reduces morbidity or mortality more than intermittent hemodialysis in patients with acute renal failure.

Amino acid losses during CVVH or CVVHD are influenced by the permeability characteristics of the filter membrane, the ultrafiltration and dialysis flow rates, and the rate of amino acid infusion, which will influence the plasma amino acid concentrations. Approximately 4 to 7 g/day of amino acids are removed with CVVH. The 24-hour amino acid losses with CVVH or CVVHD are roughly similar to the losses during a single hemodialysis treatment, which averaged roughly 8.0 ± 2.8 (SD) and 9.0 ± 2.7 g in two studies of patients undergoing maintenance hemodialysis with high-flux dialysis.

Estimation of Net Protein Degradation and Nitrogen Balance

The UNA is a simple, inexpensive, and accurate measurement of net protein breakdown (i.e., the difference between protein synthesis and degradation). Because urea is the major nitrogenous product of protein and amino acid metabolism, the UNA usually is closely correlated with total nitrogen output. UNA may be calculated as follows:

(1) UNA (g/day) = Urinary urea nitrogen (g/24 hr) + Dialysate urea nitrogen (g/24 hr) + Change in body urea nitrogen (g/24 hr)

(2): Change in body urea nitrogen (g/24 hr) = $(SUN_f - SUN_i$, g/24 hr) × (BW_i, kg) × (0.60 L/kg) + $(BW_f - BW_i$, kg/24 hr) × (SUN_f, g/L) × (1.0 L/kg)

where *I* and *f* are the initial and final values for the period of measurement; *SUN* is serum urea nitrogen (g/L; *BW* is body weight (kg); 0.58 is an estimate of the fraction of body weight that is body water (which is essentially the volume of distribution of urea in the body); and 1.0 is the volume of distribution of urea in the weight gain or loss, which is assumed to be due to change in body water. The total body water for individuals of a given weight, height, and gender may be estimated from various nomograms and equations that were developed for normal individuals. For patients with ARF, the estimated proportion of body weight that is water may be increased if they are edematous or lean and/or decreased if they are obese or very young. These techniques are somewhat limited because it is often difficult to accurately estimate the total body weight of a sick patient with ARF. Changes in body weight during the 1- to 3-day period of measurement of UNA generally can be assumed to be due entirely to changes in body water.

In patients undergoing hemodialysis or intermittent peritoneal dialysis, dialysate collection is cumbersome; UNA may be calculated during the interdialytic interval. Urea kinetic modeling may also be used to estimate the UNA. Instruments that automatically and serially measure dialysate urea during the hemodialysis procedure are available and should give more precise measurements of urea losses into dialysate.

In patients receiving CVVH or CVVHD, UNA may be determined from measurements of urea in serum, urine, and hemofiltrate or hemodialysate effluent and body weights at the beginning and end of the period of measurement as indicated in equations 1 and 2. For patients undergoing CVVH, urea in hemofiltrate can be substituted for that in dialysate. The urea output in hemofiltrate or dialysate can be estimated by measurement of urea in periodic samplings of the effluent and multiplying these concentrations by the total volume of the effluent.

Data obtained from patients with chronic renal failure indicate that total nitrogen output may be estimated from UNA as follows:

$$\text{(3)} \quad \text{Total nitrogen output (g/24 hr)} = 1.192\ \text{UNA (g/24 hr)} + 1.27$$

If the individual is in approximately neutral nitrogen balance, the UNA will also correlate with nitrogen intake. In our experience, the relation between UNA and dietary nitrogen intake in clinically stable nondialyzed patients with chronic renal failure is as follows:

$$\text{(4)} \quad \text{Dietary nitrogen intake (g/24 hr)} = 1.204\ \text{UNA (g/24 hr)} + 1.74$$

If both nitrogen intake and UNA are known, nitrogen balance can be estimated from the difference between the nitrogen intake and nitrogen output estimated from the UNA.

RECOMMENDED NUTRITIONAL THERAPY

Goals of Nutritional Therapy

The small numbers of patients studied in clinical trials of nutritional support in ARF do not demonstrate that this therapy reduces morbidity or mortality. Thus goals for nutritional therapy are currently directed at improving nutritional and metabolic surrogates. Three goals for nutritional therapy of patients with ARF are proposed: (a) to reduce negative protein balance and preserve or restore normal body composition, (b) to improve the patient's physiology and biochemistry, and (c) to normalize, to the extent consistent with the aforementioned goals, the altered chemical composition of plasma and tissues in ARF patients, particularly with regard to serum mineral levels, hydrogen ion concentrations, and potentially toxic metabolites.

Experimental evidence in patients with ARF supports the likelihood that these goals can be achieved with nutritional therapy. Moreover, research in sick nonuremic humans and animals support the feasibility of attaining these goals with nutritional therapy. Because hypercatabolism and malnutrition are associated with diminished wound healing, impaired immune function, and enhanced morbidity and mortality, it is not unlikely that nutritional therapy may reduce the risk of these adverse outcomes in patients with ARF.

Selection of Modality for Nutritional Support (Tables 83.1 and 83.2)

It is considered safest and most beneficial to provide nutrients by eating if patients are able to ingest foods. Nutritional supplements may be used to augment food intake, if necessary. Table 83.1 lists some oral supplements that are particularly designed or are commonly used for ARF patients. If patients cannot eat, tube or enterostomy feeding should be considered. Parenteral nutrition should be used only if nourishment through the intestinal tract is not safe and practical.

Energy Intake

Energy requirements for ARF patients are largely determined by the same factors as for individuals who do not have renal failure; these include weight, age, sex, associated diseases, and physical activity, if any. The patient with ARF who appears to be acutely ill is likely to have increased energy expenditure and to be hypercatabolic. Whether ARF per se affects energy expenditure or requirements is not known. Evidence suggests that if ARF itself alters energy expenditure, it has much less effect than that of superimposed illnesses. If energy balance is not maintained, patients almost always will be in negative protein balance. Moreover, the energy requirements to maintain protein balance appear to increase when nitrogen intake is low. Energy requirements can be assessed by indirect calorimetry, if available, multiplying the measured energy expenditure by 1.25. Alternatively, the Harris-Benedict equations,

TABLE 83.1. Nutrient Composition of Several Oral and Enteral Preparations Useful for Treatment of Acute Renal Failure

	Low-Protein/Amino Acid Supplements			High-Protein Supplements			No Protein
	Suplena (Ross)	Amin-Aid[a,b] (McGaw)	Travasorb Renal Diet[a,b] (Clintec)	Nephro (Ross)	Isocal HCN (Mead Johnson)	Magnacal (Sherwood)	Polycose (Liquid) (Ross)
Protein (g/100 ml)	3.0	1.94	2.3	7.0	7.5	7.0	0
Calories (kcal/ml)	2.0	1.96	1.35	2.0	2.0	2.0	2.0
Calorie Sources (%)							
Protein	6	4	6.9	14	15	14	0
Carbohydrate	51	74.8	81.1	43	40	50	100
Fat	43	21.2	12.0	43	45	36	0
Osmolality (mOsm/kg H_2O)	615	700	590	635	690	590	900
Electrolytes (mg/dl)							
Sodium	79	<34	N/A	83	80	100	70
Potassium	112	<23	N/A	106	170	125	6
Phosphorus	73	0	0	69	100	100	3
Calcium	139	0	0	137	100	100	20
Magnesium	21	0	0	21	40	40	N/A
Trace elements	Present	Absent	Absent	Present	Present	Present	Absent
Multivitamins	Present	Absent	Present	Present	Present	Present	Absent

[a] Amino acid composition (g/100 g of amino acids): *Amin-Aid,* leucine, 16.69; methionine, 16.69; phenylalanine, 16.69; valine, 12.14; lysine, 12.00; isoleucine, 10.62; threonine, 7.59; tryptophan, 3.79; histidine, 3.79. *Travasorb Renal Diet,* leucine, 9.24; methionine, 8.74; phenylalanine, 7.49; valine, 11.48; lysine, 6.87; isoleucine, 7.74; threonine, 5.74; tryptophan, 2.50; histidine, 6.49; arginine, 7.99; proline, 5.74; glycine, 5.37; alanine, 8.49; serine, 5.37; tyrosine, 0.75.

[b] No protein, only free amino acids, are provided in Amin-Aid and Travasorb.

N/A, information not available.

TABLE 83.2. Typical Composition of Total Parental Nutrition Infusates for Patients with Acute Renal Failure[a,b]

Nutrients	Final Concentration or Daily Intake	
Dextrose monohydrate (500 ml of 70%)	g/L	350
Amino acids (AA)		
Essential and nonessential (500 ml of 8.5%–10.0% AA) or	g/kg/day	1.0–1.2
Essential (500 ml of 5% AA)	g/kg/day	0.30–0.50
Energy (approx)	kcal/L	1339–1365
	(kcal/kg/day)	(30–45)
Electrolytes[c]		
Sodium[d]	mEq/L	40–50
Chloride[d]	mEq/L	25–35
Acetate[d]	mEq/L	35–40
Potassium	mEq/day	≤40
Calcium	mEq/day	10
Magnesium	mEq/day	8
Phosphorus	mmol/day	8
Iron	mg/day	2
Vitamins		
Vitamin A[e]	USP units/day	See text
Vitamin D	USP units/day	See text
Vitamin K[f]	mg/wk	7.5
Vitamin E	IU/day	10
Niacin	mg/day	20
Thiamin HCl (B_1)	mg/day	2
Riboflavin (B_2)	mg/day	2
Pantothenic acid	mg/day	10
Pyridoxine HCl (B_6)	mg/day	10[g]
Ascorbic acid	mg/day	60
Biotin	μg/day	60–100
Folic acid	mg/day	0.8–1.0
Vitamin B_{12}	μg/day	4

[a] For patients who are not very wasted, are not hypercatabolic (i.e., UNA <5 g/day), are not undergoing dialysis, and will not receive TPN for more than 2 or 3 weeks, 0.30 to 0.50 g/kg per day of the nine essential amino acids may be given. For patients who are more catabolic (i.e., UNA ≥5 g/day), are undergoing hemodialysis (particularly for 2 weeks or more), or are very wasted, about 1.0 to 1.2 g/kg per day essential and nonessential amino acids may be infused. For patients with a similar nutrition/metabolic status who are receiving CVVH or CVVHD, 1.5 to 2.5 g/kg per day of essential and nonessential amino acids may be given. Energy intake is usually maintained at 30 to 45 kcal/kg per day. Generally, 70% dextrose is used because of its greater caloric density. Lipid solutions may provide up to 30% of energy intake unless the patient has uncontrolled sepsis (see text). The 20% lipid emulsion provides the most fat and energy per milliliter of water.

[b] These nutrients are included in each bottle containing 500 ml of 5% essential amino acids or 8.5% to 10% essential and nonessential amino acids and 500 ml of 70% dextrose. The vitamins and trace elements are an exception and should be added to only one bottle per day. For any patient during a 24-hour period, the ratio of energy to amino acids in each of the containers providing the TPN solutions should be constant. Generally, the volume of the TPN solutions necessary to provide the prescribed energy and amino acid intake is about 1.5 to 2.0 L/day for patients receiving hemodialysis thrice weekly and 2.0 to 3.0 L/day for patients undergoing CVVHD.

[c] When adding electrolytes, the amounts intrinsically present in the amino acid solution should be taken into account.

[d] Refers to final concentration of electrolytes in the solution.

[e] Vitamin A probably should be avoided unless TPN is continued for more than 2 weeks.

[f] Should be given orally or parenterally and not in the TPN solution because of antagonisms.

[g] Intake of free pyridoxine, 8.2 mg/day.

which estimate basal energy expenditure (BEE), may be used as follows:

$$\text{For men: BEE} = 66.5 + (13.8 \times \text{weight in kg}) + (5.0 \times \text{height in cm}) - (6.8 \times \text{age in years})$$

$$\text{For women: BEE} = 655.1 + (9.6 \times \text{weight in kg}) + (1.8 \times \text{height in cm}) - (4.7 \times \text{age in years})$$

The BEE value derived from this equation is multiplied by an adjustment factor for associated illnesses. The following adjustments may be used: elective surgery, 1.00; peritonitis, 1.15; soft tissue trauma, 1.15; fractures, 1.20 to 1.25; mild infections, 1.00 to 1.20; moderate infections, 1.20 to 1.40; severe infections, 1.40 to 1.60; burns according to percent body surface involved: 0% to 20%, 1.00 to 1.50; 20% to 40%, 1.50 to 1.85; 40% to 100%, 1.85 to 2.05. The energy expenditure modified by these adjustment factors is then increased by 25% to account for individual variability, physical activity, and the possibly greater needs of maintaining nitrogen balance with low nitrogen intakes. Thus the energy requirement may be estimated as follows:

$$\text{Energy requirement} = \text{Estimated BEE for healthy individuals} \times \text{Adjustment for clinical state} \times 1.25$$

Generally, the energy requirements for ARF patients are between 30 and 45 kcal/kg of adjusted body weight per day. Adjusted body weight (ABW) is estimated as follows:

$$ABW = BW_{ef} + [(SBW - BW_{ef}) \times 0.25]$$

where standard body weight (SBW) is the median weight of a normal person of the same gender, height, skeletal frame size, and age range as the individual in question, as determined from the NHANES II data, and BW_{ef} is the individual's actual edema-free body weight. When nutritional intake is expressed per kilogram of body weight, this always refers to the adjusted body weight.

The higher energy intakes (i.e., 40 to 45 kcal/kg per day) are generally prescribed for patients who are severely ill, are not very obese, and have a high UNA that exceeds nitrogen intake (i.e., patients are in negative nitrogen balance). Energy intakes above 45 kcal/kg per day are virtually never administered because there appears to be no nutritional advantage to the patient, and complications of carbon dioxide retention, fatty liver, obesity, and excessive water intake (to provide the intravenous solutes) become more common with higher energy intakes.

Because ARF patients are often unable to excrete a water load, glucose is often administered as a 70% solution, which provides 2.38 kcal/ml (3.4 kcal/g of dextrose monohydrate). Amino acids provide about 3.5 kcal/g. Lipid emulsions, which are available in 10% (1.0 kcal/ml) and 20% (2.0 kcal/ml) solutions, are often given as the 20% solution. Although only a few grams per day of lipids are necessary to prevent essential fatty acid deficiency, many physicians infuse up to 30% or 40% of calories as lipids to approximate a more normal fuel mixture and to reduce the large dextrose load. Lipids may be admixed with dextrose and amino acids in the same container (three-in-one solutions) and infused over 12 to 24 hours. The three-in-one solutions are more economical to prepare and administer to the patient.

Several studies suggest that infusion of lipid emulsions may transiently impair reticuloendothelial system function, possibly by overwhelming its phagocytic capacity, and may also reduce host resistance. A prudent approach to reduce this possibility is to transiently withhold lipid infusions from patients who have a potentially overwhelming infection or are at high risk for developing such an infection (e.g., a patient with septicemia or an acute perforation of the colon). Also, it would seem prudent to infuse lipid emulsions over 12 to 24 hours to prevent marked increases in plasma lipids and to reduce the likelihood of overwhelming the phagocytic capacity of the reticuloendothelial system. Several studies suggest that omega-3 fatty acids may enhance immune function and host resistance. Oral but not intravenous solutions of omega-3 fatty acids are currently available. Research is needed to assess whether these compounds will have similar effects in patients with ARF.

Protein and Amino Acids

For patients who have a low UNA (i.e., 4 to 5 g/day or less), are not markedly malnourished, and are not undergoing dialysis, an oral or enteral intake or a regimen of parenteral nutrition may be prescribed that is low in nitrogen, that is, 0.30 to 0.50 g/kg per day of essential amino acids but no more than 20 to 30 g/day total, 0.60 g dietary protein/kg per day, or 0.60 g of intravenous essential and nonessential amino acids/kg per day. Larger quantities of essential amino acids, without nonessential amino acids, are not prescribed because of the possibility of causing dangerous amino acid imbalances. If 0.60 g protein/kg per day is prescribed, at least 60% of the protein should be of high biologic value (e.g., animal protein). These regimens usually will maintain neutral or only slightly negative nitrogen balance and will minimize the rate of accumulation of nitrogenous metabolites. Hence, dialysis therapy may be minimized or avoided. The most urea-sparing regimen provides about 0.30 to 0.50 g essential amino acids/kg per day. It generally should be used only for up to 2 or 3 weeks because of its low nitrogen content and the lack of evidence as to its safety over longer periods.

For patients who have a UNA greater than 4 to 5 g/day, are malnourished, are undergoing dialysis therapy, or require nutritional support for longer periods, nutritional therapy is determined in part by the type of renal placement therapy available to the patient. To match the nitrogen output of these patients, their nitrogen intake will be so great that there generally will be a high generation rate of urea and other nitrogen metabolites; this will usually lead to a need for dialysis therapy. If the ARF patient is given hemodialysis treatments at least 3 days per week, it is necessary to feed or infuse the patient with about 1.0 to 1.2 g/kg per day of protein or amino acids. Patients undergoing CVVH or CVVHD appear to tolerate increased amino acid and water loads more effectively because of the greater weekly clearances. With similar amino acid intakes, peak SUN levels tend to be lower with CVVH or CVVHD than with hemodialysis. If blood levels of metabolites become excessive, patients receiving CVVH or CVVHD can be treated with regular hemodialysis as well. With CVVH or CVVHD, amino acid or protein intake can be increased further, usually to levels that are commonly recommended for hypercatabolic patients who do not have renal failure, 1.5 to 2.5 g/kg per day. The nutritional formulations for patients receiving this quantity of amino acids should contain both essential and nonessential amino acids to prevent imbalances.

Most patients with ARF who are receiving nutritional support should be prescribed either 1.0 to 1.2 g/kg per day or 1.5 to 2.5 g/kg per day of amino acids or protein with intermittent hemodialysis or CVVH or CVVHD, respectively. The larger nitrogen intakes may reduce the negative nitrogen balance of the patient. Usually, peritoneal dialysis is not sufficiently efficient for treatment of such patients unless it is employed daily with rapid exchanges; also, many ARF patients in need of nutritional support do not have healthy abdominal cavities that are necessary for peritoneal dialysis. If ARF persists for more than 2 or 3 weeks, patients undergoing regular dialysis therapy usually are treated as maintenance dialysis patients and are given 1.1 to 1.2 g/kg per day if they receive hemodialysis or 1.2 to 1.5 g/kg per day if they are treated with chronic peritoneal dialysis.

TPN solutions high in branched-chain amino acids may enhance protein balance in acutely stressed catabolic patients without renal failure. However, the degree of improvement in nitrogen balance is modest. Thus such solutions are not routinely used for ARF patients. In postoperative patients receiving TPN, an intravenous infusion of the salt complex of α-ketoglutamate and ornithine is reported to decrease UNA and improve nitrogen balance. Further experience with this compound is necessary before it can be recommended for patients with ARF.

Water and Minerals

The water, mineral, and alkali needs of ARF patients vary greatly because of the marked heterogeneity of their clinical states. Hence, the recommended intake from enteral (Table 83.1) or TPN solutions (Table 83.2) must be considered tentative. Abnormalities in water, serum electrolyte concentrations, and acid–base status in ARF patients receiving TPN are much more common than in intensive care unit patients given TPN who do not have ARF. This difference is not abolished with hemodialysis therapy. Thus careful and sophisticated management of fluid and electrolyte intake is essential, and one cannot rely solely on dialysis treatment to prevent or correct fluid and electrolyte disorders in ARF.

The nutritional intake for acutely uremic patients must be reevaluated carefully each day and sometimes more frequently because these patients may undergo rapid changes in their metabolic and clinical status. The total daily water intake necessary to provide this recommended nutrient intake by TPN, using concentrated solutions, is about 1,700 to 2,000 ml and is almost always within 1,500 to 2,500 ml/day. This water load will often compel patients to receive dialysis or hemofiltration therapy. As indicated earlier, patients receiving CVVH or CVVHD are usually able to handle large water or electrolyte load more efficiently.

If a serum electrolyte concentration is increased, it may be beneficial to reduce or withhold intake of that mineral at the onset of nutritional therapy. Patients must be monitored carefully because hormonal and metabolic changes, which often occur with initiation of nutritional support, may cause serum chemistries to fall rapidly. This is especially likely to occur for serum potassium and phosphorus. Conversely, a mineral deficit may indicate a need for greater-than-usual intake of that element. Again, metabolic changes can lead to rapid repletion and a rise in serum levels. The combination of the altered metabolic milieu and a high dextrose intake in ARF patients predisposes to hyperglycemia. Crystalline zinc insulin may be administered directly to the patient or added to TPN solutions; about 1.0 to 2.5 units of regular insulin per 25 g of dextrose are often sufficient.

Vitamins

The vitamin needs of ARF patients have not been well investigated. The estimated vitamin requirements are largely based on data obtained from studies of patients with chronic renal failure. The daily requirements for most water-soluble vitamins are similar to the Recommended Dietary Allowances for normal individuals. Exceptions are vitamin B_6 (pyridoxine HCl), for which 10 mg/day are recommended, and folic acid, for which 800 to 1,000 μg/day are recommended. Vitamin C is not given in amounts greater than the Recommended Dietary Allowances for adults (60 mg/day) because it can be converted to oxalate, which will accumulate in patients with renal failure.

Although vitamin K is a fat-soluble vitamin, deficiencies have been observed in individuals without renal failure who were not eating and receiving antibiotics postoperatively. Presumably, suppression of vitamin K–synthesizing bacteria in the intestinal tract and the absence of exogenous intake of vitamin K were responsible for the development of vitamin K deficiency. Vitamin

K supplements of about 10 mg/wk are therefore given routinely to ARF patients receiving TPN or enteral nutrition, unless this amount is already present in the enteral preparation.

In patients with chronic renal failure, serum vitamin A levels are elevated, and even small increments above the Recommended Dietary Allowances for vitamin A (e.g., 1.5 to 3 times the Recommended Dietary Allowance) may cause toxicity. Because most patients with ARF receive TPN for only a few days, it is unlikely that deficiency of this fat-soluble vitamin will occur. Therefore we do not routinely give ARF patients vitamin A supplements. If patients require nutritional support for more than 2 weeks, we provide only the Recommended Dietary Allowance for vitamin A, 800 and 1,000 μg retinol equivalents/day, respectively, for women and men. Vitamin D is fat soluble, and vitamin D stores should not become depleted during a few days or weeks of TPN. However, the turnover of the most active form of vitamin D, 1,25-dihydroxycholecalciferol, is much faster. The requirement for this vitamin D analog in acute renal failure is not yet well defined.

POTENTIAL NEW TREATMENT MODALITIES

Several groups of investigators have examined the possibility of administering nutrients in hemodialysate or peritoneal dialysate. These techniques may provide sufficient quantities of amino acids and minerals. However, they do not deliver adequate calories and therefore should be considered to be a method for delivering nutritional supplements.

In experimental animal models of ARF, certain growth factors may enhance the rate of recovery of renal function. This has been observed for insulinlike growth factor-1 (IGF-1), epidermal growth factor, and hepatocyte growth factor. Most experience with the use of growth factors in ARF has been obtained with IGF-1. IGF-1 has also been shown to decrease UNA and suppress degradation and increase synthesis of protein in epitrochlearis muscle from rats with ischemic ARF. Unfortunately, studies with recombinant human IGF-1 (rhIGF-1) treatment for sick patients with ARF living in intensive care units has not shown benefits. In one study, treatment of ARF patients with atrial natriuretic peptide infusions was observed to increase their creatinine clearance in comparison to control ARF patients given standard care. However, further studies have not confirmed a benefit to atrial natriuretic peptide in patients with ARF. It is likely that the discrepancy between the benefits observed in animals with ARF given these growth factors and the lack of effect in patients with ARF treated with these compounds is due to the complex clinical condition of the patients. The patients with ARF given rhIGF-1 often had multiple illnesses, including disorders that caused acute inflammatory states. Patients often were septic and may have had episodes of hypotension. In contrast, in the experimental animals that displayed a response to growth factors, the ARF was usually uncomplicated. It would seem of value to examine why patients with ARF did not respond to rhIGF-1 and whether a modification of growth factor therapy could lead to more favorable outcomes.

Selected Readings

Bellomo R et al. A comparison of conventional dialytic therapy and acute continuous hemodiafiltration in the management of acute renal failure in the critically ill. *Renal Failure* 1993;15:595–620.

This paper described experience with nutritional therapy in patients with ARF receiving continuous venovenous hemofiltration with dialysis.

Hirschberg R, Kopple JD, Lipsett P, et al. Multicenter clinical trail of recombinant human insulin-like growth factor I in patients with acute renal failure. *Kidney Int* 1999;55:2423–2432.

This paper describes the results of a clinical trial of treatment with recombinant human insulin-like growth factor-1 for patients with ARF living in an intensive care unit. The study showed no benefit to the use of rhIGF-1 for the treatment of these patients.

Kopple JD. The Rhoads lecture: the nutritional management of the patient with acute renal failure. *J Parent Enter Nutr* 1996;20:3–12.

This manuscript reviews the experience with nutritional therapy for patients with ARF.

Mehta RL. Therapeutic alternatives to renal replacement for critically ill patients in acute renal failure. *Semin Nephrol* 1994;14:64–82.

This manuscript also discusses the use of nutritional therapy for patients with ARF receiving continuous venovenous hemofiltration with or without dialysis.

PART 2
Chronic Renal Failure

Joel D. Kopple

EFFECT OF DIETARY INTAKE ON THE RATE OF PROGRESSION OF RENAL FAILURE

Mechanisms of Progression

Physicians have known for many decades that patients with chronic renal disease who have sustained a substantial loss of glomerular filtration rate (GFR) often continue to lose renal function inexorably until they develop end-stage renal failure. Although the rate of progression of renal failure varies greatly among patients, in many individuals, the decline in kidney function is rather linear. The percentage of patients with chronic renal disease who will progress to end-stage renal failure is not known, but it seems likely that most patients who sustain a loss of GFR of 50% or greater will show continued progression of renal failure. Renal failure may progress because of continued activity of the underlying renal disease or because of superimposed disorders such as obstruction hypertension, kidney infection, nephrotoxic medicines, hypercalcemia, or hyperuricemia. However, in many instances, the progression continues even after the initial cause of the renal disease seems to have disappeared. Moreover, the continued progression of renal failure may occur when no associated causes of impaired renal function are identified. Several theories have been advanced to explain this phenomenon, and these are discussed in Chapter 67, Part 2.

Historically, dietary protein restriction was used to reduce uremic toxicity. In the first half of the twentieth century, a number of research studies in rats indicated that protein restriction could retard progression of renal failure. The experimental design of these studies was often faulty. Studies in humans with renal disease also were not well controlled, and the results were inconsistent and did not clearly show a benefit of dietary therapy on progression of renal failure.

In the 1970s and 1980s, research in both humans and rats indicated that dietary control can retard the rate of progression of renal failure in many renal diseases. In rats, several models of renal insufficiency were studied. These included surgical removal of the upper and lower poles of one kidney or ligation of about two-thirds to three-fourths of the arteries to one kidney; in both models, contralateral nephrectomy was performed. In some cases, experimental glomerulonephritis was created. In these animal models, diets low in protein and/or phosphorus retard or prevent progression of renal failure. In addition, a diet low or high in certain fats may retard progressive renal damage. Moreover, administration of prostaglandins may affect the progression of chronic renal disease in animals. The mechanisms underlying the progression of renal failure are discussed in Chapter 67, Part 3.

HUMAN STUDIES ON THE EFFECT OF DIETARY THERAPY ON PROGRESSION OF CHRONIC RENAL FAILURE

From the mid-1970s to the present, many dietary studies in humans with chronic renal insufficiency have indicated that a low intake of dietary protein and phosphorus is effective in retarding the rate of progression of renal failure. Some evidence indicates that a low protein and phosphorus intake may each act separately to slow progressive renal failure.

The earlier studies of this question in humans generally suffered from one or more major defects in experimental design, including small sample size, inadequate or absent control groups, poor documentation of the patients' actual intake, and imprecise methods of measuring renal function. Newer clinical trials have used more effective research protocols. These latter studies generally compared a low-protein, low-phosphorus diet providing either about 0.40 to 0.60 g protein/kg body weight per day or about 0.28 g protein/kg per day supplemented with essential amino acids or ketoacids to a more liberal diet containing approximately 1.0 g protein/kg per day and more phosphorus or to an ad libitum diet.

The very-low-protein diet providing about 0.28 g/kg per day (e.g., about 16 to 25 g protein per day) is supplemented with 10 to 20 g/day of the nine essential amino acids or of mixtures of several essential amino acids, several nonessential amino acids, and ketoacid or hydroxyacid analogs of other essential amino acids. The ketoacid or hydroxyacid analog is structurally identical to its corresponding essential amino acid, except the amino (NH_2) group attached to the second (α) carbon of the amino acid is replaced with a keto group or hydroxy group, respectively.

The ketoacid and hydroxyacid analogs can be transaminated *in vivo* to the respective amino acids, although a proportion of the analogs are degraded rather than transaminated. Because the ketoacids and hydroxyacids lack the nitrogen-containing amino group on the α carbon, these compounds provide the patient with a lesser nitrogen load. Because they are degraded in the body, they should engender fewer waste products that will accumulate in renal failure. Ketoacid analogs of the branched chain amino acids, especially of leucine, may be particularly likely to promote protein anabolism, possibly by decreasing protein degradation. Hence it is possible, but not yet demonstrated, that these ketoacids may play a beneficial role in maintaining protein mass in patients with renal failure.

The largest and most intensive examination of whether dietary control will retard the rate of progression of renal disease was the Modification of Diet in Renal Disease (MDRD) Study that was funded by the National Institutes of Health. This project investigated, in an intention-to-treat analysis, the effects of three levels of dietary protein and phosphorus intakes and two blood pressure management goals on the progression of chronic renal disease. A total of 840 adults with various types of renal disease, but excluding insulin-dependent diabetes mellitus, were divided into two study groups according to their GFR.

In study A, 585 patients with a GFR, measured by radiolabeled iothalamate clearances, of 25 to 55 ml/1.73m^2 per minute were examined. Patients were randomly assigned to either a usual-protein, usual-phosphorus diet (1.3 g/kg standard body weight per day of protein and 16 to 20 mg/kg per day of phosphorus) or to a low-protein, low-phosphorus diet (0.58 g/kg per day of protein and 5 to 10 mg/kg per day of phosphorus) and also to either a moderate or strict blood pressure goal (mean arterial blood pressure 107 mm Hg [113 mm Hg for those 61 years of age or older] or 92 mm Hg [98 mm Hg for those 61 years of age or older]). Study B included 255 patients with a baseline GFR of 13 to 24 ml/1.73m^2 per minute. Patients were randomly assigned to the low-protein, low-phosphorus diet or to a very-low-protein, very-low-phosphorus diet (0.28 g/kg per day of protein and 4 to 9 mg/kg per day of phosphorus) with a ketoacid–amino acid supplement (0.28 g/kg per day). They were also randomly assigned to either the moderate or strict blood pressure control groups, as in study A. Adherence to the dietary protein prescription in the different diet groups was good.

For the participants in study A, those prescribed the low-protein diet had significantly faster declines in GFR during the first 4 months than those assigned to the usual-protein diet. Thereafter, the rate of decline of the GFR in the low-protein, low-phosphorus group was significantly slower than in the group fed the usual-protein, usual-phosphorus diet. Over the course of the entire treatment period, there was no difference in the overall rate of progression of renal failure in the two diet groups. However, it is likely that the initial greater fall in GFR in the patients prescribed the low-protein diet may reflect a hemodynamic response to the reduction in protein intake rather than a greater rate of progression of the parenchymal renal disease. This might in fact be beneficial, reflecting a reduction of intrarenal hyperfiltration and intrarenal hypertension. If this explanation is correct, and it is not certain that it is correct, the subsequently slower rate of progression of disease after the first 4 months of dietary treatment is consistent with a beneficial effect of this intervention in renal disease. In study B, the very-low-protein group had a marginally slower decline of GFR than the low-protein group; the average rate of decline did not differ significantly between the two groups ($P = .066$).

In a secondary retrospective analysis of the MDRD Study in which the decrease in GFR was correlated with the actual quantity of protein ingested, there was a slower rate of loss of GFR and longer time before starting maintenance dialysis therapy in individuals who actually ingested 0.70 to 0.75 g protein/kg per day or less. This interpretation must be qualified because it is subject to the limitations of a retrospective analysis.

The following factors concerning the MDRD Study may have limited the likelihood of demonstrating that low-protein diets retard progression of renal failure. First, the very-low-protein ketoacid–amino acid supplemented diet was not compared with a usual protein or phosphorous intake. Moreover, the mean duration of treatment in the MDRD Study, 2.2 years, was rather short. If the trend toward slower progression of renal failure in the low-protein diet groups that was present at the termination of the MDRD Study had persisted for a longer follow-up period, statistically significantly slower progression would have been observed with the 0.60 g/kg protein diet in study A and the very-low-protein, ketoacid–amino acid supplemented diet in study B. Many patients assigned to each diet in the MDRD Study showed no progression of kidney disease. Also, a disproportionately large number of patients had adult polycystic kidney disease, which may be less responsive to dietary therapy.

Three meta-analyses of clinical trials evaluated the effects of low-protein and, in some studies, low-phosphorus diets on the rate of progression of kidney failure or the development of end-stage renal disease (ESRD). The three meta-analyses each evaluated a somewhat different series of clinical trials, and only two of the meta-analyses included the MDRD trial. Two meta-analyses concluded that low-protein diets delay the onset of renal replacement therapy by about 23% or 47%, and a third meta-analysis indicated that such diets retard the rate of progression of renal failure by about 7%. One meta-analysis also indicated that low-protein diets also retard progression in patients with insulin-dependent diabetes mellitus. This latter analysis was less definitive because much smaller numbers of patients were analyzed; in two of the trials, there was no randomized, concurrent control group, and the key endpoints were less precise.

Some studies suggest that vegetarian diets providing soy protein may retard progression of chronic renal failure more effectively than diets of similar protein content that contain animal protein. The mechanisms of such an effect is not known, but it may be related to the lower content and different composition of fats in the vegetarian diet. This latter diet is reported to improve the serum lipid profile in patients with chronic renal disease and nephrotic syndrome. The effect of dietary protein restriction is also discussed in Chapter 67, Part 3.

NUTRITIONAL ALTERATIONS IN NEPHROTIC SYNDROME

Nephrotic syndrome is characterized by urinary protein excretion of at least 3.5 g/day in adults or 40 mg/hr/m^2 body surface in children, low serum albumin concentrations, high serum levels of cholesterol and other fats, and edema. Patients with nephrotic syndrome often develop protein malnutrition and debility because they have large urinary protein losses and their appetite is often poor. Certain vitamins and most trace elements are protein bound in plasma, and nephrotic patients are at risk for developing deficiencies of these nutrients because the binding proteins are excreted in the urine. Vitamin D deficiency has been reported in nephrotic patients and is caused by urinary losses of vitamin D and its binding protein. The metabolic consequences of nephrotic syndrome are discussed in Chapter 39, Part 2.

Both protein-restricted diets and angiotensin-converting enzyme (ACE) inhibitors reduce proteinuria in nephrotic patients. Studies in animals indicate that diets appropriately restricted in protein may not decrease serum albumin levels or albumin pools because there is a reduction in urinary protein excretion. However, treating nephrotic patients with both an ACE inhibitor, which may decrease proteinuria, and a higher-protein diet, to increase protein synthesis, has been suggested as the most effective way to maintain a more normal albumin mass in these individuals. This hypothesis has been demonstrated to be correct in one study in nephrotic rats but has not yet been extensively tested in nephrotic patients.

NUTRITIONAL AND METABOLIC CONSEQUENCES OF CHRONIC RENAL FAILURE

Chronic renal failure causes pervasive nutritional and metabolic disorders that may affect virtually every organ system. These abnormalities are reviewed briefly.

Clinical, Nutritional, and Metabolic Disorders

Chronic advanced renal failure causes a complex set of disorders that are due to the marked reduction in the excretory, endocrine, and metabolic functions of the kidney and that collectively engender the syndrome of uremia. The many symptoms of uremia include weakness, a feeling of ill health, insomnia, fatigue, loss of appetite, nausea, vomiting, weight loss, diarrhea, itching, muscle cramps, hiccups, sallow skin, twitching or jerking of the extremities, fasciculations, tremors, emotional irritability, and decreased mental concentration and comprehension (see Chapter 34). A characteristic fetid breath is often present. The sodium and water disturbances associated with renal failure can lead to congestive heart failure and hypertension or, if excessive sodium depletion occurs, reduction in extracellular fluid volume and a fall in blood pressure. Altered serum concentrations of other electrolytes and acidosis can occur and can have profound and life-threatening effects on the physiologic processes and metabolism of the body. Most of these clinical and metabolic disorders can be controlled or prevented with dietary therapy or dialysis. When untreated, uremia can lead progressively to lethargy, loss of consciousness, coma, convulsions, and death.

Chronic advanced renal failure causes pervasive alterations in the absorption, excretion, or metabolism of many nutrients. These disorders include the accumulation of metabolic products of protein metabolism; a decreased ability of the kidney either to excrete a large sodium load or to conserve sodium avidly when sodium intake is restricted; impaired renal ability to excrete water, potassium, calcium, magnesium, phosphorus, trace elements, acids, and other compounds; a retention of phosphorus; decreased intestinal absorption of calcium and possibly iron and certain amino acids; and in animal studies, decreased absorption of intestinal riboflavin, folate, and vitamin D_3. There is a high risk for developing certain vitamin deficiencies, particularly vitamin B_6, vitamin C, folic acid, and the most potent known form of vitamin D, 1,25-dihydroxycholecalciferol [$(1,25\text{-OH})_2 D_3$]. The patient with chronic renal failure is also likely to accumulate certain potentially toxic chemicals, such as aluminum, that normally are ingested in small amounts and excreted in the urine (see Chapter 68, Part 2).

Medicinal therapy may adversely affect nutrient metabolism in renal failure. The excessive intake of aluminum from the ingestion of aluminum phosphate binders may predispose to aluminum toxicity. Anticonvulsant medicines may cause deficiencies of vitamin D and folic acid; hydralazine, isoniazid, and other medicines may cause vitamin B_6 deficiency.

Uremia is also a polyendocrinopathy, and many of the metabolic and clinical manifestations of uremia are caused by endocrine disorders. Many hormone concentrations are elevated in renal failure, particularly those of the peptide hormones, because of the impaired ability of the kidney to degrade peptides. These include parathyroid hormone (PTH), glucagon, insulin, growth hormone, prolactin, luteinizing hormone, often follicle-stimulating hormone (FSH), and gastrin. Increased secretion of some hormones, such as PTH, insulin, and prolactin, may contribute to elevated plasma levels. Chronically uremic patients have an altered thyroid hormone pattern that is similar to the euthyroid sick syndrome, but hypothyroidism is not common (see Chapter 74, Part 4). Of the hormones elaborated by the kidney, plasma erythropoietin and 1,25-dihydroxycholecalciferol are reduced, and plasma renin activity may be increased, normal, or decreased. Serum insulinlike growth factor-1 (IGF-1) is usually reported to be normal in renal failure, but there is resistance to the activity of IGF-1 as well as of insulin. In malnourished patients with chronic renal failure, serum IGF-1 is reduced. There is increased sensitivity to the actions of glucagon, which is reversed by hemodialysis, although hyperglucagonemia persists. These effects on insulin and glucagon contribute to the mild glucose intolerance that is often present in chronic renal failure.

Impaired actions of hormones in uremia may be due to increased levels of inhibitory compounds in serum or tissues, downregulation of receptor numbers, or postreceptor defects in the signal transduction system. Cytosolic calcium participates in certain cell signalling systems. Elevated basal cytosolic calcium, induced by hyperparathyroidism, appears to be one of the postreceptor signal transduction disorders induced by chronic renal failure and may contribute to IGF-1 resistance and impaired insulin secretion.

The ability of the failing kidney to synthesize or metabolize many compounds, including amino acids, is impaired. In chronic renal insufficiency, the diseased kidney displays reduced catabolism of glutamine, impaired synthesis of alanine, and decreased conversion of arginine to citrulline, glycine to serine, and amino groups to ammonium.

Many products of metabolism accumulate in renal failure; many of these are derived from amino acids and proteins. Most of these compounds accumulate as the result of decreased excretion, although in some instances, enhanced synthesis or impaired degradation by the diseased kidney or other organs plays a role (See Chapter 68, Part 4). Altered gastrointestinal function may affect nitrogen metabolism in uremic patients. The gastrointestinal tract metabolizes urea, uric acid, creatinine, and choline and synthesizes or releases from larger molecules dimethylamine, trimethylamine, ammonia, sarcosine, methylamine, and methylguanidine. The gut metabolism or synthesis of many of these compounds is increased in chronic renal failure, possibly because of the rise in the quantity of intestinal bacterial flora. Quantitatively, the most important end-product of nitrogen metabolism is urea. In a clinically stable patient with chronic renal failure who eats at least 40 g of protein per day, the net quantity of urea nitrogen produced each day is equal to about 80% to 90% of the daily nitrogen intake.

In nondialyzed chronically uremic patients, maintenance hemodialysis (MHD) patients, and chronic peritoneal dialysis (CPD) patients, there is a high incidence of type IV hyperlipoproteinemia with elevated serum triglyceride levels, a low serum high-density lipoprotein (HDL) cholesterol, and elevated serum low-density lipoprotein (LDL) and intermediate-density lipoprotein (IDL). Plasma triglyceride, LDL cholesterol, and apolipoprotein B concentrations tend to be higher in CPD patients than in those undergoing MHD. CPD patients often have abnormally increased serum total cholesterol levels. Patients with chronic renal failure, including maintenance dialysis patients, often display high serum concentrations of lipoprotein (a) [Lp(a)] (i.e., greater than 30 mg/dl). Also, in chronic renal failure, there are alterations in the concentration and/or composition of certain lipoproteins, with an abnormal proportion of individual lipids and altered structure of some apolipoproteins. Production of triglycerides generally is normal, but the metabolic clearance is impaired. Many of these lipid disorders, including increased serum Lp(a) and LDL cholesterol levels and low serum HDL cholesterol are associated with a high risk for coronary artery atherosclerosis, cerebrovascular arteriosclerosis, or stenosis of saphenous vein bypass grafts. Detailed discussion of lipid abnormalities in patients with chronic renal disease is found in Chapter 74, Part 2, and in those with nephrotic syndrome is found in Chapter 39, Part 2C.

There are abnormal concentrations of a number of plasma and intracellular amino acids as well as their metabolites. Indeed, the altered plasma amino acid pattern in chronic renal failure is pathognomonic for this condition. Many plasma sulfur amino acid concentrations are altered. Of greatest concern are the increased plasma homocysteine concentrations, which occur in roughly 85% of maintenance dialysis patients and which are also associated with an increased risk of atherosclerosis and coronary artery disease (see Chapter 68, Part 3).

With the institution of dietary therapy or treatment with hemodialysis or peritoneal dialysis, blood levels of many metabolic products that accumulate in uremic plasma decrease and the patient may experience clinical improvement. MHD or peritoneal dialysis enables patients to live for many years with essentially no renal function. Despite such improvement, however, many clinical and metabolic disorders may persist or even progress. These include (a) type IV hyperlipidemia, elevated serum Lp(a), and other disorders of lipid metabolism; (b) increased plasma homocysteine; (c) hypertension—this theoretically is reversible, but in fact is usually present; (d) a high incidence of cardiovascular disease; (e) osteodystrophy with disordered bone architecture, osteoporosis, or osteomalacia (aluminum toxicity often contributes to the osteomalacia); (f) anemia—this is correctable in most patients with sufficient quantities of erythropoietin, iron, and folic acid; (g) impaired immune function and decreased resistance to infection; (h) mildly impaired peripheral and central nervous system function; (i) muscle weakness and atrophy; (j) frequent occurrence of viral hepatitis; (k) sexual impotency and infertility; (l) generalized wasting and malnutrition; (m) a general feeling of ill health or emotional depression; and (n) poor rehabilitation.

Underlying comorbid conditions, such as diabetes mellitus, may also adversely affect the patient and may be progressive. All of the foregoing problems do not seriously affect every patient, and many patients with chronic renal failure, including those undergoing maintenance dialysis, lead full and productive lives. Most of these complications can be aggravated by poor nutritional intake and improved with good nutrition.

The Syndrome of Protein-Energy Malnutrition

Virtually every study of the nutritional status of nondialyzed patients with advanced chronic renal failure and patients undergoing MHD or CPD indicates that the patients often have protein and/or energy malnutrition (Table 83.3). Evidence includes decreased relative body weight (i.e., the patient's body weight divided by the weight of normal people of the same age, height, sex, and skeletal frame size), or body mass index (BMI), skinfold thickness (an estimate of total body fat), arm muscle mass, and total body nitrogen and potassium, as well as low growth rates in children. There are decreased serum concentrations of many proteins, including albumin, prealbumin, transferrin, and low muscle alkali-soluble protein. The plasma amino acid pattern, which is pathognomonic for renal failure, also has many similarities to that found in malnutrition. The findings of malnutrition are sometimes observed in nondialyzed patients with chronic renal failure but are more prevalent in patients undergoing MHD or CPD. Not every dialysis patient has evidence of these disorders. The prevalence of protein-energy malnutrition in different reports varies from about 18% to 75%, with an average value of roughly 40%. Protein-energy malnutrition in chronic dialysis patients is usually mild to moderate. About 6% to 8% of dialysis patients have evidence of severe malnutrition. It is important to recognize that in addition to protein-energy malnutrition, patients with chronic renal failure are at higher risk for malnutrition of iron, zinc, and certain vitamins, particularly vitamin B_6, vitamin C, folic acid, 1,25-dihydroxycholecalciferol, and possibly carnitine.

Causes of Protein-Energy Malnutrition

There are many causes for protein-energy malnutrition in patients with chronic renal failure. Probably most important is inadequate dietary protein and energy intake; this is particularly the case for energy intake. The low dietary intake is mainly due to anorexia. This is usually caused by uremic toxicity, acute or chronic illnesses, and emotional depression. The effects of acute superimposed illnesses on the patient's ability to eat or to accept tube feeding also reduce nutrient intake. In addition, the diet

TABLE 83.3. Evidence for Protein-Energy Malnutrition in Patients with Advanced Chronic Renal Failure or End-Stage Renal Disease

Anthropometry, Body Composition, and Isotope Dilution Studies[a]	Biochemistry[a]
Decreased	Total protein
Body weight	Albumin
Height (children)	Prealbumin
Growth (children)	Transferrin
Body fat (skinfold thickness)	Prealbumin
Fat-free solids	Urea (predialysis)
Intracellular water	Creatinine (predialysis)
Muscle mass (mid-arm muscle	Cholinesterase
circumference)	Insulinlike growth factor-1
Total body potassium	*Plasma*
(nondialyzed patients)	Leucine
Total body nitrogen (chronic	Isoleucine
peritoneal dialysis patients)	Total tryptophan
Total albumin mass, synthesis,	Valine
and catabolism	Tyrosine
Valine pools (nondialyzed	*Muscle*
patients)	Alkali soluble protein
Creatinine appearance	RNA:DNA ratio
Diet	Valine
Low energy intake	Tyrosine
Low protein intake	**Decreased**
	Serum
	Total protein
	Urine
	Creatinine excretion
	Normal to Increased
	Plasma
	Total nonessential amino acids
	Glycine

[a]Patients with chronic renal failure may have normal values for these parameters, but statistical comparisons indicate that the measurements are often abnormal in these individuals. For any of these measures (excepting nutrient intake), causes other than impaired nutritional intake, such as inflammation, hypercatabolic illnesses, or reduced meat intake (for creatinine measures), could contribute to the abnormal values.

prescribed in renal failure, which is low in protein and other nutrients and which may be difficult to prepare or may be unpalatable, can lead to a low nutrient intake, and of particular importance, low energy intake. In some studies of maintenance dialysis patients, serum albumin concentrations correlate with normalized protein nitrogen appearance (nPNA).

Patients with chronic renal failure have a high incidence of superimposed acute or chronic catabolic illnesses. In this regard, evidence suggests that many patients undergoing maintenance dialysis therapy may suffer from chronic inflammatory disorders. The most important findings in support of this thesis are that serum concentrations of a number of inflammatory cytokines and proteins, such as tumor necrosis factor-α, interleukin-1, C-reactive protein, and serum amyloid A protein, are elevated in maintenance dialysis patients. Elevated serum C-reactive protein is a predictor of mortality in these individuals. Some of the inflammatory cytokines can induce anorexia and stimulate protein catabolism. Elevated serum C-reactive protein has also been associated with coronary artery disease in the general population. This association may be due to enhanced proliferation of fibroblasts and smooth muscle cells in coronary arteries in response to inflammatory stimuli. Thus it has been postulated that many maintenance dialysis patients are in a state of chronic inflammation. Chronic inflammation may induce protein-energy malnutrition both by engendering anorexia and by enhancing the catabolic rate and also may increase the mortality rate by promoting coronary artery disease and possibly by engendering protein-energy malnutrition. In this regard, epidemiologic studies indicate that some of the reduction in serum albumin levels in maintenance dialysis patients can be predicted by elevated serum C-reactive protein. It is also possible that malnutrition may predispose to the development of an inflammatory state by predisposing the patient to infection or other chronic illnesses. Thus at least some of the relationship between low serum albumin or other indicators and high mortality may, in fact, be caused by the effects of chronic inflammation on clinical outcome. These theories, although attractive, are still based largely on epidemiologic evidence and await more definite research to establish their veracity.

Another cause of protein-energy malnutrition is the nutrient losses caused by the dialysis procedure itself. Hemodialysis and peritoneal dialysis remove many biologically valuable compounds, including nutrients. MHD treatment with low-flux dialyzers removes about 6 to 8 g of amino acids when patients are postabsorptive (fasting) and about 8 to 10 g when patients are postprandial. Approximately 2 to 3 g of peptides or bound amino acids are also removed. In two studies, routine hemodialysis with high-flux membranes was reported to remove 8.0 ± 2.8 (SD) g and 9.3 ± 2.7 g of amino acids from patients, respectively. During the sixth reuse of high-flux polysulfone hemodialyzers with bleach and formaldehyde reprocessing, amino acid losses are reported to be 12.2 ± 4.4 g.

In normoglycemic individuals, about 15 to 25 g of glucose may be removed if glucose-free dialysate is used. When the hemodialysate contains 200 mg/dl of glucose (180 mg/dl of anhydrous glucose), there is a net absorption of approximately 10 to 12 g of glucose with each dialysis. Typically, little protein is lost during hemodialysis.

About 2.0 to 3.0 g/day of free amino acids are removed during continuous ambulatory peritoneal dialysis (CAPD). In our experience, 8.8 ± 0.5 (SEM) g/day of total protein and 5.7 ± 0.4 g/day of albumin are lost into the dialysate with CAPD. Other studies describe similar findings. During an intermittent peritoneal dialysis treatment of about 36 hours' duration, about 22 g of total protein, including 13 g of albumin, are removed. With mild peritonitis, the quantity of protein removed during CAPD increases to about 15.1 ± 3.6 g/day; protein losses can rise markedly with severe peritonitis, and we have observed peritoneal protein losses as high as 100 g/day before initiating therapy. Water-soluble vitamins are removed by both hemodialysis and peritoneal dialysis. The vitamin losses can easily be replaced by food intake and vitamin supplements, but in patients with poor nutritional intake, such losses may cause vitamin deficiency.

Hemodialysis also increases net protein breakdown. This appears to be due to activation of the complement cascade system, which is primarily activated by release of interleukin from leukocytes. Activation of the complement cascade, in turn, stimulates release of catabolic cytokines, including tumor necrosis factor-α, and activation of proteolytic enzymes derived from granulocytes. This catabolic stress is particularly likely to occur when bioincompatible dialyzer membranes are used, such as Cuprophan, and can be mitigated with the use of dialyzers made from more biocompatible materials.

Patients with renal failure sustain blood losses. Because blood is a rich source of protein, these losses may contribute to protein depletion. The blood losses are caused by frequent blood drawing for laboratory testing; occult gastrointestinal bleeding, which is common in renal failure; and sequestration of blood in the hemodialyzer and blood tubing.

Other possible but less well-established causes of protein-energy malnutrition include (a) altered endocrine activity, particularly resistance to insulin and IGF-1, hyperglucagonemia, hyperparathyroidism, and deficiency of 1,25-dihydroxycholecalciferol; (b) endogenous uremic toxins; (c) exogenous uremic toxins, such as aluminum; and (d) loss of metabolic functions of the kidney. Because the kidney is a metabolic organ that synthesizes or degrades many biologically valuable compounds, including certain amino acids, the loss of these activities in kidney failure could possibly disrupt the body's metabolism and promote wasting.

Relationship Between Nutritional Status and Clinical Outcome

The great interest in the nutritional status of patients with chronic renal failure and those undergoing maintenance dialysis is due to the strong correlation between nutritional intake or nutritional status and morbidity and mortality in these individuals. Several investigators have shown an inverse relationship between dietary protein consumption, as determined by the patient's urea nitrogen appearance (UNA) or average serum urea nitrogen (SUN) level, and morbidity and mortality. Moreover, a striking inverse relationship exists between the predialysis serum concentrations of albumin, prealbumin, creatinine, and cholesterol; the body weight adjusted for height or body mass index; and the degree of malnutrition as determined by the subjective global assessment and the mortality rate in these patients. These studies were not prospective with randomized assignment to different nutritional intakes, and it is likely that the patients' underlying illnesses and inflammatory status contributed to both their high mortality and the low protein intake or other indicators of protein-energy malnutrition. Indeed, as indicated earlier, markers of inflammation, such as serum C-reactive protein, also correlate both with mortality rates and with protein-energy nutritional status. Nonetheless, the data are consistent with the thesis that poor nutrient intake and malnutrition adversely affect prognosis in patients undergoing MHD or CPD.

DIETARY MANAGEMENT OF CHRONIC RENAL DISEASE AND CHRONIC RENAL FAILURE

A recommended plan for nutrient intake is given in Table 83.4 for patients with chronic renal failure who are not undergoing dialysis therapy as well as for patients undergoing MHD or CPD. The following text explains this approach to the dietary management of these patients.

General Principles of Dietary Therapy

The widespread metabolic and nutritional disorders, frequent occurrence of protein-energy malnutrition, and evidence that diet may retard the progression of renal failure indicate that nutritional management is a critical aspect of the treatment of chronic renal failure. The three goals of dietary therapy are (a) to maintain good nutritional status, (b) to prevent or minimize uremic toxicity and the metabolic derangements of renal failure and, (c) to retard or stop the rate of progression of renal failure.

Adherence to specialized diets is difficult and stressful for most patients and their families. Generally, it requires patients to undergo a major change in their behavior patterns and to forsake many of their traditional sources of daily pleasure. The patient must procure special foods, prepare special recipes, usually forego or severely limit intake of favorite foods, and often eat foods that are not as desirable. Demands are made on the time, effort, and emotional support system of the family or close associates. Therefore it is incumbent on the physician not to prescribe radical changes in dietary intake without a clear indication that such changes may be beneficial to the patient. To ensure successful dietary therapy, patients with renal failure must undergo extensive training in the principles of nutritional therapy and the design and preparation of diets, and they need continuous encouragement regarding dietary adherence. These patients must receive repeated retraining with regard to their nutritional therapy. When nutritional intake is not carefully monitored, patients tend to adhere poorly to dietary prescriptions. They may eat too little of some essential nutrients rather than too much.

A team approach to dietary management may improve adherence to the dietary therapy as well as to other aspects of the medical regimen. The team should include the physician, dietitian, close family members or friends, nursing staff, and where available, psychiatrists or social workers. Diet plans should be designed specifically for the individual tastes of the patient. A problem-oriented approach to dietary compliance can be very effective. At each visit, the physician should monitor dietary intake and discuss the results with the patient.

The physician must strongly support the dietitian's efforts to train and counsel the patient and to obtain dietary compliance. Generally, the patient's spouse or other close relatives or friends should work closely with the patient to provide moral support and to assist with acquisition and preparation of foods. To promote adherence to the diet, the entire medical team should assume an energetic, positive, and sympathetic approach. Research indicates that these techniques can enable many patients to attain acceptable levels of dietary compliance.

At least two cross-sectional studies indicate that many clinically stable patients with chronic renal disease begin to display spontaneous reductions in dietary energy and protein intake when the GFR decreases to 35 to 50 ml/min/1.73m^2. At a GFR of approximately 35 ml/min/1.73m^2 (e.g., a serum creatinine concentration averaging roughly 2.3 mg/dl in men and 2.1 mg/dl in women), serum albumin and transferrin concentrations and body weight, mid-arm muscle area, and percentage of body fat also begin to show declines. It should be emphasized that frank malnutrition has not been observed in clinically stable populations with these levels of renal function. On the other hand, individuals commencing maintenance dialysis therapy have a high prevalence of protein-energy malnutrition.

Evidence suggests that chronically uremic patients are at greatest risk for protein energy malnutrition during the period when the GFR falls below 10 to 15 ml/min and when the patient is beginning maintenance dialysis therapy. The nutritional status of patients at the onset of chronic dialysis treatment appears to be a strong predictor of their nutritional status 1 to 3 years later. Moreover, nutritional status at the onset of maintenance dialysis therapy is a strong predictor of mortality risk during the course of such treatment. Hence, particular effort should be made to prevent malnutrition as the patient approaches the time when dialysis should be instituted and during the first few weeks of chronic dialysis therapy. Such effort should be directed toward maintaining good nutritional intake during this period, rapidly instituting therapy for supervening illnesses, and maintaining good nutritional intake during such illnesses. Evidence for deteriorating nutritional status should lead to prompt corrective action.

Patients with advanced renal failure are at particular risk for inadequate energy intake. The prescribed diets, in comparison to the food intakes of the general population, are often marginally low in some nutrients, such as protein and phosphorus,

TABLE 83.4. Recommended Nutrient Intake for Nondialyzed Patients with Chronic Renal Failure and Patients Undergoing Maintenance Hemodialysis or Chronic Peritoneal Dialysis

	Chronic Renal Failure[a]	Maintenance Hemodialysis or Chronic Peritoneal Dialysis (CPD)[b]
Protein	0.55–0.60 g/kg/day ≥0.35 g/kg/day of protein of high biologic value If a patient will not accept the above diet or is unable to maintain an adequate energy intake with such a diet, an intake of up to 0.75 g/kg/day with ≥0.35 g/kg/day of protein of high biologic value may be prescribed	**Maintenance Hemodialysis[b]** 1.2 g/kg/day; ≥50% protein of high biologic value **Chronic Peritoneal Dialysis** 1.2–1.3 g/kg/day; ≥50% protein of high biologic value; CPD patients may be given up to 1.5 g/kg/day
Energy[c]	35 kcal/kg day; 30–35 kcal/kg/day for individuals ≥60 years; if the patient's relative body weight is >120% or the patient gains unwanted weight, lower energy intakes may be prescribed	
Fat (% of total energy intake)[d,e]	30	30
(Polyunsaturated: saturated fatty acid ratio[e,f]	1.0 : 1.0	1.0 : 1.0
Cholesterol	≤300 mg/day	≤300 mg/day
Carbohydrate[f]	Rest of nonprotein calories	
Total fiber intake[e]	20–25 g	20–25 g
Minerals	*Range of Intake*	
Sodium	1,000–3,000 mg/day[f]	750–1,000 mg/day[g]
Potassium	40–70 mEq/day	40–70 mEq/day
Phosphorus	5–10 mg/kg/day[h]	8–17 mg/kg/day[h]
Calcium	1,400–1,600 mg/day[i]	1,400–1,600 mg/day[i]
Magnesium	200–300 mg/day	200–300 mg/day
Iron	≥10–18 mg/day[j]	sufficient iron to maintain serum iron at 30%–40% saturation and serum ferritin at 100–800 μg/dl
Zinc	15 mg/day	15 mg/day
Water	Up to 3,000 ml/day usually 750–1,500 ml/day as tolerated[g]	
Vitamins	*Diets to Be Supplemented with These Quantities*	
Thiamin	1.5 mg/day	1.5 mg/day
Riboflavin	1.8 mg/day	1.8 mg/day
Pantothenic acid	5 mg/day	5 mg/day
Niacin	20 mg/day	20 mg/day
Pyridoxine HCl	5 mg/day	5 mg/day
Vitamin B_{12}	3 μg/day	3 μg/day
Vitamin C	60 mg/day	60 mg/day
Folic acid[k]	5–10 mg/day	5–10 mg/day
Vitamin A	No addition	No addition
Vitamin D	See text	See text
Vitamin E	15 IU/day	15 IU/day
Vitamin K	None[l]	None[l]

[a] Glomerular filtration rate above 5 ml/1.73 m^2/min and below about 75 ml/1.73 m^2 (see text).
[b] Protein intake for chronic peritoneal dialysis (CPD) patients who are not malnourished should be about 1.2 to 1.3 g/kg day.
[c] This includes energy intake from dialysate in the CPD patients.
[d] Refers to percentage of total energy intake (diet plus dialysate); if triglyceride levels are markedly elevated, the percentage of fat in the diet may be increased to about 40% of total calories to reduce carbohydrate intake; otherwise, 30% of total calories is strongly preferred.
[e] These dietary recommendations are considered less crucial than the others, unless hyperlipidemia is present (see text).
[f] Should be primarily complex carbohydrates, if tolerated by the patient.
[g] Can be higher in CPD patients or in those nondialyzed patients with chronic renal failure and hemodialysis patients who have greater urinary losses.
[h] Phosphate binders (calcium carbonate, acetate or citrate, aluminum carbonate, or hydroxide or sevelamer hydrochloride) are often needed as well.
[i] Dietary intake usually must be supplemented to provide these levels.
[j] 10 mg/day for males and nonmenstruating females; ≥18 mg/day for menstruating females.
[k] These quantities of folate are prescribed to reduce plasma homocysteine levels in patients with hyperhomocysteinemia.
[l] Vitamin K supplements may be needed for patients who are not eating and who are receiving antibiotics.

and high in others, such as calcium. Because of the high prevalence of cardiovascular disease in patients with advanced renal failure, the patient's serum lipid profile (e.g., serum total cholesterol, LDL cholesterol, HDL cholesterol, and triglycerides) and possibly plasma homocysteine concentrations should be monitored periodically.

In general, to maintain good dietary compliance and to monitor fluid and electrolyte disorders and clinical and nutritional status, patients with advanced renal failure should be seen every 1 to 2 months by the physician and dietitian. Patients with slowly progressive mild or moderate renal insufficiency sometimes may be seen less frequently.

Is There a Role for Early Dialysis?

A number of studies indicate that patients who have protein-energy malnutrition at the time that they begin maintenance dialysis therapy are more likely to have more comorbid events and shortened survival. This has led some investigators to suggest that dialysis therapy should be inaugurated earlier, when the GFR is higher. There are no randomized, prospective controlled clinical trials that have examined whether there are benefits to early dialysis therapy or at what level of renal function dialysis treatment should be inaugurated. Advocates of this approach often make the qualification that if patients are asymp-

TABLE 83.5. Recommended Measures for Monitoring Nutritional Status of Maintenance Hemodialysis and Chronic Peritoneal Dialysis Patients

Category	Measure	Minimum Frequency of Measurement
I. Measurements that should be performed routinely in all patients	• Predialysis or stabilized serum albumin	• Monthly
	• Percentage of usual postdialysis (MHD) or postdrain (CPD) body weight	• Monthly
	• Percentage of standard (NHANES II) body weight	• Every 4 months
	• Subjective global assessment (SGA)	• Every 6 months
	• Dietary interview and/or diary	• Every 6 months
	• Normalized protein nitrogen appearance (nPNA)	• Monthly MHD; every 3–4 months CPD
II. Measures that can be useful to confirm or extend the data obtained from the measures in category I	• Predialysis or stabilized serum prealbumin	• As needed
	• Skinfold thickness	• As needed
	• Mid-arm muscle area, circumference, or diameter	• As needed
	• Dual-energy x-ray absorptiometry	• As needed
III. Clinically useful measures, which, if low, might suggest the need for a more rigorous examination of protein-energy nutritional status	• Predialysis or stabilized serum	• As needed
	- Creatinine	
	- Urea nitrogen	• As needed
	- Cholesterol	• As needed
	• Creatinine Index	• As needed

Reprinted with permission from the NKF-DOQI Clinical Practice Guidelines for Nutrition in Chronic Renal Failure. *Am J Kidney Dis* 2000;35(Suppl 1):S1–S122.
CPD, chronic peritoneal dialysis; MHD, maintenance hemodialysis.

tomatic and adhere carefully to a high-energy, low-protein diet, the need for dialysis therapy may be postponed. However, in practice, it is uncommon to recommend early dialysis and ignore the role for nutritional management.

Several arguments support the importance of nutritional management for patients with progressive chronic renal insufficiency. First, all three published meta-analyses indicate that low-protein diets may delay the need for dialysis therapy. Second, many studies show that most patients with chronic renal failure will maintain neutral or positive protein balance with high-energy diets providing about 0.60 g protein/kg per day. Third, as indicated previously, spontaneous reductions in energy intake may occur when the GFR is 35 ml/min/1.73 m^2 body surface area or higher, which is a much greater GFR than is currently recommended for early dialysis. Fourth, there is a need to regulate the dietary intake to prevent deficiencies or excessive body burdens of many other nutrients in patients with chronic renal failure. These nutrients include sodium, water, phosphorus, calcium, magnesium, and a number of vitamins. Fifth, the intake of energy and, often, protein of maintenance dialysis patients is often below the recommended amounts. Although nutritional status is reported to improve in some malnourished patients after they begin maintenance dialysis therapy, roughly 40% of prevalent maintenance dialysis patients show evidence for protein and/or energy malnutrition. Thus maintenance dialysis therapy is not necessarily a solution for low nutrient intake or malnutrition.

The gross 1-year mortality rate for maintenance dialysis patients in the United States is approximately 23%, the quality of life of patients is often impaired when they are undergoing maintenance dialysis, and maintenance dialysis is costly. It could be argued, therefore, that patients should not be placed on maintenance dialysis treatment until they have demonstrated an inability to either comply with a high-energy, low-protein diet or they have begun to demonstrate deterioration on such diets.

On the other hand, the recommended dietary protein intake of 0.60 g/kg per day, although adequate, is marginal, and some patients may display nutritional deterioration on these diets. Thus it is recommended that patients with advanced chronic renal failure be encouraged to ingest high-energy, low-protein diets. If these patients agree to undergo such diets, they should receive intensive nutritional counseling initially, and periodic assessment of their nutritional status (Table 83.5). If deterioration in protein-energy nutritional status begins to occur and there is no obvious cause other than low nutrient intake, energy intake should be increased to the recommended levels and protein intake should be increased up to about 0.70 to 0.75 g protein/kg per day. If the patient's nutritional status does not improve after attempting to increase energy and/or protein intake and there is no obvious cause other than low nutrient intake, maintenance dialysis therapy should be inaugurated or a renal transplant performed. The National Kidney Foundation Dialysis Outcome Quality Initiative (NKF DOQI) Clinical Practice Guidelines on Nutrition in Chronic Renal Failure expresses this view: "In patients with chronic renal failure (e.g., GFR < 15-20 mL/min) who are not undergoing maintenance dialysis, if protein-energy malnutrition develops or persists despite vigorous attempts to optimize protein and energy intake and there is no apparent cause for malnutrition other than low nutrient intake, initiation of maintenance dialysis or a renal transplant is recommended." Maintenance dialysis or renal transplantation should be performed if other signs of chronic uremia, such as pericarditis, neuropathy, or profound malaise, occur.

Nutritional Evaluation of Patients with Chronic Renal Failure

Because of the propensity for chronic renal failure patients to ingest suboptimal quantities of nutrients (especially calories), their high incidence of malnutrition, and the adverse consequences of malnutrition, routine nutritional monitoring of these individuals is recommended. No single measure of nutritional status provides a complete overview, and a panel of measures is recommended. Nutritional evaluation for nondialyzed individuals with chronic renal failure (GFR less than 20 ml/min) should include assessment of dietary intake by dietary interviews and diaries and measurement of nPNA (protein equivalent of total nitrogen appearance normalized to a function of body weight) and evaluation of body composition by serum albumin and by edema-free actual body weight, percentage of normal body weight (from the NHANES II database), and/or subjective global assessment. These recommendations are consistent with the NKF DOQI Nutrition Clinical Practice Guidelines.

For MHD or CPD patients, nutritional status should be assessed routinely by the nPNA (obtained monthly with hemodialysis and every 3 to 4 months for peritoneal dialysis), dietary interviews and/or diary (every 6 months), serum albumin (monthly), percentage of usual postdialysis (hemodialysis) or postdrain (peritoneal dialysis) body weight (monthly), percentage of standard (NHANES II body weight (every 4 months), and subjective global assessment (every 6 months). Other measures can be useful to confirm or extend these data and include serum prealbumin and cholesterol, body mass index, more anthropometric assessments (skinfold thickness; mid-arm muscle area, circumference, or diameter; dual-energy x-ray absorptiometry and creatinine index). These recommendations are also consistent with the NKF DOQI Nutrition Guidelines.

Divalent ion and bone status assessment should include serum PTH, calcium, phosphorus, and magnesium and bone radiology, densitometry, or biopsy (see Chapter 77). Iron status assessment should include serum iron, percentage of iron-binding capacity, and ferrites.

Urea Nitrogen Appearance and the Serum Urea Nitrogen:Serum Creatinine Ratio

The control of protein intake is pivotal to the nutritional management of patients with acute or chronic renal failure. Hence one must accurately monitor nitrogen intake. Fortunately, this is possible for most patients. Those who are in nitrogen balance should have a total nitrogen output equal to nitrogen intake minus about 0.5 g nitrogen per day for unmeasured losses from growth of skin, hair, and nails and from sweat, respiration, flatus, and blood drawing. For clinical purposes, a slightly positive or negative balance does not substantially alter the use of the nitrogen output to estimate intake. If patients are in very positive or negative balance, such as from pregnancy or severe infection, nitrogen output may not reflect intake. However, it is usually readily apparent to the clinician whether the patient is in very positive or negative balance and whether the nitrogen output will reflect intake.

The measurement of total nitrogen output is too laborious and expensive to be widely applied for clinical uses. However, because urea is the major nitrogenous product of protein and amino acid degradation, the UNA can be used to estimate total nitrogen output and hence nitrogen intake. *UNA* refers to the amount of urea that appears or accumulates in body fluids and all outputs, such as urine, dialysate, and fistula drainage. The term *UNA* is used rather than *urea production* or *generation* because some urea is degraded in the intestinal tract; the ammonia released from urea is largely transported to the liver and converted back to urea. Thus the enterohepatic urea cycle leads to an increase in absolute urea synthesis but has little effect on serum urea levels or total nitrogen economy, and this cycle can be ignored without compromising the accuracy of the UNA for estimating total nitrogen output or intake. This offers an important advantage because the recycling of urea cannot be measured without costly and time-consuming isotope studies.

UNA is calculated as follows:

$$\text{(1)}\quad \text{UNA (g/day)} = \text{Urinary urea nitrogen (g/day)} + \text{Dialysate urea nitrogen (g/day)} + \text{Change in body urea nitrogen (g/day)}$$

$$\text{(2)}\quad \text{Change in body urea nitrogen (g/day)} = (\text{SUN}_f - \text{SUN}_i,\ \text{g/L/day}) \times \text{BW}_i(\text{kg}) \times (0.60\ \text{L/kg}) + (\text{BW}_f - \text{BW}_i,\ \text{kg/day}) \times \text{SUN}_f(\text{g/L}) \times (1.0\ \text{L/kg})$$

where i and f are the initial and final values for the period of measurement, *SUN* is serum urea nitrogen (grams per liter), *BW* is body weight (kilograms), 0.60 is an estimate of the fraction of body weight that is water, and 1.0 is the volume of distribution of urea in the weight that is gained or lost.

The estimated proportion of body weight that is water may be increased in patients who are edematous or lean and decreased in individuals who are obese or very young. Changes in body weight during the 1- to 3-day period of measurement of UNA are assumed to be due entirely to changes in body water. In patients undergoing hemodialysis, the UNA may be estimated during the interdialytic interval and then normalized to 24 hours. Alternatively, UNA may be calculated by urea kinetic techniques for hemodialysis patients (see Chapter 84, Part 1A). Two pool models for urea kinetic measurements that take into account delays in equilibration of endogenous urea pools during hemodialysis will give more accurate results for both the UNA method described here and the urea kinetic technique. A newer instrument that serially measures urea in the dialysate outflow provides an accurate method for calculating UNA. The 24-hour dialysate urea concentration can be readily measured in CAPD or CCPD patients. Measurement of total protein as well as urea in peritoneal dialysate may give more accurate measurements of total nitrogen output and hence dietary protein intake.

In our experience, the relationship between UNA and total nitrogen appearance (TNA) in patients with chronic renal failure not undergoing dialysis is as follows:

$$\text{(3)}\quad \text{TNA (g/day)} = 0.97\ \text{UNA (g/day)} + 1.93$$

The UNA can be used to estimate the PNA (protein equivalent of total nitrogen appearance). For nondialyzed patients with chronic renal failure not undergoing dialysis this equation is as follows:

$$\text{(4)}\quad \text{PNA (g/day)} = 6.06\ \text{UNA (g/day)} + 12.1$$

If the individual is more or less in neutral nitrogen balance, the UNA also will correlate closely with nitrogen intake. Equation 4 describes our observed relationships between UNA and dietary nitrogen intake in clinically stable, nondialyzed, chronic renal failure patients.

$$\text{(5)}\quad \text{Dietary nitrogen intake (g/day)} = 0.69\ \text{UNA (g/day)} + 3.3$$

When both nitrogen intake and UNA are known, nitrogen balance can be calculated from the difference between nitrogen intake and nitrogen output estimated from the UNA. If the patient is markedly anabolic, such as in pregnancy or in a young person with anorexia nervosa who is being refed, equation 5 will underestimate nitrogen intake. In patients who have large protein losses (e.g., from nephrotic syndrome or peritoneal dialysis) or who are acidemic and have sufficient kidney function to excrete large quantities of ammonia, equations 3, 4, and 5 will underestimate both nitrogen output and nitrogen intake. In most circumstances, however, these conditions are not present, and the UNA provides a powerful tool for monitoring nitrogen output and intake or for estimating balance. Other investigators have described similar approaches to monitoring nitrogen intake and output.

The ratio of the SUN to serum creatinine also correlates fairly closely with dietary protein or amino acid intake in nondialyzed patients with chronic renal failure. This relationship can be used to estimate the recent daily intake of these patients. Although the SUN:serum creatinine ratio is not as precise as the UNA and is influenced by a number of clinical factors, it is easy and inexpensive to measure. For clinically stable, nondialyzed, chronically uremic patients, this ratio can also be used to estimate the level at which the SUN will stabilize for any given dietary protein intake and GFR.

RECOMMENDED NUTRIENT INTAKES

Protein

GFR Greater Than 70 ml/min/1.73 m²

There is almost no information concerning the most desirable dietary protein and phosphorus prescription for patients with chronic renal disease and mild impairment in renal function. Indeed, almost all of the studies of the effect of low-protein diets on the rate of progression of renal failure have examined patients with moderately advanced to advanced renal failure (i.e., serum creatinine 2.5 mg/dl or greater). It is recommended that protein (and phosphorus) intake be restricted for patients with a GFR greater than 70 ml/min/1.72 m² only if there is evidence that renal function is continuing to decline. In this situation, the patient is treated as indicated in the next paragraph.

GFR 25 to 70 ml/min/1.73 m²

At present, it is the author's policy to discuss with the patient the evidence that low-protein, low-phosphorus diets may retard progression or delay the need for dialysis therapy and to indicate that the data, although not definitive, are sufficiently convincing to justify prescription of a protein- and phosphorus-restricted diet. If the patient agrees to dietary therapy, he or she is offered a diet providing about 0.60 g protein/kg per day, of which at least 0.35 g/kg per day is high biologic value protein to ensure a sufficient intake of the essential amino acids. This quantity of protein should maintain neutral or positive nitrogen balance, and for many patients, it should not be excessively burdensome. Ketoacid preparations are not available in the United States for therapeutic use.

GFR Less Than 25 ml/min/1.73 m²

At this level of renal insufficiency, the potential advantages to using a low-protein, low-phosphorus diet becomes more compelling. First, at this degree of renal failure, potentially toxic products of nitrogen metabolism begin to accumulate in substantial quantities. The low-protein diet will generate less potentially toxic nitrogenous compounds. Second, because the low-protein diet generally contains less phosphorus and potassium, the intake of these minerals can be lowered more readily with this diet (see later sections on recommended phosphorus and potassium intakes). Third, some patients with chronic renal insufficiency eat too little protein rather than too much. Specific training and encouragement to follow a prescribed diet may increase the likelihood that the patient will not ingest too little protein. Patients should be prescribed 0.60 g protein/kg per day with at least 0.35 g/kg per day of high biologic value protein (Table 83.4). This diet will generally maintain neutral or positive nitrogen balance as along as energy intake is not deficient (Table 83.4) and should generate a low UNA. The protein content of this diet should be increased by 1.0 g/day of high biologic value protein for each gram of protein excreted in the urine each day.

Exceptions to These Recommendations

For individuals with a GFR less than 70 ml/min/1.73 m² who will not accept a diet providing 0.60 g protein/kg per day or who are not able to maintain an adequate dietary intake with such a diet, up to 0.70 to 0.75 g protein/kg per day may be prescribed. The NKF DOQI Nutrition Guidelines make a similar recommendation for nondialyzed chronic renal failure patients with a GFR less than 25 ml/min/1.73 m². When the GFR falls below 5 ml/min/1.73 m², there is no conclusive evidence that patients fare as well with low-nitrogen diets as with regular dialysis therapy and higher protein intakes. Because these patients are at high risk for malnutrition, it is recommended that maintenance dialysis or renal transplantation be inaugurated at this time even if patients have no signs of uremia or nutritional deterioration.

Maintenance Hemodialysis

There are few studies of dietary protein requirements in patients undergoing MHD, and most of these studies were carried out using dialyzers and schedules of dialysis therapy that are no longer in use. It is apparent that maintenance dialysis patients have increased dietary protein requirements, probably because of the removal of amino acids and peptides by the dialysis procedure and because hemodialysis appears to stimulate protein catabolism, particularly when it is conducted with less biocompatible dialyzer membranes. Most of the nitrogen balance studies suggest that MHD patients probably require about 1.0 to 1.2 g protein/kg per day. Moreover, clinical outpatient experience with this level of protein intake indicates that patients ingesting 1.0 to 1.2 g protein/kg per day maintain nitrogen balance and tolerate this level of protein intake well, particularly if energy intake is high. Because many MHD patients show evidence of protein wasting, a protein intake of 1.2 g/kg per day is recommended as safe. To ensure adequate intake of essential amino acids, at least half of the dietary protein should be of high biologic value. These recommendations are consistent with the NKF DOQI Nutrition Guidelines.

Chronic Peritoneal Dialysis

Blumenkrantz and co-workers studied protein and mineral balances in eight clinically stable men undergoing CAPD who participated in 13 metabolic balance studies of 14 to 33 days' duration in a clinical research center. Patients were fed diets that provided an average of 0.98 or 1.44 g protein/kg per day. Total energy intake (diet plus dialysate glucose) was 41.3 ± 1.9 and 42.1 ± 1.2 kcal/kg per day with the low- and high-protein diets, respectively. Peritoneal dialysate total daily protein losses averaged about 9 g (Table 83.6). Nitrogen balance, adjusted for changes in body urea nitrogen but not for unmeasured losses, was + 0.35 ± 0.83 g/day with the protein diet of 1.0 g/kg and + 2.94 ± 0.54 g/day with the higher protein intake. These differences are not statistically significant. Only the latter diet was significantly different from zero, even if nitrogen balances were adjusted by about 1.0 g/day for losses through skin, respiration, flatus, and blood sampling. There was a curvilinear relationship between dietary protein intake and nitrogen balance in the 13 studies. Nitrogen balance rose as protein intake increased until protein intake was 1.09 g/kg per day. At this level, balance was significantly positive. As dietary protein increased above this level, there was no further increment in nitrogen balance.

These findings are similar to those of other investigators who reported neutral to positive nitrogen balance in seven of eight CAPD patients who were fed about 1.2 g protein/kg per day. Neutral or positive nitrogen balance was also found in five

TABLE 83.6. Serum Proteins and Dialysate Protein Losses in Eight Men Undergoing Continuous Ambulatory Peritoneal Dialysis

	Serum Proteins[a]	Protein Losses[b] per 24 hr
Total Protein	6.6 ± 0.1[c] g/dl	8.8 ± 0.5 g
Albumin	3.5 ± 0.1 g/dl	5.7 ± 0.4 g
Transferrin	228 ± 11 mg/dl	333 ± 22 mg
IgG	1.41 ± 0.12 g/dl	1.25 ± 0.20 g
IgA	220 ± 18 mg/dl	173 ± 21 mg
IgM	234 ± 36 mg/dl	71 ± 18 mg
C3	107 ± 6 mg/dl	70 ± 7 mg
C4	32 ± 2 mg/dl	21 ± 2 mg

[a]Grand mean of values from 13 metabolic balance studies in eight men fed 1.0 or 1.4 g protein/kg/day. Data were obtained periodically during the course of study with each diet.

[b]Losses of each protein into dialysate over 24 hours were measured on 110 occasions in the 8 patients.

[c]Mean ± standard error.

Adapted with permission from Blumenkrantz MJ, et al. Protein losses during peritoneal dialysis. *Kidney Int* 1981;19:593.

patients undergoing CAPD who were ingesting lower-protein diets that provided 0.71 to 0.96 g protein/kg per day, but feces were not collected. Short-term (10- to 14-day) balance studies were carried out in 10 patients undergoing CAPD who were fed diets containing 0.76 to 1.07 g protein/kg per day. Total energy intake was about 29 kcal/kg per day. Nitrogen balance, adjusted for unmeasured losses, was positive in all patients. However, there was a positive correlation between protein intake and nitrogen balance in these patients.

There are virtually no studies that have directly examined dietary protein requirements for patients undergoing other types of CPD (e.g., continuous cyclic or nocturnal peritoneal dialysis). Because the protein and amino acid losses with other types of CPD are probably similar to CAPD losses, the dietary protein requirements probably should be similar to that of CAPD patients. Based on these foregoing considerations, it seems prudent to prescribe 1.2 to 1.3 g protein/kg per day to CPD patients. Unless the patient has demonstrated adequate protein nutritional status with a diet providing 1.2 g protein/kg per day, 1.3 g protein/kg per day should be prescribed. As with hemodialysis patients, at least 50% of the daily protein intake of CAPD patients should be of high biologic value. Patients undergoing CPD who are protein depleted may be prescribed up to 1.5 g protein/kg per day. In most CPD patients, SUN levels and uremic toxicity should be controlled adequately with this protein intake, although there may be a need in some patients to increase the number of dialysate exchanges or at least the volume of dialysate outflow.

Some nephrologists describe MHD or CPD patients who have dietary protein intakes of about 0.9 g/kg per day and who do not appear protein depleted and lead physically active, rehabilitated lives. These observations have raised questions as to whether the foregoing recommended dietary protein intake may be excessive for CPD patients. Several comments may be pertinent in this regard. First, the number of CAPD patients carefully studied with protein intakes between 0.90 and 1.30 g/kg per day is small, and conclusions concerning dietary protein needs therefore are rather imprecise. On the other hand, the concept of dietary allowances presupposes that to ensure a sufficient nutrient intake for virtually all individuals within a given population, the recommended allowance must be greater than the actual requirement for a large proportion of that population. Thus, if the recommended dietary protein allowance is 1.2 to 1.3 g/kg per day, it is to be expected that many patients will tolerate lower protein intakes without developing protein depletion. However, at present, there is no method that will identify in advance, under the conditions of clinical practice, which patients can safely ingest lower levels of protein. Hence, to be safe, the patients should be prescribed the recommended dietary allowance, an especially relevant consideration given the high incidence of protein malnutrition in CAPD patients. Finally, subtle forms of malnutrition are particularly difficult to detect. The recommended protein intakes may provide some protection against mild forms of protein malnutrition.

It has been shown that patients classified as high peritoneal transporters by the peritoneal equilibration test lose more protein and amino acids than those classified as low transporters (e.g., typical 24-hour losses in high versus low transporters: albumin, 4.9 ± 2 (SD) versus 3.2 ± 1 g/day, $P < .03$, total free amino acids, 15.4 ± 4 versus 10 ± 4 mmol/day, $P = .002$). The high transporters have also been shown to have lower serum albumin levels. The difference in protein and amino acid losses with high versus low transporters, however, is not great. Dietary protein intakes of 1.2 to 1.3 g/kg per day should provide sufficient amounts of protein and amino acids to compensate for the increased peritoneal losses if the endogenous synthetic function for serum proteins is normal.

Energy

In nondialyzed, chronically uremic patients and patients undergoing MHD, energy expenditure, measured by indirect calorimetry, appears to be normal or near normal during resting and sitting, following ingestion of a standard meal, and with defined exercise. However, in one study, resting energy expenditure measured by direct calorimetry was increased by about 7% in MHD patients. The effect of a hemodialysis treatment on energy expenditure is uncertain. Resting energy expenditure in one study in CPD patients was normal.

Nitrogen balance studies in nondialyzed, chronically uremic patients ingesting 0.55 to 0.60 g protein/kg per day indicate that the amount of energy intake necessary to ensure neutral or positive nitrogen balance is approximately 35 kcal/kg per day. In clinically stable patients undergoing MHD who ingested 1.13 ± 0.02 (SEM) g protein/kg per day, nitrogen balance studies and anthropometric measurements indicate that about 35 kcal/kg per day may be necessary to maintain body weight and protein mass. On the other hand, virtually every study of the dietary habits of nondialyzed, chronically uremic patients and MHD patients indicates that their mean energy intakes are lower than this level, usually about 24 to 27 kcal/kg per day. The finding that decreased body fat is one of the more prominent alterations in nutritional status in nondialyzed patients with advanced chronic renal failure and patients undergoing maintenance hemodialysis supports the contention that these patients require more energy than they usually ingest.

Energy requirements in CPD patients have not been as systematically evaluated. Many patients undergoing CAPD tend to gain body fat and weight, probably due to the glucose uptake and the attendant surges in plasma insulin that accompany the dialysate exchanges. The quantity of glucose absorbed from CAPD is reported to vary between 78 and 316 g/day. There appears to be a close correlation between the quantity of glucose instilled into the peritoneal cavity and the quantity of glucose absorbed, particularly when the dwell time of the dialysate is kept constant. In any individual patient, the daily rate of glucose absorption with the same dialysis regimen is rather constant.

It is currently recommended that nondialyzed, chronically uremic patients and patients undergoing MHD or peritoneal dialysis ingest at least 35 kcal/kg per day (Table 83.4). Individuals 60 years old or older, who tend to be more sedentary, may be prescribed 30–35 kcal/kg per day. These recommendations are the same as the NKF DOQI Nutrition Guidelines. Patients who are obese with an edema-free body weight greater than 120% of desirable body weight may be treated with lower calorie intakes. Some patients, particularly those with more mild renal insufficiency and young or middle-aged women, may become obese on this energy intake or may refuse to ingest the recommended calories out of fear of obesity. These individuals may require a lower energy prescription.

As indicated previously, energy (and protein) intake seems to decrease when the GFR falls to about 25 to 38 ml/min/1.73 m^2. Thus, when the GFR decreases to this level, to prevent malnutrition, it is important to monitor dietary intake and to treat inadequate intakes, even in clinically stable healthy appearing adults. This level of GFR may be associated with a serum creatinine as low as 1.8 to 2.5 mg/dl in an adult patient.

Many high-calorie foodstuffs that are low in protein, sodium, and potassium are commercially available. The renal dietitian can recommend these products as well as other low-protein, high-calorie foods that can be prepared easily at home.

Lipids: Prevention of Cardiovascular Disease

There are a number of reviews of the causes for the abnormal serum lipids and lipoproteins in chronic renal failure and MHD patients. Because these alterations may contribute to the high incidence of atherosclerosis and cardiovascular disease in uremic patients, attention has been directed toward reducing serum triglycerides and LDL cholesterol and increasing HDL cholesterol. Elevated serum triglyceride levels in uremia appear to be caused primarily by impaired catabolism of triglyceride-rich lipoproteins. Also, because diets for renal failure patients are usually restricted in protein, sodium, potassium, and water, it is often difficult to provide sufficient energy intake without resorting to a large intake of purified sugars that may increase triglyceride production. Activities of plasma and hepatic lipoprotein lipase and lecithin cholesterol acyltransferase (LCAT) are reduced. CPD, which provides a glucose load, appears to promote a further increase in serum triglycerides and cholesterol.

Serum triglycerides may be lowered by feeding a diet in which the carbohydrate content is reduced to about 35% of total calories. However, this requires the dietary fat to be increased to about 55% of total calories. The evidence that high cholesterol and fat intakes enhance the risk for arteriosclerotic vascular disease indicates that such a diet is inadvisable, particularly because hypertriglyceridemia is a weak risk factor for arteriosclerotic heart disease. Omega-3 fatty acids (e.g., eicosapentaenoic acid and docosahexaenoic acid, which are found in fish oil) lower serum triglycerides and have more variable effects on serum LDL cholesterol and HDL cholesterol. Fish oil also decreases platelet aggregation and appears to exert antiinflammatory effects, and omega-3 fatty acids may enhance immune function. Low-fat diets and lipid-lowering medicines retard the rate of progression of renal failure in animal models. Some research suggests that omega-3 fatty acids may lower the progression of renal failure in renal transplant patients. A preponderance of studies suggest that omega-3 fatty acids given as fish oil may retard the rate of progression of IgA nephropathy. Abnormal carnitine metabolism has been implicated as a cause of hypertriglyceridemia in chronic renal failure. However, the many studies of treatment of hypertriglyceridemia with carnitine in patients with chronic renal failure are split between those that show carnitine lowers serum triglycerides and those that show no change or, rarely, a rise in serum triglycerides with carnitine intake.

Ingestion of activated charcoal may lower serum cholesterol and triglycerides in chronically azotemic rats. Clofibrate also lowers serum triglycerides in uremic patients, but because of the altered pharmacokinetics of this drug in renal failure patients, there is a substantial risk of developing myopathy or other toxicities. The phosphate-binding gel, sevelamer hydrochloride (RenaGel, Genzyme), also lowers serum LDL cholesterol and total cholesterol by as much as 23% to 35%.

Hydroxymethylglutarate coenzyme A (HMG-CoA) inhibitors suppress cholesterol synthesis; lower serum levels of total cholesterol, LDL cholesterol, and certain apolipoproteins; and increase serum HDL cholesterol. HMG-CoA reductase inhibitors exert these effects in individuals with chronic renal failure and also those with nephrotic syndrome. The reduction in serum LDL cholesterol and in apolipoprotein B100 in these individuals averages roughly 30%, and the rise in serum HDL cholesterol averages about 10%. This is the most optimal lipid profile effect of any lipid-lowering medicine.

Evidence suggests that end-stage renal disease is associated with oxidant stress and often with a state of chronic inflammation, both of which may promote arteriosclerotic, atherosclerotic, and proliferative vascular disease. These findings have raised questions as to whether intake of a health-enhancing diet or of antioxidant medicines, such as vitamin E or ascorbic acid, may be of particular value for patients with chronic renal failure or nephrotic syndrome. There are no data indicating that the chronic intake of antiinflammatory medicines prevents vascular disease in chronic renal failure.

At present, we encourage nondialyzed patients with chronic renal failure and maintenance dialysis patients to ingest the National Cholesterol Education Program (NCEP) I diet. This diet provides no more than 30% of total calories from fat, less than 10% of total calories from saturated fat, and 300 mg/day or lower of cholesterol. Patients are encouraged to ingest up to five servings of vegetables or fruits each day, depending on their ability to tolerate the potassium level. It is our current policy to treat hypertriglyceridemia by dietary modification only when serum triglycerides are more than slightly elevated (e.g., at least 100 to 200 mg/dl above the upper given limit of normal). In this situation, patients are strongly encouraged to ingest a high proportion of their carbohydrates as complex carbohydrates. These modifications often lower the palatability of the diet; therefore the patient's total energy intake must be monitored closely to ensure that it does not fall. With high serum triglyceride values that are unresponsive to dietary therapy, clofibrate or other fibric acid analogs may be tried cautiously. L-carnitine at about 500 to 1,000 mg/day for chronic renal failure patients or L-carnitine at 10 to 20 mg/kg per day at the end of each dialysis three times weekly for hemodialysis patients may be tried if hypertriglyceridemia is severe and unresponsive to these treatments. Dietary fat intake may be increased, but not to above 40% of total calories, if serum triglyceride levels remain markedly elevated (e.g., 1,000 mg/dl or greater) despite triglyceride-lowering medicines. Hypercholesterolemia may be treated with a hydroxymethylglutarate coenzyme A (HMG-CoA) inhibitor in addition to a step I or step II American Heart Association diet.

There is no established treatment for low serum concentrations of HDL in uremic patients, although a small amount of red wine (one glass per day), exercise, and HMG-COA reductase inhibitors may increase these levels. It should be emphasized that there are almost no long-term data on the effects of dietary fat, carbohydrate, fruits or vegetables, antioxidant intake, obesity, or a change in serum lipid levels on the clinical course of patients with specific renal diseases, nephrotic syndrome, renal failure, or a renal transplant. Treatment of hyperhomocystinemia, a finding in about 85% of MHD patients, is discussed in the following section. The recommendations given here are largely based on epidemiologic data or long-term clinical trials in populations without renal disease. Effective therapy for elevated Lp(a) levels is not as yet available.

Carbohydrates

Patients should be encouraged to eat complex rather than purified carbohydrates to reduce triglyceride synthesis and to improve glucose tolerance if it is abnormal.

Carnitine

Carnitine is a naturally occurring compound that is essential for life. It is both synthesized in the body and ingested. Carnitine facilitates the transfer of long-chain (more than 10 carbon) fatty acids into muscle mitochondria. Because fatty acids are the major fuel source for skeletal and myocardial muscle at rest and during mild to moderate exercise, this activity is considered necessary for normal skeletal and cardiac muscle function.

MHD and CPD patients display low serum free carnitine and, in some studies, low skeletal muscle free and total carnitine levels; in addition, serum and, in some reports, muscle acylcarnitines (fatty acid–carnitine compounds) are increased, and serum total carnitine (i.e., acylcarnitines plus free carnitine) is normal. The low serum and skeletal muscle free carnitine levels have led some investigators to postulate that many maintenance dialysis patients are carnitine deficient. Such a deficiency could be due to impaired synthesis of carnitine *in vivo,* reduced dietary intake of carnitine, and removal of carnitine by dialysis. However, the weekly loss of free carnitine by dialysis is approximately equal to the normal weekly urinary excretion of carnitine, and the administration of oral or intravenous carnitine usually does not lead to a sudden change in the patient's clinical status. These findings raise the possibility that a simple deficiency of carnitine is not the cause of carnitine disorders in maintenance dialysis patients. Patients with chronic renal insufficiency not in need of dialysis treatment have normal or even increased plasma levels of free carnitine and acylcarnitine. These findings provide some support for the thesis that removal of carnitine by dialysis and/or impaired renal synthesis may account for the low plasma free carnitine concentrations in maintenance dialysis patients. Other theories are that increased concentrations of acylcarnitines interfere with normal actions of carnitine physiology and that the accumulation of toxic organic compounds may increase the requirement for carnitine that is necessary to bind with these compounds, thereby detoxifying them.

A number of clinical trials in patients with chronic renal failure, particularly those undergoing maintenance dialysis therapy, suggest that carnitine may provide clinical benefits. The types of improvement that have been described in randomized, prospective studies include increased physical exercise capacity, reduced intradialytic symptoms of skeletal muscle cramps or hypertension, or improvement in quality of life and overall global sense of well-being. A decrease in predialysis serum urea, creatinine, and phosphorus; an increase in mid-arm muscle circumference; and in short term studies, more positive nitrogen balance have also been reported; the mechanisms responsible for these effects are not clear, particularly with regard to changes in the predialysis serum chemistries. Other studies, usually nonrandomized, suggest that carnitine may increase hematocrit or reduce the erythropoietin requirement to maintain a given hematocrit, reduce cardiac arrhythmias, and improve ventricular function in maintenance dialysis patients.

Many nephrologists remain unconvinced by the published results of carnitine benefits. The reasons are that a number of the studies were not well designed (e.g., not prospective and randomized or not double-blinded), the results were not consistent in all studies, the outcome measures were often soft or difficult to quantify precisely, and it seems that patients may not respond to carnitine treatment for up to several months. Nonetheless, the preponderance of studies that have used certain measures appear to show benefits. Also, L-carnitine appears to be a safe agent.

Until more definitive studies are available, it is the author's policy to use L-carnitine for patients who satisfy both of the following conditions: (a) disabling or very bothersome skeletal muscle weakness or cardiomyopathy, skeletal muscle cramps or hypotension during hemodialysis treatment, severe malaise, or anemia refractory to erythropoietin therapy with no obvious cause other than renal failure or uremia itself, and (b) the aforementioned conditions do not respond to more standard treatment. The patient is given a 3- to 6-month trial of L-carnitine (up to 9 months for refractory anemia). If there is no measurable improvement in symptoms by the end of the treatment period, the carnitine therapy is discontinued. L-carnitine may be administered orally, intravenously, or into dialysate. Oral L-carnitine is less expensive, but intestinal absorption is somewhat unpredictable in nonuremic individuals and has not been examined in patients with chronic renal failure. Clearly some ingested carnitine is absorbed in patients with chronic renal failure. Until more information is available, intravenous carnitine may be a more reliable method of treatment, at least for initiating treatment. The optimal dose of carnitine is not defined. Some workers use a carnitine dose of 20 mg/kg at the end of each hemodialysis, three times weekly.

Sodium

Normally, the renal tubules reabsorb more than 99% of the filtered sodium. As renal insufficiency progresses, both the glomerular filtration and the fractional reabsorption of sodium fall progressively. Thus many patients with renal failure are able to maintain sodium balance with a normal sodium intake. In both normal individuals and people with chronic renal failure, only about 1 to 3 mEq/day of sodium are excreted in the feces, and in the absence of visible sweating, only a few milliequivalents per day of sodium is lost through the skin. Despite the adaptive reduction in the renal tubular reabsorption of sodium, patients with advanced renal failure may be unable to excrete the quantity of sodium ingested, and they may develop edema, hypertension, and congestive heart failure. This syndrome is particularly likely to occur when the GFR is below 4 to 10 ml/min. When congestive heart failure, nephrotic syndrome, or advanced liver disease complicates renal insufficiency, the propensity for sodium retention is increased. In renal failure patients, hypertension often is more easily controlled when they are sodium restricted, and hypertension may be accentuated by an increased sodium intake, probably because of expanded extracellular fluid volume and possibly due to altered intracellular electrolyte composition within arteriolar smooth muscle cells that increase contractility. With a decreased ability to excrete sodium or an expanded extracellular fluid volume, restriction of sodium and water intake and the use of diuretic medications may be necessary.

Nondialyzed patients with chronic renal failure often have an inability to conserve sodium normally. A low sodium intake may not be sufficient to replace urinary and extrarenal sodium losses, and the patient may develop sodium depletion; a decrease in extracellular fluid volume, blood volume, renal blood flow; and a further reduction in GFR (i.e., prerenal insufficiency superimposed on chronic renal failure). Volume depletion may be difficult to recognize. Unexplained weight loss or reduction in blood pressure may be signs of volume depletion. If the nondialyzed patient with chronic renal failure does not have evidence of fluid overload, hypertension, or heart failure, he or she may be cautiously given a greater sodium intake to determine whether the GFR can be improved slightly by extracellular volume expansion.

Usually, when sodium balance is well controlled, the thirst mechanism will regulate water balance adequately. However, when the GFR falls below 2 to 5 ml/min, the risk of overhydration increases, and water intake should be controlled independently of sodium to prevent overhydration. In patients with diabetes mellitus, hyperglycemia may also increase thirst and enhance positive water balance. For patients with far-advanced renal failure whose total body water is considered appropriate (as indicated by normal or near normal blood pressure, absence of edema, and normal serum sodium), urine volume may be a good guide to water intake; the daily water intake should equal the urine output plus approximately 500 ml to replace insensible losses.

In most nondialyzed patients with advanced renal failure, a daily intake of 1,000 to 3,000 mg (40 to 130 mEq) of sodium and 1,500 to 3,000 ml of fluid will maintain sodium and water balance. The requirement for sodium and water varies markedly, and each patient must be managed individually. Patients undergoing MHD or peritoneal dialysis are often oliguric or anuric. For hemodialysis patients, sodium and total fluid intake generally should be restricted to 1,000 to 1,500 ml/day and 700 to 1,500 mEq/day, respectively. Because sodium and water can be removed easily with CAPD or other forms of CPD, a more liberal salt and water intake is usually allowed. By maintaining a larger dietary sodium and water intake, the quantity of fluid removed from the patient and hence the daily dialysate outflow volume can be increased. This may be advantageous, because with CPD, the daily clearance of small- and middle-sized molecules is directly related to the volume of dialysate outflow. Thus, for some CPD patients, a higher sodium and water intake (e.g., 6 to 8 g/day of sodium and 3 L/day of water) may enable the patient to use more hypertonic glucose exchanges to increase the dialysate outflow volume, thereby increasing dialysate clearances and glucose and energy uptake from dialysate. This treatment may be undesirable for obese or hypertriglyceridemic patients because the greater use of hypertonic glucose exchanges will increase their glucose load. Also, there is the potential disadvantage that some patients may become habituated to high salt and water intakes; if they change to hemodialysis therapy, they may have difficulty in curtailing their sodium and water intake.

In nondialyzed, chronically uremic patients or patients undergoing maintenance dialysis who are not anuric and who gain excessive sodium or water despite attempts at dietary restriction, a potent diuretic, such as furosemide, may be tried to increase urinary sodium and water excretion.

Potassium

The kidney normally is the major vehicle for potassium excretion. In renal failure, potassium retention may occur and cause fatal hyperkalemia. Three factors may counteract this side effect of renal failure: First, when the urine volume is approximately 1,000 ml/day or greater, the tubular secretion of potassium per unit GFR tends to increase, and therefore the renal potassium clearance does not fall as markedly as the GFR. Second, in both nondialyzed patients with chronic renal failure and MHD and CPD patients, the fecal excretion of potassium increases, probably because of enhanced intestinal secretion. Third, potassium intake tends to fall as a result of anorexia and also in response to dietary counseling.

Thus patients with chronic renal failure usually do not become hyperkalemic unless there is (a) excessive intake of potassium; (b) acidemia, oliguria, or hypoaldosteronism (e.g., secondary to decreased renin secretion by the diseased kidney or renal tubular resistance to the actions of aldosterone); (c) catabolic stress; or (d) possible hypoinsulinism or use of medicines such as potassium-sparing diuretics, nonsteroidal antiinflammatory drugs, ACE inhibitors, and β-receptor blockers; (e) digitalis toxicity; and (f) constipation. Patients with chronic renal failure and those undergoing maintenance hemodialysis should generally receive no more than 70 mEq of potassium per day.

Magnesium

In nondialyzed patients with chronic renal failure and in maintenance dialysis patients, there is a net absorption of about 40% to 50% of ingested magnesium from the intestinal tract (net absorption is the difference between dietary intake and fecal excretion). Because the absorbed magnesium is excreted primarily by the kidney, hypermagnesemia may occur in renal failure patients. The restricted diets of uremic patients are low in magnesium (usually about 100 to 300 mg/day for a 40-g protein diet), and the patients' serum magnesium levels are therefore usually normal or only slightly elevated unless the patient takes substances that are high in magnesium content, such as magnesium-containing antacids and laxatives. Nondialyzed, chronically uremic patients require about 200 mg/day of magnesium to maintain neutral magnesium balance. The optimal dietary magnesium allowance for the dialysis patient has not been well defined. Experience suggests that when the magnesium content is about 1.0 mEq/L in hemodialysate or 0.50 to 0.75 mEq/L in peritoneal dialysate, a dietary magnesium intake of 200 to 300 mg/day will maintain the serum magnesium at normal or only slightly elevated levels.

Calcium

Nondialyzed patients with chronic renal failure and patients undergoing maintenance dialysis therapy have an increased dietary requirement for calcium because they have vitamin D deficiency and resistance to the actions of vitamin D. These abnormalities, which are discussed in greater detail in Chapters 13, Part 11, and 77, impair the intestinal absorption of calcium. The risk of calcium deficiency in these patients is enhanced because the diets prescribed for uremic patients are almost always low in calcium. Foods high in calcium content are usually high in phosphorus (e.g., dairy products) and are therefore restricted for uremic patients. For example, a 40-g protein diet generally provides only about 300 to 400 mg/day of calcium, whereas the recommended dietary allowances for healthy, nonpregnant, nonlactating adults is about 800 to 1,200 mg/day.

Balance studies indicate that nondialyzed, chronically uremic patients usually require about 1,200 to 1,600 mg/day of calcium for neutral or positive calcium balance. Total daily calcium intake (diet plus supplement) should therefore be maintained at about 1,400 to 1,600 mg/day (Table 83.4). Thus the low-protein diets should be supplemented with about 1,000 to 1,400 mg/day of elemental calcium. As indicated earlier, slightly higher intakes (1,000 to 2,000 mg/day) of elemental calcium may be given as calcium carbonate and calcium acetate to bind phosphate in the intestinal tract. Calcium citrate should not be used in combination with aluminum compounds because such combinations may increase intestinal aluminum absorption and cause acute encephalopathy. To prevent calcium phosphate deposition in soft tissues, the supplemental calcium should not be given unless the serum phosphorus concentration is normal or near normal (i.e., 5.5 mg/dl or lower). Frequent monitoring of serum calcium also is important because hypercalcemia may develop, particularly if serum phosphorus falls to low normal or low levels. Patients undergoing MHD or peritoneal dialysis may need 1.0 g/day of supplemental calcium even though there is net calcium uptake from dialysis. The treatment of hyperphosphatemia in patients with chronic renal failure and the supplementation of calcium to these patients are also discussed in Chapter 77.

In CAPD patients, the calcium uptake from dialysate is inversely correlated with the serum concentration of total calcium and ionized calcium. It has been reported that in CAPD patients, there was net absorption of calcium from dialysate that averaged 84 mg/day. On the other hand, other investigators showed that calcium losses averaging 77 mg/day occurred in CAPD patients who had elevated serum ionized calcium (greater than 5 mg/dl) and calcium uptake of 44 mg/day in patients with low serum ionized calcium (below 4.4 mg/dl). The more hypertonic the peritoneal dialysate, the greater the dialysate outflow volume and the larger the calcium losses; it was found that a net calcium uptake of 9.8 mg per exchange with 1.5% dextrose and net calcium loss of 21 mg per exchange with 4.25% dextrose occurred. Other studies also found that calcium balance was usually neutral or positive when dietary calcium intake was 720 mg/day or greater. Based on these observations, CAPD patients should probably be given a total dietary calcium intake (diet plus dietary supplement) of about 800 to 1,000 mg/day.

The calcium content is 40% for calcium carbonate, 25% for calcium acetate, 21% for calcium citrate, 18% for calcium lactate, and 8% for calcium gluconate. In general, calcium chloride should not be given to chronically uremic patients because of its acidifying characteristics. Because calcium preparations may contain phosphorus and other ingredients, it is advisable to ascertain the composition of any new calcium preparation before it is taken by a patient with renal insufficiency. Treatment with 1,25-dihydroxycholecalciferol will decrease the daily calcium requirement by enhancing intestinal calcium absorption.

Phosphorus and Phosphate Binders

The rationale for controlling dietary phosphorus and the use of gastrointestinal binders of phosphate to prevent and treat hyperphosphatemia, a high serum calcium–phosphorus product, calcium phosphate deposition in soft tissue, and hyperparathyroidism are discussed in Chapters 77. This section considers the prescription of dietary phosphorus intake and phosphate binders. In renal failure patients, a large dietary phosphorus intake can lead to a high plasma calcium–phosphorus product with increased risk of calcium and phosphate deposition in soft tissues. Also, animal and human studies suggest the possibility that a low phosphorus intake may reduce the rate of progression of renal failure in individuals with chronic renal disease.

There are little data concerning the optimal level of phosphorus restriction for retarding progressive renal failure or for minimizing or preventing hyperparathyroidism; the latter could be achieved by reducing dietary phosphate in proportion to the reduction in GFR. It is recommended that in both nondialyzed and dialyzed patients, the morning fasting serum phosphorus concentrations be maintained, if possible, within the normal range. Because there is a rough correlation between the protein and phosphorus content of the diet, it is much easier to reduce phosphorus intake if a lower-protein diet is used.

For patients who have a GFR between 25 and 70 ml/min/1.73 m^2 or who have a higher GFR with a progressive loss of renal function, 5 to 10 mg phosphorus/kg per day may be prescribed with the diet of 0.55 to 0.60 g protein/kg per day. These individuals generally are not given phosphate binders unless the serum phosphorus levels rise above normal. For nondialyzed patients with a GFR below 25 ml/min/1.73 m^2 who are prescribed a diet of 0.55 to 0.60 g protein/kg per day, the phosphorus intake generally can be decreased to about 5 to 10 mg/kg per day, although this may increase the burdensomeness of the diet, particularly at the lower end of this range of phosphorus intake. Without phosphate binders, there is a net intestinal phosphate absorption (diet minus fecal phosphorus) of roughly 60% of the phosphorus intake. Therefore this level of dietary phosphorus restriction usually will not maintain normal serum phosphorus levels in patients with a GFR under about 15 ml/min, even with a substantial reduction in the renal tubular reabsorption of phosphorus. Hence, phosphate binders are also used. The recommended phosphorus intake for MHD, CAPD, or CCPD patients is about 17 mg/kg per day or less. This higher upper limit was chosen because with their greater protein intakes, dialysis patients cannot readily ingest less phosphorus without making the diet too restrictive. Maintenance dialysis patients almost always require phosphate binders to prevent hyperphosphatemia.

Traditionally, the two most commonly used phosphate binders have been aluminum carbonate and aluminum hydroxide. Usually, two to four 500-mg capsules taken three to four times per day are needed. Larger doses may be used if necessary. Evidence that aluminum-induced osteomalacia and other toxicities may be caused by the intake of aluminum phosphate binders (see Chapter 68, Part 2) has led nephrologists to use calcium salts to bind phosphate. Calcium carbonate, calcium citrate, and calcium acetate have been used for this purpose. Of these three compounds, calcium acetate may have the greatest binding affinity to phosphate and may be more effective at lowering serum PTH. Intestinal calcium absorption may or may not be lower with calcium acetate. However, calcium acetate appears to cause more symptoms such as nausea, diarrhea, and constipation. This may be the cause of poorer compliance described with calcium acetate tablets. Hypercalcemia is reported to be less common with calcium acetate as compared with calcium carbonate. Calcium citrate enhances the intestinal absorption of aluminum and should not be given with aluminum salts. Calcium binders should be taken in divided doses with meals and should not be prescribed if the serum phosphorus level is very high in order to prevent precipitation of calcium and phosphate in soft tissues. Thus hyperphosphatemic patients may be treated with an aluminum binder of phosphate until serum phosphorus falls to normal or near normal. At that time, the regimen may be changed to a calcium binder.

Aluminum and probably iron toxicity can cause a syndrome of low bone turnover that has been referred to as *aplastic bone disease* and that is characterized by low serum PTH levels, decreased bone osteoblasts, and markedly reduced bone turnover (see Chapters 68, Part 2, and 77). The large intakes of calcium binders, which are used to control serum phosphorus levels and in clinical practice may exceed 3 to 5 g/day of elemental calcium, may also potentially cause calcium deposits in soft tissues. It has been suggested that the large calcium intake from dietary calcium supplements or dialysate may also cause this syndrome of low bone turnover. This is mediated to suppression of blood levels of PTH to less than 65 pg/ml (immunoradiometric [IRMA] assay). Normally, patients should probably not receive more than about 2.0 g/day of elemental calcium to prevent excessive calcium. Because amino acid and ketoacid formulations do not contain phosphorus, one advantage of very-low-protein diets supplemented with these preparations was the greater ease with which the phosphorus intake could be reduced, often to as low as 4 to 6 mg/kg per day. At present, there is no well-defined safe lower limit for the serum phosphorus level in renal failure patients. Experience suggests that if the fasting serum phosphorus level is maintained above the lower limit of normal, patients will not develop phosphate depletion. More research is required to ascertain whether this view is correct.

A new calcium-free and aluminum-free phosphate binder polymer, sevelamer hydrochloride (RenaGel, Genzyme), has recently become available for routine clinical use. This is a hydrogel of cross-linked polyallylamine, is resistant to digestive degradation, and is not absorbed from the gastrointestinal tract. Two to four capsules of sevelamer hydrochloride with each meal appears to be roughly as effective as calcium- and aluminum-containing phosphate binders and does not provide a calcium or aluminum load. Sevelamer hydrochloride also has the benefit of lowering serum total cholesterol and LDL cholesterol. It is generally well tolerated.

Trace Elements

A number of factors in renal failure patients tend to either increase or decrease the body burden of certain trace elements. Many trace elements are excreted primarily in the urine, and with renal failure, they may accumulate. Elements such as iron, zinc, and copper, which are protein bound, may be lost in excessive quantities when there are large urinary protein losses (e.g., in nephrotic syndrome). Excessive uptake or losses of trace elements may also occur during dialysis therapy depending on their relative concentrations in plasma and dialysate and the degree of binding to protein or red cells. Hemodialysance of copper, strontium, zinc, and lead, for example, which are largely bound to plasma proteins or red cells, should be minimal. Hemodialysis or hemodiafiltration may remove some trace elements if the dialysate concentrations are sufficiently low (e.g., bromide and zinc). Zinc may be taken up and copper lost from peritoneal dialysate. Because many trace elements are bound avidly to serum proteins, they may be taken up by blood against a concentration gradient when present in even small quantities in dialysate. These observations provided part of the justification for purifying dialysate water before use (e.g., the reverse osmosis and ion exchange systems).

Protein-calorie malnutrition, by lowering serum concentrations of proteins that bind trace elements, may decrease the serum levels of a number of these elements. Occupational exposure or pica may increase the burden of some trace elements. Therapeutic doses of trace elements may be administered through dialysis, as has been done for zinc. The effect of the altered dietary intake of the uremic patient on body pools of trace elements is unknown. Oral iron supplements are often given to patients who are iron deficient or, as a routine treatment, for patients who have a propensity to develop iron deficiency (e.g., individuals who frequently have marginal or low serum iron, percentage of iron-binding capacity, or ferritin levels).

Assessment of trace element burden in renal failure patients is difficult because the binding protein concentrations may be decreased, thereby lowering serum trace element levels, and the binding characteristics of these proteins may be altered in renal failure. Also, red cell concentrations of trace elements may not reflect levels in other tissues. Trace element supplementation should be undertaken with caution because impaired urinary excretion and poor dialysance of trace elements increase the risk of overdosage.

Dietary requirements for trace elements have not been well defined in uremic patients. Iron deficiency is common, particularly in MHD patients, because intestinal iron absorption is sometimes impaired, there are often substantial blood losses, iron may bind to the dialyzer membrane, and the erythropoietin-induced rise in hemoglobin concentrations may deplete the body's iron stores. Indeed, the iron requirements increase during the time when erythropoietin therapy is initiated and hemoglobin concentrations rise. Ferrous sulfate (300 mg three times per day 30 minutes after meals) may be used. Patients with a chronic need for iron supplements sometimes require only one or two iron doses per day. Some patients develop anorexia, nausea, constipation, or abdominal pain with ferrous sulfate; sometimes, these individuals will tolerate other iron compounds better, such as ferrous fumarate, gluconate, or lactate. Patients who are intolerant to oral iron supplements or who have iron deficiency may be best treated with intramuscular or intravenous iron. Increased body burden of iron or aluminum in hemodialysis or CAPD patients may be reduced by infusion of deferoxamine, which is dialyzable. Care must be taken because deferoxamine may promote infection, particularly mucormycosis. Injections of erythropoietin with repeated phlebotomy is another method for removing excess body iron.

Although the zinc content of most tissues is normal in renal failure patients, serum and hair zinc usually are reported to be low and red cell zinc increased. In nondialyzed, chronically uremic patients, the fractional urinary excretion of zinc is increased; however, because the GFR is reduced, total urinary excretion of zinc may be decreased. Fecal zinc is increased, and a dietary zinc intake greater than the recommended dietary allowance may be necessary to maintain normal body zinc pools. Further studies are needed to confirm this. Some reports indicate that dysgeusia, poor food intake, and impaired sexual function, which are common problems of uremic patients, may be improved by giving patients zinc supplements. Other studies, however, have not confirmed this. Intestinal absorption of zinc is not affected by administration of 1,25-dihydroxycholecalciferol.

The finding that serum selenium is low in dialysis patients has raised the question of whether selenium supplements are indicated. This question is of particular importance because selenium participates in the defense against oxidative damage of tissues, which may be increased in renal failure. Further research will be necessary to resolve this issue.

Vitamins

Chronically uremic patients are reported to have a high incidence of vitamin deficiencies. These are due to several factors. First, in renal failure, 1,25-dihydroxycholecalciferol production is impaired by the diseased kidney. Second, vitamin intake is often decreased in uremic patients because of anorexia and reduced food intake. Intercurrent illnesses, which occur frequently in chronically uremic patients, also impair food intake. Many foods that are high in water-soluble vitamins are often restricted for renal failure patients because of the elevated protein and potassium content of these foods; the diets prescribed for nondialyzed chronic renal failure and maintenance dialysis patients often contain less than the recommended daily allowances for certain water-soluble vitamins. Third, renal failure appears to alter the absorption, metabolism, or activity of some vitamins. Animal studies indicate that intestinal absorption of riboflavin, folate, and vitamin D_3 is impaired in renal failure. The metabolism of folate and pyridoxine appears to be abnormal in chronic renal failure. Fourth, certain medicines interfere with the intestinal absorption, metabolism, or actions of vitamins. Fifth, water-soluble vitamins can be dialyzed.

On the other hand, vitamin B_{12} deficiency is uncommon in chronic uremia because the daily requirement for this vitamin is small (e.g., 3 μg/day) for normal nonpregnant, nonlactating adults; the body stores large quantities of this vitamin; and even though vitamin B_{12} is water soluble, it is protein bound in plasma and hence poorly dialyzed. There is a report of low serum vitamin B_{12} concentrations in 19 of 60 MHD patients; the serum vitamin B_{12} concentrations tended to fall progressively with the months of dialysis treatment, and serum vitamin B_{12} levels correlated directly with nerve conduction velocities, which improved with ingestion of large quantities of B_{12}. Another study reported low serum vitamin B_{12} levels in four hemodialysis patients, only one of whom demonstrated an intestinal absorption defect for vitamin B_{12}. Their hematocrit levels improved after receiving vitamin B_{12} injections. The explanation for these two discrepant reports of low serum vitamin B_{12} levels in maintenance hemodialysis patients is not known.

Vitamin deficiencies have been observed with particular frequency for 1,25-dihydroxycholecalciferol, folic acid, vitamin B_6, vitamin C, and to a lesser extent, other water-soluble vitamins. Blood folate concentrations were reported to be decreased in patients undergoing MHD who did not take folic acid supplements. Several investigators found normal serum or red blood cell folate concentrations in patients undergoing MHD. However, although the mean plasma or red cell values may be normal in some patients, a substantial number of patients have deficient levels. In addition, several investigators found hypersegmentation of polymorphonuclear leukocytes in these patients that decreased after administration of folate supplements.

Some investigators noted that the reticulocyte count and hematocrit rose when patients undergoing MHD were given folic acid supplements. We have observed normal serum folate concentrations in virtually all patients undergoing MHD who receive 1.0 mg/day of supplemental folic acid. Higher folate levels have been reported in hemodialysis patients as compared with controls, but the folate intake and type of dialysis were not indicated. Dietary folic acid requirements increase in patients with chronic renal failure during the time when they commence erythropoietin therapy and sustain a major rise in their hemoglobin levels.

Plasma homocysteine is increased in nondialyzed chronic renal failure patients as well as in about 80% to 85% of MHD and CPD patients. This issue is of considerable importance because elevated plasma homocysteine is associated with a high incidence of occlusive vascular disease (see Chapter 68, Part 3). Vitamin B_6 is a cofactor for cystathionine synthetase, which catalyzes the conversion of methionine to cystathionine, and for cystathionase, which converts cystathionine to cysteine. Pyridoxine HCl in general does not lower plasma homocysteine in individuals with chronic renal failure. On the other hand, folic acid supplements will often decrease plasma homocysteine concentrations in nondialyzed chronic renal failure and maintenance dialysis patients, although not to normal values. The folate metabolite tetrahydrofolic acid is necessary for the remethylation of homocysteine to reform methionine. The lowest dosage of folic acid associated with the maximum lowering effect on plasma homocysteine is about 5 to 10 mg/day.

There are substantial losses of vitamin C into dialysate. Low plasma and leukocyte ascorbic acid concentrations may occur in patients undergoing hemodialysis who were not receiving supplemental vitamin C. Clinical signs suggestive of mild scurvy have been described in several MHD patients with very low ascorbic acid concentrations. Administration of ascorbic acid orally or into the dialysate prevented negative vitamin C balance during hemodialysis.

Many workers find evidence for low plasma or red blood cell vitamin B_6 concentrations in subjects undergoing MHD or CPD who do not take supplemental vitamin B_6. Activation coefficients of erythrocyte transaminase enzymes (i.e., the activity of the enzyme divided into the activity of the same enzyme after the vitamin B_6 cofactor pyridoxal-5-phosphate is added to the assay) are not uncommonly elevated in patients undergoing MHD who do not receive supplemental vitamin B_6, indicating that these subjects are deficient in vitamin B_6. Improvement in the activation coefficient during hemodialysis has been reported, suggesting that there might be an inhibitor of vitamin B_6 in uremic sera that is removed by dialysis. Low stimulation ratios in mixed lymphocyte cultures from these patients have been reported. Pyridoxine hydrochloride supplements improve several parameters of immune function in hemodialysis patients, including lymphoblast formation. These observations suggest that vitamin B_6 deficiency, which is known to cause abnormal immunologic function, may be one cause of the altered immune response in uremic patients. Interestingly, serum glutamate–oxaloacetate transaminase activity is reduced in renal failure. This effect appears to be related to vitamin B_6 activity, possibly due to a uremic inhibitor in serum.

Plasma oxalate levels are elevated in renal failure. Increased plasma oxalate appears to be largely due to impaired urinary excretion, although large doses of vitamin C (ascorbic acid), a precursor of oxalate, may increase oxalate production. Glyoxylate, a metabolic precursor of oxalate, may also be transaminated to form glycine. Vitamin B_6 is a cofactor for the enzyme that catalyzes this step. Indeed, vitamin B_6 deficiency increases urinary oxalate excretion in rats with experimental renal insufficiency as well as in normal individuals. In patients with chronic renal failure, some studies indicate that treatment with large doses of pyridoxine HCl decreases plasma oxalate levels, although not to normal values. Other clinical trials have not been able to confirm these results.

Pyridoxine hydrochloride (5 mg/day) produced a normal red cell erythrocyte glutamate–pyruvate transaminase activation index in nondialyzed, clinically stable, chronically uremic patients, and 10 mg/day of pyridoxine hydrochloride normalized this index in stable MHD patients and in chronically uremic individuals with superimposed infections.

Despite the water solubility of riboflavin, thiamine, pantothenic acid, and biotin, plasma concentrations of these vitamins are usually not decreased in patients undergoing MHD. It is possible that losses of these vitamins into hemodialysate are offset by the lack of urinary excretion in these patients. Low plasma niacin concentrations have been reported in some patients receiving maintenance dialysis therapy. However, these findings were not confirmed in patients receiving 7.5 mg/day of supplemental nicotinic acid. Low thiamine and, in some patients, thiamine and pyridoxine have been found in patients prescribed low-protein diets.

Serum retinol-binding protein and vitamin A are increased in renal failure patients. Elevated liver vitamin A was described in two patients with chronic renal failure, although other investigators could not confirm elevated vitamin A levels in solid tissues. Moreover, even relatively small supplements of vitamin A [i.e., 7,500 to 15,000 IU/day (about 1,500 to 3,000 retinal equivalents per day)] appear to cause bone toxicity and hypercalcemia in some patients. Normal, low, and increased plasma or red cell vitamin E (α-tocopherol) levels have been described in nondialyzed chronic renal failure or MHD patients. Vitamin E deficiency may cause oxidative injury to tissues. Vitamin K deficiency is uncommon. Patients who do not eat (and hence do not ingest foods containing vitamin K) and who are receiving antibiotics that suppress intestinal bacteria for extended periods may require supplemental vitamin K to prevent deficiency of this vitamin.

Vitamin levels were measured in 10 CAPD patients who apparently were eating an unrestricted protein diet and not receiving vitamin supplements. These measurements showed that plasma vitamin B_1 (thiamine), vitamin B_6, folic acid, and vitamin C were frequently reduced. Plasma vitamin B_2 and B_{12} were normal, although vitamin B_{12} levels tended to decline with time in patients who did not receive supplements of this vitamin. Dietary intake of several vitamins, including vitamin A, vitamin B_1, vitamin B_6, vitamin B_{12}, and nicotinamide, was often reduced below the recommended allowances for normal adults. Other investigators have reported low serum folic acid levels in CAPD patients. In CPD patients not receiving supplements, other investigators have found a high incidence of low or normal plasma folate levels, low vitamin B_1, vitamin B_6, and vitamin C. Reduced plasma vitamin E was found in 13% of CPD patients, whereas increased plasma vitamin E levels were found by others.

The nutritional requirements for most vitamins are not well defined in renal failure patients, and it is likely that they will be modified in the future. There is evidence that in addition to vitamin intake from foods, the following daily supplements of vitamins will prevent or correct vitamin deficiency (Table 83.4): pyridoxine hydrochloride, 5 mg in nondialyzed patients and 10 mg in MHD or CPD patients; folic acid, 5 to 10 mg; and the recommended daily allowance for normal individuals for the other water-soluble vitamins. A supplement of only 60 mg/day of vitamin C (the recommended daily allowance) is advised because ascorbic acid can be metabolized to oxalate. Large doses of ascorbic acid have been associated with increased plasma oxalate levels in renal failure patients. Oxalate is highly insoluble, and there is substantial concern that high plasma oxalate concentrations can lead to precipitation in soft tissues, including the kidney, possibly causing further impairment in renal function in the nondialyzed patient with renal insufficiency.

Supplemental vitamin A is not recommended because serum levels are increased and there appears to be a high risk of vitamin A toxicity with supplements. It is unclear whether vitamin E supplements are necessary. Additional vitamin K is not needed unless the patient is not eating and receives antibiotics that suppress intestinal bacteria that synthesize vitamin K. Recommendations for vitamin D intake are given in Chapter 77.

Alkalinizing Agents

Nondialyzed patients with advanced renal failure often develop metabolic acidosis associated with an increased anion gap because the kidney's ability to excrete acidic metabolites is impaired. In the earlier stages of chronic renal failure, and occasionally with advanced renal failure, hyperchloremic metabolic acidosis may also be caused by excessive renal losses of bicarbonate. Ingestion of low-nitrogen diets may prevent or decrease the severity of the acidosis because the endogenous generation of acidic products of protein metabolism will be reduced. Because the rate of acid production is usually normal or below normal in clinically stable patients with chronic renal failure, alkalinizing medicines are usually very effective for preventing or treating the acidosis. Research indicates that metabolic acidosis may engender protein and amino acid catabolism and net protein and bone loss.

Calcium carbonate (5 g/day) may correct mild acidosis, provide needed calcium, and reduce intestinal phosphate absorption. If the acidosis is more severe, sodium bicarbonate or citrate may be administered orally or intravenously. If the nondialyzed, chronically uremic patient is not oliguric and is not particularly likely to develop edema, sodium is usually readily excreted when it is given as sodium bicarbonate. Because the exact level of acidemia at which net protein loss or bone reabsorption is stimulated is not well defined, it would seem prudent to prevent any degree of chronic acidemia. Therefore alkali therapy should probably be initiated if the arterial pH is below 7.35 or the serum bicarbonate is less than 22 mEq/L. In general, oral treatment may be administered with sodium bicarbonate or citrate salts. Before implementing alkali therapy, it must be ascertained that the low serum bicarbonate is not a compensatory response to chronic respiratory alkalosis. If acidosis is severe and is not controlled by the foregoing measures, hemodialysis or peritoneal dialysis may be used.

Fiber

Studies in normal individuals suggest that a high dietary fiber intake may lower the incidence of constipation, irritable bowel syndrome, diverticulitis, and neoplasia of the colon; in addition, it may improve glucose tolerance. In patients with chronic renal failure, a high dietary fiber intake also may reduce SUN by decreasing colonic bacterial ammonia generation and enhancing fecal nitrogen excretion. Because it seems reasonable that the benefits of a high dietary fiber intake in normal people would also occur in nondialyzed patients with chronic renal failure and in maintenance dialysis patients, a high dietary fiber intake of 20 to 25 g/day is recommended.

PRIORITIZING DIETARY GOALS

The number and magnitude of the changes in the dietary intake for chronically uremic patients are so great that if they were all presented to the patient at one time, the patient could become demoralized and lose his or her motivation to comply with the diet. We therefore prioritize goals for dietary treatment. Usually, we emphasize the importance of controlling the protein, phosphorus, sodium, energy, potassium, and magnesium intake as well as the need to take calcium and vitamin supplements. On the other hand, unless the patient has a lipid disorder that carries a high risk of atherosclerotic disease, the recommended quantity and types of dietary carbohydrate, fat, and fiber are discussed with the patient, but adherence to these dietary guidelines is not strongly emphasized. If the patient has complied well with the other, more critical elements of dietary therapy; has a specific lipid disorder that may benefit from dietary therapy; or has expressed an interest in modifying fat, carbohydrate, or fiber intake, the modification of the dietary intake of these latter nutrients is explored more intensively with the patient.

Dietary Therapy for the Nephrotic Syndrome Patient

Nephrotic syndrome is characterized by proteinuria (more than 3.5 g/24 hr), lipiduria, hypoalbuminemia, hypercholesterolemia, and edema, which can be massive. Serum total proteins may decrease markedly, from 7 to 8 g/dl to as low as 4 to 5 g/dl, and the resultant fall in plasma oncotic pressure promotes extravascular movement of fluid, sodium retention, and edema formation. Two narrow transverse white bands (Muehrcke's lines) may occur in the fingernails in association with severe hypoproteinemia.

Serum triglycerides; phospholipids; and apoproteins B, CII, CIII, and E are increased, whereas apoproteins AI and AII are normal. Plasma lipoprotein [LP(a)] is elevated. Both LDL and very-low-density lipoprotein (VLDL) may be increased. There is increased serum cholesterol ester transfer protein (CETP) and decreased catabolism of LDL apolipoprotein, at least by the more typical receptor pathway. These metabolic changes contribute to the elevated LDL cholesterol and frequently observed low HDL cholesterol levels. Hypercholesterolemia, hypertriglyceridemia, increased LDL cholesterol and VLDL-cholesterol, increased CETP and LP(a), and low HDL cholesterol all are risk factors for an increased incidence of atherosclerotic cardiovascular disease and cerebrovascular disease in nephrotic patients. It has been suggested that the altered serum lipid pattern in nephrotic syndrome may accelerate the progression of renal failure. Altered membrane lipid composition and oxidant injury of the kidney and also erythrocytes have been described.

It has been reported that protein-restricted diets providing less than 30% of calories from fat, less than 200 mg/day of cholesterol, and an abundant amount of polyunsaturated fatty acids, with 10% of calories from linoleic acid, resulted in a reduction in serum total and LDL cholesterol and a decrease in proteinuria in nephrotic patients. A vegetarian soy-based low-protein diet may reduce proteinuria and hyperlipidemia in nephrotic patients. Reduction in serum lipids by the HMG-CoA reductase inhibitor simvastatin is reported to cause a partial remission in nephrotic syndrome in patients.

Low serum protein levels are caused by enhanced urinary protein excretion and by degradation of the increased quantity of filtered protein in renal tubular cells. Also, albumin synthesis may be increased, normal, or decreased, depending at least partly on the adequacy of dietary protein intake. Massive proteinuria may occur (e.g., up to 40 g/24 hr or more of protein) and may be incapacitating or life-threatening. Serum levels of many biologically active proteins, including clotting factors and inhibitors, are reduced because of enhanced excretion and renal degradation; the clinical importance of these effects are not well defined. However, low plasma concentrations of clotting inhibitors may contribute to the frequency of renal vein thrombosis in nephrotic syndrome.

The vitamin D analogs 25-hydroxycholecalciferol and 1,25-dihydroxycholecalciferol are bound to an α-like globulin and may be lost in urine in nephrotic syndrome. In experimental nephrosis, intestinal absorption of vitamin D appears to be normal. Evidence of vitamin D deficiency with low serum 25-hydroxycholecalciferol and 1,25-dihydroxycholecalciferol, decreased ionized and total calcium, and bone disease has been found in patients with nephrotic syndrome. Others have reported normal serum vitamin D levels and no bone disease. There is loss of organic iodide and thyroxine in the urine in nephrotic syndrome, although hypothyroidism is probably not present. Also, there may be increased urinary losses of trace elements bound to proteins such as zinc, copper, and iron. These losses may cause nutritional deficiencies.

The severity of nutritional disorders in patients with nephrotic syndrome varies greatly; in the author's experience, patients with nephrotic syndrome are not infrequently wasted and debilitated to a degree that is disproportionate to their renal insufficiency. This is particularly common in patients with more massive proteinuria. The causes of wasting and debility are large urinary protein losses, anorexia, the urinary losses of vitamins and trace elements that are protein bound in plasma, glucocorticoid and/or cytotoxic therapy, and the frequent incidence of infections that result from such treatment.

A high-protein diet providing up to 2.3 g protein/kg per day has been reported to improve nutritional status, if uremia is not present. The findings that low-protein diets may retard progression of renal failure and reduce proteinuria have prompted a reexamination of the use of low-protein diets in this disorder. Some investigators fed isocaloric diets providing 0.8 and 1.6 g protein/kg per day to nephrotic patients. These studies showed that with the lower protein intake, urine albumin, renal albumin clearance, and fractional urinary albumin excretion decreased. Serum albumin concentrations and plasma albumin mass were actually greater with the low-protein diet, although total albumin mass did not differ with the two diets. Soy-protein diets also reduced proteinuria.

In rats and humans with proteinuria or nephrotic syndrome, converting enzyme inhibitors may reduce but not abolish the proteinuria. The addition of converting enzyme inhibitor medicines seems to allow protein intakes to be increased modestly without increasing urinary protein losses, thereby increasing the likelihood of nutritional repletion. Reduction of proteinuria is an important goal because large urine protein losses are a risk factor for more rapid progression of renal failure. Long-term studies have not demonstrated whether these lower protein intakes will prevent or correct protein malnutrition; this problem is complicated by the difficulty of assessing protein nutrition in nephrotic patients.

It is our policy to prescribe for patients with nephrotic syndrome diets that provide 0.70 or 0.80 g protein/kg per day. The higher value would be prescribed for patients with more severe proteinuria. At least 0.35 g/kg per day of the protein should be of high biologic value. This diet should be supplemented with 1.0 g of protein of high biologic value for each gram of urine protein excreted each day. Intake of energy and minerals in general is prescribed as described for patients with chronic renal insufficiency. ACE inhibitors or, if they are not tolerated, angiotensin II antagonists are routinely added to reduce proteinuria. An American Heart Association step I diet may benefit lipid metabolism, although, by itself, it probably will not lower serum lipids. Hypercholesterolemia also may be treated with HMG-CoA reductase inhibitors. Phosphorus intake may need to be liberalized if the protein intake is much greater than 0.70 g/kg per day. For nephrotic individuals with a reduced GFR, the phosphorous binder sevelamer hydrochloride not only may lower serum phosphorous concentrations but also may reduce serum LDL cholesterol and total cholesterol. Diuretics are often used, and sodium is restricted because of edema and the tendency to retain sodium. When sodium is restricted adequately, thirst will usually regulate water intake to prevent the development of substantial hyponatremia. Vitamin supplements should provide the normal daily allowances for the fat-soluble vitamins, including vitamin D, as well as the water-soluble vitamins.

For patients with moderate or advanced renal insufficiency, 1,25-dihydroxycholecalciferol (0.25 to 0.50 μg/day) probably should be substituted for vitamin D_3 or cholecalciferol. The potential benefits of administering trace elements have not been established, although for patients with large amounts of proteinuria, iron, zinc, copper, and probably other trace element supplements should be given. Good blood pressure control is essential. More studies are needed to examine these questions as well as the use of medicines and diet to treat hyperlipidemia and hypercholesterolemia in nephrotic syndrome.

Selected Readings

Bergstrom J, Lindholm B. Malnutrition, cardiac disease, and mortality: an integrated point of view. *Am J Kidney Dis* 1998;32:834–841.

This paper reviews the evidence for inflammation as a cause of mortality, particularly from cardiovascular disease in patients with advanced chronic renal failure. The authors review evidence indicating that malnutrition and chronic inflammation may each contribute to cardiovascular disease and mortality and that malnutrition and inflammation may each promote the other.

Fouque D, Laville M, Boissel JP, et al. Controlled low protein diets in chronic renal insufficiency: meta-analysis. *BMJ* 1992;304:216–220.

This paper addresses whether dietary protein restriction retards the rate of progression of renal failure in patients with chronic renal disease. The meta-analysis indicates that dietary protein restriction delays the onset of maintenance dialysis treatment.

Kasiske BL, Lakatua JD, Ma JZ, et al. A meta-analysis of the effects of dietary protein restriction on the rate of decline in renal function. *Am J Kidney Dis* 1998; 31:954–961.

This paper addresses whether dietary protein restriction retards the rate of progression of renal failure in patients with chronic renal disease. The meta-analysis indicates that dietary protein restriction reduces the rate of decrease in the GFR.

Kopple JD. Dietary protein and energy requirements in ESRD patients. *Am J Kidney Dis* 1998;32:S97–S104.

This paper reviews the dietary energy and protein needs of MHD and CPD patients. Evidence on which the recommended protein and energy intakes are based is discussed.

Kopple JD, Greene T, Chumlea WC, et al. Relationship between nutritional status and GFR: results from the MDRD study. *Kidney Int* 2000;57:1688–1703.

This cross-sectional analysis of more than 1,700 patients with chronic renal disease indicates that protein and energy intake and protein-energy nutritional status deteriorates as the GFR decreases below 55 ml/min/1.73 m^2.

Kopple JD, Zhu X, Lew NL, et al. Body weight-for-height relationships predict mortality in maintenance hemodialysis patients. *Kidney Int* 1999;56:1136–1148.

This is one of several studies indicating that in MHD patients, body weight adjusted for height is associated with a high risk for 12-month mortality.

Lowrie EG, Lew LN. Death risk in hemodialysis patients: the predictive value of commonly measured variables and an evaluation of death rate differences between facilities. *Am J Kidney Dis* 1990;15:458–482.

This seminal study was the first comprehensive analysis of the relationship between measurements of nutritional status and mortality rates in MHD patients.

National Kidney Foundation Dialysis Outcomes Quality Initiative (NKF-DOQI) Clinical Practice Guidelines for Nutrition in Chronic Renal Failure. *Am J Kidney Dis* 2000;35(Suppl 1):S1–S122.

These NKF-DOQI Clinical Practice Guidelines examine the evidence concerning the validity of the methods for assessing protein-energy nutritional status and the recommendations for dietary protein and energy intake for patients undergoing MHD or CPD and patients with advanced chronic renal failure. Practice guidelines are offered based on the evidence and expert opinion.

Obrador GT, Pereira B. Early referral to the nephrologist and timely initiation of renal replacement therapy: a paradigm shift in the management of patients with chronic renal failure. *Am J Kidney Dis* 1998;31:398–417.

This is a small meta-analysis indicating that in patients with advanced chronic renal failure, late referral to a nephrologist is associated with an increased risk of mortality.

Pedrini MT, Levey AS, Lau J, et al. The effect of dietary protein restriction on the progression of diabetic and nondiabetic renal diseases: a meta-analysis. *Ann Intern Med* 1996;124:627–632.

This paper addresses whether dietary protein restriction retards the rate of progression of renal failure in patients with chronic renal disease. The meta-analysis indicates that dietary protein restriction delays the onset of maintenance dialysis treatment.

CHAPTER 84

Dialysis Therapy

PART 1
Hemodialysis
A: Kinetics of Hemodialysis

Thomas A. Depner

The word *kinetic* means movement, which for hemodialysis is the movement of solutes driven by the diffusive forces of molecular concentration gradients created by the dialyzer. The dialyzer is essentially a semipermeable membrane, located outside the body, that separates a flowing stream of blood from a flowing stream of dialysate and is permeable to solutes that accumulate in patients with renal failure. The unwanted solutes in the blood diffuse down their concentration gradients across the membrane and are eliminated in the dialysate, whereas larger particles and vital solutes, such as the blood proteins, are retained.

SOLUTE REMOVAL DURING HEMODIALYSIS

The immediate goal of therapeutic dialysis is to eliminate diffusible solutes, whereas the ultimate goal is to reduce the levels of these solutes in the patient. Solutes retained in patients with renal failure are collectively known as *uremic toxins,* many of which are compounds found in normal urine. Accumulation of these toxins in the patient causes the uremic syndrome or uremia, a nearly uniform set of symptoms and signs common to patients with renal failure, independent of the cause. The signs and symptoms of uremia are the toxic effects of retained solutes. Proof of this statement is found in the therapeutic success of dialysis, which ameliorates uremia by removing solutes. Moreover, the toxins responsible for the life-threatening aspects of uremia must be relatively low in molecular weight because they are removed by hemodialysis membranes derived from cellulose that have a relatively low cutoff at approximately 10,000 D. We can also conclude, based on the patients' frequent requirement for hemodialysis treatments, that generation of these toxins is relatively rapid.

Removing uremic toxins by dialysis lowers their concentrations in the blood and presumably in the patient as a whole. Blood levels therefore should correlate directly with toxicity and inversely with the effectiveness of dialysis. Numerous classes of compounds and several hundred individual compounds have been identified in the serum of uremic patients but unfortunately no single compound stands alone as a target for removal, the level of which correlates with the severity of uremia or the adequacy of dialysis. In addition, the most abundant organic compounds to accumulate, such as urea and creatinine, have little toxicity. Studies in patients with acute and chronic renal failure during the 1970s showed that the uremic syndrome could be ameliorated without removing urea, which was added to the dialysate to prevent its removal.

Physicians were therefore left without a good method for monitoring the adequacy of dialysis in their patients until the mid-1980s, when an analysis of the U.S. National Cooperative Dialysis Study (NCDS) showed that outcome correlated closely with the effective dialyzer urea clearance. Although it was well recognized that urea is not very toxic, and that urea levels in the patient correlate poorly with outcome, the dialyzer urea clearance, when averaged over the entire dialysis treatment, was an effective marker for the adequacy of dialysis. The clearance of urea presumably reflects the clearance and removal of more toxic compounds that, probably in concert, account for the uremic syndrome. This indirect approach of using a clearance instead of a toxin level to quantifying dialysis has prevailed, partially because it is easy to measure, as shown in the following section. Standards were soon developed for patients treated three times per week.

Precise laws of thermodynamics that are based on statistic probability define the behavior of dissolved solutes. Temperature-dependent random motion of molecules always takes the path of least resistance, which is in the direction of lower concentration. A concentration gradient is therefore a force that causes net vectorial movement of solutes in solution. The dialyzer makes use of these forces to move solutes out of the blood compartment, thereby lowering their concentrations in the patient. A semipermeable membrane is not necessary for diffusive movement of solute, but it reduces or eliminates convective movement (see discussion of filtration following) and provides an opportunity to select the solutes that are allowed to diffuse. Fortunately, for dialysis, the more desirable solutes are larger and the more vital small solutes can be added to the dialysate inexpensively. This basic principle, removal of small toxic compounds and retention of larger desirable compounds, was a fortuitous empiric discovery that is largely responsible for the success of therapeutic dialysis.

DIALYSIS KINETICS

Removal Rate Versus Clearance

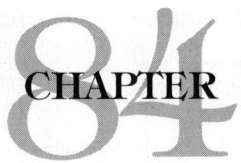

Solute removal, either by filtration or by dialysis, is proportional to the solute concentration (a first order process). Therefore *clearance*, which is the removal rate divided by the concentration, is a more meaningful expression of the dialysis or filtration process itself because it tends to be constant, independent of concentration:

$$K_D = \text{Removal rate}/C_B \quad (1)$$

where K_D is the dialyzer clearance and C_B is the blood concentration. Because the removal rate and C_B have a common element (the amount of solute), the expression of clearance simplifies to a flow and can be conceptualized as the blood volume per minute that is completely purged of solute. Despite the fall in concentration during hemodialysis, this virtual flow remains constant because the rate of removal falls proportionately. First-order processes such as dialysis are always better expressed as a clearance than a removal rate.

DIALYSANCE

Static dialysis is self-limiting because the solute concentration gradient dissipates with time causing the clearance to fall. Because the rate of solute movement across the membrane is proportional to the driving force, dividing the rate of solute removal by the solute gradient yields a more constant expression of the dialyzer effect called *dialysance* (D).

$$D = \text{Solute removal rate}/(C_{\text{blood}} - C_{\text{dialysate}}) \quad (2)$$

Dialysance is a more precise index of dialysis but for modern, single-pass dialysis, it is equivalent to clearance, therefore the dialysance concept has been deemphasized. When defining dialysance and clearance, the dialyzer is considered an inaccessible black box, so the only measurable concentrations are those of the dialysate and blood entering or exiting the device. Because the entering dialysate concentration is zero for single-pass dialysis, clearance and dialysance are equal.

Dialyzer K_0A

The most important factors that determine the *intrinsic clearance* of a dialyzer for a particular solute are the *membrane porosity*, membrane area, and the solute size. Membrane and solute charge also play a role for some solutes. Membrane porosity depends on the effective pore diameter, length, distribution, and geometry of the pores. The intrinsic clearance, known as K_0A, is the product of membrane permeability and area and is essentially the maximum clearance possible for a given membrane and solute. It is important to note that permeability (and therefore K_0A) is solute specific.

During dialysis the membrane becomes a more complex barrier to diffusion due to the effect of unstirred layers of solvent at the membrane borders. Efforts to reduce these layers by creating turbulent flow on the dialysate side of the membrane have improved solute clearance. The currently most popular hollow fiber geometry of modern dialyzer membranes maintains maximum flow velocity on the interior blood side of the membrane, minimizing these boundary effects. On the dialysate side, however, higher flow rates have recently been shown to increase K_0A, in part by reducing the unstirred layer effect.

Effect of Blood and Dialysate Flow

For simple diffusion in static solutions, dialysis is self-limiting because it causes the concentration gradient, which is the driving force for dialysis, to fall. To counteract this effect, the solutions on either side of the membrane can be set in motion. Under these conditions, in addition to K_0A, the rate of solute

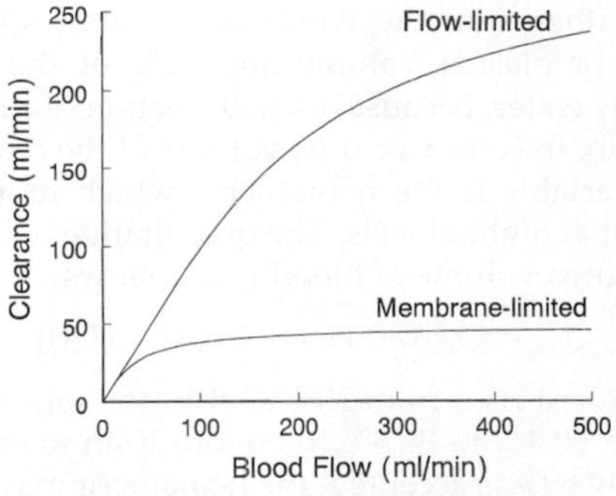

Figure 84.1. Flow-limited versus membrane-limited clearance. The relationship between dialyzer blood flow and clearance is steeper for solutes that pass easily through the membrane *(top graph)*. For less permeable solutes *(bottom graph)*, clearance reaches a plateau as the solute gradient across the entire membrane reaches a maximum. Beyond this point, clearance is not affected by delivering more solute (at the same concentration) to the membrane.

diffusion across the membrane is determined by the flow rates of blood and dialysate, which have predictable effects on the dialyzer clearance. For countercurrent flow [blood flow (Q_B) in opposite direction to dialysate flow (Q_D)], which is the most efficient flow orientation, the dialyzer clearance (K_D) is a function of flow and K_0A:

$$K_D = Q_B\left[\frac{e^{K_0A\frac{(Q_D-Q_B)}{(Q_DQ_B)}} - 1}{e^{K_0A\frac{(Q_D-Q_B)}{(Q_DQ_B)}} - \frac{Q_B}{Q_D}}\right] \quad (3)$$

Equation 3 is derived from consideration of solute mass balance along the dialyzer membrane assuming that the mean driving force is the log mean concentration gradient:

$$\text{Log mean gradient} = (\Delta C_1 - \Delta C_2)/\ln[(\Delta C_1/(\Delta C_2)] \quad (4)$$

ΔC_1 is the concentration gradient across the membrane at one end of the dialyzer and ΔC_2 is the concentration gradient at the other end. Figure 84.1, which is a graph derived from equation 3 shows that for highly permeable dialyzers and highly diffusible solutes, flow is the major determinant of clearance (flow-limited clearance). For less-permeable dialyzers and relatively poorly diffusible solutes, solute clearance is minimally affected by flow (membrane-limited clearance).

Expressions of Dialyzer Clearance

Equation 1 is an expression of *instantaneous clearance*, a snapshot of clearance at one point in time, and is directly measurable. Instantaneous clearance can be measured either on the blood side or on the dialysate side because the solute removal rate must be the same on either and the denominator in equation 1 is always the blood concentration. Equation 3 gives the *prescribed clearance*, which is the predicted instantaneous clearance based on previous measurements of membrane K_0A and flow rates of blood and dialysate. Predicting the clearance with equation 3 eliminates the need to measure solute concentrations but its accuracy depends on the accuracy of the dialyzer K_0A and flow measurements. Equation 3 also does not include the ultrafiltration component of clearance, which must be added (see following).

A distinction should also be made between *whole blood clearance* and *blood–water clearance*. Because a significant proportion of blood volume consists of protein and red cell membranes that exclude many solutes, the delivery of urea and other aqueous solutes to the dialyzer is actually determined by the blood–water flow (Q_{Bw}) rather than the whole blood flow (Q_b). Approximately 93% of plasma volume and 72% of the erythrocyte cell volume is water. Because a small fraction of urea is bound to hemoglobin, the effective urea volume of the red cell is 80%. The major variable is the hematocrit, which reduces blood–water content at higher levels. The quantitative relationship for the effective urea volume of blood is as follows:

$$Q_{Bw} = Q_B[0.80 \cdot \text{Hct} + 0.93(1 - \text{Hct})] \quad (5)$$

As the hematocrit rises from 20% to 40%, the ratio $Q_{Bw}:Q_B$ falls slightly, from 90.4% to 87.8%, therefore if an average ratio of approximately 89% is accepted, the hematocrit may be ignored. Urea diffuses extremely rapidly across the red cell membrane, so rapidly that during the short transit of blood through the dialyzer, no disequilibrium between red cell and plasma can be demonstrated. For other solutes (e.g., creatinine) that do not diffuse as rapidly as urea into and out of the red cell, the effective dialyzable volume flowing through the dialyzer is considerably lower than the urea volume. Postdialysis blood must be allowed to sit for a period of time to allow creatinine to equilibrate across the red cell membrane before separating the plasma. To avoid this delay, which is more than 1 hour for creatinine, dialyzer creatinine clearance is best measured on the dialysate side.

Clearance is also often *normalized* to the size of the patient; for the creatinine clearance of native kidneys, *body surface area,* is conventionally used, whereas for the urea clearance of a dialyzer, *body water volume*, equal to the urea distribution volume, is more popular. Although scaling of native renal function follows body surface area more closely, the two indices of body size are comparable in adults and, as will be shown below, urea volume is a much more convenient denominator for normalizing intermittent urea clearance. Recently, large population studies of dialysis outcome that are very sensitive to the dialysis dose have detected small statistical differences in outcome (worse) for small patients compared with large patients. These differences may be due, in part, to the use of volume instead of surface area as the denominator for the prescription, which provides proportionately more dialysis for larger patients.

More useful than either the measured or predicted instantaneous clearance is the average clearance during a single dialysis, often called the *integrated clearance*. When normalized to body water volume (V) and averaged for the entire dialysis, the integrated clearance can be expressed as Kt/V (the origin of Kt/V will be discussed in more detail in a following section).

As discussed in the following, the patient can be considered as a second dialyzer connected in series with the artificial kidney, allowing clearance to be expressed as the *patient clearance*. Patient clearance is the removal rate divided by the mean concentration in the patient and is always lower than the dialyzer clearance.

FLUID REMOVAL DURING DIALYSIS

Nearly all patients gain fluid between hemodialyses and the few who do not usually have significant native kidney function. The excess fluid is removed by applying a hydrostatic pressure gradient (the *transmembrane pressure* or TMP) across the membrane during dialysis treatments. Removal occurs when either a positive pressure is applied on the blood side or a negative pressure (subatmospheric) is applied on the dialysate side. Within the range of filtration rates used clinically, the relationship between ultrafiltration and TMP is linear. The slope shown in Fig. 84.2 is called the *ultrafiltration coefficient*, expressed in ml/hr/mm pressure gradient. Note that the intercept in Fig. 84.2 is approximately 20 mm Hg. This represents the plasma oncotic pressure that counteracts the applied TMP and must be overcome before any filtration occurs.

Effect of Ultrafiltration on Clearance

The required ultrafiltration that must accompany each treatment can augment the diffusive clearance, but the magnitude of the increase is less than one might expect. In the absence of dialysis, the convective clearance from ultrafiltration is simply the ultrafiltration rate (e.g., 17 ml/min for a filtration rate of 1 L/hr). Simultaneous dialysis reduces the contribution of ultrafiltration to clearance, rendering it negligible as the fractional extraction of the particular solute approaches 100%. This is reasonable because more than 100% removal is impossible no matter how much ultrafiltration accompanies the treatment. The effect of ultrafiltration (Q_f) on clearance can be approximated as follows:

$$K_d = K_{d0} + Q_f(1 - K_{d0}/Q_b) \quad (6)$$

where K_{d0} is the dialyzer clearance with no ultrafiltration.

When filtration and dialysis occur at the same location in the membrane, the contribution of ultrafiltration to clearance is still less than predicted by equation 6 because unidirectional bulk movement of solvent across the membrane reduces the concentration gradient that drives diffusion.

For equation 6, the concentration of solute in the filtrate is assumed to be identical to blood water, which technically means that the *sieving coefficient* for the solute/dialyzer is 1.0. For larger

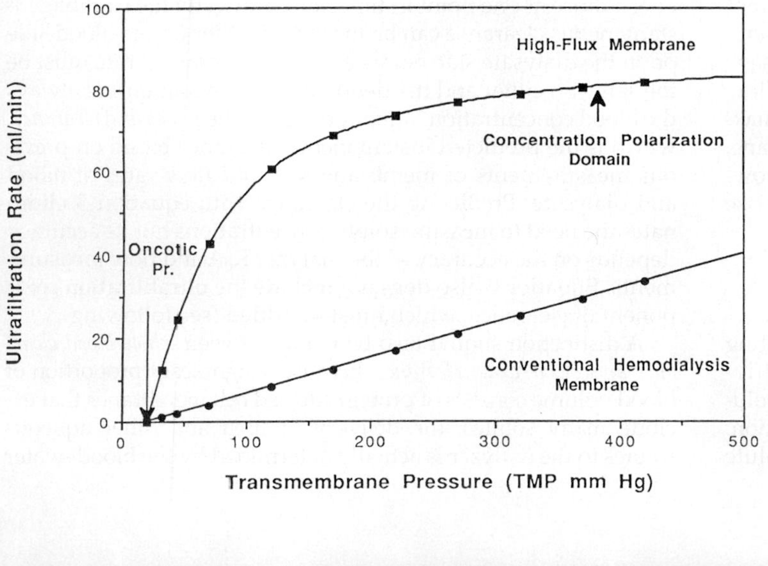

Figure 84.2. Filtration: a comparison of standard and high-flux membranes. The relationship between the ultrafiltration rate and transmembrane pressure is linear for conventional membranes and curvilinear for high-flux membranes. The plateau of the high-flux curve is caused by concentration polarization.

molecular-weight compounds, the sieving coefficient is often considerably lower, further reducing the effect of ultrafiltration on clearance.

FILTRATION THROUGH HIGH-FLUX MEMBRANES

As the ultrafiltration rate rises above the usual clinical range, the membrane is altered by nonfilterable solutes that are pushed toward the membrane surface by convective forces. Because it cannot pass through the membrane, a solute with a low sieving coefficient accumulates, creating a higher concentration at the membrane surface. This build up of poorly filterable solute is called *concentration polarization*. It effectively reduces the ultrafiltration rate, causing the curvilinear relationship between the filtration rate and TMP shown in the upper graph of Fig. 84.2. It also reduces the permeability of the membrane by adding a layer of larger molecules through which the smaller diffusible solutes must move before passing through the membrane.

Modern high-flux membranes require precise and accurate minute-to-minute control of ultrafiltration because their high ultrafiltration coefficients can cause dangerously rapid fluid removal or fluid gain. Control is achieved by using volumetric servomechanisms that remove fluid by precisely balancing inflow and outflow to the dialyzer, eliminating the need for the dialysis technician to control TMP. Even if no net filtration is desired, the high permeability of the membranes and ordinary perfusion pressures cause filtration to occur proximally balanced by backfiltration distally in the dialyzer as shown in Fig. 84.3. The consequences of this internal filtration and backfiltration have not been thoroughly explored but could be beneficial because filtration improves the clearance of larger molecules. Earlier concerns about backfiltration causing exposure of the patient to endotoxin have not been substantiated.

NATIVE KIDNEY FUNCTION

The dialyzer differs from the native kidney that begins the processing of blood, not by diffusion but by filtration. The net effect is similar, but native kidney function, even when inadequate to sustain life, appears to add more to the dialyzer clearance than is apparent from comparison with solute clearances. The additional benefit may simply result from the continuous nature of native kidney clearance or from additional renal tubular effects that are independent of filtration.

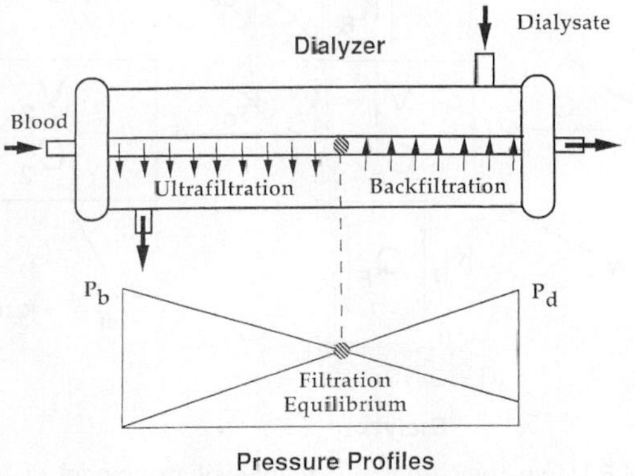

Figure 84.3. High-flux membranes can theoretically cause backfiltration as shown by this schematic. The blood and dialysate pressure profiles along the length of a single hollow fiber are shown below the dialyzer. The crossover point is the location along the fiber where filtration ends and backfiltration begins.

TABLE 84.1. Causes of Dialysis Underdelivery

Vascular access recirculation
Poorly calibrated or nonoccluding blood pumps
Low prepump pressure in the blood line
Shortened time on dialysis without compensating for disequilibrium
Dialyzer variance (e.g., bad lot of dialyzers)
Loss of surface area from reuse

MEASUREMENT OF KT/V

As noted previously, Kt/V is an integrated fractional clearance expressed per dialysis so that it can be used to compare dialysis treatments among patients of differing sizes. Its real value and its popularity as a measure of dialysis derive from its dependence on the fractional fall in urea concentration during dialysis. To illustrate this, consider a patient who behaves as a single pool, who dialyzes without any fluid removal, and who has negligible urea generation during the procedure. In such an uncomplicated dialysis, the end concentration of urea (C) can be expressed as an exponential function of the beginning concentration (C_0):

$$C = C_0 e^{-Kt/V} \qquad (7)$$

Equation 7 describes a simple, single exponential decline in urea concentration with time, analogous to pharmacokinetic models of drug metabolism and elimination. Log transformation of both sides of the equation yields the following:

$$Kt/V = \ln(C_0/C) \qquad (8)$$

Equation 8 shows that the desired yardstick for dialysis, Kt/V, can be calculated from the ratio of predialysis to postdialysis blood urea nitrogen (BUN) without knowledge of K, t, or V. The result is an effective delivered clearance, more useful to the clinician than the prescribed clearance obtained by combining the three elements K, t, and V. If the three elements are available, however, comparison of Kt/V obtained by the two different methods provides additional information that can be used for troubleshooting dialysis equipment and the patient's vascular access device. The discrepancy is almost always an under delivery of prescribed Kt/V, which can be caused by one or more of the problems listed in Table 84.1.

FORMAL UREA MODELING

In the example patient discussed previously, urea generation as well as the change in the patient's body fluid content during and between dialyses were ignored. If these variables are included in the model, the solution is more complex:

$$d(V \cdot C)/dt = G - (K_D + K_R)C \qquad (9)$$

K_D and K_R are the dialyzer and native kidney–urea clearances respectively. V is the patient's urea volume that is considered to be equivalent to total body water, and G is the urea generation rate that is presumed to be constant. Integration of equation 10 gives a better, although more complex, expression of urea concentration during and between dialyses:

$$C = C_0\left(\frac{V + Bt}{V}\right)^{-\left(\frac{K+B}{B}\right)} + \left(\frac{G}{K + B}\right)\left(1 - \left(\frac{V + Bt}{V}\right)^{-\left(\frac{K+B}{B}\right)}\right) \qquad (10)$$

V_0 is the volume of urea distribution predialysis, K during dialysis is the sum of $K_D + K_R$, K between dialyses is K_R, and B is the rate of fluid gain between or during dialyses (negative during dialysis). The single compartment, variable-volume model of urea kinetics uses equation 10 inversely to calculate V and G from C_0 and C.

Note that modeling urea concentrations using equation 10 as described previously is possible only for intermittent dialysis in which urea concentrations change significantly from the beginning to the end of the treatment. Thus intermittent treatment, although less efficient than continuous treatment (see the following), is easier to analyze because it requires only two blood samples to calculate V, G, Kt/V, and net protein catabolic rate (PCR) (see the following). To measure these parameters in patients treated continuously or in patients with native kidney function requires collection of dialysate or urine as well as blood.

PROTEIN CATABOLISM FROM UREA KINETICS

Modeling urea kinetics between dialyses provides a measure of the urea generation rate (G). Although G makes a minor but significant contribution to intradialysis urea kinetics, it is the major determinant of urea concentration between dialyses; thus applying the model to the intradialysis and the interdialysis intervals simultaneously allows more accurate calculations of V and G as well as Kt/V and PCR. Furthermore, by extrapolating the kinetics to an entire week, generating a profile of urea concentration as shown in Fig. 84.4, the requirement for drawing blood from the patient can be reduced to a single predialysis and a single postdialysis sample.

PATIENT KINETICS: RESISTANCE TO SOLUTE MOVEMENT WITHIN THE PATIENT

As blood with its lowered concentration of dialyzable solutes returns from the dialyzer to the patient, a concentration gradient forms within the patient that favors movement of these solutes from the patient's tissues into the blood. In this sense, the patient becomes another hemodialyzer with reversed movement of solutes into the blood (Fig. 84.5). This aspect of dialysis received limited attention until the application of high-efficiency dialyzers augmented and highlighted its effects (see following discussion of disequilibrium). Like the hemodialyzer, the patient dialyzer is also limited by both flow and cell membrane permeability (see following discussion of effects of blood flow and cardiopulmonary recirculation) but a significant concentration gradient within the patient forms only for those solutes that are removed by the dialyzer.

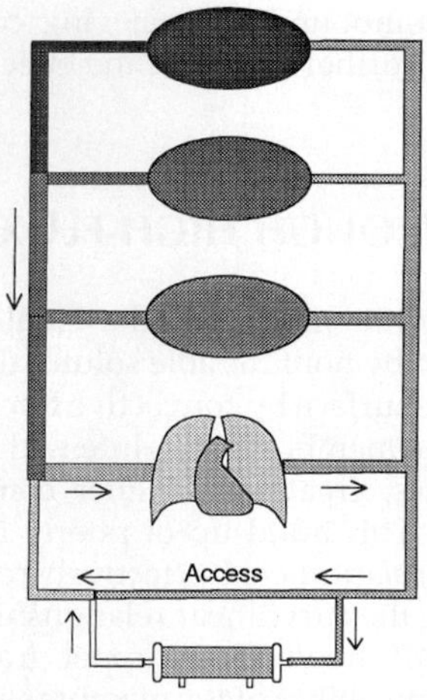

Figure 84.5. Flow-dependent disequilibrium. Regional differences in blood perfusion of organs and tissues causes solute concentrations in the blood entering the dialyzer to fall *(lighter shades)* below that predicted by the single-compartment model. Dialyzer clearance is not affected but solute removal falls and the overall efficiency of the dialysis is reduced.

Diffusion-Dependent Disequilibrium

The classic two-compartment model shown in Fig. 84.6 attributes solute disequilibrium to diffusive resistance between intracellular and extracellular body compartments. For some, especially larger or highly charged solutes, the cell membrane can be considered a uniform resistance to diffusion that fits this model.

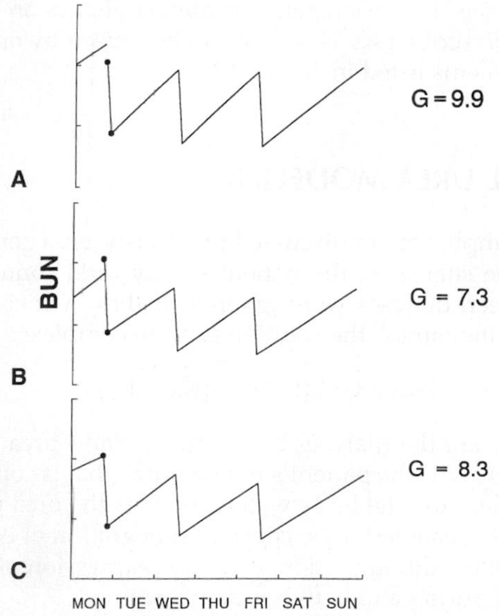

Figure 84.4. A 2-BUN computerized method for determining G. The computer searches (**A** and **B**) for a value of G that causes the calculated predialysis BUN at the end of the week to match the measured predialysis BUN **(C).** (Reproduced with permission from Depner TA, Cheer A. Modeling urea kinetics with two vs. three BUN measurements. A critical comparison. *ASAIO J* 1989;35:499–502.)

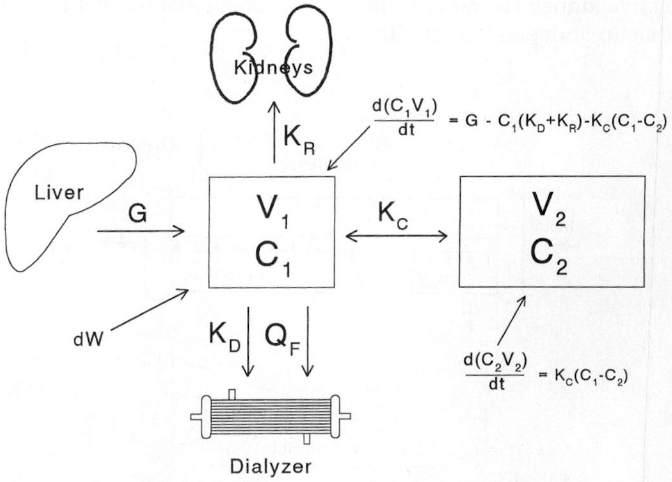

Figure 84.6. Two-compartment, variable-volume model of urea mass balance. V_1 and V_2 correspond to the extracellular and intracellular body water compartments respectively. K_C is the intercompartment mass transfer coefficient. See text for explanation of equation symbols. (Adapted with permission from Depner TA. *Prescribing hemodialysis: a guide to urea modeling.* Boston: Kluwer Academic Publishers, 1991.)

Application of the model assuming the usual 2:1 ratio for intracellular to extracellular volume usually predicts measured urea concentrations well, and at least one study of muscle biopsies obtained during dialysis found higher intracellular urea concentrations, supporting this model. However, the classic model cannot explain blood urea concentrations measured within the first 10 minutes after starting dialysis and differences in urea concentrations measured simultaneously within the blood compartment during dialysis.

Flow-Dependent Disequilibrium

The flow model of urea disequilibrium shown in Fig. 84.5 also accurately predicts urea concentrations during and immediately following dialysis but this model also fits the early concentrations and accounts for the simultaneous differences in blood compartment concentrations that the classic model fails to predict. Flow-dependent disequilibrium results from differences in regional perfusion of tissues. The model predicts that organs with relatively high blood flow, such as the liver and brain, will maintain lower solute concentrations during dialysis than organs such as the skin and muscle that are less well perfused at rest.

Because diffusion is not a part of flow-dependent disequilibrium, molecular size and charge have no influence. Large and small molecules exhibit the same magnitude of flow-dependent disequilibrium. However, because molecular size apparently does affect the magnitude of disequilibrium for many solutes, the actual solute gradients that have been observed during hemodialysis most likely result from a combination of these two mechanisms.

Regardless of the mechanism for disequilibrium and the postdialysis urea rebound, the equilibrated, postdialysis BUN provides a more realistic measure of Kt/V than the immediate postdialysis value. When the equilibrated value is used to calculate Kt/V using either formal modeling or one of the simplified formulas, the result is a measure of the patient clearance (see previous discussion), or eKt/V. Population studies have shown that eKt/V can be predicted from the treatment time:

$$\begin{aligned} \text{eKt/V} &= \text{spKt/V} - 0.6\text{K/V} + 0.03 \\ &= \text{spKt/V}(1 - 0.6/\text{t}) + 0.03 \end{aligned} \tag{11}$$

eKt/V is a virtual clearance for which no standards have been set, thus it is not widely used.

OTHER YARDSTICKS OF DIALYSIS

Some centers monitor the total volume of blood processed during dialysis as a measure of dialysis adequacy. This volume is easily measured with each dialysis, can be automated, and does not require expensive blood tests, computer software, or mathematic analysis. However, as a sole indicator of dialysis adequacy, the total volume of blood processed is highly prone to error because it cannot identify a failing dialyzer or access recirculation or blood pump errors that reduce the efficiency of dialysis. In addition, because the extraction ratio for urea and other easily dialyzed solutes is a function of blood flow, omitting consideration of flow adds an additional element of error. Calculating or modeling Kt/V from measured values of the predialysis and postdialysis BUN can eliminate all of these errors. However, after the prescription for achieving a satisfactory Kt/V has been established, automated monitoring of the processed blood volume during each treatment provides an extra insurance that the patient will not be dismissed early.

Similarly, after obtaining the predialysis (C1) and postdialysis (C2) BUN, some have attempted to avoid formal modeling and the more complicated equations by calculating the urea reduction ratio (URR):

$$\text{URR} = (\text{C1} - \text{C2})/\text{C1} \tag{12}$$

This parameter is a mathematic equivalent of Kt/V when no urea generation or volume changes occur during hemodialysis:

$$\text{URR} = 1 - e^{-\text{Kt/V}} \tag{13}$$

However, because fluid removal is necessary during most dialyses, URR can vary considerably for the same Kt/V and, in contrast to Kt/V, URR offers no specific recipe for correcting an inadequate prescription (e.g., by a quantitative increase in t or K). The most significant effort required for determining Kt/V is measuring the predialysis and postdialysis BUN. Once obtained, the additional effort to calculate Kt/V (instead of URR) using modern calculators and computers is trivial.

Because analysis of solute kinetics on the blood side is complex, as noted previously, and is an indirect measure of dialysis, analysis of the dialysate has been recommended as a more-direct measure. This approach eliminates concerns about disequilibrium and rebound because the postdialysis sampling is not required. Instead, dialysate solute removal must be assessed by collecting the total dialysate volume, by a stream-splitting technique, or by continuous analysis of the effluent dialysate stream. This approach requires an analyzer that can accurately measure low dialysate solute concentrations and usually requires an immediate analysis of the dialysate in the dialysis center, thus its use has been limited.

To enable large population studies and allow a more-direct calculation of Kt/V from the predialysis and postdialysis BUN, simplified formulas have been developed to approximate the results of formal urea modeling. The most widely used is the second-generation formula developed empirically by Daugirdas:

$$\frac{K \cdot t}{V} = -\ln(R - 0.008 \cdot t)4 - 3.5 \cdot R)\frac{\Delta \text{BW}}{\text{BW}} \tag{14}$$

DEPENDENCE OF DIALYSIS EFFICIENCY ON THE FREQUENCY OF TREATMENT

For continuous dialysis, the rate of removal correlates with the degree or completeness of removal. If the rate is increased the solute level will fall, and the level will rise if the rate is decreased. For intermittent dialysis, the treatment time and frequency of treatments are additional variables that modify the effectiveness of a removal rate. If the rate is increased and the treatment time is proportionally reduced, the removal is less complete. If the rate and time per week are kept constant but the frequency per week is increased, removal is increased and average solute levels fall. The efficiency of intermittent dialysis depends on its frequency because intermittent dialysis is intrinsically self-limiting. Two specific causes can be invoked. First, the mean solute concentration during a single intermittent treatment, even for a perfect solute that distributes in a single compartment, is lower than the true arithmetic mean and is closer to the logarithm mean. If the concentration were to fall linearly, then intermittent dialysis would be as efficient as continuous dialysis. Second, solute disequilibrium causes the concentration to fall even further during dialysis, increasing the difference between the arithmetic mean and the actual mean.

Efforts over the past 10 years to speed up the removal rate and to shorten dialysis time have reduced the cost and inconvenience of regular dialysis treatments but have generated a new set of complications that are just beginning to be appreciated. To achieve the same average solute levels, the weekly clearance must be higher for intermittent treatments and even higher for short intermittent treatments. This helps to explain the difference in weekly standards that have been empirically derived for continuous peritoneal dialysis versus hemodialysis (see the following section, Standards). In addition to solute disequilibrium, intermittent dialysis also contributes to fluctuations in fluid balance, which are better recognized as a complication. Oscillations in the patient's extracellular volume contribute to hypertension between dialyses and to hypotension during dialysis.

The effect of intermittence on clearance can be quantitated as the *continuous equivalent of intermittent clearance* (EKR). This measure of dialysis, which can be expressed as an unadjusted clearance (K) or as a normalized clearance (e.g., EKR·t/V) simply equates solute removal with solute generation assuming a weekly steady state of nitrogen balance:

$$EKR_{urea} = (\text{urea removal})/(\text{mean urea concentration}) \quad (15)$$
$$= G/TAC$$

Both G and time-averaged urea concentration (TAC) can be measured by applying formal urea modeling to a predialysis and a postdialysis BUN.

STANDARDS FOR HEMODIALYSIS ADEQUACY

For the most commonly prescribed frequency—three treatments per week—standards have been established based on results of the National Cooperative Dialysis Study (NCDS) extrapolated to modern dialysis methods. The extrapolation is not based on controlled data but is rather a consensus derived from observations by numerous investigators and the collective clinical experience. The minimum Kt/V for thrice weekly hemodialysis has been set at 1.2 per dialysis and the recommended target at 1.3 to 1.4 per dialysis to guarantee that the majority of patients will remain above the minimum. This approach is justified by results of cross-sectional studies showing a correlation between mortality and Kt/V that appears to reach a plateau at the 1.2 Kt/V level. An ongoing, randomized, interventional study, sponsored by the National Institutes of Health (NIH), is currently investigating the potential benefit of raising the dose further [the Hemodialysis (HEMO) Study].

SUMMARY

Models of solute kinetics have helped to explain the complexity of solute removal during dialysis and have given us insight into the generation and distribution of these solutes, but analysis of urea kinetics is no longer an isolated pursuit of dialysis investigators. Modeling is routinely used as a clinical tool in many dialysis centers to measure and prescribe hemodialysis. Kinetic analysis allows each prescription to be tailored to the individual patient's needs based on the patient's size and the available equipment. From analysis of urea kinetics, dialysis is prescribed as a clearance, independent of urea generation and of urea concentration in the body. This avoids the vicious cycle that can develop from reliance on the BUN as the sole indicator of dialysis need and is currently accepted as the best surrogate measurement of toxin levels in patients with end-stage renal disease.

Selected Readings

Borah MF, Schoenfeld PY, Gotch FA, et al. Nitrogen balance during intermittent dialysis therapy of uremia. *Kidney Int* 1978;14:491–500.
This paper describes the original metabolic balance study that established the relationship between urea generation and net protein catabolism in patients with end-stage renal disease. The findings of this exhaustive study have been used for the past 20 years to convert measured or modeled urea appearance to the equivalent of net protein catabolism.

Colton CK, Lowrie EG. Hemodialysis: physical principles and technical considerations. In: Brenner BM, Rector FC, Jr., eds. *The kidney*. Philadelphia: Saunders, 1981:2425–2489.
This textbook chapter describes many of the fundamental properties of diffusion and dialysis and their application to clinical dialysis.

Daugirdas JT. Second generation logarithmic estimates of single-pool variable volume Kt/V: an analysis of error. *J Am Soc Nephrol* 1993;4:1205–1213.
This paper describes an explicit equation for estimating Kt/V. The equation was derived empirically by measuring Kt/V using formal urea modeling in a large number of patients and then choosing the mathematic expression that fit the data best.

Depner TA. *Prescribing hemodialysis: a guide to urea modeling*. Boston: Kluwer Academic Publishers, 1991.
This textbook is devoted to urea kinetic modeling that describes its use as a tool for prescribing hemodialysis and assessing nutritional status in end-stage renal disease patients maintained with hemodialysis. It describes the many variables and pitfalls of urea modeling and includes details about single-pool and double-pool models.

Depner TA, Beck GJ, Daugirdas JT, et al. Lessons from the Hemodialysis (HEMO) Study: an improved measure of the actual hemodialysis dose. *Am J Kidney Dis* 1999;33:142–149.
This paper describes the methods used by investigators in the National Institutes of Health–sponsored HEMO Study to evaluate the effect of dialyzer Kt/V and membrane flux on patient outcome. It includes a definition and extensive comparison of eKtV with single-pool Kt/V.

Gotch FA. Kinetic modeling in hemodialysis. In: Nissenson AR, Fine RN, Gentile DE, eds. *Clinical dialysis*, 3rd ed. Norwalk, CT: Appleton and Lange, 1995:156–188.
This is a meticulous review of the various models used for urea kinetic modeling. It includes a critical evaluation of the techniques by which urea models have been clinically validated.

Gotch FA, Sargent JA. A mechanistic analysis of the National Cooperative Dialysis Study (NCDS). *Kidney Int* 1985;28:526–534.
This is the cornerstone paper describing the correlation of patient morbidity in the NCDS with Kt/V. It justified the use of Kt/V as a criterion for prescribing hemodialysis and demonstrated the error of using the blood urea nitrogen alone as the sole measure of patient outcome.

Lowrie EG, Laird NM, Parker TF, et al. Effect of the hemodialysis prescription on patient morbidity: report from the National Cooperative Dialysis Study. *N Engl J Med* 1981;305:1176–1181.
This is the original report from the NCDS announcing the primacy of controlling the patient's serum urea concentration as compared with controlling dialysis treatment time as the determinant of morbidity in patients dialyzed three times per week. The reader was also cautioned not to restrict dietary intake of protein and other nutrients.

Lowrie EG, Lew NL. Death risk in hemodialysis patients: the predictive value of commonly measured variables and an evaluation of death rate differences between facilities. *Am J Kidney Dis* 1990;15:458–482.
This is a descriptive report and analysis of mortality in more than 10,000 patients that included multiple clinical and laboratory parameters. Striking correlations with mortality were found for serum albumin, serum creatinine, and the dose of dialysis. Other parameters showed more complex relationships with mortality.

National Kidney Foundation–Dialysis Outcomes Quality Initiative. Clinical practice guidelines for hemodialysis adequacy. *Am J Kidney Dis* 1997;30:22–63.
This report lists an important set of clinical guidelines representing the work of several committees working with the National Kidney Foundation in the United States who surveyed the literature and polled clinicians to establish the best clinical practice methods. The guidelines are based on both evidence and opinion but are clearly labeled in each case.

Schneditz D, Kaufman AM, Polaschegg HD, et al. Cardiopulmonary recirculation during hemodialysis. *Kidney Int* 1992;42:1450–1456.
This report is one of the first descriptions of flow-dependent urea disequilibrium developing during hemodialysis. It helped to explain several kinetic phenomena that previously puzzled investigators who encountered errors when attempting to measure access recirculation and when attempting to predict urea concentrations both early in dialysis and early in the rebound phase postdialysis.

B: Vascular Access for Hemodialysis

Steve J. Schwab and David W. Butterly

Hemodialysis is a lifesaving procedure for patients with end-stage renal disease (ESRD), acute renal failure, and certain intoxications. Hemodialysis in any of these situations requires repeated reliable access to the central circulation capable of providing rapid extracorporeal blood flow. Ideal vascular access should be readily accessible, capable of providing rapid blood flow, and resistant to thrombosis and infection. Double-lumen vascular catheters serve this need well in the setting of acute renal failure and intoxications requiring dialysis. Unfortunately, in chronic maintenance hemodialysis this repeated reliable access to the circulation remains the weakest link in the provision of adequate dialysis to our patients.

In humans, access-related problems account for a large number of hospital days, frequent procedures, and significant morbidity and mortality in the ESRD population. Frequent thrombosis and infections lead to a large percentage of the hospitalizations in patients on maintenance hemodialysis. Additionally, it is well established that inadequacies in the delivery of dialysis may contribute to long-term poor outcome in the ESRD population. This failure to deliver adequate treatment is most often due to access malfunction, consequently increasing the long-term morbidity by decreasing the delivered dose of dialysis. In addition, infections of hemodialysis access not only lead to loss of vascular access, but may even constitute a life-threatening clinical problem.

In economic terms, maintenance of access is extraordinarily expensive, conservatively accounting for nearly $1 billion in expenditures annually. Managed care organizations planning for possible capitation estimate the maintenance of vascular access accounts for 25% to 33% of the total ESRD cost. In the latest report of the United States Renal Data System (USRDS), it was estimated that care of vascular access approaches $8,000 per patient year and placement and maintenance of vascular access represents an estimated 17% to 25% of hospital stays. Accordingly, the effective management of vascular access has emerged as not only an important issue in the morbidity and mortality of the patient with ESRD, but also one with tremendous economic implications.

This chapter reviews the types of vascular access available to the clinician for both acute and chronic hemodialysis. The problems associated with placement of vascular access and strategies to maintain long-term access patency are reviewed in detail.

VASCULAR ACCESS FOR ACUTE HEMODIALYSIS

Temporary angioaccess is frequently required in the setting of acute renal failure, acute intoxications, and in the ESRD patient who may lose their chronic dialysis access to thrombosis or infection. This access to the circulation is most often furnished by coaxial dual-lumen vascular catheters (Fig. 84.7A). These catheters are generally made of polymers such as polyurethane, polyethylene, or polyfluoroethylene. All of these polymers are relatively rigid at room temperature to allow easy insertion but soften at body temperature to minimize the risk of vessel trauma or laceration. Of the available polymers, polyurethane is reported to be the most flexible and least thrombogenic. These catheters all have dual lumens arranged coaxially or side by side as shown in Fig. 84.7. To minimize recirculation, the venous and arterial ports are spaced 2 to 3 cm apart (Fig. 84.7B).

These catheters are usually inserted at the bedside over a guidewire using a modified Seldinger technique. In most instances the availability of portable ultrasound devices to aid cannulation of central veins have dramatically decreased insertion complications (Fig. 84.8). For relatively short-term treatments or in patients with significant pulmonary pathology, in whom pneumothorax may be catastrophic, the femoral vein is the site of choice. The femoral vein is cannulated immediately below the inguinal ligament. Inadvertent femoral artery puncture occurs frequently, but with manual compression this is rarely problematic. Other complications of femoral vein cannulation include femoral vein thrombosis, retroperitoneal hemorrhage, and arteriovenous fistula formation. Patients with femoral vein catheters must remain on bedrest for the duration of catheter use. It has been recommended that femoral catheters be at least 19 cm long so that the catheter will rest in the inferior vena cava and minimize recirculation. Catheters in the femoral vein are the most prone to infection, therefore sites should be rotated every 3 to 5 days.

Insertion of a catheter in the internal jugular position lessens the risk of infection and can be used for 2 to 3 weeks before site rotation, making this a good option for the patient who may need access of an intermediate duration. The right internal jugular vein provides the straightest path to the atrium and is the neck site of choice. Either the anterior approach between the heads of the sternocleidomastoid or the posterior approach is acceptable. The risk of both carotid cannulation and pneumothorax is somewhat lower with the posterior approach. There is a higher risk of insertion complications than with femoral site use, but the overall complication rate is lower than with subclavian insertion, and in experienced hands the risk of pneumothorax is still less than 1%.

Insertion at the subclavian carries the highest insertion risk. Laceration of the subclavian artery cannot easily be compressed manually and can lead to hemothorax or other serious bleeding complication. The subclavian vein also carries the highest risk for pneumothorax, averaging 1% to 5%. Finally, prior subclavian vein cannulation has been strongly associated with subclavian

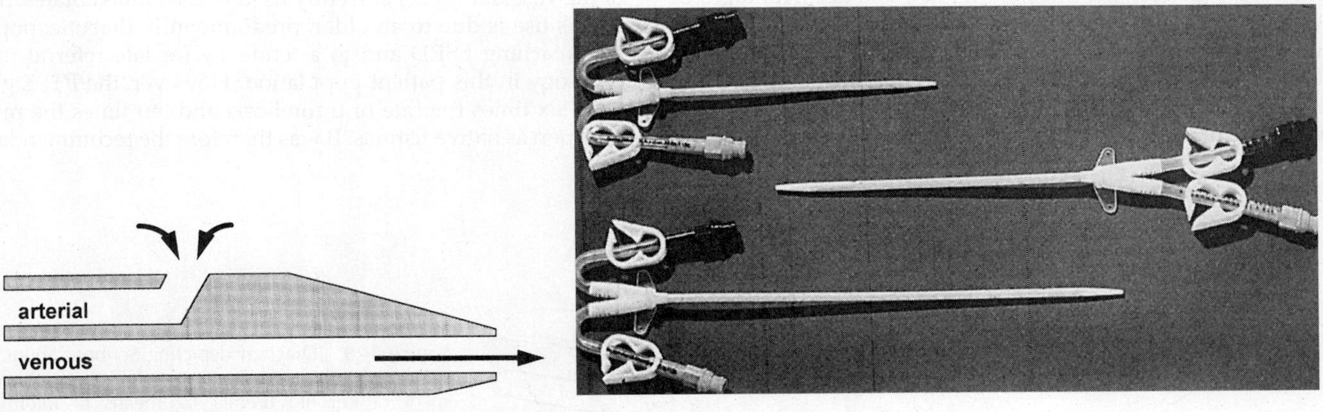

Figure 84.7. **A:** Typical hemodialysis catheter tip with separation of arterial and venous ports. **B:** An array of available hemodialysis catheters. (Reprinted with permission Fan PY. Acute vascular access: new advances. *Adv Renal Repl Ther* 1994;I:2, 90–98.)

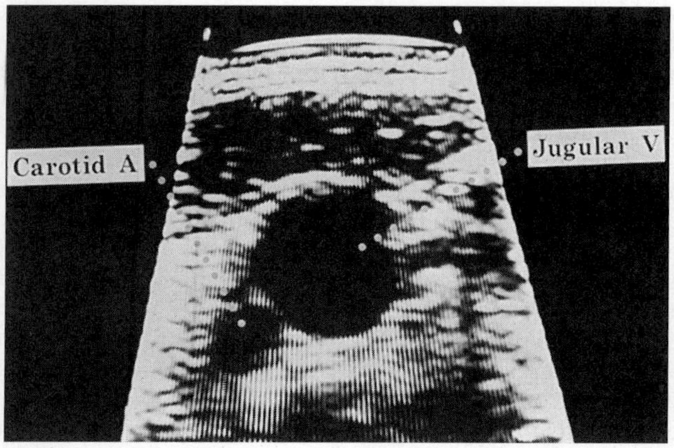

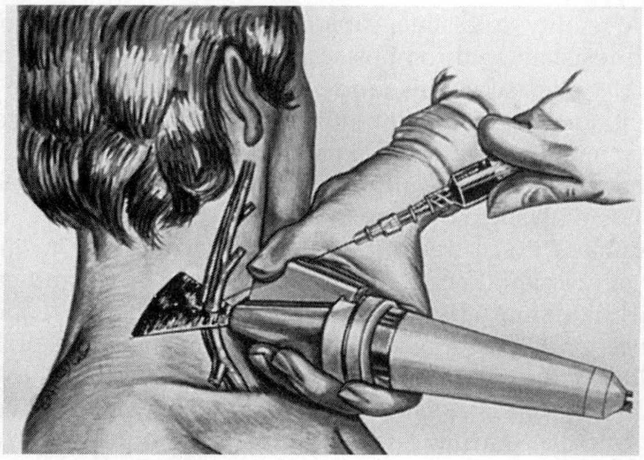

Figure 84.8. Ultrasound image (**A**) and guided cannulation (**B**) of internal jugular vein. (Reproduced with permission from Dymax Corporation, 271 Kappa Drive, Pittsburgh, PA 15238.)

vein stenosis, which can potentially eliminate the possibility of further access in the ipsilateral arm. This approach should therefore be avoided in any patient with coagulopathy, in patients with serious pulmonary pathology, and in any patients in whom future long-term dialysis is a possibility. In these situations other sites should be chosen preferentially and subclavian catheter use should be minimized.

VASCULAR ACCESS FOR CHRONIC HEMODIALYSIS

Scribner Shunts

Hemodialysis at its inception required venous and arterial cut downs for each individual treatment, which quickly depleted the patient of any viable access sites. Therefore dialysis was only a reasonable alternative for the treatment of patients with a short episode of acute renal failure. It was not until 1960, when Belding Scribner described the more durable external "Scribner" shunt, that dialysis for those with chronic failure became a reality. The Scribner Shunt is an externalized silastic shunt connected by a short Teflon cannula that was immediately usable after placement. It was typically placed in the radial artery with return through the cephalic vein (Fig. 84.9). For dialysis, the extracorporeal circuit was hooked directly to the arterial line with return via the forearm vein line. When not in use, the lines were reconnected with a short Teflon bridge. For patients with no upper extremity access, the shunt could be alternatively placed in the lower extremity. The disadvantages of these devices was that they thrombosed regularly, requiring frequent embolectomy and were prone to infection. The lifespan of the Scribner Shunt was only about 6 months due to intimal hyperplasia. Placement also frequently rendered the vessel unusable for future vascular access. Consequently, Scribner Shunts have been supplanted by other modalities and are largely of historic interest. The early 1990s saw a rebirth in the use of these devices for CAVH in the intensive care unit (ICU) patient with acute renal failure, however with greater CVVH-D use, Scribner Shunts are again used only rarely.

Primary Arteriovenous Fistulas

The first described and still the access of choice is the autologous radio cephalic fistula described by Brescia and Cimino in 1966. This is created with either a side-to-side or end-to-side anastomosis of the radial artery to the cephalic vein in the distal forearm as shown in Fig. 84.10. The major disadvantage of these accesses is that they typically take a minimum of 2 months to mature and have a high rate of early failure. An early failure rate of approximately 25% should be anticipated. Once mature, however, these have the highest rate of trouble-free service. Because they are created without synthetic material, they are resistant to both infection and thrombosis. For patients without suitable forearm sites, primary fistulas can be created in the upper arm by anastomosis of the brachial artery to either the cephalic or the basilic vein. The National Kidney Foundation Dialysis Outcome Quality Initiative on Hemodialysis Vascular Access (NKF-DOQI) considered primary arteriovenous fistulas (AVFs) to be superior to all other modes of vascular access. They defined the radio-cephalic AVF as the access of first choice followed by brachial-cephalic AVFs.

Despite the many advantages of primary AVFs, synthetic polytetrafluoroethylene (PTFE) grafts make up more than 80% of the vascular access currently used in the United States. Some of this use is due to an older, predominantly diabetic, population reaching ESRD and to a tendency for late referral to nephrology in this patient population. However, the PTFE grafts have six times the rate of thrombosis and ten times the rate of infection as native fistulas. It was therefore the recommendation

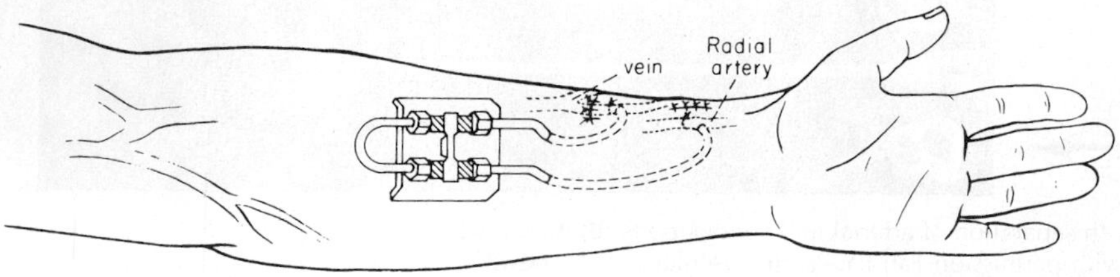

Figure 84.9. Diagram depicting Scribner Shunt. (Reproduced with permission from Schreiner GE. The treatment of chronic uremia by means of intermittent hemodialysis: a preliminary report. *Trans Am Soc Artif Int Org* 1960;VI:113.)

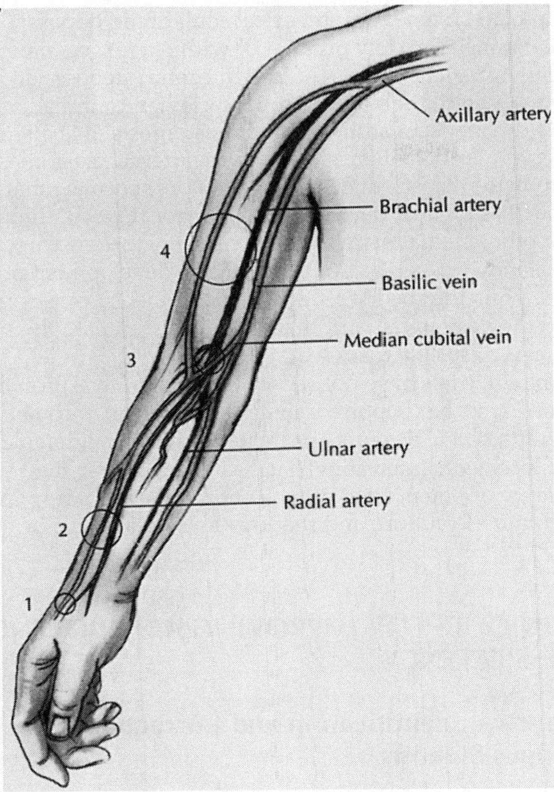

Figure 84.10. Four possible anastomotic sites for creation of arteriovenous fistulas in the upper extremity. (Reproduced with permission from Haisch CE, Cerilli J. Vascular access procedures for renal dialysis. In: Sabiston DC, ed. *Textbook of surgery*. Philadelphia: WB Saunders, 1997:431.)

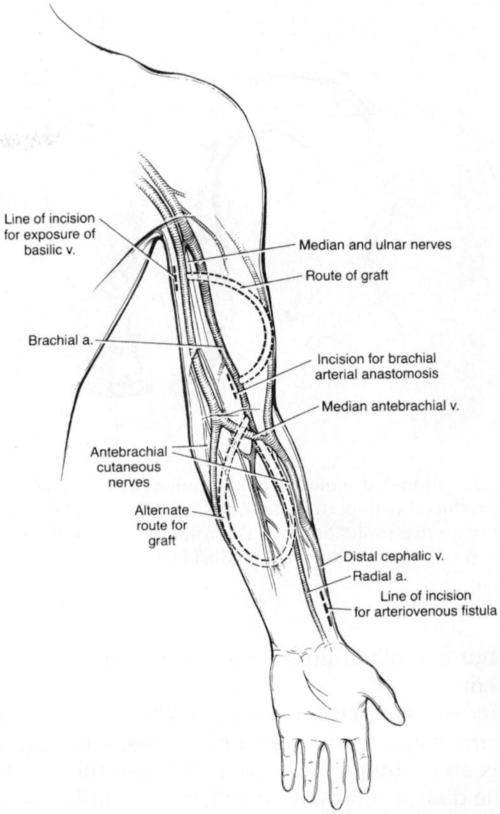

Figure 84.11. Possible sites for PTFE interposition grafts in the upper extremity. (Reproduced with permission from Stickel D. Renal dialysis procedures. In: Sabiston DC, ed. *Atlas of general surgery*. Philadelphia: WB Saunders, 1994:94.)

of the NKF-DOQI guidelines that we should increase the overall use of primary fistula with the goal that half of all new dialysis patients will have attempts at primary fistula placement, with 40% of prevalent patients maintained on dialysis via a primary fistula. Early referral, avoidance of venous cannulation in the nondominant arm, patient education, and placement of primary fistula in patients well before the anticipated initiation of dialysis will do much to improve the percentage of patients with primary AVF.

Synthetic Arteriovenous (AV) Graft

Synthetic internal fistulas, generally referred to as *arteriovenous (AV) grafts* can be placed in many sites in the upper or lower extremities in most patients, even in those with less than ideal arterial and venous anatomy. This ease of use and multiple possible insertion sites and relatively short maturation time have made these grafts the most used form of chronic vascular access in use in the United States, despite a lower patency rate than native AVFs.

Autogenous saphenous vein grafts and bovine heterografts were used briefly but were less durable than synthetic PTFE grafts, and have consequently fallen into disuse. PTFE grafts are usually placed in the forearm in a loop or straight configuration (brachial or radial artery to antecubital vein) or in the upper arm (brachial artery to basilic vein) as shown in Fig. 84.11. For patients with limited vascular access these can be placed in the chest (axillary artery to jugular or axillary vein) and in the leg (femoral artery to vein). The advantage of these grafts is the short maturation time and the multiple potential access sites for needle placement. Although 3 to 4 weeks maturation is ideal, they often can be used in as little as 2 weeks. The overwhelming disadvantage is the propensity for venous outflow stenosis and subsequent thrombosis. Unassisted patency rates of 30% to 70% at 1 year are the rule. Cumulative patency rates of 50% at 3 years are seen at most centers. Techniques for improving access patency are discussed subsequently.

Cuffed Tunneled Catheters

Although initially intended as temporary access, soft, cuffed tunneled catheters have come into long-term use for patients without viable peripheral vascular access (Fig. 84.12). The design of these devices has increased their use beyond that of acute access catheters. Improved survival on hemodialysis has increased the number of patients without peripheral access and thus has increased the use of these catheters. In addition, initiation of dialysis in an older, diabetic population prone to peripheral vascular disease has likewise increased our reliance on cuffed catheters. These catheters are typically placed with ultrasound guidance to aid insertion, using fluoroscopy to ensure appropriate catheter tip placement. Failure to place the tip of theses soft catheters at the atrial caval junction or just inside the atrium will compromise their blood-flow capability. Unlike acute catheters, the soft material and larger lumens of these catheters allow more central placement while reducing thrombosis and vessel-puncture risk. There is typically a long tunnel, along with a felt or other cuff to minimize migration of bacteria down the outer surface of the catheter. These catheters are usually placed in the internal jugular position, but alternatively can be placed in the subclavian, the femoral, and even in the inferior vena cava in patients with no alternative access. Blood-flow rates of 400 to 500 ml/min are achievable with some catheter

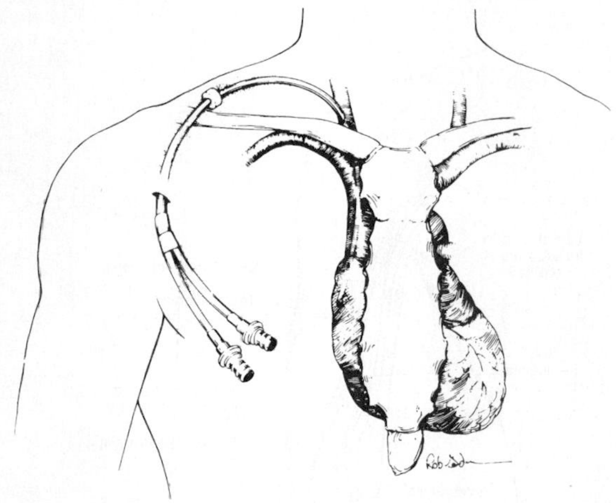

Figure 84.12. Tunneled, cuffed double-lumen sialistic catheter ("Perm-Cath") (Reproduced with permission from Schwab SJ, Buller GL, McCann RL, et al. Prospective evaluation of a Dacron cuffed hemodialysis catheter for prolonged use. *Am J Kidney Dis* 1988;11:166–169.)

designs, but low blood-flow rates due to catheter malfunction are frequent.

Catheter survival has ranged from 30% to 65% at 1 year. Infection is the major reason for catheter loss. Thrombosis of the catheter is also a frequent occurrence. Often this can be remedied in the dialysis unit with instillation of urokinase at a volume calculated to fill the lumen of the catheter. Patients not responsive to this maneuver may have a surrounding fibrin sheath that can be removed with a goose-neck snare by vascular radiology or with a more prolonged infusion of urokinase. The NKF-DOQI has specific recommendations. The rate of bacteremia and resultant complications due to these catheters, along with the frequent low dialysis–blood flow and resultant complications under dialysis are such that the long-term use of these catheters should be discouraged. The best use of these catheters is as a bridge to the development of more suitable long-term access with either a fistula or graft. They do, however, serve a role in the patient with steal syndrome or severe cardiomyopathy and congestive heart failure in whom peripheral vascular access may not be attainable. Management of bacteremia in cuffed tunneled catheters will be discussed in the following section.

BIOLOGY OF ARTERIOVENOUS ACESS FAILURE

The leading cause of AV access failure is failure to correct a thrombotic event. These thrombotic events are mediated in more than 85% of instances by a venous outflow stenosis. These outflow stenoses ultimately impede access flow until thrombosis occurs. In AV grafts, access flows of less than 600 ml/min are associated with access thrombosis. More than 60% of the stenoses in AV grafts occur within 4 cm of the vein graft anastomoses, with the remainder occurring at areas of vein bifurcation, at venous valves, and at areas of vessel trauma such as central vein cannulation sites. The consensus is that venous stenosis is caused by endothelial injury and subsequent smooth muscle fibrosis and hyperplasia in areas of flow turbulence (response to injury hypothesis).

The pathology of these lesions is remarkably uniform. The lesions typically demonstrate intimal hyperplasia with proliferation of vascular smooth muscle and extracellular matrix deposition. Unlike typical atherosclerotic lesions, there is absence of macrophages, foam cells, and extracellular lipid deposits. These lesions characteristically occur at or within a few centimeters of the vein graft anastomosis. Although central stenoses do occur, particularly in the setting of prior subclavian cannulation, they usually do not occur at the arterial anastomosis. It is interesting that equally turbulent areas such as the arterial anastomosis are not prone to stenosis, making investigators speculate that mitogens such as platelet-derived growth factor (PDGF), thromboxane, or other mediators released at venipuncture sites upstream of the stenosis may play some role in the development of these lesions. Thus the theory reflects that turbulence causes the injury to the vessel wall and that mitogens stimulate the hyperplasia and dysplasia cascade.

Although trials have not shown any benefit to aspirin use, at least one trial has reported some reduction in thrombosis in new grafts when patients are treated with dipyridamole after graft placement. Interestingly it has been shown that dipyridamole is a potent inhibitor of fibromuscular dysplasia in smooth muscle culture and that this hyperplasia can be stimulated by PDGF.

TECHNIQUES FOR IMPROVING ARTERIOVENOUS ACCESS PATENCY

Prospective Identification and Correction of Venous Stenosis

Venous stenoses repaired before a thrombosis occurs provide a much better cumulative AV access patency than access stenoses repaired once thrombosis has occurred. Not only should prospective identification and stenosis treatment lead to increased longevity of the access but should also lead to fewer missed treatments due to access thrombosis and decreased use of emergency rooms and other expensive inpatient services due to loss of viable access. The authors therefore believe such an approach will not only prove best for patient care but also most cost effective. Multiple prospective and retrospective American and European trials have confirmed these hypotheses. The vascular access NKF-DOQI considered prospective detection and correction of hemodynamically significant access stenoses to be one of the key areas for improving access patency. Table 84.2 shows prospective indicators for detection of venous stenoses that have been validated.

Physical Examination

Careful examination of the fistula is an inexpensive, underused tool to identify the patient with graft problems. Simple inspec-

TABLE 84.2. Methods for Prospective Identification of Vascular Access Stenoses

Physical examination
Arm edema
Absence of thrill or change in quality of bruit over graft
Prolonged bleeding after dialysis
Venous dialysis pressures
Dynamic venous pressure
Static venous pressure
Access recirculation
Urea recirculation
Non–urea-based methods of recirculation
Access blood flow
Ultrasound dilution
Doppler ultrasonography

tion of the graft and physical examination is helpful in identifying patients with access stenosis. The presence of edema in the arm after graft placement is common. However, when edema fails to resolve or appears *de novo,* this may be an indicator of central venous stenosis. It has also been demonstrated that the presence of a thrill at the arterial, mid, and venous segments of the graft is associated with fistula flows of more than 450 ml/min. A pulse without thrill suggests lower flows and should prompt further evaluation. Auscultation of the graft is also clinically useful. Generally, the pitch of the bruit should diminish as one moves further from the arterial anastomosis. Because a stenosis will result in increased velocity of blood through the area of the stenosis, this will result in an increase in the intensity of the bruit over this area. Digital compression of the graft between the arterial and venous needles during dialysis will effectively short circuit the recirculation pathway. Thus in AV grafts with high recirculation, compression will lead to an increase in venous pressure and a fall in arterial pressure. In addition, episodes of prolonged bleeding after dialysis can be indicative of venous outflow stenosis. Therefore in patients in whom prolonged bleeding cannot be explained by excessive anticoagulation, fistulogram to rule out venous stenosis should be obtained.

Venous Dialysis Pressures

Venous dialysis pressures are readily available to the rounding physician, are inexpensive, and were the first screening tool rigorously studied as a means of screening for venous outflow stenoses. Venous dialysis pressures must be checked in a uniform manner to be predictable and are an indirect measure of access flow. The venous dialysis pressure is affected by needle size, needle position, dialysis machine, dialysis tubing, and blood flow. Although venous dialysis pressures have been demonstrated to be predictive of stenosis at low blood-flow rates of 200 ml/min, the positive predictive value is lost at higher blood flows. Thus dynamic venous pressures need to be measured during the first few minutes of each treatment before increasing to peak blood flow (QB). Static venous pressure using the technique developed by Besarab (dialysis pressure measured at extracorporeal QB 0 ml/min) is more predictive than dynamic venous pressure because it eliminates many of the variables associated with dynamic pressure false positives. Venous pressure measurements are most predictive for outflow stenoses close to the vein graft anastomoses and are less reliable for stenoses further upstream where collateral circulation may allow decompression of the pressure. Despite these limitations venous dialysis pressure, when followed carefully and combined with access correction either with angioplasty or surgical revision, has been found to significantly increase cumulative AV access patency. However, pressure is a relatively late predictor of impending thrombosis and corrective measures must be rapidly used (less than 10 days) to prevent thrombosis. Direct measures of access flow have become practical and are more precise and predictive than access pressures.

Recirculation

Recirculation is defined as the volume of blood that has crossed the dialyzer and is recirculated directly through the extracorporeal circuit again rather than returning to the systemic circulation. Urea recirculation is defined by the following formula:

$$\%\ \text{Recirculation} = (\text{Peripheral} - \text{Arterial})\ \text{BUN}/(\text{Peripheral} - \text{Venous})\ \text{BUN} \times 100$$

Recirculation of blood during the dialysis procedure occurs when the blood-pump speed exceeds the fistula blood flow, when the needles are reversed, or when dialysis needles are too close together. To minimize this, it is recommended that needles be placed no closer together than 4 cm when possible. Direct recirculation of dialyzed blood through the extracorporeal circuit cuts down on the efficiency of the dialysis treatment. The first indication of this phenomenon may be a decrease in the delivered dose of dialysis or Kt/V. Recirculation is generally a very late indicator of venous stenosis, because of the degree of stenosis required to allow recirculation to occur.

The three-needle, peripheral-vein method of determining recirculation, previously considered the gold standard, is calculated from blood taken simultaneously from the arterial and venous ports of the dialyzer along with a peripheral specimen drawn from the contralateral extremity. During dialysis, disequilibrium can occur such that the arterial inflow blood urea nitrogen (BUN) is not equal to the peripheral venous specimen, which leads to overestimation of the recirculation. This method tends to overestimate access recirculation in an unpredictable manner and requires unnecessary venipuncture. The three-needle method of determining recirculation consequently should no longer be used.

The stop-flow or slow-flow method of determining the peripheral BUN was thus devised to decrease the problem with arteriovenous disequilibrium. In this method, QB is slowed to 50 ml/min for 20 to 30 seconds. The "peripheral" BUN is then drawn from the arterial circuit. Arterial and venous samples are collected as before. Under these conditions the peripheral BUN should more accurately reflect inflow BUN. Despite this, recirculation rates will average from 5% to 10% even in the absence of recirculation.

New non–urea-based methods for determining access recirculation have been developed. These techniques involve indicator dilution or conductivity tracer methods. The results of these studies has demonstrated that recirculation is the exception rather than the rule with the true incidence of recirculation much lower than previously suspected. As one would predict, recirculation should not occur unless access flow is less than dialysis circuit flow or QB. Because blood flows of this magnitude are not currently used in clinical practice, true recirculation is not seen until access dysfunction is quite advanced, with flows less than 500 ml/min. The average recirculation by these methods in well-functioning grafts was zero and values greater than this were seen with reversal of needles or low-access blood flow.

There is some debate in the literature regarding the exact level of urea recirculation that should prompt further investigation for stenosis, but the current NFK-DOQI guidelines recommend that any value more than 10% should lead to further investigation. The amount of recirculation when the needles are reversed is substantial, usually more than 20%. Reversal of needles is particularly common with new grafts. Thus recirculation rates in this range should prompt investigation into this. When using one of the non–urea-based methods, any recirculation at all should prompt further investigation.

Measurement of Access Flow

Venous dialysis pressure and recirculation are both indirect indicators of access flow. Direct determinations of access flow are now emerging as the most accurate method for detecting stenosis. This has been most carefully validated by measuring access flow with the use of ultrasound dilution. Devices for measuring access flow and recirculation by the use of ultrasound dilution of a saline bolus are readily available and relatively inexpensive if one considers that only one machine per hemodialysis unit is required (Fig. 84.13). It is clear that access flow of less than 600 ml/min in PTFE grafts rapidly leads to access thrombosis. In addition, decrements of more than 15% when flow is

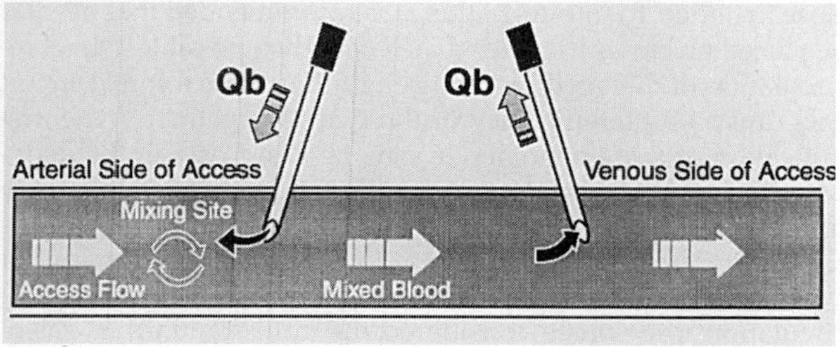

Figure 84.13. Diagram of ultrasound dilution technique used for determining access flow with reversal of arterial and venous needles. (Reproduced with permission from Transonic System Inc., Ithaca, NY 14850.)

less than 1,000 ml/min are equally predictive of access failure. The use of monthly flow measurements appears adequate for predictive purposes. It is the authors' belief that direct measurement of access flow will make all non–flow-measurement, access-screening indicators obsolete.

The use of Doppler to measure access flow and to determine the site of stenoses is attractive. However, prospective studies have shown Doppler flow measurements to be very observer and machine dependent. The NKF-DOQI panel was unable to endorse the technique until validating studies are performed.

TREATMENT OF VENOUS STENOSIS AND ACCESS THROMBOSIS

Hemodynamically significant stenosis, once detected, must be treated to avoid thrombosis and graft loss. No firm data indicate that correcting a venous stenosis not associated with a hemodynamic correlate is of any clinical benefit. If hemodynamic parameters (access flow, venous dialysis pressure) do not return to normal after angioplasty, the patient should be referred for surgical revision.

Angioplasty has become the procedure of choice for anatomically suitable venous stenosis as shown in Fig. 84.14. Mean primary patency of angioplasty treatment of a hemodynamically significant venous outflow stenoses not associated with a thrombotic event is approximately 6 months. This patency rate following angioplasty of outflow stenoses falls to less than 40% at 3 months if associated with an access thrombosis. This highlights the need for prospective treatment of outflow stenoses if angioplasty is to be used as a primary treatment modality. The reason for these significant differences in patency after treatment probably relates to the degree stenosis. There is emerging evidence that access thromboses are associated with near total lumen stenosis, whereas lesions detected earlier are typically 50% to 70% of the lumen. The less favorable results with angioplasty in these instances is expected. In contrast, surgical revision of outflow stenoses seems to be equally effective independent of the degree of stenosis. Mean primary patency at our institution is approximately 6 months. The use of endovascular stents in most studies has not been shown to be of any additional benefit to angioplasty alone except in the case of central vein stenosis in which surgical salvage is often not possible.

Once thrombosis has occurred, surgical thrombectomy, pharmicomechanical thrombolysis, or mechanical thrombolysis may be used. The latter two procedures have the advantage that a fistulogram is performed after flow is restored and venous stenosis can be corrected immediately with angioplasty. In pharmicomechanical thrombolysis, two hook-shaped catheters are introduced into the graft in a crossed fashion as shown in

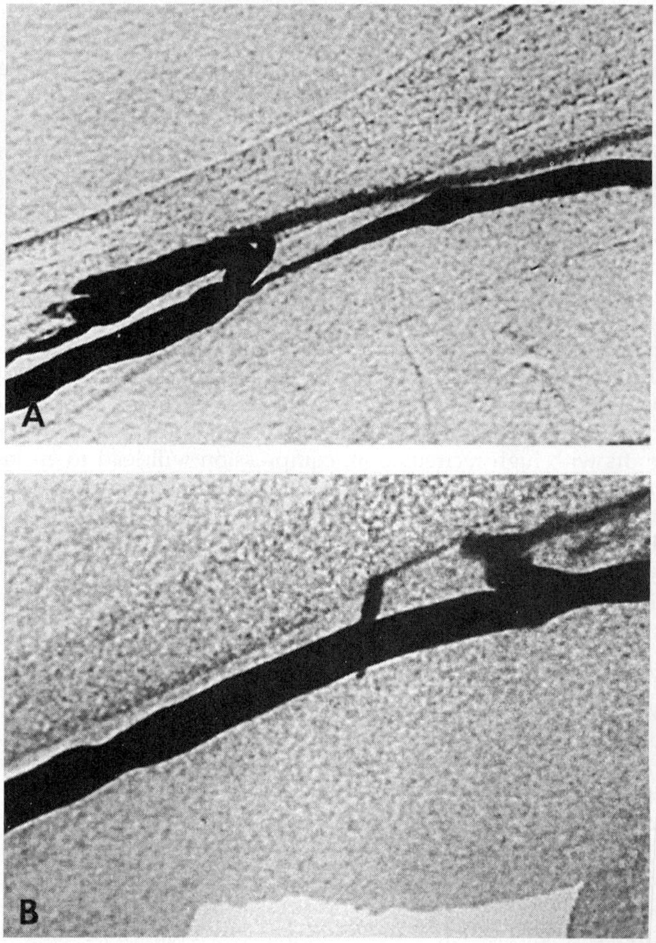

Figure 84.14. Stenosis of outflow vein before **(A)** and after **(B)** angioplasty. (Reproduced with permission from Beathard GA. The treatment of vascular access graft dysfunction. *Adv Renal Repl Ther* 1994;I:2, 131–147.)

Fig. 84.15. Urokinase is sprayed into the clot under high pressure and the clot is lysed by both mechanical and pharmacologic means. After flow is restored, venous stenosis can be approached by angioplasty. This usually can be done in 1 to 2 hours, is performed as an outpatient procedure, and the graft is immediately usable for hemodialysis. Retrospective trials have shown thrombolysis to be of equal efficacy to surgical embolectomy. Mechanical thrombolysis is a newer technique using either special clot-macerating devices or high-pressure saline and appears to yield equivalent results. Complications have included bleeding and ischemia of the ipsilateral limb due to distal embolization. With thrombolysis, small clots are undoubtedly being relapsed into the circulation traveling to the lungs. There have been case reports of septic emboli, but clinically apparent pulmonary emboli are rare.

Surgical treatment of a thrombosed AV graft is accomplished with the use of a balloon embolectomy catheter after a small incision is made in the access. It is essential to perform imaging immediately after thrombectomy to identify outflow stenoses. If necessary, a short jump graft or a patch graft can be performed to bypass venous outflow obstruction (Fig. 84.16). This allows continued use of the access and obviates the need for temporary access. Surgical revision has the longest primary patency rate but has the disadvantage of requiring hospitalization and often extends the access up the arm, taking away future access options. When treatment of access thrombosis does not ad-

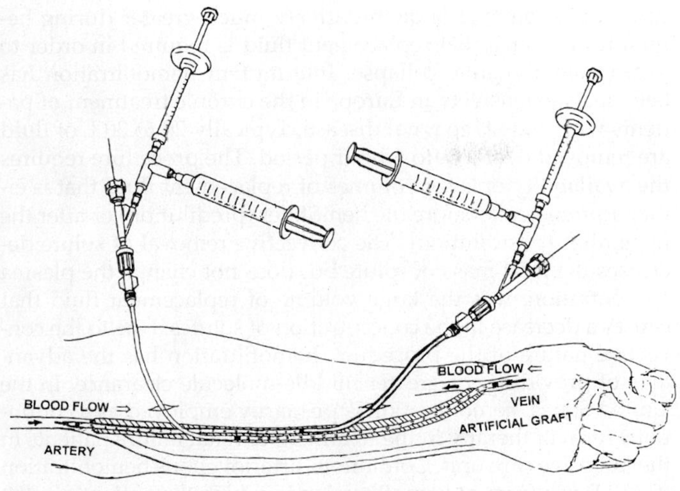

Figure 84.15. Technique for pulsed-spray thrombolysis. (Reproduced with permission from AngioDynamics Incorporated, Queensbury, NY 12804.)

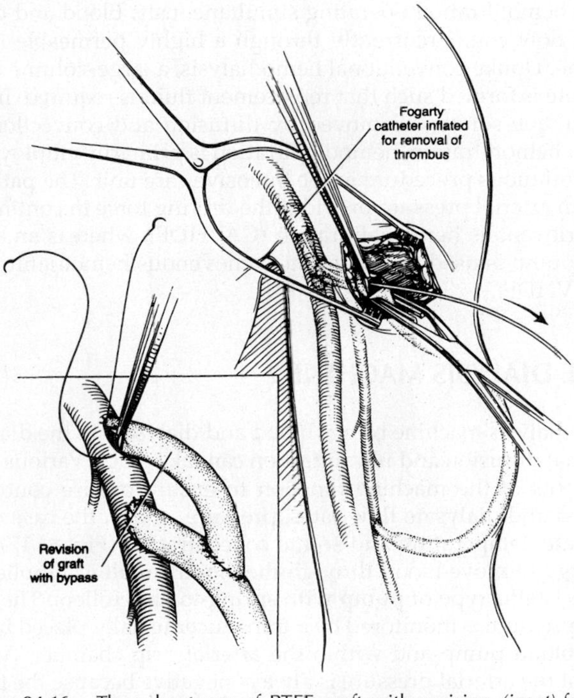

Figure 84.16. Thrombectomy of PTFE graft with revision *(inset)* for venous stenosis. (Reproduced with permission from Stickel D. Renal dialysis procedures. In: Sabiston DC, ed. *Atlas of general surgery* 1994.)

dress the presence of an underlying stenosis, there is a greater than 90% chance that rapid rethrombosis will occur. Therefore surgical embolectomy should be followed by fistulogram to assess for stenoses. Detection and revision of stenoses before thromboses is correlated with better outcomes than waiting for thrombosis to occur.

Access Infections

Infections are the primary cause of cuffed catheter loss and the second-leading cause of graft loss after thrombosis, accounting for 15% to 20% of graft failure. The majority of infections are due to Gram-positive organisms, generally *Staphylococcus aureus* or *S. epidermidis.* The recent prospective study by Marr and coworkers showed that in cuffed catheters, the rate of infection is 1 per 250 patient catheter days. Twenty two percent developed serious complications including endocarditis, osteomyelitis, and death. Attempts to salvage the catheter with intravenous antibiotics alone was successful in only a small minority. In contrast, intravenous antibiotic therapy combined with guidewire exchange has had a much higher (80%) success rate if the catheter tunnel track is uninvolved.

Infection involving a PTFE graft usually requires removal of all or part of the graft in addition to antibiotic therapy to achieve a cure. Primary AV fistulas are only rarely infected and can generally be managed with antibiotics alone.

Pseudoaneurysm

Pseudoaneurysms of PTFE grafts develop as progressive damage of the graft material leads to the inability to seal puncture sites. Therefore these occur at the site of repeated needle puncture in grafts. Dialysis staff should be educated to routinely rotate the venipuncture sites to minimize this complication. Once these complications occur, needle insertion at the site of the aneurysm should be avoided. Thrombosis or bleeding from skin erosion may result. Surgical repair of the aneurysms should be undertaken when they expand rapidly, compromise the overlying skin, become infected, or exceed twice the diameter of the remainder of the graft.

Distal Ischemia

Distal ischemia or steal is a relatively uncommon complication and occurs more often with PTFE grafts than with primary AVF due to the higher initial blood flow in the former. This occurs in the setting of severe peripheral vascular disease due to shunting of blood through the access and away from the dependent extremity. This results in diminished or absent pulses, extremity coolness, and paraesthesia. Sometimes, these symptoms may occur only with dialysis. Ischemic symptoms may improve with time as distal collaterals develop. However, PTFE banding or access ligation performed emergently is necessary in severe cases.

Cardiovascular Complications

Vascular access–related cardiac decompensation is a relatively rare event, particularly given the frequency of cardiomyopathy in the ESRD population. These patients are reported to be at particularly high risk for decompensation if fistula flow exceeds 20% of cardiac output. This generally occurs in primary AVFs rather than PTFE grafts. In such cases, banding the access to reduce flow may result in improved cardiac function but frequently results in thrombosis of the graft. The authors have occasionally had to ligate access grafts in patients with severe cardiomyopathy and hypotension with resultant improvement clinically. These patients should preferentially be selected for peritoneal dialysis or hemodialysis with a permanent catheter.

Selected Readings

Berkoben M, Schwab SJ. In: *Nissenson textbook of dialysis hemodialysis vascular access* (in press).

Authoritative, well-referenced review of all aspects of vascular access.

Feldman HI, Kobrin S, Wasserstein A. Hemodialysis vascular access morbidity. *J Am Soc Nephrol* 1996;7:523–535.

Recent review well-detailed on the magnitude of vascular access complications and morbidity in clinical practice.

Marr KA, Sexton DJ, Conlon PJ, et al. Catheter related bacteremia and outcome of attempted catheter salvage in patients undergoing hemodialysis. *Ann Intern Med* 1997;127:275–280.

Details large experience with management of permanent catheter infections and unlikely prospects of permanent catheter salvage.

National Kidney Foundation. Dialysis Outcomes Quality Initiatives: clinical practice guidelines for vascular access. National Kidney Foundation Supplement, October 1997.

Extensively referenced. Detailed guidelines for optimal management of vascular access.
Schwab SJ. Nephrology forum: vascular access. *Kidney Int* 1998 (in press).
Detailed review of pathology of vascular access failure and long-term morbidity associated with graft loss. Includes detailed discussion of strategies for prospective identification of venous stenoses.

C: Dialyzers, Dialysates, and Delivery Devices

Biff F. Palmer

Hemodialysis is a life-sustaining procedure for the treatment of patients with end-stage renal disease. In the setting of acute renal failure the procedure provides for the rapid correction of fluid and electrolyte abnormalities that pose an immediate threat to the well-being of the patient. In the setting of chronic renal failure, hemodialysis results in a dramatic reversal of uremic symptoms and helps to improve the functional status of the patient and to increase patient survival. This chapter will discuss the various devices available that are employed in the extracorporeal treatment of renal failure patients. A discussion of dialysis membranes and dialysate composition will also be provided.

TYPES OF EXTRACORPOREAL THERAPY

Various modalities are available for the process of extracorporeal blood purification. Intermittent hemodialysis is the most common procedure used for the treatment of patients with acute or chronic renal failure. Hemodialysis is a diffusive-based form of therapy in which a semipermeable membrane separates the blood compartment from a dialysate compartment. Solute flux across the membrane is determined by the concentration gradient. For example, urea will diffuse from the blood to the dialysate such that the total body mass of urea and plasma concentration will decline during the course of the procedure. Conversely, the concentration gradient for bicarbonate favors diffusion from dialysate to blood such that the plasma bicarbonate concentration will rise during the procedure. This method of solute removal is most efficient for small molecular-weight substances with large concentration gradients.

Fluid removal during hemodialysis is achieved by the process of ultrafiltration. This is accomplished by creating a transmembrane pressure gradient across the dialysis membrane. During ultrafiltration there is additional removal of solute from the blood by the process of solvent drag or convection. In comparison with diffusion, the process of convection favors the removal of higher molecular-weight solutes and therefore provides for better clearance of middle molecules. Although ultrafiltration is most commonly performed simultaneously with dialysis, it can also be a stand-alone procedure. This can be accomplished by establishing a transmembrane pressure across the membrane in the absence of dialysate flow. Fluid removal will be in proportion to the pressure gradient and solute removal will be restricted to that which occurs by solvent drag.

Hemofiltration is a form of extracorporeal therapy in which blood flows through a hemofilter that contains a membrane characterized by large pores. Because there is no dialysate flow, solute removal solely occurs by the process of convection. In contrast to ultrafiltration performed with a conventional dialyzer, fluid removal is quantitatively much greater during hemofiltration such that replacement fluid is required in order to avoid hemodynamic collapse. Intermittent hemofiltration has been used extensively in Europe in the chronic treatment of patients with end-stage renal disease. Typically 20 to 30 L of fluid are removed over a 3- to 6-hour period. The procedure requires the availability of large volumes of replacement fluid that is either administered before the hemofilter (predilution) or after the hemofilter (postdilution). The convective removal of solute decreases the total mass of solute but does not change the plasma concentration. It is the large volume of replacement fluid that causes a decrease in the concentration of solutes. Due to the convective nature of the procedure, hemofiltration has the advantage of providing for greater middle-molecule clearance. In the United States, hemofiltration is primarily employed as a continuous form of therapy in the treatment of renal failure patients in the intensive care unit. Continuous arteriovenous hemofiltration (CAVH) is a form of hemofiltration in which the patient's mean arterial pressure provides the driving force for the procedure. Continuous venovenous hemofiltration (CVVH) differs in that an external pump serves as the pumping mechanism.

Hemodiafiltration refers to the combination of hemodialysis and hemofiltration operating simultaneously. Blood and dialysate flow countercurrently through a highly permeable membrane. Unlike conventional hemodialysis, a large-volume ultrafiltrate is formed such that replacement fluid is required. In this technique solute is removed by diffusion and convection. As with hemofiltration, hemodiafiltration is primarily employed as a continuous procedure in the intensive care unit. The patient's mean arterial pressure provides the driving force in continuous arteriovenous hemodiafiltration (CAVHDF), whereas an external pump is used in continuous venovenous hemodiafiltration (CVVHDF).

THE DIALYSIS MACHINE

The dialysis machine brings blood and dialysate to the dialyzer so that diffusion and ultrafiltration can take place. Various components of the machine function to ensure precise control of blood and dialysate flow rates, pressure, and in the case of dialysate, temperature and solute concentration (Fig. 84.17). The energy to move blood through the blood circuit is supplied by a peristaltic type of pump with spring-loaded rollers. The arterial pressure is monitored by a transducer usually placed before the blood pump and within the arterial drip chamber. At this point the arterial pressure is always negative because the blood pump applies suction on the blood across the opening of the access needle. The arterial-pressure monitor guards against excessive suction on the vascular-access site. Common causes of excessively negative pressure include poor arterial pull due to an improperly placed needle, a poorly functioning temporary-access device, and kinking of the tubing between the access and pressure monitor. The pressure beyond the blood pump is positive. A venous pressure transducer is present after the dialyzer usually within the venous drip chamber. Causes of elevated venous pressures include clotting or kinking of the venous line or venous side of a temporary-access device or a stenosis in the venous limb of an arteriovenous loop graft. A sudden fall in the venous pressure occurs if the venous line disconnects. Upper and lower alarm limits are set for both arterial and venous pressures. An air detector is typically placed on the venous drip chamber and functions to prevent foam or air that may have entered the extracorporeal circuit from being infused into the patient. When air is detected, an occlusion clamp located beyond the detector closes the venous return line and the blood pump stops.

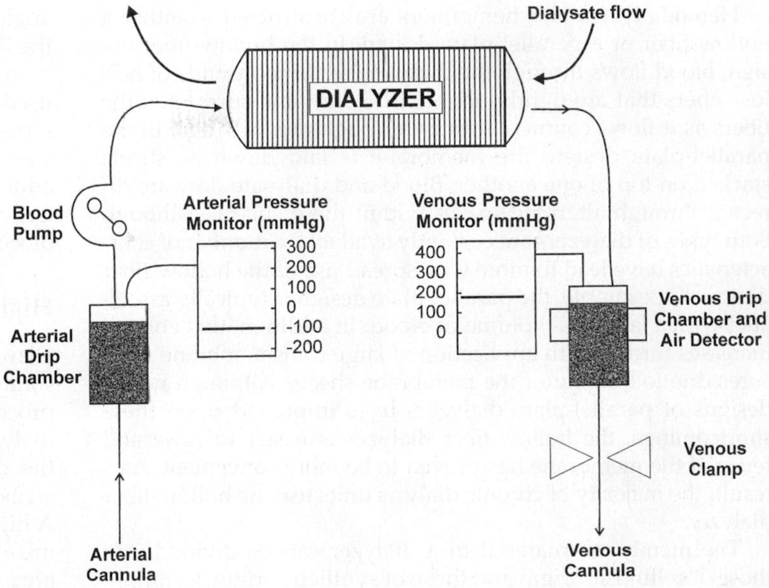

Figure 84.17. The principle components of the blood circuit in a conventional dialysis machine.

The dialysate flows through the dialyzer and into a drain in a single-pass arrangement (Fig. 84.18). As discussed in the following section, the production of dialysate is continuous and is achieved with a proportioning device that mixes a bicarbonate and an acid concentrate with purified water. The final composition of the dialysate is monitored by continuous measurement of the conductivity. Because the primary solutes in the dialysate are electrolytes, the degree of concentration of dialysis solution will be reflected by its electrical conductivity. The temperature of the dialysate is regulated and is set between 35° and 37°C. Purposely lowering the dialysate temperature to 35°C has been shown to provide more hemodynamic stability in hypotensive-prone patients. A bloodleak detector monitors the clarity of the dialysate effluent such that membrane ruptures or minor blood leaks in the dialyzer are detected.

A sorbent regenerative dialysis system exists that enables a treatment to be performed with only 6 L of total dialysate as compared with more than 100 L used with other systems. The ability to use such a small volume of dialysate is achieved by directing the dialysate effluent through a sorbent cartridge in which the dialysate is regenerated. Chemicals within the cartridge function to convert urea to CO_2, sodium bicarbonate and water, while adsorbing uremic and nonuremic toxins. Although once used as a delivery device in home hemodialysis, this system is being phased out due to cost and an inability to provide adequate dialysis on a chronic basis.

HEMODIALYZERS AND HEMOFILTERS

The hemodialyzer is the component in the dialysis circuit in which all diffusion and ultrafiltration takes place. Blood and dialysate typically flow countercurrently through the dialyzer, entering and exiting the structure by way of dedicated ports. Within the dialyzer the blood and dialysate compartments are separated by a semipermeable membrane. A hemofilter that is used in the process of hemofiltration also provides an inlet and outlet for blood flow but lacks a flow pathway for dialysate. Rather, a single outlet exists for removal of formed ultrafiltrate.

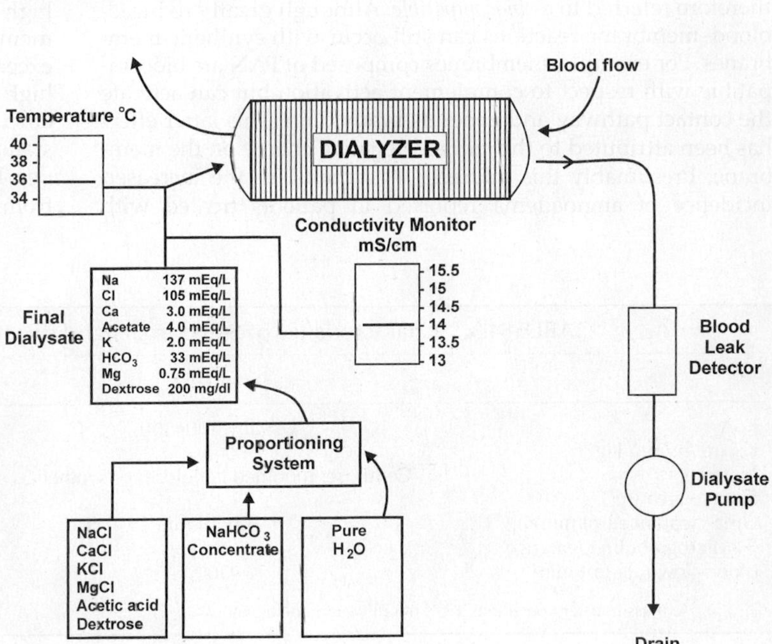

Figure 84.18. The principle components of the dialysate circuit in which bicarbonate serves as the buffer source.

Hemodialyzers and hemofilters are constructed in either a hollow-fiber or a parallel-plate design. In the hollow-fiber design, blood flows through the dialyzer inside thousands of hollow fibers that are tightly bound. The dialysate surrounds the fibers as it flows countercurrently through the cartridge. In the parallel-plate design, the membrane is laid down as sheets stacked on top of one another. Blood and dialysate flow are directed through alternate spaces within these sheets. Although both types of dialyzers are currently available, a number of characteristics have lead to more widespread use of the hollow-fiber design. For example, the parallel-plate design is typically associated with a larger fill volume of blood. In addition, this volume increases further with application of large transmembrane pressures due to bulging of the membrane sheets. Although newer designs of parallel-plate dialyzers have improved upon these shortcomings, the hollow-fiber dialyzer is easier to rinse and reuse of the membrane has proven to be more convenient. As a result, the majority of chronic dialysis units use the hollow-fiber dialyzer.

The membrane material in a dialyzer can be divided into those of cellulosic origin and those of synthetic origin. Cellulose membranes, derived from processed cotton, are the most commonly used membranes in hemodialysis. Unsubstituted cellulose membranes are composed of repetitive polysaccharide units that contain free hydroxy groups. The large number of hydroxy groups contributes to the hydrophilicity of the membrane. This latter characteristic has been associated with a greater degree of blood–membrane interaction or bioincompatibility such as complement activation. The potential deleterious effects of biocompatibility is discussed in detail in Chapter 84, Part 1D. In order to lessen the degree of hydrophilicity and improve biocompatibility, substituted cellulose membranes have been developed. One such example is a cellulose-acetate membrane in which a large number of the hydroxy groups are bonded to acetate. The membrane can also be modified in order to enhance the diffusive and ultrafiltration properties. An example of this modification is the addition of copper ammonia to cellulose to form a cuprammonium cellulose membrane (Cuprophan).

Synthetic membranes can be composed of any one of several materials not to include cellulose. Materials used to make synthetic membranes include polysulfone, polymethylmethacrylate (PMMA), and polyacrylonitrile (PAN). Synthetic membranes are associated with much less complement activation and are therefore referred to as *biocompatible.* Although greatly reduced, blood–membrane reactions can still occur with synthetic membranes. For example, membranes composed of PAN are biocompatible with respect to complement activation but can activate the contact pathway and generate bradykinin. This latter effect has been attributed to the surface negative charge on the membrane. Presumably this interaction accounts for the increased incidence of angioedema reported in patients treated with angiotensin-converting enzyme inhibitors and dialyzed against the PAN containing AN-69 membrane.

A combination of cellulose and synthetic material can also be used in the generation of a membrane. This hybrid has been referred to as a *cellulosynthetic membrane.* Hemophane is the trade name for a membrane in which a tertiary amino compound is added to liquefied cellulose during the manufacturing process. Cellulosynthetic membranes offer the advantage of increased biocompatibility as compared with a cellulose membrane alone.

High-Efficiency and High-Flux Membranes

Dialysis membranes vary in regards to the permeability of solutes and water. The clearance of solutes during the dialysis procedure are influenced by various factors such as blood and dialysate flow rate and the size of the molecule. Properties of the dialysis membrane that influence clearance are best described by the mass transfer coefficient (KoA) of the membrane. A high KoA membrane is characterized by features that maximize contact between blood and dialysate. A thin, large–surface area membrane with wide pores will be associated with a greater urea clearance as compared with a membrane without these features. When the KoA value of the membrane is greater that 700 the membrane is classified as a high-efficiency membrane. High-efficiency dialyzers can be cellulosic-based or synthetic membranes.

Water flux across the membrane is determined by the transmembrane pressure and the permeability of the membrane. Water permeability of the dialysis membrane is directly related to pore size and is described by the ultrafiltration coefficient (KUf). The KUf is described as the number of milliliters of ultrafiltrate formed per hour per mm Hg pressure (ml/hr per mm Hg) applied across the membrane. Dialysis membranes with a KUf of greater than 15 ml/hr per mm Hg have high water permeability and are referred to as *high-flux dialyzers.* Use of a high-flux membrane requires an ultrafiltration control system that can tightly regulate the rate of ultrafiltrate formed because small errors in the transmembrane pressure will result in large errors in the amount of fluid removed. High-flux membranes are most commonly made of synthetic material although the cellulose triacetate membrane has a KUf of 30 ml/hr per mm Hg and is considered high flux.

The major difference between a high-flux membrane and a high-efficiency membrane is the KUf (Table 84.3). Both types of membranes have similar urea clearances and KoA values that exceed 700. In this respect, all high-flux membranes are also high efficiency. The reverse, however, is not true. Whereas high-efficiency membranes typically have KUf values greater than a standard dialyzer (usually between 10 and 12 ml/mm Hg per hour), the KUf of high-flux membranes usually range from 30 to 60 ml/hr per mm Hg. The porous nature of these

TABLE 84.3. Characteristics of Standard, High-Efficiency, and High-Flux Dialysis Membranes

	Standard	High Efficiency	High Flux
KoA	Usually 300–500	>700	>700
K_{UF} (ml/hr/mm Hg)	3–8	Usually 10–12	>15
Material	Cellulose, modified cellulose, or synthetic	Modified cellulose or synthetic	Mostly synthetic
Surface area (m^2)	<1.5	1.7–2.0	1.7–2.0
Urea clearance (ml/min)	<200 ml/min	>200	>200
β_2-Microglobulin clearance	No	No	Yes
Blood-flow rate (ml/min)	~300	400–500	400–500

KoA, mass transfer coefficient; KUf, ultrafiltration coefficient.

membranes allow for greater middle-molecule clearance (molecular-weight solutes between 1,500 and 5,000) and better clearance of β_2-microglobulin (more than 20 ml/min). Whether these characteristics of a high-flux membrane actually translate into a long-term clinical benefit is currently being examined in the National Institutes of Health–sponsored hemodialysis study.

Reuse of Membranes

Reprocessing of dialysis membranes is practiced in the majority of chronic dialysis facilities. After the completion of the dialysis procedure the membrane is rinsed thoroughly with water. In some instances the membrane is then treated with a cleaning solution such as bleach. The dialyzer is then filled with a disinfecting agent and stored until the next procedure. The most commonly used disinfecting agents are formaldehyde, peracetic acid, and glutaraldehyde. Before the next treatment, the dialyzer is rinsed and tested to ensure that the disinfectant is completely removed. In addition to cost savings, reuse of dialyzers is associated with increased biocompatibility and a decreased incidence of first-use syndromes. The improved biocompatibility is particularly evident with cellulose membranes and is thought to be related to coating of the membrane by serum proteins. The first-use syndrome is an acute anaphylactoid type of reaction that occurs within the first several minutes of hemodialysis. This syndrome, which is now referred to as a *type 1 reaction,* is not related to complement activation but rather is due to sensitization to ethylene oxide, a compound used in the sterilization of dialyzers during the manufacturing process. Extensive rinsing of a new dialyzer before use can markedly reduce the incidence of this reaction.

Reprocessing of dialyzers requires extensive monitoring to ensure sterility, adequate removal of reprocessing chemicals, and maintenance of structural and functional integrity of the membrane. In order to detect loss of membrane surface area due to capillary occlusion, measurement of fiber-bundle volume needs to be performed. When the volume falls to less than 80% of the original value, the membrane should be discarded. Pressure tests on both blood and dialysate compartments are essential to ensure membrane integrity. Many centers no longer use bleach in the initial steps of the reuse procedure because bleach can alter the characteristics of some dialysis membranes in a deleterious way. For example, reprocessing of polysulfone dialyzers with bleach and formaldehyde increases the permeability of the membrane, resulting in increased protein loss and enhancing the possibility of endotoxin transfer from contaminated dialysate.

DIALYSATE COMPOSITION

Dialysate Water

During the dialytic procedure patients are exposed to a large volume of water that passes through the dialyzer. In order to avoid exposing the patient to bacterial and chemical contaminants, water for the dialysate is purified in a series of steps involving filters, exposure to ion exchange resins and activated charcoal, and reverse osmosis. This process provides for the removal of aluminum, which has been linked to the development of a low bone turnover state, anemia, and dementia as well as removal of copper and chloramine, both of which can cause hemolytic anemia. A maximum of 200 colony-forming units/ml in water purified for dialysis and 2,000 colony-forming units/ml in dialysate is currently permitted by the Association for the Advancement of Medical Instrumentation. The importance of water purification was recently highlighted by a report linking the development of acute liver failure in a group of dialysis patients to microcystins, toxins produced by Cyanobacteria found in the reservoir water used in dialysate solutions.

Dialysate Sodium

In the early days of hemodialysis, the dialysate sodium concentration was deliberately set low in order to avoid the problems of chronic volume overload such as hypertension and heart failure. As volume removal became more rapid because of shorter dialysis times, symptomatic hypotension emerged as a common and often disabling problem during dialysis. It soon became apparent that changes in the serum sodium concentration, and more specifically changes in serum osmolality, were playing a role in the development of this hemodynamic instability. A decline in plasma osmolality during regular hemodialysis favors a fluid shift from the extracellular space to the intracellular space, thereby exacerbating the volume-depleting effects of dialysis (Fig. 84.19). With the advent of high-clearance dialyzers and more efficient dialysis techniques, this decline in

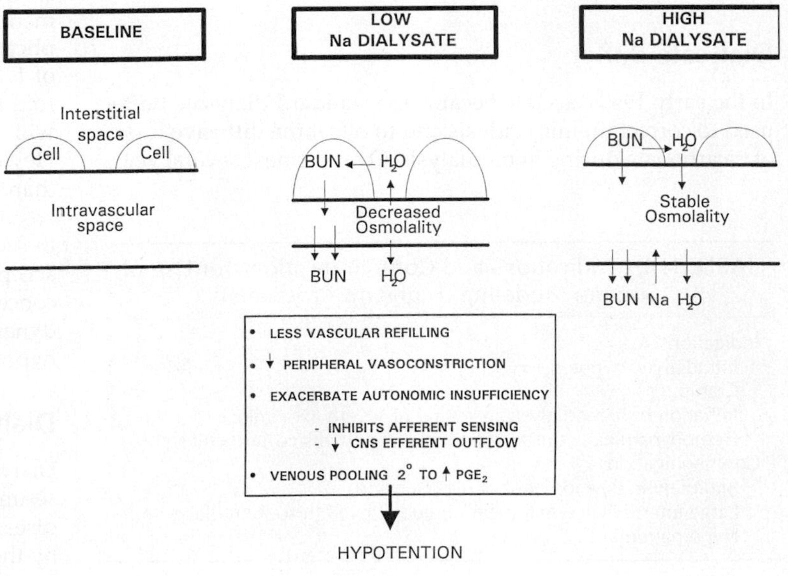

Figure 84.19. Use of a low sodium dialysate is more commonly associated with intradialytic hypotension as a result of several mechanisms. The drop in serum osmolality as urea is removed leads to a shift of water into the intracellular compartment preventing adequate refilling of the intravascular space. A high sodium dialysate helps minimize the development of hypoosmolality allowing for better refilling of the intravascular compartment. Other potential mechanisms whereby a low sodium dialysate contributes to hypotension are indicated.

plasma osmolality becomes more apparent as solute is more rapidly removed. Use of a low dialysate sodium concentration would tend to further augment the intracellular shift of fluid as plasma tends to become even more hyposmolar consequent to the movement of sodium from plasma to dialysate. The use of a higher dialysate sodium concentration (more than 140 mEq/L) has been among the most efficacious and best-tolerated therapies for episodic hypotension. The high sodium concentration prevents a marked decline in the plasma osmolality during dialysis, thereby protecting the extracellular volume by minimizing osmotic fluid loss into the cells.

There has been interest in varying the concentration of sodium in the dialysate throughout the procedure in order to minimize the potential complications of a high sodium solution and yet retain the beneficial hemodynamic effects. A high dialysate sodium concentration is used initially with a progressive reduction toward isotonic or even hypotonic levels by the end of the procedure. This method of sodium control allows for a diffusive sodium influx early in the session in order to prevent the rapid decline in plasma osmolality due to the efflux of urea and other small molecular-weight solutes. During the remainder of the procedure, when the reduction in osmolality accompanying urea removal is less abrupt, the dialysate sodium level is set at a lower level, thereby minimizing the development of hypertonicity and any resultant excessive thirst, fluid gain, and hypertension in the interdialytic period.

This method of sodium variation often referred to as *sodium modeling* offers little advantage over a constant dialysate sodium of between 140 and 145 mEq/L in most chronic renal failure patients. However, in certain patients, sodium modeling may be of benefit (Table 84.4). Patients with far-advanced renal insufficiency are often deliberately dialyzed so as to decrease the urea concentration slowly over the course of several days in order to avoid the development of the dialysis disequilibrium syndrome. The use of a high-/low-sodium dialysate in these patients, who often have extremely high urea concentrations, may minimize fluid shifts into the intracellular compartment and thus decrease the tendency for neurologic complications. Sodium modeling may also be beneficial in those patients who suffer frequent side effects while on dialysis such as intradialytic hypotension, cramping, nausea, vomiting, fatigue, and headache. In such patients, the modeling protocol can be individually tailored in order to minimize increased thirst, weight gain, and hypertension. Combining dialysate sodium profiling with a varying rate of ultrafiltration may provide additional benefit in particularly symptomatic patients.

Dialysate Buffer

In the early 1960s, acetate became the standard dialysate buffer used to correct uremic acidosis and to offset the diffusive losses of bicarbonate during hemodialysis. Over the next several years reports began to accumulate linking routine use of acetate with cardiovascular instability and hypotension during dialysis. As a result, bicarbonate-containing dialysate began to reemerge as the principal dialysate buffer especially as advances in biotechnology made the use of bicarbonate dialysate less expensive and less cumbersome to use. Widespread use of high-efficiency and high-flux dialysis has also lead to increased use of bicarbonate-containing dialysate because the increased clearance associated with these procedures would allow the rate of acetate influx to exceed the maximal rate of metabolism such that acid–base balance could not be maintained.

The current use of a bicarbonate dialysate requires a specifically designed system that mixes a bicarbonate and an acid concentrate with purified water (Fig. 84.18). The acid concentrate contains a small amount of acid, either lactic or acetic acid, and all the calcium and magnesium. The exclusion of these cations from the bicarbonate concentrate prevents the precipitation of magnesium and calcium carbonate that would otherwise occur in the setting of a high bicarbonate concentration. During the mixing procedure, the acid in the acid concentrate will react with an equimolar amount of bicarbonate to generate carbonic acid and carbon dioxide. The generation of carbon dioxide causes the pH of the final solution to fall to approximately 7.0 to 7.4. The acidic pH as well as the lower concentrations present in the final mixture allow for calcium and magnesium to remain in solution.

For the most part, the bicarbonate concentration used in most dialysis centers is set at 33 to 35 mmol/L and is rarely adjusted. Emphasis is now being placed on individually adjusting the dialysate bicarbonate concentration to maintain the predialysis tCO_2 concentration of more than 23 mmol/L. Increasing evidence suggests that correction of chronic acidosis is of clinical benefit in terms of bone metabolism and nutrition. In some patients supplemental oral bicarbonate therapy will be required to achieve this goal.

TABLE 84.4. Indications and Contraindications for Use of Sodium Modeling (High/Low Programs)

Indications
Intradialytic hypotension
Cramping
Initiation of hemodialysis in setting of severe azotemia
Hemodynamically unstable patient (as in intensive care unit setting)
Contraindications
Intradialytic development of hypertension
Large interdialytic weight gain induced by high sodium dialysate
Hypernatremia

Dialysate Calcium

To avoid negative calcium balance as well as potentially suppress circulating parathyroid hormone, the dialysate calcium concentration is typically set at 3.0 to 3.5 mEq/L (1.5 to 1.75 mmol/L). This concentration is equal to or slightly greater than the ionized concentration in the serum of most patients. As a result, there is net calcium absorption in most patients during the procedure. As the use of calcium carbonate as phosphate binders has progressively replaced the use of aluminum compounds, the development of hypercalcemia has become more common. This complication has been further exacerbated by the widespread use of $1,25(OH)_2$ vitamin D to reduce circulating levels of parathyroid hormone. In order to avoid hypercalcemia, some patients will require a lower calcium concentration in the dialysate. However, when using dialysate calcium concentrations less than 1.5 mmol/L, one needs to monitor the patients closely to ensure that negative calcium balance does not develop and that inducible parathyroid hormone (iPTH) levels remain in an acceptable range. In addition, lowering the dialysate calcium concentration can potentially lead to a worsening of hemodynamics during the dialysis procedure, particularly in a hypotensive-prone patients (Table 84.5).

Dialysate Potassium

Dialysis assumes a major role in the maintenance of a normal serum potassium concentration in patients with end-stage renal disease. The removal of excess potassium by dialysis is achieved by the use of a dialysate with a lower potassium concentration

TABLE 84.5. Effects of Altering the Electrolyte Concentration in the Dialysate

Dialysate component		Advantage	Disadvantage
Na:	Increased	More hemodynamic stability Less cramping	Dipsogenic effect, increased interdialytic weight gain, ? chronic hypertension
	Decreased (rarely used)	Less interdialytic weight gain	Intradialytic hypotension and cramping more common
Ca:	Increased	Suppression of PTH, promotes hemodynamic stability in HD	Hypercalcemia with vitamin D and high dose calcium-containing phosphate binders, ? contribution to adynamic bone disease
	Decreased	Permits greater use of vitamin D and calcium-containing phosphate binders	Potential for negative calcium balance, stimulation of PTH, slight decrease in hemodynamic stability
K:	Increased	Less arrhythmias in setting of digoxin or coronary heart disease, ? improved hemodynamic stability	Limited by hyperkalemia
	Decreased	Greater dietary intake of K with less hyperkalemia, ? improvement in myocardial contractility	Increased arrhythmias (ramped dialysate K ideal, lessens transcellular gradient), may exacerbate autonomic insufficiency
HCO_3:	Increased	Corrects chronic acidosis, thereby benefits nutrition and bone metabolism	Postdialysis metabolic alkalosis
	Decreased	Less metabolic alkalosis	Potential for chronic acidosis
Mg:	Increased	? Less arrhythmias, ? hemodynamic benefit	Potential for hypermagnesemia
	Decreased	Permits greater use of magnesium-containing phosphate binders, which in turn permits reduced dose of calcium binders and results in less hypercalcemia	Symptomatic hypomagnesemia

HD, hemodialysis; PTH, parathyroid hormone.

so that a gradient-favoring potassium movement from plasma to dialysate is achieved. The dialysate concentration needs to be individualized but is commonly set at 2 mEq/L. A potassium-free dialysate can be used in the treatment of a hyperkalemic patient but only for the first 1 to 2 hours of the procedure. After this time the dialysate should be increased to at least 1 mEq/L in order to avoid the development of arrhythmias, which can be precipitated by a rapid fall in the serum potassium concentration. A potassium concentration of 3 to 4 mEq/L may be indicated in patients with a normal or low predialysis serum potassium concentration or in those patients receiving digoxin.

The rate of potassium removal is largely a function of the predialysis concentration. The higher the initial plasma concentration, the greater the plasma-to-dialysate gradient and hence the greater the potassium removal. As a result, the plasma potassium concentration can be expected to fall rapidly in the early stages of dialysis, but as the plasma concentration falls, potassium removal becomes less efficient. Because potassium is freely permeable across the dialysis membrane, movement of potassium from the intracellular space to the extracellular space appears to be the limiting factor that accounts for the smaller fractional decline in potassium concentration at lower plasma potassium concentrations. After the completion of a standard dialysis there is an increase in the plasma concentration of potassium of approximately 30%, which occurs over 4 to 5 hours. This "rebound" is thought to be due to continued exit of potassium from the intracellular space to the extracellular space in an attempt to reestablish the intracellular–extracellular potassium gradient.

Approximately 80 to 100 mEq of potassium is removed during a typical dialysis session. This amount exhibits considerable variability and is influenced by changes in acid–base status, changes in tonicity, changes in glucose and insulin concentration, and catecholamine activity. During dialysis there is net addition of base to the extracellular space, which promotes cellular uptake of potassium and therefore attenuates the removal of potassium during dialysis. With routine dialysis the change in blood pH is of small magnitude and the effect on potassium removal is not profound. By contrast, dialysis in patients who are acidotic will result in less potassium removal because potassium is shifted into cells as the serum bicarbonate rises. Insulin is known to stimulate the cellular uptake of potassium and can therefore influence the amount of potassium removal during dialysis. The use of a glucose-free dialysate is associated with greater amounts of potassium removal as compared with patients treated with a glucose-containing bath. A glucose-free dialysate leads to less stimulation of insulin and, as a result, the amount of potassium accessible for dialysate removal is increased. β-Adrenergic stimulation is known to shift potassium into cells and lower the extracellular concentration. Because inhaled beta stimulants have been reported to be effective in the acute treatment of hyperkalemia, such therapy before dialysis may lower the total amount of potassium removed during the dialytic procedure.

Dialysate Magnesium

The usual concentration of magnesium in the dialysate is 0.5 to 1.0 mEq/L. There has been interest in using magnesium-containing compounds as a phosphate binder in order to minimize the development of hypercalcemia associated with the use of calcium-containing phosphate binders and vitamin D. The use of oral magnesium has necessitated the use of a low magnesium dialysate concentration so as to avoid the development of hypermagnesemia.

Selected Readings

Allon M, Shanklin N. Effect of albuterol treatment on subsequent dialytic potassium removal. *Am J Kidney Dis* 1995;26:607–613.

Administration of β agonists is one of several factors that can stimulate potassium movement into the intracellular compartment and as a result decrease the total amount of potassium available for dialytic removal.

Graham K, Reaich D, Channon S, et al. Correction of acidosis in hemodialysis decreases whole-body protein degradation. *J Am Soc Nephrol* 1997;8:632–637.

Raising the dialysate bicarbonate concentration to 40 mmol/L was effective in correcting the chronic acidosis of hemodialysis patients. The higher predialysis bicarbonate concentration was beneficial in terms of protein turnover, suggesting that optimal correction of acidosis may improve the long-term nutritional status of dialysis patients.

Himmelfarb J, Tolkoff Rubin N, Chandran P, et al. A multicenter comparison of dialysis membranes in the treatment of acute renal failure requiring dialysis. *J Am Soc Nephrol* 1998;9:257–266.

A multicenter study of patients with acute renal failure requiring dialysis comparing the use of biocompatible and bioincompatible membranes. Use of the biocompatible membrane was associated with both improved patient survival and recovery of renal function.

Kaplan A, Halley S, Lapkin R, et al. Dialysate protein losses with bleach processes polysulphone dialyzers. *Kidney Int* 1995;47:573–578.

A study illustrating how reprocessing of certain dialyzers can change the baseline characteristics of the membrane potentially leading to an adverse clinical effect.

Levin A, Goidstein M. The benefits and side effects of ramped hypertonic sodium dialysis. *J Am Soc Nephrol* 1996;7:242–246.

Sodium modeling and rates of ultrafiltration individually tailored to symptomatic dialysis patients can markedly improve symptoms such as cramps, lightheadedness, and fatigue.

Palmer, BF. Dialysate composition in hemodialysis and peritoneal dialysis. In: Henrich WL, ed. *Principals and practice of dialysis* 2nd ed. Baltimore: Williams and Wilkins, 1999:22–40.

A review of the latest literature dealing with dialysate composition in both hemodialysis and peritoneal dialysis.

Ronco C, Bellomo R. Continuous renal replacement therapy: evolution in technology and current nomenclature. *Kidney Int* 1998;53(Suppl 66):S166–S164.

An overview of continuous renal replacement therapy in which the often confusing nomenclature is nicely clarified.

D: Membrane Biocompatibility

Gerald Schulman and Raymond M. Hakim

For more than 400,000 patients worldwide, hemodialysis is a lifesaving procedure, although it may also be associated with potentially life-threatening side effects. Many of these side effects are a direct consequence of the nature of the dialysis procedure itself. Thus changes in electrolyte composition may produce arrhythmias, and rapid ultrafiltration may lead to hypotensive episodes. However, it has become increasingly clear that significant adverse events may occur during the interaction of blood with the membrane of the artificial kidney.

Hemodialysis is not a simple diffusive process with blood and dialysis separated by an inert semipermeable membrane. Indeed, the biocompatibility of the dialysis procedure, broadly defined, involves not only the dialysis membrane but variables such as the format of the membrane (parallel plate or hollow fiber), the type of anticoagulation, the nature of the dialysate (composition and temperature), water treatment, and reuse of membranes (Table 84.6). However, the most closely studied phenomena have been the side effects due to interactions between components of blood and the hemodialysis membrane. Rarely, these interactions may lead to dramatic symptoms that can be life threatening. More often they are mild, but it should be remembered that these interactions occur repetitively during each dialysis session, and over time may also result in adverse consequences. The direct consequence of blood–membrane interaction is the initiation of an inflammatory response.

TABLE 84.6. Hemodialysis and Biocompatibility

Membrane
Biomaterial
Permeability
Dialysate
Anticoagulant
Method of exchange
Convection
Diffusion
Rate of exchange
Blood flow
Time

TABLE 84.7. Activated Systems During Hemodialysis

Humoral pathways
Complement
Coagulation
Contact pathway
Leukocytes
Neutrophils
Monocytes
Lymphocytes
Platelets
Red cells

It was recognized in 1968 that profound but transient neutropenia occurred during hemodialysis. This neutropenia could be reproduced in rabbits by the administration of plasma that had been exposed to cellulosic dialysis membranes. Heat-inactivated plasma did not produce neutropenia, suggesting that the complement system might be mediating the phenomenon. This was confirmed when components of the complement system could be directly measured, indicating activation via the alternative pathway of complement. Cellulose membranes were the only type for many years. Because of its tensile strength and its ability to be molded into a number of different formats, cellulose membranes served as the backbone of hemodialysis treatments until the late 1970s. Although data from the United States Renal Data System (USRDS), the dialysis registry for the United States, suggests that the use of cellulosic membranes is declining in the United States, their relatively low cost has led to their continued use for maintenance hemodialysis worldwide.

This initial set of observations has led to a rapidly expanding body of information over the ensuing years, demonstrating that virtually all of the major cellular and humoral components of blood may interact to a variable extent with different hemodialysis membranes (Table 84.7 and Fig. 84.20). The sum of these interactions can be considered to reflect the degree of biocompatibility associated with hemodialysis.

HUMORAL PATHWAYS

The dialysis membrane is capable of activating the coagulation cascade, contact pathway (kallikrein-kininogen), and the complement system. During contact of blood with the dialysis membrane, several protein-mediated and cellular pathways are activated. The first such interaction described was one between the membrane and the complement system. Because of its widespread, direct systemic effects as well as its influence on the cellular components of blood, complement activation has served as an important index of bioincompatibility. The polysaccharide components of the cellulosic dialysis membrane makes it a trigger for the activation of complement via the alternative pathway. Unlike the classical pathway, which is activated by immune complexes, the more primitive alternative pathway is activated by surface structures such as the cell walls of bacteria

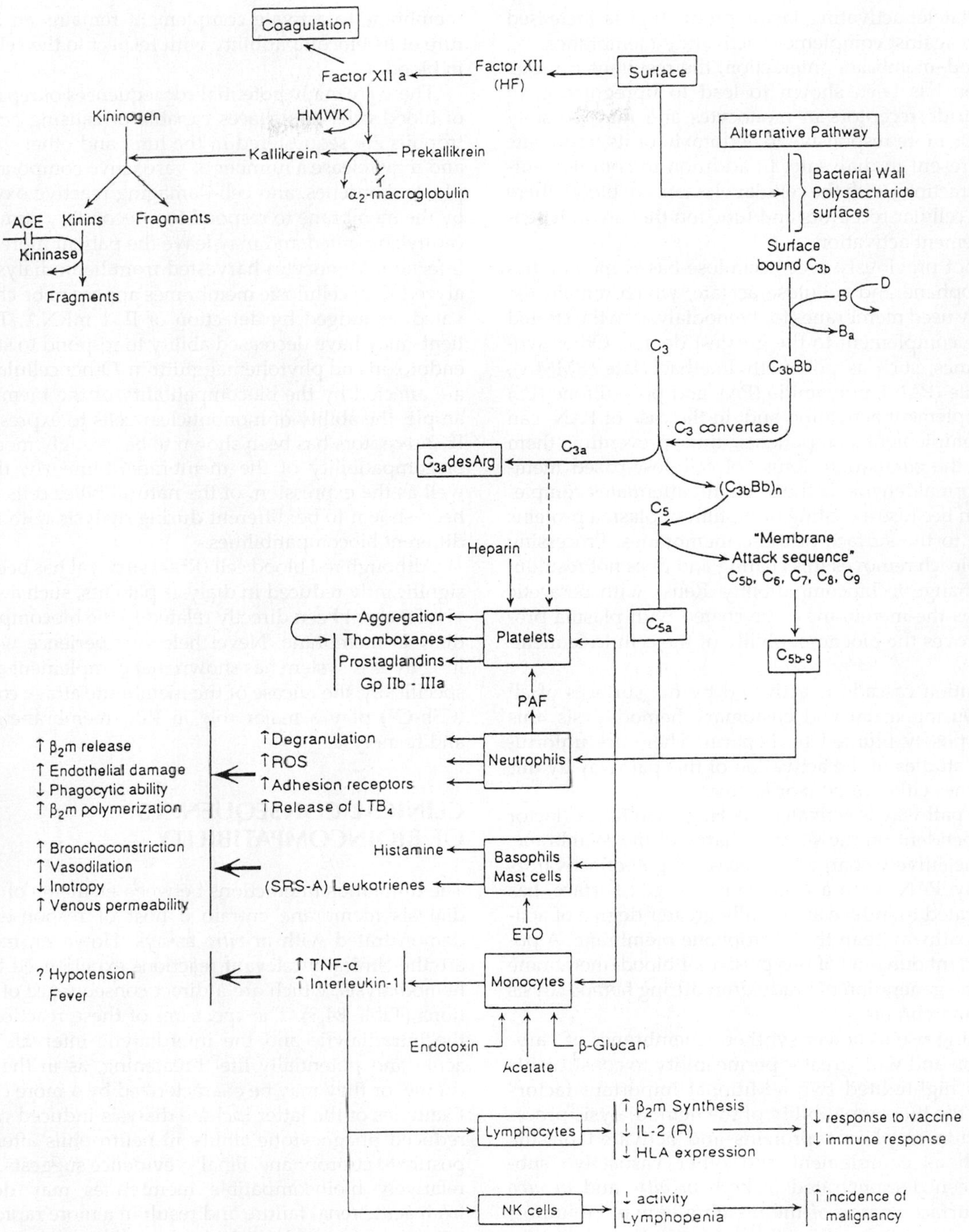

Figure 84.20. Interrelation between humoral and cellular components of blood following activation by artificial surfaces. ACE, angiotensin-converting enzyme; β_2m, β_2-microglobulin; C_{5b-9}, membrane attack complex; ETO, ethylene oxide; Gp IIIb-IIIa, platelet receptor; HF, Hageman factor; HMWK, high-molecular-weight kininogen; IL-2, interleukin 2; LTB_4, leukotriene B_4; NK, natural killer cell; PAF, platelet-activating factor; ROS, reactive oxygen species; SRS-A, slow releasing substance-anaphylaxis; TNF-α, tumor necrosis factor-α.

or the dialysis membrane. Activation of complement leads to the generation of the anaphylatoxins C3a and C5a and the membrane attack complex C5b-C9. Although these activated components are rapidly inactivated by plasma factors, there is activation of neutrophils and monocytes via complement receptors.

The result of complement interaction with neutrophils following activation by cellulosic membranes leads to expression of adhesion surface receptors, degranulation and release of intracellular enzymes, and the elaboration of reactive oxygen species. Cytokines produced following the interaction of complement products with monocytes also may produce biologic effects. Platelets also participate in blood–membrane interactions. There is rapid platelet turnover in hemodialysis patients. Release of eicosanoids from platelet membrane during dialysis have been reported. In addition, platelet-leukocyte aggregates have been shown during hemodialysis against cellulosic membranes. Hydrogen peroxide is formed as a consequence of these platelet-neutrophils aggregates after exposure to cellulosic membranes. Platelet-activating factor production is increased during dialysis against complement-activating membranes.

During blood–membrane interaction, the resultant complement activation has been shown to lead to upregulation of lipopolysaccharide receptors in monocytes and may possibly make these cells more responsive to endotoxin or its fragments that may be present in dialysate. In addition to complement-associated interactions with the cellular elements of blood, there are changes in cellular receptors and function that are independent of complement activation.

New (i.e., not previously used) cellulose-based membranes made of cuprophane and cellulose acetate, which remain the most frequently used membranes for hemodialysis in the United States, activate complement to the greatest degree. Other synthetic membranes, such as polymethylmethacrylate (PMMA), polyacrylonitrile (PAN), polyamide (PA), and polysulfone (PS) cause less complement activation and, in the case of PAN, can bind active complement components, thus preventing them from entering the circulation. Reuse of cellulose-based membranes, with formaldehyde as the sterilant, attenuates complement activation because a coating or biofilm of plasma proteins becomes fixed to the surface of these membranes. Processing that includes bleach removes this coating and does not result in a significant change in biocompatibility. Reuse with peracetic acid also allows the membrane to be coated with plasma proteins and improves the biocompatibility of the cellulosic membrane gradually.

The coagulation cascade is activated by the surfaces of all membranes. During usual and customary hemodialysis, this cascade is purposely blunted by heparin. There are unfortunately too few studies of the activation of this pathway by different membranes either *in vitro* or *in vivo*.

The contact pathway is activated via Hageman factor (factor XII) and is dependent on the surface charge of the membrane. In particular, negatively charged surfaces are potent activators of this pathway. PAN, with a negatively charged surface, has been demonstrated to induce an initially greater degree of activation of this pathway than the cuprophane membrane. A potentially important outcome of this particular blood–membrane interaction is the generation of bradykinin during hemodialysis with the PAN membrane.

The increasing use of newer synthetic membranes of varying composition and with greater permeability to constituents of plasma has highlighted two additional important factors that modulate the biocompatibility of the hemodialysis procedure. Adsorption of plasma proteins and activated plasma products, such as complement and other vasoactive substances, has been demonstrated in both *in vitro* and *in vivo* models. The surface charge of the membrane may be important, because significant adsorption of complement occurs with PAN but not with cuprophane or PS membranes. The second attribute of the newer synthetic membranes is related to greater pore size. Thus activation products (e.g., peptides) that result from blood–membrane interactions may be cleared during the hemodialysis treatment.

CELLULAR COMPONENTS

Neutrophils, monocytes, lymphocytes, red cells, and platelets are influenced by contact with the membrane. Properties intrinsic to the cuprophane dialysis membrane may act independently of complement to cause cell activation [e.g., synthesis of interleukin 1 messenger ribonucleic acid (IL-1 mRNA) by monocytes], but complement-activation products greatly enhance the mRNA synthesis of these cytokines. Thus the ability of the membrane to activate complement remains an important feature of its biocompatibility with respect to the cellular elements in blood.

There are many potential consequences of repeated exposure of blood cells to surfaces capable of causing activation. Neutrophils are sequestered in the lung and other vascular organs and may release a number of vasoactive components, for example, leukotrienes, and cell-damaging reactive oxygen activated by the membrane to respond to a secondary stimulus is significantly abrogated and may leave the patient more susceptible to infection. Monocytes harvested from hemodialysis patients dialyzed with cellulosic membranes appear to be chronically activated, as judged by detection of IL-1 mRNA. Thus these patients may have decreased ability to respond to stimuli, such as endotoxin and phytohemagglutinin. Other cellular systems also are affected by the biocompatibility of the membrane. For example, the ability of mononuclear cells to express high-affinity IL-2 receptors has been shown to be strongly modulated by the biocompatibility of the membrane. Similarly, the activity, as well as the expression, of the natural killer cells (NK cells) has been shown to be different during dialysis with membranes of different biocompatibilities.

Although red blood cell (RBC) survival has been shown to be significantly reduced in dialysis patients, such a shortened survival has not been directly related to the biocompatibility of the dialysis membrane. Nevertheless, experience with the heart–lung bypass system has shown that complement activation and, specifically, the release of the membrane attack complex (MAC) (C5b-C9) play a major role in RBC-membrane fragmentation and hemolysis.

CLINICAL CONSEQUENCES OF BIOINCOMPATIBILITY

The numerous interactions between elements of blood and the dialysis membrane entrain a host of responses that can be demonstrated with *in vitro* assays. However, more important are the clinically relevant reactions experienced by patients on hemodialysis, which are a direct consequence of these interactions (Table 84.8). The spectrum of these reactions spans both the intradialytic and the interdialytic interval. They may be acute and potentially life threatening, as in the first-use syndrome, or they may be characterized by a more chronic course. Examples of the latter include dialysis-induced catabolism and reduced phagocytotic ability in neutrophils after repeated exposure to cuprophane. Finally, evidence suggests that the use of relatively bioincompatible membranes may delay recovery from acute renal failure and result in a more rapid loss of residual renal function in end-stage renal disease.

The First-Use Syndrome

The *first-use syndrome* is a rare reaction occurring in 1 in 60,000 to 100,000 hemodialysis treatments. It is characterized by a constellation of symptoms and signs, including urticaria, cough, chest and back pain, shortness of breath, and hypotension, usu-

TABLE 84.8. Clinical Correlates of Bioincompatibility
Hypersensitivity
Infection
β_2-Microglobulin
Malnutrition
Renal function

ally within the first 15 to 20 minutes of hemodialysis. In its most fulminant form, it is similar to a full anaphylactic reaction and can result in cardiac arrest and death. It is seen most commonly when cuprophane dialyzers are used for the first time. This reaction may be mediated by IgE antibodies induced by ethylene oxide that has been used as a sterilant for the cuprophane dialyzers before their use. However, patients subject to this reaction have also been shown to generate much higher-activated complement products and at an earlier point in the treatment following exposure to cuprophane than patients who do not experience this reaction. This suggests that the complement system is implicated in some of these reactions as well.

A similar syndrome has been reported in patients dialyzed against PAN membranes and reused PS membranes. As mentioned previously, bradykinin is generated during contact with PAN membranes. Converting enzyme is a kinase and can inactivate bradykinin. The inhibition of this enzyme by angiotensin-converting enzyme (ACE) inhibitors may lead to elevated levels of bradykinin with resultant symptoms, such as hypotension and bronchospasm, accounting for the response seen with PAN membranes, particularly in those patients who are receiving ACE inhibitors.

Infection

Infection accounts for 21% of the deaths in all hemodialysis patients and for as much as 40% of the deaths in those individuals who have been on maintenance hemodialysis for an extended period of time. Although there are many causes of white cell dysfunction in the hemodialysis population, evidence is mounting that patients undergoing hemodialysis with bioincompatible membranes suffer a greater incidence of infection compared with those dialyzed against the more biocompatible synthetic membranes. A procedure that repeatedly induces defects in neutrophil function would be expected to place the patient at increased risk of infection.

An additional problem arises from lymphopenia, with CD4 cells sometimes approaching levels seen in patients infected with human immunodeficiency virus (HIV). Although the cause of the lymphopenia is undoubtedly multifactorial, the hemodialysis membrane has been shown to have an effect on NK cell function. These cells have the ability to spontaneously lyse target cells without deliberate prior sensitization and are important in providing resistance to viral infections and destroying tumor cells. When hemodialysis patients who had been dialyzed against PMMA membranes are switched to new cuprophane membranes, NK cell function deteriorates. This may explain, in part, why hemodialysis patients demonstrate immune defects and have a higher incidence of malignancy. Repeated bouts of production of hydroxyl radicals may also have oncogenic potential.

β_2-Microglobulin

Several lines of evidence suggest that chronic blood–membrane interactions are responsible for the development of bone and joint disease due to β_2-microglobulin–associated amyloidosis. β_2-Microglobulin deposits lead to symptoms such as carpal tunnel syndrome, painful lesions in long bones, and arthropathy in patients who have been on hemodialysis for more than 5 years. By 15 years of maintenance hemodialysis, many patients will be affected by this disorder. The incidence of β_2-microglobulin is greater in patients undergoing dialysis against complement-activating cellulosic membranes. The release of this substance from mononuclear cells following contact with cellulosic membranes is greater than release following contact with more biocompatible membranes. In a prospective study period of 18 months of a cohort of hemodialysis patients dialyzed with either complement-activating membranes or the biocompatible synthetic PMMA membrane showed that the levels of β_2-microglobulin in the group dialyzed with the cellulosic membrane were significantly higher than in patients treated with the PMMA membrane. The finding suggests that the polymerization of β_2-microglobulin is enhanced in the presence of activated neutrophils and provides a pathogenic mechanism for the higher levels and the increased incidence of arthropathy in patients dialyzed against complement-activating membranes.

Reuse of the dialysis membrane has the potential of impacting on the biocompatibility of the membrane both with respect to the removal of β_2-microglobulin as well as the loss of plasma components such as albumin. Because formaldehyde- and glutaraldehyde-reuse methods involve the use of bleach, the high-flux synthetic membranes may become more permeable to large molecules with multiple reuses. β_2-Microglobulin removal is enhanced with reuse, but there is also the possibility that essential plasma factors may also be removed. On the other hand, reuse of the hemodialyzer with peracetic acid–hydrogen peroxide decreases the permeability to larger molecules including β_2-microglobulin. Reuse of the membrane must be a factor with respect to its biocompatibility. Detailed discussion of the issue of β_2-microglobulin and amyloid in dialysis patients is found in Chapter 84, Part 1E.

Nutritional Status

Emerging evidence indicates that the nutritional status of the hemodialysis patient can be influenced by the biocompatibility of the membrane. Cytokines, such as IL-1, may be released from cells activated during dialysis with cuprophane. The elaboration of these proinflammatory substances may be responsible for a wide range of metabolic events, including protein catabolism. It has also been shown that for any given dose of dialysis, as determined by urea kinetics, protein intake by the patient increases to a greater extent in patients dialyzed with PAN membranes compared with those patients dialyzed with cuprophane membranes. Preliminary evidence suggests that increasing the dose of dialysis to levels that can be achieved only with the synthetic membranes translates into higher serum albumin levels, an important marker of nutritional status. Although the influences on nutrition undoubtedly are multifactorial, dialysis with cellulosic membranes results in numerous systemic adverse events involving the humoral and cellular components of blood, and these reactions have the potential for influencing nutritional status. In addition, the reduction in proinflammatory cytokines and acute-phase reactants by the use of biocompatible membranes may also impact on hepatic synthesis of albumin and improve albumin levels.

Acute Renal Failure

The implication that reactions occurring as a result of bioincompatibility are truly systemic in nature has led to a realization that vascular beds other than the lung may be affected. Several studies have suggested that treatment of acute renal failure by hemodialysis may prolong its course. Hemodynamic perturbations, which arise as the result of the treatment itself, may be responsible for this observation. However, other investigations suggest that dialysis membrane–induced complement activation may be implicated in the protracted course of acute tubular necrosis.

Acute tubular necrosis has been induced in rats by bilateral renal artery occlusion. Chronic exposure of the rats to cuprophane following such injury resulted in prolongation of the course of renal failure compared with animals exposed to PAN. A similar prolongation was seen in animals with acute tubular necrosis chronically exposed to zymosan, a substance known to activate complement as well. Reminiscent of the leukosequestration seen in the pulmonary vasculature on exposure to cuprophane, an increased number of neutrophils were seen in the renal parenchyma. The presence of infiltrating neutrophils in the kidney suggests that they may be playing a role in mediating further injury. Studies in humans with acute renal failure in the intensive care unit, matched for APACHE scores, demonstrated earlier recovery of renal function in those patients dialyzed with biocompatible membranes. Transplant patients with primary graft dysfunction also recover renal function when biocompatible membranes are used.

Morbidity and Mortality of Dialysis Patients

The effect of the biocompatibility of hemodialysis membranes on morbidity and mortality has not been examined in a prospective manner. However, there are retrospective studies that suggest that membrane biocompatibility does indeed impact on morbidity and mortality. In two groups of patients of comparable age, 9,000 dialysis sessions were reviewed. The patients dialyzed against cellulosic membranes were hospitalized for an average of 6.1 ± 1.1 days/patient/year compared with 2.1 ± 0.5 days/patient/year for those dialyzed against polyacrylonitrile membranes, a significant difference. Another study, in which multivariate analysis was adjusted for a variety of comorbid conditions, demonstrated that the annual mortality was 7% for patients dialyzed against the biocompatible synthetic membrane, polysulfone, compared with 20% for patients dialyzed against cellulosic membranes ($P < .001$). In a random sample of 6,000 patients from the USRDS, the mortality of patients treated with cellulosic, semisynthetic, and synthetic membranes was examined. The mortality of patients dialyzed against the latter two classes of membranes was 25% less than patients dialyzed against the cellulosic membranes. However, such a difference was not seen in an Italian study of 380 patients with 2 years of follow-up.

Loss of Residual Renal Function

Rapid loss of residual function has been noted in patients with chronic renal failure who are initiated on hemodialysis as compared with those who are initiated on peritoneal dialysis. A preliminary study using renal ablation in rats has demonstrated that glomerular filtration rate declines more rapidly in rats exposed to zymosan or cuprophane compared with animals exposed to PAN membranes. These experiments suggest additional clinical implications for the treatment of renal failure and implicate bioincompatible membranes and complement activation in causing adverse effects in the native kidney during hemodialysis.

Selected Readings

Bommer J, Wilhelmls OH, Barth HP, et al. Anaphylactoid reactions in dialysis patients: role of ethylene oxide. *Lancet* 1985;21:1382–1384.

An early report of the role of ethylene oxide in hypersensitivity reactions of dialysis patients.

Cheung AK, Henderson LW. Effects of complement activation by hemodialysis membranes. *Am J Nephrol* 1986;6:81–91.

Excellent review of the role of complement activation.

Craddock PR, Fehr J, Dalmasso AP, et al. Hemodialysis leukopenia: pulmonary vascular leukostasis resulting from complement activation by dialyzer cellophane membranes. *J Clin Invest* 1977;59:879–888.

The original article describing the effects of complement activation and hypersensitivity reactions to dialysis membranes.

Guiterrez A, Alvestrand A, Wahren J, et al. Effect of *in vitro* contact between blood and dialysis membranes on protein catabolism in humans. *Kidney Int* 1990; 38:487–494.

An important study that describes the role of the membrane in protein catabolism during blood–membrane interactions.

Hakim RM. Hemodialysis membrane biocompatibility. *Kidney Int* 1993;44:484–494.

An extensive review of the subject of biocompatibility.

Hakim RM, Breillatt J, Lazarus JM, et al. Complement activation and hypersensitivity reactions to dialysis membranes. *N Engl J Med* 1984;311:878–882.

Discussion of the role of complement in hypersensitivity reactions in different dialysis populations.

Hakim RM, Fearon DT, Lazarus JM, et al. Biocompatibility of dialysis membranes: effects of chronic complement activation. *Kidney Int* 1984;26:194–200.

Review of the kinetics of complement activation and the effects of chronic complement activation.

Hakim RM, Held PJ, Stannard DC, et al. Effect of the dialysis membrane on mortality of chronic hemodialysis patients. *Kidney Int* 1996;50:566–570.

A study based on data from the United States Renal Data System suggesting that the use of biocompatible membranes lowers mortality.

Hakim RM, Wingard RL, Parker RA. Effect of the dialysis membrane in the treatment of patients with acute renal failure. *N Engl J Med* 1994;331:1338–1342.

A randomized, prospective study in which survival of patients with acute renal failure dialyzed against biocompatible membranes was superior to the survival of those dialyzed against bioincompatible membranes.

Kant KS, Pollack VE, Cathey M, et al. Multiple use of dialyzers: safety and efficacy. *Kidney Int* 1981;19:728–738.

Report on the morbidity of hemodialysis patients treated with new and reused dialyzers.

Kaplow LS, Goffinet JA. Profound neutropenia during the early phase of hemodialysis. *JAMA* 1968;203:1135–1137.

The first description of the profound neutropenia seen with hemodialysis.

Parker TF, Wingard RL, Husni L, et al. Effect of the membrane biocompatibility on nutritional parameters in chronic hemodialysis patients. *Kidney Int* 1996;49: 551–556.

A randomized, prospective study in which survival of patients with acute renal failure dialyzed against biocompatible membranes was superior to the survival of those dialyzed against bioincompatible membranes.

Schulman G, Fogo A, Gung A, et al. Complement activation retards resolution of acute ischemic renal failure in the rat. *Kidney Int* 1991;40:1069–1074.

A study that suggests that parenchymal injury results from complement activation during hemodialysis.

Vanholder R, Ringoir S, Dhondt A, et al. Phagocytosis in uremic and hemodialysis patients: a prospective and cross-sectional study. *Kidney Int* 1991;39:320–327.

A description of white cell dysfunction and infection risk as a function of bioincompatibility.

E: β_2-Microglobulin Amyloidosis

Charles van Ypersele de Strihou and Michel Jadoul

β_2-Microglobulin amyloidosis (Aβ_2M) has emerged during the last 15 years as a specific complication of long-term uremia. It is observed mainly in patients on dialysis and exceptionally in patients with long-standing chronic uremia before the onset of renal replacement therapy.

PATHOLOGY

The histologic diagnosis of Aβ_2M rests on the positivity of deposits by Congo red staining with characteristic birefringence and immunostaining with a specific anti-β_2M antiserum. Aβ_2M has a strong affinity for peripheral joints and vertebrae. Its

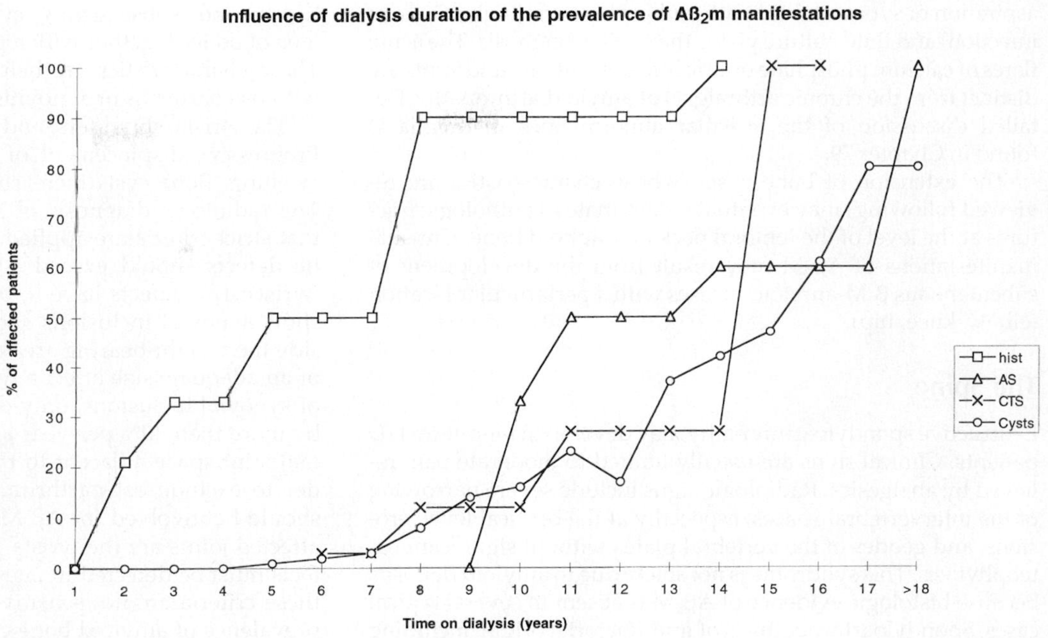

Figure 84.21. –□– Histologic articular Aβ_2M. (Data derived from Jadoul M, Garbar C, Noel H, et al. Histologic prevalence of β_2-microglobulin amyloidosis in hemodialysis: a prospective postmortem study. *Kidney Int* 1997; 51:928–932.) –△– Histologic systemic Aβ_2M. (Data derived from Miaata T, Jadoul M, Kurokowa K, et al. Beta-2 microglobulin in renal disease. *J Am Soc Nephrol* 1998;9:723–735.) –X– Operated carpal tunnel syndrome. (Data derived from van Ypersele de Strihou C, Jadoul M, Malghem J, et al., and the working party on dialysis amyloidosis. Effect of dialysis membrane and patient's age on signs of dialysis-related amyloidosis. *Kidney Int* 1991;39:1012–1019.) –○– Radiologic bone cysts. (Data derived from van Ypersele de Strihou C, et al. *Kidney Int* 1991;39:1012–1019.)

prevalence, assessed in pathologic studies, increases with dialysis duration (Fig. 84.21). It is much higher than suspected on clinical grounds; up to 20% to 30% of patients are affected within 2 to 3 years of hemodialysis (HD), and more than 90% beyond 7 years of HD, both in peripheral joints and spine. Distribution is uneven among joints; sternoclavicular joints and cervical vertebrae are more frequently involved than shoulders or dorsal vertebrae.

Deposits appear first in the cartilage and extend subsequently to the synovia, the joint capsules, and the attached tendons. Initially paucicellular deposits are eventually surrounded by macrophages. This latter stage often includes marginal bone erosions with the eventual formation of *para*-articular cysts filled with fibrous tissue and Aβ_2M.

The initial paucicellular Aβ_2M deposits are asymptomatic, whereas the late deposits invaded by macrophages are often associated with arthralgias. Infiltration of capsules and tendons may be initially evaluated and followed by ultrasonography. *Para*-articular bone defects are probably the first step leading to the development of typical bone cysts visible on radiographs.

Aβ_2M is also found in the vessels of various organs. Deposits are usually minute and asymptomatic. Rarely, after more than 10 years of HD, they expand and result in various symptoms determined by their location (Fig. 84.21). A review of all postmortem reports of systemic Aβ_2M shows preferential involvement of some organs: heart, 80%; gastrointestinal tract, 78%; lungs, 59%; liver, 41%; kidneys, 33%; and, more rarely, spleen, 5%.

CLINICAL PRESENTATIONS

The Carpal Tunnel Syndrome

The carpal tunnel syndrome (CTS) is usually the first manifestation of Aβ_2M. Its prevalence becomes clinically significant after more than 7 years of HD, and reaches ≈ 100% after more than 20 years (Fig. 84.21). Clinical characteristics are similar to those reported in nonuremic patients. Paresthesias of the palmar surface of the first three to four fingers develops with eventual sensory and motor loss as well as wasting of the thenar muscles. Pain typically exacerbates at night and during HD sessions. After several months, symptoms tend to become bilateral. Electromyography confirms the diagnosis. The differential diagnosis should consider uremic neuropathy and cervical root compression.

Surgery is often required to release the median nerve. The material removed during surgery contains mainly fibrous tissue and, in approximately 70% of the cases, β_2M amyloid deposits. Absence of Aβ_2M deposits in 30% of patients may be ascribed either to sampling problems or to the fact that Aβ_2M is not the only etiology of the CTS in HD patients: the vascular access and microcrystalline wrist arthritis have been incriminated; furthermore, the CTS is not uncommon, especially in middle-age women. Aβ_2M-related CTS should be strongly suspected in long-term (more than 7 years) HD patients, especially when its symptoms are associated with chronic arthralgias.

Peripheral Joints

The prevalence of arthralgias rises with HD duration. In a large series, shoulder pain and stiffness are noted as early as 5 years after HD onset and affect 50% and 100% of patients after 13 and 19 years HD, respectively. Arthralgias, initially insidious, follow a chronic, progressive course with bilateral involvement, starting usually in the shoulders and extending later to the hips, knees, and wrists. Joint mobility becomes restricted. Associated chronic tenosynovitis of the finger flexors causes mobility restriction, pain, and palmar swelling, and, in some patients, trigger fingers.

Joint effusions may develop and are usually of the low-inflammatory type unless hemarthrosis occurs as observed in a minority of patients. Synovial fluid aspiration may yield small synovial fragments in which β_2M-amyloid deposits may be recognized.

The differential diagnosis of arthralgias in HD patients includes infection, microcrystalline deposits of calcium phosphate or uric acid, and erosive enthesopathy associated with severe hyperparathyroidism. Monoarticular involvement suggests infection or microcrystalline deposition. Yet, septic arthritis may be polyarticular in HD patients, with low-grade or no fever. Needle aspiration of synovial fluid with leukocyte count (high in case of infection) and fluid culture yields the correct diagnosis. The acute flares of calcium phosphate or uric acid deposits around joints are distinct from the chronic arthralgias of amyloid arthropathy. Detailed discussion of the articular abnormalities in uremia is found in Chapter 79.

The extension of bone cysts (whose characteristics are reviewed following) may eventually culminate in pathologic fractures at the level of the femoral neck or scaphoid bone. Unusual manifestations of Aβ_2M may result from the development of subcutaneous β_2M-amyloid masses with a periarticular location (elbow, knee, hip).

The Spine

Destructive spondyloarthropathy may develop in long-term HD patients. Clinical signs are usually limited to moderate pain relieved by analgesics. Radiologic signs include severe narrowing of the intervertebral spaces, especially at the cervical level; erosions; and geodes of the vertebral plates without significant osteophytosis. This syndrome is not solely due to amyloid deposits because histologic evidence of Aβ_2M is absent in several typical cases. Spondyloarthropathy is of multifactorial origin, including age, mechanical stress, and/or severe hyperparathyroidism.

Destructive spondyloarthropathy should be differentiated from infectious discitis, whose clinical presentation is usually more acute with fever and increased serum C-reactive protein level. Magnetic resonance imaging shows normal disc signals in T1 and T2 sequences in destructive spondyloarthropathy, in contrast to the low-T1, high-T2 signals in infectious discitis.

Other unusual spinal complications are directly related to the presence of Aβ_2M masses in the epidural space and joints of the cervical spine, especially the atlanto-occipital joint. They include subacute or acute neurologic compression with quadriparesis, occipital nerve neuralgia, and pathologic fractures at the C1-C2 junction resulting from the extension of amyloid bone cysts.

Systemic (Nonosteoarticular) Manifestation

The small, vascular β_2M deposits detected in various organs are asymptomatic. Rarely, in very long-term HD patients, they expand and produce symptoms such as heart failure with pulmonary hypertension, gastrointestinal tract bleeding, bowel perforation, infarction or pseudoobstruction, chronic diarrhea, macroglossia, or lingual nodules. In the latter cases, HD duration exceeded 12 years.

DIAGNOSIS

Histology

In patients with gross clinical evidence of joint effusion, joint puncture with histologic examination of the collected fluid may reveal Aβ_2M (+) synovial fragments. In a small series of seven patients, the sensitivity of this test reaches 87%. Biopsy of joint tissues is usually unavailable in patients suspected of Aβ_2M. Biopsies of nonosteoarticular structures such as subcutaneous fat and rectum have proven insensitive.

Skeletal Radiograph

The radiologic pattern in Aβ_2M is similar to that observed in osteoarticular AL amyloidosis. It includes, first, swelling of soft tissues and, subsequently, cystic defects in the juxtaarticular area of bones together with a preserved or widened joint space. These characteristics are helpful in the differential diagnosis with osteoarthritis or synovitis.

The wrists, shoulders, and hips are preferentially involved. Progressive displacement of fat pads reflects the soft-tissue swelling. Bone cysts increase in size and number over time. The radiologic diagnosis of Aβ_2M is very specific, provided that strict criteria are applied. The diameter of individual cystic defects should exceed 10 mm (hip, shoulder) or 5 mm (wrist). The defects have to be located outside areas prone to show synovial inclusions such as the femoral neck and outside the weight-bearing area of the acetabulum. When defects of an adequate size affect a weight-bearing area or usual sites of synovial inclusions, only defects whose diameter increases by more than 30% per year are considered significant. A normal joint space adjacent to the bone defect is required in order to exclude osteoarthritic bone cysts. At least two joints should be involved for Aβ_2M to be diagnosed. When the two affected joints are the wrists, at least two significant bone defects must be detected in one of them. Although very specific, these criteria are not sensitive in the detection of Aβ_2M. The prevalence of amyloid bone cysts increases with HD duration (Fig. 84.21).

Ultrasonography

Capsulosynovial ("soft tissue") swelling precedes the development of bone cysts in Aβ_2M. Technical developments of joint ultrasonography (US) now permit an accurate assessment of the thickness of capsules and tendons. Ultrasonography has thus become a promising, more sensitive tool for Aβ_2M diagnosis.

A thickness of the supraspinatus tendon (rotator cuff) of more than 8 mm and of the femoral neck capsule of more than 7 mm strongly suggests Aβ_2M.

To be reliable, ultrasonographic evaluation of joints should take notice of several pitfalls. Measurements should be perpendicular to the bone surface, outside irregularities of bone outline. Anechogenic effusions should not be confused with tissue thickening. Of note, transient thickening may be observed in case of tendinitis or synovitis. Preliminary studies report a 79% to 100% sensitivity and 100% specificity for ultrasonographic evaluation.

SAP and β_2-Microglobulin Scintigraphy

SAP Scintigraphy

SAP, a nonfibrillar plasma glycoprotein synthesized by the liver, binds in a noncovalent way to almost all types of amyloid fibrils. This avidity has been used in scintigraphic studies with I^{123}-SAP in the various types of human amyloidosis.

In HD patients, SAP scintigraphy is poorly sensitive in the detection of hip or shoulder deposits but more reliable for wrist and knee deposits. Its specificity is disputed because splenic uptake is observed in up to 30% of long-term HD patients despite the rarity of histologic evidence of splenic Aβ_2M. The diagnostic significance of SAP scintigraphy is further limited by the fact that SAP binds to all types of amyloid. In elderly patients, it does not discriminate among Aβ_2M and other amyloidoses including those associated with age.

SAP scintigraphy has been advocated in order to quantify the amount of deposited amyloid. As yet, little histologic evidence supports this claim, an unsurprising conclusion when the difficulties related to histologic quantitation and the variable sensitivity of the scintigraphic method are taken into consideration. At present, SAP scintigraphy remains a research tool.

β_2-Microglobulin Scintigraphy

β_2M labeled by I^{131} has also been used in scintigraphic studies. Sensitivity for the detection of large amyloid deposits appears excellent; tracer enrichment has been demonstrated in resected amyloid tissue and isolated amyloid fibrils. Specificity is also adequate because no uptake has been documented in short-term HD patients or HD patients with inflammatory conditions. Aβ_2M scintigraphic images appear reproducible. The test is more sensitive than clinical or radiologic signs of Aβ_2M. The diagnostic value of β_2M scintigraphy for small, incipient amyloid deposits remains to be documented. Unfortunately β_2M scintigraphy cannot be used in patients with a significant renal function, because β_2M is readily excreted by the kidney.

I^{131}-labeled β_2M scintigraphy entails a substantial radiation exposure. ^{111}Indium-DTPA–labeled β_2M lowers this risk, allows easier labeling, and provides better optical resolution and stable images. Histologic validation of indium-β_2M scintigraphy is now required. The use of β_2M scintigraphy remains limited because the β_2M used in the procedure is derived from human urine with an attendant risk of viral contamination.

RISK FACTORS

Several risk factors for the development of Aβ_2M have been identified. The prevalence of both histologic evidence and clinical signs of Aβ_2M increases with duration of dialysis and age at the onset of therapy. There is evidence that dialysis with high-flux, noncomplement-activating membranes such as polyacrylonitrile (AN69) and (high-flux) polysulfone retards the onset of symptomatic Aβ_2M when compared with low-flux, complement-activating membranes such as cuprophane. By contrast, dialysis modality [hemodialysis, hemofiltration, or continuous ambulatory peritoneal dialysis (CAPD)] does not influence the risk of Aβ_2M. A single-center study has recently reported that the prevalence of Aβ_2M clinical signs has fallen substantially between 1988 and 1996. This observation raises the intriguing, as yet unconfirmed, hypothesis that other factors such as dialysate purity may play a role.

PATHOPHYSIOLOGY

β_2-Microglobulin Retention

Long-term β_2M retention is a prerequisite for the development of Aβ_2M, although no critical threshold has been demonstrated. No dialysis modality is able to clear the daily endogenous production of β_2M despite elevated plasma levels. The resulting accumulation of β_2M over the years probably accounts for the effect of dialysis duration on Aβ_2M prevalence. The higher removal rate of β_2M by high-flux rather than by low-flux membranes slows the accumulation of β_2M and might contribute to the delay of symptomatic Aβ_2M reported with polyacrylonitrile or polysulfone membranes. There is at present no evidence that low-flux, complement-activating membranes accelerate the onset of clinical β_2M by increasing β_2M production above that of high-flux, noncomplement-activating membranes.

β_2-Microglobulin Modification

Serum β_2M levels are not significantly different in patients with and without Aβ_2M. This finding, taken together with the observation that *in vitro* formation of β_2M fibrils requires very demanding experimental conditions, suggests that β_2M has to be modified to generate amyloid fibrils.

Advanced glycoxidative end-product (AGE) modification of β_2M has been demonstrated in β_2M-amyloid deposits. Some of the AGE adducts of β_2M such as pentosidine have the ability to cross-link proteins and might contribute to the formation of fibrils. Furthermore, *in vitro* evidence demonstrates that AGE-modified β_2M is endowed with chemotactic power, attracts monocytes, and stimulates derived macrophages to secrete proinflammatory cytokines. It also stimulates bone resorption with the eventual formation of bone cysts. Advanced glycoxidation may thus also contribute to the transformation of clinically silent Aβ_2M deposits, devoid of monocytes, into symptomatic Aβ_2M masses surrounded by macrophages.

Presence of Enhancing Factors

The identification of a variety of coprecipitants such as antiproteases in β_2M-amyloid deposits raises the hypothesis that factors modifying the local microenvironment may enhance β_2M-fibril formation.

The preferential accumulation of β_2M in osteoarticular tissues appears linked with the biochemical composition of such tissues and, in particular, with collagen type and the presence of highly sulphated glycosaminoglycans (especially keratan sulphate). Advanced glycoxidation of collagen also enhances its binding capacity for β_2M. Both factors are age dependent and might also account for the effect of patient age at the onset of dialysis on the development of Aβ_2M.

PREVENTION AND TREATMENT OF β_2-MICROGLOBULIN AMYLOIDOSIS

Prevention

Prevention relies at present on enhanced dialytic removal of β_2M by high-flux membranes. Whether drugs inhibiting advanced glycoxidation such as aminoguanidine are able to delay Aβ_2M remains to be tested.

Medical Treatment

Chronic arthralgias are best treated by paracetamol/dextropropoxyphene because nonsteroidal antiinflammatory drugs entail a substantial risk of gastrointestinal tract complications in fragile patients. Intraarticular steroids are helpful when a single joint is painful, but their transient effectiveness and the risk of infectious complications limit their long-term usefulness. If first-line therapies fail, low-dose oral prednisone (0.1 mg/kg per day) may prove effective.

Small, uncontrolled, and up until now, unconfirmed studies have reported a subjective improvement of arthralgias of a few patients switched from cuprophane HD to CAPD or high-flux HD with or without inclusion of a selective β_2M-adsorbent cartridge in the blood circuit.

Surgical Treatment

In patients with CTS, early surgery is recommended because the relentless course of Aβ_2M may otherwise lead to serious, irreversible neuromuscular impairment. It may be performed either classically or endoscopically, although experience with the latter procedure in HD patients remains limited. Recurrences should be rare if the surgeon is experienced and removes meticulously the tissue compressing the nerve.

Severe shoulder arthralgias have benefited at least transiently from various endoscopic or surgical procedures. These include

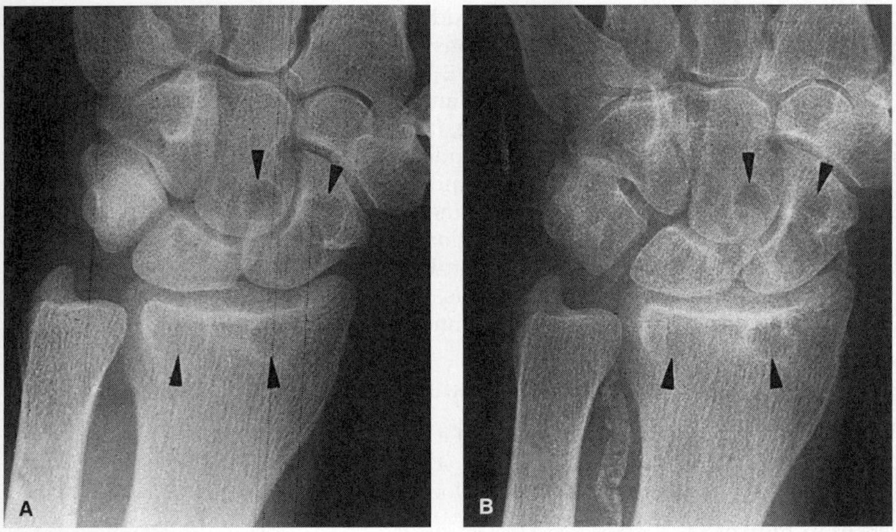

Figure 84.22. **A:** Multiple bone cysts in the left wrist and distal radius *(arrowheads)* at the time of renal transplantation. **B:** Unchanged aspect, 15 years later despite a normal graft function.

endoscopic resection of the coracoacromial ligament or arthroscopic synovectomy of the shoulder, open surgery with curettage of humeral cysts, and ceramic implantation together with resection of hypertrophied synovium and masses. More information on the long-term follow-up of such interventions is needed. Pathologic femoral fractures or spinal cord compression require joint prosthesis or vertebral fusion, respectively.

Renal Transplantation

Curative treatment by renal transplantation should be urgently considered in all patients with symptomatic Aβ_2M who are suitable candidates. Successful transplantation results in a striking, almost immediate improvement of Aβ_2M joint symptoms. Although this beneficial short-term effect has been ascribed to the high doses of steroids, it lasts in the long term despite the reduction and, sometimes, the interruption of steroid treatment. Progression of Aβ_2M deposits is stopped as demonstrated by the lack of progression of typical amyloid bone cysts (Fig. 84.22).

Regression of Aβ_2M deposits after transplantation remains a controversial issue. On the one hand, radiologic bone cysts do not regress after a 15-year follow-up (Fig. 84.22). Furthermore, histologic evidence of Aβ_2M is still detectable up to 10 years after a successful transplantation. Both observations argue against regression. On the other hand, the fall of labeled SAP uptake, 3 to 5 years after a successful transplantation, has been interpreted as evidence of significant Aβ_2M regression. Reconciliation of both views will probably require an alternative approach.

Selected Readings

Hou FF, Chertow GM, Kay J, et al. Interaction between β_2-microglobulin and advanced glycation end products in the development of dialysis related-amyloidosis. *Kidney Int* 1997;51:1514–1519.

The demonstration that unmodified β_2M binds more avidly in vitro to collagen-AGE than to unmodified collagen. This may account for the age effect in Aβ_2M.

Koch KM. Dialysis-related amyloidosis. *Kidney Int* 1992;41:1416–1429.

A good description of a patient with multiple typical Aβ_2M-related complications. Thorough discussion of the main therapeutic considerations.

Miyata T, Jadoul M, Kurokawa K, et al. Beta-2 microglobulin in renal disease. *J Am Soc Nephrol* 1998;9:723–735.

A thorough, up-to-date review with special emphasis on the role of AGEs in Aβ2M.

Tan SY, Irish A, Winearls CG, et al. Long term effect of renal transplantation on dialysis-related amyloid deposits and symptomatology. *Kidney Int* 1996;50: 282–289.

A longitudinal study by SAP scintigraphy, demonstrating a decrease in SAP uptake after renal transplantation.

van Ypersele C, Drüeke TB. *Dialysis amyloid.* Oxford: Oxford University Press, 1996:282.

A multiauthored monograph covering all aspects of Aβ_2M. Including, of special note, a thorough clinical description of the Aβ_2M arthropathy (by T. Bardin), a detailed presentation of the radiologic aspects of Aβ_2M (by B. Maldague et al.), a well-documented discussion of β_2M metabolism (by R. Deppisch et al.), and a review of the prevention and treatment of Aβ_2M (by C. van Ypersele and M. Jadoul).

F: Individualized Hemodialysis Treatment Regimens

Eduardo K. Lacson, Jr., and William F. Owen, Jr.

Methods of Measuring Dialysis Dose

There are more than 300,000 patients with end-stage renal disease (ESRD) in the United States; approximately 210,000 patients use hemodialysis as their primary treatment modality. Since the 1960s, the initial therapeutic goal has evolved from maintaining survival into improving morbidity, decreasing mortality rates, and enhancing the quality of life. Clearly the hemodialysis prescription is merely one facet of the complex management for ESRD and alone is insufficient to return the patient to normal health. However, the hemodialysis prescription is one of the most actionable components of care that is within the purview of the nephrologist.

METHODS FOR MEASUREMENTS OF DIALYSIS DOSE

An incomplete understanding of the pathobiology of uremia has led to multiple standards being proposed to measure dialysis dose and thus define adequate dialysis. Numerous compounds accumulate in ESRD and it is unclear which toxic solutes account for the morbidity. Because urea is easily measured and products of protein metabolism correlate with symptoms, it is used as a surrogate for the putative "uremic" toxins. The National Cooperative Dialysis Study (NCDS) is the landmark validation of intradialytic urea clearance and interdialytic urea accumulation rate as dialysis-associated measures of outcome. For the NCDS, small solute clearance was represented by the weekly time-averaged concentrations (TAC) of urea and larger molecular solute clearance was represented by dialysis treatment time. In a two by two factorial design, four groups of patients were followed for at least 6 months with hospitalization as the endpoint of the study. The patient group randomized to short dialysis time and higher TAC of urea had the worst morbidity, whereas groups with lower TAC of urea had fewer hospitalizations irrespective of the dialysis time. Subsequent outcome studies have linked other measures of urea clearance with mortality.

Using data from the NCDS, a subsequent mechanistic analysis examined the fractional urea clearance as a function of its distribution volume (Kt/V). The Kt/V is a pharmacokinetic construct based on the assumption that (a) urea is generated into and cleared from a single pool (sp), effectively intracellular and plasma water, and (b) urea clearance follows first-order elimination during the dialysis session, without significant intradialytic urea generation. In its most fundamental operational interpretation, K represents the clearance by the dialyzer membrane (liters/minute), t is the duration of the dialysis treatment session (minutes), and V represents the volume of distribution of urea (liters). The spKt/V can be determined from a single hemodialysis treatment using predialysis and postdialysis patient weight and blood urea nitrogen (BUN) levels, actual duration of the dialysis session, and the actual measured dialyzer clearance.

The double pool or equilibrated (eKt/V) measure of dialysis dose has been proposed in an attempt to account for the observed postdialysis urea rebound phenomenon as well as significant intradialytic urea generation. The eKt/V assumes that urea is generated in an intracellular compartment separated by the biologic cell membrane and equilibrates with the extracellular plasma water. The latter compartment is effectively cleared of urea during the dialysis procedure and is often limited by the movement of urea from the intracellular to the extracellular compartments. The gradient and equilibration rate are also affected by the actual blood flows into and out of these urea-rich cellular tissues. The eKt/V can be derived from the spKt/V using regression formulae (Daguirda's formula) or actual measurement of the equilibrated BUN at approximately 30 minutes after the dialysis procedure. The eKt/V can vary from 0.2 to 0.6 spKt/V units over the entire range of patient V.

The preferred method of calculating spKt/V is formal urea kinetic modeling (UKM). Computational software is required to generate the mandatory iterative solution to two equations solving for end dialytic urea distribution volume and interdialytic urea generation rate. Formal UKM is recommended for measuring the delivered dose of hemodialysis. Unlike other measures of dialysis dose, UKM permits the generation of hemodialysis prescriptions, calculation of the protein catabolic rate, and checks for errors in the measurement of the delivered dose of hemodialysis. However, because of the inherent complexity of the calculation and requirement for new software, not all nephrologists are willing or able to integrate formal UKM into their hemodialysis units.

An alternative method to calculate the spKt/V is to extrapolate this value from the predialysis and postdialysis BUN, the change in the patient's weight, and the duration of dialysis. A logistic regression formula (Daugirda's formula II) uses these components to measure solute removal by diffusive and convective transport. However, unlike formal UKM, this extrapolation of spKt/V does not provide error analysis and flexibility in establishing a hemodialysis prescription.

The urea reduction ratio (URR) is calculated by dividing the difference between the predialysis and postdialysis BUN concentration by the predialysis BUN concentration. The URR is the fractional removal of urea by diffusion in a single hemodialysis session. It does not account for the impact of ultrafiltration volume (convective clearance), is not prescriptive, and does not permit error analysis. However, URR has no less predictive power for patient mortality than Kt/V.

TARGETS FOR DIALYSIS DOSE

The interpretation of an adequate dose of hemodialysis has evolved as the goals of dialysis therapy advanced over the last 30 to 40 years. It has shifted from being the minimum amount of dialysis needed to sustain life, to the maximal amount of dialysis that can be supported by limited resources, provided in the most efficacious yet cost-effective manner, and translated into optimal survival, decreased hospitalizations, and improved quality of life. Therefore the operational definition of adequate hemodialysis dose has shifted toward intermediate outcomes. Unfortunately, no outcome studies have established an optimal hemodialysis dose. The current benchmarks for dialysis dose are derived from an evidence-based review of the existing literature with a consensus of best practice (when data are lacking). The National Kidney Foundation-Dialysis Outcomes Quality Initiative (NKF-DOQI) Clinical Practice Guideline for Hemodialysis Adequacy was published in 1997. The guideline recommended a *minimum* (in lieu of adequate) delivered hemodialysis dose of spKt/V in excess of 1.2 or URR in excess of 65%. Some investigators advocate even higher minimum doses of hemodialysis but these suggestions are not supported by adequate study design. Outcome-based target values for the eKt/V have not been established.

ELEMENTS OF THE HEMODIALYSIS PRESCRIPTION

In order to arrive at a specific hemodialysis regimen, the nephrologist has to consider both clearance (K) and time (t) modified according to a patient's volume of distribution (V) of urea. The V is inherent to the patient, so it is not readily actionable. Therefore the focus is the Kt product. Although the impact of t on outcome independent of spKt/V is uncertain, very few patients should be on hemodialysis for less than 3 hours unless the eKt/V is followed, too. Therefore beyond the limitations set on t, the urea clearance K can be manipulated by the choice of dialysis membrane, blood-flow rate, and dialysate-flow rate to achieve adequate spKt/V.

Membrane Characteristics

The surface area, pore size and configuration, thickness, and membrane charge and composition impact on the solute diffusivity. For any given dialyzer, the membrane's efficiency for a number of solutes including urea (representing small solutes) and vitamin B_{12} or β_2-microglobulin (representing larger solutes) is quantitated as the mass transfer coefficient (KoA). Functionally, this value is converted to K by the inclusion of two other factors: blood flow (range 200 to 500 ml/min) and dialysate flow (500 to 1,000 ml/min). KoA values are usually derived from *in vitro* studies using water instead of blood and are prone to machine calibration (flow rate) variance as well as the effect of cardiopulmonary recirculation. Therefore the KoA and consequently the derived K, are usually lower *in vivo*.

The dialyzer membrane also has an ultrafiltration coefficient (KUf) denoting the amount of ultrafiltrate formed per mm Hg of transmembrane pressure. Values greater than 8 ml/hr/mm Hg will require machines with special ultrafiltration controls to prevent massive fluid removal over short periods of time. Dialyzers with KUf values greater than 15 to 20 ml/hr/mm Hg are usually referred to as *high-flux dialyzers,* which allow substantial solvent drag. Similar to KoA, the *in vitro* KUf measurements are usually lower than *in vivo* measurements by 5% to 30%. Patients with low clearance rates despite adequate blood and dialysate flows may benefit from a switch to high-flux dialysis. The potential contribution of pore size and convective clearance can be substantial. Increased total solute clearance of as high as 10% to 20% for patients with large interdialytic weight gain (more than 4 kg) is not uncommon. The added benefit of improved clearance of larger-molecular-weight solutes is unknown.

Blood Flow

The clearance of solutes during dialysis may be functionally defined as the volumetric removal of solute from the patient's blood and is dependent on the blood flow into the dialyzer. The K of dialyzers can be maximized with blood flows of more than 300 ml/min, especially when using the high-efficiency and high-flux dialyzers. Higher blood flows permit better solute clearance, albeit not proportionally so. However, demanding more inflow than is permitted by the vascular access will increase blood recirculation, therefore limiting clearance. For example, a venous catheter can provide blood-flow rates of 200 to 450 ml/min but recirculation increases markedly at flows of more than 350 ml/min. Most primary and prosthetic arteriovenous fistulae can provide blood-flow rates of 350 to 550 ml/min when functioning adequately. Such internal vascular-access devices are the preferred hemodialysis access. Large-bore needles (15 gauge) may facilitate higher blood-flow rates.

Dialysate Flow

A similar functional relationship exists for the dialysate flow and diffusive clearance of solute from the blood. Therefore another way to improve the diffusion process is to increase the dialysate-flow rate. Using a high-efficiency dialyzer with adequate blood-flow rates (in excess of 300 ml/min), clearance may be augmented by 5% to 10% when dialysate-flow rate is increased from 500 to 800 ml/min. This is effected by an increase in KoA.

INDIVIDUALIZED HEMODIALYSIS PRESCRIPTION

The minimum hemodialysis dose for the majority of adult patients is well defined, and it is the responsibility of the nephrologist to ensure that the patients receive at least a delivered spKt/V of 1.2 or a URR of 65%. However, because of the inherent variability of the measurement, it is recommended that the target dose of hemodialysis should be at least a spKt/V of 1.3 and a URR of 70%. Having selected the target spKt/V, the next step in prescribing hemodialysis is determining the patient's V from anthropometric measures such as those described by Humes, Watson, or Chertow that incorporate variables such as weight, height, gender, and/or age. For a given V, an appropriate combination of dialysis membrane, achievable blood-flow rate, and dialysate-flow rate is selected to generate a prescribed K. The choices are usually impacted by the nephrologist's experience, hemodialysis unit options and operating costs, and the patient's condition and preference. Nomograms are available to aid in decision making. It then becomes a matter of arithmetic to solve for t once spKt/V, K, and V are determined.

The advantage of using formal UKM then becomes apparent because the nephrologist can attempt various combinations among the aforementioned treatment parameters to arrive at the desired spKt/V. In contrast, a more protracted manipulation of these parameters (based on a trial-and-error methodology) to achieve the desired hemodialysis dose is required when using the URR.

SPECIFIC CONSIDERATIONS FOR SPECIAL POPULATIONS

Specific factors elaborated in the following section may be considered when individualizing the hemodialysis prescription.

Residual Renal Function

Patients with residual renal function (RRF) may contribute substantial interdialytic solute and fluid removal to supplement delivered hemodialysis dose [such that there are patients with residual glomerular filtration rate (GFR) in excess of 5 ml/min who may tolerate twice weekly dialysis]. A simple arithmetic transformation of GFR to spKt/V is not physiologically accurate. Therefore UKM is needed to account for RRF in the dialysis prescription. It is common for dialysis patients to lose RRF with increasing vintage, and the decline is not always predictable. Therefore it is recommended to increase the frequency of serial monitoring for RRF and hemodialysis dose in these patients. Unless such monitoring is available, these patients are better served with thrice weekly dialysis sessions and target delivered spKt/V of at least 1.2 without inclusion of solute clearance from RRF.

Diabetes

There is no consensus from the available evidence that higher target dialysis dose is required in diabetic patients.

Patients with Large V

There is difficulty in reaching target spKt/V in patients with a large V, especially in those weighing more than 80 kg. Despite maximal available K (using high-flux/high-efficiency dialyzer with blood flows of 500 ml/min and dialysate flows of 800 ml/min) and tolerable t (5 hours in a compliant patient), some fail to reach spKt/V of 1.2 or greater. Because these patients often have large interdialytic weight gains, they benefit from increased fluid removal and enhanced convective solute clearance. This contribution to total solute clearance will not be appreciated by units relying solely on URR. In addition, the added survival advantage of improved nutrition, reflected by an expanded V, may provide decreased sensitivity to dialysis dose. It is recommended that the same minimum dialysis dose should be attempted in these patients up to the limits of patient preference and cost.

Race and Gender

The current evidence indicates improved age-adjusted survival for Asian-Americans, African-Americans, and women for similar dialysis doses compared with Caucasians and men. Although biologic differences may explain some of these differences in outcome, the beneficial impact of adequate nutrition may play a deciding role. The measure of dialysis dose, Kt/V, attempts to normalize solute clearance ($K \times t$) with V, a nutritional surrogate. The independent effect of Kt and V on survival confounds their mathematical coupling to measure dialysis dose. However, there is no evidence that a lower minimum hemodialysis dose is acceptable for all races and genders.

Dialyzer Reuse

The practice of dialyzer reuse is prevalent in more than 85% of centers in the United States with the motivation primarily being economic. Multiple outcome studies have shown inconsistent adverse outcomes associated with reuse. The variable findings may be a consequence of unappreciated decrements in KoA, and therefore reduced Kt/V. Some analyses have shown that reuse may decrease the delivered dialysis dose despite adherence to the standards for dialyzer reuse established by the by the Association for the Advancement of Medical Instrumentation. If no other reasons for inadequate hemodialysis dose can be appreciated, dialyzer reprocessing techniques should be reviewed.

Selected Readings

Lacson E, Wish JB. Hemodialysis adequacy. In: Henrich WL, ed. *Principles and practice of dialysis*, 2nd ed. Baltimore: Williams & Wilkins, 1999:99–113.

This chapter contains an overview of the issues involved in the determination of hemodialysis adequacy, including a critique of the National Cooperative Dialysis Study. It provides a discussion of barriers to adequate delivery of dialysis.

Lau TW, Owen WF. Hemodialysis adequacy. In: Brady HR, Wilcox CS, eds. *Therapy in nephrology and hypertension: a companion to Brenner and Rector's The Kidney*. Philadelphia: WB Saunders, 1999:535–550.

This chapter contains a detailed discussion of the technical aspects of measuring the dialysis dose. It provides a comprehensive review of the dose formulae and troubleshooting techniques.

Lowrie EG, Chertow GM, Lew NL, et al. The urea (clearance × time) product (Kt) as an outcome based measure of hemodialysis dose. *Kidney Int (in press).*

This study examines the weakness of current measures of dialysis dose associated with the mathematic linkage of Kt/V, and demonstrates that Kt and V are independent predictors of mortality. It provides a possible explanation for race and gender differences in mortality relative to measured dose of dialysis.

Lowrie EG, Laird NM, Parker TF, et al. Effect of hemodialysis prescription on patient morbidity: report from the National Cooperative Dialysis Study. *N Engl J Med* 1981;305:1176–1181.

This is the landmark, randomized, intervention trial that established the role of small solute clearance as a valid measure of adequate dialysis dose.

National Kidney Foundation's Dialysis Outcomes Quality Initiative's clinical practice guidelines for hemodialysis adequacy. *Am J Kidney Dis* 1997;30(Suppl 2):15–66.

This comprehensive literature analysis offers evidence-based recommendations of best clinical practice. It is the basis of current clinical performance measures for hemodialysis adequacy.

Owen WF, Lew NL, Liu Y, et al. The urea reduction ratio and serum albumin concentration as predictors of mortality in patients undergoing hemodialysis. *N Engl J Med* 1993;329:1001–1006.

This study validates the importance of nutrition as a stronger predictor of mortality than dialysis dose.

Parker TF. Trends and concepts in the prescription and delivery of dialysis in the United States. *Semin Nephrol* 1992;12:267–275.

Thoughtful review of the process involved in the prescription and delivery of dialysis.

Sehgal AR, Snow RJ, Singer ME, et al. Barriers to adequate delivery of hemodialysis. *Am J Kidney Dis* 1998;31:593–601.

This is a contemporary, population-based cohort study that quantifies the impact of patient- and dialysis-related technical factors on the inadequate delivery of dialysis. Specific variables for intervention are identified.

G: *Morbidity and Mortality in Hemodialysis*

Morrell M. Avram and Rajanna Sreedhara

Morbidity and mortality of hemodialysis patients are influenced by demographic profiles, comorbid clinical conditions that are present at the onset of dialysis, and the effects of the dialysis therapy itself. The median age of new end-stage renal disease (ESRD) patients continues to increase worldwide; the median age of patients beginning ESRD therapy in 1996 in the United States was 60 years. Advanced age, diabetic status, cardiac disease, and poor nutritional status negatively impact on the morbidity and mortality of patients. In addition, the dose of dialysis, membrane type, quality of water and of reprocessing procedures, type of dialysis delivery system, the physician and dialysis team support, and patient compliance all have the potential to influence morbidity and mortality.

DATA FROM THE UNITED STATES

Detailed information on the incidence, prevalence, treatment modality, morbidity, and mortality of ESRD patients in the United States has been made possible by the creation of the United States Renal Data System (USRDS) in 1988. The data are reported annually and are now readily available via the Internet at http://www.med.umich.edu/usrds/. Because the Medicare system does not achieve complete reporting of patient data before day 90 on hemodialysis, the USRDS defines the incident cohort to consist of those patients whose ninety-first day of therapy occurred during each specific year, and calculated death rates in 1-year increments from day 90. Caution must therefore be exercised in interpreting the Annual Data Reports because the death rate in the first 90 days is known to be higher than in the reminder of the first year.

From the latest available data released in 1998, the unadjusted mortality rate in the first year for the 1995 cohort in the United States was 23 per 100 ESRD patient-years at risk. The adjusted (for age, race, gender, and diabetic status) first-year death rate for all dialysis patients has progressively decreased from 36.3 per 100 patient-years at risk for the 1985 cohort to 24.6 per 100 patient-years at risk for the 1995 cohort. Diabetic ESRD patients have shown a greater decline in first-year death rates than nondiabetics over this time period, resulting in identical unadjusted 1-year survival probability of diabetic ESRD patients and patients with ESRD due to hypertension. Adjusted 2-year (62.7% for the 1994 cohort) and 5-year (29.3% for the 1991 cohort) survival rates of ESRD patients have also shown consistent improvement since 1985.

Despite the modest declines in death rates, the remaining life expectancy of dialysis patients remain significantly lower, between 17% and 39% for those of the age-, sex-, and race-matched U.S. population. The inclusion of healthier transplanted patients in the all ESRD calculations yields longer life expectancies compared with the dialysis-only calculations, especially in the younger age groups that have higher rates of transplantation. For patients older than age 70, the remaining life expectancy for all ESRD is about the same as that for dialysis-only patients, because transplants are much less frequent in these older age groups.

Age, Race, and Gender

As noted previously, the mean and median age of incident ESRD patients continues to increase in the United States. Death rates for 44- to 64-year-old patients are almost 2-fold higher than for 20- to 44-year-old patients. Death rates for patients 65 years and older are almost twice as high as for 44- to 64-year-old dialysis patients. The most consistent and greatest improvement in survival for dialysis patients has been seen in the younger-adult age ranges (20 to 44 years). First-year death rates for this age group decreased from 27.8 per 100 patient years at risk in 1985 to 10.2 per 100 patient years at risk in 1995. In the 45- to 64-year age group, the first-year death rate decreased from 29.4 to 17.2 per 100 patient years at risk; and in the 65- to 74-year age group, the death rate decreased from 40.4 to 30.3 per 100 patient years at risk in the same time interval (1985–1995). For pediatric ESRD patients (0 to 19 years), death rates have decreased from 20.1 per 100 patient years at risk in 1985 to 3.6 per 100 patient years at risk in 1995.

African-American dialysis patients in general have greater remaining life expectancies for all ages when compared with whites. However, there has been a consistent improvement in first-year mortality rates for white ESRD patients since 1985, except in 1987. Therefore the difference between African-American and white patient 1-year death rates has decreased from 12.3 to 4.6 per 100 patient years at risk between the 1985 and 1995 incident cohorts. There has also been a substantial improvement in survival for patients of other races since 1985, although the year-to-year trend has not been as consistent as it has been for white or African-American patients, in part because of random fluctuations due to small counts of patients.

There has generally been an improvement in survival for both males and females in each cohort since 1985. Until 1993, females had lower adjusted mortality at 1 year than males for each incident cohort. From 1985 through 1988 the difference was approximately 5 deaths per 100 patient years. This difference decreased to about 2 deaths per 100 patient years for the period 1989 through 1992. In the 1993, 1994, and 1995 cohorts the death rates have been similar for males and females (25.1 and 23.9 per 100 patient years, respectively, in the 1995 cohort).

Etiology of End-Stage Renal Disease

The proportion of diabetic ESRD patients in the United States has increased from 31.2% in 1988 to 40.6% in 1995. Both hospitalization rates and death rates for diabetic patients are higher than those for nondiabetics (see following discussion). Long-term studies have also confirmed increased mortality in diabetic ESRD patients (Fig. 84.23). The high morbidity and mortality among diabetic patients is largely related to their predialysis comorbidity such as increased prevalence of cardiac disease (30% to 60% higher prevalence of concentric left ventricular hypertrophy, ischemic heart disease, and heart failure). Diabetic patients are also at increased risk of malnutrition, peripheral vascular disease, and infection. As noted previously, there has been a greater improvement in the survival rates of diabetic ESRD patients over the past decade than in nondiabetic ESRD patients.

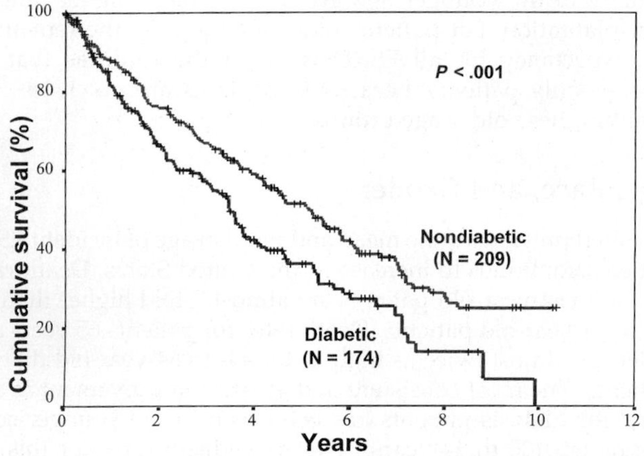

Figure 84.23. Observed survival in nondiabetic and diabetic hemodialysis patient (n = 383).

Five-year patient survival is best with chronic glomerular diseases and polycystic kidney disease and is intermediate with hypertension-induced renal disease.

DATA FROM OUTSIDE THE UNITED STATES

Whereas the USRDS collects data on more than 90% of ESRD patients in the United States, the response rate in the European Dialysis and Transplant Association (EDTA) registry is significantly less (approximately 65% to 75%). This underreporting may affect the accuracy of the information. Like in the United States, the mean age and the proportion of diabetic ESRD patients in Europe also continues to rise. The number of deaths in 1996 per 1,000 living patients in the EDTA registry on renal replacement therapy on December 31, 1996 was 120.

The Lombardy Regional Dialysis and Transplantation Registry was started in 1982 in Italy and has provided more complete information about ESRD patients in the region. Detailed comparisons have been made between patients in this registry against patients in the United States who started renal replacement therapy in 1986 and 1987. The unadjusted mortality risk for patients in the Lombardy registry was 56% lower than U.S. patients. However, when adjusted for demographic and comorbid conditions, the decrement in relative death risk was less pronounced (29% lower relative risk of death).

Adjusted survival in the first years of renal replacement therapy in Japan shows a 17% improvement at 1 year and 23% at 2 years for 45- to 64-year-old dialysis patients over the United States. However, this must be evaluated in the back drop of significantly lower transplantation rates in Japan (one-tenth the transplantation rate of the United States). The latest data from the Australia–New Zealand registry shows death rates of 15.6 per 100 patient years in Australia. The International Dialysis Outcomes and Practice Patterns Study (I-DOPPS) is ongoing to prospectively investigate the relationship between hemodialysis practice patterns and the outcomes of mortality, hospitalization, and the quality of life by collecting data relating to 3,000 hemodialysis patients randomly selected from 100 participating dialysis units in the United States, the United Kingdom, France, Italy, Spain, Germany, and Japan.

Several explanations have been proposed for the increased mortality rate of ESRD patients in the United States: (a) acceptance of patients for maintenance dialysis in the United States who are relatively older and/or have more comorbidity than patients in other countries; (b) failure to deliver an adequate dose of dialysis; (c) prevalent practice in the United States of dialyzer reuse that may expose hemodialysis patients to toxic chemicals and/or to dialyzers with decreased clearance; (d) failure in the United States to adequately meet the nutritional needs of hemodialysis patients; (e) differences in reporting to registries in other countries, completeness, accuracy of relevant patient comorbidity and outcomes; and (f) differences in transplantation rates. As noted previously, there has been a progressive decline in death rates in the United States since 1985. A possible explanation for the decline in mortality in the United States may be changes made in dialysis therapy. During this time period the renal provider community has given increasing attention to the dose of dialysis that is delivered to hemodialysis patients. In addition, there have been changes in dialysis equipment, including a shift from cellulosic to synthetic hemodialysis membranes and improved connection devices for peritoneal dialysis. The use of erythropoietin also began during this period. As improvements in delivered care continue to spread through the com-

TABLE 84.9. Selected Total Hospital Admissions by Diagnostic-Related Groups (DRG) for 1996 (One DRG Code Per Admission)

Description	Type	DRG Code(s)	Admissions
Noncardiac Vascular Procedures			
Other vascular procedures	P	478	31,030
Other circulatory system OR procedures	P	120	19,515
Amputation for circulatory system disorders	P	113, 114	8,329
Cardiac Procedures			
Coronary bypass	P	106, 107	1,852
Permanent cardiac pacemaker implant	P	115, 116	1,320
Other cardiovascular procedures	P	110, 112	4,286
Cardiovascular-Related Medical Admissions			
Acute MI, discharged alive	M	121, 122	3,570
Acute MI, expired	M	123	1,069
Circulatory disorders except acute MI, with cardiac catheter	M	124, 125	4,307
Heart failure and shock	M	127	22,721
Cardiac arrest, unexplained	M	129	301
Peripheral vascular disorders	M	130	3,962
Atherosclerosis	M	132	3,493
Cardiac arrhythmia and conduction disorders	M	138	4,853
Angina pectoris	M	140	2,171
Syncope and collapse	M	141	1,527
Chest pain	M	143	2,502
Other circulatory system diagnoses	M	144	16,200
Pulmonary edema and respiratory failure	M	087	2,915
Infections			
Respiratory infections and pleurisy	M	079, 089	12,032
Septicemia	M	416, 417	11,908
Cellulitis	M	277	2,654
OR procedure for infectious and parasitic diseases	P	415	4,344
Gastrointestinal			
Gastrointestinal hemorrhage	M	174	7,261
Esophagitis and other digestive disorders	M	182	8,251
Other			
Cerebrovascular and nerve disorders	M	014, 015, 018	10,049
Nutritional and miscellaneous metabolic disorders	M	296	9,835
Respiratory system diagnosis with ventilator support	M	475	2,742

Data from United States Renal Data System. *USRDS 1998 annual data report*. Bethesda, MD: The National Institutes of Health, National Institute of Diabetes and Digestive and Kidney Diseases, 1998.

M, medical; MI, myocardial infarction; OR, operating room; P, procedure.

munity of renal providers, there may be continued improvements in survival across the nation.

MORBIDITY

In the United States, total hospital admission rate in hemodialysis patients for 1994 through 1996 was 1.94 per patient year at risk (2.27 for diabetics, and 1.76 for nondiabetics). The total hospital days per patient year at risk was 15 days per hemodialysis patient (18 days for diabetics, and 13 days for nondiabetics). Younger patients tend to have less hospitalization. Selected total hospital admissions by diagnosis-related groups are shown in Table 84.9. Vascular access–related problems account for the highest number of in-hospital procedures in hemodialysis patients. Cardiovascular diseases and infections are the most common medical causes of hospitalization among hemodialysis patients. The total spending for ESRD in 1996 in the United States was $14.6 billion.

CAUSES OF DEATH

Cardiovascular Diseases

Cardiovascular diseases account for approximately 50% of deaths in hemodialysis patients (Table 84.10). The incidence of cardiac death is five to ten times higher than that of age-matched general population. The predominant cause of cardiac death is cardiac arrest (sudden death) of uncertain etiology,

TABLE 84.10. Death Rates by Cause of Death and Diabetes in Hemodialysis Patients in the United States (Per 1,000 Patient Years at Risk)
Year group: 1994–1996, at risk until death, transplantation, or end of year

	All	(%)	Diabetic	(%)	Nondiabetic	(%)
All Causes	227	100	259.6	100	201.9	100
Cardiovascular	**109.7**	**48.3**	**134.8**	**51.9**	**93**	**46.1**
Acute myocardial infarction	19.8	8.7	25.8	9.9	16	7.9
Atherosclerotic heart disease	8.5	3.7	10.6	4.1	7.1	3.5
Cardiomyopathy	9	4.0	9.1	3.5	8.7	4.3
Cardiac arrhythmia	13	5.7	16.1	6.2	11	5.4
Cardiac arrest	43.1	19.0	53.6	20.6	36.2	17.9
Pulmonary edema	2.2	1.0	2.3	0.9	2	1.0
Cerebrovascular disease	12.4	5.5	16.1	6.2	10.1	5.0
Valvular heart disease	1.7	0.7	1.2	0.5	1.9	0.9
Infections	**29.8**	**13.1**	**34.7**	**13.4**	**26.4**	**13.1**
Septicemia	21.4	9.4	27.7	10.7	17.4	8.6
Pulmonary infection	5.2	2.3	5.1	2.0	5.2	2.6
Viral infection	0.3	0.1	0.3	0.1	0.3	0.1
Acquired immunodeficiency syndrome	1.9	0.8	0.3	0.1	2.7	1.3
Other infection	1	0.4	1.3	0.5	0.8	0.4
Other causes	**59.1**	**26.0**	**59.1**	**22.8**	**57.8**	**28.6**
Hyperkalemia	4.2	1.9	5.2	2.0	3.7	1.8
Pericarditis	0.3	0.1	0.3	0.1	0.3	0.1
Cachexia	2.2	1.0	2.2	0.8	2.2	1.1
Gastrointestinal hemorrhage	2.4	1.1	2.2	0.8	2.4	1.2
Other hemorrhage	1.9	0.8	1.3	0.5	2.1	1.0
Malignant disease	8.1	3.6	4.8	1.8	9.7	4.8
Other cause	26	11.5	26.4	10.2	25.2	12.5
Unknown cause	14	6.2	16.7	6.4	12.2	6.0
Information missing	**28.5**	**12.6**	**30.8**	**11.9**	**25.1**	**12.4**
Years at risk	428,173		146,856		273,765	
Patients	562,152		199,616		351,772	

Data from United States Renal Data System. *USRDS 1998 annual data report.* Bethesda, MD: The National Institutes of Health, National Institute of Diabetes and Digestive and Kidney Disease, 1998.

with myocardial infarction accounting for only one-fifth of cardiac deaths. Cardiovascular deaths are observed at all ages in the hemodialysis population and, when expressed as a percentage of total deaths, increase only modestly, from 35% to 49%, when patients younger than 20 years are compared with those older than 65 years.

Cardiovascular disease in dialysis patients is observed at an earlier age than in the general population. In addition to increased incidence, the rate of deterioration of cardiac disease is also higher among dialysis patients. The probability among dialysis patients of requiring hospitalization for a myocardial infarction or angina is 10% per year. Admission for pulmonary edema also occurs with a probability of 10%.

A prospective, multicenter Canadian study of 433 patients followed for a mean of 41 months demonstrated a high prevalence of cardiac diseases at the onset of ESRD therapy: 31% of patients had heart failure, 19% angina, 14% coronary artery disease, 8% peripheral vascular disease, and 7% arrhythmias. Echocardiographic abnormalities were even more frequent: 74% of patients had left ventricular hypertrophy, and 15% systolic dysfunction. In this study, age, diabetes, heart failure, peripheral vascular disease, and systolic dysfunction independently predicted death in all time frames. Coronary artery disease was associated with a worse prognosis in patients with heart failure at baseline. High left ventricular cavity volume and mass index were independently associated with death after 2 years. It has been reported that left ventricular hypertrophy correlates positively with age and systolic blood pressure, and negatively with the duration of hemodialysis therapy and hematocrit. A USRDS study of new and established dialysis patients also showed that cardiac disorders were already present in a large fraction of patients when they began dialysis. Similar data has been reported for patients in most registries.

The prognosis is poor for patients with congestive heart failure unresponsive to optimization of volume status. Under these conditions, 2-year survival rates have been reported as low as 33% (as opposed to 80% in those without heart failure). Although it is difficult to distinguish on clinical grounds alone, slightly more than half of the patients with congestive heart failure have dilated cardiomyopathy by echocardiographic analysis, with the rest having hypertrophic-hyperkinetic disease.

In a study of 34,189 dialysis patients who were hospitalized for a first myocardial infarction after the initiation of renal replacement therapy (years of study, 1977 to 1995), the overall mortality rates were 59.3% within 1 year, 79.3% within 2 years, and 89.9% within 5 years. In this study, 29% of myocardial infarctions occurred within 1 year of initiation of dialysis and 52% within 2 years. Patients who were older or had diabetes had higher mortality than patients without these characteristics. These numbers are in contrast to the general population, whose cardiovascular death rates have declined recently. In addition to antecedent disease, three additional factors common in dialysis patients may promote the development of coronary disease and enhanced cardiovascular mortality: (a) hypertension, which is present in approximately 80% of patients at the onset of dialysis and, with effective fluid control, in approximately 25% to 30% at the end of the first year; (b) left ventricular hypertrophy, due to both hypertension and to chronic anemia; and possibly, (c) hyperlipidemia.

The specific role that hemodialysis *per se* contributes to cardiovascular disease remains to be elucidated because substantial irreversible cardiac disease is already present on entry to the dialysis program. In fact, only a minority of patients develop cardiomyopathy after starting dialysis therapy. Of those patients in whom cardiac function deteriorates, frequent changes in blood volume (due to interdialytic weight gain), high blood flow through dialysis fistulas, recurrent metabolic changes as a result of blood–membrane interactions, and dialysis-related hypoxia may play a role in promoting cardiovascular disease. Other hemodynamic/metabolic derangements of uremia, such as anemia, hypertension, state of secondary hyperparathyroidism, calcium phosphate deposition in tissues, aluminum and iron overload, β_2-microglobulinemia, hyperlipidemia, and such abnormalities in endothelial growth factors as advanced glycosylation end-products, also have potential adverse effects on cardiovascular morbidity. Cardiac disease in uremic patients is discussed in detail in Chapter 70, Part 2.

Lipid Abnormalities

The primary finding in chronic renal failure and dialysis is hypertriglyceridemia; the total cholesterol concentration is usually normal (probably reflecting malnutrition in these patients). The elevation in triglyceride levels is due to diminished clearance. Both an alteration in the composition of circulating triglycerides (which become enriched with apolipoprotein C-III) and, perhaps later, reductions in the activity of lipoprotein lipase and hepatic triglyceride lipase may contribute to the decrease in triglyceride removal. Secondary hyperparathyroidism and retained circulating lipase inhibitor may be responsible for diminished hepatic lipase and lipoprotein lipase activity. Other major lipid/abnormalities include a modest decline in high-density lipoprotein (HDL) cholesterol, elevated plasma levels of lipoprotein(a), marked reduction in hepatic clearance of postprandial chylomicron remnants, and increased oxidative modification of low-density lipoprotein (LDL) cholesterol. The hyperlipidemia of uremia is discussed in detail in Chapter 74, Part 2.

Dietary modification may be helpful for the hypertriglyceridemia of chronic renal failure; drug therapy is not usually given. The fibric acids, such as clofibrate and gemfibrozil, are most effective in lowering triglyceride levels. There is, however, no proven long-term benefit of drug therapy and these agents are associated with an increased risk of rhabdomyolysis in the presence of renal failure. In the infrequent patient with hypercholesterolemia, a 3-hydroxy-3-methyl-glutaryl-coenzyme A (HMG-CoA) reductase inhibitor can effectively and safely (at least in the short term) lower the plasma cholesterol concentration to or near acceptable levels. Two additional therapeutic modalities that have been evaluated are erythropoietin, which is commonly given to treat the anemia of chronic renal failure, and high-flux hemodialysis. Erythropoietin appears to have a modest hypolipidemic effect, lowering total cholesterol and triglyceride levels by 7% to 10%. The lipid-lowering effects of high-flux hemodialysis may be due to removal of inhibitors of lipoprotein lipase or decreased production of reactive oxygen species and other cytoactive products of complement activation, thus decreasing the oxidation of LDL (see following discussion).

Peripheral Vascular Disease

Atherosclerosis is common in hemodialysis patients and results in cardiac, neurologic, and peripheral vascular disease. Vascular disease results in hospitalization for bypass surgery as well as amputation, but also contributes substantially to morbidity resulting from poorly healing wounds, especially in the extremities of diabetic patients. Soft-tissue calcification exacerbates the vascular disease associated with some patients undergoing dialysis. The etiology of atherosclerosis is multifactorial and may relate to hypertension, lipid abnormalities, parathyroid hormone (PTH), and the type of dialysis membrane used. Patients with ischemic renal disease, most of whom tend to have severe generalized atherosclerotic vascular disease burden, have the highest cardiovascular morbidity and mortality: twice the mortality risk of patients with other renal diseases (excluding diabetes mellitus).

Cerebrovascular Disease

Cerebrovascular accidents (CVAs) also remain a common cause of morbidity in these patients. Death rates from CVAs declined in the 1980s due to improved antihypertensive therapy. Still, cerebrovascular diseases contributed to 5.5% of deaths in dialysis patients from 1994 to 1996. It has been suspected that CVAs may be under-reported as a cause of death due to withdrawal from dialysis that may happen after a patient suffers stroke.

Intracranial hemorrhage occurs more commonly in the hemodialysis population than in the general population because of uremic platelet dysfunction, the high prevalence of hypertension, and the requirements for anticoagulation during treatment. Aluminum-related encephalopathy is much less common than in the past with the use of water treatment systems that produce aluminum-free dialysate and with the avoidance or reduction of aluminum-containing phosphate binders. Uremic polyneuropathy or encephalopathy is related to neglected uremia or inadequate dialysis and should be less common with the timely initiation of treatment and appropriate monitoring of dialysis delivery. The restless leg syndrome is a vexing manifestation of uremic neuropathy that is more prevalent among diabetics. Burning dysesthesia of the feet caused by thiamin deficiency should be prevented by the routine replacement of water-soluble vitamins removed by the hemodialysis process.

Infection

Infection accounts for 20% of all deaths in the 20- to 44-year age group, but for only 14% and 12% of deaths in the 45- to 64-year and 65-years-and-older age groups, respectively. These figures may be an underestimation because a detailed chart analysis of causes of death suggested that infection may account for up to 40% of the deaths in this patient population, particularly in younger age groups. Infections also cause a significant number of hospitalizations among both hemodialysis and peritoneal dialysis patients. Exposure to infectious agents can potentially occur in the hemodialysis setting but, additionally, fundamental abnormalities in the phagocytic system including defects in cellular immunity, neutrophil function, and complement activation exist in the uremic patient. A number of factors have been reported to affect immune status, including iron stores, PTH, phosphorus, and membrane biocompatibility. Infections are usually due to common bacterial pathogens (e.g., *Staphylococcus aureus*) and are often related to the vascular access. Septicemia makes up more than 75% of the infection category.

Other Causes

Withdrawal from and withholding of dialysis may be responsible for as much as 20% of deaths in dialysis patients. There usually appears to be a proximate reason to consider foregoing dialysis. As an example, reasons for foregoing dialysis noted on the USRDS death notification form in order of declining percentage in 1991 and 1992 were: (a) failure to thrive (42%); (b) medical complications (35%); and (c) dialysis access failure (4%). Certain comorbid conditions are also frequently present near the time of withdrawal, including diabetic gastropathy, neuropathy, the need for surgery, neoplastic disease, neurologic deterioration, worsening quality of life, and increasing pain. In addition, dialysis is sometimes begun as a therapeutic trial in an attempt to improve an extremely poor quality of life; it is subsequently discontinued if no improvement occurs. For some patients, the reason for withdrawal is simply the overall burden that long-term dialysis places on their lives.

One to four percent of deaths in dialysis patients are attributable to malignancy. Previous studies have suggested an increased risk of certain malignancies in the dialysis population compared with the general population. Although this may be due to the effect of uremia or a side effect of dialytic therapy, the USRDS Case Mix studies found a diagnosis of malignancy in 9% of patients at initiation of therapy, suggesting that acceptance of patients with malignancy is not uncommon. Detailed discussion on cancer and uremia is found in Chapter 81.

ROLE OF DIALYSIS PRESCRIPTION AND DELIVERED DIALYSIS DOSE

Several lines of evidence suggest that the high mortality rate in the United States may be due to the decreased dose of delivered dialysis. The landmark in experimental dialysis studies, the National Cooperative Dialysis Study (NCDS), was reported in 1983. The study quantified the dose of dialysis and its correlation with patient outcomes. The NCDS used the time-averaged concentration of urea, a measure of the average weekly blood urea concentration, as a marker for the dose of dialysis delivered in patients whose dietary intake was strictly maintained between 0.8 and 1.4 g/kg/day. In the setting of this defined protein intake, groups of high (BUN 110 to 130 mg/dl) or low (BUN 60 to 80 mg/dl) time-averaged concentrations of urea were achieved by varying urea clearance by manipulating blood-flow rate, dialysate-flow rate, and/or the surface area of the dialyzer. Under these conditions, poor urea clearance was associated with increased risk of medical complications or hospitalizations. Second in importance only to a low urea clearance was a low value of protein catabolic rate (PCR), a surrogate for dietary protein intake, although there were few observations of adequate dialysis delivery in this group. Furthermore, because PCR was not a truly independent variable, the NCDS data did not allow conclusions regarding whether therapeutic manipulations of PCR affected patient outcome.

A later evaluation of the NCDS data introduced the concept of fractional urea clearance, Kt/V, where K represents the urea clearance of the dialyzer obtained from the manufacturer (milliliters/minute), t represents the time on dialysis (minutes), and V represents the distribution space of urea (in milliliters, which is approximately equal to the total body water). When Kt/V and PCR were related to adverse effects in the NCDS patient population, practical guidelines for the kinetic prescription of dialysis were defined that continue to serve as the basis for the application of urea kinetic modeling as performed today. In this reanalysis of the NCDS data, it was suggested that poor medical outcome was a discontinuous step function of Kt/V, with Kt/V less than 0.9 associated with a poor outcome relative to treatments with Kt/V 0.9 to 1.5. Others, however, have argued that medical outcome is a continuous function of Kt/V, with an asymptotic decrease in dialysis failure as dialysis dose is increased to Kt/V more than 1.0.

Extrapolating from the NCDS data to current dialysis practice is difficult for several reasons. The NCDS was performed before the widespread dissemination of current hemodialysis technologies such as ultrafiltration control, bicarbonate dialysate, variable dialysate sodium programming, and biocompatible dialysis membrane. Furthermore, demographic and comorbidity characteristics of patients in the NCDS differed significantly from the current ESRD patients. For example, diabetics and patients over the age of 70 were excluded from the NCDS. Finally, morbidity, and not mortality, was the principal outcome.

The complicated calculation of the Kt/V requiring the use of advanced mathematics had retarded its acceptance and widespread use. However, computer software programs are now commonly available. When supplied with simple clinical information such as predialysis and postdialysis weights, ultrafiltration volume, hematocrit, and predialysis and postdialysis blood urea nitrogen (BUN), these programs will perform the necessary computations and print the Kt/V, PCR, and other data in a readable format that can be used to alter the dialysis prescription if necessary. Furthermore, the newest hemodialysis machines have built-in computers that gather and store clinical data during dialysis such as blood pressure, blood-flow rate, dialysis-flow rate, nursing entries of body weight, and the like.

Another measure of dialysis that has been used by several investigators is the urea reduction ratio (URR). The URR is one minus the ratio of the postdialysis over predialysis BUN expressed in percentages. Several investigators have shown correspondence between Kt/V and URR, whereas some have shown a mathematic relationship.

Both of the aforementioned approaches to the scientific prescription of dialysis use urea as a surrogate marker to assess (Kt/V or URR) the adequacy of treatment. The rationale is based on the observations that urea is easily measured and well studied and, like several potential uremic toxins, is a product of protein metabolism. Urea has the additional advantage of serving as a marker of net protein metabolism, which allows for the quantitation of protein intake in the noncatabolic patient. However, it must be pointed out that urea by itself may not be a uremic toxin.

There are several reports of single center, multicenter, and registry studies to assess the mortality risk by dose of dialysis. In a prospective study of 130 patients in a single, outpatient dialysis center, the dose of dialysis (Kt/V) was increased from 0.82 to 1.33 over 4 years. The gross annual mortality rate in the dialysis unit decreased from 22.8% in 1988 to 9.1% in 1991. Even when changes in patient characteristics were accounted for by the measurement of standardized mortality rate (SMR), there was a striking decrease in the mortality rate, from 1.03 in 1988 to 0.61 in 1991. In addition, the number of hospital days per patient year also declined from 15.2 days/patient/year in 1988 to 10.3 days/patient/year in 1991.

Others analyzed retrospectively the demographic characteristics, mortality rate, duration of hemodialysis, serum albumin concentration, and URR in 13,473 patients treated from October 1, 1990, through March 31, 1991. As compared with patients with URR of 65% to 69%, patients with values below 60% had a higher risk of death during follow-up (odds ratio, 1.28 for URR of 55% to 59% and 1.39 for URR below 55%). Fifty-five percent of the patients had URR below 60%. In this study the duration of dialysis by itself was not predictive of mortality. The serum albumin concentration was a more powerful (21 times greater) predictor of death than URR, and 60% of the patients had serum albumin concentrations predictive of an increased risk of death (values below 4.0 g/dl). The odds ratio for death was 1.48 for serum albumin concentrations of 3.5 to 3.9 g/dl and 3.13 for concentrations of 3.0 to 3.4 g/dl. Diabetic patients had lower serum albumin concentrations and URR than nondiabetic patients. More recently, these investigators have reported that the effects of dialysis dose on survival may be different across demographic features such as gender and race.

A special study of the USRDS (the Case Mix Adequacy Study [CMAS]) evaluated more than 2,300 patients who were alive on December 31, 1990, selected randomly from 347 dialysis units to assess the effects of delivered dialysis dose on patient mortality. All of these patients had been on hemodialysis for at least 12 months (so chosen to minimize the impact of residual renal function). Demographic data, anthropometric measures, comorbidity profile, and laboratory markers of nutrition and dialysis adequacy were collected. Mean delivered Kt/V was 1.10 and URR was 60.1%. After adjusting for 21 covariates, a 5% increase in URR was associated with an 11% lower mortality risk, whereas a 0.1 unit increase in Kt/V was associated with a 7% lower mortality risk. Kt/V and URR correlated with each other ($r = 0.96$). In the analysis of comorbidity, statistically significant and quantitatively notable effects on mortality included age, race, diabetes, nutritional status (both undernourished and serum albumin), inability to ambulate, congestive heart failure, coronary heart disease, cerebrovascular disease, peripheral vascular disease, and chronic obstructive pulmonary disease. In addition, it was reported that at Kt/V values more than 1.3 and URR values more than 70%, the impact of dialysis dose on mortality may be less striking. In this CMAS, the effect of dialysis dose was even more prominent in diabetic hemodialysis patients (i.e., Kt/V and mortality had steeper slopes for diabetic than for nondiabetic patients). Also, each skipped dialysis treatment led to 8% reduction in monthly Kt/V and accounted for a 14% increase in mortality risk (i.e., the effect of a missed treatment was almost twice the linear effect).

Studies in both Germany and the United States have documented the relationship between shorter dialysis time and poorer outcome. Patients dialyzed fewer than 3.5 hours three times per week have approximately twice the mortality risk compared with patients dialyzed 4 or more hours three times per week. Thus time on dialysis may have an independent effect on patient survival even with adequate URR or Kt/V because of differential effects of time on small versus large molecular clearance during dialysis.

Studies comparing survival for new ESRD patients accepted for hemodialysis between 1982 and 1987 have found striking geographic differences. Five-year survival rates for patients beginning renal replacement therapy in 1982 were 61%, 59%, and 40% for Japan, Europe, and the United States, respectively. These differences were particularly significant for patients who were 60 years or older and did not appear to be based solely on differences in acceptance or transplantation rates for these populations or on a higher proportion of elderly or diabetic patients in the United States, because when adjusted for age and diabetes, the 5-year survival rate in Japan was 54% and in Europe, 48%. It must be pointed out that the mortality rates in the United States have progressively improved since 1985 and the differences may be much less at the present time than previously reported.

When European and U.S. ESRD patients were compared using data from 1986 to 1988, dialyzers selected in Europe had at least 20% larger surface areas, and dialysis time was nearly 25% greater than in U.S. patients (Table 84.11). The median extracorporeal blood-flow rate for the U.S. population was 250 ml/min. Although data for blood-flow rate were not available from the European registry given the larger dialyzer size and longer dialysis treatment time, even blood-flow rates of 160 ml/min would have resulted in a larger dose of dialysis than was typical for the United States. In fact, there is little reason to believe that European blood-flow rates were different from those prescribed in the United States. Thus it is almost certain that the prescribed dose of dialysis was substantially higher in Europe than in the United States in 1986 to 1988. It is hypothesized that the higher mortality of dialysis patients in the United States occurred, in large part, because of a lower dose of delivered dialysis. This view is now supported by numerous observations linking low doses of delivered dialysis with poor patient outcome as detailed previously.

TABLE 84-11. Comparison of European Dialysis and Transplantation Association (EDTA) and U.S. Dialysis Prescriptions[a]

	EDTA	United States
Dialyzer surface area (m^2)	1.20	0.97
Prescribed dialysis (hr/wk)	11.3	9.0
Extracorporeal blood flow (ml/min)	N/A	250
Prescribed urea clearance per week (L)	132	101

[a] Median data 1986–1988. Dialyzer reuse was 10% in EDTA and 72% in U.S. patients. Average body weight and body mass index were similar in EDTA and U.S. patients.

Abstracted from Held PJ, Blagg CR, Liska DW, et al. The dose of hemodialysis according to dialysis prescription in Europe and the United States. *Kidney Int* 1992; 42:S16–S21.

The best dialysis survival estimates of any program or registry were reported from France, with a 15-year survival rate of 65% in 445 patients followed from 1970 through 1990 in Tassin (Fig. 84.24). These patients, who were dialyzed more intensively than at any other center (Kt/V of 1.67), also had a high incidence of full rehabilitation and most of them were rendered normotensive with aggressive fluid removal and without antihypertensive medications.

Since the 1980s, technologic advances, such as bicarbonate-based dialysate and volumetric ultrafiltration control, have permitted these dialyzers to be used to allow appropriate dialysis delivery despite reductions in dialysis time. The use of highly efficient, larger–surface area dialyzers is increasing in the United States. A special study of the USRDS revealed the delivered dose of dialysis (Kt/V) in the United States for December 1993 was between 1.18 and 1.32 depending on the region of the country. This represents a significant increase over the previous Kt/V of 0.97 for 1986 to 1988.

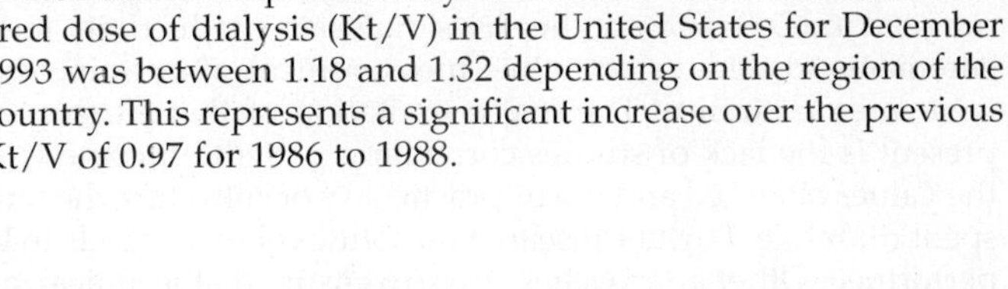

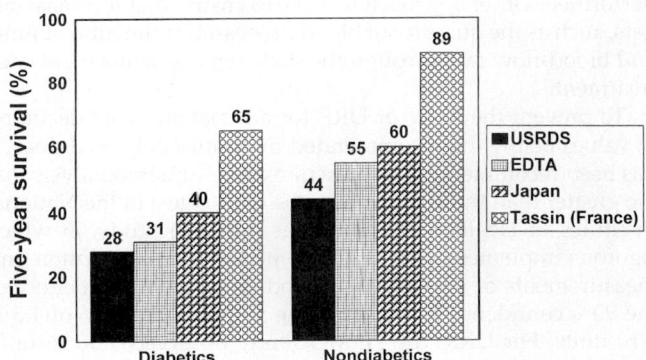

Figure 84.24. Five-year survival of ESRD patients by geographic distribution. (Data from Held PJ, Brunner F, Odaka M, et al. Five-year survival for end-stage renal disease patients in the U.S., Europe, and Japan 1982–1987. *Am J Kidney Dis* 1990;15:451–457; and Charra B, Calemard E, Ruffet M, et al. Survival as an index of adequacy of dialysis. *Kidney Int* 1992;41:1286–1291.)

Not all patients receive their prescribed dose of hemodialysis. Some studies have suggested that only 50% of ESRD patients in the United States actually receive their prescribed hemodialysis dose. There are many reasons for the failure to deliver the prescribed dialysis dose. Among the most common are differences between *in vitro* and *in vivo* dialyzer clearances of urea, individual variation in total body water when compared with demographic estimates, inaccurate assessment of effective treatment time (during which diffusion occurs at the prescribed blood- and dialysate-flow rates), vascular access recirculation, and laboratory or blood sampling errors. The timing of the postdialysis BUN is a critical variable that impacts significantly on the measured dose of delivered dialysis (Kt/V or URR). Within 2 minutes after dialysis, both access and cardiopulmonary recirculations dissipate, and the differences in arterial and venous BUN concentrations are largely resolved. Most studies have recommended that the postdialysis sample be measured between 1 and 5 minutes after dialysis or during slow-flow phase but before the lines have been flushed with saline, which can acutely lower the BUN by dilution. Other factors leading to less-than-prescribed delivered dose of dialysis include inadequate dialyzer reprocessing leading to poor dialyzer clearance, dialyzer clotting, and blood-pump/dialysate-flow calibration errors. Because of the plethora of variables that adversely affect the delivered dose of hemodialysis, the deliberate targeting of a delivered Kt/V of 1.2 or a URR of 65% will result in a significant number of hemodialysis sessions in which the Kt/V or URR falls below these threshold values.

Although urea kinetic modeling represents the current state-of-the-art of dialysis prescription, it is performed only on a monthly basis. Thus the measurement of delivered dialysis occurs, at best, during 1 of 13 treatments per month. If the modeled treatment is not representative of the other treatments due to one or more of the aforementioned multiple causes that may affect delivered dialysis dose at each treatment, the usefulness of modeling will be seriously weakened. In an attempt to achieve an improved assessment of delivered dialysis on a per-treatment basis, several new techniques are under development or already available. One approach uses the direct analysis of dialysate urea to provide an estimate of dialysis delivery ("solute removal index"), and another uses dialysate conductivity measurements to achieve an online measurement of effective dialyzer urea clearance. The major limitation of this measure at present is the lack of studies correlating patient outcome with the values obtained and the impracticality of collecting the total spent dialysate. Further research on solute removal needs to be performed. Other approaches strive to ensure that technical targets, such as the quantity of blood processed, a function of time, and blood-flow rate through the dialyzer, are achieved at each treatment.

To prevent the Kt/V or URR for any patient from declining to values below the recommended minimum delivered dose, it has been recommended to prescribe doses of hemodialysis that are greater than these minimum-desired values. In the National Institutes of Health's Hemodialysis (HEMO) Study, in which rigorous implementation of the hemodialysis prescription and measurements of the dose of hemodialysis have been effected, the 90% confidence interval for the single-pool Kt/V of 1.3 is 0.10 units. For URR, the HEMO Study observed a 90% confidence limit of 4%. Therefore the Hemodialysis Adequacy Work Group of the National Kidney Foundation (see following discussion) recommends that the prescribed minimum Kt/V be 1.3 and the minimum target URR, 70%. Furthermore, the work group recommends that the delivered dose of hemodialysis should be measured at least once a month in all adult and pediatric hemodialysis patients. The frequency of measurement may have to be increased if the patient is noncompliant, or when blood-flow problems, treatment interruptions, or changes in the dialysis prescription occur.

Despite these observations, the optimal level of hemodialysis remains undefined. Most of the aforementioned studies were retrospective in design and ignored the wide variation in dialysis delivery. The previously noted HEMO Study is an ongoing, prospective, randomized trial evaluating the effects of two well-defined and carefully maintained dialysis prescriptions on survival; its results will be available in the year 2002.

In March of 1995, the National Kidney Foundation-Dialysis Outcomes Quality Initiative (NKF-DOQI) was established with the primary objective to improve patient outcomes and survival by providing recommendations for optimal clinical practices, thereby increasing the efficiency of patient care and positively impacting patient outcomes. The project proposed to achieve this goal by subjecting the literature on pertinent clinical issues to structured review and developing evidence-based clinical practice guidelines. In addition to some of the guidelines on hemodialysis adequacy noted previously, NKF-DOQI has several other guidelines in the areas of hemodialysis, peritoneal dialysis, anemia, and vascular access. The reader is strongly urged to review these guidelines, which were published in 1997 by the National Kidney Foundation of the United States.

ROLE OF DIALYZER MEMBRANES

Efficiency

The efficiency of the dialyzer generally refers to the clearance of urea and is a function of the urea mass transfer coefficient (KoA), which is determined by the dialyzer's blood–membrane surface area, membrane characteristics, and dialyzer geometry. High-efficiency dialyzers generally have urea clearance of more than 200 ml/min and can achieve the desired small-molecule clearance in a shorter period of time than with conventional dialyzers. Although a rapid reduction in serum osmolarity has been reported to cause a disequilibrium state characterized by central nervous system symptomatology, this is an uncommon consequence of high-efficiency treatment except for cases in which predialysis urea is inordinately elevated. Fluid removal with short dialysis can result in intradialytic hypotension, particularly when intravascular refilling is inadequate relative to the ultrafiltration rate, but many other factors play a role in dialysis-induced hypotension. High dialysate sodium concentration, bicarbonate-based dialysate, volumetric ultrafiltration control, high dialysate calcium concentration, and low dialysate temperature all are used to promote hemodynamic stability during rapid fluid removal and are usually adequate to minimize symptomatic hypotensive episodes. However, in some instances, a consequence of rapid dialysis may be failure to achieve the lowest possible target weight. Under these conditions, blood pressure may be less well controlled than with longer treatments.

Flux

The U.S. Food and Drug Administration (FDA) defines a high-flux membrane as one with an ultrafiltration coefficient of more than 8 ml/hr/mm Hg. Although this defines water permeability, the definition does not characterize membrane permeability (sieving coefficient). Conventional cellulosic membranes remove an insignificant fraction of substances with molecular weights of more than 2,000 D. Thus a better working definition for high-flux membranes would be those membranes that remove substances with a molecular weight of more than 10,000 D. Removal may occur by diffusion, convection, or adsorption. Small-molecule removal is also excellent and, in fact, is enhanced by the increase in convective transport resulting from the simultaneous ultrafiltration and back filtration of dialysate that is a feature of open membranes. Although high-flux membranes differ in their sieving capacity (or ability to absorb large molecules), they all possess sieving properties closer to those of the normal kidney than conventional membranes. Currently available membranes can efficiently remove molecules of at least the molecular weight of β_2-microglobulin (11,900 D). Some membranes may even remove substances with a molecular weight of 60,000 Daltons, similar to the normal kidney, which excretes and/or catabolizes substances, particularly proteins, with molecular weights in that range.

High-flux membranes in common use [acrylonitrile, polysulfone, polyamide, and polymethylmethacrylate (PMMA)] can remove approximately 40% of β_2-microglobulin production per treatment. Cellulosic membranes do not remove β_2-microglobulin. The major clinical implication with respect to the use of high-flux membranes may be to delay the onset of carpal tunnel syndrome and bone cysts in patients on dialysis. Bone cysts have been described as occurring in 23% and 11% and carpal tunnel syndrome in 30% and 13% of patients dialyzed with cellulosic and high-flux membranes, respectively, for the same number of years.

Dialysis with high-flux membranes may be associated with an increase in HDL and a decrease in triglyceride levels of the patients compared with dialysis with conventional membranes. High-flux dialysis may increase lipoprotein lipase activity by removing inhibitors of the enzyme. Several studies have also suggested that increased hematocrit:erythropoietin dose ratio in patients treated with PMMA and polysulfone may be related to the removal of an inhibitor of erythropoiesis (molecular weight, 1,000 to 10,000). N-terminal PTH (molecular weight, more than 3,000) and advanced glycosylation end-products may also be removed during dialysis with high-flux membranes; the biologic significance of these processes is unclear.

Removal of anaphylotoxins (C3a and C5a) represents a meeting point between permeability and biocompatibility in that a high-flux membrane may remove the products of complement activation before they can exert their adverse effects. Removal (by convection or adsorption) of these substances has been demonstrated with polysulfone, acrylonitrile, polyamide, and polyacrylonitrile (PAN) membranes. The clinical significance is that biocompatibility is, in part, a consequence of membrane permeability. If this phenomenon applies to other aspects of biocompatibility, such as cytokine production, a number of biologic effects of the latter may be ameliorated. Included among these effects are activation of neutrophils with reduced response to infection and oxidation of lipoprotein, T-cell dysfunction, polymorphonuclear phagocytic dysfunction, and impaired granulocyte superoxide production.

The dosage of medications may also be different with high-flux dialysis. For example, vancomycin is not removed by conventional hemodialysis; however, high-flux dialysis with cellulose triacetate, polysulfone, or PAN membranes removes approximately 15% to 20% of body vancomycin stores. This leads to a one-third reduction in plasma vancomycin levels that is rapidly reversed by redistribution of vancomycin out of the cells.

BIOCOMPATIBILITY

Interaction of the dialysis membrane with the components of blood has the potential to induce an inflammatory response and to lead to numerous long-term clinical sequelae that are in part determined by the degree of membrane biocompatibility. A biocompatible membrane (BCM) has traditionally been defined as "one that elicits the least amount of inflammatory response in patients exposed to it." Membrane compatibility may impact on recovery from acute renal failure, the rate of loss of residual renal function, infections, hyperlipidemia, progression of atherosclerosis, dialysis-related amyloidosis, nutritional state by its effects on protein catabolism, red-cell survival, and myriad other aspects affecting morbidity and mortality in hemodialysis patients. Detailed discussions on the histocompatibility of dialysis membranes and their effects on the patients are found in Chapter 84, Parts 1D and 1E.

Oxidized LDL has been shown to induce the formation of intimal foam cells, the precursors of the atherosclerotic lesion. Studies have shown increased levels of derivatives of oxidized LDL, such as malonaldehyde, in hemodialysis patients, and particularly so in patients dialyzed with unmodified cellulosic membranes. It has been proposed that increased production of reactive oxygen species and other cytoactive products of complement activation may favor the oxidation of LDL and may have a role in the progression of atherosclerosis and coronary artery disease in hemodialysis patients. Because of decreased complement activation with BCM compared with conventional membranes, dialysis with BCM may be associated with decreased cardiovascular mortality in hemodialysis patients (see the following discussion).

Survival, dialysis adequacy, and the biocompatibility of hemodialysis membrane all seem to be closely interrelated. In the CMAS, patients dialyzed with either modified cellulose or synthetic (high- or low-flux and more biocompatible) membranes had a lower mortality rate than those treated with cellulosic nonbiocompatible membranes (relative risk of mortality was 0.72). One possible contributing factor to this difference other than biocompatibility was that patients dialyzed with either modified cellulosic or synthetic membranes received more intensive dialysis than those dialyzed with nonbiocompatible membranes (Kt/V of 1.14 versus 1.07, $P < .01$). Another report of the CMAS evaluated the relationship between membrane type (unmodified cellulose versus modified cellulose or synthetic) and specific causes of death. In this report 62% of the more than 4,000 patients studied were dialyzed with unmodified cellulose, whereas the remaining 38% were dialyzed with either modified cellulose or synthetic membranes. Modified cellulose or synthetic membranes were associated with a 31% lower risk for death from infection ($P = .03$) and a 26% lower risk for death from coronary artery disease ($P = .07$) after adjusting for a large number of demographic variables, comorbidity, and treatment parameters. In this report, several deaths from coronary artery disease may have been misclassified as "other cardiac" causes because of the way in which death notification was reported to the USRDS. For example, cardiac arrest, which accounted for nearly 18% of all deaths, was classified as "other cardiac" even though the majority of these patients may have had coronary artery disease. Therefore the true effect of the membrane type on cardiac death may be even higher and statistically significant. Furthermore, when the analysis was confined to patients whose Kt/V was measured, the relationship between membrane type and death from coronary artery disease was stronger and statistically significant. As noted previously, high-flux synthetic membranes have various favorable effects on lipid metabolism in hemodialysis patients. A retrospective, uncontrolled study with a prolonged follow-up (1968 to 1994) of more than 800 patients from Japan also confirms the benefits of biocompatibility on hemodialysis patients' mortality and morbidity. In this study, patients who were dialyzed with high-flux membranes or those who were switched from a conventional membrane to a high-flux membrane had lower risk of mortality and β_2-microglobulin-associated morbidity.

Dialyzer Reuse

Because of the relatively high cost of high-performance membranes, reuse is an economic necessity in the United States when these membranes are used. According to a 1992 annual report from the Centers for Disease Control and Prevention (CDC), 72% of the surveyed chronic hemodialysis units in the United States reprocessed dialyzers regularly, affecting 78% of hemodialysis patients. Most centers have automated techniques for dialyzer reprocessing. The number of reuses from a single dialyzer varies widely among patients and dialysis units. In one study evaluating a large number of dialysis centers, the average number of reuses was 13. Reuse is not commonly practiced in Europe (only 10% of patients were on reused dialyzers in 1988) and it is not permitted in Japan. There are three major concerns with reuse: the risk of infection, biochemical and immunologic effects, and loss of performance with impairment in clearance and/or ultrafiltration.

Risk of Infection

Pyrogenic dialyzer reactions are manifested by fever, chills, myalgia, nausea, and hypotension. These reactions can occur when endotoxins (usually from a contaminated water supply) enter the bloodstream. In addition, nontuberculous mycobacteria are frequently found in tap water and are much more resistant to chlorine than *Pseudomonas aeruginosa* and other Gram-negative bacteria. *Mycobacteria* resistant to 2% formaldehyde have been isolated from as many as 83% of dialysis unit water samples and deaths in two dialysis units have been attributed to dialysis-acquired *Mycobacterium chelonei* infection. Since these outbreaks, the CDC has recommended the use of 4% formaldehyde for at least 48 hours during reprocessing.

Many studies have shown dialyzer reuse to be a safe procedure when performed according to accepted standards and practices. The Health Care Financing Administration (HCFA) requires all dialysis centers that reprocess dialyzers in the United States to comply with the Association for the Advancement of Medical Instrumentation (AAMI) guidelines as a condition for reimbursement. Additional regulations may be imposed by city, county, or state health departments. Several comparative and double-blind, randomized clinical trials have not shown an increased risk of pyrogenic reactions with dialyzer reuse. These findings implicate a contaminated water supply as the cause of the pyrogenic reaction. Contaminated water used in the reprocessing of a dialyzer can contaminate the dialyzer even in the presence of germicides because bacteria can be trapped in areas where the germicide cannot penetrate. Pressures generated during dialysis can open the trapped areas, releasing viable bacteria. There may be a greater risk of infection in centers in which the dialyzer headers are removed during reprocessing. In 1998, AAMI water quality standards were changed to lower acceptable bacterial counts and endotoxin levels in water.

There is at present no evidence that dialyzer reuse is associated with viral hepatitis or human immunodeficiency virus (HIV) transmission to patients or dialysis personnel if appropriate guidelines are followed. To minimize any risk, dialyzers should be handled with universal precautions and dialyzers from hepatitis B surface antigen–positive patients should be reprocessed and stored in a separate area. Dialyzers from patients with sepsis or acute hepatitis should not be reused. In comparison, there are no CDC recommendations against dialyzer reuse in hepatitis C– or HIV-infected patients.

Biochemical and Immune System Effects

Cuprophane dialyzers can be rendered biocompatible by reuse, an effect that is presumably due to membrane coating by serum proteins. Removal of this protein coat that can occur during reprocessing with bleach will return the membrane to its previous complement-activating state. At least one study using cuprophane dialyzers rendered more biocompatible after reuse has shown an improvement in peak expiratory flow rate when compared with new cuprophane dialyzers.

Loss of Performance

There are negligible effects on urea, creatinine, and phosphorus removal with cellulose membranes. However, one report measured Kt/V for urea during dialysis with a low (mean fourth reuse) and a high (mean fourteenth reuse) number of reuses. The Kt/V was significantly lower in the high number reuse treatment (1.05 versus 1.10 early in the sequence). Ultrafiltration may fall slightly after reuse with a mixture of peracetic acid, acetic acid, and hydrogen peroxide (PAM, Renalin) and increase after reuse with bleach and formaldehyde.

Germicide Exposure

There is continuing concern about possible adverse effects to germicide exposure with reuse. Patients and even dialysis staff may have allergic reactions to formaldehyde. Some patients may develop antibodies to formaldehyde; the clinical importance of these antibodies is unknown. Another potential complication is an anaphylactoid reaction that, in one study, was documented in 10 patients treated with reprocessed dialyzers sterilized with PAM; these reactions appeared to be more frequent in patients taking angiotensin-converting enzyme (ACE) inhibitors. These general problems have led to the search for other modalities to reprocess dialyzers, including heat disinfection. One reported a favorable experience using heat disinfection for Fresenius polysulfone dialyzers. Although this process is somewhat more expensive (approximately $6.85 versus $5.35 for bleach and formaldehyde), it has the significant advantage of avoiding the problems with chemical disinfection noted previously. One disadvantage is that the number of reuses with heat disinfection will probably be less than with chemicals, due primarily to casing deterioration.

Effects of Reuse on Patient Mortality

Data collected in 1986 suggested that the mortality of patients in units reusing dialyzers was lower than that of comparable patients in units that did not reuse. However, much of the early mortality data relating to reuse were established when formaldehyde was used as the chemical germicide. A large study (the Urban Institute study) evaluated the mortality associated with dialyzer reprocessing using PAM or glutaraldehyde compared with formaldehyde or nothing. This study prospectively evaluated two cohorts of patients (66,097 patients from 845 units in 1989 and 857 units in 1990), 81% of whom were treated with reprocessed dialyzers. Patient comorbidity was not controlled. The major findings of this study were as follows. For low-flux dialyzers, reuse was associated with increased overall mortality (13% with PAM, $P < .001$ and 17% with the use of glutaraldehyde, $P = .01$). However, different findings were noted in the subset of hospital-based outpatient units using low-flux dialyzers in which mortality was lower with PAM reuse and unchanged with glutaraldehyde reuse compared with nonreuse hospital units, suggesting that the germicidal agent is not the only issue and but the quality of the reprocessing technique may contribute to increased mortality as well. The use of PAM was also associated with an 11% increase in hospitalization rates. On the other hand, there was no increase in mortality associated with the use of formaldehyde. In addition, the results were quite different with high-flux dialyzers. In the dialysis units that used predominantly high-flux dialyzers, mortality was somewhat lower in units reusing high-flux dialyzers with PAM (r = 0.89) or glutaraldehyde (r = 0.79) and similar with formaldehyde (r = 0.98) when compared with units using non-reprocessed low-flux dialyzers. The study was not controlled for the quality of the reuse process, the adequacy of dialysis, or other unmeasured center effects. Thus it is premature to speculate about the significance of this report. In another study comparing the survival of patients dialyzed in free-standing dialysis units with hospital-based dialysis units, it was found that reuse with PAM in free-standing units was associated with a higher mortality than was reuse with formaldehyde or no reuse. Current recommendations stress careful review of reuse procedures and scrupulous attention to manufacturers' recommendations when these germicides are used.

In summary, dialyzer reuse appears to be a safe and cost-effective procedure for high-flux dialyzers. Reprocessing these expensive dialyzers may ensure their availability to more patients and have a positive impact on patient morbidity and mortality in the future. The use of heat disinfection as an alternative to the chemical process is promising and needs further investigation.

ROLE OF NUTRITION

Protein-energy malnutrition is widespread in hemodialysis patients. Subjects from the NCDS reported a mean caloric intake 31% less than the recommended intake of 35 kcal/kg. Dietary-protein intake was less than 0.8 g/kg/day in 23% of patients. Body fat and muscle stores were reduced. The prevalence of malnutrition in a typical patient mix is, if anything, likely to be greater than that in the NCDS population. Depending on the method used to define malnutrition, the condition may be present in as many as 40% to 70% of patients on dialysis.

In the NCDS, low protein intake was second only to low dose of dialysis in predicting poor clinical outcome. In large patient studies, a low predialysis BUN is a marker for a low-protein intake and has been reported to correlate with poor patient outcome. In a stable (noncatabolic, nonanabolic) dialysis patient, quantitation of protein intake can be achieved by measuring the PCR as determined by interdialytic net urea appearance. Urea appearance rate is proportional to PCR under these conditions and may be determined by urea kinetic analysis or by direct quantitation of dialysate urea. In the NCDS, a PCR of less than 0.8 g/kg body weight was associated with a high risk of treatment failure. In a subgroup of NCDS patients with a mean PCR of 0.63 g/kg per day, hospitalization rate and mortality rate were far greater than in subgroups with 0.93, 1.02, and 1.29 g/kg per day protein intake.

In a large, cross-sectional study of more than 12,000 hemodialysis patients by Lowrie and colleagues, the death risk for patients increased exponentially as serum albumin concentration decreased. The adjusted mortality risk of patients with serum albumin concentrations between 4.00 and 3.51, 3.50 and 3.01, 3.00 and 2.51, and less than 2.50 was, respectively, 2.2, 6.7, 10.7, and 18.5 times that of a reference group with albumin concentrations of more than 4.00 g/day. In nearly 3,400 patients beginning hemodialysis in 1986 and 1987 who were studied by the USRDS (the Case Mix Severity Study), there was an inverse correlation between serum albumin level and mortality. Further, patients labeled as undernourished had higher relative risk of death (r = 1.34, $P < .0001$).

We reported a 7-year prospective analysis of nearly 250 hemodialysis patients in two urban dialysis centers. Patients with albumin less than 3.5 g/dl at enrollment had more than twice the mortality risk of those with albumin more than 4.0 g/dl even after adjustments were made for age, race, and diabetic status. Patients with lower creatinine (less than 9 mg/dl) at enrollment also had increased mortality risk compared with those with higher creatinine levels (more than 12 mg/dl). Indeed, differences in patient survival by baseline albumin and creatinine with life-table analyses persist even when patients were followed for up to 11 years.

Whether there is a mathematical link between Kt/V and PCR because they are both calculated from similar parameters is a subject of debate. The relationship between the dose of dialysis and protein intake was demonstrated in a small group of hemodialysis patients in whom the intensity of dialysis was increased by enhancing dialysis time, blood flow, and/or membrane surface area. As the Kt/V rose from 0.82 to 1.32 over a 3-month period, there was a concurrent elevation in PCR from 0.81 to 1.02 g/kg per day. The rise in PCR was indicative of increased protein intake (and better nutrition) due, presumably, to improved appetite. A second group in which the dialysis regimen was unchanged had no increase in either Kt/V or PCR. In a single dialysis center study wherein the average Kt/V was increased from 0.82 to 1.33 over a period of 4 years, in addition to improved patient survival and decreased hospitalization days, there were associated increases in protein catabolic rate from 0.83 to 1.0 and in plasma albumin concentration from 3.5 to 3.9 g/dl. Thus enhanced nutrition may have contributed to the improvement in survival.

The most readily treatable cause of malnutrition in many patients is inadequate dose of dialysis, which can lead to anorexia and decreased taste acuity. Patients with a minimally acceptable Kt/V (e.g., 1.0 to 1.2 for hemodialysis) and a low mid-week BUN may appear well dialyzed on paper. However, many such patients are underdialyzed, with poor protein intake being responsible for the low BUN. This problem has led to the appreciation that protein intake must be considered when evaluating the adequacy of dialysis. Thus estimation of the PCR, as index of protein intake, is a routine part of management of a chronic dialysis patient. However, it should be remembered that the PCR is only valid as a measure of protein intake in the patient in neutral nitrogen balance.

Even in the well-dialyzed patient a number of factors can impair nutrition: (a) loss of nutrients in the dialysate; protein and amino acid losses as high as 20 grams in one hemodialysis has been reported with polysulfone dialyzers reused with bleach; (b) dietary restrictions making food less palatable and the restriction of fluid intake to minimize intradialytic weight gain may lead to a concurrent decrease in caloric intake; (c) the dialysis procedure itself may be catabolic especially with the use of conventional, nonbiocompatible membranes; (d) persistent, mild metabolic acidosis may enhance protein degradation and amino acid oxidation; (e) gastroparesis (by slowing gastric emptying); (f) some medications, such as phosphate binders, can impair nutrient absorption; antihypertensive medications, particularly calcium channel blockers, may interfere with gastrointestinal function; and (g) serum levels of leptin, a hormone that induces satiety via effects on the hypothalamus, may be increased due to reduced clearance. Other causes include depression and socioeconomic factors.

There are no studies that analyze morbidity and mortality in patients in whom interventions were directed specifically to increase serum albumin controlling for the dose of dialysis. However, preliminary reports indicate that long-term trends in serum albumin and serum cholesterol are strong independent predictors of survival. In a prospective evaluation of hemodialysis patients over 7 years with monthly measurements of nutritional markers (albumin, creatinine, and cholesterol), if the slope of serial albumin measurements over the duration of the study was positive, the mortality risk decreased by 75% compared with patients with no improvement in the slope of albumin. Positive trend in cholesterol was also associated with decreased relative risk of mortality in this study.

As noted previously, another marker of nutritional status at the time of dialysis initiation is the plasma creatinine concentration. The creatinine level reflects muscle mass as well as renal function. Thus a patient requiring dialysis at a lower-than-usual plasma creatinine concentration has a reduced muscle mass and may be malnourished. Data from the USRDS are also consistent with this hypothesis because the late mortality rate was increased in patients with a plasma creatinine concentration below 10 mg/dl at the start of dialysis. Other markers of malnutrition also may prove useful, including the plasma concentrations of prealbumin, transferrin, somatomedin C, and cholesterol. In patients treated with continuous ambulatory peritoneal dialysis, for example, low serum prealbumin concentrations (less than 30 mg/dl) have been associated with increased mortality risk. A similar finding has been shown with maintenance hemodialysis patients as well. The nutritional management of patients with chronic renal failure and those on dialysis is addressed in Chapter 83, Part 2.

ROLE OF VASCULAR ACCESS

Vascular access dysfunction is the most common complication encountered in the care of ESRD patients maintained on long-term hemodialysis. Studies indicate that 0.5 to 1 episode of thrombosis per patient year of dialysis is not uncommon. In 1986, Medicare ESRD patients had approximately 30,000 vascular access–related hospital admissions (with a median duration of 7 days each) constituting 17.4% of all hospital stays in this population. As shown in Table 84.11, the number of vascular access–related hospitalizations has increased constituting nearly 25% of all admissions among these patients. When outpatient procedures related to access dysfunction are considered, the prevalence of access-related problems is even higher.

The preferred permanent vascular access is the creation of a native arteriovenous (AV) fistula because of superior patency rates. However, 80% of hemodialysis patients in the United States have polytetrafluoroethylene (PTFE) prosthetic grafts for vascular access probably due to changing demographics of ESRD patients (increasing proportion of diabetics, elderly, and females). Thrombosis of the PTFE grafts is the most common complication encountered in the care of chronic hemodialysis patients. Thrombosis of AV grafts can occasionally be attributed to mechanical factors such as hypotension, decreased cardiac output, or prolonged AV access compression, and at times to a hypercoagulable state. However, neointimal hyperplasia and stenosis at or distal to the venous anastomosis appear to be associated with almost 80% of patients with PTFE graft thrombosis. Platelet activation has been proposed to play an important role in the development of neointimal hyperplasia and several studies have been performed to assess the efficacy of antiplatelet agents in the prolongation of patency of vascular grafts.

Complications from the placement of an AV fistula include ipsilateral distal hypoperfusion as a result of shunting of arterial blood from the hand. The so-called steal syndrome is particularly prominent in patients with severe peripheral vascular disease. Carpal tunnel syndrome also has been reported to occur more frequently on the side of the dialysis access. Construction of an AV fistula flow may result in cardiac decompensation when fistula flow is high relative to cardiac output (more than 20%) when and cardiac reserve is limited.

Acute dialysis access includes placement of a temporary dialysis catheter in the femoral vein using the Seldinger technique. Generally, a double-lumen dialysis catheter is placed for the duration of a single hemodialysis treatment and then removed. Under some circumstances, however, a catheter can be secured and left in place for several days. Infectious complications are minimized when catheters are removed after a single use. Internal jugular, dual-lumen catheters placed in the right atrium are the preferred route of placement if temporary access is needed and if catheters are to remain in place for multiple dialysis sessions. Dual-lumen catheters designed with a Dacron cuff to be placed with an exit site tunneled through the skin have resulted in fewer infectious complications and are useful when temporary access is needed for prolonged use. Subclavian catheters have been used for acute dialysis but have resulted in a high incidence of subclavian vein stenosis with upper extremity edema, or poor access function following ipsilateral AV fistula construction. Exit-site infections may occur with a frequency of 6% to 8%, and bacteremia may occur with a frequency of 4% to 9% with noncuffed catheters, with lesser rates of infection with cuffed catheters placed under optimal conditions. Transient malfunction of temporary catheters usually can be resolved with the instillation of urokinase or, in the case of a noncuffed catheter, replacement over a guidewire. Detailed discussion of vascular access of hemodialysis is provided in Chapter 84, Part 1B.

HYPERTENSION

Hypertension is common in dialysis patients and is an important factor in the pathogenesis of cardiovascular disease in these patients. Hypertension may be more important than cigarette smoking or hyperlipidemia in influencing the rate of coronary artery disease. However, the presence of hypertension in incident patients in the USRDS Case Mix study and hypertension in prevalent patients is not correlated with subsequent mortality.

In a substantial number of patients, removal of excess fluid volume will normalize blood pressure and even allow discontinuation of antihypertensive medications. Adequate fluid removal depends on both the technical ability to remove excess fluid and on the patient's tolerance to the fluid removal rate. Shorter dialysis necessitates more rapid fluid-removal rates, which is more likely to induce episodes of hypotension that are treated with fluid administration. The net effect is that the patient may not achieve dry weight, leading to persistent volume expansion, hypertension, and possible deterioration in left ventricular function. These complications may contribute to the high and increasing cardiac mortality in dialysis patients. In those instances in which shorter time produces difficulties with respect to fluid removal, the duration of the dialysis session must be increased. The issue of hypertension in patients with renal failure and those treated with dialysis is discussed in detail in Chapter 70, Part 3.

AMYLOIDOSIS

Amyloidosis represents the most crippling complication of ESRD and is related to the accumulation and tissue deposition of β_2-microglobulin. It severely limits lifestyle and rehabilitation of long-term dialysis patients. Advanced age, 10 or more years of dialysis, and low-flux, nonbiocompatible membranes increase the risk of developing secondary amyloidosis. The clinical syndromes are now well described and include bone cysts and pain, as well as carpal tunnel syndrome. Conventional cellulosic membranes are impermeable to β_2-microglobulin, and the permeability of cellulose acetate membranes to this compound is variable. Synthetic membranes with high-flux characteristics provide significant dialyzer clearance of β_2-microglobulin. The clearance of β_2-microglobulin varies in different membranes with differences in sieving properties and adsorbence and, possibly, by β_2-microglobulin generation as a result of blood–membrane interactions. A retrospective analysis of the radiologic signs of dialysis-induced amyloidosis and carpal tunnel syndrome reported a lower incidence of disease in patients undergoing treatment with PAN membrane, a high-flux membrane, than in those treated with cellulosic membranes. However, it is not likely that high-flux membranes can eliminate dialysis-induced amyloidosis entirely, because removal cannot completely keep up with the production rate. High-flux treatment can delay the development of disease and may reduce symptoms but cannot reverse established lesions. Several other clinical studies demonstrate the relative benefits of high-flux and biocompatible membranes on morbidity related to dialysis-related amyloidosis. These issues are discussed in greater detail in Chapter 84, Part1E.

INTRADIALYTIC MORBIDITY AND MORTALITY

Hypotension

Intradialytic symptoms and signs occur largely as a result of acute perturbations of physiology in patients, many of whom have underlying illnesses that prevent adequate compensation for those hemodynamic changes. Hypotension may be the most common problem observed during dialysis. The incidence is lower with longer dialysis periods and low ultrafiltration rates and in patients with intact cardiovascular and autonomic nervous systems. Consequently, hypotension is more common in noncompliant, diabetic, and older patients. A fall in blood pressure during dialysis is usual. Factors involved in excessive decreases include inadequate refilling of the blood volume from extracellular and intracellular compartments during ultrafiltration, inadequate vasoconstriction because of autonomic nervous system impairment, and vasodilation because of heat gain from dialysate. Dialysis-induced differences in intracellular and extracellular osmotic pressure usually play a small role. Dialysis prescription factors that may influence blood pressure adversely include high rates of ultrafiltration, low dialysate sodium concentration, use of acetate dialysate, low dialysate calcium, high dialysate temperature settings, and the use of nonbiocompatible dialyzer membranes. Controlled ultrafiltration systems and the widespread use of bicarbonate dialysate have reduced the frequency of symptomatic hypotensive episodes. Development of thermal balance–control systems combined with on-line measurement of blood volume changes that can feed back and alter ultrafiltration rate may contribute to decreased frequency of intradialytic hypotension. Muscle cramps may also relate to hemodynamic changes during dialysis in that the symptoms occur in the context of reduced intracellular volume and reduction in muscle perfusion. Use of quinine sulfate may alleviate muscle cramps in some hemodialysis patients.

Dialyzer Reactions

Dialyzer reactions refer to all of the abnormal sequelae resulting from the interaction between blood constituents and the hemodialysis membrane. There are two types of reactions: type A and type B. In the past, these reactions were grouped under the term *first-use syndrome* because they primarily occurred with new dialyzers. Type A reactions are estimated to occur in approximately 4 of every 100,000 dialysis treatments. They usually begin in the first few minutes of dialysis, immediately after the return of blood from the dialysis circuit to the patient; in occasional cases, however, the onset is delayed for up to 30 minutes into the treatment. Mild episodes may be associated with a variety of symptoms such as itching, urticaria, flushing, cough, sneezing, wheezing, abdominal cramps, diarrhea, headache, back and chest pain, nausea, vomiting, fever, and chills. More severe reactions lead to dyspnea, a sense of impending doom, and hypotension, potentially resulting in cardiac arrest and death. Patients with an allergic diathesis and eosinophilia appear to be predisposed to this type of reaction. Type A reactions are probably caused by leachable substances from the dialyzer or by contamination with bacterial peptides. A classic cause of this type of reaction is ethylene oxide, which is used to sterilize hollow-fiber dialyzers. Reactions to ethylene oxide, which are now uncommon, occur exclusively during the first use, usually when there has been inadequate rinsing of the dialyzer before use. IgE antibodies directed against ethylene oxide are present in some cases, particularly in those with more severe reactions, and may also lead to a greater degree of complement activation and interleukin-2 production after exposure to a cuprophane membrane.

A high incidence of anaphylactoid reactions is also seen when ACE inhibitors are used in patients treated with high-flux hemodialysis using PAN dialyzers. In one study 57% of patients treated with an ACE inhibitor and dialyzed with a PAN membrane developed anaphylactoid reaction, whereas none of the 71 patients taking an ACE inhibitor but dialyzed with other membranes had any reaction. These membranes appear to act by increasing the rate of kinin generation. Contact of blood with a dialysis membrane leads to binding of Hageman factor (factor XII) and circulating complexes of high-molecular-weight kininogen with prekallikrein. Activation of prekallikrein by Hageman factor results in the formation of kallikrein, which cleaves bradykinin from kininogen. Activation of this process is facilitated by a negatively charged surface (like the PAN membrane) that induces conformational changes in Hageman factor. The ensuing enhancement of bradykinin production is generally well tolerated unless the patient is taking an ACE inhibitor. ACE is also a kininase. Thus blocking converting enzyme prevents inactivation of bradykinin, thereby raising bradykinin levels as much as 20- to 30-fold and increasing the likelihood of an anaphylactoid reaction. A recent report suggests that calcium level in the dialysate may also play a role in kinin function.

The association of anaphylactoid reactions with bleach-reprocessed but not formalin-reprocessed PAN dialyzers is also consistent with the importance of surface activation of Hageman factor. Hypochlorite (bleach), a strong oxidizing agent, removes the protein coat from the used dialysis membranes and is therefore likely to activate Hageman factor. On the other hand, formaldehyde fixes the protein layer on the surface, thereby reducing the chance for further activation of the Hageman factor.

When a patient develops type A reaction, the dialysis treatment should be immediately stopped without returning the blood to the patient. The patient is then treated, depending on the severity of the symptoms, with antihistamines, steroids, epinephrine, bronchodilators, and/or pressors. Type A reactions can usually be prevented by proper rinsing of the dialyzer, adequate sterilization techniques for the dialysis machine, reuse of the dialyzer, and avoiding PAN membranes in patients treated with an ACE inhibitor. Sterilization of the dialyzer with gamma irradiation or steam and pretreatment with antihistamines and/or steroids may be necessary during the first use in patients with a previous history of a type A reaction. Reuse of the dialyzer with proper sterilization techniques prevents most reactions, probably because the dialyzer membrane is coated with proteins from the patient plasma. However, reprocessing of nonbiocompatible membranes with bleach strips the protein coat deposited during the first clinical use of the membrane and permits a blood–membrane interaction similar to that with a new dialyzer.

Type B reactions are more common but less severe than type A reactions. They occur in 3% to 5% of patients dialyzed with new cellulosic membranes. The most common symptoms are chest and back pain, dyspnea, nausea, vomiting, and hypotension. Anaphylaxis is extremely rare. In contrast to type A reactions, symptoms are delayed, typically beginning within the first 15 to 30 minutes of the dialysis treatment, but occasionally much later, and they generally improve with continuation of the dialysis treatment. Type B reactions are believed to be mediated by complement activation by cellulosic membranes. The free hydroxyl groups on the dialysis membrane activate the alternative pathway of complement, leading to neutrophil activation and subsequent sequestration in the pulmonary circulation. These changes are frequently associated with marked and transient neutropenia, followed subsequently by an increased number of immature neutrophils (bands) appearing in the circulation, returning the neutrophil count to predialysis values by 1 hour. Animal studies have shown that the neutropenia is almost entirely explained by the sequestration of neutrophils in the pulmonary capillary bed. Furthermore, the timing of activation of the complement parallels the changes in leukocyte count. C3a formation begins immediately after blood is exposed to a new cuprophane dialyzer; maximal plasma C3a levels are seen at 15 minutes and return to normal values within 10 minutes of completing dialysis.

Cellulose acetate dialyzers appear to possess only about one-half the complement-activating property of new cuprophane dialyzers, whereas PAN membranes induce minimal complement activation and do not lead to leukopenia. Synthetic polysulfone membranes are able to activate the complement pathway but the complement products are then adsorbed, thereby blunting their effect. In contrast to the transient release of C3a and C5a, ongoing generation of the terminal-complement components (C5b-9) continues throughout the dialysis session and possibly for several hours afterward. The terminal-complement components are able to activate mononuclear cells to release various cytokines, such as tumor necrosis factor and interleukin-1. This may contribute to other complications associated with hemodialysis such as enhanced tissue catabolism, a greater risk of infection, increased β_2-microglobulin generation, and perhaps more rapid loss of residual renal function.

The treatment of type B reactions is typically supportive, because the symptoms characteristically resolve as dialysis is continued. The syndrome can be minimized or prevented by reuse of the dialyzer, which reduces complement activation and leukopenia by 90%. This protective effect is thought to result from coating of the free hydroxyl groups by plasma proteins. In some cases, it may be necessary to change to a more biocompatible membrane to relieve symptoms.

Hypoxia

A fall in arterial P_{O_2} ranging from 5 to 40 mm Hg resulting in hypotension and/or angina and their sequelae is observed frequently in dialysis patients, particularly in those with compromised cardiopulmonary function. The major reasons for hypoxemia are hypoventilation caused by CO_2 loss into the dialysate, seen particularly with acetate dialysate, and by membrane-induced complement activation with white blood cell sequestration in the lungs and decreased pulmonary diffusing capacity. Appropriate choice of membrane, dialysate composition, and when appropriate in frail individuals, oxygen supplementation can alleviate the problem.

Arrhythmias

Arrhythmias are particularly common in patients receiving digitalis, especially in the presence of alkalosis, hypocalcemia, hypokalemia, and myocardial disease. Contributory factors include high rates of ultrafiltration, hypotension, and hypoxemia. Digitalis may provoke arrhythmias in the presence of low-potassium dialysate, but this point is controversial. Although accurate diagnosis of the particular arrhythmia is vital, the potential harm produced by the arrhythmia must be balanced by the problems of pharmacologic or electrical intervention. Where possible, higher dialysate potassium may be prescribed to ameliorate cardiac arrhythmias. A careful follow-up of potassium levels is mandatory to avoid dangerously high or low values.

Seizures

Seizures occurring during or immediately after dialysis are rare. They may be caused by neuromuscular instability associated with severe uremia and by the effects of dialysis itself, such as dialysis disequilibrium, rapid acid–base changes, hypoxemia, intracranial bleeding, acute increases or decreases in blood pressure, or dialytic removal of anticonvulsants. Some drugs, such as meperidine, result in poorly dialyzable metabolites that are epileptogenic.

Fatigue

Fatigue is a common complaint after a dialysis treatment and may relate to hypovolemia following ultrafiltration. The symptoms usually resolve over several hours as reequilibration of body fluid occurs. In some patients, however, symptoms may last for a longer time and may relate to membrane-induced cytokine production (e.g., interleukin 1 and tumor necrosis factor). Biocompatible membranes may prove helpful in these circumstances.

Human and Mechanical Errors

Human and mechanical errors during the dialysis procedure may contribute to intradialytic morbidity and mortality. Exposure to incorrectly prepared dialysate can occur if the wrong concentrate or combination of concentrates is used (e.g., acid and acid instead of acid and bicarbonate). This also may occur if dialysate mixing fails or the conductivity monitor is defective. Under these conditions, marked acid–base and electrolyte changes can occur. Air embolus can occur if air is sucked into the prepump tubing segment during dialysis. However, the air detector, if armed, should immediately stop dialysis from proceeding. Air can also enter the patient because of user error when blood is returned at the end of dialysis. Any break in the continuity of the dialysis line downstream from the blood pump can result in a variable loss of blood to the environment. A decrease in venous pressure should trigger stoppage of the blood pump if alarm limits have been properly set by the user. A loss of structural integrity of the dialyzer with blood loss into the dialysate should be recognized by a properly functioning blood-leak detector. Poor heparinization can result in clotting of the blood in the extracorporeal circuit. Excessive fluid removal can follow incorrect prescription by the user or by a malfunctioning ultrafiltration control. The latter should be detected by the transmembrane pressure monitor if appropriately set.

Death

Death may occur during dialysis as a result of acute cardiovascular events, such as arrhythmia, myocardial infarction, or stroke. Heparinization during treatment may exacerbate an expanding subdural hematoma, and electrolyte changes may promote cardiac arrhythmias. The hemodynamic stress of treatment, particularly if hypotension occurs, may precipitate cardiac ischemia when cardiac blood flow is borderline. Mechanical complications, such as air embolism or improper dialysate solutions (with failure of safety alarms), rarely can result in death on treatment. Use of improperly treated water, such as may occur when exhaustion of deionizers is not detected, may result in toxic levels of substances such as fluoride.

Use of Temporary Catheters

The use of temporary venous catheters in the internal jugular vein, subclavian vein, or femoral vein for dialysis may be associated with bleeding, hematoma, pneumothorax, and infection (especially if the catheter is left in place for long durations). A precipitous fall in hematocrit in a patient who underwent femoral catheterization for hemodialysis should alert the physician to the possibility of a retroperitoneal hematoma. Subcutaneous tunneling of the catheter into internal jugular or subclavian vein decreases the incidence of infection thus prolonging the life of the catheter. The reader is strongly urged to note that subclavian catheterization must be avoided as much as possible because subsequent stenosis may severely affect vascular access in the ipsilateral upper extremity.

Selected Readings

Avram MM. Dialysis in diabetic patients: three decades of experience, from 1964 to 1997. In: Friedman EA, L'Esperance FA, eds. *Diabetic renal-retinal syndrome.* Dordrecht, The Netherlands: Kluwer Academic Publishers, 1998: 67–78.

Earliest experience of dialysis in diabetic patients.

Avram MM, Mittman N, Bonomini L, et al. Markers for survival in dialysis: a seven-year prospective study. *Am J Kidney Dis* 1995;26:209–219.

Analysis of baseline demographic and nutritional indicators (albumin, creatinine, cholesterol, prealbumin) on survival in hemodialysis and peritoneal dialysis.

Bloembergen WE, Hakim RM, Stannard DC, et al. Relationship of dialysis membrane and cause-specific mortality. *Am J Kidney Dis* 1999; 33:1–10.

This USRDS report from the Case Mix Adequacy Study evaluates the relationship between the dialysis membrane type (specifically biocompatibility) and the cause of death in a national random sample of more than 4,000 hemodialysis patients.

Depner TA. *Prescribing hemodialysis: a guide to urea modeling.* Boston: Kluwer Academic Publishers, 1991.

An excellent, detailed review of urea kinetics and their practical application.

Gotch FA, Sargent JA. A mechanistic analysis of the National Cooperative Dialysis Study (NCDS). *Kidney Int* 1985;28:526–534.

Quantification of dialysis therapy (Kt/V) and its relation to morbidity.

Hakim RM. Clinical implications of hemodialysis biocompatibility. *Kidney Int* 1993; 44:484–494.

A review of clinical implications of blood–membrane interactions in hemodialysis patients.

Hakim RM, Breyer J, Ismail N, et al. Effects of dose of dialysis on morbidity and mortality. *Am J Kidney Dis* 1994;23:661–669.

A prospective study of the effects of increasing the dose of dialysis in a single, university-affiliated, outpatient dialysis center.

Held PJ, Blagg CR, Liska DW, et al. The dose of hemodialysis according to dialysis prescription in Europe and the United States. *Kidney Int* 1992;42:S16–S21.

Demonstrates reduced dose of prescribed dialysis in the United States when compared with European prescriptions.

Held PJ, Brunner F, Odaka M, et al. Five-year survival for end-stage renal disease patients in the U.S., Europe, and Japan 1982–87. *Am J Kidney Dis* 1990;15:451–457.

Comparative mortality statistics in different countries.

Held PJ, Levin NW, Bovbjerg RR, et al. Mortality and duration of hemodialysis treatment. *JAMA* 1991;265:871–875.

Shortened time with conventional dialysis treatment, a surrogate for less delivery of dialysis, is associated with increasing mortality rate.

Held PJ, Port FK, Wolfe RA, et al. The dose of hemodialysis and patient mortality. *Kidney Int* 1996;50:550–556.

A special study of USRDS to evaluate the effect of the dose of dialysis measured as Kt/V and URR on patient mortality. A large number of demographic, anthropometric, comorbidity, and laboratory measures of nutrition and adequacy were included in the analyses.

Herzog CA, Ma JZ, Collins AJ. Poor long-term survival after acute myocardial infarction among patients on long-term dialysis. *N Engl J Med* 1998;17: 799–805.

A study to assess long-term survival after a first acute myocardial infarction (n = 34,189) after the initiation of renal-replacement therapy among patients in the United States who were receiving long-term dialysis during the period from 1977 to 1995.

Locatelli F, Vecchio LD, Manzoni C. Morbidity and mortality on hemodialysis. *Nephron* 1999;80:380–400.

Review of morbidity and mortality in hemodialysis with special emphasis on data from Europe.

Lowrie EG, Lard NM. Cooperative dialysis study. *Kidney Int* 1983;23:S1–S122.

The first federally funded and a landmark clinical trial of hemodialysis therapy.

National Kidney Foundation-Dialysis Outcome Quality Initiative's Clinical Practice Guidelines. New York: National Kidney Foundation, 1997.

The National Kidney Foundation has published guidelines for several important clinical issues in the management of hemodialysis and peritoneal dialysis patients. These guidelines are based on the best literature available at the time and evaluated rigorously by expert work groups. The areas covered in the initial set of guidelines are hemodialysis adequacy, peritoneal dialysis adequacy, management of anemia, and management of vascular access.

Owen WF, Lew NL, Liu Y, et al. The urea reduction ratio and serum albumin concentrations as predictors of mortality in patients undergoing hemodialysis. *N Engl J Med* 1993;329:1001–1006.

Describes the complex relationship among mortality, serum albumin concentration, and dialysis dose in a large, well-studied patient population.

Parfrey PS, Hargett JD. *Cardiac dysfunction in chronic uremia.* Boston: Klewer Academic Publishers, 1992.

An excellent, detailed review of cardiac disease in the dialysis patient population.

United States Renal Data System. *USRDS 1998 annual data report.* Bethesda, MD: The National Institutes of Health, National Institute of Diabetes and Digestive and Kidney Diseases, 1998.

A comprehensive compilation of data related to U.S. patient survival and causes of death.

H: Dialysis of Special Groups of Patients

Claude Jacobs

An optimal delivery of renal replacement therapies (RRT) for infants or young children, pregnant women, very old patients, or in populations who are made fragile by multiple extrarenal complications, as is the case for many diabetic patients, requires a specific approach and adapted treatment strategies, which are reviewed in this chapter.

DIALYSIS AND PREGNANCY

Maintenance dialysis may have to be initiated in some women who become pregnant in an advanced stage of chronic renal failure (CRF) to reduce the adverse effects of the uremic environment both to mother and fetus, and to permit a better control of fluid overload and blood pressure as well as a higher caloric and protein intake. In these patients, the likelihood of giving birth to a surviving infant is good. In contrast, the reversal of a rapid deterioration of renal function during pregnancy, which could have precipitated the start of dialysis, is only rarely observed after termination of pregnancy.

Pregnancy remains a rather rare event among women who undergo maintenance hemodialysis (HD) or peritoneal dialysis (PD). Uremia-induced perturbations of the hypothalamus-pituitary axis, anovulatory cycles, reduced sexual function, and elevated concentrations of prolactin and leptin all contribute to the reduced fertility documented in dialysis patients of childbearing age. However, improved dialysis methods and strategies, along with a more generalized use of recombinant human erythropoietin (rh-EPO) account for an increase in fertility among women on dialysis treatment. The true incidence of conception in dialysis patients is difficult to estimate. Most single-center studies report only successful outcomes; losses of pregnancy before clinical confirmation also contribute to underreporting. The diagnosis of pregnancy in dialysis patients remains difficult in many cases. Urine pregnancy tests are unreliable, and borderline elevation of serum concentration of β-human chorionic gonadotropin may be misleading. The positive diagnosis and stage of gestation thus rests mainly on the results of ultrasonography.

Surveys conducted in several countries have yielded conception rates ranging from 0.3% per 100 patient-years in Belgium, to 2.2% in HD patients and 1.1% in PD patients among 6,230 women age 44 years or younger treated in the United States between 1992 and 1995. In Saudi Arabia between 1985 and 1990, 7.3% of married women age 50 years or younger became pregnant while being treated with HD. The frequency of conception is reported as two to three times higher in HD than in PD patients, the reason(s) for this difference remains unclear thus far. Successful pregnancy rates have improved notably in recent years: birth of a live infant is reported in 40% to 55% of pregnant dialysis women in the United States, in 60% of cases in the Belgian series, and in 71% of pregnancies in a review including 55 cases published since 1990. Successful outcomes are favored by the maintenance of some residual renal function and increased delivery of dialysis during gestation. Spontaneous abortions and stillbirths account for the majority of pregnancy losses. Moreover, 8% to 15% of live-birth infants are reported to die in the neonatal period. The majority of infants born to dialysis-treated women are indeed preterm, with a gestational age at delivery in the 30.5- to 32.4-weeks range and a birth weight averaging 1.6 kg. Congenital abnormalities are not reported as being more frequent than in the general population. On the other hand, the incidence of polyhydramnios is markedly increased, due to the osmotic diuresis induced by the high blood urea concentration delivered to the fetal kidneys with normal renal function.

The management of pregnancy in dialyzed women requires a close, multidisciplinary cooperation involving nephrologists, obstetricians, neonatologists, and nutrition specialists. The experience accumulated to date is greater with HD than with PD, and both procedures are safe during pregnancy. If HD is used, the number of sessions has to be augmented up to 5 to 6 per week, with minimal heparinization, bicarbonate buffer, and slow ultrafiltration rate. The global objective is to avoid the need for too much fluid removal and the occurrence of subsequent hypotensive episodes. The most common dialysis guideline is to maintain the predialysis blood urea nitrogen (BUN) under 50 mg/dl. Maternal dry weight and weight gain need frequent reevaluation according to changes in fetal weight, which is best estimated through repeat ultrasound determinations. Special attention has to be focused on serum electrolytes (potassium, calcium) and acid–base balance with specific adjustments to be made in the composition of the dialysis fluid mainly to avoid hypokalemia, alkalosis, hypocalcemia, or hypercalcemia. Use of PD has shown little difficulty in the placement of catheters and a low rate of peritoneal infections. In late pregnancy, the volume of the exchanges has to be reduced and their frequency increased. Like in other nonpregnant PD patients, the maintenance of some residual renal function is highly beneficial for a satisfactory control of clinical, nutritional, and metabolic parameters. If indicated, cesarean delivery can be performed through an extraperitoneal route to preserve the integrity of the peritoneal membrane. PD is thereafter resumed with small volumes 2 or 3 days after delivery. Frequent fetal monitoring aims at detecting uteroplacental and fetal circulation disturbances. Heart rate monitoring, Doppler assessment of uterine and umbilical arteries, and ultrasound examinations to check fetal growth are mandatory technical procedures for ensuring a safe development and outcome of pregnancy.

Development or aggravation of hypertension are frequent complications in pregnant women on maintenance dialysis. Careful assessment of fluid balance may be insufficient for adequate control of blood pressure, rendering administration of antihypertensive medications necessary. α-Methyldopa still remains the drug of first choice, followed by labetalol and hydralazine. Experience with several varieties of calcium channel blockers is more limited. β-Blockers may provoke episodes of fetal bradycardia, neonatal hypoglycemia, or respiratory depression. The use of angiotensin-converting enzyme (ACE) inhibitors and angiotensin II–receptor antagonists are firmly contraindicated in pregnancy because of their adverse effects on the fetus. Intravenous administration of hydralazine or labetalol is recommended in case of hypertensive emergencies. Malnutrition should be prevented through a high caloric supply (35 to 40 g/kg per day), with a daily protein intake of 1.6 to 1.8 g/kg along with a supplementation of water-soluble vitamins and calcium.

Anemia usually worsens during pregnancy, making blood transfusions often necessary when rh-EPO is not available. When possible, the use of rh-EPO is highly recommended, aiming at reaching a target hematocrit ranging between 32% and 35%. rh-EPO requirements usually increase by approximately 50% in pregnant women. No rh-EPO–associated teratogenicity has been documented. rh-EPO does not cause aggravation of maternal hypertension or polycythemia in the infants. rh-EPO therapy requires carefully monitored intravenous iron administration, because oral iron is largely ineffective due to poor intestinal absorption. Monitoring of iron status is performed with serial measurements of serum ferritin, transferrin saturation, and the determination of the percentages of hypochromic red cells or reticulocytes. Prematurity is the major cause of morbidity in infants born to dialyzed women. Treatment of premature labor remains debated between advocates of the use of magnesium salts, β-adrenergic agonists, and nonsteroidal antiinflammatory drugs, the latter carrying the risk of inducing neonatal acute renal failure and premature closure of the ductus arteriosus.

The negative opinion that prevailed among nephrologists regarding pregnancy in women with advanced-stage renal insufficiency or treated with maintenance dialysis is evolving toward a less pessimistic view. The constant improvement of the global management of dialysis patients together with the beneficial effects of the administration of rh-EPO contribute to render conception and outcome of pregnancy less rare and less risky to mother and infant than a decade ago. Birth control measures, mainly with oral contraceptives, are indicated for dialyzed women who remain sexually active, have regular menstrual periods, and do not want to conceive. On the other hand, (successful) childbearing in some instances can be considered as one of the goals to be achieved by young, dialyzed women rather than an unwanted event, provided that the safety of the mother and the best chances of survival and normal development of the infant are ensured by a close follow-up through a highly qualified, multidisciplinary medical environment.

DIALYSIS IN CHILDREN

In addition to ensuring survival, one of the major goals of RRT in children with end-stage renal disease (ESRD) is to strive for achievement of normal physical growth, good education, and social integration. These objectives are best met by successful renal transplantation, therefore dialysis methods should be considered for most children as the shortest possible, temporary therapeutic bridge before transplantation. The consensus on this issue is well demonstrated by the fact that 37% of the 5,155 children taken on RRT in the United States between 1992 and 1996 were transplanted within the first year after start of dialysis, compared with only 8.7% of the patients age 20 to 64 years at the time dialysis was initiated.

Data on the age-adjusted incidence rates of pediatric patients starting RRT for ESRD in the United States for the period between 1994 and 1995 show a steady increase with age, whereas the overall incidence rate in the population age 0 to 19 years [according to the definition of the pediatric population adopted by the United States Renal Data System (USRDS)] was 15 per million population (PMP); it was only 9 PMP in the youngest age group (0 to 4 years), 8 PMP in children age 5 to 9 years, and rose up to 14 PMP and 15 PMP in patients age 10 to 14 and 15 to 19 years, respectively.

In all age groups, the incidence rates were greater for boys than for girls, reflecting the higher incidence in boys of congenital disorders, including obstructive uropathies and renal dysplasia. Among the countries reporting to the European Dialysis and Transplant (EDTA) Registry, the acceptance rate in 1994 onto RRT of new patients age 15 years or younger ranged between 3 PMP in Germany, 6 PMP in Italy and France, 7 PMP in the United Kingdom, 11 PMP in Finland, and 13 PMP in Belgium. However these figures suffer from important underreporting; only 224 of 2,855 centers known to the registry by the end of 1992 have reported treating children younger than 15 years, and only 90 centers considered themselves specialized pediatric centers. Among 5,155 new children and adolescents taken onto RRT in the United States between 1992 and 1996, primary glomerulonephritis (GN) and cystic, hereditary, and/or congenital diseases accounted for 31.7% and 24.4% of renal failures, respectively, followed by interstitial nephritis/pyelonephritis (19.8%). Focal segmental GN was the most commonly identified type of GN (31%). Lupus nephritis was most common in females (75% of 257 cases) and interstitial nephritis more common in males (63% of 558 cases). This distribution of causes of ESRD is in sharp contrast with that observed in the adult population. Cystic, hereditary, and/or congenital diseases prevail in the 0- to 4-year-old age group, and GN and collagen diseases are becoming the leading causes of ESRD in the older groups of children (adolescents). This distribution of primary renal diseases in U.S. children is very similar to that reported for the pediatric population treated in the countries contributing to the EDTA Registry in 1993.

The indications for initiation of dialysis therapy in children, like in adults, rest on an intelligent combined evaluation of biochemical data together with clinical manifestations of intolerance to advanced-stage uremia. According to the National Kidney Foundation–Data Outcomes Quality Initiative (NKF-DOQI) Clinical Practice Guidelines for initiation of dialysis set forward for adult patients, which can be reasonably be extended to the pediatric population, dialysis should be initiated when the renal Kt/V urea falls below 2.0, which corresponds to a residual creatinine clearance ranging between 9 and 14 ml/min/1.73 m^2. Moreover, dialysis should be started in case of persistent, diuretic-treatment–resistant fluid overload, uncontrolled hyperkalemia, hyperphosphatemia or acidosis, or overt clinical signs or symptoms of malnutrition. Both HD and PD are efficacious methods for treating ESRD in children. The selection of a dialysis modality has to take into account the individual requirements of each child. Therefore the treatment facilities caring for children should provide HD as well as PD and participate in an active transplantation program. Currently in North America as well as in the European countries, virtually all infants receive PD, whereas an equal percentage of older children and adolescents receive HD and PD. Among 1,427 children less than 15 years of age followed in specialized pediatric centers in Europe (78% of all children reported to the EDTA registry in 1994), 21% underwent PD, 23% HD, and 56% had a functional renal graft. Automated PD (APD) using a cycler is the preferred PD method for children because, being performed nightly, it offers better day-time availability for educational and other activities, less risk of abdominal infectious complications [due to less connections than conventional continuous ambulatory peritoneal dialysis (CAPD)], and optimized depurative performances. The first and prominent difficulty encountered with HD treatment in children is the creation and maintenance of an efficient vascular access, which requires the cooperation of expert, dedicated vascular surgeons familiar with microsurgery techniques. Construction of a vascular access has to be performed preferably several months before the estimated date of initiation of HD, particularly in young children. Both arteriovenous fistulas and subcutaneous vascular grafts are used for permanent angioaccesses, according to the patient's available vascular bed and surgical preferences. Percutaneously inserted central venous catheters (using internal jugular, subclavian, or femoral veins) may be a temporary solution, either in emergency situations or if a renal transplantation is scheduled very shortly after initiation of dialysis.

Several components of the dialysis equipment have to be adapted to the childrens' weight and size. The volume of the extracorporeal circuit should be approximately the same as the child's body surface area (BSA). A bicarbonate-buffered (optimally sterile, pyrogen-free) dialysate with an adjustable sodium concentration (140 mmol/L being standard, and sodium profiling being programmed if appropriate); smooth, volumetrically controlled fluid removal; and use of dialyzers equipped with biocompatible membranes may contribute to short- and long-term improved safety and tolerance of HD treatment in the pediatric population. The modalities of dialysis prescription and assessment of dialysis adequacy in children are to this date mainly derived from studies performed in the adult dialysis population. It can be reasonably postulated that the target doses of dialysis for children should at least meet, or even exceed to some extent, the guidelines recommended for adults. The evaluation of PD adequacy should be based on repeat measurements (every 3 months) of both peritoneal and renal residual creatinine clearances. The progressive loss of residual renal function must be compensated for by changes in the number or volume of daily dialysate exchanges, with the target of reaching a weekly total creatinine clearance of at least 60 L/1.73 m^2. Extrapolation to children of the NKF-DOQI guidelines elaborated for adult PD patients (i.e., weekly Kt/V urea of at least 2.0) is also reasonable, although a method for determining total body water (V) specifically in children has yet to be validated. Increased efficacy of PD can be obtained either by increasing the volume or the number of daily dialysate exchanges according to patients' tolerance and peritoneal membrane transport characteristics. Like in adult patients, urea kinetic modeling can also be used for prescribing HD in children. In the absence of available data specific for the pediatric population, the recommended HD dose for children should be at least equal to, or even higher than, that recommended for adults (e.g., single-pool Kt/V urea of 1.3

or more at each dialysis session). Some authors have proposed to assess dialysis adequacy using a "solute removal index," which normalizes the removal to the solute content in the body at the beginning of a dialysis treatment. This mode of calculation offers a more accurate comparison of efficiency between continuous and intermittent dialysis therapies than the conventional Kt/V urea index.

As in adults, HD or PD are only part of the overall treatment of uremia in children. Malnutrition is particularly detrimental for growth, especially in infants less than 2 years old and in adolescents. Children treated with either mode of dialysis should receive an energy supply of at least 100% of the daily recommended allowance (DRA) for age, 44 to 55 kcal/kg per day for an adolescent boy, 40 to 50 kcal/kg per day for an adolescent girl. Persistent anorexia may preclude the regular intake of such high-caloric and protein-rich (2 to 3 g/kg per day of protein) diets, making supplemental nasogastric or even gastrostomy feeding mandatory. The contributions of nutritionists and of expert pediatric dieticians are absolutely essential. An optimal management of renal osteodystrophy is crucial to ensure, as close as possible, normal growth. This implies adequate control and management of acid–base balance and normal intact parathyroid hormone (PTH), serum calcium, and phosphate levels. Oral calcium supplementation, oral or intravenous administration of vitamin D derivatives, and non–aluminimum-containing phosphate binders are used with indications similar to those recommended in adults. Regular radiographic assessment for bone age and detection of signs of renal osteodystrophy should be performed at least at yearly intervals. Efficient treatment of anemia with rh-EPO is highly beneficial, eliminating the need for most blood transfusions and improving greatly the overall quality of life. Administration and monitoring of rh-EPO therapy are quite similar to that used in adult patients, with rh-EPO being started when the hematocrit falls below 30% and a target hematocrit being approximately 36%. These criteria may evolve in the future according to results that will come out from several studies currently in progress in dialysis populations whose hematocrit is raised with rh-EPO to closer-to-normal values. At present, the required rh-EPO doses in children range between 100 and 200 U/kg/week, administered subcutaneously in PD patients and intravenously or subcutaneously in HD patients.

Providing adequate growth and thus preventing the future handicap of severe statural deficit in adulthood is a prominent goal assigned to the nephrologic teams caring for children with ESRD. Growth failure is all the greater in children whose renal insufficiency has developed in the early years of life. The causes involved in the growth retardation of uremic children are multifold, including the type of renal disease, renal osteodystrophy, metabolic acidosis, anemia, psychosocial factors, and dysfunctions of the growth hormone (GH)–insulinlike growth factor-1 (IGF-1) axis. Advances made in the pathophysiology of the disorder of the GH–IGF-1 axis in advanced-stage uremia have opened the way for the use of rh-GH for treating growth retardation in nondialyzed and dialyzed children. "Catch-up" growth with rh-GH in children with already short stature at the start of dialysis [defined as a height standard deviation score (SDS) worse than −1.88] may not be constantly achievable, stressing the necessity for early, predialysis treatment of growth retardation with rh-GH. Furthermore, the changes in height velocity and SDS require higher doses of rh-GH during dialysis treatment. The potential benefits of rh-GH treatment seem to be somewhat lower in children whose spontaneous growth velocity was superior to 6 cm/yr. Despite the well-documented, beneficial effects of rh-GH therapy for promoting growth in children treated with dialysis, only a small minority of them are currently treated, particularly few of those are dialyzed in nonspecialized pediatric centers. In 1994, among 123 European pediatric centers, 50% to 60% of them used rh-GH for treating growth retardation, whereas this percentage amounted to only 11% to 13% in nonspecialized centers. A large survey conducted in 140 centers treating children with ESRD in the United States, Canada, Mexico, and Costa Rica (NAPRTCS research group) showed that in 1997 only 15% of the children who met the previously designated criteria for growth retardation were actually receiving rh-GH.

Serious psychosocial and emotional difficulties are often experienced by dialyzed children and their families. Optimally integrated medical and psychosocial care is thus mandatory for those patients, which is best achieved in specialized pediatric nephrologic centers that can provide efficient support not only from specially qualified medical and nursing staffs but also from the standing cooperation of a working team. This team should include dietician, social worker, psychologist/psychiatrist, and teaching staff for providing education opportunities for children during their time spent on dialysis treatments.

The survival rates of the children treated with dialysis have to be interpreted, taking into account the high proportion of children who can benefit from a kidney transplant within a short period of time after initiation of RRT: among 2,639 incident pediatric patients treated in the United States in 1991 through 1993, 63% of those age 0 to 9 years and 67% of those age 10 to 19 years had a functioning transplant at 2 years after the start of RRT, a much higher proportion than that recorded in corresponding adults age 20 to 44 years, in whom the percentage was only 29%. For the year 1995, the mean time from first ESRD service to living-donor transplantation in the United States was 291, 137, and 290 days for children age 5 to 9 years, 10 to 14 years, and 15 to 19 years, respectively. Mean time to first cadaveric transplantation was 443, 387, and 576 days for patients in the same age groups. The waiting time was shortest for very young children (0 to 4 years), 238 days.

In 1996 the annual death rate was 44.3 per 1,000 patient-years at risk in dialyzed children 0 to 14 years old and 28.2 in those 15 to 19 years old. By comparison, the death rates were 3.2 and 8.6 per 1,000 patients at risk in transplanted children of the same age groups. The most frequent causes of death reported during the 1994 to 1996 period in dialyzed patients 0 to 19 years old were, in decreasing order, cardiac arrest (cause unknown), septicemia, cardiomyopathy, and cardiac arrhythmia. Overall, in the United States in 1994, the 2-year survival probabilities in children treated by dialysis age 5 to 9 years, 10 to 14 years, and 15 to 19 years were 92.4%, 96.1%, and 94.1%, respectively, and 90.7%, 74.9%, and 78.5% at 5 years. Five-year survival probabilities after living-donor transplantation ranged between 94.6% and 98.5% according to age groups and was 95.4% for 0- to 19-year-old patients who received a cadaveric kidney. These figures strongly plead for a renal transplant to be offered to the pediatric population as soon as possible after reaching ESRD. Preemptive transplantation for children has progressively increased in recent years and this strategy of treatment should certainly be encouraged, particularly for the pediatric population.

DIALYSIS IN VERY OLD PATIENTS

There is currently no universal consensus for the definition of "elderly people." A 65-year age limit is widely recognized in many countries for designating elderly people on social, professional, or administrative grounds. In many people, "old age" cannot be strictly identified with chronologic age; it may actually be better defined as "a state of mind." This is particularly important for people with a chronic illness in whom the will to survive plays a key role in the success or failure of a life-long, demanding treatment for which their personal, active contribution is permanently required as is, for example, the case in patients treated with chronic PD. Similar difficulties and complications can be encountered during long-term dialysis treatment in patients age 40 to 75 years, depending on their past history or the presence of comorbid, extrarenal diseases. To highlight some of the problems more specifically related to aging in dialysis patients, it seems appropriate to concentrate on "truly old" patients, defined by an age of at least 75 years at start of dialysis treatment.

In the United States, among the 73,091 patients who where newly taken on RRT in 1996, 19.8% were age 75 or older, whereas this group of patients accounted only for 8.6% and 16.9% of the incident ESRD patients recorded in 1985 and 1990, respectively. The point prevalence on December 31, 1996 of patients 75 years and older treated for ESRD was 12.9% of the 283,932 patients alive at that date, whereas it was 7.5% and 9.7% on December 31, 1985 and 1990, respectively. By the end of 1996, 89.3% of the 36,635 ESRD patients age 75 years or older treated in the United States underwent center HD, 6.8% CAPD/CCPD (continuous cycling peritoneal dialysis), and 1.4% were on home HD. These percentages have not changed notably compared with data collected in December 1988, with center HD, PD, and home HD accounting for, respectively, 88.6%, 8.1%, and 1.3% of patients age 75 or older treated by that time. It seems worthwhile to mention that a functioning renal transplant was reported on December 31, 1996 in 408 patients age 75 to 79 years, in 59 patients age 80 to 84 years, and even in 10 patients age 85 years or older. Among the 51,097 incident patients older than 75 years taken onto RRT in the United States during the period between 1993 and 1996, the most common underlying renal disease was nephropathy due to hypertension (45.3%) followed by diabetes (25.8%), thus in reverse order with the distribution observed in the younger population with ESRD. Glomerulonephritis accounted only for 8.1% of cases. Altogether, these three causes amounted to 79.5% of all new old patients taken onto RRT during this 4-year time span.

Both HD and PD are suitable options for very old patients. Apart from each patient's clinical condition, the choice between the two methods has to take into account his or her cognitive and psychologic status, familial and social environment, and acceptance or refusal either to RRT itself or toward the mode and location of dialysis, in-center or home. Besides technical reasons that would preclude the use of PD, such as previous intraabdominal surgery, repeat episodes of peritoneal infection, or poor peritoneal membrane performances, HD remains the sole mode of therapy for patients who are unable to perform self-care and/or who have no support available from a spouse, relatives, or other caregivers to assist them for their daily requirements. Vascular access for HD is best achieved with an arteriovenous fistula because arteriovenous grafts, especially if they are placed in proximal segments of the limbs, may provoke arterial steal syndromes favored by preexisting atherosclerotic lesions and distal ischemic gangrenous lesions. Satisfactory results can be obtained for prolonged periods with the use of percutaneously placed internal jugular vein catheters, if an internal vascular access is very difficult to construct or keep patent.

The general guidelines recommended for applying dialysis techniques to very old patients are similar in many ways to those set forth for other groups of frail patients, such as children or diabetics. Because of frequent vascular instability, HD sessions should be performed very smoothly with a slow, volumetric-controlled, fluid removal bicarbonate dialysate with a minimal and adjustable sodium concentration of 140 mmol/L to avoid hypotensive episodes, which can precipitate the occurrence of angina, myocardial infarction, or cerebrovascular accidents. Addition of glucose to the dialysate (up to 200 mg/dl) may be helpful for better tolerance and provides some caloric supply. Intradialytic supply of amino acids or other nutritional components/mixtures may also be indicated in malnourished patients. PD should be considered as the first-line mode of treatment primarily for patients with coronary heart disease, arrhythmias, or peripheral vascular disease. PD is also preferred for patients whose residences are distant from a dialysis center and who wish to preserve optimally their personal and family lifestyle. Moreover, PD is a rescue method for patients who cannot tolerate HD for some medical or logistic reason(s). PD techniques have become very diversified, from conventional three to four daily exchanges, to nightly automated PD performed with a cycler, completed if necessary with one or two daily exchanges. PD treatment can thus be tailored to an individual patient's medical and personal requirements, and can be rendered safer, more efficient, and more tolerable in the long term. Despite all the advantages offered by PD, this mode of therapy remains stagnant (or even slightly decreasing) in elderly patients. This is probably more often due to familial or environmental difficulties suffered by many isolated, depressed, and economically disadvantaged patients than to technical problems related to PD per se.

Whichever dialysis method is used, close attention should be given to avoid underdialysis. Biochemical values alone may be misleading for an adequate dialysis prescription: low values of BUN may be due to low protein intake, and low serum creatinine concentrations may result from the reduced muscle mass. Insufficient delivery of dialysis dose with HD may result from vascular access problems or early ending of dialysis sessions in case of multiple hypotensive episodes. In case of a marked shortage of in-center dialysis facilities, elderly patients are often the first category of patients for whom the number of weekly sessions will be reduced. PD patients are also exposed to underdialysis either through personal or familial noncompliance with the dialysis regimen, or by medical inaccurate evaluation of qualitative/quantitative dialysis efficiency, particularly by lack of adjustment of the number or volume of daily dialysate exchanges according to the reduction over time of the patients' residual renal function. Malnutrition, which greatly enhances the risk of infectious complications, is very common in all dialysis patients. Anorexia, with a specific loss of taste for meat; depression; and low financial resources frequently associated with clinical problems (autonomic dysfunction, adverse effects of medications on digestive motility) are often implicated in the development of severe malnutrition. Active support from a dietician/nutritionist team is essential for counselling the patients and their families for adequate caloric and protein intake. Correction of anemia with rh-EPO with a target hematocrit set around 33% to 36% usually greatly improves physical performances and an overall feeling of well-being. Not to be overlooked are also the precautions to be taken regarding the prescription and monitoring of drugs such as antihypertensives, analgesics, hypnotics, and some classes of antibiotics, because even slight overdosage may induce particularly harmful cardiovascular, neurologic, or psychiatric complications.

No unequivocal conclusion can be drawn from the papers published in the literature over the past 15 years on the respective superiority in terms of morbidity/mortality of HD or PD for the ESRD population in general, at least in the 5 years following start of RRT, and this holds true for the very old patients as well. Optimal management of elderly patients requires that a fully integrated HD plus PD program be available in the treatment facility, because a switch to an alternative mode of RRT may become necessary for many of them according to modifications in their physical or mental status that may occur over time or to changes in their sociofamilial environment that, for example, may render institutionalization mandatory. Results in terms of survival may vary greatly between single-center experiences and data collected in large national or international registries. Multiple biases in patient-selection policies, differences in technical options or degree of expertise and in the sophistication or availability of dialysis equipment, and positive or negative influences of sociocultural and environmental factors all contribute to the difficulties of providing sound and objective answers concerning the most appropriate mode of treatment for very old ESRD patients as well as for an objective and flawless assessment of the results on morbidity and mortality.

According to the most recent USRDS data, the 5-year survival probability for patients age 75 years and older who started dialysis in the United States in 1991 was 11.35%. At first glance, this figure did not differ much from that reported for patients of the same age group who started dialysis 4 years earlier and who had a survival probability of 9.9% at 5 years. However, during this relatively short period of time, the age distribution of these very old patients has markedly changed: the patients age 80 or older who were newly taken on dialysis in 1991 increased by 107% since 1987 (2,669 and 1,403, respectively) and those age 85 and older have increased by 120% (1,085 versus 493). The impact on survival of the comorbidities present in this oldest category of patients is of utmost importance. It should also be reasonably stated that dialysis therapy *per se* cannot grant immortality, a reality that some patients' families have difficulty understanding. On the other hand, more satisfactory results are reported in several single-center studies: a 30% 2-year survival rate was achieved in 30 consecutive patients age 83 ± 3 years who started dialysis in France in 1995 and 1996. The mean survival time on dialysis in a series of 47 patients over age 80 who began dialysis in Germany after 1990 was 28.8 months. Survival rates of 73.6%, 59.6%, and 45% at 1, 2, and 3 years, respectively, were reported in a series of 213 elderly patients treated in French centers with PD. Cardiac arrest, acute myocardial infarction, and septicemia are among the leading causes of death in elderly dialysis patients. More specific to this age group is the high death rate due to withdrawal from dialysis. Approximately 17% of the dialysis patients who died in the United States in 1991 and 1992 had withdrawn from dialysis before death of any cause. Death rates preceded by (not necessarily due to) withdrawal was about three times higher in white patients age 65 or older than in patients of the same race in the 45- to 64-year age range. Withdrawal from dialysis was more commonly recorded in males, whereas no significant difference was found between deaths associated with withdrawal in diabetics versus nondiabetics, or in patients treated with HD or PD. Among the older age groups of patients, chronic failure to thrive was the leading reason for withdrawal from dialysis.

Taking an upper age limit as a selection criterion for excluding or withdrawing older patients from RRT is currently widely rejected by the medical community in most of the countries where dialysis facilities are commonly available. Nevertheless, given the increasing pressure and restrictions in health care funding, which are implemented nowadays even in economically well-developed countries, the political and ethical debate on priorities, or in other words, "rationing in health care," focuses in many instances on the issue of the unlimited provision of very expensive treatments such as dialysis for patients who have a rather limited expectancy of survival and for whom RRT offers often only a poor quality of life. Actually, the decision to institute, continue, or end dialysis therapy should continue to take into account the global situation of each individual patient, whose assessment should prevail over any national or regional purely economic arguments. The complexity of medical and/or psychosocial problems encountered in some patients may generate highly emotional reactions among families and/or medical and nursing staff when facing the decision of excluding or ending dialysis therapy in the presence of social isolation, severe debilitation, or dementia. Applying a demanding life-supporting therapy for the sole objective of extending the duration of life, regardless of its "quality," may become questionable on medical and ethical grounds. If clearly expressed, particularly through advanced directives, the patient's own wishes for refusing to begin or continue dialysis should be extensively considered, while being careful not to make irreversible decisions for someone who may suffer a transient depressive episode that could subside within a short period of time with the aid of adequate family or social support. In profoundly demented or severely debilitated patients, the decision for withholding dialysis should preferably be a consensual one, based on a full agreement between the medical team and the patients' families.

DIALYSIS IN DIABETICS

The continuously "rising tide" of ESRD patients with diabetic nephropathy is well documented in all of the epidemiologic reports on renal diseases published in the developed countries. In the United States, the incidence rate of new diabetic patients taken onto RRT soared from 43 PMP in 1987 up to 117 PMP in 1996 (172% increase). Diabetics accounted for 30.4% of all the incident patients who commenced RRT in 1987 and they were 42.3% in 1996. In the European countries, the incidence rates of ESRD diabetic patients remained at a lower rate than in the United States as had been the case in earlier years, amounting to 17.6 PMP in France in 1995, 20.2% in Denmark in 1997, and 15.3% in the Netherlands in 1996. Thirty-three percent of the new patients taken on dialysis in Japan in 1996 were diabetic, versus 21% in 1986. In Australia in 1997, diabetics accounted for 21.4% of the incident dialysis patients. A much higher percentage was recorded in neighboring New Zealand, where diabetics represented 40% of all new patients taken on RRT.

The distinction between the types of diabetes present in patients with ESRD is not assessed with precision in the majority of the published reports. The classical distribution between type 1 (insulin-dependent) and type 2 (non–insulin-dependent) does not reflect the accurate status of many patients, who are not really insulin dependent, but only insulin requiring, because oral hypoglycemic agents have been previously withdrawn at a more or less advanced stage of renal insufficiency. Data from the Australia and New Zealand Dialysis and Transplant Registry are thus particularly informative, showing that among the 314 new diabetic patients taken on RRT in 1997, 45% were non–insulin-requiring type 2, 36.3% insulin-requiring type 2, and only 18% really insulin-dependent type 1 patients. In New Zealand, during the same year 51% of the incident diabetics taken on RRT were non–insulin-requiring type 2 patients. Overall, the non–insulin-dependent patients constitute the vast majority of the diabetic patients taken on RRT. During the years 1994 to 1996, only 13.2% of the diabetic patients who commenced RRT in the United States were younger than 45 years, 43.4% were age 45 to 64 years, and 30.6% belonged to the 65- to 84-year age group.

The prevalence of diabetic patients alive on RRT in the United States increased from 107 PMP in December 1987 up to 346 PMP in December 1996. Diabetics accounted for, respectively, 21.1% and 32.4% of all the U.S. patients alive on RRT on these dates. In the European countries, the prevalence rates in 1992 and 1993 ranged between 109 PMP in Sweden, 44.6 PMP in Spain, 40.3 PMP in France, and 35.4 PMP in Italy. Data available for Japan indicate that in 1994, diabetics accounted for 18.2% of the whole population receiving RRT, whereas they were 8.5% in 1984. Among the 93,601 diabetics alive on RRT in the United States by the end of 1996, 70.2% were treated with center HD, 10.4% with CAPD/CCPD, 0.7% with home HD, and 17.8% benefited from a functioning renal transplant. At the same date, among the 194,014 nondiabetic patients, 56.8% were on center dialysis, 9.3% on CAPD/CCPD, 0.8% on home HD, and 32% had functioning renal transplant. In Japan, in 1994, diabetics accounted for 19.5% of the patients treated with extracorporeal techniques and for 14% of those treated with PD.

It has become widely accepted that combined pancreas and kidney transplantation is the real method of choice for treating insulin-requiring or insulin-dependent diabetic patients with ESRD. Unfortunately this method will remain, at least for some time, available only for a minority of patients, due to the pyramid of ages of diabetic patients, frequent comorbidities precluding organ transplantation, and shortage in organ donors. Over the past 10 years the controversies on a clear superiority of CAPD/CCPD over HD as the preferential techniques for diabetics continue, not only on survival criteria but also in terms of their respective efficiency for controlling the medical and metabolic disturbances of uremia and on the frequency and gravity of treatment-induced morbidities, psychologic tolerance, and quality of life. The debate has become all the more complex as important technical advances have been made for PD, in terms of novel dialysis-fluid compositions, connectology, and measurements of dialysis adequacy, which have all rendered PD safer and better adaptable to a wider group of patients than was the case 10 years ago.

The reasons for privileging PD over HD more specifically in diabetic patients are preservation of blood vessels for vascular access and a better hemodynamic stability, which is highly desirable because the frequency of hypotensive episodes is frequently augmented by disorders of the autonomous nervous system. A better and prolonged preservation of the residual renal function contributes, among other advantages, to a higher amount of sodium removal and, hence, an easier control of blood pressure. Less blood loss related to dialysis technique reduces the amount of rh-EPO required for maintaining a satisfactory hematocrit level. CAPD (but not APD) allows the intraperitoneal administration of insulin, a more physiologic method than the subcutaneous route, resulting in a lower degree of hyperinsulinemia, a more stable blood glucose control, and an amelioration of the lipoprotein profiles, which is considered beneficial for the prevention of the extension of atherosclerotic complications. In spite of all these advantages, PD cannot be considered as the universally best method for treating diabetics with ESRD. The incidence of abdominal complications (peritonitis episodes, infections of catheter exit sites) is estimated in many studies as being no more frequent than in nondiabetics. Malnutrition, mainly protein deficiency aggravated by the protein loss in the dialysate, is in fact one of the major causes of complications in diabetics on PD, who are submitted to multiple dietary restrictions and who are frequently anorectic, this being aggravated by the sensation of abdominal filling and the glucose uptake from the dialysate. Profound and prolonged hypoalbuminemia is the most widely recognized marker reflecting this poor nutritional status, and should entail discontinuation of PD and an at least temporary transfer to HD. A transfer to HD has to be made in quite a number of patients who develop a "burn-out" syndrome after a variable period of time of PD treatment, or in case of difficulties arising among the patient's social environment.

In all single-center, national or international studies published over the past 10 years, the survival rates in diabetic patients treated for ESRD is reported lower by 20% to 25% compared with age-adjusted, nondiabetic patients. These comparisons however are frequently flawed, due to the more frequent and more severe comorbidities present in diabetics at the start of dialysis treatment, which are unequally taken into account in the various Cox proportional hazard models and other statistical tools used in studies of different sizes and origins. The widely pessimistic statements can be tempered somewhat by the improvement of the results recorded for diabetic ESRD patients during the last decade. The first-year mortality rate for diabetics treated with (all) dialysis methods in the United States (all ages combined) has decreased from 46 per 100 patient-years in 1985 down to 26.8 per 100 patient-years in 1995. The 5-year probability of survival for incident diabetics taken on dialysis in the United States in 1981 and 1991 increased from the dismal figure of 14.8% to the more favorable figure of 29.3%. Several comparisons of survivals yielded by HD and PD in diabetic patients based either on large multicenter surveys or on single-center, retrospective data have to be interpreted with great caution due to heterogeneity between the populations of investigated patients regarding comorbidities at the start of dialysis, differences in patient-selection–transfer-withdrawal of treatment policies, technical options, and degree of expertise of the medical and nursing staffs.

A comprehensive and sophisticated analysis based on data collected by the USRDS in more than 55,000 U.S. diabetic patients treated during the period extending from 1987 to 1993 showed that, on average, the 1-year death rates among diabetics treated with PD were higher than those treated with HD. However, further analyses indicated that the higher risks of death were concentrated in females and in patients older than 50 years. Patients under the age of 50 treated with PD had, in fact, a significantly lower risk of death than those treated with HD. In an Italian series of 731 diabetic patients accepted for dialysis between 1983 and 1992, the survival rate was 82% at 1 year and 28% at 5 years. The relative risk of death of the patients on PD versus those on HD was not significantly different after having taken into account the patients' age and comorbid conditions. In our own series of 110 diabetic patients taken on PD between 1978 and 1995, the actuarial survival rate at 4 years was 30%, almost identical to that recorded in 337 nondiabetic patients treated with PD during the same period (29%). These results may be related to earlier transfer to HD if complications occur on PD and also because more diabetic patients are successfully transplanted.

In the United States as well as in the European series of diabetic patients treated with dialysis, the causes of death are mainly of cardiac and infectious origin. Early transfers from PD to HD in case of repetitive peritonitis episodes, overt malnutrition, or psychologic intolerance should contribute to reduce the deaths due to infections or cachexia. Severe cardiac, cerebral, or peripheral vascular complications, especially when associated with other heavily disabling or distressing comorbidities, may lead more often in diabetics than in other categories of ESRD patients to discussing withdrawal from RRT.

A fully integrated PD–HD transplantation program is actually mandatory for providing each ESRD diabetic patient with the therapeutic choice initially best adjusted to his or her overall situation, bearing in mind that for most of them it will change several times over the years either by organ transplantation for the younger cohort or by temporary or definitive transfers from PD to HD and vice versa for the majority of older patients who are not candidates for transplantation or who have to return to dialysis after transplant failure.

Selected Readings

Hou S. Pregnancy in chronic renal insufficiency and end-stage renal disease. *Am J Kidney Dis* 1999;33:235–252.

A comprehensive review of the management of pregnancy in women treated with either dialysis methods or renal transplantation including prepregnancy counselling and postdelivery follow-up.

Latos DL. Chronic dialysis in patients over age 65. *J Am Soc Nephrol* 1996;7: 637–646.

This paper well describes the technical, psychosocial, and ethical issues that are specific for a rapidly growing part of the dialysis-treated population.

Marcelli D, Spotti D, Conte F, et al. Prognosis of diabetic patients on dialysis: analysis of Lombardy Registry Data. *Nephrol Dial Transplant* 1995;10: 1895–1900.

Description of the clinical profile, course of treatments, and outcome in 731 diabetic patients taken onto dialysis therapy in Lombardy, Italy between 1983 and 1992.

United States Renal Data System. *USRDS 1998 annual data report.* Bethesda, MD: National Institutes of Health, National Institute of Diabetes and Digestive and Kidney Diseases, 1998.

The indispensable gold standard for demographic and epidemiologic information on ESRD.

Vonesh EF, Moran J. Mortality in end-stage renal disease: a reassessment of differences between patients treated with peritoneal dialysis and hemodialysis. *J Am Soc Nephrol* 1999;10:354–365.

A sophisticated analysis on the subject based on data collected by the USRDS annual reports over the period from 1987 to 1993.

Waradi BA, Alexander SR, Watkin S, et al. Optimal care of pediatric end-stage renal disease in children. *Am J Kidney Dis* 1999;33:567–583.

This current state-of-the-art article on the subject encompasses very comprehensively the clinical, technical, psychosocial, and educational problems encountered in children with ESRD.

PART 2
Peritoneal Dialysis
A: Kinetics of Peritoneal Dialysis

Robert A. Mactier, Ramesh Khanna, and Karl D. Nolph

In peritoneal dialysis, solutes and water are transported between peritoneal capillary blood and repeated infusions of commercially produced dialysis solutions into the peritoneal cavity. Transcapillary transport therefore should provide net removal of water and solutes in the drained dialysate effluent. The efficiency of peritoneal dialysis is dependent on the sustained efflux of fluid and solutes across the visceral and parietal peritoneum, which may be considered as a biologic, reusable, complex semipermeable membrane. Optimal clinical application of modern techniques of peritoneal dialysis requires an understanding of the mechanisms of transperitoneal solute transport and osmotic-induced ultrafiltration.

ANATOMY OF PERITONEAL DIALYSIS

Effective Peritoneal Blood Flow

Although the absolute peritoneal blood flow rate is not known, CO_2 gas diffusion studies in humans have implied that the effective peritoneal blood flow rate is at least 70 ml/min. Under resting conditions, not all peritoneal capillaries are perfused and, consequently, vasodilator drugs can increase peritoneal capillary flow and/or the number of capillaries perfused. It has been estimated that perfused capillaries underlie only 0.5% of the total surface area of the peritoneum.

Peritoneal Membrane

The peritoneum is a continuous membrane that invests the visceral organs, forms the mesentery that connects loops of bowel, and reflects over and covers the inner surface of the abdominal wall. The cavity so enclosed normally contains only a small amount of isosmotic fluid, usually less than 100 ml. The inner surface of this membrane is a layer of flattened cells with numerous microvilli (the mesothelium) supported by its basement membrane and underlying interstitium. The peritoneal interstitium contains blood vessels and lymphatics interspersed between extracellular fluid and a gellike matrix within collagen fibers, fibroblasts, and fat. The surface area of the peritoneum in adults is estimated to be 1 to 2 m^2 and almost equates with body surface area.

Solutes and water transfer across the peritoneum by intercellular, transcytoplasmic, and vesicular mechanisms. At least six major anatomic resistance sites for solute and water transport from the peritoneal capillaries to the peritoneal cavity have been identified (Fig. 84.25). These resistance sites may be summarized as follows:

R_1 fluid films within the capillary lumen
R_2 endothelium
R_3 endothelial basement membrane
R_4 interstitium
R_5 mesothelial layer
R_6 fluid films within the peritoneal cavity

Dialysate Flow Rate

At least 2 L of dialysis solution can be instilled into the peritoneal cavity of most adult patients without causing discomfort or symptoms related to increased intraperitoneal pressure. The dialysate flow rate is governed by the infusion volume and the total exchange time, and either may be adjusted as needed. In intermittent peritoneal dialysis (IPD), dialysate flow rates of 40 ml/min are readily achieved by rapid cycling with the assistance of an automated machine, whereas in continuous ambulatory peritoneal dialysis (CAPD), flow rates with four exchanges per day are frequently only 7 ml/min. Continuous flow meth-

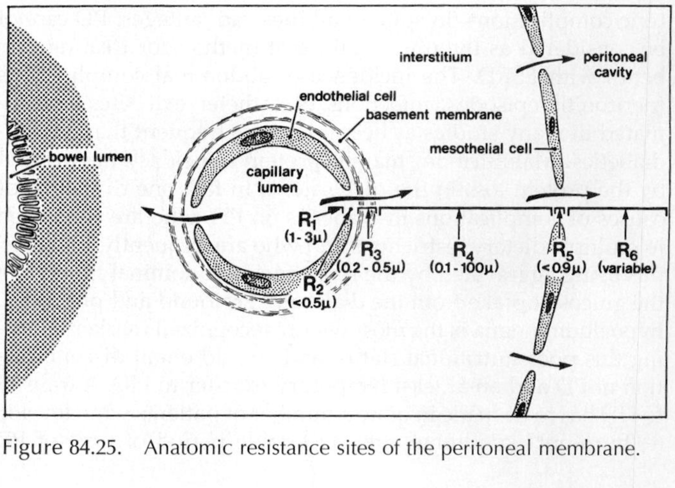

Figure 84.25. Anatomic resistance sites of the peritoneal membrane.

ods using double-lumen or twin catheters can provide higher dialysate flow rates for IPD, but rates greater than 100 ml/min are often associated with abdominal pain. Infusion dialysate volumes may be increased until intraperitoneal pressure approaches 18 cm H_2O before vital capacity is reduced by more than 20% or fluid absorption rates are increased. Average-size adults can usually accommodate infusion volumes of 2.5 L before the measured intraperitoneal pressure exceeds 18 cm H_2O.

Peritoneal Cavity Lymphatics

The subdiaphragmatic surface of the peritoneum contains specialized end lymphatics called *stomata,* which is the major site of absorption of intraperitoneal particles, cells, colloids, and isosmotic fluid. Peritoneal lymph flow rates in malignant and hepatic ascites are reported to be at least 50 ml/hr provided there is no obstruction or dysfunction of the diaphragmatic or mediastinal lymphatics. The intraperitoneal volumes of dialysate used in peritoneal dialysis also ensure constant contact of fluid with the subdiaphragmatic peritoneum and increase intraperitoneal pressure. Thus convective flow into the peritoneal lymphatics and submesothelial tissues in peritoneal dialysis results in continuous fluid loss from the peritoneal cavity at approximately 1 ml/min, which significantly reduces net transperitoneal water and solute transport during long-dwelling exchanges.

Comparison with Hemodialysis

In contrast with peritoneal dialysis, the standard blood flow rate in hemodialysis is at least 200 ml/min and all of the blood channels are perfused and in close proximity to dialysate flowing in the opposite direction at a rate of 500 ml/min or greater. The internal diameter of the individual fibers of a hollow-fiber dialyzer is 200 ± 30 μm, which is much greater than that of the biologic capillary of the peritoneal membrane. Although peritoneal capillary wall thickness is approximately one-tenth of cellulose fibers, the functional pore area of capillary endothelium is estimated to be 0.2%, which is less than the percentage of effective pore area of the mesh of fibrils in synthetic membranes. Intercellular gaps between endothelial cells may be 40 A or greater in diameter, whereas the "pore" diameter of cuprophane membranes is almost 20 A. Thus the peritoneal capillaries have a relatively high mean-pore diameter but low pore density in comparison with hemodialysis membranes. Even though the calculated surface areas of peritoneal and hemodialysis membranes are similar at 1 to 2 m², the area of the peritoneum involved in mass transfer is much lower because of perfusion–dialysate flow mismatching.

PHYSIOLOGY OF PERITONEAL DIALYSIS

Ultrafiltration (Convective Mass Transfer)

Water Flux

Hydraulic permeability to water (L_P) is an intrinsic property of all membranes. The water flux rate (J_W) across the peritoneal membrane is equal to the product of membrane area (A), hydraulic permeability in ml/min/cm² mm Hg, and the sum of the osmotic and hydrostatic transmembrane pressure gradients ($\Delta\pi + \Delta P$). Thus water flux rate may be expressed as follows:

$$J_W = A\,L_P\,(\Delta\pi + \Delta P)$$

In peritoneal dialysis, ultrafiltration is osmotic induced ($\Delta\pi$) and the predominant crystalloid osmotic pressure gradient is produced by the glucose concentration of standard dialysis solutions. The net ultrafiltration rate is maximal at time zero and decreases exponentially as the glucose concentration gradient is dissipated by a combination of transmembrane glucose absorption and dilution by the ultrafiltrate (Fig. 84.26). It is not established whether the glucose concentration gradient is transcapillary or transmesothelial or both. However, because the mesothelium does not prevent glucose absorption, and water flux decreases with hyperglycaemia, the transcapillary osmotic gradient is likely to be the most important.

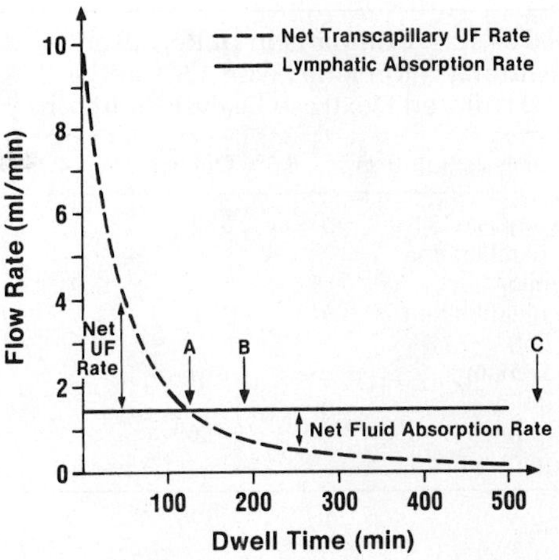

Figure 84.26. Net ultrafiltration (UF) and fluid absorption rates during a representative 2.5% dextrose exchange. *Arrow A* represents maximum intraperitoneal volume when net UF is zero. *Arrow B* depicts crystalloid osmotic equilibrium, and *arrow C* represents glucose equilibrium.

The intraperitoneal volume continues to increase until a maximum is reached when the net transcapillary ultrafiltration rate has reduced to equal the transperitoneal absorption rate into the lymphatics and submesothelial tissues (point A in Figs. 84.26 and 84.27). After peak ultrafiltration volume is reached, transcapillary efflux continues at a slow rate until crystalloid osmotic equilibrium is approached later in the dwell time (point B in Figs. 84.26 and 84.27). Net absorption begins when the transperitoneal fluid absorption rate exceeds the transcapillary ultrafiltration rate and thereafter averages 40 ml/hr.

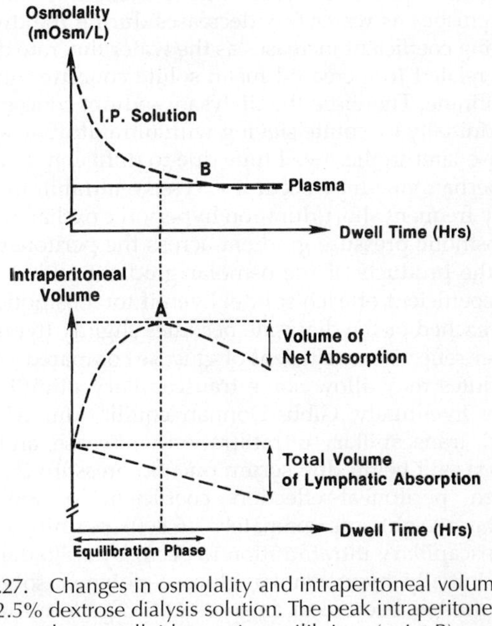

Figure 84.27. Changes in osmolality and intraperitoneal volume after infusion of 2.5% dextrose dialysis solution. The peak intraperitoneal volume *(point A)* precedes crystalloid osmotic equilibrium *(point B).*

TABLE 84.12. Comparison of Representative Net Ultrafiltration Rates with 1.5% and 4.25% Hydrated Dextrose Dialysis Solutions

Dextrose Dialysis Solution	1.5% Dextrose	4.25% Dextrose
Osmolality (mOsm/L)	332	477
Maximum ultrafiltration rate (ml/min)	12	17
Maximum ultrafiltration volume (ml)	331	1028
Time of maximum volume (min)	140	247
Fluid absorption rate (ml/min)	− 0.68	− 0.87

For any given patient on peritoneal dialysis, an increase in the osmolality of the dialysate results in a higher initial ultrafiltration rate, a greater peak in intraperitoneal volume, prolongation of the time until crystalloid equilibrium is achieved, and delay until net intraperitoneal fluid absorption begins (Table 84.12). In addition, hypertonic glucose dialysis solutions have a vasodilator effect on the peritoneal microcirculation, which tends to increase transmembrane hydrostatic pressure and promote ultrafiltration before osmotic equilibrium is approached.

Solute Sieving

Solute transport occurs with water flux by solvent drag. The peritoneal membrane offers greater resistance to accompanying solutes than to water so that the concentration of solutes in the ultrafiltrate is less than in plasma water. The membrane resistance to convective transfer of solutes is indicated by the solute-sieving coefficient (S), which is the ratio of solute concentrations in ultrafiltrate to plasma water, or by the osmotic reflection coefficient (σ), which is almost equal to 1-S. Hence convective solute flux is the product of water flux, sieving coefficient, and mean transmembrane–solute concentration (C_S). That is:

$$J_S = J_w (1 - \sigma_S) C_S$$

The contribution of convective mass transfer to solute transport diminishes as water flux decreases during the dwell time. The sieving coefficient increases as the water flux rate decreases, perhaps related to increased mean solute concentration within the membrane. Therefore the dialysate sodium concentration is reduced initially by solute sieving with ultrafiltration and tends to increase later in the dwell time due to diffusion. For this reason, hypernatremia may occur if excessive ultrafiltration is sustained by frequent short-duration hypertonic exchanges.

The osmotic pressure gradient across the peritoneum is the sum of the products of the osmolar gradient and osmotic reflection coefficient of each solute. Even if total osmotic equilibrium is reached or the dialysate becomes slightly hypoosmolar, the higher reflection coefficient of glucose compared with other small solutes may allow some transcapillary ultrafiltration to continue. Eventually, Gibbs-Donnan equilibrium will be approached, transcapillary ultrafiltration will cease, and venular absorption will begin due serum oncotic pressure (Fig. 84.26). The high peritoneal-reflection coefficient of polyglucose (molecular weight approximately 16,800) permits sustained, slow transcapillary ultrafiltration to occur by colloidal osmosis with an initially hypoosmolar glucose–polymer solution and polyglucose has been used as an osmotic agent in dialysis solutions to achieve net ultrafiltration after long-dwell exchanges.

Diffusive Mass Transfer

In the absence of ultrafiltration, solutes transfer across the peritoneum in a direction to discharge their concentration gradients. Other than buffer anion, calcium, and glucose or alternative osmotic agents, the direction of solute movement is from blood to dialysate. Magnesium also diffuses from blood to the dialysis solution if low-magnesium dialysate formulations are infused. The diffusive mass transfer rate of free solutes is equal to the product of membrane permeability (P_S), effective membrane area (A), and solute concentration gradient (ΔC). That is:

$$J_S = P_S \, A \, \Delta C$$

Membrane permeability is dependent on solute size (molecular weight), charge, and configuration. The concentration gradient for diffusion is maximum near completion of installation of dialysate and decreases exponentially as solute equilibrium with extracellular fluid is approached. At the point of equilibrium diffusion will cease. The effective membrane area (pore area) for each solute is unknown and therefore membrane permeability × area are considered together in studies of peritoneal diffusive transport.

Interrelation of Convection and Diffusion

Convective and diffusive mass transfer are interdependent. Ultrafiltration enhances the diffusive component of transport of solutes other than buffer anion, calcium, and osmotic agent by:

1. Maintaining the concentration gradient by solute sieving
2. Shortening the length of the diffusive path by reducing blood and dialysate fluid films

In contrast, diffusion limits ultrafiltration because of absorption of glucose or alternative low-molecular-weight osmotic agents. If the permeability of the peritoneal membrane to glucose increases, the osmolar gradient is dissipated more rapidly and the osmotic pressure generated at any given glucose osmolar gradient is reduced because of the lower osmotic-reflection coefficient. Rapid glucose absorption diminishes cumulative ultrafiltration by reducing the time and osmolar gradient for transcapillary fluid flux and thus permits net absorption to commence earlier in the dwell time. High peritoneal transport for glucose is the major cause of poor peritoneal-ultrafiltration capacity (type 1 membrane failure).

Peritoneal Backfiltration

Solute and water transport in peritoneal dialysis are modified by absorption into the peritoneal cavity lymphatics and submesothelial tissues. Although interstitial lymphatics underlie approximately 4% of the calculated surface area of the peritoneum, their low flow rate suggests that their role in solute exchange is minor. Because transperitoneal transport occurs via pathways through the interstitium, the ultrafiltration that is observed in peritoneal dialysis must overcome the resorptive capacity of the interstitial lymphatics. Alternatively, some ultrafiltrate may come from the interstitial lymphatics subsequent to the osmotic effects of interstitial glucose. Absorption by the subdiaphragmatic lymphatics is cumulative from the beginning of the dwell time (Fig. 84.27) and is the major site of backfiltration from the peritoneal cavity. In effect, the drain volume is equal to the infusion volume plus total net transcapillary ultrafiltration minus cumulative backfiltration during the dwell time, assuming that the residual volume remains constant. Observed (net) ultrafiltration equates with total transcapillary ultrafiltration minus cumulative backfiltration by bulk flow into the peritoneal lymphatics and submesothelial tissues.

Comparison with Hemodialysis

Fluid flux in hemodialysis is induced by the transmembrane hydrostatic pressure gradient and remains nearly constant during dialysis. Peritoneal permeability to solutes decreases linearly with the logarithm of solute molecular weight, whereas permeability of cuprophane and cellophane membranes decreases more rapidly and curvilinearly with the logarithm of solute molecular weight. The peritoneum is more permeable to larger solutes than the aforementioned hemodialysis membranes but produces greater solute sieving of small solutes with ultrafiltration. This apparent paradox has been explained by the heteroporosity of the peritoneal membrane and a three-pore model of peritoneal transport. The three-pore model of transperitoneal transport in peritoneal dialysis proposes that water removal, which is dependent primarily on the crystalloid osmotic pressure gradient derived from small solutes such as glucose or alternative osmotic agents, occurs via aquaporin-mediated transcellular pores (r <0.8 nm) and small pores (r = 4.0 to 6.0 nm), whereas water removal, which is dependent on the colloid osmotic pressure gradient derived from macromolecules such as polyglucose or albumin, occurs across both the small and large (r >20 nm) pores. Thus ultrafiltration and solute sieving are assumed to occur via transcellular and small pores and ultrafiltration without sieving and solute diffusive transport are restricted to the small and large pores.

Unlike single-use hemodialysis membranes, the peritoneum is a composite biologic "membrane" that is subjected to chronic reuse and it is established that peritoneal membrane transport may change with time on peritoneal dialysis. In contrast, the solute clearances and ultrafiltration characteristics of hemodialysis membranes are predictable for given conditions and vary only within the limits of quality control during manufacture.

EFFICIENCY OF PERITONEAL DIALYSIS

Indices of Efficiency of Peritoneal Dialysis

The net removal of solute per unit time is measured by the mass transfer rate, which in peritoneal dialysis is calculated as follows:

$$\frac{(\text{Drain volume} \times \text{Drain solute concentration}) - (\text{Infused volume} \times \text{Infused dialysate solute concentration})}{\text{Total cycle time}}$$

The mass transfer rate is a function of peritoneal permeability and area, net ultrafiltration, and the blood-to-dialysate concentration gradient, which is influenced by cycle timing and infusion volume. Mass transfer is considered to be affected negligibly by the effective peritoneal blood flow rate unless this is reduced markedly as in hypovolemic or cardiogenic shock. Net solute-removal rates are not a good index of membrane permeability and area because they depend on ultrafiltration and the blood solute concentration.

The instantaneous clearance rate (dialysance) is highest at the beginning of an exchange, when the blood-to-dialysate concentration gradient is maximum and no ultrafiltration has yet occurred. Derivations of this rate called the *mass transfer area coefficient (MTAC)* correct for net ultrafiltration but neglect solute mass transfer, which occurs during dialysate instillation. However, because the MTAC of each solute is independent of dialysate flow rate, ultrafiltration rate, blood solute concentration, and peritoneal blood flow rate, it is primarily a function of the peritoneal diffusive permeability and effective membrane area for the solute. Peritoneal permeability and membrane area cannot be evaluated separately because the effective membrane area for each solute is unknown. If the effective membrane area for two solutes is assumed to be the same their dialysance (MTAC) ratio will reflect their relative membrane permeability. Using this approach indicates that the permeability of the peritoneum to solutes is a function of solute size and the MTAC has been extrapolated to equal 333.6 (molecular weight)$^{-0.561}$. The MTAC for small solutes increases almost linearly as the infusion volume rises from 0.5 to 2.0 L and by less than 10% as the infusion volume increases further between 2 and 3 L. The peak MTAC for urea in average-size adults is achieved with infusion volumes of approximately 2.5 L and therefore 2.5-L infusion volumes should be used more commonly in prescribing peritoneal dialysis regimens. It has also been shown that the MTAC for small solutes is greater with supine than upright posture.

Dialysate to plasma (D/P) solute concentration ratios measured during standardized peritoneal dialysis exchanges (peritoneal equilibration test [PET]) are a more useful clinical index of peritoneal permeability × area. The equilibration curves relating dialysate/plasma creatinine ratios and sequential/initial dialysate-glucose concentration ratios to the dwell time (time 0, 2, and 4 hours) exhibit wide interpatient variation within the peritoneal dialysis population and reference ranges divided into high, high-average, low-average, and low transport are now established (Fig. 84.28).

The net ultrafiltration volume shows greatest interindividual variation after a hypertonic (4.25%) hydrated dextrose exchange. Hypertonic cycles have therefore been advocated for assessing the ultrafiltration characteristics of the peritoneal membrane and the peritoneal equilibration test uses 2.5% rather than 1.5% hydrated dextrose solutions. The PET is helpful in selecting and modifying the patient's individual peritoneal dialysis prescription and is especially useful in investigating patients with poor ultrafiltration capacity or inadequate small-solute clearances.

Factors Influencing Efficiency of Peritoneal Dialysis

Effective Peritoneal Blood Flow

Although indirect evidence suggests that peritoneal capillary blood is the major source of solutes and water removed during peritoneal dialysis, maximum clearances of small solutes are not determined primarily by peritoneal blood flow. Irrespective of the peritoneal dialysis technique, urea clearances do not usually exceed 30 ml/min even though the effective peritoneal blood flow rate is several-fold greater. Conversely, reduced urea clearances have been observed only if shock or systemic vascular disease were extremely severe.

Membrane Resistances

Microcirculatory permeability (pore size) and effective pore area are important determinants of large-solute clearances. Vasodilators increase dialysate protein clearances by 100% and urea clearances by 20%, most likely due to increased pore area. Limited pore area would explain why small-solute clearances are not altered greatly by changes in blood or dialysate flow provided that these flow rates are at least twice the urea clearances.

Interstitial and stagnant dialysate fluid–film resistances (Fig. 84.25) are the major limit to small-solute clearances. The interstitial solute path is a relatively long distance for diffusion, and transport may be impaired further by the resistance of the mucopolysaccharide and collagenous matrix. Vigorous mixing of the dialysate in an *in vitro* simulation of peritoneal dialysis using a hollow-fiber dialyzer in stagnant dialysate improved urea clearances presumably by reducing stagnant dialysate–film resistances.

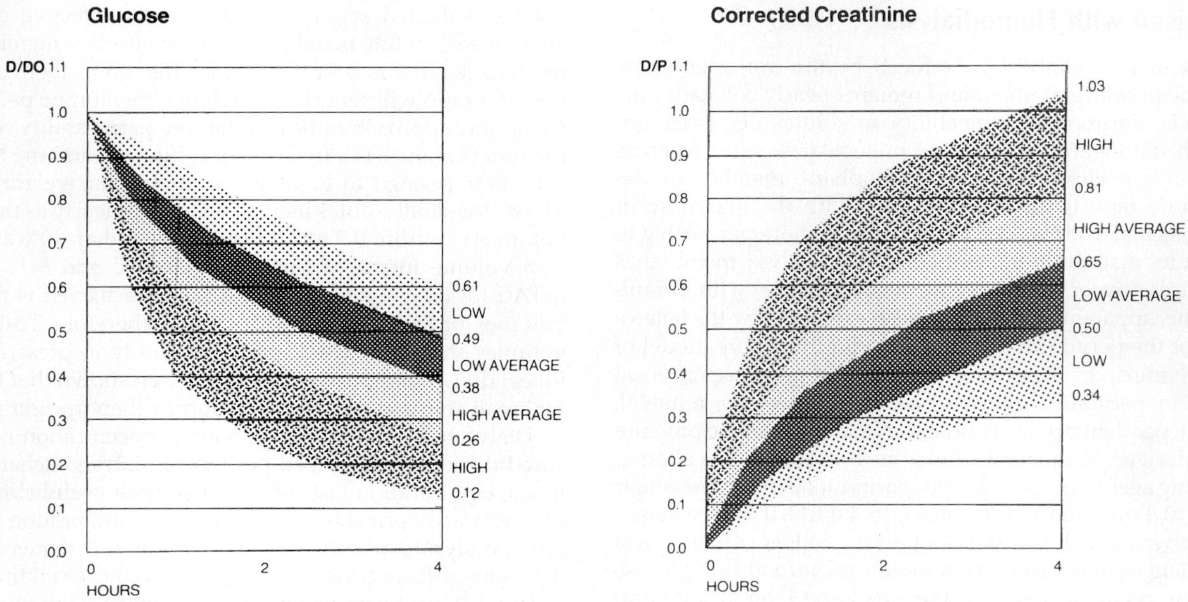

Figure 84.28. Dialysate to plasma (D/P) creatinine concentration ratios and dwell/initial (D/D_0) dialysate glucose concentration ratios during standardized 4 hour exchanges using 2 L of 2.5% dextrose dialysis solution. (Reproduced with permission from Twardowski ZJ. Clinical value of standardised equilibration tests in CAPD patients. *Blood Purif* 1989;7:95–108.).

Peritonitis and long-term peritoneal dialysis lead to loss of the mesothelial layer, which has been associated with increased dialysate glucose absorption, loss of ultrafiltration capacity, and greater dialysate protein losses (higher peritoneal permeability × area).

Dialysis Solutions and Flow Rate

Hypertonic dextrose dialysis solutions increase solute mass transfer by inducing greater ultrafiltration, solvent drag, and solute diffusion. Hypertonic dextrose and buffer anion have an additive vasodilator effect on the peritoneal microcirculation that persists for several exchanges after the dialysate osmolality is reduced. Vasodilation is near maximal with hypertonic dextrose solutions and the addition of vasodilators causes mainly venodilation and venular hyperpermeability, which produces unwanted dialysate protein losses.

At dialysate flow rates greater than 4 L/hr urea clearances plateau at around 30 ml/min. With lower flow rates, clearances decrease due to loss of solute concentration gradients during the dwell time. However, rapid cycling leads to loss of exchange time during infusion and draining of dialysate. The time allowed for drainage may be limited in rapid cycles using an automated machine because 83% of the total potential drain volume with 2-L exchanges occurs in the first high outflow period (mean ± SD = 5.6 ± 2.3 min). Nevertheless, the most efficient dwell time to optimize urea clearances with 2 L of 1.5% dextrose dialysis solution is approximately 44 minutes. Tidal or reciprocating peritoneal dialysis modalities that leave an intraperitoneal reservoir volume obviate this problem. Increasing the dialysate infusion volume augments solute clearances proportionately with the resultant increase in dialysate flow rate. Hence solute clearances in peritoneal dialysis are determined primarily by the lowest of the following:

1. Effective peritoneal blood flow
2. Mass transfer area coefficient of the solute
3. Dialysate flow rate

Backfiltration into Lymphatics and Submesothelial Tissues

Backfiltration of fluid by bulk flow from the peritoneal cavity diminishes net ultrafiltration and solute clearances and, if transcapillary transport decreases, this contribution will become relatively more important. If backfiltration is elevated significantly, ultrafiltration and solute clearances will decrease even if transcapillary transport is within normal limits. Indirect measurements of backfiltration of fluid from the peritoneal cavity have been calculated from the rate of disappearance of marker macromolecules added to the infused dialysis solution and average more than 1 ml/min in adult patients. This method estimates the upper limit of true lymphatic flow from the peritoneal cavity and indicates the magnitude of backfiltration of fluid during peritoneal dialysis. Measurements of the rate of plasma appearance of radiolabeled macromolecules that have been added to the infused dialysate have estimated that the lower limit of true lymphatic flow is 0.3 ml/min. Although the quantitation of actual lymphatic flow rates remains uncertain, the continuous backfiltration of dialysate at a low rate during peritoneal dialysis makes an important contribution to loss of ultrafiltration and solute clearances in long-dwell exchanges.

Enhancement of Peritoneal Dialysis Efficiency

Not all of the aforementioned variables of peritoneal dialysis efficiency are amenable to manipulation. Practical measures to improve dialysis efficiency depend on whether increased solute clearances and/or net ultrafiltration are required. Small-solute clearances may be enhanced by increasing the volume and/or number of exchanges (dialysate flow rate). When more than four exchanges per day are prescribed, most patients will prefer to employ an overnight-exchange device or an automated machine overnight [automated peritoneal dialysis (APD)]. Net ultrafiltration may be increased by shortening the exchange time to capture maximum ultrafiltration or by increasing the osmolality and/or volume of dextrose exchanges. The former strategy in

TABLE 84.13. Comparison of Solute Clearance Rates in Intermittent Peritoneal Dialysis, Continuous Ambulatory Peritoneal Dialysis, and Hemodialysis

Dialysis Modality	IPD		CAPD		HD	
Solute (MW)	ml/min	L/wk	ml/min	L/wk	ml/min	L/wk
Urea (60)	25	60	7	70	150	108
Vitamin B_{12} (1,355)	8	19	4	42	17	12
Inulin (5,500)	5	12	2.6	26	5.5	4

CAPD, continuous ambulatory peritoneal dialysis; HD, hemodialysis; IPD, intermittent peritoneal dialysis; MW, molecular weight.

CAPD requires the patient to perform more exchanges each day or to leave the peritoneal cavity empty overnight (daytime ambulatory peritoneal dialysis [DAPD]). For long-dwell exchanges (at least 8 hours dwell time), net ultrafiltration may be achieved using glucose–polymer solutions instead of 4.25% dextrose dialysis solutions. Intraperitoneal drug therapy is not currently of clinical benefit. Large-solute clearances can be increased with vasodilators, but is not advised because high-dialysate protein losses are also observed.

It is important to emphasize that peritoneal dialysis prescriptions should be individualized and the aforementioned equilibration curve (PET) data are useful adjuncts to standard clinical and laboratory parameters in deciding the preferred dialysis prescription for each patient.

Comparison with Hemodialysis

Representative values of solute clearances for IPD (40 hr/week), CAPD (4 exchanges/day), and hemodialysis with cuprophane and cellophane membranes (12 hr/week) are shown in Table 84.13. Weekly small-solute clearances with IPD are inadequate and this dialysis modality is no longer used routinely as a chronic mode of therapy. The low small-solute clearances with CAPD are compensated for by dialysis being performed continuously. The weekly clearances of larger solutes are greater with continuous techniques of peritoneal dialysis. The peritoneum behaves as a membrane with lower effective membrane pore area but pore size is greater than standard hemodialysis membranes. CAPD results in steady-state body metabolite concentrations being maintained at the level at which their rate of generation is matched by renal and dialysate removal rates. This absence of transcellular dysequilibrium with CAPD is a potential advantage over hemodialysis.

Urea clearance is blood flow limited in hemodialysis, membrane-resistance limited (interstitial and dialysate fluid–film resistances) in IPD, and dialysate flow limited in CAPD.

Individualized Prescription of Peritoneal Dialysis

A prospective, noninterventional study of new CAPD patients has shown better survival rates in patients receiving higher total (peritoneal and residual renal) weekly urea and creatinine clearances. The National Kidney Foundation–Dialysis Outcome Quality Initiative (NKF-DOQI) guidelines recommend a target total weekly Kt/V urea of at least 2.0 and total weekly creatinine clearance of at least 60 L/1.73m^2 body surface area. Higher target small-solute clearances are advised for intermittent modalities of peritoneal dialysis such as nocturnal intermittent peritoneal dialysis (NIPD). In addition in automated peritoneal dialysis, urea clearances may be augmented more readily than creatinine clearances because dialysate/plasma urea equilibrates more rapidly than creatinine during short-duration exchanges. It is noteworthy that a weekly creatinine clearance of 60 L/week represents only 5.9 ml/min of creatinine clearance. In the Canusa study, residual renal function at the beginning of CAPD averaged 4 ml/min and declined to approximately 1.0 to 1.5 ml/min 2 years after peritoneal dialysis commenced. Thus peritoneal prescriptions need to be individualized and adjusted with time on dialysis to allow for interpatient and intrapatient variation in the following:

1. Peritoneal transport characteristics
2. Body size
3. Ultrafiltration requirements
4. Residual renal function

In general, CAPD patients and high-average peritoneal transport rates, as assessed by a PET performed at least 4 to 6 weeks after beginning peritoneal dialysis when peritoneal transport rates have stabilized, may maximize small-solute clearances and net ultrafiltration using short-duration dextrose dialysate exchanges. CAPD patients with low-average peritoneal transport rates can optimize small-solute clearances using longer dwell times and the highest-tolerated infusion volumes. Some patients using four CAPD exchanges of 2 L/day will be unable to achieve the aforementioned target weekly small-solute clearances and/or to obtain adequate peritoneal ultrafiltration to maintain fluid balance if they become oligoanuric. Kinetic modelling and clinical measurement of small-solute clearances on peritoneal dialysis indicate that *anuric* patients will need modification of their dialysis prescription to increase infusion volumes and/or perform CAPD or APD using five or more exchanges per day if they are to achieve the aforementioned target small-solute clearances. The small group of anuric patients who have both large body size (body surface area of more than 2 m^2) and low peritoneal transport rates may need to change to hemodialysis to achieve the previously mentioned weekly small-solute clearance rates.

EVALUATION OF LOSS OF ULTRAFILTRATION IN PERITONEAL DIALYSIS

Apparent or true loss of peritoneal ultrafiltration capacity is observed in approximately 30% of CAPD patients after 5 years. Identification of the underlying etiology serves as a further clinical application of peritoneal dialysis kinetics. It is important to exclude apparent causes of ultrafiltration loss such as excessive fluid intake or loss of residual urinary output. Mechanical catheter malfunction due to either catheter outflow obstruction or catheter displacement should be suspected if there is a sudden

TABLE 84.14. Peritoneal Equilibration Curve Data in Peritoneal Dialysis Patients with Different Causes of Loss of Ultrafiltration

Etiology of Reduced Net UF	Dialysate/Plasma Creatnine Concentration	Sequential/Initial Glucose Concentration	Decrease in Dialysate Sodium at 1 Hour
Type 1 membrane failure	↑	↓	↓
Type 2 membrane failure	↓	↑ or N	↓
Type 3 membrane failure	N	N	N
Intraperitoneal fluid loculation	↓	↑	↓

N, normal; UF, ultrafiltration.

reduction in drain volumes. Other causes of poor peritoneal ultrafiltration alter peritoneal dialysis kinetics as predicted from their effects on solute and water flux (Table 84.14), and comparison with previous PET results may enable these causes to be differentiated. The majority of patients with poor ultrafiltration capacity have reduced cumulative transcapillary ultrafiltration due to high peritoneal transport rates, rapid absorption of dialysate glucose, and early loss of the transperitoneal glucose–osmotic gradient (type 1 membrane failure). The reduction in water flux into the peritoneal cavity in type 1 membrane failure is indicated by a loss of the transient decrease in dialysate sodium concentration during the first 2 hours of the dwell time (Table 84.14). Rarely decreased transcapillary ultrafiltration may be due to loss of effective membrane area in patients with extensive peritoneal adhesions or sclerosing peritonitis (type 2 membrane failure). Ultrafiltration failure also occurs in patients with well-preserved transcapillary ultrafiltration who have high rates of backfiltration of fluid into the peritoneal lymphatics and submesothelial tissues (type 3 membrane failure). Such patients will have no evidence of a dialysate leak after performing an abdominal computed tomography scan with intraperitoneal contrast. This investigation helps exclude patients who have an external dialysate leak into abdominal scars that is not manifested clinically by abdominal wall edema. Although the kinetics of ultrafiltration failure in peritoneal dialysis are better understood, the underlying pathophysiologic changes within the peritoneal membrane remain uncertain. Sustained vasodilation of the peritoneal microcirculation, loss of proteoglycans on the mesothelial surface, loss of microvilli, reduced glycerophospholipids on the mesothelial surface, and glycation of structural proteins with resultant tanning of the peritoneum have been postulated as underlying mechanisms of loss of ultrafiltration capacity.

Selected Readings

Brandes JC, Packard WJ, Watters SK, et al. Optimization of dialysate flow and mass transfer during automated peritoneal dialysis. *Am J Kidney Dis* 1995;25:603–610.

This paper characterizes the drainage time profile during peritoneal dialysis exchanges and describes the effect of posture on small-solute mass transfer area coefficients in peritoneal dialysis.

Churchhill D, Taylor D, Keshaviah P, et al. Adequacy of dialysis and nutrition in continuous peritoneal dialysis: association with clinical outcomes. *J Am Soc Nephrol* 1996;7:198–207.

This prospective observational study of new patients on CAPD demonstrates that patient survival is correlated with total weekly small-solute clearances.

Durand PY, Chanliau J, Gamberoni J, et al. APD: clinical measurement of the maximal acceptable intraperitoneal volume. *Adv Perit Dial* 1994;10:63–67.

This paper demonstrates that the intraperitoneal volume correlates positively with hydrostatic intraperitoneal pressure and negatively with vital capacity.

Ho-dac-Pannekeet MM, Atasever B, Struijk DG, et al. Analysis of ultrafiltration failure in peritoneal dialysis patients by means of standard permeability analysis. *Perit Dial Int* 1997;17:144–150.

This paper evaluates the prevalence and etiology of ultrafiltration failure in peritoneal dialysis patients using standardized study dialysis exchanges with dextran 70 as a volume marker.

Keshaviah P, Emerson PF, Vonesh EF, et al. Relationship between body size, fill volume, and mass transfer area coefficient in peritoneal dialysis. *J Am Soc Nephrol* 1994;4:1820–1826.

This paper shows that the mass transfer area coefficient for small solutes increases almost linearly as fill volume is increased from 0.5 to 2.0 L and by less than 10% as infusion volumes are increased between 2 and 3 L. The peak mass transfer area coefficient for urea for average-size adults was observed with fill volumes around 2.5 L.

Mactier RA, Khana R, Twardowski ZJ, et al. Contribution of lymphatic absorption to loss of ultrafiltration and solute clearances in CAPD. *J Clin Invest* 1987;80:1311–1316.

This paper shows the negative influence of continuous backfiltration of fluid into the peritoneal lymphatics and submesothelial tissues on net ultrafiltration and small-solute clearances in peritoneal dialysis.

Mactier RA, Twardowski ZJ. Influence of dwell time, osmolality, and volume of exchanges on ultrafiltration and solute mass transfer in peritoneal dialysis. *Semin Dial* 1988;1:40–49.

This review evaluates the factors that are important clinically in determining the efficiency of peritoneal dialysis.

Nolph KD, Miller FN, Rubin J, et al. New directions in peritoneal dialysis concepts and applications. *Kidney Int* 1980;18:S111–S116.

This paper discusses the major resistance sites of the peritoneum to solute and water transport in peritoneal dialysis.

Nolph KD, Popovich RP, Ghods AJ, et al. Determinants of low clearances of small solutes during peritoneal dialysis. *Kidney Int* 1978;13:117–123.

This review discusses the variables that limit solute clearances in peritoneal dialysis.

Twardowski ZJ. Clinical value of standardised equilibration tests in CAPD patients. *Blood Purif* 1989;7:95–108.

This paper reviews the practical use and applications of the peritoneal equilibration test in peritoneal dialysis.

B: Techniques, Indications, and Complications of Peritoneal Dialysis

Ram Gokal

Peritoneal dialysis (PD) has now become an established form of renal replacement therapy for end-stage renal failure (ESRF). In the 1960s and 1970s PD was used predominantly to manage patients in acute renal failure and a limited number of patients on intermittent peritoneal dialysis (IPD); at times this was a holding procedure for hemodialysis (HD) therapy. However, the introduction in 1976 of continuous ambulatory peritoneal dialysis (CAPD) transformed this situation. The use of PD has risen dramatically over the last 2 decades. Currently, more than 110,000 patients are on PD, comprising roughly 15% of the total world dialysis population. Importantly, there has also been a dramatic improvement in outcomes of patients undergoing PD. Patient survival is now recognized to be at least as good as with HD. Retention of patients on PD still lags behind that of HD but here again there have been dramatic strides in improving the outcome, which is related to the innumerable advances and innovations in the technology of PD, provision of an adequate prescription and the means to deliver it, and a reduction in some of the complications inherent to the technique of PD. In addition, indications and contraindications for the use of PD are better recognized, as is the role of PD as an integrated modality in delivering total renal care for a patient in ESRF. Indeed PD is no longer regarded as an inferior therapy and adds to the armamentarium available to the nephrologist in managing these patients.

TECHNIQUES

The technical aspects of PD include access to the peritoneal cavity, the composition of the dialysis solution, the various dialysis machines and systems, and the prescription.

Peritoneal Access

The key to successful chronic PD is permanent and safe access to the peritoneal cavity. Despite improvements in catheter survival over the last few years, catheter-related complications still occur causing significant morbidity and permanent change to HD in up to 20% of all patients who need such a change.

Peritoneal Catheters

An ideal catheter provides reliable and rapid dialysate flow rates without leaks or infections. The Tenckhoff catheter is still the most often used catheter, but a variety of catheter modifications and improvements (Fig. 84.29) have been introduced to try to minimize complications. The standard two-cuff, straight Tenckhoff catheter is still the most widely used access device because it satisfies the needs of most patients and there is no conclusive evidence that any other catheter is superior. The commonly used catheters are standard one or two cuffs, straight or coiled Tenckhoff catheters, the Swan-neck catheters, and the Toronto Western Hospital catheter. The intraperitoneal portion is either straight or coiled, the latter probably allows for better flow, less inflow pain, and less propensity for catheter migration and omental wrapping. It is now recognized that the subcutaneous tract and the exit need to be directed caudally to minimize exit-site and tunnel infections, and catheters with a preformed bend, eliminating the resilient force or "shape memory" of straight catheters, are gaining wider acceptance. Swan-neck catheters were designed to diminish cuff extrusions and catheter migration associated with straight catheters implanted in arcuate tunnels. Randomized studies comparing the Swan-neck catheter with straight Tenckhoff catheters without a preformed bend showed a lower probability for the first exit infection with the Swan-neck catheter but the survival was not

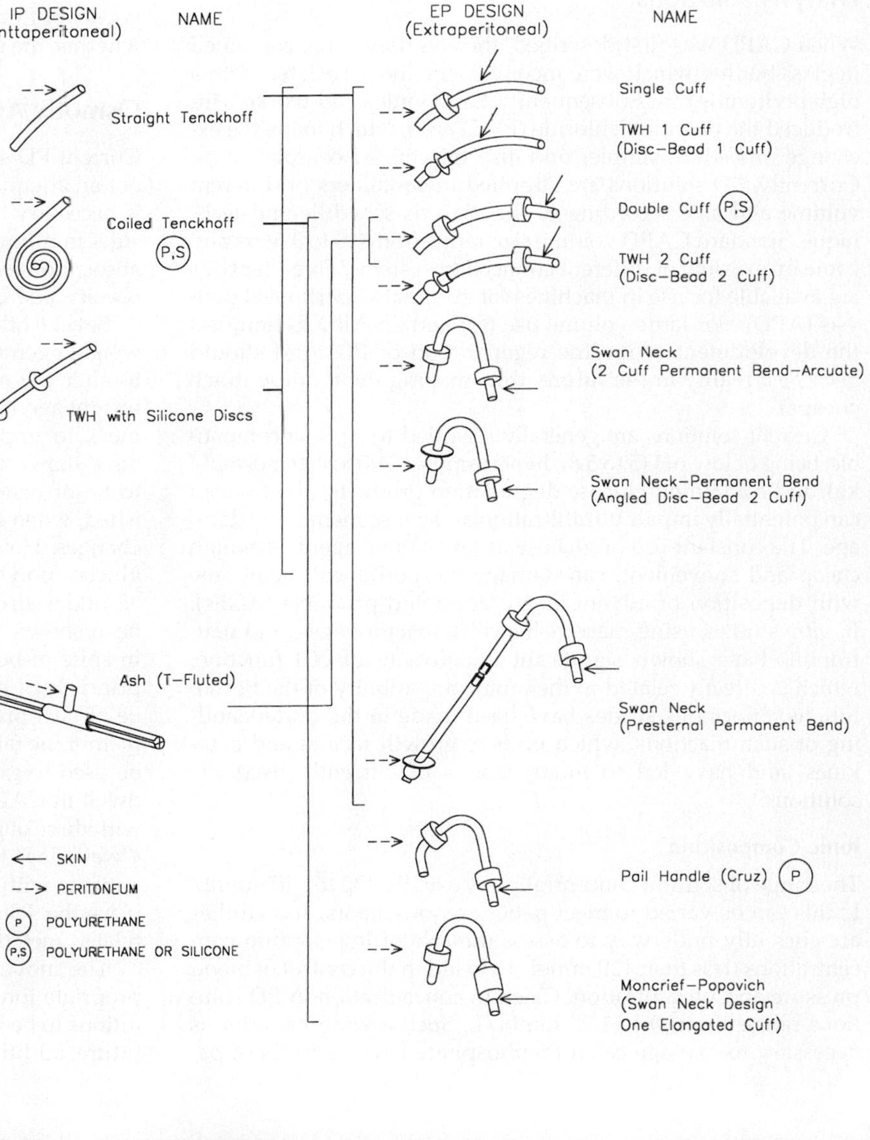

Figure 84.29. Currently available chronic peritoneal catheters showing combinations of intraperitoneal and extraperitoneal designs. (Reproduced with permission from Gokal R, Alexander SR, Ash S, et al. Peritoneal catheters and exit-site practices toward optimum peritoneal access: 1998 update. *Perit Dial Int* 1998;18:11–33.)

different. Several other studies have confirmed this finding. In a recent report from the Adhoc Committee on peritoneal catheters, it was recommended that double-cuff catheters are preferable to single cuff; a downward-directed exit decreases the risk of catheter-related peritonitis and therefore catheters allowing for this (Swan neck, Pail handle) are advantageous.

In terms of catheter insertion, various techniques are available and related to the types of catheters. In general, implantation needs to be performed by a competent and experienced operator in a planned manner. Peritoneal entry should be lateral (deep cuff in or below the rectus musculature) or paramedian to give good deep-cuff fixation and to minimize the risks of herniation and fluid leaks. The deep cuff should be placed in the musculature of the anterior abdominal wall or in the preperitoneal space. In addition, the subcutaneous cuff should be located near the skin surface and at a distance of at least 2 cm from the exit site. The exit site should be facing downward or directed laterally.

Various surgical techniques (surgical, blind insertion using a Tenckhoff trocar, blind placement using a Seldinger technique, use of minitrocar and peritoneoscopy, and the Moncrieff/Popovich technique) are all used. The surgical insertion is still the most common approach, with most procedures performed under local anesthesia. Catheters used for acute renal failure are semirigid and mounted on a stylet. These can be inserted easily and quickly and used for one or few sessions in hospitalized patients.

Dialysis Solutions

When CAPD was first described, the solutions were contained in glass bottles, which were inconvenient and associated with a high peritonitis rate. Subsequently, Oreopoulos and workers introduced the polyvinylchloride (PVC) bags, which made the exchange procedure simpler and also minimized complications. Currently, PD solutions are supplied in containers of different volume and size according to the dialysis schedule and technique. Standard CAPD volume size range from 0.5 to 3 liters and come in a variety of different connection systems. Five-liter bags are available for use in machines for automated peritoneal dialysis (APD). For large-volume use (for certain APD techniques) the development of on-line regeneration of PD fluid should become a reality in the future, thus making the therapy much cheaper.

Current solutions are generally regarded to be bioincompatible, being of low pH (5 to 5.8), hyperosmolar (340 to 490 mosmol/kg), and containing glucose degradation products, all of which can potentially impair ultrafiltration and cause membrane damage. The constant use of glucose as an osmotic agent, although cheap and convenient, can damage the peritoneal membrane with deposition of advanced glycation end-products (AGEs). *In vitro* studies using mesothelial cells, macrophages, and neutrophils have shown significant impairment of cell function, which is directly related to the bioincompatibility of the PD solutions. Enormous strides have been made in the understanding of such reactions, which involve growth factors and cytokines, and have led to modifications of currently used PD solutions.

Ionic Composition

The range of sodium concentration is usually 132 to 140 mmol/L; this can be varied to meet patient requirements, and studies are currently underway to assess the role of low-sodium concentrations (less than 120 mmol/L) to aid in the control of blood pressure and ultrafiltration. Calcium concentration in PD solutions ranges from 0 to 1.75 mmol/L. Such a wide variation is necessary to manage calcium–phosphate balance in these patients, especially because the use of aluminium-containing phosphate binders has been replaced by calcium-containing salts. The varied PD solution calcium concentrations allow a more rational use of vitamin D and calcium salts to treat hyperparathyroidism. The lower calcium concentration minimizes the risk of hypercalcemia, which is associated with the adynamic bone lesion, an entity commonly seen in CAPD patients.

The best dialysis buffer to correct uremic acidosis is the naturally occurring one—bicarbonate. Unfortunately, it has been impossible to use bicarbonate because calcium reacts with bicarbonate to make an insoluble salt. To overcome this problem of insoluble calcium-salt precipitation, double-chambered bags have been developed; one chamber contains the acid and the other contains bicarbonate solution, which are mixed just before inflow into the peritoneal cavity. This is likely to replace the currently used lactate (35 to 40 mmol/L), which has to be metabolized in the liver. Use of bicarbonate or bicarbonate/lactate mixtures is associated with good correction of acidosis, decrease in the infusion pain associated with the low pH, high osmolality lactate solutions, and *in vitro* studies, showing a degree of normalization of the adverse cellular reactions related to the previous bioincompatible solutions. Another cation that might replace lactate as a buffer is pyruvate, and early *in vitro* work shows considerable promise. Recently, modification of the sterilization process (prepared by separating glucose from the rest of the fluid components during heat sterilization to produce a two-compartment bag) has resulted in an increase in the pH (about 6.3), a decrease in glucose degradation products, and some clinical benefits. The extended experiences with these newer buffered solutions with higher pH are awaited to see whether the early promise from initial results is fulfilled.

Osmotic Agents

Current PD solutions use varying concentrations of glucose to obtain adequate ultrafiltration. However, for long-dwell PD, as is necessary for CAPD, its rapid and continuous absorption results in a limited ultrafiltration capacity. Furthermore, glucose absorption leads to metabolic complications of hyperlipidemia, obesity, and damage to the mesothelial cells.

Several other osmotic agents have been tried—low-molecular-weight agents (fructose, sorbitol, xylitol, amino acids, glycerol), to alter the metabolic profile of glucose, and large-molecular-weight agents (polypeptides, dextran, gelatin and glucose polymer), to improve the ultrafiltration profile. Only two agents have shown any clinical benefit. Amino acids have been shown to be of benefit in patients who are protein-calorie malnourished, when used to replace one or two of the four glucose exchanges. However, it is unlikely to replace glucose totally. The glucose polymer, icodextrin, has now had extensive clinical trials and is also available commercially in Europe. This agent has been shown to produce sustained ultrafiltration over 12 hours in spite of being isosmotic to uremic plasma (it works on the principle of colloid osmosis). This solution has been shown to be of advantage in patients who are losing ultrafiltration from membrane failure, and anecdotal evidence suggests that it could be used to extend therapy time on PD when used for the long dwell in CAPD on a daily regimen of one exchange combined with three of glucose. It has also been used for the daytime dwell ("wet" day) to enhance fluid and solute removal (especially in patients with a hyperpermeable membrane) in APD and to replace the 3.86% glucose solution at night (to minimize glucose-related metabolic and membrane changes).

The move to more biocompatible solutions and use of appropriate ionic and osmotic agent combinations will allow solutions to be modified to meet appropriate clinical needs. In the future, additives to the PD solutions (antioxidants, procysteine, gluthatione, glycosaminoglycans, soluble omega 3 fatty acids) may make it possible to alter cardiovascular, metabolic, and adequacy profiles, thereby improving the outcomes in PD patients. The solution modifications are expensive to develop and therefore are costly; it would be pertinent for industry to produce solutions that are within the reach of all patients.

Peritoneal Dialysis Systems

The original standard CAPD system entailed an exchange procedure, the first step of which was the drainage of PD effluent from the peritoneal cavity into the constantly attached empty bag, then detaching this drained bag and connecting to a new solution bag (critical step with potential for bacterial contamination), and finally draining the new fluid by gravity into the peritoneal cavity. This increased the potential of any contamination, at the time of the exchange, to be passed into the peritoneal cavity. Italian workers in the early 1980s introduced the disconnect or Y system, whereby the first maneuver following a connection was to drain the fluid from the peritoneal cavity into an empty bag, thereby flushing out any contamination introduced at the time of making the connection. There is now universal acceptance and use of the disconnect systems, which are available in several formats, but all using the "flush before fill" principle. Some incorporate a disinfectant in the "Y" piece as originally introduced by the Italians. In addition to this, other sterilization techniques (ultraviolet light, heat) are available and try to minimize the risk of infection. Devices are available to aid patients with manual dexterity problems and those that are blind. All of these innovations have certainly reduced the risk of peritonitis considerably.

There has been enormous progress in APD delivering systems. The more recent variety of PD cyclers that are used in the various APD prescriptions have sophisticated computerized programs with time- and volume-controlled delivery of fluid, providing active control of fluid balance. In addition, they are very user friendly, safe, compact, and portable. These developments have allowed better patient care by matching the dialysis prescription to the patients' clinical, social, and personal needs and have led to APD being the fastest growing dialysis modality. Further details of this are given in Chapter 84, Part 2D.

Peritoneal Dialysis Prescription and Methods

In arriving at a particular prescription for an individual patient one needs to take into account the fixed components that impact on prescription (residual renal function, peritoneal membrane permeability, and size of the patient) and the variable components of dialysate volume, dwell times, and the number of exchanges. Because it is difficult to modify the fixed variables (other than increasing the prescription to compensate for declining residual renal function), a prescription will therefore entail modifications of the variable components to arrive at a regimen that provides for adequate solute and fluid removal to meet clinical and patient lifestyle needs and maintain reasonable quality of life. The hope is that the decided-upon prescription will enhance outcomes.

The initial setting of a PD prescription is outlined in Fig. 84.30, which is a flow diagram used to arrive at a prescription using the various factors (peritoneal permeability, residual renal function, size, dwell times, fill volume, number of exchanges) to meet adequacy and nutritional targets. The prescription is then modified by regular monitoring of dose of dialysis, fluid status, and clinical well being. Various guidelines have emerged outlining targets to be attained for various PD regimes [e.g., in the United States, the National Kidney Foundation–Dialysis Outcomes Quality Initiative ([NKF-DOQI)].

The various regimens and methods for daily PD are indicated in Fig. 84.31. Standard CAPD involves three to five exchanges per day of varying volume. This is the only manually performed PD therapy. Various APD variants have emerged and are shown in Fig. 84.31. These range from IPD performed in acute or chronic patients three times a week in sessions of 24 hours exchanging 20 to 60 L of dialysis fluid to the more sophisticated ones. The latter involve continuous cycling peritoneal dialysis (CCPD), which originally entailed three exchanges during the night and one during the day—a reversal of the CAPD regimen; nightly intermittent peritoneal dialysis (NIPD), with rapid exchanges during the night with the abdomen kept dry during the day—"dry day"; nightly PD plus two exchanges during the day to allow for increased solute and fluid clearance (NIPD with "wet day," also called *higher-dose CCPD*); and tidal peritoneal dialysis (TPD), in which 40% to 60% of the volume introduced in the first cycle is left in the abdomen and

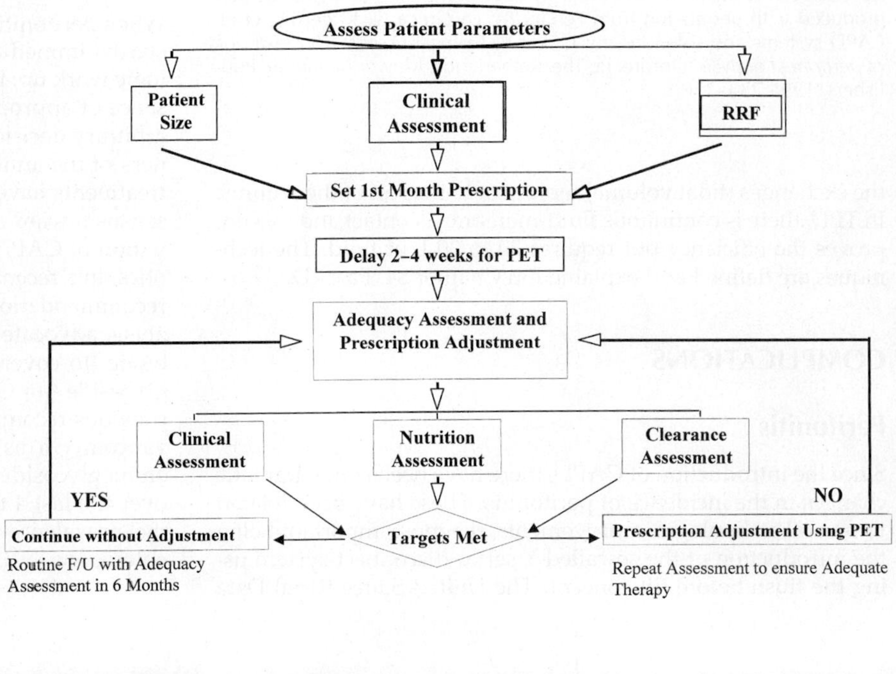

Figure 84.30. An overview of prescription management for peritoneal dialysis. PET, peritoneal equilibration test.

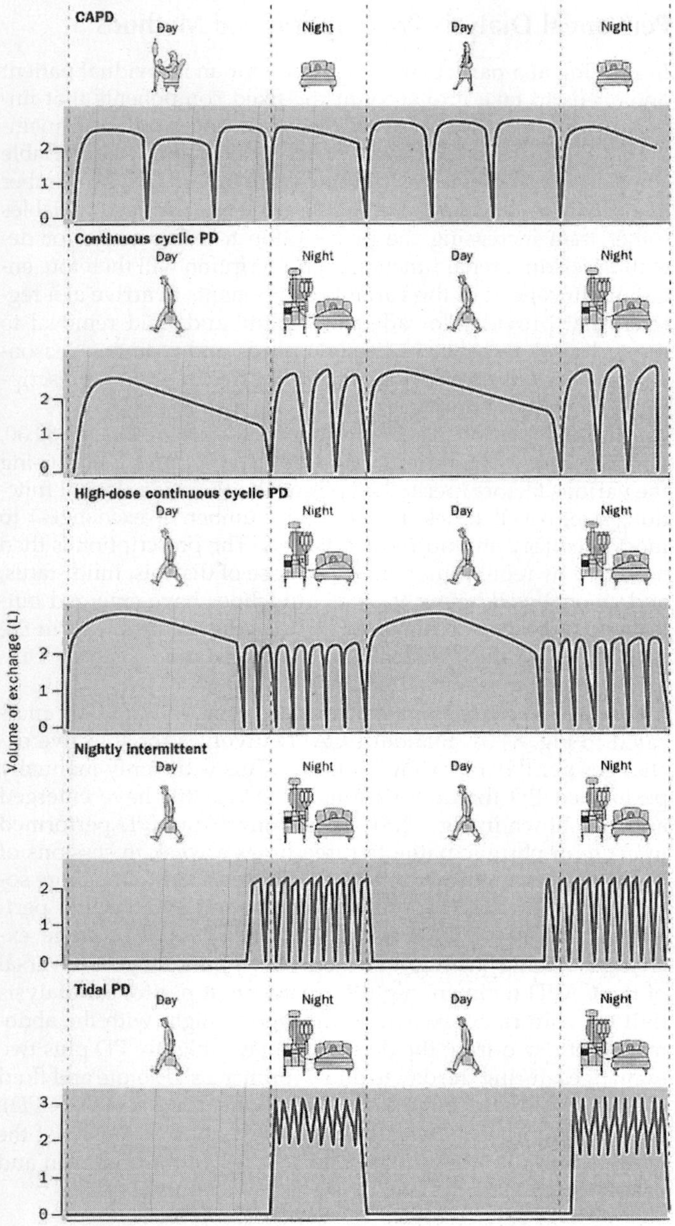

Figure 84.31. Different methods of daily PD. The *top figure* indicates the standard CAPD regimen. All others represent various APD regimens. (Reproduced with permission from Feriani M, La Greca G, Kriger FL, et al. CAPD systems and solutions. In: Gokal R, Nolph KD, eds. *The textbook of peritoneal dialysis.* Dordrecht, The Netherlands: Kluwer Academic Publishers, 1994:233–270.)

the exchanges (tidal volume) replace only the rest of the volume. In TPD, there is continuous fluid-membrane contact and this improves the efficiency but requires 20 to 30 L of fluid. The techniques are defined and explained in Chapter 84, Part 2D.

COMPLICATIONS

Peritonitis

Since the introduction of CAPD, there have been some dramatic changes in the incidence of peritonitis. These have been related to several technologic improvements, the most important being the introduction of the so-called Y set or disconnect system using the flush before fill concept. The United States Renal Data System (USRDS) reported in 1992 that the time to first peritonitis of patients on Y set was 20.6 months compared with the standard connection system in which it was 11.4 months. Many other factors are important in diminishing the incidence of peritonitis, including adequate patient training, appropriate infrastructure to support a PD program, good patient compliance, and catheter care.

Definitions, Signs, and Symptoms

Diagnosis of peritonitis requires the presence of two of the following criteria in any combination: (a) presence of organisms on Gram stain or subsequent culture, (b) cloudy fluid (white cell greater than 100/mm; greater than 50% neutrophils), or (c) symptoms and signs of peritoneal inflammation. Relapse is defined as recurrence of an episode of peritonitis caused by the same genus/species that caused the immediately preceding episode occurring within 4 weeks of completion of the antibiotics used. Cloudy dialysate effluent is almost invariably present, whereas abdominal pain is present in approximately 80% to 95% of cases. Gastrointestinal symptoms, chills, and fever are present in up to 25% of the cases, whereas abdominal tenderness accompanies the symptoms in three-fourths of the cases.

Pathogenesis of Peritonitis

Contamination at the time of peritoneal dialysis exchange is still a major cause of peritonitis. Approximately 15% to 20% of peritonitis episodes are secondary to catheter infections. Peritonitis due to Gram-negative organisms are generally considered to be enteric in origin, probably due to transcolonic migration of bacteria. Microorganisms causing peritonitis are now well defined, with up to 70% being Gram-positive (coagulase negative staphylococci account for up to 25%, *Staphylococcus aureus* up to 15% of episodes). Gram-negative organisms account for up to 25% of episodes with 20% of episodes being culture negative.

The clinical course of peritonitis is variable. It is estimated that there is an incubation period of 24 to 48 hours from touch contamination to development of overt symptoms. During this period, any bacterial invasion will result in clinical peritonitis unless it is overcome by an adequate host-defense response. There is therefore a constant battle in the peritoneal cavity between invading microorganisms (which goes on repeatedly through the various portals of entry—catheter intraluminal, extraluminal, transcolonic, hematogenous) and the host-defense mechanisms.

Treatment of Peritonitis

When peritonitis occurs in patients on PD, treatment should be started immediately after completion of appropriate microbiologic work up; however, treatment has to be initiated in the absence of appropriate diagnostic information. Therefore certain arbitrary decisions have to be made regarding the appropriateness of the antibiotic treatment. Several protocols of antibiotic treatments have been proposed and there is an increasing consensus toward a standardized approach combining the continuation of CAPD with intraperitoneal administration of antibiotics. In a recent update of the PD-related peritonitis treatment recommendations, the Advisory Committee on Peritoneal Dialysis advocated use of a first-generation cephalosporin antibiotic (to cover for Gram-positive organisms) and an aminoglycoside (for Gram-negative cover). This was a reversal of the previous recommendation in 1993, which advocated the use of vancomycin as a first-line blind therapy combined with an aminoglycoside. This change has become necessary because, over the last 4 to 5 years, there has been a dramatic increase in the prevalence of vancomycin-resistant organisms, especially enterococci (VRE).

For the initial empiric antibiotic selection, a first-generation cephalosporin with an aminoglycoside given intraperitoneally (IP) is used (Fig. 84.32). It is now recognized that antibiotics can be given as a single dose overnight with good efficacy. Treatment is modified once culture and sensitivity results are known. For Gram-positive microorganisms, if the culture reveals an enterococcus, the cephalosporin is replaced with ampicillin (125 mg/L); the aminoglycoside may be continued with one exchange per day based on sensitivity testing. If the organism is *S. aureus*, its sensitivity will dictate further therapy changes. If it is sensitive to the cephalosporin, the aminoglycoside should be discontinued; if the clinical response is less than desired, rifampin (600 mg/day) is added orally to the IP cephalosporin. The use of rifampin in areas with a high prevalence of tuberculosis cannot be advocated. If the *S. aureus* is methicillin resistant (MRSA), rifampin should be added and the cephalosporin should be changed to clindamycin or vancomycin (2 g IP every 7 days). For coagulase negative staphylococci, which are methicillin resistant (MRSE), one needs to consider changing to vancomycin if there is no clear improvement. For culture-negative peritonitis episodes, the cephalosporin and aminoglycosides are continued such as for initial empiric therapy. Experience would indicate that if the patient is clinically improving up to 4 to 5 days and there is no suggestion of Gram-negative organisms on Gram stain, only the cephalosporin should be continued for the duration of therapy (usually 2 weeks).

Gram-negative microorganisms are difficult to manage especially if *Pseudomonas aeruginosa* is isolated. Their management is outlined in Fig. 84.33. The decision to discontinue the aminoglycoside and continue with general cephalosporin will be guided by *in vitro* sensitivity testing. For fungal organisms, the general practice is for immediate catheter removal, although few reports suggest that cure can be obtained with prolonged causes of antifungal agents.

Most patients with peritonitis will show considerable clinical improvement within 2 days of starting antibiotics. At 96 hours, if patients have not shown definitive clinical improvement a reevaluation of the clinical status is essential. One should be cognisant of potential intraabdominal or gynecologic pathologies, presence of unusual pathogens (mycobacteria, fungi, fastidious organisms), or catheter-related or tunnel infections. In these situations it is almost mandatory to remove the catheter. For anaerobic bacteria or peritonitis from polymicrobial organisms with fecal contamination, catheter removal and surgical exploration should be considered.

Possible Course and Outcome in Peritonitis

It should be possible, in up to 80% of cases, to achieve complete cure without having to resort to catheter removal. Persistent symptoms beyond 96 hours can occur in approximately 10% to 30% of episodes, with relapsing peritonitis being a feature in approximately 10% to 15% of episodes. Catheter removal is necessary in up to 15% of cases and death is reported in about 1% to 3% of cases. Peritonitis results in marked increase in peritoneal protein losses and transient decrease in ultrafiltration, and over time with long-term PD, there can be an increase in solute transport and loss of ultrafiltration with the development of a hyperpermeable membrane. Although the changes in a peritoneal membrane are usually transient and related to peritonitis, peritoneal fibrosis (often referred to as *sclerosing peritonitis*) may result from severe episodes, or from a cumulative effect of multiple episodes or episodes later in the course of PD.

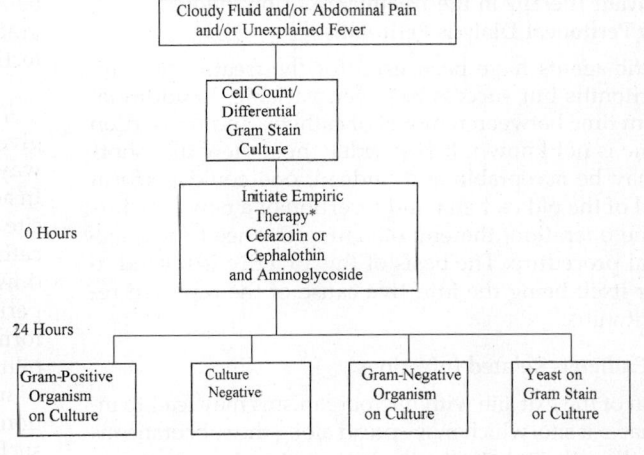

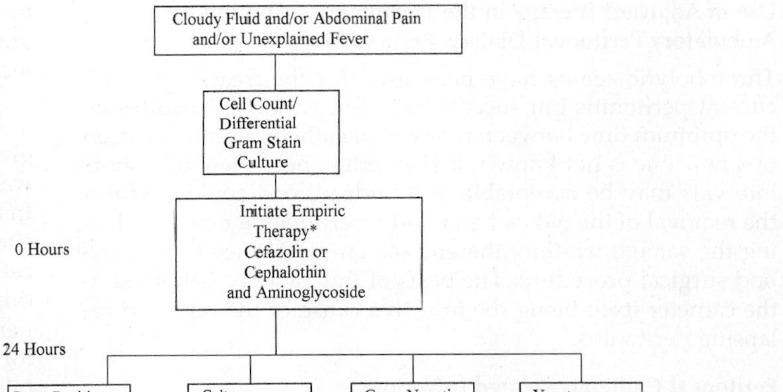

Empiric Therapy

Agent	Continuous Dose	Intermittent Dose (in 1 exchange/day)	
		Residual urine output (mL/day)	
		Anuria (<500)	Non-anuria (>500)
cefazolin or cephalothin	500 mg/L load, then 125 mg/L in each exchange	500 ug/L (or 15 mg/kg)	increase dose by 25%
gentamicin netilmicin	8 mg/L load then 4 mg/L in each exchange	0.6 mg/kg body weight	1.5 mg/kg initial loading dose
amikacin	25 mg/L load then 12 mg/L in each exchange	2 mg/kg body weight	5 mg/kg initial loading dose

Figure 84.32. Initial assessment and therapy of a patient presenting with peritonitis. The dose is related to residual renal function. (Reproduced with permission from Keane WF, Alexander SR, Bailie GR, et al. Peritoneal dialysis–related peritonitis treatment recommendations: 1996 update. *Perit Dial Int* 1996;16:557–573.)

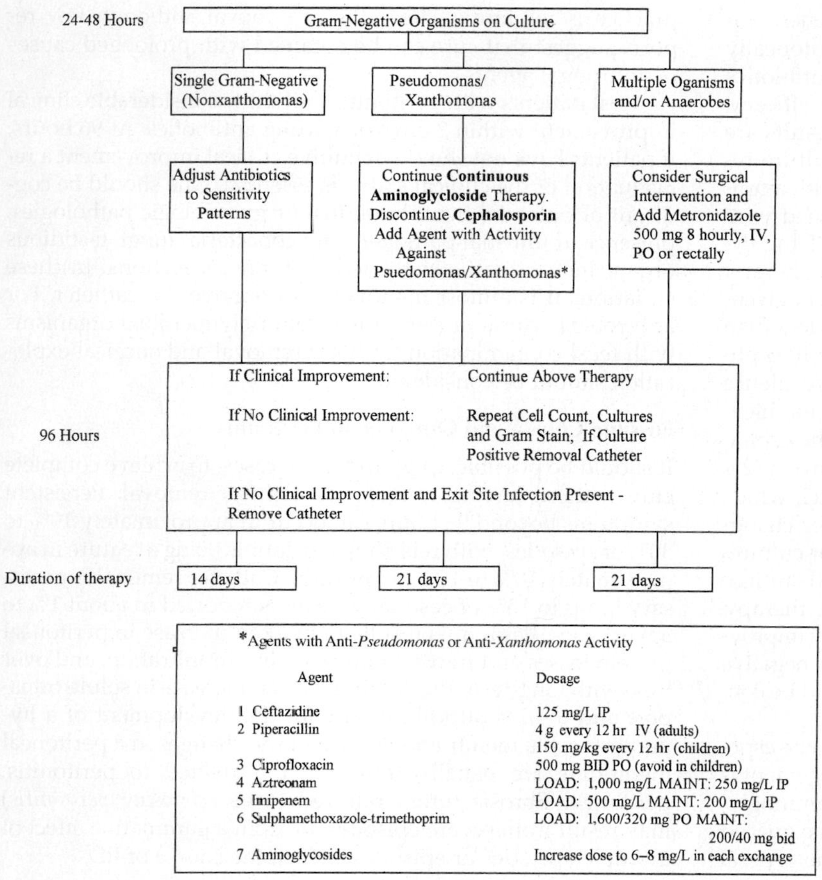

Figure 84.33. Treatment of Gram-negative peritonitis after identification on Gram stain or culture. *Choice of treatment should always be guided by sensitivity patterns. (Reproduced with permission from Keane WF, Alexander SR, Bailie GR, et al. Peritoneal dialysis–related peritonitis treatment recommendations: 1996 update. *Perit Dial Int* 1996; 16:557–573.

Use of Adjuvant Therapy in the Treatment of Continuous Ambulatory Peritoneal Dialysis Peritonitis

Thrombolytic agents have been used for the treatment of recurrent peritonitis but success has been variable. In addition, the optimum time between removal of catheter and reinsertion of a new one is not known. It is a widely held view that short intervals may be acceptable and, indeed, one could perform the removal of the old catheter and insertion of a new one during the same operation, thereby obviating the need for a second surgical procedure. The basis of this practice is related to the catheter itself being the infective cause of the repeated relapsing peritonitis.

Peritoneal Catheter–Related Infections

Colonization of the exit site with microorganisms may lead to infection of that exit site, which may spread along the subcutaneous pathway of the catheter between the inner cuff and subsequently to the peritoneum. Catheter infections, a term that includes both exit-site and tunnel infections, will occur at a rate of 0.6 episodes per year. *S. aureus* and *P. aeruginosa* are the most common and serious catheter infections because they are difficult to resolve and frequently result in peritonitis leading to catheter loss.

Exit-Site Infection. Exit-site infection is defined as a purulent drainage at the peritoneal catheter exit site with surrounding erythema, tenderness, exuberant granulation tissue, and edema. It can be acute (if less than 4 weeks duration) or chronic (if greater than 4 weeks duration). The latter may be a result of an untreated or inadequately treated acute infection, in which case pain and erythema are frequently absent. The equivocal exit site is defined as a purulent and/or bloody drainage only in the sinus that cannot be expressed outside, accompanied by the regression of epithelium and the occurrence of slightly exuberant granulation tissue in the sinus. This represents a low-grade infection. Management of these exit-site cuff/tunnel infections is shown in Table 84.15.

Prevention of Exit-Site and Tunnel Infections. Antibiotics given at the time of catheter insertion have been identified as a way to decrease catheter-related peritonitis in animal studies. In addition, catheter immobilization, proper location of the exit site, sterile wound care immediately after placement of the catheter, and minimizing trauma are all recommended. The downward or lateral-pointing exit site is associated with low peritonitis rates, and exit-site or tunnel infections and the preformed catheters (Swan neck, Pail handle) show a lower probability for the first exit-site infection. Recently, the identification of nasal carriage of *S. aureus* as a risk factor for exit-site infections and peritonitis provides us with the means of preventing such infections. Several protocols have been shown to be effective in preventing *S. aureus* catheter infection by eradicating nasal carriage. Treatment with intranasal mupirocin, oral rifampin, or mupirocin to the exit site as part of routine daily care have all been shown to be effective. Rifampin is not recommended but the use of mupirocin at the exit site seems to be appropriate and easy to administer. Rates of *S. aureus* exit-site infections are approximately 0.3 to 0.4 episodes a year and, with a prophylaxis, this reduces to less than 50%.

Catheter Malfunction, Hernias, and Fluid Leaks

The most important noninfectious complications during PD are abdominal wall–related hernias, leakage of dialysis fluid, and inflow and outflow malfunction of the catheter.

Before PD treatment is started, all significant abdominal wall–related hernias should be corrected. With the presence of 2 to 3 L of dialysate in the abdominal cavity, there is an in-

TABLE 84.15. Treatment Schedule and Management Plan for Each Category of Exit-Site Appearance

	Equivocal Infection	Acute Infection	Chronic Infection	Cuff Infection
Evaluation	Culture and sensitivities on periexit smear Gram stain	Culture and sensitivities on exudate Gram stain	Culture and sensitivities on exudate Gram stain	Palpation of cuff and tunnel Culture and sensitivities and Gram stain of exudate (spontaneous or after-pressure on cuff) Ultrasound of cuff/tunnel
Initial therapy	Cauterize slightly exuberant granulation tissue Topical mupirocin	Cauterize slightly exuberant and exuberant granulation tissue First-generation cephalosporin for Gram-positive organisms; quinolone for Gram-negative organisms; vancomycin for MRSA	Cauterize slightly exuberant and exuberant granulation tissue If initial therapy: first-generation cephalosporin for Gram-positive organisms; quinolone for Gram-negative organisms; vancomycin for MRSA If previously treated: add synergistic drug or change antibiotic according to culture and sensitivities	Cauterize slightly exuberant and exuberant granulation tissue Initial antibiotic therapy based on Gram-stain results
48 hours	Change to Neosporin or gentamycin ointment if Gram-negative organisms on culture	Adjust therapy according to culture and sensitivities	Adjust therapy according to culture and sensitivities	Adjust antibiotic according to culture and sensitivities
Follow-up	If no improvement in 2 weeks, change to systemic antibiotic based on initial culture and sensitivities Continue therapy 7 days past achieving a good appearance Response to systemic antibiotic therapy is excellent, with cure occurring in almost all instances	Evaluate weekly; reculture if no improvement Substitute another appropriate antibiotic or add a second, synergistic antibiotic; use rifampicin as a second antibiotic for staphylococcal infections Most acute infections respond favorably to therapy; continue to treat for 7 days after achieving a good appearance If accompanying peritonitis, consider catheter removal	Evaluate every 2 weeks; reculture every 2 weeks if no improvement on appropriate therapy If infection recurs repeatedly after achieving a good appearance: 1. Consider chronic antibiotic suppression 2. If no improvement after a month of treatment, suspect cuff infection and treat as such If accompanying peritonitis, remove catheter	Reevaluate every 2 weeks; reculture monthly If no remission: 1. consider cuff shaving; 2. consider catheter replacement If accompanying peritonitis, remove catheter

Reproduced with permission from Gokal R, Alexander SR, Ash S, et al. Peritoneal catheters and exit sites practices toward optimal peritoneal access: 1998 update. *Perit Dial Int* 1998;18:11–33.
MRSA, methicillin-resistant *Staphylococcus aureus.*

creased intraabdominal pressure, and all preexisting hernias will become worse during PD treatment. The most frequently occurring hernias during PD are insertional, umbilical, and inguinal. Significant hernias should primarily be repaired surgically and, following repair, intermittent PD may be continued postoperatively using low volumes in a supine position.

Leakage of peritoneal fluid is related to catheter implantation technique, trauma, and/or patient-related anatomic abnormalities. It can occur early (less than 30 days) or late (more than 30 days) after implantation and can have different clinical manifestations depending on whether the leak is external or subcutaneous. Early leakage is usually external, appearing as fluid through the wound or the exit site. Subcutaneous leakage may develop at the site of an incision and entry into the peritoneal cavity and the exact site of the leakage can be determined with computed tomography (CT) after infusion of 2 L of dialysis fluid containing radiocontrast material. Therapy usually entails a period off PD during which the patient, if in need of dialysis, is maintained on HD or intermittent small-volume supine PD. For recurrent leaks, surgical repair is essential. Leakage of fluid into the subcutaneous tissue is sometimes occult, difficult to diagnosis, and may present as diminished drainage, which might be mistaken for ultrafiltration failure. CT and abdominal scintography may identify the leak.

Outflow and/or inflow obstruction are the most frequently observed early events within 2 weeks of the catheter implantation, although these complications can be seen later during PD-related complications such as peritonitis. It is important to differentiate between the various causes, which include the following: (a) mechanical obstruction (tip migration, kink in external tubing), (b) constipation, and (c) catheter blockage. One-way outflow obstruction is the most frequent problem, characterized by poor flow and failure to drain the peritoneal cavity. Both intraluminal factors (blood clot, fibrin) or extraluminal factors (constipation, occlusion of catheter holes from pressure exerted by adjacent organs or omental wrapping, catheter-tip dislocation out of the true pelvis, incorrect catheter placement at implantation) are common causes. Depending on the cause, appropriate therapy entails laxatives, heparinized saline flushes, urokinase instillation in the catheter, fluoroscopy and manipulation (using a stiff wire or stylet manipulation combined with a whiplash technique), revision, and replacement.

PERITONEAL MEMBRANE CHANGES: LOSS OF ULTRAFILTRATION

Anatomic Changes

The normal peritoneal membrane consists of mesothelium, which on the surface has a profuse mantle of microvilli. Entangled within these are lamellar bodies, containing phospholipid lubricant released from the underlying mesothelium, which rests on a thin, but readily visible basement membrane. This separates the submesothelial layer consisting of collagen fibers, ground substance, and capillaries.

The peritoneum undergoing PD usually does react to changes in response to the new environment; this consists of reactive proliferation of the mesothelium and decrease in the microvillus projections, and in the submesothelium there is a variation of ground substance and collagen fibers with a degree of disorganization. There is also thickening of the peritoneal interstitium and basement membrane reduplication both in the mesothelium as well as in the capillary. Such changes have been identified to occur secondary to the unphysiologic composition of the dialysis solution and also to the direct action of glucose and glucose degradation products, which bring about the aforementioned AGE-related changes in the peritoneal membrane. Some of the changes are diabetiform in nature, there is also deposition of AGE products as early as 3 months after dialysis, diabetiform alterations of peritoneal microvessels, and neovascularization as seen in diabetic retinopathy with deposition of collagen IV. Case-controlled studies have also shown that peritoneal sclerosis occurs in patients in whom the sclerosis is related to greater glucose exposure. Other factors that are important in the changes described previously are acute intraperitoneal inflammation related to peritonitis; chronic inflammatory reaction mediated through the process of dialysis, whereby there is activation of peritoneal macrophages; increase in the number of neutrophils; intraperitoneal production of bioactive substances promoting inflammation [interleukin (IL)-1, IL-8]; and peritoneal fibrosis [transforming growth factor-β (TGF-β)], as well as peroxidation of the peritoneum. To maintain membrane integrity, more physiologic solutions need to be introduced and peritonitis needs to be minimized.

Changes to the peritoneal membrane have been described with time on dialysis, physiologically reflected in a hyperpermeable membrane. Membrane changes vary but can progress eventually to peritoneal sclerosis, which is a rare event (less than 1%); there are defined ultrastructural changes associated with peritoneal sclerosis.

Physiologic Considerations

There is now greater understanding of the physiology of peritoneal dialysis, which appears to correlate with the aforementioned anatomic findings. Fluid and solute removal is now thought to occur through defined pathways and structures in the peritoneal membrane enshrined in the three-pore model of permselectivity. This describes three different "pores"—transcellular (radius less than 0.5 nm), small pore (radius 40 to 60 nm), and large pore (more than 200 nm). The small pores (which, anatomically, are interendothelial slits) represent the dominant transcapillary pathway for small water-soluble solutes and water. Across these pores the so-called Starling equilibrium is established and hydrostatic pressure usually outweighs the effective colloid osmotic pressure. Transcellular pores are now recognized to be the water channel aquaporin, in which there is maximal effect of crystalloid osmotic pressure. The large pores may represent the pathway for lymph flow and hydrostatic pressure may dominate here. Transcapillary ultrafiltration induced by glucose not only occurs through the small-pore system but also through transcellular pores, which allow the transport of water but not of solutes. The transcellular water channel has been identified to be present in the mesothelial cells and the peritoneal microvasculature. The contribution of the ultrasmall pores to the total transport of water can roughly be judged from the sieving of sodium, that is, the decrease of the dialysate sodium concentration that occurs during the initial phase of the dialysis dwell using 3.86% glucose concentration. The minimum sodium concentration is usually reached after 30 to 60 minutes.

Physiologically, an important way of assessing peritoneal function is by using the peritoneal equilibration test (PET), which gives a crude idea of the peritoneal membranes' functional capacity to ultrafilter. The greater the permeability, the less is the crystalloid osmotic pressure and therefore ultrafiltration will be of short duration. Solute clearance is excellent in these circumstances. More extensive information can be obtained using the standard permeability analysis (SPA) in which the transport of serum proteins and the kinetics of fluid transport are also determined. Because the peritoneal transport of serum protein is hindered in a size-selective way, protein clearances are not only determined by the surface area of the membrane, that is, the number of pores available, but also by the size of the large pores, that is, the intrinsic permeability. The latter can be characterized by the selectivity index. This is expressed as the peritoneal restriction coefficient, a high value for which indicates low permeability. The relationship between membrane characteristics and parameters of solute transport are now well defined, which include parameters to assess mesothelial and interstitial abnormalities as well as vascular abnormalities. The former can be looked at using the cancer antigen, CA125, which declines as mesothelial mass decreases, and the latter can be assessed in terms of ultrafiltration failure by looking at various peritoneal-solute and fluid-transport markers.

Ultrafiltration Failure

Net ultrafiltration failure is the most important transport abnormality in long-term CAPD. Based on clinical symptoms its prevalence has been reported to increase from 3% after 1 year on CAPD to approximately 30% after 6 years. Recently, evidence has been obtained that net ultrafiltration less than 400 ml after a 4-hour dwell using a 3.86% glucose is probably a good definition of ultrafiltration failure. Both recurrent peritonitis and exposure to dialysis fluids have been suggested as pathogenetic factors in the development of morphologic and functional alterations of the peritoneal membrane during long-term CAPD. The peritoneal membrane is a tenacious anatomic structure that seems to recover well after infective and inflammatory insults; there is some evidence that continued exposure to these insults may delay this recovery and recovery may also be incomplete. However, it is likely that serious peritoneal infections caused by microorganisms such as *P. aeroginosa* and *S. aureus* may contribute to alteration of a more permanent nature in the peritoneal membrane.

Ultrafiltration failure is associated with a large vascular peritoneal surface area, a highly effective peritoneal lymphatic absorption, and impaired aquaporin channel-mediated water transport. The diagnosis of this can be made using either a PET or SPA as shown in Fig. 84.34. Diagnosis of membrane failure should

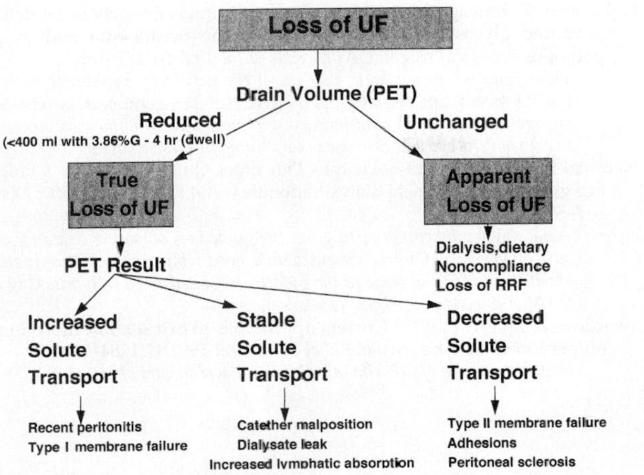

Figure 84.34. Management of patient with loss of ultrafiltration. The PET (peritoneal equilibration test) can be replaced with the SPA (see text for details).

be considered in the presence of fluid overload and symptoms of inadequate solute removal. Type 1 membrane failure with the permanent loss of ultrafiltration capacity is linked with high transporter status (hyperpermeable membrane) and is the initial stage of membrane damage; this may subsequently lead to type 2 membrane failure associated with sclerosing encapsulating peritonitis, peritoneal adhesions, and peritoneal sclerosis.

Improvement of peritoneal function can be brought about by minimizing glucose exposure, peritoneal rest (use of glucose-free dialysate), use of icodextrin, and by using large dialysate volumes in patients who have effective high peritoneal lymphatic absorption. In patients who have ultrafiltration failure associated with signs of structural membrane abnormalities (such as impaired sodium sieving and low dialysate CA125 levels), the temporary discontinuation of PD or transfer to HD are the only options. In patients with ultrafiltration failure, icodextrin use is of advantage and has been shown to extend therapy time on PD. In the future, not only will the development of physiologic solutions help, but a better control of intraperitoneal inflammatory reactions by enhancement of natural homeostatic mechanisms (intraperitoneal glycosaminoglycans, antioxidant therapy) may well be of value.

INDICATIONS AND CONTRAINDICATIONS FOR PERITONEAL DIALYSIS

Indications and contraindications for PD are shown in Table 84.16, which looks at conditions that favor patients going on to either HD or PD.

Contraindications

There are very few absolute contraindications to the use of PD. Most of these relate to inadequate peritoneal surface area in order to perform adequate PD. There are a number of relative contraindications, which include colostomy, ileostomy, hernias, and polycystic kidney disease. Prior abdominal aneurysm surgery is also a relative contraindication. Care needs to be taken in prescribing PD in patients with severe obstructive lung disease, peripheral vascular disease, and diverticulosis of the bowel. Another absolute contraindication is inability of the patient or spouse and caregivers to perform CAPD in a home or nursing environment. The patient must have the capacity and understanding of PD and self-care requirements for the therapy to succeed at home.

Indications

Peritoneal dialysis can be used to manage most patients with end-stage renal disease (ESRD), except those with absolute contraindications. It is a treatment particularly well suited to those patients in whom vascular access is going to be a major problem, with poor cardiovascular reserve, in diabetics, children, the elderly, and those that live a long distance away from a center. The use of APD, rather than HD, in children is now the norm.

The selection of a dialytic modality is influenced by several considerations other than medical and social ones. It is felt that in a population of ESRD patients, 15% to 20% will have good clinical indications for HD, a similar percentage for PD. The majority of patients however would manage adequately on either therapy. The choice then depends on local factors, facilities, physician bias, and most important of all, patient choice. De-

TABLE 84.16. Medical and Psychologic Factors Favoring Peritoneal Dialysis and Hemodialysis

HD Preferred	Do Well on Either Therapy	PD Preferred
Severe inflammatory bowel disease	**In-center HD-Oriented**	Unstable CV disease
Homeless	Dependent lifestyle	Vascular access problem
Incapable of self-care dialysis	Active diverticulitis	Age
Unsuitable peritoneum or abdomen	Ischemic renal disease	Children (younger than 5)
Severe psychotic disorder	APKD	Elderly
	Recurrent hernias	Diabetes mellitus
	Ileostomies	Distance from center
	Severe pulmonary disease	
	CAPD-Oriented	
	Independent lifestyle	
	Vascular access problems	
	Diabetes mellitus	
	APD-Oriented	
	Hyperpermeable membrane	
	Social support	

APD, automated peritoneal dialysis, APKD, adult polycystic kidney disease; CHPD, continuous ambulatory peritoneal dialysis; CV, cardiovascular; HD, hemodialysis; PD, peritoneal dialysis.

pending on social, home, and work conditions, the patient and the family would choose the therapy that would best suit their psychosocial makeup.

A future indication for peritoneal dialysis may be to accomplish "healthy/early" start as has been advocated in the NKF-DOQI guidelines. In this situation, PD may be positively indicated; with reasonable residual renal function, there is less need for dialysis clearance and therefore a reduced number of exchanges would suffice. These are gradually increased as the residual renal function declines. The use of icodextrin, which allows for long-dwell PD, may be an apt way to implement this recommendation.

Selected Readings

Coles G. Have we underestimated the importance of fluid balance for survival of PD patients? *Perit Dial Int* 1997;17:321–326.
Editorial on the importance of maintaining proper fluid balance in PD patients. It is believed that PD patients are "chronically fluid overloaded" and greater emphasis is necessary on this aspect of achieving adequacy. Adverse fluid status is linked with poor cardiovascular outcomes in dialysis patients.

Feriani M, La Greca G, Kriger FL, et al. CAPD systems and solutions. In: Gokal R, Nolph KD, eds. *The textbook of peritoneal dialysis.* Dordrecht, The Netherlands: Kluwer Academic Publishers, 1994:233–270.
This is a comprehensive chapter review on the ever-increasing complex exchange systems, automated PD cyclers, and the connectology. It also addresses the wide area of PD fluid composition in terms of electrolyte content, osmotic agents, and acid–base status using the newer bicarbonate-based solutions.

Gokal R. New strategies for peritoneal dialysis solutions. *Nephrol Dial Transplant* 1997;12(suppl 1):74–77.
This review outlines the recent developments in peritoneal fluid composition, which are linked with better understanding of peritoneal membrane physiology, role of glucose in membrane damage, and the development of a hyperpermeability.

Gokal R, Alexander SR, Ash S, et al. Peritoneal catheters and exit-site practices toward optimum peritoneal access: 1998 update. *Perit Dial Int* 1998;18:11–33.
This is a report from the Internation Society of Peritoneal Dialysis. It provides guidelines on the management of all aspects of peritoneal access (Catheter types, insertion, outcomes, exit-site care, treatment of catheter-related infections). It is comprehensive with a good bibliography.

Hendriks PM, Ho-dac-Pannekeet MM, van Gulik TM, et al. Peritoneal sclerosis in chronic peritoneal dialysis patients: analysis of clinical presentation, risk factors, and peritoneal transport kinetics. *Perit Dial Int* 1997;17:136–143.
This study analyzes the clinical features of peritoneal sclerosis in a group of PD patients and compares this with a control group. The likely risk factors appear to be severe peritonitis, glucose use. Treatment of the advanced cases of sclerosis appears to be conservative.

Holmes CJ. Biocompatibility of peritoneal dialysis solutions. *Perit Dial Int* 1993; 13:88–94.
Biocompatibility of PD solutions is an important area of research, aimed at preserving peritoneal membrane integrity, which is so important in longevity of PD therapy. In vitro studies are conclusive in showing that bioincompatibility has an adverse impact on cell function; convincing clinical evidence to support this is still lacking.

Keane WF, Alexander SR, Bailie GR, et al. Peritoneal dialysis–related peritonitis treatment recommendations: 1996 update. *Perit Dial Int* 1996;16:557–573.
This outlines the latest guidelines for the diagnosis and treatment of PD-related infections—peritonitis and exit site. It incorporates the changes resulting from the emergence of vancomycin-resistant enterococci.

Kopple JD, Barnard D, Messana J, et al. Treatment of malnourished CAPD patients with an amino acid–based dialysate. *Kidney Int* 1995;47(4):1148–1157.
The role of amino acid–based PD solution in the treatment of malnutrition in CAPD patients is established by this carefully conducted study, performed in metabolic wards. It shows a positive nitrogen balance and improvement in other simple measure of nutrition when one to two exchanges of this solution are used daily.

Krediet R, Ho-dac-Pannekeet MM, Smit W, et al. Peritoneal dialysis: how to improve peritoneal permeability or function. *Adv Nephrol Necker Hosp* 1997;27: 167–188.
A review on the current thinking on peritoneal membrane physiology, methods of accurately measuring peritoneal function, and means to improve dysfunction (hyperpermeability, loss of ultrafiltration, peritoneal sclerosis) with the use of novel solutions (icodextrin) and avoidance of glucose.

Mistry CD, Gokal R, Peers E, and the Midas Study Group. A randomised multicentre clinical trial comparing isosmolar dextrin 20 with hyperosmolar glucose solutions in continuous Ambulatory peritoneal dialysis (CAPD): a 6 month study. *Kidney Int* 1994;46:496–503.
A prospective, randomized, controlled trial on the efficacy and safety of icodextrin-containing PD fluid, used for the long overnight dwell. It showed that the icodextrin had superior ultrafiltration as compared with the glucose-based solution, with so toxic side effects from its use over 6 months.

Nakayama M, Kawaguchi Y, Yamada K, et al. Immunohistochemical detection of advanced glycosylation end-products in the peritoneum and its possible pathophysiological role in CAPD. *Kidney Int* 1997;51:182–186.
This study on morphologic changes of the peritoneal membrane with time on CAPD shows progressively more AGEs in the peritoneal membrane. These changes are correlated with increasing permeability, and by association, decreasing ultrafiltration. Glucose use is implicated in these changes.

National Kidney Foundation–Dialysis Outcomes Quality Initiative. Clinical practice guidelines peritoneal dialysis adequacy. *Am J Kidney Dis* 1997;30(suppl 3): S67–S136.
A milestone publication setting out the guidelines on solute clearance as a measure of adequacy. Clearly set out with a good bibliography. There is still debate about the validity of some of the guidelines, stated to be so but lacking evidence (Kt/V and weekly creatinine clearance).

Twardowski ZJ, Prowant BF. Current approaches to exit site infections in patients on peritoneal dialysis. *Nephrol Dial Transplant* 1997;12:1284–1295.
Editorial on care of exit-site infections and overall care of exit sites.

C: Continuous Ambulatory Peritoneal Dialysis

Rosario Maiorca and Giovanni C. Cancarini

Continuous ambulatory peritoneal dialysis (CAPD), an innovative kind of peritoneal dialysis (PD), was proposed by Popovich and Moncrief in 1976. These authors, basing on the urea kinetic modelling, demonstrated that a peritoneal perfusion of 2 L dialysis fluid, five times a day, 7 days a week, ensured sufficient blood purification. However, CAPD became an acceptable dialysis modality only when plastic bags instead of glass bottles were introduced as fluid containers by Oreopoulos. This change resulted in decreasing the high incidence of peritonitis to one episode every 10 to 12 patient-months. Later, in the 1980s, the introduction of Y set and double bag further reduced the incidence of peritonitis to about one episode every 3 years, thus removing one of the main obstacles to the penetration of CAPD.

TECHNICAL ASPECTS

Solutions Available for Continuous Ambulatory Peritoneal Dialysis

Composition

The solute contents of peritoneal dialysis fluid (Table 84.17) have partially changed with increased experience. The concentration of sodium ranges from 132 to 140 mmol/L, lower than in the plasma water, in order to avoid excessive sodium removal and possible hypotension, or to avoid excessive sodium increase due to the membrane-sieving effect under the highest glucose concentrations.

For the majority of CAPD patients, no potassium is contained in the dialysis solution. This allows the removal of approximately 38 to 48 mmol of potassium per day, an amount generally sufficient to maintain stable serum potassium concentrations. Patients with low food intake may need the use of one or more bags with 2 mmol/L of potassium. Only very few patients who have very low food intake or diarrhea need one or more bags with a potassium concentration of 4 mmol/L.

The usual concentration of calcium in the bags is 1.75 mmol/L. This gives a calcium balance positive with a 1.5 g/dl dextrose solution, neutral with 2.5 g/dl dextrose, and negative with

TABLE 84.17. Composition of the Peritoneal Dialysis Fluids Commercially Available

Sodium (mmol/L)	132–140
Potassium (mmol/L)	0–4
Calcium (mmol/L)	1.00–1.75
Magnesium (mmol/L)	0.25–0.75
Lactate (mmol/L)	35–40
Chloride (mmol/L)	101–107
Dextrose (g/dl)	1.36–4.25
pH (pH units)	5.0–5.5
Osmolality (mOsm/kg)	340–507

4.25 g/dl dextrose, because the more hypertonic the solution, the greater the amount of calcium removed with the ultrafiltration volume. The wider use of oral calcium salts as phosphate binders has increased the risk of transient hypercalcemic peaks, which has suggested the use of solutions with a lower calcium concentration (i.e., 1.25 mmol/L).

Uremic patients are hypermagnesemic, thus the use of low-magnesium PD fluids are suggested, from 0.25 to 0.75 mmol/L. The lower concentration is indicated for patients given magnesium salt as phosphate binders.

The buffer contained in the currently available PD solution is lactate. Acetate, used in the first years of CAPD was abandoned after the demonstration of its association with ultrafiltration loss. The standard solutions contain racemic lactate, that is, half L-lactate and half D-lactate. After absorption, L-lactate is metabolized by lactate dehydrogenase and D-lactate by an aspecific dehydrogenase. The rate of metabolism is sufficiently rapid to prevent the elevation of lactacidemia. However, because lactate is metabolized mainly in the liver, patients with severe hepatic failure may present dangerous hyperlactacidemia. The substitution of pyruvate for lactate has been suggested, in consideration of its reduced negative effects on cellular anaerobic glycolysis; however, the long-term safety of pyruvate for the peritoneal membrane remains to be demonstrated. Both lactate and pyruvate generate the physiologic buffer, bicarbonate. Bicarbonate cannot be introduced in PD solutions as such, because in the presence of calcium it precipitates as calcium carbonate. A two-chambered bag has been proposed, which allows maintenance of bicarbonate separated from calcium and dextrose until the time of use, when the separating, frangible seal is crushed and the bag contents are mixed. This procedure, besides avoiding calcium–carbonate precipitation, permits the maintenance of the acidic compartment at a pH low enough to reduce the formation of dextrose degradation products during heat sterilization. The efficacy and the safety of this solution have been demonstrated in recent clinical trials. However, in such conditions, the complete substitution of lactate by bicarbonate requires a high concentration of bicarbonate (38 to 39 mmol/L) that, in turn, needs a high P_{CO_2} concentration to remain in solution, and this may cause abdominal pain at fluid infusion. For this reason, a new formulation with a mixture of bicarbonate and lactate (bicarbonate 25 mmol/L plus lactate 15 mmol/L) has been tested and has proven to be safe and effective in a 2-month study. Long-run studies are, currently, in progress. Such a solution does not remove bicarbonate from the blood when it is in the normal ranges, and tends to correct situations of low and high bicarbonatemia. Moreover, it reduces the risk of hyperlactacidemia, even in patients with hepatic failure. But the main advantage of bicarbonate-based solutions is in their physiologic pH, approximately 7.4. In the lactate-based fluids, the low pH, approximately 5.0 to 5.5, has extensively proven negative effects on the viability of mesothelial and polymorphonuclear cells and on macrophages. Because many papers have suggested a synergistic negative effect of low pH and lactate, this new solution might have beneficial effects on peritoneal viability and defense mechanisms.

Dextrose is added to the solution to oppose the blood oncotic pressure and to obtain adequate water ultrafiltration. However, dextrose has many disadvantages. It requires a low pH to reduce the appearance of glucose degradation products during heat sterilization. The high concentration of dextrose needed (from 13.6 to 42.5 times the normal plasma concentration) can lead to protein glycosylation, which may affect the structure and the function of many peritoneal components. The observed duplication of the peritoneal capillary basal membrane, similar to that seen in diabetic microangiopathy, and a structural change of the peritoneal membrane, known as *tanned peritoneum,* have been suggested to be the consequence of the high concentration of dextrose. The search for new osmotic agents in substitution for dextrose has been extensive and has included the use of both low-molecular-weight solutes and polymers. Thus far, few of them have entered clinical use; those that have are glycerol, a mixture of amino acids, and polyglucose. Glycerol has a molecular weight approximately half that of dextrose, thus it is rapidly absorbed. Amino acids, besides being osmotic agents also act as nutritional supplements, which is particularly useful for patients with low protein intake. However, they cannot be used in more than one or two bags a day (the concentration of amino acids is 1.1 g/dl) in order to avoid an excessively high nitrogen load and the development of acidosis; the latter impairs protein synthesis and negatively affects the deposition of calcium on the bone crystallization surface. Glucose polymers, a mixture of polymers with different molecular weights, thanks to their larger molecular size, are absorbed slowly from the peritoneal cavity and allow a sustained ultrafiltration flow even during long-indwelling periods. The polymer solution has an osmolality of 286 mOsm/kg, which is much lower than that given by the lowest dextrose concentration (340 mOsm/kg); nevertheless, thanks to its poor absorption, it allows higher ultrafiltration volumes at lower rates but sustained over time. The curves of the ultrafiltration volume given by glucose and polyglucose are quite different (Fig. 84.35); the glucose being more effective during short-indwelling periods and polyglucose during longer ones. A negative effect of polyglucose is the trend toward the plasma accumulation of maltose and maltotriose, which increase the plasma osmolality. For this reason the use of no more than one bag a day is recommended.

Inflow Volume

PD solutions are available in bags of different volumes ranging from 1 to 3 L to meet the peritoneal capacity of each patient. The

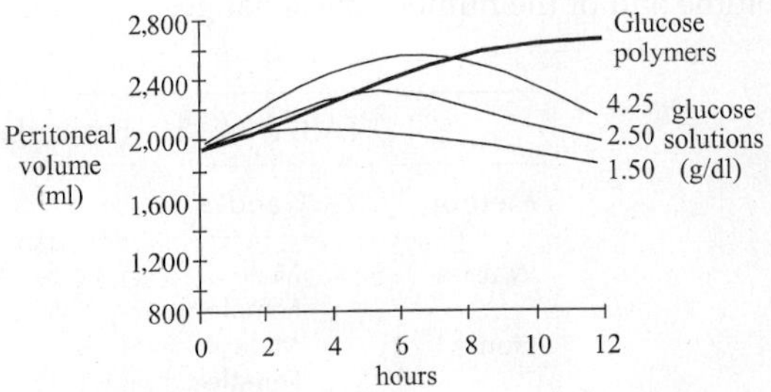

Figure 84.35. Changes in peritoneal volume over time with glucose polymers and different concentrations of glucose.

patient can administer the required volume by weighing the bag or, when using a double-bag system, by pouring part of the fresh solution into the drainage bag.

Connection Systems and Catheters

This topic has been discussed in Chapter 84, Part 2B. It is important to remark here that the important improvements in this field have made possible a strong reduction in the incidence of peritonitis and have boosted the clinical use of CAPD. The fear of causing peritoneal damage by using disinfectants within the connection has been shown to be justified only for chlorhexidine, the use of which has been associated with sclerosing encapsulating peritonitis. The clinical complication due to these devices, mainly peritonitis, have been described in the previous section.

Dialysis Schedule

There is no general agreement on the right time to initiate dialysis. Some authors suggest starting when residual renal Kt/V reaches the limit of 2.0, but an impairment of the nutritional status, a difficult ECV control, and a low diet compliance constitute indications to start dialysis. At the start of PD treatment, when defining the amount of dialysis adequate for the patient, a few factors must also be taken into account: the residual renal function (RRF); the ECV status; and the patient's social needs, including his or her quality of life.

An interval of 2 weeks between the introduction of the catheter and the start of CAPD ("break-in" period) is generally considered sufficient to allow the healing of the surgical wound. It is preferable to start with low inflow volumes the first days (i.e., 1,500 ml) and then to progressively increase up to volumes compatible with the patient size. If low-glucose solutions are used, there is the risk of insufficient or negative ultrafiltration. Monitoring the daily ultrafiltration volume, body weight, presence or absence of edema, and blood pressure helps to choose the right concentration of glucose to regulate ECV.

The contribution of the RRF to blood purification and ECV control generally permits the usage of three bags a day during the first weeks or months. Sometimes, a different schedule can help patients become accustomed to the new lifestyle: four bags a day for 6 days, with a dry day a week, or a dry abdomen for part of the day (i.e., to allow the children to play and the adults to do some physical exercise). However, such a *trade-off* is acceptable only for a limited period of time and in the presence of adequate RRF, because one should not forget that the original urea kinetic study of Popovich and Moncrief required *continuous* peritoneal dialysis. Loop diuretics can help control the fluid balance during the day free of dialysis. The use of diuretics has been recommended also to reduce the need for hypertonic bags, and the negative effect of the same on the peritoneal membrane.

The progressive reduction of RRF can inadvertently lead to inadequate dialysis. Frequent checking (every 3 to 4 months) of the indices of adequacy allows a timely adjustment of the inflow volume and of the number of exchanges.

CLINICAL ASPECTS

Adequacy and Residual Renal Function

Dialysis patients suffer high morbidity related to both uremia and dialysis modality and have a mortality much higher than the normal population. One critical point is whether these poor results can be partly attributed to an inadequate dose of dialysis administered. Until the early 1980s, the dose of dialysis was defined according to the clinical assessment, mainly based on the appearance of signs and symptoms known to be related to the uremic status. Since then, many efforts have been made to define one or more parameters measuring the dose of dialysis delivered and able to predict patient morbidity and mortality. The main progress in this field has been obtained by the National Cooperative Dialysis Study in the United States, and following studies. An important contribution has been the definition of the Kt/V parameter for hemodialysis. Kt/V is the ratio between the amount of plasma cleared from its urea content by the dialyzer (K = urea clearance of the filter in ml/min; t = duration of dialysis, in minutes) and the volume of distribution of the urea (V, measured in ml and equivalent to the total body water). Similar studies were carried out, later, in peritoneal dialysis. In this modality, two indices have been proposed: urea Kt/V and normalized weekly creatinine clearance (WCC). Because PD patients maintain a residual renal function for a long period of time, both Kt/V and WCC must be calculated by adding the renal clearance to the peritoneal clearance. Such a procedure implies that peritoneal clearance and renal clearance are equivalent, but this has not been demonstrated thus far.

Calculation of Kt/V in Continuous Ambulatory Peritoneal Dialysis

The patient must collect and measure the daily total peritoneal drainage and urine volume. The needed blood sample can be taken at any time of the collection period, because it is assumed that serum urea changes minimally during the day. The peritoneal and the renal clearances are calculated with the well-known Kt/V formula, as described in the previous paragraph. The sum of the two clearances gives the total clearance per minute, and from this the clearance per week. To calculate V, many formulas have been suggested, but all of them only approximate the true water content. One suggests to calculate V as 58% of the body weight; in another, V is 60% of the body weight for men and 55% for women. We suggest to use one of the formulas indicated in Table 84.18 that take into account both weight and height, and which, in adults, shows a better relationship with the isotopically measured total body water.

Calculation of Weekly Creatinine Clearance in Continuous Ambulatory Peritoneal Dialysis

Also this calculation requires the collection of the daily peritoneal drainage, the urine output, and a blood sample. The clearance formula is the same. Two main points must, however, be remembered: first, the creatinine concentration measured in

TABLE 84.18. Formulas for the Calculation of Total Body Water

Method	Gender	Formula
Watson	Male	V = 2.447 + 0.3362 × weight + 0.1074 × height − 0.09516 × age
	Female	V = − 2.097 + 0.2466 × weight + 0.1069 × height
Hume	Male	V = − 14.012934 + 0.296785 × weight + 0.192786 × height
	Female	V = − 35.270121 + 0.183809 × weight + 0.344547 × height

Note: V in liters, weight in kg, height in cm, and age in years.

the peritoneal effluent must be corrected for the interference due to its very high dextrose concentration; second, the renal clearance must be calculated as a mathematic mean of urea clearance and creatinine clearance, to adjust for the tubular secretion of creatinine. The two clearances (peritoneal and renal) are then summed and the result is multiplied by the 10,080 minutes in a week. The weekly clearance is then normalized to the body surface area (BSA), in analogy to what is usually done for the creatinine renal clearance. The BSA is calculated by the formula of Du Bois and Du Bois:

$$\text{BSA (m}^2) = 0.007184 \times \text{weight (kg)}^{0.425} \times \text{height (cm)}^{0.725}$$

For a correct calculation of both Kt/V and WCC, the patient should be free of edema and have no limb amputations. Some formulas allow adjustment for these conditions.

Targets of Dialysis Dose

Few studies are available currently to define the adequate targets. According to the guidelines forwarded by the National Kidney Foundation–Dialysis Outcome Quality Initiative (NKF-DOQI), a dose (peritoneal plus renal clearance) equivalent to Kt/V 2.0/week for urea and to 60 L/week/1.73 m² BSA for creatinine clearance should be adequate and is associated with better survival and lower morbidity. In the case of discrepancy between the two indices, it would be advisable to achieve the minimum target with both of them because there is no evidence that either of them better represents adequate blood purification.

Adjustment of the Dialysis Dose

In the case of inadequate dialysis dose, an attempt to increase it can be made by either increasing the number of exchanges or the volume per exchange or both. The following formula of the peritoneal dialysis clearance for a solute "a" (PCla) suggests the practical possibilities to increase the peritoneal clearance:

$$\text{PCla} = \frac{\text{Da} \times \text{Vd}}{\text{Pa} \times 1440}$$

or

$$\text{PCla} = \frac{\text{Da}}{\text{Pa}} \times \frac{(\text{Vi} \times \text{NoE} + \text{VUF})}{1440}$$

where Da is the concentration of "a" in dialysis fluid, Vd is the daily peritoneal effluent, Pa is the plasma concentration, 1,440 is the minutes in a day, Vi is the inflow volume of each exchange, NoE is the number of exchanges per day, and VUF is the daily ultrafiltration volume. The first term of the formula is the D/P ratio for a defined molecule and can change according to the number of exchanges per day and the duration of the indwelling times. However it depends, for each patient, on the permeability and surface area of the peritoneal membrane. The use of drugs for the pharmacologic manipulation of its permeability has been suggested by many studies, but has not yet entered clinical use, thus inflexibility remains an intrinsic limit for the peritoneal membrane. The only possible variations are in the volumes exchanged for each bag and in the number of bags. Usage of large volumes raises the risk of hernias, leakage, and hemorrhoids, and also increases the intraperitoneal hydrostatic pressure, thus partially neutralizing the dialysate osmotic pressure and reducing the ultrafiltration volume.

Increasing the number of exchanges has a negative impact on the quality of life. Moreover, the increase from four to five exchanges per day does not increase the total clearance of 25%, because each indwelling period becomes shorter and consequently the D/P value becomes lower.

A larger use of hypertonic bags (with 3.86 or 4.25 g/dl dextrose) increases ultrafiltration volume (UFV) and peritoneal clearance, and allows freer water intake. On the other hand, high-dextrose concentrations favor protein glycosylation, with a negative impact on the membrane function. When any attempt to increase the CAPD dose fails, the change to automated peritoneal dialysis (APD) or to hemodialysis must be seriously considered.

Clinical Assessment

On clinical grounds, providing an adequate dialysis is much more than dialyzing with a sufficient dose of dialysis. Many other factors must also be taken into consideration, such as ECV and arterial blood pressure control, acid–base equilibrium, anemia, nutrition, calcium/phosphate metabolism, and so on.

Many patients have a good control of the acid–base status, that is, 25 to 27 mmol/L venous bicarbonate concentration (or 26 to 28 mmol/L of total CO_2), with 40 mmol/L lactate PD solutions. In those using 35 mmol/L lactate, supplements of sodium bicarbonate are often necessary. The administration of sodium bicarbonate, however, increases sodium load, stimulating thirst and fluid assumption, and increasing the daily ultrafiltration demand.

The correction of acidosis in dialysis patients has not been sufficiently stressed in the past years. Acidosis stimulates protein catabolism, inhibits protein synthesis, and negatively affects bone-surface crystallization. It follows that a patient whose acidosis is not adequately corrected may become malnourished even on an adequate dialysis dose.

The prevention of the hyperparathyroidism with low-phosphate diets and phosphate binders must start early in patients with renal insufficiency, and continue on dialysis. The risk of aluminum accumulation (with consequent bone disease, anemia, and risk of brain toxicity) has progressively led to the substitution of aluminum-containing phosphate binders with calcium carbonate and calcium acetate. These salts, when given during meals, bind food phosphate and prevent its absorption and, if given far from meals, they act as calcium supplements and are useful in hypocalcemic patients. Hyperparathyroidism can be prevented and ameliorated by using oral Calcitriol, or intravenous in appropriate doses. The risk of hypercalcemia, due to the use of Calcitriol and/or an excessive amount of calcium salts can be prevented by using dialysis solutions with low-calcium concentrations.

The anemia of uremia is, in PD patients, less severe than in hemodialysis patients, thanks to the absence of blood loss in the extracorporeal circulation and, probably, to better dialysis of solutes inhibiting hemopoiesis. Doses of rhEPO of 4,000 to 8,000 units per week permit the achievement of the suggested hematocrit target of 32% to 36%. Patients unable to reach these values must be checked for inadequate dialysis, iron deficiency, aluminum overload, or other associated diseases.

Hypertension is frequent in PD patients, and some of its major causes are ECV expansion, activation of renin-angiotensin-aldosterone system, decreased synthesis of antihypertensive prostaglandins, and other hormonal abnormalities. Many antihypertensive drugs can be used, but all of them have some unwanted side effects: β-blockers have been indicated as possible promoters of peritoneal sclerosis; calcium antagonists can increase the peripheral edema induced by the peritoneal fluid pressure on the iliac veins; clonidine gives "dry mouth," which increases the water intake; and ACE inhibitors may reduce the effect of rhEPO. Patients must be trained to moderate salt and fluid intake and to reach a correct balance of dialysis fluid, to limit the antihypertensive medication that can be given as an association of low doses of different drugs.

Complications of Continuous Ambulatory Peritoneal Dialysis

Local Complications

The local complications of PD have been discussed in Chapter 84, Part 2B.

Systemic Complications

Malnutrition. During PD, part of the dextrose in the peritoneal solution is absorbed and enters the blood circulation. The dextrose absorbed accounts for approximately 70% of the amount present in the bag. It also increases with the length of the indwelling time and may reach more than 80% during the night exchange. On CAPD, continuous glucose absorption has many effects. It reduces appetite, which is often already poor due to dysgeusia, increased abdominal pressure, uremic gastroenteropathy, and, in the elderly, masticatory problems. The loss of appetite generally has no effect on the carbohydrate intake, being compensated for by the peritoneal absorption of dextrose, but it does negatively affect protein intake, because in these conditions meat foods become particularly less attractive.

Moreover, the peritoneal filter enables the passage of amino acids and proteins from blood to dialysate. The daily removal accounts for 5 to 12 g of protein and 1 to 4 g of amino acids per day, and protein loss increases to 15 to 20 g during peritonitis episodes. Patients having the peritoneal permeability in the highest range lose more proteins and are at higher risk of developing malnutrition. Reduced protein intake and removal of amino acids and proteins with the peritoneal drainage can lead to protein malnutrition. This status might be masked by a contemporary increase in the body fat content, which might disguise the decrease in lean body mass.

The importance of the nutritional status has been supported by many studies showing that serum albumin concentration at the start or during PD is one of the major factors correlating with patient survival and morbidity. Preventing malnutrition is one of the most challenging problems of PD. Many tools are available to assess nutritional status and its change over time. Serum levels of prealbumin, albumin, transferrin, pseudocholinesterase, and G immunoglobulins are the most common indices of protein synthesis. The serum concentration of these proteins is not a timely index of protein intake, but some of them with shorter half-lives, such as prealbumin, are more sensitive indicators. Protein nitrogen appearance (PNA), more often referred to as *protein catabolic rate (PCR),* consists in the measurement of the peritoneal and renal nitrogen excretion. From this value it is easy to calculate the protein intake, which can also be obtained by recording dietary intake for some days. Many formulas have been suggested to calculate PNA (Table 84.19), and some of them also take into account protein and amino acid peritoneal loss. Nitrogen appearance derives from protein intake and from body protein breakdown. It follows that to avoid erroneous estimates, patients must be metabolically stable and unaffected by intercurrent diseases. Anthropometric measurements and subjective global assessment (SGA) may be of further help but are subjected to interobserver variability. Bioimpedance has been repeatedly proposed, but its reliability in PD patients has not been validated thus far.

TABLE 84.19. Formulas Used to Calculate Protein Nitrogen Appearance (PNA) in Peritoneal Dialysis Patients

Author, Years	Formula
Blumenkrantz MJ, 1985	6.25 × (0.93 × UNA + 5.47)
Teehan BP, 1985	6.25 × (UNA + 1.81 + 0.031 × BW)
Randerson DH, 1991	10.76 × (UNA × 0.69 + 1.46)
Bergstrom J, 1993	19 + (7.62 × UNA)

BW, body weight; UNA, urea nitrogen appearance that is the sum of the daily urea nitrogen amount eliminated in dialysate and urine.

In case of malnutrition, an accurate medical history is the first step, to rule out masticatory deficiency, diseases affecting the digestive tract, social causes opposing correct food intake, and possible side effects of medications. The second step is to verify that the dialysis dose is adequate, because protein nitrogen appearance, thus protein intake, is closely related to the amount of dialysis delivered up to Kt/V values of 2.0 to 2.2. Higher dosages of dialysis seem to be inefficacious in giving further increases in protein intake. The third step consists of assessing whether the uremic acidosis is adequately corrected by either dialysis alone or oral supplementation of alkali. Acidosis stimulates protein catabolism and inhibits protein synthesis. Protein supplementation is not effective in increasing the protein pool if there is acidosis; in such a situation the result would only be an increase in blood urea nitrogen. Finally, a diet analysis must be done, to evaluate if the protein intake is adequate. Diet counselling should also attempt to obtain a balance among the different nutrients. A protein intake of 1.0 to 1.2 g/kg body weight is generally recommended for adult patients, but many of them are unable to reach this target. Pediatric patients need more proteins to grow. Very old patients probably need less protein intake, but reliable data on this topic have not been provided.

The whole energy intake, too, has great influence on nutritional status because, if it is low, amino acids are metabolized to produce energy and are not available for protein synthesis. The recommended energy intake is approximately 35 kcal/kg of body weight and is the sum of the food intake and of the peritoneal absorption of dextrose. Doing exercise, avoiding constipation, and taking care of food tastes are useful ways to increase the energy intake. Moving the time of bag exchange to after the meal may prevent the first-hour glucose load that switches the appetite off.

When all these ways have been tried and failed, a nitrogen supplementation must be considered. Oral supplementation with proteins or amino acids is effective, but patient compliance can be low due to the large number of tablets to consume. There is, on the other hand, better compliance to the use of peritoneal dialysis solution containing 1.1 g/dl of amino acids. In a standard 2-L bag there are 22 g of amino acids, 60% to 80% of them are absorbed and give about 15 g of nitrogen compounds (i.e., more than 0.2 g/kg of body weight in a 70-kg patient). A possible side effect of this solution is acidosis, which can negate the wanted effect, but, if checked, can be corrected. Many patients improve their protein nutrition with one such bag per day; other patients may need two bags per day, but, in this case, much attention must be paid to both acidosis and blood urea nitrogen concentration. The amino acid solution should be used immediately after a meal, because an adequate energy intake will favor protein synthesis.

Peritonitis and other infectious and catabolic diseases and use of steroids need accurate monitoring of the nutritional status, not forgetting that their detrimental effects on nutrition can take long periods to fully disappear.

Dyslipidemia. The continuous glucose load in CAPD stimulates the secretion of insulin. Its consequent high peripheral serum concentration is one of the causes of the hypertriglyceridemia, which appears in 60% to 80% of CAPD patients. The rise in serum concentration of triglycerides is often seen after a few weeks or months on CAPD and is proportional to both the serum triglyceride concentration before CAPD and the daily glucose absorption from the dialysate. A rapid and major increase in serum triglyceride concentration may be the first sign of diabetes mellitus type II, previously undiagnosed and revealed by the continuous glucose load. Very-low-density lipoproteins (VLDL) are generally increased and apolipoprotein B has a major increase. Thus as in hemodialysis (HD), CAPD seems unable to correct the so-called uremic dyslipoproteinemia (e.g., hypertriglyceridemia and increased serum lipoproteins). A mild increase in serum cholesterol concentrations is often present with reduced concentration of high-density lipoprotein cholesterol (HDL-C) and apolipoprotein A (apoA) and increased concentrations of low-density lipoprotein cholesterol (LDL-C). Besides the glucose load, other factors are involved in the pathogenesis of uremic dyslipidemia: loss of apoA in the peritoneal effluent and a reduced activity of hepatic lipase and lipoprotein lipase, which lead to reduced removal of triglycerides. Furthermore, CAPD patients show higher concentrations of serum lipoprotein (a) than HD patients, a well-known risk factor for atherosclerotic disease. Serum triglycerides and cholesterol maximally increase during the first year of CAPD, and in many patients they subsequently decrease, reaching values not much different from those before the start of CAPD. This might depend on some kind of adaptation to the glucose load or to changes in diet.

All the lipid abnormalities on CAPD may play an atherogenic role. Actually, death from cardiovascular disease is not different on CAPD and HD, in spite of the lack, on CAPD, of the negative cardiovascular effects of HD: hyperkinetic circulation due to the arteriovenous fistula and repeating rapid changes in ECV, electrolyte concentrations, and acid–base status.

The correct patient diet should contain unsaturated fatty acids and very few saturated fatty acids. Foods rich in, or supplemented with, omega 3-polyunsatured fatty acids can be of some help in improving the lipid abnormalities. Attention must be paid to reduce the fluid intake in order to reduce the use of hypertonic bags, which cause greater dextrose load. Moreover, patients should stop drinking alcohol and should exercise regularly. In the case of failure of these measures, therapy with statins [inhibitors of the 3-hydroxy-3-methyl-glutaryl-coenzyme A (HMG-CoA) reductase] should be considered.

On the other hand, a spontaneous fall in the levels of triglycerides and cholesterol below the normal range may be one of the signs of malnutrition, and in HD patients low cholesterol level is associated with increased mortality. In these cases, a complete reevaluation of clinical status, adequacy of dialysis, and diet should be made, with adequate intervention.

Indications and Contraindications of Continuous Ambulatory Peritoneal Dialysis

Indications and contraindications of PD have been discussed in Chapter 84, Part 2B. Once PD treatment is selected, the next choice is the modality of PD, which can be based on the peritoneal compliance and permeability, as well as on the patient's clinical and social aspects.

The ambulatory characteristics of CAPD enable the patient to pursue his or her daily activities, but the upright position increases the intraabdominal pressure and consequently the risk of hernias, leakage, and hemorrhoids. It follows that an accurate evaluation of possible hernias and an estimation of the fluid capacity of the peritoneal cavity must be performed before catheter implantation. Wide peritoneal adhesions or large polycystic kidneys can reduce the peritoneal capacity so much that it makes the dialysis inadequate, once the residual renal function is lost. Patients with severe cardiac failure, who do not tolerate the rapid ECV changes of the hemodialysis treatment, take advantage of the electrolyte and extracellular volume stability on CAPD. Cirrhotic patients with severe liver failure who suffer from hypotension during the hemodialysis sessions often improve when treated with CAPD.

Another limit for PD may come from the peritoneal permeability. Patients with wide adhesions or high body size may not reach the targets of dialysis adequacy that are inversely proportional to the body weight and surface area. In these cases, the peritoneal equilibration test (PET), which studies the peritoneal transport pattern, helps to foresee whether that patient will be able to continue on CAPD once the residual renal function disappears. PET must be performed a few weeks (4 or 8, according to different authors) after catheter implantation, when, after the surgical operation, a steady state is reached.

Special Groups of Patients

Children

PD enables the treatment of uremic neonates in whom the preparation of a vascular access is difficult and extracorporeal treatment is not easy to perform. In infants, PD is the method of choice because it can be performed at home, without venipuncture, and with a better ECV, hence cardiovascular and electrolyte stability. It allows less dietary restrictions, which are not well tolerated by children. There are, however, contraindications to PD. Besides those in adults, in children they are often related to the small peritoneal cavity, urinary or intestinal diversion, prune-belly syndrome, or other diseases involving either the cavity or the wall of the abdomen. The volume of dialysis solution must be tailored to the body size and varies from 10 ml/kg of body weight in the first days, to 30 to 40 ml/kg of body weight when the break-in period has ended.

The introduction of APD has further increased the use of PD, and APD is now the preferred dialysis modality for children. It is performed at night, in order to leave a free day for school attendance and play, and to reduce the negative psychologic impact of the illness.

In children, much attention must be paid to the diet, which has to warrant an energy and protein intake per kg of body weight higher than in adults, for the growth. The problem of slower growth in uremic children, unsolved by PD alone, has received important support by the use of recombinant human growth hormone (rhGH), which gives excellent results on PD.

Failure of the peritoneal catheter is frequent in children, mainly due to the presence of a larger omentum that entraps the catheter. Omentectomy is, hence, recommended in all cases by some authors, or in the case of catheter failure by others. The incidence of infections, peritonitis, and exit-site infection is reported to be higher in children than in adults, but very often it has a favorable outcome.

When PD seems to be unable to ensure an adequate dialysis or when its complications are too frequent, the transfer to HD must be done without delay to avoid further negative effects on outcome and growth. Kidney transplant is the treatment of choice in children, and many data from the literature support the same graft and patient survival of those previously treated with PD as those on HD.

Elderly

Many factors influence the choice of the dialysis modality for elderly uremics and, among them, cardiovascular status is important. Old patients often suffer from cardiovascular senescence and acquired cardiopathies, with myocardiosclerosis, atherosclerosis, and/or ischemic coronary disease. They may have diastolic and, sometimes, systolic dysfunction, arrhythmias, angina and myocardial infarction, and impaired sympathetic response to fluid removal and orthostasis. In these patients, the hyperkinetic circulation induced by the arteriovenous fistula is usually badly tolerated. Moreover, the rapid changes in ECV, in serum electrolyte concentration, and in acid–base status (characteristic of HD) frequently cause intradialytic hypotension and postdialytic arrhythmias. All considered, in the elderly in the presence of cardiomyopathy, a smooth, continuous therapy such as CAPD is preferable to HD.

On the other hand, protein malnutrition is more frequent in the elderly, and the protein intake might be insufficient to the metabolic needs in a situation of protein and amino acid peritoneal loss. The peritoneal glucose load might reduce the already decreased tolerance to carbohydrates, which is typical of the elderly. Moreover, the risk of peritonitis and exit-site infection might increase, due to the increased susceptibility to infection in the elderly. Finally, decreased muscle mass and tone might increase the risk of hernias.

Home therapy presents with some difficulties in many elderly due to visual or handling impairment and to psychic depression, and often they require the help of a relative to perform CAPD. However, the evolving changes in social customs, even in countries with traditionally strong family solidarity, have progressively reduced the availability of a family helper. When elderly people are admitted to nursing homes, the role of the family partner may be substituted by trained nurses, who may find PD easier to perform than HD.

Elderly survival has not been found to be significantly different in CAPD and HD patients in many single-center and multicenter studies. Some national registries, such as the United States Renal Data System (USRDS), have found a reduced life expectancy on CAPD, others (Canadian Registry) have found the opposite. The differences might depend on the different experiences with either modality, on number or quality of risk factors taken into account, on different criteria or time period of patient enrollment, and on statistic analysis incident versus prevalent patient or "intention to treat" versus historic analysis. Moreover, some socioeconomic aspects might play a role: public or private health service, family and social solidarity, kind of reimbursement of the treatment, and use of drugs (e.g., EPO).

Dropout from CAPD is less frequent in elderly patients than in young patients, because often they do not live long enough to experience loss of peritoneal permeability and other complications, and they less easily accept a change in dialysis modality.

Patients with Congestive Heart Failure

Congestive heart failure refractory to diuretics can be a rational indication for CAPD or APD. In these patients, dialysis must often be started earlier, and sometimes much earlier than usual, in order to control the volume overload no longer possible pharmacologically, and PD is preferable to HD for its better cardiovascular stability.

Patients with very low-ejection fractions and who are waiting for heart transplantation may benefit from this method for some time. In the first weeks or months, one or two bags per day can be sufficient. Ultrafiltration should be performed preferably during the night when the reabsorption of edema, favored by the recumbent position, may worsen fluid overload. With increases in time, however, patients undergo a progressive, irreversible reduction of the residual renal function, which forces an elevation in the number of bags exchanged per day.

Diabetics

The percentage of patients suffering from diabetic nephropathy varies, in different countries, from 15% to 35% of the patients accepted for chronic renal replacement therapy and is higher in Northern Europe and the United States. Diabetic nephropathy is the main cause of end-stage renal disease (ESRD) in North America and the second in Europe, Japan, Australia, and New Zealand. Thus any dialysis modality must be prepared to treat this group of patients.

Many of the complications of diabetes may take advantage from CAPD. Cardiomyopathy and orthostatic hypotension related to autonomic neuropathy may all benefit from the continuity of CAPD. Retinopathy can be favored by the lack of anticoagulation. Serum potassium concentrations and acid–base status are continuously corrected. The gastrointestinal effects of autonomic dysfunction, which can lead to malnutrition, can take advantage from the peritoneal glucose absorption. On the other hand, the continuous glucose load can impair glycemic control, and hyperlipemia can accelerate atherosclerosis and negatively affect both peripheral and cerebral vasculopathy.

Attempts to change the osmotic agents in PD has not brought about a satisfactory solution thus far. Glycerol-containing solutions have been used. They allow a better control of glycemia, but the ultrafiltration volume is lower due to the lower molecular weight of glycerol, and the caloric load is similar to that of glucose. The use of different osmotic agents, such as amino acids or polyglucose, is possible for only one bag a day, because amino acids favor acidosis and polyglucose hyperosmolality. However, the latter can improve metabolic control by reducing the need for hypertonic dextrose solutions.

The possibility to introduce insulin into the peritoneal cavity was the main factor that brought about the widest use of CAPD in diabetics during the 1980s. The entry of insulin into the portal circulation, the decrease of peripheral insulin concentration with positive effects on the lipid profile, and the administration of insulin simultaneously to the peritoneal load of dextrose were claimed as factors favoring the metabolic control of diabetes. Thus far no data give evidence that these metabolic advantages bring real clinical benefits, and the peritoneal way of insulin administration has been abandoned by several centers due to its increased risk of causing peritonitis. Moreover, a few patients show the so-called malignant omentum syndrome characterized by entrapment of insulin in the omentum, with inefficacy of even high doses of intraperitoneal insulin in obtaining glycemic control. Finally, subcapsular liver steatosis has been found only in CAPD diabetics treated with intraperitoneal insulin.

All outcome studies have shown that diabetics have higher mortality and higher morbidity than nondiabetics, irrespective of the dialysis modality. On the contrary, there is no full agreement on the comparative efficacy of CAPD and HD on patient and technique survival at different ages. The different results might depend on many factors, including patient selection and dialysis adequacy. Attempts to adjust for such differences with statistic analyses may fail because of limitations linked to the methodology used or the number of patients, thus the casualties observed, the insufficient or different evaluation of risk factors, and the length of follow-up.

The infectious complications of PD (e.g., peritonitis and exit-site infections) have similar incidences in diabetics and nondiabetics, therefore the highest hospitalization rates of diabetics depend on the complications of diabetes itself. When infectious complications occur, glycemic control may become difficult, especially during peritonitis in which peritoneal inflammation increases the rate and quantity of glucose absorbed.

Today there is no clear indication for the dialysis modality in diabetics. Often the choice seems influenced more by the contraindications than by specific indications for each modality. Therefore diabetics with cardiovascular instability or with vascular-access problems are addressed by CAPD, whereas those with poor metabolic control and hyperlipemia are addressed by HD. Other factors that can affect the choice of the modality are the ability to perform self-dialysis, the presence or the absence of visual and handling impairment, the availability of a partner, the distance from the facility, and patient compliance. The benefit of early dialysis in diabetics, mainly with peritoneal dialysis, which preserves residual renal function for a longer time than HD, has been asserted but not clearly demonstrated and defined.

CAPD has shorter technique survival than HD in all patients and this is true also in diabetics, and one must be ready to change modality when PD complications do not allow for safe treatment, without wasting precious time.

Selected Readings

Advisory Committee on Peritonitis Management of the International Society for Peritoneal Dialysis. Peritoneal dialysis-related peritonitis treatment recommendations: 1996 update. *Perit Dial Int* 1996;16:557–573.

Diagnosis, treatment, and course of peritonitis during peritoneal dialysis are clearly discussed and shown in useful flow charts.

Canada-USA (CANUSA) Peritoneal Dialysis Study Group. Adequacy of dialysis and nutrition in continuous peritoneal dialysis: association with clinical outcomes. *J Am Soc Nephrol* 1996;7:198–207.

Multicenter prospective study analyzing the relationship between dialysis dose and mortality and morbidity. Although it analyzes only new patients with residual renal function, and for a short period, its conclusions appear to be correct because they have been confirmed by other papers.

Gokal R, Alexander S, Ash S, et al. Peritoneal catheters and exit-site practices toward optimum peritoneal access: 1998 update.

Evidence-based guidelines and consensus-based recommendations on the following topics about the peritoneal dialysis catheter: choice, insertion, postoperative care, chronic exit-site care, and diagnosis and treatment of exit-site and tunnel infections.

Gokal R, Khanna R, Krediet R, et al. *Textbook of peritoneal dialysis*, 2nd ed. Dordrecht, The Netherlands: Kluwer Academic Publishers, 2000.

Many authors, leaders in the field of peritoneal dialysis, have contributed to this book that analyzes in depth all the aspects, both technical and clinical, of peritoneal dialysis.

Maiorca R, Brunori G, Zubani R, et al. Predictive value of dialysis adequacy and nutritional indices for mortality and morbidity in CAPD and HD patients. A longitudinal study. *Nephrol Dial Transplant* 1995;10(12):2295–2305.

A single-center, prospective study comparing dialysis dose in hemodialysis and peritoneal dialysis and its effect on patient outcome. Its results suggest that a target of as much as 1.96 of urea Kt/V a week must be reached.

National Kidney Foundation–Dialysis Outcomes Quality Initiative (NKF-DOQI). Clinical practice guidelines for peritoneal dialysis adequacy. New York: National Kidney Foundation, 1997.

This book contains practice guidelines about initiation of dialysis, measurement of peritoneal dialysis dose, assessment of nutritional status, adequacy of dialysis dose, and indications and contraindications for peritoneal dialysis. A wide list of references enables the reader to find easily papers that have analyzed specific topics in depth.

D. Automated Peritoneal Dialysis

Jose A. Diaz-Buxo

The term *automated peritoneal dialysis (APD)* is used to describe all modalities of peritoneal dialysis (PD) that use a mechanical device to automatically perform the procedure. Attempts at automating the PD procedure date back to the 1960s, when Tenckhoff used large containers of dialysis solution and mechanical devices to provide infusion of dialytic solution by gravity, clocks to control the duration of the cycle phases, and mechanical occluders to direct solution flow. APD offers several advantages: (a) minimal patient involvement, making nocturnal dialysis possible and freeing the patient during the day; (b) convenient for children and disabled patients in need of partner assistance; (c) makes possible the use of large volumes of solution for high-flow dialysis; (d) reduces the cost of solutions by using larger-volume containers; and (e) helped control the high incidence of peritonitis initially experienced with manual PD.

The current cyclers are designed to deliver a specific volume of dialysis solution into the peritoneal cavity and allowed to dwell for a predetermined length of time, followed by drainage of the effluent. Modern cyclers are very simple and reliable. The typical procedures consist of connecting the peritoneal catheter to the device line, entering the prescription into a computerized program, and activating the cycler. The program contains the specified number of cycles, volume of infusion, length of dwell and drainage, type of solution to be used, and a variety of safety parameters. Once activated, the cycler effects the exchanges automatically and continuously monitors the procedure. At the end of the session, the patient manually disconnects from the cycler and is free from any mechanical devices or procedures until the next session.

Approximately 33,000 patients in the United States and 110,000 patients worldwide undergo peritoneal dialysis. During the past several years, APD use has shown a significant increment, with more than 40% estimated to use some modality of APD in the United States. This positive trend is likely due to the realization that higher doses of delivered therapy are necessary for larger patients and those without residual renal function (RRF).

KINETIC AND PHYSICAL CONSIDERATIONS

Three techniques of PD exist as defined by their flow patterns: intermittent, tidal, and continuous. For intermittent flow, a specific volume of solution is instilled into the peritoneal cavity, allowed to dwell, and followed by complete drainage of the solution (Fig. 84.36A). Examples of the intermittent technique are intermittent PD (IPD), nocturnal intermittent PD (NIPD), continuous ambulatory PD (CAPD), continuous cyclic PD (CCPD), and PD Plus (which uses a single catheter).

In tidal flow, a specific volume of solution is instilled into the peritoneal cavity and allowed to dwell, followed by alternative drainage of a fraction of the solution and infusion of a similar volume. Total drainage is performed at the end of the procedure (Fig. 84.36B). A single catheter is used.

During continuous flow, a specific volume of solution is instilled into the peritoneal cavity followed by a continuous

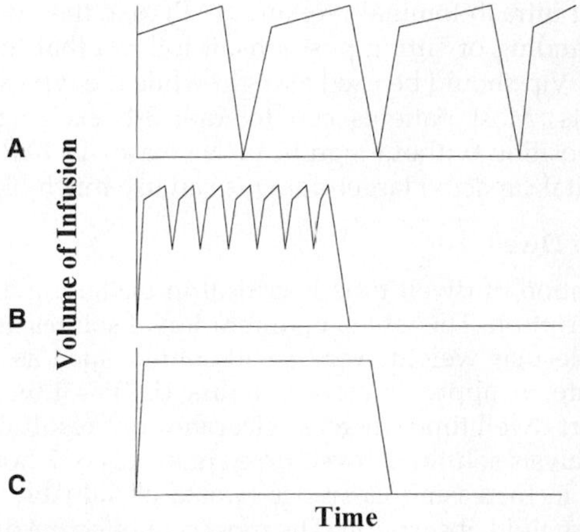

Figure 84.36. Techniques of peritoneal dialysis: (**A**) intermittent, (**B**) tidal, and (**C**) continuous flow. See text for discussion.

inflow that is matched by a continuous outflow of dialysate over a specific period of time using two catheters. At the end of the procedure, the peritoneal cavity is completely drained (Fig. 84.36C).

All three techniques have been applied to modalities of APD. Each modality uses a different combination of cycle dwell time, infusion volume, dialysate flow rate, and total dialysate volume. In addition, some modalities are used mostly at night with the patient supine, others occur during the day when the patient is ambulatory, and most are used continuously. These variations affect the efficiency of the therapy, both in terms of solute removal and ultrafiltration. Thus it is important to understand the effect of each of these variables on clearance and ultrafiltration in order to optimize therapy according to the patients' needs and to take full advantage of the flexibility offered by APD.

Dialysate Flow Rate

An increase in dialysate flow rate (DFR) is a most effective way to increase the clearance of small solutes. In practice this is accomplished by performing frequent, short-lasting exchanges. Solute transport is accelerated by maximizing the concentration gradient between plasma and dialysate (diffusion) and by increasing ultrafiltration (i.e., convective transport). However, high DFR has the disadvantages of being costly and inefficient at very high flows due to limitations in solution flow using intermittent techniques. In other words, when the DFR exceeds approximately 2 L/hr, the solution transit time, or nondialytic time, increases to the point of becoming inefficient.

Exchange Volume

An optimal exchange volume (Vip) is the most critical and efficient manner of enhancing PD therapy. A strong relationship exists between mass transfer area coefficient (MTAC) and Vip. This correlation remains linear over a wide range of Vip, but is affected by patient size. It was found that the Vip associated with peak MTAC increased with increasing body surface area (BSA). The mechanisms by which Vip may increase efficiency of PD are the increase in solute concentration gradient between plasma and dialysate (D/P) and a possible increase in effective membrane surface area.

Patient Position

Using the same Vip, the MTAC in the supine position has been shown to be significantly higher than in the ambulatory, upright position. This finding is consistent with previous observations suggesting an increase in effective peritoneal surface area in the supine position, higher urea and creatinine clearances, and higher portal blood flows in the supine position. Because a higher Vip is better tolerated in the supine position by generating lower intraabdominal pressure (IAP) than the same volume in the standing or sitting positions, it follows that the highest-tolerated Vip should be used at night while the typical APD patient rests. Most patients can tolerate 3-L exchanges in the supine position without significant increases in IAP or reduction in vital capacity; larger patients can use much higher Vips.

Length of Dwell

Optimization of dwell time is critical in designing an efficient PD prescription. The rate of equilibration of solutes depends on their molecular weight. Very small solutes such as urea fully equilibrate in approximately 4 hours (D/P = 1.0). Therefore very short dwell times increase clearance but result in waste of costly dialysis solution. Dwell times in excess of 7 hours are ineffective in increasing clearance (waste of valuable time) and may cause fluid absorption. The most cost-effective dwell times are in the range of 4 to 6 hours.

Catheter Flow Rate

Good catheter function affects the efficiency of PD by reducing the solution transit time or nondialytic time. Under conditions of low DFR, such as CAPD or APD with few exchanges, the effect is minimal because the ratio of transit time to total dialysis time (24 hours) is very low. However, as DFR increases the catheter flow rate becomes critical.

Increasing DFR and shortening dwell time mostly affect the clearance of solutes with relatively low molecular weight such as urea and creatinine. These maneuvers do not have much influence on the removal of so-called middle molecules, whose clearance is mostly dependent on time and peritoneal surface area. Therefore using continuous modalities and larger Vip increase clearance of larger molecules. Finally, larger solute removal is also favored by convective transport (high ultrafiltration). Large proteins are mostly transported by convection as evidenced by increased protein losses with the use of more hypertonic solutions. The relative roles of small-solute and middle-molecule clearance in preventing uremic complications remain controversial. However, a good correlation between urea kinetic parameters and clinical outcome has been reported among patients undergoing PD with and without RRF.

Peritoneal Transport Rate

Peritoneal transport rates (PTRs) have been classified according to the rate of equilibration of small solutes between plasma and dialysate (D/P) or the rate of glucose absorption from the peritoneal solution (D/D_0) (the ratio of glucose concentration in dialysate at 4 hours to the concentration of glucose in dialysate immediately after infusion). For practical purposes, we will use Twardowski's initial classification.

High transporters can attain better clearances with CAPD due to their faster solute equilibration; however, they are less likely to achieve adequate ultrafiltration. The use of more frequent, shorter exchanges characteristic of intermittent APD modalities may achieve acceptable clearances and ultrafiltration in these patients.

APD Modalities

IPD/NIPD

The intermittent modalities of PD can be performed daily (NIPD) or several times weekly (IPD). The typical prescription uses short and frequent automated exchanges, usually lasting 30 to 60 minutes. Total therapy time is 8 to 12 hours. The procedure is otherwise similar to CCPD, but the peritoneal cavity is maintained dry during the day. The total dialytic time is significantly shorter than with continuous therapies and therefore solute clearance diminishes as the solute molecular weight increases.

CCPD. CCPD is based on the same principles as CAPD but is provided in an automated manner with the assistance of a cycler. CCPD can be considered a virtual day–night reversal of the CAPD technique, with all the short exchanges occurring at night and the prolonged exchange during the day. The preparation of the equipment and the connection between the permanent peritoneal catheter and the cycler line take place just before the patient retires at night. After the last dialysate infusion in the morning, the catheter can be disconnected and capped in a sterile environment. Otherwise, the catheter can be clamped with a disposable device that provides complete and irreversible occlusion of the cycler line, and thereafter the line can be cut with unsterile scissors. The latter procedure can be performed by practically every patient and saves time and the cost of sterile supplies.

The typical adult prescription consists of three to five nocturnal cycles lasting 2 to 3 hours each, a dialysate volume of 2 to 3 L, and dialysate glucose concentrations between 1.5% and 4.25%. The cycler is programmed to deliver the final or diurnal cycle after the last nocturnal cycle using hypertonic dialysate and a volume of 1.5 to 2.0 L as tolerated by the patient.

Modifications in the volume of the dialysate exchange are necessary in children. Children generally require four to six nocturnal cycles over a 10-hour period and a diurnal cycle using volumes of 1.2 L/m^2. The specific volume of the exchange must be individualized according to tolerance.

The automated nature of the procedure allows great flexibility in terms of dialysate flow and ability to manipulate dialysate volume and dwell time. A significant number of pediatric patients and most infants undergoing dialysis are actually on CCPD. Other groups that have benefited from this therapy are patients unable to effect manual exchanges because of visual or neuromuscular impairment, those patients unwilling or unable to interrupt their daytime schedule for dialysate exchanges, patients requiring reductions in dialysate exchange volume during the day due to complications arising from increased intraabdominal pressure, and patients requiring increased small molecular solute clearance.

Hybrid Forms of CAPD/CCPD (PD Plus)

In an attempt to enhance clearances and provide adequate doses of PD to large anuric patients, new forms of therapy combining automated cycles and manual diurnal cycles have been developed. These modalities incorporate all the aforementioned principles to improve solute removal. PD Plus uses a simple cycler capable of handling up to 18 L of dialysis solution. The simplified cycler functions are to (a) provide a limited number of automated cycles (4 to 6); (b) allow selection of a "last bag option"; (c) make possible a manual fill from the system during the day (pause exchange); (d) warm the solutions to body temperature; and (e) automatically drain the effluent. This system uses large containers of dialysis solution (5 L), thus reducing the total cost of therapy. Because most exchanges occur at night, the Vip can be increased when the patient is supine. An additional manual diurnal exchange increases efficiency, improves ultrafiltration and results in the use of less hypertonic glucose solutions. This therapy offers prescription flexibility and maintains a steady concentration of solutes and continuous ultrafiltration.

The main disadvantage of PD Plus is the need for a manual exchange during the day. However, this single exchange is much less time consuming than the four manual exchanges characteristic of CAPD. A variation of PD Plus is the use of CAPD with the addition of a single automated exchange at night, using a cycler with limited capabilities. Although this system is more efficient than CAPD, it still requires significant patient involvement with multiple diurnal exchanges and the use of a mechanical device at night.

The current goals of PD adequacy are to provide a weekly Kt/V in excess of 2.0 and/or a creatinine clearance (K_{Cr}) of 60 L/1.73 m^2 or more. Large patients with minimal RRF are unable to achieve these goals with CAPD. However, more than 90% of anuric patients are expected to achieve the Kt/V goal and 70% can attain the K_{Cr} guideline with PD Plus using 15 L/day.

Tidal Peritoneal Dialysis

Tidal peritoneal dialysis (TPD) consists of maintaining a reserve volume of dialysate that remains constant in the peritoneal cavity and a tidal volume that continuously flows into and out of the peritoneal cavity. TPD requires a cycler that is volume rather than time controlled. The rationale for this technique is the potential improvement in clearances through better mixing of dialysate and reduction of the stagnant dialysate films along the peritoneal membrane. The superiority of this technology remains controversial at best and the high dialysate flows and increase in cost associated with this technique have hindered its growth. Several clinical experiences have failed to show better clearances of small solutes when compared with NIPD if Vip, DFRs, and total dialysate volume are controlled. The higher cost associated with larger volumes of solution is difficult to justify in the absence of conclusive evidence of superior clearances.

Continuous Flow Peritoneal Dialysis

In the 1960s, a new PD technique (recirculation PD) was introduced. Two PD catheters were used to provide a continuous flow of dialysate. The peritoneal cavity was filled with fresh solution to a predetermined Vip. Thereafter, a continuous flow of 100 to 200 ml/min was maintained using regenerated effluent. The effluent was regenerated using a conventional hemodialysis system with twin-coil dialyzers. The efficiencies of this continuous flow peritoneal dialysis (CFPD)-recirculation system were compared with IPD in controlled clinical studies. Clearances of urea, creatinine, and urate during CFPD were directly related to DFR. At rapid DFR they doubled or tripled over those observed with IPD. The improved clearances obtained with this system are probably related to (a) high DFR; (b) maintenance of a large Vip; and (c) reduction of stagnant layers of dialysate in contact with the peritoneal membrane due to the turbulence created by high flows of dialysate. More recent experiments in normal dogs, using CFPD, IPD, and TPD have also shown that CFPD can provide significantly higher urea clearances in the range of 32 ml/min when the DFR is kept at 6 L/hr. These results suggest that practically all patients, regardless of size or renal function, could achieve the suggested adequacy goals with CFPD. Furthermore, such therapy could improve the quality of life of many patients by reducing the present cycling time required by other modalities of APD. In addition, the constant flow of fresh dialysate will maintain a high osmotic gradient, augmenting ultrafiltration and allowing the use of lower glucose concentration in the solution.

The major disadvantage of CFPD is the need for very large volumes of solution and their associated cost. Several potential solutions to this problem are being explored. The on-line production of sterile dialysis solution by means of reverse osmosis–treated water and a proportioning system to mix dialysate concentrate and water has been used in the past. Those systems are relatively complex, require much maintenance, and are costly. Another solution is regeneration of spent peritoneal dialysate by means of a sorbent cartridge or the use of hemofilters. The latter has the additional advantage of providing flexibility of dialysis solution formulation because the bicarbonate, calcium, and sodium concentrations can be varied by the hemodialysis equipment. A third possibility is the reuse of spent peritoneal dialysate. Because the uremic solute concentration is very low after a single pass through the peritoneal cavity using very high DFRs, the peritoneal effluent could be effectively used a second or third time using a simple, inexpensive cycling device. However, the efficiency of the process diminishes as the concentration of uremic toxins increases in the dialysate. Another disadvantage of CFPD is the need for two peritoneal catheters or a single catheter with a double lumen. The two internal lumens should maintain considerable separation to avoid recirculation of dialysate. Such catheters are not readily available, but should not constitute a significant barrier to the development of CFPD. Further clinical investigation is needed to confirm the apparent benefits of this regimen.

MODALITY SELECTION

The success of any dialytic therapy depends on matching the prescription to the individual patient's metabolic needs and selecting a modality that provides a good quality of life. Compromises are often necessary in order to satisfy the patient's preference, but we must always keep in mind that quality of life frequently depends on physical health. Therefore every effort should be made to provide adequate therapy.

The use of algorithms and computerized kinetic modeling programs can facilitate the formulation of the PD prescription and the feasibility of using a certain modality of therapy. The basic determinants of dose are: patient size, RRF, and PTRs. With these three pieces of information, a prescription can be formulated to achieve the adequacy goals.

The patient's lifestyle, preferences, and phobias must be considered in therapy selection. In many cases, it is possible to achieve the therapeutic goals with various modalities, thus allowing patient satisfaction and adequate dose. It is also imperative to assess the patient's ability to perform self-therapy and to identify a committed relative or helper if assistance with procedures is necessary. Based on these considerations the following selection guidelines can be offered for the three clinically available modalities of APD.

NIPD

NIPD should be mostly reserved for patients with high-transport peritoneal characteristics who can achieve adequate ultrafiltration and clearances with this therapy, but are unable to ultrafilter with continuous APD. Because of the intermittent nature of this therapy, the adequacy goals for NIPD should be adjusted to a weekly Kt/V in excess of 2.2 and a K_{Cr} in excess of 60 L. Occasionally, elderly patients with low body mass or RRF who are dependent on partners for their dialytic procedures may also benefit from NIPD.

CCPD

CCPD has the advantages of providing continuous dialysis, with limited demands on the patient or partner and schedule flexibility. The maximum tolerated Vips are recommended for the nightly cycles. Lower volumes can be used during the day, especially in patients suffering from complications related to high IAP, such as low back pain, gastroesophageal reflux, herniae, and uterine prolapse. CCPD allows total freedom from procedures during the day for work or recreation. Most children can enjoy adequate dialysis administered by parents or guardians with minimal effort. The most frequent reason for CCPD selection among diabetic patients has been blindness or neuromuscular disability requiring the assistance of a partner. With the use of the simple disconnection procedure, most of these patients require assistance only in the evening for initial connection to the cycler. In addition, the incidence of peritonitis associated with CCPD is among the lowest reported with any modality of PD. CCPD is particularly effective among patients with low-average transport who may benefit from the higher Vip during the night and fair ultrafiltration during the long diurnal cycle.

PD Plus

The main indication of PD Plus and other hybrid PD modalities is in the treatment of large anuric patients. The prescription can be modified to accommodate most patients' ultrafiltration and dialytic needs. The relative uniformity of dwell times allows steady ultrafiltration and solute removal, important in the treatment of unstable cardiovascular patients and diabetics using intraperitoneal insulin.

COMPLICATIONS OF APD

The complications of APD are essentially the same as those of CAPD. Therefore only those complications characteristic of these modalities of therapy or those with a significantly different incidence are discussed in this section.

Peritonitis remains the most frequent complication of APD, yet the incidence of peritonitis in APD patients has been significantly lower than that observed for CAPD, especially in the adult population. Table 84.20 summarizes the incidence of peritonitis for adults in various centers with CAPD and CCPD using the standard spike technique and the newer Y sets. CCPD and Y sets have invariably shown some of the lowest rates of peritonitis.

Several characteristics of APD may explain the reduced rate of peritonitis. The fact that all connections for CCPD, NIPD, and TPD take place only once per day in the home may allow better aseptic control, improved concentration, the possible use of a partner, and less stress on the patient and the partner. The number of actual connections can be reduced by using larger-volume dialysate containers, thus minimizing the potential risk of intraluminal contamination. Dialysate outflow following a connection may play an important role in lowering the rate of peritonitis by reducing the concentration of bacteria at the connecting site. The extremely low rate of peritonitis obtained with double-bag CAPD systems that use a flow sequence similar to that of CCPD suggests that flushing the connecting site may help reduce peritonitis. Finally, it is possible that the long diurnal dwell of CCPD and the "dry day" of NIPD improve peritoneal host–immune defenses by allowing repopulation of the peritoneal resident macrophages. We have observed peritoneal cell counts as high as 200 cells/mm^3 at the end of the diurnal cycle of CCPD, compared with counts consistently lower than 50 cells/mm^3 at the end of a 3-hour dialysate dwell. Prolongation of dwell time has also been shown to enhance macrophage function as well as effluent opsonic activity, thereby providing improved host defense.

Aside from the lower rate of peritonitis, recent reports have also shown a lower rate of catheter exit-site infection with CCPD. CAPD patients using the spike system have the highest rates of catheter infections at 1.2 episodes per year, followed by CAPD patients using the Y set at 0.8 episodes per year, whereas CCPD patients have the lowest rates at 0.5 episodes/year. It has been suggested that reduced catheter exit-site trauma from disconnect systems such as CCPD and Y-set CAPD lower catheter exit-site infection rates.

Other catheter-related complications are also common to both CAPD and CCPD. Early pericatheter leaks are mostly influenced by surgical catheter placement techniques or nutritional state. However, disconnect techniques should somewhat

TABLE 84.20. Incidence of Peritonitis for Adult Patients in Various Series

Reference[a]	CCPD	CAPD (spike) Episodes/Year	CAPD (Y set)
Diaz-Buxo, et al.	0.48	1.41	ND
Rottenbourg, et al.	0.50	1.03	0.52
de Fijter, et al.	0.60	ND	1.20
Holley, et al.	0.30	1.30	0.50

[a] For specific references see Diaz-Buxo JA. Is continuous ambulatory peritoneal dialysis adequate long term therapy for end-stage renal disease? A critical assessment. *J Am Soc Nephrol* 1992;3:1039–1048.

CAPD, continuous ambulatory peritoneal dialysis; CCPD, continuous cyclic peritoneal dialysis; ND, no data reported.

reduce these complications by reducing the amount of trauma to the catheter and allowing better healing. Catheter obstruction is more common with IPD, probably because of the accumulation of fibrin strands in the peritoneal cavity during the interdialytic period. One-way obstruction (ball-valve effect) is also more frequent with IPD than with continuous PD (CPD). We have not seen a difference in catheter-related complications between CAPD and CCPD.

Abdominal and inguinal hernias have become a relatively common complication of CPD, affecting as many as 30% of patients on CAPD. In our experience with CCPD, 9% of the patients develop hernias and 15% develop late pericatheter fluid leaks during the first 2 years of observation. Because both of these complications are most likely due to increased abdominal pressure during the day, we have opted for reduction of the diurnal dialysate volume to 20 ml/kg body weight. The incidence of hernias is now 2%, a figure comparable with our previous experience with IPD.

TREATMENT OF DIABETIC PATIENTS

Diabetics make up approximately 34% of the end-stage renal dialysis population in the United States. Insulin-dependent patients can be instructed in intraperitoneal insulin administration and regular blood sugar determinations using a glucometer. The gradual transition from subcutaneous insulin injection to intraperitoneal administration should be monitored closely while the patient is in the hospital and during the training period. In our experience, most patients have required two to three times the total dose previously administered subcutaneously for good control of glycemia. Most patients use 50% of the dosage for the long diurnal cycles and 50% equally divided among the dialysate containers used for nocturnal cycles. There is significant interpatient variation in these requirements; therefore regular blood sugar determinations are mandatory while the precise insulin prescription is being determined.

Although intraperitoneal administration of insulin is convenient and perhaps more physiologic than subcutaneous administration, the use of subcutaneous insulin injections with multiple dosage or with the use of an insulin pump have shown equally satisfactory control of glycemia. There are potential advantages and disadvantages for both methods of insulin administration, and no consensus of opinion has been achieved regarding the best methodology. For additional discussion of the use of intraperitoneal insulin in diabetic patients treated with PD, the reader is referred to Chapter 84, Part 2C.

The demands for higher PD dosages dictated by clinical experience and theoretic constructs during recent years, the larger number of patients on long-term therapy who have lost all renal function, and the increasing number of patients with comorbid conditions have resulted in a higher use of APD and have stimulated the search for more effective PD therapy. Advances in electronics, computer science, biomaterials, and membrane technology will likely allow the use of more efficient modalities of PD, such as CFPD, in the not-too-distant future. This technology will likely provide the means to use more physiologic solutions associated with lower complications and a lower cost of therapy. Although peritonitis remains an important complication of PD in general, its incidence has diminished significantly during the last decade. APD is partially responsible for this improvement. The greatest challenge for future investigation is the prolongation of peritoneal membrane function and the provision of therapy that is simple and convenient enough to improve patient compliance. APD promises to help fulfill these requirements.

Selected Readings

de Fijter CWH, Verbrugh HA, Oe LP, et al. Peritoneal defense in continuous ambulatory versus continuous cyclic peritoneal dialysis. *Kidney Int* 1992;42: 947–950.

Preliminary results of an ongoing, prospective, randomized study comparing CAPD Y sets with CCPD on incidence of peritonitis and peritoneal host defense.

Diaz-Buxo JA. CCPD is even better than CAPD. *Kidney Int* 1985;28:S26–S28.

Description of the kinetics of CCPD, summarizing the clinical experiences with a large patient population and comparing the significant differences between CCPD and CAPD.

Diaz-Buxo JA. Current status of continuous cyclic peritoneal dialysis (CCPD) [Editorial]. *Kidney Int* 1989;9:9–14.

Clinical experience with CCPD, modifications of the technique, and recent developments.

Diaz-Buxo, JA. Enhancement of peritoneal dialysis: the PD Plus concept. *Am J Kidney Dis* 1996;27:92–98.

Discussion of the principles for enhancement of PD therapy and their practical applications.

Holley JL, Bernardini J, Piraino B. Continuous cycling peritoneal dialysis is associated with lower rates of catheter infections than continuous ambulatory peritoneal dialysis. *Am J Kidney Dis* 1990;16:133–136.

Compares the rates of catheter-related infection in CAPD and CCPD patients.

Keshaviah P, Emerson PF, Vonesh EF, et al. Relationship between body size, fill volume, and mass transfer area coefficient in peritoneal dialysis. *J Am Soc Nephrol* 1994;4:1820–1826.

Describes the relationship between BSA, Vip, and MTCA in PD.

Twardowski ZJ, Prowant BF, Nolph KD, et al. High volume, low frequency, continuous ambulatory peritoneal dialysis. *Kidney Int* 1983;23:64–70.

A report illustrating the effects of peritoneal dialysate volume on intraabdominal pressure and multiple cardiopulmonary parameters. The information is valuable when considering selection of different peritoneal dialysis regimens for specific patients.

Warady BA, Alexander S, Hossli S, et al. The relationship between intraperitoneal volume and solute transport in pediatric patients. *J Am Soc Nephrol* 1995;5: 1935–1939.

Multicenter study to determine the relationship between intraperitoneal volume and solute transport in children.

E: Morbidity and Mortality

John Moran and Edward Vonesh

The major reason for an interest in the mortality and morbidity associated with peritoneal dialysis (PD) is to allow the nephrologist to advise new dialysis patients about the better therapy modality for them to commence. Thus one is asking an "intent-to-treat" question: "What is the best initial dialysis modality for this patient that will produce the best long-term outcome?" The difficulties in answering this question are manifold.

First, there are no randomized, prospective studies comparing outcomes in hemodialysis (HD) and PD, and it is highly unlikely that there ever will be. The two major modalities—center HD and home PD—are so dissimilar that most patients will select one or the other for "nonmedical" reasons, such as fear of performing their own therapy, unwillingness to travel to the center for treatment three times per week, and so forth, and thus refuse to enter a randomized study.

Many other factors bedevil any discussion of morbidity and mortality in PD and comparisons with HD. The most important of these is that the standard of care in both modalities is constantly changing and outstripping data collection. Examples of such changes include the recognition of the importance of adequacy of therapy (which in HD, preceded by some years that in PD), the introduction of erythropoietin, the use of biocompatible membranes in HD, the widespread use of high-efficiency, short-duration HD, the introduction of twin-bag disconnect systems for continuous ambulatory peritoneal dialysis (CAPD), the rapidly increasing proportion of PD patients using continuous cycling peritoneal dialysis (CCPD), and the recognition of the importance of residual renal function (RRF) in achieving adequate clearances in PD. Changes in the patient population, with ever-increasing numbers of patients with diabetes and other comorbid conditions that increase morbidity and mortality, and an increasing number of elderly patients further complicate the application of even the most recently published literature to current practice.

An important factor to be considered when examining the morbidity and mortality in PD is the *center effect*. There are many centers throughout the world that use PD only for patients who are unsuitable for HD or have "failed" HD, usually because of vascular access problems. These centers will have only a small number of PD patients and will not develop either the experience or the infrastructure for optimum results with PD. Furthermore, in many countries a high percentage of patients are on PD because of a limitation of HD facilities or funding. One therefore must not assume that because these countries have a wide experience with PD that they are getting the best possible results with the modality.

Two types of studies in the literature attempt to look at outcomes in dialysis. One is of large registries, either national or regional. The other is based on review of patients from one or, at most, a few centers. Most of these latter studies suffer from short follow-up and limited patient numbers, and hence poor statistic power. They are usually retrospective studies and are never randomized. Because of these limitations, only one well-documented series is discussed here, that from the Brescia group (Italy). This group has published a detailed series of papers outlining their changing practices in both PD and HD and comparing the results obtained with each modality. The mortality of patients commencing either PD or HD in this center between 1991 and 1996 was identical, with a 36% 5-year survival rate. Analysis of baseline comorbidities showed the groups to be similar in the two groups. This Brescia group has paid particular attention to delivering adequate therapy in both modalities. Three national registries that provide up-to-date patient data as well as complete or almost complete patient reporting will be discussed.

UNITED STATES RENAL DATA SYSTEM

In a widely discussed article from the United States Renal Data System (USRDS) examining a cohort of patients prevalent in 1987 to 1989, it was reported that there was a 19% higher death rate in PD patients and a 38% higher death rate in diabetic patients on PD compared with HD patients. These findings caused deep concern in the nephrology community and caused many nephrologists, especially in the United States, to question PD as a therapy. However more recent cohorts of patients from the USRDS show a much different picture, for at least two reasons. First, the cohort of patients chosen for study showed the worst results for PD relative to HD, with subsequent cohorts showing much smaller differences in mortality between the two modalities. Second, when analyses that examine diabetic and nondiabetic patients are performed separately, it is found that among period-prevalent patients (that is, current plus new patients) there is no clinically significant difference in mortality between PD and HD in nondiabetics, whereas the excess mortality in diabetics on PD is seen only in older diabetics, and especially in females. For younger diabetics, the mortality risk for patients on PD is a significantly *lower*. Most importantly, when the analysis is restricted to purely incident (new) patients (the "gold standard" for epidemiologic research), nondiabetic patients receiving PD had a significantly lower mortality than those receiving HD. Among incident diabetics on PD, those under the age of 55 years had a significantly better survival compared with patients on HD, whereas among those over the age of 55 years, only females showed a higher death rate. Parenthetically, it is interesting that the nephrology community has absorbed the message that there is a higher mortality for the older diabetic patient on PD, but has largely ignored the message that there is a higher mortality for younger diabetics on HD.

A caveat that must be kept in mind when drawing conclusions from the USRDS data is that a study including 821 patients has shown that the accuracy of the Medical Evidence Report (Form 2728), which the USRDS relies on for collecting comorbidities at the initiation of dialysis, is disturbingly poor. For example, the sensitivity of recording congestive heart failure, coronary artery disease, and myocardial infarction was only 52%, 51%, and 42%, respectively. However, there were only two conditions in which a significant difference in sensitivity between HD and PD patients was seen; myocardial infarction (HD 27%, PD 58%) and insulin dependence (HD 70%, PD 84%). Therefore one would assume that survival comparisons of PD versus HD based on the USRDS would remain valid.

CANADIAN ORGAN REPLACEMENT REGISTER

The Canadian Organ Replacement Register (CORR) has reported strikingly different results from those initially reported from analysis of USRDS. Using a similar method of analysis (Poisson regression), there was a markedly reduced relative risk of death for incident patients on PD compared with those on HD (0.73, 95% confidence interval: 0.68 to 0.78) in patients commencing dialysis between 1990 and 1994 and followed for a maximum of 5 years. Factors controlled for included age, primary renal diagnosis, center size, and predialysis comorbid conditions. These results held true for both diabetics and nondiabetics, and for all age groups. The increased mortality on HD compared with PD was concentrated in the first 2 years of follow-up, but the mortality curves did not cross until after 36 months. This study confirms that when incident patients are studied there is an overall survival advantage for patients treated with PD. A further publication from the CORR shows that there has been a continuous and marked improvement in mortality rates for patients treated with PD in Canada during the period from 1981 to 1996. This decreased mortality was observed for all causes of death, including cardiovascular disease (37.7% of deaths) and peritonitis (3.5% of all deaths). Clearly the reduction in cardiovascular mortality made a far greater contribution to the decreased mortality than the reduction in peritonitis deaths.

A report of data on 822 patients from 11 Canadian centers suggests that the lower mortality in PD patients shown in the CORR reports (of which these patients are necessarily a subset) is no longer demonstrable when a more detailed adjustment for comorbidities present at the initiation of dialysis is carried out. This study shows that, following such adjustment, the mortality rates associated with the two modalities in this group of patients become equal.

It should also be noted that in the Canadian–USA (CANUSA) study of PD there was a significantly lower mortality in the Canadian studies centers compared with the U.S. centers. The 2-year survival for Caucasian patients was 77% in Canada and 55% in the United States. This survival difference was not explained by any of the parameters examined, including age, gender, functional status, insulin-dependent diabetes mellitus, severity of cardiovascular disease, adequacy of dialysis, and RRF. The prevalence of PD in the study centers was 48% in

Canada and 22% in the United States, whereas the incidence of new dialysis patients in 1992 was 100 per million population in Canada compared with 211 per million in the United States. These differences may partly explain the disparity in the outcomes; lower patient compliance in the United States may also be a factor.

AUSTRALIA AND NEW ZEALAND DIALYSIS AND TRANSPLANT REGISTRY

The annual Australia and New Zealand Dialysis and Transplant Registry (ANZDATA) reports generally show little difference in mortality rates between patients treated with PD and those treated with HD, but the mortality rate on PD has been somewhat higher than that on HD. There was an insignificant difference in the diabetic patient death rate for PD or HD. In earlier reports, the death rate among young and middle-age diabetics using HD was higher, but more recently it has decreased to levels similar to PD. Data covering the period between 1994 and 1998 show that PD patients have a consistently higher number of comorbid conditions including all types of vascular disease; thus in Australia and New Zealand there seems to be negative selection of patients toward PD.

CHANGES IN RELATIVE DEATH RATES WITH PERITONEAL DIALYSIS AND HEMODIALYSIS WITH TIME ON DIALYSIS

The findings of the more recent analyses of patient cohorts from the USRDS, which contain incident as well as prevalent patients, show an improved mortality for PD patients compared with HD patients, which suggests that the mortality rates for the two modalities may alter, especially relative to each other, with time on dialysis. A number of studies have confirmed that the mortality for PD patients is lower in the first 1 to 3 years after the patient commences maintenance dialysis but thereafter becomes higher. It is likely that this phenomenon is related to loss of RRF, an important contributor to the adequacy of PD. Another study has supported this hypothesis; RRF was similar in survivors and nonsurvivors at the initiation of PD, but fell at a significantly higher rate in nonsurvivors than in survivors. Now that the need to individualize the patient's dialysis prescription in order to ensure (and to continue to ensure) adequate dialysis as RRF falls has been generally recognized, this late mortality should decrease.

An alternative explanation for the better survival on PD in the first years after commencing dialysis is that patients who select or are directed toward PD have fewer and/or less severe comorbidities. However, the available data look only at the number of comorbid conditions, not their severity. There is evidence from Wave 2 of the USRDS Dialysis Morbidity and Mortality Study that HD patients have more comorbid conditions. Data from Canada, discussed previously, suggest that HD patients have more comorbid conditions at the initiation of dialysis, whereas data from ANZDATA suggest that it is PD patients in Australia who have a higher number of comorbid conditions. In the earlier cohorts of patients from the Brescia study, there were more comorbidities in the PD patients, but more recent cohorts had equal numbers of comorbidities at the commencement of maintenance dialysis. Thus one can find variations in practice that lead to patients with more comorbidities being placed on either PD or HD.

TECHNIQUE SURVIVAL

All studies show a lower technique survival for PD compared with HD, and this equates with a major imbalance in the number of transfers between the therapies—there are many more transfers from PD to HD than vice versa. The major causes of technique failure in PD are peritonitis, often associated with Tenckhoff catheter exit-site or tunnel infection, inadequate dialysis as RRF declines, ultrafiltration failure, and patient preference, usually related to "burn-out." The major cause of transfer from HD to PD is failed vascular access. The Brescia group has documented the cause and incidence of transfer from PD to HD over many years.

PERITONEAL TRANSPORT CHARACTERISTICS AND MORTALITY IN PERITONEAL DIALYSIS

Several studies have now shown that patients who have the most rapid transport across the peritoneal membrane have a higher morbidity and mortality. This may be related to poor ultrafiltration with consequent hypervolemia and hypertension or to excessive protein losses in the dialysate leading to malnutrition. Alternatively, it may be due to high glucose absorption leading to poor appetite or to excess cardiovascular risk due to hyperlipidemia. Interestingly, rapid peritoneal transport may be an acquired phenomenon in the PD patient; there was a progressive rise with time on PD in the dialysate to plasma creatinine concentration ratio measured during the conventional peritoneal equilibration test (PET). It is important to note that high transporters constitute only 10% to 15% of prevalent PD patients. Until this problem is better understood such patients should be treated with APD to ensure adequate ultrafiltration, or they may be better treated with HD.

HOSPITALIZATION RATES

Most studies comparing hospitalization within centers show that PD patients have more hospital days per year than HD patients. However, the difference has steadily decreased as peritonitis rates have fallen with the introduction of twin-bag disconnect systems. The USRDS 1997 report shows that hospital admission rates are very similar for both modalities, but does not provide data on hospital days per year. A study examining the costs of treatment with HD and PD found that hospitalization was much less in PD patients during the year of the study (1994); the days per year hospitalized in this large, multicenter U.S. group were 4.12 days for PD patients compared with 9.00 days for HD patients.

CONTROVERSIES AND UNANSWERED QUESTIONS

Controversy in medicine arises when there are insufficient data to resolve an issue. There has indeed been much controversy since the publication of the landmark USRDS article in 1995 raised concerns regarding the relative mortality rates between HD and PD. However, it is now clear that the rates are very similar overall, with an early survival advantage for PD and, in some studies, a later (more than 2 years after the initiation of dialysis) advantage for HD.

Some questions require further research. Why does this switch in mortality rates occur? Is it related to loss of RRF, and can it be prevented by increasing the PD prescription? Why is there a higher mortality in PD patients with the most rapid peritoneal transport? Why, in the United States, do older female diabetics have a higher mortality on PD, whereas younger diabetics of both sexes have a higher mortality on HD?

Although these questions remain to be answered, it must be understood that, for example, the relative risk of PD versus HD in female diabetics of 1.18 translates into an absolute 3% difference in 1-year survival (74% versus 77%). Therefore "nonmedical" or "social" factors are and should be far more important in determining the choice of modality for a particular patient. Such factors include the capacity of the center to provide the therapy, the relative skill and experience (and enthusiasm) of the center for each modality, the willingness of the patient to be responsible for his or her therapy, the distance from the patient's home to the center, and many more.

It is good clinical practice to offer PD as a modality choice to any patient unless there are *specific* contraindications. Indeed it might be said that PD is the initial therapy of choice for all patients commencing maintenance dialysis.

Selected Readings

Bloembergen WE, Port FK, Mauger EA, et al. A comparison of mortality between patients treated with hemodialysis and peritoneal dialysis. *J Am Soc Nephrol* 1995;6:177–183.

A study of United States Renal Data System data, which raised doubts about the mortality rates of patients treated with peritoneal dialysis (PD) compared with those treated with hemodialysis (HD), and was therefore invaluable in focusing the attention of the nephrology community. This study is now obsolete by more recent reports that give a more accurate and up-to-date picture.

Cancarini GC, Brunori G, Zani R, et al. Long-term outcomes of peritoneal dialysis. *Perit Dial Int* 1997;17(Suppl 2):S115–S118.

The latest of a series of detailed reports describing the changing practices and results from one center for both PD and HD over nearly 2 decades.

Churchill DN, Thorpe KE, Vonesh EF, et al. Lower probability of patient survival with continuous peritoneal dialysis in the United States compared with Canada. Canada-USA (CANUSA) Peritoneal Dialysis Study Group. *J Am Soc Nephrol* 1997; 8:965–971.

A subanalysis of the CANUSA study, which demonstrates a significantly higher mortality in the four U.S. study centers than in the ten Canadian centers.

Churchill DN, Thorpe KE, Nolph KD, et al. Increased peritoneal membrane transport is associated with decreased patient and technique survival for continuous peritoneal dialysis patients. Canada-USA (CANUSA) Peritoneal Dialysis Study Group. *J Am Soc Nephrol* 1998; 9:1285–1292.

Another subanalysis of the CANUSA study data, which demonstrate that the most rapid peritoneal transport rates are associated with a higher mortality.

Collins AJ, Hao W, Xia H, et al. Mortality risks of CAPD/CCPD and hemodialysis. Submitted for publication.

An analysis of the USRDS data, which confirms and extends the findings reported by Vonesh and Moran. This study is particularly valuable because it includes only incident patients.

Davies SJ, Phillips L, Russell GL. Peritoneal solute transport predicts survival on CAPD independently of residual renal function. *Nephrol Dial Transplant* 1998; 13:962–968.

An important article that shows that nonsurvivors on PD are characterized by a more rapid loss of residual renal function and a progressive rise in peritoneal transport rates.

Fenton SS, Schaubel DE, Desmeules M, et al. Hemodialysis versus peritoneal dialysis: a comparison of adjusted mortality rates. *Am J Kidney Dis* 1997;30: 334–342.

A report from the Canadian Organ Replacement Register (CORR) showing much lower mortality rates for all groups of patients on PD than for HD in Canada; this difference is concentrated in the first 2 years of dialysis.

Heaf J. CAPD adequacy and dialysis morbidity: detrimental effect of a high peritoneal equilibration rate. *Ren Fail* 1995;17:575–587.

An important article that describes the relationship between dialysis adequacy and peritoneal transport rate and morbidity in PD.

McMurray SD, Miller J. Impact of capitation on free-standing dialysis facilities: can you survive? *Am J Kidney Dis* 1997;30:542–548.

A detailed examination of the costs of caring for HD and PD patients and the factors generating those costs.

Vonesh EF, Moran J. Mortality in end-stage renal disease: a reassessment of differences between patients treated with hemodialysis and peritoneal dialysis. *J Am Soc Nephrol* 1999;10:354–365.

An examination of USRDS patient cohorts from 1987 to 1993, which indicates that there is little or no overall difference in mortality between patients on HD and PD. When different subsets of patients are examined there is no significant difference for nondiabetic patients, an excess mortality for diabetics age less than 50 years on HD, and an excess mortality for female diabetics on PD.

PART 3

Continuous Renal Replacement Therapy

Miles H. Sigler and Brendan P. Teehan

The use of slow continuous therapy to treat critically ill patients with acute renal failure is increasing in popularity. As experience has been gained in the use of slow continuous therapy, there has been an inclination for more frequent use of the combined diffusion convection therapies (continuous venovenous hemodialysis) as opposed to the purely convection-based therapies (continuous arteriovenous hemofiltration), which were the first slow therapies to be described. However, both approaches are still used depending on clinical circumstances. Several technical variations distinguish the slow therapies from one another, but they all have in common simplicity of operation and slow removal of solute and water over a prolonged period of time. The most commonly used therapies are (a) continuous venovenous hemodialysis or continuous venovenous hemodiafiltration (CVVHD), (b) continuous arteriovenous hemodialysis (CAVHD), (c) continuous venovenous hemofiltration (CVVH), (d) continuous arteriovenous hemofiltration (CAVH), and (e) continuous arteriovenous ultrafiltration (CAV-U, also called SCUF).

CONTINUOUS VENOVENOUS HEMODIALYSIS

Rationale

Most critically ill patients with acute renal failure have precipitating comorbidities, such as septicemia, myocardial infarction, gastrointestinal bleeding, and acute respiratory distress syndrome, which render the patient hemodynamically unstable and prone to hypotension. This, in turn, may make conventional high-efficiency intermittent hemodialysis technically difficult to accomplish. Many of these patients are catabolic, requiring a high urea clearance to control azotemia. The potential advantages of CVVHD in this setting are outlined in Table 84.21.

TABLE 84.21. Advantages of Continuous Renal Replacement Therapies (CVVHD) in Treating Intensive Care Patients

1. Hemodynamically well tolerated; minimal change in plasma osmolality
2. Better control of azotemia and electrolyte and acid–base balance; corrects abnormalities as they are evolving; steady-state chemistries
3. Highly effective in removing fluid (pulmonary edema, acute respiratory distress syndrome)
4. Facilitates administration of parenteral nutrition and obligatory intravenous medications (i.e., pressors, inotropes) by creating unlimited "space" through continuous ultrafiltration
5. Procedure technically simple; reliable machinery

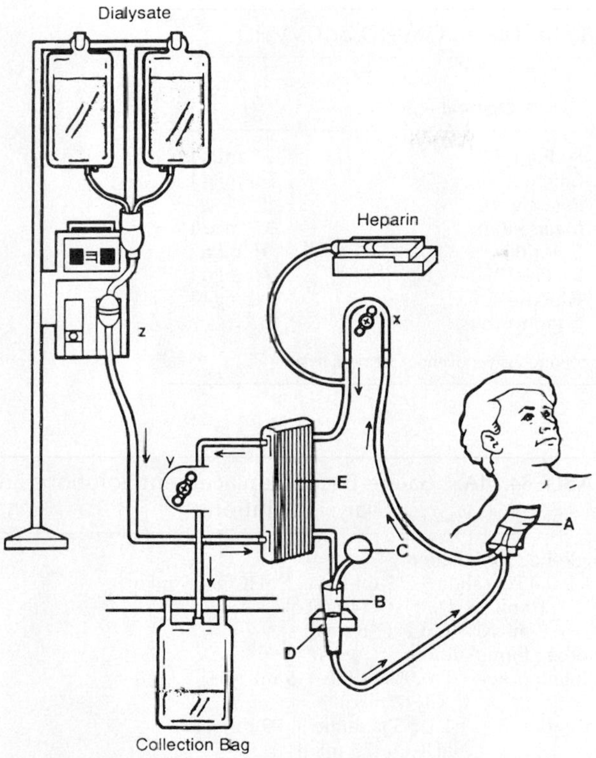

Figure 84.37. The circuit for continuous venovenous hemodialysis (CVVHD). **A:** Double-lumen subclavian vein access (internal jugular and femoral veins could also be used). **B:** Venous air trap. **C:** Venous pressure monitor. **D:** Air detector. **E:** Hemodialyzer. **X:** Roller blood pump. **Y:** Dialysate outflow pump. Although pump *X* and *Y* are shown separately, the BSM 22 pump has them mounted together and electrically coordinated. **Z:** Dialysate inflow pump. (Reproduced from Sigler M, Teehan BP. In: Nissensan AR, Fine RN, eds. *Dialysis therapy,* ed 2. Philadelphia: Hanley and Belfus, 1993:144.)

Maintenance of hemodynamic stability and control of fluid balance are the major advantages. CVVHD has the potential for providing the highest cumulative clearances in a 24-hour period compared with any of the blood cleansing techniques currently in use. The circuitry is pictured in Fig. 84.37.

Procedure

The blood is accessed through a large central vein (i.e., subclavian, internal jugular, or femoral) using a dual-lumen venous catheter and pumped through a hemodialyzer at 100 to 150 ml/min and then back into the patient. Sterile dialysis fluid is slowly pumped countercurrent to blood flow through the dialysis compartment at 12 to 15 ml/min, which is approximately 2% to 3% of the conventional dialysate inflow rate. Small-molecule diffusive clearance (on average about 15 ml/min) and ultrafiltration (yielding about 4 ml of convective clearance) occur, yielding a combined convective and diffusive clearance of approximately 18 to 20 ml/min, which is less than 10% of the conventional intermittent hemodialysis urea clearance. However, because the process is continuous, the cumulative 24-hour clearance is comparable to, if not greater than, conventional dialysis. Therefore this procedure is particularly effective in patients with high urea generation rates. Ultrafiltration rates are kept low (3 to 5 ml/min) only to offset obligatory fluid intake, 3 to 5 L/day. The lower ultrafiltration rate, as opposed to the high filtration rates in the convective-based therapies, is less prone to induce hypotension in a hemodynamically unstable patient.

Technical Points

Venous Blood Access

The advantages of venous access are (a) minimum delay, an 11.5-Fr, 15-cm long, dual-lumen catheter can be inserted by a treating physician; (b) avoidance of arterial cannulation with potential distal ischemic (occlusive and atheroembolic) complications and bleeding; (c) the pump ensures high, constant blood flow rate; (d) the patient can sit in a chair during treatment; and (e) there is minimal risk for large local hematoma on removal of the access catheter. The disadvantages of venous access are (a) a risk of exit-site infections and catheter-induced bacteremia if the catheter is left in for more than 5 days (11%) and (b) subclavian vein thrombosis and stenosis. Femoral or internal jugular venous access is preferred.

Choice of Hemofilter and Blood Lines

Originally, a flat-plate pediatric hemodialyzer, surface area 0.5 m^2, with an acrylonitrile and sodium-methallyl-sulfonate copolymer membrane was used for CAVHD. The current name for that device is Hemospal AN69S. The flat-plate geometry confers a low resistance to blood flow, which makes it ideal for a pumpless system such as CAVHD. It also has high diffusivity, high hydraulic permeability, and good dispersion of dialysate and blood. With the advent of pump-assisted CVVHD, there are various flat-plate and hollow-fiber hemodialyzers that are of comparable efficiency (Table 84.22). They all allow almost com-

TABLE 84.22. Dialyzer Membrane Data

Membrane Material	Type	Model No.	Surface Area
Cuprophane	Flat plate	Lundia IC-5H CGH Medical Inc., Denver, CO	1.1m^2
Polysulfone	Hollow fiber	F-8 Fresenius AG, Bad Homburg, Germany	1.8 m^2
	Hollow fiber	Renaflo HF-500 Renal Systems, Minneapolis, MN	0.5 m^2
Acrylonitrile, methallyl, sulfonate	Hollow fiber	Multiflow 60 CGH Medical Inc., Denver, CO	0.6 m^2
copolymer	Flat plate	Hemospal AN695 CGH Medical Inc., Denver, CO	0.5 m^2

TABLE 84.23. Dialysate Composition (mEq/L) for Use in CAVHD or CVVHD

Baxter CAVHD Dialysis Fluid		Dianeal (1.5%)	
Sodium	140 mEq/L	Sodium	132 mEq/L
Calcium	3.5 mEq/L	Calcium	3.5 mEq/L
Potassium	2.0 mEq/L	Potassium	—
Magnesium	1.5 mEq/L	Magnesium	0.5 mEq/L
Chloride	117 mEq/L	Chloride	96 mEq/L
Lactate	30 mEq/L	Lactate	40 mEq/L
Dextrose	100 mg/dl	Glucose (anhydrous)	1300 mg/dl

CAVHD, continuous arteriovenous hemodialysis; CVVHD, continuous venovenous hemodialysis.

plete diffusion equilibrium of blood solute with dialysate. Thus the ratio of solute concentration of dialysate effluent (C_{Do}) to incoming plasma (C_{Bi}) is 0.8 to 1.0. In effect, there is almost complete saturation of dialysate with low-molecular-weight blood solute. Because of the propensity for cellulosic membranes to activate complement, as well as various cytokine pathways, they are not recommended for dialysis patients with acute renal failure.

Dialysis Solutions

Five-liter bags of commercially prepared sterile peritoneal dialysis solutions are used in continuous hemodialysis (Dianeal, Baxter). Because the sodium concentration in Dianeal is 132 mEq/L, 10 ml of hypertonic (23.4%) sodium chloride (4 mEq/ml) is added to raise the sodium concentration to the physiologic range of 140 mEq/L. Table 84.23 lists the concentrations of solutes in commercially available dialysis solutions used in both CVVHD and CAVHD. Increasing the dialysate dextrose concentration from 1.5% to 2.5% or 4.25% results in an uptake of glucose from dialysate amounting to 1,300 to 2,300 kcal/day. Because of the rapid dissipation of the dialysate to blood glucose concentration gradient, increasing the concentration of glucose to 4.25% does not result in increased osmotic removal of fluid from the blood compartment. Sterile solutions are used because filtration of dialysate into blood can occur, although this has not been demonstrated convincingly in plate dialyzers. Phosphate clearance in CVVHD is high, and phosphate replacement often is necessary after several days of therapy. Serum calcium must also be monitored. The high glucose load from the dialysate may also contribute to the hypophosphatemia.

There has been a trend toward the use of bicarbonate-based dialysate (either commercially prepared or made on site) and alternative dialysate formulation to compensate for citrate anticoagulation methods. Although both of these approaches are quickly becoming standard procedures, comparative data exist only for dialysis patients with concomitant liver failure where bicarbonate is better tolerated than lactate (Dianeal, Baxter) dialysate. A recipe for compounding a bicarbonate-saline dialysate and the resulting composition are outlined in Tables 84.24A and 84.24B. Bicarbonate also forms insoluable salts when in solution with calcium and magnesium. Therefore bicarbonate-based dialysate and replacement solutions should be prepared just before use.

In the two-bag method, the bags of 0.9% saline with added calcium are alternated with bags of 0.45% saline with added bicarbonate. Magnesium is given parenterally as needed and serum calcium and magnesium are monitored every 12 hours.

Dialysis Solution Inflow and Outflow Rate

In CVVHD and CAVHD, the dialysate becomes 100% saturated with urea at dialysate inflow rates up to 28 ml/min and blood flows of 100 to 150 ml/min. Thus the dialysate outflow rate in milliliters per minute will equal the extracorporeal plasma urea clearance. The dialysate outflow rate, in turn, is the sum of the dialysis inflow rate plus the plasma ultrafiltration rate. Because dialysate flow rate determines in large part the urea clearance, it is first necessary to know how much urea clearance is required to control plasma urea nitrogen at a given urea nitrogen generation rate. Once the required clearance is calculated, the dialysis solution inflow and outflow rates can be determined. Several concepts related to urea nitrogen generation and urea clearance can be reviewed at this point.

Definition and Determination of Urea Nitrogen Generation Rate. The urea nitrogen generation rate is the rate at which urea nitrogen is being produced by the body. The urea nitrogen generation rate is directly dependent on the rate at which ingested proteins and amino acids are broken down, as well as the rate of breakdown of endogenous body proteins. A method of calculating the urea nitrogen generation rate is described in Table 84.25. The method makes the assumption that all of the

TABLE 84.24A. Saline-Based Replacement Solutions and Dialysis Solutions

Single-bag formulation
- 1 L 0.45% saline + 35 ml 8.4% NaHCO (35 mEq)
- + 10 ml 23.4% NaCl (40 mEq)
- + 2 ml 10% $CaCl_2$ (2.8 mEq)

Two-bag formulation
- Solution A: 1 L 0.9% saline + 5 ml 10% $CaCl_2$ (7 mEq)
- Solution B: 1 L 0.45% saline + 75 ml 8.4% $NaHCO_3$ (75 mEq)

TABLE 84.24B. Composition of Saline-Based On-Site Formulated Bicarbonate Replacement Solutions

	One-Bag Formulation (can also be used as dialysis fluid)	Two-Bag Formulation
Volume	1.05 L	2.08 L
Na^+	145 mEq/L	147 mEq/L
Cl	114 mEq/L	114 mEq/L
HCO_3^-	33 mEq/L	36 mEq/L
Ca^{2+}	2.7 mEq/L	3.4 mEq/L
Mg^{2+}		

urea nitrogen in the body is dissolved in the total body water (approximately 60% of lean body weight). The urea nitrogen concentration in the total body water is reflected by the plasma level. Thus the increase in body urea nitrogen over a given period can be calculated by multiplying the change in the plasma urea nitrogen concentration that occurs by the estimated urea nitrogen distribution volume. Any losses of urea nitrogen must also be accounted for as described in Table 84.25. The urea nitrogen generation rate in intensive care patients commonly ranges from 5 g/day to more than 20 g/day. For example, consider the case of an anuric, 70-kg, septic surgical patient with acute renal failure generating urea nitrogen at 20 g/day, as determined by using the method described in Table 84.25. How much dialysis clearance (and, hence, how much dialysate inflow) is necessary to maintain the blood urea nitrogen (BUN) at 70 dl?

1. Convert 20 g urea nitrogen per day to mg/min

$$G_u = \text{urea nitrogen generation} = \frac{20{,}000}{1{,}440} = 13.9 \text{ mg/min}$$

At steady state, urea nitrogen generation rate (G_u) equals urea nitrogen removal rate.

2. Thus

$$G_u = \text{urea nitrogen removal rate}$$

$$G_u = \text{plasma urea clearance} \times \text{plasma urea concentration}$$

$$\frac{G_u \text{ (mg/min)}}{\text{Plasma urea concentration (mg/ml)}} = \text{plasma urea clearance}$$

3. To simplify, we assume no residual renal function. Assume that we desire a steady-state plasma urea concentration of 70 mg/dl. Therefore

$$\frac{13.9 \text{ mg/min}}{0.70 \text{ mg/ml}} = \text{plasma clearance} = 20 \text{ ml/min}$$

or 28.8 L/day of plasma clearance is required to maintain BUN at 70 mg/dl.

Once the clearance required to maintain the BUN at a given level in the presence of a given urea generation rate is determined (i.e., 20 ml/min), the dialysate inflow can be determined as follows. In CVVHD and CAVHD, the concentration of urea in effluent dialysate is approximately the same as its concentration in plasma entering the dialyzer. Therefore the amount of effluent exiting the dialysate compartment in milliliters per minute is numerically equal to the dialyzer clearance in milliliters per minute. If, in the example given, we desire to remove 6 L of body fluid in 24 hours, or approximately 4 ml/min, by plasma ultrafiltration to offset the daily obligatory fluid intake, the required dialysate inflow rate is computed as follows: 20 ml/min (total urea clearance required and equal to total dialysate effluent) minus 4 ml/min desired ultrafiltration rate (or 4 ml convective clearance) equals 16 ml/min diffusive urea clearance, which is achieved by 16 ml/min dialysate inflow rate.

TABLE 84.25. Calculation of the Urea Nitrogen Generation Rate

1. Determine the plasma urea nitrogen level at two time points, usually about 24 hr apart.
2. Estimate the total body water at each of these time points. The total body water can be estimated at 60% of the lean, dry body weight plus the estimated amount of edema fluid.
3. Calculate the total body urea nitrogen at each of the time points, assuming that the concentration of urea nitrogen in the total body water is equal to the plasma level.
4. Subtract the total body urea nitrogen content at the first time point from that at the second time point to determine the change in total body urea nitrogen content during the measurement period.
5. Calculate or estimate any other urea nitrogen losses during the measurement period. These losses represent urea nitrogen that was produced during the measurement period but was not reflected by an increase in the plasma urea nitrogen concentration. The most important losses will be via urine and via dialysate or ultrafiltrate if dialysis or hemofiltration was performed. Add the amount of urea nitrogen lost to the environment to the change in total body content urea nitrogen from step 4.
6. Correct all measurements for a 24-hr period if the measurement period was over a shorter or longer time interval.

Modified from Sigler M, et al. In: Daugirdas J, Ing T, eds. *Handbook of Dialysis*. Boston: Little Brown & Co, 1994.

Anticoagulation

Anticoagulation in the continuous therapies is achieved in much the same manner whether the technique is CVVHD, CVVH, CAVH, or CAVHD. Clotting within the dialyzer or lines in the system is the most difficult technical issue in using the continuous therapies. Prolonged anticoagulation, which is required in continuous therapy, constitutes a theoretic risk of bleeding. On the other hand, insufficient anticoagulation results in premature clotting and ineffective, expensive therapy.

Heparin Anticoagulation. Assuming normal baseline coagulation studies, the dialyzer is primed with a bolus of 2,000 IU of heparin at the start of the procedure. A solution of 1,000 IU of heparin per milliliter of saline is infused at a rate of 500 IU/hr into the arterial line leading into the dialyzer if the baseline partial thromboplastin time (PTT) is normal (Fig. 84.37). This start-up dose is simply a first-order approximation because heparin sensitivity varies widely in accordance with a host of factors. These include the thrombogenicity of the dialyzer membrane, the hemodynamics of the patient, the associated comorbidities, the intrinsic heparin sensitivity, and the coagulation status of the patient. Although a dose of 10 IU/kg per hour was suggested originally, this has not been found to be a helpful guideline. Rather, a heparin anticoagulation protocol as indicated in Table 84.26 is instituted and revised on the basis of 6-hour coagulation studies (PTT as indicated in Table 84.26). Although anticoagulation is continuous, there is no evidence that bleeding in the continuous therapies is more prevalent than it is in conventional intermittent hemodialysis. If heparin must be omitted because the patient is actively bleeding or may have heparin-induced thrombocytopenia, a clotting strategy is used. This consists of increasing dialysate inflow from 1 L/hr to approximately 2 L/hr. The higher dialysate flow rate will increase the total dialyzer clearance to at least 2 L/hr, which would compensate for the anticipated loss of clearance as the unheparinized dialyzer slowly clots. When no heparin is used, most dialyzers will clot within 8 hours or sooner, even with saline predilution up to 500 ml/hr. A sign of early clotting occurs

TABLE 84.26. Heparin Anticoagulation Protocol for CVVHD and CAVHD

2,000 IU heparin in arterial line; start with 500 IU/hr constant infusion
PTT arterial and venous[a] every 4 hr
If arterial PTT >45 seconds, decrease heparin by 100 IU/hr
If venous PTT <65 seconds, increase heparin by 100 IU/hr only if arterial PTT <45 seconds
Maintain arterial PTT 40 to 45 seconds
If arterial PTT <40 seconds, increase heparin by 100 IU/hr

CAVHD, continuous arteriovenous hemodialysis; CVVHD, continuous venovenous hemodialysis; PTT, partial thromboplastin time.
[a] "Venous" refers to the line exiting the dialyzer and returning to the patient via the femoral internal jugular or subclavian vein.

when the ratio of dialysate fluid urea nitrogen/plasma urea nitrogen is less than 0.8. When the ratio is less than 0.6, clotting is imminent. However, this ratio may have inherent inaccuracies. When a prospective analysis of fiber-bundle clotting was conducted, the correlation of the ratio was poor. This is thought to be due to an excess of membrane surface area available in low-efficiency system. Thus the system continues to operate at close-to-maximal efficiency despite a significant clotting-related decrement in total fiber-bundle volume available for solute exchange.

Regional anticoagulation with heparin and protamine neutralization has been tried and has been moderately successful. Regional citrate anticoagulation also has been tried and appears to hold promise. Figure 84.38 depicts a technique for regional citrate anticoagulation. Citrate is infused into the dialyzer, complexing calcium and thus preventing the blood from clotting as it courses through the dialyzer. Four percent trisodium citrate, which contains 140 mmol citrate and 320 mmol sodium/L (Baxter Corp.), is infused prefilter at approximately 170 ml/hr, depending on blood flow rate, in order to maintain the postfilter-activated clotting time (ACT) at 200 to 250 seconds. Physiologic (0.9%) saline is used as replacement fluid because the net ultrafiltration rate in this system is 400 to 600 ml/hr. A special dialysate solution (Fig. 84.38) is prepared that is low in sodium (to offset the hypertonic sodium citrate infusion) and does not contain calcium or potential alkali (lactate). Calcium is replaced via a separate central venous catheter using a solution of 20 ml of 10% calcium chloride added to 250 ml of 0.9% saline infused at 40 ml/hr. Using citrate anticoagulation, filter life was prolonged as compared with heparin anticoagulation, and bleeding with citrate CAVHD was not encountered. Heparin-induced thrombocytopenia can be managed with this technique. Further details of this method have been published by Mehta and colleagues. Prostacyclin and low-molecular-weight heparin also have been used as anticoagulants, but the data supporting their use are limited.

Pumps

CVVHD requires the use of a blood pump system, which increases the complexity of the procedure as compared with the original pumpless, slow continuous procedures, such as CAVH. However, the assumption is made that the advantages of the pumped system outweigh the disadvantages of increased complexity. The roller pumps most commonly used with CVVHD are the Prizma (Gambro, Denver, CO) and the Baxter pump (Baxter Corp., Deerfield, IL). There is a slight difference between the two systems. With the Prizma system, the entry dialysate flow rate is set and ultrafiltration is accomplished by varying the dialysate outflow rate. Because total solute clearance is based on total dialysate outflow, varying the ultrafiltration parameter will lead to variations in solute clearance. With the Baxter system, ultrafiltration is accomplished by varying the dialysate inflow rate at a fixed outflow rate, thus maintaining constant solute clearance. In addition, the Prizma system is module-based and only allows for a fixed product, whereas the Baxter system is component-based and allows for variations in equipment. Recently, Fresenius has modified the 2008H standard hemodialysis delivery system for CVVHD. This provides online bicarbonate dialysate, programmed, volumetric ultrafiltration, continuous blood pressure monitoring, and low, variable dialysate flow rates.

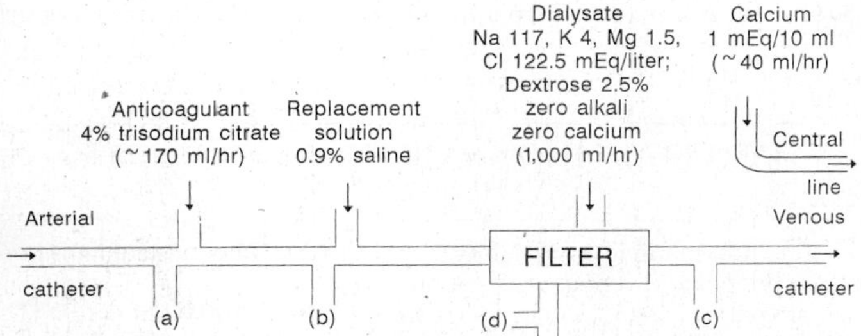

Figure 84.38. Circuit diagram for citrate CAVHD. Sampling parts are marked (*a*) peripheral, (*b*) prefilter, (*c*) postfilter, and (*d*) ultrafiltrate. (Reproduced from Mehta R, McDonald BR, Aquilar MM, et al. Regional citrate anti-coagulation for continuous arteriovenous hemodialysis in critically ill patients. *Kidney Int* 1990;38:976–981.)

TABLE 84.27. Approximate Dosage Adjustments of Antibiotics in Acute Renal Failure While on CAVHD and CVVHD[a]

Antibiotic	Adjustment
Cefuroxime	500–700 mg q12hr
Ceftazidime	1 g q24hr
Tobramycin	Loading dose followed by 60–80 mg/24 hr
Gentamicin	Loading dose followed by 80–100 mg/24 hr
Ciprofloxacin	200 mg q8hr
Vancomycin	1 g q48hr

[a] Blood levels should also be measured if possible.

Compensating for Removal of Therapeutic Drugs by Continuous Venovenous Hemodialysis

Because of the high 24-hour cumulative clearances, therapeutic drugs (antibiotics and pressors) and nutritional agents (crystalline amino acids in total parenteral nutrition [TPN] solution) may be excessively removed. Table 84.27 lists the approximate dosage adjustments of antibiotics in acute renal failure patients being treated with CVVHD or CAVHD. Total amino acids are removed in the amount of 12 g/24 hr when infused at 60 to 100 ml/hr in standard parenteral nutrition solutions. Significant quantities of pressors do not appear to be removed.

CONTINUOUS ARTERIOVENOUS HEMODIALYSIS

Rationale

CAVHD is essentially the same slow dialysis procedure as CVVHD except that the patient's arterial pressure is used to propel the blood through the extracorporeal circuit rather than a pump. This is achieved by cannulating the femoral artery. Spontaneous arterial blood flows of 90 to 150 ml/min are obtained routinely in patients with mean arterial pressures of 80 mm Hg. Lower mean pressures will sometimes deliver adequate blood flows as well. The circuitry is depicted in Fig. 84.39.

Technical Points

Blood Access

Using commercially available kits (Medcomp and Vas Cath), the femoral artery is cannulated 2 cm below the inguinal ligament using the percutaneous Seldinger technique. A special 5-Fr catheter mounted on a dilator is inserted over the guidewire into the femoral artery. The catheter is designed for CAVHD and CAVH with a single hole at the end of the catheter and no side holes. Thus if the tip of the catheter is outside the vessel, there will be little or no blood return. The femoral vein is cannulated in the same manner. Both are sutured in place, and povidone-iodine dressing is applied. Transparent dressings are

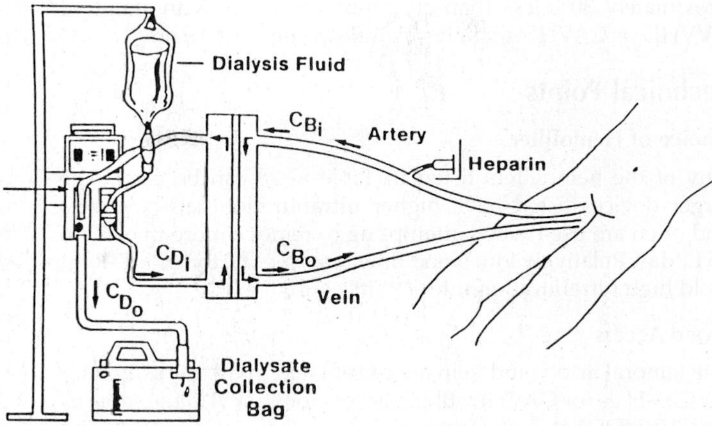

Figure 84.39. Circuitry for continuous arteriovenous hemodialysis (CAVHD). Dialysate infusion pump is a dual-channel I-MED Gemini PC-II. One channel infuses dialysate (C_{Di}, and the other channel pumps dialysate out (C_{Do}) into the dialysate bag. The outflow rate can also be controlled by gravity drainage alone. (Reproduced from Sigler M, Teehan B. In: Glassock RJ, ed. *Current Therapy in Nephrology and Hypertension*. St. Louis: Mosby Year Book, 1992:282.)

avoided because they trap moisture and they are conducive to exit-site infections. Before femoral artery cannulation, Doppler-audible foot pulses should be present, with no vascular bruits over the femoral artery. The cannulated leg must be monitored constantly for signs of ischemia or atheroemboli. The patient must remain in bed, with a femoral artery catheter in place. Complication rates of femoral artery hemorrhage and obstruction are approximately 5% to 6%. Scribner shunts are now rarely used because of poor blood flow, a tendency to clot, and a tendency to become infected.

Choice of Equipment

The choices of hemofilters, dialysis solutions, and dialysis inflow rates in CAVHD are the same as for CVVHD. If flat-plate dialyzers are used, flow through the blood compartment is first established before dialysate is pumped in and the dialysate outflow port is unclamped to allow the blood channel to expand.

The pump used to infuse dialysate can be an I-MED Gemini PC-II dual-channel infusion pump. One channel infuses the dialysate countercurrent to blood flow at 800 ml/hr. The dialysate is pumped out through the other channel of the Gemini PC-II into a Foley catheter bag at a rate greater than the inflow rate (inflow is usually 1 L/hr) to remove enough fluid to offset the obligatory fluid and parenteral nutritional intake (Fig. 84.40). In some cases of polyuric acute renal failure, an alternative to actively pumping dialysate fluid out is to allow the spent dialysis fluid to flow out by gravity into the collection bag, which is placed about 40 cm below the level of the dialyzer. The net ultrafiltration rate can be varied by changing the distance of the collection bag below the level of the dialyzer. Intakes and outputs are recorded hourly, as in CVVHD. If higher dialysate inflow rates are needed to increase urea clearance, a second I-MED Gemini PC-II pump can be used.

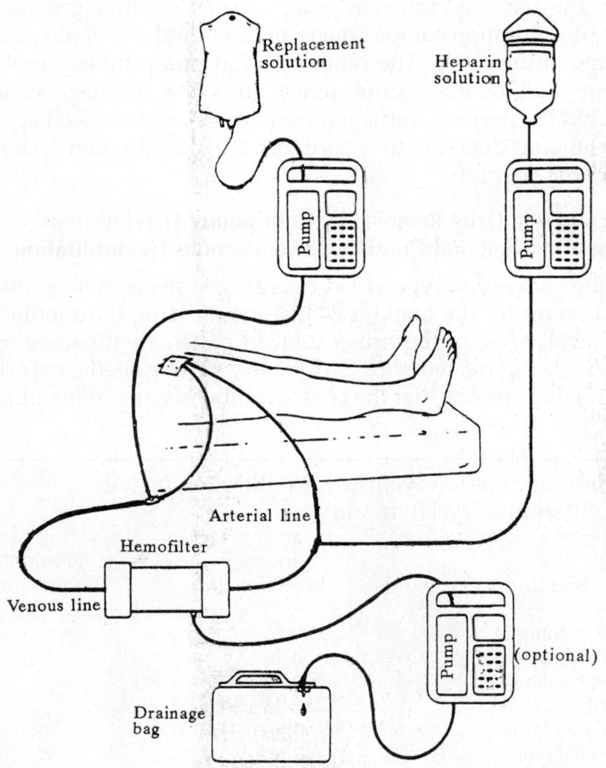

Figure 84.40. The circuit for continuous arteriovenous hemofiltration (CAVH). The two-pump method is illustrated, with intravenous infusion pumps used to control both the infusion rate of replacement solution and the rate of ultrafiltration. Replacement solution is shown infused into the venous line (postdilution mode). The third pump is used for heparin infusion. (Reproduced from Swann S, Paganini EP. *Acute continuous renal replacement therapy*. Hingham, MA: Martinus Nijhoff, 1986:61.)

CONTINUOUS ARTERIOVENOUS HEMOFILTRATION AND CONTINUOUS VENOVENOUS HEMOFILTRATION

Rationale

CAVH historically was the first of the slow continuous therapies described by Kramer. It is a purely convection-based blood cleansing technique as compared with the combined diffusion convection systems used in CVVHD and CAVHD. As blood flows through the hemofilter, a transmembrane pressure gradient between the blood compartment and the ultrafiltrate compartment causes plasma water to be filtered across the highly water-permeable plastic membrane. As the plasma water crosses the membrane, it conveys small and large molecules across the membrane and thus cleanses the blood. This ultrafiltrate must be replaced by a balanced electrolyte solution infused either before or after the hemofilter into the blood line. Typically, 10 to 15 L of fluid is removed isosmotically, and approximately 8 to 12 L of replacement solutions are infused per day. The circuitry for CAVH is depicted in Fig. 84.40. CVVH is essentially the same procedure as CAVH except that the blood access is venous and a pump is therefore required to circulate the blood. The blood circuitry for CVVH is similar to that of CVVHD (Fig. 84.37), except that the dialysate component of the circuitry is omitted. Twenty-four-hour small-molecule clearances achieved with CAVH are approximately 30% less than clearances achieved with standard CVVHD or CAVHD at dialysate inflow rates of 1 L/hr.

Technical Points

Choice of Hemofilter

Any of the hemofilters listed in Table 84.28 can be used. The larger devices listed have higher ultrafiltration capacity rates and often are used when attempting to remove more than 10 to 15 L/day. Relatively low blood flow rates (i.e., 80 to 100 ml/min) yield high ultrafiltration rates (10 ml/min).

Blood Access

The femoral artery and vein are cannulated in the same manner for CAVH as for CAVHD. Blood access for CVVH is the same as for CVVHD; that is, the internal jugular, femoral, or subclavian venous routes can be used. Scribner shunts are rarely used now that the pump-assisted venovenous alternatives are available.

Replacement Fluid

Several types of replacement fluid can be used, depending on patient requirements. The sodium concentration should be in the range of 140 mEq/L in most cases. Lactate, acetate, or bicarbonate concentration should average 30 to 40 mEq/L, depending on the patient's acid–base status. Calcium and magnesium cannot be added to the same fluid container with bicarbonate because precipitation of calcium or magnesium carbonate may occur.

Predilution Versus Postdilution

Replacement fluid can be infused either into the arterial blood line leading to the hemofilter (predilution) or into the venous blood line leaving the hemofilter (postdilution). The standard method is postdilution. However, when using postdilution at high fluid-removal rates (more than 10 L/day), the blood in the hemofilter can become very concentrated as its water is rapidly removed, leading to difficulty in obtaining adequate ultrafiltration and to increased resistance in the blood flow pathway (which can lead to clotting). The problem can be solved by diluting the blood with replacement fluid before it reaches the hemofilter (predilution). The disadvantage of predilution is that the ultrafiltrate in the hemofilter is then generated from blood diluted with replacement fluid and therefore contains a lower concentration of waste products. The loss of efficiency is not great, however, because at the usual flow rates, the urea concentration of ultrafiltrate obtained from the blood replacement fluid mixture will be 75% to 90% of the plasma value. We recommend using predilution whenever it is desired to remove more than 10 L/day. Predilution is also performed if the baseline blood viscosity is relatively elevated (e.g., if the hematocrit is greater than 35%).

Deciding on the Amount of Continuous Arteriovenous Hemofiltration to Prescribe

The conceptual basis for determining the amount of CAVH to prescribe is essentially the same as that used in prescribing for CVVHD or CAVHD. First, the urea generation rate must be determined, as outlined in Table 84.25, and second, the desired steady-state BUN level must be determined. The calculation is then made, as outlined in the section on CVVHD, to obtain a constant clearance that would maintain the desired steady-state BUN. The clearance in milliliters per minute is converted to liters per 24 hours. Because the concentration of solute (urea) in the ultrafiltrate is the same as in the plasma, the plasma extracorporeal clearance that will be necessary to maintain the BUN at a desired level will be equal to the ultrafiltration rate, assuming there is insignificant remaining renal function. Hence, if the calculated required clearance is 15 L/day, the ultrafiltration volume should also be 15 L/day. The ultrafiltration rate in CAVH is controlled by the gravity method or the two-pump method. In the gravity method, the line leading from the ultrafiltration port of the filter is connected directly to the drainage bag, which is kept below the patient. The distance that the drainage bag is located below the level of the hemofilter determines the negative pressure in the ultrafiltrate compartment. Raising or lowering the bag determines the negative pressure or siphon effect and, hence, the ultrafiltration rate. For each centimeter that the collection bag is below the hemofilter, 0.74 mm Hg negative pressure is exerted. The two-pump method (Fig. 84.40) is used to obtain higher ultrafiltration rates (15 to 20 L/day). One infusion pump is interposed in the ultrafiltration line leading to the drainage bag. An ultrafiltration rate is dialed in on the pump, and the activated infusion pump creates negative pressure in the ultrafiltration compartment, pulling fluid out of the plasma at the desired rate. The other infusion pump infuses replacement fluid in the venous return line. The drainage volume should be carefully measured periodically and checked against the amount dialed in to ensure that the ultrafiltration system is working properly.

Therapeutic Drug Removal by Continuous Arteriovenous Hemofiltration and Continuous Venovenous Hemofiltration

In the convection-type blood cleansing systems, it is necessary to account for the amount of therapeutic drug (i.e., antibiotic) removal. Most of the drugs used in patients with acute renal failure being treated with CAVH have sieving coefficients close to 1, which means that the concentration of drug in the ultrafil-

TABLE 84.28. Selected Hemofilters in Current Use for Continuous Arteriovenous Ultrafiltration (CAV-U) and Continuous Arteriovenous Hemofiltration (CAVH) in Adults

Type	Source	Brand	Membrane	Surface Area (m^2)	Priming Volume (ml)
PP	Hospal	Hemospal AN69S	Acrylonitrile	0.50	60
HF	Asahi	PAN-50—P	Polyacrylonitrile	0.50	50
HF	Amicon	Diafilter-10	Polysulfone	0.20	25
HF	Amicon	Diafilter-20	Polysulfone	0.25	27
HF	Fresenius	Ultraflux-400	Polysulfone	0.50	48
HF	Gambro	FH-55	Polyamide	0.60	43
HF	Gambro	FH-66	Polyamide	0.60	43
HF	Renal systems	HF-250	Polysulfone	0.25	27
HF	Renal systems	HF-500	Polysulfone	0.50	39

Modified from Sigler M, et al. In: Daugirdas J, Ing T, eds. *Handbook of Dialysis*. Boston: Little Brown & Co, 1994.
HF, hollow-fiber hemofilter; PP, parallel-plate hemofilter.

trate is similar to that in plasma water. Thus if 10 L of ultrafiltrate per day are removed, the amount of drug removed based on the ultrafiltrate or plasma level can be estimated and that amount readministered to the patient. Heparin anticoagulation in CAVH and CVVH is achieved in the same manner as in CAVHD and CVVHD. Citrate anticoagulation cannot be recommended for CVVH or CAVH at this time.

SLOW CONTINUOUS ULTRAFILTRATION

In some patients with acute renal failure requiring intensive care, a major problem is fluid overload rather than uremic toxicity. Despite the fluid overload, such patients must continue to receive intravenous fluids to convey life-sustaining pressors, antibiotics, and parenteral nutrition. Slow continuous ultrafiltration (SCUF) removing 3 to 4 ml/min of plasma water (4,300 to 5,700 ml/day) helps to create the space to accommodate this obligatory fluid intake. Filtration is achieved by using the technique of CVVH or CAVH but maintaining the filtration rate at a much lower level. No replacement fluid is needed in this modality.

EFFECT OF CONTINUOUS THERAPIES ON MORBIDITY AND MORTALITY IN ACUTE RENAL FAILURE

The mortality rate in patients with acute renal failure and multiorgan failure being treated in the intensive care unit remains high at 75% to 95%. This dismal prognosis is attributable to the severity of the comorbidities that precipitated the acute renal failure. Under these circumstances, it might be difficult to demonstrate a favorable effect of any dialytic intervention. However, a retrospective study by Bellomo and coworkers comparing clinical outcome related to the use of conventional intermittent dialysis versus acute continuous hemodialysis in critically ill patients with acute renal failure showed that continuous slow dialysis is beneficial.

Several studies have indicated that the total dialysis dose delivered to a patient with acute renal failure may be an important factor in determining outcome. If this can be substantiated by prospective controlled trials, then the use of continuous renal replacement therapies would be favored over intermittent dialysis modalities because a much greater dialysis dose can be delivered by continuous method of dialytic therapy.

Another area of great interest is the severity of disease scoring to help predict outcomes and to accurately stratify patients for prospective comparative studies. Several such scoring systems are available for use. Patient data can be entered via the internet (www.bio.ri.ccf.org/ar) and acute renal failure severity score obtained.

The treatment of acute renal failure by extracorporeal methods, including continuous renal replacement, is undergoing close scrutiny from both the financial and the outcome perspectives. Well-designed and executed prospective trials that critically evaluate the role of continuous renal replacement therapy in the treatment of acute renal failure still need to be carried out. Patients most likely to benefit from such therapy are those with intermediate disease severity scores. Patients with acute renal failure accompanied by severe multiorgan failure do poorly despite any form of dialysis therapy. Patients with acute renal failure and few or no complications or co-morbid conditions seem to do as well with conventional intermittent dialysis as with continuous renal replacement therapy.

Selected Readings

Bellomo R, Mansfield D, Rumble S, et al. Acute renal failure in critical illness. Conventional dialysis vs acute continuous hemodiafiltration. *ASAIO J* 1992;38: M654–M657.

Analyzes the clinical outcome in critically ill patients with acute renal failure. Analysis shows that patients with certain degrees of illness severity (APACHE scores) may be benefited by continuous versus intermittent dialysis.

Bosch JP. Continuous arteriovenous hemofiltration (CAVH): operational characteristics and clinical use. *Nephrol Lett* 1986;3:15–26.

Describes in more detail the indications for CAVH besides acute renal failure and the determinants of ultrafiltration rate. Also describes the clinical problems encountered and the relationship of urea generation and the quantity of ultrafiltration required to maintain a given blood urea nitrogen (BUN).

Mehta R, McDonald BR, Aquilar MM, et al. Regional citrate anticoagulation for continuous arteriovenous hemodialysis in critically ill patients. *Kidney Int* 31990;8:976–981.

Seminal article on the use of citrate in CAVHD. Compares and describes regional citrate anticoagulation with heparin anticoagulation.

Sigler MH, Teehan BP. In: Nissenson AR, Fine RN, Gentile DE, eds. *Continuous arteriovenous hemodialysis [CAVHD] in clinical dialysis,* ed 2. Norwalk, CT: Appleton & Lange, 1990:720–734.

An in-depth, how-to description of the technique of CAVHD and the unique solute transport characteristics of CAVHD. Also a quantitative comparison of CAVHD versus conventional intermittent dialysis and acute peritoneal dialysis. In addition, there is a description of the integration of total parenteral nutrition with CAVHD.

Sigler MH, Teehan BP, Van Valkenburgh D. Solute transport in continuous hemodialysis: a new treatment for acute renal failure. *Kidney Int* 1987;32:562–571.

Seminal article describing rates of small-molecular-weight solute transport in relation to blood flow and ultrafiltration rate. Describes the additive effects of diffusive and convection clearance.

CHAPTER 85

Drugs in Renal Failure

PART 1
Pharmacokinetics of Drugs and the Effects of Renal Failure

Ralph E. Cutler and Steven C. Forland

The kidney is a major organ involved in the elimination of drugs. Not unexpectedly, the frequency and severity of drug reactions may be more common in patients with renal failure. Therefore understanding the basic principles and various processes controlling the clearance of drugs from the body under normal conditions and during renal failure is of importance.

GENERAL PHARMACOKINETIC PRINCIPLES

Although the concentration of a drug or its metabolites at its receptor site may correlate best with a response, no convenient assay of this type is available in humans. Because all drugs do not distribute instantaneously and homogeneously throughout body tissues, and because the site of drug action may not be in immediate contact with the tissue or fluid being sampled, predicting serum drug concentrations or pharmacologic effect at any given time is complex. To facilitate this, mathematic models are used to predict what is occurring over time.

Pharmacokinetic Models

The simplest model is the one-compartment system (Fig. 85.1), which depicts the body as a single space or volume into which the drug is absorbed and distributed instantaneously and homogeneously. This model is useful in describing the kinetics of many things, primarily those that are rapidly distributed throughout the body. It also may adequately describe the kinetics of elimination when renal failure is present for drugs that are eliminated mainly by the kidney.

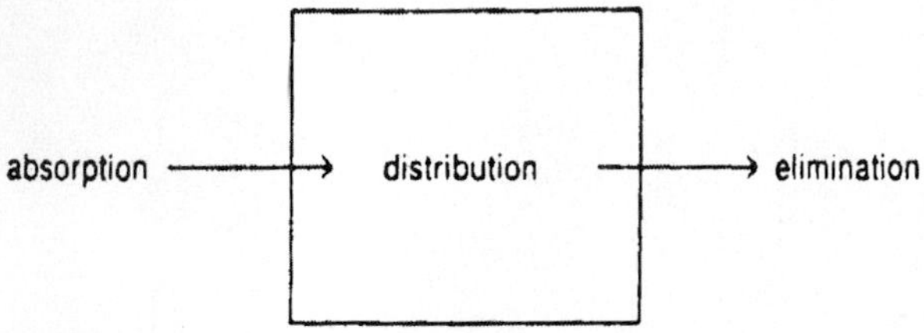

Figure 85.1. A model of the one-compartment system.

Although the one-compartment model is mathematically and conceptually simple, it does not accurately portray the time versus plasma concentration curve of most drugs. The two-compartment model is a better predictor of the plasma concentration over time. The model (Fig. 85.2) consists of (a) a central compartment (blood and highly perfused tissues that rapidly equilibrate with the drug) into which the drug is initially distributed and (b) a peripheral compartment into which the drug distributes at a slower rate.

Elimination is generally assumed to occur from the central compartment, because major organs of elimination usually fit the criteria of tissues included in this compartment. As the concentration of drug in the central compartment falls, redistribution occurs from the peripheral compartment back into the central compartment. It must be remembered that these compartments are conceptual and do not necessarily correspond to actual body fluid compartments.

Although pharmacokinetic models are useful for predicting plasma concentrations and pharmacodynamics of drugs, many pharmacologists are using model-independent techniques to analyze pharmacokinetic data. This approach avoids the assumptions of model compartments. The model-independent system consists of fitting the plasma versus time data to an equation

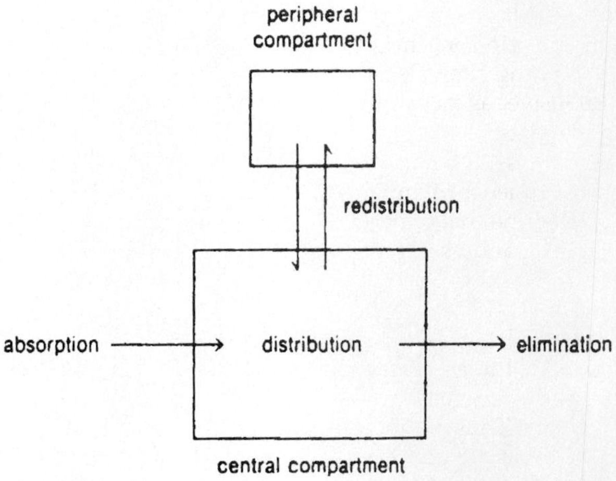

Figure 85.2. A model of the two-compartment system.

with the least number of exponentials, as well as obtaining the area under the plasma concentration versus time curve and the area under the first moment (product of serum concentration and time) versus time curve. Kinetic parameters, such as volume of distribution (V_d), total body clearance, and bioavailability, are calculated directly from these measurements.

Absorption

Bioavailability may be defined broadly as the amount of a drug that is absorbed following administration. Before drugs have systemic effects, they must be absorbed into the body and possibly metabolized into their active form. The oral route is the most frequent route of administration. It is also the route that gives rise to the most complex kinetics. A number of factors influence the absorption and bioavailability of orally administered drugs. These factors include the physicochemical characteristics of the drug, the formulation of the drug product, its interaction with other substances in the gastrointestinal tract, transport across the gastrointestinal mucosa, biotransformation by the liver (first-pass effect), and various other patient characteristics.

Distribution

Each drug is dispersed throughout the body in a characteristic manner. At equilibrium, the extent of distribution is defined as that volume of fluid into which the drug appears to distribute with a concentration equal to that in plasma. This concept assumes that the body acts as a single container or compartment with respect to the drug. This apparent V_d is useful in calculating the amount of drug in the body when the concentration (C) of drug in plasma is known or in predicting the plasma concentration following absorption of a given dose [f represents fractional absorption of dose (D)].

$$C = \frac{f \times D}{V_d} \tag{1}$$

The apparent V_d for any agent is relatively constant, but it may vary widely among patients and also may vary in the same patient at different times. A number of factors, such as body size, obesity, gender, physical stress, thyroid function, renal function, cardiac output, age, protein binding, and presence of other drugs, affect it.

One of the consequences of renal failure is a decrease in the ability of plasma proteins to bind certain drugs. This is especially true for acidic drugs existing as anions in blood, but occasionally may be true for cationic drugs (organic bases) as well. Available data suggest that the decreased protein binding of drugs in uremia may be caused by several factors, such as competitive displacement from normal binding sites, a reduction in binding protein concentration, or synthesis of proteins with reduced binding sites. Because these mechanisms are not mutually exclusive, all may exist, but with varying intensity in different patients.

An increase in the apparent V_d of the drug is a pharmacokinetic consequence of impaired plasma protein binding. Gilbaldi formulated the mathematic relationship between the apparent V_d of a drug and its degree of binding in blood as follows:

$$V_d = V_B + V_T\,(F_B/F_T) \tag{2}$$

where V_d is the apparent volume of distribution; V_B and V_T are the actual volumes of water in blood and tissues, respectively; and F_B and F_T are the fractions of free drug in blood and tissues, respectively. Thus an increase in the free fraction of drug in blood without a proportional increase in the free fraction in tissue would produce an *increase* in the apparent V_d. Such a relationship is seen with several drugs as noted in Table 85.1.

TABLE 85.1. Effect of Renal Failure on Volume of Distribution

Drug	Volume of Distribution, L/kg — Normal	Renal Failure
Increased		
Bretylium	3.6	4.5
Cefoxitin	0.16	0.26
Dicloxacillin	0.08	0.18
Phenytoin	0.64	1.4
Decreased		
Digoxin	7.3	4
Ethambutol	3.7	1.6
Pindolol	2.1	1.1

Digoxin, ethambutol, and pindolol represent examples of decreased tissue binding in renal failure (Table 85.1). Unfortunately, information on tissue binding in patients with renal failure is not available for most drugs.

Elimination

Concept of Body Clearance

The concept of clearance also can be applied to organs other than the kidney. The sum of all the individual organ (renal hepatic, pulmonary, and others) clearances of a drug is the body clearance. Because plasma is usually sampled for drug assays, body clearance is often referred to as *plasma clearance* (Cl_p). In this discussion, body clearance is simply expressed as the sum of the renal clearance (Cl_r) and the nonrenal clearance (Cl_{nr}), such that:

$$Cl_p = Cl_r + Cl_{nr} \tag{3}$$

Nonrenal (Metabolic) Clearance

Although some drugs are entirely eliminated by the kidney, undergoing little metabolism, most drugs undergo biotransformation to metabolites that are then excreted. Renal failure may alter the biotransformation rate of drugs and thus the excretion of polar metabolites in urine. The usual pathways of drug metabolism include oxidation, reduction, hydrolysis, and synthesis. Although extensive studies of drug metabolism in uremia have not been performed, there is evidence to suggest that some of these metabolic pathways are impaired (Table 85.2).

On the other hand, some observations show that oxidation of certain drugs may be accelerated. The mechanism of enhanced oxidation of drugs in renal failure has not been elucidated but may be related to a decrease in plasma protein binding or induction of oxidative enzymes. Consequently, drug metabolism may be normal, accelerated, or retarded by uremia. Of equal

TABLE 85.2. Effect of End-Stage Renal Disease on Metabolic (Nonrenal) Clearance

Increased	Unchanged	Decreased
Bumetanide	Acetaminophen	Acyclovir
Phenytoin	Clonidine	Captopril
	Codeine	Cefotaxime
	Insulin	Cilastatin
	Isoniazid	Cimetidine
	Metoprolol	Cortisol
	Theophylline	Procainamide

TABLE 85.3. Pharmacologic Activity of Metabolites

Parent Drug	Metabolite	Pharmacologic Activity of Metabolites
Codeine	Morpinie-6-glucuronide	Possibly more active than parent compound; may contribute to prolong narcotic effect in renal failure patients.
Meperidine	Normeperidine	Less analgesic activity than parent, but more CNS stimulatory effects. Avoid in renal failure.
Procainamide	*N*-acetyl procainamide	Distinct antiarrhythmic activity, the mechanism of which is different from that of the parent compound.
Propoxyphene	Norpropoxyphene	Less analgesic activity than parent but more cardiotoxicity. Avoid in renal failure.
Theophylline	1,3-Dimethyl uric acid	Cardiotoxicity has been demonstrated.

CNS, central nervous system.

importance also may be the effect of drug–drug interactions on drug metabolism, either enhancing or retarding biotransformation by competitive inhibition.

When chronic drug treatment is given in renal failure, both the parent agent and/or its metabolite(s) may accumulate. Some metabolites have been reported to have significant adverse effects (Table 85.3).

Renal Clearance

Entry of drugs into urine occurs by means of a combination of glomerular filtration and tubular transport. Glomerular filtration is unidirectional and permits entry of any dissociated or undissociated drug molecules that are not bound plasma proteins and are small enough to penetrate the glomerular wall. In contrast, tubular transport is bidirectional. Many organic acids and bases are both secreted and reabsorbed by carrier-mediated processes located principally in the S3 segment of the proximal tubule (see Chapter 7, Part 4). Protein binding apparently has little effect on tubular secretion except when the drug has a low affinity for the carrier-mediated transport system. Tubular transport mechanisms have a limited capacity, as do drug-metabolizing systems in the liver. Glomerular filtration of a drug is not subject to this limitation. As the concentration of an unbound drug in plasma increases, there is a linear increase in the amount filtered. Clearly, this is an advantage for the elimination of a drug by the kidney.

Two basic processes govern the reabsorption of drugs from glomerular filtrate: passive diffusion and active transport. Drug reabsorption by active transport has not been studied extensively for most agents. The marked reduction in the volume of filtrate caused by tubular reabsorption of sodium chloride and water creates a large concentration gradient favoring the passive reabsorption of certain drugs, assuming that the membrane is sufficiently permeable and that adequate contact time of the agent with the membrane is available. Hence, an increasing urine flow rate by osmotic diuresis could reduce passive diffusion and increase renal excretion.

Nonionic diffusion is a special variety of passive diffusion. Because most drugs are weak acids or bases, they exist in a mixture of ionic and nonionic forms, depending on the pK_a of the drug and the pH of the urine. Because the nonionic form is more lipid soluble, it shows higher cellular permeability and diffuses at a faster rate toward a site of lower concentration, thereby favoring reabsorption. Hence, weak acids (low pK_a), such as aspirin, will be in a nonionized form of acid urine. An elevation of urine pH will increase the ionized form, retard reabsorption, and increase renal excretion. The acceleration of urinary drug excretion by alterations in urine pH can thus be used if (a) the pK_a of the drug lies within the usual range of urine pH, (b) the glomerular filtration rate (GFR) is not significantly impaired, and (c) the drug is mainly excreted by the kidney and exhibits minimal nonrenal elimination. Both salicylates and phenobarbital have shown such characteristics. Movement of these molecules generally proceeds readily because the diffusible (nonionized) fraction of most organic drugs is sizable and may be increased by appropriate acidification or alkalinization of the urine, depending on the pK value of the drug. Thus the urinary excretion of such drugs as acetylsalicylic acid (pK 3.5) and probenecid (pK 3.3) is increased by alkalinization of the urine.

PHARMACOKINETIC PROPERTIES OF DRUGS

Tables 85.4 to 85.12 give useful data for evaluating both the effects of end-stage renal disease (ESRD) on the overall pharmacokinetics of drugs and the impact of 4 hours of conventional hemodialysis. Many drugs that became available before 1970 were not always studied in renal failure. Nonetheless, an approximation of the kidney as a significant route of drug elimination is made by knowledge of the percentage of drug excreted unchanged in the urine of healthy subjects, and such data are included in Tables 85.4 to 85.12.

The dialyzability of drugs is, in part, inversely related to the degree of plasma protein binding and V_d. Drugs with high plasma protein binding and large apparent V_d are therefore not eliminated rapidly by dialysis. However, the rate of hemodialysis clearance does not give a full picture of drug removal during hemodialysis. A better measure of significant removal by this route is the fraction of the body drug load that is eliminated during routine hemodialysis. Only large fractional removal (e.g., more than 20%) of drugs requiring a high steady-state plasma concentration require postdialysis dosing.

Dialysis of Drugs

The increase in plasma clearance of drugs that may occur with dialysis is symbolically represented as follows:

$$Cl_p = Cl_r + Cl_{nr} + Cl_d \qquad (4)$$

where Cl_d is the dialyzer clearance of any drug.

A drug with a low molecular weight (less than 500) and with minimal plasma protein binding may have a dialysis clearance between 15 and 100 ml/min. However, other characteristics of

(Text continued on p. 1580.)

TABLE 85.4. Pharmacokinetic Properties of Antiinfective Drugs in Normal Adults and Those with End-Stage Renal Disease

Drug Name	Apparent Volume of Distribution (L/kg)	Terminal Half-Life (hr)		F_0	Plasma Clearance (ml/min)		Excreted in Urine Unchanged[a] (%)	Plasma Protein Bound[a] (%)	Hemodialyzer Clearance (ml/min)	Drug Removal During 4 Hr of Hemodialysis		
		Normal	ESRD		Normal	ESRD				Dialysis	Nondialysis	Total
Antifungal Drugs												
Amphotericin B[b]	4	1–15 days	1–15 days	1	—	—	2–5	90–95	NS	NS	—	—
Fluconazole	0.71	32	98	0.3	—	—	80	11	—	45	—	40–50
Flucytosine	0.7	5	85	0.07	113	7	76–107	4	110	41	3	44
Griseofulvin	1.6	14	20	0.7	95	65	1	—	—	—	—	—
Itraconazole	—	38	38	1.0	—	—	<1	99.8	NS	NS	—	NS
Ketoconazole	1.9	8[c]	8[c]	1.0	210	210	<1	99	NS	NS	30	30
Miconazole	21	24	24	1.0	700	700	<1	92	NS	NS	—	NS
Terbinafine	13.5	11–16	—	—	1246	—	—	—	—	—	—	—
Antiparasitic Drugs												
Amoscanate	—	20 days	—	1.0	—	—	<1	80	—	—	—	—
Chloroquine	200	12 days	—	0.5[d]	722	—	55	55	NS	NS	—	—
Diethylcarbamazine	3.2	12	—	0.5	193	—	50	<5	—	—	—	—
Ivermectin	0.67	28	—	1.0	—	—	0	93	—	—	—	—
Levamisole	1.5	4–5	—	1.0	333	—	<5	—	—	—	—	—
Mebendazole	1.2	1.1	—	1.0	1050	1050	<1	—	—	—	—	—
Mefloquine	6–50	20 days	—	0.9	25	—	1–9	98	NS	—	—	NS
Oxamniquine	—	2	—	1.0	—	—	2	—	—	—	—	—
Suramin	0.5	42 days	—	0.5[d]	—	—	>90	99.7	NS	NS	—	—
Antitubercular Drugs												
Cycloserine	—	10	—	—	—	—	60–70	0	—	—	—	—
Ethambutol	1.6	3	10	0.3	435	130	50–65	20–30	50	9	23	32
Ethionamide	—	3	9	0.3	—	—	1	10	—	—	—	—
Isoniazide	0.60	1[e]	4	0.3[e]	485[e]	120	7[e]	1–10	50	18	44	62
Isoniazid[f]	—	3[f]	4	0.8[f]	160[f]	—	37[f]	1–10	50	—	—	—
Pyrazinamide	0.7	10	—	—	—	—	4–14	17	—	—	—	—
Rifabutin	9	16–69	—	—	—	—	10	71	—	—	—	—
Rifampin	0.93	4	4	1.0	215	215	5–15	60–90	NS	—	—	—
Antiviral Drugs												
Acyclovir	0.6	2–3	20	0.1	300	25	60–90	15	82	36	11	46
Amantadine	4.5	24	9 days	0.1	306	20	90	—	67	5	1	6
Didanosine	0.8	1.5	4.5	0.3	800	231	55	<5	—	5	30	35
Famciclovir (prodrug)												
Penciclovir	—	2	>18	0.15	—	—	—	—	—	—	—	—
Foscarnet	0.43	4.5	85	0.05	152	—	87	17	80	—	—	—
Ganciclovir	0.47	2–4	40	0.1	208	16	91–100	1–2	68	—	—	50
Indinavir	—	1.8	—	—	—	—	10	60	—	—	—	—
Lamivudine	1.4	9	21	0.43	377	—	—	—	—	—	—	—
Nelfinavir	—	4	—	1.0	—	—	1	98	NS	NS	—	—
Ritonavir	0.4	4	—	1.0	147	—	3.5	98	NS	NS	—	—
Saquinavir	10	—	—	—	1330	—	<3	97	NS	NS	—	—
Zalcitabine	0.5	2	—	—	—	—	75	<4	—	—	—	—
Zidovudine	1.4	1.1	1.4	0.8	1500	727	13–19	30	63	—	—	—
GATZ	—	0.9	29–94	—	—	—	—	—	91	—	—	—

(Continued)

TABLE 85.4. *(Continued)*

Drug Name	Apparent Volume of Distribution (L/kg)	Terminal Half-Life (hr) Normal	Terminal Half-Life (hr) ESRD	F_0	Plasma Clearance (ml/min) Normal	Plasma Clearance (ml/min) ESRD	Excreted in Urine Unchanged[a] (%)	Plasma Protein Bound[a] (%)	Hemodialyzer Clearance (ml/min)	Drug Removal During 4 Hr of Hemodialysis: Dialysis	Nondialysis	Total
Aminoglycosides												
Amikacin	0.25	2.5	70	0.04	90	3	81–98	<10	18	21	4	25
Gentamicin	0.24	2	60	0.03	95	2	80–90	<10	24	29	2	31
Kanamycin	0.23	2	80	0.03	95	2	84–90	<10	25	31	2	33
Netilmicin	0.25	2	40	0.06	88	5	90–100	<10	30	33	5	38
Streptomycin	0.26	2.5	80	0.03	85	3	41–87	35	22	25	3	28
Tobramycin	0.23	2.5	60	0.04	80	3	80–90	<10	27	32	3	35
Carbapenem												
Imipenem	—	1	1	1	205	205	22	13–21[g]	—	—	—	—
With cilastatin	0.31	1	4–5	0.3	238	54	50–70	13–21[g]	67	41	33	74
Meropenem	0.25	1	10	0.1	250	25	59–79	2	81	—	—	70
Cephalosporins												
Cefaclor	0.24	0.8	2.8	0.3	240	69	—	24	60	39	45	84
Cefadroxil	0.26	1.5	17	0.09	142	10	88–93	20	35	35	10	45
Cefazolin	0.14	1.8	27	0.07	60	5	80–90	70–85	10	21	10	31
Cefixime	0.1	4	13	0.3	119	36	40	65–70	NS	NS	—	NS
Cefmenoxime	0.17	1	8	0.1	2	0.2	80	43–75	—	—	—	16–51
Cefmetazole	0.16	1	24	0.04	126	5	85	85	—	—	—	60
Cefonicid	0.11	5	70	0.07	18	1	88	98	3	5	2	7
Cefoperazone	0.22	1.8	2.9	0.8	100	78	20–30	65–90	62	—	—	—
Cefotetan	0.15	3.7	35	0.1	39	4	60–75	78–91	—	—	—	—
Cefotaxime	0.28	1	2.5	0.4	322	135	40–60	36	81	35	58	93
Desacetylcefotaxime	—	1.3	15	0.09	—	—	—	—	[h]	—	—	—
Cefoxitin	0.30	0.9	22	0.04	290	12	80–90	50–60	—	—	—	—
Ceftazidine	0.24	2	25	0.07	130	7	76–100	10–17	25–50	40	7	47
Ceftizoxime	0.40	1.4	35	0.04	190	6	72	31	—	—	—	—
Ceftriaxone	0.09	6–9	12–57	0.5	15	8	40–65	85–95[g]	NS	NS	—	—
Cefuroxime	0.20	1.3	20	0.07	140	15	95–100	33	—	—	—	—
Cephalexin	0.26	0.8	20	0.04	263	10	90–98	10–15	70	57	8	65
Cephapirin	0.23	0.6	2	0.3	310	93	50–70	44–54	—	17	66	83
Cephradine	0.31	1.0	12	0.08	323	20	78–96	8–20	—	—	—	—
Penicillins												
Amoxicillin	0.2	1	9	0.1	160	25	50–70	15–25	23	27	29	56
Ampicillin	0.48	1.2	14	0.09	325	30	50–90	16–20	46	25	17	42
Cloxacillin	0.15	0.6	0.8	0.8	220	115	62–78	85–95	NS	NS	—	—
Dicloxacillin	0.20	0.7	1.0	0.7	225	160	73–90	97	NS	NS	—	—
Mezlocillin	0.2	1	3.6	0.3	250	50	45–70	16–42	50	46	39	85
Nafcillin	0.32	0.5	1.2	0.4	520	215	35–40	90	NS	NS	—	—
Oxacillin	0.21	0.5	1	0.5	335	170	40–55	93	NS	NS	—	—
Penicillin G	0.18	0.7	13	0.05	205	10	75–90	65	12	19	16	35
Piperacillin	0.21	1	3.3	0.3	188	57	50–70	21	50	39	44	83
Ticarcillin	0.21	1.2	11	0.1	140	15	90–100	45	35	39	17	56

TABLE 85.4. *(Continued)*

Drug Name	Apparent Volume of Distribution (L/kg)	Terminal Half-Life (hr)		F_0	Plasma Clearance (ml/min)		Excreted in Urine Unchanged[a] (%)	Plasma Protein Bound[a] (%)	Hemodialyzer Clearance (ml/min)	Drug Removal During 4 Hr of Hemodialysis		
		Normal	ESRD		Normal	ESRD				Dialysis	Nondialysis	Total
Quinolones												
Ciprofloxacin	2.8	3–4	17	0.3	652	300	40	40	NS	NS	—	—
Enoxacin	2.9	6.5	30	0.2	433	83	26–72	—	—	—	—	—
Grepafloxacin	5	16	16	1	32	50	6	—	—	—	—	—
Levofloxacin	1.1	7	76	0.09	—	—	80	24–38				
Lomefloxacin	—	8	45	0.2	271	31	65–70	—	—	—	—	—
Norfloxacin	—	3–7	7–9	0.5	—	—	33–40[i]	15	NS	NS	—	—
Ofloxacin	1.2	6–7	>50	0.1	234	44	72–99	30	—	—	—	—
Trovafloxacin	1.3	10–12	10–12	1	99	99	10	76	NS	NS	—	NS
Sulfonamides												
Sulfamethoxazole	0.36	10	35	0.3	30	10	16–33	60–68	16	13	8	21
Sulfisoxazole	0.20	6	12	0.5	30	15	50–70	40–90	—	—	—	—
Tetracyclines												
Demeclocycline	1.8	12	50	0.2	121	29	40–50	75–91	—	—	—	—
Doxycycline	0.7	20	20	1	29	29	15–35	80–93	NS	NS	NS	NS
Minocycline	0.4	18	16	1	40	40	5–15	75	NS	NS	NS	NS
Tetracycline	1.5	9	80	0.1	131	14	48–60	25–65	—	—	—	—
Miscellaneous												
Azithromycin	32	68	—	—	630	—	11–14	7–51[g]	NS	NS	NS	NS
Aztreonam	0.2	1.8	7.2	0.3	80	22	60–70	56–60[j]	—	—	—	50
Chloramphenicol	0.9	3	5	0.6	245	147	5–10	25–60	NS	—	—	—
Clarithromycin	3.5	2–7[g]	—	—	400–1,100[g]	—	36[i]	42–72	—	—	—	—
14-Hydroxyclarithromycin	4.3	5–9[g]	—	—	—	—	—	—	—	—	—	—
Clavulanic acid	0.39	1	2.9	0.3	170–260	27–48	22	88	—	—	—	—
Clindamycin	0.7	2.3	4	0.6	250	150	10–28	94	NS	—	—	—
Erythromycin	0.57	2	5	0.4	310	90	15	73–93	NS	—	—	—
Loracarbef	—	1	32	0.03	—	—	90–100	25	—	—	—	—
Metronidazole	0.7	7	7	1	82	82	20	20	—	—	—	—
Nitrofurantoin	0.5	0.3	1	0.3	1360	408	30–50	60	60	12	84	96
Sulbactam	0.25	1	21	0.05	250	—	73–89	—	—	—	—	—
Teicoplanin	0.75	6 days	—	—	10	—	99	90	—	—	—	—
Trimethoprim	2	13	25	0.5	125	65	80–90	40–70	100	15	10	25
Vancomycin	0.47	7	240	0.03	55	2	90–100	10	NS	NS	—	—

[a] In normal adults.
[b] Reported by one investigator.
[c] The plasma concentration-time curve is biphasic with an initial phase half-life of 1.5 to 2 hours and a terminal phase half-life of 8 hours.
[d] Dosage modification felt unnecessary despite change in F_0.
[e] Rapid acetylators.
[f] Slow acetylators.
[g] Concentration dependent.
[h] Half-life decreased from 14 to 3 hours during dialysis.
[i] Data based on oral dosing.
[j] Decreased to 30% in ESRD.
ESRD, end-stage renal disease; NS, no significant removal, but actual clearance unknown.

TABLE 85.5. Pharmacokinetic Properties of Antiarthritic Drugs in Normal Adults and Those with End-Stage Renal Disease

Drug Name	Apparent Volume of Distribution (L/kg)	Terminal Half-Life (hr)		F_0	Plasma Clearance (ml/min)		Excreted in Urine Unchanged[a] (%)	Plasma Protein Bound[a] (%)	Hemodialyzer Clearance (ml/min)	Drug Removal During 4 hr of Hemodialysis		
		Normal	ESRD		Normal	ESRD				Dialysis	Nondialysis	Total
Allopurinol	0.6	5	5	1	245	245	10	<10	—	—	—	—
Oxypurinol	—	24	—	—	—	—	<10	100	—	—	—	—
Aspirin	0.2	2–19[a]	2–19[b]	—	9–85[b]	9–85[b]	5–85[c]	73–94	30	33	22	55
Colchicine	2.1	0.3	0.7	0.4	5650	2420	20–50	<10	NS	NS	—	—
Diclofenac	0.15	1.5	1.5	1.0	80	80	<1	99	NS	NS	—	—
Diflunisal	7.5	11[b]	115	0.09	8	2	<5	99	NS	NS	—	—
Etodolac	0.36	7	—	—	48	—	<1	99	NS	NS	—	—
Fenoprofen	0.15	3	—	1	70	—	<5	>90	NS	NS	—	—
Ibuprofen	0.18	3	3	1	49	49	<5	>90	NS	NS	—	—
Indomethacin	1	5	5	1	163	163	10–20	>90	NS	NS	—	—
Ketoprofen	0.1	3	—	—	70	—	<5	99	NS	NS	—	—
Ketorolac	0.2	5	10	0.5	—	—	50–60	—	—	—	—	—
Meclofenamate	—	3	—	—	—	—	<5	>90	NS	NS	—	—
Nabumetone[d]	0.79	23	40	0.5	26	—	50	>99	NS	NS	—	—
Naproxen	0.12	14	14	1	7	7	<10	>99	NS	NS	—	—
Oxaprozin	0.19	23	—	—	2	—	<1	>99	NS	NS	—	—
Piroxicam	0.14	50	50	1	2	2	<5	99	NS	NS	—	—
Probenecid	0.13	4–17[b]	—	—	15	—	4–13	75	NS	NS	—	—
Salsalate	0.2	1	—	—	—	—	<1	73–94	20[e]	33[e]	22[e]	55[e]
Sulindac	—	8	—	—	—	—	<20	>93	NS	NS	—	—
Sulindac sulfide	—	16	—	—	—	—	<1	>90	NS	NS	—	—
Tolmetin	0.12	1	—	—	100	—	20	>99	NS	NS	—	—

[a] In normal adults.
[b] Dose dependent.
[c] Excretion variable and dependent on dose and urine pH.
[d] Parent drug inactive; values refer to the active metabolite, 6-methoxy-2-naphthylacetic acid.
[e] Calculated as salicylate.
ESRD, end-stage renal disease; NS, no significant removal, but actual clearance unknown.

TABLE 85.6. Pharmacokinetic Properties of Anticoagulant and Antihistamine Drugs in Normal Adults and Those with End-Stage Renal Disease

Drug Name	Apparent Volume of Distribution (L/kg)	Terminal Half-Life (hr)		F_0	Plasma Clearance (ml/min)		Excreted in Urine Unchanged[a] (%)	Plasma Protein Bound[a] (%)	Hemodialyzer Clearance (ml/min)	Drug Removal During 4 Hr of Hemodialysis		
		Normal	ESRD		Normal	ESRD				Dialysis	Nondialysis	Total
Anticoagulants												
Heparin	0.06	1[b]	1.5	1	50	30	50[c]	>90	NS	NS	—	—
Warfarin	0.11	33	30	1	3	3	<1	97	NS	NS	—	—
Antihistamines: H_1-Receptor Antagonists												
Acrivastine	0.7	2.5	—	—	—	—	65	50[d]	—	—	—	—
Astemizole	—	22	—	—	—	—	0	97	NS	NS	NS	NS
Cetirizine	0.7	8	25	0.3	—	—	86	93	NS	NS	—	9
Chlorpheniramine	2.5	13	300	0.4	155	7	<10	72	NS	NS	—	—
Diphenhydramine	3.7	5	—	—	575	—	1	85	NS	NS	—	—
Fexofenadine	5.6	14	25	0.6	—	—	<11	65	—	—	—	—
Loratadine	—	13	—	—	—	—	0	97	NS	NS	NS	NS
Antihistamines: H_2-Receptor Antagonists												
Cimetidine	0.81	2	5	0.4	330	132	45–75	13–25	50	15	39	54
Famotidine	1.4	3	24	0.1	337	47	65–80	17	NS	NS	—	6–16
Nizatidine	1.3	1.6	5.3	0.3	665	233	63	30	35	7	44	51
Ranitidine	1.8	2	10	0.2	727	150	69	15	100	15	23	38
Proton Pump Inhibitors												
Lansoprazole	—	1.5	1	1	—	—	0	97	NS	NS	NS	NS
Omeprazole	0.35	0.5–1	0.6	1	600	562	<1	95	NS	NS	NS	NS

[a] In normal adults.
[b] Increases with dose: 100 U/kg = 1.0 hour; 200 U/kg = 1.5 hours; 400 U/kg = 2.5 hours.
[c] Usually excreted as a metabolite; unchanged drug appears in doses only.
[d] Concentration dependent.
ESRD, end-stage renal disease; NS, no significant removal, but actual clearance unknown.

TABLE 85.7. Pharmacokinetic Properties of Antineoplastic and Immunosuppressive Agents in Normal Adults and Those with End-Stage Renal Disease

Drug Name	Apparent Volume of Distribution (L/kg)	Terminal Half-Life (hr)		F_0	Plasma Clearance (ml/min)		Excreted in Urine Unchanged[a] (%)	Plasma Protein Bound[a] (%)	Hemodialyzer Clearance (ml/min)	Drug Removal During 4 Hr of Hemodialysis		
		Normal	ESRD		Normal	ESRD				Dialysis	Nondialysis	Total
Azathioprine	0.6	3	50	0.6	—	—	10	30	—	—	—	—
Bleomycin	0.35	4	>21[b]	<0.2	71	<13	50–80	1	—	—	—	—
Carboplatin	0.25	6	—	0.06	112	0.7	32[c]	15–24	—	—	—	—
Cisplatin	0.5	0.5[c]	—	—	17	—	27–45	>90	NS	NS	—	—
Cyclophosphamide	0.64	6.5[c]	6.5	1	56	56	21–45	13	78	—	—	—
Cyclosporine	4.3	19	17	1	182	205	<1	90	NS	NS	NS	NS
Cytarabine	2.6	2	—	1	—	—	6	15	—	—	—	—
Etoposide	0.4	6	19	0.3	43	13	20–60	94	NS	NS	—	—
Doxorubicin	20–30	30	—	1	850	—	<15	80–85	NS	NS	—	—
Fluorouracil	0.63	0.3	—	—	514	—	20	—	—	—	—	—
Mycophenolate	4	17	—	—	193	—	<1	97	NS	NS	NS	NS
Melphalan	0.7	1.3	—	—	350	—	12	90	NS	NS	—	—
Methotrexate	0.64[d]	10[e]	64	0.2	52	5	76–80	50–70	30–74	—	—	—
Mitomycin	0.54	0.7	—	—	367	—	—	—	—	—	—	—
Mitoxantrone	14–94	40–200	—	—	358	—	<7	>95	NS	NS	—	—
Tacrolimus	0.9	21	—	—	47	—	<1	75–99	NS	NS	NS	NS
Tamoxifen	20	18	—	—	50	—	0	>98	NS	NS	NS	NS
Vincristine	8.6	1.8	—	—	126	—	12	75	—	—	—	—

[a] In normal adults.
[b] Data on one person with Cl_{cr} = 11 ml/min.
[c] For carboplatin itself, total platinum species are 50% to 75%; only free circulating platinum species appear to possess cytotoxic properties.
[d] Volume of distribution reduced to 0.42 L/kg in ESRD.
[e] Following high-dose treatment.
ESRD, end-stage renal disease; NS, no significant removal, but actual clearance unknown.

TABLE 85.8. Pharmacokinetic Properties of Cardiovascular Drugs in Normal Adults and Those with End-Stage Renal Disease

Drug Name	Apparent Volume of Distribution (L/kg)	Terminal Half-Life (hr)		F_0	Plasma Clearance (ml/min)		Excreted in Urine Unchanged[a] (%)	Plasma Protein Bound[a] (%)	Hemodialyzer Clearance (ml/min)	Drug Removal During 4 Hr of Hemodialysis		
		Normal	ESRD		Normal	ESRD				Dialysis	Nondialysis	Total
Antianginal and/or Hypotensive Drugs												
Acebutolol	1.4	8.8	7.5	1	827	—	12	11–19	43	4	83	87
Diacetolol	—	11	32	0.3	—	—	—	—	40	—	—	—
Amiodipine	21	43	43	1	—	—	5–10	98	NS	NS	NS	NS
Atenolol	1.2	5.5	73	0.07	176	13	85–100	<5	29–39	9	3	12
Benazepril	—	—	—	—	—	—	<1	97	NS	NS	NS	NS
Benazeprilat	—	10	—	—	—	—	20	95	NS	6	—	—
Betaxolol	6	14–22	30	0.7	327	200	16	55	NS	—	—	—
Bisoprolol	2.9	11	24	0.5	250	130	55	30–40	NS	NS	—	—
Captopril	3	1.9	35	0.05	1277	69	50	25–30	120	12	7	19
Carteolol	4	3–7	—	—	735	—	63	—	—	—	—	—
Carvedilol	1.7	8	—	—	—	—	<1	96	NS	NS	NS	NS
Clonidine	3.2	8	40	0.2	315	65	50	20–40	NS	—	—	—
Diltiazem	5.3	4	3.4	1	1400	1400	2	80–85	—	—	—	—
Doxazosin	1.5	20	—	1	119	—	<1	98	NS	NS	NS	NS
Enalapril	—	—	—	—	—	—	18	—	—	—	—	—
Enalaprilat	—	11[b]	130[c]	0.2	—	—	43	<60	40	—	—	55[d]
Esmolol	3.2	0.2	—	—	19950	—	<1	—	—	—	—	—
Felodipine	10	9	9	1	800	800	<1	100	NS	NS	NS	NS
Fosinopril	—	—	—	—	—	—	<1	—	—	—	NS	—
Fosinoprilat	0.14	12	17	0.7	32	22	50	95–100	NS	NS	—	—
Guanabenz	5	4	—	—	—	—	<1	90	NS	NS	NS	NS
Guanethidine	60	120	245	0.5	400	200	35–50	0	NS	—	—	—
Hydralazine	1.6	3	>16	0.2	431	<80	3–14	87	NS	—	—	—
Isradipine	3	8	—	—	1400	—	0	95	NS	NS	—	—
Labetalol	5.6	7	13	0.7	1700	1198	<5	50	31	1	39	40
Lisinopril	1.8	13	>180	0.07	1167	<82	95	0	40	—	—	50[d]
Losartan	—	1.8	—	—	—	—	4	99	NS	NS	—	—
E-3174 (metabolite)	—	7	—	—	—	—	7	—	—	—	—	—
Methyldopa	0.69	2	5	0.4	280	104	24	0	—	—	—	—
Metropolol	4.5	3.5	4	1	1000	1000	3–10	12	NS	—	—	—
Minoxidil	2.5	4.2	4	1	588	588	10	0	48	4	54	58
Nadolol	2	10–14	45	0.2	—	—	70	20–30	46–102	7–16	3–6	13–21
Nicardipine	0.64	0.8–1.7	—	1	560	—	<0.3	99	NS	NS	—	—
Nifedipine	1.4	2	2.6	1	1100	1100	—	90–95	3–8	<1	93	93
Nimodipine	1.6	1.7–7	22	0.1	8925	923	<1	—	—	—	—	—
Penbutolol	—	26	—	0.9	—	—	<10	>95	NS	NS	—	—
Pindolol	2	3–4	3–5	0.7	538	400	35	40–60	—	—	—	—
Prazosin	0.94	3	3	1	255	255	<10	97	NS	NS	—	—
Propranolol	3	3.5	3.5	1	695	695	0	93	NS	NS	—	—
Quinapril	—	1	1	1	—	—	—	—	—	—	—	—
Quinaprilat	0.4	2	20	0.1	140	14	28	97	NS	NS	NS	NS
Ramipril	—	—	—	—	—	—	<2	73	—	—	—	—
Ramiprilat	—	15	—	—	77	—	39	56	—	—	—	—
Reserpine	1.7	60	185	0.3	23	7	1	40	—	—	—	—
Terazosin	—	12	—	—	—	—	12	—	—	—	—	—
Timolol	3.5	3.5	3.5	1	650	650	20	10	NS	NS	—	—
Valsartan	0.24	7.5	—	—	37	—	10	94	NS	NS	NS	NS
Verapamil	5	3.7	3.8	1	1000	1000	3	90	27	2	49	51

(Continued)

TABLE 85.8. *(Continued)*

Drug Name	Apparent Volume of Distribution (L/kg)	Terminal Half-Life (hr)		F_0	Plasma Clearance (ml/min)		Excreted in Urine Unchanged[a] (%)	Plasma Protein Bound[a] (%)	Hemodialyzer Clearance (ml/min)	Drug Removal During 4 Hr of Hemodialysis		
		Normal	ESRD		Normal	ESRD				Dialysis	Nondialysis	Total
Antiarrhythmic Drugs												
Adenosine	—	5 sec	—	1	—	—	0	—	—	—	—	—
Amiodarone	66	25 days	—	1	140	—	<1	96	NS	NS	NS	NS
Bretylium	7	7–8	105	0.07	725	35	77	0–1	NS	—	—	—
Cibenzoline	4.5	7	22	0.3	700	224	60–70	60	—	—	—	—
Disopyramide	0.48	7	30	0.2	59	13	40–60	5–65[d]	30	18	8	26
Flecainide	8.7	14–26	9–58	0.6	567	357	10–50	40	NS	1	NS	—
Lidocaine	1.2	2	2	1	606	606	<10	66	NS	NS	—	—
Mexiletine	5–6	5–9	22	0.3	846	200	<10	<1	NS	NS	—	—
Moricizine	4	1.4	—	1	1400	—	<1	95	NS	NS	—	—
Procainamide	2	2	8	0.3	810	200	40–54	15	65	9	28	37
NAPA	1.5	6	42	0.1	200	29	59–89	10	97	19	6	25
Propafenone	3	2.4[e]	2.8	1	860	1029	<1	77–95	—	—	—	—
Quinidine	2	6	6	1	270	270	10–50	80–85	<10	1	37	38
Tocainide	3.2	11–14	17–43	0.5	182	100	38	10–15	25	3	10	13
Cardiotonic Agents												
Amrinone[g]	1.4	4.4	—	—	280	—	10–40	35–49[h]	—	—	—	—
Amrinone[i]	1.4	2	—	—	616	—	10–40	35–49[h]				
Digitoxin	0.5	145	200	0.7	3	2	8–30	90[h]	NS	NS	—	—
Digoxin	7.1[j]	36	100	0.4	160	35	>90	20–30	20	1	2	3
Milrinone	0.35	0.8	3.2	0.25	400	28	80	70	—	—	—	—

[a] In normal adults.

[b] Serum time curve for enalaprilat is biexponential; the initial phase of 11 hours, which correlates with drug accumulation on chronic dosing; terminal phase has a half-life of 30–35 hours and may represent binding to plasma angiotensin-converting enzyme.

[c] Based on AUC data; patients with Cl_{cr} <60 ml/min eliminate enalaprilat at a significantly slower rate. Patients with ESRD who are receiving hemodialysis may have therapeutic serum concentrations of enalaprilat 96 hours following a single oral dose of enalapril.

[d] Binding is concentration dependent.

[e] Half-life as short as 2.4 hours in fast metabolizers to as long as 32 hours in slow metabolizers.

[f] Patients with PVCs.

[g] Slow acetylators.

[h] Binding is 86% to 89% in ESRD.

[i] Fast acetylators.

[j] V_d = 4.2 L/kg in patients with moderate to severe renal failure.

AUC, area under the curve; Cl_{cr}, creatinine clearance; ESRD, end-stage renal disease; NAPA, *N*-acetylprocainamide; NS, no significant removal, but actual clearance unknown; PVCs, premature ventricular contractions; V_d, volume of distribution.

TABLE 85.9. Pharmacokinetic Properties of Central Nervous System Drugs in Normal Adults and Those with End-Stage Renal Disease

Drug Name	Apparent Volume of Distribution (L/kg)	Terminal Half-Life (hr)		F_0	Plasma Clearance (ml/min)		Excreted in Urine Unchanged[a] (%)	Plasma Protein Bound[a] (%)	Hemodialyzer Clearance (ml/min)	Drug Removal During 4 Hr of Hemodialysis		
		Normal	ESRD		Normal	ESRD				Dialysis	Nondialysis	Total
Analgesics												
Acetaminophen	1	2	2	1	400	400	2–3	10–21[b]	120	19	64	83
Codeine	3.5–6[c]	4	19[d]	0.5	1050	770	<1	7	—	—	—	—
Hydromorphone	2.9	2.4	—	—	1050	—	6	—	—	—	—	—
Meperidine	4.5	3–7	3–7[e]	1	840	840	2	40–60	—	—	—	—
Methadone	3.6	25	—	—	126	—	4	60–90	NS	NS	NS	NS
Morphine	3.2	3	3[f]	1	860	—	10–12	35	—	—	—	—
Pentazocine	6	4	4	1	1330	—	<5	50–75	—	—	—	—
Propoxyphene	16	16	16[g]	1	959	959	1–5[g]	80	NS	NS	NS	NS
Anticonvulsant Drugs												
Carbamazepine	1.1	15	—	1	59	—	1	70–80	NS	NS	NS	NS
Clonazepam	2	25	—	1	65	—	2	47–82	NS	NS	NS	NS
Ethosuximide	0.7	60	—	—	10	—	20	0	—	—	—	—
Felbamate	0.8	21	—	—	35	—	45	23	—	—	—	—
Gabapentin	0.8	6.5	—	—	112	—	80	0	—	—	—	—
Lamotrigine	1.2	23	60	—	—	—	10	40–60	—	—	—	17
Phenytoin	0.57[h]	18	9	2[i]	25	125	5	87–93	0	NS	NS	NS
Primidone	0.6	12	—	1	40	—	1	0	—	—	—	30
Topiramate	0.7	21	—	—	25	—	60	13	—	—	—	—
Valproic acid	0.2	14	—	1	7	—	2	90	NS	NS	NS	NS
Antiemetic Drugs												
Metoclopramide	3.4	3	14	0.2	916	196	20	—	—	—	—	—
Granisetron	2.5	10	—	1	440	—	12	65				
Ondansetron	2.3	10	—	1	650	—	7	75	—	—	—	—
Psychotherapeutic Drugs												
Amitriptyline	—	25	—	—	—	—	—	96	NS	NS	—	—
Chlordiazepoxide	0.3	10	—	1	25	—	0	86–93	NS	NS	—	—
Chlorpromazine	—	15	—	—	—	—	—	90	NS	NS	—	—
Desipramine	—	17	—	—	—	—	—	69–76	NS	NS	—	—
Diazepam	0.74[j]	20	20	1	35	90	1	98	0	—	—	—
Fluoxetine	20–40	3	—	1	672	—	2–5	94	NS	NS	—	—
Haloperidol	23	14	—	—	1330	—	—	90	NS	NS	—	—
Imipramine	—	10	—	—	—	—	—	86–96	18	—	—	—
Lithium carbonate	0.79	30	640	0.05	20	0	89–98	0	150	48	—	—
Nortriptyline	21	23	—	1	740	—	1–4	94	NS	NS	—	—
Sertraline	76	23	—	—	2060	—	<1	99	NS	NS	NS	NS
Sedative/Hypnotics												
Chloral hydrate[k]	6	8	—	—	600	—	—	70–80	120	—	—	—
Ethchlorvynol	2.8	25	—	—	90	—	—	30–50	64	—	—	—
Flurazepam	—	75	—	—	—	—	—	—	NS	NS	—	—
Meprobamate	0.75	10	—	—	60	—	10–20	0–20	60	—	—	—

(Continued)

TABLE 85.9. *(Continued)*

Drug Name	Apparent Volume of Distribution (L/kg)	Terminal Half-Life (hr)		F_0	Plasma Clearance (ml/min)		Excreted in Urine Unchanged[a] (%)	Plasma Protein Bound[a] (%)	Hemodialyzer Clearance (ml/min)	Drug Removal During 4 Hr of Hemodialysis		
		Normal	ESRD		Normal	ESRD				Dialysis	Nondialysis	Total
Sedative/Hypnotics—cont'd												
Methaqualone	6	35	—	—	140	—	—	80	23	—	—	—
Pentobarbital	0.99	22	22	1	36	36	—	66	—	—	—	—
Phenobarbital	0.75	70	100	0.7	9	6	—	25–60	80	—	—	—
Secobarbital	1.42	25	—	—	4.6	—	—	70	NS	NS	—	—

[a] In normal adults.
[b] Concentration dependent.
[c] Increased to 7.3 L/kg in ESRD.
[d] Active metabolites: morphine and morphine glucuronides.
[e] Normeperidine, a metabolite, accumulates in renal failure.
[f] The active glucuronide metabolite accumulates during renal failure.
[g] Norpropoxyphene, a cardiotoxic metabolite, accumulates in renal failure; negligible urinary excretion of parent drug but 20% to 25% of metabolite.
[h] V_d in uremia is 1.4 L/kg body weight.
[i] Fractional clearance is greater than normal in ESRD but dosing is unchanged because of an increase in active unbound drug.
[j] V_d in uremia is 2.2 L/kg body weight.
[k] Data are for the metabolite trichlorethanol.
ESRD, end-stage renal disease; NS, no significant removal, but actual clearance unknown; V_d, volume of distribution.

TABLE 85.10. Pharmacokinetic Properties of Diuretic Drugs in Normal Adults and Those with End-Stage Renal Disease[a]

Drug Name	Apparent Volume of Distribution (L/kg)	Terminal Half-Life (hr)		F_0	Plasma Clearance (ml/min)		Excreted in Urine Unchanged[b] (%)	Plasma Protein Bound[b] (%)	Hemodialyzer Clearance (ml/min)	Drug Removal During 4 Hr of Hemodialysis		
		Normal	ESRD		Normal	ESRD				Dialysis	Nondialysis	Total
Acetazolamide	0.3	8	—	—	30	—	90	70–90	—	—	—	—
Amiloride	17	21	100	—	700	—	49	40	—	—	—	—
Bumetanide	0.15	0.9	1.9	0.5	129	73	66	93	3	3	79	82
Chlorthalidone	0.1	47	—	—	—	—	65	75	NS	NS	NS	NS
Furosemide	0.12	0.5	1.4	0.4	162	105	40–95	95	NS	NS	—	—
Hydrochlorothiazide	0.83	2.5	—	—	343	—	>95	58	—	—	—	—
Indapamide	0.36	15	15	1	20	20	7	76	NS	NS	—	—
Metolazone	—	8	—	—	—	—	—	90	NS	NS	—	—
Spironolactone	—	19	—	1	—	—	1	98	NS	NS	—	—
Torsemide	0.27	3.5	—	—	—	—	20	>99	NS	NS	—	—
Triamterene	13.4	4.2	—	—	4410	—	52	61	—	—	—	—

[a] For organic acid diuretics (e.g., acetazolamide, thiazides, "loop" diuretics, chlorthalidone), natriuresis is dependent on the amount of drug in tubular lumen so that an *increase* in dose is required as renal function decreases. Agents affecting potassium transport (amiloride, spironolactone, triamterene) are best avoided in renal failure.

[b] In normal adults.

ESRD, end-stage renal disease; NS, no significant removal, but actual clearance unknown.

TABLE 85.11. Pharmacokinetic Properties of Antidiabetic Drugs in Normal Adults and Those with End-Stage Renal Disease

Drug Name	Apparent Volume of Distribution (L/kg)	Terminal Half-Life (hr)		F_0	Plasma Clearance (ml/min)		Excreted in Urine Unchanged[a] (%)	Plasma Protein Bound[a] (%)	Hemodialyzer Clearance (ml/min)	Drug Removal During 4 Hr of Hemodialysis		
		Normal	ESRD		Normal	ESRD				Dialysis	Nondialysis	Total
Acarbose	0.32	3[b]	—	1	600	—	<2	15	—	—	—	—
Acetohexamide	0.2	2[c]	30	0.07	80	5	—	65–90	—	—	—	—
Chlorpropamide	0.18	33	65	0.5	4	2	20	60–90	—	—	—	—
Glipizide	0.16	3–7	—	1	52	—	3–10	92–99	NS	NS	—	—
Glyburide	0.3	10–16	—	1	35	—	0	99	NS	NS	—	—
Metformin[d]	—	1.5–6.2	—	—	—	—	90	<1	—[e]	—	—	—
Tolazamide	—	7	—	—	—	—	—	—	—	—	—	—
Tolbutamide	0.2	6	6	1	27	27	—	80–95	NS	NS	—	—
Troglitazone	18	16–34	—	1	—	—	3	99	NS	NS	—	—

[a] In normal adults.
[b] Terminal half-life may be longer but has not been determined because of assay insensitivity.
[c] Half-life of active metabolite is 5 hours.
[d] Drug should not be used in patients with significant renal insufficiency (serum creatinine >1.5 in men and >1.4 in women).
[e] Drug can be removed and acidosis corrected with hemodialysis, but measurable clearances and fractional removal of the drug has not been reported.
ESRD, end-stage renal disease; NS, no significant removal, but actual clearance unknown.

TABLE 85.12. Pharmacokinetic Properties of Miscellaneous Drugs in Normal Adults and Those with End-Stage Renal Disease

Drug Name	Apparent Volume of Distribution (L/kg)	Terminal Half-Life (hr)		F_0	Plasma Clearance (ml/min)		Excreted in Urine Unchanged[a] (%)	Plasma Protein Bound[a] (%)	Hemodialyzer Clearance (ml/min)	Drug Removal During 4 Hr of Hemodialysis		
		Normal	ESRD		Normal	ESRD				Dialysis	Nondialysis	Total
Antilipemic Drugs												
Atorvastatin	—	14	—	1	—	—	2	98	NS	NS	—	—
Clofibrate	0.12[b]	8.6	80	0.1	11	2	32	96	<10	—	—	—
Gemfibrozil	0.14	1	1	1	260[c]	260[c]	<1	97	NS	NS	—	—
Lovastatin	—	1.4	—	—	770	—	<1	95	NS	NS	—	—
Pravastatin	0.46	1.8	—	—	245	—	47	46	—	—	—	—
Simvastatin	—	1.9	—	—	542	—	<1	94	NS	NS	—	—
Hemorrheologic Agents										—	—	—
Pentoxifylline	2.5	3.4	—	1	1333	—	0	—	—	—	—	—
Spasmolytic										—	—	—
Theophylline	0.45	8.7	7.3	1	46	67	<10	60	70	30	28	58
Antimigraine Agents												
Sumatriptan	2.4–3.3	2	—	—	1120	—	22	14–21	—	—	—	—
Dermatologic												
Isotretinoin	—	10–36[d]	—	1	—	—	—	—	—	—	—	—
	—	9[e]	—	1	—	—	0	99	NS	NS	—	—

[a] In normal adults.
[b] V_d is 0.22 L/kg in uremic patients.
[c] Plasma clearance after oral ingestion.
[d] Single dose.
[e] Multiple doses.
ESRD, end-stage renal disease; NS, no significant removal, but actual clearance unknown; V_d, volume of distribution.

the drug, such as its apparent V_d, the rapidity of its transport between body fluid spaces, and the extent of metabolism or excretion from nonrenal sources, also must be considered. For example, if the apparent V_d is very large (more than 1 L/kg body weight), only a small fraction of the drug is available in the plasma for elimination by dialysis. For most drugs, the distribution from plasma into extravascular tissues is rapid and greatly exceeds dialysis clearance. However, a long distribution time indicates that withdrawal of the drug from tissue stores during dialysis may be more rate limiting than dialyzer clearance.

In the end, the additive effect of dialysis clearance on overall drug elimination may be trivial unless it can increase plasma clearance by at least 100% or more (Tables 85.4 to 85.12). Because few drugs have a dialysis clearance exceeding 100 ml/min, the removal of body stores of a drug by dialysis will be significant only when the combined renal (residual function) and nonrenal clearance is less than 150 ml/min. Procainamide is a useful example to illustrate this point. In ESRD, the residual renal clearance is trivial (less than 5 ml/min), but the drug continues to be acetylated at a rapid rate and is cleared from the plasma at a rate of 250 ml/min. However, the kidney principally excretes its metabolite, *N*-acetylprocainamide (NAPA), and its nonrenal removal from plasma is only 30 ml/min. Both agents are active antiarrhythmic drugs and are hemodialyzable, procainamide at a rate of 65 ml/min and NAPA at 97 ml/min. During 4 hours of hemodialysis, removal of procainamide by dialysis is trivial (9%) compared with plasma clearance by biotransformation (28%). However, hemodialysis removal of NAPA is more than threefold its plasma clearance and hence a very significant source of elimination of this metabolite.

Where appropriate data are available, the fraction of drug removed during 4 hours of hemodialysis is included in Tables 85.4 to 85.12. The values reported were calculated using the following equations:

$$\text{Nondialysis removal} = \frac{Cl_{esrd}}{Cl_d + Cl_{esrd}} \times \left[1 - e - \left(\frac{Cl_d + Cl_{esrd}}{V_d}\right) \times t\right] \quad (5)$$

$$\text{Removal by dialysis} = \frac{Cl_d}{Cl_d + Cl_{esrd}} \times \left[1 - e - \left(\frac{Cl_d + Cl_{esrd}}{V_d}\right) \times t\right] \quad (6)$$

$$\text{Total removal} = \text{nondialysis removal} + \text{removal by dialysis} \quad (7)$$

where Cl_d is the hemodialyzer clearance of drug and Cl_{esrd} is the plasma clearance in ESRD and includes elimination from nonrenal sources and residual renal excretion. Nondialysis removal refers to the fraction of drug removed by nonrenal and residual renal routes during the time of dialysis. For the data in Tables 85.4 to 85.12, time (t) is set at 4 hours, a common interval for hemodialysis.

Although dialysis may be a significant route of elimination for some drugs, it is critical to remember that any nonrenal removal or residual renal function may exert a marked effect on the total amount of drug eliminated during treatment because of the long interdialytic interval. Thus plasma clearance of any drug during dialysis treatment must be considered separately from its clearance during the interdialytic interval. Furthermore, because the scheduling and duration of dialysis treatment are selected on clinical grounds alone, it is difficult to predict the plasma concentration for any drug without using pharmacokinetic principles. To make such predictions, however, it is necessary to have data concerning dialyzer clearance, as well as the usual pharmacokinetic data. Unfortunately, few quantitative studies during dialysis have been made with most commonly used drugs.

PREDICTION OF BODY CLEARANCE OF DRUGS IN RENAL FAILURE

It is impossible to predict accurately the pharmacokinetic parameters of a drug in an individual patient. This determination can only be made by measuring drug concentration in plasma in each patient as a function of time. However, a reasonable estimate of the plasma clearance of a drug in azotemic patients can be made if the renal and plasma clearances of the drug in persons with normal renal function are known. Such estimates are based on the assumption that the nonrenal clearance (plasma clearance minus renal clearance) of the drug is not affected by renal disease and that the degree of reduction of the renal clearance is proportional to the GFR estimated by the endogenous creatinine clearance, as shown in the following equation:

$$GFR = \alpha \times Cl_{cr} \quad (8)$$

where α is a proportionality constant. Therefore the plasma clearance in Equation 3 can be symbolically rewritten as follows:

$$Cl_p = (\alpha \times Cl_{cr}) + Cl_{nr} \quad (9)$$

There are problems with the assumptions cited. Nonrenal clearance may be subject to pronounced interindividual variation and may be affected by renal disease. Also, the apparent V_d of a drug may be modified by renal disease. Such estimates are approximations and are unsuitable for use in patients with variable renal function. Despite these limitations, the approach is reasonable for a first estimate of drug dosage. This estimate should then be refined on the basis of information obtained from monitoring plasma drug concentration during treatment and, where possible, from an assessment of the patient's clinical response.

Dosing Nomograms and Renal Function

Referring to the relationships described in Equation 3, plasma clearance could be of three forms: (a) mainly renal, (b) mainly nonrenal, or (c) a combination of both renal and nonrenal (Fig. 85.3). Gentamicin represents a drug that is eliminated almost exclusively by renal clearance; doxycycline is excreted mainly by nonrenal routes, and changes in renal function do not exert any effect on its plasma clearance; and cloxacillin undergoes both renal and nonrenal elimination. Note that the intercept of the various dosing lines with the ordinate represents the nonrenal rate of removal in functionally anephric patients.

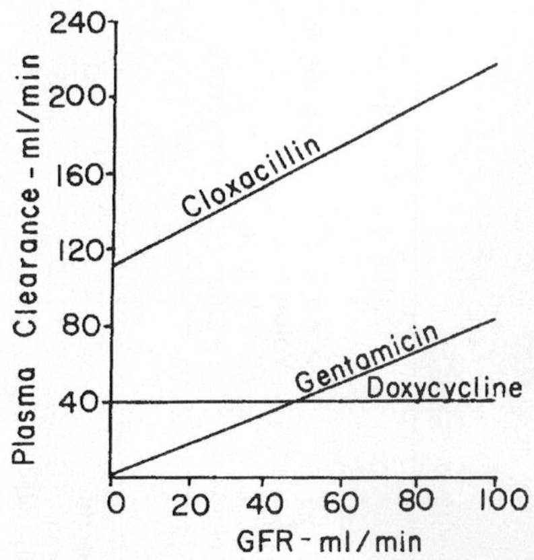

Figure 85.3. The relationship between plasma clearance and glomerular filtration rate (GFR) for cloxacillin, gentamicin, and doxycycline. Note that the elimination of doxycycline is independent of renal function, and cloxacillin has a large nonrenal clearance.

The spectrum of plasma clearance of drugs is large and depends on the major routes of elimination and the functional state of these routes. For drugs with substantial renal elimination, dosage calculations must be individualized when renal failure is present. Grouping the degree of renal dysfunction into mild, moderate, and severe categories, with suggested dosage adjustment modifications for each group, is often used. Although this approach is simple, it does not enhance an understanding of the drug kinetics underlying these suggestions. Therefore a system that is reasonably simple and enhances a comprehension of the pharmacokinetic principles is chosen for discussion here.

For patients in whom renal function is compromised, dosing nomograms (Fig. 85.4) have been developed to help achieve the usual therapeutic plasma concentrations of a drug. To simplify the estimating process, a graphic estimate is made of a specific drug plasma clearance in relation to the degree of renal failure that is currently present. The nomogram is based on changes in the plasma clearance fraction, F, as a linear function of the creatinine clearance. F is called the *plasma clearance fraction* because it describes the plasma clearance as a fraction of the mean plasma clearance in subjects with normal renal function (Cl in excess of 75 ml/min).

$$F = \frac{Cl_r + Cl_{nr}}{Cl_p} \tag{10}$$

In the anuric or functionally anephric patient ($Cl_r = 0$ ml/min), the plasma clearance fraction is called F_0 and is calculated as follows:

$$F_0 = \frac{Cl_{nr}}{Cl_p} \tag{11}$$

In the subject with normal renal function, F = 1.

Because of these relationships, a dosing line for a specific drug is constructed by drawing a line between its F_0 value on the left ordinate and F = 1 at the right upper corner of the nomogram (Fig. 85.4). The point of intersection between the patient's creatinine clearance and the dosing line indicates, at the left ordinate, the estimated plasma clearance fraction, F, for the drug in this patient. The values of F, for various drugs calculated according to Equations 9 and 11, and other useful pharmacokinetic data, are listed in Tables 85.4 to 85.12.

Example. This question might be asked: How much change must be made in the maintenance dose or dosing interval for erythromycin in a patient with a creatinine clearance of 30 ml/min?

Calculation of the fractional value, F, will give the answer to that question. First, turn to Table 85.4 and find the F_0 value. For erythromycin, this number is 0.40. This indicates that the Cl_p in

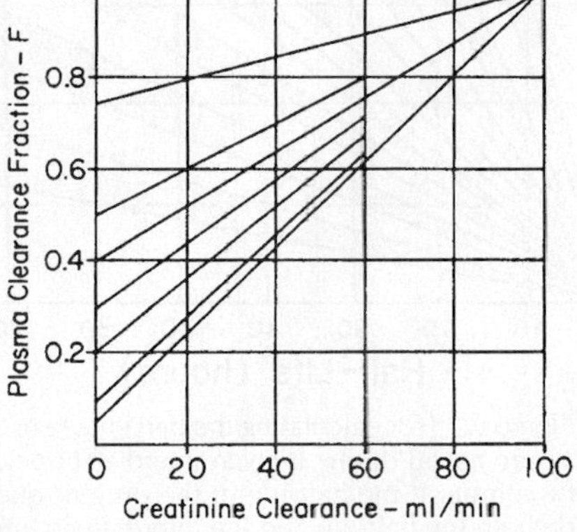

Figure 85.4. Nomogram for the graphic determination of the individual plasma clearance fraction, *F*, of drugs in patients with renal failure. Use of nomogram explained in the text.

an anephric patient is 40% of that seen in patients with normal renal function. Thus 40% of erythromycin plasma clearance occurs through nonrenal routes. The value 0.40 is plotted on the left ordinate of the dosing nomogram (Fig. 85.4). This point is then connected with a line to the right upper corner of the nomogram. Next, the current stable creatinine clearance is found on the abscissa, in this case, 30 ml/min. The point of intersection between this patient's Cl_{cr} and the dosing line for erythromycin, as read on the ordinate, is the individual clearance rate fraction, F, in this patient. The number in this case is 0.58. This indicates that the plasma clearance for erythromycin in an average patient with a Cl_{cr} of 30 ml/min is 58% of that in a patient with a Cl_{cr} of 100 ml/min. Further use of this value in dosage modification is illustrated in a subsequent section.

Estimation of Creatinine Clearance

Serum creatinine is used as a predictor of creatinine clearance to avoid difficulties and inaccuracies with direct measurement. In principle, a reciprocal relationship between serum creatinine and the creatinine clearance is expected if its endogenous production and metabolism are constant. However, production and metabolism are dependent on body muscle mass, gender, age, and disease. Nonetheless, several formulas and nomograms have been reported to predict creatinine clearance from serum creatinine concentrations without the necessity of collecting urine. One such formula (Cockcroft and Gault) is as follows:

$$Cl_{cr} = \frac{(140 - Age)\ (Body\ weight)}{72 \times \text{Serum creatinine}} \tag{12}$$

Age is expressed in years, weight in kilograms, serum creatinine in mg/dl, and creatinine clearance in ml/min. Although the formula was developed from data in adult men, it may be used for women provided the estimated creatinine clearance is reduced by 15%.

This relationship between the creatinine clearance and the serum creatinine concentration is *not valid and should not be used in the following circumstances:* (a) acute renal failure or unstable renal function, (b) patients receiving dialysis, and (c) abnormalities of muscle mass, such as cachexia, muscular dystrophies, trauma, and rhabdomyolysis. In these situations, the actual creatinine clearance should be measured.

PRINCIPLES OF DOSAGE MODIFICATION

A very precise modification of the dosage regimen clearly is not important for drugs that have minor or insignificant adverse effects or are cleared rapidly by nonrenal routes. Also, no mathematic formula will prevent adverse effects when a drug is very toxic, especially if the therapeutic versus toxic margin is small. In such cases, only clinical knowledge of the possible adverse effects and pharmacokinetics of the drug, along with repeated clinical observation and measurements of plasma levels, will prevent undesirable effects.

Ideally, modification of the dosage regimen should produce serum concentrations as close as possible to those observed in normal subjects. Unfortunately, such a goal is impossible except in the case of continuous intravenous therapy. In addition, quite often the basic pharmacologic properties of the drug are not well understood in patients with normal kidney function and less so in patients with renal insufficiency. Thus uncertainties usually exist about the relative importance of the drug peak and trough concentrations and the duration of blood concentration necessary to obtain reasonably effective and safe pharmacologic effects. With these important reservations in mind, the following methods of modifying drug dosage regimen in renal insufficiency are presented.

Clinically, two dosing goals are potentially useful: (a) to reach the same maximum and minimum blood levels or (b) to achieve a similar amount of drug in the body during a given dosage interval (i.e., a similar drug residence time) for both normal and renal failure patients. Independent of the approach used, the desired effect can be approximated by the usual three types of dosage modification: (a) increase of dosage intervals without changing the dose, (b) reduction of the dose without changing the frequency of administration, or (c) a combination of both interval and dosage modification.

The best approach for dosing modification of an individual drug will be determined by numerous factors, such as the dosage form, the pharmacologic characteristics of the drug, the severity of the renal disease, and last but not least, the sophistication of the clinician in pharmacokinetics.

Use of Dosing Nomogram

A general dosing nomogram (Fig. 85.4) can be used to modify a normal dosage regimen in stable renal failure. Four arithmetic values are required for calculation: (a) the normal dosage regimen; (b) the fractional elimination rate in anuria, F_0; (c) the current creatinine clearance; and (d) the elimination rate fraction, F, for the current Cl_{cr}.

Example. What changes might be made in the dosage regimen for gentamicin in a 60-year-old patient weighing 75 kg with a serum creatinine of 4 mg/dl?

Step 1. The normal dosage regimen would be to give 1 to 2 mg/kg every 8 hours; 1 mg/kg × 75 kg = 75 mg every 8 hours.

Step 2. The F_0 value (Table 85.4) for gentamicin is 0.03. This value is located on the left side of the nomogram and is connected with a straight line to the right upper corner of the nomogram.

Step 3. The current Cl_{cr} is estimated as follows:

$$Cl_{cr} = \frac{(140 - 60)(75)}{72 \times 4} = 21 \text{ ml/min} \quad (13)$$

Step 4. The point of intersection of a Cl_{cr} of 21 ml/minute with the dosing line for gentamicin is F = 0.24.

Based on these values, the following modifications are possible:

1. Change the usual dosing interval: 8 hours/0.24 = 33 hours.
2. Change the maintenance dose: 75 mg × 0.24 = 8 mg.
3. Change the rate of administration: 75 mg/8 hours × 0.24 = 2.3 mg/hour or 27 mg/12 hours.

In this patient, an initial loading dose of 75 mg (1 mg/kg) could be followed by any of the suggested modifications. Modification of the dosing interval (method 1) is the most common technique used for aminoglycoside drugs in renal failure because it appears to be the safest. Altering the dosing interval gives high peaks and low troughs because most of the drug is excreted before the next dose is given. Thus the risk of ototoxicity and nephrotoxicity from high sustained tissue and plasma concentrations of gentamicin may be lessened.

Changing the maintenance dose of aminoglycoside drugs with method 2 or the rate of administration with method 3 gives a plateau effect with moderate oscillation of the plasma concentration around the mean. This technique *may* be (not proven) more therapeutically effective but also may be more toxic. However, for certain agents such as the antiarrhythmic and anticonvulsant drugs, the maintenance of a relatively constant plasma concentration is desirable, and if drug modification is needed, dosage or rate modification rather than interval changes should be made.

Dosage Modification During Dialysis Treatment

Drug removal in patients during dialysis theoretically can be predicted by the relationship shown in Equation 3. There are at least two general areas of consideration in determining a dose: pharmacokinetic and pharmacodynamic. Drugs with short half-lives in ESRD relative to their dosing interval are usually administered in the same doses as in patients with normal renal function. For example, acetaminophen with a half-life of 8.3 hours in ESRD is given every 4 to 6 hours, as is customary in patients without renal failure. For agents with a long half-life of 24 hours or more, it is most convenient to make the dosing interval coincide with the end of each dialysis treatment when hemodialysis or intermittent peritoneal dialysis is used. If significant removal occurs during intermittent dialysis, supplemental doses are required to replace those lost during both the interdialytic interval and the dialysis procedure. With continuous ambulatory peritoneal dialysis (CAPD), drug removal is slow and low. Dosage modifications with CAPD are best made assuming that the patient has a removal rate comparable with a GFR of 10 ml/min and using the dosage nomogram in the manner already described.

When supplemental doses of an agent are required following intermittent dialysis, it is necessary to first determine the amount of drug eliminated between doses. This usually includes the loss during the interdialytic interval plus losses during the dialysis treatment. The first step is a calculation of the amount of loss occurring during the interdialytic interval. This is easily estimated with Fig. 85.5. The half-life in ESRD (Tables 85.4 to 85.12) is located on the abscissa and a vertical line is extended until it intersects with a horizontal line extending from the ordinate, representing the time since the last dose, excluding the dialysis interval. The closest diagonal line to this intersection represents the approximate amount of drug that is eliminated during the interdialytic interval.

As an example, consider captopril with a half-life in ESRD of about 35 hours (Table 85.8). With a typical interdialytic interval of approximately 44 hours, Fig. 85.5 indicates a loss of between 56% and 62% of body stores. If dialysis was not done,

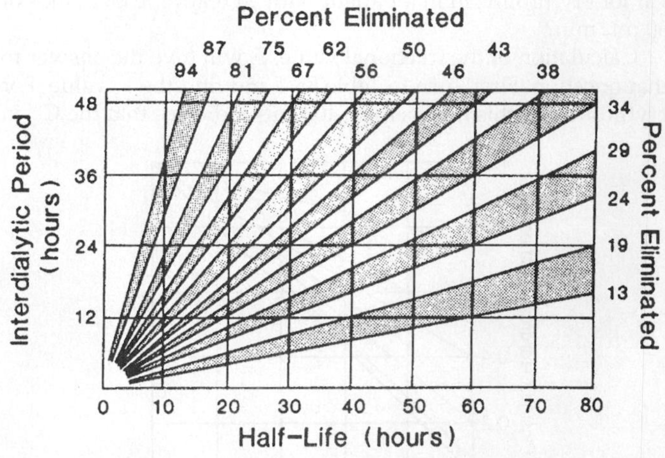

Figure 85.5. Nomogram for calculating the percentage of the body stores of a drug that are removed during a given interdialytic interval based on the half-life of the drug. If the half-life of the drug in question exceeds 80 hours, divide both the half-life and the interdialytic interval by 2 and use the nomogram in the usual way. An explanation for use of the nomogram is given in the text.

a dose of approximately 60% of the initial dose would replenish body stores. Four hours of hemodialysis removes approximately 19% of the drug that is present at the time of hemodialysis. Because approximately 60% of the dose was eliminated during the interdialytic interval before hemodialysis, leaving only 40% in the body, hemodialysis will remove 19% of this 40%, or an additional 8%. Thus a postdialysis dose of approximately 68% of the initial dose would restore body stores of this drug.

Once the pharmacokinetic estimates of the loss are calculated, a clinical decision is made about an acceptable fluctuation in body stores or plasma concentration of the administered drug. This decision determines the frequency of the interdialytic dose and whether postdialysis supplementation is necessary. Pharmacokinetic data and conventional dosing intervals when renal function is normal are extremely important. For example, isoniazid has a half-life of between 1 and 3 hours when renal function is normal and is administered every 24 hours. In ESRD, the half-life of isoniazid increases to 4 hours, but a conventional dosing interval can still be used because six half-lives occur between doses and 98% of the drug is eliminated. Although hemodialysis removes a substantial amount of isoniazid, 62% in 4 hours, removal is not greater in 24 hours than occurs when renal function is normal. Therefore in an adult with ESRD, a reasonable dosing regimen for isoniazid would be 300 mg given once daily. On a dialysis day, the dose would be given at the end of hemodialysis.

Another example is cotrimoxazole (trimethoprim-sulfamethoxazole), which is dosed every half-life (every 12 hours) when renal function is normal. In ESRD, the half-life of trimethoprim and sulfamethoxazole increase to about 25 hours and 35 hours, respectively. Although there is a slight accumulation (approximately 32%) of sulfamethoxazole above that expected in patients with normal renal function if a customary dose of cotrimoxazole is administered every 24 hours, accumulation of trimethoprim should be similar to that in normal subjects, and dialysis removal every other day should drop sulfamethoxazole accumulation to an acceptable concentration.

For drugs with known therapeutic ranges, such as anticonvulsants and some antiarrhythmics, the dosing interval can be determined by matching the percentage fall in serum concentration with the percentage lost, using Fig. 85.5. The dosing interval is found by drawing a horizontal line across to the ordinate (dosing interval) from the point where a vertical line from the abscissa, at the drug half-life, intersects with the diagonal bar corresponding to the percentage fall in plasma concentration. In some cases, the dosing interval may be inconvenient. Here again, clinical judgment is necessary in adjusting the dose, as well as the dosing interval, using F_0 to arrive at a regular dosing interval.

Selected Readings

Brater DC. *Drug use in clinical medicine,* 6th ed. Indianapolis, IN: Improved Therapeutics, Inc., 1993.

An excellent small booklet with useful data on the kinetics of drugs in renal failure, cirrhosis, and heart failure, with suggestions for therapy.

Cockcroft DW, Gault MH. Prediction of creatinine clearance from serum creatinine. *Nephron* 1976;16:31–47.

One of the earliest descriptions of the correlation of serum creatinine with measured creatinine clearance.

Dettli I. Elimination kinetics and dosage adjustment of drugs in patients with kidney disease. *Prog Pharmacol* 1977;1:1–34.

A classic, detailed description of a simplified scheme for modifying dosage in renal failure. The major emphasis is on principles and concepts.

Gibson TP. Problems in designing hemodialysis drug studies. *Pharmacotherapy* 1985;5:23–29.

A discussion of the best techniques for obtaining reliable pharmacokinetic data in dialysis patients.

Kroh UF, Holl TJ, Steinhdauber W. Management of drug dosing in continuous renal replacement therapy. *Semin Dial* 1996;9:161–165.

Review of the factors involved in the process of drug removal during continuous renal replacement, a technique often used instead of intermittent hemodialysis in acute renal failure.

Lam YW, Banerji S, Hatfield C, et al. Principles of drug administration in renal insufficiency. *Clin Pharmacokinet* 1997;32:30–57.

A recent review of the pharmacologic principles involved in drug modification in renal insufficient patients. Extensive reference list.

Swan SK. Pharmacologic approach to renal insufficiency. In: Dale DC, Federman DD, eds. *Scientific American medicine.* (Nephrology) 1998.

A brief update on drug use in renal failure, with specific suggestions regarding dosage modification.

PART 2
Use of Drugs in Renal Failure

George R. Aronoff and Michael E. Brier

Introduction

Uremia effects every organ system in the body. The kidney is the major regulator of the internal fluid environment, and the physiologic changes associated with renal disease have pronounced effects on the pharmacology of many drugs. Changes in the absorption, distribution, metabolism, and excretion of drugs and their active or toxic metabolites are frequent in patients with impaired renal function. Furthermore, renal impairment is often superimposed on underlying problems, such as hypertension, diabetes, and heart disease. These comorbidities compound the complexity of drug management.

Several factors have led to an increased number of patients with impaired renal function. Patients with chronic diseases that decrease renal function live longer because of improved management of their underlying diseases. We now provide chronic renal replacement therapy to patients with advanced age, diabetes mellitus, and coronary artery disease. Because renal function decreases with age, and patients older than the age of 65 years make up the most rapidly growing patient group for which special understanding of drug disposition is important.

The application of continuous extracorporeal renal replacement with new dialysis membranes and devices, and the widespread use of intermittent and continuous peritoneal dialysis enhance the need for detailed understanding of drug transport across biologic and artificial membranes. This chapter provides a rational schema of pharmacotherapy for patients with decreased renal function and for those on dialysis. It describes some of the biochemical and physiologic effects of uremia on drug disposition, and the effects of dialysis on drug and metabolite removal.

Patient Assessment

A careful history and physical examination is essential for appropriate pharmacotherapy of patients with kidney disease. Medication history and drug-related allergy or toxicity are important in the initial evaluation of patients with impaired renal function. Dialysis patients average more than eight concurrent medications and suffer three times the incidence of adverse drug events as patients with normal renal function. Preventing potential drug interactions before choosing a drug regimen may reduce adverse drug events.

Before initiating drug therapy, a specific diagnosis should be established. This approach decreases the chances of untoward drug interactions by minimizing polypharmacy. Therapeutic choices should be individualized such that one drug is used to treat several conditions. For example, an angiotensin-converting enzyme (ACE) inhibitor used to lower blood pressure in a hypertensive patient can also improve heart failure and slow the progression of diabetic glomerulosclerosis.

Determination of an appropriate loading dose requires an assessment of hydration status because the extracellular fluid volume determines the distribution volume of many drugs. Edema or ascites increases the volume of distribution of water-soluble drugs, while dehydration contracts this volume. A usual loading dose of a water-soluble drug given to an edematous patient will result in potentially subtherapeutic effect, whereas dose-related toxicity may occur in dehydrated patients. After the state of hydration is determined, an appropriate adjustment to the recommended loading dose can be made.

Accurate drug dosing also requires measurements of body height and weight. Ideal body weight (IBW) can be a guide for dosing obese patients. For men, IBW is 50 kg plus 2.3 kg for each inch over 5 feet. For women, IBW is 45.5 kg plus 2.3 kg for each inch over 5 feet. Many clinicians use the average of the measured body weight and the IBW as the value on which to base drug doses.

Liver impairment has a substantial effect on drug therapy in patients with renal disease by limiting alternative pathways for drug and metabolite elimination. Finding the stigmata of liver disease is a strong indication of the need to further decrease drug doses in patients with renal impairment.

Measurement of Renal Function

The glomerular filtration rate (GFR) determines the rate and extent of drug and metabolite elimination by the kidneys, even for drugs primarily excreted by tubular secretion. However, the serum creatinine measurement also reflects muscle mass. Serum creatinine measurements within the normal range will not accurately estimate renal function in elderly or debilitated patients. In such patients, the use of standard drug doses may result in serious overdose and toxic drug or metabolite accumulation.

The Cockroft and Gault equation relates the serum creatinine measurement to the patient's age, body mass, and gender, as follows:

$$Cl_{Cr} = \frac{(140 - \text{age}) \times \text{Body weight in kg} \times (0.85 \text{ if female})}{72 \times \text{SrCr in mg/dl}}$$

where Cl_{Cr} is the creatinine clearance (ml/min) and *SrCr* is the serum creatinine (mg/dl).

When renal function is unstable, the serum creatinine does not reflect the clearance rate. Oliguric patients usually have a creatinine clearance of less than 5 ml/min.

Dialysis patients may have residual renal function that contributes to the elimination of drugs and their metabolites. Residual renal function decreases over time, but depends on the level of renal function present at the initiation of renal replacement therapy and the underlying renal disease. Most dialysis patients lose any remaining renal function during the first year after they start dialysis.

Serum creatinine measurements alone should never be used to estimate intrinsic renal function in dialysis patients. Estimating residual renal function in nonoliguric dialysis patients is difficult, because the serum creatinine reflects the adequacy of dialysis and muscle mass, as well as residual glomerular filtration. Because creatinine clearance measurements do not accurately estimate the GFR in patients with renal failure requiring dialysis, the determination of renal function requires measurement of the plasma clearance rate of radioisotopes or other markers of glomerular filtration such as iothalamate or iohexol.

Medications may interfere with laboratory measurements of renal function. Drugs can falsely increase or decrease the measurement of serum creatinine concentration, urea nitrogen, and uric acid, and alter urine color or urine protein concentration.

Drug Dosing Calculations

When the physical examination suggests that a patient with renal impairment has a normal extracellular fluid volume, an initial drug dose equal to the dose given to a patient with normal renal function should produce therapeutic drug concentrations rapidly. A loading dose of any drug can be calculated from the following expression:

$$\text{Loading Dose} = V_d \times \text{IBW} \times \text{Cp}$$

where V_d is the drug's volume of distribution (L/kg), *IBW* is the patient's ideal body weight (kg), and *Cp* is the desired steady-state plasma drug concentration.

For subsequent drug doses, the fraction of the normal dose recommended for a patient with renal failure can be calculated as follows:

$$\text{Df} = t_{1/2} \text{ normal}/t_{1/2} \text{ renal failure}$$

where *Df* is the fraction of the normal dose to be given, $t_{1/2}$ *normal* is the elimination half-life of the drug in a patient with normal renal function, and $t_{1/2}$ *renal failure* is the elimination half-life of the drug in a patient with renal failure. To maintain the normal dose interval in patients with renal impairment, the amount of each dose, following the loading dose, can be determined from the following relationship:

$$\text{Dose in renal impairment} = \text{Normal dose} \times \text{Df}$$

The resulting dose is usually given at the same dose interval as that for patients with normal renal function. This method is effective for drugs with a narrow therapeutic range and a short plasma half-life. Figure 85.6 illustrates plasma concentrations following an initial loading dose and reduction of the individual doses.

Prolonging the dose interval in dialysis patients is a convenient method to reduce drug dosage. This method is particularly useful for drugs with a broad therapeutic range and long plasma half-life. If prolonging the dose interval, rather than decreasing the individual doses, is desirable, the dose interval in renal impairment can be estimated from the following expression:

$$\text{Dose interval in renal impairment} = \text{Normal dose interval/Df}$$

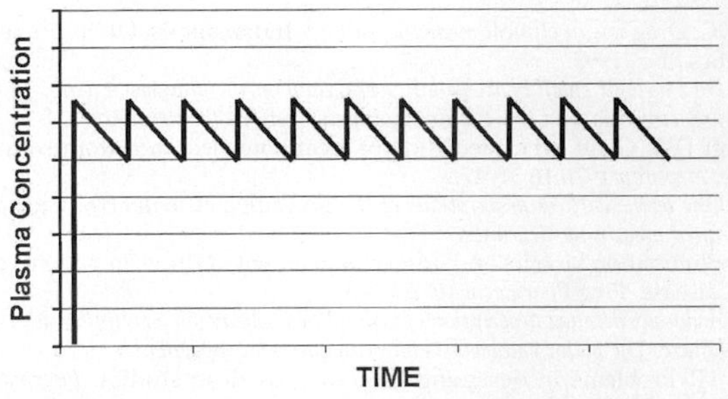

Figure 85.6. Plasma concentrations following a normal loading dose and reduced maintenance doses. This approach avoids high-peak and low-trough concentrations and is best for drugs with a narrow range between the therapeutic and toxic concentrations.

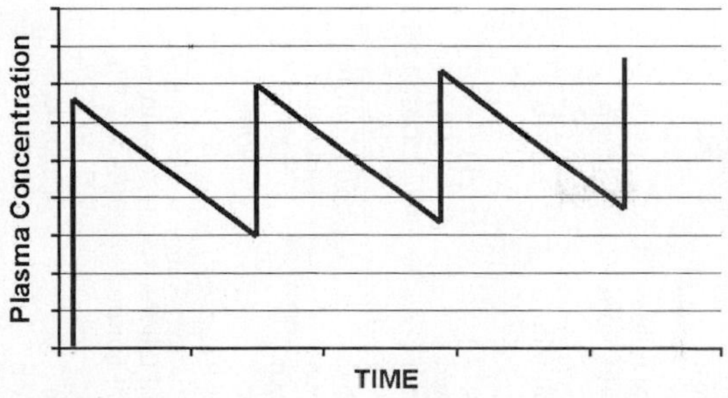

Figure 85.7. Plasma concentrations following a normal loading dose and repeated normal doses at a prolonged dose interval. Higher-peak and lower-trough concentrations result.

If the range between therapeutic and toxic levels is too narrow, either potentially toxic or subtherapeutic plasma concentrations result. The resulting plasma concentrations from prolonging the dose interval in an individual with impaired renal function are shown in Fig. 85.7.

Combining dose reduction and interval prolongation is a practical and convenient approach. The dosage is modified by multiplying the usual daily maintenance dose by the dose fraction. Once the average daily dose is calculated, it can be divided into convenient dosing intervals. The decision to extend the dosing interval beyond a 24-hour period should be based on the need to maintain therapeutic peak or trough levels. The dosing interval may be prolonged if the peak level is most important. When the minimum trough level must be maintained, it is preferable to modify the individual dose or use a combination of dose and interval methods to determine the correct dosing strategy. Drugs removed by dialysis and given once daily should be given after the dialysis treatment.

SPECIFIC DRUG CLASSES IN PATIENTS WITH RENAL FAILURE

Analgesics

Hepatic metabolism illuminates most commonly used analgesics. They require little does reduction for patients with renal insufficiency. Saturable, nonlinear excretion complicates salicylate elimination kinetics. Because of the hemorrhagic diathesis in patients with severe renal failure and the variability of salicylate elimination, avoid large doses of aspirin in patients with severe renal failure. Narcotic analgesics produce sedation that may be more profound in patients with renal insufficiency. The clinician must carefully titrate the doses of these drugs and use the smallest effective doses for the shortest possible time. Meperidine requires special care. The primary metabolite, normeperidine, has little analgesic activity, accumulates in patients with renal failure, and may decrease the seizure threshold. Reports document similar less frequent effects with morphine and its metabolite, normorphine. Although meperidine and morphine can be used in patients with severe renal failure, repetitive doses should be avoided.

Antihypertensive and Cardiovascular Agents

Hypertension and coronary heart disease occur frequently in patients with impaired renal function. Antihypertensive and cardiovascular agents are the most commonly prescribed drugs in patients with renal disease. Narrow therapeutic range and individual variability in drug response complicate the use of these drugs. As indicated in Table 85.13, some of these drugs or their metabolites accumulated in patients with renal insufficiency. Abnormalities of drug binding to plasma proteins increase free drug at receptor sites, enhancing both drug efficacy and toxicity.

The relationship between renal drug limitation and the cardiovascular system is well established. Drugs may alter their own elimination rate or their effect on the kidneys by improving cardiac output and effective renal blood flow. For example, patients with decompensated congestive heart failure may be resistant to diuretics. If natriuresis can be initiated, the subsequent improvement in cardiovascular function can increase response to the diuretic. Thus the effect of cardiovascular drugs may also vary for individual patients as cardiac function changes.

The use of antiarrhythmic agents requires particular care. Because toxicity may appear as the arrhythmia that the drug is intended to correct, recognition of toxicity may be delayed. Inappropriate increases in antiarrhythmic dose may be fatal. Monitoring other electrocardiographic evidence of toxicity, for example, prolonged QT interval or widening of the QRS complex, may be essential for proper diagnosis. Procainamide presents particular difficulty in patients with renal dysfunction. If elimination it is slowed by renal failure, the excretion of its primary metabolite, *N*-acetylprocainamide (NAPA), also depends on kidney function. The parent drug and metabolite appear to have different antiarrhythmic spectrums and elimination rates. Avoiding procainamide in patients with renal impairment would seem prudent, but this approach is often not practical. Careful monitoring is essential, and measurement of drug and metabolite levels may be helpful.

The kidney eliminates many antihypertensive agents. The wide variability of drug response makes it necessary that the response of blood pressure to dose be monitored for individual patients. Steady-state drug levels are usually not achieved until after the drug has been given for a least three to four half-lives.

Diuretics remain an essential part of antihypertensive therapy. They can be grouped into two categories based on their clinical use. The potassium-sparing diuretics may produce hyperkalemia in patients with creatinine clearances lower than 30 ml/min and should be avoided in these patients. The remaining diuretics are organic acids and need to reach the tubular lumen to be active. In patients with impaired real function, endogenous organic acids accumulate and compete with diuretics for secretion into the tubular lumen. Consequently, as renal function decreases, large doses of diuretics are required. As glomerular filtration falls, the thiazides become ineffective. However, large doses of loop diuretics may still produce diuresis. In patients with renal insufficiency, diuretic-induced dehydration may result in further loss of renal function. Unless patients require diuresis for substantial peripheral edema or congestive heart failure, hypertension in patients with decreased renal function should be managed to avoid unnecessary volume contraction. Each of the antihypertensive drugs listed in Table 85.13 can be toxic. In general, the adverse effects are related to the pharmacologic effect and can be avoided by careful dose titration. The development of newer, effective antihypertensive agents allows more individualized therapy. In choosing an antihypertensive agent, one should understand the altered homeostatic mechanisms in patients with impaired renal function.

When blood pressure is appropriately lowered in hypertensive patients with renal insufficiency, a transient decrease in renal function may occur. As hypertensive microvascular changes improve, renal function should increase. In some cases, dialysis may be needed temporarily. If renal function decreases with antihypertensive therapy and does not improve, drug-related nephrotoxicity or other potentially reversible causes should be considered.

(*Text continued on p. 1596.*)

TABLE 85.13. Dose Adjustment for Drugs Frequently Used in Patients with Renal Failure

Drug	Half-Life (hr) Normal/Renal Failure	Protein Binding (%)	Volume of Distribution (L/kg)	Method	Renal Failure Dose	Dose After Hemodialysis	Dose During CAPD	Dose During CRRT
Acarbose	3–9/Prolonged	15	0.32	D	Avoid	Unknown	Unknown	Avoid
Acebutolol	7–9/7	20	1.2	D	30% to 50%	None	None	50%
Acetazolamide	1.7–5.8/Unknown	70–90	0.2	I	Avoid	Unknown	Unknown	Avoid
Acetohexamide	1–1.3/Unchanged	65–90	0.21	I	Avoid	Unknown	None	Avoid
Acetohydroxamic acid	3.5–5/15–23	Unknown	Unknown	D	Avoid	Unknown	Unknown	Unknown
Acetaminophen	2/2	20–30	1–2	I	q8h	None	None	q6h
Acetylsalicylic acid (Aspirin)	2–3/Unchanged	80–90	0.1–0.2	I	Avoid	Dose after dialysis	None	q4–6h
Acrivastine	1.4–2.1/Unknown	50	0.6–0.7	D	Unknown	Unknown	Unknown	Unknown
Acyclovir	2.1–3.8/20	15–30	0.7	D,I	2.5 mg/kg q24h	Dose after dialysis	Dose for renal failure	3.5 mg/kg/day
Adenosine	<10 sec/Unchanged	0	?	D	100%	None	None	100%
Albuterol	2–4/4	7	2–2.5	D	50%	Unknown	Unknown	75%
Alcuronium	3–3.5/16	40	0.28–0.36	D	Avoid	Unknown	Unknown	Avoid
Alfentanil	1.4–2/Unchanged	88–95	0.3–1.0	D	100%	Unknown	Unknown	100%
Alfentanil	1–3/Unchanged	88–95	0.3–1	D	100%	NA	NA	NA
Allopurinol	2–8/Unchanged	<5	0.5	D	25%	½ dose	Unknown	50%
Alprazolam	9.5–19/Unchanged	70–80	0.9–1.3	D	100%	None	Unknown	NA
Alteplase (tPA)	0.5	Unknown	0.1	D	100%	Unknown	Unknown	100%
Altretamine	7/Unknown	Unknown	Unknown	D	Unknown	Unknown	Unknown	Unknown
Amantadine	12/500	60	4–5	I	q7d	None	None	q48–72h
Amikacin	1.4–2.3/17–150	<5	0.22–0.29	D,I	20% to 30% q24–48h	⅔ normal dose after dialysis	15–20 mg/L/day	30% to 70% q12–18h
Amiloride	6–8/10–144	30–40	5–5.2	D	Avoid	NA	NA	NA
Amiodarone	14–120 days/Unchanged	96	70–140	D	100%	None	None	100%
Amitriptyline	24–40/Unchanged	96	6–36	D	100%	None	Unknown	NA
Amiodipine	35–50/50	>95	21	D	100%	None	None	100%
Amoxapine	8–30/Unknown	90	Unknown	D	100%	Unknown	Unknown	NA
Amoxicillin	0.9–2.3/5–20	15–25	0.26	I	q24h	Dose after dialysis	250 mg q12h	NA
Amphotericin	24/Unchanged	90	4.0	I	q24–36h	None	Dose for renal failure	q24h
Amphotericin-B colloidal dispersion	24–30/? Unchanged	90	4.0	I	q24–36h	None	Dose for renal failure	q24h
Amphotericin-B lipid complex	19–45/? Unchanged	90	1.7–3.9	I	q24–36h	None	Dose for renal failure	q24h
Ampicillin	0.8–1.5/7–20	20	0.17–0.31	I	q12–24h	Dose after dialysis	250 mg q12h	q6–12h
Amrinone	2.6–8.3/Unknown	20–40	1.3–1.6	D	50% to 75%	Unknown	Unknown	100%
Anistreplase	1.2	Unknown	.08	D	100%	Unknown	Unknown	100%
Astemizole	20 day/Unchanged	97	Unknown	D	100%	Unknown	Unknown	NA
Atenolol	6.7/15–35	3	1.1	D,I	30% to 50% q96h	25–50 mg	None	50% q48h
Atovaquone	55–77/Unknown	99	Unknown		Unknown: 100%	Unknown: None	Unknown	Unknown
Atracurium	0.3–0.4/Unchanged	82	0.15–0.18	D	100%	Unknown	Unknown	100%
Auranofin	70–80 day/Unknown	60	Unknown	D	Avoid	None	None	None
Azathioprine	0.16–1/Increased	20	.55–0.8	D	50%	Yes	Unknown	75%
Azithromycin	10–60/?	8–50	18	D	100%	None	None	None
Azlocillin	0.8–1.5/5–6	30	0.18–0.27	I	q8h	Dose after dialysis	Dose for renal failure	q6–8h
Aztreonam	1.7–2.9/6–8	45–60	0.5–1.0	D	25%	0.5 g after dialysis	Dose for renal failure	50% to 75%
Benazepril	22/30	95	0.15	D	25% to 50%	None	None	50% to 75%
Bepridil	24–48/24–48	Unknown	Unknown		Unknown	None	None	Unknown
Betamethasone	5.5/Unknown	65	1.4	D	100%	Unknown	Unknown	100%
Betaxolol	15–20/30–35	45–60	5–10	D	50%	None	None	100%
Bezafibrate	2.1/7.8	95	0.24–0.35	D	25%	Unknown	Unknown	50%

TABLE 85.13. *(Continued)*

Drug	Half-Life (hr) Normal/Renal Failure	Protein Binding (%)	Volume of Distribution (L/kg)	Method	Renal Failure Dose	Dose After Hemodialysis	Dose During CAPD	Dose During CRRT
Bisoprolol	9–13/18–24	30–35	3	D	50%	Unknown	Unknown	75%
Bleomycin	9/20	Unknown	0.3	D	50%	None	Unknown	75%
Bopindolol	4–10/Unchanged	Unknown	2–3	D	100%	None	None	100%
Bretylium	6–13.6/16–32	6	8.2	D	25%	None	None	25% to 50%
Bromocriptine	3/Unknown	90–96	Unknown	D	100%	Unknown	Unknown	Unknown
Brompheniramine	6/Unknown	Unknown	12	D	100%	Unknown	Unknown	NA
Budesonide	2–2.7/Unknown	88	4.3	D	100%	Unknown	Unknown	100%
Bumetanide	1.2–1.5/1.5	96	0.2–0.5	D	100%	None	None	NA
Bupropion	10–21/Unknown	82–88	27–36	D	100%	Unknown	Unknown	NA
Buspirone	2–3/5.8	95	5.0	D	100%	None	Unknown	NA
Busulfan	2.5–3.4/Unknown	3–15	1.0	D	100%	Unknown	Unknown	100%
Butorphanol	2–4/Unknown	80	9–11	D	50%	Unknown	Unknown	NA
Capreomycin	2	Unknown	Unknown	I	q48h	Give dose after HD only	None	q24h
Captopril	2–3/21–32	25–30	0.7–3	D,I	50% q24h	25% to 30%	None	75% q12–18h
Carbamazepine	24 single; 4–6 chronic dosing	75	0.8–1.6	D	100%	None	None	None
Carbidopa	2/Unknown	Unknown	Unknown	D	100%	Unknown	Unknown	Unknown
Carboplatin	6/Increased	15–24	0.23–0.28	D	25%	½ dose	Unknown	50%
Carmustine	1.5/Unknown	Unknown	3.3	D	Unknown	Unknown	Unknown	Unknown
Carteolol	7/33	20–30	4.0	D	25%	Unknown	None	50%
Carvedilol	5–8/5–8	95	1–2	D	100%	None	None	100%
Cefaclor	1/3	25	0.24–0.35	D	50%	250 mg after dialysis	250 mg q8–12h	NA
Cefadroxil	1.4/22	20	0.31	I	q24–48h	0.5–1.0 g after dialysis	0.5 g/day	NA
Cefamandole	1/6–11	75	0.16–0.25	I	q12h	0.5–1.0 g after dialysis	0.5–1.0 g q12h	q6–8h
Cefazolin	2/40–70	80	0.13–0.22	I	q24–48h	0.5–1.0 g after dialysis	0.5 g q12h	q12h
Cefepime	2.2/18	16	0.3	I	q24–48h	1.0 g after dialysis	Dose for renal failure	Not recommended
Cefixime	3.1/12	50	0.6–0.11	D	50%	300 mg after dialysis	200 mg/day	Not recommended
Cefmenoxime	0.8–1.3/6–12	43–75	0.27–0.37	D,I	0.75 g q12h	0.75 g after dialysis	0.75 g q12h	0.75 g
Cefmetazole	1.2/21	75	0.18	I	q48h	Dose after dialysis	Dose for renal failure	q24h
Cefonicid	4/17–59	96	0.09–0.18	D,I	0.1 g/day	None	None	None
Cefoperazone	1.6–2.5/2.9	90	0.14–0.20	D	100%	1 g after dialysis	None	None
Ceforanide	3/25	80	0.17	I	q24–48h	0.5–1.0 g after dialysis	None	1.0 g/day
Cefotaxime	1/15	37	0.15–0.55	I	q24h	1 g after dialysis	1 g/day	1g q12h
Cefotetan	3.5/13–25	85	0.15	D	25%	1 g after dialysis	1 g/day	750 mg q12h
Cefoxitin	1/13–23	41–75	0.2	I	q24–48h	1 g after dialysis	1 g/day	q8–12h
Cefpodoxime	2.5/26	26	0.6–1.2	I	q24–48h	200 mg after dialysis only	Dose for renal failure	NA
Cefprozil	1.7/6	40	0.65	D,I	250 mg q24h	250 mg after dialysis	Dose for renal failure	Dose for renal failure
Ceftazidime	1.2/13–25	17	0.28–0.4	I	q48h	1 g after dialysis	0.5 g/day	q24–48h
Ceftibuten	1.5–2.7/22	70	0.2	D	25%	300 mg after dialysis only	Dose for renal failure	50%
Ceftizoxime	1.4/35	28–50	0.26–0.42	I	q24h	1 g after dialysis	0.5–1.0 g/day	q12–24h
Ceftriaxone	7–9/12–24	90	0.12–0.18	D	100%	Dose after dialysis	750 mg q12h	100%
Cefuroxime axetil	1.2/17	35–50	0.13–1.8	D	100%	Dose after dialysis	Dose for renal failure	NA
Cefuroxime sodium	1.2/17	33	0.13–1.8	I	q12h	Dose after dialysis	Dose for renal failure	1 g q12h
Celiprolol	4–5/5	Unknown	Unknown	D	75%	Unknown	None	100%
Cephalexin	0.7/16	20	0.35	I	q12h	Dose after dialysis	Dose for renal failure	NA

(Continued)

TABLE 85.13. *(Continued)*

Drug	Half-Life (hr) Normal/Renal Failure	Protein Binding (%)	Volume of Distribution (L/kg)	Method	Renal Failure Dose	Dose After Hemodialysis	Dose During CAPD	Dose During CRRT
Cephalothin	0.5–1/3–18	65	0.26	I	q12h	Dose after dialysis	1 g q12h	1 g q8h
Cephapirin	0.4/2.5	45–60	0.22	I	q12h	Dose after dialysis	1 g q12h	1 g q8h
Cephradine	0.7–1.3/6–15	10	0.25–0.46	D	25%	Dose after dialysis	Dose for renal failure	NA
Cetirizine	7–10/20	93	0.4–0.6	D	30%	None	Unknown	NA
Chloral hydrate	7–14/Unknown	70–80	0.6	D	Avoid	None	Unknown	NA
Chlorambucil	1/Unknown	Unknown	0.86	D	Unknown	Unknown	Unknown	Unknown
Chloramphenicol	1.6–3.3/3–7	45–60	0.5–1.0	D	100%	None	None	None
Chlorazepate	39–85/36	Unknown	1.3	D	100%	Unknown	Unknown	NA
Chlordiazepoxide	5–30/Unchanged	94–97	0.3–0.5	D	50%	None	Unknown	100%
Chloroquine	2–4/5–50 days	50–65	Large	D	50%	None	None	None
Chlorpheniramine	14–24/Unknown	72	6–12	D	100%	None	Unknown	NA
Chlorpromazine	11–42/Unchanged	91–99	8–160	D	100%	None	None	100%
Chlorpropamide	24–48/50–200	88–96	0.09–0.27	D	Avoid	Unknown	None	Avoid
Chlorthalidone	44–80/Unknown	76–90	3.9	I	Avoid	NA	NA	NA
Cholestyramine	Not absorbed	None	None	D	100%	None	None	100%
Cibenzoline	7/22	50	4–5	D,I	66% q24h	None	None	100% q12h
Cidofovir	2.5/Unknown	<6	0.3–0.8	D	Unknown	Unknown	Unknown	Unknown
Cilastin	1/12	44	0.22	D	Avoid	Avoid	Avoid	Avoid
Cilazapril	40–50/>60	Unknown	0.5–0.8	D,I	10% to 25% q72h	None	None	50% q24–48h
Cimetidine	1.5–2/5	20	0.8–1.3	D	25%	None	None	50%
Cinoxacin	1.2/12	63	0.25	D	Avoid	Avoid	Avoid	Avoid
Ciprofloxacin	3–6/6–9	20–40	2.5	D	50%	250 mg q12h (200 mg if IV)	250 mg q8h (200 mg if IV)	200 mg IV q12h
Cisapride	7–10/Unchanged	98	2.4	D	50%	Unknown	Unknown	50% to 100%
Cisplatin	0.3–0.5/Unknown	90	0.5	D	50%	Yes	Unknown	75%
Cladribine	7–14/Unknown	Unknown	50–80	D	Unknown	Unknown	Unknown	Unknown
Clarithromycin	2.3–6/?	70	2–4	D	50% to 75%	Dose after dialysis	None	None
Clavulanic acid	1/3–4	30	0.3	D	50% to 75%	Dose after dialysis	Dose for renal failure	100%
Clindamycin	2–4/3–5	60–95	0.6–1.2	D	100%	None	None	None
Clodronate	13/Increased	36	0.25	D	Avoid	Unknown	Unknown	Unknown
Clofazimine	10–70 days (?)/Unknown	Unknown	Unknown		Unknown: 100%	Unknown: None	Unknown: None	Unknown
Clofibrate	15–17.5/30–110	92–97	0.14	I	Avoid	None	Unknown	q12–18h
Clomipramine	19–37/Unknown	97	Unknown	D	Unknown	Unknown	Unknown	NA
Clonazepam	18–50/Unknown	47	1.5–4.5	D	100%	None	Unknown	NA
Clonidine	6–23/39–42	20–40	3–6	D	100%	None	None	100%
Codeine	2.5–3.5/Unknown	7	3–4	D	50%	Unknown	Unknown	75%
Colchicine	19/40	31	2.2	D	50%	None	Unknown	100%
Colestipol	Not absorbed	None	None	D	100%	None	None	100%
Cortisone	0.5–2/3.5	90	Unknown	D	100%	None	Unknown	100%
Cyclophosphamide	4–7.5/10	14–20	0.5–1	D	75%	0 dose	Unknown	100%
Cycloserine	0.5	Unknown	0.11–.26	I	q24h	None	None	q12–24h
Cyclosporine	3–16/Unchanged	96–99	3.5–7.4	D	100%	None	None	100%
Cytarabine	0.5–3/Unchanged	13	2.6	D	100%	Unknown	Unknown	100%
Dapsone	20–30/Unknown	70–90	1–1.5		Unknown	Unknown: None	Dose for renal failure	Unknown
Daunorubicin	18–27/Unknown	Unknown	Unknown	D	100%	Unknown	Unknown	Unknown
Delavirdine	5.8	98	0.5		Unknown	Unknown	Unknown	Unknown
Desferrioxamine	6/Unknown	Unknown	2–2.5	D	100%	Unknown	Unknown	100%
Desipramine	18–26/Unknown	92	10–50	D	100%	None	None	NA
Dexamethasone	3–4/Unknown	70	0.8–1	D	100%	Unknown	Unknown	100%
Diazepam	20–90/Unchanged	94–98	0.7–3.4	D	100%	None	Unknown	100%
Diazoxide	17–31/30–60	>90	0.2–0.3	D	100%	None	None	100%

TABLE 85.13. *(Continued)*

Drug	Half-Life (hr) Normal/Renal Failure	Protein Binding (%)	Volume of Distribution (L/kg)	Method	Renal Failure Dose	Dose After Hemodialysis	Dose During CAPD	Dose During CRRT
Diclofenac	1–2/Unchanged	>99	0.12–0.17	D	100%	None	None	100%
Dicloxacillin	0.7/1–2	95	0.16	D	100%	None	None	NA
Didanosine	0.6–1.6/4.5	<5	1.0	I	q24–48h	Dose after dialysis	Dose for renal failure	Dose for renal failure
Diflunisal	5–20/62	>99	0.1–0.13	D	50%	None	None	50%
Digitoxin	144–200/210	94	0.6	D	50% to 75%	None	None	100%
Digoxin	36–44/80–120	20–30	5–8	D,I	10% to 25% q48h	None	None	25% to 75% q36h
Dilevalol	8–12/19–30	75	25	D	100%	None	None	Unknown
Diltiazem	2–8/3.5	98	9–10	D	100%	None	None	100%
Diphenhydramine	3.4–9.3/Unknown	80	3.3–6.8	D	100%	None	None	None
Dipyridamole	12/Unknown	99	2.4	D	100%	Unknown	Unknown	NA
Dirithromycin	30–44/Unknown	15–30	>10		100%	None	Unknown	100%
Disopyramide	5–8/10–18	54–81	0.8–2.6	I	q24–40h	None	None	q12–24h
Dobutamine	2 min/Unknown	Unknown	0.25	D	100%	Unknown	Unknown	100%
Doxacurium	1.2–1.6/3.7	28–34	0.12–0.22	D	50%	Unknown	Unknown	50%
Doxazosin	16–22/16–22	98	1–1.7	D	100%	None	None	100%
Doxepin	8–25/10–30	95	9–33	D	100%	None	None	100%
Doxorubicin	35/Unchanged	80–85	21.5	D	100%	None	Unknown	100%
Doxycycline	15–24/18–25	80–90	0.75	D	100%	None	None	100%
Dyphylline	1.8–2.3/12	<3	0.8	D	25%	⅓ dose	Unknown	50%
Enalapril	11–24/34–60	50–60	Unknown	D	50%	20% to 25%	None	75% to 100%
Epirubicin	35/35	80–85	10–40	D	100%	None	Unknown	100%
Erythromycin	1.4/5–6	60–95	0.6–1.2	D	50% to 75%	None	None	None
Esmolol	7–15 min/Unchanged					None	None	Unknown
Estazolam	8–24/Unknown	93	Unknown	D	100%	Unknown	Unknown	NA
Ethacrynic acid	2–4/Unknown	90	0.1	I	Avoid	None	None	NA
Ethambutol	4/7–15	10–30	1.6–3.2	I	q48h	Dose after dialysis	Dose for renal failure	q24–36h
Ethchlorvynol	10–20	35–50	3–4	D	Avoid	None	None	NA
Ethionamide	2.1	30	Unknown	D	50%	None	None	None
Ethosuximide	35–55/Unchanged	10	0.6–0.9	D	100%	None	Unknown	Unknown
Etodolac	5–7/Unchanged	>99	0.4	D	100%	None	None	100%
Etomidate	4–5/Unchanged	75	2–4.5	D	100%	Unknown	Unknown	100%
Etoposide	4–8/19	74–94	0.17–0.5	D	50%	None	Unknown	75%
Famciclovir	1.6–2.9/10–22	<25	1.5	I	50% q48h	Dose after dialysis	Unknown	Unknown
Famotidine	2.5–4/12–19	15–22	0.8–1.4	D	10%	None	None	25%
Felodipine	10–14/21–24	99	9–10	D	100%	None	None	100%
Fenoprofen	2–3/Unchanged	>99	0.1	D	100%	None	None	100%
Fentanyl	2.5–3.5/Unchanged	79–87	2–5	D	100%	Unknown	Unknown	100%
Fexofenadine	14/19–25	70	Unknown	I	q24h	Unknown	Unknown	q12–24h
Flecainide	12–19.5/19–26	52	8.4–9.5	D	50% to 75%	None	None	100%
Fleroxacin	13/21–28	20	1.1–2.4	D	50%	400 mg after dialysis	400 mg/day	NA
Fluconazole	22/Unknown	12	0.7	D	100%	200 mg after dialysis	Dose for renal failure	100%
Flucytosine	3–6/75–200	<10	0.6	I	q24h	Dose after dialysis	0.5–1.0 g/day	q16h
Fludarabine	7–12/24	Unknown	5–40	D	50%	Unknown	Unknown	75%
Flumazenil	0.7–1.3/Unknown	40–50	0.6–1.1	D	100%	None	Unknown	NA
Flunarizine	17–18 day/Unknown	99	43–78	D	100%	None	None	None
Fluorouracil	0.1/Unchanged	10	0.25–0.5	D	100%	Yes	Unknown	100%

(Continued)

TABLE 85.13. *(Continued)*

Drug	Half-Life (hr) Normal/Renal Failure	Protein Binding (%)	Volume of Distribution (L/kg)	Method	Renal Failure Dose	Dose After Hemodialysis	Dose During CAPD	Dose During CRRT
Fluoxetine	24–72/Unchanged	94.5	12–42	D	100%	Unknown	Unknown	NA
Flurazepam	47–100/Unchanged	Unknown	3.4	D	100%	None	Unknown	NA
Flurbiprofen	3–5/Unchanged	99	0.1	D	100%	None	None	100%
Flutamide	4–6/Unknown	Unknown	Unknown	D	100%	Unknown	Unknown	Unknown
Fluvastatin	0.5–1/Unknown	Unknown	0.42	D	100%	Unknown	Unknown	100%
Fluvoxamine	12–15/Unchanged	77	25	D	100%	None	Unknown	NA
Foscarnet	3/Prolonged (up to 100 hr)	17	0.3–0.6	D	6 mg/kg	Dose after dialysis	Dose for renal failure	15 mg/kg
Fosinopril	12/14–32	95	0.15	D	75% to 100%	None	None	100%
Furosemide	0.5–1.1/2–4	95	.07–0.2	D	100%	None	None	NA
Gabapentin	5–7/132	Unbound	0.7	D,I	300 mg qd	300 mg load, then 200–300 mg		300 mg q12–24h
Gallamine	2.3–2.7/6–20	30–70	0.21–0.24	D	Avoid	NA	NA	Avoid
Ganciclovir	3.6/30	Unknown	0.47	I	q48–96h	Dose after dialysis	Dose for renal failure	2.5 mg/kg/day
Ganciclovir-oral				D,I	500 mg q48–96h	Dose after dialysis	Dose for renal failure	NA
Gemfibrozil	7.6/Unchanged	97–99	Unknown	D	100%	None	Unknown	100%
Gentamicin	1.8/20–60	<5	0.23–0.26	D,I	20% to 30% q24–48h	0 normal dose after dialysis	3–4 mg/L/day	30% to 70% q12h
Glibornuride	5–12/Unknown	95	0.25	D	Unknown	Unknown	Unknown	Avoid
Gliclazide	8–11/Unknown	85–95	0.24	D	Unknown	Unknown	Unknown	Avoid
Glipizide	3–7/Unknown	97	0.13–0.16	D	100%	Unknown	Unknown	Avoid
Glyburide	1.4–2.9/Unknown	99	0.16–0.3	D	Avoid	None	None	Avoid
Gold sodium thiomalate	250 day/Unknown	95	5–9	D	Avoid	None	None	Avoid
Griseofulvin	14/20	Unknown	1.6	D	100%	None	None	None
Guanabenz	12–14/Unknown	90	10–12	D	100%	Unknown	Unknown	100%
Guanadrel	4–10/19	20	11.5	I	q24–48h	Unknown	Unknown	q12–24h
Guanethidine	120–140/Unknown	<5	Unknown	I	q24–36h	Unknown	Unknown	Avoid
Guanfacine	12–23/15–25	65	4–6.5	D	100%	None	None	100%
Haloperidol	10–19/Unknown	90–92	14–21	D	100%	None	None	100%
Heparin	0.3–2/Unchanged	>90	0.06–0.1	D	100%	None	None	100%
Hexobarbital	3.5–4/Unknown	65	1.1	D	100%	None	Unknown	NA
Hydralazine	2–4.5/7–16	87	0.5–0.9	I	q8–16h	None	None	q8h
Hydrocortisone	1.5–2/Unknown	Unknown	Unknown	D	100%	Unknown	Unknown	100%
Hydroxyurea	Unknown	Unknown	0.5	D	20%	Unknown	Unknown	Unknown
Hydroxyzine	14–20/Unknown	Unknown	19.5	D	Unknown	100%	100%	100%
Ibuprofen	2–3.2/Unchanged	99	0.15–0.17	D	100%	None	None	100%
Idarubicin	36–70/Unknown	Unknown	Unknown		Unknown	Unknown	Unknown	Unknown
Ifosfamide	4–10/Unknown	Unknown	0.4–0.64	D	75%	Unknown	Unknown	100%
Iloprost	0.3–0.5	Unknown	0.7	D	50%	Unknown	Unknown	100%
Imipenem	1/4	13–21	0.17–0.3	D	25%	Dose after dialysis	Dose for renal failure	50%
Imipramine	12–24/Unknown	96	10–20	D	100%	None	None	NA
Indapamide	14–18/Unchanged	76–79	0.3–1.3	D	Avoid	None	None	NA
Indinavir	1.8/Unknown	60	Unknown		Unknown	Unknown	Dose for renal failure	Unknown
Indobufen	6–7/27–33	>99	0.18–0.21	D	25%	Unknown	Unknown	NA
Indomethacin	4–12/Unchanged	99	0.12	D	100%	None	None	100%
Insulin	2–4/Increased	5	0.15	D	50%	None	None	75%
Ipratropium	1.6/Unknown	Unknown	4.6	D	100%	None	None	100%
Isoniazid	0.7–4/8–17	4–30	0.75	D	50%	Dose after dialysis	Dose for renal failure	Dose for renal failure
Isosorbide	0.15–0.5/4	72	1.5–4	D	100%	10–20 mg	None	100%

TABLE 85.13. *(Continued)*

Drug	Half-Life (hr) Normal/Renal Failure	Protein Binding (%)	Volume of Distribution (L/kg)	Method	Renal Failure Dose	Dose After Hemodialysis	Dose During CAPD	Dose During CRRT
Isradipine	1.9–4.8/10–11	97	3–4	D	100%	None	None	100%
Itraconazole	21/25	99	10	D	50%	100 mg q12–24h	100 mg q12–24h	100 mg q12–24h
Kanamycin	1.8–5/40–96	<5	0.19–0.23	D,I	20% to 30% q24–48h	⅔ normal dose after dialysis	15–20 mg/L/day	30% to 70% q12h
Ketamine	2–3.5/Unchanged	Unknown	1.8–3.1	D	100%	Unknown	Unknown	100%
Ketanserin	14–19/25–35	95	3–6	D	100%	None	None	100%
Ketoconazole	1.5–3.3/3.3	99	1.9–3.6	D	100%	None	None	None
Ketoprofen	1.5–4/Unchanged	99	0.11	D	100%	None	None	100%
Ketorolac	4–6/10	>99	0.13–0.25	D	50%	None	None	50%
Labetalol	3–9/Unchanged	50	5.6	D	100%	None	None	100%
Lamivudine	5–11/20	36	0.83	D,I	25 mg qd (50 mg first dose)	Dose after dialysis	Dose for renal failure	50–150 mg qd (full first dose)
Lamotrigine	25–30/Unknown	0.55	0.9–1.3	D	100%	Unknown	Unknown	100%
Lamotrigine	18–30/Unchanged	40–60	1.2	D	100%	Unknown	Unknown	Unknown
Lansoprazole	1.3–2.9/Unchanged	>98	Unknown	D	100%	Unknown	Unknown	Unknown
Levodopa	0.8–1.6/Unknown	5–8	0.9–1.6	D	100%	Unknown	Unknown	100%
Levofloxacin	4–8/76	24–38	1.1–1.5	D	25% to 50%	Dose for renal failure	Dose for renal failure	50%
Lidocaine	2–2.2/1.3–3	60–66	1.3–2.2	D	100%	None	None	100%
Lincomycin	4–5/10–20	70–80	0.31–0.6	I	q12–24h	None	None	NA
Lisinopril	30/40–50	0–10	0.13–0.15	D	25% to 50%	20%	None	50% to 75%
Lispro Insulin	1/Prolonged	Unknown	0.26–0.36	D	50%	None	None	None
Lithium carbonate	14–28/40	None	0.5–0.9	D	25% to 50%	Dose after dialysis	None	50% to 75%
Lomefloxacin	8/44	15	1.8–3.1	D	50%	Dose for renal failure	Dose for renal failure	NA
Loracarbef	0.8–1.3/32	25	0.3–0.4	I	q3–5d	Dose after dialysis	Dose for renal failure	q24h
Lorazepam	5–10/32–70	87	0.9–1.3	D	100%	None	Unknown	100%
Losartan	3/4–6	30	0.4	D	100%	Unknown	Unknown	100%
Lovastatin	1.1–1.7/Unchanged	>95	Unknown	D	100%	Unknown	Unknown	100%
Low-molecular-weight heparin	2.2–6/3.6–5	Unknown	0.06–0.13	D	50%	Unknown	Unknown	100%
Maprotiline	48/Unknown	Unknown	Unknown	D	100%	Unknown	Unknown	NA
Meclofenamic acid	3/Unchanged	>99	Unknown	D	100%	None	None	100%
Mefenamic acid	3–4/Unchanged	Unknown	Unknown	D	100%	None	None	100%
Mefloquine	15–33 days/Unknown	98	20		Unknown	Unknown	Unknown	Unknown
Melphalan	1.1–1.4/4–6	90	0.6–0.75	D	50%	Unknown	Unknown	75%
Meperidine	2–7/7–32	70	4–5	D	50%	Avoid	None	Avoid
Meprobamate	9–11/Unchanged	0–30	0.5–0.8	I	q12–18h	None	Unknown	NA
Meropenem	1.1/6–8	Low	0.35	D,I	250–500 mg q24h	Dose after dialysis	Dose for renal failure	250–500 mg q12h
Metaproterenol	2–6/Unknown	10	7.6	D	100%	Unknown	Unknown	100%
Metformin	1–5/Prolonged	Negligible	1–4	D	Avoid	Unknown	Unknown	Avoid
Methadone	13–58/Unknown	60–90	3–6	D	50% to 75%	None	None	NA
Methenamine mandelate	4/Unknown	Unknown	Unknown	D	Avoid	NA	NA	NA
Methicillin	0.5–1/4	35–60	0.31	I	q8–12h	None	None	q6–8h
Methimazole	3–6/Unchanged	None	0.6	D	100%	Unknown	Unknown	100%
Methotrexate	8–12/Increased	45–50	0.76	D	Avoid	None	None	50%
Methyldopa	1.5–6/6–16	<15	0.5	I	q12–24h	250 mg	None	q8–12h
Methylprednisolone	1.9–6/Unchanged	40–60	1.2–1.5	D	100%	Yes	Unknown	100%
Metoclopramide	2.5–4/14–15	40	2–3.4	D	50%	None	Unknown	50% to 75%

(Continued)

TABLE 85.13. *(Continued)*

Drug	Half-Life (hr) Normal/Renal Failure	Protein Binding (%)	Volume of Distribution (L/kg)	Method	Renal Failure Dose	Dose After Hemodialysis	Dose During CAPD	Dose During CRRT
Metocurine	3.5–5.8/11.3	70	0.42–0.57	D	50%	Unknown	Unknown	50%
Metolazone	4–20/Unknown	95	1.6	D	100%	None	None	NA
Metoprolol	3.5/2.5–4.5	8	5.5	D	100%	50 mg	None	100%
Metronidazole	6–14/7–21	20	0.25–0.85	D	50%	Dose after dialysis	Dose for renal failure	100%
Mexiletine	8–13/16	70–75	5.5–6.6	D	50% to 75%	None	None	None
Mezlocillin	0.6–1.2/2.6–5.4	20–46	0.18	I	q8h	None	None	q6–8h
Miconazole	20–24/Unchanged	90	Large	D	100%	None	None	None
Midazolam	1.2–12.3/Unchanged	93–96	1.0–6.6	D	50%	NA	NA	NA
Midodrine	0.5/Unknown	Unknown	Unknown		Unknown	5 mg q8h	Unknown	5–10 mg q8h
Miglitol	3–5/Prolonged	Unknown	Unknown	D	Avoid	Unknown	Unknown	Avoid
Milrinone	1/1.5–3	Unknown	0.25–0.35	D	50% to 75%	Unknown	Unknown	100%
Minocycline	12–16/12–18	70	1.0–1.5	D	100%	None	None	100%
Minoxidil	2.8–4.2/Unchanged	0	2–3	D	100%	None	None	100%
Mitomycin C	0.5–1/Unknown	Unknown	0.5	D	75%	Unknown	Unknown	Unknown
Mitoxantrone	23–40/Unknown	75	200–300	D	100%	Unknown	Unknown	100%
Mivacurium	1.5–3	Unknown	0.1	D	50%	Unknown	Unknown	Unknown
Moricizine	2/3	95	>5.0	D	100%	None	None	100%
Morphine	1–4/Unchanged	20–30	3.5	D	50%	None	Unknown	75%
Moxalactam	2.3/18–23	35–59	0.18–0.4	I	q24–48h	Dose after dialysis	Dose for renal failure	q12–24h
Nabumetone	24/Unchanged	>99	0.11	D	100%	None	None	100%
N-Acetylcysteine	2.3–6/Unknown	50	0.33–0.47	D	75%	Unknown	Unknown	100%
N-Acetylprocainamide	6–8/42–70	10–20	1.5–1.7	D,I	25% q12–18h	None	None	50% q8–12h
Nadolol	19/45	28	1.9	D	25%	40 mg	None	50%
Nafcillin	0.5/1.2	85	0.35	D	100%	None	None	100%
Nalidixic acid	6/21	90	0.25–0.35	D	Avoid	Avoid	Avoid	NA
Naloxone	1–1.5/Unknown	54	3	D	100%	NA	NA	100%
Naproxen	12–15/Unchanged	99	0.1	D	100%	None	None	100%
Nefazodone	2–4/Unchanged	99	0.22–0.87	D	100%	Unknown	Unknown	NA
Nelfinavir	1.8–3.4/Unknown	Unknown	Unknown		Unknown	Unknown	Unknown	Unknown
Neostigmine	1.3/3.0	None	0.5–1.0	D	25%	Unknown	Unknown	50%
Netilmicin	1–3/35–72	<5	0.16–0.30	D,I	10% to 20% q24–48h	⅔ normal dose after dialysis	3–4 mg/L/day	20% to 60% q12h
Nevirapine	40/?	60	1.2–1.4	D	Unknown	Unknown	Unknown	Unknown
Nicardipine	5/5–7	98–99	0.8	D	100%	None	None	100%
Nicotinic acid	0.5–1/Unknown	Unknown	Unknown	D	25%	Unknown	Unknown	50%
Nifedipine	4–5.5/5–7	97	1.4	D	100%	None	None	100%
Nimodipine	1–2.8/22	98	0.9–2.3	D	100%	None	None	100%
Nisoldipine	6.6–7.9/6.8–9.7	99	2.3–7.1	D	100%	None	None	100%
Nitrazepam	18–36/Unknown	Unknown	Unknown	D	100%	Unknown	Unknown	NA
Nitrofurantoin	0.5/1	20–60	0.3–0.7	D	Avoid	NA	NA	NA
Nitroglycerine	2–4 min/Unchanged	Unknown	2–3	D	100%	Unknown	Unknown	100%
Nitroprusside	<10 min/<10 min	0	0.2	D	100%	None	None	100%
Nitrosourea	Short/Unknown	Unknown	Unknown	D	25% to 50%	None	Unknown	Unknown
Nizatidine	1.3–1.6/5.3–8.5	28–35	0.8–1.3	D	25%	Unknown	Unknown	50%
Norfloxacin	3.5–6.5/8	14	<0.5	I	Avoid	NA	NA	NA
Nortriptyline	25–38/15–66	95	15–23	D	100%	None	None	NA
Ofloxacin	5–8/28–37	25	1.5–2.5	D	25% to 50%	100 mg BID	Dose for renal failure	300 mg/day
Omeprazole	0.5–1/Unchanged	95	Unknown	D	100%	Unknown	Unknown	Unknown
Ondansetron	2.5–5.5/Unchanged	75	2	D	100%	Unknown	Unknown	100%
Orphenadrine	16/Unknown	Unknown	Unknown	D	100%	Unknown	Unknown	NA
Ouabain	21/60–70	40	Unknown	I	q36–48h	None	None	q24–36h

TABLE 85.13. *(Continued)*

Drug	Half-Life (hr) Normal/Renal Failure	Protein Binding (%)	Volume of Distribution (L/kg)	Method	Renal Failure Dose	Dose After Hemodialysis	Dose During CAPD	Dose During CRRT
Oxaprozin	50–60/Unchanged	>99	0.2	D	100%	None	None	100%
Oxatomide	20/Unknown	91	Unknown	D	100%	None	None	NA
Oxazepam	5–10/25–90	97	0.6–1.6	D	100%	None	Unknown	100%
Oxcarbazepine	8–9/Unknown	40	0.7–0.8	D	100%	Unknown	Unknown	Unknown
Paclitaxel	9–30/Unknown	Unknown	30–60	D	100%	Unknown	Unknown	100%
Pancuronium	1.7–2.2/4.3–8.2	70–85	0.15–0.38	D	Avoid	Unknown	Unknown	50%
Paroxetine	10–16/30	95	13	D	50%	Unknown	Unknown	NA
PAS	1.0	15–50	0.11–24	D	50%	Dose after dialysis	Dose for renal failure	Dose for renal failure
Penbutolol	22/24	>95	Unknown	D	100%	None	None	100%
Penicillamine	1.5–3/Increased	80	Unknown	D	Avoid	⅓ dose	Unknown	Avoid
Penicillin G	0.5/6–20	50	0.3–0.42	D	20% to 50%	Dose after dialysis	Dose for renal failure	75%
Penicillin VK	0.6/4.1	50–80	0.5	D	100%	Dose after dialysis	Dose for renal failure	NA
Pentamidine	29/118	69	55–462	I	q48h	None	None	None
Pentazocine	2–5/Unknown	50–75	5	D	50%	None	Unknown	75%
Pentobarbital	18–48/Unchanged	60–70	1.0	D	100%	None	Unknown	100%
Pentopril	2–3/10–14	60	0.8	D	50%	Unknown	Unknown	50% to 75%
Pentoxifylline	0.8/Unchanged	None	2.4–4.2	D	100%	Unknown	Unknown	100%
Perfoxacin	10/15	25–43	2.0	D	100%	None	None	100%
Perindopril	5/27	20	0.6–0.8	D	50%	25% to 50%	Unknown	75%
Phenelzine	1.5–4/Unknown	Unknown	Unknown	D	100%	Unknown	Unknown	NA
Phenobarbital	60–150/117–160	40–60	0.7–1	I	q12–16h	Dose after dialysis	½ normal dose	q8–12h
Phenylbutazone	50–100/Unchanged	99	0.09–0.17	D	100%	None	None	100%
Phenytoin	24/Unchanged	90	1.0	D	100%	None	None	None
Pindolol	2.5–4/3–4	50	1.2	D	100%	None	None	100%
Pipecuronium	2.3/4.4	Unknown	0.31	D	25%	Unknown	Unknown	50%
Piperacillin	0.8–1.5/3.3–5.1	30	0.18–0.30	I	q8h	Dose after dialysis	Dose for renal failure	q6–8h
Piretanide	1.4/1.6–3.4	94	0.3	D	100%	None	None	NA
Piroxicam	45–55/Unchanged	>99	0.12–0.15	D	100%	None	None	100%
Pllcamycin	2/Unknown	Low	Unknown	D	50%	Unknown	Unknown	Unknown
Pravastatin	0.8–3.2/Unchanged	Unknown	Unknown	D	100%	Unknown	Unknown	100%
Prazepam	36–200/36	Unknown	Unknown	D	100%	Unknown	Unknown	NA
Prazosin	2–3/2–3	97	1.2–1.5	D	100%	None	None	100%
Prednisolone	2.5–3.5/Unchanged	Saturable	2.2	D	100%	Yes	Unknown	100%
Prednisone	2.5–3.5/Unchanged	Saturable	2.2	D	100%	None	Unknown	100%
Primaquine	4–7/Unknown	Unknown	3–4		Unknown	Unknown	Unknown	Unknown
Primidone	5–15/Unchanged	20–30	0.4–1	I	q12–24h	⅓ dose	Unknown	Unknown
Probenecid	5–8/Unchanged	85–95	0.15	D	Avoid	Avoid	Unknown	Avoid
Probucol	23–47 day/Unknown	Unknown	Unknown	D	100%	Unknown	Unknown	100%
Procainamide	2.5–4.9/5.3–5.9	15	2.2	I	q8–24h	200 mg	None	q6–12h
Promethazine	9–12/Unknown	Unknown	Large	D	100%	Unknown	Unknown	100%
Propafenone	5/Unknown	>95	3.0	D	100%	None	None	100%
Propofol	3–4.5/Unchanged	Unknown	3.0–14.4	D	100%	Unknown	Unknown	100%
Propoxyphene	9–15/12–20	78	16	D	Avoid	None	None	NA
Propranolol	2–6/1–6	93	2.8	D	100%	None	None	100%
Propylthiouracil	1–2/Unchanged	80	0.3–0.4	D	100%	Unknown	Unknown	100%
Protriptyline	54–98/Unknown	92	15–31	D	100%	None	None	NA
Pyrazinamide	9/26	5	0.75–1.3	D	Avoid	Avoid	Avoid	Avoid
Pyridostigmine	1.5–2/6	Unknown	0.8–1.4	D	20%	Unknown	Unknown	35%
Pyrimethamine	80/Unchanged	27	2.9	D	100%	None	None	None

(Continued)

TABLE 85.13. *(Continued)*

Drug	Half-Life (hr) Normal/Renal Failure	Protein Binding (%)	Volume of Distribution (L/kg)	Method	Renal Failure Dose	Dose After Hemodialysis	Dose During CAPD	Dose During CRRT
Quazepam	20–40/Unknown	95	Unknown	D	Unknown	Unknown	Unknown	NA
Quinapril	1–2/6–15	97	1.5	D	75%	25%	None	75% to 100%
Quinidine	6/4–14	70–95	2–3.5	D	75%	100–200 mg	None	100%
Quinine	5–16/Unchanged	70	0.7–3.7	I	q24h	Dose after dialysis	Dose for renal failure	q8–12h
Ramipril	5–8/15	55–70	1.2	D	25% to 50%	20%	None	50% to 75%
Ranitidine	1.5–3/6–9	15	1.2–1.8	D	25%	½ dose	None	50%
Reserpine	46–168/87–323	96	Unknown	D	Avoid	None	None	100%
Ribavirin	30–60/Unknown	0	9–15	D	50%	Dose after dialysis	Dose for renal failure	Dose for renal failure
Rifabutin	16–69/Unchanged	71–89	8.2–9.3		100%	None	None	Unknown
Rifampin	1.5–5/1.8–11	60–90	0.9	D	50% to 100%	None	Dose for renal failure	Dose for renal failure
Ritonavir	3/Unknown	98–99	0.4		Unknown	Unknown	Unknown	Unknown
Saquinavir	12/?	98	10		Unknown	Unknown	Unknown	Unknown
Secobarbital	20–35/Unknown	44	1.5–2.5	D	100%	None	None	NA
Sertraline	24/Unchanged	97	25	D	100%	Unknown	Unknown	NA
Simvastatin	Unknown	>95	Unknown	D	100%	Unknown	Unknown	100%
Sodium valproate	6–15/Unchanged	90	0.19–0.23	D	100%	None	None	None
Sotalol	7.5–15/56	<1	1.3	D	15% to 30%	80 mg	None	30%
Sparfloxacin	15–20/38.5	35–55	4.5	D,I	50% q48h	Unknown	Unknown	50% to 75%
Spectinomycin	1.6/16–29	5–20	0.25	D	100%	None	None	None
Spironolactone	10–35/Unchanged	98	Unknown	I	Avoid	NA	NA	Avoid
Stavudine	1.0–1.4/5.5–8	<1	0.5	D,I	50% q24h	Dose after dialysis	Unknown	Unknown
Streptokinase	0.6–1.5/Unknown	Unknown	0.02–0.08	D	100%	NA	NA	100%
Streptomycin	2.5/100	35	0.26	I	q72–96h	½ normal dose after dialysis	20–40 mg/L/day	q24–72h
Streptozotocin	0.25/Unknown	Unknown	0.5	D	50%	Unknown	Unknown	Unknown
Succinylcholine	3/Unknown	Unknown	Unknown	D	100%	Unknown	Unknown	100%
Sufentanil	1–2/Unchanged	92	1.7–5.2	D	100%	Unknown	Unknown	100%
Sulbactam	1/10–21	30	0.25–0.5	I	q24–48h	Dose after dialysis	0.75–1.5 g/day	750 mg q12h
Sulfamethoxazole	10/20–50	50	0.28–0.38	I	q24h	1 g after dialysis	1 g/day	q18h
Sulfinpyrazone	2.2–5/Unchanged	>95	0.06	D	Avoid	None	None	100%
Sulfisoxazole	3–7/6–12	85	0.14–0.28	I	q12–24h	2 g after dialysis	3 g/day	NA
Sulindac	8–16/Unchanged	95	Unknown	D	100%	None	None	100%
Sulotroban	0.7–3/9–39	Unknown	Unknown	D	10%	Unknown	Unknown	Unknown
Tamoxifen	18/Unknown	>98	20	D	100%	Unknown	Unknown	100%
Tazobactam	1/7	22	0.21	D	50%	⅓ dose after dialysis	Dose for renal failure	75%
Teicoplanin	33–190/62–230	60–90	0.5–1.2	I	q72h	Dose for renal failure	Dose for renal failure	q48h
Temazepam	4–10/Unknown	96	1.3–1.5	D	100%	None	None	NA
Teniposide	6–10/Unknown	99	0.2–0.7	D	100%	None	None	100%
Terazosin	9–12/8–12	90–94	0.5–0.9	D	100%	Unknown	Unknown	100%
Terbutaline	3/Unknown	15–25	0.9–1.5	D	Avoid	Unknown	Unknown	50%
Terfenadine	16–23/Unknown	97	Unknown	D	100%	None	None	NA
Tetracycline	6–10/57–108	55–90	>0.7	I	q24h	None	None	q12–24h
Theophylline	4–12/Unchanged	55	0.4–0.7	D	100%	½ dose	Unknown	100%
Thiazides	6–8/12–20	40	3.0	D	Avoid	NA	NA	NA
Thiopental	3.8/6–18	72–86	1–1.5	D	75%	NA	NA	NA
Ticarcillin	1.2/11–16	45–60	0.14–0.21	D,I	1–2 g q12h	3 g after dialysis	Dose for renal failure	1–2 g q18h
Ticlopidine	24–33/Unknown	98	Unknown	D	100%	Unknown	Unknown	100%
Timolol	2.7/4	60	1.7	D	100%	None	None	100%
Tobramycin	2.5/27–60	<5	0.22–0.33	D,I	20% to 30%	⅔ normal dose	3–4 mg/L/day	30% to 70%

TABLE 85.13. *(Continued)*

Drug	Half-Life (hr) Normal/Renal Failure	Protein Binding (%)	Volume of Distribution (L/kg)	Method	Renal Failure Dose	Dose After Hemodialysis	Dose During CAPD	Dose During CRRT
					q24–48h	after dialysis		q12h
Tocainide	14/22–27	10–20	3.2	D	50%	200 mg	None	100%
Tolazamide	4–7/Unknown	94	Unknown	D	100%	Unknown	Unknown	Avoid
Tolbutamide	4–6/Unchanged	95–97	0.1–0.15	D	100%	None	None	Avoid
Tolmetin	1–1.5/Unchanged	>99	0.1–0.14	D	100%	None	None	100%
Topiramate	19–23/48–60	9–17	0.6–0.8	D	25%	Unknown	Unknown	50%
Topotecan	4–6/Prolonged	Unknown	40	D	25%	Unknown	Unknown	50%
Torsemide	2–4/4–5	97–99	0.14–0.19	D	100%	None	None	NA
Tranexamic acid	1.5/Unknown	3	Unknown	D	10%	Unknown	Unknown	Unknown
Tranylcypromine	1.9–3.5/Unknown	Unknown	Unknown	D	Unknown	Unknown	Unknown	NA
Trazodone	6–11/Unknown	89–95	1–2	D	Unknown	Unknown	Unknown	NA
Triamcinolone	1.9–6/Unchanged	Unknown	1.4–2.1	D	100%	Unknown	Unknown	100%
Triamterene	2–12/10	40–70	2.2–3.7	I	Avoid	NA	NA	Avoid
Triazolam	2–4/Unchanged	85–95	Unknown	D	100%	None	None	NA
Trihexyphenidyl	10/Unknown	Unknown	Unknown	D	Unknown	Unknown	Unknown	Unknown
Trimethadione	12–24/Unknown	None	Unknown	I	q12–24h	Unknown	Unknown	q8–12h
Trimethoprim	9–13/20–49	30–70	1–2.2	I	q24h	Dose after dialysis	q24h	q18h
Trimetrexate	4–22/Unknown	95	0.6 (10–31 L/m²)	D	Unknown	Unknown	Unknown	Unknown
Trimipramine	24/Unknown	90–96	31	D	100%	None	None	NA
Tripelennamine	3–4.5/Unknown	Unknown	10	D	Unknown	Unknown	Unknown	NA
Triprolidine	5/Unknown	Unknown	Unknown	D	Unknown	Unknown	Unknown	NA
Tubocurarine	0.5–4/5.5	30–50	0.22–0.39	D	Avoid	Unknown	Unknown	50%
Urokinase	Unknown	Unknown	Unknown	D	Unknown	Unknown	Unknown	Unknown
Valacyclovir				D,I	0.5 g q24h	Dose after dialysis	Dose for renal failure	Unknown
Vancomycin	6–8/200–250	10–50	0.47–1.1	D,I	500 mg q48–96h	Dose for renal failure	Dose for renal failure	500 mg q24–48h
Vecuronium	0.5–1.3/Unchanged	30	0.18–0.27	D	100%	Unknown	Unknown	100%
Venlafaxine	4/6–8	27	6–7	D	50%	None	Unknown	NA
Verapamil	3–7/2.4–4	83–93	3–6	D	100%	None	None	100%
Vidarabine	1.5/Unknown	25	0.7	D	75%	Infuse after dialysis	Dose for renal failure	100%
Vigabatrin	5–7/13–15	None	0.8	D	25%	Unknown	Unknown	50%
Vinblastine	1–1.5/Unknown	75	13–40	D	100%	Unknown	Unknown	100%
Vincristine	1–2.5/Unknown	75	5–11	D	100%	Unknown	Unknown	100%
Vinorelbine	20–40/Unknown	15	75	D	100%	Unknown	Unknown	100%
Warfarin	34–45/Unchanged	99	0.15	D	100%	None	None	None
Zafirlukast	10/Unchanged	99	Unknown	D	100%	Unknown	Unknown	100%
Zalcitabine	1–2/>8	<4	0.54	I	q24h	Unknown	Unknown	Unknown
Zidovudine	1.1–1.4/1.4–3	10–30	1.4–3	D,I	100 mg q8h	Dose for renal failure	Dose for renal failure	100 mg q8h
Zileuton	2.3/Unchanged	>90	2.3		100%	None	Unknown	100%

Method refers to changing the dose (D) or the dose interval (I). Percentages are the percent of the dose for normal renal function. NA is listed for drugs where dosing is not applicable during renal replacement therapy. CAPD, continuous ambulatory peritoneal dialysis; CRRT, continuous renal replacement therapy.

The choice of cardiac glycosides in patients with renal insufficiency is controversial. The kidneys excrete digoxin. Digoxin doses should be reduced substantially for patients with even modest decreases in renal function. Because the liver excretes digitoxin, only patients with severe renal impairment require dosage reduction. However, digitoxin's long half-life makes toxicity with this drug potentially more serious. Both drugs have a smaller volume of distribution in patients with renal insufficiency, making calculation of the appropriate loading dose more difficult. When digitalization can be done gradually, a small loading dose followed by reduced maintenance doses should be given.

Antimicrobial Agents

Dosage reduction that results in ineffectively low plasma concentrations is the greatest danger in prescribing antimicrobial agents for patients with renal impairment. Although some antimicrobial agents have a narrow therapeutic index, many are relatively nontoxic. These drugs have a great difference between therapeutic and toxic plasma concentrations. The aminoglycoside antibiotics have a narrow therapeutic range. They are eliminated almost exclusively by glomerular filtration, and accumulation may cause nephrotoxicity and ototoxicity. Patients on aminoglycoside therapy require precise dose reduction, drug level monitoring, and carefully repeated measurements of renal function.

Antimicrobial therapy in patients with renal disease begins with an attempt to isolate the causative organism. Uremic patients with serious infections may not have elevated temperatures. Uremic symptoms or the effects of dialysis may mask nonspecific symptoms of infection. Because patients with renal insufficiency are more likely to have adverse effects from antimicrobial therapy than are patients with normal renal function, culture documentation of bacterial infection is essential. When patients are seriously ill, the clinician should choose antimicrobial therapy empirically only after exhaustive attempts to isolate specific pathogens.

The choice of antimicrobial agents includes consideration of potential toxicity and the consequences of inadvertent drug or metabolite accumulation. Side effects, which are rarely seen in patients with normal renal function, occur more often in patients with renal failure. For example, seizures from β-lactam accumulation are rare in patients with sufficient kidney function to prevent drug accumulation, but they may occur in patients with renal impairment, when large doses are given. Although nephrotoxicity in patients with renal insufficiency may result in overt uremia, a decrease in renal function of as much as 50% from aminoglycoside nephrotoxicity may go unnoticed in patients with normal kidney function. A similar change in patients with creatinine clearances less than 20 ml/min might precipitate the need for dialysis.

The clinician should consider the accumulation of metabolic waste products in patients with impaired excretory capacity. The antianabolic effects of tetracycline may cause an increase in the blood urea nitrogen. Drugs that increase metabolic load should be avoided.

The kidneys eliminate antimicrobial agents. For most of these drugs, detailed kinetics studies in patients with renal impairment have led to detailed dosing guidelines. However, the derived suggestions are appropriate for the average patient and are only a starting point for individualization of therapy. To reach therapeutic plasma drug levels rapidly, the initial dose of antimicrobial agents for patients with impaired renal function should be the same as that for patients with normal renal function. If substantial edema or ascites is present, a larger initial dose may be necessary. Conversely, dehydrated or severely debilitated patients may require smaller initial doses.

No controlled clinical trials have compared the relative efficacy of modifying drug dose in renal insufficiency by decreasing the individual doses or by increasing the dose interval. When subsequent doses need to be decreased because of diminished renal function, the dose for most antimicrobial agents should be modified by prolonging the dose interval. Because the wide therapeutic range of these drugs allows higher peak levels without toxicity and lower trough levels without loss of efficacy, the dose interval often may be extended to 24 hours or more. Extension of the dose interval is more convenient and less expensive. When the clinical situation permits, outpatient parenteral antimicrobial therapy may be given.

To eliminate the risk of ineffectively low drug concentrations in seriously ill patients, the dose interval should not be extended beyond 24 hours. In such patients, a decrease in the individual doses combined with prolonging the dose interval maintains safe, therapeutic drug levels. This combined approach results in therapeutic efficacy, convenience, and cost savings.

Because there is often a direct relation between plasma levels and antimicrobial efficacy or toxicity, drug levels should be measured. Generally, three or four doses should be given before levels are measured to ensure that steady-state concentrations have been established. For some drugs, both maximum and minimum concentrations are relevant. Peak levels are most meaningful when measured after rapid distribution has occurred. Minimum plasma drug concentrations should be measured immediately before the next dose is given. These trough levels are measures of elimination and reflect more closely the potential drug accumulation in patients with renal failure. Drug level monitoring is particularly important in patients with unstable renal function.

Anticonvulsants

Generalized major motor seizures occur in patients with uremia. Phenytoin is one of the most commonly used drugs for such seizures. Phenytoin absorption is slow and erratic, hepatic metabolism is concentration dependent and saturable, and its distribution and elimination vary. In addition, phenytoin protein binding is decreased and distribution volume increased in renal failure. With any given total plasma level, the concentration of active, free drug will be higher in uremic patients than in patients with normal renal function. Most clinical laboratories measure the total serum drug concentration; thus a low total phenytoin level in a patient with renal failure should not necessarily be misinterpreted as subtherapeutic.

Physical findings such as a nystagmus may be helpful in deciding not to increase the dose. Seizures are also a manifestation of phenytoin excess, and small dosage increases may result in disproportionately large increases in the serum drug level. Dosage increments should be small, sufficient time should be allowed for the patient to reach steady-state drug levels, and measurements of free serum phenytoin concentration should be taken frequently in uremic patients who are not responding to therapy.

Nonsteroidal Antiinflammatory Drugs

Adverse effects of nonsteroidal antiinflammatory drugs (NSAIDs) can be the result of either the pharmacologic action of prostaglandin synthesis inhibition or direct hypersensitivity. Prostaglandins are important in maintaining renal vasodilation and in ensuring adequate renal blood flow. NSAIDs are potent inhibitors of renal prostaglandin synthesis, resulting in the renal arterial vasoconstriction, decreased renal blood flow, and reduced GFR.

Prostaglandins are also important for maintaining fluid and electrolyte homeostasis. Reduction in glomerular filtration allows increased tubular reabsorption. Decreased prostaglandin production increases tubular chloride reabsorption in Henle's loop and increases the effect of antidiuretic hormone on the distal tubule. These effects may lead to salt and water retention. In addition, renin generation is diminished. The result is a decrease in plasma aldosterone production that can lead to potassium retention and hyperkalemia in patients with decreased renal function. Adverse effects of NSAIDs are more clinically apparent in patients with decreased effective circulating fluid volume. Thus patients with congestive heart failure, chronic liver disease, chronic renal failure, dehydration, or hemorrhage are at increased risk of adverse effects.

Acute renal failure characterized by proteinuria or the nephrotic syndrome is consistent with a hypersensitivity reaction. Discontinuing treatment with the NSAID results in the gradual disappearance of proteinuria and a return toward normal renal function.

Sedatives, Hypnotics, and Psychiatric Drugs

Psychotherapeutic drugs are commonly given to patients with renal disease to relieve anxiety and depression. Excessive sedation is the most common adverse effect in patients with renal insufficiency. Because malaise, somnolence, and encephalopathy are common uremic symptoms, recognition of the adverse drug reactions may be delayed.

Benzodiazepines are often used to treat emotional stress associated with decreasing renal function in patients on dialysis, although the efficacy of chronic benzodiazepine treatment has been questioned. Members of this class are generally safer than other antianxiety agents, and short-term administration is effective. Active polar metabolites of these compounds normally excreted by the kidneys are likely to accumulate in patients with renal impairment and produce enhanced, prolonged sedation. Because of the potential for drug or metabolite accumulation, the chronic use of long-acting benzodiazepines should be discouraged in patients with decreased renal function.

Phenothiazines and tricyclic antidepressants can produce excessive sedation. Patients taking these drugs may also exhibit anticholinergic effects, orthostatic hypertension, confusion, and extrapyramidal symptoms.

Lithium carbonate has become an increasingly prescribed antidepressant. The drug is excreted by the kidneys and has a narrow therapeutic range. Careful dosage reduction and plasma lithium level monitoring are required in patients with impaired or unstable renal function. Hemodialysis has been used in cases of lithium overdose. Although lithium is effectively removed by dialysis, a rebound increase in plasma levels is common after hemodialysis, and repeated treatments or continuous renal replacement therapy maybe required.

DRUG REMOVAL BY DIALYSIS

Hemodialysis removes drugs from plasma by diffusion across the dialysis membrane. Diffusion proceeds from higher concentrations in the plasma to lower concentrations in the dialysate. The drug, the dialysis procedure, and the patient influence the rate and extent of drug removal by dialysis. Drugs smaller than 500 D readily cross standard dialysis membranes. Dialysis does not remove drugs that are more than 90% protein bound or drugs with large volumes of distribution. Porous membranes, used for continuous renal replacement therapies, allow the filtration of much larger drugs. Because hemodialysis removes drugs by diffusion, large surface-area dialyzers, increasing the blood flow rate, increasing the dialysate flow rate, and lengthening the duration of the treatment, increase the amount of drug removed. The following relationship estimates the hemodialysis clearance of a drug:

$$Cl_{HD} = Cl_{urea} \times (60/MW_{drug})$$

where Cl_{HD} is the drug's clearance by hemodialysis, Cl_{urea} is the clearance of urea by the dialyzer, and MW_{drug} is the molecular weight of the drug. The urea clearance for most standard dialyzers is approximately 150 ml/min.

The efficiency of drug removal by peritoneal dialysis is much less than that during hemodialysis. Drug removal by peritoneal dialysis is most effective for smaller-molecular-weight drugs, drugs that are not extensively bound to serum proteins, and drugs distributed in the extracellular fluid. The rate and extent of small-molecular-weight drug removal depends on the volume of peritoneal dialysate exchanged. In general, if a drug is not removed by hemodialysis, it will not be removed by peritoneal dialysis.

Table 85.13 lists drugs commonly used in dialysis patients and the appropriate dosage adjustments. Suggestions for reducing the individual doses, prolonging the dose interval, or a combination of the methods are included. Recommendations for supplemental doses following hemodialysis and during continuous ambulatory peritoneal dialysis (CAPD) are listed.

When medications are added to peritoneal dialysate, drug transport across the peritoneal membrane is unidirectional. The addition of drugs to peritoneal dialysate results in high drug concentrations in the dialysis fluid relative to the blood. Although peritoneal dialysis does not rapidly remove drugs, many are well absorbed when placed in peritoneal dialysate because of the resulting large concentration gradient between the dialysate and the blood.

The rate and extent of drug removal by continuous renal replacement therapies (CRRT) depends on the drug's molecular weight, membrane characteristics, blood flow rate, and the addition of dialysate to the extracorporeal circuit. Molecular weight effects drug removal by diffusion during dialysis more than during convection during CRRT because of the large pore size of membranes used for CRRT. Because most drugs are less than 1,500 D, drug removal by CRRT does not depend greatly on molecular weight.

A drug's volume of distribution and binding to serum proteins are the most important factors determining removal by CRRT. Drugs with a large volume of distribution are highly tissue bound and not accessible to extracorporeal circuit in quantities sufficient to result in substantial removal by CRRT. Even if the extraction across the artificial membrane is 100%, only a small amount of a drug with a large volume of distribution is removed. A volume of distribution greater than 0.7 L/kg substantially decreases CRRT drug removal.

Drug protein binding also determines how much is removed during CRRT. Only unbound drug is available for elimination by CRRT. Protein binding of more than 80% is a substantial barrier to drug removal by convection or diffusion.

During continuous hemofiltration, a filtration rate of 10 to 30 ml/min is achieved. The addition of diffusion by continuous dialysis adds 15 to 20 ml/min. Therefore continuous dialysis and continuous hemofiltration together provide a drug clearance of 10 to 50 ml/min.

The use of porous membranes and high blood flow rates during routine hemodialysis has blurred the distinction in drug removal among renal replacement therapies. Little data are available on drug removal by these techniques. Results from studies in chronic, stable hemodialysis patients are often extrapolated to make dosing recommendations for patients with acute renal failure or those treated with very high-flux dialysis. Underestimating drug removal in these circumstances risks ineffective therapy.

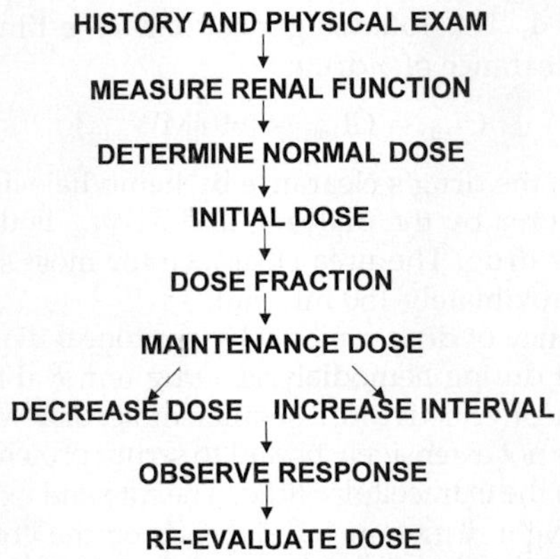

Figure 85.8. A practical schema for drug dosing in dialysis patients.

DRUG LEVEL MONITORING

Plasma drug concentrations guide drug therapy when the relationship between drug levels and efficacy or toxicity is known. These measurements are most important for drugs with a narrow therapeutic range. They may also be useful when drug level–related pharmacologic effects are difficult to measure.

If a loading dose is not given, three or four doses of the drug should be administered before serum levels are measured. This approach ensures that a steady-state serum concentration has been established. For some drugs, both maximum and minimum concentrations are relevant. Peak levels are most meaningful when measured after rapid drug distribution has occurred. Conversely, minimum concentrations are usually measured just before giving the next scheduled dose. A practical schema for drug prescribing in patients with renal impairment is shown in Fig. 85.8.

Patients with renal disease are heterogeneous and their response to drug therapy is variable. Dosage nomograms, drug tables, and computer-assisted dosing recommendations provide guidelines for an initial drug administration in patients with decreased renal function. Individualizing the dose regimen for each patient requires continuing evaluation of the therapeutic response for drug efficacy and toxicity.

Selected Readings

Aronoff GR, Berns JS, Brier ME, et al., eds. *Drug prescribing in renal failure. Dosing guidelines for adults.* 4th ed. Philadelphia: American College of Physicians, 1999.

Contains drug dosing data in renal failure on more than 450 drugs and a brief discussion of drug dosing considerations for major classes of drugs

Matzke GR, Frye RF. Drug administration in patients with renal insufficiency. Minimising renal and extrarenal toxicity. *Drug Saf* 1997;16(3):205–231.

Describes pharmacotherapeutic principles and approaches to enhance the safety of drugs in patients with renal insufficiency.

Preston SL, Briceland LL, Lomaestro BM, et al. Dosing adjustment of 10 antimicrobials for patients with renal impairment. *Ann Pharmacother* 1995;29(12):1202–1207.

Describes a program of creatinine clearance–based dosage adjustment of 10 renally eliminated antimicrobial agents and discusses the utility of such a program in a hospital setting. A good example of pharmacokinetic monitoring as a method of quality assurance.

Swan SK, Bennett WM. Drug dosing guidelines in patients with renal failure. *West J Med* 1992;156(6):633–638.

Discusses the metabolism and excretion of many drugs and their pharmacologically active metabolites in patients with impaired renal function.

SECTION X

Renal Transplantation

CHAPTER 86

Immunology and Genetics of Transplantation

Alan M. Krensky and Carol Clayberger

The immune system developed to combat infectious organisms. Cellular and humoral mechanisms are responsible for recognition and destruction of non-self while leaving self intact. These same mechanisms are involved in tumor surveillance and transplant rejection. When an organ from one individual of a species is transplanted into a genetically different individual of the same species (allografting), the foreign graft is recognized and destroyed. The major target antigens on the allograft are the human leukocyte antigens (HLA). The major effectors responsible for graft rejection are antibodies made by B lymphocytes, soluble mediators made by a variety of immune cells, and T lymphocytes. This chapter reviews the immune response and genetics relevant to transplant rejection.

HUMAN LEUKOCYTE ANTIGENS

The human leukocyte antigens are encoded on chromosome 6 (Fig. 86.1). They consist of class I molecules, HLA-A, -B, and -C; class II molecules, HLA-DR, -DP, and -DQ; and other "class III" molecules involved in the immune response.

Class I molecules are composed of a 44,000 molecular weight heavy chain that is noncovalently associated with a 12,000 molecular weight light chain, β_2-microglobulin. The light chain is monomorphic within humans, but the heavy chain is highly polymorphic. Serologic analysis with alloantibodies identifies at least 18 HLA-A, 35 HLA-B, and 8 HLA-C alleles, whereas molecular sequencing of cloned genes identifies at least 94 HLA-A, 208 HLA-B, and 52 HLA-C alleles. The function of HLA class I molecules is to present endogenous antigens, such as viral proteins, as peptides to CD8+ T cells (Fig. 86.2). Many of these T cells are cytolytic, capable of killing a cell that expresses a foreign peptide in the context of self-HLA or a foreign HLA class I molecule.

HLA class II molecules are composed of a 34,000 molecular weight α chain associated with a 29,000 molecular weight β chain. Although both chains are polymorphic, most of the polymorphism is in the β chain. Only one HLA-DR α chain sequence (encoded by two different alleles) has been identified, but serologic analysis reveals at least 14 HLA-DR β chains and 6 HLA-DQ β chains. In stark contrast, there are at least 230 HLA-DR β and 32 HLA-DQ β chains by sequence analysis. Class II molecules present exogenous antigens, soluble proteins such as tetanus or diptheria toxin, to CD4+ T helper cells (Fig. 86.2). Additional genes important to the immune response in general and antigen presentation in particular are also found among the class II genes (Fig. 86.1). TAP genes encode for *t*ransporters of *a*ntigen *p*resentation. These proteins form structures that transport antigenic peptides from the cytoplasm to the endoplasmic reticulum, where they associate with HLA antigens. Large multifunctional protease (LMP) genes encode proteins that form the proteasome, a large molecular weight structure in the cytoplasm that is responsible for cleavage of large proteins into smaller peptides. Constituent proteins of the proteasome are polymorphic, and there may be differences between individuals in the peptides generated in the cytoplasm as well as the ability of peptides to bind to different HLA alleles.

Class III antigens are encoded between HLA classes I and II (Fig. 86.1). They include complement proteins, such as C2, C4, and factor B (Bf); cytokines, such as TNF-α, and heat shock proteins (Hsp 70; not shown in the figure).

The function of HLA antigens is to present antigenic peptides. Class I molecules tend to bind peptides of 7 to 8 amino acids tightly in a central groove, whereas class II molecules bind

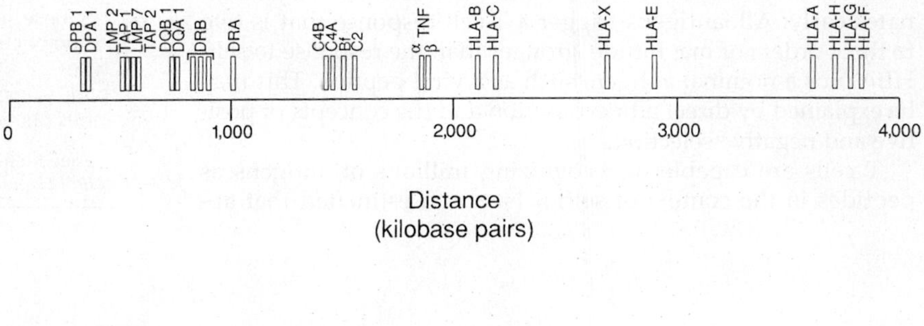

Figure 86.1. Genomic organization of the human Major Histocompatibility Complex (HLA). For details see text and Krensky AM, Clayberger C. Structure of HLA molecules and immunosuppressive effects of HLA derived peptides. *Int Rev Immunol* 1996;13:173–185. (Reproduced with permission from Krensky AM. The HLA system, antigen presentation and processing. *Kidney Int* 1997;51:S3.)

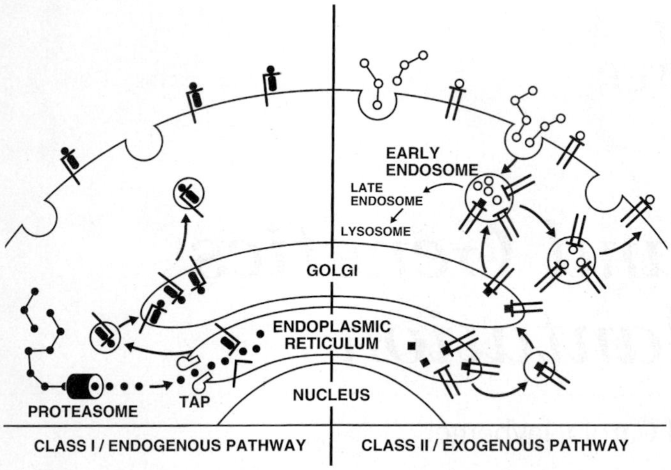

Figure 86.2. Antigen presentation pathways. The figure compares intracellular trafficking of the HLA class I and class II pathways. HLA class I molecules generally bind endogenous antigens. Proteins are degraded to peptides in cytosolic proteasomes and/or by other mechanisms. These peptides are delivered to the endoplasmic reticulum (ER) via transporters. Peptide, HLA class I heavy chain and β_2-microglobulin form a complex in the ER and are exported to the Golgi, and eventually to the cell surface. In contrast, HLA class II molecules generally bind exogenous antigens that enter through endosomal/lysosomal pathways. HLA class II α and β chains associate with invariant chain in the ER. A nonameric form exits the ER, through the Golgi, and into an early endosome. There, the invariant chain is degraded, leaving a "CLIP" fragment in the groove. Peptides from the extracellular space taken up by endocytosis are targeted to the "compartment for peptide loading" where antigenic peptides replace CLIP in the groove. Mature heterotrimeric molecules are transported to the cell surface. Details are provided in Noessner E, Krensky AM. HLA and antigen presentation. In: Tilney NL, Strom TB, Paul LC, eds. *Transplantation biology: cellular and molecular aspects.* New York: Lippincott-Raven Press, 1996:31.1–31.13. (Reproduced with permission from Krensky AM, Clayberger C. Structure of HLA molecules and immunosuppressive effects of HLA derived peptides. *Int Rev* Immunol 1996;13:176.)

longer peptides, typically 8 to15 amino acids in length, that may bulge out more in the middle and hang out of the ends of the antigen presentation groove. Most of the polymorphisms lie along the antigen presentation grooves. These amino acid differences determine which peptides can bind to a given HLA allele. It benefits the species to bind as many different peptides as possible so that the species will not succumb to a single new infectious invader. Transplant rejection is the result of these polymorphisms and the fact that T lymphocytes recognize differences in HLA sequences, triggering the immune response.

The Alloantigen

The nature of the alloantigen is complex. There are at least two mechanisms by which T lymphocytes can recognize HLA molecules (Fig. 86.3). Direct allorecognition involves T-cell recognition of whole non–self-HLA molecules. In contrast, indirect allorecognition involves recognition of non–self-HLA peptides in the context of self-HLA. The relative importance of these two pathways remains controversial. Nevertheless, certain characteristics of the alloresponse suggest that the direct pathway dominates early: Alloantigens trigger a T-cell response that is two to three orders of magnitude stronger than the response to self-HLA plus a nominal antigen, such as a viral peptide. This may be explained by direct allorecognition and the concepts of positive and negative selection.

T cells are capable of recognizing millions of antigens as peptides in the context of self; it has been estimated that approximately 10^{13} different $\alpha\beta$ and 10^{17} different $\gamma\delta$ T-cell receptor (TCR) sequences are possible). There is a natural affinity between T cells and HLA molecules, but because there is no *a priori* genetic relationship between a given HLA type and the T-cell repertoire, this "relationship" must be learned. Development of T-cell specificity occurs in the thymus by both positive and negative selection. T cells with very high affinity for self-HLA are potentially autoreactive and are deleted from the repertoire by negative selection. T cells with very low affinity are not selected and die. Only those T cells with intermediate affinity for self-HLA plus peptides are positively selected and enter the periphery as mature T lymphocytes. Thus selection results in only those cells with "proper" affinity entering into the bloodstream and peripheral organs. In transplantation, a given T cell may for the first time interact with an HLA allele for which it has high natural affinity but for which it was not deleted in the thymus. Therefore these high-affinity interactions may account for the strength of direct allorecognition. Alternatively, non–self-HLA may mimic self-HLA plus a non-self peptide. In addition, the density of alloantigens on the transplant may contribute to the strength of the alloresponse. Finally, the role of peptide in the groove in allorecognition is still unclear. Rammansee et al showed that allogeneic T cells can recognize HLA molecules in a variety of patterns (Table 86.1).

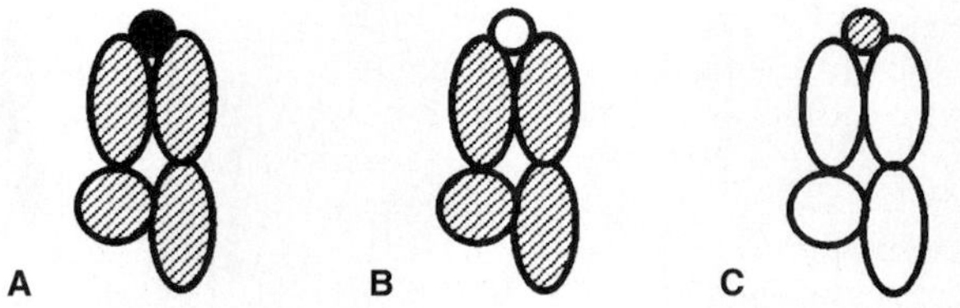

Figure 86.3. Direct and indirect allorecognition. Alloantigen can be recognized in distinct forms. In direct recognition, allogeneic HLA is recognized regardless of the peptide bound in the groove **(A)** or as allogeneic HLA plus a particular peptide **(B)**. In indirect recognition, self HLA presents allogeneic peptides **(C)**. For details see Krensky AM, Clayberger C. The nature of allorecognition. *Curr Opin Nephrol Hypertens* 1993;2:898–903.

Role of HLA Matching in Clinical Transplantation

The benefits of HLA matching in living related transplantation are clear even in the cyclosporine era. Although current 1-year graft survival statistics for sibling transplants are similar regardless of HLA matching, longer term transplant survival is highly correlated with the degree of matching. Recipients of a 2- haplotype match enjoy a graft half-life of 25 years compared with 16 years for a 1-haplotype match and 11.9 years for a 0-haplotype match.

The effect of HLA matching in cadaveric transplantation is more controversial. The impact of HLA-DR matching appears

TABLE 86.1. Molecular Nature of Alloantigen Recognized by T Lymphocytes

HLA molecules with no peptide present (empty)
HLA molecule with peptide present but peptide is irrelevant to the response
Specific peptide is necessary but may be expressed with several HLA types
Peptide is specific for the HLA type (faithfully HLA dependent)
Various peptides suffice

See Krensky AM, Clayberger C. The nature of allorecognition. *Curr Opin Nephrol Hypertens* 1993;2:898–903 for details.

to be most important during the first 5 months posttransplant. This may correspond to the importance of donor antigen presenting cells (APCs; "passenger leukocytes") during this time period. In the Collaborative Transplant Study of Opelz and colleagues of approximately 10,000 patients treated with cyclosporine, there was a 17% better 1-year graft survival rate in recipients matched for HLA-B and HLA-DR compared with those mismatched for these antigens. The 1996 United Network for Organ Sharing (UNOS) data revealed that poorly matched kidneys gave lower graft survival rates whether they were shared or used locally. Current UNOS policy involves sharing of zero mismatch (0MM) cadaver kidneys nationwide. One to six antigen-mismatched kidneys are distributed within the local Organ Procurement Organization (OPO) based on the time on the waiting list and ABO compatibility.

Serologic Cross-Matching

Another important consideration in recipient selection is the presence of antibodies reactive with the donor's HLA antigens. Therefore a serologic cross-match is performed immediately before transplantation. Standard technique involves incubation of recipient serum with donor T or B lymphocytes in the presence of rabbit complement and measurement of lymphocyte lysis. Cytotoxic antibodies directed against donor class I antigens (a positive T-cell cross-match) is an absolute contraindication to transplantation because of the very high risk of hyperacute rejection. In contrast, a positive B-cell cross-match, indicating antibodies against donor class II antigens, is not as highly associated with hyperacute rejection, but does carry a 10% to 20% graft survival disadvantage. A variety of newer techniques are able to detect even lower levels of donor specific antibodies in recipient serum, but data as to how to use this information are limited. Patients who are highly sensitized to foreign HLA antigens as a result of previous blood transfusions, prior transplantation, or pregnancies are more likely to have a positive cross-match and will generally wait longer for a transplant.

Minor Transplant Antigens

In addition to the HLA molecules encoded within the major histocompatibility complex, there are minor histocompatibility (miH) antigens that can target rejection in the absence of MHC differences. More than 30 minor systems have been described, largely in rodents. Typically, minor antigens are limited in their polymorphism and are presented as peptides in the context of self-MHC to T lymphocytes. It has been difficult to develop serologic reagents that are specific for small peptides, necessitating the use of cell proliferation or cytotoxicity assays to identify them. Some examples of bona fide miH in humans include mitochondrial proteins (which are only inherited from the mother) and H-Y antigens (expressed by males but not females).

THE ALLORESPONSE

Regardless of the precise molecular nature of alloantigen, it triggers T lymphocytes to start the non-self response (Fig. 86.4). CD4+ helper T lymphocytes recognize foreign HLA on the graft, in draining lymph nodes, and in the context of self-antigen-presenting cells (monocytes, B lymphocytes, dendritic cells). The antigen receptor on T lymphocytes (TCR) recognizes HLA plus peptide. There are two types of T-cell receptors: the common α, β heterodimers and the uncommon (less than 10%) γ, δ T-cell receptors. The α, β TCR is the most important in transplant rejection and it is still unclear what role if any γ, δ T-cell receptors have in this process.

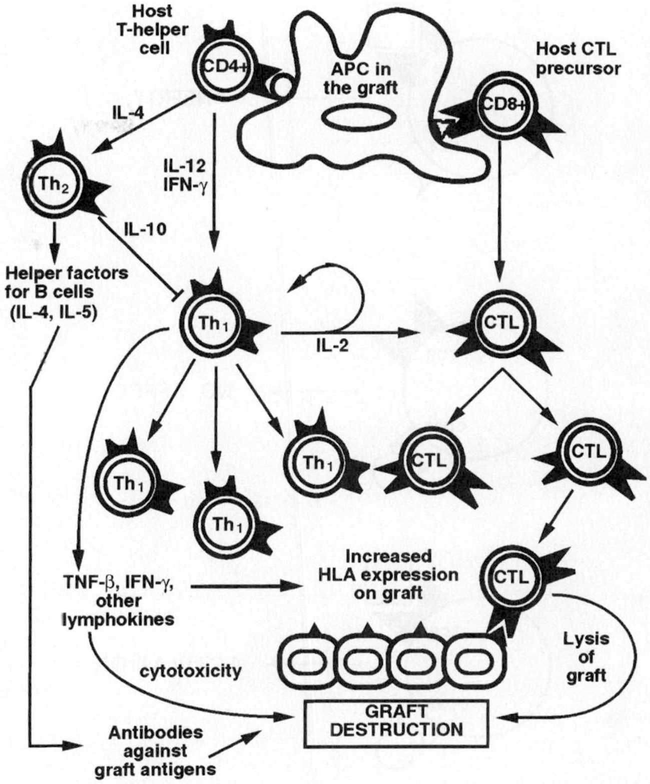

Figure 86.4. Simplified scheme of cellular and molecular events underlying transplant rejection. For details see Krensky AM, Weiss A, Crabtree G, et al. Mechanisms of disease: T lymphocyte–antigen interactions in transplant rejection. *N Engl J Med* 1990;322:510–517.

Costimulation

Engagement of the TCR with its specific peptide antigen-HLA complex is not sufficient to activate a T cell. Schwartz et al showed that "two signals" were required (Fig. 86.5). The TCR provides the first signal, but other cell surface receptor–ligand interactions are required to provide the second signal. If only the first signal is provided, the T cell enters into a nonresponsive state called *anergy*. If both signals are provided, the T cell is activated to differentiate and divide, expressing lymphokines and cell surface molecules that both regulate the immune response and mediate effector function. Several receptor-ligand pairs may provide the second signal (Table 86.2), but the best studied to date is the interaction between CD28 and CD152 (CTLA4) on the T cell with CD80 (B7-1) and CD86 (B7-2) on the antigen presenting cell (monocyte, B lymphocyte, dendritic cell, and so on). CD28 is expressed constitutively on 95% of resting CD4+ T cells and 50% of CD8+ T cells, and its expression increases on T-cell stimulation. CTLA4 is normally expressed in very low levels by peripheral blood lymphocytes but is markedly upregulated after activation. B7-1 expression is induced on B cells by a variety of signals including engagement of cell surface immunoglobulin (Ig) by antigen or CD40 by its ligand, CD40L. B7-2 is constitutively expressed. Engagement of CD28 with either B7-1 or B7-2 leads to T-cell activation. Engagement with CTLA4 with these same two ligands leads to a damping of the immune response. Mice that do not express CTLA4 because of gene disruption (CTLA4 knockout) develop

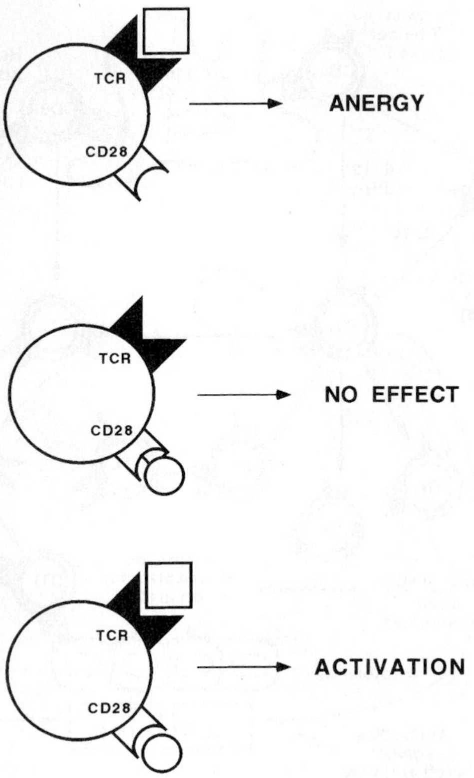

Figure 86.5. T-cell activation requires two signals. Signalling through both the T-cell receptor and the CD28 costimulatory receptor are required for optimal activation of naive T cells. Signalling through the T-cell receptor alone results in anergy, a state of unresponsiveness. Signalling through CD28 alone has no known effect. For details see Sayegh MH, Turka LA. The role of T cell costimulatory activation pathways in transplant rejection. *N Engl J Med* 1998;338:1813–1821.

TABLE 86.2. Selected Second Signals Involved in T-Cell Activation

Receptor-Ligand Pair	Biologic Action
CD28 - B7-1 (CD80)	Costimulation
CD28 - B7-2 (CD86)	Costimulation
CTLA4 - B7-1, B7-2	Suppression
CD40 - CD40 ligand (CD154)	Costimulation
LFA-1 - ICAM-1,2,3,4,5	Leukocyte adherence, migration, activation
CD2 - CD58 (LFA-3)	Leukocyte adhesion
VLA-4 - VCAM	Leukocyte adherence, migration, activation

ICAM, intracellular adhesion molecule; LFA, lymphocyte function–associated antigen; VCAM, vascular cell adhesion molecule; VLA, very late antigen.
LFA-1 = CD11a, CD18; ICAM-1 = CD54; ICAM-2 = CD102; CTLA4 = CD152.

a disorder characterized by unrestricted lymphocyte proliferation and death.

T-Cell Response

Once a T-cell receptor engages its specific peptide-HLA target and a second signal is provided via costimulation, the T cell is activated. A series of biochemical events at the cell surface are followed by a cascade of sequential gene activation in the nucleus (Fig. 86.6). Intracellular calcium levels rise dramatically, due to both an influx of extracellular calcium and release of calcium from intracellular stores. Phosphatidyl inositol signaling pathways and tyrosine kinases are activated, and protein kinase C translocates from the cytoplasm to the cell membrane. These early changes at the plasma membrane are followed by changes in the nucleus. For instance, invariant sequences of the TCR complex interact with *src* family members, *lck* and *fyn*, and are phosphorylated. The coreceptors CD4 and CD8 bind *lck* through a common cysteine-containing motif, bringing *lck* into proximity with the TCR. In a separate but related pathway, vav phosphorylation activates the ras signal transduction system. Ras, a guanosine triphosphate (GTP) binding protein with GTPase activity, interacts with Raf-1, a serine-threonine kinase, which regulates a cascade of other kinases including Mek and MAP (mitogen activated protein) kinases. These events lead to c-fos and c-jun transcription factor binding to the IL-2 promoter. Along with the nuclear factor of activated T cells (NF-AT), these factors promote the transcription of new genes, including IL-2. Interleukin-2 induces proliferation and differentiation of the T cell that produces it (autocrine stimulation) and nearby cells (paracrine stimulation). Numerous other lymphokines and cytokines are produced, including γ-interferon, which induces both *de novo* and increased expression of HLA class II antigens, which in turn amplify the stimulation. Chemokines (chemoattractant cytokines), adhesion molecules, growth and differentiation factors, and effector molecules are produced (Table 86.3).

CD4+ Helper T Cells. CD4+ T cells initiate specific immunity by recognizing antigenic peptides bound to MHC class II molecules on B cells or other antigen-presenting cells, such as dendritic cells and macrophages and secreting soluble proteins, such as interleukin (IL)-2, IL-4, and interferon (IFN)-γ that are collectively referred to as cytokines (Fig. 86.4). These cytokines "help" in the activation and differentiation of other lymphoid cells, hence the designation of CD4+ T cells as "helper" T cells.

$CD4^+$ helper T cells can be divided into two mutually exclusive subsets. These subsets can be distinguished by the particular cytokines they produce, the lymphocytes they affect, and the types of pathogen to which they respond. Th_1 cells produce cytokines such as IL-2, IFN-γ, and tumor necrosis factor-α/β, while Th_2 cells produce IL-4, IL-5, IL-6, IL-10, and IL-13. Th_1 cells induce the differentiation of IgG_{2a} antibody-producing B cells, whereas Th_2 cells induce differentiation of IgG_1 and IgE-producing B cells. Th_1 cells mediate delayed type hypersensitivity (DTH), while Th_2 cells activate eosinophils and mast cells. Th_1 cells are beneficial in response to leishmaniasis, leprosy, viruses, and allergy, while Th_2 cells are beneficial in arthritis, autoimmunity, helminth infection, and pregnancy. In humans, a Th_0 subset has also been described. These cells can produce various combinations of both Th_1 and Th_2 cytokines.

Th_1 and Th_2 cells derive from a common precursor. Differentiation into Th_1 versus Th_2 cells is determined by the particular cytokines in the microenvironment of the developing cell. Th_2 cells differentiate in the presence of IL-4 whereas Th_1 cells differentiate in the presence of IL-12 and IFNγ. The source of these cytokines is still controversial, but in some cases, $\gamma\delta$ T cells and natural killer (NK) cells provide IL-4 early in an immune response while phagocytes produce IL-12 in response to certain pathogens.

Cytolytic T lymphocytes. $CD8^+$ T lymphocytes that recognize peptide/HLA class I antigens can, in the presence of cytokines such as IL-2 made by T helper cells, differentiate into cytolytic T lymphocytes (CTL). Once fully differentiated, CTL can kill targets by at least two distinct pathways. The first pathway, called *granule exocytosis,* involves the regulated directional

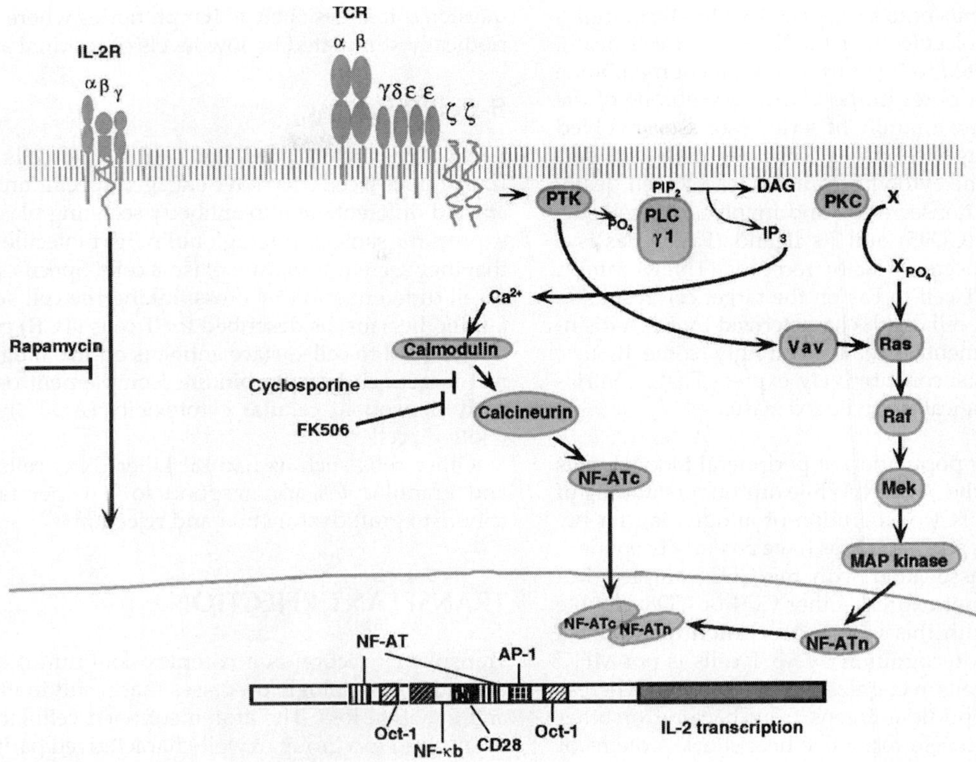

Figure 86.6. Simplified scheme of T-cell activation. Occupation of the T-cell receptor initiates a cascade of intracellular signals, ultimately resulting in gene transcription. IP3, inositol 1,4,5-trisphosphate; NF-AT_c, nuclear factor of activated T cells cytosolic form; NF-AT_n, nuclear factor of activated T cells nuclear form; PIP_2, phosphatidylinositol 4,5-bisphosphate; PKC, protein kinase C; PLC, phospholipase C; PTK, protein tyrosine kinase. Sites of inhibition by the immunosuppressive drugs cyclosporine, FK506, and rapamycin are shown. For details see Cantrell D. T cell antigen receptor signal transduction pathways. *Annu Rev Immunol* 1996;14:259–274.

TABLE 86.3. Selected T-Cell Activation Molecules (Chemokines, Lymphokines, Adhesion Molecules, Effector Molecules)

Molecule	Biologic Function
Chemokines	
RANTES	Chemoattractant for monocytes, T lymphocytes, etc.
MCP 1-4	Chemoattractant for monocytes, T lymphocytes, etc.
MIP-1α, β	Chemoattractant for monocytes, T lymphocytes, etc.
Lymphokines	
Interferon-γ	Broad activation and differentiation factor
IL-2	T-cell proliferation and differentiation (growth factor)
IL-4	Broad proliferation and differentiation (growth factor) favors TH2 cells
IL-10	T-cell proliferation and differentiation (growth factor) favors TH2 cells
IL-12	T-cell proliferation and differentiation (growth factor) favors TH1 cells
IL-15	T-cell proliferation and differentiation (growth factor)
Adhesion molecules	
LFA-1 (CD11a, CD18)	Interacts with ICAMs
CD2	Interacts with LFA-3 (CD58)
ICAM-1 (CD54)	Interacts with LFA-1
VLA-4 (CD49d)	Interacts with VCAM-1, same as α4 integrin
Effector molecules	
Perforin	Complement 9-like pore-forming protein
Granzymes	Serine esterases involved in cytolysis, apoptosis
Granulysin	Saposinlike cytolytic molecule
Fas Ligand	Interacts with Fas (CD95) to induce cell death (apoptosis)

ICAM, intercellular adhesion molecule; IL, interleukin; LFA, lymphocyte function-associated antigen; MCP, monocyte chemoattractant protein; MIP, macrophage inflammatory protein; RANTES, regulated upon activation, normal T cell expressed and secreted; VCAM, vascular cell adhesion molecule; VLA, very late activation antigen.

release of granular contents onto a target cell. Cytolytic granules contain a number of molecules that mediate target cell death. Perforin is a protein related to C9 of the complement membrane attack complex. It forms pores in the plasma membrane of the target cell. Granzymes are a family of serine esterases involved in the degradation of target cell DNA. Together, these and perhaps other proteins in the cytolytic granules lead to cell death. The second pathway is nonsecretory and involves the cell surface interaction of Fas (CD95) and its ligand (FasL). Fas is a member of the tumor necrosis factor receptor (TNFR) family. Binding of FasL on the T cell to Fas on the target cell results in apoptosis (programmed cell death characterized by DNA disintegration and cell fragmentation). Interestingly, some tissues, such as cornea and testis, constitutively express FasL, contributing to their immunologically privileged status.

γδ T Cells. A minor population of peripheral blood T cells (less than 10%) express the γδ TCR. While our understanding of the rules governing γδ TCR recognition of antigen lag far behind that of the αβ TCR, some features have recently been identified. The γδ TCR is associated with the CD3 complex, but many of these cells do not express either CD4 or CD8 (double negative). Consistent with this is the observation that, with a few exceptions, antigen recognition by γδ T cells is not MHC restricted. Some γδ T cells recognize intact proteins, whereas others recognize nonpeptidic antigens from bacteria or other pathogens. γδ T cells can also recognize heat shock proteins or phosphorylated alkyl, carbohydrate or nucleotide residues. Thus γδ T cells recognize an overall structure, rather than the antigenic peptide and MHC complex recognized by αβ T cells.

Delayed-Type Hypersensitivity Responses. Delayed-type hypersensitivity (DTH) is a cell-mediated immune response in which an activated mononuclear phagocyte (macrophage) is the ultimate effector cell. DTH is a primary immune defense against intracellular bacteria such as *Listeria monocytogenes* and mycobacteria. It can also be induced by sensitization to chemicals or environmental antigens or by intradermal injection of microbial antigens, e.g., purified protein derivative (PPD) from *Mycobacterium tuberculosis* in presensitized or vaccinated individuals. DTH is initiated when CD4+ or CD8+ T cells recognize MHC associated antigenic peptides and produce inflammatory cytokines such as IL-2, TNF, and IL-8. Within a few hours, neutrophils accumulate at postcapillary venules at the site, but by 12 hours, T cells and macrophages replace the neutrophils. These T cells produce additional inflammatory cytokines, including IFN-γ, which activate the macrophages. The endothelial cells lining the postcapillary venules swell and fibrinogen leaks from the blood vessels into the surrounding tissue, where it is cleaved to fibrin. Deposition of fibrin, plus the infiltrating T cells and macrophages, cause the tissue to become swollen and hard. Induration is obvious by about 18 hours and peaks by 24 to 48 hours. The activated macrophages eliminate the antigen, leading to resolution of the response.

T-Cell Memory. In most cases, the immune response to foreign antigens has distinct short- and long-term phases. Immediately following the primary antigenic challenge, specific effector T cells rapidly expand and destroy the pathogen. Most effector cells are relatively short lived and are eliminated at the end of the primary immune response. However, some of these cells are spared and develop into memory cells. Subsequent challenge with the same antigen leads to a more rapid and effective response because of both an increase in the precursor frequency of antigen-specific T cells and increased sensitivity to antigen. Memory T cells are small resting cells that may be sequestered in areas such as lymph nodes where they can be periodically stimulated by low levels of residual antigen.

B-Cell Response

Some of the factors produced by T-helper cells (IL-4, IL-5, and IL-6) induce B cells that have engaged specific antigen to proliferate and differentiate into antibody secreting plasma cells. B cells express the same immunoglobulin (Ig) molecule on their surface that they secrete as mature plasma cells. Specific antigen triggers B-cell differentiation by cross-linking the cell surface receptors (antibodies) just as described for T cells (TCR) previously. Antibodies bind to cell surface antigens on the allograft and can direct target cell lysis by binding complement or directing antibody dependent cellular cytotoxicity (ADCC) mediated by K ("killer") cells.

Other cells such as natural killer (NK) cells, macrophages, and granulocytes also respond to T-helper factors and contribute to graft dysfunction and rejection.

TRANSPLANT REJECTION

Transplant rejection is a complex continuum of immunologic and nonimmunologic processes that result in graft dysfunction and eventual loss. The aforementioned cellular and molecular events lead to a group of well-characterized pathologic and clinical patterns of rejection. This classification affects our understanding of the pathogenesis and therapy of different states.

Hyperacute Rejection

Almost immediate rejection of vascularized allografts is the result of preexisting donor-specific antibodies, including those against ABO blood group and HLA antigens. In hyperacute rejection, antibodies bind to the endothelium, activate complement, and cause concomitant coagulation and chemotaxis. Within 12 hours of transplantation, fibrin and platelet thrombi are evident within capillaries, and there is a prominent neutrophilic infiltrate. By 12 to 18 hours there is more diffuse thrombosis, with involvement of arterioles, interstitial edema, and cortical infarction. Routine cross-matching procedures have largely eliminated the occurrence of hyperacute rejection from clinical practice.

Acute Vascular Rejection

Fibrinoid necrosis of arterial beds characterizes this type of accelerated rejection, which occurs within 30 to 90 days after transplantation and typically progresses to graft loss within 1 to 6 months. Lesions are characterized by fibrinoid necrosis of the media and fibrin-platelet thrombosis of the lumens. Prominent interstitial edema and hemorrhage, tubular necrosis, and foci of cortical infarction are characteristic features. Tubulointerstitial mononuclear cell infiltrates may be present. This type of rejection is probably caused by preexisting donor-specific antibodies that are present at levels below the limit of detection by standard T-lymphocyte cross-matching but that are identifiable by flow cytometry.

Acute Cellular, Tubulointerstitial, and Vascular Rejection

Perivenular and periglomerular lymphocytes and macrophages are characteristic of this type of rejection. Mononuclear cells infiltrate the interstitium and tubular epithelium, often associated with edema and occasionally with extravasation of erythrocytes.

Tubular lumens dilate, the brush borders disappear, and dead epithelial cells can be found within the tubular lumens as the basement membrane becomes denuded. Subendothelial infiltrates may also be present, indicating vascular involvement. Rarely, the process involves the entire vessel wall, resulting in inflammatory necrotizing vasculitis.

Chronic Rejection

Long-term graft survival has not improved despite major improvement in 1-year graft survival (Fig. 86.7). Although 1-year graft survival is 95% for living-related transplants and 90% for cadaveric transplants in our center, the half-life for cadaveric transplants remains constant at approximately 7 years. The major cause of graft loss is now chronic rejection, a combination of immunologic, hemodynamic, and social (compliance) factors.

Several potential risk factors have been associated with chronic rejection. Immunologic factors correlating with chronic rejection include poor HLA matching (especially for HLA-DR) and high frequency of acute rejection episodes. There is a lower rate of chronic rejection in grafts from living-related rather than cadaveric donors, and this difference increases over time. Cytomegalovirus infection in the recipient is associated with chronic rejection. Nonimmunologic factors, including ischemia and reperfusion injury, have immunologic consequences, including increased expression of HLA-DR and accessory molecules, like lymphocyte function-associated antigen-1 (LFA-1) and intercellular adhesion molecule-1 (ICAM-1). Another major factor is extremes of donor age. Transplantation of pediatric kidneys into adults, female kidneys into large males, and kidneys from older donors or blacks (with fewer nephrons) into whites all result in lower than average graft survival, suggesting that the ratio of initial functioning nephrons to body mass may be an important determinant. Although there is a great deal of discussion as to the relative importance of immunologic and nonimmunologic factors in this process, such a duality is not physiologically relevant because of the continual interplay of such factors. Chronic rejection is dynamic and multifactorial.

Chronic rejection is characterized by chronic vascular and fibroobliterative changes. The vascular lumen is narrowed by

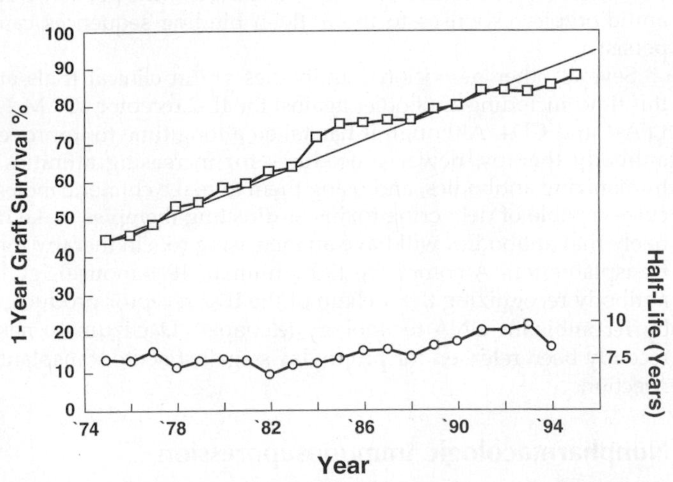

Figure 86.7. Better early graft survival has not decreased the risk of late graft loss. Despite progressive improvement in 1-year graft survival rates (>80%), the rate of failure of kidney allografts has remained constant at approximately an 8-year half-life. For details see Hata Y, Ozawa M, Takemoto SK, et al. HLA matching in clinical transplants. *Clin Transpl* 1996; Cecka JM, Terasaki PI, eds. UCLA Tissue Typing Laboratory. Los Angeles, 1997: 381–396. (This figure was prepared by and a gift from C.B. Carpenter and E. Milford, Harvard University.)

cellular myofibroproliferation, although the media is typically normal. The fibrous tissue and subendothelial spaces contain lymphocytes and macrophages. These vascular lesions can be associated with tubular atrophy, interstitial fibrosis and glomerular capillary collapse. So-called chronic transplant glomerulopathy is characterized by double and multicontoured capillary walls, the result of mesangial interposition and replication of the endothelial cell basal lamina. Immunofluorescence may show linear and granular deposits of immunoglobulin and complement along the capillary walls and peritubular capillaries.

Periglomerular and perivascular macrophages secrete fibrogenic cytokines, including platelet derived growth factor (PDGF) and transforming growth factor (TGF)-β. Increased expression of IL-1, tumor necrosis factor (TNF), IL-6, and ICAM-1 have also been associated with chronic rejection. Glomerulosclerosis and arterial obliteration contribute to hypertension, causing remaining glomeruli to hyperfilter and eventually fibrose, leading to further chronic functional deterioration. To date, the only effective therapy for chronic rejection is retransplantation, although there is hope that new drugs like rapamycin may slow fibroproliferation and that the combination of angiotensin-converting enzyme (ACE) inhibitors, protein restriction, and control of systemic hypertension can slow functional decline.

PHARMACOLOGY OF TRANSPLANT REJECTION

Drugs

The mainstays of current immunosuppressive therapies are corticosteroids and calcineurin inhibitors (cyclosporine and FK506). Azathioprine is increasingly being replaced by mycophenolate mofetil. A new drug with considerable promise is rapamycin. (The use of these drugs in the management of transplant recipients is discussed in detail in Chapter 88, Part 2.)

Corticosteroids

Corticosteroids have numerous immunologic effects and are potent inhibitors of transplant rejection. At low doses they prevent rejection and at higher doses they can reverse rejection. Corticosteroids bind to specific receptors which in turn bind response elements for key genes. They block the transcription of IL-1, TNF, and IL-6 in accessory cells and of IL-2 in T lymphocytes. They also block the expression of important chemokines, including IL-8, MCP-1, and RANTES, interfering with recruitment of inflammatory cells. In high doses, steroids cause lympholysis. The use of steroids is limited by the myriad of associated side effects, including infections, glucose intolerance, growth retardation, bone disease, delayed wound healing, hypertension, and psychologic disturbances.

Calcineurin Inhibitors

Cyclosporine and FK506 (tacrolimus), the two most potent immunosuppressives in use, are related in their mechanism of action. They block T-cell activation by binding to cytoplasmic receptors called immunophilins. Cyclosporine binds to cyclophilins and FK506 binds to FK-binding proteins (FKBP). These drug-receptor complexes in turn bind to calcineurin, a phosphatase required for regulated expression of the IL-2 and other genes. Transcription factors, including a component of the nuclear factor of activated T lymphocytes (NFAT), must be dephosphorylated by calcineurin to translocate from the cytoplasm to the nucleus. When NFAT does not move to the nucleus, IL-2 transcription and T-cell activation do not occur. Both drugs are highly potent immunosuppressives that have revolutionized solid-organ transplantation. However, the use of both drugs is limited by nephrotoxicity. In addition, cyclosporine can cause hepatotoxicity, hyperkalemia, hypertension, gingival hypertrophy, neurotoxicity, and hirsutism. Deleterious side effects of FK506 include neurotoxicity, impaired glucose tolerance, and hypertension.

Nucleic Acid Synthesis Inhibitors

Azathioprine, mycophenolate mofetil, mizoribine, and brequinar block T- and B-cell proliferation by inhibiting nucleotide biosynthesis. Azathioprine, a derivative of 6-mercaptopurine, disrupts both RNA and DNA synthesis by interfering with the synthesis of adenine and guanine nucleotides. Mycophenolate mofetil and mizoribine inhibit the *de novo,* but not the salvage, pathway of purine synthesis. Brequinar is a noncompetitive inhibitor of dihydroorotate dehydrogenase in the *de novo* pathway of pyrimidine synthesis. Mycophenolate mofetil, mizoribine, and brequinar are reported to be more selective antiproliferative agents than azathioprine is. In early clinical studies, mycophenolate mofetil (Cellcept) appears to significantly decrease the incidence of acute rejection episodes when used in place of azathioprine in otherwise standard protocols. The major side effects of azathioprine are neutropenia and thrombocytopenia, megaloblastic anemia, interstitial pneumonitis, hepatotoxicity, and malignancy. Mycophenolate mofetil is also myelotoxic, causing hypochromic anemia, leukopenia, and thrombocytopenia, as well as diarrhea, constipation, nausea, and vomiting.

Rapamycin

Rapamycin (sirolimus) is a macrolide, like FK506, and also binds to FKBPs, but it does not block cytokine gene transcription. Rather, it inhibits signal transduction by IL-2 and other growth factors. Rapamycin binds to FKBP12 and the target of rapamycin (TOR), which has sequence homology to the catalytic domain of a PI-3 kinase subunit. It blocks cell cycle progression from G1 to S by inhibiting cyclin-dependent kinases and a series of downstream events. Rapamycin and FK506 are pharmacologic antagonists (both bind FKBP12), while cyclosporine and rapamycin appear to act synergistically (binding to different immunophilins). Rapamycin may have added advantages in inhibition of vascular rejection due to its antiproliferative effects on smooth muscle cells and fibroblasts. It can cause diabetes in rats but not in primates, and it is reported to be less nephrotoxic than cyclosporine.

Antibodies

Antibodies recognize antigens with high affinity on the allograft and have the capacity to target various effector mechanisms, including complement and antibody-dependent cellular cytotoxicity (ADCC). For these reasons, they may prove useful for immunotherapy of transplantation.

Polyclonal Antibodies

Polyclonal antilymphocyte or antithymocyte globulins have been used to prevent or reverse allograft rejection since the 1960s. These reagents are generated by immunizing animals with human lymphoid or thymic cells and purifying the resultant antisera to obtain isolated gamma globulin fractions. These reagents contain a heterogeneous group of antibodies, only some (if any) of which are specific for effector T cells involved in transplant rejection. Nevertheless, lymphocytes coated with such antisera are removed from the peripheral blood via the reticuloendothelial system and complement-mediated lysis. In addition, these antibodies may block lymphocyte function at the cell surface and may induce suppressor cell populations. Because each preparation varies in its constituent antibodies, efficacy and side effects are variable. Side effects include increased risk of infection and malignancies, thrombocytopenia, neutropenia, serum sickness, glomerulonephritis, and anaphylaxis.

Monoclonal Antibodies

Many of the limitations of polyclonal antibodies can be overcome with monoclonal preparations. Kohler and Milstein received the Nobel Prize for describing methods to generate essentially unlimited quantities of antibody of a single specificity. Mice are immunized and their immune cells (spleen or lymph node) harvested and immortalized by fusion with a suitable B-cell myeloma that has been selected for inability to grow in a selection media (supplemented with hypoxanthine, aminopterin, and thymidine). Only murine B cells fused to the myeloma will survive in the selection media. They can then be cloned, characterized, and maintained indefinitely. OKT3 is an FDA-approved monoclonal antibody used for therapy of transplant rejection. OKT3, which recognizes a chain of the CD3 complex, blocks T-cell receptor function (blockade, inhibition), clears TCRs from the T-cell surface (internalization, shedding), and/or clears T cells from the peripheral blood (depletion). Peripheral blood T lymphocyte counts fall transiently, and reappearing T cells fail to express the TCR complex until OKT3 treatment is stopped. OKT3 therapy is effective for both induction therapy and reversal of rejection.

The main side effect of OKT3 therapy is a flulike syndrome resulting from cytokine release. In addition to fever, chills, and rigors, less frequently occurring complications include aseptic meningitis, renal insufficiency, and pulmonary edema. These symptoms are greatly alleviated by premedication with steroids and antihistamines. Viral infections and lymphoproliferative disease occur at an increased frequency when OKT3 is used. Human antimouse antibodies (HAMA), which neutralize the antibody's efficacy, are typically produced after the first use. Concurrent immunosuppression can decrease the incidence of HAMA, but development of "humanized" antibodies has largely overcome this problem. Antibodies are engineered such that the vast majority of the molecule is human, and only the antigen-specific combining region sequences are derived from mouse. This decreases the antibody response to the murine portion, but antiidiotypic responses to the antigen binding sequences can persist.

Several other monoclonal antibodies are in clinical trials at this time, including antibodies against the IL-2 receptor, ICAM-1, LFA-1 and CD4. Although it has taken a long time to improve antibody therapy, newer procedures for increasing affinities, humanizing antibodies, and using them to make chimeric molecules capable of delivering toxins or directing therapies make it likely that antibodies will have an increasing role in therapy for transplantation. A composite (90% human, 10% mouse) IgG1 antibody recognizing the α chain of the IL-2 receptor produced by recombinant DNA technology (Zenapax, Daclizumab) has recently been released for prophylaxis against acute transplant rejection.

Nonpharmacologic Immunosuppression

Plasmapheresis, splenectomy, total body irradiation (TLI), and blood transfusions historically have been used as adjuvant therapies for transplantation. All these modalities are infrequently used today. Plasmapheresis does not appear to be generally applicable. Splenectomy and total lymphoid irradiation are associated with the risk of overwhelming sepsis. Although blood transfusions were efficacious in the precyclosprine era, differences in outcome have disappeared in the modern immunotherapy era. Some of these therapies, particularly blood transfusions and TLI, may prove useful in protocols for induction and maintenance of tolerance.

Combination Therapy

Because the various immunotherapies just listed inhibit rejection at different points and by different mechanisms, combination therapies can provide additive or even synergistic immunosuppression without added toxicity. In addition, by decreasing individual doses (sparing), toxicities can be further reduced. For these reasons, current protocols involve administration of three or four different drugs in combination.

TOLERANCE

To date, antirejection therapies have been directed at generalized blockade or suppression of the immune response. Broad-based immunosuppression leaves the patient at risk for opportunistic infections and secondary tumors. Therefore it might be easier to work with the immune system rather than against it to achieve tolerance, an active state of antigen-specific nonresponsiveness. Tolerance can be readily induced in a variety of animal models and occurs spontaneously in some humans who receive transplants. Despite a detailed understanding of the mechanisms leading to experimental tolerance, it has been exceedingly difficult to induce and maintain tolerance in clinical practice. Nevertheless, experimental protocols with the potential to obtain tolerance are under clinical evaluation.

The immune system must discriminate self from non-self, destroying harmful invaders or mutations, while leaving self intact. Owen first showed that antigen-specific nonresponsiveness was an active state in his studies of freemartin cattle (in twin cattle sharing a common maternal placenta *in utero*). Bovine twins sharing a common placenta are hematologic chimeras as adults and fail to reject the sibling's cells as foreign. This "experiment" of nature led Burnet to hypothesize a "critical period" in development during which the fetus learns to discriminate self from non-self. Others showed that freemartins accepted grafts from their cotwin while rejecting third-party transplants. This led to a series of experiments in which immunologic tolerance was induced by the transplantation of donor tissues during the critical period in neonates. These seminal observations showed that the immune response could be manipulated in a positive manner to accept transplants and laid the foundation for modern transplant immunobiology.

Immunologic tolerance can result from a number of different possible mechanisms, the three most important being clonal deletion, anergy, and suppressor cells. In clonal deletion, all T lymphocytes capable of recognizing a particular MHC/peptide complex are deleted from the repertoire. This is likely to be important in early education to self versus non-self in the fetus. It has been shown that mice that expressed a particular MHC class II molecule, I-E, deleted all T cells with a particular receptor, Vβ7. Anergy, by contrast, does not involve deletion of T cells. Antigen-specific T cells are present in the periphery but cannot respond. Engagement of the T-cell receptor in the absence of costimulatory signals induces anergy.

Other experimental systems that can result in anergic T cells depend on the dose of antigen and its route of entry. At very high or low antigen doses, there is no immune response. These situations have been termed "high" and "low" zone tolerance. Antigens provided orally tend to induce tolerance while antigens presented via the lungs, skin, or blood are more likely to be immunogenic. Finally, suppressor cells explain the phenomenon of "infectious tolerance" first reported by Gershon and Kondo. They found that T lymphocytes from a tolerant animal could be transferred to a second naive animal, inducing tolerance. They coined the term *suppressor cells* to explain this phenomenon. Although it has proved difficult to grow suppressor cells *in vitro* and to characterize their mechanism of action, it is clear that there are regulatory cells *in vivo* that are capable of downregulating an immune response. This is in contrast to the proinflammatory role of helper T cells.

Recent progress with new drugs, costimulatory molecules, HLA-derived peptides, and cord blood, bone marrow, and blood cell transfusions suggest that immunologic tolerance may be achievable in transplant recipients in the near future.

XENOTRANSPLANTATION

Despite the progress in understanding the immunologic basis of transplant rejection and acceptance, the number of candidates for organ transplantation continues to rise. At present there are more than 30,000 people waiting for renal transplants in the United States. One approach to the shortage of suitable organs is xenotransplantation, the transplantation of organs from other species into humans. The immunologic barriers to xenotransplantation, however, are even greater than those to allotransplantation. Nevertheless, much progress has been made in this area over the past decade. The first immunologic barrier to xenotransplantation is hyperacute rejection mediated by naturally occurring antibodies. These antibodies bind to and activate complement, resulting in rapid death of the graft. Currently, pigs are the leading candidate donors for human transplants. Pigs are appropriate in size, and there are fewer disease and ethical concerns than for primate donors. However, a large fraction of naturally occurring human antibodies react with a carbohydrate determinant, Gal α 1-3Gal, expressed on pig, but not human, cells. Gal α 1-3Gal antibodies can be transiently removed from the recipient's serum by absorption or by administration of blocking peptides or carbohydrates. An alternate approach has been to breed pigs that no longer express the Gal α 1-3Gal epitope for use as donors. Complement activity can be modulated by specific inhibitors or modulation of cell-associated regulatory proteins like decay accelerating factor (DAF, CD55) or membrane inhibitor of reactive lysis (CD59).

Once hyperacute rejection is overcome, acute vascular rejection, characterized by endothelial damage and intravascular coagulation, can occur. This form of rejection appears to be mediated not only by xenoreactive antibodies and complement, but also by cellular components. T lymphocytes (and perhaps NK cells) recognize foreign MHC across species. Analogous to allotransplants, either direct recognition of the foreign MHC or indirect allorecognition of foreign MHC peptides in the context of self HLA can take place. Because direct xenogeneic responses are weaker than alloresponses probably secondary to incompatibility of accessory molecule interactions, there is every reason to believe that they can be easily overcome. On the other hand, the "indirect" pathway is formidable in xenotransplantation. Foreign peptides from other species can be presented by donor HLA, giving rise to a strong and destructive cellular response. Of particular interest in xenotransplantation is the phenomenon of accommodation. If the hyperacute and acute xenogeneic immune responses can be overcome by depletion of antidonor antibodies, the recipient often accommodates to the foreign graft—that is, the graft survives even when pathogenic antibodies are reintroduced. Collectively, recent progress gives hope to the eventual transplantation of organs from other species, although several immunologic hurdles remain. However, social issues and infectious diseases are perhaps bigger problems than the immune response. These include animal rights issues and the potential for zoonoses transmitted from other species to humans.

CONCLUSION

The short-term outcome of renal transplantation is excellent because of progress in organ procurement, tissue typing, clinical care, and immunosuppression. Nevertheless, current approaches involving immunosuppression leave patients at risk for opportunistic infections, secondary tumors, and other side effects. Although the development of more specific immunosuppressive agents remains an area of active research and development, the ultimate goal of transplantation biologists remains the achievement of antigen-specific nonresponsiveness or tolerance. Such tolerance is routinely obtained in animal systems and occasionally in clinical practice, but we still do not understand how to reproducibly induce and maintain tolerance in the clinics. When this is possible, transplantation will be a true cure for kidney failure.

Selected Readings

Cantrell D. T cell antigen receptor signal transduction pathways. *Ann Rev Immunol* 1996;14:259–274.

Discusses the role of T-cell receptor signal transduction pathways linking cell surface interactions with nuclear targets (transcription factors) that control the expression of cytokine genes.

Davis MM, Boniface JJ, Reich Z, et al. Ligand recognition by αβ T cell receptors. *Ann Rev Immunol* 1998;16:523–544.

Provides details about T-cell receptor structure and function.

Goral S, Helderman JH. The evolution and future of immunosuppression in renal transplantation. *Semin Nephrol* 1997;17:364–372.

Details the mechanism of action and clinical importance of the major immunosuppressive drugs and monoclonal antibodies.

Hata Y, Ozawa M, Takemoto SK, et al. HLA matching in clinical transplants. In: Cecka JM, Terasaki PI, eds. *Clinical transplants 1996.* Los Angeles, UCLA Tissue Typing Laboratory, 1997:381–396.

This annual review of clinical transplant data provides a summary of United Network for Organ Sharing and other registries and databases.

Koskinen P, Lemstrom K, Hayry P. Chronic rejection. *Curr Opin Nephrol Hypertens* 1996;5:269–272.

Reviews the current understanding of the risk factors, pathogenesis and prevention of chronic renal allograft rejection.

Krensky AM, Clayberger C. The nature of allorecognition. *Curr Opin Nephrol Hypertens* 1993;2:898–903.

Reviews what is known about the nature of alloantigen.

Krensky AM, Clayberger C. Prospects for induction of tolerance in renal transplantation. *Pediatr Nephrol* 1994;8:772–779.

Highlights progress in understanding immunologic tolerance with special attention to prospects for the induction and maintenance of clinical transplant tolerance.

Krensky AM, Clayberger C. Structure of HLA molecules and immunosuppressive effects of HLA derived peptides. *Int Rev Immunol* 1996;13:173–185.

Describes HLA structure and function.

Krensky AM, Weiss A, Crabtree G, et al. Mechanisms of disease: T lymphocyte-antigen interactions in transplant rejection. *N Engl J Med* 1990;322:510–517.

Describes the cellular and molecular events involved in T-lymphocyte–mediated transplant rejection.

Nelson PJ, Krensky AM. Chemokines, lymphocytes, and viruses: what goes around, comes around. *Curr Opin Immunol* 1998;10:265–270.

Updates the structure and function of the growing family of chemokines and their receptors.

Noessner E, Krensky AM. HLA and antigen presentation. In: Tilney NL, Strom TB, Paul LC, eds. *Transplantation biology: cellular and molecular aspects.* New York: Lippincott-Raven Press, 1996:31.1–31.13.

Details antigen presentation pathways.

Platt JL. New directions for organ transplantation. *Nature* 1998;392:S1–7.

Reviews new approaches to organ transplantation with details about xenotransplantation.

Sayegh MH, Turka LA. The role of T cell costimulatory activation pathways in transplant rejection. *N Engl J Med* 1998;338:1813–1821.

Reviews costimulatory molecules and signal transduction pathways relevant to transplant rejection.

Simpson E, Roopenian D, Goulmy E. Much ado about minor histocompatibility antigens. *Immunol Today* 1998; 19:108–112.

Summarizes the First International Symposium on Minor Histocompatibility Antigens, highlighting current knowledge about minor histocompatibility loci located outside the MHC (major histocompatibility complex).

Solez K, Afrouzian M, Pakasa N, et al. Renal transplant biopsy: what does it tell? *Curr Opin Nephrol Hypertens* 1997;6:538–543.

Highlights recent breakthroughs which have increased the value of renal biopsies in the management of renal transplant patients.

CHAPTER 87

Selection and Preparation of Donors and Recipients for Renal Transplantation

William E. Braun

LIVING DONORS

Kidneys from living-related donors (LRD) and, with increasing frequency, from living-unrelated donors (LURD) now account for approximately 24.7% and 4.5% of the 12,000 renal transplants being performed annually in the United States. Because the median waiting time for a cadaveric kidney in the United States is nearly 2 years, a kidney from a living donor may offer a much earlier opportunity for transplantation and sometimes avoid the need for dialysis. Both LRD and LURD kidneys have a reduced frequency of delayed graft function and rejection, as well as higher short- and long-term patient and graft survival (Table 87.1).

In simplified terms, a potential living donor should be freely willing and able to donate a kidney. The donor should be mentally competent, of legal age, and should provide a consent to donate that is well-informed, voluntary, and free of coercion. Although the consensus is that the best donors are usually found among members of the recipient's immediate family, most centers now accept emotionally related but genetically unrelated living donors, usually a spouse; these transplants commonly achieve allograft success rates of about 90% at 1 year and 82% to 87% at 3 years (Table 87.1). The commercial exchange of live donor organs is prohibited by law in the United States.

Risks for Living Kidney Donors

The perioperative mortality rate for live kidney donation is approximately 3 per 10,000 (0.03%); the major complication rate is 4.4 ± 3.5%. Usually within a week after donating one of two normal kidneys, a donor's remaining kidney will have a glomerular filtration rate (GFR) approximately 70% to 75% of the previous total GFR for both kidneys. The prenephrectomy GFR is the primary predictor of postnephrectomy GFR, with age being a secondary independent factor. Compensatory changes in absolute GFR are smaller for older donors, but the percentage increase in GFR is not significantly different from that in younger donors. Kidney donation from healthy living donors up to about 65 or 70 years of age may be safe if the prenephrectomy GFR is above 75 ml/min/1.73m^2. However, there is debate about a definite level of renal function to use as an absolute cutoff point. In kidney donors who become pregnant, pregnancy is generally uncomplicated for the mother and fetus if there have been both normal renal function and a normotensive course before pregnancy.

Follow-up of living donors more than 20 years after kidney donation has shown mild increases in proteinuria but at a clinically insignificant level and higher blood pressures without a significantly increased frequency of hypertension. These findings have not shown a tendency to progress to renal failure. Nevertheless, a small number of kidney donors have developed renal failure, primarily from *de novo* renal disease in a solitary kidney. Kidney donors should be advised that they ought to have periodic follow-up blood pressure checks, urinalyses, and serum creatinine determinations as well as prompt attention to any health issue.

Medical Evaluation

Before initiating an extensive medical investigation, a preliminary evaluation may disclose features that would preclude or create a higher risk for transplantation, such as significant pulmonary, cardiovascular, or hepatic disease, a history of malignant disease possibly even within 5 years, diabetes mellitus, hypertension, nephrolithiasis, proteinuria, hematuria, pyelonephritis, obesity, and infections such as tuberculosis, viral hepatitis, HIV, and Creutzfeldt-Jakob disease. When an LRD is being considered, it is important to have the most accurate possible diagnosis of the recipient's original kidney disease to gain

TABLE 87.1. Graft Survival Rates for Kidney Transplants According to Donor Relationship

Donor	Number	1-Year (%)	2-Year (%)	3-Year (%)
Parent	3,709	90.3	85.8	81.4
Offspring	1,534	88.4	85.8	82.3
Sibling	6,960	92.6	89.6	86.0
Other	594	90.1	86.0	82.2
Spouse	416	89.7	85.4	82.4
Cadaver	47,010	80.6	74.8	69.0

Reproduced with permission of the UNOS Scientific Registry; and adapted from First MR. Expanding the donor pool. *Semin Nephrol* 1997;17:373–380.

a more complete picture of the recipient's potential for disease recurrence, being mindful that the same disease may exist in the donor. Renal diseases with a significant possibility of recurrence in the recipient include focal segmental glomerulosclerosis, IgA nephropathy, Henoch-Schönlein purpura, membranoproliferative glomerulonephritis type II, hemolytic uremic syndrome, fibrillary glomerulonephritis, oxalosis, and diabetic nephropathy. Familial diseases that may require special investigation to ensure that the LRD does not have the same disease include: Alport's syndrome, autosomal-dominant polycystic kidney disease, diabetes mellitus, Fabry's disease, hemolytic uremic syndrome, IgA nephropathy, oxalosis, systemic lupus erythematosus, and familial renal cell carcinoma. Rarely, a renal biopsy may be necessary to clarify the potential donor's renal condition.

If there are no obvious reasons from the initial history for excluding a donor, the simplest next step is to obtain the red blood cell types of the potential donor and recipient and establish that there is ABO compatibility between them. Incompatibility for ABO red blood cell types is, except with complex and infrequently used pretransplantation treatment protocols (intensive plasma exchange of the recipients to remove isohemagglutinins), a contraindication to transplantation. Whether or not the recipient is known to have anti-HLA antibody (panel reactive antibody, PRA) from testing the recipient's pretransplant serum specimens, it is necessary to perform a cross-match between the recipient's serum and the donor's T and B lymphocytes. If a positive cross-match occurs against the donor's T lymphocytes, then the transplant is contraindicated. For a repeat renal transplant, if the cross-match is positive against the donor's B lymphocytes, that transplant may also be subject to a high risk of hyperacute or accelerated rejection (Table 87.2).

Depending on circumstances relating to the donor and the varying procedures at different transplant centers, the preliminary evaluation just described may be performed before the complete history, physical, and laboratory evaluations are undertaken, or at the same time if the donor is only available for a brief time. It is appropriate that the donor evaluation be conducted by medical persons other than those responsible for the recipient's care.

A full history, physical examination, and extensive laboratory evaluations are used to complete the donor evaluation, and though they may vary somewhat from center to center, will generally include complete blood cell count (CBC) and differential white blood cell count, complete metabolic profile, phosphorus, magnesium, uric acid, lipid profile, ALT, hemoglobin A_1C, hepatitis profile, IgM and IgG antibodies for cytomegalovirus, tests for Epstein-Barr, herpes simplex, and zoster viruses, HIV antibody, urinalysis (with examination of the urine sediment by a nephrologist), urine culture, ECG, chest x-ray evaluation, stool for occult blood, 24-hour urine protein and creatinine analysis, creatinine clearance, iothalamate GFR, and renal angiography. Abnormal findings on the renal angiogram may preclude transplantation (e.g., renal cell carcinoma), require experienced transplant surgeons (e.g., multiple renal arteries or renal artery aneurysm), yield suboptimal results (e.g., unilaterally small kidneys in the range of 9.7 to 11.0 cm), or carry the possibility of recurrent vascular disease following transplantation (e.g., recurrent fibromuscular dysplasia).

CADAVER DONOR

Cadaver donors are the major source of kidneys for transplantation. However, there is a far greater demand for than supply of cadaver organs. Nevertheless, since 1993 there has been an increase of approximately 20% in the number of organ donors in the United States, largely as a result of intensified public and professional education that has permitted the use of "expanded criteria donors" (ECD).

Overall, a cadaver donor may be considered ideal, generally acceptable, or ECD (also known as "marginal"). A donor may be designated ECD because of extremes of age, a history of certain diseases, level of renal function, abnormalities of gross or microscopic renal anatomy, and factors relating to renal perfusion and renal preservation (Table 87.3). From 1988 to 1992, the percentage of cadaveric donors older than 55 years of age more than doubled from 5.4% to 10.7%. When graft outcomes are compared between the optimal donor age group (18 and 34 years) and an ECD group older than 65 years of age, the 1-year and 3-year graft survivals are decreased from 83.9% and 73.4%, respectively, to 69.8% and 52.5%, respectively. These data from

TABLE 87.2. Sensitization Risk Factors for a Repeat Renal Transplant Recipient

- Prior graft survival time (PGST) <3 months when cause by rejection
- Positive flow cytometry cross-match [negative complement–dependent cytotoxicity (CDC) cross-match] when associated with PGST <3 months caused by rejection
- Remote-positive, current-negative CDC crossmatch, combined with repeat mismatched HLA antigen
- Positive B-lymphocyte cross-match that becomes negative after platelet absorption[a]
- Repeat mismatched HLA-DR antigen, even with a negative B-lymphocyte cross-match

[a] Because platelets have only class I, and not class II HLA antigens, absorption of serum with platelet removes class I anti-HLA antibodies and eliminates a positive cross-match caused by them but does not negate a positive cross-match caused by class II anti-HLA antibodies.

Reproduced with permission from the American College of Physicians, Medical Knowledge Self-Assessment Programs, 1998.

TABLE 87.3. Cadaver Donor

	Ideal	Expanded Criteria Donor (ECD)[a]
Age (yr)	18–34	>55 or <5
History of:		
Hypertension	Negative	Positive
Diabetes mellitus	Negative	Positive
Atherosclerosis	Negative	Positive
CDC high risk	Negative	Positive
HCV antibody	Negative	Positive
Renal function		
Serum creatinine (mg/dl)	<1.4	>1.8
Proteinuria	Negative	Positive
Oliguria	Negative	Positive
Vasopressors	Negative	High-dose, prolonged use
Renal anatomy		
Gross	Normal	Variety of vascular, ureteral, or other abnormalities, horseshoe kidney, en-bloc kidney
Microscopic	Normal	Significant nephrosclerosis, glomerulosclerosis, and interstitial fibrosis
Preservation		
Warm ischemic time (min)	<1	>10
Cold ischemic time (hr)	<12	>42

[a] The definition of ECD may vary from center to center, and the features given here are only general guidelines.

cadaver donors older than 65 years of age showing a 14% lower 1-year graft survival and a 21% lower 3-year graft survival are strikingly different from the results of living donors over 65 years of age, in whom the 1-year graft survival is only 2% lower, and the 3-year graft survival only 6% lower than the ideal age group of 18 to 34 years. The causes for the reduced allograft survival in older cadaver donors are generally believed to be attributable to already established senescent changes (varying degrees of arteriolonephrosclerosis, glomerulosclerosis, and interstitial fibrosis), progressive deterioration of already compromised kidneys with time, the morbid condition of cadaver donors, and additional ischemic injury accentuating the functional significance of these lesions.

Unavoidably, the criteria for cadaver donor acceptance vary among transplant centers, and the responsibility for a final decision about any particular donor will be made by the transplant team. In certain cases, particularly for the older donor, it may be necessary to do a wedge biopsy of each kidney to determine the extent of arteriolonephrosclerosis, glomerulosclerosis, and interstitial fibrosis. Although patients with primary renal diseases are generally unacceptable donors, it should be noted that there are thus far five types of renal diseases in the donor that seem to have disappeared after transplantation. These include four recipients of donors with relatively early reversible lesions of diabetic nephropathy, two recipients of a donor with type I membranoproliferative glomerulonephritis, two recipients of a donor with minimal change disease, several recipients of kidneys with IgA nephropathy that do, however, seem to be more susceptible to rejection episodes, and the recipients of kidney donors with the hepatorenal syndrome. When an ECD kidney is to be used, there should be informed consent of the recipient who should have an understanding of the risks, benefits, and alternatives for such a transplant.

Because about 98% of actual cadaveric organ donors originate in the intensive care unit (ICU), it is the primary area for early donor identification. Most donors are recognized within 24 hours in the ICU, but about 20% of potential donors die in less than 6 hours and 50% in less than 24 hours. Usually, brain death protocols are being considered while consent for donation is being sought from the next-of-kin. The discussion of possible organ donation should be done separately from the condolences expressed to the family members about the imminent death of their loved one. The dying person may have actually completed an organ donor card that should establish the patient's personal intentions for organ donation. Legislation to ensure that every potential donor family has the question of organ donation placed before them (required request or routine referral) has not fulfilled expectations, probably because most forms of the law initially mandated that the hospital administration be responsible for this duty, rather than the organ procurement organizations (OPOs) whose members specialize in this area.

Another complexity has been introduced into organ donation, namely, the use of non–heart-beating donors (NHBD). NHBD may occur in an uncontrolled or controlled situation. An uncontrolled NHBD may either unexpectedly succumb to cardiac death in the hospital or suffer cardiac death shortly after arrival in the emergency department. If consent for organ donation has already been obtained, the donor may be rushed to an operating room or have core cooling done through the femoral artery until the operating room is available. Kidneys obtained in this way are more likely to be marginal or unacceptable for transplantation.

A controlled NHBD is a more complex situation. In such a case, a ventilator-dependent potential donor whose further treatment is futile has all life support discontinued because of the patient's own prior intentions and the family's request; a brain death protocol is not involved. In the operating room the ventilator is discontinued, the patient is monitored for the occurrence of death, and subsequently the donated organs are rapidly removed. The moral and ethical issues of various steps and procedures in such organ procurement have not been resolved to everyone's satisfaction. From the areas of the country in which this type of organ donation has been used, the survival rate at 1-year was 83%, not significantly different from the 86% for grafts obtained from heart-beating donors.

RECIPIENT EVALUATION

Patients with irreversible renal failure who are competent and express a desire to have a renal transplant should be thoroughly evaluated to determine the risks and benefits that the procedure offers for them as well as a comparison with treatment alternatives. Potential risk factors for transplant recipients include cardiovascular disease, active or recent malignancy, active or potentially life-threatening infection, viral hepatitis and other liver diseases, pulmonary disease, gastrointestinal disease, recurrent renal disease, presence of urinary tract abnormalities, hyperparathyroidism, older age, obesity, a variety of psychosocial issues, and histocompatibility issues and the degree of sensitization to HLA antigens expressed as the percent panel reactive antibody (%PRA).

Cardiovascular Diseases

Coronary Heart Disease

Coronary heart disease (CHD) is the primary cause of mortality after renal transplantation. It is essential to identify not only those patients who have had symptomatic CHD (previous myocardial infarction, angina pectoris), but also those who are asymptomatic but have developed a high risk profile for CHD (Fig. 87.1). This latter group of asymptomatic patients may be identified by using (a) weighted criteria developed in the Framingham study based on increasing age, male gender, high levels of total cholesterol, low levels of high-density lipoprotein HDL cholesterol, level of systolic blood pressure, and presence or absence of diabetes mellitus, smoking, and left ventricular hypertrophy (LVH) by the EKG; (b) criteria developed from evaluating both symptomatic and asymptomatic renal transplant candidates (presence of type 1 diabetes mellitus, angina pectoris, congestive heart failure, age 50 years of age or older, and an abnormal ECG exclusive of LVH); or (c) criteria developed exclusively from diabetic candidates for renal transplantation in whom age 45 years of age or older was a high risk factor and in whom the combination of an age of 45 years or younger, duration of diabetes mellitus less than 25 years, smoking history less than 5 pack/years, and the absence the ST-T wave changes on ECG defined a low-risk group. Patients who have symptomatic CHD and are therefore already exhibiting ischemia may be considered candidates for coronary angiography. Asymptomatic high risk patients would usually be studied initially with a noninvasive procedure to elicit possible ischemic changes (Fig. 87.1). The choice of the appropriate noninvasive test will depend on whether the patient can perform an exercise-based stress test or should have a pharmacologically mediated stress test evaluating either coronary perfusion or wall motion abnormalities. If significant CHD is found, then a judgment can be made as to the use of percutaneous transluminal coronary angioplasty (PTCA), stent placement, atherectomy, or coronary artery bypass grafting (CABG). Patients with severe LVH and diffuse three-vessel disease not amenable to bypass surgery would not be kidney-only transplant candidates because of their poor prognosis.

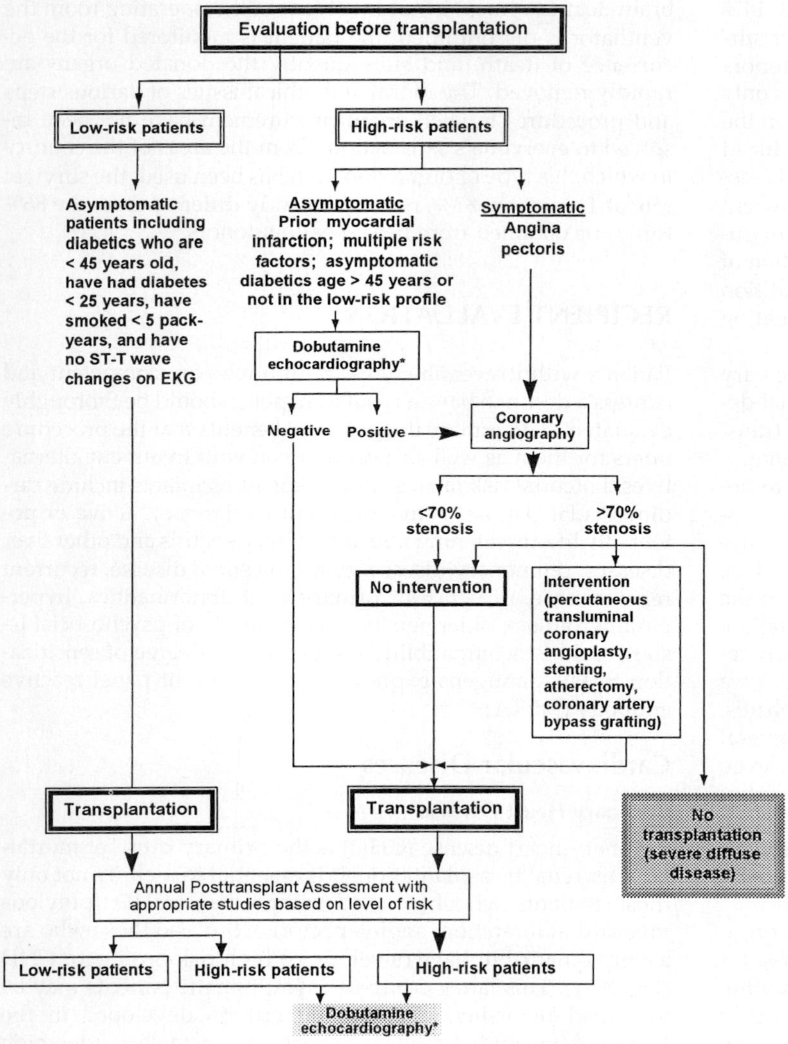

Figure 87.1. Algorithm for detecting and treating coronary artery disease in renal transplant candidates and recipients. The inclusion of dobutamine echocardiography in this algorithm is not intended to exclude other appropriate noninvasive tests, as described in the text. The combination of clinical, noninvasive, and angiographic findings determines both current coronary artery status and future monitoring requirements, depending on whether the patient is at high-risk of low-risk for coronary artery disease.* Because of the lack of uniform results from center to center, other noninvasive tests, such as exercise or dipyridamole thallium scanning, may be useful. (Reproduced with permission Braun WE, Morwick TH. Coronary artery disease in renal transplant recipients. *Cleve Clin J Med* 1994; 61:370–385.)

Cerebrovascular Disease

Cerebrovascular disease should be sought on the physical examination by nonsimultaneous palpitation of the carotid arteries and auscultation for bruits. If a bruit is identified from the carotid arteries (the transmission of sounds from a large AV fistula or an aortic stenosis murmur may make interpretation difficult), then duplex ultrasonography of the carotid arteries is recommended. If the degree of stenosis is 80% or more, carotid endarterectomy is recommended.

Patients with autosomal-dominant polycystic kidney disease (ADPKD) have an overall frequency of intracranial aneurysm (ICA) of approximately 12%. A positive family history of an ICA or subarachnoid hemorrhage (SAH) in conjunction with ADPKD increases the frequency of an ICA in the patient to about 24%, whereas a negative family history decreases it to approximately 5%. Patients with a family history of ADPKD and ICA, and patients with ADPKD who have neurologic symptoms that suggest an ICA are usually screened for an ICA with a magnetic resonance angiogram (MRA) as the initial study.

Peripheral Vascular Disease

Because of the increasing number of diabetics and elderly patients presenting as transplant candidates, careful evaluation of the peripheral vascular system, particularly the lower extremities, is mandatory. In addition, the iliac arteries may need to be studied because of the placement of the renal transplant artery anastomosis in that arterial system.

Malignancy

Transplant candidates with a previously treated malignancy need careful evaluation to ensure that they are free of recurrent disease and have had an appropriate disease-free interval before transplant immunosuppressive therapy is begun. The general guidelines for management of renal transplant recipients who have had a preexisting malignancy are (a) a 2-year recurrence-free interval after treatment is justified for most neoplasms; (b) more than a 2-year interval may be necessary for most malignant melanomas, breast and colorectal carcinomas, and nonfocal prostate cancer; and (c) no waiting period may be necessary for *in situ* carcinoma, incidentally discovered renal cell carcinoma, and possibly small single-focus neoplasms or low-grade bladder and basal cell skin cancer.

Infection

Active infection is generally a contraindication to renal transplantation. A thorough history and physical examination may uncover sources of infection such as dental abscess, perirectal abscess, or chronic cellulitis at a dialysis access site. Peritoneal dialysis-related peritonitis within a 3- or 4-week period is also generally a contraindication to transplantation. Careful attention needs to be directed to individuals who may have tuberculosis or HIV. Patients who are serologically negative for exposure to cytomegalovirus (CMV), Epstein-Barr virus (EBV), and herpes varicella zoster virus (VZV) are at the greatest risk for severe primary infections with the specific virus after transplantation.

Viral Hepatitis and Liver Disease

The presence of abnormal liver function tests, HBsAg, HBeAg, hepatitis C antibody, symptoms or history of hepatobiliary disease, ingestion of potentially hepatotoxic drugs, and alcohol abuse need further investigation before transplantation. Two of the most common problems are the presence of HBsAg or HCV antibody. In one major North American study, HBsAg-positive patients who had undergone renal transplantation had higher morbidity and mortality rates than patients who remained on dialysis. However, another major study from France showed no significant difference between HbsAg-positive and HbsAg-negative patient mortality rates after transplantation. The most recent study of over 800 renal transplant patients has shown 10 year graft survivors of 55 ± 6% in 128 HBsAg-positive patients, 65 ± 5% in 216 anti-HCV antibody positive patients, and 80 ± 3% in 490 patients without HBsAg or anti-HCV antibody ($p<0.001$). Chronic HBV infection without cirrhosis is a definite risk but not a contraindication to renal transplantation. Because liver function tests typically underestimate the severity of viral hepatitis, a liver biopsy may be necessary to determine whether cirrhosis is present. If it is, the patient may be best managed by continuation of dialysis or possibly a combined liver/kidney transplant. Renal transplant recipients with HCV have a 3.3-fold increase in overall mortality and a 9.9-fold increase in deaths from liver disease or sepsis. If treatment with interferon-alpha is planned, it should be done before transplantation because of the risk of irreversible rejection being induced by interferon-alpha after transplantation. About 50% of patients with HBV or HCV have normalization of elevated liver enzymes and clearance of virus from the serum at the end of treatment with interferon-alpha. Among those showing a response to interferon-alpha the response is sustained in most patients with HBsAg but only about 20% of those with HCV. Lamivudine, a nucleoside analog that interferes with reverse transcriptase, has been shown in studies to reduce HBV DNA to undetectable levels with sustained response in about 20%. Ribavirin is also being studied for the treatment of hepatitis C.

Pulmonary Disease

Respiratory symptoms or a history of asthma or smoking should be evaluated by pulmonary function studies, and a smoking cessation program should be instituted for smokers. The forced expiratory volume may be the best predictor of postoperative respiratory complications. The principles that apply to the standard preoperative evaluation of a patient also apply to transplantation, with special attention given to the possibilities of tuberculosis, fungal disease, and acute bacterial and viral Infections.

Gastrointestinal Disease

Two of the most common gastrointestinal diseases seen in transplant patients are colonic disease, usually diverticulitis, and peptic ulcer disease. If a potential transplant recipient has had recurrent bouts of acute diverticulitis and has severe diverticular disease demonstrated on a barium enema or CT scan of the pelvis and abdomen, then a partial colectomy should be considered. If signs or symptoms of active peptic ulcer disease are confirmed by radiography or endoscopy, appropriate medical therapy should be instituted and a response demonstrated before proceeding with transplantation. Specific tests for *Helicobacter pylori* should be included so that the necessary combination therapy for this causative agent can be used.

Renal Disease Prone to Recurrence

Patients with renal disease prone to recur following transplantation should be fully informed of that possibility. Although recurrent disease may affect approximately 25% to 30% of renal allografts, it accounted for the loss of less than 5% of allografts. However, the rate of graft loss is increasing with longer graft survival. Glomerulopathies that have had a particularly rapid pretransplant course in the native kidneys generally are more prone to have an adverse course after transplantation. Diseases prone to recurrence after renal transplant (discussed in detail elsewhere) include diabetic nephropathy, focal segmental glomerulosclerosis, fibrillary glomerulonephritis, hemolytic uremic syndrome, IgA nephropathy, Henoch-Schönlein purpura, oxalosis, and type II membranoproliferative glomerulonephritis. Although Alport syndrome is not subject to recurrence in a renal allograft, up to 33% of patients with Alport syndrome may have linear IgG staining on the glomerular basement membrane after transplantation, an indication that they have made an anti-GBM antibody in response to the normal basement membrane antigens of the transplanted kidney, and a small percentage of these have severe allograft damage.

Urinary Tract Abnormalities

If a patient has voiding symptoms, known or suggested genitourinary tract abnormalities, or is older than 65 years of age, a voiding cystourethrogram is usually required. If the test results are abnormal, or if the results are normal but there is a history of recurrent urinary tract infections, then renal ultrasonography, CT studies, cystoscopy, or retrograde pyelography may be indicated. If one of these tests shows abnormal results, there may be an indication for native kidney nephrectomy. If nephrectomy would not improve the condition, then bladder dysfunction is the probable cause, and either ureteral diversion or intermittent self-catheterization should be considered. Pretransplant nephrectomies are usually recommended for patients with significant reflux that may be associated with recurrent urinary tract infections, polycystic kidneys that are so massive that they do not allow space for the transplant or have areas suspicious for neoplasm or infected cyst, renal calculus disease with infection, and renal carcinoma, but only rarely for patients with massive proteinuria and debilitating nephrosis, or uncontrolled malignant hypertension.

Hyperparathyroidism

Patients with symptomatic secondary hyperparathyroidism, usually in the form of bone pain, fractures, ectopic calcification, or otherwise unexplained hypercalcemia with marked elevations of intact parathyroid hormone should be seriously considered for sub-total parathyroidectomy. Aluminum toxicity may present a similar picture and needs careful consideration.

Older Age

Elderly potential transplant candidates, usually 60 to 75 years of age, require especially careful evaluation for comorbid diseases as well as the relative rehabilitation potential offered by transplantation compared with dialysis. In particular, the presence or absence of CHD, cerebrovascular disease, and peripheral vascular disease, should be clearly defined. An occult malignancy is an unavoidable consideration, particularly when findings as mundane as mild anemia, subtle weight loss, unexplained back pain, or a chronic cough are encountered.

Although patients older than 75 years of age are usually treated almost exclusively with dialysis, occasionally an exceptionally fit patient may still be a transplant candidate. The patient and allograft survival rates in the cyclosporine era are nearly comparable to those for younger patients up to about 3 years posttransplantation, but then begin to fall below those levels. Graft loss in elderly transplant recipients is more often due to death than to allograft-related problems. The most common causes of death in elderly transplant recipients remain cardiovascular disease and infection related to immunosuppressive therapy. Because the elderly have lower immune competence and decreased hepatic enzyme levels, lower doses of immunosuppressive therapy may be feasible.

Obesity

A body mass index above 30 kg/m^2 is associated with an increased frequency of delayed graft function, postoperative complications, and decreased patient and allograft survival rates. Often transplantation should be postponed until the patient has achieved adequate weight reduction.

Psychosocial Issues

Patients with psychosocial problems will require in-depth evaluation for evidence of cognitive impairment, alcohol or drug abuse, psychiatric illness, or history of noncompliance with medications, scheduled tests, or dialysis treatments. When there has been a history of alcohol or drug abuse, supervised abstinence should be documented.

Hematologic Abnormalities

An increasing number of harmful prothrombotic factors have been reported in renal transplant recipients and may need to be considered in selected cases. These abnormalities include high-titer cold agglutinins, anti-cardiolipin antibodies, coagulation disorders affecting the protein C system (Factor V Leyden mutation, protein S or protein C deficiency, lupus anticoagulant), and prothrombin gene mutations.

HISTOCOMPATIBILITY MATCHING

Because an extensive discussion of the HLA system is given elsewhere, just a few salient points will be made here. A living-related donor-recipient pair can have tissue typing studies of the family (genotyping) that identify the genetic unit of HLA antigens (haplotype) inherited from each parent. One haplotype is received from each parent and includes one antigen from each of the class I (HLA-A, -B, and -Cw) and class II (HLA-DR, -DQ, and -DP) series of HLA antigens. Transplants from an LRD should be described according to the number of matched (or mismatched) haplotypes; namely, 2, 1, or 0. Among full siblings the chances for a 2-, 1-, or 0-haplotype match are 25%, 50%, and 25%, respectively. Parental donors are typically 1-haplotype matches, although in rare situations, parents with shared haplotypes may actually be HLA-identical to an offspring. An HLA-identical (2-haplotype match) sibling may still be ABO incompatible and unable to be used as a donor. Allograft survival rates at 1 and 3 years for 2-haplotype matched sibling (HLA-identical) recipients are approximately 97% and 93% and superior to those of 1- and 0-haplotype matched kidneys that have similar survivals at 1 and 3 years of 93% and 85%, respectively. The point in time when allografts functioning at 1 year have a 50% reduction in survival ($t^1/_2$) is about 26 to 36 years for 2-haplotype and 15 years for the 1- and 0-haplotype–matched kidneys that have similar outcomes.

Because full tissue typing of both the donor's and the recipient's families is not usually performed for LURD transplants, matching for these individuals is based on the same principle as for cadaver donors; namely, counting either the number of HLA antigens matched between the donor and recipient (6 to 0) or the number of HLA antigens mismatched (0 to 6) when judged against the HLA antigens that the donor presents. A study of 2,281 LURD transplants found a significant correlation between the number of HLA-A, -B and -DR mismatches and the 5-year transplant success rate ($P < .0001$). The additional finding of a higher than expected number of zero HLA-DR mismatches suggested that a prospective effort for HLA matching was apparently being made.

For cadaver transplants, the best success rates are achieved with 6-antigen matched (or 0-antigen mismatched) allografts that have 1- and 3-year graft survivals of about 89% and 83%, respectively. The world's largest renal transplant registry, the Collaborative Transplant Study (CTS), also has reported a progressive decline in cadaver allograft survivals with increasing numbers of HLA antigen mismatches so that allografts with 6-antigen mismatches have lower 1- and 3-year survivals of 80% and 68%, respectively. For reasons that are as yet unclear, HLA-DR mismatches have a more marked effect on 1-year, and HLA-A mismatches a more pronounced effect on 5-year allograft survivals. When the recipient is sensitized and has more than 50% PRA, HLA mismatching has an even more pronounced adverse effect on allograft survival. Repeat renal transplants have special presensitization considerations (Table 87.2).

In the United States, cadaver kidneys are allocated according to a point system democratically developed by the transplantation community and administered by the United Network for Organ Sharing (UNOS). This system is based primarily on the quality of HLA antigen matching or the absence of antigen mismatching, the level of recipient sensitization (PRA), length of waiting time, and whether the recipient is in the pediatric age group. These criteria are periodically revised.

Selected Readings

First MR. Expanding the donor pool. *Semin Nephrol* 1997;17:373–380.

This is a very informative synopsis of current trends in kidney donation, such as the increase in living unrelated and extended criteria cadaver donors and their outcome.

Kasiske BL, Ramos EL, Gaston RS, et al. The evaluation of renal transplant candidates: clinical practice guidelines. Patient Care and Education Committee of the American Society of Transplant Physicians. *J Am Soc Nephrol* 1995;6:1–34.

The evaluation of potential renal transplant recipients has been made clearer and safer by this comprehensive set of guidelines, developed by highly experienced transplant physicians.

Kasiske BL, Ravenscraft M, Ramos EL, et al. The evaluation of living renal transplant donors: clinical practice guidelines. Ad Hoc Clinical Practice Guidelines Subcommittee of the Patient Care and Education Committee of the American Society of Transplant Physicians. *J Am Soc Nephrol* 1996;7:2288–2313.

A highly experienced group of transplant physicians has provided a valuable set of guidelines for evaluating potential living kidney donors.

Pereira BJ, Levey AS. Hepatitis C virus infection in dialysis and renal transplantation. *Kidney Int* 1997;51:981–999.

The enigma of hepatitis C in renal transplant recipients is being unraveled by the careful studies of Dr. Pereira and co-workers who now report the increased overall and liver-related mortality of patients with hepatitis C.

Cecka JM, Terasaki PT, eds. *Clinical transplants 1999.* Los Angeles: UCLA Tissue Typing Laboratory, 1999.

This annual publication provides not only the current results of the United Network for Organ Sharing (UNOS) renal transplants, but also an interesting collection of other human transplant studies.

CHAPTER 88

Renal Allograft Dysfunction

PART 1
Clinical Manifestation and Diagnosis

Chris N. Fotiadis, Mahendra V. Govani, and J. Harold Helderman

Despite all the efforts of tissue typing laboratories and transplant nephrologists to avoid the immunologic response to the foreign antigens contained within the renal allograft, rejection remains the most important cause of graft loss. It is important to emphasize that allograft dysfunction is not synonymous with allograft rejection. Indeed, the differentiation of the various causes of allograft dysfunction, both early and late in the posttransplant course, represent critical points in the overall management of transplant recipients. The nephrologist providing care for transplant recipients should be intimately familiar with the various causes of allograft dysfunction and be able to recognize the advantages and limitations of various diagnostic tests utilized to achieve precision in determining which of many possible processes are responsible for alterations in graft function. For the sake of convenience, the evaluation of allograft dysfunction can be divided into early posttransplant phases (less than 3 months following transplantation) and late posttransplant graft dysfunction (3 months to many years following transplantation).

EARLY POSTTRANSPLANTATION GRAFT DYSFUNCTION

Following renal transplantation, the allograft may demonstrate a variety of functional patterns: (a) immediate function with achievement of a nadir serum creatinine within the first posttransplant week; (b) initial urine flow with delayed clearance; (c) primary nonfunction with delayed recovery and; (d) persistent nonfunction. These categories of function are influenced by events that occur before transplantation; as well as factors inherent to the transplant recipient and donor. The common causes of early graft dysfunction are listed in Table 88.1.

Acute Tubular Necrosis

Primary renal dysfunction following transplantation, commonly referred to as delayed graft function (DGF), occurs in 10% to 50% of allografts. Most cases of DGF are related to *acute tubular necrosis* (ATN) of the transplanted kidney, and the two terms are often used interchangeably although a masked immune-mediated dysfunction is possible. It is generally manifested as oliguria and lack of decline in serum creatinine; however, some patients may

TABLE 88.1. Early Allograft Dysfunction: Less Than 3 Months After Transplant Surgery

Acute tubular necrosis
Ischemic/reperfusion injury
Hypovolemia
Excessive diuresis
Hemorrhage
Third spacing
Gastrointestinal losses
Urologic complications
Urine leak
Obstruction
Bladder catheter obstruction
Ureteral obstruction
Bladder outlet obstruction
Vascular complications
Hemorrhage
Renal artery thrombosis
Renal vein thrombosis
Renal artery stenosis
Calcineurin inhibitor nephrotoxicity (cyclosporine and tacrolimus)
Vasoconstriction
Thrombotic microangiopathy
Other nephrotoxicity
Aminoglycosides
Nonsteroidal antiinflammatory drugs
Acyclovir
Amphotericin
Angiotensin-converting enzyme inhibitors
Radiocontrast
Infection
Sepsis
Pyelonephritis
Cytomegalovirus infection
Recurrent renal disease
Focal segmental glomerulosclerosis
Hemolytic uremic syndrome
Glomerulonephritis
Acute rejection
Humoral
Hyperacute
Accelerated
ABO incompatibility
Cellular
Interstitial
Vascular

TABLE 88.2. Risk Factors for Delayed Graft Function

Donor factors
Age (<5 or >50)
Pre-existing disease (hypertension and cardiovascular disease)
Cause of death (cardiovascular versus traumatic)
Hypotension
Nephrotoxic agents (contrast, antibiotics, and vasopressors)
Disseminated intravascular coagulation (DIC)
Nonbeating heart donation
Prolonged warm and cold ischemic time
Trauma to renal vasculature at harvest
Intraoperative factors
Prolonged anastomotic time
Renal artery vasospasm
Intraoperative hypotension
Negative intraoperative fluid balance
Recipient factors
Prior failed transplants
Postoperative hypotension and hypovolemia
Peripheral vascular disease
Early high-dose cyclosporine
Early OKT3 use

TABLE 88.3. Risk Factors for Graft Thrombosis

Younger recipient age
Membranous glomerulopathy
Diabetic nephropathy
Atherosclerosis
Hypercoagulable state
Female or pediatric donor
Multiple graft vessels
Prolonged ischemic time
Intimal trauma of graft vessels
Perioperative hemodynamic instability
Cyclosporine
OKT3
Hyperacute rejection
Vascular rejection

have brief periods of urine formation and then develop oliguria, while others will remain nonoliguric but lack significant clearance. DGF is usually limited to cadaver transplants; its occurrence in live donor transplants is exceptional and almost always portends a serious surgical complication. Multiple factors have been identified which contribute to the development of this lesion in the renal allograft (Table 88.2). Awareness of the presence of these factors allows the astute nephrologist to predict the functional pattern that will be achieved by the renal allograft almost immediately after transplantation.

Posttransplant ATN increases the risk of both acute rejection and graft loss. Its occurrence has been shown to reduce 1-year graft survival by 20% to 30%, compared with allografts with immediate normal graft function. Long-term renal allograft survival is also impaired: 85% versus 60% 5-year survival for cadaver grafts experiencing neither DGF nor acute rejection versus those sustaining both injuries has been reported. The adverse effect of delayed graft function on long-term allograft survival is likely a reflection of its association with acute rejection. ATN is reported to increase the frequency of acute rejection by 10% to 25%. However, ATN has little effect on survival if no rejection occurs.

There is substantial evidence to indicate that the association of ATN with acute rejection is an antigen-driven, immune-mediated process and not merely a consequence of delayed recognition of the rejection event in an oliguric transplant. Ischemic injury induces a stereotypic inflammatory response. Injured parenchymal cells increase expression of class I and class II HLA molecules as a consequence of the up-regulation of multiple cytokines and growth factors within the allograft; such as, interferon-α (IFN-α), IL-2, IL-10, and transforming growth factor-β (TGF-β). This cytokine response is of long duration, lasting up to 5 weeks after a single insult. Ischemic injury has also been shown to attract macrophages to the allograft and increase class II HLA expression on passenger donor macrophage/dendritic cells. Last, there is evidence that costimulatory and adhesion molecule expression is upregulated within the ischemically injured allograft. Thus the nonspecific injuries sustained by the transplanted kidney before and at the time of implantation can provoke a cascade of events that results in T-cell recognition and the onset of rejection within the allograft.

Several interventions have been attempted to prevent or mitigate ATN in the renal allograft. Volume expansion of the recipient, mannitol, furosemide, and interarterial or systemic calcium antagonist are commonly administered at the time of transplantation. Experimental approaches have included the use of urodilantin, atrial natriuretic peptide, insulin-like growth factor, free radical scavengers, prostaglandins, IL-8, anti-LFA-1, and anti-ICAM-1.

Restoration of renal function in the ATN course generally occurs within 2 weeks, although it may take as long as 6 weeks after transplantation, particularly in older recipients or those receiving older donor kidneys. With persistent oliguria, or nonoliguric allograft dysfunction of prolonged duration, aspiration needle biopsy or core needle biopsy of the kidney may be necessary to differentiate the process of ATN from other causes of early posttransplant graft dysfunction (see discussion of rejection below). Radionuclide imaging may also be helpful in differentiating ATN from rejection (Table 88.3).

Posttransplant Hypovolemia

Posttransplant *hypovolemia* may be a cause of impaired renal function, particularly in patients who have had excessive blood loss, postoperative third-spacing, or have been maintained at or near dry weight while on pretransplant dialysis. Central venous or pulmonary artery wedge pressure monitoring can be useful in the early detection of the hypovolemic state and a "fluid challenge" with crystalloid or colloid solution is often used. For patients with immediate allograft function, fluid balance can often be maintained by replacing urine volume plus 30 ml of dextrose and normal saline solution per hour. Diuretics should be used judiciously in the early posttransplant period. If there is no response to diuretics in the allograft with DGF within the first 6-12 hours of the transplant, it is best to refrain from further use until clearance is established. Excessive diuretic usage, along with volume losses related to vomiting and diarrhea (frequently caused by the side effects of medications used in transplantation) are common causes of hypovolemia and allograft dysfunction.

Urologic Complications

There are a variety of *urologic complications* that may impair renal function in the early posttransplant period. *Urine leakage* occurs in 3% to 10% of recipients, almost exclusively at the site of the vesicoureteric anastomosis. The leakage may result from undue tension created by a short ureter, by distal ureteral ischemia, or as a consequence of injury engendered by rejection episodes. It generally occurs early, within the first month after transplant surgery, presenting with pain and swelling over the graft site, fever, elevated serum creatinine, oliguria, cutaneous urinary drainage, and frequently, sepsis. Ultrasonography reveals a peritransplant fluid collection in 60% to 70% of such cases. Nuclear renography with delayed imaging can detect most leaks, particularly in patients with good function and large disruptions. Antegrade pyelography is the optimal study, because it provides superior diagnostic sensitivity and anatomic definition to assist in planning surgical revision. A percutaneous diverting nephrostomy combined with antegrade ureteral stenting can close up to 87% of leaks but is often complicated by sepsis. Surgical correction is the preferred treatment modality. The most common approaches are revision of the ureteroneocystostomy or donor-to-recipient pyeloureterostomy.

Urinary obstruction in the early postoperative phase is most often caused by a blood clot in the bladder-catheter drainage system. This usually resolves with careful flushing with saline solution or replacement of the catheter. Continuous saline flushing of the bladder in a grossly hematuric patient following transplantation will often prevent this complication.

The next most common urinary tract complication is *ureteral obstruction*. The majority of lesions occur at the distal ureter and may present at any time following transplantation. Obstruction during the early postoperative period may be caused by edema of the ureter, blood clots, hematoma in the wall of the distal ureter, or malrotation and kinking of the ureter. Late onset obstruction is generally the result of scarring from chronic ischemia with fibrosis, or extrinsic compression usually by a lymphocele. Clinically ureteral obstruction presents with oliguria, sepsis, local pain over the graft site, or a gradual rise in serum creatinine. The diagnosis is confirmed by ultrasonography, nuclear renography, or antegrade pyelography. Pyelography is the most accurate method for anatomically defining the location and degree of obstruction. The obstruction can initially be managed with percutaneous nephrostomy to allow recovery of renal function. The preferred approach to definitive correction is surgical, with revision ureteroneocystostomy as the most common procedure. Percutaneous transluminal dilatation is also effective with a reported success rate of 70% to 80%. (Urologic complications in the renal transplant recipient are discussed in Chapter 89, Part 2.)

Vascular Complications

Vascular complications are among the most serious postoperative events that can impair allograft function. Anastomotic *hemorrhage* is potentially the most life-threatening of these complications. Both the arterial and venous anastomosis are at risk. Mycotic aneurysms, perianastomotic infection, or excessive tension on the transplant vessels are responsible for most cases. The symptoms of hemorrhage may include a palpable mass at the graft site, intense graft site pain, or back pain radiating to the flank, accompanied with a falling hematocrit level and symptoms of vascular collapse. Prompt exploration for control of the hemorrhage is essential to preserve the patient's life. Attempts to repair the anastomosis are generally futile, and nephrectomy is the most prudent course of action. Despite prompt surgical attention, the mortality rate can be as high as 50%.

Nonanastomotic postoperative bleeding is the more common hemorrhagic complication. Most cases are related to uremic coagulopathies, unappreciated small host or torn donor hilar vessels, or anticoagulation for preoperative hemodialysis or prevention of graft thrombosis in a high-risk patient. Symptoms are generally the same as those for anastomotic hemorrhage, though often without the same degree of vascular instability. The diagnosis can be confirmed by ultrasonography or by a radiolucent halo on radionuclide scans. Early exploration is indicated to evacuate most large hematomas before they occlude arterial supply or obstruct the ureter. Although smaller hematomas usually resolve spontaneously, they remain a potential site for bacterial colonization.

Renal Graft Thrombosis

Renal graft thrombosis, arterial or venous, is another devastating vascular complication after kidney transplantation. It usually occurs early in the posttransplant course, most often within the first 2 weeks. Except in exceptional circumstances when urgent thrombectomy is employed rapidly, the graft is usually lost, accounting for 30% to40% of early graft failures. Arterial thrombosis may be complete or only involve a segment of the renal vasculature. Graft thrombosis may be accompanied by morbid and potentially life-threatening events, such as graft rupture, hemorrhage, thromboembolic complications, and sepsis. The overall incidence rate is between 0.5% and 6.2% in most reported series, with arterial thrombosis accounting for one-third and venous thrombosis two-thirds of cases.

The typical clinical presentation is sudden onset oliguria or anuria with deterioration of graft function, and, in the case of renal vein thrombosis, hematuria and graft pain. Extensive venous thrombosis may involve the iliac veins and lead to ipsilateral swelling of the lower extremity. In cases of delayed graft function diagnosis is particularly difficult and delays in recognition are the rule. Radionuclide imaging may disclose absence of blood flow to all or a portion of the kidney. Duplex Doppler scanning and arteriography can be used to confirm the diagnosis. Several risk factors have been identified (Table 88.4). One study identified the following high-risk factors after multivariate analysis: diabetic nephropathy, hemodynamic instability of the recipient, and technical surgical problems. Postoperative anticoagulant therapy can reduce the risk of graft thrombosis, but at the risk of increased bleeding complications.

Renal Artery Stenosis

Transplant *renal artery stenosis* (RAS) is the last of the major vascular complications that can impair allograft function. The incidence of this complication varies from 1-22%, depending on the modality used to identify this lesion. A report employing serial color Doppler ultrasonography detected RAS in 12% of cases. The most frequent presentation is severe hypertension with or without allograft dysfunction that becomes apparent 3 months to 2 years after transplantation. Angiotensin-converting enzyme (ACE) inhibitors may produce severe hypotension and rapid deterioration in allograft function if administered in such patients.

The presence of a bruit may be of little diagnostic value because of the lack of sensitivity and specificity of this finding. Most stenoses develop at or near the vascular anastomosis. It is believed that most stenoses are the result of intimal injury either to the donor or recipient vasculature, with subsequent intimal hyperplasia and stenosis. Captopril isotopic renography is not of sufficient sensitivity and specificity to be of value in diagnosis.

Ultrasonography is highly sensitive but has a reported specificity of only 75%. Spiral CT scanning can provide satisfactory

TABLE 88.4. Late Allograft Dysfunction: More Than 3 Months After Transplant Surgery

Mechanical: Obstruction (ureteral stenosis, stone, lymphocele, transplant artery stenosis)
Infections: Pyelonephritis, cytomegalovirus
Cyclosporine and tacrolimus nephrotoxicity
Recurrent primary disease (diabetes, oxalosis, glomerulonephritis, hemolytic syndrome)
Chronic rejection

three-dimensional reconstruction of vessels, avoids arterial puncture, and requires less intravenous contrast medium than conventional angiography does, but has not been as rigorously studied as the other diagnostic modalities. The diagnostic gold standard remains angiography. The recent development of CO_2 angiography has reduced the risk of contrast nephropathy and hypersensitivity reactions and may replace standard angiography as the preferred diagnostic modality. Hemodynamically significant stenoses (greater than 70% stenosis, pressure gradient above 15 mm Hg) are likely to impair allograft function and are associated with substantial risk of long-term graft loss. Management has evolved, with percutaneous transluminal balloon renal angioplasty (PTRA) supplanting surgery as the intervention of first choice in appropriately selected cases. The efficacy of PTRA is estimated to be 75% to80% in the most experienced centers. Restenosis occurs in 10% to 33% of cases. The role of renal artery stents is undefined at this time. Patients who have unsuccessful angioplasty, or stenoses that are very severe or inaccessible to PTRA, may require surgical intervention. Surgical techniques include resection and revision of the anastomosis, saphenous vein bypass graft of the stenotic segment, or localized endarterectomy. Surgery carries a significant risk of graft loss (15% to 20%), ureteral injury (10% to 15%), and mortality (5%). Correction rates for surgery range from 60% to 90%.

The *calcineurin inhibitors*, cyclosporine and tacrolimus, are potentially nephrotoxic and commonly induce allograft dysfunction in the early posttransplant period. The toxicity of these agents is most commonly related to a dose-dependent, reversible arteriolar vasoconstriction; less commonly, they can cause hemolytic-uremic syndrome associated with thrombotic microangiopathy and allograft dysfunction. The nephrotoxicity of these agents is most often seen in the early posttransplant period as a result of the higher doses required during this interval to prevent acute rejection. Prolonged administration of these agents has been associated with interstitial fibrosis and arteriolar vasculopathy. Nephrotoxicity of calcineurin inhibitors can be reduced by careful monitoring of blood levels and by the concomitant use of calcium channel-blocking agents. Agents that interfere with the metabolism of these agents may enhance nephrotoxicity (erythromycin, ketoconazole, diltiazem). The vasoconstrictive effects of the calcineurin inhibitors, together with the reduced renal reserve of the allograft, enhances the nephrotoxicity of other potentially injurious agents, even in allografts with near-normal function; such as aminoglycosides, amphotericin, acyclovir, (NSAIDs), ACE-inhibitors and radiocontrast agents.

Infection

Infection can be associated with allograft dysfunction in the early posttransplant period. A postoperative fever associated with graft dysfunction requires a thorough and complete evaluation for infection, because prompt recognition and appropriate antimicrobial therapy may be life saving and intensification of immunosuppression may be very hazardous. Genitourinary (GU) infections are quite common in the renal transplant population and can result in renal allograft dysfunction when cystitis is complicated by graft pyelonephritis or systemic sepsis. There are multiple risk factors for the development of bacterial colonization and subsequent infection of the bladder in this patient population, including impaired bladder emptying related to neurogenic bladder (most commonly in diabetic patients) or bladder outlet obstruction secondary to prostate hypertrophy or urethral strictures, congenital or acquired anatomic anomalies of the GU system (particularly pediatric patients), bladder catheters, and ureteral stents.

The high frequency of ureteral reflux into the transplanted kidney, as high as 50%, predisposes to pyelonephritis and subsequent allograft dysfunction. Fever, leukocytosis, pyuria, bacteruria, and graft tenderness are the typical manifestations of this complication. Other common bacterial infectious complications that, when associated with systemic infection and volume depletion, can lead to allograft dysfunction include diverticulitis or diverticular abscesses and cholecystitis. Patients with polycystic kidney disease, diabetes, and advanced age are at particular risk for these complications. Immunosuppression, particularly high-dose steroids, may mask the signs of intraabdominal infection, often delaying diagnosis until systemic sepsis supervenes. Cytomegalovirus (CMV) infection may also evoke transient allograft dysfunction weeks to months after engraftment. There are a variety of disease processes involving the kidney that have been linked to CMV infections; specifically, CMV inclusion disease associated with glomerular and interstitial pathologic conditions, immune complex nephritis, immunotactoid glomerulopathy, glomerular vascular rejection, and the precipitation of acute cellular rejection. Thus any episode of fever associated with allograft dysfunction, particularly in the first 6 months posttransplant, should prompt an investigation for CMV infection.

Recurrent Renal Disease

Recurrent renal disease is an uncommon cause of graft loss, even more so in the early posttransplant period. Several studies estimate a rate of recurrent disease of 3.5% in 5 years. Nevertheless, there are a few primary renal disease that can recur quite early following renal transplantation with potentially devastating consequences. *Focal and segmental glomerulosclerosis* is reported to recur in 25% to 50% of allografts. There are certain high-risk groups with reported rates of recurrence up to 75%: pediatric patients (younger than 3 years of age) and those with prior recurrence within an allograft, those with mesangial expansion on native kidney biopsy, or those who had rapid progression to end-stage renal disease. Fifty percent to 75% of allografts are lost to recurrence within 2 years of diagnosis. If recurrence is recognized early before significant sclerosis is present as demonstrated on biopsy, plasmapheresis may be of benefit in inducing remission. *Hemolytic-uremic syndrome* can also recur within the first few months of transplantation. Recurrence rates are 12% to 25%, most often in those with the atypical, non–diarrheal-associated syndrome. The disease is often limited to the allograft, but it can provoke a systemic flare of the syndrome, even in those who have had inactive disease for prolonged periods. Cyclosporine or tacrolimus probably increases the risk of recurrence, and it is often necessary to withdraw the immunosuppressive agent and institute intensive plasmapheresis to control the disease. It is estimated that 50% of allografts are lost to recurrence. Finally, some forms of *glomerulonephritis* may recur within the early posttransplant period—most notably, membranoproliferative glomerulonephritis, lupus nephritis, and crescentic glomerulonephritis. Recurrence risk is greatest if the disease has been active within 6 to 12 months of transplantation.

Allograft Rejection

Allograft rejection is becoming an increasingly less common cause of graft dysfunction in the early posttransplant period. Recent advances in immunosuppressive therapy over the last 5 years have significantly reduced rates of acute rejection from 50% to 60% to 25% to 30%. The immunosupressive agents that have accounted for much of this decline are mycophenolate mofetil (Cellcept), tacrolimus (FK506), and the monoclonal anti-IL-2 receptor antibodies, Xenepax and Simulec. Rapamycin is another immunosuppressive agent, currently in phase 3 clinical trials, that holds promise in significantly reducing rates of acute rejection. The new microemulsion of cyclosporine, Neoral, has also been demonstrated to reduce rates of rejection as a result of its improved bioavailability compared with the older formulation, Sandimmune. These advances and several others on the horizon hold the promise of eliminating acute rejection as a significant cause of graft loss and hopefully will translate into improved long-term allograft survival.

Acute rejection is slightly more common in cadaver compared with living donor organ recipients. Approximately two-thirds to three-fourths of rejection episodes occur within the first month, and 90% to 95% of rejection episodes will occur within the first three months. More than 85% of first rejection episodes can be reversed by appropriate therapy and both mycophenolate mofetil and tacrolimus have demonstrated effectiveness in reversing many of the once resistant and/or recurrent forms of acute rejection. Risk factors for acute rejection episodes include lower cyclosporine dosage and blood levels, pretransplant immunization as indicated by the presence of panel reactive antibodies and positive B-cell cross-matches, young recipient age and HLA mismatching. Graft rejection episodes have a deleterious effect on long-term graft function and are the most potent risk factor for chronic allograft nephropathy.

Rejection episodes in the early posttransplant period can be classified into three different types based on the temporal relationship to surgery.

Hyperacute Rejection

Rejection occurring in minutes or hours following transplant surgery is called *hyperacute rejection.* This type of rejection is caused by binding of performed antibodies to their respective antigens within the allograft. In the modern era of transplantation, hyperacute rejection is rare because of meticulous testing (highly sensitive T-cell cross-matches) for preformed cytotoxic IgG antibodies in the recipient directed to donor HLA class I antigens. These antibodies bind quickly to the vascular endothelium of the graft and destroy it within minutes to hours. Similar events are involved in the hyperacute rejection of xenografts, although the antibodies may be binding to non-HLA antigens. Activation of complement and lysis of endothelial and renal parenchymal cells are likely to be involved in this reaction. Hyperacute rejection may also occur as a result of ABO incompatibility.

Grossly, the transplanted kidney looks cyanotic and flaccid. On microscopic examination, widespread microvascular thrombi, platelet aggregates, and neutrophilic infiltrates are seen. Sometimes there is little alteration in renal morphology suggesting a bland ischemia. At the present time, no treatment is successful, and prevention is the mainstay of management. Failure to recognize hyperacutely rejected kidneys may ultimately lead to graft rupture and massive hemorrhage. In hyperacute rejection, there is immediate nonfunction, and radionuclide imaging will fail to demonstrate graft perfusion (Table 88.3).

Accelerated Rejection (Delayed Hyperacute Rejection)

Accelerated rejection usually occurs in a few days (5 to 7 days) after transplantation. Humoral or cellular immune mechanisms are involved in this type of rejection. It can be divided into four different subtypes based on pathogenesis: (a) a vascular type of rejection related to undetected but low levels of preformed cytotoxic IgG antibodies in the recipient to donor HLA class I antigens (false-negative cross-match); (b) a vascular type of rejection caused by antibodies directed to HLA class II antigens; (c) a vascular type of rejection caused by antibodies directed to donor vascular endothelial cells, this type of rejection is mostly seen in HLA-identical, mixed leukocyte culture nonstimulatory living related donor transplant recipients; and (d) a cellular type of rejection caused by a primed T-cell response, this type of accelerated rejection may be seen in living-related donor transplants following donor-specific transfusions. Morphologically, accelerated rejection may appear similar to hyperacute rejection; however, there may be more tubular interstitial infiltrates. Endothelial cell injury, interstitial hemorrhage, and glomerular ischemia are common. The vascular types of rejection related to preformed antibodies are difficult to treat. Intensive plasma exchange combined with intravenous polyvalent immunoglobulin therapy may be occasionally successful. The cellular type of accelerated rejection can be treated with similar success as for acute rejection and by the same reagents.

Acute Cellular Rejection

Because untreated acute rejection leads to graft loss and up to 90% of acute rejections are reversible, prompt and accurate diagnosis is extremely important. In the cyclosporine era, the classic constitutional inflammatory clinical features of acute rejection, such as fever, chills, graft tenderness, and enlargement, described in the early days of transplantation, are often not present. It is usually manifested by evidence of graft dysfunction characterized by an abrupt rise in blood urea nitrogen and serum creatinine levels, occasionally associated with oliguria. Importantly, there is evidence that 50% or more of allografts within the first 3 months of transplantation will demonstrate histologic evidence of acute rejection in the absence of decline in renal function (subclinical rejection), often histologically as severe as those with overt evidence of allograft dysfunction. Transplants with subclinical rejection have poorer long-term outcome than those with normal histology. In addition, those that were empirically treated, despite stable renal function at the time of biopsy, had reductions in the severity of chronic rejection on follow-up biopsy, although there was no difference in functional outcome. These data underscore the importance of immune-mediated inflammatory events in determining long-term outcome and the need for improved means of detecting such immunologic processes, as well as the need for intensive immunosuppression in the early posttransplant period and meticulous attention to compliance and adequacy of the regimen used. The advances in immunosuppression over the last 5 years may further reduce the likelihood that acute rejection will be apparent clinically, thereby mitigating any long-term benefit to allograft outcome, if better means for detecting allorecognition are not realized.

It is always important to exclude other causes of graft dysfunction such as obstruction, hypovolemia, delayed acute tubular necrosis, arterial and venous complications, and bacterial or viral infections. Calcineurin inhibitor nephrotoxicity may also be difficult to separate from allograft rejection. Analysis of cyclosporine or tacrolimus concentration and a therapeutic trial of reduction in the dose may help in distinguishing acute rejection from the diagnosis of calcineurin inhibitor nephrotoxicity. Ultrasonography usually excludes obstruction, and Doppler flow analysis or radionuclide imaging helps to assess the integrity of vascular supply.

For the definitive diagnosis of acute rejection, renal transplant biopsy of the kidney has been employed as the gold standard. In experienced hands, a fine-needle aspiration biopsy of the kidney is highly sensitive in making the diagnosis of acute cellular rejection. Aspirated cells can be studied not only for their morphologic features but also for their expression of cell surface markers, such as HLA-DR, and their synthesis of factors activated by rejection, such as tumor necrosis factor, interferon, and adhesion molecules. Cell flow cytometry is currently being used to further increase the diagnostic accuracy and reduce the difficulty and cost of this procedure, making it more broadly available in clinical practice. Also efforts are underway to employ PCR technology to quantitatively assessing the expression of mRNA for proinflammatory cytokines to further refine the diagnostic utility of fine-needle aspirates.

Core renal biopsy remains as the mainstay of diagnosis in many centers. Morphologically, acute cell-mediated rejection is characterized by interstitial edema, cortical mononuclear and eosinophilic infiltration and lymphocytic tubulitis. The criteria for diagnosis and classification of allograft rejection by morphologic terms have been agreed on and are referred to as the Banff Classification. The standard histologic means of evaluating core needle biopsies has been augmented with immunohistologic staining for markers of acute rejection. The best studied are the adhesion molecules ICAM-1 and VCAM-1. Increased staining of ICAM-1 in renal tubular cells and VCAM-1 staining in vascular locations are strongly correlated with acute rejection and can differentiate cyclosporine toxicity from rejection. Also, PCR analysis of core biopsies for expression of granzyme B (a cytotoxic attack molecule produced by cytotoxic T cells) and the proinflammatory cytokines IL-2 and IL-10 is significantly correlated with acute rejection, and application of this technique may improve the diagnostic yield of the core biopsy.

Another technique employed in the diagnosis of acute rejection is urine cytology. Urine flow cytometry with immunohistochemical analysis of the cells for the presence of HLA-DR, ICAM-1, CD3 (a cell-surface marker for T cells), and the IL-2 receptor has an estimated sensitivity of greater than 90% for the diagnosis for acute rejection. Increases in the urinary excretion of C5A have also shown utility in diagnosing acute rejection with estimated diagnostic accuracy of 81% with the increment in urine excretion preceding the clinical diagnosis of rejection by 1.6 days. Finally, increases in serum ICAM-1 levels are correlated to acute rejection and changes in levels often precede the overt manifestations of rejection by several days.

LATE POSTTRANSPLANT ALLOGRAFT DYSFUNCTION

Late posttransplant allograft dysfunction is arbitrarily defined as deterioration in graft function appearing 3 or 4 months following initial surgery. The common causes are given in Table 88.4.

Mechanical Causes of Late Graft Loss

Most causes of urinary tract obstruction in the transplanted kidney occur in the early time period. Uncommonly, obstructive uropathy occurs in the chronic setting; this has been well described in the literature. First, it must always be recognized that whatever disorder can occur in native nontransplanted kidneys can also occur in the renal transplant, thus patients with a propensity to form urinary stones have had obstruction to nephrolithiasis occur in the transplant as well. Particularly related to the transplantation event are obstructions from the uncommon late development of a lymphocele or, more frequently, usually in the context of rejection, ureteric stenosis. In evaluating renal dysfunction in this chronic period, urinary tract obstruction must first be ruled out usually with sonographic imaging before more ominous diagnoses are entertained. Vascular complications have been more common in the past, but with newer techniques of transplant artery anastomosis, these have become rare. Patients presenting with the late onset of hypertension and progressive renal dysfunction occasionally associated with a new perigraft bruit should have this complication entertained. Newer methods of imaging, such as magnetic resonance angiography or color flow Doppler ultrasonography, have been useful in diagnosis. The appearance of acute renal failure or abrupt reduction in glomerular filtration after use of an ACE inhibitor, antihypertensive agent, or an angiotensin-receptor blocker may be a clue to the presence of this mechanical problem of late dysfunction.

Infection

Unique transplant-related infections become progressively uncommon over time in a successful renal transplant. Indeed, after 1 year, unless patients are retreated for acute transplant rejection, the majority of the infections that renal transplant recipients develop are community acquired. In the brief window of time between 3 and 6 months after surgery, two important categories of infection are both transplant related and may be the cause of allograft dysfunction. *Acute urinary tract infections* often associated with frank transplant pyelonephritis can lead to substantial allograft dysfunction with symptoms that may resemble allograft rejection such as fever, graft swelling and tenderness, high ultrasound resistive indices, and elevated serum creatinines. Pyuria rather than mononuclear infiltration of the urine associated with the presence of bacteria is a clue. Biopsy and even aspiration biopsy with culture is the definitive diagnostic maneuver. *Cytomegalovirus* infection may also appear in this 3- to 6-month window in the renal transplant recipient. The most common syndrome resembles a fever of unknown origin, with fever malaise, leukopenia, pancytopenia, myalgia, and occasional renal dysfunction. Additional organ manifestations of CMV can include pulmonary infiltrates with potential hypoxia, hepatitis, and frank renal involvement. This viral infection is associated with certain high-risk transplant recipients. Because a donor kidney from a patient who has been infected with CMV in the past transfers the infection, the recipient who has never been infected and is immunologically unprotected is at the highest risk for a frank CMV clinical infection. In this setting, prophylactic antiviral therapy has been shown to be helpful. Most recently the most effective prophylaxis is now thought to be hyperimmune serum, or intravenous ganciclovir. There is evidence that high-dose oral ganciclovir is also effective. Because the state of immunosuppression predicts susceptibility to CMV infection, patients with multiple or frequent rejections treated with high-dose immunosuppression such as either monoclonal or polyclonal antilymphocyte antibodies may also be treated with prophylactic antiviral therapy. CMV may also involve the kidney itself reducing transplant function. Some even believe that CMV glomerulonephropathy should be considered in rare cases of CMV infection. Finally, CMV infection can upregulate the appearance of major histocompatibility complex (MHC) antigens in the kidney, adhesion molecules, and other immunoactants, which can tip the balance between immunosuppression and rejection leading to frank immunologic rejection and renal dysfunction a possibility that must be kept in mind when appropriate therapy of the CMV infection has not reversed renal dysfunction.

Calcineurin Inhibitor Chronic Nephropathy

The calcineurin enzyme inhibitor immunosuppressants cyclosporine and tacrolimus are associated with chronic renal dysfunction. In the setting of extrarenal transplantation, such dysfunction occurs in the native kidneys. Paradoxically this dysfunction can also occur in the renal transplant. Acute calcineurin inhibitor toxicity can always confound the interpretation of late renal dysfunction and is frequently associated with elevations in the cyclosporine or tacrolimus blood levels above the upper limits of the empirically derived therapeutic window. Stable renal transplant recipients who are taking newly prescribed concomitant medications that alter the metabolic handling of either of the calcineurin inhibitors may have sudden increases in blood level associated with acute nephrotoxicity and renal dysfunction. Careful attention to concomitant medications, especially to newly described agents, must be paid in interpretation of late allograft dysfunction. A more chronic variety of toxicity has also been described with intrarenal fibrosis, often in a classic intermittent or striped pattern. This form occurs more commonly in patients with extrarenal transplantation, but can occasionally occur in individual renal transplant recipients. Some have argued that blood levels of these important immunosuppressant agents have been kept improperly too low to forestall smoldering acute and ultimately chronic rejection out of fear of potential chronic nephrotoxicity related to the drugs. For cyclosporine, in patients not consuming other medications that confound metabolic handling of the molecule, a dose of about 4 mg/kg/day has been shown to avoid chronic nephrotoxicity and acute rejection episodes in the majority of patients. For patients with inexorable cyclosporine nephrotoxicity, attempts may be made at converting the patient to the macrolide calcineurin inhibitor, tacrolimus. The reverse is also true.

RECURRENT PRIMARY DISEASE

Certain disorders culminating in end-stage renal disease recur in the transplant at a high rate and may be relative contraindications to organ transplantation such as the metabolic defect leading to *oxalosis*. In oxalosis recurrence is inescapable, especially during periods of reduced glomerular filtration. Some have attempted to address oxalosis by performing a double transplant of liver and kidney simultaneously. Other systemic diseases also recur at rates acceptable for engraftment but must be kept in mind in the interpretation of late renal dysfunction. Morphologic changes of diabetic glomerulopathy are well described in renal transplant recipients, appear to occur at a more rapid tempo than *de novo* disease, and may be forestalled by tight glucose control or even pancreatic transplantation. The atypical form of *hemolytic uremic syndrome* also recurs in transplant patients; the rate is felt to be increased in patients receiving either cyclosporine or tacrolimus therapy. Recurrence rates have been described between 25% and 50% with no clinical predictors, except for recurrence in a first transplant lost to that condition when a retransplant is being contemplated. Certain glomerular diseases are known to recur, some culminating in the loss of the allograft.

It was well recognized in the era of identical twin transplantation that renal dysfunction in a setting in which organ transplant rejection was immunologically impossible could be ascribed to recurrent glomerular diseases. One strategy to avoid recurrent glomerular disease in immune-mediated glomerulonephritis has been to wait until evidence of immune activity has ceased before contemplating transplantation. Recurrence rates are relatively high for patients with *IgA nephropathy* (up to 50%) and those with *membranoproliferative glomerulonephritis* (especially type I) but rarely is the cause of renal allograft dysfunction or loss. On the other hand, recurrent *idiopathic focal* and *segmental glomerulosclerosis*, thought to be related to an intrinsic circulating factor leading to diminished permselectivity, substantial proteinuria, and mesangial injury leading to glomerulosclerosis, is more common and can occur within minutes of the establishment of the transplant arterial anastomosis. Recently, plasmapheresis in general and with specific protein A columns has been shown to ameliorate the proteinuria of recurrent transplant focal sclerosing glomerulonephritis without altering the long-term decline in renal function. Some forms of glomerulonephritis have been felt to rarely recur such as that of systemic *lupus erythematosus*. More recently estimates of increased incidence of this disorder recurrent in the transplant have been reported especially in patients who persist in forming anti-DNA antibodies or who have low serum complements at the time of transplantation. In all of these disorders a transplant renal biopsy is required to differentiate renal dysfunction from allograft rejection of the acute or chronic variety.

CHRONIC REJECTION

Chronic allograft rejection is the most common cause of late renal allograft dysfunction. It has immunologic and nonimmunologic mechanisms that are causally related, such as the degree of match, the adequacy of immunosuppression, the number of rejection episodes, the presence of hypertension, and the presence of delayed graft function. Clinical features include slowly progressive and inexorable renal dysfunction associated with proteinuria and hypertension morphologically associated with interstitial fibrosis, tubular atrophy, arteriolopathy, and in some cases, glomerulosclerosis. Splitting and rarefaction of the basement membrane and mesangial interposition associated with interstitial fibrosis defines a subset of patients with chronic rejection often accompanied by the nephrotic syndrome, called *transplant glomerulopathy*. The importance of interstitial mononuclear cell infiltrates particularly those of monocyte-macrophages, the release of profibrotic cytokines, the presence of smoldering rejection leading to enhanced matrix formation, growth factor development, and scar formation are considered important in the development of the immunologic causes of chronic rejection. Newer forms of acute immunosuppressive medications in study have been shown to ameliorate experimental forms of chronic rejection and will be tested in the clinic.

Alternately enhanced immunosuppression in patients found to have smoldering rejection by protocol biopsy or analysis of fibrotic cytokine genes by reverse transcriptase polymerase chain reaction and inhibition of the link between these cytokines and matrix formation with the use of such agents as the HMG-CoA reductase inhibitor drugs or angiotensin receptor blockers or ACE inhibitors are also being studied. In any case, the core renal biopsy remains the gold standard means for discerning the diagnosis of chronic rejection coupled to imaging studies to rule out mechanical problems along with the potential use of fine needle aspiration either for gene analyses or for the discovery of infection within the allograft.

Selected Readings

Amante AJM, Kahan BD. Technical complications of renal transplantation. *Surg Clin North Am* 1994;74(5):1117–1131.

Well-written and concise review of technical/surgical aspects of renal transplantation.

Azuma H, Tilney NL. Immune and nonimmune mechanisms of chronic rejection of kidney allografts. *J Heart Lung Transplant* 1995;14:136–142.

Best review of the topic by investigators who have primary experience as well as a review of the data.

Bakir N, Sluiter WJ, Plueg RJ, et al. Primary renal graft thrombosis. *Nephrol Dial Transplant* 1996;11:140–147.

Excellent original paper on the impact of graft thrombosis on renal transplantation.

Bennett WM, deMattos AM, Meyer MM, et al. Chronic CSA nephropathy: the Achilles' heel of immunosuppressive therapy. *Kidney Int* 1996;50:1089–1100.

Excellent review of the importance and meaning of calcineurin inhibitor nephrotoxicity.

Fervenza FC, Lafeyette RA, Alfrey EJ, et al. Renal artery stenosis in kidney transplants. *Am J Kidney Dis* 1998;31:142–148.

Concise review of impact of this problem on renal transplantation.

Paulakis M, Strehlau J, Lipman M, et al. Use of intra-graft gene expression in the diagnosis of kidney allograft rejection. *Transplant Proc* 1996;28:2019–2021.

Concise review on this emerging area of research in renal transplantation.

Ramos EL. Recurrent diseases of the renal allograft. *J Am Soc Nephrol* 1991;2: 109–121.

Best review of this topic extant.

Rubin RH. Infectious complications of renal transplantation. *Kidney Int* 1993;44: 221–236.

Recent iteration of Rubin's encyclopedic experience with this topic.

Shoskes DA, Halloran PF. Delayed graft function in renal transplantation: etiology, management and long-term significance. *J Urol* 1996;155:1831–1840.

A comprehensive review on the impact of delayed graft function on renal transplantation.

Suthanthiran M, Strom TB. Mechanisms and management of acute renal allograft rejection. *Surg Clin North Am* 1998;78:77–93.

Well-written monograph on this subject by two of the leading researchers in the field.

PART 2
Prevention and Treatment
A: Glucocorticoids and Azathioprine

Mary G. McGeown and James F. Douglas

Glucocorticoids (steroids) and azathioprine, used together, were the first drugs to achieve prolonged graft survival in human kidney transplantation. During the early 1950s, cadaver kidneys were transplanted in humans by Küss and Dubois in Paris, and by Murray, Holden, and Hume in Boston, using small doses of adrenocorticotropic hormone (ACTH) or cortisone. A few functioned briefly but there were no longer-term survivors.

In 1958, Dameshek and Schwartz reasoned that the anticancer drug, 6-mercaptopurine (6MP), might be used in the treatment of aplastic anemia and leukemia. They soon afterward reported that rabbits treated with this drug showed little reaction to foreign protein. In 1960 and 1961, Hopewell in London, Murray and colleagues in Boston, and Küss in Paris used 6MP as the immunosuppressive agent for human kidney transplants without success. Then Küss reported prolonged survival of a kidney from an unrelated donor, the recipient receiving 6MP and intermittent prednisone, as well as irradiation. Meanwhile Calne, working in Murray's laboratory, tested derivatives of 6MP, including azathioprine. In dogs, the new drug proved to be immunosuppressive and less toxic than the parent drug. Murray and Calne went on to use azathioprine in human kidney transplants; the third attempt succeeded, and despite rejection episodes, functioned for 2 years. In 1962, Goodwin reported that steroid injections reversed several rejection episodes in a mother-to-child transplant; the child later died of sepsis.

Steroids and azathioprine were soon in general use for human kidney transplantation. Despite troublesome side effects, careful dosage allowed a high quality of life for many recipients. Used in combination, they set a standard against which more recent regimens must be measured and are still widely used for long-term immunosuppression.

GLUCOCORTICOIDS (STEROIDS)

Steroids dominate in the treatment of acute rejection and are the backbone of most induction and maintenance regimens. However, there is only limited consensus regarding how they should best be used. This is probably because of the therapeutic dilemma posed by their evident effectiveness and equally clear toxicity. Protocols vary widely between centers and a tendency to overdose persists, particularly in the early posttransplant period.

Mechanism of Action

Steroids reversibly block the expression of T-cell– and antigen-presenting cell (APC)–derived cytokines and cytokine receptors. Their hydrophobic structures allow them to diffuse easily into cells and bind to specific cytoplasmic receptors.

The resulting complexes move to the nucleus, where they attach to deoxyribonucleic acid (DNA) elements, inhibiting the transcription of cytokine genes. Steroids also prevent the migration to the nucleus of transcription factors central to the induction of genes encoding a wide range of cytokines. In addition, they inhibit the synthesis of cytokines after their genes have been transcribed into messenger ribonucleic acid (mRNA). By these mechanisms they have been shown to block the expression of the T-cell– and APC-derived cytokines, interleukin-1 (IL-1), IL-2, IL-3, IL-6, tumor necrosis factor-α (TNF-α), and interferon-γ (IFN-γ). This multiple interference in every element of the T-cell activation process underlies their profound immunosuppressive, antiinflammatory, and hormonal actions as well as their potential for toxicity.

Steroids have a number of nonspecific immunosuppressive effects. High doses block production of IL-1 (endogenous pyrogen), causing the antipyretic effect of immunosuppression. They also lead to a marked increase in total white blood cell count (often triggering fears of infection), but with a redistribution of lymphocytes back into lymphoid tissue. The whole inflammatory process is strongly suppressed by inhibition of many chemotactants, permeability factors, vasodilators, and other mediators.

Pharmacology and Pharmakinetics

Prednisone and its derivative, prednisolone, are almost completely absorbed, with peak plasma levels occurring within 2 hours. Inactive hepatic metabolites are mostly excreted in the urine along with a small amount of unchanged drug. Plasma half-life is 2 to 4 hours, although lymphokine inhibition persists for up to 24 hours; thus the immune response can be controlled just as effectively by a single morning dose as by divided doses. This also results in significantly less endogenous steroid suppression, provided that slow-release preparations are avoided. Methylprednisolone, the main intravenous agent, behaves similarly. Steroid metabolism is delayed in age and in liver disease. It is impaired by some drugs, including oral contraceptives and ketoconazole, which increase plasma levels. Enzyme-inducing drugs, such as barbiturates, phenytoin, and rifampicin, have the opposite effect. In the absence of useful assays, dose changes are usually made empirically. Renal insufficiency does not significantly change dose requirements.

Removal by dialysis has not been shown.

Therapeutic Use

The Precyclosporine Era

High-dose steroids with azathioprine were widely used for induction and postgraft treatment. These led to a high rate of complications. However, low-dose regimens were found to be just as effective, with a much lower morbidity and mortality. Azathioprine and low-dose steroids were used for the long-term treatment of many successfully transplanted patients dating from the end of the 1960s. In Belfast, we gave 200 mg of hydrocortisone intravenously in the surgical theater as soon as the intravenous infusion was set up, followed by azathioprine 5 mg/kg of body weight. Neither drug can be safely withdrawn or, in the case of steroids, reduced much below the equivalent of 10 mg/day. Alternate-day maintenance dosing with a steroid has been shown to minimize side effects without significantly increasing the risk of rejection.

The Cyclosporine Era

Steroids in varying doses continue to be used for induction, reversal of acute rejection, and long-term maintenance. A typical induction regimen consists of methylprednisolone (1 to 2 g) daily, given intravenously for several days, followed by an oral dose tapering to 20 to 30 mg at 2 weeks and further reducing to 5 to 10 mg at 1 year; this becomes the long-term maintenance dose. It should be noted that considerably more steroid is given in most cyclosporine protocols than was found necessary in the Belfast azathioprine regimen. Graft function is carefully monitored at each downward step.

Acute rejection (preferably biopsy proven) is treated with short courses of high-dose steroids. Pulses of methylprednisolone (1 to 2 g) for 3 to 5 days are the rule, but oral doses starting from as little as 120 mg/day of prednisolone have been used in some centers. Up to 80% of first rejections are successfully reversed, often within 48 hours. Later rejection episodes often respond, but with a lower success rate and with increased risk of side effects. Steroid-resistant rejection is usually treated with alternative agents following further biopsy evaluation. There is no evidence that higher-dose antirejection therapy with steroids improves graft survival, which makes it logical to adopt a policy of restraint, particularly if multiple agents are being used.

The Belfast regimen of prednisolone 20 mg (with azathioprine 3 mg/kg, both given orally) from the day following transplantation, and an antirejection protocol of prednisolone 200 mg, falling stepwise to the baseline dose within 15 days, is as effective as more aggressive policies. Low-dose maintenance steroid therapy is widely used. Although it is clear that cyclosporine and other "steroid-sparing" drugs allow more scope for dose reduction, ideas differ regarding the acceptable minimum.

Complications, Avoidance, and Withdrawal

The complications associated with steroid therapy are well known. Those of significance in transplantation are listed in Table 88.5. Infections (opportunistic or otherwise) are the most serious complication, and at one time accounted for at least 30% of deaths in transplant patients. The adoption of low-dose steroid regimens greatly reduced this risk but did not eliminate it.

Individual response to steroids varies considerably, possibly as a result of differences in tissue-receptor distribution and in steroid metabolism. The persistence of cardiovascular disease, as the main threat to recipient survival has stimulated efforts either to avoid the use of steroids from the outset (except for cases of acute rejection) or to withdraw steroids at a later time from suitable patients. At first, avoidance took the form of cyclosporine monotherapy, but it now can consist of various combinations using such drugs as azathioprine, tacrolimus, and mycophenolate mofetil. Although achievable, avoidance carries an increased risk of acute rejection, and the prospect of toxicity induced by cyclosporine and other immunosuppressants. Steroid withdrawal is associated (as is avoidance) with lower blood pressure, better control of diabetes, and lower cholesterol levels—all clinically desirable. However, withdrawal also leads to an increased rate of acute rejection, higher rates of impaired graft function, and reduced overall graft survival. Steroids should not usually be withdrawn within 6 months of grafting. Compelling potential advantages should be present, with few or no counterbalancing immunologic risks.

TABLE 88.5. Main Side Effects of Steroid Therapy

Increased risk of infection
Polyphagia and obesity
Cushingoid features
Fluid retention
Hypertension
Osophagitis, gastritis, peptic ulceration
Glucose intolerance
Adrenopituitary suppression
Growth suppression in children
Avascular necrosis of bones and joints
Osteoporosis
Posterior polar cataract
Hyperlipidemia
Emotional problems
Psychosis (manic-depressive)
Acne

Patients most likely to benefit are those with reduced bone mass (especially older women at risk for osteoporosis), diabetic patients, and others at increased risk of infection or cardiovascular disease.

In children, steroids tend to be well tolerated and promote prolonged graft survival. However, they also induce prolonged growth suppression, and such children may already be stunted in growth. Contributory factors may be reduced levels of growth hormone and somatomedin, renal phosphate wasting, and impaired calcium absorption. Recombinant growth hormone appears to improve prepubertal growth in children with transplants, without significantly affecting graft function. It may be of benefit to counteract the effect of steroids on growth.

Withdrawal of steroids may be difficult in cases of donor-recipient mismatching. Caution and intensive monitoring should be used in second or later transplant patients, in highly mismatched grafts, and in patients with impaired graft function. Adequate alternative immunosuppression is essential, usually with cyclosporine. Azathioprine without steroids is insufficient on its own but may be combined with cyclosporine.

The value of newer agents such as tacrolimus and mycophenolate mofetil may be considerable. Late steroid withdrawal does not decrease the incidence of such complications as posterior polar cataracts, avascular bone necrosis, or osteoporosis. The incidence of these complications correlates best with total steroid load, which is a consequence of early high dosage.

AZATHIOPRINE

Azathioprine, a precursor of 6MP, was synthesized by Burroughs Wellcome in their New Jersey laboratories in 1960. After finding it had immunosuppressant activity in dogs, Calne and Murray went on to use it in human cadaveric transplantation.

Mechanism of Action

Azathioprine converts (*inter alia*) to 6MP, which in turn is metabolized to thionucleotides. These inhibit purine synthesis and thereby block most T-cell functions, preventing primary antibody production. Unlike cyclosporine, azathioprine is unable to prevent gene activation, but its metabolites are able to impede DNA replication and T-cell proliferation, RNA transcription and protein production, the formation of adenosine triphosphate (ATP) and cyclic adenosine monophosphate (cAMP), and the synthesis of adhesion molecules. Azathioprine delays the rapid proliferation of cells in the bone marrow and lymphoid tissue, particularly lymphocytes and neutrophils. Although acting through partial conversion to 6MP, it is a more effective immunosuppressant in some experimental animals.

Pharmacology and Pharmakinetics

Azathioprine is rapidly and fully absorbed when given orally, significant amounts appearing in the blood in 15 minutes. It is quickly distributed to all tissues, and within 4 hours conversion to 6MP is virtually complete, although most of the drug remains either unchanged or is converted to other metabolites. Intravenous administration does not increase bioavailability. Azathioprine is mainly eliminated the urine, 10% of the dose being excreted unchanged after 24 hours along with 50% as metabolite. We have found that dose reduction is advisable when renal function is impaired, although some regard this as unnecessary.

Dosage and Therapeutic Use

Before the introduction of cyclosporine, azathioprine in combination with steroids was used for induction and long-term maintenance therapy. It does not significantly affect established immune responses and is not useful in reversing acute rejection. A typical daily dose is 2 to 3 mg/kg. Many patients from the precyclosporine era have excellent long-term graft function. In the Belfast experience, on a regimen of azathioprine and low-dose steroids, 45% of 350 first cadaver grafts actually had a functioning graft 10–26 years later. The dose of azathioprine may be slowly reduced with time to minimize side effects, but cannot be withdrawn completely. Nor can steroids be withdrawn, because azathioprine alone is insufficient to prevent rejection. Its role in cyclosporine-based regimens is somewhat curtailed. It is useful as induction before graft function is established, and it may also form part of multiple-drug maintenance regimens, when lower, less toxic doses are used. A number of studies have failed to show a clear advantage to these regimens. Conversion from cyclosporine to azathioprine maintenance therapy is possible, but great care is necessary to avoid late acute rejection. Gradual change after a period on triple therapy appears to be the best policy. Nephrotoxicity, gum hypertrophy, hirsutism, and cost are the main reasons for conversion from cyclosporine.

Azathioprine may be combined with cyclosporine or tacrolimus as maintenance therapy after steroid withdrawal. Among newer drugs with similar immunosuppressive actions, mycophenolate mofetil, used instead of azathioprine in various combinations, appears to be more effective in reducing the incidence and severity of acute rejection, and in controlling refractory rejection. It may also achieve better graft function and survival than azathioprine, but further evidence is needed.

Azathioprine is converted to inactive 6-thiouric acid by xanthine oxidase. Allopurinol, given for the prevention of acute gout attacks in hyperuricemia, inhibits this enzyme and prolongs azathioprine activity. Where possible, the drugs should not be given together. However, azathioprine is associated with a 30% increase in plasma uric acid levels, and their use in combination may be unavoidable. In such circumstances, the dose of azathioprine should be reduced by 50% or more, while starting allopurinol at a dose of 100 mg/day.

Side Effects of Azathioprine

The unwanted effects of azathioprine are shown in Table 88.6. Bone marrow suppression is manifested by leukopenia, thrombocytopenia, and/or macrocytic anemia. Toxicity is dose related, but patient sensitivity varies considerably. Frequent (at least twice weekly) blood cell count monitoring is necessary after first use of the drug, particularly if doses of more than 2 mg/kg are used. With mild depression of the blood cell count, reduction in dose and vigilant attention to the blood cell count may be sufficient, but severe leukopenia requires suspension of the drug, which can be reintroduced at a lower dose after the white blood cell count becomes normal. Leukopenia predisposes to opportunistic viral infections but may also be a consequence of such infection.

Leukopenia is not a marker for immunosuppressive effect. Careful differential diagnosis is essential. Cover with other agents such as cyclosporine can now be used until the blood cell count recovers. Bone marrow suppression is most common during the first weeks after commencing azathioprine, but occasionally is seen for the first time after many years of use. Hepatotoxicity and cholestatic jaundice have been reported but are rare; some earlier cases may have been caused by unrecognized hepatitis C infection.

In common with other cytotoxic agents, azathioprine increases the incidence of malignancies, particularly lymphoma, sarcoma (including Kaposi's sarcoma), liver and kidney tumors, and carcinoma (skin, lip, and cervix). Exposure to direct sunlight greatly increases the risk of skin lesions and all patients must be made aware of this. The overall risk of malignancy is much greater than that of the general public, especially where azathioprine has been used with other cytotoxic drugs. Regular appropriate screening and treatment for early tumours is mandatory. (A detailed discussion of malignancy in transplant recipients is found in Chapter 89, Part 6.)

Azathioprine has been superseded as a mainline immunosuppressant drug for organ transplantation. Despite the manifest advantages of the modern era's more potent drugs, it still has a place in adjunctive therapy in certain circumstances, as described previously. In the Belfast experience the incidence of malignant neoplasms is less in patients treated with azathioprine and low dose steroid than that in patients treated with cyclosporine.

Its great disadvantage is that it is insufficient on its own and must be given with a steroid or one of the modern drugs. However, many patients still survive from the late 1960s and 1970s who are fit and with grafts that function well, who never received cyclosporine or any form of antilymphocyte serum. It could be argued that azathioprine's toxic side effects are, if anything, less than those of cyclosporine, and it is certainly less expensive. In countries where cost is a consideration, it may still have a place.

TABLE 88.6. Main Side Effects of Azathioprine After Transplant Surgery

Increased risk of infection (mainly viral)
Bone marrow suppression
Leukopenia
Thrombocytopenia
Macrocytic anemia
Increased risk of neoplasia
Lymphoma
Sarcoma
Kaposi's sarcoma
Carcinoma: skin, lip, cervix, liver, kidney
Hepatotoxicity
Pancreatitis
Allopurinol interaction
Alopecia

Selected Readings

Hricik DE, Almawi WY, Strom TB. Trends in the use of glucocorticoids in renal transplantation. *Transplantation* 1994;57:979–989.
A comprehensive and still relevant review, emphasizing issues of steroid dosage, avoidance, and withdrawal.

Keown P, Hayry P, Mathew T, et al. (Executive Committee, the Tricontinental Mycophenolate Mofetil Renal Transplantation Study Group). A blinded randomized clinical trial of mycophenolate mofetil for the prevention of acute rejection in cadaveric renal transplantation. *Transplantation* 1996;61:1029–1037.
In this report, mycophenolate mofetil reduced the incidence and severity of acute rejection when contrasted with azathioprine in comparable patient groups, with lower rates of treatment failure. Differences persisted throughout the first year after transplant surgery.

Laine J, Krogerus L, Sarna S, et al. Recombinant growth hormone treatment. Its effect on renal allograft function and histology. *Transplantation* 1996;61:898–903.
In this group's experience, recombinant growth hormone improved growth in prepubertal children after transplant surgery without significantly affecting graft function or the histologic picture.

McGeown MG. Immunosuppression. In: McGeown MG, ed. *Clinical management of renal transplantation.* Dordrecht: Kluwer Academic Publications, 1992:201–209.
A full account of the Belfast low-dose steroid regimen of the 1960s and 1970s, the demonstration of excellent graft survival with low complication rates, and a comprehensive survey of the author's clinical practice.

McGeown MG, Clark C. Results of renal transplantation five to twenty-six years after surgery, using azathioprine and low-dose prednisolone as sole immunosuppression. In: Cecka JM, Terasaki PI, eds. *Clinical transplants* 1996;265–270.
Describes the results for a single center over a prolonged period in patients never treated with cyclosporine.

Radcliffe PJ, Dudley CRK, Higgins RM, et al. Randomised controlled trial of steroid withdrawal in renal transplant recipients receiving triple immunosuppression. *Lancet* 1996;348:643–648.
Late steroid withdrawal was feasible in stable patients and has potentially beneficial metabolic effects; but a substantial proportion showed a reduction in graft function.

B: Cyclosporine and Tacrolimus

Hamid Shidban and Robert Mendez

CYCLOSPORINE

Cyclosporine was extracted from the fungus *Tolypocladium inflatum Gams,* which was obtained from soil samples in Norway in 1969. The discovery of the immunologic activity of the compound by Borel led to trials in clinical renal transplantation. Since its approval for clinical use, cyclosporine has become the central component of most immunosuppressive regimens and has improved the survival of all types of allografts.

The clinical use of cyclosporine is complicated by its uncertain bioavailability, narrow therapeutic range, complex pharmacokinetic and pharmacodynamic interaction, and important intrinsic toxicity. This chapter reviews the current approach to cyclosporine therapy, and the principal complications arising from its use.

Mechanism of Action

There has been a considerable increase in published information about the action of cyclosporine within the cell at a molecular level. Some studies suggest that cyclosporine may downregulate antigen presentation, and thereby impede the recognition of foreign major histocompatibility complex (MHC) antigens. There is no evidence that cyclosporine significantly decreases the costimulatory action of the macrophage or the production of macrophage-driven cytokines such as interleukin-1 (IL-1) at either the mRNA or peptide level. Complete inhibition of the mixed lymphocyte reaction (MLR) by cyclosporine has been demonstrated in several species, including humans. The generation of cytotoxic lymphocytes in the MLR is prevented by cyclosporine, but once generated, cyclosporine has no effect on their cytotoxic activity.

The main action of cyclosporine is directed against the T lymphocyte, predominantly $CD4^+$ subset, where it exerts discrete effects at the membrane, cytosolic, and nuclear levels. This effect on the T-helper cell prevents the production of lymphokines, specifically IL-2. Within the membrane, cyclosporine inhibits early steps of phospholipase A_2-dependent phospholipid metabolism and reduces membrane potential. Cyclosporine is a prodrug and acts by binding to the cytosolic receptor protein, cyclophilin. Cyclophilins belong to a group of ubiquitous and abundant intracellular proteins with isomerase activity called *immunophilins.* The cyclosporine–cyclophilin complex is the active drug. The complex engages and inhibits a calcium-dependent serine phosphatase, calcineurin. Inhibition of calcineurin, which is integral to the Ca^{2+}-dependent mechanisms, prevents or reduces the activation of several calcineurin-dependent transcription factors, including the nuclear factor of activated T cell (NFAT). These factors are essential in the activation of the transcription of genes for T-cell cytokines such as IL-2, IL-4, tumor necrosis factor-α (TNF-α), interferon γ (IFN-γ), and CD40 ligand. Identification of calcineurin as the target of cyclosporine has permitted the direct measurement of calcineurin activity in the leukocytes of cyclosporine-treated patients. It has been shown that even at peak cyclosporine levels, calcineurin activity is not completely inhibited.

Cyclosporine-treated renal transplant patients have 50% less calcineurin activity in their peripheral blood leukocytes (PBL) than controls, despite blood cyclosporine levels that would be completely inhibitory *in vitro.* This discrepancy regarding the effect of cyclosporine is due to the partitioning of cyclosporine in blood to irrelevant binding sites. The partial inhibition of calcineurin activity in PBL of cyclosporine-treated patients is consistent with both the immunosuppressive effect of cyclosporine and the lack of immunodeficiency side effects. Inhibition of T-helper cells by cyclosporine also allows the uninhibited generation of suppressor T lymphocytes, which implies that T-suppressor cells are relatively resistant to cyclosporine. Activation of costimulatory pathway also leads to IL-2 production and IL-2 receptor expression, which is resistant to cyclosporine. Although, in general cyclosporine has not been thought to inhibit the function of B lymphocytes, some studies demonstrated a cyclosporine-sensitive subpopulation of T- independent B lymphocytes in mouse.

Cyclosporine inhibits cytokine-dependent alterations in the endothelial venules and blocks dynamic upregulation of MHC determinants that occur under the influence of IFN-γ, TNF-α, and other inflammatory cytokines. In this manner, cyclosporine acts to decrease both lymphocyte migration and accumulation within the graft and clustering of T cells necessary for interaction between graft antigen and T-cell receptor. Cyclosporine is generally most effective in preventing rejection when administered from time of engraftment. When administration is delayed, there is progressive reduction in the protective effect to the point at which cyclosporine is no longer able to prevent graft loss during the process of rejection.

Clinical Pharmacology

The original proprietary formulation of cyclosporine (Sandimmune) and now microemulsion formulation (Neoral), as well as other generic cyclosporine products, all contain cyclosporine, a neutral, water-insoluble, cyclic 11–amino acid polypeptide.

Cyclosporine is administered either through continuous intravenous infusion or orally, usually twice a day. A more frequent dose schedule may be needed in children, or in patients receiving other drugs that affect the metabolism of cyclosporine.

Sandimmune is an oil-in-water macroemulsion; it is absorbed when oil droplets are emulsified by bile salts or digested by pancreatic enzymes to release the drug. Biopharmaceutical limitations of Sandimmune that produce blood level variability have been overcome with the Neoral microemulsion formulation. Neoral has self-emulsifying properties and spontaneously forms a microemulsion in the aqueous fluids of the gastrointestinal (GI) tract; endogenous bile salts are not required for absorption. Cyclosporine microemulsion (Neoral) displays a 33% higher oral bioavailability than Sandimmune in end-stage renal disease patients, confirming findings observed in healthy volunteers and in organ transplant recipients. Neoral improves the extent of cyclosporine precipitation and enhances the permeability of the cyclosporine molecule across the GI mucosa.

Cyclosporine absorption from Neoral likely occurs by various mechanisms, including diffusion across the tight cellular junctions, or through the Peyer's patches. Cyclosporine is absorbed from the GI tract into enterocytes in the upper small intestine. Many factors can affect cyclosporine absorption including food intake, bile flow, gastrointestinal motility, and disorders of absorptive surface. Food has been reported to both delay and impair or, paradoxically, to increase the absorption of the cyclosporine. Delayed gastric emptying and intestinal dysmotility caused by autonomic neuropathy of diabetes mellitus lead to erratic and impaired cyclosporine uptake. Similarly, accelerated transit during diarrhea may decrease absorption of cyclosporine. Absorption of cyclosporine appears to be affected by the duration of therapy, and an increase in bioavailability of up to 50% has been observed in renal transplant patients during the first 3 months after transplantation. This may reflect an alteration in the mechanism of cyclosporine transport, a change in distribution and binding of cyclosporine and metabolites, or a resolution in the enteropathy accompanying chronic renal disease.

Cyclosporine is transported in the blood mainly by red cells and plasma proteins, and less than 5% of cyclosporine remains free. Partitioning between red cells and plasma is inversely related to hematocrit. In plasma, cyclosporine is primarily bound to lipoproteins. It has been postulated that low-density lipoprotein (LDL) serves as a carrier for cyclosporine, facilitating delivery to the immunocompetent cell and transport to metabolic sites via the LDL-receptor pathway. Cyclosporine distributes readily across most biologic membranes but does not readily cross the blood–brain barrier, and drug concentrations are low in the cerebrospinal fluid, brain, and spinal cord. Placental transfer of cyclosporine is low in humans, but significant concentrations of cyclosporine accumulate in breast milk. To protect the developing neonatal immune system, breastfeeding is contraindicated in transplant recipients.

Metabolism of cyclosporine occurs predominantly in the liver and bowel, under the influence of the cytochrome P450 III gene family. More than 25 metabolites have now been documented in human blood, bile, and urine. A coding system has been developed for metabolite designation based on the molecular position of metabolic biotransformation. The first oxidation products of cyclosporine are the primary metabolites M1, M9, and M4N. Further oxidation of these compounds then produces a second group of metabolites such as M19, M49, or M4N9. All metabolites are considered less immunosuppressive than unchanged cyclosporine.

There is considerable interindividual variation in the bioavailability of cyclosporine (i.e, 1% to 67%, with an average of 30%). Drug clearance rates vary from 2 to 32 ml/min/kg; and the average time to peak blood concentration after oral administration is from 1 to 8 hours, with a mean of 3.8 hours. The drug has a half-life that varies from 4 to 34 hours. Clinical data suggesting that approximately three-fourths of interpatient variability of cyclosporine can be attributed to variation in liver CYP3A4 activity and variation in expression of P-glycoprotein in small bowel enterocytes.

Cyclosporine elimination is increased approximately 40% in children and is slower in older patients. Females appear to clear cyclosporine more slowly than males, reflecting partly the accumulation of drug in body fat. Obese patients show higher blood levels than nonobese subjects when cyclosporine is administered according to actual body weight, but not when the administered dose is adjusted for ideal body weight. Cyclosporine is eliminated primarily by biliary excretion, with a median of 6 to 8 hours. Clearance of cyclosporine is significantly impaired in patients with liver disease, and elimination time may be prolonged 4-fold or more. Longer dosing intervals or substantial reduction in dosage are therefore necessary in the presence of hepatic dysfunction. By contrast, renal excretion represents a minor pathway of elimination, accounting for approximately 6% of total body clearance in humans, and renal failure does not alter cyclosporine clearance.

The microemulsion formulation of cyclosporine facilitates inception of oral therapy in *de novo* renal transplant recipients, although patients generally show poor absorption of Neoral for the first 2 days postoperatively. Thereafter they show rapid recovery and therapeutic drug levels after day 3. The rapid postoperative recovery of drug absorption represents the first advantage of the new microemulsion formulation. Furthermore, therapeutic drug levels are achieved more quickly after Neoral administration for recipients with limited absorption of Sandimmune formulation. Greater drug exposure with Neoral is likely to reduce incidence of rejection, a second advantage of the new formulation. The third advantage of Neoral over the Sandimmune formulation is the reduced variation observed in a crossover study of stable renal transplant recipients who received both formulations. Serial pharmacokinetic profiles between 90 days and 5 years after transplantation showed a correlation between the occurrence of chronic rejection episodes and a highly variable drug exposure. Thus a fourth potential benefit of Neoral may be that because of the reduced variation in drug exposure, therapy with this new formulation will reduce the occurrence of chronic allograft rejection.

Drug Interactions

A broad range of drugs, including anticonvulsants, antibiotics, antimycotics, calcium channel blockers, adrenal steroids, and other medications interfere with the metabolism of cyclosporine. Interaction may occur at the levels of drug absorption, disposition, metabolism, or elimination and may increase or decrease cyclosporine concentration (Table 88.7). Phenytoin produces a rapid decline in blood cyclosporine concentration, which can persist for several weeks after the drug is discontinued. Phenobarbital and carbamazepine exert similar but smaller dose-related effects. All three drugs are potent inducers of the cytochrome P450 enzyme system in the gut and liver. Interaction increases presystemic metabolism of cyclosporine thus reducing bioavailability, and accelerates hepatic metabolism, which increases systemic clearance. Valporic acid exhibits no clinically important interaction and may be substituted in this situation.

Rifampicin is a known inducer of microsomal enzymes and causes a pharmacokinetic interaction similar to that of phenytoin. A variety of other agents including nafcillin, isoniazid, and sulphonamide-trimethoprim have been reported to decrease cyclosporine concentrations *in vivo*. Erythromycin is perhaps one

TABLE 88.7. Drug Interactions with Cyclosporine

Decreased Blood Level Resulting from Increased Hepatic and/or Gastrointestinal Metabolism
Phenytoin
Phenobarbital
Carbamazepine
Isoniazid
Rifampicin
Nafcillin
Trimethoprim-sulfamethoxazole?
Increased Blood Levels Resulting from Decreased Hepatic and/or Gastrointestinal metabolism
Ketoconazole
Erythromycin
Clarithromycin
Diltiazem[a]
Verapamil[a]
Nicardipine[a]
Glucocorticoids (high dose-intravenous)
Grapefruit juice (naringin)
Metoclopramide
Fluvoxamine
Nefazodone
Acetazolamide?
Fluoroquinolones?
Increased Renal Toxicity (No Change in Metabolism)
Amphotericin B
Melphalan
Aminoglycosides
Trimethoprim-sulfamethoxazole
Nonsteroidal antiinflammatory agents
Radiocontrast agents

[a] Although blood levels of cyclosporine may increase, nephrotoxicity may not occur because these agents protect the kidney.

of the most potent and well-recognized antibiotics interacting with cyclosporine, and causes a twofold to fivefold increase in cyclosporine levels. Although clarithromycin, one of the newer macrolide antibiotics, has the same inhibitory effect on the CYP3A activity, azithromycin does not have a significant interaction with cyclosporine metabolism. The antifungal agent, ketoconazole, is another potent inhibitor of cyclosporine metabolism, often producing acute nephrotoxicity caused by a rapid rise in cyclosporine levels. The mechanism of interaction is related to concentration-dependent inhibition of microsomal enzyme activity demonstrated both *in vitro* and *in vivo*.

The influence of calcium channel blockers is particularly important in view of prevalent use of these agents in the management of posttransplant cardiovascular disease and hypertension. The combination of cyclosporine with the calcium channel blocker, diltiazem, has proved to be beneficial in reducing the incidence of nephrotoxicity and graft rejection. Diltiazem is a competitive inhibitor of cyclosporine metabolism in the liver. Pharmacokinetic studies have shown that the increased bioavailability of cyclosporine, when combined with diltiazem, could better be explained by the inhibition of GI CYP enzymes than by the inhibition of its hepatic metabolism. CYP enzymes are 25% more active in the liver and 200% more active in the small intestine of females than of males. The higher intestinal CYP activity explains the gender-specific modifications of cyclosporine pharmacokinetics after coadministration of the CYP enzymes inhibitor. Enzyme inhibition is dose dependent and starts with dosages of diltiazem as low as 10 mg/day. A lesser effect has been reported with verapamil and nicardipine, whereas nifedipine or nitrendipine have no significant influence. The effects of newer calcium channel blockers, such as amlodipine, have not been well studied. Clinical consequences of this drug interaction are mitigated by the protective effects of calcium channel blocker on the renal microvasculature, so that renal blood flow and glomerular filtration remain unchanged or even increase despite a rise in cyclosporine levels.

The newer antidepressants, including fluvoxamine and nefazodone, could increase the cyclosporine level by inhibiting cytochrome P450 isoenzymes. Drug interactions also occur with other agents including acetazolamide, alcohol, colchicine, fluoroquinolones, and nonsteroidal antiinflammatory agents, but these are clinically less important and not well established. Administration of high-dose intravenous methylprednisone (more than 3 mg/kg per day) may slightly increase cyclosporine trough levels. Grapefruit juice contains naringin, the flavonoid that gives grapefruit its distinctive taste and is thought to be responsible for inhibiting cyclosporine metabolism. Some agents may augment renal toxicity of cyclosporine without influencing its metabolism; these include amphotericin B, aminoglycosides, trimethoprim-sulfamethoxazole, nonsteroidal antiinflammatory agents, and radiocontrast agents.

Clinical Transplantation

Cyclosporine has been a major advance in renal transplantation. It has reduced the frequency and severity of acute graft rejection, improved the immediate and-long term clinical outcome of transplantation, liberalized recipient selection criteria, and decreased the stringency of histocompatibility matching required. Furthermore, it has reduced hospitalization time and procedural costs, enabling patients to be discharged earlier following surgery. Finally, the use of cyclosporine has improved the expectation of health and the opportunity for rehabilitation following renal transplantation. As a result, kidney transplantation is now the treatment of choice for most patients with end-stage renal failure, particularly children and young adults. Over the last 20 years, cyclosporine has been used clinically in a variety of combinations that differ according to each institution's protocol, clinical course, and time following transplantation.

Cyclosporine has been used alone or in combination with other immunosuppressive drugs, including prednisone, azathioprine, or mycophenolate, and in combination with sirolimus in clinical trials. The optimal combination remains uncertain, and introduction of newer and more potent drugs with different mechanisms of action expands the possibility of different combinations. Monotherapy is the least common protocol, used almost exclusively in certain European centers. In this protocol, cyclosporine is commenced at a dose of 10 to 12 mg/kg per day.

In an Italian multicenter trial, 354 recipients of cadaveric renal transplant were randomized to receive cyclosporine alone versus double or triple therapy. Hyperimmunized patients [panel reactive antibody (PRA) more than 50%] and patients with acute rejection or oliguria within the fifth posttransplant day were excluded from the study. Patients on cyclosporine alone received higher doses compared with the other group. Although there was significantly more acute rejection in patients receiving cyclosporine alone than in other groups, the 4-year graft and patient survival were not significantly different among the three groups. The mean creatinine clearance was slightly lower in the cyclosporine-alone group. Acute rejection was the most frequent reason for adding steroids in patients on monotherapy, and only about half could be maintained on cyclosporine alone. Monotherapy in patients with no acute rejection provided excellent results without side effects related to steroid therapy.

Dual- or triple-therapy regimens with prednisone and either azathioprine or mycophenolate are more widely employed, forming the basis for treatment in more than half the centers currently performing renal transplantation. In this protocol, cyclosporine is commenced at 8 to 10 mg/kg per day. Sequential therapy in which cyclosporine administration is delayed by using a short introductory course of antilymphocytic globulin or monoclonal antibody is used predominantly in North America during the early postoperative phase following renal transplantation, when absorption of cyclosporine is unpredictable. This approach, although not unequivocally superior, might reduce the risk of inadequate immunosuppression at a critical time when rejection is most likely, and this also avoids the toxic effect of cyclosporine on the newly transplanted organ. The dose of cyclosporine is gradually reduced during the first few months after transplantation as immunologic adaptation occurs in both host and graft.

Acute graft rejection occurs in approximately 45% of patients receiving cyclosporine immunosuppression. Combination of cyclosporine with mycophenolate has been able to decrease the rejection rate close to 20%. Acute rejection usually indicates that the total immunosuppression is inadequate, and the dose of cyclosporine needs to be increased to achieve a blood level at the higher limit of target range.

Neoral has improved the ability to achieve and maintain desired blood levels. Cyclosporine levels will now be more predictable from each dose, facilitating titration of levels into the desired target range. Initial clinical trials comparing Neoral with Sandimmune show improved pharmacokinetics with faster absorption, increased C_{max}, and increased area under the concentration-time curve (AUC). In addition, Neoral reduced interpatient and intrapatient variability in the pharmacokinetic parameters. This has made the relationship between dose, trough level, and AUC directly proportional for Neoral. An analysis of 2-year, double-blind data from two groups of *de novo* renal transplant recipients confirmed the safety and the tolerability of Neoral compared with Sandimmune. Conversion from Sandimmune to Neoral in stable renal transplant recipients has also been shown to be safe and tolerable. Headache, dyspepsia, and vomiting were seen more frequently after conversion, and diminished with dose reduction.

In a study of 302 patients with stable renal allografts, the 1:1 conversion from Sandimmune to Neoral was accompanied by substantial dose reduction of 16% after the 6-month observation period. In another study, 345 patients were switched from cyclosporine to Neoral, and 35% of patients showed a rising serum creatinine level, which was improved on dose reduction. Patients on higher doses (more than 300 mg/day) of Sandimmune required much closer monitoring than those on lower doses. The accumulated data from a broad range of pharmacokinetic studies of Neoral indicate that it offers substantially improved consistency of oral absorption compared with Sandimmune, with modest increase in oral bioavailability, and its use may improve the clinical value of trough blood concentration monitoring. Other studies found not only that higher cyclosporine AUC is predictive of lower risk for rejection, but also that lower AUC is predictive of increased incidence of acute rejection, and Neoral with higher and more reliable bioavailability might improve efficacy as well. Converting patients from Sandimmune to Neoral is accomplished by giving the same dose the patient is taking to produce therapeutic cyclosporine blood levels. It is recommended that before conversion to Neoral, cyclosporine trough level, serum creatinine, and blood pressure be measured, then repeated 4 to 7 days after conversion.

Because of concern about potential for progressive renal injury as well as the cost of drug and the high incidence of undesirable side effects, cyclosporine withdrawal has been attempted by many groups in different trials after renal transplantation. The results of cyclosporine withdrawal studies are controversial and proved to be either beneficial, deleterious, or equivocal. The timing of withdrawal is variable in different studies, ranging from 3 months up to 2 years. In a large trial, the Collaborative Transplant Study, patients who discontinued cyclosporine during the first year after transplantation had a 5-year graft survival rate that was 11% lower than that of patients who continued treatment with cyclosporine. In the 10-year follow-up results of an Italian, multicenter, controlled trial on 108 recipients of cadaveric renal transplantation, although the patient survival rate was the same between the cyclosporine group and the azathioprine group (89% versus 83%), graft survival was significantly better in the cyclosporine group (56% versus 35%). In a meta-analysis of randomized and nonrandomized studies of early cyclosporine withdrawal, no difference was found in short-term graft survival between patients discontinuing cyclosporine and those remaining on cyclosporine; however, the risk of acute rejection was statistically significant in the cyclosporine-withdrawal group. Because of the potential for late immune-mediated graft loss, cyclosporine withdrawal does not seem to be appropriate in stable renal transplant patients also receiving azathioprine and prednisone. Most patients should be maintained on a cyclosporine dose of 3 to 5 mg/kg per day.

Monitoring of Immunosuppression

Pharmacokinetic monitoring of immunosuppressive treatment is an important therapeutic asset. It provides an accurate assessment of the absorption, distribution, and metabolism of cyclosporine. Routine trough level monitoring of whole blood is required for effective clinical management of patients prescribed cyclosporine. Very low, very high, or variable trough blood levels of cyclosporine are associated with reduced long-term graft survival. Three factors may explain the imperfect correlation between trough level and clinical events: variable pharmacodynamic effects at given drug concentrations; failure to obtain properly timed trough level blood samples, which results in modest but not insubstantial differences between measured concentration and the true trough level; and a poor correlation between the single time point trough level and the actual drug exposure. High-performance liquid chromatography (HPLC), although regarded as the prototype-specific assay, is a manual technique with compromised applicability. Cyclosporine monitoring has been facilitated in the clinical setting with the introduction of various monoclonal immunoassay methods: radioimmunoassay (RIA); fluorescence polarization immunoassay (FPIA), and enzyme immunoassay (EMIT), which has the potential for application to various automated analyzers. FPIA offers advantages of simplicity, rapidity, and technical accuracy with minimal technologic expertise. In pregnancy, several physiologic changes occur that could alter the pharmacokinetics of drugs. Cyclosporine whole-blood levels tend to decline during pregnancy from prepregnancy levels in the majority of patients receiving the same dose. Correlation analysis between individual timed samples and AUC determinations revealed that Neoral requires significantly less frequent blood monitoring for prediction of total drug exposure than does Sandimmune.

Therapeutic monitoring is useful for interpretation of acute events, but is less helpful in distinguishing the cause of chronic organ dysfunction. Trough levels of cyclosporine in whole blood are normally maintained at 200 to 400 ng/ml in the first 3 months after transplantation. Graft rejection occurs predominantly with trough cyclosporine concentrations below 200 ng/ml, whereas renal toxicity occurs with cyclosporine levels maintained above this range. Aggressive reduction in cyclosporine dosage after the first 3 months progressively narrows the therapeutic operating range of whole blood to 100 to 150 ng/ml. This, coupled with decrease in severity of late rejection or renal toxicity, and lack of precision in distinguishing between the two, limits the specificity, sensitivity, and predictive value of simple trough level monitoring. Pharmacokinetic monitoring of the area under the time/activity curve at steady state provides a more accurate index of the biologic effect of cyclosporine, and limited sampling strategies have been developed to facilitate this approach.

Side Effects

The side effects of cyclosporine involve almost all organ systems and in general reflect the dose and duration of treatment. Cyclosporine has little effect on bone marrow, although a mild anemia is seen in most patients receiving the drug, and may reflect inhibition of IL-3 or erythropoietin production. At normal therapeutic concentrations, cyclosporine causes no change in leukocyte or platelet numbers or function.

Hypertrichosis and trichomegaly have been documented in the literature; these conditions appear in 10% to 50% of patients receiving cyclosporine. The hair growth–stimulating effect of cyclosporine is observed in both normal and pathologic conditions of hair growth, such as alopecia areata. Blood concentrations of sex hormones and sex hormone–binding globulin are generally normal. Available evidence suggests cyclosporine induces resting follicles to enter an active growth phase, but the exact mechanism of the hair growth–stimulating effect of cyclosporine is unknown. Gingival hyperplasia occurs in approximately 21% to 35% of renal transplant patients and may be related to increased metabolism of testosterone within the affected tissue. The effect of cyclosporine on calcium homeostasis might also reducing the collagenolytic activity of the fibroblasts. Penicillin, metronidazole, and azithromycin appear to be useful in the treatment of cyclosporine-induced gingival hyperplasia. Effectiveness of these antibiotics has led to the belief that overgrowth of anaerobic bacteria might be one of the causes of gingival hyperplasia. Other drugs, such as phenytoin, nifedipine, and diltiazem, may accentuate the effect of cyclosporine. Both hypertrichosis and gum hypertrophy gradually resolve within a few months after withdrawal of the drug.

Avascular bone necrosis, previously a frequent and crippling complication attributed to the use of glucocorticoid, now occurs in less than 2% of renal transplant recipients treated with cyclosporine. Cyclosporine does not retard bone growth but has an important effect on skeletal remodeling, causing osteoporosis with a loss of trabecular volume. Patients receiving cyclosporine often demonstrate a high-turnover osteoporotic state when bone histologic examination is performed. This may contribute to the bone loss following renal and, more particularly, nonrenal transplantation.

Peripheral tremor and hyperesthesia of the hands and face occur following initiation of cyclosporine treatment and are usually transient and dose related. Headache is common and may be severe, persistent, or recurrent but often responds to treatment with propranolol. Subtle organic mental disorders may present as anxiety, lethargy, memory loss, insomnia, and sleep-wake reversal. Although seizures, drowsiness, confusion, hallucinations, visual disturbances, and mental changes have also been reported, most neurologic sequelae resolve following a reduction in dose or discontinuation of cyclosporine.

Cyclosporine can cause increased incidence of thromboembolic complications. The pathogenesis of hemostatic disturbances and thrombotic complications in kidney transplant recipients treated with cyclosporine, despite many years of research, is not fully understood. Kidney transplant recipients who are receiving cyclosporine show decreased fibrinolytic activity, hyperfibrinogenemia, and elevated levels of von Willebrand's factor (vWF) and lipoprotein-a (Lpa), indicative of a prothrombotic state. An increased level of vWF may be a marker of chronic vascular endothelial injury and may have important implications when there is preexisting vascular disease, such as diabetes mellitus or atherosclerosis.

Hypertension occurs in 70% to 90% of recipients on cyclosporine. Hypertension is often associated with elevated blood cyclosporine levels or impaired renal allograft function resulting from cyclosporine nephrotoxicity. Suppression of plasma renin and aldosterone activity occurs, and tubular insensitivity to aldosterone inhibits potassium excretion. Posttransplant hypertension in patients receiving cyclosporine is frequently severe and resistant to therapy. Angiotensin-converting enzyme (ACE) inhibitors are of limited efficacy and may exacerbate the hyperkalemia. Calcium channel inhibitors are more effective and simultaneously minimize cyclosporine nephrotoxicity. β-Blockers and other direct vasodilators are often used in a formal stepped-care approach, if required.

Cyclosporine is directly hepatotoxic, although liver toxicity is normally mild and dose related. Acute hepatotoxicity occurs in up to 20% of patients within the first 2 months after renal transplantation and is characterized by a mild, transient increase in serum bilirubin levels and a disproportionate rise in ALT:AST ratio. Chronic hepatotoxicity occurs later in the graft course and may be associated with an increased incidence of cholelithiasis.

Despite the beneficial impact of the widespread use of cyclosporine on graft survival, nephrotoxicity is one of the major side effects that seem related to the vascular toxicity of cyclosporine. The precise mechanism underlying cyclosporine nephrotoxicity remains unclear. Morphologic and functional studies in animals and humans have suggested that increased arteriolar resistance with a predominant afferent arteriolar vasoconstriction is the major mechanism accounting for the acute reduction in glomerular filtration rate (GFR) when cyclosporine is given. Vasoconstriction might be a result of a local effect of cyclosporine on renal blood vessels or of a systemic effect of cyclosporine A on circulating and neural factors. It has been suggested that vasoactive humoral substances, including angiotensin II, prostaglandin, endothelin, and adenosine, mediate the renal vascular effects of cyclosporine, but the role of these substances is uncertain. Cyclosporine-induced renal vasoconstriction impairs the capacity of the glomeruli to respond with afferent arteriolar dilation. The mechanism underlying normal renal functional reserve could be mediated by prostaglandins. Cyclosporine could impair this response either specifically by its cyclooxygenase inhibitor effect or nonspecifically by its influence on the afferent arteriolar tone.

Acute cyclosporine nephrotoxicity, which occurs in more than 30% of patients within the first 6 months after renal transplantation, has three forms: delayed initial graft function, thought to be caused by the propensity of cyclosporine for exacerbating renal ischemic injury; acute reversible impaired graft function, which improves with cyclosporine dose reduction; and less commonly, an acute arteriopathy, usually affecting the afferent arterioles, which may be associated with thrombotic microangiopathy, characterized by thrombocytopenia, red cell fragmentation, hyperbilirubinemia, and acute graft failure. Acute microangiopathic vasculopathy often resolves following temporary withdrawal of cyclosporine, although plasma exchange with fresh-frozen plasma may be required in cases with systemic involvement. The hallmark of chronic cyclosporine nephropathy is based on the demonstration of vascular lesions in the afferent arteriole. These vascular lesions are not necessarily dose related and in some patients can be observed with doses as low as 2 to 4 mg/kg. Chronic cyclosporine nephrotoxicity is characterized by tubulointerstitial fibrosis in a striped pattern, and degenerative hyaline changes in the walls of afferent arteriolar-size blood vessels. These findings usually are associated with some degree of renal dysfunction. It is possible that cyclosporine-induced injury may play a role in chronic allograft failure that is caused predominantly by chronic rejection.

Chronic cyclosporine nephropathy may be more common in the native kidney, and progression to dialysis is reported in up to 5% of heart and liver transplant recipients. Although it has been suggested that renal denervation protects the transplanted kidney, recent studies have shown that renal denervation does not protect against chronic cyclosporine nephropathy. Despite many years of cyclosporine-based immunosuppression in renal transplant recipients, the long-term renal safety of this compound has not been documented in a prospective study.

Abnormalities in lipoproteins are common after renal transplantation, in part because of the effects of cyclosporine. Moreover, lipid abnormalities have been reported to correlate with both cardiovascular disease (CVD) and chronic rejection. In the absence of large multicenter primary or secondary intervention trials, there is no proof that lipid abnormalities cause CVD in renal transplant patients. However, it is reasonable to assume that the beneficial effects of antilipemic therapy on CVD found in the general population may be applicable to renal transplant recipients. Cyclosporine-treated patients may have an increased risk of side effects (myopathy) if their hyperlipidemia is managed with 3-hydroxy-3-methyl-glutaryl-coenzyme A (HMG-CoA)–reductase inhibitors.

Several groups have reported that hyperuricemia is a common metabolic consequence of cyclosporine therapy, occurring in 55% to 80% of renal transplant patients. Despite this high prevalence of hyperuricemia, gouty arthritis occurs in only 4% to 28% of these patients. The pathophysiology of hyperuricemia is multifactorial. Renal insufficiency causes the renal retention of urate by modifying several steps in urate excretion, including impairment of renal handling of urate as a result of a tubular abnormality and the use of diuretics. Colchicine is effective in the treatment of acute episodes of arthritis, but its long-term use is limited by GI or bone marrow toxicity. There are several reports about the myotoxic potential of colchicine. Renal insufficiency, which favors the accumulation of colchicine during the treatment of gout, increases the risk of myopathy. The combination of cyclosporine and colchicine has been shown to potentiate myopathy. Muscular symptoms improve after colchicine withdrawal.

TACROLIMUS (FK506)

Tacrolimus is one of the relatively new agents approved for use in the prevention of graft rejection in kidney transplantation. It is a macrolide antibiotic derived from *Streptomyces tsukubaensis.* Tacrolimus is a potent immunosuppressive medication and has been tested both *in vitro* and *in vivo* in several multicenter clinical trials in the United States, Europe, and Japan.

Mechanism of Action

The mode of action of tacrolimus is very similar to that of cyclosporine and binds to an immunophilin, FK-binding protein (FKBP) in the cytoplasm. There are many different intracellular FKBPs, but tacrolimus binds to FKBP-12, and this complex then interacts with a calcium-calmodulin–dependent phosphatase called *calcineurin.* The tacrolimus/FKBP complex, once bound to calcineurin, prevents activation of the enhanced region and hence its transcription. Calcineurin has two subunits, the catalytic calcineurin A and the regulatory calcineurin B, which must bind the calcium-calmodulin complex to be functional after T-cell activation. Like cyclosporine, the interaction of tacrolimus-immunophilin complex with calcineurin is the crucial step in suppressing the transduction of the T-cell–receptor signal. Because the immunophilins and calcineurin appear to be broadly distributed in diverse cells and tissues, the effects of tacrolimus and cyclosporine in various tissues depend on the relative cell concentrations of these substances immunophilins and calcineurin. A high calcineurin/immunophilin ratio may reduce the sensitivity to these types of immunosuppressants. In this manner, tacrolimus inhibits the secretion of a number of cytokines by activated T cells, including IL-2, -3, -4, -5, and -7, IFN-γ, TNF-α, granulocyte-macrophage colony–stimulating factor (GM-CSF), and CD40 ligand. It also inhibits generation of cytotoxic T cells and T-cell–dependent B-cell activation.

Tacrolimus has no effect on IL-10 transcription, CD28, or the protein kinase pathway of T-cell activation. It also modulates cyclic AMP (cAMP)–dependent signaling and decreases activities of cAMP-responsive element binding protein. These actions could modulate immunosuppressive properties of the drugs and may be involved in diabetogenic and nephrotoxic effects. In experimental studies of renal allografts in rat, dog, and baboon, tacrolimus has been shown to be very effective in suppressing rejection at doses 10 to 100 times less than that of cyclosporine, resulting in prolonged survival.

Tacrolimus may differ from cyclosporine with regard to the effects on TGF-β. Whereas cyclosporine increases the synthesis of TGF-β in various cells, including T lymphocytes and endothelial and renal cells, tacrolimus may selectively block the function of the TGF-β receptors. TGF-β acts as an immunosuppressant and thus inhibits cell proliferation. However, a sustained elevation of TGF-β may stimulate smooth muscle proliferation and activate the endothelin gene, which may contribute to fibrinogenesis and development of chronic allograft rejection.

Pharmacokinetics and Dosage

The size and the physicochemical properties of the tacrolimus molecule are responsible for its limited absorption from the GI tract and mean bioavailability of approximately 20%, although there is a large variability in the absorption rate with a range of 4% to 89%. In most patients, maximum plasma or blood concentrations are reached after about 1 hour. In contrast to cyclosporine, bile flow is not an essential prerequisite for the absorption of tacrolimus. Both the rate and extent of absorption of tacrolimus are reduced when given with food. It is therefore advisable to administer tacrolimus at least 1 hour before or 2 hours after a meal. Once tacrolimus is absorbed, it is disproportionately distributed between red blood cells and plasma. In plasma, tacrolimus binds strongly to serum albumin and α1-acid glycoprotein.

Dose-finding studies in kidney graft recipients have shown good correlation between tacrolimus dose and resulting trough blood levels [enzyme-linked immunosorbent assay (ELISA) method]. This suggests that trough concentration of tacrolimus is a good indicator of systemic exposure and may be used for therapeutic drug monitoring.

Tacrolimus undergoes hepatic metabolism and biliary excretion of the mother compound and its metabolites. Only approximately 5% of the drug is eliminated through the kidney. The main metabolic pathway of tacrolimus involves demethylation and hydroxylation. The enzyme system involved is the hepatic cytochrome P450 3A4. Metabolites retain some immunosuppressive activity, but only small amounts can be detected in the blood, which may increase in case of severe hepatic dysfunction, wherein dose adjustment may be necessary.

In the concentration-ranging trial of tacrolimus, the occurrence of toxicity increased significantly with increasing whole blood level. Conversely, the likelihood of rejection decreased significantly with increased whole blood level. The target range of whole blood levels of 5 to 15 ng/ml was associated with optimal efficacy and minimal toxicity. The recommended initial dose of tacrolimus to reach target level is 0.2 mg/kg per day in two divided doses. In general, oral doses of tacrolimus need to be three to four times greater than the intravenous doses to achieve comparable drug exposure. African-American patients may require higher dosages of tacrolimus than white or Asian patients. In a U.S. multicenter trial, African-American patients required a 37% mean higher dose of tacrolimus than white patients to achieve comparable blood concentrations. Clearance of tacrolimus appears to be higher in children than in adults; therefore children require higher milligram-per-kilogram doses of the drug.

Monitoring Immunosuppression

Therapeutic drug monitoring is essential for dosing to obtain an optimal risk-benefit ratio. Although measuring AUC is a more reliable parameter for the pharmacologic effectiveness of drugs, trough levels in whole blood and plasma have been used in different centers to monitor tacrolimus. Whole blood is the preferred medium because of 10 to 30 times higher concentrations of tacrolimus in red blood cells.

Several assays are available for quantifying tacrolimus levels in blood and plasma. ELISA is a nonspecific assay, because the polyclonal antibody employed cross-reacts with tacrolimus metabolites. This method has a limit of quantification in plasma of 100 ng/L and a higher limit of approximately 1 μg/L in blood. The semiautomated microparticle enzyme immunoassay (MEIA) has also been used for monitoring tacrolimus in whole blood only. This method is also nonspecific, and its limit of quantification is currently 5 μg/L. High-pressure liquid chromatography coupled with mass spectrometry (HPLC-MS) is the most accurate, sensitive, and specific assay for determining tacrolimus concentrations in blood and has a limit of quantification of 0.2 μg/L. This method can separately quantify the parent compound and its metabolites.

The Pro-Trac ELISA is a new, commercially available immunoassay for therapeutic drug monitoring of tacrolimus. The limits of detection by this assay is stated to be 0.5 μg/L and the results generated by this method were comparable with those obtained using MEIA or HPLC-MS. Therefore this assay seems to be a useful alternative for tacrolimus blood level measurement.

Therapeutic target ranges for tacrolimus have not been clearly defined. Levels of 20 ng/ml or more are frequently associated with toxicity, and therapeutic target ranges of 10 to 25 ng/ml in early clinical trials were probably excessive. The lower limit required to prevent organ rejection is unknown. Most U.S. centers have adopted a therapeutic range of 5 to 15 ng/ml for liver transplant patients. The therapeutic range for kidney transplant patients is most likely somewhat higher, requiring trough levels of 10 to 20 ng/ml to reduce the risk of organ rejection while minimizing the risk of toxicity.

Drug Interactions

Tacrolimus is metabolized mainly by the cytochrome P450 3A4 enzyme system; thus as with cyclosporine, potential drug interactions are numerous with tacrolimus. Although few drug interaction studies have been performed with tacrolimus, coadministration of drugs that inhibit or induce the enzyme may influence the metabolism of tacrolimus. Drugs that potentially interact with the tacrolimus metabolism are mainly the same as those interacting with cyclosporine (Table 88.7).

There is also potential for additional impairment of renal function when tacrolimus is coadministered with compounds such as the amino glycosides, and similarly, neurotoxicity may be enhanced with drugs such as ganciclovir.

A pharmacokinetics study performed on 18 stable renal transplant patients receiving tacrolimus and mycophenolate showed minimal effect of mycophenolate on tacrolimus pharmacokinetics. However, patients receiving mycophenolate displayed significantly higher levels (AUC) of mycophenolic acid than those receiving cyclosporine, suggesting specific inhibition of the conversion of mycophenolic acid to mycophenolic acid-glucuronide (MPAG) in tacrolimus-treated patients. These studies in renal transplant patients suggest that tacrolimus in combination with mycophenolate result in a greater degree of immunosuppression than may be anticipated.

Clinical Transplantation

Tacrolimus is an established immunosuppressive agent for primary and rescue therapy in renal transplant recipients. As a primary immunosuppressive drug, tacrolimus is more effective than cyclosporine (Sandimmune), but it has yet to be shown that it is more potent than the microemulsion cyclosporine (Neoral) and that it decreases the rate of chronic rejection. The 1-year actuarial graft survival of more than 90% has been reported in most of the studies. In a U.S. multicenter trial, although there were no graft and patient survival differences between the two groups, rejection was less frequent and histopathologically less severe in tacrolimus-treated patients compared with the cyclosporine-treated group.

Combinations of tacrolimus with mycophenolate as maintenance immunosuppressive therapy has been reported in both retrospective and prospective trials. In a report dealing with the experience with tacrolimus and mycophenolate without induction therapy in cadaveric renal transplant recipients, acute rejection was observed in 26% of the triple-therapy group and in 42% of tacrolimus and corticosteroid group. The rejection rate has been even lower when antibody-induction therapy was added to the protocol. In a retrospective study, the incidence of biopsy-proven acute rejection within the first 6 months after transplant was 8% in triple-therapy patients and 21% in the double-therapy group. The markedly lower incidence of acute rejection in tacrolimus-mycophenolate-glucocorticoid patients is attributed to the synergistic effect of these two potent immunosuppressive drugs and antibody-induction therapy.

Despite improvement in the cyclosporine era, renal allograft survival in African-Americans remains inferior compared with white recipients. Tacrolimus in combination with mycophenolate was found to be highly effective in preventing rejection episodes in African-American recipients of cadaveric renal allografts. In a small series, this combination could decrease the rejection rate to 17% compared with 62% rejection rate with cyclosporine-azathioprine. A larger series with longer follow-up will be needed to confirm this superior outcome.

Tacrolimus showed no significant teratogenic activity in the chromosomal aberration test and successful pregnancies with minimal complications have been reported in both kidney and kidney–pancreas transplant patients receiving tacrolimus.

Patients with kidney disease demonstrate substantial health-related quality of life (QOL) improvement after transplantation. Compared with cyclosporine, patients on tacrolimus have better QOL improvement by having less rejection and fewer physical-appearance side effects, including facial hirsutism and gingival hyperplasia.

Tacrolimus has been used as a primary immunosuppressive agent in a variety of clinical settings, from a small single-center trial to large, prospective, multicenter trials. Protocols for tacrolimus as primary immunosuppression or as rescue therapy varied depending on the type of graft, and many included glucocorticoids with and without azathioprine and, less frequently, an antilymphocyte agent. The conventional formulation of cyclosporine has been used in all the comparison trials.

Early trials in renal transplantation from Pittsburgh involving 240 recipients of cadaver kidneys demonstrated 1-year graft survival of 74%, with an acute rejection episode rate of close to 50%. Compared with the cyclosporine group there were no differences in graft survival, although the rejection rate and need for antibody therapy were lower in the tacrolimus-treated group. Steroids were reduced rapidly and discontinued in 44% of the patients during the first year. In the Japanese clinical trials, double therapy with tacrolimus and steroids in 104 patients demonstrated a 95% 3-year graft survival in living-related donor transplants and 80% in cadaver kidney transplants, with 35% incidence of reversible acute rejection.

A prospective trial of tacrolimus and steroids versus tacrolimus-azathioprine-prednisone in 397 recipients of renal allografts demonstrated 1-year actuarial graft survival rates of 90% and 88% and rejection episodes rates of 55% and 45%, respectively. Although there were fewer rejection episodes in the triple-therapy group, the difference was not statistically significant. The longer follow-up of this study demonstrated an overall 3-year graft survival rate of 80%. Overall, 69% of patients who had functioning grafts were taken off prednisone therapy; additionally, in 38% of patients antihypertensive agents were discontinued. The incidence of infection and new-onset diabetes was equal in both groups. In two large, prospective, randomized, multicenter trials conducted in Europe and the United States, the 2-year patient and graft survival rates were 94% and 84% for the tacrolimus-treated group and 95% and 85% for cyclosporine-treated group, respectively. All patients in the U.S. study also received an antilymphocyte antibody agent. The overall 1-year actuarial rate of acute rejection episodes was 28% for tacrolimus and 46% for cyclosporine. Fewer tacrolimus than cyclosporine recipients experienced moderate or severe acute rejection episodes and required antilymphocyte therapy.

Chronic rejection rates did not differ significantly between tacrolimus and cyclosporine recipients in the European group. More patients receiving cyclosporine than those receiving tacrolimus needed to be switched to alternative treatment. However, the higher number of patients were switched from cyclosporine to tacrolimus therapy rather than vice versa as a result of rejection as a complicating factor in comparative randomized trials. Several studies demonstrated that 70% to 85% of refractory acute rejection episodes in renal allograft recipients on a cyclosporine-based regimen could be salvaged by conversion to tacrolimus. This approach provides prompt and effective reversal of refractory rejection, good long-term allograft function, and balanced immunosuppression with respect to recurrent rejection. Although there was no correlation with allograft histology stratified by Banff criteria and the response to tacrolimus, recipients with more severe histologic rejection episodes and higher serum creatinine levels at the time of conversion showed a poorer response.

Higher rates of infectious complications have been observed in rescue trials; these were mainly related to a higher dose of tacrolimus. In a German study, 31 patients converted to tacrolimus from cyclosporine after biopsy-proven acute rejection that was refractory to pulse steroids. In this study, a lowered dose of tacrolimus (0.1 to 0.15 mg/kg per day) rather than that which had been previously used (0.3 mg/kg per day) with antiviral and antibacterial prophylaxis could reduce complications without impact on the success rate of rescue therapy.

The Pittsburgh group reported a 74% salvage rate with 30 months of follow-up in 169 patients with refractory rejection. The majority (85%) of patients had failed prior treatment with antilymphocyte preparations. The grafts with chronic rejection without any acute component did not benefit from tacrolimus conversion. The remarkable degree of similarity in the results of two independent U.S. trials provides convincing evidence that tacrolimus therapy is an attractive alternative to glucocorticoid and antilymphocyte antibody preparation in the treatment of refractory renal allograft rejection.

Side Effects

Early information concerning side effects associated with tacrolimus were obtained from experience with liver transplantation. The Japanese FK506 trial and the U.S. multicenter study have also contributed to our information. Major side effects are neurotoxicity, diabetogenicity, nephrotoxicity, and GI symptoms. Hyperkalemia, hypomagnesemia, and hyperuricemia have also been reported. Cardiac symptoms such as chest pain, palpitations, and abnormal ECG results have been reported in 18% of recipients.

The incidence of posttransplant diabetes mellitus (PTDM) has been shown in earlier trials to be significantly higher in tacrolimus-treated recipients than in cyclosporine-treated patients during the first year. The initial incidence ranged from 6% to 28% and the final incidence from 1.4% to 12.0%, with a reversibility of 37% to 83%. The U.S. multicenter trial showed a higher incidence of PTDM in African-American patients than in white recipients. The diabetogenicity of tacrolimus appears to be related to a reversible effect of the drug on islet cells. FKBP is present in islet cells, and decreased insulin gene transcription and secretion, possibly via interruption of the calcium-dependent signaling pathway, have been demonstrated experimentally.

The decrease of insulin secretion is reversible when tacrolimus therapy is discontinued. A direct correlation of PTDM with tacrolimus trough level and steroid dosage has been demonstrated. In a randomized, prospective trial of stable renal transplant recipients, conversion of immunosuppression from cyclosporine to maintenance-dose tacrolimus showed no new cases of diabetes. There were no differences in glycemic control, Hgb A1C level, or fasting blood glucose between tacrolimus-treated and cyclosporine-treated recipients.

Nephrotoxicity in kidney transplant recipients receiving tacrolimus is very similar to that seen in patients receiving cyclosporine posttransplant, ranging from 17% to 44% in different studies. Although the exact mechanism of tacrolimus nephrotoxicity is not well defined, in the rat model it has been shown that inactivation of calcineurin in renal tissue by tacrolimus will increase calcium influx into the cell through dihydropyridine-sensitive calcium channels. Because the main ionic carrier in vascular smooth muscle is calcium, the result in this tissue would be vasoconstriction.

An experimental model of tacrolimus nephrotoxicity in sodium-depleted rats has been developed that is characterized by reduced GFR and structural damage to the proximal tubule, accompanied by interstitial fibrosis. It appears that sodium depletion is critical for development of tacrolimus-induced progressive tubulointerstitial fibrosis, associated with macrophage influx and remarkable increase in plasma-renin activity. These animal data provide suggestive evidence for a renin-angiotensin system–dependent mechanism in chronic nephrotoxicity of tacrolimus.

The nephrotoxicity of tacrolimus has been divided into functional and structural categories. The morphologic findings, including mitochondrial changes, tubular microcalcification, and nonisometric foamy vacuolization of the straight and convoluting portions of proximal tubules. Vacuoles consisted of enlargement of endoplasmic reticulum and secondary lysosomes. More serious tacrolimus nephrotoxicity can cause arteriolar hyalinosis, degeneration of vascular smooth muscle cells, and diffuse interstitial fibrosis. Tacrolimus can also cause microvascular injury in human renal allografts. Glomerular capillary and arteriolar fibrin thrombi have been reported in 1% of the renal transplant recipients by the Pittsburgh group. Although hemolytic uremic syndrome has been reported in patients receiving tacrolimus, it has also been used in patients who developed hemolytic uremic syndrome during cyclosporine therapy without recurrence of the syndrome. Nephrotoxicity is usually associated with higher levels of tacrolimus and improves with dose reduction. In the Japanese multicenter trial of renal transplantation, nephrotoxicity was reported in 20% of the patients, and although there was a correlation between the drug level and nephrotoxicity, some patients' tacrolimus levels were normal.

Decreased renal blood flow initiates acute effects, usually within the first 7 days. Chronic effects may be evident as early as 30 days after initiation of treatment. Nephrotoxicity is characterized by increased serum creatinine levels, decreased GFR, and reduced renal blood flow. The renal tubular effect that occurs independent of decreased GFR results in impaired secretion of uric acid and reduced fractional excretion of sodium, potassium, lithium, and phosphate as well as hyperkalemia and diminished reabsorption of bicarbonate. Hyperuricemia has been reported in 15% and hyperkalemia in 25% to 67% of recipients. The mechanisms responsible for hyperkalemia are not well understood, but an effect of tacrolimus on mineralocorticoid secretion and activity on renal tubules have been proposed. Sodium-losing nephropathy has also been reported by the Japanese group. These sodium-losing states were spontaneously restored to normal values in a short period without any reduction of the tacrolimus dosage.

It is known that tacrolimus alters magnesium metabolism in animals and in patients with normal renal function following liver transplantation. In sodium-depleted rats treated with tacrolimus, the lower urinary osmolality and inappropriately high fractional excretion of magnesium suggest a tacrolimus-mediated physiologic defect in urinary concentrating capacity and magnesium transport in the medullary thick ascending limb. These appear to alter the renal capacity to conserve magnesium, which may be related to its tubulotoxic action.

The effect of tacrolimus on magnesium metabolism was studied in 11 patients after renal transplantation. There was a significant decrease in serum magnesium levels during tacrolimus treatment, and hypomagnesemia developed in 9 of the patients. The amount of daily renal magnesium excretion was normal, but fractional magnesium excretion was extremely high compared with healthy control subjects.

Neurologic side effects are common and range from relatively minor symptoms such as tremor, insomnia, and nightmares, to major problems such as dysphasia, confusion, psychosis, encephalopathy, and coma. In the European tacrolimus study, tremor was reported in 35%, insomnia in 24%, and headache in 20% of patients. Other neurologic complications are relatively rare.

Severe neurotoxicity occurs relatively infrequently in pediatric renal transplant patients who are subsequently treated with tacrolimus. The most common symptoms have been myalgia and tremors in 50% of patients, followed by fatigue in 38% of the recipients.

Hyperlipidemia is a significant management issue after renal transplantation. Tacrolimus has been shown to have less adverse effect on the lipid profile than other immunosuppressive agents. Most studies, including data from our center, demonstrate that hypercholesterolemia is almost three times less prevalent in tacrolimus-treated than in cyclosporine-treated patients. Levels of triglycerides have also been reported to be significantly lower in some studies, although this has not been confirmed by others. There are no differences in high-density lipoprotein (HDL) cholesterol; however, the concentration of LDL cholesterol, the independent risk factor Lp(a), was lower in tacrolimus-treated patients.

It appears that tacrolimus has no inhibitory effect on the metabolism of fatty acids. This indicates that tacrolimus offers some advantage in patients with cardiovascular risk factors. In a randomized, prospective study of stable renal transplant patients with hypercholesterolemia, conversion from cyclosporine to tacrolimus was reported to be safe and resulted in lower levels of serum cholesterol, LDL, and apolipoprotein B. Although the rate of hirsutism and gum hyperplasia are significantly lower in tacrolimus-treated patients, alopecia has been reported in 10% of recipients.

Selected Readings

Barone G, Chang CT, Choc MG, et al. The pharmacokinetics of a microemulsion formulation of cyclosporine in primary renal allograft recipients. *Transplantation* 1996;61:875–880.

The Neoral Study Group report on pharmacokinetics of microemulsion formulation.

Bennet WM, De Mattos A, Meyer MM, et al. Chronic cyclosporine nephropathy. *Kidney Int* 1996;50:1089–1100.

An excellent review of chronic cyclosporine nephrotoxicity.

Beveridge T, Calne RY. Cyclosporine in cadaveric renal transplantation. *Transplantation* 1995;59:1568–1570.

A report of 10- year follow-up of the European multicenter trial.

Chueh SC, Kahan BD. Pretransplant test-dose pharmacokinetic profiles: cyclosporine microemulsion versus corn oil-based soft gel capsule formulation. *J Am Soc Nephrol* 1998;9:1–13, 1998.

An excellent pharmacokinetic review of different cyclosporine formulations.

Cole E, Keown P, Landsberg D, et al. Safety and tolerability of cyclosporine and cyclosporine microemulsion during 18 months of follow-up in stable renal transplant recipients. *Transplantation* 1998;65(4):505–510.

A report of clinical study of stable renal transplant recipients on cyclosporine microemulsion.

Jordan ML, Naraghi R, Shapiro R, et al. Tacrolimus rescue therapy for renal allograft rejection—five year experience. *Transplantation* 1997;63:223–228.

An excellent study of the effect of tacrolimus as a rescue therapy in kidney rejection.

Kahan BD. Pharmacokinetic considerations in the therapeutic application of cyclosporine in renal transplantation. Reduced inter- and intrasubject variability in cyclosporine pharmacokinetics in renal transplant recipients treated with a microemulsion formulation in conjunction with fasting, low-fat meals, or high-fat meals. *Transplant Proc* 1996;28:2143–2146.

Kahan BD, Dunn J, Fitts C, et al. *Transplantation* 1995;59:505–511.

Keown P, Landsberg D, Halloran P, et al. A randomized, prospective multicenter pharmcoepidemiologic study of cyclosporine microemulsion in stable renal graft recipients. *Transplantation* 1996;62:1744–1752.

These three articles provide an excellent review of the pharmacokinetic and pharmacoepidemiologic study of the cyclosporine microemulsion in renal transplantation.

Laskow DA, Vincenti F, Neylan JF, et al. An open-label, concentration-ranging trial of FK506 in primary kidney transplantation. *Transplantation* 1996;62:900–905.

Mayer AD, Dmitrewsky J, Squifflet JP, et al. Multicenter randomized trial comparing tacrolimus (FK506) and cyclosporine in the prevention of renal allograft rejection. *Transplantation* 1997;64:436–443.

Neylan JF, for the FK506 Kidney Transplant Study Group. Racial differences in renal transplantation after immunosuppression with tacrolimus versus cyclosporine. *Transplantation* 1998;65:515–523.

These three articles review the results of multicenter trials of tacrolimus in renal transplant recipients.

Noble S, Markham A. Cyclosporin: a review of the pharmacokinetic properties, clinical efficacy and tolerability of a microemulsion-based formulation (Neoral). *Drugs* 1995;50:924–941.

A basic review of the cyclosporine pharmacokinetics.

Pirsch JD, Miller J, Deierhoi MH, et al. A comparison of tacrolimus (FK506) and cyclosporine for immunosuppression after cadaveric renal transplantation. Transplantation 1997;63:977–983.

An excellent review of tacrolimus in cadaveric renal transplantation.

Ritschel WA. Microemulsion technology in the reformulation of cyclosporine: the reason behind the pharmacokinetic properties of Neoral. *Clin Transplantation* 1996;10:364–373.

A review article to define the pharmacokinetic properties of Neoral.

Smith SR, Minda SA, Samsa GP, et al. Late withdrawal of cyclosporine in stable renal transplant recipients. *Am J Kidney Dis* 1995;26(3):487–494.

This article reviews the risks involved in late withdrawal of cyclosporine.

Spencer CM, Goa KL, Gillis JC. Tacrolimus: an update of its pharmacology and clinical efficacy in the management of organ transplantation. *Drugs* 1997;54(6): 925–975.

A basic review of tacrolimus pharmacology and efficacy in renal transplantation.

Woodle ES, Thistlethwaite JR, Gordon JH, et al. A multicenter trial of FK506 (tacrolimus) therapy in refractory acute renal allograft rejection. *Transplantation* 1996;62:594–599.

This article reviews the significant impact of tacrolimus in refractory acute rejection.

C: Mycophenolate Mofetil

Bryan N. Becker and Hans W. Sollinger

Immune responses arise in a microenvironment that favors their occurrence, with antigen presentation, costimulation, cytokine release from activated T cells, and subsequent nucleotide synthesis. Each step is a potential target for immunosuppressive regimens that are designed to prolong graft function in solid-organ transplant recipients. Most immunosuppressive drugs can be categorized based on their mechanism of action in the context of these events. For example, some commonly used immunosuppressive medications act specifically on T cells (e.g., cyclosporine and tacrolimus).

Nucleotide synthesis represents another ready target. Since the introduction of azathioprine, it has become apparent that antimetabolite medications can provide additional immunosuppressive benefits. Their pharmacologic and immunosuppressive actions are linked to their antimetabolite effects as well as inhibition of the humoral component of the immune system. The development of mycophenolate mofetil (MMF) (Fig. 88.1), the next generation of immunosuppression-focused antimetabolite medications, represents a significant advance for the role of such medications in solid-organ transplantation.

BACKGROUND AND MECHANISM OF ACTION

Mycophenolic acid (MPA) is a weak organic acid that was originally isolated as fermentation product of *Penicillium stoloniferum* and named by Alsberg and Black in 1913. Florey and colleagues later noted that it had antifungal and antibiotic activity. Although its effectiveness as an antibiotic agent was poor, interest in MPA as an antineoplastic and immunosuppressive agent led to a number of investigations. MPA's questionable efficacy in early trials, an increased incidence in latent viral infections in MPA-treated patients, and its possible carcinogenicity resulted in discontinuation of many of these studies. However, *in vitro* investigations by Allison and others continued to stimulate enthusiasm for MPA's immunosuppressive potential. They analyzed the *de novo* and salvage purine biosynthesis pathways in various cell types and noted that lymphocytes required a fully functional *de novo* pathway for purine biosynthesis and cell proliferation (Fig. 88.2).

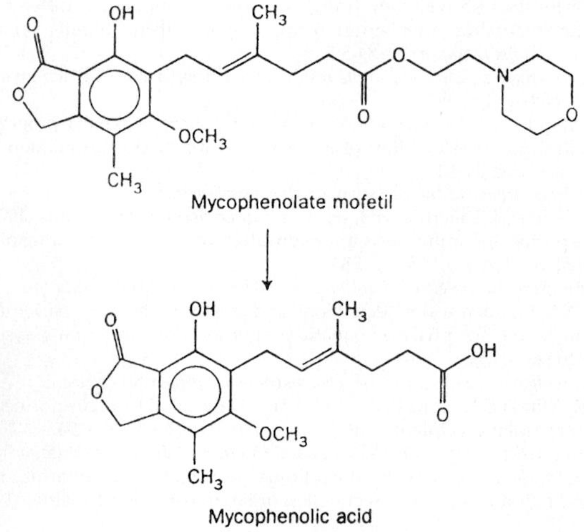

Figure 88.1. Mycophenolate mofetil, the prodrug of mycophenolic acid. Mycophenolate mofetil is the morpholinylethyl ester of mycophenolic acid. (Reproduced with permission from Lipsky JJ. Mycophenolate mofetil. *Lancet* 1996;348:1357.)

In human lymphocytes, adenosine monophosphate (AMP) and adenosine diphosphate (ADP) inhibited 5-phosphoribosyl-1-pyrophosphate (PRPP), whereas guanosine monophosphate (GMP), guanosine diphosphate (GDP), and guanosine trisphosphate (GTP) activated PRPP. Inosine monophosphate (IMP), the branch point for purine nucleotide synthesis, can be converted to adenosine or guanosine nucleotides. MPA inhibits inosine monophosphate dehydrogenase (IMPDH), blocking the conversion of inosine-5-phosphate and xanthine-5-phosphate to guanine nucleotides by serving as a replacement for the nicotinamide portion of the nicotinamide adenine dinucleotide (NAD) cofactor and a catalytic water molecule. Cell types that rely predominantly on *de novo* purine biosynthesis (e.g., lymphocytes) thus are singularly more susceptible to the effects of MPA.

IMPDH is expressed intracellularly as a constitutive (type I IMPDH) and an inducible enzyme (type II IMPDH). Interestingly, the type II isoform is approximately five times more susceptible to the inhibitory effect of MPA than the type I isoform. IMP levels increase as IMPDH is inhibited, leading to adenosine and deoxyadenosine nucleotide accumulation and a concomitant decrease in guanosine and deoxyguanosine nucleotides. This downregulates lymphocyte IMPDH activity, PRPP and DNA polymerase activity, and ultimately, limits lymphocyte proliferation without significantly affecting neutrophils and their phagocytic and bactericidal activity.

MPA is lipid soluble. Chemically modifying MPA to produce an ester form, MMF, enhances the drug's oral bioavailability. This allowed for further investigations that established MMF's additional mechanisms of action. It inhibits T-cell and B-cell proliferative responses to calcium-dependent, T-cell–dependent, and T-cell–independent mitogens. It also inhibits lymphocyte proliferative responses to alloantigenic stimuli and antigen-specific antibody responses in memory B cells. Furthermore, MPA abrogates mitogenic responses in fibroblasts and endothelial cells, inhibits mixed lymphocyte reactions, and decreases glycosylation of adhesion molecules and/or their ligands.

PHARMACOKINETICS

MMF undergoes complete oral absorption and is rapidly hydrolyzed by esterases to MPA before it is converted to an inac-

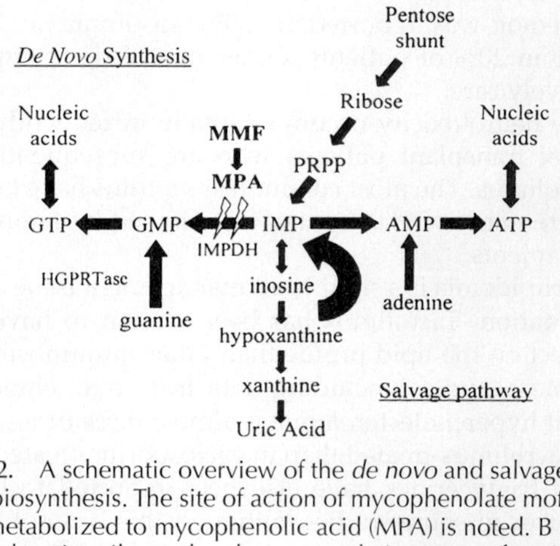

Figure 88.2. A schematic overview of the *de novo* and salvage pathways of purine biosynthesis. The site of action of mycophenolate mofetil (MMF) after it is metabolized to mycophenolic acid (MPA) is noted. B and T lymphocytes rely primarily on the *de novo* as their source of purine nucleotides for DNA and RNA synthesis.

tive glucuronide metabolite (MPA-glucuronide). MPA is lipid soluble and therefore can easily penetrate cells in contrast to its glucuronide metabolite. However, by virtue of the enterohepatic circulation and the expression of β-glucuronidase in gastrointestinal epithelia, MPA-glucuronide can be deglucuronidated and MPA can be freely reabsorbed.

The drug is renally excreted with tubular secretion contributing to its clearance. Chronic renal insufficiency reduces this clearance and, as such, plasma MPA-glucuronide accumulates. Doses therefore should be limited to 2 g/day or less in individuals with chronic renal dysfunction.

MMF's pharmacologic activity is directly related to free MPA plasma concentrations, a finding of importance because MPA is extensively bound to serum albumin. An increasing number of clinical investigations have focused on the relationship between plasma MPA–area under the concentration time-curve (AUC) and the drug's efficacy and toxicity. Studies to date, however, have not demonstrated significant relationships between plasma MPA-AUC and any untoward effects.

A number of medications can potentially interact with MMF. Food reduces and delays peak MPA plasma concentrations for up to an hour. Magnesium- and aluminum-containing antacids decrease the maximum concentration (C_{max}) and AUC. Tacrolimus given concomitantly with MMF can increase MPA-AUC. However, cyclosporine does not appear to interact with MMF.

Any medication that affects the enterohepatic circulation also can reduce MPA levels, including resins such as cholestyramine. Conversely, compounds that compete for renal tubular secretion, for example, acyclovir or probenecid, may inhibit MPA-glucuronide elimination and increase their own concentrations as well as the AUC for MPA-glucuronide. Obviously, coadministration of highly protein-bound drugs, such as furosemide, can displace MPA from serum albumin and increase free drug levels. Given the extent of protein binding by MPA, it is not surprising that hemodialysis is relatively ineffective in removing MPA or MPA-glucuronide.

MMF IN CLINICAL USE

Any discussion of MMF and its clinical use has to start with investigations that examined the use of MPA for psoriasis in the late 1970s. In several open-label trials and in a double-blind, placebo-controlled trial, oral MPA therapy proved efficacious in reducing or clearing psoriatic skin lesions. However, enthusiasm for MPA subsided. Yet, with the development of MMF there was renewed interest in MPA, this time for use as an immunosuppressive to prevent another predominantly T-cell–mediated phenomenon, renal transplant rejection.

MMF initially was investigated in a phase I study that examined eight different MMF dosing schedules (100 to 3,500 mg/day) in renal transplant patients. MMF was given in combination with cyclosporine, prednisone, and antilymphocyte globulin. MMF in doses of more than 2 g/day was associated with a significant reduction in acute rejection episodes and courses of muromonab CD3 or prednisone therapy for acute rejection.

PROPHYLAXIS AGAINST ACUTE RENAL ALLOGRAFT REJECTION

MMF was evaluated as prophylaxis against acute renal allograft rejection in three randomized, double-blind investigations. In all three studies, MMF was administered as 1,000 mg or 1,500 mg twice daily. Study endpoints for each investigation included biopsy-proven rejection, graft loss, death, or lack of response to therapy for any other reason.

The European Mycophenolate Mofetil Cooperative Study Group was a placebo-controlled MMF trial. Four-hundred-and-ninety-one first or second cadaveric renal transplant recipients culled from 20 European transplant centers were enrolled. All patients received corticosteroid and cyclosporine without induction therapy. Patients were randomized to three groups: placebo (n = 166); MMF 2,000 mg/day (n = 165); and MMF 3,000 mg/day (n = 160). At 6 months, the placebo arm had a 56% treatment failure rate compared with 30.3% in the MMF 2,000 mg/day group ($P \leq .001$) and 38.8% in the MMF 3,000 mg/day group ($P \leq .001$). The placebo group also had a higher rate of biopsy-proven rejection (46.4%) compared with rates of 17% and 13.8% in the MMF 2,000 mg/day and 3,000 mg/day groups, respectively. Furthermore, MMF reduced the need for additional antirejection medications. Greater than 17% of the placebo patients required multiple courses of glucocorticoid therapy compared with 4.2% in the MMF 2,000 mg/day and 5.0% in the MMF 3,000 mg/day groups. Antilymphocyte agents were also used less frequently in the MMF-treated patients.

The U.S. Renal Transplant Mycophenolate Mofetil Study Group investigation was undertaken at 14 sites. Primary cadaveric transplant recipients were enrolled and given cyclosporine, steroids, and induction therapy with antithymocyte globulin. The study compared patients who received azathioprine 1 to 2 mg/kg per day with patients who received MMF 1,000 to 1,500 mg twice daily. The azathioprine group had a 47.6% treatment failure rate at 6 months compared with 31.1% ($P = .0015$) for the 2,000 mg/day and 31.3% ($P = .0021$) for the 3,000 mg/day MMF groups. Biopsy-proven rejection was also more common in the azathioprine group (38%) compared with 19.8% in the 2,000 mg/day and 17.5% in the 3,000 mg/day MMF groups. In addition, antilymphocyte sera use was more frequent in the azathioprine group (20.1%) versus the MMF 2,000 mg/day (10.3%) and MMF 3,000 mg/day (5.4%) groups and azathioprine-treated patients required more courses of bolus glucocorticoid therapy.

The Tricontinental Mycophenolate Mofetil Renal Transplantation Study Group was the third of the large MMF trials and included 21 sites in Australia, Europe, and Canada. Five-hundred-and-three primary or second cadaveric renal transplant recipients were enrolled. All patients were treated with cyclosporine, corticosteroid therapy, and either azathioprine (100 to 150 mg/day) or MMF (2,000 to 3,000 mg/day) without induction therapy. The azathioprine-treated patients had a 50% treatment failure rate at 6 months compared with 38.2% in the MMF 2,000 mg/day ($P = .0287$) and 34.8% in the MMF 3,000 mg/day ($P = .0045$) groups. Biopsy-proven rejection was present in 35.5% of the patients taking azathioprine versus 19.7% in the MMF 2,000 mg/day and 15.9% in the MMF 3,000 mg/day patient groups. Azathioprine-treated patients in this study, similar to the U.S. Study, also received more courses of bolus glucocorticoids and antilymphocyte therapy.

These three studies solidified the efficacy of MMF in renal transplantation as prophylaxis against acute rejection. In each study, MMF-treated patients had significant reductions in rates of treatment failure compared with non–MMF-treated patients. Importantly, MMF treatment also appeared to reduce the number of courses of bolus glucocorticoid therapy as well as use of antilymphocyte globulin in the treatment of rejection episodes. Follow-up data from the International Mycophenolate Mofetil Renal Transplant Study Groups further highlighted the important beneficial effect of MMF (Table 88.8). Pooling the analyses of the three aforementioned studies demonstrated that MMF at 2,000mg/day or 3,000 mg/day resulted in a significant reduction in acute rejection episodes over a 12-month period compared with treatment with placebo or azathioprine and a slight but not statistically significant improvement in graft survival

TABLE 88.8. First Biopsy-Proven Rejection or Treatment Failure During First 12 Months After Transplantation Excluding Routine Biopsies in Patients Treated With Mycophenolate Mofetil (MMF), Placebo, or Azathioprine

	Placebo/ Azathioprine	MMF 2,000 mg/day	MMF 3,000 mg/day
Patients enrolled	498	505	490
First biopsy-proven rejection (%)	203 (40.8)	100 (19.8)	81 (16.5)
Grade I	84 (16.9)	50 (9.9)[a]	41 (8.4)[a]
Grade II	92 (18.5)	41 (8.1)	30 (6.1)
Grade III	27 (5.4)	9 (1.8)	10 (2.0)
Patients with biopsy-proven rejection or treatment failure (%)	268 (53.8)	186 (36.8)[b]	194 (39.6)[b]

Biopsy-proven rejection was indicated by core biopsy using Banff severity more than 1.

[a] $P < .001$ for pair-wise comparisons (MMF 2,000 mg/day or 3,000 mg/day versus placebo/azathioprine) with competing risk analysis using proportional hazards regression and 97.5% confidence intervals.

[b] $P < .002$

Adapted from Halloran P, Mathew T, Tomlanovich S, et al. for the International Mycophenolate Mofetil Renal Transplant Study Groups. Mycophenolate mofetil in renal allograft recipients. *Transplantation* 1998;63:45.

rates. Other studies suggest that MMF may be even more effective in preventing acute rejection in combination with tacrolimus, but larger prospective analyses comparing this combination with MMF plus cyclosporine will be necessary to formally answer this question.

RESCUE THERAPY FOR ACUTE RENAL TRANSPLANT REJECTION

MMF also was compared with high-dose glucocorticoid therapy as treatment for refractory acute renal allograft rejection. Patients with biopsy-proven acute cellular rejection were treated with MMF 1,500 mg twice daily or high-dose intravenous methylprednisolone 5 mg/kg for 5 days with a taper to 20 mg/day or the patient's baseline dose subsequent to at least 7 days of antilymphocyte agent therapy. Seventy-seven patients received MMF; 73 patients received intravenous methylprednisolone. At 6 months, 14.3% of the MMF-treated patients had either died or lost their grafts compared with 26% of the high-dose corticosteroid-treated patients. This is not a statistically significant difference. These percentages increased to 18.2% for the MMF-treated patients versus 31% for the steroid-treated patients by 12 months ($P = .042$). Biopsy-proven or presumed rejection and treatment failure occurred in 64.4% of the glucocorticoid-treated patients and in 39% of the MMF-treated patients ($P = .001$).

An expanded, multicenter, open-label trial was performed in 75 renal transplant recipients with biopsy-proven rejection unresponsive to at least one course of antilymphocyte globulin or muromonab CD3 as well as patients with recurrent rejection who could not tolerate additional courses of these agents. Oral MMF dosing (2,000 or 3,000 mg/day) was begun within 48 hours of the biopsy results with concomitant cyclosporine and prednisone treatment. Successful rescue long term, defined as stabilization or improvement in renal function, was evident in 69% of the patients. The rescue rate for patients with Scr less than 4.0 mg/dl was 79% versus a 52% rescue rate in individuals with a Scr more than 4 mg/dl.

MMF IN CHRONIC RENAL TRANSPLANT REJECTION

The reduction in acute rejection episodes in each of the three aforementioned trials raised the possibility that MMF could be protective against chronic transplant rejection. In a 3-year follow-up analysis for the International Mycophenolate Mofetil Study Group, MMF use marginally reduced the rate of graft loss at 3 years compared with azathioprine treatment (MMF 3,000 mg/day, 84.8%; MMF 2,000 mg/day, 81.9%; azathioprine, 80.2%). It should be noted that these data represented a secondary outcome point for this study that was neither designed or powered at its outset to detect differences in graft survival at 3-year follow-up.

MMF IN LIVER AND CARDIAC TRANSPLANTATION

MMF with cyclosporine or tacrolimus extended hepatic allograft survival in dogs and in a hamster-to-rat liver xenograft model. Thus MMF has been investigated in liver transplantation as well. In one study of 23 liver transplant patients with persistent acute rejection, substitution of MMF for azathioprine led to resolution or improvement of the rejection in 21 patients. MMF also was given in combination with tacrolimus and prednisone to 38 liver transplant recipients in a nonrandomized trial with 6-month follow-up. MMF use reduced tacrolimus dosing requirements without an increased incidence of rejection. In a large, retrospective study, MMF 2,000 mg/day during the first 3 months after liver transplantation combined with tacrolimus and a standard steroid taper reduced the incidence of acute liver allograft rejection and again allowed for a tacrolimus dose reduction, thereby limiting drug-induced nephrotoxicity.

MMF has also been used in cardiac transplantation as a substitute for azathioprine in patients with mild cellular rejection but no allograft dysfunction. Small, uncontrolled trials suggested that MMF was efficacious in persistent or refractory rejection in cardiac transplantation and more effective than azathioprine in such instances. A recent multicenter, randomized trial also analyzed MMF for primary prevention of rejection in cardiac transplantation. MMF treatment was beneficial in terms of survival and in reducing rates of rejection, providing further evidence for MMF as an adjunct immunosuppressive medication in cardiac transplantation.

MMF IN PANCREAS TRANSPLANTATION

In animal models, MMF, alone and in combination with cyclosporine, prolonged islet allograft function and pancreas allograft survival. MMF has only recently been studied in humans as immunosuppressive therapy for simultaneous kidney–pancreas allografts. Single-center studies have suggested that MMF was more effective than azathioprine in preventing biopsy-proven acute rejection in simultaneous kidney–pancreas (SKP) transplantation. For example, data from the University of Wisconsin demonstrated a marked reduction in biopsy-proven renal allograft rejection in MMF-treated SKP recipients (MMF, 31% versus azathioprine, 75%; $P = .0001$). Moreover, 2-year pancreas graft survival also was significantly better with MMF treatment (95% versus azathioprine, 83%; $P = .016$).

Again, taking advantage of the effect that tacrolimus boosts MPA levels, additional studies have examined the combination of tacrolimus plus MMF in pancreas transplantation (SKP, pancreas-after-kidney, and pancreas alone). In these studies, patients received quadruple sequential induction immunosuppression, predominantly with antithymocyte globulin. These data also highlight the effectiveness of this combination with a significant reduction in acute rejection episodes in the first year following transplant.

MMF IN NONTRANSPLANT SETTINGS

Glomerular Disease

Animal studies suggested that MMF limited renal damage in certain models of glomerular disease. Astute clinicians extrapolated these findings to the clinical setting and have used MMF in select cases for the treatment of lupus nephritis, Wegener's granulomatosis, microscopic polyangiitis, IgA nephropathy, membranous nephropathy, minimal-change disease, and focal segmental glomerulosclerosis. Dosages of 750 mg to 1,000 mg twice daily were used in uncontrolled fashion along with glucocorticoids in some instances. MMF effectively suppressed proteinuria and stabilized serum creatinine in the majority of these cases, although follow-up has been less than 1 year in each. In another series, MMF (approximately 1,000 mg/day) used in combination with prednisone significantly decreased proteinuria and improved serum creatinine values in 12 patients with severe lupus nephritis treated at the University of North Carolina and at Ohio State University. These anecdotal data suggest that MMF had short-term clinical efficacy potentially in certain subsets of glomerular disease and may have steroid-sparing effects as well. Larger controlled trials will be necessary to determine its true efficacy in this setting.

Other Diseases

MMF has been evaluated in open-label studies in dosages ranging from 1,000 to 4,000 mg/day in patients with refractory rheumatoid arthritis. These studies yielded variable results with a reduction in numbers of painful and swollen joints. In other studies, MMF reduced rheumatoid factor titers and induced improvement in overall symptomatology in daily doses of 2,000 mg/day.

As mentioned previously, MPA in doses ranging between 3,000 mg/day and 4,000 mg/day has been used for the treatment of psoriasis with documented improvement in symptoms and skin lesions. Case reports and small case series have also described MMF as adjunct therapy for bullous pemphigoid and ulcerative colitis with some benefit.

SIDE EFFECTS

Although the adverse effects of MMF vary greatly, the vast majority are mild and seldom necessitate discontinuing the drug. The three large, randomized, renal allograft rejection prophylaxis trials provide a compilation of the major toxicities and adverse events associated with MMF (Table 88.9). The most commonly reported side effects with a dosage of 2,000 mg/day were gastrointestinal (diarrhea, abdominal pain, nausea, dyspepsia, gastroenteritis, and vomiting). In addition, hematologic side effects (leukopenia, anemia, thrombocytopenia, and pancytopenia) as well as opportunistic infections [cytomegalovirus (CMV) viremia, CMV invasive disease, herpes simplex, and *Candida*] have been noted with MMF treatment. Interestingly, MMF may have a unique anti-*Pneumocystis carinii* effect despite the increased risk for other opportunistic infections during treatment. All of these side effects were reported more frequently in patients who took 3,000 mg/day. In addition, reports of MMF-associated pulmonary toxicity have occurred as well. In this regard, it is notable that more than 5% of patients in one MMF trial suffered from noninfectious respiratory side effects during treatment. Other trials of MMF in renal allograft recipients, other solid-organ transplant patients, and nontransplant patients have described all of the aforementioned adverse drug effects as well as pancreatitis, CMV colitis, and severe gastrointestinal bleeding.

TABLE 88.9. Major Adverse Reactions Reported with Mycophenolate Mofetil Use

Systemic	
	Fatigue, edema, fever
Hematologic	
	Leukopenia, anemia, thrombocytopenia,
Gastrointestinal	
	Diarrhea, nausea and vomiting, gastrointestinal bleeding, abdominal cramping
Genitourinary	
	Urinary tract infections, frequency, urgency, dysuria
Respiratory	
	Respiratory tract infection, bronchitis, dyspnea, pharyngitis
Infectious	
	Increased incidence viral infections (cytomegalovirus, herpes simplex, herpes zoster)

Nephrotoxicity, neurotoxicity, and hepatotoxicity are infrequent with MMF, and long-term safety data suggest that side effects may be less frequent with a longer duration of therapy. Neurologic side effects such as fatigue, headache, tinnitus, and disturbed sleep patterns usually are not significant enough to warrant discontinuation of therapy. Patients with gastrointestinal side effects often respond to either a dose division to three or four times/day or a dosage reduction before discontinuing the drug. Hematologic side effects generally reverse within 1 week of discontinuing MMF.

MMF has been shown to be teratogenic in rats and rabbits. It is also excreted in rat milk. To date, no studies examining MMF administration to pregnant women or MMF excretion in breast milk have been published; MMF should not be given to pregnant women.

DOSAGE AND ADMINISTRATION

MMF is currently available in 250 mg and 500 mg tablets. Because of the variability in absorption and metabolism in the early postoperative period, an intravenous form of MMF has been developed. This formulation has been evaluated as a 2-hour infusion twice daily in the early postoperative period (first 5 days). In preliminary studies, mean AUC and C_{max} for intravenous MMF were 29% and 20% greater than that obtained by oral administration. Hypertension was the most common adverse event reported with intravenous MMF use.

The usual initial dosage in renal transplant recipients is 1,000 mg orally twice daily. In patients with a glomerular filtration rate less than 25 ml/min/1.73 m^2 outside of the immediate post-transplant period, dosages of more than 2,000 mg/day should be avoided. However, no dosage reduction is necessary in patients with delayed graft function. Dosages should be held or reduced in patients with significant neutropenia (absolute neutrophil count less than $1.3 \times 10^3/mm^3$).

Dosage and use in pediatric patients have not been well defined. A dose of 46 mg/kg/day has been reported in children undergoing renal transplantation. Optimal dosages in heart and liver transplant recipients also remain to be determined.

Nevertheless, 2,000 mg/day appears to be an adequate initial dose in these transplant settings.

Due to the potential teratogenic effects of MMF, opening or crushing the capsules is not recommended. However, in certain clinical situations, such as pediatric administration or administration through a nasogastric tube, the capsules are often opened. Although no reports of harm to caregivers administering MMF have been published, inhalation of the powder and physical contact with the agent should be avoided.

COST-EFFECTIVENESS OF MMF

Cost is always of concern with any new medication, and MMF is expensive, with an average wholesale price (AWP) in the United States of $1.875 per 250 mg capsule. This corresponds to a yearly maintenance cost of $5,475 for a dosage of 2,000 mg/day. In contrast, generic azathioprine, the drug that MMF most frequently replaces in immunosuppressive regimens, has an AWP in the United States of $1.166 per 50-mg tablet, representing a yearly cost of $851 to $1,277 for a dosage of 100 to 150 mg/day.

However, the cost-effectiveness of MMF therapy has to take into account its demonstrated efficacy in reducing treatment failures, acute rejection episodes, and use of antilymphocyte and bolus glucocorticoid therapy. Sullivan and coworkers examined the cost-effectiveness of MMF in the first year after primary cadaveric renal transplant, analyzing data from the U.S. Renal Transplant Mycophenolate Mofetil Study Group. They determined that patients treated with MMF were likely to have lower rejection-related treatment costs and lower dialysis and graft failure costs despite higher additional immunosuppression costs. They calculated that MMF was cost-effective, with first-year costs averaging $27,807 versus control azathioprine costs of $29,158. The long-term potential cost-effectiveness of MMF, especially as it may relate to conditions other than renal transplantation remains to be determined.

Selected Readings

Eckhoff DE, McGuire BM, Frenette LR, et al. Tacrolimus (FK506) and mycophenolate mofetil combination therapy versus tacrolimus in adult liver transplantation. *Transplantation* 1998;65:180–187.

A large, retrospective case series that demonstrated the efficacy of the tacrolimus–mycophenolate mofetil combination in liver transplantation.

European Mycophenolate Mofetil Cooperative Study Group. Placebo controlled study of mycophenolate mofetil combined with cyclosporin and corticosteroids for prevention of acute rejection. *Lancet* 1995;345:1321–1325.

A multicenter European trial that evaluated mycophenolate mofetil as prophylaxis against acute renal transplant rejection in a placebo-controlled trial that included 491 primary and secondary cadaveric renal transplant recipients. Patients received induction antibody therapy in this trial.

Gruessner RWG, Sutherland DER, Drangstveit MB, et al. Mycophenolate mofetil in pancreas transplantation. *Transplantation* 1998;66:318–323.

A two-part analysis demonstrating the benefit of the mycophenolate mofetil plus tacrolimus combination in pancreas–kidney, pancreas-alone and pancreas-after-kidney transplantation in a single-center case series and in a matched-pair analysis using International Pancreas Transplant Registry data.

Halloran P, Mathew T, Tomlanovich S, et al. for the International Mycophenolate Mofetil Renal Transplant Study Groups. Mycophenolate mofetil in renal allograft recipients. *Transplantation* 1998;63:39–47.

A pooled analysis of three phase III randomized, double-blind, multicenter clinical trials that focused on graft loss, patient death, incidence, and treatment of rejection and graft function at 1 year following transplant.

Kobashigawa J, Miller L, Renlund D, et al. A randomized active-controlled trial of mycophenolate mofetil in heart transplant recipients. *Transplantation* 1998;66:507–515.

A prospective, randomized, multicenter, double-blind study that demonstrated the effectiveness of mycophenolate mofetil in preventing acute rejection and reducing mortality during the first year following cardiac transplantation.

Simmons WD, Rayhill SC, Sollinger HW. Preliminary risk-benefit assessment of mycophenolate mofetil in transplant rejection. *Drug Saf* 1997;17:75–92.

A complete early overview of mycophenolate mofetil combining summaries of in vitro data and clinical efficacy data.

Sintchak MD, Fleming MA, Futer O, et al. Structure and mechanism of inosine monophosphate dehydrogenase in complex with the immunosuppressant mycophenolic acid. *Cell* 1996;84:921–930.

An intricate study that used x-ray crystallography to define the structure of inosine monophosphate dehydrogenase and the site of action of mycophenolic acid.

Sollinger HW for the U.S. Renal Transplant Mycophenolate Mofetil Study Group. Mycophenolate mofetil for the prevention of acute rejection in primary cadaveric renal allograft recipients. *Transplantation* 1995;60:225–232.

A prospective, randomized, multicenter trial that compared mycophenolate mofetil with azathioprine as prophylaxis against acute renal transplant rejection. All patients were treated with quadruple sequential induction immunosuppression. Mycophenolate mofetil (2 g/day or 3 g/day) significantly reduced the incidence of acute rejection.

Tricontinental Mycophenolate Mofetil Renal Transplantation Study Group. A blinded, randomized clinical trial of mycophenolate mofetil for the prevention of acute rejection in cadaveric renal transplantation. *Transplantation* 1996;61:1029–1037.

A multicenter, randomized trial that included patients from Europe, Canada, and Australia. It enrolled 503 patients who were randomized to azathioprine or mycophenolate mofetil treatment with cyclosporine and corticosteroids following renal transplantation. Notably, induction antibody therapy was not used in this trial.

D: Antilymphocyte Antibodies

V. Ram Peddi and M. Roy First

The three phases of immunosuppressive therapy after transplantation are (a) induction of immunosuppression immediately following transplantation, when potent therapy is required to prevent acute rejection and facilitate acceptance of the allograft; (b) maintenance immunosuppression is the long-term therapy, which should be substantial enough to prevent allograft rejection, but at the same time preserve host-defense mechanisms against infections; and (c) treatment of an established acute rejection episode. Antilymphocyte antibodies are ideally suited for use as induction immunosuppressive agents and for the treatment of acute rejection. They have been available for use as immunosuppressive agents since the late 1960s. All early forms of antilymphocyte antibodies were polyclonal, which are made by injecting human lymphocytes into horses, goats, rabbits, or sheep. Polyclonal immunoglobulins represent a heterogeneous group of antibodies, only a minority of which are specific to T cells. They also often cross-react with other body tissues such as endothelium. In contrast to polyclonal antibodies, a monoclonal antibody is highly specific, recognizing a single antigen epitope. They have a greater potency at lower doses, and have a more predictable and consistent effect. Monoclonal antibodies may be directed at cell-surface receptors such as CD3/T-cell–receptor (TCR) complex and interleukin-2 receptor (IL-2R), or against adhesion molecules.

POLYCLONAL ANTILYMPHOCYTE AGENTS

Polyclonal antibodies against human lymphoid tissue are obtained by injecting a variety of animals with human lymphoid cells such as peripheral blood lymphocytes, thymocytes, or B-cell lymphoblasts. The resulting immune serum is purified to obtain the γ-globulin fraction. Harvesting of the polyclonal antibodies can be performed regularly without harm to the animal. Preparations of antibodies used clinically include antilymphocyte and antilymphoblast globulin (ALG), antithymocyte globulin (ATG), and antilymphocyte serum (ALS) obtained from horses, rabbits, goats, or sheep. Polyclonal immune globulins represent a heterogeneous group of antibodies only a minority of which are specific to the T cell. The remainder consists of antibodies against other antigens that already exist as part of the animal repertoire, and to the many different molecules on the injected human lymphocytes. Several mechanisms of action have been proposed to explain the immunosuppressive effect of polyclonal antibodies. These include (a) complement-mediated cell lysis, (b) clearance of lymphocytes by opsonization and subsequent phagocytosis by macrophages, and (c) antibody-dependent cell-mediated cytolysis. Polyclonal antibody treatment induces marked lymphocyte depletion, which persists during the entire treatment period. The number of circulating T cells will gradually increase after the cessation of treatment, and they reach pretreatment levels in 1 to 6 weeks, with major variability among patients. Each polyclonal antilymphocyte preparation varies in its constituent antibodies. Because of this unpredictable antibody mixture and batch-to-batch variability, treatment responses and side effects are variable between the different preparations. The most common side effects (Table 88.10) are fever and chills, which usually occur after the administration of the first few doses. This is believed to be due to the release of cytokines during T-cell lysis; however, these symptoms are not as severe as the cytokine-release syndrome induced by muromonab-CD3 (OKT3). More severe reactions include the development of skin rashes, hypotension, acute respiratory distress, and anaphylaxis. Polyclonal antibodies often cross-react with antigens on unrelated cells including red blood cells, platelets, and body tissues such as endothelium, resulting in side effects such as granulocytopenia, thrombocytopenia, arthralgia, serum sickness, phlebitis, and immune complex glomerulonephritis. Because these agents severely impair the cell-mediated immunity, patients are prone to develop opportunistic infections and posttransplant malignancies, especially posttransplant lymphoproliferative disorders (PTLD) (discussed further in Chapter 89, Part 6). Administration of polyclonal antibodies requires 4 to 6 hours using a central venous catheter or a peripheral vein with a high flow rate. Earlier studies have shown a significant improvement in graft survival in patients receiving a polyclonal antibody for induction together with azathioprine and steroids. Historically, the use of these agents has been particularly valuable as induction therapy, especially for patients with delayed graft function who may be more sensitive to the nephrotoxic effects of the calcineurin inhibitors, cyclosporine or tacrolimus. With polyclonal antibody induction, institution of calcineurin inhibitors can be delayed until good graft function has been obtained. Antibody induction is also valuable in other immunologic high-risk patients such as pediatric patients, African-American recipients, previously sensitized patients, repeat transplants, and combined kidney and pancreas transplant recipients. However, with the advent of mycophenolate mofetil, several centers are now using this agent as a primary immunosuppressive agent and have eliminated antibody induction therapy for patients with immediate graft function. With the introduction of anti–IL-2 monoclonal antibodies (daclizumab and basiliximab), several centers are using these agents for induction in patients with delayed graft function and in other immunologically high-risk patients. Polyclonal antilymphocyte agents have also been used successfully in the treatment of steroid-resistant rejection episodes.

TABLE 88.10. Side Effects of Polyclonal Antilymphocyte Agents

Fever and chills
Skin rashes
Hypotension
Acute respiratory distress
Anaphylaxis
Granulocytopenia and thrombocytopenia
Arthralgia and serum sickness
Phlebitis
Immune complex–mediated glomerulonephritis
Opportunistic infections
Posttransplant lymphoproliferative disease

Atgam, an equine polyclonal ATG prepared by immunizing horses with human thymocytes, is the only polyclonal agent approved for use in organ transplant recipients in the United States. The daily dose of Atgam is 10 to 15 mg/kg administered as an intravenous infusion over a period of 4 to 6 hours for 7 to 14 days. Because of the possibility of anaphylactic reactions with Atgam, intradermal skin testing has been recommended. Thymoglobulin is a purified immunoglobulin solution that is produced by the immunization of rabbits with human thymocytes. It has been approved for use in Europe for several years, and is expected to be approved for use in the United States in the relatively near future. Thymoglobulin is administered in a dose of 1.5 mg/kg/day over a period of 4 hours for 7 to 14 days. It consists of antibodies specific for T-cell epitopes including CD2, CD3, CD4, CD8, CD11a, CD18, CD25, human leukocyte antigen [HLA]-DR, and HLA class I. Clinical studies have demonstrated that Thymoglobulin is an effective immunosuppressive agent for the prophylaxis and treatment of acute rejection in allograft recipients. Lymphoglobuline and thymoglobuline are the respective horse and rabbit polyclonal antibodies approved for use in Europe.

In a double-blind, randomized, multicenter, phase III clinical trial, Thymoglobulin was compared with Atgam for the treatment of acute rejection episodes after renal transplantation. A total of 163 patients were enrolled in the study in 29 U.S. transplant centers. Patients were stratified based on the severity of rejection according to the Banff classification of the kidney biopsy specimen, to receive a 7- to 14-day course of either Thymoglobulin (1.5 mg/kg per day) or Atgam (15 mg/kg per day). The primary end point of the study was a successful response defined as a return of the serum creatinine level to or below baseline (day 0 value). Successful response was seen in 88% of Thymoglobulin-treated patients versus 76% of the Atgam-treated patients (P = .027). In each Banff rejection severity category, there was a tendency toward improved response in the Thymoglobulin-treated group when compared with the Atgam-treated group. In addition, recurrent rejection occurred less frequently in Thymoglobulin-treated patients when compared with Atgam-treated patients. Thymoglobulin use was associated with a significantly greater depletion of CD2+, CD3+, CD4+, and CD8+ cells, indicating that the superior T-cell depletion may be responsible for the lower rate of recurrent rejection. A single-center, randomized, double-blind study compared Thymoglobulin with Atgam induction for 7 days in mismatched living-donor or cadaveric renal transplant recipients. This study reported an acute rejection rate of 4.2% with Thymoglobulin and 25% with Atgam (P = .014) at a mean follow-up of 14 months. In addition to less frequent rejection episodes, Thymoglobulin patients also had less severe rejections, less cytomegalovirus (CMV) disease, fewer serious adverse events, but more frequent leukopenia. Although polyclonal antibodies are effective for the treatment of acute rejection, in most instances the monoclonal antibody, OKT3, has tended to supersede the use of polyclonal antibodies.

MONOCLONAL ANTIBODIES

The technology for the production of monoclonal antibodies was described by Köhler and Milstein in 1975, and led to the award of the Nobel Prize for medicine in 1984. The procedure combines the fusion of myeloma cells with immunized spleen cells to produce a hybridoma. This fusion provides the benefits of linking the immortality of the myeloma cell with the antibody production and secretion of the immunized spleen cell. An inbred laboratory mouse is injected with a specific antigen; antibody-producing B lymphocytes from the animal's spleen are harvested and fused with immortal myeloma cells *in vitro*, in the presence of polyethylene glycol, which promotes fusion. The newly created hybridomas are screened for antibody activity. Cells with positive activity are placed into separate culture wells and cloned. The desired hybridomas are then either frozen for future use or are cultured for the production of monoclonal antibody. This process occurs by mass tissue culture or by intraperitoneal inoculation into immunodeficient mice, where they form tumors that produce large amounts of ascitic fluid containing the monoclonal antibody. This highly specific antibody against a single antigenic determinant is then purified and sterilized before use in humans. Because each hybridoma is derived from a single antibody-producing B cell, all antibodies produced by the hybridoma are identical. Until the introduction of anti–IL-2R antibodies, muromonab-CD3 (OKT3) was the only monoclonal antibody in widespread use. Prophylactic use of monoclonal antibodies for induction therapy has been shown to decrease the incidence of acute rejection episodes. OKT3 is also highly effective in reversing acute rejection episodes.

MUROMONAB-CD3 (OKT3)

OKT3 is a murine monoclonal antibody of the IgG_{2a} subclass, specifically directed against the epsilon portion of the CD3 receptor on the surface of the human T cells. The CD3 molecule is closely associated with the TCR. This complex plays a vital role in T-cell function. Antigen recognition by the TCR results in signal transduction via the CD3 molecule and subsequent T-cell proliferation and activation of cytotoxic cells. OKT3 inhibits the CD3/TCR complex, inactivating lymphocytes. After the first dose, OKT3-bound CD3+ cells are opsonized and removed from circulation by the reticuloendothelial system. A decrease in the number of CD3+ T cells occurs during OKT3 therapy, but after cessation of therapy the cell counts return to pretreatment levels. T cells appearing during OKT3 treatment are either coated with the administered antibody or their CD3/TCR is modulated, thus preventing antigen recognition by the CD3+ cells. As a result, the T cells are made immunologically incompetent and they cannot be activated to participate in the immune response against the allograft.

The successful clinical use of OKT3 for the treatment of acute renal allograft rejection was first reported in 1981. The initial multicenter, randomized, prospective study using OKT3 for the treatment of acute rejection reported a rejection reversal rate of 94%, which was significantly better than the 75% reversal rate obtained with steroid treatment. The 1-year graft survival rate for the OKT3-treated group was 62%, as compared with 45% for the steroid-treated group. This study was performed in the precyclosporine era. Following this initial study, numerous similar experiences have been reported with OKT3 in reversing primary and steroid-resistant acute renal allograft rejection, as well as acute vascular rejection. Given the observation that acute rejection is associated with poor long-term graft survival, several centers have employed OKT3 as first-line treatment for Banff grades IIa, IIb, and III acute rejection episodes. Rejection reversal rates of up to 98%, with 1-year post-OKT3 graft and patient survival rates of 87.5% and 95.5%, respectively, have been reported when OKT3 was used as first-line therapy for the treatment of acute rejection episodes.

OKT3 has also been used for induction therapy. Strategies have varied regarding the prophylactic administration of OKT3. It has been used in high-risk patients, such as retransplant recipients, or highly sensitized recipients of first allografts, and in patients with delayed graft function in order to avoid early cyclosporine or tacrolimus exposure. In a multicenter trial comparing OKT3 induction plus triple therapy versus triple therapy with steroids, azathioprine, and cyclosporine, OKT3 prophylaxis significantly decreased the percentage of patients developing rejection (51% versus 66%, $P = .032$), increased the time from transplantation to the first rejection episode (46 days versus 8 days, $P = .014$), and reduced the number of rejection episodes per patient (0.82 versus 1.14, $P = .014$). In addition, a greater percentage of rejection episodes in the OKT3 group were responsive to steroid therapy. Although the 2-year graft and patient survival rates were better in the OKT3 group, they were not statistically significant. In a subsequent analysis of this data, patients were stratified according to the cold ischemia time (24 hours or less versus more than 24 hours). This study revealed that the beneficial effects of OKT3 were mainly observed in patients with prolonged cold ischemia time. In the group with cold ischemia of 24 hours or less, although the mean number of rejection episodes per patient were lower in the OKT3 patients than in the cyclosporine patients, this difference did not reach statistical significance (0.81 ± 0.12 versus 1.06 ± 0.12, $P = .113$ at 1-year and 1.05 ± 0.13 versus 1.15 ± 0.12, $P = .578$ at 5 years). In contrast, in patients with cold ischemia more than 24 hours, OKT3 induction resulted in (a) significantly lower mean number of rejections per patient compared with cyclosporine induction, both at 1-year (0.87 ± 0.11 versus 1.35 ± 0.14, $P = .008$), and at 5 years (1.07 ± 0.12 versus 1.49 ± 0.15, $P = .032$), and (b) significantly better graft survival compared with patients receiving cyclosporine induction both at 2 years (84% versus 64%) and at 5 years (71% versus 56%) after transplantation. In all study patients, there was a nonstatistically significant trend toward higher graft survival rates in the OKT3 group compared with the cyclosporine group (85% versus 75% at 2 years and 73% versus 66% at 5 years $P = .182$).

The most common side effect of OKT3 is the *cytokine release syndrome*, which typically begins 30 to 60 minutes after the administration of the first few doses and may last for several hours. This syndrome is characterized by fever, chills, tremor, nausea, vomiting, diarrhea, headache, myalgia, chest pain and tightness, and wheezing (Table 88.11). This syndrome is believed to be mediated by a massive systemic release of cytokines—tumor necrosis factor-α (TNF-α), interferon-γ (INF-γ), and IL-2 by the activated T cells. OKT3 causes reversible renal dysfunction, also believed to be mediated by high levels of circulating cytokines,

TABLE 88.11. Side Effects of OKT3

Fever, chills, tremors, myalgia
Nausea, vomiting, diarrhea
Chest pain, wheezing
Acute pulmonary edema
Headache, photophobia, aseptic meningitis
Cytokine nephropathy
Opportunistic infections
Posttransplant lymphoproliferative disease
Human antimouse antibody formation precluding further use

thus termed *cytokine nephropathy*. A number of approaches have been used in an attempt to minimize or avoid the cytokine-release syndrome. These include premedication with high-dose methylprednisolone 1 hour before the first dose of OKT3, indomethacin, pentoxifylline, antihistamine, and antipyretics. Severe pulmonary edema may develop in patients who are fluid overloaded before OKT3 administration. It is therefore essential to assess the volume status of the patient before initiating OKT3 treatment and to diurese or dialyze as indicated. Because OKT3 therapy significantly impairs the cell-mediated immunity, patients are prone to develop opportunistic infections and post-transplant malignancies. The usual adult dose of OKT3 for the treatment of acute rejection is 5 mg/day for 7 to 14 days. Some centers have found a lower dosage of 2.5 mg/day to be effective when used for induction therapy.

Production of human antimouse antibodies has profoundly influenced the development of protocols of how OKT3 has been used. Results from the Ortho Multicenter Transplant Study Group revealed that 80% of patients treated with OKT3 5 mg/day for 14 days developed an anti-OKT3 antibody response either during or after the second week of treatment. Concurrent immunosuppressive therapy in this study consisted of azathioprine 25 mg/day and prednisone 0.5 mg/kg per day. In view of this high rate of antibody formation, OKT3 use was often withheld until all conventional forms of reversing rejection had failed. However, several subsequent studies have reported that with the addition of cyclophosphamide or cyclosporine to a regimen of azathioprine and prednisone, or increasing the azathioprine to full dose in conjunction with prednisone, the antibody formation rate has been significantly lowered to 26% to 39%. The anti-OKT3 response consists of both IgM and IgG antibodies with approximately 70% of patients exhibiting an IgM response and 50% developing an IgG response. The antibodies are further characterized as antiidiotypic or antiisotypic in specificity. The antiidiotypic antibody reacts specifically with the idiotypic determinants of OKT3. These determinants are unique to OKT3 and are absent in other IgG_{2a} molecules. The antiisotypic antibody reacts with all murine IgG_{2a} immunoglobulins, even without anti–T-cell specificity, but not with non-IgG_{2a} immunoglobulins. However, only the IgG antibodies that are antiidiotypic in specificity inhibit the ability of OKT3 to bind to T cells. The antiisotypic or IgM antiidiotypic antibodies have not been shown to neutralize the efficacy of OKT3 treatment. Phase II studies are being performed using a humanized form of OKT3 in an attempt to overcome this problem.

Immunologic monitoring plays an essential role in the treatment of patients receiving OKT3. Monitoring can be accomplished by three methods. The most commonly used method is a flow cytometric determination of the lymphocyte subsets to monitor depletion of CD3+ lymphocytes from the peripheral blood. The absolute number of CD3+ cells should remain depressed throughout OKT3 treatment. The guidelines for the number of CD3+ cells varies from less than $10/mm^3$ to less than $50/mm^3$ in different studies. A second method is monitoring OKT3 serum levels by either enzyme-linked immunosorbent assay, flow cytometry, or a cartridge-based enzyme immunoassay. The recommended sample is a 24-hour trough level of plasma or serum for all methods. Studies have shown that OKT3 concentrations in excess of 800 ng/ml are associated with *in vitro* blocking of TCR function. *In vivo*, following a 5-mg/day dose of OKT3, relatively low serum OKT3 levels (less than 800 ng/ml) occur during the first 2 to 3 days of OKT3 therapy. These low levels are related to the drugs binding to the CD3 receptor. After the third dose of OKT3, trough serum concentrations exceed 800 ng/ml and remain at this level until discontinuation of treatment. Serum concentrations become undetectable within 48 hours of discontinuation, owing to the short half-life of OKT3, which is approximately 18 hours. The third modality of immune monitoring is the determination of anti–OKT3-antibody titer, which is useful in patients in whom retreatment with OKT3 may be necessary. Previous OKT3 treatment does not preclude OKT3 reuse. However, it is important to know the patient's antibody status before and during reuse. OKT3 therapy can be reinstituted successfully in patients who are antibody negative or have a low titer (1:100 or less) anti-OKT3 antibody following their first course of OKT3. These patients have rejection reversal rates that are equivalent to those obtained with primary therapy. However, in patients with low-titer antibodies it may be necessary to increase the dose of OKT3 during reuse to overcome the antibody response and achieve depletion of all CD3+ cells. Reappearance of CD3+ cells and fall in serum OKT3 levels during OKT3 therapy are associated with increasing antibody formation. Patients who have a high-titer antibody response (in excess of 1:1000) should be treated with immunosuppressants other than OKT3.

Anti–Interleukin-2 Receptor Antibodies

IL-2 is a cytokine responsible for the growth and proliferation of activated T cells. During an immune response, IL-2 exerts its effects on the T lymphocyte by binding to the IL-2R on the surface of the antigen-activated T lymphocyte. The IL-2R is composed of three distinct membrane components, which are the α chain (T-cell activation antigen [TAC], IL-2Rα, or CD25), β chain (IL-2Rβ, CD122), and the γ chain (IL-2Rγ, CD132). Most resting T, B, and natural killer (NK) cells express IL-2Rβ and IL-2Rγ but not IL-2Rα. IL-2Rα is expressed only on activated T cells. In combination with IL-2Rβ and IL-2Rγ, it forms a receptor complex with high affinity for IL-2. The predominant role of the IL-2 and IL-2R in lymphocyte proliferation and the selective expression of the α chain of the IL-2R on activated lymphocytes led to the identification of IL-2Rα as a potential target for monoclonal antibody therapy. Murine monoclonal antibodies directed against IL-2Rα have been developed and used both in the prevention and treatment of acute rejection after renal transplantation. In a randomized study of 100 primary cadaver renal transplant recipients, the immunosuppressive effect of 33B3.1, a rat monoclonal antibody against the human IL-2Rα, was compared with that of a rabbit polyclonal antithymocyte globulin. It was shown that 33B3.1 was as effective as ATG in the prevention of renal allograft rejection, with fewer infections and side effects. Subsequently, a similar randomized study in combined kidney and pancreas transplant recipients showed a significantly higher rejection rate in patients treated with 33B3.1 monoclonal antibody as compared with rabbit polyclonal ATG. However, in 3-month and 36-month patients, kidney and pancreas actuarial survival rates were similar in the two groups. In another randomized, prospective trial, recipients of primary cadaver allografts were randomized to receive either anti-Tac, another anti–IL-2R monoclonal antibody, in combination with low-dose cyclosporine (4 mg/kg per day), prednisone, and azathioprine or conventional triple therapy with cyclosporine (8 mg/kg per day), prednisone, and azathioprine. A significant reduction in early rejection episodes, and a significant delay in the time to the first rejection episode was noted in the anti-Tac–treated patients. However, there was no difference in the actual or actuarial patient or graft survival between the groups. A pilot study in patients with ongoing acute rejection episodes treated with 33B3.1 anti–IL-2R monoclonal antibody concluded that 33B3.1 therapy was ineffective and the results inconsistent in the treatment of an established acute rejection episode. Anti-Tac and 33B3.1 elicited strong host antimouse and antirat responses primarily of the antiidiotypic

TABLE 88.12. Comparison of Basiliximab and Daclizumab

	Basiliximab (Simulect)	Daclizumab (Zenapax)
Nature	Chimeric (mouse variable region with human constant region)	Humanized [murine hypervariable regions, rest of the molecule (90%) is human]
Mechanism of action	Blocks the binding of IL-2 to its receptor	Blocks the IL-2 pathway by binding to the Tac-subunit of the IL-2 receptor
Half-life	7.2 days	20 days
Saturation	36 days	120 days
Affinity	More (9 × 10^9 mol/L)	Less (3 × 10^9 mol/L)
Recommended adult dosing schedule	20 mg within 2 hours before and 20 mg 4 days after transplantation	Five doses of 1 mg/kg; first dose given within 24 hours before transplantation and four remaining doses at intervals of 14 days
Adverse reactions	Similar to placebo	Similar to placebo
*Results**		
Biopsy-confirmed acute rejection	29.8% versus 44% with placebo (P = .012)	22% versus 35% with placebo (P = .03)
Graft survival	87.9% versus 86.6% with placebo (P = .591)	95% versus 90% with placebo (P = .08)
Patient survival	95.3% versus 97.3% with placebo (P = .293)	98% versus 96% with placebo (P = .51)

*Data from Nashan B, Moore R, Amlot P, et al. Randomized trial of Basiliximab versus placebo for control of acute cellular rejection in renal allograft recipients. *Lancet* 1997;350:1193–1198; Vincenti F, Kirkman R, Light S, et al. Interleukin-2-receptor blockade with Daclizumab to prevent acute rejection in renal transplantation. *N Engl J Med* 1998;338:161–165.

type. The clinical effectiveness was also limited by a short circulating half-life. These shortcomings have been overcome by the development of two engineered anti–IL-2Rα antibodies, basiliximab (a chimeric product) and daclizumab (a humanized product), which have been approved recently for prophylaxis against acute rejection in renal transplant recipients. Table 88.12 compares the features of these two anti–IL-2R monoclonal antibodies.

Basiliximab

Basiliximab is a chimeric (human and mouse) monoclonal antibody of the $IgG_{1\kappa}$ isotype. It is a glycoprotein obtained by continuous culture fermentation of a murine-myeloma cell line, genetically engineered to express plasmids containing the human heavy- and light-chain constant region genes and mouse heavy- and light-chain variable region genes encoding the RT5 antibody that binds selectively and with high affinity to IL-2Rα on activated T cells. It has a half-life of 7.2 days. In adult patients, the recommended regimen is two doses of 20 mg each administered as an intravenous infusion over 20 to 30 minutes through a central or peripheral venous catheter. The first 20 mg dose is given within 2 hours before transplantation. The second dose is given 4 days after transplantation. Two multicenter, randomized, double-blind, placebo-controlled phase III studies using basiliximab have been completed. In the European/Canadian study 21 centers participated. There were 190 intent-to-treat patients in the basiliximab arm, and 186 intent-to-treat patients in the control arm. The incidence of biopsy-confirmed acute rejection 6 months after transplantation was 29.8% in the basiliximab group compared with 44% in the control group (P = .012). The occurrence of steroid-resistant first rejection episode that required antibody therapy was significantly lower in the basiliximab group (10% versus 23.1%, P <.001), and the graft loss at 12 months posttransplantation was comparable in the two groups. The incidence of infection and other adverse events was similar in the two groups. The results of the trial performed in the United States were similar to those obtained in the European/Canadian study. Similar reductions in the first rejection episode (35% versus 52%, P = .002 at 6 months and 38% versus 55%, P = .001 at 12 months) and fewer rejection episodes requiring treatment with augmented immunosuppression other than steroids (25% versus 42%, P = .001) were seen in the basiliximab group. Basiliximab was well tolerated and there was no evidence of cytokine-release syndrome in either study. Antiidiotypic antibodies were detected in 1 of 246 patients treated with basiliximab.

Daclizumab

Daclizumab is a genetically engineered, humanized IgG_1 monoclonal antibody that is produced by recombinant DNA technology. It binds specifically to the α chain of the IL-2R. In a randomized, double-blind, multicenter, phase III trial, daclizumab was compared with placebo. All patients received triple-drug-combination therapy with azathioprine, prednisone, and cyclosporine. Daclizumab (1.0 mg/kg body weight) was administered intravenously before transplantation and followed by once every other week, for a total of five doses. Patients randomized to daclizumab had a lower incidence of biopsy-confirmed acute rejection in the first 6 months after transplantation compared with patients receiving placebo (22% versus 35%, P = .03). In addition, the time to the first rejection episode was significantly prolonged (73 ± 59 versus 30 ± 27 days, P = .008), and the mean number of rejection episodes per patient were significantly lower in the daclizumab group (0.3 versus 0.6, P = .01). There was a decrease in the number of patients requiring antilymphocyte agents for the treatment of rejection in the daclizumab group (8% versus 14%, P = .09). There was no significant difference in the reported adverse events between the two groups, in particular, no concomitant increase in infectious complications or cancers in the daclizumab-treated group was noted. Daclizumab also reduced the acute rejection rate when compared with placebo in combination with dual immunosuppressive therapy of prednisone and cyclosporine (28% versus 47%, P = .001). The safety and efficacy of daclizumab in combination with mycophenolate mofetil and steroids in the absence of calcineurin inhibitors is being studied in a prospective, multicenter trial. Preliminary data from the first 50 patients revealed that acute rejection occurred in 13 patients (26%). The histologic severity of the acute rejection was Banff grade I in 7 patients, and Banff grade IIb in 6 patients. Calcineurin inhibitors were initiated in all patients with acute rejection. Although the idea of maintenance immunosuppression without nephrotoxic calcineurin inhibitors is appealing, long-term graft survival data are required before this regimen can be widely adopted.

MONOCLONAL ANTIBODIES IN EXPERIMENTAL USE

Several monoclonal antibodies have been used in experimental preclinical and clinical studies. Some of the more notable monoclonal antibodies are reviewed briefly here.

Anti–T-Cell Receptor Antibodies

Monoclonal antibodies against the α and β chains of TCR have been produced and tested in clinical trials. They include BMA 031, which is an IgG_{2b} mouse antihuman antibody, and T10B9.1A-31, which is a murine IgM monoclonal antibody.

BMA 031 has been used for the prevention and treatment of allograft rejection as well as graft-versus-host disease following allogeneic bone marrow transplantation. It is directed against a monomorphic part of the human TCR. After the first dose, BMA 031 induces rapid depletion of the CD3+ T cells. However, by the tenth day of therapy, pretherapeutic levels of CD3+ cells appear in the circulation. BMA 031 induces an intense and early sensitization that neutralizes its therapeutic activity. In contrast to OKT3, it does not cause the first-use syndrome despite high levels of TNF, which are seen 1 hour after the first dose of BMA 031. A Scandinavian two-center study using 50 mg of BMA 031 given daily for 7 days to 25 renal transplant recipients with biopsy-proven, steroid-resistant rejection, reported reversal or partial reversal of the rejection episode in all patients. However, 84% of the patients experienced repeat rejections 3 to 46 days after the last dose of BMA 031, requiring treatment with methylprednisolone or rabbit ATG. Graft loss at 1 year was seen in 28% of patients, including two patients with a functioning graft who died of an infection.

T10B9.1A-31 is a nonmitogenic monoclonal antibody that detects an epitope on the α and β chains of the TCR. It does not induce production of cytokines IL-2, interferon-γ, and TNF-α, and therefore does not cause significant first-dose reactions. Phase II clinical trials have demonstrated that T10B9.1A-31 is as effective as OKT3 in reversing acute renal allograft rejection, with fewer untoward effects, less cytokine nephropathy, and fewer serious infections. Human antimouse antibody development was similar to that of OKT3. There was no cross-reactivity with OKT3 in patients treated with T10B9, and there was only 9.7% cross-reactivity to T10B9 in patients treated with OKT3. The main disadvantage of T10B9.1A-31 is the relatively short half-life requiring administration every 8 hours. Interest in this antibody has diminished because of its short half-life.

Anti-CD4 Monoclonal Antibodies

CD4 is expressed on approximately 65% of peripheral TCRαβ+ T cells. CD4+ T cells react predominantly with the class II major histocompatibility complex (MHC) molecules on the antigen-presenting cells. Therefore the CD4 molecule is essential to the early immunologic process involved in allograft rejection, and thus it has become a target for the development of monoclonal antibodies. Interest in clinical transplantation is focused on the potential use of nondepleting anti-CD4 antibodies largely because depletion of CD4+ T cells may lead to prolonged periods of nonspecific immunosuppression. Administration of anti-CD4 monoclonal antibody as the sole immunosuppressive agent has been shown to prolong the survival of skin, cardiac, and renal allografts in rodent and nonhuman primate models. OKT4A is a murine antihuman monoclonal antibody of the IgG_{2a} subclass. In a phase I study, treatment with OKT4A (0.5 mg/kg for 12 days) in addition to combination therapy with cyclosporine, prednisone, and azathioprine was associated with a 2-year graft survival of 95%. Acute rejection occurred in 37% of patients within 3 months after transplantation. A human antimouse antibody response of more than three times pretreatment levels was observed in 84% of patients. OKT4A was well tolerated without first-dose side effects. Detectable OKT4A serum levels and more than 90% CD4-receptor saturation were achieved in almost all patients. There was no evidence of CD4 T-cell depletion. Other anti-CD4 monoclonal antibodies that have been studied include the murine antibodies, Leu-3A and BL4, which interact with distinct epitopes of the CD4 molecule.

Anti–T-12 Monoclonal Antibodies

Anti–T-12 is a mouse monoclonal antihuman antibody that is directed to a lymphocyte-differentiation antigen expressed on mature postthymic cells. In a clinical study, 19 patients with acute renal allograft rejection were treated with anti–T-12 antibody. Seven patients had a reversal of the rejection episode, four patients an equivocal response, and eight failed to respond. Treatment failures were related to the presence of alloantibody-mediated vasculitis. Because of unsatisfactory results, interest in this antibody has declined.

Monoclonal Antibodies Against Adhesion Molecules

Adhesion molecules play an important role in the cell-to-cell interactions pertinent to allograft ischemia, inflammation, and immunity. The role of adhesion molecules during the development of the inflammatory infiltrate that leads to allograft destruction is an area of major interest. Leukocyte function–associated antigen (LFA-1), which belongs to the β2 integrin family, plays an essential role in the adhesion of leukocytes to endothelial cells and to a variety of targets on immunocompetent cells. LFA-1 promotes adhesion through specific interaction through its ligands, intercellular adhesion molecules (ICAM)-1, -2, and -3. LFA-1 is expressed on most leukocytes. ICAM-1 is weakly expressed on resting endothelium, and is induced by activation with IL-1 and TNF. Anti–LFA-1 monoclonal antibodies have been effective in preventing graft rejection following bone marrow transplantation; however, in kidney transplantation, it was unable to reverse ongoing acute rejection episodes. In a multicenter, randomized, open trial in France, a monoclonal antibody directed against the α chain of LFA-1 (Odulimomab) was compared with rabbit ATG as part of a quadruple sequential protocol in 101 patients receiving a first kidney transplant. Anti–LFA-1 or ATG were administered for 10 days after transplantation. The incidence of acute rejection was not significantly different between the groups (36% with anti–LFA-1 versus 35% with ATG). Rejection episodes occurred more often during the induction phase in the anti–LFA-1 group; 11% of patients experienced rejection before day 10 in this group. Actual graft survival at 12 months was similar in the two groups (92% in the anti–LFA-1 group, and 90% in the ATG group). The incidence and severity of infections were comparable in the two groups. Fifty-nine percent of the patients in the anti–LFA-1 group developed IgM or IgG antibodies to the monoclonal antibody after day 15. The need for posttransplantation dialysis was reduced in the anti–LFA-1 group (19% versus 35% for ATG), although the difference was not statistically significant. The authors concluded that the reduced need for dialysis was due to a protective effect of anti–LFA-1 antibody against reperfusion injury. Anti–ICAM-1 murine monoclonal antibody, BIRR1, has been shown to prolong graft survival as a sole immunosuppressive agent in monkeys.

A phase I trial with anti–ICAM-1 monoclonal antibody in a series of 18 kidney transplant recipients who received cadaver-donor renal allografts at high-risk for delayed graft function, reported that BIRR1 was associated with significantly less delayed graft function and rejection in patients with adequate serum levels. However, to date, data from clinical trials using an anti–ICAM-1 monoclonal antibody are limited. In the mouse model, injection of a combination of anti–LFA-1 and anti–ICAM-1 antibodies completely blocked allograft rejection, and indefinite survival of cardiac allografts was obtained after only a 7-day treatment course. This combination, which appears to have a synergistic effect in an animal model, has not been tested in a human trial.

Costimulatory Signals and Fusion Proteins

T cells require two signals for activation. The first is recognition of antigens through the TCR. The second signal is an antigen-independent signal mediated by the interaction of the T-cell surface receptor, CD28, with the B7 ligand. In addition, the CD40 molecule on the antigen-presenting cell (APC), which binds to CD40 ligand (CD40L) on the activated T cell, also appears to provide costimulation to T cells. Studies of T-cell activation have shown that TCR stimulation by itself not only fails to lead to proliferation, but in the absence of a costimulatory signal, induces anergy (a state of unresponsiveness even to appropriate stimuli that persists for several weeks) in the T cell. Selective inhibition of T-cell costimulation using the B7-specific fusion protein, CTLA4-Ig, has been shown to induce long-term allograft survival in rodents. Antibodies preventing the interaction between CD40 and its T-cell–based ligand, CD40L, have been shown in rodents to act synergistically with CTLA4-Ig. In primates, brief induction courses of CTLA4-Ig or CD40L-specific monoclonal antibody, 5C8, alone significantly prolonged rejection-free survival (20 to 98 days). Two of the four animals treated with both agents experienced extended (more than 150 days) rejection-free allograft survival without the need for chronic immunosuppression. This therapeutic approach shows great promise for the achievement of specific acquired immunologic tolerance in organ allotransplantation, the "holy grail" of transplant biology.

SUMMARY

Antilymphocyte antibodies provide effective immunosuppression in organ transplant recipients. They are useful for induction of immunosuppression and treatment of rejection episodes, and have proven to be superior to corticosteroids in these situations. Antilymphocyte antibodies reduce the risk of acute rejection when used for induction therapy, and when used for the treatment of an acute rejection episode, they reverse rejection and improve graft survival. These agents, however, may have several disadvantages. They cause profound immunosuppression and make the transplant recipient prone to serious bacterial, viral, and fungal infections, and for posttransplant lymphoproliferative disorder. They may cause other serious side effects, including the cytokine-release syndrome. Antilymphocyte antibodies may induce a host antibody response that limits further use of the antibody. In addition, this treatment is expensive and adds substantially to the overall cost of transplantation. The optimal use of antilymphocyte antibodies in renal transplantation is not established, and protocols for their use vary considerably among the transplant centers. Additional studies comparing polyclonal antilymphocyte agents and the newer monoclonal antibodies such as the anti–IL-2R antibodies as induction agents in high-risk transplant recipients are clearly warranted.

Selected Readings

Abramowicz D, Norman DJ, Vereerstraeten P, et al. OKT3 prophylaxis in renal grafts with prolonged cold ischemia times: association with improvement in long-term survival. *Kidney Int* 1996;49:768–772.

This study is a long-term analysis of data from patients enrolled in two randomized, prospective trials of induction therapy with OKT3. It concludes that patients receiving organs with long cold ischemia times strongly benefit with OKT3 prophylaxis.

Cosimi AB, Burton RC, Colvin RB, et al. Treatment of acute renal allograft rejection with OKT3 monoclonal antibody. *Transplantation* 1981;32:535–539.

This is the first report of the successful use of OKT3 for the treatment of acute rejection episodes. It depicts the clinical course of the renal allograft patient treated with OKT3 monoclonal antibody.

Gaber AO, First MR, Tesi RJ, et al. Results of the double-blind, randomized, multicenter, phase-III clinical trial of Thymoglobulin versus Atgam in the treatment of acute graft rejection episodes after renal transplantation. *Transplantation* 1998;66:29–37.

Thymoglobulin with Atgam for the treatment of acute rejection episodes after renal transplantation. Successful response was significantly better in Thymoglobulin-treated patients.

Kamath S, Dean D, Peddi VR, et al. Efficacy of OKT3 as primary therapy for histologically confirmed acute renal allograft rejection. *Transplantation* 1997;64:1428–1432.

Single-center study with use of OKT3 as first-line treatment for the treatment of acute rejection episodes. Rejection reversal rate of 98%, with 1-year post-OKT3 graft and patient survival rates of 87.5% and 95%, respectively, are reported.

Masroor S, Schroeder TJ, Michler RE, et al. Monoclonal antibodies in organ transplantation: an overview. *Transplant Immunol* 1994;2:176–189.

This paper presents an overview of the various monoclonal antibodies that are being used either experimentally or clinically for the prophylaxis and treatment of acute rejection episodes.

Nashan B, Moore R, Amlot P, et al. Randomized trial of Basiliximab versus placebo for control of acute cellular rejection in renal allograft recipients. *Lancet* 1997;350:1193–1198.

This is a phase III study to assess the effects of prophylactic treatment with basiliximab. The incidence of biopsy-confirmed acute rejection 6 months after transplantation was 29.8% in the basiliximab group compared with 44% in the control group. No clinically relevant safety or tolerability concerns were reported with basiliximab use in this study.

Norman DJ, Kahana L, Stuart FP Jr, et al. A randomized clinical trial of induction therapy with OKT3 in kidney transplantation. *Transplantation* 1993;55:44–50.

This study compares the safety and efficacy of OKT3 for induction therapy with that of conventional therapy administered to cadaveric renal allograft recipients. OKT3 patients had significantly fewer rejection episodes, longer time to the first rejection episode, and fewer recurrent rejection episodes.

Ortho Multicenter Transplant Study Group. A randomized clinical trial of OKT3 monoclonal antibody for acute rejection of cadaveric renal transplants. *N Engl J Med* 1985;313:337–342.

This multicenter randomized prospective study using OKT3 for the treatment of acute rejection reported a rejection reversal rate of 94%, which was significantly better than the 75% reversal rate obtained with steroid treatment.

Schroeder TJ, First MR, Hurtubise PE, et al. Immunologic monitoring with Orthoclone OKT3 therapy. *J Heart Transplant* 1989;8:371–380.

This article reports the antibody formation rate, lymphocyte subset data, and OKT3 serum concentrations in transplant recipients treated with OKT3. Immunologic monitoring during and after OKT3 use and re-treatment with OKT3 are discussed.

Schroeder TJ, First MR. Monoclonal antibodies in organ transplantation. *Am J Kidney Dis* 1994;23:138–147.

This article is an extensive review of the monoclonal antibodies that have been used in organ transplantation.

Vincenti F, Kirkman R, Light S, et al. Interleukin-2-receptor blockade with Daclizumab to prevent acute rejection in renal transplantation. *N Engl J Med* 1998;338:161–165.

In this phase III trial, daclizumab was compared with placebo. Patients randomized to daclizumab had a lower incidence of biopsy-confirmed acute rejection in the first 6 months after transplantation compared with patients receiving placebo. There was no significant increase in the reported adverse events with daclizumab use.

E: Other Approaches

Thomas Waid

In the 1990s, the antirejection drug armamentarium was substantially augmented. Tacrolimus is becoming more widely used in kidney and kidney–pancreas transplantation and mycophenolate mofetil is replacing azathioprine at many centers with rates of acute allograft rejection episodes of 20% or less being reported. The transplantation community has become less concerned about early graft survival and more concerned about refractory or recurrent rejection and the difficult problem of chronic rejection and graft loss. Conditioning the patient's immune system into a state of specific unresponsiveness undoubtedly prolongs graft survival. Immunologic tolerance, the indefinite survival of a nonidentical transplanted allograft in the absence of ongoing immunosuppressive therapy while maintaining an otherwise normal host immune system, is a highly desirable but as yet unrealized goal. Until this goal can be achieved, blood and/or bone marrow transfusions and immunosuppressive drugs will continue to be the cornerstone of transplantation immunosuppression. This chapter addresses alternative therapies, some established and some experimental, that may emerge in the near future. Finally, the current state-of-the-art of tolerance induction will be briefly mentioned.

BLOOD TRANSFUSION AND BONE MARROW INFUSION

The increased survival of allografts brought about by cyclosporine-based immunotherapy continues to lead many programs away from the deliberate pretransplantation blood transfusion protocol; however, optimum success is still achieved when transfusions are employed. Studies from the Netherlands have demonstrated improved 5-year kidney and heart graft survivals in patients receiving at least one transfusion from a blood donor who is matched for one of the recipient's human leukocyte antigen–reaction of degeneration (HLA-DR) antigens. Matching of at least one HLA-DR locus between the recipient and donor is required, raising the possibility that the suppressive phenomenon is a process in response to HLA-restricted antigen presentation. These patients seem to have fewer cytotoxic T-lymphocyte cell precursors. In a study of 213 patients at the University of California, the role of random blood transfusions in augmenting cyclosporine immunosuppression, 1-year graft survival is reported to be as follows: 0 transfusions, 64% ± 8%; 1 to 5 transfusions, 78% ± 4%; and 6 to 10 transfusions, 97% ± 3%. At 2 years in 183 patients the distribution is similar: 56% ± 8%, 77% ± 4%, and 92% ± 3%, for 0, 1 to 5, and 6 to 10 transfusions, respectively.

Donor-specific transfusions (DST) result in improved graft survival in one haplotype-matched (one HLA-DR mismatched) and zero haplotype-matched donor-recipient pairs in living-related donor transplantation (LRDT). Administration of a 200-ml aliquot of donor-specific blood infused three times at 2-week intervals during which time the recipient is screened for panel reactive antibodies (PRA) will eliminate a potential donor if sensitization occurs in the recipient. If no sensitization occurs, DST can enhance the 2-year graft survival of one haplotype-mismatched transplantation from 65% to 95%, with the additional benefits of fewer posttransplant rejection episodes and less total steroid dose. Random transfusions also improve survival of one haplotype mismatches in LRDT and reduce the risk of developing donor-specific antibodies. Random blood units are also used in protocols for recipients of cadaveric allograft; however, heightened awareness of the dangers of hepatitis C, human immunodeficiency virus (HIV), and cytomegalovirus (CMV), and the improved graft survival in the cyclosporine era, has dampened the enthusiasm for transfusion protocols in the majority of transplant centers. As yet, the mitigating effects of transfusions with the actions of newer immunosuppressive drugs such as tacrolimus and mycophenolate mofetil remain unknown.

Bone marrow infusion is an additional way of introducing donor hematopoietic cells into a recipient in the setting of immunosuppressant conditioning. The goal is that of developing chimerism, or the acceptance of a number of donor lymphoid cells that circulate and persist unscathed in the host. If only a scant number of cells is accepted, the term *microchimerism* is used. The persistence of alloantigen on the graft is needed to maintain the tolerant state. T lymphocytes of donor origin that suppress the immune response have also been identified as mediators and are known as *veto cells*. In a search for mechanisms that promote chimerism as a step in developing tolerance, blood transfusion and bone marrow infusion are gaining interest. With current technology it is possible to harvest stem cells from peripheral blood. Introducing chimerism through stem-cell infusion warrants investigation.

ANTIGEN PRESENTATION AND CELL SIGNALING

Antigen presentation occurs after transplantation and is highly T-lymphocyte (T-cell) dependent; therefore immunosuppressant drugs must directly or indirectly control the T-cell response. We now conceptualize a three-signal model of the immune response starting with antigen presentation by antigen presenting cells (APC) to the T-cell–receptor complex (TCR), which activates the calcium-dependent calcineurin pathway required for cytokine gene transcription and cytokine expression (signal 1, antigen presentation). TCR stimulation by itself does not cause T-cell proliferation; indeed, in the absence of costimulation it induces T-cell anergy. Costimulation occurs when CD28 on the T cell engages its ligand on the APC, such as B7-1 (CD80) and B7-2 (CD86), which then augments and stabilizes mRNA and enhances cytokine gene transcription (signal 2, costimulation). An additional pathway of costimulation is mediated through the CD40 molecule on APCs and the CD40 ligand (CD40L, CD154) on activated T cells. It appears that the CD40L-mediated costimulation can substitute for CD28 signals, preventing T-cell anergy and promoting immune responses. Finally, there is signaling due to activated T cells engaging cytokine receptors and activating signal-transduction pathways leading to cell division (signal 3, cytokine engagement). This is known as the *TOR (target of rapamycin) pathway*. Following the message delivered by these three signals, the cell begins *de novo* synthesis of purine and pyrimidine nucleotides, which in turn allows it to enter the cell cycle and proliferate (Fig. 88.3). As previously discussed, cyclosporine and tacrolimus (see Chapter 88, Part 2B) inhibit calcineurin-dependent signaling. Anti-CD3 monoclonal antibodies (Chapter 88, Part 2D) block antigen presentation to the TCR as one of their actions. These drugs preferentially interfere with the calcium-dependent pathway (signal 1). The newer immunosuppressive drugs are more likely to allow antigen presentation (signal 1), but to inhibit costimulation (signal 2) or to inhibit the TOR pathway (signal 3), the calcium-independent pathways. Because antigen presentation without costimulation may lead to anergy, blockade of costimulatory signals becomes an attractive alternative to the current immunosuppression paradigm of signal 1 blockade. Furthermore, blocking the more distal calcium-independent pathways provides additive and/or alternative immunosuppression to the calcineurin inhibitors. These investigational agents are both chemical and biologic and will be discussed later.

Chemical Agents

Sirolimus (rapamycin) is a 31-membered lactone macrolide antibiotic. It binds to the immunophilin FK binding-protein

12 (FKBP12), yet it affects a different site in the signal transduction pathway. Sirolimus blocks interleukin-2 (IL-2)–mediated signal transduction (signal 3), whereas tacrolimus and cyclosporine prevent the transcription of IL-2 mRNA. The sirolimus–FKBP12 complex does not inhibit calcineurin as does the tacrolimus–FKBP complex and does not inhibit T-cell cycle progression from G0 to G1. It appears that the sirolimus–FKBP complex inhibits a kinase (p70s6 kinase) that increases the protein synthetic activity of the s6 ribosomal protein and prevents T cells from progressing from G1 to S phase of the cell cycle. Sirolimus interferes with calcium-independent signaling pathways in T and B lymphocytes (Fig. 88.3); therefore although sirolimus inhibits T-cell activation caused by antigenic stimulation sensitive to cyclosporine and tacrolimus inhibition (signal 1, calcium-dependent pathway), it also inhibits cyclosporine–tacrolimus–resistant pathways such as stimulation of T cells by IL-2, IL-4, IL-6 and by blocking CD28 (signal 2)-mediated events. Sirolimus also possesses anti–B-lymphocyte activity and at much higher concentrations there is inhibition of lymphocyte-activated killer (LAK) cells, natural killer (NK) cells, and antibody-dependent, T-cell–mediated cytotoxicity (ADCC).

The antiproliferative effects of sirolimus are not limited to the cells of the immune system. Growth factor–induced cell proliferation of fibroblasts, endothelial cells, smooth muscle cells, and hepatocytes is inhibited by sirolimus. In animal studies, there appears to be less transplant coronary arteriopathy in sirolimus-treated recipients of heart allografts. Furthermore, sirolimus appears to be efficacious in preventing chronic rejection, perhaps due to its inhibition of rejection and suppression of growth factor–stimulated arterial smooth muscle proliferation.

The pharmacokinetics of sirolimus have been evaluated, and the half-life in humans is more than 60 hours with 97% of the drug being contained within erythrocytes and leukocytes. High-performance liquid chromatography (HPLC) is the best method to assess blood levels, with a sensitivity of 1 mg/L.

Unlike cyclosporine and tacrolimus, sirolimus does not cause diabetes in nonhuman primates and does not cause renal insufficiency or significant hypertension; however, thrombocytopenia and hyperlipidemia remain clinically significant problems.

Sirolimus first entered into a phase III clinical trial in 1997. This prospective, randomized, double-blind, multicenter trial compared the safety and efficacy of sirolimus with azathioprine added to an immunosuppressive regimen of cyclosporine and glucocorticoids in the prophylaxis of acute rejection. A total of 719 patients were stratified by center (n = 38) and race (23% African-American; 77% non–African-American). Within 48 hours of transplantation, patients were randomly assigned to one of three treatment groups: sirolimus 2 mg/day, sirolimus 5 mg/day, azathioprine 2 to 3 mg/kg per day along with cyclosporine and glucocorticoids. At 210 days, the overall graft and patient survival for the first 450 patients was 97% and 98%, respectively. The rates of acute rejection were as follows: sirolimus 2 mg/

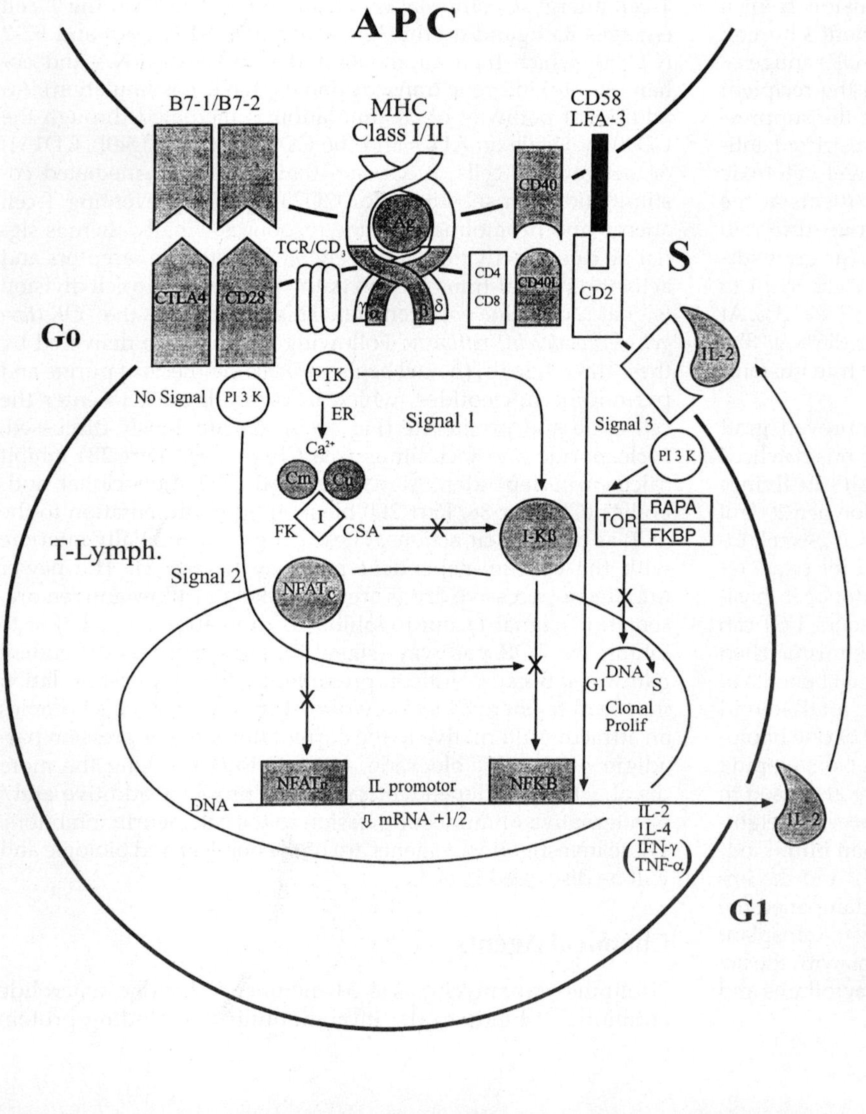

Figure 88.3. T-cell activation by 3 signals: *(1)*, Signal 1, presentation of antigenic peptide to the TCR leads to calcineurin activation and induction of cytokine genes. *(2)*, Signal 2, costimulation as a result of CD28 engaging the B7 family synergizing with signal 1 to induce cytokine production by downregulating inhibitory factor IκBa, a cytosolic protein that prevents nuclear translocation of DNA-binding protein, NFκB. *(3)*, Signal 3, interaction between cytokine (IL-2) and its receptor leading to cell cycling and division through the TOR pathway. Ag, antigen; APC, antigen-presenting cell; cm, calmodulin; cu, calcineurin; CSA, cyclosporine; ER, endoplasmic reticulum; FK, tacrolimus; FKBP, FK binding-protein 12; I, immunophilin; IκB, inhibitor κB; NFAT, nuclear factor of activated T cells; NFκB, nuclear factor κB; PI-3K, phosphatidyl inositol 3′ OH kinase; PTK, protein tyrosine kinase; RAPA, sirolimus; TCR, T-cell–receptor complex; TOR, target of rapamycin.

day, 15%; sirolimus 5 mg/day, 10%; azathioprine/cyclosporine, 24%. The incidence of viral infection was similar in all groups. Based on these promising results, sirolimus was released by the Food and Drug Administration for chemical use for the prevention of renal allograft rejection in 1999.

SDZ RAD (RAD) is a new immunosuppressant related to sirolimus. The introduction of a 2-hydroxyethyl moiety at position 40 of sirolimus increases the polarity of the molecule in an attempt to improve its pharmacokinetic properties. The half-life of RAD is 25 hours, shorter than that of sirolimus in humans. This is probably due to a more rapid systemic clearance despite improved intestinal absorption compared with sirolimus. In recent studies, oral absorption was calculated at 40% for RAD and at 14% for sirolimus. The first-pass clearance of the orally absorbed compounds was 71% and 56% for RAD and sirolimus, respectively. Despite RAD and cyclosporine sharing the cytochrome P450–3A4 metabolic pathway, there was no effect on the steady-state pharmacokinetics of concurrently administered cyclosporine, and the immunosuppressive efficacy of RAD was maintained.

RAD seems to ameliorate the proliferative responses of vascular and bronchial smooth muscle cell in response to injury or chronic rejection. In a double-blind, placebo-controlled, ascending-dose study initiated to evaluate the safety and tolerability of a 4-week course of RAD administered as once-daily doses of 0.75, 2.5, or 7.5 mg in stable renal transplant patients, the toxicities of RAD, myelodepression, and hyperlipidemia were determined to be similar to those of sirolimus. RAD-treated patients also displayed dose-related increases in gastrointestinal and infectious complications; however, these toxicities reversed within 2 weeks. Phase III studies for the *de novo* administration of RAD are ongoing.

Leflunomide (LFM) is an isoxazole compound that originated from an antiinflammatory drug development program at Hoescht-Marion-Roussel (Aventis) pharmaceuticals. In animal studies, LFM has been shown to prevent autoimmune diseases in rodents and chronic graft versus host disease (GVHD) in mice, and to delay the onset of acute rejection of tissues and organ allograft in rodents, dogs, and nonhuman primates. LFM inhibits the formation of xenophile antibodies, prolongs the survival of xenografts, and, additionally, arrests chronic rejection. There have been no human trials of LFM to date other than a pharmacokinetics trial in stable renal allograft recipients.

LFM is a prodrug that is metabolized by the intestinal mucosa and perhaps the liver to an active malononitrilamide form known as *A77 1726.* This molecule inhibits both T- and B-lymphocyte proliferation with a more pronounced effect on the B cell. Although the exact mechanism of action remains to be elucidated, the following is known: (a) At high drug concentrations, A77 1726 inhibits CD3/TCR–induced tyrosine phosphorylation of T lymphocytes; (b) it inhibits tyrosine phosphorylation in murine T-lymphocyte clones after IL-2 stimulation; (c) the activity of tyrosine kinase p56 lck and p59 fyn is inhibited; and (d) there is inhibition of transcription of the early response genes fos and c-jun. A77 1726 does not inhibit IL-2 receptor (IL-2R) expression in response to antigenic stimulation, suggesting a site of action interrupting the signaling between CD3/TCR and protein kinase C activation.

In addition, LFM (A77 1726) may have an effect on nucleotide biosynthesis. The administration of the pyrimidines/cytidine and uridine, but not purine nucleotides, in preparations of Jurkat T lymphocytes treated with A77 1726 antagonized the inhibitory properties of the drug. More specifically, the addition of 2′ deoxycytidine was able to antagonize the antiproliferative effects of A77 1726, but a similar antagonism could be produced neither by thymidine nor 2′ deoxyuridine addition. Deoxycytidine is a substrate for both deoxythymidine triphosphate and deoxycytidine triphosphate, both DNA precursors; thymidine and 2′ deoxyuridine are metabolized only to deoxythymidine triphosphate. Failure of the latter two nucleosides to antagonize the antiproliferative effects of A77 1726 could be due to the inhibition of tyrosine kinase, the enzyme common to the metabolic phosphorylation of both DNA precursors (Fig. 88.4). Thus it would appear that not only does LFM and its active compound inhibit pyrimidine biosynthesis, but like sirolimus it inhibits growth factor–initiated signal transduction.

Unfortunately, the parent compound, LFM, has an extremely long half-life of approximately 150 hours, making dosing adjustments difficult. Currently, work is under way to develop malonitrilamide compounds with more favorable pharmacokinetic profiles for use in the future.

Brequinar sodium is a 4-quinoline carboxylic acid analog. It is known to be a reversible, noncompetitive inhibitor of the enzyme dihydroorotate dehydrogenase, and thereby inhibits the *de novo* pathway of pyrimidine synthesis (Fig. 88.4). Unlike purine synthesis in which the *de novo* pathway predominates in lymphocytes, the salvage pathway is the primary pathway for pyrimidine nucleotide synthesis in activated T cells. The *de novo* pathway becomes critically important when salvage pathways substrates become limited and the intracellular pools of uridine triphosphate (UTP), cytidine triphosphate (CTP), deoxythymidine triphosphate (dTTP), and deoxycytidine triphosphate (dCTP)

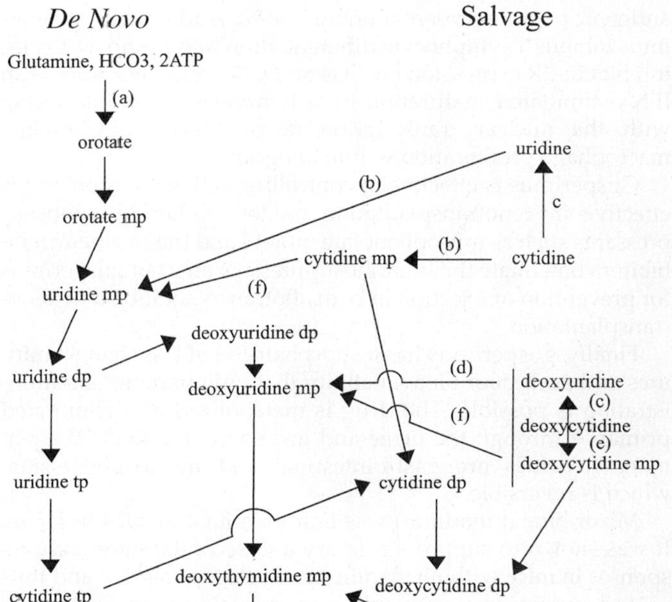

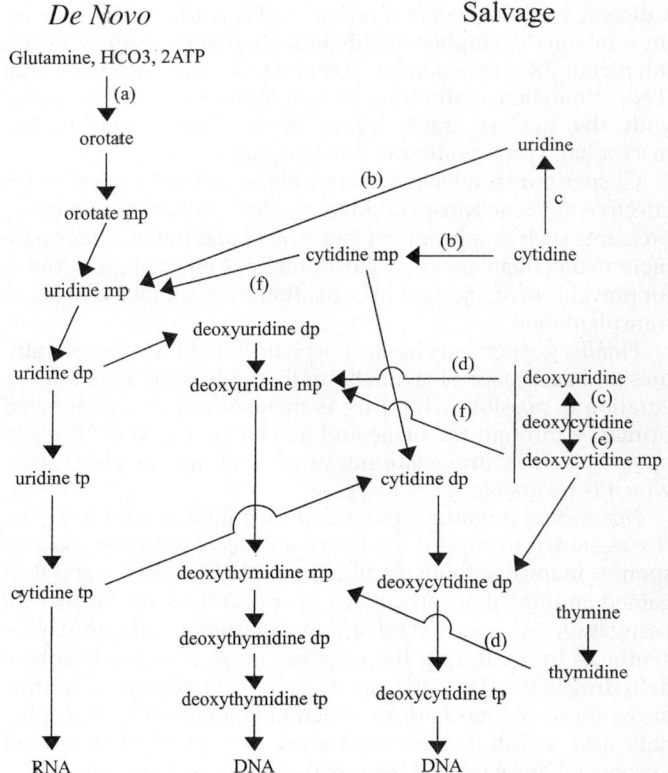

Figure 88.4. Biosynthetic pathway of pyrimidine nucleotides. The antiproliferative effects of A77 1726 are not reversed by thymidine nor 2′ deoxyuridine, both of which are transformed into deoxythymidine triphosphate. Inhibition of thymidine kinase by A77 1726 is a possible mechanism. Additionally, dihydroorotate dehydrogenase is inhibited by A77 1726 and by brequinar sodium, blocking the *de novo* synthesis of uridine monophosphate. dp, diphosphate; mp, monophosphate; tp, triphosphate. Enzymes: (a), dihydroorotate dehydrogenase; (b), uridine-cytidine kinase; (c), deoxycytidine deaminase; (d), thymidine kinase; (e), deoxycytidine kinase; (f), d cmp deaminase.

are depleted in lymphocytes. Because brequinar inhibits both T- and B-lymphocyte proliferation, it is likely that both the salvage and *de novo* pathways must be fully functional for normal lymphocyte proliferation.

Brequinar has been shown to prolong survival of heart, small bowel, liver, and kidney allografts in rats, with some recipients developing donor-specific antigenic tolerance. Brequinar was determined to be as potent an immunosuppressant as sirolimus in a mouse-heart allograft transplantation model; however, the antirejection effects are less striking in larger animals including nonhuman primates.

Unfortunately brequinar is toxic, producing thrombocytopenia, leukopenia, and diarrhea. Increasing the dosing interval from 24 to 48 hours lessens the clinical toxicity; however, the drug is not currently being developed further by the pharmaceutical company that first synthesized it.

Gusperimus was the result of a screening effort in an attempt to discover new anticancer drugs. Because it inhibited murine leukemia cells, further investigations were initiated, demonstrating its immunosuppressive properties. In 1994, the drug was approved for treatment of rejection in Japan.

The mechanisms of action of gusperimus on T and B lymphocytes and antigen-presenting cells are not well understood. Gusperimus binds to a cytosolic protein in the heat-shock protein family called Hsc 70, and analogs of gusperimus, which do not bind to Hsc 70, are not immunosuppressive. Because heat-shock proteins have a peptide-binding groove similar to that of major histocompatibility complex (MHC) class I molecules, it is possible that gusperimus competes for this site and disrupts antigenic peptide presentation by Hsc 70. Additionally, gusperimus inhibits T-lymphocyte differentiation into cytotoxic T cells, inhibits IL-2R expression on CD4 and CD8 cells, interferes with IFNγ-stimulated maturation of B lymphocytes by interfering with the nuclear transcription factor NFκB, and inhibits macrophage proliferation within allografts.

Gusperimus is effective in controlling active rejection and is effective in xenotransplantation models. Other immunosuppressants such as mycophenolate mofetil and the calcineurin inhibitors potentiate the immunosuppressive effect of gusperimus for prevention of rejection in both allotransplantation and xenotransplantation.

Finally, gusperimus has a short half-life of less than 30 minutes and such poor bioavailability that only parenteral administration is possible. The drug is metabolized and eliminated primarily through the urine and less so via the liver. The primary toxicities are gastrointestinal and myelosuppression, which is reversible.

Mizoribine (brendinin) was first identified in 1974 in Japan. It was shown to suppress primary and secondary antibody responses in mice without significant myelosuppression and thus gained an immediate advantage over azathioprine. Further investigation revealed that mizoribine interfered with purine biosynthesis by inhibiting the enzyme, inosine monophosphate dehydrogenase (IMPDH), in the *de novo* pathway of purine biosynthesis. Its mechanism of action is identical to mycophenolic acid, which is approved for use in the United States and Europe, whereas mizoribine remains approved only in Japan.

Mizoribine is more immunosuppressive and less hepatotoxic and myelotoxic than is azathioprine. Mizoribine is also more cyclosporin and steroid sparing than azathioprine. It does not interrupt early G_1 events after T-lymphocyte stimulation such as mRNA elaboration and IL-2 synthesis, and expression is seen in cells treated with the drug. Rather, mizoribine appears to interrupt progression of the cell cycle from G_1 to S.

The toxicity of mizoribine is increased in declining renal function, producing higher plasma levels of the drug. In dog studies, hemorrhagic and erosive enteritis have been seen and there is a degree of myelosuppression as there is with mycophenolate, which may require a dosage adjustment. Because mycophenolate mofetil is approved for use in the United States and Europe, it is unlikely that mizoribine will be developed outside Japan unless some clear advantage over the former can be shown. Thus far there appears to be none.

FTY720, unlike any other immunosuppressant drug as yet discussed, possess the unique mechanism of affecting lymphocyte trafficking. Administration of FTY720 results in a marked reduction of peripheral blood lymphocytes due to cell emigration to lymph nodes and Peyer's patches. There is no effect on circulating neutrophils and monocytes, keeping host resistance intact.

FTY720 appears to be synergistic with cyclosporine and sirolimus, prolonging allograft survival *in vitro*. There are reports that FTY720 induces lymphocyte apoptosis *in vivo* in rats and reverses active rejection in rat-liver allografts. In addition, there is evidence that the agent affects the expression of adhesion molecules on lymphocyte surfaces.

Total Lymphoid Irradiation and Local Allograft Irradiation

Total lymphoid irradiation (TLI) is an effective immunosuppression technique. Usually, a dose of 800 to 2,000 cGy [centi Gray; 1 Gray (Gy) equals 100 rad] is administered in 80 to 100 cGy fractions. TLI has been administered to patients in addition to antilymphocyte globulin, steroids, and cyclosporine, or bone marrow infusion. Although bone marrow infusion enhances the effect of TLI, the best results appear to occur when cyclosporine is administered concurrently. TLI has been used successfully as a conditioning regimen for living-related transplantation; however, it is not effective for cadaveric transplantation in that it requires too much time to deliver adequate doses.

Local graft irradiation is an option in patients not responding to immunosuppressive manipulation. In this scenario, the patient is treated with 150 cGy every other day for a total dose of 450 cGy (some centers use up to 600 cGy). Methylprednisolone 500 to 1,000 mg is administered before the first radiation fraction and on the nonradiation days.

Photopheresis

Photopheresis is a unique therapy that is currently approved for the treatment of cutaneous T-cell lymphoma (mycosis fungoides). It requires the administration of a compound, 8-methoxypsoralen (8-MOP). When 8-MOP is photoactivated by ultraviolet light it binds with the pyrimidine bases of DNA in nucleated cells, preventing their replication. When these cells are reinfused into transplanted patients, the immune system is stimulated against these cells and circulating clones of the treated cells. There also appears to be apoptosis of the photoactivated cells. The procedure requires that blood be removed from the patient, which is then heparinized and collected in the photopheresis unit. The white cells are separated by centrifugation, exposed to ultraviolet light, and then returned to the patient. The plasma and erythrocytes are also returned to the patient having never been irradiated.

A group in Italy reported two patients with multiple rejection episodes after transplantation refractors to steroids and OKT3 responding to photopheresis. Each patient received two weekly treatments followed by two treatments at 2-week intervals during the second and third months, and then monthly treatments for 3 months. Steroids were reduced to 8 mg daily in both patients following photopheresis. Photopheresis has been useful in treating refractory rejection in heart and lung transplantation as well as treating GVHD and may be more widely used in the future.

Tolerance

This chapter began with a brief statement on donor-specific tolerance and it is fitting that it should end with a discussion of the same. Inducing a state of tolerance or allospecific immune unresponsiveness that leads to indefinite engraftment even upon withdrawal of immunosuppression remains a desirable but elusive goal in humans. As we determine more information about altering antigen recognition and blocking costimulatory signals, tolerance becomes more realistic.

The basic mechanisms of T-lymphocyte tolerance are as follows: clonal deletion, anergy, and suppression. Clonal deletion involves the physical elimination of T lymphocytes in the thymus and is the basis of central or thymic-derived tolerance. T-lymphocyte death can occur only in the periphery by activation of programmed cell death through fas protein (CD95) or by the loss of survival genes. Anergy, the state of specific immune unresponsiveness, occurs when a T lymphocyte fails to become activated and proliferate in response to antigenic exposure. As stated previously, T-lymphocyte activation requires not only antigen and T-cell–antigen receptor (TCR) engagement, but also a costimulatory signal. Antigen recognition without costimulation results in T-lymphocyte anergy. Suppression is the ability of cells from tolerative animals to suppress the antigen-specific immune response of the host after adoptive transfer. Cytokine-mediated suppression (IL-4, IL-10) from a predominance of T-helper type 2 (Th2) cells and "veto" (CD3−/CD8+) cells may help maintain tolerance, the latter by the selective destruction of allospecific-host T-lymphocytes precursors. The result of veto cell action appears to be peripheral clonal deletion or anergy maintained despite the addition of IL-2–positive or functional APCs. Microchimerism, the permanent persistence of a small number of donor-origin hematopoietic cells in a recipient, may provide a continuous stimulus by secreting soluble MHC molecules. It may also be the result of tolerance due to the inability of tolerant animals to remove donor cells via immune responses.

Tolerance may be induced by the following strategies: formation of bone marrow chimeras, inhibition of antigen recognition, inhibition of costimulation, inhibition of adhesion molecules, use of synthetic peptide, and acquired thymic tolerance. The infusion of donor bone marrow into immunosuppressed recipients can induce tolerance possibly through suppressor cell (Th2 or veto cell) formation or through the development of microchimerism. Clonal deletion is the proposed mechanism. Inhibition of antigen recognition by anti-CD3 and anti-CD4 antibodies has been tolerogenic in animals; however, human data have been disappointing. In this case, production of anergy is the presumed mechanism. Inhibition of costimulatory signals required for T-lymphocyte activation and of prevention of T-cell anergy induction appears to be useful in promoting tolerance. The blockade of CD28/B7 ligation by CTLA4Ig fusion protein and antibody against CD40 ligand (anti-CD154) allows recognition of antigen and still results in anergy, due to deletion and suppression via Th2 switching. Adhesion-molecule inhibition disrupts the ability of the T lymphocyte to adhere to cellular targets. Interruption of intercellular adhesion molecule-1 (ICAM-1) and its ligand, leukocyte function–associated antigen-1 (LFA-1), inhibits costimulation in response to this ligation. Graft survival has been prolonged in mice and in primates when this pathway is inhibited. Anergy may be produced by anti–ICAM-1 and anti–LFA-1 antibodies; clinical trials are ongoing. Finally, synthetic peptides that correspond to highly conserved regions of MHC class I and class II molecules can immunomodulate T-lymphocyte responses. Anergy and suppression occur.

Tolerance may yet become a clinical reality; however, considerable investigation is necessary. Current immunosuppressive regimens using signal 1 inhibitors such as cyclosporine and tacrolimus may actually abrogate tolerance, and withholding such agents would be unethical due to their current success in transplantation practice. Only well-designed clinical trials that minimize the clinical risk to the transplanted patient while optimizing currently recognized tolerogenic strategies will provide future direction in this area.

Selected Readings

Blackman M, Kappler J, Murrade P. The role of the T-cell receptor in positive and negative selection of developing T-cells. *Science* 1990;248:1335–1341.
This is a good review of the role of the T-cell–receptor complex's influence on T-cell populations.

Cao WW, Kao PN, Chao AC, et al. Mechanisms of the antiproliferative action of leflunomide. *J Heart Lung Transplant* 1995;14:1016–1030.
The authors review the proposed mechanism of action of leflunomide, a possible future antirejection medication.

Chow B, Saper V, Strober S. Renal transplant patients treated with total lymphoid irradiation show specific unresponsiveness to donor antigens in MLR. *J Immunol* 1987;130:3746–3752.
The authors review total lymphoid irradiation as an adjunct immunosuppressant or possible conditioning modality.

Dorsch S, Roser B. Suppressor cells in transplantation tolerance: identification and probable mode of action of chimeric suppressor T-cells. *Transplantation* 1982; 33:525.
The authors present a good review of the known mechanisms of suppressor T cells on immune recognition.

Kahan BD. New immunosuppressive drugs—pharmacologic approaches to alter immuno regulation. *Ther Immunol* 1994;1:33–44.
This paper is a good review of newer immunosuppressive agents, their kinetics, and potential use.

Morris RE. Commentary on new xenobiotic immunosuppressants for transplantation: where are we, how did we get here, where are we going? *Clin Transplant* 1993;7(1):138–146.
This is an excellent review of new immunosuppressants with xenotransplantation in mind.

Morris RE. Mechanisms of action of new immunosuppressive drugs. *Kidney Int* 1996;53(suppl):S26–S38.
This is an excellent review of new immunosuppressant agents.

Murgia MG, Jordan S, Kahan BD. The side effect profile of sirolimus. A phase I study in quiescent cyclosporine-prednisone treated renal transplant patients. *Kidney Int* 1996;49:209–216.
The authors state their findings after treating stable renal transplant patients with rapamycin (sirolimus).

Schuler W, Sedruni R, Coltens S, et al. SDZ RAD, a new rapamycin derivative. *Transplantation* 1997;64:36–42.
This is an early study of a rapamycin derivative with a similar immunosuppressant mechanism but a shorter duration of action.

Sehgal SN. Rapamune (sirolimus, rapamycin): an overview and mechanism of action. *J Therap Drug Monitor* 1995;17:660–665.
This is an excellent review of the known mechanisms of action (TOR inhibition) of sirolimus.

Suthanthiran M, Morris RE, Strom TB. Immunosuppressants: cellular and molecular mechanism of action. *Am J Kid Dis* 1996;28:159–172.
This is an excellent broad-spectrum review of current immunosuppressive therapy.

Thomas JM, Verbanc KM, Thomas FT. The veto cell mechanism in transplant tolerance. *Transplant Rev* 1991;5:209229.
This is a good review of cellular tolerating mechanisms with emphasis on the role of veto cells.

Yoo EK, Rook AH, Elenitsas R, et al. Apoptosis induction by ultraviolet light and photochemotherapy in cutaneous T-cell lymphoma: relevance to mechanism of therapeutic action. *J Invest Derm* 1996;107:235–242.
This paper discusses proposed mechanisms of photochemotherapy in attenuation of T-cell responses.

Zimmerman JJ, Kahan BD. Pharmacokinetics of sirolimus in stable renal transplant patients after multiple oral dose administration. *J Clin Pharmacol* 1997;37: 405–415.
This is a good review of kinetics of sirolimus after administration to stable renal transplant recipients.

CHAPTER 89

Complications of Renal Transplantation

PART 1
Infections in Renal Transplant Recipients

Nina E. Tolkoff-Rubin and Robert H. Rubin

Because of advances in a wide variety of disciplines over the past 3 decades, renal transplantation has become the most effective means of rehabilitating patients with end-stage renal disease. Thus at many centers, more than 90% 1-year allograft and more than 95% patient survival are now being achieved following unrelated-donor renal transplantation. Despite this success, infection still occurs in more than two-thirds of transplant recipients and remains the leading cause of death in this patient population. A number of factors combine to pose particular challenges to the clinician in preventing and treating infection in the transplant patient:

1. The combination of life-long immunosuppressive therapy, the presence of an organ that differs from the recipient at both major and minor histocompatibility loci, and the occurrence of infection with a group of agents (particularly viruses) that are both modulated by the immunosuppressive therapy being administered and are themselves immunomodulating has created a series of clinical syndromes and effects that are unprecedented in human biology and medicine. ***Infection and rejection, the two most important barriers to successful transplantation, are closely intertwined, linked both by the immunosuppressive therapy required and by the similar array of cytokines, chemokines, and growth factors elaborated during the course of both processes.***
2. The potential sources of infection for the transplant patient are many: endogenous, environmental, the allograft itself, and the wide array of pathogens that circulate in the general community.
3. Because the immunosuppressive therapy necessary to prevent and treat rejection will also suppress the inflammatory response to microbial invasion, the signs and symptoms of infection will usually be muted until late in the clinical course. As a result, the microbial burden will be increased and clinical disease will often be further advanced at the time of diagnosis. Because the survival of transplant patients with infection is usually related to how quickly an etiologic diagnosis is made and therapy instituted, great skill and attention to detail is required on the part of the transplant clinician in recognizing early, often occult, signs of infection.
4. Because the consequences of clinical infection in these patients can be so devastating, the emphasis should be on infection prevention. Hence, *the therapeutic prescription for the transplant patient should be regarded as having two components: an immunosuppressive program to prevent and treat rejection; and an antimicrobial program, which is closely linked to the nature and intensity of the immunosuppressive program, to make it safe.*

RISK OF INFECTIONS IN THE TRANSPLANT RECIPIENT

The risk of infection in the renal transplant patient is largely determined by the interaction of three factors: (a) the occurrence of *technical/anatomic mishaps* that result in devitalized tissue, fluid collections, and the prolonged requirement for indwelling drains, catheters, endotracheal tubes, and vascular access devices that compromise the integrity of the primary mucocutaneous barriers to infection; (b) the *epidemiologic exposures* the patient encounters; and (c) the individual's *net state of immunosuppression.* As far as the first of these is concerned, it should be emphasized that there is no more unforgiving form of surgery than that performed in immunosuppressed individuals, and attention must be paid not only to the operation itself, but also to the management of the wound, intravascular access, endotracheal tube, and drainage catheters in the perioperative period. In particular, skin maceration by tape, prolonged venous access with central lines, indwelling bladder catheters, and aspiration pneumonia must be assiduously avoided.

The epidemiologic exposures of importance for the transplant patient can be divided into two general categories: those occurring in the community and those occurring within the hospital. The community exposures of particular importance include the following: the geographically restricted systemic mycoses (blastomycosis, coccidioidomycosis, and histoplasmosis); tuberculosis; *Strongyloides stercoralis;* and such respiratory viruses as influenza, respiratory syncytial virus, parainfluenza, and the adenoviruses. As far as the mycoses and tuberculosis are concerned, three patterns of disease may be observed: reactivation of an old, dormant focus of infection, with secondary dissemination; progressive primary infection, with primary dissemination; and superinfection on new exposure to the pathogen, again with a significant risk of dissemination. In each case, immunosuppression attenuates the host response, thus amplifying the extent of infection and the opportunity for disseminated disease.

In the case of *S. stercoralis,* this parasite can remain asymptomatically in the gastrointestinal tract for decades. With the initiation of immunosuppressive therapy, life-threatening disease of two types ensues: a hyperinfestation syndrome characterized by hemorrhagic pneumonia and hemorrhagic enterocolitis; and a disseminated strongyloidiasis syndrome, in which the organism migrates throughout the body, often accompanied by Gram-negative bacilli from the gut and therefore the frequent clinical presentation of disseminated strongyloidiasis as Gram-negative bacteremia or meningitis unresponsive to appropriate antibacterial therapy. Because of the gravity of these syndromes, transplant candidates with history of residence in regions where *Strongyloides* is present should be screened serologically (routine screening of stool specimens for ova and parasites has a sensitivity of less than 20% for this organism), with the presence of circulating antibody triggering preemptive therapy with thiabendazole or ivermectin before transplant.

Community-acquired respiratory virus infection is a particular problem in transplant patients, with a higher rate of viral pneumonia, pulmonary superinfection with a variety of pathogens, and need for hospitalization than what is observed in the general population. Unfortunately, other than attempts to avoid exposures, strategies for dealing with this category of infection are less than satisfactory; indeed influenza vaccination, although recommended, is less effective than in the nonimmunosuppressed host, and antiviral therapy remains unsatisfactory for these infections.

As important as community exposures are to the transplant patient, exposures within the hospital to such organisms as *Aspergillus* species, *Legionella* species, and such Gram-negative bacilli as *Pseudomonas aeruginosa* are even more important. In these cases nosocomial exposures to contaminated air or potable water can occur either in a domiciliary or nondomiciliary pattern. The term *domiciliary* is employed to describe the circumstance in which the exposure occurs on the ward where the patient is housed and often there is the clustering of several cases in time and space to suggest the presence of a clinically important environmental hazard; the term *nondomiciliary* is employed to describe the circumstance in which the exposure occurs in a central location such as an operating room or a radiology suite where a patient is taken for an essential procedure; such environmental hazards are often difficult to recognize because of the lack of clustering of cases on a single ward. Nondomiciliary exposures and outbreaks are actually more common than domiciliary, and constant surveillance is necessary to identify such hazards.

An increasing problem for transplant patients is the person-to-person transmission within the hospital of such emerging pathogens as methicillin-resistant *Staphylococcus aureus,* vancomycin-resistant enterococci, highly resistant Gram-negative bacilli, and fluconazole-resistant *Candida* species. These organisms are not infrequently transmitted on the hands of medical personnel and, although a problem throughout the hospital, have a special impact on the transplant patient. Accordingly, active surveillance for nosocomial hazards, assiduous handwashing, the institution of stringent infection-control measures when a problem is identified, and appropriate antibiotic use is essential in the care of these compromised hosts. We have likened transplant, and other immunosuppressed, patients to "sentinel chickens" that will be affected by any excessive traffic in microorganisms that exists in their environment.

The net state of immunosuppression is a complex function determined by the interaction of a number of factors: the dose, duration, and temporal sequence of immunosuppressive therapy; the presence or absence of leukopenia, breaches in the mucocutaneous barriers, and such metabolic abnormalities as uremia, protein-calorie malnutrition, and, perhaps, hyperglycemia; and the presence of infection with one or more of the immunosuppressing viruses such as cytomegalovirus, Epstein-Barr virus, the hepatitis viruses, the human immunodeficiency virus, and, perhaps, human herpesvirus-6. Although immunosuppressive therapy is the dominant determinant of the net state of immunosuppression, two statistics drawn from our own transplant experience illustrate the multifactorial nature of this function: transplant patients with a serum albumin less than 2.8 g/dl have a 10-fold increase in the risk of life-threatening infection; 90% of opportunistic infections occur in patients with preexisting viral infection; indeed, the 10% exceptions are almost invariably a clue to the presence of a significant environmental hazard and resulting exposure.

The interaction between the net state of immunosuppression and the environmental exposures should be regarded as a semiquantitative one: if the net state of immunosuppression is minimal, then only an overwhelming exposure will cause disease; conversely, if the net state of immunosuppression is great, then minimal exposure to commensal organisms may cause disease.

TIMETABLE OF INFECTION

Following renal transplantation and the initiation of the standard regimens of immunosuppression that are used today, the patient is subject to a stereotyped pattern of infections at different time points; that is, an infectious disease syndrome such as pneumonia can occur at any time in the posttransplant course, but the etiology of the pneumonia is different at different times. This "timetable of infection" (Fig. 89.1) is useful in three different ways: in the differential diagnosis of the individual patient with an infectious disease syndrome; as an infection control tool because exceptions to the timetable usually connote an unrecognized environmental hazard and exposure; and as the basis for designing cost-effective, targeted antimicrobial preventative strategies. The posttransplant course is conveniently divided into three time periods, each with a different pattern of infection. These time periods are as follows:

1. *First Month Posttransplant:* There are three causes of infection in this time period: (a) infection that was present before transplant and not eradicated before transplantation, a circumstance to be avoided if at all possible; (b) infection conveyed by the allograft that was seeded from the donor or in the harvesting procedure; and (c) the same bacterial or candidal infections of the surgical wound, lungs, urinary tract, or vascular access that occur in any individual undergoing comparable surgery, with the consequences often greater in transplant patients. Although great effort should be expended to avoid the first two of these, because these infections can be catastrophic (particularly the presence of bloodstream infection in the donor or recipient, which can infect the vascular anastomosis, causing a mycotic aneurysm at risk for rupture), the last category accounts for more than 95% of infections in this time period. The leading factor in the pathogenesis of this class of infection is the technical skill with which the surgery and postoperative care is accomplished. Thus infection in this time period is best prevented

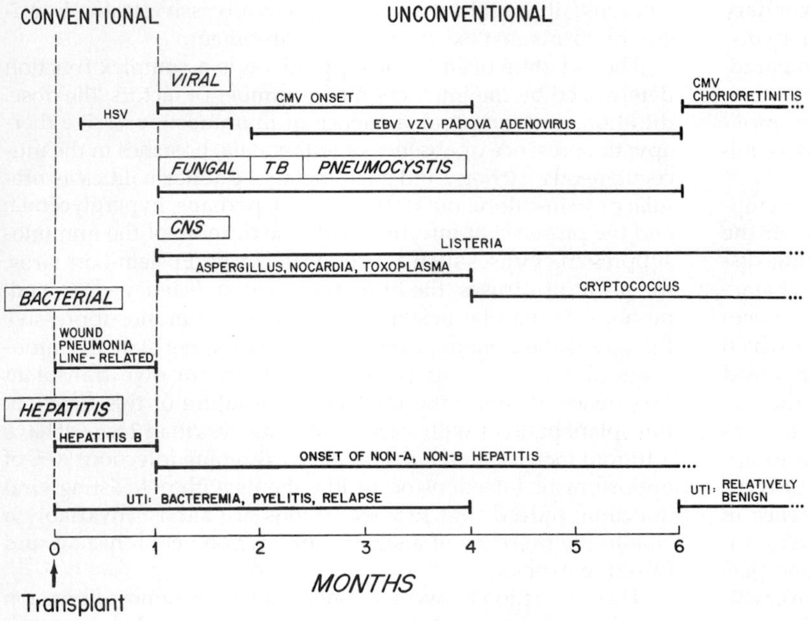

Figure 89.1. Timetable for the occurrence of infection following renal transplantation. (Reproduced with permission from Rubin RH, Wolfson JS, Cosimi AB, et al. Infection in the renal transplant recipient. *Am J Med* 1981;70:405–411.)

by technically impeccable surgery and a brief course of perioperative antibiotics (e.g., a single dose of cefazolin). Noteworthy by their absence in this time period, when daily doses of immunosuppressive drugs are at their highest, are opportunistic infections, unless an unusually intense exposure occurs. This observation emphasizes that it is the sustained effect of immunosuppressive therapy that is important, not the daily dose.

2. *One to Six Months Posttransplant:* In this time period there are two major categories of infection: (a) symptomatic viral infection, particularly with cytomegalovirus, Epstein-Barr virus, and, perhaps, human herpesvirus-6; and (b) opportunistic infection due to such organisms as *Pneumocystis carinii, Listeria monocytogenes,* and *Aspergillus* species, which occur without an undue exposure, due to the effects of sustained immunosuppression and the presence of immunomodulatory viral infection. Accordingly, infection during this time period is best prevented with the proper use of antiviral strategies especially aimed against cytomegalovirus, which itself accounts for 70% of febrile episodes during this time period; a low-dose trimethoprim-sulfamethoxazole prophylaxis (which effectively eliminates *Pneumocystis, Listeria, Nocardia,* and, perhaps, *Toxoplasma,* infection), and ensuring quality of the air the patient breathes (including the use of HEPA filters when necessary) are useful measures.
3. *More than Six Months Posttransplant:* Patients more than 6 months posttransplant can be divided into three general categories, with differing risks of infection: (a) the 80% of patients with good allograft function on maintenance doses of immunosuppression who resemble the general community, with the major problems being due to community-acquired respiratory viruses and urinary tract infection; (b) the 10% of patients with chronic viral infection, particularly with hepatitis B and C viruses and who are at major risk for progressive organ dysfunction and/or viral induced malignancy; and (c) the 10% of patients with a poor result from transplantation; that is, poor graft function and a history of excessive exposure to immunosuppression (the "chronic ne'er-do-wells") who are at the highest risk of any transplant patient for disseminated opportunistic infection (due to such species as *Cryptococcus neoformans, Pneumocystis carinii, Nocardia asteroides, Aspergillus* species, and the geographically restricted systemic mycoses). The chronic ne'er-do-wells merit lifetime trimethoprim-sulfamethoxazole prophylaxis and, possibly, fluconazole prophylaxis. In addition, consideration should be given to the possibility of stopping immunosuppression and returning to dialysis.

INFECTIONS OF PARTICULAR IMPORTANCE IN THE RENAL TRANSPLANT RECIPIENT

Herpes Viruses

The human herpesviruses—cytomegalovirus (CMV), Epstein-Barr virus (EBV), herpes simplex viruses 1 and 2 (HSV-1 and HSV-2), varicella-zoster virus (VZV), and human herpesviruses-6, -7, and -8 (HHV-6, -7, and -8) are the most important group of pathogens affecting the transplant recipient. These DNA viruses share several characteristics that make them particularly effective pathogens in this patient population; discussion of some of these characteristics follows:

1. *Latency:* All human herpesviruses exhibit the property of latency; once infected with the virus, one stays infected for life (the laboratory marker for this being the presence of circulating antibody to the virus, seropositivity), with the potential for reactivating the virus in response to certain stimuli. Among these stimuli are proinflammatory cytokines (particularly tumor necrosis factor [TNF]) and certain immunosuppressive agents such as antilymphocyte antibodies and cytotoxic drugs, but not cyclosporine, tacrolimus, or prednisone—these last drugs will amplify the level of any replicating virus that is present.
2. *Cell Association:* All the herpesviruses are highly cell associated, meaning that transmission between individuals requires intimate contact, blood transfusion, or transplantation of a latently infected allograft. Systemic dissemination of the virus within the individual patient occurs via infected cells, rendering humoral immunity inefficient and cell-mediated immunity essential. The key host defense against these viruses is virus specific, major histocompati-

bility complex–restricted cytotoxic T cells (i.e., the aspect of host defense most inhibited by current immunosuppressive regimens).

3. *Direct and Indirect Effects of the Herpesviruses:* The clinical effects of the herpesviruses on the transplant recipient can be divided into two general categories: the *direct* production of infectious disease syndromes; and the *indirect* effects of cytokines, chemokines, and growth factors elaborated in response to viral replication. Possible indirect effects of these viruses are of three types: a global immunosuppressive effect that predisposes to opportunistic superinfection with a variety of fungal and bacterial pathogens, a role in the pathogenesis of allograft injury, and a role in the pathogenesis of certain forms of malignancy (Table 89.1).

Cytomegalovirus

CMV is the single most important microbial pathogen identified in transplant patients. Three patterns of transmission of CMV are recognized: (a) *Primary infection,* in which latently infected cells from a seropositive donor are transmitted to a seronegative recipient (D+R−), with 60% of these individuals becoming ill; more than 90% of the time, the cells are within the allograft, whereas in the remainder, the virus is transmitted in viable leukocytes in blood products; (b) *reactivation infection,* in which endogenous latent virus of a seropositive individual reactivates after transplantation (D−R+), with 10% to 20% of these individuals becoming ill; and (c) *superinfection,* in which the allograft donor and recipient are both seropositive (D+R+), but the virus that reactivates is of donor origin, with 20% to 30% of these individuals becoming ill. Clinical illness here is used to mean the direct infectious disease consequences of CMV replication. In addition, asymptomatic viral replication is not uncommon with each of these patterns of infection. An important unanswered question is whether such asymptomatic replication has significant indirect consequences on the allograft recipient.

Intravenous ganciclovir at a dose of 5 mg/kg twice daily (with dosage decrease for renal dysfunction) for 2 to 3 weeks (ideally, until viremia is cleared, as assessed by antigenemia or quantitative polymerase chain reaction assay) is more than 90% effective in treating symptomatic disease. Relapses occur in approximately 60% of patients with primary infection, and in approximately 15% of those who are seropositive. This can be decreased by following the intravenous therapy with oral ganciclovir at a dose of 1 gram thrice daily for 3 months. A variety of approaches to the prevention of CMV disease have been taken, including hyperimmune globulin, high-dose oral acyclovir, and oral valacyclovir. The approach we advocate, using a combination of intravenous and oral ganciclovir, as well as viremia monitoring, is delineated in Table 89.2.

Epstein-Barr Virus

EBV is an occasional cause of a mononucleosis syndrome in transplant recipients. However, its major effect is its role in the pathogenesis of posttransplant lymphoproliferative disease (PTLD). Current concepts of the pathogenesis of this process suggest that EBV replication in the oropharynx results in the infection, transformation, and immortalization of B cells—the first step in the development of lymphoproliferative disease. In nonimmunosuppressed adults (more than 95% of whom are seropositive for EBV), a very active surveillance mechanism based on virus-specific cytotoxic T cells eliminates these transformed B cells. In the transplant patient, antilymphocyte antibody therapy increases the level of EBV replication, and both cyclosporine and tacrolimus are potent inhibits of the surveillance mechanism, thus making possible the development of PTLD. Risk factors for PTLD include primary EBV infection, high-dose immunosuppression (particularly with cyclosporine, tacrolimus, and/or antilymphocyte antibodies), and previous symptomatic CMV disease (which increases the risk of PTLD 7- to 10-fold).

The clinical features of PTLD can include one or more of the following: unexplained fever, tonsillitis, gastrointestinal bleeding, obstruction or perforation, hepatocellular dysfunction, focal brain disease, lymphadenopathy, and even invasion of the allograft. Some patients will respond to a cessation of immunosuppression; the optimal therapy of the remainder is still unclear. Far better would be the prevention of this condition, perhaps with antiviral therapy whenever immunosuppression is

TABLE 89.1. Direct and Indirect Effects of Herpesviruses on the Renal Transplant Recipient[a]

Virus	Direct Effects	Indirect Effects
Cytomegalovirus	Fever, mononucleosis, pneumonia, gastrointestinal ulceration, hepatitis (encephalitis)	Predisposes to opportunistic superinfection; allograft injury; increases risk of PTLD 7- to 10-fold
Epstein-Barr Virus	Mononucleosis, PTLD	Predisposes to opportunistic superinfection; PTLD
Varicella-Zoster Virus	Primary: disseminated visceral disease Reactivation: dermatomal zoster	???
Herpes Simplex Virus	Mucocutaneous ulceration (CNS, disseminated infection)	???
Human Herpesvirus-6	Fever, mononucleosis, ? (hepatitis, encephalitis)	? predisposes to opportunistic superinfection; ? allograft injury; synergy with CMV
Human Herpesvirus-7	????	????
Human Herpesvirus-8	????	Kaposi's sarcoma

[a] Unusual effects are placed in parentheses.
CMV, cytomegalovirus; CNS, central nervous system; PTLD, posttransplant lymphoproliferative disorder.

TABLE 89.2. Preventative Strategies Directed Against Cytomegalovirus (CMV) Employed at the Massachusetts General Hospital[a]

High Risk Patients
1. *Patients at risk for primary infection:* (donor seropositive, recipient seronegative): intravenous ganciclovir 5 mg/kg/day for 7 days, followed by oral ganciclovir 1 g three times a day for 3 months
2. *CMV seropositive patients treated with antilymphocyte antibodies for rejection:* intravenous ganciclovir 5 mg/kg/day during the antilymphocyte antibody therapy, followed by oral ganciclovir 1 g three times a day for 3 months
3. *Prevention of symptomatic relapse in patients with symptomatic primary infection:* intravenous ganciclovir 5 mg/kg twice daily until viremia is cleared (e.g., 3 weeks), followed by oral ganciclovir 1 g three times a day for 4 months
Lower Risk Patients
1. *CMV seropositive patients not receiving antilymphocyte antibody therapy:* oral ganciclovir 1 g three times a day for 3 months or No prophylaxis, but weekly viremia monitoring by polymerase chain reaction or antigenemia assays, with preemptive therapy (intravenous ganciclovir 5 mg/kg twice daily for 2 weeks) given for asymptomatic viremia

[a] All transplant recipients should receive CMV seronegative or leukocyte-free blood products when red cell or platelet transfusions are necessary. Ganciclovir dosages are modified in the face of renal dysfunction.

intensified. Further discussion on PTLD is found in Chapter 89, Part 6.

Varicella-Zoster Virus

Reactivation VZV infection, causing dermatomal zoster, occurs in approximately 10% of transplant patients. Unlike the situation in lymphoma patients, visceral dissemination rarely occurs in the transplant patient, and treatment with oral famciclovir or valacyclovir is quite effective. In contrast, primary VZV is a devastating disease in this patient population, causing pneumonia, encephalitis, hepatitis, pancreatitis, disseminated intravascular coagulation, and gastrointestinal ulcerations. This requires early recognition and high-dose intravenous acyclovir therapy (10 mg/kg every 8 hours, with dosage decreases for renal dysfunction). It is our policy to check every transplant candidate's VZV antibody status before transplant, and to administer the varicella vaccine to seronegative individuals, documenting seroconversion in response to the vaccine. Any posttransplant patient who is seronegative should receive prompt administration of zoster immune globulin on exposure to this virus, again with close clinical follow-up to document protective efficacy.

Herpes Simplex Virus

HSV infection in the transplant recipient is almost invariably mucocutaneous reactivation infection (orolabial, usually caused by HSV-1, and anogenital, usually caused by HSV-2). Occasional cases of aseptic meningitis due to these viruses can occur, but both encephalitis and disseminated visceral HSV infection are quite rare in these patients. Although the severity of attacks and the number of recurrences are both greater than in the general population, herpetic infection in the transplant patient responds quite well to oral acyclovir, 200 mg five times per day, for 7 to 14 days. Although anti-HSV prophylaxis does work, our preference is to design prophylactic programs aimed primarily at CMV and EBV, knowing that virtually any antiviral program effective for these two viruses will also be effective in preventing HSV.

Human Herpes Viruses-6, -7, -8

These herpesviruses have only recently been described, and their precise role in the transplant patient is still being defined. At present, the most information is available on HHV-6, which has been linked to such infectious disease syndromes as unexplained fever, mononucleosis, bone marrow dysfunction, and encephalitis. Most provocative data are suggesting that HHV-6 may play a role in the pathogenesis of allograft dysfunction, and that dual infection with HHV-6 and CMV may cause significantly worse disease than either by itself. HHV-7 replication can be demonstrated in transplant recipients, but the clinical effects are still unclear. HHV-8 has been linked to the pathogenesis of Kaposi's sarcoma, a tumor that is far more common in transplant patients than in the general population.

Hepatitis Viruses

Both hepatitis B and hepatitis C (HBV and HCV) can have an important effect on the transplant patient. The primary acquisition of HBV at the time of transplant carries a high risk of acute hepatic failure, and it is fortunate that with modern screening of potential donors that this is now a rare event *provided an appropriate blood sample (not diluted by transfused blood) is tested.* Potential donors who are HBsAg positive should be avoided; kidneys from donors who are HBsAb or HBcAb positive can be safely transplanted with minimal risk of HBV transmission. The bigger issue with HBV is the appropriate approach to HBV carriers with chronic renal failure, because posttransplant immunosuppression will markedly increase the level of viral replication. Untreated HBV infection in the transplant patient carries a more than 50% risk of cirrhosis and/or hepatocellular carcinoma at 10 years posttransplant. The advent of chronic lamivudine therapy in these patients has been a significant advance, although escape drug-resistant mutants may emerge after 12 to 15 months of therapy. Fortunately, other drugs (such as lobucavir) effective against HBV are in development, and it is likely that a multidrug regimen akin to that used in acquired immunodeficiency syndrome (AIDS) will be the standard of care in a relatively short period.

With the improved control of HBV in dialysis patients, HCV has become the major cause of chronic liver disease in transplant patients. Chronic hepatic dysfunction due to HCV occurs in 5% to 15% of renal transplant recipients, with 15% to 25% of these individuals developing cirrhosis and/or hepatocellular carcinoma at 10 years posttransplant. The most effective therapy currently available for HCV infection posttransplant is the combination of interferon and ribavirin, although sustained remission with this program is observed in the minority of patients. HCV is effectively transmitted by transplantation of organs from an anti-HCV–positive donor, with a transmission efficiency of approximately 50% (these are the ones harboring replicating virus in their blood). There is, however, considerable controversy regarding whether such donors should be used, because primary HCV infection acquired by this route usually does not cause difficulty in the first 5 to 7 years posttransplant. Uncommonly, a more accelerated form of liver disease is encountered, as well as cryoglobulinemia resulting in membranoproliferative glomerulonephritis in the allograft. Our policy is to reserve allografts from anti-HCV–positive donors for elderly patients, highly sensitized patients, and those with an emergent need for transplantation because of lack of dialysis access; the use of such kidneys in children is avoided. Further discussions on this topic and on the issue of liver disease in transplant recipient are found in Chapter 89.

Fungal Infection

Fungal infections in the renal transplant patient can be divided into two major categories: the geographically restricted systemic mycoses such as blastomycosis, coccidioidomycosis, and histoplasmosis; and the opportunistic fungi (most commonly *Candida* species, *Aspergillus* species, and *Cryptococcus neoformans*). With the exception of candidal infection, all of these have a pulmonary portal of entry, with the subsequent potential for systemic dissemination. A variety of clinical syndromes should suggest the possibility of noncandidal infection: unexplained fever, unexplained nonproductive cough, focal nodularity or infiltrate on chest radiograph, and sites of metastatic infection (most commonly the skin, the central nervous system, and the bones and joints). Early diagnosis is essential in treating these infections and requires an aggressive biopsy approach to unexplained focal abnormalities. Amphotericin B remains the cornerstone of primary therapy for these infections with fluconazole providing a far less toxic alternative in the management of cryptococcosis.

Candidal infection is primarily a mucocutaneous process, with breaks in the integrity of these surfaces permitting bloodstream invasion and dissemination. Whereas mucocutaneous infection (skin, pharynx, or esophagus) usually responds to topical therapy with nystatin or clotrimazole, bloodstream infection always requires systemic therapy with amphotericin or fluconazole. A particular problem in renal transplant patients, especially those with impaired bladder emptying, is the development of obstructing fungal balls at the ureterovesical junction (with ascending infection, pyelonephritis, and dissemination). Because of the difficulty in managing this entity, we advocate aggressively treating even asymptomatic candiduria with systemic antifungal therapy such as fluconazole, or the combination of low-dose amphotericin and flucytosine.

URINARY TRACT INFECTION

Before the advent of effective prophylaxis, urosepsis was the most common form of life-threatening bacterial infection observed in the transplant recipient, with an overall incidence of 30% to 60%. In the first 6 months posttransplant, in particular, there is a high risk of transplant pyelonephritis and bacteremia, even in the absence of instrumentation or technical problems with the transplant. In the late period, more than 6 months posttransplant, unless a urologic abnormality such as a stone or a stricture is present, most urinary tract infections are unassociated with pyelonephritis and are easily treated. Most transplant groups now employ prophylaxis with either low-dose trimethoprim-sulfamethoxazole or a fluoroquinolone, which has essentially eradicated urosepsis, for a minimum period of 6 to 12 months posttransplant.

PRINCIPLES OF ANTIMICROBIAL THERAPY IN THE TRANSPLANT RECIPIENT

The cornerstone of immunosuppressive programs today is the calcineurin antagonists cyclosporine and tacrolimus. Both may be affected by antibiotics, either their metabolism (the key step in the metabolism of both drugs is via hepatic P450-linked enzymes) or in the production of synergistic nephrotoxicity (Table 89.3). Knowledge of these interactions should affect both the choice of antibiotics (e.g., β-lactams instead of aminoglycosides and fluconazole instead of amphotericin whenever possible) and the dosing of the immunosuppressive agents.

TABLE 89.3. Interactions of Antimicrobial Agents with Cyclosporine and Tacrolimus

1. Upregulation of the metabolism of cyclosporine and tacrolimus, resulting in decreased blood levels, lower than expected immunosuppressive effect, and an increased risk of allograft rejection. Examples: rifampin, nafcillin, and isoniazid.[a]
2. Downregulation of the metabolism of cyclosporine and tacrolimus, resulting in increased blood levels, greater than expected immunosuppressive effect, an increased susceptibility to infection, and an increased risk of drug-induced nephrotoxicity. Examples: macrolides (erythromycin, azithromycin, and clarithromycin) and azoles (ketoconazole, itraconazole, and fluconazole).[a]
3. Idiopathic interaction with cyclosporine and tacrolimus to produce an accelerated and more severe form of nephrotoxicity. Examples: aminoglycosides, amphotericin, vancomycin, high-dose trimethoprim-sulfamethoxazole, and high-dose fluoroquinolones.[b]

[a] These effects usually begin 5 to 14 days after initiating or discontinuing the antimicrobial agent and can be managed by careful monitoring of cyclosporine blood levels and then making appropriate dosage adjustments following both the initiation and completion of therapy.

[b] These effects are idiosyncratic, can occur with the first dose of the antimicrobial agent, and cannot be managed by monitoring cyclosporine levels.

The three different modes in which antimicrobial drugs can be used follow:

1. A *therapeutic* mode, in which antimicrobial agents are administered to treat established disease.
2. A *prophylactic* mode, in which nontoxic antimicrobial agents are administered to all individuals to prevent an infection that is both common enough and important enough to merit such an approach.
3. A *preemptive* mode, in which antimicrobial agents are administered to a subgroup of patients before the appearance of clinical disease. This is predicated on the use of a laboratory marker or patient characteristic that identifies that subgroup of individuals with the highest risk of serious disease at a time when antimicrobial intervention would be maximally effective in aborting the disease process.

Because of the emphasis on infection prevention in transplant patients, there is particular attention to the use of prophylactic and preemptive strategies in these patients.

Selected Readings

Basgoz N, Preiksaitis J. Post-transplant lymphoproliferative disorder. *Infect Dis Clin North Am* 1995;9:901–923.
A complete review of pathogenesis, clinical manifestations, and management.

Fishman JA, Rubin RH. Infection in organ-transplant recipients. *N Engl J Med* 1998;338:1741–1751.
A complete review of the most important infections occurring in organ transplant recipients and their clinical management and prevention.

Hadley S, Karchmer AW. Fungal infections in solid organ transplant recipients. *Infect Dis Clin North Am* 1995;9:1045–1074.
A comprehensive summary of the epidemiology, pathogenesis, and clinical management of this important class of infection in organ transplant recipients.

Rubin RH. Infectious disease complications of renal transplantation. *Kidney Int* 1993;44:221–236.
A detailed review of the clinical consequences of infection in the renal transplant recipient.

Terrault NA, Wright TL, Pereira BJG. Hepatitis C infection in the transplant recipient. *Infect Dis Clin N Amer* 1995;9:943–964.
A balanced view of a controversial subject.

PART 2

Surgical Complications of Transplant Recipients

Robert Mendez and Arturo Martinez

Improved renal allograft success rates seen in the 1980s, related in large part to improved immunosuppressive medications such as cyclosporine, have made renal transplantation the treatment of choice for patients with end-stage renal disease. In 1997, the United Network of Organ Sharing (UNOS) noted that more than 45,000 people are on the waiting list, with one new patient added every 20 minutes. Unfortunately, organ procurement has reached a plateau during the past several years, making organ access even more difficult at a time of increased need. These circumstances have led to two major situations that impact the incidence of surgical complications, namely, the liberalization of recipient criteria as more individuals desire transplantation, and secondly, the expansion of organ-donor criteria to less pristine donors. With the scenario of more difficult recipient patients being transplanted and progressively more fragile and marginal kidneys being used, it becomes even more imperative that surgical techniques in both organ retrieval and allograft implantation is accomplished with great precision. In addition, postoperative care must be given maximum attention. This short review will cover the surgical complications and outline their treatment.

VASCULAR COMPLICATIONS

Arterial stenosis occurs in approximately 1% of transplant recipients. The causes of renal artery stenosis (RAS) include not only mechanical kinks or twists, but also reaction to suture placement material, intimal injury from the perfusion canula, intimal hyperplasia, arterial narrowing with external iliac arterial placement, acquired extraluminal fibrosis, and native renal artery disease (i.e., atherosclerosis, fibromuscular disease, polyarteritis nodosum). The development of new onset hypertension that is difficult to control is a clue to a possible renovascular problem. At times, the differential diagnosis of chronic rejection is difficult to ascertain. Thomas Hefty correctly points out that the presence or absence of a bruit over the graft is of no diagnostic significance. Similar problems can occur with segmental ischemia or thrombosis in patients with multiple renal arteries.

Doppler ultrasonography and spiral magnetic resonance images can ascertain certain lesions, although the most accurate diagnosis is made by renal angiogram. Treatment can be accomplished many times by angioplasty with exploration, and revascularization may be necessary, although the incidence of graft loss (±30%) is high especially in cadaveric allografts with compromised function. Renal vein thrombosis may be due to several factors: (a) ligation of an accessory renal vein that is too large; (b) narrowing of the renal vein lumen from repair of branch vessel leaks; (c) venous lacerations at the time of retrieval, especially with right renal vein lesions during retrieval of the liver; and (d) as a complication of the extension of a deep venous thrombosis.

Perhaps the most serious vascular complication is stump blow out following a transplant nephrectomy. This usually occurs only in an infected field. Simple ligation of the allograft vessels with graft removal in the face of an abscess is usually insufficient, requiring excision of the foreign material, and oversewing of the vessels or a venous path are the preferred treatments.

Right vein syndrome can be addressed in cadaveric allografts by simply lengthening the renal vein by the width of the vena cava as described by John Barry, or use of a venous patch for extension. Also of great benefit is to ligate all the branches of the internal iliac vein, in order to mobilize the external iliac vein as much as possible.

Lastly, renal transplantation can cause vascular compromise distally to the ipsilateral leg. This can occur from a raised intimal internal flap due to improper suture placement, trauma to the artery during vascular occlusion, atheroemboli from dislodged plaque, and vascular steal in a patient with severely compromised distal runoff.

RENAL COMPLICATIONS

Calyceal Fistulas

Calyceal fistulas usually occur secondary to partial infarction of renal tissue caused by the ligation of an accessory renal artery, and/or due to large wedge biopsies usually taken on marginal kidneys. This latter situation usually occurs on the bench where an inadvertent opening of the calyx is not as readily apparent. Most of the time, accessory renal arteries can be ligated if they are in the upper or middle pole areas and supply less than 10% of the kidney. However, if there is slightly higher than 10% renal parenchymal involvement, infarction of the parenchyma and calyx of that area may lead to necrosis and calyceal fistulization. With lower pole accessory arteries, calyceal and renal pelvic necrosis can occur and also cause pelvic-calyceal fistulization. Diagnosis of this event can be accomplished by both analysis of perinephric fluid, which will accumulate, or by nuclear scan techniques. Treatment can be accomplished by either heminephrectomy or wedge excision of the necrotic tissue with meticulous closure of the calyx by 4.0 Vicryl suture and approximation of parenchymal tissue with surgical pledgets and 2.0 chromic mattress sutures. Drainage with an internal ureteral stent is also recommended along with perinephric closed-suction drainage. The incidence of calyceal disruption or pelvic-calyceal fistulization is less than 1% in most series.

Goldblatt Kidney Phenomenon

A Goldblatt kidney phenomenon can occur when subcapsular hemorrhage develops following thrombosis of a small cortical vessel. This can ultimately lead to cortical necrosis and loss of the allograft if the tamponade is not quickly relieved. Duplex ultrasonography and nuclear renography are the best modalities to diagnose the severe complications in the clinical setting of severe hypertension, anuria, and a falling hematocrit. Surgical intervention is mandatory. Capsulotomy and meticulous hemostasis is the treatment of choice. Partial nephrectomy may also be curative, and lastly, if cortical necrosis is extensive, a nephrectomy is indicated.

Renal Cortical Abscesses

Renal cortical abscesses develop from hematogenous seeding. Ascending infections are from occult mechanical problems in a cadaveric donor. An aggressive systematic approach to this serious problem will minimize patient morbidity and preserve allograft function. First, broad spectrum antibiotics should be instituted immediately. Next, urinary obstruction should be relieved with a ureteral stent or percutaneous nephrostomy. The abscess should be aspirated for culture and drained percutaneously if possible. Having managed the acute problem, the etiology of the abscess may then be pursued. Frequently, treatment may necessitate open drainage or partial or total nephrectomy.

Renal Allograft Rupture

Spontaneous allograft rupture most commonly occurs secondary to accelerated acute rejection and may be life threatening. Immediate surgical intervention is necessary and, most commonly, allograft nephrectomy is required. In this day of histocompatibility excellence, this occurrence is rare but is still seen. Allograft rupture resulting from other causes such as renal vein thrombosis or partial kinking of the renal vein can, at times, be treated more conservatively with renal vein thrombectomy and/or correction of the renal deformity. Review of the literature demonstrates a rather dismal result at attempted salvation with less than 30% salvaged in those particular instances.

Renal Calculi

Calculi within a transplanted kidney is not a rare event in as much as secondary hyperparathyroidism is known to continue in 30% to 50% of patients receiving transplants. In addition, a high percentage of patients continue to be or become hyperuremic, predisposing them to stone formation. In our series of more than 2,000 patients, 2 Staghorn calculi were found, ranging from 1 to 7 years postoperatively. Diagnosis is frequently made by the presence of recurrent urinary tract infections, hematuria, and, at certain times, oliguria, as well as on radiographic studies. Therapy should be attempted to remedy the cause of the calculi by either metabolic therapy and/or relief of any obstructive pathology that exists. Removal of the stone can presently best be afforded by endourologic technique. Endoscopic therapy and stone extraction must be accompanied by ureteral stent placement, and also wound drainage; however, persistent calyceal fistulization or pyelocutaneous fistulization is a significant risk.

Renal Carcinoma

It is well documented that immunosuppression in the previously uremic individual predisposes significantly to the development of malignancies. Although most of these consist of skin cancers and lymphomas, occasional renal cell carcinoma is encountered in transplantations. More commonly however, it is found to be retained in native allografts where acquired renal cystic disease has been shown to develop especially in individuals on long-term hemodialysis. Transitional cell carcinoma has also been reported and both malignancies have been associated with hematuria, whereas cases have also been reported in which it is believed the tumor has been transplanted within the kidney at onset. Therapy should only be radical nephrectomy and immediate cessation of immunotherapy. Urothelial tumors, if occurring within the bladder, may be approached in the routine manner as that of nontransplanted individuals. However, if they occur within the transplanted kidney or ureter, a nephrectomy is indicated.

URETERAL COMPLICATIONS

By far the most common surgical complications seen in renal transplant recipients are those associated with ureteral problems. Ureteral complications have been reported from 3% to 27% by numerous experienced transplant centers. The most common cause is terminal ureteral necrosis with leak. This event is most commonly associated with ischemic damage to the ureter at the time of donor nephrectomy and more commonly seen in living-donor nephrectomies than in cadaveric-donor nephrectomies. Its event is accompanied by oliguria, ureteral cutaneous fistulization, and perinephric fluid collection with azotemia, and at times, hydronephrosis. Occasionally, hematuria may also be seen. Attempts at more conservative therapy with antegrade ureteral stent placements have been experienced as unrewarding and prompt and immediate surgical exploration with either reimplantation of the ureter or a ureteroureterostomy or ureteropyelostomy is the treatment of choice. Ureteral stent should be placed at the time of surgical repair and left indwelling for a minimum of 3 weeks. Attention should be paid to generous excision of the ureter to fresh-bleeding and tissue viability with spatulated ends being accomplished in a ureteroureterostomy. When the aforementioned recommendations for the development of extra vesicoureteral implants are followed, ureteral complications are noted to be significantly less. Upwards of 90% of ureteral complications occur the first 6 weeks following transplantation. It can be seen in a delayed fashion following acute rejection episodes. It is well known now that acute rejection episodes not only effect parenchymal tissue but also have a profound effect on the ureter as well, causing ischemia, edema, and at times, necrosis. Other forms of ureteral stenosis and obstruction can also occur due to implantation. This may occur due to greater tightening the extra vesicle tunnel, or to kinking of the ureter upon establishing the intravesical tunnel. At times, the kidney of the donor has double and triple ureters. Under these circumstances, some degree of compromise of vascularization of the terminal part of the ureter can cause one or two fistulae to occur. Separate reimplantation of these ureters should then be accomplished and/or the effected ureter reestablished in continuity with a ureteroureterostomy of the native ureter. It has been our experience that native nephrectomies are not required with the necessary use of the native ureter for a ureteroureterostomy. Native nephrectomies have only been required in less than 1% of those cases in our series. Significant other ureteral events also can occur, such as ureteral calculi, which can be removed endoscopically, either retrograde or antegrade. Another rare complication previously seen has been double-luminal ureteral stent migrations requiring endourological antegrade retrieval.

In the case of en bloc pediatric kidney implantation, ureteral necrosis may occur, compromising both ureters if they have been spatulated together. For this reason, sequential ureteroneocystostomies is the preferred method of implantation by the author.

BLADDER COMPLICATIONS

Most significant bladder complications can be obviated by careful urologic evaluation of the patient before transplantation. If there are any symptoms, historic problems, or findings noted on physical examination of the lower genitourinary system, or history of infections, further urologic evaluation of the potential recipient should be pursued, to include, at minimum, urine cultures, urinalysis, and a voiding cystourethrogram. Depending on any abnormalities found, further urologic evaluation should then ensue. Postoperatively, perhaps the most common complication that occurs is a vesicle fistula. It is our custom to close any bladder opening in a three layer manner using absorbable 4.0 Vicryl sutures on the mucosal layer in a running fashion, following by a 2.0 running Vicryl suture on the muscularis layer with a third embrocating layer of muscularis and adventitia with another 2.0 suture. A Foley catheter should be left in place for 4 to 5 days if a formal cystotomy is made. If the transplant team uses the extravesical ureteral implantation, the bladder catheter #18 may only be left in for 2 to 3 days. At times, hematuria will be seen and cystoscopy may be indicated under those situations. Most of the time, a minimal bladder leak can be treated conservatively with prolonged catheterized drainage and a suprapubic closed suction drainage. If after a 2- to 3-week period a closure has not occurred, a formal exploration, excision, and closure of the bladder in a three-layer manner can be accomplished as mentioned previously. On rare occasions, a foreign object or calculus may be seen in the bladder and this can usually be treated transurethrally.

PENIS

Preputial Phimosis

Preputial phimosis is a condition in which the penile foreskin is unable to be retracted. This condition is usually a preexisting problem seen especially in diabetic males with a history of recurrent balanitis. Treatment includes good diabetic control, hygiene, and circumcision.

A more common occurrence is the development of a paraphimosis during the urethral catheter insertion. This is an iatrogenic problem in which the foreskin, after being retracted to insert the urethral catheter, is not reduced at the end of the procedure. Paraphimosis causes strangulation of the glans penis and severe edema of the foreskin. Reduction of the foreskin in the vast majority of patients can be achieved by "stuffing" the glans penis back through the preputial ring. A dorsal slit incision of the prepuce may sometimes be necessary. Priapism can occur from intrapelvic trauma or from impaired venous outflow, but this is a rare complication.

URETHRAL INJURIES

Urethral problems at the time of transplant can easily be avoided by a careful voiding history at the time of transplant evaluation. Any patient with a history of voiding difficulty undergoes evaluation with a voiding cystourethrogram. The study will uncover potential urethral problems such as a urethral stricture. The latter may make catheterization very difficult. Ideally, this is treated at the time of transplant with dilation or internal urethrotomy. Preoperative correction is recommended only in patients who will have native urine output to prevent restenosis from a "dry anastomosis."

IMPOTENCE

Although a majority of men are impotent due to their uremia, chronic dialysis, and multiple antihypertensive medications, more than 50% will have return of normal potency following successful transplantation. There is a 65% chance of vasculogenic impotence if both internal iliac arteries have been used, whereas only 10% have vasculogenic impotence after the first transplant. Because of this, young men and diabetics are revascularized using the external iliac artery with an end-to-side anastomosis preserving the circulation to the internal iliac artery.

For men who develop impotence, we recommend treatment only after 9 to 12 months posttransplant. By this time, immunosuppression has been reduced to a stable minimum and the patient's physiologic and psychologic condition is stable. Workup should be undertaken as with any other patient, with a careful sexual history and hormonal profile. Transplant patients can be successfully treated with vasoactive agents such as intracorporeal injection of papaverine, phentolamine, and prostaglandin E_2, as well as penile prosthesis and external vascular constrictor devices. The new drug Viagra has recently been shown to be successful in the treatment of both organic and psychogenic impotency.

PROSTATE

Prostatitis

Prostatitis can occur in any male with prolonged urethral catheter drainage. The catheter facilitates retrograde migration of perineal organism into the urethra, prostate, and bladder. The catheter may also obstruct the outflow of prostatic effluent. Since the advent of the extravesicle ureteroneostomy (Lich-Gregoir procedure), urethral catheters are left in place for much shorter time periods (less than 4 days), therefore making this is a rare complication. Patients present with frequency, urgency, dysuria (especially a prolonged ache at tip of penis), and, rarely, urinary retention. Patients should be treated aggressively with broad-spectrum antibiotics avoiding aminoglycosides.

With the exception of renal tumors from acquired cystic disease in end-stage renal disease patients, there is no increased risk of urologic tumors in transplant patients. Therefore transplant recipients should have routine prostate malignancy monitoring as with the normal population with determination of serum prostate-specific antigen (PSA) in patients over the age of 40 to 45 years and TRUS prostate biopsy dictated by the digital rectal examination (DRE). Patients diagnosed with treatable prostate cancer should be approached in the same manner as nontransplanted males with normal renal function. Cessation of immunosuppressive therapy is not advocated by the author in individuals whose PSA remains zero. With recurrent or palliative therapy, immunosuppression is simply dropped to levels at which allograft function is not impaired.

WOUND

The transplantation operation is performed via a right or left oblique lower quadrant incision to enter the retroperitoneal space. The peritoneal envelope is reflected superior-medially exposing the vessels. Superficial cellulitis may be a manifestation of a deeper problem or may be related to long-term use of skin staples or sutures. Superficial seromas rarely cause significant problems but one must rule out a urine leak before dismissing their importance. Seromas can be very troublesome for the patient requiring drainage and gauze packing, until the drainage ceases. Our current regimen is to do a two-layer closure of the subcutaneous fat and place the patient in an abdominal binder (corset) to obliterate the potential superficial space. It is our practice to leave a closed suction drainage system for the first few days after the operation.

FASCIAL NECROSIS AND DEHISCENCE

Fascial necrosis and dehiscence are major complications that are multifactorial in etiology and relate to poor vascular supply to the superficial external oblique fascia. Of the last 100 transplants performed at our institution, 4 cases of early fascial dehiscence have occurred in diabetic patients who were less than 1 week following the operation. One occurred because of a chronic cough caused by the use of an angiotensin-converting enzyme (ACE) inhibitor in a young, nondiabetic male. A clue to this serious complication is heralded by a serous effluent from the wound. Repair is performed by reexploring the entire wound and suturing the muscular-fascial layers with interrupted "Figure of 8" (Sneed-Jones) monofilament, nonabsorbable sutures. The patients are then also required to use their corset for 1 month.

NERVE INJURY

Ilioinguinal, Genitofemoral, Femoral Nerves

Because of the oblique nature of the incision, the morbidity of neurologic complications tend to be minimal, but the frequency is high. The most common neurologic deficit experienced by the patient is anesthesia (rarely hypesthesia) of the skin, superior medial to the incision, medial thigh, and lateral scrotum in men. Conservative management of this is warranted because new nerve growth will occur over the proceeding months from the uninvolved cutaneous nerve roots. Hypesthesias are treated with ilioinguinal nerve blocks (lidocaine or Marcaine with steroids) or nerve ablations with phenol or alcohol. Occasionally, nerve entrapment may occur during closure requiring exploration and neurolysis.

The genitofemoral nerve and femoral nerve are rarely permanently damaged during renal transplantation because of their lateral and deep location, respectively. However, significant damage can occur during a complicated transplant nephrectomy, or with transplantation in a previously operated iliac fossa. More commonly, one sees a temporary neuropraxia secondary to traction on the nerve from the self-retaining detractor used for exposure. The patient experiences anesthesia (and hypesthesias) on the anterior portion of the thigh below the inguinal crease with injury to the genitofemoral nerve.

Of greater concern and morbidity is a traction injury to the femoral nerve ("transplant leg"). Patients experience global weakness of the involved leg. Failure to recognize this injury postoperatively may inadvertently lead to the patients falling when they get up for the first time. Early physical therapy, transfer precautions, and ambulatory aids (cane, walker) promote a speedy recovery. There have been no reported cases of permanent nerve damage. Full recovery is expected in 1 to 8 weeks.

BOWEL INJURIES

Bowel injuries are rare during renal transplant. Complications that can occur are serosal tears of the colon during mobilization of the peritoneum, herniation of bowel contents through a small peritoneal opening, and puncture of the bowel during wound closure. Early recognition and repair is required to prevent a catastrophic outcome.

With the advent of percutaneous surgery, additional injuries can be encountered during antegrade percutaneous access to the renal pelvis. This injury can usually be avoided by using ultrasound-guided puncture of the kidney and by staying inferior-lateral to the skin incision where the kidney is retroperitoneal. If the bowel is inadvertently perforated, appropriate broad-spectrum antibiotics are instituted and the tube or needle is simply removed.

LYMPHOCELE

Lymphoceles arise from two sources in the transplant wound. One from the lymphatic vessels, which are cut during the preparation of the iliac vessels, and the second from the transplanted kidney. Every effort is made to prevent their occurrence by ligating the lymphatic channels before transplantation. Lymphoceles are common, but they are only clinically significant in less than 5% of transplants.

Regardless of the etiology, treatment of lymphoceles is only indicated for a painful mass in the abdomen, urinary or vascular obstruction, and infection. The classic mode of therapy is open marsupialization of the lymphocele sack transabdominally. Laparoscopic marsupialization have been reported with good results. The diagnosis is usually made with increased creatinine and an ultrasound showing a medial fluid collection and hydronephrosis. Other modes of treatment include percutaneous drainage with or without installation of sclerosing agents such as iodine and tetracycline. These may be successful; however, if recurrence occurs formal surgical intervention is required.

Selected Readings

Barry JM, Lemmers MJ. Patch and flap techniques to repair right renal vein defects caused by cadaver liver retrieval for transplantation. *J Urol* 1995;153(6): 1803–1804.

Authors describe two techniques that allow right renal vein extension and prevent renal vein stenosis if the cephalic portion of the renal vein has been amputated when the liver is separated from the kidneys during multiple organ retrieval. These techniques were successfully used in eight cadaveric kidney transplant recipients.

Fernandez AT, Minana LB, Fraile GB, et al. Renal transplantectomy. *Arch Esp Urol* 1996;49(10):1079–1091.

Renal transplantation is currently the treatment of choice for most patients with end-stage renal failure; however, approximately 35% present failure of graft function within 5 years posttransplantation. The need for graft removal, which is infrequently discussed in the literature, and the surgical techniques employed are discussed. Literature is reviewed with special reference to the indications for graft removal and the different surgical techniques employed. Like other authors, approach is to leave the graft in site with or without low doses of corticosteroids. Transplant nephrectomy is reserved for the symptomatic cases. For cases requiring nephrectomy less than 3 months posttransplantation, the use of extracapsular approach is recommended; thereafter the use of the subcapsular technique is recommended.

Mendez R, Berne T, Silcott G, et al. Management of multiple renal arteries in renal transplantation. *Urology* 1974;3:409.

Several options of managing multiple renal arteries are described. Coarctation end to side of smaller vessels to main renal artery and individual anastomosis of individual vessels. The physics of blood flow are described.

Naraghi RM, Jordan ML. Surgical complications. In: *Renal transplantation*. Appleton & Lange, 1997:269–297.

PART 3
Metabolic and Endocrine Abnormalities After Renal Transplantation

Michael M. Friedlaender
and Mordecai M. Popovtzer

Endocrine and metabolic abnormalities are not unusual in renal transplant recipients. The most frequently encountered are those involving the skeletal system and mineral homeostasis, lipid and glucose metabolic defects, renal tubular acidosis, and erythrocytosis.

BONE AND MINERAL METABOLISM

Successful renal transplantation is the only treatment that can truly correct the many factors, shown in Fig. 89.2, that cause the osteodystrophy and disturbed mineral metabolism in renal failure patients. The clinical features and extent of the correction process depend on the quality of function of the new kidney and also on the severity and duration of the disturbances before transplantation. Specific problems in the field of mineral metabolism in the renal transplant recipient include secondary hyperparathyroidism, hypercalcemia and hypophosphatemia, and posttransplant bone disease, which includes immunosuppression-related bone disease and avascular necrosis.

Secondary Hyperparathyroidism

A decrease in the blood levels of parathyroid hormone (PTH) occurs after successful renal transplantation. This is due partly to the excretion of the C-terminal fragment of PTH, which accumulates in the uremic patients, and partly to reduction in PTH secretion induced by the normalization of serum calcium levels and of $1,25(OH)_2D$ metabolism. However, a large segment of renal transplant recipients with good renal function may continue to have elevated blood levels of PTH, thus being in a state of persistent secondary hyperparathyroidism. These patients may have normocalcemia or hypercalcemia. There are at least three documented complications of persistent secondary hyperparathyroidism in renal transplant recipients: (a) hypercalcemia, (b) aseptic necrosis of the head of the femur (see Chapter 79), and (c) ulcerations and gangrene of extremities (see Chapter 77). This latter complication responds well to subtotal parathyroidectomy; and the latter should be considered in patients who develop the earliest signs of aseptic necrosis or tissue necrosis.

Hypercalcemia and Hypophosphatemia

Hypercalcemia

The clinical manifestations of hypercalcemia after transplantation may be of several forms; it may appear soon after the transplant procedure (*immediate hypercalcemia*); it may become evident several months later (*delayed hypercalcemia*); and it may be transient or persistent.

The possible mechanisms for the rise in serum calcium include reversal of bone resistance to circulating PTH, mobilization of soft-tissue calcium deposits, hypophosphatemia, and, in particular, the adequate activation of 1α-hydroxylase in the new kidney by PTH, which restores to normal the production of $1,25(OH)_2D_3$, especially in the absence of hyperphosphatemia. The excessive levels of circulating PTH in chronic renal failure give rise to posttransplant phosphaturia and transient hypercalcemia, which are seen not infrequently; the incidence of the latter varies from 15% to 35%. In some patients the rise in serum calcium is more insidious, occurring after several weeks or months and persisting. These features would appear to be related to the "mass" of parathyroid tissue at the time of transplantation. Hypertrophied glands may involute spontaneously, but the feedback "setpoint" for the inhibition of PTH secretion may persist at higher serum calcium levels for many years. Possible mechanisms for persisting posttransplant hyperparathyroidism are shown in Table 89.4. Normalization of reduced $1,25(OH)_2D_3$ binding to its receptors, which occurs in the uremic state, has been reported in kidney transplant recipients. However, it is unclear if this also occurs in the hyperplastic regions of the parathyroid. It has also been suggested that the normal serum $1,25(OH)_2D_3$ levels after renal transplantation may be inappropriately low both for the raised levels of circulating PTH and for the low-normal posttransplant serum phosphate levels. Higher levels of $1,25(OH)_2D_3$ may be expected to stimulate $1,25(OH)_2D_3$ receptor expression and to decrease the expression of the PTH gene. Indeed cautious administration of calcium and $1,25(OH)_2D_3$ or its analogs to nonhypercalcemic posttransplant patients has been shown to have beneficial effects on both raised PTH levels and on bone mineral density. Renal dysfunction or the addition of nephrotoxic drugs may be expected to exacerbate deficiency of $1,25(OH)_2D_3$. In uremia, decreased expression of the calcium-sensing gene occurs and the decrease is reversed by $1,25(OH)_2D_3$. Whether this occurs after renal transplantation is under investigation. PTH gene expression may be further stimulated by corticosteroid administration.

Mild persisting hypercalcemia has not been shown to be deleterious except in patients with poorly functioning grafts. Elective parathyroidectomy may be indicated in patients, particularly if serum calcium remains higher than 12 mg/dl or in those with persisting bone pain, renal impairment, nephrolithiasis, calciphylaxis, pancreatitis, and psychiatric abnormalities. Because recent monitoring of reduced bone-mineral density after renal transplantation has suggested close correlation with elevated PTH levels, there may be an indication to be more aggressive in controlling elevated PTH levels.

Hypophosphatemia

Hypophosphatemia is usually secondary to PTH-induced phosphaturia. However, other causes may be operative as well. These

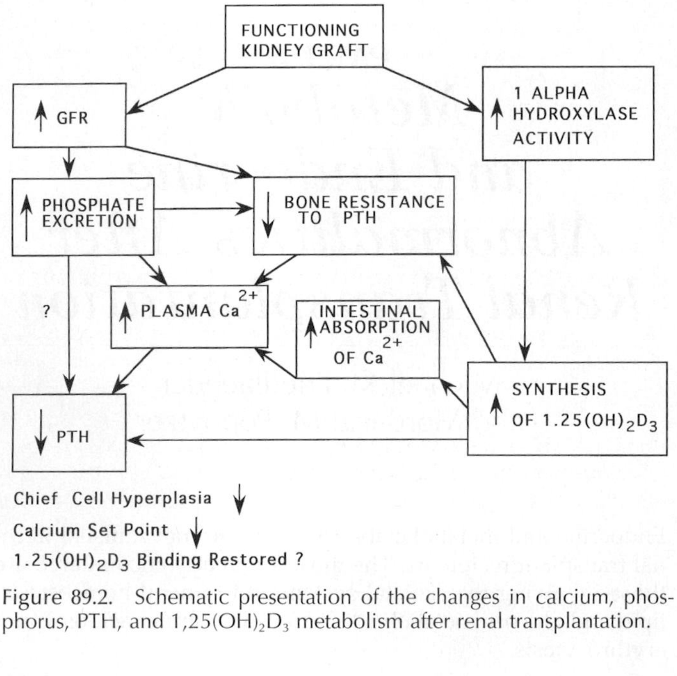

Figure 89.2. Schematic presentation of the changes in calcium, phosphorus, PTH, and $1,25(OH)_2D_3$ metabolism after renal transplantation.

TABLE 89.4. Possible Mechanisms for Persisting Hyperparathyroidism After Successful Renal Transplantation

Increased parathyroid "mass"
Reduced binding of $1,25(OH)_2D_3$ in hyperplastic tissue
Inappropriately "low" serum $1,25(OH)_2D_3$ levels
Decreased calcium-sensing receptor gene expression
Corticosteroid-induced increase in PTH gene expression

PTH, parathyroid hormone.

include postoperative osmotic diuresis and extracellular volume expansion; routine posttransplant antacid therapy, which reduces gastrointestinal phosphate reabsorption; and therapy with steroids or drugs, such as acyclovir, which cause phosphaturia. Posttransplant renal PTH-independent phosphate leak has also been described. Though hypophosphatemia is rarely a symptomatic problem and resolves spontaneously, early transplant series reported some cases of hypophosphatemic osteomalacia.

Posttransplant Bone Disease

Two major transplant-related bone problems are avascular necrosis and the direct effects of immunosuppressive agents.

Necrosis of Femoral Head

The incidence of avascular necrosis (previously 7% to 29%) appears to have declined in recent years, probably as a result of better understanding and treatment of dialysis osteodystrophy and also as a consequence both of the steroid-sparing effect of cyclosporine and the treatment of acute rejection crises with antilymphocytic globulins rather than massive intravenous steroid therapy. The lack of close correlation of steroid dose to avascular necrosis has been emphasized by some authors. Children receiving the same cumulative dose of steroids for nephrotic syndrome have a much lower incidence of avascular necrosis than age-matched transplant recipients, and the risk of avascular necrosis is correlated to alkaline phosphatase levels at the time of transplantation. Thus factors other than cumulative steroid dosage are probably also involved. Whether steroids cause fat-cell swelling with increased intraosseous pressures in the femoral head or hypercoagulability and fat emboli in osseous blood vessels is unclear.

Evidence also exists that a state of persistent secondary hyperparathyroidism plays an important pathogenic role in the development of necrosis of the femoral head. Indeed the incidence of the latter in transplant recipients with secondary hyperparathyroidism and hypercalcemia is six times higher than in those with normal levels of PTH and normocalcemia.

Use of isotope scanning or nuclear magnetic resonance (NMR) has been shown to be valuable in early diagnosis but, although they decrease pain, the net long-term results of diminished weight bearing or decompression procedures are disappointing, and total hip replacement may be required in some patients.

It should be mentioned that "painful legs syndrome," which is a transient phenomenon of unknown cause in the early weeks after transplantation, has also been ascribed to microfractures in the long bones or epiphyses. It has been reported to respond to reduction of high blood cyclosporin A levels and to administration of calcium channel blockers.

Immunosuppression-Related Bone Disease

Corticosteroids induce osteoporosis, especially in trabecular bone of the axial skeleton, by direct osteoblast inhibition, by reduction in gastrointestinal calcium absorption, and also by increasing bone resorption. Longitudinal studies of vertebral bone-mineral density have shown an 8.8% decrease within 18 months of transplantation, mostly occurring within the first 6 months and being associated with increased fractures. These changes, which may be reversible in patients with well-functioning grafts, have been correlated with the total cumulative dose of steroids, with the number of steroid-treated acute rejection episodes, and also with the evolution of secondary hyperparathyroidism after transplantation. Age and nutrition at the time of transplantation, obesity, diabetes mellitus, female sex, menopausal state, hypogonadism, and immobility are contributory factors to this form of posttransplant bone disease.

The contribution of cyclosporine to this problem is unclear. Levels of bone Gla protein (osteocalcin), a marker for bone formation secreted by osteoblasts, have been reported to be increased by cyclosporine therapy and to be reduced by prednisone, suggesting that cyclosporine may have a protective effect. Although cyclosporine causes high-turnover osteopenia in rats, there is no evidence that this occurs after renal transplantation in humans. Of the other immunosuppressive agents, only tacrolimus (FK506), but not sirolimus (rapamycin), Imuran (azathioprine), or Cellcept (mycophenolate mofetil) appears to have similar bone effects to cyclosporine. In practice, the steroid-sparing effect of these agents has undoubtedly contributed to a reduced incidence of symptomatic posttransplant bone disease.

Two further bone complications are occasionally seen after renal transplantation. Low-turnover aluminum bone disease of dialysis has been found to be improved with much reduced aluminum staining, as evidenced by bone biopsy results 1 year after successful transplantation and without correlation to pretransplant or posttransplant PTH status. Progression of dialysis-related amyloid osteodystrophy is also halted by successful renal transplantation.

Strategies to reduce the incidence of posttransplant bone disease are largely preventive and include reduction of steroid dose and optimization of treatment to prevent renal osteodystrophy before transplant. Follow-up of serial bone-mineral densities is useful. Judicious calcium supplementation, perhaps with $1,25(OH)_2D_3$ or one of its analogs, together with hormone replacement and perhaps addition of the newer biphosphonates that inhibit bone resorption, may all become part of routine posttransplant therapy in the future.

Nephrocalcinosis and Renal Calculi

Nephrocalcinosis and renal calcium stones may be encountered infrequently in renal transplant recipients. The pathogenesis of these abnormalities is not known, but secondary hyperparathyroidism, hypercalcemia, distal renal tubular acidosis, and urinary tract infection may be contributory factors.

HYPERLIPIDEMIA

The wide range of reported prevalence of posttransplant hyperlipidemia is 16% to 72% and partly reflects differences in the study time points after transplant. Hyperlipidemia is variously affected by medications, graft function, the presence of proteinuria, glucose intolerance, obesity, age, and gender. Increased triglyceride and total cholesterol levels are common as are increases in both very-low-density lipoprotein (VLDL) and low-density lipoprotein (LDL) cholesterol. High-density lipoprotein (HDL) cholesterol is near normal or even low. The changes are most significant in the first months after transplantation and tend to improve after the first year. This probably reflects subtle changes in several of the multifactors causing lipid abnormalities in these patients, in particular dose reduction in medications such as corticosteroids and cyclosporine, which appear to be independent factors causing hypercholesterolemia. Cyclosporine may decrease postheparin lipolytic activity, increase lipoprotein (a) levels, interfere with LDL binding to receptors, or alter lipid metabolism indirectly by causing glucose intolerance, reduced bile-acid synthesis, or decreased renal function. Tacrolimus and sirolimus probably have similar properties. The close relationship of hyperlipidemia to cardiovascular disease has also been demonstrated in posttransplant populations. This and the growing evidence that progression of renal disease is accelerated in the presence of hyperlipidemia has prompted some workers to adopt an aggressive approach to these lipid abnormalities. Dietary therapy is always appropriate but steroid dose reduction, alternate-day steroids, or conversion from steroids and/or cyclosporine to azathioprine must be carefully weighed against the risk of precipitating graft rejection. Closely monitored therapy with low doses of 3-hydroxy-3-methyl-glutaryl-coenzyme A (HMG-CoA) reductase inhibitors and/or clofibrate have also been successful. Both these agents may cause rhabdomyolysis and the risk is increased when they are used in combination, used in patients receiving cyclosporine, and if renal function is reduced. Because cyclosporine is lipophilic, close monitoring of blood levels is advisable if lipid-reducing therapy is instituted. Some delay in treatment is thus advisable in nonextreme cases of hyperlipidemia because, as noted, lipid levels tend to decrease with time.

GLUCOSE INTOLERANCE

Glucose intolerance is not unusual after transplantation, occasionally requiring inordinately high-dose insulin therapy for its control. With reduction in steroid dose, these problems usually become easily manageable. Subclinical glucose intolerance is still verifiable in many patients even on low-dose glucocorticoid therapy, which causes peripheral insulin resistance. Despite previous *in vitro* and animal observations to the contrary, newer studies have failed to confirm a clinically important effect of cyclosporine on pancreatic β-cell function. Tacrolimus-treated patients may have an increased incidence of diabetes mellitus.

Older patients, especially males with strong demographic and genetic predisposing factors, may show less tendency for remission of the diabetes. Diabetic nephropathy, occurring within a few years, has been reported in some of these patients.

GOUT

The incidence of gouty arthritis may have increased since the introduction of cyclosporin A, perhaps related to a specific effect on tubular handling of uric acid, or to reduced glomerular filtration rate (GFR), and/or to increased use of diuretics in cyclosporine-treated patients. Allopurinol therapy should be used with care. Azathioprine metabolism is reduced by coadministration of allopurinol. The dosage of azathioprine must therefore be reduced.

HORMONES

Clinical *thyroid* dysfunction is unusual in chronic renal failure. Low free and total triiodothyronine levels normalize after successful renal transplantation. *Adrenal* suppression may be a complication of long-term steroid therapy. However, Addisonian crises under stress are rare, and newer publications have found no evidence that supplemental high-dose steroid therapy is necessary for renal allograft recipients receiving 5 to 10 mg prednisone daily. Isolated hypoaldosteronism has been described soon after renal transplantation and may cause severe hyperkalemia. This condition is transient unless it is part of a systemic infiltrative disease such as amyloidosis, which may cause chronic adrenal insufficiency and necessitate mineralocorticoid replacement therapy. Hyporeninemic hypoaldosteronism has also been described, perhaps reflecting early transient damage to the new kidney graft.

Cyclosporine may induce a dual interference with renin-aldosterone system. It both reduces aldosterone secretion and blunts the renal response to aldosterone. In this regard, it is of interest that drugs such as ketoconazole and diltiazem may further aggravate this complication by increasing the half-life of cyclosporine.

Disturbances in *sex hormones* also normalize after renal transplantation, in particular, there is return of the normal pulsatile release of gonadotrophins. This may thus restore to normal the receptor downregulation seen in uremic patients who have more sustained gonadotrophin release.

Studies on growth abnormalities after renal transplantation in children suggest that the pulsatile secretion of *growth hormone* is not normalized and that glucocorticoids, apart from their catabolic effects, blunt insulinlike growth factor-1 production. Treatment with recombinant human growth hormone to improve growth velocity has shown promise.

Plasma levels of *atrial natriuretic peptide* (ANP) are raised in patients with chronic renal failure, decreasing during hemodialysis and ultrafiltration. After transplantation, the high levels also decrease to normal over 7 to 10 days, parallel to the improvement in the function of the kidney, to falling fractional excretion of urinary sodium, and to plasma and urine cyclic guanosine monophosphate (cGMP) levels. The trial use of ANP to improve immediate renal function has not been shown to have any long-term benefits.

ERYTHROCYTOSIS

In chronic renal failure, endogenous erythropoietin levels are low in relation to the degree of anemia. The new kidney produces an early peak in erythropoietin level that is unrelated to graft function and causes little or no hemopoietic response. A later peak occurs after 2 weeks, which is more sustained and is related to resolution of anemia. Up to 30% of patients show posttransplant erythrocytosis that, in most cases, is related to persistent inappropriate high-normal serum levels of erythropoietin and that may necessitate elective venesection if the hematocrit is more than 55%. Theophylline, an adenosine antagonist, blocks erythropoietin production but is poorly tolerated. Both ACE inhibitors and angiotensin II–receptor blockers have been shown to reduce posttransplant erythrocytosis. Previously suggested, rarer causes of erythrocytosis include acute and chronic rejection, transplant renal artery stenosis, hydronephrosis, and overuse of diuretics.

RENAL TUBULAR ACIDOSIS AND TUBULAR TRANSPORT DEFECTS

Distal renal tubular acidosis, proximal tubular dysfunction (phosphaturia, glucosuria, and aminoaciduria), and hyperchloremic acidosis after renal transplantation were first reported in 1967. Since then, several urinary acidification defects have been encountered in renal transplant recipients. These include proximal renal tubular acidosis, distal renal tubular acidosis (complete and incomplete), and/or reduced ammonia excretion. These acidification defects may occur separately or simultaneously. The incidence of these abnormalities is difficult to assess, but they are not uncommon. They may be more frequent in cadaveric renal transplantation.

The proximal renal tubular acidosis may be mild or severe and is thought to be due to proximal bicarbonate wasting induced by excess blood levels of PTH and/or hypophosphatemia or phosphate depletion. This type of acidification defect usually occurs in the early posttransplant period when blood levels of PTH are highest and those of phosphorus are lowest.

Proximal renal tubular acidosis usually disappears with time as the blood levels of PTH and phosphorus return toward normal.

Distal renal tubular acidosis may become evident at any time after renal transplantation. It may be transient or permanent and complete or incomplete (detected only after an acid load). The pathogenesis of distal renal tubular acidosis is not completely understood but may be related to acute tubular necrosis, acute rejection, and/or immunologic insults to the distal tubules. Hyperchloremic acidosis has been frequently noted before acute rejection. Hyperchloremic acidosis was observed during pregnancy in renal transplant recipients and reversed after delivery. The clinical manifestations and the diagnosis of the various types of renal tubular acidosis are discussed in Chapter 20, Part 5. Hyperkalemic, hyperchloremic renal tubular acidosis (type IV) has been observed in renal transplant recipients treated with cyclosporine. The drug may cause suppression of plasma-renin activity and aldosterone (hyporeninemic hypoaldosteronism) and/or reduced renal tubular sensitivity to aldosterone. Hyperkalemia has also been noted without renal tubular acidosis.

Proximal tubular transport defects have been observed in transplant recipients. These include phosphaturia, bicarbonaturia, glucosuria, aminoaciduria, and/or uricosuria. Occasionally, the patient may have the full manifestations of Fanconi's syndrome.

CATARACT

Posterior capsule cataracts are very common in renal transplant recipients, and in a series of 312 patients, 52 (16%) developed this complication. In another series of adult patients, the incidence of cataracts was 34%. Among 69 children, cataracts were present in 44 (59%) after renal transplantation. The cataracts may be unilateral or bilateral, usually appear within the first 6 months after transplantation, and are thought to be due to glucocorticoid therapy. The lens changes are usually mild but can be severe enough to cause significant visual impairment requiring surgical removal of the cataract. They are encountered less frequently since the introduction of cyclosporine and the reduction in the glucocorticoid dose in the management of the transplant recipients.

Selected Readings

Bromberg JS, Alfrey EJ, Barker CF, et al. Adrenal suppression and steroid supplementation in renal transplant recipients. *Transplantation* 1991;51:385–390.

A study in 40 renal allograft recipients during significant physiologic stress failed to show evidence of functional adrenal suppression.

Chatterjee SN, Friedler RM, Berne TV, et al. Persistent hypercalcemia after successful renal transplantation. *Nephron* 1976;17:1–7.

Observations on the prevalence of hypercalcemia, persistent secondary hyperparathyroidism, and aseptic necrosis of the femoral head in 60 renal transplant recipients followed for up to 6 years.

Epstein S. Post-transplantation bone disease: the role of immunosuppressive agents and the skeleton. *J Bone Min Res* 1996;11:1–7.

A short review of the possible mechanisms and the effects of posttransplant immunosuppression on bone mineral density.

Julian BA, Laskow DA, Dubovsky J, et al. Rapid loss of vertebral mineral density after renal transplantation. *N Engl J Med* 1991;325:544–550.

Dual and single photon absorptiometry, bone histomorphometry, serum biochemistry, and vitamin D levels followed for 18 months after 20 successful renal transplants from living donors.

Keane WF. Derangement of lipid metabolism and its management in renal transplant patients. *Min Elect Metab* 1997;23:166–169.

A good, short, updated review.

Massari PU. Nephrology forum. Disorders of bone and mineral metabolism after renal transplantation. *Kidney Int* 1997;52:1412–1421.

An excellent review on the subject.

Massry SG, Preuss HG, Maher JF, et al. Renal tubular acidosis after cadaver kidney homotransplantation. *Am J Med* 1967;42:284–292.

The first report of a detailed study in a renal transplant recipient demonstrating renal tubular acidosis.

Noordzij TC, Leunissan KML, Van Hoof JP. Renal handling of urate and the incidence of gouty arthritis during cyclosporine and diuretic use. *Transplantation* 1991;52:64–67.

A survey of the incidence and predictive factors for gout in 85 cadaver kidney recipients.

Wilson DR, Siddiqui AA. Renal tubular acidosis after kidney transplantation. *Ann Intern Med* 1973;79:352–361.

A study of the spectrum of renal tubular acidosis in 32 renal transplant recipients.

PART 4
Gastrointestinal Complications

William J.C. Amend, Jr.

Although a variety of gastrointestinal complications continue to be noted in renal transplant recipients, the types and frequencies of these various disorders have changed over the past 30 years of clinical renal transplantation. Table 89.5 illustrates those factors that have altered the prevalence of these abnormalities. More than half of patients with end-stage renal failure are now over 50 years old. Many of these patients are now eligible for renal transplantation. Age-related "usual" prevalence of colonic carcinomas, for instance, have been noted and represent new types of renal transplant gastrointestinal complications. In addition, given the greater success and longer time of follow-up in currently transplanted patients, routine screening and concern for usual gastrointestinal neoplasms (gastric, pancreatic, colonic, and rectal carcinomas) is now necessary. These types of neoplasms are noted to have only a slight increase in incidence compared with the age-matched general population (versus the posttransplant lymphomas). With longer posttransplant follow-ups, however, more surveillance for solid gastrointestinal tumors might be warranted.

Concurrent diseases are also an important contributor to the presence of posttransplant gastrointestinal disorders. This is especially noted in diabetic recipients who have higher incidences of ischemic bowel complications or intestinal motility disorders. Because diabetic patients now make up 25% to 30% of renal transplant populations, it is to be expected that these gastrointestinal complications might be noted more frequently.

In addition, 15% to 20% of transplant recipients may have had preceding chronic peritoneal dialysis [continuous ambulatory peritoneal dialysis (CAPD) or continuous cyclic peritoneal dialysis (CCPD)] therapy. Posttransplant gastrointestinal problems in previously peritoneally dialyzed patients also include intestinal adhesions and mesenteric intussusception owing to

TABLE 89.5. Factors Affecting Posttransplant Gastrointestinal Complications

1. Older transplanted population
2. Long duration of posttransplant follow-up
3. Concurrent diseases (e.g., diabetes)
4. Preceding peritoneal dialysis
5. Steroid-sparing regimens
6. Newer immunosuppressive agents (e.g., tacrolimus, mycophenolic acid)

peritoneal fibrotic bands. This is especially a problem if the peritoneal dialysis treatment has been of long duration or has been associated with multiple bouts of peritonitis. Because the renal transplant is usually extraperitoneal in location (in patients older than 12 to 16 years of age), intraabdominal mechanical obstructive problems were formerly unusual in hemodialyzed patients. Peritoneal dialysis has slightly increased these complication in the past 10 years. A severe process, idiopathic sclerosing peritonitis, can present with bowel obstruction, malnutrition, and pain and is associated with progression and a high mortality rate.

An important factor relating to the changing frequencies of various posttransplant gastrointestinal complications has been alterations of the immunosuppressive drugs. Since the widespread use of cyclosporine, there has been a marked reduction in glucocorticoid usage in both the early and late posttransplant periods. Many patients are even treated with steroid-free regimens or with alternate-day steroid dosages. This has had a profound effect in reducing gastric and colonic bleeding and perforation complications. Newer drugs such as tacrolimus and mycophenolic acid have been reported to have a higher prevalence of nonspecific epigastric complaints (pain and eructation) and diarrhea (up to 30%). These functional gastrointestinal conditions usually reverse with dosage modifications. However, they do complicate the management of postrenal transplant patients in that they can confuse the differential diagnoses from other more serious gastrointestinal conditions.

Most of the gastrointestinal disorders occur in the first year posttransplant and may account for 20% to 30% of rehospitalizations. These sorts of patients are markedly affected by gastrointestinal fluid losses, and often have severe "prerenal" renal failure and states of poor immunosuppressive drug bioavailability.

PRETRANSPLANT EVALUATION

The patient's pretransplant gastrointestinal history must be carefully noted. Patients with active epigastric symptoms should be evaluated by endoscopy and treated, especially if there is associated gastrointestinal bleeding. Treatment against *Heliobacter pylori* has markedly reduced both pretransplant and posttransplant peptic ulcer morbidity. This has precluded the use of pretransplant peptic ulcer surgical therapy in almost all patients. Patients, however, are given prophylactic H_2-blockers with lowered steroid regimens in the first 6 months following transplantation.

Diverticular disease is more common in those uremic patients with certain concurrent diseases such as polycystic kidney disease, older dialysis patients, and/or patients with moderate constipation (usually resulting from reduced luminal water content and the frequent use of constipating phosphate-binding agents or resins). Patients who have had diverticulitis should have a careful pretransplant assessment possibly including a prophylactic subtotal colectomy if there is a history of perforation or fistulous tracts. It is not clear if the presence of diverticular disease, *per se,* mandates a pretransplant partial colectomy. Although the majority of diverticula are noted in the distal colon in most patients with diverticulosis, the vast majority of posttransplant colonic perforations actually occur in the proximal and transverse colon. Pretransplant identification of high-risk, uremic patients by barium enema would still be useful so that the clinician would have a high index of suspicion for colonic complications should there be any bowel symptoms after transplantation.

In the pretransplant evaluation process, patients should be given information regarding these gastrointestinal complications so that they can be fully informed about these potential posttransplant problems. In addition, screening tests, such as colonoscopy and/or serial tests for occult blood in stool, should be considered in patients at higher risk (i.e., those with a family or personal history of cancer, abdominal symptomatology, and older potential transplant recipients).

ESOPHAGEAL DISORDERS

Posttransplant esophageal conditions can be classified by those that occur in the early and late posttransplant periods. Symptoms of dysphagia, singultus (hiccups), or frank upper gastrointestinal bleeding in the first 3 to 6 months after transplantation require prompt investigation usually with endoscopy. Both cultures and biopsies must be obtained to look for infective versus peptic reflux conditions. Infectious causes include *Candida albicans* (often with a positive oropharyngeal examination), cytomegalovirus (CMV) (usually with an associated febrile illness), and *Herpesvirus hominis* (often with severe chest pain). Patients with postoperative acid reflux conditions usually have pretransplant symptoms or history suggesting this disorder. Infectious causes occasionally coexist and often occur following intensification in immunosuppression (with antithymocyte globulin or high-dose steroids). Prophylactic regimens of fluconazole for 1 month and acyclovir or ganciclovir for 3 to 6 months have reduced the incidence of both *Candida* and CMV esophagitis. Treatment for these esophageal infections currently includes the following:

Candida: ketoconazole 200 mg/day orally for 2 to 3 weeks; occasionally a low-dose, short course of systemic amphotericin is needed (0.2 to 0.7 mg/kg total dose)
CMV: ganciclovir 1.25 to 5 mg/kg per day for 14 to 21 days
Herpesvirus hominis: acyclovir 5 mg/kg intravenously every 8 hours for 7 to 10 days

During ketoconazole therapy, reductions and close follow-up of cyclosporine and tacrolimus trough levels are necessary because the blood levels of the drugs usually rise. In addition, viscous Xylocaine and narcotic analgesics are usually given for symptomatic relief.

In long-term posttransplant patients, symptoms suggestive of hiatal hernia with reflux can be seen in older patients, especially in those patients with underlying polycystic kidney disease. Antacids, H_2-blockers, metoclopramide, and head elevation at night are useful therapies. Dysphagia in the late posttransplant setting should arouse concerns not regarding infection as much as other conditions (e.g., neoplasms).

GASTRODUODENAL DISORDERS

Peptic ulcer disease still represents a significant problem with renal transplant recipients with an impact not only on graft survival but also on patient mortality. Although this complication accounted for 20% to 40% of gastrointestinal disorders in the precyclosporine era, it is less frequently noted now because of reduced steroid dosages, prophylactic antiulcer regimens of H_2-blockers and/or intensive antacids, pretransplant or posttransplant *H. pylori* therapy, and possibly selective pretransplant surgical prophylactic procedures for peptic ulcer disease. The latter continues to occur in 2% to 5% of renal transplant patients and often has associated hemorrhage. Whether this, plus glucocorticoids and other factors such as uremia-associated hypergastrinemia and/or secondary hyperparathyroidism, put these patients at an excess risk is hard to determine. At higher risk are elderly patients, patients with a pretransplant history of peptic ulcer disease, patients with recent rejection (and augmented immunosuppressive dosages), and patients with recent systemic infections. Important measures to reduce patient morbidity include prompt, endoscopically guided diagnosis (and endoscopically guided therapeutic monitoring); aggressive medical management with antacids, H_2-blockers, antibiotics, and/or sucralfate; and appropriate surgical intervention with oversewing of the bleeding ulcer when necessary. In these latter instances, more definitive antiulcer surgery may be delayed until the critical condition of the patient has improved.

Posttransplant gastritis may be diffuse or localized to the cardia and prepyloric regions of the stomach. It formerly was termed *Cushing's ulcers* and often was noted in situations of stress as occurs with concurrent sepsis, uremia, and/or allograft rejection. As with peptic ulcer disease, its incidence in the posttransplant setting may be less in recent years because of reduced overall steroid dosages. Other factors important in reducing the incidence of gastritis include improved attention to nutrition (pretransplant and posttransplant), lessened degrees of transplant hyperparathyroidism, and interventions for smoking curtailment. It often is manifested by upper gastrointestinal hemorrhage. Endoscopic evaluation is necessary because many of these cases are not idiopathic but represent erosive CMV gastroduodenitis. In this circumstance, viral cultures are often negative and the diagnosis is determined only by mucosal biopsy specimens showing characteristic intranuclear viral inclusions in multinucleated giant cells. Treatment for this condition includes ganciclovir 1.25 to 5 mg/kg per day for 14 to 21 days in addition to H_2-blockers or sucralfate. In the idiopathic gastritis cases, treatment resembles that for peptic ulcer disease with the use of H_2-blockers, antacids, and/or sucralfate, and blood transfusions as necessary. Emergency gastrectomy is unusual.

PANCREATIC DISORDERS

In the later posttransplant period (more than 1 year following transplantation), patients may be at risk to develop acute pancreatitis. This may be on a viral (CMV) or drug (azathioprine/steroid) basis and can affect approximately 1% of such patients. Many dialysis and transplant patients have associated gallstones. These are often of the pigmented, bilirubin variety, yet these do not appear to be associated with cases of posttransplant pancreatitis. Usual evaluation is necessary, however, to exclude biliary tract disease with obstruction. Endoscopic, retrograde-guided cholangiopancreatography may reveal the need for sphincterotomy during such patient's care. Despite conservative management, mortality may approach 50%.

INTESTINAL DISORDERS

Motility Abnormalities

Serious motility problems may occur following renal transplantation and are usually noted in the first postoperative week. These are termed *pseudoobstruction* or *acute colonic ileus* and manifest in the initial postoperative period as constipation, serious abdominal distension, and massive but nontoxic dilation of the colon on abdominal x-ray examination but with air detected to the rectosigmoid area (i.e., not mechanical obstruction). Risk factors include uremia, postoperative bedrest and analgesics, older age, prednisone dosage, and preceding use of postoperative potassium-binding resins (enema or oral preparations). Some have suggested that the allograft itself may impact on this syndrome with a mild "vascular steal" producing brief, segmental colonic dysmotility. The dilation of the cecum can reach 8 to 12 cm in diameter in some affected patients. This condition must be treated promptly to avoid colonic perforation. Treatment includes carefully performed colonoscopy for bowel decompression; fluoroscopically guided, low-volume Hypaque enemas (if colonic material is present and partially obstipating); and rarely surgery. Postoperative enemas, early postoperative ambulation, and avoidance of postoperative binding regimens (e.g., aluminum hydroxide, potassium-exchange resins) are necessary to limit this problem.

Motility problems are usually frequently noted in the diabetic recipients with gastroparesis or intestinal dysmotility. This is treated with the usual motility agents such as metoclopramide, cisapride, or erythromycin. Erythromycin will interact with both cyclosporine and tacrolimus and produce higher drug levels. The newer microemulsion forms of cyclosporine have better bioavailability, as does tacrolimus, in these sorts of patients than the original cyclosporine preparation.

Colonic Perforation

Colonic perforation is a significant complication that occurs rarely but carries a high mortality rate (70% to 90%). It may occur at any time in the posttransplant follow-up, but usually occurs in the first 1 to 2 months postoperatively. Most patients (60%) with this disorder have a ruptured diverticula, hence older patients and patients with polycystic kidney disease or a history of diverticulitis are at particular risk and should be especially followed. Other risks include high steroid dosage, early postoperative constipation/distension, and recent boosts of antirejection therapy. Most of these postoperative colonic perforations involve the proximal or transverse colon, whereas the most severe diverticula noted in patients with pretransplant barium enemas are in the distal/sigmoid colon. Hence, as mentioned previously, it is not clear whether pretransplant surgical prophylaxis with subtotal colectomy would eliminate this posttransplant complication.

Importantly, this is a difficult complication to accurately diagnose. Fever, diarrhea, abdominal pain, and leukocytosis usually occur. The immunosuppressant drugs may mask symptoms, but more importantly they mask signs and delay clinical diagnosis. The abdominal examination is often benign. Free perforations are more common than walled-off processes, so standard (and repeated) roentgenographic examinations are needed. Abdominal computed tomography scans with contrast are also helpful. A two-stage colectomy/diverting colostomy procedure is required with extensive use of antibiotics. Rarely, these perforations are associated with opportunistic infection, but this should be evaluated as well with attention to preoperative and intraoperative culture and pathologic specimens. This is especially important to rule out coexisting CMV disease.

Colitis

Colitis is a relatively frequent condition, occurring in 1% to 1.5% of postrenal transplant patients. The most common type is *ischemic colitis,* in half the cases. Such patients have abdominal pain, fever, and lower gastrointestinal hemorrhage. It occurs more frequently in patients with atherosclerotic risk factors (older age patients, diabetes, smokers, and those patients with a significant hypertensive history) and can occur months to years postoperatively. The use of glucocorticoids may make the colonic mucosa more vulnerable to mild intestinal ischemia. In addition, it is suggested that the allograft circulation, using the hypogastric artery, causes a blood-volume redistribution and steals some flow from colonic collateral circulation, thus leading to reduced vascular perfusion of the colon. Diagnostic barium enema shows "thumb printing" and colonoscopy is necessary for diagnosis. The mortality of such patients is high (70% to 80%), especially if massive bleeding or perforation occurs. Treatment is conservative with such antibiotics and transfusions, but these patients may require subtotal and/or total colectomy. It appears that embolization or locally perfused vasopressin is not helpful in such circumstances.

A second form of posttransplant colitis is that associated with *diverticulitis* (0.7% incidence). This is treated as usual, can occur at any time following transplantation, and is noted in older patients and patients with polycystic kidney disease and/or with a preceding history of diverticulitis. Usually, patients have pain more than bleeding, but complications of perforation and/or massive bleeding can occur.

Localized colitis with shallow ulcers may be seen with either ischemia or nonspecifically with constipation, but if it is diagnosed in the first half-year following transplant, *infectious colitis* should be suspected. If recent antibiotics have been given, and there is diarrhea, abdominal cramping, and abdominal pain with a negative clinical examination, *Clostridium difficile* may be present with pseudomembranous colitis. If routine testing for *C. difficile* enterotoxin is positive, therapy with metronidazole (500 mg three times daily for 1 week) or vancomycin (125 mg four times daily for 1 week) should be provided. Colonoscopy in this condition will reveal scattered cheesy exudative lesions, which are round to ovoid and predominantly affect the left colon.

On further workup, diagnostic tests for infections associated with colitis should be employed. Besides cultures (which are helpful with *Shigella*, *Candida*, and tuberculosis), colonoscopic mucosal biopsies are necessary (especially in situations involving CMV or varicella-virus colitis). The most frequent cause of infectious colitis in this group of patients is CMV. Colonoscopy in these cases reveals diffuse, small, shallow ulcers with some vesicle formation. Such patients need to be carefully followed up for intestinal perforation and/or bleeding. Administration of ganciclovir (1.25 to 5 mg/kg per day for 21 days) and other conservative therapy may allow patients to avoid surgery. If moderate massive bleeding occurs in association with opportunistic infection colitis, mortality may approach 90%.

Appendicitis

Appendicitis can occur and is noteworthy only that it occurs in an older patient population (40 to 50 years old versus the usual appendicitis risk population of 15 to 25 years of age). It may be difficult to diagnose, especially confusing when the renal allograft is also located in the right iliac fossa.

NEOPLASMS

Neoplasia in transplant recipients is discussed in detail in Chapter 89, Part 6. Here, we will only refer to gastrointestinal neoplasia. Some neoplastic processes occur excessively in patients receiving immunosuppression and can affect 1% to 2% of the renal transplant patients long term. The malignancy of note is the posttransplant lymphoproliferative disorder, which progresses from a polyclonal lymphoproliferation to a monoclonal B-cell type of lymphoma. There is some suggestion that this is related to an oncogenic effect of Epstein-Barr virus in such patients. The lymphomas can involve the gastrointestinal system in approximately 25% of such cases. They usually occur in the first 2 years of follow-up and especially affect patients with higher amounts of posttransplant immunosuppression. The prognosis is poor if the gastrointestinal tract is involved.

Another condition that can excessively occur in transplant patients is Kaposi's sarcoma even in human immunodeficiency virus (HIV)-negative transplant recipients. If Kaposi's sarcoma is limited to mucocutaneous areas, resolution and cure have been described with curtailment of posttransplant immunosuppressants. Many patients, however, have Kaposi's sarcoma lesions affecting the gastrointestinal system as well (visceral Kaposi's sarcoma). In such circumstances, immunosuppressive reductions do not improve survival, with gastrointestinal bleeding and infection being terminal problems. We now understand that this sarcoma may be of an infectious origin [human herpesvirus-8 (HHV-8)]. Further follow-up with the use of antivirals in transplant patients with gastrointestinal Kaposi's sarcoma will be important.

Lastly, Bowen's disease (perianal carcinoma *in situ*, a squamous carcinoma variant) can occasionally be noted in renal transplant patients. Transplant patients, as well, have an excessive frequency of various other cutaneous malignancies.

Importantly, gastrointestinal malignancies do occur in the posttransplant setting, and common malignancies (such as gastric, pancreatic, and colonic) should be more frequently recognized now that older patients with longer posttransplant follow-up are being seen. Gastric or colonic malignancies can be difficult to detect, especially in a patient with massively enlarged polycystic kidneys and polycystic liver. Routine internal medicine principles in follow-up and screening are necessary. If such malignancies are noted, review with the transplant center regarding the continued use of immunosuppression may be helpful. In the case of solid tumor malignancies, there is little evidence to date to suggest that complete curtailment of immunosuppression will importantly improve patient survival.

Selected Readings

Alexander JA, Brouillette DE, Chien M, et al. Infectious esophagitis following liver and renal transplantation. *Dig Dis Sci* 1988;33:1121–1126.

Approaches to the diagnosis and management of esophageal infections in renal transplant recipients.

Komorowski RA, Cohen EB, Kauffman HM, et al. Gastrointestinal complications in renal transplant recipients. *Am J Clin Pathol* 1986;86:161–167.

Good review of the variety of gastrointestinal complications in this patient population. Good pathologic descriptions.

Rao V. Posttransplant medical complications. *Surg Clin North Am* 1998;78:113–132.

Posttransplant gastrointestinal complications are reviewed in the setting of other multisystemic posttransplant complications.

Soderdahl G, Tyden G, Groth CG. Incidence of gastrointestinal complications following renal transplantation in the cyclosporine era. *Transplant Proc* 1994;26: 1771–1772.

Two brief reports emphasizing reductions in gastrointestinal morbidity following cyclosporine use.

Tokot Y, Zeytunlu M, Kilic M, et al. Gastrointestinal complications in renal transplantation. *Transplant Proc* 1996;28:2351–2352.

A good description of gastrointestinal complications after transplantation.

Troppmann C, Papalois BE, Chiou A, et al. Incidence, complications, treatment, and outcome of ulcers of the upper gastrointestinal tract after renal transplantation during the cyclosporine era. *J Am Coll Surg* 1995;180:433–443.

Nice review demonstrating a reduced incidence of gastric ulcers in renal transplant patients during the cyclosporine era.

PART 5
Liver Disease in Renal Transplant Recipients

Khaled Selim and Neil Kaplowitz

Liver disease is an important cause of morbidity and mortality among renal transplant recipients. In a survey of 2,041 renal transplant patients reported in the literature, 16% were found to manifest abnormal liver function tests. In a prospective study of 785 patients who received renal transplants, 37% presented

TABLE 89.6. Mortality From Liver Failure in Long-Term Renal Allografts Recipients

Study	Year	Observation Period (yr)	Total Deaths	Percent of Total Deaths from Hepatic Failure
Kirkman et al. (Boston)	1982	>5	33	21%
Sengar et al. (Ottawa)	1989	>10	16	25%
Rao et al. (Minneapolis)	1989	>10	11	36%
LeFrancois et al. (Lyon)	1987	>10	7	57%

Adapted from Rao VK, Anderson WR. Liver disease after liver transplantation. *Am J Kidney Dis* 1992;19(5):497.

with evidence of liver dysfunction in the posttransplant period; of these, 23% were classified as having acute disease (i.e., liver test abnormalities reverted to normal or patient died within 6 months of the onset of the disease). The remaining 14% had chronic liver disease as defined by persistent liver test abnormalities longer than 6 months.

As many as 28% of long-term survivors of renal transplants die because of liver failure. The exact figure for mortality from acute liver failure is unknown; however, it seems to be quite low. In contrast, chronic liver disease progressing to hepatic failure is the leading cause of death in late survivors of renal transplantation, which ranges from 21% to 57% in different series (Table 89.6).

ETIOLOGY

Many factors may contribute to liver dysfunction in renal transplant recipients depending on whether it is acute or chronic liver disease.

Acute Liver Disease

In addition to hepatitis B virus (HBV) and hepatitis C virus (HCV) infection, causes of acute liver dysfunction include viral infection such as cytomegalovirus (CMV), herpes simplex, varicella, and Epstein-Barr virus (EBV). Drugs used in the posttransplant period (e.g., azathioprine, cyclosporine) may be hepatotoxic and are important factors in posttransplant liver dysfunction. Usually, acute liver disease remits as patients recover from viral infection or the offending medication is discontinued.

The incidence of acute hepatitis B in renal transplant recipients is becoming increasingly low because of the isolation of patients with hepatitis B and end-stage renal failure in dedicated independent dialysis units. The exact incidence of clinical acute hepatitis C is unknown; however, it is infrequent. To our knowledge there are no reported cases of fulminant hepatitis C.

Chronic Liver Disease

The main causes of chronic liver disease in renal transplant recipients are the same as in the community, namely hepatitis B and C and alcohol abuse in addition to iron overload due to multiple blood transfusions before transplantation, especially in the era before erythropoietin therapy.

DIFFERENTIAL DIAGNOSIS OF ACUTE LIVER DISEASE

CMV hepatitis is not uncommon in renal transplant recipients in the early posttransplant period (few weeks). It manifests with fever, chills, leukopenia, and a high level of aminotransferases in the absence of jaundice. The disease is usually self-limited with good prognosis. In cases of disseminated CMV, especially if complicated with opportunistic infections, acute liver failure may ensue.

Herpes simplex virus hepatitis is serious, but fortunately rare. It should be suspected in patients with severe mucocutaneous herpes and acute hepatitis. Immunosuppression can reactivate latent infection.

Varicella zoster hepatitis is also rare in renal transplant recipients and can be severe in immunosuppressed graft recipients who may present with pneumonitis and/or meningoencephalitis together with confluent hemorrhagic rash. Prognosis is poor.

Patients presenting with fever, lymphadenopathy, and hepatitis should raise the suspicion of EBV infection. Hepatitis usually resolves as patients recover from viral infection.

Drug toxicity is an important cause of hepatic dysfunction in renal transplant recipient and should be considered in differential diagnosis in every case.

Azathioprine, a 6-mecaptoprine derivative, can cause hepatic injury in up to 40% of all recipients. A review of 320 heart transplants revealed a 9% incidence of azathioprine-related hepatotoxicity, which necessitated discontinuation of the drug. Azathioprine causes mainly intrahepatic cholestasis, which manifests by jaundice, pruritus, dark urine, and acholic stool, and usually occurs 3 weeks to 6 months after initiating the therapy. Liver enzymes are moderately elevated and alkaline phosphatase is always high. Azathioprine hepatotoxicity, which is dose dependent, develops when doses exceed 2 mg/kg/day, or with lower doses in previously diseased liver. The prognosis is good when the drug is discontinued. However, progressive irreversible cholestasis may rarely occur, despite discontinuing azathioprine, resulting in liver failure a few weeks later. Chronic use of azathioprine has been implicated in inducing venoocclusive disease, peliosis hepatis, nodular regenerative hyperplasia, and sinusoidal fibrosis.

Cyclosporine can cause dose-dependent cholestatic hepatic dysfunction characterized by increases in serum bile acids and bilirubin, but with little or no increase in aminotransferases. Studies in humans have demonstrated inhibition of bile acid transport without any evidence of cell necrosis. It usually appears in the first weeks after renal transplant when high doses of cyclosporin are used. Prognosis is good with lower doses.

MANAGEMENT OF ACUTE HEPATIC DYSFUNCTION IN RENAL TRANSPLANT RECIPIENTS

The management of acute hepatic dysfunction in renal transplant recipients depends mainly on identification of the potential etiology. Thorough drug history and elimination of hepatotoxic drugs is essential. Appropriate serologic tests for hepatitis B, C, and A; CMV (in blood, urine, and saliva); EBV; and herpes simplex should be performed. Because antibody response is altered in immunosuppressed renal transplant recipients, a high index of suspicion based on history and clinical presentation in conjunction with appropriate laboratory tests should help in reaching the correct diagnosis of viral hepatitis. Thus if hepatitis B or C is suspected, HBV DNA (deoxyribonucleic acid) and HCV RNA (ribonucleic acid) by polymerase chain reaction (PCR), rather than serology, may be needed for definitive diagnosis. In cases of cholestasis, it is advisable to obtain an ultrasound or computed tomography to rule out infiltrative or metastatic disease as well as biliary tract obstruction.

Ganciclovir has been used for prophylaxis and treatment of CMV with good results. Acyclovir is the treatment of choice for both herpes simplex and varicella zoster hepatitis.

DIFFERENTIAL DIAGNOSIS OF CHRONIC LIVER DISEASE

Clinical and Biochemical Manifestation

The classical signs and symptoms of liver disease such as jaundice, pruritus, ascites, edema, and encephalopathy are usually absent in immunosuppressed renal transplant recipients, except in the rare case of fulminant hepatic failure or when the patient develops end-stage liver disease. Not only are the clinical findings sparse but also the biochemical abnormalities are subtle and show only mild to moderate rise in transaminases, which fluctuate during the posttransplant course.

Liver Histology

Despite the subtle clinical and biochemical findings in renal transplant recipients with liver disease, histologic progression to cirrhosis occurs in many of these patients. In one series, during a mean follow-up of 5 years, death from hepatic failure ensued in 26% of patients with histologic evidence of chronic persistent hepatitis, compared with 64% with chronic active hepatitis and 55% with hemosiderosis. In these patients, liver disease progressed to cirrhosis. None of the patients with morphologic diagnosis of fat metamorphosis or chronic portal triaditis died from hepatic failure or developed cirrhosis.

CHRONIC HEPATITIS B

The natural history of HBV infection in renal transplant recipients differs from that in the dialysis population as well as from the general population. This is because immunosuppressed renal transplant recipients fail to mount adequate immune response to viral infections. They have less than 1% conversion of hepatitis B surface antigen (HBsAg) to anti-HBs as compared with 20% and 85% in dialysis patients and the general population, respectively. Several studies have demonstrated that HBV infection is associated with more severe hepatic dysfunction in renal transplant patients as compared with dialysis patients. This is manifested by accelerated progression of liver disease to cirrhosis as well as increased frequency of hepatocellular carcinoma with substantial increase in the morbidity and mortality in renal transplant recipients. This increase in morbidity and mortality has cautioned against renal transplant in HBV-infected patients and implies that chronic hemodialysis may offer a better long-term outcome.

Immunosuppression not only impairs the immune response but is also responsible for reactivation of previously quiescent HBV infection as evidenced by increase in viral replication, reappearance of HBsAg in anti-HBs positive patients, and detection of HBV DNA in patients who were negative for HBsAg and HBV DNA before transplant. These findings suggest that immunosuppression amplifies even minimal residual HBV infection.

The absence of hepatitis B e antigen (HBeAg) or HBV DNA in sera of renal transplant recipients may decrease the likelihood of hepatic decompensation but does not exclude it. The advent of the sensitive PCR testing has demonstrated that even a minute pretransplantation viral level can be associated with HBV reactivation.

The progression of HBV-related liver disease to extensive liver fibrosis and ultimately cirrhosis in renal transplant recipients occurs in the absence of extensive hepatocellular necrosis or inflammation. This may explain the lack of a significant rise of the aminotransferase level often observed. It is noteworthy that sudden discontinuation of immunosuppressive therapy in these patients can result in very severe or even fulminant hepatitis. This is due to the high viral load in previously immunosuppressed individuals who become immunocompetent after discontinuation of immunosuppressive therapy.

The effect of HBV infection on graft survival following renal transplantation is not clear. Some data suggest that the presence of HBsAg or even HBV DNA in serum delays renal graft rejection, whereas anti-HBs was associated with early graft rejection.

Management

There is no clear evidence that reducing immunosuppressive therapy is of benefit in ameliorating the course of hepatitis B in renal transplant recipients. However, in histologic study of liver disease in HBsAg-positive renal recipients receiving cyclosporine over a mean follow-up of 43 months, the liver disease was mild. This was attributed to the reduction in doses of prednisone and azathioprine when cyclosporine was added.

Recombinant alpha-interferon has an immunomodulating effect and carries, at least theoretically, the risk of graft rejection and is not recommended outside controlled clinical trials. Newer antiviral medication (e.g., Lamivudine) may be beneficial but this is yet to be seen.

Recommendation of Renal Transplantation in Hepatitis B Virus–Infected Patients

The decision to perform renal transplantation in HBV-infected patients should be restricted to those who have histologically mild disease, for example, chronic persistent hepatitis. Although absence of HBeAg and HBV DNA does not preclude reactivation of HBV infection after transplant, it is advisable that both markers be negative before transplant. Patients should be informed about the possibility of deterioration of their liver disease even if they manifest the favorable criteria mentioned previously.

HEPATITIS D (DELTA HEPATITIS)

Hepatitis D virus (HDV) occurs only in the presence of HBV infection. Infection can be either simultaneous (coinfection) or may be acquired in the presence of chronic hepatitis B (superinfection). In North America, HDV infection is most commonly found in intravenous drug abusers. It usually results in severe hepatitis.

HDV infection is a rare event in renal transplant recipients, but should be considered in any patient with rapidly deteriorating hepatitis B. Diagnosis is based on detection of antibody to HDV.

CHRONIC HEPATITIS C

The prevalence of hepatitis C in the renal transplant population varies between 10% and 30% in various studies. This range may simply reflect significant variation in geographic prevalence of HCV infection. Most of these patients acquired the infection while on dialysis. Duration of dialysis, number of blood transfusions, retransplantation, and intravenous drug abuse are recognized risk factors for acquiring HCV before transplantation. Nonetheless, transmission of hepatitis C by organ transplantation from the HCV-infected donor has been clearly documented with variable though high transmission rate ranging from 56% to 97%. These differences in transmission rate can be explained in part by differences in organ preservations. Pulsatile perfusion with modified Belzer's perfusate has been shown to reduce viral load in the kidney and HCV RNA in the perfusate by 99% after several hours of pulsatile perfusion. Others suggest that perioperative blood transfusion or variability of virulence according to HCV genotype may account for transmission of HCV via the graft.

Outcome

The natural history of HCV in renal transplant patients is not well established. However, neither patient survival nor graft tolerance was affected in 10-year follow-up with or without biochemical evidence of hepatitis. HCV viremia as tested with PCR persists in virtually all HCV-positive patients after transplantation. It is worth understanding that the presence of HCV RNA may be the only clue of HCV infection, as shown by test positivity in 2% to 9% of transplanted patients who did not have anti-HCV antibodies by second-generation tests [enzyme-linked immunosorbent assay (ELISA) 2].

There is insufficient data in the literature about the evolution of liver disease in HCV-positive transplant patients to draw firm conclusions. However, at least 50% of these patients exhibit uncomplicated clinical courses with normal transaminases in 5-year follow-up. Normal transaminases do not exclude hepatopathy in HCV-positive patients. In fact as many as half of patients with histologic evidence of chronic liver disease have normal transaminases. In addition, there is no correlation between HCV titre and biochemical abnormality.

Other factors that contribute to the severity of HCV-related liver injury include HCV genotype, alcohol abuse, and coinfection with HBV and HCV. There are at least six different genotypes of HCV. Many studies have demonstrated that not only disease progression but also responsiveness to interferon therapy is determined by HCV genotype. There is also a theoretic risk of HCV genotype coinfection via infected organ with different HCV genotype.

HCV infection causes more severe liver injury in alcoholics possibly due to alcohol-induced enhancement of viral replication. The progression of liver disease is more rapid and the risk for development of hepatocellular carcinoma is higher among alcoholics. Hence, patients with HCV infection are strongly encouraged to abstain from all alcoholic beverages.

Also, coinfection with HBV and HCV has been found to be more prevalent in renal transplant recipients with suggestion of more aggressive disease. However, more studies using the more sensitive PCR testing method rather than serologic markers are needed to confirm this finding.

Effect of Immunosuppression

It is likely that posttransplantation immunosuppression activates viral replication. Quantitative HCV RNA measured by PCR significantly increased 1 year after transplantation. The effect of the long-term maintenance immunosuppression on the course of HCV disease remains unclear.

Management

As in HBV infection in kidney transplant recipients, interferon treatment carries the risk of inducing or facilitating graft rejection; also, its efficacy has not been proven in immunosuppressed patients. Hence, its use should be restricted to clinical trials.

The issue of transplantation of kidneys from HCV-positive organ donors has been debatable. Most centers avoid transplantation of kidneys from HCV-positive donors to negative recipients. Some authors suggest using positive HCV allografts in HCV RNA–positive recipients.

Anti-HCV–positive patients before kidney transplantation should have a PCR test for HCV RNA and a liver biopsy for histologic staging regardless of the transaminases level.

Patients with minimal-change or chronic persistent hepatitis are suitable for transplant. However, for those with more aggressive disease or early cirrhosis, there are insufficient longitudinal follow-up data that permit the determination of whether such patients should be transplanted or remain on dialysis. Some authors suggest a trial of interferon before transplantation for those with active disease, but again safety and efficacy of interferon in patients with end-stage renal disease has yet to be determined.

As for HCV-positive transplant recipients, every effort should be made to minimize immunosuppressive therapy. Perhaps the use of cyclosporine as maintenance monotherapy could be useful.

HEMOSIDEROSIS

Hemosiderosis is a frequent cause of chronic liver disease in renal transplant recipients. In one series, hemosiderosis was demonstrated in 12.7% of liver biopsy specimens of transplant recipients with chronic liver disease who had no evidence of iron deposition before renal transplantation. During a mean follow-up of 5 years, death from hepatic failure occurred in 55% of patients with hemosiderosis.

Multiple blood transfusions before transplantation, especially before the era of erythropoietin therapy, is probably the major etiologic factor. However, unrecognized viral hepatitis or alcoholic liver disease, which is associated with increased hepatic iron deposition, could be the cause.

In patients with histologic evidence of hemosiderosis, intermittent phlebotomies are the treatment of choice and carry good prognosis if initiated early. If significant hepatic fibrosis is established, the disease will progress to cirrhosis despite depletion of hepatic iron.

Selected Readings

DeLeve LD, Kaplowitz N. Mechanisms of drug-induced liver disease. *Gastroenterol Clin North Am* 1995;24:787–810.

An in-depth review of drug-induced liver disease.

Martin P, Friedman LS. Chronic viral hepatitis and the management of chronic renal failure. *Kidney Int* 1995;47:1231–1241.

An excellent comprehensive discussion of chronic viral hepatitis in chronic renal failure and kidney transplant recipients.

Pereira BJG, Milford EL, Kirdman RL, et al. Transmission of hepatitis C virus by organ transplantation. *N Engl J Med* 1991;325:454–460.

An important article about transmission of hepatitis C virus (HCV) by organ transplantation.

Rao VK, Anderson WR. Liver disease after liver transplantation. *Am J Kidney Dis* 1992;19(5):496–501.

An overview of the scope of liver diseases in renal transplant recipients.

Rostaing L, Izopet J, Baron E, et al. Preliminary results of treatment of chronic hepatitis C with recombinant interferon alpha in renal transplant recipients. *Nephrol Dial Transplant* 1995;10(Suppl 6):93–96.
A description of the outcomes of interferon treatment in renal allograft recipients.
Roth D. Hepatitis C virus infection and the renal allograft recipient. *Nephron* 1995; 71:249–253.
A useful article on the transmission and diagnosis of HCV infection in renal allograft recipients.

PART 6
Neoplasms in Renal Transplant Recipients

Israel Penn

Prolonged or heavy immunosuppressive therapy used in transplantation is complicated by the development of an unusual assortment of malignancies. This chapter is based on 10,667 patients with 11,359 types of cancers that arose *de novo* after transplantation, who were reported to the Cincinnati Transplant Tumor Registry (CTTR) up until May 1998. The patients included 8,665 renal allograft recipients; 1,116 cardiac; 521 hepatic; 176 bone marrow; 101 pancreatic; 48 pulmonary; 34 combined heart–lung; 4 upper abdominal organ cluster transplants; and 2 small bowel transplant recipients.

INCIDENCE OF TUMORS

Overall there was a threefold to fivefold increased risk of malignancies compared with age-matched controls in the general population. Table 89.7 indicates the types of cancers that are increased in transplant patients. The common cancers that are seen in the general population (carcinomas of the lung, breast, prostate, and colon, and invasive uterine cervical carcinomas) show no increase. If nonmelanoma skin cancers and *in situ* carcinomas of the cervix are excluded from the 11,359 malignancies, as they are from most cancer statistics, we then observe a variety of tumors in transplant patients that are uncommon in the general population: lymphomas, 24% versus 6%; lip cancers, 6.2% versus 0.3%; Kaposi's sarcoma, 5.7% versus a negligible incidence; carcinomas of the kidney, 5.1% versus 2.4%; carcinomas of the vulva and perineum, 3.5% versus 0.5%; hepatobiliary tumors, 2.2% versus 1.1%; and sarcomas (excluding Kaposi's), 1.8% versus 0.6% (Table 89.7).

TABLE 89.7. Epidemiologic Frequency of Common Tumors Found in Transplant Patients

Type of Cancer	Fold Increase
Skin cancer	4–21
Lip cancer	29
Carcinomas *in situ* of uterine cervix	14–16
Non-Hodgkin's lymphoma	29–49
Kaposi's sarcoma (KS)	400–500
Hepatobiliary carcinomas	30
Carcinomas of vulva and anus	100
Renal carcinomas	2–3
Sarcomas (excluding KS)	2–3

ETIOLOGY OF TUMORS

Though many factors are probably etiologic, two play a key role. Depressed immunity *per se* impairs the body's ability to cope with cancers caused by various carcinogens such as sunlight or oncogenic viruses. Infections with potentially oncogenic viruses are common in immunosuppressed patients. Epstein-Barr virus (EBV) infection may contribute to the development of non-Hodgkin's lymphomas, some cases of Hodgkin's disease, and some leiomyosarcomas; papillomavirus infections contribute to carcinomas of the cervix, vulva, perineum, and possibly other skin areas; and hepatitis B or C virus contribute to hepatocellular carcinomas. Kaposi's sarcomas is strongly linked to infection by human herpesvirus-8 (HHV-8), also known as the *Kaposi's sarcoma–associated virus.*

CLINICAL FEATURES OF POSTTRANSPLANT TUMORS

The tumors affected a relatively young group of people whose average age at the time of transplantation was 42 years (range 8 days to 80 years). Forty percent were younger than 40 years of age at the time of transplantation. Sixty-six percent were male, in keeping with the 2:1 ratio of male to female patients who undergo renal and cardiac transplantation.

The incidence of malignancy increases with the length of follow-up after transplantation. An Australasian study of 6,596 patients showed that the percent probability of developing cancer following renal transplantation from cadaver donors 24 years after operation was 66% for skin cancers, 27% for nonskin cancers, and 72% for any type of neoplasm. These exceptional figures must be interpreted with caution because most tumors were skin cancers (which are very common in Australia) and the number of 24-year survivors was small. Nevertheless, they emphasize the need to follow transplant patients indefinitely.

Certain tumors appeared at fairly distinct intervals after transplantation. In contrast with other known oncogenic stimuli in man, which often take 15 to 20 years or more before they cause clinical lesions, cancers were diagnosed a relatively short time after transplantation. Kaposi's sarcoma was first to appear at an average of 21 (range 1 to 225.5) months after transplantation. Lymphomas appeared at an average of 34 (range 0.25 to 305.5) months after transplantation. Carcinomas of the vulva and perineum appeared at the longest time after transplantation at an average of 113 (range 1 to 289) months. The average time of appearance of all tumors was 63 (range 0.25 to 305.5) months.

Cancers of the Skin and Lips

Cancers of the skin and lips were the most common and comprised 4,269 of the 11,359 malignancies (38%) (Table 89.8).

The prevalence of cutaneous tumors increases with the length of follow-up after transplantation, as demonstrated by an Australasian study of 6,596 cadaveric renal allografts who showed a linear increase in the prevalence of skin cancer, reaching 66% at 24 years posttransplantation. Similarly, a Dutch study showed a 10% prevalence of nonmelanoma skin cancer in renal transplant recipients at 10 years posttransplantation, rising to 40% after 20 years.

Skin cancers in transplant patients showed some unusual features compared with similar lesions in the general population. Basal cell carcinomas outnumber squamous cell carcinomas in the general population by a ratio of 5 to 1. But the opposite was true in transplant recipients in whom squamous cell

TABLE 89.8. *De Novo* Tumors in Organ Allograft Recipients[a]

Type of Neoplasm	No. of Tumors
Cancers of skin and lips	4,269
Lymphomas	1,910
Carcinomas of the lung	635
Kaposi's sarcoma	451
Carcinomas of uterus (cervix 352; body 66; unspecified 5)	423
Carcinomas of the kidney (host kidney 345; allograft kidney 38; unspecified 22)	405
Carcinomas of colon and rectum	386
Carcinomas of the breast	353
Carcinomas of the head and neck (excluding thyroid, parathyroid, and eye)	313
Carcinomas of the vulva, perineum, penis, scrotum	278
Carcinomas of urinary bladder	246
Carcinomas of prostate gland	225
Metastatic carcinoma (primary site unknown)	224
Leukemias	201
Hepatobiliary carcinomas	185
Sarcomas (excluding Kaposi's sarcoma)	142
Carcinomas of thyroid gland	134
Cancers of stomach	132
Testicular carcinomas	84
Carcinomas of pancreas	82
Miscellaneous tumors	281
TOTAL	11,359

[a] There were 10,667 patients of whom 647 (6.1%) had two or more distinct tumor types involving different organ systems. Of these, 43 patients each had 3 separate types of cancer and 1 had 4.

carcinomas outnumbered basal cell carcinomas by 1.8 : 1. In the general population, these types of skin cancer occur mostly in people between 60 and 80 years of age, but the average age of transplant patients was 30 years younger. In addition, the incidence of multiple skin cancers in this worldwide collection of patients (present in at least 43%) was remarkably high and was similar to that seen among the general population living only in areas of copious sunlight. Several individuals each had more than 100 skin cancers. Malignant melanomas comprised 5% of skin cancers in contrast with an incidence of 2.7% in the general population of the United States.

Some conditions that are common in transplant patients can closely resemble skin cancers. They include warts, hyperkeratoses, and keratoacanthomas. If there is any suspicion of malignancy one should biopsy the questionable areas. Lip cancers may also pose diagnostic problems because they frequently are atypical, and appear as superficial ulcers that do not have an indurated base and rolled everted edge. Occasionally, two superficial lip cancers may occur simultaneously. It is advisable to biopsy all lip ulcers that persist for more than 1 month except during the early posttransplant period when herpetic ulcers are common.

Lymphomas and Lymphoproliferations

Of a total of 1,910 lymphomas in the CTTR (Table 89.8) less than 3% were cases of Hodgkin's disease, whereas it comprises 9% of lymphomas in the general population. Similarly, myeloma comprised almost 4% of posttransplant lymphomas compared with 18% in the general population. The bulk of the posttransplant lymphomas (1,782) were non-Hodgkin's lymphomas, which comprised 93% of lymphomas compared with 73% in the general population.

Morphologically, most non-Hodgkin's lymphomas and lymphoproliferations were classified as immunoblastic sarcomas, reticulum cell sarcomas, microgliomas, or large cell lymphomas. Because many lesions occupied the ill-defined "no-man's land" between infection and neoplasia, the term *posttransplant lymphoproliferative disorder (PTLD)* is now frequently used, and this term will be used in the remainder of this chapter. Of those studied immunologically, 85% arose from B lymphocytes, whereas 15% were T-cell lymphomas. PTLDs differed from their counterparts in the general population in several respects. Whereas extranodal involvement occurs in 24% to 48% of patients with non-Hodgkin's lymphomas in the community at large, it was present in 70% of transplant patients with PTLD. In the general population, approximately 1% of non-Hodgkin's lymphomas affect the brain parenchyma, whereas in organ transplant patients 21% involved the central nervous system (CNS), usually the brain, in which the lesions were frequently multicentric in distribution. Spinal cord involvement was rare. Another notable feature was that in 53% of patients with CNS involvement, the lesions were confined to this site, whereas in the general population cerebral lymphomas are frequently associated with lesions in other organs.

A remarkable finding was the frequency of either macroscopic or microscopic allograft involvement, which occurred in 23% of patients with PTLD. In some individuals with renal, cardiac, or hepatic allografts, the lymphomatous infiltrate was misdiagnosed as rejection when biopsies, performed because of allograft dysfunction, were studied microscopically. This resulted in erroneous therapeutic decisions as immunosuppressive therapy was intensified, whereas a major treatment of PTLD is reduction of dosage.

The genome of EBV has been isolated for more than 90% of PTLDs but some tumors showed no evidence of the virus despite the use of sensitive molecular probes. EBV is believed to cause a spectrum of lesions ranging from benign polyclonal B-cell hyperplasia on one hand to frank monoclonal B-cell lymphomas on the other.

The clinical presentation of PTLD was extremely variable. Some patients were completely asymptomatic or presented with a picture resembling infectious mononucleosis. Other presenting features included fever, night sweats, upper respiratory infection, weight loss, diarrhea, abdominal pain, lymphadenopathy, and tonsillitis. Tonsillar enlargement was sometimes so marked that emergency tracheostomy was necessary. Because the gastrointestinal tract was frequently involved, a common presentation was acute perforation of an intestinal lesion causing peritonitis. Less commonly, gastrointestinal bleeding or intestinal obstruction was the presenting feature.

At times patients, presented with lung lesions, or a renal mass or a mass in another organ. Occasionally the presentation imitated allograft rejection and the diagnosis was made by finding an atypical lymphoblastic infiltrate in a biopsy specimen. Some patients presented with a confusing picture of disseminated sepsis and multiple organ failure and the diagnosis was made only at autopsy examination.

A possible CNS lymphoma should be suspected whenever a transplant patient develops neurologic symptoms. A thorough workup is necessary and may include examination of the cerebrospinal fluid, computerized axial tomography, electroencephalography, radionuclide brain scan, cerebral angiography, and magnetic resonance imaging. Such tests help to exclude other causes of neurologic symptoms in these patients such as hypertensive encephalopathy, meningitis, brain abscess, or intracranial bleeding.

The outcomes were studied in 1,324 patients with PTLD. Of these, 217 patients (16%) had no treatment, and the tumor was discovered at autopsy in 104 of them (48%). It is a matter of concern that so many patients died without treatment, either because the diagnosis was missed or was made too late for effective therapy to be started. No data regarding therapy were available in 61 other patients. Treatment was given to 1,045 patients of whom 394 (38%) had complete remissions. In 68 of these recipients (17%), the only treatment used was reduction or cessation of immunosuppressive therapy.

Kaposi's Sarcoma

The frequent occurrence of Kaposi's sarcoma in transplant recipients was in marked contrast with its incidence in the general population of the United States (before the acquired immunodeficiency syndrome [AIDS] epidemic started), where it comprised only 0.02% to 0.07% of all neoplasms. Its high incidence in this worldwide collection of patients is comparable to that seen in tropical Africa, where Kaposi's sarcoma occurs with greatest frequency, and where it makes up 3% to 9% of all tumors. It is striking that the number of transplant patients with Kaposi's sarcomas (451) in the CTTR exceeds those with carcinomas of the colorectum (386) or breast (353) (Table 89.8). Apart from individuals with AIDS, who frequently have Kaposi's sarcoma, there is probably no other series in which the number of Kaposi's sarcoma exceeds either of these two common cancers, except possibly in tropical Africa where Kaposi's sarcomas occurs frequently and colon cancer is rare.

Kaposi's sarcoma affected males and females in a 3:1 ratio, but far less than the 9:1 to 15:1 ratio seen with Kaposi's sarcoma in the general population. Kaposi's sarcoma was most common in transplant patients who were Arab, African-American, or of Greek, Italian, Jewish, or Turkish ancestry.

Transplant-related Kaposi's sarcoma was rare in children. Only a small percentage tested positive for the human immunodeficiency virus (HIV).

Fifty-eight percent of 446 patients, in whom the distribution of lesions was known, had nonvisceral Kaposi's sarcoma confined to the skin, conjunctiva, or oropharyngolaryngeal mucosa, and 42% had visceral disease that involved mainly the gastrointestinal tract, lungs, and lymph nodes but also affected other organs. Of 260 patients with nonvisceral disease, the lesions were confined to the skin in 255 patients (98%) and to the mouth or oropharynx in 5 (2%). The 186 patients with visceral disease had no skin involvement in 44 instances (24%), but 8 of them (4%) had oral involvement, which provided a readily accessible site for biopsy and diagnosis of the disease. Of those with nonvisceral involvement, 142 (55%) had complete remissions after treatment. Interestingly, 35% of these remissions occurred when the only treatment was a drastic reduction of immunosuppressive therapy. In patients with visceral disease, only 56 of 186 patients (30%) had complete remissions. However, 32 of the 56 remissions (57%) occurred in response to reduction or cessation of immunosuppressive therapy only. Fifty-four percent of patients with visceral Kaposi's sarcoma died. Of the deaths, 75 of the 101 patients (74%) died of the malignancy per se.

Of 39 kidney allograft recipients, in whom renal function was recorded following reduction or cessation of immunosuppressive therapy, 21 lost their allografts to rejection, 2 had impaired function, and 16 retained stable function.

The physician should suspect Kaposi's sarcoma whenever a transplant patient presents with reddish-blue macules or plaques in the skin or oropharyngeal mucosa, or apparently infected granulomas that fail to heal. If the diagnosis is confirmed, a comprehensive workup is needed to exclude internal visceral involvement.

Carcinomas of the Uterus

Carcinomas of the cervix occurred in 10% of the women with posttransplant malignancies. *In situ* lesions comprised at least 70% of cases (Table 89.8). Two epidemiologic studies suggest a 14- to 16-fold increased incidence of *in situ* cervical carcinoma; however, the small numbers of cases reported to the CTTR suggest that many cases are being missed. To avoid this error every postadolescent female organ transplant recipient should have regular pelvic examinations and cervical smears.

Carcinomas of the Vulva and Perineum

Carcinomas of the vulva, perineum, scrotum, penis, perianal skin, or anus comprised 3.5% of posttransplant malignancies (Table 89.8). Females outnumbered males by 2.6% in contrast with most other posttransplant cancers in which males outnumbered females by more than 2:1.

One-third of patients had *in situ* lesions. A disturbing feature is that patients with invasive lesions were much younger (average age 42 years) than their counterparts in the general population, whose average age is usually between 50 and 70 years. More than 40% of transplant patients with these neoplasms gave a preceding history of condyloma acuminatum. Female patients sometimes exhibited a "field effect" with cancerous involvement not only of the vulva but also of the vagina and/or uterine cervix.

Renal Carcinomas

A striking feature was that 99 of the 405 patients (24%) had incidentally discovered renal cancers, mostly renal cell carcinomas. These were found during workup for other disorders, at nephrectomy for hypertension or other reasons, during operation for some other disease, or at autopsy examination.

Unlike most other posttransplant malignancies that arose as complications of immunosuppressive therapy, many renal carcinomas were related to the underlying kidney disease in renal allograft recipients, but no explanation is available for 29 carcinomas that occurred in 25 cardiac and 4 liver allograft recipients. Most cancers in renal recipients developed in their own diseased kidneys, although 39 (10%) appeared in renal allografts, from 2 to 258 (average 75) months after transplantation. Nine of the 39 tumors (23%) were diagnosed within 2 years of transplantation. It is possible that they may have been present in the allograft at the time of transplantation but were small enough to escape notice.

Two predisposing causes of renal carcinomas were identified. Analgesic nephropathy was the underlying indication for transplantation in 29 of 366 (8%) transplant patients with carcinomas of their own diseased kidneys. This disorder is known to cause malignancies, mostly transitional cell carcinomas, in various parts of the urinary tract. This is borne out in the CTTR series in which 17 of 29 (59%) patients with analgesia-related renal carcinomas had similar tumors elsewhere in the urinary tract.

Another predisposing cause of cancers in renal transplant recipients is acquired cystic disease (ACD) of their own kidneys. It occurs in 30% to 95% of patients receiving long-term hemodialysis, and is complicated by renal adenocarcinoma, which is increased 30- to 40-fold over its incidence in the general population. With a successfully functioning transplant, ACD tends to regress and, theoretically, the risk of developing carcinoma is reduced. However, cases of persistent ACD and development of renal cell carcinoma have been reported in patients with successfully functioning renal allografts. The precise incidence of ACD-related carcinomas in renal transplant recipients is not known.

Hepatobiliary Tumors

Most cases (73%) in the CTTR (Table 89.8) were hepatomas and, in a substantial number, there was a preceding history of hepatitis B infection. Since hepatitis C screening became available, increasing numbers of hepatomas related to chronic hepatitis C infection are being reported.

Sarcomas (Excluding Kaposi's Sarcoma)

The majority of sarcomas involved the soft tissues or visceral organs, whereas cartilage or bone involvement was uncommon. Of the 142 sarcomas, the major types were fibrous histiocytoma (26 cases), leiomyosarcoma (22), fibrosarcoma (12), hemangiosarcoma (12), rhabdomyosarcoma (11), mesothelioma (9), liposarcoma (7), synovial sarcoma (6), and miscellaneous sarcomas (37).

RELATIONSHIP TO INDIVIDUAL IMMUNOSUPPRESSIVE AGENTS

Successful maintenance of prolonged allograft function requires continuous therapy with powerful immunosuppressive agents that impair lymphocyte function. In the pioneering years of transplantation, immunosuppressive therapy consisted of two agents, azathioprine (or occasionally cyclophosphamide) and prednisone, supplemented at some centers by a brief course of antilymphocyte globulin (ALG) or antithymocyte globulin (ATG). During the past 15 years, cyclosporine was, in large part, responsible for the dramatic improvement in the results of transplantation. The immunosuppressive armamentarium was also broadened by the introduction of various monoclonal antilymphocyte antibody preparations (of which OKT3 is the most widely used) for short-term administration (days to weeks) to prevent or treat rejection. More recent additions include tacrolimus and mycophenolate mofetil. The introduction of these new agents caused changes in therapy so that three, four, or even five drugs were given to some patients over a short time span. An undesired side effect of such intense immunosuppression was a disproportionately high incidence of those malignancies that occur during the early months after transplantation, mostly PTLDs. The most commonly used immunosuppressive measures in the present series are shown in Table 89.9. A glance at the table suggests disproportionately high usage of cyclosporine and monoclonal antilymphocyte antibodies in patients who developed lymphomas compared with nonlymphomatous tumors. However, cyclosporine was rarely used alone, but was usually part of triple-therapy regimens including azathioprine and prednisone. Similarly, monoclonal antibodies were never used alone but were most commonly added to regimens using triple therapy, or, less commonly, quadruple therapy (with ALG or ATG added), and, least frequently, double therapy (cyclosporine and prednisone). Experience with tacrolimus and mycophenolate mofetil is limited but, thus far, the pattern of neoplasms observed has mimicked that seen soon after cyclosporine therapy was first introduced when a disproportionate number of PTLDs was observed.

TREATMENT OF POSTTRANSPLANT CANCERS

When treating cancers in organ allograft recipients, one must emphasize that some neoplasms demonstrate more aggressive behavior than do similar malignancies in nontransplant patients. Early tumors are curable with local therapy provided that their growth has not given them adequate vascular access. Once this has been obtained, the host's depressed immune system is believed to permit greater-than-normal survival of cancer cells in the bloodstream. The result is more rapid tumor dissemination and demise of the host than would be expected in a setting of immunocompetence.

In managing patients with premalignant skin lesions or early cancers, a useful treatment is a 6-week course of topical 5-fluorouracil cream applied twice daily. This destroys many premalignant lesions and even very superficial carcinomas. This treatment is rapidly being replaced by topical use of 0.05% tretinoin cream (a retinoid). This is effective in treating warts and keratoses in organ allograft recipients and perhaps may inhibit cutaneous carcinogenesis.

TABLE 89.9. Most Common Immunosuppressive Measures Used

Agent	All Patients[a]	% of Patients	Patients with Lymphomas[b]	% of Patients	Patients with Nonlymphomas	% of Patients[c]
Prednisone	10,396	97	1,768	93	8,628	98
Azathioprine	9,242	87	1,492	78	7,750	88
Cyclosporine	5,670	53	1,258	66	4,412	50
Antilymphocyte globulin (ALG) or antithymocyte globin (ATG)	3,020	28	653	34	2,367	27
Monoclonal antilymphocyte antibodies (mainly OKT3)	944	9	440	23	504	6
Splenectomy	836	8	113	6	723	8
Local irradiation of the allograft	747	7	108	6	639	7
Cyclophosphamide	458	4	111	6	347	4
Actinomycin	201	2	41	2	160	2
Total body irradiation	118	1	70	4	48	0.5
Tacrolimus	117	1	68	4	49	0.6
Mycophenolate Mofetil	42	0.4	24	1	18	0.2

[a] 10,667 patients
[b] 1,907 patients; includes 128 patients with Hodgkin's disease, multiple myeloma, or plasmacytoma.
[c] 8,760 patients

In patients with numerous skin cancers, some dermatologists advocate reduction of immunosuppressive therapy in individuals with long-term stable graft function. The reduction consists of progressive discontinuation of azathioprine in patients receiving triple therapy. Some dermatologists give oral retinoids to reduce the frequent recurrences. Experience is limited thus far, but one must be aware of side effects including elevated serum lipids, hepatic intolerance, mucocutaneous xerosis, hair loss, and skeletal abnormalities. Treatment of skin tumors includes surgical excision, cryosurgery, chemosurgery, or radiation therapy. *In situ* carcinomas of the uterine cervix are managed by simple hysterectomy, cervical conization, or cryotherapy.

Localized PTLD may be successfully excised or treated with radiation therapy. A significant proportion of more extensive lesions have regressed, partially or completely, after reduction or cessation of immunosuppressive therapy. In particular, in recipients with widespread, or extensive, or potentially life-threatening PTLD, all immunosuppression should be stopped except for a minimal dose of prednisone, until all evidence of neoplasm has disappeared. Allograft rejection may not occur or may evolve slowly in chronic fashion, because many of these patients have been very heavily immunosuppressed and a long time may elapse before they regain immunocompetence. Once PTLD has regressed, immunosuppressive therapy should be resumed in small doses and then gradually increased to maintenance levels that, however, should be lower than those given before the appearance of PTLD.

Often PTLD responds to multimodality therapy, which may include excision, radiation therapy, reduction of immunosuppression, acyclovir or ganciclovir administration to combat an associated EBV infection, and treatment with interferon-α. Other treatments that may be beneficial include infusion of IgG, administration of monoclonal antibodies directed against B cells, infusion of donor T lymphocytes, and administration of lymphokine-activated killer (LAK) cells. Chemotherapy is usually reserved for patients who do not respond to other measures.

Localized Kaposi's sarcoma responds well to excision, radiation therapy, or intralesional injections of chemotherapeutic agents such as bleomycin. More extensive lesions may respond to reduction or cessation of immunosuppressive therapy. Interferon-α is another useful treatment in some patients with widespread Kaposi's sarcoma. Kaposi's sarcoma also responds well to chemotherapy using agents such as vincristine, vinblastine, bleomycin, or etoposide. Attainment of complete remissions frequently requires use of various combinations of the aforementioned treatments.

Cancers other than those mentioned previously should be treated by standard surgical, radiation, or chemotherapeutic modalities. As mentioned previously, one option in treating posttransplant tumors is reduction or cessation of immunosuppressive therapy. The value of this approach is borne out by experience with inadvertently transplanted cancers, some of which regressed completely following cessation of immunosuppressive therapy and removal of a renal allograft. As previously stated, cessation or reduction of immunosuppressive therapy, when used by itself, resulted in a substantial number of complete remissions of PTLD and Kaposi's sarcoma. However, such treatment has rarely caused regression of epithelial tumors. A drawback of this treatment is that it may precipitate allograft rejection with return of renal allograft recipients to dialysis therapy, but nonrenal allograft recipients may die of this complication. For example, this treatment caused impaired function or allograft loss from rejection in 21 of 39 renal recipients treated for Kaposi's sarcoma. Similarly, in a series of 14 renal recipients whose PTLD was treated (among other methods) by reduction or cessation of immunosuppression, 8 of 12 survivors lost their allografts.

In patients requiring systemic cytotoxic therapy of widespread cancers, we must remember that most agents depress the bone marrow. It is therefore prudent to stop or reduce the administration of azathioprine, cyclophosphamide, or mycophenolate mofetil dosage during such treatment to avoid severe bone marrow depression. Because most cytotoxic drugs have immunosuppressive side effects, satisfactory allograft function may persist for prolonged periods. Treatment with prednisone may be continued because it is an important component of many cancer chemotherapy protocols. Many patients, particularly with PTLD, are already heavily immunosuppressed, therefore chemotherapeutic agents should be used with caution because some patients have died of overwhelming infections following their use. When using cytotoxic therapy in renal transplant recipients, or in nonkidney recipients who have impaired renal function, one should avoid, if possible, the use of nephrotoxic agents such as cisplatin.

Alpha-interferon has been used to treat some patients with Kaposi's sarcoma or non-Hodgkin's lymphomas, or other cancers. Interferon is a potent immune modulator that increases membrane expression of class I antigens of the major histocompatibility complex, T-cell–mediated cytotoxicity, and natural killer cell function. It may therefore stimulate rejection. However, conflicting findings have been reported following its use in renal allograft recipients. A review of the literature suggests that small doses may be safe but large doses may precipitate rejection.

PROGNOSIS OF POSTTRANSPLANT TUMORS

Most skin cancers are merely a nuisance, although a few may require mutilating procedures in their management. However, a disturbing feature is the aggressive behavior of some skin cancers, mainly squamous cell carcinomas. In the general population, skin cancers seldom metastasize and cause fatalities. Those that do so are usually malignant melanomas. In striking contrast, lymph node metastases occurred in 5.7% of transplant patients with skin cancers. Of 242 such patients, 178 had squamous cell carcinomas, 41 malignant melanomas, 22 Merkel's cell tumors, and one a basal cell carcinoma. Even more worrying is that almost 5% of patients died of their skin cancers. Of 209 deaths, 126 were from squamous cell carcinomas, 62 from malignant melanomas, 17 from Merkel's cell tumors, and 4 from basal cell carcinomas. As indicated previously, 38% of patients with PTLD can expect to have a complete remission, provided that treatment is started in a timely fashion. As regards Kaposi's sarcoma, the prognosis of patients with visceral involvement is much worse than in those with nonvisceral disease because 40% of the former patients died of their disease, which rarely caused fatalities in patients with nonvisceral disease. Although many patients with cancers of the vulva and perineum have responded well to local or extensive excisions of their lesions, 12% have succumbed from metastases despite abdominoperineal resections or radical vulvectomies.

As regards the remaining malignancies, deaths occurred mainly from high-grade carcinomas or sarcomas.

PREVENTION OF POSTTRANSPLANT TUMORS

The level of immunosuppressive therapy should be kept as low as is compatible with good allograft function. Renal transplant physicians and surgeons have learned by bitter experience that it is foolhardy to persist with intense immunosuppressive therapy in the face of repeated or persistent rejection. Rather, they have found it safer to discontinue immunosuppression and return the patient to dialysis therapy until he or she has recovered sufficiently to attempt another transplant procedure. In dealing with severe rejection of a nonrenal allograft, the transplant team does not have the means to provide long-term artifical support should it fail, and in consequence, tends to give high doses of immunosuppressive agents to salvage the graft. One may try to replace a failing liver or cardiac allograft before the patient develops complications of heavy immunosuppression, but the shortage of donors frequently precludes timely retransplantation.

Although the overall risk for the development of cancer in renal transplant recipients is small, it is vitally important to follow patients indefinitely. All postadolescent female patients require regular pelvic examinations and cervical smears to diagnose cervical or vulvar lesions at an early stage. Any untoward symptoms should be thoroughly investigated keeping in mind the most common neoplasms. Because cancers in transplant patients are often mistaken for other disorders, any suspicious areas should be biopsied, if accessible.

It may be possible to prevent the development of some malignancies. Administration of hepatitis B vaccine to dialysis and transplant patients may prevent the development of hepatitis and the associated hepatocellular carcinomas. In addition, avoidance of excessive sun exposure, wearing of protective clothing, and the use of sunscreen applications or tretinoin or other retinoids may prevent skin tumors. Use of barrier methods of contraception may prevent the development of condyloma acuminatum. Early eradication of this disorder possibly may prevent the development of carcinomas of the vulva, perineum, and uterine cervix.

As in the case with many other neoplasms, prevention of posttransplant lymphomas entails avoidance of overimmunosuppression. Ideally, dosage of immunosuppressive agents should be kept at low levels that are able to prevent rejection and maintain good allograft function. In particular, one should try to avoid the use of multiple agents given over a short time period and prolonged or repeated courses of potent antilymphocyte antibody preparations. When courses of intense immunosuppressive therapy are necessary, many physicians use acyclovir or ganciclovir or related antiviral agents as prophylaxis against EBV. On theoretic grounds they may not be as effective as they are virustatic rather than virucidal, and they act only on the linear form of the virus and not on the circular (latent) form that is important in the development of PTLD. There are no prospective, randomized controlled studies to test the efficacy of prophylactic acyclovir or ganciclovir administration. However, a recent study showed that ganciclovir or acyclovir given preemptively, during administration of antilymphocyte agents, reduced the incidence of PTLD to 1 in 198 consecutive recipients, compared with a historic control group in which 7 of 179 recipients developed this disorder. Antiviral prophylaxis is especially important when transplanting organs from EBV-positive donors into EBV-negative recipients, most of whom are children.

Acknowledgment

The author wishes to thank his many colleagues throughout the world who have generously contributed data concerning their patients to the CTTR.

Selected Readings

Barrett WL, First R, Aron BS, et al. Clinical course of malignancies in renal transplant recipients. *Cancer* 1993;72:2186–2189.
A study that demonstrates a more aggressive course of some posttransplant cancers compared with the behavior of similar malignancies in the general population.

Hanto DW. Classification of Epstein-Barr virus-associated posttransplant lymphoproliferative diseases: implications for understanding their pathogenesis and developing rational treatment strategies. *Annu Rev Med* 1995;46:381–394.
An analysis of patients with PTLD with subdivision into categories according to morphology and immunopathology and determining prognosis and treatment.

Kedda M-A, Margolius L, Kew MC, et al. Kaposi's sarcoma-associated herpesvirus in Kaposi's sarcoma occurring in immunosuppressed renal transplant recipients. *Clin Transplant* 1996;10:429–431.
An analysis of several South-African transplant patients who had Kaposi's sarcoma and, in whom, the newly discovered virus was demonstrated in the lesions.

Naiesnik MA, Starzl TE. Epstein-Barr virus, infectious mononucleosis, and posttransplant lymphoproliferative disorders. *Transplant Sci* 1994;4:61–79.
A detailed analysis of the types of lymphomas and lymphoproliferation that occur posttransplantation, treatment of the disorders, and the role of EBV in their development.

Penn I. Why do immunosuppressed patients develop cancer? In: Pimentel E, ed. *CRC Critical reviews in oncogenesis.* Boca Raton: CRC, 1989;1:27-52.
A detailed description of the types of de novo cancer that occur in immunosuppressed patients and detailed analysis of possible etiologic factors.

Penn I. The problem of cancer in organ transplant recipients: an overview. *Transplant Sci* 1994;4:23–32.
A review of cancers that occur in transplant patients in three settings: (a) transmission of cancer from donors with malignancies, (b) cancers presenting before transplantation, and (c) de novo cancers occurring after transplantation.

Penn I, Porat G. Central nervous system lymphomas in organ allograft recipients. *Transplantation* 1995;59:240–244.
A review of 289 organ allograft recipients with posttransplant lymphomas, mainly involving the brain, with details regarding prognosis and treatment.

Penn I. Kaposi's sarcoma in transplant recipients. *Transplantation* 1997;64:669–673.
A review of the clinical features, distribution, treatment, and prognosis of Kaposi's sarcoma with emphasis on racial or ethnic groups who are most likely to develop this problem.

Penn I. Primary kidney tumors before and after renal transplantation. *Transplantation* 1995;59:480–485.
An analysis of several hundred patients with renal carcinomas with guidelines regarding timing of transplant following treatment of preexisting cancers. Also discussion of contributory causes of posttransplant renal cancers.

Sheil AGR, Disney APS, Mathew TH, et al. De novo malignancy emerges as a major cause of morbidity and late failure in renal transplantation. *Transplant Proc* 1993;25:1383–1384.
A report from the Australian and New Zealand Transplant Registry summarizing the types of cancers seen in that area of the world.

Starzl TE, Najaesnik MA, Porter KA, et al. Reversibility of lymphomas and lymphoproliferative lesions developing under cyclosporine-steroid therapy. *Lancet* 1984;1:583–587.
The first report in the world literature of regression of PTLD after reduction of immunosuppressive therapy. One of the seminal articles in the management of this disorder.

PART 7
Hypertension Following Renal Transplantation

Robert S. Gaston and John J. Curtis

As therapeutic advances have reduced the number of immunologic graft losses, greater attention has turned to the impact of nonimmunologic events, such as hypertension. The latter is an important risk factor for accelerated atherosclerosis, now the most common cause of death among transplanted patients. In addition, hypertensive recipients are at significantly increased risk of late allograft failure. Appropriate diagnosis and therapy of hypertension is thus a significant component of the long-term management of renal transplant recipients.

CHARACTERISTICS AND CAUSES (TABLES 89.10 AND 89.11)

Hypertension is a common finding after renal transplantation, at one time or another afflicting more than two-thirds of recipients.

TABLE 89.10. Causes of Posttransplant Hypertension

Intrinsic
Delayed graft function
Acute rejection
Chronic rejection
Cyclosporine nephropathy—chronic
Recurrent primary renal disease
Extrinsic
Native kidneys
Immunosuppressive medications
Cyclosporine
Tacrolimus
Corticosteroids
Transplant renal artery stenosis
Hypercalcemia

The severity of posttransplant hypertension tends to be mild to moderate, and hypertensive crises are relatively rare. Factors usually predicative of essential hypertension (e.g., age, gender, race) are less likely to be associated with posttransplant hypertension; likewise, there is little relationship to the primary renal disease of the recipient. However, severe hypertension before transplantation imparts significant risk afterward, and the greatest risk of posttransplant hypertension occurs in recipients with retained native kidneys and/or whose allograft was of cadaveric origin.

Unlike essential hypertension, with its poorly understood and sometimes obscure pathogenesis, hypertension in a renal transplant recipient often reflects the interplay of several definable, potentially correctable, variables. These pathogenetic factors may be conveniently grouped as residing either intrinsic or extrinsic to the allograft (Table 89.10). In hypertensive animals undergoing cross-transplantation experiments, the contribution of the transplanted kidney to hypertension in the recipient is dominant: hypertension travels "with the kidney." Unless there is some impairment in renal function, under most circumstances the renal pressure-natriuresis relationship should act to normalize blood pressure. Accordingly, whether posttransplant hypertension reflects the presence of intrinsic or extrinsic pathogenetic variables, it likely is maintained via the common mechanism of impaired renal allograft function.

PATHOGENESIS

Intrinsic Impairment of Allograft Function

Intrinsic causes of posttransplant hypertension reflect renal allograft dysfunction as a primary event. In a patient with delayed graft function early after transplantation, the pathogenesis of hypertension resembles that associated with chronic renal failure—elevated systemic pressures due to renin production from diseased native kidneys (and/or the allograft), and absence of renal excretory capacity. Such patients require careful management of volume status and timely dialysis and, in most cases, continuation of previous antihypertensive medications.

After satisfactory allograft function has been established, hypertension can reflect immunologic processes occurring within the transplanted kidney. In both acute and chronic rejection, hypertension has a similar pathogenesis: a poorly functioning kid-

TABLE 89.11. Causes, Characteristics, and Management of Posttransplant Hypertension

Cause	Clinical Characteristics	Management
Delayed graft function	Oliguria, volume excess	Dialysis as indicated Antihypertensive medication Monitor for acute rejection
Acute rejection	Declining GFR Fever with tender, swollen graft	Diagnosis by isotope renogram, fine needle aspirate, or core biopsy High-dose corticosteroids Antilymphocyte agents
Cyclosporine or tacrolimus toxicity, acute	Dose-related, reversible Mild to moderate azotemia Elevated hepatocellular enzymes Tremor, edema	Monitor blood levels Reduction of cyclosporine or tacrolimus dose Must exclude acute rejection
Cyclosporine toxicity, chronic	Slowly progressive azotemia Minimal proteinuria Biopsy—vascular disease with "striped" interstitial fibrosis	May respond to cyclosporine dose reduction Difficult to separate from chronic rejection Antihypertensive medications
Chronic rejection	Slowly progressive azotemia Mild to nephrotic-range proteinuria Biopsy—fibroobliterative arterial lesions, glomerular sclerosis, interstitial fibrosis	Antihypertensive medications HMG-CoA reductase inhibitors ACE inhibitors
Transplant renal artery stenosis	Severe, refractory hypertension with progressive decline in graft function ACE inhibitor may exacerbate decline in GFR	Diagnosis: Captopril renography, angiography Treatment: Angioplasty, surgery
Recurrent or *de novo* glomerulonephritis	Nephrotic-range proteinuria Slowly progressive decline in graft function (can remain stable)	Variable response to specific intervention (e.g., steroids, plasmapheresis) Antihypertensive medications (especially ACE inhibitors)
Native kidneys	May exacerbate hypertension at anytime posttransplant	Nephrectomy should be limited to the patient with refractory hypertension and excellent allograft function

ACE, angiotensin-converting enzyme; GFR, glomerular filtration rate; HMG-CoA, 3-hydroxy-3-methyl-glutaryl-coenzyme A.

ney, with activation of the renin-angiotensin axis and impairment of renal excretory capacity. There is sodium retention and volume expansion. In acute rejection, a decline in glomerular filtration rate (GFR) is accompanied by increased renal vascular resistance (RVR) and reduced renal plasma flow (ERPF). Angiotensin blockade attenuates these changes, implying a key role for angiotensin-mediated vasoconstriction in the process. However, in the milieu of an acutely rejecting allograft, other vasoactive substances also contribute to the altered hemodynamics. Cytokines (e.g., interleukin-2, interferon-γ, tumor necrosis factor-α), integral components of the rejection response, stimulate release of the vasoconstrictor, endothelin, and the vasodilator, nitric oxide, and may also modulate prostaglandin production. The contribution of these inflammatory mediators to altered renal hemodynamics is emphasized by the response of hypertension to appropriate antirejection therapy. Administration of high-dose corticosteroids, which may exacerbate hypertension in other situations, often results in its prompt amelioration in the setting of acute rejection.

Chronic rejection defines a clinical syndrome characterized by gradual loss of allograft function, proteinuria, and, in most cases, hypertension. Histologically, there is allograft vasculopathy, with interstitial fibrosis and ischemic glomerular changes. The pathogenesis of chronic rejection is not well understood, but likely reflects the confluence of both immunologic and nonimmunologic events. In chronic rejection, the gradual onset of renal impairment is again accompanied by reduced ERPF and increased RVR. These hemodynamic changes reflect both chronic vasculopathy and angiotensin-mediated vasoconstriction. Again, loss of excretory function contributes to volume expansion. Unlike acute rejection, renal impairment in this scenario reflects structural as well as functional changes, and is most often not reversible.

Recurrence of renal diseases within the allograft is not uncommon, particularly in recipients with a primary glomerulopathy (e.g., IgA nephropathy, membranoproliferative glomerulonephritis type II, focal glomerulosclerosis) as the original cause of chronic renal failure. In these patients, hypertension evolves along with the recurrent disease, worsening as allograft function declines. In the special case of recurrent, or *de novo*, hemolytic uremic syndrome, severe hypertension, a complication that may occur with greater frequency under cyclosporine-based immunosuppression, may herald the onset of clinical disease.

Extrinsic Impairment of Allograft Function

In the absence of overt allograft dysfunction, other factors may adversely impact blood pressure control. Prominent among these is the contribution of retained native kidneys. Hypertension is less common in allograft recipients who have previously undergone bilateral native kidney nephrectomy. Likewise, native kidney nephrectomy (either medical or surgical) "cures" hypertension in many patients after a successful transplant. Before cyclosporine, diseased native kidneys were perhaps the major factor contributing to posttransplant hypertension in recipients with otherwise normal allograft function. In these patients, there was persistent elevation of plasma renin activity (PRA), increased RVR, and salt intake did not influence blood pressure responses. Because converting enzyme inhibition and native kidney nephrectomy both reduced PRA and RVR, as well as arterial pressure, activation of the renin-angiotensin system appears to have been a key pathogenetic event.

Soon after the introduction of cyclosporine in the early 1980s, its association with nephrotoxicity and hypertension was recognized. For many patients with excellent graft function, cyclosporine is now the prime factor responsible for posttransplant hypertension. Clinically, cyclosporine is associated with hypertension in at least two settings. The first is more acute, presenting as a dose-related elevation in blood pressure, often accompanied by elevated cyclosporine levels and azotemia, and responding to either reduction or withdrawal of cyclosporine dosing. The second syndrome is a more chronic, relatively irreversible nephropathy associated with prolonged cyclosporine use, even in the absence of elevated blood levels of cyclosporine. Although cyclosporine dose reduction may improve blood pressure control, renal function often remains impaired due to scarring and vasculopathy within the allograft, and hypertension persists.

In multiple studies, cyclosporine has been found to be a potent vasoconstrictor. *In vitro*, a direct vasoconstricting effect on vascular smooth muscle has been demonstrated. Activation of both sympathetic pathways and the renin-angiotensin axis, as well as stimulation of thromboxane and/or inhibition of vasodilatory prostaglandins have also been proposed. Other studies have focused on the roles of transforming growth factor-β (TGF-β) and endothelin.

Despite substantial efforts to separate the underlying immunosuppressive efficacy of cyclosporine from its renal and vascular toxicities, it now appears that the two are inalterably intertwined. Cyclosporine exerts its immunosuppressive effect by inhibiting calcineurin-dependent pathways of lymphocyte activation. These same molecular mechanisms may contribute to its potent vasoconstrictive effects. As cyclosporine inhibits transcription of inflammatory cytokines such as interleukin-2 and interferon-γ, transcription and production of another cytokine, TGF-β, is upregulated in lymphocytes as well as other cell lines. TGF-β is a potent inducer of both endothelin and angiotensin production, which, in turn, may actually mediate cyclosporine's vasoconstrictive effects, potentiating hypertension. Endothelin is the most potent vasoconstrictor yet discovered, and the renal vasculature, particularly the afferent arteriole, is rich in endothelin receptors. *In vitro* studies have documented enhanced sensitivity of the afferent arteriole to endothelin-mediated vasoconstriction. Cyclosporine also directly stimulates endothelin production from cultured endothelial and mesangial cells; both antiendothelin antibodies and antagonism of the endothelin receptor abolish cyclosporine-induced vasoconstriction. Perhaps via a direct toxic effect on vascular endothelium, cyclosporine also inhibits secretion of the vasodilator, nitric oxide. Thus a substantial body of evidence links TGF-β, endothelin, and cyclosporine-related hypertension. Ultimately, ischemic changes within the allograft, along with TGF-β–related fibrous tissue proliferation, may produce the chronic scarring associated with long-term cyclosporine administration.

Although increased plasma endothelin levels have also been documented in humans receiving cyclosporine, a secondary mechanism may be operative as well. Cyclosporine reduces ERPF, increases RVR, and reduces GFR. These changes result in enhanced urea reabsorption and sodium retention. Furthermore, most human studies have found relative suppression of plasma levels of renin and angiotensin, with hypertension that is responsive, rather than refractory, to salt restriction. Thus in humans, these data indicate that cyclosporine-associated hypertension reflects a combination of renal and systemic vasoconstriction, reduced renal blood flow, increased proximal tubular reabsorption of sodium, and volume expansion. Although not as extensively investigated, the newer immunosuppressant, tacrolimus, appears to exhibit similar effects, particularly at higher dosages.

Outside the transplant setting, pharmacologic doses of corticosteroids exacerbate hypertension. In the absence of cyclosporine, alternate-day prednisone was associated with less hypertension than daily administration of similar steroid doses. Even in the presence of cyclosporine, discontinuation of prednisone may reduce blood pressure in some patients. Corticosteroids appear to be synergistic with cyclosporine in enhancing salt reabsorption. Nonetheless, corticosteroids are probably not a major factor contributing to hypertension in recipients of nonrenal solid organ transplants, and few consider prednisone doses of 5 to 15 mg/day as a major cause of hypertension after kidney transplantation. Posttransplant hypercalcemia may be associated with hypertension.

Transplant Renal Artery Stenosis

Stenotic lesions of the transplant renal arterial circulation may account for as many as 5% of cases of posttransplant hypertension. In contrast to most patients with hypertension after a kidney transplant, the elevated blood pressures that accompany transplant renal artery stenosis (TRAS) are often severe and refractory to therapy. TRAS most commonly presents as severe hypertension associated with a mild (or profound) reduction in renal function. Although a bruit is often evident over the allograft, such a finding is nonspecific and of little diagnostic significance.

Recipients of kidneys with multiple arteries and from pediatric donors are at greater risk of developing this complication. Stenosis occurs most commonly at the site of vascular anastomosis, although occasional patients will demonstrate lesions proximal to the allograft, such as in the common iliac artery. Most cadáveric kidneys are harvested with a cuff of aorta (Carrel patch) attached to the proximal renal artery; the cuff is then sewn into the external iliac artery in an end-to-side fashion. Stenotic lesions resulting from this technique are rare. However, end-to-end anastomoses (renal to hypogastric artery) and end-to-side anastomoses (renal to external iliac) performed without a Carrel patch (as in kidneys from living donors) are more likely to become problematic.

The physiology is similar to the one-kidney Goldblatt model—volume-mediated hypertension, with suppression of renin. However, the introduction of diuretic therapy often stimulates plasma renin activity. In this setting, GFR is preserved by angiotensin-mediated efferent arteriolar vasoconstriction. Converting enzyme inhibition may thus provoke a precipitous decline in GFR when administered to the patient with TRAS, and can result in overt renal failure. This phenomenon is usually reversible, however, and may be of diagnostic value as a screening test in the recipient suspected of having TRAS.

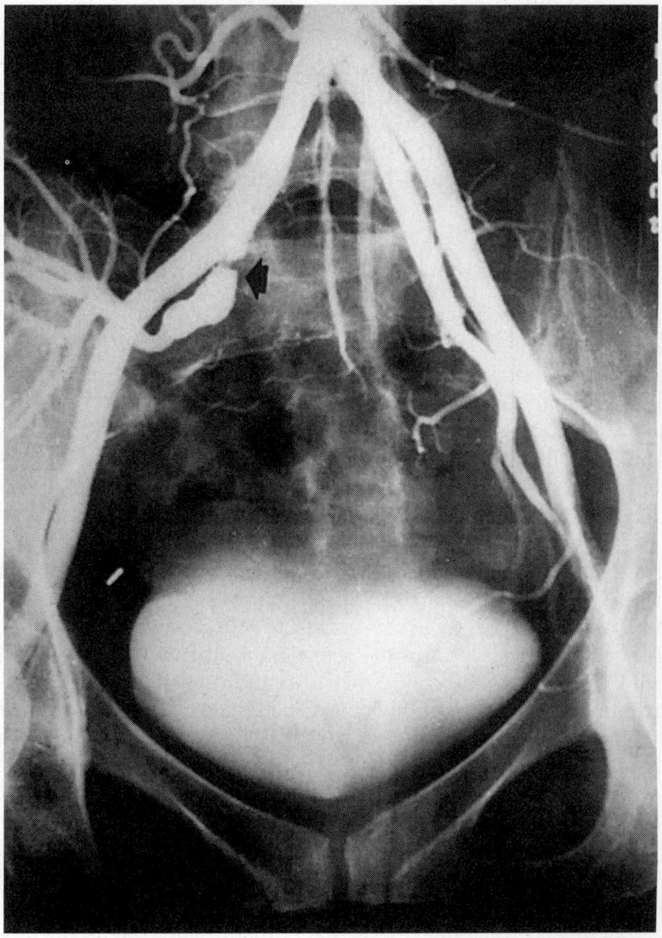

Figure 89.3. Arteriographic study of iliac and transplant renal arteries in a patient with transplant renal artery stenosis (TRAS). Lesion is located at site of vascular anastomosis with poststenotic dilation.

DIAGNOSIS

In the evaluation of hypertension after kidney transplantation, the first challenge is to elicit a potentially correctable cause. The time that has elapsed after a transplant may influence the likelihood of any particular cause contributing to posttransplant hypertension. For instance, immediately following transplantation, delayed graft function may cause hypertension by both volume- and renin-dependent mechanisms. After good graft function is established, acute rejection can be heralded by either new onset or worsening of hypertension. In addition, with risk of acute rejection greatest during the first 3 months posttransplant, blood cyclosporine levels are usually maintained highest in this period, and acute cyclosporine toxicity may precipitate worsening hypertension. Beyond 6 months posttransplant, the risk of acute rejection diminishes. At that time, in the recipient with *de novo* or worsening hypertension beyond 6 months, other causes, such as cyclosporine toxicity, chronic rejection, or TRAS, should be suspected. Finally, retained native kidneys may contribute at any time.

With this timetable in mind, initial diagnostic efforts should be directed toward evaluating allograft function, including measurement of GFR and urinary protein excretion. Cyclosporine or tacrolimus dosing should be carefully optimized, although across-the-board decreases in cyclosporine run the risk of precipitating acute rejection. If deterioration in graft function is documented, biopsy may be necessary to distinguish the precise cause.

Late onset of hypertension, particularly in a previously stable recipient, may indicate TRAS. In such patients, a brief, closely supervised "challenge" with an angiotensin-converting enzyme (ACE) inhibitor may be a useful screen for hemodynamically significant stenosis. In a patient who develops renal dysfunction after addition of an ACE inhibitor, further evaluation for TRAS may be in order. Although a captopril renal isotope scan may be of some assistance in this regard, ACE inhibitor–induced acute renal failure at our center generally results in diagnostic angiography. A substantial percentage of such patients are found at angiography to have significant TRAS, and usually respond to angioplasty or surgical revascularization (Fig. 89.3).

THERAPY

In the hypertensive recipient with stable allograft function, medical management aimed at normalizing blood pressure (mean arterial pressure of 95 mm Hg or less) is the goal. Current therapeutic approaches are based largely on theoretic considerations regarding the pathophysiology of posttransplant hypertension. Foremost among these is the role of cyclosporine-induced renal vasoconstriction in precipitating hypertension. As one might expect given our understanding of its pathogenesis, endothelin antagonists have proved extremely effective experimentally in attenuating cyclosporine-related hypertension. However, because these drugs are not yet available for clinical use, calcium channel blockers (CCBs) have become the agents of choice for many transplant physicians. *In vitro*, these agents have been shown to attenuate both cyclosporine- and endothelin-induced vasoconstriction. In human studies, CCBs lower renal vascular resistance and prevent the acute deterioration in ERPF and GFR that accompanies peak cyclosporine blood levels. Others have suggested that CCBs might enhance immunosuppression, prevent delayed graft function, and improve GFR in cyclosporine-treated allograft recipients.

Significant differences exist among currently available CCBs regarding effects on cyclosporine metabolism. The nondihydropyridine derivatives verapamil and diltiazem, along with the dihydropyridine nicardipine, interfere with hepatic metabolism of cyclosporine and tacrolimus, increasing blood levels by 40% to 50%. Although some have found this interaction to be beneficial in achieving higher cyclosporine levels and improved graft function, for many patients immunosuppressive management becomes more complex—dosing of the CCB and cyclosporine must be altered concurrently. Amlodipine may increase cyclosporine levels by 10% to 15%, an increment that usually is well tolerated and not of clinical significance. Nifedipine and isradipine exert little if any effect on cyclosporine blood levels. CCBs are generally well tolerated in this population. However, peripheral edema is not an infrequent complication, and there is also a link between CCB therapy and worsening of gingival hyperplasia.

Diuretics have come into disfavor in the treatment of essential hypertension, primarily due to a potential adverse effect on lipids. However, in light of the volume expansion and salt sensitivity that usually accompanies posttransplant hypertension in the cyclosporine- or tacrolimus-treated recipient, there is a role for sodium restriction and/or diuretic therapy in its management. Although salt restriction may pose less medical risk, we have rarely found it to be adequate in achieving or enhancing blood pressure control. Thus in patients who respond to a CCB with suboptimal blood pressure control or worsening edema, addition of diuretic therapy may be beneficial. In this setting, a loop diuretic (furosemide or bumetanide) is usually required to achieve adequate natriuresis. Although thiazide-type diuretics may also be effective, these agents may increase the risk of hyperuricemia and/or hypercalcemia. Potassium-sparing diuretics may exacerbate cyclosporine-induced hyperkalemia, and are not commonly used.

In the past, ACE inhibitors have been used sparingly in renal allograft recipients due to concerns regarding acute renal failure, hyperkalemia, and anemia. However, these agents are effective antihypertensives, and studies have documented a clear beneficial impact on renal hemodynamics in most patients, along with the potential for prolongation of allograft function. Posttransplant erythrocytosis is a complication seen most often in stable recipients with well-functioning grafts, and usually responds to ACE inhibitor therapy. Favorable experience with ACE inhibitors for this indication has tended to alleviate concerns regarding potential side effects. In the hypertensive patient with an elevated hematocrit, ACE inhibitors are probably the agents of choice. In other settings, particularly in the early posttransplant period, they may be of benefit, but should be used cautiously. Angiotensin-receptor antagonists (losartan, valsartan) appear to be safe alternatives to ACE inhibitors in transplant recipients, and achieve similar results.

There appear to be no distinct advantages or disadvantages associated with the use of other antihypertensive agents. Vasodilators (hydralazine, minoxidil), β-blockers (propranolol, atenolol), central agonists (clonidine), and α-antagonists (prazosin, doxazosin) are all useful in the appropriate setting. The combination of diuretic, β-blocker, and vasodilator (furosemide, propranolol, hydralazine) may be particularly effective for some patients, and is relatively inexpensive. The use of minoxidil is usually reserved for refractory hypertension; intense sodium retention with this agent demands concurrent use of potent diuretic therapy.

If posttransplant hypertension proves refractory to standard therapies as noted previously, TRAS should be considered. When TRAS is demonstrated, it appears that surgical repair offers the best hopes for both immediate and long-term cure (92% and 82%, respectively). However, angioplasty may be successful in as many as three-fourths of patients, with long-lasting remissions in the majority. Most transplant physicians would thus offer angioplasty as a first intervention, particularly for those patients with distal lesions. Proximal stenosis or stenosis at the vascular anastomosis may more frequently require surgical intervention. If TRAS is excluded, in the patient with well-preserved allograft function and no evidence of rejection, bilateral native kidney nephrectomy should be considered. Unfortunately, there is no diagnostic study that accurately predicts who will, or will not, benefit from this not inconsequential operation. However, with currently available medications, native kidney nephrectomy is rarely indicated solely for blood pressure control.

Selected Readings

Cosio FG, Falkenhain ME, Pesavento TE, et al. Relationships between arterial hypertension and renal allograft survival in African-American patients. *Am J Kidney Dis* 1997;29:419–427.

This retrospective analysis documents the importance of preexisting hypertension on the subsequent clinical course in renal allograft recipients, and the influence of hypertension after transplantation on outcome in a high-risk subgroup of patients.

Curtis JJ, Luke RG, Dubovsky E, et al. Cyclosporine in therapeutic doses increases renal allograft vascular resistance. *Lancet* 1986;2:477–479.

This study reported the effects of cyclosporine on renal hemodynamics in 14 patients taken off cyclosporine at 8 to 12 months posttransplant. Renal blood flow increased by 40% due to a decline in renal vascular resistance, documenting the reversibility of cyclosporine-induced renal vasoconstriction.

Curtis JJ, Luke RG, Jones P, et al. Hypertension in cyclosporine-treated renal transplant patients is sodium dependent. *Am J Med* 1988;85:134–138.

Characterization of posttransplant hypertension in the cyclosporine era, comparing the responsiveness of 30 recipients on and off cyclosporine with salt restriction and converting enzyme inhibition. Only the cyclosporine-treated recipients lowered blood pressure on a low-salt diet.

Kasiske BL, Guijarro C, Massy ZA, et al. Cardiovascular disease after renal transplantation. *J Am Soc Nephrol* 1996;7:158–165.

A cogent analysis of risk factors, including hypertension, that predispose transplant recipients to cardiovascular disease. Significant variables include age, gender, tobacco use, hyperlipidemia, diabetes, and hypertension.

Kirk AD, Jacobson LM, Heisey DM, et al. Posttransplant diastolic hypertension: associations with TGFβ, endothelin, and renin transcription. *Transplantation* 1997;64:1716–1720.

This clinical trial uses histologic specimens obtained from transplant renal biopsies to examine the relationship between these mediators and hypertension in human renal allograft recipients.

Lanese DM, Conger JD. Effects of endothelin receptor antagonist on CsA-induced vasoconstriction in isolated rat renal arterioles. *J Clin Invest* 1993;91:2144–2149.

This study explores the role of the vasoconstrictor, endothelin, in mediating cyclosporine-induced vasoconstriction in an in vitro model.

Ruggenenti P, Perico N, Mosconi L, et al. Calcium channel blockers protect transplant patients from cyclosporine-induced daily renal hypoperfusion. *Kidney Int* 1993;43:706–711.

A study of renal hemodynamics in cyclosporine-treated renal allograft recipients that elegantly delineates the theoretic basis underlying use of calcium antagonists in posttransplant hypertension.

PART 8
The Lung in Renal Transplant Recipients

Gordon R. Bernard, Florence L. Watts, and Kenneth L. Brigham

The multitude of insults dealt to the pulmonary circulation during dialysis, transplant surgery, and the long posttransplant period of immunosuppression often results in confusing and serious lung lesions. Because of the profound immunosuppression required for transplantation, radiologic and clinical clues to diagnosis based on characteristic host responses become obscure. Thus mere history, physical examination, and chest radiograph are no longer reliable; instead, tissue diagnosis becomes imperative. Immunosuppression further complicates the situation by requiring more immediate intervention for infectious etiologic conditions.

DIFFUSE BILATERAL PULMONARY INFILTRATES

The most common cause of diffuse bilateral pulmonary infiltrates in the posttransplant period, sometimes called *transplant lung,* is pulmonary edema. The use of the Swan-Ganz flow-directed pulmonary artery catheter for the direct measurements of pulmonary artery and pulmonary wedge pressure is a very helpful diagnostic tool. When such measurements are not available, the chest x-ray examination can be used to differentiate various forms of pulmonary edema from other causes of diffuse infiltrates (Table 89.12). There is a correlation between distribution of blood flow and the various forms of pulmonary edema. Studies have shown that the distribution of pulmonary blood flow in patients with cardiac failure tends to be "inverted" from a primarily basilar distribution to a primarily apical distribution, whereas patients with overhydration and/or renal failure have a primarily homogeneous or "balanced" pulmonary blood flow. Patients with increased permeability pulmonary edema were found to have a distribution of blood flow that is a combination of normal and balanced. It was also established that the distribution of pulmonary edema is homogeneous in cardiac failure patients, central in patients with overhydration or renal failure, and patchy when edema is secondary to increased capillary permeability. Patients receiving anti–T-cell antibody (e.g., OKT3) for induction therapy are prone to develop pulmonary edema secondary to increased capillary permeability especially if they are volume expanded. Other clinical methods of estimating volume status are notoriously unreliable in patients who have recently had surgery, have various degrees of renal and cardiac dysfunction, and may have low serum protein levels because of malnutrition and protein wasting. Because this diffuse pulmonary infiltrate is often associated with respiratory failure and can be confused with diffuse infection, rapid diagnosis is imperative. Although pulmonary edema is more common, the differential diagnosis includes, first and foremost, infection because the early diagnosis and treatment are of such importance (Table 89.13).

Pulmonary edema in the immediate posttransplant period is most commonly caused by fluid accumulation resulting from excessive fluid intake combined with inadequate diuresis, often caused by inadequate graft function. Complicating this is the fact that many transplant patients are hypoproteinemic because of inadequate protein intake and high-dose glucocorticoid therapy to prevent graft rejection. If one studies the Starling forces that normally act to keep the lung dry (i.e., maintaining the proper balance between plasma and interstitial oncotic pressure and microvascular pressure), it is readily apparent why pulmonary edema is so common in these patients. Many patients respond well to volume reduction, but a few do not.

The cases of pulmonary edema that do not respond to volume reduction have given rise to confusion about the nature of the edema. If the measurement of plasma proteins and pulmonary vascular pressures does not explain the pulmonary edema in light of the Starling equation, the diagnosis of noncardiogenic (increased permeability) pulmonary edema should be entertained. In its most severe form, noncardiogenic pulmonary edema is usually referred to as the *acute respiratory distress syndrome,* which can be catastrophic in its manifestation, requiring intensive care and mechanical ventilation. On the other hand, less severe diffuse lung injury resulting from any of several com-

TABLE 89.12. Radiographic Features of Pulmonary Edema[a]

	Type of Pulmonary Edema		
	Cardiac	Renal	Injury
Heart size	Enlarged	Enlarged	Not enlarged
Vascular pedicle	Normal or enlarged	Enlarged	Normal or reduced
Pulmonary blood flow distribution	Inverted	Balanced	Normal or balanced
Pulmonary blood volume	Normal or increased	Increased	Normal
Septal lines	Not common	Not common	Absent
Peribronchial cuffs	Very common	Very common	Not common
Air bronchogram	Not common	Not common	Very common
Lung edema, regional distribution (horizontal axis)	Even	Central	Peripheral
Pleural effusions	Very common	Very common	Not common

[a] Each factor listed has been shown to have statistic significance in determining which type of edema is present.
Reproduced with permission from Milne ENC, Pistolesi M, Miniati M, et al. The radiologic distribution of cardiogenic and noncardiogenic edema. *AJR* 1985;144:879–894.

TABLE 89.13. Causes of Diffuse Pulmonary Infiltrates in the Transplant Patient

Diffuse infections, usually opportunistic
Pneumocystis pneumoniae
Cytomegalovirus
Miliary tuberculosis
Disseminated fungal infection
Diffuse lung injury
Sepsis
Massive transfusions
Aspiration
Anti–T-cell antibody (OKT3)
Volume overload (crystalloid, blood)
Heart failure
Pulmonary drug reaction
Extension of the underlying disease to include the lungs

TABLE 89.14. Common Causes of Pleural Effusion in the Renal Transplant Patient

Volume overload
Heart failure
Uremic pleuritis
Bacterial pneumonia
Pulmonary embolus

plications of renal transplantation (e.g., massive blood transfusion, sepsis, aspiration) can be so mild that only supplemental oxygen is required. The course of this form of pulmonary edema is unpredictable but is usually relatively long, often lasting several weeks. Excessive diuresis of the patient is not recommended because of potential deleterious effects on cardiac output and renal perfusion; instead, the patient should be maintained at a low-normal volume status.

Pleural effusion is also a common finding in the posttransplant period (Table 89.14). The most common cause is volume overload, and thus it should respond to fluid restriction and diuretics. However, effusions should be sampled to determine whether they are transudates or exudates because this will have a bearing on the therapeutic approach. Exudates must be taken much more seriously and demand specific diagnosis.

Early diagnosis of diffuse lung infiltrates in the immunocompromised host is crucial because of the usually good response to therapy begun promptly after onset and the dire effects of delayed diagnosis and therapy.

PULMONARY EMBOLI

A diagnosis that is not frequently considered in the transplant patient but is an important cause of death in the posttransplant period is pulmonary emboli. These are most likely to occur in the first 2 to 3 weeks after surgery and can sometimes be complicated by superinfection of the infarcted area. Superimposed infection of pulmonary emboli is more common in the immunocompromised patient. The incidence of pulmonary emboli has declined because of better surgical technique and earlier mobilization of the patients postoperatively, but interestingly, an increase in thromboembolic events has been noted with the use of cyclosporine. In young, otherwise healthy patients, pulmonary infarction is rare and chest x-ray findings will be subtle, or more often absent, but gas exchange may suddenly deteriorate with marked hypoxemia and hyperventilation (respiratory alkalosis). The diagnosis will rest on a high clinical suspicion along with a high probability ventilation-perfusion lung scan. However, if the scan is equivocal and suspicion of embolus is still high, the patient should undergo pulmonary arteriography, especially if there is a contraindication to anticoagulation therapy.

PULMONARY INFECTION

Pulmonary infection is a greater problem in renal transplantation than in uremia alone. The stage is set by having an immediately postoperative patient who is frequently azotemic and is receiving high-dose glucocorticoids and immunosuppressive drugs. The diagnosis of these infections is difficult because the manifestation of the various infections is seldom classic and the organisms involved are pathogens seldom seen in the normal host. Also, renal transplant recipients are prone to secondary infections, especially if their primary infection is cytomegalovirus (CMV) pneumonia, possibly because of its ability to further suppress T-cell–mediated immunity. Secondary infections carry an extremely high mortality rate, exceeding 95% in some institutions. Whether this is due to patient selection (i.e., the more compromised patients are the ones more likely to develop multiple infections) or whether other factors are involved is not known. However, there are clues to the correct diagnosis of the pulmonary infection, including time from transplantation, type of onset (acute, subacute, or chronic), character and extent of radiographic changes, and magnitude of hypoxemia.

The length of time from kidney transplantation can be a guide to the likely invading organism (Table 89.15). In the first month after transplantation, postsurgical bacterial infection is the most common. From 1 to 4 months following transplantation, opportunistic infections predominate, with CMV being the most likely cause of pneumonia, particularly in those institutions that use antilymphocyte serum. That opportunistic infections occur most frequently in this period is not surprising because this is the time of greatest suppression of host immunity. This is also the most likely period for secondary infections to

TABLE 89.15. Causes of Pneumonitis After Renal Transplantation, Correlated with Time After Transplantation

Less than 1 month
Aspiration
Bacteria
Wound infection or intravascular line colonization
1 to 4 months
Cytomegalovirus
Herpes simplex
Varicella zoster
Pneumocystis carinii
Aspergillus
Zygomycetes
Nocardia
Mycobacteria
Adenovirus
Greater than 4 months
Cryptococcus
Pneumocystis
Legionella

Reproduced with permission from Wilson WR, Cockerill FR, Rosenow EC. Pulmonary disease in the immunocompromised host: second of two parts. *Mayo Clin Proc* 1985;60:610–631.

occur, especially in association with CMV pneumonia and pulmonary emboli. *Pneumocystis carinii* is the most common secondary invader in CMV pneumonia. Either of these two infections is likely to cause serious gas exchange abnormalities marked by severe hypoxemia. In the late posttransplant period, a combination of conventional and opportunistic infections occurs depending on whether the patient has good renal function with minimal immunosuppression or rejection requiring increased immunosuppression.

Further discussion is warranted regarding some of the infections described. *Pneumocystis* pneumonia often appears as steroid immunosuppression is being tapered, possibly because of enhanced host response to the organism. In fact, the use of glucocorticoids as supplemental treatment for *Pneumocystis* pneumonia is now recommended for this infection when it occurs in patients immunocompromised by the acquired immunodeficiency syndrome. Tuberculosis is usually not seen in transplant patients unless there has been previous exposure as determined by history or the tuberculin skin test. When possible, this test should be applied before the transplant because glucocorticoids are known to suppress a positive test. Even so, the incidence of false-negative results in normal patients is approximately 20%, even in uremia. If the skin test is positive, it is generally recommended that the patient receive isoniazid for at least 1 year. It is not clear whether treatment beyond 1 year is useful. Pneumococcal pneumonia is also at least partially preventable in the postoperative period through the use of pneumococcal polyvalent vaccine.

The patient most likely to die of infection after renal transplantation is one who has received repeated large doses of glucocorticoids to reverse rejection or who has had recurrent episodes of leukopenia and frequent minor infections. The use of alternate-day rather than daily glucocorticoids is possibly helpful in reducing this risk. The day steroids are administered is marked by neutropenia, monocytopenia, and lymphocytic suppression, whereas these findings are reversed on the day steroids are not administered.

The chest x-ray examination is a useful qualitative tool in the setting of renal transplantation and infection. The common radiographic findings of pathogens found in transplant patients are listed in Table 89.16. Normal chest x-ray findings usually rule out pulmonary parenchymal infection. However, early in the course of infection, especially with *P. carinii* or miliary tuberculosis, the radiograph changes can be very subtle.

An etiologic diagnosis in this syndrome of diffuse pulmonary infiltrates should be pursued vigorously because early treatment significantly reduces morbidity and mortality. Although cardiogenic pulmonary edema can be ruled out by measurement of pulmonary capillary wedge pressure with a Swan-Ganz catheter, it is not as easy to diagnose infections. Sputum, if available, should be the first step in the workup. Unfortunately, sputum culture alone does not make the diagnosis. Results of the culture must be interpreted in the light of the chest radiograph, sputum Gram staining, and the clinical manifestations. In addition, transbronchial lung biopsy through the fiberoptic bronchoscope along with bronchial brushings and washings can provide useful information. Occasionally, percutaneous lung aspiration with a small-gauge, thin-walled needle is an appropriate and relatively simple procedure when infection is suspected. Bronchoalveolar lavage has been demonstrated as an effective tool for diagnosing pulmonary infiltrates in the renal transplant patient if the lesions are secondary to infection. Bronchoalveolar lavage does not appear to be adequate in diagnosing immunosuppressive drug toxicity, which is another important cause of diffuse pulmonary infiltrates in this population. Transtracheal aspiration can be beneficial when one suspects an anaerobic infection, because this procedure avoids the problem of contamination of oropharyngeal secretions. The highest yield procedure is the open lung biopsy, with a diagnostic yield of 95% or more and with the additional advantage that it can give a more rapid diagnosis than other techniques. Some reports suggest that complications are less and results better than with the less invasive procedures described previously. On the other hand, some reports demonstrate a relatively low yield from open biopsy (in some, less than 60% of the biopsies resulted in a specific diagnosis). When other standard, less invasive procedures are employed first and found to be nondiagnostic, the percentage of positive (specific) biopsies may decrease even more. Figure 89.4 shows an algorithm for the approach to the immunosuppressed nonneutropenic transplant patient as proposed by a National Institutes of Health Conference Committee.

In summary, pulmonary infiltrates and deterioration in gas exchange in the renal transplant recipient pose a challenge to the physician, but clinical tools can provide an accu-

TABLE 89.16. Differential Diagnosis of Fever and Pulmonary Infiltrates in the Renal Transplant Patient, According to Roentgenographic Abnormality and Pace of Illness[a]

	Etiology According to Pace of Illness	
Chest Radiograph Abnormality	Acute	Subacute-Chronic
Focal or multifocal	Bacterial, thromboembolic (pulmonary edema)	Fungal, nocardial (tuberculous)
Diffuse	Pulmonary edema	Viral, pneumocystis (fungal)
Nodular	(Bacterial, pulmonary edema)	Fungal, nocardial
Peribronchovascular	Pulmonary edema (bacterial)	Viral, pneumocystis
Consolidation	Bacterial, thromboembolic (pulmonary edema)	Fungal, nocardial (viral)

[a] Unusual causes of a process are placed in parentheses. An acute illness is one developing and requiring medical attention in a matter of a few hours (less than 24 hours). A subacute chronic process develops over several days to weeks.

Reproduced with permission from Ramsey PG, Rubin RH, Tolkoff-Rubin NE, et al. The renal transplant patient with fever and pulmonary infiltrates: etiology, clinical manifestations, and management. *Medicine (Baltimore)* 1980;59:206–222.

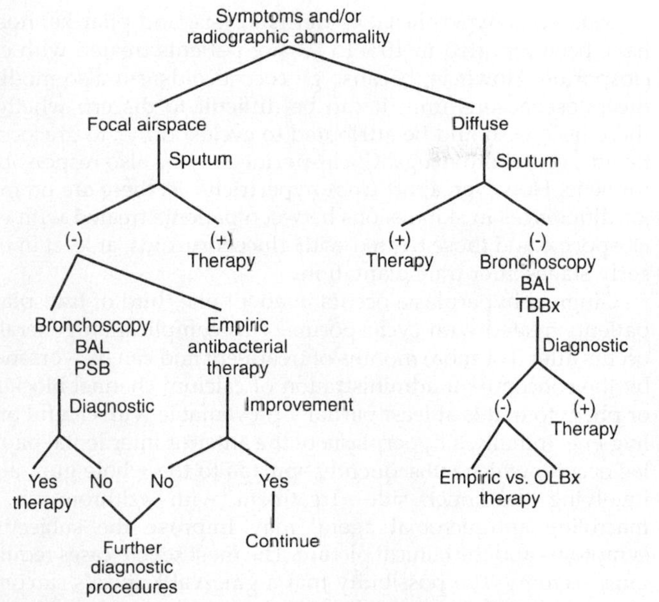

Figure 89.4. Approach to the diagnosis of respiratory disease in the immunosuppressed nonneutropenic patient. BAL, bronchoalveolar lavage; OLB_x, open lung biopsy; PSB, protected specimen brush; TBB_x, transbronchial biopsy. [Reproduced with permission from Shelhamer JH, Toews GB, Mosur H, et al. Respiratory disease in the immunosuppressed patient. *Ann Intern Med* 1992;117(5):415–431.]

rate diagnosis such that appropriate therapy can be instituted early, resulting in a reduction in morbidity and mortality. Details of the treatment of various specific pulmonary infections in renal transplant recipients are provided in Chapter 89, Part 1.

Selected Readings

Consensus statement for use of corticosteroids as adjunctive therapy for *Pneumocystis* pneumonia in AIDS. *N Engl J Med* 1990;323(21):1500–1504.

This article summarizes several clinical trials conducted for the purpose of determining whether corticosteroids are useful in Pneumocystis pneumonia. Although restricted to patients with AIDS, this article is important to the issue of renal transplantation because Pneumocystis pneumonia is a known complication of this immunocompromised state. The rationale and guidelines for therapy are presented.

Milne ENC, Pistolesi M, Miniati M, et al. The radiologic distinction of cardiogenic and noncardiogenic edema. *AJR* 1985;144:879–894.

An interesting and useful paper reviving the notion that cardiogenic and noncardiogenic pulmonary edema can be differentiated on the basis of chest radiographic findings. Simple clues to look for in the evaluation are listed, along with the data to substantiate the sensitivity and specificity of this technique.

Ramsey PG, Rubin RH, Tolkoff-Rubin NE, et al. The renal transplant patient with fever and pulmonary infiltrates: etiology, clinical manifestations, and management. *Medicine (Baltimore)* 1980;59:206–222.

A large, retrospective study of 227 renal transplant patients admitted to Massachusetts General Hospital between 1966 and 1978. It establishes pulmonary disease as the most important single cause of mortality (more than 50%). Pulmonary diseases are classified into several categories aside from infectious causes, and outcome as well as new approaches aimed at reducing mortality are discussed.

Shelhammer JH. Diagnostic approach. In: Shelhammer JH, moderator. NIH Conference: respiratory disease in the immunocompromised patient. *Ann Intern Med* 1992;117:415–431.

Excellent review of infectious and noninfectious complications in patients who are severely immunocompromised. The authors provide an in-depth discussion of host defense factors, disease categories of most concern, timing of typical complications, and general principles of management.

Uranga RM, Simmons RL, Kjellerstrand CM, et al. Pathogenesis of "transplant lung": interstitial pulmonary edema. *Ann Surg* 1973;178:573–577.

Review of the cases of 13 patients who developed pulmonary infiltrates after renal transplantation; includes discussion of the differential diagnosis and therapy of the underlying conditions.

Vanrenterghem Y, Roels L, Lerut T, et al. Thromboembolic complications and haemostatic changes in cyclosporin-treated cadaveric kidney allograft recipients. *Lancet* 1985;1:999–1002.

Description of the incidence and nature of thromboembolic complications of cyclosporine therapy compared with a retrospective analysis of this type of complication in transplant patients in the precyclosporine era. Several possible explanations are suggested for the increased incidence of thromboses in the cyclosporine group.

Wilson WR, Cockerill FR, Rosenow EC. Pulmonary disease in the immunocompromised host: second of two parts. *Mayo Clin Proc* 1985;60:610–631.

Discussion of the clinical approach to the immunocompromised host, including renal transplant recipients, categorizing the likely infecting agent according to the type of immunologic defect. Further attention is given to the epidemiologic factors involved in such infections.

Young JA, Hopkin JM, Cuthbertson WP. Pulmonary infiltrates in immunocompromised patients: diagnosis by cytological examination of bronchoalveolar lavage fluid. *J Clin Pathol* 1984;37:390–397.

A report of the findings of bronchoalveolar lavage in 26 immunocompromised patients, 16 of whom had severe renal disease or transplant. Bronchoalveolar lavage can provide rapid diagnosis in 93% of such cases.

PART 9
The Skin in Renal Transplant Recipients

Claudio Ponticelli and Fabio Zorzi

The prolonged use of glucocorticoids, calcineurin inhibitors, and antimetabolite agents can expose the transplant patient to the development of various cutaneous lesions, which may be divided into iatrogenic changes, infections, and precancerous and cancerous lesions (Table 89.17). In this chapter we will not deal with malignant lesions, which are covered in Chapter 89, Part 6.

TABLE 89.17. Abnormalities of the Skin and Its Appendages in Renal Transplant Recipients

Iatrogenic complications
Steroid-related lesions
Fat maldistribution
Bateman's purpura
Acne
Erythrosis and rosacea
Striae rubrae
Hair growth
Azathioprine-related lesions
Changes in color and texture of hair
Cyclosporine-related lesions
Hypertrichosis
Sebaceous hyperplasia
Epidermal cysts
Pilar keratosis
Gum hyperplasia
Hyperpigmentation
Bullous lesions
Vegetative lesions
Infections
Mycotic
Viral
Bacterial
Infestations
Miscellaneous
Porokeratosis
Malakoplakia
Precancerous and cancerous lesions

IATROGENIC COMPLICATIONS

Glucocorticoid-Related

Most patients given protracted glucocorticoid therapy develop abnormalities in fat distribution, resulting in the typical cushingoid appearance, with facial and neck fullness, buffalo hump, increased supraclavicular and suprasternal fat, and truncal obesity. Bateman's purpura is also a frequent complication particularly in patients given glucocorticoids for years. It consists of irregular purpuric areas that develop spontaneously or after minor trauma, mainly on the extensor surfaces of the hands, forearms, and legs often with spontaneous star-shaped pseudoscars. The most frequent skin problem is acne, which is usually dose related and may be worsened by the concomitant use of cyclosporine. Acne occurs early on the cheeks, forehead, chin, and chest. Rarely the lesions may progress to nodularcystic transformation (acne conglobata). Doxycycline (100 mg daily) may be effective in reducing acne. Severe cases can be successfully treated with isotretinoin or acitretin, a second-generation retinoid used also for progressive solar keratoses, widespread warts, or recurrent skin malignancies. The severity of acne tends to decrease as the doses of glucocorticoids are reduced. Striae rubrae are wide and violaceous stripes, mainly located over the abdomen, thighs, and buttocks. Facial erythrosis and rosacea can occur. Finally, the skin of glucocorticoid-treated patients can become atrophic and friable. Topical retinoic acid at concentrations ranging from 0.01% to 0.05%, may reverse this complication even if the patients often complain of irritation. Ammonium lactate 6% to 12% creams are usually more tolerated. Some patients have an increased hair growth mainly on face and back.

The glucocorticoid-related lesions are particularly frequent in the initial posttransplant period, when higher dosages of glucocorticoids are used. In the long term, some lesions may spontaneously disappear. However, some 40% of patients still maintain a cushingoid appearance in spite of the low dosage of prednisone, whereas teleangiectases, ecchymoses, and skin atrophy tend to develop or to aggravate after 10 or more years. It must be reminded that cyclosporine and glucocorticoids are both metabolized by cytochrome P450. This may cause some retention of both drugs, with consequent appearance of glucocorticoid-related side effects even when low doses of glucocorticoids are used.

Azathioprine

Thinning of the hair and scalp hair loss can occur in patients treated with azathioprine. The drug appears also to be responsible for changes of color or texture of the hair. Actinic keratoses may occur in azathioprine-treated patients particularly after extensive sunlight exposure. Little information is available about the effects, if any, of mofetil mycophenolate.

Cyclosporine

The skin is one of the principal sites of accumulation of cyclosporine. The drug, which is highly lipophilic, may partly be eliminated through the sebaceous glands. This could explain the frequent pilosebaceous lesions observed in cyclosporine-treated patients.

Approximately 30% to 70% of patients given cyclosporine suffer from hypertrichosis, characterized by thick and pigmented hair appearing over the trunk, back, shoulder, arms, neck, forehead, helices, and malar areas. Alopecia has also been described. This includes alopecia areata and universalis. Accelerated male-pattern balding may occur. Skin hyperpigmentation and bullous or vegetative lesions have also been reported in cyclosporine-treated patients.

Sebaceous hyperplasia, epidermal cysts, and pilar keratosis have been reported in 10% to 20% of patients treated with cyclosporine. However, because glucocorticoids can also modify the pilosebaceous unit, it can be difficult to discern whether these lesions should be attributed to cyclosporine, to glucocorticoids, or to both drugs. Cyclosporine may be also responsible for acne. However, apart from hypertrichosis, there are no major differences in skin lesions between patients treated with cyclosporine and those treated with glucocorticoids, at least in the early stages after transplantation.

Gingival hyperplasia occurs in about one-third of transplant patients treated with cyclosporine. This complication generally occurs after 3 or more months of treatment and can be worsened by the concomitant administration of calcium channel blockers or phenytoin. It is at least partially preventable with careful oral hygiene. Initially, a hyperplasia of the anterior interdental papillae occurs, which subsequently spreads to the whole gum also involving the inner side. Treatment with azithromycin, a macrolide antimicrobial agent, may improve the subjective symptoms and the clinical picture. The most severe cases require gingivectomy. The possibility that a gingival Kaposi's sarcoma may mimic a cyclosporine-related gingival hyperplasia should be taken into account.

In spite of the similar mechanism of inhibition of calcineurin, tacrolimus gives less skin abnormalities and does not cause gingival hyperplasia. Cases of alopecia have been reported in patients treated with tacrolimus. Whether hair loss had to be attributed to tacrolimus *per se* or to the concomitant use of glucocorticoids is still uncertain.

INFECTIONS

Mycotic Infections

Mycotic infections account for approximately half of the mucocutaneous infections observed in transplant patients. Candidiasis of the mouth and intertriginous areas of the skin is frequent in the early posttransplant period when the immunosuppression is more vigorous. Oral rinsing with sodium bicarbonate, nystatin, or other antifungal agents may be helpful in preventing this complication.

Infections due to dermatophytes (i.e., ringworm-causing fungi) become increasingly frequent in the late posttransplant period. Their clinical appearance is often atypical due to the lack of the erythematosus changes.

Pityriasis versicolor, caused by Pityrosporon ovale/orbiculare, a dimorphic (yeast-mycelial) lipophilic yeast is the prevalent infection, affecting approximately 20% of transplant patients. This complication can involve large areas of the trunk and flexural zones. The same fungus can also cause an acneiform eruption consisting of bland or mildly erythematosus follicular papules and pustules over the shoulders, chest, upper back, and arms *(Pityrosporum folliculitis)*.

Primary cutaneous aspergillosis is rare. It is characterized by painful erythematous plaques, and sometimes cellulitis. Disseminated aspergillosis may produce cutaneous lesions such as papulae and pustules or subcutaneous nodules. Nocardiosis may also present with particularly painful subcutaneous nodules, which are easy to biopsy. Generalized cryptococcosis may cause erythema nodosumlike deep nodules, whereas primary cutaneous cryptococcosis may appear as nodular, pustular, or ulcerative lesions or as abscesses. Phycomycosis of the sinuses may manifest as a facial cellulitis, and nocardiosis with cutaneous pustules. Dissemination of previously localized pathogenic agents, such as *Histoplasma capsulatum,* leads to erysipelas-like lesions. Early cutaneous histoplasmosis consists of painless diffuse swelling of the affected areas, whereas older lesions are represented by multiple draining ulcers.

Cutaneous chromomycosis is characterized by scaly papules that progress to verrucous nodules or ulcerating plaques. It is caused by pigmented fungi that are common saprophytes growing in soil, vegetation, and wood. Dermal alternaria infection is manifested by fleshy papules and nodules, smooth and firm, spreading centrifugally, with an elevated crusted border and a central area slightly depressed and atrophic.

Viral Infections

Herpes simplex causes multifocal, extensive, and hemorrhagic lesions (Fig. 89.5). Ulcers of the mouth and the perioral, perigenital, and perianal skin can also occur. Herpes zoster lesions are frequently gangrenous and hemorrhagic, which usually do not extend to other areas. However, atypical herpetic infection may also cause disseminated ulcerative or necrotic skin. The administration of acyclovir is mandatory for patients with severe lesions.

Varicella can occur in transplant patients, and can have a life-threatening course. Children awaiting a renal transplant should receive specific vaccine to prevent this complication. If varicella develops, immunosuppression should be reduced and even stopped in the most severe cases. Specific immunoglobulin infusion may improve the prognosis.

Cutaneous manifestation caused by cytomegaloviruses are exceptional. These consist of exanthema with vasculitis, hyperpigmented nodules and plaques, vesicobullae, and buccal and perineal ulcerations.

Oral hairy leukoplakia, a typical Epstein-Barr virus lesion mostly observed in patients affected by acquired immunodeficiency syndrome, has been also reported in human immunodeficiency virus (HIV)-negative transplant recipients.

Warts and condylomata caused by human papilloma virus are frequent in long-term functioning transplant patients. They develop on sun-exposed areas, mainly in light-skinned patients but may be so widespread as to constitute general verrucosis. This is seen especially in long-term transplant patients. Both ultraviolet light exposure and immunosuppressive treatment decrease the number of epidermal antigen-presenting Langerhans cells, which are important for cutaneous immunosurveillance. Topical keratolytic agents or retinoic acid are the treatments of choice.

Lesions similar to epidermodysplasia verruciformis (an inherited precancerosis characterized by several, widespread viral warts and pityriasis versicolorlike lesions) may be seen. They are caused by oncogenic human papilloma viruses. Extensive diffusion of condylomata acuminata or of molluscum contagiosum can also occur in renal transplant recipients.

Bacterial Infections

Bacterial infections are usually trivial in the early period after transplantation, being represented almost exclusively by folliculitis. However, subcutaneous abscesses, erysipelas, and impetigo, caused by Gram-positive cocci, may develop in the long-term period. Cutaneous infections caused by atypical mycobacteria are often manifested as a spreading cellulitis around joints.

Miscellaneous Lesions

Disseminated actinic porokeratosis is frequent, up to 10% in transplant patients. It is caused by a proliferation of an abnormal clone of epidermal cells and clinically is characterized by annular lesions surrounded by a raised keratotic ring histologically constituted of a column of parakeratotic cells (Fig. 89.6).

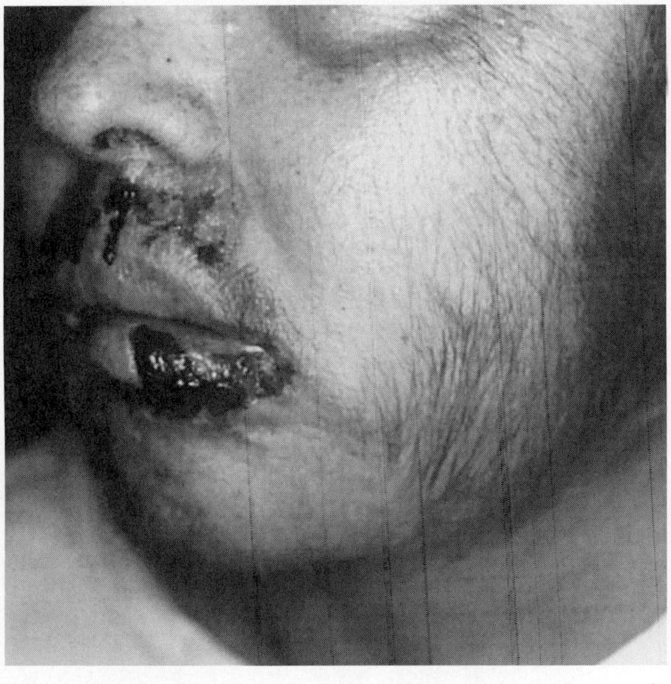

Figure 89.5. Herpes simplex: Erosions and brownish hemorrhagic scabs on the lips and perioral skin.

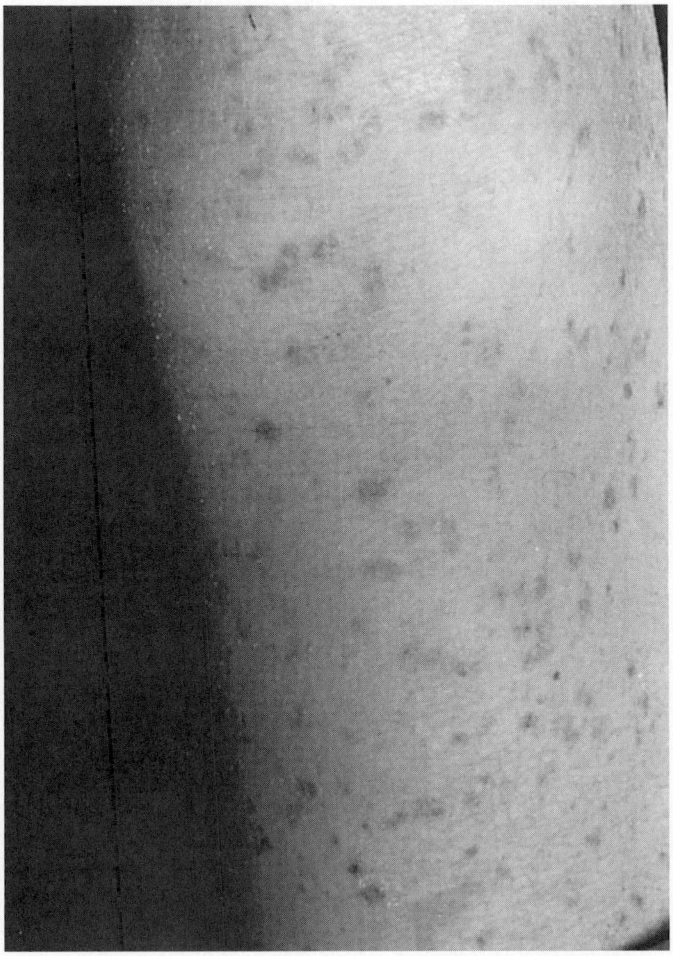

Figure 89.6. Disseminated superficial actinic porokeratosis: Multiple small lesions, characterized by a brownish atrophic area surrounded by a whitish, keratotic ring, arising on the limbs.

The disease carries the potential risk of squamous cell epithelioma. However in transplant patients this has never been reported, even in large series.

Norwegian scabies is characterized by thick-crusted plaques occurring in wide areas of the skin. Chronic urticaria may be a cutaneous manifestation of an intestinal infestation, such as giardiasis. Malakoplakia, the term meaning soft plaque, is an immunodeficiency disease in which macrophages fail to phagocytose and digest bacteria adequately. It has been observed in the skin and subcutaneous tissues adjacent to the transplant scar. Histologically, one can find in the skin large foamy histiocytes with basophilic inclusion bodies (so-called Michaeli-Gutmann bodies), which are considered to represent abnormal degradation of bacteria and are pathognomonic for this disease. The origin of this disorder remains unknown, although there is some evidence suggesting a possible role of Gram-negative enteric bacilli. In transplant patients, the disease is related to drug-induced immunosuppression.

Selected Readings

Barba A, Tessari GB, Boschiero L, et al. Renal transplantation and skin diseases: review of the literature and results of a 5-year follow-up of 285 patients. *Nephron* 1996;73:131–136.

A review of cutaneous lesions observed in a large series of transplant patients.

Bencini PL, Montagnino G, De Vecchi A, et al. Cutaneous manifestations in renal transplant recipients. *Nephron* 1983;34:79–83.

A review of dermatologic lesions observed in a large series of transplant patients.

Bunney MH, Benton EC, Barr BB, et al. The prevalence of skin disorders in renal allograft recipients receiving cyclosporin A compared with those receiving azathioprine. *Nephrol Dial Transplant* 1990;5:379–382.

A retrospective study showing that apart from hypertrichosis, which was more frequent in cyclosporine-treated patients, there was no difference in skin tumors, infections, and other cutaneous disorders between patients receiving cyclosporine or azathioprine.

Euvrard S. Cutaneous complications in renal transplant recipients. *Eur J Dermatol* 1991:1:171–184.

An excellent discussion of the skin complications in transplant patients.

Shuttleworth D, Philpot CM, Salaman JR. Cutaneous fungal infection following renal transplantation: a case control study. *Br J Dermatol* 1987;117:585–590.

A study of skin infections in renal transplant recipients.

CHAPTER 90

Renal Transplantation in Specific Diseases

Miroslaw Smogorzewski

Renal transplantation is an acceptable form of therapy for most end-stage renal disease (ESRD) patients, and for children and young adults, it is a treatment of choice. The primary disease that leads to ESRD is an important factor in patient and graft survival after transplantation. Unfortunately, the information on primary disease is not always available. Furthermore, the diagnosis is not precise in as many as one-third of the patients undergoing transplantation. Four major data sources are available for analysis of various aspects of renal replacement therapy. These include United States Renal Data System (USRDS), United Network of Organ Sharing (UNOS) Scientific Registry, North American Pediatric Renal Transplantation Cooperative Study (NAPRTCS), and European Dialysis and Transplantation Association Registry. The accuracy of the data depends heavily on the collection methods. Table 90.1 presents the diagnosis of original disease in patients receiving transplants between 1987 to 1995 according to NAPRTCS and UNOS Scientific Registry. These combined data from hundreds of centers allow the analysis of the impact of various causes of ESRD on patient and graft survival. Unfortunately, the diagnosis of many diseases is not well documented as suggested by the low percentage of biopsy use in the children presented in Table 90.1. The other sources of information are the reports from numerous centers regarding their experience in kidney transplantation in various diseases. These analyses are more focused, more critical, and use stricter criteria for diagnosis of primary disease, but they are encumbered with a selection bias.

The decision whether to perform renal transplantation in a patient with a specific disease must be based on the following factors: (a) the potential patient and kidney survival after transplantation, (b) the risk of recurrence of original disease, and (c) any special operative, metabolic, and systemic problems that exist. The standard for success of transplantation in various disorders is usually measured against the results in the chronic glomerulonephritis group. Such a comparison must be adjusted for age, sex, gender, source of kidney (cadaver or live donor), and other factors that may affect the outcome. This selection of modality of renal replacement therapy must also depend on the comparison of the success of the transplantation with regular dialysis treatment. Usually, these two modalities are mutually, but not exclusively, interdependent, although patients with certain diagnosis will have better prognosis while on dialysis or may require dialysis for a period of time before transplantation, whereas others will greatly benefit from immediate or even preemptive transplantation.

The assessment of the risk of recurrence is a difficult task despite the volume of information available. Strict criteria for diagnosis of recurrence of the primary disease in the allograft require: (a) complete diagnosis of disease in native kidney by biopsy evaluation, which includes light microscopy, immunofluorescence, and ultrastructural studies; (b) finding the same disease in the allograft kidney biopsy specimen; and (c) assurance that this disease was not present in the allograft at the time of transplantation. The recurrent disease can be categorized into the glomerular or nonglomerular forms, and the glomerular disease can be further divided into primary and secondary glomerulopathies. The glomerulopathy in the transplanted kidney may also be the result of the *de novo* glomerulonephritis, preexisting disease in the donor allograft, and drugs used after transplantation. Transplant glomerulopathy associated with acute or chronic rejection can also resemble some recurrent diseases, especially type I membranoproliferative glomerulonephritis. The recurrent diseases as a whole have an overall incidence of less than 10% to 20% and account in adults for approximately 4%, and in children for 7% of all allograft failure. However the frequency of graft loss due to recurrent glomerulonephritis is increased in grafts from living donors compared with grafts from cadaveric donors (16.2% versus 4% at 5 years). In patients with glomerulonephritis undergoing kidney transplantation, the recurrence rate of glomerular disease is in the range of 10% to 30%. Our knowledge of the mechanism regarding the reasons certain diseases reoccur commonly after transplantation is incomplete. It is very likely that similar immunologic mechanisms that have been responsible for injury of the native kidney are operating after transplantation. This suggestion is supported by the finding that circulating anti–glomerular basement membrane (GBM) antibodies may lead to recurrence of anti-GBM nephritis. In addition, sera from patients with recurrent focal segmental glomerulosclerosis (FSGS), when injected in rats, increased protein excretion, suggesting the presence of humoral factor in the recipient that predisposes to development of proteinuria and FSGS.

Clearly the recurrence of systemic diseases such as amyloidosis, systemic sclerosis, and monoclonal gammopathies is due to the persistence of the primary disease after kidney transplantation. Also, metabolic products such as oxalate in patients with oxalosis can accumulate in allograft. In this chapter, the attempt will be made to piece together the information available on renal transplantation for specific diseases. The reader is also referred to the chapters covering each disease.

TABLE 90.1. Diagnosis of 3,673 Children Who Received Transplants from January 1, 1987 (NAPRTCS) and 88,747 Adult and Pediatric Patients Who Received Transplants Between January 1990 and December 1997 (UNOS Scientific Registry 1998)

NAPRTCS Data				UNOS Scientific Registry Data		
Diagnosis	N	%	No. Bx%[a]	Diagnosis	N	%
Obstructive uropathy	605	16.4	55	IDDM	16,434	18.5
Aplastic/dysplastic kidney	603	16.5	66	Chronic GN (unspecified)	12,299	13.8
Focal segmental glomerulosclerosis	426	11.6	3	Hypertensive nephrosclerosis	10,874	12.2
Reflux nephropathy	209	5.7	56	Glomerulonephritis (specified)		
Systemic immunologic disease	174	4.7	7	Focal glomerulosclerosis	3,160	3.5
Chronic glomerulonephritis	160	4.4	28	IgA nephropathy	2,368	2.7
Congenital nephrotic syndrome	103	2.8	5	Membranous GN	1,213	1.4
Syndrome of agenesis of abdominal musculature	112	3.0	48	Idiopathic/postinfectious crescentic GN	582	0.7
Hemolytic uremic syndrome	101	2.7	33	Membranoproliferative GN type I	461	0.5
Polycystic kidney disease	100	2.7	36	Membranoproliferative GN type II	65	0
Medullary cystic disease/juvenile nephrophthisis	94	2.6	27	Anti-GBM	247	3.1
Cystinosis	92	2.5	48	Nephritis (unspecified)	1,681	1.9
Pyelonephritis/interstitial nephritis	84	2.3	28	Polycystic kidney	6,846	7.7
Membranoproliferative GN type I	84	2.3	2	NIDDM	4,325	4.9
Renal infarction	75	2.0	47	Systemic lupus erythematosis	2,754	3.1
Familial nephritis	83	2.3	2	Malignant hypertension	1,971	2.2
Idiopathic crescentic GN	65	1.8	0	Chronic pyelonephritis/reflux nephropathy	1,792	2.0
Membranoproliferative GN type II	37	1.0	0	Hypoplasia/dysplasia	1,044	1.2
Oxalosis	29	0.8	25	Retransplant	1,311	1.5
Membranous nephropathy	23	0.6	0	Alport's syndrome	1,173	1.3
Wilms' tumor	22	0.6	0	Acquired obstructive nephropathy	1,158	1.3
Drash syndrome	20	0.5	0	Wegener's granulomatosis	322	0.4
Sickle cell nephropathy	5	0.1	50	Hemolytic uremic syndrome	324	0.4
Diabetic nephropathy	4	0.1	0	Medullary cystic disease	269	0.3
Other	203	5.5	30	Cyclosporine toxicity	199	0.2
Unknown	160	4.4	62	Analgesic nephropathy	169	0.2
				Other	10,914	12.3
				Not reported	4,792	8.3

UNOS data based on OPTN/Scientific Registry data as of March 31, 1998.

[a] Renal biopsy or nephrectomy confirmation of primary diagnosis (%) from NAPRTCS from *Pediatr Nephrol* 1993;7:711–720.

(Reproduced from Wardy, BA, Hebert D, Sullivan EK, et al. Renal transplantation, chronic dialysis, and chronic renal insufficiency in children and adolescents. The 1995 annual report of the North American Pediatric Renal Transplant Cooperative Study. *Pediatr Nephrol* 1997;11:49–64.)

Bx, renal biopsy; GBM, glomerular basement membrane; GN, glomerulonephritis; IDDM, insulin-dependent diabetes mellitus; NAPRTCS, North American Pediatric Renal Transplant Cooperative Study; NIDDM, non-insulin-dependent diabetes mellitus; UNOS, United Network of Organ Sharing.

SYSTEMIC VASCULAR DISEASES (TABLE 90.2)

Diabetes Mellitus

The number of patients with ESRD treated by renal replacement therapy because of diabetes mellitus is continually increasing, especially during the 1980s and 1990s. According to the 1998 USRDS annual report, the 1996 incidence of diabetes was 42.3%, and prevalence was 32.5% of total Medicare ESRD patients.

Both insulin-dependent diabetes mellitus (IDDM, type I) and non–insulin-dependent diabetes mellitus (NIDDM, type II) can cause renal failure. It seems that the risk of developing renal failure for type I and type II diabetes is similar and the clinical picture following the onset of overt diabetic nephropathy in the two types of patients is not very different. It has been estimated that approximately 95% of all patients with diabetes have NIDDM, and the majority of ESRD diabetic patients are type II. In contrast to that, according to the UNOS Scientific Registry, 98% of diabetic patients receiving a first-time transplant between 1987 and 1992 had type I diabetes. It changed significantly between 1994 and 1998. Data from the same source show that between 1994 and 1997, 35% of diabetics with transplanted kidney were type II. At the end of 1996 in the United States, approximately 17.8% of ESRD diabetic patients had a functioning transplant, 70.8% were treated by hemodialysis, and 10.4% by peritoneal dialysis. Since 1998, one-third of kidney transplants performed in this population is accompanied by transplantation of the pancreas.

It is difficult to compare the survival rate of the patients treated by different modalities because of the patient and center selection bias. In general, significant improvement in the 1-year survival rate of diabetic patients treated by dialysis was noticed, but the 5-year survival was only 26.5% for a 1991 cohort. Selected centers reported that 50% of patients with end-stage diabetic nephropathy survived 5 years while receiving hemodialysis. Patient survival for cadaveric-transplant recipients (1-year survival close to 91% and 5-year survival approximately 66%) is clearly better than for patients receiving dialysis therapy.

Type I diabetic patients are potential candidates either for kidney transplant alone (KTA) or simultaneous pancreas–kidney transplantation (PKT), whereas type II diabetics generally receive renal graft only.

Data from the University of Minnesota support a choice of kidney transplantation over dialysis. Five-year survival in diabetic patients treated with kidney transplantation was 82% to 84% for those age 15 to 44 as compared with 25% to 35% for the same age group treated by dialysis. Also with newer immunosuppressive protocols, 1- and 6-year graft survival was similar in diabetic and nondiabetic kidney transplant recipients. Living-donor transplant recipients had a better outcome. Retransplantation in diabetic patients has led to successful function less often. Death, most commonly caused by cardiac disease or infection,

TABLE 90.2. Renal Transplantation in Patients with Systemic Diseases

Disease	Graft Survival[a] 1 Year	Graft Survival[a] 3 Years	Graft Survival[a] 5 Years	Clinical % of Recurrence	Histologic Findings Mimic Rejection	Graft Loss Resulting From Primary Disease	Comments
Vascular diseases							
Diabetes mellitus type I	83%	73%	61%	Rare early, late in 100%	No	5%	Graft failure resulting from diabetes mellitus usually after 8 to 10 years.
Diabetes mellitus type II	88%	73%	51%	? Most likely as in Type I	No	?	
Systemic lupus erythematosus	81%	70%	60%	1%–2%	No	2%–3%	Recurrence may occur during the time of systemic activity.
Hemolytic uremic syndrome	74%	59%	47%	13%–46%	No	10%–77%	Precipitated factors should be avoided; atypical form has worse prognosis.
Wegener's granulomatosis/ systemic vasculitis	88%	79%	70%	Rare, but reported	Yes	Rare	Good response to increased dose of steroids and cyclophosphamide.
Henoch-Schönlein purpura	83%	74%	55%	10%	No	10%–20%	Wait for 6 to 12 months after disappearance of skin purpura.
Systemic sclerosis	66%	61%	48%	Rare, but reported	No		Relatively high; some patients may recover kidney function during the first 6 months on dialysis.
Deposition disorders							
Oxalosis	70%	57%	51%	100%	No	30%	Liver–kidney transplantation is now recommended; better graft survival of kidney transplant alone was recently reported.
Cystinosis	86%	76%	76%	None	No	None	
Amyloidosis	78%	70%	53%	5%–30%	No	?	Higher morbidity and mortality, especially during first year after transplantation.
Renal carcinoma	89%	79%	54%		No	?	
Wilms' tumor	83%	83%	70%	10%–20%	No	?	Wait at least 2 years after remission before transplantation.
Multiple myeloma	?			High	No	?	High rate of infections.
Miscellaneous conditions							
Fabry's disease	85%	72%	62%	None	No	None	
Sickle cell anemia	81%	58%	45%	High	No	High	Heterozygous living-related donors should not be used.

[a] Based on UNOS OPTN/Scientific Registry data as of April 26, 1999. Data are presented as Kaplan-Meir graft survival rates for transplants performed: 1988–1997 for the kidneys obtained from cadaver donors. Results for kidneys obtained from living donors are 5% to 15% better depending on primary diagnosis and status of the recipients.

remains the most frequent cause of renal graft failure for diabetic recipients; chronic rejection is the third most common cause. Patients' rehabilitation and quality of life are better after kidney transplant but a higher rate of deterioration of eyesight (38% versus 12%) and more frequent requirement for amputation (31% versus 13%) have been reported in diabetic transplant patients as compared with those receiving dialysis.

Better overall results of kidney transplantation as a modality of treatment for diabetic ESRD patients are partially related to patient selection. Transplanted patients are younger, more likely to be type I, and with less microvascular and macrovascular pathology. Since 1998, simultaneous PKT is performed in the United States in one-third of diabetic recipients. Because there is an increased risk associated with PKT versus KTA, healthier uremic diabetic patients are generally selected for PKT. Three years after either PKT or KTA, kidney function and patients and grafts survival are similar in both groups. Improvement in the quality of life and slight improvement in peripheral and autonomic neuropathy, nephropathy, gastropathy, and cardiac function were reported after PKT.

Despite euglycemia, there is little improvement in established retinopathy and progression of peripheral vascular disease is very frequent. Twenty percent to thirty percent of PKT patients had amputations during 5-year follow-up; similar or lower numbers were reported for KTA.

Diabetic candidates for kidney transplantation require careful evaluation. Significant stenosis of one or more coronary arteries was seen in 25% to 40% of symptomatic diabetic patients screened with coronary angiography before renal transplantation. Aggressive attempts to screen diabetic transplant candidates, especially those older than 35 years of age, for cardiovascular disease including coronary angiography are strongly advised. If significant coronary arteries lesions exist, they should be treated by angioplasty or bypass before the transplantation.

Diabetic nephropathy will recur in the transplanted kidney. During the first 2 years after transplantation, no significant changes are observed in the kidney biopsy; but after that, the kidney shows GBM thickening and mesangial expansion, changes typical for diabetic nephropathy, and by 4 years hyalinization of afferent and efferent arterioles is present. Clinically recurrent diabetic nephropathy manifested as proteinuria and slow deterioration of allograft function with graft loss seen after 10 years in 5% of the patients.

De novo posttransplant diabetes mellitus, which occurs in 2.5% to 20% of allograft recipients treated with steroids and calcineurin antagonists (tacrolimus, cyclosporine), is associated with impaired long-term survival and function of the kidney. Complications similar to those in non–transplant-associated diabetes mellitus may develop, hence, tight glycemic control is advised.

A successful pancreas transplant alone in a patient with moderate diabetic nephropathy due to type 1 diabetes will result in reversal of the clinical and histologic manifestations of diabetic nephropathy.

Systemic Lupus Erythematosus

Most extrarenal manifestations of systemic lupus erythematosus (SLE) can be controlled by immunosuppressive therapy, but renal failure remains an important cause of morbidity and mortality. More than 1.3% of patients treated with renal replacement therapy in the United States had ESRD related to lupus nephritis. In the early days of kidney transplantation, there was a fear that this immune complex disease may frequently recur and lead to graft loss. However, after satisfactory results were reported in 1975 by the Advisory Committee to the Renal Transplant Registry, patients with ESRD secondary to SLE are considered as good candidates for renal transplantation. During the period between 1988 and 1997, approximately 3,195 renal transplants were performed in the United States in patients with SLE. One-year graft survival in these patients was 84%, comparable to the general transplant population, but 5-year graft survival (64%) was slightly lower than expected. It was suggested that autoantinuclear or other antibodies undetected before transplantation by standard screening could be responsible for the higher rejection rate and this poorer outcome. It is generally recommended that clinical manifestations of SLE should be quiescent on small doses (less than 10 mg/day) of steroids and serologic parameters to be normal or stable before transplantation. Also SLE patients should be screened for antiphospholipid antibodies and, once positive, they should be considered for anticoagulation therapy to prevent thrombotic events. The recurrence rate of SLE in transplanted kidney was believed to be in the range of 1% to 2%. A report from University of California–San Francisco, which specifically focused on recurrence in lupus nephritis, challenges this view. Ninety-seven SLE recipients had a total of 106 transplanted kidneys from 1984 to 1996. The frequency of lupus nephritis during the follow-up (mean 4.8 years) was 8.5% and four (3.8%) kidneys were lost due to recurrence. In addition, eight patients lost their grafts secondary to complications of antiphospholipid syndrome.

Some authors suggested the positive correlation between pretransplant and posttransplant positive antinuclear antibodies and an elevated anti–double-stranded deoxyribonucleic acid (DNA) titer and disease recurrence rate, but others reported poor correlation between clinical and serologic activities of disease and the likelihood of recurrence. The data accumulated at this point do not suggest that longer dialysis time in seropositive patients will prevent these recurrences. The histologic and immunofluorescence patterns of recurrent lupus nephritis in renal allograft are usually the same as original glomerulonephritis. Most of the reported cases have been successfully treated with an increased dose of immunosuppression.

Hemolytic Uremic Syndrome

Hemolytic uremic syndrome (HUS) is a common cause of ESRD in children (approximately 5% of all cases) but may also occur in adults at all ages. It is an etiologically heterogeneous entity, characterized by microangiopathic hemolytic anemia, thrombocytopenia, and acute renal failure.

Shiga toxin (verotoxin)–associated HUS is usually described as classical, sporadic or epidemic, commonly diarrhea-associated form that occurs mainly in children. More than 95% of patients with this form of HUS will recover from acute renal failure. Those who reach ESRD, when transplanted, usually will not have recurrence. None of 18 children with classical HUS reported from Argentina had recurrence.

The idiopathic (atypical) form of HUS carries a worse prognosis, a higher mortality rate, and an increased (up to 50%) incidence of ESRD. Patients with this form of HUS have, after kidney transplantation, high recurrence rate (13% to 46%) and high incidence of graft loss (10% to 77%). Six-month and 1-year posttransplant graft survival are 5% to 8% less than in other glomerular diseases. The outcome of 24 patients who received 36 transplants at the University of Minnesota between 1972 and 1999 demonstrated recurrent HUS in 14 grafts in 11 patients. Nine of those patients had atypical HUS and the majority of episodes took place within 2 months after transplantation. Eleven grafts were lost despite intensive treatment, including plasmapheresis and plasma infusion.

Rarely, HUS is inherited in autosomal-recessive or autosomal-dominant modes. The former one affects mainly children, whereas the latter occurs in adults of the same family. The risk for recurrence, presenting a clinical picture similar to the atypical HUS, is high. HUS recurred in six of the seven adults with autosomal-recessive inheritance 2 weeks to 6.5 years after transplantation, regardless of the allograft source.

De novo HUS after renal transplantation is commonly associated with the use of cyclosporine, tacrolimus, and OKT3 or antilymphocyte globulin (ALG) for the treatment of acute rejection. Reduction of the dose of cyclosporine A or withdrawal of the drug leads, in the majority of patients, to recovery of kidney function. Specific immunosuppressive agents may provoke recurrence in an individual patient, but overall contribution of these drugs to recurrent HUS is small.

There are no markers for HUS recurrence. Preventive measures include: a delay of transplantation until acute presentation of the disease is burn-out; caution in the use of cyclosporine, tacrolimus, OKT3, and ALG; and avoidance, during the second transplantation, of the medication associated with the loss of the first graft because of HUS recurrence. The family-related donation of the kidney is not recommended.

Therapeutic approaches to HUS after transplantation are essentially the same as those used for primary HUS, although there are no controlled trials to evaluate the efficacy of plasmapheresis and fresh-frozen plasma infusion in patients after transplantation. Despite that, these treatments are frequently used together with modification of immunosuppressive drugs.

WEGENER'S GRANULOMATOSIS AND MICROSCOPIC POLYANGITIS

The most common forms of kidney involvement in systemic vasculitis are Wegener's granulomatosis and microscopic polyangiitis. They are strongly associated with the presence of antineutrophilic cytoplasmic antibodies (ANCA). Most patients with untreated Wegener's granulomatosis are positive for cytoplasmic (C)-ANCA with the specificity against proteinase 3 (PR3) of neutrophils granules. Approximately 80% of patients with microscopic polyangiitis have either C-ANCA or perinuclear (P)-ANCA, with most having P-ANCA (antibodies against myeloperoxidase, MPA-ANCA). Both Wegener's granulomatosis and microscopic polyangiitis are presented as narcotizing crescentic glomerulonephritis on kidney biopsy. Wegener's granulomatosis has, in addition, granulomatous vasculitis of respiratory tract and less frequently typical granulomas in the renal tissue. Current immunosuppressive (cyclophosphamide and glucocorticoids) treatment improves the outcome of these diseases, but eventually more than 150 ESRD patients every year are admitted for renal replacement therapy in the United States because of Wegener's granulomatosis/polyangiitis. Of these, 40 to 50 patients have kidney transplantation every year. The 3-year survival rate on hemodialysis was approximately 58% to 62% and 5-year survival was 27% to 47% for Wegener's granulomatosis/periarteritis nodosa patients. The success of transplantation is difficult to assess, but during the period of 1988 to 1997, 5-year patient survival was 85% and 1-year graft survival was 90.5%. Five-year graft survival was 72%. There is a general agreement that transplant outcome is similar to that of controls. Seven of eight patients reported from a single center were alive with a functioning graft 40 to 128 months after transplantation. The usual immunosuppressive regimen (without cyclophosphamide) is used in the posttransplant period. There are more than 20 cases of recurrence of Wegener's granulomatosis in the allograft together with classic upper respiratory tract presentation. The recurrence rate was, on average, 22% in four single centers reporting a total of 79 patients. The time of recurrence after transplantation ranged from 2 weeks to 89 months. One case had ureteral stenosis resulting from necrotizing granulomas. Kidney biopsy results show both vasculitis and necrotizing glomerulonephritis consistent with Wegener's granulomatosis. The recurrent Wegener's granulomatosis/microscopic polyangiitis can be treated successfully with an increased dose of steroids and cyclophosphamide. Cyclophosphamide can be considered a permanent addition to the immunosuppressive protocol. The usefulness of the screening for ANCA titer in these patients before and after transplantation is not clear. Relapse of the vasculitis occurred both in patients with positive and negative ANCA before transplantation. Presence of ANCA should not preclude transplantation, provided the disease is clinically inactive, but patients with high or rising titer of ANCA may have increased rates of relapse.

Henoch-Schönlein Purpura

Henoch-Schönlein purpura (HSP) has a relatively high rate of recurrence in the allograft kidney, especially in children. Allograft biopsy specimens of HSP children were positive for IgA in 75% to 88% of the cases reported from France. The clinically detectable recurrence rate is probably less than 10%. The clinical features of HSP may appear immediately after transplantation, but were described as late as 20 months after transplantation. The typical picture includes hematuria, proteinuria, joint pain, and, more rarely, purpura with progressive deterioration of the allograft function. Overall graft loss is 10% to 20% but may be much higher if purpuric skin lesions are present. It is of interest that most of the clinically significant recurrences occur in those cases in which the kidneys were obtained from living-related donors. This may imply a genetic predisposition in the pathogenesis of HSP. It is advised to wait at least 12 months after the disappearance of purpura before attempting transplantation.

Progressive Systemic Sclerosis

Systemic sclerosis is characterized by widespread skin fibrosis and obliterative vascular lesions with frequent (20% to 40%) kidney involvement. Renal failure is usually due to scleroderma renal crisis (SRC) associated with accelerated or malignant hypertension, rapidly progressive renal insufficiency, microangiopathic hemolysis, and consumptive thrombocytopenia. Aggressive use of angiotensin-converting enzyme (ACE) inhibitors can halt renal deterioration, but if treatment is started late, when severe kidney failure is already present, dialysis may be required temporarily or permanently. Approximately 150 new patients per year are admitted in the United States for renal replacement therapy with systemic sclerosis. Only 4% to 5% received a transplanted organ during the first year. Three-year survival with dialysis was approximately 35% in one study of 311 patients. A high proportion of the patients who continued with dialysis for at least 3 months have been able to completely discontinue dialysis 5 to 18 months later if they maintain therapy with ACE inhibitors.

Successful kidney transplantation can lead to disappearance of the clinical features of SRC, but in 3 of 13 patients the graft was lost from recurrence. Patients who are recommended for transplantation should be clinically stable with absence of active visceral systemic sclerosis. Those with severe cardiac, pulmonary, and gastrointestinal involvement may be at high risk of complications. It is also prudent to wait at least 6 months on dialysis because some patients may recover their kidney function with dialysis. Improvement in skin thickening and in other nonrenal manifestations such as Raynaud's syndrome may occur after transplantation.

DEPOSITION DISEASES (TABLE 90.2)

Cystinosis

Children with nephropathic cystinosis, without treatment, will develop ESRD between 7 and 10 years of age. Chronic dialysis and transplantation pose no greater problems in children with cystinosis than in other children. Cells of transplanted kidney have normal transport of cysteine out of the lysosome, so the graft is not affected by the recurrence of the disease. Cysteine can accumulate in infiltrating monocytes and interstitial cells but does not generate the symptoms of proximal tubular dysfunction, such as Fanconi's syndrome. Data from the European Registry collected after 1985 show 5-year survival rates of 60% and 70% in children depending on whether grafts were from cadaver donors (150 patients) or from living-related donors (33 patients). These results are not different from those in noncystinotic patients. Similar results were reported by NAPRTCS in 1995. Patients with cystinosis do not have increased incidence of bacterial, viral, or fungal infections. Unfortunately, transplantation does not prevent progression of the disease in the nonrenal tissue such as eyes and the nervous, endocrine, and respiratory systems, and does not improve the growth rate of the recipients. Treatment with cysteamine may change this posttransplant course similar to the change in natural course of disease in children treated early with cysteamine.

Oxalosis (Primary Type 1)

Primary hyperoxaluria type 1 (PH1) is an autosomal-recessive disease, caused by a deficiency of the liver-specific enzyme, alanine (glyoxylate aminotransferase), with widespread tissue accumulation of calcium oxalate, nephrocalcinosis, and progressive renal insufficiency.

The early experience of kidney transplantation in PH1 was disappointing, and many authors considered oxalosis as an absolute contraindication for transplantation. European experience of 96 patients who received first allograft transplants from 1965 to 1986 shows that after 3 years, only 23% of living-donor and 17% of cadaver-donor transplants survived. The use of a protocol, which includes intensive pretransplant hemodialysis, hydration, intravenous pyridoxine, low oxalate and ascorbic acid diet, and phosphate and magnesium supplementation, as well as the optimal conditions for immediate graft function, significantly improved the results. In one center, four of eight children had graft survival 6.5 to 10.5 years after transplantation with good kidney function and no evidence of renal oxalate deposition. Renal transplantation alone should be performed when GFR approaches 20 ml/min/1.73 m^2, because oxalate retention increases rapidly as GFR falls below this level and systemic oxalosis develops.

Liver transplantation offers the possibility to correct the enzyme deficiency and can be used either before ESRD develops or as a combined liver–kidney transplant after kidney failure. The largest series of 87 liver transplant (67 simultaneously with kidney) in 80 patients was reported from 30 European centers. Following transplantation performed between 1989 and 1997, 1-, 2-, and 5-year patient survival were 88%, 80%, and 72%, respectively, and graft survival rates were 82%, 78%, and 62% at the same time intervals. Patients who stayed on dialysis less than 2 years before transplantation and were without marked systemic oxalosis had better survival. Based on this experience, the following guidelines have been suggested based on kidney function: GFR, 25 to 60 ml/min/1.73 m^2, orthotopic liver transplantation if disease is undergoing aggressive course; GFR, 25 ml/min./1.73 m^2, plan for early hepatorenal transplant; GFR 10 ml/min/1.73 m^2, immediate hepatorenal transplant preceded by intensive hemodialysis and/or hemofiltration.

A survey of transplantation for PH1 patients less than 55 years of age in the United States shows that between 1984 and 1996, there were 61 patients who had kidney transplant alone, 31 had hepatorenal transplant, and 35 were dialyzed only. Overall patient survival rate was 80% of those with kidney allograft alone, 78% with hepatorenal transplant, and 46% for nontransplant patients. The data support the notion that transplantation represents a good option for ESRD patients with PH.

Amyloidosis

Amyloidosis is the second most common metabolic disorder causing ESRD. It accounts for 0.3% of all patients treated by renal replacement in the United States and 2% of those treated in Australia. In the Middle East, it is one of the most common causes of uremia because of the high incidence of familial Mediterranean fever (FMF). Two large series of transplant patients with amyloidosis have concluded that transplantation can be performed with acceptable results. Overall, early mortality was high, survival rate of the patients was 79% at 1 year, 65% at 5 years, and 43% at 10 years; however, graft survival at 1 year was 74%, at 5 years 62%, and at 10 years 41%. Patients with primary (AL) amyloidosis did as well as those with the secondary (AA) form. Infectious complications accounted for 61% and cardiovascular complications caused 17% of all deaths. Recurrent AA amyloid deposition in renal allografts has been shown in 21% of all patients with FMF, in 10% to 15% of patients transplanted with rheumatologic disease, and in 14% transplanted with chronic infections, but not all of the patients had undergone kidney biopsy. Fewer than 10% of the patients suffered from graft amyloidosis, and only 5% lost graft because of that. Colchicine in a dose higher than 1 mg/24 hours was used in the posttransplant period in FMF and was effective in protecting the graft from amyloidosis.

Renal transplantation is the treatment of choice of dialysis-related β_2-microglobulin amyloidosis. Immediate improvement of joint symptoms occurs after transplantation and has been ascribed to immunosuppressive medication. Progression of β_2-microglobulin deposits is halted, but no regression of bone cysts was noticed and amyloid depositions were present in the bone even after 10 years of successful transplantation.

MALIGNANCY AND RENAL TRANSPLANTATION

Kidney transplantation in patients with ESRD caused by malignancy was successfully used in patients with primary renal neoplasm (renal cell carcinoma and nephroblastoma), in a small group of patients with monoclonal gammopathies and multiple myeloma, and very rarely in cases of chronic leukemia or lymphoma. In most of these cases the malignancy was believed to be cured. Disseminated malignancy either in the donor or the recipient is uniformly recognized as a contraindication to kidney transplantation. Patients with localized malignancy who have been successfully treated and remain free of disease for at least 5 years can be regarded as acceptable. The exception to this is patients with primary brain tumors who could be a donor at any time.

Nephroblastoma (Wilms' tumor) is the malignancy most often requiring renal replacement therapy in childhood secondary to bilateral nephrectomy, radiation, or chemotherapy. After 2 years of remission of Wilms' tumor, achieved with surgical removal and chemotherapy, the risk of recurrence or metastasis is small, and renal transplantation can be safely performed at this time. Metastasis in children transplanted before 2 years of remission and septicemia were the two major causes of mortality in this population. In a few reports, children with kidney allografts were followed 1 to 25 years after transplantation without recurrence of nephroblastoma.

For 257 patients with ESRD and renal carcinoma treated by dialysis, the 1-year survival was 63% and 3-year survival was 38%. The recurrence rate for renal carcinomas treated before transplantation and reported to the Cincinnati Transplant Tumor Registry was 1 of 72 (1%) in patients with incidentally discovered tumor and 61 of 222 (27%) for patients with symptomatic lesions. The same data suggest that patients with asymptomatic, early discovered tumors may undergo transplantation without a waiting period, whereas patients with symptomatic lesions should wait at least 2 years without evidence of recurrent tumor before transplantation can take place.

Multiple myeloma is the most common malignancy in adults leading to ESRD and accounts for more than 500 patients admitted every year for renal replacement therapy in the United States. The prognosis for 1-year survival with dialysis for these patients is 56%, and 30-month survival is only 34%. Renal transplantation has been used in few patients, and results are discouraging. Frequently, the diagnosis of multiple myeloma is made retrospectively after kidney transplantation. Among those treated for multiple myeloma before transplantation, the recurrence rate was more than 60%. In a recent review of 13 patients with multiple myeloma, six patients died from sepsis with fungal pathogens in three cases. Eight of these 13 allografts had recurrence of myeloma nephropathy with light-chain deposits present in the kidney. It must be noted that six patients survived more than 3 years. The presence of monoclonal gammopathy without evidence of multiple myeloma or macroglobulinemia is now termed *monoclonal gammopathy of undetermined significance (MGUS)*. This diagnosis can be made only after intensive screening for myeloma. Most patients with MGUS will remain stable indefinitely without treatment; however, some of them will evolve to myeloma, amyloidosis, or macroglobulinemia. MGUS can develop in patients during dialysis therapy. The follow-up for 3 to 9 years of four patients who were transplanted with this syndrome shows that two patients developed smoldering myeloma, and in two others monoclonal component remained stable. They do not experience more rejection nor more infectious complications than other transplanted patients. It can be concluded that MGUS is not a contraindication for transplantation, but patients must be carefully followed for development of overt myeloma.

OTHER SYSTEMIC DISORDERS

Fabry's Disease (Table 90.2)

Fabry's disease is a rare X-linked, recessive disorder of glycosphingolipid metabolism resulting from deficiency of α-galactosidase. Renal failure usually occurs in the third or fourth decade of life. The early transplant experience was disappointing. Many of these patients died of sepsis, pulmonary hemorrhage, and thrombosis. It was found that transplanted kidney is not a sufficient source of missing enzyme, but good graft function provides better excretion and less ceramide accumulation. Recent UNOS data show that kidney transplantation is a good modality of renal replacement therapy for these patients. Three-year graft survival was 80%, and low incidence of infectious complications was also noted. The reported recurrences occurred 6 to 14 years posttransplant. The use of living-related donors should be considered with caution because they could be heterozygous for the defective enzyme gene and their kidney can be more prone to develop excessive accumulation of glycosphingolipid deposits.

Sickle Cell Syndrome (Table 90.2)

Patients with sickle cell diseases, which include sickle cell anemia (S-S), sickle cell trait (S-A), and sickle cell combined with hemoglobinopathies disease (S-C, S-Thal, S-D), are infrequently candidates for transplantation despite the fact that between 1992 and 1996 there were 345 new cases of ESRD caused by sickle cell nephropathy. It is difficult to give an absolute recommendation with regard to the type of replacement therapy in these patients. The national survey of 110 centers in the United States in 1984 revealed 45 transplants in 40 patients with sickle cell disease; 13 with sickle cell (S-S) anemia, 27 with sickle cell trait. Patient mortality was 12% in the first year and 1-year graft survival was 82% in living-donor transplant recipients and 62% in cadaveric transplant recipients. Twelve patients (7 of them had S-S disease) experienced sickle cell crisis after transplantation. The author concluded that transplantation is not contraindicated in patients with a sickle cell disease.

Analysis of the outcome in 82 (81 had HbSS) end-stage sickle cell nephropathy patients transplanted from 1984 to 1996 shows similar 1-year cadaveric graft survival (78%) to age-matched controls (77%), but inferior 3-year graft survival (48% versus 60%). The mortality was higher in sickle cell patients than in the control group, but there was a trend toward improved survival in transplant recipients compared with their dialysis-treated, wait-listed counterparts.

Single-center reports are less optimistic. Sickle cell crisis occurred in five of eight patients within 6 months after transplantation, and four allografts were lost as a result of sickling. Two more kidneys were removed for irreversible rejection. Two recipients died from severe sickle cell crisis and only two of eight patients had a functioning kidney graft beyond 1 year. In addition, few case reports stress the complexity of posttransplant patient care in sickle cell disease. Nonetheless, it is clear that transplantation should be available for the patients with sickle cell anemia with ESRD. Preparation of the patient before surgery with transfusions of normal blood and concurrent use of hydroxyurea to increase HbF production may reduce the frequency of crisis. Rewarming the kidney immediately before revascularization and avoidance of relative hypoxia in the immediate postoperative period are recommended. The commonly accepted principles apply to the treatment of sickle cell crisis after transplantation. One case report suggested recurrence of sickle cell nephropathy in the graft 3.5 years after transplantation.

RENAL TRANSPLANTATION IN SPECIFIC GLOMERULONEPHRITIDES (TABLE 90.3)

Membranoproliferative Glomerulonephritis

Both membranoproliferative glomerulonephritis (MPGN) type I (with subendothelial deposits) and MPGN type II (dense-deposit disease) recur in transplanted kidney. Type I MPGN has a recurrence rate that varies from a low of 9% to a high of 53%, with an average of 30%. Some of these rates may be an overestimation because the light microscopy features of classic double contours of GBM may also be present in transplant glomerulopathy associated with chronic rejection.

The differential diagnosis of these two diseases is based on the finding of extensive immune complex deposition of IgG in the mesangial and subendothelial space and large well-developed

TABLE 90.3. Renal Transplantation in Patients with Glomerulonephritis

Type of GN	Frequency of Recurrence: Morphologic	Frequency of Recurrence: Clinical	Clinical Manifestation	Graft Loss Resulting From Recurrence	Comments
Membranoproliferative GN					
Type I	20%–30%	20%–30%	Proteinuria, hematuria, nephrotic syndrome	10%–40%	May resemble transplant glomerulopathy.
Type II	50%–100%	50%–100%	Nonnephrotic range proteinuria	10%–20%	Higher graft loss if crescents present in biopsy specimen.
Focal segmental glomerulosclerosis	20%–30%	20%–30%	Nephrotic syndrome leading to graft failure	10%–20%	Patients with malignant course of FSGS, younger than 6 years of age, and recurrence in the prior allograft are at higher risk; early diagnosis and plasma exchange may be helpful.
Membranous GN	4%–10%	4%–10%	Proteinuria without deterioration of graft function	2%	Prognosis worse if accompanied by chronic rejection.
IgA nephropathy	25%–50%	20%–40%	Proteinuria and hematuria	1%–10%	High risk for recipients of living donors.
Anti-GBM disease	10%–50%	5%	Low-grade proteinuria	3%	Avoid transplantation for 3 to 12 months after anti-GBM antibodies are negative.

FSGS, focal segmental glomerulosclerosis; GBM, glomerular basement membrane; GN, glomerulonephritis.

dense deposits with distinct edges in type I MPGN. In chronic transplant glomerulopathy, the deposits are of low-density material, have irregular outlines, and do not contain IgG. Clinically, patients have proteinuria and/or hematuria, leading to nephrotic syndrome and early graft failure. The C3 serum level is not helpful in establishing diagnosis or for the evaluation of the progress of the disease. Various types of treatment including plasma exchange failed to decrease proteinuria and to prevent the graft loss, although antiplatelet treatment stabilized kidney function according to one report.

Type II MPGN has a histologic recurrence rate of electron-dense material in the basement membranes of the transplant as high as 50% to 100%. Clinical recurrence is less common, and manifests as proteinuria, usually not in the nephrotic range, within the first year after transplantation. Graft failure will occur in 10% of patients. One report, however, shows graft loss in 50% of the patients. Males and patients with nephrotic-range proteinuria and more aggressive disease in native kidney showing extensive crescent formation had recurrence of dense-deposit disease early after transplantation and developed graft failure within 1 year. In most of the patients with type II MPGN after successful transplantation, C3 nephritic factor activity disappears and C3 levels return to normal values.

Focal And Segmental Glomerulosclerosis

Focal and segmental glomerulosclerosis (FSGS) is one of the most common glomerular diseases leading to ESRD, particularly in children, and has the highest rate of recurrence in the renal allograft. European Pediatric Registry data collected between 1971 and 1990 show that of 152 children with FSGS, 29% had recurrence of the disease after the first transplantation and half of these recurrences were noted within the first month after transplantation. Only seven children received the second graft, and six of them developed nephrotic syndrome once again. The first cadaver graft survival for 1, 2, and 3 years in children with FSGS was 8% less than with other forms of glomerulonephritis. NAPRTCS registry (1987 to 1992) recorded 168 transplants in children with FSGS and analyzed 132 transplanted kidneys in 127 patients. The recurrence rate was 20.5% but was lower in African-Americans than in whites and Hispanics. The pretransplant therapy (cyclophosphamide or cyclosporine), age at the time of transplantation, sex, and degree of human leukocyte antigen (HLA) mismatch did not differ between children with and without recurrences. Newer analysis of 379 children with FSGS and kidney allograft confirm the increased risk for graft failure during the first 2 years posttransplant (25.4% and 41.1% of grafts from living donors and cadavers donors, respectively, were lost). Recurrent FSGS was a cause of graft failure in 22.5%. Patients who lost their graft due to rejection without evidence of recurrence of FSGS were likely to have excellent results with subsequent allograft. The risk of recurrence is increased in patients younger than the age of 15 years, in those with rapid course of disease, and in those with evidence of mesangial proliferation in the native kidney or in the graft if the first graft was lost due to FSGS relapse. Indeed, in children less than 5 years of age the recurrence rate is approximately 50% and once the recurrence developed in the first graft there is an increased chance (60% to 80%) for subsequent recurrences in the second graft as well. Patients with recurrent disease are also more likely to have episodes of acute renal failure and acute rejection. Data from centers with mixed transplant populations of children and adults with FSGS support the higher frequency of recurrence in those younger than 15 years and older than 60 years of age. Heavy proteinuria and graft failure are the features of recurrent FSGS. Proteinuria is usually in the nephrotic range, and may appear immediately or in the few weeks after transplantation. Microscopic hematuria and hypertension are also common. Eventually half of these patients will lose their graft because of FSGS, but some of them may have a long and benign course.

De novo collapsing glomerulopathy has been described in five patients, four of whom have been treated with anti–intercellular adhesion molecule (anti-ICAM) monoclonal antibody. The clinical presentation was similar to the previously reported *de novo* FSGS without collapsing features, including new onset of proteinuria between 4 month and 2 years after transplantation and deterioration of kidney function.

Treatment of recurrent FSGS with ACE inhibitors may delay onset of renal failure. None of the immunosuppressive protocols described until now, including cyclosporine, have prevented FSGS, and these therapeutic modalities have been useful in the treatment of recurrence. Plasmapheresis or immunoadsorption of plasma on columns containing protein A or sheep antihuman immunoglobulin can reduce (although transiently) albuminuria, most likely by removing factor(s) altering permeability of GBM. The future of these techniques and their value in the treatment of FSGS are not clear. However, aggressive plasmapheresis for about 2 weeks started early in the recurrence led to remission lasting more than 1 year in 11 of 15 patients. One study suggested a strong correlation between the high level of the factor(s) increasing permeability of filtration barrier before transplantation and the rate of recurrence, but other studies did not confirm these findings.

Membranous Glomerulonephritis

Membranous glomerulonephritis (MGN) has a relatively low incidence (4% to 7%) of recurrence in the kidney allograft, although higher rates have been reported. It seems that *de novo* MGN is at least two to three times more common than recurrent MGN. In patients with an unknown form of primary glomerulopathy, it is difficult to make a definite diagnosis of recurrent versus *de novo* MGN, because both entities cannot be differentiated in allograft biopsy specimens. Usually, recurrent MGN manifests as a nephrotic-range proteinuria within the first year after transplantation. The prognosis is relatively poor. Eight of 13 patients reported in sufficient detail progressed to end-stage renal failure in 6 months to 10 years. In other series, 30% of the affected patients lost their graft as a result of MGN. Immunosuppressive regimens after transplantation did not modify the frequency of the recurrence of MGN and no therapeutic benefits were achieved by additional administration of high-dose steroids. The therapeutic approach can be similar to the one used for idiopathic MGN, including cytotoxic drugs if moderate to severe nephrotic syndrome and declining renal function are observed. Another option is to use ACE inhibitors to reduce proteinuria and its consequences. The recurrence rate is significantly greater in the living-related donor group than in the cadaveric group. It was suggested that living-related transplant should be used with caution in these patients.

De novo membranous glomerulopathy was described in patients with a wide variety of causes of ESRD, including anti-GBM glomerulonephritis, FSGS, Alport's syndrome, autosomal-dominant polycystic kidney disease, and diabetic nephropathy, with the prevalence approximately 2% and incidence increasing with time of follow-up (from 0% to 5.3% over 8 years). The association of hepatitis C virus (HCV) infection and *de novo* MGN was observed in a transplant population with high (20%) prevalence of HCV in Spain. All patients had normal complement, negative cryoglobulin, and rheumatoid factors. Clinical features of *de novo* MGN are similar to recurrent MGN but occurs later with a mean time to initial recurrence of 21 months after transplantation. Prognosis is relatively poor, with 5-year graft survival of 49%. It is partly determined by chronic rejection, which is present at the same time in the allograft.

IgA Nephropathy

IgA nephropathy is recognized as a disease with frequent recurrence in the allograft. Berger followed 32 recipients with IgA nephropathy with routine biopsy at 6 months and 2, 4, and 10 years after transplantation. Recurrent mesangial IgA deposits were observed in 17 patients and initially occurred 3 months to 4 years after transplantation. The amount of deposits increased during the early period but was stable thereafter. Other studies show recurrence in the allograft biopsy specimen in 13% to 59% of the selected patients. Higher rates were found in patients with longer follow-up, suggesting continued rise in the prevalence of recurrence over time.

Clinical recurrence is usually seen as microscopic hematuria and minimal proteinuria. The course of disease is insidious, similar to primary IgA nephropathy. It has been assumed that recurrence of IgA nephropathy carries small risk for graft loss. Indeed, in most earlier observations the loss of graft in IgA recipients because of the recurrence was in the range of 1%. Cumulative data from six single centers published between 1994 and 1998 from Australia, Europe, and the United States change this perspective. Of 247 allograft recipients with primary diagnosis of IgA nephropathy followed for a period of 3 to 183 months (mean approximately 60 months), 81 patients (33%) had clinical presentation of IgA disease with biopsy-proven recurrence, and 25 recipients (10.1%) lost their graft secondary to recurrence. Most patients who lost an allograft had a severe form of the disease in their native kidney and few cases with rapidly progressive course have been reported. At least three studies suggest that living-related donor transplants are associated with a higher rate of recurrence than cadaver grafts, but this point remains to be confirmed and, in accepted practice, it is suggested that living-related donors not be discouraged.

In the absence of a confirmed diagnosis in the native kidney, IgA deposits in the graft can also be due to *de novo* nephropathy, or IgA deposits can be present in the donor kidney before transplant. Disappearance of the IgA deposits in donor kidney after transplantation within 2 to 4 weeks have been reported in eight cases.

The results of kidney transplantation in ESRD patients caused by IgA nephropathy are at least as good as in other diseases. Data from the University of California–Los Angeles (UCLA) and UNOS Kidney Transplant 1992 file show a higher (87% versus 80% at 1 year and 76% versus 60% at 5 years) graft survival rate in IgA patients as compared with other patients with other primary disease. This high graft survival in IgA nephropathy patients was associated with high pretransplant levels of IgA antibodies to HLA class I molecules.

Anti–Glomerular Basement Membrane Disease

Anti-GBM disease with pulmonary and renal involvement (Goodpasture's disease) or without overt pulmonary hemorrhage (anti-GBM antibody–associated nephritis) accounts for less than 1% of glomerulonephritis causing ESRD. The common practice is to delay transplantation for 3 to 12 months after the onset of disease, particularly when rapidly progressive renal failure was the clinical manifestation, and until circulating anti-GBM antibody level falls to low or undetectable values. Pretransplant bilateral nephrectomy is no longer recommended.

The risk of clinical recurrence of disease is low, but renal biopsy specimens may show linear anti-GBM deposits in as many as 50% of patients. The interpretation of isolated discovery of anti-GBM antibody by immunofluorescence microscopy must be approached with caution, and absence of nonspecific linear staining by other serum protein must be proved before diagnosis of anti-GBM disease can be established. Less than 20% of those with anti-GBM staining in the kidney will develop clinically significant anti-GBM disease.

Recurrence of the disease is usually immediate after transplantation and patients have proteinuria and hematuria. Circulating anti-GBM antibodies levels are usually high. Graft loss is rare, and plasmapheresis together with cyclophosphamide may be of help. Identical twins should receive immunosuppressive therapy after transplantation to avoid the recurrent disease.

Idiopathic Crescentic Glomerulonephritis

There are no large series reporting of transplantation associated with idiopathic crescentic glomerulonephritis. Earlier reports did not distinguish this disease from anti-GBM nephritis or from some form of MPGN. Few reports from the last decade describe relatively high recurrence rates of idiopathic crescentic glomerulonephritis after transplantation. But the true rate appears to be lower, because only 1 of 80 cases in the Australian series with idiopathic crescentic glomerulonephritis failed because of recurrent disease. In nonimmunosuppressed twins, a correlation was found between the rapidity of the development of the original disease and rapidity of recurrence in the allograft.

HEREDITARY AND CONGENITAL RENAL DISEASE

Autosomal-Dominant Polycystic Kidney Disease

Polycystic kidney disease is responsible for 4% to 10% of ESRD in the United States, Europe, and Australia. All modalities of renal replacement therapy are appropriate therapeutic choices. Approximately 20% of autosomal-dominant polycystic kidney disease (ADPKD) patients receive transplants during the first year of dialysis, a percentage similar to chronic glomerulonephritis patients with ESRD. The results of kidney transplantation in ADPKD patients are very similar to those of other nondiabetic patients. With current immunosuppressive protocols, patient survival at 1 and 5 years are 95% and 85%, respectively, and allograft survival is 85% for 1 year and 70% for 5 years. Posttransplant erythrocytosis requiring treatment was reported in 14% of ADPKD recipients compared with 4% in the control population.

The common question in patients with ADPKD is whether to perform nephrectomy before transplantation. Studies have shown both increased and decreased morbidity and mortality in ADPKD patients who undergo pretransplant nephrectomy. Especially at risk for the surgery are patients with a very large polycystic kidney. The current practice may vary, but most of the centers reserve nephrectomy to the cases with suspected malignancy, severe hematuria, recurrent urinary tract infection, and when the size of the polycystic kidney precludes future allograft placement. Screening guidelines in transplant patients for other-than-kidney organ involvement in ADPKD are the same as for predialysis patients. In addition, patients with ADPKD do appear to have a higher risk for complicated diverticulitis and may need colonic screening. Polycystic liver disease can cause massive hepatomegaly, venous flow obstruction, hemorrhage into cysts, intrahepatic fibrosis, ascites, and severe pain. Some of these patients who may benefit from combined liver–kidney transplantation. DNA testing by genetic linkage analysis can be used in case ultrasonography is inconclusive in selection of potential living-related kidney donors.

Alport's Syndrome

In 1982, a 15-year-old male with Alport's syndrome who developed anti-GBM antibodies and lost the kidney allograft 5 months after transplantation was described. This antibody, as well as monoclonal antibodies against Goodpasture antigen, did not react with the kidney GBM of another Alport's syndrome patient. It was hypothesized that introduction of kidney with normal GBM antigenic epitopes had immunized this patient.

Molecular genetic studies identify two major forms of Alport's syndrome: an X-linked dominant form due to mutation of COL4A5 locus (Xg22) affecting α5 collagen IV carboxyterminal noncollagenous [α5(IV) NC1] chain and an autosomal-recessive form due to mutation at COL4A3 or COL4A4 locus on chromosome 2. GBM of males with X-linked Alport's syndrome and of patients with autosomal-recessive Alport's syndrome express α1(IV) and α2(IV) chains but usually lack of expression of α3(IV), α4(IV), and α5(IV) chains. These nonexpressed chains of collagen IV are recognized as foreign in the newly transplanted kidney and can be a target of immune response by the host. Studies show that the α5(IV) NC1 was the primary target in 9 of 12 patients with Alport's syndrome who developed posttransplant anti-GBM disease, whereas sera from one patient was binding to both α5 and α3(IV) NC1 and from two patients was bound predominantly to α3(IV) NC1.

Only a small number of patients with Alport's syndrome will have anti-GBM antibodies in the blood after transplantation, and frequently anti-GBM antibodies are detected in sera without consequences to the allograft. Linear anti-GBM staining in the allograft is detected in approximately 15% of Alport's syndrome transplant patients without nephritis. On the other hand, standard anti-GBM assays are not a reliable way to exclude diagnosis. Currently, biopsy evidence of glomerulonephritis with positive immunofluorescence is the only way to make diagnosis of *de novo* anti-GBM nephritis. Clinically significant anti-GBM glomerulonephritis in these patients is relatively rare (3% to 5%), and does not seem to modify significantly survival rate of the transplanted kidney in patients with Alport's syndrome as a group, but may be a catastrophic event for affected individuals who developed nephritis. Data of NAPRTCS show that of 26 patients who developed anti-GBM nephritis, 23 were males, all patients where deaf, and all reached ESRD before age 30. Seventy-five percent of grafts failed, usually within a few weeks to a month after diagnosis, and treatment with plasmapheresis and cyclophosphamide had limited benefit. Anti-GBM nephritis has recurred in seven of eight patients who had a second transplant.

Although routine evaluation of the blood for anti-GBM antibodies in Alport's recipients may not be cost effective, it is important to check blood and tissue for anti-GBM antibodies whenever allograft function deteriorates. In this early period, disease may respond to appropriate therapy with plasma exchange and cyclophosphamide. Patients who lost their first allograft because of anti-GBM nephritis are more likely to develop the same disease in subsequent transplants. DNA testing can be used in the detection of an asymptomatic female carrier, which is crucial in view of kidney donation.

Congenital Nephrotic Syndrome

Congenital nephrotic syndrome (CNS) is a hereditary disorder manifested in infants as massive proteinuria, edema, and ascites during their first 3 months of life. Aggressive medical management, especially nutritional support and treatment of infection, improves infant survival during the first 2 years. Renal replacement therapy is typically required in the third year of life. Frequently, bilateral nephrectomy is performed, even before end-stage renal failure, to eliminate proteinuria to allow the growth necessary for renal transplantation procedure.

NAPRTCS registry has 132 transplant recipients with CNS; 78 living-related and 54 cadaver donor transplants between 1987 and 1997. At the time of analysis there was a graft failure rate of 20.5% and 50.0%, respectively, which was attributed mainly to renal vascular thrombosis and patients death due to infection. These complications were largely avoided in CNS children in Finland by anticoagulation from 3 to 4 weeks of age with warfarin and prompt treatment of bacterial infections.

Since the first report in 1973 from the University of Minnesota, more than 54 transplants have been performed in 38 children with CNS in this center. The average age at the time of transplantation was 3 years and for retransplantation was 7.1 years. The actual graft survival at 5 years was 62%, not different than other pediatric recipients. Sixteen children had second or third transplants. Rejection was the most frequent cause of graft loss. These results are probably better than in the other United States centers, partly because of the overall good experience in transplantation in children younger than 5 years of age at this center, but also because 90% of the kidney allografts were from living donors. There has been no recurrence of CNS, although three cases of steroid-dependent/steroid-resistant nephrotic syndrome have been reported. Six of 28 children with CNS of Finnish type who received transplant in Finland developed steroid-resistant nephrotic syndrome with histologic features resembling to some extent those of transplant glomerulopathy. The recurrence of CNS however, could not be definitely excluded. The response of proteinuria to steroids or cyclophosphamide was poor, with total remission in two patients and partial remission in one patient. Children with good renal function after transplantation have demonstrated improvement in growth, and the majority had a normal social life.

OUTFLOW PROBLEMS AND PYELONEPHRITIS

The overall results in patients with obstructive uropathy who received a kidney transplant do not seem to differ from those obtained in patients with glomerulonephritis. However, urologic disorders may affect the recipient and the graft. Patients with reflux nephropathy have a high rate of recurrence of urinary tract infection, which is difficult to control with antibiotic prophylaxis. They may require native nephrectomy, usually after transplantation.

Abnormalities in the bladder and urethral anatomy and function must also be carefully assessed before transplantation. A voiding cystourethrogram should be performed in patients with diabetic neuropathy, and history of bladder dysfunction, and recurrent urinary tract infections. Whenever possible, the implantation of a ureter into the native bladder is preferred. A small bladder may develop normal compliance after transplantation. Patients with an unusable urinary bladder may present a special technical problem because of the need for an ileal bladder, which should be constructed before transplantation. The rate of infection and stone formation is high with the use of an ileal bladder requiring external drainage or repeated catheterization, but the overall patient and graft survival is not different from patients with an intact urinary tract. In some patients with neurogenic bladder or with other voiding abnormalities, the clean intermittent self-catheterization may be the best solution.

Older men with prostate hypertrophy may develop outflow tract obstruction following the transplantation surgery and require an indwelling bladder catheter until the resection of the prostate.

Pyelonephritis is less frequently reported as a cause of ESRD. In fact, only 0.8% of allograft recipients in UNOS 1992 data had this diagnosis. The success of transplantation in these patients is slightly better than in patients with glomerulonephritis. There was no significant difference in patient survival whether or not prior bilateral nephrectomy was performed. Urinary tract infection is a common problem and occurs in 75% of all patients without antibiotic prophylaxis after renal transplantation, but it is usually asymptomatic and not associated with deterioration in renal function.

ANALGESIC NEPHROPATHY

Analgesic nephropathy may be responsible for a variable percentage of the causes of ESRD depending on geographic location. This entity seems to be rare in the United States, but is still high, with decreasing prevalence in the last decade, in Australia and some European countries. In one of the series from Berlin, Germany, 30% of patients receiving hemodialysis and 17% of transplanted patients had ESRD resulting from analgesic nephropathy. The 5-year patient and graft survival rate (89% and 54%, respectively) were not different from those reported for patients with other renal diseases, despite the fact that patients with analgesic nephropathy were older. Six percent of the recipients continued taking analgesics and had positive urine for this drug after transplantation. They also had a ten times higher rate of urothelial carcinoma (3.7% versus 0.32%) than those with other renal disease, despite that the routine cytoscopy and retrograde pyelography before transplantation were negative. The *de novo* development of analgesic lesions in the transplanted kidney is unlikely because 20 years of analgesic abuse is usually required to develop this disease. Two cases of papillary necrosis in allograft kidney possibly caused by analgesic abuse have been reported.

HYPERTENSIVE NEPHROSCLEROSIS

Hypertensive nephrosclerosis is an important cause of ESRD and accounts for one-third of ESRD in African-Americans in the United States, and 5% to 10% of ESRD in whites in Europe and the United States has been attributed to essential hypertension. Approximately 10% of kidney allograft patients have hypertensive nephrosclerosis. Graft outcome is not significantly worse for whites with nephrosclerosis than for those with other diseases, but African-Americans, especially males, had only 50% graft survival 3 years after transplantation. These results have not changed significantly since the 1990s.

RENAL TRANSPLANTATION IN ELDERLY PATIENTS

The ESRD population in the United States is progressively older, as shown by the increased percentage of patients 65 years or older (40% in 1989, 53% in 1993, and 60% projected in the year 2000). Over the last decade, the success of transplantation in patients over the age of 65 years has improved because of better patient selection screening as well as the use of cyclosporine and lower doses of steroids. One-year cadaveric renal transplantation patient survival rates range between 80% and 90% and 5-year survivals are 70%. Graft survival rate is 85% at 1 year, and 5-year graft survival rate is in the range of 55% to 60%. Death with a functioning graft is the main cause of graft loss in

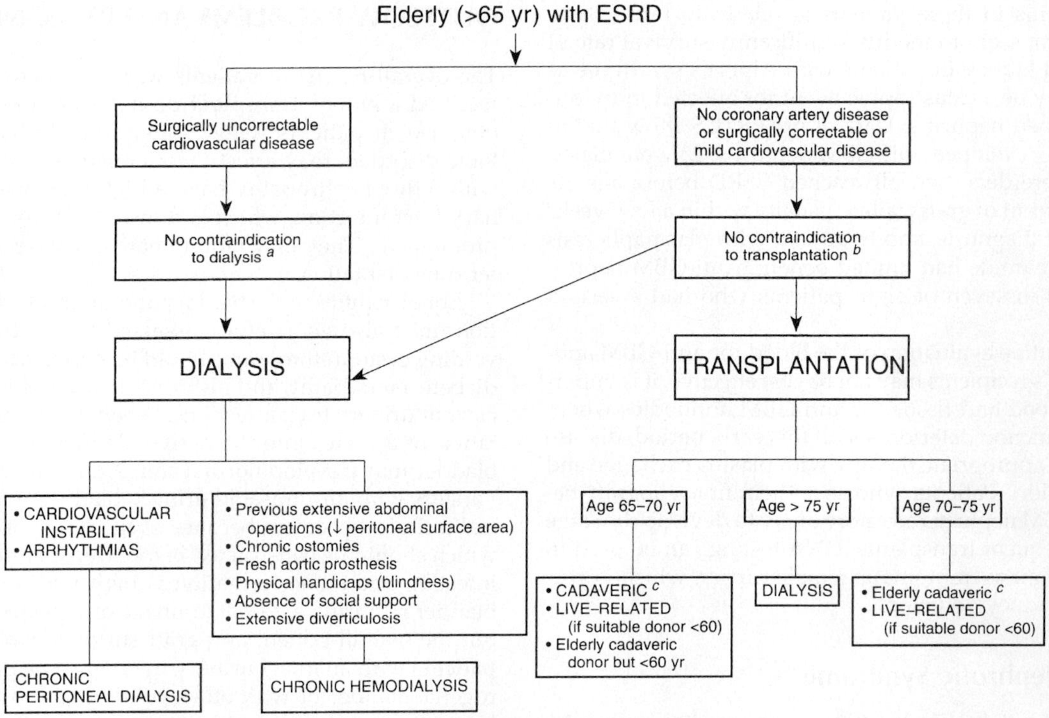

Figure 90.1. Algorithm for selection of treatment modality for geriatric ESRD patients. **A:** Alzheimer's disease, metastatic malignancy (except multiple myeloma), and advanced liver disease. **B:** Recent or metastatic malignancy, severe extrarenal disease (cardiac, liver, pulmonary), and psychiatric illness. Some centers may be more liberal in allocating cadaveric transplants to the elderly than others. (Reproduced with permission from Ismail N, Hakim RM, Helderman JH. Renal replacement therapy in elderly. Part II. Renal transplantation. *Am J Kidney Dis* 1994;23:1–15.)

the elderly patient. In several studies, graft loss rate was close to 50% as a consequence of death. The leading causes of death are infections and cardiovascular events.

The immune response changes with aging. B-cell function is usually preserved but T-cell–mediated cytotoxicity; interleukin-2 (IL-2) production and IL-2 receptor expression; immunity against viral, bacterial, and fungal infections; and recognition of self-major histocompatibility complex (MHC) are diminished in the elderly. This may contribute to the finding that elderly patients have fewer episodes of rejection and may require less aggressive but still adequate immunosuppression. Infections occurred mostly during the first 6 months after transplantation, at the time of higher immunosuppression, and they account for almost 50% of patient deaths. Smaller doses of cyclosporine can be used because elderly patients have reduced activity of hepatic P-450 microsomal enzymes. Steroids can be tapered more rapidly, and intensive use of OKT3 and antilymphocyte globulin should be avoided.

The frequency of cardiovascular events depends on the selection of recipients. In a very select group of patients, cardiac causes accounted for 10% of patient death, in an unselected group it may be as high as 58%. Nondiabetic patients older than 55 years even without symptoms should undergo extensive evaluation to rule out significant cardiac dysfunction and coronary artery disease. Most centers use noninvasive cardiac evaluation. Cardiac catheterization and correction of the underlying disease should be achieved in symptomatic patients with a positive stress test before transplantation is attempted. Patients with diabetes should be subject to a more rigorous approach, as discussed previously.

Dialysis therapy in elderly patients is equally effective as transplantation, but the quality of life is usually better after successful transplantation. The algorithm presented in Fig. 90.1 seems to be useful in selecting the type of renal replacement therapy for these patients. Life expectancy of an individual patient should also be considered in choosing the optimal therapy. From the perspective of cadaver-organ shortage, the allocation of cadaveric kidney to the patients 70 years and older is a controversial issue and an ethical dilemma.

Selected Readings

Allen A, Pusey CH, Gaskin G. Outcome of renal replacement therapy in antineutrophil cytoplasmic antibody–associated systemic vasculitis. *J Am Soc Nephrol* 1998;9:1258–1263.

Extensive discussion of current literature and retrospective analysis of 59 patients with vasculitis (including 22 transplants) from Hammersmith Hospital, London, United Kingdom.

Becker BN, Ismail N, MacDonnell RC, et al. Renal transplantation in the older end stage renal disease patients. *Semin Nephrol* 1996;16:352–362.

A good summary on the role of kidney transplantation in the treatment of ESRD in the elderly and how to evaluate and select allograft recipients of older age.

Clinical Transplants 1997, Cecka MJ, Terasaki PI, eds. The Regents of the University of California. Los Angeles, California, 1998.

This volume and previous edition are a good source of information based on data acquired by the United Network of Organ Sharing and published each year by UCLA Typing Laboratory.

Davision AM, Johnston PA. Allograft membranous nephropathy. *Nephrol Dial Transpl* 1992;7:114–118.

A review article on the membranous nephropathy, both current and de novo, in kidney allograft.

Goldfarb DA, Neuman HPH, Penn I, et al. Results of renal transplantation in patients with renal cell carcinoma and von Hippel-Lindau disease. *Transplantation* 1997;64: 1726–1729.

Outcome of 32 patients with von Hippel-Lindau disease and kidney transplantation after treatment of renal cell carcinoma.

Jamieson NV. The results of combined liver kidney transplantation for primary hyperoxaluria (PHI) 1984-1997. The European PH1 transplant registry report. *J Nephrol* 1998;11(S-1):36–41.

Analysis of data from the European registry of hepatorenal transplantation for primary hyperoxaluria.

Kasiske BL, Ramos EL, Gaston RS, et al. The evaluation of renal transplant candidates: clinical practice guidelines. *J Am Soc Nephrol* 1995;6:1–34.

Comprehensive guidance developed by the American Society of Transplant Physicians based on literature published until December 1994 and on the author's opinion.

Kotanko P, Pusey CD, Levy JB. Recurrent glomerulonephritis following renal transplantation. *Transplantation* 1997;63:1045–1052.

Latest, in-depth review of the problem of recurrent diseases in renal transplantation and source of older but important references.

Miller RB, Burke BA, Schmidt WJ, et al. Recurrence of haemolytic uraemic syndrome in renal transplant: a single-center report. *Nephrol Dial Transplant* 1997; 12:1425–1430.

The analysis of data form University of Minnesota, where 24 HUS patients received 36 transplants between May 1972 and December 1994. Recurrence of HUS in the allograft was confined almost entirely to patients with atypical form of HUS. Recurrence was not more frequent in patients receiving a CsA or ALG, but only 8 patients received CsA as an initial immunosuppressive agent.

Ojo AO, Govaerts TC, Schmouder RL, et al. Renal transplantation in end-stage sickle cell nephropathy. *Transplantation* 1990;67:291–295.

Retrospective analysis of the USRDS and the UNOS data of 82 patients with end-stage sickle cell nephropathy and kidney transplant.

Schwarz A, Offerman G, Keller F. Analgesic nephropathy and renal transplantation. *Nephrol Dial Transplant* 1992;7:427–432.

Analysis of the results of renal transplantation in analgesic nephropathy in one European transplantation center.

Stone JH, Amend WJC, Criswell LA. Outcome of renal transplantation in ninety-seven cyclosporine-era patients with systemic lupus erythematosus and matched controls. *Arthritis Rheum* 1998;41:1438–1445.

Discussion of long-term results of kidney transplantation in patients with systemic lupus erythematosus.

United States Renal Data System. *USRDS 1998 annual data report.* Bethesda, MD: The National Institutes of Health, National Institute of Diabetes and Digestive and Kidney Diseases, 1998.

Report of United States Renal Data System, which is based on data obtained from the Health Care Financing Administration. One of the goals of the publication is to develop and analyze the data on the effect of various modalities of treatment by disease and patient group categories.

Wardy BA, Hebert D, Sullivan EK, et al. Renal transplantation, chronic dialysis, and chronic renal insufficiency in children and adolescents. The 1995 annual report of the North American Pediatric Renal Transplant Cooperative Study. *Pediatr Nephrol* 1997;11:49–64.

This report presents data on 5,197 children and adolescents registered voluntarily, from 123 centers in the United States, Canada, Mexico, and Costa Rica.

CHAPTER 91

Renal Transplantation in Children

Amir Tejani and Richard N. Fine

The United States Renal Data System (USRDS) data show that of approximately 11,900 renal transplants performed in adults and children in the United States annually, living-related donation accounts for more than 28% of the cases. In 1987, 40% of all transplants performed in children were from a living-donor (LD) source; by 1991, the figure had risen to 53%, and since 1995, LDs accounted for approximately 50% of all pediatric renal transplants. Parents compose 85% of LDs, and mothers compose the majority of parental donors, but contrary to public perception, fathers do account for 44%. Interestingly, both parents donate equally to sons and daughters. Due to the fact that children most often have siblings who are children too (under 18 years), the North American Pediatric Renal Transplant Cooperative Study (NAPRTCS) registry records only 182 transplants between siblings. Of these, 97 grafts were from donors under the age of 21 years. Because donation from a minor is usually unauthorized in the United States, a review of the NAPRTCS registry identified only 10 living donors under 18 years of age, of which nine were transplants between siblings and one was from parent to child. In recent years there has been a substantial interest in living-unrelated donation in the adult transplant literature because the graft outcome of these kidneys has been shown to be better than that of cadaver source kidneys. The NAPRTCS has identified 38 instances of living-unrelated donation in a special study encompassing 5,362 transplants from 1987 through 1997. Of the 38 living-unrelated recipients, 23 (61%) were male, 30 were white (79%), 8 were younger than 6 years, and 20 were older than 12 years. Contrary to the concept that living-unrelated donation occurs only in extreme circumstances, for 29 of the 38 recipients this was the primary transplant. A more detailed inquiry observed that, of the 38 donors, 22 were nonbiologic parents, and a family friend was the donor in 10 of the cases.

Because the percentage of living donation was as low as 41% in the years of 1987 and 1988, cadaver donors (CD) form the bulk of pediatric kidney transplants performed in the United States since 1987. The majority of cadaver kidneys are recovered from adult donors. In the early years there was a tendency to preferentially place kidneys recovered from infants into infant recipients, with disastrous consequences for patient and graft survival as will be shown later in this chapter. As a result of widespread dissemination of these data, there has been a marked change in the practice. From 1987 through 1990, the percentage of CDs older than 10 years ranged from 59% to 68%. From 1991 through 1994, these percentages ranged from 78% to 88%. Before 1991, children less than 2 years of age comprised 3.2% of CDs. In 1991, no pediatric recipient received a kidney from a cadaver donor under 2 years of age; from 1992 to 1994, only 1% of the kidneys recovered and used in children came from this age group, and in 1995 and 1996, there were no such kidneys used in children.

PRIMARY DIAGNOSIS

In previous years it was difficult to obtain an accurate analysis of the diagnoses leading to end-stage renal disease (ESRD), but with the large database of the NAPRTCS it is now possible to determine the percentages of each disease category by age at the time of transplantation as well as by gender and race. In reviewing 4,329 transplants, the most common congenital diagnoses are obstructive uropathy and aplastic/hypoplastic/dysplastic kidneys, each representing about 16% of the patients. Among glomerular disorders, focal segmental glomerulosclerosis (FSGS) is the most common; in the decade of 1987 to 1996, 516 children received a renal transplant for FSGS. The primary diagnosis also varies with the racial background of the recipient. Overall in the NAPRTCS registry, Caucasian children account for 64% of all recipients; however for FSGS, Caucasian children only account for 50%. Similarly for systemic immunologic disease, Caucasian children account for only 54% of the patients, whereas for hemolytic uremic syndrome, Caucasian children account for 82% of the patients receiving a transplant. Table 91.1 depicts the primary diagnoses by gender and race of 4,329 children who have received a transplant in North America since 1987, as well as the percentage of biopsy-proven diagnoses. It is important to observe that the biopsy confirmation of the primary diagnosis was made in 95% of FSGS, in 93% of systemic immunologic diseases, and in 91% of congenital nephrotic syndrome patients. These are figures usually not seen in data on primary diagnosis of the adult recipients. The information regarding primary diagnosis becomes critical in predicting graft survival as well as recurrence of the original disease, as discussed later.

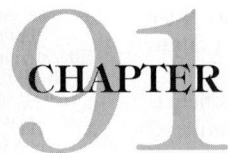

TABLE 91.1. Index Transplant Sex and Race Distribution, by Primary Renal Diagnosis

Diagnosis	N (4329)	% (100)	% Biopsied (60)	% Male (60)	% Caucasian (64)
Obstructive uropathy	711	16.4	38	87	70
Aplastic/hypoplastic/dysplastic kidneys	693	16.0	31	61	67
Focal segmental glomerulosclerosis	516	11.9	95	58	50
Reflux nephropathy	242	5.6	38	42	74
Systemic immunologic disease	212	4.9	93	32	54
Chronic glomerulonephritis	187	4.3	76	37	47
Syndrome of agenesis of abdominal musculature	124	2.9	48	97	65
Congenital nephrotic syndrome	120	2.8	91	48	68
Hemolytic uremic syndrome	120	2.8	59	59	82
Polycystic kidney disease	117	2.7	61	49	77
Medullary cystic disease/juvenile nephronophthisis	105	2.4	68	54	84
Cystinosis	101	2.3	54	51	87
Familial nephritis	101	2.3	79	76	60
Membranoproliferative glomerulonephritis type I	98	2.3	98	46	57
Pyelonephritis/interstitial nephritis	93	2.1	76	46	71
Renal infarct	82	1.9	43	52	80
Idiopathic crescentic glomerulonephritis	72	1.7	97	33	67
Membranoproliferative glomerulonephritis type II	43	1.0	100	49	72
Oxalosis	31	0.7	74	61	90
Drash syndrome	27	0.6	100	52	67
Membranous nephropathy	27	0.6	96	74	59
Wilms' tumor	26	0.6	92	50	88
Sickle cell nephropathy	9	0.2	56	56	0
Diabetic glomerulonephritis	5	0.1	100	40	20
Other	265	6.1	70	57	60
Unknown	202	4.7	34	54	38

(Adapted with permission from Feld LG, Stablein DM, Firush BA, et al. Transplantation in children from 1987-1996. *Pediatric Transplantation* 1997;1:146–162.)

AGE AT THE TIME OF TRANSPLANTATION

It is generally accepted that transplantation before 6 months of age or to a patient whose weight is below 6 kg is hazardous. From 1987 to 1996, 60 transplants were performed in children younger than 12 months. Of these, six transplants were performed in children between 3 to 5 months, 18 were performed in children between 6 to 8 months, and 33 were performed in children between 9 to 11 months of age. Because infants and adolescents have different risk factors for both patient and graft survival, we divide all children into five age groupings: 0 to 2 years (younger than 2 years of age), 2 to 5 years (younger than 6 years of age), 6 to 12 years (younger than 13 years of age), 13 to 17 years (younger than 18 years of age), and 18 to 21 years of age. It has been suggested that children 0 to 5 years have a more robust immune response and are therefore at higher risk for graft failure. In 1987, 25% of all transplants were performed in children 0 to 5 years of age, whereas in 1994, the same age group accounted for 16%, and in 1995 the figure was 17%. Whether the decreased number of transplants in this group is due to an awareness of their vulnerability or to more optimum dialysis has not been established.

INDICATIONS AND CONTRAINDICATIONS FOR TRANSPLANT IN CHILDREN

All children reaching ESRD are considered to be candidates for a transplant. In certain situations the definition may be confusing, but for practical purposes, patients who are dialysis-dependent are ESRD patients. Dialysis dependent is defined as being on dialysis for longer than 30 days. This would exclude patients who have suffered an episode of acute reversible renal failure. The definition of dialysis-dependent patients as candidates for transplantation is inadequate in pediatrics, however, because a significant number of children receive a preemptive kidney transplant without ever having been on dialysis. In a review of 4,329 children transplanted from 1987 through 1996, the NAPRTCS noted that 1,064 (25%) of the patients had never received maintenance dialysis.

Preemptive Transplantation

Because preemptive transplantation is a modality generally reserved for children, the NAPRTCS has conducted a special study to determine the frequency and outcome of this therapy. From 1987 through 1992, 26% of the patients were registered as preemptive transplantation. The study compared data of those recipients who had been on maintenance dialysis versus patients who had no previous dialysis. Of 2,213 primary grafts during that time period, 1,150 (52%) were from a LD source, whereas for the preemptive group 70% were recipients of a live-related kidney. For the dialysis group, 58% were male, whereas the preemptive group had 68% males. The racial distribution was also different: Caucasians represented 64% in the dialysis group, versus 78% of those receiving a preemptive transplant. The frequency of preemptive transplantation was not different from regular transplants between the various age groupings. A primary argument against preemptive transplants has been that without the rigors of prior dialysis, compliance will be poor and the children will promptly lose their grafts. To determine whether this hypothesis was correct, graft survival was compared between the two groups, which was not different at 1 or 4 years. When causes for graft loss were analyzed, the preemptive group did not have a higher incidence due to noncompliance. The NAPRTCS also surveyed the motive for preemptive transplantation and determined that the primary reasons were parents' desire to avoid dialysis (34%) and the nephrologists' recommendations (18%). Desire for improved growth was considered a contributory factor in 50% of the patients. This study was carried out in 1992; since then the percentage of children receiving a preemptive transplant has remained constant.

Contraindications for Transplantation

There are no absolute contraindications for transplantation, except for human immunodeficiency virus (HIV)-induced nephropathy. The concern of further immunosuppressing an already compromised host makes HIV a contraindication, however most children who develop HIV nephropathy succumb to the systemic ravages of the virus, either before or very shortly after reaching ESRD status. Another relative contraindication is a preexisting malignancy. There have been 26 children with Wilms' tumor who have received a kidney transplant and no recurrences have been reported. Potential for recurrence of the original disease is of major concern and will be discussed later. With successful combined liver and kidney transplantation oxalosis, which used to be an absolute contraindication due to a high incidence of recurrence, is not currently a contraindication.

PRETRANSPLANT BLOOD TRANSFUSIONS

In the precyclosporine era, blood transfusions were shown to have a beneficial effect on graft outcome, but their effect has diminished in recent years. The beneficial effect of pretransplant transfusions in children was demonstrated by French studies, as well as data from the Terasaki registry. In the past donor-specific transfusions were also given to children. Early results from such studies suggested better graft survival; however, more prolonged follow-up showed no benefit, and the practice of donor-directed transfusions has now been abandoned in pediatric renal transplantation.

The role of random pretransplant transfusions in improving graft survival is still unclear. In 1992, the NAPRTCS, in a study of 1,667 transplants of which 57% were of CD origin, did not observe any beneficial or detrimental effect of pretransplant blood transfusions. However subsequently, in 1993 with a larger patient pool of 2,033 patients, 55% of whom were recipients of a CD kidney, a deleterious effect of pretransplant transfusion was obvious. For LD source transplants, the use of five or more prior transfusions was a relative risk (RR) factor with a value of 1.8. By 1995, the use of prior transfusions was a risk factor for CD source transplants as well, and the use of five or more transfusions had a value of 1.3 for graft loss. The 1996 NAPRTCS report, which analyzed 4,714 transplants, shows greater than five transfusions to have an RR of 1.7 for LD graft failure, and 1.3 for CD graft failure. A special analysis indicated that less than five transfusions may be beneficial. Although the exact number is not clear, some centers routinely give two transfusions before the transplant.

HISTOCOMPATIBILITY ISSUES

In renal transplantation, two histocompatibility systems are used for matching: the ABO blood group and the human leukocyte antigen (HLA) system. The donor should be ABO- compatible with the recipient. In the past when ABO-incompatible renal transplants were performed inadvertently, they uniformly resulted in hyperacute rejection. In recent years however, successful ABO-incompatible transplants have been performed. The NAPRTCS registry reports 11 transplants across the ABO-compatibility barrier, and a special analysis revealed that such transplants are successful if the recipient's anti-A titer is low.

HLA Matching Results in Children

For cadaver source transplants, the NAPRTCS registry indicates a 2-DR mismatch graft failure rate at 4 years after transplant of 32%, compared with 25% with a 0-DR mismatch. Comparative figures for LD kidneys are not significant at 13% and 17%, respectively. There is also a 10% better graft survival at 4 years among CD recipients with a zero HLA-B mismatch, compared with two mismatches.

INDUCTION THERAPY

In an attempt to improve graft survival, prophylactic use of anti–T-cell antibody has been in vogue for quite some time. The rationale for this practice is to preempt the development of the first rejection, which is injurious to long-term graft survival. Unfortunately the studies reporting successful use of T-cell antibody were all performed in adults, although retrospective data from the NAPRTCS do show a beneficial effect. In a review of LD transplants, 5-year graft survival was 81% in 1,041 patients who received T-cell antibody therapy compared with 75% in 1,399 patients who did not. Similar figures for CD kidneys were 66% in 1,423 T-cell antibody–treated patients, compared with 56% in 1,034 patients who did not receive T-cell antibody. A major problem of these data is that two different types of T-cell antibody were used. In the early years, a polyclonal antibody prepared from horse serum and designated as MALG (Minnesota antilymphocyte globulin) was used, whereas in more recent times a monoclonal antibody directed at subsets of T cells, called *OKT3,* has been employed.

The polyclonal antibody currently available is antithymocyte globulin (Atgam-Upjohn), which, due to the sclerosing nature of the solution, is given intravenously through a central catheter for 10 to 15 days. The dose used is 15 mg/kg, and calcineurin inhibitors (cyclosporine or tacrolimus), which form the mainstay of maintenance immunosuppression, are withheld during the administration of the T-cell antibody. The monoclonal antibody, OKT3, is administered into a peripheral vein for 10 days at a dose of 5 mg for older children and 2.5 mg for children weighing less than 30 kg. Calcineurin inhibitors are also withheld during the use of OKT3. A major problem with these induction therapies is the potential for the development of superimposed infections, such as cytomegalovirus (CMV) disease, and the high potential for the development of malignancy. These issues are of paramount importance in pediatric transplantation, and therefore a major multicenter, prospective, randomized trial, sponsored by the National Institutes of Health, is currently underway in the United States. This trial, being conducted in more than 20 pediatric centers, will test the safety and efficacy of OKT3 in both LD and CD recipients.

If T-cell antibody is not chosen for induction therapy, one of the calcineurin inhibitors may be used instead. Currently, there are two such drugs, cyclosporine and tacrolimus, which have similar mechanisms but act at different sites to inhibit calcineurin. The induction dosing for these drugs is described in the following section.

MAINTENANCE IMMUNOSUPPRESSION

Cyclosporine

Cyclosporine was first used in renal transplantation by Calne in 1978. The initial experience was followed by controlled trials in the United States, Canada, and Europe, all of which showed a significant improvement in graft survival over the then existing therapies. The drug was licensed in the United States in 1983, and has been the mainstay of solid-organ transplantation for more than 15 years. There have been no controlled trials in children, but over the years of use, a large body of information regarding its dosing and side effects has accumulated. In the NAPRTCS database of more than 5,000 children transplanted since 1987, 85% are maintained on cyclosporine at varying doses.

Induction Dose

For induction purposes cyclosporine is given intravenously in a dose of 165 mg/m^2 daily for children under 6 years of age, and 4.5 mg/kg daily in children older than 6 years. The dose for younger children is calculated in square meter format because they metabolize the drug differently. The drug is preferably given in a continuous infusion over a 24-hour period starting intraoperatively. If practicality precludes a continuous infusion, the drug should be administered in three divided doses daily. Induction therapy using intravenous cyclosporine should be continued only for 48 hours and then substituted with oral cyclosporine. The recommended oral dose for children under the age of 6 years is 500 mg/m^2 daily, administered in three divided doses; for children over the age of 6 years, it is 15 mg/kg daily, administered in two divided doses. These doses are higher than those prescribed for adults because experience has determined that the drug is metabolized more rapidly in children.

Maintenance Dose

Because of the inherent nephrotoxicity of the drug, dose adjustments are constantly necessary. Data from the NAPRTCS show that at 1 year posttransplant, the mean cyclosporine dose varies from 5.6 to 8 mg/kg. It has also been demonstrated that higher maintenance doses prevent graft rejection. Among cadaver kidney recipients the rate of rejection was 16% in those receiving doses higher than 8 mg/kg at 1 year posttransplant, compared with 24% in those receiving less than 6 mg/kg daily. The difficulty of maintaining constant dosing has led to methods of measuring cyclosporine blood levels. Either high pressure liquid chromatography (HPLC) or fluorescence polarization immunoassay (FPIA) techniques are used. Drug adequacy is considered to be a range of 100 to 200 ng/ml HPLC whole-blood trough level, or 200 to 450 ng/ml TDX whole-blood levels for patients more than 3 months posttransplant. Higher levels are necessary in the first 3 months.

Side Effects

The primary concern with the use of cyclosporine is its nephrotoxicity. A major concern in children is the hypertrichosis and facial dysmorphism. A worrisome side effect in children is gingival hypertrophy, seen more often with higher doses and in the presence of poor dental hygiene.

Tacrolimus

Pediatric use of this drug in renal transplantation is limited; data from the NAPRTCS show that less than 15% are being maintained on tacrolimus at 1 year posttransplantation.

Dosage

Due to the limited experience in children, dosing regimens have not been established. One method is to initiate use at 0.1 mg/kg per 24 hours as a continuous infusion, with a switch to oral therapy within 2 to 3 days. Oral doses should not exceed 0.15 mg/kg twice daily and should be reduced to 0.1 mg/kg as the maintenance dose. Blood monitoring is necessary as with cyclosporine, and target whole-blood trough levels, measured by an enzyme-linked immunosorbent assay (ELISA), should be maintained around 15 to 20 μg/L.

Side Effects

Because of the similar mode of action, all the side effects of cyclosporine therapy are also seen with tacrolimus. The nephrotoxic effect is similar. It is claimed that the hypertrichosis and the dysmorphic features noted with cyclosporine are not seen to the same extent. A major drawback for the use of tacrolimus in pediatric renal transplantation has been the concern for the development of diabetes, because in the Japanese renal study one-third of the patients developed hyperglycemia requiring insulin therapy.

Adjunct Therapy

The calcineurin inhibitors are the primary immunosuppressants. Azathioprine, steroids, and mycophenolate mofetil (MMF) are three drugs used for adjunct therapy. The mechanism of action and side effects of these drugs are described first, and then a dosing scheme is presented.

Azathioprine

Azathioprine is a purine analog, prevents interconversion among the precursors of purine synthesis, and results in inhibition of both DNA and RNA synthesis. For pediatric patients, the drug is given in the dose of 1 to 2 mg/kg per day. Higher dosages should be closely monitored for myelosuppression.

In the early years of transplantation, azathioprine was routinely used in all transplant recipients; when cyclosporine became available it was still widely used as an adjunct drug. In 1989 and 1990, 80% of pediatric patients in the NAPRTCS registry were receiving azathioprine, but as more familiarity is established with MMF, the use of azathioprine will probably taper off to an historic relic.

Mycophenolate Mofetil

Like azathioprine, MMF blocks purine synthesis, but by inhibiting inosine, monophosphate dehydrogenase purine synthesis is blocked *de novo*, and because lymphocytes rely on *de novo* purine synthesis, this drug targets lymphocytes primarily. *In vitro* studies have demonstrated its ability to inhibit proliferative responses in both T and B cells. Because of limited information, the drug is not yet widely accepted in pediatric renal transplantation. As of 1996, the NAPRTCS registry noted that only 6.5% of patients were being maintained on MMF.

Glucocorticoids

The first successful use of glucocorticoids in renal transplantation was in 1960. The 1997 annual report of the NAPRTCS shows that 96% of children with a functioning graft are maintained on prednisone. The numerous mechanisms of action of glucocorticoids lead to side effects and toxicities. The important concern in children is growth retardation. Studies have shown that doses in excess of 8.5 mg/day will impair normal growth. The dosage is usually high in the immediate posttransplant period, about 2 mg/kg per day, with a gradual reduction to approximately 0.2 to 0.3 mg/kg per day within a 6-month to

1-year period. Because of the multiple side effects of maintenance glucocorticoid therapy, attempts have been made to withdraw glucocorticoids altogether, reported both in adult and pediatric literature. These attempts have been made both in LD and CD kidney recipients. Unfortunately, in the absence of a surrogate marker for hyporesponsiveness, identification of children who would not develop a rejection episode after glucocorticoid withdrawal is impossible. Additionally, in the absence of a controlled trial it is difficult to tease out the role of glucocorticoids withdrawal in triggering the rejection episode. Unless the newer drugs make steroid withdrawal possible, a compromise may be the use of alternate-day steroid therapy, which appears to reduce the growth-inhibiting effect without unduly increasing rejection episodes.

Sirolimus (Rapamycin)

Sirolimus is a macrolide antibiotic that has completed Phase-3 trials in both the United States and Europe. The drug was approved in 1999 for use in the United States. Dosing for children has not been established.

Newer Monoclonal Antibodies for Prophylactic Therapy

Two such monoclonal antibodies are entering the clinical armamentarium. Monoclonal antibodies can be directed with targeted selectivity against predetermined components of the immune system and hence offer a strong possibility for manipulation of the immunologic events that occur during rejection. Simulect (basiliximab) is an anti–interleukin-2 (IL-2) receptor chimeric monoclonal antibody for acute rejection immunoprophylaxis. It is administered in two doses: a 20-mg infusion on day 1 and another 20-mg infusion on day 4, posttransplant. Significant improvement in the number of acute rejections is observed. A similar humanized anti-Tac monoclonal antibody (daclizumab) is administered in five doses at biweekly intervals, and has shown significant improvement in reducing the number of acute rejections. There is limited pediatric experience in the use of these monoclonal antibodies, but considering that they have very few side effects, they will likely supplant the older monoclonal antibodies, such as OKT3, for prophylactic therapy.

ALLOGRAFT REJECTION

Frequency and Management of Various Types of Rejection

Hyperacute Rejection

Hyperacute rejection is the result of specific recurrent antidonor antibodies against HLA, ABO, or other antigens. Irreversible rapid destruction of the graft occurs. Histologically there is glomerular thrombosis, fibrinoid necrosis, and polymorphonuclear leukocyte infiltration. In the early years of transplantation, when the HLA matching techniques were not well advanced, hyperacute rejection was common but now, in most centers, it is an historic rarity. The latest data from the NAPRTCS show the incidence of hyperacute rejection to be less than 1% (9 of 4,712 transplants) during the 1990s. The primary therapeutic concern is the necessity for surgical removal of the allograft.

Acute Rejection

Accurate information regarding the incidence and outcome of acute rejection in pediatric renal transplantation is available from the NAPRTCS data. These data consider a rejection episode to have occurred when a patient is treated with antirejection therapy. In a review of 6,193 rejection episodes over a 10-year study, 2,540 episodes occurred in 2,520 LD transplants (rejection ratio 1:1), and 3,653 episodes occurred in 2,520 CD transplants (rejection ratio 1:32). In the early weeks posttransplant, the rejection patterns are identical. At days 15, 30, and 45, 21%, 29%, and 35% of LD patients, and 21%, 39%, and 48% of CD patients have a rejection. Overall, half of all transplant recipients have a rejection episode by day 137. By the end of the first year posttransplant, 49% of LD and 63% of CD patients have had one or more rejection episodes. These rejection rates are higher than those generally observed in adult patients. Risk factors for cadaver source transplants include the absence of prophylactic T-cell antibody therapy and donor age less than 5 years. Risk factors for living-related source transplants are the absence of T-cell antibody and one DR mismatch. In an earlier study, the NAPRTCS noted that when reviewed by age-group rejection ratios, time to first rejection and the mean number of rejection episodes were not different; however, for the initial rejection episode, recipients less than 6 years of age had significantly increased irreversible rejections leading to graft loss. To determine whether irreversible rejections in younger children are due to their heightened immune response, a multicenter study is currently underway. In this study surveillance biopsies are performed in all children under 6 years of age on days 5 and 12 posttransplant and analyzed for the immune mediators of rejection.

Diagnosis of Acute Rejection. Rejection is suspected when there is decreasing urinary outflow and a rising serum creatinine. In the past, classical signs of acute rejection included fever and graft tenderness. Under cyclosporine and prophylactic T-cell antibody therapy however, these signs are rarely seen, thus early evidence of graft dysfunction should initiate concern. The differential diagnosis consists of ureteric obstruction, renal vascular compromise from stenosis, and an infectious process. To rule out anatomic obstruction, an ultrasound is performed. Obstruction can be the result of perirenal fluid collection, a large lymphocele, hematoma, or rarely, an abscess. An isotopic renal scan, using a radionuclide such as mertiatide (MAG3), is a helpful tool in establishing the diagnosis. Rejection is suggested by rapid uptake of the tracer by the kidney but a delayed excretion. Unfortunately radionuclide scans cannot distinguish between a rejection episode and cyclosporine toxicity; a definitive diagnosis requires a renal biopsy.

Renal Biopsy. With light sedation and under ultrasound guidance, the renal biopsy procedure is relatively easy and safe. In the past some centers shied away from performing a biopsy for the diagnosis of rejection because of the fear of serious side effects, particularly in the early transplant course. However recent data evaluating more than 150 pediatric biopsies, including some in intraperitoneal kidneys and many performed during the first week posttransplantation, have demonstrated a very low risk. A major factor in reducing postbiopsy bleeding is the use of a BIOPTY GUN and a small (18 gauge) rather than the standard (15 gauge) needle.

Treatment of Acute Rejection. Standard treatment of an episode of acute rejection is intravenous methylprednisolone in a single daily dose of 20 mg/kg (maximum dose: 1 g) for three consecutive days. Most grade I and grade II rejections will respond to steroid therapy. Steroid-resistant rejection episodes are treated with T-cell antibody, either the monoclonal OKT3, or the polyclonal antithymocyte globulin (ATG). OKT3 is administered in the dose of 2.5 mg for children with a body weight of 30 kg, and 5 mg for children more than 30 kg for 10 days. Polyclonal antibody is given in the dose of 15 mg/kg, through a central venous catheter, for 10 to 14 days depending on the white cell and platelet count, because it will deplete all formed elements in the blood system. It is advisable to maintain the white cell count above 2,000 mm^3 and the platelet count above 20,000 mm^3. Both antibodies have several side effects. Of concern are the first-dose symptoms of OKT3 due to cytokine release. This is clinically observed as fever with chills, and rarely, as pulmonary edema. Defervescents, such as acetaminophen, should be given every 4 hours and the administration of the antibody should be preceded an hour before with a bolus dose of 500 mg of methylprednisolone. Respiratory compromise, in the form of fluid extravasating into the pulmonary capillary bed, is only seen in patients with fluid overload. Due to the sudden onset of acute rejection many patients have abruptly reduced urine output. Dialytic fluid removal must be carried out before the administration of OKT3 in patients whose body weight exceeds 3% of their baseline. Precautions against the polyclonal antibody (ATG) therapy, which may set up an anaphylactic reaction, consist of using 500 mg of methylprednisone with the infusion of the antibody and administration of an antihistaminic, such as diphenhydramine (Benadryl), 30 minutes before drug administration.

Reversibility of Acute Rejection. NAPRTCS data observe that among LD kidneys 55% of rejection episodes are completely reversed, 40% are partially reversed, and 5% end in graft failure. Similar figures for CD kidneys are 48%, 45%, and 7%, respectively. As noted previously, when stratified by age, young transplant recipients more frequently have irreversible rejection episodes. Ten percent of acute rejections among infants receiving a LD kidney end in graft failure, compared with 4% for older children. For CD kidneys, the rate of graft failure in infants is 15%, compared with 7% for older children. Complete reversibility percentages decrease with repeat acute rejections, averaging approximately 63% and 57%, respectively, for LD and CD sources following the first rejection, and 47% and 36% following the third episode.

Chronic Rejection

The gradation from acute to chronic rejection is gradual, however many biopsies may show features of both, and characteristic vascular changes of chronic rejection may be seen as early as 10 days posttransplant. The clinical picture is that of gradually declining renal function together with varying degrees of proteinuria and hypertension. The clinical condition is also referred to as *transplant glomerulopathy.* An ongoing controversy exists regarding whether the changes seen in chronic rejection are immune mediated, are ischemic in nature, or are nonimmunologic injury due to hyperfiltration. Data in children have shown clearly that acute rejection is a predictor of chronic rejection. In a study of 1,699 LD and 1,795 CD patients, the NAPRTCS noted acute rejection was a relative risk (RR) factor for chronic rejection (RR = 3.1), and multiple acute rejections increased this risk to 4.3. Late acute rejections are also clinical correlates of chronic rejection. If acute rejection is the most critical element in the genesis of chronic rejection, then similar immune mechanisms could be mediating chronic rejection. One possible explanation would be that in patients who go on to develop chronic rejection, the immune mediators of acute rejection, such as granzyme B, perforin, and Fas ligand, are expressed in a more robust fashion and are quantitatively different from the responses of an acute rejection that does not lead to chronic rejection. Alternatively, the immune mediators of chronic rejection may be qualitatively different from those associated with an acute episode. Data has emerged to show that the multifunctional cytokine transforming growth factor-β ($TGF-β_1$), with fibrogenic properties, is present in biopsy tissue of patients with chronic rejection. These issues are pertinent because currently there is no effective therapy and if immune mediators could be identified that are amenable to intervention by newer immunosuppressives, chronic rejection could be controlled.

Management of Chronic Rejection. Symptomatic therapy is currently the only available tool. Hypertension should be controlled and the proteinuria may occasionally respond to angiotensin-converting enzyme (ACE) inhibitors, however the renal function will continue to decline. In children, chronic rejection has an additional burden because decreased renal function will result in deceleration of growth. It is in this context that prevention of chronic rejection by early aggressive therapy in patients who have had an episode of acute rejection may be rewarding. The use of newer immunosuppressives may be beneficial. One such agent may be sirolimus, which has only limited effect on cytokine production; however, it blocks proliferative responses to a variety of cytokines. It also inhibits proliferation of cultured smooth muscle cells stimulated with basic fibroblast growth factor and platelet-derived growth factor. Its ability to block smooth muscle cell proliferation would be of particular interest in blocking obliterative vascular changes. A multicenter trial of the ability of this drug to control the interstitial fibrosis and inhibit the expression of $TGF-β_1$ messenger RNA in biopsy tissue of children with acute rejections is currently underway.

GRAFT SURVIVAL

Pediatric renal centers reporting graft survival show varying results. Due to the fact that these are small numbers, such data are not representative of the pediatric transplant population at large. In order to get a proper population mix representing gender, age, and racial diversity, we have used the NAPRTCS annual reports. The data shown here are derived from 4,714 transplants performed in 73 participating centers from 1987 through 1996.

A total of 1,170 graft failures occurred among 4,714 (25%) transplants. This includes 117 patients who lost two or more grafts, seven subjects who had three graft failures, and one with four graft failures. Of initial transplants 1,045 of 4,329 (24%) failed, whereas 125 of 386 (32%) subsequent transplants had graft failure. Of the failures, 908 (78%) were returned to dialysis, and 48 (4%) were retransplanted at the time of failure. Table 91.2 provides the distribution of graft failure causes. With increased length of follow-up, chronic rejection continues to increase in importance; it is now the most common cause of graft failure. Overall, 50% of graft failures are caused by rejection, with chronic rejection accounting for 28% and acute rejection accounting for 18%. Recurrence of original disease as a cause of graft failure was observed 80 times (focal segmental glomerulosclerosis, 38; membranoproliferative glomerulonephritis type II, 7; oxalosis, 10; hemolytic uremic syndrome, 7; chronic glomerulonephritis, 5; and others, 13). Vascular thrombosis remains as a major cause of failure, and 204 graft failures were attributed to primary nonfunction, vascular thrombosis, or miscellaneous technical causes. These data suggest that such problems will occur in 4.3% of pediatric transplants.

Estimated (actuarial) graft survival for index transplants at 1, 2, and 5 years for LD kidneys is 90%, 86%, and 76%, respectively, and for CD kidneys it is 80%, 73%, and 60%. Table 91.3 shows actuarial 4-year graft survival for selected transplant characteristics for both LD and CD kidneys. A primary function of graft survival data is to establish risk factors. Relative risks

TABLE 91.2. Causes of Graft Failure

Cause	Index Graft Failures n = 1045	(%)	Second[a] Graft Failures n = 125	(%)	Total Graft Failures n = 1170	(%)
Vascular thrombosis	126	(12.1)	23	(18.4)	149	(12.7)
Miscellaneous technical	18	(1.7)	3	(2.4)	21	(1.8)
Primary nonfunction	32	(3.1)	2	(1.6)	34	(2.9)
Hyperacute rejection, less than 24 hr	9	(0.9)	3	(2.4)	12	(1.0)
Accelerated acute rejection, 2–7 days	32	(3.1)	6	(4.8)	38	(3.2)
Acute rejection	191	(18.3)	18	(14.4)	209	(17.9)
Chronic rejection	299	(28.6)	31	(24.8)	330	(28.2)
Renal artery stenosis	11	(1.1)	0	(0.0)	11	(0.9)
Infection/discontinue meds	23	(2.2)	2	(1.6)	25	(2.1)
Cyclosporine toxicity	9	(0.9)	0	(0.0)	9	(0.9)
(De Novo) kidney disease	4	(0.4)	2	(1.6)	6	(0.5)
Patient discontinued meds	26	(2.5)	1	(0.8)	27	(2.3)
Malignancy	12	(1.2)	1	(0.8)	13	(1.1)
Recurrence of original disease	65	(6.2)	15	(12.0)	80	(6.8)
Death	113	(10.8)	12	(9.6)	125	(10.7)
Other	75	(7.2)	6	(7.8)	81	(6.9)

[a]Seven patients had 3 graft failures, one patient has had 4 failures. (Adapted with permission from Feld LG, Stablein DM, Firush BA, et al. Transplantation in children from 1987-1996. *Pediatric Transplantation* 1997;1:146–162.)

TABLE 91.3. Graft Failure Summary, by Allograft Source and Transplant Characteristics

	Live Donor Number	Live Donor (% Failure)	Live Donor Prob. 4-Yr. Function	Cadaver Donor Number	Cadaver Donor (% Failure)	Cadaver Donor Prob. 4-Yr. Function
Total						
	2,133	(17.3)	.789	2,194	(30.7)	.644
Sex						
Male	1,310	(17.9)	.79	1,268	(29.4)	.67
Female	823	(16.5)	.79	926	(32.5)	.61
Race						
Caucasian	1,551	(15.9)	.81	1,222	(30.1)	.67
African-American	245	(28.2)	.65	450	(32.9)	.54
Hispanic	275	(15.3)	.82	353	(32.0)	.63
Other	59	(20.3)	.78	166	(27.1)	.67
Prior Transplant						
No	2,028	(17.3)	.72	1,859	(28.8)	.67
Yes	89	(20.2)	.69	308	(43.8)	.53
Prior Dialysis						
No	722	(14.3)	.82	271	(22.5)	.74
Yes	1,411	(18.9)	.77	1,922	(31.9)	.63
Recipient Years						
0–1	181	(20.4)	.75	75	(50.7)	.45
2–5	355	(19.2)	.79	308	(31.5)	.68
6–12	750	(16.9)	.81	765	(30.0)	.68
13–20	847	(16.3)	.77	1,046	(29.5)	.61
Donor Years						
0–5	NA			367	(43.3)	.55
6–10	NA			237	(33.3)	.63
>10	NA			1,559	(27.0)	.67
Cold Time (hrs)						
≤24	NA			1,294	(29.0)	.65
>24	NA			841	(34.0)	.62

(continued)

TABLE 91.3. *(Continued)*

	Live Donor			Cadaver Donor		
	Number	(% Failure)	Prob. 4-Yr. Function	Number	(% Failure)	Prob. 4-Yr. Function
Machine Preservation						
No	NA			1,811	(29.7)	.65
Yes	NA			298	(38.6)	.59
HLA-A Mismatch						
0	355	(16.4)	.78	186	(29.0)	.66
1	1,653	(17.6)	.79	881	(31.4)	.64
2	145	(16.6)	.72	1,127	(30.4)	.65
HLA-B Mismatch						
0	258	(14.0)	.81	182	(22.5)	.73
1	1,698	(17.7)	.79	758	(29.0)	.67
2	177	(18.6)	.67	1,254	(32.9)	.62
HLA-DR Mismatch						
0	349	(13.2)	.85	232	(25.9)	.72
1	1,491	(18.4)	.78	965	(30.0)	.66
2	293	(17.1)	.73	997	(32.5)	.61
Pre-Operative Immunotherapy						
No	893	(15.0)	.80	NA		
Yes	1,237	(19.1)	.78	NA		
Native Nephrectomy						
No	1,496	(16.6)	.80	1,718	(29.5)	.66
Yes	632	(19.2)	.77	470	(35.5)	.59
Lifetime Transfusions						
0	795	(13.8)	.81	488	(22.8)	.67
1–5	949	(15.5)	.81	930	(25.4)	.70
>5	355	(29.6)	.71	734	(42.1)	.57
ATG/ALG or OKT3 Early Administration						
No	1,232	(19.6)	.77	939	(36.0)	.60
Yes	901	(14.2)	.82	1,255	(26.8)	.68

(Adapted with permission from Feld LG, Stablein DM, Firush BA, et al. Transplantation in children from 1987-1996. *Pediatric Transplantation* 1997;1:146–162.)
ALG, antilymphocyte globulin; ATG, antithymocyte globulin; HLA, human leukocyte antigen; NA, not available.

of graft failure are derived using Cox proportional hazards regression models. For LD kidneys the risk factors are African-American race (RR = 2), more than five prior transfusions (RR = 1.7), and absence of HLA-B matches (RR = 1.6). Treatment with T-cell antibody is associated with significantly increased graft survival (RR = 0.73). A similar risk-factor analysis for CD kidneys is presented in Table 91.4. The risk factors are similar with additional hazards such as young recipient age, young donor age, and prolonged cold ischemia time. The use of T-cell antibody improves graft survival just as it does for LD kidneys. Some factors that increase the relative risk of cadaver graft failure in children, such as recipient age, are integral to pediatrics; others such as recipient race, the degree of HLA matching, and prior transplantation are factors that cannot be easily manipulated. Improvement in cadaver allograft survival rates, however, can be achieved by judicious choice of donors, pretransplant management, manipulation of induction therapy, and optimal immunosuppressive therapy.

TABLE 91.4. Proportional Hazards Analysis for Cadaver Donor Transplants

	Relative Risk	*P* Value
Recipient age <2 years	2.25	<.001
Donor age <6 years	1.37	.001
Prior transplant	1.39	.001
No ATG/ALG/OKT3 early administration	1.32	<.001
>5 lifetime transfusions	1.33	.001
No HLA-B match	1.24	.001
No HLA-DR match	1.19	.03
Annual cohort 1987 versus 1992	1.46	<.001
African-American race	1.24	.03
Prior dialysis	1.30	.07
Cold ischemia time >24 hr	1.15	.08

(Adapted with permission from the NAPRTCS 1996 Annual Report.)
ALG, antilymphocyte globulin; ATG, antithymocyte globulin; HLA, human leukocyte antigen.

GROWTH FOLLOWING TRANSPLANTATION

A major distinguishing feature of pediatric from adult recipients is the need for children to grow. The growth failure observed in children at the time of transplantation is multifactorial, however the primary cause is the reduction of growth hormone secretion. The problem begins insidiously early in renal failure. The NAPRTCS recently observed, in an analysis of 1,768 children with a glomerular filtration rate of less than 75 ml/min/m^2, that more than one-third were short statured [height deficit of 2 standard deviation score (SDS)]. Nutritional factors, metabolic acidosis, hypocalcemia, and anemia were contributory factors. It has been amply demonstrated that chronic renal insufficiency beginning in infancy leads to permanent reduction in growth potential. Growth retardation continues in children on a dialysis regimen, whether the mode of dialysis is peritoneal or hemodialysis. For several years it has been suggested that a functioning transplant would enable the child to achieve catch-up growth. Before the establishment of the NAPRTCS, single-center data were of limited value because no long-term follow-up was provided. As graft survival has improved, the quality of life posttransplantation has become the crucial question. The Achilles heel of posttransplant rehabilitation continues to be the growth of children with a functioning graft. Individual center studies have adopted a variety of techniques, such as discontinuation of prednisone, alternate-day steroid therapy, or the use of recombinant human growth hormone. These studies, although providing useful information, deal with small selected populations, and unless the natural history of posttransplant growth is known the impact of these studies becomes marginalized.

Studies from the NAPRTCS have tracked growth posttransplantation longitudinally, using the same cohort for at least 5 years. In these studies, height data was analyzed at 2 years, again at 3 years, and repeated at 54 months posttransplantation. The height deficit was −2.41 in the first study, −2.46 in the second evaluation, and −2.29 at the end of the third study period. Children in the first study had an improvement in height SDS of +0.18, of +0.16 in the second period, and of +0.11 in the third period. When improvement in height deficit was evaluated by donor source, no differences were noted between living-related and cadaver donor recipients. Analysis of height SDS by race revealed that, whereas for Caucasian children a steady improvement was noted during the second and third periods, there was an actual deceleration of growth for African-American and Hispanic children. Only the initial height deficit and recipient age are independent predictors of improved height posttransplantation. Catch-up growth, defined as an improvement of 1 SDS, was seen only in children 0 to 1 year of age. Overall catch-up growth was seen in only 47% of children between the ages of 2 and 5 years. For children over the age of 5 years, who form 72% of the study cohort, little catch-up growth was noted.

These studies on long-term growth posttransplantation are disappointing, however they do focus on mechanisms that prevent growth despite a milieu with normal renal function and production of growth hormone. It has been known for several years that steroids used for immunosuppressive therapy will inhibit growth. It has also been demonstrated that glucocorticoids affect growth hormone secretion. Measurements of pulsatile and pharmacologically stimulated hormone release reveal that steroids play an inhibitory role. Attempts to convert patients to alternate-day steroid therapy have shown improvement in growth, however catch-up growth is only seen in patients completely withdrawn from glucocorticoids. Numerous uncontrolled studies have shown that steroids can be withdrawn from children posttransplantation, however acute rejection tends to occur shortly afterward in many of these patients. There is no immune marker that can identify patients who are hyporesponsive and can safely undergo steroid withdrawal. An alternative method of attaining catch-up growth posttransplantation would be the use of growth hormone. Recombinant human growth hormone is not approved for use in children posttransplantation, however numerous uncontrolled studies have shown its ability to accelerate growth.

Selected Readings

Baqi N, Tejani A. Maintenance immunosuppression regimens. In: Tejani A, Fine RN, eds. *Pediatric renal transplantation.* New York: Wiley-Liss, 1994.

This chapter is an in-depth review of posttransplant immunosuppression, deals with drug action mechanism, provides dosing information, and discusses drug toxicity and methods to ameliorate them.

Feld LG, Stablein DM, Fivush BA, et al. Renal transplantation in children from 1987–1996: The Annual Report of the North American Pediatric Renal Transplant Cooperative Study (NAPRTCS). *Pediatr Transplant* 1997;1:146–162.

This report involves 4,329 transplants from 130 centers of the NAPRTCS and provides information on long-term graft survival extending to 6 years posttransplant. It analyzes rejection episodes and growth patterns as well.

Fine RN, Tejani A, Sullivan EK. Preemptive renal transplantation in children. A report of the North American Pediatric Renal Transplant Cooperative Study (NAPRTCS). *Clin Transplant* 1994;8:474–478.

This study reviews the data on children who undergo preemptive transplantation without prior dialysis and analyzes the results of a survey conducted in all the participating centers of the NAPRTCS to identify the factors that lead to recommendation to proceed directly to transplantation.

McEnery P, Arbus G, Stablein DM, et al. Renal transplantation in children. *N Engl J Med* 1992;2:S258–S263.

This is the first multicenter data on pediatric renal transplantation in the United States and Canada. The data are provided from 56 participating centers of the NAPRTCS and describes the demography of children receiving a renal transplant and their outcome.

Tejani A, Fine RN, Alexander SR, et al. Factors predictive of sustained growth in children posttransplantation. *J Pediatr* 1993;122:397–402.

This study reviews the growth posttransplantation in 300 children who have a functioning renal allograft at 2 years posttransplantation and analyzes the factors that would be predictive of catch-up growth. The data are derived from 72 participating centers of the NAPRTCS.

Tejani A, Sullivan EK, Fine RN, et al. Steady improvement in renal allograft survival among North American children. A five-year appraisal by the North American Pediatric Renal Transplant Cooperative Study (NAPRTCS). *Kidney Int* 1995;9:S61–S65.

This study deals with 1,641 cadaver donor transplants performed from 1987 to 1994 and observes that the 1-year graft survival of the 1991 cohort is 10 percentage points better than that of the 1987 cohort and analyzes the factors that led to this improvement.

CHAPTER 92

Outcome of Renal Transplantation

J. Michael Cecka

Renal transplantation has become the treatment of choice for many patients with end-stage renal disease. A successful renal transplant can take away the burden of dialysis and return the patient to a relatively unencumbered life. However, achieving maximal rehabilitation for the patient requires prolonged survival of both the patient and the graft with minimal complications due to the surgery or to the lifetime of immunosuppressive medications that are currently needed to sustain the transplanted kidney. It may also require a long wait, because transplantation is unique among surgical procedures because its availability is limited to the number of human kidneys that are donated for transplantation. Since the first successful renal transplant, which was performed in 1954 in Boston, more than 400,000 kidney transplants have been done. Although none of the original recipients is still alive today, in 1998 at least 70 patients were alive with a transplanted kidney that had survived more than 30 years. All but 15 of these known long-term survivors had received their transplanted kidney from a close relative. For the more than 11,000 patients who were transplanted in the United States during 1996, the 1-year patient and graft survival rates were 96% and 89%, respectively.

More than 70% of renal transplants depend on kidneys from individuals who are brain dead and whose relatives agreed to donate the organs of the deceased (cadaveric donor). The 1-year graft survival rates following cadaver-donor renal transplantation have improved from less than 50% before 1975 to more than 87% of transplants performed since 1994. Figure 92.1 traces the improvement in the results of first cadaveric renal transplants performed in the United States and reported to the UCLA Transplant Registry (before 1988) and to the United Network for Organ Sharing (UNOS) Scientific Renal Transplant Registry (since October 1987). These large transplant registries and several others are an important resource because they have been maintained throughout the development of transplantation and they catalog the progress that has been made in this field. Most of the results for this chapter are based on data reported to the UNOS Registry for all renal transplants performed at more than 250 transplant centers in the United States since 1991.

Many different factors have contributed to the improving graft survival rates over the years. The improved patient survival rates between 1974 and 1986 reflect better treatment of comorbid disease, better selection of appropriate patients for transplantation, and better control of serious complications after the transplant. Rising graft survival rates have resulted from more powerful immunosuppression as well as ancillary progress in immunologic screening, infection prophylaxis, and treatment of rejection episodes. The introduction of cyclosporine A (CsA) in 1984 resulted in a 15% improvement in graft survival rates over the subsequent 2 years and ushered in the modern era of transplantation. These advances have resulted in better survival rates in the first year, but progress in changing the rate of late graft loss has been slower. Long-term graft survival is reflected in the plot of annual graft half-lives. These represent a constant failure rate, which is established between 3 to 9 months after transplantation. Graft half-lives—that is, the number of years on average that grafts that survived the first year will continue to function—remained constant at about 7.5 years until the mid-1990s. Some of the factors that influence the long- and short-term survival of kidney transplants are listed in Table 92.1 and are discussed in more detail later in this chapter.

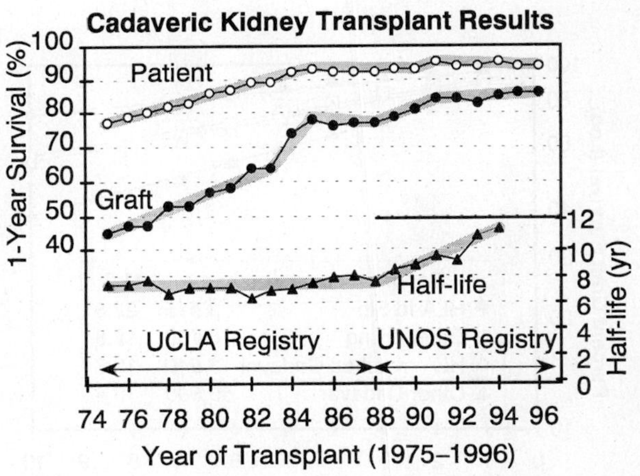

Figure 92.1. Improvements in the 1-year patient and kidney graft survival rates and graft half-lives for transplants performed in the United States since 1974. Most of the results that are described in this chapter are based on transplants performed between January 1991 and December 1996 and reported to the United Network for Organ Sharing (UNOS) Scientific Renal Transplant Registry.

TABLE 92.1. Factors That Influence Short- and Long-Term Kidney Graft Survival

First Year	Long-Term (1–5 years)
Donor relationship	Donor age
Transplant center	Recipient race
Donor death	Transplant center
Sensitization	Recipient sex
Transplant year	Donor relationship
Histocompatibility	Donor death
Cold ischemia	Histocompatibility
Graft number	Recipient age

Abbreviated with permission from Cecka JM, Terasaki PI, eds. *Clinical Transplants 1996.* Los Angeles: UCLA Tissue Typing Laboratory 1997.

GRAFT SURVIVAL RATES AFTER RENAL TRANSPLANTATION (FIG. 92.2)

Two factors that have a strong influence on long-term survival are the relationship between the patient and the kidney donor and the degree of tissue compatibility. The best graft survival rates are achieved when the donor is an HLA-identical sibling [i.e., one who inherited the same chromosome that encodes the major histocompatibility (HLA) antigens from each parent as the recipient]. The 1-year and projected 10-year graft survival rates for HLA-identical sibling transplants were 96% and 73%, respectively, with a graft half-life of more than 20 years. Kidneys transplanted from other living donors had the second best survival rates (91% and 56% at 1 and 10 years, respectively). The half-life for HLA-mismatched living-donor kidneys (13 years) was only about half that for HLA-identical siblings. Cadaver kidneys that had no HLA antigens mismatched to the recipient also provided better short- and long-term results than HLA-mismatched cadaver kidneys. The results of the well-matched cadaver-donor transplants were nearly the same as those for HLA-mismatched living-donor kidneys. Unfortunately, transplanting histocompatible kidneys usually is not an option. On average, only one in four siblings is HLA identical and the enormous polymorphism of the HLA system makes good matches among genetically unrelated individuals very rare indeed. Even though the HLA types of all patients on the national waiting list (36,000 patients at the end of 1997) are searched to find a match for each cadaver donor, fewer than 20% of cadaver kidneys are transplanted to an HLA-matched recipient.

Many other factors influence the results of kidney transplants, certainly more than are listed in Table 92.1, and many that would be difficult to simplify for inclusion in a large-scale analysis. To eliminate some of the complexity, the analyses that follow are based on the results of first cadaver-donor transplants performed between January 1991 and December 1996 in the United States. These transplants cover a relatively stable period in terms of 1-year graft and patient survival rates as can be seen in Fig. 92.1, but a period of improving long-term outcomes and a period during which many advances in immunosuppression have been made.

PATIENT CHARACTERISTICS THAT INFLUENCE TRANSPLANT OUTCOME

Recipient's Age (Fig. 92.3)

The recipient's age is an important factor in the outcome of renal transplants. As might be expected, older patients have the poorest graft survival rates because of their shortened life expectancy. In fact, only about two-thirds of patients over age 60 survive 5 years after their transplant. Relatively few transplants in this age group fail because of graft rejection. The majority result from patient death caused by cardiovascular disease. At the other age extreme, very young children present special technical challenges and tend to have increased mortality in the early postoperative period. However, when they survive this early high-risk period, young children have the best long-term survival as judged from their superior graft half-lives. Teenage patients tend to have poor long-term graft survival that is not associated with any increased mortality risk and may reflect difficulties in maintaining adequate immunosuppression.

Recipient's Race (Fig. 92.4)

Patient survival does not differ among the different racial groups. However, there are significant differences in graft survival rates associated with the recipient's race. Poorer graft survival rates

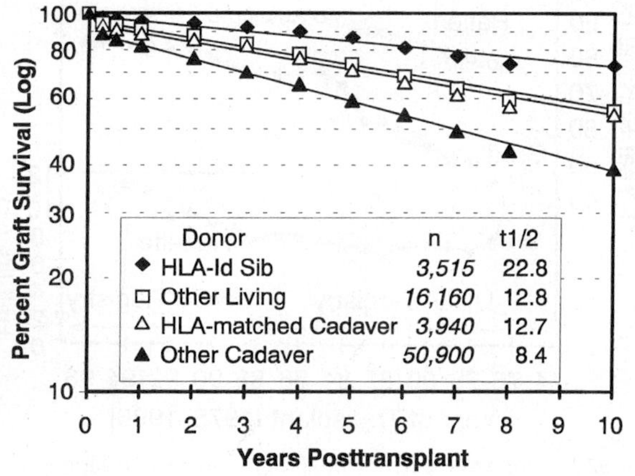

Figure 92.2. Actuarial graft survival rates for patients receiving kidney grafts according to the donor source and tissue match. (Reproduced with permission from Cecka JM, Terasaki PI, eds. *Clinical Transplants 1997.* Los Angeles: UCLA Tissue Typing Laboratory, 1998:2.)

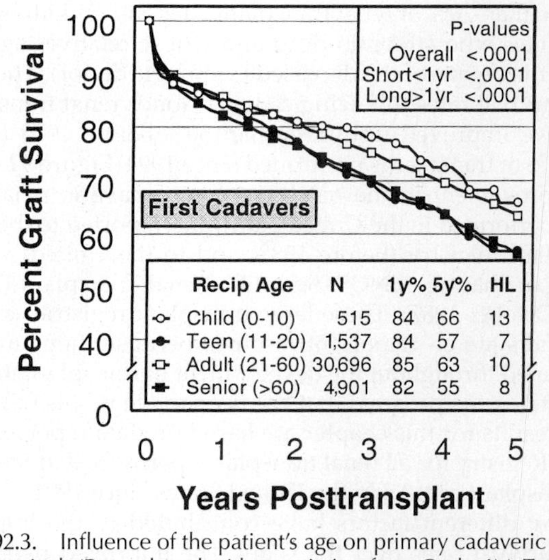

Figure 92.3. Influence of the patient's age on primary cadaveric renal allograft survival. (Reproduced with permission from Cecka JM, Terasaki PI, eds. *Clinical Transplants 1997.* Los Angeles: UCLA Tissue Typing Laboratory, 1998:346.)

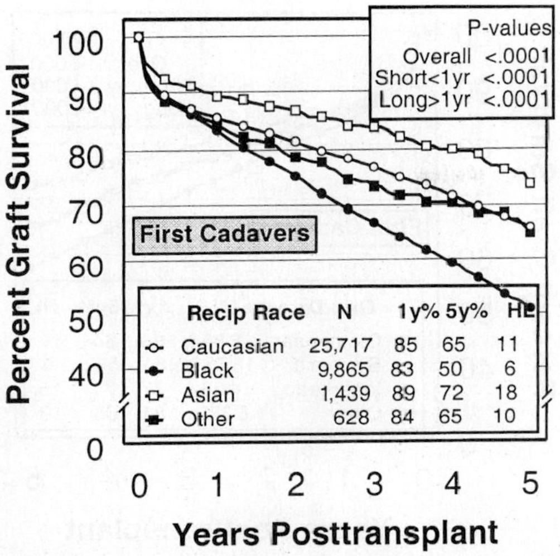

Figure 92.4. Racial differences in transplant success rates. (Reproduced with permission from Cecka JM, Terasaki PI, eds. *Clinical Transplants 1997*. Los Angeles: UCLA Tissue Typing Laboratory, 1998:344.)

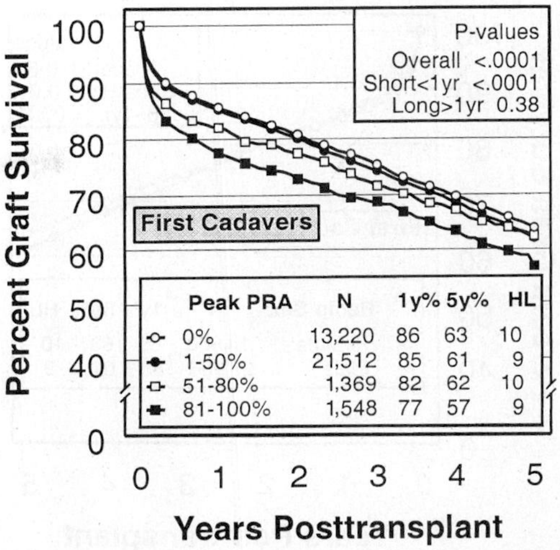

Figure 92.5. The effect of sensitization on the outcome of first cadaveric renal transplants. PRA, panel reactive antibody. (Reproduced with permission from Cecka JM, Terasaki PI, eds. *Clinical Transplants 1997*. Los Angeles: UCLA Tissue Typing Laboratory, 1998:354.)

among African-Americans than whites have been observed consistently. Although there is no survival difference during the first year, the rate of graft loss among African-Americans after 1 year is nearly double that of whites. Several mechanisms have been offered to explain this difference, ranging from genetic differences in immune responsiveness and tissue compatibility to socioeconomic differences. Each of these probably plays some role, although reports that African-Americans who had private insurance tended to have better outcomes than whites whose transplant was funded primarily through Medicare or Medicaid suggest that socioeconomic factors must play a strong role in the racial differences in success rates. Asian patients have higher graft survival rates than whites or other racial groups. This observation casts some doubt about whether racial histocompatibility differences between the donor and recipient play a key role in explaining racial differences in outcomes. It would be as difficult to find well-matched Asian donors for Asian recipients as it is to find well-matched African-American donors for African-American recipients because the majority of donors are white.

Sensitization (Fig. 92.5)

Patients who have been previously exposed to allogeneic tissue, most commonly as a result of pregnancies (the fetus expresses paternal HLA antigens), blood transfusions, or prior transplantation may develop immunity to certain tissue antigens. Patients awaiting transplant are regularly screened for the presence of circulating antibodies against panels of lymphocytes from individuals who are representative of the local-donor pool (panel reactive antibody [PRA]). Circulating anti-HLA antibodies that react with antigens expressed on the donor kidney cause hyperacute rejection. This is an immediate and massive destruction of the kidney characterized by infiltrating polymorphonuclear cells, platelet thrombi, and necrosis and is usually irreversible. A positive crossmatch test using fresh serum from the patient and lymphocytes from the potential donor prevents transplantation in the face of destructive antibodies, and hyperacute rejection is extremely rare today as a result. Screening for sensitization against a cell panel also provides an estimate of the likelihood that a patient will be transplanted with any donor that becomes available. When a patient has antibodies reactive with 50% of panel lymphocytes, for example, the chance of a positive crossmatch is 50% with each new donor. Broadly reactive circulating antibodies cause long delays for patients awaiting a transplant because the antibodies will react with most donors. The median waiting time for broadly sensitized patients who were put on the waiting list in 1991 was more than 6 years, and some may never be transplanted for lack of a suitable donor. The best donors for these sensitized patients are those with HLA antigens similar to their own. In fact, about half of the transplanted patients who had more than 80% panel reactive antibodies received a well-matched kidney.

Immunologic memory may also result from previous exposure to foreign HLA antigens and can cause accelerated rejection. Even when antidonor antibodies are not detected by the crossmatch test, broadly sensitized patients have poorer graft survival rates than those who are not sensitized (Fig. 92.5). The effect of sensitization is evident in the early posttransplant period consistent with an accelerated response. There is no apparent long-term influence of sensitization on graft survival.

Recipient's Sex (Fig. 92.6)

The recipient's sex has very little influence on the survival of renal transplants. There is a small, but statistically significant, advantage for females, which begins to show after about 3 years. This advantage is more pronounced among older patients. There is no evidence to suggest that a male H-Y antigen acts as an important transplantation antigen as has been shown in animal studies and suggested in human liver transplantation. In fact, women who receive male donor kidneys have somewhat better outcomes than those who receive female donor kidneys or than men who are transplanted with female donor kidneys.

Some important differences that can affect the likelihood of receiving a transplant are linked to recipient sex. Females are more often sensitized as a result of previous pregnancies, and the production of anti-HLA antibodies may be increased by blood transfusions. Although approximately 43% of kidney transplant candidates are women, they comprise only 39% of recipients. More than two-thirds of transplants between spouses are from wives donating to their husbands, and although there may be cultural and practical influences that bias the direction of these transplants, wives may also be excluded from receiving their husband's kidney because they have made antibodies to his HLA antigens.

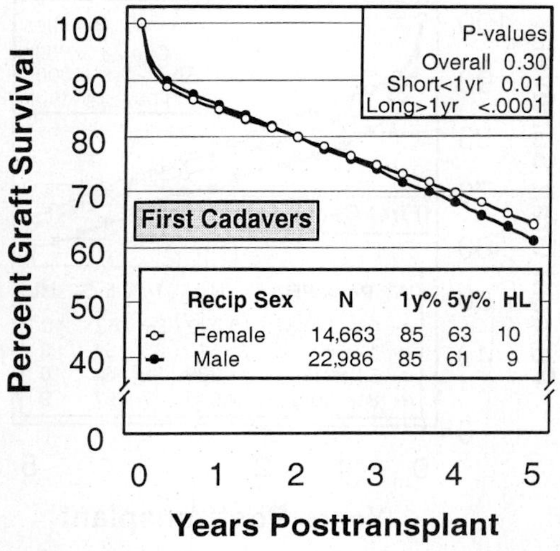

Figure 92.6. Minor differences in long-term primary graft survival associated with the recipient's sex. (Reproduced with permission from Cecka JM, Terasaki PI, eds. *Clinical Transplants 1997*. Los Angeles: UCLA Tissue Typing Laboratory, 1998:342.)

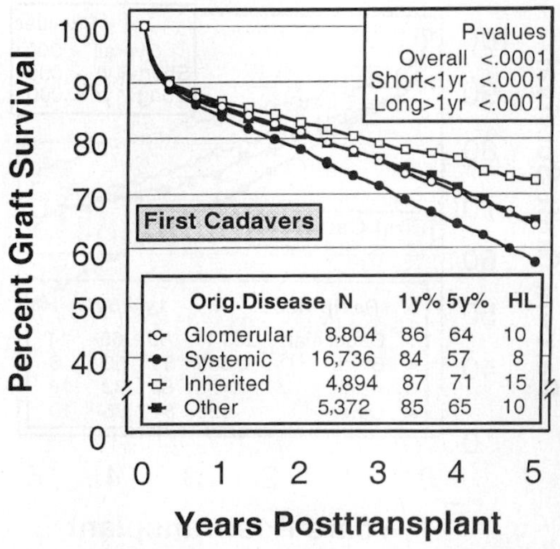

Figure 92.7. Results of first cadaver transplants according to the type of end-stage renal disease. (Reproduced with permission from Cecka JM, Terasaki PI, eds. *Clinical Transplants 1997*. Los Angeles: UCLA Tissue Typing Laboratory, 1998:352.)

Recipient's Disease (Fig. 92.7)

Among the major diseases that cause end-stage renal failure, diabetes stands out as the most problematic. With their concomitant vascular disease and particularly coronary artery disease, diabetics generally have had lower long-term patient survival rates. During the period between 1994 and 1996, diabetics comprised approximately 30% of the patients waiting for renal transplants and about one-fourth of the recipients. In Fig. 92.7, diabetics were included among those with other systemic diseases (primarily hypertensive nephrosclerosis) who had similar graft survival rates. By controlling the underlying systemic disease, results have improved. But extensive evaluation is required when considering these patients for transplantation.

During the past 4 years, almost half of transplanted diabetic patients received a simultaneous pancreas transplant. These multiorgan recipients were not included in the analysis of Fig. 92.7, nor in other figures included in this chapter. Diabetic recipients of a simultaneous pancreas–kidney (SPK) transplant have slightly higher graft survival rates at 1 year and a 40% longer half-life (14 years compared with 10 for kidney alone) than diabetic patients who receive a kidney without a pancreas. Although SPK transplants eliminate insulin dependence in approximately 80% of cases over the first 3 years, it is difficult to attribute their better long-term graft survival solely to the success of the pancreas graft. These patients generally receive stronger courses of immunosuppressant therapy and are selected to receive an SPK transplant. The SPK recipients are more often younger and healthier patients and fewer are minorities than diabetics who receive a kidney only.

Patients with inherited diseases (polycystic disease, medullary cystic disease, Alport's syndrome, renal dysplasia, prune belly, and others) tend to have better graft survival rates because of the relative lack of comorbid disease. Other primary disease groups have similar outcomes, intermediate between the systemic and inherited disease groups. Disease recurrence is not commonly cited as a cause of graft failure, although the progression may be slow in the transplanted kidney. Focal sclerosis commonly recurs in children. IgA nephropathy recurs in the transplanted kidney of up to one-third of these patients and has been implicated in substantial graft loss beginning at about 5 years after renal transplantation when it does reappear.

Recipient's Health Status (Fig. 92.8)

Patients who are sufficiently debilitated by disease that they require hospitalization before their transplant have the poorest prognosis after transplantation, as expected. These patients have an increased mortality risk during the first year after transplantation. Using work as a surrogate for health, patients who were able to work or attend school full time before their transplant had slightly better outcomes in the first year and long-term than those who were unable to engage in full-time occupation or who were homebound before their transplant. Comorbid disease and conditions such as hypertension, coronary artery or peripheral vascular disease in the patient may have a significant effect on mortality risk. These conditions are more common among older patients and the transplant success can be improved by treating and controlling vascular disease before transplantation. Other factors such as peptic ulcer disease with gastrointestinal bleeding, chronic active granulomatous disease

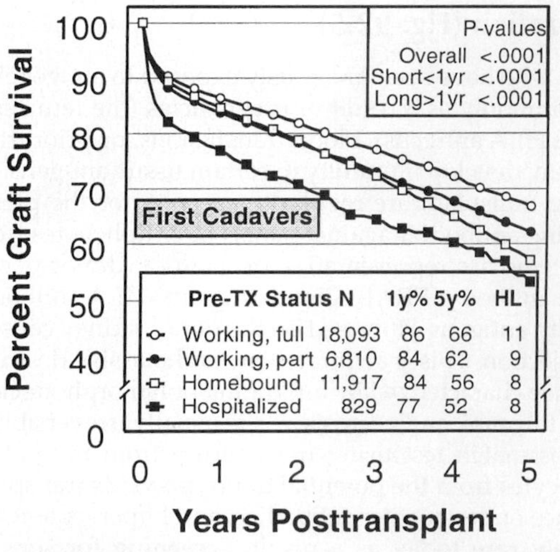

Figure 92.8. The effect of the recipient's pretransplant health status on the results of first cadaver transplants. (Reproduced with permission from Cecka JM, Terasaki PI, eds. *Clinical Transplants 1997*. Los Angeles: UCLA Tissue Typing Laboratory, 1998:350.)

(tuberculosis, histoplasmosis, coccidioidomycosis), colonic diverticular disease, pancreatitis, lower urinary tract obstruction and infections, bleeding disorders, and psychiatric illness can also affect the outcome. Viral infections (cytomegalovirus, Epstein-Barr, and hepatitis B or C) may become active in the immunosuppressed patient, and the risk for preexisting malignancy to recur is also heightened by long-term immunosuppression.

DONOR CHARACTERISTICS THAT INFLUENCE TRANSPLANT OUTCOME

Tissue Compatibility (Fig. 92.9)

The role of HLA compatibility between the donor and recipient in the success of renal transplants has been a controversial issue, and one that continues to be debated. The HLA antigens of the donor that differ from those of the recipient are the major targets of rejection reactions. Analyses of first cadaver transplants (Fig. 92.9) show that transplants with none of the HLA-A,-B, or -DR locus antigens mismatched between the donor and recipient have significantly better outcomes than grafts with 1 to 2 antigens mismatched. Graft survival rates decline with increasing numbers of HLA-antigen mismatches. The difference between the best and most poorly matched transplants is approximately 10% after 5 years. The incidence of early rejection episodes also correlates with the number of HLA-antigen mismatches, and this relationship affects the cumulative immunosuppression the patient receives to treat rejection, the number of days of hospitalization required, and the transplant costs.

The debate about the relative importance of HLA matching to transplant outcome often hinges on the observation that the survival differences between grafts with 1 to 2 or 3 to 4 mismatches are not large and frequently cannot be demonstrated in a single transplant center's analysis of its own results. Reports of unexpectedly high graft survival rates among recipients of poorly HLA-matched living-donor transplants have further fueled the discussion. Although the superior results for HLA-identical sibling donor grafts are rarely contested, the survival rates of transplants between genetically unrelated spouses and other donors who are not HLA matched are essentially the same as the results of transplants between family members who share one HLA haplotype (parent-to-child, child-to-parent, one haplotype-matched siblings). As noted in cadaver donor transplants, the incidence of early rejection episodes correlates well with the degree of HLA mismatch among living donors, but the rejections often are sufficiently mild or are detected early enough that they can be treated successfully.

Histocompatibility is one of a very few factors that can be used prospectively to improve long-term graft survival rates. The graft half-life for HLA-identical sibling transplants is nearly double that for other living-related donor grafts. This means that after the first year, these well-matched transplants will survive twice as long as other living-donor grafts on average. Although the difference is not quite as large for recipients of first cadaver transplants, the half-lives suggest that HLA-matched grafts will survive 30% longer than those from donors with more than three HLA-A, -B, or -DR antigens mismatched with the recipient. Because of these potential gains in short- and long-term survival and because there is an advantage for sensitized patients to receive an HLA-matched kidney, HLA compatibility is one of the criteria considered in allocating cadaver kidneys. UNOS coordinates shipping of cadaver kidneys to completely HLA-matched recipients anywhere in the country to facilitate their transplantation. But even in local areas for kidneys that are not completely matched, candidates move up in their ranking if they are more HLA compatible with the donor.

Donor Age (Fig. 92.10)

The quality of the grafted tissue is a key to the long-term success of renal transplants. The role of donor factors in graft outcome has become prominent in recent years. As automobile safety has improved through the use of seat belts and air bags and more cyclists and others wear protective helmets, the number of donors whose deaths resulted from head trauma has steadily declined. These donors were most often younger individuals. More and more older donors now are being accepted, often with cerebrovascular deaths. In 1988, just more than 2% of the cadaver kidneys transplanted came from donors over age

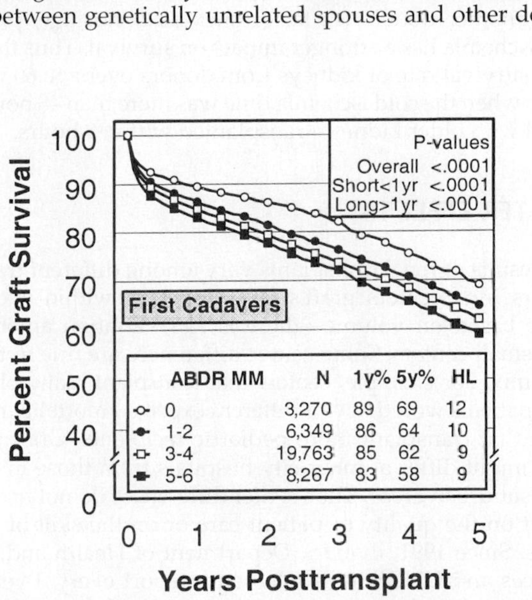

Figure 92.9. The effect of HLA-A, -B, and -DR antigen mismatches between the donor and recipient on first cadaver transplant survival rates. ABDR MM, number of A, B, DR mismatches. (Reproduced with permission from Cecka JM, Terasaki PI, eds. *Clinical Transplants 1997.* Los Angeles: UCLA Tissue Typing Laboratory, 1998:372.)

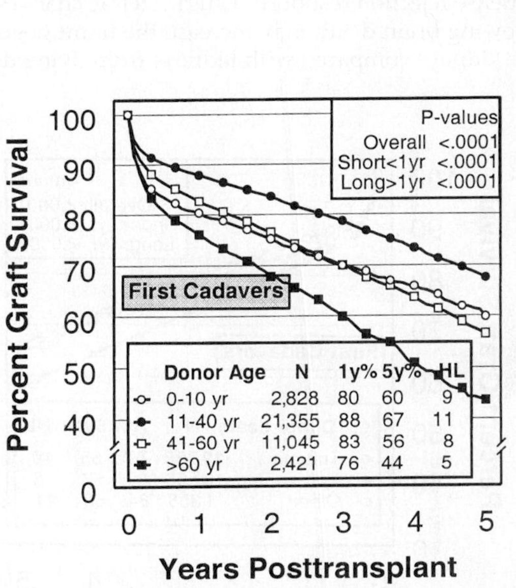

Figure 92.10. Actuarial survival of first transplants according to the cadaver donor's age. (Reproduced with permission from Cecka JM, Terasaki PI, eds. *Clinical Transplants 1997.* Los Angeles: UCLA Tissue Typing Laboratory, 1998:360.)

60, whereas in 1996 nearly 8% were from older donors. Approximately 80% of those were from donors who died from stroke. Aged kidneys have fewer functioning nephrons and probably are more susceptible to ischemic or immunologic injury than younger kidneys. More than half of the kidneys transplanted from donors over age 60 were lost within 5 years. Figure 92.10 shows that even using kidneys from donors age 41 to 60 resulted in lower graft survival rates than could be obtained with kidneys from donors age 11 to 40. More detailed analyses have revealed that long-term graft survival begins to decline with donors over age 45. Obviously age is only a general predictor of donor quality. Most centers biopsy kidneys from older or otherwise marginal donors to estimate the fraction of sclerosed glomeruli and to look for vascular problems.

Transplanting very young donor kidneys, particularly the very small kidneys from children less than 2 years old, is technically challenging and some prefer to transplant them *en bloc*. With cadaver kidneys in short supply, however, there is debate about whether these kidneys can be used successfully for two recipients. Paradoxically, very small kidneys do not fare as well when transplanted to children as when they are transplanted to adults. Although kidneys from very young children have the same number of functioning nephrons as young adult kidneys, a rejection episode that might be tolerated by an adult kidney can devastate the small kidney. It is preferable to transplant very small donor kidneys into a small adult rather than to a young child.

Cause of Donor Death (Fig. 92.11)

The cause of donor death also influences graft outcome, even when the donor is younger. Kidneys from donors who had non-trauma (cerebrovascular, cardiovascular) deaths had poorer early outcomes than those from trauma donors. Whether this difference is related to underlying disease, donor treatment before death, donor management, or other factors is not established.

Interestingly, evidence from animal models have shown that kidneys from brain-dead animals are rejected more quickly than those from anesthetized control animals. In these models, adhesion molecules were expressed on vascular endothelium and glomeruli of brain-dead but not control animals resulting in a more intense rejection response. Thus systemic changes that occur following brain death may increase the immunogenicity of cadaver kidneys compared with kidneys from living donors.

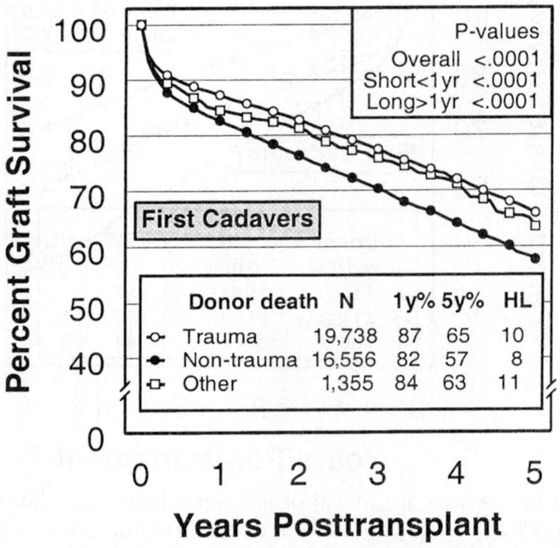

Figure 92.11. The cause of donor death and outcome of first transplants. (Reproduced with permission from Cecka JM, Terasaki PI, eds. *Clinical Transplants 1997*. Los Angeles: UCLA Tissue Typing Laboratory, 1998:364.)

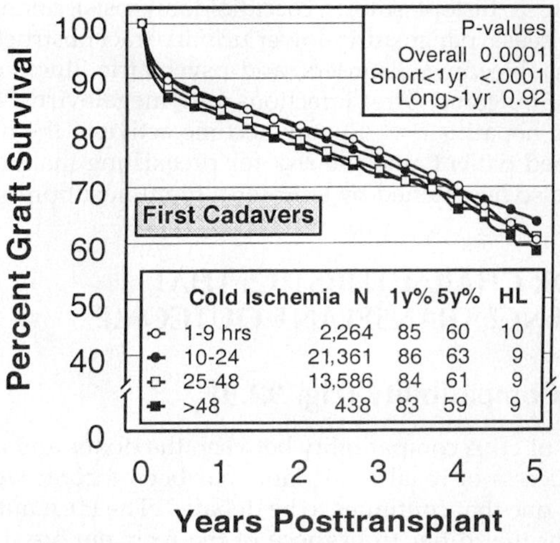

Figure 92.12. The effect of cold ischemia time on first cadaver transplant survival rates. (Reproduced with permission from Cecka JM, Terasaki PI, eds. *Clinical Transplants 1997*. Los Angeles: UCLA Tissue Typing Laboratory, 1998:366.)

Cold Ischemia Time (Fig. 92.12)

Cadaver kidneys may be subjected to ischemic damage during procurement, storage, or reanastomosis in the recipient. Warm ischemia during the procurement is rare because the organs are precooled and, unless there is a technical problem with the surgery, the anastomosis time is minimal. Cold storage time can vary widely depending on whether the kidney is shipped to a distant center for transplantation or unforeseen complications arise in placing the kidney with a local recipient. The incidence of delayed graft function increases significantly with prolonged cold ischemia time; however, the effect on graft survival is relatively small. Kidneys transplanted within 9 hours had an 85% 1-year graft survival rate compared with 83% for those stored more than 48 hours. There is no clear correlation between longer cold ischemia and long-term graft survival. When combined with another donor risk factor such as donor age, prolonged cold ischemia has a stronger impact on survival. Thus the 1-year graft survival rate of kidneys from donors over age 60 was 20% lower when the cold ischemia time was more than 48 hours compared with older kidneys transplanted within 9 hours.

CENTER EFFECTS

The results of renal transplants vary among different transplant centers. Most centers' graft survival rates fall within an expected range based on volume—there is less variation among large than small centers. Some center differences are due to their patient mix. For example, centers that transplant many older diabetic patients would have a different expected mortality rate than those that transplant more pediatric recipients. Graft survival rates might differ at inner-city hospitals from those in middle-class suburban areas. Thus center differences do not necessarily reflect on the quality of patient care or on the skill of the surgeons. Since 1991, the U.S. Department of Health and Human Services and UNOS have released a report every 3 years containing graft and patient survival rates at each transplant center in the United States. After adjusting for several patient demographic factors, each center's actual survival rates are compared with those expected according to their patient mix. The 1997 report showed that approximately 10% of kidney transplant centers had graft survival rates significantly lower than expected and a similar percentage had higher than expected survival rates. Thus there were differences among centers that were not accounted for by the patient characteristics used to create a level playing field in these analyses. Moreover, a good center performance when measuring 1-year graft survival rates did not guarantee good long-term survival at that center. Clearly, there are different skills involved in posttransplant care during the first year and later. But different patient mix factors can influence long-term survival than affect the first year results (Table 92.1). Changes in the health care system have also begun to present challenges in long-term care and follow-up of some transplant recipients. Maintenance of expensive immunosuppressive regimens over long periods of time may cause financial hardship and lead to inappropriate discontinuation of medication and thereby to graft loss secondary to rejection.

EVENTS DURING THE EARLY POSTTRANSPLANT PERIOD THAT INFLUENCE TRANSPLANT OUTCOME

Delayed Graft Function (Fig. 92.13)

Whether or not the graft functions well in the immediate posttransplant period has an important effect on short- and long-term graft survival. In Fig. 92.13, the patient's need for dialysis within the first week after the transplant was used as a surrogate for delayed graft function (DGF). Delayed function complicates the ability to detect rejection early and may result in more immunosuppression to cover the period of DGF. It is also more difficult to detect nephrotoxicity of the drugs when the kidney does not have good function. But DGF can reflect damage to the kidney either because of aging, ischemic damage, or damage associated with brain death or donor management before organ procurement, as well. These underlying causes of DGF may be the primary cause of poor long-term survival notwithstanding additive effects of immunologic assault or nephrotoxicity. The fraction of first cadaver kidneys that have delayed graft function did not change substantially between 1988 to 1992 and 1994 to 1996. The graft half-life improved among recent transplants that had good early function, but for those that did not function well, the long-term prognosis was similar to that for transplants performed in the earlier period.

Rejection Episodes (Fig. 92.14)

Rejection episodes that occur during the initial transplant hospitalization are associated with lower 1-year graft survival rates but have only a modest effect on long-term survival rates. Changes in the immunosuppressive drugs available for transplant recipients have reduced the incidence of these early rejection episodes by more than half. During the period 1988 to 1990, approximately 30% of first transplant recipients had experienced early rejection episodes compared with 12% of those transplanted between 1994 and 1996. The survival rates for those who had rejection episodes were similar during both periods in Fig. 92.14, suggesting that the more severe rejections may have not been ameliorated by the newer immunosuppressants.

Quality of Graft Function

The impact of early graft function and of rejection on subsequent graft survival are somewhat controversial. Some report that early rejection episodes are the strongest predictor of subsequent rejections and of chronic rejection, whereas others find that rejections in the absence of DGF have little effect on long-term graft survival. The results of analyses from different centers may be confounded by issues of donor quality and how successfully rejections were treated. The quality of graft function that is achieved after recovery from DGF or from a treated episode of rejection is the best indicator of subsequent graft survival.

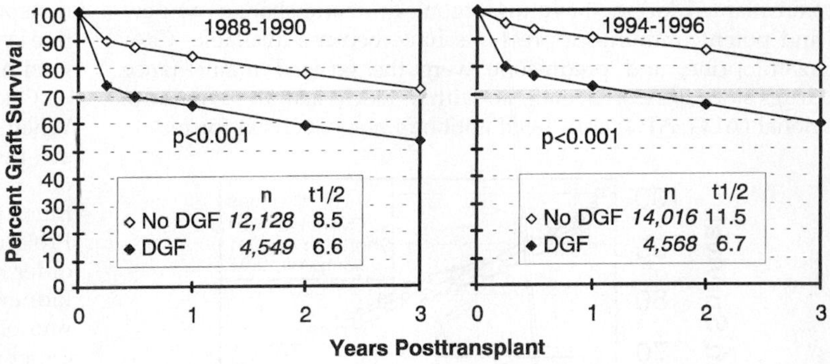

Figure 92.13. Delayed graft function after cadaveric transplantation—a similar effect in two eras. DGF, delayed graft function. (Reproduced with permission from Cecka JM, Terasaki PI, eds. *Clinical Transplants 1997.* Los Angeles: UCLA Tissue Typing Laboratory, 1998:8.)

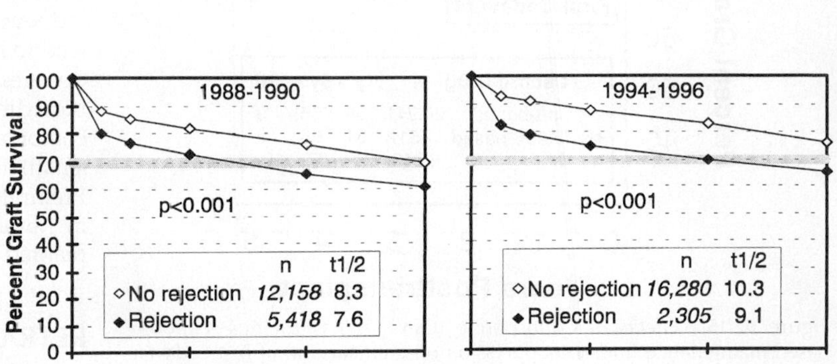

Figure 92.14. The effect of acute rejection episodes during the initial transplant hospitalization on subsequent graft survival in two eras. (Reproduced with permission from Cecka JM, Terasaki PI, eds. *Clinical Transplants 1997.* Los Angeles: UCLA Tissue Typing Laboratory, 1998:8.)

TABLE 92.2. Causes of Graft Failure During the First Year and Among Transplants That Survived More Than 1 Year

	First Year	Long-Term (1–5 yr)
Graft failures	(n = 5,570)	(n = 3,816)
Rejection		
Hyperacute	<1%	0
Acute	26%	6%
Chronic	11%	37%
Noncompliance	2%	4%
Thrombosis	11%	<1%
Primary failure	6%	0
Technical	<1%	0
Recurrence	1%	3%
Death	25%	40%

Based on first cadaver donor transplants between January 1991 and December 1996.

CAUSES OF GRAFT FAILURE (TABLE 92.2)

Approximately one-fourth of first cadaver grafts that fail during the first year are lost to acute rejection episodes. Patient deaths within the first posttransplant year account for another 25%. It is often difficult to determine the degree to which these early deaths are related to the transplant; some early postoperative deaths result from infections or complications of the surgery. These early deaths tend to occur more frequently in very young or very old patients. After the first year, death is the leading cause of graft failure, comprising 40% of late graft losses. These late deaths are primarily cardiovascular deaths of older transplant recipients. Chronic rejection is the second leading cause of graft failure after the first year.

IMMUNOSUPPRESSION (FIG. 92.15)

Strategies to prevent allograft rejection and ensure survival of the transplanted kidney have undergone dramatic changes as new and potent immunosuppressants have become available. CsA, azathioprine, and prednisone were the favored maintenance drugs since 1984, often coupled with monoclonal (OKT3) or polyclonal (ALG, ATG) anti–T-cell antibody reagents used for induction during the immediate posttransplant period. Since the introduction of mycophenolate mofetil in the United States in July 1995, there has been a rapid conversion from azathioprine, and many centers also have begun replacing CsA with tacrolimus (FK506), which was approved for use in kidney transplant recipients in 1997. The use of antibody prophylaxis or induction therapy has declined as these newer combinations have substantially reduced the incidence of early rejection episodes. Preliminary results suggested a graft survival advantage for patients receiving FK506 as a study drug, but the results shown in Figure 92.15 indicate that the results with CsA and FK506 are now very similar.

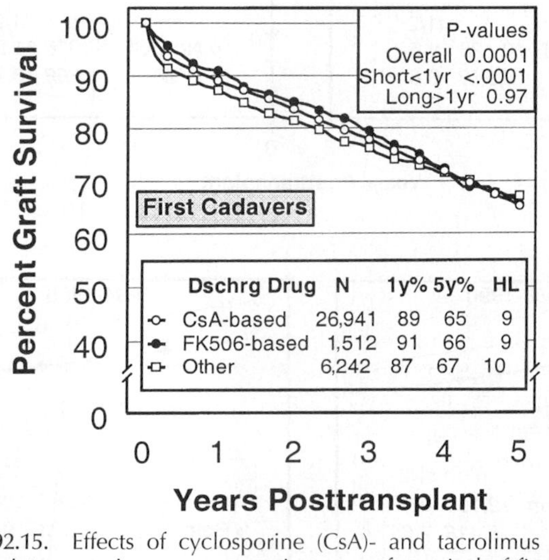

Figure 92.15. Effects of cyclosporine (CsA)- and tacrolimus (FK506)-based maintenance immunosuppression on graft survival of first cadaver transplants. (Reproduced with permission from Cecka JM, Terasaki PI, eds. *Clinical Transplants 1997*. Los Angeles: UCLA Tissue Typing Laboratory, 1998:374.)

PATIENT COMPLIANCE

Long-term graft survival is dependent on patient compliance. Transplantation requires a lifelong commitment to immunosuppressive drugs and patients who take their medications erratically or who stop taking them are at risk for acute rejection or low-grade chronic rejection. The incidence of noncompliance is often difficult to measure because of the need to rely on self-reporting by the patient. Chronic noncompliance may be detected by measuring drug levels, by monitoring usage, or by inference from compliance with clinic visits or other parameters. Most successful transplant programs make a concerted effort to educate patients about their drug regimens before the transplant.

CHRONIC GRAFT DYSFUNCTION

The slow deterioration of renal function after many months or years was generally referred to as *chronic rejection*. However, data suggest that this may not always be an immunologically mediated process. There is no doubt that the transplanted kidney can be slowly damaged by inflammation or the action of antibodies that can cause endothelial changes. However, there is growing evidence that limited renal mass, ischemic injury, and nonspecific inflammatory responses can also lead to a destructive cycle of renal injury. The pathologic aspects of immune and nonimmune injury can be very similar.

One example of limited renal mass is the older donor kidney. When older kidneys are transplanted to younger patients, they are more often rejected than when they are transplanted to older patients. Similarly, survival of older donor kidneys is much poorer when they are transplanted to sensitized patients. Prolonged cold ischemia time results in much lower survival of older kidneys. These observations may be linked if older donor kidneys have less reserve and are less likely to recover from immunologic assaults or ischemic injury than younger kidneys. Other problems may arise from placing small female or pediatric kidneys in very large patients. Extreme mismatches in size may lead to hyperfiltration injury or to nephrotoxicity (because drug dosages are tailored to the patient's size). There is disagreement regarding the deleterious effects of size mismatches, but the combinations of very old kidneys and young recipients or very small kidneys and large recipients have generally been avoided. Preliminary results using two kidney transplants in animals and in humans have supported the concept that increased transplanted renal mass relative to body mass is beneficial.

RETRANSPLANTATION (FIG. 92.16)

One of every five candidates for a renal transplant in 1996 was a previous transplant recipient whose graft had failed. Each

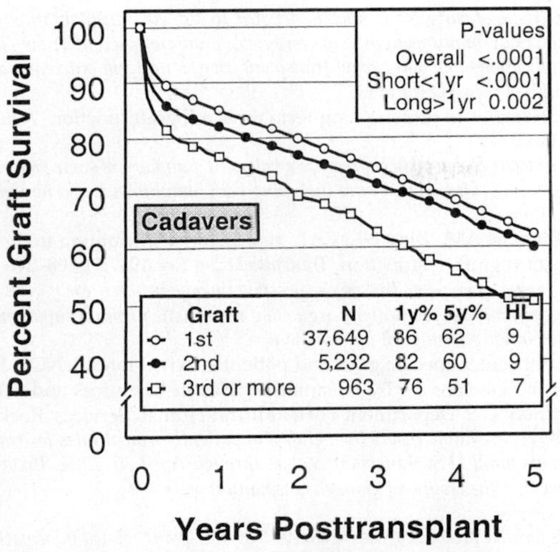

Figure 92.16. Results of retransplantation using cadaver kidneys. (Reproduced with permission from Cecka JM, Terasaki PI, eds. *Clinical Transplants 1997*. Los Angeles: UCLA Tissue Typing Laboratory, 1998:340.)

year approximately 14% of cadaver kidneys are transplanted to patients with one or more prior graft failures. The discrepancy between the percentages of waiting and retransplanted patients is because these patients are often broadly sensitized to HLA antigens from their failed transplant and must wait longer for a compatible donor. Despite the use of sensitive crossmatch tests to exclude donors whose HLA antigens could serve as targets for recipient antibodies, retransplanted patients have lower graft survival rates than recipients of first transplants. The survival difference between primary and repeat transplants is established within the first 3 months, suggesting that antidonor antibodies sometimes may escape detection and cause early damage to the graft or that underlying cellular immunity has been established that can result in accelerated or severe acute rejection even under high levels of immunosuppression. Thereafter, the survival curves for first and second transplants are nearly parallel. Multiply retransplanted patients have poorer short- and long-term graft survival rates.

QUALITY OF LIFE

Renal transplantation probably does not restore "normal" life to the recipient, however, a majority of studies have found that the patients' perceptions are that their transplant improved their life. Dialysis can be disruptive for patients who work or attend school and removing the need for dialysis can be liberating. The long-term changes that result from transplantation and immunosuppression may also affect the patient's quality of life and consequently their compliance. Continued studies of quality of life long after the transplant may yield key insights into patients' attitudes and help improve long-term survival rates. Quality-of-life issues are also an important consideration in determining who can most benefit by receiving a cadaver kidney transplant.

THE CADAVER-DONOR SHORTAGE

The success of renal transplantation has resulted in increased demand and a rapid growth in the number of patients who are placed on the waiting list. The number of waiting patients increased from about 13,000 in 1988 to more than 36,000 in 1996. The number of cadaver kidneys donated each year has remained remarkably stable at approximately 8,000 kidneys (4,000 donors). This acute shortage of organs for transplantation has extended the median waiting time for a kidney transplant from 400 days (1.1 years) in 1988 to 824 days (2.3 years) in 1994. For patients who joined the waiting list in 1995, fewer than half had been transplanted in 1997, when these median waiting times were calculated.

The kidney shortage has had a profound impact on the practice of transplantation. There is increasing pressure to expand the limits of donor acceptability. A growing usage of older donor kidneys is an obvious example. The oldest cadaver kidney transplanted to date came from an 82-year-old donor. A history of hypertension or diabetes no longer automatically excludes a donor. A few centers have transplanted both kidneys from a marginal donor to a single recipient in order to increase the renal mass with good early success. Kidneys from donors whose hearts have stopped beating have also been used by some centers. The number of living-donor transplants has doubled during the past 10 years, and the largest increases have been in the number of transplants from offspring to their parents and transplants between spouses and other genetically unrelated individuals.

LIVING-UNRELATED DONOR TRANSPLANTS

The results of living-unrelated donor transplants have been very good despite their HLA incompatibility. Their 1-year graft survival rates and transplant half-life are 91% and 15 years, respectively. These results are comparable with those for transplants from genetically related family members who share one HLA chromosome with the recipient. The unexpectedly high graft survival rates of living-unrelated donor transplants have been variously attributed to the uniform health of the donor kidney, more potent immunosuppression, and strong support from the donor, improving compliance. Because approximately two-thirds of living-unrelated transplants are performed between spouses in the United States, the donor and recipient live together, which often is not the case when the donor is a first-degree relative.

Although exposing healthy living donors to the risks of major surgery is a serious concern for the transplant community, morbidity and mortality have been minimal. Very few deaths (less than 0.1% according to survey results) have been identified among a large number of living donors. Serious complications have been reported in approximately 2% of cases (depending on what is considered serious) and minor complications range between 8% to 50% (primarily infections). In the interest of completeness, most of the studies of donor morbidity and mortality have included very old cases and, in newer data on living donations, the incidence of complications may be declining with improved patient care and surgical technique. Long-term complications of uninephrectomy also seem to be rare, but there have been anecdotal reports of donors who developed end-stage renal disease and required dialysis. The risks to the living donor are not trivial, however, and the risks must be explained to potential donors. Careful evaluation of the potential living donor is critical to ensure that the donor has two healthy kidneys and has no underlying medical problems that could lead to complications after nephrectomy as well as to determine the suitability of the kidney for donation.

A patient who has a healthy, compatible, and highly motivated donor, whether a blood relative or someone who is otherwise emotionally related can be transplanted under optimum conditions for both the patient and donor with excellent results. For those patients who have this option, prolonged waiting for a cadaver organ can be avoided and more cadaver organs will be available for those who do not have a motivated spouse or relative.

Selected Readings

Cecka JM. In sickness and in health . . . high success rates of kidneys transplanted between spouses. *Transplant Rev* 1996;10:216–224.

This review article covers the literature on unrelated living-donor transplants and includes supplementary data from the UNOS Registry on recent U.S. experience with kidney transplants between spouses.

Cecka JM, Terasaki PI, eds. *Clinical Transplants 1997.* Los Angeles: UCLA Tissue Typing Laboratory, 1998.

This book contains registry and single-center reports of transplant results for kidneys and other organs. The chapter from which most of the figures for this chapter were taken includes tables for each figure with graft survival rates stratified by several recipient, donor, and transplant characteristics. An extensive review of literature on immunosuppression is interesting and provides more than 300 references.

Dew MA, Switzer GE, Goycoolea JM, et al. Does transplantation produce quality of life benefits? *Transplantation* 1997;64:1261–1273.

A review of more than 200 quality-of-life studies on transplant recipients including results from nearly 7,000 kidney transplant recipients led these authors to conclude that there are distinct quality-of-life benefits to transplantation. In addition to some interesting insights, a table of studies, with the author and year, is provided.

Rao VK. *Surgical clinics of North America: renal transplantation*, vol 8. Philadelphia: WB Saunders, 1998.

This issue of Surgical Clinics is devoted to kidney transplantation. It includes chapters on immunosuppression, surgical, immunologic, infectious, and medical complications following renal transplantation, long-term outcomes, and the economics of transplantation.

Velosa JA. Strategies to prolong long-term renal allograft function. *Transplantation Rev* 1998;12:1–13.

This recent review article presents a balanced summary of some factors that affect long-term graft survival rates including both immunologic and nonimmune complications.

Waaga AM, Rocha AM, Tilny NL. Early risk factors contributing to the evolution of long-term graft dysfunction. *Transplantation Rev* 1997;11:208–216.

This review article addresses the possible linkage between early graft injury and late graft failure. The authors argue that inadequate nephron supply may be a key factor in long-term graft dysfunction.

1997 Report of center specific graft and patient survival rates, UNOS, Richmond, VA and the Division of Transplantation, Health Resources and Services Administration, U.S. Department of Health and Human Services, Rockville, MD.

This seven-volume report lists graft and patient survival rates for transplant recipients at all U.S. transplant centers through April 30, 1994. Two volumes are devoted to the results of kidney transplantation.

www.unos.org

This website provides access to a wealth of transplant-related information and statistics from the United Network for Organ Sharing.

CHAPTER 93

Xenotransplantation of the Kidney

Jeffrey L. Platt

Xenotransplantation, once called *heterotransplantation,* refers to the transplantation of tissues or organs between individuals of different species. Xenotransplantation is of current interest as a potential solution to the severe and worsening shortage of kidneys available for transplantation into patients with end-stage renal failure, and to the very long waiting time for those kidneys that do become available. Xenotransplantation also provides a model system in which to evaluate the pathogenesis and treatment of vascular disease, because vascular disease is a cardinal manifestation of the rejection reaction seen in renal xenografts. Although clinical xenotransplantation of the kidney is not currently practiced, even as an experimental procedure, recent progress in overcoming rejection of renal xenografts has encouraged the view that renal xenotransplantation may eventually find widespread application. Accordingly, this chapter will review the current understanding of immunology, pathophysiology of renal xenotransplantation, and therapeutic approaches that may become vital to the clinical success of xenotransplants.

HISTORY OF XENOTRANSPLANTATION

The field of organ transplantation owes its inception to a technical advance—the development of the vascular anastomosis. When experiments by Carrel and Guthrie demonstrated that the kidneys could be harvested from one animal and successfully implanted into another animal, some enthusiasm developed for trying this new technique as a treatment for patients with renal failure. However, it was not clear how a kidney or any organ could be harvested from a deceased person because there was no generally accepted definition of biologic death. It was reasoned by some that because some of the cells of the kidney or of other organs are found to be alive after the heart ceases beating, the organs could not be removed from a human cadaver. The only way, then, that organs might be obtained in an ethical manner would be to procure them from animals rather than humans. Accordingly, the first attempts, by Ullman and Jaboulay, to connect the circulation of patients with renal failure to healthy kidneys involved the use of kidneys obtained from animals. These xenografts performed in 1906 and the few others attempted in subsequent years exhibited only momentary function. Because of these failures, the 5 decades that followed brought only a few attempts at transplanting animal organs into humans.

With the advent of immunosuppressive therapy, however, the era of clinical renal transplantation began in earnest. The demand for kidneys grew, but in the absence of laws defining brain death, organs could still not be readily obtained from cadavers. This shortage of human donors sparked renewed interest in xenotransplantation. Thus in the early 1960s, Reemtsma transplanted kidneys harvested from chimpanzees into patients with renal failure. Some of these xenografts suffered repeated and very severe rejection reactions and some of the patients experienced frequent, life-threatening infections, results notably less successful than kidney allotransplants. Still, some of the patients survived for months, the longest for 9 months, with the kidney xenografts as the only source of renal function. When the advent of brain-death laws increased the opportunities to obtain human kidneys, interest in xenotransplantation waned once again.

The recent years have brought renewed interest in the use of animal—particularly pig—kidneys for transplantation into humans. This interest stems in large part from the severe shortage of human donor organs and from the prolonged waiting time for obtaining organs. This interest is also sparked by recent advances in understanding the molecular basis of xenograft rejection and the ability to apply genetic engineering to address at least some of the immune hurdles. Interest in xenotransplantation may also stem from the idea that in some limited cases, an animal kidney might be less susceptible than a human kidney to recurrence of disease or destruction by immune reactions such as those directed against allogeneic major histocompatibility complex (MHC).

THE SPECIES USED AS A SOURCE OF XENOGRAFTS

It might be intuitive that the best source of a kidney xenograft would be an animal that is phylogenetically close to the recipient. Thus recent attempts to xenotransplant the kidney involved chimpanzees and baboons as the xenograft source. However, nonhuman primates are only available in small numbers and there is concern that such transplants might introduce lethal

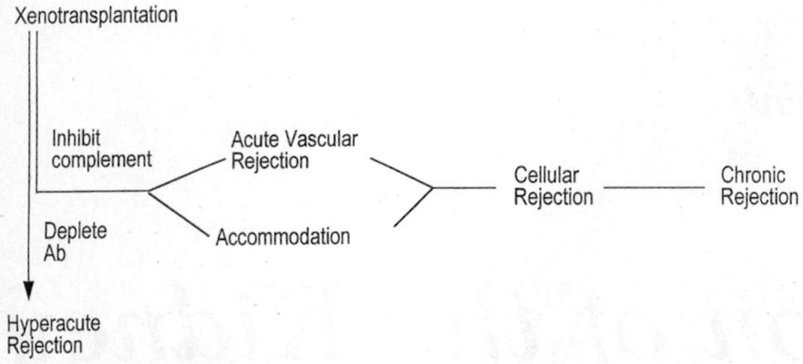

Figure 93.1. The biologic responses to xenotransplantation. A porcine kidney transplanted into a human would be subject to one or more of the several immunologic reactions listed in the figure. A xenogeneic kidney transplanted into an unmanipulated recipient would be expected to undergo hyperacute rejection. Hyperacute rejection can be avoided by depleting antidonor antibodies or inhibiting complement. If hyperacute rejection is avoided, the graft becomes subject to acute vascular rejection. Acute vascular rejection can sometimes be avoided by depletion of antidonor antibodies or treatment with high dosages of cyclophosphamide. If anti-donor antibodies are depleted from the recipient, the graft may also undergo accommodation, a condition in which acute vascular rejection does not occur despite the presence of anti-donor antibodies in the circulation of the recipient. If acute vascular rejection is avoided, the graft may undergo cellular rejection or chronic rejection.

viruses into human populations. Consequently, most investigators now favor the use of nonprimates, especially the pig, rather than primates as a source of organs. The transplantation of organs from phylogenetically disparate animals, such as the pig, has proven very difficult however, because of severe immunologic and biologic hurdles. These hurdles are summarized in Fig. 93.1 and in the text that follows.

THE IMMUNOLOGIC HURDLES TO XENOTRANSPLANTATION

Hyperacute Rejection

A kidney of one species transplanted into a phylogenetically disparate species is subject to hyperacute rejection. Hyperacute rejection of xenografts, like hyperacute rejection of allografts, destroys the newly transplanted organ within minutes to a few hours. It is characterized histologically by interstitial hemorrhage and thrombosis, the thrombi consisting predominantly of platelets (Fig. 93.2). Combinations of donor-recipient species in which hyperacute rejection occurs with regularity, such as pig-to-human, are called *discordant;* combinations of species in which hyperacute rejection is not generally observed, such as chimpanzee-to-human, are called *concordant.*

Hyperacute rejection of a pig kidney by a human would be triggered by binding of "natural antibodies" to the endothelial lining of graft blood vessels. Natural antibodies are present in the circulation of all immunocompetent humans without a known history of sensitization to the corresponding antigen. Those natural antibodies that recognize the cells of foreign species are called *xenoreactive natural antibodies.* The xenoreactive natural antibodies in humans that would trigger the hyperacute rejection of porcine kidney predominantly recognize Galα1-3Gal, a sugar synthesized by lower mammals. Although a human serum may contain both IgM and IgG antibodies specific for Galα1-3Gal, IgM antibodies specific for Galα1-3Gal would seem to be of greater importance in the pathogenesis of hyperacute rejection. Binding of xenoreactive IgM antibodies causes activation of the complement system and it is the complement system that mediates the rejection reaction.

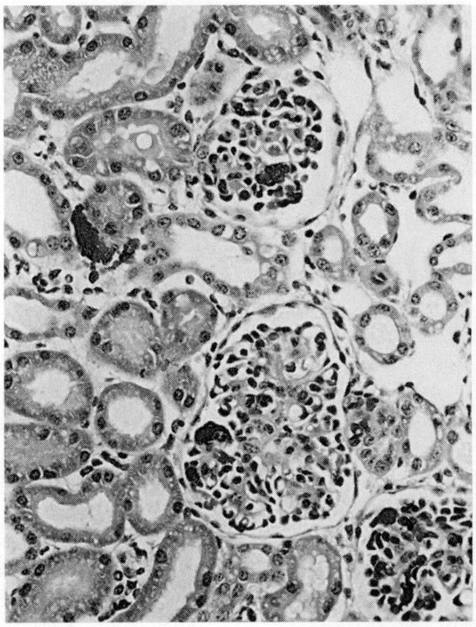

Figure 93.2. Pathologic picture of hyperacute rejection. A pig kidney transplanted into a baboon is undergoing hyperacute rejection. Hyperacute rejection is characterized by the formation of platelet thrombi and interstitial hemorrhage; several platelet thrombi are apparent in the glomeruli. A small focus of interstitial hemorrhage adjacent to a distal tubule can be seen. Magnification × 325.

Susceptibility of a xenograft to hyperacute rejection is especially great because the xenograft has limited ability to control the activation of the complement system of disparate species. This failure of complement control stems from failure of complement regulatory proteins, such as decay-accelerating factor (DAF) and CD59 expressed on the surface of cells in the xenograft, to inhibit activation of the recipient's complement cascade (Fig. 93.2). So important is this factor in the susceptibility of a xenograft to hyperacute rejection that hyperacute rejection does not occur if the pig organs express low levels of human complement regulators, as can be achieved by the development of pigs transgenic for the genes encoding the human proteins. Because the expression of human-complement regulatory proteins in a pig kidney averts hyperacute rejection but the presence of these proteins in a human kidney does not prevent hyperacute rejection of kidneys in presensitized subjects, it is likely that that humoral reaction of allografts, which generally involves anti-HLA (human leukocyte antigen) antibodies, is more severe than the humoral reaction causing hyperacute rejection of pig kidneys. Consistent with this concept are studies suggesting that the humoral reactions leading to hyperacute rejection of xenografts are analogous to the reactions occurring in the transplantation of kidneys across an ABO barrier, a circumstance in which hyperacute rejection occurs only infrequently.

How does the activation of complement in a xenograft or in an allograft cause the devastating picture of hyperacute rejection? A model for the pathogenesis of hyperacute rejection is shown in Fig. 93.3. Recent studies have suggested that the development of hyperacute rejection requires assembly of terminal complement complexes, because graft recipients with inherited deficiencies of C6 do not reject grafts hyperacutely and because the blockade of complement at the level of C5 or C8 prevents injury to rat hearts perfused with human blood. It might be thought therefore that hyperacute rejection results from complement-mediated lysis of endothelial cells. However, ultrastructural studies of hyperacutely rejecting organs gener-

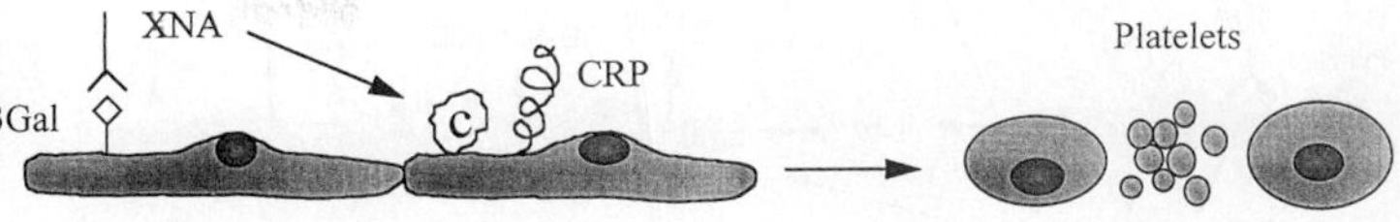

Figure 93.3. Pathogenesis of hyperacute rejection. Hyperacute rejection of a kidney xenograft is initiated by binding of xenoreactive natural antibodies (XNA) to endothelial cell antigens (in a pig the major antigen is Galα1-3Gal). XNA binding triggers activation of complement (C). Complement activation is amplified because pig complement regulatory proteins (CRP) in endothelial cell membranes fail to inhibit complement. Complement activation on endothelium causes loss of vascular integrity (rounding of endothelial cells), which in turn causes platelet aggregation and hemorrhage, as seen in Fig. 93.2.

ally reveal that the endothelial cells are viable early in the development of the lesion and hyperacute rejection may occur even if assembly of the membrane attack complex is inhibited. The development of hyperacute rejection thus would seem to reflect noncytotoxic effects of complement on endothelium. Among these effects may be the formation of gaps between endothelial cells, leading to loss of the endothelial barrier and antithrombotic functions, and the loss from endothelium of heparan sulfate, a protein–polysaccharide conjugate responsible for such endothelial functions as barrier formation to protein and cell efflux and anticoagulation.

Hyperacute rejection was once thought to be the preeminent hurdle to transplanting animal organs into humans. Research in the last decade has shown, however, that hyperacute rejection of xenografts can be prevented by interfering with antibody binding to the graft or by inhibiting activation of the complement system. Inhibition of antibody binding is generally achieved by depletion of xenoreactive antibodies from the graft recipient. Such depletion can be accomplished by perfusion of the recipient's blood through columns bearing Galα1-3Gal as an immunoabsorbent. One potential alternative to the depletion of xenoreactive antibodies is the genetic engineering of donor animals to bring about a lowering of antigen expression. Various approaches to accomplishing this goal have been recently reviewed (see Selected Readings).

Hyperacute rejection can also be prevented by inhibition of complement. Complement can be inhibited by administration of such agents as cobra venom factor or soluble complement receptor type 1 to the xenograft recipient. Although quite effective at preventing hyperacute rejection, the inhibition of complement in this way might impair host defense against infectious microorganisms. Accordingly, several alternative strategies have been pursued. One method involves the administration of gamma globulin, which actually diverts active complement proteins away from endothelial cell surfaces (the same mechanism may account for the efficacy of gamma globulin in the treatment of idiopathic thrombocytopenic purpura). Another method involves the use of organs from transgenic animals that express human proteins that inhibit complement reactions on cell surfaces as discussed previously. The complement regulatory proteins such as DAF and CD59 normally prevent inadvertent cellular injury arising during the course of complement activation, but these proteins function in a species-restricted fashion. Organs from transgenic pigs expressing human DAF and CD59 have been shown to prevent hyperacute rejection (Fig. 93.2).

Acute Vascular Xenograft Rejection

If hyperacute rejection is averted, a kidney xenograft is subject to "acute vascular xenograft rejection" (sometimes called *delayed xenograft rejection*) (Fig. 93.1). Acute vascular rejection is characterized pathologically by endothelial swelling, focal ischemia, and inflammation, with diffuse intravascular coagulation often beginning within 24 hours of transplantation and destroying the graft over a period of days to weeks (Fig. 93.4). Acute vascular xenograft rejection is now widely viewed as a major barrier to clinical application of xenotransplantation.

Acute vascular rejection of xenografts, like acute vascular rejection of allografts, appears to be initiated by the action of xenoreactive antibodies on graft endothelium (Fig. 93.5). Following exposure to porcine tissues or organs, the synthesis of xenoreactive antibodies, particularly those specific for Galα1-3Gal, increases and that increase coincides with the time that acute vascular rejection would be observed. Removal of antibodies from the circulation of xenograft recipients and/or inhibition of antibody synthesis by treatment with cytotoxic agents delays or averts acute vascular rejection. Also, a very similar type of rejection in concordant xenografts and allografts is associated with the development or administration of antidonor antibodies. These antibodies may be specific for donor MHC antigens. It would seem not unlikely that antibodies specific for donor MHC antigens will also be found in xenograft recipients, in which case they might also cause acute vascular rejection.

Another potential mechanism for acute vascular xenograft rejection involves the action on the graft of host leukocytes and platelets. This concept is supported by studies documenting the presence of inflammatory cells and platelets in organs with acute vascular xenograft rejection. Further evidence is the finding that

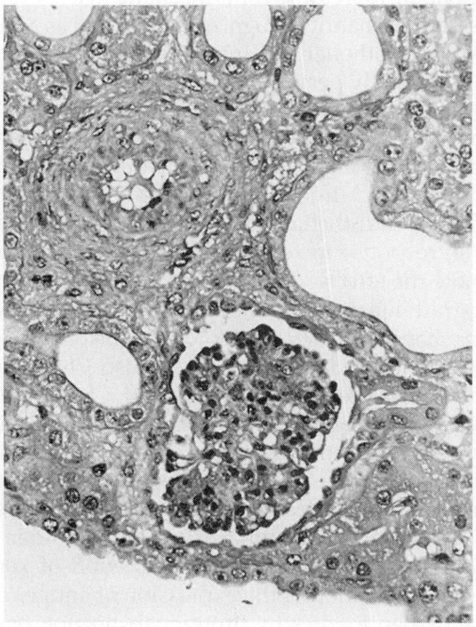

Figure 93.4. Pathologic picture of acute vascular rejection. A porcine kidney expressing human decay-accelerating factor and CD59, which inhibit complement, was transplanted into a baboon. The kidney underwent acute vascular rejection over the ensuing 10 days. Acute vascular rejection is characterized pathologically by ischemia, formation of fibrin thrombi (see glomerulus and artery), and endothelial injury, which can be seen in the artery.

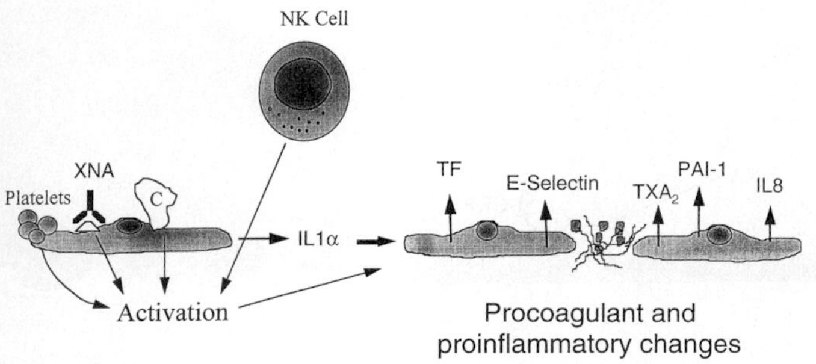

Figure 93.5. Pathogenesis of acute vascular rejection. Anti-donor antibodies may directly perturb endothelial cells or trigger activation of complement (C). Stimulation of endothelial cells by complement leads to synthesis of IL-1α, which activates endothelial cells. Direct stimulation of endothelial cells by anti-donor antibodies or by platelets or natural killer (NK) cells may do likewise. Activation of endothelial cells leads to expression of procoagulant molecules such as tissue factor (TF) and plasminogen activator inhibitor type I (PAI-1) and proinflammatory molecules such as E-selectin and IL-1β. Antidonor antibodies may also serve as ligands for natural killer (NK) cells, macrophages (MØ), and other inflammatory cells bearing Fc receptors. These changes in turn cause intravascular coagulation, ischemia, and inflammation, the hallmarks of acute vascular rejection.

xenograft survival is prolonged by treatment of recipients with antibodies that inhibit the function of inflammatory cells. The involvement of natural killer (NK) cells in acute vascular xenograft rejection may be especially troublesome, because receptors for MHC class I, which usually downregulate NK cell function, may fail to recognize xenogeneic MHC. Still unclear is whether the presence of the cells constitutes an underlying cause of graft destruction or a response to tissue injury.

Regardless of the initiating events, acute vascular rejection is thought to result from the activation of endothelial cells in the xenograft, which leads to procoagulant and proinflammatory changes in endothelium. Endothelial cell activation might be caused by one or more of several mechanisms. As xenoreactive antibodies predominantly recognize Galα1-3Gal as N-linked substitutions on endothelial cell integrins, binding of these antibodies might directly perturb the function of endothelial cells or deliver signals leading to endothelial cell activation. Antibody binding might also lead to formation of the membrane attack complex on porcine endothelial cells leading to *de novo* synthesis of interleukin (IL)-1α, which in turn acts as an autocrine factor stimulating endothelial activation. Xenoreactive antibodies produced in response to xenotransplantation, particularly IgG, may promote the effector functions of NK cells, which may mediate xenograft injury, as described in the following. Nonimmunologic mechanisms such as biological incompatibilities between the donor and recipient may also contribute to the development of acute vascular xenograft rejection. For example, porcine thrombomodulin fails to interact effectively with human thrombin to activate protein, raising the possibility that a xenograft may be excessively susceptible to thrombosis.

Various therapeutic strategies might be applied to the problem of acute vascular rejection. Interventions under investigation revolve around two strategies: depletion of xenoreactive antibodies and alteration of the expression of antigen. Depletion of xenoreactive antibodies by immunoabsorption or use of cytotoxic therapy to inhibit antibody production has been used successfully as an investigational tool to study acute vascular rejection. Another, more enduring approach to depleting xenoreactive antibodies involves the induction of immunologic tolerance. Although still at an investigational level, tolerance to carbohydrate antigens has been induced by the generation of mixed hematopoietic chimerism. Alteration in the expression of antigen, focusing especially on Galα1-3Gal, has been undertaken. For example, some groups have developed transgenic pigs expressing α1,2-fucosyltransferase, an enzyme that competes with α1,3-galactosyltransferase (the enzyme that catalyzes synthesis of Galα1-3Gal) for catalyzing the termination of certain carbohydrates. Instead of Galα1-3Gal, cells in the transgenic pigs synthesize H antigen, which is not a target of xenoreactive antibodies. Other genetic approaches to decreasing expression of this antigen have been recently reviewed.

Yet another way of dealing with acute vascular rejection may be the establishment of accommodation. Accommodation is a condition first recognized from the analysis of ABO-incompatible kidney allografts in which depletion of antidonor antibodies from the graft recipient brought about enduring graft survival even when antidonor antibodies later returned to the circulation. Accommodation might thus result from a change in xenoreactive antibodies or a change in the antigens they recognize and/or an acquired resistance of endothelium to humoral injury.

Cellular Immune Responses to Xenotransplantation

Xenotransplantation clearly leads to elicited cellular immune responses; however, the extent to which these responses differ from the responses to allotransplantation and the need for novel therapies is still uncertain. Xenografts of free tissues such as pancreatic islets and hepatocytes can survive and function in highly disparate recipients (e.g., human-to-mouse) treated with conventional immunosuppressive therapy. However, pig renal xenografts seem to engender immune responses more intense than those seen in allografts.

How the xenogeneic cellular immune response might differ from the allogeneic response and why it might be more powerful is summarized in Figure 93.6. Surprisingly, T cells respond poorly to stimulation by xenogeneic cells in conventional mixed leukocyte cultures. This poor response is thought to reflect a limited ability of T cells to recognize xenogeneic cells "directly"—that is, recognizing the intact foreign cell rather than the anti-

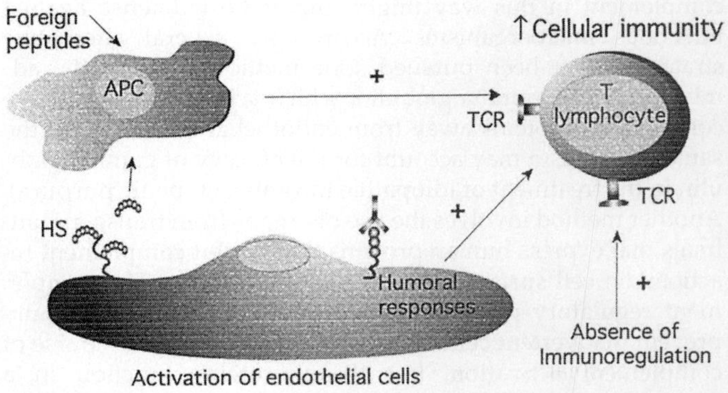

Figure 93.6. Mechanisms that might amplify T-cell–mediated immune responses to a xenotransplant. Four mechanisms are illustrated. First, a diversity of antigens taken up and presented by recipient antigen presenting cells (APC) might stimulate a diverse and therefore intense T-cell response. Second, the release of immunomodulatory factors, such as heparan sulfate (HS) from endothelium owing to humoral immunity leads to activation of antigen-presenting cells. Third, the inflammatory products of endothelial cells and the activation of endothelial cells promotes activation and migration of T cells. Fourth, failure of the recipient's T cells to interact directly with the transplant prevents the development of down-regulatory immunoregulation. (Adapted with permission from Platt JL. New directions for organ transplantation. *Nature* 1998;392(Suppl):11–17.)

gens of such cells taken up and presented by autologous antigen presenting cells. This limitation was once thought to reflect a bias of the T-cell repertoire toward recognition of allogeneic versus xenogeneic MHC; however, other studies have shown that human T cells can recognize disparate MHC directly and that the limitations in the *in vitro* responses reflect rather impaired interaction of CD4 and CD8 with xenogeneic MHC and costimulation by xenogeneic cells. Whereas some interpreted the limited *in vitro* responses to xenogeneic stimulation as evidence that cellular immunity to a xenograft might be diminished, the author has suggested an alternative view: that the limited response predicts diminished immune regulation and thus contributes to a more severe reaction, as suggested in Fig. 93.6.

In contrast to the limited cellular immune responses *in vitro* discussed previously, the cellular immune response to kidney xenografts is often quite vigorous. It was observed that frequent and severe episodes of cellular rejection occur in porcine kidneys transplanted into baboons. Cellular immune responses to xenografts might be amplified by the availability of an enormous variety of foreign peptides and by the presence of cytokines and other agonists as a byproduct of humoral reactions. Another factor may be a relative failure of T-cell regulation across species.

Whether cellular rejection of xenografts will respond to treatment by current immunosuppressives is uncertain. Rejection in the pig-to-baboon kidney xenografts of Alexandre et al. responded only partly to infusions of high doses of corticosteroids. Administration of higher doses of the immunosuppressive drugs in current use would seem to pose an inordinate risk of opportunistic infection in the patient with a renal transplant, especially if dialysis is an alternative. In this situation, the development of more specific or less toxic immunosuppressive agents or preferably the induction of immunologic tolerance may be needed for widespread application of kidney xenotransplantation.

One approach to tolerance induction across species is the development of mixed hematopoietic chimerism, as mentioned previously, by reconstituting the recipient's immune system with both recipient and donor hematopoietic stem cells. Tolerance might also be induced by the transplantation of donor thymus leading to the development of a tolerant T-cell repertoire. Yet another approach involves the infusion of small amounts of donor hematopoietic stem cells generating "microchimerism"; this approach has shown promise in rodents. Various other methods for generating allogeneic tolerance might work in the xenotransplant setting provided that the graft is protected from destruction by the humoral immune responses as discussed previously.

Chronic Rejection of Xenotransplants

Whether or to what extent kidney xenotransplants will be subject to chronic rejection like allotransplants is not established. If chronic rejection has an immunologic basis, it can be anticipated that the condition would be more severe in xenotransplants than in allotransplants. However, xenotransplantation offers the opportunity to readily replace the failing graft and potentially to address the problem through genetic engineering.

Physiologic Hurdles to Xenotransplantation of the Kidney

The critical issue in considering xenotransplantation of the kidney is whether a xenograft can replace the function of the native kidneys. There is limited but fairly persuasive experimental work addressing this question for pig-to-primate renal xenografts. Alexandre et al. established more than a decade ago that if rejection of a kidney xenograft is averted temporarily with plasma exchange to remove antidonor antibodies and high doses of immunosuppression, a pig kidney could support a primate physiologically for a period of 2 to 3 weeks. Recently, Sablinski et al. confirmed the ability of the pig kidney to maintain the fluid and electrolyte balance of a nonhuman primate for a period of nearly 2 weeks; however, the limiting factor in these experiments, as in Alexandre's, was the extreme susceptibility of such kidneys to rejection. White and colleagues announced that they were able to prevent rejection of porcine kidneys expressing human DAF in nonhuman primates for periods exceeding 2 months. In these limited studies, as in others, the fluid and electrolyte homeostasis of the primate was maintained by the pig kidney, suggesting that a pig kidney might provide physiologic fluid and electrolyte support under clinical conditions. Two questions yet to be resolved, however, are the extent to which the porcine kidney will support human hematopoiesis and the extent to which the porcine kidney will regulate blood pressure within the normal range. The author's own preliminary studies indicate that hypertension is not a significant feature of pig-to-primate xenotransplantation.

The Infectious Risk

Interest in xenotransplantation has been tempered by consideration of the possibility that a xenograft could introduce infectious agents into the recipient leading to the development of disease. Nephrologists and transplant surgeons have grappled with this problem in allotransplantation and are accustomed to weighing the risk of infection against the benefit anticipated for the patient. In the case of xenotransplantation it might be expected that most, if not all, serious infections can be prevented by rigorous screening of potential donor animals. In the case of xenotransplantation, however, there is the additional fear that the transplant might transmit a novel pathogen to the general population, inducing an epidemic. Concern has been vehemently expressed with respect to the use of baboons as donors. Although such concerns are generally thought to be less justified for pigs, the recent discovery that a pig endogenous retrovirus might be able to infect human cells in culture has brought this into more immediate focus. Current investigations in various centers are aimed at determining whether the pig endogenous retrovirus can infect humans and in so doing cause disease, and if it infects human graft recipients, whether it might become infectious for others in the population.

In determining the extent to which an infectious agent might pose a risk to the public health, one salient consideration is whether the agent is likely enter the human population by other means, in which case xenotransplantation is unlikely to be the exclusive vehicle for entry. For example, while the transmission of influenza virus by a xenotransplant is a theoretic concern, it is obvious that such a virus will infect humans by other means and that xenotransplants are unlikely to be the source of an epidemic. At present, there is no agent known that could only be transmitted by a xenograft and by no other means.

CONCLUSION

Interest in xenotransplantation has always stemmed from an urgent need to develop a plentiful supply of organs and tissues for clinical transplantation. A plentiful supply of kidneys would allow the planning of transplant procedures and the elimination of preservation injury. It would reduce the waiting time for transplantation and allow the ready replacement of transplanted organs that fail due to chronic rejection, recurrence of the original disease, or other problems. Xenotransplantation in particular would allow the intensive screening of donors and application of presurgical treatments that are not feasible using human transplants. Xenotransplantation would also allow the genetic engineering of the donor animals to reduce the severity of rejection or overcome other problems. Despite all of the advantages, xenotransplantation had seemed only a distant prospect until recent studies illuminated the molecular basis for xenograft rejection. Understanding some of the factors contributing to rejection has allowed the development of novel and highly specific strategies for dealing with xenograft rejection, which have brought about greater optimism that xenotransplantation of the kidney and other organs may be attainable in the near future. In fact, early clinical trials are underway using tissue xenografts as treatment for Parkinson's disease and diabetes. It can be hoped that as this chapter comes to press, early trials on the clinical xenotransplantation of the kidney will likewise occur.

Acknowledgments

I thank Patricia Rowe for critical comments, and the National Institutes of Health for supporting my work in this area.

Selected Readings

Alexandre GPJ, Gianello P, Latinne D, et al. Plasmapheresis and splenectomy in experimental renal xenotransplantation. In: Hardy MA, ed. *Xenograft 25.* New York: Elsevier Science Publishers, 1989:259–266.

This paper reports results of pig kidney transplants in baboons.

Cooper DKC, Kemp E, Platt JL, et al. *Xenotransplantation: the transplantation of organs and tissues between species.* Berlin: Springer-Verlag, 1997.

This book provides a comprehensive survey of progress in experimental xenotransplantation.

Platt JL. *Hyperacute xenograft rejection.* New York: RG Landes, 1995.

This book provides background information on the history and the immunology of xenotransplantation. It also summarizes results of kidney transplants between species.

Platt JL. New directions for organ transplantation. *Nature* 1998;392(Suppl):11–17.

This paper reviews the current status of xenotransplantation and potential application of genetic engineering of donor animals.

Sablinski T, Latinne D, Gianello P, et al. Xenotransplantation of pig kidneys to nonhuman primates: I. Development of the model. *Xenotransplantation* 1995;2:264–270.

This paper reports results of pig kidney transplants in baboons.

Sachs DH, Sablinski T. Tolerance across discordant xenogeneic barriers. *Xenotransplantation* 1995;2:234–239.

Some would argue that the clinical application of xenotransplantation will require induction of immunologic tolerance. The subject of tolerance in xenotransplantation is reviewed in this paper.

SECTION XI

Clinical Procedures and Techniques

CHAPTER 94

Hemodialysis and Hemoperfusion in the Management of Drug Intoxication

A.R. Amir and James F. Winchester

Clinical toxicology is an important discipline that intervenes with exposures to variable drugs, chemicals, or naturally occurring substances. Acute toxic exposure can be accidental (environmental, occupational, or therapeutic error) or intentional (suicidal or abuse).

In the United States, the American Association of Poison Control Center Toxic Exposure Surveillance System (AAPCC-TESS) reported 2.19 million cases of human poisoning in 1997 with 786 fatalities. This reflects an increase of 3.7% in reported poison exposures from 1996 to 1997. Although children younger than 6 years were responsible for the majority of poisonings (52.5%), they comprised just 3.2% of fatalities. The following were important observations: 59.8% of deliberate exposures occurred in females during warmer months; 60% of fatalities occurred between the age of 20 and 50 years, the majority of which were intentional; and a single substance was implicated in 88.6% of reports. Most of the reported exposure cases occurred at home and were managed there (74.9%). Decontamination and supportive care with the use of specific antidotes were the mainstay of therapy in the majority of patients. Hemodialysis and hemoperfusion were used in 1,015 patients to enhance drug elimination (Table 94.1). It is also worth noting that overdoses of acetaminophen, aspirin, tricyclic antidepressants, and cardiovascular medications were responsible for most of the fatalities (44.9%).

TABLE 94.1. Treatment Provided to Intoxicated Patients Reported to the American Association of Poison Control Centers (1997)

Treatment	Number of Cases
Decontamination	1,442,541
Specific antidotes	25,120
Alkalinization (with or without diuresis)	6,702
Hemodialysis	927
Hemoperfusion	55
Other extracorporeal procedure	33
Transplantation	20

Data adopted from the 1997 AAPCC-TESS report. Litovitz TL, Klein-Schwartz W. Annual report of the American Association of Poison Control Centers Toxic Exposure Surveillance System. *Am J Emerg Med* 1998;16:443–497.

Alcohol, analgesics, and antidepressants were responsible for 50% of adolescent deaths. This chapter highlights the variable methods of decontamination and drug elimination with the main emphasis on the role of extracorporeal methods of detoxification.

THE ROLE OF CLINICAL ASSESSMENT AND LABORATORY EVALUATION IN THE POISONED PATIENT

Obtaining a history of intoxication may be difficult, particularly in psychiatric patients or trauma victims. Impaired level of consciousness may preclude obtaining any information about the type, the amount, and the route of intoxication. On the other hand, patients may be reluctant to admit a history of drug abuse. Symptom complexes or toxic syndromes may give clues to undetermined poisoning (Table 94.2). Listing medications with recognition of adverse drug reactions and possible drug interactions may determine the etiology of confusion in an elderly patient.

The validity of a diagnostic test depends on its ability to confirm a diagnosis and/or exclude others. It may also help to determine the severity of intoxication. Therefore a basic diagnostic test to determine end-organ toxicity should include not only a comprehensive drug screen, but also baseline serum electrolytes with blood urea nitrogen (BUN), serum creatinine, blood glucose, and an electrocardiogram. Certain classes of toxins may have characteristic laboratory abnormalities, laboratory toxidromes, as seen with substances causing metabolic acidosis or sodium channel blockade (e.g., cyclic antidepressants, procainamide, quinidine, flecainide, cocaine, diphenhydramine). A high osmolal gap (more than 25 mOsm/kg), in the presence of high anion gap metabolic acidosis and in the absence of a history suggestive of lactic or ketoacidosis, may strongly point toward methanol or ethylene alcohol intoxication. Ethanol and isopropyl alcohol ingestion may cause an osmolal gap in the absence of significant metabolic acidosis. Quantitative serum drug levels probably are more helpful than simple qualitative urinary drug screen, because a negative screen does not rule out intoxication.

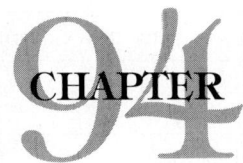

TABLE 94.2. Examples of Symptom Complexes or Toxidromes

Toxidrome Complex	Consciousness	Pupils	Other	Possible Toxic Agents
Anticholinergic	Agitation, hallucination	Dilated	Fever, flushing Dry skin	Atropine, Jasmine weed, Antihistamine
Cholinergic	Coma	Pinpoint	Fasciculations Bradycardia Salivation Lacrimation	Organophosphate insecticide Carbamates, nicotine
Extrapyramidal	Wakefulness	No changes	Dystonia, akathisia opisthotonos	Haloperidol
Opioid	Coma	Pinpoint	Hypothermia Hypotension	Opiates, Lomotil, Darvon, Pentazocine
Phenothiazine	Coma	Pinpoint	Arrhythmia Hypotension	Phenothiazine
Salicylates	Semicoma, agitation	No changes	Diaphoresis Fever, tinnitus Alkalosis (early) Acidosis (late)	Salicylates Wintergreen oil
Sedatives/ hypnotic	Coma	Dilated	Hypothermia Decrease reflexes Hypotension	Sedatives Barbiturates
Sympathomimetic	Agitation, hallucinations	Dilated	Seizures Diaphoresis Tremor Tachycardia Hyperreflexia Acidosis	Cocaine Theophylline Caffeine Amphetamine
Uremia	Coma	No changes	Uremic frost Uremic fetor Acidosis Hyperkalemia	(Uremia)

Modified from Haddad LM, Shannon MW, Winchester JF. *Clinical management of poisoning and drug overdose,* 3rd ed. Philadelphia: WB Saunders, 1998.

MANAGEMENT OF THE INTOXICATED PATIENT

In resuscitating an intoxicated patient, attention should be directed toward adequate airway and ventilatory support, as well as adequate cardiac circulatory support with frequent monitoring of vital signs, preferably with cardiac and pulse oximetry. Naloxone should be given to the comatose patient, along with 100 mg thiamine intravenously and 50 ml of 50% dextrose. Seizures can be aborted with a short-acting benzodiazepine (lorazepam or diazepam). Seizures induced by isoniazid or anticholinergic drug overdoses can be managed by pyridoxine and physostigmine, respectively. General anesthesia may be required to control theophylline-induced seizures.

Decontamination can be achieved by dilution, use of activated charcoal, cathartic or ipecac syrup, bowel irrigation, and gastric lavage. Induced emesis via ipecac in oral ingestion has fallen out of favor, because many clinical trials failed to show any improvement in outcome when compared with the use of activated charcoal alone. Gastric lavage can be omitted when dealing with adults after acute oral overdose and with those who present shortly after intoxication or show signs of severe intoxication. Cathartics are no longer routinely being used because, for some drugs, absorption is increased. On the other hand, activated charcoal currently is the most useful agent for the prevention of drug absorption. With few exceptions, activated charcoal adsorbs most ingested drugs and chemicals (Table 94.3). Multiple-dose activated charcoal (MDAC) has been shown to enhance the clearance of a number of drugs (Table 94.4). MDAC is thought to produce its beneficial effect by interrupting the enterohepatic circulation of drugs and by binding to any drug that enters the gut lumen from the circulation. MDAC is given orally or via a nasogastric tube with a loading dose of 1.0 g/kg, followed by a continuous infusion intragastrically of 0.2 g/kg per hour. The duration of infusion depends on the clinical status and the patient response.

TABLE 94.3. Substances That Poorly Adsorb to Activated Charcoal

Alcohols (ethanol, methanol, isopropyl alcohol, acetone)
Metals and inorganic minerals (sodium, potassium, bromide, borates, lead, iron, iodine)
Corrosives

TABLE 94.4. Drugs Studied with Multiple-Dose–Activated Charcoal (MDAC) in Humans

Amitriptyline	(Doxepin)	Piroxicam
Carbamazepine	(Imipramine)	Quinine
(Chlorpropamide)	Meprobamate	Salicylates
Cyclosporine	Methotrexate	Sotalol
Dapsone	Nadolol	Theophylline
Diazepam	Nortriptyline	(Tobramycin)
Digoxin	Phenobarbital	Valproic acid
(Diltiazem)	Phenytoin[a]	(Vancomycin)

[a] Mixed effectiveness.
( ) Not effective.
Modified from Chyka PA: Multiple dose activated charcoal and enhancement of systemic drug clearance: Summary of studies in animals and human volunteers. *J Toxicol Clinical Toxicol,* 1995;33:399–405.

TABLE 94.5. Active Drug Elimination Techniques

Forced diuresis with pH manipulation
Multiple doses of activated charcoal, cholestyramine, kayexalate
Peritoneal dialysis
Hemodialysis
Sorbent hemoperfusion
Hemofiltration
Plasma exchange and exchange transfusion
Hemoperfusion and hemodialysis with chelating agents
Continuous hemodiafiltration and hemoperfusion
Cerebrospinal fluid drainage and replacement
Toxin-specific antidotes

Active Drug Elimination Techniques

Elimination of any toxic compound depends on the drug's specific kinetics and the modality by which detoxification is being attempted. High endogenous drug clearance renders detoxification unnecessary, whereas a high volume of distribution renders the drug unavailable for detoxification. Enhanced elimination will be accepted as a modality of intervention if total body clearance of a toxin can be increased by at least 30%. Methods for enhancing elimination of toxic compounds are listed in Table 94.5.

Forced Diuresis with pH Manipulation

In the kidney, drug excretion involves three main processes: glomerular filtration; tubular secretion via organic anion transporters in the straight segment of the proximal tubule; and passive distal tubular reabsorption. Most drugs are either weak acids or bases that exist in the nonionized or ionized form. The nonionized molecules are lipid soluble and diffuse across cell membranes. Increasing the pH of the tubular fluid increases the degree of ionization of weak acids and hence reduces tubular reabsorption. The reverse applies to weak bases. For the drug to respond to urinary pH alteration, it has to have low protein binding, a (pKa) in the appropriate range, and be confined to the extracellular fluid compartment. Elimination of a weak acid by the kidney is increased in alkaline urine if the pKa of the drug is 3.0 to 7.5. For weak bases, elimination is increased if the pKa of the drug is 7.5 to 10.5.

Because forced diuresis following the administration of large volumes of fluids with or without diuretics can be complicated by hyponatremia, hypokalemia, and water intoxication with pulmonary edema and cerebral edema, accurate measurements of patient intravascular volume status and perhaps hemodynamics by means of Swan-Ganz catheter are required. Urine output and urine pH along with serum electrolytes should be monitored every 1 to 2 hours initially, and frequently thereafter.

Alkaline diuresis is initiated by using 1 L of 0.75 normal saline in 5% dextrose with 25 mEq/L of bicarbonate (½ ampoule of sodium bicarbonate), to which appropriate amounts of potassium are added. The rate of infusion is adjusted initially to maintain a urine flow of 300 to 500 ml/hr and a pH in the range of 7.5 to 8.5. Mannitol or frequent furosemide boluses are given when necessary to maintain the urine flow rate. Alkaline diuresis is suitable for phenobarbital poisoning when the plasma level exceeds 10 mg/dl; barbital, when the plasma level exceeds 10 mg/dl; and salicylates, when the plasma level exceeds 50 mg/dl. In moderate salicylate intoxication, administration of alkali alone without excessive fluid may have the same efficacy without the risk of volume overload. Urinary alkalinization with or without diuresis is also used to enhance renal methotrexate elimination and to protect the kidneys from the toxic effect of myoglobin in severe rhabdomyolysis.

On the other hand, forced acid diuresis increases excretion of amphetamines, fenfluramine, phencyclidine, strychnine, and quinidine. Urinary acidification is no longer recommended because it is usually complicated by systemic metabolic acidosis and does not significantly enhance removal of toxic substances. It is still considered for treatment of resistant amphetamine overdose cases that do not respond to diazepam or chlorpromazine. Urinary acidification is contraindicated in renal or hepatic insufficiency and in myoglobinuria. Acidification is achieved by using an intravenous preparation of L-arginine, lysine, or ammonium chloride (4 g every 2 hours orally or intravenously). One liter of normal saline in 5% dextrose is infused over 1 to 2 hours, to which 10 g of arginine or lysine hydrochloride is added. The dose is adjusted to maintain urinary pH at approximately 5.5 to 6.5. Although ascorbic acid has been used as an acidifying agent (75 mg/kg/day in divided doses), its effect has been questioned. It failed to acidify the urine in human subjects. Ascorbic acid prevents urinary alkalinization by urease inhibition rather than acidification.

Extracorporeal Techniques of Detoxification

In 1913, Abel, Rowntree, and Turner constructed the first hemodialyzer and demonstrated that salicylate could be removed. In 1951, Doolan and colleagues demonstrated that salicylate was more efficiently removed by hemodialysis than by spontaneous processes. However, it was not until 1955 that Schreiner and associates reported the first successful use of hemodialysis in a patient intoxicated with aspirin. Since then peritoneal dialysis and hemodialysis have been used in the management of several poisoning cases.

The decision to use an extracorporeal therapy depends on the evaluation of both patient- and drug-related factors (Table 94.6). The use of bicarbonate hemodialysis is useful in treating acid–base disorders and counteracts the delayed metabolic derangements seen in poisoning with salicylate, methanol, and ethylene glycol. It is also useful in removing their active toxic metabolites (formic acid and oxalate, respectively). In the following section we will discuss the different extracorporeal methods of detoxification.

Peritoneal Dialysis. Compared with hemodialysis and hemoperfusion, peritoneal dialysis is a relatively inefficient method of detoxification because drug removal is slow, and sufficient blood flow to achieve a high drug clearance cannot be

TABLE 94.6. Factors That Mandate the Use of Extracorporeal Techniques for Detoxification

Patient-Related Factors
Severe clinical deterioration despite intensive supportive therapy.
Underlying medical conditions that complicate intoxication outcomes (e.g., heart failure, chronic obstructive pulmonary disease).
Impairment of normal drug-excretion routes, as in hepatic or renal failure.
The development of coma-related complications, such as aspiration pneumonia or sepsis.
Drug-Related Factors
Documented lethal plasma levels of ingested toxins.
Intoxication with agents that have active toxic metabolites or delayed rebound effects.

TABLE 94.7. Factors That Increase Drug Dialyzability

Drug Properties	Dialysis Properties
Molecular weight <500 D	Large membrane surface area
High water solubility	High-flux membrane
Small volume of distribution	High dialysate flow rate
Low nonrenal clearance	High blood flow rate

accomplished. Because of the molecular weight of most drugs (300 D), the maximum drug clearance that can be achieved by peritoneal dialysis is 10 to 15 ml/min (50% less than urea clearance). Nevertheless, peritoneal dialysis can be useful for rewarming in hypothermic patients and as the initial therapy in patients awaiting hemodialysis or hemoperfusion. Elimination of a drug via peritoneal dialysis is optimized if the drug has low molecular weight, is water soluble, has low protein binding, and has a low volume of distribution.

Hemodialysis. Hemodialysis is recommended for a wide variety of intoxications, in severely poisoned patients. Factors that increase drug dialyzability include those related to specific drug properties and to the physical properties of the dialysis provided (Table 94.7). Drugs with low molecular weight and a small volume of distribution (less than 1 L/kg) are most suitable for removal by hemodialysis. With little exception (e.g., acetylsalicylic acid), most drugs with high protein-binding affinity are poorly dialyzed. Lipophilicity of a drug indicates a large volume of distribution, and therefore is inaccessible for hemodialysis. On the contrary, drugs that are water soluble are more readily removed by aqueous dialysate. Although lipid-soluble drugs were removed with soybean oil hemodialysis (lipid dialysis) in the past, this technique was abandoned when modern high-flux dialyzers were introduced. Hemoperfusion is preferred for highly lipid-soluble drugs.

Some of the dialyzer characteristics that favor drug removal by hemodialysis include the type of the dialysis membrane, its surface area, and both the blood and the dialysate flow rates. The newer high-flux, biocompatible, more permeable membranes (such as polysulphone and polyacrylonitrile) can remove larger-molecular-weight substances. The greater the surface area of the dialyzer, the greater the amount of the drug removed. The effect of hemodialysis on drug removal is determined by the dialyzer clearance (CL_{HD}), as calculated by the following equation:

$$CL_{HD} = Q \times [(C_a - C_v)/C_a]$$

where Q is the blood flow rate, C_a is the arterial (inlet) concentration of the drug, and C_v is the venous (outlet) concentration of the drug.

It is essential to remember that the total clearance of any drug during hemodialysis is the sum of the dialyzer clearance and the endogenous clearance of the drug for an individual patient. It is also important to consider the redistribution phenomenon after dialysis when determining the amount of the drug removed. A list of drugs and chemicals removed with hemodialysis are shown in Table 94.8.

Hemodialysis should be used whenever the intoxicated patient suffers concomitantly from renal failure or has developed significant volume overload, electrolytes, or acid–base disorders. Hemodialysis is preferred for small molecules such as lithium and for compounds that produce delayed metabolic effects, such as salicylates, methanol, and ethylene glycol. Lithium concentrations may rebound after hemodialysis un-

TABLE 94.8. Drugs and Chemicals Removed with Hemodialysis

Antimicrobials/	**Antiviral/**	**Barbiturates**
Anticancer	**Antifungal**	
		Amobarbital
Ampicillin	Acyclovir	Aprobarbital
Amoxicillin	Amantadine	Barbital
Azlocillin	Famciclovir	Butabarbital
Carbenicillin	Foscarnet	Cyclobarbital
Clavulanic Acid	Ganciclovir	Pentobarbital
(Cloxacillin)	Fibavirin	Phenobarbital
(Floxacillin)	Valacyclovir	Quinalbital
Mecillinam	Zalcitabine	(Secobarbital)
Mezlocillin	Zidovudine	
(Nafcillin)		**Nonbarbiturate**
Penicillin	Fluconazole	**Hypnotics, Sedatives,**
Piperacillin	Flucytosine	**Tranquilizers,**
Temocillin	Itraconazole	**Anticonvulsants**
Ticarcillin	(Chloroquine)	
	Quinine	Carbamazepine
(Cefaclor)		Carbromal
Cefadroxil	**Cardiovascular**	Chloral hydrate
Cefamandole		(Chlordiazepoxide)
Cefazolin	Acebutolol	(Diazepam)
Cefixime	Atenolol	(Diphenylhydantoin)
Cefmenoxime	Benazepril	(Diphenylhydramine)
(Cefonicid)	Bretylium	Ethinamate
(Cefoperazone)	Captopril	Ethchlorvynol
Ceforanide	(Diazoxide)	Ethosuximide
(Cefotaxime)	(Digoxin)	Gallamine
Cefotetan	Fosinopril	Glutethimide
Cefotiam	Labetalol	(Heroin)
Cefoxitin	(Lidocaine)	Meprobamate
Cefroxadine	Lisinopril	(Methaqualone)
Cefulodin	Metoprolol	Methsuximide
Ceftazidime	Methyldopa	Methyprylon
(Ceftriaxone)	N-acetylprocainamide	Paraldehyde
Cefuroxime	Nadolol	Primidone
Cephacetrile	Propranolol	Valproic Acid
Cephalexin	Practolol	
Cephaloridine	Procainamide	**Alcohols**
Cephalothin	Quinapril	
(Cephapirin)	Quinidine	Ethanol
Cephradine	Ramipril	Ethylene glycol
	Sotalol	Isopropanol
Amikacin	Tocainide	Methanol
Dibekacin		
Fosfomycin	**Metals, Inorganics**	**Others**
Gentamicin		
Kanamycin	(Aluminum)*	Aminophylline
Neomycin	Arsenic	Aniline
Netilmicin	(Copper)*	Borates
Sisomicin	(Iron)*	(Chlorpropamide)
Streptomycin	Lead	Chromic Acid
Tobramycin	Lithium	Cimetidine
(Vancomycin)	(Magnesium)	Folic Acid
	(Mercury)*	Mannitol
Aztreonam	Potassium	Methylprednisone
Cilastin	Phosphate	Sodium Citrate
Imipenem	Sodium	Theophylline
	Strontium	Thiocyanate
Bacitracin	(Tin)	Ranitidine
Colistin	(Zinc)	
	Bromide	**Solvents, Gases**
Moxalactam	Chloride	
(Chloramphenicol)	Iodide	Acetone
Ciprofloxacin	Fluoride	Camphor
(Clindamycin)		Carbon Monoxide
(Erythromycin)	**Antidepressants**	(Carbon Tetrachloride)
Metronidazole		(Eucalyptus Oil)
Nitrofurantoin	(Amitriptyline)	Thiols
Ofloxacin	Amphetamine	Tolune
Sulfonamides	Isocarboxazid	Trichloroethylene
Tetracycline	MAO-inhibitors	
Cycloserine	(Pargyline)	**Plants, Animals,**
Isoniazid	(phenelzine)	**Herbicides,**
(Azathioprine)	(Tricyclics)	**Insecticides**
Cyclophosphamide		
5-fluorouracil		Alkyl Phosphate
(Methotrexate)		(Organophosphates)
		Paraquat

( ), not well removed; ( )*, removed with chelating agent.

less dialysis is prolonged and/or repeated. Hemodialysis with ethanol-enriched, bicarbonate-based dialysate is used in treating acute methanol or ethylene glycol intoxication.

Sorbent Hemoperfusion. Hemoperfusion is the direct contact of blood with sorbent particles incorporated in plastic housings. This process was introduced by Muirhead and Reid in 1948 to remove uremic toxins. Schreiner, in 1958, used a lactated anion-exchange resin column to remove pentobarbital in an uremic patient. The study was complicated by pyrogenic reaction, thrombocytopenia, and hemolysis. It was not until 1964 that Yatzidis introduced the first usable activated charcoal device for removal of poisons and other solutes. In the early 1970s, Chang and associates introduced a more biocompatible polymer-coated charcoal hemoperfusion device. Nonionic resin hemoperfusion was introduced by Rosenbaum, who showed that nonionic polystyrene resin (XAD 4) was useful in lipid-soluble poisons, such as glutethimide, methyprylon, and short-acting barbiturates. It was shown that coated charcoal hemoperfusion was successful in treating a range of intoxications and gave drug clearance values exceeding those with hemodialysis. The circuitry used for hemoperfusion is similar to hemodialysis with the exception of not having a blood-warming apparatus (only used in hypothermic patients). Anticoagulation with heparin is necessary. Heparin requirements are slightly higher than for hemodialysis and are slightly higher for resin (10,000 units) than for charcoal hemoperfusion (6,000 units).

Typical sorbents are activated carbons (charcoals), ion exchange resins, or nonionic macroporous resins. Activation is induced by controlled oxidation to increase charcoal surface area and porosity. Removal of circulating toxins is related to the avidity of the charcoal to adsorb toxins rather than diffusion as in hemodialysis. It removes both polar (e.g., salicylates and methotrexate) and nonpolar drugs and their metabolites. On the other hand, nonionic resin (XAD 4—no longer available in United States) has high affinity to adsorb organic solutes and nonpolar, lipid-soluble drugs (glutethimide, meprobamate, methaqualone, theophylline) (Table 94.9).

Although nonionic resins adsorb lipid-soluble drugs more efficiently than charcoal sorbent, they bind with less energetic forces resulting in more reversible binding. In general, hemoperfusion is instituted with a column that contains between 100 and 300 g of activated charcoal or 650 g of polystyrene resin (Table 94.10). The adsorptive capacity of the cartridge is reduced over time due to deposition of cellular debris and blood proteins. Therefore the cartridge is changed every 6 to 8 hours. Prolonged hemoperfusion treatment is not usually necessary. Thrombocytopenia (often a 30% reduction) is commonly associated with the use of hemoperfusion, and usually normalizes in 24 to 48 hours. Transient leukopenia (often 10% reduction) probably due to complement activation also occurs and rarely predisposes to infection. Hypoglycemia, hypocalcemia, and trace mineral losses have also been reported infrequently.

TABLE 94.9. Drugs and Chemicals Removed with Hemoperfusion

Antimicrobials/ Anticancer	**Antidepressants**	**Metals, Inorganics**
(Adriamycin)	(Amitriptyline)	(Aluminum)*
Ampicillin	(Imipramine)	(Iron)*
Carmustine	(Tricyclics)	
Chloramphenicol		**Solvents, Gases**
Chloroquine	**Barbiturates**	
Clindamycin		Carbon Tetrachloride
Dapsone	Amobarbital	Ethylene Oxide
Doxorubicin	Butabarbital	Trichloroethanol
Gentamicin	Hexobarbital	
Isoniazid	Pentobarbital	**Others**
(Methotrexate)	Phenobarbital	
Thiabendazole	Quinalbital	Aminophylline
	Secobarbital	Cimetidine
Analgesics	Thiopental	(Fluoroacetamide)
	Vinalbital	(Phencyclidine)
Acetaminophen		Phenols
Acetylsalicylic Acid	**Nonbarbiturate Hypnotics, Sedatives, Tranquilizers**	(Podophyllin)
Colchicine		Theophylline
D-propoxyphene		
Methylsalicylate		**Plants, Animals, Herbicides, Insecticides**
Phenylbutazone	Carbromal	
Salicylic Acid	Chloral Hydrate	
	Chlorpromazine	
Cardiovascular	(Diazepam)	Amanitin
	Diphenhydramine	Chlordane
Digoxin	Ethchlorvynol	Demeton Sulfoxide
(Disopyramide)	Glutethimide	Dimethoate
N-acetylprocainamide	Meprobamate	Methylparathion
Procainamide	Methaqualone	Nitrostigmine
Quinidine	Methsuximide	Organophosphates
Flecainide	Methyprylon	Phalliodin
	Promethazine	Paraquat
		Parathion

( ), not well removed; ( )*, removed with chelating agent.

In general, coated-charcoal hemoperfusion devices cause less complications than all other charcoal-sorbent forms. Hemoperfusion should be reserved for lipid-soluble drugs such as barbiturates, and for nonhypnotic sedatives and tranquilizers, digoxin, theophylline, and *N*-acetylprocainamide (NAPA). A comparison of the relative efficiency of hemodialysis and hemoperfusion in the removal of various agents is illustrated in Tables 94.11 and 94.12.

Plasma Exchanges and Exchange Transfusion. Plasma exchange refers to the removal of large quantities of plasma (usually 2 to 5 L) from a patient and replacement by either fresh-frozen or stored plasma. Plasmapheresis is different from plasma exchange in which solutions other than plasma are used as replacement fluids. This technique was initially introduced in the 1950s and widely used thereafter for treatment of varieties of medical conditions in which circulating factors were thought to be contributing to their pathogenesis. Both techniques have been

TABLE 94.10. Types of Hemoperfusion Devices Available Worldwide

Manufacturer	Device	Amount of Sorbent Type	Sorbent
Braun	XR-004	XAD-4 resin	350 g
Chang-collodion	ACAC	Merck charcoal	300 g
Gambro	Adsorba	Norit	100 or 300 g
NMC	Hemocart	Petroleum-based charcoal	140 g
Organon-Teknika	Hemopur 260	Norit-extruded charcoal	260 g
Smith and Nephew	Hemocol or Haemocol	Sutcliffe Speakman charcoal	102 or 300 g

TABLE 94.11. Plasma Drug Extraction with Different Hemodialysis/Hemoperfusion Devices[a]

Drug	Charcoal Hemodialysis	Coated or Uncoated Hemoperfusion	Resin Hemoperfusion
Acetaminophen	0.4	0.5	0.7
Acetylsalicylic acid	0.5	0.5	—
Carbromal	0.31	0.55	1
Digoxin	0.2	0.3–0.6	0.4
Ethchlorvynol	0.32	0.7	1
Glutethimide	0.16	0.65	0.8
Paraquat	0.5	0.6	0.9
Phenobarbital	0.27	0.5	0.85
Theophylline	0.5	0.7	0.75
Tricyclics	0.35	0.35	0.8

[a] Calculated for BFR 200 ml/min.

TABLE 94.12. Plasma Concentrations of Common Poisons in Excess of Which Hemodialysis (HD) or Hemoperfusion (HP) Should Be Considered

Drug	Serum Concentration (μg/ml)	Method of Choice
Glutethimide	40	HP
Lithium	3.5 mEq/L[a]	HD
Meprobamate	100	HP
Methaqualone	40	HP
Methanol	50	HD
Paraquat	0.1	HP > HD
Salicylates	800	HD
Phenobarbital	100	HP > HD
Theophylline	400	HP > HD
Trichloroethanol	50	HP > HD

[a] Although hemodialysis is indicated with plasma lithium concentration of more than 2.5 mEq/L in symptomatic patients or in those who have renal insufficiency.

used infrequently in the treatment of intoxications and their roles remain unclear. They are predominantly used in intoxication with drugs that have high protein-binding affinity and are poorly dialyzable (as with chromic acid and chromate poisoning). Also they are used when hemolysis and methemoglobinemia have complicated the poisoning (sodium-chlorate poisoning).

Hemoperfusion and Hemodialysis with Chelating Agents. In dialysis patients, aluminum and iron intoxication can be treated with deferoxamine in conjunction with hemoperfusion or dialysis (hemodialysis or peritoneal dialysis). The goal is removal of deferoxamine–aluminum complex with clinical improvement in anemia, renal osteodystrophy, encephalopathy, and hemosiderosis. During hemodialysis, metal removal may be enhanced with certain chelating agents, such as *N*-acetylcysteine or cysteine. On the other hand, removal of mercury and thallium by hemoperfusion appears modest at best.

Continuous Hemodiafiltration and Hemoperfusion. Because of their low efficacy, continuous therapies are rarely indicated in the treatment of drug intoxication. However, they are beneficial in combination with hemodialysis or hemoperfusion for substances with slow diffusion from tissue, large volumes of distribution, or delayed cell-membrane transport. The use of continuous hemoperfusion therapy was found to be simpler, safer, more effective, and less expensive than the conventional hemoperfusion. With continuous arteriovenous hemoperfusion (CAVHP), blood is accessed through the femoral artery, pumped through a hemoperfusion cartridge, and returned via the femoral vein to the patient. The systemic blood pressure is the driving force, delivering a blood flow rate of 90 to 150 ml/min.

With continuous venovenous hemodiafiltration (CVVHD) or hemoperfusion (CVVHP), access is readily obtained by a dual-lumen catheter inserted into a central vein. Here a blood pump is used to provide adequate blood flow (100 to 200 ml/min) or to create sufficient transmembrane pressure (TMP). The hemoperfusion cartridge may need to be changed every 4 hours to prevent saturation. Continuous therapies have been used for intoxication with methotrexate and procainamide. Continuous hemodiafiltration with an increased dialysate flow to 4 L/hr is an effective alternative to intermittent hemodialysis for the treatment of lithium poisoning. The long treatment time and gradual removal of intracellular lithium completely avoids the postdialysis rebound.

Immunoadsorption. Specific adsorption of immune proteins on antigen-coated or antibody-coated carrier particles in hemoperfusion columns have been developed, allowing the specific removal of antibodies or drugs. Monoclonal antidigoxin antibodies covalently coupled to agarose polyacrolein microsphere beads have been used with success in digoxin overdose in humans. The role of this technique remains to be defined.

Selected Readings

Chow MT, Di Silvestro VA, Yung CY, et al. Treatment of acute methanol intoxication with hemodialysis using an ethanol-enriched, bicarbonate-based dialysate. *Am J Kidney Dis* 1997;30:568.

A very important article that determines the utility of using ethanol-enriched, bicarbonate-based dialysate in treating acute methanol intoxication.

Chyka PA. Evaluation of a porcine model to study repeat-dose activated charcoal therapy. *Vet Hum Toxicol* 1993;35:367.

A useful article that demonstrates the role of multiple doses of activated charcoal in treatment of poisoning.

Haddad LM, Shannon MW, Winchester JF, eds. *Clinical management of poisoning and drug overdose*, 3rd ed. Philadelphia: WB Saunders, 1998:175–188.

A comprehensive text on approaches and general and specific management of various poisons.

Hylander B, Kjellstrand CM. Prognostic factors and treatment of severe ethylene glycol intoxication. *Intensive Care Med* 1996;22:546.

A collaborative study featuring certain prognostic factors that determine outcome in patients with ethylene glycol intoxication.

Jambou P, Levraut J, Favier C, et al. Removal of methotrexate by continuous venovenous hemodiafiltration. *Contrib Nephrol* 1995;116:48.

An excellent study that determines the use of continuous renal replacement therapy in treating methotrexate overdose.

Krik M, Pace S. Pearls, pitfalls, and updates in toxicology. *Emerg Med Clin North Am* 1997;15:427.

Interesting review of some common pitfalls in clinical toxicology. It also provides an update in the emerging role of N-acetylcysteine and some other new antidotes.

Litovitz TL, Klein-Shwartz W. Annual report of the American Association of Poison Control Centers Toxic Exposure Surveillance System. *Am J Emerg Med* 1998;16:443.

The most up-to-date survey of poisoning incidence in the United States and an appreciation of current practices in the field of intoxication.

Ohning BL. Continuous nasogastric administration of activated charcoal for the treatment of theophylline intoxication. *Pediatr Pharmacol* 1986;5:241.

The cornerstone study that established the unmistakable role of activated charcoal in managing acute theophylline intoxication.

Pond SM, Lewis-Driver D, Williams G. Gastric emptying in acute overdose: prospective randomised controlled trial. *Med J of Aus* 1995;163:345.

A reference study that clearly demonstrates the importance of activated charcoal in managing acute intoxicated patients and has defined the role of gastric emptying in the treatment of such cases.

Shannon MW. Comparative efficacy of hemodialysis and hemoperfusion in severe theophylline intoxication. *Acad Emerg Med* 1997;4:674–678.

A standard study that determines the efficacy of hemoperfusion over hemodialysis in the treatment of theophylline intoxication.

CHAPTER 95

Plasmapheresis

Andre A. Kaplan

RATIONALE

Therapeutic plasma exchange (TPE) is a technique designed for the removal of large-molecular-weight substances such as pathogenic autoantibodies, immune complexes, cryoglobulins, myeloma light chains, endotoxin, and cholesterol-containing lipoproteins. The basic premise is that removal of these substances will promote the reversal of the pathologic processes related to their presence. Other potential benefits for TPE include an unloading of the reticuloendothelial system, stimulation of lymphocyte clones to enhance cytotoxic therapy, and the possibility of reinfusing large volumes of plasma without the risk of intravascular volume overload.

For TPE to be a rational choice as a blood purification technique, at least one of the following conditions should be met:

1. The substance to be removed is sufficiently large (in excess of 15,000 D) in order to make other purification techniques unacceptably inefficient (i.e., hemofiltration or high-flux dialysis).
2. The substance to be removed has a comparatively prolonged half-life, so that extracorporeal removal provides a therapeutically useful period of diminished serum concentration.
3. The substance to be removed is acutely toxic and resistant to conventional therapy, thus the rapidity of extracorporeal removal is clinically indicated.

The removal of pathogenic autoantibodies offers an example. Considering that the natural half-life of IgG is approximately 21 days and assuming that an immunosuppressive agent could immediately halt production (unlikely), the serum levels would still be 50% of the initial values for at least 21 days after initiating therapy. Such a delay might be unacceptable in the presence of a very aggressive autoantibody such as that involved with Goodpasture's syndrome.

COMPLICATIONS

The most common complications are citrate-induced paresthesias, muscle cramps, and urticaria (Table 95.1). Serious complications are reported at a rate of 0.025% to 0.2% and include life-threatening anaphylactoid reactions that are most commonly associated with the use of plasma-containing replacement fluids (e.g., fresh-frozen plasma, purified protein fraction). The overall incidence of death is 0.05% but some of these "treatment-associated" deaths were in patients with severe preexisting conditions and the treatment itself may not have been the precipitating factor.

Anaphylactic Reactions to Protein-Containing Replacement Fluids

Large volumes of fresh-frozen plasma (FFP) from many different donors (four to five donors per liter) increase the risk of anaphylactoid reactions. Patients with severe and repetitive reactions to FFP can be pretreated with ephedrine, prednisone, and diphenhydramine. Our own protocol prescribes oral doses of 50 mg of prednisone given 13 hours, 7 hours, and 1 hour before the treatment, combined with 50 mg of diphenhydramine

TABLE 95.1. Complications of Plasmapheresis

Symptom	Percentage
Urticaria	0.7–12
Paresthesias	1.5–9
Muscle Cramps	0.4–2.5
Dizziness	<2.5
Headaches	0.3–5
Nausea	0.1–1
Hypotension	0.4–4.2
Chest pain	0.03–1.3
Arrhythmia	0.1–0.7
Anaphylactoid reactions	0.03–0.7
Rigors	1.1–8.8
Hyperthermia	0.7–1.0
Bronchospasm	0.1–0.4
Seizure	0.03–0.4
Respiratory arrest/pulmonary edema	0.2–0.3
Myocardial ischemia	0.1
Shock/myocardial infarction	0.1–1.5
Metabolic alkalosis	0.03
DIC	0.03
Central nervous system ischemia	0.03–0.1
Hepatitis	0.7
Hemorrhage	0.2
Hypoxemia	0.1
Pulmonary embolism	0.1
Access Related	
Thrombosis/hemorrhage	0.02–0.7
Infection	0.3
Pneumothorax	0.1
Mechanical	0.08–4

Data extracted from more than 15,000 treatments.

Adapted with permission from Mokrzycki MH, Kaplan AA. Therapeutic plasma exchange: complications and management. *Am J Kidney Dis* 1994; 23:817.

DIC, disseminated intravascular coagulation.

and 25 mg of ephedrine given 1 hour before the treatment. In the event of a severe life-threatening reaction (e.g., laryngeal edema), 0.3 to 0.5 ml of epinephrine should be available for subcutaneous administration.

Depletion Syndromes

Intensive replacement of plasma with albumin will yield a depletion coagulopathy as evidenced by marked elevations of the prothrombin times and partial thromboplastin times. Thus the patient with a recent renal biopsy or with significant pulmonary hemorrhage may benefit from substituting 1 to 2 L of FFP as the replacement fluid toward the end of the procedure (each unit of FFP is approximately 200 to 250 ml). One potential complication with FFP (14% citrate by volume) is the development of metabolic alkalosis because the infused citrate will produce bicarbonate, the excretion of which may be limited by concurrent renal failure. This alkalosis may also occur if citrate is used as the anticoagulant during the procedure, as is commonly done with centrifugal apheresis equipment.

TPE will also induce a substantial lowering of serum immunoglobulin levels, a condition that may predispose to or exacerbate an intercurrent infection. If the infection is severe, a single infusion of immunoglobulin (100 to 400 mg/kg) will partially replenish antibody levels that were reduced by the exchanges. Continued apheresis will eventually deplete these infused immunoglobulins.

RENAL INDICATIONS FOR THERAPEUTIC PLASMA EXCHANGE

Anti–Glomerular Basement Membrane Antibody–Mediated Disease (Goodpasture's Syndrome)

Despite the existence of only one, randomized, controlled study of plasma exchange as an adjunct to immunosuppressive therapy for antiglomerular basement membrane (GBM) antibody–mediated glomerulonephritis, the available data are generally in agreement that plasma exchange is useful in providing a more rapid decline in anti-GBM antibody, a lower posttreatment serum creatinine level, and a decreased incidence of end-stage renal disease (ESRD). TPE has also been found to have a beneficial effect on the course of severe pulmonary hemorrhage in this disease. The best correlation with a positive renal outcome is the initiation of therapy before the onset of severe renal impairment. Avoidance of ESRD is uncommon if treatment is begun after serum creatinine exceeds 7 mg/dl. Some patients presenting with severe renal impairment have responded to therapy if the presentation is very acute or if there are signs of associated vasculitis and anti–neutrophil cytoplasmic antibodies (ANCA). In a study of 889 cases of rapidly progressive glomerulonephritis, 67 patients were positive for anti-GBM antibodies in whom 20 (30%) were also positive for ANCA.

TPE is prescribed to provide a rapid lowering of the anti-GBM antibody and as a means of reducing the serum concentrations of other potentially detrimental inflammatory mediators, such as complement. Immunosuppression with steroids, cyclophosphamide, or azathioprine is essential as a means of slowing the production of the anti-GBM antibody and decreasing the inflammatory response. The recommended initial prescription is 14 daily 4-L exchanges. Further plasmapheresis may be unnecessary if serum creatinine levels have decreased and there is a marked decline in serum anti-GBM antibody titers. In contrast, continued apheresis may be required if antibody titers are still elevated.

Crescentic, Rapidly Progressive Glomerulonephritis (Not Associated With Anti-GBM Antibody)

Treatment of rapidly progressive glomerulonephritis (RPGN) often involves steroids and some form of immunosuppressive regimen. TPE has been investigated as a means to hasten the removal of pathogenic autoantibodies, immune complexes, and other inflammatory mediators such as complement and fibrinogen. In general, TPE has been a relatively safe but costly addition to more conventional treatment regimens. This added expense should be viewed in the context of the eventual long-term cost of maintenance dialysis for those patients whose outcome will terminate with ESRD.

Despite favorable uncontrolled reports, the results of four randomized, controlled studies failed to demonstrate a generalized benefit for TPE in the treatment of non–anti-GBM–associated RPGN when added to standard immunosuppressive therapy. Nonetheless, in all of these studies, subset analysis reveals that TPE was found to be beneficial for those patients presenting with severe disease or dialysis dependency (Table 95.2). As an example, in one study, 48 patients with crescentic glomerulonephritis without anti-GBM disease and other well-defined vasculitides, systemic lupus erythematosus (SLE) and Henoch-Schönlein purpura were excluded. The clinical diagnoses were that of Wegener's granulomatosis, microscopic polyarteritis, and idiopathic RPGN (ANCA values not reported). In 25 patients, plasma exchange was initiated with five 4-L exchanges in the first week with a subsequent mean total of 9 treatments per patient (range 5 to 25). Prednisolone, cyclophosphamide, and azathioprine were administered to all 48 patients. Results revealed no outcome difference in those patients in which treatment was initiated when serum creatinines were less than 500 μmol/L (5.8 mg/dl). Of those patients who were originally dialysis dependent, however, 10 of 11 receiving TPE recovered renal function, whereas only 3 of 8 in the non-TPE group recovered to a similar degree ($P = .04$). Thus the results of this study and three

TABLE 95.2. Controlled Trials of TPE for Patients with Severe or Dialysis Dependent RPGN[a]

Trial	Index of Severity	TPE	No TPE
Mauri et al. 1985	Creatinine >9		
Initial creatinine (number of pts.)		13.5 (6)	13.1 (5)
Creatinine after 3 years		8.7[b]	13.4
Glockner et al. 1988	Dialysis dependent		
Initial creatinine (number of pts.)		7.4 (8)	9.2 (4)
Creatinine after 6 months		1.7[b]	5.5
Pusey et al. 1991	Dialysis dependent		
Initial number of pts. on dialysis		11	8
Pts. off dialysis at 12 months		10[c]	3
Cole et al. 1992	Dialysis dependent		
Initial number of pts. on dialysis		4	7
Pts. off dialysis at 12 months		3	2

All studies had concomitant treatment with steroids and immunosuppressive agents.

[a] Subset analysis, most patients with "idiopathic" RPGN, creatinine values in mg/dl.

[b] = $P < .05$ with day 0, [c] = $P < .05$ TPE versus no TPE, pts = patients, TPE = therapeutic plasma exchange.

Modified from Kaplan AA. Therapeutic apheresis 1997;1:255–259.

RPGN, rapidly progressive glomerulonephritis; TPE, therapeutic plasma exchange.

other controlled trials supports the use of TPE in RPGN only in those patients presenting with severe renal failure or dialysis dependency.

Renal Failure in Multiple Myeloma

After a reasonable diagnostic evaluation to rule out other common causes of myeloma-associated renal failure, including a therapeutic trial of hydration, patients with myeloma-associated renal failure and elevated *serum* levels of free light chains may have myeloma "cast nephropathy." The enhanced removal of light chains by TPE, in conjunction with a proper antineoplastic regimen (usually steroids with melphalan or cyclophosphamide), has been demonstrated to provide a more likely return of renal function and a better overall survival. In a randomized, controlled trial of 29 patients with mean pretreatment serum creatinine levels of 11 mg/dl, 13 of 15 patients treated with plasmapheresis (3 to 4 L of plasma exchanged on 5 consecutive days) had substantial return of renal function (to a mean creatinine of 2.6 mg/dl) within 2 months, whereas improvement occurred in only 2 of 14 treated without plasmapheresis.

Well-established renal failure considered to be due to cast nephropathy may respond less dramatically, but a combination of TPE and chemotherapy has been successful if treatment is initiated before the onset of oligoanuria. Renal biopsy to determine the density of cast formation may be useful as a guide to predict an eventual response to TPE.

IgA Nephropathy and Henoch-Schönlein Purpura

The removal of circulating IgA complexes by plasma exchange has been advocated as a maintenance strategy for the management of IgA-related disease but current treatment modalities such as fish oil and angiotensin-converting enzyme (ACE) inhibitors have eclipsed TPE as a treatment option for chronic, progressive IgA nephropathy.

The usefulness of TPE as a treatment for acute disease remains unresolved. There are seven case reports in which RPGN was successfully treated with TPE alone, without concomitant immunosuppression. Although there is no randomized, controlled trial for evaluation, the available data suggest a possible beneficial effect of TPE in the treatment of IgA-associated RPGN. A reasonable initial prescription would be to perform TPE thrice weekly for 3 weeks and then once weekly.

Focal Segmental Glomerulosclerosis: Recurrence Posttransplant

It has been estimated that 15% to 55% of all patients with ESRD secondary to focal segmental glomerular sclerosis (FSGS) will have a rapid recurrence of proteinuria after renal transplantation. Some of these patients may have a circulating protein that is capable of increasing glomerular permeability to albumin. The protein has been characterized to have a molecular weight of less than 100,000 Daltons and is therefore not an immunoglobulin. Nonetheless, a trial of immunoadsorption using a regenerating protein A column (ostensibly designed for the removal of three of subclasses of IgG) was capable of transiently lowering the level of proteinuria in patients with recurrent FSGS after transplantation. In a subsequent report, standard plasma exchange was performed in patients soon after the recurrence of proteinuria in the immediate posttransplant period. Patients were treated with plasma exchange equaling 1.5 plasma volumes for 3 consecutive days followed by every-other-day treatments for a total of nine exchanges. Six of nine patients treated within 1 week of the onset of proteinuria had a mean reduction in urinary protein from 11.5 to 0.8 g/day; with at least one patient maintaining normal allograft histology for up to 27 months after treatment. Two patients relapsed and then responded to a repeat course of plasmapheresis. Two of the three nonresponders (as opposed to one of six responders) already had glomerular hyalinosis on renal biopsy. The authors concluded that plasma exchange is likely to be effective in the treatment of recurrent FSGS if therapy is initiated promptly after the initiation of proteinuria and there is no significant hyalinosis on preplasmapheresis biopsy.

Renal Allograft Rejection

The assumed role of cytotoxic antibodies as mediators of acute vascular rejection has prompted several attempts to employ plasma exchange as a means of enhancing antirejection therapy. Unfortunately, at least two controlled trials of TPE for acute vascular rejection did not find this treatment to be useful. In contrast, others added cyclophosphamide to the standard methylprednisolone pulse therapy and found that the addition of three to seven plasmapheresis treatments for antibody-associated rejection resulted in a more rapid decline in antihuman leukocyte antigen (anti-HLA) antibodies, a greater improvement in renal function, and an improved graft survival. These episodes of acute rejection, however, were not typical because the mean interval between transplantation and the onset of rejection was 11 months. There are no trials of TPE for acute rejection in the cyclosporine era.

Several recent publications have suggested a role for photopheresis in the treatment of acute and recurrent renal allograft rejection, a situation that may mirror the encouraging reports, suggesting a role for this technique in the management of heart transplant rejection.

The Transplant Candidate with Cytotoxic Antibodies

High levels of preformed cytotoxic antibodies against donor ABO, HLA class I, and perhaps other antigens preclude successful real transplantation because of the risk of hyperacute rejection. Despite the theoretic risk of *de novo* resynthesis after transplantation, several investigators have attempted to manage this problem by the use of protein A columns for the immunoadsorption of plasma reactive antibodies (PRA). Some investigators prescribed an average of 6 immunoadsorbent treatments to lower PRA levels but results were hampered by a high *de novo* rate of resynthesis. Nonetheless, with the concomitant administration of cyclophosphamide and prednisolone, 7 of 12 patients were transplantable with a graft survival of 86%. Others reported that four of five hypersensitized patients undergoing this procedure had successful transplants with stable serum creatinines for up to 34 months.

It should be noted that these treatments were performed with a device allowing for the continued regeneration of the protein A columns resulting in a substantial lowering of PRA levels. This device is not currently available in the United States and should not be confused with the Prosorba protein A column, which has a very limited immunoadsorbent capability.

Despite the potential usefulness of this approach, the limited amount of available data would lead one to conclude that this aggressive and unconfirmed protocol should not be attempted outside of a well-designed experimental study.

Cryoglobulinemia

There has never been a randomized, controlled study of plasmapheresis for cryoglobulinemia, but numerous successful case reports, uncontrolled studies, and the opinions of the most experienced investigators have led to a general consensus that TPE is a useful adjunct for the treatment of severe, active disease as manifested by progressive renal failure, coalescing purpura, or advanced neuropathy.

In general, TPE is performed in conjunction with the administration of steroids and immunosuppressive agents, but the implication of hepatitis C viral infection as an etiologic factor for mixed "essential" cryoglobulinemia suggests that immunosuppressive agents may be detrimental and it may be time to reconsider their use. Indeed, ourselves and others have witnessed the rapid resolution of nephritic renal failure and severe purpuric lesions with TPE alone, without the concomitant use of steroids or immunosuppressive agents.

A reasonable plasmapheresis prescription is to exchange one plasma volume three times weekly for 2 to 3 weeks. The replacement fluid can be 5% albumin, which must be warmed to prevent precipitation of circulating cryoglobulins. Selective removal techniques can be used to eliminate or minimize the need for replacement fluid.

There is evidence that interferon-α can lead to a reduction in circulating cryoglobulin levels and clinical remission. Unfortunately, disease activity can recur after discontinuation of interferon. Considering the delayed onset of clinical response to the reinitiation of interferon, TPE can be useful as the initial, immediate therapy for these exacerbations.

THROMBOTIC THROMBOCYTOPENIC PURPURA AND HEMOLYTIC UREMIC SYNDROME

Thrombotic Thrombocytopenic Purpura

Thrombotic thrombocytopenic purpura (TTP) is a syndrome characterized by thrombocytopenia, microangiopathic hemolytic anemia, neurologic abnormalities, fever, and renal dysfunction. There is currently a general agreement in the literature that plasma exchange with replacement by FFP or cryosupernatant is the treatment of choice. Before the use of plasmapheresis, mortality with TTP was as high as 90%.

The pathogenesis of the microthrombotic lesions of TTP are only incompletely understood, and it remains unclear whether the major factor in the pathogenic platelet aggregation is the presence of a procoagulant factor or the absence of an antithrombotic factor. As a result, controversy remains whether treatment should be aimed at removing the procoagulant(s) or replacing the antithrombotic factor(s). Translating this controversy to available treatment options, it is still unresolved whether plasma exchange or plasma infusion is the best treatment for TTP.

In the largest controlled trial of its type, 102 patients were randomized to receive either plasma exchange with FFP or plasma infusion alone (the Canadian Apheresis group). All patients also received aspirin and dipyridamole. Because plasma infusion alone was limited by the onset of intravascular volume overload, the patients receiving plasma exchange received three times the amount of plasma. At 6 months, the remission rate and survival rate was statistically higher in the group receiving plasma exchange (78% versus 31% remission, and 78% versus 50% for survival). Unfortunately, the results of the aforementioned trial do not answer the question of whether plasma exchange is more beneficial than plasma infusion alone, because the plasma-exchange group received more plasma than the infusion group.

In general, plasma exchange *with FFP replacement* is performed daily until the platelet count is normalized and hemolysis has largely ceased, as evidenced in part by a LDH level below 400 and the disappearance of schistocytes on the peripheral blood smear. On average, 7 to 16 daily exchanges are required to induce remission. The recommended volume to be exchanged is 1.5 times the estimated plasma volume for the first three treatments followed by one plasma volume exchanges thereafter. There is an early relapse rate of approximately 40% with decreases in platelet counts occurring in a mean of 5 days.

It has been suggested that the infusion of large amounts of von Willebrand's factor (vWF) in the FFP may promote further platelet aggregation. Thus in patients resistant to an initial trial of TPE treatments, the use of cryosupernatant may be preferable because vWF is largely removed in the cryoprecipitate.

TTP in Pregnancy

The differential diagnosis of thrombocytopenia in pregnancy includes chronic TTP, hemolytic uremic syndrome (HUS), intermittent thrombocytopenic purpura, preeclampsia with HELLP syndrome (hemolysis, elevated liver enzymes and thrombocytopenia), and Evan's syndrome. Considering the dismal prognosis of TTP in pregnancy before the initiation of plasma manipulations (1of 27 maternal survivors after 2 years, only 7 of 25 fetal survivors) and the clear superiority of TPE in the nonpregnant patients, plasma exchange is also the treatment of choice for TTP during pregnancy.

Hemolytic Uremic Syndrome in Adults

Distinction between adult HUS and TTP can be difficult but may be possible when a clear etiologic agent can be identified, such as the association of HUS with the verotoxin produced by *Escherichia coli* O157-H7, or by the presence of certain inciting drugs such as cyclosporine, mitomycin, cisplatinum, quinine, or oral contraceptives or associated diseases (SLE, carcinoma). In contrast with HUS in children, the prognosis of HUS in the adult is poor, with an estimated mortality between 25% and 50% and an incidence of ESRD of up to 40% in the remaining survivors. A review combining TTP and HUS found that dialysis was required in 11 of 68 cases. Of these 11, four expired during hospitalization but five of the remaining seven were able to come off dialysis after a period ranging between 4 and 120 days. The authors suggest that the poorer renal outcome was obtained before the general use of TPE. Considering the difficulty in distinguishing adult HUS from TTP and the similarity in their pathology and mortality, it would seem prudent to approach the treatment of HUS in a similar fashion as with TTP (i.e., the early and intensive initiation of plasma exchange).

Mitomycin-Induced, Cancer-Associated HUS

An exceptional situation may exist in the context of mitomycin-induced, cancer-associated HUS, in which plasma perfusion over the Prosorba protein A column has been reported to be more effective than standard plasma exchange. In an uncontrolled trial of 11 patients with this condition, protein A immunoadsorption was found to be successful in nine patients, with a stabilization of progressive renal failure achieved in six of these nine.

Recurrent HUS in Renal Transplantation

Recurrent HUS in patients having received a renal transplant after losing renal function to an original episode of HUS is a well-documented problem. In the differential diagnosis of HUS in the renal transplant patient is acute vascular rejection of the allograft, cyclosporine, FK506, or antilymphocyte antibody nephrotoxicity and malignant hypertension. An extensive review of the literature revealed 19 reports describing 68 cases and suggested that TPE remains an efficacious treatment but the end points for terminating the treatments are not well defined.

HUS in Children

HUS is a major cause of acute renal failure in the pediatric population and often follows an episode of bloody diarrhea as a result of infection with a verotoxin-producing *E. coli* (type O157-H7). The prognosis with supportive therapy is generally good, but there remains a small percentage of patients suffering strokes or significant renal failure. There have been no randomized, controlled trials of plasma exchange as a therapy for childhood HUS. Retrospective analysis and anecdotal reports, however, suggest that TPE may be beneficial in limiting the incidence of significant renal damage in those children considered to be at particularly high risk, such as those who present without a diarrheal prodrome or those older than 5 years of age. Children with significant central nervous system involvement may also benefit from plasma exchange. Successful TPE prescription for children older than 5 years of age is reported to be a median of 4.5 TPE treatments (range 3 to 10) with a median of 1 L of plasma exchanged per session (range 200 to 2,000 ml).

Systemic Lupus Erythematosus

Despite early reports suggesting a positive effect of plasma exchange on severe lupus nephritis, several randomized, controlled trials could not document any therapeutic benefit of TPE. The largest and most recent of these involved the randomization of 86 patients with severe lupus nephritis. All 86 received similar conventional therapy with prednisone and cyclophosphamide, whereas 40 of these 86 underwent plasma exchange three times weekly for the first 4 weeks of treatment. Despite a more rapid decline in double-stranded DNA titers, 25% in the TPE-treated group developed renal failure as compared with only 17% in those not receiving TPE. Thus the weight of the currently available evidence suggests that standard regimens of TPE are not beneficial as a general adjunct to conventional immunosuppressive therapy for lupus nephritis. TPE may still be useful for the treatment of lupus-associated TTP, for the treatment of symptoms associated with the lupus anticoagulant, or as a means of controlling the disease during pregnancy when cytotoxic agents are undesirable.

Of pending interest are the results of an ambitious international trial that was designed to take advantage of a proposed apheresis-induced antibody rebound. The protocol involves the withdrawal of cytotoxic and steroid therapy, 3 days of TPE followed by 3 days of pulse cyclophosphamide with up to 6 months of oral dosing. The rationale is that pathogenic lymphocytes will be stimulated during the postpheresis period, thus being more susceptible to subsequent cyclophosphamide therapy. There were 170 patients enrolled, and the trial has been completed but official results have yet to be published.

Lupus Anticoagulant, Anticardiolipin Antibodies, and the Antiphospholipid Antibody Syndrome

The lupus anticoagulant and the anticardiolipin antibody are antiphospholipid antibodies that are associated with the development of recurrent arterial and venous thromboses, thrombocytopenia, recurrent fetal loss, and, on occasion, renal disease. Systemic coagulation can result in multiple organ involvement and the "catastrophic antiphospholipid syndrome." An analysis of more than 1,000 patients with SLE found a 34% frequency for the lupus anticoagulant and a 44% frequency for the anticardiolipin antibody. Nonetheless, 65% of patients with antiphospholipid antibodies (APA) do not have lupus or a lupus-like disease. In this group, the most common associations are with other autoimmune diseases, certain drugs (chlorpromazine, procainamide, hydralazine), and neoplastic disorders. Considering that the lupus anticoagulants are IgG, IgA, or IgM antibodies, several investigators have used TPE as a means of treating the disorder. TPE has been reported to be successful for the removal of APA in order to avoid spontaneous abortion and recurrent fetal loss and for the management of the catastrophic antiphospholipid syndrome (CAPS).

Although the majority of patients with SLE-associated nephritis and APA will have renal disease compatible with the standard World Health Organization (WHO) classification of lupus nephritis, there will be a small subset whose glomerular pathology is associated with intraglomerular thrombi characteristic of a thrombotic microangiopathy. In an in-depth study of the different types of APA and lupus nephritis, intraglomerular thrombi were associated with IgG APA. Anecdotal reports of TPE for removal of APA have been successful and, despite the paucity of information, if APAs are associated with an intraglomerular thrombotic microangiopathy, the available data do suggest the possibility of improving renal outcome with the successful lowering of the APA levels. Actual prescription of TPE will depend on the individual patient presentation, but a reasonable schedule is three to five treatments over a 7-day period.

Scleroderma

Two separate reports have described the coexistence of scleroderma and a particular type of normotensive, normoreninemic renal disease (i.e., not compatible with scleroderma renal crises) in which the patients were positive for ANCA. In both of these reports, TPE seemed to offer clinical benefit.

Vasculitis

Polyarteritis nodosa (PN) associated with hepatitis B infection has been successfully treated with vidarabine and TPE. During the first 3 weeks of treatment, 14 TPE treatments were performed, followed by three sessions per week for 2 weeks then two sessions per week for 2 weeks. Vidarabine was given by continuous infusion at 15 mg/kg/day for 7 days, then 7.5 mg/kg/day for 14 days. During subsequent weeks, TPE was performed once or twice a week. In 18 of 25 patients, the treatment was effective. Although unsubstantiated by a randomized, controlled trial, this type of antiviral/TPE approach is particularly appealing for hepatitis B–associated PN because it avoids the use of steroids or immunosuppressive agents that may facilitate viral replication and the development of a chronic hepatitis B virus infection. Another study by the same authors replaced vidarabine with interferon-α, an equally appealing approach.

TPE for the Treatment of Intoxications Involving Renal Failure

As a general rule, TPE is only an efficient blood purification treatment for those poisons or drugs that have a high percentage of protein binding and a relatively modest volume of distribution (less than 0.6 L/kg). An example is cisplatin, which is 90% protein bound and has a volume of distribution of 0.5 L/kg and for which TPE has been employed for treating accidental, massive overdose. Occasionally, TPE may be useful as a means of treating the results of intoxication, as in the rapid removal of free hemoglobin in the case of massive hemolysis such as induced by intoxications with arsine (Coombs' positive hemolytic anemia), sodium chlorate (methemoglobinemia), or the mushroom, *Paxillus involutus.* TPE has also been used for the removal of nephrotoxins related to several other mushrooms, such as *Amanita phalloides, Amanita verna,* and *Cortinarius.*

Selected Readings

Agarwal A, Mauer SM, Matas AJ, et al. Recurrent hemolytic uremic syndrome in an adult renal allograft recipient: current concepts and management. *J Am Soc Nephrol* 1995;6:1160–1169.

Exhaustive literature review of recurrent hemolytic uremic syndrome (HUS) in the renal transplant recipient.

Artero ML, Sharma R, Savin VJ, et al. Focal segmental glomerulosclerosis in renal transplants. *Am J Kidney Dis* 1994;23:574–581.

Therapeutic plasma exchange (TPE) for the treatment of recurrent focal segmental glomerular sclerosis (FSGS) in the early posttransplant period.

Coppo R, Basolo B, Roccatello D, et al. Plasma exchange in primary IgA nephropathy and Henoch-Schönlein syndrome nephritis. *Plasma Ther Transfus Technol* 1985;6:705–723.

Primary data and literature review describing the use of TPE as a treatment for IgA nephropathy.

Gianviti A, Perna A, Caringella A, et al. Plasma exchange in children with hemolytic-uremic syndrome at risk of poor outcome. *Am J Kidney Dis* 1993;22:264–266.

Retrospective analysis of TPE for the treatment of HUS in children. Defines high-risk patients likely to benefit.

Kaplan AA. *A practical guide to therapeutic plasma exchange.* Malden, MA: Blackwell Science Inc., 1999.

Extensive review of technical aspects and clinical indications for TPE. Exhaustively referenced.

Lewis EJ, Hunsicker LG, Lan SP, et al., & the Lupus Nephritis Collaborative Study Group. A controlled trial of plasmapheresis therapy in severe lupus nephritis. *N Eng J Med* 1992;326: 1373–1379.

Prospective, randomized, controlled trial of TPE in the treatment of diffuse proliferative lupus nephritis.

Madore F, Lazarus J M, Brady HR. Therapeutic plasma exchange in renal disease. *J Am Soc Nephrol* 1996;7:367–386.

Exhaustive literature review of the use of TPE in renal disease. State of the art.

Mokrzycki MH, Kaplan AA. Therapeutic plasma exchange: complications and management. *Am J Kidney Dis* 1994;23:817–827.

Extensive literature review involving more than 15,000 treatments. Detailed discussion of the mechanisms of complications and guidelines for their avoidance and management.

Pusey CD, Rees AJ, Evans DJ, et al. Plasma exchange in focal necrotizing glomerulonephritis without anti-GBM antibodies. *Kidney Int* 1991;40:757–763.

Randomized, controlled study of TPE for vasculitic-related glomerulonephritis.

Rock GA, Shumak KH, Buskard NA, et al. Comparison of plasma exchange with plasma infusion in the treatment of TTP. *N Eng J Med* 1991;325:393–397.

A prospective, randomized, controlled trial involving 102 patients comparing TPE using FFP replacement with FFP replacement alone.

Ross CN, Gaskin G, Gregor-Macgregor S, et al. Renal transplantation following immunoadsorption in highly sensitized recipients. *Transplantation* 1993;55: 785–789.

Small series describing outcome of renal transplantation after lowering of plasma reactive antibodies (PRA) with immunoadsorption.

Savage CO, Pusey CD, Bowman C, et al. Antiglomerular basement membrane antibody-mediated disease in the British Isles 1980–1984. *Br Med J* 1986;292: 301–304.

Extensive experience with the treatment of antiglomerular basement membrane (anti-GBM) disease.

Zucchelli P, Pasquali S, Cagnoli L, et al. Controlled plasma exchange trial in acute renal failure due to multiple myeloma. *Kidney Int* 1988;33:1175–1189.

Prospective, controlled trial of TPE for the treatment of "cast nephropathy."

CHAPTER 96

Renal Biopsy

Richard J. Glassock and Shaul G. Massry

Renal biopsy has become an established part of the diagnostic and prognostic methods available to the nephrologist. Several procedures have been devised to obtain renal tissue. This chapter focuses on percutaneous renal biopsy, which is performed under local anesthesia.

Open surgical biopsy under general or spinal anesthesia is performed only occasionally: when the patient is deemed unsuitable for the percutaneous approach (comatose or very uncooperative and agitated), when the patient has a single kidney, or when a greater amount of renal tissue is needed for study.

A technique involving transvenous renal biopsy has been introduced that can be performed safely when other techniques are difficult or contraindicated (such as massive obesity or coagulation disturbances). In this technique, a biopsy device similar to that used in cardiac biopsy is inserted into a peripheral vein (jugular or femoral), and the device is guided into the renal vein and ultimately wedged into a peripheral location where the biopsy specimen is taken. Bleeding, if it occurs, is confined to the kidney. A satisfactory specimen usually can be obtained, although considerable experience is required to obtain success rates comparable with those of percutaneous needle biopsy of the kidney. At present, this technique is used in few centers that possess the specialized equipment and skill.

Thin-needle aspiration of the cellular elements of the renal tubules and interstitium is widely used to evaluate the status of renal allografts. Using special stains and reagents, this technique has shown great promise in diagnosis of acute tubular necrosis, allograft rejection, and cyclosporine nephrotoxicity, but more definitive evaluation of renal parenchymal disease requires a core of tissue rather than disassociated parenchymal and infiltrating cells. Nevertheless, the technique is simple, easily learned, and safe. Repetitive samples can be obtained with relative ease, thus offering the opportunity for serial observations.

Percutaneous biopsy of the kidney was first performed in the 1950s, but it did not become popular as a diagnostic procedure until the reports of Iversen and Brun and of Muehrcke, Kark, and associates were released. The Vim-Silverman needle was introduced in 1953 and was later modified by Franklin to provide a better core of renal tissue and more reliability. Initially, the renal biopsy was performed with the patient in the sitting position, but the prone position is now used except in late pregnancy. The localization of the kidney was at first done by intravenous urography and measurements, but image-intensified fluoroscopy or ultrasonography is now used for this purpose.

Renal biopsies are seldom diagnostic of a specific disease entity, but rather they provide information on morphologic alterations in the glomeruli, tubules, interstitium, and vasculature that are useful in helping to assess prognosis and guide therapy.

TABLE 96.1. Renal Diseases That May Be Diagnosed By Renal Biopsy

Glomerular and Vascular Diseases
Diabetic nephropathy
Amyloidosis
Light- and heavy-chain disease
Fibrillary/immunotactoid glomerulopathy
Dense deposit disease
Macroglobulinemia
Cryoimmunoglobulinemia
Goodpasture's disease
IgA nephropathy
Henoch-Schönlein purpura
Systemic lupus erythematosus (seldom)
Collageno-fibrotic glomerulopathy
Lipoprotein glomerulopathy
Alport's syndrome
Fabry's disease
Nail-patella syndrome
Lecithin-cholesterol acyltransferase deficiency nephropathy
Thin basement membrane nephropathy
HIV-associated nephropathy
Thrombotic thrombocytopenic purpura
Cholesterol-embolic nephropathy
Tubulointerstitial Diseases
Oxalosis
Cystinosis
Sarcoidosis
Lead nephropathy
Myeloma kidney

HIV, human immunodeficiency virus.

Lesions that are diagnostic of a specific disease entity are limited to those listed in Table 96.1.

INDICATIONS FOR RENAL BIOPSY

It is not possible to provide a list of indications for renal biopsy that will cover the myriad of clinical circumstances in which examination of renal tissue possibly or definitely contributes to patient management, but a few broad comments and suggestions seem appropriate. Certainly, the performance of a renal biopsy should be guided by the individual clinical situation and by careful balancing of potential risks and benefits. Experience and technical skills of the physician performing the biopsy are prerequisites for submitting the patient to the procedure.

Table 96.2 summarizes a variety of clinical situations in which performance of a renal biopsy might be considered. Although universal agreement on these indications could not be obtained, they represent our views and most likely those of a substantial segment of the nephrology community. Undoubtedly, these indications will be modified as additional data become available.

We continue to believe that a renal biopsy should be performed in adults with nephrotic syndrome in whom the cause is not evident after thorough clinical and laboratory evaluation (idiopathic nephrotic syndrome). Although some may propose that empiric glucocorticoid therapy *before* biopsy is appropriate based on group statistical data and decision analysis theory, we recommend that renal biopsy be performed before embarking on an empiric course of glucocorticoids, at least in adults (16 years and older). There are several reasons for this approach: (a) In experienced hands, renal biopsy is safe (one biopsy-related death and two major bleedings requiring surgery occurred in 3,061 biopsies, giving a prevalence of serious complications of 0.03% and 0.06%, respectively). (b) Lesions that are not helped by glucocorticoid therapy or for which such treatment might be harmful, such as amyloidosis, occur in as many as 10% of older adults with otherwise idiopathic nephrotic syndrome. (c) Knowledge of the nature of the lesion may be required for future decisions about the use of adjunctive therapy, such as cyclophosphamide, cyclosporine, or plasma exchange. (d) Examination of the renal tissue may provide useful information on (i) prognosis (IgA nephropathy, focal sclerosis), (ii) potential risks for complications (e.g., renal vein thrombosis and other thromboembolic phenomena in membranous glomerulonephritis), (iii) the presence of a disorder that was not suspected clinically and that may respond to specific therapy (κ-chain glomerulopathy), and (iv) the risk of recurrent disease should the patient become a candidate for renal transplantation.

TABLE 96.2. Indications for Renal Biopsy
Most Useful
Idiopathic nephrotic syndrome in adults *before* empiric therapy
Idiopathic nephrotic syndrome in children unresponsive to glucocorticoids
Rapidly progressive renal failure caused by glomerulonephritis
Evaluation and follow-up of collagen disease, predominantly systemic lupus erythematosus with proteinuria, abnormal urine sediment, or reduced renal function
Glomerular proteinuria of unknown cause accompanied by abnormal urine sediment or quantitative persistent proteinuria of more than 1.0 g/day
Persistent or recurrent glomerular hematuria accompanied by proteinuria, irrespective of the amount
Evaluation of renal allotransplant for rejection, cyclosporine nephrotoxicity, prolonged nonfunction, or recurrent disease[a]
Acute renal failure of unknown cause with normal kidney size and without obstruction
Possibly Useful
Isolated persistent or recurrent glomerular hematuria without proteinuria
Isolated glomerular proteinuria of less than 3.5 g/day with normal urine sediment
Slowly progressive tubulointerstitial disease
Unexplained renal failure with normal kidney size
Kidney disease in pregnancy
Evaluation of possible glomerular heredofamilial disorders (Alport's syndrome, thin basement membrane disease, Fabry's disease)
Diabetic nephropathy, especially in non–insulin-dependent diabetes mellitus, in the absence of retinopathy or in the presence of active urine sediment
Not Useful
End-stage renal disease with small kidneys
Polycystic kidney disease
Malignant hypertension
Hepatorenal syndrome
Infectious acute tubulointerstitial disease (acute pyelonephritis)

[a] By fine-needle aspiration.

Because of the high likelihood of glucocorticoid-responsive lesions underlying the nephrotic syndrome in children—particularly those younger than 10 years of age with normal C3 component of complement, a benign urinary sediment, and highly selective proteinuria—a renal biopsy could be deferred until a course of empiric glucocorticoid therapy has been administered. Renal biopsy only of those children who are unresponsive to an initial course of glucocorticoids would be recommended to identify potential responsiveness to adjunctive therapy with cyclophosphamide (minimal lesion disease) and for prognostic reasons (focal sclerosis, membranoproliferative glomerulonephritis).

In our opinion, patients with rapidly declining renal function in whom urinary tract obstruction has been excluded, in whom normal renal size has been documented by ultrasonography, and whose urinary sediment is indicative of glomerulonephritis should undergo renal biopsy without delay to categorize the pathologic basis of the renal disease. However, in patients who have rapidly progressive glomerulonephritis, pulmonary hemorrhage, and high blood levels of antiglomerular basement membrane (GBM) antibody (Goodpasture's disease) or with high levels of anti–neutrophil cytoplasmic antibody (vasculitis), appropriate therapy could be initiated without a renal biopsy.

The role of renal biopsy in the evaluation and follow-up of collagen vascular disease, including systemic lupus erythematosus (SLE), is controversial. However, studies have shown that clinical and serologic findings may not be predictors of underlying histology and that glomerular, tubulointerstitial, and vascular alterations may be useful markers of prognosis and potential responsiveness to therapy. Therefore we continue to recommend renal biopsy in patients with SLE for (a) the initial evaluation of patients with definite signs of renal involvement (proteinuria, hematuria, abnormal renal function), (b) the patient with established renal disease who has a rapidly worsening urinary sediment and renal function or recent onset of the nephrotic syndrome, and (c) the patient with advanced renal failure (serum creatinine more than 3 mg/dl) and normal kidney size, to assess the potential for reversal of renal failure. *We do not recommend renal biopsies in patients with SLE without clinical or laboratory evidence of renal involvement.*

The overall value of renal biopsy in patients with non–nephrotic range proteinuria with or without an accompanying abnormal urinary sediment is uncertain. Although it is arbitrary, we prefer to limit biopsy to those patients who excrete more than 1.0 g/day of protein of glomerular origin or to those in whom the proteinuria is accompanied by abnormal urinary sediment, mainly dysmorphic hematuria. We adopt this approach because of the likelihood of finding a lesion that can be categorized in a way that will be useful therapeutically or prognostically. Such information would be particularly useful in younger patients contemplating marriage, education, career change, or insurance application.

The management of persistent or recurrent hematuria of glomerular origin (dysmorphic hematuria) without proteinuria is not likely to be clarified by renal biopsy. However, the adverse prognostic connotation of hematuria accompanied by significant proteinuria (more than 1.0 g/dl) would constitute an indication for renal biopsy.

Renal biopsy has a clear and unquestioned role in the evaluation of renal allograft disorders, although the technique of fine-needle aspiration cytology may be used as a substitute under certain conditions to discriminate between acute rejection and cyclosporine nephrotoxicity. Patients with acute renal failure and prolonged oliguria in whom obstruction has been excluded and who have two normal-sized or enlarged kidneys should be considered candidates for renal biopsy.

On occasion, slowly progressive renal failure in a patient suspected of having a tubulointerstitial disease may be an indication for a renal biopsy. Sarcoidosis involving the kidney and a drug-induced hypersensitivity are examples of such a clinical setting. Patients with unexplained renal failure and normal-sized kidneys are also candidates for renal biopsy.

Renal biopsy is seldom performed during pregnancy, and if at all possible, it is better to defer biopsy until after pregnancy is concluded. Nonetheless, with acute onset of a particularly debilitating disease (such as severe nephrotic syndrome in the first trimester), a renal biopsy followed by appropriate therapy may be indicated. Renal biopsy occasionally may be indicated in a pregnant woman to diagnose a heredofamilial disease, such as Alport's syndrome or Fabry's disease, to facilitate genetic counseling.

Patients with diabetes mellitus, whether insulin dependent or non–insulin dependent, constitute a particular problem in deciding whether to perform a renal biopsy, because in most of these patients the apparent renal disease is consequent to diabetic nephropathy. However, when renal disease appears early in the course of diabetes mellitus, abnormal urinary sediment is present, or proliferative or background retinopathy is absent, a renal biopsy is appropriate to identify a nondiabetes-related lesion.

Renal biopsy is not useful in evaluating small, shrunken kidneys with advanced azotemia, cystic kidney disease, hepatorenal syndrome, or acute bacterial infection.

Once a renal biopsy has established a diagnosis of a clinicopathologic entity, it is seldom necessary to consider a follow-up or repeat biopsy. However, an abrupt change in clinical course, such as the emergency of rapidly progressive renal failure, can signal an important morphologic transition requiring new, more intensive, or a change in therapy. When nephrotoxic agents such as cyclosporine are used, serial renal biopsies may be required to monitor the potential side effects of therapy. Occasionally, repeat renal biopsies may be a help in deciding whether to discontinue therapy in the face of progressive disease. The conversion of a steroid-responsive to a steroid-nonresponsive form of idiopathic nephrotic syndrome also may indicate the need for a repeat biopsy.

CONTRAINDICATIONS

There is only one *absolute* contraindication to percutaneous renal biopsy: an uncorrectable, clinically overt, bleeding disorder likely to result in postbiopsy hemorrhage. Percutaneous renal biopsy could be performed in patients with bleeding disorders after correction with appropriate therapy.

The relationship of laboratory tests of bleeding diatheses to risks of postbiopsy bleeding is uncertain. For example, although advanced renal failure is accompanied by platelet dysfunction and prolonged bleeding time, percutaneous renal biopsy often can be accomplished safely in this setting. If desired, an infusion of desmopressin (DDAVP) several hours or conjugated estrogens several days before the biopsy may normalize the bleeding time in patients with renal failure. However, we do not use this procedure routinely. Modest thrombocytopenia (100,000 to 150,000/mm^3) is not a contraindication to renal biopsy, although severe thrombocytopenia (less than 50,000/mm^3) would be. If renal tissue is urgently needed for diagnosis, fresh platelet infusion may be given before the biopsy is performed.

Relative contraindications to percutaneous renal biopsy include solitary kidney, uncooperative patient, active renal infection, renal vasculitis with aneurysms, hydronephrosis, uncorrected volume depletion, and uncontrolled severe hypertension. Repletion of extracellular fluid volume and control of hypertension will allow the safe performance of the biopsy in the latter instances.

COMPLICATIONS

The incidence of complications of percutaneous renal biopsy varies according to the experience of the individual performing the procedure, the general condition of the patient, and the presence or absence of relative contraindications. Thus it is difficult to provide an exact value for the risk of a complication in any particular patient. *Microscopic hematuria* is often present, postbiopsy, but gross hematuria occurs only occasionally. *Perirenal hematomas* probably occur in nearly all patients and are easily detected by ultrasonography or computed tomography (CT) scan, the latter being more sensitive. These hematomas are usually small and resolve without sequelae. In 200 consecutive percutaneous renal biopsies, we found no correlation between the size of the perirenal hematoma and major bleeding with the results of various coagulation tests. Pain following the renal biopsy is variable. A mild, dull, aching sensation in the biopsy area is common. More prolonged pain should be a cause for concern and may indicate an expanding perirenal hematoma or urinary obstruction from clots.

Perirenal bleeding and/or gross hematuria sufficient to require blood transfusion occurs in 1 in 200 to 500 biopsies. Surgery for correction of postbiopsy hemorrhage may be required in less than 1 in 1,000 biopsies, and death related to biopsy is rare (less than 1 in 3,000 biopsies). Mild to moderate postbiopsy hemorrhage can be managed by bed rest, observation, and blood transfusion if necessary. Severe and massive bleeding may require surgical intervention. Angiographic localization with balloon or clot occlusion of a bleeding vessel has also been used successfully.

Arteriovenous fistula may develop in up to 10% of patients undergoing renal biopsy. These fistulas often are asymptomatic but occasionally may be the source of persistent hematuria. A persistent bruit over the kidney following a biopsy is pathognomonic of arteriovenous fistula, but this is seldom observed. Renal arteriography is required for definitive diagnosis. Occlusion of fistula during arteriography may be necessary for a large fistula or for the control of bleeding.

Other complications include calyceal fistula and rupture of the kidney. Occasionally, other organs may be inadvertently biopsied, including the pancreas, spleen, liver, or small intestine. Improper renal localization procedure may lead to accidental biopsy of the aorta or renal artery, with disastrous consequences.

TECHNICAL ASPECTS OF THE PROCEDURE

In addition to obtaining an informed consent, the physician should carefully review the patient's history for bleeding manifestations. Although a coagulation screen (prothrombin time, partial thromboplastin time, platelet count, and bleeding time) is not absolutely necessary for the ordinary patient, it should be performed if a bleeding abnormality is suspected. The hematocrit should be measured, and urinalysis should be done before renal biopsy as a reference for the postbiopsy values. The location and size of both kidneys should be assessed. Ultrasonography is sufficient for this purpose. In the exceptional patient for whom ultrasonography may not be unequivocally adequate, a radionuclide scan or intravenous urography may provide the answer.

Either kidney may be selected for biopsy, but many physicians prefer the right kidney. It is usually not necessary to type or crossmatch for blood transfusion except in small children, when the hematocrit is reduced or when the bleeding risk is increased. The patient should be relaxed and cooperative but not overly sedated. Prebiopsy sedation and analgesia need only be provided for the markedly anxious individual.

Biopsy is performed with the patient in the prone position in a well-lighted room, using image-intensification fluoroscopy or with ultrasound guidance. The former procedure requires an intravenous infusion of a radiocontrast medium, beginning half an hour before the biopsy. We prefer ultrasound guidance to avoid the use of contrast media, which may be nephrotoxic in some patients.

The patient is comfortably positioned in the prone position with a firm support under the midabdomen. The site where the biopsy needle will be inserted is marked with indelible ink, using the ultrasound or x-ray image of the kidney in midinspiration to deep inspiration as a guide. The outer side of the lower pole of the kidney is the preferred site for the biopsy. The patient is then draped, and the skin is prepared with an antiseptic (Betadine). The needle insertion site is anesthetized with a local anesthetic (lidocaine). A small incision is made with a pointed scalpel to facilitate insertion of the biopsy trocar. The biopsy site down to the surface of the kidney is anesthetized using a 6-inch, 21-gauge needle. The biopsy trocar (Vim-Silverman needle modified by Franklin, Travenol Tru-Cut disposable needle, or a semiautomatic spring-loaded device) is inserted through the incision site. For the Vim-Silverman needle, the trocar containing the obturator is advanced superiorly and medially toward the biopsy site, with the patient holding the breath in midinspiration to deep inspiration. In between the advancement of the trocar, the patient should be allowed to breathe quietly, and the operator should not restrain the movement of the trocar. Once the capsule of the kidney is reached, the trocar tip is advanced a few millimeters into the kidney substance while the patient holds the breath. The success of this penetration is ascertained by the movement of the trocar with breathing. The obturator is removed, and the patient is allowed to take a few quiet breaths while the lumen of the unrestrained trocar is inspected for bleeding. If blood does not appear in the trocar lumen, the cutting needle is inserted and advanced into the trocar until it rests on the surface of the kidney. Resistance to further advancement of the cutting needle is a sign of its proper position. The patient is allowed to take several quiet breaths with the trocar unrestrained. The patient is then asked to take a breath and hold it until instructed to breathe again. During breath-holding, the cutting needle is quickly advanced into the substance of the kidney, and the trocar is advanced in a rotating manner over the cutting needle to the same depth.

The trocar and the cutting needle are removed from the patient in unison. The cutting needle is removed from the trocar, and the renal tissue is carefully extracted from the tip of the needle with a minimum of manipulation. If possible, a second core of tissue is obtained by repeating the procedure. The renal tissue is submitted for light, immunofluorescence, and electron microscopic studies. A sample could also be reserved for microdissection and molecular biology study if possible. If renal tissue is not obtained with two or three puncture attempts, the biopsy procedure should be abandoned.

Immediately after the termination of the biopsy procedure, local pressure should be exerted on the biopsy site by the operator, and the patient's pulse and blood pressure should be obtained. The patient should then lie quietly in the supine position for at least 8 to 12 hours. Blood pressure and pulse should be monitored every 15 minutes for the first hour, hourly for 4 hours, and then every 4 hours until discharge from the hospital or the ambulatory surgery unit, 12 to 24 hours following the biopsy. Hematocrit should be measured 8 to 12 hours after biopsy and at discharge. All voided urine should be examined for gross and microscopic hematuria. Gross hematuria, persistent pain, or a significant drop in hematuria requires CT scan of the renal area to detect the presence and size of a hematoma. Occasionally, an arteriogram may be required for detection of an arteriovenous fistula.

The patient should be advised not to engage in running, contact sports, horseback riding, or strenuous exercise for at least a week after discharge from the hospital. He or she should be asked to report immediately gross hematuria, pain, colic, or orthostatic dizziness.

A semiautomatic, spring-driven biopsy device has become quite popular (Biopty). This device uses a narrower needle (18 gauge) than the Vim-Silverman or Tru-Cut device, and therefore less tissue is obtained. The needle attached to the automated device in the cocked position is introduced into the renal parenchyma under *direct* real time ultrasound guidance. (This requires a skilled operator and a specialized ultrasonic probe.) When properly placed in the kidney, the device is manually activated, and the biopsy specimen is taken by rapid, programmed movement of the cutting needle and its sheath. Satisfactory results are obtained almost as frequently as with other techniques, and bleeding risk may be less because of the smaller needle size and the rapid sampling time (less than 1 second). In our view, the performance of renal biopsy using the percutaneous technique should remain in the purview of nephrologist. However some nephrologists do not have the opportunity to perform renal biopsies frequently enough to maintain their skill (less than 6 per year). Under these circumstances, such nephrologists should seek the help of more experienced nephrology colleagues or interventional radiologists who have acquired the skills for performing renal biopsy.

In cooperative patients with no significant risk factors and an experienced operator, it is possible to safely perform renal biopsies with limited periods of prebiopsy and postbiopsy observation. Patients should be examined and observed prebiopsy to be sure no contraindications exist (e.g., very high blood pressure, vomiting, uncooperative behavior).

Follow-up postbiopsy can be as short as 8 hours, which would permit biopsy in an ambulatory surgery center or equivalent, providing the biopsy procedure itself was not difficult or complicated *and* the patient is compliant, cooperative, free of excessive risk of complications, and understands the risks of shorter postbiopsy observation periods. Otherwise, hospitalization with a 24-hour postbiopsy observation period would be the safest alternative.

The procedure for biopsy of a transplanted kidney is simpler and safer. The kidney in the transplant recipient lies in an extraperitoneal location in the pelvis. The kidney is thus superficial and easily palpable and does not move with respiration. Sedation is not required. The skin and the subcutaneous tissue overlying the upper pole of the kidney are infiltrated with local anesthesia. A cut is made in the skin with a sharp scalpel, and the biopsy needle is advanced slowly until it meets the surface of the kidney. This distance is about 1 to 2 cm. The resistance to further advancement is appreciable once the needle meets the surface of the kidney. The biopsy material is obtained as previously described. Postbiopsy precautions are similar to those described. Concealed bleeding may dissect into the retroperitoneal space and may result in compression of the veins draining the ipsilateral leg, thus leading to edema.

Selected Readings

Burstein D, Karbet S, Schwartz M. The use of the automated core biopsy system in percutaneous renal biopsies. A comparative study. *Am J Kidney Dis* 1993; 22:545–552.

A comparison of standard and automated renal biopsy techniques.

Donavan KL, Thomas DM, Wheeler DC, et al. Experience with a new method for percutaneous renal biopsy. *Nephrol Dialysis Transplant* 1991;6:731–733.

A good description of the automated needle biopsy: real true ultrasound technique.

Harry P. Transplant aspiration cytology: background and current applications. In: Kreis H, Diaz D, eds. *Renal transplant cytology.* Milan: Wichtg, 1984.

An excellent description of technique and applications of a fine-needle aspiration biopsy of the kidney.

Mal F, Meyrier A, Collord P, et al. The diagnostic yield of transjugular renal biopsy: experience in 200 cases. *Kidney Int* 1992;41:445–449.

A description and evaluation of the transvenous method of renal biopsy.

Parrish AE. Complications of percutaneous renal biopsy: a review of 37 years experience. *Clin Nephrol* 1992;38:141–146.

An excellent summary of renal biopsy complications by an experienced clinician.

Tisher CL. Clinical indicators for renal biopsy. In: Tisher CL, Brenner BM, eds. *Renal pathology with clinical and functional correlations*, 2nd ed. Philadelphia: JB Lippincott, 1994:75–84.

An excellent overview with an extensive list of references.

CHAPTER 97

Use of the Urethral Catheter

Joel Gelman and Jacob Rajfer

Catheterization of the urinary bladder is one of the most common procedures performed in the hospital environment. In fact, it has been estimated that approximately 10% to 15% of all hospitalized patients will require the insertion of an indwelling catheter sometime during their hospitalization. These figures do not account for those patients who are placed on intermittent catheterization regimens. There are many reasons for the high usage of bladder catheterization in the hospital population. It is easy to perform, regarded as a relatively benign procedure for the amount of information obtained, and sometimes used as a convenience by nurses and physicians in the care of some patients. However, in contrast to its simplicity and potential benefit in draining the urinary tract while accurately measuring the urinary output, bladder catheterization is well known to be the major cause for nosocomial infections that carries with it the potential for developing some life-threatening complications such as urinary tract infection and septicemia. Approximately 40% of all nosocomial infections are catheter-associated urinary tract infections. The onset of catheter-related complications then requires treatment with antibiotics, and this usually prolongs hospitalization. Consequently, it is both cost-effective and good medical practice to use a urethral catheter only when it is indicated and not as a convenience to the medical personnel. Yet, catheterization is essential when accurate hourly urine output must be measured in the patient requiring intensive care. Furthermore, failure to catheterize the patient with a distended bladder may lead to overdistension and damage to the protective lining in the adjacent mucosal layer of the bladder. This protective lining of the bladder mucosa is partially composed of glycosaminoglycans, and loss of these substances is thought to predispose the bladder to a variety of disturbances, in particular the development of cystitis. In this chapter we will review certain indications for the use of the urethral catheter, the complications that may arise with its use, and the recommended method of inserting the urethral catheter.

INDWELLING CATHETERIZATION

There are five major indications for the use of an indwelling catheter: (a) when urine output must be accurately monitored continuously in the intensive care setting, (b) to provide chronic drainage of the bladder in a patient who is totally incontinent when other treatment options fail or are contraindicated, (c) as a stent following prostate or urethral surgery, (d) in patients who are in urinary retention, and (e) in the management of traumatic bladder injuries to allow spontaneous healing. Most of the patients who are chronically managed with an indwelling catheter are elderly or incapacitated by a neurogenic disorder such as multiple sclerosis, cerebral vascular accident, or traumatic cord injury. However, a decision to indefinitely manage a patient with an indwelling catheter should be made only after a careful urologic evaluation that often includes a urodynamic study and consideration of all alternatives. For example, a patient with a contracted neurogenic bladder secondary to a spinal cord injury may be a candidate for bladder augmentation (using bowel) with intermittent catheterization or continent cutaneous diversion. The use of these newer surgical procedures allows many patients with neurogenic bladders to now be free of indwelling catheters and urine collection devices. In the chronically debilitated male patient without retention, overflow incontinence, or other impairment of bladder storage and emptying, external condom drainage may be substituted for an indwelling catheter. If a catheter is left indwelling, it should be changed every 2 to 6 weeks because of the potential for calcium encrustations on the catheter that may provide a nidus for calculus formation, urinary tract infection, or obstruction of the lumen of the catheter. In the patient whose urinary output is being observed, such as the postoperative surgical patient, the catheter should ideally not be left in for more than 14 days, again because of the associated bacterial colonization and propensity for infectious complications after this time period. If possible, intermittent catheterization should be substituted for an indwelling catheter in any patient who is likely to require prolonged bladder catheterization. For patients undergoing urethral reconstruction or prostatectomy or those patients who have sustained traumatic bladder disruption, a catheter is rarely left indwelling for more than 21 days. If possible, these indwelling catheters should be made of silastic or silicone materials, which are inert, in lieu of the traditional latex catheters, which may be very irritable to the urethra and lead to urethritis.

INTERMITTENT CATHETERIZATION

Intermittent catheterization, as the name implies, refers to the periodic evacuation of the bladder by the intermittent placement of a catheter into the bladder. Intermittent catheterization is an accepted mode of therapy for the neurogenic bladder, in that it prevents bladder distension and eliminates the bacterial colonization that occurs with an indwelling catheter. Intermittent catheterization can be performed by the patient (intermittent self-catheterization) or by an attendant in a hospital setting. In order for an individual to perform intermittent self-catheterization, functional upper extremities are a must.

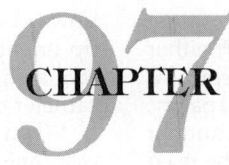

Because of the excellent long-term results of intermittent catheterization, it is now common to attempt to convert either pharmacologically (anticholinergic medication) or surgically, a spastic (uninhibited bladder contractions) or low-capacity, high-pressure bladder to an atonic bladder so that intermittent catheterization instead of an indwelling catheter may be used for bladder evacuation.

Intermittent catheterization should be performed regularly during the day so that bladder distention does not occur. This is important because over distension may lead to damage of the protective layer of the glycosaminoglycans on the bladder lumen. All the urine in the bladder should be drained each time intermittent catheterization is performed because of the propensity of the urinary tract to become infected in the presence of a residual urine.

TECHNIQUE OF CATHETERIZATION

When the decision is made to use a catheter, the smallest catheter that can provide adequate drainage should be used. Usually in an adult, a No. 16 French (Fr) catheter is adequate. Large sizes should only be used initially when there is some special justification, such as following transurethral prostatectomy when the catheter is used to drain blood clots out of the bladder. In order to prevent contamination of the bladder and the catheter collecting system, the catheter should be inserted aseptically using sterile technique. To accomplish this, it is necessary for the catheter to be connected aseptically to the connection system before inserting the catheter. The genitalia should be cleaned with an antibacterial agent such as pHisoHex or a povodine-iodophor solution, and adequate lubrication should be used. The catheter should be passed gently. The injection of a lubricant containing viscous lidocaine into the urethra before insertion of the catheter often facilitates passage of the catheter in comparison with the application of lubrication to the tip of the catheter alone. Lubrication within the urethra is increased and this facilitates passage of the catheter. Furthermore, pain in response to catheterization may result in contraction of the external striated urethral sphincter. The anesthetic effects of the lidocaine prevent the voluntary contraction of the external sphincter, and this facilitates passage of the catheter through the sphincter. The catheter should be advanced as far as possible into the bladder. A good indicator of proper catheter placement is urine output following insertion of the catheter. If the patient is dehydrated or anuric, or if lubricant is within the lumen of the catheter, urine output may not be observed initially. In this situation, the bladder should be irrigated gently with 50 to 100 ml of saline using a 60 cc catheter-tipped "Toomey" syringe. If "what goes in doesn't come out," it is unlikely that the catheter is in the bladder and may be in the prostatic urethra. The catheter balloon should never be inflated when the position of the catheter is uncertain. Following insertion, the catheter balloon is inflated with saline, and the catheter should be properly secured to prevent unnecessary movement and traction on the urethra at the level of the bladder neck. In males, care should be taken to prevent the catheter from exerting pressure on the glans penis, because this can lead to pressure necrosis and erosion of the glans, especially ventrally.

Occasionally, the physician or attendant fails to catheterize the bladder because the catheter will not advance through the posterior urethra. In the older man with bladder outlet obstruction secondary to benign prostate hypertrophy, a small-bore catheter may lack the rigidity to pass the occlusive prostate. In this situation, a larger catheter (20 to 24 Fr) may be needed. Alternatively, a Coudé catheter can be passed. This catheter has an upward curvature at the distal aspect, and is passed with the tip oriented upward (cephalad). The urethra normally curves cephalad along the proximal aspect, and the use of the Coudé catheter can facilitate passage through the prostatic urethra.

When the aforementioned catheters do not pass with relative ease, one should not attempt to force the catheter past the point of resistance. Instead, urologic assistance is advised. The most common reason for inability to pass a catheter is inexperience. This is not to say that there may not be other causes of difficulty in performing catheterization, such as the presence or creation of a false passage within the urethra, trauma to the urethra from inflation of a catheter balloon in the urethra, a markedly enlarged and obstructive prostate, or a urethral stricture. When a small or large catheter cannot be placed, the reasonable next step may be cystoscopy. When the urethra is patent, and a false passage and/or marked prostate enlargement appears to be the cause of failure of the catheter to pass, it may be possible for a guide wire to be placed cystoscopically, where the catheter (with a hole at the tip) can be placed over the guide wire. When a urethral stricture is diagnosed or suspected, management in the past often consisted of sequential urethral dilation with filiforms and followers (which are progressive dilators), then placement of the catheter. This approach is traumatic and represents an invasive treatment before a definitive diagnosis of the length and location of the stricture. In most cases, a definitive diagnosis should be made before treatment is undertaken because an alternative such as elective open urethral reconstruction may be best for the patient long term. When immediate catheterization is needed to relieve urinary retention in the presence of a urethral stricture, urologic placement of a percutaneous suprapubic tube is usually the treatment of choice.

All collection systems should be sterile and of the closed type. Any disruption to the integrity of the catheter and collection system must be considered contamination, and in certain institutions, is just cause for replacement of the catheter and drainage system. Poorly functioning or obstructed catheters should be replaced. The flow of urine from the bladder through the catheter should be "downhill." To accomplish this, the collection bag should always be lower than the level of the bladder. When the collection bag is emptied, disposable gloves should be worn. A fresh pair of gloves should be used for each patient when more than one catheterized patient shares a hospital room, because cross-contamination from one catheterized patient to another by medical personnel has been shown to be a mode of transmission of infectious organisms. Ideally, an iodophor solution should be used to cleanse the drainage tube before and after emptying of the bag. The drainage bag should not be disconnected from the catheter to drain the bag and should not be allowed to touch the collecting receptacle. The drainage bag should always be emptied from the bottom.

If for some reason the integrity of the collection system is violated, such as when irrigating the catheter, sterile technique must be used at all times. When a sample of urine for analysis is obtained from the catheter, it should be aspirated from the sampling port on the catheter, or when a port is not present, a 25-guage needle is introduced into the catheter after the catheter is cleansed with an iodophor solution. Finally, catheters that are left indwelling for long periods of time should be changed every 4 to 6 weeks because of encrustations on the catheter. Silicone or silastic catheters may lessen any chance of encrustations on the catheter and subsequent obstruction.

In the hospital environment, intermittent catheterization can be performed under sterile conditions, but this is certainly not necessary. It appears that proper hygiene is the only requirement to perform this procedure, and indeed this is the way intermittent catheterization is performed in the nonhospital setting. The hands should be washed, and the catheter, either a sterile one or one that has been rinsed off with water, is placed gently into the urethra. Lubrication should be used to facilitate its passage. In the female patient, the labia are held apart, whereas in the male patient, if a foreskin is present it is usually retracted over the glans. The catheter is placed into the bladder and the urine is drained completely. The catheter is removed slowly in order to drain any residual urine, because retention of urine may promote bacterial growth and development of a symptomatic urinary tract infection. In the individual with a high bladder neck, the only catheter that may easily pass into the bladder is the Coudé catheter. Once the catheterization is performed, the patient may place the catheter in a plastic bag after rinsing it off gently with tap water. It can be used again later that day and again rinsed off following its use. Catheters that are reused should be sterilized by being placed in boiling water at the end of the day.

COMPLICATIONS

The placement of an indwelling catheter into the bladder in a patient with sterile urine will almost unequivocally result in bacteriuria if left in long enough. Before the advent of closed drainage systems, the incidence of bacteriuria was almost 100% within 96 hours after the catheter was inserted. With the use of closed drainage systems, approximately 50% of patients develop bacteriuria by 2 weeks. In most patients, catheter-related bacteriuria is totally asymptomatic and usually resolves following catheter removal and/or antibiotic therapy. However, in some patients, the bacteriuria may proceed to clinical cystitis, acute pyelonephritis, and possibly Gram-negative septicemia. The use of prophylactic antibiotics in patients with an indwelling catheter in an effort to avoid bacterial colonization should be condemned because a resistant strain of organisms is likely to emerge.

The urinary tract is the most common site of nosocomial infections, and it is not surprising that the most common pathogens associated with nosocomial urinary tract infections are the Gram-negative organisms. These are the enteric organisms that inhabit the perineal skin and urethra. The pathogens responsible for nosocomial urinary tract infections in descending incidence are *Escherichia coli*, enterococci, yeast, *Pseudomonas*, and *Klebsiella* (Table 97.1). Therefore in empirically treating the symptomatic upper urinary tract or systemic infection complicating urethral catheterization, adequate coverage of these organisms should be instituted and this may involve the use of aminoglycosides, a drug effective against enterococci such as ampicillin, and/or, possibly, an antifungal agent.

TABLE 97.1. Distribution of Pathogens in Nosocomial Urinary Tract Infections

Organism	Isolates (%)
Escherichia coli	29
Enterococci	13
Yeast	13
Pseudomonas	9
Klebsiella	8
Coagulase—*Staphylococcus*	5
Proteus	4
Enterobacter	4
Citrobacter	3
Other	12

In addition to these infectious complications, the urethral catheter may in male patients lead to the development of epididymitis, bacterial prostatitis, urethral strictures, and urethral fistulae. Epididymitis is usually secondary to the bacteriuria associated with the indwelling catheter, and it is not unusual for an epididymitis in this setting to proceed to septicemia. Treatment may involve surgical epididymectomy if antibiotic therapy fails to control the infection. Urethral strictures are believed to be secondary to traumatic insertion or urethritis induced by the indwelling catheter. It has been shown that latex catheters are more irritative to the urethra than silastic or silicone catheters, and consequently, in a patient who requires an indwelling urethral catheter for longer than 1 week, it is recommended that either a silastic or silicone catheter be used. Urethral fistulas rarely develop, and in certain instances the catheter has been known to cause pressure necrosis of the urethra.

The development of bacteriuria in the patient on intermittent catheterization may not be harmful. Some investigators think that asymptomatic bacteriuria is insignificant in patients on intermittent catheterization and does not require any antibiotic therapy. The organisms that are usually cultured from patients on intermittent catheterization are those of the normal skin and perineal flora. Some studies have shown that the route of bacterial entry into the urinary tract of catheterized patients differs by gender. In women, the majority of bacteria entering the urinary tract emanate from the rectal flora, colonize the periurethral area, and subsequently enter the urinary tract. In men, infections often occur via the intraluminal route. However, periurethral migration of bacteria into the bladder is also considered to be a cause of urinary tract infection in men.

The presence of a urinary tract anatomic abnormality, such as hydronephrosis, may predispose patients with a neurogenic bladder to urinary tract infections and pyelonephritis, and hence treatment of these patients with prophylactic antibiotics may be recommended. Prophylaxis for intermittent catheterization usually involves therapy with nitrofurantoin, which is primarily excreted into the urine and has a low level of bacterial resistance. There are some data to suggest that trimethoprim-sulfasoxazole in small doses may also be effective prophylaxis, but evidence of bacterial resistance to this drug combination has been reported.

The sequelae of urinary tract infections in patients with neurogenic bladder are stones, vesicoureteral reflux, bladder fibrosis, hydronephrosis, epididymitis, and prostatitis. Care should be taken during intermittent self-catheterization not to introduce hair into the bladder with the catheter because it may be a nidus for calculus formation within the bladder.

URETHRAL CATHETER SYSTEMS

Over the years, it became apparent that when the urethral catheter was allowed to drain into collecting systems that were not sealed to the catheter, there was an unacceptably high incidence of bacteriuria with its resultant morbidity and mortality. Although the incidence of bacteriuria in such an open collecting system can be minimized with antibacterial agents, it has been shown that such therapy, although eliminating susceptible organisms, permits the emergence of fungi and other resistant bacteria. The bacteria have been shown to multiply in the collection device and then ascend into the bladder either through the lumen of the catheter or between the catheter and the urethra.

In an attempt to minimize bacterial colonization of the bladder during catheterization, a variety of solutions have been used to rinse the bladder in hope that the bacteria can be eradicated. Acetic acid (0.25%) is one such solution that has undergone limited therapeutic trials. For acetic acid to be effective, the pH of the bladder contents must be kept below 5.0 and to accomplish this, constant pH monitoring of the urinary drainage is required. In addition to this continued monitoring, which may be difficult to accomplish on the hospital ward, acetic acid may cause severe vesical irritation, which may preclude its use. Another solution that has been used to irrigate the bladder includes a mixture of neomycin and polymyxin. This irrigant solution, like acetic acid, is usually run through the bladder by a three-way indwelling catheter as a continuous irrigation. Although initial studies using open drainage systems suggested that the use of this irrigant in patients with short-term bladder catheterization resulted in a decrease in bacteriuria, it later became apparent that there was no significant difference in the incidence of bacteriuria between patients who used this neomycin-polymyxin irrigant and those who did not. In the latter group of patients, the closed drainage system was used, and it is believed that the decrease in bacteriuria seen in these patients was due to the closed drainage system and not to the irrigating solutions. Again, as with acetic acid, the bacteriuria in patients who use neomycin-polymyxin irrigation is usually caused by resistant strains of organisms. Other observations suggest that the instillation of 30 ml of 3% hydrogen peroxide periodically into the urethral catheter drainage bag may be effective in decreasing the incidence of catheter-induced bacteriuria.

It is obvious that the optimum method of continuously draining the urinary bladder is through a sterile closed drainage system that is hooked up aseptically to a urethral catheter. The incidence of bacteriuria when using the closed drainage system is significantly less than for the open system, and for this reason, systemic antibiotics are usually not used in a closed drainage system. However, if this closed drainage system is broken by disconnecting the drainage tube to the catheter, the incidence of bacteriuria approaches that occurring with the open drainage system.

Intermittent catheterization in the home environment is best conducted with either inexpensive rubber catheters that can be resterilized (by boiling water) or disposable plastic catheters. Newer catheters that are coated with substances that provide lubrication when exposed to water are now being developed and marketed. The objective with self-catheterization is to achieve bladder emptying with a catheter that can be easily and atraumatically inserted.

Ongoing investigative efforts are attempting to develop ways to decrease the incidence of complications associated with catheterization of the bladder. For example, it has been shown that catheter encrustation and blockage is often associated with Proteus colonization. The bacteria form crystalline biofilms, and there is associated deposition of the divalent cations along the catheter. The development of new urease inhibitors and catheter materials or coatings that resist biofilm formation may prevent catheter encrustation. Other studies are directed toward the development of antimicrobial-coated catheters that will prevent periurethral bacterial migration.

Selected Readings

Bronsema DA, Adams JR, Pallares R, et al. Secular trends in rates and etiology of nosocomial urinary tract infections at a university hospital. *J Urol* 1993;105: 414–416.

A review of the current pathogens associated with nosocomial urinary tract infections. Data from this study appear in Table 97.1.

Lapides J, Diokno AC, Silber SJ, et al. Clean, intermittent self-catheterization in the treatment of urinary tract disease. *J Urol* 1972;107:458–461.

A classic early study of the special role of self-catheterization in patients with bladder dysfunction.

Morris NS, Stickler DJ. Encrustation of indwelling urethral catheters by *Proteus mirabilis* biofilms growing in human urine. *J Hosp Infect* 1998;39(3):227–234.

One of several recent studies that seek to find ways to prevent infectious complications of catheterization.

Stamm WE. Catheter-associated urinary tract infections: epidemiology, pathogenesis, and prevention. *American J Med* 1991;91(suppl 3B):65S–71S.

Recent review of infections associated with bladder catheterization.

Warren JW. Catheter-associated urinary tract infections. *Infect Dis Clin North Am* 1997;11(3)609–622.

Recent review of infections associated with bladder catheterization.

CHAPTER 98

Bone Biopsy

Marie-Claude Monier-Faugere, M. Chris Langub, and Hartmut H. Malluche

Renal failure produces changes in mineral metabolism, which affect bone structure, turnover, and cellular characteristics. When patients reach end-stage renal failure and require chronic maintenance dialysis, nearly all of them have abnormal bone histology. Improved dialytic therapy has increased survival rates of patients on dialysis, but the resultant increased duration of dialysis has led to a rise in renal osteodystrophy, a metabolic bone disease associated with uremia that can produce fractures, bone pain, and deformities late in the course of the disease. Therefore prevention and early treatment of renal osteodystrophy are critical. To date, bone biopsy is the most powerful and informative diagnostic tool to provide important information on the precise type of renal osteodystrophy affecting patients, the degree of severity of the lesions, and the presence and amount of aluminum deposition in bone.

Bone biopsies have been used for research purposes to assess the effects of new therapies on bone. Newer technologies such as the methods of *in situ* hybridization histochemistry and immunohistochemistry are providing the means to study local biomolecules that play a role in bone metabolism.

This chapter presents an overview of bone biopsy techniques, discusses indications for and clinical applications of bone biopsy, and reviews the research implications of *in situ* hybridization histochemistry and immunohistochemistry.

BONE BIOPSY TECHNIQUES

Prerequisites for Bone Biopsies

Labeling of Bone. The first prerequisite for an informative bone biopsy is a proper *in vivo* labeling with specific, nontoxic, time-spaced bone markers before the biopsy. Antibiotics from the tetracycline family are used because they have spontaneous fluorescence (Fig. 98.1) and bind to actively forming bone surfaces. With labeling, the level of bone turnover and rate of bone formation can be determined, and possible mineralization abnormalities can be identified. A double labeling technique is best, although the schedule is somewhat more complicated for patients than one prolonged, single administration. Double labeling provides information on mineralization rate and bone formation and differentiates between a mineralization defect and active mineralization.

In most cases, the first label is administered for 2 days followed by an 8- to 15-day free interval. Anything fewer than 8 days lessens the distinction between labels, particularly in the case of a mineralization defect. Anything more than 15 days may artificially increase the number of single labels because the number of forming sites being completed or started will probably increase. During the 2 to 4 days after the free interval, the patient takes a second course of antibiotics. Bone biopsy is then performed 4 to 6 days after the last administration of tetracycline. During this delay, the tetracycline becomes slightly buried within mineralized osteoid and thus does not leach out. If the bone biopsy is delayed more than 10 days after the last label, however, the first label may have undergone resorption and the labels will not correspond to active formative sites.

In an emergency, labeling can be shortened to a 1-day-on, 6-days-off, and 1-day-on schedule with a single dose of oral tetracycline per day (1.0 to 1.5 g of tetracycline or 600 to 900 mg of Declomycin). Gastrointestinal side effects may be greater with this approach.

Using two labels with different colors ensures accurate assessment of the mineralization rate. Tetracycline hydrochloride has a light yellow fluorescence and demeclocycline hydrochloride has a yellow-orange fluorescence. With the use of only one type of tetracycline, the two labels can merge in states of low bone turnover and be unrecognizable as a double label. For patients with normal renal function, dosages of tetracycline hydrochloride and Declomycin are usually 500 mg and 300 mg three times per day, respectively. For patients with impaired

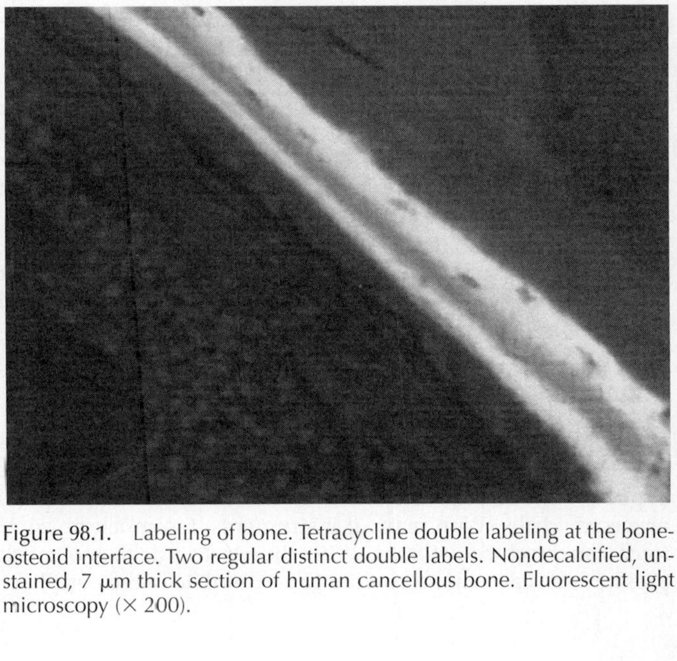

Figure 98.1. Labeling of bone. Tetracycline double labeling at the bone-osteoid interface. Two regular distinct double labels. Nondecalcified, unstained, 7 μm thick section of human cancellous bone. Fluorescent light microscopy (× 200).

renal function, dosages should be reduced to 500 mg and 300 mg two times per day.

Problems Encountered with Labeling. Physicians should stress the importance of labeling to patients who are scheduled for bone biopsies. If a patient does not take the pills as prescribed, the bone sample may lack fluorescent labels or show evidence of only one label. Intestinal absorption of tetracycline and thus its uptake by bone is decreased when a patient takes it with meals or with antacids. Also, the pathologist may have difficulty interpreting a slide if the patient has previously been taking tetracycline antibiotics. Patients usually tolerate double tetracycline labeling well, but some side effects may occur, such as photosensitivity, vomiting, and allergic reactions.

Obtaining the Bone Sample

Obtaining a representative bone sample that will yield sufficient information is a major prerequisite. Therefore the biopsy specimen must contain an adequate amount of cortical and deep cancellous bone to establish a diagnosis. Of equal importance is specimen quality. It should be free of artifacts; that is, no broken or fractured cortex or trabecules, no compressed trabecular bone, no bone marrow hemorrhage, and no damage to cells caused by heat produced during the drilling process. Obtaining a sample of optimal quantity and quality depends on the bone biopsy instrument employed and the operator's skill and experience.

Bone Biopsy Sites

The optimum site for the bone biopsy is the anterior iliac crest. The operator can reach it easily, it does not require extensive surgery (as is needed for rib biopsies), and it is associated with fewer postoperative complications. Local forces known to affect regional bone remodeling, such as direct weight bearing or tension and forces exerted by muscle pull, are minimized at the anterior iliac crest. Moreover, normal values are easier to collect, and comparisons between iliac crest values correlate well with vertebrae, tibiae, and femora.

Iliac crest bone biopsies can be obtained in a vertical or horizontal direction. The biopsy obtained with the vertical approach allows good assessment of cortical bone (superior table), subcortical cancellous bone, and deep cancellous bone. Although the biopsy obtained with the horizontal approach provides information on the inner and outer cortices, the thickness of the iliac bone limits sample size.

Coefficients of variance for routinely used histomorphometric parameters in iliac crest bone samples show no difference in cancellous bone volume between sections of vertical and horizontal biopsies. These samples include those taken from the left or right, anterior or posterior, horizontal or vertical, and superior or inferior iliac crest. All other histomorphometric parameters are significantly higher in vertical biopsies except for lower trabecular thickness because the specimen includes more and deeper cancellous bone.

Bone Biopsy Instruments

One goal of the bone biopsy procedure is to obtain a bone sample of the desired size with minimal surgical invasiveness. Types of bone biopsy instruments available are manual trochars or electric drills. With manual instruments, too much physical force can produce artifacts. With the electric drill, too much pressure can cause bone powder to accumulate in the periphery of spongy bone. Also, heat artifacts of bone cells can result from drilling speeds that are too high.

For qualitative and quantitative bone histology, anterior iliac crest bone samples of 0.4 to 0.5 cm diameter and 2.5 to 3.5 cm length taken vertically, or 0.8 cm diameter taken horizontally, are usually sufficient. We conducted a comparative study of established electric-drill techniques and the manual Jamshidi needle while performing vertical anterior iliac crest bone biopsies (with 3 mm and 5 mm diameter, respectively) on 14 patients suffering from various metabolic bone disease. The anterior and posterior samples obtained from alternately using both instruments showed that even though there was relatively little difference in terms of quality between samples, results of the osteoclast surface/bone surface did not correlate and the mineral apposition rate was different. This indicates that bone samples of 3 mm inner diameter provided by the Jamshidi technique do not provide the same useful information as those derived from 5 mm samples. Based on this study, we cannot support the use of the relatively noninvasive and inexpensive Jamshidi technique for routine diagnostic bone biopsies.

A novel electric drill (Straumann Medical, Waldenburg, Switzerland) performs like the established electric drill with the addition of a one-step drilling and extraction procedure, which shortens the surgical time for performing bone biopsies. This improves patients' acceptance of the procedure. Also, the use of disposable drill bits decreases infection risks, avoids problems with dull drill bits, and eliminates the risk of breakage of drill bits that accompanies frequent resharpening.

Potential Complications of Bone Biopsies

Complications from bone biopsies can include pain, hematoma, wound infection, and, rarely, neuropathy. However, studies show that horizontal or transiliac and vertical or superior biopsies of the anterior iliac crest result in very small morbidity and no mortality as a result of the procedure. The operator's experience is important in minimizing morbidity and in obtaining an adequate specimen. Use of newer techniques should further decrease any complications. Patient reports of pain range from none to moderate and, rarely, severe.

Mineralized Bone Histology

Processing bone biopsy samples requires four steps: fixation and dehydration, embedding, sectioning, and staining.

Fixation and Dehydration. To preserve bone tissue and cells in the most lifelike condition, the bone sample should be immersed in the fixative as soon as possible after the biopsy. Room temperature ethanol is the best fixative for routine mineralized bone histology. It does not leach calcium from bone within several weeks of exposure. Formalin is a stronger fixative but tends to leach out calcium, tetracycline, and aluminum. Osmium tetroxide, although a good fixative, promotes contrasts in cellular structures and stains tissue.

After 24 to 48 hours of ethanol immersion, depending on sample size, the specimen is ready for thorough dehydration. This step is very important because the commonly used embedding media are not miscible with water. For optimal dehydration, bone samples should be passed through fresh absolute ethanol at least five times, 24 hours each time. A recently developed tissue processor using a microwave and heat sink (to reduce microwave irradiation) is available; it greatly shortens the time necessary to fix, dehydrate, and penetrate bone samples (Straumann Medical, Waldenburg, Switzerland).

Embedding. For good section quality, methyl methacrylate is among the most useful embedding medium. It approximates the hardness of bone; it penetrates the bone specimen quickly without causing artifacts such as bubbles; it is nontoxic, nonflammable, and adjustable in hardness for final cutting; and solvents are available for dissolving it after cutting.

Sectioning. Special microtomes equipped with carbide edges or diamond knifes are used for cutting bone samples (Mikrom, Heidelberg, Germany). Several factors determine the number of sections to be cut. One factor is the number of different stains that will be used. The number of sections also depends on the amount of cancellous or cortical bone available in the bone sample. The smaller the bone sample, the higher the number of histologic sections. The third factor is the reproducibility of the quantitative method employed. To cover variation within the block, several sets of serial sections taken at different depths within the block should be obtained. Serial sections within one set allow quantitation of dynamic parameters of bone on the closest section (3 μm) to the one used to measure static parameters.

Staining. The flotation staining technique is less revelatory than staining after mounting sections on slides. Sections initially sealed on the slides can be very thin, and careful removal of plastic before staining provides excellent cellular details for bone cells and especially bone marrow cells. The most valuable and frequently used staining techniques to discriminate between calcified bone and uncalcified matrix are the modified Masson-Goldner trichrome stain, the solochrome cyanine stain, and von Kossa's stain. Special stains are also available for differentiation or for further classification.

Techniques to document aluminum accumulation in bone include measuring aluminum content of bone by atomic absorption spectrophotometry, histochemical staining to identify aluminum at the mineralization front or at other sites, and energy-dispersive x-ray analysis (EDAX). Although EDAX is very sensitive and specific for aluminum, it does not allow assessment of the exact severity and extent of aluminum deposition in bone. Determining bone aluminum content accurately estimates the magnitude of the aluminum load in bone. However, it cannot discriminate between aluminum embedded within mineralized bone or at the mineralization front or in bone marrow.

Two histologic staining techniques are available to detect aluminum on bone slides. The aurin-tricarboxylic acid method, which stains aluminum deposits as red bands, is very specific (Fig. 98.2). However, because the human eye is less sensitive to red than to other colors, deposits of light intensity are sometimes difficult to see. To recognize light aluminum deposits, bone slides need to be examined with green filter and under fluorescent light. With the solochrome azurin method, aluminum deposits appear dark purple-blue and are easily recognized at the mineralization front and within bone. The disadvantage to this method is that nonspecific staining can be seen at the edge of bone sections and when artifacts disrupt trabeculas.

Histopathologic changes associated with aluminum accumulation in bone correlate better with the extent of stainable bone aluminum at the mineralization front than with results of direct measurements of total aluminum content in bone. Therefore stainable bone aluminum is more useful than measurement of bone aluminum content to assess a patient's aluminum-related bone disease.

To detect abnormal amounts of iron in bone, the modified Gomori method provides the best results because of its high specificity for iron. The Congo red stain detects amyloid deposits, which can be viewed under polarized light microscopy.

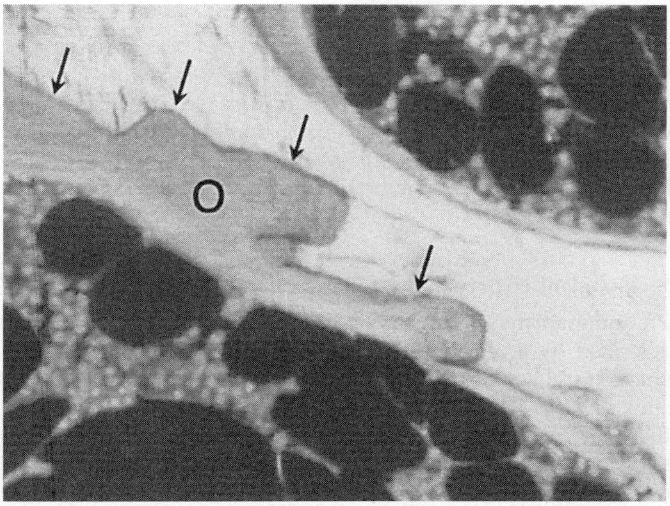

Figure 98.2. Aluminum deposits in bone *(arrows)*. Stainable bone aluminum at the osteoid (O)-mineralized bone (MB) interface, that is, the mineralization front. Nondecalcified, 3 μm thick section of human iliac bone (aurin-tricarboxylic acid stain; × 200).

Qualitative and Quantitative Evaluation of Bone

Qualitative and quantitative evaluations of the bone sample constitute the final steps in processing a bone biopsy. Pathologists must use their best judgment in diagnosing the underlying bone disease through microscopic examination of mounted sections of bone and bone marrow. The final decision may be based on qualitative or quantitative assessment of bone sections. Individuals who perform these evaluations must be well trained and have considerable experience in bone morphometry.

Qualitative assessment consists of such factors as the suitability of a biopsy for morphometric analysis, the amount of sample needed, where histologic structures should be measured, and what elements to evaluate.

With quantitative evaluation, numerical values are assigned to the various elements constituting bone. Potential differences between groups of patients or normal individuals or changes occurring after treatment can then be statistically evaluated. Compared with earlier techniques for statistical evaluation, the semiautomatic computerized method introduced by us greatly reduced the time required to measure surface, thickness, volume, and profile count of bone. Software programs developed for use with the semiautomatic method are all reliable for calculating areas and counts, but some differences exist in computation of lengths, thus affecting all parameters. A software must be chosen that automatically avoids this problem. Advantages to the computerized-assisted histomorphometric analysis of bone also include many means of data verification, and the data obtained can be automatically transferred to any statistical software, thus avoiding entry error.

Fully automated image analyzers are available, greatly reducing the time required to evaluate bone slides. Although they assess parameters of bone structure, they are not yet reliable in discriminating such elements as cellular details, detecting woven versus lamellar bone, and recognizing erosion surface. However, complete automatic analysis of bone may be possible in the future, with improved video cameras, staining techniques, and computerized image analysis capabilities.

TYPES OF RENAL OSTEODYSTROPHY

Despite a mostly common initial pathogenic pathway, renal osteodystrophy is not a uniform bone disease. The forms of renal osteodystrophy comprise (a) predominant hyperparathyroid bone disease, (b) low turnover bone disease including osteomalacia and adynamic bone disease, and (c) mixed uremic osteodystrophy. Transformation from one form to another can occur.

Predominant Hyperparathyroid Bone Disease

Predominant hyperparathyroid bone disease (PHBD) is characterized by a marked increase in bone turnover. Irregularly shaped trabeculas display numerous abnormal remodeling sites (Fig. 98.3), and an unusually high number of bone cells that are irregular in arrangement and shape. Deep, irregular resorption cavities often dissect or tunnel the trabeculas. Numerous enlarged osteoclasts contain multiple nuclei with prominent nucleoli.

Osteoblast's shape changes from cuboidal to polygonal or spindled shaped. Nuclei containing several nucleoli lose their polarity and occupy random positions within the cytoplasm of osteoblasts. The usual palisadelike monolayer of osteoblasts can be replaced by atypical multilayered arrangements of cells with variable orientation toward the bone surface (from parallel to perpendicular). These morphologic osteoblast abnormalities are accompanied by profound disturbances of their function. Osteoid surface and volume increase, and an osteoid seam can thicken because of collagen overproduction. The resulting osteoid is primarily of the woven, irregular type. Because collagen fibers accumulate toward the bone surfaces and are deposited between osteoblasts and toward the bone marrow, peritrabecular and bone marrow fibrosis results. In advanced cases, fibrosis replaces bone marrow entirely, reflecting the irregular activity of osteoblasts in which the regular activity of individual cells is decreased. Numerous irregular osteocytic lacunae within woven osteoid and mineralized bone result from the increased number of osteoblasts entrapped in bone, and the mineral apposition rate and the extent and number of mineralizing sites are notably increased. Calcium deposition in woven osteoid proceeds diffusely, irregularly, and incompletely. Findings of thick osteoid seams and diffuse, irregular tetracycline uptake in woven bone are sometimes mistakenly diagnosed as osteomalacia.

A marked increase in bone turnover often leads to cancellization of the cortical bone. This causes a net decrease in cortical bone volume most evident in the appendicular skeleton. PHBD usually presents with high bone volume, but malnutrition, immobilization, or other causes can markedly reduce bone volume. Also, areas of high bone mass may be adjacent to pseudocysts consisting primarily of hyperplastic or fibrotic bone marrow. In any case, bone strength cannot be equated with high bone volume in PHBD patients because the irregular trabeculae may lose their proper three-dimensional architecture and connectivity. Also, the poorly mineralized trabeculae consist mainly of mechanically deficient woven bone with a propensity to fracture. This disease creates a particularly fragile fracture-prone bone; thus the use of the term *osteosclerosis* is inappropriate.

Low Turnover Bone Disease

Representing the other end of the spectrum from PHBD, low turnover uremic osteodystrophy is marked by a profound decrease in active remodeling sites. Certain features reflect a marked decrease in osteoblastic activity, and there are few osteoclasts and osteoblasts. Most of the trabecular bone is covered by lining cells. Usually only a few thin single labels of tetracycline are observed. Other characteristics include predominantly lamellar bone structure, few active bone formation sites, and markedly reduced mineralizing surfaces.

In low turnover uremic osteodystrophy, the number of bone-forming and bone-resorbing cells is dramatically reduced and bone formation and mineralization are significantly decreased. This type has two subgroups: low turnover osteomalacia (LTOM) and adynamic renal bone disease (ABD). These two histologic subgroups can be identified by the sequence of events leading to a decline in the number and/or activity of the osteoblasts. LTOM is characterized by an accumulation of unmineralized matrix in which a diminution in mineralization precedes or is more pronounced than the inhibition of collagen deposition (Fig. 98.4). Although bone volume/tissue volume may vary, mineralized bone volume is always low.

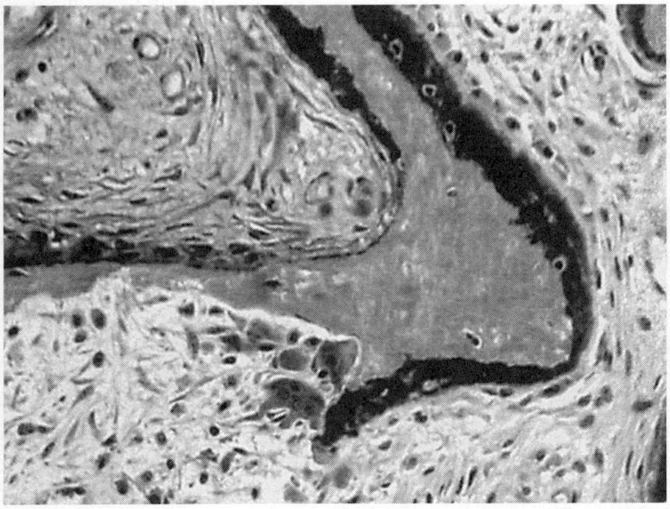

Figure 98.3. Predominant hyperparathyroid bone disease. High fraction of trabecular surface covered by osteoid seams. High osteoid-osteoblast interface. High bone-osteoclast interface with appearance of deep resorption lacuna. Marrow fibrosis. Nondecalcified, 3 μm thick section of human iliac bone (modified Masson-Goldner stain; × 200).

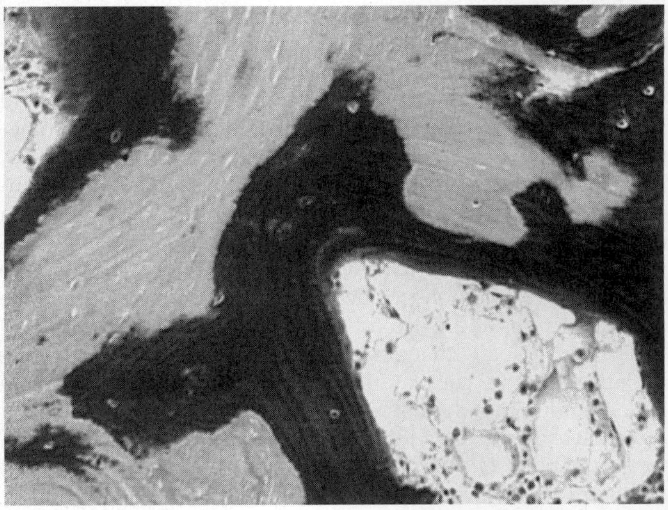

Figure 98.4. Low turnover osteomalacia. Increase in osteoid volume. Wide osteoid seams. Absence of osteoblasts and resorption surface. Nondecalcified, 3 μm thick section of human iliac bone (modified Masson-Goldner stain; × 125).

In LTOM, unmineralized bone makes up a sizable portion of trabecular bone volume. The increased lamellar osteoid volume results from the presence of wide osteoid seams that cover much of the trabecular surface. The occasional presence of woven bone buried within the trabeculas indicates past high bone turnover. Osteoclasts, when present, are usually seen within trabecular bone or at the small fraction of trabecular surface left without osteoid coating.

With ABD, bone volume is frequently reduced. Reduced mineralization is coupled with a parallel decrease in bone formation. ABD is characterized by few osteoid seams (Fig. 98.5).

Mixed Uremic Osteodystrophy

Mixed uremic osteodystrophy (MUO) is caused primarily by defective mineralization with or without increased bone formation and by increased parathyroid hormone (PTH) activity on bone, features that may coexist in varying degrees in different patients. Bone volume/tissue volume is extremely variable and depends on a dominant pathogenic cause. Other features include increased numbers of heterogeneous remodeling sites and usually an increase in osteoclasts. Active foci with numerous cells, peritrabecular fibrosis, and woven osteoid seams coexist with adjacent lamellar sites with a more reduced activity. Therefore greater production of lamellar or woven osteoid causes the accumulation of osteoid with normal or increased thickness of osteoid seams (Fig. 98.6). Although active mineralizing surfaces are often present in woven bone with higher mineralization rate and diffuse labeling, mineralization surfaces may be low in lamellar bone with a low mineral apposition rate.

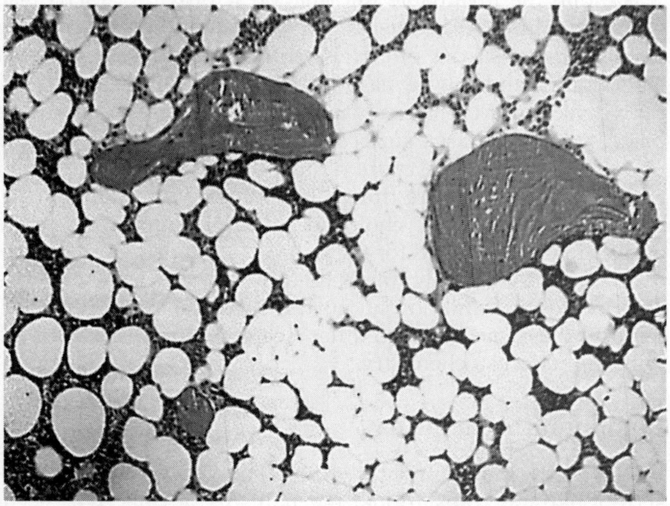

Figure 98.5. Adynamic bone disease. No accumulation of osteoid. Absence of bone formation of resorption. Nondecalcified, 3 μm thick section of human iliac bone (modified Masson-Goldner stain; × 125).

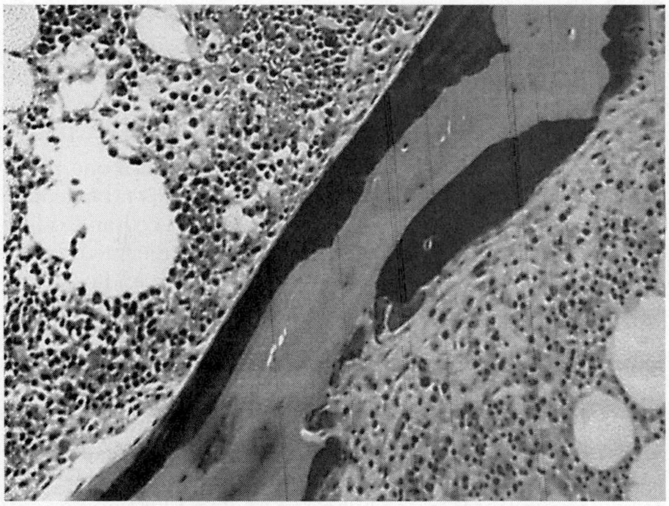

Figure 98.6. Mixed uremic osteodystrophy. Increased fraction of trabecular surface covered by osteoid. Mean thickness of osteoid seams is increased, resulting in high osteoid volume. Increased extent of trabecular surface exhibiting resorption lacunae filled with or void of osteoclast. Nondecalcified, 3 μm thick section of human iliac bone (modified Masson-Goldner stain; × 7.5).

EVOLUTION OF RENAL OSTEODYSTROPHY

In the past, diversity in bone lesions was partly attributed to aluminum toxicity in bone. The major sources of contamination with aluminum in end-stage renal disease (ESRD) patients are aluminum-containing phosphate binders and high aluminum content of water and dialysate. High morbidity and mortality accompany severe aluminum intoxication, and deferoxamine (DFO) chelation, though efficient, is not without risks (Chapter 68, Part 2). Therefore efforts were made to develop tests capable of diagnosing this disease. Determining serum levels of aluminum before and after DFO treatment, alone or in association with serum PTH, proved useful, but only in those patients with high baseline serum aluminum levels who showed a marked increase after DFO challenge and had low serum PTH levels. Therefore bone biopsies were the only unequivocal means to establish aluminum accumulation in bone and determine the type of renal osteodystrophy.

Today, aluminum dialysate content is under better control, and aluminum-containing phosphate binders have largely been replaced with calcium salts. To overcome parathyroid gland overactivity, therapeutic regimens ensuring better control of serum calcium and phosphorus levels and correction of calcitriol deficiency are also widely used.

In a study in which we analyzed the changing pattern of renal osteodystrophy in 2,248 patients over 13 years (from 1983 to 1995), distribution of the four histologic forms varied. MUO was found in the majority of patients over the years, but a slight decrease was seen in 1990 and 1995. PHBD was observed in a large number of patients in 1983, but decreased constantly until 1988, then increased gradually to reach a level in 1995 similar to the one found in 1983. LTOM incidence decreased progressively over the 13 years of the survey. The number of patients with ABD, which was first diagnosed in 1984, increased until the late 1980s, then stayed approximately the same. The trends for patients on hemodialysis and peritoneal dialysis were similar for the four histologic groups. However, peritoneal dialysis patients consistently exhibited more histologic signs of ABD and fewer signs of PHBD than did hemodialysis patients.

Between 1983 and 1984, the number of biopsied patients positive for aluminum increased from approximately 40% to approximately 60%, remained stable until 1992, then tended to decrease. In 1995, however, approximately 25% of the biopsies analyzed still showed aluminum in bone. Patients with low bone turnover, either LTOM or ABD, showed higher aluminum deposition than patients with other forms of renal osteodystrophy, and this did not change with time. More patients with stainable aluminum of more than 30% were in the LTOM, ABD, and MUO groups than in the PHBD group. From 1984 to 1995, bone aluminum accumulation decreased within each histologic group, and in 1995 aluminum accumulation was mostly seen in patients with MUO and ABD.

In spite of newer therapeutic strategies, however, aluminum accumulation has not completely disappeared, and dialyzed patients still present with PHBD, MUO, and ABD. Available evidence shows that low bone turnover has both histologic and clinical relevance. Patients with this abnormality were found to have abnormal calcium homeostasis, higher incidence of fractures, more bone pain, delayed healing, and higher morbidity and mortality than did patients exhibiting other histologic abnormalities.

CLINICAL APPLICATIONS

Nephrologists must determine a patient's level of bone turnover to apply the correct therapy. Serum PTH levels measured with radioimmunometric assay are commonly used to assess bone turnover in dialyzed patients. Although these levels have been found to be more sensitive than the previously employed radioimmunoassays, there is still no consensus regarding the serum level of PTH that reflects normal bone turnover in ESRD patients. A recent study in our laboratory found that serum PTH levels between 65 and 450 pg/ml, seen in the majority of dialysis patients, are unpredictive of the underlying bone disease. Because bone biopsies provide a sensitive measurement of bone changes, they more accurately determine the type of renal osteodystrophy and can indicate potential aluminum accumulation in dialyzed patients. Bone biopsies also allow tailored therapeutic measures. The extent of aluminum deposits at the bone-osteoid interface and the level of bone turnover determine the optimal duration of chelation therapy. The higher the extent of stainable aluminum at the bone surface and the lower the bone turnover, the longer the duration of chelation therapy. For instance, with ABD, aluminum accumulation over 70% of the trabecular surface may require more than a year of chelation therapy. Aluminum deposits of approximately 30% of the bone surface associated with marked secondary hyperparathyroidism may disappear in several months. Practitioners generally agree that chelation therapy should be initiated when stainable aluminum is at 30% or more of the bone surface.

If the biopsy shows no significant deposits of aluminum, the degree of bone turnover will help the practitioner determine the route, aggressiveness, and length of calcitriol therapy. Severe hyperparathyroidism with marked bone marrow fibrosis is an indication for high doses of intravenous calcitriol if the calcium–phosphorus product can be controlled. A bone biopsy can predict whether there will be high resistance to intravenous calcitriol at the needed massive doses. In this case, parathyroidectomy may be necessary. The severity of the effect of secondary hyperparathyroidism on bone may also indicate the extent of the postparathyroidectomy "hungry bone syndrome" and allow preventive measures such as the preoperative injection of calcitriol to avoid postsurgical hypocalcemia. In patients with mild to moderate increase in bone turnover with or without mineralization defect, the doses of oral or intravenous calcitriol and duration of therapy may be adjusted to avoid the development of ABD. In case of ABD, calcitriol therapy is not desirable because of the risk of inducing hypercalcemia and extraosseous calcifications.

A bone biopsy establishes the precise relationships between serum indices of calcium metabolism and bone lesions. This enhances the interpretation of longitudinal follow-up of noninvasive parameters while the patient is undergoing a particular therapy.

MOLECULAR BONE HISTOLOGY

In situ hybridization histochemistry (ISHH) and immunohistochemistry (IHC) are two powerful methodologies used to investigate bone cell metabolism.

In Situ Hybridization Histochemistry

ISHH applied to bone sections reveals cellular sources and differential gene expressions of the specific biomolecules involved in bone metabolism (i.e., cytokines, matrix proteins, and receptor species). Through the use of a sequence of complementary ribonucleic acid (RNA) probes labeled with a reporter molecule, ISHH can detect cellular nucleic acids. ISHH can also evaluate the actual content of specific nucleic acids in the volume of a single cell. With ISHH, the relationship between gene expression and cell number and activity can be analyzed directly in the bone microenvironment.

Despite the invaluable information it provides, ISHH also has several limits that must be kept in mind when interpreting results. The sensitivity of ISHH is difficult to assess in different laboratories, and low levels of RNA gene expression may escape detection if the corresponding autoradiographic signal is dispersed over a large surface of the section or is masked by background. Therefore caution must be used before important biologic conclusions are drawn from negative results. Finally, specificity relies on the choice of suitable sequences of probe and stringency adopted for the hybridization procedure. Moreover, ISHH reveals only intracellular RNA transcripts and does not provide information about the subsequent steps of protein synthesis and extracellular secretion unless associated with immunohistochemistry.

Immunohistochemistry

IHC is highly complementary to ISHH in that it links the transcriptional and translational mechanisms of cells. IHC accurately assesses the metabolic state of bone cells by visualizing protein production. Although the technique of IHC is well established in soft tissue, its use with hard tissue such as bone is relatively new. Therefore researchers using IHC must be particularly careful to ensure a reliable and reproducible outcome.

Information Derived From Molecular Histology

Researchers have demonstrated that factors believed to play important roles in regulating bone turnover are expressed in bone cells. ISHH has documented expression of bone matrix proteins, including type I collagen, osteocalcin, and osteopontin. These proteins are associated with cell-to-cell and cell-to-mineralized matrix adhesion. ISHH has also documented changes in biologic activity measured by type I collagen and osteopontin messenger RNA (mRNA) expression in bone cells. The vitamin D receptor, which plays an important role in regulating bone turnover, has been shown to be expressed in bone cells through ISHH.

We used histomorphometric and ISHH techniques to document expressions of the cytokine interleukin-6 (IL-6) and its receptor IL-6R in renal osteodystrophy patients. IL-6 is believed to be a significant factor in bone remodeling. Our findings indicate that IL-6 and IL-6R are intricately involved in osteoclastic bone resorption.

Although molecular histology is still in its beginnings, its value has been clearly established. The continuing development of more efficient, economical methods will lead to its routine use as a morphologic tool in the study of bone.

CONCLUSION

Bone biopsies are presently much more widely used for diagnosis and research than they have been in the past. However, traditional constraints continue to be perceived because of the procedure's invasiveness and cost, potential pain for the patient, delays between the biopsy and pathology reports, lack of specialized centers with expertise to interpret bone samples, lack of technical training, and limited understanding of the information provided by the results.

Efforts to minimize these constraints have included improved instrument design and biopsy techniques and more intensive and detailed training of clinicians and pathologists. Advances in bone sample processing have resulted in faster turnaround time between bone biopsy and availability of histologic results. This has enhanced the value of bone biopsy in routine patient care. Also, bone morphometrists have adopted a uniform and simple nomenclature for bone histomorphometric parameters, and nonmorphometrists can now better understand bone biopsy results. The establishment of the International Society for Bone Morphometry has increased the number of individuals involved in bone morphometry.

Alternatives to the bone biopsy continue to be pursued. The search for noninvasive serum or bone markers that predict bone turnover, mineralization status, bone aluminum accumulation, and cellular abnormalities has resulted in improved methods to determine serum levels of various calciotropic hormones, isolation of proteins and enzymes from bone, and development of commercially available assays. However, these alternatives have not proven to be specific or sensitive enough to effectively determine the potential value of a specific therapeutic regimen.

Selected Readings

Malluche HH, Faugere MC. Renal bone disease 1990: an unmet challenge for the nephrologist. *Kidney Int* 1990;38:193–211.

Current knowledge, unresolved problems, and future directions in the field of renal osteodystrophy.

Malluche HH, Faugere MC. *Atlas of mineralized bone histology.* New York: Karger; 1986.

Detailed and illustrated description of bone biopsy techniques, mineralized bone histology, bone histomorphometry, indications for bone biopsies, and information derived from bone biopsies in metabolic bone diseases and related bone abnormalities.

Malluche HH, Meyer W, Sherman D, et al. Quantitative bone histology in 84 normal American subjects. Micromorphometric analysis and evaluation of variance of iliac bone. *Calcif Tissue Int* 1982;34:449–455.

Normal values for histomorphometric parameters of bone structure, bone formation, bone resorption, and bone dynamics. Assessment of variance of these parameters in left versus right iliac crests, anterior versus posterior, and superior versus inferior portions of the iliac bone in normal humans.

Malluche HH, Monier-Faugere MC. The role of bone biopsy in the management of patients with renal osteodystrophy. *J Am Soc Nephrol* 1994;4:1631–1642.

Detailed description of requirements and indications for bone biopsies. Impact of the information derived from mineralized bone histology on the management of patients with end-stage renal failure.

Monier-Faugere MC, Langub MC, Malluche HH. Mineralized bone histology in normal and uremic states. In: Bushinsky DA, ed. *Renal osteodystrophy.* Philadelphia: Lippincott-Raven, 1998:49–87.

Present understanding on bone metabolism at the tissue, cellular, and molecular levels. Principles and nomenclature of bone morphometry and their applications to renal osteodystrophy.

Monier-Faugere MC, Malluche HH. Trends in renal osteodystrophy: a survey from 1983 to 1995 in a total of 2248 patients. *Nephrol Dial Transplant* 1996; 11:111–120.

Evolution of clinical and histologic forms of renal osteodystrophy in a large series of patients with end-stage renal disease. In particular, emergence of adynamic bone disease and analysis of its risks factors.

CHAPTER 99

Shock-Wave Lithotripsy

Matthew D. Dunn and Jeffry L. Huffman

Perhaps one of the greatest contributions that technology has provided in medicine over the last 20 years is in the treatment of urinary calculi. The management of stone disease has evolved from primarily open stone surgery to endoscopic management to completely noninvasive therapy. With the development of shock-wave lithotripsy (SWL) as a modality to fragment urinary stones, the majority of patients with stone disease can now be managed in an outpatient setting. This has further led to decreased morbidity, hospitalization time, anesthetic requirements, and overall cost, which obviously pleases a growing managed care–based industry.

SWL was introduced in the early 1980s and although modifications have taken place, the same basic tenets still apply. Lithotripsy has its roots in military research by the German aerospace company, Dornier. After noticing the damage from shock waves to aircraft and crew members in military tanks, a program to further study the effects of shock waves was developed. This required developing artificial methods of reproducing shock waves. Intense research in the 1970s by Chaussy led to the realization that focused shock waves capable of fragmenting stones could be delivered to the kidney without untoward effects to surrounding tissues. Studies in which human stones were transplanted into dog kidneys demonstrated the ease with which stones could be easily fragmented. Also, the small fragments generated could be passed from the urinary collecting system. Dornier created the first lithotripsy machine, which successfully treated the first human in 1980. The first commercially available machine was Dornier's HM3 lithotripter in 1984. This machine became very successful and, although it has stimulated the creation of many different types of newer lithotripters, it is still considered by many to be the gold standard for SWL today.

FEATURES OF LITHOTRIPSY DEVICES

Although a variety of lithotripter machines are available, they all produce the same effect—that is, they generate shock waves. The method of shock-wave generation is what characterizes them. All machines ultimately focus these waves at a distant focal point where the stone lies. The most potent lithotripter machine to this date is still the Dornier HM3 because of its relatively high peak pressures and large focal volumes. It allows greater energy delivery than any other lithotripsy machine and as such is very efficient in fragmenting stones.

Basic features shared by all SWL machines include an energy source to generate the shock waves, a mechanism of focusing the shock wave to a distal site (F2), a coupling medium that in most cases is water, and an in-line imaging system to localize the stone.

The delivery of shock waves from an external source requires an efficient mechanism to transmit the shock wave to the stone without losing energy. The early machines such as the Dornier HM3 use the water bath as the coupling medium to facilitate transmission of shock waves without impedance. Newer generation machines have localized the water medium in a water cushion directly over the shock head, obviating the need for patient immersion in a water bath.

The imaging system for stone localization has evolved as well. The initial SWL machines and most machines today use biplanar fluoroscopy for stone localization. Subsequent generations began using in-line ultrasound imaging, and certain newer machines have even combined both. Both modalities can image stone fragmentation in real time. The advantage of ultrasound is decreased radiation exposure to the patient and easier localization of radiolucent stones such as uric acid stones. Stones located within the kidney are easily identified with ultrasound. Ureteral stones are more difficult to detect with ultrasound because of overlying bowel gas. Fluoroscopy is far superior to ultrasound in imaging stones located in the ureter.

METHODS OF SHOCK-WAVE LITHOTRIPSY

Electrohydraulic Lithotripters

The energy most commonly used for SWL today is electrohydraulic. Shock waves are created by a spark-gap electrode within a liquid medium. Current applied to the electrode results in a spark that vaporizes water at its tip. Sudden expansion of water creates shock waves that permeate the surrounding water medium. These waves are reflected toward a focal point where the stone would be located. Tissues in the path of the shock waves proximal to this focal point are not as effected because the waves have not converged.

Piezoelectric Generators

Piezoelectric energy uses small ceramic discs lining a reflector. When activated with a high-voltage current they rapidly expand, generating a shock wave in a surrounding fluid medium. The configuration of each ceramic disc is such that shock waves from each disc converge at a focal point, thus providing a focused shock wave able to fragment a stone.

Electromagnetic Lithotripters

Electromagnetic energy devices use water-filled shock tubes with a thin, metallic membrane associated with an electromagnetic coil. An electric current applied to the coil causes the membranes to repel, resulting in shock waves that are focused by a reflector to a distal focal point.

Microexplosive Generator

Microexplosive energy is rarely used. This modality employs a small, lead-azide pellet within an ellipsoid reflector to generate shock waves. The safety of lead azide has come into question because of its explosive nature.

The initial machines such as the Dornier HM3 usually require general anesthesia because of the significant amount of pain produced. The goals of newer generation SWL machines have been to maximize stone fragmentation while at the same time minimizing pain and trauma to surrounding structures. Thus the anesthetic requirements for SWL depend on the actual device used. By enlarging the shock-wave aperture, a wider shock-wave entry at the skin level is realized and less pain results. Therefore the newer generation machines have minimized anesthetic requirements, relying on light sedation and, in some cases, even a topical anesthetic cream. The disadvantage is that this results in a narrower focal volume, which requires better accuracy localizing the stone precisely in the path of the shock wave.

In general, the newer generation of lithotripters have also been less powerful. Of the newer machines, the authors use the Siemens Lithostar, which, although not as powerful as the HM3, strikes a better balance between stone fragmentation and minimal anesthetic needs.

Mobile lithotripsy machines are becoming increasingly popular, increasing the availability of SWL to a wider patient population. These machines, however, are less powerful than their stationary predecessors with the disadvantage of less-efficient stone fragmentation.

INDICATIONS

Lithotripsy has been employed for the treatment of all urinary stones from the renal calyces to the bladder, although with varying degrees of success. The effectiveness of SWL depends on several variables: stone location, size, and composition. Other important variables include the presence of urinary obstruction and anatomic abnormalities, which may effect stone passage.

For stones within the kidney, one can expect approximately a 90% success rate after SWL. Middle- and upper-pole calyceal stones have an improved success rate over lower-pole stones with lithotripsy. This results from the dependent position and poorer drainage of the lower pole. Ureteral stones, especially in the proximal ureter between the ureteropelvic junction and sacroiliac joint, enjoy excellent success rates after SWL. Fragmentation of middle and distal ureteral stones are less predictable. Because of the bony pelvis, patients require different positioning (usually in the prone position), which may not be possible with certain lithotripsy machines. Stone visualization may also be difficult. As a result, success rates are more varied but still have been reported as high as 80%. Distal ureteral stones also may be treated with SWL but are more reliably treated with ureteroscopic extraction. Successful treatment of bladder stones has been reported with SWL when applied in the prone position. Unfortunately, this does not address the possibility of bladder outlet obstruction, which may be the etiology of stone development. Likewise, the majority of these stones can be easily managed endoscopically, allowing simultaneous management of prostatic or urethral pathology.

There is an inverse relationship between stone size and stone-free rates after lithotripsy. Regardless of location, the larger the stone burden, the less successful SWL becomes. Stones greater than 2 cm will have lower stone-free rates than smaller stones and will often require subsequent procedures for residual fragments. This includes either repeat SWL, percutaneous nephrolithotomy, or ureteroscopy. It is recommended that stones less than 2 to 2.5 cm be treated with SWL as first-line therapy. Larger stones are best managed endoscopically either with percutaneous nephrolithotomy or ureteroscopy. SWL can be used to rid smaller residual fragments that remain after the aforementioned procedures.

Stone composition is another important variable in the effectiveness of SWL. The majority of urinary stones are composed of calcium oxalate, which can exist in a dihydrate or monohydrate form. The dihydrate form of calcium-oxalate stones is relatively "soft" and responds well to SWL, whereas the monohydrate form is much harder and requires more energy to break up, often breaking up into large fragments. As a result, calcium-oxalate–monohydrate stones have a lower stone-free rate than the dihydrate counterpart when managed with SWL. Uric acid stones respond well to lithotripsy but pose a problem in that they are radiolucent stones and can be difficult to visualize. Ultrasound can easily identify renal stones but less so in the ureter. This problem can be resolved by injecting contrast media either intravenously or directly into the collecting system, outlining the stone as a filling defect when imaged fluoroscopically. Struvite, or magnesium-ammonium-phosphate stones, are "soft" stones and respond well to SWL. Perhaps the most difficult stones to treat with lithotripsy are cystine stones. The disulfide bond between the amino acid residues is relatively resistant to shock waves. Unless they are small stones, they are best treated by percutaneous nephrolithotomy or ureteroscopy.

Previously, lithotripsy was used for fragmenting biliary stones. Because of the high incidence of gallstones, it was anticipated that this may be a viable nonoperative mode of management. However, interest waned once success rates did not match that of renal lithotripsy rates. Likewise laparoscopic cholecystectomy brought forth a better minimally invasive method of management. Another potential use for SWL is in orthopedics to facilitate the treatment of nonunion bone fractures, although long-term benefits are unknown.

EFFECTS ON RENAL FUNCTION

The impact of SWL on renal function has been documented in animal studies, which have demonstrated acute and chronic changes to the renal parenchyma. The pathologic changes described include intraparenchymal hemorrhage and chronic renal fibrosis. SWL may affect renal tubular function in that reversible nephrotic-range proteinuria has been demonstrated. Animal studies in pigs have demonstrated temporarily reduced glomerular filtration rate (GFR), renal blood flow (RBF), and urine flow rates in shocked kidneys immediately after SWL as well as diminished renal plasma flow (RPF) to the contralateral kidney, signifying that hemodynamics may be impaired in both kidneys. Vasospasm has been suggested as the cause of this phenomenon because this effect can be attenuated by administering verapamil.

Effects on developing kidneys have been studied in animals as a model to identify potential effects on children. SWL applied to immature rabbit kidneys caused histologic changes including interstitial fibrosis, tubular atrophy, glomeruli destruction, capsular thickening, perivascular fibrosis, and mild arteriole-wall thickening. These changes were proportional to the number of shocks given. However, despite these permanent histologic changes, renal growth and function were not significantly affected.

Damage to surrounding tissues have likewise been reported and include pulmonary contusion, submucosal intestinal hematomas, and liver petechiae. Fortunately, these are rarely of any clinical significance. Shock waves delivered directly to ovaries in rats also show no significant effects. Nevertheless, because animal data may not extrapolate to human data, it is still recommended not to use SWL for distal ureteral stones in women of reproductive age.

CONTRAINDICATIONS

Because of the previously described effects of SWL on various organ systems, absolute and relative contraindications have been developed. Most studies evaluating harmful effects were performed on animals, which may not necessarily extrapolate to humans. As experience with SWL develops, the list of contraindications is diminishing, leading to an expanded use of lithotripsy for more patients. A comprehensive review of the literature regarding the contraindications to SWL has helped to clarify absolute from relative contraindications. For example, patients with calcified aortic and renal aneurysms who were initially never considered candidates, appear to suffer no harmful effect from SWL. Nevertheless, as a point of caution, guidelines have been developed for patients with calcified aneurysms. It is suggested that asymptomatic patients with renal artery aneurysms less than 2 cm and aortic aneurysms less than 5 cm may be treated. However, the stone should be more than 5 cm from the aneurysm to minimize the pressure generated at the aneurysm site. Despite these recommendations there have been no adverse effects of SWL on calcified aneurysms to date.

Patients with pacemakers no longer pose a contraindication for SWL. Because the majority of pacemakers are away from the stone target, most patients suffer no undue effect. However, as a point of caution, it is recommended that a cardiologist experienced in pacemaker management be available for these patients in that rare case that a pacemaker may fail. Defibrillators pose more of a problem because they are usually implanted in the subcutaneous tissues of the abdomen, thus they are potentially closer to the focal point of the shock wave. However, in data from available studies, there appears to be no harm to the device if treating a contralateral stone. In these patients, a polystyrene shield was used to protect the device from shock waves. In general, it is recommended that patients with defibrillators have their device checked after SWL to confirm no electrophysiologic disruptions.

At present, the only absolute contraindications are pregnancy and irreversible coagulopathies. As such, all bleeding disorders should be corrected before treatment. Patients on anticoagulant therapy with heparin, warfarin (Coumadin), aspirin, or nonsteroidal antiinflammatory drugs should consider discontinuation of this therapy for an appropriate time interval before treatment.

Relative contraindications include untreated hypertension, distal ureteral urinary obstruction precluding the successful passage of stone fragments, and active urinary tract infections. Because the long-term effects to the ovary are unknown, it is recommended to avoid SWL to distal ureteral stones in women of reproductive age.

COMPLICATIONS

SWL is generally a well-tolerated procedure with low morbidity and mortality rates. In a series evaluating 62,000 patients, the mortality rate of SWL was reported as 0.02%. Most patients will have gross hematuria, which is usually mild and transient, resolving within 24 hours. The most common postlithotripsy complication is perirenal or intrarenal hematoma. The incidence has been reported as high as 20% to 25%, although clinically significant hemorrhage is rarely seen (less than 1%). The most consistent risk factors for this complication are unrecognized bleeding disorders and preexisting hypertension. Indeed, the majority of clinically significant hematomas have occurred in patients who had unrecognized or untreated coagulopathies. Fortunately, the usual course of these hematomas is spontaneous resolution within 2 years. Other factors implicated in predisposing to bleeding complications include active urinary tract infection, obesity, and a higher number of shock waves delivered to the kidneys.

Steinstrasse, which literally means "stone street" in German, refers to the collection of stone fragments that become lodged distally in the ureter. A larger stone fragment may become lodged distally allowing smaller fragments to accumulate behind, giving its characteristic radiographic appearance. Treatment of steinstrasse is dependent on the clinical condition of the patient. If the patient is asymptomatic, observation with hydration can be used. The presence of pain and an associated infection indicated by fever and leukocytosis necessitate drainage of the kidney either by stent placement or percutaneous nephrostomy placement. Persistent steinstrasse may be cleared ureteroscopically.

The renal trauma resulting from SWL has initially stimulated concern regarding the development of hypertension, and indeed several studies reported new onset of hypertension as a complication of SWL. However, newer studies have disputed this finding. One study suggests that a certain subset of patients may be at risk of developing hypertension after SWL. Patients older than 60 years had a significantly increased risk; at 26 months follow-up of this group of patients, almost half ultimately developed hypertension. Overall, the majority of studies to date show no increased risk of post-SWL hypertension.

Selected Readings

Chaussy CG. ESWL: past, present, and future. *J Endourol* 1988;2:97–105.

This general overview of SWL focuses on indications, contraindications, and complications of SWL. Other nonurologic applications of SWL are briefly discussed, as are future applications in research.

Janetschek G, Frauswcher F, Knapp R, et al. New onset hypertension after extracorporeal shock wave lithotripsy: age related incidence and prediction by intrarenal resistive index. *J Urol* 1997;158:346–351.

This study followed 57 patients for more than 2 years after SWL to investigate the relevance of elevated resistive index levels and the incidence of new onset hypertension. The data showed that lithotripsy caused an immediate increase in the resistive index in 75% of patients older than 60 years with 45% of these patients developing new onset hypertension. They also demonstrated a strong positive correlation between pathologic resistive index levels and blood pressure.

Kaji DM, Xie HU, Hardy BE, et al. Extracorporeal shock wave lithotripsy on renal growth, function, and arterial blood pressure in an animal model. *J Urol* 1991; 146:544–547.

To study the long-term bioeffects of SWL on an immature animal, 30 young rabbits underwent a unilateral nephrectomy and subsequent SWL to the remaining kidney. When compared with a control group who received no shock waves, there was no significant change in animal growth, renal growth, and renal function from SWL. Permanent histologic renal changes were noted, with severity proportional to the number of shocks given.

Lingeman JE. Extracorporeal shock wave lithotripsy: development, instrumentation, and current status. *Urol Clin North Am* 1997;24:185–211.

This comprehensive review discusses the origins of SWL and the evolution of technology that has led to today's machines.

Martin TV, Sosa EV. Shock-wave lithotripsy. In: Walsh RC, Retik AB, Vaughan ED, et al., eds. *Campbell's urology.* Philadelphia: WB Saunders Company, 1998: 2735–2752.

This chapter gives a thorough review of all aspects of SWL, including the various energy sources used as well as indications, contraindications, complications, and a review of the literature regarding results of lithotripsy. Other applications for SWL are briefly discussed.

Streem S. Contemporary clinical practice of shock wave lithotripsy: a reevaluation of contraindications. *J Urol* 1997;157:1197–1203.

This comprehensive review article evaluates the recent literature regarding absolute and relative contraindications of SWL. A critical review of the basic scientific and clinic studies refute previous empiric assumptions that certain concurrent conditions, such as aortic aneurysms and pacemakers, preclude SWL. Most patients with these conditions can be safely treated and problems circumvented with appropriate preparation. Pregnancy remains the only absolute contraindication.

Teh LC, Aslan P, Preminger GM. What's new in shock wave lithotripsy? *Contemp Urol* 1997;Oct:26–36.

This review article describes the various energy sources and mechanisms used in today's lithotripsy machines.

Venkatesh K, Streem S. Long-term radiographic and functional outcome of extracorporeal shock wave lithotripsy induced perirenal hematomas. *J Urol* 1995; 154:1673–1675.

In this study, 19 patients with SWL-induced perirenal hematomas were followed to determine the radiologic and functional outcome. The majority of hematomas resolved spontaneously within 2 years without clinically evident adverse effects on blood pressure or renal function.

Willis LR, Evan AP, Connors BA, et al. Effects of extracorporeal shock wave lithotripsy to one kidney on bilateral glomerular filtration rate and PAH clearance in minipigs. *J Urol* 1996;150:1502–1506.

This provides a systematic assessment of the acute effects of SWL on renal hemodynamics in an animal model. Shock waves delivered to one kidney resulted in alterations in glomerular filtration rate and renal plasma flow to both kidneys. The effect was attenuated with verapamil, suggesting vasoconstriction as the etiology for this bilateral effect.

SECTION XII

Laboratory Procedures and Techniques

CHAPTER 100

Urinalysis

Gavin J. Becker and Kenneth F. Fairley

Examination of the urine is among the least invasive of all commonly performed investigations, yet it can be extremely informative, particularly in patients with renal disease. To obtain the most information the urine must be collected in an appropriate manner and be examined promptly and carefully; the result also has to be interpreted intelligently, in context with the clinical condition. This full process is best dealt with by the nephrologist caring for the patient. In this chapter we will focus on the practical rather than the theoretical aspects of diagnostic urinalysis.

METHODS OF COLLECTION OF URINE

The manner of collection varies with the form of urinalysis to be performed.

Clean Voided Specimen

The most frequently used form of urinalysis is the testing of a freshly voided specimen of urine using plastic strips to which chemically impregnated paper indicator squares are attached. These indicator strips, commonly called *dipsticks,* are useful in screening for a variety of normal and abnormal urinary characteristics. They are used routinely by primary care physicians and on all patients at the time of hospital admission. More specific or sensitive tests, particularly in patients with suspected or known renal disease, often require a more carefully collected urinary specimen. A clean-voided specimen is usually adequate for tests of urinary biochemistry and, if combined with an estimate of urinary creatinine concentration, can also be used to assess the excretion rate of solutes. This is particularly useful in patients who are considered unreliable in collecting 24-hour urine specimens.

Midstream Specimen of Urine

For urine microscopy and culture techniques a carefully collected midstream specimen of urine (MSU) is the preferred sample in most instances. A moderately full bladder is required.

In males, the foreskin, if present, should first be retracted. The glans is then gently washed with cotton wool swabs soaked in water or saline solution. The patient then begins voiding, and after passing at least 200 ml, moves the container into the stream to collect a sample of 100 to 200 ml.

In females, the technique is more difficult, and contamination with vulval or vaginal cells and bacteria occurs more commonly. The patient must hold the labia apart with the first and second fingers of one hand while gently washing the internal labia and meatus from front to back with water- or saline-soaked cotton wool swabs. With the labia still held apart, the patient passes approximately 200 ml of urine before moving a container into the stream to collect 100 to 200 ml of urine.

Preferably this is performed with the patient watching the stream, to ensure a clear passage into the container. This may be easier if the patient sits facing the back of the toilet bowl; the procedure may require nursing assistance and can be very difficult if the patient is obese, pregnant, or is physically or mentally handicapped. In such patients, particularly when the presence of pus cells or bacteria is of critical concern, it may be necessary to collect either an open-ended catheter specimen or suprapubic aspirate. Occasionally patients who find it difficult to perform a clean MSU in the sitting position find that they can do so by standing in the shower cubicle with the legs astride. In other cases, a nurse may be able to help collect a specimen with the patient in the Trendelenburg position.

Open-Ended Catheter Specimen

In females, when there is a concern about contamination by cells or bacteria suspected to come from the vagina or vulva, a specially designed open-ended catheter can be used. This is invaluable in preventing the need to collect costly repeat MSU specimens until a "clean" sample is obtained (Fig. 100.1).

The important features of the catheter are its narrow diameter (14 F) to reduce trauma and a blunt tip with an open end to allow thorough flushing of urethral contents through the catheter. It is inserted to just enter the internal sphincter of a moderately full bladder, 200 ml of urine is allowed to drain freely into a kidney dish, flushing urethral secretions from the catheter, then 20 ml is collected for examination. The catheter is then removed and the patient is asked to void immediately to clear any introduced organisms from the bladder.

Iatrogenic urinary infection is extremely uncommon following the use of this type of catheter as described previously. It has been shown that this technique gives results many times more sensitive bacteriologically than midstream specimens, is devoid of the potential for causing traumatic hematuria that commonly accompanies a sidehole catheter, and yields bacterial counts similar to those achieved by suprapubic aspiration, at least to as low as 500 colony-forming units (cfu) per milliliter or less. Colony counts below this level can represent contamination, and a repeat or suprapubic catheter specimen should be obtained.

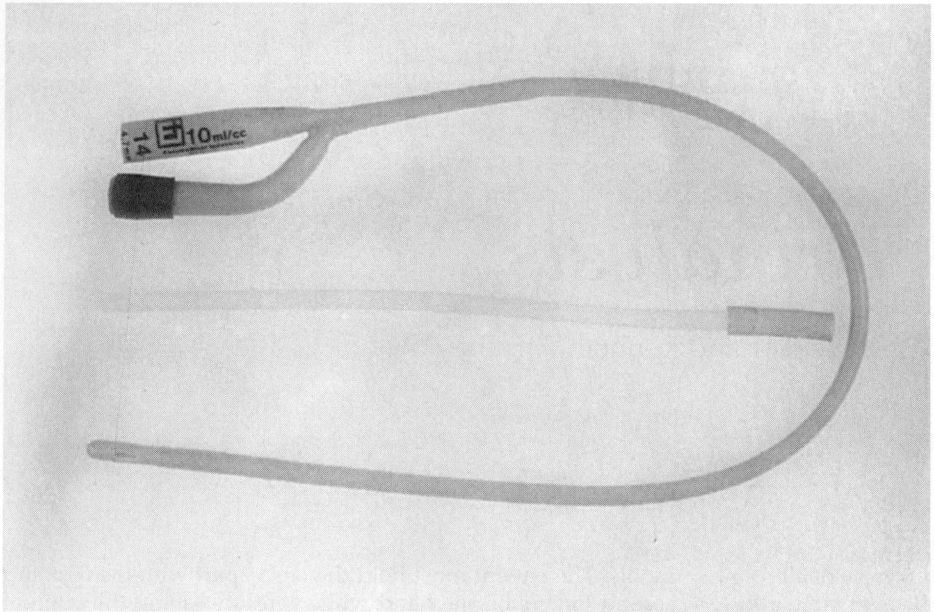

Figure 100.1. Open-ended catheter for collection of urine compared with conventional Foley catheter for urinary drainage.

Suprapubic Aspiration of Urine

The bacteriologic gold standard for diagnosis of urine infection is suprapubic aspiration of the urine. This procedure is often used in infants and occasionally in adults, particularly when low colony counts of bacteria have been detected in midstream urine specimens and urine infection is suspected. It is also the preferred technique when bacterial species with fastidious growth requirements (e.g., *Mycoplasma* species) are being sought.

The major prerequisite is that the bladder be very full. Preferably, this should be allowed to occur in a normal fashion, without forced diuresis, thus avoiding urinary dilution, which will interfere with interpretation because of reduced concentration of urinary bacteria and particles and possible lysis of cells and casts. The fullness of the bladder can be confirmed by percussion and by application of pressure suprapubically, because this will usually cause the patient to wince if the bladder is distended sufficiently.

The skin is prepared with aqueous chlorhexidine or povidine iodine and sterile gloves are donned. A lumbar puncture needle (in infants, a smaller needle) is quickly inserted through the anterior abdominal wall about 2 cm above the pubic symphysis. It will enter the bladder at a depth of about 3 to 5 cm in adults (Fig. 100.2). On withdrawal of the stylet, the urine will usually flow out, a syringe is attached, and 20 ml of urine is aspirated and discarded. Next a second syringe is used to collect 20 ml for microscopy and culture. The patient is sent to empty the bladder, thus obliterating the needle tract. An MSU performed at this stage is often useful for comparison, because it helps gauge the patient's capacity to perform an uncontaminated MSU. For practical purposes, the finding of any bacteria in a suprapubic aspirate, no matter how low the colony count, is sufficient to make the diagnosis of bacteriuria, though theoretically bacteria might be also derived in a retrograde manner from the urethra. To enable very low colony counts to be detected, the laboratory must plate out a larger volume of urine than is usual for routine MSU cultures; therefore it is imperative that the laboratory be aware that low colony counts are to be sought. Urine collected by suprapubic aspiration is therefore the most accurate method for diagnosing and quantifying bladder bacteriuria and is very helpful in excluding contamination by anything other than lower tract red cells. Transient macroscopic hematuria is a surprisingly rare complication, and red blood cell counts are often very similar in count to those found in midstream specimens, suggesting that contamination by bladder wall red cells is usually minimal.

In experienced hands, when the procedure can be guaranteed to be carried out swiftly and with minimal discomfort, we recommend that local anesthetic *not* be used, because it causes more discomfort than the procedure itself. For less experienced operators and in patients who have had previous lower ab-

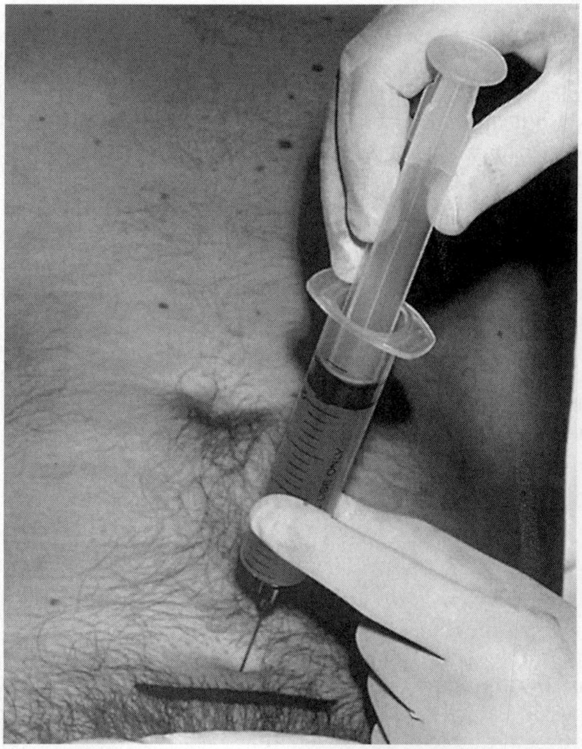

Figure 100.2. Suprapubic aspiration. The upper margin of the pubic symphysis is marked on the skin.

dominal surgery, the technique can be made safer by the use of ultrasonographic guidance to the site of the bladder.

Twenty-Four-Hour and Timed Urine Collection

For the accurate determination of chemical excretion rates a timed 24-hour collection of urine is required. After voiding and discarding the urine at a defined time, usually 8:00 AM, the patient collects all urine voided until the same time the next day, when a final voided urine is passed and collected. Refinements include overnight urine collection; this is sometimes useful in metabolic stone disease, because the urinary crystalloids are usually at their maximum concentration overnight. The simultaneous measurement of urinary creatinine excretion is used to judge the likelihood of a full 24-hour collection having been obtained, because the daily excretion of creatinine is relatively constant in any patient, assuming stable renal function, diet, and metabolism. The measurement of the urinary creatinine concentration is also very useful to allow calculation of the amount of any substance excreted per milligram of creatinine, as has been mentioned with the use of clean-voided samples. This refinement is particularly helpful in children, in whom performing a 24 hour collection is difficult.

URINALYSIS WITH REAGENT STRIPS

Reagent strips for convenient office or ward urinalysis are being increasingly refined; these are currently available for assessment of urine pH, protein, blood or hemoglobin, specific gravity, nitrite, and leukocytes, as well as other chemical constituents not germane to this chapter, such as glucose, ketones, bilirubin, and urobilinogen. The usefulness of these strips should not be underestimated. Dipstick analysis of any sample of urine should always accompany urine microscopy. Although the strips vary in detail between manufacturers, the following comments apply generally.

Urine pH

Urine pH is measurable in the range of 5 to 9 pH units with the use of reagent strips. A high urinary pH is persistently found in patients with type I renal tubular acidosis, in patients who maintain vegetarian diets, and often in the presence of urine infection with *Proteus* species or other urea-splitting organisms. Red blood cells lyse more quickly in alkaline urine, as do hyaline and other urinary casts. Alkaline urine may precipitate phosphate crystals, which will obscure the sediment for microscopy.

Acid urine is a usual finding in patients with uric acid stones, metabolic acidosis, and high-protein diets. Uric acid and cystine crystals are more commonly found in acidic urine.

Urine pH should be monitored as part of the surveillance of patients being treated with urinary alkalinizing agents to manage uric acid or cystine stone disease.

Protein

Screening for urinary protein is one of the most important methods for detecting significant renal disease. It is performed using dipsticks that incorporate the protein-sensitive dye tetrabromophenol buffered at pH 3. These are far more sensitive to albumin than to globulins, Bence Jones protein, Tamm-Horsfall protein (uromucoid), or hemoglobin; hence a negative result does not rule out the presence of these proteins. False-positive results can occur in very alkaline urine, in the presence of some antiseptics and detergents, and if the strips are held in the urine stream, which may wash out the buffer.

Dipsticks give a semiquantitative estimate of urinary albumin in the approximate range of 300 mg/L (1+ proteinuria) to 20 g/L (4+ proteinuria); hence with nephrotic-range proteinuria the reading will usually be 3+ proteinuria (3 g/L) or more. Normal adults excrete less than 80 mg of albumin per day; thus their urine should read as negative, although in highly concentrated or alkaline urine a trace reading may be found.

In early diabetes, microalbuminuria, defined as 20 to 200 μg/min of albumin excretion (30 to300 mg/24 hr), has been shown to predict subsequent clinical nephropathy and mortality. This concentration is below or at the lowest level of sensitivity of conventional dipsticks. Accordingly, dipstick testing using immunochemical methods for detecting albumin in a concentration range of 20 to 200 μg/L has been developed, and this method is now widely used to screen diabetics for microalbuminuria. Because false-positive test results occur and the albumin excretion rate (AER) is highly variable, it is necessary to confirm positive results on several occasions using AER calculated from 24-hour urine collections. Similarly positive test results for protein using conventional dipsticks should be confirmed and the absolute proteinuria determined in 24-hour urine collections, usually with simultaneous creatinine excretion and creatinine clearance.

Older methods for bedside testing for proteinuria, such as precipitation with sulfosalicylic or trichloracetic acid or boiling with a drop of acetic acid, are now rarely used. Bence Jones (light chain) proteinuria can be detected by traditional coagulation at 50° to 60°C and redissolving on boiling; however, this technology is obsolete and is less sensitive and less specific than immunochemical testing for light chains after urinary concentration, as is performed in laboratories.

Hemoglobin and Blood

These reagent patches detect hemoglobin, myoglobin, and methemoglobin and give a speckled reaction in the presence of intact red blood cells. The test is equally sensitive to myoglobin and hemoglobin—an important consideration in acute renal failure when myoglobinuria, glomerular bleeding, and traumatic hematuria are all possibilities.

False-positive results may also occur when oxidizing agents such as microbial peroxidases produced by some urinary pathogens, or the disinfectants hypochlorite or hydrogen peroxide, are present. High concentrations of ascorbic acid due to oral supplements and use of the drug captopril may reduce the sensitivity.

The test is therefore best interpreted in association with the findings with urine microscopy, bearing in mind that red cell lysis may occur rapidly if the urine is dilute, when a positive test result for hemoglobin yet a low count of urinary red cells may be found. Contamination with blood from menses can occur, or red cells may be caused by trauma in catheterized patients or too-energetic periurethral cleansing (particularly in postmenopausal women).

In most circumstances these reagent patches are both specific and sensitive and are complementary to microscopy. In routine use the strips are reasonably reliable in detecting red blood cells once the concentration reaches approximately 2×10^4/ml, close to the normal range as determined by phase-contrast microscopy. The quantitation range is approximately 2×10^4 to about 10^5 red cells/ml, well short of macroscopic hematuria (Table 100.1).

The relationship between the hemoglobin and protein estimates is helpful in distinguishing glomerular from nonglomerular disease. If one assumes a red blood cell count (RBC)

TABLE 100.1. Comparison of Urinary Erythrocyte Concentration as Determined by Reagent Strip Stick and with Phase-Contrast Microscopy in 706 Patients

Concentration	$0–10^4$	$10^4–10^5$	$>10^5$
0	428	37	1
Trace	56	76	1
1+	4	24	2
2+	0	15	9
3+	1	12	31
4+	1	0	8
Total no. of patients	490	164	52

of 5×10^{12}/L, a hematocrit of 45% and a plasma protein concentration of 80 g/L, then 1 ml of blood contains 5×10^9 red cells and 55% of 80 g (i.e., 44 mg of protein). The effect of 1 ml of whole blood in a bladder volume of 1 L would be to raise the red blood cell count to 5×10^6 cells/ml, with consequent macroscopic hematuria, yet only elevate the urine protein concentration by 44 mg/L (i.e., not into the abnormal range). Accordingly, the presence of more than a trace of protein in urine that is not showing macroscopic hematuria suggests that protein is being excreted in amounts proportionately greater than red cells—the most likely cause of this combination being glomerular disease, although it can also occur with urine infection (Fig. 100.3).

When urine appears dark red-brown, yet there is no heavy hematuria on dipstick testing, other causes of the red-brown discoloration must be considered (Table 100.2). Incidentally, other urinary discolorations that can be disconcerting in clinical practice and are relatively common include the orange urine caused by fluorescein after fluorescein angiography of the eye, and the blue urine seen after methylene blue is given for surgical reasons, such as preoperatively before a parathyroidectomy.

Specific Gravity and Osmolarity

Osmolality, an index of the number particles per kilogram of water, is the scientifically accurate expression of urine concentration, usually determined by measurement of depression of the freezing point of the solution. In clinical practice this is rarely employed, except in studies addressing the urinary concentrating mechanisms of the kidney. It is too difficult for routine urinalysis; however, some assessment of urinary concentration should be performed whenever quantitative urine microscopy is undertaken. Specific gravity (SG) can now be measured by reagent strip (between about 1.000 and 1.030), by clinical hydrometer, or by the refractive index method using a refractometer.

A hydrometer is a comparatively clumsy instrument that requires a much larger volume of urine than the much simpler reagent strips. In addition, reagent strips are not sensitive to heavy molecules such as sugar, radiocontrast media, or very high protein concentrations, as is the hydrometer. Refractometers calibrated to read SG require only a drop of urine and are not too expensive for most laboratories performing routine urinalysis.

An assessment of the urinary concentration is required to estimate the effect of dilution of the urine on counts of cells and sediments and the likelihood that red cell lysis has occurred.

TABLE 100.2. Causes of Red-Brown Dark Urine

- Endogenous pigments
  - Hemoglobin
  - Myoglobin
  - Methemoglobin
  - Bile (jaundice)
  - Porphyrins (porphyria)
  - Homogentisic acid (alkaptonuria, on standing)
- Melanin (disseminated melanoma)
- Exogenous pigments
  - Foods
    - Beetroot
    - Rhubarb
    - Food dyes
  - Drugs
    - Rifampicin
    - Phenolphthalein
    - Pyridium

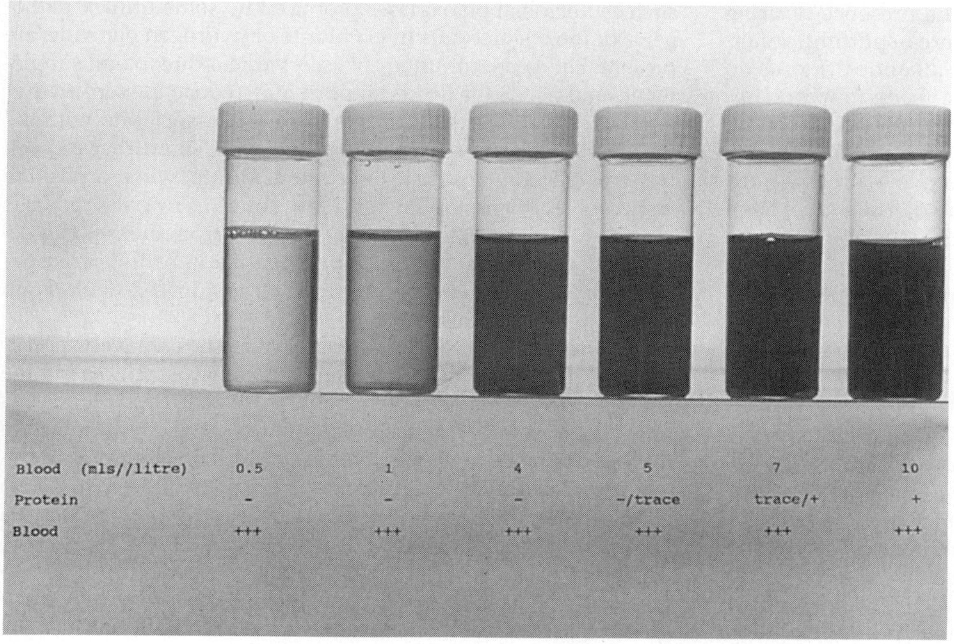

Figure 100.3. The result of adding whole blood to saline. The saline is macroscopically bloody with 1 ml/L of blood, but proteinuria is not detectable by reagent strip till 5 to 10 ml/L is added. (See Color Figure 100.3.)

Red cells start to lyse at an SG below 1.012, and there is severe lysis once SG falls below 1.009. We have found in the same patient a sixfold reduction in urinary red cell counts when the urinary SG was less than 1.006 compared with when the urine SG was greater than 1.015. Lysis is the most common of the several possibilities to be considered when the urinary reagent strip for blood reads very positive, yet few cells are found. Myoglobinuria and hemoglobinuria secondary to intravascular hemolysis are two other important causes of blood on dipstick testing with disproportionately few red cells on microscopy. When the urine SG is less than about 1.015, cast formation is reduced.

Urinary SG is also useful in assessment of acute oliguric renal failure when this index of renal concentrating capacity is very quickly measurable, helping to distinguish between prerenal renal failure and established acute tubular necrosis.

When assessing the urine concentration, a reasonable working relationship between osmolality and SG is that at osmolality 40 mOsm/kg the SG is approximately 1.001, at 600 mOsm/kg the SG is 1.015, and at 1,200 mOsm/kg the SG is approximately 1.030.

Leukocyte and Bacteria-Nitrite Tests

Although reagent strips for leukocytes are available, they are not widely used and are not very sensitive. Positive results generally indicate pyuria, but contamination with a vaginal discharge can cause false-positive results.

Most *Enterobacteriaceae* convert urinary nitrate to nitrite. Nitrite-detecting reagent strips are usually positive when these organisms are present in the urine in concentrations exceeding 10^5 colony-forming units per milliliter. The test results may be negative if there is infection with non–nitrate-converting bacteria, such as Gram-positive organisms or *Pseudomonas* species, if the urine has not been retained in the bladder for at least 4 hours to allow bacterial nitrite conversion or if there are high urinary levels of ascorbic acid.

Leukocyte and nitrite tests have found a place mainly in the follow-up of patients who are prone to recurrent urine infection, particularly children with vesicoureteric reflux.

URINE MICROSCOPY

Few clinical tests in nephrology are as potentially informative yet as frequently inadequately performed as urine microscopy. Ideally, an MSU specimen collected first thing in the morning or at a time when the patient is likely to have concentrated urine is examined immediately or at least within a few hours of collection. For maximum yield the urine should be examined in a counting chamber of 0.2 mm depth using a phase-contrast microscope before (for red cell and white cell counts) and after concentration by centrifugation (for casts and other particles usually found in low concentration). Polarized light is a very useful option, particularly to identify urinary fat particles and to characterize crystals.

If there is delay and cooling of the urine before microscopy, crystals can form and obscure the view of other sediments, cells and casts can lyse, and ultimately bacteria can grow. Urine can be stored at 4°C overnight and still be useful for diagnostic microscopy, although obscuring urate or amorphous phosphate crystals are an occasional problem. Urate crystals will dissolve if the urine is heated to 37°C. Although a water bath is recommended, we often just hold the test tube containing the urinary precipitate under a running warm water tap to redissolve the crystals. Amorphous phosphates can be cleared by adding one or two drops of 1N hydrochloric acid. This time constraint on urinary microscopy can be very inconvenient and particularly interferes with teaching and with obtaining a second opinion when one is unsure of the findings. We have found that if the urine sediment is resuspended in 0.5% glutaraldehyde or 4% formaldehyde in phosphate-buffered saline solution, the cells, casts, and crystals maintain their morphologic characteristics for up to 4 weeks at room temperature. Unfortunately, the potentially simpler technique of directly adding fixative to the urine often results in a dense precipitate, probably resulting from denaturing of the urinary proteins.

A counting chamber is essential for accurate quantitative assessment of cells and casts. With a glass slide and coverslip the urine depth can vary significantly, even between different areas on the same slide, and counting cells per high-powered field (cells/HPF) is thus extremely inexact, especially at about 2 cells/HPF, which can represent anything between 10^2 and 10^5 cells/ml. A Fuchs-Rosenthal counting chamber is particularly suitable for microscopic urinalysis and is no more difficult to use than a slide and coverslip. Because the counting chamber is reused, whereas the slides are discarded with each use, the counting chamber is probably cheaper in the long term than using disposable slides.

Centrifugation (we centrifuge 10 ml of urine at 3,000 rpm for 5 minutes and resuspend in 0.5 ml) has the advantage of concentrating the urinary sediment but has the disadvantage of unpredictably reducing the cell count, with up to 50% of red cells remaining suspended or depositing on the test tube wall. Resuspension should be performed very gently to avoid disintegration of fragile casts. Uncentrifuged urine is therefore best for counting cell numbers, although if there are low cell numbers, large numbers of "squares" in the Fuchs-Rosenthal chamber have to be counted for a statistically valid result (Table 100.3). In clinical practice, however, once a count is in the midnormal range or below, further numerical precision is unimportant to diagnosis. A centrifuged sediment is best for searching for casts, erythrophagocytes, oval fat bodies, and cystine crystals, because these are usually rather sparse in uncentrifuged urine, and often gives a better impression of red cell heterogeneity, because many cells will be seen in the same field.

Phase-contrast microscopy accentuates the interfaces of surfaces of slightly differing refractive indexes. Accordingly, it enhances the ability to rapidly see and identify cells and casts, many of which might be missed with bright-light microscopy, and is by far the preferred method for urinary microscopy. If a phase-contrast microscope is not available, some enhancement of the edges of cells and casts can be obtained by lowering the condenser until maximal refringence of the cell edge is obtained. Alternatively, there are a variety of stains that can be used, but none match the convenience, speed, and accuracy of phase-contrast illumination.

TABLE 100.3. White and Red Cell Counts Should Be Established by Counting at Least 50 Cells, or the Cells in Five Large Squares of a Modified Fuchs-Rosenthal Counting Chamber, on Unspun Urine

	Spun[a]			Unspun
5 Large squares	X	50	X	1,000
2 Large squares	X	100	X	2,000
1 Large square	X	250	X	5,000
8 Small squares	X	500	X	10,000
4 Small squares	X	1000	X	20,000
1 Small square	X	4000	X	80,000

[a] Method: 10 ml spun at 3000 rpm, 5 minutes, resuspend sediment in 0.5 ml.

A valuable technique for accentuating the shape of nuclei in leukocytes and epithelial cells involves placing a drop of glacial acetic acid against the edge of the coverslip. As it diffuses into cells, cytoplasmic granules clear, allowing the nuclei to be seen more clearly, hence positive identification of polymorphonuclear leukocytes. Immunohistochemical techniques have been employed to further dissect cell and cast types in the urine, but these techniques are beyond the scope of this chapter and routine laboratory practice.

The urine is examined for cells, casts, crystals, and other particulate matter.

Erythrocytes

Red cells in the urine vary considerably in appearance. The general pattern of red cell morphology gives a good indication of their likely site of origin (Figs. 100.4 and 100.5).

Cells that originate from sites distal to the papillary ducts are influenced uniformly by the physical properties of the urine, all being changed toward a common end-point; accordingly, they are relatively homogenous in appearance. The appearance of cells in isotonic urine of neutral pH is similar to the biconcave disks seen in peripheral blood, while hypertonic urine can result in crenated cells (Fig. 100.6). In acid urine the hemoglobin steadily leeches from cells, resulting eventually in dehemoglobinized cell ghosts (Fig. 100.7). Because the physical and chemical properties of the urine may change while the cells are in the urinary tract, it is possible to have two or even three populations of cells. However, if more than three populations are seen, the most likely explanation is that cells are present that have originated from within the nephron.

When the erythrocytes originate from within the nephron, usually the glomulus, each cell traverses its own relatively

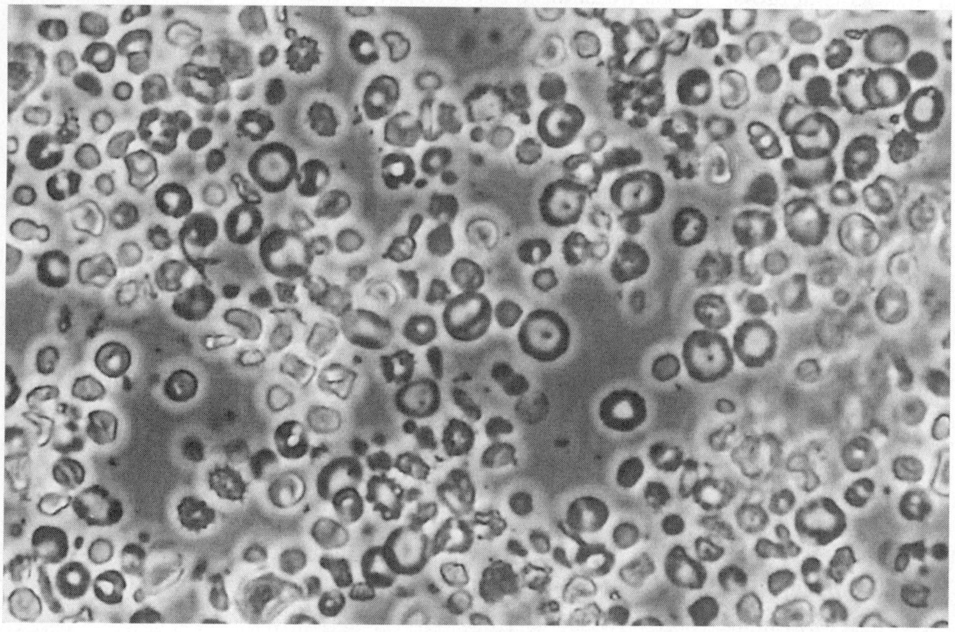

Figure 100.4. Phase-contrast microscopic appearance of heavy glomerular hematuria with a wide variety of cell shapes and sizes. (See Color Figure 100.4.)

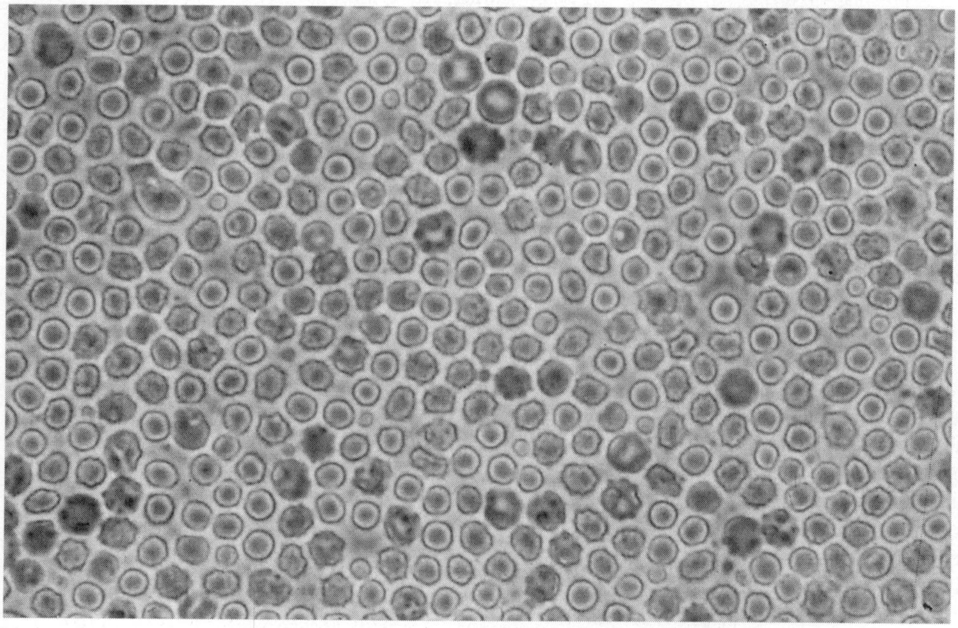

Figure 100.5. Phase-contrast microscopic appearance of lower tract hematuria (bladder tumor). The cells are of similar sizes and appearance, except for a very occasional dysmorphic cell. (See Color Figure 100.5.)

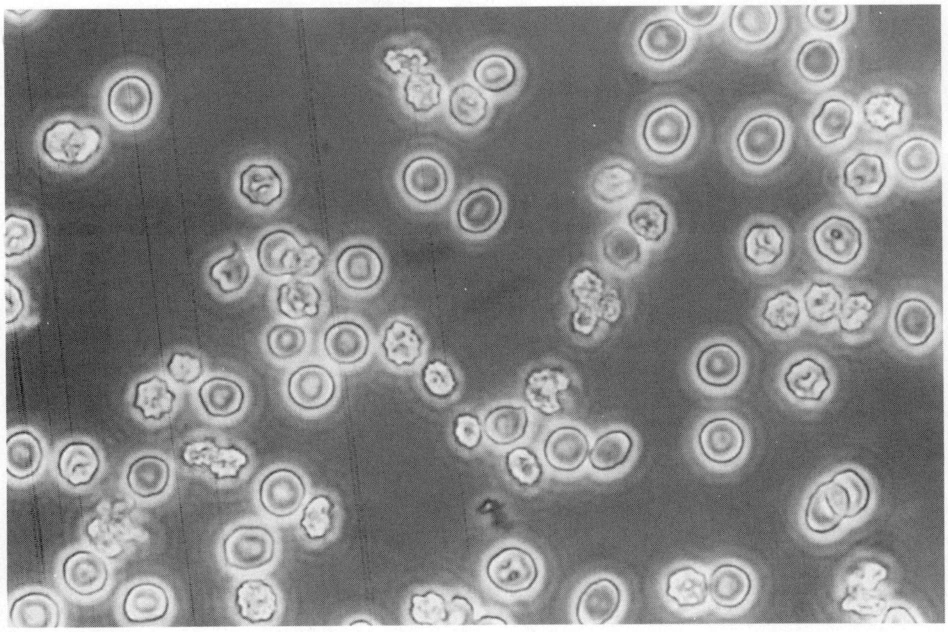

Figure 100.6. Lower tract bleeding with two populations of cells, with one population crenated.

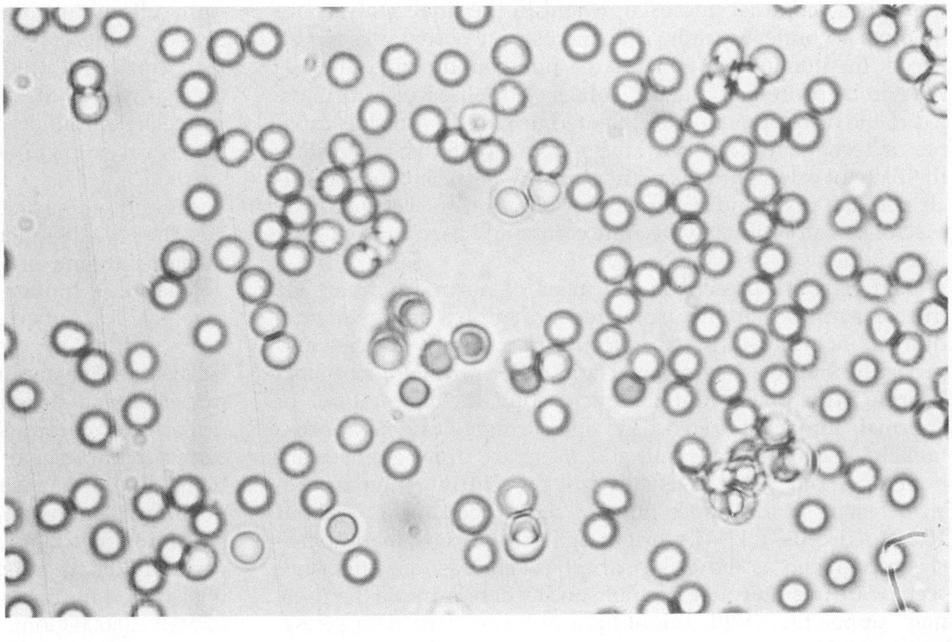

Figure 100.7. Lower tract bleeding with dehemoglobinized ("ghost") cells.

unique series of environments as it passes through the tubule of that nephron. It is also probable that passage through a damaged basement membrane is traumatic to the cell resulting in more bizarre cell shapes. Red blood cells range in age from 1 to 120 days, and it is probable that cells nearing the end of their lifetime are more susceptible to damage by osmotic and other forces. Accordingly, the cells vary markedly in size, shape, and hemoglobin content. Biconcave disks, crenated cells, ghost cells, and a variety of cells of bizarre appearance, particularly those with a "budding yeast"-like or "Mickey Mouse ears" appearance may be seen (Fig. 100.8). Because most nephron bleeding occurs from the glomerulus, we have called this dysmorphic pattern *glomerular* and the more homogeneous pattern *nonglomerular*.

The use of urinary morphologic evaluation to differentiate glomerular bleeding from nonglomerular causes of urinary tract bleeding (such as with tumors and calculi) is very specific mean, but its efficacy depends on a trained observer and intelligent interpretation of the result in light of other abnormalities in the deposit as well as clinical and laboratory findings. It cannot be overemphasized that one should consider the overall pattern, not the presence of small numbers of any particular cell type, when deciding whether the bleeding is glomerular or nonglomerular.

The heterogeneity of cell types has been confirmed by automated blood-cell analyzers, which show that glomerular bleeding is associated with a much wider distribution of cell size and generally smaller cells than nonglomerular bleeding; a variety of techniques, including electron microscopy and flow cytometry, have been used to detail the bizarre cell shapes seen. Both techniques, however, are more difficult and time consuming

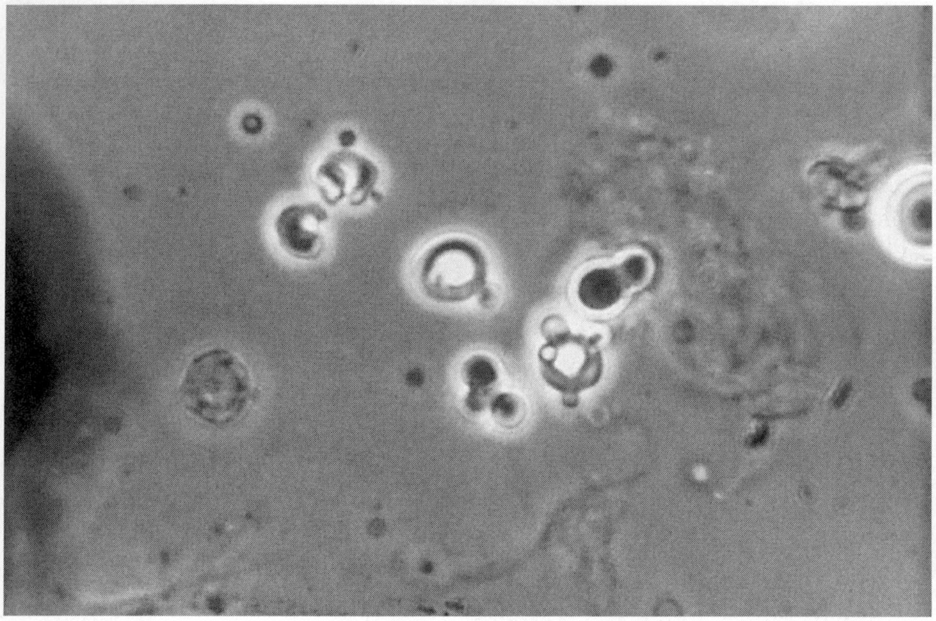

Figure 100.8. Bizarre appearance of urinary red cells in glomerular bleeding, including blebs from cell surface, giving "Mickey Mouse ears" appearance.

than phase-contrast microscopy, and in the final analysis are no more accurate, assuming the microscopic observer is experienced. In situations in which large numbers of urine samples have to be processed, the difficulties with observer error have led to the development of automated urinalysis, which is capable of recognizing not only the red cell patterns, suggesting their site of origin, but also other urinary particles, such as nucleated cell casts and bacteria, and one can predict that such machines will ultimately become commonly used in urinalysis laboratories.

Red cells are present in the urine of normal individuals; the concentration in the urine, depending on a variety of conditions, including urinary concentration, recent exercise and probably the presence of fever and other physiologic disturbances. With phase-contrast microscopy the upper limit of "normal" for urinary red cells in uncentrifuged urine is approximately 15,000 red cells/ml, and these are of a "glomerular" pattern. About 30% are usually lost by centrifugation and resuspension, so the upper limit in centrifuged urine is about 10,000 red cells/ml. With bright-light microscopy many particles recognized as red cells with phase-contrast are either not seen or are misinterpreted as nonspecific debris; hence the "normal" upper limit with bright-light is lower than with phase-contrast microscopy.

The importance of the distinction of glomerular from nonglomerular hematuria is that this simple test can help guide further investigation. Nonglomerular bleeding requires a traditional urologic workup, such as with cystoscopy and renal imaging, whereas if glomerular bleeding is present, a renal biopsy will probably be the appropriate final diagnostic test if further investigation is required.

As with all investigations, however, there are important caveats. First, the test must be interpreted in the context of the clinical situation. In the urine of some patients with IgA nephropathy there may be up to about 30% of well-hemoglobinized red cells of a nonglomerular pattern, raising the possibility in older patients of dual pathologic conditions. In acute crescentic and poststreptococcal glomerulonephritis sometimes there is a majority of uniform cells, but if dysmorphic cells are counted they are always present in high numbers, and there is usually abundant other evidence of glomerular disease, with red cell and other abnormal casts. The reason for the large number of uniform cells in these diseases is unclear. Although excessive numbers of glomerular red cells are rarely seen in patients with urologic causes of bleeding, when there are two or three populations as well as the usual admixture of up to 15,000 glomerular red cells per milliliter, the distinction from glomerular bleeding can be very difficult. Often a repeat specimen will clarify the issue.

Second, some patients will have more than one cause of bleeding. Neither glomerular bleeding (as with IgA or thin basement membrane diseases) nor urologic bleeding (as with stones, neoplasm, or trauma) is so uncommon that these cannot occur together. To further complicate the issue, patients with malignancy will not uncommonly demonstrate evidence of glomerular disease. The important rule is not to let the pattern of urinary red cells stand alone in assessment of the patient; a good reason urinary microscopy should be performed by the clinician concerned, because he or she is most aware of the balance of probabilities. In our hands the specificity of the test is about 93%, both in glomerular and nonglomerular disease.

Although counts greater than 15,000 glomerular red cells per milliliter are outside the usual range in normal individuals, the isolated finding of a urinary red cell count of up to approximately 50,000 glomerular red cells per milliliter, in the absence of any clinical renal abnormality, impaired renal function or proteinuria, is not generally regarded as an indication for renal biopsy, because the likelihood of finding a cause requiring treatment is low, most patients having either mild mesangial proliferation, thin basement membrane disease, or mild IgA nephropathy.

Finally, contaminant red cells of lower tract morphology will almost invariably be found in the urine of menstruating women, unless the urine is very carefully collected by an experienced patient using a fresh tampon. Accordingly in this situation, urine microscopy for cell type is best deferred until after menstruation or at least should be interpreted with great care. Lower tract red cells in such specimens are usually ignored.

Leukocytes

In normal urine leukocytes are far less frequently seen than erythrocytes are. As with red cells and casts, many laboratories still express leukocyte counts in terms of cells per high-powered

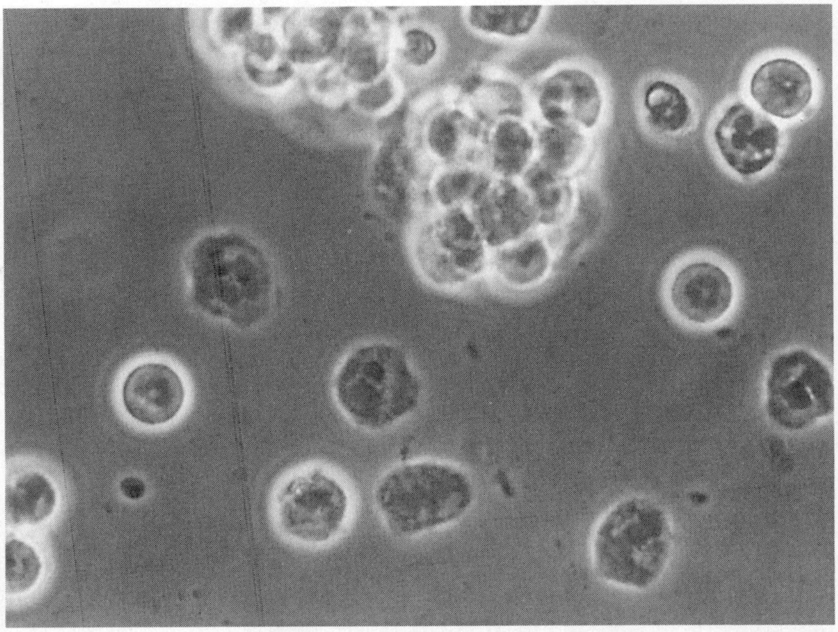

Figure 100.9. Leukocytes in infected urine. In dilute urine the leukocyte nuclei may be visible. Leukocyte clumps and bacterial rods can also be seen.

field (cells/HPF) in a centrifuged urinary sediment, although the gross inaccuracy of this, particularly in the range 1 to 3 cells/HPF, is widely acknowledged. If there are 4 or more cells/HPF, pyuria is definitely present. Using phase-contrast microscopy and a counting chamber, we have found that the upper limit of the normal value for the urinary leukocyte concentration is 2,000 cells/ml in a properly collected midstream urine sample. In urine collected by suprapubic aspiration from normal control subjects of both sexes and varying ages, the count does not commonly exceed 1,000 cells/ml, indicating that leukocytes are present in very low counts in the bladder urine of healthy persons.

Leukocytes are slightly larger than red cells and have a characteristic granular cytoplasm, particularly in urine of high SG; in urine of low SG the granules are less dense, and the nuclear shape may be occasionally seen with phase-contrast microscopy (Fig. 100.9). The characteristic multilobed nuclei are much more clearly seen if glacial acetic acid is diffused under the coverslip, as previously mentioned. This can be particularly useful in distinguishing these cells from renal tubular cells, which have a rounded nucleus and are slightly larger, but also have a granular cytoplasm. More formally, a Prescott-Brodie stain for cytoplasmic peroxidase will label leukocytes and not tubular cells; however, this stain is potentially carcinogenic and hence is not recommended for routine use.

The main reason for assessing leukocyturia relates to the diagnosis of bacterial urine infection. In patients with symptomatic urine infection (acute cystitis or pyelonephritis), leukocyturia is almost always present. The absence of pyuria should result in serious reconsideration of the diagnosis.

On the other hand, leukocyturia may be found, yet bacteriuria may not be detected. This once had great significance in the diagnosis of renal tuberculosis, because this bacterium has slow, fastidious growth requirements, resulting in so-called sterile pyuria. Presently a variety of other conditions are more commonly the cause of culture-negative leukocyturia. In patients with urinary symptoms and culture-negative leukocyturia the most likely diagnosis is still bacterial urinary infection, with failure to culture or recognize the bacteriuria. A common reason for this is failure to realize that low numbers of bacteria in the urine can represent genuine infection. It has been found that nearly 50% of women with symptomatic coliform infection, as proven by analysis of a suprapubic aspiration or a catheter specimen, have less than 10^5 colony-forming units (cfu) per milliliter in a midstream specimen. Indeed, some patients with proven bladder bacteriuria have as few as 10 cfu/ml in the suprapubic aspirate.

Tuberculosis bacillus is not the only organism that is difficult to grow and yet causes urinary infection. Anaerobic bacteria, *Mycoplasma* species and *Ureaplasma* species are examples of other organisms that may cause pyuria and symptoms; these require specialized culture techniques for their growth. *Gardnerella vaginalis* commonly colonizes the bladder in pregnancy but requires suprapubic aspirate or a catheter specimen to confirm its presence.

Bacteria may be present in the bladder, yet will not grow in culture if the patient has taken an antibacterial agent, or a disinfectant or soap has been used to clean the periurethral area and has contaminated the urine specimen, thus interfering with subsequent culture of the organism.

In acute allergic tubulointerstitial nephritis, leukocytes are often found in the urine in large numbers, and commonly a substantial proportion are eosinophils. The latter are best identified by staining with Hansel's or Wright's stains, although the sensitivity and specificity of eosinophiluria for acute interstitial nephritis is very low. Renal tubular cells may be seen when there is significant tubular damage and may be confused with leukocytes unless acetic acid is added, as described previously.

High counts of leukocytes may also be found in the urine when there are other anatomic abnormalities such as calculi, renal papillary necrosis, interstitial cystitis, and polycystic disease. In such cases covert infection or infection with fastidious organisms such as *Ureaplasma urealyticum* may be present and should be sought. Suprapubic aspiration and the culture of larger volumes of urine may be necessary to detect organisms in low concentrations.

An interesting observation in many patients with glomerulonephritis (especially those with systemic lupus erythematosus, membranoproliferative disease, and crescentic nephritis) is the presence of large numbers of leukocytes in the urine, along with the usual red cells, casts, and protein. It is unknown whether these leukocytes are derived from the glomeruli, where they are often seen in renal biopsy tissue, or from the accompanying tubulointerstitial nephritis, which is virtually always found in severe proliferative glomerulonephritis. Their presence does, however, seem to reflect the activity of the disease.

The most common, and therefore an important misleading cause of excessive numbers of leukocytes in the urine, is contamination of the midstream specimen. The presence of large numbers of squamous epithelial cells, vaginal debris, and even spermatozoa are the hallmarks on microscopy of contamination in females, where the pus cells are derived from the vagina and vulva. A few squames are occasionally seen in urine collected by suprapubic aspiration, as the area of the trigone has a squamous lining. In males, failure to retract the foreskin can lead to contamination of the urine with leukocytes and squames. Most urinary infections are caused by a single organism, about 5% by two of the common urinary pathogens and less than 2% by three or more organisms. Multiple organisms grown from the MSU therefore usually suggests contamination.

In males, prostatitis may also need to be considered. This can only be accurately diagnosed by the technique described by Stamey. A series of specimens is collected for microscopy and microbial colony counting during a single emptying of the bladder. First the initial 5 ml of the stream is collected (urethral bacteria) then the midstream specimen (bladder bacteria). Voiding is then interrupted and prostatic massage performed. If there is any expressed secretion, it is collected for culture (prostatic bacteria). Finally, the first 5 ml of urine passed after prostatic massage is collected (prostatic bacteria). In prostatitis the colony count in the prostatic secretion and postprostatic massage specimens are higher than in the MSU unless there is concurrent active bladder infection, making differentiation difficult.

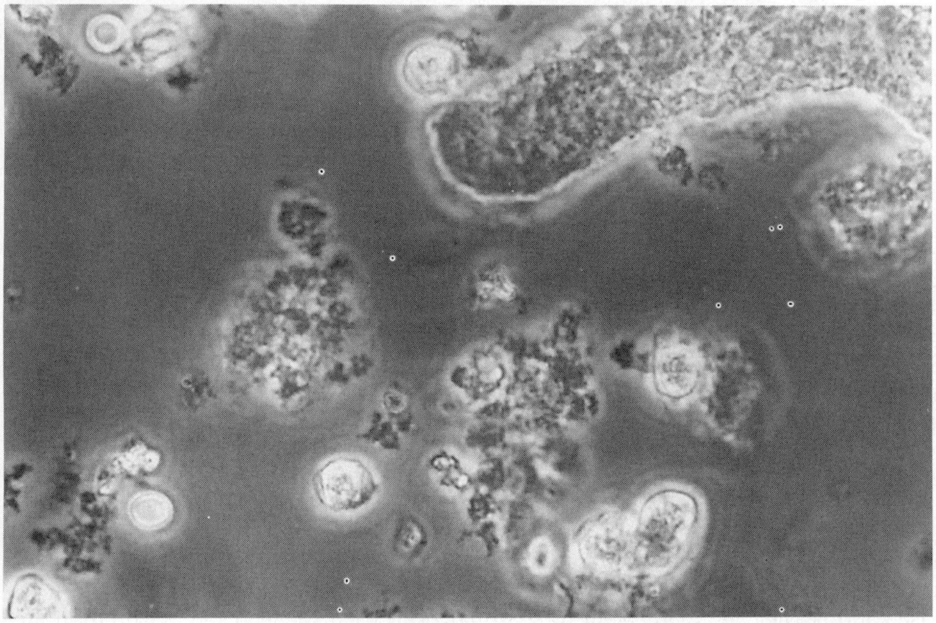

Figure 100.10. Renal tubular cells in the urine of a patient with acute tubular necrosis resulting from rhabdomyolysis. A granular cast and tubular debris are also present.

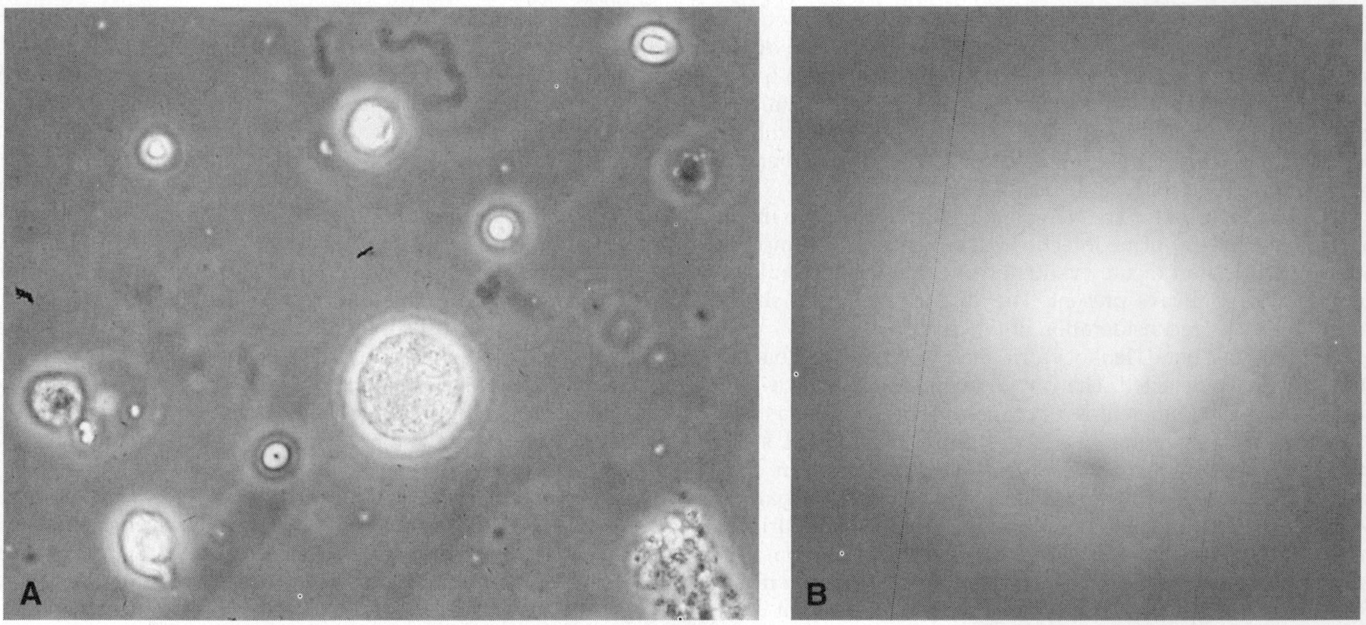

Figure 100.11. Oval fat body. A tubular cell packed with lipid droplets **(A)**, which exhibit birefringence under polarized light **(B)**. (Courtesy of Bilal Jamil, M.D.) (See Color Figure 100.11A.)

Renal Tubular Epithelial Cells

Renal tubular cells are not normally present in the urine in any quantity, but they can be present in large numbers when there is tubular damage from any cause. A little larger than leukocytes, tubular cells have a granular cytoplasm and rounded nucleus that can be seen more clearly if glacial acetic acid is added. Usually in acute tubular necrosis these cells are accompanied by granular debris and casts (Fig. 100.10). This urinary appearance can be very helpful when assessing patients with acute renal failure.

Occasionally, tubular cells with intracellular inclusions may be seen. Oval fat bodies or "brown bodies" (cells full of cholesterol esters) may be seen in the nephrotic syndrome and less commonly with other forms of glomerulonephritis especially as renal failure supervenes. The fat is easily identified with polarized light microscopy when birefringent particles, some of which may exhibit a "Maltese cross" appearance, are seen (Fig. 100.11). Similar cells are occasionally in the urine of patients with prostatitis. With glomerular bleeding erythrophagocytosis can occur (Fig. 100.12); this is a very useful finding, because this has the same significance as that of red cell casts.

Squamous and Transitional Epithelial Cells

Large, flat cells with rounded nuclei may be derived from the bladder or urethra when there is irritation resulting from infection, instrumentation, or vaginal cell contamination (Fig. 100.13). Vaginal squames are usually polygonal, which easily distinguishes them from the smaller, rounded transitional uroepithelial cells. If large numbers of squamous cells are seen in urine collected from females, the cells can usually be assumed to reflect

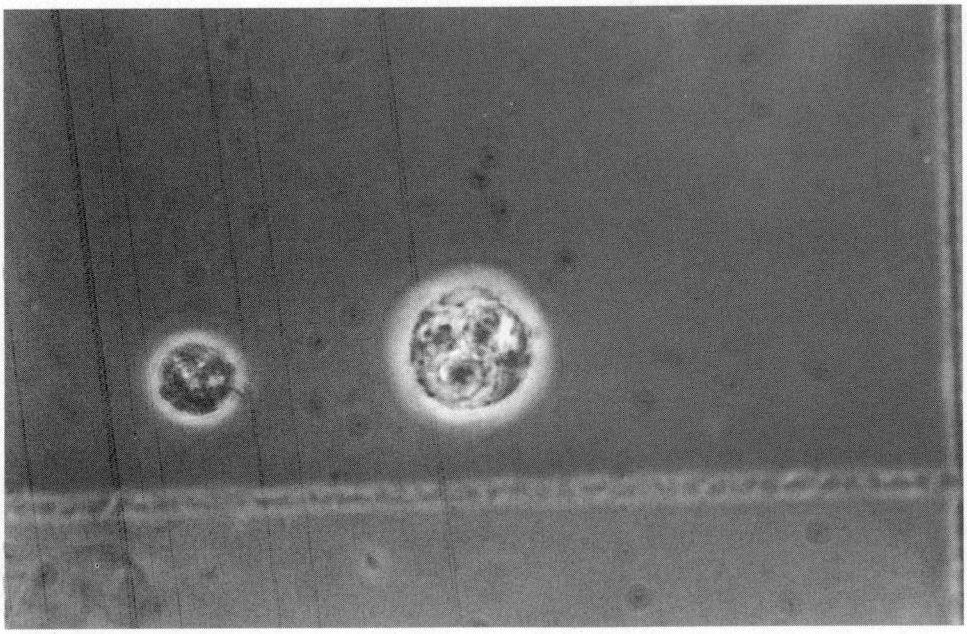

Figure 100.12. A renal tubular cell containing a phagocytosed erythrocyte, diagnostic of nephron bleeding. (See Color Figure 100.12.)

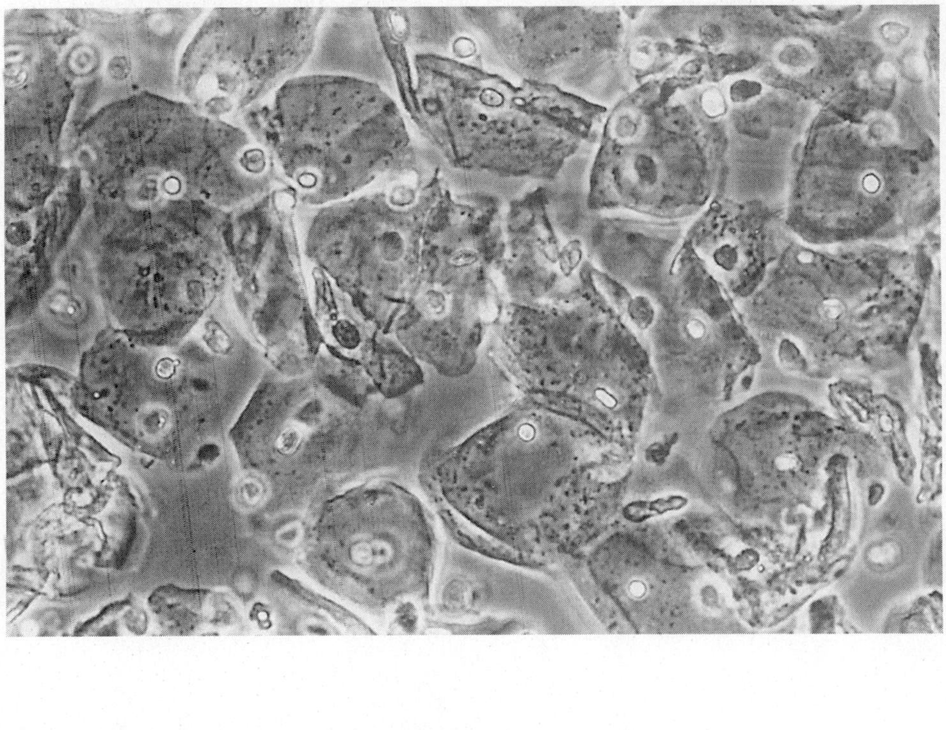

Figure 100.13. Dense, squamous epithelial cells in the midstream urine from a female patient, indicating contamination of the midstream specimen by vaginal-vulval contents.

contamination with vaginal contents. This is particularly relevant to the diagnosis of urinary infection, because moderate counts of mixed bacteria in such urine can usually be ignored.

Urinary Casts

Urinary casts are formed by the aggregation of Tamm-Horsfall glycoprotein with other proteins in the renal tubules. They have a cylindrical structure, with size and shape reflecting the tubular lumen in which they have formed. Entrapment of other tubular contents leads to various types of cast, each distinguishable under the microscope.

Hyaline Casts

Hyaline casts are composed mainly of Tamm-Horsfall glycoprotein, have a homogeneous, clear, colorless appearance (Fig. 100.14), and are often difficult to see without phase-contrast microscopy. Hyaline casts and hyaline casts containing granules are found in small numbers in the urine of normal sedentary persons. Many factors can increase the excretion of hyaline casts, including concentrated urine, fever, exercise, and diuretic administration. With loop diuretic administration counts as high as 10,000/ml can be seen. They are preserved in acid urine, tend to dissolve in alkaline urine, and rarely form when the urinary SG is low. If there are no precipitating factors, such as fever, exercise, or diuretic intake, it is unusual to see more than 100 hyaline casts per milliliter of urine unless there is an underlying renal abnormality.

Immunofluorescent studies have shown various immunoglobulins contained in hyaline casts in patients with glomerulonephritis and monoclonal gammopathies; however, such techniques have little application in clinical practice.

Red Cell Casts

The most diagnostically useful casts are those in which red cells are seen (Fig. 100.15). These can vary from those containing only a few cells, to casts composed virtually entirely of erythrocytes. Red cell casts are diagnostic of nephron (presumably glomerular) bleeding. High counts of red cell casts rarely occur in the absence of severe, often crescentic, glomerular disease.

Degraded red cells may also be present, resulting in pigmented granular casts. If recognized, these have the same diagnostic connotations as red cell casts. Hemoglobin and myoglobin casts, with pigmented granules, may be indistinguishable and occur with hemoglobinuria or myoglobinuria.

Leukocyte Casts

Cylinders of densely packed leukocytes indicate acute or chronic inflammation of the renal parenchyma, usually caused by infection. Their presence should lead to careful investigation for bacteriuria. Occasionally, leukocyturia can accompany glomerulonephritis, particularly active membranoproliferative, lupus, or poststreptococcal nephritis. In such cases leukocyte casts may be seen, and they are thus not specific to pyelonephritis.

Granular Casts

Many casts have a granular appearance (Fig. 100.10), which is usually thought to be the result of breakdown of cells within the hyaline matrix. These may still be occasionally identifiable as degraded red cells, tubular epithelial cells, or polymorphs if some intact cells, cell membranes, or pigments are still present. Normal serum proteins can aggregate in hyaline casts; hence hyaline casts with fine granules may be seen in normal urine.

Broad, Waxy, and Convoluted Casts

Very long, wide, or convoluted casts are not seen in normal individuals under normal conditions. Broad casts (Fig. 100.16) are usually of hyaline type and are probably formed in hypertrophied tubules or occur because of slow urine flow through collecting ducts. They are found in patients with acute or chronic renal failure or in patients with diseases associated with focal nephron damage and hypertrophy, such as reflux nephropathy or medullary cystic disease.

Sometimes casts are highly refractile so-called waxy casts, with sharp ends and even cracks along their sides (Fig. 100.17).

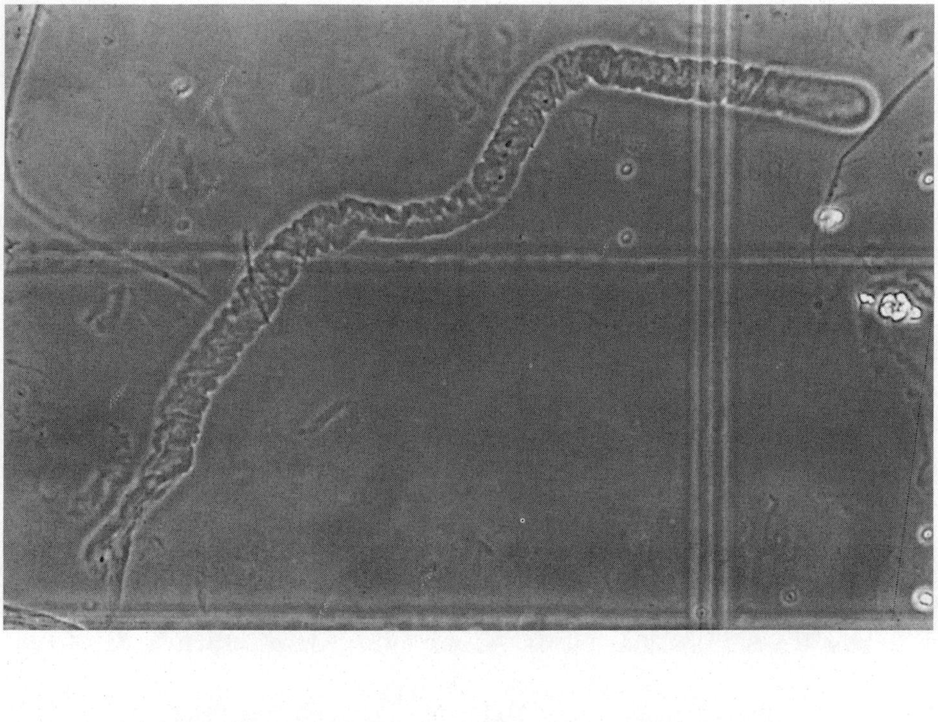

Figure 100.14. A long, thin hyaline cast.

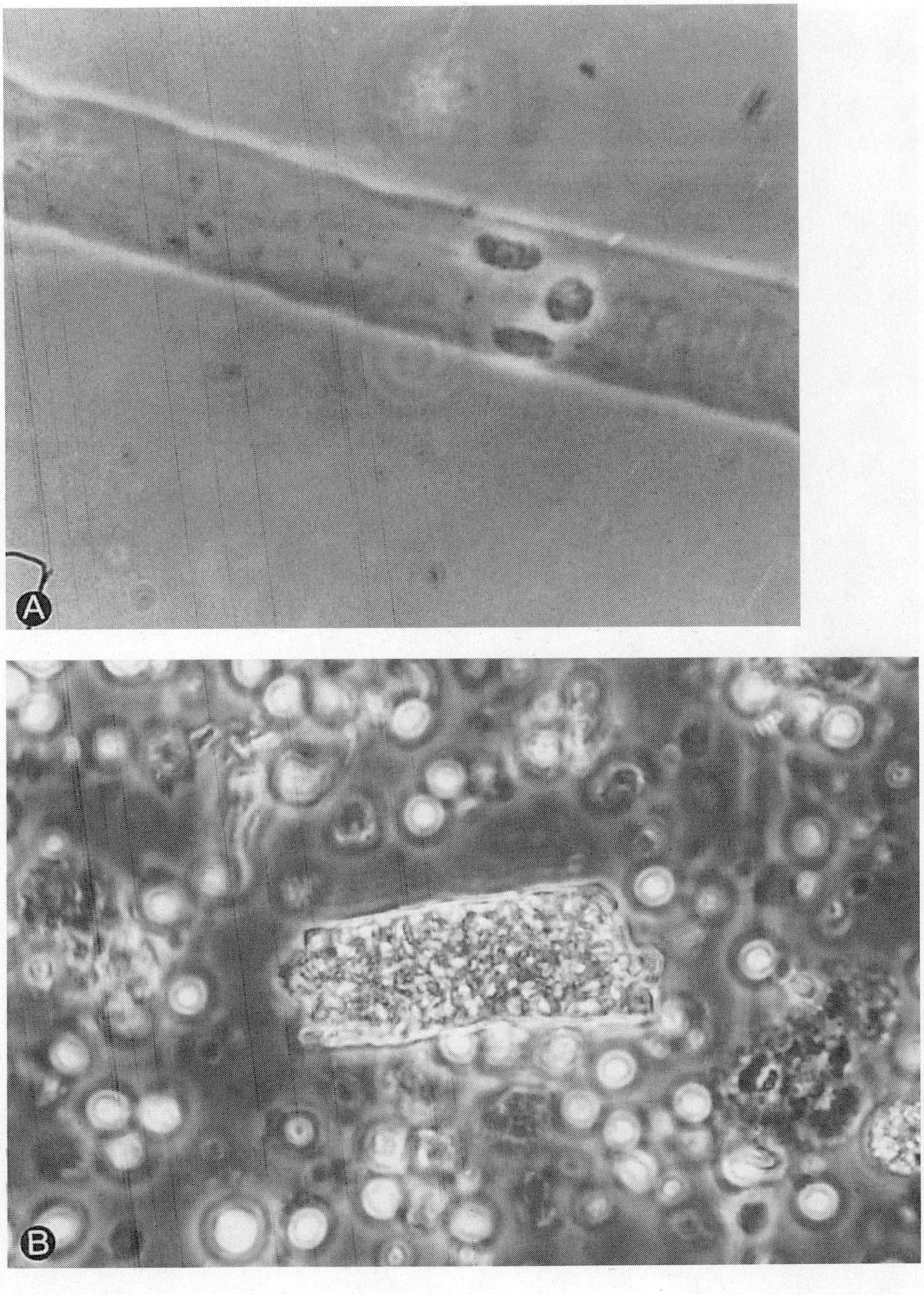

Figure 100.15. Red cell casts. **A:** Sparse red cells incorporated into a hyaline cast. **B:** Red cells densely incorporated into cast.

These are easily seen with bright-light illumination, and their significance is unknown. As with broad casts, they do not occur in normal urine and usually reflect renal damage.

Other Inclusions

Fat globules incorporated in casts may be seen in many types of nephritis. High counts are particularly found in patients with nephrotic syndrome and hyperlipidemia, especially with membranous glomerulonephritis. These may also occur in reflux nephropathy, membranous lupus nephritis, focal and segmental hyalinosis and sclerosis, moderately advanced IgA disease, and some familial glomerulonephritis. The fat may be identified by polarized light microscopy (Figs. 100.17 and 100.18).

Crystals, often identifiable by polarized light microscopy, can occasionally be incorporated in casts. These may be endogenous crystals, particularly calcium oxalate or other substances. The drug triamterene, particularly, produces a dramatic appearance in casts in an acid urine.

Renal Tubular Epithelial Cell Casts

These casts are composed of tightly packed renal tubular epithelial cells. They are not found in normal urine but are usually present in large numbers when there is acute tubular necrosis, along with free renal tubular cells and granular debris and casts. Other causes of tubular damage including acute glomerulonephritis can also sometimes result in these casts appearing in the urine.

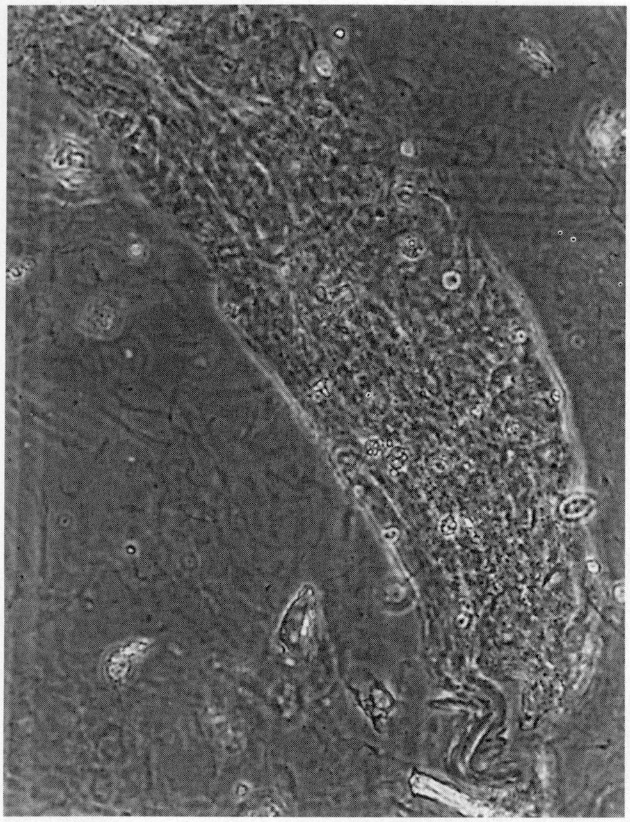

Figure 100.16. Broad hyaline cast with some granularity from a patient with medullary cystic disease.

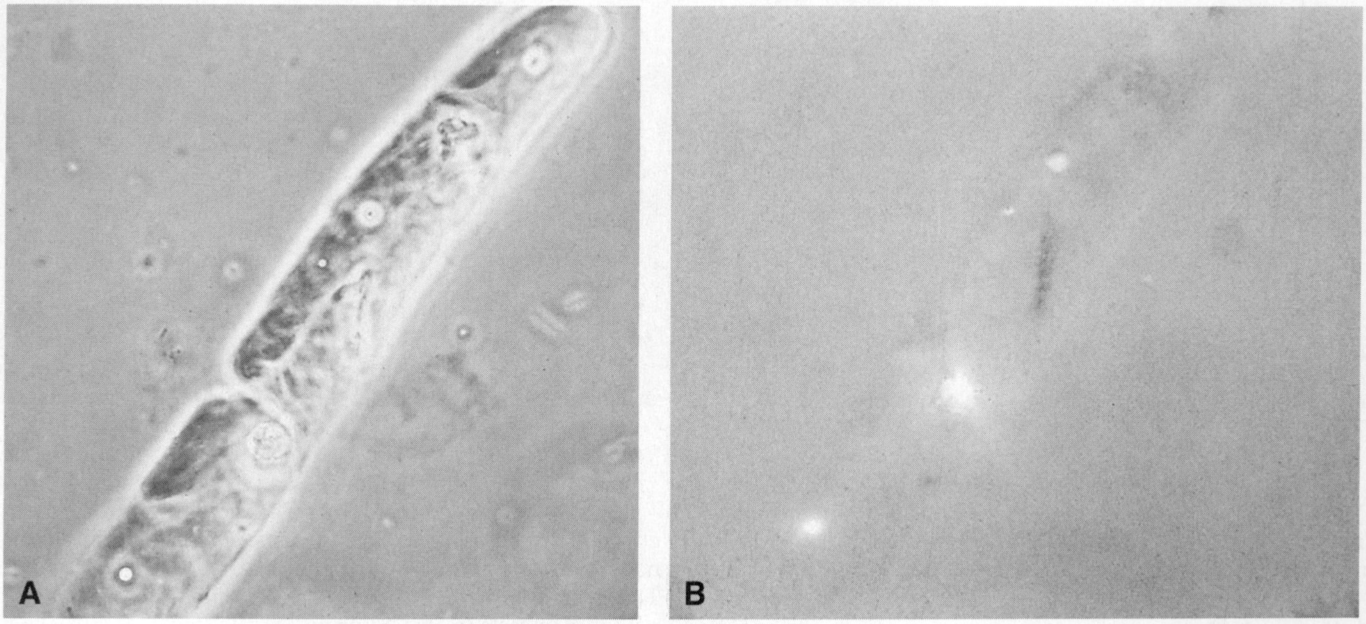

Figure 100.17. **A:** Dense waxy cast with characteristic clefts. **B:** Inclusions are shown by polarized light to be birefringent fat particles. (Courtesy of Bilal Jamil, M.D.)

Mixed Casts

Often hyaline casts will include more than one type of inclusion. Hence casts with different cells throughout the cast, or different cells at different ends of the cast, can be seen (Fig. 100.19). Occasionally, a small cast of one cell type may be seen included in a larger cast of a different type from lower in the nephron. Bacteria may occur in casts. If seen, bacterial casts are pathognomonic of renal parenchymal infection.

Fat Particles

Fat particles in the urine are largely composed of cholesterol esters, thought to be formed by tubular metabolism of urinary

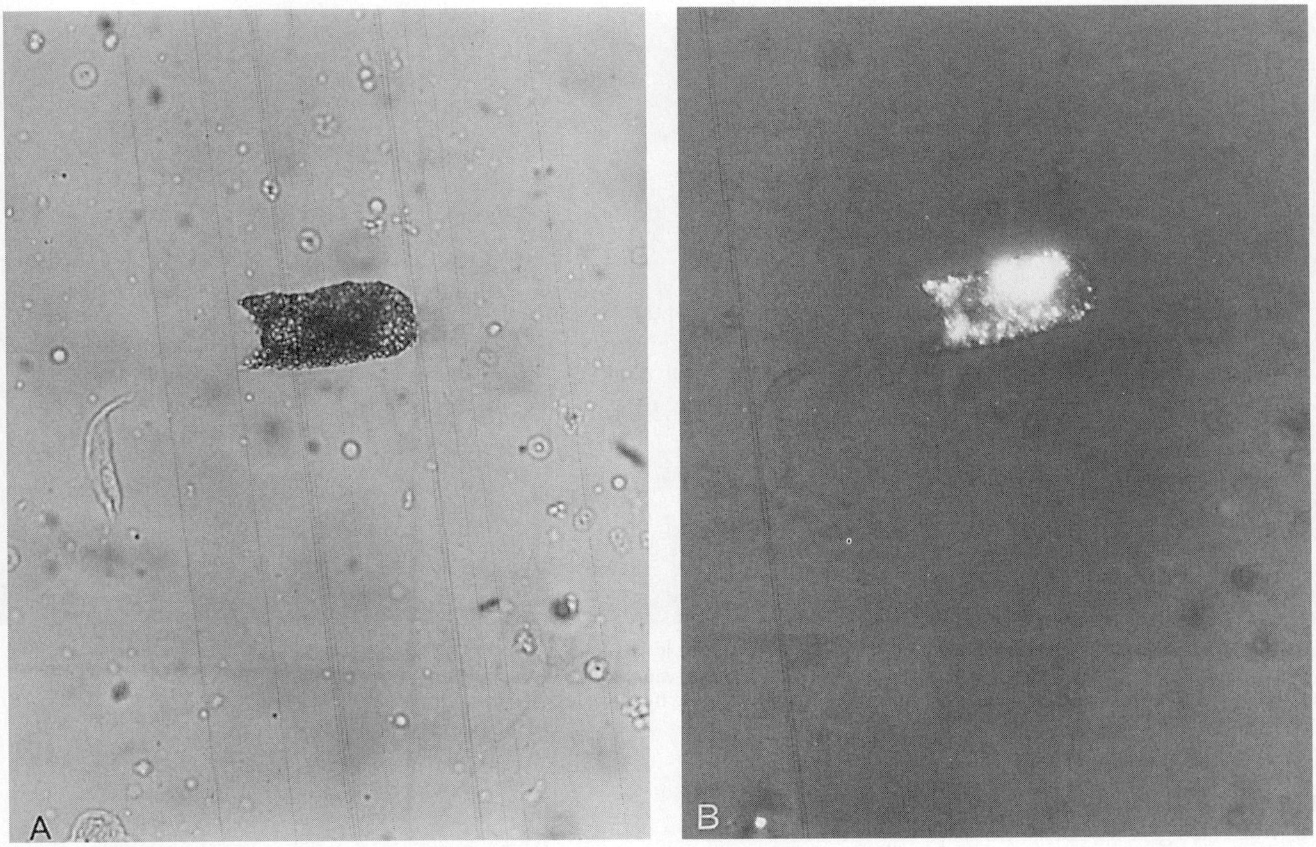

Figure 100.18. **A:** A granular cast containing fat particles under phase-contrast microscopy. **B:** With polarized light microscopy fat particles exhibit birefringence.

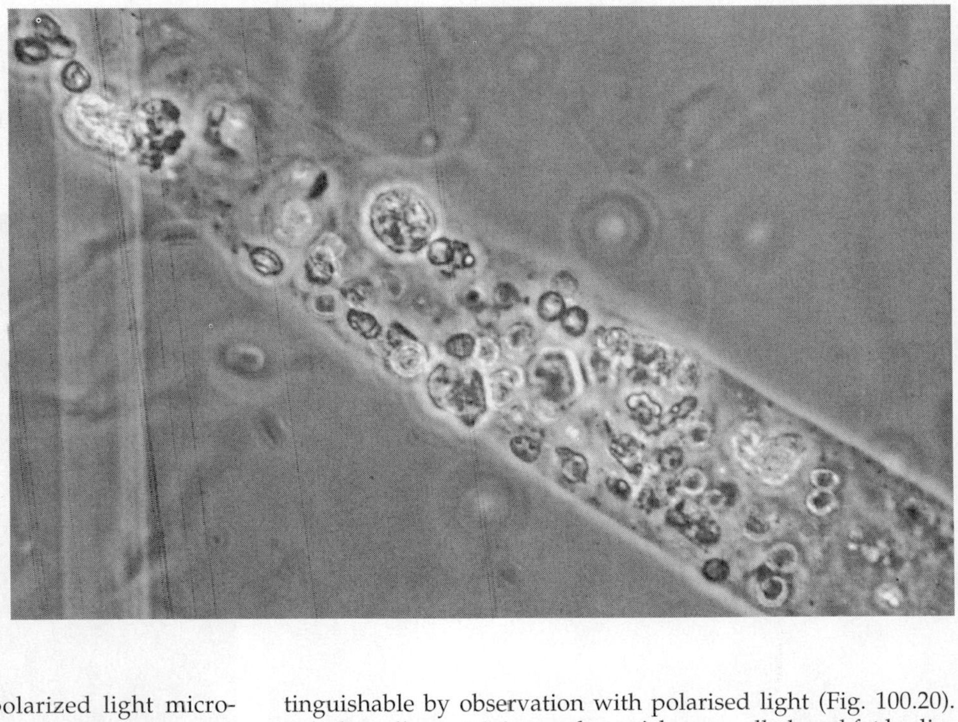

Figure 100.19. Mixed cast containing red cells and tubular epithelial cells. (See Color Figure 100.19.)

lipoprotein. They are identifiable by polarized light microscopy where a characteristic "Maltese cross" appearance may be seen and occur in most types of glomerulonephritis. Fat particles are not found in normal urine, except following strenuous exercise.

Free fat particles (spherulites) vary widely in size. They are perfectly spherical and can resemble red cells and only be distinguishable by observation with polarised light (Fig. 100.20). Tubular cells containing such particles are called oval fat bodies or brown bodies (Fig. 100.11) and are most commonly seen in the nephrotic syndrome. They are also occasionally seen in crescentic glomerulonephritis and IgA glomerulonephritis when function is deteriorating, as well as in many other types of glomerulonephritis.

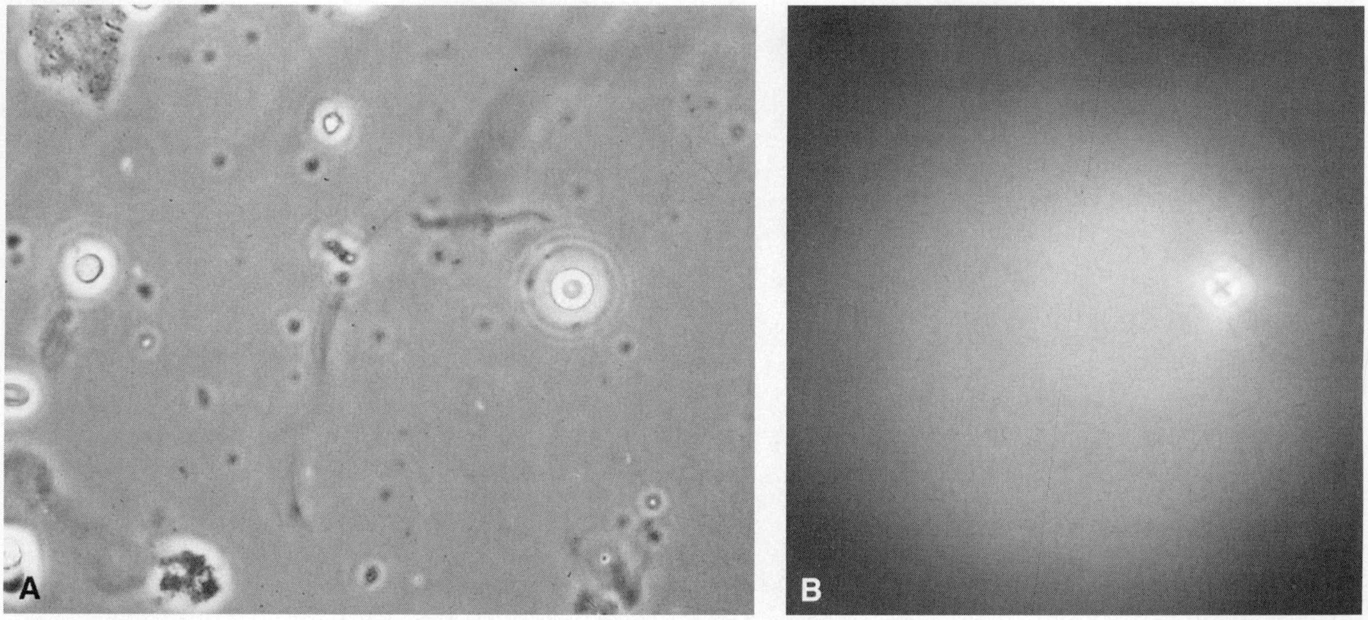

Figure 100.20. **A:** Free fat particle under phase-contrast microscopy. It is spherical and except for a more crisp outline, it could be confused with a red cell. Red cells of varying shape and size are also seen. **B:** Under polarized light, the fine fat particle is clearly identifiable by the "Maltese cross" birefringence. (Courtesy of Bilal Jamil, M.D.) (See Color Figure 100.20A.)

In Fabry's disease the urine contains particles of sphingolipid, which also give a Maltese cross appearance with polarized light microscopy. As free particles they are less perfectly spherical than free fat bodies (Fig. 100.21). There are often tubular cells packed with these particles (Mulberry cells) or sphingolipid laden casts (Fig. 100.22). The sphingolipid particles can be further identified by electron microscopy, when the laminated "myelin bodies" characteristic of lipid storage disease are seen.

Fat can be also identified by Sudan III stains, and if there are large amounts of fat particles that do not have polarized spherulites, contamination of the urine by ointments or unclean collection containers should be suspected.

Crystals

A variety of crystals may be seen in normal and disease states. Because most can form in normal urine, depending on the diet and the concentration and pH of the urine, except for cystine crystals they are uncommonly diagnostic in themselves.

Urate Crystals

Urate crystals form an amorphous background in acid urine, and when present in large numbers, they can interfere with urine microscopy. This is particularly likely if the urine is highly concentrated, is allowed to cool, or is refrigerated

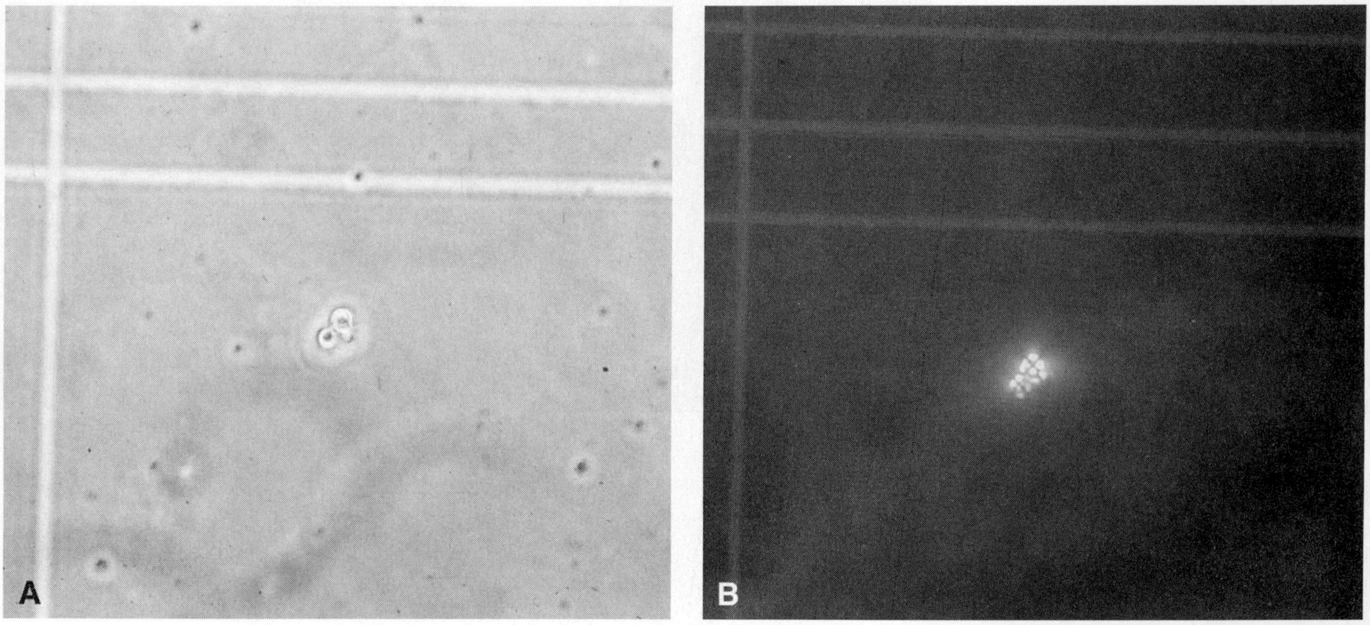

Figure 100.21. In Fabry's disease, sphingolipid particles are seen as irregularly rounded under polarised light **(A)** and have "Maltese cross" birefringence under polarised light **(B)**. (Courtesy of Bilal Jamil, M.D.)

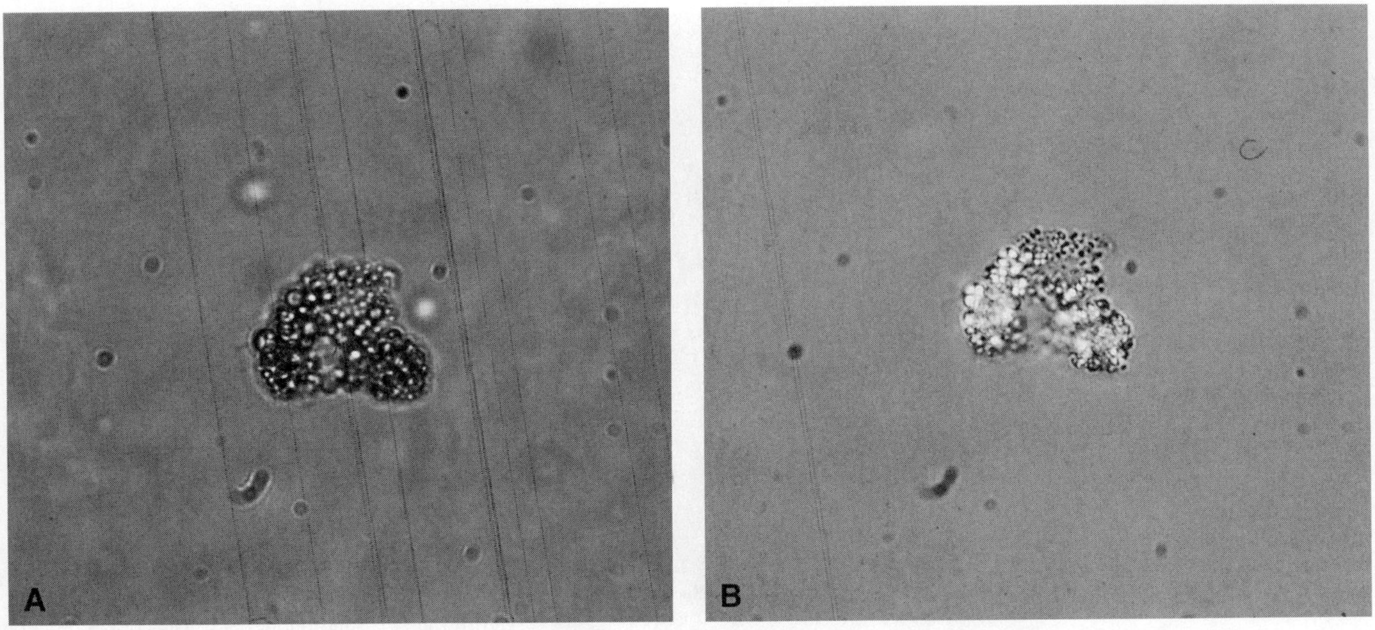

Figure 100.22. **A:** Tubular cell packed with sphingolipid "mulberry cell" is seen with phase-contrast microscopy in urine from a patient with Fabry's disease. **B:** With polarised light the multiple birefringent particles are revealed. (See Color Figures 100.22A and 100.22B.)

before being studied. Identifiable uric acid crystals may be diamond-, needle-, or rhombic-shaped (Fig. 100.23). They are sufficiently commonly seen as to be of little diagnostic value. Gentle warming of the urine toward 37°C will usually dissolve amorphous urates allowing visualization of the rest of the sediment. Uric acid crystals appear multicolored in polarized light, with the colors changing as the polarizer is rotated.

Amorphous Phosphate

In alkaline, normal urine amorphous phosphate crystals can similarly interfere with microscopy (Fig. 100.24) but can be cleared by adding dilute hydrochloric acid, as previously mentioned.

Calcium Oxalate Crystals

Calcium oxalate crystals occur in several shapes but are most easily recognized when they form small, octahedral, "envelope-like" shapes. They shine brightly in polarized light.

Triple Phosphate Crystals

Triple phosphate crystals may occur in normal alkaline urine or in patients with renal-infection (triple phosphate) stones. They form a variety of shapes, resembling coffin lids or quartz crystals.

Cystine Crystals

Cystine crystals are virtually diagnostic of the metabolic disorder cystinuria. They are perfect hexagons and may occur

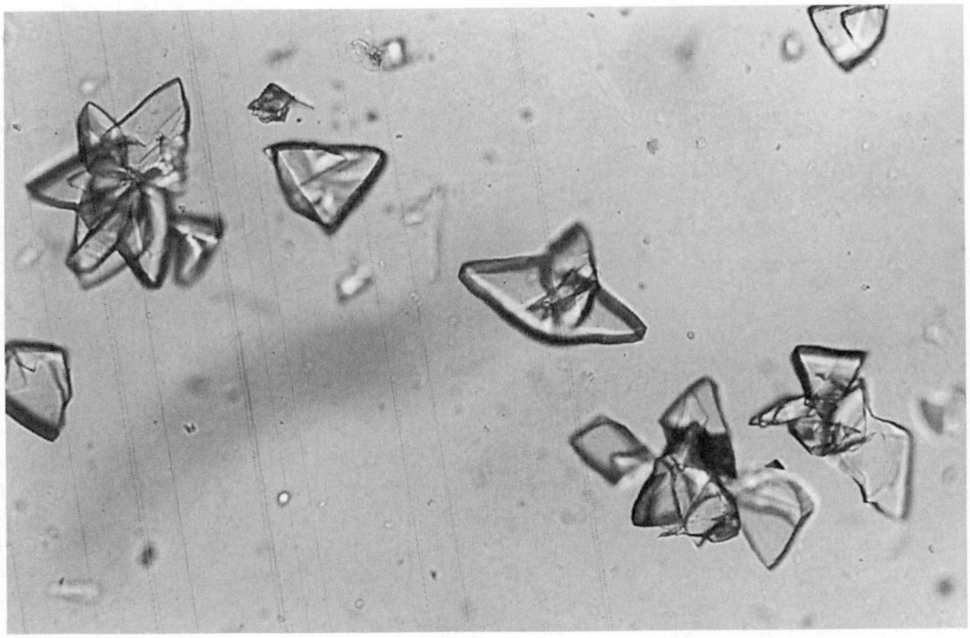

Figure 100.23. Uric acid crystals.

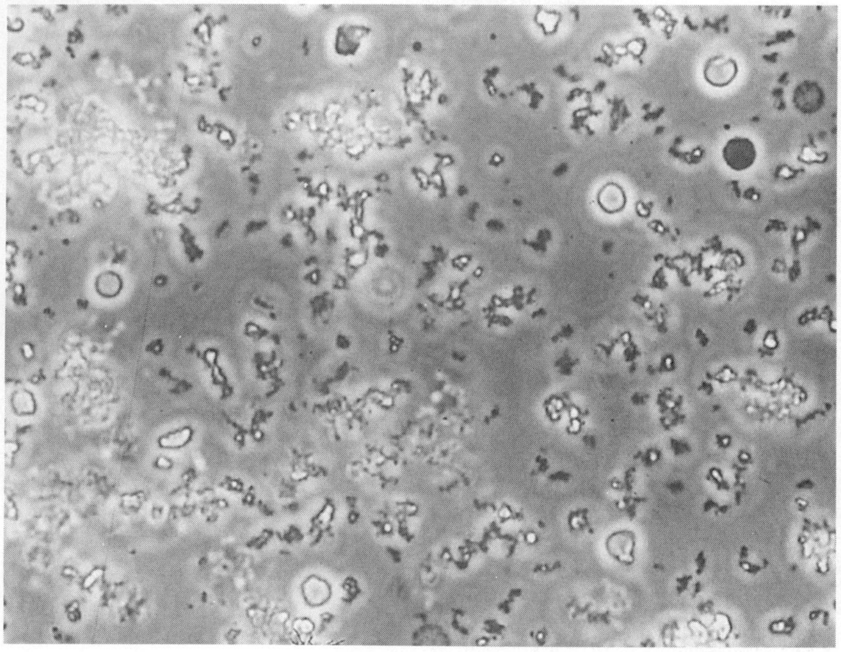

Figure 100.24. Amorphous phosphate crystals obscuring urinary sediment.

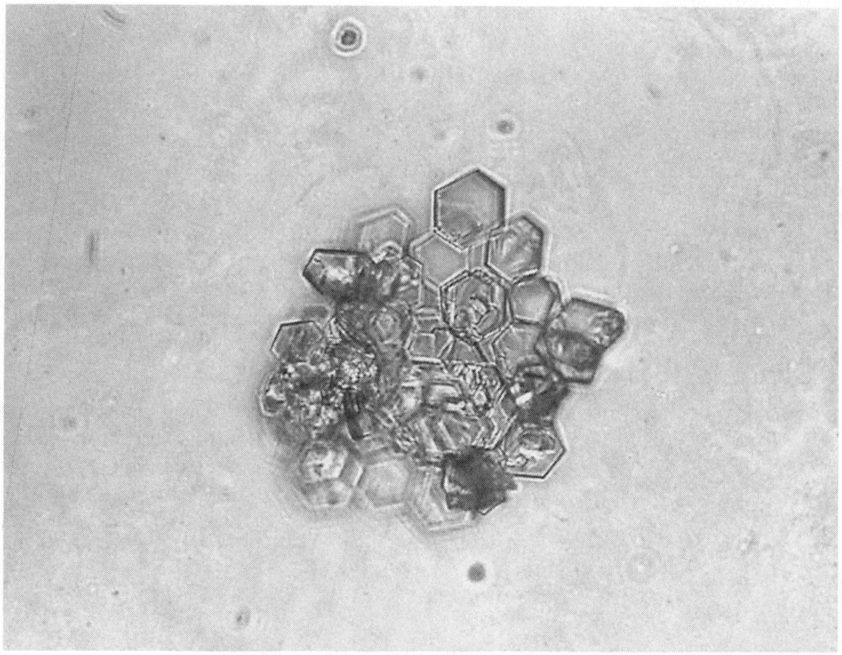

Figure 100.25. Cystine crystals. Typical hexagonal "benzine ring" crystals when seen in the urine are diagnostic of cystinuria.

alone as flat plates or as overlapping crystals of varying sizes (Fig. 100.25); they are, like uric acid, multicolored in polarized light.

URINE MICROSCOPY IN RENAL DISEASE

Glomerulonephritis

The major urinary microscopic findings in glomerulonephritis are of glomerular hematuria, red cell casts, abnormal complex casts, and fat particles.

In crescentic glomerulonephritis of any type, large numbers of glomerular red cells, usually exceeding 10^6 RBC/ml of urine, are seen. Large numbers of red cell casts are usual, and tubular and granular casts may also be found. Fat particles are very commonly found if sought. Moderate to heavy proteinuria is usually present concurrently.

In all forms of proliferative glomerulonephritis, glomerular red cells are usually found in numbers varying from under 10^5 to over 10^6 RBC/ml. If there is little or no associated proteinuria or casts, mild IgA nephropathy of thin basement membrane disease should be suspected.

In thin basement membrane disease the usual red cell count is 100,000 to 250,000/ml, although higher counts may be seen. Red cell casts are infrequent, strings of red cells are often present, and urinary protein excretion rarely exceeds 0.25 g/day. In IgA disease the number of red cells mirrors activity, and in quiescent disease urine microscopy is not clearly distinguishable from thin-basement membrane disease. With increasing activity a wide range of red cell counts to over 10^6/ml may be seen, and of these up to about 30% may be well hemoglobinized homogenous red cells, with the rest varying in morphologic structure. The reason for the large admixture of homogenous red cells is unknown. Proteinuria varies greatly with disease activity, often 2 to 3 g/day in progressive and advanced disease.

In membranous glomerulonephritis the red cell count is usually about 50,000 red cells/ml, but characteristically there are fat particles in large numbers, including free fat, casts full of fat particles, and oval fat bodies, with very few casts of other types. This is usually associated with heavy proteinuria, not necessarily in the nephrotic range.

The wide variety of renal pathologic changes that can occur in systemic lupus erythematosus is reflected by the variety of abnormalities that may be found in the urinary sediment. The presence of casts of all types, shapes, and sizes is called *telescoped sediment,* most commonly seen in lupus nephritis, but occasionally in other glomerular diseases. In lupus there may be large numbers of glomerular red cells and red cell casts—the higher the number, the more florid the proliferative and crescentic changes found. A high leukocyte count, not caused by urinary infection, is also a marker of more florid damage. In membranous lupus nephritis the red cell count usually exceeds 10^5 red cells/ml, and the rest of the deposit is similar to that found in idiopathic membranous nephritis, with free fat, casts containing fat, and oval fat bodies.

Patients with chronic tubulointerstitial diseases may have urine that appears normal microscopically, but if there is active inflammation, commonly leukocytes, renal tubular cells, and granular and tubular epithelial casts and debris are present. Proteinuria may indicate development of the progressive lesion of focal and segmental glomerulosclerosis and is an indication of poor prognosis.

In acute tubular necrosis from any cause, the urine usually contains many tubular cells, along with granular casts, tubular cell casts, and tubular cell debris in a wide variety of sizes and shapes. If the cause is acute tubulointerstitial nephritis, large numbers of leukocytes are also usual; eosinophils may be found, but this is neither a positive nor a specific finding. The absence of abnormal sediment in a patient with renal failure suggests either chronic renal failure or a prerenal cause not yet resulting in tubular necrosis.

Selected Readings

Birch DF, Fairley KIF, Becker G, et al. *A colour atlas of urine microscopy*. London: Chapman & Hall, 1993.

A clinically oriented text and atlas of urinary microscopy.

Birch DF, Fairley KIF, Whitworth JA, et al. Urinary erythrocyte morphology in the diagnosis of glomerular hematuria. *Clin Nephrol* 1983;20:78–84.

A paper describing the technique of identifying glomerular bleeding by phase-contrast microscopy of urinary red cells.

Brody LK, Salladay JR, Armbruster K. Urinalysis and the urinary sediment. *Med Clin North Am* 1971;55:243–266.

An early and important description of the advantages of phase-contrast microscopy in urinalysis.

Fairley KIF, Birch DF. Hematuria: a simple method for identifying glomerular bleeding. *Kidney Int* 1982;21:105–108.

A paper describing the technique of identifying glomerular bleeding by phase-contrast microscopy of urinary red cells.

Fogazzi GB. Crystalluria: a neglected aspect of urinary sediment analysis. *Nephrol Dial Transplant* 1996;11:379–387.

A detailed review of crystalluria, incorporating phase-contrast and polarized microscopy including discussion of the clinical relevance of a wide variety of urinary crystals.

Gilbert RE, Akdeniz A, Jerums G. Semi-quantitative determination of microalbuminuria by urinary dipstick. *Aust NZ J Med* 1992;22:334–337.

The usefulness of one of the immunochemical dipstick (Micral-Test, Boehringer Mannhein, GmbH Mannheim, Germany) was examined, with the finding of high sensitivity but a high level of fake positives, particularly at the threshold value of 20 mg/L when compared with radioimmunoassay.

Ginsberg JM, Change BS, Matarese RA, et al. Use of single voided urine samples to estimate quantitative proteinuria. *N Engl J Med* 1983;309:1543–1546.

The use of the urinary protein/creatinine ratio in the assessment of proteinuria.

Hyodo J, Kumano K, Naga M, et al. Analysis of urinary red blood cells of healthy individuals by an automated urinary flow cytometer. *Nephron* 1997;75: 451–457.

Describes a purpose designed urinary cytometer that distinguishes glomerular from nonglomerular hematuria, as well as identifying leukocytes epithelial cells, casts, and bacteria.

Kubota H, Yamabe H, Ozawa K, et al. Mechanism of urinary erythrocyte deformity in patients with glomerular disease. *Nephron* 1988;48:338–339.

A paper investigating the genesis of the glomerular pattern of urinary red cell morphology.

Loh EH, Keng VW, Ward PB. Blood cells and red cell morphology in the urine of healthy children. *Clin Nephrol* 1990;34:185–187.

Urinary red cell excretion in normal children.

Murphy BF, Fairley KF, Birch DF, et al. Culture of mid catheter urine collected via an open-ended catheter: a reliable guide to bladder bacteriuria. *J Urol* 1984; 131:19–21.

A description of the open-ended catheter technique for obtaining urine samples as an alternative to suprapubic aspiration in adult women.

Nolan CR, Anger MS, Kelleher SP. Eosinophiluria—a new method of detection and definition of the clinical spectrum. *N Engl J Med* 1986;315:1516–1519.

An assessment of Hansel's stain to detect eosinophiluria.

Rath B, Turner C, Hartley B, et al. What makes red cells dysmorphic in glomerular hematuria? *Pediatr Nephrol* 1992;6:424–427.

A paper investigating the genesis of the glomerular pattern of urinary red cell morphology.

Ruffing KA, Hoppes P, Blend D, et al. Eosinophils in urine revisited. *Clin Nephrol* 1994;41:163–166.

Using both Wright's and Hanser's stains to detect eosinophils, the sensitivity, specificity and positive predictive value of eosinophiluria for diagnosis in acute interstitial nephritis were found to be low.

Segasothy M, Fairley KF, Birch DF, et al. Immunoperoxidase identification of nucleated cells in urine in glomerular and acute tubular disorders. *Clin Nephrol* 1989;31:281–291.

Monoclonal antibody staining used to distinguish renal tubular cells and leukocytes and hence to differentiate between crescentic and noncrescentic nephritis and acute tubular necrosis and interstitial nephritis.

Stamm WE, Wagner KF, Amsel R, et al. Causes of the acute urethral syndrome in women. *N Engl J Med* 1980;303:410–415.

The relative values of quantitative assessment of leukocytes and bacteriuria in the diagnosis of urine infection in dysuric women.

Tanaka M, Kitamoto Y, Sato T, et al. Flow cytometric analysis of hematuria using fluorescent antihemoglobin antibody. *Nephron* 1993;65:354–358.

Describes a technique for using a flow cytometer to identify glomerular hematuria by the different size distribution of red cells, and their surface irregularity.

Tomita M., Kitamoto Y., Nakayama M., et al. A new morphological classification of urinary erythrocytes for differential diagnosis of glomerular hematuria. *Clin Nephrol* 1992;37:84–89.

A description of some of the bizarre red cell shapes that can occur with glomerular hematuria.

CHAPTER 101

Quantitative and Qualitative Measurements of Urinary Protein

Sharon G. Adler

The earliest recorded observations relating proteinuria with renal disease include those of Hippocrates (circa 500 BC), who noted that foamy urine indicated disease of the kidneys, and those of Rufus of Ephesus (circa AD 100), who recognized an association between edema and small, scarred kidneys. These observations appear to have been lost to physicians and were subsequently rediscovered during the Renaissance. A qualitative assessment of proteinuria was described by Dekkers (1648–1720), who reported that heated acidified urine "coagulates." Although Dekkers did not associate this phenomenon with the development of edema, almost 100 years later this relationship was suggested by Cotugno (1736–1822). Cruickshank (1745–1800) reported that diabetic but not cirrhotic edema was associated with proteinuria, and Blackall in 1818 noted that syphilis and mercury intoxication were associated with proteinuria. Wells (1757–1818) made the first attempt to quantitate proteinuria and proposed that urinary protein was caused by a leakage of serum proteins into urine as a result of a renal defect. Wells expressed his results as urine-to-serum protein ratios, rather than in absolute amounts of urine protein. It was Bright (1789–1858), however, who stressed a causal relation between edema, proteinuria, and contracted kidneys. Bright's contributions included the utilization of biochemical data, such as 24-hour urine protein excretion rates and urine and blood urea nitrogen measurements, in the standard evaluation of patients with renal disease. Later workers described variants of "benign proteinuria," including Matur, who in 1837 reported the functional proteinuria associated with fever, and Leube and Moxon, who in 1878 first discovered orthostatic proteinuria. Major developments in the understanding of proteinuria during the twentieth century have included the role of the tubule in the pathogenesis of low-molecular-weight proteinuria, the mathematical modeling of glomerular ultrafiltration, the effects of glomerular hemodynamics on perm-selectivity and filtration, and the toxic effects of proteinuria on tubular structure and function.

Normal adults excrete less than 150 mg of protein per day in urine, with the majority falling between 30 and 130 mg/day. Healthy children excrete less than 140 mg of protein/m^2 of body surface area per day in urine. One-third of physiologic proteinuria is albumin. Most of the remaining two-thirds is globulin, some of which is derived from serum. Small amounts of κ (2.4 mg) and of λ (1.5 mg) light chains are excreted per day in normal subjects. Approximately 10 to 60 mg of urinary protein may be secreted by the uroepithelium. Tamm-Horsfall protein is a glycoprotein secreted into urine by the cells of the thick ascending limb of Henle's loop. It is the major matrix material of urinary casts. Other renal-derived antigens, such as proximal renal tubule brush border antigens, are also found in trace amounts in normal urine. Abnormal proteinuria is generally classified by one of two systems, one based on pathogenesis (Table 101.1) and the other based upon clinical manifestation (Table 101.2). The pathogenetic mechanisms and the clinical approach to the evaluation of these varieties of proteinuria are discussed in Chapter 32.

TABLE 101.1. Pathogenic Classification of Abnormal Proteinuria

Altered glomerular function
Altered tubular function
Diminished tubular reabsorption
Enhanced tubular secretion
Overload proteinuria (prerenal proteinuria)
Addition of proteins not derived from plasma ultrafiltration or tubular secretion (tissue proteinuria)

TABLE 101.2. Clinical Classification of Abnormal Proteinuria

Constant proteinuria
Nephrotic range (>3 g/day)
Nonnephrotic range (<3 g/day)
Inconstant proteinuria
Benign physiologic (functional)
Fever, pneumonia, seizures, congestive heart failure, exercise, hypothermia, emotional stress, severe lordosis, angiotensin II, or epinephrine infusion
Intermittent proteinuria—abnormal proteinuria in >70% of randomly obtained specimens
Orthostatic proteinuria—fixed proteinuria with upright posture but minimal or absent with recumbency

URINE COLLECTION

Depending on the clinical need, urinary protein may be measured by qualitative, semiquantitative, or quantitative procedures. The 24-hour urine collection is the traditional urine sample provided to laboratories for quantitative measurements of protein excretion, but spot morning urine protein:creatinine

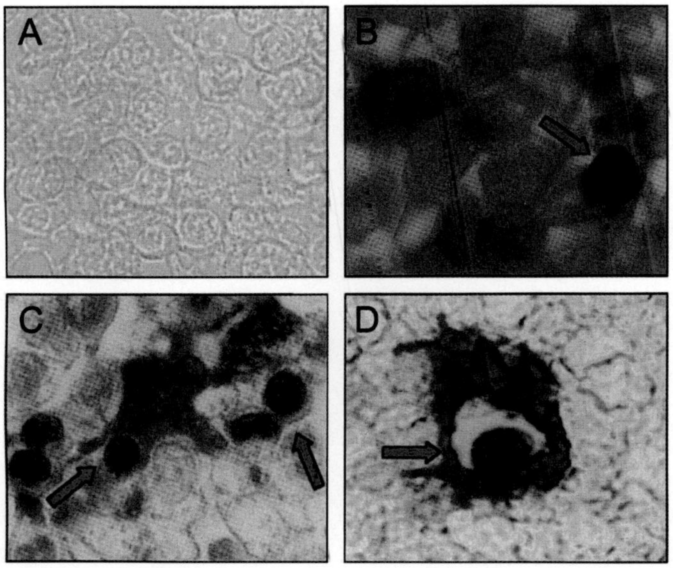

Color Figure 72.2. Regulation of erythropoiesis by apoptosis and phagocytosis of apoptotic erythroblasts. Photomicrographs of normal bone marrow show unstained control **(A)**, immature erythroblast (*arrow*) undergoing apoptosis **(B)**, and apoptotic immature erythroblasts undergoing ingestion by a neighboring macrophage (**C** and **D**). Erythropoietin blocks Fas/Fas-ligand mediated phagocytosis. (Reproduced with permission from De Maria R, Testa U, Luchett L, et al. Apoptotic role of Fas/Fas ligand in the regulation of erythropoiesis. *Blood* 1999;93:796–803.)

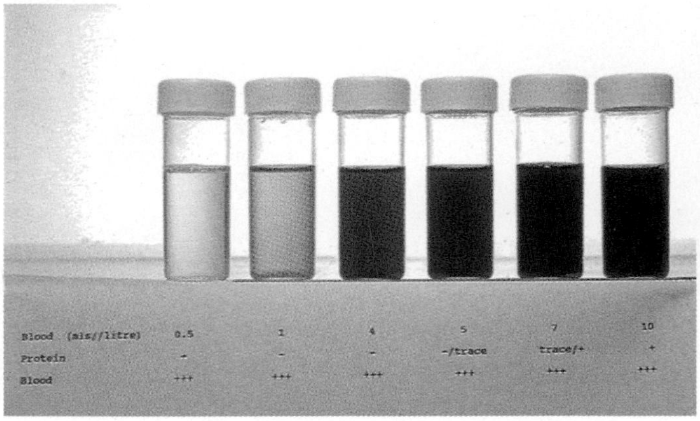

Color Figure 100.3. The result of adding whole blood to saline. The saline is macroscopically bloody with l ml/L of blood, but proteinuria is not detectable by reagent strip till 5 to10 ml/L is added.

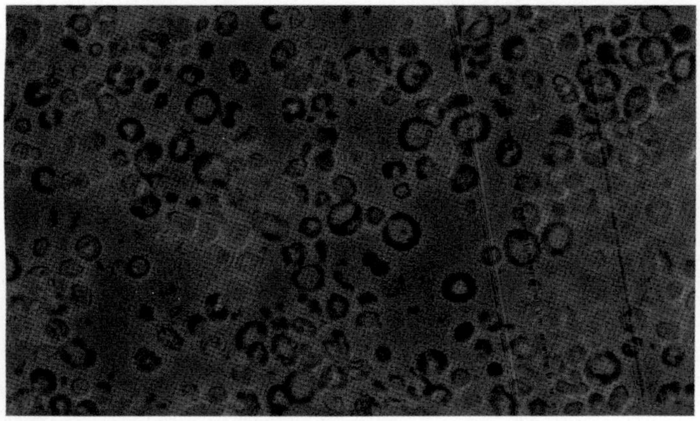

Color Figure 100.4. Phase-contrast microscopic appearance of heavy glomerular hematuria with a wide variety of cell shapes and sizes.

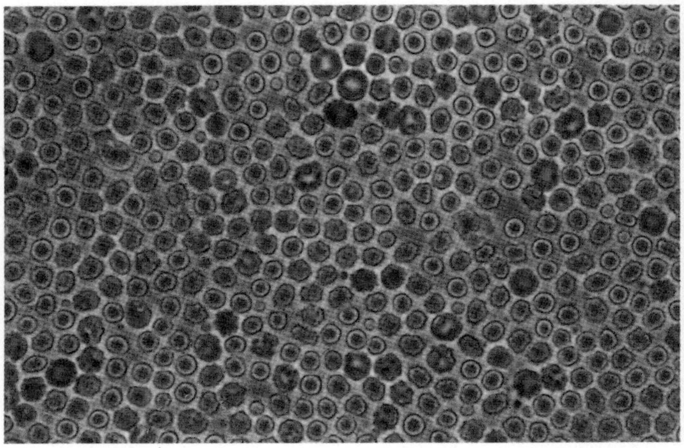

Color Figure 100.5. Phase-contrast microscopic appearance of lower tract hematuria (bladder tumor). The cells are of similar sizes and appearance, except for a very occasional dysmorphic cell.

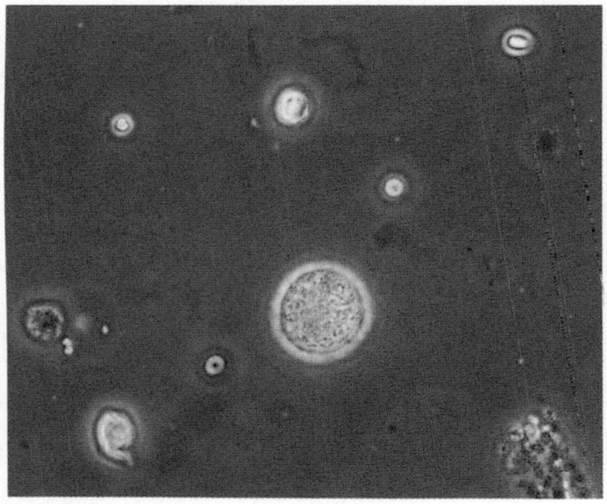

Color Figure 100.11A. Oval fat body. A tubular cell packed with lipid droplets. (Courtesy of Bilal Jamil, M.D.)

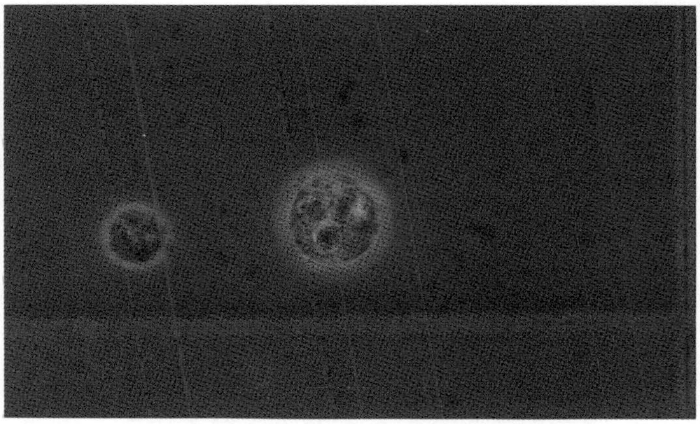

Color Figure 100.12. A renal tubular cell containing a phagocytosed erythrocyte, diagnostic of nephron bleeding.

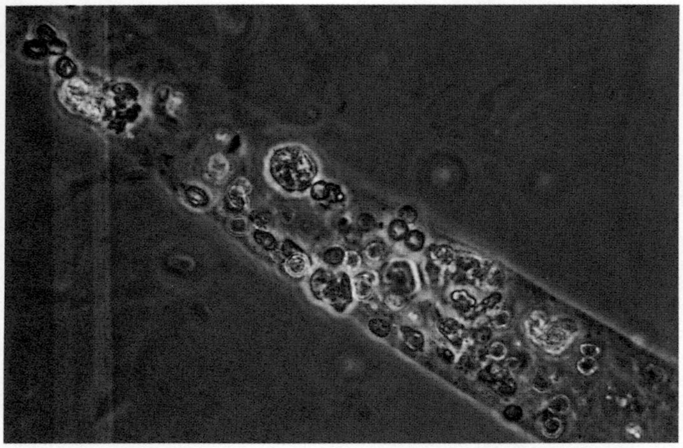

Color Figure 100.19. Mixed cast containing red cells and tubular epithelial cells.

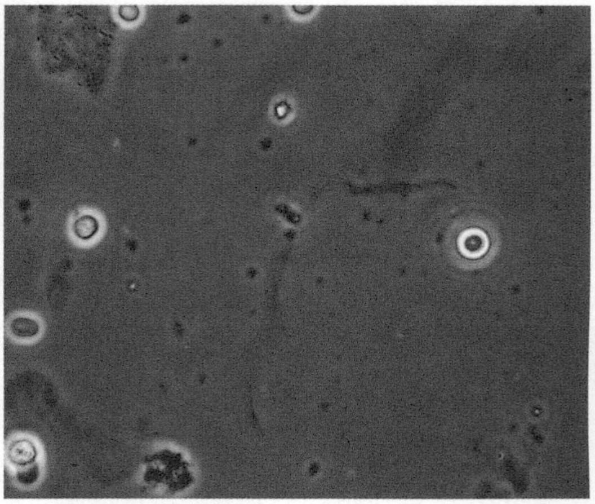

Color Figure 100.20A. Free fat particle under phase-contrast microscopy. It is spherical and except for a more crisp outline, it could be confused with a red cell. Red cells of varying shape and size are also seen. (Courtesy of Bilal Jamil, M.D.)

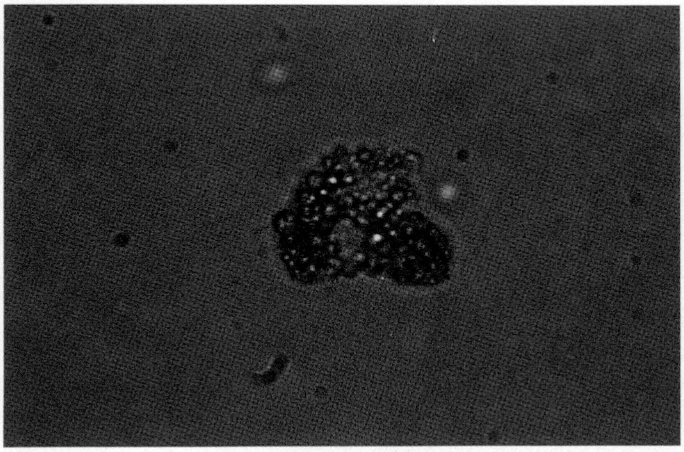

Color Figure 100.22A. Tubular cell packed with sphingolipid "mulberry cell" is seen with phase-contrast microscopy in urine from a patient with Fabry's disease.

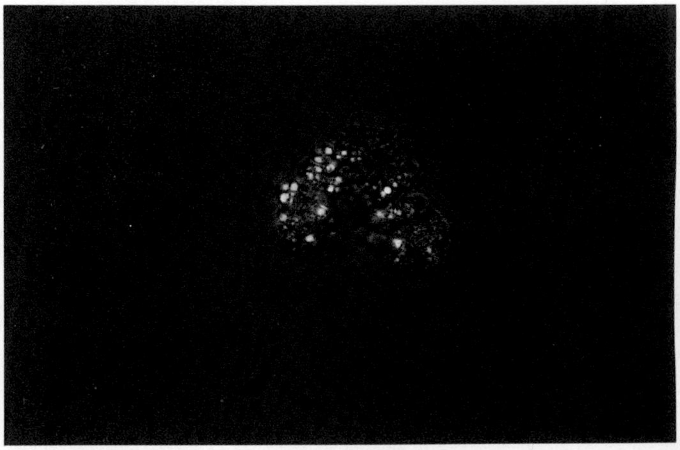

Color Figure 100.22B. Tubular cell packed with sphingolipid "mulberry cell" is seen with phase-contrast microscopy in urine from a patient with Fabry's disease. With polarized light the multiple birefringent particles are revealed.

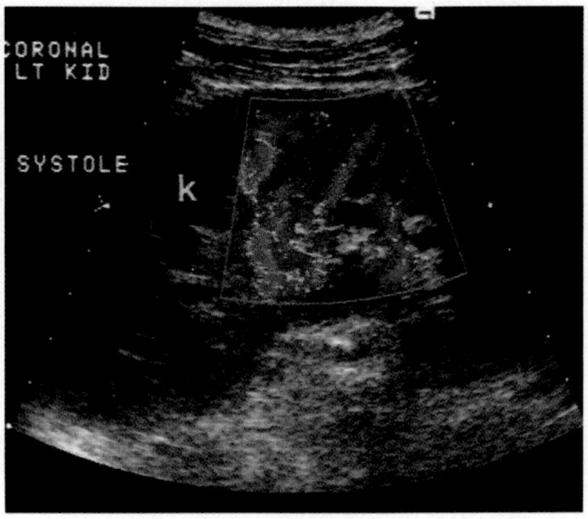

Color Figure 106.3A. Normal renal color Doppler sonogram. Coronal color flow Doppler image of the left kidney (*k*). Intrarenal systolic phase.

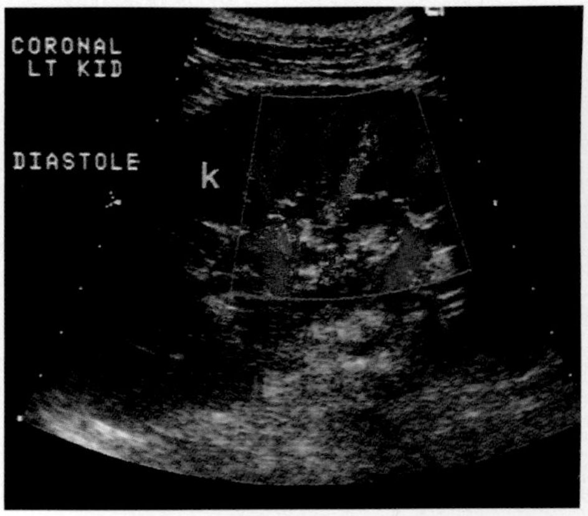

Color Figure 106.3B. Normal renal color Doppler sonogram. Coronal color flow Doppler image of the left kidney (*k*). Intrarenal diastolic phase.

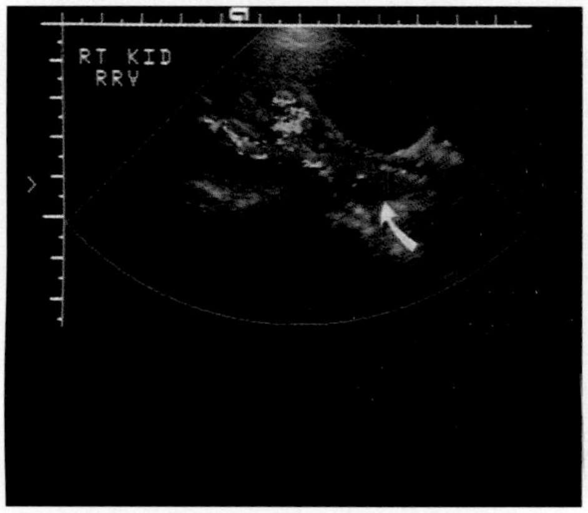

Color Figure 106.3C. Normal renal color Doppler sonogram. Transverse color flow Doppler image of the right kidney. Normal flow. *Curved arrow* indicates right renal vein.

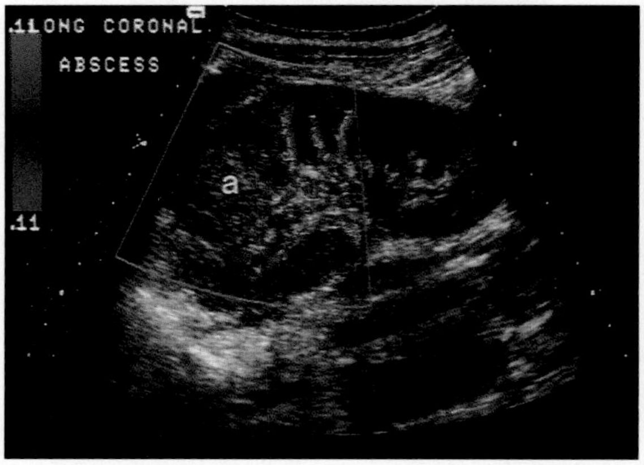

Color Figure 106.32. Renal abscess. Coronal color flow Doppler image of the left kidney. The homogeneous hyperechoic renal abscess (*a*) has no demonstrable internal vascular flow.

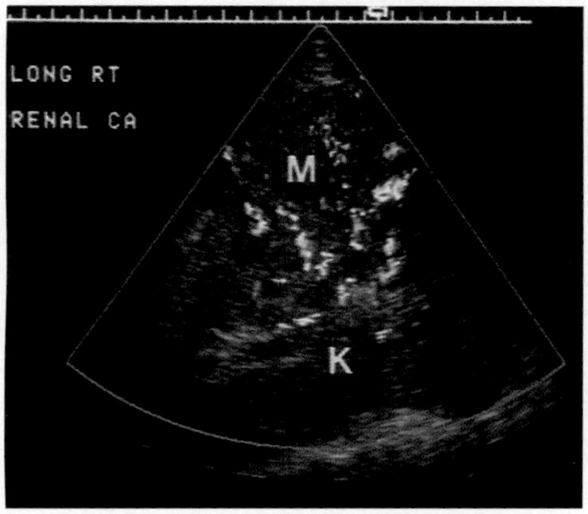

Color Figure 106.52A. Spectrum of renal cell carcinoma vascularity. Longitudinal oblique gray-scale Doppler image of the right kidney. There is no evidence of increased blood flow into the tumor. L, liver; R, right kidney; T, renal cell carcinoma.

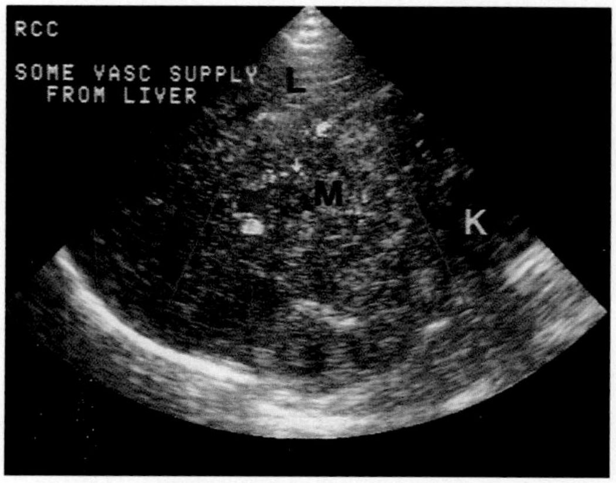

Color Figure 106.55. Renal cell carcinoma invading adjacent liver. Longitudinal color Doppler image of the right kidney and liver. The renal cell carcinoma has invaded the liver and is parasitizing the hepatic vasculature. The *arrow* denotes vascular flow from the liver to the mass. K, right kidney; L, liver; M, mass-renal cell carcinoma.

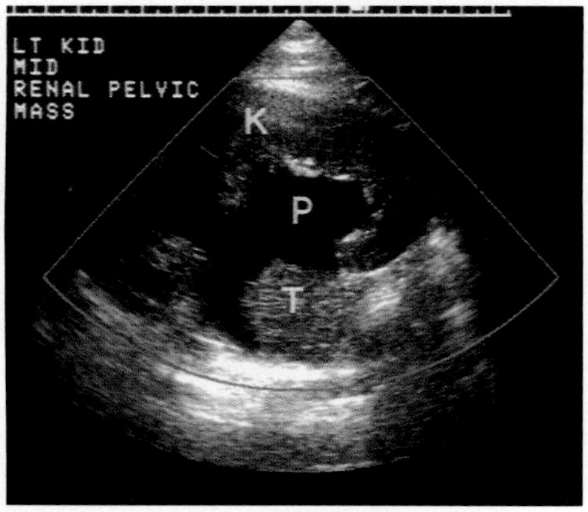

Color Figure 106.57. Transitional cell carcinoma. Longitudinal color flow Doppler image of the left kidney. The homogenous hyperechoic tumor is free of demonstrable vascular flow. It is partially obstructing the renal pelvis. K, left kidney; P, dilated renal pelvis; T, transitional cell carcinoma (tumor).

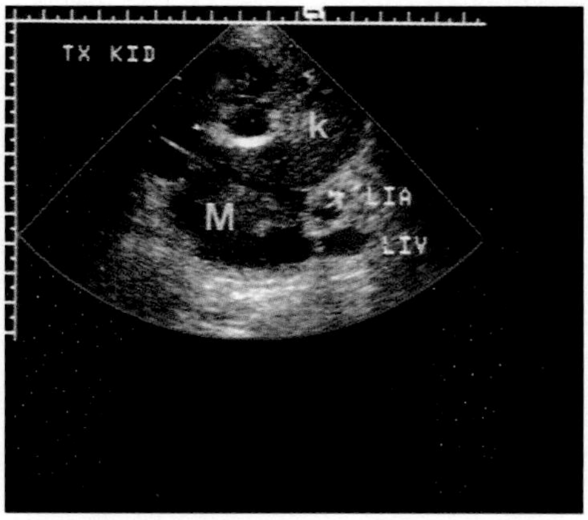

Color Figure 106.68. Posttransplant perirenal hematoma. Transverse color flow Doppler image of the transplanted kidney in the left pelvis. The heteroechoic mass (*M*) adjacent to kidney is a hematoma. There is no Doppler signal within the clot. k, transplant kidney; LIA, left iliac artery; LIV, left iliac vein.

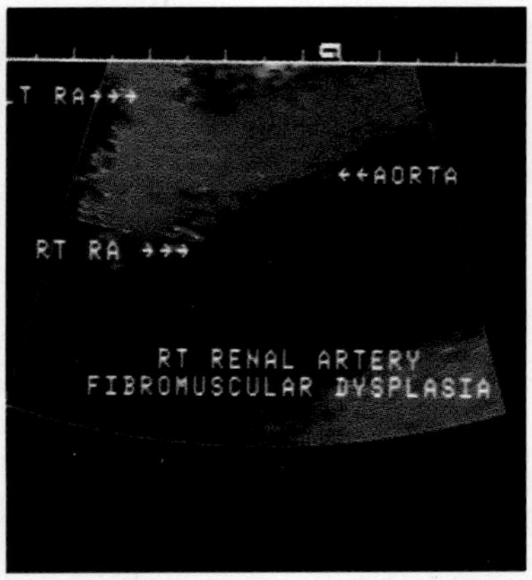

Color Figure 106.75A. Fibromuscular dysplasia of the renal artery. Longitudinal color flow Doppler image of the renal arteries at their origin. Stenosis of the proximal right renal artery secondary to fibromuscular dysplasia. LT RA, left renal artery; RT RA, right renal artery with stenosis.

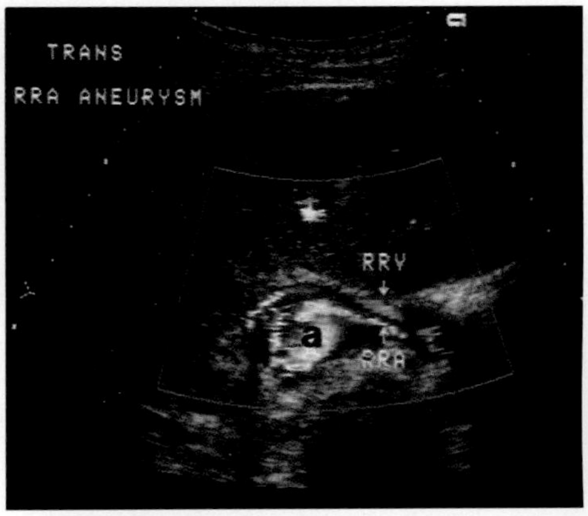

Color Figure 106.76. Renal artery aneurysm. Transverse color flow Doppler image of the right kidney. Aneurysm with increased arterial flow in a young patient with hypertension. a, aneurysm; RRV, right renal artery.

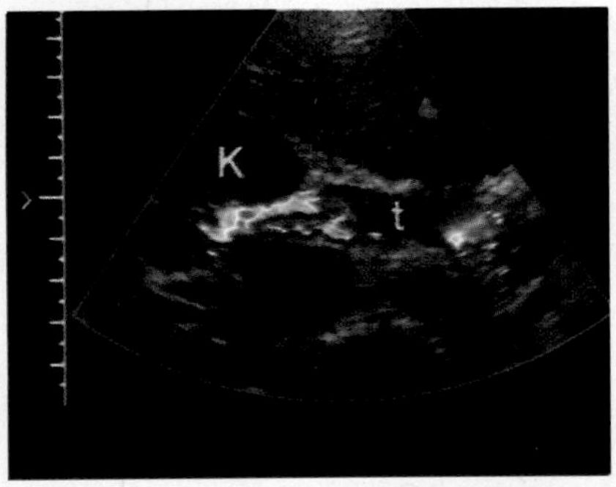

Color Figure 106.78A. Renal vein thrombosis. Transverse color flow Doppler image of the right kidney. Partial obstruction of flow in the vein by a thrombus. The patient has nephrotic syndrome. *K*, right kidney; *t*, renal vein thrombus.

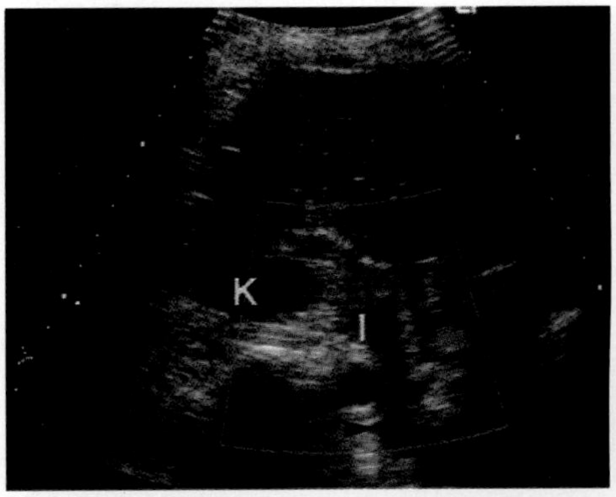

Color Figure 106.78B. Renal vein thrombosis. Renal vein and inferior vena cava thrombus. Transverse color flow Doppler image of the right kidney and inferior vena cava. Left renal vein clot extends into the inferior vena cava. Flow in the right renal vein is normal. The patient has nephrotic syndrome. The *arrowhead* denotes left renal vein with a clot. I, inferior vena cava (with clot); K, right kidney.

ratios are fast becoming a substitute for the 24-hour urine sample in the assessment of proteinuria. For the traditional method, the patient is instructed to collect all urine for a 24-hour period; usually the 24-hour collection period begins in the morning when the patient arises. The first voided specimen of the first morning is discarded, and the patient is asked to note the time. For the next 24 hours, all excreted urine is saved in the collection vessel, including any voided specimens occurring during the night. The patient is then instructed to awaken the following morning at the same time as the previous day, when the collection first began. The first voided specimen of the second morning should be collected and saved at the same time that the first voided specimen was discarded the day before. Ordinarily, quantitation of both the 24-hour protein and creatinine excretion is requested. In any given patient whose diet, renal function, and muscle mass remain constant, 24-hour urine creatinine excretion also remains approximately constant. Because of this, the latter serves as a measure of completeness of the 24-hour collection. The average man excretes 16 to 26 mg of creatinine per kilogram of ideal body weight per day; the average woman excretes 12 to 24 mg of creatinine per kilogram of ideal body weight per day. In aged individuals, urinary creatinine excretion may decline to 8 to 15 mg/kg of ideal body weight.

In patients suspected of having orthostatic proteinuria, 24-hour urine collections should be divided into two separate specimen bottles. The collection should proceed as described above, with the first morning specimen discarded. All subsequent urine collected during the course of the patient's daily activities should be collected in the first specimen container. After retiring for the evening, the patient should be instructed to remain in bed until the end of the collection period the next morning. Urine collected in the morning should be placed in the second specimen container and represents urine produced during recumbency. A comparison of supine and upright proteinuria can then be made. Patients with nocturia in whom this test is deemed necessary should be encouraged to void with the use of a bedpan or bedside urine collection container to avoid ambulation during the nighttime collection.

The timed 24-hour urine specimen is inconvenient to collect, and there are often difficulties in assessing the completeness of collection. For these reasons, some investigators have examined the utility of measuring the protein-to-creatinine ratio of random "spot" morning urine samples as a semiquantitative measure of proteinuria. This collection technique is rapidly becoming the standard collection technique in place of the 24-hour urine specimen in separating nephrotic-range from nonnephrotic-range proteinuria and also for following the clinical responsiveness of patients undergoing therapy for proteinuric states. A value greater than 3 mg protein/mg creatinine indicates nephrotic-range proteinuria. Available data have shown that the protein/creatinine ratio correlates with absolute and log-transformed 24-hour urine protein values ($P = .0001$ and $P < .0001$, respectively). The degree of proteinuria by this measure correlates with the rate of loss of renal function and is a risk factor for progression to end-stage renal disease.

The detection of small increases in urinary albumin excretion (more than 15 to 30 μg/min) in patients with insulin-dependent diabetes (incipient diabetic nephropathy) suggests the presence of early diabetic kidney disease and is highly predictive of the development of subsequent overt diabetic nephropathy. However, nonspecific factors may also induce small increments in proteinuria that might confound the prognostic usefulness of this test. Therefore, to maximize the prognostic accuracy of microalbuminuria, the following recommendations regarding urine collection have been suggested. Timed, overnight urine collections (preferably two or three) should be obtained. An overnight collection minimizes the contribution of an erect posture to albumin excretion. The patient should have adequate glycemic and blood pressure control during the collection, should avoid exercise, and the urine should be sterile. The patient should have no condition, other than diabetes, which may cause proteinuria. Urinary albumin is then usually measured by radial immunodiffusion, radioimmunoassay, or enzyme-linked immunosorbent assay (ELISA). Under these carefully controlled conditions, the presence of microalbuminuria identifies patients with insulin-dependent diabetes who are at high risk for developing overt diabetic nephropathy. In patients with adult-onset diabetes mellitus, the detection of microalbuminuria correlates better with cardiovascular and cerebrovascular disease than it does with nephropathy. Microalbuminuria may now also be detected using commercially available dipsticks which are more sensitive than those utilized for the standard urinalysis.

URINARY PROTEIN MEASUREMENT

Semiquantitative Measures of Proteinuria

Ideally, screening tests for proteinuria should be sensitive enough to identify low levels of abnormal proteinuria, but not so sensitive that normal low levels of proteinuria are detected and erroneously interpreted to be pathologic. The most commonly used semiquantitative test for proteinuria is the standard dipstick method, with a sensitivity of 10 to 30 mg/dl for albumin. The protein dipstick is a reagent stick impregnated with a color indicator, usually bromphenol blue, which is yellow at pH 3. Between pH 5 and 7, the indicator binds albumin and the color changes in proportion to the concentration of albumin in the urine. The dipstick is much less sensitive for detection of globulins, including low-molecular-weight proteins and light chains and may thus be falsely negative in the presence of tubular proteinuria, multiple myeloma, and overflow proteinuria because of the predominance of nonalbumin proteins in these conditions. Translation of the results of the dipstick method as an indicator of the amount of protein excreted requires knowledge of urine volume; 1+ proteinuria corresponds to 30 mg/dl protein and 4+ proteinuria indicates greater than 300 mg/dl. The dipstick proteinuria may also be falsely negative in the presence of very dilute urine. The dipstick method may falsely indicate abnormal proteinuria in the presence of a highly concentrated urine, in urine with a pH higher than 8, in the presence of phenazopyridine, or in urine contaminated with antiseptics such as chlorhexidine or benzalkonium (Table 101.3). An alternative

TABLE 101.3. Semiquantitative Studies for Proteinuria—False-Positive and False-Negative Results

	Method	
	Dipstick	Turbidometric
Concentrated urine	False +	False +
Dilute urine	False −	False −
Urine pH >8	False +	False −
Contamination with antiseptics	False +	No effect
Tolbutamide metabolites	No effect	False +
Penicillins, cephalosporins (massive doses)	No effect	False +
Sulfisoxazole metabolites	No effect	False +
Phenazopyridine	False +	No effect
Radiographic contrast media	No effect	False +

means of assessing proteinuria semiquantitatively depends on protein precipitation by sulfosalicylic, trichloroacetic, or nitric acids or by heat and acetic acid. Turbidity is measured on a semiquantitative scale. These latter methods tend to be much more sensitive than the dipstick method for detecting proteinuria as low as 3 to 5 mg/dl. False-positive results are more common. Such false-positive results occur when testing highly concentrated urines with radiocontrast agents, sulfonamide and tolbutamide metabolites, and high concentrations of penicillins or cephalosporins. False-negative results may be seen in the presence of highly buffered alkaline urine or highly dilute urine. Despite their relative lack of specificity, one advantage of the turbidometric measures is that they are more sensitive than the dipstick method to nonalbumin proteins in the urine, including globulins and glycoproteins. Therefore a discrepancy between the dipstick method and the turbidometric methods suggests the presence of proteinuria characterized primarily by nonalbumin proteins. The finding of significant proteinuria by precipitation methods not confirmed by dipstick would require further studies to rule out the presence of multiple myeloma or other lesions leading to tubular proteinuria.

Quantitative Measures of Proteinuria

The most common procedures for quantitating proteinuria in clinical laboratories in the United States are the turbidometric methods, with quantitation by a photometer or nephelometer. Proteinuria may also be quantitated by ultraviolet spectrophotometry at 210 nm, the wavelength at which albumin and globulin display similar absorbance. Ultraviolet spectrophotometry offers enhanced precision of measurement compared with protein precipitation methods, but it is less sensitive and more time-consuming. The biuret method of measuring proteinuria depends on a color change occurring in the presence of alkaline copper sulfate and the biuret compound, quantitated spectrophotometrically at 557 nm. The biuret assay is more sensitive but more labor intensive than turbidometric methods. The micro-Kjeldahl method for measurement of protein nitrogen is the most accurate; however, it is expensive, tedious, and time-consuming and is therefore reserved for research purposes.

Qualitative Measures of Proteinuria

The qualitative aspects of abnormal proteinuria can be studied by the identification of specific proteins or classes of proteins using a variety of methods, including electrophoresis on cellulose acetate or polyacrylamide, immunoelectrophoresis in agarose gel, radial or double immunodiffusion, radioimmunoassay, and ELISA. Many of these methods may be readily adapted to provide quantitative information (e.g., densitometric scanning). Such techniques are particularly helpful for characterizing the pathogenetic mechanisms for abnormal proteinuria. The identification of a monoclonal paraprotein in urine would suggest overflow proteinuria, such as in multiple myeloma or primary amyloidosis. The presence of a high β_2-microglobulin excretion relative to albumin excretion would indicate a tubular origin of the proteinuria. The specific detection of small quantities of albumin (microalbuminuria) may be useful in the evaluation of early stages of diabetic nephropathy. In addition, microalbuminuria appears to be a general risk factor for cardiovascular and cerebrovascular mortality and morbidity, not just in diabetics, but also in the general population. This may suggest the utility of microalbuminuria as a marker for generalized endothelial dysfunction.

The specific immunologic measurements of fibrinogen or fibrin degradation products (fibrinopeptide A), complement proteins (C3 or C4), or tubular glycoproteins may be of clinical value in specific disorders such as crescentic glomerulonephritis (elevated excretion of fibrin degradation products), Alport's syndrome (elevated excretion of a fragment of C3), or acute tubular necrosis (elevated excretion of proximal renal tubular brush border antigen). The presence of the terminal component of complement [membrane attack complex (MAC)] in the urine may correlate with disease activity in membranous nephropathy.

A rapidly growing literature also demonstrates the presence of growth factors, cytokines, and extracellular matrix and albumin fragments in the urine of patients with proteinuria, and numerous studies have been performed to demonstrate that these products may be toxic to the tubulointerstitium. The interaction of these proteins with tubular cells are thought to mediate, at least in part, the tendency for progressive renal dysfunction in patients with proteinuria. Finally, experimental evidence suggests that specific proteins may be found in urine as markers of genitourinary malignancy.

PROTEIN SELECTIVITY

Calculation of a ratio of urinary clearances of several proteins, often referred to as *protein selectivity,* has been used to assess the degree of damage to the glomerular permeability barrier (Chapter 4). This can be accomplished by simultaneous measurement of the serum and urine concentrations of several proteins of differing molecular size (e.g., IgG and transferrin). The selectivity index is then calculated as $(U_{IgG}/P_{IgG}) \div (U_{transferrin}/P_{transferrin})$, where *U* and *P* represent the concentration of protein in urine and plasma, respectively. Values of less than 0.1 for this ratio indicate highly selective proteinuria and thereby less severe glomerular damage.

Fractional IgG clearance has also been used to indicate the extent of disruption of the glomerular permselectivity barrier (see Chapter 4). This is determined by measuring the urine and plasma concentrations of IgG and inulin. Fractional IgG clearance is then calculated as $(U_{IgG}/P_{IgG}) \div (U_{inulin}/P_{inulin})$. Values of less than 0.001 for this ratio indicate highly selective proteinuria.

Selected Readings

Bruzzi I, Benigni A, Remuzzi G. Role of increased glomerular protein traffic in the progression of renal failure. *Kidney Int* 1997;62:S29–S31.
An overview of the pathogenetic role that proteinuria plays in the progression of chronic renal insufficiency.

Grimm RH Jr, Svendsen KH, Kasiske B, et al. Proteinuria is a risk factor for mortality over 10 years of follow-up. MRFIT Research Group: Multiple Risk Factor Intervention Trial. *Kidney Int* 1997;63:S10–S14.
Epidemiologic study demonstrating a relationship between proteinuria and vascular disease in nondiabetic subjects.

Ruggenenti P, Gaspari F, Perna A, et al. Cross-sectional longitudinal study of spot morning urine protein:creatinine ratio, 24-hour urine protein excretion rate, glomerular filtration rate, and end-stage renal failure in chronic renal disease in patients without diabetes. *Br Med J* (Clinical Research Edition) 1998;316:504–509.
In this study of 177 patients with nondiabetic glomerular disease, the efficacy of ramipril on the course of progression of renal disease was assessed. The study analyzed the correlation of spot protein:creatinine ratios to the more traditional 24-hour urine measurements, and correlated the spot values to renal outcomes. There was good correlation between the spot and 24-hour urine collection methods; the spot measurement of proteinuria was a reliable predictor of prognosis.

Scherberich JE. Urinary proteins of tubular origin: basic immunochemical and clinical aspects. *Am J Nephrol* 1990;10:43–51.
A review of the pathophysiology, differential diagnosis, and laboratory methods for the identification of proteinuria caused by tubulointerstitial disorders.

Stephenson JM, Kenny S, Stevens LK, et al. Proteinuria and mortality in diabetes: the WHO Multinational Study of Vascular Disease in Diabetes. *Diabetic Med* 1995;12:149–155.
An epidemiologic study demonstrating a relationship between proteinuria and vascular disease in diabetic subjects.

Walker KV, Ward KM, Mahan JD, et al. Current concepts in proteinuria. *Clin Chem* 1989;35:755-765.
Comprehensive review of the pathophysiology of proteinuria, including differential diagnosis and laboratory methodologies for the study of proteinuric states. The emphasis is on glomerular proteinuria.

CHAPTER 102

Biochemical Investigations of Urine

Nosratola D. Vaziri and Charles J. Kaupke

The chemical composition of urine changes in a variety of renal and extrarenal disorders. Thus identifying and monitoring these biochemical alterations may provide an insight into the nature, severity, site, or even prognosis of the underlying process. Glomerular proteinuria, Bence Jones proteinuria, and various urinary changes associated with renal tubular disorders have been discussed elsewhere in text. This chapter reviews the urinary excretion of various fibrin(ogen) fragments, coagulation and related proteins, selected enzymes of renal and extrarenal origin, β_2-microglobulin, and kallikrein in health and disease.

URINARY FIBRIN(OGEN) FRAGMENTS AND COAGULATION FACTORS

Activation of the coagulation system has been implicated in the pathogenesis of a variety of renal diseases. For instance, fibrin deposition in the renal vasculature is thought to play an important role in the genesis of renal lesions in microangiopathic disorders. Similarly, fibrin deposition within Bowman's space may contribute to epithelial cell proliferation in crescentic glomerulonephritides. Fibrin(ogen)-related antigens have been demonstrated by immunofluorescent microscopy within the glomerular capillary walls and lumina as well as in the mesangium in numerous renal diseases, including hemolytic uremic syndrome, systemic sclerosis, malignant nephrosclerosis, and renal allograft rejection. Although the cause-and-effect relationship between these changes and the associated renal lesions remains uncertain, measurement of various fibrin(ogen) fragments in serum and urine may provide useful information as to the disease activity. Moreover, various circulating fibrin(ogen) fragments and coagulation proteins may pass through glomerular capillary walls and appear in the urine.

Products of Fibrin(ogen)olysis

Degradation of fibrin(ogen) by plasmin yields a group of compounds called *fibrin(ogen) degradation products* (FDP). Sequential proteolytic digestion of fibrinogen or fibrin monomer by plasmin produces fragments X (Mr = 250,000), Y (Mr = 155,000), D (Mr = 85,000), and E (Mr = 50,000), whereas solubilization of cross-linked fibrin by plasmin produces fragments D-dimer (Mr = 170,000) and E. Presence of D-dimer is therefore indicative of formation of cross-linked fibrin and its subsequent lysis by plasmin. Some or all of these fragments are usually found in the urine of patients with various glomerulopathies. Urinary clearance of these compounds is inversely proportional to their molecular size in highly selective proteinuria, such as minimal change glomerulopathy in children. In contrast, patients with nonselective proteinuria fail to exhibit such proportionality.

The origin of urinary FDP is varied. It may include filtration of circulating FDP through damaged glomeruli, breakdown of fibrin deposits in the glomerular lesions, or degradation of filtered fibrinogen in the renal tubules. It should be noted that intact fibrinogen (Mr = 340,000) is generally undetectable in the urine of patients with various glomerulopathies. As noted earlier, presence of D-dimer in the urine indicates the formation of cross-linked fibrin and its subsequent degradation by plasmin at some renal or extrarenal site. Determination of the urinary clearance of D-dimer and its comparison with clearance of IgG, whose molecular weight approximates that of D-dimer, appears to be helpful in differentiating renal and extrarenal processes. A clearance of D-dimer to clearance of IgG ratio of less than 1 suggests mere filtration of these compounds in the damaged glomeruli, whereas a ratio greater than 1 suggests additional quantities originating from the kidney (e.g., fibrin deposits in the glomerular lesions). Accordingly, the ratio of the clearance of D-dimer to IgG is usually less than 1 in minimal change nephrotic syndrome and more than 1 in crescentic glomerulonephritis, acute glomerulonephritis, membranoproliferative glomerulonephritis, and Henoch-Schönlein purpura, suggesting renal deposition of fibrin in the latter conditions. It should be noted that there is no consistent correlation between the presence of D-dimer and other FDP in the urine and demonstrable immunoreactive fibrin deposits (on immunofluorescent microscopy) in renal tissue. However, the degree of urinary FDP excretion does correlate with the disease activity, and serial determinations are useful in following the course of the pathologic process.

Urinary FDP excretion rises in the presence of urinary tract infection. The reported rise is greater with pyelonephritis than with lower urinary tract infection and is more pronounced in acute than in chronic infections. In addition, urorenal tumors have been shown to increase urinary FDP. Urinary FDP excretion is elevated during the first 2 weeks after renal transplantation. In addition, acute graft rejection is associated with a rise in urinary FDP. This finding, however, is not of special value, because it appears in parallel with various other clinical and conventional laboratory manifestations of acute rejection. Nonetheless, serial measurements have been used to assess the response to therapeutic measures.

All fibrin(ogen) degradation fragments are immunoreactive with antisera against fibrinogen. Employing this property, a variety of immunologic assays, including radial immunodiffusion and latex agglutination, have been developed for determining total FDP. In addition, individual fragments can be quantitated by electrophoretic separation of the immunoadsorbed material.

Fibrinopeptide A

Fibrinopeptides A and B are small peptides (Mr = 2000) cleaved by thrombin from the N-terminal portions of alpha- and beta-chains of fibrinogen to form fibrin monomers. Consequently, the presence of these peptides denotes active fibrin formation, and as such, plasma fibrinopeptide A (FPA) determination is commonly used to diagnose thrombotic events and monitor the response to anticoagulant therapy. FPA is normally filtered in the glomeruli and is readily excreted in the urine. Because of the short plasma half-life of FPA (3 to 5 minutes), its urinary excretion is a more reliable indicator of *in vivo* coagulation than is plasma FPA. In fact, elevated urinary FPA excretion has been shown in peripheral arterial disease, aortic aneurysm, and severe coronary artery disease in the absence of frank thrombosis. Measurement of urinary FPA is of value in the diagnosis of renal vein thrombosis and other thromboembolic events in nephrotic syndrome, in which it can serve as a useful tool for evaluation of response to anticoagulation therapy. Sensitive radioimmunoassays are available for the measurement of the urine and plasma FPA.

Coagulation Factors and Related Proteins

Various coagulation factors and inhibitory proteins may be lost in the urine in patients with heavy proteinuria. This can result in deficiency states that may be associated with either bleeding diathesis or hypercoagulability.

Urinary excretion and deficiency of factor XII (Mr = 76,000) occurs with considerable frequency in nephrotic syndrome. Although acquired factor XII deficiency leads to prolongation of partial thromboplastin time, it is not associated with bleeding diathesis. Factor XII deficiency may paradoxically contribute to thrombogenic diathesis in nephrotic syndrome. Urinary factor XII can be determined by immunoelectrophoresis.

Heavy urinary losses of factor IX (Mr = 55,400) leading to its deficiency and bleeding complications have been reported in several patients with severe nephrotic syndrome. Presence of factor IX in the urine was suspected by demonstration of factor IX–like procoagulant activity.

Factor VII (Mr = 53,000) may be lost in the urine of patients with nephrotic syndrome. On rare occasions, this can cause a deficiency state and severe bleeding complications. Urinary factor VII can be measured by radioimmunoassay. Prothrombin (Mr = 69,000 to 74,000) is also lost in the urine of patients with nephrotic syndrome. Immunodiffusion or immunoelectrophoresis can be used to measure prothrombin antigen in the urine.

Antithrombin III (Mr = 63,000) deficiency and its urinary excretion is common in the nephrotic syndrome. Immunodiffusion or immunoelectrophoresis can be used to measure antithrombin III in the urine. Antithrombin III deficiency is thought to be the main determinant of thromboembolic complications in nephrotic syndrome.

Patients with the nephrotic syndrome may lose significant quantities of plasminogen (Mr = 82,000) in the urine. This can lead to a reduced plasma level of this important protein. Urinary plasminogen can be measured by immunodiffusion.

URINARY ENZYMES

Since the initial report by Rosalki and Wilkinson in 1959 of increased urinary lactic dehydrogenase (LDH) in patients with renal disease, many investigations have been carried out to study urinary enzymes in a variety of renal and urinary tract disorders. So far, more than 40 different urinary enzymes have been studied. Urinary enzymes may originate from several different sources: (a) enzymes released from the leukocytes, erythrocytes, or bacteria in the urine; (b) enzymes liberated from the renal parenchyma; (c) enzymes originating from the bladder and urinary tract; and (d) filtered plasma enzymes escaping removal by the proximal tubules. With regard to the fourth group, enzymes with Mr greater than 60,000 are poorly filtered in normal glomeruli. However, they are partially filtered in patients with glomerular proteinuria. In contrast, lower molecular weight enzymes, such as various amylase isoenzymes (Mr = 45,000) as well as lysozyme and ribonuclease, are partially filtered in glomeruli. Like other proteins, the filtered enzymes are removed by the proximal tubules and only the fraction escaping removal appears in the urine. In the absence of renal and glomerular dysfunction, changes in the urinary excretion of the circulating enzymes reflect the rates of their release into the plasma. For instance, plasma and urinary amylase levels increase in acute pancreatitis. However, urinary amylase excretion is normal in patients with hyperamylasemia caused by increased protein-bound amylase (macroamylasemia). This is a consequence of the large size of the amylase-protein complexes, which precludes their filtration in the glomeruli.

Urinary enzymes originating in the kidney have received greater attention than those of extrarenal origin, primarily because of their potential utility as a marker for renal parenchymal injury. In fact, the presence of certain enzymes or isoenzymes in the urine may help to determine the site and even the nature of the lesion within the kidney and urinary tract. For instance, elevated urinary LDH_1 and LDH_2 isoenzymes in a child with urinary tract infection suggests bladder and lower urinary tract involvement, while elevation of LDH_4 and LDH_5 isoenzymes suggests renal involvement. Likewise, increased levels of LDH_4, LDH_5, carbonic anhydrase, and aspartate aminotransferase (AST or SGOT), which are primarily located in the cortex (proximal and distal convoluted tubules), tend to denote cortical lesions. In contrast, increased urinary alanine aminotransferase (ALT or SGPT) may be indicative of a medullary process. In general, gluconeogenic enzymes, beta-glucosidase, catalase, glutathione-S-transferase, and brush border enzymes (alkaline phosphatase, alanine aminopeptidase) are present in the proximal tubules, whereas glycolytic enzymes are found in the distal nephron. It should be noted that while under most circumstances, presence of significant quantities of these and other large molecular size enzymes in the urine represents their exclusive urorenal origin, this is not always the case. For instance, release into the circulation of large quantities of such enzymes from other organs in the presence of glomerular lesions can lead to their appearance in the urine. This should be considered in interpretation of the urinary enzymes. Also, the release of every enzyme does not necessarily denote cell damage or death. For instance, lysosomal enzymes may enter the urine without cell destruction. Likewise, parts of the brush border and its enzymes may be lost reversibly without cell death. In contrast, however, release of mitochondrial and cytosolic enzymes is often indicative of cell death. Because of the normal turnover of tubular epithelial cells, small amounts of the constituent enzymes are normally detectable in the urine.

To date, tests of urinary enzymes have received limited acceptance and utility in clinical practice and have largely remained as investigative tools because of a number of problems: (a) variations of urinary enzymes are nonspecific and as such do not allow definitive diagnosis of specific renal lesions; (b) standardization of the laboratory methods has been lacking and substantial differences are often found between values obtained by different laboratories; c) before functional assays, it is often necessary to remove various enzyme inhibitors and chromogens usually present in the urine, but this is not necessary when immunologic methods or electrophoretic separation are used; (d) the urinary excretion of enzymes often shows considerable circadian variation; and (e) the tests are often costly and not readily available in most clinical laboratories. Despite these and other limitations, measurement of urinary enzymes, when considered in conjunction with clinical and other laboratory data, may serve as a valuable adjunct in the diagnosis of a number of urorenal disorders. In addition, regular monitoring of certain urinary enzymes may allow early detection of renal transplant rejection or drug nephrotoxicity before these complications could be ascertained from clinical and routine laboratory findings. This may enable the physician to take remedial measures before extensive tissue damage occurs. Tests of various urinary enzymes have been found useful in the diagnosis of acute tubular necrosis, renal transplant rejection, drug nephrotoxicity, renal and urinary tract neoplasms, and differentiation of pyelonephritis from cystitis in children and renal parenchymal damage from bladder disorders in paraplegic patients. However, presently the most reliable indication for these tests is in drug evaluation for potential nephrotoxicity in normal subjects and experimental animals. Changes of a selected number of urinary enzymes associated with some of the above conditions were considered above.

Alanine Aminopeptidase

Alanine aminopeptidase (AAP) is a brush border enzyme that, because of its large molecular size (Mr = 240,000), is not normally filtered in the glomeruli. Therefore the presence of AAP in the urine primarily reflects its release from the proximal tubular epithelial cells. Moreover, because the brush border surface proteins are readily detached with minimal insult, measurement of urinary AAP can detect early stages of toxicity. Urinary excretion of AAP rises in a variety of conditions associated with proximal tubular stress or injury, such as toxic and ischemic acute tubular necrosis, urorenal neoplasms, acute renal transplant rejection, severe jaundice, acute glomerulonephritis, and acute pyelonephritis. Thus elevated urinary AAP is a nonspecific finding. However, the test is an excellent tool for evaluation of potential drug nephrotoxicity. Urinary AAP rises after administration of radiocontrast agents. The reported increase is greater in patients with preexisting renal disease than in those with normal kidneys, and correlates with the dose and osmolality of the compound employed. Likewise, urinary AAP has been used to assess the nephrotoxicity of aminoglycoside antibiotics, *cis*-platinum, and lithium salts. Urinary AAP rises tremendously following administration of *cis*-platinum. The pattern of the reported increase within 4 days after administration of a single dose appears to be of predictive value for the future course of renal injury. The abnormal enzymuria ceases by day 3 in the majority of patients, who will show no significant renal insufficiency. However, persistent elevation of urinary AAP and presence of epithelial cell fragments in the urinary sediment herald subsequent development of acute or even chronic renal failure.

Urinary AAP excretion has been shown to correlate with the urine output. Therefore, the test underestimates the degree of tubular damage in oliguric patients. Urinary AAP excretion rises in individuals receiving aminoglycoside antibiotics. However, it should be noted that a variety of conditions (such as sepsis, the effects of recent surgery, use of cytotoxic drugs, and hypotension) are often present in patients requiring aminoglycosides, and these can independently cause an increase in urinary enzymes. Consequently, in such patients it is difficult to separate the effects of these antibiotics on urinary enzymes from the effects of the above conditions. Because of the loss of renal parenchyma, urinary AAP excretion is subnormal in patients with end-stage renal disease and in those with irreversible renal allograft failure. In contrast, urinary AAP rises in acute graft rejection either before, simultaneously with, or after the appearance of the usual clinical and laboratory findings.

N-Acetyl-Glucosaminadase (NAG)

N-acetyl-β-glucosaminidase is a hydrolytic enzyme (Mr = 130,000 to 140,000) that acts on glycosyl compounds and is widely distributed in various tissues. In the kidney it is primarily located in the lysosomal fraction and to a much lesser extent in the microsomal fraction of the tubular epithelial cells. It can be accurately measured by an automated fluorometric technique. When refrigerated, the enzyme is stable in the urine for several days. Its concentration in renal tissue is much greater than that found in the urinary tract, and because of its relatively large molecular size, it is not filtered in the glomeruli. Therefore urinary NAG is primarily tubular in origin except when glomerular proteinuria is present, in which NAG may also appear in the urine by filtration. Normally the rate of urinary NAG excretion is relatively constant with little circadian variation and is similar in men and women. For these reasons, NAG has been widely used in the assessment of drug nephrotoxicity, renal transplant rejection, and a variety of other renal disorders. Increased urinary NAG has been reported to precede the appearance of clinical and conventional laboratory manifestations of acute rejection in renal transplant recipients with stable graft function. Therefore serial determinations of urinary NAG has been recommended in the early posttransplant period. Urinary NAG rises with ultrafiltration in the absence of renal injury. Therefore, the test is not a reliable tool in transplant recipients undergoing dialysis. The issue is further complicated in patients receiving cyclosporine, which is widely used as the main immunosuppressant after renal transplantation. Cyclosporine is nephrotoxic and is capable of damaging proximal tubules and the thick ascending limb Henle's loop. As such, cyclosporine nephrotoxicity is associated with increased urinary excretion of various enzymes including NAG. Consequently, measurement of urinary enzymes is not of value in differentiating cyclosporine nephrotoxicity from acute rejection, the two most common causes of graft dysfunction.

Urinary NAG excretion rises in a variety of renal and urinary tract disorders, including acute tubular necrosis, pyelonephritis, glomerulonephritis, obstructive uropathy, bladder carcinoma, nephrotic syndrome, and nephrotoxic injury. Thus the measurement lacks specificity, although it is helpful in monitoring the disease activity. Urinary NAG is of considerable value in the assessment of drug nephrotoxicity in normal volunteers or experimental animals when other causes of enzymuria are lacking.

β-Glucuronidase

β-Glucuronidase is a lysosomal enzyme whose urinary excretion rises in a variety of active renal diseases, including acute tubular necrosis, active glomerulonephritis, heavy proteinuria, acute pyelonephritis, transplant rejection, renal cell carcinoma, and nephrotoxic injury. Increased urinary β-glucuronidase is a nonspecific finding, although it is a useful tool in the assessment of the severity of renal damage and monitoring of the disease activity.

Glutathione S-Transferase Alpha

Glutathione S-transferase alpha (GST-alpha) displays selective localization only to the proximal tubular epithelium. As such, this enzyme may serve as a sensitive indicator of damage to the proximal tubule. GST-alpha is excreted in large amounts in cyclosporine toxicity and cadmium exposure.

Ligandin

Ligandin is a cytosolic protein (Mr = 46,000) that is capable of binding many substances, including various organic anions (e.g., drugs, carcinogens, hormones, hippurates), and as such is thought to be involved in organic anion transport. In addition, ligandin is a major glutathione-S-transferase, which catalyzes the conjugation of its ligands to the sulfhydryl group of reduced glutathione. It is present in the renal tubular epithelial cells, intestinal mucosa, and hepatocytes and plays a major role in elimination of many toxic compounds. In humans, ligandin is found in the proximal tubules and thick ascending limb of Henle's loop, whereas it is confined to the proximal tubules in rats and rabbits. Because of its cytosolic localization, presence of ligandin in the urine may denote cell destruction. It can be measured by both immunologic and enzymatic assays.

Ligandinuria has been produced in experimental animals using mercuric chloride, potassium dichromate, gentamicin, and cis-platinum. In every instance the peak enzymuria corresponded with the peak in serum creatinine concentration. Likewise, presence of ligandin in the perfusate used to preserve donor kidneys is correlated with the posttransplant acute tubular necrosis syndrome. Mild increases in urinary ligandin excretion have also been shown following intravascular administration of large quantities of radiocontrast material but not with smaller doses. Similarly, increased urinary ligandin has been found following ischemic injury to the kidneys. As expected, appearance of liganduria coincides with the occurrence of cell injury.

Lactic Dehydrogenase

Lactic dehydrogenase is a cytosolic enzyme that is present in all organs and is nearly uniformly distributed along the nephron and urinary tract. Urinary excretion of LDH is a nonspecific finding and occurs in a variety of diverse conditions such as acute glomerulonephritis, acute tubular necrosis, renal allograft rejection, chronic glomerulonephritis, urorenal carcinomas, and urinary tract infection, to mention a few. In addition, lysis of erythrocytes in patients with hematuria can increase urinary LDH. Measurement of LDH isoenzymes in the urine can be helpful in differentiating lower urinary tract infection from pyelonephritis in children, in whom the distinction is difficult. Accordingly, increased urinary LDH isoenzymes 4 and 5 are indicative of kidney infection, while elevated urinary isoenzymes 1 and 2 suggest cystitis. Similarly, urinary LDH isoenzyme determination has been used in the assessment of patients with spinal cord injury and associated neuropathic bladder dysfunction, with and without urinary tract infection. Bladder overdistension in these patients may be associated with increased urinary LDH isoenzymes 1 and 2, while renal involvement with reflux, infection, or calculi may increase urinary isoenzymes 4 and 5.

In summary, increased urinary enzyme excretion, while nonspecific, is often a sensitive indicator of renal injury and disease activity. Various brush border enzymes such as alanine aminopeptidase and gamma-glutamyltranspeptidase are released in the urine with minimal tissue injury. In contrast, increased urinary excretion of lysosomal enzymes such as *N*-acetylglucosaminidase, β-glucuronidase, and arylsulfatase A denotes more severe injury, while elevated urinary content of cytosolic enzymes such as ligandin may reflect severe damage or cell necrosis. Considerable difficulty exists as to the choice of suitable reference parameters for urinary enzymes. Expression of the activity or concentration of urinary enzymes per unit of volume is highly unreliable because of wide variability in urine output. Likewise, use of the rate of excretion per unit time is subject to circadian rhythm and interindividual variations based on age, sex, and size of the patient. Although urinary creatinine is an acceptable reference parameter in the presence of stable renal function, it is not reliable in the absence of steady-state glomerular filtration rate. Unfortunately, this provision is often lacking in many patients requiring such tests. In such circumstances, expression of urinary enzymes per volume or unit time may be acceptable, particularly if serial measurements are obtained.

As noted earlier, urinary excretion of most enzymes shows a substantial circadian rhythm both in health and disease. Therefore, urine collection periods should be kept constant when possible, especially if serial determinations are intended.

β_2-Microglobulin

β_2-Microglobulin (β_2M) is a globular protein (Mr = 11,800) consisting of a single peptide chain whose structure is strongly homologous with the constant domain region of the immunoglobulins. β_2M constitutes the light chain of class I major histocompatibility antigens (HLA) and as such is a membrane component of all cells expressing HLA antigens. Thus β_2M is synthesized and released by nearly all human cells and is detectable in virtually all body fluids, including serum (about 2 mg/dl), saliva, synovial fluid, and urine. Functionally, β_2M is thought to be responsible for the control of biosynthesis and/or expression of HLA heavy chain, which in turn determines HLA specificity. β_2M can be readily measured by solid-phase radioimmunoassay. It is highly susceptible to bacterial degradation as well as spontaneous proteolysis in an acidic environment. Consequently, alkalinization of urine (pH of approximately 5.8) and addition of an antimicrobial agent to the urine specimen may be necessary to achieve accurate results.

In normal adults, less than 0.1% of the filtered β_2M appears in the urine (370 μg/24 hr). However, in normal neonates, fractional excretion of β_2M is considerably higher and gradually declines as a function of gestational and postnatal age. Glomerulotubular balance for β_2M is established at a fetal age of 35 weeks, and fractional excretion of β_2M can be used as a measure of renal tubular maturation in neonates. Urinary excretion of β_2M is usually unaltered during normal pregnancy; however, it increases by threefold to fourfold in preeclampsia and returns to normal within several days postpartum.

Like other small molecular weight proteins, β_2M is normally filtered in the glomeruli. More than 99% of the filtered β_2M is removed by pinocytosis and degraded by lysosomal enzymes in the proximal tubules. Therefore disorders of proximal tubules result in increased urinary β_2M excretion due to failure of reabsorption (Table 102.1). β_2M production rises in a variety of conditions, including disseminated malignancies, particularly those of B-lymphocytic origin (e.g., multiple myeloma, chronic lymphocytic leukemia, and Waldenström's disease); inflammatory disorders associated with polyclonal lymphocyte activation (e.g., Sjögren's disease, rheumatoid arthritis, sarcoidosis, systemic lupus erythematosus, and hepatitis); acquired immunodeficiency syndrome (AIDS); and liver cirrhosis.

Urinary β_2M excretion rises as early as 1 to 2 days after the institution of therapy with aminoglycosides. This is consistent with the known toxic effects of these antibiotics on proximal tubules. While the histologic changes, increased urinary β_2M excretion, and enzymuria occur in most cases, only a portion of the aminoglycoside-treated patients develop significant renal in-

TABLE 102.1. Conditions Associated with Increased Urinary β_2-Microglobulin Excretion Resulting from Failure of Renal Reabsorption

Fanconi's syndrome
Cystinosis
Bartter's syndrome
Wilson's disease
Sickle cell nephropathy
Chronic cadmium poisoning
Balkan nephropathy
Preeclampsia
Renal transplantation
Drug toxicity
Analgesic nephropathy
Hypokalemic nephropathy
Diabetic nephropathy
Upper urinary tract infection

sufficiency. Prospective studies have revealed that most patients destined to develop renal insufficiency excrete more than 50 mg of β_2M per day for several days before the rise of serum creatinine concentration. However, the reverse is not always true, because fewer than 50% of patients exhibiting heavy β_2M excretion develop acute renal failure. Nonetheless, early occurrence of marked urinary β_2M excretion denotes a high risk for subsequent development of azotemia. It should be noted that the magnitude of β_2-microglobulinuria declines commensurate with the rise in serum creatinine, due to reduced filtered load of β_2M.

Despite increased serum β_2M concentrations (averaging six times the normal values), urinary excretion of β_2M is reportedly normal in hepatorenal syndrome. In fact, β_2M excretion has been shown to rise considerably with improvement of renal function following placement of a LeVeen shunt in a patient with hepatorenal syndrome. For this reason, measurement of urinary β_2M may be a useful test for differentiating hepatorenal syndrome from other causes of renal insufficiency in patients with liver disease. However, the test may not be helpful when severe jaundice is present because the latter increases β_2M excretion in hepatorenal syndrome.

Ordinarily, urinary β_2M excretion is increased in renal transplant recipients to several times the normal values. This is often superimposed on a sharp rise a few days prior to the onset of clinically discernible acute rejection. For this reason, regular monitoring of urinary β_2M during the high risk period has been recommended by some investigators.

URINARY KALLIKREINS

Kallikreins are serine proteases that convert inactive kininogens to kinins. The effects of kinins on the kidney include renal vasodilatation, natriuresis, and diuresis. Based on molecular weight, antigenicity, and substrate specificity, two major types of kallikreins have been recognized: the plasma form (Mr = 120,000), which is present in an inactive form (prekallikrein), and the tissue or glandular type (Mr = 30,000), which is produced by various organs, including the kidneys, intestines, pancreas, and salivary and sweat glands. Minute quantities of tissue-type kallikrein from salivary glands and pancreas normally enter the circulation and can be detected in human serum (10 ng/ml). Because of its large molecular size, circulating prekallikrein is not filtered in normal glomeruli, although some filtration may occur in the nephrotic syndrome. Small quantities of circulating tissue-type kallikrein are normally filtered by the glomeruli but are totally removed in the proximal tubules. In fact, the kallikrein found in the urine is primarily produced and added to the urine by distal tubules. Urinary and serum kallikreins can be measured by radioimmunoassay. The normal urinary kallikrein excretion averages 130 μg/24 hr. The physiologic role of the renal kallikrein-kinin system is discussed in detail in Chapter 13, Part 4. Our comments in this chapter will be restricted to the changes of urinary kallikrein in various pathophysiologic conditions (Table 102.2).

Urinary kallikrein excretion correlates inversely with sodium intake and directly with potassium intake. In addition, water loading lowers urinary kallikrein excretion. Most conditions associated with elevated aldosterone levels, including primary hyperaldosteronism and Bartter's syndrome, show increased urinary kallikrein excretion. Urinary kallikrein is usually but not always reduced in patients with hypertension and may even be undetectable in those with renal vascular hypertension. Moreover, a large epidemiologic study has revealed that families with low mean urinary kallikrein excretion tend to exhibit higher blood pressures than those with normal kallikrein excretion. Interestingly, in the United States, urinary kallikrein excretion is significantly lower in the African-American population, which is more prone than the white population to hypertension. Urinary kallikrein excretion may be normal or reduced in patients with chronic renal failure. However, the amount excreted

TABLE 102.2. Changes in Urinary Kallikrein Excretion in Various Physiologic and Pathologic Conditions

Increased
Physiologic
Decreased dietary sodium
Increased dietary potassium
Water loading
Winter season; morning
Pathologic
Hyperaldosteronism
Primary
Bartter's syndrome
Exogenous mineralocorticoid
Cirrhosis without renal failure
Pheochromocytoma
Drug-related
Diuretics
Acetazolamide
Furosemide
Bumetanide
Thiazides
Decreased
Physiologic
Increased dietary sodium
Reduced dietary potassium
Summer season; evening
Pathologic
Anti-GBM disease
Cirrhosis with renal failure
Uninephrectomy
Essential hypertension[a]
Renovascular hypertension
Chronic renal failure
Renal transplantation
Allograft rejection
Drug-related
Amiloride

[a] Urinary kallikrein is significantly lower in the African-American population, which has a higher incidence of hypertension than the white population.
GBM, glomerular basement membrane.

per milliliter of glomerular filtrate in both chronic and acute renal failure is greatly increased.

Patients with advanced hepatic cirrhosis and functional renal insufficiency show a reduction in renal production and urinary excretion of kallikrein, whereas those without renal insufficiency have normal or increased kallikrein excretion. It may also be increased in diabetic patients with normal renal function during periods of poor glycemic control, which is reversible with adequate glycemic control.

Unilateral nephrectomy leads to a significant reduction in urinary kallikrein excretion, which is not fully reversed by subsequent hypertrophy of the remaining kidney and near normalization of glomerular filtration rate. This observation may be of interest in view of recent reports of the increased incidence of hypertension in kidney donors. Interestingly, renal transplant recipients tend to have even lower urinary kallikrein excretion than their uninephrectomized donors. This may be of relevance in the genesis of hypertension in renal transplant recipients.

The effect of acute rejection and posttransplant acute tubular necrosis syndrome on urinary kallikrein excretion has been debated. Although both conditions appear to further lower urinary kallikrein, acute tubular necrosis is thought to be associated with a greater reduction than that observed with acute rejection.

MARKERS OF BONE METABOLISM

Increased bone formation and resorption (bone turnover) results in a rise in urinary excretion of various bone-derived enzymes, byproducts of bone matrix synthesis, and bone breakdown products. These biochemical markers are of use in the diagnosis and evaluation of bone diseases (especially osteoporosis), in population studies, and for monitoring the responses to hormones and drugs in clinical studies. In population studies, biochemical measurements may predict rates of bone loss and occurrence of fractures. However, they are less useful in diagnosis and management of individual patients because of considerable biologic and analytical variation in their measurements.

The most sensitive markers of bone formation include the immunoassay for human osteocalcin recognizing the intact molecule and its major proteolytic fragment, bone alkaline phosphatase, and several peptides derived from type I procollagen.

The most useful markers of bone resorption are breakdown products of type I collagen such as hydroxyproline. Assays for hydroxyproline are cumbersome, and results are not bone-specific, as hydroxyproline is also derived from the diet. Therefore recent interest has focused on collagen products that are more specific to bone, including galactosyl hydroxylysine, and the collagen cross-links pyridinoline and deoxypyridinoline. Total urinary excretion of pyridinoline crosslinks measured by high pressure liquid chromatography is currently the most accurate marker available for the noninvasive clinical assessment of osteoporosis. The new immunoassays recognizing either the free pyridinoline cross-links or pyridinoline cross-linked–type I collagen peptides in urine may improve the assessment of risk of osteoporotic fractures in postmenopausal women, particularly when used in combination with bone mass measurement. In addition, the test can be used to monitor the efficacy of antiresorption therapy.

ISOPROSTANES

Isoprostanes belong to a class of biologically active products of arachidonic acid metabolism of potential relevance in vascular disease. They are formed *in vivo* primarily by nonenzymatic lipid peroxidation. Enhanced urinary excretion of 8-iso-$PGF_{2\alpha}$ has been described in association with cardiac reperfusion injury and with cardiovascular risk factors, including cigarette smoking, diabetes mellitus, and hypercholesterolemia. Besides providing a likely noninvasive index of lipid peroxidation in these settings, measurements of specific F_2isoprostanes in urine may provide a sensitive biochemical end point for dose-finding studies of natural and synthetic inhibitors of lipid peroxidation. The biologic effects of 8-iso-$PGF_{2\alpha}$ *in vitro* suggest that it and other eicosanoids may contribute to the functional consequences of lipid peroxidation. However, it is not yet clear as to whether the *in vitro* observations are applicable to the *in vivo* settings.

Selected Readings

Davey PG, Cowley DM, Geddes AM, et al. Clinical evaluation of β_2-microglobulin, muramidase and alanine aminopeptidase as markers of gentamicin nephrotoxicity. *Contrib Nephrol* 1984;42:100–106.

This study reports on the patterns of urinary excretion of β_2-microglobulin, muramidase and alanine aminopeptidase in a group of gentamicin-treated patients. The results are compared with those of a control group, which consisted of patients with hypotension, septicemia, major surgery, or those receiving cytotoxic agents, who were not receiving aminoglycosides. They found alanine aminopeptidase (but not muramidase or β_2M) to be a good marker of acute tubular necrosis in both groups, without providing a distinction between ATN induced by gentamicin and that produced by other insults.

Elias AN, Correon G, Vaziri ND, et al. The pituitary-gonadal axis in experimental nephrotic syndrome in male rates. *J Lab Clin Med* 1992;120:949–954.

This paper describes an acquired hypogonadism in nephrotic rats caused by abnormal urinary losses of testosterone along with its binding protein.

Mondorf AW. Urinary enzyme markers of renal damage. In: Whetton A, Neu HC, eds. *The aminoglycosides—microbiology, clinical use and toxicology.* New York: Marcel Dekker, 1982:283–301.

This chapter provides an in-depth review of changes in urinary alanine aminotransferase associated with aminoglycoside administration.

Scherberich JE. Urinary proteins of tubular origin: basic immunochemical and clinical aspects. *Am J Nephrol* 1990;10(Suppl 1):43–51.

This paper provides a comprehensive and well-referenced examination of brush border enzymes in a variety of renal disorders.

Sherman RL, Drayer DE, Leyland-Jones BR, et al. N-acetyl-13-glucosaminidase and beta-2-microglobulin—their urinary excretion in patients with renal parenchymal disease. *Arch Intern Med* 1983;143:1183–1185.

This paper demonstrates that urinary excretion of NAG and β_2-microglobulin is elevated in patients with various renal parenchymal diseases, including membranous nephropathy, membranoproliferative glomerulonephritis, focal glomerulosclerosis, obstructive pyelonephritis, nephrosclerosis, and minimal-change disease. Higher urinary NAG and β_2-microglobulin were found in patients with progressive renal disease than in those with stable renal disease of the same nature and severity.

Tolkoff-Rubin NE, Rubin RH, Bonventre JV. Noninvasive renal diagnostic studies. *Clin Lab Med* 1988;8:507–525.

A review of low-molecular-weight proteins and urinary enzymes in diagnosis of renal disorders.

Vaziri ND. Nephrotic syndrome and coagulation and fibrinolytic abnormalities. *Am J Nephrol* 1983;3:1–6.

A review of various coagulation abnormalities in the nephrotic syndrome, with reference to the urinary excretion of factors IX and VII in this condition.

Vaziri ND. Endocrinological consequences of the nephrotic syndrome. *Am J Nephrol* 1993;13:360–364.

This paper provides a review of the published studies on the effects of nephrotic syndrome on plasma level, urinary excretion, regulation and metabolism of various protein and protein-bound hormones.

Vaziri ND, Gonzales EV, Barton CH, et al. Factor XII and its substrates, fibronectin, fibrinogen and alpha-2-antiplasmin in plasma and urine of patients with nephrosis. *J Lab Clin Med* 1991;117:152–156.

This paper reports on altered plasma concentration of several coagulation factors and their urinary excretion in nephrotic syndrome. In addition, the paper provides a summary of the information on the effect of nephrotic syndrome on plasma concentration and urinary excretion of various other coagulation and related proteins.

Zhou XJ, Vaziri ND. Erythropoietin metabolism and pharmacokinetics in experimental nephrosis. *Am J Physiol* 1992;263:F812–F815.

This paper describes altered erythropoietin metabolism and regulation primarily caused by its abnormal losses in the urine of rats with nephrotic syndrome and to a lesser extent its expanded distribution volume and inappropriately decreased biosynthesis. The paper also provides a summary of other examples of endocrine disorders attributed to excessive urinary losses of protein or protein-bound hormones in nephrotic syndrome.

CHAPTER 103

Evaluation of Renal Function

Ira W. Reiser and Jerome G. Porush

Undoubtedly, the most important parameter in assessing renal function is determination of the glomerular filtration rate (GFR). The GFR represents the rate at which an ultrafiltrate of the plasma is formed by the glomeruli and is indicative of the functional renal mass. Using either an endogenously produced or exogenously administered substance that is unbound by serum proteins, freely permeable through the glomerular capillaries and not reabsorbed, metabolized, synthesized, or secreted by the renal tubules, an accurate estimation of GFR may be obtained. The urinary excretory rate of such a substance [the product of the urine concentration of the substance (U) and urine flow rate (V)] divided by the plasma concentration of the substance (P) expresses the virtual amount of plasma cleared of the substance (in milliliters per minute or liters per 24 hours) and represents the GFR.

Inulin, a 5,200-D uncharged fructose polymer, fulfills the above criteria, making it an extremely accurate marker for estimating GFR; it represents the gold standard by which other filtration markers are judged. The performance of an inulin clearance is extremely impractical, however, because it generally requires the intravenous infusion of inulin to maintain a steady-state plasma level. To obviate the need for a constant infusion, some investigators have used a single injection of inulin followed by measuring either its urinary or plasma clearance for determining the GFR. The results of urinary clearances of inulin, when performed in this manner, have been similar to those obtained with constant infusions of inulin. Unfortunately, timed and complete urine collections, which may necessitate urinary bladder catheterization to ensure complete voiding, are still required. Measurement of plasma clearance of inulin following a single injection eliminates the need for urine collection but results in overestimation of the GFR at all levels of renal function when compared with its urinary clearance. Although a correction factor may be used to arrive at a GFR that is in good agreement with those achieved with conventional urinary clearances, its reliability has only been proved in subjects with a GFR in the range of 28 to 124 ml/min/1.73 m^2. In addition, multiple plasma samples are generally necessary, and laboratory facilities capable of measuring and analyzing inulin are required. For these reasons, other modalities for measuring GFR are frequently employed in clinical practice.

SERUM CREATININE AS A MEASURE OF GFR

Creatinine is an endogenous substance produced within muscle cells by the nonenzymatic conversion of creatine and phosphocreatine. In normal subjects consuming a stable diet, the daily creatinine generation varies little and represents the conversion of 1.6% to 1.7% of the total body creatine. Because creatinine has a low molecular weight and is not protein bound in the plasma, it is freely filtered at the level of the glomerulus. For these reasons, it would appear that creatinine offers an excellent potential substitute for inulin in estimating GFR. However, its use as a marker for GFR has many limitations and shortcomings; variation in the generation of creatinine poses a significant limitation in its utility as an index of GFR. Although the GFR is known to decrease with advancing age (after age 30), the serum creatinine (Scr) may not increase, because production of creatinine declines as muscle mass decreases. Moreover, renal failure itself is associated with a reduction in creatinine generation. In addition to the creatinine produced by muscle, approximately 30% of the daily creatinine pool is derived from ingested meat, which contains approximately 3.5 to 5.0 mg creatine/g. A variable amount of this creatine (18% to 65%) is converted to creatinine with cooking. Thus both the muscle mass and quantity of ingested meat in addition to the urinary clearance will determine the level of the Scr.

Although neither metabolized nor synthesized by the kidney, creatinine, unlike inulin, is variably secreted by the proximal tubule of the nephron, probably via the same transport mechanism as other organic cations. Tubular secretion of creatinine in normal subjects may constitute 10% to 40% of the total creatinine excreted in the urine and may increase to 50% to 60% in subjects with renal disease. The tubular secretion of creatinine is known to be blocked by phlorizin, an inhibitor of proximal tubular transport, as well as by many commonly used medications such as cimetidine, trimethoprim, triamterene, amiloride, and probenecid (a drug secreted by the anionic pathway in the proximal tubule). With inhibition of the tubular secretion of creatinine, the Scr concentration will increase as the total renal clearance of creatinine is diminished; however, the GFR will remain unaltered. In addition to tubular secretion, tubular reabsorption of creatinine may also take place when urine flow rates are markedly diminished (less than 0.5 ml/min), possibly by simple passive diffusion across intact tubular and urinary tract epithelium.

Although creatinine is primarily excreted by the kidney, extrarenal excretion of creatinine does occur as the result of degradation by the intestinal flora. In subjects with normal renal function, the extrarenal metabolism of creatinine is negligible. With progressively decreasing renal function, however, extrarenal excretion of creatinine progressively increases and, as a consequence, may negate the expected increase in the Scr concentration.

Aside from these metabolic considerations, the methodology by which creatinine is measured poses another obstacle to its use as a marker of GFR. Creatinine is usually measured by a colorimetric assay utilizing the reaction which occurs between creatinine and alkaline picrate (Jaffe's reaction). Although simple to perform and widely used, a major drawback of this assay stems from an overestimation of creatinine, because noncreatinine chromogens such as glucose, protein, acetoacetate, pyruvate, uric acid, fructose, and ascorbic acid may account for up to 20% of the color reaction during assays of either the plasma or serum. Measurement of these noncreatinine chromogens will lead to an overestimate of the plasma or serum creatinine but will not appreciably alter the urinary creatinine measurement so that the GFR will be artificially lowered. In addition to these substances, many cephalosporins, most notably cephalothin, cefazolin, cefoxitin, and cefamandole, may also produce a colorimetric reaction with picrate and falsely increase the Scr concentration. Other analyses that measure the true creatinine have been devised to circumvent this problem. The two most frequently employed are the autoanalyzer and the creatinine imidohydrolase (Ektachem) methods. The former method distinguishes creatinine from noncreatinine chromogens by the rate at which the colorimetric reaction takes place. With this method only bilirubin levels greater than 5 mg/dl affect the creatinine measurement and may decrease the concentration by 0.1 to 0.5 mg/dl. The Ektachem method uses the enzymatic reaction of creatinine with creatinine imidohydrolase to form ammonia and N-methylhydantoin. Although this procedure is accurate, both a markedly elevated blood sugar and the antifungal agent 5-flucytosine are known to interfere with the assay (the former falsely lowers and the latter falsely elevates the creatinine concentration). Regardless of the method chosen to measure creatinine, a wide range of variability exists between simultaneously repeated measurements within the same subject, in addition to the problems noted with each assay, which further impairs the usefulness of the Scr in estimating GFR; for example, an increase in the measured Scr from 0.7 to 1.0 mg/dl (both within the normal range) could correspond to a significant change in actual renal function (30% decrease) but could represent only assay variability.

In view of the foregoing, it is apparent that the Scr may be variably independent of the absolute renal function, making it a less than an ideal marker of GFR. Only when there is a constant rate of creatinine generation, tubular secretion, and extrarenal metabolism will the Scr accurately reflect the true GFR. These conditions, however, are frequently not met clinically and, as such, the use of the Scr alone as a measure of renal function is not reliable. Furthermore, as seen in Fig. 103.1, which depicts the relationship between the Scr and inulin clearance, Scr may remain within the normal range despite a reduction in GFR of 60% or greater.

For any given Scr, it is possible to estimate the creatinine clearance (Ccr). For this purpose nomograms have been derived that incorporate the age, gender, and body size of a subject eliminating some of the inherent difficulties described. The most commonly used nomogram is that devised by Cockcroft and Gault:

$$\text{Ccr} = \frac{(140 - \text{Age}) \times \text{Weight (kg)}}{\text{Scr (mg/dl)} \times 72} \text{ (men)}$$

$$\text{Ccr} = \frac{(140 - \text{Age}) \times \text{Weight (kg)}}{\text{Scr (mg/dl)} \times 85} \text{ (Women)}$$

These formulas are only applicable when a steady state of creatinine balance exists and, unfortunately, will overestimate Ccr when total body weight is significantly greater than the lean body mass. Furthermore, after deriving the Ccr in this manner, the same problem will exist with regard to its relationship to GFR, as noted. This will be particularly true for debilitated subjects, as well as those with reduced renal function.

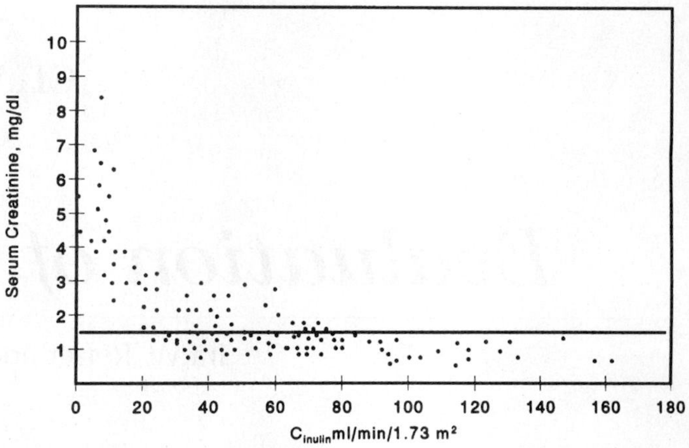

Figure 103.1. The relationship between serum creatinine and inulin clearance in subjects with glomerular disease. The horizontal line represents the upper limit for serum creatinine concentration (1.4 mg/dl) (Reproduced with permission from Levey AS. Measurement of renal function in chronic renal disease. *Kidney Int* 1990;38:171.).

CREATININE CLEARANCE AS A MEASURE OF GFR

To obviate the unpredictability of the creatinine load in a given subject, the determination of the Ccr will provide a better estimate of GFR than the Scr. Ccr is generally performed by determining the total creatinine excreted in a finite period of time (usually 24 hours) and obtaining a single Scr at the end of the collection period or averaging two values taken before and on completion of the urine collection. Because the creatinine excretion is dependent on glomerular filtration and tubular secretion, the relationship between the true GFR, as determined by inulin clearance, and Ccr will not be linear. When determining the Ccr, it is essential to know the method used to determine the Scr, because this will have an impact on the Ccr's accuracy. In individuals with normal renal function and using the Jaffe reaction to measure the Scr, the Ccr will closely approximate a simultaneously determined inulin clearance, because the percentage of creatinine excreted by tubular secretion is similar to, and negated by, the percentage of noncreatinine chromogens measured in the serum by this colorimetric assay. With renal failure, however, this fortuitous relationship no longer exists, because tubular secretion of creatinine assumes a greater percentage of the excreted load, and the percentage error reflected by the noncreatinine chromogens diminishes as the Scr increases. Under these circumstances the Ccr will overestimate the GFR. When assays for true creatinine are used instead, the Ccr will uniformly exceed simultaneously obtained inulin clearances at all levels of GFR because of tubular secretion. As shown in Table 103.1, the greatest absolute difference between inulin and creatinine (true) clearances occurs when the GFR is in the range of 40 to 80 ml/min/1.73 m², while the ratio of the Ccr to inulin clearance is greatest when the GFR is less than 40 ml/min/1.73 m². When tubular secretion is inhibited by cimetidine, which has been examined in a variety of renal diseases, the Ccr will more closely approximate the inulin clearance.

TABLE 103.1. Relationship of Observed Clearances of Inulin and Creatinine and Derived Values for Serum Creatinine at Various Levels of Renal Function[a]

Range of GFR (ml/min/1.73m^2)	>80	40–80	<40
Number of patients examined	42	50	81
Inulin clearance (ml/min/1.73m^2) (mean ± S.D.)	113 ± 5	60 ± 1	22 ± 1
Creatinine clearance (ml/min/1.73m^2) (mean ± S.D.)	134 ± 7	94 ± 4	42 ± 2
Absolute difference between mean creatinine clearance and mean inulin clearance (ml/min/1.73m^2)	21	34	20
Ratio of mean creatinine clearance to mean inulin clearance	1.16	1.57	1.92
Derived serum creatinine (mg/dl)[b]	0.9	1.3	2.9
Derived serum creatinine assuming no tubular secretion (mg/dl)[c]	1.1	2.0	5.5

[a]Data are from 171 patients with glomerular disease. (Reproduced with permission from Levey AS, Perrone RD, Madias NE. Serum creatinine and renal function. *Annu Rev Med* 1998;39. © 1988 by Annual Reviews, Inc.)

[b]Values for serum creatinine are derived from observed values for creatinine clearance and an assumed constant value for urinary creatinine excretion of 1,730 mg/day.

[c]Values for serum creatinine are derived from observed values for inulin clearance and an assumed constant value for urinary creatinine excretion of 1,730 mg/day.

Creatinine clearances are also hampered by the inherent difficulties that arise in obtaining complete and accurate timed urine collections. The adequacy of a 24-hour urine collection may be judged by comparing the total amount of creatinine excreted to that anticipated for a subject based on their daily production of creatinine. For this purpose, it is generally assumed that men will excrete approximately 20 to 25 mg/kg of body weight per day and women 15 to 20 mg/kg of body weight per day. These estimates, however, are not applicable to the elderly (older than 60 years of age) in whom the progressive loss of muscle mass leads to a reduction in creatinine production. In these subjects a more appropriate estimate is achieved by using formulas that incorporate the age: creatinine excretion will be approximately 28.2 − (0.172 × age) mg/kg per day in men and 21.9 − (0.115 × age) mg/kg per day in women.

Errors in the collection process may be mitigated by performing multiple serial urine collections of shorter duration (1 or 2 hours) during periods of water diuresis following a water load and obtaining a Scr at the midpoint of each collection. Performed in this manner, the collection process can be supervised, a more representative value of Scr will be obtained, and a more accurate Ccr can be determined; however, many of the shortcomings that have been described in using Scr as a marker of GFR will still pertain.

BLOOD UREA NITROGEN AS A MEASURE OF GFR

Urea, which is mainly synthesized in the liver, primarily represents the end product of dietary protein metabolism. Following its generation, the kidney is the predominant site of urea excretion. The renal handling of urea is complex and depends greatly on the rate of urine formation. Because urea has a low molecular weight, is not protein bound, and is uncharged, it is freely filtered at the level of glomerulus. Following its filtration, approximately 40% to 50% of the filtered load of urea is reabsorbed by the proximal tubule regardless of the state of hydration of the subject. It is at the level of the medullary collecting duct that the state of hydration has an impact on urea handling. During antidiuresis (presence of antidiuretic hormone [ADH]), urea permeability within this nephron segment is enhanced and as a consequence, only 35% to 40% of the total filtered urea load is excreted. In contrast, during states of water diuresis (absence of ADH), urea permeability in the distal nephron is negligible and the ratio of urea clearance to GFR may achieve values as high as 0.55–0.65. When renal function is markedly impaired (GFR less than 20 ml/min/1.73 m^2), however, the state of hydration has little bearing on the renal handling of urea.

Aside from the state of hydration, urea plasma concentration also depends on both nitrogen load and metabolism. With a large nitrogen load resulting from increased protein intake, enhanced catabolic rates (infection, trauma), or suppression of anabolism (as seen with corticosteroid administration or tetracycline therapy), the blood urea nitrogen (BUN) level will increase. Similarly, a decreased catabolic rate or a reduction in dietary protein ingestion will result in a lowering of the BUN. In addition, severe parenchymal liver disease and myxedema may also result in reduction of the BUN because of a decrease in urea synthesis.

From the aforementioned, it is evident that the BUN is a poor marker of GFR. Nevertheless, the BUN may be clinically useful, particularly when the renal handling of urea is understood. Acute deterioration of renal function associated with a decreased urine flow rate, as occur with volume contraction, renal ischemia, or early obstructive uropathy may result in an increase in the blood urea nitrogen (BUN)/Scr ratio (normally 10:1) to two to three times normal. This disproportionate increase of the BUN compared with the Scr may provide the diagnostic clue to these causes of renal insufficiency. In subjects with advanced renal failure (GFR less than 15 ml/min/1.73 m^2), the mean of the creatinine and urea clearances will approximate the true GFR as determined by inulin. This fortuitous finding is explained by the fact that at this level of renal function the urea clearance will underestimate the GFR (because of tubular reabsorption) to approximately the same extent that the creatinine clearance will overestimate the GFR (due to tubular secretion).

SERUM CYSTATIN C AS A MEASURE OF GFR

Cystatin C, a nonglycosylated 13-kD basic protein of the cystatin superfamily of cysteine protease inhibitors, is an endogenous product of nucleated cells. Cystatin C is produced at a constant rate, is unaltered by inflammatory conditions or diet, and is almost exclusively cleared from the circulation by glomerular filtration. As a consequence, its serum concentration may serve as a suitable marker of GFR. In the past, easy and rapid methods of quantification of cystatin C serum levels were unavailable, and as a result its usefulness as a marker of GFR unfulfilled. However, the determination of cystatin C concentration can now be performed quickly and accurately with a particle enhanced immunoturbidimetric assay. This technique measures the serum cystatin C concentration through changes in the absorbance signal that are produced by the agglutination of cystatin C with microparticles covalently covered with antibodies to cystatin C. The precision of the assay has been shown to be excellent (with intraassay and interassay variability of less than 3% and less than 5%, respectively, across the assay range) and to be unaffected by many of the factors that can interfere with Scr determinations. When compared with Scr, cystatin C levels correlate better with GFR, particularly in subjects with normal or moderately reduced renal function, and appear to be a more sensitive marker for detecting early reductions in GFR.

RADIONUCLIDE, NONRADIOACTIVE IOTHALAMATE AND RADIOCONTRAST MEDIA MEASUREMENTS OF GFR

Several radionuclides are currently available to measure GFR. The most frequently used radioisotopes in the United States are ^{125}I-iothalamate (and ^{131}I- iothalamate) and diethylenetriaminepenta-acetic acid (DTPA) chelated to ^{99m}technetium (^{99m}Tc), whereas in Europe ethylenediaminetetra-acetic acid (EDTA) chelated to ^{51}Cr is the radionuclide of choice (not commercially available in the United States). In general, these radioisotopes are almost entirely cleared by glomerular filtration so that their disappearance from the plasma can be used as a measure of GFR. Although none has been shown to be as accurate as inulin, they are frequently used and highly desirable because of their relative ease of application and because of the accuracy and reproducibility with which they can be measured. Clearances of these radioisotopes may be obtained using standard renal clearances after either a bolus intravenous or subcutaneous injection, requiring the usual timed plasma and urine collections. Although the GFR obtained in this fashion is precise and parallels those obtained with inulin over a wide range of renal function, the usual problems of urine collection remain. As a consequence, the GFR is more frequently obtained by measuring the rate of disappearance of the radioactive tracer from the plasma after either continuous intravenous or bolus infusion. The bolus or single-shot technique is preferred, because it obviates the need for a continuous infusion as well as the maintenance of a constant blood level of the radionuclide. The GFR measured with this technique is derived from the plasma disappearance of the tracer determined by obtaining timed plasma concentrations (two or more specimens) over a 2- to 6-hour period following its administration, using either a one compartment method (where the tracer is assumed to be present only within the plasma volume) or two compartment method (where the tracer is assumed to be distributed in both the plasma and extracellular fluid space). Although repeated measurements are precise with little coefficient of variation, the GFR obtained by plasma clearance with each radioisotope is not as accurate as those obtained by their renal clearance. Plasma clearances will uniformly overestimate GFR and exceed simultaneous renal clearances of the radioisotope by 5 to10 ml/min. Because the renal clearance of ^{51}Cr EDTA is 5% to 15% less than that of simultaneously measured inulin clearances (possibly the consequence of tubular reabsorption, plasma protein binding or *in vivo* dissociation of the chelate) the plasma clearance of ^{51}Cr EDTA is similar to the renal clearance of inulin, DTPA or iothalamate. Although two or more plasma samples are generally required with these agents, the use of a single plasma sample drawn 2 to 4 hours after their administration has also been used for determining GFR. In general, this method is less precise than when multiple plasma samples are taken, particularly in those subjects with a GFR less than 30 ml/min.

As renal uptake of these radionuclides is directly proportional to GFR, direct renal scintagraphic measure of the radioisotope (DTPA primarily has been studied) in the 1- to 3-minute interval following its injection will also permit the determination of the GFR. With this technique, urine or blood samples are not required, a study can be completed within minutes and the percent contribution of each kidney to the total GFR may be obtained. Although highly reproducible, quick, and less tedious to perform, errors may occur using this method because of inaccuracies in background subtraction of counts and estimation of renal depth, particularly in pediatric patients, resulting in inaccurate measurement of GFR. Indeed, of all the methods using radionuclides for the measurement of GFR, this is the least precise.

Although the use of radiolabeled compounds provides an excellent and simple means for measuring GFR, they require special handling, storage, and disposal, and may be contraindicated in pregnant women or nursing mothers. To obviate the need for radioactive agents, both renal and plasma clearances of nonradioactive iothalamate have been used to measure GFR. The simplest method for determining the renal clearance uses a single timed urine sample and two plasma samples. Following the subcutaneous administration of nonradioactive iothalamate, the concentration of iothalamate in the samples is determined by capillary electrophoresis, a technique that separates molecules on the basis of their electrophoretic mobility within capillary tubes. When performed in this fashion, the renal clearance has been shown to correlate well with those simultaneously obtained with isotopic iothalamate with a coefficient of variation of less than 3%. The plasma clearance of nonradioactive iothalamate, as determined by high-performance liquid chromatography, is performed in a manner similar to that previously described for the radionuclides following a single intravenous injection of unlabeled iothalamate. With this methodology, the plasma clearance of unlabeled iothalamate has been shown to be reproducible and reliable and to correlate well with the simultaneously obtained ^{51}Cr EDTA plasma clearance over a wide range of GFR.

In addition to radionuclides and nonradioactive iothalamate, nonionic iodinated contrast media (iohexol, iopentol) have been used to measure GFR, as these agents are primarily excreted by glomerular filtration. The plasma clearance of the contrast agent is determined using the same principle of plasma disappearance as discussed above (one or two compartment methods), by measuring the iodine concentration present in timed plasma samples. In the past, up to 50 ml of contrast medium was used during urography and the iodine concentration was determined by x-ray flourescence of plasma samples. When performed in this manner, both functional and morphologic information can be obtained simultaneously. Unfortunately, this technique poses a risk for contrast-induced nephrotoxicity in subjects with reduced renal function (Ccr below 25 ml/min). Recently, newer methods for measuring iohexol have been developed (high-performance liquid chromatography and capillary electrophoresis) and have allowed as little as 2 to 5 ml of this contrast agent to be administered specifically for the purpose of measuring GFR. Although two plasma samples are needed when the volume of distribution cannot be estimated from anthropometric data (weight, height, age, and sex), a single appropriately timed sample is generally sufficient for defining the slope of the elimination curve of this agent and for allowing an accurate determination of GFR, which correlates well with those obtained with multiple plasma samples. In addition, an accurate determination of GFR may even be obtained in those subjects with advanced renal failure (Ccr of 2 to 25 ml/min). In these subjects, the timing of the plasma sample is adjusted to account for the slow elimination of the contrast agent from the extracellular space, and the sample is taken at a time when the agent has declined to approximately half of its initial concentration in the semilog elimination curve. For this purpose, the estimated GFR (corrected to a BSA of 1.73 m^2) is used to predict the appropriate timing of the plasma sampling. These agents, used extensively in Scandinavia, have been shown to correlate well with simultaneously obtained ^{51}Cr EDTA or ^{99m}Tc DTPA plasma clearances. Furthermore, these contrast media have been shown to be well tolerated, they have a low side effect profile, and they do not alter the GFR during their administration.

ASSESSMENT OF THE PROGRESSION OF RENAL FAILURE USING THE RECIPROCAL OR LOGARITHM OF THE SERUM CREATININE CONCENTRATION

After bilateral renal injury, further functional and structural deterioration usually proceeds despite the fact that the initiating insult may cease to exist. This period has been called the *phase of progression* and has been thought to occur at a constant rate for each individual subject, regardless of the inciting injury. Many investigations have found that a linear relationship exists between the reciprocal (or logarithm) of the Scr concentration and the rate of decline in the Ccr in most subjects with chronic renal failure. By plotting the reciprocal of the Scr concentration (Y axis) versus time (X axis), the rate of decline in renal function may be derived by the slope of the line. A change in the slope has been assumed to represent a change in the natural progression of the renal failure, and also may provide a method by which to determine whether a decrease in disease progression has been achieved by a particular therapeutic intervention. Unfortunately, the linearity of the reciprocal of Scr over time has been widely debated and questioned. As previously described, the Scr concentration reflects not only changes in the GFR, but will also be affected by changes in creatinine generation, as well as by the tubular secretion and extrarenal metabolism of creatinine. Thus the validity of the reciprocal of the Scr concentration would be subject to question unless the creatinine generation, tubular secretion, and extrarenal metabolism of creatinine were constant throughout the time course of a subject's renal failure. Because these variables are usually not constant, the 1/Scr versus time slope will not provide an absolute guide by which to measure the rate of decline in GFR or to assess deviations in this rate. Nevertheless, this slope can provide a reasonable approximation of the time required for a particular subject to reach end-stage renal disease, and changes in the slope may be clinically useful, as noted above. For the purpose of clinical studies designed to address the impact of therapeutic interventions in arresting or slowing disease progression, a more accurate measurement of GFR may be necessary. Methods for the assessment of progression of renal failure are discussed in detail in Chapter 67, Part 1.

CLINICAL ESTIMATES OF RENAL BLOOD FLOW

Measurements of renal blood flow (RBF) are infrequently needed in clinical nephrology. When necessary, however, an estimate of RBF may be derived from the rate of renal clearance of a marker that during its first pass through the kidney is totally extracted from the plasma. The renal clearance of such a marker, under these circumstances, will represent the renal plasma flow (RPF). RBF may then be obtained by simply dividing the measured RPF by [1-Hct].

The plasma clearance of *p*-aminohippurate (PAH) is the most widely used method in clinical practice for determining RPF. PAH clearance by the kidney occurs by both glomerular filtration and tubular secretion (primarily the latter), and, although variable from subject to subject, renal extraction approaches 90% at low plasma concentrations. Because not all of the RBF perfuses the major site of PAH secretion (pars recta of the proximal tubule), the measured RPF will underestimate the true RPF and is called the *effective RPF* (ERPF). In addition to this factor, PAH extraction may be reduced as a result of diminished proximal tubular secretion as a result of renal disease, drugs such as probenecid or by increases in RBF. In these instances the ERPF may significantly underestimate the actual RPF and only by measuring the PAH concentration in the renal venous plasma (to obtain the true extraction) will a more accurate estimate of RPF be obtained. Unfortunately, PAH clearances require the continuous infusion of PAH, the maintenance of a steady state plasma PAH level, as well as timed urine and blood sampling and are, therefore, cumbersome to perform.

A suitable alternative to the urinary clearance of PAH may be obtained by the plasma clearance of ^{131}I-hippuran, a radionuclide isotope with a similar structure and properties as PAH, but with a slightly lower renal extraction (other radionuclides such as mercaptoacetyltriglycine [MAG_3] chelated to ^{99m}Tc are also available for this purpose). Following the injection of a known quantity of ^{131}I-hippuran, the ERPF is calculated based on the tracer's rate of disappearance from the plasma over time. Either a one- or two-sample plasma clearance method may be used to calculate the ERPF. With the two-sample method, blood is obtained at 30 and 40 minutes after injection of the ^{131}I-hippuran and the concentration of the radionuclide determined, while in the one-sample method blood is obtained only at 44 minutes after injection. Although both techniques provide similar results, only the two-sample clearance technique provides reliable results in the pediatric age group or in those subjects with significant extravascular fluid collections (ascites, edema). Finally, the same factors that reduce proximal tubular secretion of PAH, as previously discussed, are applicable to these radionuclides, and thus the ERPF derived under those situations will similarly significantly underestimate RPF.

ERPF may also be measured by external counting of radioactivity of the kidneys after radionuclide administration. Although obviating the need for blood sampling, this method provides a less accurate estimate of ERPF as compared with the plasma clearance techniques.

In addition to these methods, other noninvasive techniques for measuring RBF have been developed. These include the use of ultrasound with echo-Doppler duplex scanning of the renal artery, phase-contrast cine magnetic resonance imaging, positron emission tomography (PET) after the first pass extraction of ^{82}Rb in the kidney, and finally, extrarenal measurement of the ^{81}Rb/^{81m}Kr ratio following intravenous infusion of ^{81}Rb. This latter method takes advantage of the rapid decay of ^{81}Rb to ^{81m}Kr that occurs in the kidney and the rate of clearance of ^{81m}Kr, which is directly dependent on the RBF. Because these techniques are quite sophisticated and are not universally available, and because large standard errors exist with the ultrasonographic determination of RBF, their clinical utility remains to be determined.

CLINICAL ESTIMATION OF THE CAPACITY TO DILUTE AND CONCENTRATE URINE

A full exploration of the mechanisms by which the kidney dilutes and concentrates the urine is beyond the scope of this chapter and is described in detail in Chapters 8 and 15, Part 1. Derangements in water homeostasis are frequently encountered in clinical nephrology and as a consequence, assessing the ability to dilute or concentrate the urine remains an important function for the clinician. Measurement of urine and plasma osmolalities is the central focus of this discussion. Although a fair approximation of the serum osmolality may be derived from the concentration of its major solutes (sodium and potassium with their corresponding anions, urea and glucose), similar formulas when used to calculate urine osmolality are imprecise, and thus direct measurements are needed.

The osmolality of a solution is determined by either the decrement in freezing point or the increment in vapor pressure of the solution as compared with that of distilled water. The osmolality is directly proportional to the number of particles in the solution and is not influenced by the size, charge, or density of the particles; thus 1 mmol of glucose will be isoosmotic with that of 1 mmol of sodium. Osmometers, which measure the freezing point depression or increment in vapor pressure of a solution, provide precise results, but because they are not always readily accessible in clinical practice, the specific gravity or the refractive index (RI) is more commonly used.

The specific gravity (the weight of a solution as compared with that of an equal volume of distilled water) and RI (the ratio of the speed of light through air to that of light through a solution) of urine, as measured by a hydrometer or refractometer, respectively, are not only dependent on the number of particles in solution, but also on the size and density of the particles (the latter less so with RI). As a consequence, a solution of glucose equimolar to that of a solution of sodium will have a greater measured urine concentration. Furthermore, high urine concentrations of protein, glucose, or exogenous solutes, such as mannitol or radiocontrast media, will significantly decrease the reliability of these methods as a measure of urine osmolality. In the absence of these substances, however, the correlation between specific gravity or RI and osmolality is quite good. In general, a specific gravity of 1.000 to 1.001 approximates an osmolality of 50 mOsm/kg H_2O; a specific gravity of 1.010 approximates an osmolality of 300 mOsm/kg H_2O; and a specific gravity of 1.020 approximates an osmolality of 800 mOsm/kg H_2O or greater. When significant proteinuria or glycosuria is present, the error introduced in the specific gravity measurement may be eliminated by lowering the observed specific gravity by 0.003 units for each g/dl of urine of either substance. Much less is known about the quantitative relationship of RI to osmolality; however, it appears that an RI of 44 roughly corresponds to an osmolality of 400 mOsm/kg H_2O and an RI of 134 is equivalent to an osmolality of 1300 mOsm/kg H_2O.

Urine specific gravity may also be determined with urine dipsticks. This method is based on the principle that as the concentration of solutes increases in the urine a corresponding increment in the concentration of salts will occur. These salts react with the reagents on the strip, inducing pH changes that result in a color change of the dipstick. Because this method measures only the concentration of ions in the urine, high concentrations of nonionic substances (glucose, urea) will go unmeasured and the urine concentration will be underestimated. In addition, the specific gravity measured in a highly alkaline urine (pH above 6.5) or a urine with a large concentration of protein will be inaccurate with this method.

ASSESSMENT OF URINE DILUTION

Because a random urine osmolality or specific gravity only reflects the dilution or concentration of urine at one particular moment in time, other methods are needed in order to assess the kidney's capacity to handle a water load. A frequently used concept for this purpose is that of free water clearance (C_{H_2O}), which is the hypothetical volume of urine that is excreted free of solute. C_{H_2O} is derived from the formula:

$$C_{H_2O} = V - C_{osm} \text{ or } V - \frac{(U_{osm} \times V)}{P_{osm}}$$

where V represents urine volume, C_{osm} the urine osmolar clearance, U_{osm} the urine osmolality, and P_{osm} the plasma osmolality. C_{H_2O} is dictated by the GFR, the osmotic load that must be excreted, the presence or absence of ADH, and by the minimal achievable urine osmolality, and provides an indirect method of quantifying the diluting capacity. Whenever the capacity to excrete water is exceeded, retention of water will occur and dilution of the fluid spaces of the body will ensue.

The following examples will help illustrate this concept. If two subjects with similar plasma osmolalities (300 mOsm) and minimal achievable urine osmolalities (50 mOsm/kg H_2O) but differing solute loads to excrete (600 mOsm versus 300 mOsm) are compared, the subject with the higher osmolar load could excrete it in 12 L of urine ($50 \times 12 = 600$) and have a C_{H_2O} of 10 L in 24 hours, whereas the other could only have a maximum urine volume of 6 L ($50 \times 6 = 300$) and a C_{H_2O} of 5 L. Thus the first subject will require ingestion of more than 12 L of water (twice that of the latter) before water retention and dilution will occur. Similarly, two subjects with identical osmolar loads to excrete (600 mOsm) but different minimal achievable urine osmolalities (150 versus 50 mOsm/kg H_2O) will have different capacities to handle a water load before dilution occurs (4 L versus 12 L). Because C_{H_2O} is also proportional to the GFR, the capacity to handle a water load is impaired in subjects with chronic renal disease despite the fact that their ability to maximally dilute the urine may be preserved.

Diluting capacity is assessed by measuring both urine output and urine osmolality in a 3-hour period following the rapid oral administration of water (45 minutes) at the rate of 20 ml/kg of body weight. In normal subjects more than 50% of the water load is excreted within 3 hours, and the urine will attain an osmolality of 80 mOsm/kg H_2O or a specific gravity of 1.002 or less. Because of the relatively low diagnostic yield to risk ratio, however, water loading is seldom done in clinical practice. Rather, it is more important to recognize the appropriateness of an observed urine osmolality than it is to know the maximum diluting capacity. When true serum hypoosmolality coexists with a urine that is not maximally dilute, it is clear that a defect in the diluting process is present, and as a result no formal studies need be undertaken.

ASSESSMENT OF URINE CONCENTRATION

As previously discussed, a random evaluation of urine osmolality or specific gravity will not convey information regarding the maximal concentrating capacity of a subject. However, if a randomly collected urine has an osmolality greater than or equal to 800 mOsm/kg H_2O or a specific gravity greater than or equal to 1.020 in the absence of substances known to falsely elevate these measurements, it may be concluded that the individual's urine-concentrating capacity is normal.

Assessment of the kidney's ability to concentrate the urine becomes important when evaluating subjects with polyuria. The polyuria that arises from an osmotic diuresis generally results in a urine that is isoosmolar, with a total solute excretion in excess of the usual 500 to 800 mOsm/day seen in normal subjects. Formal assessment of the urine concentrating ability is required to distinguish the major causes of polyuria with a concomitant low urine osmolality, as seen with diabetes insipidus (complete central, partial central, nephrogenic) and psychogenic polydypsia.

The maximal urinary concentrating capacity may be assessed in a polyuric subject by fluid restriction for approximately 12 to 16 hours with a concomitant loss of approximately 3% of body weight. During the fluid deprivation, care must be taken to ensure against excessive dehydration, and the subject should be monitored to prevent surreptitious water ingestion.

TABLE 103.2. Anticipated Response to Fluid Deprivation Followed by Vasopressin in Patients with Hypotonic Polyuria

	Urine Osmolality After Dehydration (mOsm/kg H_2O)	Change in Urine Volume and Osmolality Following Vasopressin Given After Dehydration
Normal	>900	No further change.
Complete DI	<200	Urine volume is reduced and osmolality increased markedly but does not approach normal maximal osmolality.
Partial DI	<500	Urine volume is reduced and osmolality is increased by 20%–30%.
Nephrogenic DI	<300	Urine volume unchanged; osmolality remains low.
Compulsive water drinking	600–800	No further change in urine volume. Osmolality may rise but by less than 10%.

DI, diabetes insipidus

Normal subjects will generally achieve a urine osmolality of 1000 ± 200 mOsm/kg H_2O (specific gravity of 1.025 ± 0.005) following fluid restriction. If this urine osmolality (specific gravity) is not achieved, the response to the intravenous administration of 5 units of aqueous vasopressin is noted and used to distinguish the causes of the polyuria. Table 103.2 depicts the results of water deprivation and the subsequent response to vasopressin for each potential cause of dilute polyuria. In subjects with compulsive water drinking the maximum urine osmolality achieved following fluid deprivation will be submaximal as compared with that of normal subjects as a consequence of a washout of the medullary interstitium. In addition, as the endogenous level of ADH will be increased by the water deprivation and volume contraction, essentially no further increment in urine osmolality will be observed following exogenous vasopressin administration. With complete central diabetes insipidus the maximal urine osmolality achieved is generally hypotonic to plasma (although with severe dehydration isotonic or slightly hypertonic urine may be found), whereas with partial central diabetes insipidus the urine will be hypertonic following dehydration. In both forms of central diabetes insipidus the response to exogenous vasopressin will result in a decrease in urine volume and an increase in urine osmolality. These results are in contrast with those seen in subjects with nephrogenic diabetes insipidus, in whom the urine osmolality following fluid restriction is low and remains unaltered after this dose of exogenous vasopressin. Finally, when the serum sodium concentration, serum osmolality, and body weight remain unchanged during fluid deprivation, a diagnosis of surreptitious water ingestion is supported. The diagnostic utility of the water deprivation test is further improved by measuring plasma ADH levels. Together, these tests offer a sound approach by which to evaluate the causes of dilute polyuria.

Other methods that require less severe water deprivation, have been advocated for assessing maximal urine concentration. These generally require only an overnight restriction of fluid (approximately 8 hours) and thus avoid prolonged fluid deprivation and its potentially serious side effects in polyuric subjects. Following overnight fluid restriction, 4 μg of 1 desamino-8-arginine vasopressin (DDAVP) is administered subcutaneously and the urine osmolality measured over the ensuing 3 to 6 hours. As the response to DDAVP is inversely related to age, the results must be interpreted accordingly. Further discussion on this topic is found in Chapter 26.

CLINICAL ASSESSMENT OF URINE ACIDIFICATION

The avid reabsorption of bicarbonate (HCO_3^-) in the proximal tubule and the secretion of hydrogen ions (H^+) in the distal tubule constitute the normal renal response to the development of metabolic acidosis. Because an increase in ammoniagenesis is central to this renal response, most of the H^+ secretion will be in the form of (NH_4^+). In subjects with metabolic acidosis and severe acidemia, a defect in the distal urinary acidification process is thought to be present whenever the urine pH (as measured by a pH electrode) is found to be "inappropriately" high (higher than 5.5). The use and reliance on the urine pH in this manner, however, may lead to an erroneous conclusion unless the entire urine acidification process is fully understood. In subjects who are chronically acidemic, ammoniagenesis is stimulated. As a result of excess ammonia production relative to H^+ secretion in the distal nephron, the urine pH will increase as the urinary concentration of NH_4^+ increases. This contrasts to the scenario in which normal subjects are rendered acidotic following an acute ammonium chloride (NH_4Cl) load (0.1 g/kg bw), which leads to a relative excess of H^+ secretion compared with NH_3 in the collecting duct (in this setting ammoniagenesis has not been primed) and the urinary concentration of NH_4^+ increases as the urine pH declines to less than 5.3 in urine samples collected 6 to 8 hours after NH_4Cl administration. Thus, when a renal acidification defect is suspected, other tests in addition to the urine pH are required.

From the above it is clear that extrarenal causes of metabolic acidosis may be distinguished from renal causes based on the amount of NH_4^+ excreted in the urine. In the former, the NH_4^+ concentration will be greater than 100 mM/L, while in the latter, a low NH_4^+ concentration (usually below 40 mM/L) will be found. As the urinary concentration of NH_4^+ is difficult to measure in most clinical laboratories, the NH_4^+ concentration may be estimated by calculating the urine anion gap ($[Na^+ + K^+] - Cl^-$). As urinary Cl^- is the major anion which accompanies NH_4^+ in the urine (the exception being when there is an increase in unmeasured non-Cl^- anions such as ketones), the presence of a negative urine anion gap will signify abundant NH_4^+ in the urine, while a positive gap will, in contrast, imply minimal urinary NH_4^+ excretion and suggest the presence of an alteration in the renal acidification process. In the absence of a urine anion gap ($[Cl^-] = [Na^+ + K^+]$) the NH_4^+ concentration is approximately 80 mM/L and represents the excretion of NH_4^+ with sulfates, phosphates and organic anions. Thus, the presence of a urine anion gap of −50 will reflect the net excretion of approximately 130 mM of NH_4^+. Although the urine anion gap provides a semiquantitative measure of NH_4^+ excretion, it should be emphasized that it may underestimate NH_4^+ excretion whenever increased unmeasured anions (i.e. ketones) accompany NH_4^+. The presence of increased unmeasured NH_4^+ should be suspected whenever a significant urine osmolal gap (the difference between the actual urine osmolality and the calculated urine osmolality) exists, which should be calculated when the clinical situation points to this possibility.

When faced with a non–anion gap metabolic acidosis of renal origin and a urinary NH_4^+ excretion <40 mM, a useful approach to identifying the urinary acidification defect is outlined in Fig. 103.2. The response to HCO_3^- administration represents the initial diagnostic step. For this purpose, either 0.9 M sodium bicarbonate can be given intravenously at a rate of 2 to 3 ml/min after administering a 100 to150 mEq bolus or an oral sodium bicarbonate load of 0.5 to 2.0 mEq/kg may be given with 500 ml of water. As proximal renal tubular acidosis is manifested by both an impaired ability to reabsorb HCO_3^- as well as by reduced NH_4^+ excretion, a reduced threshold for proximal HCO_3^- reabsorption will be exposed following the HCO_3^- load. The distal nephron H^+ secretory capacity will be insufficient to reclaim the excess HCO_3^-, and, as a consequence, the urine pH will be alkaline (pH above 7.0) while the plasma HCO_3^- remains abnormally low. If the plasma HCO_3^- normalizes following the HCO_3^- load, the urine-to-blood P_{CO_2} difference is examined during the HCO_3^- infusion while the urine pH is maintained alkaline (pH above 7.5). In normal subjects, alkalinization of the urine to this level is associated with a P_{CO_2} of the urine approximately 30 mm Hg greater than that of blood. This difference between the urine and blood P_{CO_2} is attributed to H^+ secretion in the distal nephron. Subjects with a classic distal renal tubular acidosis will manifest a urine P_{CO_2} similar to that of blood, indicating that there is either deficient H^+ secretion or that a voltage-dependent defect is present. By contrast, a defect in the permeability of the tubular membrane to secreted H^+ (backleak) is associated with a normal urine-to-blood P_{CO_2} difference. In subjects with markedly impaired urinary concentrating capacity, the urinary P_{CO_2} is always low because of a low urinary HCO_3^- concentration; therefore this approach cannot be applied unless the urine HCO_3^- excretion is increased.

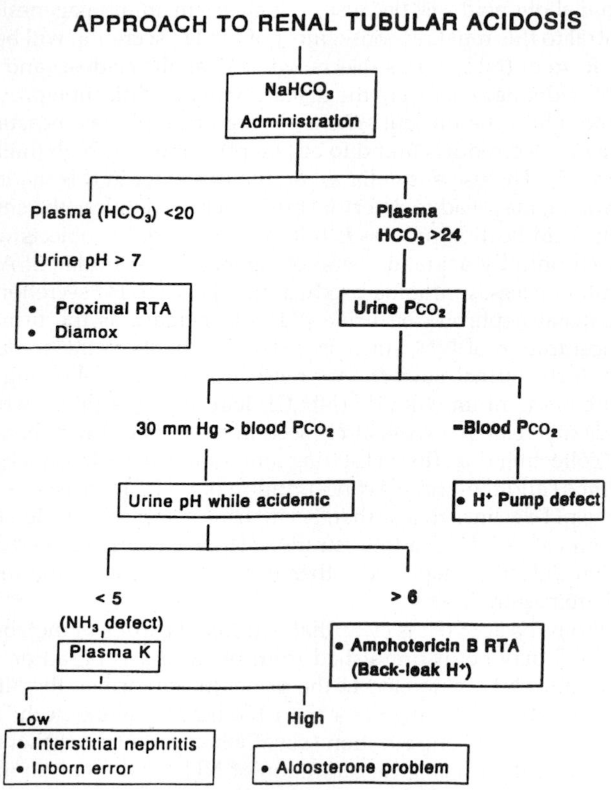

Figure 103.2. A clinical approach to identifying the urinary acidification defect in a subject with a non–anion gap metabolic acidosis of renal origin. (Reproduced with permission from Goldstein MB, Levin A. Insights derived from the urine in acid-base disturbances. *AKF Nephrol* [Letter]. 1989;6:22.)

In children, the determination of the urine-to-blood P_{CO_2} difference may also be assessed with the use of oral acetazolamide rather than with alkalinization with sodium bicarbonate. Studies performed in pediatric subjects have shown no significant differences between oral acetazolamide (17 mg ± 2 mg/kg) and oral sodium bicarbonate loading (2.5 mEq/kg) with respect to their effects on urinary pH, HCO_3^- concentration, plasma P_{CO_2}, and the urine-to-blood P_{CO_2} difference, nor in their ability to distinguish disturbances in distal acidification resulting from a H^+ secretory defect. Because acetazolamide is more palatable than bicarbonate and shortens the testing time, it is the preferable approach in this age group.

Other tests in addition to HCO_3^- loading are available to the clinician to help distinguish between the distal acidification defects of secretory or permeability (backleak) origin. With infusions of either sodium sulfate (0.5 L of 4% sodium sulfate administered intravenously over 40 to 60 minutes) in subjects avidly retaining sodium (following administration of 1 mg of fludrocortisone the night before) or neutral phosphate (0.2 M in 180 ml saline infused intravenously at 1 ml/min for 3 hours) the distal delivery of poorly reabsorbable anions will increase and result in acidification of the urine to a pH below 5.5 with the former infusion and a normal urine-to-blood P_{CO_2} difference with the latter infusion in those subjects without a H^+ secretory defect. Finally, the response to a single dose of either furosemide or bumetamide may also be used to differentiate between these two defects of distal acidification. Following the oral administration of either agent, there will be decreased tubular reabsorption of Na^+ and Cl^- in the thick ascending limb of Henle and increased delivery of these solutes to the cortical collecting duct. As a result, $Na^+:H^+$ exchange will increase and the presence of urinary Cl^- in this segment will further increase the lumen negative potential difference. Thus in subjects with an intact H^+ secretory process the urine will become more acidic and the pH will decrease to less than 5.5.

If the urine-to-blood P_{CO_2} difference is found to be normal, then the distinction between a distal tubular acidification defect caused by backleak (permeability defect) from decreased ammoniagenesis (as may occur in subjects with hyperkalemia, renal failure or severe tubulointerstitial disease) may be made by the examination of the urine pH while the patient is acidemic. A urine pH greater than 6.0 implies a permeabililty defect, while a very low urine pH suggests that there is decreased availability of NH_3 in the collecting duct (in the presence of normal H^+ secretion but deficient NH_3 production, net H^+ secretion will be limited as a consequence of a higher tubular lumen H^+ concentration). The plasma serum potassium concentration will further help discriminate these latter subjects with hypoaldosteronism (high plasma K^+) from those with decreased ammoniagenesis resulting from other causes in which a low plasma K^+ is found.

Although the algorithm in Fig. 103.2 and the tests outlined above are useful in distinguishing many of the renal tubular acidification defects which exist, it must be remembered that subjects may have mixed defects (as seen in severe tubulointerstitial disease) in which H^+ secretion and NH_3 availability are both deficient. These subjects may have a low urine pH (below 5.3), an abnormal urine-to-blood P_{CO_2} difference, as well as an abnormally low NH_4^+ excretion rate. A thorough knowledge of the principles used to identify these acidification defects, however, will enable the clinician to recognize these mixed disturbances.

In addition to the above, proximal tubular acidification can also be evaluated by measuring the fractional excretion of HCO_3^-, which is usually more than 15% in subjects with proximal renal tubular acidosis.

Selected Readings

Bauer JH, Brooks CS, Burch RN. Clinical appraisal of creatinine clearance as a measurement of glomerular filtration rate. *Am J Kidney Dis* 1982;2:337–346.

Comparison of the simultaneous performance of inulin and creatinine clearances in subjects with a wide range of renal function and a description of the disparity that exists between them as a result of enhanced tubular creatinine secretion with progressive renal disease.

Blaufox MD. Procedures of choice in renal nuclear medicine. *J Nucl Med* 1991; 32:1301–1309.

A review that describes the different radiopharmaceutical agents available for the measurement of renal function and for imaging. It also provides specific recommendations for use of these radionuclides in a variety of renal disorders.

Halperin ML, Richardson RMA, Bear RA, et al. Urine ammonium: the key to the diagnosis of distal renal tubular acidosis. *Nephron* 1988;50:1–4.

This article presents a unique approach to differentiating the various forms of non–anion gap metabolic acidoses through the use of urine electrolytes, pH, P_{CO_2}, and osmolality. The concept of the urine anion gap in approximating urinary ammonium excretion is discussed.

Harrington JT, Cohen JJ. Clinical disorders of urine concentration and dilution. *Arch Intern Med* 1973;131:810–825.

Review of the regulation of water excretion; presents a clinical approach to urinary concentration and dilution defects.

Levey AS. Nephrology forum: measurement of renal function in chronic renal disease. *Kidney Int* 1990;38:167–184.

A useful review that describes the glomerular filtration rate as an index of renal function, as well as the methods used to measure it. In addition, the use of the reciprocal of the Scr as an approximation of the glomerular filtration rate in normal subjects and during progression of renal disease is discussed.

Levey AS, Perrone RD, Madias NE. Serum creatinine and renal function. *Ann Rev Med* 1988;39:465–90.

An in-depth review of creatinine, including renal handling, extrarenal metabolism, measurement, use as a marker of glomerular filtration rate, and its role in the estimate of progression of renal disease.

Nilsson-Ehle P, Grubb A. New markers for the determination of GFR: iohexol clearance and cystatin C serum concentration. *Kidney Int* 1994; 46:S17–S19.

This article highlights the utility of iohexol and cystatin C, two unique markers for glomerular filtration, and their potential role in clinical nephrology.

Perrone RD, Steinman TI, Beck GJ, et al. The Modification of Diet in Renal Disease Study. Utility of radioisotopic filtration markers in chronic renal insufficiency: simultaneous comparison of ^{125}I-Iothalamate, ^{169}Yb-DTPA, ^{99m}Tc-DTPA, and inulin. *Am J Kidney Dis* 1990;16:224–235.

A comparison of the renal clearance of various radioisotopic filtration markers with one another and with inulin in the measurement of glomerular filtration rate in normal subjects and in those with renal insufficiency.

SECTION XIII

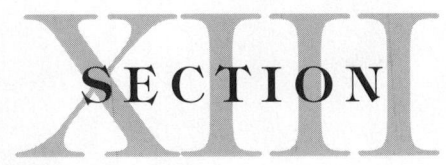

Radionuclear and Radiographic Techniques

CHAPTER 104

Assessment of Renal Anatomy and Function with Radionuclides

Joseph V. Nally, Jr. and Phillip M. Hall

Nuclear medicine techniques to evaluate the kidney and urinary tract have evolved from the pioneering studies using primitive radionuclides with handheld probe detectors to a sophisticated technology that is capable of providing important physiologic and anatomic information. Advances in the field of nuclear medicine and computer technology over the past decade have resulted in improved, clinically useful radionuclide studies to assist the clinician in the evaluation of the patient with diseases of the genitourinary tract. In this chapter, we review the principles, indications, and limitations of radionuclide renography available to today's clinician.

TECHNOLOGY

Radionuclide

A conventional radionuclide consists of two parts: (a) a compound selected to evaluate the desired function/anatomy of the organ system under study and (b) a radioisotopic label that permits detection of the radionuclide by the gamma camera. When studying the kidney and urinary tract, one obviously selects a compound that is excreted by way of the kidney. The compounds available for this purpose can be grouped into three categories (Table 104.1). The first category includes compounds that are excreted solely via glomerular filtration, such as iothalamate, diethylenetriaminepentaacetic acid (DTPA), and edetate (EDTA). The second category comprises compounds excreted via both glomerular filtration and tubular secretion, for example, *para*-aminohippurate (PAH), orthoiodohippurate (OIH), and mercaptoacetyltriglycine (MAG_3), such that their clearances serve as markers of effective renal plasma flow (ERPF). The third category comprises compounds that selectively bind to renal parenchyma, for example, 3-dimercaptosuccinic acid (DMSA), glucoheptonate (GHA), and gallium. These agents provide static imaging and renal anatomic information.

The second component of the radionuclide, the label, is equally important because it allows for accurate measurement of the entire complex. The two most commonly used labels for renography have been ^{131}I and ^{99m}Tc. The latter appears to be the better radioisotope because of its shorter half-life (approximately 6 hours), lower-energy photons (approximately 140 KeV), and superior imaging capabilities that lend themselves to computer analysis. In contrast, ^{131}I has a longer half-life (approximately 8 days), higher energy requirements (364 KeV), and poorer imaging characteristics. ^{131}I appears ideal for scintigraphic imaging, but it has not been readily available and is quite expensive. ^{125}I with low-energy photons has been used for *in vivo* and *in vitro* renal functional studies but is not suitable for scintigraphic imaging.

^{99m}Tc-MAG_3 has emerged as the radionuclide of choice for many clinical renography studies. MAG_3, a functional analog of PAH, is excreted rapidly by the kidney. ^{99m}Tc-MAG^3 appears to offer superior images of the kidney, and its diagnostic utility is being critically compared with other radionuclides for various clinical nephrologic problems. Unfortunately, ^{99m}Tc-MAG_3 is more costly than ^{99m}Tc-DTPA or ^{131}I- OIH, but the use of ^{99m}Tc-MAG_3 may become more cost-effective with appropriate scheduling to cluster the renal studies using ^{99m}Tc-MAG_3.

The radiation dose to the patient of a particular radionuclide is a function both of the physical half-life of the radioisotope and the biologic half-life of the labeled compound. For example, although the physical half-life of the tracer ^{99m}Tc is approximately 6 hours, the biologic half-life of the compound MAG_3 is less than 20 minutes because of rapid renal excretion of this compound. Thus the total radiation exposure after an injection of ^{99m}Tc-MAG_3 is relatively limited.

The radiation exposure from radionuclides commonly used for renography is given in Table 104.2. The total body radiation exposure to a patient for a ^{99m}Tc-DTPA or ^{99m}Tc-MAG_3 renal scan is about the same as from an intravenous pyelogram (IVP). Renography with 10 mCi ^{99m}Tc-DTPA results in total body exposure of 0.08 rad (0.008 rad/mCi $\times$ 10 mCi injected) or 80 millirads, compared with 60 millirads radiation exposure from a conventional IVP or 100 millirads radiation exposure from an IVP including two oblique views and two tomograms. On

TABLE 104.1 Radionuclide Compounds to Assess Kidney Function and Structure

Functional	Static Anatomic Imaging
Glomerular filtration rate	^{99m}Tc-DMSA
^{125}I-Iothalamate	^{99m}Tc-GHA
^{99m}Tc-DTPA	^{67}Ga
^{169}Yb-DTPA	
^{51}Cr-EDTA	
Effective renal plasma flow	
OIH (^{123}I or ^{131}I)	
^{99m}Tc-MAG_3	

TABLE 104.2 Radiation Absorbed Dose (rad/mCi) in Normal Individuals from Common Radionuclides for Renography

Organ	^{131}I-OIH	^{123}I-OIH	^{99m}Tc-DTPA	^{99m}Tc-MAG$_3$	^{99m}Tc-GHA	^{99m}Tc-DMSA
Kidneys	0.094	0.021	0.022	0.015	0.170	0.62
Total body	0.018	0.008	0.008	0.007	0.007	0.016
Testes	0.039	0.015	0.009	0.016	—	—
Ovaries	0.063	0.029	0.013	0.026	0.020	0.022
Bladder wall	2.14	0.47	0.14	0.480	0.800	0.28

Data from Tauxe WN, Dubovsky EV. *Nuclear medicine in clinical urology and nephrology*. Norwalk: CT: Appleton- Century-Crofts, 1985:31–37; and modified from Technescan packet insert (Mallinckrodt, Inc., St. Louis, MO).

the other hand, the radiation exposure to the ovaries from a ^{99m}Tc- DTPA renal scan (0.01 rad/mCi) is substantially less than from a conventional IVP. Nevertheless, radiation exposure with radionuclide renography is highest in the bladder and reproductive organs. Consequently, it is prudent to determine that a woman of childbearing age is not pregnant at the time of the study. All patients should be encouraged to void soon after the radionuclide study.

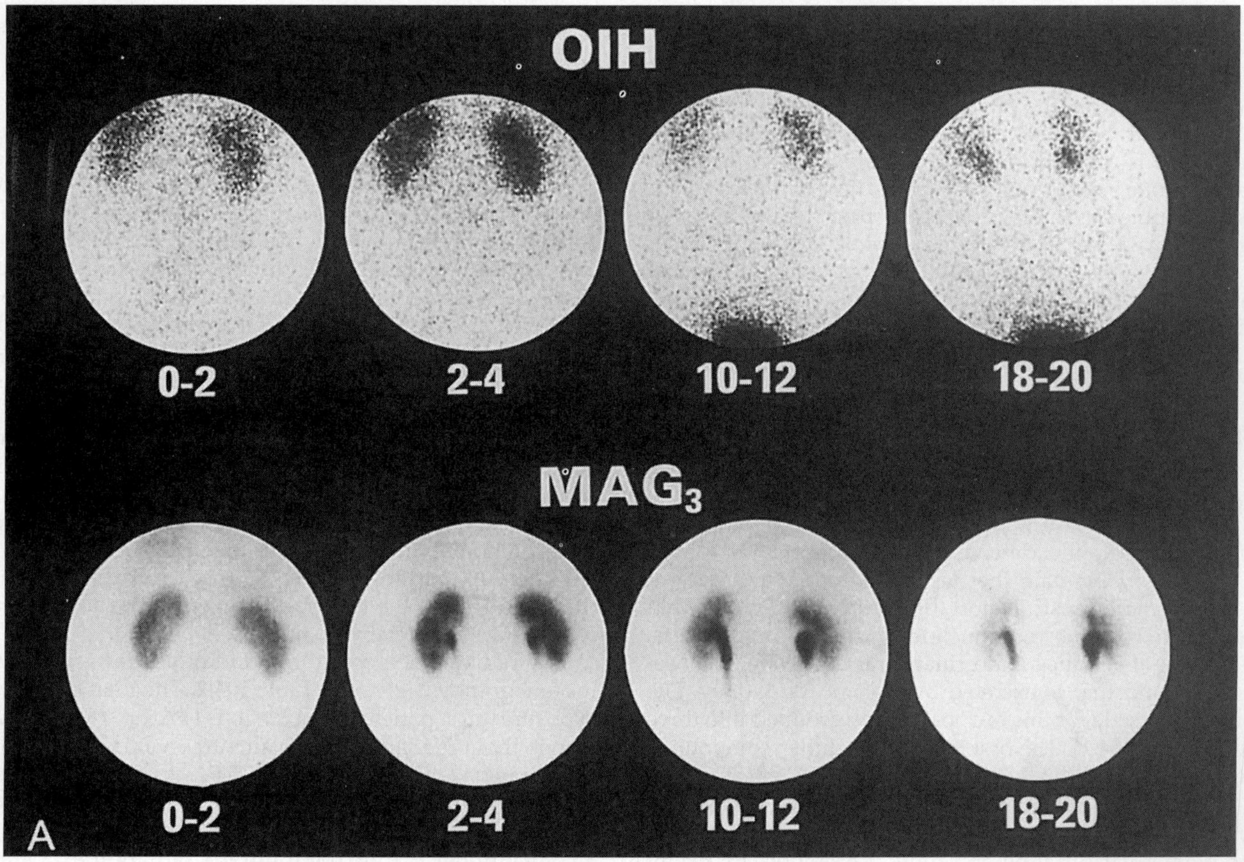

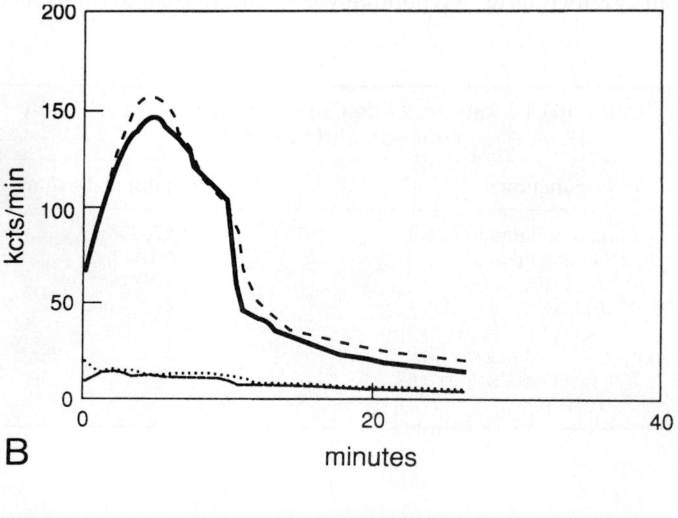

Figure 104.1. **A:** Orthoiodohippurate *(OIH)* and ^{99m}Tc-*MAG$_3$* images of a 31-year-old woman being evaluated as a kidney donor candidate. Images were obtained at 2-minute intervals in the posterior view. **B:** Time-activity curves from the same patient. (Courtesy of Andrew Taylor, Jr., M.D.)

The Gamma Camera

The gamma scintillation camera consists of a crystal that is sensitive to radiation, photomultiplier tubes (PMT) arranged to cover the crystal, and associated electronics that aid in determining the energy and special coordinates of the radiation source. The crystal emits light when radiation interacts with it, and the amount of light emitted is proportional to the energy of radiation absorbed. PMTs convert the visible light to an electronic pulse. Each pulse of energy is then displayed on a special imaging cathode ray tube as a flash of light at the correct position relative to the center of the crystal. Sophisticated computer technology coordinates the regions of uptake activity and degree of uptake.

Both scintiphotographs and time-activity curves are generated with this technology for qualitative and quantitative analysis relating to renal uptake and excretion of the radionuclide (Fig. 104.1). In addition, well counters are available in many departments for quantitating radioactivity of blood and/or urine aliquots to calculate renal clearances.

CLINICAL UTILITY OF RADIONUCLIDE STUDIES

Radionuclide studies of the kidney and urinary tract are capable of providing clinically relevant, functional information [e.g., glomerular filtration rate (GFR), ERPF] and, to a lesser extent, helpful anatomic information. The rest of this chapter focuses on the clinical utility of radionuclide studies in quantifying renal function and their role in evaluation clinical renal problems.

Quantification of Renal Function

Radionuclide studies of the kidney can provide accurate determinations of kidney function (either GFR or ERPF) using one of three general methodologies: (a) formal renal clearance studies measuring blood and urine (e.g., $C = UV/P$), (b) single-injection plasma clearances using disappearance curve techniques without urine samples, and (c) renal uptakes of radionuclides detected by the gamma camera without blood or urine sampling.

Measurement of the Glomerular Filtration Rate

Because of the complexity of the C_{In} (clearance of inulin) method and the inaccuracies of P_{Cr} and C_{Cr} as estimates of GFR, radionuclide clearance methods have been developed. These include ^{125}I-iothalamate (IOTH), ^{99m}Tc-DTPA, and ^{51}Cr-EDTA. For each of these radioisotopes, the renal clearance is predominantly via filtration. Although a small amount of tubular secretion or reabsorption occurs, its magnitude is constant through the clinical range of GFR. Several clinical studies have shown that the correlation between C_{In} and these isotopic markers is excellent. ^{125}I-IOTH and Tc-DTPA may overestimate C_{In} up to 10% in the range of GFR between 10 and 80 ml/min. Cr-EDTA underestimates C_{In}, by about 8% to 10%, between 10 and 80 ml/min. Furthermore, in patients with impaired but stable renal function, C_{IOTH} and $C_{Tc\text{-}DTPA}$ have excellent precision and reproducibility, suggesting that the small nonglomerular excretion is constant and unaffected by severe degrees of renal function impairment.

^{125}I-IOTH is an isotopically tagged triiodinated derivative of benzoic acid. Urinary clearances with this marker are safe and clinically feasible. After oral water loading (5 to 10 ml/kg) to achieve a urine flow rate of 3 ml/min (and oral Lugol's iodine to block thyroidal uptake of the isotope), 35 to 50 μC of IOTH with or without a small amount of epinephrine is administered subcutaneously in the upper arm. After allowing 60 minutes for equilibration of the isotope in the plasma, two to three timed voluntarily voided urine collections are obtained. Plasma samples are obtained before and at the end of each urine collection period. The radioactivity [counts per minute (cpm)] in plasma and urine samples is used to calculate the clearance using the standard formula.

$$C_{IOTH} = \frac{UV}{\frac{(P_1 + P_2)}{2}}$$

where *(P1 + P2)/2* is the plasma radioactivity determined by averaging the counts at the beginning and at the conclusion of the timed urinary collection (to adjust for the slightly changing plasma concentration of the isotope).

There are several reasons that this protocol is clinically useful. In addition to the excellent correlation with C_{In}, IOTH yields a low radiation dosage to the patient and technician, does not require intravenous infusions, allows same-day calculation of test results, yet has a long half-life ($t_{1/2}$) allowing flexibility regarding counting of the samples, and has high patient acceptance. Disadvantages include (a) the need to collect timed urine samples; therefore patients who are uncooperative, patients who have voiding disorders, and children are unsuitable; (b) the fact that a radioisotope is being given precludes its use in pregnancy and must be used with proper radiation safeguards in others; and (c) the infrequent but real occurrence of iodine allergy in the patient.

In our institution during the past 20 years, this method has been used in more than 10,000 patient studies. Typically, it is performed in the outpatient department and requires 3 hours of patient time and 45 minutes of technician time. In Table 104.3, the relationship between P_{Cr} and C_{IOTH} is shown in patients according to age and gender. These data demonstrate that P_{Cr} con-

TABLE 104.3 Relationship Between Iothalamate Glomerular Filtration Rate and Serum Creatinine Levels According to Age and Gender

	Mean Measured Serum Creatinine Values ±2 SD (mg/dl)[a]					
	15–30 Years		40–50 Years		60–70 Years	
GFR	M (n = 297)	F (n = 334)	M (n = 297)	F (n = 256)	M (n = 388)	F (n = 225)
10	6.6 ± 4.6	5.4 ± 3.2	5.8 ± 3.9	4.7 ± 2.5	4.6 ± 3.5	5.1 ± 3.2
25	3.0 ± 1.3	2.6 ± 1.9	3.0 ± 1.6	2.4 ± 1.2	2.6 ± 1.7	2.2 ± 1.5
50	1.8 ± 0.9	1.4 ± 0.6	1.7 ± 0.7	1.4 ± 0.5	1.6 ± 0.	1.3 ± 0.5
100	1.2 ± 0.4	0.9 ± 0.3	1.2 ± 0.4	0.9 − 0.3	1.1 ± 0.4	0.9 ± 0.3

[a] Serum creatinine values done on SMA Technicon. Glomerular filtration rate values in units of ml/min/1.73 m^2.
Data were taken from 4,000 glomerular filtration rate tests performed at the Cleveland Clinic Foundation.
M, males; F, females.

centrations within or slightly above the normal range may represent significant reductions in GFR, especially in the patient who is older and has a smaller lean body mass. On the other hand, it must be remembered that, especially for serum creatinine levels between 1.0 and 2.0 mg/dl, there is a broad overlap of the patient subpopulations defined by normal and reduced GFRs. Based on patients having GFR determinations at our institution, the serum creatinine levels at which 10%, 50%, and 90% of patients demonstrate abnormally low GFRs are, for men, 1.1, 1.5, and 1.8 mg/dl, respectively, and, for women, 0.7, 1.1, and 1.6 mg/dl, respectively. This study also documents that the levels of P_{Cr} often considered to represent moderate azotemia actually indicate advanced renal failure.

Accuracy and reproducibility of the C_{IOTH} method have been excellent. In 12 patients with a GFR between 5 and 103 ml/min, a mean C_{IOTH} of 57.9, and a C_{In} of 57.6, the regression coefficient was 0.992. In 17 patients (GFR range 28.7 to 121.7 ml/min) who had three consecutive clearance periods, the median coefficient of variation was 9.2%. In 20 subjects, a minimum of five separate C_{IOTH} studies were performed over several weeks to months. In these patients, whose P_{Cr} level did not vary by more than the error of the P_{Cr} method and whose range of GFR was 17.1 to 129.0 ml/min, the median coefficient of variation was 11.5%. The intratest and intertest precision is similar to those obtained with C_{In}.

GFR also can be measured using TC-DTPA. This isotope, a chelation complex formed from the reaction of DTPA with sodium pertechnetate-99 (^{99m}Tc), is a gamma emitter with a half-life of 6.02 hours. As stated previously, GFR measured with this isotope compares favorably with C_{In}, overestimating true GFR by 5% to 10%. There are several considerations in its choice as a clinical test. The short half-life limits patient radiation exposure but requires prompt counting of samples. Chelation of the ^{99m}Tc to the DTPA must be performed and the isotope must be checked for radiochemical purity within 1 hour of intravenous administration of the 0.5 mCi dose. Thereafter, just as with C_{IOTH}, timed urine collections with plasma sampling before and after are obtained. $C_{Tc\text{-}DTPA}$ is calculated in a fashion similar to that for C_{IOTH} using the formula C = UV/P. Because the isotope dose has higher radioactivity than an iothalamate dose, shielding of samples and syringes and other more stringent radiation safety precautions are required for personnel.

GFR may be estimated accurately by plasma disappearance methodology, using the two-compartment model of Saperstein to equate the plasma disappearance curves of selected radionuclides with the GFR. Comparative studies of the plasma disappearance versus formal clearance methodologies suggest a good correlation, such that the former technique should be valid for clinical practice and research. The plasma disappearance technique offers the advantage of avoiding urinary collection, yet it remains time-consuming, requiring data collection for 30 to 240 minutes.

Other studies have suggested that a third methodology using the renal uptake of Tc-DTPA from the first to third minutes after injection (factored for amount of injected dose, patient's body size and kidney depth, and a derived constant) closely approximates the whole-body GFR and that of each kidney. The following formula was derived.

$$\mathrm{GFR} = \left(\frac{\dfrac{\mathrm{RK} - \mathrm{Bkg}}{e^{-\mu x}}}{\text{Preinjection counts}} + \frac{\dfrac{\mathrm{LK} - \mathrm{Bkg}}{e^{-\mu x}}}{\text{Post injection counts}} \right) \times 100(9.81270) - (6.82519)$$

where *RK* represents the right kidney counts, *Bkg* represents the background counts, *LK* represents the left kidney counts, μ is the linear attenuation coefficient of Tc-DTPA in soft tissues (0.153), and x is kidney depth in centimeters.

Using this renal uptake technique, the study of Gates noted an excellent correlation (r = 0.99) with creatinine clearance, with excellent reproducibility. This technique conveniently requires only 6 minutes of imaging time and does not require sampling of blood or urine.

Unfortunately, these observations have not been reproduced with such a high degree of precision by others. An analytic review suggests that there may be a standard error of approximately 15% to 20% or approximately 12 to 20 ml/min of GFR using the Tc-DTPA and gamma camera technique. On balance, it appears that measuring GFR using either formal clearance studies or plasma disappearance techniques is more accurate and reproducible than the methodology of renal uptake of radionuclides. Computer software programs using the Tc-DTPA and gamma technique are now available commercially to nuclear medicine departments. Before accepting these programs for routine clinical use, validation within one's institution against an accepted marker of GFR is advised.

Measurement of Effective Renal Plasma Flow

The three previously described methods for quantifying GFR apply equally well to determining ERPF and renal blood flow. OIH and MAG_3, structural analogs of PAH, are extracted nearly completely from the renal artery blood, such that their clearance serves as an accurate approximation of ERPF. Although structurally similar, OIH does not behave quantitatively like PAH because of modest protein binding of OIH in the serum. However, good correlation between formal clearances of PAH and tracer amounts of ^{131}I-OIH and ^{99m}Tc-MAG_3 has been obtained. Unfortunately, these formal clearance studies remain cumbersome. Estimation of ERPF using the single-injection plasma disappearance of ^{131}I-OIH has been developed and appears to have an excellent correlation with formal clearance studies. In fact, the methodology has been simplified to permit a single blood sample at 44 minutes postinjection using the following formula:

$$\mathrm{ERPF\ (ml/min)} = 1126.20\,[1\text{-}e^{-0.0080\,(V_{44}\ -7.80)}]$$

where *V* represents the counts of the injected dose divided by counts in 1 L of plasma at 44 minutes. More recently, a similar plasma disappearance technique (including a single-sample blood sample protocol) has been reported for Tc-MAG_3, with excellent correlation with OIH studies.

For more than a decade, the third method of estimating ERPF of each kidney (i.e., renal uptake of ^{131}I- OIH) has been advocated. Unfortunately, this technique produces variable results and is not as reliable as plasma disappearance techniques. Nonetheless, just as for GFR measurements, computer software is being made available to nuclear medicine departments for clinical estimation of renal blood flow. Again, potential users should validate the technique within their own institution before accepting it for either clinical or research purposes.

Overall, quantitative assessment of renal function using gamma camera techniques appears to be potentially advantageous because it is fast and convenient and does not require sampling of blood or urine. In addition, it offers the advantage of quantitating individual kidney function to serially evaluate renal disease with asymmetric involvement (e.g., renal artery stenosis, obstructive uropathy, reflux nephropathy). Unfortunately, the technology is not sufficiently precise to advocate its widespread clinical use. In the interim, a reasonable estimate of individual (split) kidney function may be calculated by determining total GFR by clearance or plasma disappearance techniques (i.e., ^{125}I-IOTH or ^{99m}Tc-DTPA) and factoring the result by the percentage of left and right renal uptake determined by camera renography.

Clinical Evaluation of Nephrologic and Urologic Disorders

Acute Renal Failure. In evaluating the patient with acute renal failure (ARF), the goal is to discover a potentially reversible or treatable cause of the renal dysfunction. The question exists: "What questions can a renal scan answer accurately to help in clinical decision making?" With ARF secondary to acute tubular necrosis (ATN), there is a marked derangement of renal function, with only a mild to modest decrement in renal blood flow. Theoretically, this would be recognized as markedly abnormal excretion with preserved renal perfusion, as assessed by the early phases of the Tc-DTPA or Tc-MAG_3 study. However, this adds little specific information for the clinician. With marked oligoanuria and a question of whether there are any renal perfusion problems (e.g., vascular thrombosis, infarction, emboli), the early phases of the Tc-DTPA or Tc-MAG_3 study may demonstrate renal perfusion, and the renogram may noninvasively demonstrate the presence or absence of functioning renal tissue. However, in typical ATN cases, radionuclide renography usually plays a minor role in the clinical evaluation of the patient.

Obstructive Uropathy. In the setting of ARF, the anatomic information from a renal ultrasound examination is extremely helpful in determining the presence or absence of urinary tract obstruction. The renal ultrasound has a sensitivity of approximately 90% to 95%, with a specificity of 70%. However, the renal ultrasound offers anatomic information but not functional information. It is possible to have a dilated, atonic collecting system resulting in some impairment of renal function without having true obstruction. In contrast, retroperitoneal fibrosis may cause ARF secondary to obstruction, but the renal ultrasound may not demonstrate hydronephrosis. In these situations, renography (^{99m}Tc-DTPA, ^{99m}Tc- MAG_3, or ^{131}I-OIH) may be useful in demonstrating the degree of renal dysfunction in conjunction with a dilated collecting system.

In contrast to the renographic pattern for a normal collection system (Fig. 104.2A), the usual renographic pattern with obstruction is a progressive accumulation of the radionuclide within the renal pelvis that is unable to be excreted (Fig. 104.2B). Studies with the furosemide renogram suggest that true urinary tract obstruction can be differentiated from an atonic, nonobstructed collecting system. The furosemide renogram may add more specific renal functional information in patients with an atonic but nonobstructed collecting system, that is, a patient with previous urologic surgery or a partially obstructing stone. In this setting, a conventional renogram (^{99m}Tc-DTPA, ^{99m}Tc-MAG_3, or ^{131}1-OIH) is begun, and then furosemide [0.5 mg/kg IV (maximal dose 40 mg)] is administered after 15 to 20 minutes. With true obstruction (Fig. 104.2C), this accumulation of radionuclide in the obstructed renal pelvis persists despite furosemide. In contrast, the furosemide will promote passage of radionuclide from a dilated, atonic but nonobstructed renal pelvis to the bladder because of increased urine flow caused by the diuretic (Fig. 104.2B). In the neonatal population, furosemide renography is being increasingly used to address the difficult issue of surgical repair of hydroureteronephrosis (true versus functional obstruction) now being identified with prenatal ultrasonography.

Vesicoureteral Reflux. Evaluation of the patient, usually in the pediatric age group, with recurrent urinary tract infections and abnormal bladder anatomy or function requires definitive urologic diagnosis. Evaluation of bladder function using radionuclide techniques can provide important functional infor-

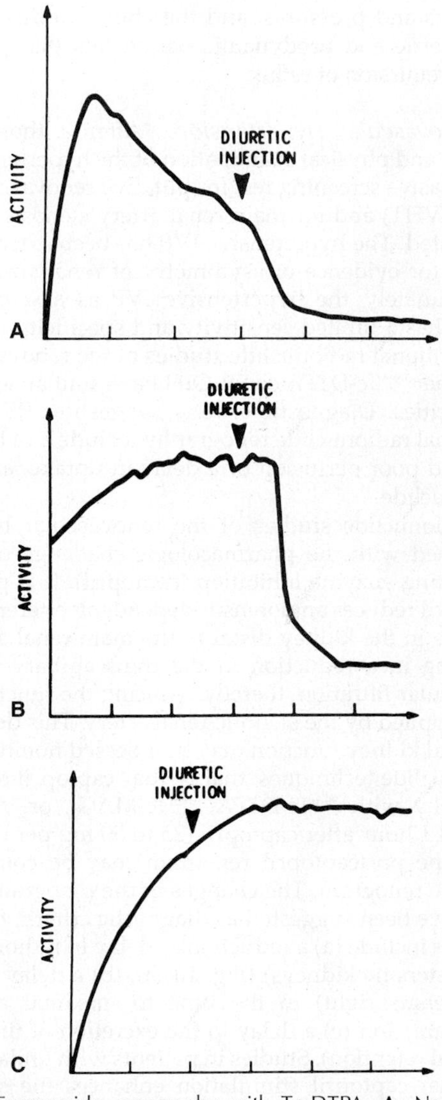

Figure 104.2. Furosemide renography with Tc-DTPA. **A:** Normal response. **B:** Dilated collecting system without true obstruction. **C:** True obstruction. See text for details. (Adapted with permission from Scharf SC, Blaufox MD. Radionuclides in the evaluation of urinary obstruction. In: Tauxe WN, Dubovsky EV, eds. *Nuclear medicine in clinical urology and nephrology.* Norwalk, CT: Appleton-Century-Crofts, 1985:191–206.)

mation using either direct or indirect cystography. Direct radionuclide cystography may be accomplished by instilling the radionuclide (^{99m}Tc-pertechnetate or ^{99m}Tc-DTPA) directly into the bladder via a Foley catheter in a fashion similar to x-ray cystography. Bladder function and the presence or absence of urinary reflux can be quantitated by analyzing scintigraphic studies and routine cystometric measurements. Urodynamic evaluation also may be accomplished. The direct radionuclide cystometrogram appears to have the same high degree of sensitivity in detecting vesicoureteral reflux as x-ray cystography, although comparative studies are limited. Indirect radionuclide cystography has been advocated, mostly in Europe. In this procedure, ^{99m}Tc-MAG_3 is administered intravenously, promptly clears through the kidneys, and fills the urinary bladder. Bladder reflux is then assessed by normal voiding. This procedure has been reported to be as effective as x-ray cystography in the detection of vesicoureteral reflux and at the same time provides an indication of split renal function. However, direct radionuclide cystography is still preferred by some because of less radiation dose, the ability to detect reflux with lower bladder volumes and pressures, and the ability to directly quantitate cystometric and urodynamic parameters that predict spontaneous remission of reflux.

Renovascular Hypertension. After a thorough medical history and physical examination of the hypertensive patient, a noninvasive screening test for putative renovascular hypertension (RVHT) and for main renal artery stenosis (RAS) may be warranted. The hypertensive IVP has been extensively used to screen for evidence of asymmetry of renal size or perfusion. Unfortunately, the hypertensive IVP as a screening test for RVHT has a limited sensitivity and specificity of 65% to 75%. Conventional radionuclide studies of the renovascular bed using either ^{99m}Tc-DTPA or ^{131}I-OIH have similar sensitivities and specificities. Diagnostic criteria suggesting RVHT from conventional radionuclide renography include a reduction in renal size and poor perfusion or a delay in uptake/excretion of the radionuclide.

Radionuclide studies of the renovascular bed have been combined with the pharmacologic challenge of angiotensin-converting enzyme inhibition (captopril). It is postulated that captopril reduces angiotensin-dependent, efferent arteriolar resistance in the kidney distal to the main renal artery stenosis, resulting in a reduction in the transcapillary forces driving glomerular filtration, thereby reducing the function of the kidney supplied by the stenotic renal artery. This decrement in individual kidney function may be assessed noninvasively using radionuclide techniques, that is, the "captopril renogram." Renography with ^{99m}Tc-DTPA, ^{99m}Tc-MAG_3, or ^{131}I-OIH is performed 1 hour after captopril (25 to 50 mg per os) administration. The postcaptopril renogram may be compared with a baseline renogram. The changes in the renogram *after captopril* that have been suggested as diagnostic criteria for renal artery stenosis include (a) a reduction or delay in radionuclide uptake of the stenotic kidneys) (Fig. 104.3), (b) a delay or asymmetry (left versus right) in the time to maximal activity of the renogram, and (c) a delay in the excretion of the radionuclide (cortical retention). Studies in patients with unilateral RAS suggest that captopril stimulation enhances the sensitivity and specificity of conventional renography and may also predict improved blood pressure control after intervention with either percutaneous transluminal renal angioplasty or renal revascularization. Existing clinical studies suggest a sensitivity of 85% to 95% and specificity of 85% to 98% for captopril renography in identifying renal artery disease in a selected hypertensive population. The postcaptopril renogram alone has been advocated by some as a single screening test for anatomic RAS and for RVHT.

Renal Transplantation. Radionuclide studies have been adapted to provide important information regarding the function and structure of the transplanted kidney. Being noninvasive, these studies may be repeated for serial evaluation, especially during the critical days and weeks following transplantation. ^{99m}Tc-DTPA and/or OIH (labeled with ^{131}I or ^{123}I) renography generally has been replaced by ^{99m}Tc-MAG_3 studies. The methodology for radionuclide renography is similar to studies in native kidneys, although selection of appropriate areas for background subtraction in the more vascular iliac fossa may represent a potential technical problem. The scintigraphs and time-activity curves may be analyzed to produce qualitative and quantitative information similar to that provided by routine radionuclide renography. Most transplant centers perform a renogram during the first day or two after transplant. For following graft function, the renogram provides baseline anatomic and functional information (independent of the serum creatinine measurement) that provides a basis for comparison with subsequent serial studies. The isolated renogram is of little value. Rather, it is the change from one renogram to another that may be helpful. Serial assessment of GFR or ERPF using radionuclide techniques is also advocated by some transplant programs.

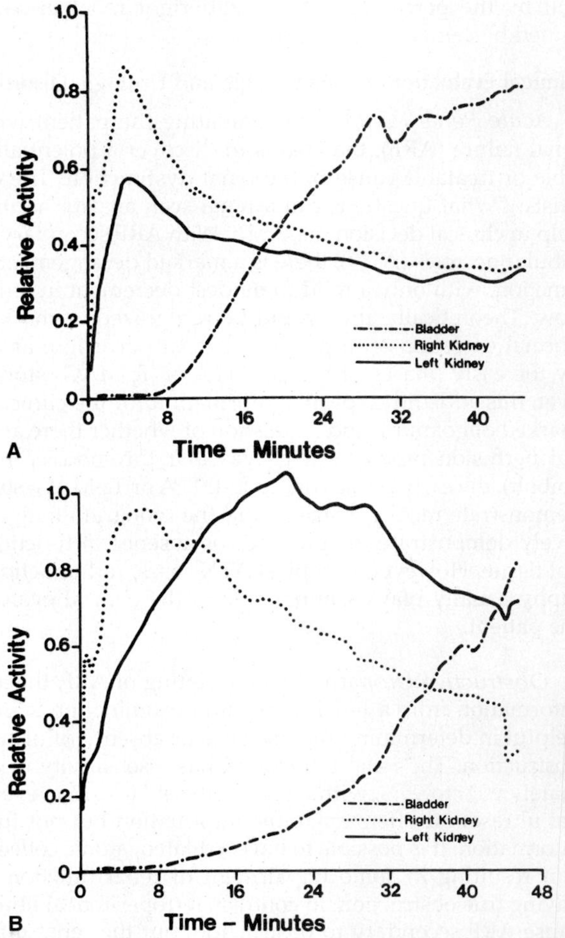

Figure 104.3. Captopril renography with ^{99m}Tc-DTPA in unilateral renal artery stenosis. **A:** Baseline study. **B:** Captopril-stimulated study. See text for details. (Reproduced with permission from Nally JV, Gupta BK, Clarke HS, et al. Captopril renography for the detection of renovascular hypertension. A preliminary report. *Cleve Clin J Med* 1988;55:311–318.)

With early graft failure, the scintigraphs may provide information about renal perfusion, vascular thrombosis, obstruction, or urinary leak with extravasation of radionuclide. Acute rejection demonstrates a marked diminution in both renal function and renal perfusion. In contrast, posttransplant ATN is often characterized by a marked disturbance in function with relatively preserved renal perfusion. Studies evaluating cyclosporine nephrotoxicity suggest that its radionuclide pattern may be similar to that of ATN. Several studies have reported that techniques involving either renal cortical perfusion indices, labeled platelets, or labeled white blood cells may be helpful in differentiating chronic rejection from cyclosporine nephrotoxicity. Unfortunately, these reports consist of small series of transplant patients and often are retrospective. Differentiating between chronic graft rejection and cyclosporine nephrotoxicity in a patient at an one point is especially difficult, even with cyclosporine levels and renal biopsy. Not surprisingly, renal scans have not resolved this diagnostic dilemma.

STATIC RENAL IMAGING

Radionuclide studies may be used to demonstrate anatomic renal abnormalities. For example, radionuclides, such as ^{99m}Tc-DMSA or GHA, are selectively taken up by the renal cortex and may identify mass lesions and help differentiate renal cysts, vascular tumors, or abscesses. In the pediatric population, serial scintigraphic imaging with ^{99m}Tc-DMSA may help delineate renal cortical scarring secondary to recurrent urinary tract infection and ureteral reflux. However, other noninvasive radiologic studies, such as an abdominal CT or renal ultrasound, provide more accurate anatomic information.

Gallium (^{67}Ga) localizes nonspecifically in the renal bed with acute inflammation and may indicate pyelonephritis and renal or perirenal abscess formation. However, specificity may vary, as gallium uptake within the kidney has been reported with interstitial nephritis and various neoplastic renal disorders, including lymphoma, leukemia, melanoma, and metastatic bronchogenic carcinoma. Gallium scanning of the kidney may have utility in evaluation of the patient with acute renal insufficiency in whom acute interstitial nephritis is suspected, because the gallium localizes to the inflammatory cells in the renal interstitium. Gallium scanning also may be useful in patients with polycystic kidney disease with an infected cyst. The infected cyst(s) may be identified and then drained percutaneously.

The clinical utility of radionuclide renography for static renal imaging obviously needs further development to provide more selective and specific diagnostic information. At present, competing radiologic modalities, such as ultrasound and CT scanning, provide acceptable diagnostic and cost-effective anatomic information about the urinary tract. Thus the major role of radionuclide renography in the clinical evaluation of renal and urologic disorders is to provide functional rather than anatomic information.

Selected Readings

Blaufox MD, Aurell M, Bubeck B, et al. Report of the Radionuclides in Nephrourology Committee on renal clearance. *J Nucl Med* 1996;37:1883–1890.

This comprehensive review presents the rationale and clinical protocols for measuring GFR and ERPF using radionuclides with the plasma disappearance, urinary clearances, and gamma camera techniques.

Dubovsky EV, Russell CD, Erbas B. Radionuclide evaluation of renal transplants. *Semin Nucl Med* 1995;XXV:49–59.

This review focuses on criteria for the selection of transplant candidates, newer techniques for the diagnosis of medical and surgical complications after transplantation, the use of new tracers (^{99m}Tc MAG_3), and new antirejection regimens.

Levey AS. Measurement of renal function in chronic renal disease. *Kidney Int* 1990;38:67–184.

Excellent review of the clinical utility of various methods for measuring renal function, including serum creatinine, creatinine clearance, and radioisotopic GFRs.

O'Reilly P, Aurell M, Britton K, et al. Consensus on diuresis renography for investigating the dilated upper urinary tract. *J Nucl Med* 1996;37:1872–1876.

This update, by one of the pioneers of diuretic renography, illustrates important concepts and practical approaches to diuretic renography.

Taylor A, Corrigan P, Russell F. Prospective validation of a single sample technique to determine technetium-99m MAG_3 clearance. *J Nucl Med* 1992;33:1620–1622.

Since ^{99m}Tc-MAG_3 is becoming the radionuclide of choice for renography, this important study validates clearance measurements of ^{99m}Tc-MAG_3 as an estimate of ERPF.

Taylor A, Nally JV Jr, Aurell M, et al. Consensus report on ACE inhibitor renography for detecting renovascular hypertension. *J Nucl Med* 1996;72:292–297.

This excellent state-of-the-art review presents the pathophysiologic concepts underlying the clinical utility of captopril renography. It also presents an up-to-date synopsis of clinical observations of captopril renography as a screening tool for renovascular

CHAPTER 105

Magnetic Resonance Imaging of the Kidney

Patrick M. Colletti

Current magnetic resonance imaging (MRI) techniques allow for faster, better quality images of the kidneys. Advantages of MRI include the following:

1. Ability to characterize normal and pathologic tissues by their appearance on various pulse sequences
2. Excellent anatomic detail in multiple planes
3. No ionizing radiation
4. Availability of glomerular contrast agents without nephrotoxicity

MRI PHYSICS

Magnetic resonance requires atoms with nuclei containing odd numbers of protons and neutrons. These possess angular momentum and act as dipoles (tiny bar magnets with north and south poles) and therefore tend to align with an external magnetic field. The atom of most abundance and of practical use in MRI is hydrogen.

Hydrogen protons placed in a strong magnetic field (MRI unit) tend to align themselves along the plane of the field (Fig. 105.1A and B). These protons wobble (precess) at a specific frequency dependant on the magnetic field strength applied. This precession results in a net magnetic vector within the patient in the direction and orientation of the main magnetic vector of the imaging unit. The deflection of this net vector and its subsequent return to the resting state are the basis of MRI signal generation.

Energy in the form of radio frequency (RF) pulses of a specific frequency and duration are applied to displace the net magnetic vector from its longitudinal, or resting state, into the transverse plane. RF is applied and received by groups of wires (coils) placed within the magnet. These coils therefore act as transmitters and receivers (Fig. 105.1C and D). With time, the deflected net magnetization vector will return to its original longitudinal orientation. This return to or regrowth of longitudinal magnetization is referred to as *T1 relaxation.* The T1 relaxation in milliseconds is the time required for it to recover 63% of its longitudinal magnetization (Fig. 105.2). Simultaneous with the regrowth of longitudinal magnetization, a second process is

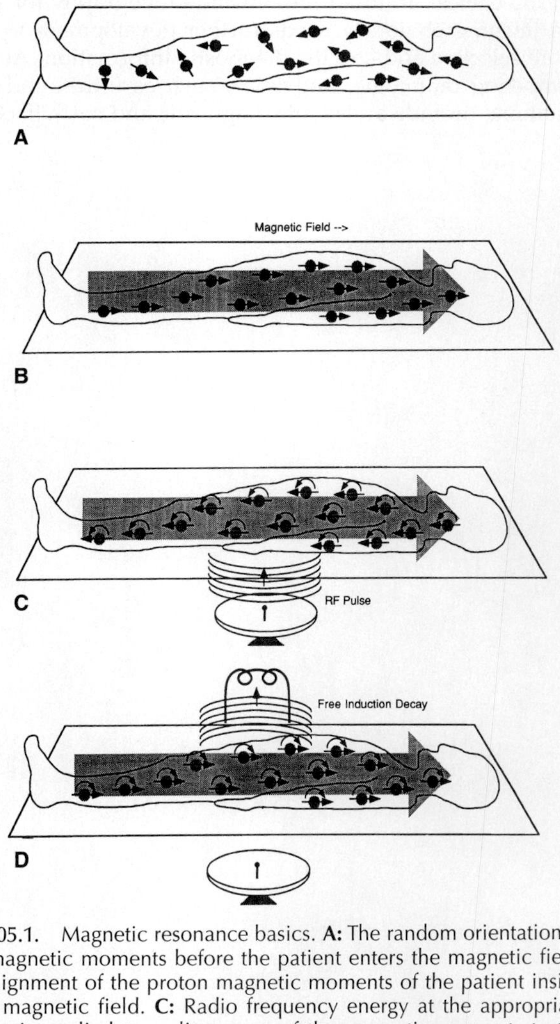

Figure 105.1. Magnetic resonance basics. **A:** The random orientation of proton magnetic moments before the patient enters the magnetic field. **B:** The alignment of the proton magnetic moments of the patient inside a strong magnetic field. **C:** Radio frequency energy at the appropriate frequency is applied to realign some of the magnetic moments to the higher energy state opposing the main magnetic field. **D:** The magnetic moments relax back to the lower energy state while giving off a characteristic radio frequency signal. This is the signal used to create magnetic resonance images.

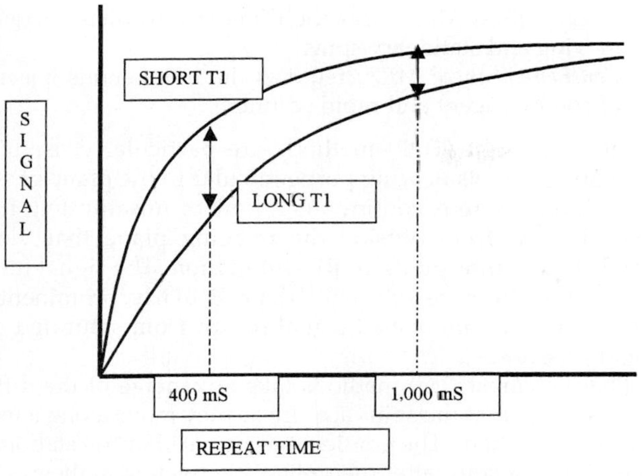

Figure 105.2. T1 relaxation effects. The longitudinal magnetization for tissues with faster longitudinal relaxation (short T1) and slower longitudinal relaxation (long T1) relax at different rates and give off different signals, depending on the repeat time. This difference may be more at a TR of 400 ms and less at a TR of 1,000 ms.

occurring. The initial RF pulse, in addition to displacing the net magnetic vector into the transverse plane, forces the majority of the precessing protons to precess together in phase. Immediately after cessation of the RF pulse, the various component magnetization vectors that form the net vector begin to be affected by the variations in magnetic field lines of flux that are present inherently in the imaging system as well as the tissue themselves. This causes the different protons to precess at varying rates. In time, more and more protons fall out of phase with each other and the net magnetization vector of the transverse plane begins to decrease in magnitude. This is *T2 relaxation.* The time required to decrease the tissues transverse magnetization to 37% of its peak value after the administration of an RF pulse in milliseconds is a tissue's T2 relaxation value (Fig. 105.3). The T1 and T2 effects work together to give a final image contrast (Fig. 105.4). The signal characteristics of different tissues are summarized in Table 105.1.

Protons placed in a magnetic field precess at a frequency that is dependent on the strength of the field and a gyromagnetic

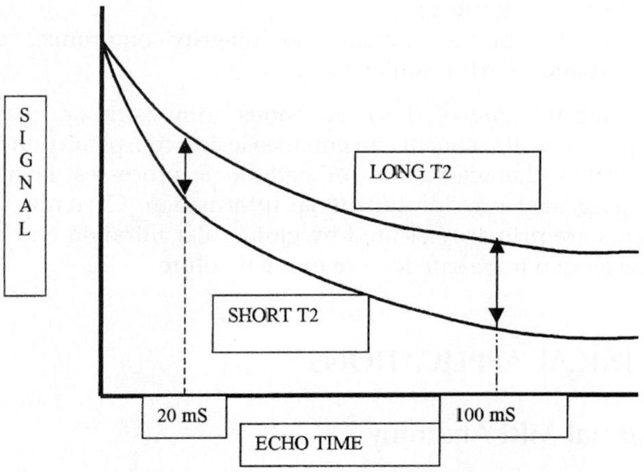

Figure 105.3. T2 relaxation effects. The transverse magnetization is less for tissues with faster (short T2) and more for slower (long T2) relaxation. Images at longer echo times (100 ms) show more differences between tissues with different T2 relaxation rates than do those at shorter echo times (20 ms).

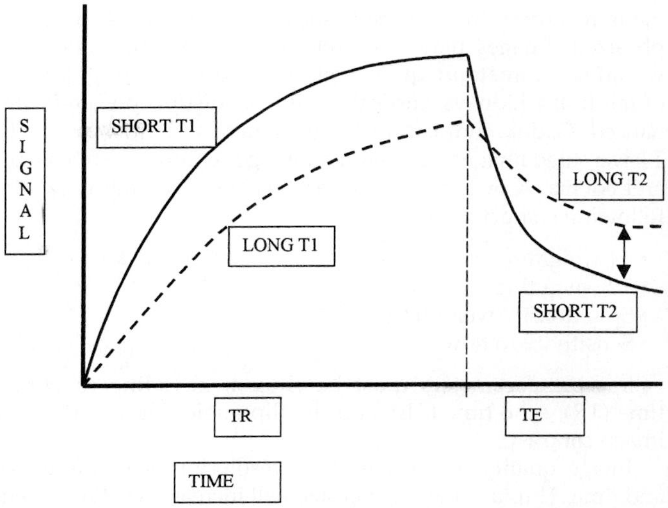

Figure 105.4. Transverse magnetization as related relative MRI signal. The combined effects on the overall signal for relatively short T1 and T2 substances versus relatively long T1 and long T2 substances depend on the TR and TE chosen.

TABLE 105.1. Tissue Magnetic Resonance Signal Characteristics

Tissue	T1-Weighted Sequence	T2-Weighted Sequence
Fat	Bright	Intermediate
Water (urine, cerebrospinal fluid, edema)	Dark	Bright
Air	Dark	Dark
Muscle	Intermediate	Intermediate
Fibrous tissue	Dark	Dark
Proteinaceous fluid	Bright	Bright
Melanin	Bright	Bright
Gadolinium	Bright	Bright
Iron	Dark	Dark

constant that is specific for each atomic nucleus. Application of a magnetic field gradient superimposed on the uniform main magnetic field results in a spectrum of precessional frequencies. This spectrum can be used to localize an imaging slice as well as to define the location of the signal returned after excitation. Selection of an imaging plane, identification of slices to be imaged, and spatial localization of the information returned from the excitation of the volume of interest requires specialized techniques. In MRI, this is accomplished by using magnetic field gradients (magnetic fields of progressively changing intensity) to increase or decrease to precessional frequency of spins in a linear fashion. This change in a spins frequency with location is used to mark its position in space. Advanced computer software and hardware techniques are then used to transform the RF energy being returned from the imaging volume (the spin echo or gradient echo) into a format that can be displayed on a screen, manipulated, and subsequently captured on film.

MRI IMAGING STRATEGIES

MRI uses preset imaging parameters to generate images with properties and attributes that best characterize the anatomy and potential disease processes to be evaluated. A decision must be made regarding the specific tissues and pathologies to be emphasized. Images may have relative T1 weighting and thus would show anatomy quite well, outlined by the bright signal of fat. In the kidneys, cortical-medullary distinction can be enhanced. Gadolinium contrast agents are also best shown with T1-weighted images. T2-weighted images emphasize free water and edema. A pulse sequence can be chosen to emphasize the following characteristics:

- T1 weighting
- T2 weighting
- Spin density weighting
- Sensitivity to flow

Specific parameters must be chosen, including repetition time (TR), echo time (TE), and the flip angle. These will affect image contrast.

Image quality is a trade-off of resolution, signal-to-noise, and time. Thus a smaller voxel size will increase resolution generally at the expense of signal to noise ratio and time. Typically, imaging times within the abdomen are from 1 second to 10 minutes, depending on the technique chosen. Obviously, faster imaging techniques can allow breath holding and motion-free studies, whereas more time-consuming sequences may yield better image contrast and resolution.

Conventional spin echo techniques consist of initial application of a 90° RF pulse of a specific frequency range and duration that displaces the magnetization vector in the slice or slab of interest into the transverse plane. Subsequently, a second 180° RF pulse is applied to rephase the component vectors of the transverse plane. A signal is generated (spin echo) that can be detected by a receiver coil. The time in milliseconds between two successive 90° pulses is the TR. The time in milliseconds between the 90° RF pulse and the generation of the spin echo is the TE. These are the most time-consuming pulse sequences, and current procedures apply multiple 180° RF pulses to acquire larger amounts of data for a given time. These so-called fast spin echo techniques can reduce acquisition time several-fold. This technique, pushed to its limit, can produce a so-called single shot fast spin echo image in 1 to 10 seconds.

Gradient echo techniques consist of the application of an RF pulse that displaces the longitudinal magnetization vector less than 90° (alpha pulse). The amount that the longitudinal vector is displaced into the transverse plane in degrees is called *a flip angle.* Subsequently, a magnetic field gradient rather than a 180° RF pulse is used to rephase the magnetization vectors in the transverse plane. The echo produced is called a *gradient echo.* These images are generally acquired more rapidly than spin echo images, and with currently available procedures, multislice abdominal examinations can be finished in a 20-second breath hold. Single, thick-slice (slab), fat-suppressed T2-weighted images can be acquired during a breath hold, in the coronal plane to create a magnetic resonance urogram.

Information can be acquired in either a two- or three-dimensional fashion. Three-dimensional (volume) acquisitions permit the imaging of smaller structures in greater detail with the retrospective division of data into slices of various orientations.

MAGNETIC RESONANCE ANGIOGRAPHY

There are three basic magnetic resonance angiography (MRA) techniques currently available:

1. *Time of flight MRA:* depends on bulk flow of spins into and out of the area being imaged
2. *Phase contrast MRA:* uses the difference in phase between moving and stationary spins
3. *Contrast-enhanced MRA:* requires the intravenous injection of contrast agent and rapid scanning

Time of flight (TOF) methods are particularly useful in evaluating vessels flowing perpendicular to the plane of slice acquisition. There is continuous inflow of unsaturated, fully relaxed spins from outside the imaging plane that yields a high signal in response to RF stimulation. The signal intensity within these vessels will be particularly prominent in contrast to the diminished signal return from saturated stationary tissues.

Phase contrast (PC) methods take advantage of the difference in phase that the spins acquire as they move along a magnetic field gradient. The gradient has no net effect on stationary spins. Moving spins alter their phases in relation to their direction and velocity of travel. This information can be manipulated to give both quantitative and directional information. PC techniques result in excellent background suppression but generally require increased imaging time and increased sensitivity to motion.

Contrast-enhanced MRA uses pulse sequences, which severely suppress nonenhanced tissue. The T1 of stationary blood is approximately 1,200 ms, whereas the T1 of contrast-enhanced blood is approximately 300 ms. With proper timing, a bolus of contrast agent within the blood vessel will markedly increase the intravascular signal. These techniques have the advantage of rapid acquisition, excellent background suppression, and excellent vascular edge demonstration.

PARAMAGNETIC CONTRAST ENHANCEMENT

Magnetic resonance contrast agents are paramagnetic. They have unpaired electrons and therefore alter the local magnetic environment of a tissue in which they accumulate. Their primary effect is T1 shortening, which results in areas of increased brightness on T1-weighted images. Beyond a certain concentration, T2-shortening effects predominate, resulting in decreased signal intensities. This effect is typically seen as a layering of signal intensities in the renal pelvis and urinary bladder after intravenous contrast administration. These so-called extracellular agents require the following three conditions for enhancement:

1. Regional perfusion
2. Capillary basement membrane integrity compromise
3. Expanded extracellular space

Static imaging of the intravenous administration of paramagnetic contrast agent can enhance lesion conspicuity and aid in further characterization of pathologic processes. Dynamic imaging may provide functional information. Currently used agents are primarily cleared by glomerular filtration and have been shown to be safe for use in renal failure.

CLINICAL APPLICATIONS

Normal MRI Anatomy

The axial plane (Fig. 105.5A) demonstrates the short axis of the kidneys and a cross-sectional view of the aorta and inferior vena cava. The axial view is analogous to the well-known cross-sections from computed tomography.

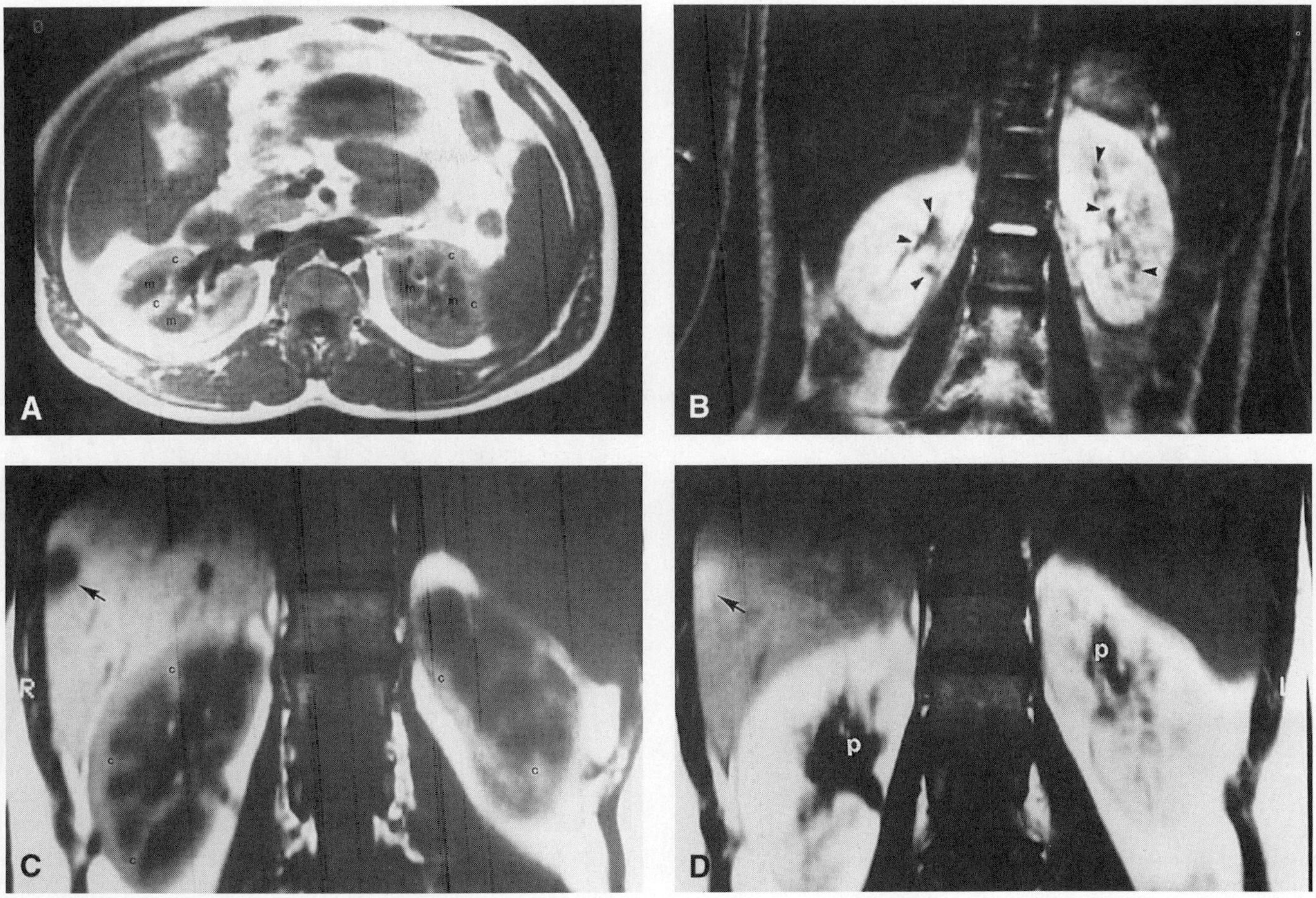

Figure 105.5. Normal kidneys. Axial T1 **(A),** TR 400, TE 20, shows the normal cortical *(c)* medullary *(m)* distinction. Coronal T2-weighted images **(B),** TR 2000, TE 100, shows the kidneys to be uniform high signal. Low-signal tubular structures *(arrowheads)* represent blood vessels. Coronal precontrast **(C)** and postcontrast **(D)** T1-weighted images, TR 400, TE 20, show that the cortical medullary distinction seen on precontrast images is lost on the postcontrast images. There is uniform enhancement of the kidneys with high signal in the cortex and medulla. The very high concentration of contrast agent in the renal collecting system *(p)* is due to extreme T2 shortening. Incidental hemangioma of the liver is noted *(arrow).*

The coronal view (Fig. 105.5B, C, and D) demonstrates urinary anatomy in a projection that is most similar to intervenous urography. Kidneys are again well shown in T1-weighted images surrounded by high signal fat. The renal cortex is generally higher in signal than the renal medulla (Fig. 105.5C). Contrast-enhanced images initially show the renal cortex dramatically, but delayed images (Fig. 105.5D) show uniformed enhancement of the kidney. There may be either a high signal or very low signal within the collecting system depending on the concentration of contrast agent. Very concentrated contrast agents cause signal reduction due to shortened T2 relaxation. Because the kidney contains a great deal of water, T2-weighted images (Fig. 105.5B) generally show uniform high signal throughout the renal parenchyma.

Renal vessels are seen as linear and serpiginous areas of signal void on spin echo images. A very bright signal is seen from the fat in the renal pelvis surrounding the lower signal of the renal collecting structures. Perinephric fat surrounds the kidney and includes the adrenal all within Gerota's fascia, which may occasionally be shown as a low-signal structure. The renal arteries may be followed to the aorta while the more anterior renal veins may be connected to the inferior vena cava. Adrenals are situated adjacent to the superior aspect of both kidneys.

Prerenal Abnormalities

Renal vascular abnormalities can now be well demonstrated with MRI and MRA. A renal vein thrombosis is easily demonstrated, as is tumor invasion into the inferior vena cava.

MRA is becoming the examination of choice for the noninvasive evaluation of renal vascular disease. Contrast-enhanced MRA is a reliable technique to demonstrate renal artery stenosis (Figs. 105.6 and 105.7).

Renal Abnormalities

Renal size may be determined with MRI in a manner similar to that used with ultrasound. Diffusely abnormal kidneys can be demonstrated, as for example with the low signal in the renal cortex in patients with myoglobinuria (Fig. 105.8). Diffuse renal disease may cause a loss of cortical medullary distinction on T1-weighted images.

Focal lesions such as nephron loss from chronic pyelonephritis (Fig. 105.9) can be well shown, as can signal space-occupying lesions such as renal angiomyolipoma (Fig. 105.10) or renal cell carcinoma (Fig. 105.11). Multifocal abnormalities such as polycystic kidneys (Fig. 105.12) are also well demonstrated as are associated cysts in other organs.

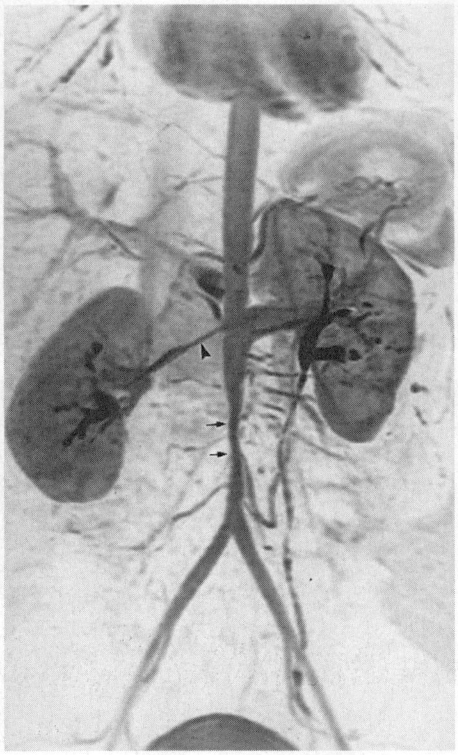

Figure 105.6. This 18-year-old female with a known history of Takayasu's arteritis presents with a blood pressure of 160/94 mm Hg. Contrast-enhanced breath-held MRA shows stenosis of the distal aorta *(arrows)* and stenosis of the right renal artery *(arrowhead).*

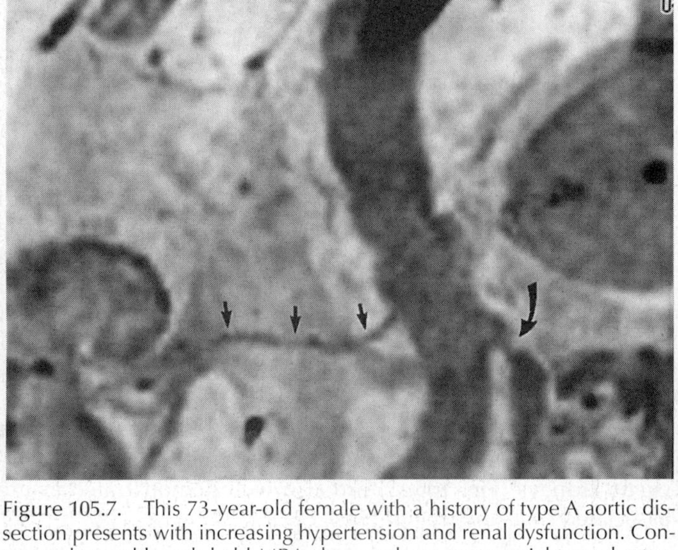

Figure 105.7. This 73-year-old female with a history of type A aortic dissection presents with increasing hypertension and renal dysfunction. Contrast-enhanced breath-held MRA shows a long, narrow right renal artery *(arrows)* and a focal stenosis in the left renal artery *(curved arrow).*

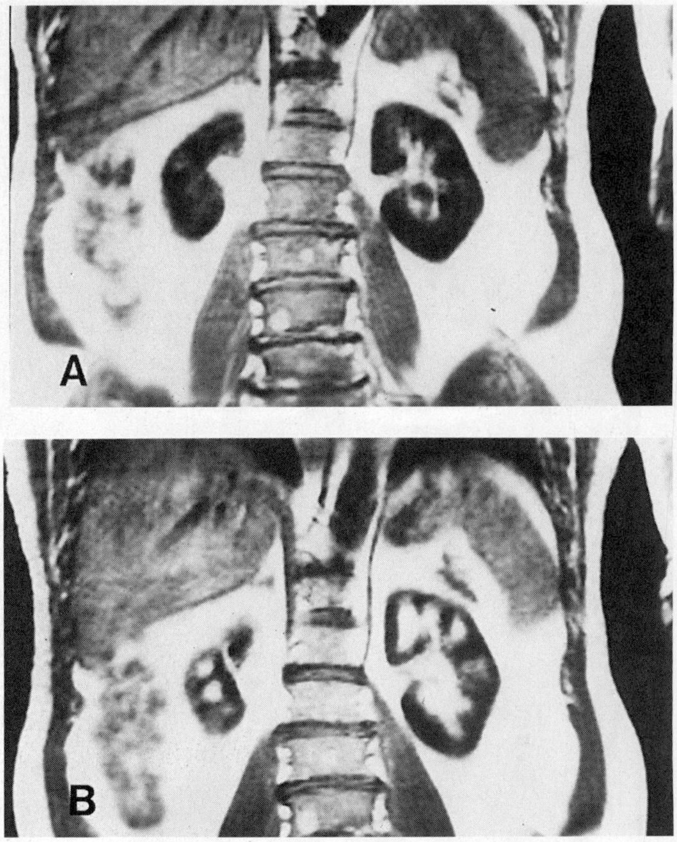

Figure 105.8. Myoglobinuria. Coronal precontrast **(A)** and postcontrast **(B)** enhanced TR 500 TE 20 T1-weighted images in a patient with very low signal renal parenchyma and loss of the corticomedullary distinction due to the very short relaxation time of the iron in myoglobin. Medullary contrast enhancement is seen in **B.**

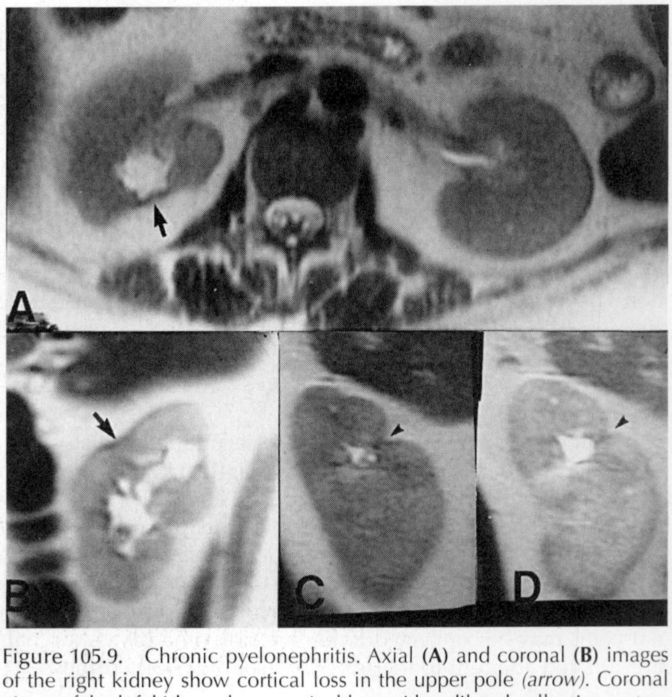

Figure 105.9. Chronic pyelonephritis. Axial **(A)** and coronal **(B)** images of the right kidney show cortical loss in the upper pole *(arrow).* Coronal views of the left kidney show cortical loss with a dilated collecting system in the upper pole *(arrowhead).*

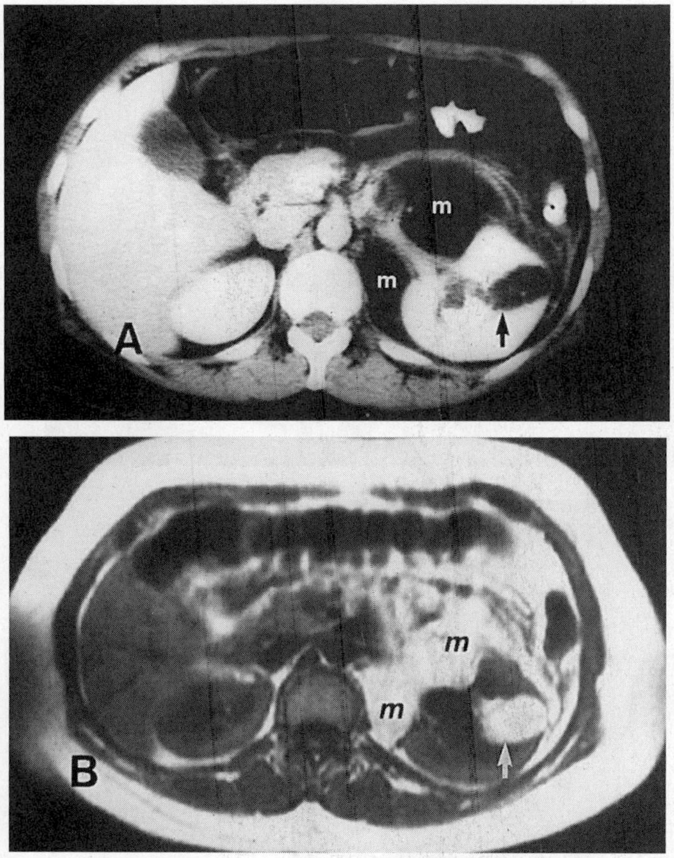

Figure 105.10. Angiomyolipoma. Computed tomography **(A)** and T1-weighted MRI **(B)**, TR 400 TE 20, images show intrarenal *(arrow)* and perirenal *(m)* masses of low attenuation on computed tomography and high signal in T1-weighted images due to their fat content.

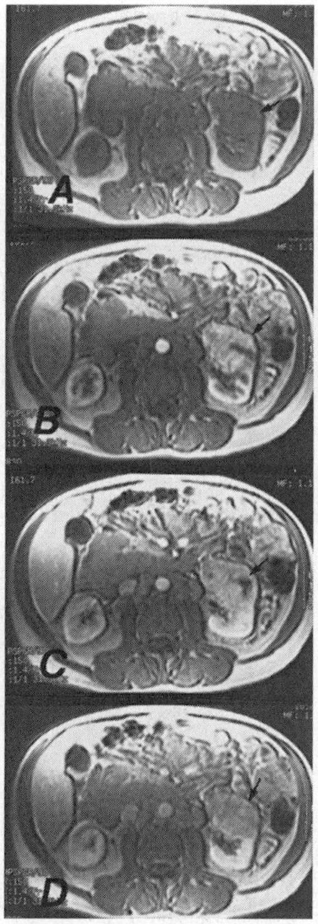

Figure 105.11. Renal cell carcinoma. Sequential contrast-enhanced spoiled GRASS images of the abdomen with breath hold during administration of contrast agent shows the sequential enhancement of the normal kidneys and the rapid enhancement of left renal mass *(arrow)*. Note that the mass enhances early with the renal cortex and medulla and washes out much more rapidly than the normal kidney.

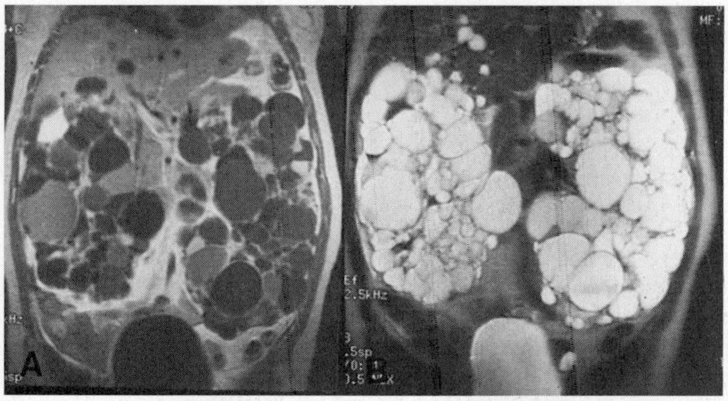

Figure 105.12. Polycystic renal disease. Coronal T1 **(A)** and T2 **(B)**, axial T1 **(C, D, F, H)**, and T2 weighted images **(E, G)** show innumerable bilateral renal cysts. Some of the cysts show high signal on T1-weighted images. These likely represent hemorrhagic cysts. Multiple liver cysts are also identified.

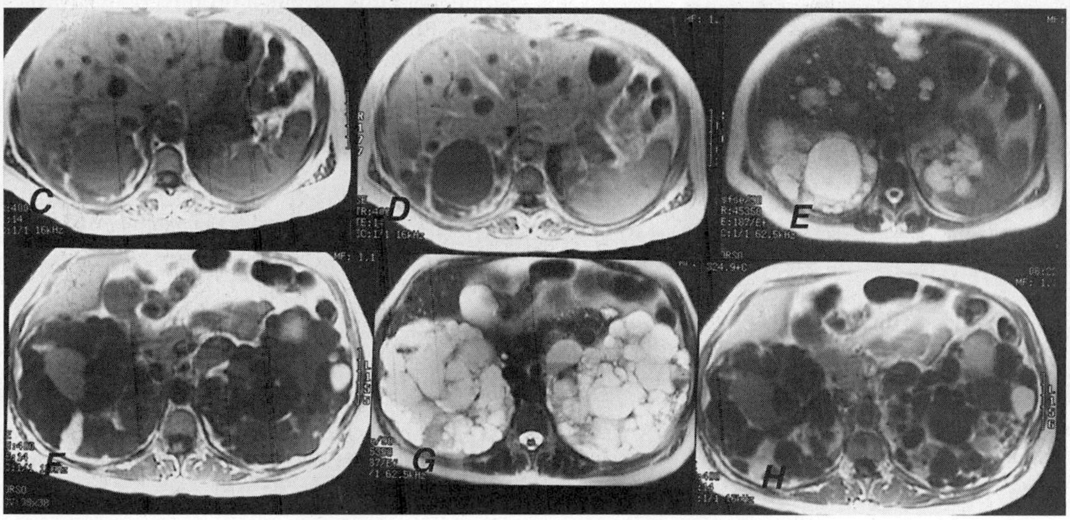

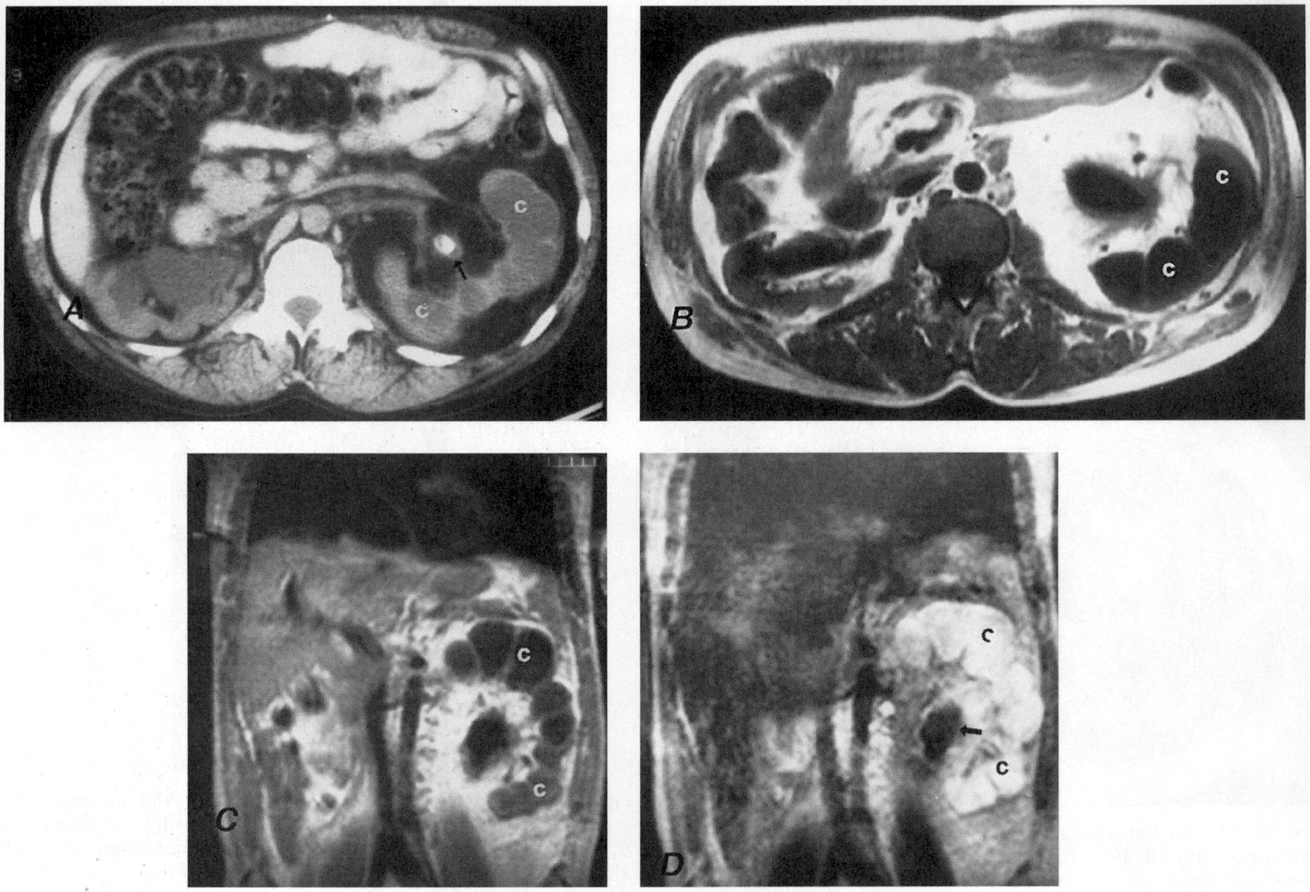

Figure 105.13. Xanthogranulomatosis pyelonephritis. Abdominal computed tomography scan with contrast (**A**) shows a calcified renal pelvis stone *(arrow)*. Axial T1-weighted image (**B**) and coronal T1 (**C**) and T2 (**D**) images show an enlarged left kidney with dilated collecting system and calices *(c)*. The renal stone is shown as a low signal in the renal pelvis on image **D.** Similar findings are noted in the right kidney.

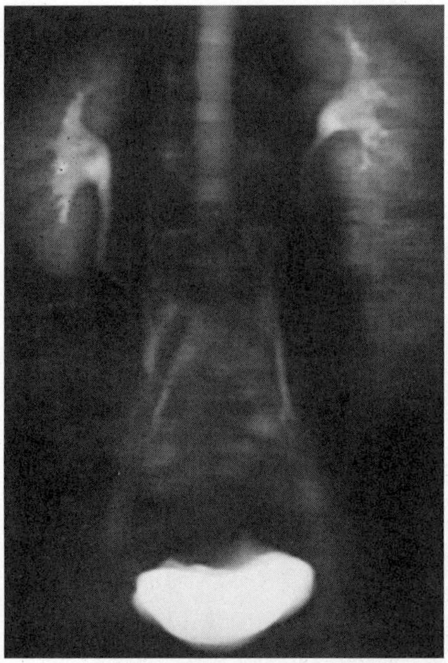

Figure 105.14. Magnetic resonance urography in a normal volunteer. High signal is noted in the collecting system and bladder in this single shot breath-held view.

Postrenal Abnormalities

Hydronephrosis is easily demonstrated with MRI (Fig. 105.13). Stones may be difficult to demonstrate with T1-weighted images, but T2-weighted images will generally be useful. Magnetic resonance urography, a new technique (Fig. 105.14), will probably be useful for demonstrating urinary stones. This may be helpful in patients with renal failure, but because most renal stones contain calcium, it is unlikely that MRI can compete with noncontrast computed tomography and even plain radiography for the demonstration of urolithiasis.

Selected Readings

Hashemi RH, Bradley WG. *MRI: the basics.* Baltimore: Williams & Wilkins, 1997.

This is an up-to-date text on the principles of MRI.

Haustein J, Niendorf HP, Krestin G, et al. Renal tolerance of gadolinium-DTPA/dimeglumine in patients with chronic renal failure. *Invest Radiol* 1992; 27(2):153–156.

Initial studies showed the safety of gadolinium DTPA in 21 patients with impaired renal function.

Kettritz U, Semelka RC, Brown ED, et al. MR findings in diffuse renal parenchymal disease. *J Magn Reson Imaging* 1996;6(1):136–144.

Although no pathognomonic features could be found, it may be helpful in the differential diagnosis of renal parenchymal diseases.

Low RN, Martinez AG, Steinberg SM, et al. Potential renal transplant donors: evaluations with gadolinium-enhanced MR angiography and MR urography. *Radiology* 1998;207(1):165–172.

This paper describes a technique for combined gadolinium-enhanced MRA, magnetic resonance urography, and magnetic resonance nephrography. Complete evaluation of renal transplant.

Prince MR, Arnoldus C, Frisoli JK. Nephrotoxicity of high dose gadolinium compared with iodinated contrast. *J Magn Reson Imaging* 1996;6(1):162–166.

This study showed the safety of high-dose gadolinium chelates compared with iodinated contrast agent; 342 patients were evaluated. High-dose gadolinium chelates are significantly less nephrotoxic than iodinated contrast. None of the patients receiving gadolinium chelate experienced renal failure. Eleven of 64 patients with iodinated contrast had contrast-induced renal failure. High-dose gadolinium chelates are significantly less nephrotoxic than iodinated contrast.

Prince MR, Schoenberg SO, Ward JS, et al. Hemodynamically significant atherosclerotic renal artery stenosis: MR angiographic features. *Radiology* 1997;205: 128–136.

The use of contrast-enhanced breath-held MRA for the evaluation of atherosclerotic renal artery stenosis is described.

Regan F, Bohlman ME, Khazan R, et al. MR urography using HASTE imaging in the assessment of ureteric obstruction. *AJR* 1996;167(5):1115–1120.

This study describes a breath-held single shot turbo spin-echo imaging in the assessment of uroteric obstruction. Perirenal fluid can be demonstrated in acute obstruction.

Rofsky NM, Bosniak MA. MR imaging in the evaluation of small renal masses. *Magn Reson Imaging Clin North Am* 1997;5(1):67–81.

Renal cell carcinoma is described.

Taylor J, Summers PE, Keevil SF, et al. Magnetic resonance renography: Optimisation of pulse sequence parameters and Gd-DTPA dose, and comparison with radionuclide renography. *Magn Reson Imaging* 1997;15(6):637–649.

Magnetic resonance renography using gadolinium DTPA compared with conventional radionuclide renography. Renograms were evaluated on the basis of time to peak signal, signal decrease after peak, and kidney function ratios.

CHAPTER 106

Diagnostic Use of Ultrasound in Kidney and Bladder

Yuri R. Parisky and Nabil A. Yassa

Ultrasound of the kidneys has become accepted as a valuable first-line diagnostic examination. In many circumstances, it has replaced intravenous pyelography as the initial diagnostic imaging examination. Today's ultrasound equipment allows the examiner to define normal anatomy, differentiate abnormal tissue or conditions, and evaluate regional perfusion in a noninvasive manner. In addition, while scanning the kidneys, the examiner can evaluate adjacent organs, such as the liver or pancreas, for potential pathology. Such a luxury is absent with the intravenous pyelogram.

BASIC PRINCIPLES AND INSTRUMENTATION

The use of ultrasound in medicine developed as an outgrowth of World War II Sound Navigation and Ranging (SONAR) technology. Diagnostic ultrasound uses sound waves, which are higher in frequency than the human ear can hear, greater than 20,000 Hertz (20,000 cycles per second). Medical sonography uses even higher frequencies of between 1 megahertz (one million cycles per second) and 15 megahertz.

Sound travels as a longitudinal waveform through regions of compression and rarefaction. It has a frequency and a wavelength, the product of which equals the speed it travels. The speed with which sound travels depends on the medium it passes through. In air, sound travels at 331 meters per second (741 miles per hour), and in human soft tissues at normal body temperature, sound travels at approximately 1,540 meters per second.

The ultrasound image is formed when a beam of sound is transmitted through tissues and is partially reflected back to the point of origin, creating what are termed *echoes.* These echoes arise from acoustic interfaces, which exist between tissues with different acoustic impedances. The interfaces may be quite large, even larger than the ultrasound beam, which results in strong echoes. This phenomenon is called *specular reflection.* Structures from which specular reflections originate are referred to as *specular reflectors* and include the renal capsule and bladder wall. When interfaces are smaller than the sound beam, nonspecular reflection occurs. These echoes are of lower amplitude and are generated, for instance, by small renal parenchymal structures. Information can be gathered only when a portion of the transmitted sound waves results in echoes. A strong reflection of sound waves close to the surface of the skin will allow no diagnostic information to be gathered from deeper tissues, while lack of acoustic impedance in fluid filled structures, such as the bladder or simple renal cyst, allows the sound beam to penetrate further, producing an image. When sound waves traverse fluid, they are attenuated less than in adjacent solid tissue, resulting in a relative increase in echoes distal to fluid containing structures. The term *increased through transmission* is used to describe this phenomenon. Use of fluid-filled structures such as the bladder or low-attenuating organs such as the liver (Fig. 106.1) to aid in imaging deeper organs, such as the adnexa or right kidney, is called *acoustic window–dependent ultrasound.*

An ultrasonic imaging device has three basic components: (a) a transducer to generate the ultrasound beam and receive the returning echoes, (b) a microprocessor-based data acquisition/signal processor, and (c) an image display system. A transducer, containing a piezoelectric crystal, which converts electrical energy into sound waves, forms the ultrasound beam. The crystal also serves as a receiver, detecting returning echoes and converting them into electrical impulses, which are processed and displayed as images.

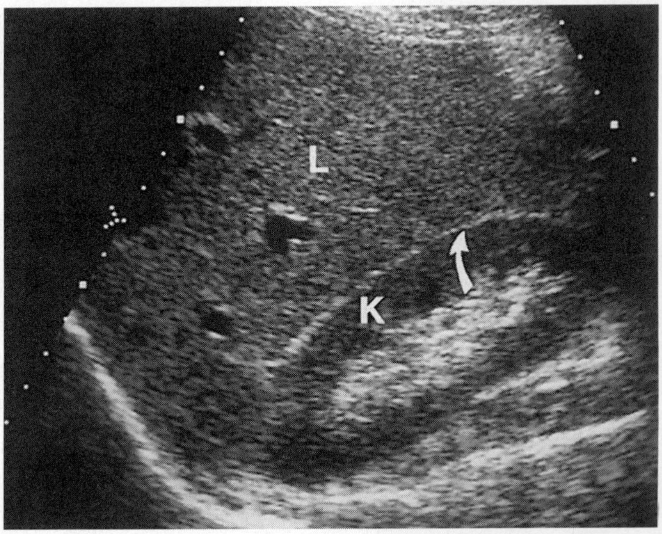

Figure 106.1. Coronal image of right kidney. The liver serves as an acoustic window in the ultrasonographic examination of the right kidney. *Curved arrow* points to the echogenic renal capsule. K, kidney; L, liver.

Modern ultrasound equipment uses a "real-time" display technique. Complete individual images are sequentially obtained and displayed in rapid sequence at a high frame rate, analogous to the process involved in motion pictures, allowing the actual motion of structures to be imaged. Arterial pulsations, cardiac contractions, and abdominal organ excursion secondary to respiration can be visualized as a result of this display technique.

Doppler ultrasound can assess venous and arterial blood flow; a technology based on the Doppler frequency shift signal. Flow velocity can be quantitatively assessed, as well as reproduced on gray-scale Doppler ultrasound images (Fig. 106.2). Arterial flow and vascular resistance in both the native and transplanted kidneys can be well demonstrated and of clinical utility in evaluating renal artery stenosis, renal vein thrombosis, renal transplant rejection, and other diseases. The Resistive Index (RI) is a means by which to quantify peripheral arterial resistance.

$$RI = \frac{\text{Peak systolic velocity} - \text{Lowest diastolic velocity}}{\text{Peak systolic velocity}}$$

Increased peripheral resistance is defined by an intrarenal RI of greater than 0.7. RI is a nonspecific indicator of disease, and its utility should be considered in the appropriate clinical context.

Renal Doppler ultrasound uses a lower frequency, usually 2 to 3 megahertz. Color Doppler ultrasound provides a computer-enhanced spectral flow pattern of the vasculature of the kidney (Fig. 106.3). This imaging modality is especially useful in detecting arteriovenous fistula and malformation, detecting thrombosis, and assessing tumor vascularity. It is also applicable in observing intravesicular ureteral jets in patients suspected of having urinary tract obstruction.

SCANNING TECHNIQUE

The benefits of using real-time ultrasound are demonstrated when it is used to scan the urinary tract. It has become a radiologic standard to obtain contiguous, sequential images at fixed intervals in orthogonal scanning planes and preserve them on film (hard copy). Appropriate notation regarding positioning and scanning parameters, along with real-time observations, should be included on representative hard copy images. Enthusiastic preservation of pathology is seldom met with criticism. Ultrasound images are displayed as white echoes on a black background (Fig. 106.4A).

Ultrasound real-time scanning can be recorded on videotape and the static images can be stored on a laser disc.

The right kidney is best imaged with the patient in supine position, using the liver as an acoustic window and obtaining longitudinal and axial images. Coronal views and views obtained along the posterior axillary line may also be used to visualize the entire right kidney. The left kidney is generally best imaged with the patient lying in a right lateral decubitus position using coronal views. Again, views obtained along the posterior axillary line may be necessary to see the kidney completely. The spleen may occasionally serve as an acoustic window. Variation in body habitus requires the ultrasonographer to be patient, persistent, and often times creative to obtain a satisfactory study. When performing an ultrasound-guided procedure, such as a renal biopsy or nephrostomy tube placement, the patient is best scanned while in the prone position and images obtained over both posterior flanks.

The bladder is best imaged when full, and that is accomplished by giving copious amounts of oral fluids before the examination or instilling saline via a urinary bladder catheter before the examination. Serial longitudinal and axial images are usually recorded at regular intervals.

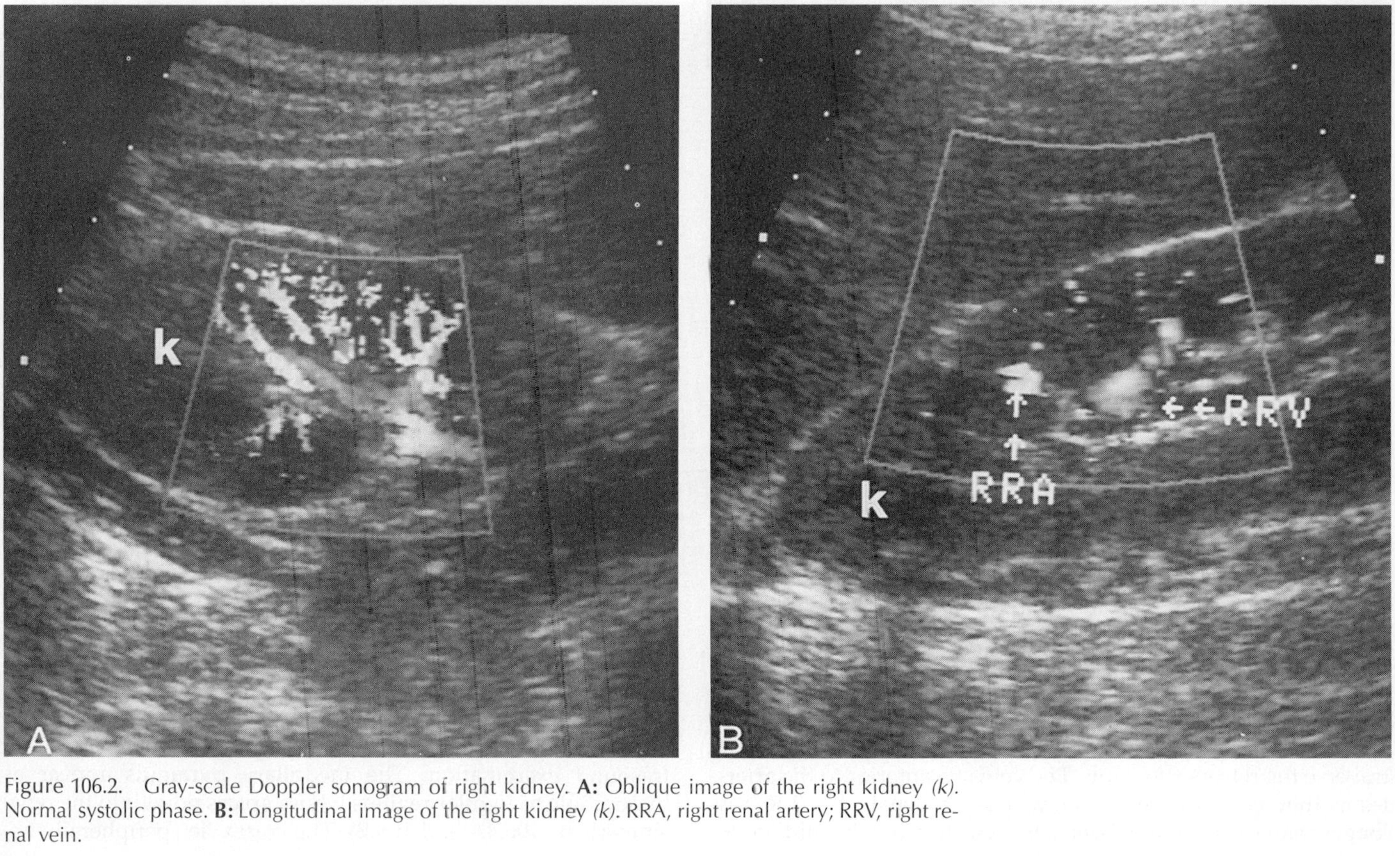

Figure 106.2. Gray-scale Doppler sonogram of right kidney. **A:** Oblique image of the right kidney *(k)*. Normal systolic phase. **B:** Longitudinal image of the right kidney *(k)*. RRA, right renal artery; RRV, right renal vein.

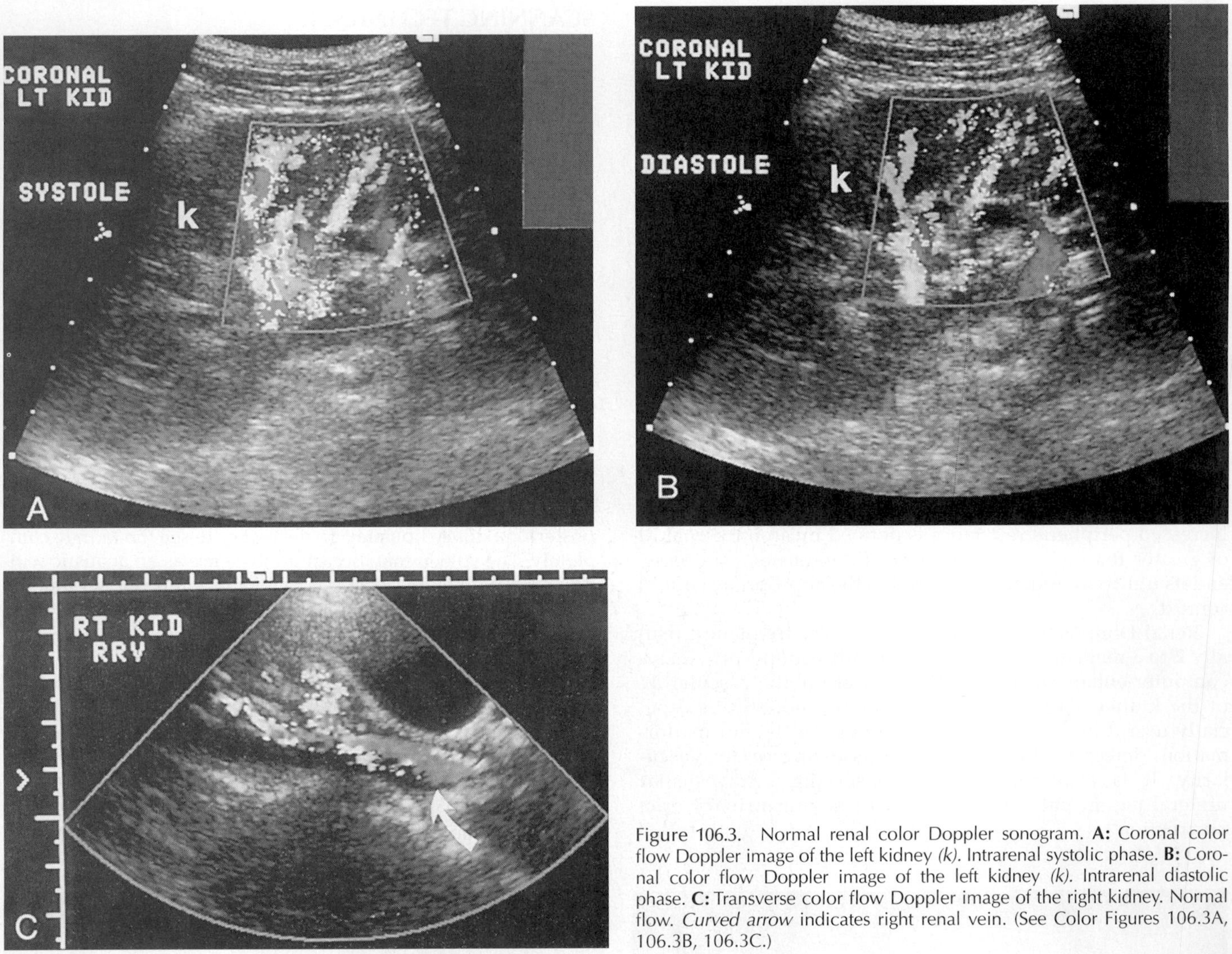

Figure 106.3. Normal renal color Doppler sonogram. **A:** Coronal color flow Doppler image of the left kidney *(k)*. Intrarenal systolic phase. **B:** Coronal color flow Doppler image of the left kidney *(k)*. Intrarenal diastolic phase. **C:** Transverse color flow Doppler image of the right kidney. Normal flow. *Curved arrow* indicates right renal vein. (See Color Figures 106.3A, 106.3B, 106.3C.)

NORMAL ANATOMY OF THE KIDNEYS

The kidneys are surrounded by Gerota's fascia, which defines the perinephric space in the retroperitoneum on either side of the spine. They are surrounded by perinephric fat, which varies in sonographic appearance from slightly less echogenic to highly echogenic compared with renal cortex. The renal capsule is most often identified as an echogenic line circumscribing the kidney (Fig. 106.1). The renal sinus, or hilum, is centrally located in the kidney and contains fat, arteries, veins, lymphatics, and the collecting system. In the normal patient, the renal hilum is predominantly echogenic due to the presence of fat, with the echogenic contour varying with the amount of fat present (Fig. 106.4A). Generally, increasing sinus fat is noted with age. Renal sinus lipomatosis (Fig. 106.5) is a normal variant manifested by greater-than-average amounts of sinus fat. Hypoechoic or anechoic tubular structures may be seen within the hilum, corresponding to fluid-filled vessels or collecting system components. Variation in kidney contour may be present. A duplicated kidney is present if cortical tissue separates the sinus fat (Figs. 106.6 and 106.7).

The renal veins and arteries can readily be identified as they traverse the retroperitoneum. The veins lie anterior to the arteries as they enter the renal hilum. The left renal vein (LRV) is longer than the right renal vein, as it has to cross the midline to empty into the inferior vena cava (IVC). Usually, the LRV crosses the midline between the superior mesenteric artery and the aorta. On occasion, the LRV is retroaortic (Fig. 106.8), circumaortic, or duplicated (Fig. 106.9). The right renal artery is usually the only artery dorsal to the IVC (Figs. 106.10 and 106.11), thus it is easier to identify than the left renal artery. Multiple arteries and veins may serve one kidney. Renal arteries branch within the kidney and are identified by color Doppler. The arcuate arteries are seen as echogenic foci at the corticomedullary junction.

A collapsed collecting system is difficult to detect within the echogenic renal hilum. When there is fullness or distension of the collecting system, as occurs with diuresis or obstruction, it can be identified as sonolucent branching structures within the hilum, which are connected to the renal pelvis. An extrarenal pelvis should not be confused with a dilated renal pelvis. For example, in pregnancy, mild collecting system dilation is expected and is more prominent on the right (Fig. 106.12). Only a short portion of the proximal ureter is normally imaged distal to the renal pelvis. If a longer portion is identified, it may be indicative of ureterectasis.

In children and many adults, components of the renal parenchyma, such as cortex and medulla, are often seen during an ultrasound examination. The medullary pyramids appear as hypoechoic triangular regions whose apices point into the renal sinus (Figs. 106.4A and 106.B). The cortex lies peripherally be-

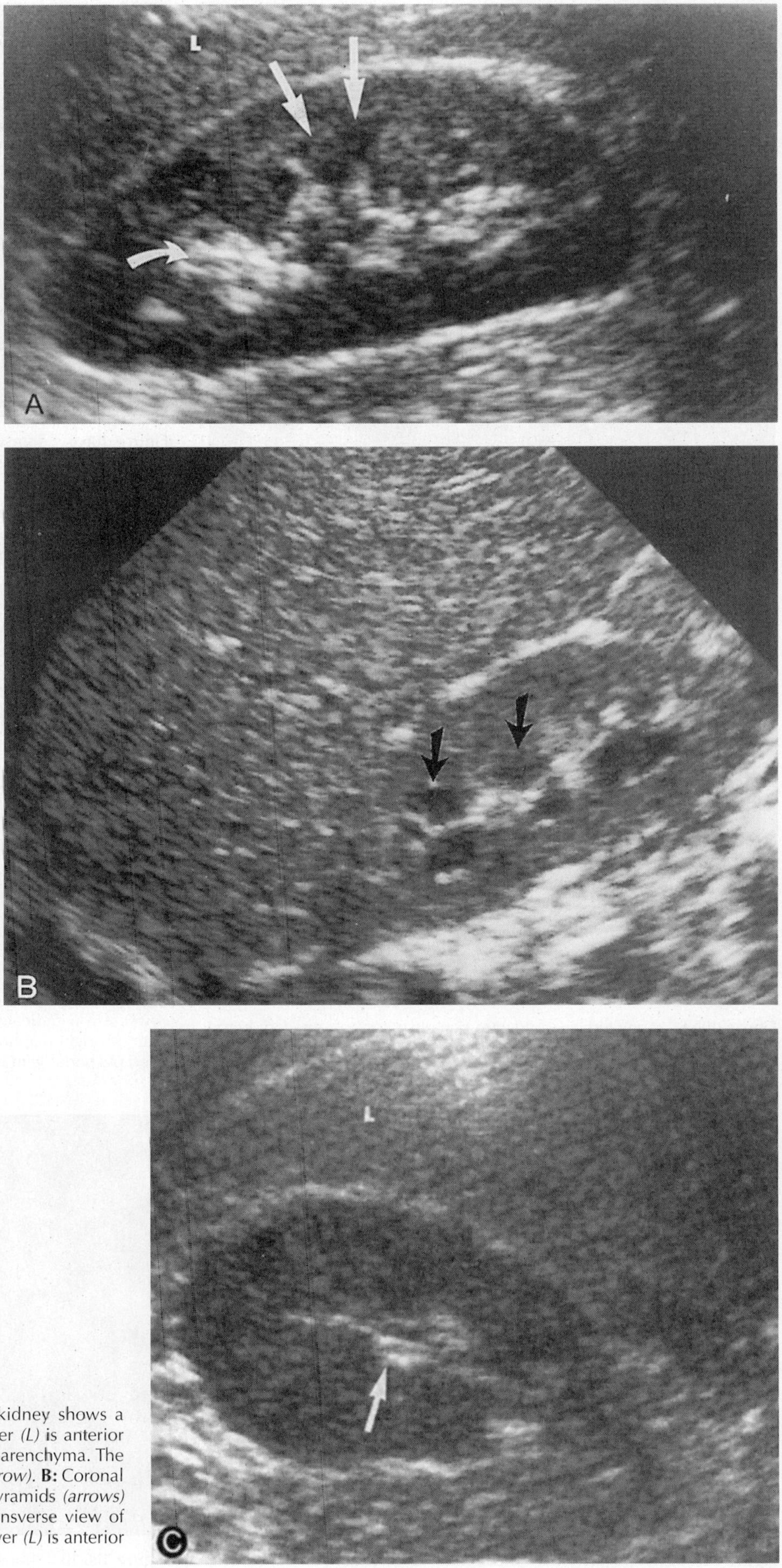

Figure 106.4. **A:** Coronal view of normal right kidney shows a triangular-shaped pyramid *(straight arrows)*. The liver *(L)* is anterior to the kidney and more echogenic than the renal parenchyma. The strongest echoes are from the renal sinus *(curved arrow)*. **B:** Coronal image of normal right kidney. Hypoechoic renal pyramids *(arrows)* should not be confused for dilated calyces. **C:** Transverse view of normal right kidney. Arrow points to renal sinus. Liver *(L)* is anterior to kidney.

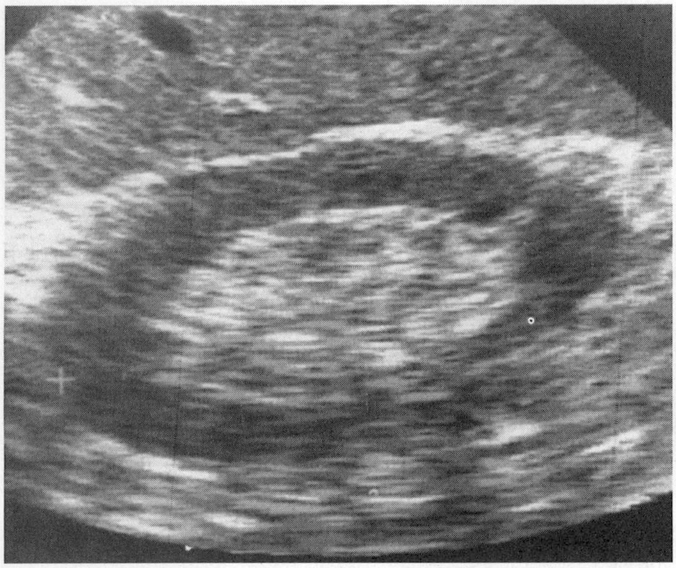

Figure 106.5. Longitudinal view of right kidney shows increased amount of renal sinus echoes caused by renal sinus lipomatosis.

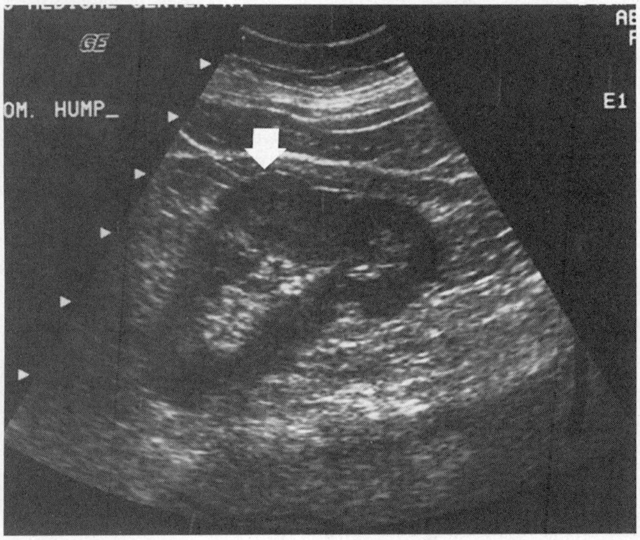

Figure 106.6. Longitudinal sonogram demonstrates a dromedary hump *(closed arrow),* a normal anatomic variant.

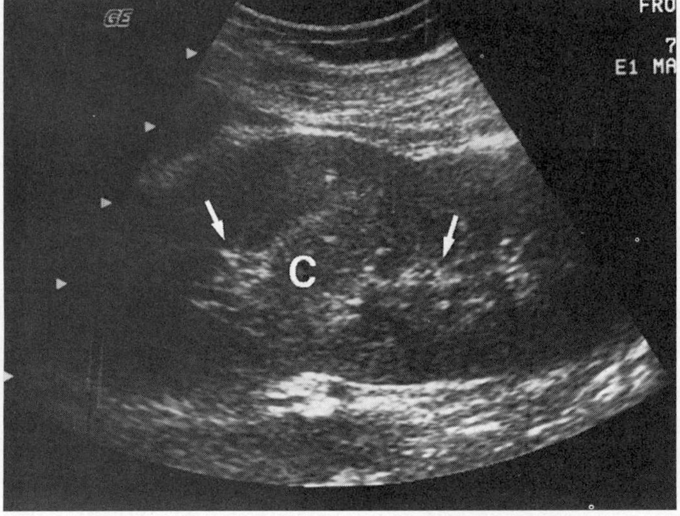

Figure 106.7. Duplicated kidney. Longitudinal sonogram of kidney with cortical tissue *(C)* separating the renal sinus fat.

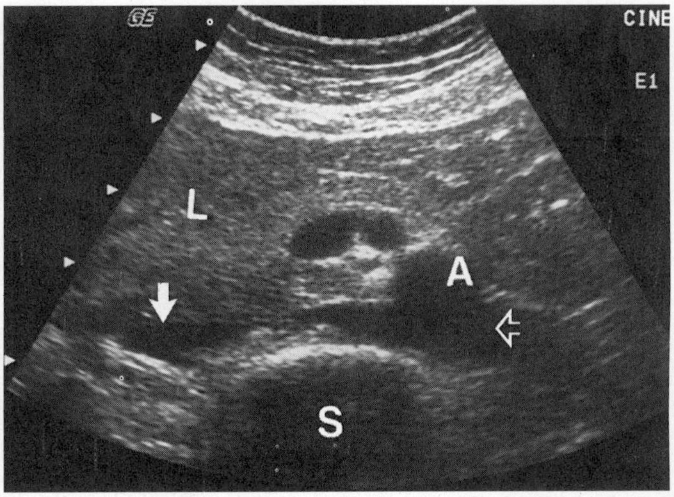

Figure 106.8. Transverse sonogram of retroaortic left renal vein *(open arrow). Closed arrow* indicates inferior vena cava. A, aorta; L, liver; S, spine.

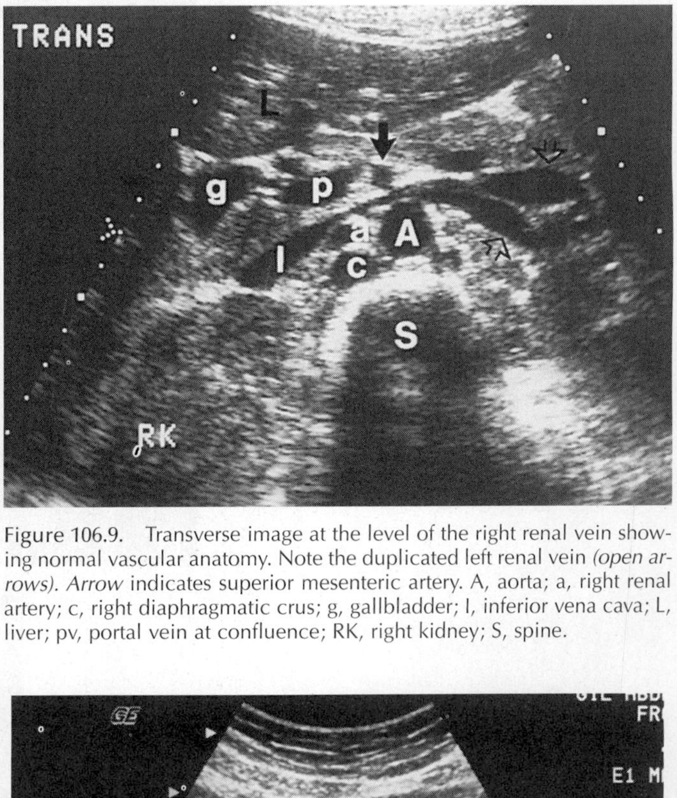

Figure 106.9. Transverse image at the level of the right renal vein showing normal vascular anatomy. Note the duplicated left renal vein *(open arrows). Arrow* indicates superior mesenteric artery. A, aorta; a, right renal artery; c, right diaphragmatic crus; g, gallbladder; I, inferior vena cava; L, liver; pv, portal vein at confluence; RK, right kidney; S, spine.

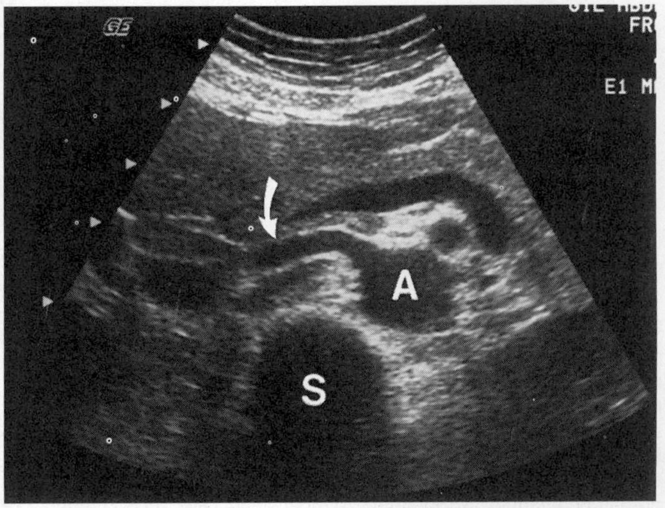

Figure 106.10. Transverse sonogram of right renal artery *(curved arrow).* A, aorta; S, spine.

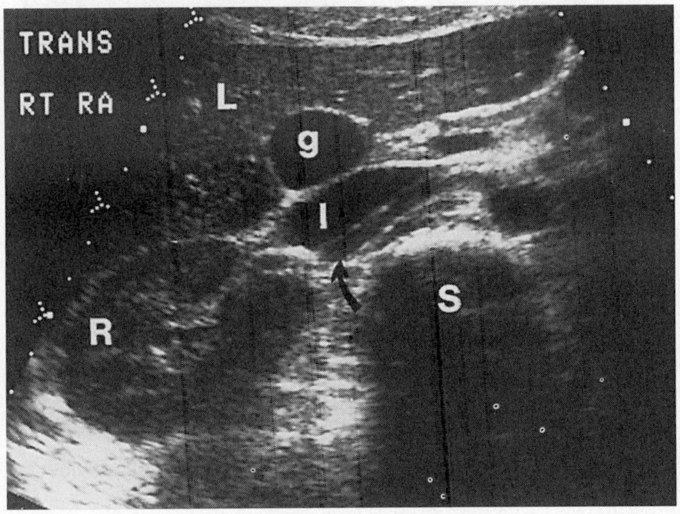

Figure 106.11. Transverse image shows right renal artery *(curved arrow)* dorsal to inferior vena cava *(I)*. g, gallbladder; L, liver; R, right kidney; S, spine.

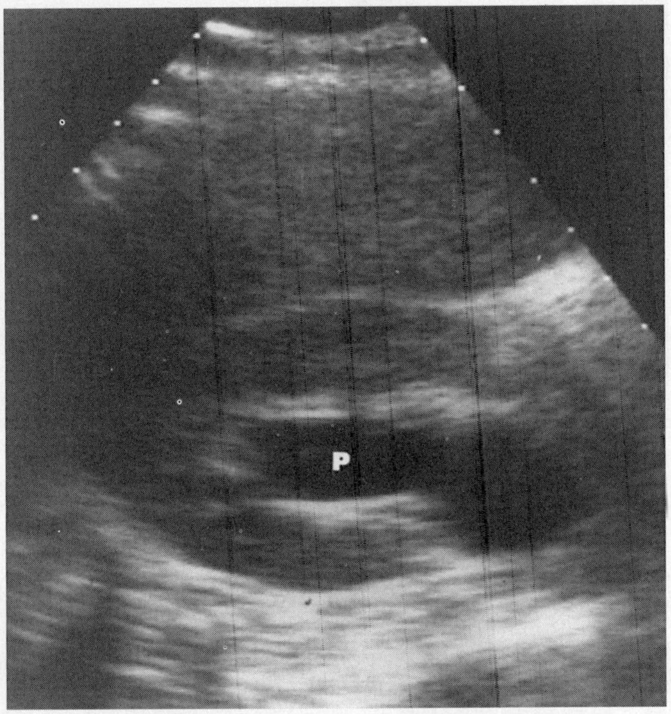

Figure 106.12. Transverse sonogram through right kidney of a pregnant patient shows mild dilation of the renal pelvis *(p)*.

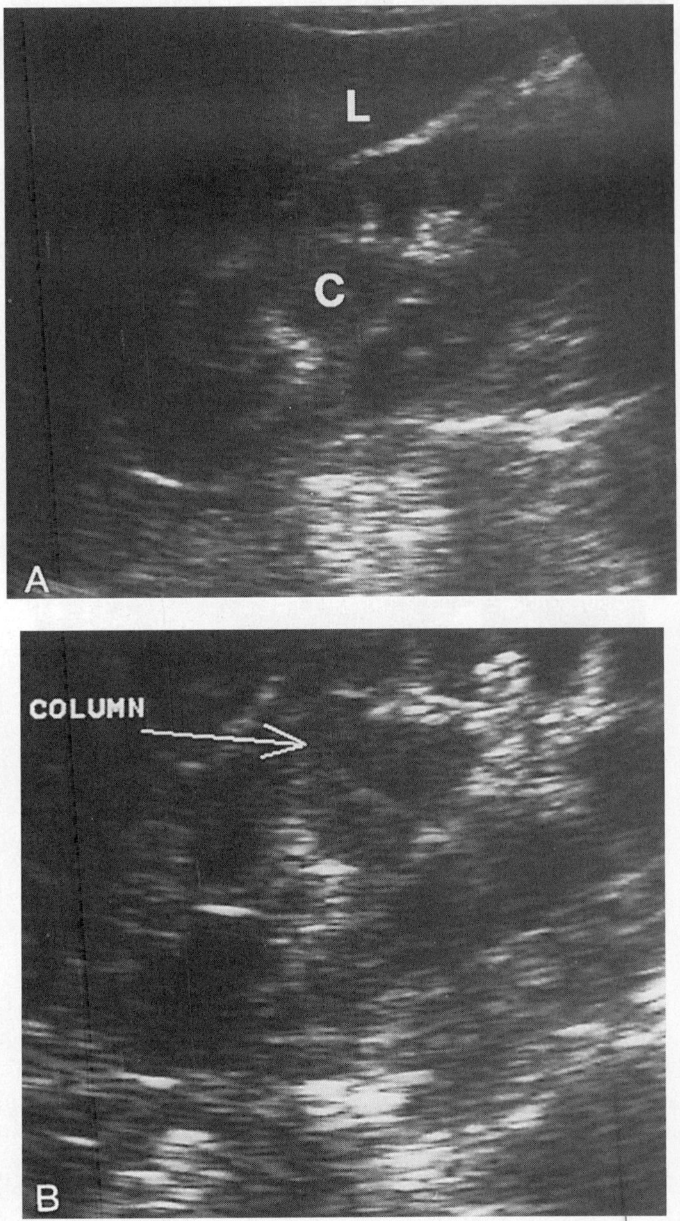

Figure 106.13. Column of Bertin. **A:** Longitudinal scan of right kidney demonstrates hypertrophied column of Bertin. Note that it is isoechoic with normal renal cortex and that it protrudes into the central sinus echoes. **B:** Longitudinal image of right kidney is technically magnified to better demonstrate the column of Bertin. C, Column of Bertin; L, liver.

tween the medulla and renal capsule, as well as between the medullary pyramids (columns of Bertin). Occasionally, a column of Bertin may be larger than usual and simulate a mass; this is known as a *pseudotumor.* The key to accurately diagnosing this presentation is noting that renal columns generally have identical texture, vascular pattern, and echogenicity as the adjacent cortex and are continuous with it; column of Bertin are usually located at the junction of the upper third with the lower two-thirds of the kidney and bulge into the sinus fat, but not externally (Fig. 106.13). If confusion as to structure persists, imaging with another modality, such as computed tomography (CT), magnetic resonance imaging (MRI), or nuclear renography, often clarifies the diagnosis. The kidneys may fuse or e ectopic in location (Figs. 106.14, 106.15, and 106.16). In the normal adult, the renal cortex gives off fine, low-level echoes and is somewhat more echogenic than the renal medulla (pyramids) (Fig. 106.4). In the neonate, the renal cortical echoes are at least as echogenic as the liver and spleen parenchyma (Fig. 106.17), this pattern occasionally persisting into adolescence. By adulthood, the renal cortex is equal to or lesser in echogenicity than the liver or spleen. In normal adults, the following spectrum of tissue echogenicity, from greater to lesser, holds true:

$$\text{Renal sinus} > \text{pancreas} > \text{liver} > \text{spleen} > \text{renal cortex} > \text{renal medulla}$$

Ultrasound is an excellent means to determine renal size. In the longest dimension, the normal right kidney is 11 cm ± 1 cm and the normal left kidney is 11.5 cm ± 1 cm. Neonatal kidneys are approximately 5 cm in their longest dimension. Between the

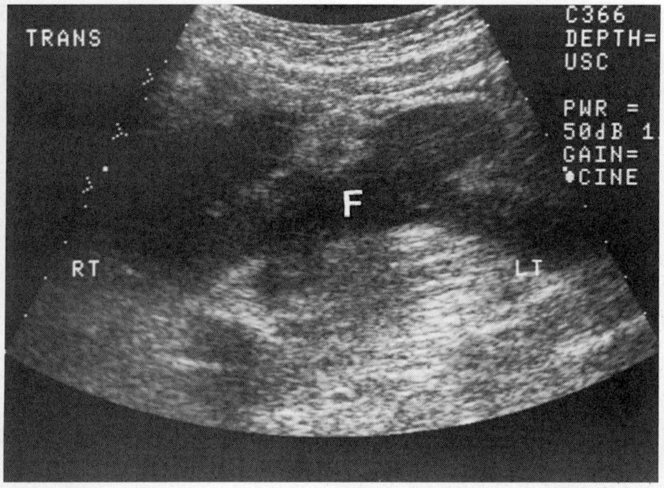

Figure 106.14. Crossed fused renal ectopia. Oblique sonogram demonstrates cortical fusion *(F)* of both kidneys.

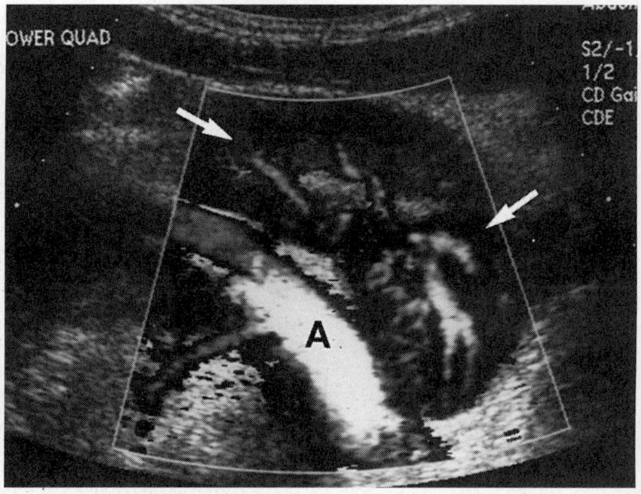

Figure 106.16. Pelvic kidney. Doppler sonogram demonstrates flow *(arrows)* in the ectopic kidney adjacent to iliac artery *(A)*.

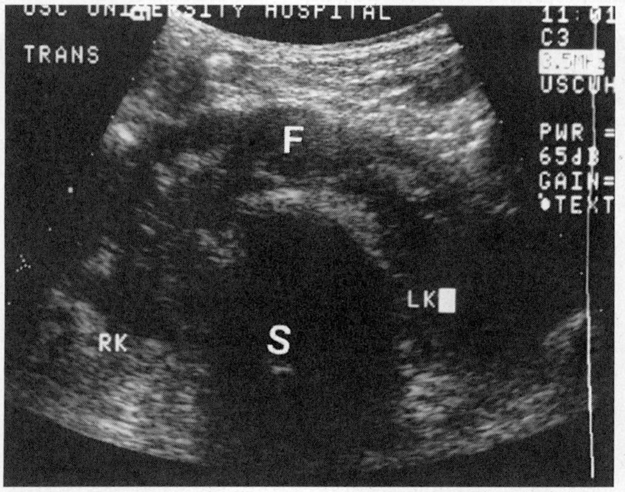

Figure 106.15. Horseshoe kidney. Transverse sonogram demonstrates midline fusion *(F)* of right and left kidney. S, Spine.

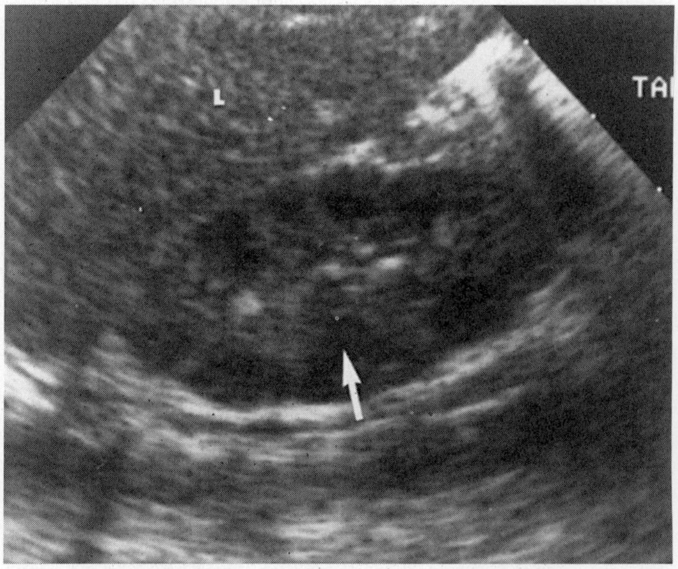

Figure 106.17. Coronal sonogram of normal right kidney in a neonate. The hypoechoic regions (one of them is marked by an *arrow*) are the medullary pyramids. The intervening regions are the cortical tissues and are of comparable echogenicity to the liver *(L)*.

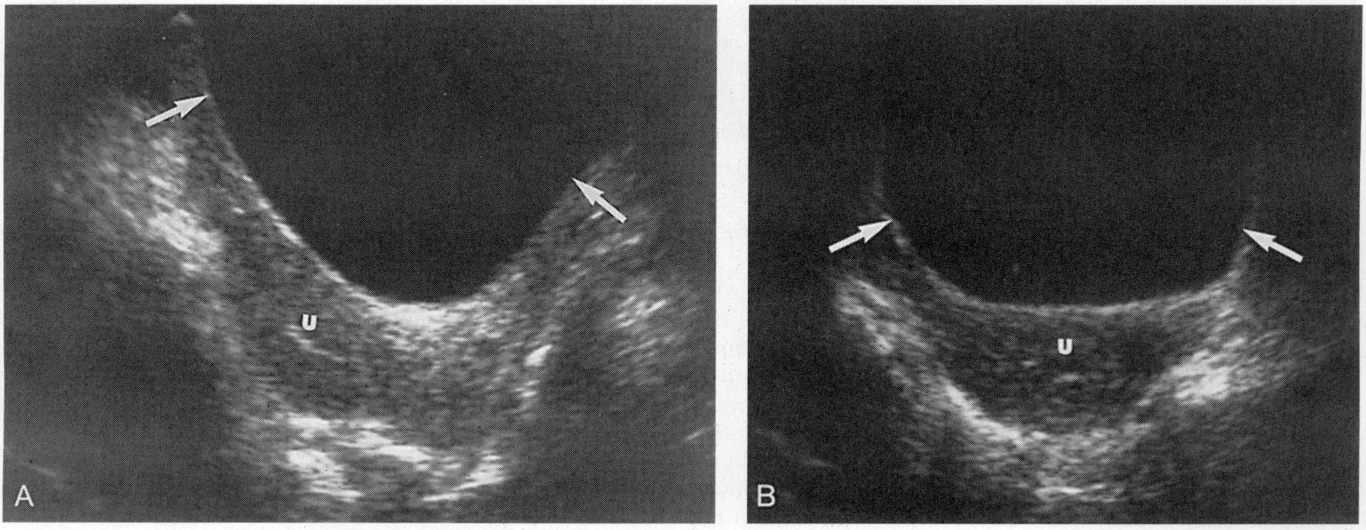

Figure 106.18. **A:** Longitudinal midline sonogram. **B:** Transverse sonogram of the normal bladder in a female. No echoes are present in the bladder and it has smooth walls *(arrows)*. The bladder is often used as an acoustic "window" to study pelvic organs such as the uterus *(U)*.

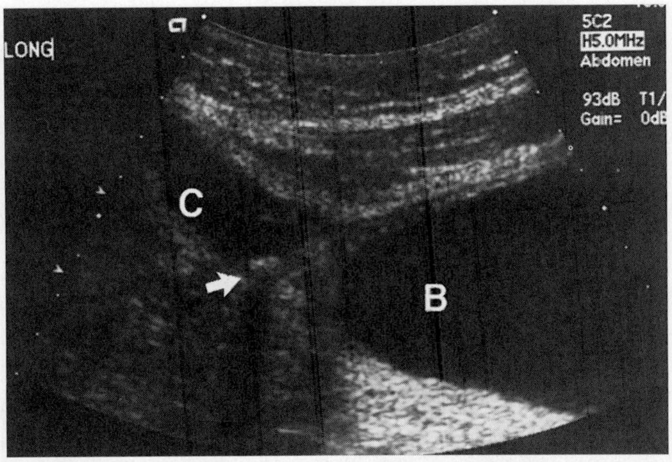

Figure 106.19. Urachal remnant with stone *(arrow)*. Longitudinal sonogram of the bladder *(B)* demonstrates a cystic *(C)* structure with an internal calculi superior to the dome of the bladder.

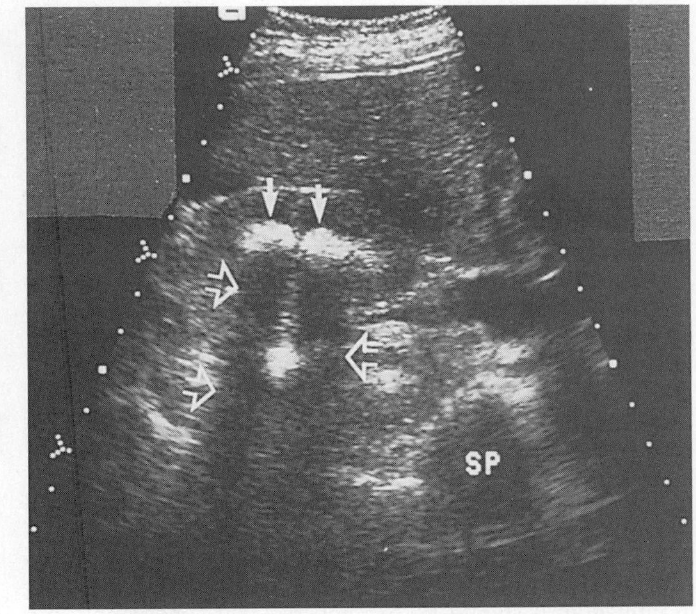

Figure 106.20. Transverse image of the right kidney. Echogenic areas *(arrows)* are dense calcium deposits within the renal parenchyma. The patient has hyperparathyroidism secondary to a parathyroid adenoma. Loss of ultrasonographic information distal to the echogenic calcium deposits is called *shadowing (open arrows)*. sp, spine.

ages of 1 and 19, the average renal length is 6.79 cm + (0.22 × age in years). When a kidney is not seen in its normal retroperitoneal location, a thorough search should be made in the entire abdomen and pelvis because ectopic kidneys can reside any of these regions (Fig. 106.16).

When the bladder is scanned transabdominally, it appears as a sonolucent pelvic structure with well-defined walls, which display through transmission of sound (Fig. 106.18). The bladder can be scanned transrectally, transvaginally, or transurethrally using special transducers. A full bladder is a useful acoustic window to study pelvic organs such as the uterus and ovaries in the female and seminal vesicles and prostate gland in the male. A urachal remnant may be seen superior to the bladder (Fig. 106.19). These pelvic organs can be imaged by endovaginal or endorectal ultrasound probes.

RENAL PARENCHYMAL DISEASE

Sonography, although not specific, is useful in suggesting the presence of renal parenchymal disease. An increase in overall renal cortical echogenicity is seen in both acute and chronic phases of renal parenchymal disorders. Differentiation among etiologies and correlation with severity of renal parenchymal diseases has remained beyond the diagnostic grasp of ultrasound. Nevertheless, recognizing the characteristic increased cortical echogenicity, which occurs with preservation of the corticomedullary junction can be helpful to the clinician. If the pattern is bilateral, consideration can be given to medical renal diseases and infiltrative diseases (leukemia or amyloidosis). Precipitation of calcium deposits in cortical nephrocalcinosis is another possibility, but generally, their presence results in greatly increased echoes (Fig. 106.20). Unilateral cortical echogenicity is uncommon; thus its presence should prompt consideration of subacute renal vein thrombosis and acute pyelonephritis.

In chronic renal failure, cortical echogenicity is related to amount of interstitial fibrosis, a nonspecific change that does not correlate well with degree of renal failure. Increased cortical echogenicity is also a nonspecific finding in acute renal failure. For instance, many disorders that cause acute renal failure exhibit increased cortical echogenicity, such as acute glomerulonephritis and lupus nephritis. An additional finding, loss of the corticomedullary junction, is also nonspecific.

Although the diagnosis of renal parenchymal disease depends primarily on laboratory tests and biopsy results, sonography continues to be applicable for these patients. A patient whose sonogram shows small, echogenic kidneys is virtually certain to have end-stage renal failure (Fig. 106.21).

Ultrasound has proven extremely useful in guiding renal biopsy, facilitating the procedure, and markedly decreasing morbidity and mortality. In the future, ultrasound tissue characterization may allow identification of specific types of parenchymal diseases. At present, the major role of sonography in the azotemic patient or patient with suspected renal disease is assessing renal size and global echogenicity, excluding obstructive uropathy, and guiding renal biopsy.

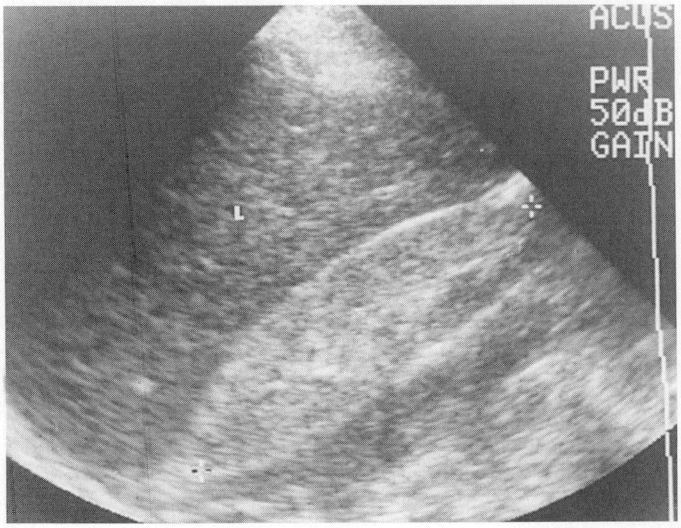

Figure 106.21. The "end-stage" kidney. The longitudinal image shows a small echogenic kidney *(between cursors)*. Note that the liver *(L)* is less echogenic than the kidney (the reverse of normal).

THE DILATED RENAL COLLECTING SYSTEM AND PELVIS

The sensitivity of sonography in detecting a dilated pelvicalyceal system approaches 100%. Although bilateral urinary obstruction accounts for fewer than 5% of all cases of renal failure, the noninvasive nature of the procedure lends itself as the technique of choice to rule out obstructive uropathy in azotemic patients. In renal insufficiency, the presence of pelvicalyceal dilation suggests an obstructive etiology. The most common cause of bilateral obstructive uropathy in an adult is a pelvic tumor; therefore the initial sonogram should include careful examination of the pelvis and bladder, as well as the kidneys and retroperitoneal regions.

Ultrasonographic findings of hydronephrosis include separation of renal sinus echoes by a sonolucent fluid-filled renal pelvis and communication of sonolucent dilated calyces and infundibula with a centrally located renal pelvis (Figs. 106.22 and 106.23). Obstruction may be functional or anatomic (Figs. 106.24 and 106.25). Longstanding obstruction results in renal parenchymal atrophy, with cortical thinning evident on sonographic examination. It should be remembered that sonography provides morphologic, not functional, information about the renal collecting system. Thus mild collecting system dilation may be seen, even though no anatomic obstruction is present. A nonobstructed, dilated collecting system may occur in one-tenth to one-fourth of patients with a dilated collecting system. Such false-positive signs may occur in structurally normal and abnormal kidneys (Table 106.1). Nonobstructive hydronephrosis can be caused by reflux. An overly distensible collecting system can be the cause for an ultrasonographic false-positive sign for obstruction. Conditions responsible for this ultrasonographic finding include the overly distended bladder, an extrarenal pelvis, increased urine production (diuresis, exuberant hydration), post-obstruction dilation, papillary necrosis, and congenital megacalyces. Cystic diseases and vascular lesions of the renal sinus, such as renal artery aneurysm, may simulate hydronephrosis. A precise sonographic examination may allow differentiation of obstructed from nonobstructed pelvicalyectasis. Color Doppler

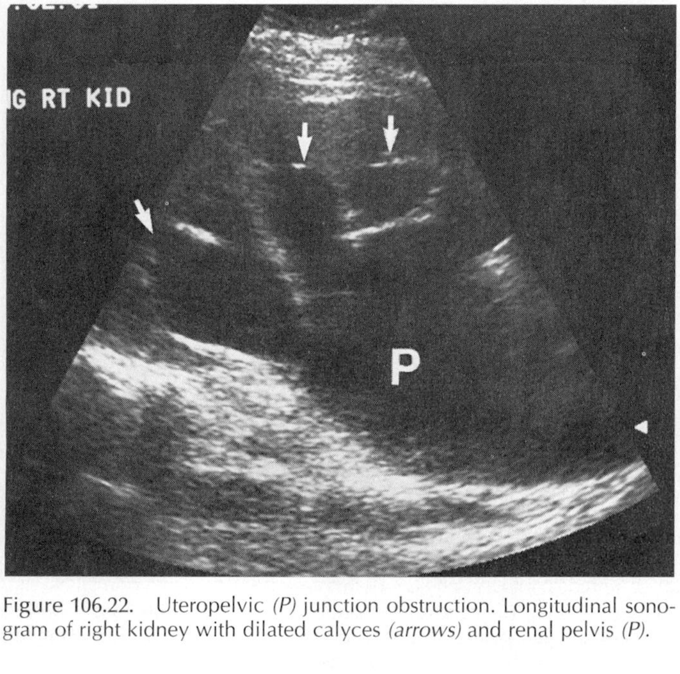

Figure 106.22. Uteropelvic *(P)* junction obstruction. Longitudinal sonogram of right kidney with dilated calyces *(arrows)* and renal pelvis *(P)*.

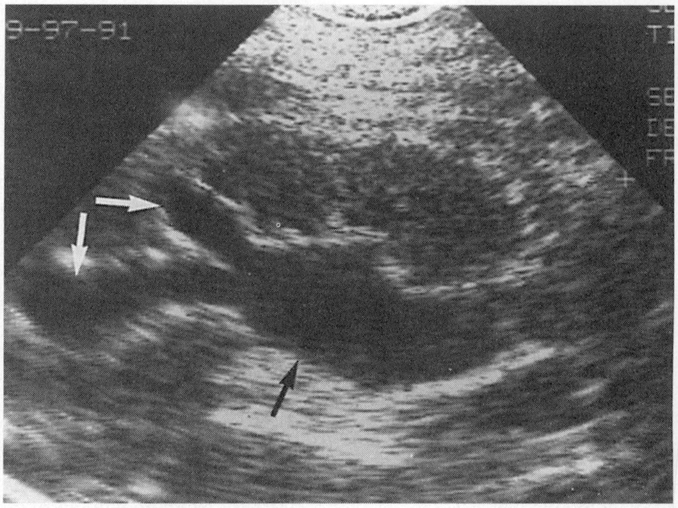

Figure 106.23. Hydronephrosis. Longitudinal sonogram of a kidney demonstrates that dilated calyces *(white arrows)* communicate with the dilated renal pelvis *(black arrow)*.

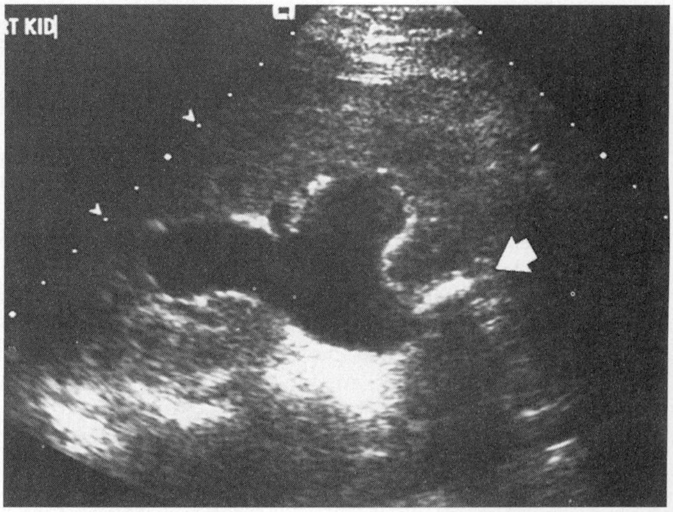

Figure 106.24. Hydronephrosis secondary to renal calculus *(arrow)*. Longitudinal sonogram of hydronephrotic right kidney.

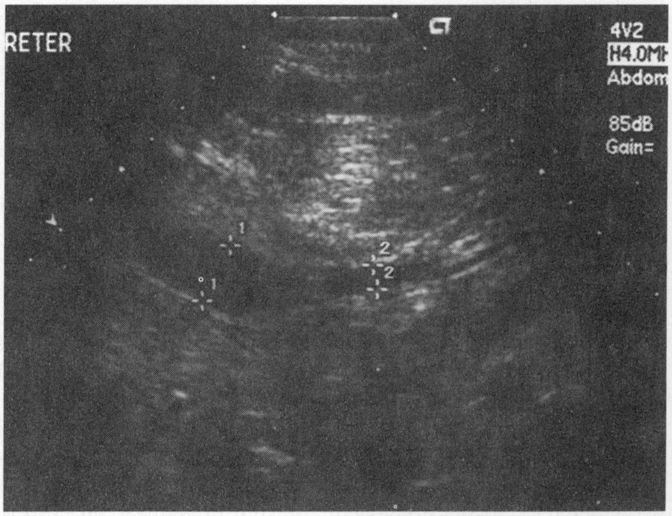

Figure 106.25. Uteropelvic junction obstruction. Longitudinal sonogram of left renal pelvis and ureter. Abrupt transition from dilated renal pelvis *(1)* to normal caliber ureter *(2)*.

TABLE 106.1 False-Positive Sonogram for Obstruction

Structurally Normal Kidney
Physiologic
Pregnancy
Full bladder
Extrarenal pelvis
Congenital megacalyces
Vesicoureteric reflux
Diuresis
Drugs
Following intravenous urography
Aggressive hydration
Diabetes insipidus
Diuretic phase of renal failure
Decreased peristalsis
Acute pyelonephritis
Postrenal transplant (immediately after surgery)
Acute or chronic transplant rejection
Structurally Abnormal Kidney
Prior hydronephrosis with subsequent relief of obstruction
Caliceal diverticula
Papillary necrosis
Chronic pyelonephritis with blunted calyces
Tuberculosis of kidney with strictured infundibulum

Modified from Amis ES Jr, Cronan JJ, Pfister RC, et al. Ultrasonic inaccuracies in diagnosing renal obstruction. *Urology* 1982;19:101–105.

can reliably exclude vascular structures, which may mimic a dilated collecting system.

The peristaltic ureteral wave in a nonobstructed system results in intermittent expulsion of urine at the ureterovesicular junction into the bladder, the so-called ureteral jet. Color Doppler imaging of the bladder may document ureteral jets, thus confirming patency.

An acutely obstructed collecting system is rarely dilated significantly, resulting in a false-negative observation. The incidence of false negatives is rare, occurring in fewer than 1% of cases. Etiology is divided into cases in which the collecting system is distensible and those in which it is not (Table 106.2). Dilated calyces may be misinterpreted as pyramids or cysts. The presence of hydronephrosis and cysts may be misdiagnosed as cysts alone. Both potential pitfalls can often be avoided by meticulous examination.

TABLE 106.2 False-Negative Sonogram for Obstruction

Distensible Collecting System
Acute obstruction (no time for distension)
Dehydration (not enough urine formed)
Ruptured calyx (decompression)
Intermittent obstruction
Partial obstruction
Staghorn calculus (stone obscures hydronephrosis)
Longstanding renal failure with superimposed obstruction
Nondistendible Collecting System
Retroperitoneal fibrosis
Tumor encasement of collecting system

Modified from Amis ES Jr, Cronan JJ, Pfister RC, et al. Ultrasonic inaccuracies in diagnosing renal obstruction. *Urology* 1982;19:101–105.

Evaluation of intrarenal arterial vascular resistance with Doppler ultrasound in the setting of obstruction has been studied. Increased resistance in distal renal arteries with concomitant pyelocalyceal dilation can be observed in acute obstruction. Limitations to this finding include elevated arterial resistance in renal parenchymal disease and refractory delay in the postobstructive renal vasculature.

Obstruction Due to Renal Calculi

The diagnosis of most renal calculi can often be made by observing their characteristic opaque density on the conventional KUB or abdominal radiograph, with or without nephrotomography. Intravenous urography or CT can confirm the presence of calculus or suspected obstruction due to renal calculus. Ultrasound is also useful in confirming the presence of calculi within the intrarenal collecting system, with some studies demonstrating a 90% detection rate. With sonography, a renal calculus appears as an echogenic focus with shadowing (no transmission of sound) distal to its location. Stones produce shadowing regardless of their composition, but size alone determines detection by ultrasound, with larger stones tending to exhibit more prominent shadowing. If no shadowing is detected, small stones can be missed. Renal parenchymal and pelvicalyceal stones are generally easy to image by sonography (Fig. 106.26). On occasion, vascular calcifications may cause a false-positive interpretation. Staghorn calculi are easily seen as well, although their size is often underestimated on ultrasound. The echogenicity and shadowing seen with Staghorn calculi may obscure concomitant collecting system dilation, resulting in a missed or false-negative diagnosis of hydronephrosis.

In most instances, the majority of the ureter is virtually obscured by gas in overlying bowel. Thus ureteral stones are rarely imaged by sonography and are noted only when they lie proximally or distally. Occasionally, during a pelvic/bladder ultrasound, an obstructing stone is seen as a shadowing echogenic focus at the ureterovesicular junction, with proximal ureteral dilation (Fig. 106.27).

Urologic management of renal calculus disease depends on ultrasound localization of calculi for extracorporeal shock wave lithotripsy (ESWL) treatment. Ultrasound guidance can also be used in performing percutaneous kidney biopsies.

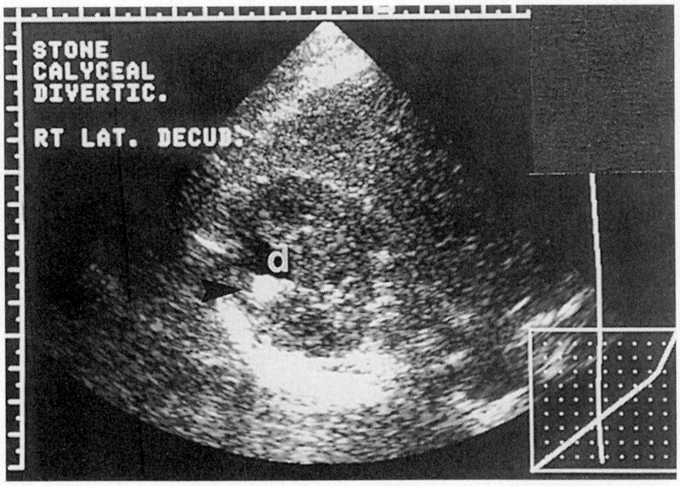

Figure 106.26. Calculus within calyceal diverticulum. Transverse image of the right kidney with the patient in right lateral decubitus position. Echogenic calculus *(arrowhead)* is in the dependent portion of the anechoic calyceal diverticulum *(d)*.

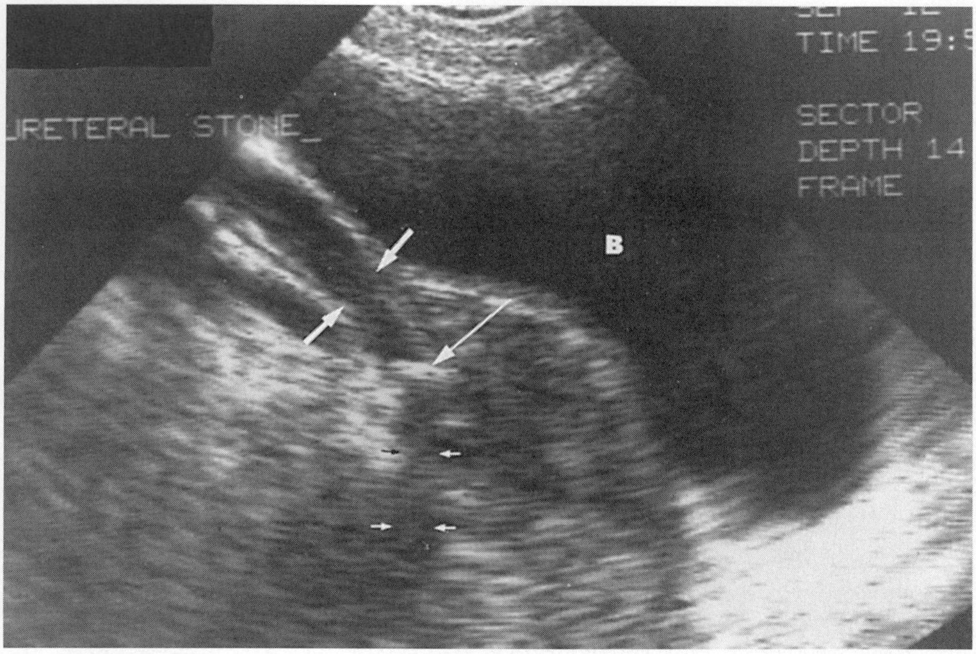

Figure 106.27. Calculus *(long thin arrow)* lodged in distal ureter *(short thick arrows)* causing obstruction. Acoustic shadowing distal to the calculus is present *(small black and white arrows)*. This is the same patient as in (Fig. 102.20). Echoes in the urinary bladder *(B)* are artifact.

INFLAMMATORY CONDITIONS OF THE KIDNEY

The kidney may become infected by the ascending route (via bladder, ureter or pyelocalyceal system) or through the circulatory system. The ascending route is the most common. Immunocompromised patients and diabetics are more prone to renal infection than healthy persons. Other risk factors for kidney infection include vesicoureteric reflux, calculus disease, obstructive uropathy, pregnancy, neurogenic bladder, and a long-standing indwelling catheter. Ultrasonographic evaluation of the kidneys in patients with suspected pyelonephritis should be performed in the following clinical settings: (a) detection of underlying pathology that may predispose the kidney to infection, such as calculi, reflux, ureteropelvic obstruction, or other anatomic anomaly, and (b) detection of complications associated with pyelonephritis-pyonephrosis or renal or perinephric abscess. Routine sonographic evaluation of the uncomplicated case of pyelonephritis is often normal.

Acute Renal Infection

There is a pathologic continuum noted in renal parenchymal infection. The degree of pyelonephritis ranges from mild to severe. When the inflammation is mild, the sonogram may be normal. Occasionally, mild renal enlargement and scattered low-level echoes (thought to represent focal edema or microabscess) may be seen. On occasion, ultrasound will reveal localized hypoechoic regions (Figs. 106.28, 106.29, and 106.30); these focal areas may have increased blood flow on color Doppler. When the inflammation is more extensive, the ultrasound shows an enlarged kidney with patchy disorganized parenchyma.

Intravenous urography may be interpreted as normal in patients with mild pyelonephritis. Although ultrasound may be more sensitive than urography, contrast-enhanced CT of the kidneys remains the most sensitive imaging modality for detection of pyelonephritis.

Acute focal bacterial nephritis (focal lobar nephronia) is a rare condition in which a focal solid mass of inflammatory tissue (infection) occurs without liquefied pus. Sonographically, a hypoechoic mass without increased through transmission of sound and without a discernible wall is seen (Fig. 106.29). This entity may prove difficult to differentiate from renal abscess by ultrasound or CT. Ultrasound- or CT-guided needle aspiration can be performed if an immediate answer is required; otherwise, the patient can be followed up with a sonogram examination. The lesion usually resolves after a course of appropriate antibiotic therapy.

Acute renal abscess is most often due to hematogenous bacterial seeding, although abscesses can occur from ascending route infections. Ultrasound examination may reveal an almost

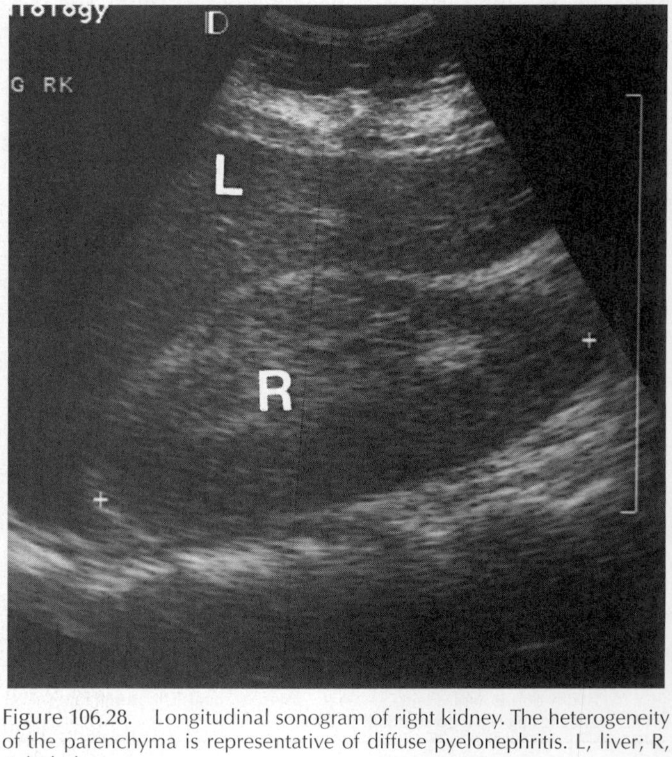

Figure 106.28. Longitudinal sonogram of right kidney. The heterogeneity of the parenchyma is representative of diffuse pyelonephritis. L, liver; R, right kidney.

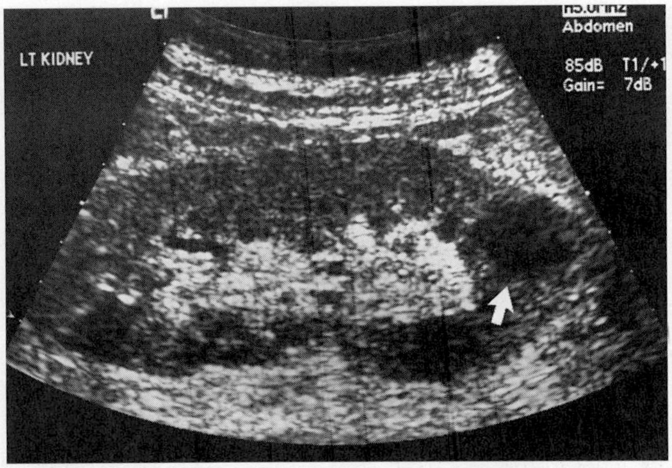

Figure 106.29. Longitudinal sonogram of left kidney with hypoechoic lesion in the lower pole represents focal pyelonephritis *(white arrow)*.

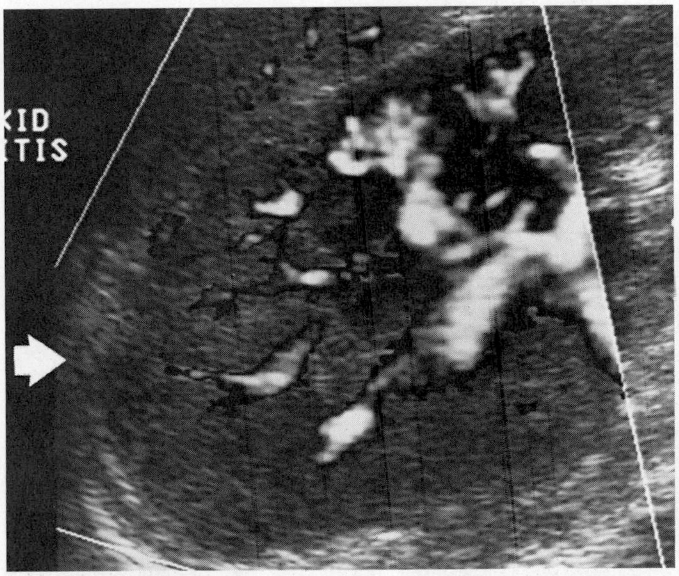

Figure 106.30. Focal pyelonephritis. Longitudinal sonogram demonstrating decreased flow *(white arrow)* in the upper pole of the kidney on color Doppler secondary to edema from inflammation.

anechoic mass with irregular walls and increased through transmission of sound. If liquefaction is incomplete, the abscess may be filled with echoes (Fig. 106.31). On occasion, the abscess may be highly echogenic (Fig. 106.32), suggesting the presence of microbubbles that occur with gas-forming organisms. Color Doppler ultrasound would demonstrate absence of vascular flow within the abscess (Fig. 106.32). A renal abscess can extend into perinephric tissues (Fig. 106.33) and beyond, including the psoas muscle (Fig. 106.34). The ultrasonographic appearance is that of a mixed or hypoechoic mass around the kidney. If a cyst becomes infected, internal echoes will be seen. A hemorrhagic cyst may present with a similar appearance.

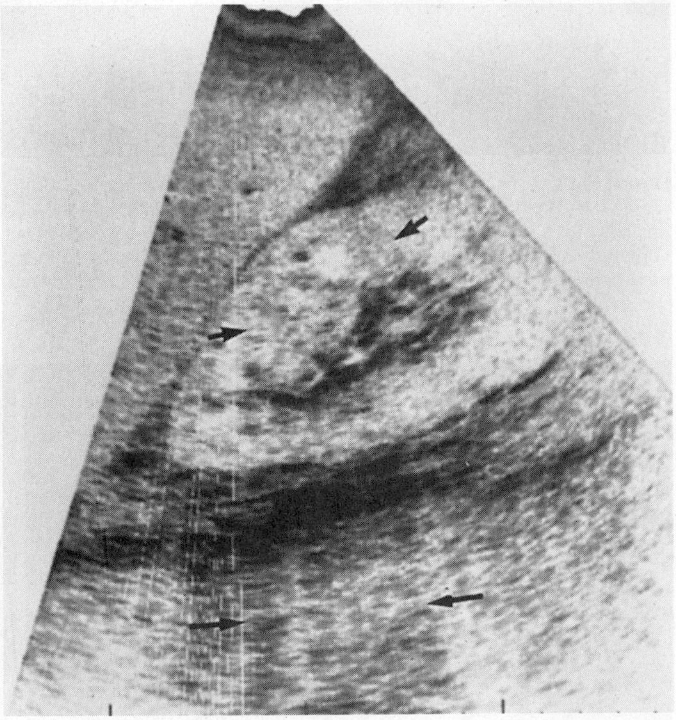

Figure 106.31. Renal abscess: Transverse image of right kidney shows a lesion with many echoes *(short arrows)* indenting the renal sinus echoes. Increased through transmission of sound is present *(long arrows)*.

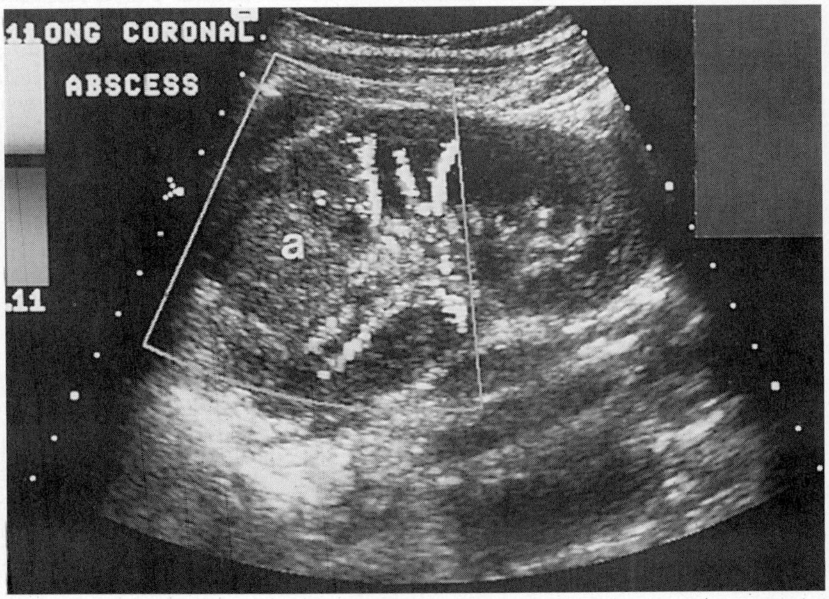

Figure 106.32. Renal abscess. Coronal color flow Doppler image of the left kidney. The homogeneous hyperechoic renal abscess *(a)* has no demonstrable internal vascular flow. (See Color Figure 106.32.)

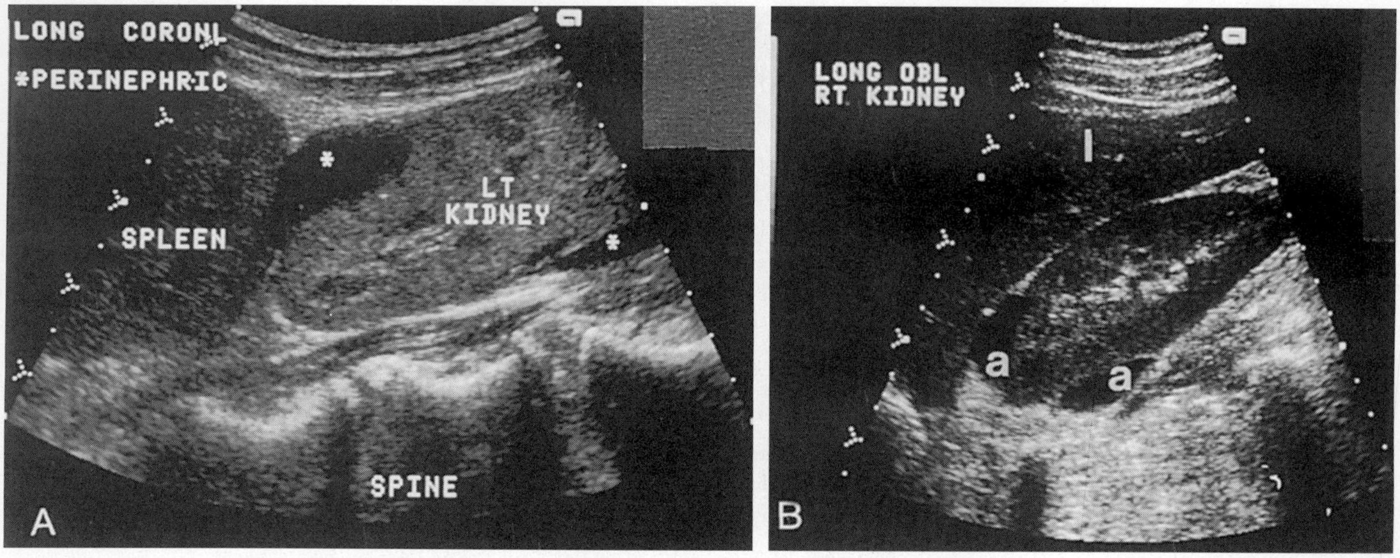

Figure 106.33. Perinephric abscess. **A:** Coronal image of the left kidney. The anechoic subcapsular abscess *(*)* deforms the renal parenchyma, as well as extends into the perinephric space. It should not be mistaken for a simple cyst. There is no posterior enhancement from "increased through transmission." **B:** Longitudinal image of the right kidney. Anechoic extracapsular collections are perinephric abscesses. a, perinephric abscess; l, liver.

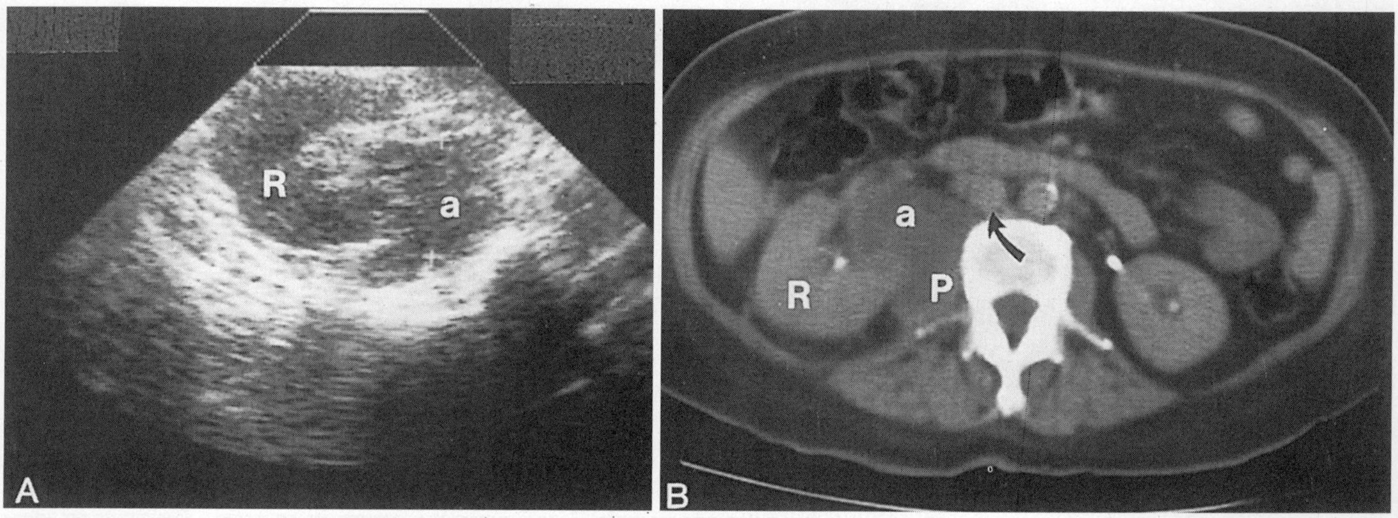

Figure 106.34. Renal abscess. **A:** Transverse image of the right kidney. Hypoechoic area medial to the kidney is an abscess extending into the adjacent psoas muscle. A, extrarenal abscess; R, right kidney. **B:** Corresponding axial CT with contrast in the same patient. Demonstration of the extrarenal abscess is superior to sonogram. *Curved arrow* indicates the inferior vena cava displaced by abscess. P, right psoas muscle with abscess (a); R, right kidney.

Emphysematous pyelonephritis is a complication of acute pyelonephritis that occurs primarily in diabetics. The disease is associated with a significant incidence of mortality. It is characterized by gas formation, usually by coliform organisms, which occurs in the collecting system, parenchyma, and retroperitoneal tissues. Ultrasound may reveal evidence of gas (echogenic foci with shadowing) in any of these locations (Fig. 106.35A), but CT is more sensitive than ultrasound in detecting its presence (Fig. 106.35B).

Subacute and Chronic Renal Infections

Subacute and chronic renal abscess results when the lesion goes untreated or is inadequately treated. The lesion is similar in appearance to an acute abscess, although the wall is thicker and may be irregular.

In chronic atrophic pyelonephritis, the renal outline is irregular, with areas of focal parenchymal loss and echogenic regions corresponding to scarring. A small echogenic kidney with irregular outlines results when involvement is more extensive.

Xanthogranulomatous pyelonephritis is an unusual chronic infection, usually related to the organism *Proteus mirabilis,* although it may be associated with other Gram-negative and staphylococcal species. Pathologically, chronically inflamed, lipid-laden histiocytes and abscess formation are noted. In a typical case, the ultrasound shows an enlarged kidney, loss of renal sinus echoes, and an obstructing calculus (echogenic focus with distal shadowing). Debris-filled hypoechoic to an-

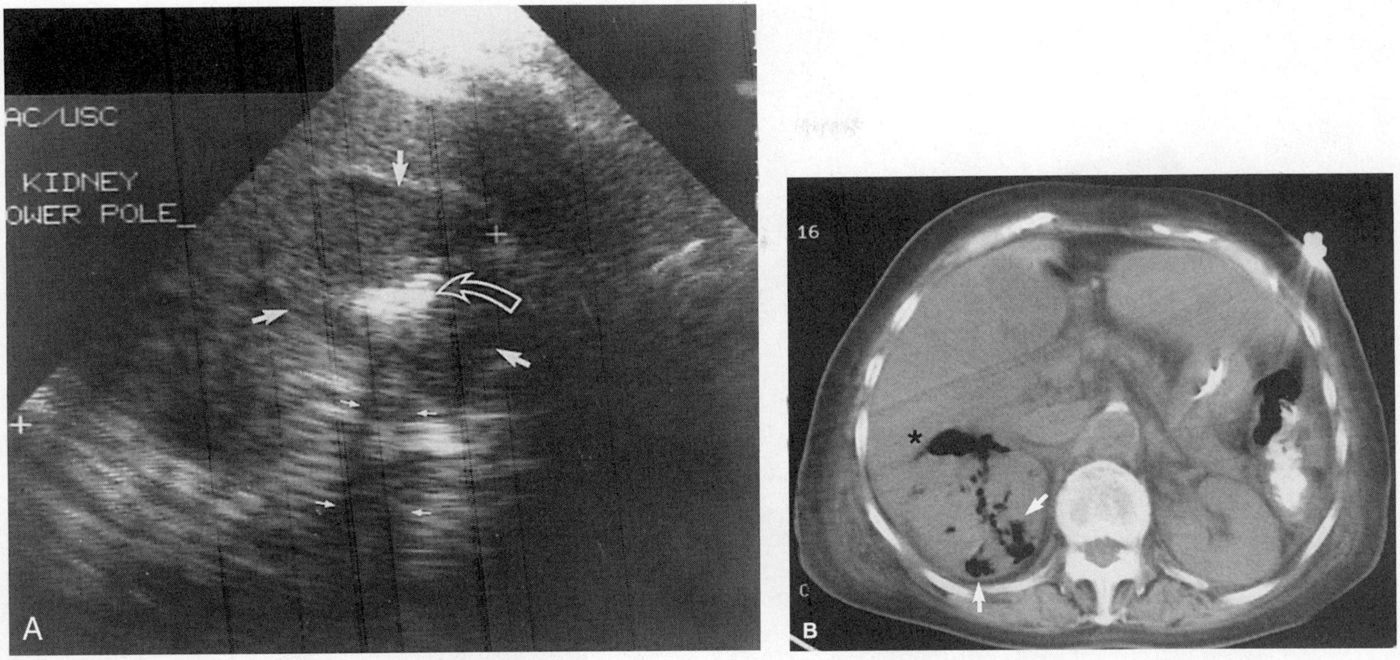

Figure 106.35. Emphysematous pyelonephritis. **A:** Transverse sonogram through lower pole of kidney *(straight arrows)* shows evidence of gas, strong echoes *(curved open arrow)*, with acoustic shadowing distal to it *(small straight arrows)*. **B:** Transverse abdominal CT scan demonstrates gas anterior to the right kidney *(*)* as well as gas within the renal parenchyma *(arrows)*.

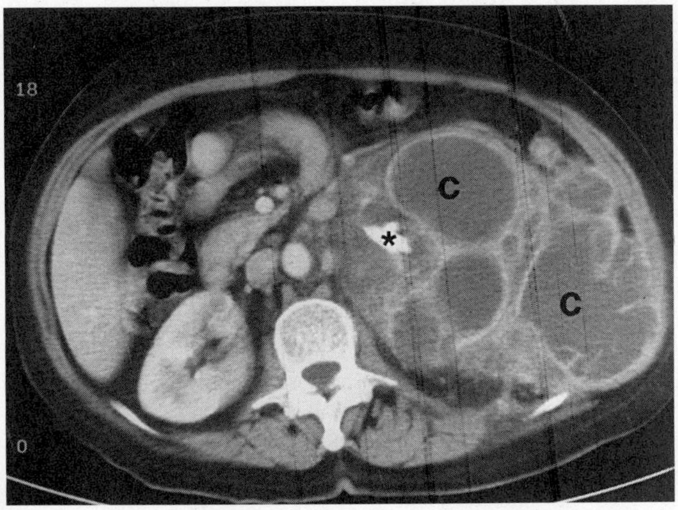

Figure 106.36. Xanthogranulomatous pyelonephritis abdominal CT scan demonstrates multiple cystic structures *(c)* within the renal fossa enhancing residual renal cortex. Ureteral calculus *(*)*.

echoic areas, with increased through transmission of sound, are noted, representing dilated calyces and/or abscesses. Xanthogranulomatous pyelonephritis may also present as a mass in the tumefactive form and may be indistinguishable from a neoplasm (Fig. 106.36). In severe cases, the inflammatory mass may extend into the perinephric space or adjacent organs and psoas muscle.

Pyonephrosis

Kidneys with pyonephrosis are often nonfunctioning when examined with intravenous urography. Ultrasound can suggest the diagnosis earlier, when a dilated collecting system filled with echoes is noted in the presence of flank pain, fever, and leukocytosis. Lack of pelvicalyceal debris can be seen in patients with pyonephrosis secondary to a distal obstructive process, thus making the differentiation between bland hydronephrosis difficult. Ultrasound can also be used to direct percutaneous aspiration of the pus-filled collecting system. It is an invaluable tool when therapeutic nephrostomy drainage is needed.

Other Infections

The potential of ultrasound for the diagnosis and treatment of renal tuberculosis and other rare inflammatory conditions of the kidney remains untapped. Ultrasound detection of pathologic changes in early renal tuberculosis is difficult, with urography and CT being more sensitive. In up to 80% of patient with early renal tuberculosis, the ultrasound examination may be normal. Focal tuberculosis renal lesions may be either hypoechoic or echogenic. Ultrasound may demonstrate calcification and changes of chronic pyelonephritis in patients with later stages of renal tuberculosis.

CYSTIC DISEASES OF THE KIDNEY

Ultrasound is unequalled in its ability to distinguish solid from cystic lesions. Differences in acoustic impedance and attenuation between solids and liquids make ultrasound ideal for this important determination.

Multicystic Dysplastic Kidney

One of the most common causes of abdominal mass in the newborn is multicystic dysplastic kidney (MCDK). In an older child, the diagnosis may be an incidental finding. This lesion is

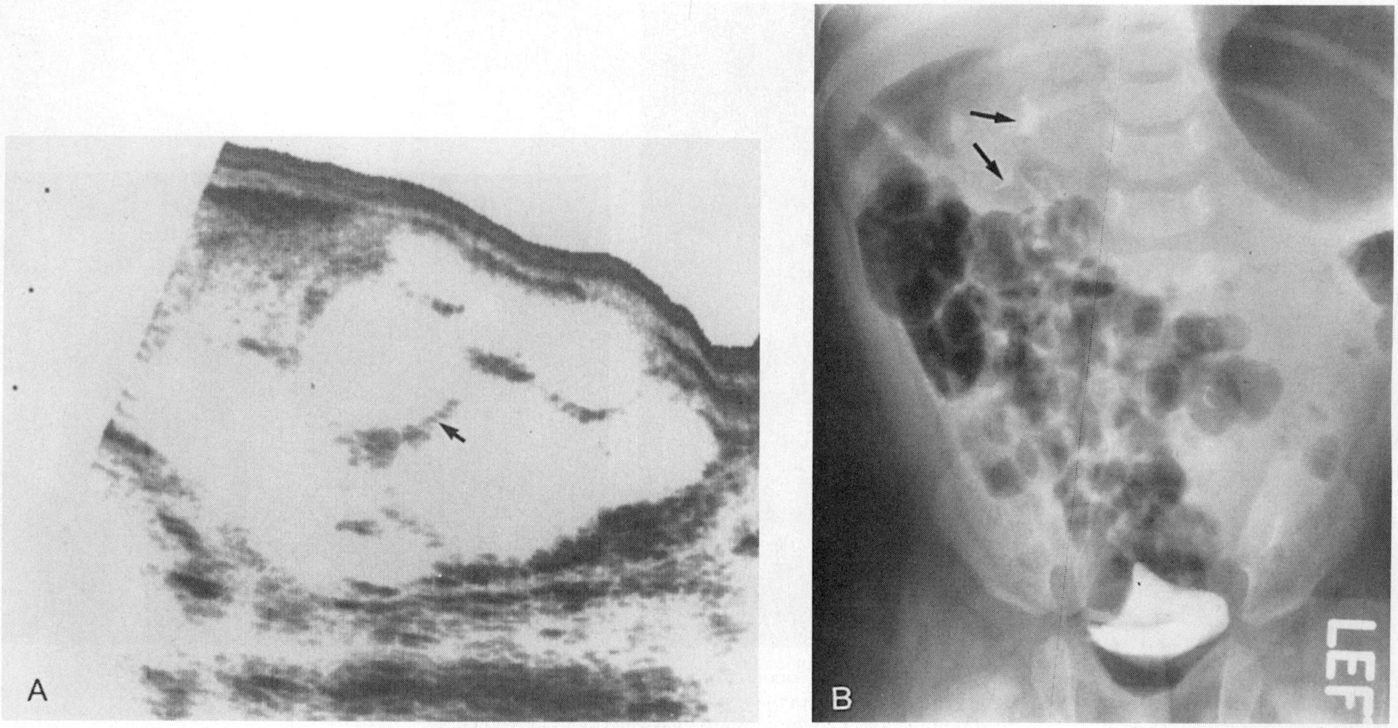

Figure 106.37. Multicystic dysplastic kidney. Intravenous urogram shows functioning right kidney excreting contrast *(arrows)* but nonvisualization of the left kidney.

associated with atresia of the renal pelvis, ureter, or both, during the metanephric stage of fetal development. The sonographic appearance is that of multiple, noncommunicating cysts of varying size, with thick septae between them and complete absence of a renal pelvis. Normal renal and ureteral tissue is unidentifiable, unless the dysplasia affects only a portion of the kidney, a rare occurrence. It is important to assess the contralateral kidney, because there is a prevalence of anomalies such as ureteropelvic junction obstruction, horseshoe kidney, and segmental ureteral disparity. MCDK is clinically insignificant if unilateral, making surgery elective. Conversely, bilateral MCDK is incompatible with life. MCDKs display no function on intravenous urography (Fig. 106.37). Unilateral hydronephrosis is the most common differential diagnostic consideration for MCDK. Hydronephrosis is easily recognizable, because dilated calyces tend to be uniform in size and communicate centrally with the dilated renal pelvis.

Autosomal-Recessive Polycystic Kidney Disease (Infantile Polycystic Kidney Disease)

The phenotypic spectrum in this inherited disorder varies from severe renal involvement in the neonate and younger child to congenital hepatic fibrosis in the older child. Thus the mode of presentation in infants is renal failure, whereas older children present with hepatic failure. Organomegaly is usually the predominant sign in the neonate, with renal enlargement occurring most frequently, followed by hepatomegaly or hepatosplenomegaly. The abnormality involves the collecting tubules, which are ectatic and 1 to 2 mm wide. Ultrasound reveals bilaterally enlarged kidneys, which are diffusely hyperechoic due to the many interfaces of ectatic tubules, and an unidentifiable corticomedullary junction (Fig. 106.38). Occasionally, a macroscopic cyst or an island of normal parenchyma may be seen. Intravenous urography shows a "streaky" nephrogram due to the presence of contrast in ectatic tubules. Prognosis is poor, with death resulting in the neonate and occasionally in the older infant and child. When a smaller percentage of renal tubules are affected, the infant may survive longer and develop systemic hypertension or portal hypertension with esophageal varices. Periportal fibrosis and bile duct ectasia are pathologically seen in the liver. The hepatic sonogram may show increased liver echogenicity and rare bile duct dilation.

Medullary Cystic Disease and Juvenile Nephronophthisis

Medullary cystic disease, unlike most autosomal-dominant disorders, affects young adults as well as children. It presents with the clinical triad of anemia, salt-losing nephropathy, and azotemia. The disorder usually involves both kidneys and is characterized by renal invasion by cysts, which vary in size from microscopic to 2 cm in diameter. Sonographically, cysts are seen in the medulla (Fig. 106.39) or at the corticomedullary junction, or they may displace fat in the renal sinus. When many small cysts are present, the medullary pyramids may appear echogenic. Small, shrunken kidneys may occur in advanced stages.

Juvenile Nephronophthisis

Juvenile nephronophthisis is an autosomal-recessive disorder seen in a younger age group than medullary cystic disease. Clinically, these patients display anemia, salt wasting, and hyposthenuria. They sometimes benefit from salt replacement. Ultrasound findings include small kidneys with loss of corticomedullary distinction and increased echogenicity. Medullary cysts may also occur.

Medullary Sponge Kidney

Medullary sponge kidney is a fairly common renal lesion (0.5% prevalence) that usually involves both kidneys. It is characterized by cystic dilation of the collecting tubules. The cystic re-

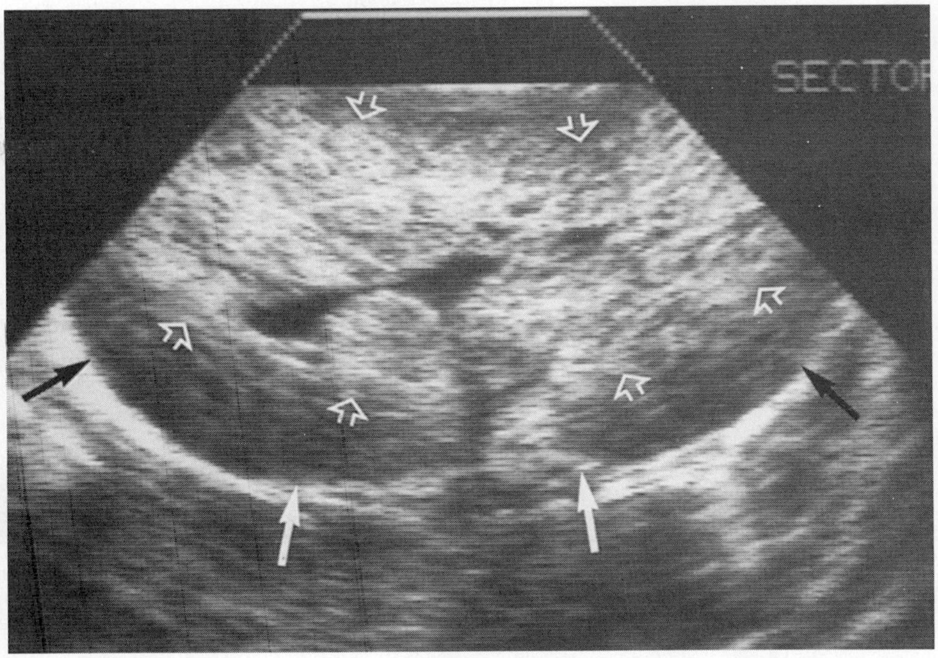

Figure 106.38. Autosomal-recessive polycystic kidney disease. Longitudinal renal scan shows an enlarged kidney *(solid arrows)* with strong echoes caused by many reflecting interfaces *(open arrows)*. The corticomedullary junction is not seen. The opposite kidney was similar in appearance.

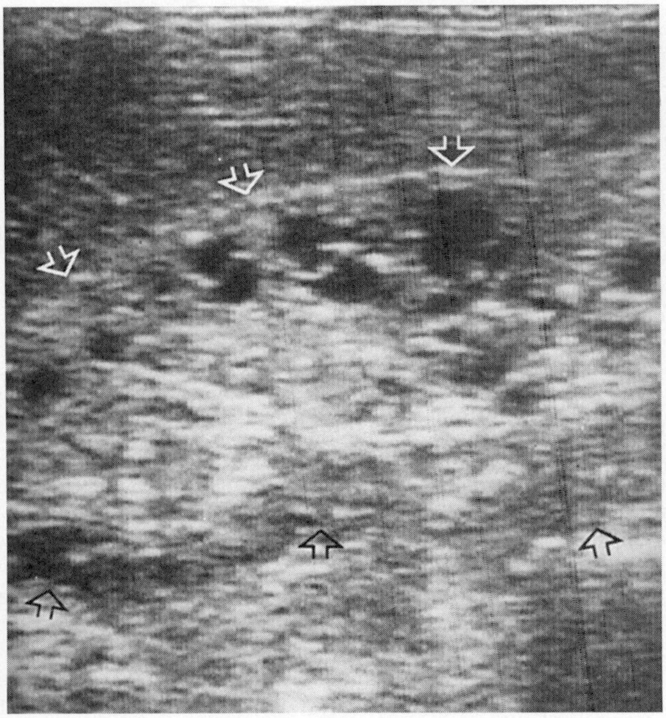

Figure 106.39. Medullary cystic disease. Longitudinal view of the kidney *(open arrows)* shows several cysts (rounded black lesions) in the medulla and at the corticomedullary junction.

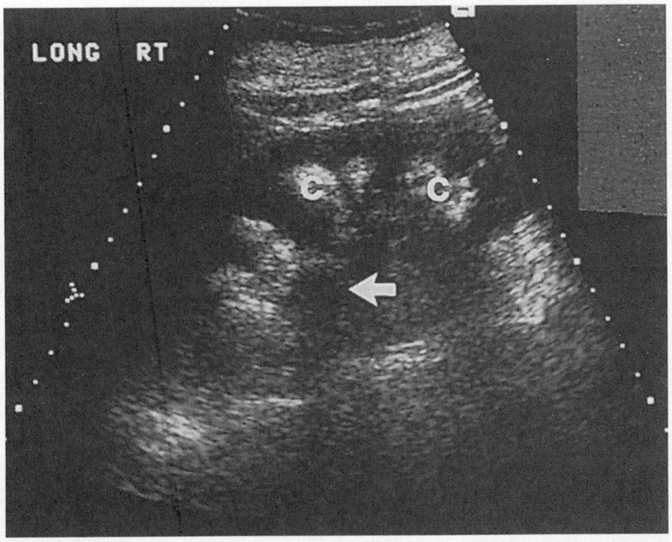

Figure 106.40. Medullary sponge kidney. Longitudinal image of the right kidney. Calculi within the dilated collected tubules are responsible for the hyperechoic renal medulla *(c)*. Note the shadowing posterior to the medulla *(white arrow)*.

gions are not well imaged by ultrasound because they are very small. Renal calculi within the dilated collecting tubules may be detected with ultrasonography (Fig. 106.40). This condition is best studied with intravenous urography.

Polycystic Kidney Disease (Autosomal Dominant)

This inherited disorder is most often discovered in adulthood during or after the fourth decade, but occasionally, it is noted earlier, sometimes in childhood. This autosomal-dominant disorder results from the same genetic abnormality as hepatic polycystic disease. The typical clinical picture is that of bilateral kidney enlargement, impaired renal function, and hypertension. There may be cysts in other organs, most commonly the liver, and rarely encountered in the pancreas and spleen. Berry aneurysms in the circle of Willis are also common in this disease. Sonography reveals bilaterally enlarged lobulated kidneys with multiple cysts of varying size (Fig. 106.41A). In contrast to simple cysts, these cysts often have irregular walls. The number of cysts in these patients varies from a few dozen to hundreds, thus resulting in massive renal enlargement. The cysts do not communicate with the renal pelvis, which allows differentiation from hydronephrosis. Liver cysts can readily be identified and often cause some hepatic enlargement (Fig. 106.41B). Sonography can also detect the presence of this disease in asymptomatic

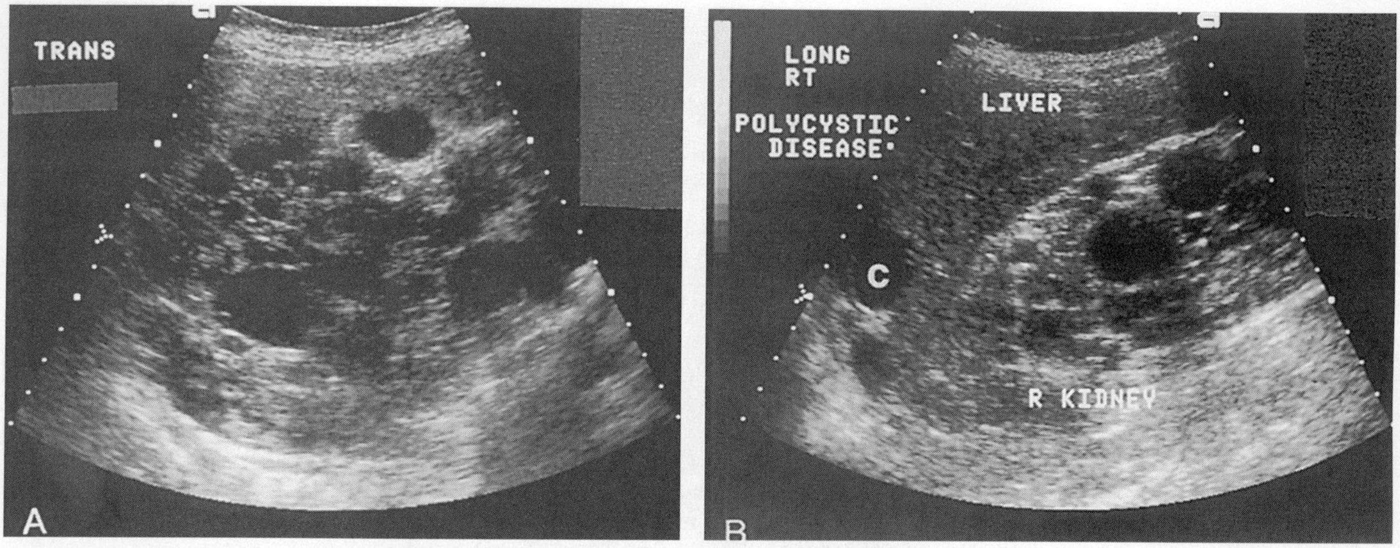

Figure 106.41. Autosomal-dominant polycystic kidney disease. **A:** Transverse image of the right kidney shows an enlarged kidney with multiple cysts (rounded black regions separated by thick walls). **B:** Longitudinal image of the right kidney. Multiple cysts within the right kidney. Note the liver cyst at the edge of the right lobe of the liver. Hepatic cysts are part of the spectrum of this disease. c, liver cysts.

patients, making it useful for genetic counseling and clinical surveillance. Complications, such as calcifications, hemorrhage into a cyst (Fig. 106.42), or cyst infection, may develop. When this occurs, sonography may show echoes within the abnormal cyst(s) and may be an invaluable aid in directing diagnostic or therapeutic cyst puncture. Cystic complications should be suspected in patients displaying focal tenderness, and careful sonography should be performed. The main differential diagnostic consideration of autosomal-dominant polycystic kidney disease is multiple simple cysts with bilateral involvement. In contrast, patients with multiple simple cysts have normal size kidneys, and the cysts are almost always less numerous and have regular margins.

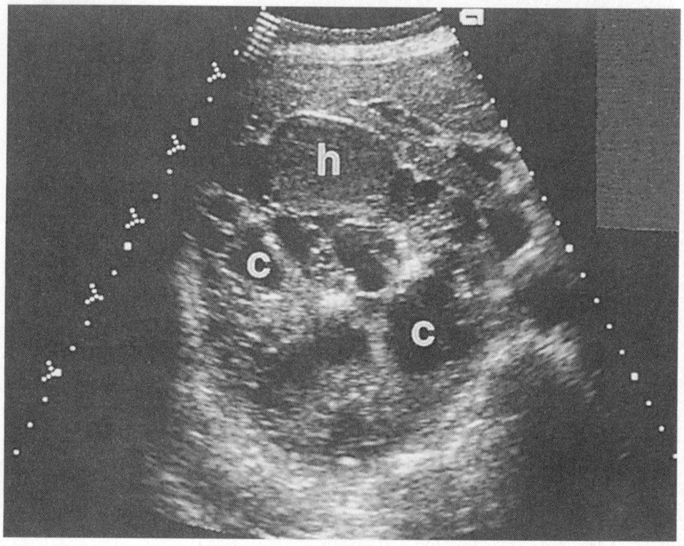

Figure 106.42. Autosomal-dominant polycystic kidney disease with a hemorrhagic cyst. Transverse image of a polycystic kidney. The relatively homogenous mass in the anterior portion of the kidney is a hemorrhagic cyst. This is not an infrequent complication of this disease. c, renal cysts; h, hemorrhagic cyst.

Simple Renal Cyst

The simple renal cyst is a benign, epithelial-lined, fluid-filled lesion of unknown etiology that occurs increasingly with advanced age. Majorities of people older than 50 years have one or more simple renal cysts. Most frequently, it is an incidental finding, with more cases being discovered due to expanded use of CT and ultrasound. Cysts usually arise in the renal cortex but can occur anywhere in the kidney. When adjacent to the renal pelvis, they are known as *parapelvic cysts.* In this location, they occasionally cause symptoms.

A simple renal cyst has the following sonographic characteristics: (a) it is anechoic, (b) there is clear definition of the posterior wall, (c) there is increased through transmission of sound distal to the cyst, (d) it is of spherical or ovoid shape, and (e) it has imperceptible walls (Fig. 106.43). Thin septa are often present and do not preclude a diagnosis of simple renal cyst. If the aforementioned diagnostic criteria are applied, sonographic diagnosis of simple renal cyst can be made with 100% accuracy. Proper diagnosis of simple cysts is important because intervention is not necessary. Care should be taken to avoid confusing multiple parapelvic cysts that lie adjacent to the renal pelvis for hydronephrosis (Fig. 106.44).

Complications such as infection or intracystic hemorrhage can develop within a simple cyst. In such a case, the patient may have flank pain and fever. Sonographically, the cyst may have internal echoes due to pus or hemorrhage (Fig. 106.45). Sometimes it is difficult to distinguish a complicated cyst from a neoplasm; thus further evaluation would be warranted. Color Doppler ultrasound may be used to document lack of vascular flow within a suspected complicated cyst. Ultrasound-guided aspiration provides an additional means to diagnose this complication. CT or MRI, in conjunction with contrast administration, may be used to resolve the more difficult cases. Mural calcification, more commonly associated with polycystic disease, occurs in 1% to 2% of simple cysts. In this presentation, there may be absence of increased through transmission of sound. In addition, acoustic shadowing may occur. A calcified cyst can be difficult to differentiate from neoplasm at times.

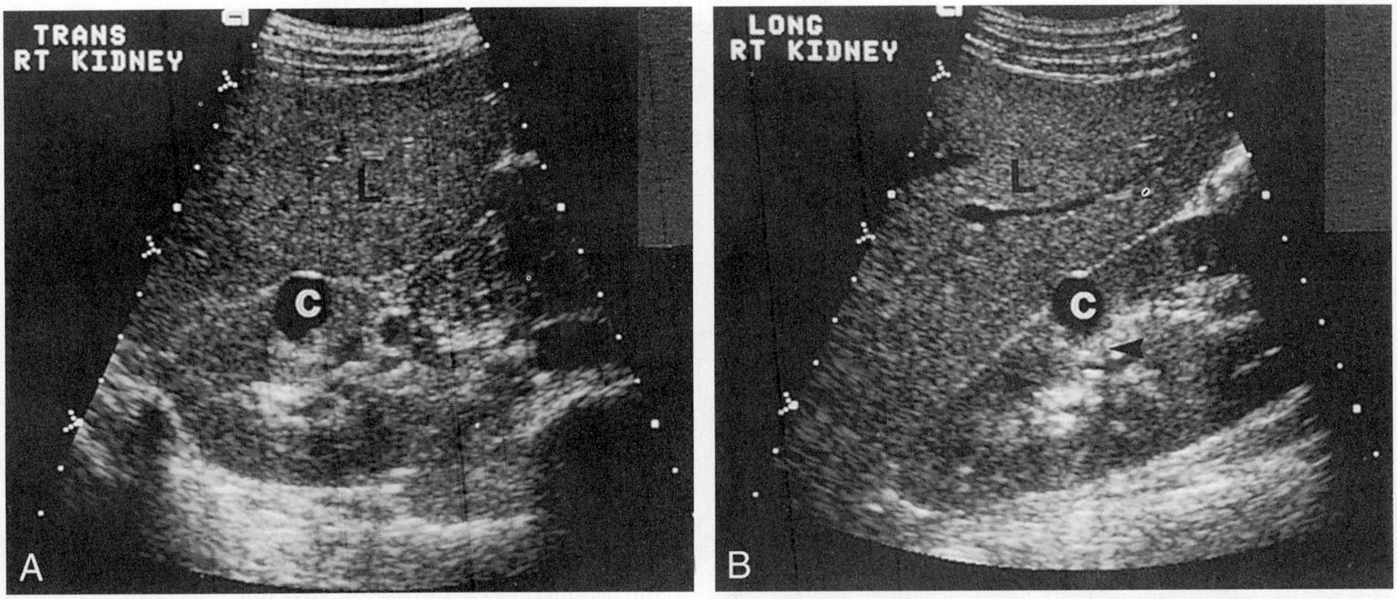

Figure 106.43. **A:** Transverse image of the right kidney. Simple cyst in the renal cortex. Note the absence of internal echoes, well-defined margins, and "increased through transmission." c, simple cortical cyst. **B:** Longitudinal image of the right kidney. c, simple cortical cyst.

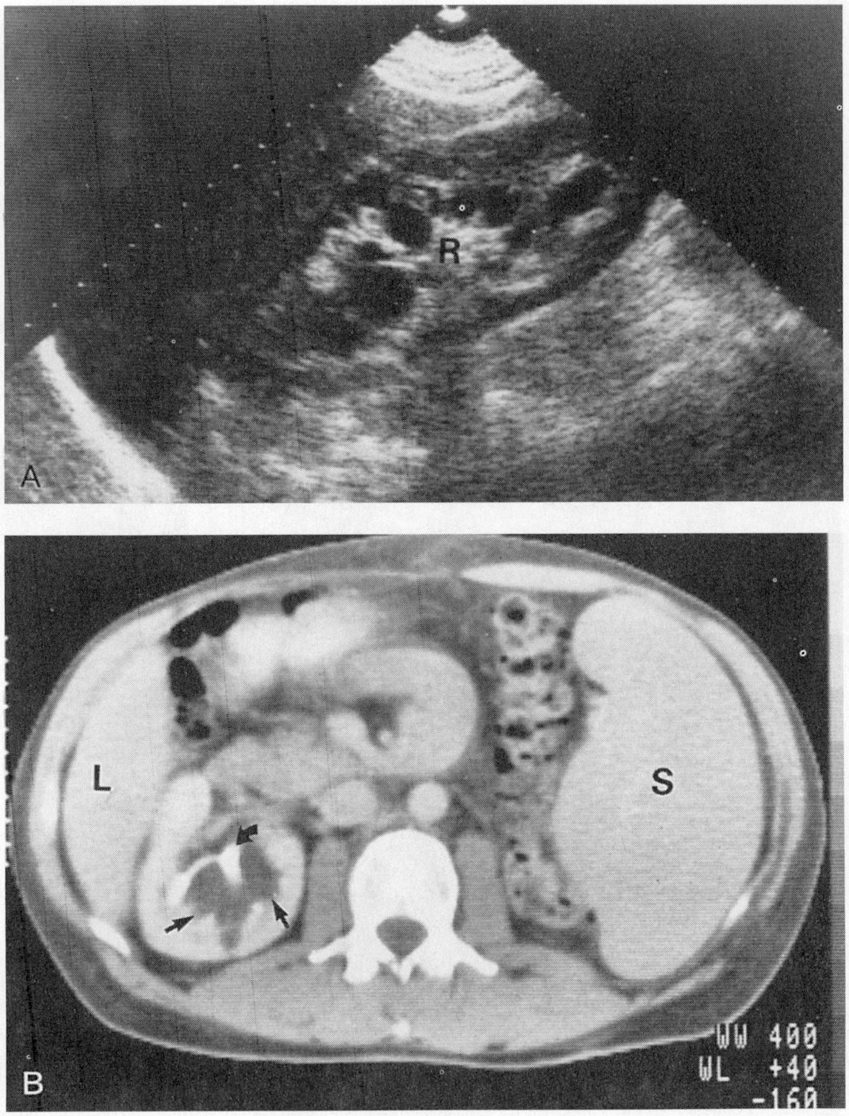

Figure 106.44. Parapelvic cysts. **A:** This transverse scan through the right kidney shows multiple sonolucent structures (rounded black structures), which are parapelvic cysts. R, renal sinus echoes. **B:** Transverse abdominal CT scan of same patient shown in **A** reveals low-attenuation structures *(straight arrows)* around the renal pelvis *(short curved arrow)* representing parapelvic cysts. The patient also has splenomegaly *(S)*. L, liver.

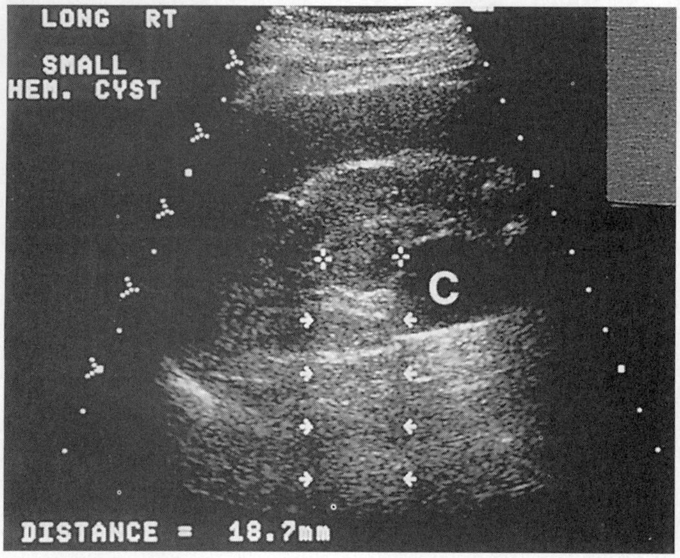

Figure 106.45. Hemorrhagic renal cyst. Longitudinal image of the right kidney. The cyst *(between the cursors)* has homogeneous midlevel internal echoes. The echoes are caused by blood. There is mild "increased through transmission" *(between the arrows)*. C, adjacent simple renal cyst.

Acquired Cystic Disease of the Kidneys

Acquired cystic disease of the kidneys occurs in patients with chronic renal failure and those treated with hemodialysis or peritoneal dialysis. Acquired cysts have been noted in native kidneys of renal transplant recipients as well. The disease is characterized by the development of bilateral small cysts, usually less than 5 mm wide, but sometimes reaching 2.5 to 3 cm. The cysts are filled with clear or hemorrhagic fluid and may arise anywhere in the kidney, but they are predominantly present in the cortex.

Sonographically, shrunken small kidneys with multiple small hypoechoic and/or anechoic lesions with increased through transmission are seen. With time, the kidneys enlarge due to cyst invasion. Patients with acquired cystic disease of the kidneys may develop renal tumors, especially renal adenoma, and less frequently renal cell carcinoma. Such a mass may be demonstrable by sonography.

In general, CT is superior to ultrasound in assessing patients with acquired cystic disease because it is more sensitive in detecting associated small cysts and small renal tumors. If a tumor developing within a cyst is less than 3 cm wide, it should be followed utilizing CT. If it is larger than 3 cm, the diagnosis of renal cell carcinoma should be considered and appropriate diagnostic measures performed.

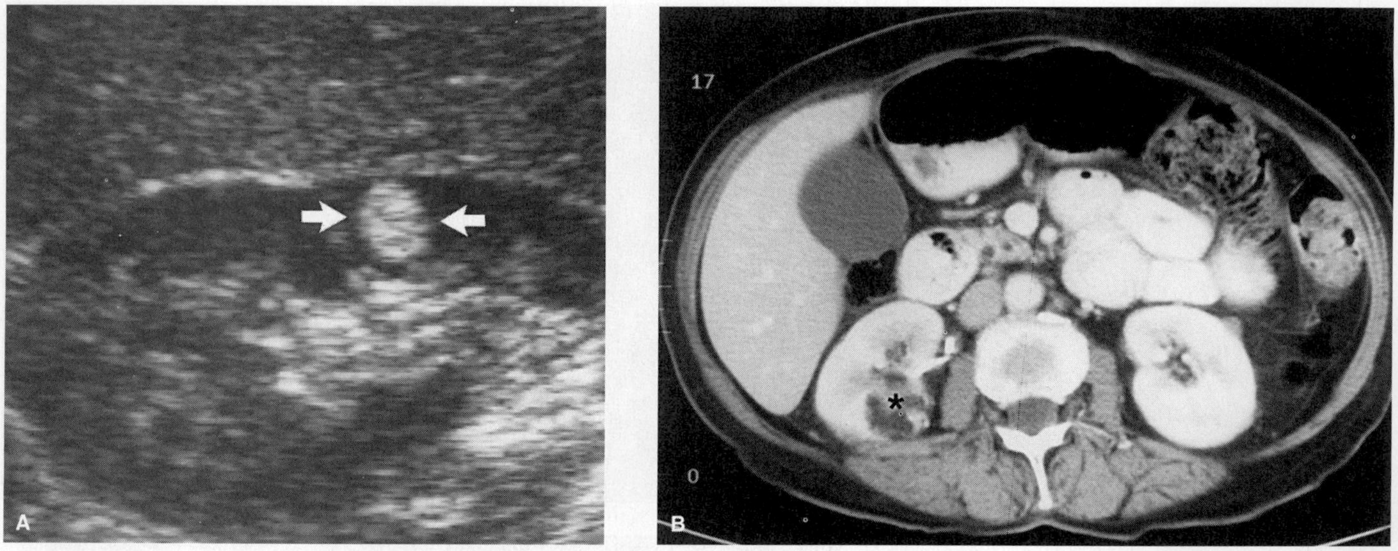

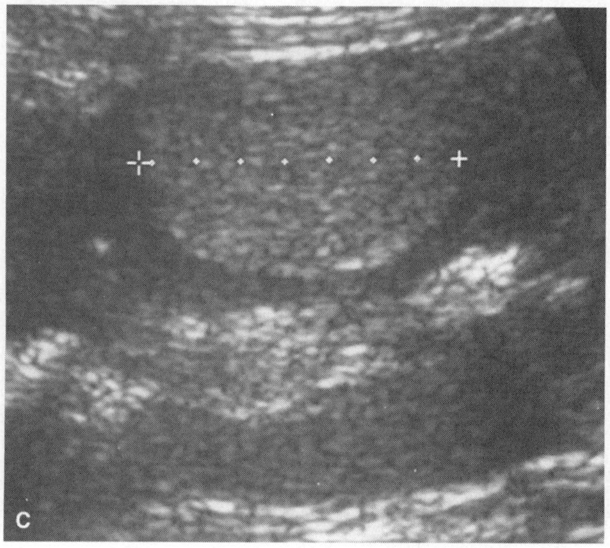

Figure 106.46. Angiomyolipoma. **A:** Transverse sonogram of the right kidney reveals an echogenic cortical mass *(arrows)*. **B:** Abdominal CT. A lesion *(*)* with fat density is seen in the posterior medial right kidney. **C:** Longitudinal sonogram kidney. Echogenic mass in the midkidney is another example of angiomyolipoma.

NEOPLASMS OF THE KIDNEY

Sonography is most useful in differentiating between solid and cystic renal masses. The sonographic characteristics of various benign and malignant renal tumors are detailed in the following sections.

Benign Renal Neoplasms

Angiomyolipoma

This tumor, as the name implies, is composed of blood vessels, smooth muscle, and fat, all in varying proportions. Clinically, there are two forms: (a) multiple bilateral renal masses commonly associated with tuberous sclerosis and (b) unilateral solitary mass, usually occurring in middle-aged women. Ultrasound typically reveals a highly echogenic mass or masses, related to the amount of fat within the tumor (Fig. 106.46A). Mixed echogenicity may be the result of intrarenal hemorrhage. Detection of a well-defined echogenic focus on renal sonography should suggest the presence of an angiomyolipoma. Because other lesions, including renal cell carcinoma, may occasionally be highly echogenic, CT should be performed to confirm the diagnosis (Fig. 106.46B). Angiomyolipomas with less fat have a complex or hypoechoic pattern. Ultrasound is less specific in this situation.

Tuberous Sclerosis

These patients have an increased incidence of renal cysts and liver hamartomas, both of which are readily demonstrated by ultrasound.

Oncocytoma

Oncocytomas are believed to be benign renal adenomas, although there is debate as to whether they constitute a separate pathologic entity. They are uncommon and occur in middle-aged and older patients. They commonly arise in the proximal or distal convoluted tubule or collecting duct. They usually present as an asymptomatic mass, but hematuria or pain may occur. The diagnosis can be suspected if a solitary, homogeneous mass with a central hyperechoic region (scar) is seen (Fig. 106.47). Oncocytomas are usually several centimeters in size. A heterogeneous ultrasound pattern is uncommon. Demonstration of a uniform density mass with central low density (scar) on CT and/or

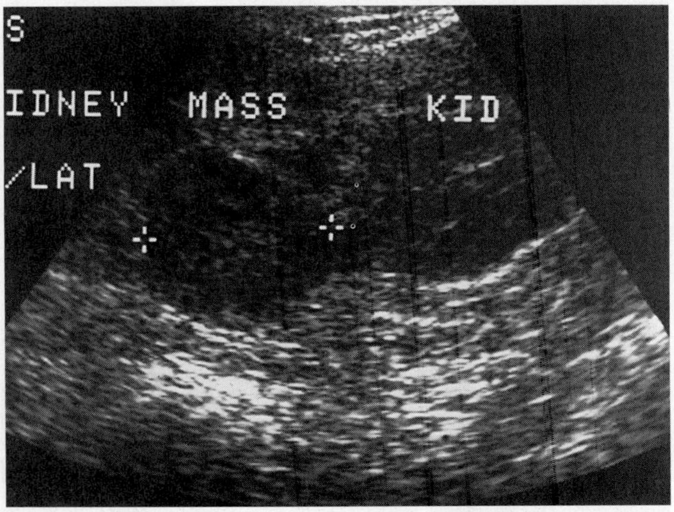

Figure 106.47. Oncocytoma. Transverse sonogram of the left kidney demonstrates a large mass *(cursor)* with a central hyperechoic region representing the central scar.

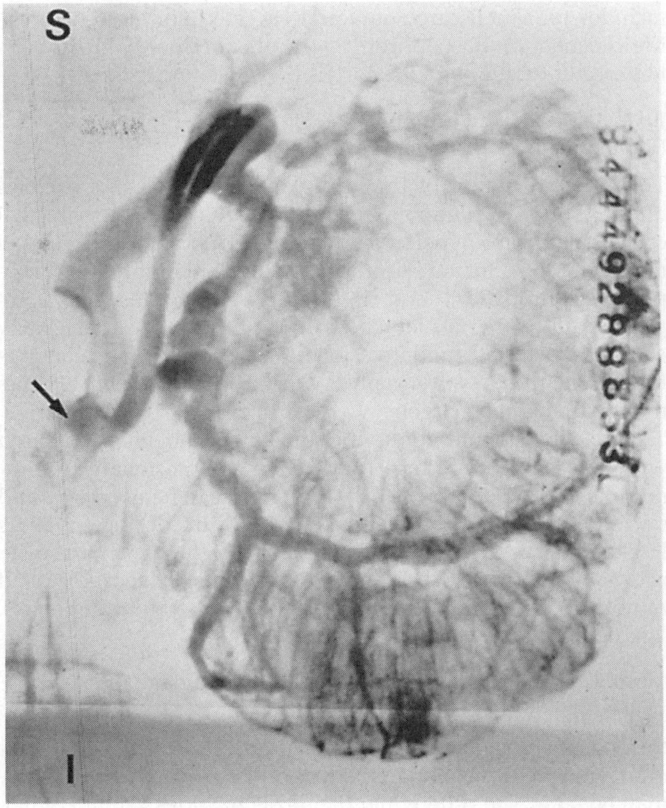

Figure 106.48. Subtraction film from a left renal arteriogram shows the classic "spoke wheel" arterial pattern. *Arrow* points to the main left renal artery. I, inferior; S, superior. (Courtesy of Neela Lamki, M.D.)

a "spoke-wheel" arteriographic pattern (Fig. 106.48) supports the diagnosis. Preoperative diagnosis of this lesion is important when renal-sparing surgery is contemplated.

Multilocular Cystic Nephroma

Multilocular cystic nephroma is a rare neoplasm that has a variety of synonyms, including multilocular renal cyst. It is usually benign and consists of noncommunicating epithelial-lined, fluid-filled locules with stroma in the septa. Occasionally, foci of Wilms' tumor or sarcoma are present in the stroma. When children develop Wilms' tumor in conjunction with this lesion, metastasis is rare; however, sarcomatous elements often metastasize.

In children, multilocular cystic nephroma usually presents as a nonpainful abdominal mass. In adults, abdominal pain and hematuria are the usual presenting symptoms. Under age 4, it is more common in males, but above that age, it has a proclivity to affect females. In females, there is a bimodal age distribution, with peaks in the 4- to 20-year-old and 40- to 50-year-old groups.

A multilocular cyst may show an abdominal mass on plain films. Intravenous urography usually shows a well-defined intrarenal mass. Rarely, the involved kidney may not function due to tumor-related obstruction of the renal pelvis. On sonography, when the cystic spaces are large enough, clustered sonolucent locules separated by septa are seen. Increased through transmission is noted distal to the locules. Occasionally, when the locules are small, a nonspecific complex renal mass will be seen.

CT usually shows a multicystic mass if the locules are large enough to be imaged. Ultrasound or CT can be used to check for recurrence in the renal bed after tumor excision if nephroblastic or sarcomatous elements were present. Differential diagnosis includes renal cell carcinoma and septated simple renal cyst. Multilocular cystic nephroma is most commonly treated by nephrectomy, although local excision is used occasionally.

Juxtaglomerular Cell Tumor (Reninoma or Hemangiopericytoma)

This is a rare tumor of the juxtaglomerular cells that excretes renin. About 50% of lesions occur in patients younger than 20. It causes significant hypertension that resolves with tumor resection. Symptoms include headaches, polydipsia, polyuria (kaliopenic nephropathy), and intermittent neuromuscular complaints due to hypokalemia. Peripheral renin level is usually elevated. Metastasis and invasion have not been reported in this tumor. The tumors are usually solitary and 2 to 3 cm in size, although they can be larger.

Typically, the tumor is sonographically echogenic compared with adjacent normal renal parenchyma. Occasionally, the tumor may be hypoechoic, which is often due to hemorrhagic and necrotic areas. With contrast-enhanced CT, this lesion enhances less-than-normal renal parenchyma. Arteriographically, the mass is usually hypovascular. Diagnosis is by clinical, laboratory, and radiologic findings, including selective renal vein renin levels. Excision of the tumor is curative.

Mesoblastic Nephroma (Fetal Renal Hamartoma)

This benign renal tumor is the most common solid renal mass in the neonate. It is usually a solitary tumor, which is fairly evenly echogenic on ultrasound. However, any pattern of echogenicity may be seen. The differential diagnosis includes Wilms' tumor.

Malignant Renal Neoplasms

Renal Cell Carcinoma (Hypernephroma, Adenocarcinoma)

Renal cell carcinoma, by far the most common primary renal malignancy, is seen in adults, chiefly occurring after age 40. There may be an increased incidence of renal cell carcinoma in patients receiving chronic dialysis with acquired cystic disease of the kidney and in patients with von Hippel-Lindau syndrome (an autosomal-dominant disorder characterized by retinal angiomas, cerebellar or spinal cord hemangioblastoma, renal cell carcinoma, renal cysts, and pancreatic cysts). Sonographically, renal cell carcinoma is seen as a hypoechoic to mixed echogenic mass (Figs. 106.49 and 106.50). Anechoic or hypoechoic regions with increased through transmission related to necrosis, hemorrhage, or tumor vascularity occurs in up to 40% of cases (Fig. 106.51). Tumor vascularity as documented on Doppler ultrasound examination may vary (Fig. 106.52). Some investigators report a correlation between echogenicity and tumor vascularity, whereas others believe no such association exists. Tumoral calcification (Fig. 106.53), which occurs in 10% to 20% of renal cell carcinomas, is seen as echogenic foci with shadowing. Some carcinomas may have a multilocular cystic appearance. Tumors

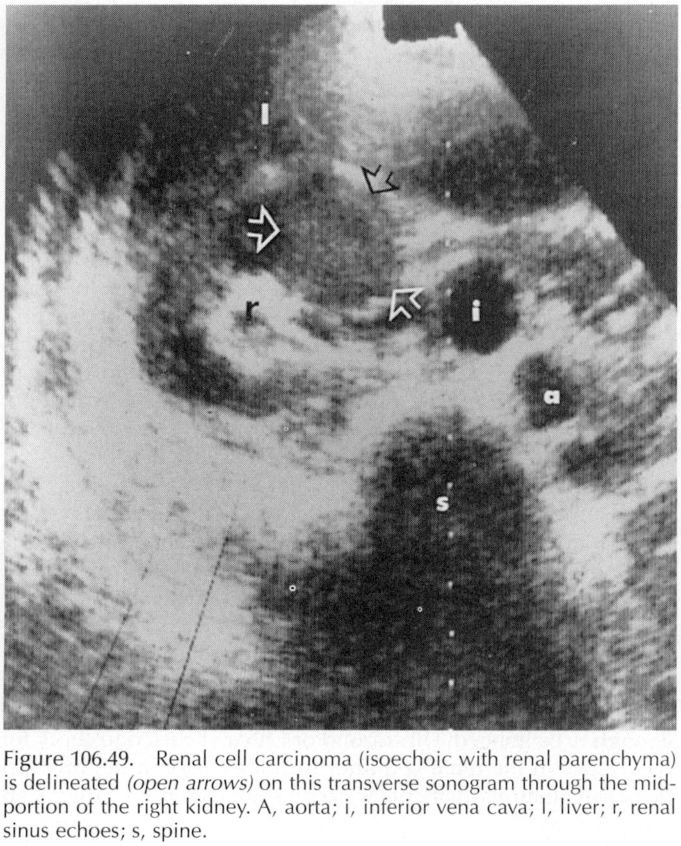

Figure 106.49. Renal cell carcinoma (isoechoic with renal parenchyma) is delineated *(open arrows)* on this transverse sonogram through the midportion of the right kidney. A, aorta; i, inferior vena cava; l, liver; r, renal sinus echoes; s, spine.

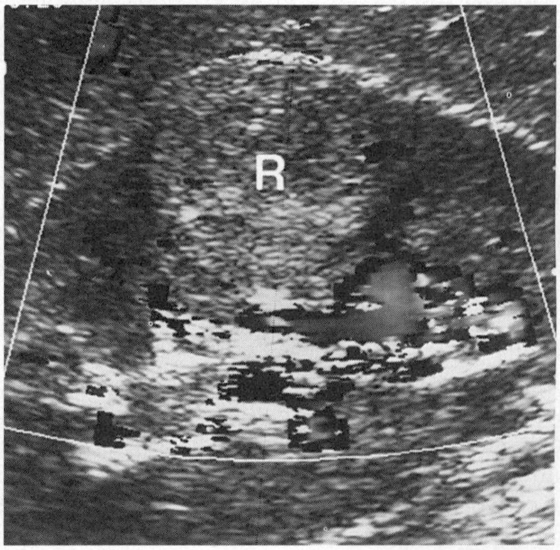

Figure 106.50. Renal cell carcinoma *(R)* (hyperechoic as compared with adjacent renal parenchyma) is delineated on this longitudinal renal sonogram. This appearance is unusual and may be confused for an angiomyolipoma because of the increased echogenicity.

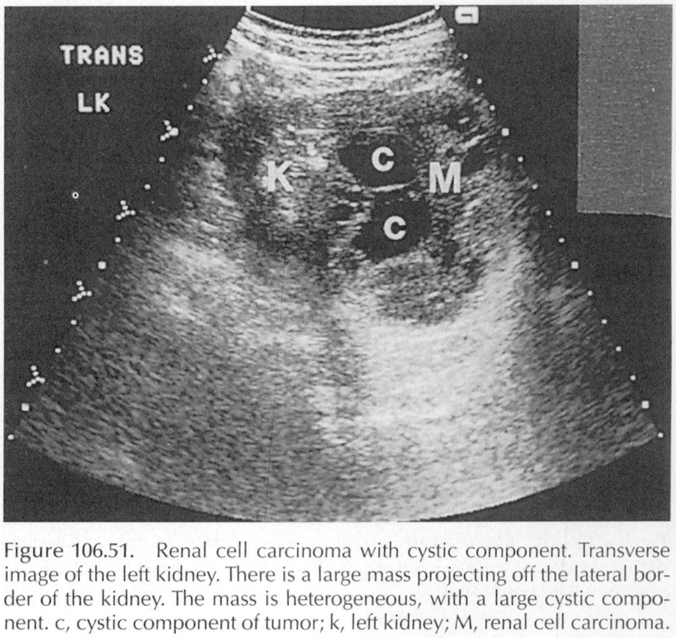

Figure 106.51. Renal cell carcinoma with cystic component. Transverse image of the left kidney. There is a large mass projecting off the lateral border of the kidney. The mass is heterogeneous, with a large cystic component. c, cystic component of tumor; k, left kidney; M, renal cell carcinoma.

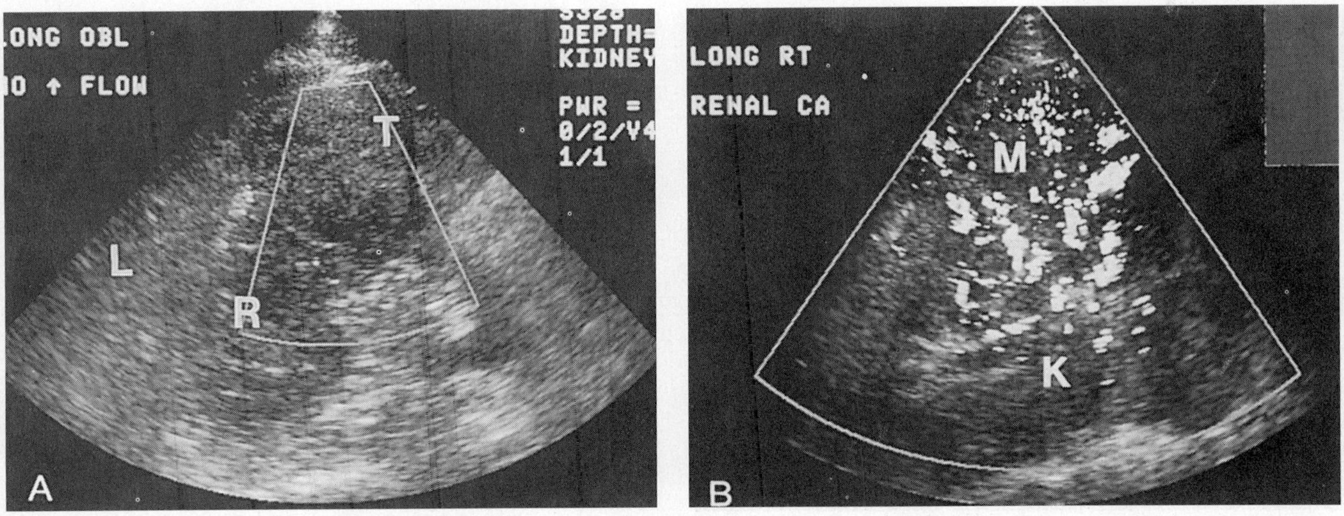

Figure 106.52. Spectrum of renal cell carcinoma vascularity. **A:** Longitudinal oblique gray-scale Doppler image of the right kidney. There is no evidence of increased blood flow into the tumor. L, liver; r, right kidney; T, renal cell carcinoma. **B:** Longitudinal color flow Doppler image of the right kidney. Increased vascular flow within a renal cell carcinoma. The mass *(M)* extends beyond the normal renal contour. K, right kidney; M, renal cell carcinoma. (See Color Figure 106.52A.)

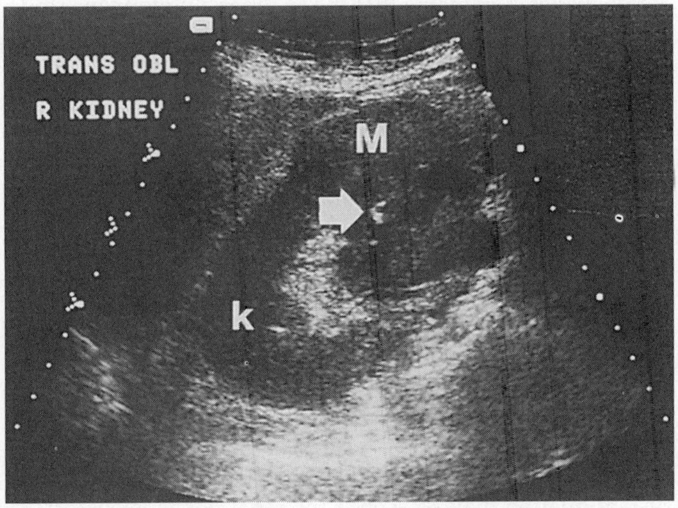

Figure 106.53. Calcifications within a renal cell carcinoma. Transverse oblique image of the right kidney. The heterogenous mass *(M)* occupying the medial inferior portion of the kidney is a renal cell carcinoma. The discrete echogenic focus within the mass is a dystrophic calcification. The *white arrow* denotes dystrophic malignant calcification. k, right kidney; M, mass-renal cell carcinoma.

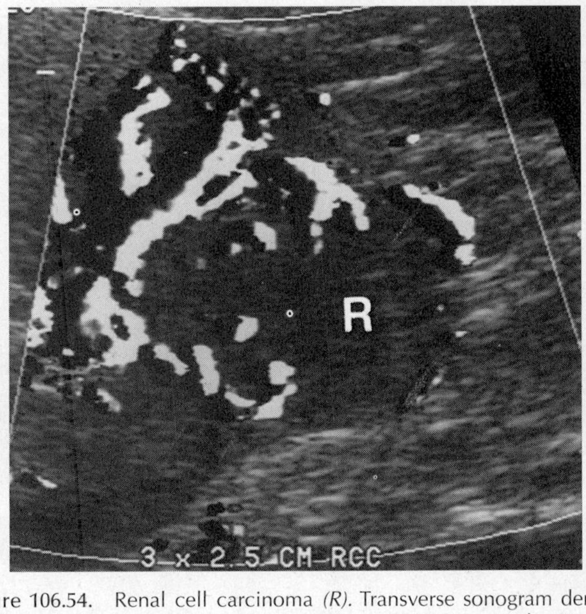

Figure 106.54. Renal cell carcinoma *(R)*. Transverse sonogram demonstrating a cortical hypoechoic mass measuring 3 × 2.5 cm. Color Doppler demonstrates minimal circumferential and internal flow.

range from well encapsulated and sharply marginated to poorly defined with infiltration of surrounding tissues (Figs. 106.54 and 106.55). Retroperitoneal lymphadenopathy, involvement of the contralateral kidney, and extension into adjacent organs such as liver or colon is sometimes seen (Fig. 106.55). When a discovered mass is suspected to be a renal cell carcinoma, a concerted effort must be made to assess the ipsilateral renal vein and inferior vena cava (Fig. 106.56). Although ultrasound may be useful in the staging of renal cell carcinoma, it is generally of lesser benefit than CT.

Urothelial Carcinoma

These renal neoplasms arise from the epithelial lining of the calyces, renal pelvis, ureters, and bladder. More than 80% of tumors arising from the collecting system and renal pelvic epithelium are transitional cell carcinomas, whereas most of the remaining 20% are squamous cell carcinomas. Adenocarcinomas of the renal collecting system and pelvis are of rare incidence. On sonography, the lesion is confined to the renal pelvis and appears relatively echogenic compared with the surrounding fluid. Hydronephrosis may be an accompanying finding (Fig. 106.57) as well as separation of the renal sinus echoes by a hypoechoic lesion. Occasionally, urothelial carcinoma presents as a bulky, infiltrating mass with low-level echoes. Renal vein invasion, although uncommon, can occur and can be visualized using ultrasound. A blood clot or nonopaque stone can mimic a renal pelvic tumor on intravenous urography; ultrasound can help differentiate these entities.

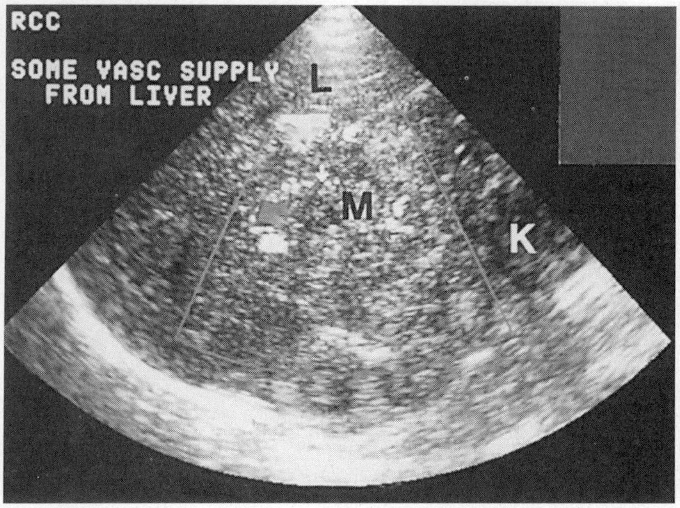

Figure 106.55. Renal cell carcinoma invading adjacent liver. Longitudinal color Doppler image of the right kidney and liver. The renal cell carcinoma has invaded the liver and is parasitizing the hepatic vasculature. The *arrow* denotes vascular flow from the liver to the mass. K, right kidney; L, liver; M, mass-renal cell carcinoma. (See Color Figure 106.55.)

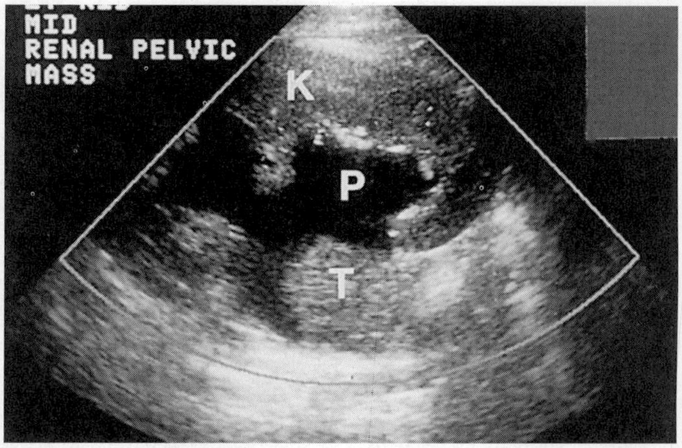

Figure 106.57. Transitional cell carcinoma. Longitudinal color flow Doppler image of the left kidney. The homogenous hyperechoic tumor is free of demonstrable vascular flow. It is partially obstructing the renal pelvis. K, left kidney; P, dilated renal pelvis; T, transitional cell carcinoma (tumor). (See Color Figure 106.57.)

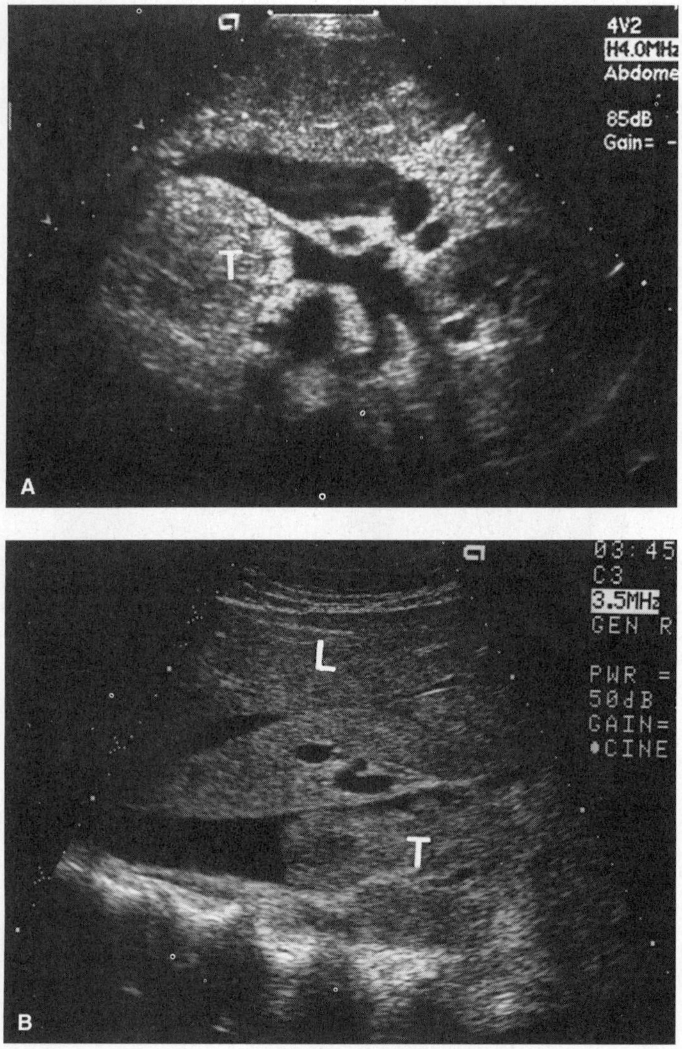

Figure 106.56. **A:** Transverse scan of the inferior vena cava showing tumor thrombus (T). **B:** Longitudinal scan of the inferior vena cava showing tumor thrombus *(T)*. L, liver.

Serial sonograms may show a change in echogenicity, size, and shape, suggesting a clot. An echogenic focus with shadowing makes it probable that the lesion is a nonopaque stone. Retrograde pyelography with a brush biopsy may be necessary for a definitive diagnosis.

Wilms' Tumor (Nephroblastoma)

Wilms' tumor is the most common abdominal neoplasm of childhood, with peak incidence at 3 years of age. It is uncommon under the age of 1 year and over the age of 8 years. Approximately 5% of patients have bilateral involvement. Nephroblastomatosis, persistence of metanephric blastema in the kidneys of infants and children, predisposes to the development of bilateral Wilms' tumor. Other congenital anomalies associated with Wilms' tumor include aniridia, Beckwith-Wiedemann syndrome, hemihypertrophy, and genitourinary tract anomalies. Sonographically, a large kidney with a solid, evenly echogenic mass is seen. A mass with a pattern of solid and cystic areas may also occur (Fig. 106.58). Cystic components are mostly due to necrosis or hemorrhage. Collecting system dilation may be seen if the renal pelvis is obstructed. Because approximately 5% of patients have bilateral tumors, it is imperative to assess both kidneys. The renal veins inferior vena cava and liver should also be examined, because tumor deposits may be seen in these locations. CT is a useful adjunct to ultrasound in patients with Wilms' tumor, because it is superior in assessing extent of disease. The differential diagnosis is mesoblastic nephroma.

Sarcomas

Kidney sarcomas arise from parenchymal mesenchymal tissues or the kidney capsule. Sarcomas account for 2% to 3% of primary malignant renal tumors. When they involve the retroperitoneum, they may be indistinguishable from primary retroperitoneal sarcomas. Leiomyosarcoma, liposarcoma, and hemangiopericytoma are the most common histologic types. To date, there are no large series describing the sonographic appearance of these tumors.

Lymphoma

Renal lymphoma may produce a solitary mass, multiple masses, or renal enlargement from diffuse infiltration (Figs. 106.59 and

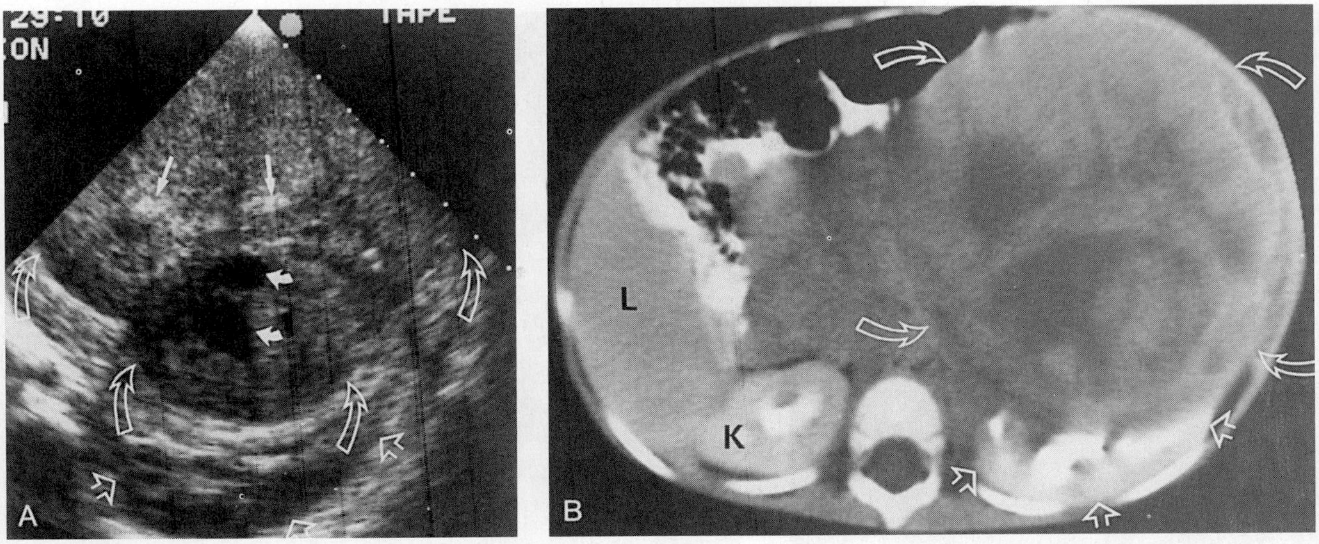

Figure 106.58. **A:** Wilms' tumor (nephroblastoma) is depicted *(curved open arrows)* on the transverse left renal sonogram. Note that it is a heterogeneous mass with hyperechoic *(straight solid arrows)* and hypoechoic *(short curved solid arrows)* components arising from the kidney. A small amount of normal renal tissue is present *(straight open arrows)*. **B:** Wilms' tumor (nephroblastoma). Transverse abdominal CT scan of patient in **A** reveals a large heterogeneous left renal mass *(curved open arrows)* that distorts the collecting system. Functioning renal tissue is present posteriorly *(straight open arrows)*. K, right kidney; L, liver.

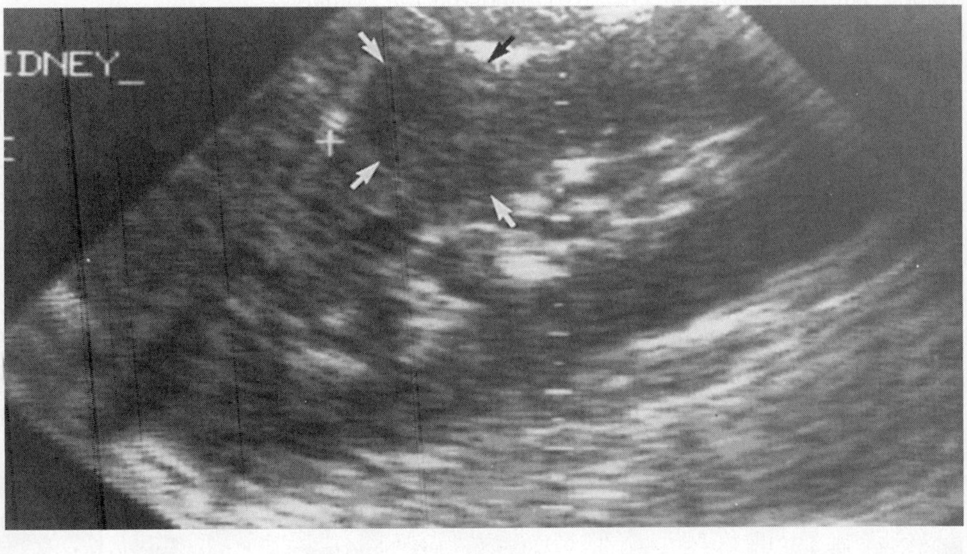

Figure 106.59. Lymphoma (focal) is seen on this transverse renal sonogram as a hypoechoic mass *(arrows)*.

106.60). Involvement of perinephric tissue is not uncommon. Primary renal lymphoma is extremely rare. Most often, renal lymphoma results from hematogenous metastasis or local extension from adjacent nodal masses. In homogeneous lymphoma, the characteristic sonographic pattern is that of a hypoechoic or anechoic mass or masses. Margins of lymphomatous masses are less sharply outlined than those of cysts. Through transmission may be seen, but it is less pronounced than that which occurs with a cyst. Discovery of a renal mass or masses with these characteristics should suggest lymphoma, especially if it coexists with retroperitoneal lymphadenopathy or hepatosplenomegaly. Multifocal lymphoma has been confused with polycystic kidney disease on ultrasound. Varying echo patterns may be seen in certain forms of lymphoma where different cellular components or fibrosis is present.

Leukemia

Renal involvement is common in all forms of leukemia, and ultrasound is the best modality to follow these patients. Sonographic findings include kidney enlargement, loss of definition and distortion of the renal sinus echoes, diffuse coarse echoes throughout the renal cortex with preservation of the renal medulla, and focal mass or masses. The kidney reverts to normal after curative chemotherapy.

Other Neoplastic Metastases

Renal metastases are commonly found in autopsy series. These tumors rarely cause symptoms, making antemortem diagnosis uncommon. They are usually discovered during staging of a primary lesion or as an incidental finding. Lung and breast

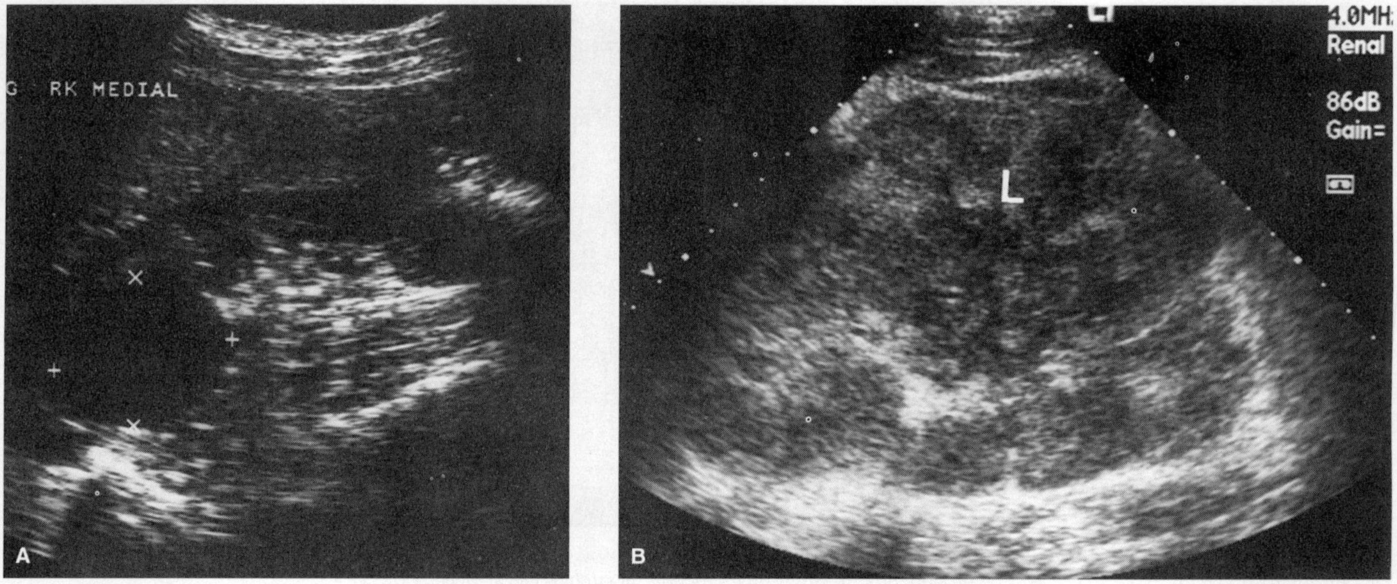

Figure 106.60. Lymphoma. **A:** Variable appearance of lymphoma may appear as a well-defined focal hypoechoic mass *(cursors in **A**)*. **B:** Variable appearance of lymphoma may appear as a heterogeneous infiltrative mass (*L* in **B**).

tissues are the most common sources of metastases. The sonographic pattern of renal metastasis depends on the primary malignancy and varies from hypoechoic to hyperechoic. On occasion, metastatic lesions invade renal veins.

THE RENAL TRANSPLANT

Ultrasound has earned a key role in evaluating renal transplant patients. Transplanted kidneys are easily imaged with ultrasound because of their relatively superficial location in the iliac fossa. Transplant-related complications include rejection, acute tubular necrosis, obstruction, infection, vascular compromise, and development of a peritransplant fluid collection. Sonographic findings in these conditions are often nonspecific; therefore correlation with clinical and laboratory data, along with other diagnostic studies, is essential to arrive at the correct diagnosis.

Normal Transplant Kidneys

Generally, the donor kidney is transplanted into the contralateral iliac fossa of the recipient. The arterial supply of the transplanted kidney is usually end-to-end anastomosis of donor renal artery to host internal iliac artery, or end-to-side anastomosis of donor renal artery to host external iliac artery. Venous drainage is usually accomplished via end-to-side anastomosis of the transplanted renal vein to the external or internal iliac vein. In the transplanted kidney, the renal pelvis and ureter are anterior to the renal artery, which in turn is anterior to the renal vein (the reverse of normal).

The donor ureter is most often anastomosed to the bladder by a ureteroneocystostomy. Typically, the transplanted kidney is ellipsoid with the anteroposterior ratio of the diameter to length varying between 0.36 and 0.54. The most echogenic portion is the renal sinus, followed by the renal cortex. Be-

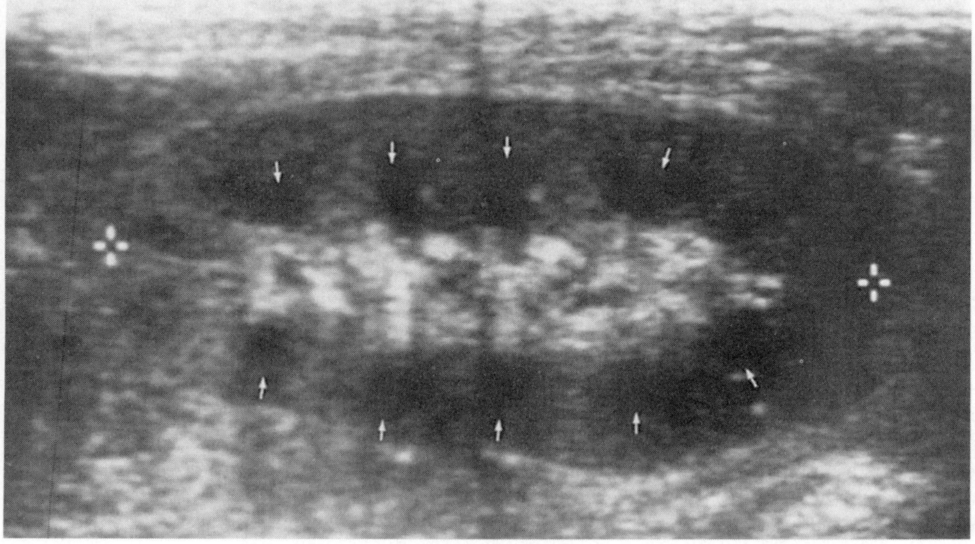

Figure 106.61. Normal transplant kidney. On this transverse image, the strong echoes in the kidney are the renal sinus echoes. The hypoechoic regions *(arrows)* are the pyramids. (Courtesy of Bharat Raval, M.D.)

cause the pyramids are hypoechoic, the corticomedullary junction is distinct (Fig. 106.61). In the immediate postoperative period, mild caliectasis is common but disappears in time. Normally, the transplanted kidney hypertrophies but maintains an ellipsoid configuration. It is important to obtain an ultrasound immediately after the renal transplant for baseline comparison.

Complications Associated with Kidney Rejection

A normal sonogram of a transplanted kidney does not exclude rejection, although in acute rejection, the kidney loses its ellipsoid shape as the anteroposterior diameter to length ratio increases, making it more globular. The parenchyma can also increase in thickness. If there is interstitial peritubular edema, the corticomedullary junction is prominent and the medullary pyramids are enlarged (Fig. 106.62). This finding can sometimes be seen in the normal adolescent and adult, as well as in acute tubular necrosis, and rarely after diuretic administration. The corticomedullary junction may be obscured if there is cellular infiltration and edema. Renal sinus echoes are decreased, or even absent, due to the decreased fat and edema (Fig. 106.63). Hypoechoic regions throughout the parenchyma may be seen.

Increased peripheral resistance, defined as greater than 0.75 or 0.90 (depending on the study), can be seen in many patients with acute transplant rejection. Elevated peripheral resistance is a nonspecific finding, occurring in patients with acute tubular necrosis, cyclosporine toxicity, renal vein thrombosis, and pyelonephritis. Transplant infarct will demonstrate absent flow on color Doppler (Fig. 106.64).

Although the sonographic appearance of chronic rejection has not been well studied, data from some investigators suggest that the transplant kidney can be diffusely hyperechoic or have increased cortical echoes (Fig. 106.65). Hypoechoic regions may be seen in the parenchyma. The kidney may decrease in size or remain unchanged.

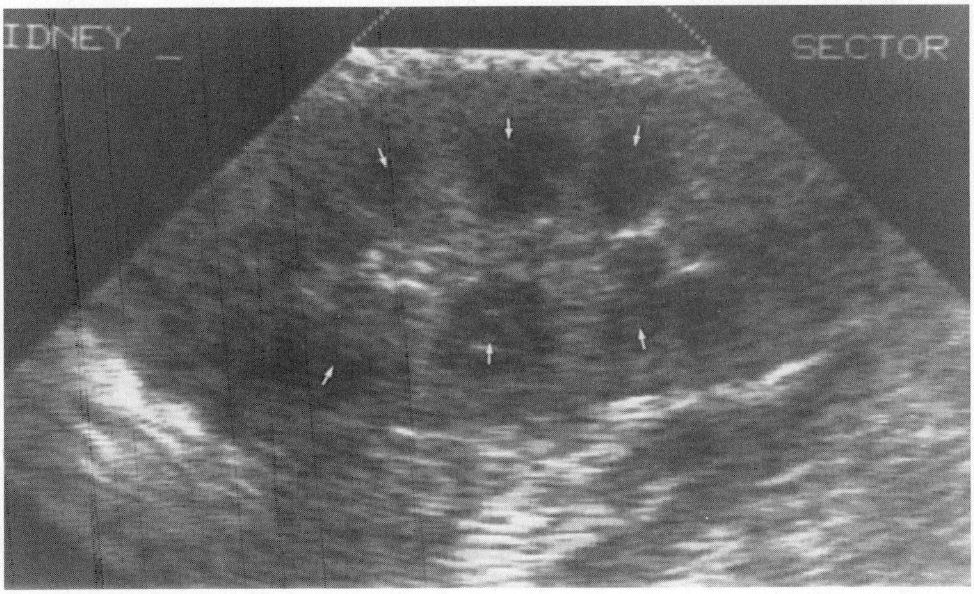

Figure 106.62. Acute rejection. Longitudinal scan of transplant kidney shows enlarged pyramids *(arrows)*.

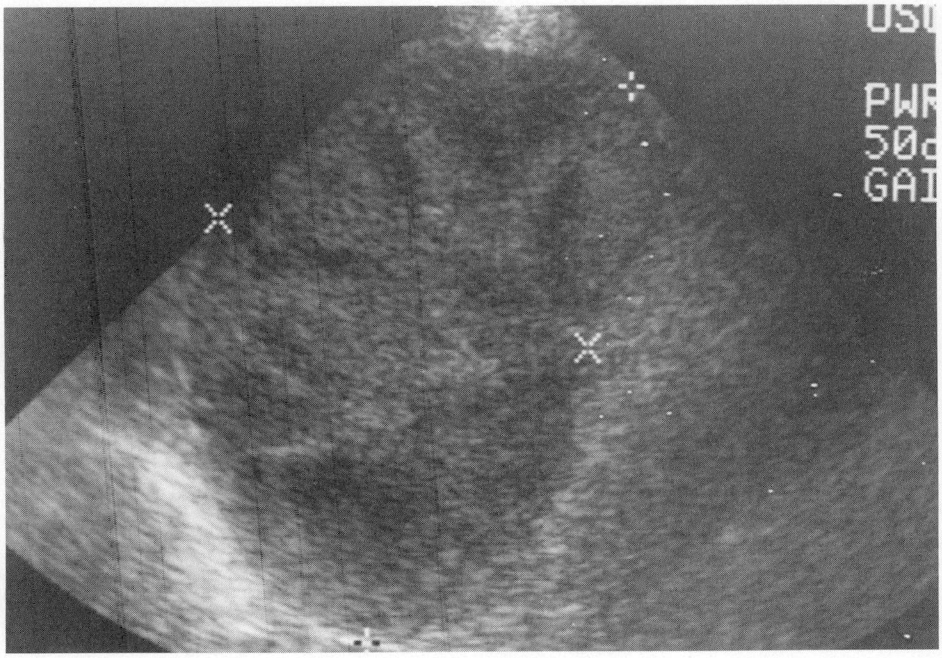

Figure 106.63. Acute rejection. Coronal sonogram of transplant kidney *(between cursors)* demonstrates obliteration of the corticomedullary junction and renal sinus echoes caused by edema (compare with normal transplant kidney in Fig. 106.61).

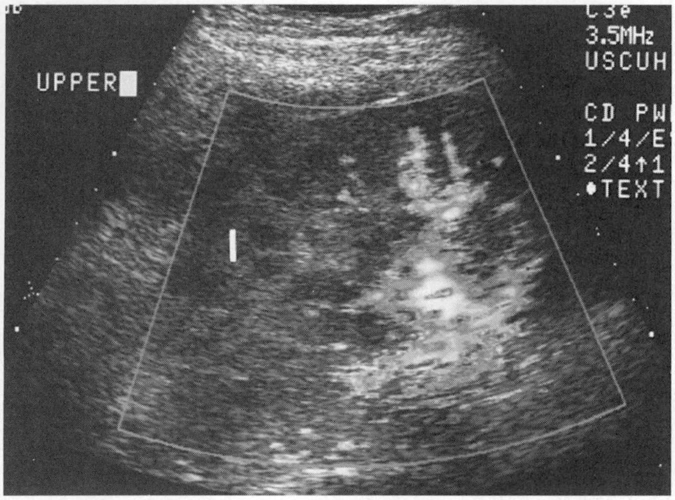

Figure 106.64. Infarct in transplant kidney. Transverse sonogram of transplant kidney demonstrates absent flow in upper pole with Doppler *(I)*.

Acute Tubular Necrosis

In acute tubular necrosis, there is usually no change in appearance of the transplant kidney from baseline. Rarely, the corticomedullary junction may be prominent and increased cortical echoes may also be identified.

Dilated Collecting System

Mild caliectasis can be present immediately after transplantation. This finding may also be seen in acute or chronic rejection without obstruction. It is important to recognize pyelocaliectasis from ureteric dilation caused by obstructive uropathy because the latter is correctable. Intrinsic causes of obstruction include calculi (Fig. 106.66), clots (Fig. 106.67), and tumor. Ureteric, ureteropelvic junction, or ureterovesicular junction strictures may develop. Finally, an adjacent peritransplant fluid collection or pelvic mass may result in obstruction of urinary flow in the ureter due to extrinsic compression. Generally, a complementary imaging study such as intravenous urography, nuclear medicine scan, or retrograde pyeloureterography is necessary to diagnose obstruction and its cause.

Vascular Lesions

Renal vein thrombosis can occur in the postoperative period. The sonographic picture includes enlargement of the transplanted kidney, hypoechoic cortex, increased thickness of the cortex, and possible obscuring of the corticomedullary junction. Because these findings may be seen in acute rejection, correlation with Doppler ultrasound or venography is necessary.

Renal artery occlusion can present as acute renal failure and have no abnormal sonographic morphologic findings. Therefore Doppler ultrasound or arteriographic correlation is necessary to make a definitive diagnosis.

Peritransplant Fluid Collection

Ultrasound is much more sensitive than intravenous urography and radionuclide scanning in detecting peritransplant fluid collection. Etiology of fluid collection includes lymphocele, urinoma, abscess, hematoma, and seroma, with overlap existing between their various sonographic appearances (Fig. 160.68); because sonographic features are not specific in fluid collection, correlation with clinical parameters is imperative. Ultrasound-guided needle aspiration is often necessary to confirm the diagnosis.

Lymphocele

A lymphocele is a collection of lymph fluid occurring quite frequently in the postoperative period. It occurs in up to 20% of renal transplant patients, usually within a few weeks after surgery. The most common location is inferior to the transplant. Lymphoceles occur when lymphatics remain ligated or are not anastomosed after ligation. On ultrasound, lymphoceles are noted as extraperitoneal fluid collections that are sonolucent, with increased through transmission of sound, and frequently contain septations. On serial sonograms, they

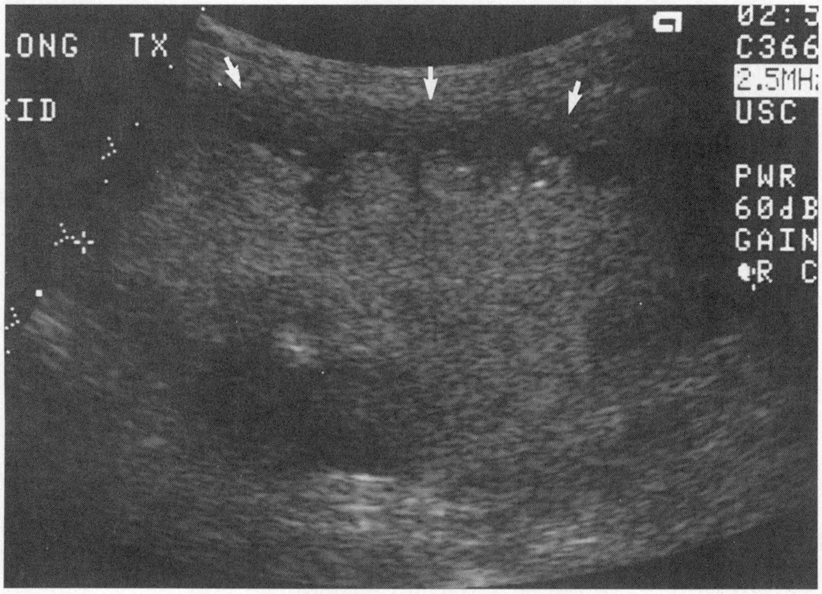

Figure 106.65. Failed renal transplant. Transverse renal sonogram shows diminished renal cortex *(arrows)* and enlarged hyperechoic central kidney.

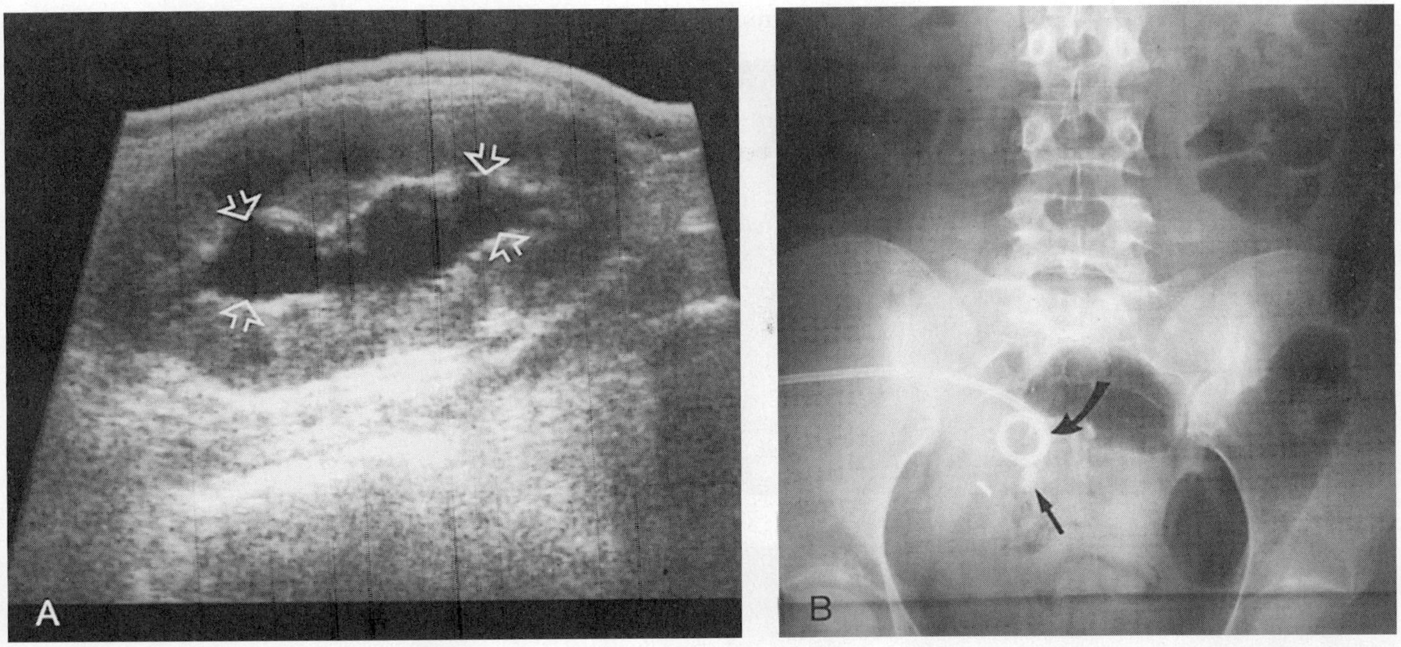

Figure 106.66. **A:** Hydronephrosis *(open arrows)* is present in this renal transplant. **B:** The cause of the obstruction was calculus *(straight arrow),* which was percutaneously extracted using sonographic guidance. A pigtail nephrostomy catheter is in place *(curved arrow)*. (Courtesy of Bharat Raval, M.D.)

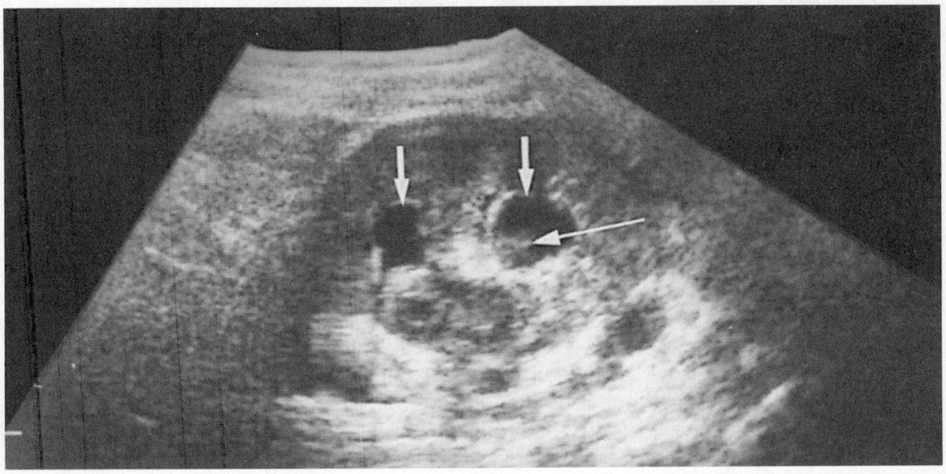

Figure 106.67. Hydronephrosis *(short arrows)* is depicted on the transverse sonogram scan of a renal transplant. The cause of obstruction was clot formation *(long arrow)* secondary to renal biopsy. (Courtesy of Bharat Raval, M.D.)

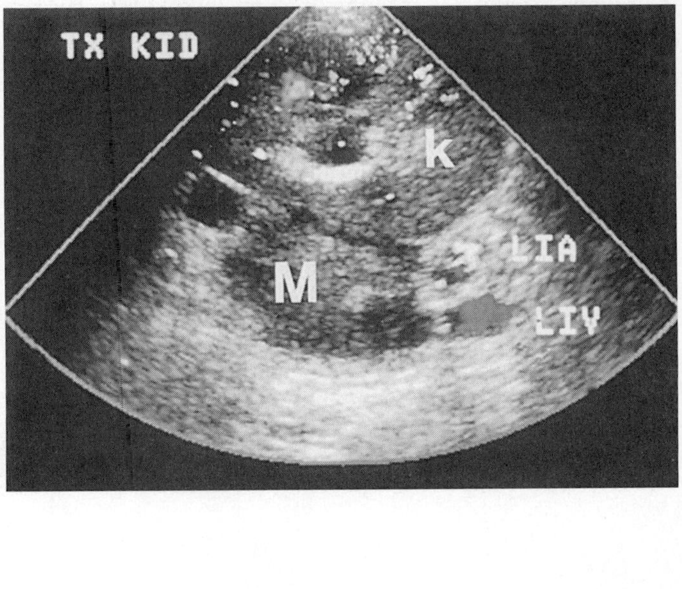

Figure 106.68. Posttransplant perirenal hematoma. Transverse color flow Doppler image of the transplanted kidney in the left pelvis. The heteroechoic mass *(M)* adjacent to kidney is a hematoma. There is no Doppler signal within the clot. k, transplant kidney; LIA, left iliac artery; LIV, left iliac vein. (See Color Figure 106.68.)

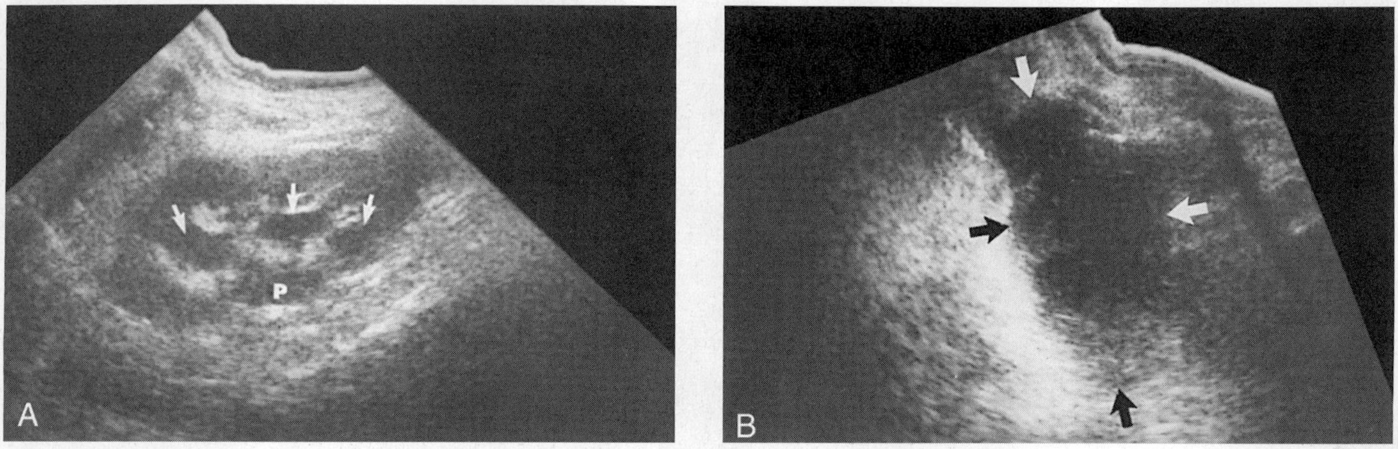

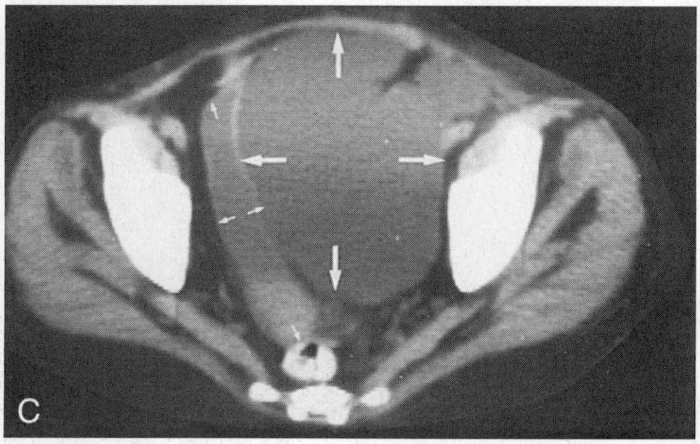

Figure 106.69. Lymphocele. **A:** Longitudinal sonogram of renal transplant 12 weeks after implantation shows hydronephrosis *(arrows)*. P, dilated renal pelvis. **B:** Longitudinal pelvic sonogram obtained after the bladder was emptied in the same patient shows a fluid collection *(arrows)* with septations representing the lymphocele. **C:** Transverse CT scan obtained through the pelvis at the time of the sonogram shows the lymphocele *(long arrows)* displacing the bladder to the right *(short arrows)*. (Courtesy of Bharat Raval, M.D.)

may be noted to gradually increase in size. When large enough, lymphoceles can cause ureteral obstruction, leading to decreased urine output (Fig. 106.69). Lower extremity venous return may be compromised, resulting in leg edema. Pressure on the bladder can cause difficulty urinating. Sonographic examination is important because clinical signs of lymphoceles can mimic rejection.

Urinoma

A urinoma usually occurs within the first 3 weeks after surgery or late in the postoperative period. It is associated with decreased urine output or urine draining through the surgical wound. The most common site of early leakage is at the ureteric anastomosis. Late development of a urinoma is generally related to closed renal injury, renal biopsy, obstructive uropathy, or urinary fistula. Sonographically, a fluid collection may be demonstrated, most commonly near the inferior renal pole. Septation is rare but may be present. Intravenous urography, radionuclide scanning, or aspiration is necessary to diagnose urinoma (Fig. 106.70).

Abscess

Abscesses and other infections frequently occur in renal transplant patients because they are immunosuppressed. The sonographic appearance of an abscess is variable. Abscesses may be partially liquefied, creating regions of increased and decreased echoes. When completely liquefied, an abscess may be cystic (Fig. 106.71). If gas-producing bacteria are present, increased echoes and "dirty" shadowing distal to the lesion may be seen.

Hematoma (Fig. 106.68)

In the acute postoperative period, a hematoma is usually due to a vascular anastomotic leak (Fig. 106.65). When it occurs later, a hematoma may be due to rejection or a complication of biopsy. On sonography, hematomas are echogenic if less than a week old and may be difficult to differentiate from peritransplant tissues if no mass effect is present. With time, they liquefy and become cystic in appearance, often with thick septations.

Seroma

This is a focal collection of serum, which results in a mass. This complication generally occurs immediately postoperatively. Sonographically, a seroma is cystic in appearance.

RENAL TRAUMA

Although ultrasound is typically not the modality of choice in evaluating the patient with renal trauma, it can be useful as a follow-up examination in patients who are managed conservatively. Intrarenal, perirenal, and subcapsular hematoma, as well as renal fracture, can be demonstrated with sonography. Depending

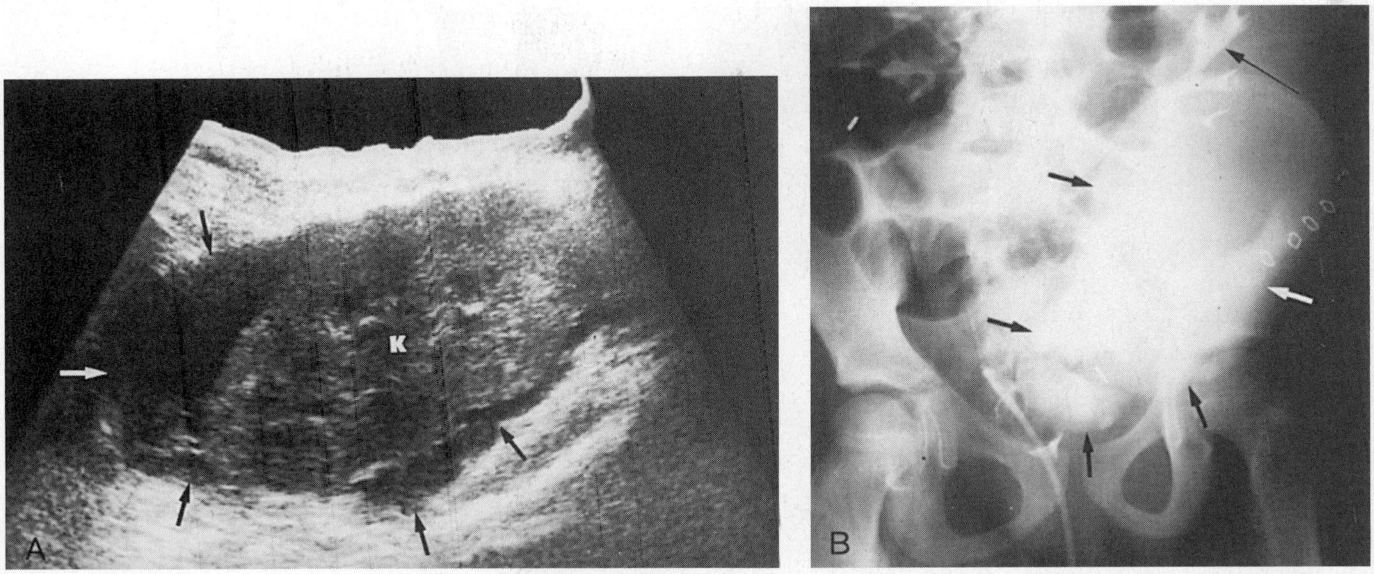

Figure 106.70. Urinoma. **A:** Fluid is present around the renal transplant *(arrows)* on this longitudinal sonogram. k, transplant kidney. **B:** Intravenous urography shows the transplant to be functioning *(long arrow)* and demonstrates leakage of contrast *(short arrows)* forming a urinoma (the cause for the fluid collection seen on the sonogram). (Courtesy of Bharat Raval, M.D.)

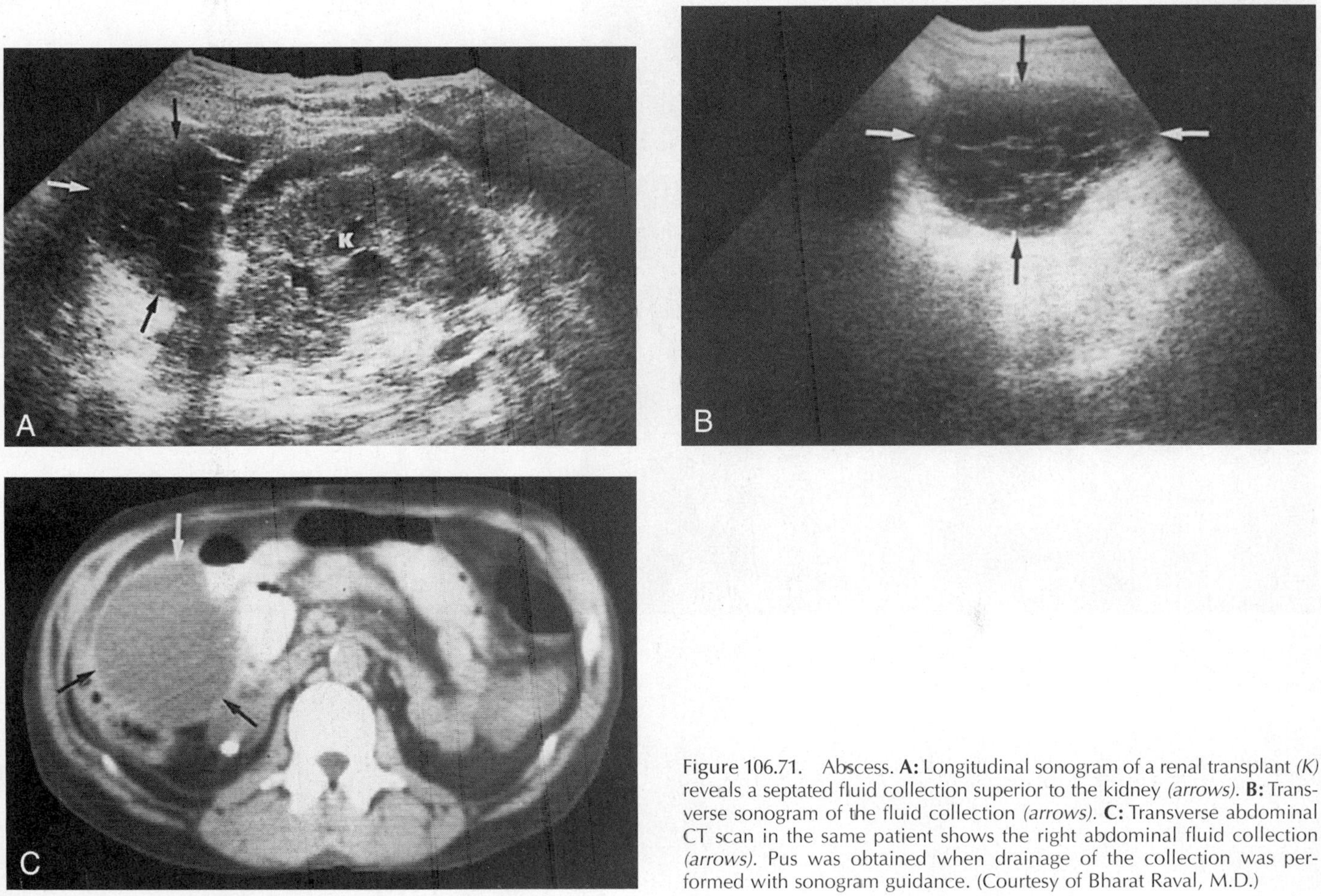

Figure 106.71. Abscess. **A:** Longitudinal sonogram of a renal transplant *(K)* reveals a septated fluid collection superior to the kidney *(arrows)*. **B:** Transverse sonogram of the fluid collection *(arrows)*. **C:** Transverse abdominal CT scan in the same patient shows the right abdominal fluid collection *(arrows)*. Pus was obtained when drainage of the collection was performed with sonogram guidance. (Courtesy of Bharat Raval, M.D.)

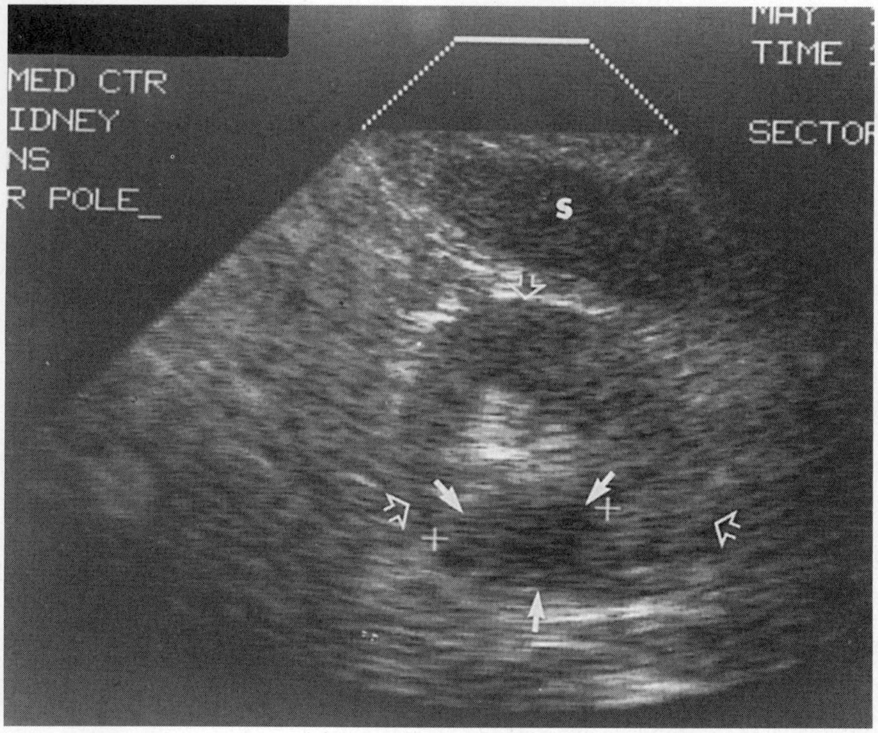

Figure 106.72. Hypoechoic intrarenal hematoma *(solid arrows)* is shown on this transverse scan through the lower pole of the left kidney *(open arrows)*. The hematoma was secondary to a closed renal biopsy. S, spleen.

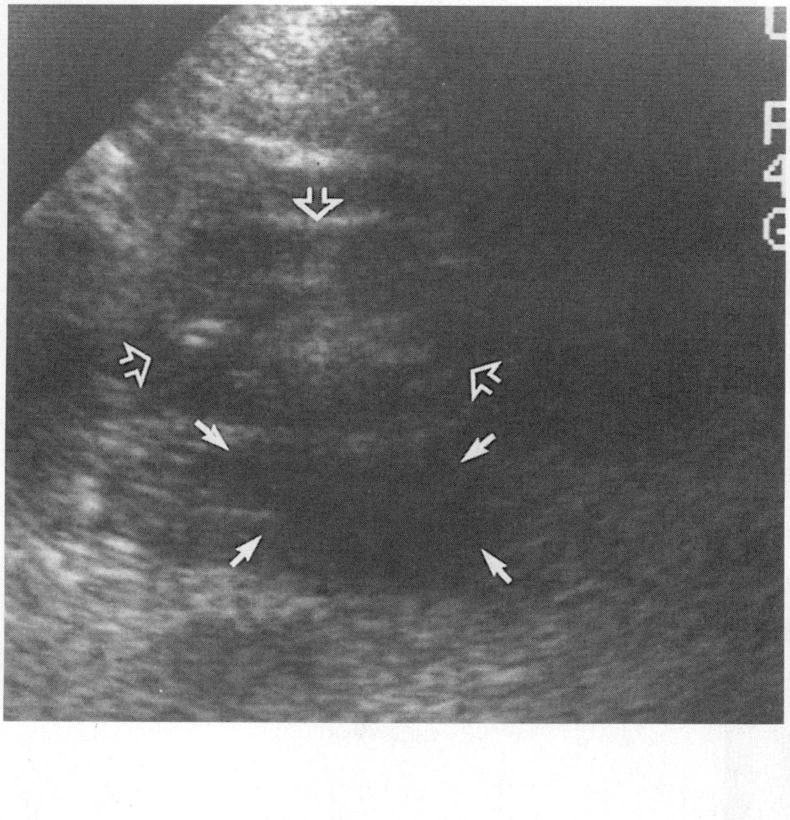

Figure 106.73. Hypoechoic perirenal hematoma *(solid arrows)* is demonstrated on the transverse sonogram of the left kidney *(open arrows)*. The cause was closed renal biopsy.

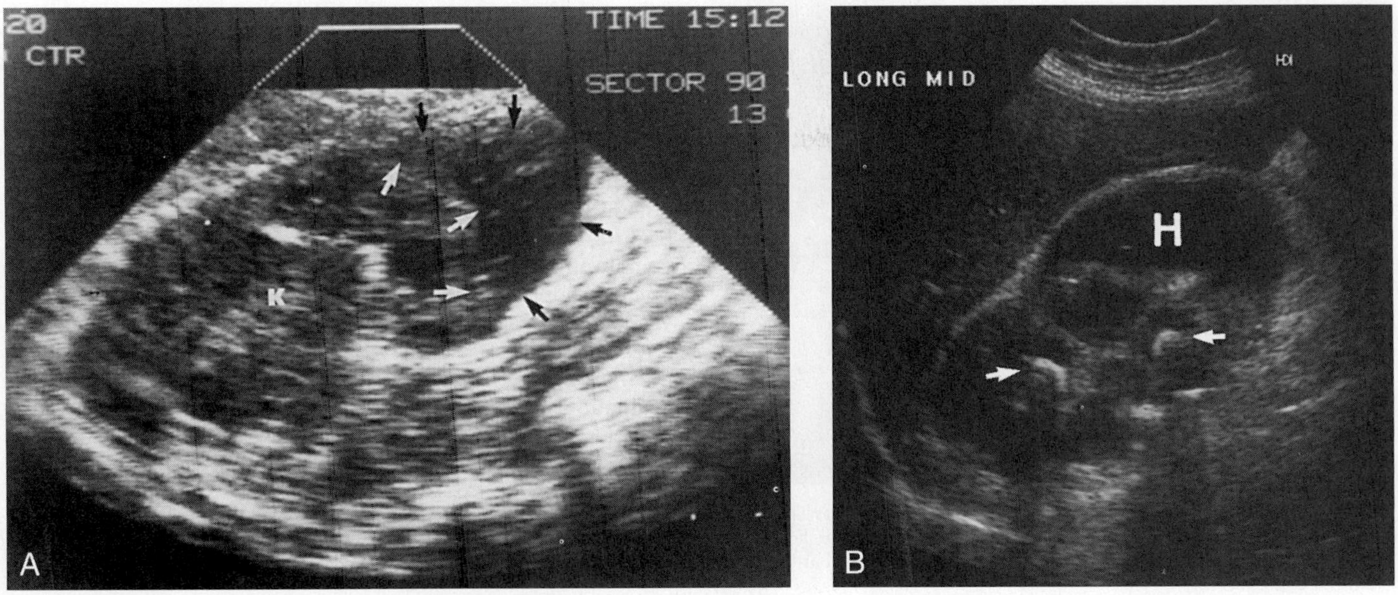

Figure 106.74. **A:** Subcapsular hematoma *(arrows)* shown on this longitudinal renal sonogram image developed after a stab wound. K, kidney. **B:** Subcapsular hematoma *(H)* as a complication of lithotripsy *(H)*. Longitudinal renal sonogram in a patient with renal calculi *(arrows)*.

on the stage of evolution of the hematoma, it may appear hypoechoic or hyperechoic (Figs. 106.72, 106.73, and 106.74).

RENAL VASCULAR DISEASE

Renal artery stenosis may result in a treatable form of hypertension, although accounting for roughly 1% of hypertension cases. Most stenoses are a result of advanced arteriosclerotic disease, with the remainder caused by fibromuscular hyperplasia (Fig. 106.75) or a number of rarer entities. Assessment of main or segmental renal artery flow is often technically difficult, predicated on demonstrating renal artery velocities, which are greater than 1.5 to 1.9 meters per second on spectral Doppler analysis. Other renal arterial lesions such as aneurysms (Fig. 106.76), pseudoaneurysms, arteriovenous

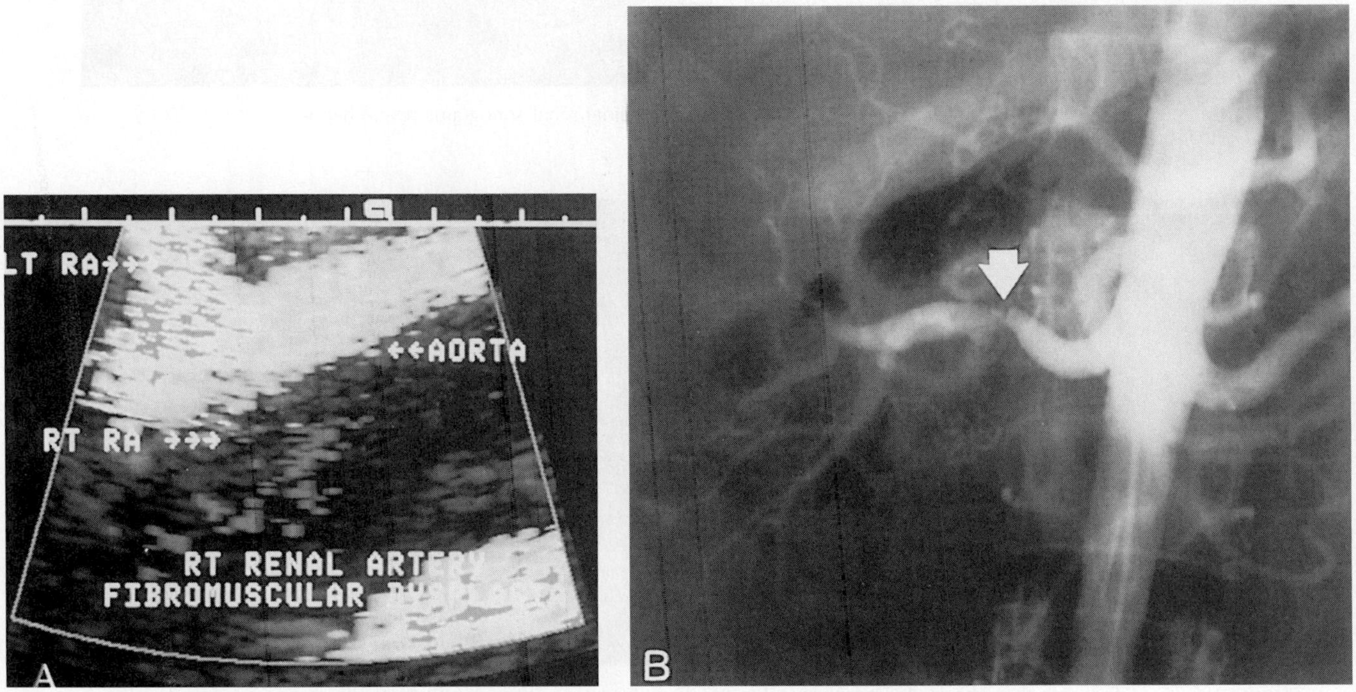

Figure 106.75. Fibromuscular dysplasia of the renal artery. **A:** Longitudinal color flow Doppler image of the renal arteries at their origin. Stenosis of the proximal right renal artery secondary to fibromuscular dysplasia. LT RA, left renal artery; RT RA, right renal artery with stenosis. (See Color Figure 106.75A.) **B:** Abdominal aortogram. *White arrow* indicates proximal right renal artery stenosis.

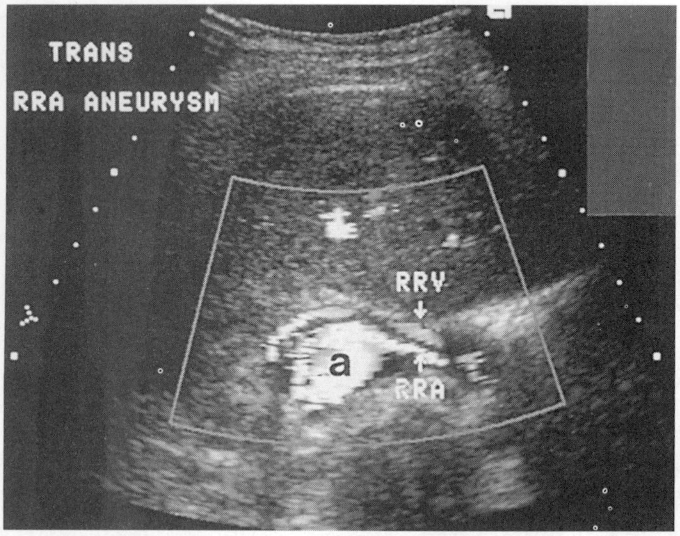

Figure 106.76. Renal artery aneurysm. Transverse color flow Doppler image of the right kidney. Aneurysm with increased arterial flow in a young patient with hypertension. a, aneurysm; RRV, right renal artery. (See Color Figure 106.76.)

malformations, or fistulae can be demonstrated with color Doppler sonography. Cortical infarcts appear as hypoechoic focal lesions with decreased arterial flow (Fig. 106.77).

Renal vein thrombosis is often a sequel to primary renal disease such as glomerulonephropathies, nephrotic syndrome, or extension of a renal malignancy into the renal vein. Rarely, renal vein thrombosis is seen in clinical settings of shock and hypovolemia (more commonly seen in the pediatric population), trauma, sepsis, or hypercoagulable conditions. Although renal vein thrombosis can be sonographically detected without benefit of color Doppler, usually as a filling defect within the anechoic vessel, the conspicuity of the thrombus, and extension into the inferior vena cava on color Doppler merits implementation of the more sophisticated ultrasound technique (Fig. 106.78). In the evaluation of patients with primary renal malignancies, color Doppler evaluation of the renal vein and inferior vena cava may be a suitable alternative to MRI, CT, or venography in staging tumor spread.

Color Doppler sonography is very useful in demonstrating renal artery occlusion, although underutilized in most clinical situations, with the exception of renal transplant patients. Seg-

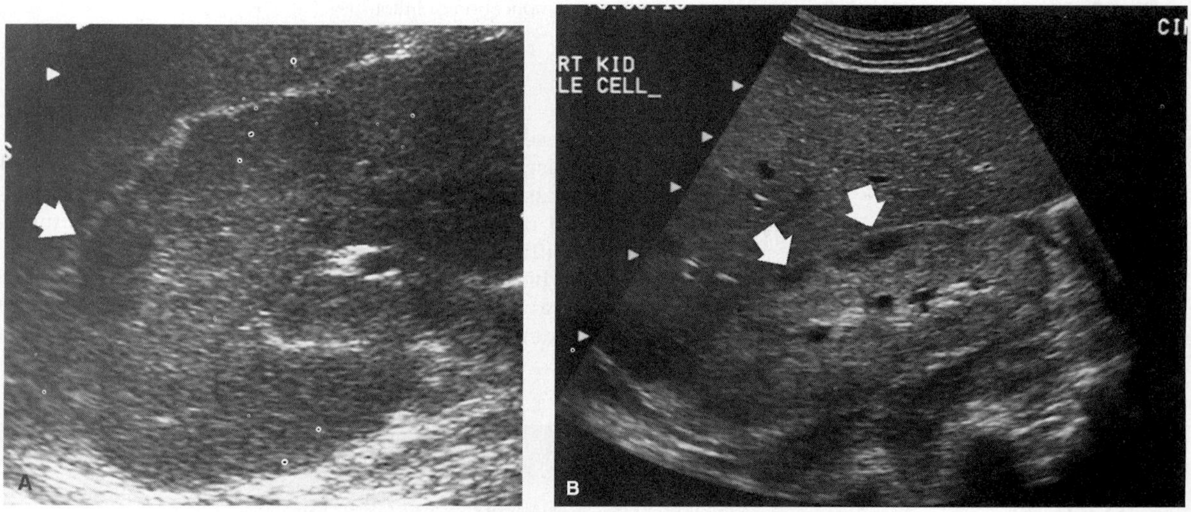

Figure 106.77. Cortical Infarct (*white arrows* on **A** and **B**). Longitudinal renal sonograms reveal hypoechoic focal areas within the renal cortex.

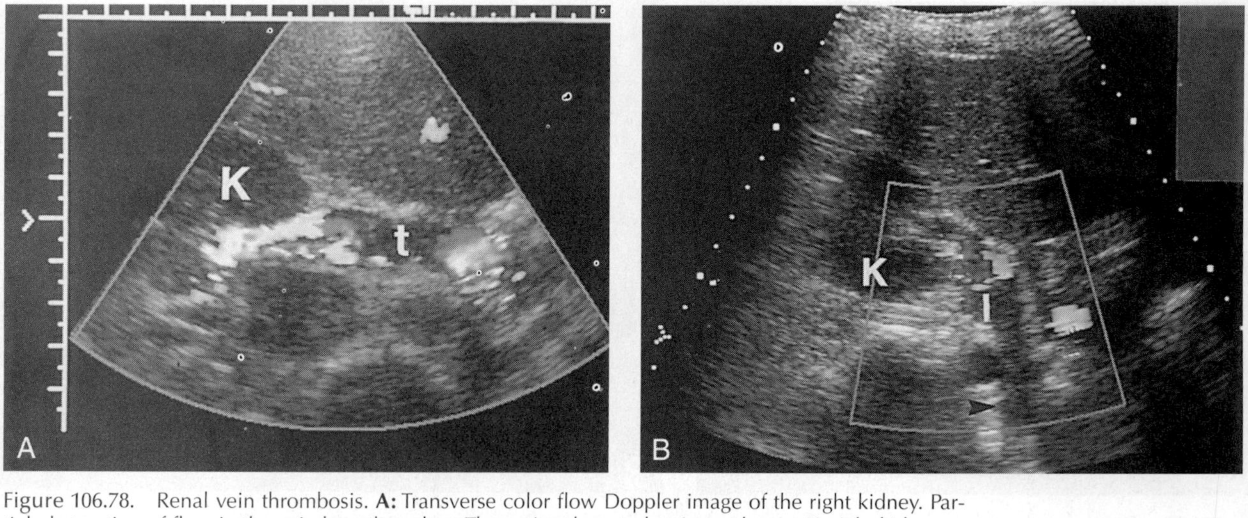

Figure 106.78. Renal vein thrombosis. **A:** Transverse color flow Doppler image of the right kidney. Partial obstruction of flow in the vein by a thrombus. The patient has nephrotic syndrome. K, right kidney; t, renal vein thrombus. **B:** Renal vein and inferior vena cava thrombus. Transverse color flow Doppler image of the right kidney and inferior vena cava. Left renal vein clot extends into the inferior vena cava. Flow in the right renal vein is normal. The patient has nephrotic syndrome. The *arrowhead* denotes left renal vein with a clot. I, inferior vena cava (with clot); K, right kidney. (See Color Figures 106.78A and 106.78B.)

mental or global renal artery occlusion is often the result of trauma, atherosclerosis, or iatrogenic injury (ligation or embolization). Other imaging modalities, CT or angiography, are more routinely used to diagnose renal arterial occlusion.

HIV INFECTION AND AIDS

Renal involvement in patients suffering from an immunocompromised state may exhibit a number of sonographic findings. AIDS-related lymphoma more commonly presents as discrete hypoechoic renal masses. Patients with disseminated *Pneumocystis* infection demonstrate diffuse punctate cortical and medullary calcifications. The calcifications create a scattered echogenic pattern. Focal coarse calcifications occasionally are seen in patients with *Pneumocystis* and may also occur in the presence of mycobacterium avium intracellulare infection. AIDS-related nephropathy progresses rapidly to renal failure and proteinuria, ultimately resulting in death. Ultrasonographic findings include renal enlargement and pronounced cortical echogenicity.

BLADDER ABNORMALITIES

Lesions of the bladder mucosa are best studied by cystoscopy. However, ultrasonic examination can be helpful in assessing invasion of perivesicular structures and fat by bladder neoplasms. In addition, other pelvic processes involving the bladder may be well demonstrated using ultrasound. For instance, in a patient with a dilated collecting system, ultrasound is recommended to evaluate the possibility of an obstructing lesion (Figs. 106.79, 106.80, and 106.81). Occasionally, bladder diverticula

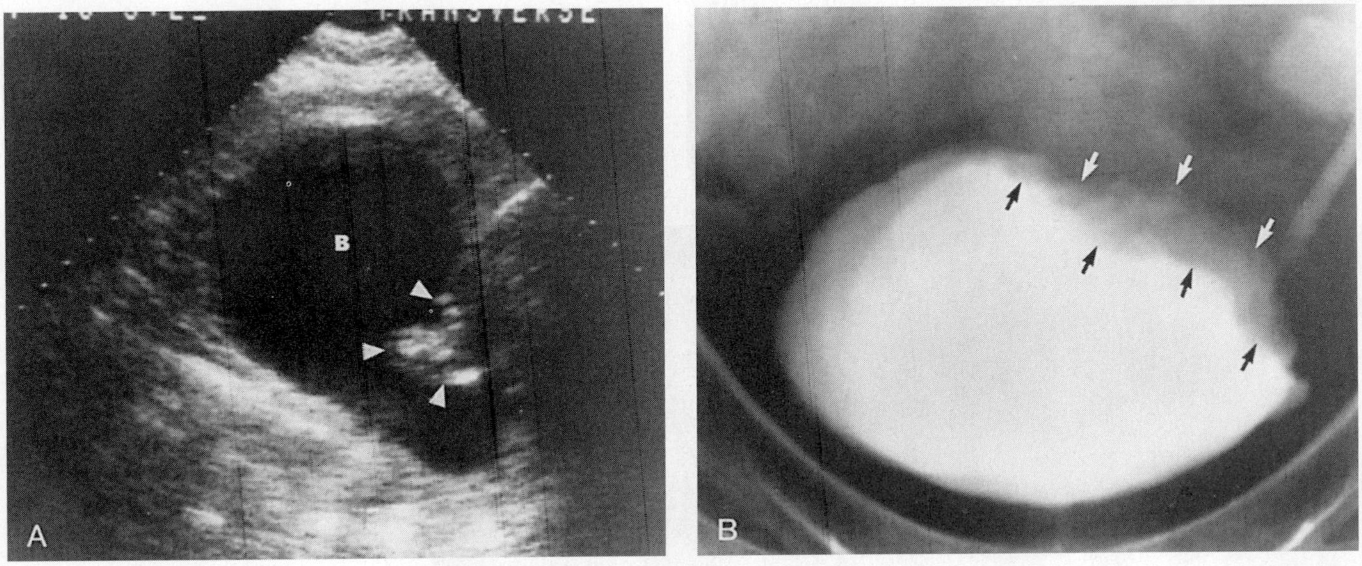

Figure 106.79. Transitional cell carcinoma. **A:** Transverse sonogram of pelvis reveals a tumor arising from the left lateral wall of the bladder *(arrowheads)*. **B:** Bladder film from intravenous urogram in same patient as in **A** shows an irregular left superolateral margin caused by the tumor *(arrows)*.

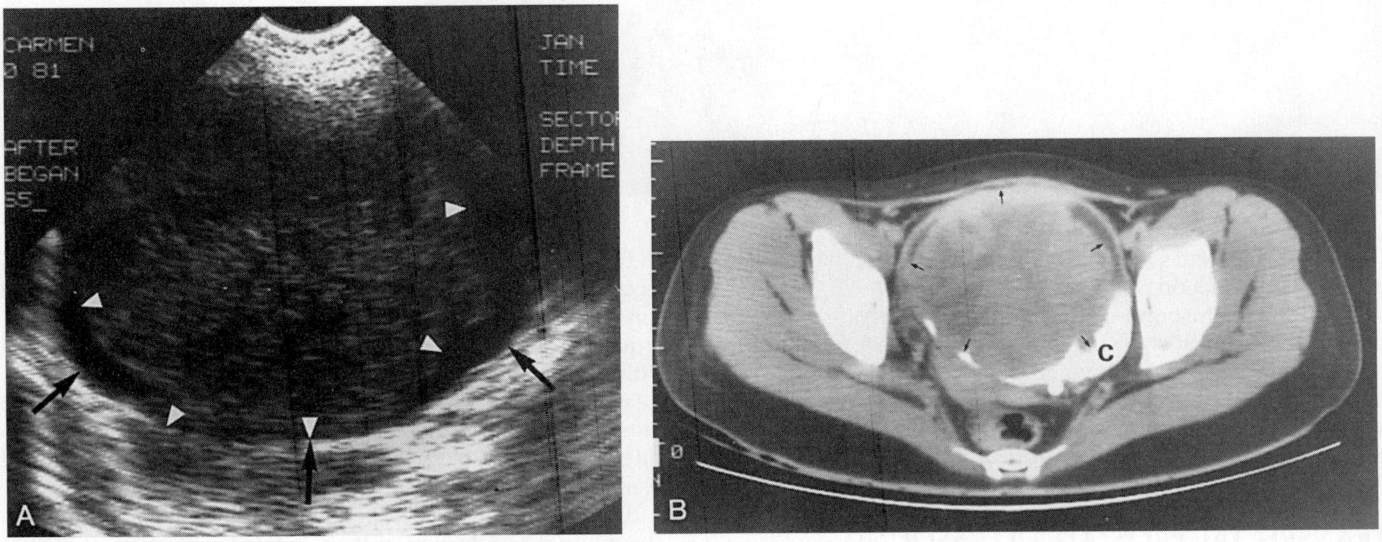

Figure 106.80. Leiomyosarcoma of the bladder. **A:** Transverse bladder sonogram shows a mass in the bladder *(arrowheads)*. There is very little space between the tumor and bladder wall *(arrows)*. This patient's kidneys both showed a dilated collecting system caused by obstruction of the ureteral orifices by the mass. **B:** Transverse pelvic CT scan shows the bladder tumor *(arrows)* equally well. *C*, Contrast in the bladder.

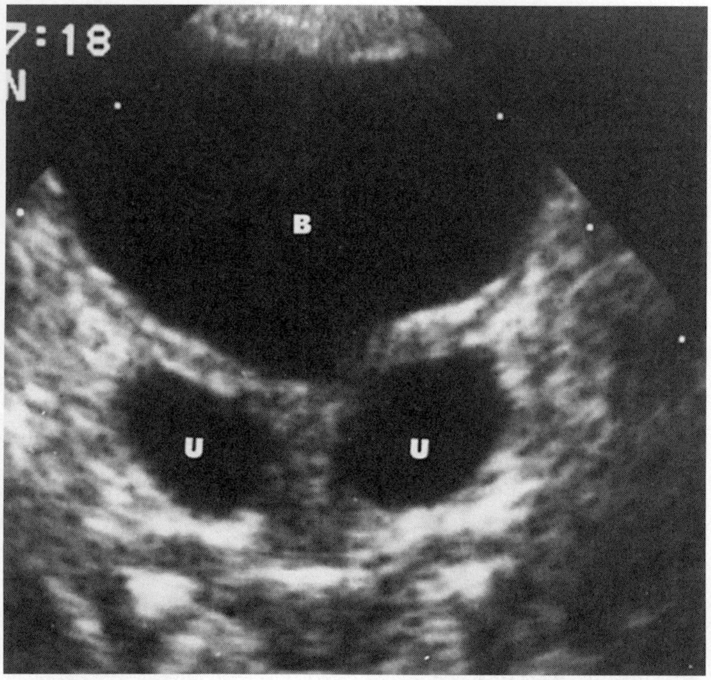

Figure 106.81. Bilateral simple ureteroceles. This patient had bilateral caliectasis. The bladder was scanned during sonographic assessment to look for a cause for the caliectasis. The transverse sonogram shows a ureterocele *(U)* on each side posterior to the bladder *(B)*.

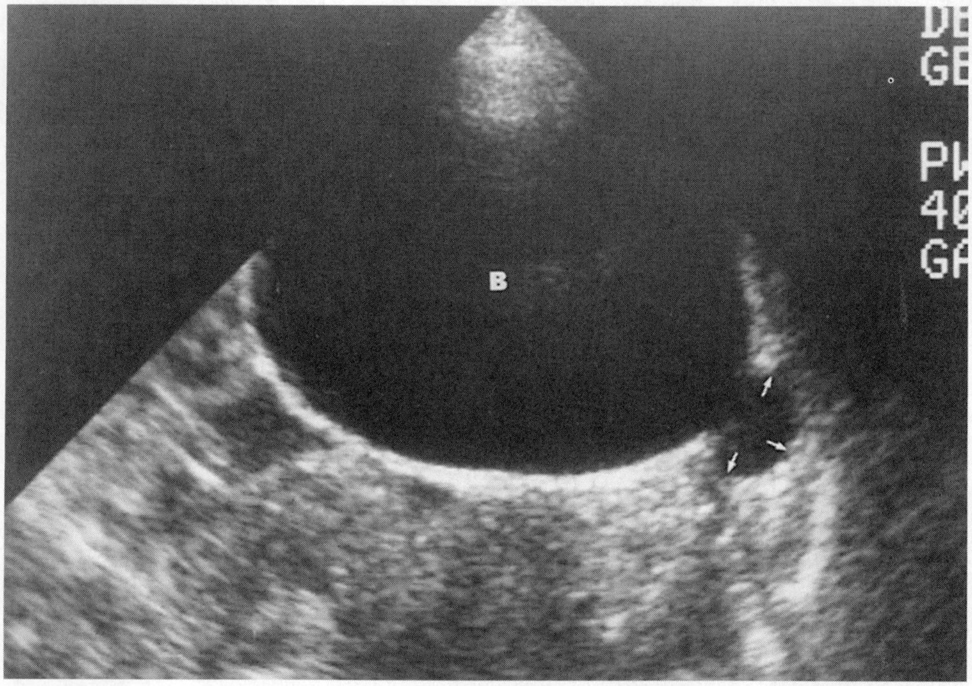

Figure 106.82. Bladder diverticulum. Transverse bladder sonogram shows a left-sided diverticulum *(arrows)*. B, bladder. (Courtesy of Bharat Raval, M.D.)

(Fig. 106.82) or stones may be discovered when evaluating bladder outlet obstruction.

Real-time ultrasound of the bladder has become useful for diagnosing urinary stress incontinence and vesicoureteral reflux, as well as assessing the neurogenic bladder. In situations in which it is undesirable to catheterize a bladder for urine volume estimation, ultrasound can be used for gross volume estimates.

TRANSRECTAL PROSTATE ULTRASOUND

The use of transrectal ultrasound (TRUS) of the prostate has increased dramatically over the past several years. The acceptance of this imaging modality is founded on several technical and clinical advances: (a) development of sophisticated transrectal linear array ultrasound transducers with short focal zones and (b) discovery of the prostate-specific antigen (PSA), a quantitatively measurable serum protein that is elevated with benign prostate hypertrophy and that significantly increases with prostate carcinoma. Selection of patients who should be examined with TRUS is based on detection of elevated serum PSA levels and/or an abnormal digital rectal examination.

The prostate is scanned in both the sagittal and axial planes. The internal architecture of the prostate is observed, as well as the adjacent seminal vesicles, bladder, and periprostatic tissue (Fig. 106.83).

The majority of adenocarcinomas occur in the peripheral zone of the prostate gland, and most of these cancers are rela-

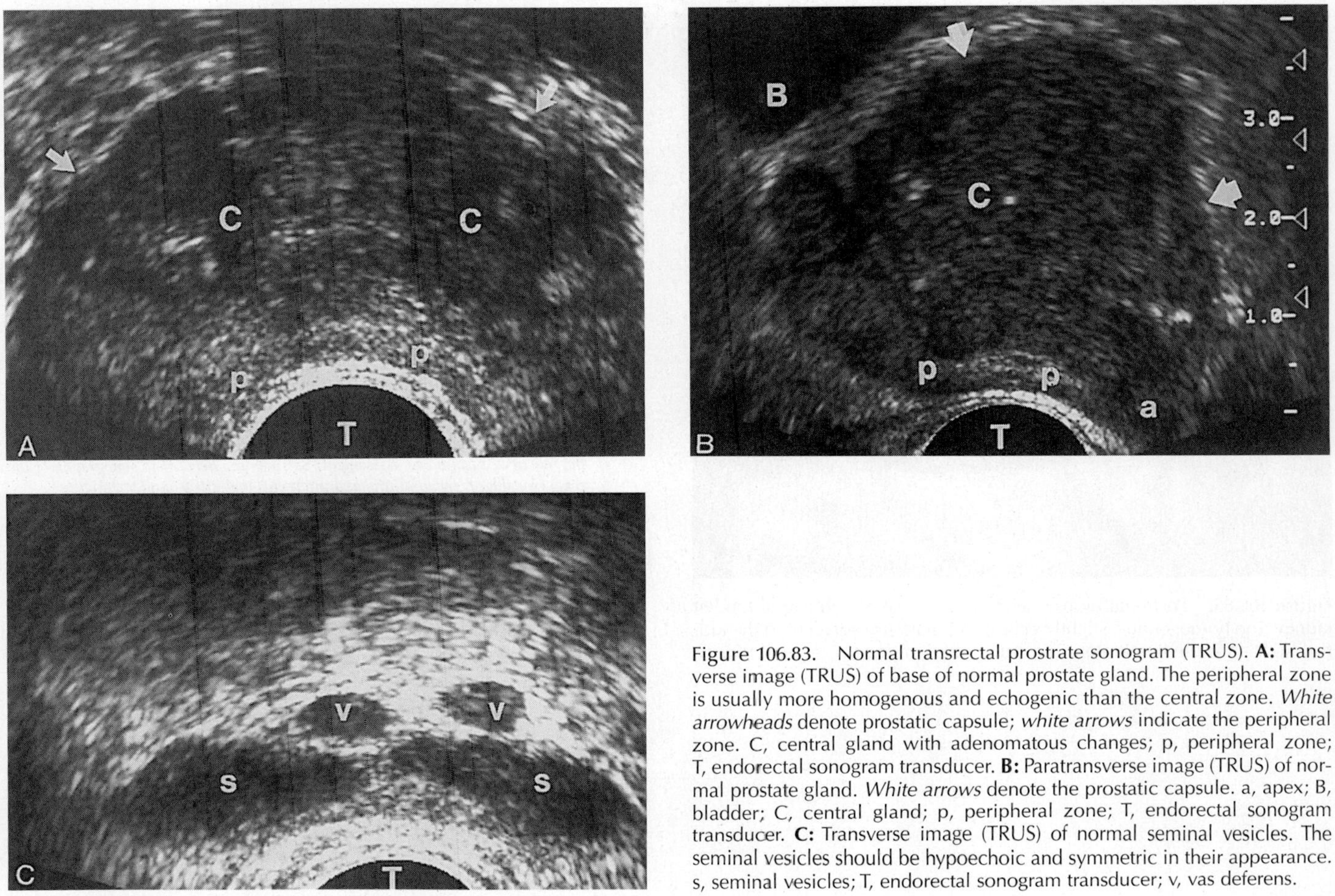

Figure 106.83. Normal transrectal prostrate sonogram (TRUS). **A:** Transverse image (TRUS) of base of normal prostate gland. The peripheral zone is usually more homogenous and echogenic than the central zone. *White arrowheads* denote prostatic capsule; *white arrows* indicate the peripheral zone. C, central gland with adenomatous changes; p, peripheral zone; T, endorectal sonogram transducer. **B:** Paratransverse image (TRUS) of normal prostate gland. *White arrows* denote the prostatic capsule. a, apex; B, bladder; C, central gland; p, peripheral zone; T, endorectal sonogram transducer. **C:** Transverse image (TRUS) of normal seminal vesicles. The seminal vesicles should be hypoechoic and symmetric in their appearance. s, seminal vesicles; T, endorectal sonogram transducer; v, vas deferens.

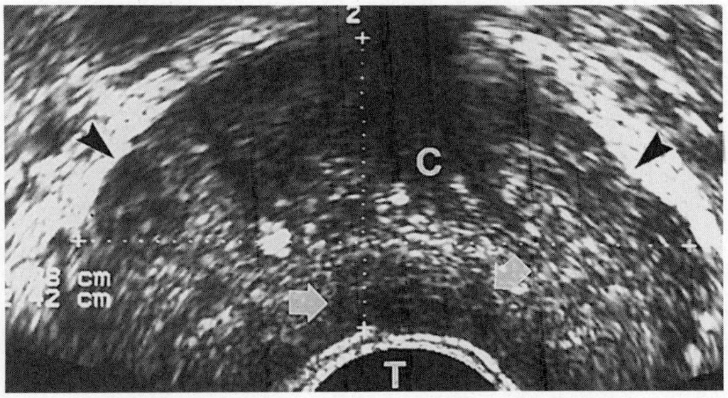

Figure 106.84. Hypoechoic peripheral zone. Transverse image (TRUS) of the base of the prostate. The peripheral zone is heterogeneous with areas of discrete hypoechogenicity. These areas are suspicious for malignancy and should be examined by biopsy. *White arrows* indicate the hypoechoic peripheral zone. The *black arrowheads* denote the prostatic capsule. C, central zone of the prostate; T, endorectal sonogram transducer.

tively hypoechoic to the adjacent prostate tissue (Fig. 106.84). Other sonographic findings suggestive of malignancy include (a) a deformed and irregular area within the gland, (b) loss of symmetry within the gland, and (c) alteration in the normal echogenic homogeneity characteristic to each respective zone within the prostate. Ultrasonographically identified suspicious areas within the prostate can be biopsied with an automated core biopsy device.

ULTRASOUND-DIRECTED INTERVENTIONAL TECHNIQUES

Ultrasound is a means of accurately localizing organs and lesions. It has been proven an excellent imaging tool for performing percutaneous renal biopsy under real time. As a result, diagnostic yield of renal biopsy has improved, while the morbidity and mortality historically associated with the procedure have declined. Much of this decline can be attributed to early ultrasonographic recognition of complications, such as bleeding (Fig. 106.85), with resultant expedition of management.

Another application of ultrasound, which is increasingly employed, is percutaneous aspiration of a renal abscess. If a suspected abscess is confirmed with the procedure, external drainage may be established at the same time.

If ultrasound reveals atypical cysts, identified by irregular walls, mural nodules, or hemorrhage, they should be further evaluated for neoplasm using skinny needle cyst puncture. This procedure can be facilitated with ultrasound guidance.

Therapeutic percutaneous nephrostomy placement under sonographic guidance is now common. Ultrasound used in conjunction with fluoroscopy decreases the amount of time required to access the collecting system compared with fluoroscopy alone. Indications for percutaneous nephrostomy include drainage of a pyonephrotic kidney, relief of obstruction to preserve renal function, diversion of urine externally to allow ureteral fistula healing, and access to the collecting system and ureter for interventional procedures such as stone retrieval, percutaneous lithotripsy, and ureteral stent placement. Patients with urosepsis and those at risk for developing it should receive antibiotic therapy before any of the aforementioned procedures.

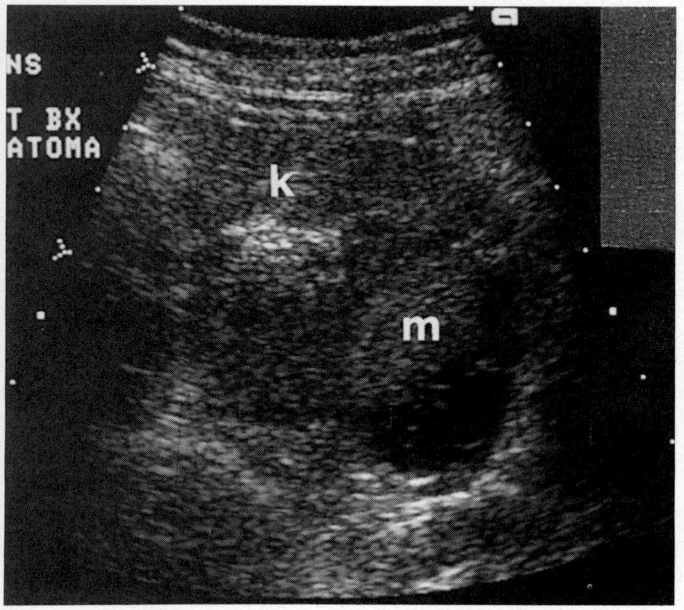

Figure 106.85. Postrenal biopsy hematoma. Transverse image of the left kidney. The homogenous, slightly echogenic mass *(m)* adjacent to the kidney *(k)* is an acute hematoma. The patient had undergone a renal biopsy.

Selected Readings

Amis ES, Hartman DS. Renal ultrasonography 1984: a practical overview. *Radiol Clin North Am* 1984;22:2:315–332.

This article provides a good overview of renal sonography. There are several useful tables that list differential diagnostic possibilities of specific renal sonographic patterns.

Coleman BG. Ultrasonography of the upper genitourinary tract. *Urol Clin North Am* 1985;12(4):633–644.

A concise review of sonography of the upper urinary tract.

Grantham JJ, Levine E. Acquired cystic disease: replacing one kidney disease with another (Editorial Review). *Kidney Int* 1985;28:99–105.

The current status of acquired cystic kidney disease is well discussed in this editorial.

Grossman H, Rosenberg ER, Bowie JD, et al. Review: sonographic diagnosis of renal cystic disease. *AJR* 1983;140:81–85.

This review article discusses ultrasound in cystic renal conditions. It has a chart showing the age distribution of the various cystic lesions. Acquired cystic kidney disease is not discussed.

Hricak H, ed. Genitourinary ultrasound. *Clin Diagn Ultrasound* 1986;18:1–179.

This is an excellent review of the spectrum of diseases affecting the kidneys and the role of ultrasound in assessment. Sections are devoted to sonography of the renal transplant, renal failure, and interventional ultrasound techniques.

Melson GL. Coordinated diagnostic imaging—kidney. *Clin Diagn Ultrasound* 1984; 14:189–219.

Ultrasound and CT findings of renal infections are covered. The role of ultrasound and CT in suspected renal infection is discussed. A practical algorithm for an imaging approach to renal infections is proposed.

Rifkin MD. Ultrasonography of the lower genitourinary tract. *Urol Clin North Am* 1985;12(4):645–647.

A concise review of sonography of the lower genitourinary tract.

CHAPTER 107

Computed Tomography of the Kidney and Urinary Tract

William D. Boswell, Jr.

Computed tomography has been known by many names, such as computerized axial tomography, computerized tomography, computer-assisted tomography, computerized transverse axial tomography, and CAT scan. *Computed tomography* (CT) is the general term used to describe the process of x-ray generated and computer-reconstructed images of a particular plane of an object.

HISTORICAL BACKGROUND

CT has been heralded as the greatest improvement in diagnostic radiology since the original discovery of x-rays by Roentgen in 1895. Independently, many investigators laid the groundwork for Sir Godfrey Hounsfield. Radon, in 1971, proved that two- or three-dimensional objects could be reconstructed from an infinite set of projections or data points. Bracewell, working in the field of radioastronomy in the 1950s, developed the principles of image reconstruction. In 1961, Oldendorf described a method for cross-sectional imaging of the brain. Cormack successfully developed a mathematically accurate method of various image processing projection methods for transverse section nuclear medicine brain scans in 1968. Sir Godfrey N. Hounsfield, working in the area of pattern recognition and information retrieval at the Central Research Laboratories of EMI, Ltd., in London, pulled together his work and that of the others and developed the first computed tomographic scanner in 1970. This work led to the first clinical application of CT in September of 1971, when a head scanner was installed at Atkinson Morley's Hospital under the direction of James Ambrose. The first whole-body scanner was developed and installed at Georgetown University Medical Center by Ledley in 1974. The field has not stopped advancing since that time. No area in radiology has changed more rapidly than the field of CT. For his outstanding work in the field and for demonstrating its unique and remarkable clinical abilities, Sir Godfrey N. Hounsfield was awarded the Nobel Prize for Medicine in 1979.

CT PHYSICS

CT is the reconstruction of an x-ray generated image by a computer that depicts a slice through an area of the body. An x-ray source, a highly collimated fanbeam, is mounted opposite a set of electronic detectors. This system rotates around the patient in a complete circle. The data collected by the detectors are transferred to a computer, which reconstructs an image. This image is then displayed on a television monitor and subsequently can be transferred to film for viewing.

The image itself is made up of many small picture elements, called *pixels*, each of which is assigned a CT number corresponding to the amount of x-rays absorbed by the object, or patient, at a particular point. The CT image is composed of a matrix of pixels, with each pixel having its own CT number. Although pixel size is usually given by its cross-sectional area, it is important to remember that the image is three-dimensional (3D), its other measurement being depth. Each slice through the object has a finite thickness depending on the width of the x-ray beam or detector collimator or both. Thus the CT number is actually the average x-ray attenuation of all the tissues within a specific volume element, called the *voxel*, which is portrayed by the pixels on the monitor.

CT numbers represent the x-ray attenuation in each voxel relative to the attenuation of water. Structures with more attenuation than water have positive CT numbers, and those with less attenuation have negative CT numbers. The CT image is sent on the television screen to have varying shade of gray. Different gray levels are assigned a range of CT numbers from which the image is the end result. Image manipulation is possible to accentuate different areas of image. Variation of the range of CT numbers at a particular gray level leads to changes in the image, a key element of the CT scanner.

The design of CT scanners has changed in the past few years. The new generation of scanners has a continuously rotating x-ray tube around the region being scanned. As the tube rotates, the patient is moved through the gantry or opening in the scanner. The data are collected as a continuous set, and subsequently the computer is instructed to reconstruct the information into slices. The data may also be retreated as a 3D-volume set and off-axis reconstructions, or volume images may be produced for viewing and diagnosis. Slice thickness can be as small as 1 mm. Resolution in the Z-axis may approach 1 mm. The radiation dose of a typical examination of the abdomen is 2 to 4 rads, comparable with that of a conventional intravenous pyelography (IVP). These state-of-the-art CT scanners are known as *spiral* or *helical scanners*.

TECHNIQUE

All examinations of the kidneys should be tailored to the particular problem being investigated. Before the beginning of the

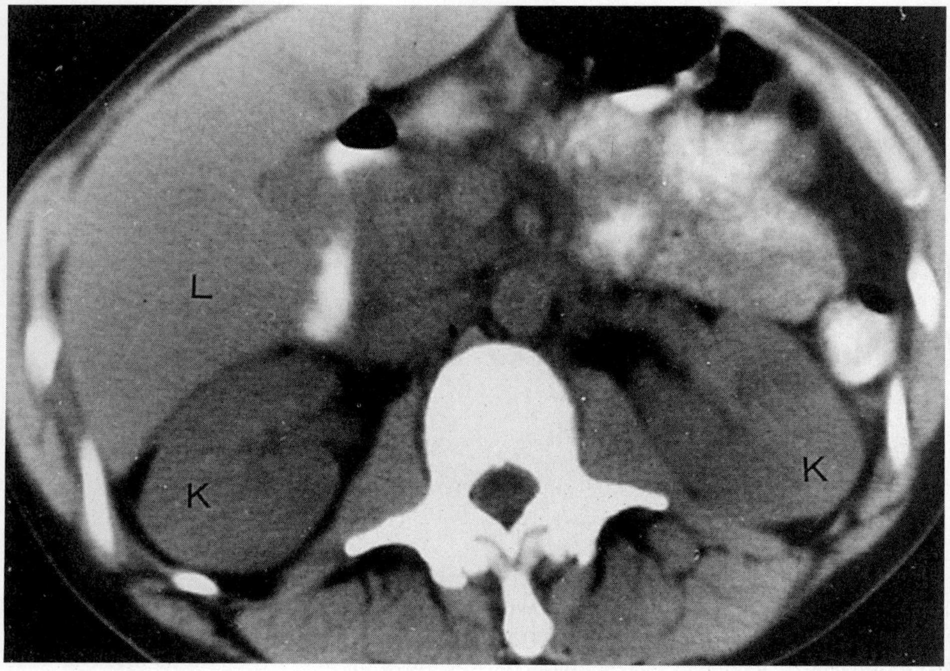

Figure 107.1. Noncontrast scan, normal kidneys. Note the uniform density of the kidneys *(K)*, which is slightly less than that of the adjacent liver *(L)*.

study, a digital/computer-generated radiography is obtained to assess the position of the kidneys and the area to be scanned. A nonenhanced study (without intravenous contrast media) is performed with 10-mm thick slices every 2 cm through the entire area of the kidney (Fig. 107.1). Usually, an enhanced study is required for complete evaluation of the kidney. As little as 25 to 30 ml of intravenous contrast may be used to provide diagnostic information, but this should be used only in extraordinary circumstances. Either nonionic, low osmolar iodinated contrast or conventional ionic, high osmolar iodinated contrast may be used for CT scans. A rapid bolus intravenous injection of 75 to 100 ml of contrast (approximately 30 g of iodine) is generally used for the enhanced scan (Fig 107.2). The contrast is injected at a rate of 3 to 4 ml/sec. Scanning begins after a slight delay of 45 to 60 seconds. The data may be collected as one complete volume set in 15 to 30 seconds, which are then reconstructed in slices or as individual slices every several seconds until the kidneys are scanned through. In the typical case, the slices are 10 mm thick, although thinner sections may be necessary at times. Scanning may also be accomplished in a manner that images are obtained in the arterial phase and venous phase of the contrast injection to assess the kidney further. 3-D volumetric images may then be generated to demonstrate the arterial and/or venous anatomy of the kidney—so-called CT angiography (CTA).

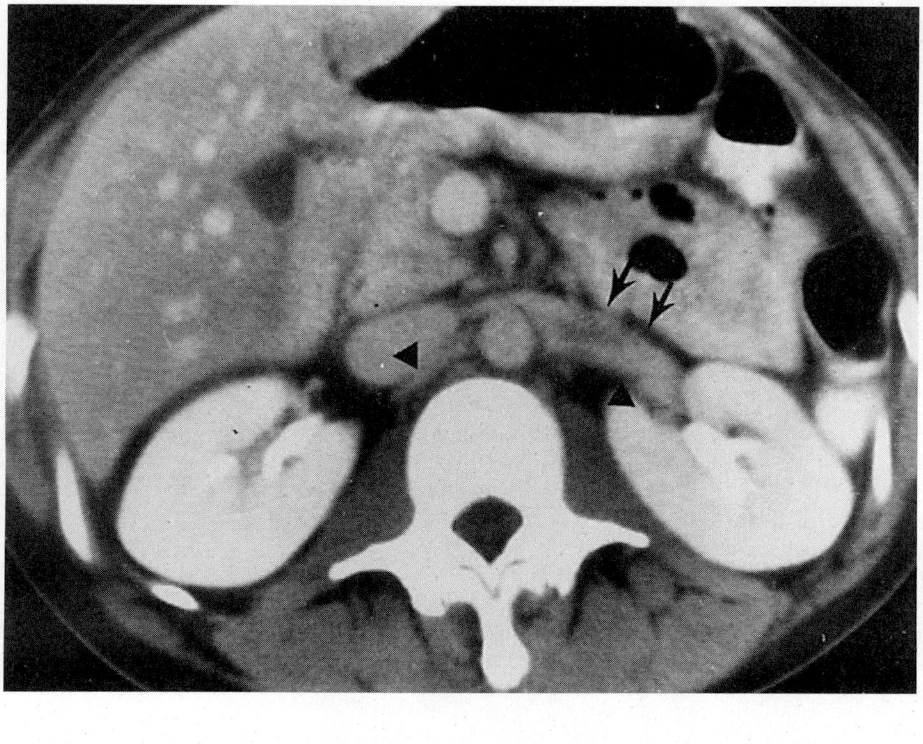

Figure 107.2. Postcontrast normal kidneys. This enhanced scan of the same patient as in Fig. 107.1 shows the marked increase in density of the kidneys when compared with the liver. Note the renal arteries *(arrowheads)* and the left renal vein *(arrows)*.

NORMAL ANATOMY

The kidneys lie in the retroperitoneum within the perinephric space. They are bounded by the anterior and posterior pararenal spaces. Because of the ability of the CT scanner to differentiate small differences in the density between one tissue and another, these compartments surrounding the kidneys frequently are well delineated. The greater the amounts of fat present in the retroperitoneum, the better the visualization of the compartments. The renal parenchyma is usually of uniform density. Before administration of any intravenous contrast material, the density of the kidneys is slightly less than that of other nearby organs, such as the liver, spleen, or aorta. The fat in the peripelvic region is usually easily identified. The unopacified calyceal system and renal pelvis are difficult to define unless there is some element of dilation. Portions of the renovascular pedicle are frequently identified.

The density of the kidneys changes markedly after administration of intravenous contrast material. With the bolus injection technique and rapid consecutive scans, one is able to discern the aorta, main renal arteries, and cortical nephrogram early (Fig. 107.3). From 5 to 10 seconds later, the renal veins and inferior vena cava will be seen. Still later, scans will show a dense nephrogram of the renal parenchyma. With rapid infusion technique, the renal parenchyma usually is uniformly dense, without corticomedullary differentiation's (Figs. 107.2 and 107.4).

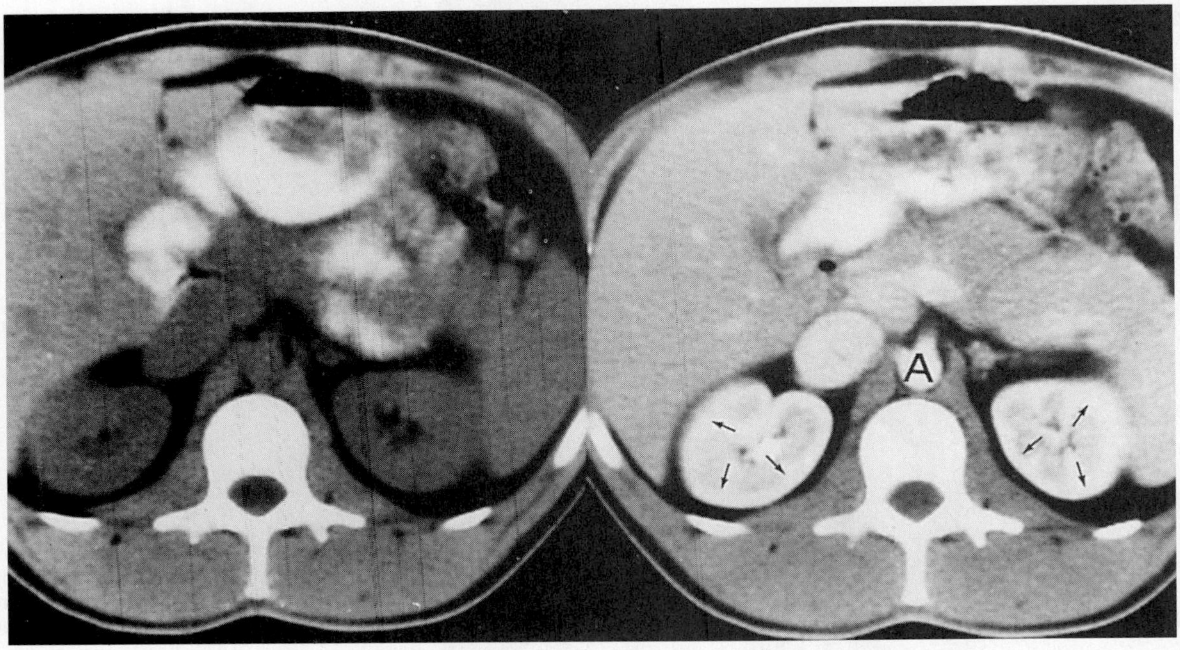

Figure 107.3. Normal kidneys following a bolus injection. On the *left* is the noncontrast scan, and on the *right* is the scan during the bolus injection. Note the aorta *(A)*, which appears dense because of the large concentration of iodine from the bolus injection. The corticomedullary junction is seen in the kidneys *(arrows)*.

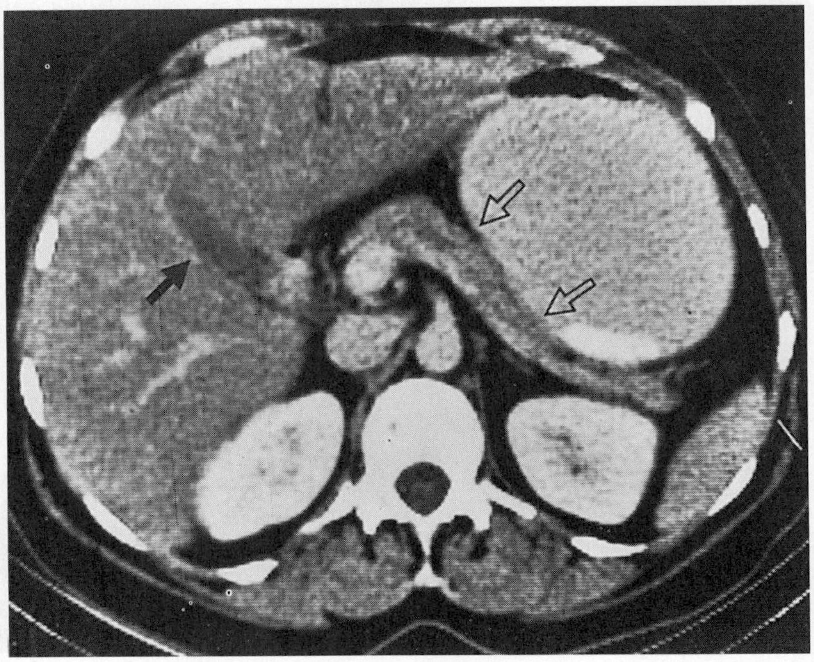

Figure 107.4. Normal kidneys after infusion. The kidneys have a uniform appearance except in the central region, where fat or contrast material in the collecting systems may be seen. Note the proximity of the pancreas to the left kidney *(open arrows)*. The gallbladder *(solid arrow)* is seen adjacent to the liver and anterior to the right kidney.

The intrarenal calyceal system and renal pelvis are well seen after contrast administration, and the ureter can usually be followed in its course to the bladder. The CT numbers of the renal parenchyma after administration of intravenous contrast material increase to greater than those of the surrounding organs because of the concentrating ability of the kidney.

As the CT scans are obtained in a transverse configuration, other organs are included on scans through the regions of the kidneys (Figs. 107.1 and 107.4). The liver and gallbladder are located anterosuperior to the right kidney. The adrenal glands are noted just superior to the top of the kidneys (Fig. 107.5). The tail of the pancreas courses above the left kidney (Fig. 107.4). The spleen is intimately situated superolateral to the left kidney. The duodenum and pancreatic head are located anteromedial to the superior pole of the right kidney. The ascending and descending colons are closely related to the lateral margins of the kidneys. The spine and psoas muscles are noted posteromedial to the kidneys.

The borders of the kidney are typically smooth except in the region of the renal hilum. Fetal lobulation is noted easily on CT scans by the regular small indentations in the cortex between the calyces (Fig. 107.6). Incidental small renal cysts are the most

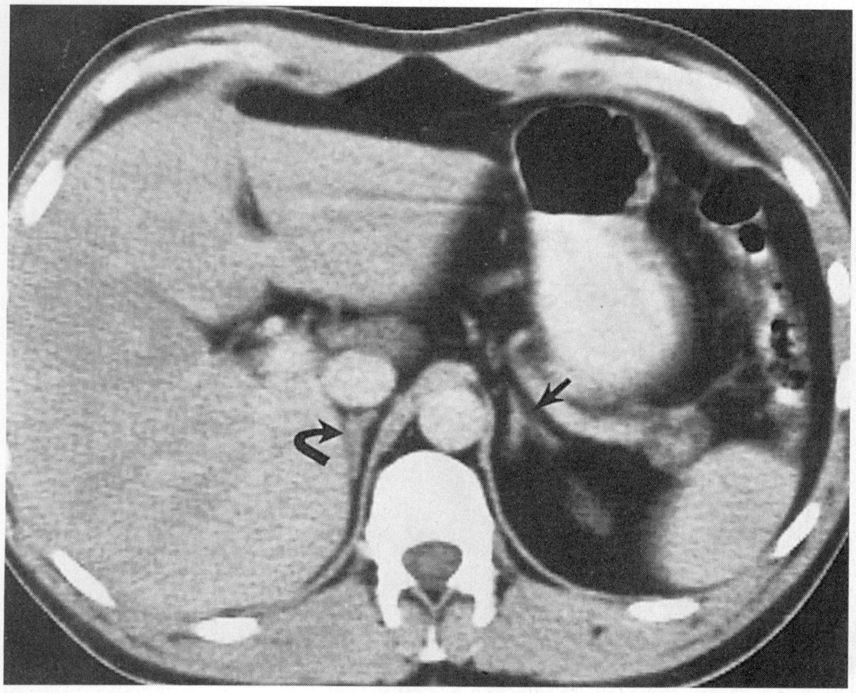

Figure 107.5. Normal adrenals. The normal adrenal glands lie cephalad to the kidneys. The right adrenal gland *(curved arrow)* is posterior to the inferior vena cava. The left adrenal gland *(arrow)* is to the left of the aorta.

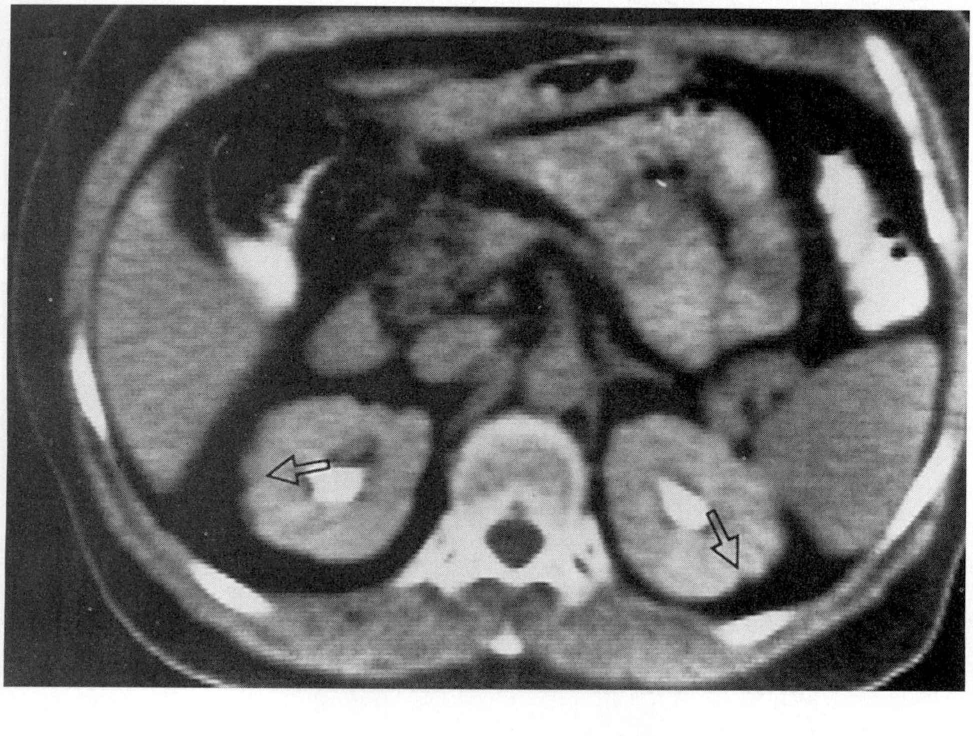

Figure 107.6. Fetal lobulation. The slight irregularity of the cortical surface of the kidneys is caused by fetal lobulation *(open arrows)*.

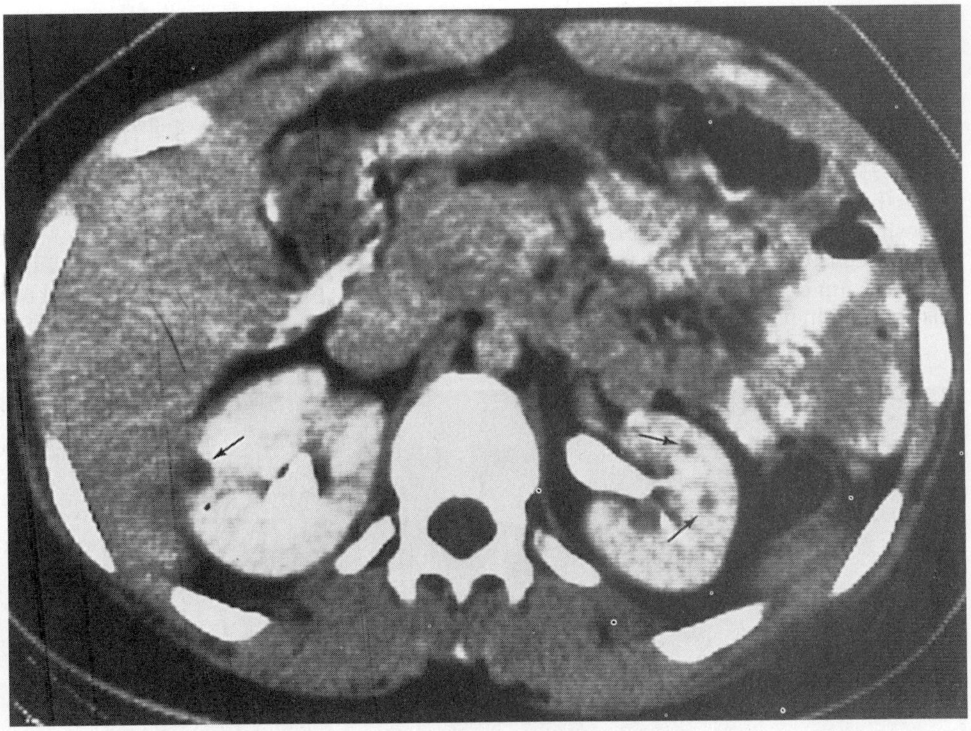

Figure 107.7. Small incidental cysts. These cysts *(arrows)* are found frequently on CT scanning. They may be located in either the medulla or the cortex.

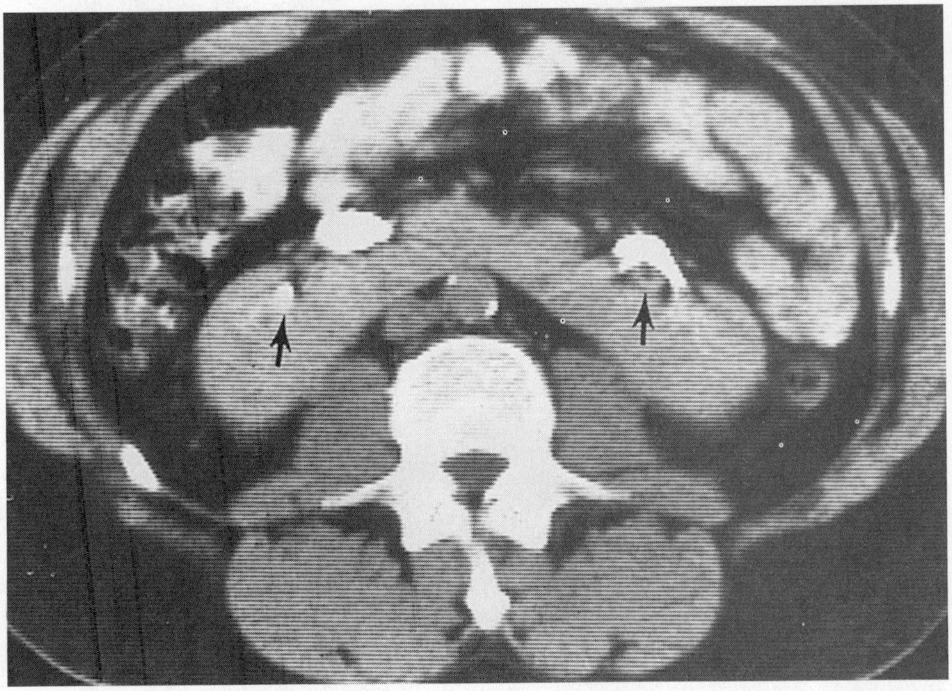

Figure 107.8. Horseshoe kidney. Note the two sets of collecting systems *(arrows)*, with the fused renal parenchyma in front of the aorta and inferior vena cava.

common abnormality seen on CT scans of the abdomen (Fig. 107.7). CT scans are able to demonstrate more renal cysts than any other imaging modality. Approximately half of all patients older than 50 will have at least one small simple renal cyst. Congenital abnormalities, such as ectopic kidneys or horseshoe kidneys (Fig. 107.8), occasionally are encountered during CT scans of the abdomen and pelvis.

Approximately 25% to 30% of all abdominal CT scans are performed for evaluation of the kidneys and surrounding retroperitoneal structures. The areas in which CT scanning has proved effective and valuable in the diagnosis of renal and urinary tract disorders are outlined in Table 107.1. CT scanning is an excellent imaging method when used in conjunction with patient information and the use of other conventional imaging modalities.

TABLE 107.1. Indications for Computed Tomography Scans

Renal axis deviation
Localization of small kidneys
Nonfunctioning kidneys
Hydronephrosis and site of obstruction
Renal stones and nonopaque filling defects
Renal trauma
Renal infections
Perinephric fluid collections
Renal masses
Renal cell carcinoma and its staging and recurrence
Suspected retroperitoneal mass or adenopathy
Evaluation of tumors of the adrenal glands, bladder, prostate, and other pelvic organs

RENAL DISORDERS

Deviation of the Renal Axis

The excellent anatomic display characteristics of CT scanning reveal the retroperitoneum with great advantage. When the axis or position of the kidneys is abnormal on an IVP, the cause is usually seen with CT scanning. The exact position in the retroperitoneum of fluid collections or masses that may cause the axis of the kidney to be changed is easily revealed with CT. Frequently, however, the cause is shown to be merely large depositions of retroperitoneal fat, which displace the kidneys anteriorly or straighten their axes (Fig. 107.9).

Localization of the Small Kidney

Although ultrasound often is used as the method of choice in evaluating the kidneys in the patient with renal failure, CT may be used when the kidneys are not found or are small and difficult to localize. The small contracted kidneys of renal failure

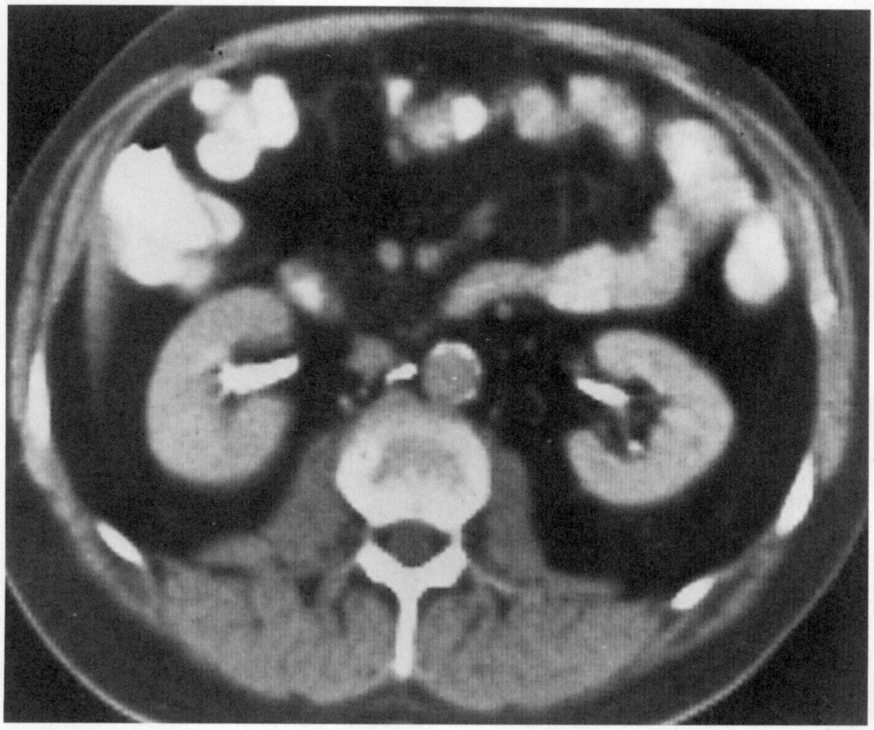

Figure 107.9. Retroperitoneal fat deviating the kidney. On the intravenous pyelogram, these kidneys appeared to be displaced laterally. The CT scan reveals only a rather large amount of retroperitoneal fat surrounding the kidneys. The kidneys are slightly more anterolaterally positioned than is normal.

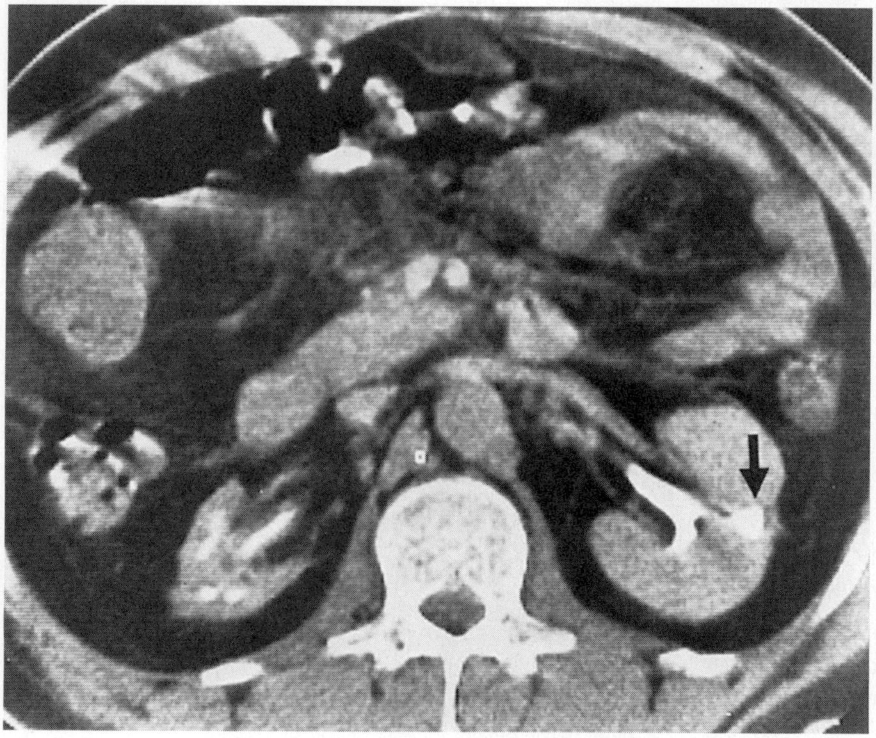

Figure 107.10. Chronic pyelonephritis and chronic renal failure. This patient with mild chronic renal failure (creatinine = 3.2 mg/dl) demonstrates a small, contracted, yet still functioning right kidney. The left kidney still shows good parenchyma. However, a cortical scar with dilated calyx is seen on the midlateral margin *(arrow)*.

usually are easily displayed with CT because of the presence of large amounts of fat in the perirenal space (Fig. 107.10). This tends to be true even in the somewhat cachectic patient. Small scarred kidneys of chronic pyelonephritis usually are easily demonstrated (Fig. 107.10). Even in the face of rather severe renal failure, small amounts of contrast media can be seen to be excreted by the kidneys, which are not visualized on conventional x-ray films.

A unilateral hypoplastic or atretic kidney also can be displayed with CT. These kidneys are often difficult to see with conventional radiographic techniques, such as intravenous urography. A small hypoplastic kidney is noted to be a miniature type of kidney with normal excretion of contrast (Fig. 107.11). The small atretic kidney may show no significant excretion of contrast. The opposite kidney generally shows compensatory hypertrophy (Fig. 107.11).

Nonfunctioning Kidneys

After intravenous urography has demonstrated a unilateral nonfunctioning or poorly functioning kidney, ultrasound generally is used as the next method of choice in evaluation of these patients. Ultrasonographic examination usually is successful in demonstrating a hydronephrotic kidney. When ultrasound fails to demonstrate the kidney or the cause for a unilateral nonfunctioning kidney, CT may be used to help in the evaluation of the cause. The obstructed kidney with hydronephrosis is easily demonstrated with CT scanning (Fig. 107.12). Vascular problems, such

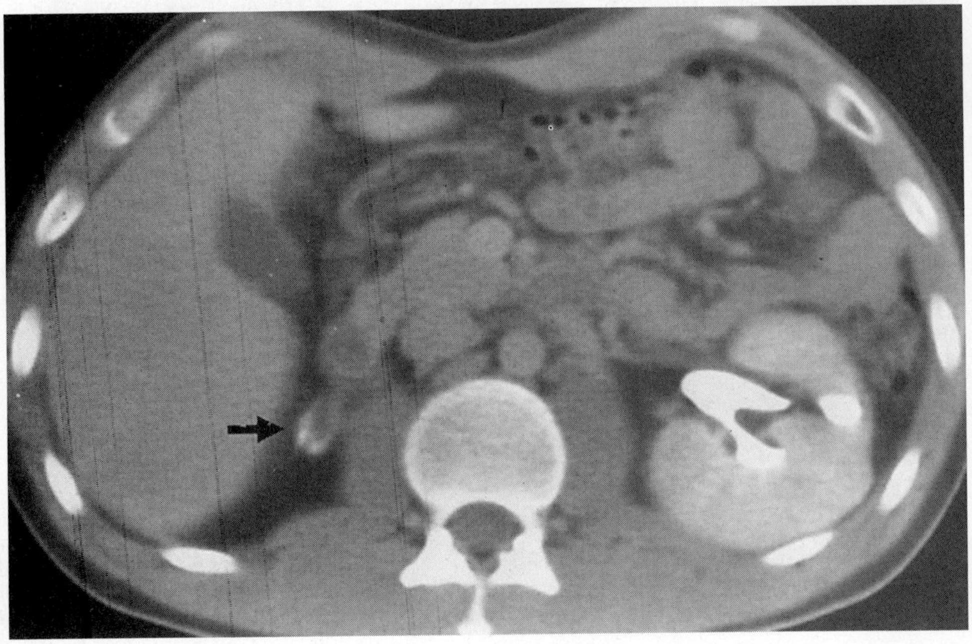

Figure 107.11. Hypoplastic kidney with hypertrophy on the opposite side. A small, smooth, functioning right kidney is identified, which is a hypoplastic kidney *(arrow)*. The left kidney is larger because of hypertrophy.

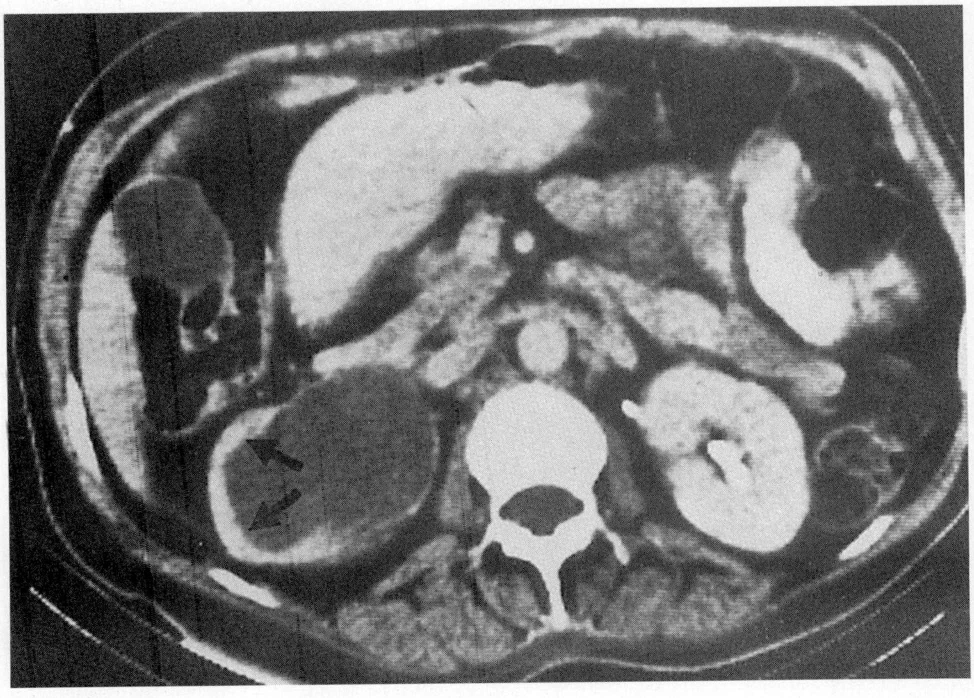

Figure 107.12. Hydronephrosis. A hydronephrotic right kidney is identified. Marked thinning of the cortex is noted *(arrows)*, with marked dilation of the renal pelvis. Little function is noted, because no contrast material is seen in the dilated collecting systems and the CT numbers are those of water. Note the normal left kidney.

as renal artery thrombosis or renal vein thrombosis (Fig. 107.13), occasionally may be noted with CT. With the advent of rapid dynamic CT scanning, the area of the renal artery and vein may be evaluated with better success. This may lead to the diagnosis with a noninvasive technique instead of angiography. Occasionally, patients with pyelonephritis will initially have a "nonfunctioning" kidney on intravenous urography. CT usually will demonstrate an enlarged swollen kidney with focal areas of decreased density because of the edema and inflammation involving the kidney (Figs. 107.14 and 107.15).

Bilaterally nonfunctioning kidneys are also best evaluated with ultrasonography, which can elucidate the reason for nonfunction, such as extrarenal or intrarenal bilateral obstruction or chronic renal failure. When ultrasound is unsuccessful in differentiating extrarenal from intrarenal causes of renal failure, CT may be helpful.

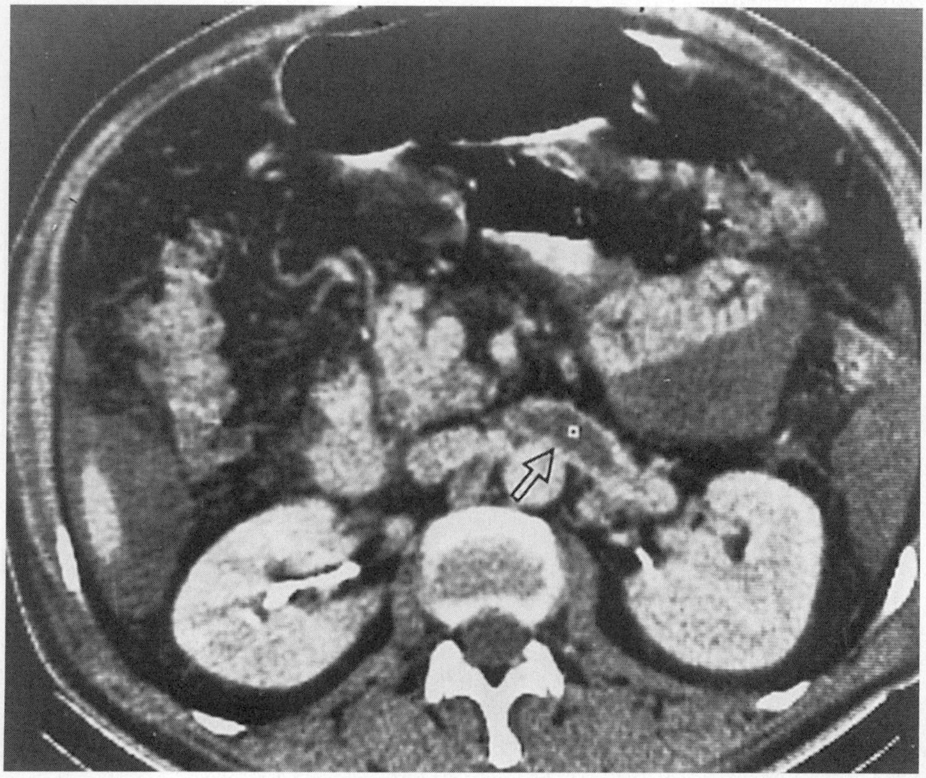

Figure 107.13. Renal vein thrombosis. A clot is identified in the left renal vein (*white box* and *arrow*) in this patient with nephrotic syndrome and renal vein thrombosis.

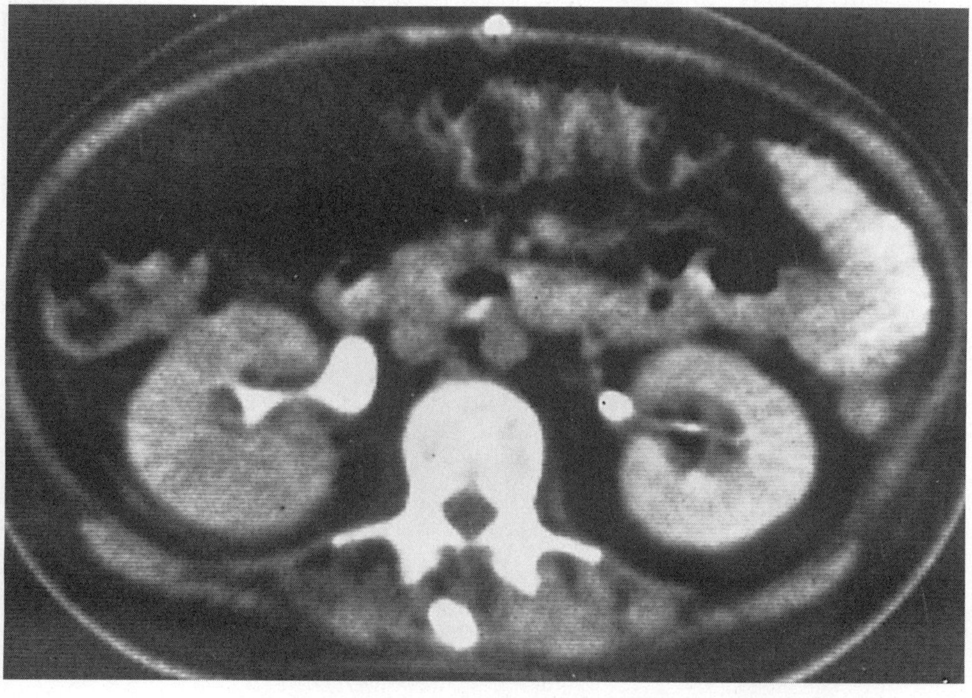

Figure 107.14. Acute pyelonephritis. The right kidney is swollen and enlarged and shows areas of decreased density compared with the normal left kidney.

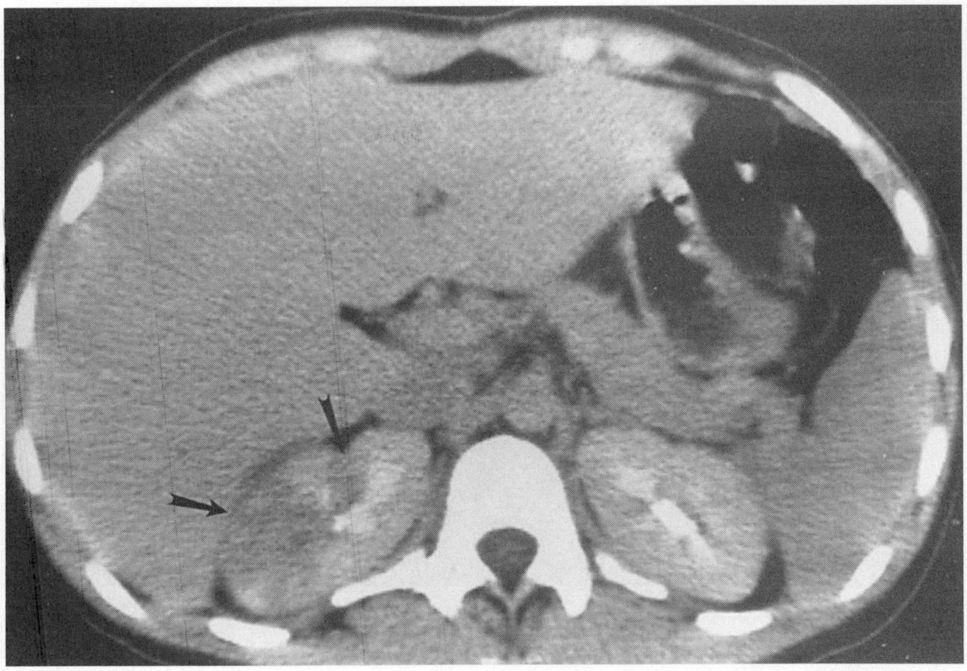

Figure 107.15. Acute pyelonephritis. Focal areas of decreased density are seen in the lateral aspect of the right kidney *(arrows)*.

Hydronephrosis and the Site of Obstruction

Conventional urography usually demonstrates the site and cause of obstruction. Ultrasonography often is used to quantitate the degree of hydronephrosis. Occasionally, the cause (e.g., stone) may even be identified. When conventional techniques and ultrasonography are unable to demonstrate the site or nature of obstruction, retrograde pyelography is usually the next diagnostic procedure. CT scanning has, to a limited extent, helped in evaluating patients who are unable to undergo retrograde pyelography or in whom it is contraindicated. A specific cause for the obstruction, such as retroperitoneal tumors, lymph nodes, or other retroperitoneal processes, is demonstrated well with CT scanning. Occasionally, an elusive stone that is difficult to identify with urography and retrograde pyelography may be demonstrated.

Renal Stones and Nonopaque Filling Defects

Although the patient with renal calculus disease is evaluated with plain films, intravenous urography, and occasionally, retrograde pyelography, CT scanning may play an increasing role in examining some of these patients. In fact, in some institutions, the use of CT scanning as the primary mode of assessing the patient with suspected renal calculi is becoming commonplace. Because of the presence of calcium in most renal stones, the CT numbers tend to be very high, in the range of 300 to 500, when compared with the renal parenchyma. These high CT numbers make even small stones (1 mm) detectable with CT scans (Fig. 107.16). In evaluating the patient with suspected renal calculi, it is important to scan the patient without the use of intravenous contrast so as not to obscure the calcific density by contrast material in the collecting system or ureter. The difficult problem of a nonopaque filling defect in the calyceal system or ureter can be evaluated with CT. Common causes of nonopaque filling defects are uric acid stones, blood clots, and transitional cell carcinomas. Because of the different CT numbers of these lesions, CT scanning has proven effective in distinguishing the specific cause of the nonopaque filling defect. Complete nonopaque uric acid stones

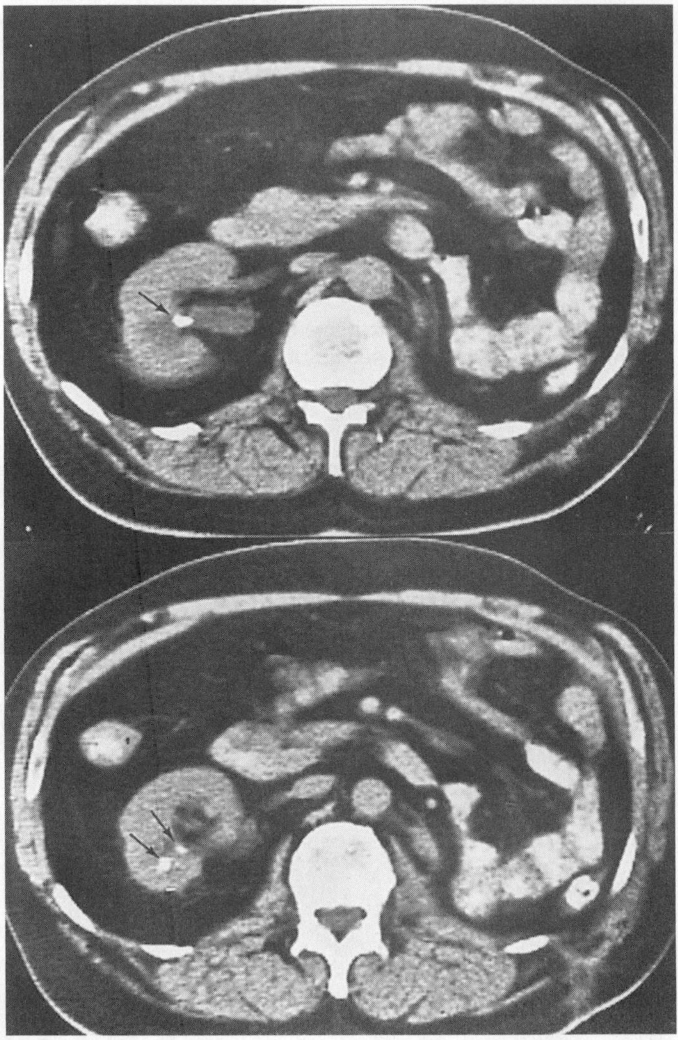

Figure 107.16. Renal calculi. Areas of increased density, renal calculi *(arrows)*, are noted in the collecting system of the right kidney. These were not identified on plain films, tomograms, or intravenous pyelography.

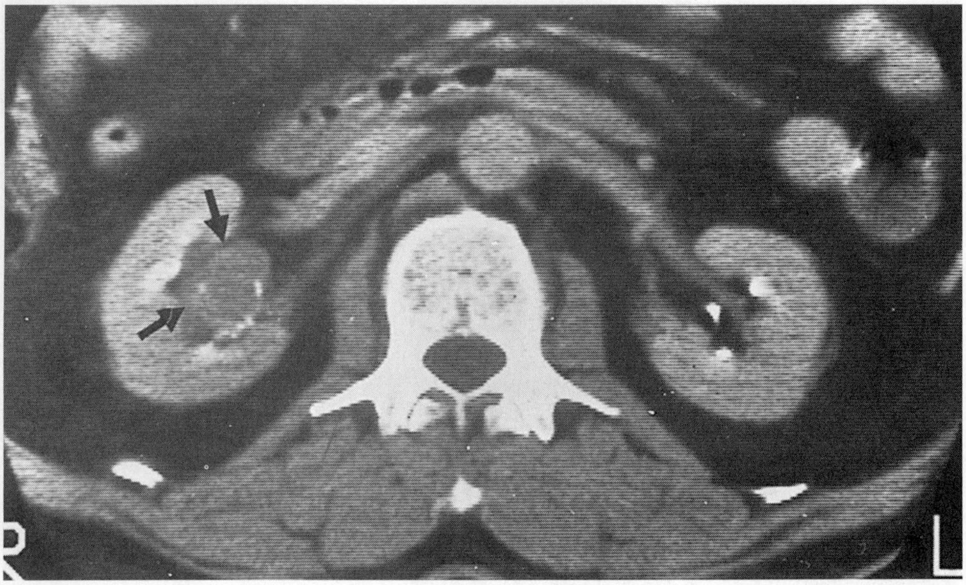

Figure 107.17. Transitional cell carcinoma. Note the mass density within the right renal pelvis *(arrows)*. It is less dense than the renal parenchyma. The contrast material in the calyces and around the mass in the renal pelvis is more dense.

have CT numbers of 50 to 80 and do not change after intravenous contrast administration. A transitional cell carcinoma has CT numbers in the range of 15 to 25 and shows an increase after intravenous contrast (Fig. 107.17). Blood clots have varying CT numbers depending on their age. They are usually in the range of 10 to 40 and show no change after the administration of intravenous contrast material. The same applies to sloughed renal papillae. Thus CT can be used to complement the conventional imaging modalities when a nonopaque filling defect is identified in the calyceal system or ureter.

Renal Trauma

In the past, patients with suspected renal trauma with or without hematuria were evaluated initially with intravenous urography, followed by angiography when abnormalities were noted. For these patients, CT scanning has proven to be the method of choice for final definitive diagnosis. CT scanning in patients with evidence of renal trauma has eliminated the need for angiography in most patients. Angiography is performed only in the patient in whom interventional procedures are contemplated, that is, embolization of a bleeding artery.

CT scans easily demonstrate intrarenal as well as external injuries. In addition, CT appears to be more accurate in distinguishing minor injuries (contusions and lacerations) from major injuries (fracture and pedicle disruption). As the whole abdomen is viewed with the CT scan, other injuries to nearby organs, such as the spleen, liver, and retroperitoneum, may be found and evaluated. The sensitivity of CT scanning permits one to document small amounts of extravasating urine or ureteral leaks. Ac-

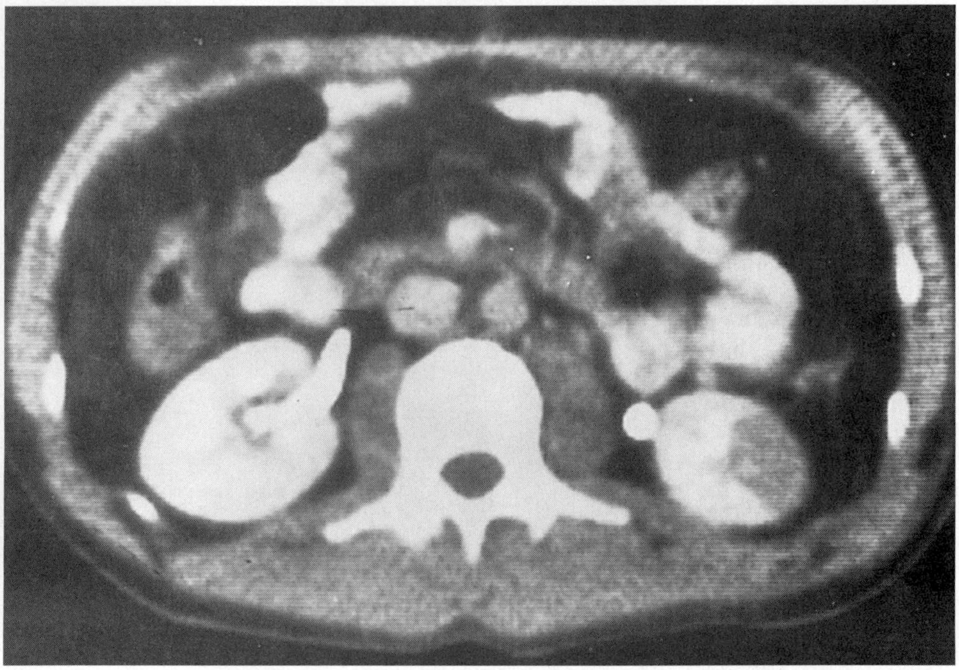

Figure 107.18. Renal contusion. A low-density region is seen in the lateral aspect of the left kidney. Angiography confirmed this to be a renal contusion.

curate demonstration of subcapsular and perirenal hematomas is easily accomplished by CT scanning.

The use of intravenous contrast material is imperative when examining the patient with renal trauma. As blood and renal tissue have similar CT numbers, contrast material is needed to increase the attenuation of the normal renal tissue to fully evaluate the extent of injury. Renal contusions and hematoma are manifested by an intact outline of the kidney with areas of decreased enhancement in the parenchyma (Fig. 107.18). Hematomas tend to be rounded, whereas contusions are more diffuse and poorly marginated (Fig. 107.19). The presence of a focal parenchymal injury with extension into the collecting system indicates a renal laceration. Extravasation of urine and contrast material is usually seen. Separation of a portion of renal parenchyma from the rest of the kidney indicates a renal fracture (Fig. 107.20). If the fracture line in the parenchyma extends into the renal pelvis or collecting system, urine will be seen to extravasate into the perirenal tissues. When the kidney is separated into multiple fragments, this is usually defined as a shattered kidney. CT scanning with contrast is able to evaluate which of the different segments will have an intact vascular system (Fig. 107.20). Catastrophic types of injuries, such as pedicle disruptions, will be shown on CT by the absence of enhancement of the parenchyma after contrast material. Even immediately after a disruption of the pedicle, collateral vessels do supply some blood flow to the capsule area of the kidney, which can be demonstrated by CT (Fig. 107.21).

Because of the excellent display characteristics in the axial plane of CT, the subcapsular and perinephric regions of the kidneys are usually well demonstrated. Perinephric (Fig. 107.19) and subcapsular hematomas are thus easily seen. Small collections that are not normally noted either with intravenous urography or angiography may be observed with CT. Subcapsular hematomas tend to deform the lateral margin of the kidney, with subsequent compression of the renal parenchyma. Perinephric hematomas spread in a more generalized fashion throughout Gerota's fascia and will tend to encapsulate the entire kidney. The size and location of the extrarenal collection, as well as the associated intrarenal injury, usually are well demonstrated with CT.

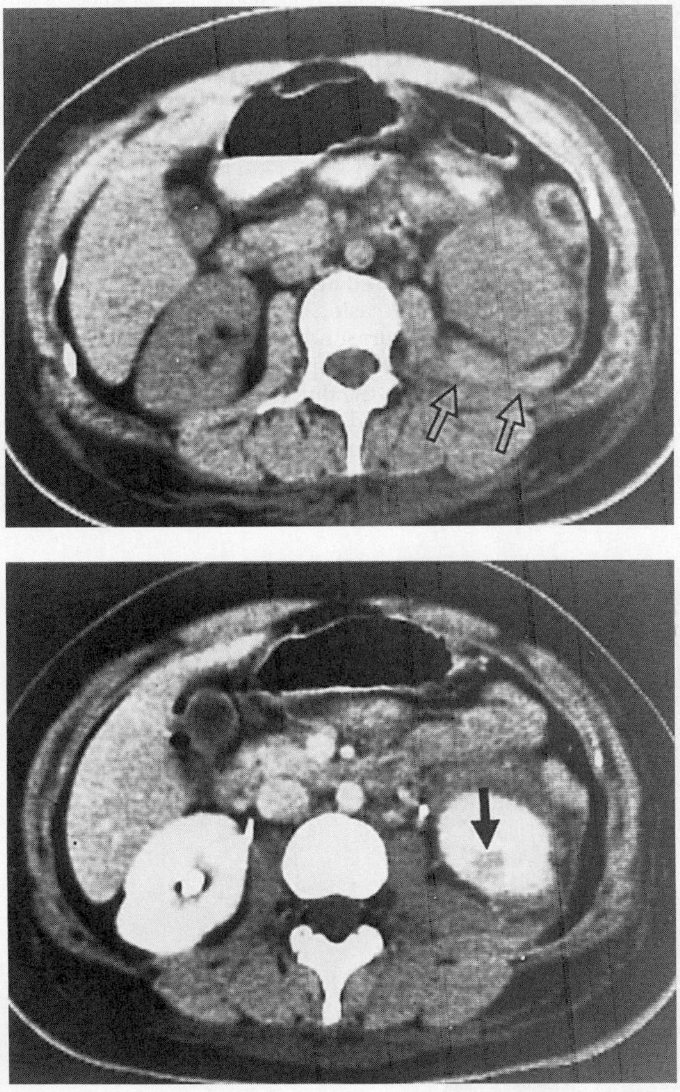

Figure 107.19. Small intrarenal hematoma and perinephric hematoma. **Top:** The unenhanced scan demonstrates a slightly irregular, normal density left kidney. A small amount of blood *(open arrows)* is seen posterior to the kidney. **Bottom:** After the infusion of intravenous contrast, a larger amount of blood is seen around the kidney, with a low-density hematoma *(solid arrow)* within the kidney.

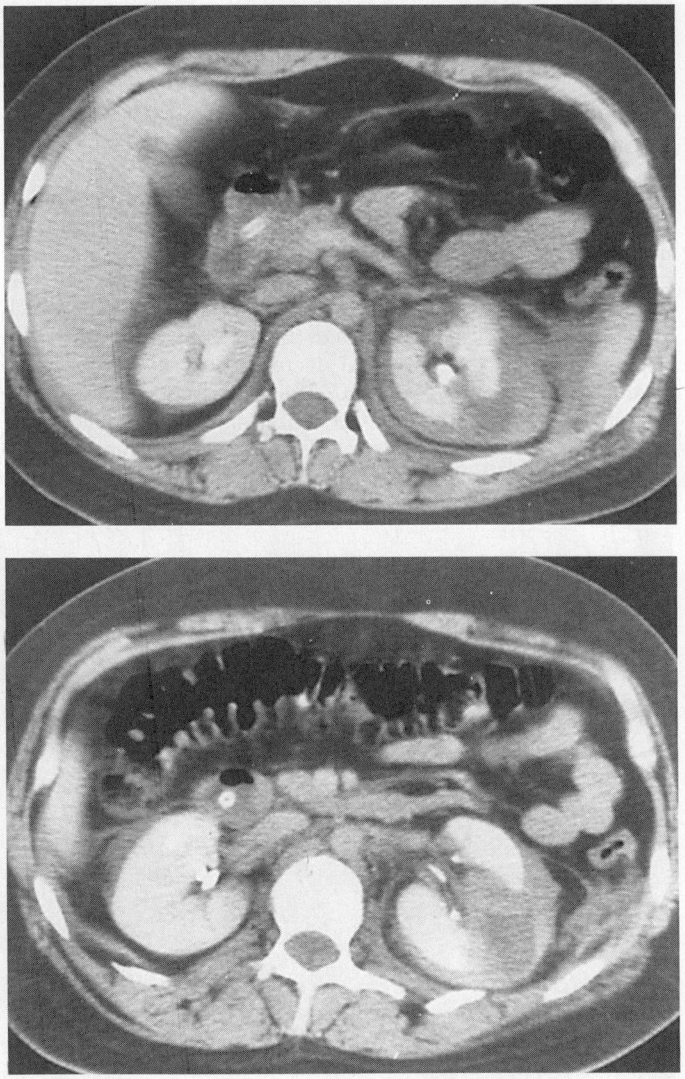

Figure 107.20. Fractured kidney. Two sections (**top** and **bottom**) through the midabdomen demonstrate a fractured left kidney with an associated perinephric hematoma. Note the fracture line separating the kidney into several parts, which continue to function and excrete contrast medium.

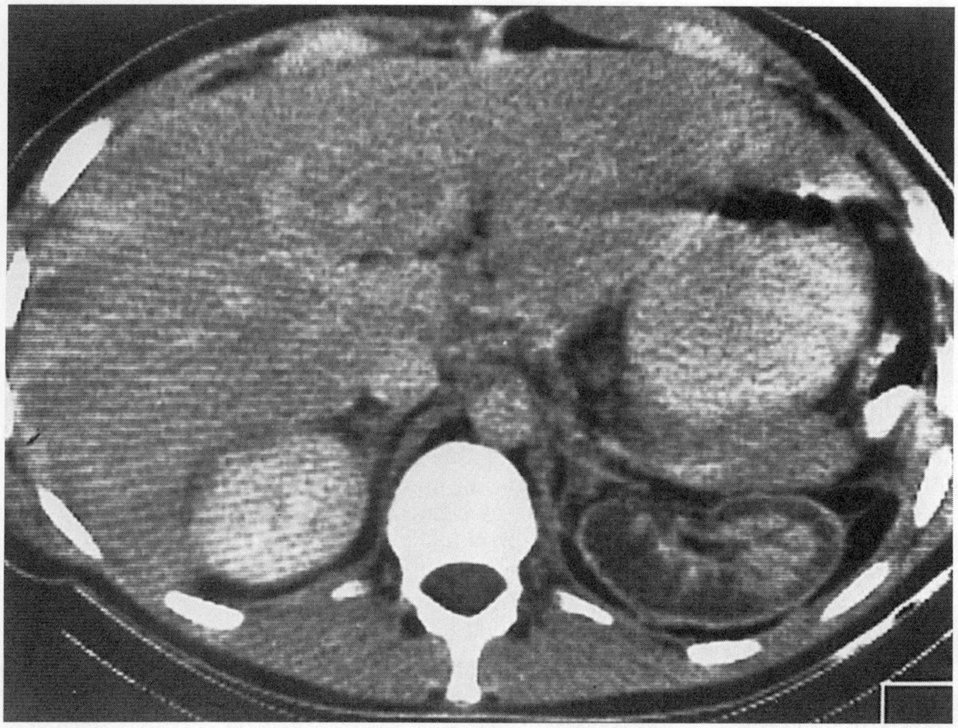

Figure 107.21. Renal artery thrombosis. Left renal artery thrombosis results in no blood flow to the left kidney. The left kidney is thus markedly decreased in density when compared with the normal right side. A small amount of collateral blood supply provides minimal blood flow to the renal capsule, which outlines the kidney.

Renal Infection

Renal infection is difficult to evaluate radiographically. The diagnosis of pyelonephritis is made using history, physical findings, and positive urine cultures. The yield of the radiographic evaluation of the patient with pyelonephritis using intravenous urography is at best poor. There are myriad findings, all of which are nonspecific. CT examination of the patient with acute pyelonephritis reveals focal areas of decreased density in the renal parenchyma (Fig. 107.14 and 107.15). More than one area of involvement in the kidney may be found. Normal-appearing areas of renal parenchyma surround the areas of decreased attenuation. These findings are consistent with the typical pathologic picture of pyelonephritis, that of a focal process.

Intrarenal abscess and renal carbuncle tend to show a more well-defined area of decreased attenuation within the renal parenchyma (Fig. 107.22). Occasionally, an associated ring of increased density is noted surrounding he lower density area of abscess. With extension into the perinephric space and formation of perinephric abscess, the fluid collection surrounding the kidney is easily demonstrated with CT. It is most important to use intravenous contrast material in these patients because the unenhanced scan in the patient with perinephric abscess often may show only what appears to be an enlarged kidney on the

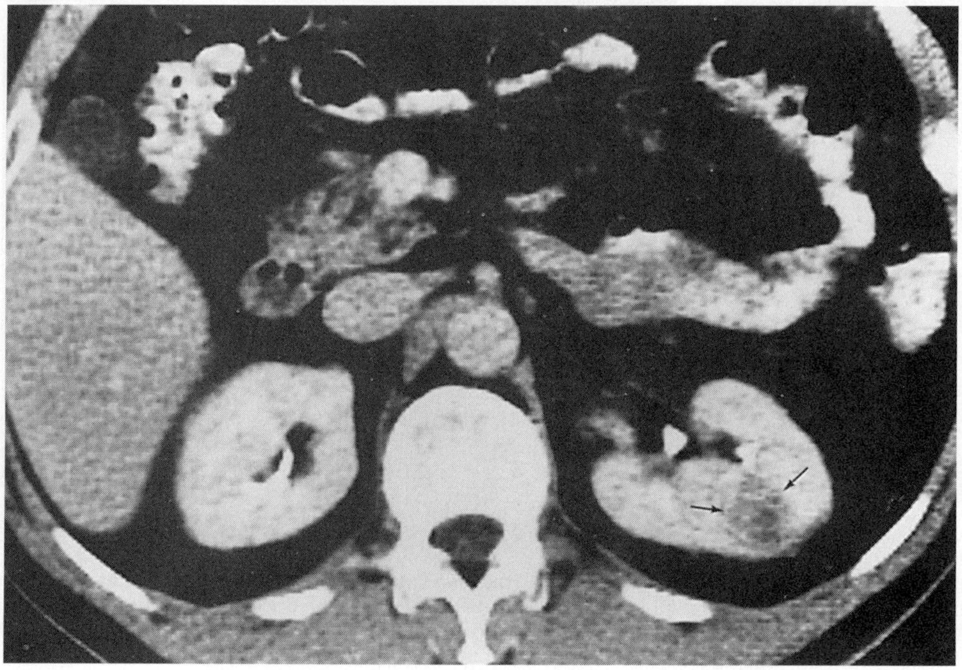

Figure 107.22. Renal abscess. A rounded but somewhat irregular area of decreased density *(arrows)* is seen on the posterolateral aspect of the left kidney. Fine-needle aspiration proved this to be an abscess.

involved side. The perinephric component is demonstrated only after administration of intravenous contrast, which produces enhancement of the kidney within the lower density perinephric abscess.

Perinephric Fluid Collections

The cross-sectional CT display of the kidney also provides images of the compartments surrounding the kidney. Anteriorly lie the anterior pararenal spaces. Surrounding the kidney is the perinephric space bordered by Gerota's fascia. Posteriorly is the posterior pararenal space. Fluid collections from pancreatitis, perforated duodenal ulcers, and other organs in the anterior pararenal space, and duodenal hematomas after direct injury may be imaged in the anterior pararenal space (Fig. 107.23). Perinephric fluid collections caused by infection, trauma, or extravasated urine are well displayed with CT (Figs. 107.19, 107.24, and 107.25). The more confined subcapsular fluid collection will show compression of renal parenchyma, whereas the perinephric collection tends to surround the entire kidney and

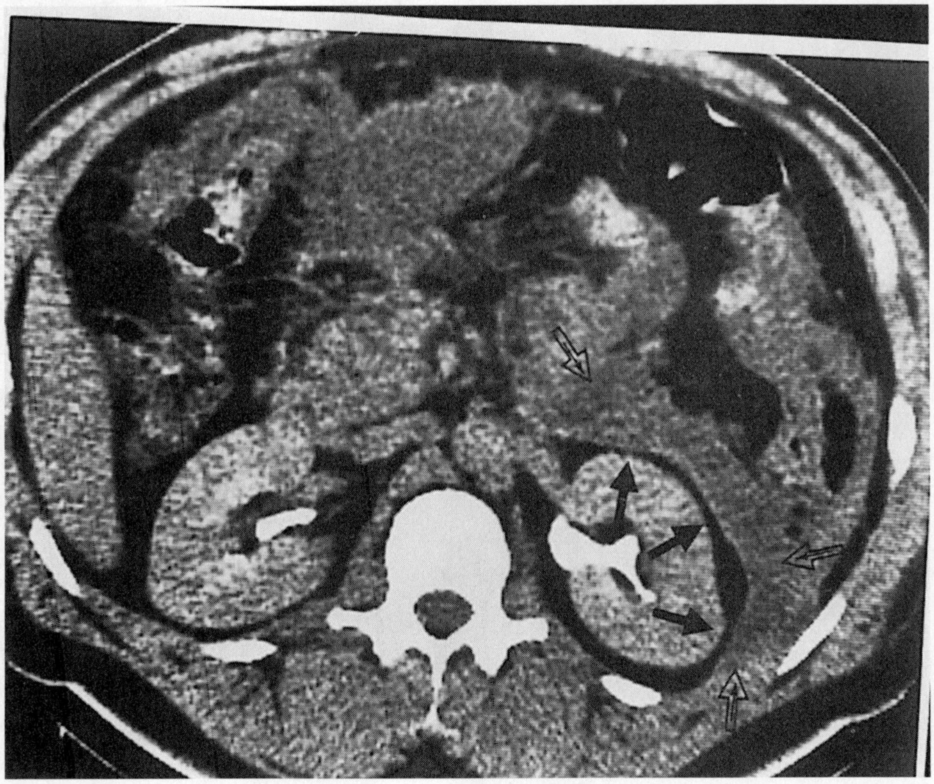

Figure 107.23. Anterior perinephric collection. A fluid density is seen in the left anterior perirenal compartment *(open arrows),* caused by pancreatitis. Gerota's fascia limits the spread of the pancreatic phlegmon into the perinephric space. *Solid arrows* indicate perinephric fat bordering the fluid collection.

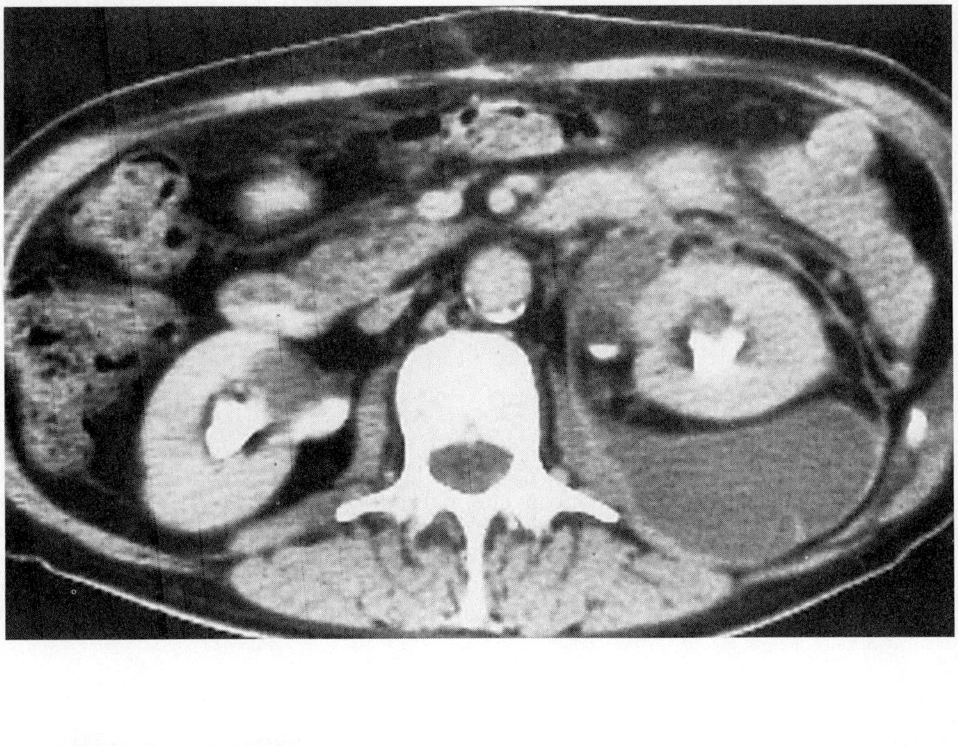

Figure 107.24. Posterior pararenal collection. This fluid collection in the posterior pararenal space is a urinoma associated with obstruction of the left kidney by a ureteral stone.

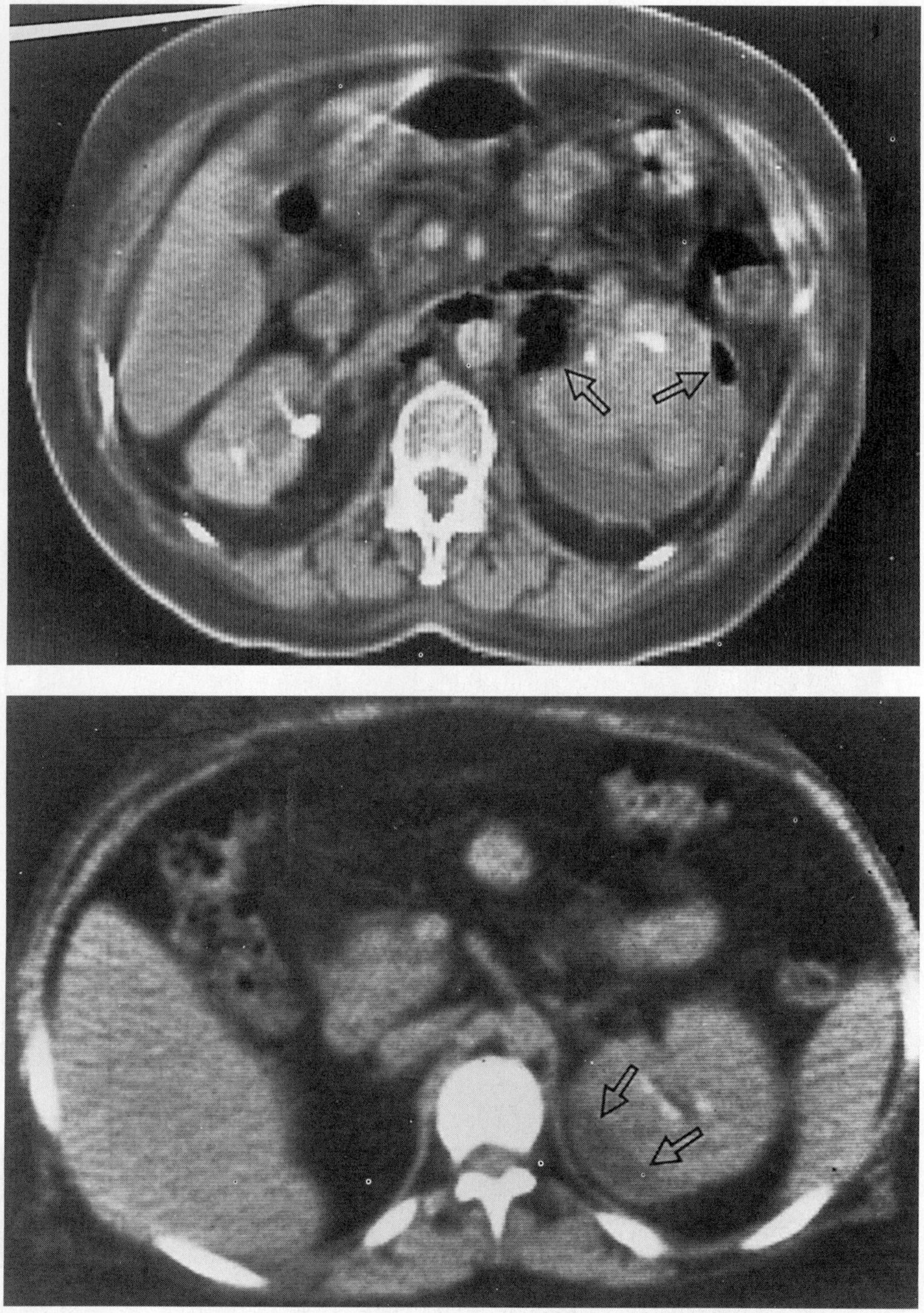

Figure 107.25. Perinephric **(top)** and subcapsular **(bottom)** abscesses. A large perinephric fluid collection is identified around the abnormal lower pole of the left kidney. Gas, diagnostic of abscess, is seen within the fluid collection *(top arrows)*. A low-density fluid collection *(bottom arrows)* deforms the medial aspect of the left kidney. This subcapsular fluid collection proved to be on abscess. No gas was noted within.

not compress the parenchyma. Posterior pararenal collections, from either infection of trauma, usually can be identified from either the anterior pararenal or perinephric spaces (Fig. 107.24). All of these fluid collections may spread inferiorly down into the pelvis.

Renal Masses

The initial detection and evaluation of patients with renal masses remain within the realm of conventional radiographic techniques, that is, intravenous urography with tomography. CT scanning is a highly sensitive means of detecting renal masses. However, it remains a secondary modality in the evaluation of these patients. It is used in conjunction with other imaging modalities, such as ultrasound, magnetic resonance imaging (MRI), and rarely angiography, to increase the specificity of the diagnosis. The approach to the patient with renal mass is provided in Chapter 33.

Renal masses are detectable with CT because of the alteration of the normal contours of the kidney. They may also be noted because the density of the mass is significantly different from the adjacent or surrounding renal parenchyma. The specific diagnosis of a renal mass depends on careful evaluation of the CT numbers, interface with surrounding tissue, presence or absence of calcification, response to intravenous contrast administration, and appearance relative to the adjacent renal parenchyma. Renal abscesses, hematomas, benign and malignant tumors, and cysts may all be evaluated with CT.

Incidental and unsuspected benign renal cysts are probably the most common abnormalities seen on CT scans of the abdomen (Fig. 107.7). Up to 50% of patients older than 50 have one or more cysts. These cysts are often 1 cm in size or smaller. CT scanning of the kidneys tends to demonstrate more renal cysts than any other radiographic method. However, large cysts are seen occasionally.

The typical renal cyst is uniform in density, with CT numbers very near that of water, that is, zero. The margins of the cyst are smooth, and there is a sharp interface with the surrounding normal renal parenchyma. No measurable thickness of the cyst wall is noted. No enhancement or significant change in the CT numbers is seen after intravenous contrast administration (Fig. 107.26).

Multiple simple cysts or polycystic kidneys can be evaluated with CT (Fig. 107.27). The extent of renal involvement with polycystic disease is frequently better appreciated with CT scanning than with other modalities. Multiple well-marginated cystic areas of varying size are seen with polycystic disease. Greater involvement of one kidney may be identified. Associated cysts in other organs, such as the liver, pancreas, or spleen, may be imaged with CT scanning.

Acquired cystic disease of the kidneys is found in patients with advanced renal failure and in those treated with chronic hemodialysis or chronic peritoneal dialysis. Bilateral cysts of varying size are found in almost all patients treated by either method for more than 3 years. Cysts are seen throughout the renal parenchyma and on the cortical surface (Fig. 107.28). Focal benign calcifications are seen not uncommonly in the cyst wall. Renal neoplasms, both adenomas and carcinomas, are found with increased frequency in these patients.

Clinical information and laboratory data often are needed in distinguishing some of the other renal masses. Renal abscess (Fig. 107.22) and hematoma (Fig. 107.19) frequently may have similar appearances. A low-density region in the kidney without distinct margination with the surrounding normal tissue and CT numbers higher than that of water may be seen with either of these entities. Intrarenal gas collections occasionally may be seen with renal abscesses. The exact age of the hematoma tends to determine the configuration and appearance within the kidney. More recent hematomas have higher CT numbers than those that are more chronic. Benign tumors of the kidney tend to take on the appearance of the structure of origin.

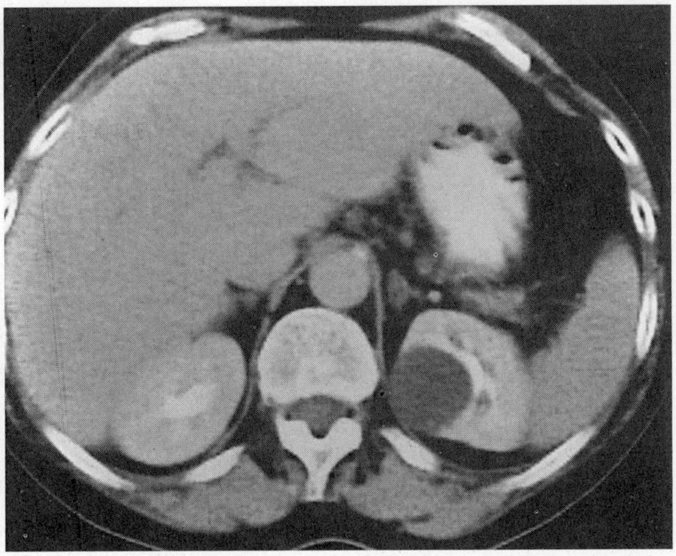

Figure 107.26. Renal cyst. A well-defined low-density renal cyst is seen on the medial aspect of the left kidney. It is uniform in density, with no discernible wall and a sharp demarcation from the adjacent normal kidney.

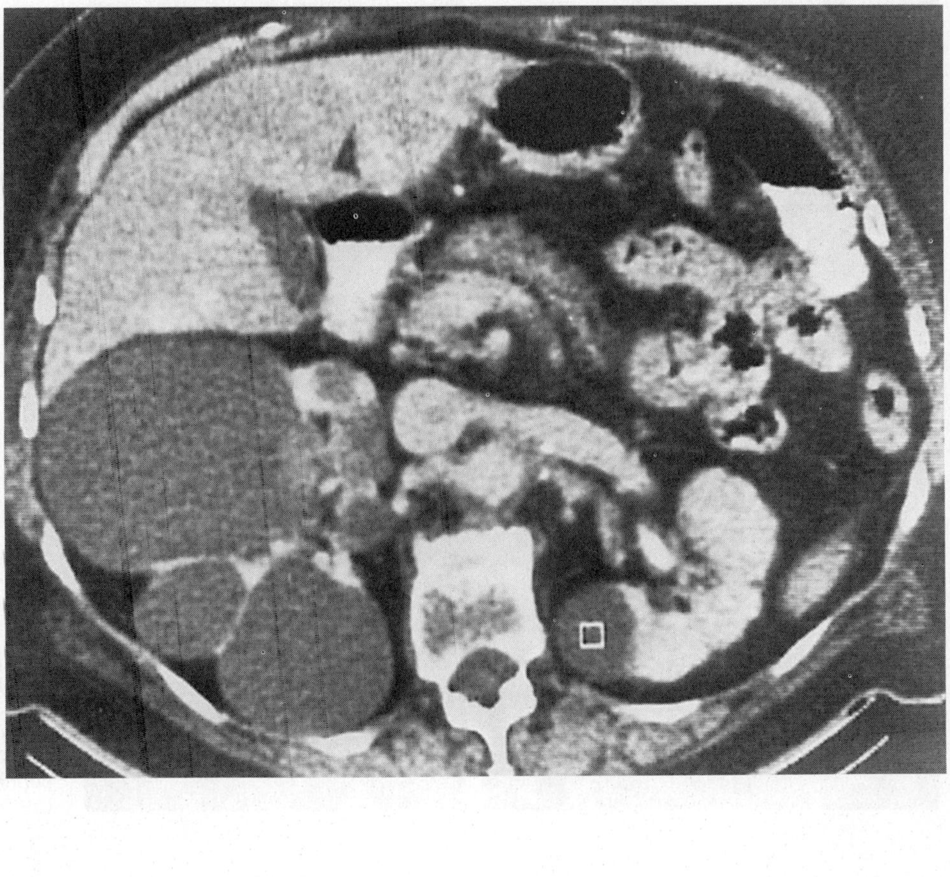

Figure 107.27. Polycystic kidneys. Note the multiple cysts in the right kidney, with little identifiable normal renal parenchyma. A moderate-sized renal cyst is noted on the medial margin of the left kidney *(white box)*, with a smaller cortical cyst noted laterally. Normal-appearing renal parenchyma remains in the left kidney, which is less severely involved than the right kidney.

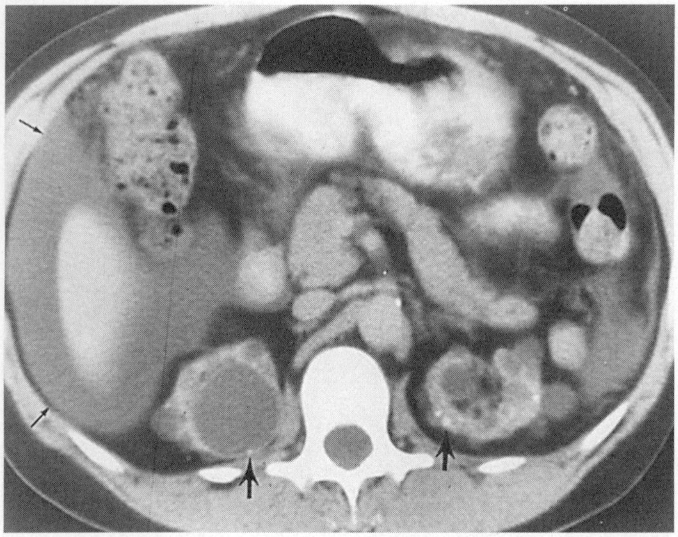

Figure 107.28. Acquired cystic disease of the kidneys. Bilateral low-density cysts are seen in both kidneys. The cysts are both medullary and cortical in location. The largest is seen in the right kidney. Small focal calcifications may be identified in cyst walls *(large arrows)*. Note fluid (dialysate) around the tip of the liver *(small arrows)*.

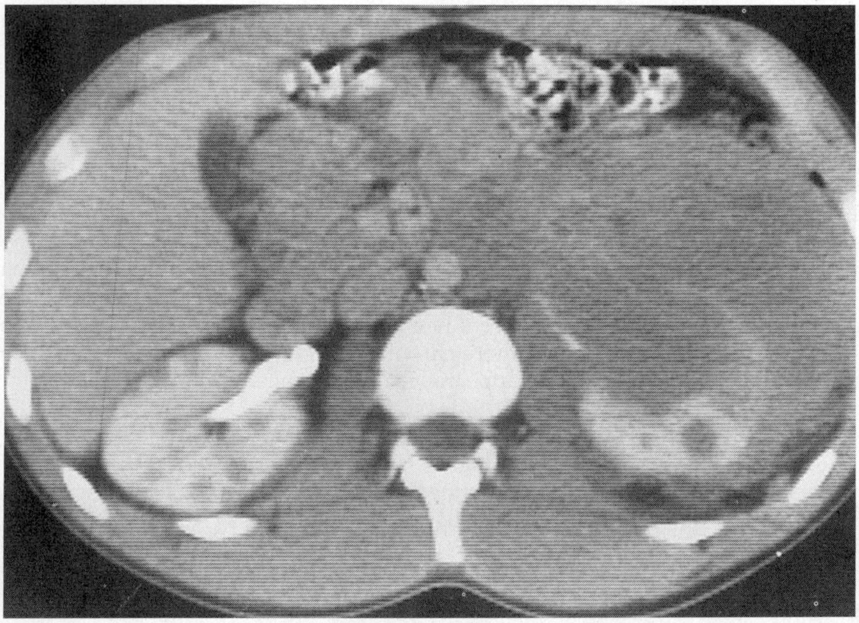

Figure 107.29. Renal lymphoma. A markedly enlarged and infiltrated left kidney is evident, with a small amount of functioning renal tissue. Multiple focal areas of involvement are seen in the right kidney.

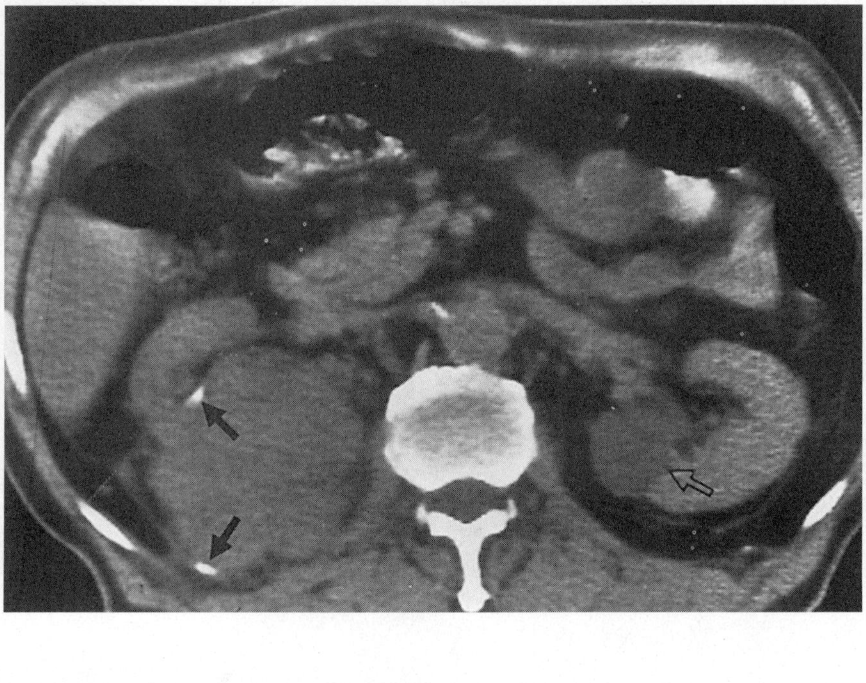

Figure 107.30. Renal cell carcinoma with calcification. This unenhanced CT scan through the midlevel of the kidneys demonstrates a lobulated mass extending off the medial and posterior aspects of the right kidney. Areas of calcifications *(solid arrows)* are noted in the periphery of the renal cell carcinoma. Note the renal cyst *(open arrow)* in the left kidney.

CT scanning in the patient with known or suspected angiomyolipoma can be extremely helpful. Because fat is present within the lesion, a relatively specific diagnosis is possible with CT. Fatty tissue will have CT numbers in a negative range, −30 to −100. These lesions are easily distinguishable from simple benign cysts and renal cell carcinoma.

Lymphoma of the kidney may be identified with CT. Several different patterns are noted. Diffuse infiltration of the renal parenchyma is the most common form (Fig. 107.29). The lymphomatous involvement is slightly less dense than the normal renal parenchyma and shows slight enhancement after intravenous contrast. Retroperitoneal masses and adenopathy are seen in conjunction with the infiltrative form. Lymphoma may occur also as a mass lesion within the kidney that is indistinguishable from renal cell carcinoma on CT. Lymph node involvement elsewhere in the body helps direct one to the proper diagnosis.

The presence of calcification within the interior of a renal mass is highly suggestive of renal cell carcinoma (Fig. 107.30). Thin, peripheral, ringlike calcification is more often seen in benign lesions, such as renal cysts. Thick, peripheral or central calcification can be seen with malignant renal lesions. The sensitivity of CT in detecting small foci of calcification may be helpful in differentiating various renal masses.

It must be remembered that CT scanning of the kidney is very sensitive in detecting renal masses but is not always specific in differentiating the various causes. Clinical history, laboratory data, and other imaging modalities, such as intravenous urography and ultrasound, may be needed in conjunction with CT to arrive at the proper diagnosis of renal mass.

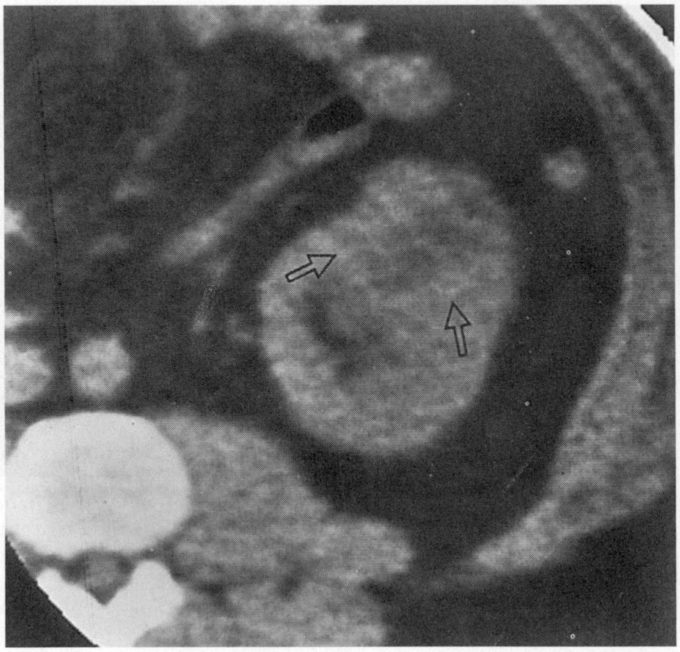

Figure 107.31. Renal cell carcinoma. This CT scan without intravenous contrast demonstrates a lobulated mass extending from the anterior aspect of the left kidney *(open arrows)*. The margins of this renal cell carcinoma are indistinct, and its density is similar to that of the adjacent normal kidney.

Renal Cell Carcinoma: Staging and Recurrence

CT scanning of the kidney is used as a complement to intravenous urography and ultrasound in the evaluation of renal cell carcinoma. The solid renal mass of renal cell carcinoma on noncontrast CT scans appears as an ill-defined, irregular area in the kidney, with CT numbers close to those of normal renal parenchyma but heterogeneous (Fig. 107.31). After the use of intravenous contrast material, there is definite enhancement of the tumor mass. However, its CT number remains less than that of the surrounding normal kidney (Fig. 107.32). With a bolus injection of contrast material and rapid scanning through the mass, there may be a transient marked increase in CT numbers, especially in the very vascular tumors. The interface with the normal kidney becomes somewhat better defined after the use

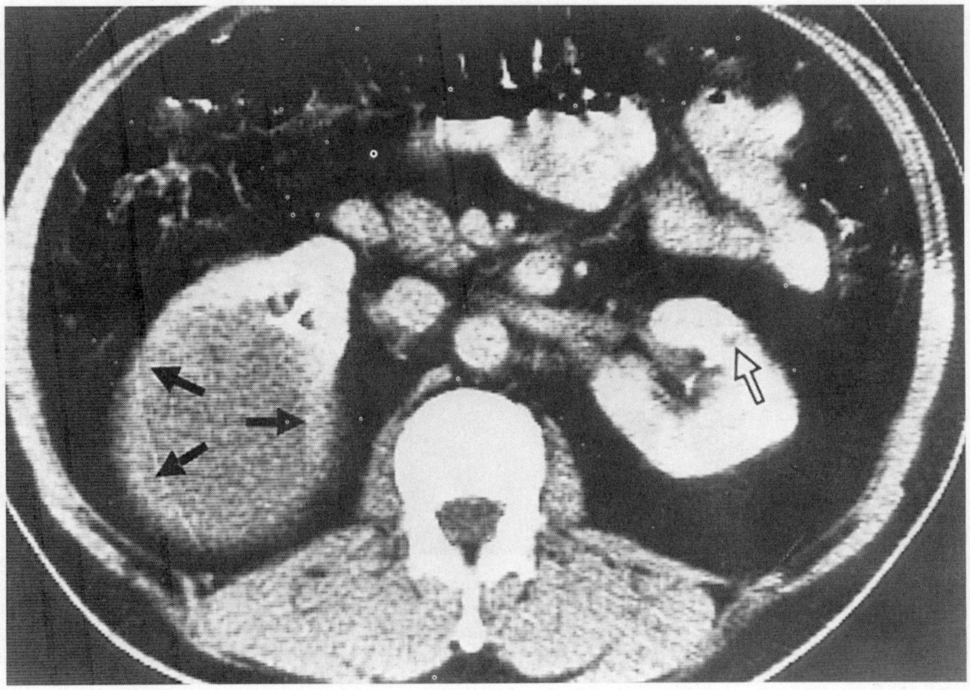

Figure 107.32. Renal cell carcinoma. With the infusion of intravenous contrast, the density difference between the normal kidney and a renal cell carcinoma becomes apparent. The large mass lesion in the right kidney has a thick wall *(solid arrows)* and a lower-density center. An incidental small renal cyst is seen in the left kidney *(open arrow)*.

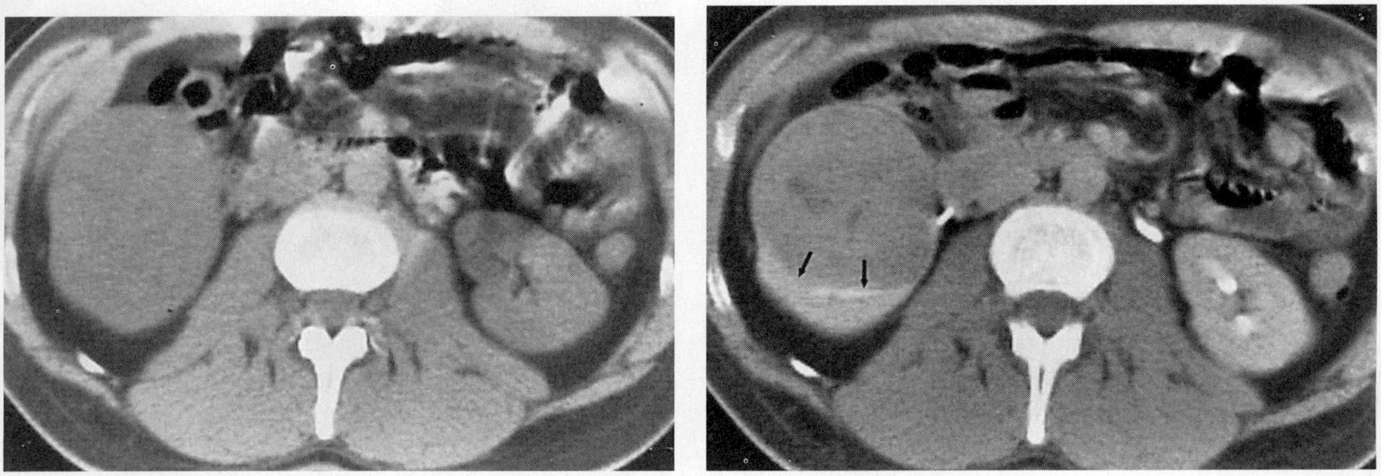

Figure 107.33. Renal cell carcinoma. The nonenhanced CT scan **(left)** demonstrates a large mass of uniform density replacing mast of the right kidney. The postcontrast CT scan **(right)** shows the clear demarcation *(arrows)* between the tumor and the thin rim of remaining normal renal tissue posteriorly.

of the contrast material but remains irregular and poorly marginated (Fig. 107.33). Wilms' tumors have a CT appearance similar to that of renal cell carcinomas.

The staging of renal cell carcinoma is important in predicting survival rates, as well as helping determine the proper surgical approach to the lesion. In a stage I carcinoma, the tumor is confined to the renal parenchyma (Figs. 107.32 and 107.33). With a stage II renal cell carcinoma, the tumor has extended beyond the renal capsule and has invaded the perinephric fat but is still within Gerota's fascia (Fig. 107.34). Both stage I and II renal cell carcinomas may be approached surgically with a retroperitoneal operation. Stage III tumors have gross involvement of the renal vein or regional lymph nodes with or without extension into the inferior vena cava (Figs. 107.35, 107.36, and 107.37). A stage IV renal cell carcinoma is defined as progression of the tumor outside Gerota's fascia, involvement of adjacent organs other than the ipsilateral adrenal, or distant metastases. An abdominal approach is needed for successful surgical intervention in stage III and stage IV renal cell carcinoma.

The imaging characteristics of CT scanning are such that the perinephric space, renal hilum inferior vena cava, and adjacent organs are well defined, so stages I to IV of renal cell carcinoma can be accurately determined. In comparing CT scanning with angiography, the conventional means of staging renal cell carcinomas, CT is found to be more sensitive and specific in detecting perinephric extension into Gerota's fascia. In determining

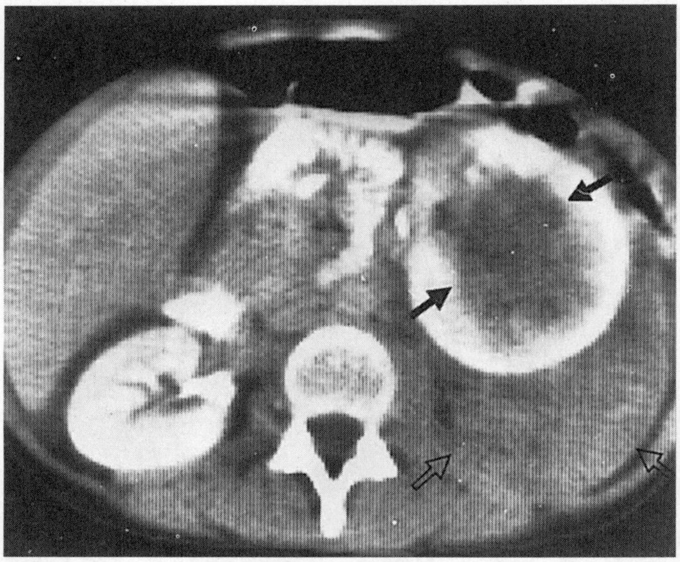

Figure 107.34. Renal cell carcinoma. This large necrotic renal cell carcinoma of the left kidney *(solid arrows)* has extended posteriorly into the perinephric space. This soft tissue mass *(open arrows)* is limited by a Gerota's fascia, and this tumor is therefore designated a stage II renal cell carcinoma.

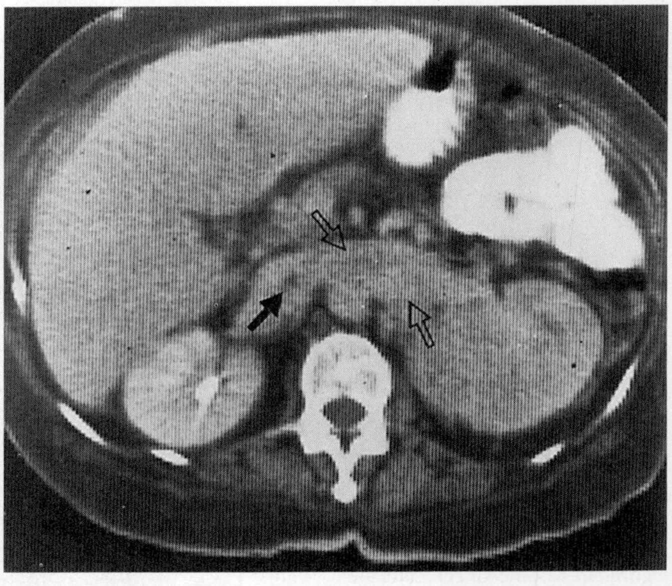

Figure 107.35. Renal cell carcinoma stage III. The renal cell carcinoma involving the medial and posterior aspects of the left kidney has extended into the renal vein and inferior vena cava. Note the low-density region in the inferior vena cava *(solid arrow)* representing tumor thrombus. The renal vein is markedly enlarged, with areas of low density within, again representing tumor thrombus *(open arrows).*

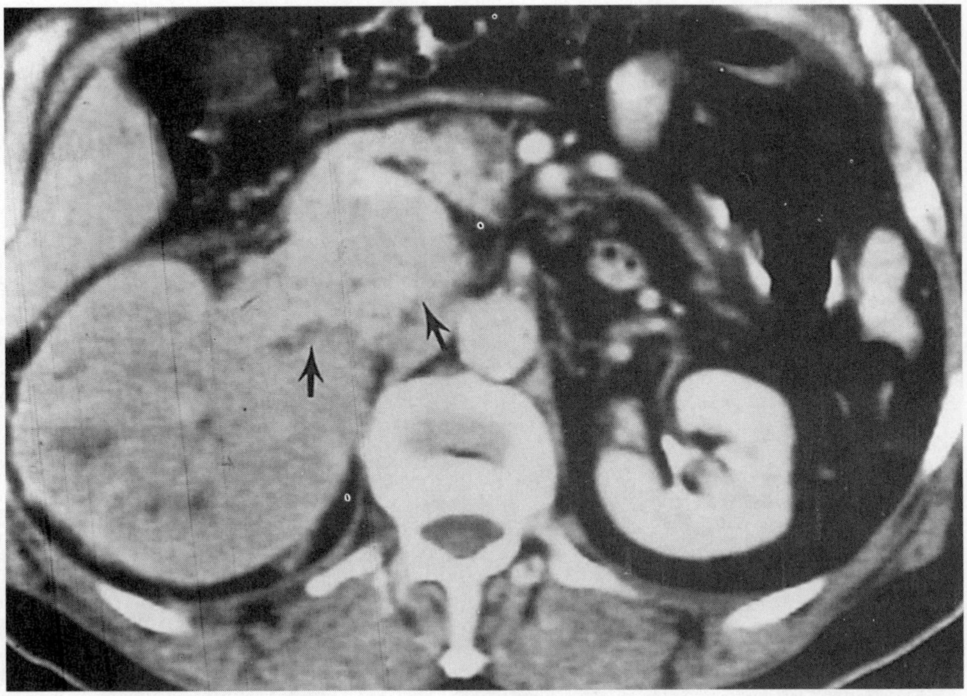

Figure 107.36. Renal cell carcinoma stage III. A large right renal cell carcinoma involves literally all of the kidney. The right renal vein is also involved, with tumor thrombus extending into the markedly enlarged inferior vena cava *(arrows)*.

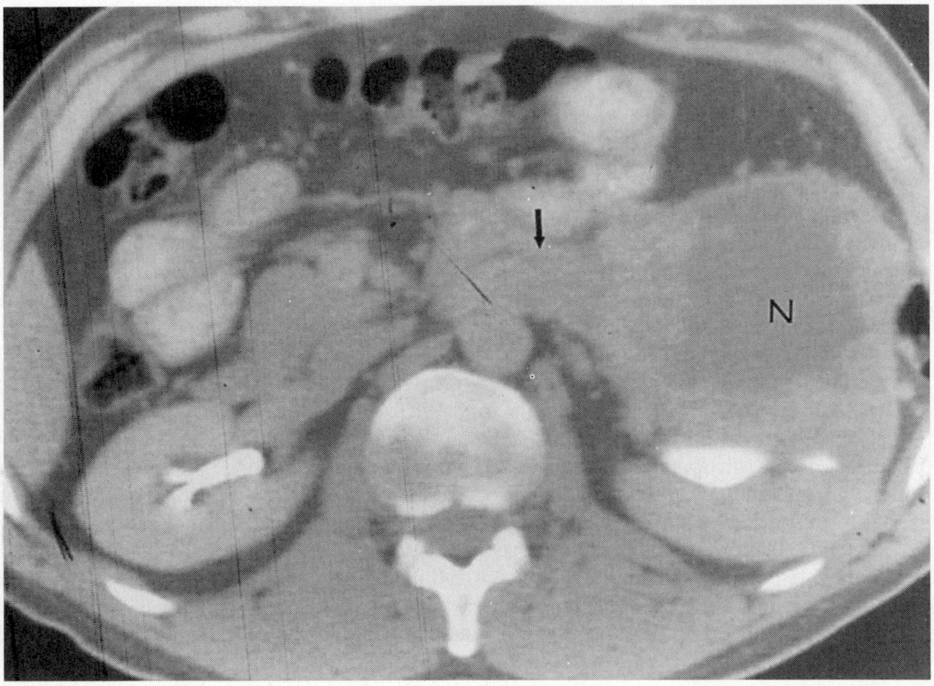

Figure 107.37. Renal cell carcinoma stage III. A large renal cell carcinoma is seen in the left kidney. The region of decreased density within the tumor represents central necrosis *(N)*. Enlargement of the renal vein is caused by tumor extension into the vein *(arrow)*.

lymph node involvement, CT scanning is more rewarding than angiography. CT and MRI are both accurate in assessing main renal vein and inferior vena cava involvement. Thus CT scanning and MRI can be used in the accurate assessment of renal cell carcinomas, and angiography is now reserved for rare cases in which a look at the detailed vascular anatomy is needed.

Although the 5-year survival rate for stage I and II renal cell carcinomas is relatively good, a large number of patients develop tumor recurrence after successful nephrectomy. Before the advent of CT scanning, there was no good means to reevaluate local recurrence in such patients. Normally, the renal bed will be empty after nephrectomy except for mild scarring in the retroperitoneum as a result of postoperative hematoma or radiation therapy in a few patients. Tumor recurrence may be suspected when a soft tissue mass is seen in the renal bed, the inferior vena cava or aorta is not seen, or the ipsilateral psoas muscle is not well defined or is abnormal (Fig. 107.38). By using CT scanning, up to one-third of patients may be found to have local recurrence of tumor within several years of surgery. With earlier detection of local recurrence by CT, long-term survival rates may be improved.

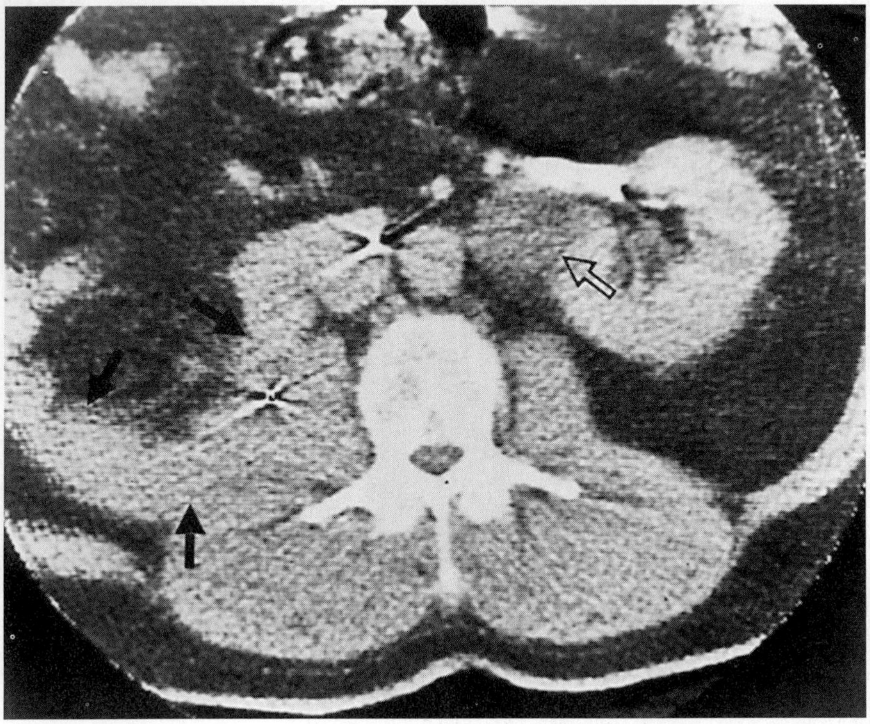

Figure 107.38. Recurrent renal cell carcinoma. A right renal cell carcinoma had been resected 4 years previously. Recurrent tumor *(solid arrows)* is now noted in the renal bed, with extension into the right psoas muscle. Note the surgical clips in the area of the recurrent renal cell carcinoma. A small, poorly defined renal cyst is noted in the left kidney *(open arrow)*.

SUSPECTED RETROPERITONEAL MASS OR ADENOPATHY

The retroperitoneal space has always been a difficult area to examine radiographically. Indirect evidence of pathologic processes in the retroperitoneum is usually obtained by plain films of the abdomen, by intravenous urography, or occasionally, during gastrointestinal radiographic studies. Masses may displace, indent, or change the relationships of various organs, that is, the kidneys, ureter, bladder, and bowel. The underlying cause is often not identifiable and only inferred from the mass effect on the retroperitoneal structures. Because of the variable position of the retroperitoneal organs, a significant retroperitoneal process may cause little or no abnormalities on conventional examinations.

The cross-sectional images obtained with CT of the abdomen and pelvis display the retroperitoneal space and its relation to the intraperitoneal space. The major structures in the retroperitoneum are easily identified and include the aorta, inferior vena cava, kidneys, ureters, bladder, psoas muscles, spine, adrenals, pancreas, and retroperitoneal portions of the bowel. The intimate relations among these structures and the potential pathways of disease spread or progression are easily observed with CT.

For the most part, retroperitoneal masses of any etiology will be demonstrated with CT scanning. Retroperitoneal tumors, benign or malignant, will cause distortion and obliteration of the normal planes within the retroperitoneum. Any or all of the retroperitoneal structures can represent the site of origin of the neoplastic process. The spread or involvement of other neighboring structures is easily documented with CT. Most tumors will appear as solid, relatively homogeneous masses in the retroperitoneum. With necrosis of the tumors, lower-density material will be seen, generally in the central region of the mass (Fig. 107.39). Small amounts of calcium deposited within the tumor generally will be seen better with CT than with conventional films. CT plays an extremely important role in the complete evaluation of these neoplasms. The cross-sectional images of CT help determine the resectability of the mass, a direct route for biopsy, or the contours of radiation therapy planning. Generally, a specific pathologic diagnosis is not possible merely from the CT appearance.

Nonneoplastic retroperitoneal processes, such as hematoma, abscess, or other fluid collections in the retroperitoneum, are seen well with CT. The CT findings of a retroperitoneal hematoma usually depend on the extent and acuteness or chronicity of the bleeding. Acute hematomas tend to have higher CT numbers and appear denser than the more chronic hematomas. The latter generally have a rim, with a relatively homogenous central area of lower attenuation. Chronic hematomas occasionally may have calcium deposits in their walls. Retroperitoneal abscesses may appear similar to chronic hematomas. However, the presence of small bubbles of gas within the abscess can help lead to this specific diagnosis (Fig. 107.40). Other fluid collections that occur in the retroperitoneum, such as urinomas, lymphoceles, or the fluid associated with pancreatitis, generally have a variable appearance depending on their specific location (Figs. 107.23 and 107.25). For the most part, however, they are low in attenuation when compared with normal soft tissue structures of the retroperitoneum.

Retroperitoneal and periaortic lymph nodes normally can be seen on CT scans of the abdomen and pelvis. The normal retroperitoneal lymph node is generally less than 1 cm in size (Fig. 107.41). Normal lymph nodes up to 1.5 cm in size are observed occasionally. With increases in the size of the nodes above 1.5 cm and increases in their number, retroperitoneal adenopathy from virtually any cause may be diagnosed with CT. The largest and most abundant nodes are usually seen with lymphomas (Fig. 107.42). The nodes may appear as discrete, round densities in the retroperitoneum. As the disease process progresses, large conglomerate masses are observed in the

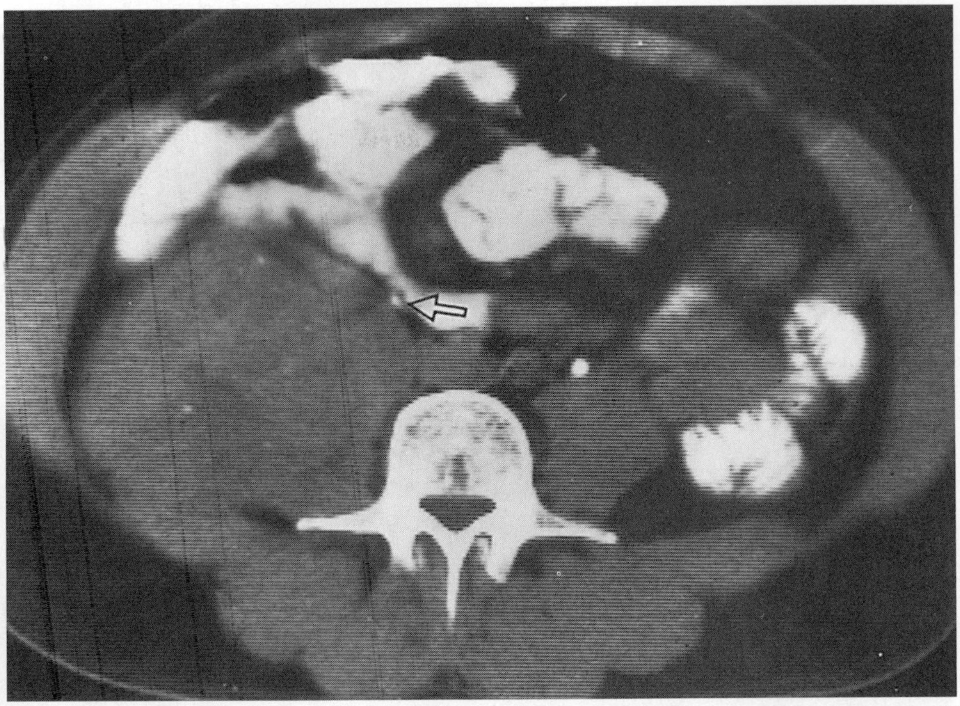

Figure 107.39. Retroperitoneal tumor. This retroperitoneal sarcoma has arisen from the region of the right psoas muscle and extends anteriorly. Small flecks of calcium are noted within the tumor. Varying areas of density are also noted. The right ureter is displaced anteriorly *(open arrow)* by the retroperitoneal sarcoma.

retroperitoneum, obliterating the normal structures and planes (Fig. 107.43). Other common causes of retroperitoneal adenopathy observed with CT are metastases from such primary sites as the testes, bladder, prostate, kidney, and pancreas. CT cannot determine the cause of retroperitoneal adenopathy. It is possible to have a normal CT scan of the retroperitoneum and still have metastatic spread to lymph nodes. This is because radiographic procedures, such as CT scanning, merely show the size and number of nodes and not the internal pathologic structure. Lymphangiography may still be helpful in the diagnosis of pathologic lesions in normal-sized retroperitoneal nodes.

The major vascular structures in the retroperitoneum, the aorta and inferior vena cava, are easily seen with CT scanning in most patients. The additional use of intravenous contrast material will highlight these areas to better advantage. Although ultrasound is the imaging modality of choice in the evaluation of abdominal aortic aneurysms, CT canning can easily display aneurysms of the abdominal aorta (Fig. 107.44). The exact luminal dimensions of the aneurysms, as well as associated findings, such as clot within the lumen or calcification within the wall, are generally well imaged. Inferior vena cava thrombosis occasionally may be imaged with CT scanning. The low-density area within the lumen of the inferior vena cava is usually diagnostic for the thrombosis.

Retroperitoneal fibrosis usually is suggested from conventional intravenous urography when there is medial deviation of

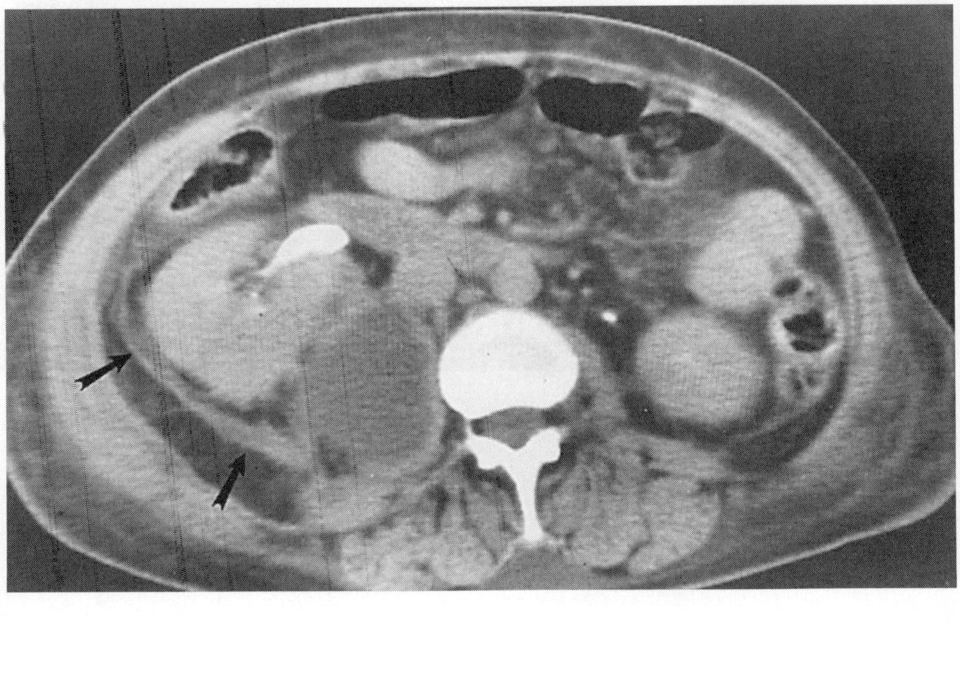

Figure 107.40. Retroperitoneal psoas abscess. A large fluid collection is seen involving the right psoas muscle. Note the normal left psoas. Thickening of Gerota's fascia *(arrows)* occurs in association with the abscess.

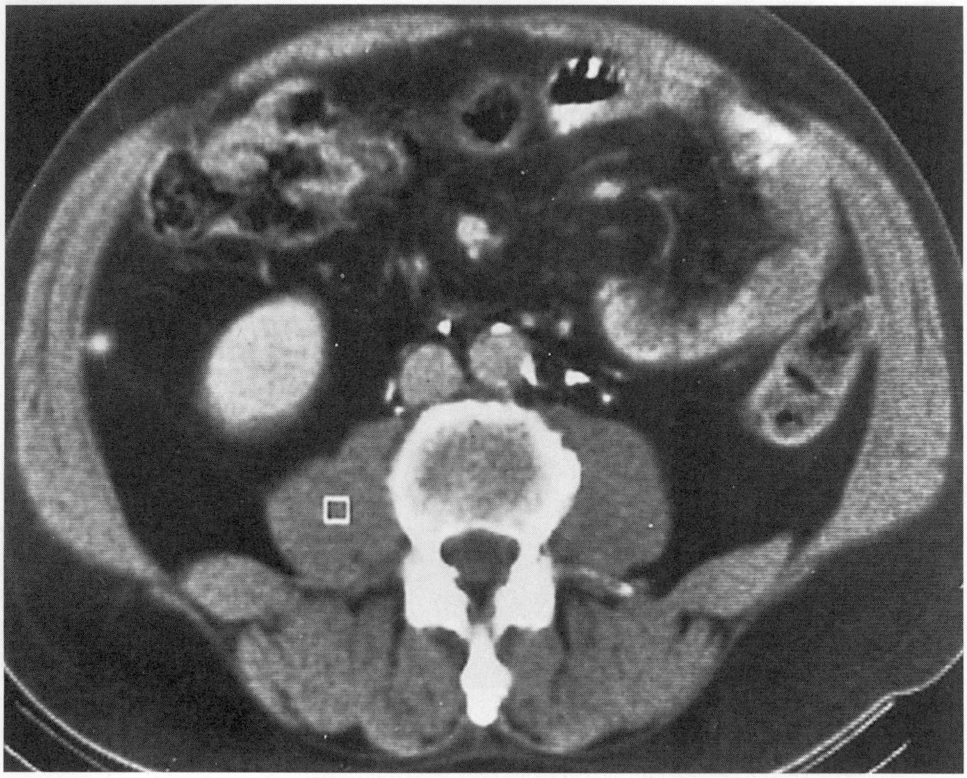

Figure 107.41. Normal retroperitoneal lymph nodes. Normal-sized (less than 1.5 cm) lymph nodes can be visualized as soft tissue densities in the paraaortic region on CT scanning. Lymphangiographic contrast material in this particular case makes the lymph nodes appear as dense structures adjacent to the inferior vena cava and aorta. The *white square* overlies the right psoas muscle.

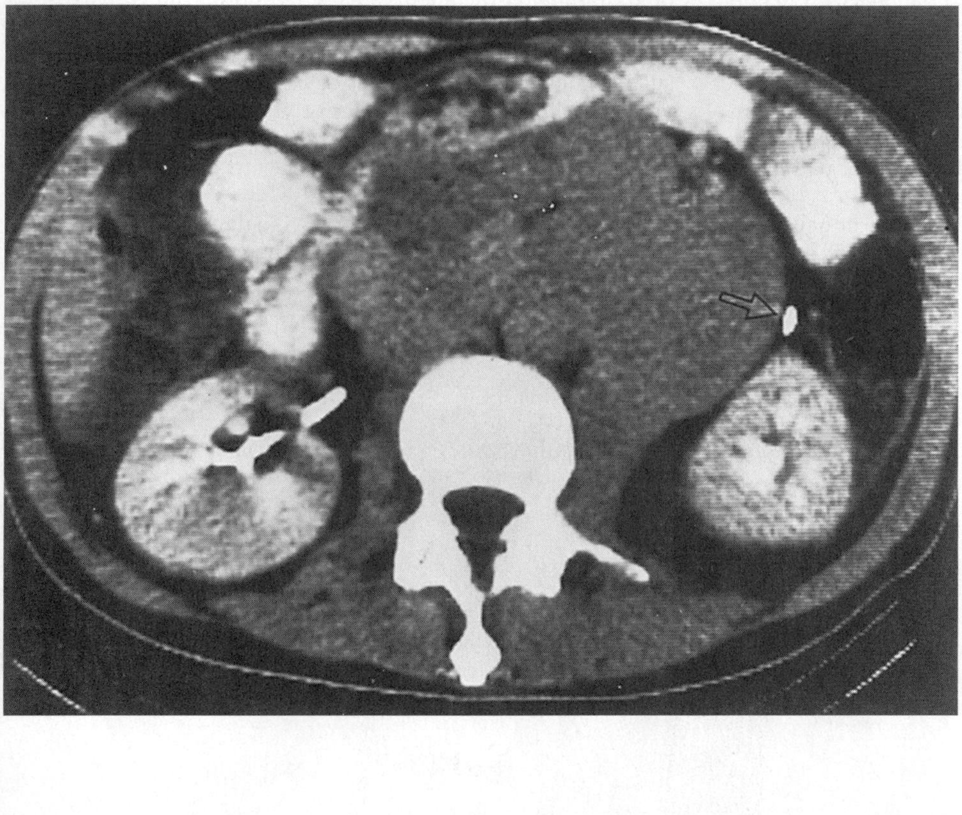

Figure 107.42. Retroperitoneal lymphadenopathy. This large conglomerate mass of retroperitoneal nodes is caused by Hodgkin's disease. Note the lateral displacement of the left ureter *(open arrow)* and anterior displacement of the contrast-filled small bowel.

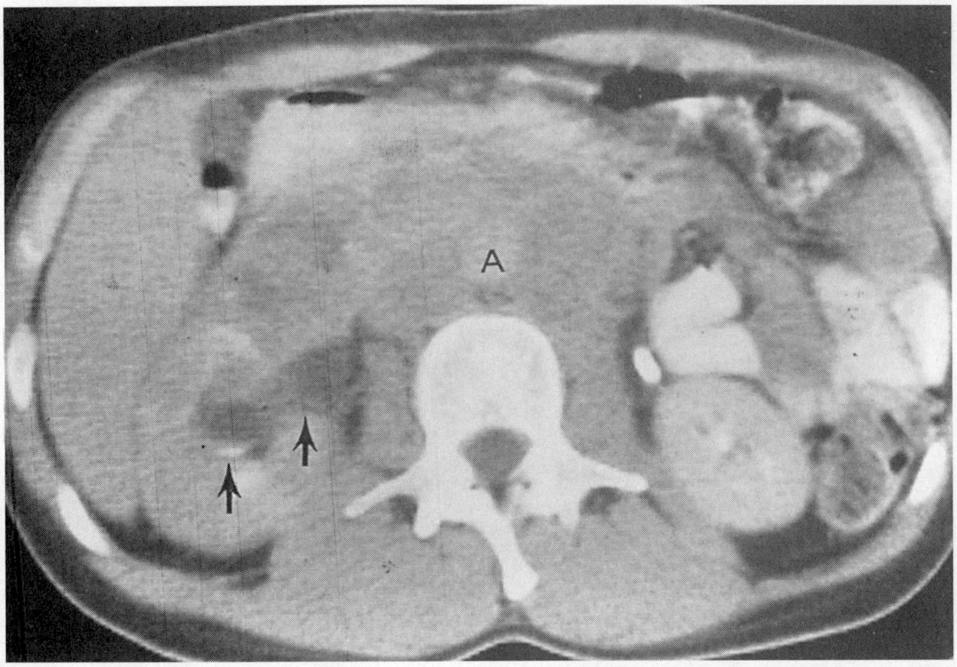

Figure 107.43. Retroperitoneal lymphadenopathy. A large soft tissue mass caused by metastatic testicular carcinoma fills the retroperitoneum, elevating the aorta *(A)* within it. Note the obstruction of the right kidney with moderate hydronephrosis *(arrows)*.

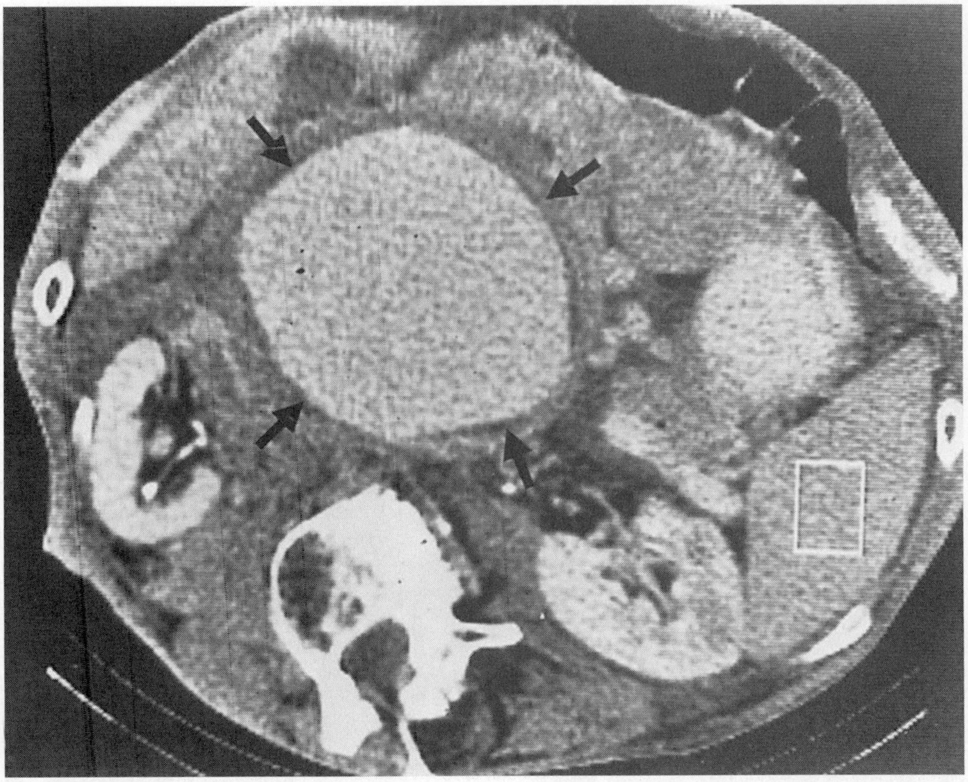

Figure 107.44. Abdominal aortic aneurysm. A large 9-cm abdominal aortic aneurysm *(solid arrows)* is noted in the midabdomen. The peculiar angulation of the vertebral body is caused by scoliosis. The kidneys are noted posteriorly. The *white box* overlies the spleen in the left side of the abdomen.

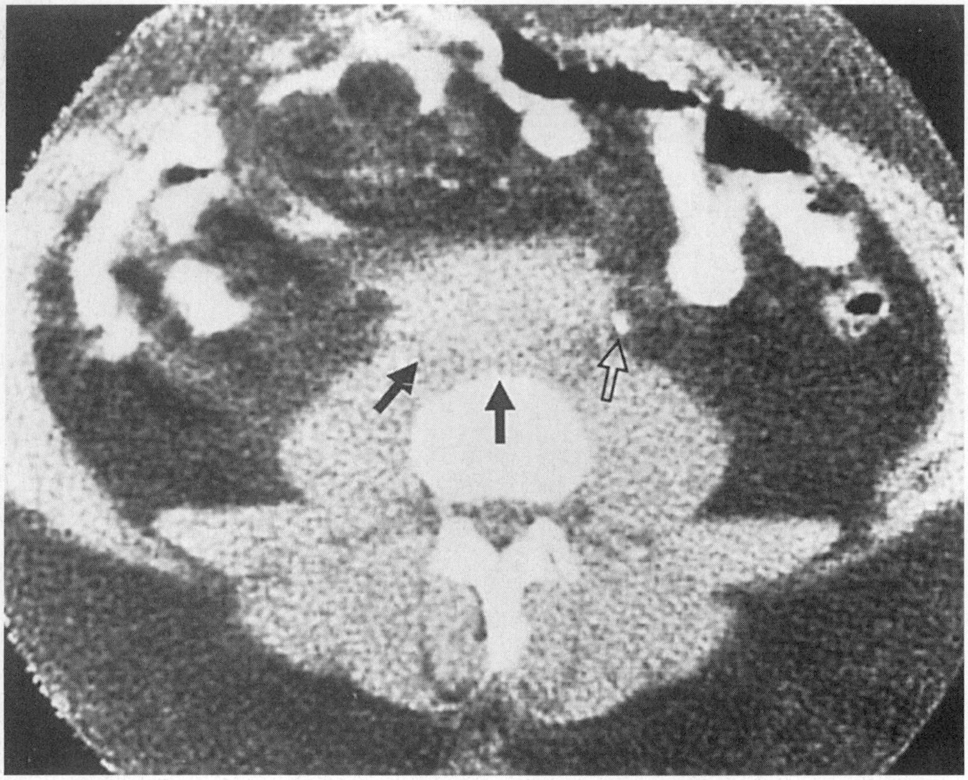

Figure 107.45. Retroperitoneal fibrosis. A large soft tissue density surrounds the aorta and inferior vena cava *(solid arrows)*. The right ureter is not visualized in the mass. The left ureter *(open arrow)* is visualized because of a ureteral stent.

the ureter and some element of obstruction. CT scanning is helpful in the evaluation of these patients by demonstrating encasement of the ureters, aorta, and interior vena cava by the fibrous tissue (Fig. 107.45). The fat planes normally present between the major retroperitoneal structures are obliterated with the fibrotic process, and a soft tissue mass is usually seen to surround the structures.

EVALUATION OF TUMORS OF THE ADRENALS, BLADDER, PROSTATE, AND OTHER PELVIC ORGANS

The adrenal glands can be visualized with CT scanning in almost all patients (Fig. 107.5). CT has provided a noninvasive

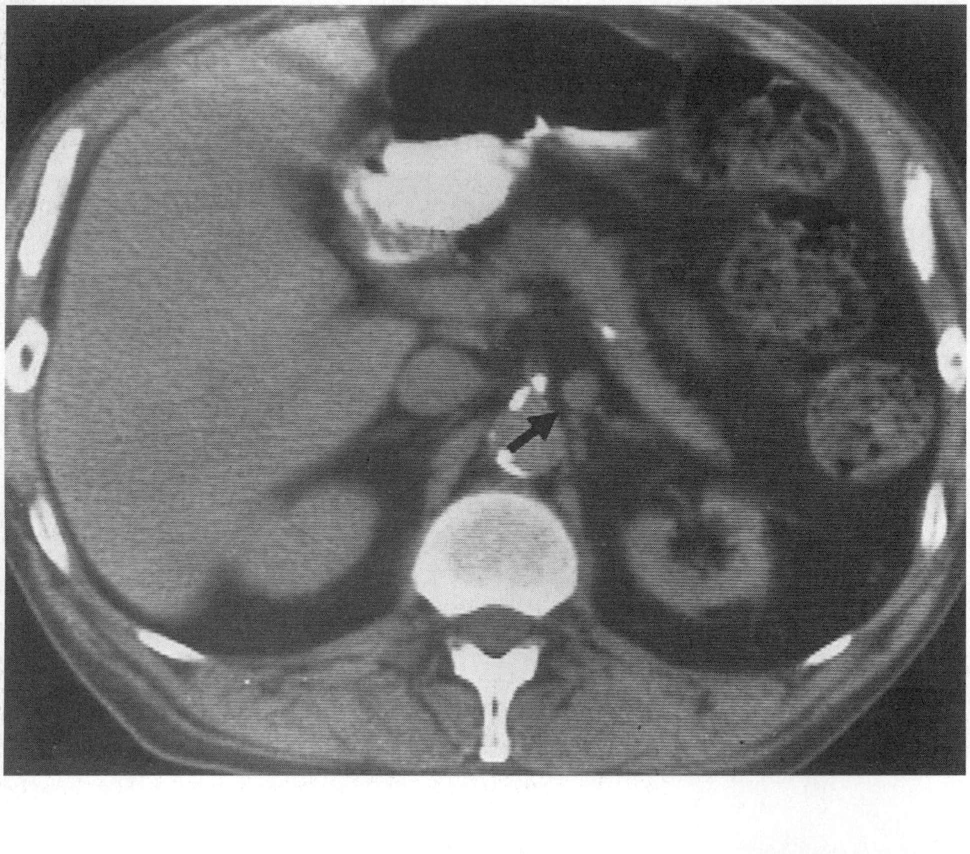

Figure 107.46. Adrenal tumor. A small, 1-cm adrenal pheochromocytoma *(arrow)* is noted in the anterior superior aspect of the left adrenal gland. It lies posterior to the pancreas and anterolateral to the aorta.

means of imaging the adrenal glands and has supplanted angiography as the method of choice in evaluating the patient with clinical signs and symptoms of adrenal tumors. CT has not, however, replaced the functional evaluation of the adrenal gland or adrenal venography and blood sampling for biochemical analysis. Masses as small as 1 cm can be detected in the adrenal gland (Fig. 107.46). The most difficult patient to assess with CT is one with suspected adrenal hyperplasia, in that the gland may appear on CT as normal in size and yet be hyperplastic. Although a mass may be identified with CT, differentiation of benign from malignant adrenal neoplasms is not always possible (Fig. 107.47). In patients with certain carcinomas having a propensity for adrenal metastasis, such as bronchogenic carcinoma, CT has proven helpful in detecting occult metastases.

Multiple imaging techniques have been used over the years in attempting to evaluate the extent of bladder neoplasms. Among these are pelvic angiography and lymphangiography, both of which are invasive and provide variable yield. The use of CT scanning in some patients with bladder carcinomas has proven helpful in staging their disease. CT is unable to differentiate the various stages of superficial lesions but can detect invasion of the tumor through the bladder wall into the perivesical fat, extension to pelvic lymph nodes or adjacent pelvic structures, or distant metastases (Fig. 107.48). Microscopic invasion into

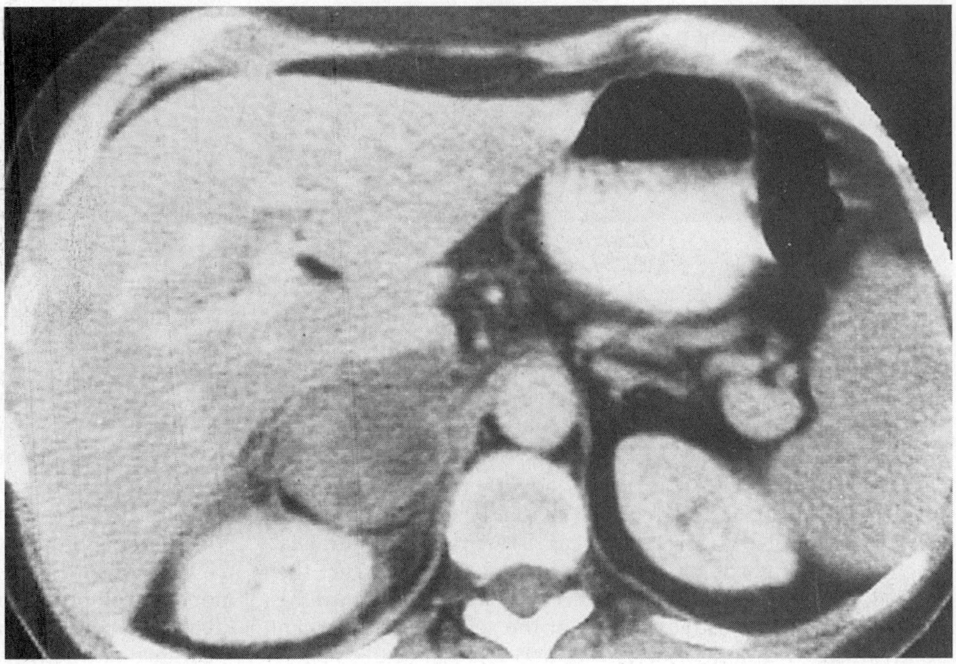

Figure 107.47. Adrenal tumor. A large, 6-cm adrenal carcinoma is seen in the right adrenal gland. Note the normal, inverted Y-shaped left adrenal gland.

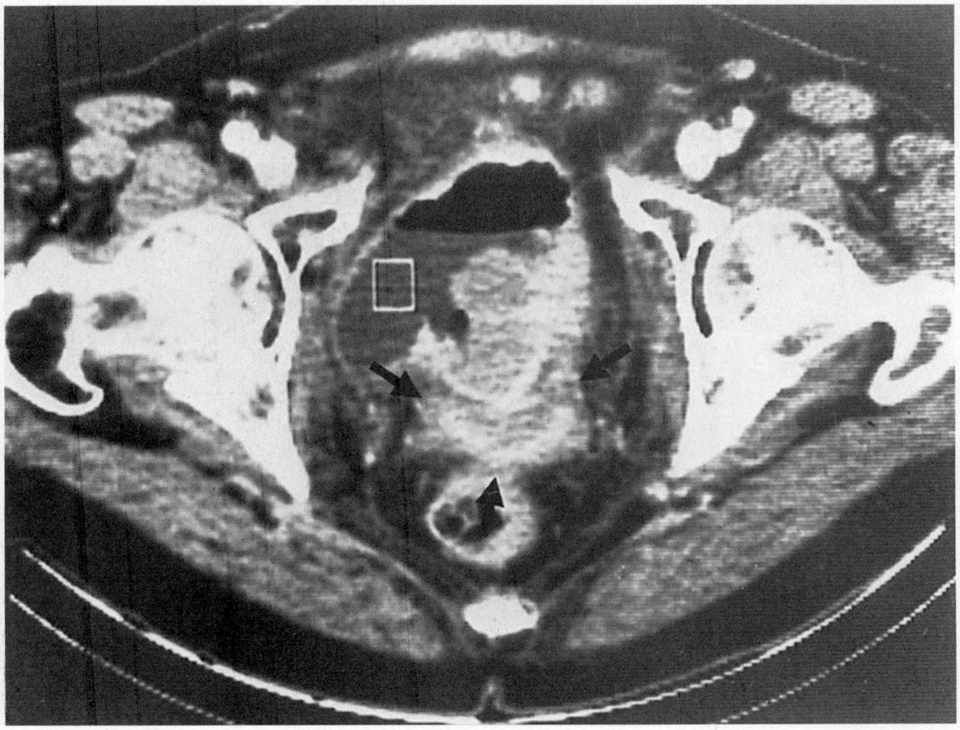

Figure 107.48. Transitional cell carcinoma of the bladder. A section through the lower aspect of the pelvis shows an air–fluid level within the bladder. Urine *(white box)* is seen adjacent to the large irregular transitional cell carcinoma. Projections of tumor into the lumen of the bladder are seen, as well as posterior extension *(arrows)* out of the bladder wall into the perivesical fat.

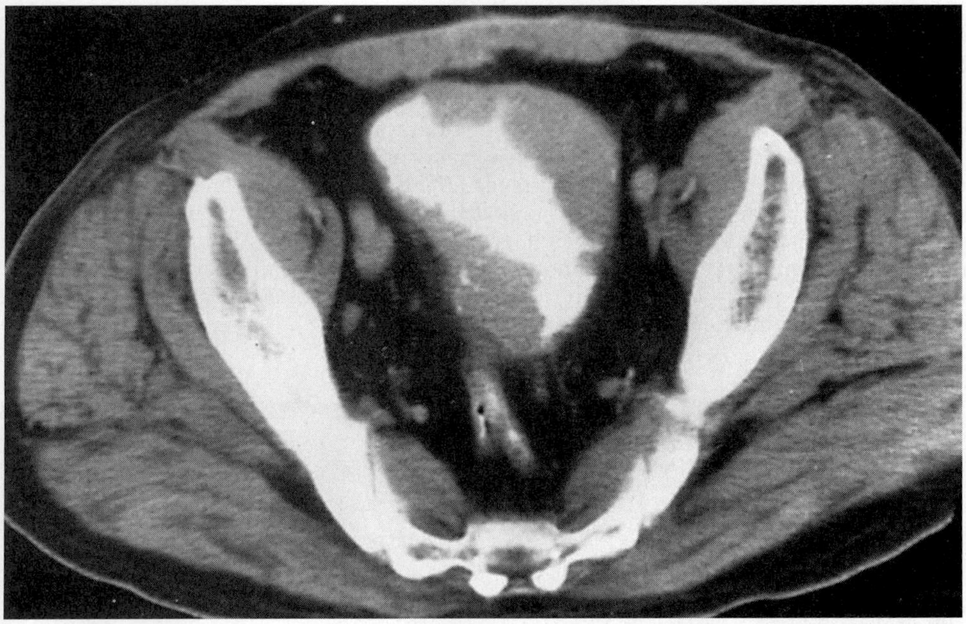

Figure 107.49. Transitional cell carcinoma of the bladder. A section through the mid-pelvis shows a large irregular mass involving both the right and left aspects of the bladder. Note the jagged contrast collection on the internal aspect of the bladder. Despite the size of the tumor, there is no obvious extension of tumor into the perivesical fat.

the perivesical fat or pelvic nodes cannot be detected and will lead to a false-negative evaluation. CT accuracy approaches 90% in differentiating superficial lesions from more invasive ones (Fig. 107.49).

In CT scans of the lower male pelvis, one is able to see in cross-section in the lower aspects of the bladder, seminal vesicles, and prostate (Fig. 107.50). Although benign prostatic hypertrophy and prostatic carcinoma cannot be distinguished by CT density alone, this procedure can be helpful in accurately staging carcinoma of the prostate. One is able to detect the extension of the tumor through the prostatic capsule into the adjacent soft tissues. Involvement of the seminal vesicles can be identified with loss of fat planes and fixation of their position (Fig. 107.51). Bladder wall involvement is better assessed cystoscopically. Metastases to pelvic nodes and extrapelvic sites can be determined with CT. The use of CT scanning for radiation therapy planning reduces the geographic misses of the treatment.

Although ultrasound is the imaging modality of choice in the initial evaluation of a suspected pelvic mass, CT scanning may add additional information in the assessment of a neoplasm of the cervix, uterus, and ovaries. One is able to establish the presence of a pelvic mass and characterize it with ultrasound, but evaluation of the extent of the lesion is often difficult. With CT, extension of the tumor into the pararectal and paravesical space can be detected. Obliteration of normal pelvic fat planes and extension to the lateral pelvic sidewalls can be determined (Fig. 107.52). Pelvic and retroperitoneal adenopathy can be identified. The site of origin may be difficult to determine with either CT or ultrasound. Even with the CT appearance and density characteristics of the mass, one cannot always distinguish benign from malignant neoplasms, such as benign uterine leiomyomas from uterine leiomyosarcomas. The diagnosis of pelvic masses is extremely important in the evaluation of female patients with unexplained progressive renal failure.

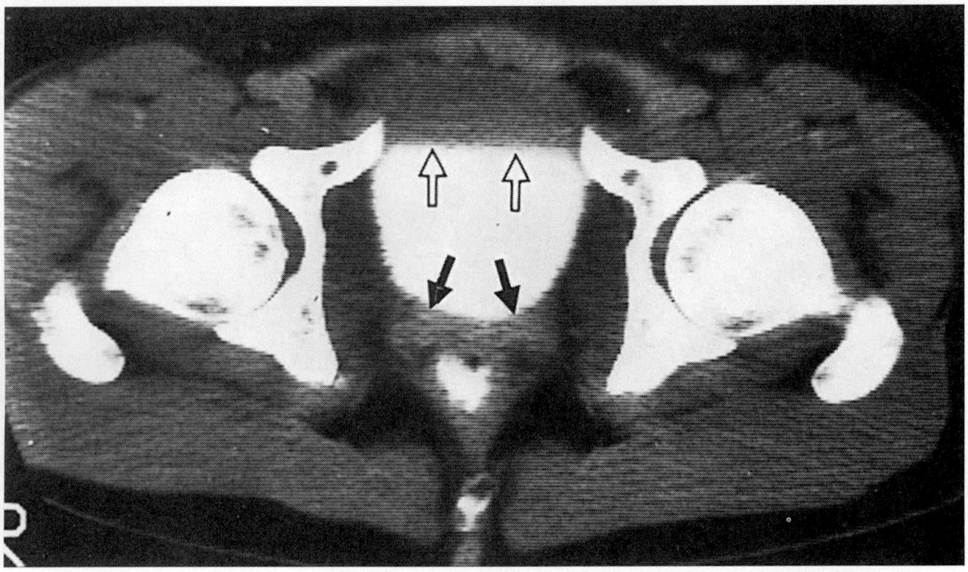

Figure 107.50. Normal low pelvis. A fluid contrast medium level *(open arrows)* is noted within the bladder. Posterior to the bladder, the seminal vesicles are noted *(solid arrows)*. More posteriorly, contrast material is seen in the rectum.

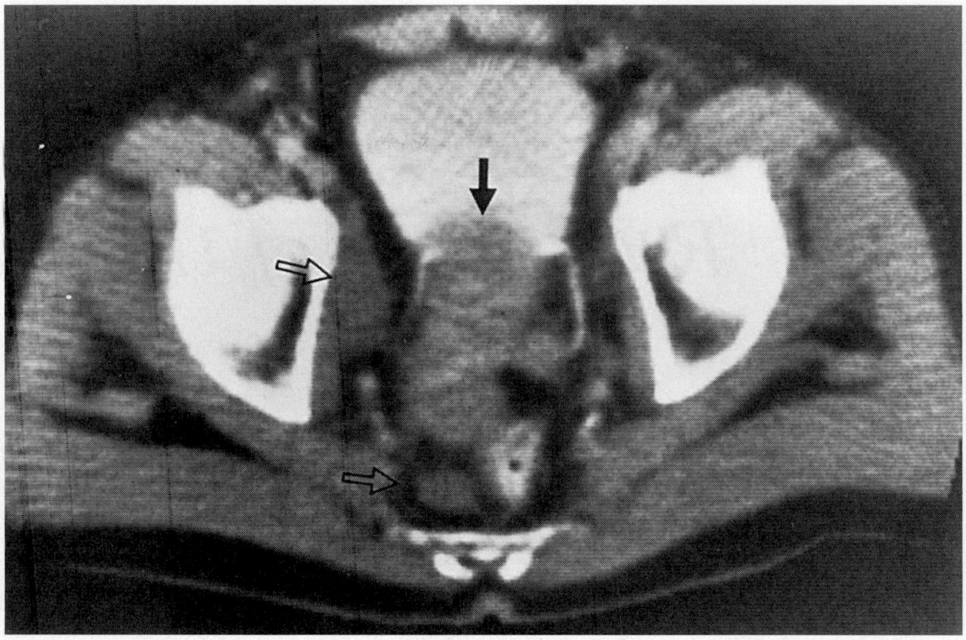

Figure 107.51. Prostatic carcinoma. A large lobulated carcinoma of the prostate is seen indenting the posterior margin of the bladder *(solid arrow)*, with posterior extension into the perirectal space. Nodal metastases adjacent to the rectum and in the right pelvic sidewall *(open arrows)* also are seen.

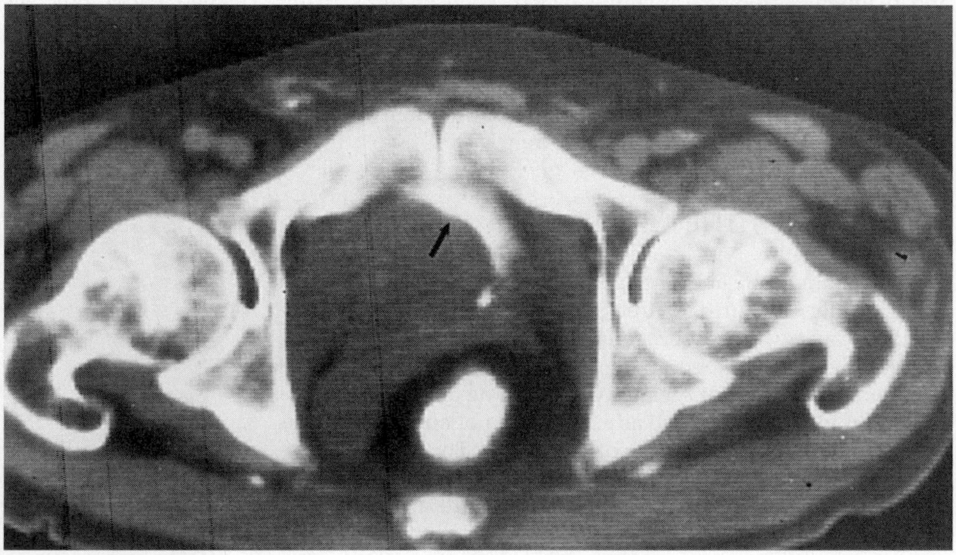

Figure 107.52. Pelvic mass. A large mass caused by squamous cell carcinoma of the cervix extends into the floor of the bladder *(arrow)*, into the right pelvic sidewall, and posteriorly into the pararectal space.

Selected Readings

Amis SE, Newhouse JH. *Essentials of uroradiology.* Boston: Little, Brown, 1991.
Straightforward general text on uroradiology.

Barbaric ZL. *Principles of genitourinary radiology,* 2nd ed. New York: Thieme Medical Publishers, 1994.
Well-organized, outline-based text with excellent drawings and illustrative images.

Dunnick NR, McCallum RW, Sandler CM. *Textbook of uroradiology,* 2nd ed. Baltimore: Williams & Wilkins, 1997.
General uroradiology text with integrated approach to the different imaging modalities—CT, ultrasound, conventional imaging, angiography, and nuclear medicine.

Fishman EK, Jeffrey RB. *Spiral CT—principles, techniques, and clinical applications.* New York: Raven Press, 1995:87–108.
CT text with explanation of spiral CT.

Kenney PJ, Lee JKT. The kidney. In: Lee JKT, Sagel SS, Stanley RJ, et al, eds. *Computed body tomography,* 3rd ed. Philadelphia: Lippincott-Raven, 1998:1087–1170.
Excellent general CT text.

Levine E. The kidney. In: Haaga JR, Lanzieri CF, Sartoris DJ, et al, eds. *Computed tomography and magnetic resonance imaging of the whole body,* 3rd ed. St Louis: Mosby, 1994:1176–1243.
General CT text.

Moss AA, Bush WH. The kidneys. In: Moss AA, Gamsu G, Genant HK, eds. *Computed tomography of the body with magnetic resonance imaging,* 5th ed. Philadelphia: WB Saunders, 1992:933–1020.
Up-to-date general text on CT with well-written chapter on the kidney.

CHAPTER 108

Radiology of the Kidney

William D. Boswell, Jr.

Many imaging modalities are available for the radiographic evaluation of the kidney. These range from the time-honored plain film of the abdomen and intravenous pyelogram to the newest means of ultrasonography, computed tomography (CT), and magnetic resonance imaging (MRI). Each of these many techniques has something to offer the physician in the evaluation of the patient's urinary tract, and they are usually complementary to one another. It is important, however, to understand the diagnostic yields and limitations of each modality so as to select the correct procedure for the patient.

PLAIN FILM OF THE ABDOMEN

The plain film of the abdomen is the first step in the evaluation of the kidney and urinary tract, as well as the rest of the abdominal cavity. This roentgenographic examination is also known as a *KUB,* or roentgenography of kidneys, ureters, and bladder. A plain film of the abdomen is done also as a preliminary examination before the administration of any intravenous contrast material or other type of procedure. This technique often affords the physician a means of evaluating the renal size by visualizing the kidneys. Because the kidneys are surrounded by fat in the perinephric space, they may be visualized on the plain x-ray film before any contrast material is given (Fig. 108.1). Also, the presence of calcifications in the kidney or collecting systems (nephrocalcinosis) (Fig. 108.2) or stones (Fig. 108.3) may be detected. Other types of renal parenchymal calcifications seen in such entities as tuberculosis or hypernephromas (Fig. 108.4) may point to the diagnosis. The plain film affords a view not only of the kidney areas but also of the rest of the abdomen and therefore may give either direct or indirect evidence of the reason for the patient's disease.

INTRAVENOUS UROGRAPHY

Intravenous urography or excretory urography or the intravenous pyelogram (IVP) is the most commonly used diagnostic radiographic procedure in evaluating the kidney and urinary tract. As the name implies, intravenous contrast material is injected into the patient, and the subsequent excretion of the contrast medium allows visualization of the urinary system. Many different contrast agents have been used over the years, all of which contained iodine. All contrast agents used in the radiologic evaluation of the kidneys and urinary tract are triiodinated benzoic acid compounds in solution. The contrast agents have been divided into groups: ionic and nonionic, or high-osmolar contrast media (HOCM) and low-osmolar contrast media (LOCM). The HOCM ionic agents have been used successfully for more than 30 years and continue to be used in the majority of cases in

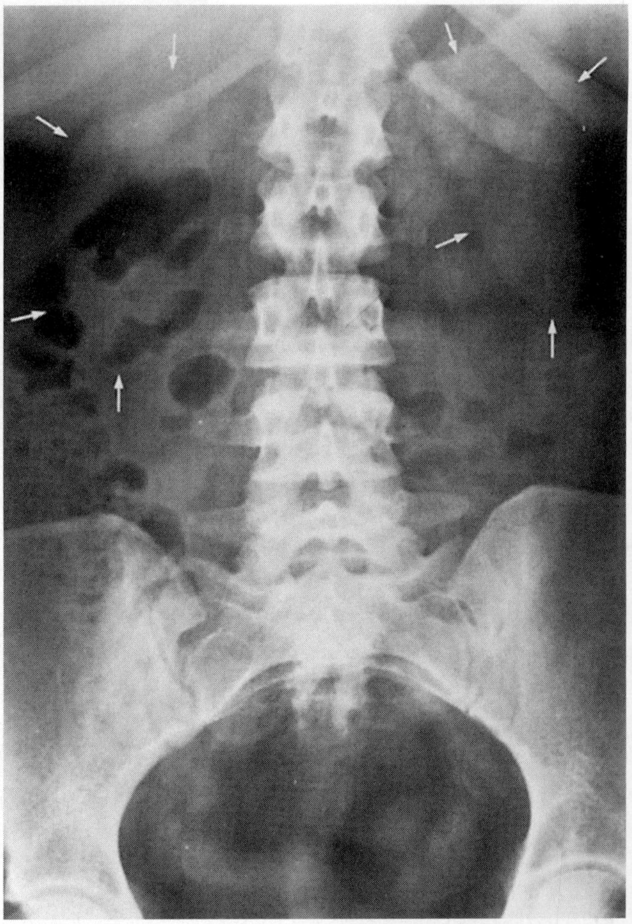

Figure 108.1. Normal plain film of the abdomen. The kidneys *(arrows)* in the upper abdomen are seen because of the presence of fat in the perinephric space. Normal amounts of gas are identified in the bowel. Normal bony structures of the lumbar spine and pelvis are noted.

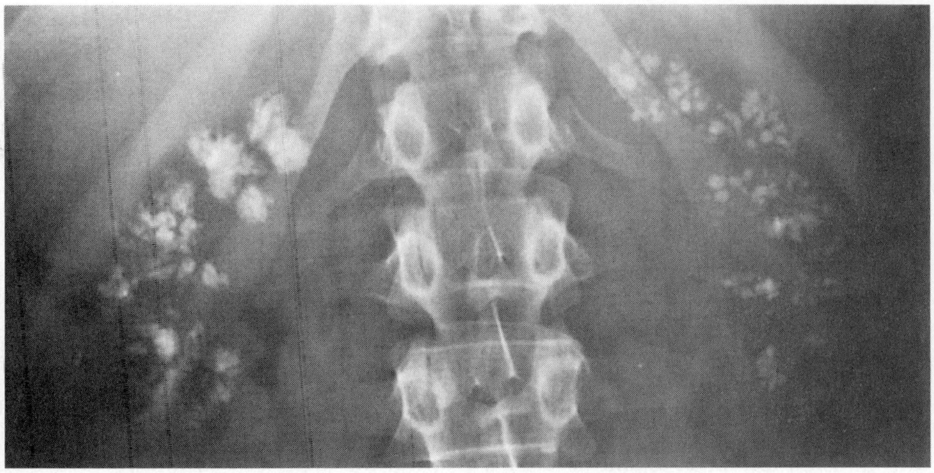

Figure 108.2. Nephrocalcinosis. Renal parenchymal calcifications are seen bilaterally in this case, resulting from renal tubular acidosis.

which iodinated contrast is required, that is, IVP and CT. The LOCM, both ionic and nonionic, have made significant inroads into conventional contrast usage since their introduction in the mid-1980s. In the area of angiography and cardiac catheterization, the LOCM are used almost exclusively. LOCM are being used increasingly for the more conventional studies as well (i.e., IVP and CT).

Most of the ionic contrast agents are HOCM. The differences among these various available ionic HOCM are slight, and these agents may be grouped into three basic categories: diatrizoates, iothalamates, and metrizoates. The compounds are water-soluble salt solutions and are hyperosmolar relative to plasma. The iodine-containing portion of the salt acts as the anion, with either sodium or meglumine as the cation. In the bloodstream, the salt is not bound to any plasma proteins to any significant extent and, as a result, passes freely through the glomerulus into the glomerular filtrate. For all practical purposes, 98% to 99% of the injected volume of the contrast material is excreted by glomerular filtration, and there is no tubular reabsorption. Thus it seems that the concentration of the contrast material within the plasma and the glomerular filtration rate (GFR) determine the amount of contrast material excreted into the collecting systems. In patients with a normal GFR, the concentration of iodine in the plasma determines the quality of the examination. Changes in tubular fluid reabsorption along the nephron affect the concentration of contrast agent within the tubular fluid and, hence, the quality of the study. Within the first 10 minutes after the injection of contrast material, approximately 12% has been cleared through the glomeruli. Within 24 hours, 94% to 100% of the contrast material has been excreted.

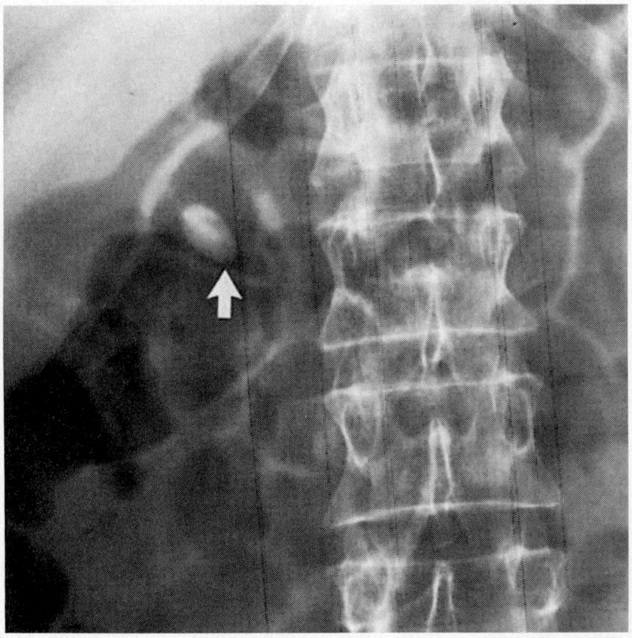

Figure 108.3. Nephrolithiasis. A single calculus *(arrow)* is seen overlying the area of the right renal pelvis. This is a right ureteropelvic junction stone.

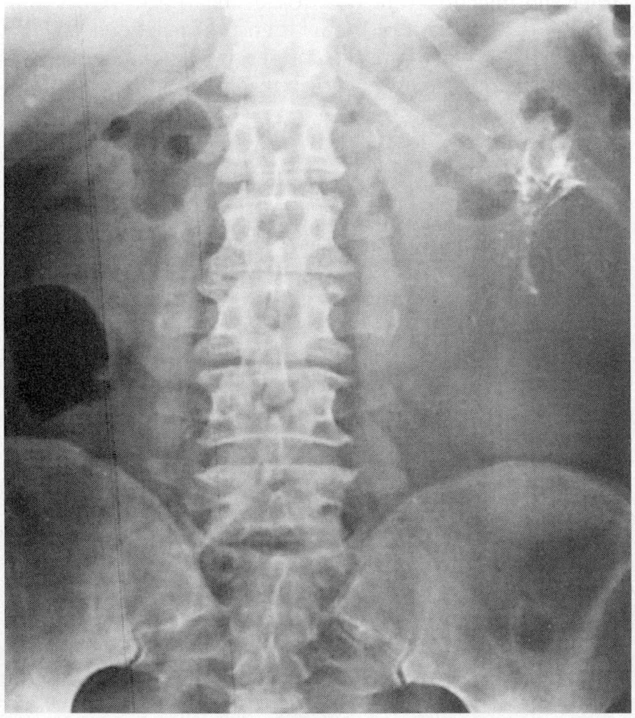

Figure 108.4. Calcification in a renal cell carcinoma. Irregular, curvilinear, and punctate calcifications are noted within a large mass on the left side of the abdomen. These calcifications are within a large hypernephroma.

The LOCM are generally nonionic compounds as well, except for ioxaglate, which is an ionic dimer. These compounds do not dissociate in solution as do the ionic contrast agents. Thus the osmolarity is reduced as well. The osmolarity of the HOCM is typically 5 to 8 times that of human plasma (300 mOsm/L). The LOCM have a higher osmolarity than human plasma but only by a factor of 2 to 3 times. These LOCM are handled in a manner similar to the HOCM by the glomerulus. As they pull less water into the tubular system, the overall concentration of iodine in the glomerular filtrate is higher, and thus, the quality of the IVP is usually slightly better.

About 25 to 40 g of iodine generally are used when performing IVPs. Using the nomenclature of the past, this would be called a *double-dose examination.* The bolus injection technique yields the highest initial plasma concentration of the contrast material and is the preferred method of contrast delivery. The drip infusion technique is still used by a few, but the highest concentrations of iodine are not obtained by this method.

Untoward responses, or reactions, can occur after the intravenous injection of any type of contrast material—LOCM, HOCM, ionic, or nonionic. Although the large majority of these reactions are minor, severe reactions and deaths from the intravenous urography do occur. In the general population, the risk for reaction from ionic HOCM is generally agreed to be approximately 5% to 6%. In patients with a history of allergies, the reaction rate approaches 10%. In patients with histories of previous reactions to contrast material, the incidence of subsequent reactions is 15% to 20%. Mild types of reactions to contrast material, such as flushing, nausea, and near-fainting, are by far the most common. These types of reactions require no treatment. Mild dermal reactions, such as urticaria, do occur and may or may not require treatment. Severe types of reactions, such as bronchospasm, laryngeal edema, seizures, arrhythmias, syncope, shock, or cardiac arrest, also can occur and obviously require treatment. These types of reactions are much less common, occurring in fewer than 1% of patients. Pretesting the patient before the examination yields little useful information. Neither the injection rate nor dosage has been clearly implicated as a determinant of the incidence of reactions. Although premedication, such as antihistamines, is administered by some physicians before the study, no controlled data are available to substantiate the advantage of use. Premedication with glucocorticoids of patients who had reactions in the past is advocated and used by many radiologists, but again no controlled studies are available to critically evaluate this treatment.

The LOCM offer a significantly lower reaction rate than the HOCM. This is true of both mild and severe reactions. It is actually safer to be an individual with an allergic history or a history of prior reaction and receive LOCM for a study than to be an individual in the general population with no allergic history and receive HOCM. The widespread use of these LOCM nonionic agents has been limited mainly by their price, which tends to be 10 to 14 times greater than that of the conventional ionic HOCM of equal iodine content.

Certain patients are at risk of developing acute renal failure (ARF) after administration of intravenous contrast material. This is discussed in detail in Chapter 47, Part 7. After the original introduction of the LOCM, it was believed that there was a lower incidence of ARF. This observation has not been substantiated, and thus it appears that LOCM and HOCM have a similar incidence of ARF in the general population and in the at-risk groups. In patients with cardiovascular disease, the sodium load from the contrast material should be recognized. This may precipitate an acute episode of congestive heart failure. The injection of contrast material into these patients may also predispose them to arrhythmias and episodes of hypotension. Patients with combined hepatic and renal failure have an increased chance of worsening of either or both because of the inability of the liver or kidney to handle the injected contrast material.

The intravenous urogram is best tailored for each individual patient. There is no universal standard as to the total numbers of films necessary. There is agreement, however, on the areas that should be examined during intravenous urography. Immediately after the injection of the contrast material, the iodine concentration within the vascular system is at its peak level. The filtered load of contrast material is thus at its highest as well. The density of the nephrogram is caused by the contrast material in the tubular system within the kidney: the greater the iodine concentration, the denser the nephrogram. During the nephrographic phase, the size and configuration of the kidney can be evaluated (Fig. 108.5). The contours of the kidney are usually well delineated, and the presence of scarring or other

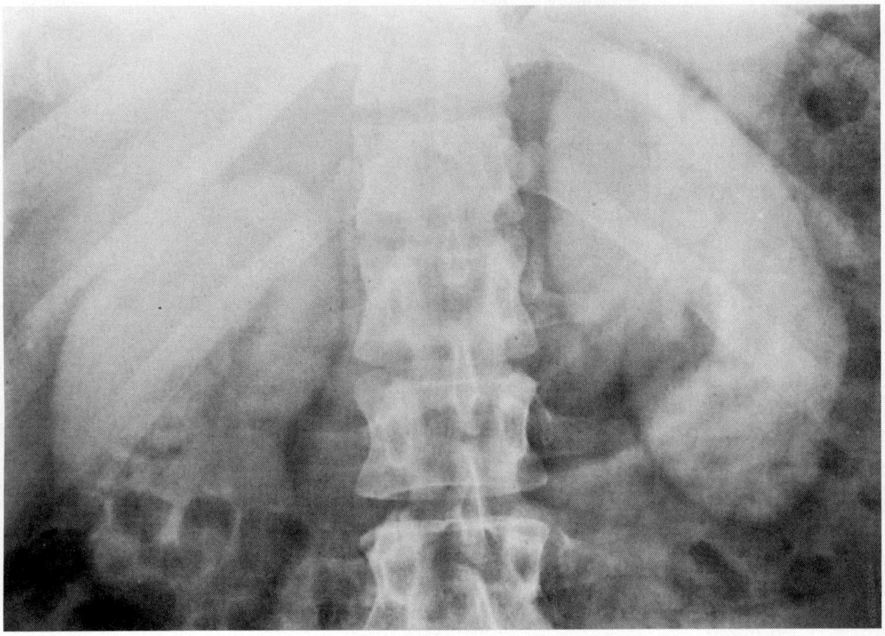

Figure 108.5. Nephrographic phase of intravenous urogram. This film obtained immediately after injection of intravenous contrast material demonstrates bilateral nephrograms. The radiodense kidneys are well seen, with smooth borders and equal size.

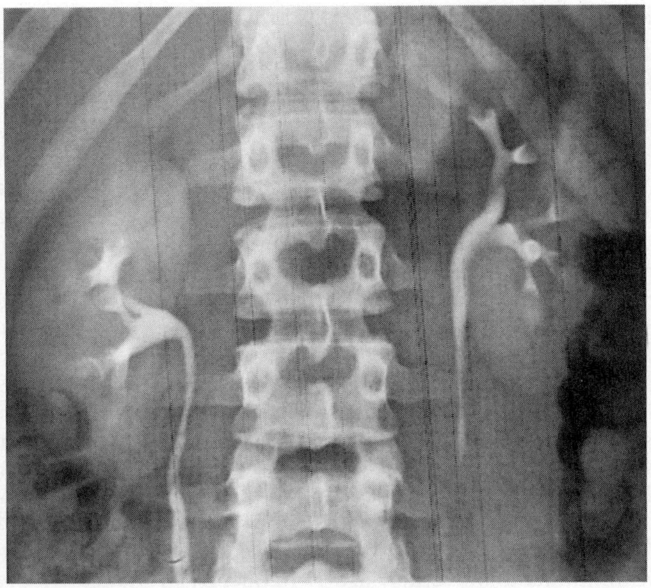

Figure 108.6. Normal intravenous pyelogram. This film obtained 5 minutes after the injection of intravenous contrast material shows excellent delineation of the calyceal elements, renal pelvis, and proximal ureters. The renal outlines are still well seen.

contour abnormalities can be detected. As the contrast material exits the tubular system into the calyces, the excretory phase of the urogram can be completed. The calyceal system is outlined in 3 to 5 minutes after the injection of contrast material but is best seen between 5 and 10 minutes (Fig. 108.6). The sharp contours of the calyces are well defined, as are the infundibula and pelvis of the kidney. The ureters are visualized after 5 minutes, many times in their entirety, especially when the double-dose examinations are performed (Fig. 108.7). The bladder is finally examined at the conclusion of the study.

Tomography is done in most studies. Tomograms give an excellent representation of the contour of the kidneys and thus help in the diagnosis of various parenchymal processes (Fig. 108.8). In addition, the architecture of the calyceal system is usually well displayed and again leads to better diagnostic accuracy. It should be emphasized that the intravenous urogram provides an anatomic study of the kidney and is not a good measure of kidney function.

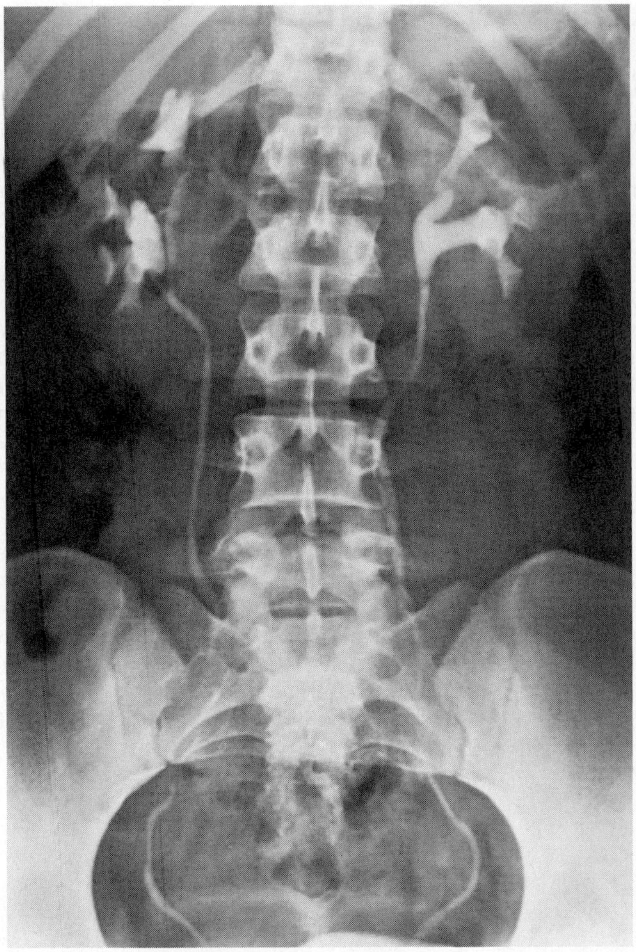

Figure 108.7. Normal intravenous pyelogram. This film was obtained 10 minutes after the injection of intravenous contrast material. The pelvocalyceal systems are well visualized, as is the entire course of the ureters bilaterally.

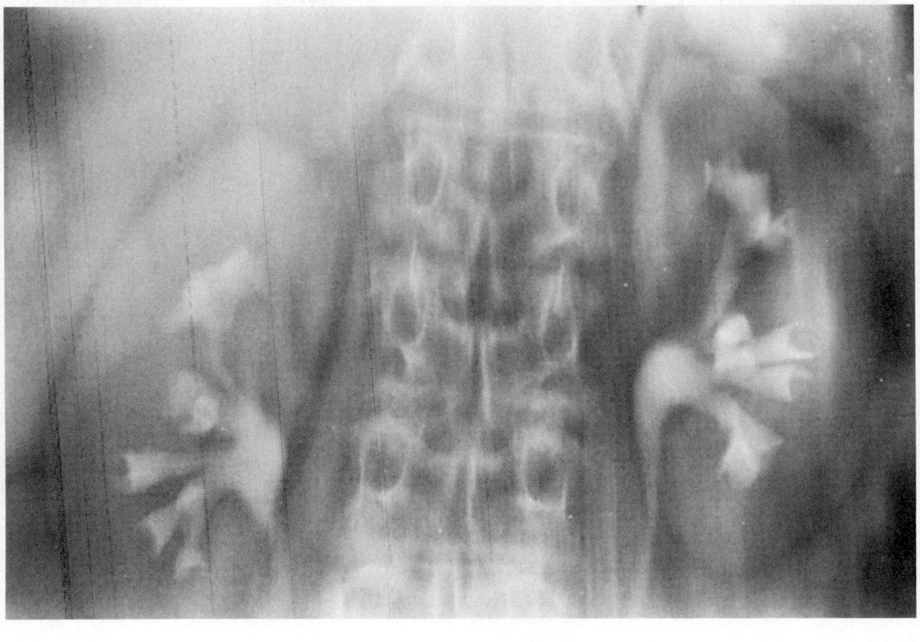

Figure 108.8. Normal intravenous pyelogram-tomogram. This tomographic film was obtained 5 to 10 minutes after the injection of intravenous contrast material. Note the excellent delineation of the renal contours, as well as the collecting systems.

RETROGRADE AND ANTEGRADE PYELOGRAMS

Retrograde Pyelogram (Fig. 108.9)

With the advent of increased dose urography and accompanying tomography, the need for retrograde pyelograms has decreased. Retrograde pyelograms involve the injection of contrast material in a retrograde manner through the distal ureter to visualize the calyceal system and renal pelvis. The study is used in patients with suspected urothelial tumors and stones when the excretory urogram is nondiagnostic. It is also used in evaluating patients with obstructing lesions for which the etiology is uncertain. The retrograde pyelogram is still used in cases of acute or oliguric renal failure in which a postrenal lesion may be suspected. The use of ultrasound evaluation in these patients has decreased the need for retrograde pyelography.

Antegrade Pyelogram

The use of the antegrade pyelogram has increased as a diagnostic and therapeutic tool. Antegrade pyelography involves the placement of a small-gauge needle into the renal pelvis, with subsequent withdrawal of urine and injection of contrast material to visualize the calyceal system, renal pelvis, and ureters. In cases of obstruction in which transient or permanent drainage is needed, percutaneous nephrostomy tubes may be inserted with little risk to the patient.

RENAL ANGIOGRAPHY AND VENOGRAPHY

Renal Angiography

Renal angiography is usually performed through a percutaneous transfemoral approach. Renal angiography provides the ultimate means of visualizing the detailed anatomy of the renal vessels and vascular architecture of the kidney. In the arterial phase of the arteriogram, the arborization of the vascular supply to the kidney is well demonstrated, with segmental, interlobar, arcuate, and interlobular branches seen (Fig. 108.10). With magnification angiography, glomerular branches occasionally can be identified. The capillary phase of the study is seen 6 to 8 seconds after the injection of contrast material (Fig. 108.11). There is usually excellent visualization of the contours of the kidney. During the study, 12 to 20 seconds after the injection, the larger renal venous branches can be visualized (Fig. 108.12). The applications for renal angiography lie in the investigation of renal vascular disease. Renal masses and renal parenchymal diseases are commonly evaluated with angiography. A patient with trauma to the kidney is also frequently evaluated with renal angiography. Both renal donors and renal transplant recipients may need to undergo angiography.

Digital subtraction angiography (DSA) uses the computerized processing of data obtained not from an x-ray film but from electronic x-ray receptors. Because of the high-contrast resolution of the x-ray receptor, the image intensifier, and the higher speed postprocessing by the computer, DSA has gained a foothold in all types of angiographic applications. Lower volumes and more dilute contrast material can be used with DSA, thus

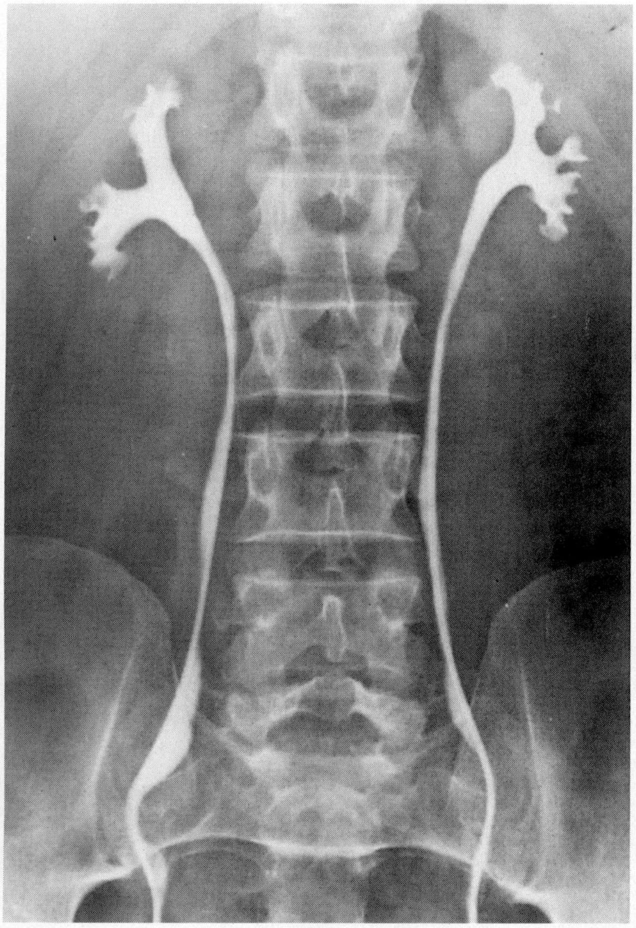

Figure 108.9. Normal retrograde pyelogram. Retrograde injection of contrast material demonstrates only the collecting systems, renal pelvis, and ureters. Note that no contrast material is within the renal parenchyma.

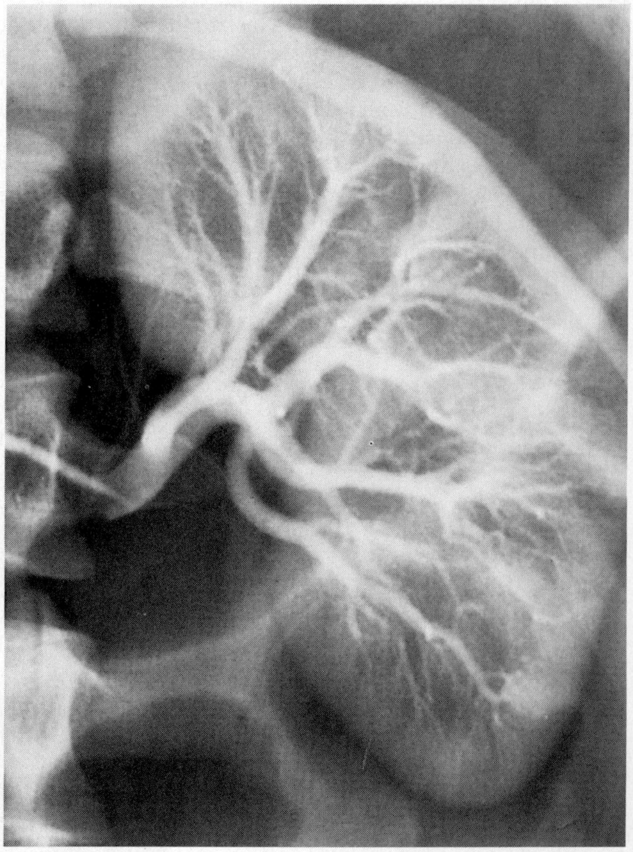

Figure 108.10. Normal selective renal angiogram: arterial phase. Note the normal arborization of the renal arterial system. Regular branching down to the arcuate level is visualized on this arteriogram.

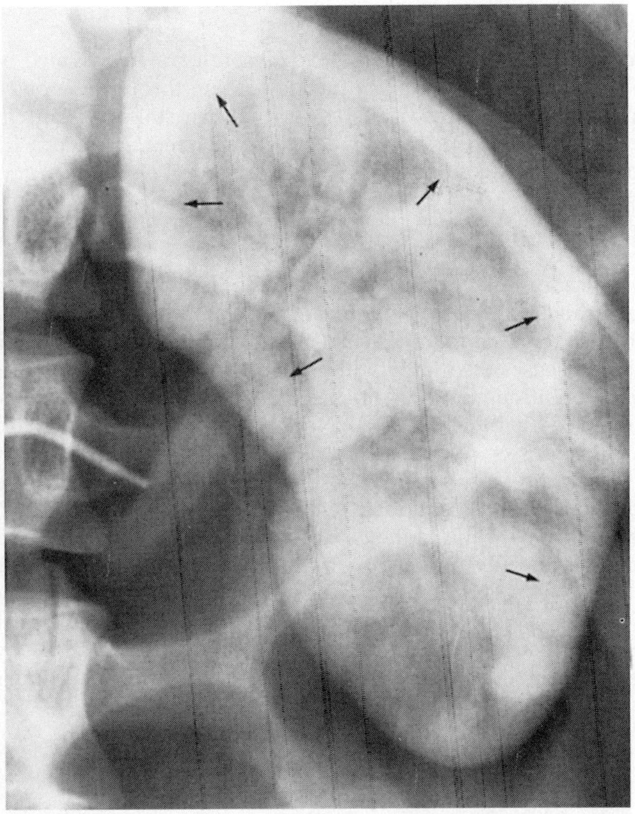

Figure 108.11. Normal selective renal arteriogram: capillary phase. Excellent delineation of the contour of the kidney is noted in this capillary phase of an arteriogram. The main renal vein is just beginning to fill. The corticomedullary junction *(arrows)* is well seen, especially in the upper pole.

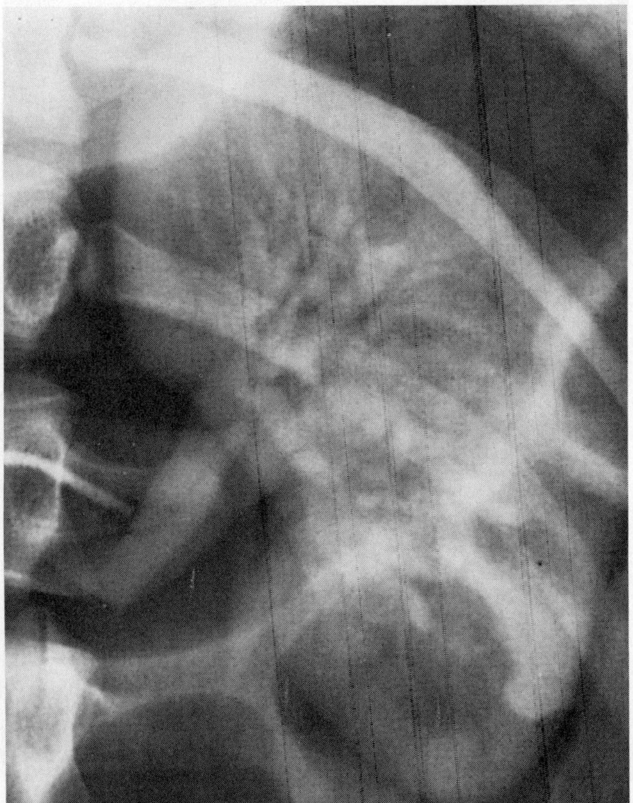

Figure 108.12. Normal selective renal arteriogram: venous phase. Intraparenchymal renal veins are seen draining into the main renal vein. The dense capillary phase has been passed.

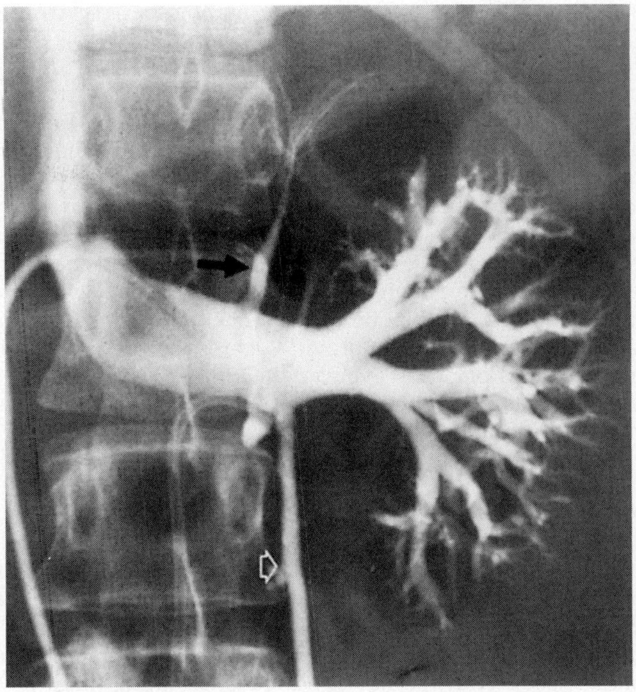

Figure 108.13. Normal renal venogram. Contrast material injected in a retrograde manner into the left renal vein demonstrates several orders of branching of the intrarenal veins. The left adrenal vein *(closed arrow)* and left gonadal vein *(open arrow)* are also seen.

leading to safer angiographic procedures. This is especially true in renal angiography, in which high concentrations of contrast material typically are injected directly into the renal artery.

The primary side effects are the same as those detailed earlier with the use of contrast media. With conventional renal angiography, the kidneys are subjected to a high concentration of contrast material for a very short period. Transitory subclinical renal failure is common. Vacuolization of cells, usually in the tubular system, secondary to the hyperosmolar contrast material is common. The use of nonionic contrast agents and DSA will make renal angiography a safer procedure.

Renal Venography (Fig. 108.13)

Renal venography is also a commonly performed procedure. The use of epinephrine-enhanced renal venogram gives excellent delineation to the intrarenal venous system. The free anastomosis of veins throughout the kidney leads to excellent visualization. The chief use of renal venography is still in the area of renal vein obstruction caused by thrombosis. However, more advances have been made in using renal venography for evaluating inflammatory versus neoplastic lesions.

RADIONUCLIDE EXAMINATIONS

The field of nuclear medicine has advanced a great deal with the application of computers and more selective radionuclides to the armamentarium of the clinician. Radionuclide examinations provide a means of assessing the function of the kidneys. With selected agents, one is able to assess the renal blood flow and glomerular or tubular function and also look for renal parenchymal abnormalities. The radionuclide examinations are better than conventional radiography in showing physiologic changes but are not as good as conventional radiographic procedures in showing anatomic changes. The various techniques and their clinical uses are discussed in Chapter 104.

ULTRASOUND

The use of ultrasonography in the evaluation of renal and urinary tract disorders is discussed in Chapter 106. It should be noted that this is a noninvasive means of evaluating the patient. No ionizing radiation is used. Ultrasound examination of the kidneys is generally considered a complementary diagnostic procedure in many cases in which the urinary tract is being investigated. It is the examination of choice in patients with renal failure who need evaluation for hydronephrosis and/or renal size. The ultrasound study provides a cross-sectional image in any number of planes to evaluate the kidney. It gives accurate measurements in evaluating the size of the kidney because no image magnification occurs.

COMPUTED TOMOGRAPHY

CT is the new dimension in radiology. CT scanning depicts the body in an axial plane or slice through the body. X-ray attenuation coefficients are related to CT numbers, generally with a range of −1,000 to +1,000 (air is equal to −1,000; water 0; and bone +1,000). With the newer scanners, scanning times have been reduced to less than 5 seconds with slice thickness as small as 1 mm. CT displays to the observer small differences in soft tissue that are not normally separable on a KUB or even at times with an IVP. Generally, when examining the kidneys, one is able to see their size and contour, calyceal elements, perinephric space, renal veins, and occasionally, the renal arteries. The aorta and inferior vena cava are well delineated, as are the other periaortic structures. The adrenals are well seen. CT usually is used as a complementary, not alternative, procedure to ultrasound. It is excellent in evaluation of retroperitoneal masses and the specific anatomic relation of the kidneys to surrounding structures. These CT diagnoses of the various renal lesions and urinary tract diseases are discussed in Chapter 103.

MAGNETIC RESONANCE IMAGING

The decade of the 1970s brought us CT, and the 1980s brought us a new diagnostic modality, MRI or nuclear magnetic resonance (NMR). MRI has the distinct feature of offering excellent anatomic detail and tissue contrast while having no known biologic hazard. Besides providing unique images and new data on tissue characteristics, MRI has the potential of assessing biochemical information in the form of spectroscopy. MRI is discussed in detail in Chapter 105.

RADIOGRAPHIC MANIFESTATIONS OF RENAL DISEASES

Many of the renal diseases are associated with a variety of radiographic manifestations. Radiology of the kidney and the urinary tract is very useful in the diagnosis of a multitude of renal disease processes. The pertinent radiographic findings of the various diseases are presented in the order in which they are discussed in this book.

Diabetes Insipidus

Lack or absence of antidiuretic hormone leads to the excretion of large volumes of hypotonic urine. As a result of the inability to adequately concentrate the urine, IVP is often of poor quality in these patients despite normal levels of serum urea nitrogen and creatinine. There is usually faint visualization of the collecting systems of the kidneys, which are passively dilated because of the large volumes of urine passing through the pelvocalyceal systems and ureters. Normal peristalsis within the ureters is lost. The urinary bladder often is overdistended, without evidence of an outlet obstruction.

Nephrocalcinosis

Calcification may occur either in the renal parenchyma or pelvocalyceal system. Nephrocalcinosis is radiographically detectable renal or parenchymal calcifications, which occur in many diseases associated with hypercalcemia or hypercalciuria or in conditions with specific lesions in the renal cortex or medulla (see Chapter 17, Part 3). Nephrolithiasis is the presence of calcifications or calculi within the pelvocalyceal system. Some disease processes my cause both nephrocalcinosis and nephrolithiasis. Hypercalcemic states tend to cause more diffuse calcifications within the kidneys. The calcifications of nephrocalcinosis are usually punctuate or stippled in character and occur bilaterally.

Specific cortical-type calcifications of nephrocalcinosis are seen in acute cortical necrosis (Fig. 108.14 and 108.15), hyperoxaluria, Alport's syndrome, and rarely, chronic glomer-

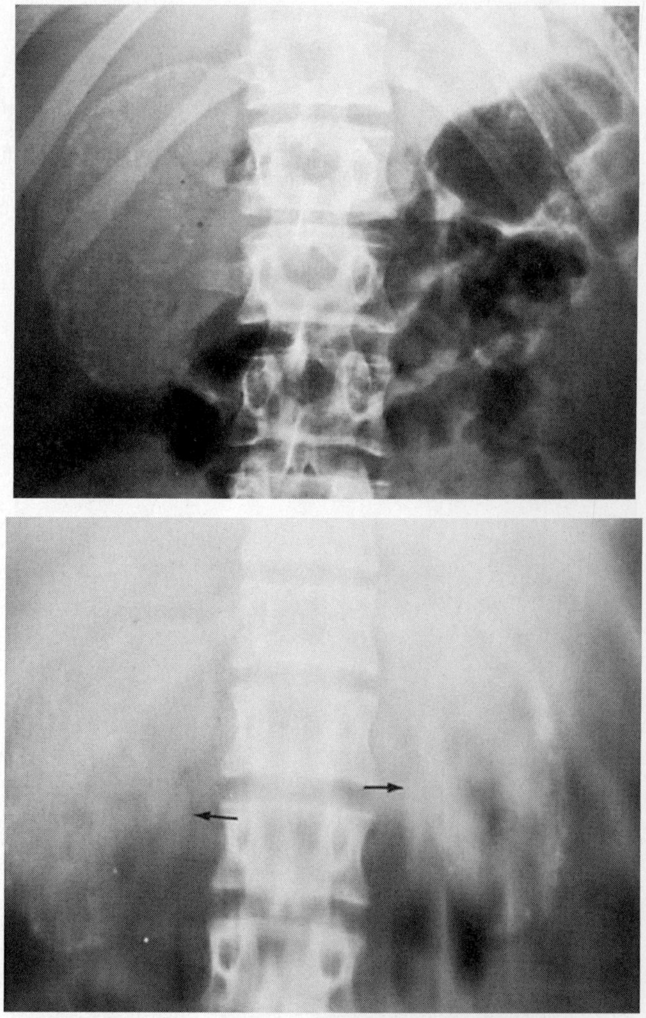

Figure 108.14. Nephrocalcinosis. A plain film of the abdomen **(top)** and a tomogram performed during an intravenous pyelogram **(bottom)** demonstrate cortical calcifications. This dystrophic calcification is relatively thin and only within the cortex. These calcifications occurred after an acute episode of cortical necrosis. Note on the nephrotomogram **(bottom)** the residual function of the kidney as evidenced by contrast material *(arrows)* in the renal pelvis bilaterally.

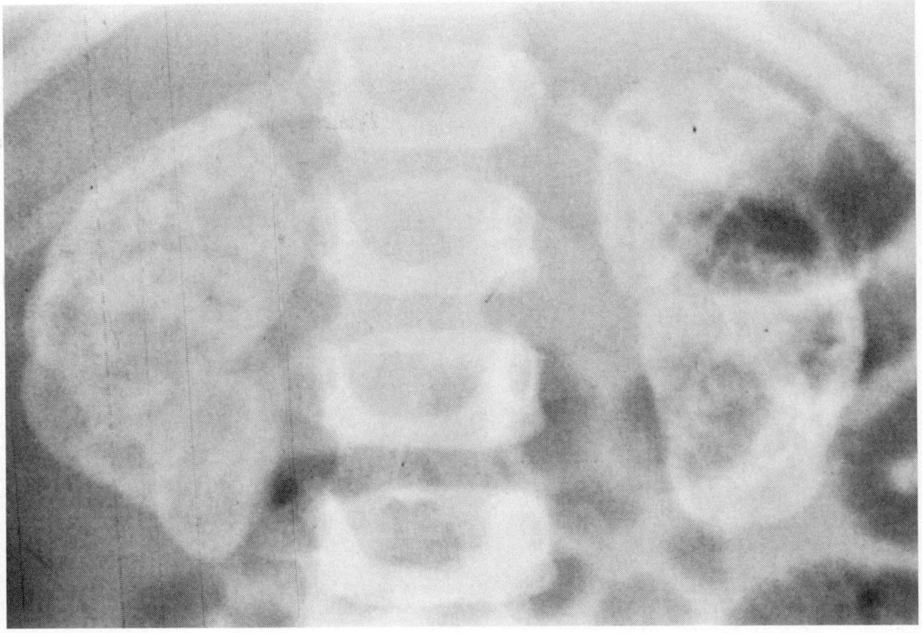

Figure 108.15. Nephrocalcinosis. Dense, cortical calcifications are seen bilaterally in this child with a history of acute cortical necrosis. The cortical calcifications are thick and circumferential.

ulonephritis. Calcification may develop in the damaged cortex after the acute episode of cortical necrosis. This dystrophic calcification is characteristically thin and tramlike in nature. In hyperoxaluria, calcium oxalate crystals are deposited within the kidney and other areas of the body, such as the heart. The diffuse stippled calcifications may occur in either the cortex or medulla or diffusely throughout the kidney. In Alport's syndrome, calcification is seen only in the cortex. Chronic glomerulonephritis is a rare cause of cortical calcifications.

Medullary calcifications are much more common than cortical calcifications. Primary hyperparathyroidism is the most common cause of the medullary form of nephrocalcinosis (Fig. 108.16). In primary hyperparathyroidism, initial intratubular deposition of calcium phosphate salts is followed by later deposition of calcium into the interstitial renal parenchyma. A papillary distribution of the calcifications frequently occurs. Small or large segments of the renal parenchyma may be involved, either unilaterally or bilaterally. Nephrolithiasis may coexist with nephrocalcinosis in patients with primary hyperparathyroidism. Other disease processes in which hypercalcemia or hypercalciuria occurs also may lead to nephrocalcinosis. These entities include hyperthyroidism, sarcoidosis, hypervitaminosis D, milk-alkali syndrome, Cushing's syndrome, idiopathic infantile hypercalcemia, immobilization, multiple myeloma, and metastatic neoplasms. The calcifications are nonspecific and punctuate and generally located in the medullary portion of the kidneys.

Distal renal tubular acidosis has evidence of nephrocalcinosis in 70% to 75% of cases. The calcifications usually are relatively uniform and distributed throughout the renal papillary areas bilaterally (Fig. 108.17).

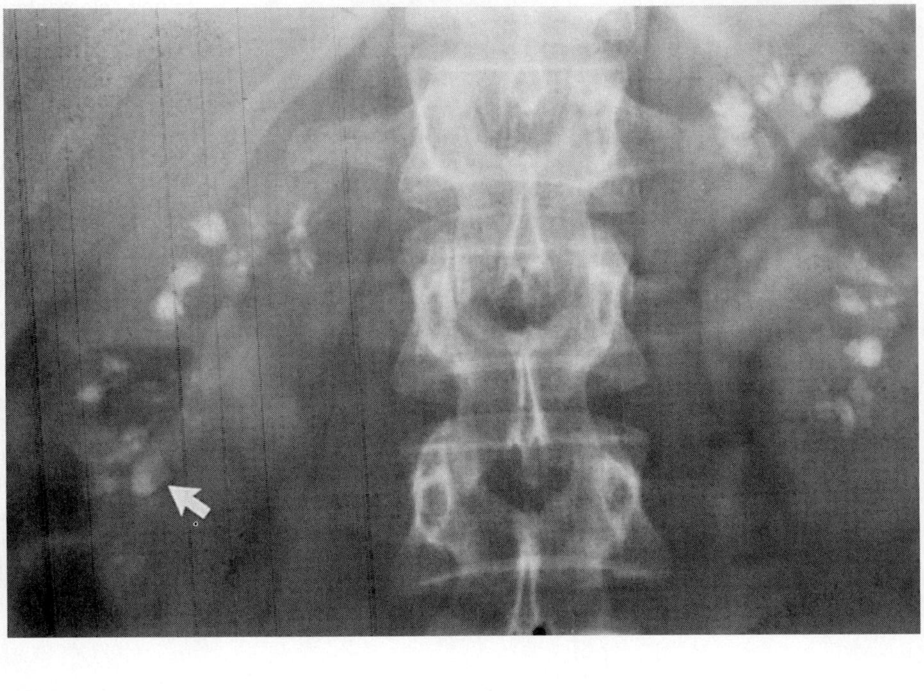

Figure 108.16. Nephrocalcinosis caused by hyperparathyroidism. Punctate, stippled calcifications are identified in the tips of the renal pyramids bilaterally. Faint opacification of the collecting systems is also identified on this intravenous pyelogram. A single renal calculus *(arrow)* is noted in the lower pole of the right kidney.

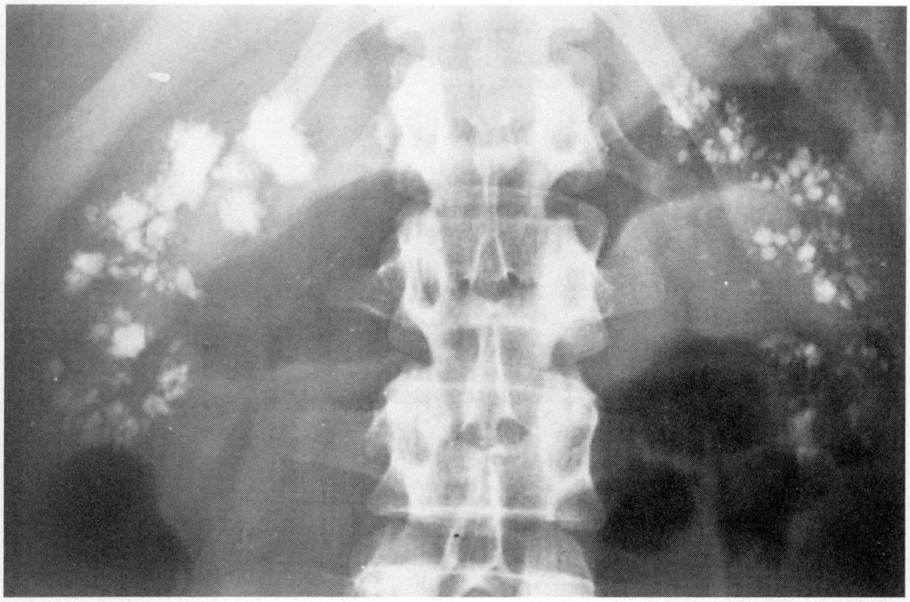

Figure 108.17. Nephrocalcinosis caused by renal tubular acidosis. Dense, bilateral calcifications are noted in the medullary portions of the kidneys.

Medullary sponge kidney (Fig. 108.18), or renal tubular ectasia, may involve only a single calyx or both kidneys completely. It is bilateral in up to 75% of cases. Small calculi form in the ectatic distal collecting tubules because of stasis. The calculi contain calcium phosphate and calcium oxalate salts. The condition is usually benign. However, the small calculi may pass into the pelvocalyceal system, resulting in the signs and symptoms of renal colic and its associated complications.

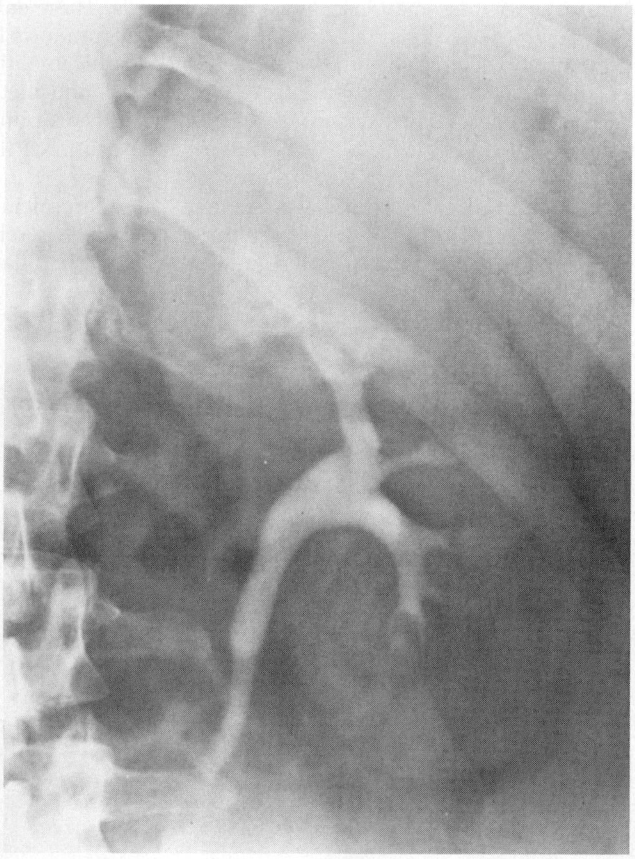

Figure 108.18. Nephrocalcinosis in medullary sponge kidney. Small calculi are present in the ectatic collecting tubules in the upper pole of this left kidney. The middle and lower pole calyces are incompletely involved with medullary sponge kidney. No calculi are identified in these calyceal elements.

Renal tuberculosis may also lead to calcifications in the medullary portion of the kidney that are indistinguishable from other forms of nephrocalcinosis (Fig. 108.19). Infection from renal tuberculosis begins in the cortex and progresses to involve the medullary area. Invasion and erosion into the collecting system subsequently result in further spread of the tuberculous infection down the ureter into the bladder. Calcification occurs in the areas of involvement and subsequently healing of renal tuberculosis. When the entire kidney is destroyed by the tuberculous process (autonephrectomy), calcification often occurs throughout the entire scarred and destroyed kidney.

Renal papillary necrosis from any cause may lead to medullary-type calcifications (Fig. 108.20). With the necrosis of the papilla and subsequent sloughing of this renal tissue into the calyx, fragments of renal tissue may be retained within the calyx and not passed down the collecting system. These retained elements may subsequently calcify and appear as medullary-type calcifications.

Glomerulonephritis

The different clinical and pathologic forms of glomerulonephritis are indistinguishable radiographically. However, the acute and chronic stages of glomerulonephritis do have separate radiographic findings. The findings on intravenous urography depend on the degree of renal impairment and the duration of the disease. The IVP may be normal in the patient with normal renal function and glomerulonephritis.

With acute glomerulonephritis, the kidneys are usually normal in size to slightly enlarged, and the calyces are normal but may be only faintly visualized if renal function is impaired (Fig. 108.21). With chronic glomerulonephritis, the renal size is smaller than normal with smooth contours, and normal faint calyces may be seen if the renal impairment is not too severe (Fig. 108.22). Ultrasonographic evaluation of the patient with glomerulonephritis usually reveals increased echoes in the parenchyma and variable size depending on the stage of the disease process.

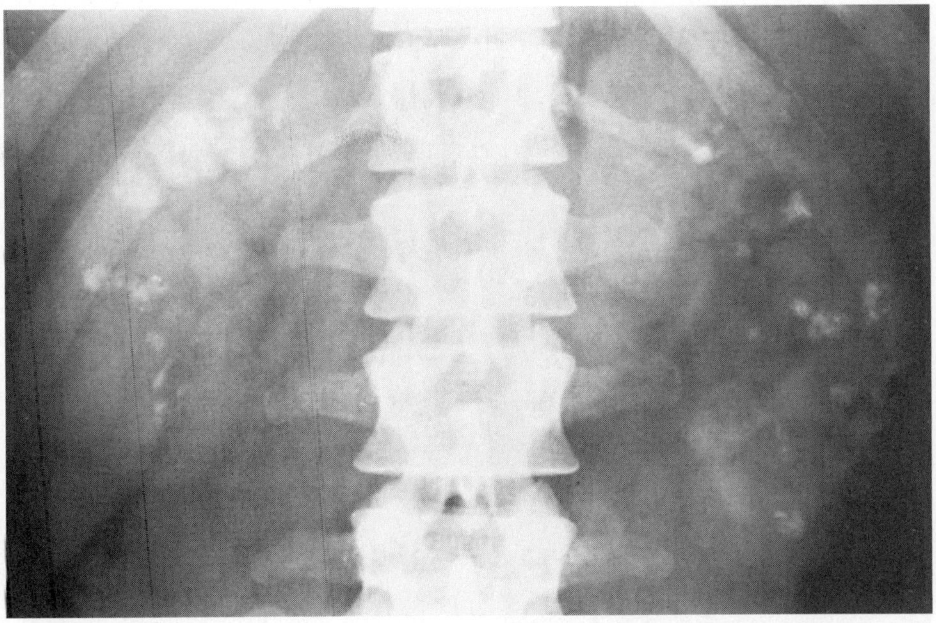

Figure 108.19. Nephrocalcinosis caused by renal tuberculosis. Conglomerate masses of calcification and more punctate calcifications are seen bilaterally in this case of relatively advanced renal tuberculosis.

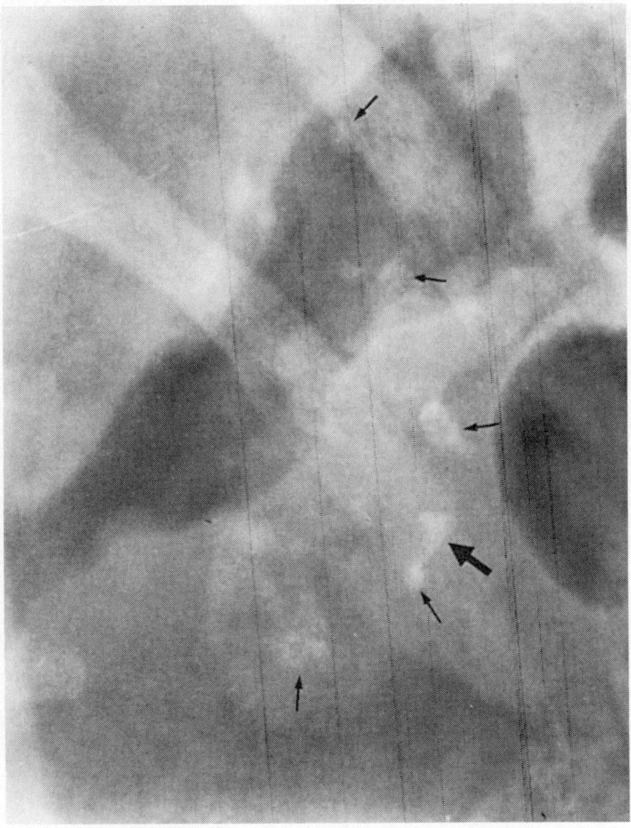

Figure 108.20. Nephrocalcinosis caused by renal papillary necrosis. Areas of irregular calcification are scattered throughout the left kidney in this case of renal papillary necrosis. The calcifications may take on a rounded form *(small arrows)* or a more triangular form *(large arrow)* in these calcified papillary remnants.

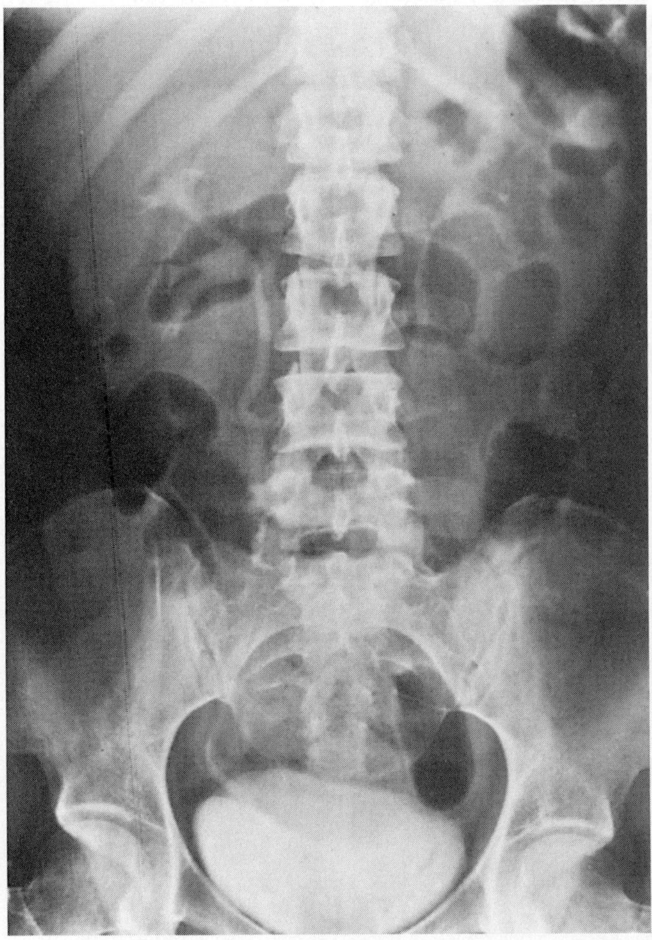

Figure 108.21. Acute glomerulonephritis. This intravenous pyelogram in a patient with acute glomerulonephritis demonstrates symmetrically enlarged kidneys with normal-appearing collecting systems bilaterally. Because there was only minimal renal impairment, the collecting systems, ureters, and bladder are well seen in this patient.

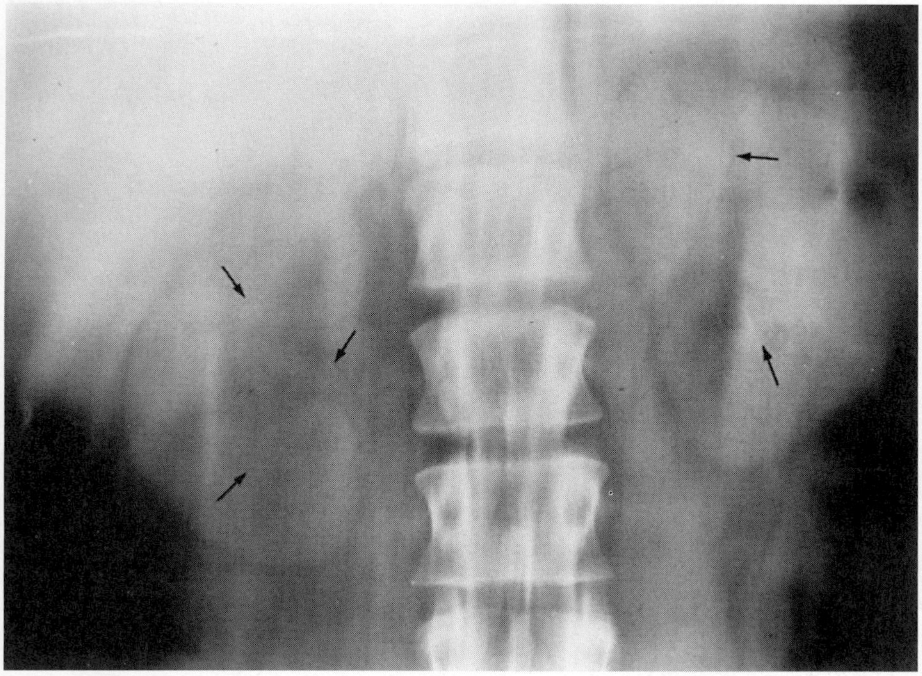

Figure 108.22. Chronic glomerulonephritis. The nephrotomogram in this patient with chronic glomerulonephritis and moderate renal impairment shows kidneys that are smaller than normal. However, the contours of the kidneys remain smooth. The collecting systems are normal but faintly seen *(arrows)* bilaterally.

The findings on angiography are usually nonspecific (Fig. 108.23). There is poor delineation of the corticomedullary junction, with some apparent thinning of the cortex itself. The angiographic findings are generally indistinguishable from those of nephrosclerosis.

Renal Vein Thrombosis

The radiographic findings in renal vein thrombosis depend on whether the process is acute or chronic. In the acute form, the intravenous urogram will usually show a large, nonfunctioning kidney (Fig. 108.24). An increase in the density of the nephrogram for up to 12 to 24 hours may be seen. Usually, little, if any, contrast material is noted in the collecting system (Fig. 108.25). Angiography usually demonstrates stretched intrarenal vessels, prolonged transit of contrast through the arterial system, decreased cortical opacification, and thus poor demarcation of the corticomedullary junction. Opacification of the renal venous system is absent. In the more chronic stages of the renal vein thrombosis, the kidney becomes smaller and atrophic with non-

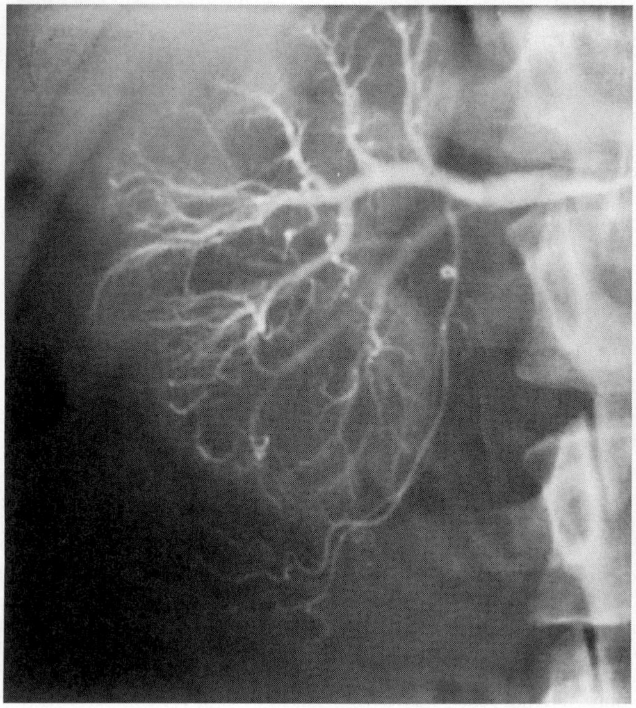

Figure 108.23. Chronic glomerulonephritis. On this selective right renal arteriogram in a patient with chronic glomerulonephritis, there is a decrease in the normal number of vessels identified, with mild tortuosity of the remaining more distal branches. The kidney itself is smaller than normal.

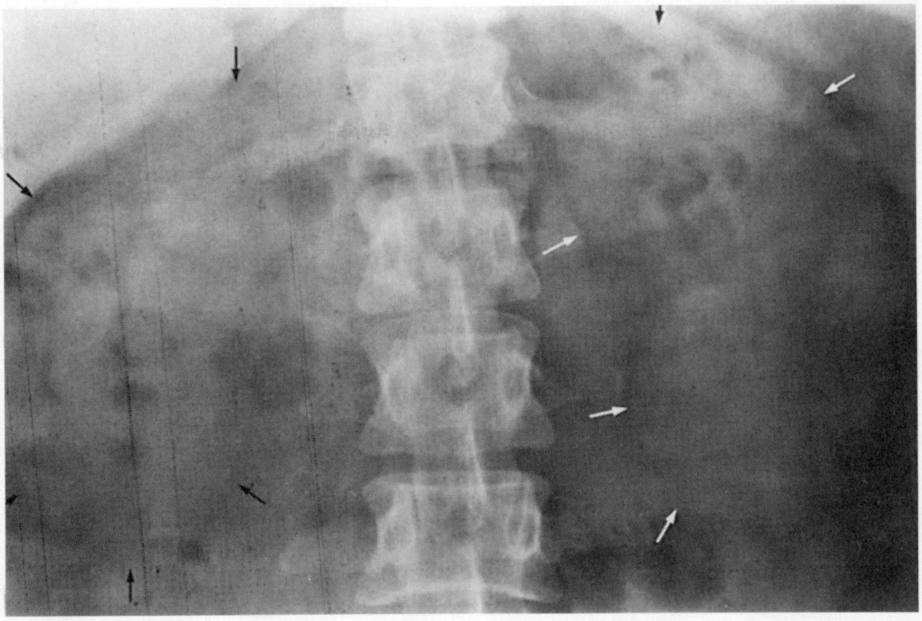

Figure 108.24. Acute renal vein thrombosis. The intravenous urogram in this patient with bilateral acute renal vein thrombosis demonstrates bilateral, slightly enlarged kidneys *(arrows)*, with no evidence of contrast excretion in the collecting systems.

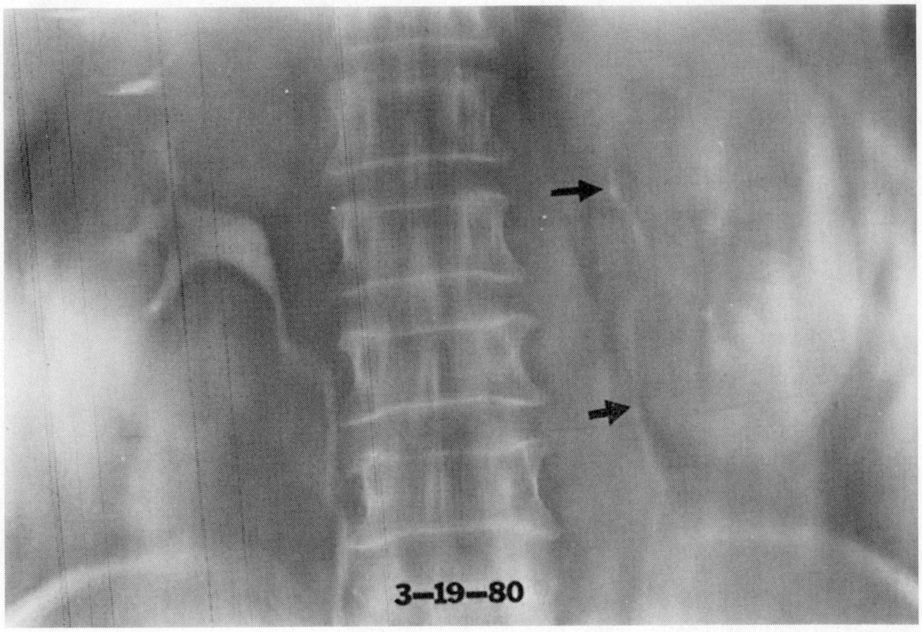

Figure 108.25. Acute left renal vein thrombosis. This tomographic section from an intravenous pyelogram shows a normal right kidney. The left kidney is enlarged, with a very small amount of contrast material identified in the area of the left renal pelvis and proximal left ureter *(arrows)*. The collecting systems are not identified because of the presence of renal parenchymal edema. Renal venography demonstrated acute left renal vein thrombosis.

function or poor function seen on intravenous urography. Renal angiography shows a renal artery with reduced caliber and again a poor nephrogram. Collateral venous channels occasionally may be seen (Fig. 108.26).

In the patient with partial renal vein thrombosis or renal vein thrombosis with a sufficient renal venous collateral system, the IVP will usually show an enlarged kidney with attenuated infundibula and calyces, as well as decreased concentration of contrast material. There may be evidence of collateral venous channels with notching of the ureter or renal pelvis (Fig. 108.27). Angiography shows some decrease in size of the main renal artery, with poor differentiation between the cortex and medulla of the kidney. Collateral venous channels may be seen.

In the chronic form of renal vein thrombosis, which is usually found in the adult, the IVP might be normal if the patient's renal function is not severely compromised (Fig. 108.28). Angiography in this setting usually reveals the underlying renal disease such as glomerulonephritis. The diagnosis of renal vein thrombosis is made with certainty by renal venography. In all cases, it is wise to perform an inferior vena cavogram before the renal venogram to note whether there is actually a thrombus in the inferior vena cava. With retrograde filling of the renal vein on renal venography, it is possible to show the extent of the thrombus as well as collateral channels (Fig. 108.26). Evidence of prior renal vein thrombosis (recannulization of the renal vein) may be shown in occasional cases.

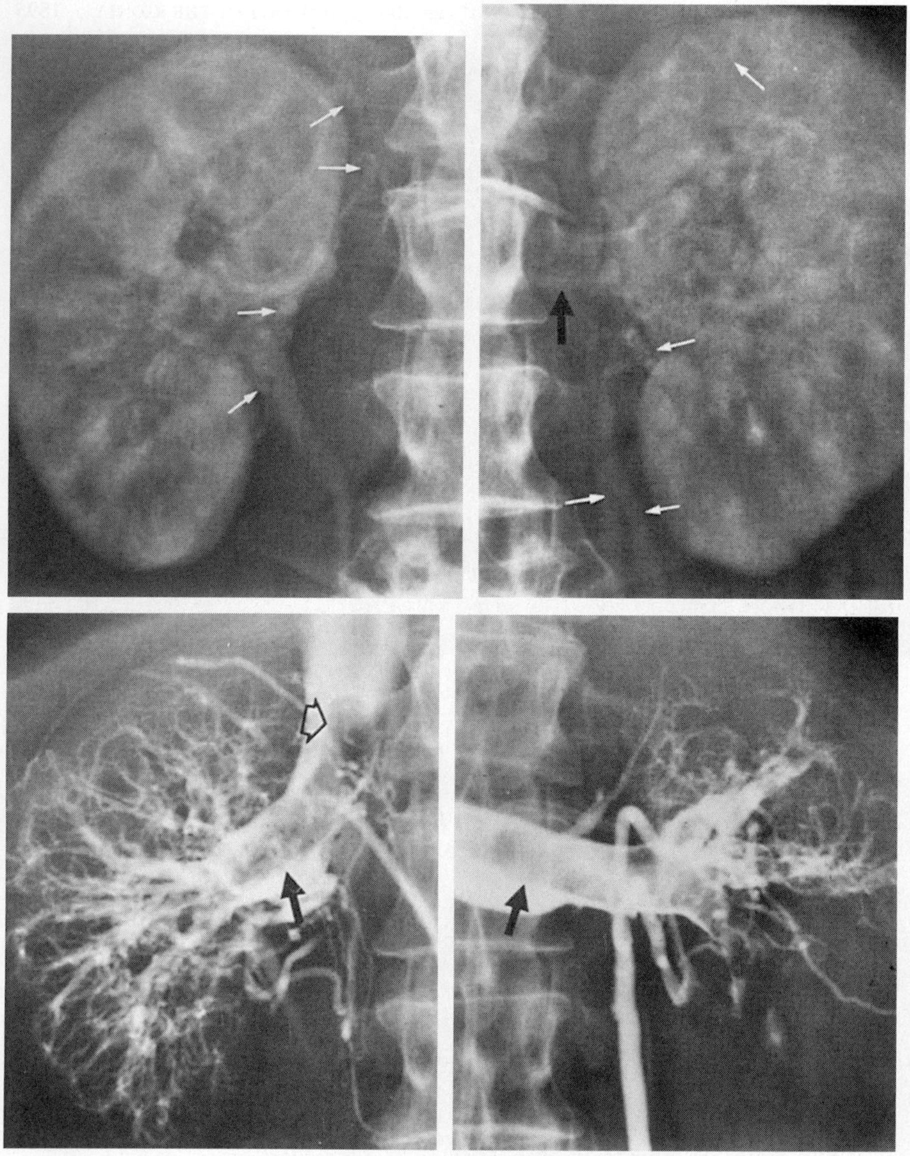

Figure 108.26. Bilateral renal vein thrombosis. **Top:** The late stage of an arteriogram demonstrates collateral venous passages in the area around the kidneys *(small arrows)*. The *larger arrow* shows actual clot within the left renal vein. **Bottom:** The selective renal venograms demonstrate thrombi within both renal veins *(solid arrows)* with extension of the right venous thrombus into the inferior vena cava *(open arrow)*.

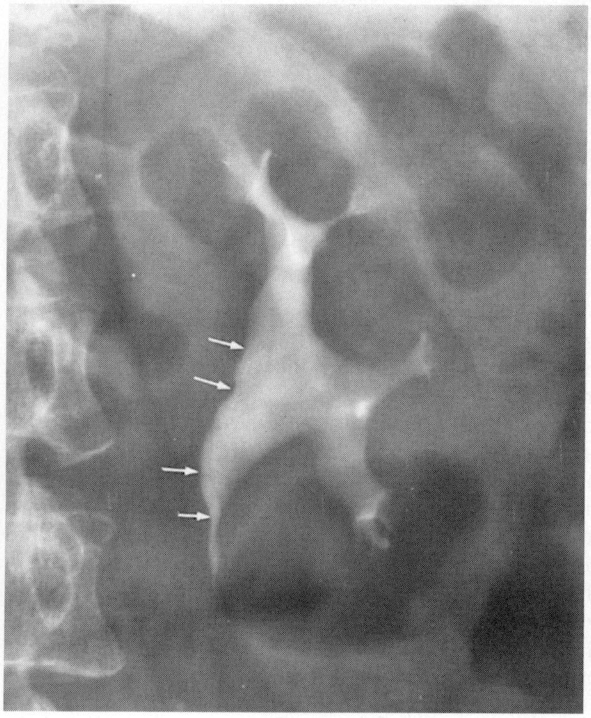

Figure 108.27. Renal vein thrombosis. Collateral venous channels cause notching of the renal pelvis and ureter *(arrows)* in this case of chronic renal vein thrombosis. A similar appearance may be seen with renal artery stenosis and collateral arterial channels in this area as well.

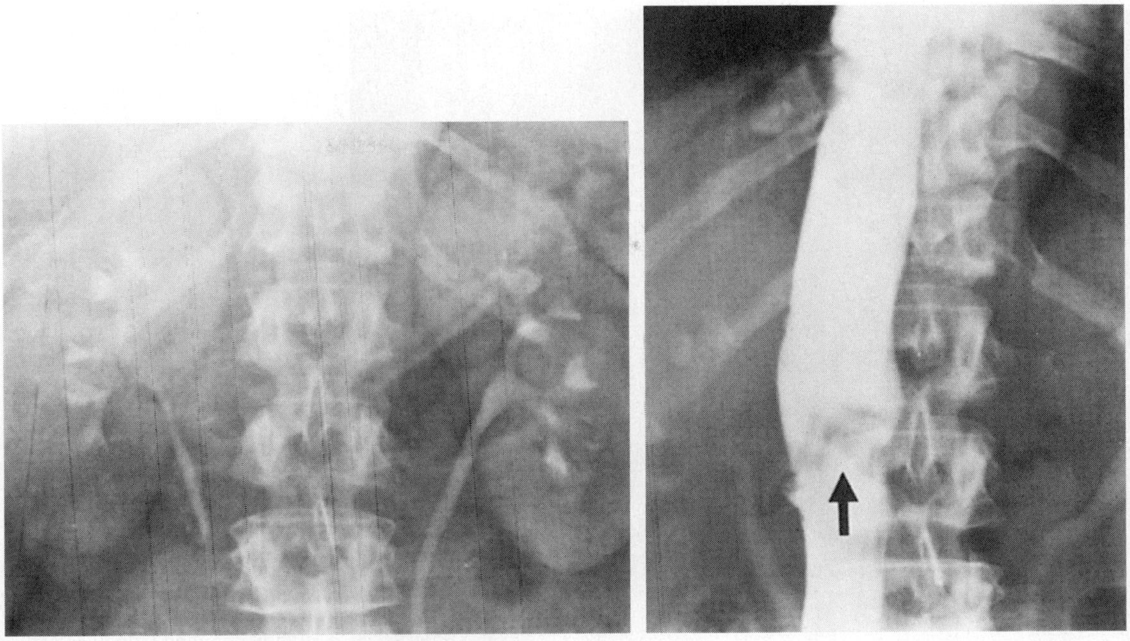

Figure 108.28. Chronic renal vein thrombosis. With adequate collateral venous drainage in chronic renal vein thrombosis, there may be a quite normal appearance to the kidneys on intravenous pyelography **(left)**. An inferior vena cavogram in this patient **(right)** demonstrates thrombus extending into the inferior vena cava *(arrow)*.

Renal Pyelonephritis

Acute Pyelonephritis

A variety of radiographic findings occur with acute pyelonephritis, most of which are relatively nonspecific. Up to 70% of patients will have an abnormal intravenous urogram.

Most patients do not require urologic investigation during the acute episode if they are responding well to antibiotic therapy. The findings on intravenous urography usually are unilateral and may be segmental (Figs. 108.29 to 108.31). These findings include renal enlargement, altered nephrogram, decreased concentration of contrast material and delay in appearance of contrast in the calyces, and attenuated or dilated calyces, renal pelvis, and ureter. Renal enlargement usually is caused by generalized edema of the kidney. The nephrogram may be absent or more frequently diminished in intensity when compared with the opposite side. The nephrogram may also be prolonged on the involved side (Fig. 108.30). Appearance of contrast material within some or all of the calyceal elements may be delayed with a slight decrease in the concentration of contrast within these calyces. Attenuated calyces may be noted in the involved area of the kidney. There also may be dilation of the collecting system and ureter because of atony or poor peristalsis. This is a form of nonobstructive dilation. The IVP will usually return to normal within 3 to 6 weeks of the episode of acute pyelonephritis. Retrograde pyelography generally is not indicated during an acute episode of pyelonephritis.

Angiography (Fig. 108.32) may appear normal in a patient with acute pyelonephritis. Renal arteriography may reveal some mild stretching of the intrarenal vessels. A decrease in the caliber of some of the visualized interlobar arteries may occur. No neovascularity is seen with acute pyelonephritis. The distribution of renal blood flow within the kidney may be mildly altered. During the nephrographic phase of the arteriogram, the nephrogram may have a diminished or inhomogeneous appearance. In addition, cortical striations may be identified during the nephrographic phase.

Chronic Pyelonephritis

The classic radiographic finding of chronic pyelonephritis is a focal cortical scar with an underlying clubbed calyx (Fig. 108.33). These focal changes involve both the cortex and medulla and

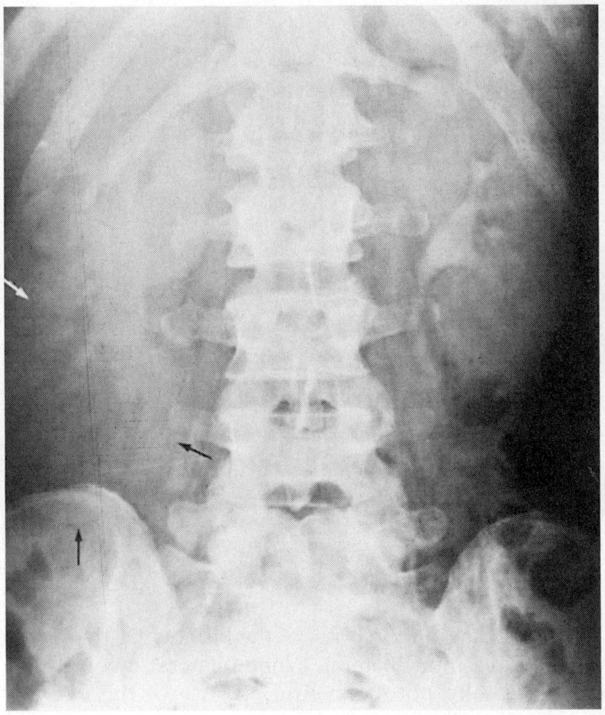

Figure 108.29. Acute pyelonephritis. The intravenous urogram in this patient with acute pyelonephritis shows a normal left kidney. There is generalized enlargement of the right kidney, with a markedly altered nephrogram. In the upper portion of the kidney, a somewhat prolonged nephrogram is seen. In the more severely involved lower pole, virtually no contrast is seen in either collecting systems or the nephrographic phase *(arrows)*.

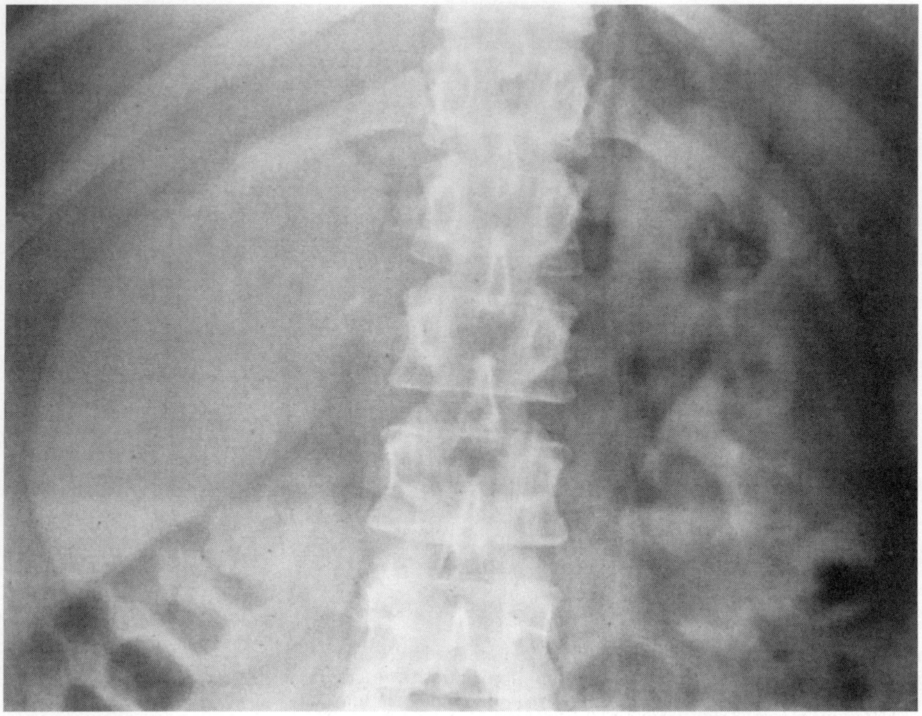

Figure 108.30. Acute pyelonephritis. This 15-minute film from an intravenous pyelogram in a patient with acute pyelonephritis shows a slightly enlarged kidney. However, a prolonged nephrogram is still present on the involved right side. No contrast material is visualized in the collecting system.

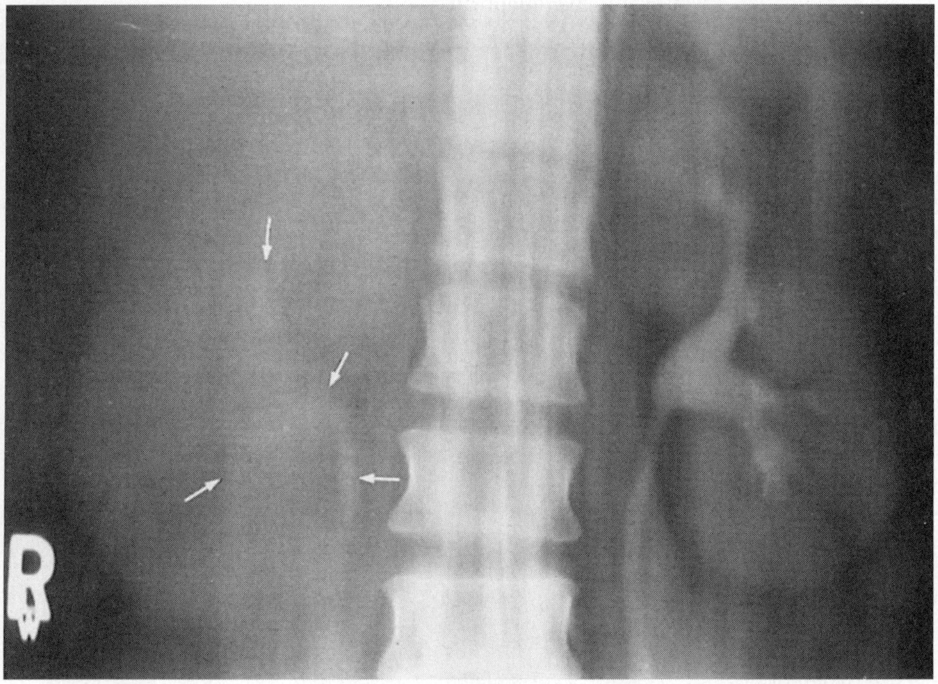

Figure 108.31. Acute pyelonephritis. This tomogram from an intravenous pyelogram in a patient with acute right pyelonephritis demonstrates a nephrogram that is slightly decreased in intensity, with faint opacification of the collecting system, renal pelvis, and right ureter *(arrows)*. A normal left kidney is seen.

are usually located in the poles of the kidney. The involvement may be unilateral or bilateral. When bilateral involvement occurs, it is usually not symmetric because of the varying involvement of each kidney and different rates of progress of the process (Fig. 108.33). The dilated clubbed calyx may extend all the way to the surface of the kidney. Intervening areas of normal cortex are often noted in chronic pyelonephritis. These areas may hypertrophy and mimic a mass within the kidney. Strictures are unusual in chronic pyelonephritis of bacterial origin but may be seen with tuberculous infection. With extensive involvement of a kidney, generalized dilation of the pelvocalyceal system may occur (Fig. 108.34). Reflux is often found during voiding cystourethrograms in patients with chronic pyelonephritis. As more and more of the kidney is destroyed and with increasing impairment of function, the calyceal system may be difficult to visualize with intravenous urography.

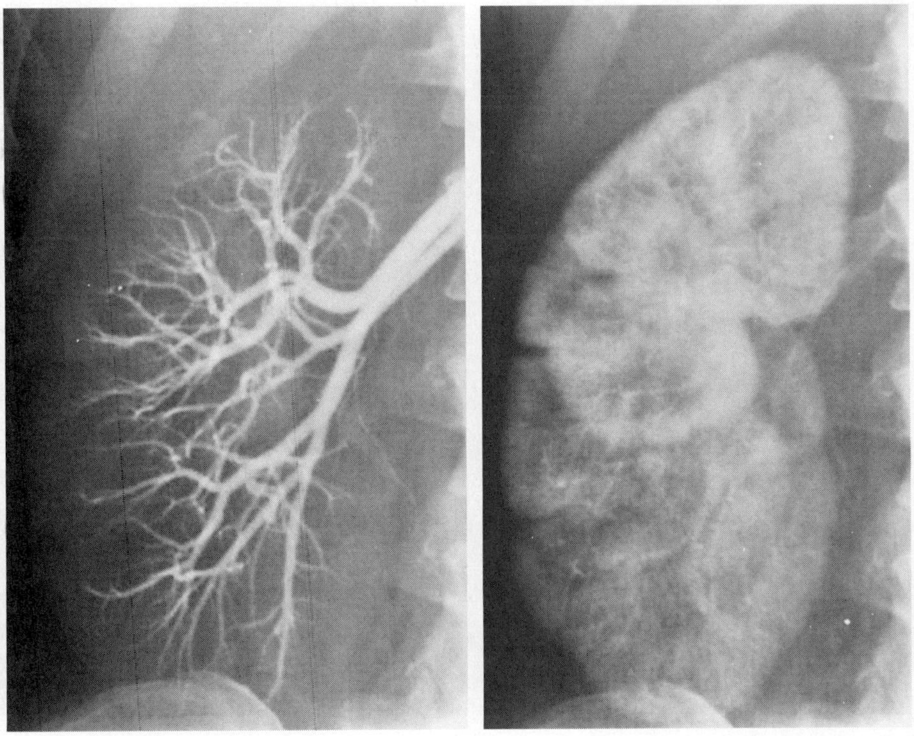

Figure 108.32. Acute pyelonephritis. **Left:** The arteriogram demonstrates mild stretching of the vessels to the middle and lower pole of the kidney. The upper pole arterial tree is essentially normal. **Right:** The late phase of the arteriogram demonstrates an altered appearance to the nephrogram, with diminished and nonhomogenous contrast appearance in the parenchyma of the lower pole.

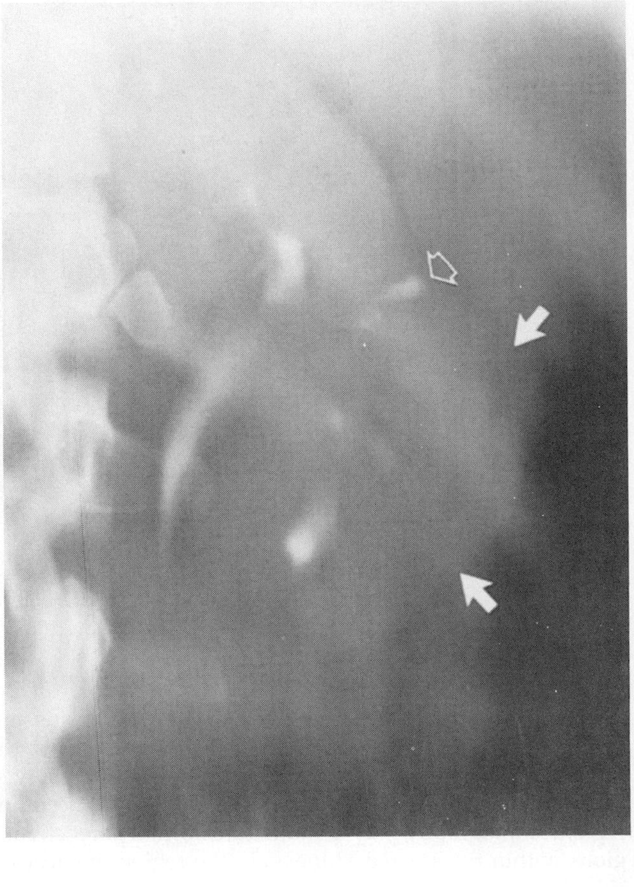

Figure 108.33. Chronic pyelonephritis. This tomogram of the left kidney during an intravenous pyelogram demonstrates a classic scar from focal pyelonephritis. There is loss of the cortex and clubbing of the underlying calyx *(open arrow)*. Just beneath the clubbed calyx, hypertrophy of a segment of normal remaining renal parenchyma is evident *(solid arrows)*.

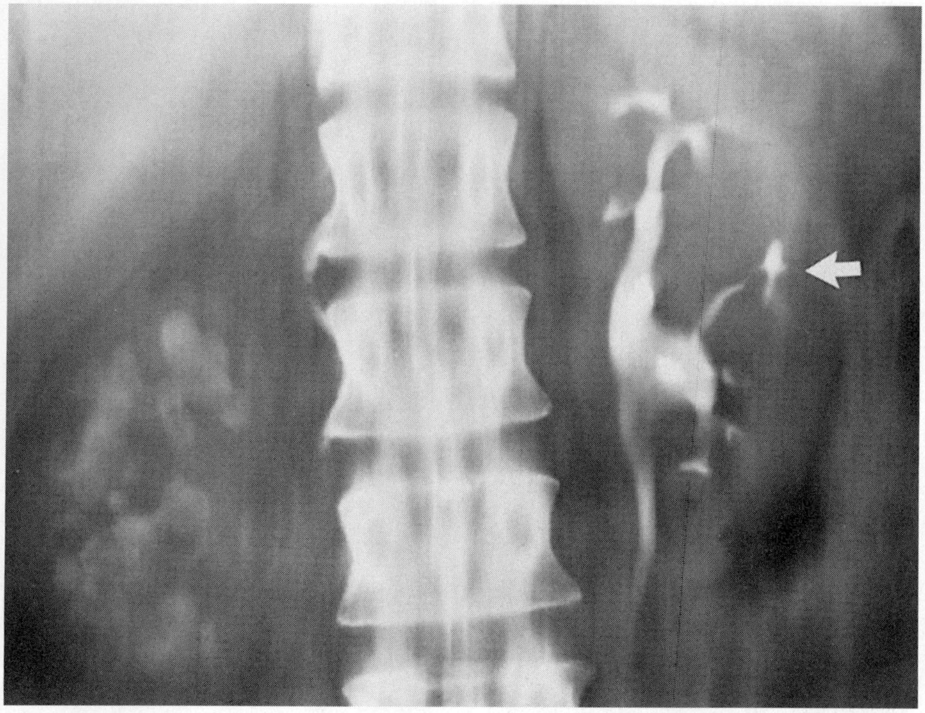

Figure 108.34. Chronic pyelonephritis. The tomographic section from an intravenous pyelogram demonstrates, in the left kidney, several areas of cortical scarring, with an underlying clubbed calyx in the midregion of the kidney *(arrow)*. The small right kidney has been extensively destroyed by pyelonephritis, leaving dilated collecting systems and little remaining cortex.

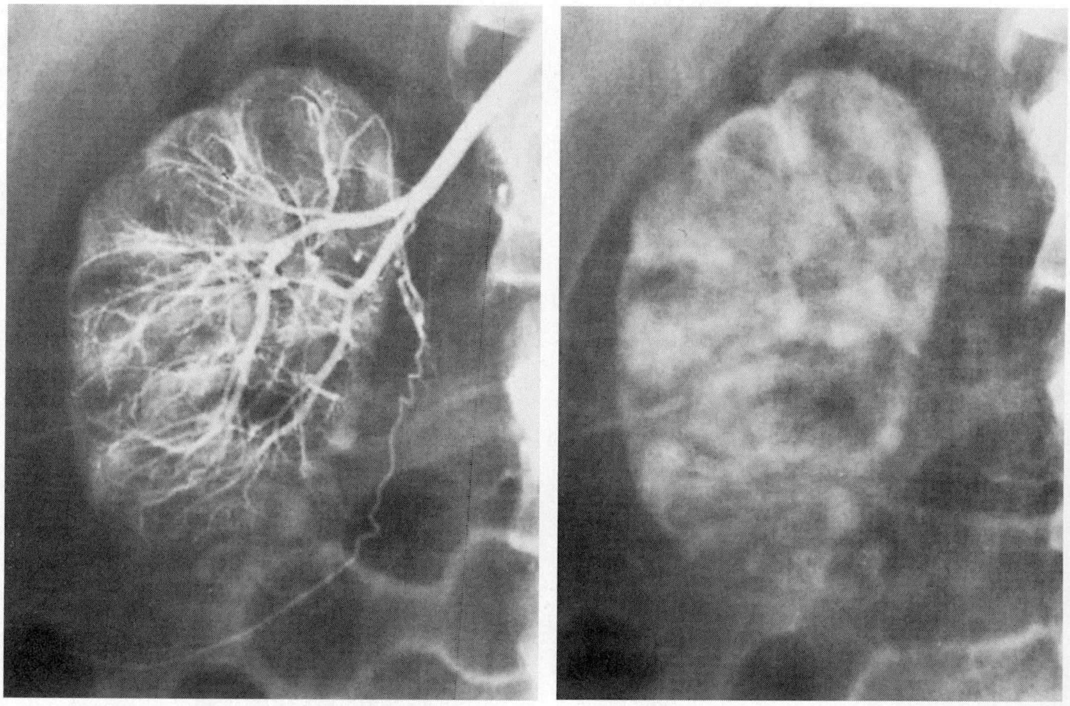

Figure 108.35. Chronic pyelonephritis. The right selective arteriogram in the arterial phase **(left)** demonstrates a small kidney with vessels much closer together and slightly irregular in caliber. In the capillary phase **(right),** there is a nonhomogenous nephrogram without definite normal regions of parenchyma remaining.

The angiographic findings in chronic pyelonephritis are relatively nonspecific (Fig. 108.35). In the regions of extensive scarring, irregular vessels that are close together are usually seen. Either an increased or decreased number of vessels occur in this region. Angiography may demonstrate normal parenchymal regions within the scarred kidneys. In the region of cortical scar and calyceal clubbing, an absent or decreased capillary phase may be identified.

Xanthogranulomatous Pyelonephritis

Xanthogranulomatous pyelonephritis is usually considered to be a complication of chronic pyelonephritis. Unilateral involvement

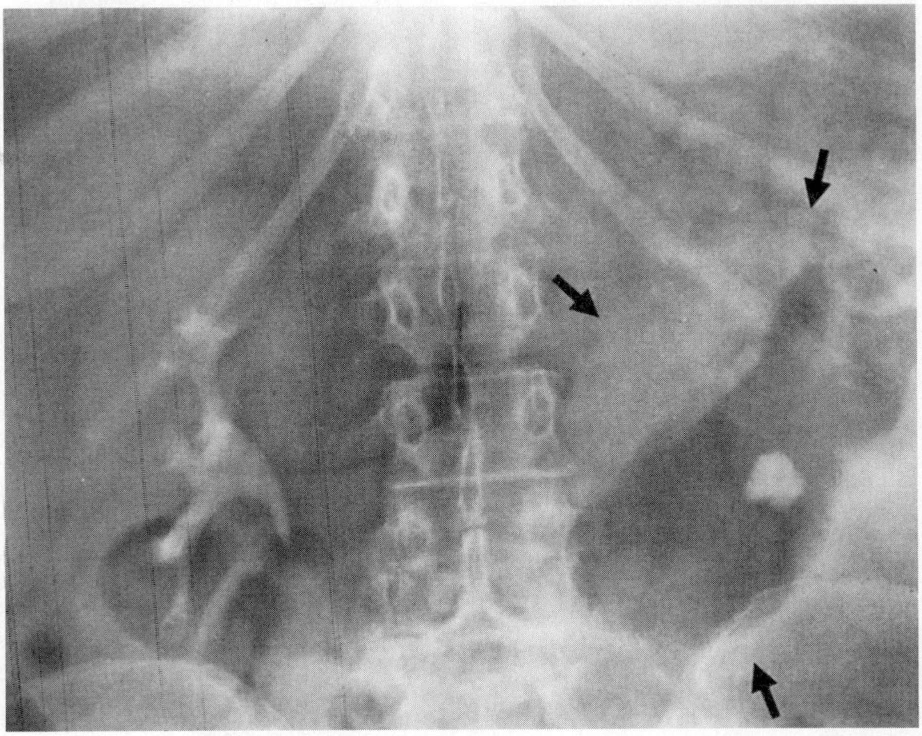

Figure 108.36. Xanthogranulomatous pyelonephritis. The intravenous pyelogram demonstrates a normal right kidney. A calcific density is identified overlying the area of the left kidney. A relatively large mass is seen in this area *(arrows)* without any identifiable collecting systems.

is most common, with a diffuse form accounting for approximately 85% of cases. The remaining 15% of cases have segmental involvement, which often appears as a mass on intravenous urography. Xanthogranulomatous pyelonephritis is much more common in females.

Radiographically (Figs. 108.36 and 108.37), a nonfunctioning or poorly functioning kidney is found in most cases. Renal calculi within the kidney may be seen. Calculi may also appear to be obstructing the kidney. Urography usually shows an enlarged and apparently hydronephrotic kidney. With segmental involvement, areas of functioning parenchyma may remain, and thus some calyces may be seen.

The angiographic findings with xanthogranulomatous pyelonephritis depend on the degree of involvement (Fig. 108.38). Stretched vessels with inflammatory vascularity may be present, giving an appearance similar to that of hydronephrosis. Varying areas of staining may be noted within the kidney. The capsular vessels are usually increased in number and caliber. An irregular and nonhomogenous nephrogram may be obtained. With the tumefactive form of xanthogranulomatous pyelonephritis, the angiogram may be difficult to differentiate from a hypovascular renal cell carcinoma or squamous cell carcinoma of the renal pelvis.

Perinephric and Renal Abscess

An intrarenal abscess is a localized collection of pus caused either by hematogenous spread of bacteria or by bacteria ascending in the urine from the bladder. Renal carbuncles are generally considered to result from a coalescence of multiple small abscesses and are caused by hematogenous spread of bacteria. Abscesses most frequently occur in diabetic patients. It is interesting to note that because of the hematogenous route of bacterial spread, urine cultures may be negative in some patients with a renal abscess. As the abscess progresses and the infection becomes more severe, perinephric extension may occur. There may also be erosion of the abscess into the

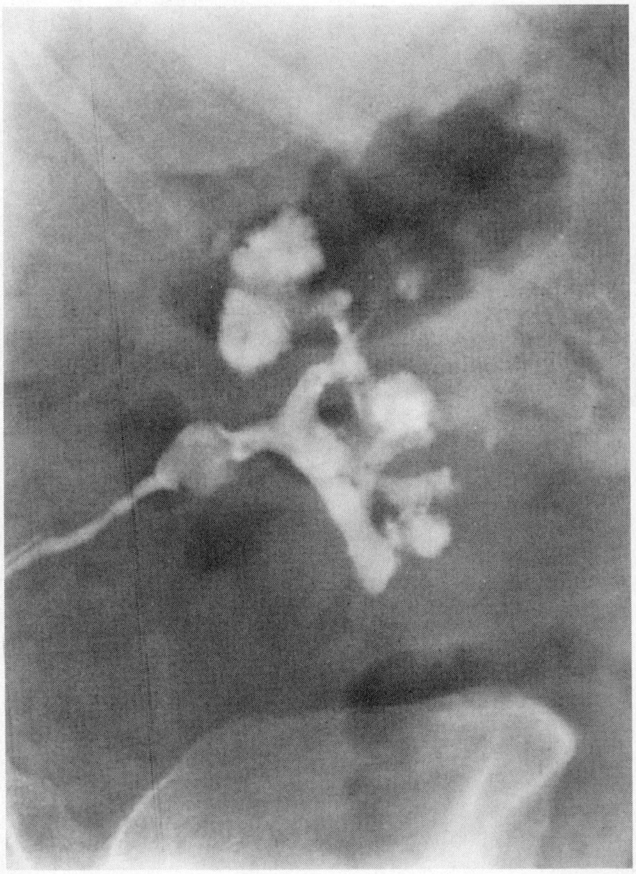

Figure 108.37. Xanthogranulomatous pyelonephritis. A retrograde pyelogram in the same patient as seen in Fig. 108.36 demonstrates the calcification to be a calculus in the left renal pelvis. Deformed, irregular, and somewhat clubbed calyces are noted. No significant hydronephrosis is identified.

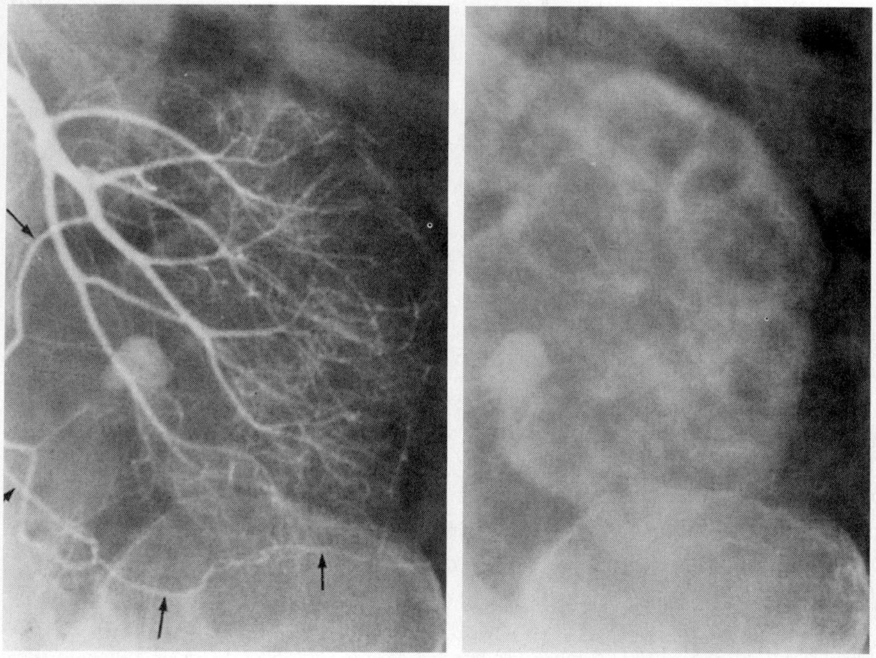

Figure 108.38. Xanthogranulomatous pyelonephritis. The angiogram of the patient noted in Figs. 108.36 and 108.37 demonstrates a somewhat enlarged kidney without identifiable normal regions **(left).** The vessels are stretched and show some irregularity consistent with an inflammatory process. A large inferior capsular vessel is present *(arrows).* In the capillary phase **(right),** there is a nonhomogenous appearance to the kidney. This entire kidney was involved with xanthogranulomatous pyelonephritis.

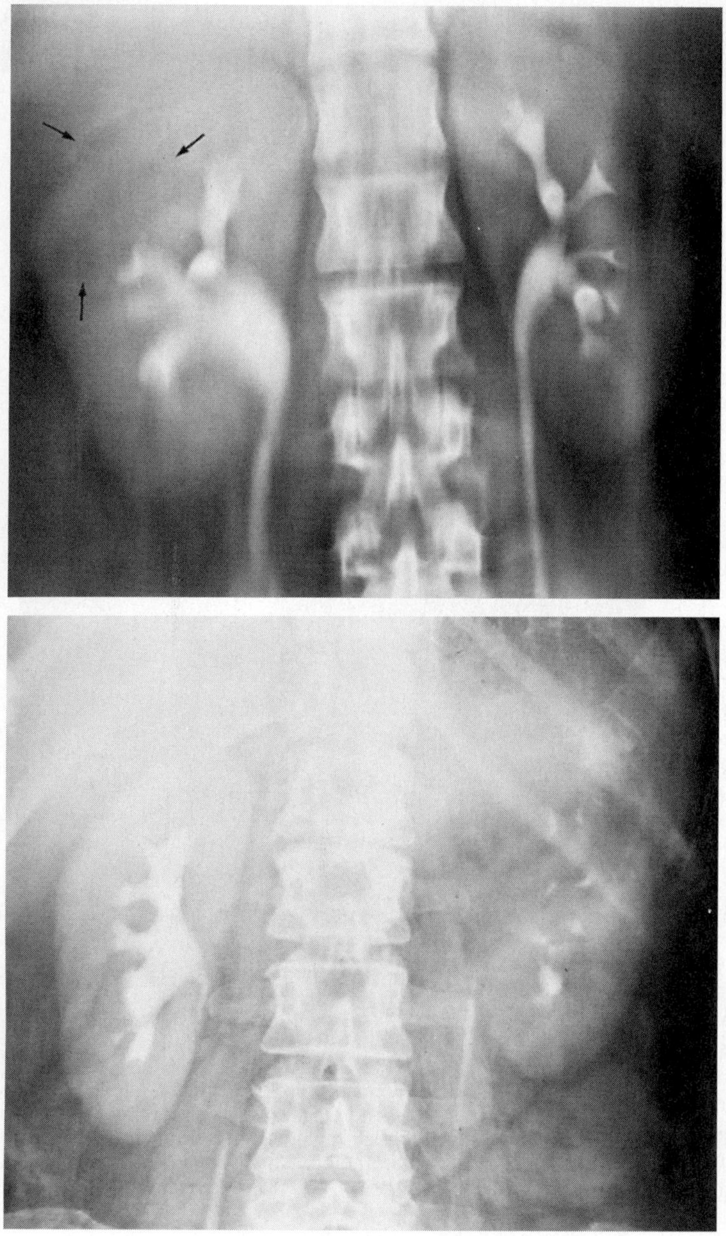

Figure 108.39. Renal abscess. **Top:** This tomographic section from an intravenous pyelogram demonstrates some deformity to the superior lateral margin of the right kidney. In addition, there is a lucency within the normally homogeneous renal parenchyma *(arrows).* The calyx to this region is poorly seen. **Bottom:** The intravenous pyelogram in this case of renal abscess demonstrates a normal right kidney with more masslike involvement of the upper and midportions of the left kidney. The medial margin of the left kidney is difficult to see. The collecting systems are stretched and somewhat displaced in the middle and upper portions of the kidney.

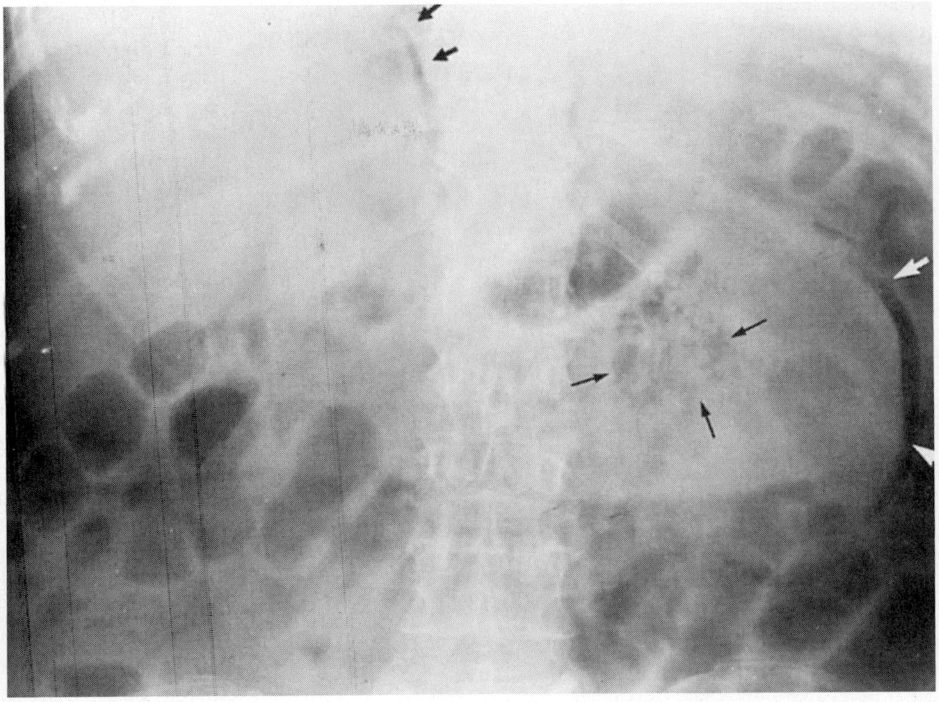

Figure 108.40. Perinephric abscess. The left kidney was extensively involved with infection that extended into the perinephric space. A masslike area is seen in the region of the left kidney, with fine collections of gas within the renal parenchyma itself *(thin black arrows)*. Gas is also seen in the left perinephric space *(white arrows)*. Because this infection extended into the anterior perirenal space and dissected superiorly, gas is also noted on the right side *(thick black arrows)*. Because gas is identifiable in both the renal parenchyma and perinephric space, this represents a case of emphysematous pyelonephritis with perinephric abscess.

pelvic calyceal system, with spontaneous decompression of the abscess.

The plain film of the abdomen may reveal an enlarged kidney or mass within the involved kidney. The psoas margin on the involved side may be poorly delineated. A reflex ileus is often noted. On intravenous urography (Fig. 108.39), poor function of the involved kidney is observed frequently. The nephrogram may show an area of lucency within. When a renal abscess occurs as a mass lesion, stretching and displacement of the calyces are sometimes observed. The margins of the mass may be poorly defined and the calyces minimally dilated displaced, poorly seen, and nonfilled. Renal calculi are occasionally seen in association with renal abscess. With perinephric extension of the abscess (Fig. 108.40), an additional mass may be noted outside the confines of the kidney.

Renal angiography (Fig. 108.41), in the patient with an intrarenal abscess will show an area of hypovascularity with displacement and spreading of the vessels around the abscess. Some inflammatory areas of neovascularity may be seen in the periphery of the abscess. No neoplastic type of neovascularity is noted with intrarenal abscesses. During the nephrographic phase of the arteriogram, the corticomedullary junction is lost in the involved area and a relatively lucent area with indistinct margins is seen. When extension into the perinephric space occurs, the number and caliber of the capsular vessels increase. The capsular vessels will be displaced away from the kidney and around the perinephric abscess. In addition, loss of the cortical nephrogram usually occurs in the region where the abscess has extended into the perinephric space. Both perinephric abscesses and intrarenal abscesses may show collection of gas on conventional radiographic studies (Fig. 108.40).

Pyohydronephrosis

Extensive destruction of the renal parenchyma because of infection and superimposed obstruction is referred to as *pyohydronephrosis*. By this stage in the cycle of renal infection, little or no function remains within the kidney. The calyceal system is usually markedly dilated and irregular and filled with pus. Plain films of the abdomen and intravenous urography usually reveal

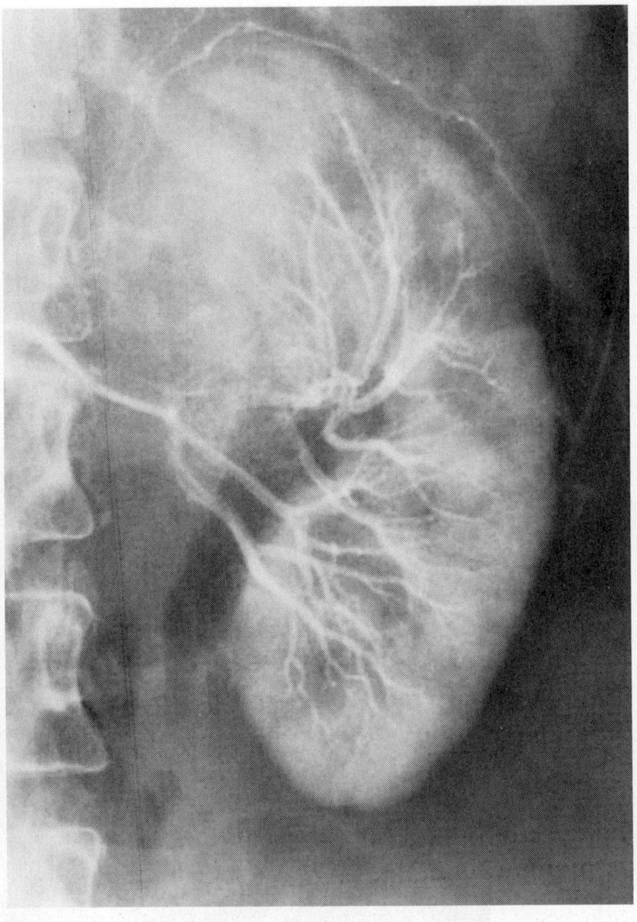

Figure 108.41. Renal abscess. The left renal arteriogram demonstrates direct displacement and some stretching of the upper pole vessels around the abscess located in the superior and medial aspects of the kidney. In addition, there is loss of a distinct margin to the medial aspect of the kidney. The region of involvement by the abscess is less dense than the more normal-appearing cortex inferiorly. A capsular vessel is seen overlying the region.

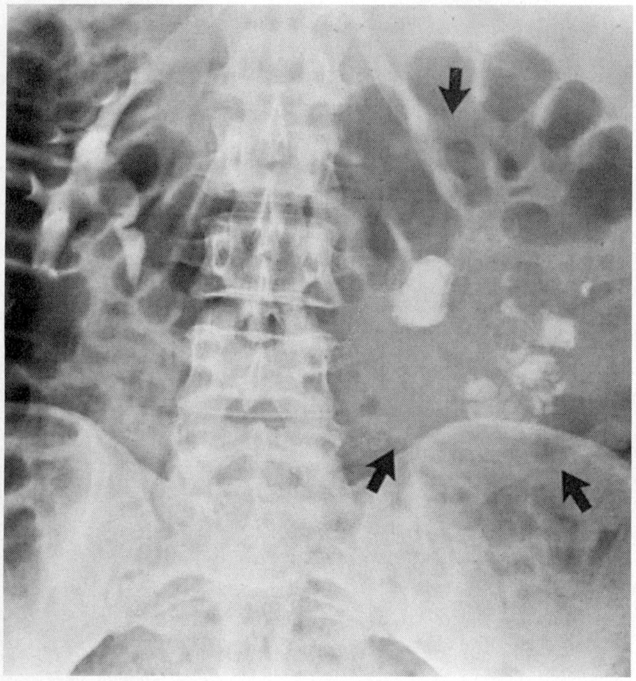

Figure 108.42. Pyohydronephrosis. A markedly enlarged left kidney is seen on this intravenous pyelogram *(arrows)*. Multiple renal calculi are seen within the kidney. No renal function is identified.

a markedly enlarged kidney (Fig. 108.42). Multiple calculi and/or a staghorn calculus may be seen. Little or no excretion of contrast material is seen during urography. A retrograde pyelogram reveals markedly enlarged calyces filled with extensive infected debris or pus. Angiography (Fig. 108.43) of pyohydronephrosis shows a renal artery that is decreased in caliber. The intrarenal vessels are stretched around large dilated calyces. Scattered areas of inflammatory neovascularity are usually noted in the markedly thinned cortex. Increased vascularity is noted also in the renal pelvic region. Occasionally, extension of the pyohydronephrosis into the perinephric space is noted, with enlarged capsular vessels displaced away from the kidney.

Tuberculosis of the Kidney and Urinary Tract

Tuberculous involvement of the kidney occurs by hematogenous spread of the tubercle bacillus. The usual site of origin is pulmonary tuberculosis. Evidence of previous pulmonary involvement is present in 70% to 75% of cases of urinary tract tuberculosis. Calcifications within the lungs and scarring in the apices are the most common findings on chest radiograph. It is uncommon for pulmonary tuberculosis to be active at the time of diagnosis of genitourinary tract tuberculosis. The renal involvement with tuberculosis is bilateral because of the hematogenous origin of the infection. Tuberculosis involvement of the ureters and bladder is most often caused by mucosal spread from renal tuberculosis through the infected urine.

The first radiographic finding of renal tuberculosis on plain films is usually evidence of calcification in the kidney (Fig. 108.19). The calcification may resemble those of nephrocalcinosis. Small dense areas of calcification involving small or large portions of the kidneys may be noted. Complete calcification of a small scarred kidney may occur. Calcification of either the

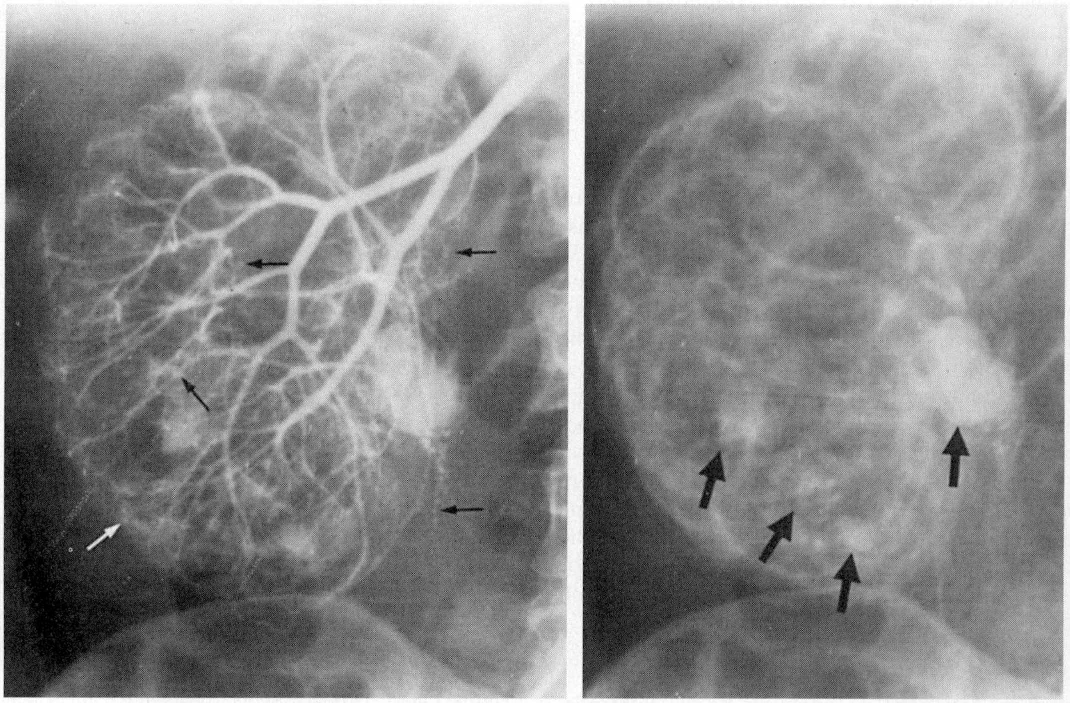

Figure 108.43. Pyohydronephrosis. The right renal arteriogram in the arterial phase **(left)** shows an enlarged kidney with extensive stretching of the arterial branches around the markedly dilated collecting systems. Areas of inflammatory vascularity are noted throughout the kidney *(small arrows)*. In the capillary phase **(right)**, the extensive hydronephrosis is noted, with calculi seen in the area of the renal pelvis and lower pole *(large arrows)*.

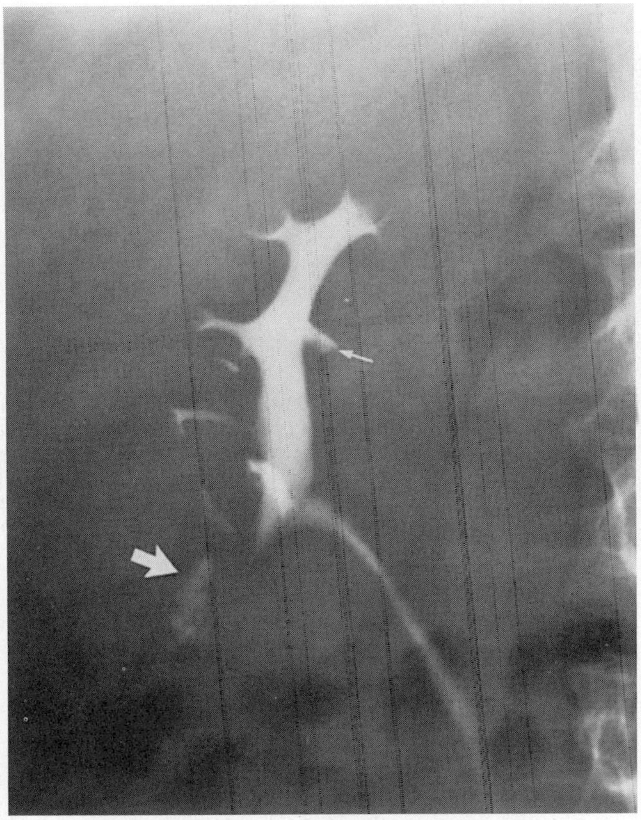

Figure 108.44. Renal tuberculosis. An intravenous pyelogram demonstrates the early changes seen in tuberculosis. In the lower pole *(large arrow)*, a fuzzy, ill-defined collection of contrast material is noted where the papillary lip has been destroyed. In the medial portion of the kidney *(small arrow)*, there is poor definition of the calyx and slight irregularity, again from tuberculous involvement.

ureter or bladder is rare in renal tuberculosis. Calcification in the prostate may occur but is difficult to distinguish from prostatic calculi.

The earliest change of renal tuberculosis seen on the IVP is usually a poorly defined calyx (Fig. 108.44). Involvement of the papillary tip results in a fuzzy, moth-eaten, and feathered appearance to the calyx on intravenous urography. Calyceal dilation may occur. A radiographic appearance resembling papillary necrosis may be noted as the disease progresses (Fig. 108.45). A single calyx may be involved, or multiple calyces in both kidneys may show radiographic findings. With cortical scarring, the process may appear similar to chronic pyelonephritis. It is unusual for tuberculosis to appear as a mass lesion, although large tuberculomas of the kidney have been reported. With disease progression, fibrosis occurs with stenoses and calyceal dilation.

Late in the course of renal tuberculosis, the kidney may take on a very bizarre appearance with alteration of the architecture of the entire kidney. An autonephrectomized kidney is a nonfunctioning kidney associated with ureteral obstruction, which is the end-stage of involvement from renal tuberculosis (Fig. 108.46). Ureteral involvement occurs by the passage of the tubercle bacillus through the urine from the kidney.

Strictures, frequently multiple, are noted (Fig. 108.47 and 108.48). The first evidence of stricture usually is seen in the distal third of the ureter. Multiple pictures of ureteral involvement have been described, including the corkscrew ureter (multiple areas of dilation and constrictions), the pipestern ureter (a long, rigid, somewhat narrowed ureter), the beaded ureter, and the ragged ureter. Calcification occasionally occurs in the wall of the ureter in the involved area. Bladder involvement is usually characterized by a thickened, small capacity, spastic bladder. The bladder lumen is usually irregular and contracted because of the extensive fibrosis (Fig. 108.49). Fistulas to other pelvic organs may be seen. With appropriate therapy, a marked improvement in the radiographic findings may occur. Marked progression of some of the findings may be seen, resulting from extensive fibrosis during healing and stricture formation. Retrograde pyelography may be helpful in demonstrating some of

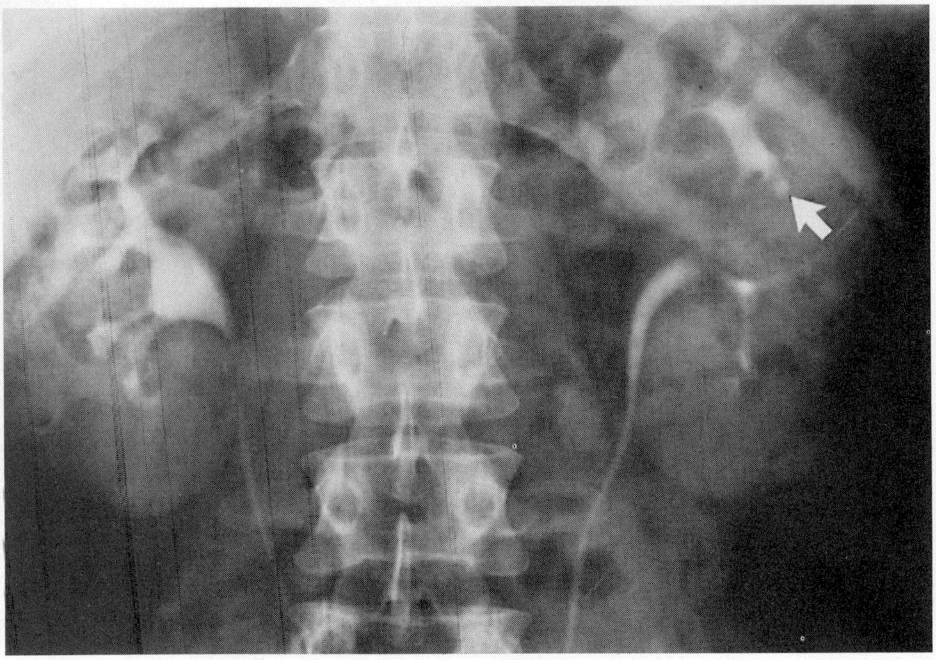

Figure 108.45. Renal tuberculosis. This intravenous pyelogram demonstrates findings resembling papillary necrosis *(arrow)* in the left kidney, caused by renal tuberculosis.

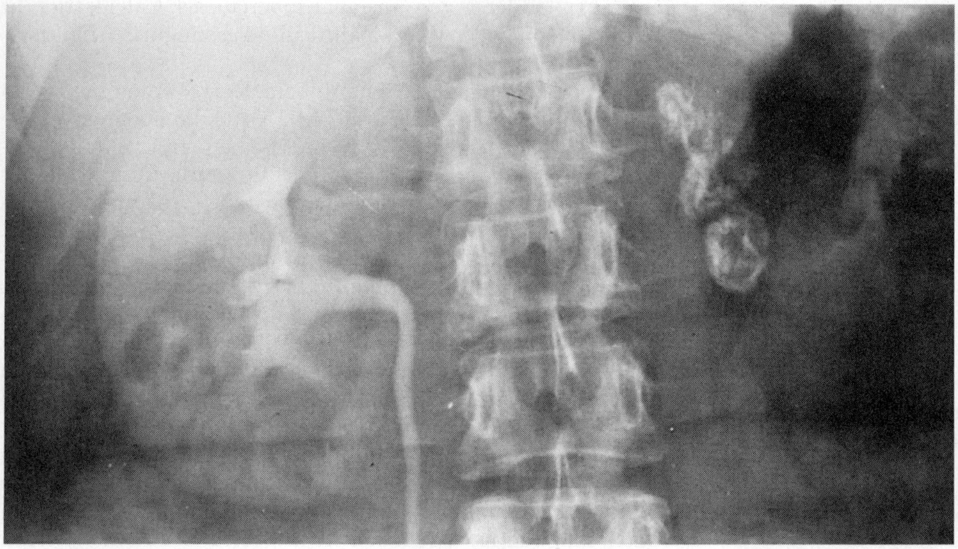

Figure 108.46. Renal tuberculosis. This intravenous pyelogram demonstrates a normal-appearing right kidney. A small, shrunken, scarred left kidney resulting from end-stage involvement with renal tuberculosis is seen. This autonephrectomized kidney is nonfunctioning and shows calcification within.

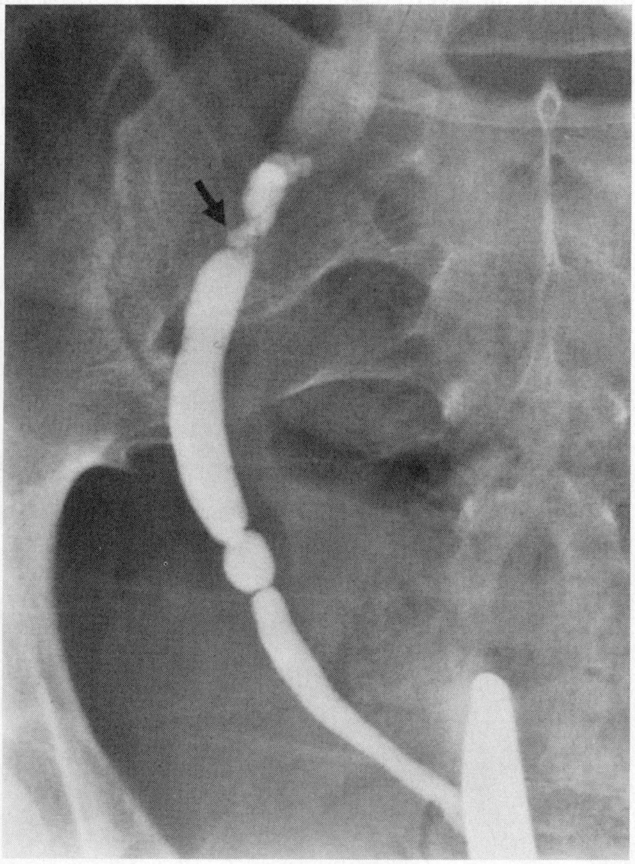

Figure 108.47. Renal tuberculosis. Ureteral involvement with renal tuberculosis is demonstrated on this retrograde pyelogram, with multiple strictures of the distal third of the ureter. The more superior strictures *(arrow)* are irregular, whereas the more inferior strictures are smooth.

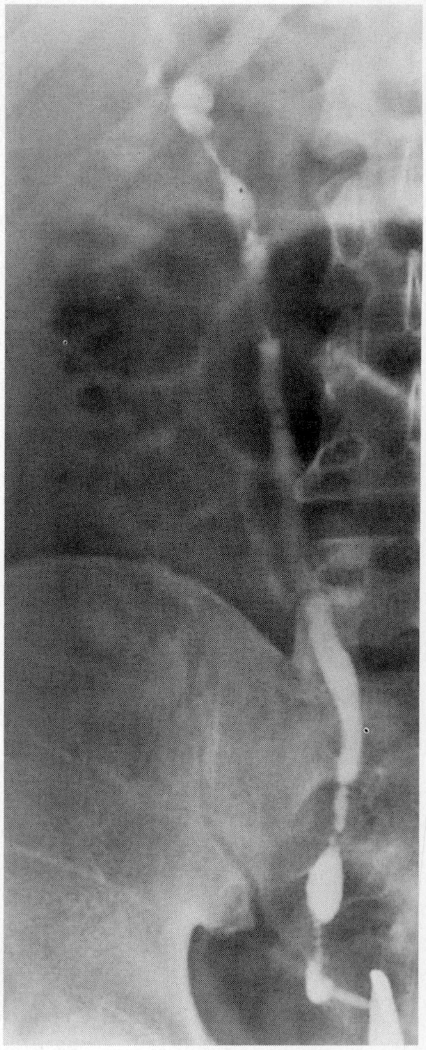

Figure 108.48. Renal tuberculosis. Extensive tuberculous involvement of the entire ureter and renal pelvis is noted on this right retrograde pyelogram. Long, as well as short, areas of stricture formation are seen in the course of the right ureter.

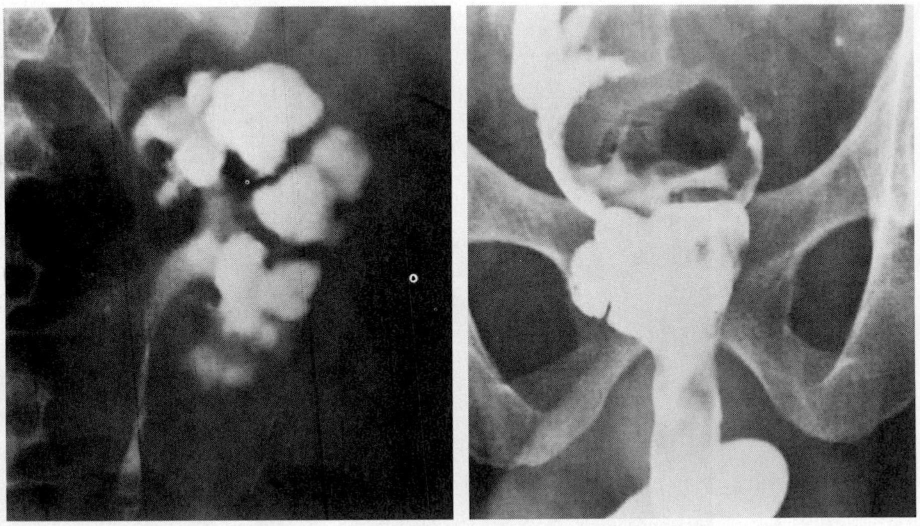

Figure 108.49. Renal tuberculosis. **Left:** Extensive involvement of the entire left kidney is seen, with irregularity and dilation of all the calyces. No normal calyx is noted. There is also early involvement of the proximal left ureter with tuberculosis. **Right:** The extension of the tuberculous process to the bladder and prostate causes this bizarre picture.

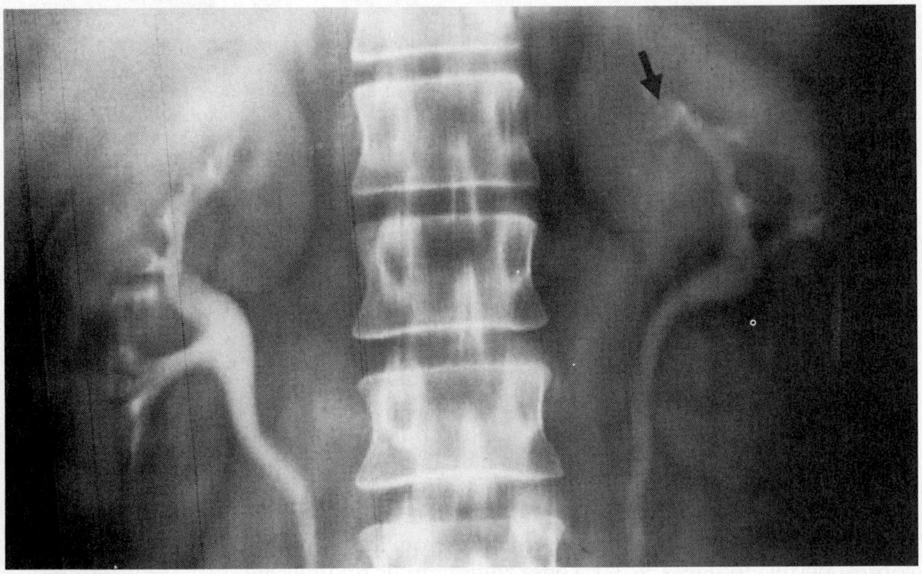

Figure 108.50. Renal tuberculosis. The tomogram from an intravenous pyelogram demonstrates some enlargement of the lower pole of the left kidney and no identifiable collecting systems in this area. This masslike appearance of the lower pole was a tuberculous abscess. In the upper pole of the left kidney *(arrow),* early changes of renal tuberculosis are evident, with a fuzzy and irregular calyx.

the findings of genitourinary tract tuberculosis in the nonfunctioning or poorly functioning kidney. Angiography has very limited use in evaluation of the patient with renal tuberculosis. The angiographic findings are nonspecific and are caused by the inflammatory process and subsequent scar formation. Angiography may be used occasionally to determine the normal areas remaining in the affected kidney. Occasionally, renal tuberculosis may appear as a mass lesion following abscess formation (Fig. 108.50).

Vaculitides

Polyarteritis nodosa is the most commonly encountered necrotizing vasculitides. The IVP is usually not helpful in evaluating these patients. Occasionally, during the nephrogram phase, small areas of renal scarring may be the only nonspecific finding. The calyces are usually normal, but they may be seen only faintly if there is significant renal impairment. Angiography is diagnostic in these patients. Multiple small aneurysms of peripheral branches of medium- and small-sized vessels are noted (Fig. 108.51). Localized areas of arterial irregularities and narrowing are commonly seen. During the capillary phase of the arteriogram, focal areas of ischemia or actual infarction may be noted. Loss of the corticomedullary junction may be seen with significant renal impairment. Retention of contrast material within the small aneurysms is occasionally noted after the contrast material has been washed out of the major renal arteries. Complications of polyarteritis nodosa, such as intrarenal hematomas and perinephric hematomas, occasionally are seen on angiography.

Findings similar to polyarteritis nodosa are found in patients who abuse methamphetamines and those who are chronically infected with hepatitis B virus. A milder form of vasculitis is seen in systemic lupus erythematosus. Aneurysm formation is not noted in systemic lupus erythematosus. Arterial irregularities, however, are seen in Wegener's granulomatosis, a necrotizing granulomatous vasculitis; arterial irregularities again may be noted by angiography. Aneurysms are unusual in these patients.

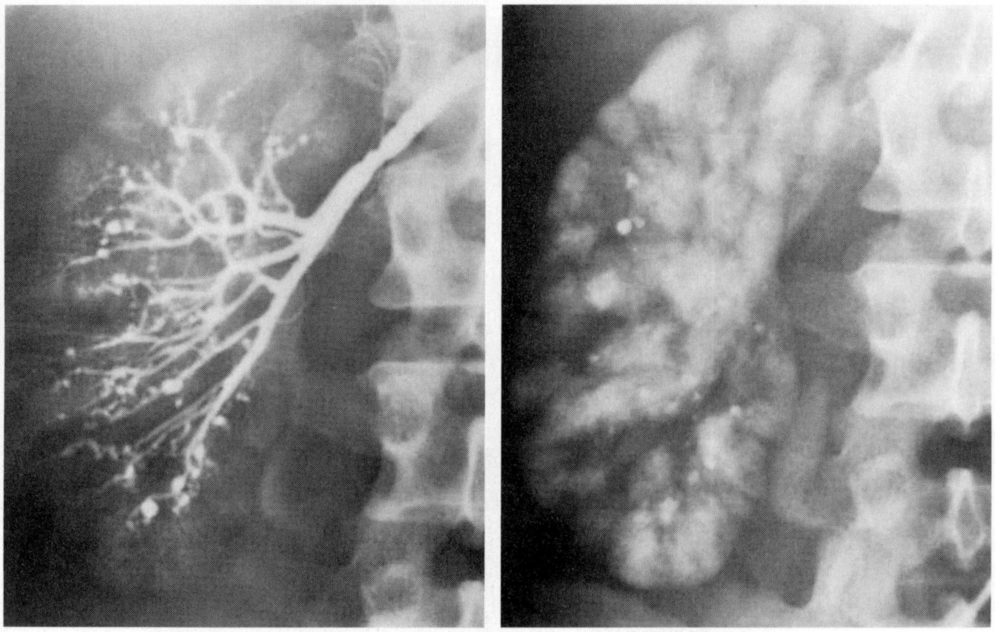

Figure 108.51. Polyarteritis nodosa. The films from an arteriogram demonstrate the findings of necrotizing vasculitis. Multiple fusiform and round aneurysms are noted in the medium and small branches of the renal arteries **(left).** During the capillary phase of the arteriogram **(right),** contrast material is retained within some of the aneurysms. The darker focal areas in the periphery of the kidney represent regions of ischemia or infarction.

Scleroderma

The renal size, shape, and outline usually are normal on intravenous urography in patients with scleroderma. The collecting systems also appear normal. With advancing disease and decreasing renal function, the kidney size may be reduced. Angiography shows minor changes of the intralobular and arcuate arteries. Areas of spasm in both segmental and main renal arteries, slow arterial flow, and loss of the corticomedullary junction may be noted. A nonhomogenous or spotted nephrogram has been described in scleroderma, resulting from the decreased cortical perfusion (Fig. 108.52). These angiographic findings are all nonspecific and are noted only in some isolated cases.

Amyloidosis

Amyloidosis may involve the kidney in both its primary and secondary forms. In either case, no specific radiographic findings are noted. The urographic findings generally depend on the degree of renal impairment (Fig. 108.53). In some cases, the amyloid accumulation produces bilaterally enlarged, smooth kidneys. The collecting systems are found to be normal, but they may be poorly visualized because of renal insufficiency. In some longstanding cases, the kidneys are actually found to be decreased in size, although the renal contour usually remains smooth. The angiographic findings in renal amyloidosis are nonspecific and of little help in establishing the diagnosis.

Sickle Cell Disease

Sickle cell disease causes abnormalities in both the medullary and cortical portions of the kidneys. Radiographic findings are encountered in patients with both SS and SA hemoglobinopathies. The renal size in sickle cell disease is usually normal,

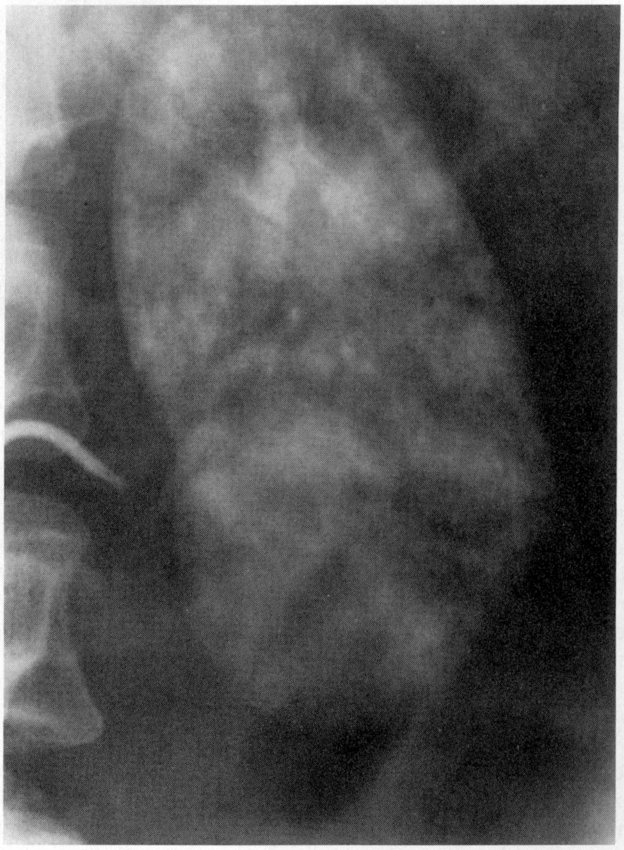

Figure 108.52. Scleroderma. This late-phase angiographic film of the left kidney demonstrates the spotted appearance to the nephrogram seen in scleroderma. The kidney is slightly small, but the contours of the kidney remain smooth and normal.

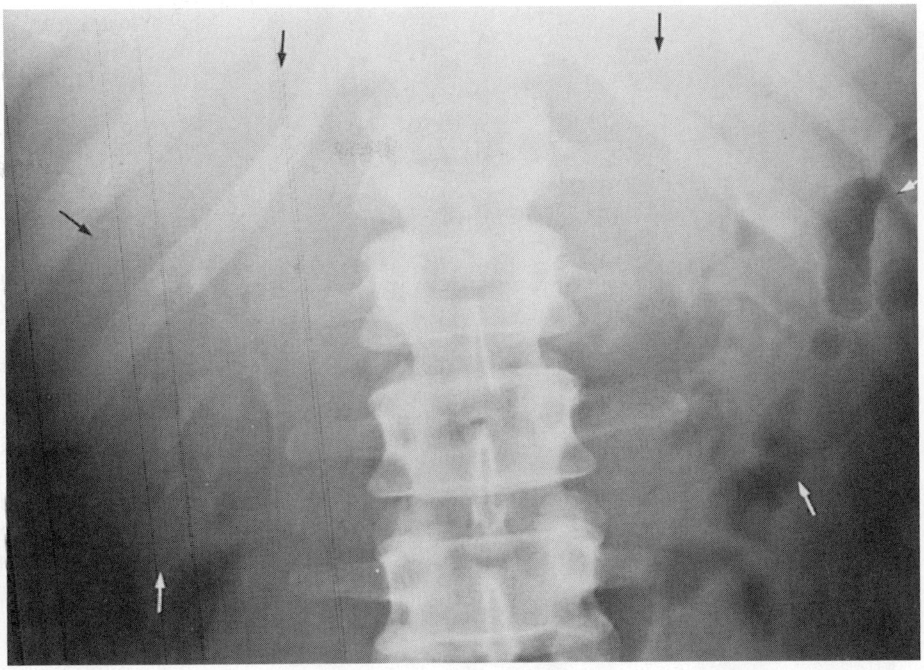

Figure 108.53. Amyloidosis. Bilateral enlarged kidneys are identified in this case of renal involvement with amyloid. Note that the contours of the kidney are smooth bilaterally *(arrows)*. Faintly opacified but normal collecting systems are seen in the kidneys.

although bilaterally enlarged kidneys may be encountered. Decreased renal size is rare and usually occurs only when renal failure is also present. IVP usually is performed in the sickle cell patient to investigate microscopic or gross hematuria. Nonionic contrast material should be used in all sickle cell patients requiring contrast. The hyperosmolar ionic contrast agents cause sickling and thus may precipitate a sickle cell crisis. The most common radiographic finding in the kidney is papillary necrosis (Fig. 108.54). The calyceal changes in the sickle cell patient are indistinguishable from other causes of renal papillary necrosis. Because of the inability to concentrate urine, there may be poor visualization of the collecting system in the IVP. The normal visualization of the calyceal system depends on adequate concentration of the contrast material within the collecting tubules. Other findings of sickle cell disease may be noted on plain films of the abdomen or during IVP. The most common abdominal radiographic finding of sickle cell disease is noted in the lumbar spine. General osteoporosis usually occurs, with coarsening of the trabeculae. In addition, the central portion of the endplate of the vertebral body is deformed, leading to a fish-mouth deformity (Fig. 108.55). Aseptic necrosis of the femoral heads may be seen in patients with sickle cell disease. Gallstones are commonly encountered. A small calcified spleen resulting from infarction may be seen in the left upper quadrant.

Diabetic Nephropathy

Nearly all diabetic patients will have some degree of change in their kidneys when the disease process is longstanding. The areas of involvement include the vascular tree, the glomerulus, and the renal papilla. Initial renal involvement in the diabetic patient tends to lead to a slightly larger than normal kidney, with normal-appearing collecting systems on intravenous urography. As the disease process progresses, the kidneys become slightly smaller than normal. The borders of the kidneys are usually smooth or may be slightly irregular because of small areas of ischemic infarction. Renal papillary necrosis may occur in the diabetic patient, especially in the presence of infection, obstruction, or both. Multiple areas of papillary involvement in both kidneys may be seen on intravenous urography. The typical cavitating lesions in the renal papillae are identified, with occasional filling defects noted within the calyces resulting from the sloughed papillae. Atheromatous narrowing of the main

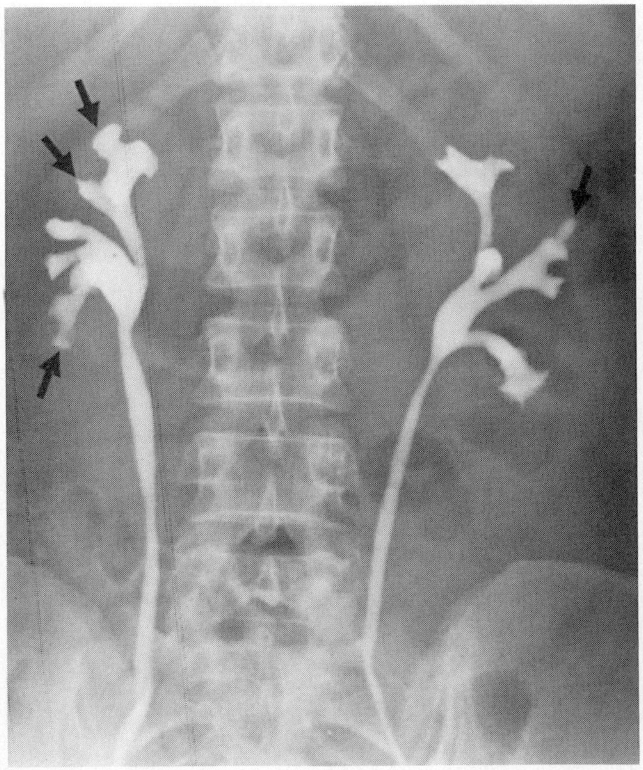

Figure 108.54. Sickle cell disease. Multiple areas of papillary necrosis *(arrows)* are present bilaterally on this retrograde pyelogram in a patient with sickle cell disease.

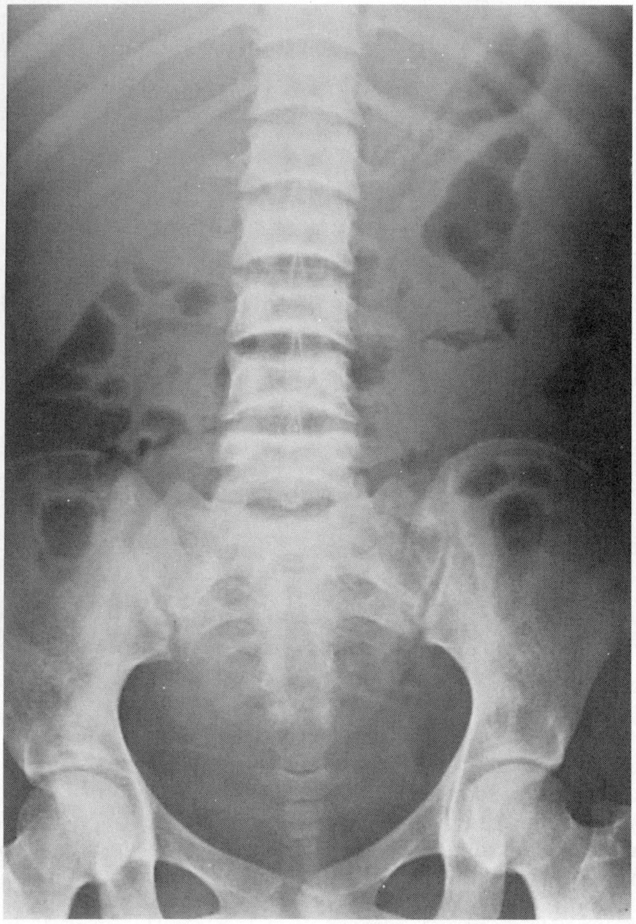

Figure 108.55. Sickle cell disease. This plain film of the abdomen demonstrates deformity of the central portion of the endplate of multiple lumbar vertebra bodies. This fishmouth deformity occurs commonly in patients with sickle cell disease.

renal artery and its segmental branches may be seen (Fig. 108.56). Diabetic patients may have renovascular hypertension because of the atheromatous narrowing of the main renal artery.

Cystic Diseases of the Kidney

Renal Dysplasia

Multicystic kidney is the most common form of renal dysplasia and is a common cause of abdominal mass in the neonate. Usually, only one kidney is affected. Focal or segmental involvement may be found. Bilateral multicystic kidneys are incompatible with life (Fig. 108.57).

The plain film of the abdomen in a patient with multicystic kidney usually reveals a large mass in the region of the flank. IVP shows this mass to be nonfunctional in that no excretion of contrast material is identified (Fig. 108.58). In addition to the congenital abnormalities that may be present in the contralateral kidney, this kidney may show some hypertrophy. The ultrasonographic appearance of a multicystic kidney is one of multiple sonolucent masses of varying size, with or without enclosed debris. Retrograde urography usually demonstrates either the complete absence of a ureter or atresia, usually in the upper third of the ureter. Angiography (Fig. 108.58) shows either a hypoplastic renal artery on the affected side or complete absence of the renal artery. When a multicystic kidney is first discovered in later life in older children or adults, the dysplastic kidney may show masses with multiple ringlike calcifications. Again, the kidney is nonfunctional. There is usually compensatory hypertrophy of the opposite kidney.

Polycystic Disease

Polycystic kidney disease is classified as infantile or adult. The radiographic findings in the infantile form include bilaterally enlarged kidneys, poor visualization of the kidneys because of impaired renal function, and a prolonged mottled nephrogram with a striated or streaky appearance (Fig. 108.59).

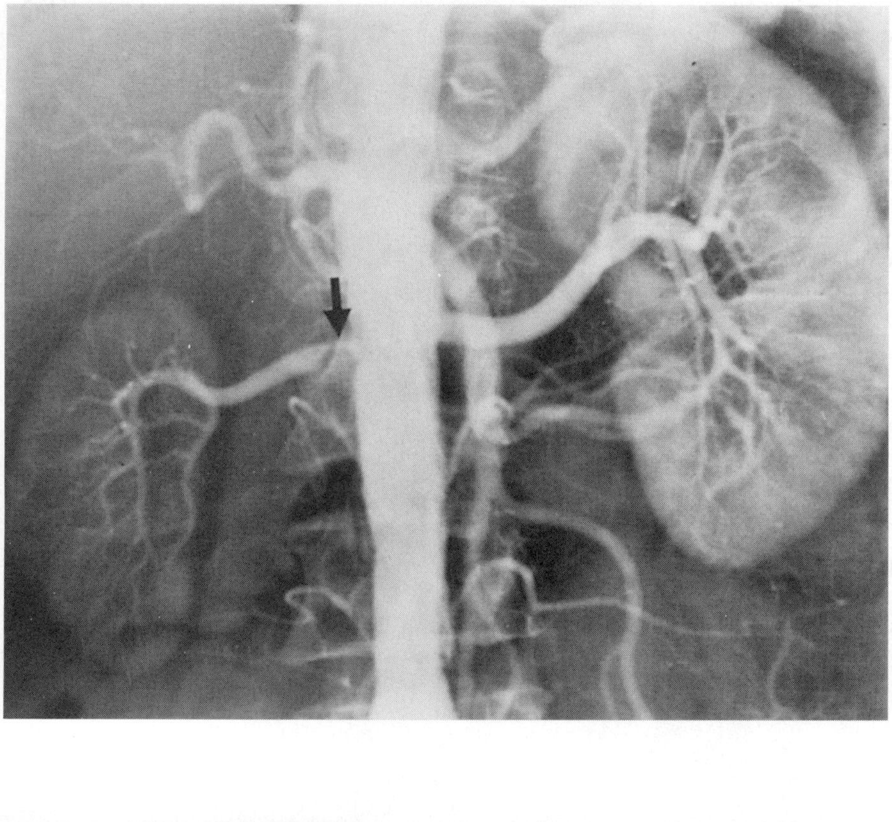

Figure 108.56. Diabetes mellitus. Extensive atheromatous narrowing of the proximal main right renal artery *(arrow)* is demonstrated in this 35-year-old diabetic patient with hypertension. Note also the small size of the right kidney when compared with the left.

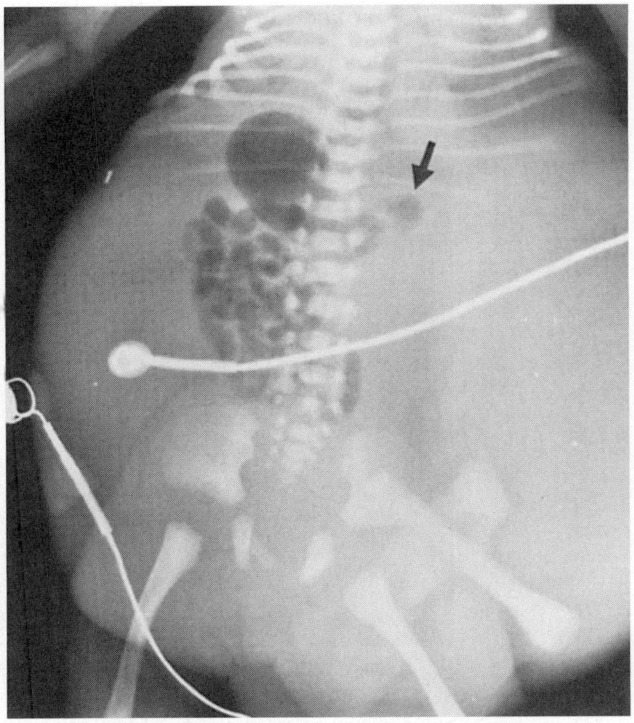

Figure 108.57. Bilateral multicystic kidneys. This newborn with multiple congenital abnormalities shows evidence of ascites, with the bowel floating centrally and huge flank masses bilaterally caused by multicystic kidneys. Note also the reversed appearance of the stomach bubble and duodenum *(arrow)* because of a situs inversus. This newborn lived only 36 hours.

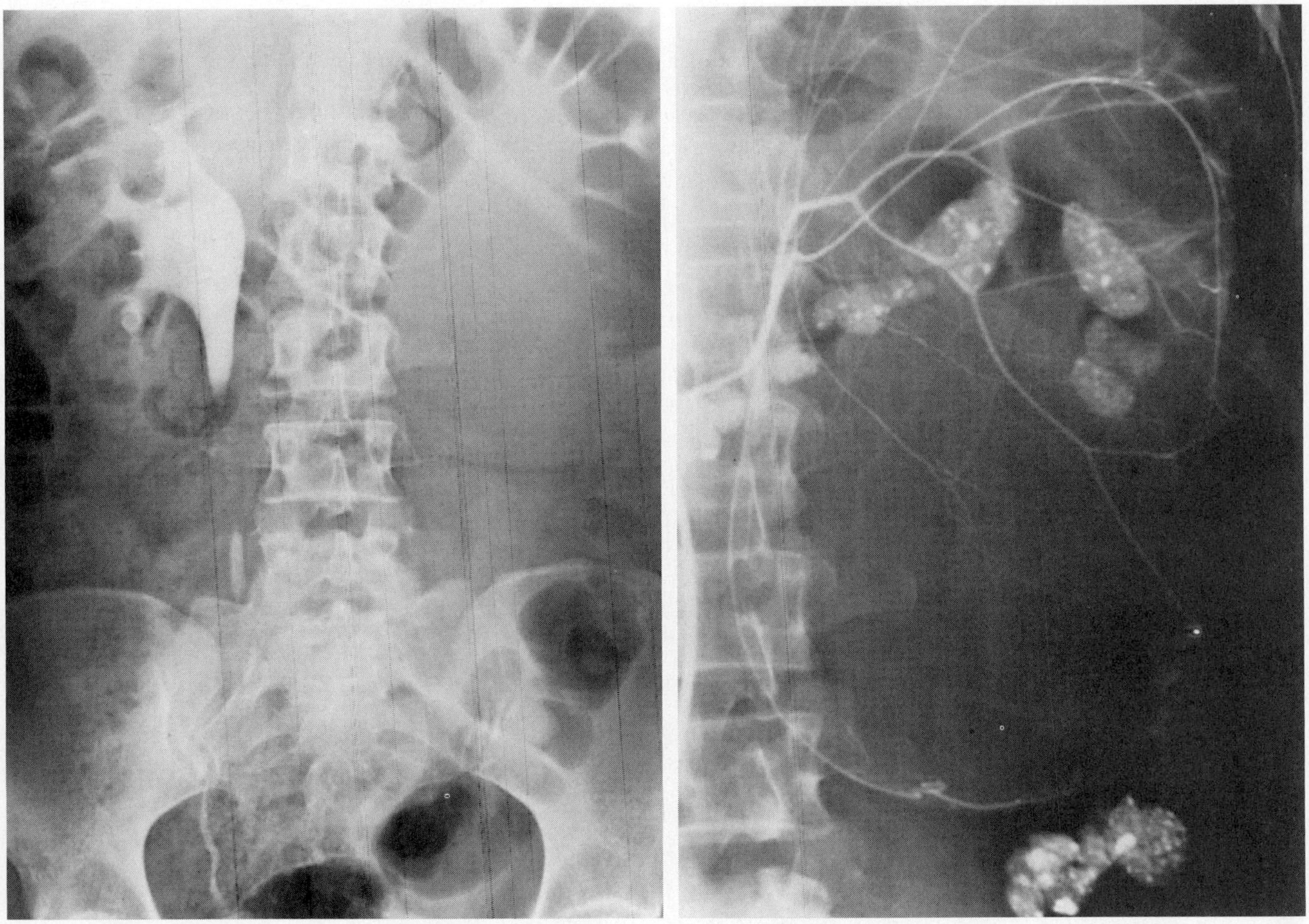

Figure 108.58. Congenital multicystic kidney. This adult had a large left-sided mass that demonstrated no excretion on an intravenous pyelogram **(left).** An attempted retrograde pyelogram showed no evidence of a ureter on the left. A selective left renal arteriogram **(right)** demonstrates a small, hypoplastic left renal artery, with extensive splaying of the remaining renal branches around the congenital multicystic kidney. No renal cortex or functioning elements are seen. The dense areas overlying the middle and lower portion of the kidney represent contrast material within the large bowel from a previous gastrointestinal study.

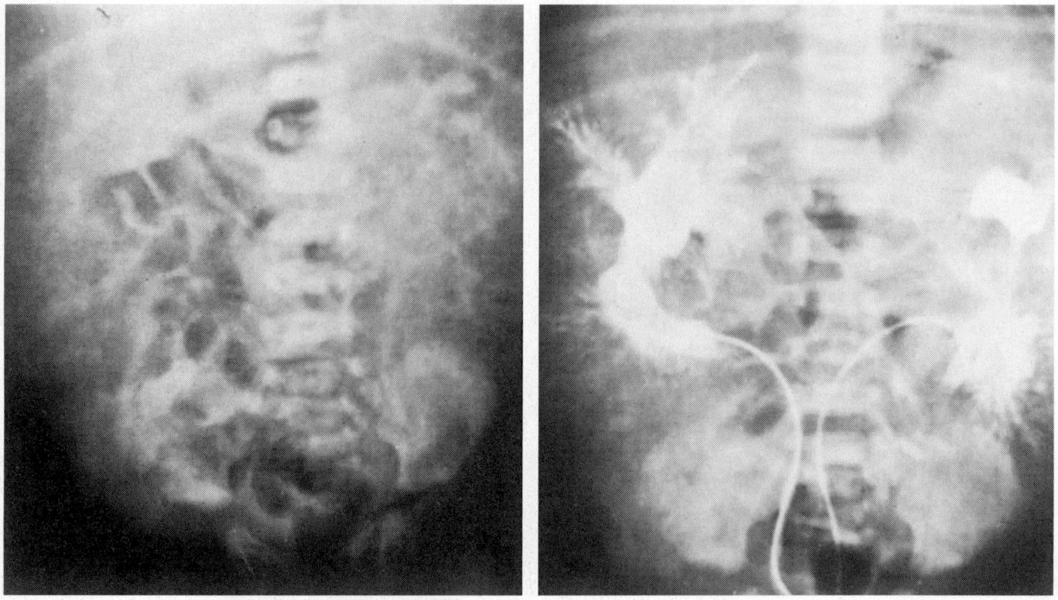

Figure 108.59. Infantile polycystic disease. **Left:** The intravenous pyelogram in this infant demonstrates a nonhomogenous nephrogram with some streaking of contrast material in the periphery. Both kidneys are markedly enlarged. **Right:** Bilateral retrograde pyelograms show contrast material refluxing into the dilated collecting tubules to the calyceal system. Again, note the marked enlargement of the kidneys.

In the adult form, the kidneys are enlarged, with a nodular or irregular contour (Figs. 108.60 and 108.61). There is extensive distortion and splaying of the calyces. The nephrogram reveals a characteristically mottled Swiss cheese appearance. Calcification in the cyst wall occasionally occurs. The ultrasonographic appearance of adult polycystic disease is relatively characteristic, with multiple sonolucent areas of varying size within the kidney. Liver cysts occasionally may be recognized by sonogra-

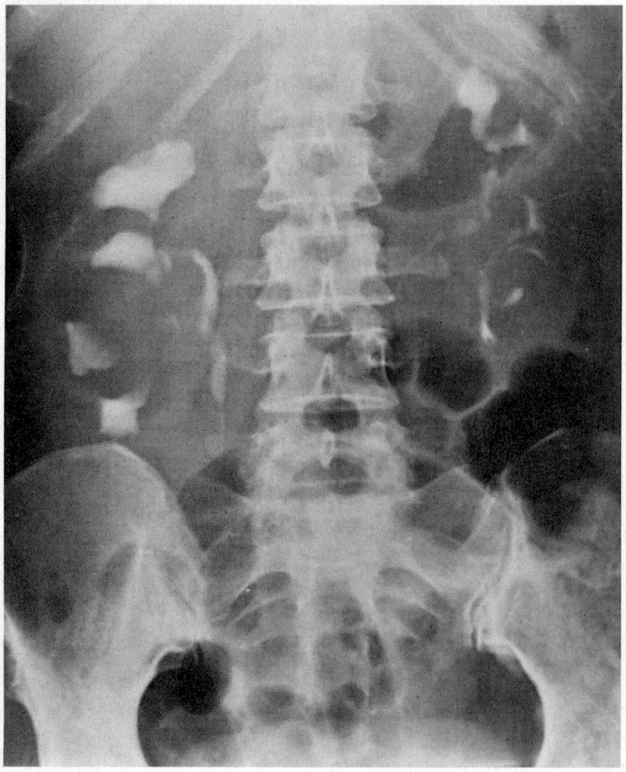

Figure 108.60. Adult polycystic disease. This film from an intravenous pyelogram shows moderately enlarged kidneys, with some displacement and splaying of the collecting systems by the cysts. The cysts in the lower poles of the kidneys cause more deformity in the calyces than those in the upper pole.

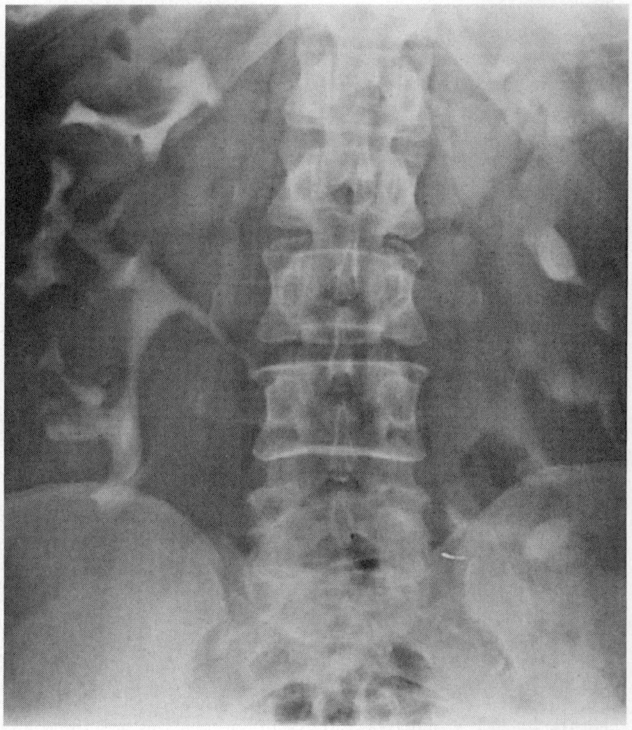

Figure 108.61. Adult polycystic disease. A film from an intravenous pyelogram in a patient with adult polycystic disease demonstrates markedly enlarged kidneys bilaterally. Distortion and splaying of the calyces are caused by the presence of multiple cysts throughout both kidneys. This demonstrates a more extensive and advanced form of polycystic disease than that seen in Fig. 108.60.

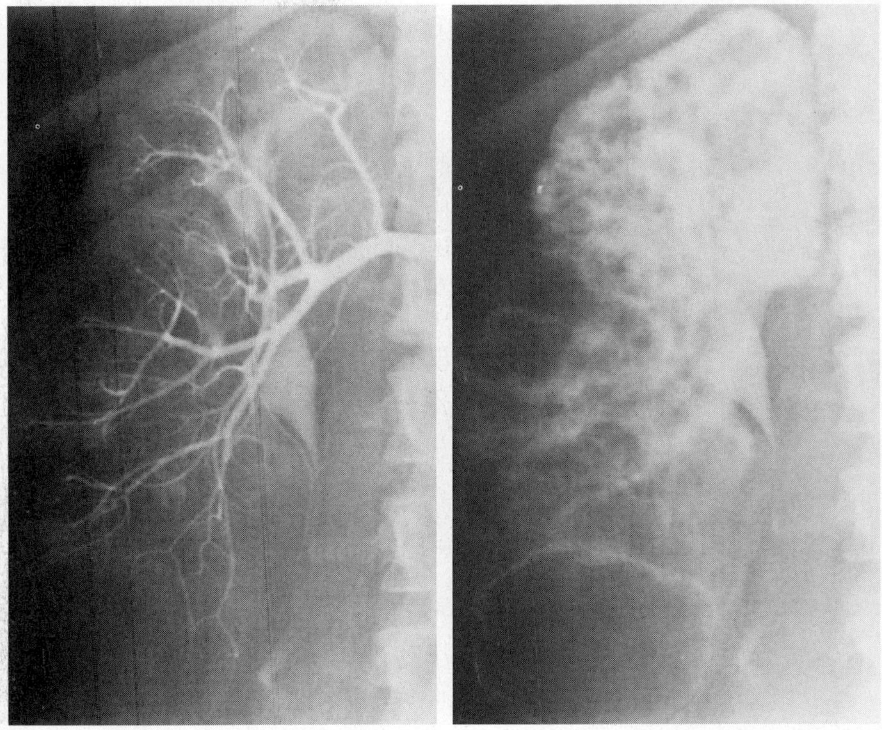

Figure 108.62. Adult polycystic disease. **Left:** The early phase, right renal arteriogram demonstrates splaying of the parenchymal branches around the cysts within the right kidney. No abnormal vascularity is noted in any of the regions of the kidney. **Right:** The capillary phase of the arteriogram shows the mottled appearance of the nephrogram, with variable-sized cysts. Small cysts are best appreciated in the upper pole of the kidney, with larger cysts being seen in the lower pole.

phy. Angiography shows displacement, stretching, and elongation of the intrarenal arteries in these enlarged kidneys (Fig. 108.62). The capillary phase of the arteriogram again shows the Swiss cheese or honeycombed appearance of the kidneys. CT scanning is again characteristic in that multiple low-density, well-circumscribed, fluid-filled structures are identified throughout both kidneys, as well as other abdominal organs.

Acquired cystic disease of the kidneys is a well-known complication of advanced renal failure and long-term dialysis. It is not imaged by conventional means (i.e., IVP). CT and ultrasound are the methods of choice to evaluate these patients.

Renal Cysts in Hereditary Syndromes

Small cortical renal cysts are occasionally associated with some hereditary syndromes. For example, in patients with tuberous sclerosis, small cortical cysts are identified in approximately 10% of cases. However, these cysts are small and usually not demonstrable by radiographic studies.

Renal Cortical Cysts

The simple renal cyst is the most commonly encountered renal mass lesion. Simple cysts are rarely found in individuals younger than 25 to 30 but are very common in those older than 50. In at least 50% of patients, single or multiple simple cysts are found at autopsy. They appear to arise frequently in the cortex. The specific cause of simple renal cysts is unknown. One to two percent may calcify with a peripheral, curvilinear type of calcification. This type of calcification is not pathognomonic because it may also be found in renal cell carcinoma. Nonperipheral calcification, however, is usually associated with renal cell carcinoma.

The radiographic findings on intravenous urography depend on the position of the cyst and the associated deformity in the rest of the kidney. The plain film of the abdomen may occasionally cause a mass overlying the area of the kidney if the cyst is quite large. The most common urographic findings are a deformity in the contour of the kidney, with associated displacement of splaying of the pelvocalyceal system. Tomography during the IVP should reveal a renal mass that is well circumscribed and lucent (Fig. 108.63). There is usually bulging to the outer contour of the kidney. The wall of the cyst should be paper thin, and a clear-cut line of demarcation between the cyst and renal parenchyma should be identified. A beaklike or clawlike deformity may be seen at the interface between the cyst and the rest of the kidney (Figs. 108.63 and 108.64). Again, calyceal displacement and splaying will be identified on tomography.

Ultrasonography of a renal mass is highly accurate in differentiating fluid-containing structures, such as renal cysts from solid masses. The ultrasonographic appearance of a renal cyst is one of a sonolucent, well-circumscribed structure with excellent through transmission of sound and demonstration of a smooth back wall.

The angiographic appearance of a simple renal cyst is that of an avascular mass (Fig. 108.64). The renal arteries are merely displaced by the cyst and do not appear abnormal or show evidence of neovascularity. The wall of the cyst, when it is seen during the capillary phase of the angiogram, is well delineated, smooth, and paper thin.

Percutaneous aspiration of a renal cyst can be undertaken with either fluoroscopic guidance or ultrasonographic localization. The aspirated fluid is usually clear or slightly amber with a low fat content, low protein, and low lactate dehydrogenase. Histologic examination shows normal-appearing cells. When the fluid is blood tinged and has a high fat content or high lactate dehydrogenase and the cells are abnormal, tumor should be suspected. Contrast material may be instilled into the cyst to reveal the smooth walls of a simple cyst (Fig. 108.65).

Medullary Sponge Kidney

Medullary sponge kidney, or renal tubular ectasia, is a noninherited developmental disorder. Ectasia and cystic dilation of

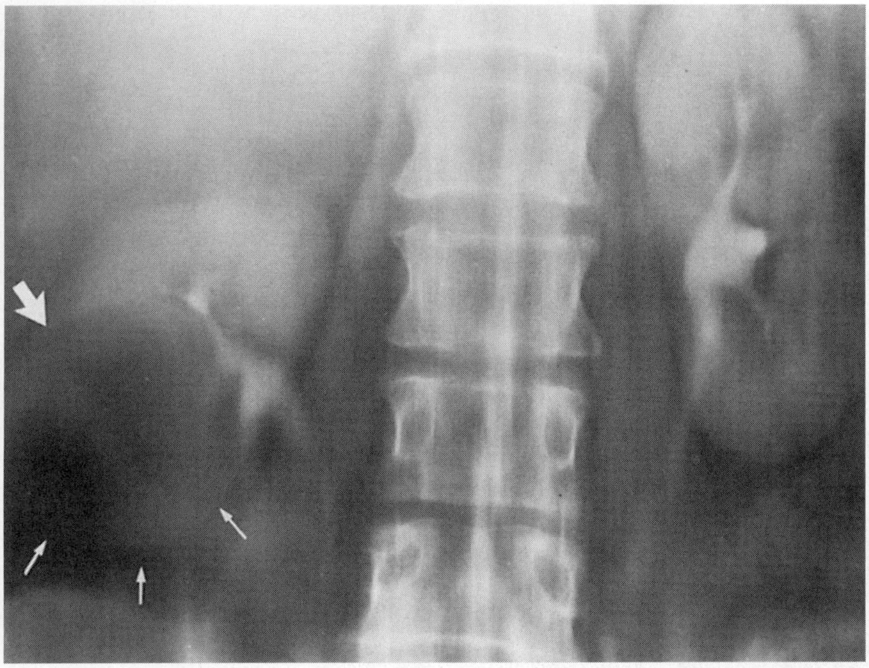

Figure 108.63. Simple renal cyst. This tomographic film from an intravenous pyelogram shows a moderate-sized cyst in the lower pole of the right kidney. There is sharp margination between the cyst and normal renal parenchyma *(large arrow)* and a pencil-thin rim *(small arrows)* characteristic of simple renal cysts.

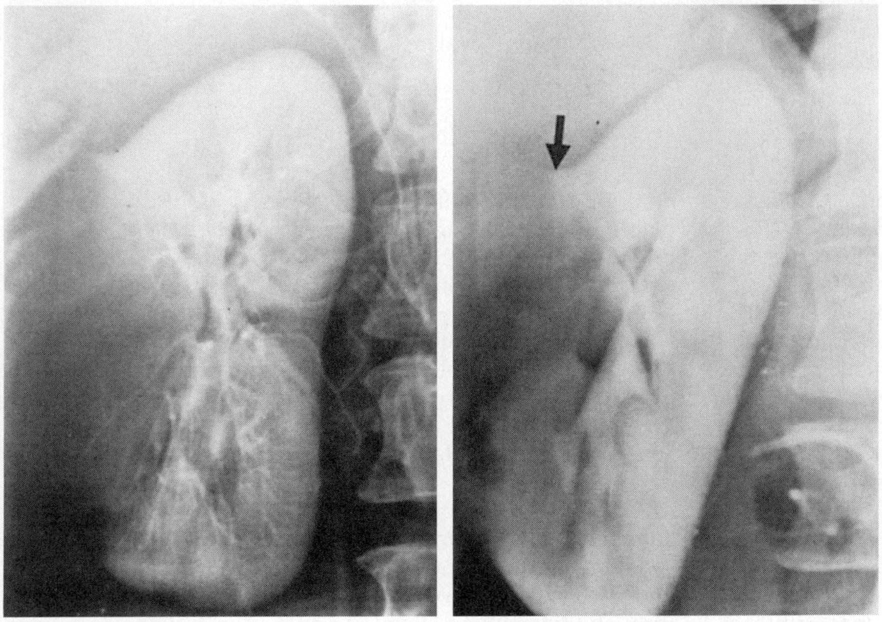

Figure 108.64. Simple renal cyst. **Left:** A mid- to late-phase arterial film from a selective right renal arteriogram demonstrates no vascularity in the region of the right renal cyst projecting from the midportion of the kidney. **Right:** The capillary phase shows the sharp break between the cyst and the normal renal parenchyma *(arrow)*.

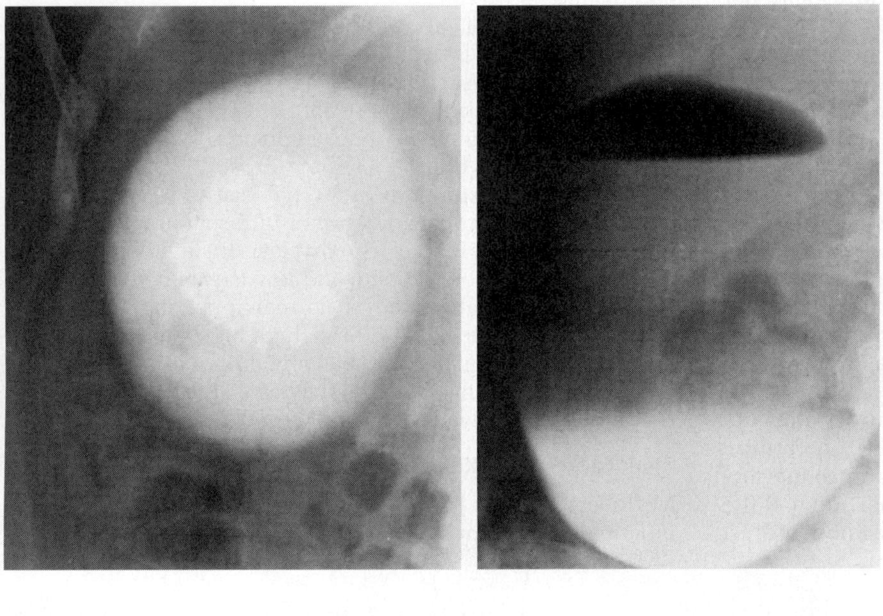

Figure 108.65. Simple renal cyst: cyst puncture. **Left:** With the patient in a supine position, contrast material is seen to outline the interior of the cyst. Pantopaque, the denser contrast material, is seen in the more central region of the cyst. **Right:** With the patient upright, the various layers of air, urine, contrast material, and Pantopaque are seen to layer out in this smooth-walled, simple renal cyst.

the distal collecting tubules occur. In most instances, the patients are asymptomatic, but the tubular ectasia predisposes to stasis, stone formation, and subsequently infection. Involvement is usually bilateral, although as few as one calyx may be involved. Radiographically, normal-sized kidneys usually are found. The extent of dilation of the collecting tubules determines the radiographic appearance. Discrete linear (brush border) or rounder collections of contrast media are seen projecting into the renal pyramid from the calyx (Fig. 108.66). In more severe cases, saccular dilations occur, which appear almost grapelike or beadlike as they extend off the calyx into the pyramid. Rarely, there is splaying or distortion of the calyces themselves. Small renal calculi may be identified in the ectatic tubules (Fig. 108.67). The calculi may eventually pass into the collecting systems of the kidney.

Medullary Cystic Disorders

Radiographic studies are not very helpful in the diagnosis of the adult or the childhood form (familial juvenile nephronophthisis) of medullary cystic disease. The intravenous urogram is nonspecific and usually shows only small areas of vague lucency in the medullary portion of the kidney. Because of the small size of the renal cysts and accompanying renal failure, the intravenous urogram is rarely helpful in the diagnosis. Renal angiography is also nonspecific, usually showing multiple small avascular masses in the medullary portion of the kidney. In addition, loss of the corticomedullary junction and a mottled nephrogram may be observed. No areas of neovascularity or abnormal vessels are noted.

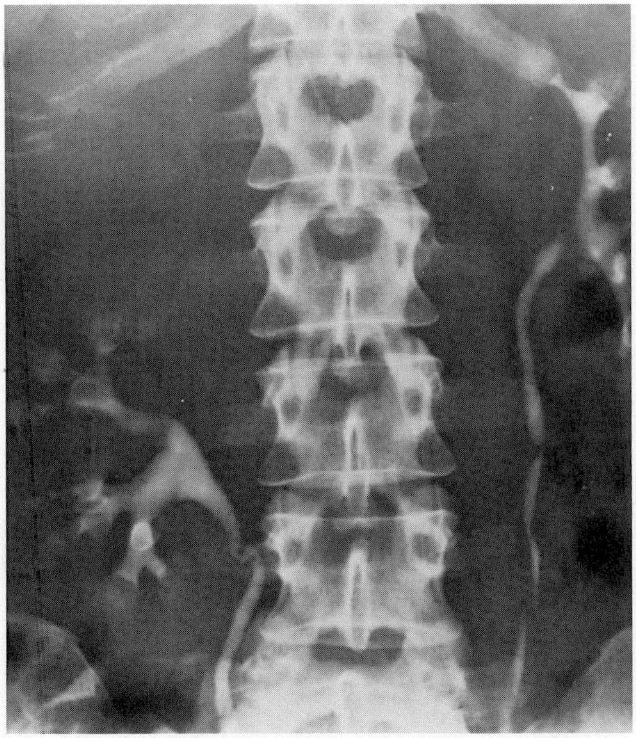

Figure 108.66. Medullary sponge kidney. On this intravenous pyelogram, discrete linear collections of contrast material are seen projecting from the normal-appearing calyces of both the right and left kidneys. This brush border appearance is characteristic of medullary sponge kidney.

Extraparenchymal Renal Cysts

Pyelogenic cysts appear as cystic structures connected to a portion of the pelvocalyceal system. Pyelogenic cysts may be termed *calyceal diverticula* or *pelvic diverticula*, depending on their site or origin. On intravenous urography, they appear as small, usually round or oval collections of contrast material connecting with the fornix of a calyx or the renal pelvis. Stasis occurs in these small diverticula, which may eventually lead to calculus formation. As a result of the calculi, infection may occur.

Parapelvic cysts are extraparenchymal cysts occurring in the region of the renal pelvis. The cysts are usually small and single but may become large and occasionally are multiple. They may result from lymphangiectasia secondary to previous infection or trauma or from an incomplete duplication anomaly. Their appearance on intravenous urography depends on their size and number. There is usually compression of the renal pelvis and infundibula (Fig. 108.68). Their appearance may be confused with that of a renal sinus lipomatosis. Ultrasonography may be used to differentiate these two conditions.

Perinephric cysts are usually collections of fluid, most frequently urine, about the kidney (Fig. 108.69). They appear to arise from leakage of urine into the perinephric space. Subsequently, fibrosis occurs with loculation of the fluid collection into a pseudocyst. The leakage of urine is usually of traumatic origin, either from obstruction or direct trauma to the kidney. The radiographic findings typically show a mass in the lucent perinephric space and may show some compression of the kidney.

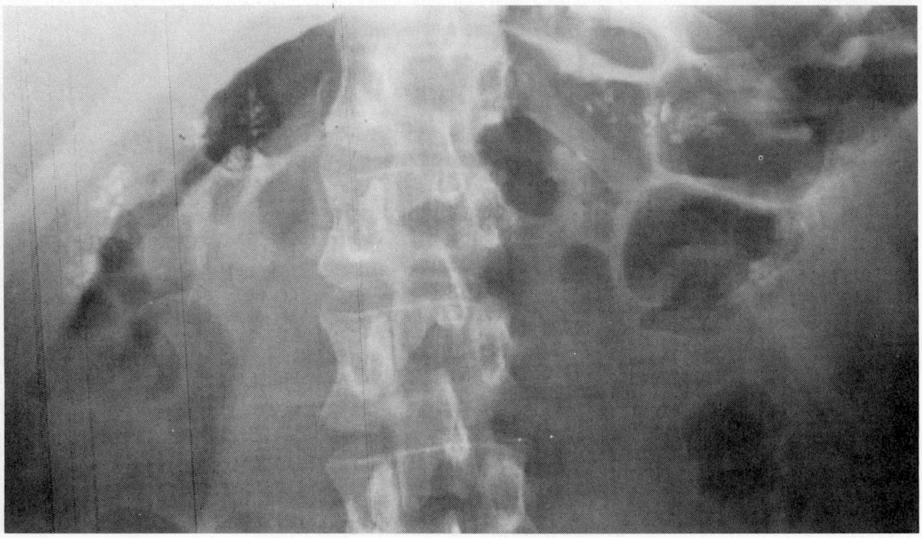

Figure 108.67. Medullary sponge kidney. Punctate calcifications are noted bilaterally in the medullary portions of the kidneys in this case of medullary sponge kidney. These discrete calculi are within the ectatic distal collecting tubules.

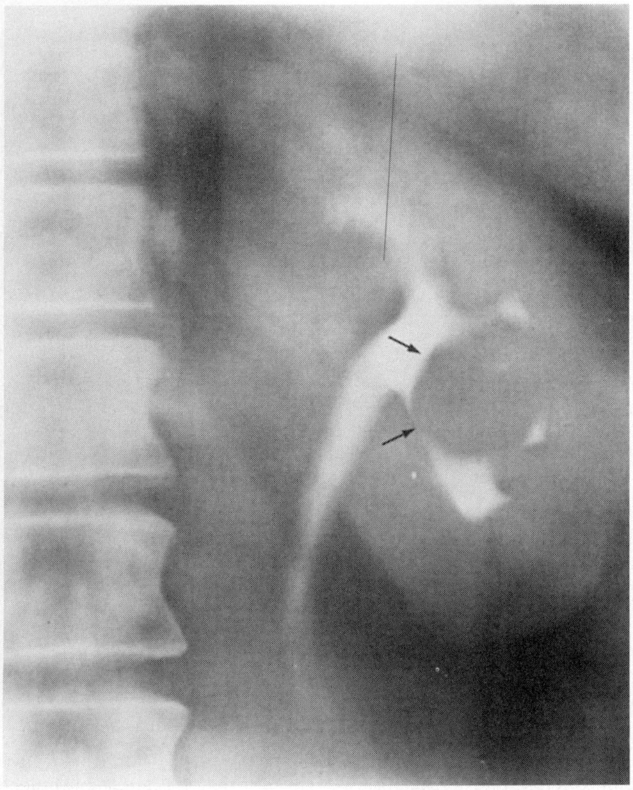

Figure 108.68. Parapelvic cyst. A single parapelvic cyst is noted on this tomogram from an intravenous pyelogram. Deformity of the lateral aspect of the renal pelvis and lower pole collecting system is caused by the presence of the cyst *(arrows)*.

Ultrasonography and CT scanning show the mass to be cystic in nature. Angiography reveals that the perinephric pseudocyst is avascular and separable from the kidney.

Sarcoidosis

The radiographic findings of sarcoidosis in the kidneys are usually related to the patient's hypercalcemia and hypercalciuria. Nephrocalcinosis and/or nephrolithiasis occur, but only rarely, in these patients. The renal size is usually normal or slightly decreased if renal insufficiency is present (Fig. 108.70).

Radiation Nephritis

The radiographic findings in radiation nephritis are nonspecific. The renal size is usually normal or reduced (Fig. 108.71). The calyceal system appears normal. If only a portion of the kidney was within the radiation field, there may be atrophy of this limited area of the kidney. Compensatory hypertrophy of the opposite kidney may occur if only one kidney was within the radiation field. This is especially true in children. Angiographic findings are extremely limited in these patients, because the changes are generally related to small vessels that are not seen with conventional angiography. Some pruning and some apparent decrease in the peripheral vasculature may occur in the more chronic forms of radiation nephritis.

Obstructive Uropathy

The term *obstructive uropathy* describes any obstructive process that causes pathologic changes, whether transient or permanent, in the urinary tract. *Hydronephrosis* is the commonly used term to describe the appearance of the urinary tract when there is any dilation of the calyces or renal pelvis. *Calyectasis, pyelectasis,* and *ureterectasis* describe anatomically the areas of dilation and involvement (calyces, renal pelvis, and ureter, respectively) by an obstructing process.

The radiographic findings depend on whether the obstruction is acute or chronic. With acute obstruction, the plain film of the abdomen usually is normal. There may be evidence of a mild ileus pattern to the bowel. The kidney involved in the obstructive process may be mildly enlarged. The cause of obstruction may be seen on the plain film, for example, a calcified renal stone (Fig. 108.3). The findings on intravenous urography are relatively classic in acute obstruction. The initial nephrogram after the injection of a contrast material is usually diminished in intensity (Fig. 108.72), but with the passage of time, the nephrogram becomes progressively more dense (Fig. 108.73). This delayed nephrogram, or obstructive nephrogram, will be seen to increase in intensity for up to several hours. Appearance of the

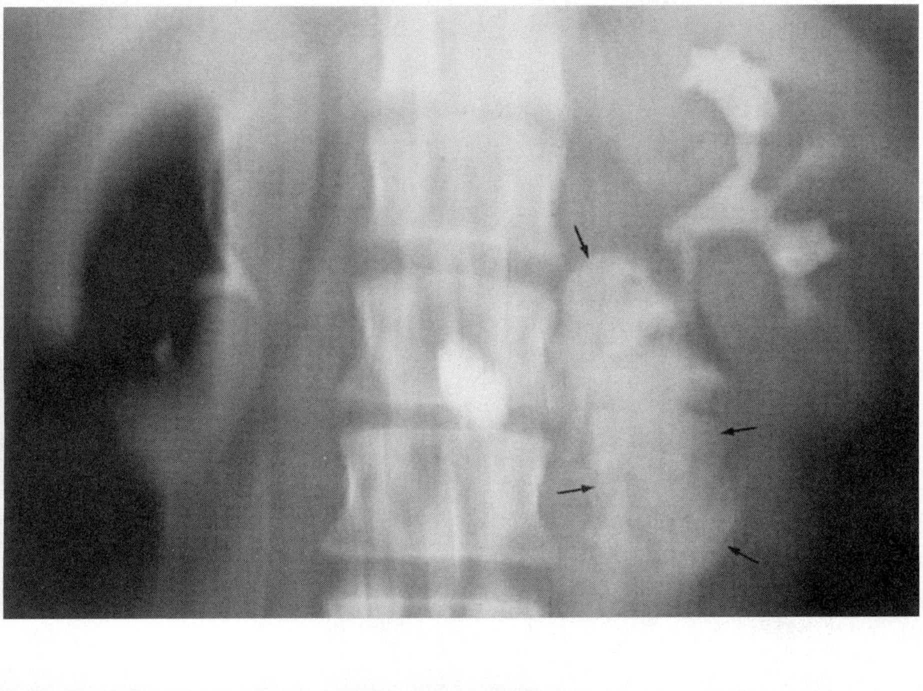

Figure 108.69. Urinoma. A tomographic film from an intravenous pyelogram shows extravasation of contrast material *(arrows)* just medial and inferior to the left renal pelvis. This urinoma resulted from a gunshot wound to the left renal pelvis and ureter. Note the bullet overlying the lumbar spine.

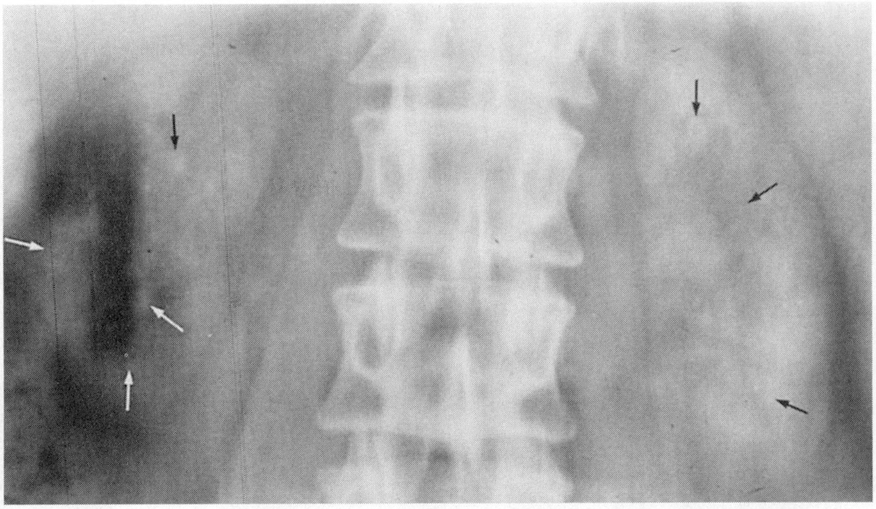

Figure 108.70. Sarcoidosis. The tomogram from an intravenous pyelogram demonstrates small kidneys bilaterally. Vague areas of calcification are seen within both kidneys *(arrows)*. Because of renal insufficiency, the collecting systems are poorly demonstrated.

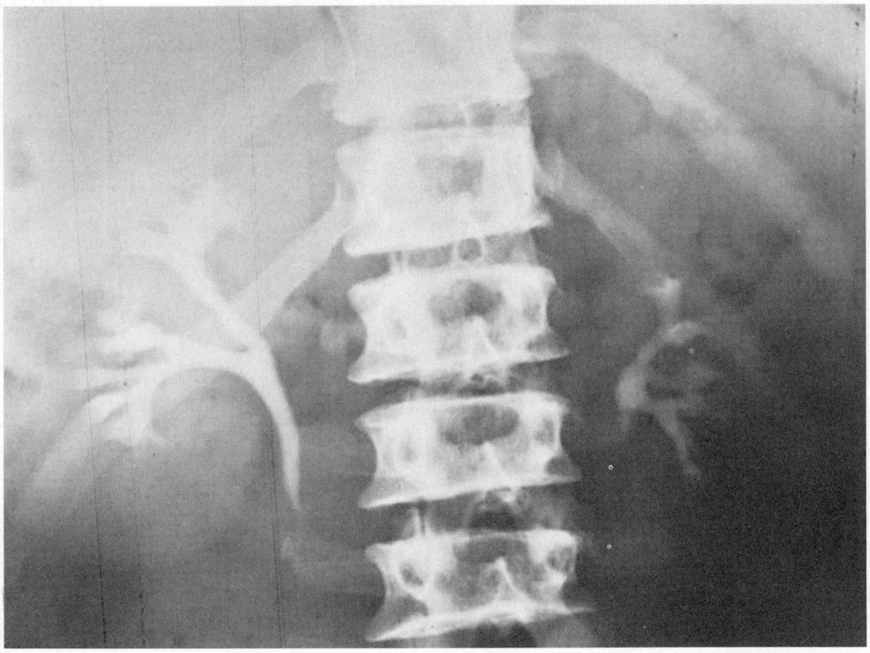

Figure 108.71. Radiation nephritis. A small left kidney is identified in this patient who had received prior radiation therapy that included the left kidney within the radiation part. The calyceal system of the left kidney appears normal, although small. Note the compensatory hypertrophy of the right kidney.

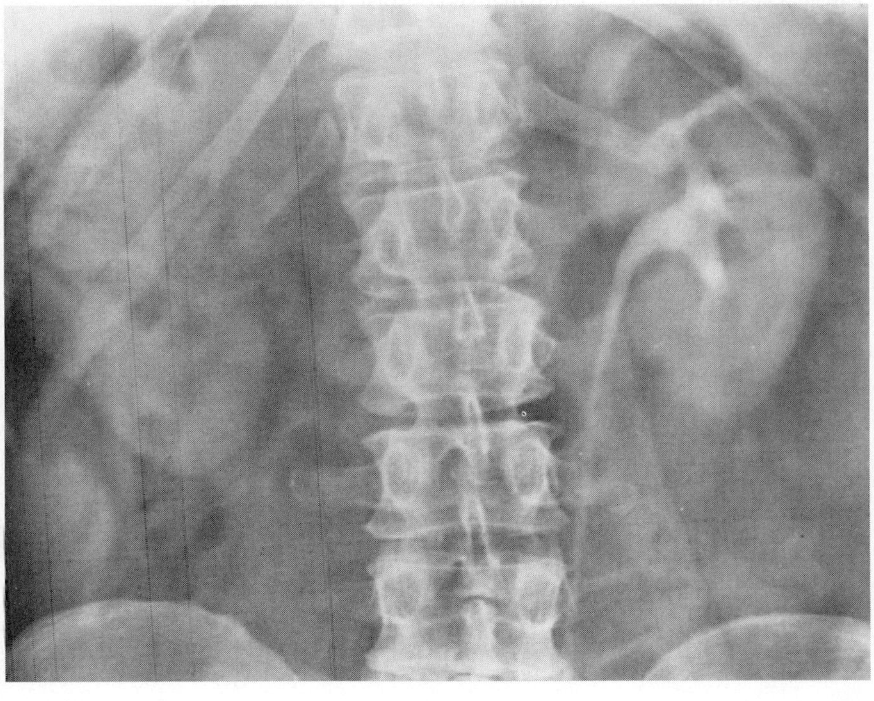

Figure 108.72. Obstructive uropathy. A diminished nephrogram is identified in the right kidney on this intravenous pyelogram. Three minutes after the injection of contrast material, the density of the right kidney is still slightly less than that of the left. Note also that contrast material is already present in the collecting system of the left kidney but not the right. This patient had an acutely obstructing distal right ureteral calculus.

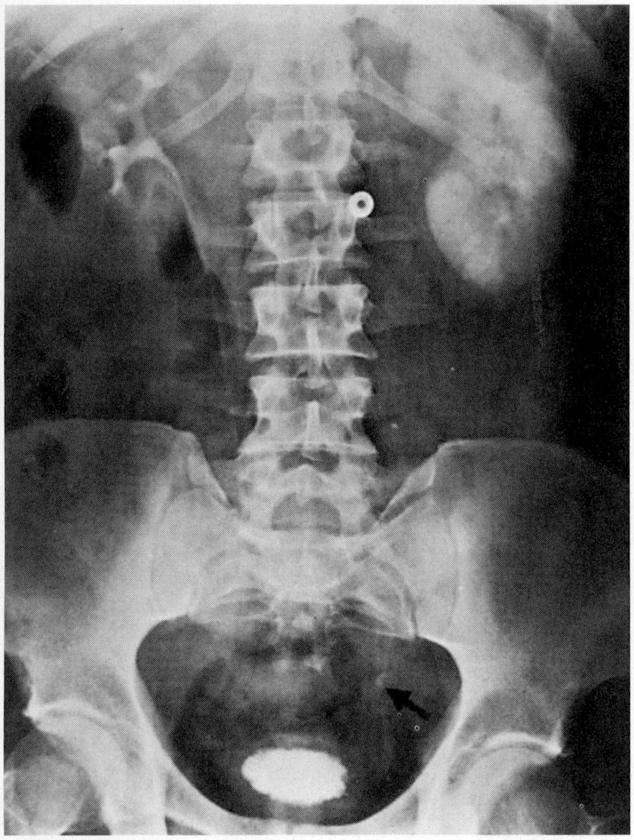

Figure 108.73. Obstructive uropathy. An obstructive nephrogram is seen on the left side of this patient with a distal left ureteral calculus *(arrow)*. This film was obtained 1 hour after the injection of intravenous contrast material. A progressively denser nephrogram was demonstrated with the passage of time. Note also that no contrast is yet visualized within the collecting system of the left kidney.

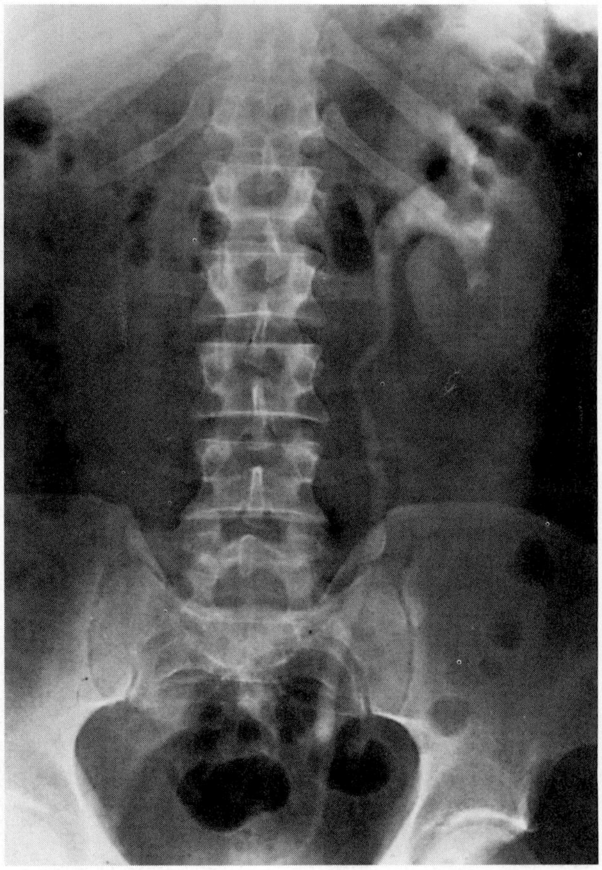

Figure 108.74. Obstructive uropathy. This 24-hour film of an intravenous pyelogram demonstrates delayed opacification and appearance time of contrast material in the left collecting system. A distal left ureteral calculus was the cause of the obstruction. There is mild dilation of the calyces, renal pelvis, and ureter on the left side. Note that contrast material is no longer visible in the normal right system.

excreted contrast material in the calyces is delayed (Fig. 108.74). The difference between the normal and obstructive kidney may be minimal, or the contrast material may not appear within the calyceal system for hours. Once there is contrast material within the calyces and ureter above the level of obstruction, these areas may remain visualized for up to 24 to 48 hours. The kidney size itself usually is increased with obstruction. If the excretion of contrast material by the obstructed kidney is not adequate to identify the site and cause of obstruction, antegrade pyelography or retrograde pyelography may be necessary to evaluate the obstruction further. With acute obstruction, mild to moderate dilation of the pelvocalyceal system occurs (Fig. 108.75). After the obstruction is relieved, the collecting systems usually revert to normal within several weeks. In acute obstruction, the ureter proximal to the site of obstruction is usually mildly to moderately dilated and has a normal, straight course. Occasionally, pyelosinus extravasation may be seen in acute obstruction (Fig. 108.76). Pyelosinus extravasation develops as a result of small ruptures within the fornices of the collecting systems. Contrast material may be seen to extravasate into the perirenal tissues during the intravenous urogram.

With chronic obstruction, extremely large masses may be seen on plain films of the abdomen. The usual status of the kidney in chronic obstruction is that of a tremendously dilated renal pelvis and collecting system (Fig. 108.77). On some occasions, the kidney may in fact be small because of extensive atrophy and reabsorption of the remaining urine. With progressive loss of function in chronic obstruction, an obstructive nephrogram

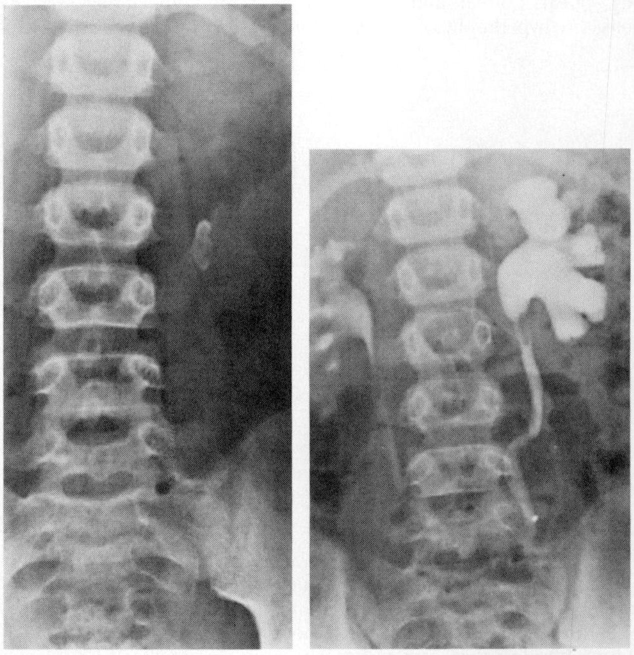

Figure 108.75. Obstructive uropathy. **Left:** A plain film demonstrates the cause of the ureteral obstruction, a left ureteral calculus. **Right:** A film from an intravenous pyelogram shows moderate dilation of the collecting systems proximal to the point of obstruction.

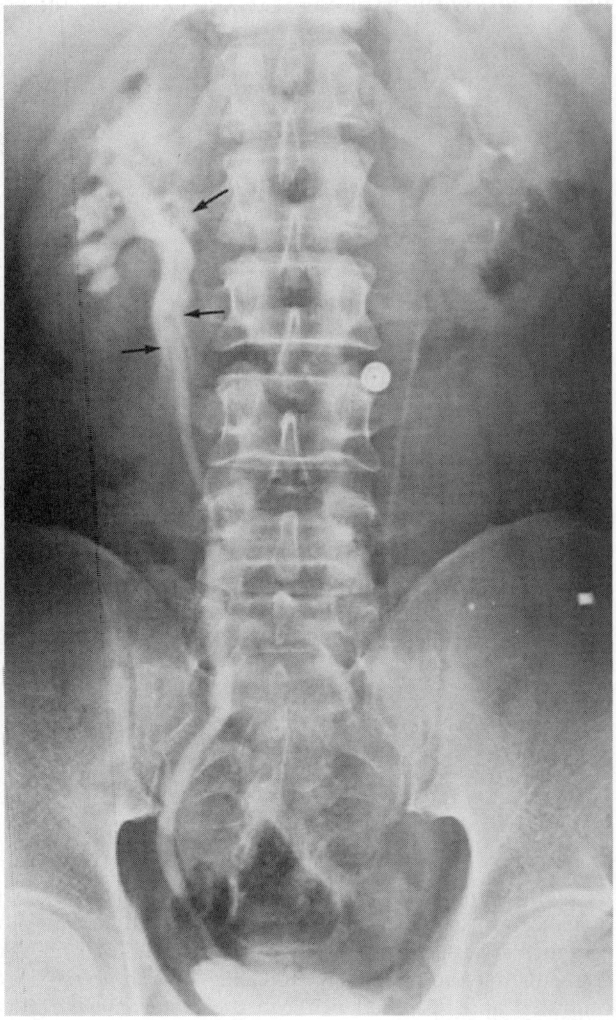

Figure 108.76. Obstructive uropathy. A distal right ureteral calculus causing acute obstruction to the right kidney leads to pyelosinus extravasation, as seen on this intravenous pyelogram. Contrast material *(arrows)* is seen outside the collecting systems and dissects along the proximal right ureter.

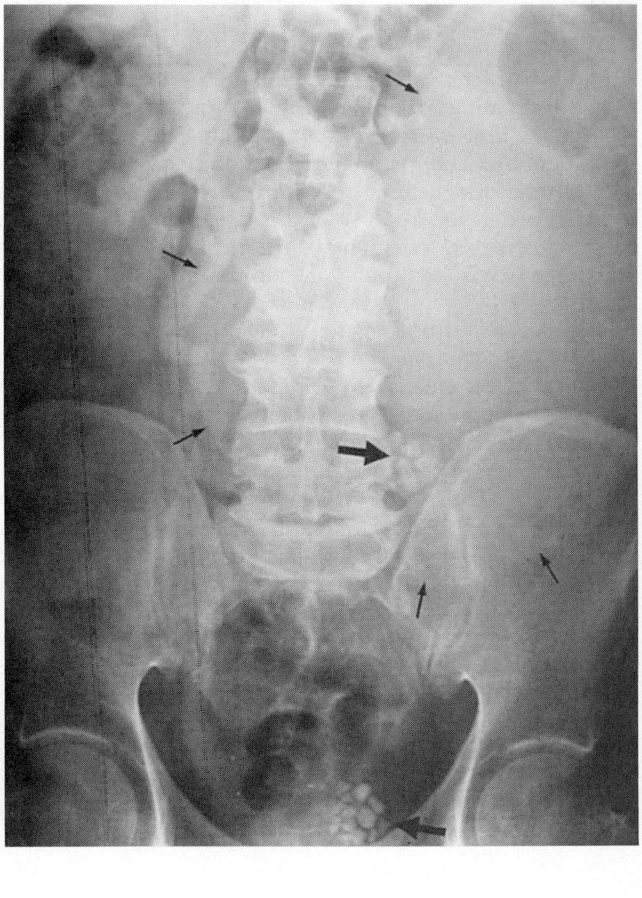

Figure 108.77. Obstructive uropathy. The intravenous pyelogram in this case of chronic bilateral obstruction (left greater than right) shows an extremely large mass on the left *(small arrows)*. Calculi, associated with the obstruction, are noted *(large arrows)* in the area of the ureteropelvic junction and the ureterovesical junction. Milder chronic obstruction on the right side causes dilation of the collecting systems and some tortuosity of the right ureter.

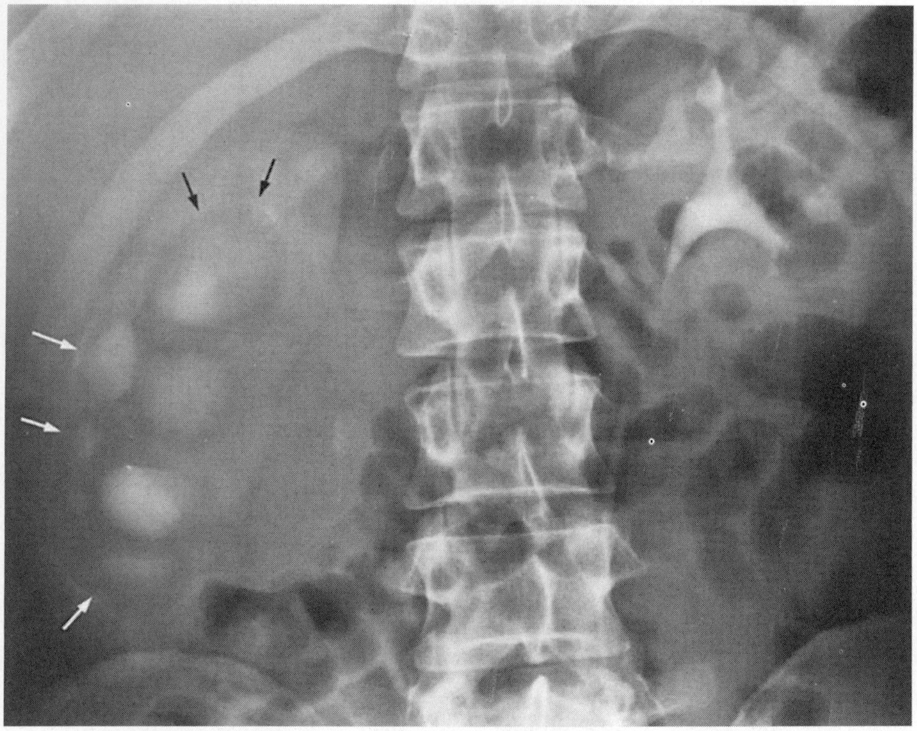

Figure 108.78. Obstructive uropathy. On this intravenous pyelogram, contrast material is just beginning to enter the dilated collecting systems in the right kidney. In the periphery of the dilated collecting systems, faint crescents *(arrows)* are noted. The crescents represent contrast material in the distal collecting tubules that is deviated by the dilated calyceal system.

may not be note with intravenous urography. Only minimal opacification of the remaining renal parenchyma may be observed. Early, as contrast material enters the collecting ducts, crescents may be noted (Fig. 108.78). These are caused by concentrated and opacified urine in the distal collecting tubules that are deviated by the dilated collecting system. The finding of crescents on intravenous urography means that some function still remains within the kidney. On lateral films, large dilated collecting systems may be noted (Fig. 108.78). If the chronic obstruction is distally located, the ureters are usually very dilated and tortuous (Figs. 108.77 and 108.79).

Delayed films, sometimes up to 24 to 48 hours after the initial injection of contrast material, are important for both acute and chronic obstruction. Because the transit time of contrast material is delayed because of the elevated intraluminal pressure in the urinary tract, it may be hours before the calyceal system, renal pelvis, and ureter are sufficiently visualized to make a diagnosis.

Direct opacification of the urinary tract involved with obstructive uropathy can be undertaken with either retrograde pyelography or antegrade pyelography (Fig. 108.79). Ultrasonographic evaluation of the obstructed urinary tract is most helpful. Assessment of the degree of obstruction and the extent of remaining renal parenchyma are easily accomplished with ultrasound. The cause of obstruction, however, may not be noted on ultrasonographic examination. CT scanning is used as a complement to other studies in evaluating the patient with obstructive uropathy. It may demonstrate a previously unknown or unsuspected cause for the obstruction.

Angiography in patients with acute obstruction may by normal. Other findings that are occasionally seen include mild to moderate enlargement of the kidney, with slight delay of transit through the renal arterial system because of increased intrarenal pressure, and edema associated with obstruction. Minimal splaying of the intrarenal arteries may occur around the mildly to moderately dilated calyces. In chronic obstruction,

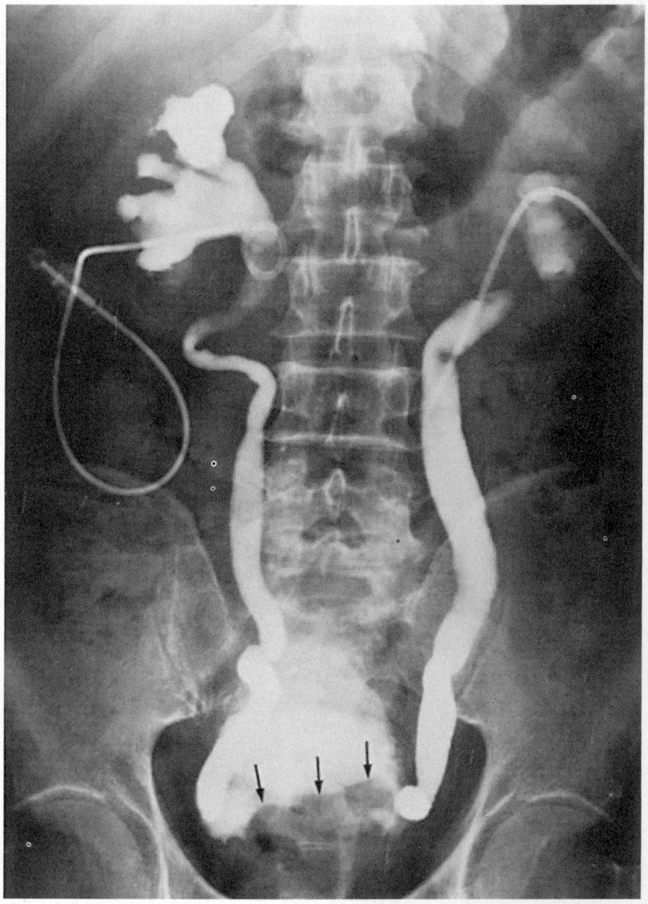

Figure 108.79. Obstructive uropathy. Bilateral percutaneous nephrostomy tubes had been placed in this patient with chronic obstruction caused by an enlarged prostate. Note the dilation and tortuosity of the ureters bilaterally. The enlarged prostate indents the base of the bladder *(arrows)*.

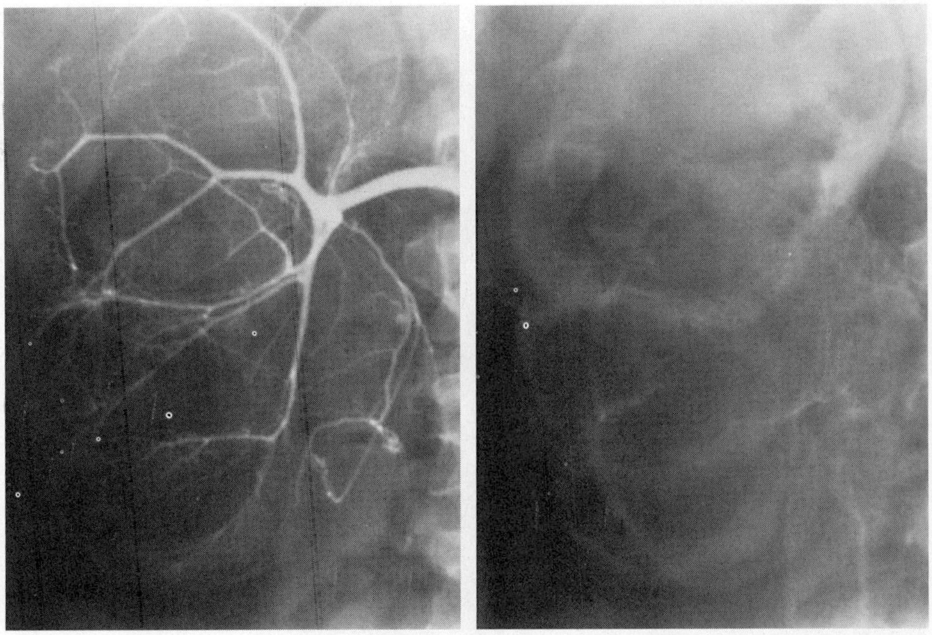

Figure 108.80. Obstructive uropathy. This selective right renal arteriogram in a patient with chronic long-standing obstruction demonstrates a main renal artery that is decreased in caliber, with extensive stretching and splaying of the intrarenal vessels around the markedly dilated calyces **(right).** The capillary phase of the arteriogram **(left)** shows only thin rims around the remaining renal parenchyma.

angiography (Fig. 108.80) generally reveals a main renal artery that is decreased in caliber. The intrarenal vessels are stretched and splayed around the markedly dilated calyces. The intrarenal vessels may appear to be elongated as they course around the dilated calyces. The kidney is usually markedly enlarged. In the capillary phase of the arteriogram, rims may be noted, showing the remaining renal tissue. Angiography in the patient with chronic obstruction may be used to assess the amount of remaining renal parenchyma to determine whether corrective surgery or nephrectomy is to be attempted.

Renal Papillary Necrosis

Renal papillary necrosis may be classified into two forms: medullary and papillary. Intravenous urography is usually the primary method used for diagnosis and evaluation of patients with suspected papillary necrosis. In patients with poor renal function, retrograde pyelography may be required to demonstrate the calyceal changes (Fig. 108.81).

In the medullary form, central necrosis occurs in the tip of the pyramid. Detachment of the necrotic papilla starts in the central region of the calyx, with the fornices of the calyx remaining intact. The resultant cavity extends from the center of the calyx and is usually round or oval. In the papillary form, necrosis occurs in a larger portion of the entire papilla. Detachment of the necrotic papilla usually begins in the region of the calyceal fornix. The resultant defect is usually triangular. A singe calyx may be involved, but because the process is usually a generalized one, the radiographic findings are generally bilateral. Various stages of the process may be seen on the same radiographic examination.

The IVP usually reveals a normal to slightly small but smooth kidneys bilaterally. Renal function is usually preserved, at least early in the course of the disease process. The earliest radiographic finding tends to be a loss of the sharp outline of the normal calyx, with slight distension of the calyces (Fig. 108.82). As the actual separation of the necrotic papillary tip begins, extravasation of contrast material will extend along the plane of separation between the still viable portion of the papilla and the

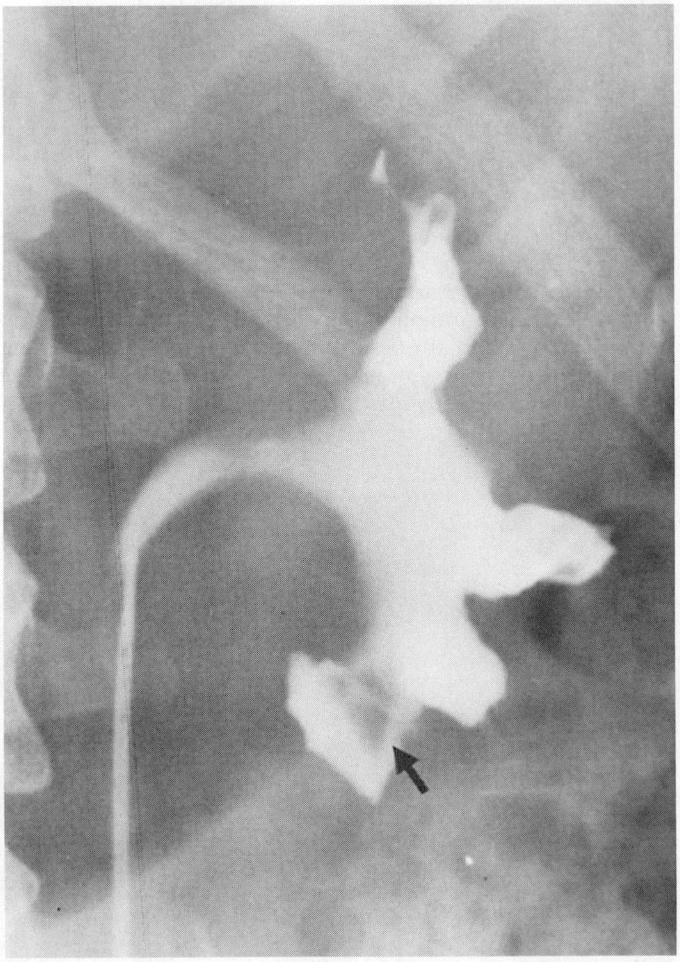

Figure 108.81. Papillary necrosis. As renal function deteriorates, retrograde pyelography may be necessary to demonstrate the changes of renal papillary necrosis. In the lower pole calyx, a sloughed, triangular papillary *(arrow)* is noted. The rest of the calyces have lost all of their normal configuration.

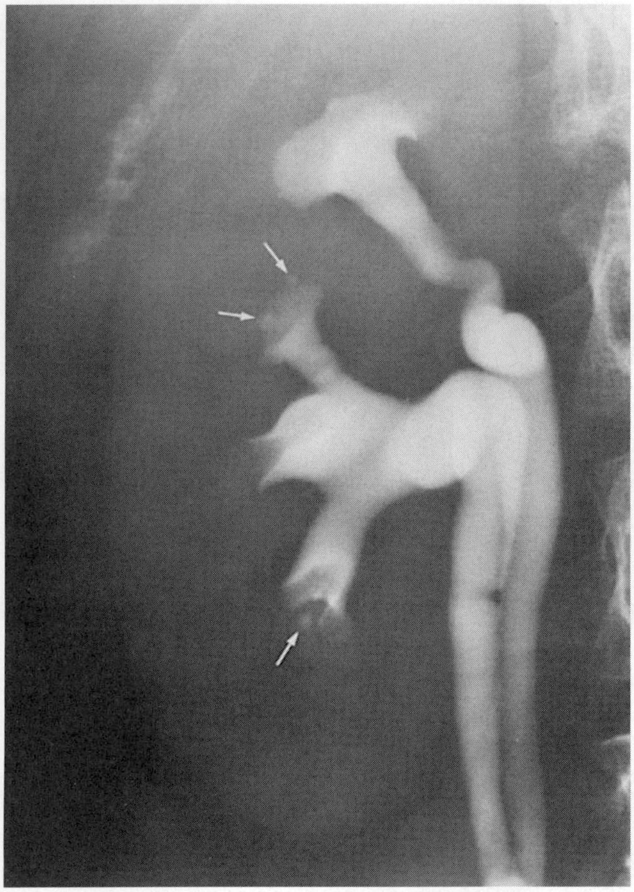

Figure 108.82. Papillary necrosis. This intravenous pyelogram demonstrates loss of the normal sharp outline of the superior pole calyx, an early sign of papillary necrosis. In the middle and lower pole calyces, a medullary type papillary necrosis is noted *(arrows)*.

necrotic sloughing tissue. After complete separation of the necrotic papillary tip, the contrast may extend in a ringlike configuration from the calyx around the sloughing papilla (Fig. 108.83). With complete separation of the necrotic segment from the tip of the renal pyramid, the tissue enters the pelvocalyceal system. It then generally fragments and is passed from the calyx into the pelvis and subsequently into the ureter and bladder. Fragments of sloughed tissue may appear as filling defects on intravenous urography (Fig. 108.84). As the fragment moves out of the area of the calyx, there is a loss of the calyceal cup (Fig. 108.85). Early, the calyx may have an irregular and ragged appearance (Fig. 108.83). In its healing stage, the calyx takes on a blunted, smooth appearance (Fig. 108.85). A portion of the sloughed material may remain sequestered within the calyx. Eventually, cal-

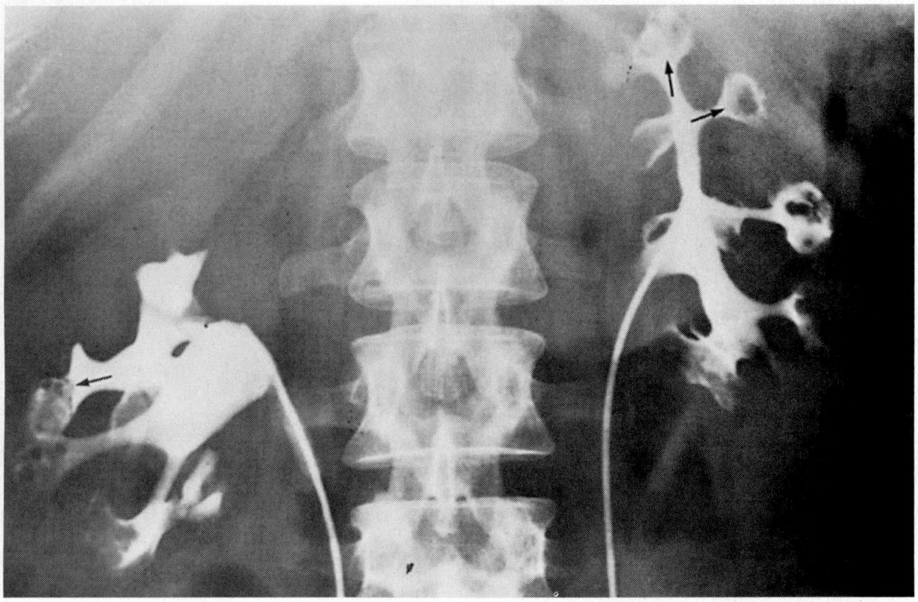

Figure 108.83. Papillary necrosis. Bilateral retrograde pyelograms demonstrate some of the classic changes in renal papillary necrosis. Ragged, irregular calyces are seen in the lower poles bilaterally. Extravasation of contrast material from the calyx around the sloughing papilla *(arrows)* forms a ringlike configuration.

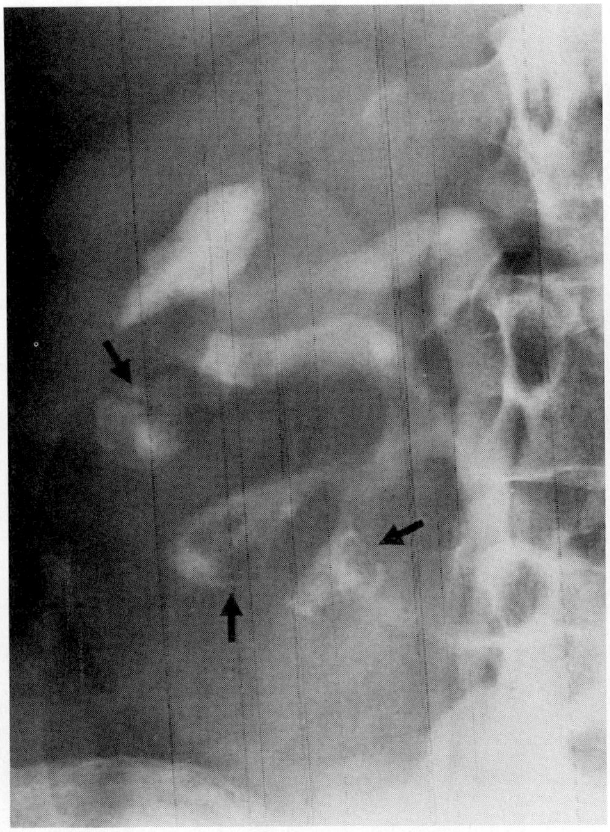

Figure 108.84. Papillary necrosis. On this intravenous pyelogram, filling defects are noted in multiple calyces *(arrows)*, representing the sloughed papillary fragments that have entered the collecting system.

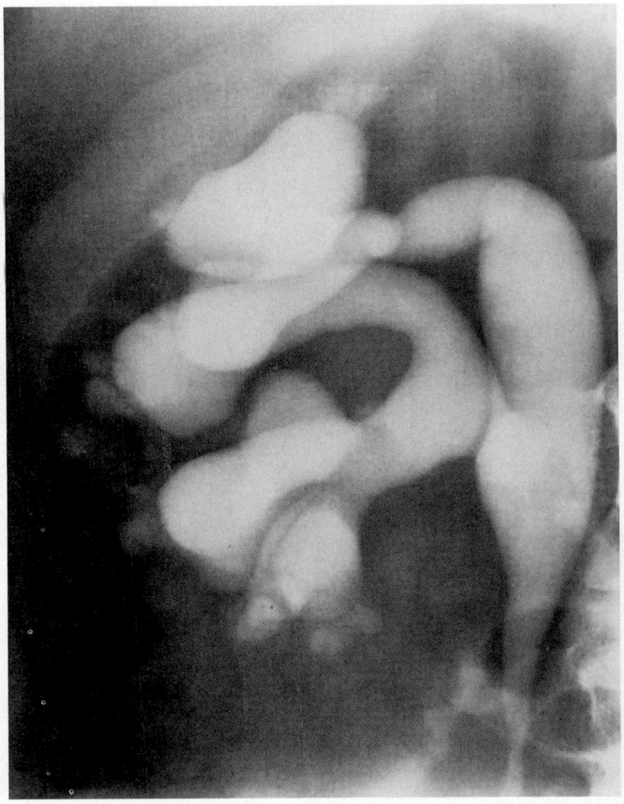

Figure 108.85. Papillary necrosis. As the acute episodes of papillary necrosis resolve, the calyces are left in a blunted condition. This film from an intravenous pyelogram also demonstrates collections of contrast material in the cavities created by the sloughed papillary elements.

cification of this tissue may result (Fig. 108.86). The end result of renal papillary necrosis is a kidney that is normal in size or slightly small, with smooth contours and blunted calyces. There are no specific angiographic features of renal papillary necrosis. The diagnosis is made from intravenous urography, occasionally with the assistance of retrograde pyelography.

Renal Artery Occlusion

Renal artery occlusion is caused by either thrombosis of the artery or embolism to the artery. The radiographic findings on plain film of the abdomen may reveal a slightly small kidney. A reflex ileus of the bowel also may be noted in acute renal artery

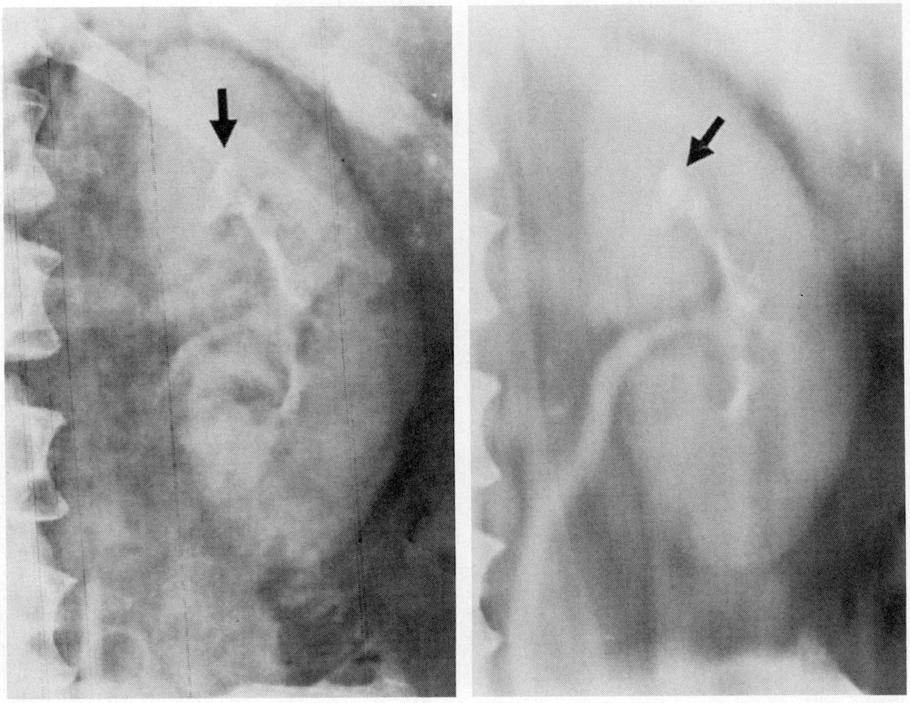

Figure 108.86. Papillary necrosis. When a fragment of renal papilla remains sequestered within a calyx, as demonstrated on this intravenous pyelogram, it may become calcified *(arrows)*.

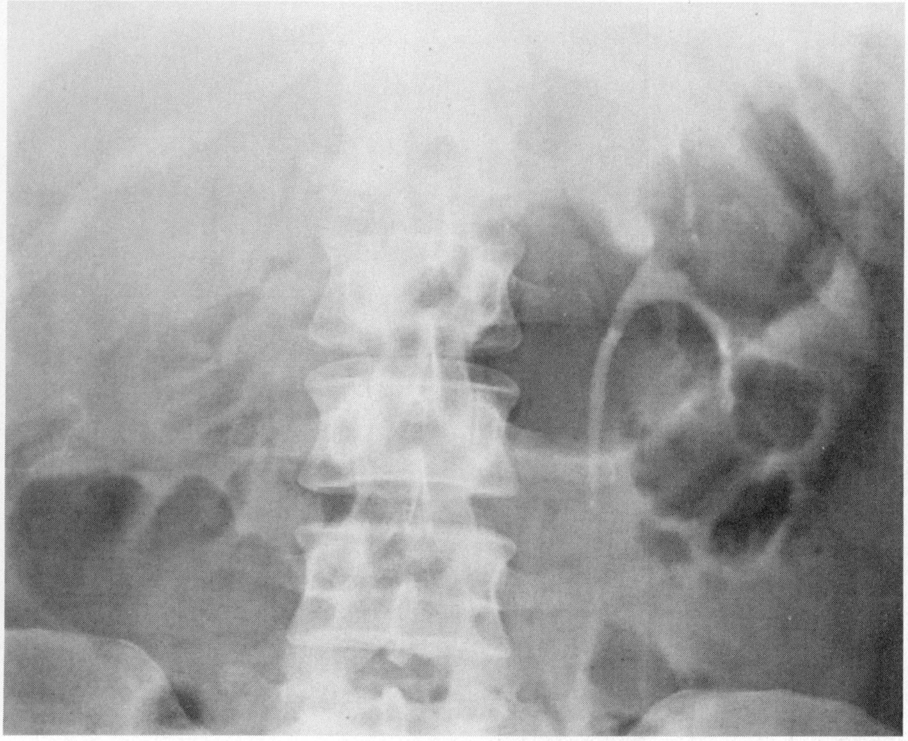

Figure 108.87. Renal artery occlusion. This intravenous pyelogram in a patient with acute renal artery occlusion demonstrates a nonfunctioning right kidney and normal-appearing left kidney.

occlusion, and the IVP usually reveals a nonfunctioning kidney (Fig. 108.87). If the occlusion is peripheral and thus segmental, only a small segmental defect may be noted in the nephrogram. However, peripheral emboli may lead to nonvisualization of the kidney of the urogram. In the acute phase, the kidney is usually slightly bigger than normal. However, as time passes, the size of the kidney progressively decreases. The retrograde pyelogram is normal in patients with acute renal artery occlusion. Angiography is diagnostic in the evaluation of the renal artery occlusion. Both renal arteries should be examined because 50% of patients may have bilateral lesions. The angiographic findings depend on whether the occlusion is complete or partial and on its location and size. Renal artery emboli usually appear as filling defects within the renal artery, with a sharp cutoff and concave border (Figs. 108.88 and 108.89). Arterial thrombosis tends to appear irregular in contour, without a

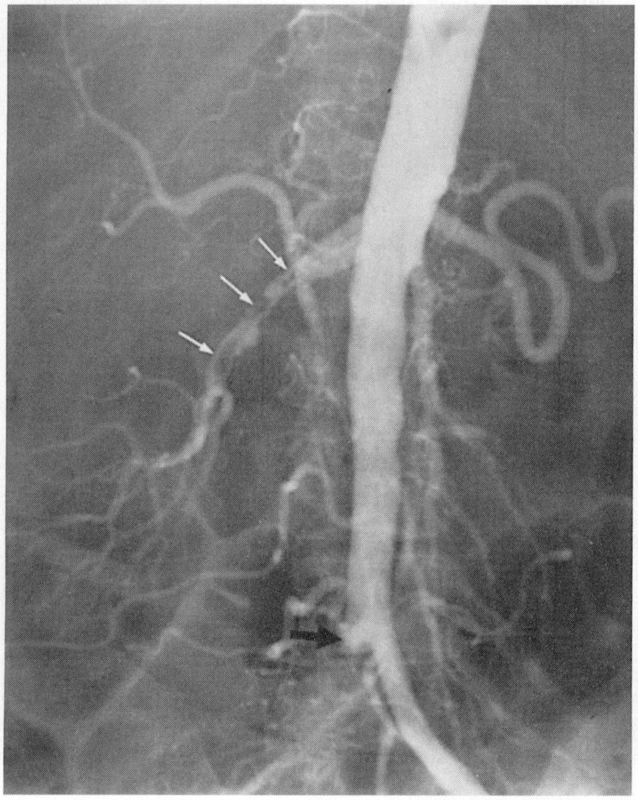

Figure 108.88. Renal artery occlusion. An abdominal aortogram reveals smooth filling defects in the right renal artery *(small arrows)* caused by emboli. A sharp cutoff of the left renal artery because of an embolus is also noted. Previous thrombosis of the right common iliac artery *(large arrow)* is evident.

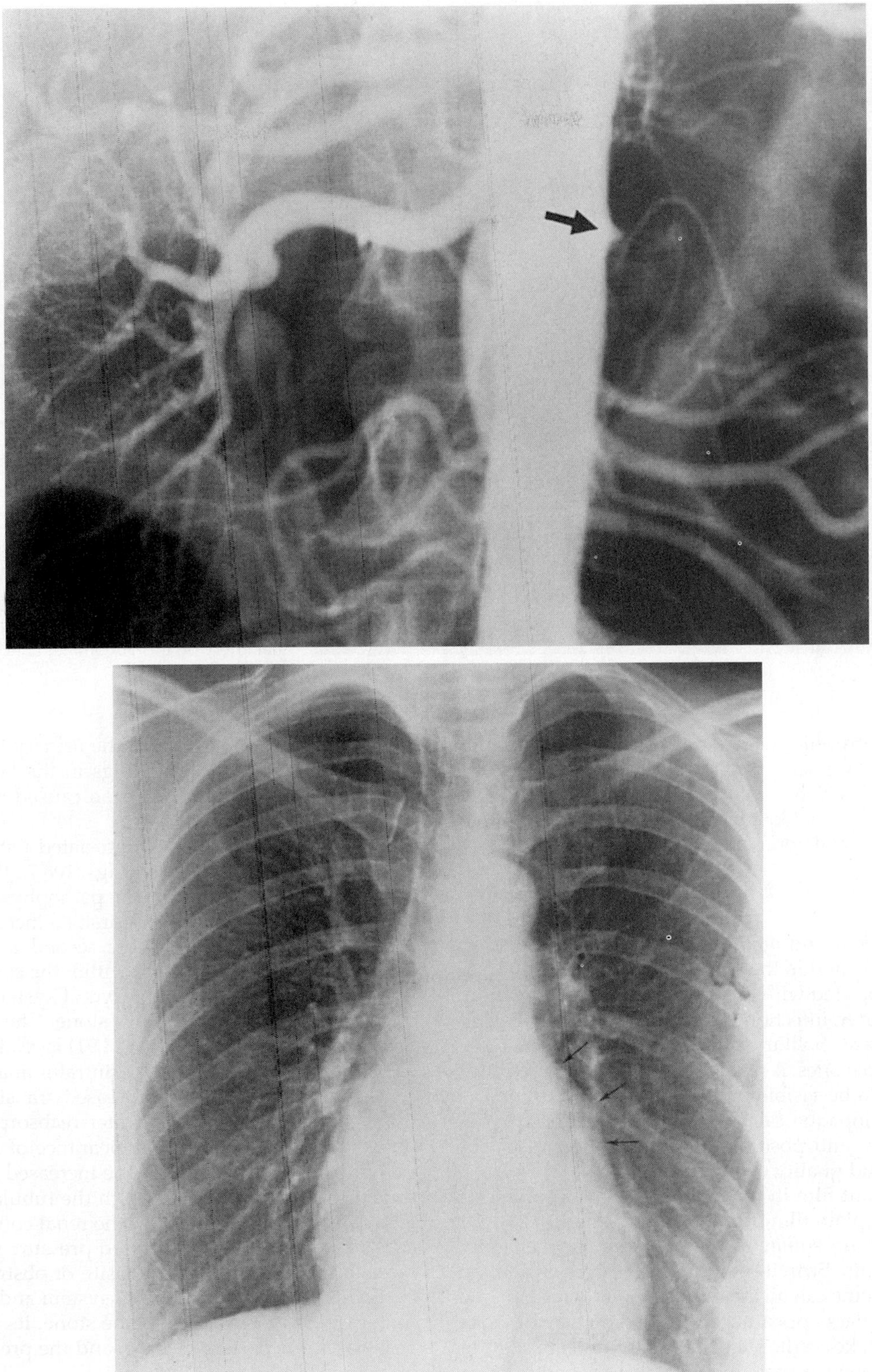

Figure 108.89. Renal artery occlusion. **Top:** An abdominal aortogram demonstrates a sharp cutoff of the left renal artery *(arrow)* caused by a renal artery embolus. **Bottom:** The source of the embolus is identified on this chest x-ray film in a patient with mitral valve disease and an enlarged left atrial appendage *(small arrows)*.

sharp cutoff (Fig. 108.90). It is difficult, however, to differentiate embolism from thrombosis in many cases in which an intraarterial filling defect is found. Emboli more frequently cause only partial occlusion of the renal artery. An intraarterial filling defect is identified angiographically, and washout of contrast material distal to a partial occlusion is slower than that in the uninvolved intrarenal arteries. In the capillary stage of the arteriogram, a peripheral defect is found in the contour of the kidney distal to the area of occlusion or partial occlusion of the artery. If the block is not relieved, the kidney eventually will

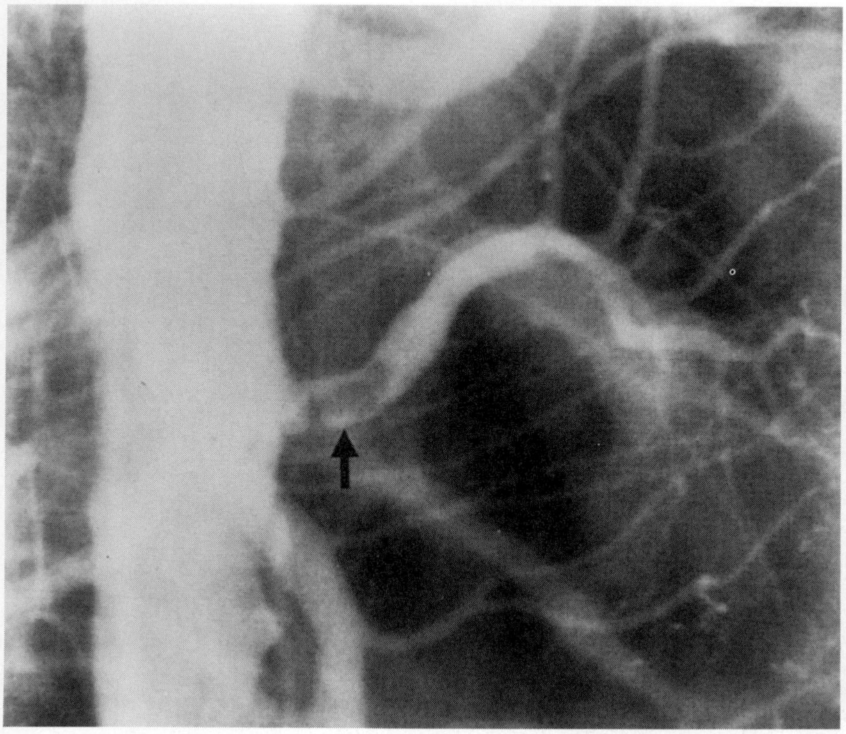

Figure 108.90. Renal artery occlusion. A thrombus, an irregular filling defect *(arrow)*, is noted in the left main renal artery on this abdominal aortogram.

become small and atrophic, with deformity of the collecting systems because of contraction. With partial resolution of the process, the kidney may be smaller than normal and show some excretion if there is adequate perfusion through both the main renal artery and collateral circulation.

Renal Calculi

The terms *nephrolithiasis* and *urolithiasis* describe calculi within the kidney specifically and in the urinary tract in general. Renal calculi are often associated with metabolic disorders, congenital anomalies of the kidney, infection, stasis, or obstruction. Calculi vary markedly in size. Solitary renal calculi are much more common than multiple ones. A renal calculus usually must be at least 2 mm in size to be visible on an optimal x-ray film. The ability to detect radiopaque calculi depends on their size, degree of opacification, and position and on the amount of obscuring bowel gas and quality of radiograph.

The most important film in the diagnosis of nephrolithiasis or urolithiasis is the plain film of the abdomen (Fig. 108.3). All urinary tract calculi are somewhat radiopaque and generally very dense and smooth. Struvite stones are less opaque and are often laminated. Cystine calculi are typically mildly radiopaque and have a ground glass appearance with radiography. Matrix concretions usually take on the shape of a calyx and are slightly radiopaque because they are covered with struvite and calcium phosphate. Uric acid stones and xanthine stones are almost completely radiolucent. However, because of the presence of such impurities as calcium oxalate and calcium phosphate, they may be seen occasionally on conventional films.

Because most renal calculi are visible radiographically, accurate localization of the calcific density depends on contrast media studies. The IVP is the method of choice for evaluation and localization of nephrolithiasis and urolithiasis. Retrograde pyelography may occasionally be necessary in the evaluation of these patients, but its role is decreasing, because large-dose intravenous urography is now the rule rather than the exception.

The presence of calculi within the urinary tract causes variable pathologic changes. The findings in the IVP are generally related to the degree of obstruction caused by the stone and its location within the urinary tract.

There are classic changes associated with acute obstruction by a calculus, as seen on IVP (Figs. 108.72 through 108.74). The radiographic findings reflect the pathophysiologic changes that occur within the urinary tract: first, an increasingly radiopaque nephrogram on the affected side, second, a delay in the appearance time of contrast material within the collecting system, and finally, dilation of the pelvocalyceal system and ureter down to the level of the obstructing stone. The increasingly dense obstructed nephrogram (Fig. 108.91) is related to the decreased GFR caused by the increased intraluminal pressure, the decreased urinary flow and increased transit time through the tubules, and the continued water reabsorption within the tubular system. The delayed appearance of contrast within the calyceal system is caused by the increased transit time of contrast material and urine through the tubular system of the affected kidney. The dilation of the renal collecting systems and ureter results from the increased pressure within the pelvocalyceal system proximal to the site of obstruction. The degree of dilation of the pelvocalyceal system and ureter is related to the degree of obstruction by the stone, its position, the acuteness or chronicity of the stone, and the presence or absence of infection.

In the radiographic evaluation of the patient with suspected calculus disease, time is an important factor. It is often necessary to obtain delayed films during the course of evaluating these patients because contrast material may not be seen in the dilated pelvocalyceal system or ureter until hours after the initial injection of contrast material (Fig. 108.91). The most common sites at which a calculus becomes lodged in the urinary tract are the areas of normal anatomic narrowing in the urinary tract, such as the ureteropelvic junction, ureterovesical junction, and the more superior aspect of the pelvis where the ureter passes over the iliac vessels.

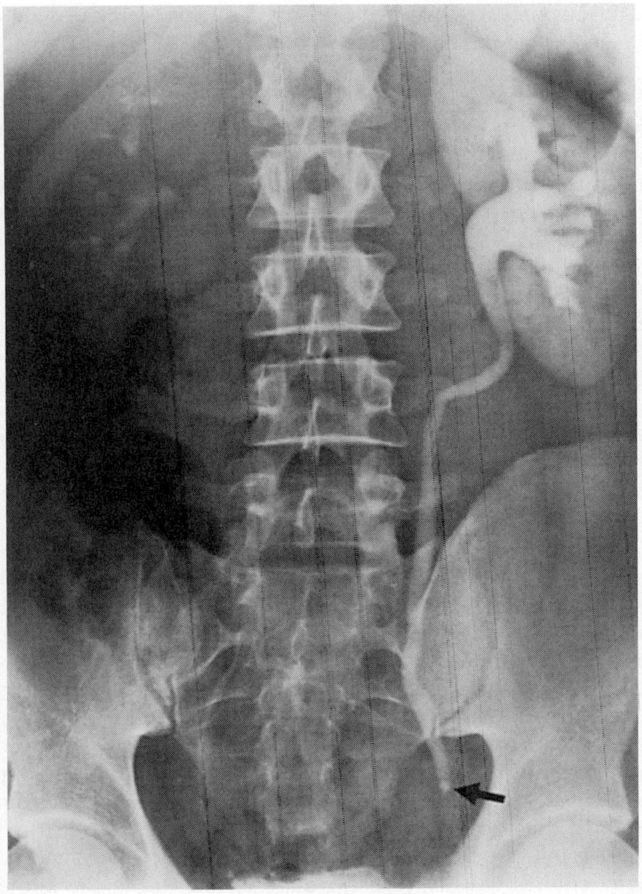

Figure 108.91. Renal calculus disease. This 12-hour delayed film from an intravenous pyelogram demonstrates a dilated left collecting system and ureter down to the point of obstruction, a small ureteral calculus *(arrow)*. Note that a dense, obstructed nephrogram still remains even 12 hours after the injection of intravenous contrast material.

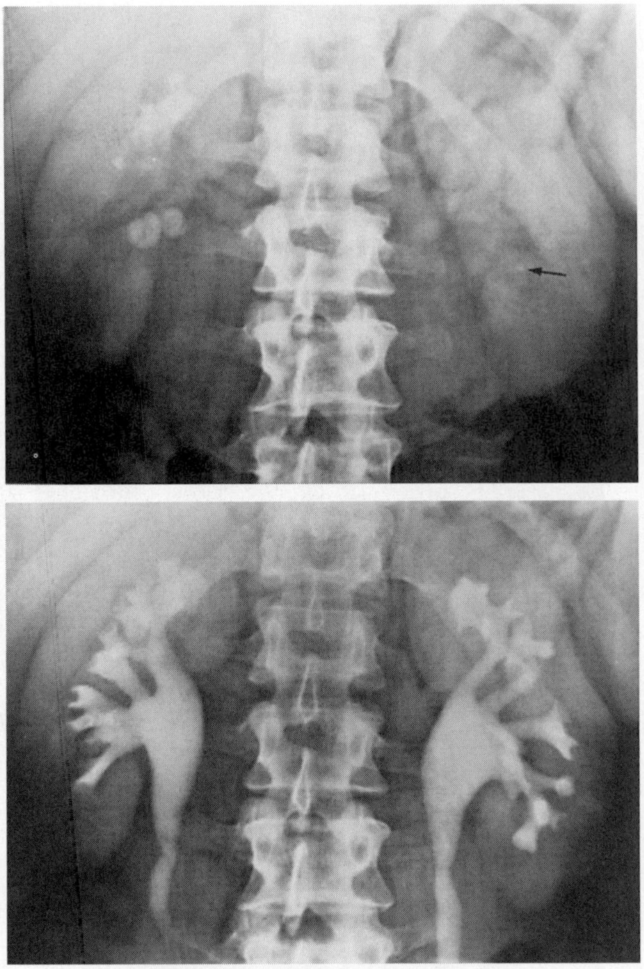

Figure 108.92. Renal calculus disease. **Top:** A plain film of the abdomen demonstrates renal calculi bilaterally. Multiple calculi are seen in the right renal pelvis and upper pole. A single small calculus is noted within the left kidney *(arrow)*. **Bottom:** After the injection of intravenous contrast material, the calculi are obscured by the contrast material that is excreted into the pelvocalyceal system.

Ureteral stones rarely cause complete obstruction of the urinary tract. When the intraluminal pressure exceeds the intravascular pressure necessary for glomerular filtration, the kidney will appear to be nonfunctioning. This phenomenon is intermittent: the intraluminal pressure waxes and wanes proximal to the site of obstruction. In general, however, the higher the grade of obstruction, the higher the intraluminal pressure within the system and thus the longer it takes for the contrast medium to reach the point of obstruction.

Calculi lying within the pelvocalyceal system occasionally may be obscured by the contrast material within the renal pelvis and calyces (Fig. 108.92). This is especially true for small renal calculi. Nonradiopaque stones may appear as a filling defect in the pelvocalyceal system or ureter (Fig. 108.93). Again, it should be remembered that most faintly opaque or nonopaque calculi are uric acid or xanthine stones.

Complications occasionally occur in association with calculus disease of the urinary tract. Pyelosinus extravasation may occur with an acute obstructing calculus (Fig. 108.76). A rapid increase in intraluminal pressure leads to small ruptures in the fornices of the calyceal elements, with extravasation of urine and contrast material into the peripelvic region. Pyelosinus extravasation is seen in approximately 2% to 5% of cases on intravenous urography. Large accumulations of contrast material may lead to formation of a urinoma (Fig. 108.69). The extravasated urine is eventually reabsorbed by the lymphatic system. A ureteral or pelvic tear is an uncommon complication of calculus disease. It usually occurs in cases of an obstructed system accompanied by chronic urinary tract infection. Ureteral structures rarely occur because of the inflammation of a passing stone. Strictures resulting from previous pyelolithotomy or ureterolithotomy are more common.

Branched or staghorn calculi form as a cast of a portion or all of the pelvocalyceal system (Fig. 108.94). Their usual composition is a combination of struvite, cystine, and uric acid. They often show laminations. Staghorn calculi may form quite rapidly, in as little as several weeks. Staghorn calculi cause variable amounts of dilation of the pelvocalyceal system. Although it is important to assess the function of a kidney with staghorn calculus, this may be difficult with intravenous urography because of the filling of the calyceal system with the staghorn calculus. The radionuclide renogram and selective renal angiography may be used for preoperative evaluation of the function that remains in a kidney with a staghorn calculus.

Renal Neoplasia

Neoplasms of the kidney may arise from either the renal parenchyma or the uroepithelium of the calyceal system or the renal pelvis. Benign and malignant tumors occur in both regions.

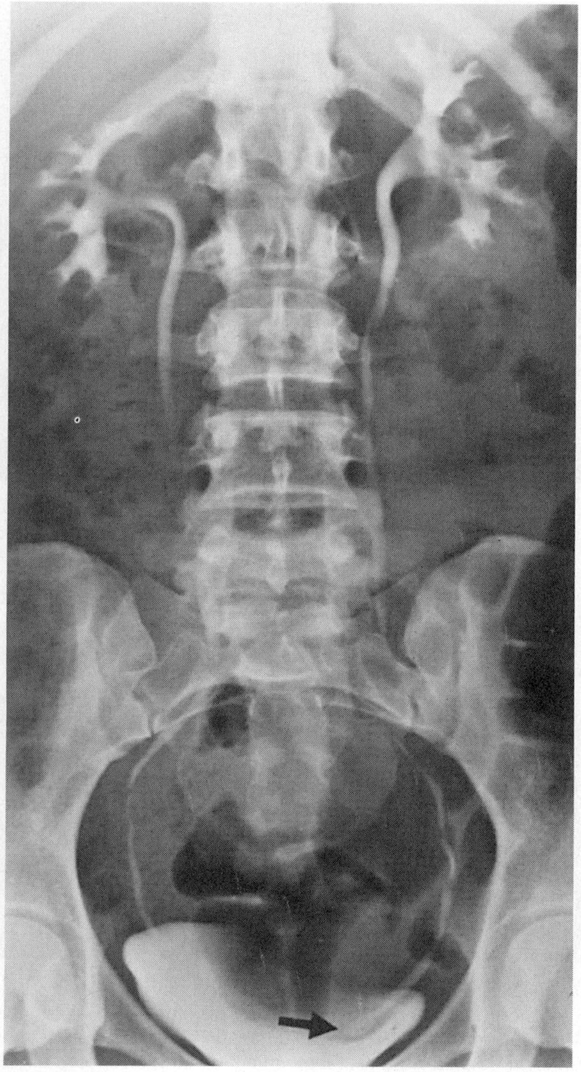

Figure 108.93. Renal calculus disease. Nonradiopaque calculi may occasionally appear as filling defects within the ureter, as noted on this intravenous pyelogram. A simple ureterocele at the distal end of the left ureter contains a nonopaque calculus causing a filling defect *(arrow)*.

Renal neoplasms have been reported during every decade of life, including the newborn.

Benign Tumors

Benign tumors of any significant size are extremely uncommon. The most common benign neoplasm is a renal adenoma. It arises from mature renal tubular cells and is almost always less than 3 cm in size. These tumors rarely cause symptoms, so their diagnosis usually is made at autopsy. They have no specific radiographic features. When detected radiographically, the renal adenoma appears as a small mass within the kidney. Angiography reveals that the vascularity may be normal and slightly increased in the area of the lesion. None of the usual features of renal cell carcinoma, such as puddling of contrast material and arteriovenous shunting, are detected with renal adenomas. Ultrasound shows a solid mass. Other benign lesions may occur but, again, are usually found only at autopsy. Lesions such as fibromas, myomas, lipomas, and hemangiomas have been reported.

Hamartomas of the kidney, angiomyolipomas, are another group of benign tumors of the kidney that are generally radiographically detectable. They are composed of different tissues, such as fat, muscle, vascular elements, and occasionally cartilage. They occur in two different groups of patients. In those with tuberous sclerosis, angiomyolipomas are usually bilateral or multiple. When multiple tumors are present, the kidney often takes on an appearance not unlike that of polycystic kidney with multiple masses. These tumors also occur in a solitary and unilateral form, usually in women in the third to fifth decades. In this group of patients, angiomyolipomas appear as a mass lesion, usually with pain and/or hematuria. Conventional x-ray studies usually reveal a mass lesion within the kidney (Fig. 108.95). Ultrasound studies show the mass as a solid, with increased echoes because of the presence of fat within the lesion. Angiography shows that angiomyolipomas are vascular lesions, indistinguishable from renal cell carcinomas (Fig. 108.96). CT in patients with angiomyolipomas is usually diagnostic, because the fat within the lesion can be detected.

Malignant Tumors

Malignant tumors of the kidney are the third most common tumors of the genitourinary system after carcinoma of the prostate and carcinoma of the bladder. As the classic presentation of

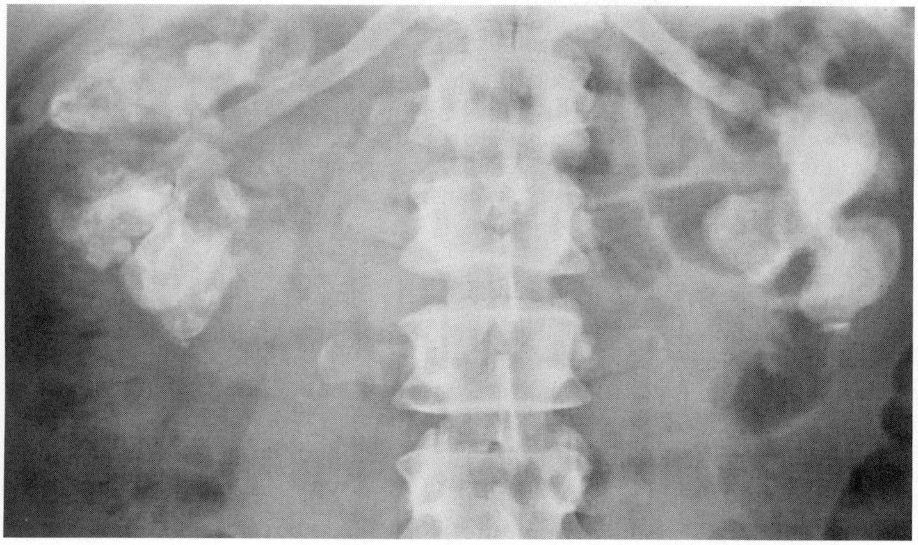

Figure 108.94. Renal calculus disease. Bilateral staghorn calculi are noted on this plain film of the abdomen. The calculi take on the form of the dilated pelvocalyceal systems.

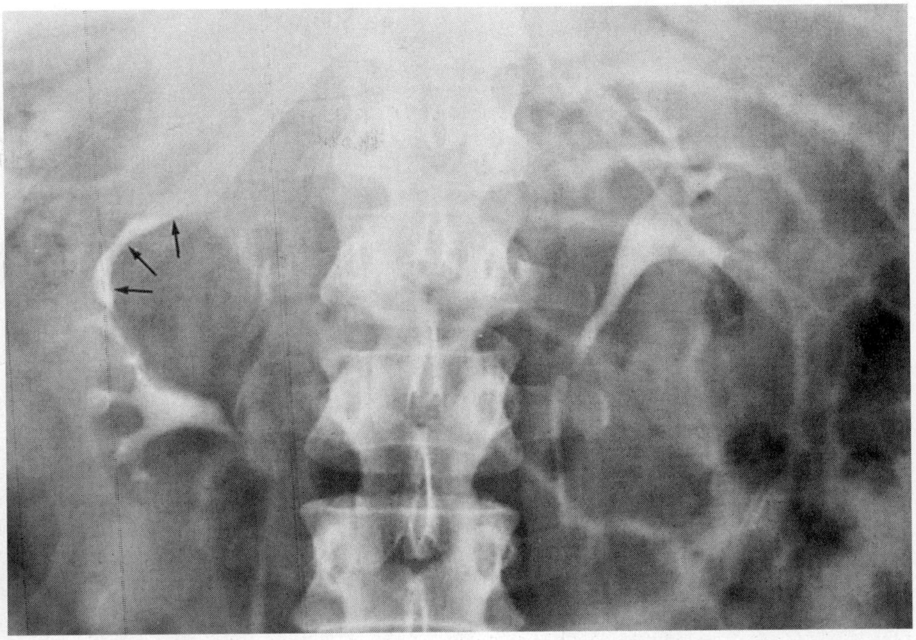

Figure 108.95. Angiomyolipoma. The intravenous pyelogram demonstrates a mass in the right upper pole of the kidney, causing displacement of the upper pole calyx *(arrows)*. Bowel gas overlies the right kidney, giving a spurious lower density appearance to the region.

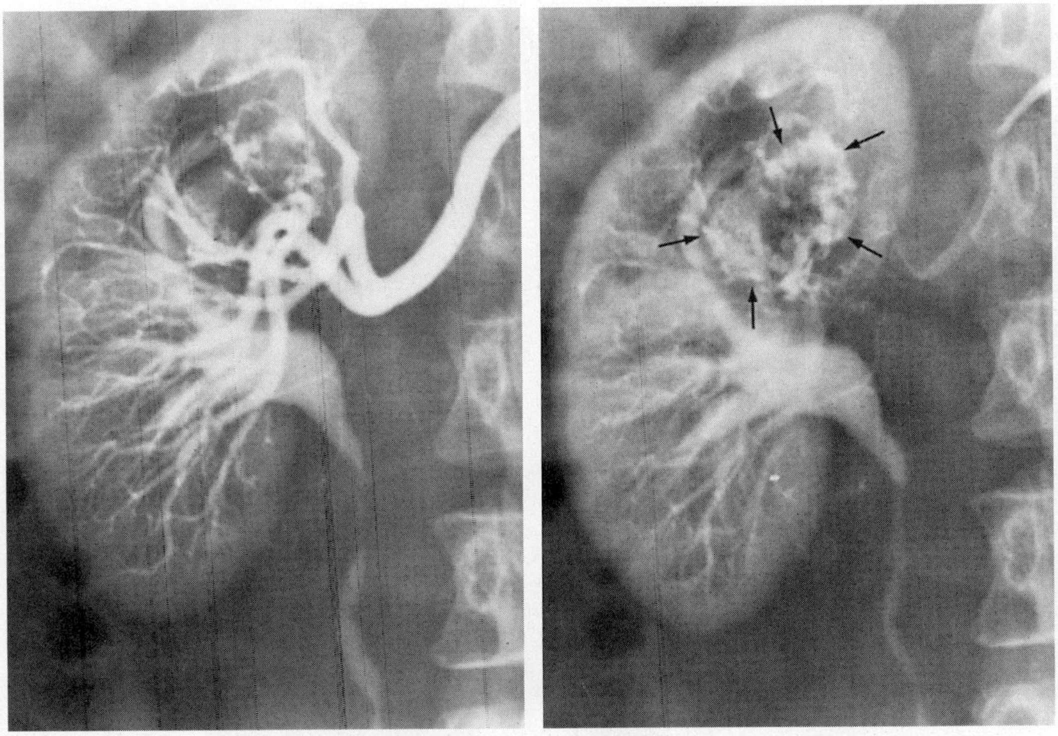

Figure 108.96. Angiomyolipoma. Selective renal angiography in the some case as in Fig. 108.95 demonstrates a hypervascular mass in the upper pole of the kidney. **Left:** Areas of neovascularity are seen within the lesion. **Right:** In the later arterial phase, areas of puddling and staining within the mass are noted ***(arrows).*** This lesion is indistinguishable from a small renal cell carcinoma.

a malignant tumor of the kidney is that of a mass lesion, the plain film of the abdomen often reveals an enlarged kidney or mass in the area of the kidney (Fig. 108.97). Ten to twenty percent of cases show evidence of calcification on the plain film (Figs. 108.4 and 108.98). Calcifications have been seen in virtually all tumors of the kidney, both benign and malignant. It should be noted that peripheral ringlike calcification does not exclude malignancy; 20% of these lesions are, in fact, malignant. Ninety percent of renal masses with central, punctuate, or mottled calcification turn out to be malignant lesions.

The IVP has been the standard x-ray examination performed in all patients suspected of having a mass lesion of the kidney. All studies should be performed with tomography (Fig. 108.99). Renal cell carcinomas generally cause distortion of the outline

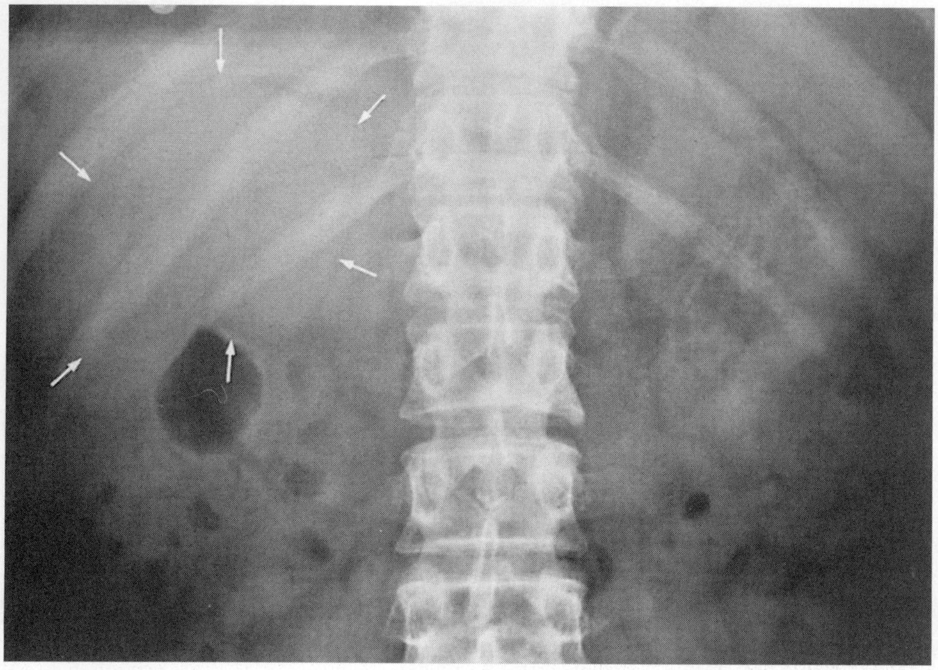

Figure 108.97. Renal cell carcinoma. This plain film of the abdomen demonstrates enlargement of the right kidney with a mass lesion in the middle and upper portions *(arrows)*. This proved to be a renal cell carcinoma on further examination.

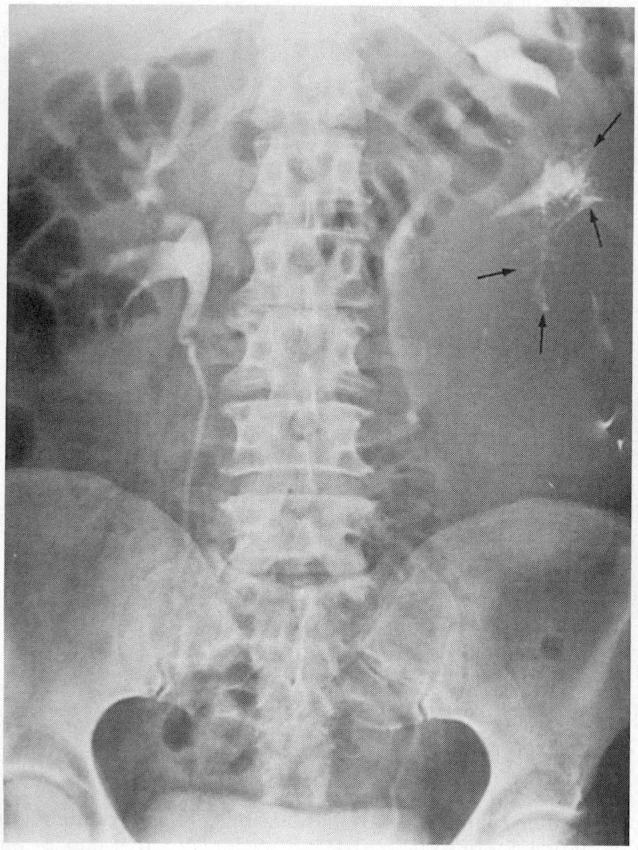

Figure 108.98. Renal cell carcinoma. On this intravenous pyelogram, there is marked enlargement of the left kidney. A mass lesion displaces the collecting systems of the middle and lower portions of the kidney. Central, somewhat curvilinear, and punctate calcifications *(arrows)* are seen in the central portion of the mass. This represents dystrophic calcification within a renal cell carcinoma.

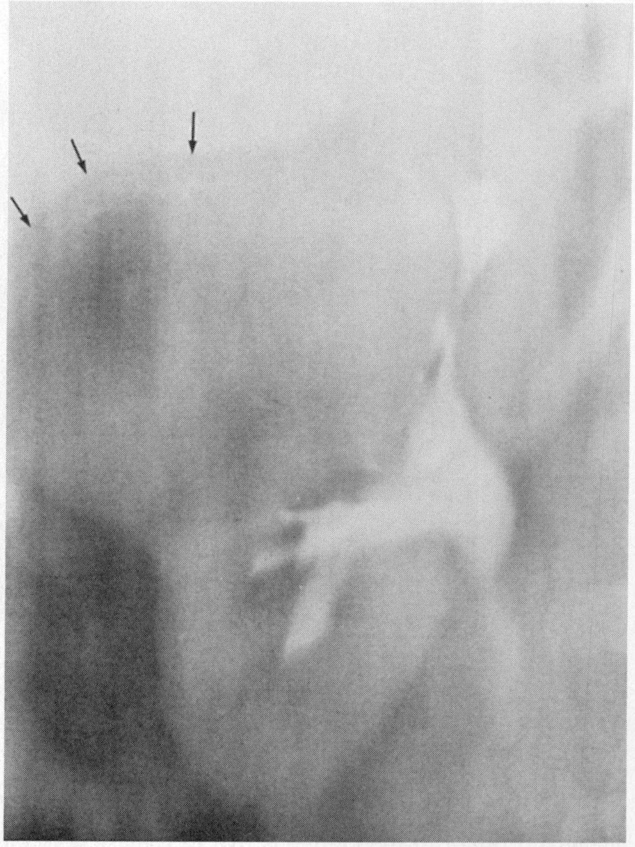

Figure 108.99. Renal cell carcinoma. On this tomographic section from an intravenous pyelogram, a large mass is seen projecting off the lateral aspect of the right kidney. The calyces in the central portion of the kidney are stretched and displaced medially. The mass itself is not low in density, and a relatively thick wall is noted superiorly *(arrows)*. No sharp line of demarcation is noted between the mass and the remaining normal portion of the kidney. Rather, these findings are of a renal cell carcinoma.

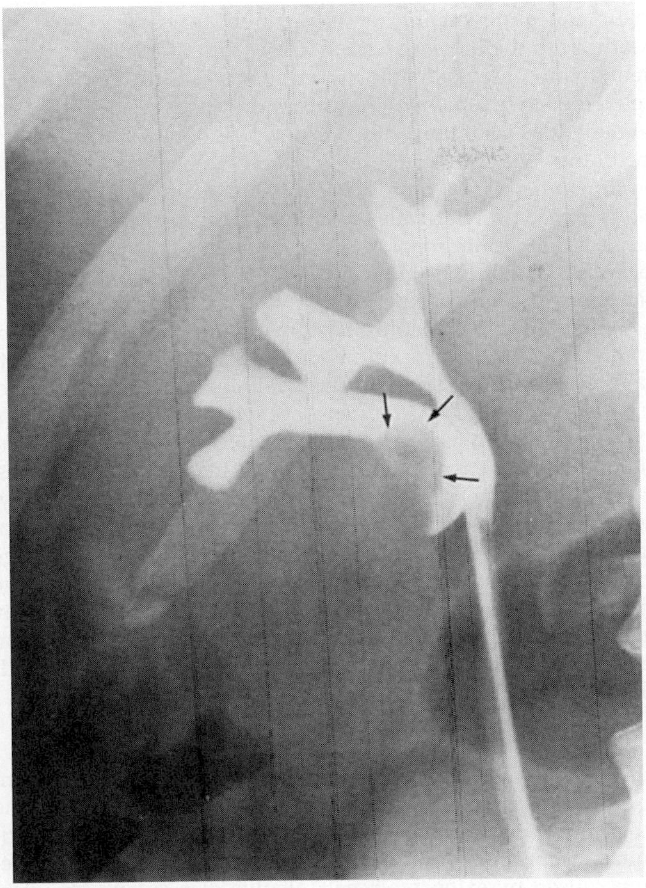

Figure 108.100. Renal cell carcinoma. This retrograde pyelogram shows a filling defect in the inferolateral aspect of the renal pelvis *(arrows)*. In addition, the lower pole calyx of this right kidney is no longer identifiable. This represents extension from a renal cell carcinoma into the renal pelvis.

of the kidney or renal enlargement. The mass density usually has an irregular junction with normal renal parenchyma. The calyces may be stretched, elongated, or obliterated by the renal mass. Although renal cell carcinomas usually appear to project beyond the normal borders of the kidney, they may extend medially to involve the renal pelvis. When there is renal pelvic extension, the renal pelvis may be narrowed or obliterated or contain an irregular filling defect that represents either tumor or blood clot (Fig. 108.100). When the IVP reveals a nonfunctioning kidney in a patient with a hypernephroma, either renal vein occlusion or complete obliteration of the renal pelvis should be suspected. The IVP is no longer the end point in diagnosis of renal cell carcinoma. Ultrasound examination of the kidney is generally performed after a mass lesion is detected. The workup of a renal mass is discussed in detail in Chapter 30. Renal cell carcinoma usually appears as a solid mass lesion with a varying complex echo pattern.

Renal cell carcinomas are hypervascular in 80% to 85% of patients. Characteristically, abnormal increased vascularity, which is irregular in caliber, and pooling or puddling of contrast material with arteriovenous shunting is seen with angiography (Figs. 108.101 and 108.102). During the capillary phase of the arteriogram, a tumor blush or stain often is seen within the tumor. Ten to fifteen percent of renal cell carcinomas are hypovascular or avascular (Fig. 108.103). These lesions usually show some small areas of abnormal vascularity in the periphery, with a thick rim and irregular interface with the normal parenchyma. Metastases from renal cell carcinoma usually have an angiographic pattern similar to that of the primary lesions within the kidney. Renal venography and examination of the inferior vena cava are extremely important in the evaluation of patients with renal cell carcinoma. Tumor thrombi may extend into the renal vein or the inferior vena cava (Fig. 108.104).

Metastatic lesions to the kidney are twice as common as primary renal cell carcinomas. Because they are usually asympto-

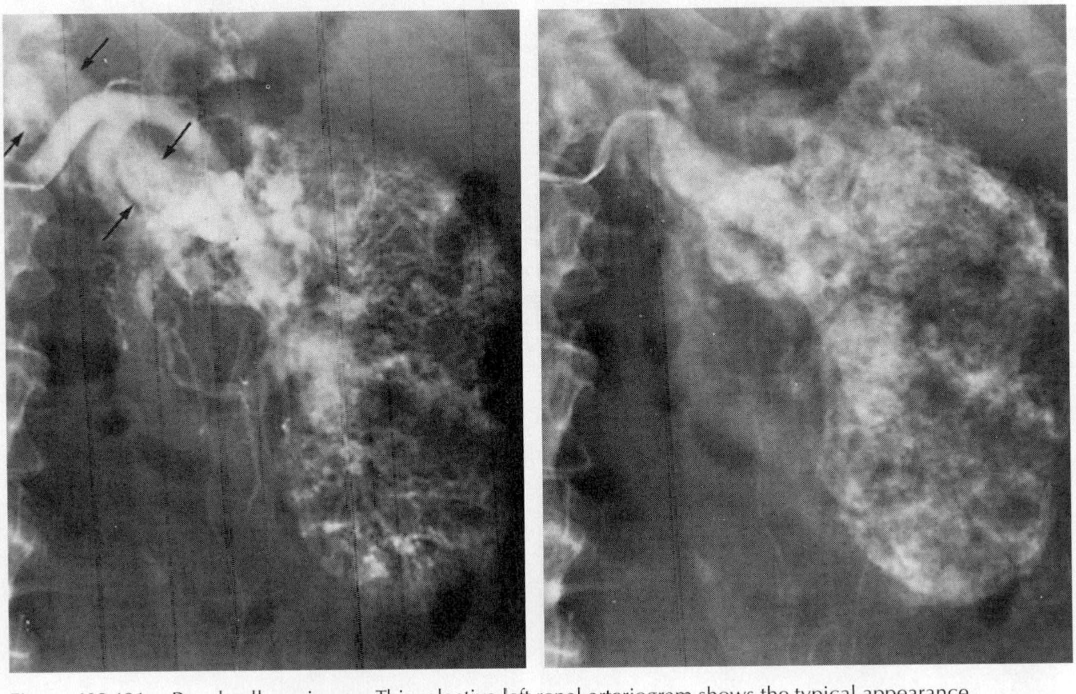

Figure 108.101. Renal cell carcinoma. This selective left renal arteriogram shows the typical appearance of a renal cell carcinoma. This hypervascular lesion shows extensive neovascularity, with vessels of varying caliber. In addition, puddles of contrast material are identified within the lesion. Arteriovenous shunting is noted **(left)** with early filling of the left renal vein *(arrows)*.

matic and quite small, they have rarely been detected before death. With the increased use of CT scanning in the cancer patient, many previously undetected metastases are being found. Leukemic involvement of the kidney may cause generalized enlargement as it infiltrates the kidney. Lymphomas may involve the kidney either by contiguous in involvement from the retroperitoneum or in a more disseminated manner. Lymphomas may appear as bilaterally symmetrical diffuse renal enlargement, as small intrarenal nodules, or even as a single primary mass lesion within the kidney. The findings on both IVP and angiography are nonspecific.

Wilms' tumor, or nephroblastoma, is the most common abdominal neoplasm of childhood. Ninety percent of the patients have a palpable abdominal mass. Although these tumors are usually unilateral, 5% to 10% may occur bilaterally. On plain film of the abdomen, a large mass is often detected in the area of the kidney. The IVP usually shows a large mass that compresses, stretches, and deforms the calyceal system (Fig. 108.105). Eighty-five to ninety percent of patients may have functioning renal parenchyma left as evidenced by urography, despite the large size of the tumor. Ultrasound in Wilms' tumor reveals a large solid mass lesion involving the kidney. Angiography is usually not necessary for diagnosis. The lesions are less vascular than most renal cell carcinomas. However, areas of staining, puddling, and arteriovenous shunting may be seen (Fig. 108.106).

Tumor of the Renal Pelvis

Although benign tumors of the renal pelvis and uroepithelium occur, they are quite rare. Transitional cell carcinomas are the most common tumors of the renal pelvis. Squamous cell carcinomas occur, but only following metaplasia of the uroepithelium caused by extensive renal calculus disease and/or infection. Involvement with transitional cell carcinoma may be multiple in up to 30% to 40% of cases.

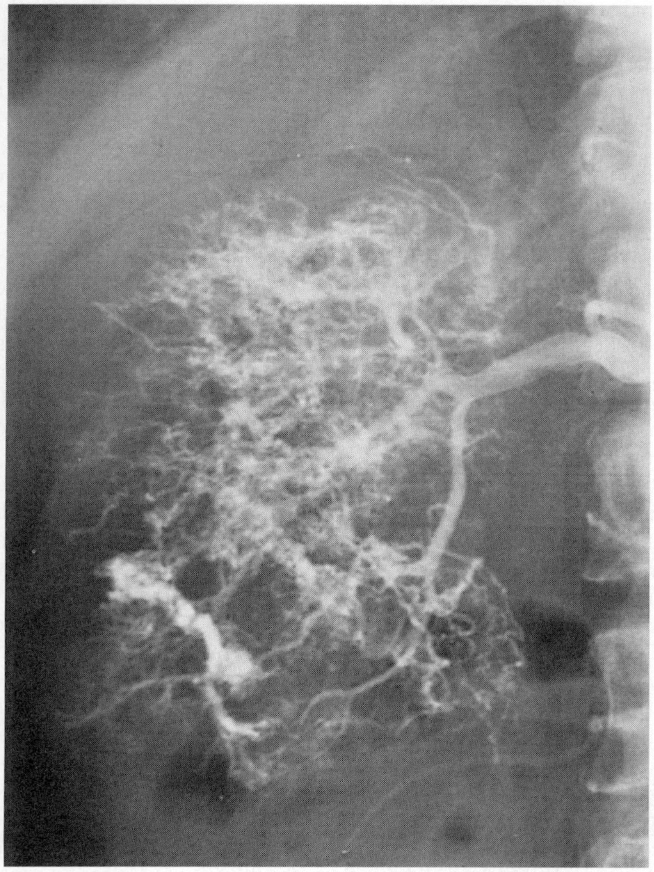

Figure 108.102. Renal cell carcinoma. An enlarged, hypervascular renal cell carcinoma has infiltrated almost the entire right kidney. Extensive areas of neovascularity and puddling of contrast material are seen within the lesion.

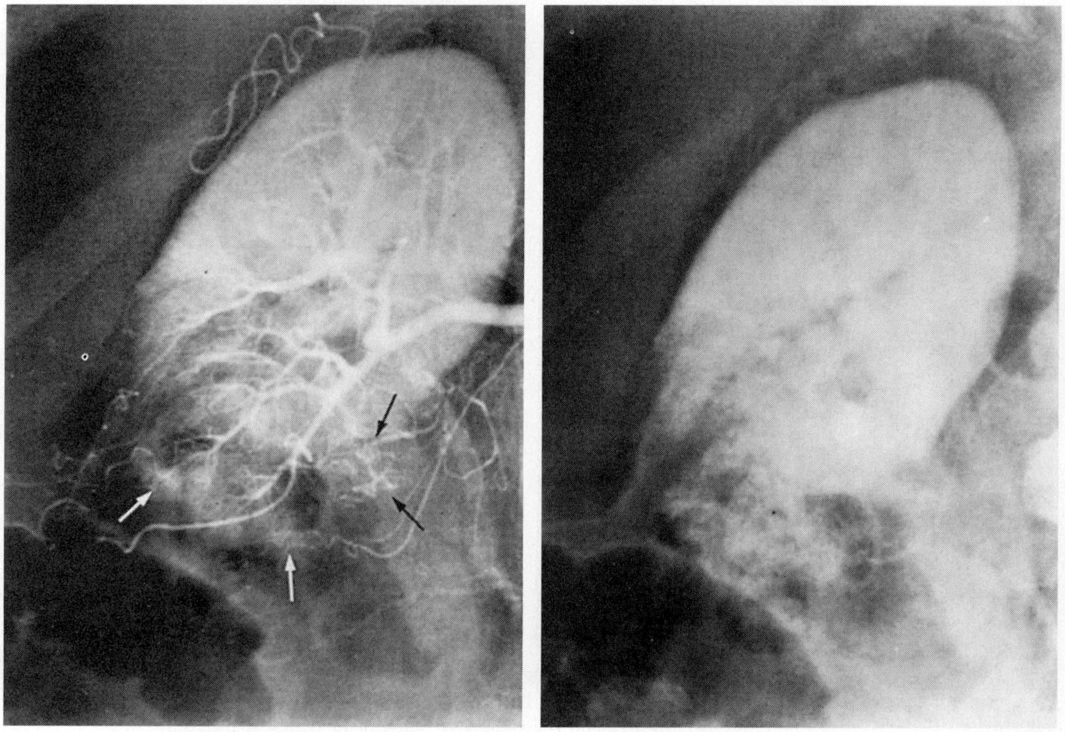

Figure 108.103. Renal cell carcinoma. A hypovascular renal cell carcinoma is seen extending off the lower pole of the right kidney. An irregular interface with the remaining normal kidney is noted on the capillary phase film **(right).** Only a few small abnormal vessels supplying the lesion are identified (**left,** *arrows*).

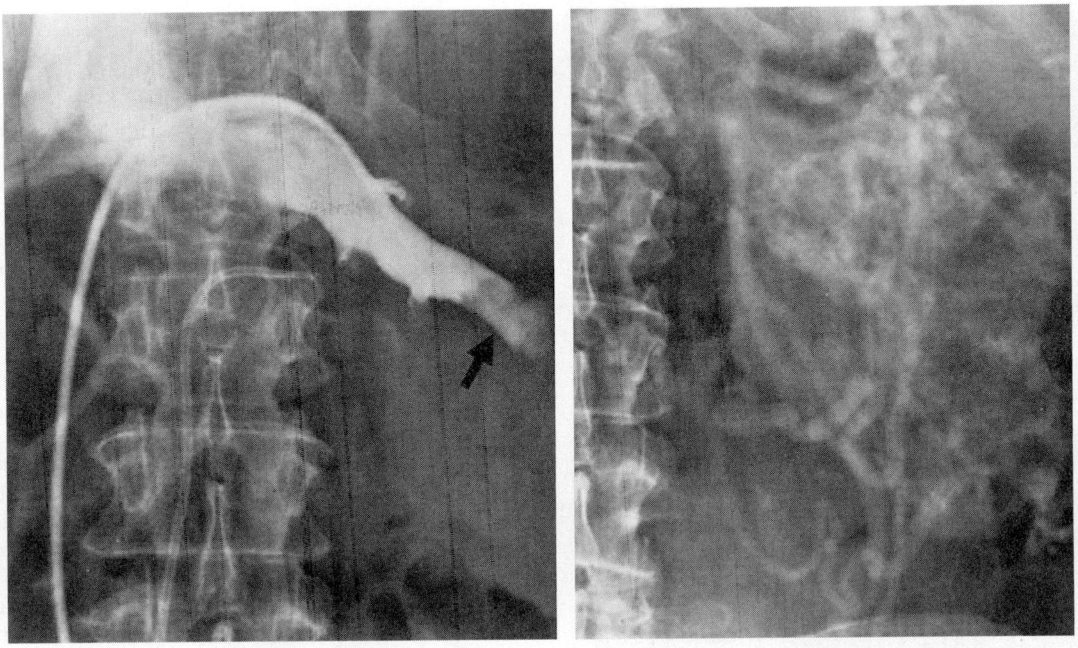

Figure 108.104. Renal cell carcinoma. **Right:** The end stage of a selective left renal arteriogram demonstrates extensive abnormal collateral venous channels surrounding the renal cell carcinoma in the lower pole of the left kidney. **Left:** A selective left renal venogram reveals the reason for the filling of the collateral venous channels to be tumor thrombus extending into the renal vein *(arrow)*.

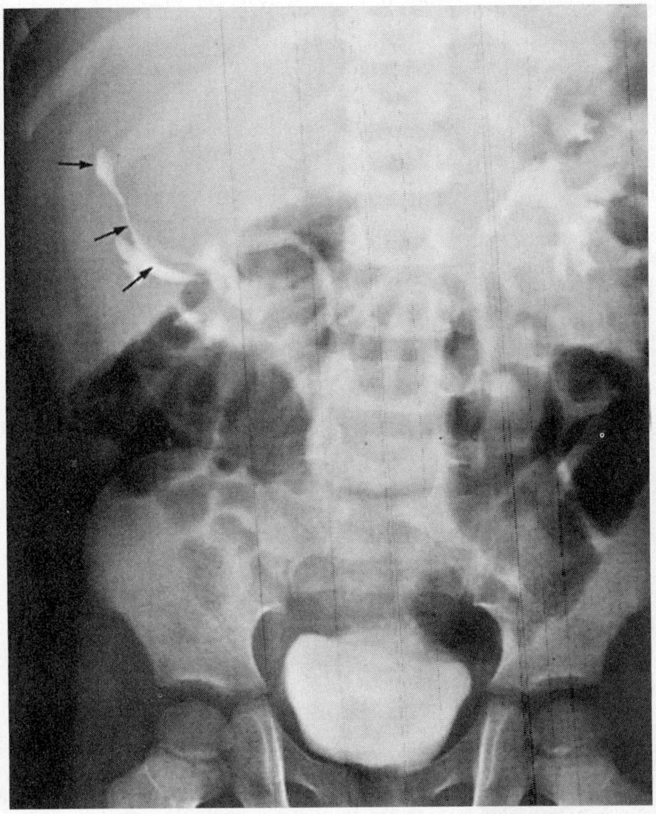

Figure 108.105. Wilms' tumor. This intravenous pyelogram performed on a child shows evidence of a large mass involving the upper pole of the right kidney, with stretching and deformity of the upper pole calyces *(arrows)*. The calyces are displaced laterally by the large mass. A normal-appearing left kidney is seen.

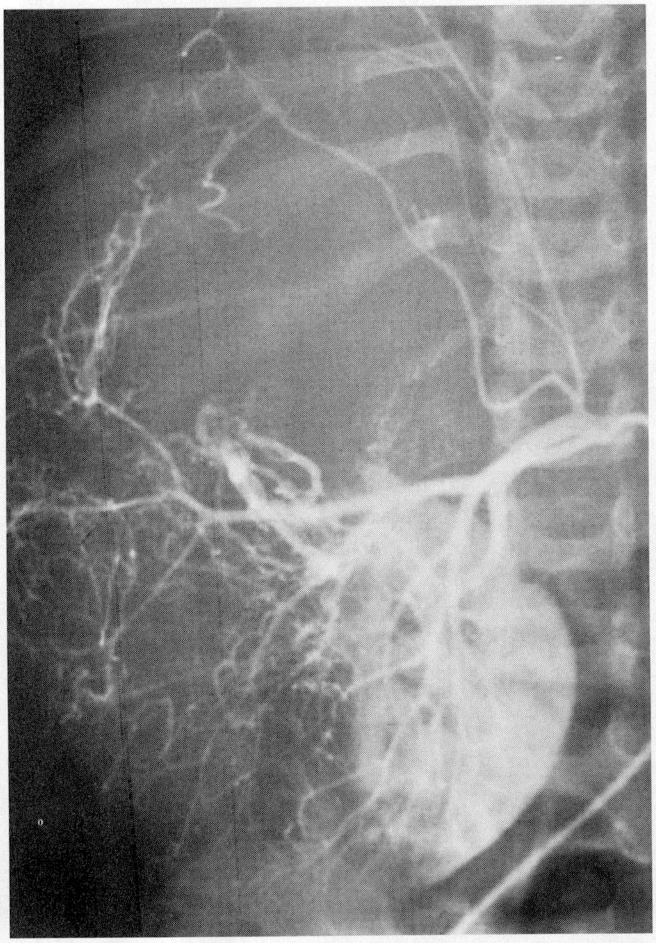

Figure 108.106. Wilms' tumor. The selective right renal arteriogram shows a hypervascular lesion involving the greater portion of the right kidney. Only a small region of normal renal parenchyma is noted inferiorly. The areas of neovascularity and puddling of contrast material are quite similar to those seen with renal cell carcinoma.

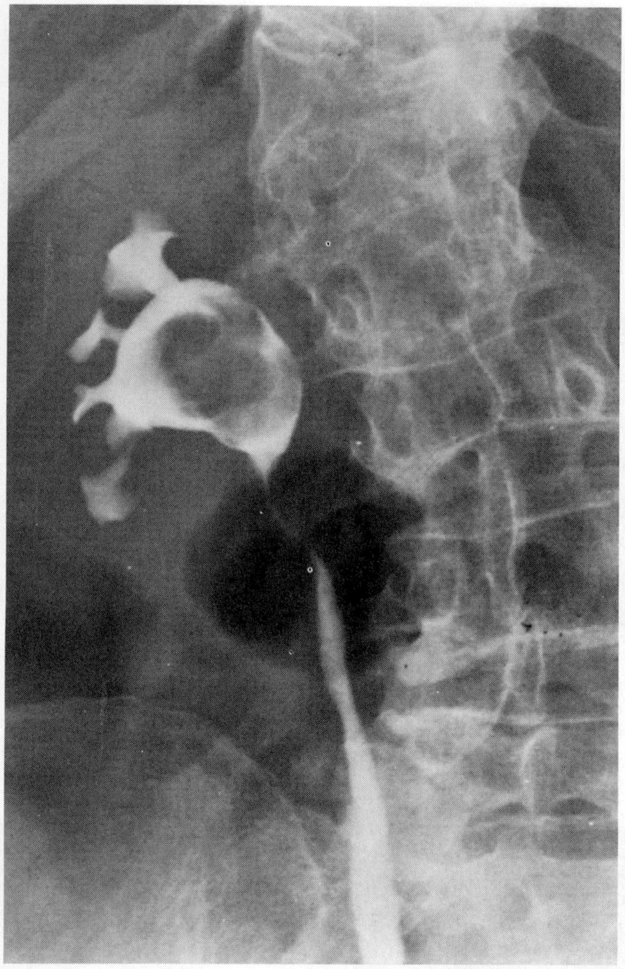

Figure 108.107. Transitional cell carcinoma. The intravenous pyelogram in this elderly patient shows large filling defect in the renal pelvis of the right kidney. The margins are somewhat irregular. It is interesting to note that although the transitional cell carcinoma is rather large and bulky, there is only mild hydronephrosis.

The IVP in transitional cell carcinoma typically shows a filling defect in the renal pelvis (Fig. 108.107). The abnormality in the renal pelvis may be either irregular or smooth. As the lesion enlarges, there may be extension into the renal parenchyma. At this point, it becomes difficult to distinguish from renal cell carcinoma. Retrograde pyelography with cytologic examination of the urine is extremely helpful in the diagnosis of renal pelvic tumors. Ultrasound, angiography, and CT scanning have as yet been of little additional help in evaluating these patients.

Renovascular Hypertension

Numerous causes for renovascular hypertension are known (see Chapter 62). Lesions may occur within the main renal artery (renal artery stenosis) or in its branches. Other causes include aneurysms of the main renal artery or its branches, traumatic stenosis of the renal artery, and embolic phenomena involving the renal arteries, both proximally and distally with subsequent infarction. Dissecting aneurysms of the abdominal aorta with resultant stenosis or occlusion of a single renal artery or its inclusion in the false lumen of the aneurysm also may lead to renovascular hypertension.

The rapid sequence, or hypertensive, IVP may be used in the evaluation of patients with suspected renovascular hypertension. The study is performed with a rapid bolus injection of intravenous contrast material and subsequent rapid filming of the renal areas at 1, 2, 3, 4, and 5 minutes after injection. After this time, the study is carried out in a more conventional manner with tomography and full films for evaluation of the ureteral system and bladder. In the classic example of renovascular hypertension caused by unilateral renal artery stenosis, the renal hypoperfusion secondary to narrowing of the main renal artery is responsible for the findings on IVP. These radiographic findings may be classified as major and minor signs. The major signs include delayed appearance of contrast material in the pelvocalyceal system, smaller renal size, increased concentration of the contrast medium, and delayed disappearance of the contrast material on the affected side.

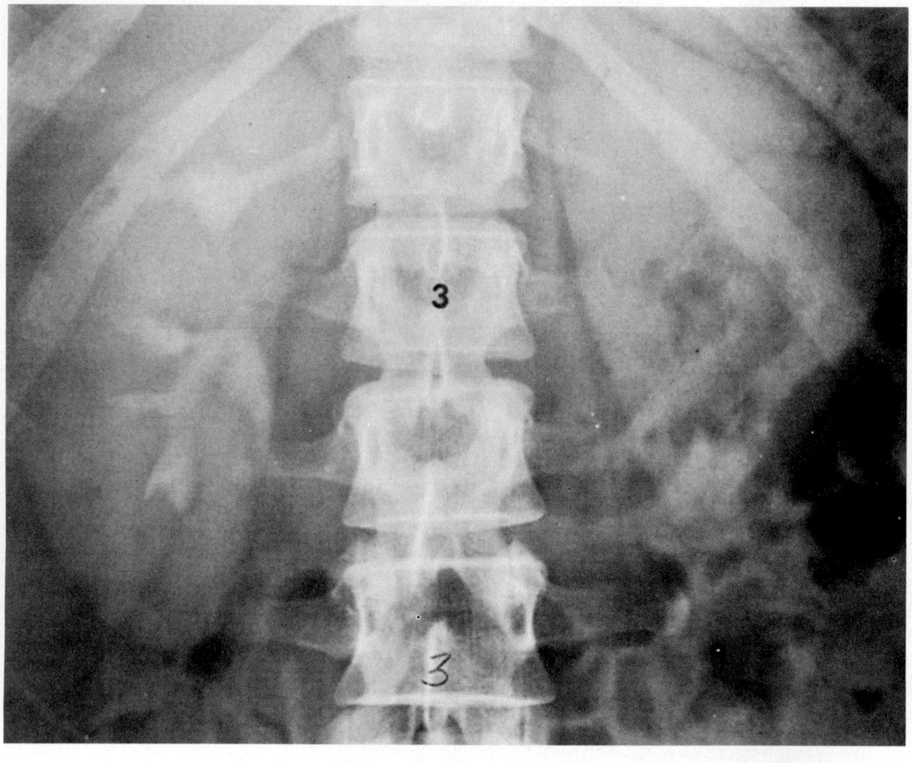

Figure 108.108. Renovascular hypertension. This 3-minute film from an intravenous pyelogram demonstrates normal excretion of contrast material from the right kidney. The left kidney, which is slightly smaller than the right, does not yet have contrast material in the collecting systems. Angiography proved this to be because of unilateral renal artery stenosis on the left side.

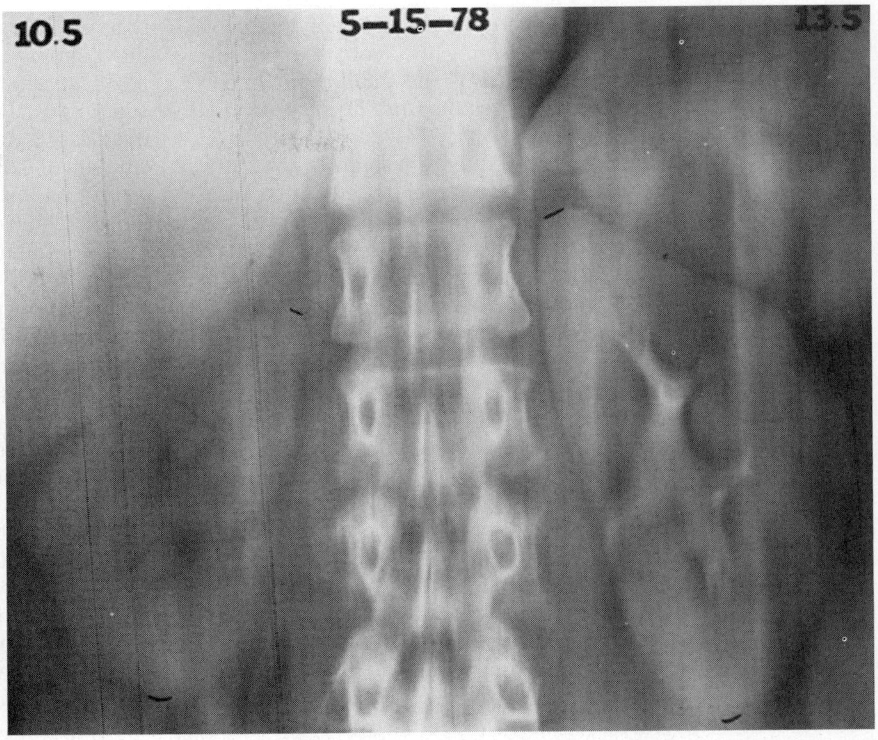

Figure 108.109. Renovascular hypertension. The tomogram from an intravenous pyelogram shows a normal-sized left kidney measuring 13.5 cm. The right kidney is 3 cm smaller, measuring 10.5 cm. There is a delay in the appearance of contrast material in the collecting systems of the right kidney. On angiography, this patient proved to have right-sided renal artery stenosis.

The delayed appearance of the contrast medium may be noted on the IVP by a 1-minute or longer difference in appearance time of contrast material in the collecting systems (Fig. 108.108). The difference in renal size is related to the decreased blood volume and diminished blood flow to the affected kidney (Fig. 108.109). Normally, the left kidney is 0.5 cm larger than the right. A significant difference in renal size is noted when the left kidney is 1.5 cm smaller than the right or when the right kidney is 2.0 cm smaller than the left. The increased concentration of contrast material on the affected side is caused by increased sodium and water reabsorption by the nephron secondary to renal hypoperfusion, as well as to increased urinary transit time. The later hyperconcentration is usually noted on 10-, 15-, or 20-minute films after the initial bolus injection of contrast material (Fig. 108.110).

The minor signs of renovascular hypertension are small-capacity collecting systems and notching of the renal pelvis or ureter on the affected side (Fig. 108.27). The minor signs of renovascular hypertension, although not specific, may help in evaluating these patients. Ureteral or pelvic notching is caused by

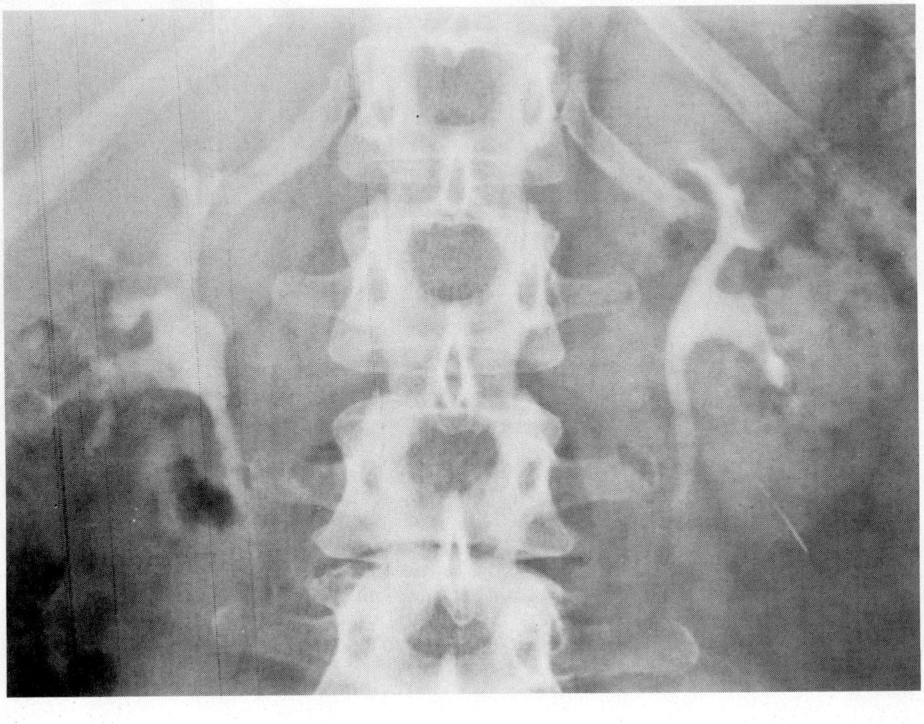

Figure 108.110. Renovascular hypertension. On this 15-minute film from an intravenous pyelogram, there is slightly greater density to the contrast material in the left pelvocalyceal system than the right. This patient was found to have unilateral renal artery stenosis involving the left renal artery.

the enlargement of collateral vessels in the area supplying blood to the kidney. The collateral vessels may be adequate to provide circulation to the kidney (Fig. 108.111). The small-capacity collecting system on the affected side results from decreased urine volume in the involved kidney.

The IVP performed in a rapid sequence fashion is not a specific test. Unfortunately, there is a large incidence of both false-positive and false-negative results. Approximately 80% of patients with unilateral renovascular disease will have an abnormal urogram. False-positive results are noted in 10% of patients with essential hypertension. False-negative results are seen in 15% to 20% of patients with unilateral renovascular disease. If the rapid sequence IVP is normal, there is still a 1% to 2% possibility of the patient's having renovascular hypertension. If the IVP gives a positive result, however, there is a 40% to 50% chance that the patient has hypertension of renovascular origin.

The arteriogram is used as the specific radiologic examination for identification of the renal arterial lesion. Unilateral renal artery stenosis caused by atherosclerosis is the most common cause of renovascular hypertension (Fig. 108.56), accounting for two-thirds of all cases. It is usually found in the elderly population, among men more frequently than among women, and particularly among smokers. The angiographically demonstrable lesion is usually in the proximal 2 cm of the main renal artery, very close to the orifice. The narrowing is usually eccentric and may be slightly irregular. Other changes of atherosclerosis may be noted in the abdominal aorta and other vessels in the abdomen.

Fibromuscular dysplasia is another lesion that leads to renovascular hypertension. The exact cause is unknown. Fibromuscular dysplasia is classified into different forms depending on the specific site of the abnormalities in the vessel wall-intima, media, or adventitia. More than two-thirds of these patients have characteristic lesions in the main renal artery. *Medial dysplasia* is the most common type, accounting for almost 95% of cases, and is further subdivided. *Medial fibroplasia* is the most common form of medial dysplasia. It usually occurs in women younger than 40, with the right renal artery being more commonly involved than the left. It tends to involve the distal portions of the main renal artery, as well as its branches. This is in contradistinction to the atherosclerotic lesion, which involves the very proximal main renal artery. The angiographic appearance of medial fibroplasia is that of a string of beads (Fig. 108.112). Aneurysms of the main renal artery alternate with areas of narrowing. *Perimedial fibroplasia* tends to occur in slightly younger women than those with medial fibroplasia, usually those younger than 30, and is the second most common type of medial dysplasia. The right renal artery is again more frequently involved than the left. Angiography demonstrates aneurysms that tend to be smaller than those of medial fibroplasia (Fig. 108.113). In addition, abundant collateral vessels tend to be present in this form of fibromuscular dysplasia. Again, the proximal portion of the main renal

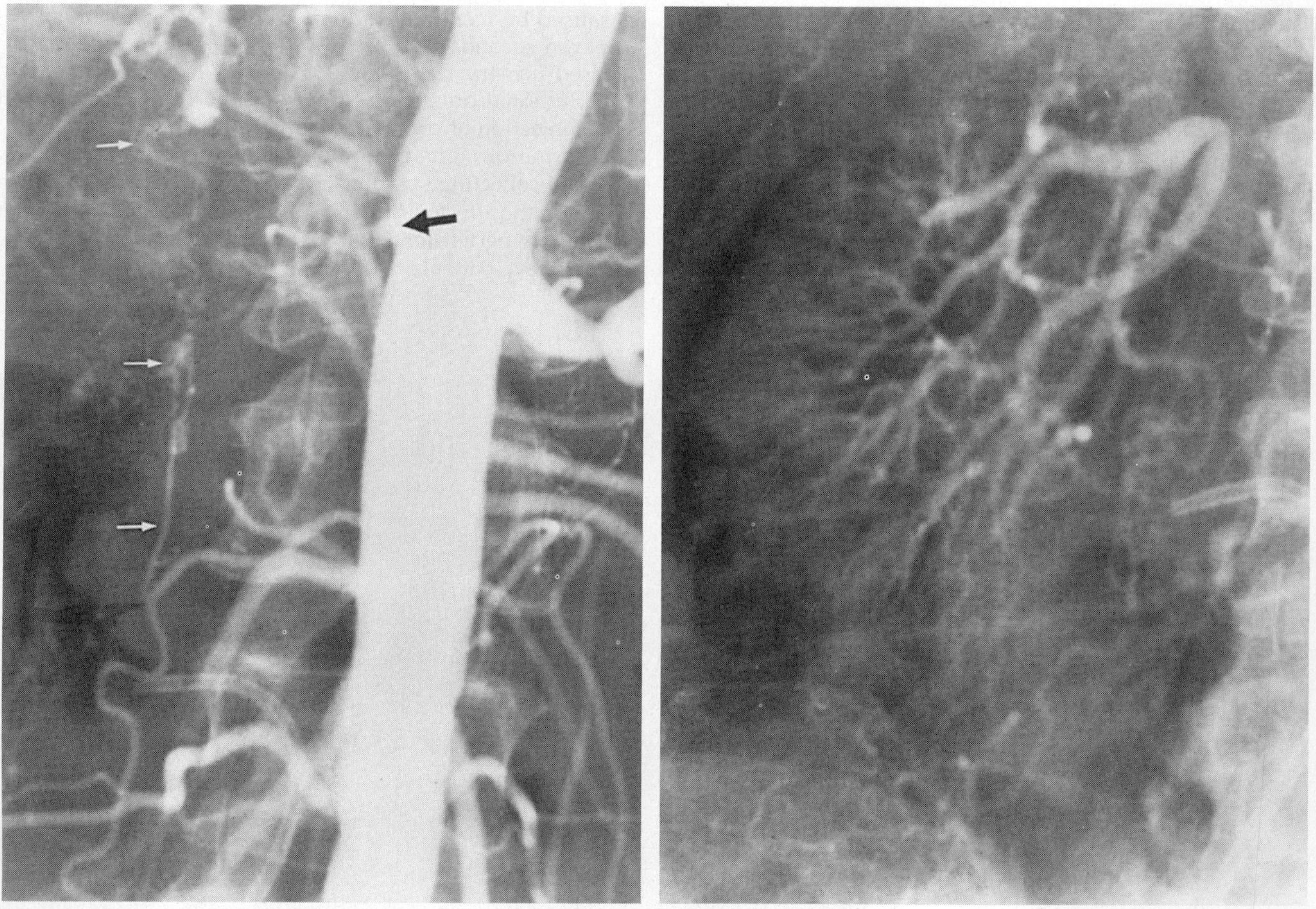

Figure 108.111. Renovascular hypertension. **Left:** Despite the complete occlusion of the right main renal artery *(large arrow)* seen in the abdominal aortogram, collateral vessels *(small arrows)*, especially from the ureteric artery and lumbar arteries, are able to supply adequate perfusion to the right kidney. **Right:** In the late phase of the abdominal aortogram, contrast material is seen filling the distal main renal artery and its parenchymal branches.

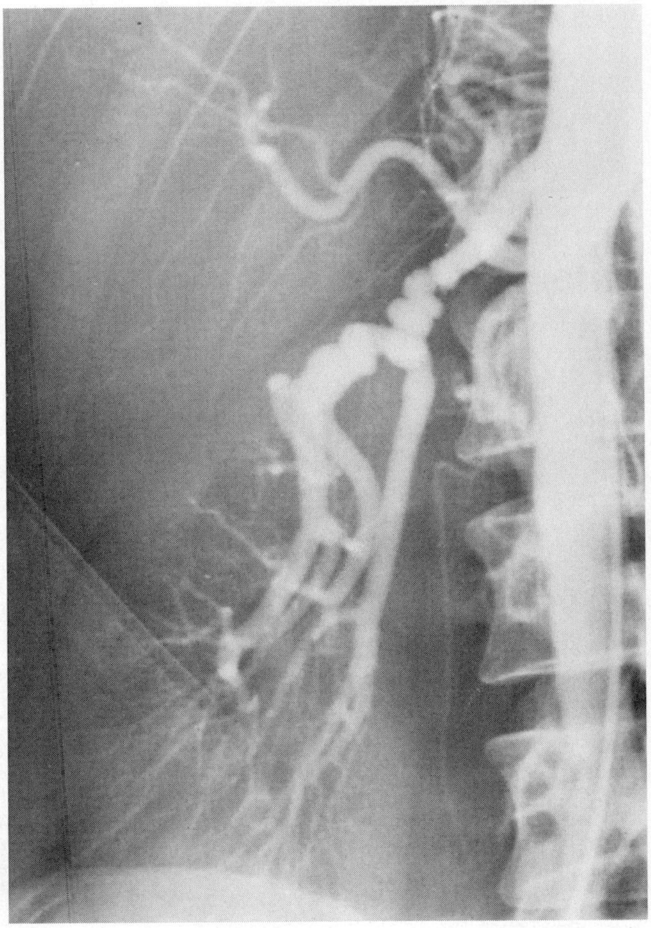

Figure 108.112. Renovascular hypertension. The typical string-of-beads appearance of the main renal artery is seen in this patient with medial fibroplasia involving the right renal artery. Note the alternating regions of narrowing and dilation of the main renal artery.

artery is spared. In *medial dissection*, a less common form of medial dysplasia, there is a longitudinal dissection of variable length that produces a fusiform type of aneurysm of the renal artery. Men and women are equally affected. Additional rare forms of fibromuscular dysplasia are noted: *intimal fibroplasia*, *medial hyperplasia*, and *adventitial fibroplasia*. Angiographically, they are indistinguishable, with concentric narrowing of the renal artery (Fig. 108.114). The midportion of the main renal

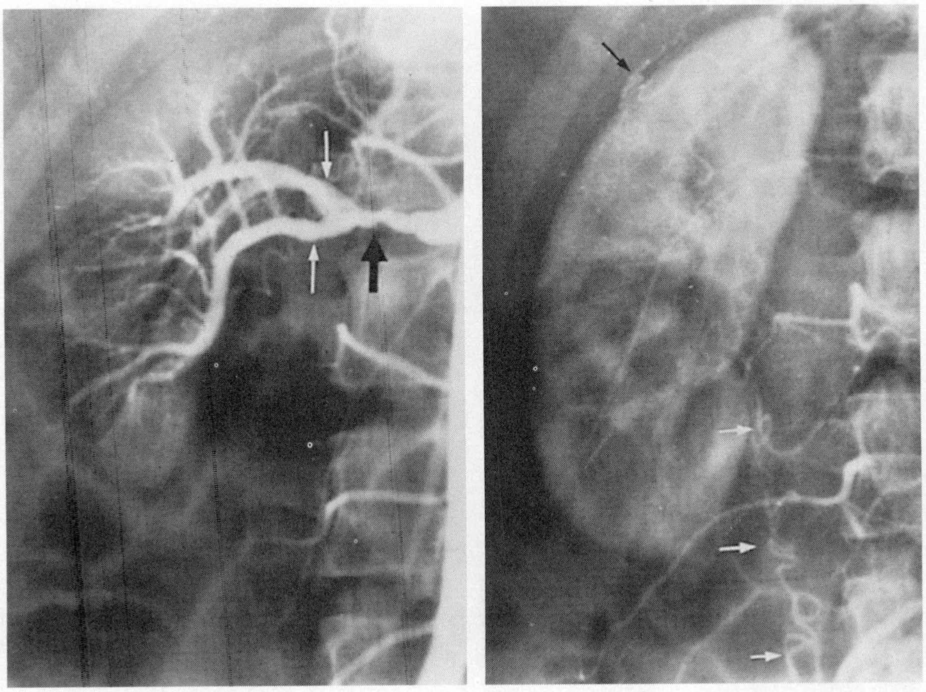

Figure 108.113. Renovascular hypertension. **Left:** The abdominal aortogram of this patient with perimedial fibroplasia shows irregular narrowing of the middle and distal aspects of the main renal artery *(large arrow)*. Dilation of the renal artery occurs after its first bifurcation *(small arrows)*. The origin of the right renal artery is normal. **Right:** A later-phase film from the abdominal aortogram shows capsular vessels and ureteric vessels *(arrows)* supplying collateral blood flow to the kidney. The presence of collateral vessels is common in perimedial fibroplasia.

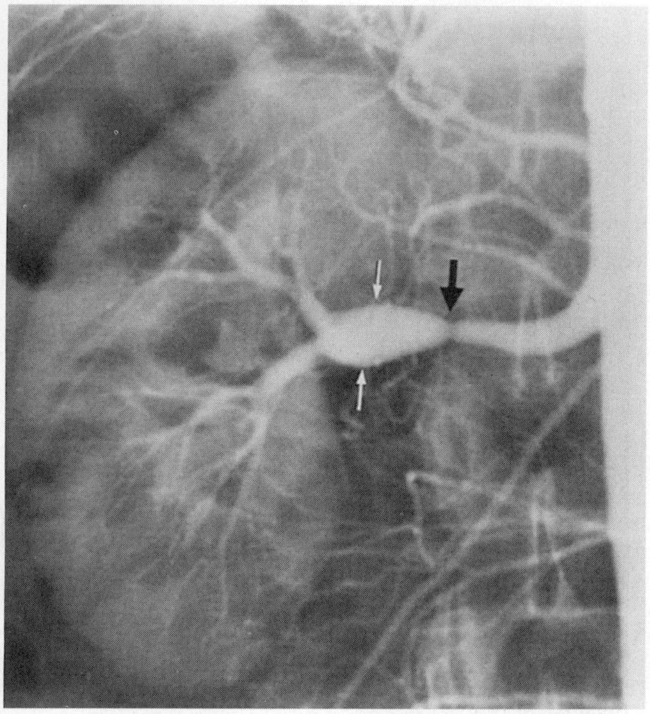

Figure 108.114. Renovascular hypertension. The abdominal aortogram demonstrates concentric narrowing of the right main renal artery *(large arrow)*, with poststenotic dilation of the renal artery *(small arrows)* beyond the area of stenosis. In this case, the cause for the narrowing was intimal fibroplasia. These findings, however, are indistinguishable from medial hyperplasia.

artery is usually the involved segment, although branch involvement may be seen as well. Intimal fibroplasia is the most common type found in childhood and often is progressive. *Periarterial fibrosis,* or *adventitial fibroplasia,* is the most uncommon form of fibromuscular dysplasia and shows angiographically a marked segmental narrowing of either the proximal or mid-renal artery. Transluminal angioplasty has become the method of choice for treatment of renovascular hypertension because of stenotic lesions caused by either atherosclerosis or fibromuscular dysplasia.

Renal artery aneurysms may be associated with renovascular hypertension (Fig. 108.115). The aneurysms may be congenital or caused by atherosclerosis, fibromuscular dysplasia, trauma, or inflammatory conditions. Approximately 25% of the aneurysms show some calcification in the wall. These calcifications are usually ringlike or at least curvilinear. Saccular aneurysms are the most common form noted. Fusiform aneurysms, poststenotic areas of dilation or aneurysm, dissecting aneurysms, or pseudoaneurysms caused by trauma are also noted. Congenital aneurysms are usually of the saccular form and occur at bifurcations. Inflammatory-related aneurysms usually are caused by collagen-vascular diseases, vasculitides, or drugs. Occasionally, mycotic aneurysms of the renal artery occur. Rupture of any type of aneurysm is rare. Neurofibromatosis may lead to either stenotic lesions of the main renal artery or aneurysms. The lesions are often multiple. Both kidneys may be involved. Any portion of the renal artery, including the orifice or branches, may be affected.

Rarely, tumors of the kidney may lead to renal-related hypertension. Juxtaglomerular cell tumors, a type of hemangiocytoma, may excrete renin. The radiographic detection of these lesions is difficult. The IVP is usually normal, and the angiogram may be normal or show a small area of hypervascularity in the cortex. Wilms' tumors rarely may be associated with hypertension as well. Large tumor bulk may lead to compression of the main renal artery, with subsequent ischemia and renin production.

Manifestations of Renal Failure

Although the primary focus in a patient with renal failure is on the kidneys, various effects on other areas of the body may be

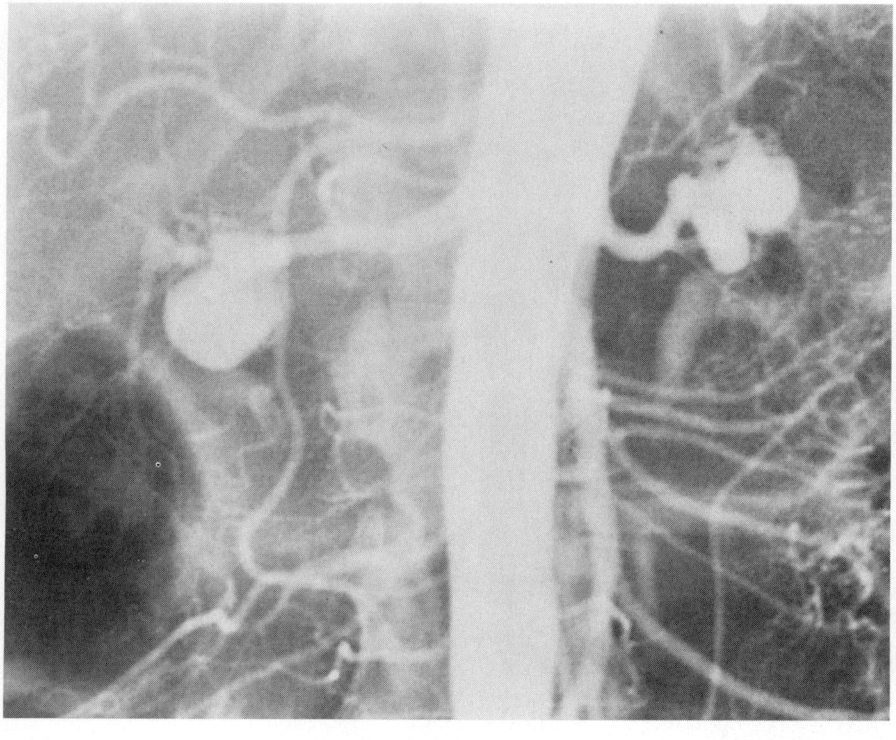

Figure 108.115. Renovascular hypertension. Bilateral congenital renal artery aneurysms are seen on this abdominal aortogram. The aneurysms are saccular in nature and are located at the bifurcations of both main renal arteries.

noted radiographically. These findings are related to the primary disease process causing the renal failure (polycystic kidney disease), the biochemical changes that occur in the renal failure (secondary hyperparathyroidism), the fluid and electrolyte problems associated with renal failure (pulmonary edema), and the drugs administered to patients with renal failure (steroid therapy).

Cardiovascular System

Episodes of pulmonary edema are common occurrences in patients with renal failure. The radiographic picture is somewhat variable depending on the specific cause of the pulmonary edema. Patients with renal failure may develop systemic hypertension and congestive heart failure. In patients with heart failure, the chest x-ray film usually reveals cardiomegaly with variable amounts of pulmonary vascular redistribution. As the left ventricle fails to pump blood adequately, the left atrial pressure increases, with subsequent pulmonary edema seen on chest radiograph (Fig. 108.116). Fluid overload and uremia may also cause a clinical picture simulating pulmonary edema. In these patients, the chest x-ray film frequently reveals pulmonary infiltrates taking the shape of a butterfly (Fig. 108.117). There is usually rapid disappearance

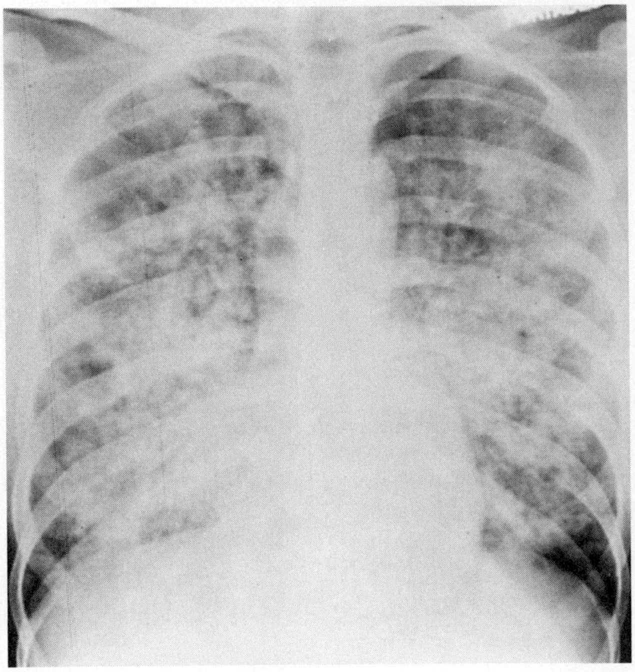

Figure 108.116. Congestive heart failure and pulmonary edema. Extensive alveolar pulmonary edema is identified bilaterally on this chest film. The alveolar edema involves all lobes of the lung and extends to the periphery. This patient with chronic renal failure recently had experienced an acute myocardial infarction.

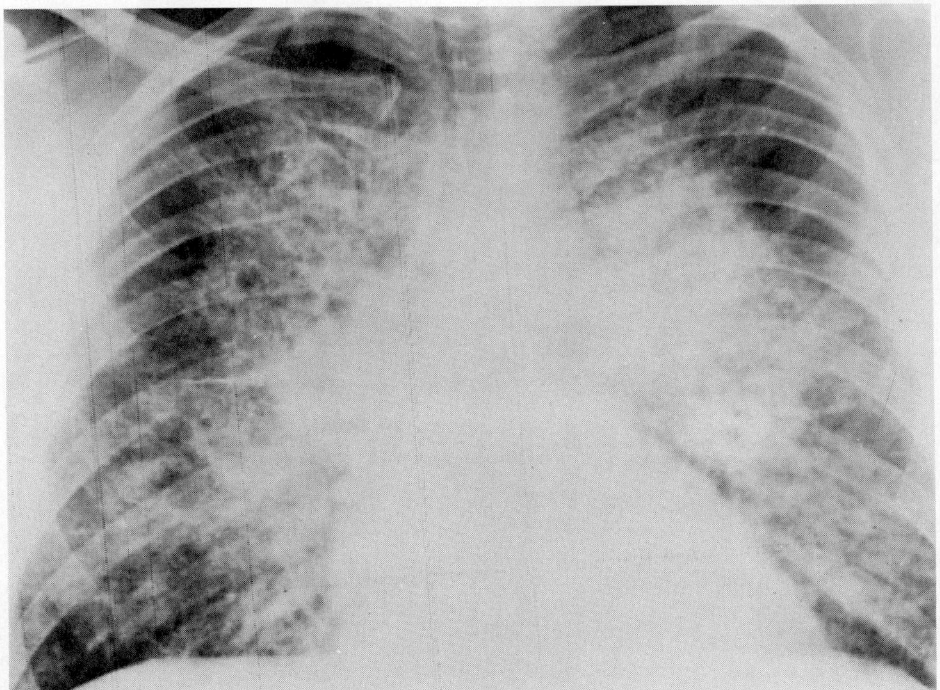

Figure 108.117. Pulmonary edema. This chest film demonstrates a typical butterfly, or bat-wing, appearance of the alveolar pulmonary edema. The alveolar fluid is distributed primarily in the parahilar region, with the periphery of the lung being spared. This pattern cleared rapidly as the patient's fluid balance was restored.

of the pulmonary edema as seen in the chest x-ray film as the uremia and fluid status are treated. Patients with chronic renal failure have an increased incidence of regular and opportunistic pulmonary infections (Fig. 108.118). Radiographically detectable pulmonary parenchymal calcifications are rarely encountered in patients with chronic renal failure (Fig. 108.119) but are more commonly discovered with ^{99m}Tc-labeled pyrophosphate scan (Fig. 108.120).

Pericarditis and pericardial effusions are commonly seen in uremic patients. On chest x-ray film, a pericardial effusion causes enlargement of the cardiac silhouette in a symmetric manner, with the end result being a large, globular, water bottle–shaped heart (Fig. 108.121). Several hundred milliliters of fluid need to be present to make the diagnosis on chest x-ray examination. Small amounts of pericardial fluid can be detected by echocardiography.

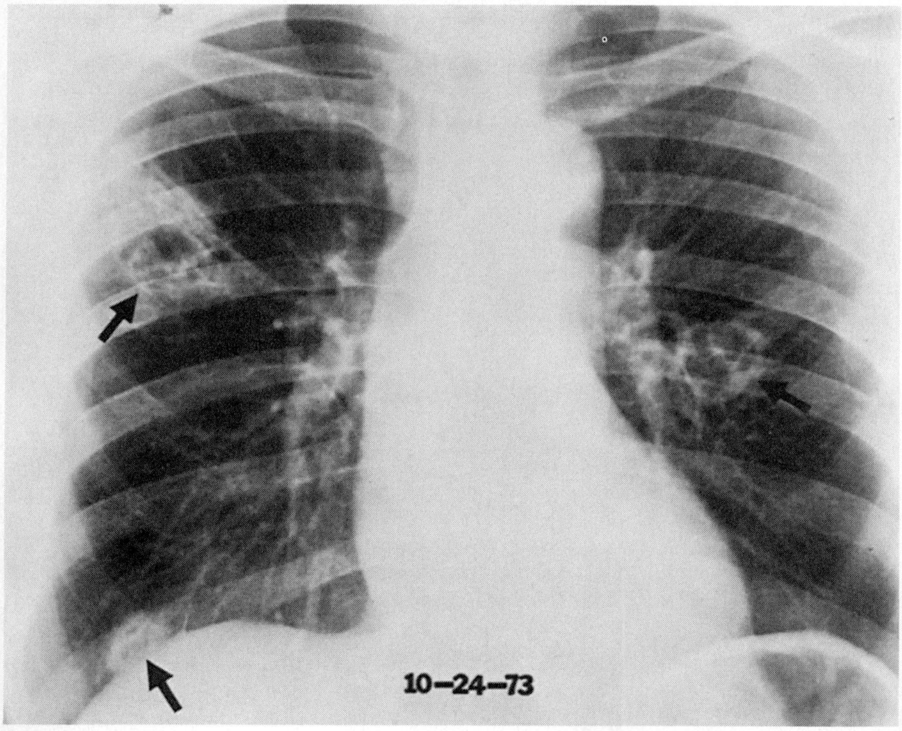

Figure 108.118. Opportunistic pulmonary infection. Bilateral cavitating lesions *(arrows)* are seen in both lungs on this chest x-ray film. The cavities were the result of a *Nocardia* infection in a patient with chronic renal failure being treated with corticosteroids.

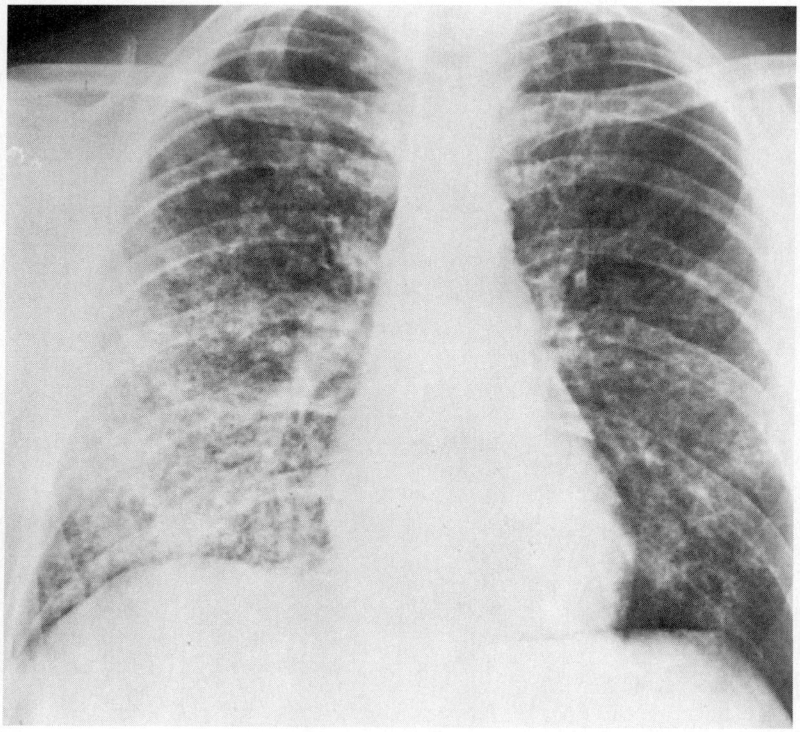

Figure 108.119. Pulmonary parenchymal calcifications. Extensive interstitial opacities of high density are noted in both lung fields on this chest film. The parenchymal calcifications occurred rapidly over a 3-month period in this patient with chronic renal failure.

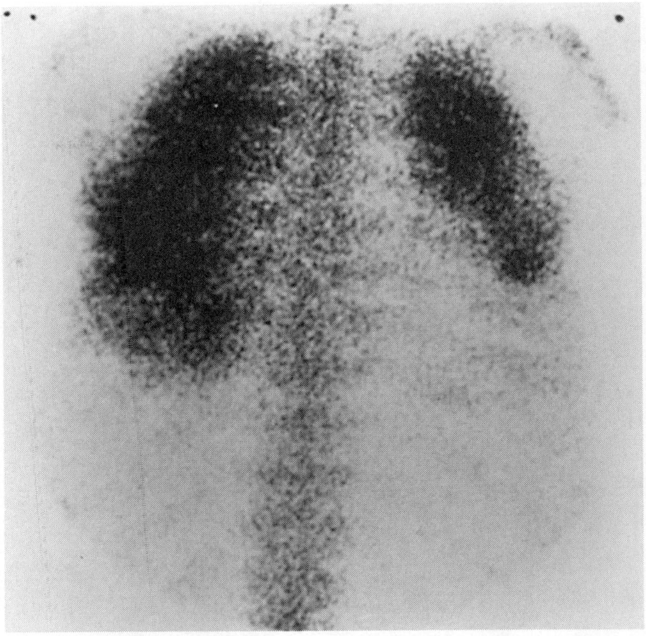

Figure 108.120. Pulmonary parenchymal calcifications. This bone scan using ^{99m}Tc-labeled pyrophosphate shows extensive uptake in the lungs bilaterally. These scan findings were noted 2 months before the changes on the chest film seen in Fig. 108.119.

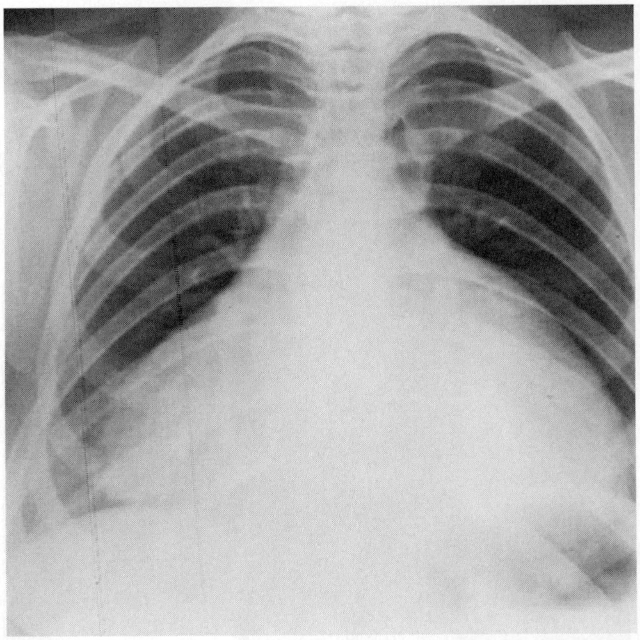

Figure 108.121. Pericardial effusion. This upright posteroanterior chest film shows a markedly enlarged cardiac silhouette, which is globular in shape. Note that there is no evidence of congestive heart failure. This pericardial effusion in a uremic patient amounted to greater than 1,000 ml.

Gastrointestinal Tract

Some renal diseases, such as polycystic kidney disease, may cause changes in the gastrointestinal tract. There is an increased incidence of hiatal hernia in patients with polycystic kidney disease (Fig. 108.122). Also, diverticula of both the small and large bowel appear to be more common in patients with polycystic kidney disease than in the general population. When the kidneys are very large, marked displacement of both the bowel and stomach may occur.

In uremic patients, there is a high incidence of hemorrhagic gastritis. It is occasionally detectable radiographically (Fig. 108.123). Mucosal edema, especially in the proximal portion of the bowel, occurs in uremic patients who are fluid overloaded (Fig. 108.124). These bowel wall changes tend to get better with improvement in fluid balance and after dialysis. In the immunosuppressed patient, monilial *Candida* esophagitis may occur (Fig. 108.125).

Bones, Joints, and Soft Tissues

The radiographic manifestations of bone disease and soft tissue calcification are shown in detail in Chapter 77 and of dialysis amyloidosis in Chapter 84, Part 1E.

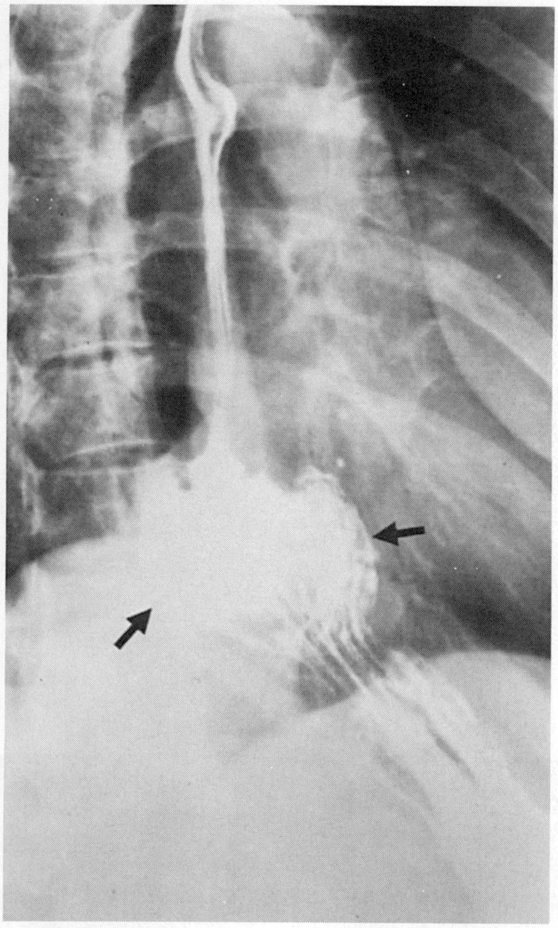

Figure 108.122. Hiatal hernia. This moderate-sized hiatal hernia *(arrows)* was discovered in a patient with polycystic kidney disease.

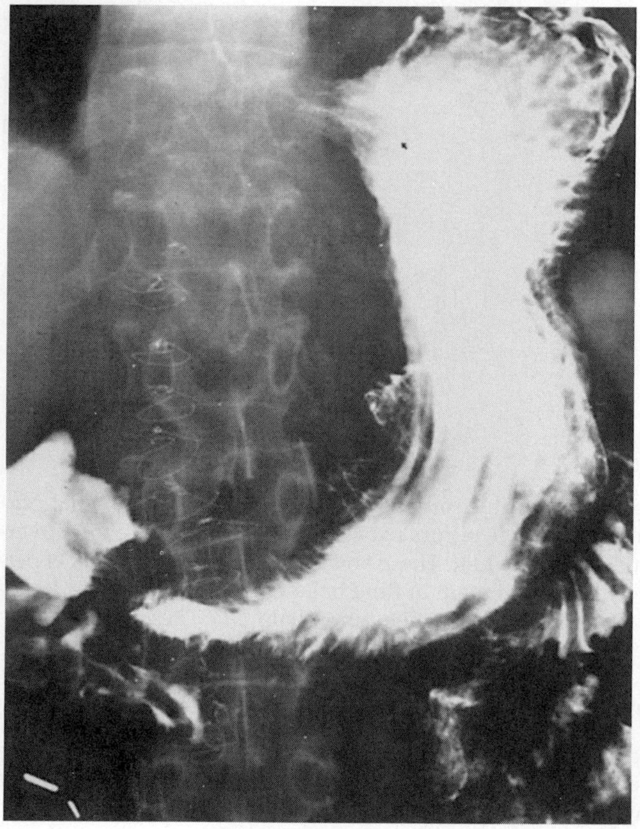

Figure 108.123. Hemorrhagic gastritis. A spiculated appearance to the distal aspect of the stomach antrum represents hemorrhagic gastritis in this patient with chronic renal failure. No distinct ulcerations are seen. However, the mucosa is extensively eroded.

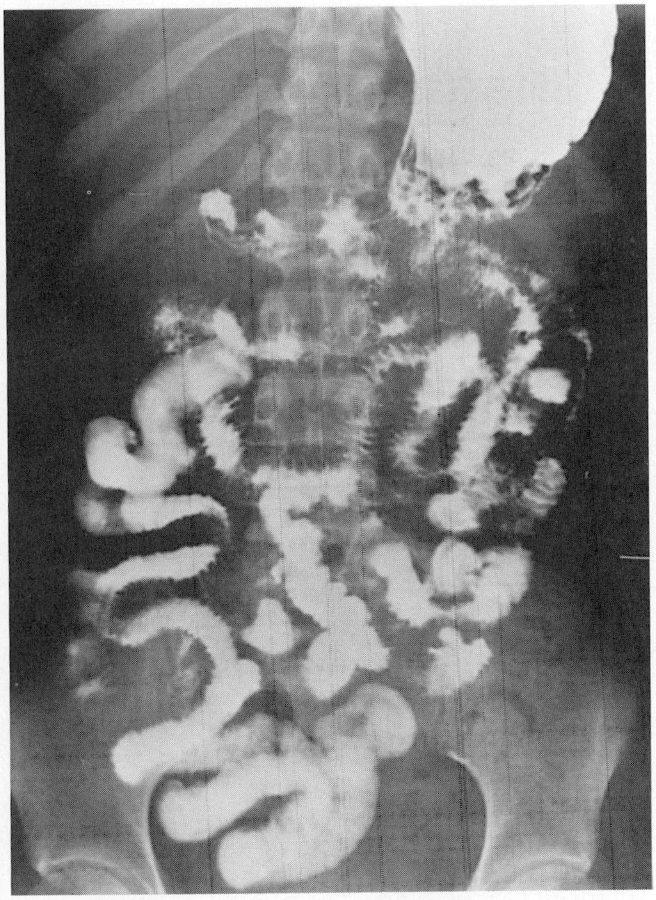

Figure 108.124. Mucosal edema. This small bowel series demonstrates mucosal thickening throughout the small bowel. Ascites is also present. This fluid-overloaded patient showed resolution of this pattern as dialysis corrected her fluid status.

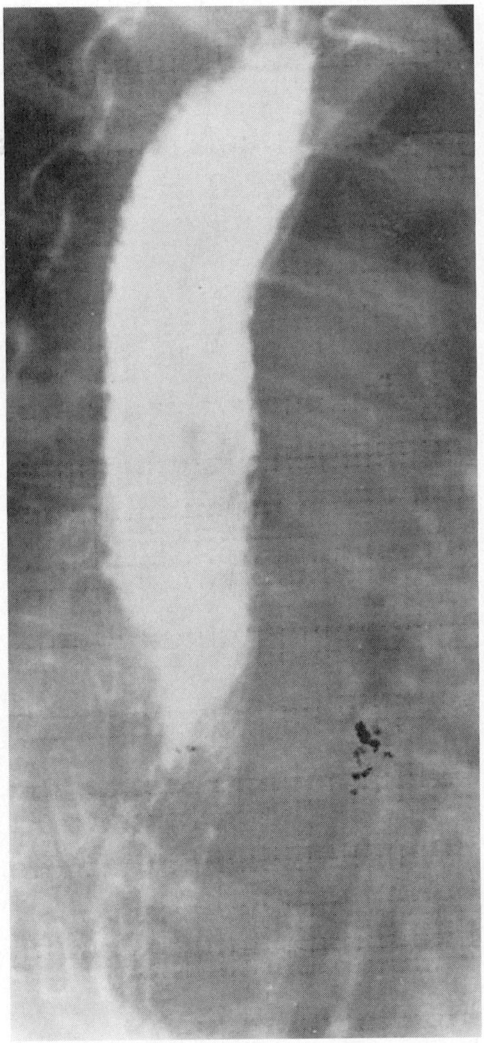

Figure 108.125. Monilial esophagitis. A markedly irregular mucosal pattern throughout the esophagus, with apparent ulcerations, is noted in this patient with chronic renal failure being treated with corticosteroids. This was caused by monilial esophagitis.

Selected Readings

Amis ES, Newhouse JH. *Essentials of uroradiology.* Boston: Little, Brown, 1991.

New look at older topics. Well-organized and readable overview.

Barbaric ZL. *Principles of genitourinary radiology.* New York: Thieme Medical Publishers, 1991.

Well-illustrated and concise text on genitourinary radiology topics. Quick reference. Covers all imaging modalities, including CT, MRI, ultrasound, and nuclear medicine.

Davidson AJ. *Radiology of the kidney.* Philadelphia: WB Saunders, 1985.

A concise, readable textbook on radiology of the kidney. It is developed in a unique manner, with a problem-oriented approach.

Dunnick NR, McCallum RW, Sandler CM. *Textbook of uroradiology.* Baltimore: Williams & Wilkins, 1991.

Comprehensive general text dealing with all areas in genitourinary radiology.

Newhouse JH, ed. Imaging and intervention in the renal fossa. *Radiol Clin North Am* 1987;22:285–460.

A concise overview of the interventional aspects of genitourinary radiology. Newer aspects of imaging are also dealt with, again in relationship to the genitourinary tract, specifically the kidney.

Ney C, Friedenberg RM, eds. *Radiographic atlas of the genitourinary tract,* 2nd ed. Philadelphia: JB Lippincott, 1981.

An extremely well-illustrated atlas that reviews all the conditions affecting the genitourinary tract, from a radiologic perspective. The illustrations, in particular, are of high quality.

Written DM, Myers GH, Utz DC. *Emmett's clinical urography,* 4th ed. Philadelphia: WB Saunders, 1977.

The classic text on radiology of the genitourinary tract. The illustrations and text are of high quality. This is basically the foundation on which all of genitourinary radiology rests.

SECTION XIV

Atlas of Renal Pathology

CHAPTER 109

Atlas of Renal Pathology

Arthur H. Cohen and Cynthia C. Nast

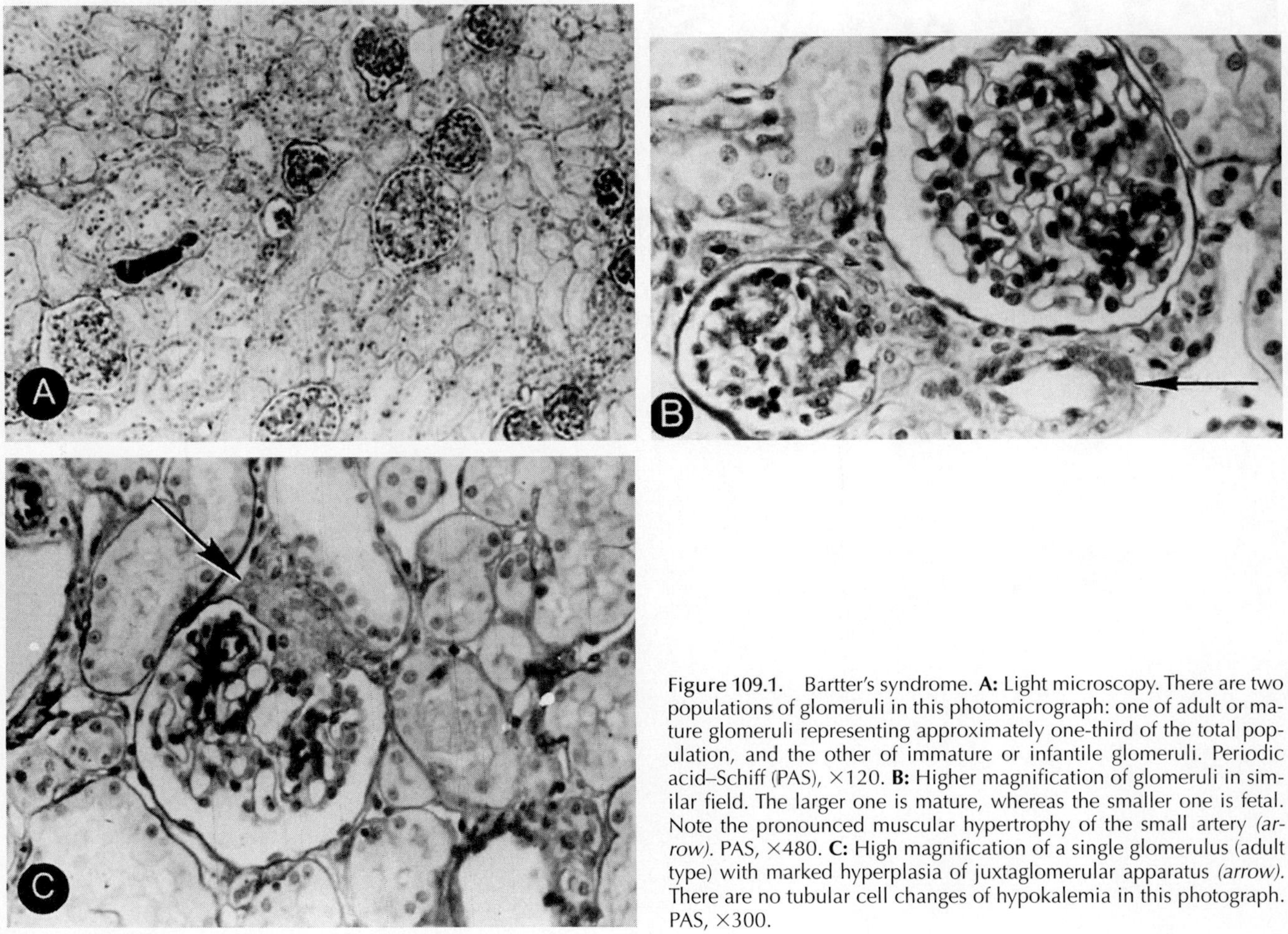

Figure 109.1. Bartter's syndrome. **A:** Light microscopy. There are two populations of glomeruli in this photomicrograph: one of adult or mature glomeruli representing approximately one-third of the total population, and the other of immature or infantile glomeruli. Periodic acid–Schiff (PAS), ×120. **B:** Higher magnification of glomeruli in similar field. The larger one is mature, whereas the smaller one is fetal. Note the pronounced muscular hypertrophy of the small artery *(arrow)*. PAS, ×480. **C:** High magnification of a single glomerulus (adult type) with marked hyperplasia of juxtaglomerular apparatus *(arrow)*. There are no tubular cell changes of hypokalemia in this photograph. PAS, ×300.

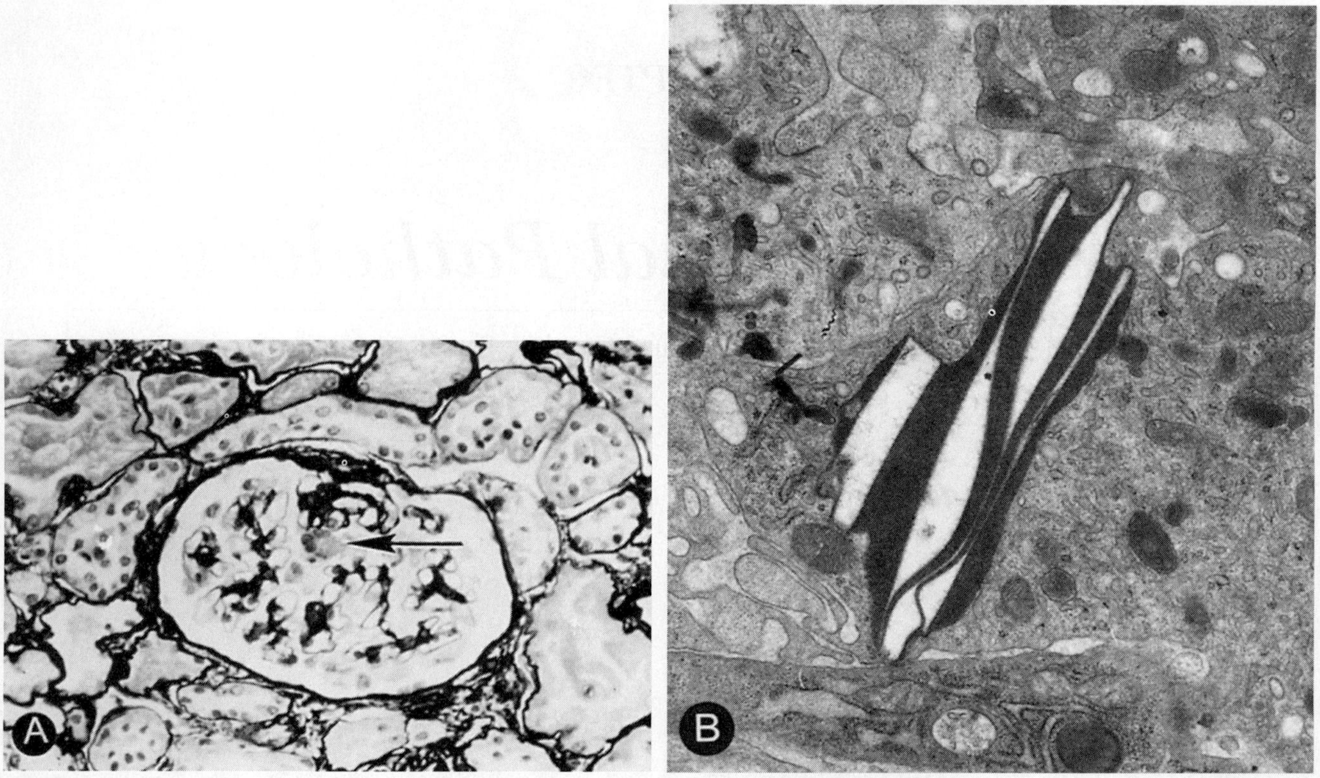

Figure 109.2. Cystinosis. **A:** Light microscopy. This glomerulus discloses one of the more characteristic light microscopic features: a visceral epithelial cell is enlarged and multinucleated *(arrow)*. Periodic acid–methenamine silver, ×300. **B:** Electron microscopy. An interstitial cell with lysosomes containing a dense precipitate within which are angular empty intracellular spaces indicative of dissolved cystine crystals. ×13,950.

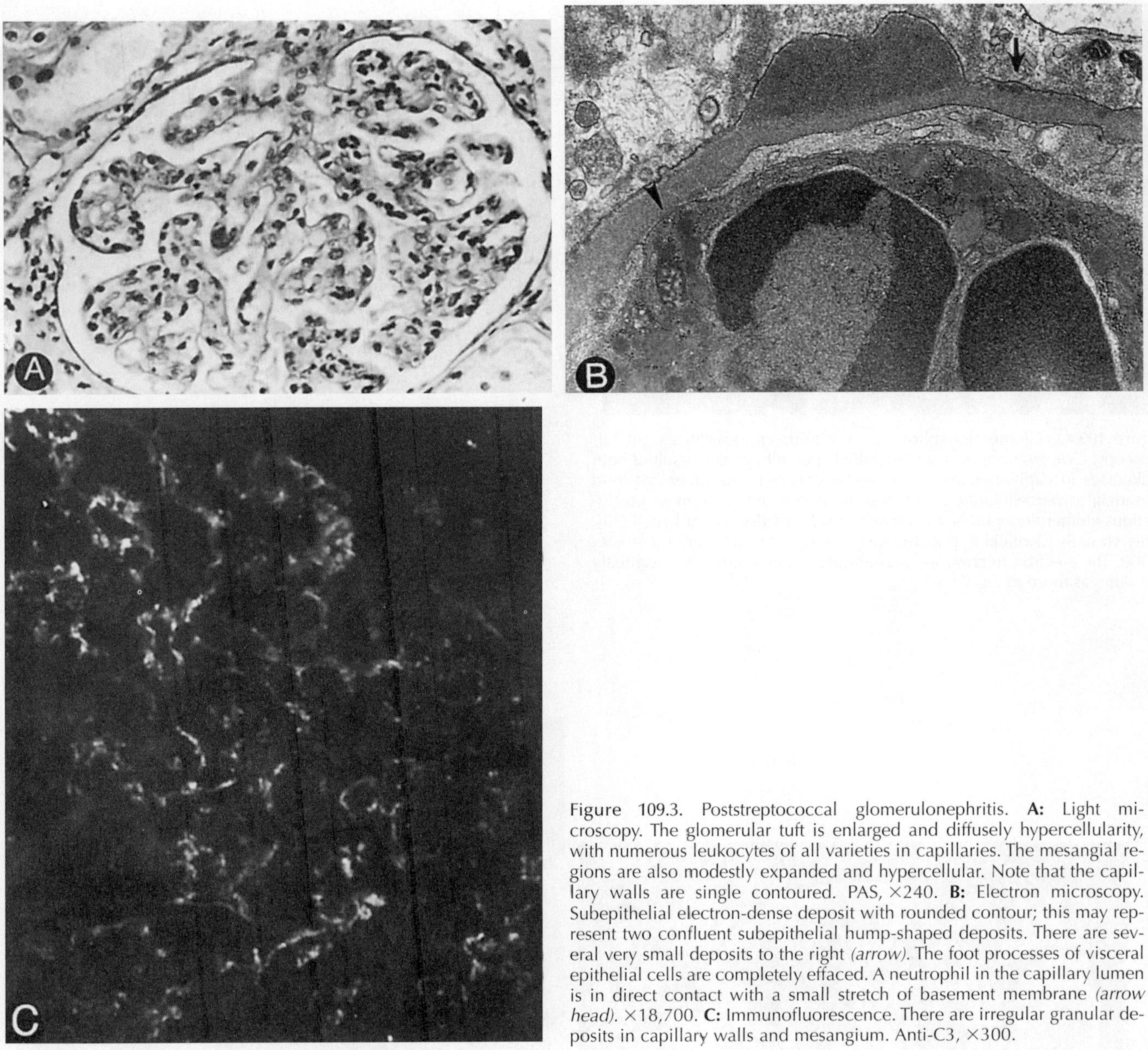

Figure 109.3. Poststreptococcal glomerulonephritis. **A:** Light microscopy. The glomerular tuft is enlarged and diffusely hypercellularity, with numerous leukocytes of all varieties in capillaries. The mesangial regions are also modestly expanded and hypercellular. Note that the capillary walls are single contoured. PAS, ×240. **B:** Electron microscopy. Subepithelial electron-dense deposit with rounded contour; this may represent two confluent subepithelial hump-shaped deposits. There are several very small deposits to the right *(arrow)*. The foot processes of visceral epithelial cells are completely effaced. A neutrophil in the capillary lumen is in direct contact with a small stretch of basement membrane *(arrow head)*. ×18,700. **C:** Immunofluorescence. There are irregular granular deposits in capillary walls and mesangium. Anti-C3, ×300.

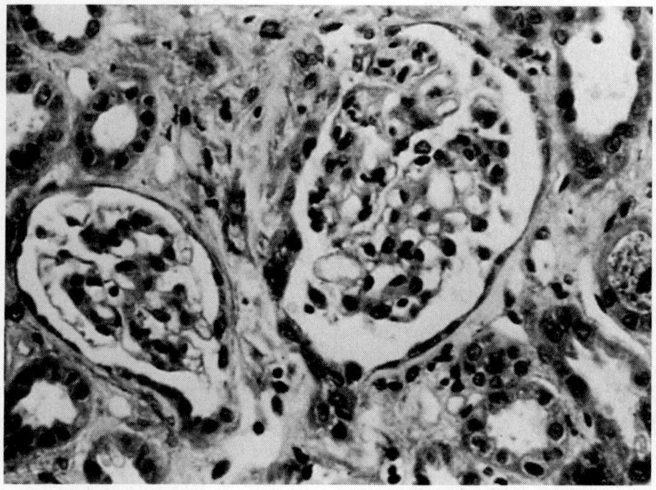

Figure 109.4. Glomerulonephritis in infectious endocarditis. Light microscopy. One glomerulus is segmentally hypercellular as a result of both leukocytes in capillaries and a segmental crescent. The other has mild mesangial hypercellularity. In this lesion, as with other forms of postinfectious glomerulonephritis, the picture may be of glomerular hypercellularity virtually identical to poststreptococcal disease. Masson's trichrome, ×300. The electron microscopy and immunofluorescence are essentially the same as those in Fig. 109.3.

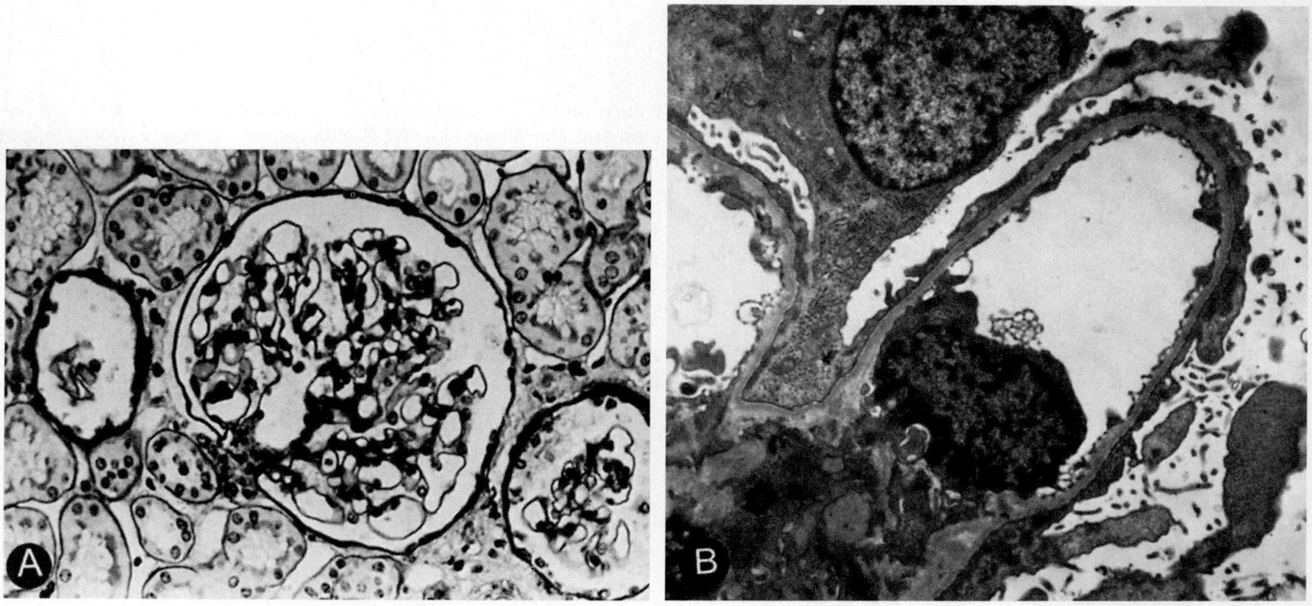

Figure 109.5. Minimal-change disease. **A:** Light microscopy. The glomeruli have a normal appearance with potent capillary lumina and thin, single-contoured capillary walls. There is no appreciable increase in cellularity. PAS, ×240. **B:** Electron microscopy. The foot processes of epithelial cells are completely effaced, resulting in a solid or near-solid cell covering over the basement membrane. There are no endothelial cell alterations. Note the complete lack of electron-dense deposits. ×5,680.

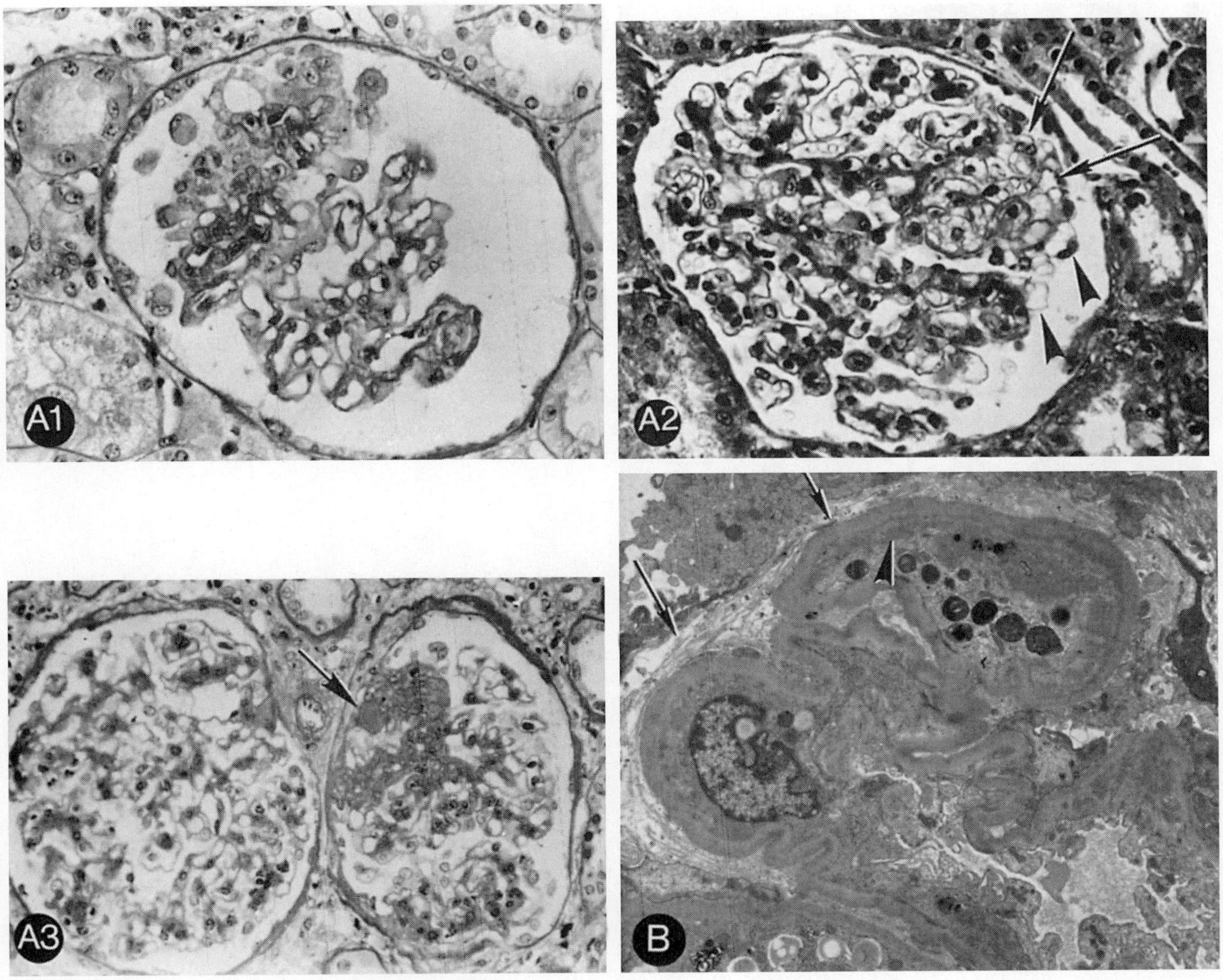

Figure 109.6. Focal and segmental glomerulosclerosis. **A1–3:** Light microscopy. **1:** Early stage of segmental glomerulosclerosis. There is segmental enlargement and increase in number of visceral epithelial cells. Each abnormal cell contains large, coarse cytoplasmic vacuoles, sometimes with protein reabsorption droplets. PAS, ×240. **2:** Slightly later stage of evaluation. Capillary lumina of the affected lobule are filled with lipid-containing cells *(arrows)*. Note the epithelial changes similar to those in **A1** *(arrowheads)*. Masson's trichrome, ×200. **3:** Late stage of segmental sclerosis. In the affected glomerulus, some capillaries are obliterated by large-protein "insudates" *(arrow)*. There is increased mesangial matrix and basement membrane material. The sclerotic segment is adherent to Bowman's capsule. Note the reduced cellularity in the abnormal segment. PAS, ×220. **B:** Electron microscopy. The uninvolved portions of glomeruli appear as minimal-change disease. The segments of sclerosis, as illustrated here, characteristically have separation of visceral epithelial cells from basement membranes; there is accumulation of thin layers of new basement membrane material alternating with pale-staining zones often containing cytoplasmic debris *(arrows)*. Note electron-dense material *(arrowhead)*, corresponding to an "insudative" lesion, on the inner aspect of the basement membrane. A remnant of a lipid-containing macrophage also occupies what is left of the lumen. ×4,000.

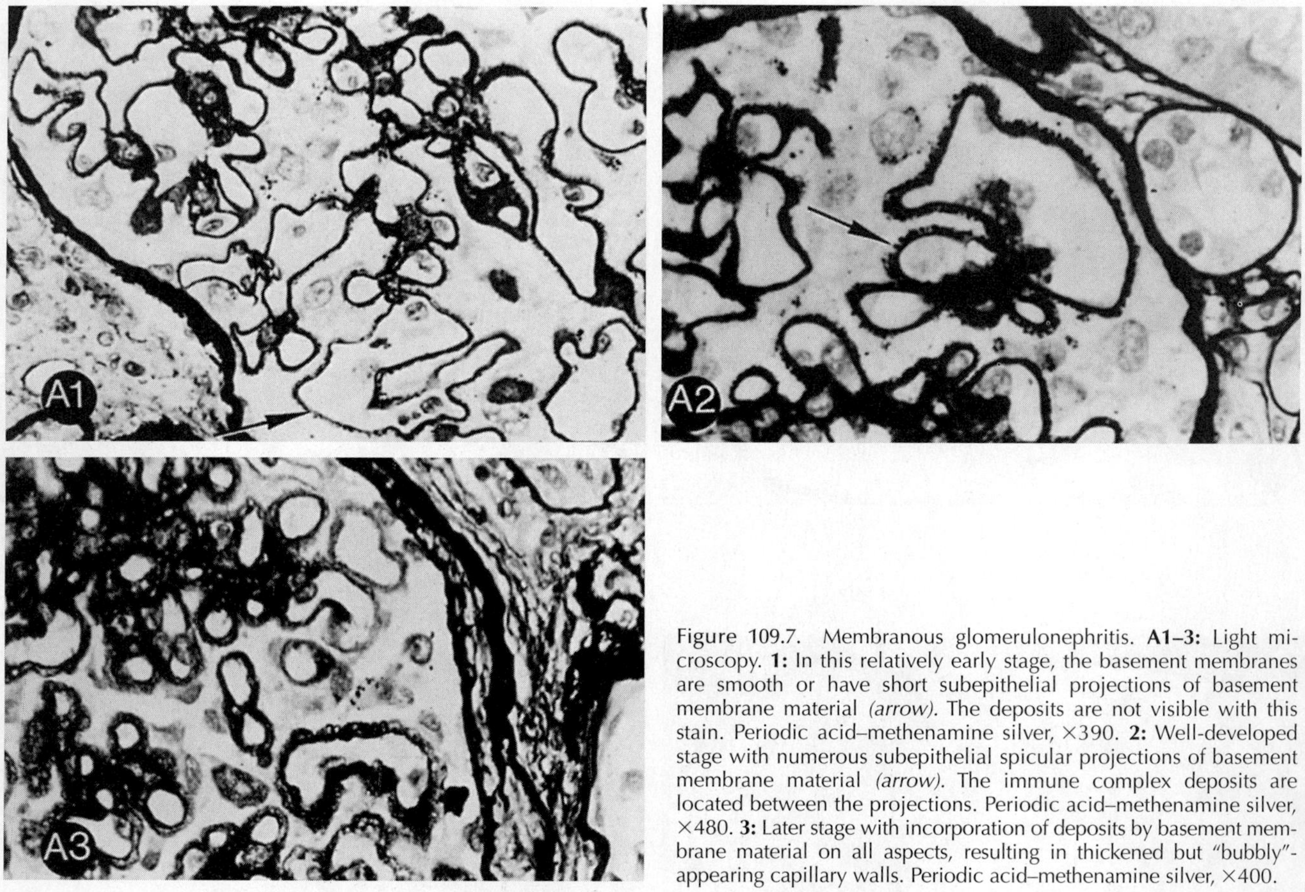

Figure 109.7. Membranous glomerulonephritis. **A1–3:** Light microscopy. **1:** In this relatively early stage, the basement membranes are smooth or have short subepithelial projections of basement membrane material *(arrow)*. The deposits are not visible with this stain. Periodic acid–methenamine silver, ×390. **2:** Well-developed stage with numerous subepithelial spicular projections of basement membrane material *(arrow)*. The immune complex deposits are located between the projections. Periodic acid–methenamine silver, ×480. **3:** Later stage with incorporation of deposits by basement membrane material on all aspects, resulting in thickened but "bubbly"-appearing capillary walls. Periodic acid–methenamine silver, ×400.

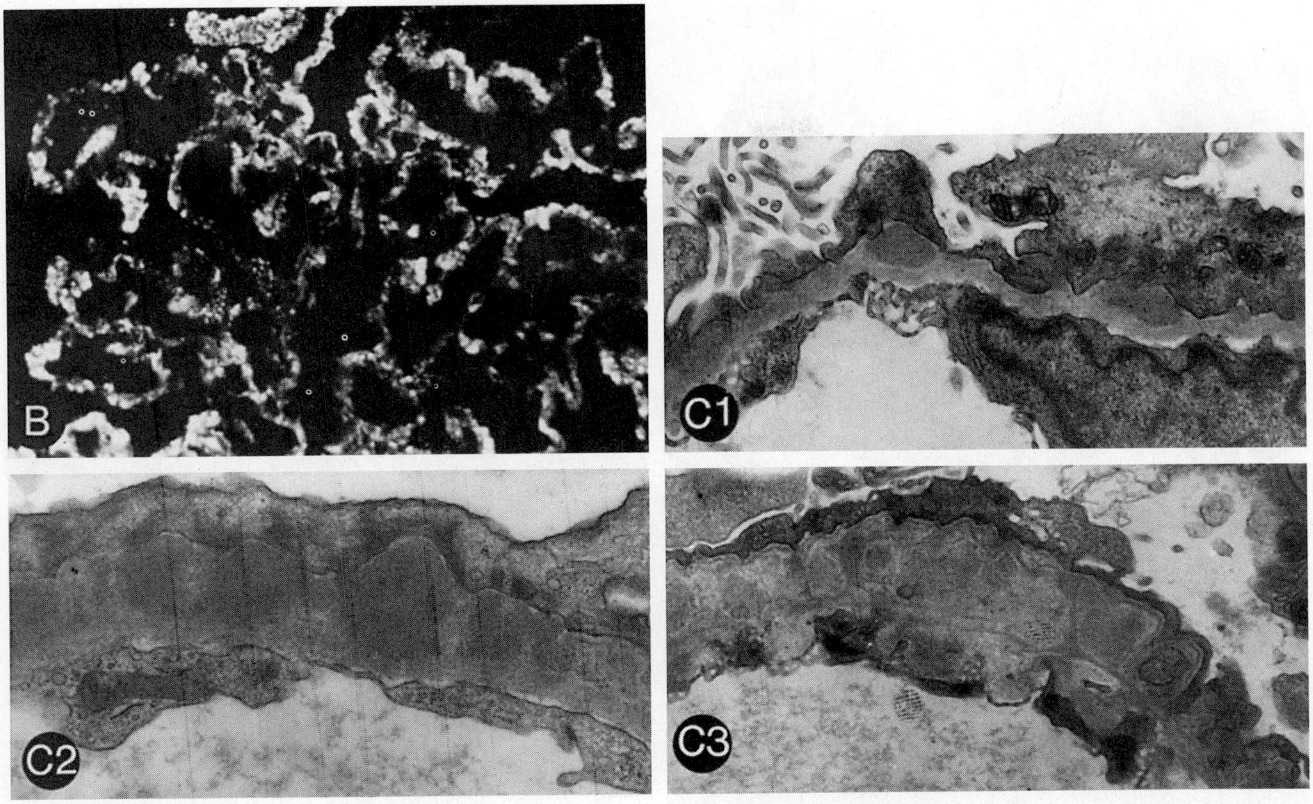

Figure 109.7 (*continued.*) Membranous glomerulonephritis. **B:** Immunofluorescence. There are uniform granular deposits along all capillary walls. This corresponds to the middle or well-developed lesion, although a similar picture may occur at almost any stage of membranous glomerulonephritis. Anti-IgG, × 480. **C1–3:** Electron microscopy. **1:** Early stage. The electron-dense deposits are small and widely separated. They initially form beneath the slit-pore diaphragms. There is virtually no alteration of basement membrane structure in association with the deposits. ×8,125. **2:** Middle stage. There are large, well-defined subepithelial electron-dense deposits with well-developed intervening basement membrane projections. Note that foot processes of epithelial cells are completely effaced. ×13,700. **3:** In this late stage, the deposits are completely surrounded by basement membrane. Many are less dense or are lucent, an indication of reabsorption. ×8,450.

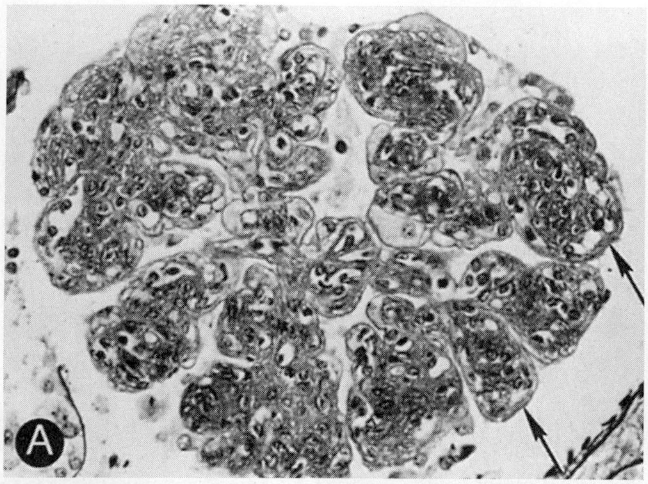

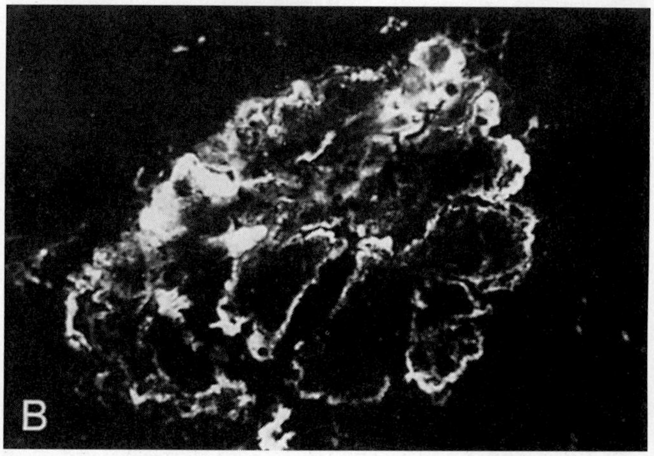

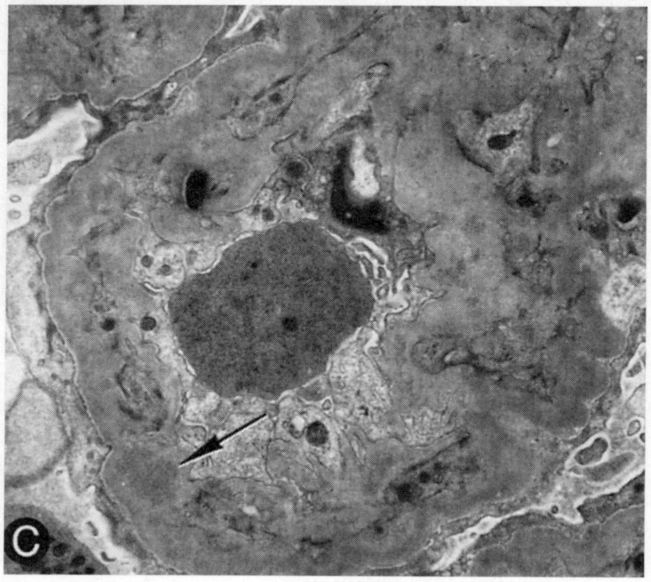

Figure 109.8. Membranoproliferative (mesangiocapillary) glomerulonephritis, type I. **A:** Light microscopy. The glomerulus is enlarged and has distinct lobular accentuation. Mesangial cellularity is increased, and there are modest numbers of leukocytes in capillary lumina. Capillary walls are thickened and have a two-layered (double-contoured) appearance *(arrows)*. PAS, ×240. **B:** Immunofluorescence. The capillary walls are stained in a discontinuous coarsely granular to linear pattern. Note the lobular appearance of the glomerulus. Anti-C3, ×300. **C:** Electron microscopy. Glomerular capillary wall showing complex abnormalities. There are six distinctive layers starting from the urinary space. Epithelial cell cytoplasm covers the original basement membrane. Immediately within are small and large electron-dense deposits *(arrow)*. The next two layers include interposed mesangial cell cytoplasm and beneath that, mesangial matrix. The endothelial cell lines the capillary lumen. The basement membrane and mesangial matrix are tinctorially the same at the light microscopic level and are responsible far the double-layered appearance. ×6,950.

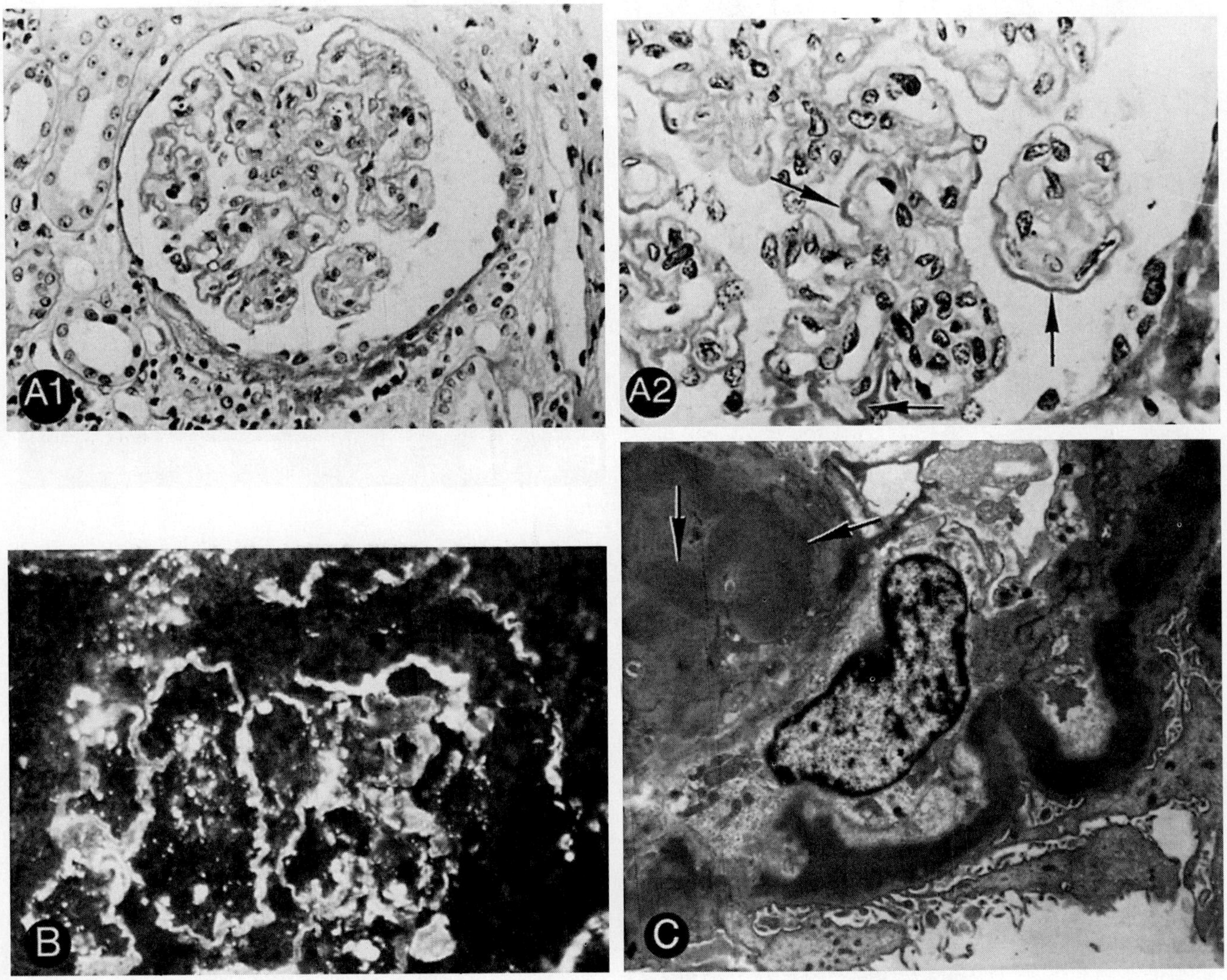

Figure 109.9. Membranoproliferative glomerulonephritis, type II (dense deposit disease). **A1–2:** Light microscopy. **1:** The glomerulus is slightly hypercellular and lobulated, and the mesangial regions are somewhat expanded. Capillary walls are thickened. PAS, ×200. **2:** This higher magnification shows many capillary basement membranes to be densely staining and thickened *(arrow)*. PAS, ×440. **B:** Immunofluorescence. The capillary walls stain in a continuous pattern; note also similar deposits along the basement membrane of Bowman's capsule. There are also isolated round mesangial deposits. Anti-C3, ×280. **C:** Electron microscopy. Dense transformation of large segments of basement membrane is depicted; note the "sausage" shape to some of the capillary wall deposits, and rounded mesangial deposits *(arrow)*. ×4,000.

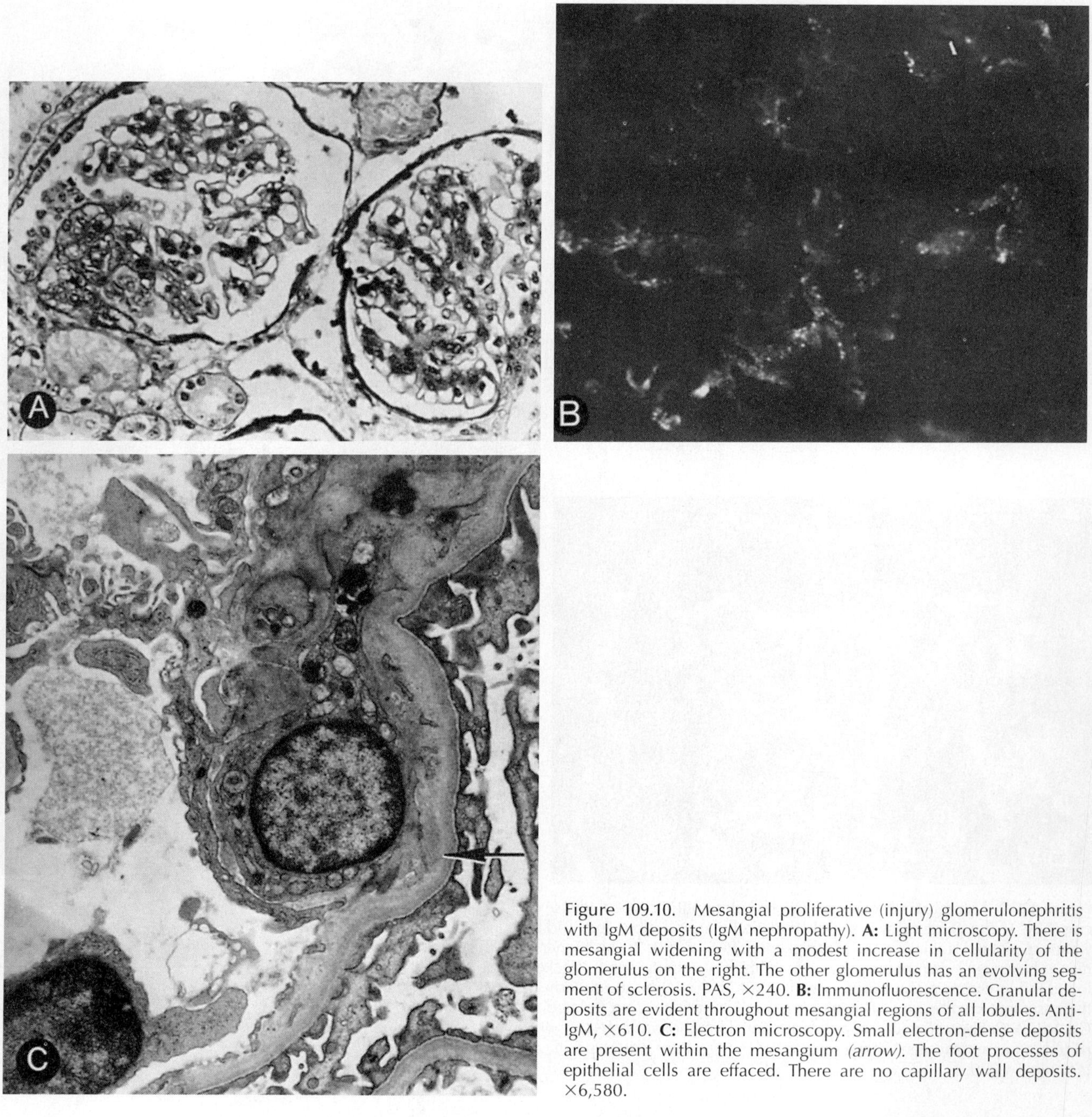

Figure 109.10. Mesangial proliferative (injury) glomerulonephritis with IgM deposits (IgM nephropathy). **A:** Light microscopy. There is mesangial widening with a modest increase in cellularity of the glomerulus on the right. The other glomerulus has an evolving segment of sclerosis. PAS, ×240. **B:** Immunofluorescence. Granular deposits are evident throughout mesangial regions of all lobules. Anti-IgM, ×610. **C:** Electron microscopy. Small electron-dense deposits are present within the mesangium *(arrow)*. The foot processes of epithelial cells are effaced. There are no capillary wall deposits. ×6,580.

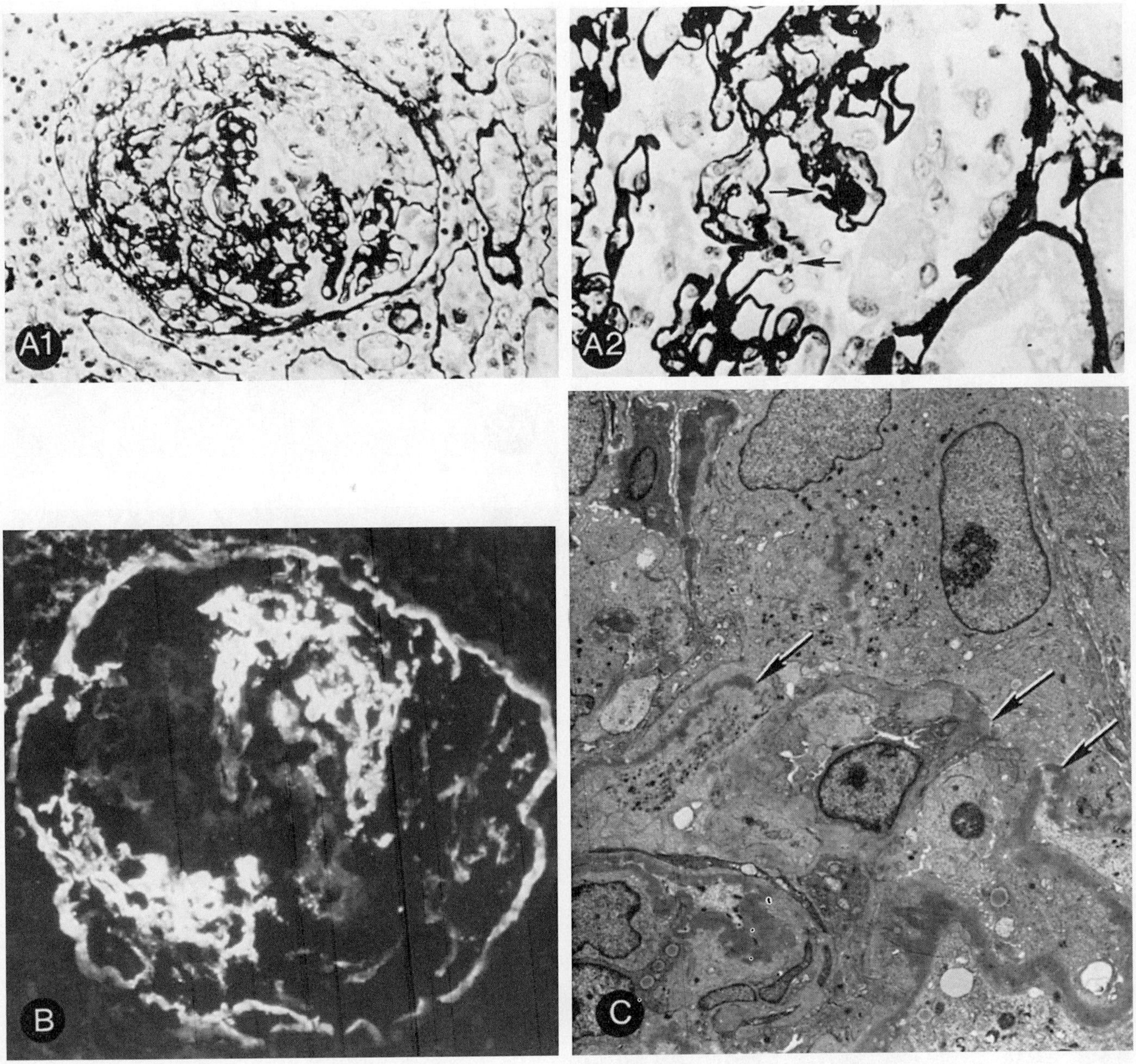

Figure 109.11. Pauciimmune crescentic glomerulonephritis. **A1–2:** Light microscopy. **1:** There is massive accumulation of cells within the urinary space. The tuft is distorted and partially compressed. Periodic acid–methenamine silver, ×300. **2:** Higher magnification of a portion of tuft from another glomerulus to demonstrate capillary wall breaks *(arrows)*. Periodic acid–methenamine silver, ×480. **B:** Immunofluorescence. Large masses of fibrin occupy the urinary space, compressing the nonstaining tuft. ×390. **C:** Electron microscopy. There are numerous capillary wall breaks *(arrows)* with adjacent cells of the crescent. ×2,500.

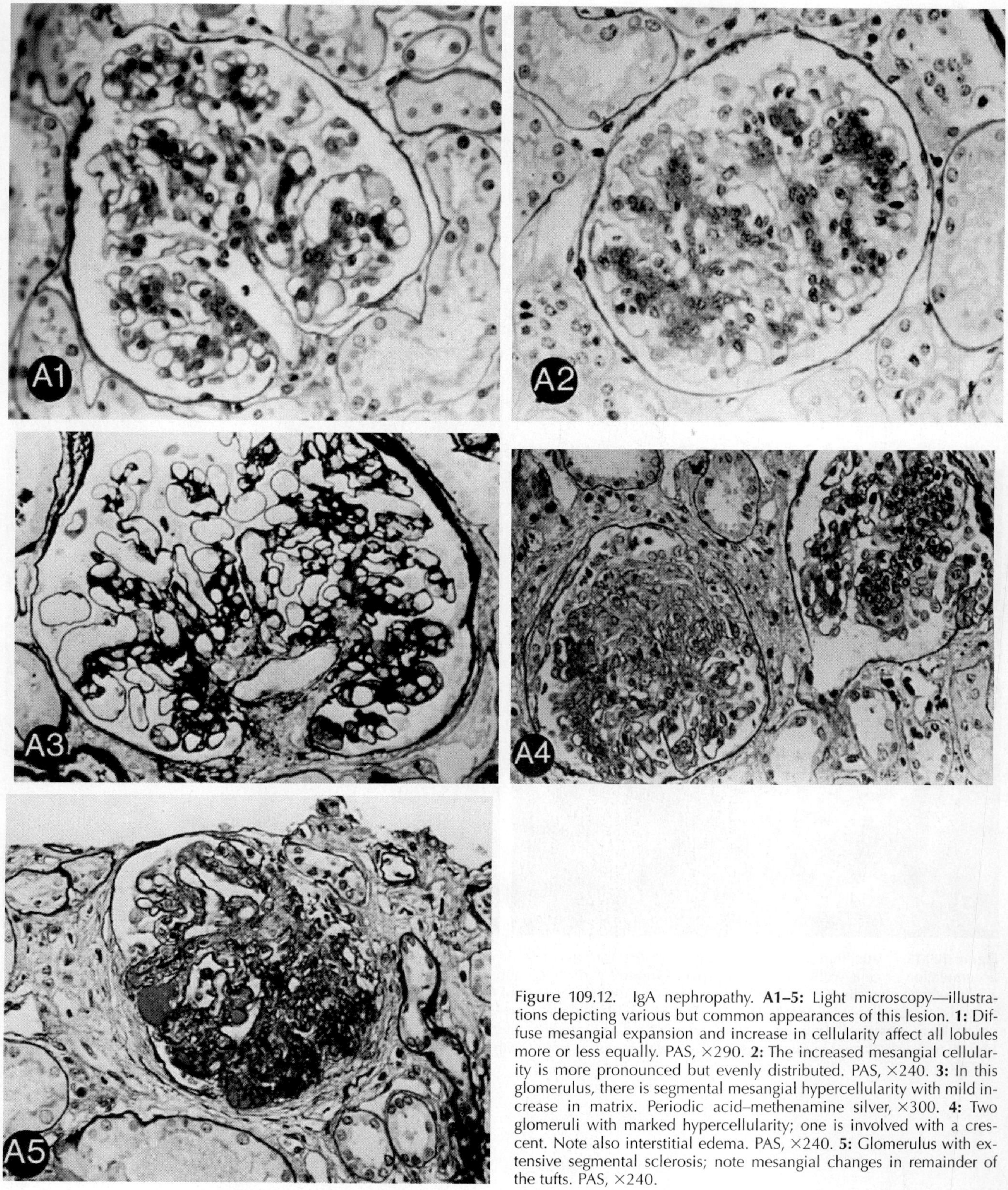

Figure 109.12. IgA nephropathy. **A1–5:** Light microscopy—illustrations depicting various but common appearances of this lesion. **1:** Diffuse mesangial expansion and increase in cellularity affect all lobules more or less equally. PAS, ×290. **2:** The increased mesangial cellularity is more pronounced but evenly distributed. PAS, ×240. **3:** In this glomerulus, there is segmental mesangial hypercellularity with mild increase in matrix. Periodic acid–methenamine silver, ×300. **4:** Two glomeruli with marked hypercellularity; one is involved with a crescent. Note also interstitial edema. PAS, ×240. **5:** Glomerulus with extensive segmental sclerosis; note mesangial changes in remainder of the tufts. PAS, ×240.

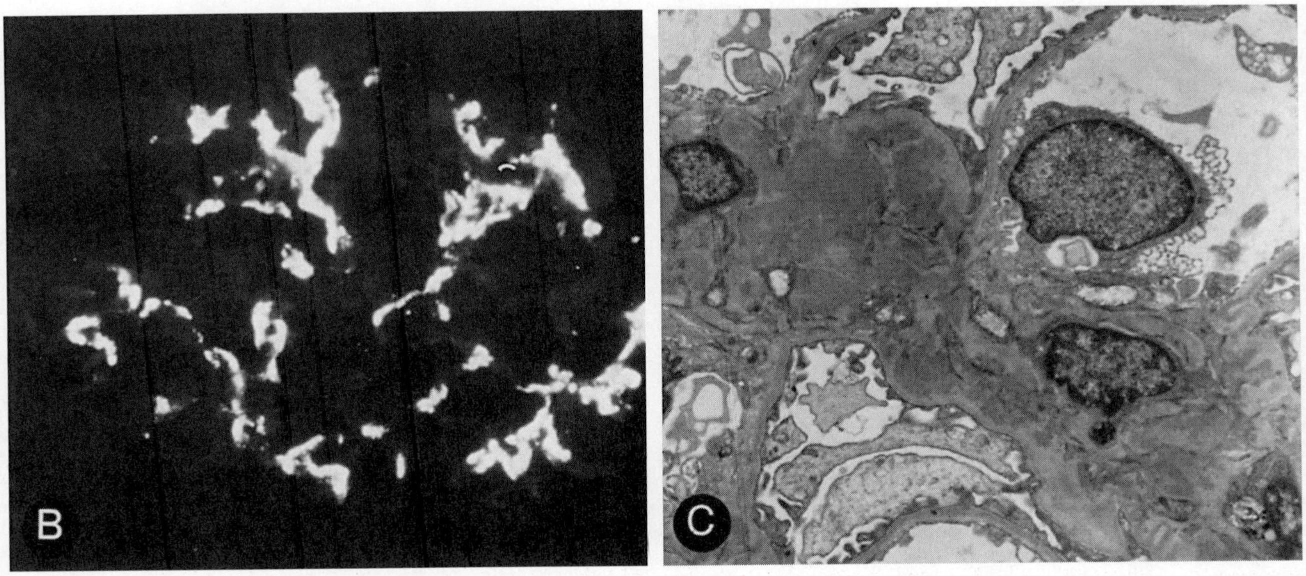

Figure 109.12 (*continued.*) IgA nephropathy. **B:** Immunofluorescence. Heavy IgA deposits are present throughout all mesangial regions in a granular to confluent granular pattern. ×400. **C:** Electron microscopy. Extremely large, prominent, and globular electron-dense deposits are present in the mesangium. ×1,775.

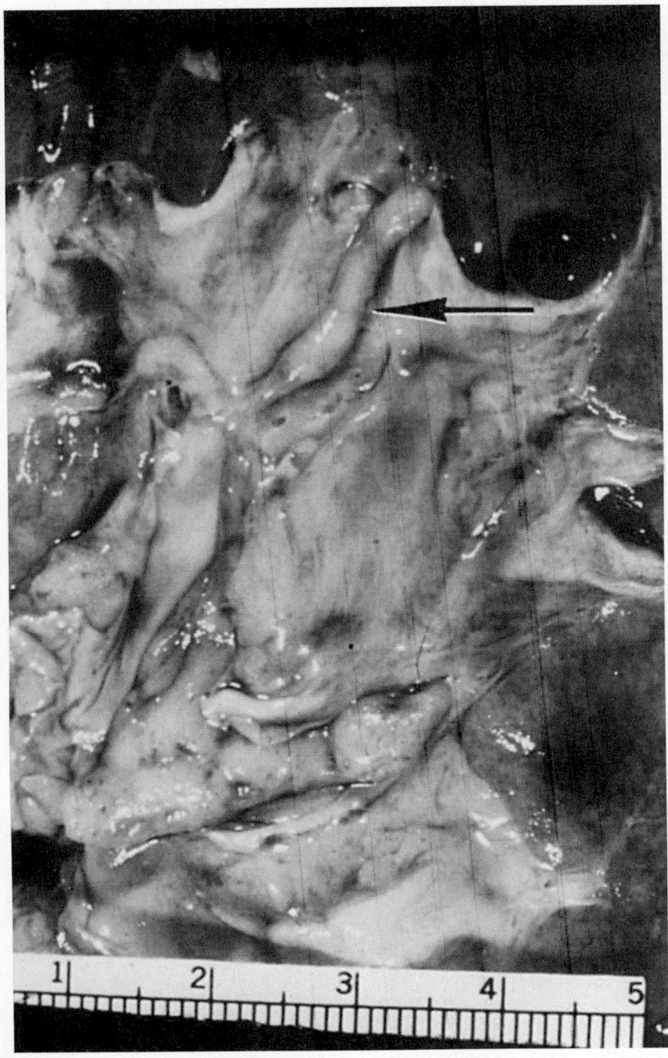

Figure 109.13. Renal vein thrombosis. This photograph of the renal hilus from a patient with membranous glomerulonephritis discloses fresh and organizing thrombi in large veins *(arrows)*.

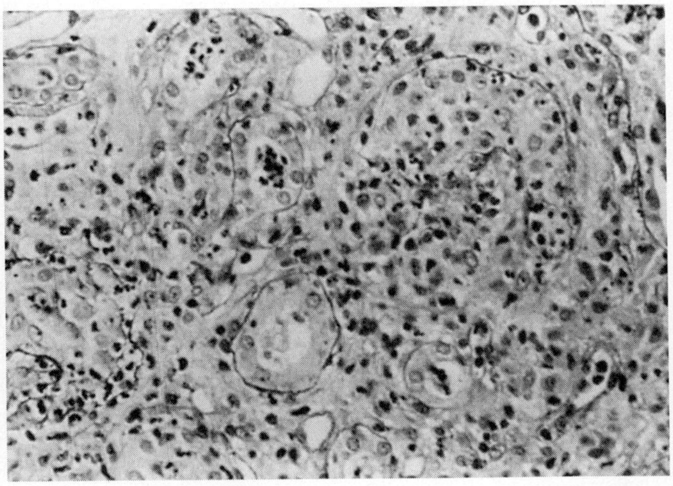

Figure 109.14. Infectious interstitial nephritis. The interstitium is edematous and infiltrated by numerous neutrophils, many of which are also in the walls and lumina of tubules. In this site, they are associated with destruction of the tubular walls. Note also that small numbers of lymphocytes, monocytes, and rare plasma cells are present in the absence of interstitial fibrosis. PAS, ×240.

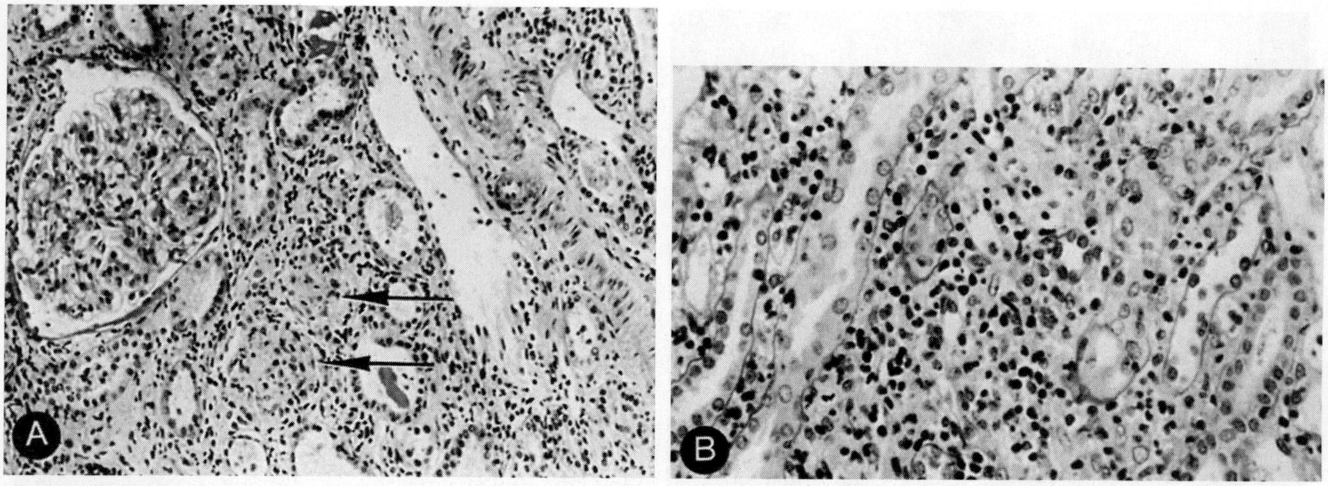

Figure 109.15. Acute drug-induced interstitial nephritis. **A:** Light microscopy. The interstitium is diffusely edematous and infiltrated by many mononuclear leukocytes and small granulomata *(arrows)*. PAS, ×120. **B:** Higher magnification of another specimen detailing interstitial edema and leukocytes; many lymphocytes are in the walls of tubules. PAS, ×300.

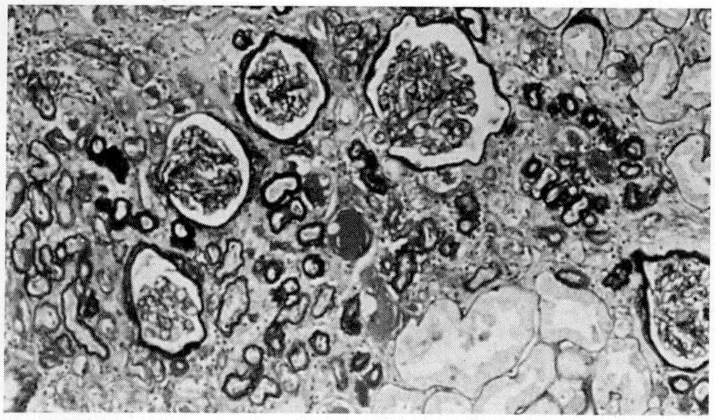

Figure 109.16. Chronic drug-induced interstitial nephritis. Light microscopy. Renal cortex several years following methicillin-induced acute interstitial nephritis. There is focal tubular atrophy with interstitial fibrosis. This is an unusual consequence of the acute lesion. PAS, ×120.

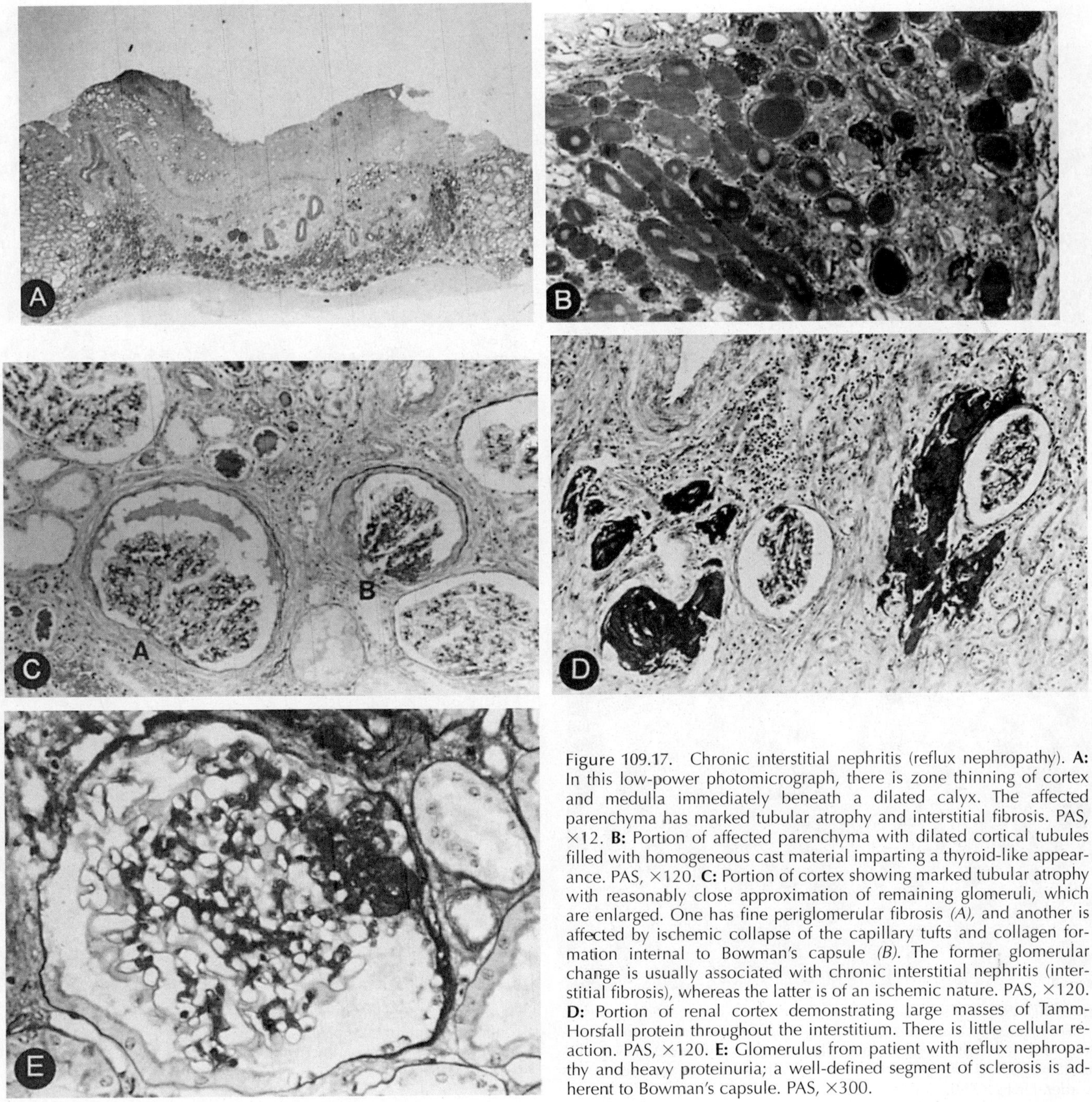

Figure 109.17. Chronic interstitial nephritis (reflux nephropathy). **A:** In this low-power photomicrograph, there is zone thinning of cortex and medulla immediately beneath a dilated calyx. The affected parenchyma has marked tubular atrophy and interstitial fibrosis. PAS, ×12. **B:** Portion of affected parenchyma with dilated cortical tubules filled with homogeneous cast material imparting a thyroid-like appearance. PAS, ×120. **C:** Portion of cortex showing marked tubular atrophy with reasonably close approximation of remaining glomeruli, which are enlarged. One has fine periglomerular fibrosis *(A)*, and another is affected by ischemic collapse of the capillary tufts and collagen formation internal to Bowman's capsule *(B)*. The former glomerular change is usually associated with chronic interstitial nephritis (interstitial fibrosis), whereas the latter is of an ischemic nature. PAS, ×120. **D:** Portion of renal cortex demonstrating large masses of Tamm-Horsfall protein throughout the interstitium. There is little cellular reaction. PAS, ×120. **E:** Glomerulus from patient with reflux nephropathy and heavy proteinuria; a well-defined segment of sclerosis is adherent to Bowman's capsule. PAS, ×300.

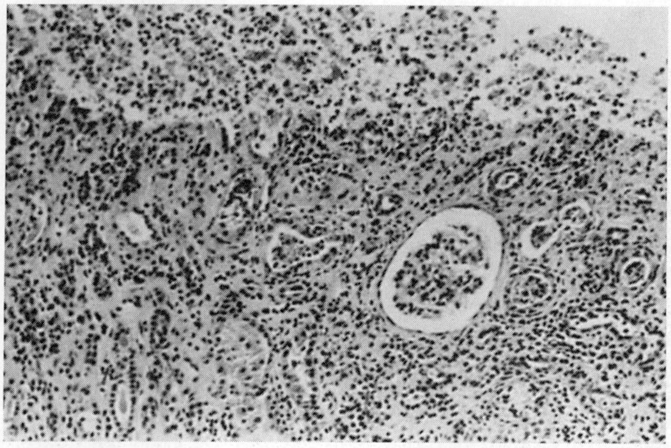

Figure 109.18. Xanthogranulomatous pyelonephritis. Light microscopy. The cortical interstitium is extensively infiltrated by leukocytes. The edge of a large abscess containing numerous "foam cells" is at the *bottom* of the photograph. Hematoxylin and eosin (H&E), ×120.

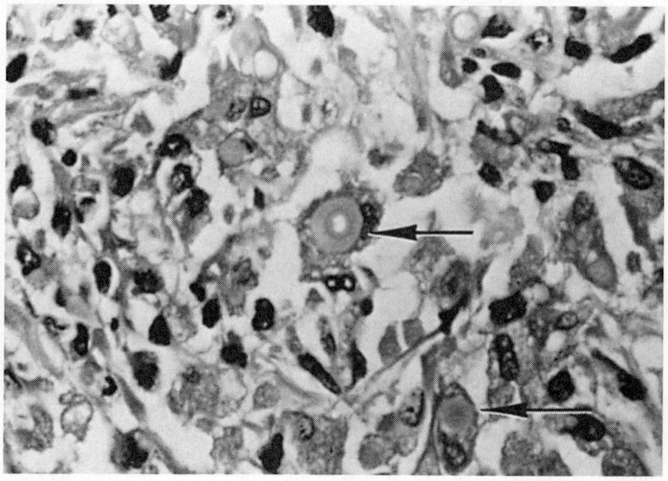

Figure 109.19. Malakoplakia. Renal parenchyma is replaced by masses of histiocytes with abundant granular cytoplasm (von Hansemann histiocytes) and cells with large intracellular calcific concretions (Michaelis-Gutmann bodies) *(arrows);* the latter are pathognomonic features of this disorder. H&E, ×750.

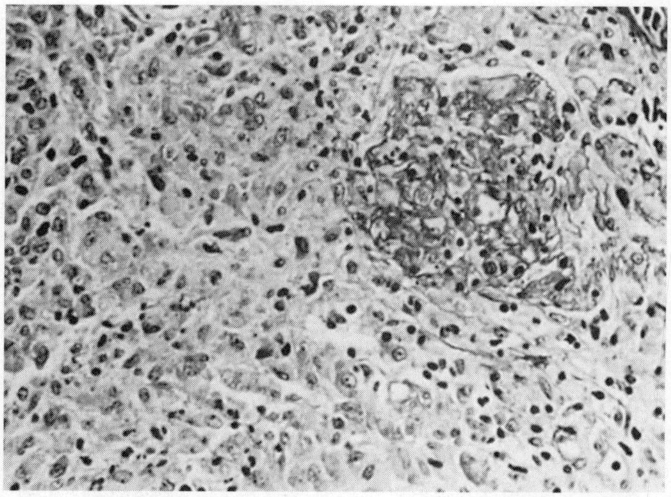

Figure 109.20. Megalocytic interstitial nephritis. This lesion is probably a variant of xanthogranulomatous pyelonephritis and malakoplakia. The interstitium is infiltrated, not only by polymorphonuclear leukocytes, lymphocytes, and monocytes, but also by large granular histiocytes. These cells may well be related to von Hansemann histiocytes of malakoplakia. PAS, ×240.

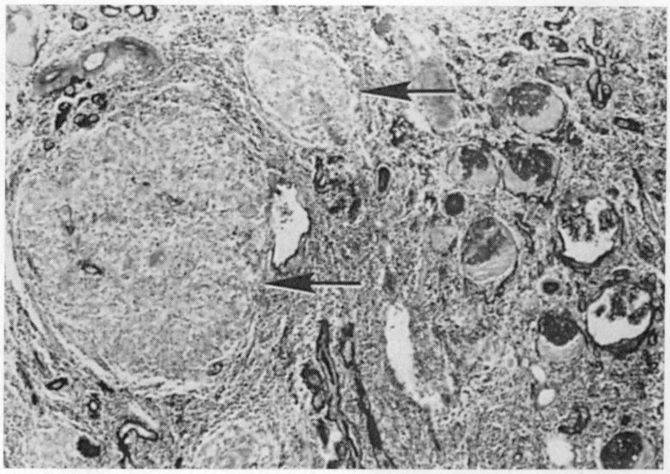

Figure 109.21. Renal tuberculosis. Light microscopy. There are large confluent granulomata *(arrows)* within the interstitium replacing considerable portions of the parenchyma. The adjacent tissue is compressed and scarred. PAS, ×48.

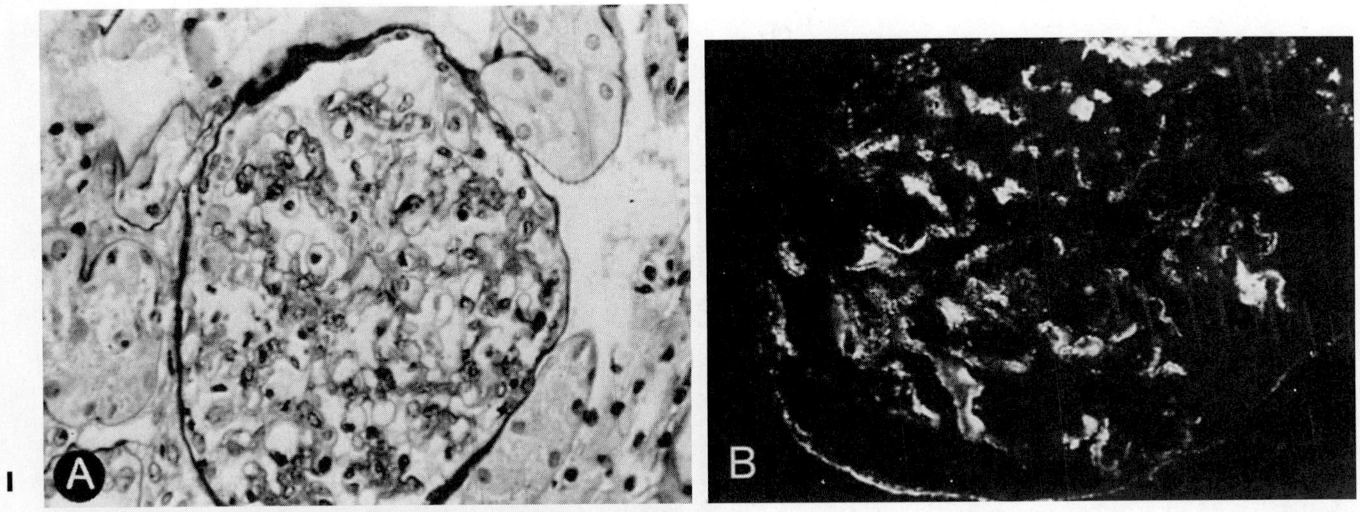

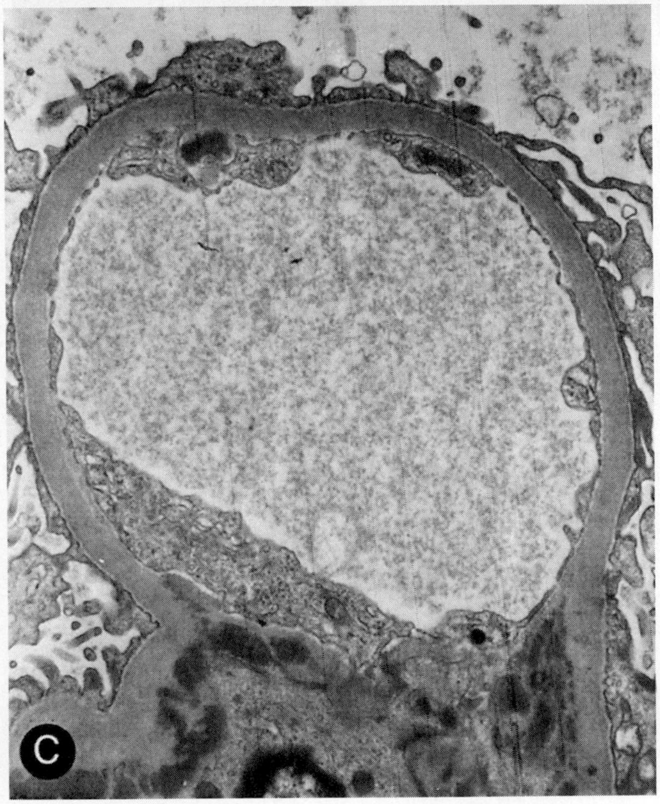

Figure 109.22. Systemic lupus erythematosus. **I:** Mesangial proliferative lupus glomerulonephritis. **A:** Light microscopy. There is mild expansion of the mesangial regions with minimal increased cellularity. Capillary lumina are largely patent, with rare circulating leukocytes. PAS, ×300. **B:** Immunofluorescence microscopy. Granular deposits are virtually limited to the mesangium. Anti-IgG, ×300. **C:** Electron microscopy. There are electron-dense deposits primarily in the mesangium. The basement membranes are normal. ×8,125.

II

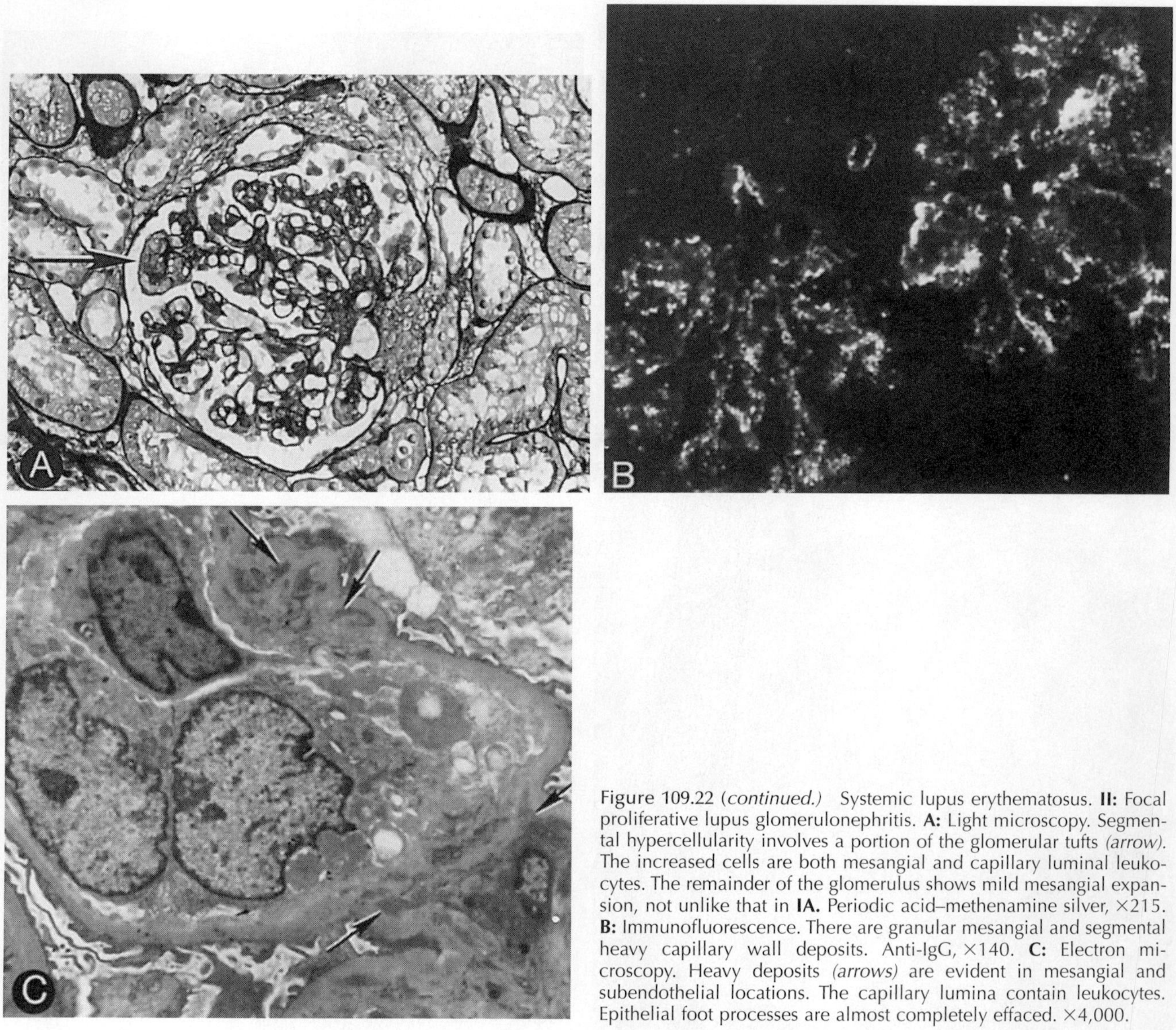

Figure 109.22 (*continued.*) Systemic lupus erythematosus. **II:** Focal proliferative lupus glomerulonephritis. **A:** Light microscopy. Segmental hypercellularity involves a portion of the glomerular tufts *(arrow)*. The increased cells are both mesangial and capillary luminal leukocytes. The remainder of the glomerulus shows mild mesangial expansion, not unlike that in **IA.** Periodic acid–methenamine silver, ×215. **B:** Immunofluorescence. There are granular mesangial and segmental heavy capillary wall deposits. Anti-IgG, ×140. **C:** Electron microscopy. Heavy deposits *(arrows)* are evident in mesangial and subendothelial locations. The capillary lumina contain leukocytes. Epithelial foot processes are almost completely effaced. ×4,000.

III

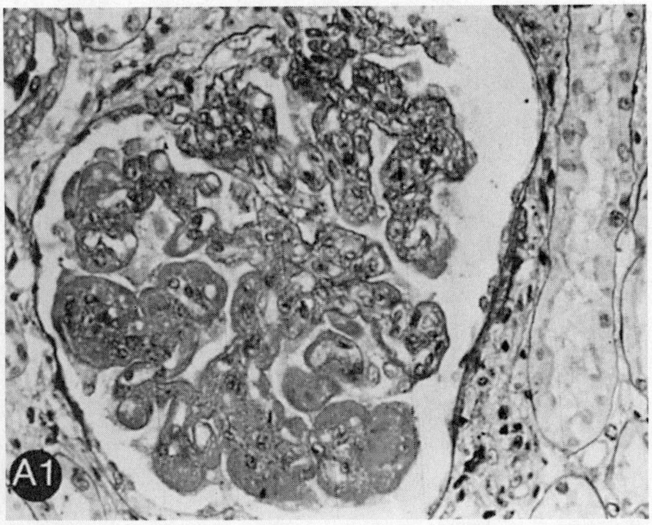

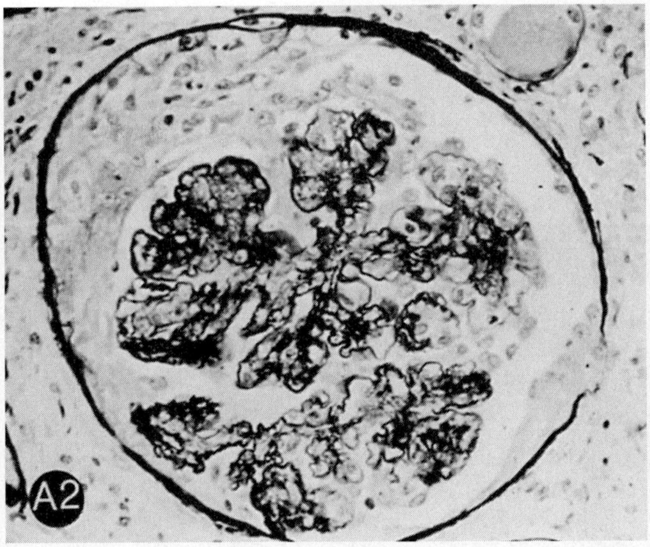

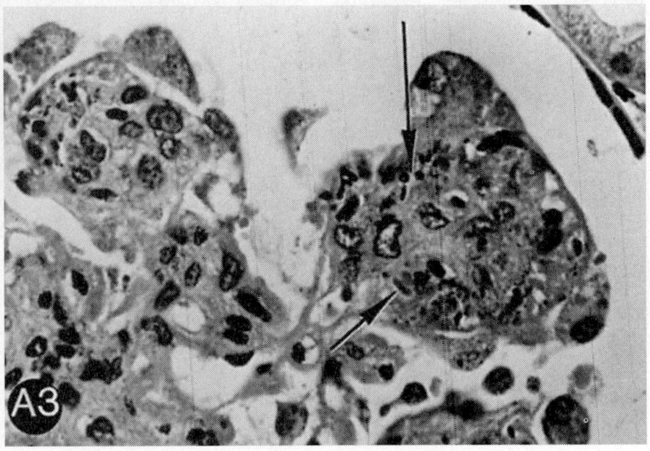

Figure 109.22 (*continued.*) Systemic lupus erythematosus. **III:** Diffuse proliferative lupus glomerulonephritis. **A1–3:** Light microscopy. **1:** This glomerulus has considerable increase in cellularity and large deposits in mesangial regions and capillary walls. This latter abnormality is the equivalent of the classically described wire-loop lesion. PAS, ×240. **2:** This photomicrograph discloses similar abnormalities to the tufts, complicated by a crescent involving a portion of the urinary space. Periodic acid–methenamine silver, ×300. **3:** High magnification of a portion of tuft, showing nuclear fragments *(long arrow)* and more pole staining hematoxylin bodies *(short arrow),* characteristic and virtually pathognomonic of systemic lupus erythematosus, although they are quite rare. H&E, ×480.

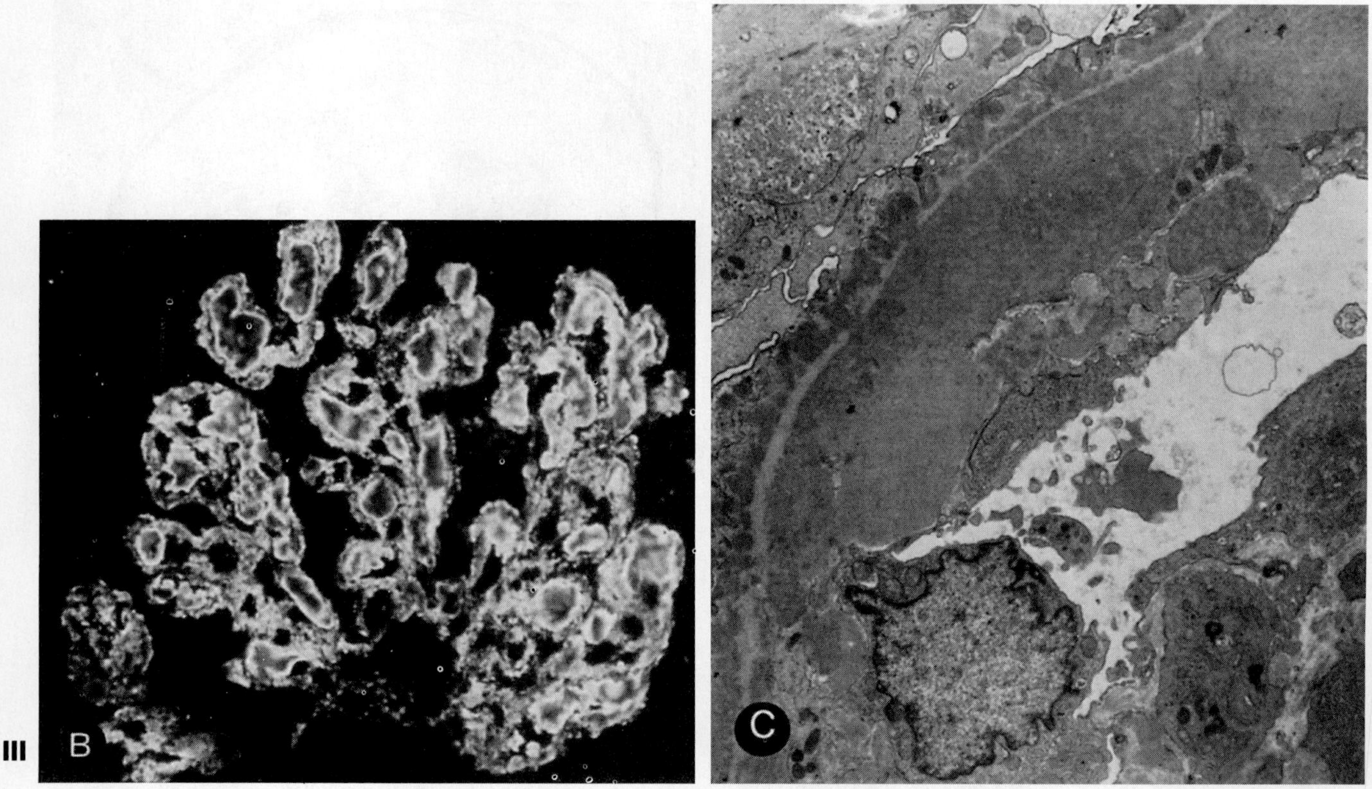

Figure 109.22 (*continued.*) Systemic lupus erythematosus. **III:** Diffuse proliferative lupus glomerulonephritis. **B:** Immunofluorescence microscopy. Heavy mesangial and capillary wall granular and confluent granular deposits. Anti-Clq, ×300. **C:** Electron microscopy. Mesangial and circumferential massive subendothelial electron-dense deposits, the latter the ultrastructural equivalent of the wire-loop lesion. There are also subepithelial deposits. ×4,000.

IV

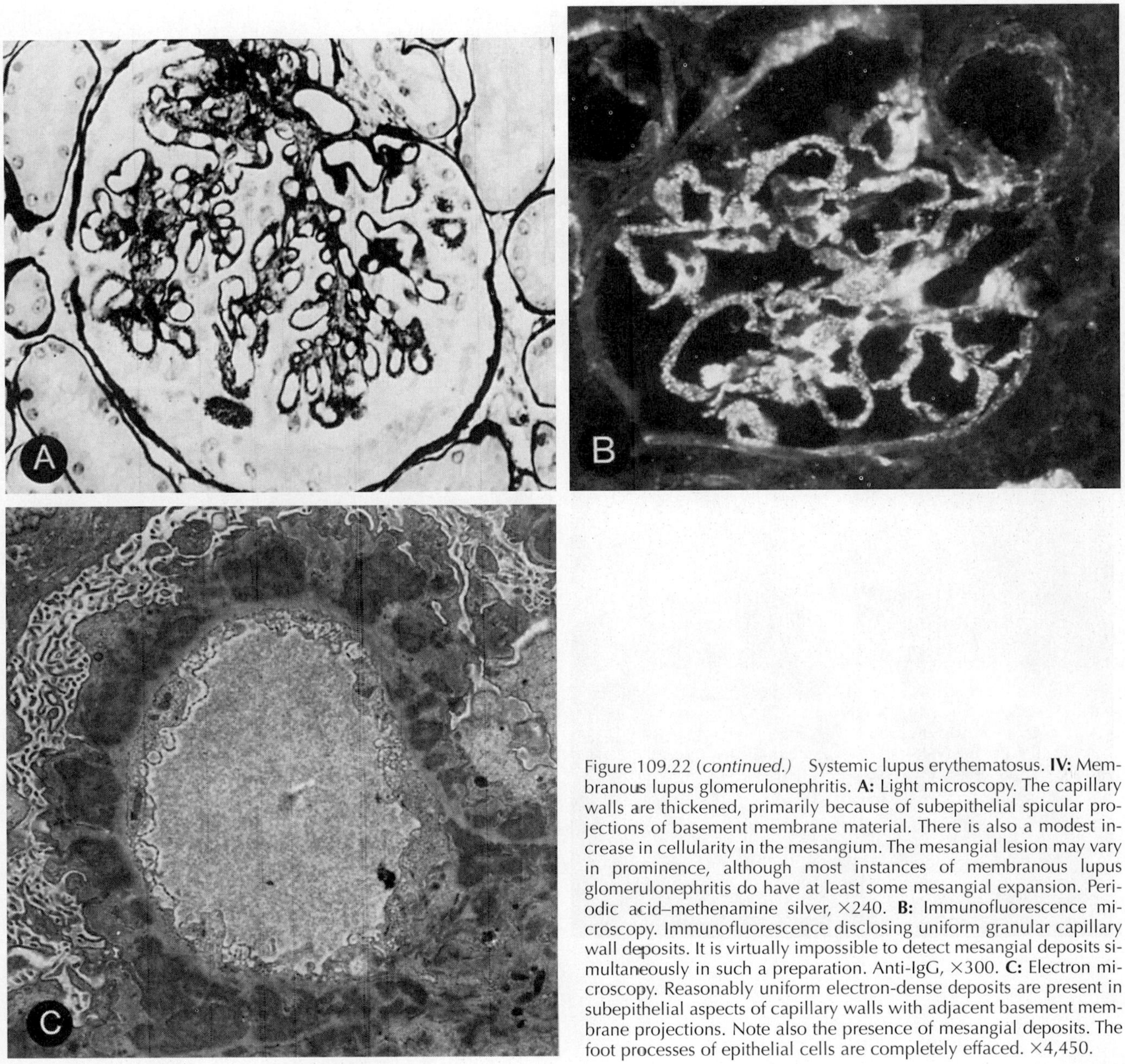

Figure 109.22 (*continued.*) Systemic lupus erythematosus. **IV:** Membranous lupus glomerulonephritis. **A:** Light microscopy. The capillary walls are thickened, primarily because of subepithelial spicular projections of basement membrane material. There is also a modest increase in cellularity in the mesangium. The mesangial lesion may vary in prominence, although most instances of membranous lupus glomerulonephritis do have at least some mesangial expansion. Periodic acid–methenamine silver, ×240. **B:** Immunofluorescence microscopy. Immunofluorescence disclosing uniform granular capillary wall deposits. It is virtually impossible to detect mesangial deposits simultaneously in such a preparation. Anti-IgG, ×300. **C:** Electron microscopy. Reasonably uniform electron-dense deposits are present in subepithelial aspects of capillary walls with adjacent basement membrane projections. Note also the presence of mesangial deposits. The foot processes of epithelial cells are completely effaced. ×4,450.

V

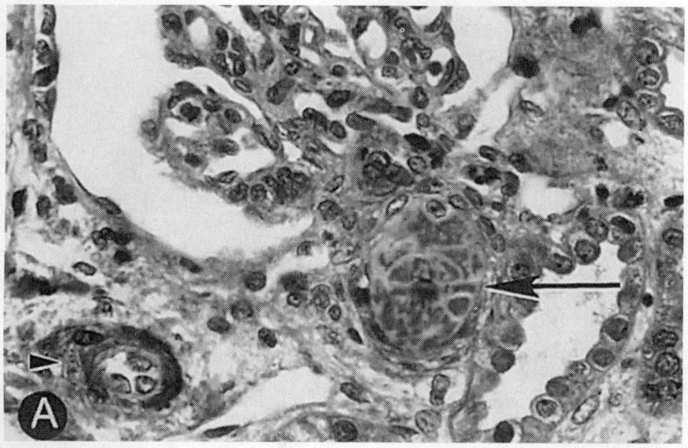

Figure 109.22 (*continued.*) Systemic lupus erythematosus. **V:** Additional lesions. **A:** Lupus vasculopathy. The arteriolar wall contains plasma protein beneath endothelial cells *(arrow);* this lesion is similar in many ways to severe essential or malignant hypertension. Compare with adjacent normal arteriole *(arrowhead).* Masson's trichrome, ×425. **B1–2:** Ultrastructural peculiarities frequently observed in lupus. **1:** Tubuloreticular structures in endothelial cells *(arrow).* ×10,875. **2:** Fingerprint organization of deposits with numerous curvilinear parallel lines; this form of deposit organization is largely limited to lupus erythematosus. ×34,000.

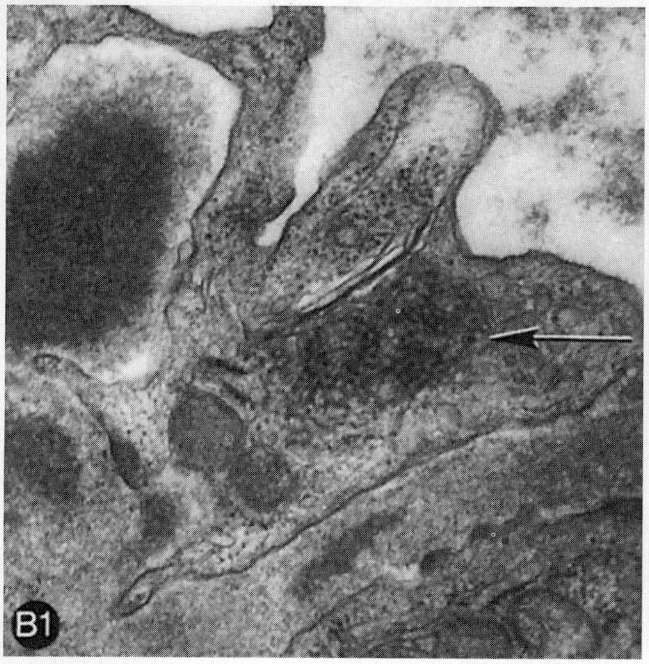

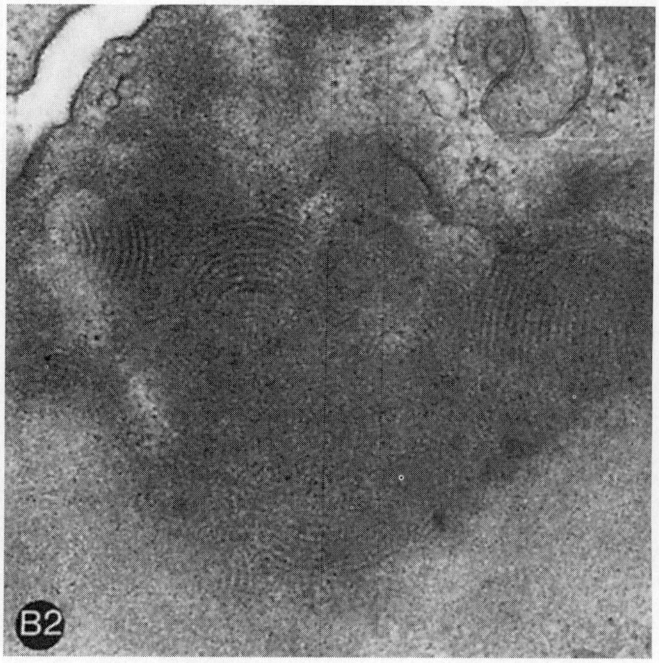

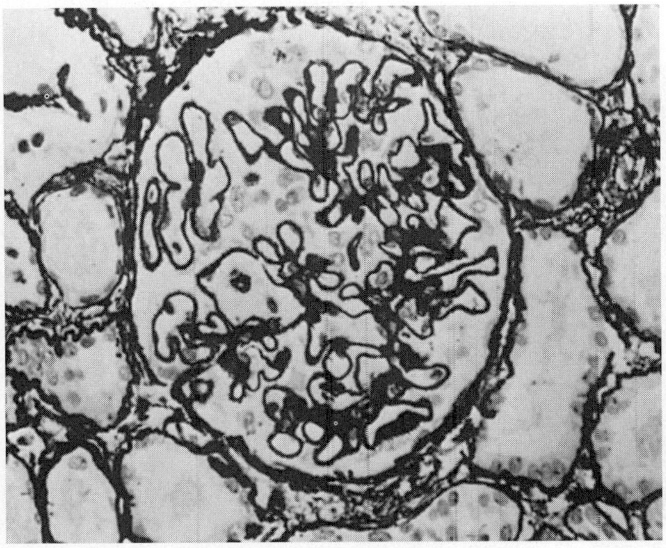

Figure 109.23. Mixed connective tissue disease. Light microscopic photograph of membranous glomerulonephritis. The changes are virtually identical to those in membranous lupus glomerulonephritis. Note the subepithelial "spikes" of basement membrane material and the widened mesangial regions. Other forms of glomerulonephritis similar to lupus also occur in mixed connective tissue disease. Furthermore, vascular lesions similar to those of progressive systemic sclerosis may also be present alone or, rarely, in conjunction with a glomerular lesion. Periodic acid–methenamine silver, ×240.

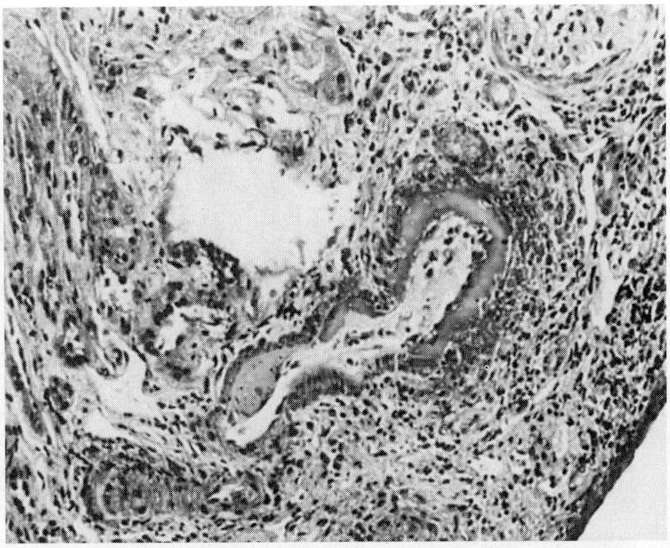

Figure 109.24. Rheumatoid arthritis. Light microscopy. A variety of glomerular, tubular, and interstitial lesions occur in rheumatoid arthritis, either as a part of the disease process or as a complication of therapy. This photomicrograph is of intrarenal arterial involvement in systemic rheumatoid vasculitis. There is "fibrinoid necrosis" of a portion of the wall, with extensive intravascular and perivascular inflammation. Masson's trichrome, ×120.

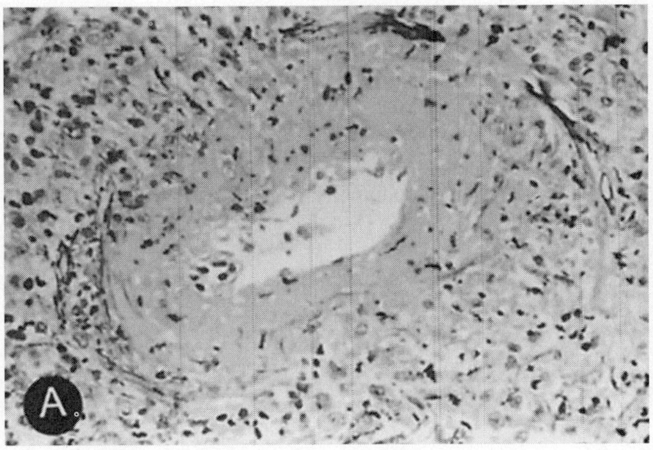

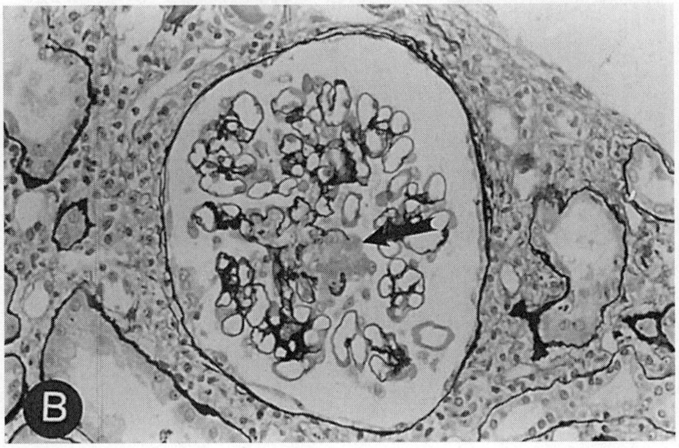

Figure 109.25. Necrotizing arteritis. Light microscopy. **A:** The arterial wall is almost completely necrotic, with deposition of "fibrinoid" material and accumulation of leukocytes. The lumen is considerably narrowed. Virtually no normal structures are left within the wall. The inflammatory process extends into the perivascular tissue. Periodic acid–methenamine silver, ×240. **B:** Glomerulus from the biopsy illustrated in **A.** There is destruction of a portion of the tuft; the capillary walls are discontinuous, and there is accumulation of cells at the site of injury and in the urinary space, indicative of early crescent formation *(arrow)*. Periodic acid–methenamine silver, ×240.

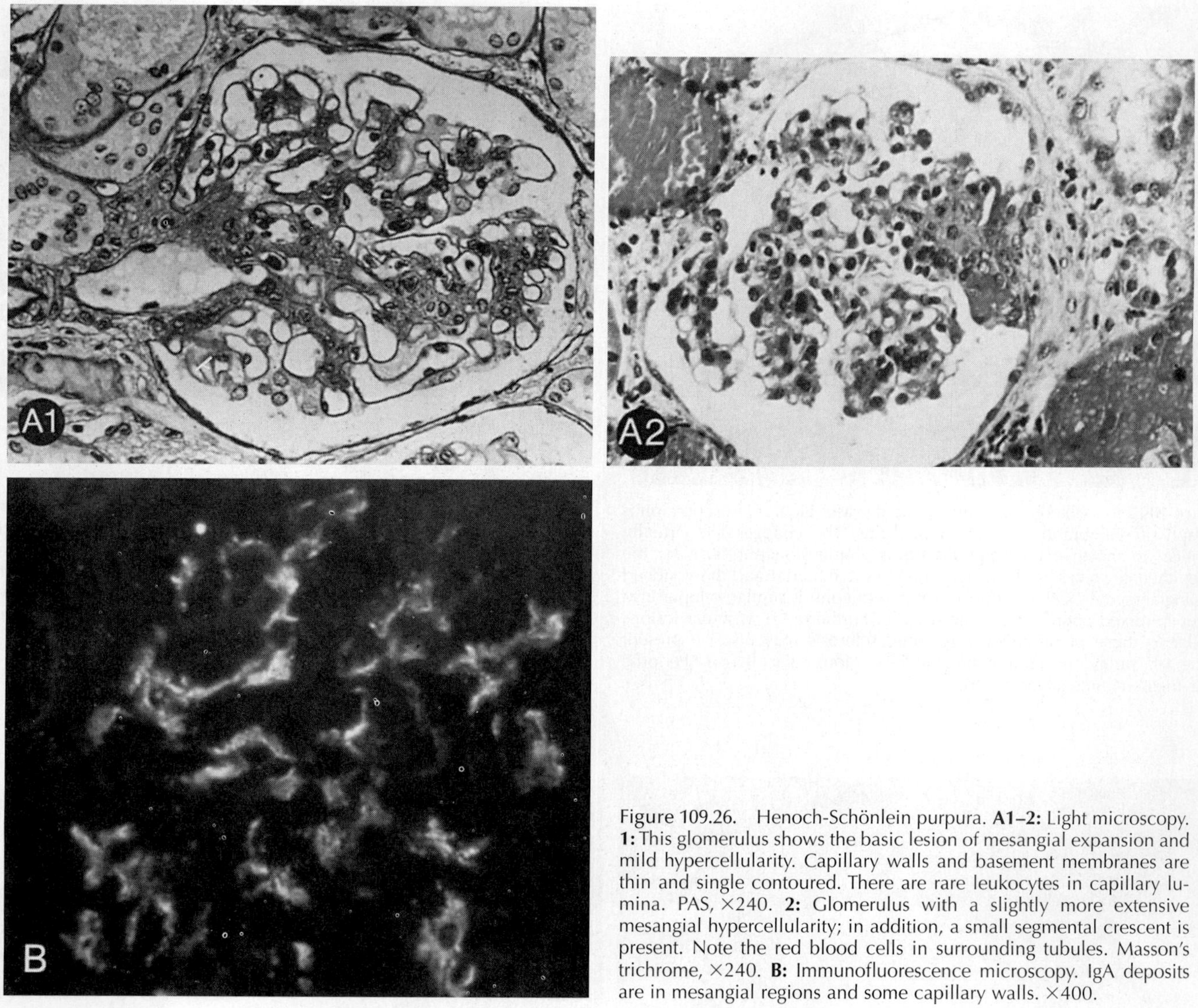

Figure 109.26. Henoch-Schönlein purpura. **A1–2:** Light microscopy. **1:** This glomerulus shows the basic lesion of mesangial expansion and mild hypercellularity. Capillary walls and basement membranes are thin and single contoured. There are rare leukocytes in capillary lumina. PAS, ×240. **2:** Glomerulus with a slightly more extensive mesangial hypercellularity; in addition, a small segmental crescent is present. Note the red blood cells in surrounding tubules. Masson's trichrome, ×240. **B:** Immunofluorescence microscopy. IgA deposits are in mesangial regions and some capillary walls. ×400.

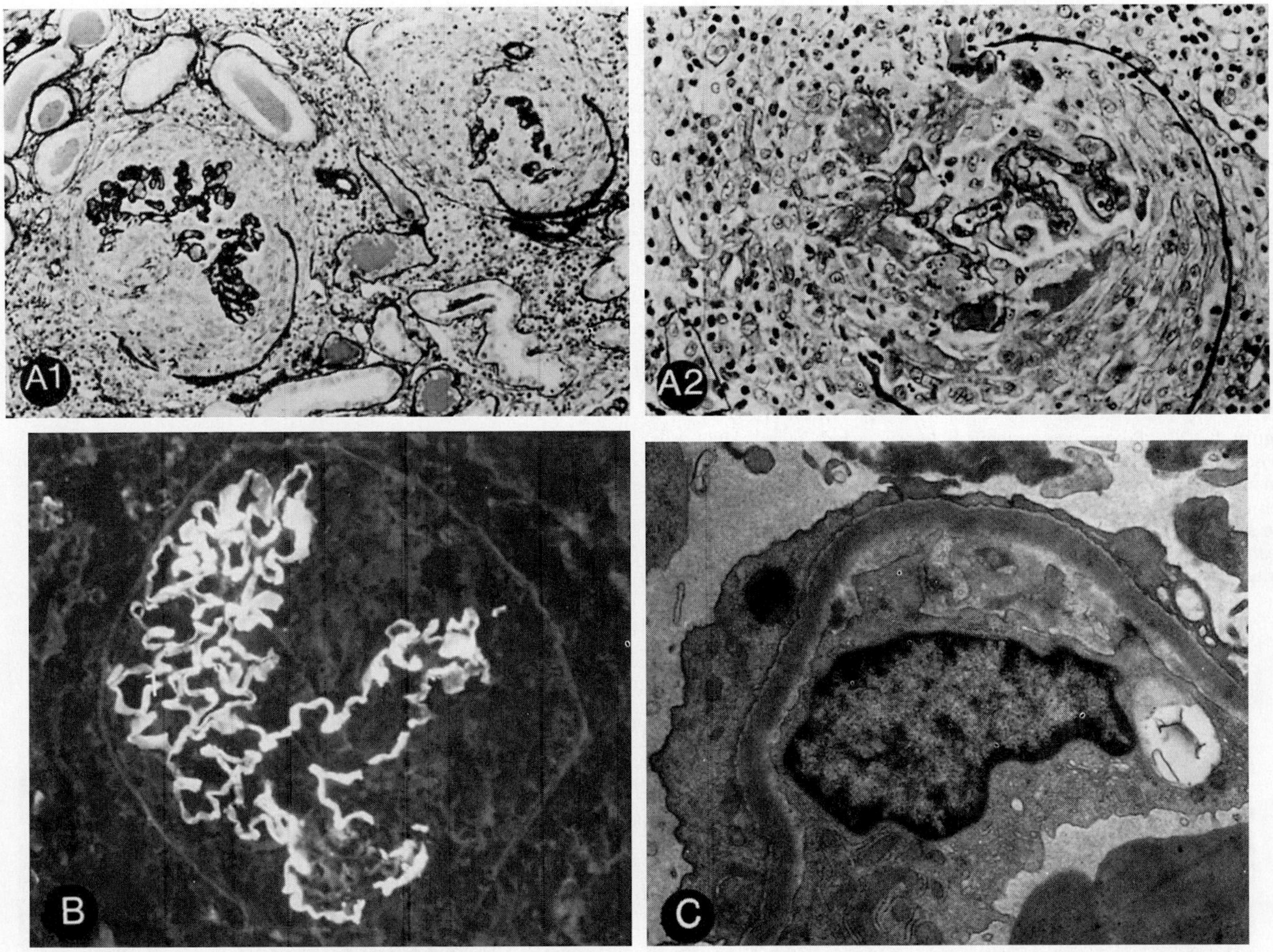

Figure 109.27. Anti–glomerular basement membrane (GBM) disease. **A1–2:** Light microscopy. **1:** This low-power photomicrograph discloses typical severe glomerular involvement. Both glomeruli have extensive circumferential cellular crescent formation, with extension of the crescentic process into the interstitium through large discontinuities in the basement membranes of Bowman's capsule. Similar breaks are also evident in capillary basement membranes. Periodic acid–methenamine silver, ×120. **2:** High magnification of glomerulus, showing the mixed nature of the cells of the crescents; most are large and mononuclear, although lymphocytes and neutrophils are also present. Note fibrin admixed with the cells. Several of the capillaries are thrombosed, and others contain leukocytes. The walls of several capillaries are discontinuous. The cells of the crescent, as well as portions of the tufts, are extruded into the interstitium through the large gap in Bowman's capsule. PAS, ×240. **B:** Immunofluorescence microscopy. Linear staining of glomerular basement membranes with antiserum to IgG. Note the distorted capillary tufts and clearly defined discontinuities. The urinary space is occupied by cells and extracellular material of the crescent. ×300. **C:** Electron microscopy. Capillary wall exhibiting prominent widened and lucent subendothelial zone; although this is not a constant feature, it probably corresponds to antibody binding. ×8,600.

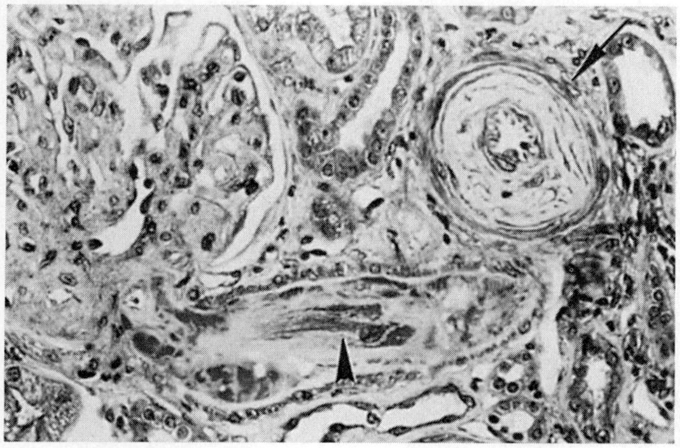

Figure 109.28. Progressive systemic sclerosis (scleroderma). Light microscopy. Typical changes are shown. The interlobular artery *(arrow)* has a narrowed lumen resulting from loose concentric accumulation of collagen and other extracellular material in the intima. The endothelial cells are swollen. A glomerular arteriole is occluded by a thrombus *(arrowhead)*. The glomerulus displays mesangial widening and mild hypercellularity. Masson's trichrome, ×240.

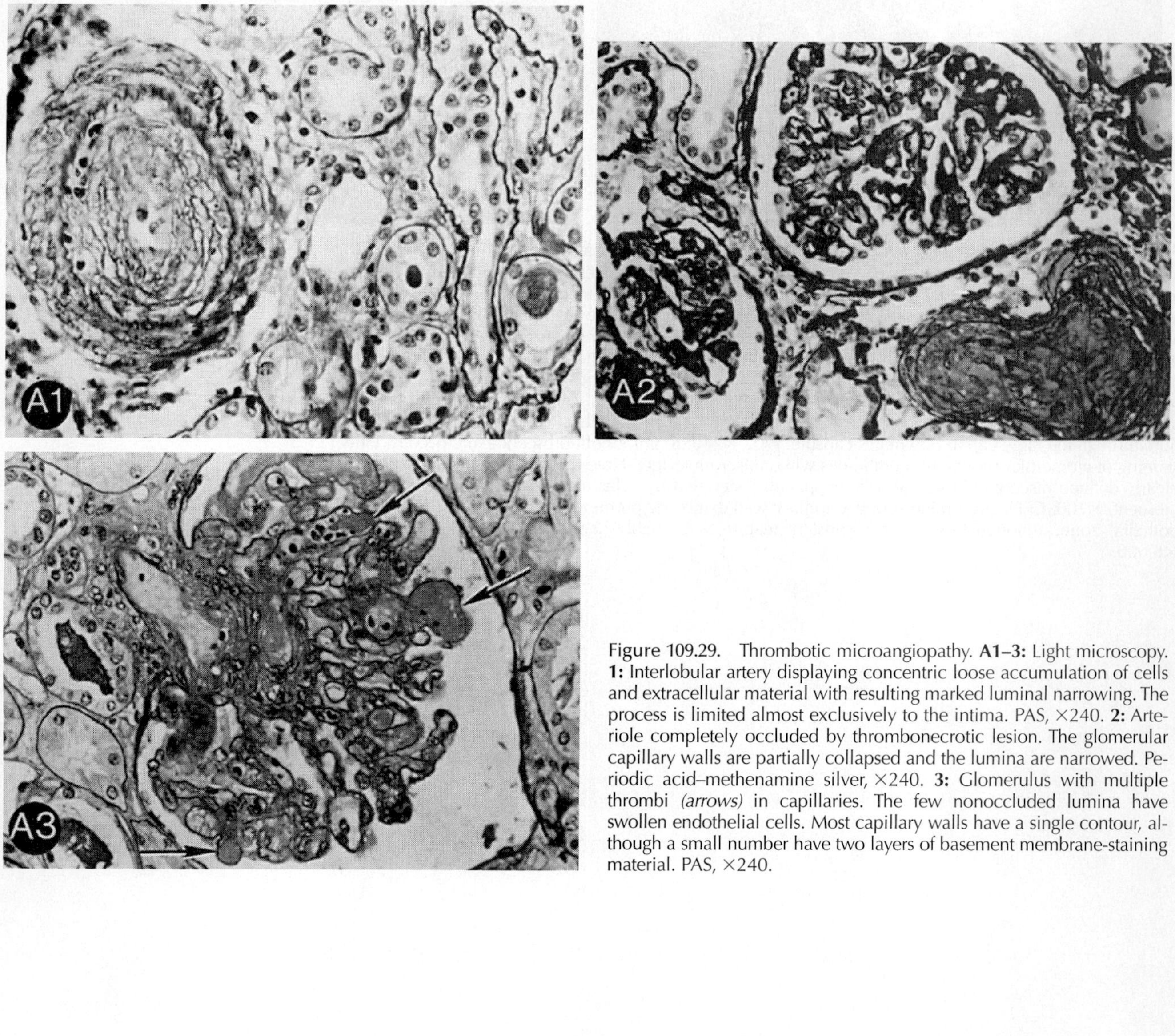

Figure 109.29. Thrombotic microangiopathy. **A1–3:** Light microscopy. **1:** Interlobular artery displaying concentric loose accumulation of cells and extracellular material with resulting marked luminal narrowing. The process is limited almost exclusively to the intima. PAS, ×240. **2:** Arteriole completely occluded by thrombonecrotic lesion. The glomerular capillary walls are partially collapsed and the lumina are narrowed. Periodic acid–methenamine silver, ×240. **3:** Glomerulus with multiple thrombi *(arrows)* in capillaries. The few nonoccluded lumina have swollen endothelial cells. Most capillary walls have a single contour, although a small number have two layers of basement membrane-staining material. PAS, ×240.

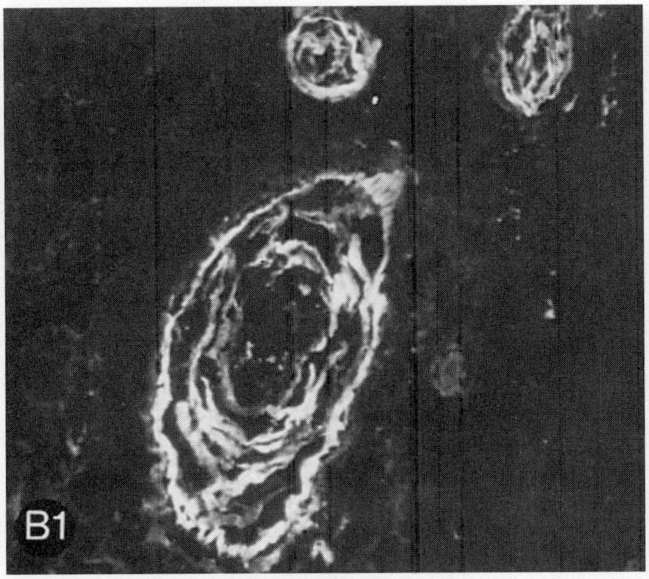

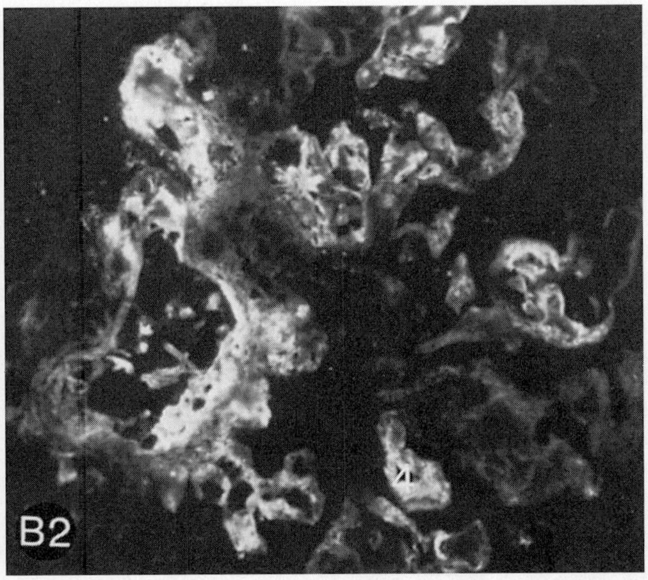

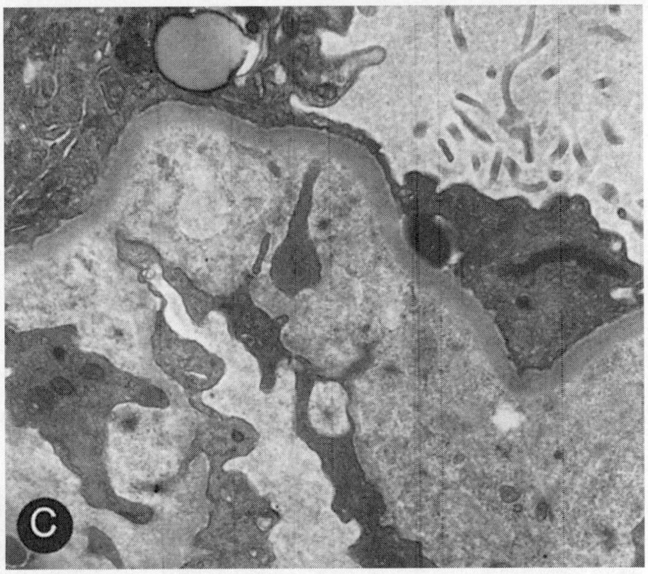

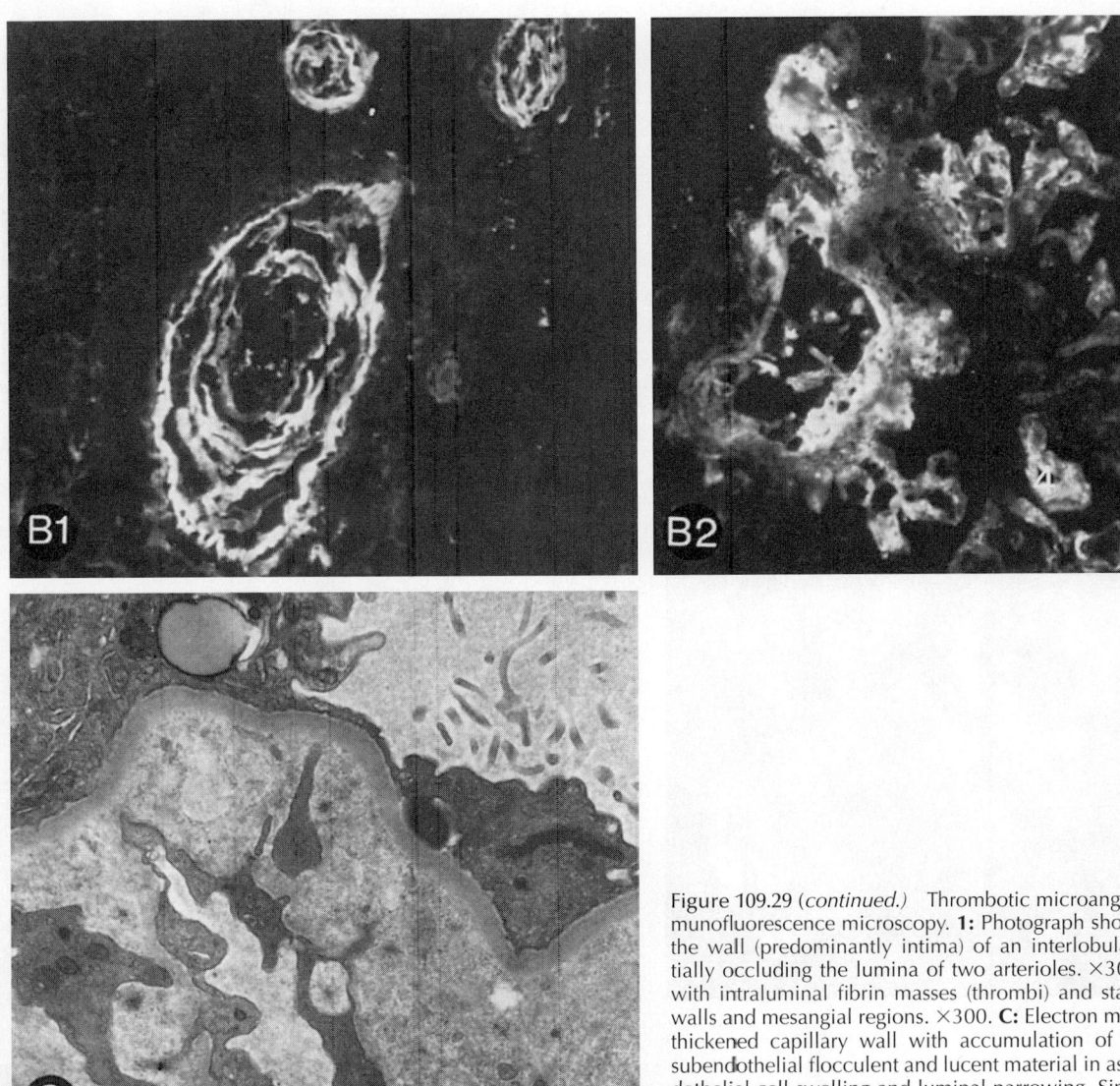

Figure 109.29 (*continued.*) Thrombotic microangiopathy. **B1–2:** Immunofluorescence microscopy. **1:** Photograph showing fibrin within the wall (predominantly intima) of an interlobular artery and partially occluding the lumina of two arterioles. ×300. **2:** Glomerulus with intraluminal fibrin masses (thrombi) and staining of capillary walls and mesangial regions. ×300. **C:** Electron micrograph. Greatly thickened capillary wall with accumulation of large amounts of subendothelial flocculent and lucent material in association with endothelial cell swelling and luminal narrowing. Similar material may also be found in the mesangium and probably represents extraluminal deposits of fibrin. ×8,000.

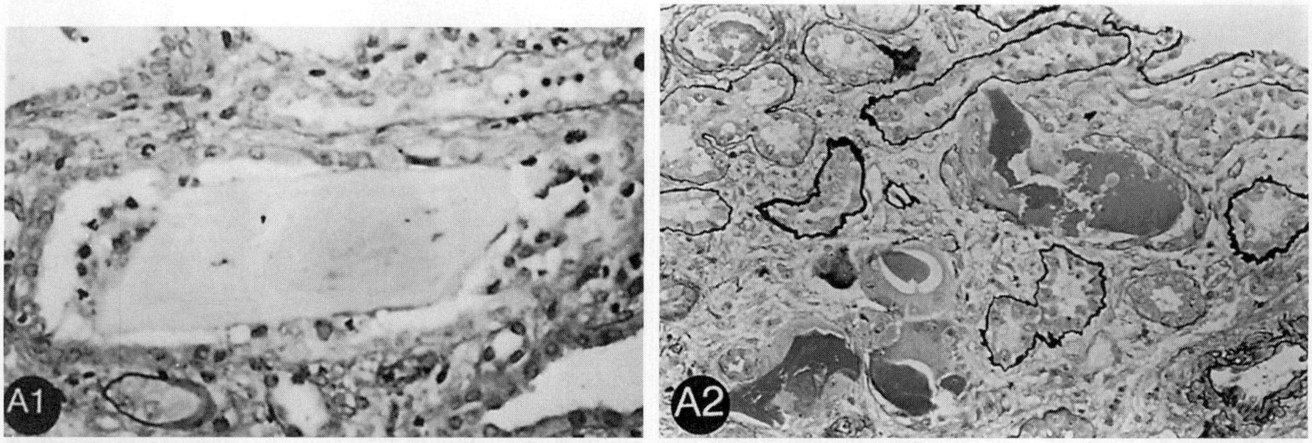

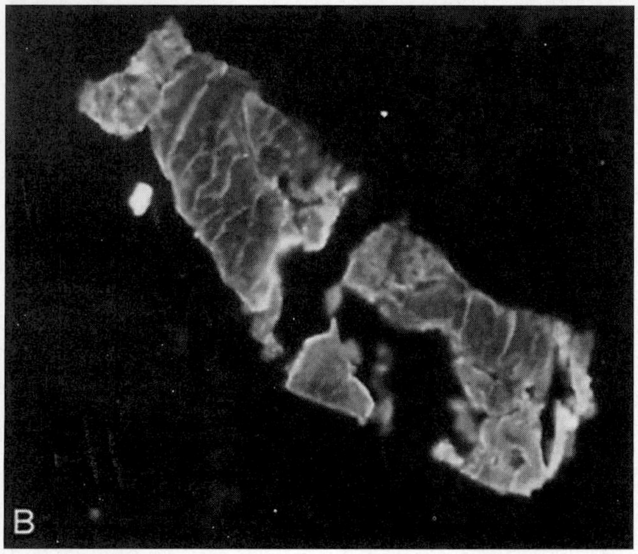

Figure 109.30. Multiple myeloma (Bence Jones cast nephropathy) **A1–2:** Light microscopy. **1:** This distal tubule contains an angulated cast surrounded by adherent leukocytes and degenerated epithelial cells. PAS, ×300. **2:** Several tubules contain densely staining fragmented casts, some of which are completely or partially surrounded by multinucleated giant cells. These affected tubules have only remnants of basement membrane. Periodic acid–methenamine silver, ×240. **B:** Immunofluorescence microscopy. Typical appearance of cost in Bence Jones cast nephropathy in which the abnormal light chain is present to a greater degree than any other protein. The cast is fractured and its periphery stains more intensely than the center. Anti-κ light chain, ×400.

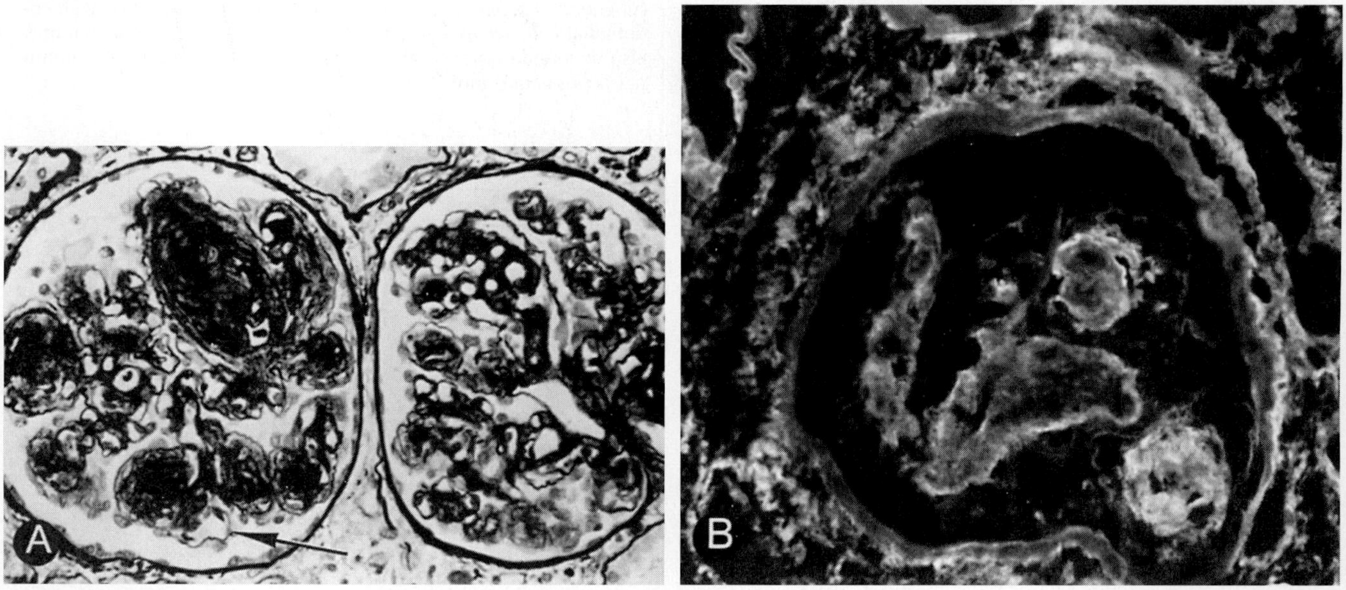

Figure 109.31. Light-chain deposit disease. **A:** Light microscopy. Two glomeruli involved to different degrees in this disorder. One has only diffuse widening of the mesangium, whereas the other is characterized by large prominent mesangial nodules. Note the early aneurysmal dilation of a capillary overlying one of the nodules *(arrow)*. Other forms of glomerular damage include various proliferative as well as crescentic patterns of injury. Periodic acid–methenamine silver, ×300. **B:** Immunofluorescence microscopy. The nodules and glomerular and tubular basement membranes stain for the abnormal light chain. The basement membrane staining is linear, whereas the nodular staining is amorphous. Anti-*κ* light chain, ×400.

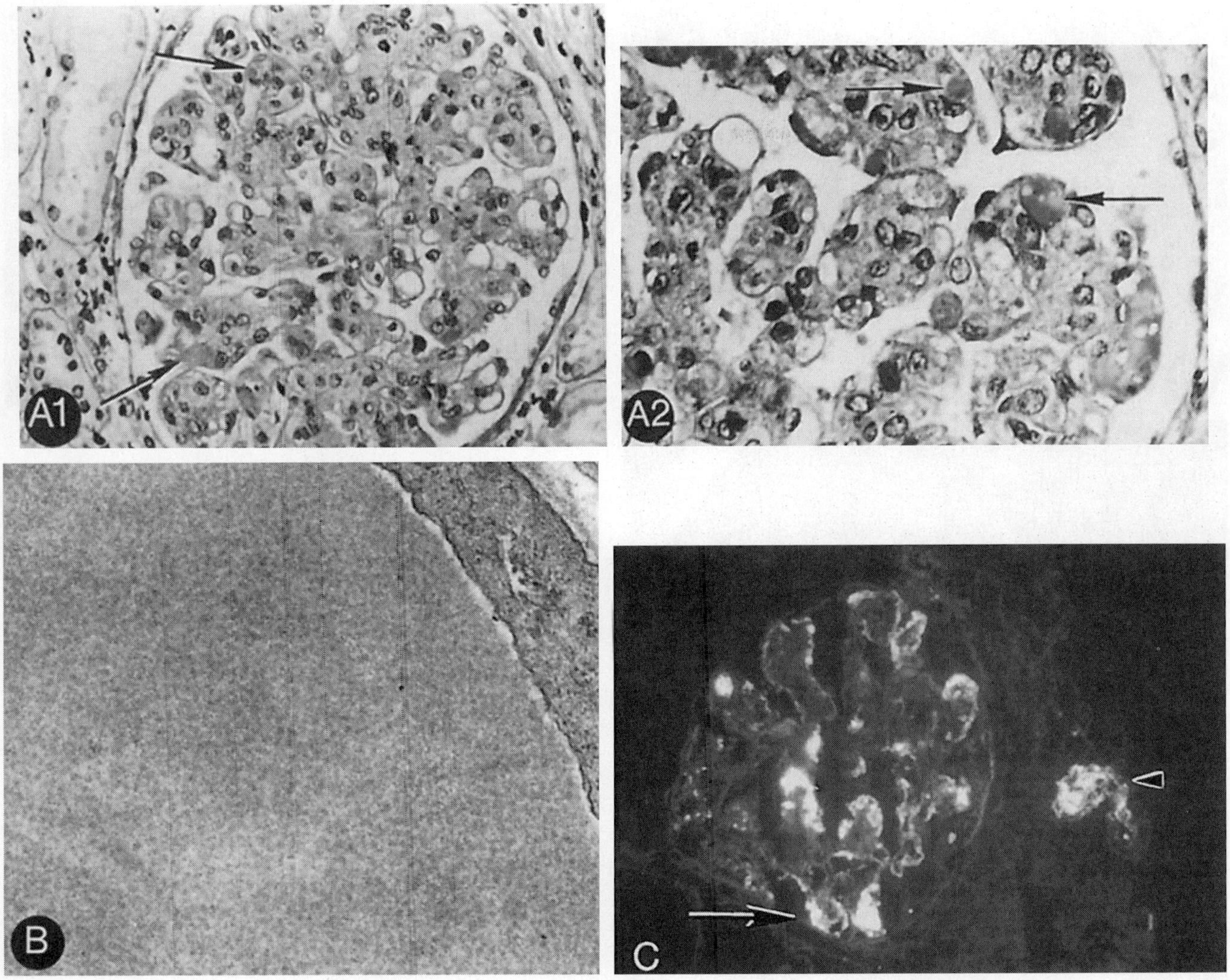

Figure 109.32. Cryoglobulinemia. **A1–2:** Light microscopy. **1:** The glomerulus is hypercellular and lobular. The increased cells are predominantly mesangial, although leukocytes are present in capillary lumina. Furthermore, there are small "thrombi" in some capillaries. The capillary walls are variably thickened *(arrows),* some with a double-contoured appearances. PAS, ×240. **2:** Higher magnification of trichrome-stained portion of glomerulus, showing luminal "thrombi" *(arrows),* representing masses of precipitated cryoglobulin. Some of these masses are also adherent to the capillary walls. There are increased cells within the mesangium. ×480. **B:** Electron microscopy. The large intraluminal mass is of medium electron density and has a crystalline to curvilinear appearance. ×35,000. **C:** Immunofluorescence. There are granular peripheral capillary wall deposits and "thrombi" in glomerular capillaries *(arrow)* and an adjacent arteriole *(arrowhead).* Anti-IgM, ×300.

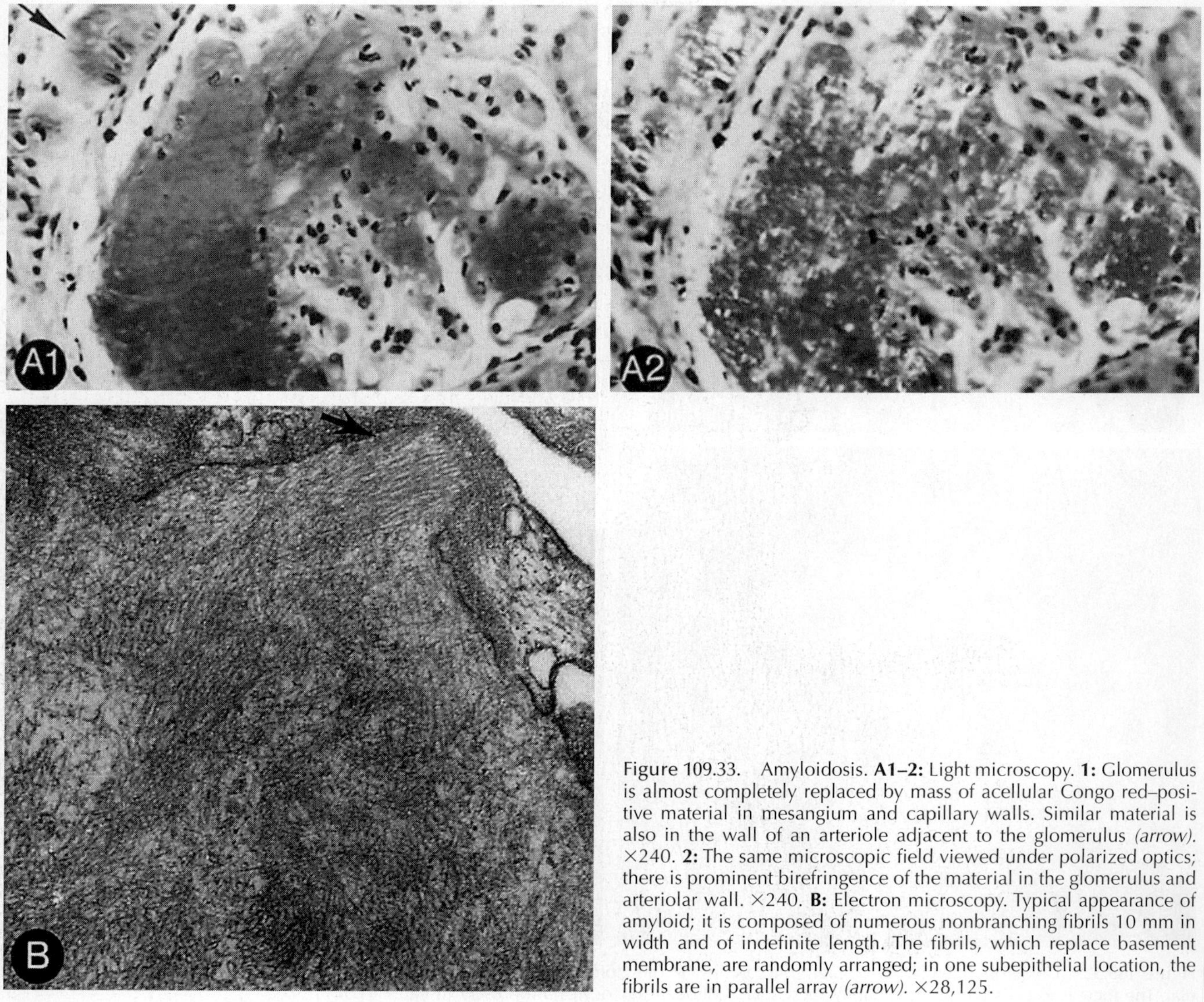

Figure 109.33. Amyloidosis. **A1–2:** Light microscopy. **1:** Glomerulus is almost completely replaced by mass of acellular Congo red–positive material in mesangium and capillary walls. Similar material is also in the wall of an arteriole adjacent to the glomerulus *(arrow)*. ×240. **2:** The same microscopic field viewed under polarized optics; there is prominent birefringence of the material in the glomerulus and arteriolar wall. ×240. **B:** Electron microscopy. Typical appearance of amyloid; it is composed of numerous nonbranching fibrils 10 mm in width and of indefinite length. The fibrils, which replace basement membrane, are randomly arranged; in one subepithelial location, the fibrils are in parallel array *(arrow)*. ×28,125.

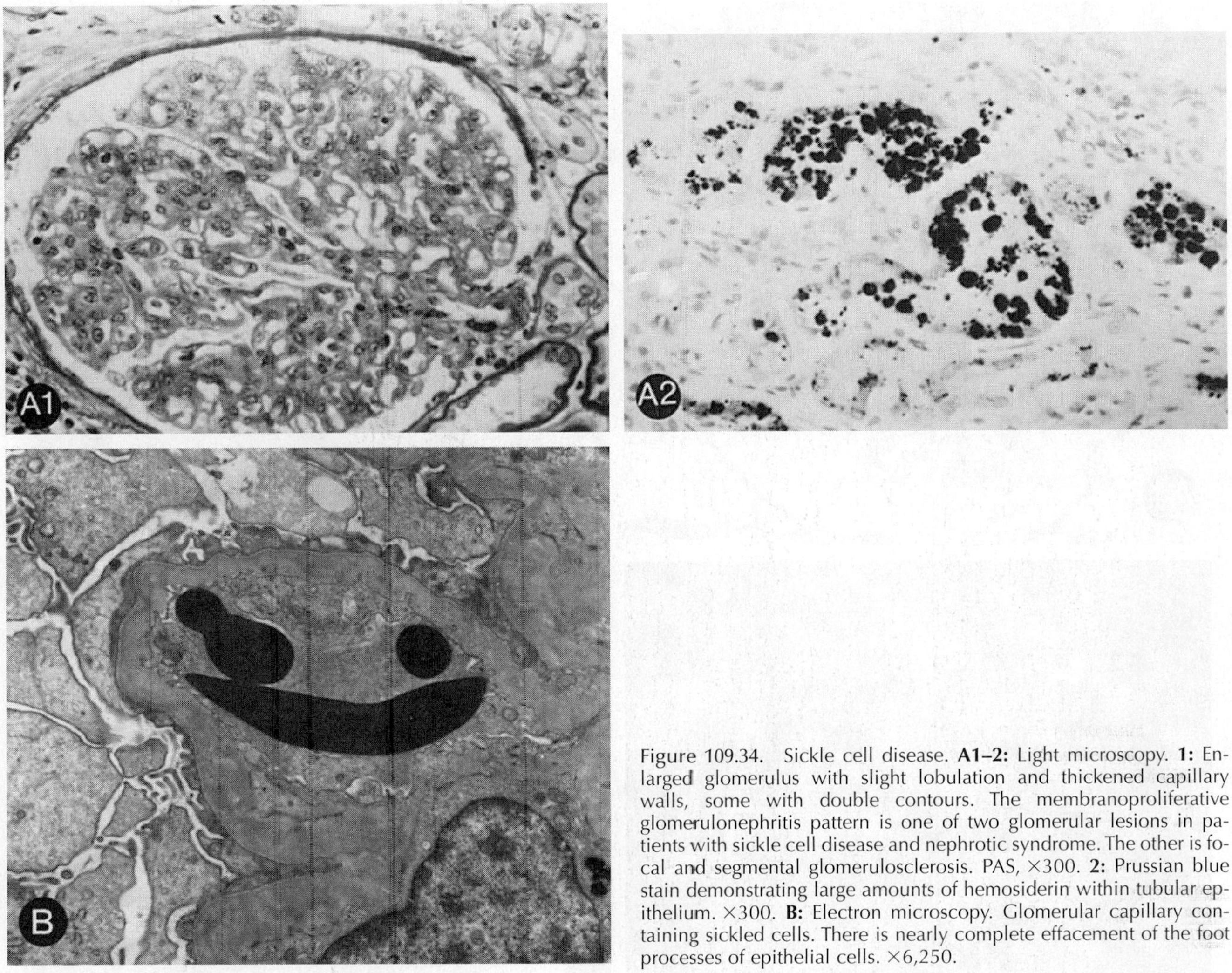

Figure 109.34. Sickle cell disease. **A1–2:** Light microscopy. **1:** Enlarged glomerulus with slight lobulation and thickened capillary walls, some with double contours. The membranoproliferative glomerulonephritis pattern is one of two glomerular lesions in patients with sickle cell disease and nephrotic syndrome. The other is focal and segmental glomerulosclerosis. PAS, ×300. **2:** Prussian blue stain demonstrating large amounts of hemosiderin within tubular epithelium. ×300. **B:** Electron microscopy. Glomerular capillary containing sickled cells. There is nearly complete effacement of the foot processes of epithelial cells. ×6,250.

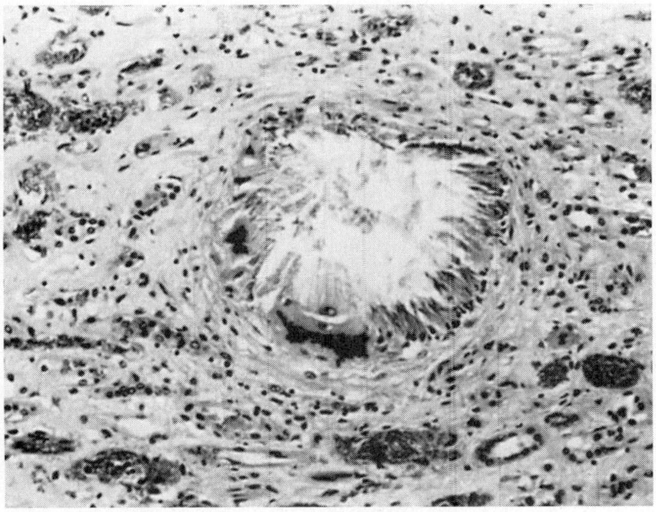

Figure 109.35. Uric acid nephropathy. Light microscopy. A mass of crystals is surrounded by mononuclear cells and giant cells within the medulla. This process probably started with precipitation of urate in a tubule, with rupture of the tubule, escape of crystals, and consequent granulomatous response. H&E, ×120.

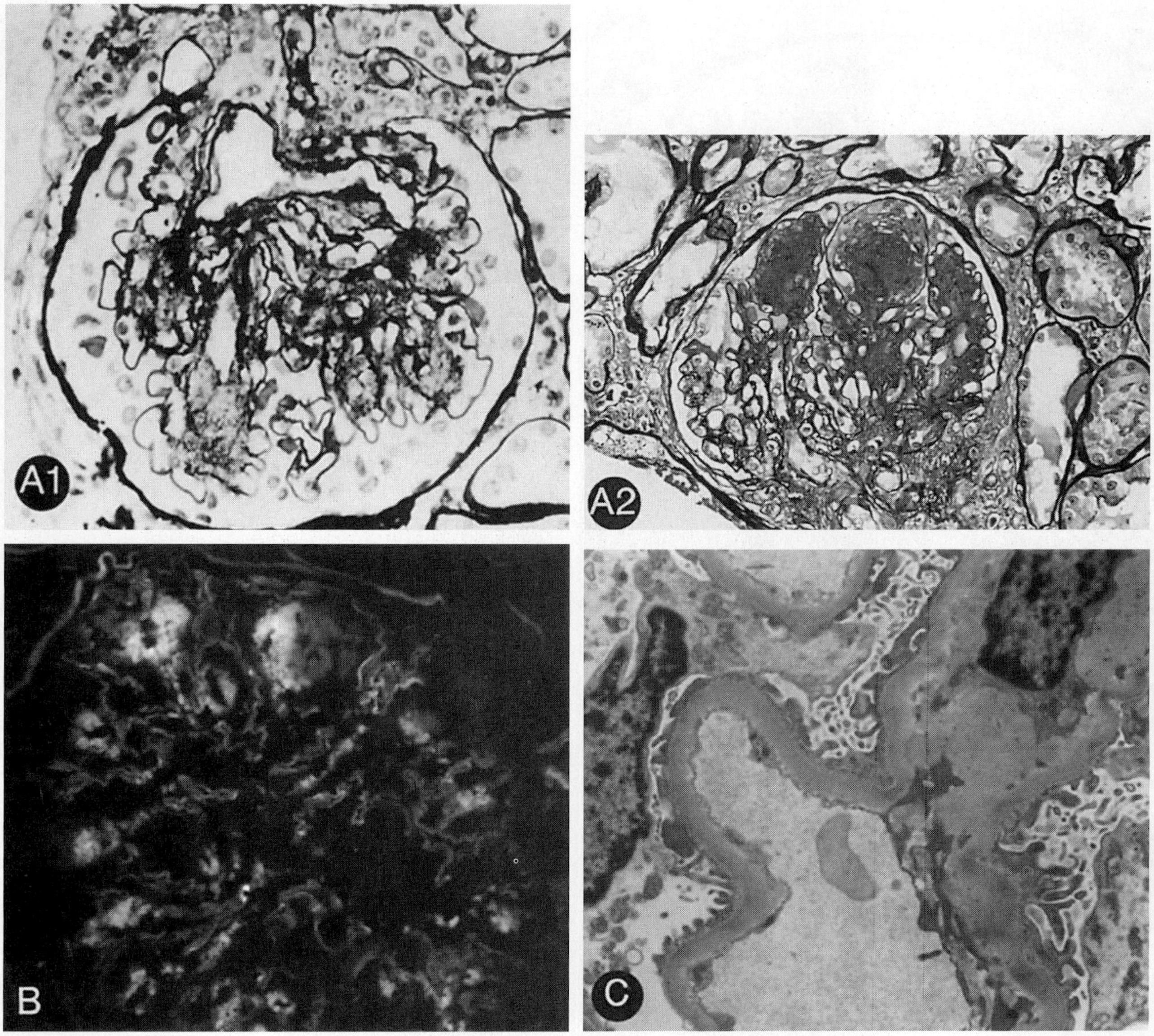

Figure 109.36. Diabetes mellitus. **A1–2:** Light microscopy. **1:** Diffuse diabetic glomerulosclerosis characterized by diffuse increase in mesangial matrix. Periodic acid–methenamine silver, ×240. **2:** Nodular glomerulosclerosis. There is a marked increase in mesangial matrix arranged in several nodules in this glomerulus. By light microscopy, this lesion and light-chain deposit disease may appear virtually identical. Compare with Fig. 109.31A. Periodic acid–methenamine silver, ×215. **B:** Immunofluorescence microscopy. Antialbumin demonstrating "pseudolinear" staining of glomerular capillary and Bowman's capsular and tubular basement membranes. ×300. **C:** Electron microscopy. Prominently thickened glomerular basement membrane and increased mesangial matrix are depicted. ×6,250.

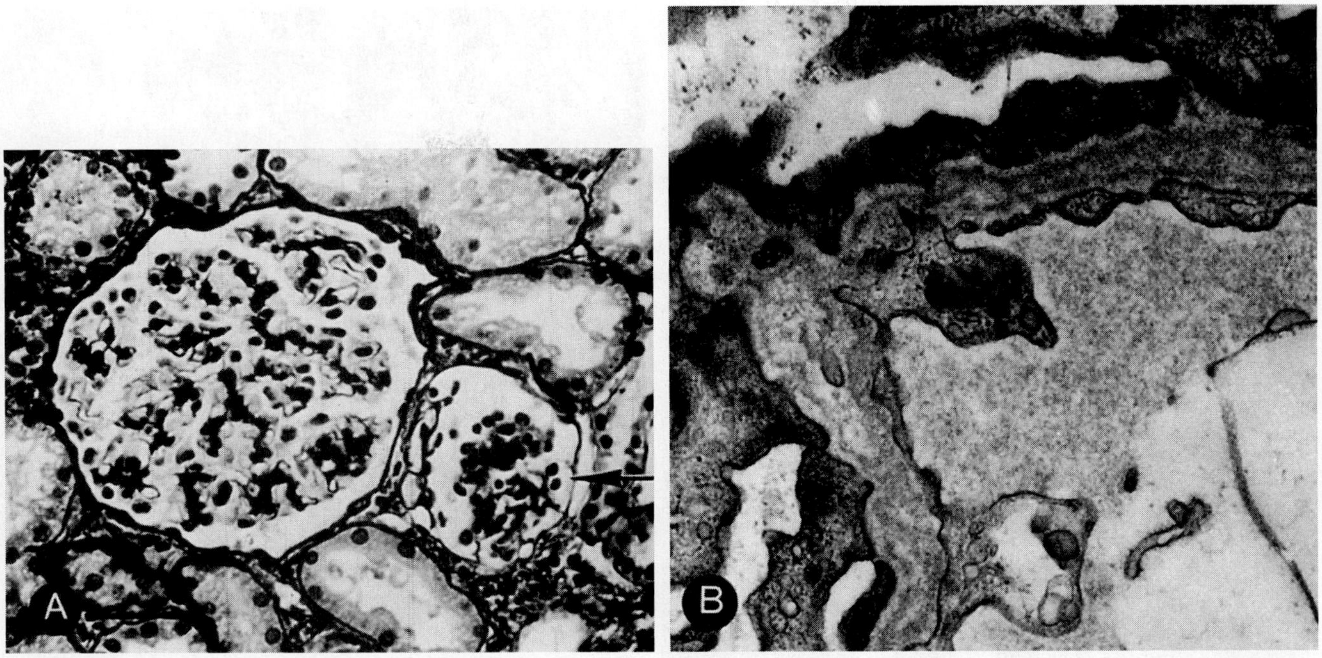

Figure 109.37. Alport's syndrome. **A:** The glomeruli are structurally normal, although there is persistence of a fetal glomerulus *(arrow)* characterized by smaller diameter capillaries and regular densely staining nuclei of visceral epithelial cells. Periodic acid–methenamine silver, ×300. **B:** Electron microscopy. In this characteristic lesion, the glomerular basement membrane is irregularly thickened with a scalloped subepithelial border; it is composed of multiple layers of medium and pole-staining material. ×20,600.

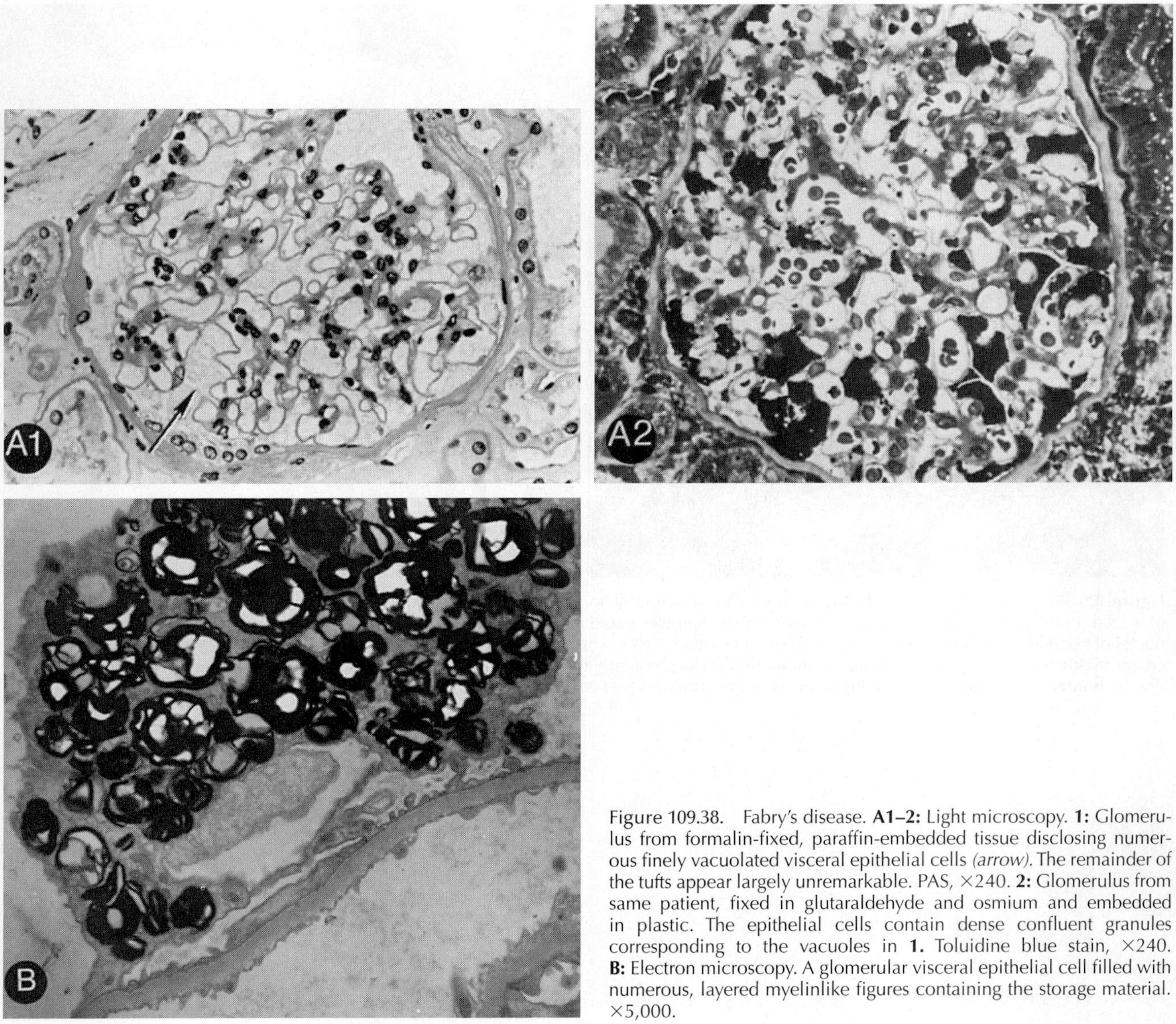

Figure 109.38. Fabry's disease. **A1–2:** Light microscopy. **1:** Glomerulus from formalin-fixed, paraffin-embedded tissue disclosing numerous finely vacuolated visceral epithelial cells *(arrow)*. The remainder of the tufts appear largely unremarkable. PAS, ×240. **2:** Glomerulus from same patient, fixed in glutaraldehyde and osmium and embedded in plastic. The epithelial cells contain dense confluent granules corresponding to the vacuoles in **1.** Toluidine blue stain, ×240. **B:** Electron microscopy. A glomerular visceral epithelial cell filled with numerous, layered myelinlike figures containing the storage material. ×5,000.

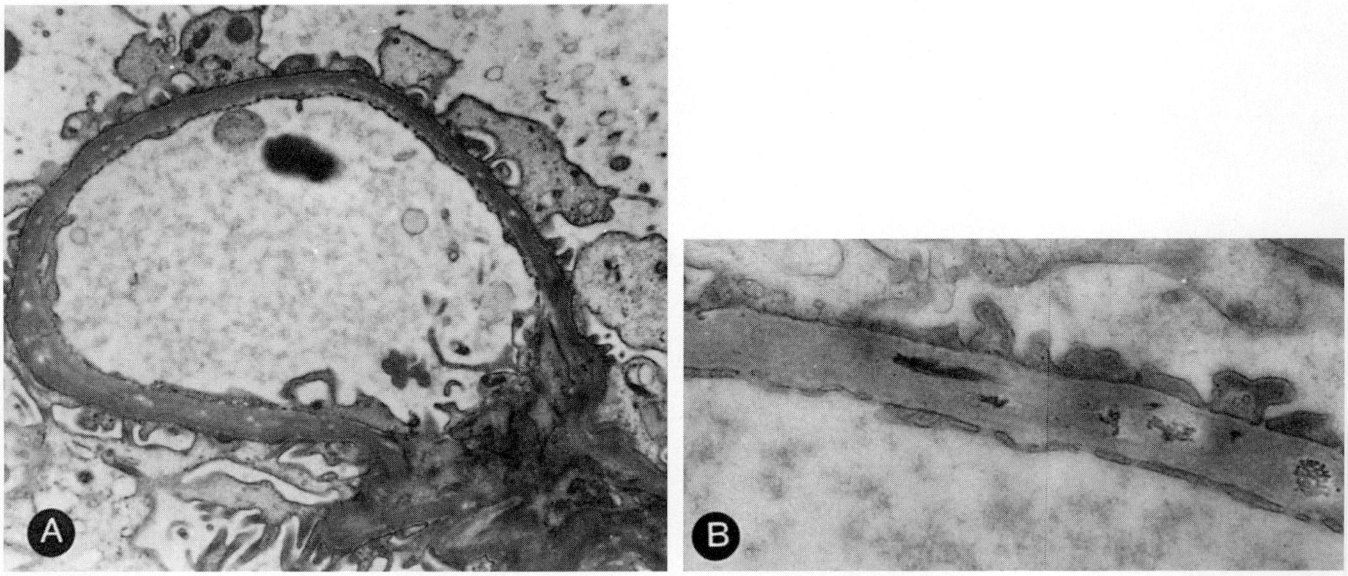

Figure 109.39. Nail-patella syndrome. **A:** Electron microscopy. Numerous lucent zones are visible throughout the thickened lamina densa of the glomerular basement membrane. ×6,250. **B:** Some glomerular capillary stained with phosphotungstic acid, indicating the presence of dense, cross-banded collagen fibrils within the abnormal areas. ×18,750.

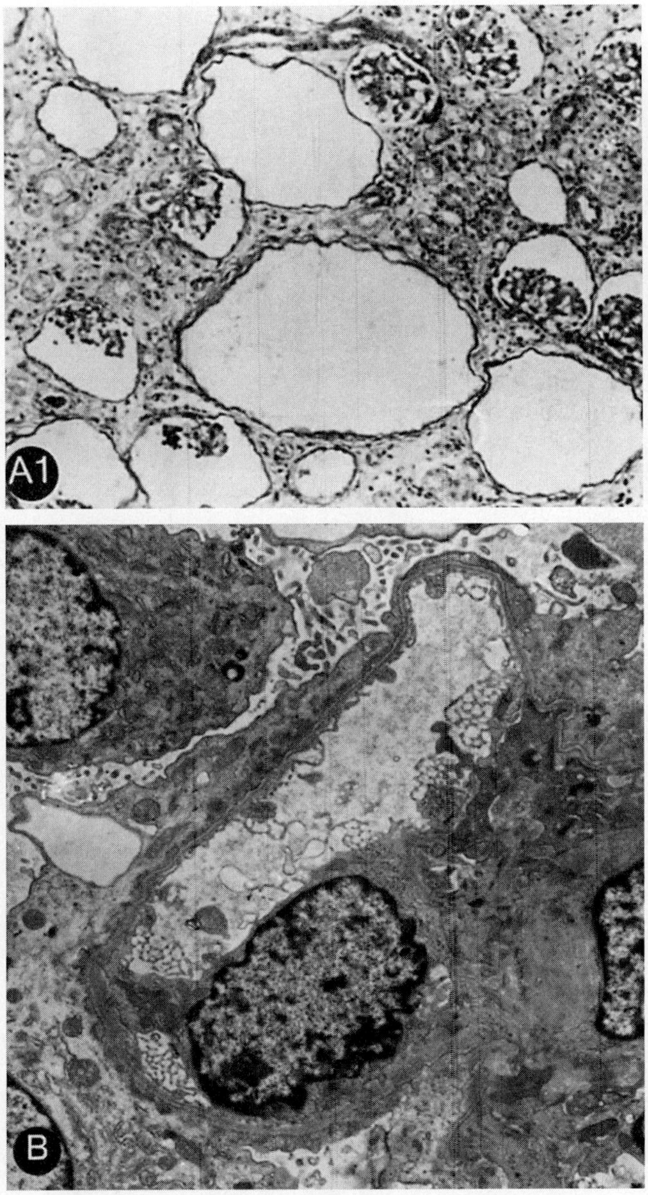

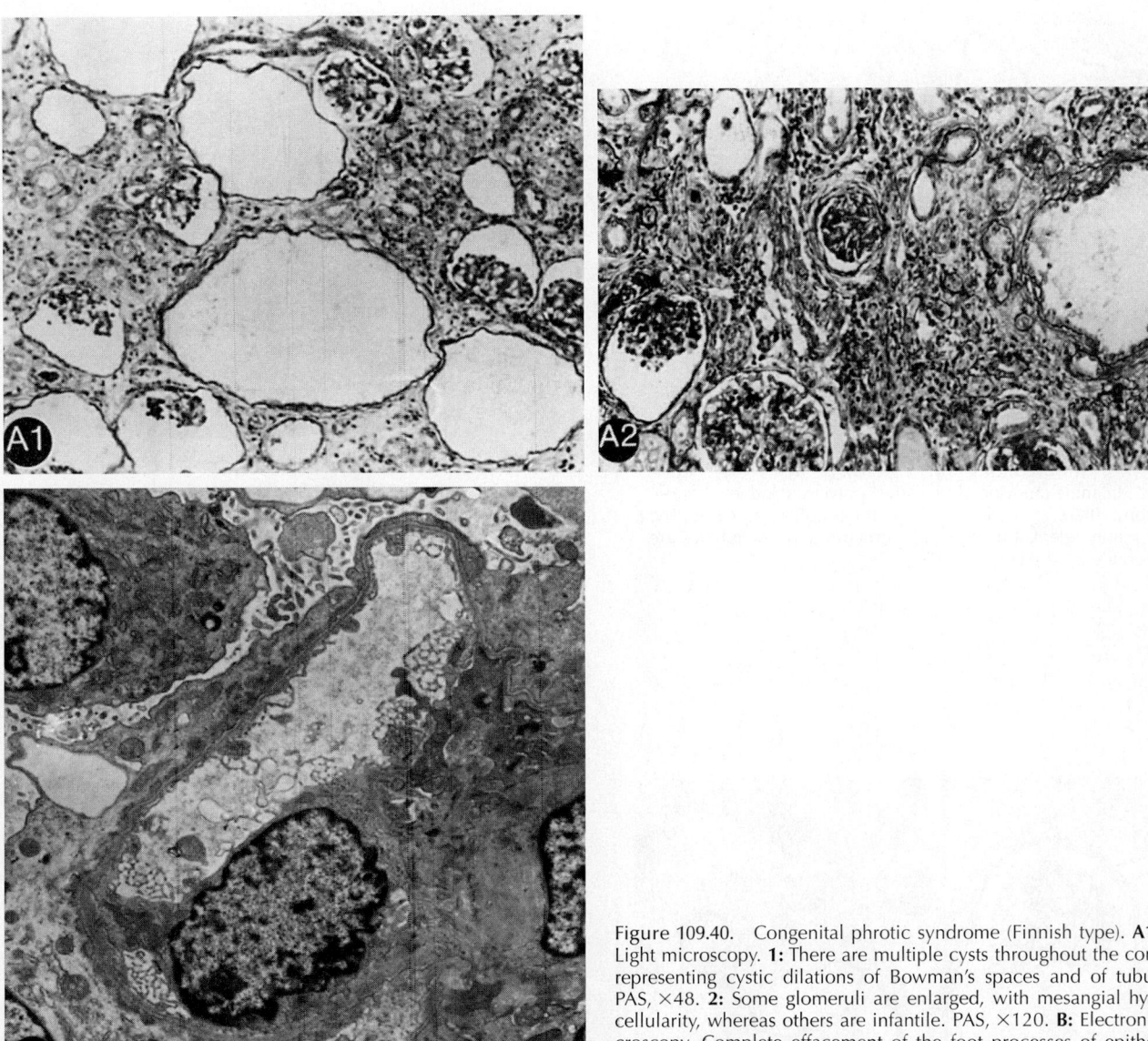

Figure 109.40. Congenital phrotic syndrome (Finnish type). **A1–2:** Light microscopy. **1:** There are multiple cysts throughout the cortex, representing cystic dilations of Bowman's spaces and of tubules. PAS, ×48. **2:** Some glomeruli are enlarged, with mesangial hypercellularity, whereas others are infantile. PAS, ×120. **B:** Electron microscopy. Complete effacement of the foot processes of epithelial cells over thin basement membranes. The latter are not abnormally thin but reflect the patient's young age. ×4,000.

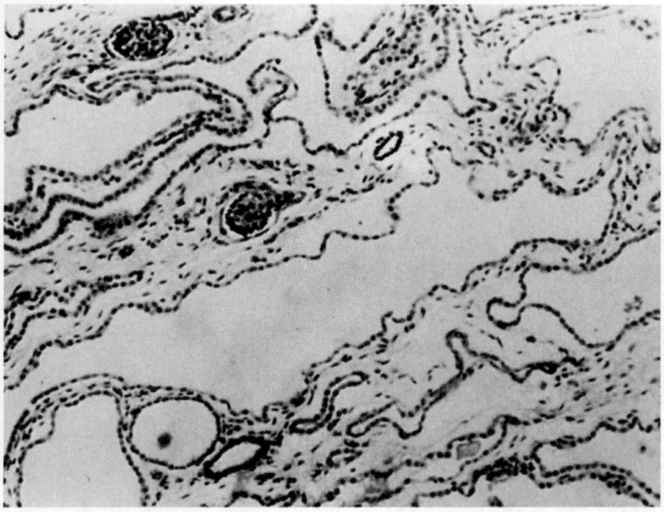

Figure 109.41. Infantile (autosomal-recessive) polycystic kidney disease. Light microscopy. There is dilation of the cortical collecting ducts. The interstitium is mildly edematous. Normal glomeruli and few tubules are present between the cysts. H&E, ×120.

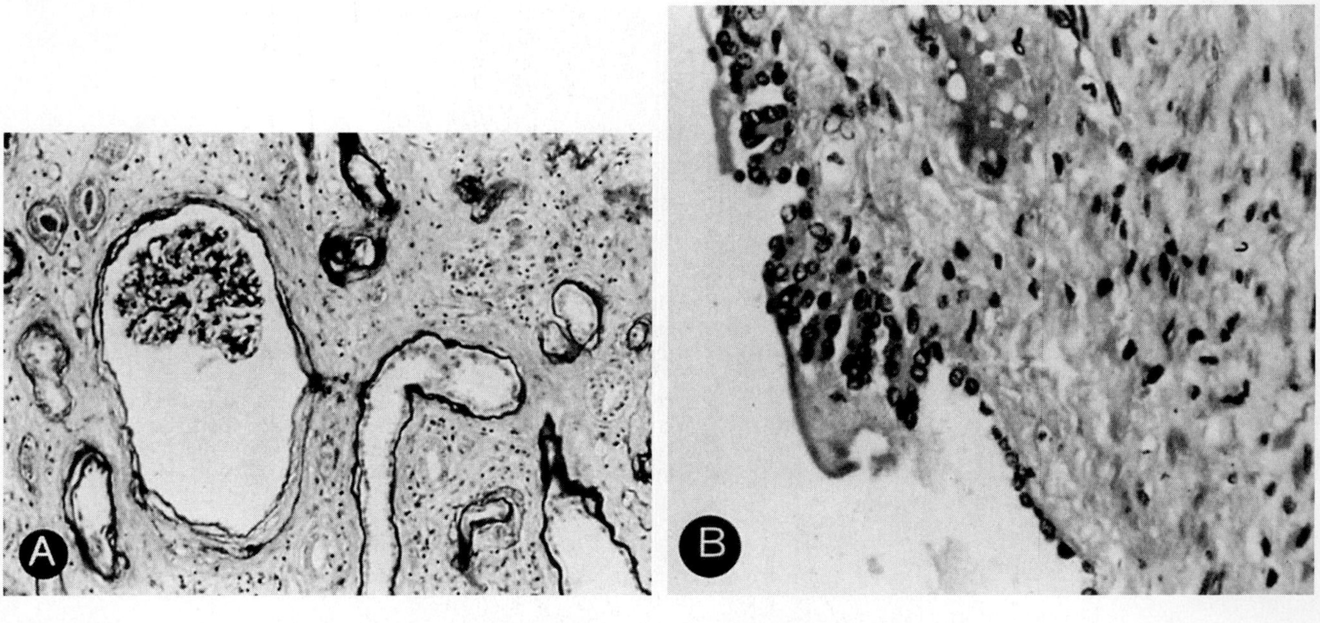

Figure 109.42. Adult (autosomal-dominant) polycystic kidney disease. **A:** Light microscopy. There are numerous cysts throughout the parenchyma, with compression atrophy of adjacent tissues. The cysts affect all segments of the nephron. This photograph shows cystic dilation of Bowman's space. PAS, ×120. **B:** Lining of one of the cysts. The epithelium is low cuboidal and is clustered as several papillary infoldings. It is thought that the papillary lesions may lead to tubular obstruction and subsequent cyst formation. H&E, ×240.

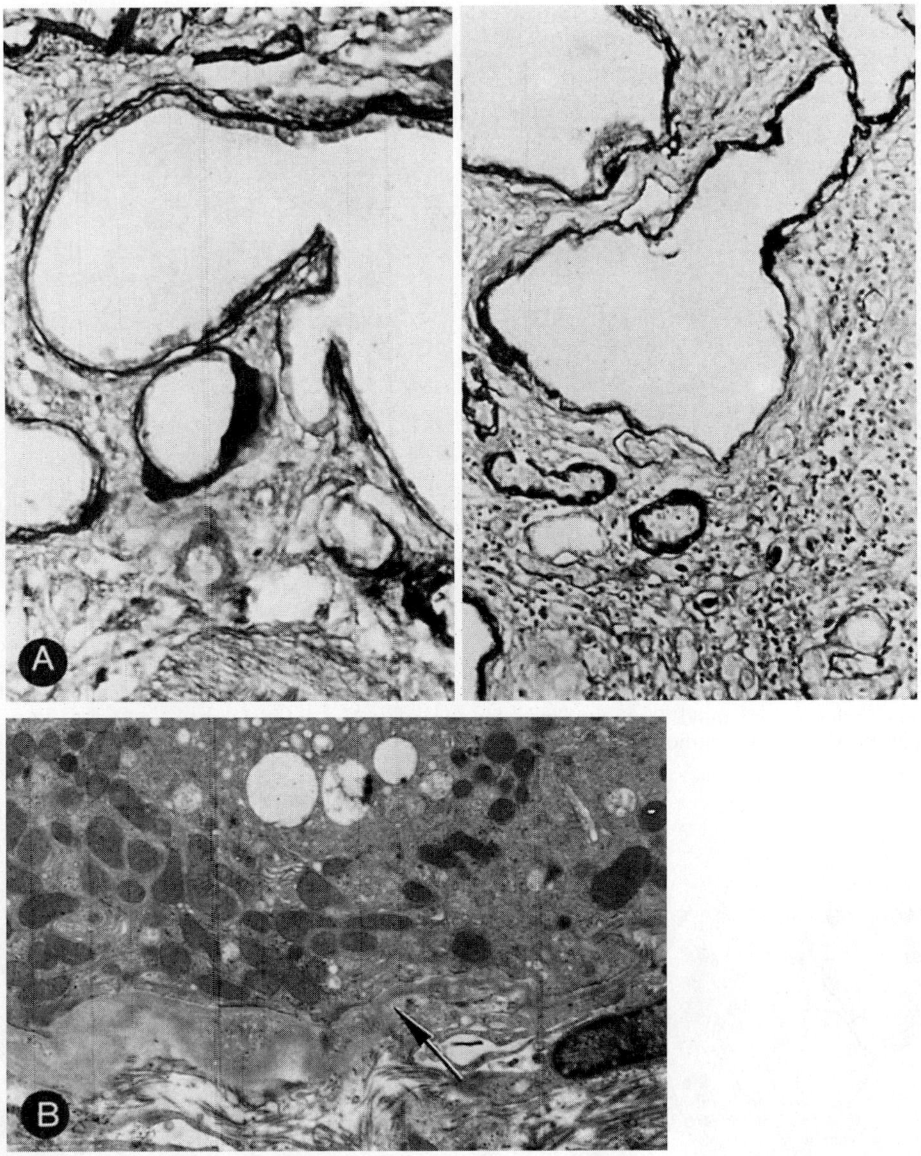

Figure 109.43. Medullary cystic disease (juvenile nephronophthisis). **A:** Light microscopy. The cysts, which are classically located at the corticomedullary junction and medulla, are often associated with interstitial fibrosis and some degree of tubular atrophy. However, as illustrated in both figures, the basement membranes of cystic as well as noncystic tubules are irregular, ranging from extremely thin to extremely thick. The dilation may be a consequence of poorly compliant basement membranes and tubular walls, as illustrated in the figure on the *left*. *Right,* PAS, ×120; *left,* PAS, ×240. **B:** Electron microscopy. The tubular basement membrane abruptly changes *(arrow)* from thick to very thin. ×13,500.

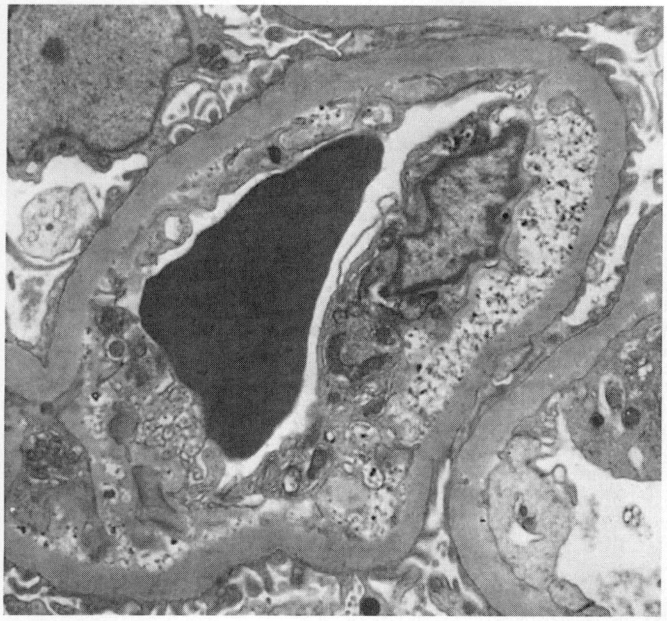

Figure 109.44. Lecithin-cholesterol acyltransferase deficiency. Electron microscopy. The typical ultrastructural features of this disorder are illustrated. There are numerous clear and lucent extracellular spaces in which dense, rounded, membranous inclusions are found. These are similar to structures in glomeruli in patients with hepatic cirrhosis. ×4,000.

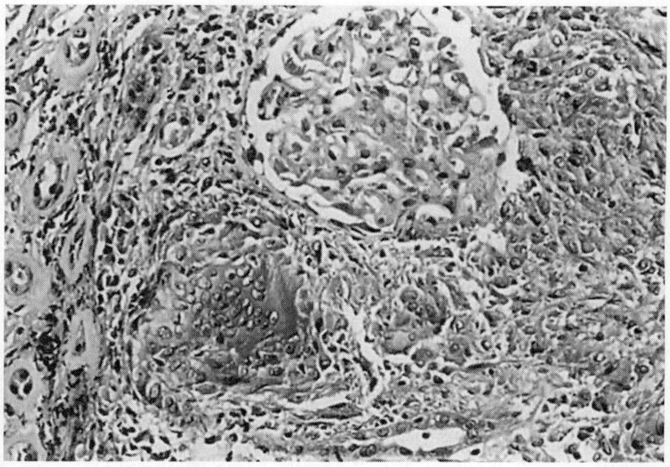

Figure 109.45. Renal sarcoidosis. Light microscopy. The interstitium contains a granuloma composed of epithelioid cells and multinucleated giant cells without necrosis. Masson's trichrome, ×215.

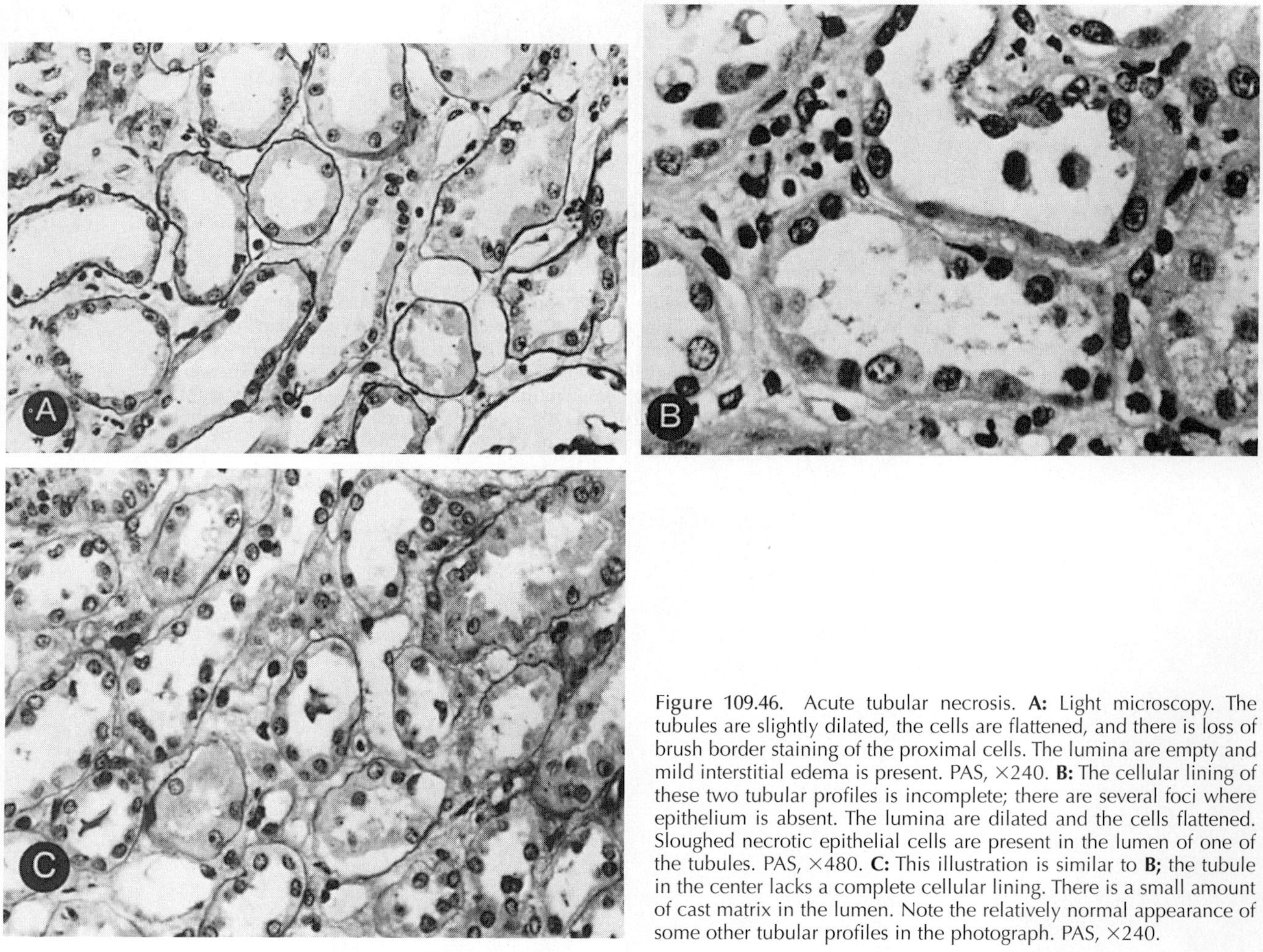

Figure 109.46. Acute tubular necrosis. **A:** Light microscopy. The tubules are slightly dilated, the cells are flattened, and there is loss of brush border staining of the proximal cells. The lumina are empty and mild interstitial edema is present. PAS, ×240. **B:** The cellular lining of these two tubular profiles is incomplete; there are several foci where epithelium is absent. The lumina are dilated and the cells flattened. Sloughed necrotic epithelial cells are present in the lumen of one of the tubules. PAS, ×480. **C:** This illustration is similar to **B;** the tubule in the center lacks a complete cellular lining. There is a small amount of cast matrix in the lumen. Note the relatively normal appearance of some other tubular profiles in the photograph. PAS, ×240.

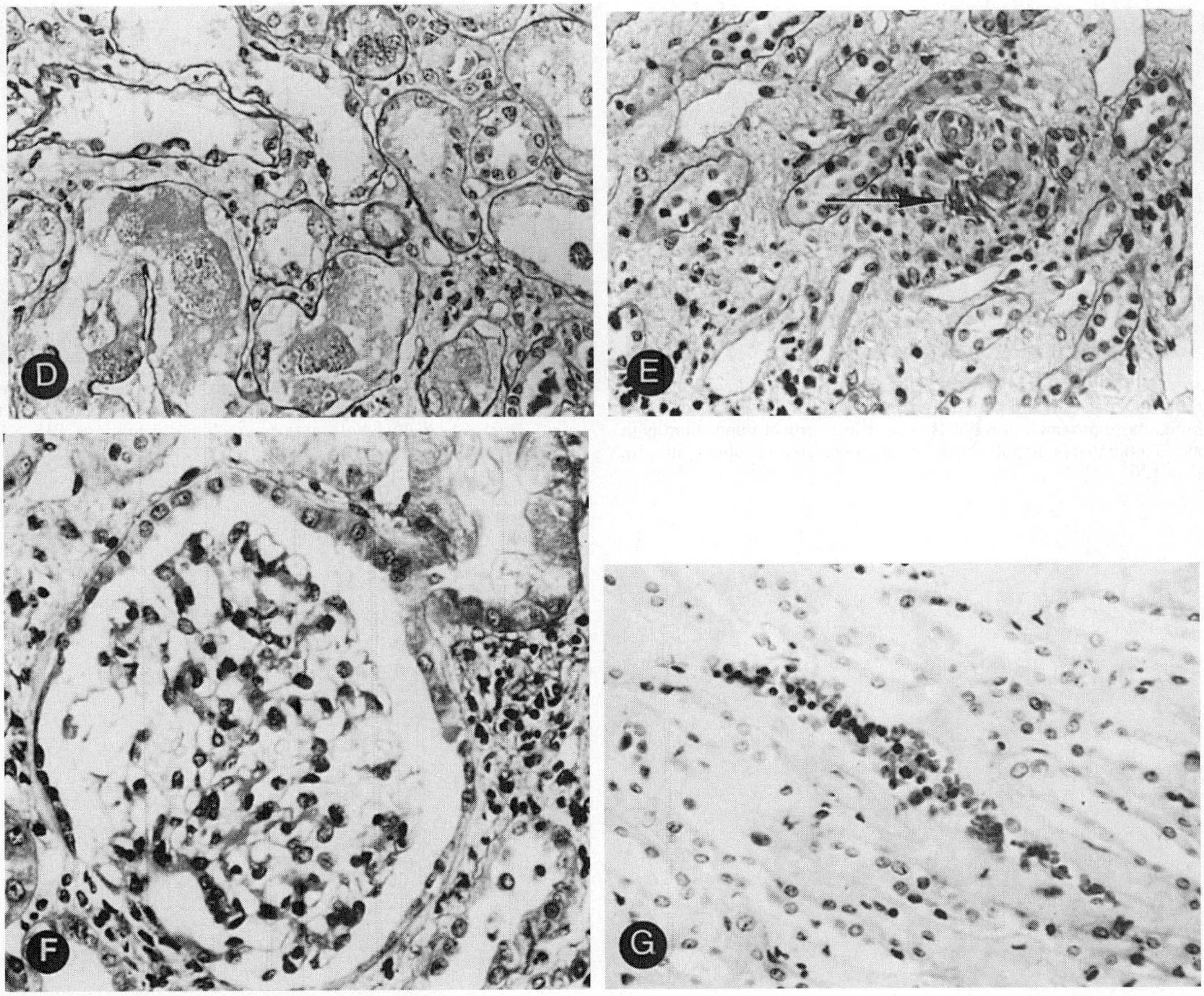

Figure 109.46 (*continued.*) Acute tubular necrosis. **D:** There is frank necrosis of cells of several tubules, with accumulation of necrotic debris within the lumina. PAS, ×240. **E:** In this illustration, a small focus of Tamm-Horsfall protein *(arrow)* is surrounded by mononuclear cells in the interstitium. This results from rupture of tubular walls consequent to necrosis, with escape of luminal contents into the interstitium. This is a relatively infrequent finding in acute tubular necrosis. PAS, ×240. **F:** In resolving phases of tubular necrosis, there may be metaplasia of the parietal epithelial cells of glomeruli. As illustrated here, the cells assume the appearance of tubular epithelium, a process known as *tubular metaplasia* or *tubularization.* Masson's trichrome, ×240. **G:** Medullary vasa recta filled with nucleated cells as well as erythrocytes. The former are predominantly lymphocytes, monocytes, and immature granulocytes, although previously they were considered to represent immature erythrocytes. This finding is commonly observed at autopsy in patients who die of the ischemic form of acute tubular necrosis. H&E, ×300.

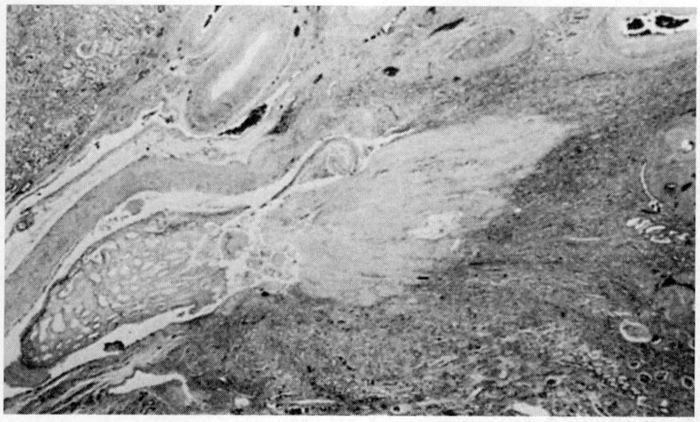

Figure 109.47. Papillary necrosis. Light microscopy. This low magnification shows a necrotic and partially sloughed papilla. The tip is separated from the more proximal portion. The overlying cortical interstitium is fibrotic, is infiltrated by lymphocytes, and has considerable tubular atrophy. H&E, ×120.

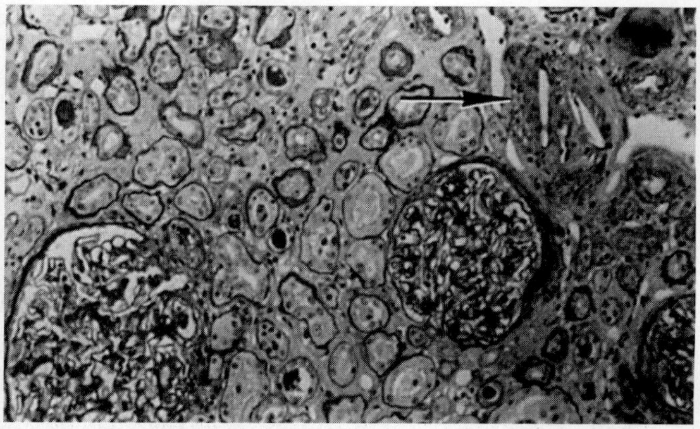

Figure 109.48. Atheromatous emboli. Light microscopy. Several empty acicular spaces are visible within the obliterated lumen of an interlobular artery *(arrow)*. Note the tubular atrophy and interstitial fibrosis. PAS, ×120.

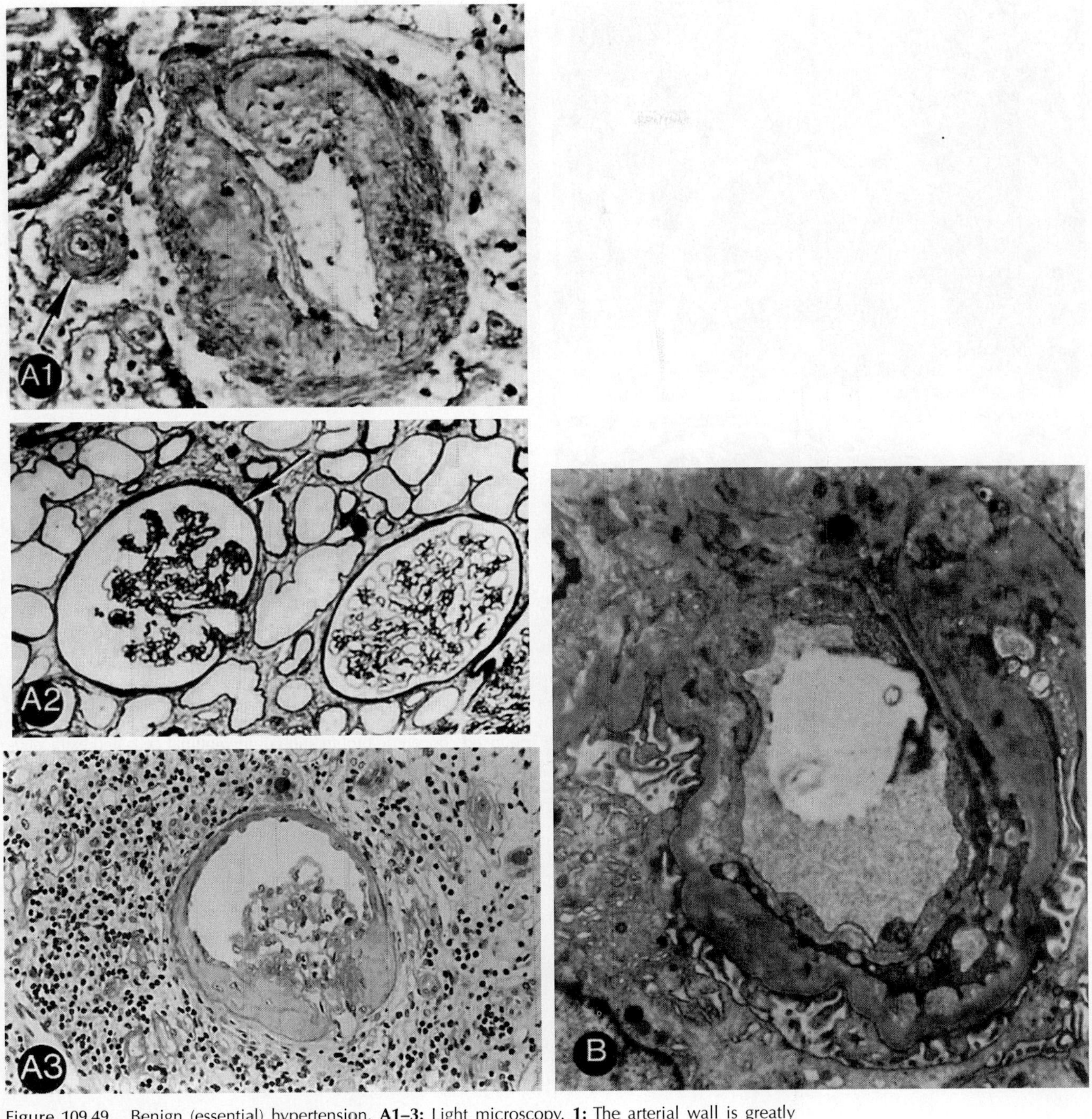

Figure 109.49. Benign (essential) hypertension. **A1–3:** Light microscopy. **1:** The arterial wall is greatly thickened, primarily because of marked intimal fibrosis resulting in luminal narrowing. Note also thickening of the arteriolar wall with accumulation of plasma protein ("hyalinization") *(arrow)*. PAS, ×240. **2:** Glomerulus exhibiting ischemic collapse of capillaries with narrowing of lumina and relative dilation of Bowman's space *(arrow)*. Compare with adjacent glomerulus lacking ischemic changes. Periodic acid–methenamine silver, ×120. **3:** Glomerulus displaying further ischemic damage. In addition to capillary collapse and solidification of the tuft, there is collagen formation internal to Bowman's capsule, growing in a collarlike fashion from the hilus. Marked tubular atrophy with interstitial fibrosis and lymphocytes is also present. PAS, ×300. **B:** Electron microscopy. Capillary wall collapse. There is interposition of mesangial cells and matrix. The foot processes of epithelial cells are nearly completely effaced. ×6,250.

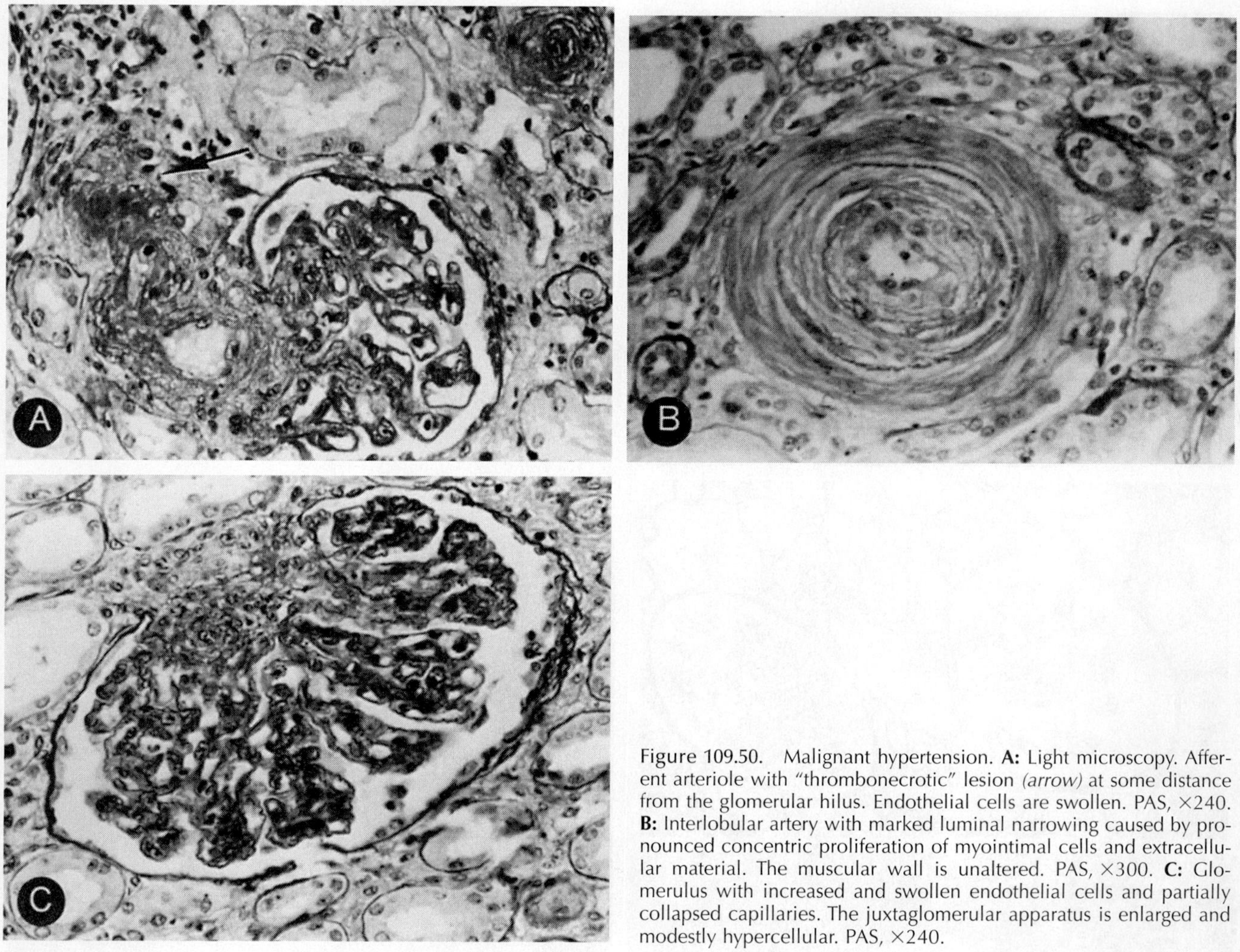

Figure 109.50. Malignant hypertension. **A:** Light microscopy. Afferent arteriole with "thrombonecrotic" lesion *(arrow)* at some distance from the glomerular hilus. Endothelial cells are swollen. PAS, ×240. **B:** Interlobular artery with marked luminal narrowing caused by pronounced concentric proliferation of myointimal cells and extracellular material. The muscular wall is unaltered. PAS, ×300. **C:** Glomerulus with increased and swollen endothelial cells and partially collapsed capillaries. The juxtaglomerular apparatus is enlarged and modestly hypercellular. PAS, ×240.

I

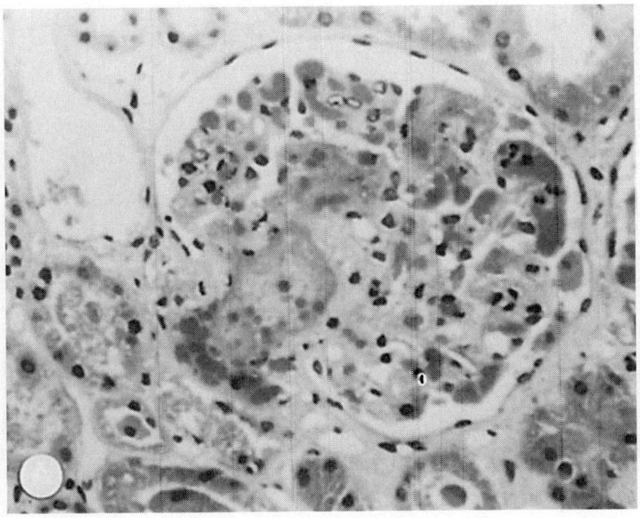

Figure 109.51. Transplant rejection. **I:** Hyperacute rejection. Almost all glomerular capillaries contain fresh thrombi, some with incorporated neutrophils. H&E, ×300. **II:** Acute rejection. **A1–3:** Routine light microscopy. **1:** There is marked edema with accumulation of mononuclear leukocytes within peritubular capillaries, throughout the interstitium and extending into the walls of tubules (tubulitis). PAS, ×240. **2:** The inflammatory infiltrate includes activated lymphocytes with smaller numbers of monocytes and plasma cells. Masson's trichrome, ×450. **3:** Interlobular artery with segmental accumulation of lymphocytes and monocytes within the lumen and beneath swollen endothelial cells. Note the presence of similar leukocytes in peritubular capillaries and interstitium in the adjacent parenchyma. PAS, ×300.

II

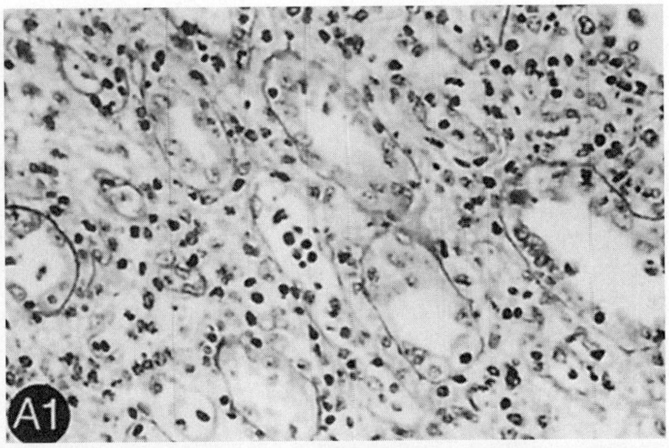

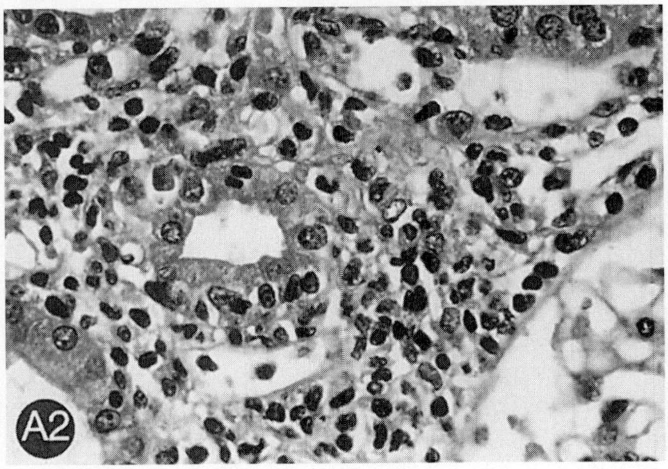

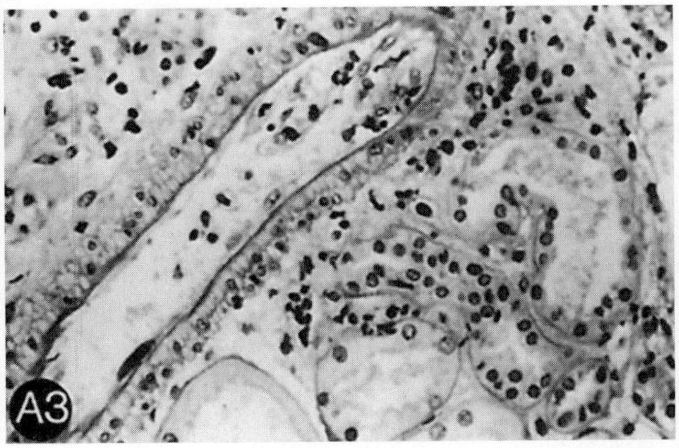

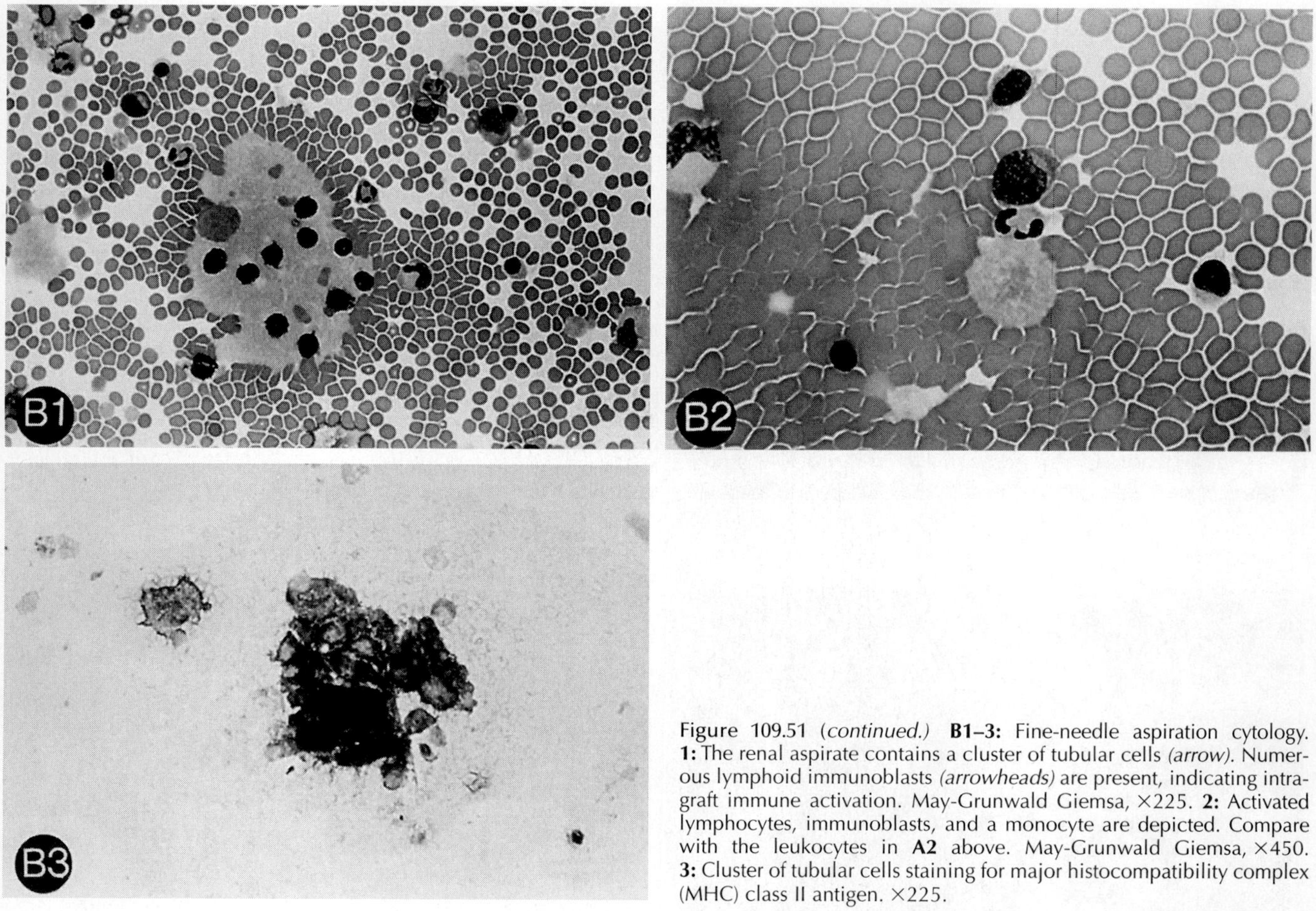

Figure 109.51 (*continued.*) **B1–3:** Fine-needle aspiration cytology. **1:** The renal aspirate contains a cluster of tubular cells *(arrow)*. Numerous lymphoid immunoblasts *(arrowheads)* are present, indicating intragraft immune activation. May-Grunwald Giemsa, ×225. **2:** Activated lymphocytes, immunoblasts, and a monocyte are depicted. Compare with the leukocytes in **A2** above. May-Grunwald Giemsa, ×450. **3:** Cluster of tubular cells staining for major histocompatibility complex (MHC) class II antigen. ×225.

III

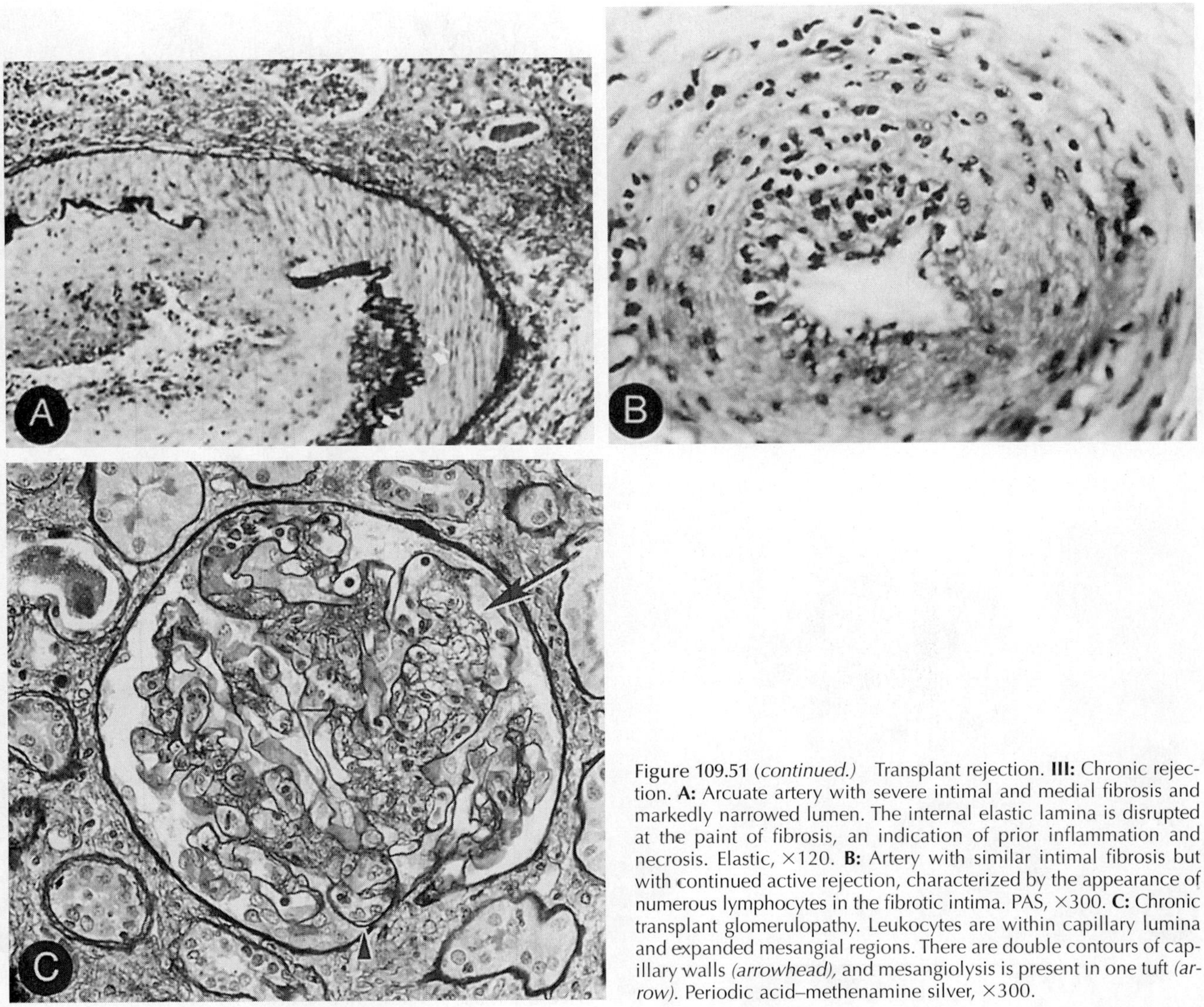

Figure 109.51 (*continued.*) Transplant rejection. **III:** Chronic rejection. **A:** Arcuate artery with severe intimal and medial fibrosis and markedly narrowed lumen. The internal elastic lamina is disrupted at the paint of fibrosis, an indication of prior inflammation and necrosis. Elastic, ×120. **B:** Artery with similar intimal fibrosis but with continued active rejection, characterized by the appearance of numerous lymphocytes in the fibrotic intima. PAS, ×300. **C:** Chronic transplant glomerulopathy. Leukocytes are within capillary lumina and expanded mesangial regions. There are double contours of capillary walls *(arrowhead),* and mesangiolysis is present in one tuft *(arrow).* Periodic acid–methenamine silver, ×300.

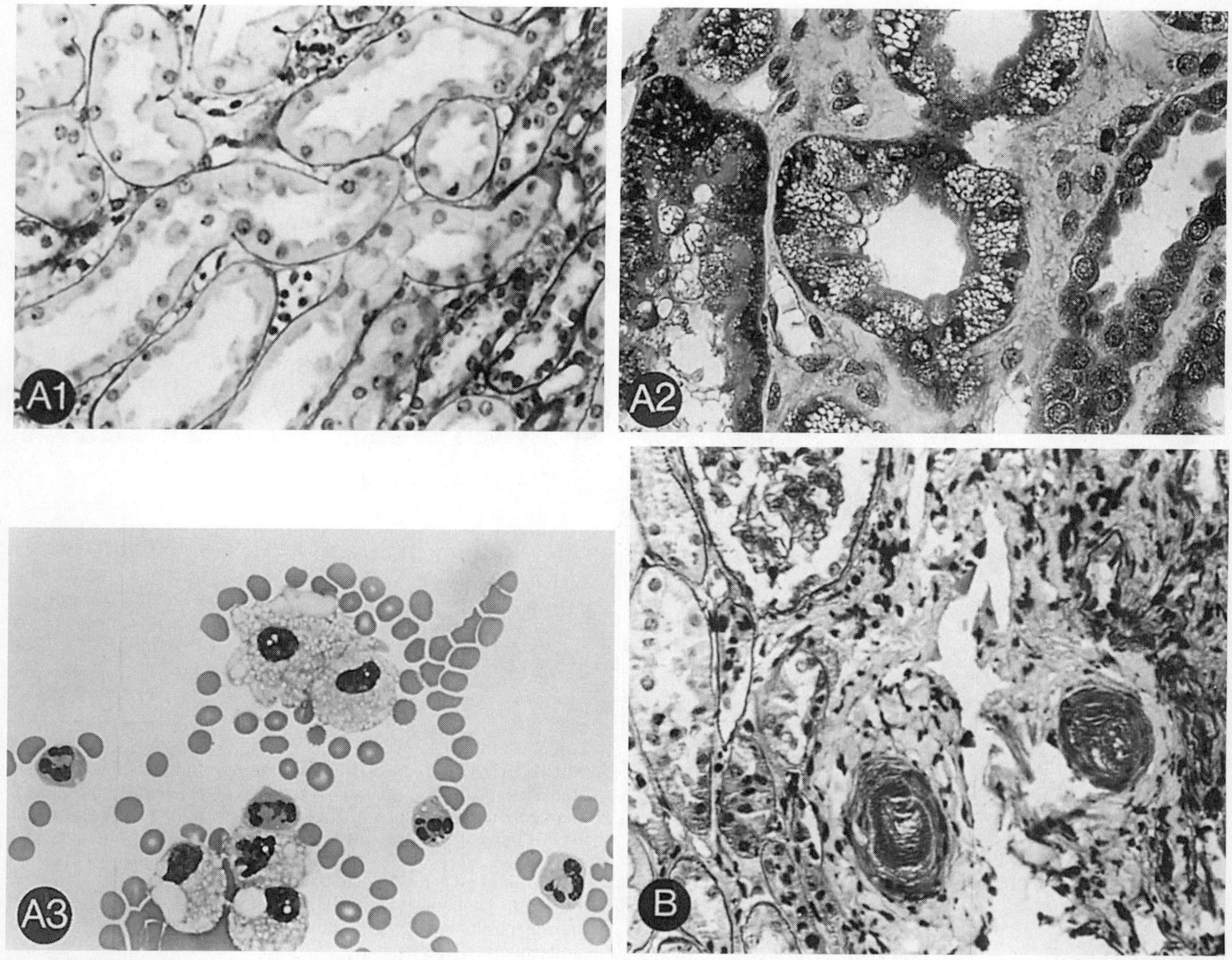

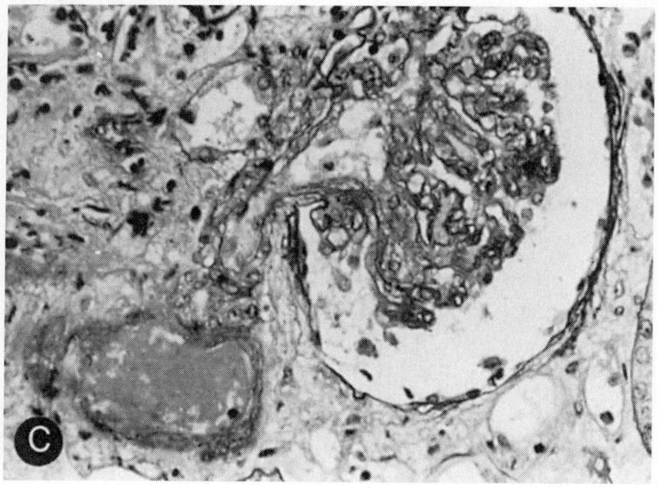

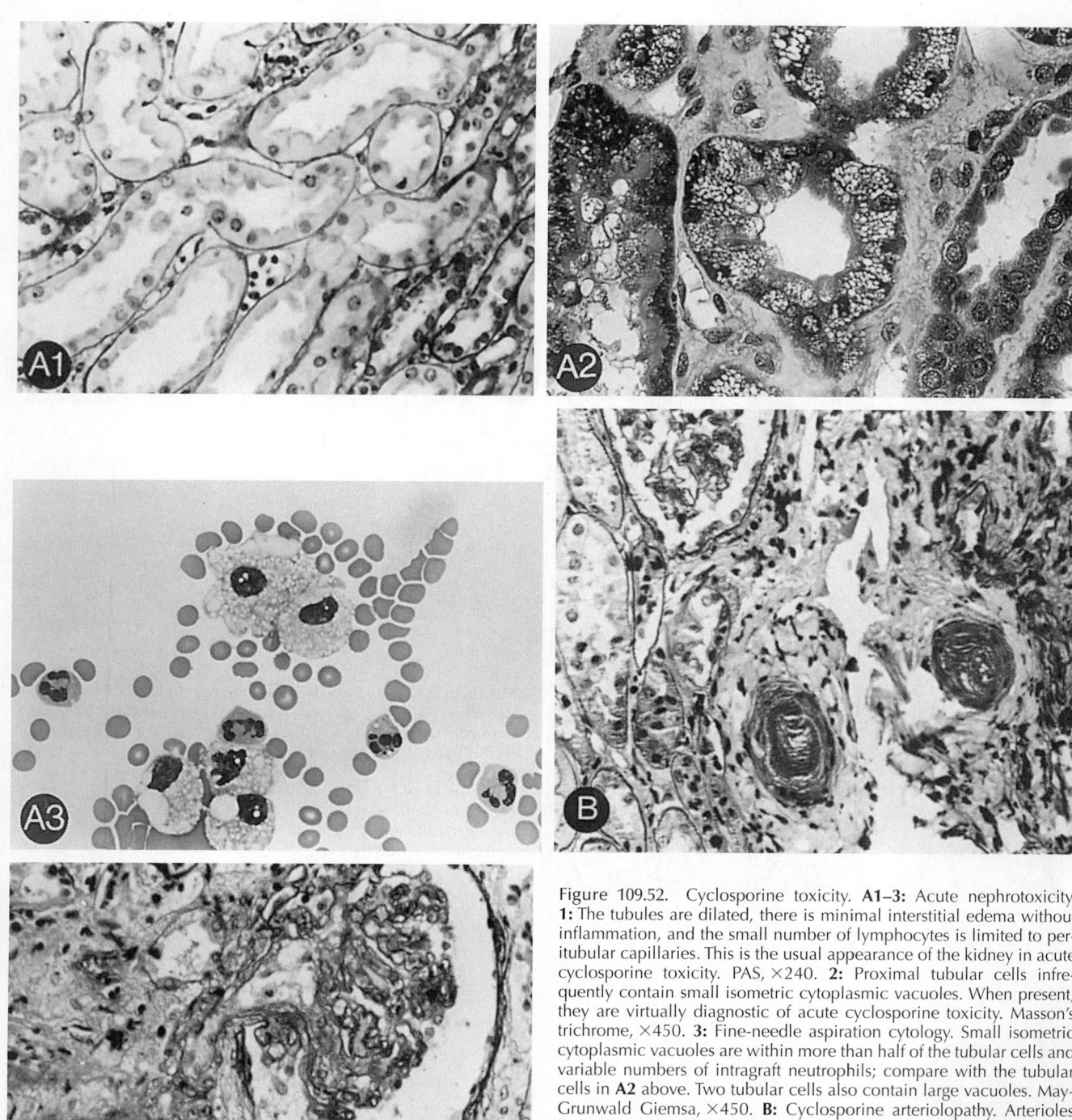

Figure 109.52. Cyclosporine toxicity. **A1–3:** Acute nephrotoxicity. **1:** The tubules are dilated, there is minimal interstitial edema without inflammation, and the small number of lymphocytes is limited to peritubular capillaries. This is the usual appearance of the kidney in acute cyclosporine toxicity. PAS, ×240. **2:** Proximal tubular cells infrequently contain small isometric cytoplasmic vacuoles. When present, they are virtually diagnostic of acute cyclosporine toxicity. Masson's trichrome, ×450. **3:** Fine-needle aspiration cytology. Small isometric cytoplasmic vacuoles are within more than half of the tubular cells and variable numbers of intragraft neutrophils; compare with the tubular cells in **A2** above. Two tubular cells also contain large vacuoles. May-Grunwald Giemsa, ×450. **B:** Cyclosporine arteriolopathy. Arterioles have prominently thickened walls because of massive accumulation of plasma protein insudates. This lesion is sometimes associated with necrosis of individual smooth muscle cells. PAS, ×240. **C:** Cyclosporine-induced thrombotic microangiopathy. The arteriole is thrombosed with glomerular endothelial swelling and capillary collapse, lesions identical to other forms of thrombotic microangiopathy. PAS, ×240.

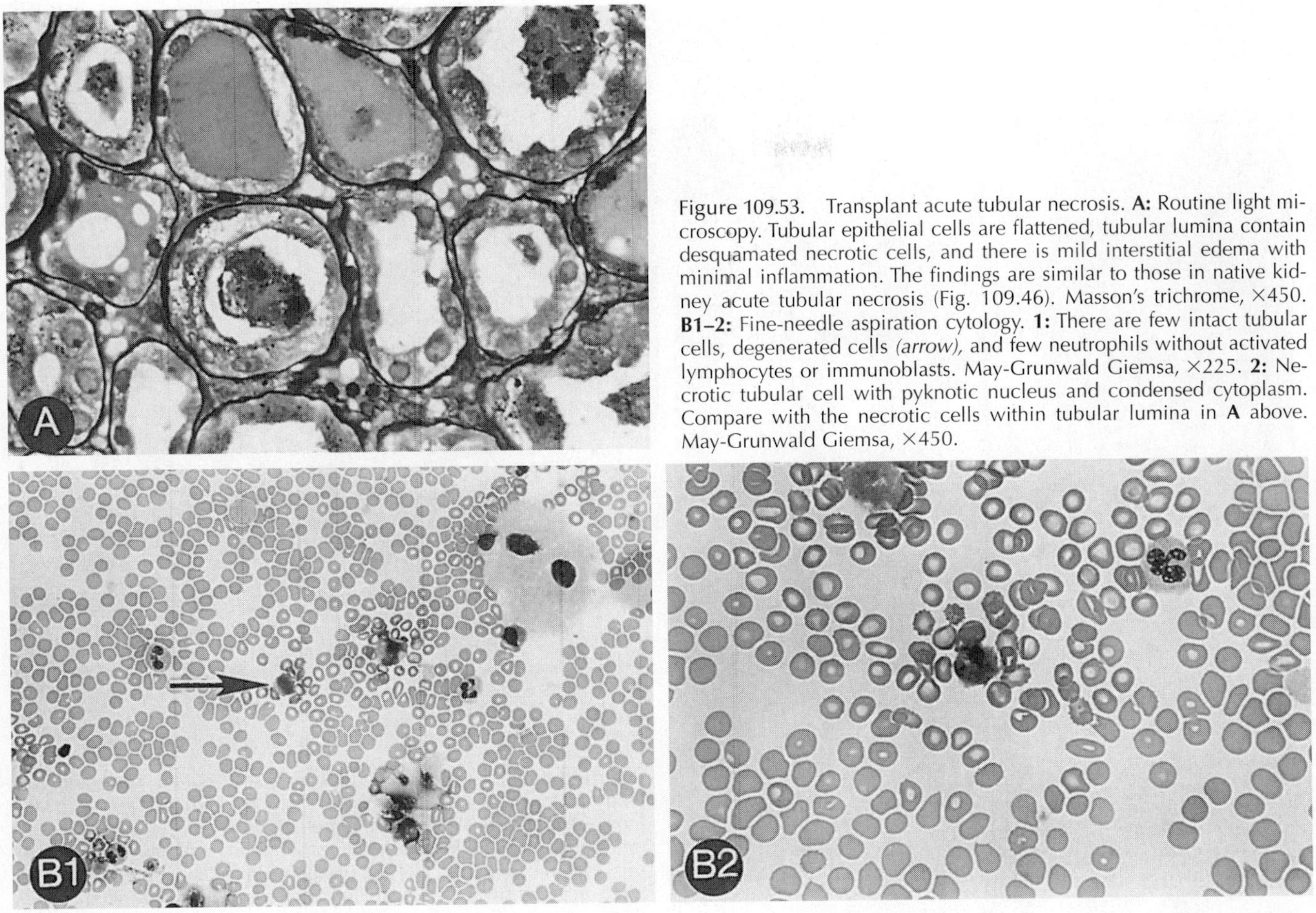

Figure 109.53. Transplant acute tubular necrosis. **A:** Routine light microscopy. Tubular epithelial cells are flattened, tubular lumina contain desquamated necrotic cells, and there is mild interstitial edema with minimal inflammation. The findings are similar to those in native kidney acute tubular necrosis (Fig. 109.46). Masson's trichrome, ×450. **B1–2:** Fine-needle aspiration cytology. **1:** There are few intact tubular cells, degenerated cells *(arrow)*, and few neutrophils without activated lymphocytes or immunoblasts. May-Grunwald Giemsa, ×225. **2:** Necrotic tubular cell with pyknotic nucleus and condensed cytoplasm. Compare with the necrotic cells within tubular lumina in **A** above. May-Grunwald Giemsa, ×450.

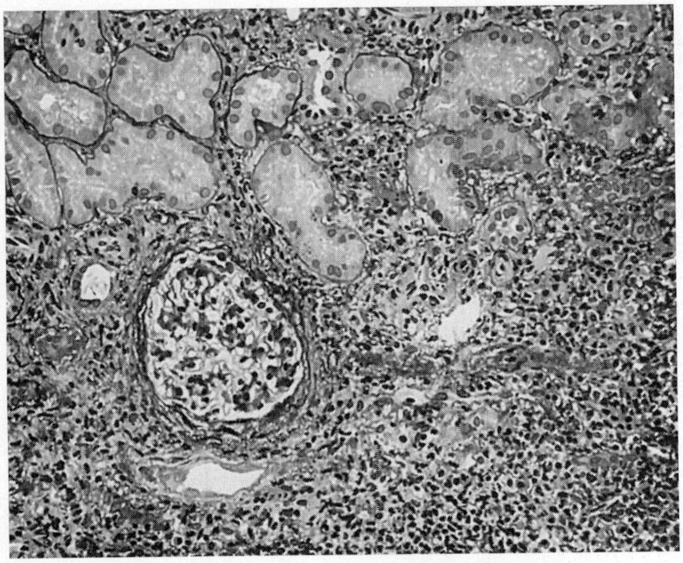

Figure 109.54. Sjögren's syndrome. Interstitial infiltrate of mononuclear leukocytes, predominantly lymphocytes and plasma cells, with focal replacement of tubules. Periodic acid–methenamine silver, ×100. (Contributed by Robert L. Winer, M.D.)

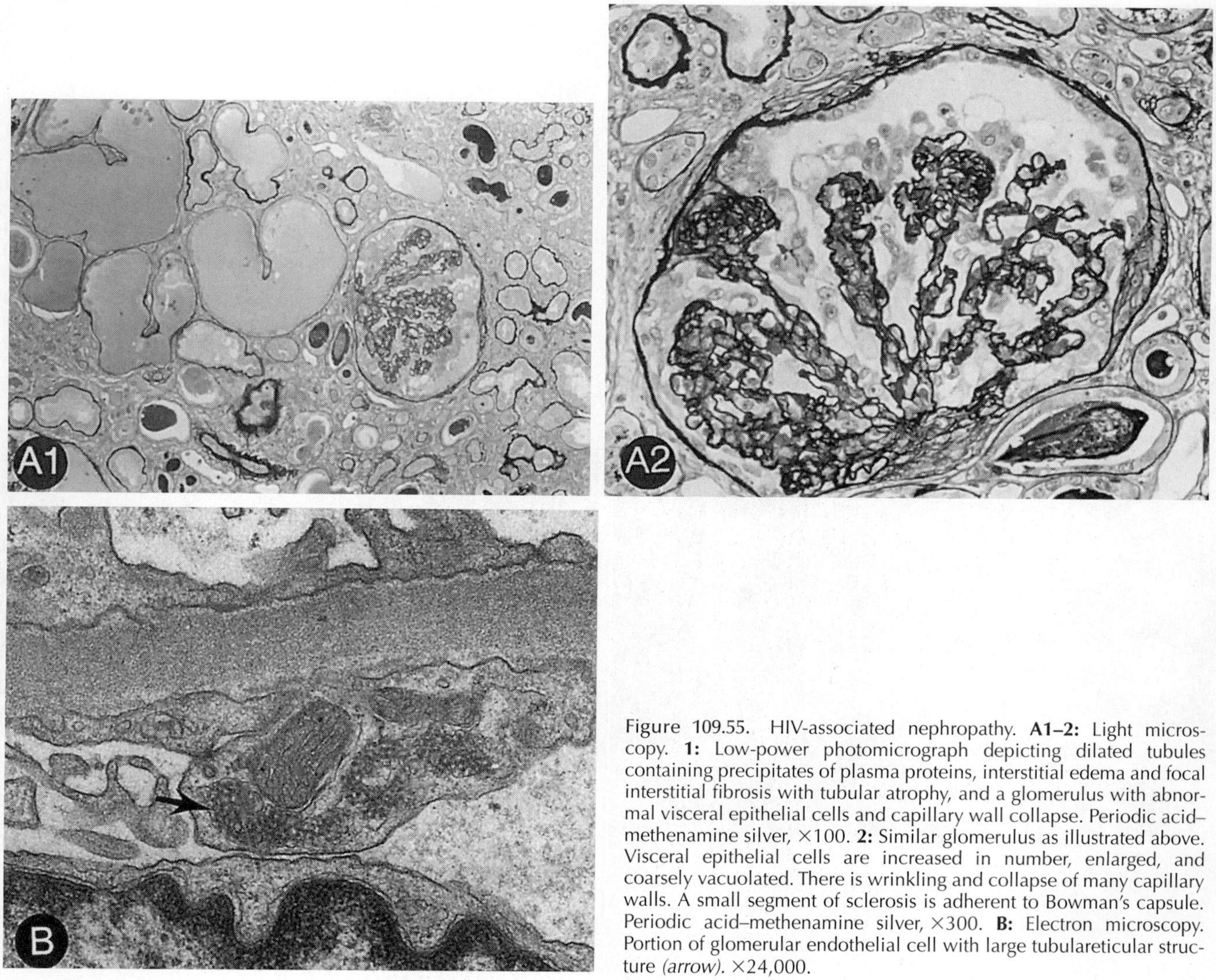

Figure 109.55. HIV-associated nephropathy. **A1–2:** Light microscopy. **1:** Low-power photomicrograph depicting dilated tubules containing precipitates of plasma proteins, interstitial edema and focal interstitial fibrosis with tubular atrophy, and a glomerulus with abnormal visceral epithelial cells and capillary wall collapse. Periodic acid–methenamine silver, ×100. **2:** Similar glomerulus as illustrated above. Visceral epithelial cells are increased in number, enlarged, and coarsely vacuolated. There is wrinkling and collapse of many capillary walls. A small segment of sclerosis is adherent to Bowman's capsule. Periodic acid–methenamine silver, ×300. **B:** Electron microscopy. Portion of glomerular endothelial cell with large tubulareticular structure *(arrow)*. ×24,000.

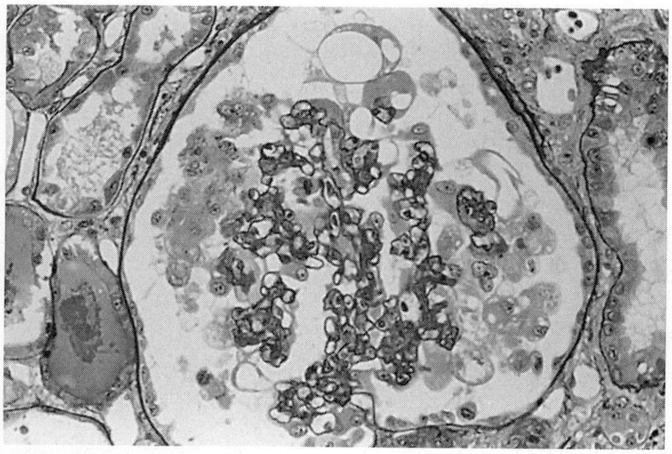

Figure 109.56. Collapsing glomerulopathy. The glomerular capillary walls are collapsed, with narrowing or obliteration of lumina. Virtually all visceral epithelial cells are enlarged and vacuolated and there is segmental hyperplasia of these cells. These abnormalities are similar to those of HIV-associated nephropathy. Periodic acid–methenamin silver, ×200.

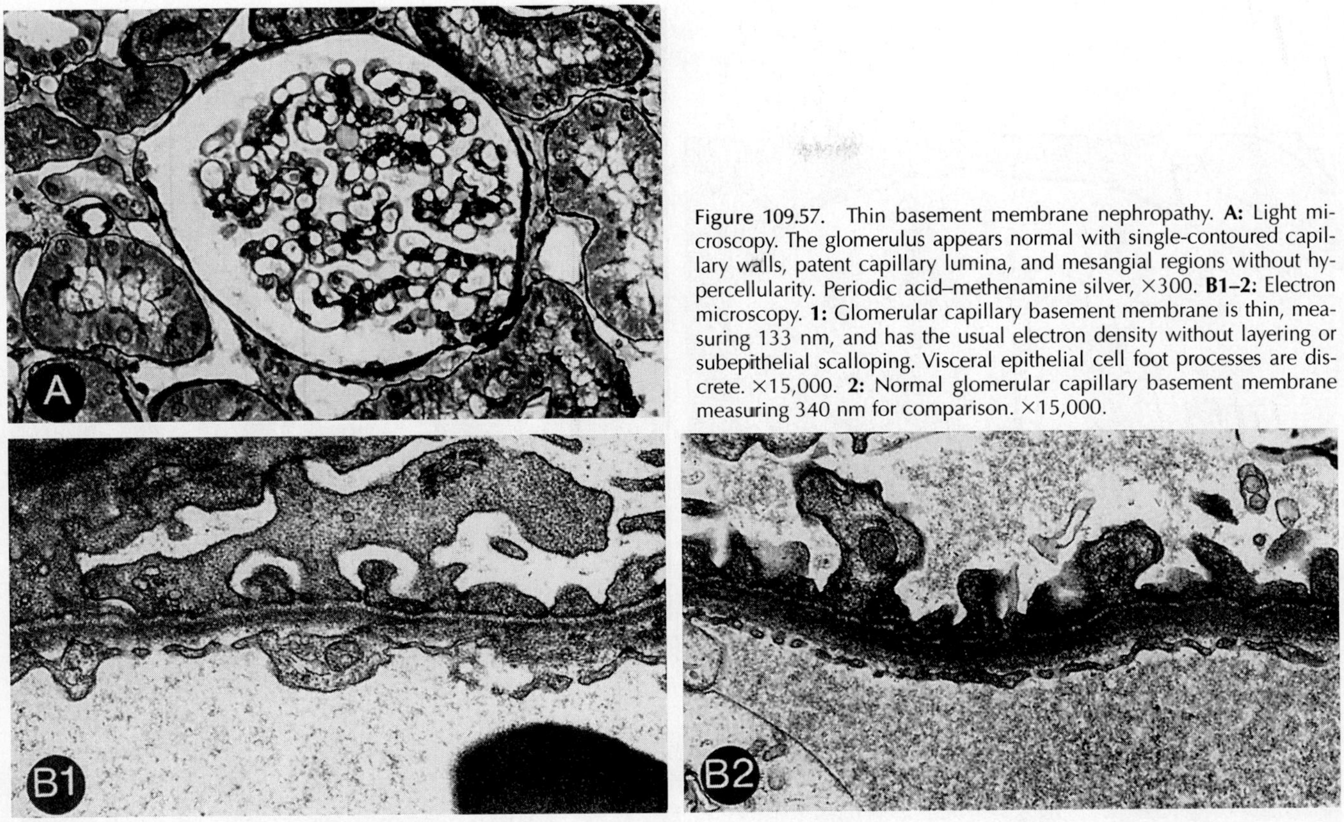

Figure 109.57. Thin basement membrane nephropathy. **A:** Light microscopy. The glomerulus appears normal with single-contoured capillary walls, patent capillary lumina, and mesangial regions without hypercellularity. Periodic acid–methenamine silver, ×300. **B1–2:** Electron microscopy. **1:** Glomerular capillary basement membrane is thin, measuring 133 nm, and has the usual electron density without layering or subepithelial scalloping. Visceral epithelial cell foot processes are discrete. ×15,000. **2:** Normal glomerular capillary basement membrane measuring 340 nm for comparison. ×15,000.

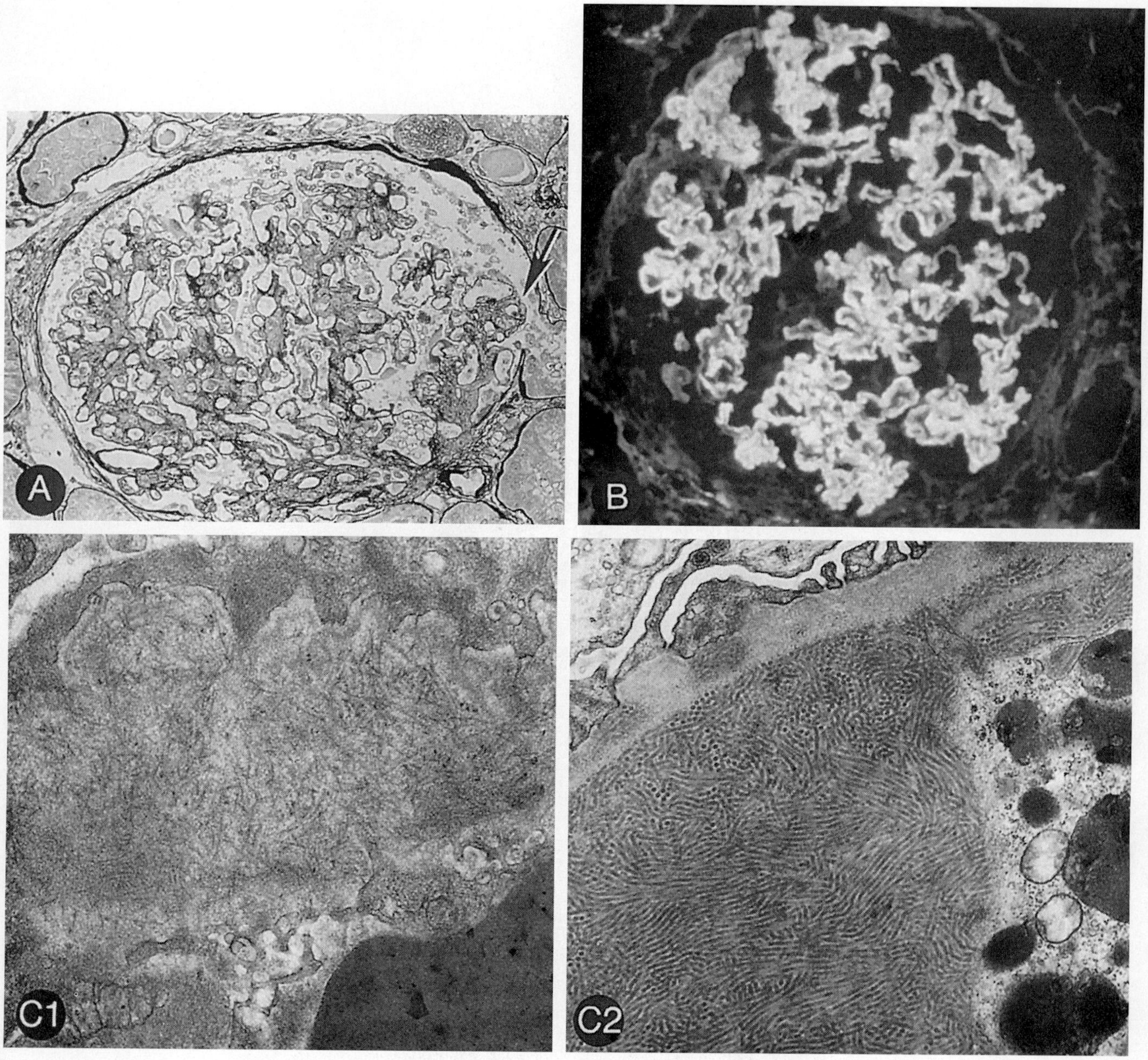

Figure 109.58. Fibrillary glomerulonephritis. **A:** Light microscopy. The glomerulus has expanded mesangial regions containing increased cells and pale-staining material. Similar material is within capillary walls, which occasionally display double contours *(arrow).* Periodic acid–methenamine silver, ×240. **B:** Immunofluorescence. Capillary walls and mesangial regions have heavy confluent granular to ribbon-like staining with anti-IgG. ×365. **C1–2:** Electron microscopy. **1:** Markedly thickened glomerular capillary wall infiltrated by fibrils measuring 12 to 15 nm in diameter, with a haphazard arrangement. Overlying epithelial foot processes are effaced. ×20,500. **2:** Widened glomerular capillary wall containing subendothelial and subepithelial deposits composed of microtubular structures with diameters of 34 to 38 nm. There is also peripheral mesangial migration and interposition. This pattern of microtubular deposition is often termed *immunotactoid glomerulopathy.* ×19,000.

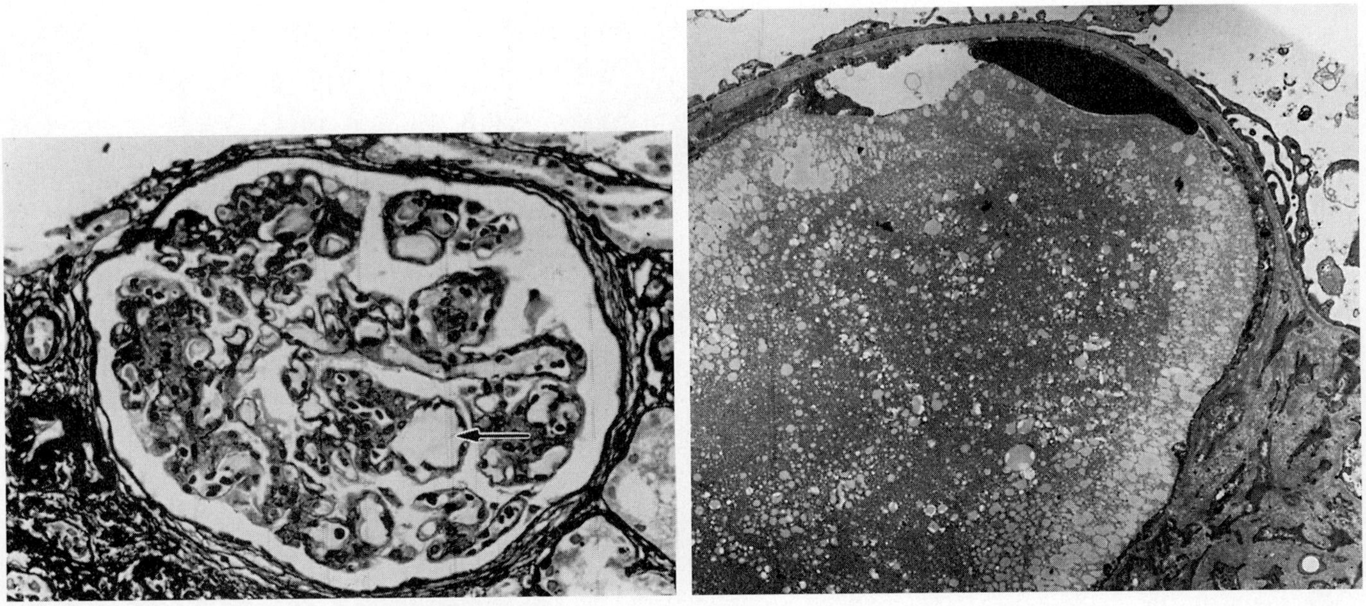

Figure 109.59. Lipoprotein glomerulopathy. **A:** Light microscopic appearance of glomerulus: some capillary lumina are dilated *(arrow)* and almost all are filled with very pale-staining material which consists of a precipitate of lipoprotein "thrombi." There is also mild segmental mesangial hypercellularity. Occasional double-contoured capillary walls are present. Periodic acid–methenamine silver, ×240. **B:** Electron microscopy of a single glomerular capillary. The lumen is filled with a lipoprotein thrombus with incorporated lipid globules. There are distortion and compression of a circulating erythrocyte in the 12 to 2 o'clock position ×(3,750).

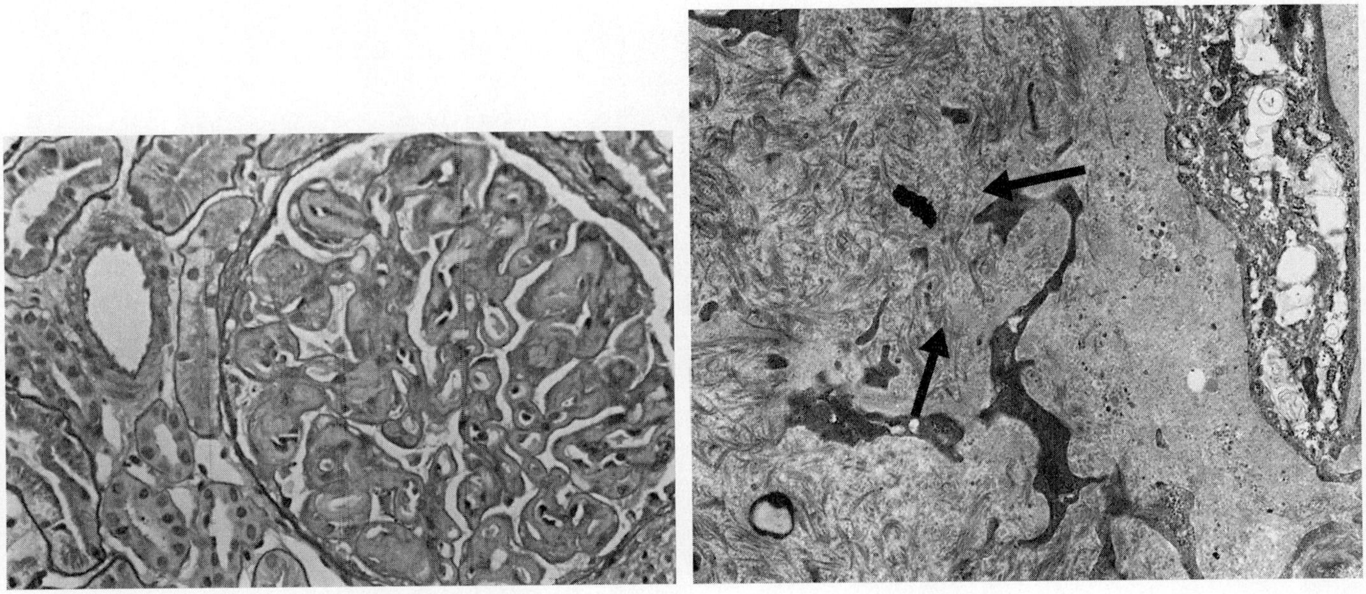

Figure 109.60. Collagen type III glomerulopathy. **A:** Light microscopic appearance of glomerulus: There are markedly thickened capillary walls and widening of mesangial regions by pale staining material representing type III collagen. Periodic acid–Schiff, ×240. **B:** Ultrastructural appearance of mesangium with numerous coarse fibrils *(arrows)* of type III collagen. At this magnification, periodicity of the fibrils cannot be appreciated. ×6,850.

INDEX

C

D

P

Q

R

S

U

W

X

Y